MEDICAL-SURGICAL NURSING

Critical Thinking for Collaborative Care

MEDICAL-SURGICAL NURSING

Critical Thinking for Collaborative Care

Donna D. Ignatavicius, MS, RN, Cm
President, DI Associates, Inc.
Hughesville, Maryland;
Former Professor,
Charles County Community College,
La Plata, Maryland

M. Linda Workman, PhD, RN, FAAN
Gertrude Perkins Oliva Professor of Oncology,
Frances Payne Bolton School of Nursing,
Case Western Reserve University,
Cleveland, Ohio

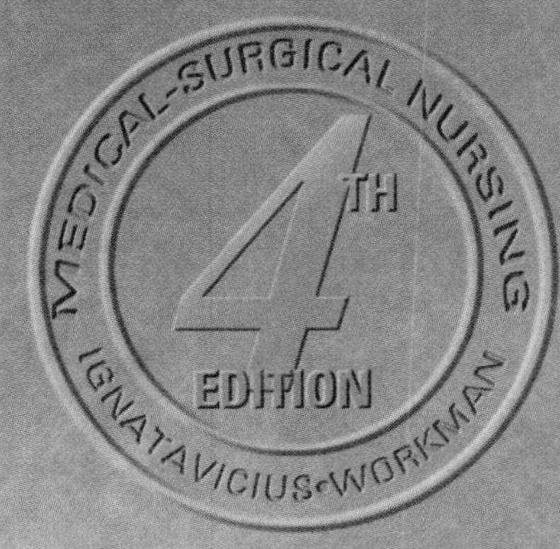

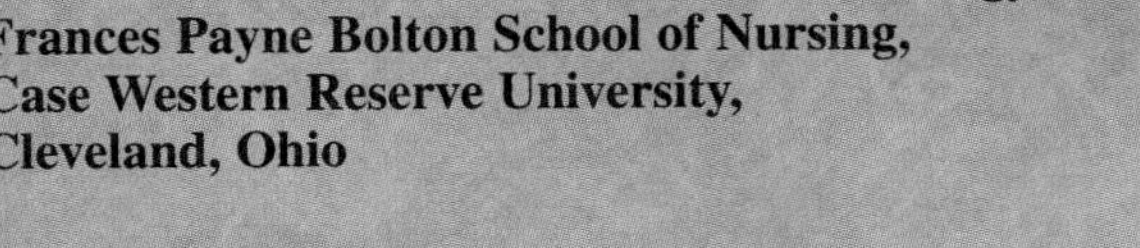

with 689 illustrations

W.B. SAUNDERS COMPANY
An Imprint of Elsevier Science
Philadelphia London New York St. Louis Sydney Toronto

W.B. SAUNDERS COMPANY
An Imprint of Elsevier Science

The Curtis Center
Independence Square West
Philadelphia, Pennsylvania 19106

NOTICE

Pharmacology is an ever-changing field. Standard safety precautions must be followed, but as new research and clinical experience broaden our knowledge, changes in treatment and drug therapy may become necessary or appropriate. Readers are advised to check the most current product information provided by the manufacturer of each drug to be administered to verify the recommended dose, the method and duration of administration, and contraindications. It is the responsibility of the licensed prescriber, relying on experience and knowledge of the patient, to determine dosages and the best treatment for each individual patient. Neither the publisher nor the editor assumes any liability for any injury and/or damage to persons or property arising from this publication.

Library of Congress Cataloging-in-Publication Data

Medical-surgical nursing: critical thinking for collaborative care / [edited by] Donna D. Ignatavicius, M. Linda Workman.—4th ed.
p. ; cm.
Rev. ed. of: Medical-surgical nursing across the health care continuum. 3rd ed. c1999.
Includes bibliographical references and index.
ISBN 0-7216-8762-8 (1 v.) — ISBN 0-7216-8763-6 (2 v. set)
1. Nursing. 2. Surgical nursing. I. Ignatavicius, Donna D. II. Workman, M. Linda. III. Medical-surgical nursing across the health care continuum.
[DNLM: 1. Perioperative Nursing. WY 161 M489 2001]
RT41 .I36 2001
610.73—dc21

2001042655

Vice President and Publishing Director: Sally Schrefer
Executive Editor: Robin Carter
Managing Editor: Lee Henderson
Project Manager: Deborah L. Vogel
Project Specialist: Jodi M. Willard
Book Designer: Teresa Breckwoldt

MEDICAL-SURGICAL NURSING: CRITICAL THINKING FOR COLLABORATIVE CARE, 4th edition

Single Volume 0–7216–8762–8
2-Volume Set 0–7216–8763–6

Printed in the United States of America.

Last digit is the print number: 9 8 7 6 5 4 3

About the Authors

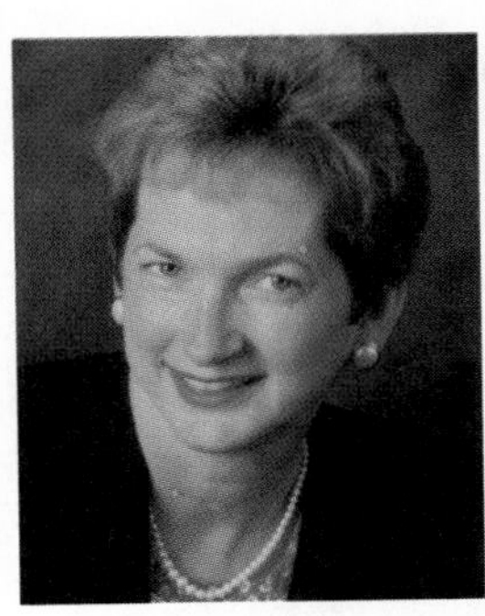

Donna D. Ignatavicius received her diploma in nursing from the Peninsula General School of Nursing in Salisbury, Maryland. After working as a staff and charge nurse in medical-surgical nursing, she became an instructor in Staff Development at the University of Maryland Medical Center. She then received her BSN from the University of Maryland School of Nursing. For 5 years she taught in several schools of nursing while working toward her MS in Nursing, which she received in 1981. Ms. Ignatavicius then taught in the BSN program at the University of Maryland for 6 years, after which she continued to pursue her interest in gerontology and accepted the position of Director of Nursing of a major skilled nursing facility in her home state of Maryland. She has been a certified gerontologic nurse since 1989 and was certified in nursing case management by the American Nurses Credentialing Center in 1998. Recently, she has taught in both diploma and associate-degree nursing programs. Through her consulting and seminar business, Ms. Ignatavicius has gained national recognition in nursing education and critical thinking. She is currently the President of DI Associates, Inc. (http://www.diassociates.com/), a company dedicated to improving health care through education and consultation.

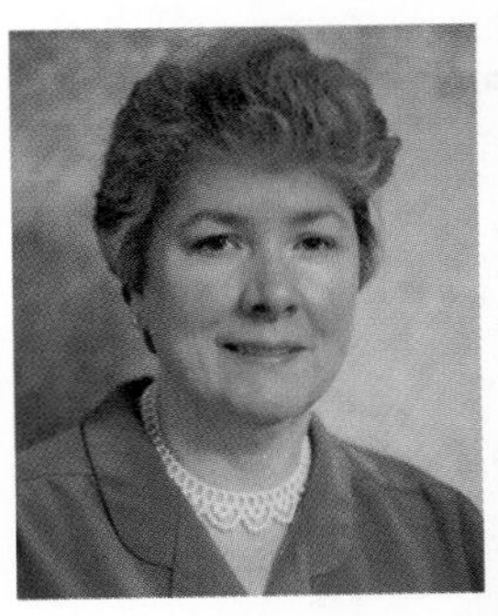

M. Linda Workman received her BSN from the University of Cincinnati College of Nursing and Health. After serving in the U.S. Army Nurse Corps and working as an Assistant Head Nurse and Head Nurse in civilian hospitals, Dr. Workman, a native of Canada, earned her MSN from the University of Cincinnati College of Nursing and Health and a PhD in Developmental Biology from the University of Cincinnati College of Arts and Sciences. Dr. Workman's 22 years of academic experience include teaching at the diploma, associate-degree, baccalaureate, and master's levels. Her areas of teaching expertise include medical-surgical nursing, physiology, pathophysiology, genetics, oncology, and immunology. Dr. Workman has been recognized nationally for her teaching expertise and was inducted into the American Academy of Nursing in 1992. She is a former American Cancer Society Professor of Oncology Nursing and is currently the Gertrude Perkins Oliva Professor of Oncology at the Frances Payne Bolton School of Nursing, Case Western Reserve University.

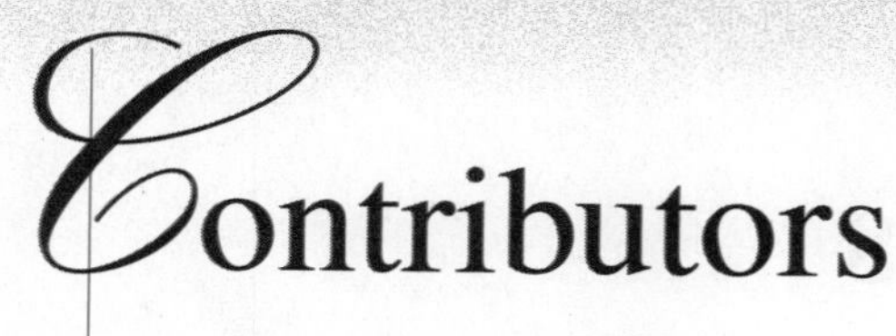

Contributors

ROBIN L. BARANOWSKI, BSN, RN
Infusion Therapy Nurse; PICC Line Specialist
Calvert Memorial Hospital
Prince Frederick, Maryland

MARCIA CHORBA, RN, MSN
Education Coordinator, Critical Care
Veterans Administration Pittsburgh Healthcare System
Pittsburgh, Pennsylvania

CAROLYN CORAZZA, BSN, RN, CWOCN
Private Practice ET Nurse
E.T. Consultants, Inc.
Rockville, Maryland

JANICE CUZZELL, MA, RN, CNS
Vice President of Staff Development
Island Health Care, Inc.
Savannah, Georgia

LUCILLE SANZERO ELLER, PhD, RN
Assistant Professor, College of Nursing
Rutgers University
Newark, New Jersey

KATHLEEN ELLSTROM, PhD, RN, CNS
Clinical Nurse Manager, Critical Care Services
Kaiser Foundation Hospitals—Riverside
Grand Terrace, California

DOROTHY J. HAMILTON, MSN, RN, CNP, CCRN
Nurse Practitioner
University Hospitals of Cleveland
Cleveland, Ohio

E. JEAN HAYES, MS, RN
Associate Professor
Purdue University—North Central
Westville, Indiana

DEBORAH H. HEATHERLY, BSN, MA
Healthcare Consultant
Moncks Corner, South Carolina

MARY KAZANOWSKI, PhD, ARNP, AOCN, CRNH
Professor, Saint Anselm College;
Palliative Care Nurse, Visiting Nurses Association Hospice
Manchester, New Hampshire

ANNE KEANE, EdD, CRNP, FAAN
Associate Professor, School of Nursing
University of Pennsylvania
Philadelphia, Pennsylvania

ELAINE BISHOP KENNEDY, EdD, RN
Professor, Nursing
Wor-Wic Community College
Salisbury, Maryland

LORI KLINGMAN, MSN, RN
UPMC Passavant Hospital
Pittsburgh, Pennsylvania

DEITRA L. LOWDERMILK, PhD, RNC, FAAN
Clinical Professor
University of North Carolina at Chapel Hill
Chapel Hill, North Carolina

ANN BUTLER MAHER, MS, RN, APNC, ONC
Family Nurse Practitioner
Sussex Family Practice
Sussex, New Jersey

JUDY MALKIEWICZ, PhD, RN
School of Nursing
University of Northern Colorado
Greeley, Colorado

ERIC MARSH, MSN, RN
Trauma Program Manager
Rainbow Pediatric Trauma Center
University Hospitals of Cleveland;
Trauma Nurse Coordinator
University Hospitals Health System
Cleveland, Ohio

JAN HOOT MARTIN, PhD, RN, GNP
Professor, School of Nursing
University of Northern Colorado
Greeley, Colorado

ELIZABETH McCLURE, MS, RN
Instructor, Adult-Health Nursing Department
University of Cincinnati College of Nursing
Cincinnati, Ohio

M. ELAINE McLEOD, MSN, APRN, BC, CDE
Clinical Nurse Specialist
Veterans Administration Tennessee Valley Healthcare System
Nashville, Tennessee

ERIN M. McMENAMIN, MSN, CRNP, AOCN
Pain Medicine Nurse Practitioner/Program Manager
University of Pennsylvania
Philadelphia, Pennsylvania

DONNA McMULLEN, RN, CWOCN
Private Practice ET Nurse
E.T. Consultants, Inc.
Rockville, Maryland

MARJORIE G. MORGAN, PhD, RN
Certified Nurse-Midwife, Certified Transcultural Nurse
South Carolina Department of Health and Environmental Control
Myrtle Beach, South Carolina

AMY NICHOLS, EdD, RN
Associate Professor, School of Nursing
San Francisco State University
San Francisco, California

REBECCA M. PATTON, MSN, RN, CNOR
Director of Nursing
Richmond Heights Hospital
University Hospitals Health System
Cleveland, Ohio

KATHLEEN OUIMET PERRIN, PhD(c), RN, CCRN
Associate Professor of Nursing
Saint Anselm College
Manchester, New Hampshire

TOMMIE WRIGHT PNIEWSKI, MSN, RN, CNAA
Associate Professor of Nursing
Hopkinsville Community College
Hopkinsville, Kentucky

ROSEMARY C. POLOMANO, PhD, RN, FAAN
Assistant Professor, Department of Anesthesiology
Penn State Milton S. Hershey Medical Center
Pennsylvania State University College of Nursing
Hershey, Pennsylvania

SUSAN M. SCHNEIDER, PhD, RN, CS, AOCN
Director, Graduate Oncology Nursing Program
Duke University
Durham, North Carolina

DEBORAH WRIGHT SHPRITZ, PhD, RN, CCRN
Assistant Professor, Department of Adult Health
University of Maryland School of Nursing
Baltimore, Maryland

JUDITH P. STURGIS, RN, BSN, CIC
Infection Control Director
Calvert Memorial Hospital
Prince Frederick, Maryland

JANICE TAZBIR, RN, MS, CCRN
Assistant Professor of Nursing
Purdue University—Calumet
Hammond, Indiana

SHIRLEY E. VAN ZANDT, MSN, MPH, CRNP
Instructor, School of Nursing
Johns Hopkins University
Baltimore, Maryland

CONSTANCE VISOVSKY, RN, PhD(c), ACNP
Research Nurse/Nurse Practitioner
Case Western Reserve University
University Hospitals of Cleveland;
Research Nurse, CHANGE Exercise Study
Frances Payne Bolton School of Nursing
Case Western Reserve University
Cleveland, Ohio

CHRIS WINKELMAN, PhD, RN, CCRN
Assistant Professor, Frances Payne Bolton School of Nursing
Case Western Reserve University
Cleveland, Ohio

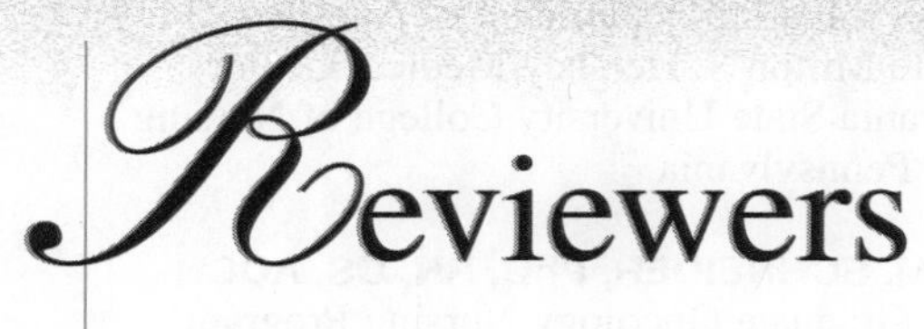

Reviewers

HELEN ADAMS, RN, MSN
Jefferson State Community College
Birmingham, Pennsylvania

MARGARET M. ANDREWS, PhD, RN, CTN
Nazareth College
Rochester, New York

CHERYL K.K. ARUGA, RN, CS, MSN, FNP
Hawaii Community College
Hilo, Hawaii

LYNN ASKEW, RN, MSN, APON
Hopkinsville Community College
Hopkinsville, Kentucky

ELLEN BARKER, MSN, RN, CNRN
President, Neuroscience Nursing Consultants
Greenville, Delaware

KATHLEEN A. BARRETT, MSN, ARNP/CNS-CS
Via Christi Regional Medical Center
Wichita, Kansas

JOYCE L. BEAVER, RN, BSN, ACLS, BCLS
Southeastern Community College,
Whiteville, North Carolina

SUZANNE K. BELTZ, PhD, RN, CS, CNS
University of Mary Hardin-Baylor
Belton, Texas

LINDA K. BENNETT, RN, CS-P, CPC
Chesapeake, Maryland

SENA J. BLICKENSTAFF, RN, BSN, CCLA, CLS, LNC
Washoe Hospital
Reno, Nevada

LARRY BOLT, RN, BSN, MED
Instructor, The Christ Hospital School of Nursing
Cincinnati, Ohio

CHERYL L. BRADY, RN, MSN
Kent State University
East Liverpool, Ohio

MICHELLE R. BUNNING, RN, MSN
Good Samaritan Hospital School of Nursing
Cincinnati, Ohio

MICHELLE BUTT, RN, BSN, MN (C)
Sunnybrook Women's College
Toronto, Ontario, Canada

REBECCA SUE CATE, RN, BSN, IHC
LDS Hospital
Salt Lake City, Utah

SHARON CHILDS, MS, CRNP-CS, ONC
Johns Hopkins University
Johns Hopkins Bayview Medical Center
Baltimore, Maryland

LAURA H. CLAYTON, RN, MSN, FNP
Shepherd College
Shepherdstown, West Virginia

DEBORAH CONAWAY, MSN, RN
Samuel Merritt College;
Kaiser Permanente Oakland Medical Center
Oakland, California

CATHERINE M. CONCERT, RN, MS, CS-FNP, CGRN
Wyckoff Heights Medical Center
Brooklyn, New York

DEBORAH DALRYMPLE, RN, MSN, CRNI
Montgomery County Community College
Blue Bell, Pennsylvania

SHARON DECKER, RN, CS, MSN, CCRN
Texas Tech University Health Sciences Center
Lubbock, Texas

SHEILA A. DUNN, RN, MSN, C-ANP
St. Louis Veterans Administration Medical Center
St. Louis, Missouri;
Belleville Clinic
Belleville, Illinois

URSULA EASTERDAY-HEITZ, RN, MSN
Consultant
Nashville, Tennessee

REBECCA S. FRUGE, RN, MN, CNS
InterAmerican University of Puerto Rico
Metropolitan Campus
San Juan, Puerto Rico

KATHLEEN A. GEIER, MS, RN, ONC
Webster Orthopaedic Medical Group/
Jackson Arthritis Center
Oakland, California

KAREN GOFF, RN, BSN
St. Joseph's Hospital of Atlanta
Atlanta, Georgia

JUDITH HALVERSON, BSN, MSN
North Idaho College
Coeur d'Alene, Idaho

CAROL HEATH, EdD, RN, CS
Sonoma State University
Rohnert Park, California

OLGA E. HENRY, BSN, MBA, RN, C
Broward Community College
Davie, Florida

LAWRENCE "BUDDY" HERRINGTON, MSN, RN
Tarrant County College
Fort Worth, Texas

MIMA M. HORNE, RN, MS, CDE
New Hanover Regional Medical Center
Wilmington, North Carolina

SUSAN J.W. HSIA, RN, PhD
Washburn University
Topeka, Kansas

CAROL A. HUNTER, RN, MSN
The Christ Hospital School of Nursing
Cincinnati, Ohio

PAULA S. JOHNSON, BSN, CCRN
Nash Health Care Systems
Rocky Mountain, North Carolina

TAMARA M. KEAR, MSN, RN, CNN
Thomas Jefferson University Hospital
Philadelphia, Pennsylvania

LEA KEESEE, RN, BSN
South Plains College
Levelland, Texas

ELAINE BISHOP KENNEDY, EdD, RN
Wor-Wic Community College
Salisbury, Maryland

NANCY L. GINDELE KRANZLEY, MS, RN
The Christ Hospital
Cincinnati, Ohio

DARLENE LACY, MSN, RNC
University of Mary Hardin-Baylor
Belton, Texas

PATRICK J. LILLEY, MBA, MSN, RN
North Central Texas College
Gainsville, Texas

BRENDA LOHRI-POSEY, RN, EdD
Wheeling Jesuit University
Wheeling, West Virginia

EDWINA A. McCONNELL, RN, PhD, ERCNA
Independent Nurse Consultant
Gorham, Maine

MARY ANN SICILIANO McLAUGHLIN, MSN, RN
Independent Nurse Consultant
Magnolia, New Jersey

MICHELLE M. MONTPAS, RN, MSN, OCN
C.S. Mott Community College
Flint, Michigan

JAY K. OBER, RN, BS, CCRN, CEN
Bay State Medical Center
United States Air Force Reserves
Springfield, Massachusetts

PATRICIA A. PALAMR, RN, BSN, CEN
Thomas Jefferson University Hospital
Philadelphia, Pennsylvania

TOMMIE W. PNIEWSKI, MSN, RN, CNNA
Hopkinsville Community College
Hopkinsville, Kentucky

JANE RENFRO, PhD, ANP (C)
Kaiser Permanente
Arlington Free Clinic
Arlington, Virginia

ANNE RATH RENTFRO, MSN, RN, CS
University of Texas at Brownsville
Brownsville, Texas

DOTTIE ROBERTS, MSN, MACI, RN, C, ONC, CNS
Penrose-St. Francis Health Services
Colorado Springs, Colorado

MARY B. SCOTT, RN, PhD, CNN
University of California—San Francisco
San Francisco, California

SUSAN SEMB, RN-CS, MSN, CDE, PHN
Sun Plus Home Health Services
San Diego, California

AMY B. SHARRON, MS, RN, CS, GNP
Roger Williams Medical Center
Providence, Rhode Island

GAIL JANET SMITH, RN, MSN
Miami Dade Community College
Miami, Florida

TERESA E. KELLY SNYDER, MN, RN
Montana State University
Missoula, Montana

CHRIS STEWERT-AMIDEI, RN, MSN, CNRN, CCRN
University of Chicago Hospitals
Chicago, Illinois

KATHLEEN G. STILLING, MS, RN, C
The Community College of Baltimore County, Essex,
Baltimore, Maryland

JUDITH P. STURGIS, RN, BSN, CIC
Calvert Memorial Hospital
Prince Frederick, Maryland

DAVID TILTON, RN, BSN, ACLS, BCLS
Western State Hospital
Tacoma, Washington

SUZANNE M. VANET, BSN, CMSN
Louis A. Johnson VA Medical Center
Clarkburg, West Virginia

CATHERINE R. VAN SON, RN, MSN
Oregon Geriatric Education Center
Portland, Oregon

NANCY CLARKE VERDIRAME, RN, BSN, MSN
Louise Obici School of Nursing
Suffolk, Virginia

JANIS WAITE, EdD, RN
St. Francis Medical Center College of Nursing
Peoria, Illinois

TERRY WOOD, RN, MSN
Jewish Hospital College of Nursing
St. Louis, Missouri

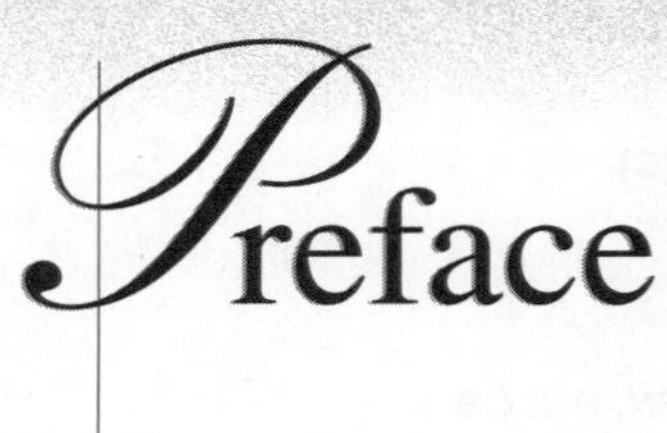

Preface

The first edition of this text, entitled *Medical-Surgical Nursing: A Nursing Process Approach,* found widespread acclaim as *the* medical-surgical nursing text of the 1990s. The second and third editions built on that achievement and further solidified the book's position as a compass for the practice of adult nursing. Now in its fourth edition, just 3 years since the previous edition, the book maps a fresh course for the future of adult nursing—a course reflected in the book's new title: *Medical-Surgical Nursing: Critical Thinking for Collaborative Care.*

This title was carefully chosen to reflect this edition's fresh emphasis on developing and enhancing critical thinking skills to help today's nursing students function in interdisciplinary teams in a variety of health care settings, including both acute care and community-based settings.

In addition to this focus on critical thinking, *Medical-Surgical Nursing: Critical Thinking for Collaborative Care,* 4th edition, provides expanded coverage of women's health issues, cultural considerations, complementary and alternative (integrative) therapies, and the special needs of older adults. Also, concepts of case management and community-based care are interwoven throughout to help the reader understand these new and growing roles and trends.

New to this edition are Critical Thinking Challenges, which are interspersed throughout the text. These case-based exercises provide a safe and effective means of practicing the on-the-spot decision making that students will face in the fast-paced world of medical-surgical nursing. Suggested answer guidelines for these Critical Thinking Challenges are provided on the book's SIMON website.

But these answer guidelines are just the beginning of the integrated multimedia learning experience provided in the fourth edition. For each of the Learning Objectives now provided at the start of each chapter, students will find corresponding Self-Assessment Questions on the SIMON website, written by co-author M. Linda Workman. Also on the SIMON site are web-based Learning Activities that correspond to the collaborative management of major diseases and disorders. These activities stimulate and validate critical thinking to help students understand and apply the material covered in the text. Internet Resources and annotated Suggested Readings are also found on the SIMON website.

CLINICAL CURRENCY AND ACCURACY

To ensure the text's currency and accuracy, we listened to the readers of the first three editions—their impressions of and experiences with the text. Based on this input, we formulated our revision plan. We assembled a team of clinical experts to revise, rewrite and, in some cases, draft entirely new chapters. We then commissioned in-depth reviews of each chapter by clinicians and instructors from across the United States and Canada and used their reviews to guide us in revising the chapters into their final form. We even enlisted the assistance of an enterostomal therapist and an infection control nurse to review every clinical chapter.

The results are reflected in the fourth edition's strong, consistent focus on critical thinking, collaborative care, pathophysiology, and community-based care; its foundation of relevant research; and its emphasis on the critical "need to know" information that nurses must master in order to provide safe, effective care based on solid scientific evidence. This base of scientific evidence is emphasized throughout the text and is highlighted in our new "Best Practice" charts.

OUTSTANDING READABILITY

With the assistance of a team of writing experts who conducted reading level analyses of each and every chapter, the fourth edition has been carefully revised from cover to cover to ensure a consistent reading level ideally suited for today's nursing students. To achieve this consistency, our writing experts evaluated the readability of the first draft of each chapter. We revised the chapters based on those results and then tested the revised chapters for readability. Those chapters that tested above our target threshold were carefully edited once again to reduce the reading level still further. These chapters were tested a third time to confirm that the editing resulted in exactly the right level of readability. The result is a med-surg text of consistently outstanding readability.

EASE OF ACCESS

To make the text as easy to use as possible, we have maintained the third edition's approach of smaller chapters of more uniform length. The fourth edition has 77 chapters, including new introductory chapters on substance abuse (Chapter 8) and cultural aspects of health (Chapter 6). Based on faculty input, we have condensed the content on stress and adaptation, body image, and sexuality—formerly separate chapters—and have incorporated this material as appropriate into other chapters.

We also have maintained the third edition's unit structure, with vital body systems (cardiovascular, respiratory, and neurologic) appearing earlier in the book. In these three units, we have continued to provide critical care content in separate chapters on managing critically ill clients with coronary artery disease, respiratory problems, and neurologic problems. To help break up long blocks of text and also to highlight key information, we have included numerous headings, bulleted lists, tables, charts, and in-text highlights. We end each chapter with a Selected Bibliography (with classic sources noted with an asterisk [*]). Key Terms are now in boldface type and are defined in the text to foster learning of need-to-know vocabulary.

A COLLABORATIVE APPROACH

As in the previous three editions, we take a collaborative approach to client care. We believe that in the real world of health care, nurses, clients, and other health care providers (including physicians, respiratory and physical therapists, advanced-practice nurses, and physician's assistants) *share* responsibility for the management of client problems. Thus we present client care in a collaborative management framework. In this framework we make no artificial distinctions between medical treatment and nursing care. Instead, under each Collaborative Management heading we cover the entire range of approaches taken by health care practitioners of all disciplines when dealing with client problems.

New to this edition are eight Concept Maps that underscore this collaborative approach. Also known as *clinical correlation maps,* these Concept Maps address eight complex health problems and visually organize the steps of the nursing process and related concepts to illustrate the relationships among disease processes, medical treatments, nursing interventions, and more. Identifying these relationships not only underscores the collaborative nature of health care but also stimulates critical thinking and fosters learning.

Although our approach is collaborative, the text is first and foremost a *nursing* text. We therefore use a nursing process approach to organize discussions of client health problems and their management. Discussions of key health problems follow a full nursing process format, with the following structure:

- Health Problem
  - Overview
    - Pathophysiology
    - Etiology
    - Incidence/Prevalence
  - Collaborative Management
    - Assessment
    - Analysis
      - Common Nursing Diagnoses and Collaborative Problems
      - Additional Nursing Diagnoses and Collaborative Problems
    - Planning and Implementation
      - Nursing Diagnosis/Collaborative Problem
        - Planning: Expected Outcomes
        - Interventions
    - Community-Based Care
      - Health Teaching
      - Home Care Management
      - Health Care Resources
    - Evaluation: Outcomes

The nursing diagnoses used in this edition are the very latest 2001-2002 NANDA-approved diagnoses, making "Iggy" the first med-surg text to incorporate the sweeping changes of NANDA's Taxonomy II.

Discussions of less common or less complex disorders, although not given this complete subhead structure, nonetheless follow the same basic format: a discussion of the problem itself (including pertinent information on pathophysiology, etiology, and incidence) followed by a section on collaborative care of clients with the disorder.

Integral to this collaborative management approach is a clear delineation of just who is responsible for what. When a responsibility is primarily the nurse's, the text says so. When a decision must be made jointly by the client, nurse, health care provider, and therapist, this is clearly stated. When different health care practitioners in different care settings might be involved in the client's care, this also is stated.

To further emphasize the nurse's role, we have integrated pertinent components of the Nursing Interventions Classification (NIC) system and the Nursing Outcomes Classification (NOC) system. These systems were developed by the Center for Nursing Classification to standardize nursing interventions and outcomes and the terminology used to describe them. Where appropriate for health problems that receive full nursing process coverage, NIC interventions are clearly identified with a NIC symbol (NIC). Selected activities associated with each identified intervention are listed in NIC Intervention Activities charts.

The expected outcomes for client care in this edition are consistent with the NOC system. However, NOC continues to be developed and refined to ensure that outcomes are evidence-based. We have therefore included outcome statements that use NOC language when appropriate, as well as other outcome statements validated empirically by clinical practice. Those statements that are particularly consistent with NOC language are identified with a NOC symbol (NOC).

ORGANIZATION

The 77 chapters of *Medical-Surgical Nursing: Critical Thinking for Collaborative Care* are grouped into 16 units. A Core Concepts Grid introduces each unit of content and highlights the essential information that the student needs to learn in the chapters that follow. These Core Concepts Grids play an integral part in linking the textbook and several of its companion publications.

Unit 1, Health Promotion and Illness, lays the foundation for the health care concepts incorporated throughout the text. Unit 2 covers important biopsychosocial concepts related to health care, including pain and rehabilitation. In addition to the new chapters on culture and substance abuse, Chapter 7 now reflects the emerging view of pain as the "fifth vital sign," and Chapter 9 has been revised to focus on end-of-life care. Unit 3 consists of six chapters on the management of clients with fluid, electrolyte, and acid-base imbalances. This unit now includes an expanded chapter on infusion therapy (Chapter 14).

Unit 4 presents the perioperative nursing content that medical-surgical nurses need to know. This content provides a solid foundation to help the student better understand the specific surgeries covered throughout the remainder of the text. Unit 5 provides core content on health problems related to immune system function. This content includes normal inflammation and the immune response, altered cell growth and cancer development, and interventions for clients with connective tissue disease, HIV infection, and other immunologic disorders, cancers, and infections. A new chapter (Chapter 23) focuses on interventions for clients with immune function excess (hypersensitivity and autoimmunity).

The remaining 11 units cover medical-surgical content by body system. Each of these units begins with an Assessment chapter and continues with one or more Interventions chapters for clients with specific health problems in that body system.

MULTINATIONAL, MULTICULTURAL, MULTIGENERATIONAL FOCUS

To reflect the increasing diversity of our society, *Medical-Surgical Nursing: Critical Thinking for Collaborative Care* takes a multinational, multicultural, and multigenerational focus. Addressing the needs of both U.S. and Canadian readers, we have included examples of trade names of drugs available in the United States and those available in Canada. A maple leaf icon (✦) identifies the Canadian trade names.

To help nurses provide quality care for clients whose cultural background differs from their own, numerous Cultural Considerations boxes highlight important aspects of culturally competent care throughout the text. A new introductory chapter on the cultural aspects of health (Chapter 6) is also included in this edition. Also new to this edition and located inside the back cover is an innovative Communication Quick Reference for Spanish-Speaking Clients. This Quick Reference helps ensure clear communication between native English speakers and the rapidly growing population of Spanish-speaking people.

Increases in life expectancy and the "graying" of the baby-boom generation add up to a steadily increasing older adult population. To help equip nurses for this challenge, the fourth edition features expanded coverage of the care of older adults. It includes a greater number of Nursing Focus on the Older Adult charts and highlights laboratory values and drug dosages typical for older clients. Charts specifying normal physiologic changes to expect in the older population are included in each Assessment chapter. In addition, Considerations for Older Adults boxes are highlighted throughout the text to emphasize key points to keep in mind when caring for these clients.

Also appearing throughout the text are Women's Health Considerations boxes, which address topics of concern to female clients and their health care providers. These in-text highlights alert the reader to gender-related differences in assessment parameters and in the incidence, severity, and treatment of common health problems.

ADDITIONAL PEDAGOGIC FEATURES

The fourth edition includes a wealth of pedagogic features to help the student quickly identify and understand key information and to serve as study aids:

- Written in "client-friendly" language, Client Education Guide charts provide the types of instructions that nurses must learn to provide to clients and their families to help them cope with life changes caused by illness.
- Laboratory Profile charts summarize important information on laboratory tests commonly ordered to evaluate health problems. Information typically includes normal ranges of laboratory values (including differences for older adults, when appropriate) and the possible significance of abnormal findings.
- Drug Therapy charts summarize important information about commonly used drugs. These charts include both U.S. and Canadian trade names, usual dosages (including dosages for older clients, as appropriate), and nursing interventions with rationales.
- Key Features charts highlight the clinical manifestations of important disorders.
- Evidence-Based Practice for Nursing boxes, provided in nearly every chapter, give synopses of recent nursing research articles and other scientific articles applicable to nursing. Each box provides a summary of the article, a brief critique, and a summary of implications for nursing practice. The goal of this feature is to help students identify the strengths and weaknesses of the research and see how research can help guide nursing practice.
- Client Care Plans and Clinical Pathways—although declining somewhat in importance in today's streamlined health care environment—remain significant tools with which the student nurse must be familiar. The fourth edition therefore includes selected examples of these care planning tools. Client Care Plans now include a distinctive icon to signal tasks that can be delegated to assistive nursing personnel.
- Focused Assessment charts serve as a convenient summary of essential assessment points for selected conditions.
- Assessment Using Gordon's Functional Health Patterns charts provide a convenient one-stop list of relevant questions to ask clients regarding the impact of health conditions on everyday function.
- Meeting Healthy People 2010 Objectives boxes suggest specific activities that nurses can undertake to promote achievement of the specific numbered objectives of the Healthy People 2010 program.
- Cost of Care: Implications for Nursing boxes provide an important financial context for medical-surgical nursing, in which nurses must increasingly understand cost factors in order to help clients work toward wellness despite financial limitations.
- Legal/Ethical Issues in Health Care boxes introduce students to some of the dilemmas they will face in the increasingly high-tech world of medical-surgical nursing.
- To help students keep pace with the constantly changing landscape of health care, each chapter concludes with a link to Online Resources—including Suggested Readings and Internet Resources—found on the book's companion SIMON website.

AN INTEGRATED MULTIMEDIA RESOURCE BASED ON PROVEN LEARNING STRATEGIES

Medical-Surgical Nursing: Critical Thinking for Collaborative Care, 4th edition, is more than a web-linked textbook. It is the hub of a comprehensive package of electronic and print publications that break new ground in the application of proven learning strategies and evidence-based educational practice. This integrated multimedia resource actively engages the student in problem-solving and critical thinking. Every effort has been made to correlate content among the text and its companion publications and to focus the content on the Core Concepts Grids developed specifically for this purpose. Unlike many textbook authors, we have personally been involved in the development of each of the companion publications to ensure consistency and cohesion between the textbook and the companion publications.

RESOURCES FOR INSTRUCTORS

Resources for instructors include an Instructor's Manual, a Test Bank, and a LectureView Image/Slide Collection.

The Instructor's Manual, written by Susan Behmke, Sharon Souter, and Donna D. Ignatavicius, continues to be a groundbreaking educational ancillary. It provides content on how to promote collaborative or cooperative learning with features never before presented in any comparable instructor's manual. It includes critical learning outcomes, suggested learning activities, and a list of supplemental resources arranged in a practical three-column format. Learning activities that involve group work are included, as are time frames for learning and strategies for promoting active learning, including aspects of teaching/learning via distance education. Supplemental resources, which foster independent exploration, include transparency masters, Internet resources, and materials from community organizations. Numerous graphic organizers—including concept maps, algorithms, team concept maps, and sequence chains—are provided to help faculty to teach students how to make connections among isolated pieces of information and to encourage them to assemble the puzzle of today's complex health care system. The focus of content is on the Core Concepts Grids, which are provided for each unit and serve as content organizers for the teaching strategies and learning activities that follow.

A high-caliber Test Bank—delivered on CD-ROM together with the LectureView—provides instructors with more than 2000 test questions. Of these 2000 questions, 900 are completely new for this edition, and each question is coded for Correct Answer, Rationale, Cognitive Type, NCLEX Client Needs Category, and Nursing Process Step. The questions, prepared by M. Linda Workman and Constance Visovsky, have been written in response to feedback from faculty to be both more challenging and more reflective of the scope of questions on the NCLEX examination. Most are application-based questions, and only about 10% are knowledge- or comprehension-level questions. Questions were written focusing on the Core Concepts Grids presented in the *Instructor's Manual*, the *Critical Thinking Study Guide*, and the textbook.

LectureView is a CD-ROM lecture resource that includes 400 full-color images from the text along with 480 text slides for projection in the classroom. This PowerPoint-compatible ancillary allows instructors to prepare customized lecture presentations with ease using their own PowerPoint software.

RESOURCES FOR STUDENTS

Resources for students include the Critical Thinking Study Guide, the Clinical Companion, and the new Virtual Clinical Excursions workbook/CD-ROM.

The newly redesigned and reformatted *Critical Thinking Study Guide* provides material to enhance learning to promote mastery of the text. Echoing one of the text's core themes, the study guide emphasizes questions aimed at *enhancing critical thinking skills*. The study guide was written by a team of authors, led by Carol Dignon, in conjunction with the *Instructor's Manual* to ensure consistency. As with the *Instructor's Manual*, its focus is on the Core Concepts Grids, which are included in the *Critical Thinking Study Guide* to help students internalize the textbook material.

The pocket-sized *Clinical Companion*, authored by Kathy Hausman with Donna D. Ignatavicius, retains the alphabetical organization that proved so popular in the first three editions. Its newly streamlined format makes it easy to find essential information in seconds. The *Clinical Companion* is a pocket-sized "Iggy" written for students going into clinicals by an author who actively supervises clinicals and who knows first-hand what students in clinicals are being asked to know about their clients.

An exciting addition to the ancillary package for this edition—and a groundbreaking learning tool in its own right—is the *Virtual Clinical Excursions* workbook/CD-ROM package. This package guides the student through a computer-generated virtual clinical environment and helps the student apply textbook content to "virtual clients" in that environment. The clinical simulations and workbook, the latter authored by Elaine Kennedy, represent the next generation of research-based learning tools that promote critical thinking and meaningful learning.

For more information on any of these innovative companion publications, contact your Harcourt Health Sciences sales representative, visit http://www.harcourthealth.com/, or call Harcourt Health Sciences Faculty Support at 1-800-222-9570.

• • •

In summary, *Medical-Surgical Nursing: Critical Thinking for Collaborative Care*, 4th edition, together with its fully integrated multimedia ancillary package, provides the tools you will need to meet the challenge of nursing in the first decade of the 21st century and beyond. The only elements that remain to be added to this package are those that you alone can provide—your diligence, your commitment, your innovation, *your nursing care*.

Donna D. Ignatavicius
M. Linda Workman

Acknowledgments

Publishing a textbook of this depth and breadth would not be possible without the combined efforts of many people. Our contributing authors once again provided consistently excellent manuscripts in a timely fashion. Our reviewers—expert clinicians and instructors from around the United States and Canada—provided invaluable suggestions and encouragement throughout the book's development.

The staff of W.B. Saunders/Harcourt Health Sciences once again provided us with crucial guidance and support throughout the planning, writing, revision, and production of the fourth edition. In particular, Executive Editor Robin Carter and Developmental Editor Jeanne Allison worked closely with us in the early stages of this edition to help us hone and focus our revision plan. Jeanne Allison and Managing Editor Lee Henderson then worked with us step by step—with wise insights from Robin Carter—to bring the fourth edition from vision to publication. Special thanks to Senior Editor's Assistant Marie Thomas, who handled the countless administrative details associated with a project of this size. She is without peer among editorial assistants.

Project Specialist Jodi Willard was a joy to work with. Her attention to detail, flexibility, and conscientiousness not only helped to make this edition the most consistently readable ever, but also made the entire production process incredibly smooth and headache-free. Thanks, too, to Copyeditor Judi Bange, who worked closely with Jodi in copyediting the entire text and supported Jodi's own work with diligence and painstaking attention to detail.

Special thanks also to Project Manager Debbie Vogel. Debbie's quiet leadership and personal commitment to the project were exemplary. Without fail, she exercised her role as collaborator and problem solver to help bring this edition to publication precisely on schedule.

Designer Teresa Breckwoldt worked tirelessly and with good humor to create a completely new interior design for this edition. Her sophisticated design treatment of this edition is easy on the eye—making long study sessions more tolerable—and it brings into appropriately sharp focus those pedagogic elements that required a distinctive look.

Thanks also to Donna Macaluso of MacArt Design and to photographer Rick Brady, whose full-color illustrations and photographs play an important part in conveying the content and context of medical-surgical nursing in the new millennium.

Our acknowledgments would not be complete without recognizing Joyce Owen, Teresa Hajdu, and other key members of the Sales and Marketing staff who helped to put this book into your hands.

Finally, we wish to thank Vice President and Nursing Editorial Director Sally Schrefer. Sally's personal leadership style creates a unique publishing environment in which authors and editors have the freedom to interact creatively to produce the best books in the field.

Donna D. Ignatavicius
M. Linda Workman

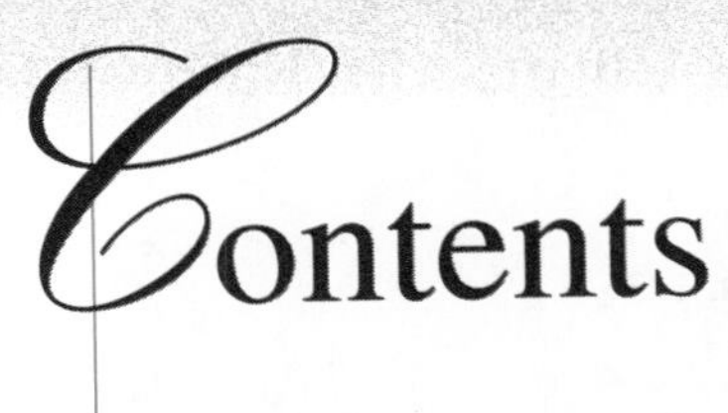

Contents

UNIT 4

MANAGEMENT OF PERIOPERATIVE CLIENTS

UNIT 5

PROBLEMS OF PROTECTION

Management of Clients with Problems of the Immune System

CHAPTER 24

Altered Cell Growth and Cancer Development, 407

M. LINDA WORKMAN

CHAPTER 25

Interventions for Clients with Cancer, 423

M. LINDA WORKMAN

CHAPTER 26

Interventions for Clients with Infection, 445

JUDITH P. STURGIS

UNIT 6

Problems of Oxygenation

Management of Clients with Problems of the Respiratory Tract

CHAPTER 27

Assessment of the Respiratory System, 467

M. LINDA WORKMAN

CHAPTER 28

Interventions for Clients Requiring Oxygen Therapy or Tracheostomy, 489

M. LINDA WORKMAN

CHAPTER 29

Interventions for Clients with Noninfectious Upper Respiratory Problems, 508

M. LINDA WORKMAN

CHAPTER 30

Interventions for Clients with Noninfectious Lower Respiratory Problems, 529

M. LINDA WORKMAN

CHAPTER 37

Interventions for Clients with Shock, 771

M. LINDA WORKMAN

CHAPTER 38

Interventions for Critically Ill Clients with Coronary Artery Disease, 789

KATHLEEN OUIMET PERRIN

UNIT 8

PROBLEMS OF TISSUE PERFUSION

Management of Clients with Problems of the Hematologic System

CHAPTER 39

Assessment of the Hematologic System, 819

M. LINDA WORKMAN

CHAPTER 40

Interventions for Clients with Hematologic Problems, 836

SUSAN M. SCHNEIDER

UNIT 9

PROBLEMS OF MOBILITY, SENSATION, AND COGNITION

Management of Clients with Problems of the Nervous System

CHAPTER 41

Assessment of the Nervous System, 871

DEBORAH WRIGHT SHPRITZ

CHAPTER 42

Interventions for Clients with Problems of the Central Nervous System: The Brain, 897

DEBORAH WRIGHT SHPRITZ

CHAPTER 68

Interventions for Clients with Burns, 1555

ERIC MARSH

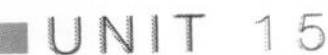
UNIT 15

Problems of Excretion

Management of Clients with Problems of the Renal/Urinary System

CHAPTER 69

Assessment of the Renal/Urinary System, 1589

CHRIS WINKELMAN

CHAPTER 70

Interventions for Clients with Urinary Problems, 1614

CHRIS WINKELMAN

CHAPTER 71

Interventions for Clients with Renal Disorders, 1642

CHRIS WINKELMAN

CHAPTER 72

Interventions for Clients with Acute and Chronic Renal Failure, 1664

CONSTANCE VISOVSKY

UNIT 16

Problems of Reproduction

Management of Clients with Problems of the Reproductive System

CHAPTER 73

Assessment of the Reproductive System, 1707

DEITRA L. LOWDERMILK

CHAPTER 74

Interventions for Clients with Breast Disorders, 1730

AMY NICHOLS • DONNA D. IGNATAVICIUS

CHAPTER 75

Interventions for Clients with Gynecologic Problems, 1751

AMY NICHOLS • DONNA D. IGNATAVICIUS

CHAPTER 76

Interventions for Male Clients with Reproductive Problems, 1782

LORI KLINGMAN

CHAPTER 77

Interventions for Clients with Sexually Transmitted Diseases, 1805

SHIRLEY E. VAN ZANDT

APPENDIXES

Guide to Special Features

CLIENT EDUCATION GUIDE

BEST PRACTICE *for*

ASSESSMENT
Using Gordon's Functional Health Patterns

CLIENT CARE PLAN

CLINICAL PATHWAY

CONCEPT MAP

COST OF CARE
IMPLICATIONS FOR NURSING

EVIDENCE-BASED PRACTICE FOR NURSING

FOCUSED ASSESSMENT *of*

Legal/Ethical Issues in Health Care

Meeting Healthy People 2010 Objectives

NIC Intervention Activities *for*

NURSING FOCUS *on the* OLDER ADULT

UNIT

1

HEALTH PROMOTION AND ILLNESS

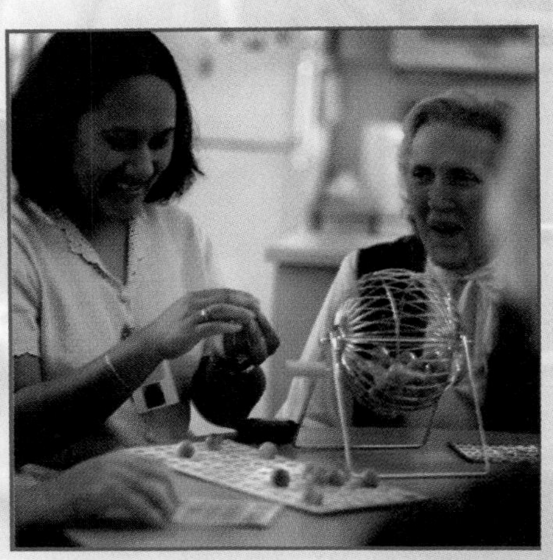

UNIT 1 Health Promotion and Illness ■ Core Concepts Grid

Critical Thinking in the Role of the Medical/Surgical Nurse	Community-Based Care	Introduction to Managed Care and Case Management	Introduction to Complementary and Alternative Therapies	Health Care of Older Adults
• **Definitions of health** • **Health promotion and protection** • **Roles** • **Teaching/learning process** • **Concept of caring** • **Practice settings** • **Nursing process**	• **Ambulatory care** • **Home care** • **Nursing home care** • **Subacute care** • **Rehabilitative care**	• **Purpose** Types • **Role of the nurse** • **Focus on outcomes** • **Case management** • **Role of case manager** • **Clinical pathways**	• **Spirituality and religion** • **Relaxation** • **Imagery** • **Music** • **Touch** • **Laughter/humor** • **Herbalism** • **Progressive muscle relaxation** • **Aromatherapy**	• **Subgroups of older adults** • **Health issues** Health promotion Nutritional needs Accidents Drug use/misuse Mental health Neglect/abuse • **Economic issues** Income Housing Other resources • **Role of gerontologic nurse**

CHAPTER 1

Critical Thinking in the Role of the Medical-Surgical Nurse

DONNA D. IGNATAVICIUS

Learning Objectives

After studying this chapter, you should be able to:

1. Compare and contrast common definitions of health.
2. Explain why some populations are more likely to experience health problems than others.
3. Differentiate the three levels of illness prevention and provide at least one example of each level.
4. Explain the purpose of Healthy People 2010.
5. Identify the major roles of the medical-surgical nurse.
6. Explain the relationship between critical thinking and evidence-based practice.
7. Describe best practice interventions for client education.
8. Describe typical health care settings in which medical-surgical nursing is practiced.
9. Identify the key components of a nursing assessment.
10. Describe the difference between a nursing diagnosis and a collaborative problem.
11. Formulate expected outcomes based on data analysis.
12. Identify best practice interventions for clinical documentation.

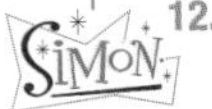

Go to http://www.wbsaunders.com/SIMON/Iggy/ for self-assessment questions related to these Learning Objectives.

The purpose of medical-surgical nursing, sometimes called adult health nursing, is to promote health and prevent illness in people from 18 to over 100 years of age. Nurses who practice medical-surgical nursing are generalists who must have a broad knowledge base to meet the needs of clients in a variety of health care settings. Rapid advances in technology, exponential increases in knowledge, and dramatic changes in the health care delivery system require that medical-surgical nurses use expert critical thinking skills to provide complex, holistic client care.

HEALTH

Beliefs about health and illness are a major feature of every known culture. How one views himself or herself as a person and as a part of the environment affects how health is defined. Health is often viewed as a continuum on which optimal wellness, at one end, is the highest level of function, and illness, at the other end, results in death (Figure 1-1). Every person is somewhere on the continuum. As a person's health state changes, his or her location on the continuum changes.

Although the term *health* is used every day, no universally accepted definition has been established. Over time, the focus and expression of health have varied depending on knowledge, theories, and beliefs. Some people view health and disease as a reward or punishment for their actions. Others consider health to be a wholeness of the body; this view is often referred to as holistic health.

Definitions of Health

A typical dictionary may define health in terms of a person's ability to function in society. Some definitions also describe health as a disease-free state or condition. Definitions such as these do not make clear what constitutes health and illness and seem to present an "either/or" situation; that is, a person is either healthy or ill.

WORLD HEALTH ORGANIZATION DEFINITION OF HEALTH

As science has progressed, the definition of **health** has evolved. One of the most commonly quoted definitions is the one presented in 1947 by the World Health Organization (WHO). WHO stated that health is "a state of complete physical, mental, and social well-being and not merely the absence of disease or infirmity" (WHO, 1947, p. 1). According to WHO, to be healthy a person must be in a state of physical, mental, and social well-being. Some health professionals

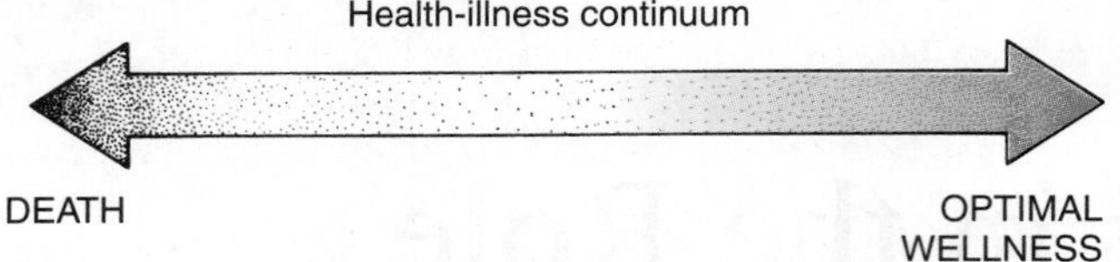

Figure 1-1 ● Common concept of health as a continuum ranging from optimal wellness at one end to illness culminating in death at the other end.

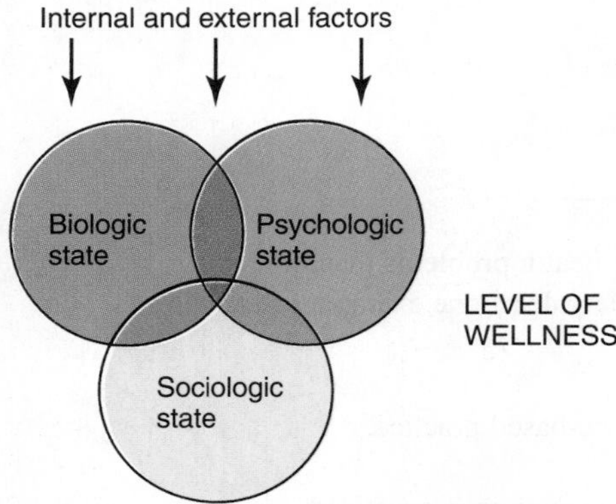

Figure 1-2 ● Textbook definition of health—a person's biologic, psychologic, and sociologic state. Internal and external factors affect a person's level of wellness.

have found this concept problematic because achieving a state of "health" seems to be an unrealistic goal. This definition does not allow for degrees of health or illness, and it fails to reflect the dynamic, ever-changing nature of health.

One concept related to health is homeostasis, or internal equilibrium or balance. When a person experiences a disturbance in homeostasis, he or she is considered to be "unhealthy." Like the WHO definition of health, this concept is losing popularity because "stasis" implies an unchanging state, and most theorists today believe that health is always changing.

SOCIOLOGIC DEFINITIONS OF HEALTH

Sociologists view health as a condition that allows for the pursuit and enjoyment of desired cultural values. Studies that have polled laypeople for their definitions of health concur that health is the absence of symptoms and a feeling of well-being. "Good health" includes the ability to carry out "normal" daily activities, such as going to work and performing household chores.

HOLISTIC HEALTH

One term often used in discussions of health and wellness is **holistic health.** The holistic view considers the body, mind, and spirit to be interrelated parts of a person's being. The concept of high-level wellness, which considers the needs of the whole person, has led to the growth of holistic health care. Holistic health focuses on promoting health and preventing illness, with an emphasis on the person's responsibility to achieve high-level wellness. There is also concern with bringing the person's mind, body, and spirit into harmony with the environment. Various integrative therapies, including alternative medicine and complementary practices, have been used for many years to promote mind-body-spirit harmony. Chapter 4 describes some commonly used therapies and how they can be incorporated into medical-surgical nursing practice.

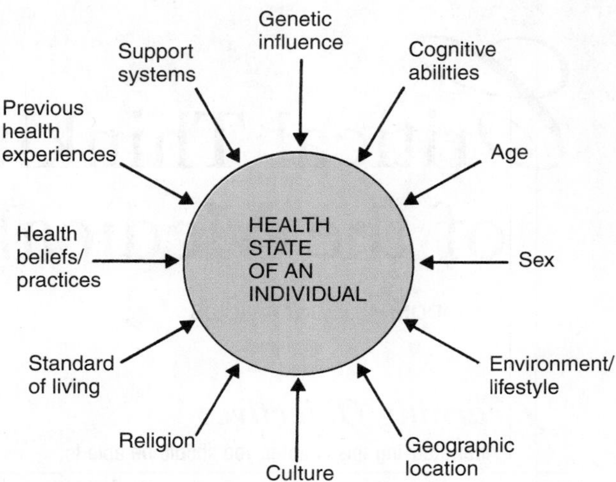

Figure 1-3 ● Multiple variables influence health and illness.

DEFINITION OF HEALTH USED IN THIS TEXT

In this text, health is defined as a person's level of wellness. This level of wellness is a process in which a person strives to attain his or her full potential. Health reflects a person's biologic, psychologic, and sociologic state (Figure 1-2). The *biologic* (physical) state refers to the structure of body tissues and organs as well as to the biochemical interactions and functions within the body. The *psychologic* state includes a person's mood, emotions, and personality. The *sociologic* (social) state involves the interaction between a person and the environment. *Spiritual health* is sometimes considered to be part of sociologic health but may be described as a separate aspect of the overall health state. Factors that affect a person's biologic, psychologic, or sociologic well-being require additional energy and alter the level of wellness.

A high level of wellness is achieved when these biopsychosocial needs are met. One of the primary functions of nursing is to assist clients in reaching this high level of wellness. It is therefore essential that nurses understand the concept of health and high-level wellness. As nurses assess clients, they must be aware of factors that affect a person's health state and must use nursing interventions to promote and maintain an optimal level of wellness (Figure 1-3).

Quality of Life

Over the past decade the concept of **quality of life (QOL)** has emerged as a broad, multidimensional description of a client's health and functional status. Cella (1994) proposed two domains for QOL measurement: subjectivity and multidimensionality. *Subjectivity* refers to clients' perceptions of satisfaction with their functional level, including activities of daily living (e.g., dressing) and independent living skills (e.g., shopping). *Multidimensionality* refers to physical, functional, emotional, and social well-being. Through her nursing research with cancer clients, Ferrell (1996) conceptualized QOL as having four domains: physical, psychological, social, and spiritual well-being.

Over the past few years, researchers have used a number of assessment tools to quantify QOL in clients with chronic diseases (Ferrell et al., 1998; Lash, 1998). Their findings can guide nurses in providing holistic care for these individuals (see the Evidence-Based Practice for Nursing box below).

HEALTH PROMOTION AND PROTECTION

Health promotion and protection refers to activities that are directed toward developing a person's resources to maintain or enhance well-being as a protection against illness. Reversing the emphasis from curing a disease to promoting health provides a more positive orientation for health care. Illness no longer needs to be the primary focus of health care. In addition, illness care is much more expensive than health promotion.

In 1990 the U.S. Department of Health and Human Services (DHHS) joined the world mission to promote health in its "Healthy People 2000" campaign. The expectation was that people would be healthier and would be practicing healthier lifestyles by the year 2000. In particular, the agenda called for health care access for everyone, a longer life expectancy, and equal life expectancy for people of all cultures. These goals have not been met. For example, some ethnic groups in the United States—especially Hispanics, African Americans, Asian Americans, and Pacific Islanders—continue to have shorter life expectancies than other groups.

"Healthy People 2010" (DHHS, 2000) has been published to revise these goals and present a more aggressive plan to improve the nation's health by focusing on health promotion practices. This plan has two overall national health goals:

- Increase quality and years of healthy life
- Eliminate health disparities among different demographic groups in the United States

The Healthy People (HP) initiative focuses on 28 areas devoted to an array of diseases, conditions, and public health challenges. Each focus area lists specific health objectives to meet by 2010. These objectives target interventions designed to reduce or eliminate illness, disability, and premature deaths. This text contains special boxes entitled "Meeting Healthy People 2010 Objectives" that list some of the key objectives from the document and the interventions that nurses can implement to help meet those national health objectives.

EVIDENCE-BASED PRACTICE FOR NURSING

What is the quality of life for clients with breast cancer?

Ferrell, B.R. et al. (1998). Quality of life in breast cancer: Part 2. Psychological and spiritual well-being. *Cancer Nursing,* 21(1), 1-9.

This qualitative research explored the psychologic and spiritual aspects of the quality of life for 21 long-term survivors of breast cancer. Examples of the subjects' sources of stress included bone marrow/stem cell transplantation, radiation, chemotherapy, breast reconstruction, hospitalization, and completion of treatment. Emotions that the subjects typically experienced were depression, fear, positive coping, increasing control/loss of control, concentration, and an improved mood since their diagnosis.

Three themes related to spirituality emerged from the data: support of spirituality, aspects of spirituality, and having an altered life. Most of the subjects believed that spirituality played an important role, giving them hope when they were uncertain.

Critique. Although the sample size is small, this exploratory research provides data for analysis regarding the quality of life for cancer survivors. For many women, the research interview allowed them to express feelings they had not previously confronted. Few studies have explored the psychologic and spiritual aspects of quality of life. Most studies have focused on the physical and social aspects.

Implications for Nursing. The information provided in this study can assist nurses in understanding the feelings experienced by clients with breast cancer. Nurses should allow clients to ventilate their feelings and support them as they balance hope with reality.

CULTURAL CONSIDERATIONS

The demographic profile of the U.S. population includes many groups that are vulnerable to multiple health problems. Three of these groups are Latinos, African Americans, and Asian Americans/Pacific Islanders.

Although the African-American population is currently the largest nonwhite ethnic group in the country, the Latino population is expected to outnumber African Americans by the year 2010. The Bureau of the Census (1997) states that 11% of the population are Latino immigrants who are identified as Spanish-speaking surnamed people of Latin America. Decreased access to health care, lack of knowledge regarding health, lifestyle choices, and environmental factors negatively affect the health of Latinos. For example, poor nutrition and lack of exercise lead to obesity, especially in Latino women. Excessive use of drugs, alcohol, and cigarettes are common health risk factors among men (Flaskerud & Kim, 1999). In view of these lifestyle factors, it is not surprising that heart disease, diabetes mellitus, cancer, human immunodeficiency virus (HIV) infection, and liver disease are much higher among Latino adults than among Caucasians.

African Americans are the most vulnerable of all populations in the United States (Davis & Curley, 1999). Nearly one third of African Americans live in poverty, compared with 11% of Caucasians. Cancer, heart disease, diabetes mellitus, and HIV infection lead to higher mortality rates among African Americans compared with Caucasians. This is partly because many African Americans lack access to health care and are reluctant to seek health promotion care, especially primary prevention and early detection (Davis & Curley, 1999).

Asian Americans and Pacific Islanders (A/PIs) currently represent between 3% and 4% of the U.S. population; that number is expected to jump to 10% by the year 2050 (Shinagawa & Jang, 1998). In 20 years the mortality rates for A/PIs with lung cancer and cardiovascular disease are expected to exceed those of other ethnic groups. In addition, the prevalence of hepatitis B and tuberculosis is higher among A/PIs than among any other ethnic group. Like Latinos, many A/PIs lack access to health care and have lifestyle and environmental factors that influence their health status.

Beliefs about health and illness for Latinos, African Americans, and A/PIs are strongly guided by religion. Chapters 4 and 6 discuss the cultural and spiritual aspects of health in more detail. In addition, Cultural Considerations are highlighted throughout this text, and research related to cultural health is presented where appropriate.

WOMEN'S HEALTH CONSIDERATIONS

Historically, women's health issues have not been studied, especially for women of color (non-Caucasian). Recent interest in women's health has shown that many women in the United States do not receive necessary health care, have many undetected and treatable problems, and experience long-lasting effects of abuse. Women of color are more likely to be poor and uninsured than are Caucasian women. All women are at serious risk for heart disease, lung cancer, and osteoporosis, but they often lack knowledge regarding how to prevent these health problems (Allen & Phillips, 1997).

Today the National Institutes of Health strongly support research on women's health. Women's health considerations are highlighted as appropriate throughout this text, and research on women's health issues is included when possible.

Several nursing theorists have developed health promotion models for nursing. One of the best-known models is that advocated by Pender. In her classic model, Pender (1987) makes a distinction between health promotion and illness prevention: Health promotion is not "health problem specific," but illness prevention (most recently called health protection) is. Pender believes that health promotion is a positive activity, whereas illness prevention is an avoidance activity.

Although this text integrates health promotion and illness prevention (health protection), it recognizes that the two concepts are somewhat different. The goal of both types of activities is to improve or maintain the client's health.

Part of the health promotion movement in nursing is reflected in the use of the term *client* rather than *patient*. The word *patient* is associated with a dependent position in a hospital, whereas the word *client* suggests an active partnership in the process of health care delivery and maintenance in any setting. Therefore *client* is the term used for the health care consumer in this text.

Practices to Promote Health

Researchers have found that certain health practices have a positive correlation with health promotion in adults. These general health practices include the following:

- Eating well-balanced meals that incorporate foods from the food pyramid, as recommended (see Figure 61-2)
- Eating moderately to maintain ideal weight and prevent obesity
- Exercising moderately on a routine schedule
- Sleeping regularly, approximately 8 hours each day
- Limiting alcohol consumption to a moderate amount
- Not smoking
- Keeping exposure to the sun to a minimum

These practices have been associated with high-level wellness regardless of sex, age, or economic status. The greater the number of these practices followed in a consistent, routine manner, the better the health state.

Practices to Prevent Illness

Illness prevention is related to health protection and maintenance. Prevention is essential to efforts to decrease the occurrence of illness. Preventive health behavior is described as a voluntary action taken by a person or group to decrease the potential or actual threat of illness and its harmful consequences. As mentioned earlier, some ethnic groups are not focused on health promotion activities, especially prevention and early detection. Throughout this text, these cultural considerations are discussed where appropriate.

People must be motivated and educated to make health-related changes. Three levels of illness prevention are summarized in Table 1-1: primary, secondary, and tertiary.

TABLE 1-1 • EXAMPLES OF HEALTH BEHAVIORS FOR THE THREE LEVELS OF ILLNESS PREVENTION

Level	Examples of Behaviors
Primary prevention	Wearing seat belts, helmets Eating well-balanced meals Not smoking Consuming no or minimal alcohol Being immunized Maintaining ideal body weight
Secondary prevention	Having yearly Papanicolaou (Pap) smear tests Performing a monthly breast or testicular self-examination Having mammograms as recommended Getting skin tests for tuberculosis screening Having routine tonometry tests to detect glaucoma
Tertiary prevention	Following a cardiac rehabilitation program Pursuing rehabilitation programs for stroke, head injury, or arthritis

PRIMARY PREVENTION

Primary prevention is used to avoid or delay the actual occurrence of a specific disease. Strategies for health maintenance raise the general level of health and well-being of a person, family, or community. Smoking cessation clinics, immunizations, the use of seat belts, and the use of helmets by motorcyclists are examples of primary prevention strategies.

SECONDARY PREVENTION

The purpose of **secondary prevention** is early detection of a disease or condition, sometimes before the signs and symptoms are evident. The emphasis is on early diagnosis and treatment as well as on intervention to prevent or limit permanent disability or death. Screening procedures such as the Papanicolaou (Pap) smear for cervical cancer and the purified protein derivative (PPD) skin test for tuberculosis are examples of secondary prevention.

TERTIARY PREVENTION

Tertiary prevention involves rehabilitation and begins when the disease or condition has stabilized and no further healing is expected, such as cardiac rehabilitation after a myocardial infarction. The goal is to return the person to the highest level of function and to prevent severe disabilities.

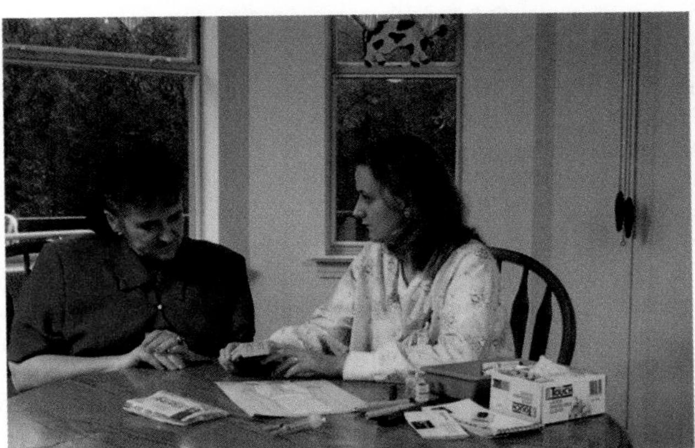

Figure 1-4 ● Medical-surgical nurses care for adult clients in various settings with such chronic disorders as diabetes mellitus. (From Harkreader, H.C. (2000). *Fundamentals of nursing: Caring and clinical judgment.* W.B. Saunders: Philadelphia.)

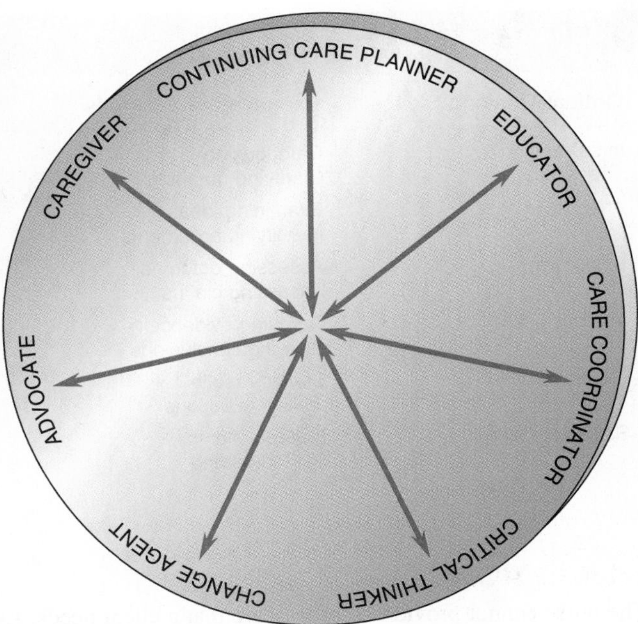

Figure 1-5 ● Major roles of the medical-surgical nurse.

Consumer Education and Awareness

Consumer education and awareness has been a major focus in an attempt to influence people and promote wellness. Information about nutrition, exercise, stress management, and routine health examinations is available at schools, work sites, and community centers, as well as in the media. This abundance of information and materials is a major resource for increasing public awareness of the need for health promotion. The Internet provides access to a vast amount of professional and public health information. See the SIMON website at http://www.wbsaunders.com/SIMON/Iggy/ for a list of commonly used websites, including the website for the complete "Healthy People 2010" document.

ROLE OF THE MEDICAL-SURGICAL NURSE

Medical-surgical nursing is one of the many specialties in nursing, yet its scope is much broader than other specialties such as cardiovascular or orthopedic nursing. In 1991, the Academy of Medical-Surgical Nurses (AMSN) was formed as the first specialty organization for this group of nurses. AMSN has published standards for medical-surgical nursing and a core curriculum. The official journal of the AMSN is *MEDSURG Nursing: The Journal of Adult Health.*

The focus of medical-surgical nursing is on the adult client with acute or chronic illness in any health care setting or on the client who is at risk for illness (Figure 1-4). Nurses who specialize in medical-surgical nursing need to have a broad knowledge of the biologic, psychologic, and social sciences because of their range of clients. The overall outcome of care is similar to that for any other specialty—the achievement of an optimal level of wellness and the prevention of illness.

Because the typical client is usually older than 65 years of age, medical-surgical nurses need a strong background in *gerontology,* or the care of older adults. In this text, charts entitled Nursing Focus on the Older Adult highlight the special nursing interventions required by this group of clients. In addition, Considerations for Older Adults are discussed as appropriate throughout this text.

As medical-surgical nursing meets changing health care needs, the expectations for providing client care expand and increase. Medical-surgical nurses assume various roles and functions within a number of health care settings (Figure 1-5). Although each role is associated with specific responsibilities, some aspects are interrelated and are common to all nursing positions and specialties.

Critical Thinker

Critical thinking, sometimes referred to as clinical reasoning or judgment, is an essential competency that all nurses need to provide quality, cost-effective client care. Alfaro-LeFevre (1999) describes critical thinking as purposeful, outcome-directed thinking that aims to make judgments based on scientific evidence rather than tradition or conjecture (guesswork). Evidence is most often the result of research, and nursing has increased its research findings on which to base its practice. The term **evidence-based practice** is often used in the profession to describe the care that nurses provide based on research and identified standards. Throughout this text, Evidence-Based Practice for Nursing boxes summarize and critique some of the most current research for medical-surgical nursing. Nursing implications are also discussed to help the nurse apply these findings to daily practice.

In their classic article, Facione and Facione (1996) discuss the relationship of critical thinking to nursing according to the 1990 consensus definition of the American Philosophical Association (APA). The APA delineated the most important critical thinking skills and subskills required for critical thinking. Medical-surgical nurses use all of these skills (Table 1-2). Critical Thinking Challenges are threaded throughout this book to help the student or licensed nurse understand the why and how of nursing and interdisciplinary client care. Additional critical thinking activities may be found at http://www.wbsaunders.com/SIMON/Iggy/.

TABLE 1-2 • ESSENTIAL CRITICAL THINKING SKILLS AND EXAMPLES OF SUBSKILLS

Critical Thinking Skill	Examples of Subskills
Interpretation	Categorizing Clarifying meaning
Analysis	Examining ideas Identifying arguments
Evaluation	Assessing outcomes Assessing claims
Inference	Querying evidence Drawing conclusions
Explanation	Stating results Justifying actions
Self-regulation	Self-examining Self-correcting

Coordinator of Care

The nurse cannot provide all of the care that a client needs. As a *care coordinator,* the medical-surgical nurse collaborates with the health care team to help the client meet expected outcomes identified as part of the interdisciplinary plan of care. Interdisciplinary clinical rounds and other methods for communication facilitate the process of planning and implementation.

Caregiver

Another role commonly associated with the medical-surgical nurse is *caregiver.* In this role, nurses assess clients, analyze collected information to determine clients' needs, develop nursing diagnoses and collaborative problems, plan care and carry out the plan with the health care team, and evaluate the care given. This process, which is referred to as the nursing process and discussed on p. 11, is used throughout this text as an organizational and practice framework.

As a caregiver, the nurse provides physical care through skills such as administering medications and performing comprehensive assessments. Some nursing tasks and activities may be delegated to assistive nursing personnel. Interventions that the nurse may delegate are indicated throughout this text and in the Client Care Plans. The nurse also implements psychosocial interventions, such as encouraging the client to discuss concerns or offering measures to reduce anxiety.

The activities performed by the nurse caregiver are often categorized as *collaborative* (interdependent) or *independent. Collaborative* functions include the following:

- Those that are mutually determined by the nurse and the physician or other health care team member, such as setting activity limitations or providing a special diet
- Those that are directed or prescribed by the health care provider (physician, nurse practitioner, or physician's assistant) but require nursing judgment to perform (e.g., administering medications)

Independent nursing functions are initiated and carried out by the nurse without direction from the health care provider. Examples include the following:

- Weighing a client
- Listening to bowel sounds
- Elevating the head of the bed to facilitate breathing

This text discusses both types of functions—collaborative and independent—in an interrelated framework under the heading *Collaborative Management.* Charts entitled Best Practice identify the most important nursing care for clients with selected health problems.

Continuing Care Planner

Because health care continues to emphasize early discharge from the hospital, nursing home, and home care, the role of the medical-surgical nurse as a continuing care planner has become increasingly important. This process involves an assessment of the client's health needs across the health care continuum. A large part of this process is health teaching and assessment of the home (or other setting to which the client is discharged) for available resources, support systems, and equipment, if needed.

Continuing care planning may be coordinated by a case manager or by a designated discharge planner employed by the agency in collaboration with the staff nurse. The discharge planner or case manager is usually a nurse or social worker. If the agency does not employ designated discharge planners, the staff nurse caring for the client is typically responsible for the continuing care planning. Throughout this text, sections entitled Community-Based Care are included to facilitate planning and describe settings in which continuing care may be needed (see also Chapter 2).

Educator

Client education is a major component of medical-surgical nursing care. In collaboration with the interdisciplinary health team, the nurse tries to improve health by facilitating client learning regarding health promotion, disease and illness, and specific treatment. As educators, nurses work with individual clients and family members or other caregivers. The role of education has become increasingly important because clients are discharged "quicker and sicker" from the hospital, subacute unit, or nursing home. Nurses often become frustrated when they feel they do not have the time they need to teach in these fast-paced settings.

THE TEACHING-LEARNING PROCESS

In collaboration with other members of the health care team, the nurse assesses the client's learning needs and barriers to learning. A client with a disease of 20 years' duration may need as much teaching as one with a newly diagnosed condition. The nurse makes no assumptions but instead assesses each client individually. The client's goals and willingness to learn are also determined. If the client has no interest in learning, the nurse waits for another time or setting before beginning client education. Chart 1-1 summarizes the most important teaching-learning principles for adults.

Teaching may occur in a spontaneous, informal manner, or it may follow a more structured, formal approach based on written teaching plans. Most facilities provide written teaching plans and tools for the interdisciplinary team to ensure that every client receives the same accurate information.

The nurse documents on the appropriate record what was taught and what the client learned (Figure 1-6). Some health care agencies use a lay version of the clinical pathway as a learning tool that outlines care in a sequential manner for the

CHART 1-1

BEST PRACTICE *for* Adult Learning

- Assess the client's goals and willingness to learn.
- Before beginning teaching, assess how the client is feeling (e.g., a client in acute pain is unlikely to learn).
- Include family and significant others in teaching as appropriate.
- Assess factors that may influence the client's ability or motivation to learn, such as educational level, socioeconomic status, and cultural background.
- Provide pictures or other types of visual aids to reinforce learning.
- Break complex information or skills into small parts until the client learns them.
- Provide the client with "hands-on" experience for psychomotor skills, and request a return demonstration by the client (e.g., insulin administration, dressing change, colostomy care).
- Provide the client with a health resource contact for follow-up questions or concerns.

client (see Developing the Collaborative Plan of Care, p. 14). In general, a summary of the teaching-learning process for each client becomes a part of the client's medical record. A copy is also given to the client or family member or significant other at discharge. EachCommunity-Based Care section within this text includes a subsection entitled Health Teaching. Client Education Guides for teaching clients are also included as appropriate throughout the text.

FACTORS AFFECTING THE TEACHING-LEARNING PROCESS

As interdisciplinary team members assess the teaching-learning needs of each client, they evaluate many factors that may enhance or impede learning. Some of the most important factors include the client's educational level, socioeconomic level, support system, age, and cultural considerations.

Educational Level

The client's educational level directly affects the nurse's plans for teaching. In the United States it is estimated that more than one third of adults do not have a high school diploma. Consequently, illiteracy in the United States is quite widespread. Therefore information written for the public should not be above the sixth-grade reading level, and it often needs to be lower.

For illiterate clients and for those with limited reading skills, the nurse uses other types of visual aids (e.g., pictures and videos). When possible, the nurse explains and interprets information for clients rather than merely offering them a booklet or instruction sheet.

Socioeconomic Level

The nurse must consider the clients' financial resources when teaching them how to care for themselves at home. For example, if a client needs to perform muscle-strengthening exercises using small weights, the nurse cannot expect the client to purchase expensive commercial weights. Instead, the nurse suggests the use of 1- or 2-pound coffee cans or bags, bags of sugar or flour, or similar household items.

Teaching-Learning Record for Insulin Self-Administration			
Client Steps	Taught/ Demonstrated (Initial)	Date	Return Demonstration (Initial)
1. Selects correct insulin type.			
2. Selects correct syringe.			
3. Cleans top of vial.			
4. Draws up correct insulin amount(s).			
5. Selects appropriate site for injection.			
6. Cleans skin with alcohol swipe.			
7. Uses 90-degree angle when injecting insulin.			

Figure 1-6 ● A sample teaching-learning record for the self-administration of insulin.

Another concern for the nurse is the cost of required medications, equipment, or supplies. Clients who do not qualify for medical assistance but work for an employer that does not provide group health insurance may not be able to afford the necessary medical items or follow-up care. As part of continuing care planning, the nurse attempts to locate resources that can provide the necessary items, such as community health organizations (e.g., American Cancer Society). Clinics that specialize in providing care for working and uninsured clients are available in some parts of the United States. Some of these clinics are nurse-managed community centers.

Support Systems

The nurse assesses the client's support systems and should include part or all of these systems in client education. Examples of support systems include families, significant others, churches, and social community clubs and organizations. In general, people tend to be more compliant with their health regimen if they have the encouragement of others. Support is particularly important if the client must follow many lifestyle restrictions. For instance, a farmer who may be accustomed to eating fried foods and red meat may find it difficult to change to a low-fat, low-sodium diet. If the farmer's wife has always been the cook in the home, the nurse includes her in the teaching process to help ensure compliance with the new dietary restrictions.

Age

Age also affects the teaching-learning process. An older adult may take longer to process information or may have visual or hearing deficits (Chart 1-2). The nurse provides small

CHART 1-2

NURSING FOCUS *on the* OLDER ADULT
Facilitating Learning

- Ensure that the client wears glasses or hearing aids if needed.
- Be sure that the area for teaching has ample lighting and minimal distraction.
- Provide most of the teaching in the morning (after breakfast), before the client becomes too fatigued.
- Speak slowly, and provide small amounts of new information at a time.
- Ask the client to repeat the information to make sure that he or she has learned it.
- Provide written information so the client can refer to it later if needed.

CULTURAL CONSIDERATIONS

The nurse considers the client's cultural background before teaching. If the client does not clearly understand the primary language, the nurse locates resources that can help with the teaching process. For example, many people who emigrated to the United States in the 1940s have attempted to retain their language and culture and not become too "Americanized." As a result, when interacting with health care professionals, they often cannot understand and need someone to interpret for them.

Another factor to consider during health teaching is the health practices of various cultures. For example, Mexican Americans, particularly those living near the Mexican border, often use *curandismo* (folk medicine) either because they cannot afford Westernized health care or because they prefer their own medical traditions. These clients may also avoid the health care system because of limitations in speaking, reading, or writing English or Spanish. The nurse also considers spiritual and religious differences. A client whose spiritual beliefs forbid taking medication is not likely to comply with instructions about drug therapy. The nurse needs to know this information so he or she can incorporate cultural beliefs and practices into the teaching-learning process.

amounts of information at a time and checks with the client before proceeding to make sure that he or she has understood. Too much information is difficult to comprehend and absorb and usually results in frustration and noncompliance.

Advocate

As a client advocate, the medical-surgical nurse assists the client and family in interpreting information from other health care team members. The nurse offers additional assistance that the client needs in making decisions about health care. Such assistance may include explaining the implications of the client's decisions and ensuring that the client receives appropriate care. For example, a client scheduled for a total knee replacement may not understand that the knee joint will be removed and replaced with a prosthesis. If the nurse determines that the client does not fully understand the operative procedure, he or she notifies the surgeon of the need for additional preoperative education. The information is reinforced even if another health team member has provided it.

Change Agent

The medical-surgical nurse serves as a change agent within the work setting and within the profession. The role of the change agent involves planning and implementing a system to change the client's health-related behaviors. In the work setting, the nurse assesses the health behaviors of the client and family and identifies those that need altering. The most important factor in this process is assessing the client's readiness to change. If the client is not ready, he or she will not comply with the change, and the nurse will be ineffective in this role.

Within the community, medical-surgical nurses serve as role models and assist consumers in bringing about changes to improve the environment, work conditions, or other factors that affect health. Nurses also work together to bring about change through legislation. For example, they provide and support legislative bills that can affect a person's health status, such as those that mandate a client's bill of rights.

THE CONCEPT OF CARING

A critical attribute for medical-surgical nurses is caring. Nurse caring has been broadly described as a process, a set of actions, and an attitude that conveys physical care and emotional concern for others. Nurses have been studying and practicing caring for many years, yet confusion remains about a precise definition of caring. Debate also continues among nursing theorists and researchers regarding the best method for measuring human caring (McCance, McKenna, & Boone, 1997; Beck, 1999).

The results of a study by Barr and Bush (1998) found four factors or broad examples of caring in critical care nurses:

- Support from colleagues (nurses they work with)
- Nurses modeling care (and caring)
- Observable client progress and positive client and family interaction
- Economic/bureaucratic factors (negative factors that nurses must overcome)

When providing client care, the nurse subjects in the study stated that listening and caring were key caring techniques. Today's medical-surgical nurses who work in hospitals often feel they do not have time to listen to or show caring toward their clients. The focus of client care is often on technical tasks rather than on outcomes or psychosocial interventions such as caring. However, in keeping with the definition of health and the role of the nurse, clients need to have their biopsychosocial needs met to promote health and prevent illness.

PRACTICE SETTINGS FOR MEDICAL-SURGICAL NURSES

Medical-surgical nurses have opportunities to provide health care in a variety of settings, including hospitals, long-term care facilities, and community-based settings (Figure 1-7). The hospital setting is described in this chapter. Chapter 2 discusses community-based settings.

Hospitals, or acute care facilities, have historically been the largest employers of nurses, with slightly more than half of all nurses working within hospitals. This percentage is declining as hospitals continue to "rightsize" and as care continues to move into the community. Few hospitals are free-

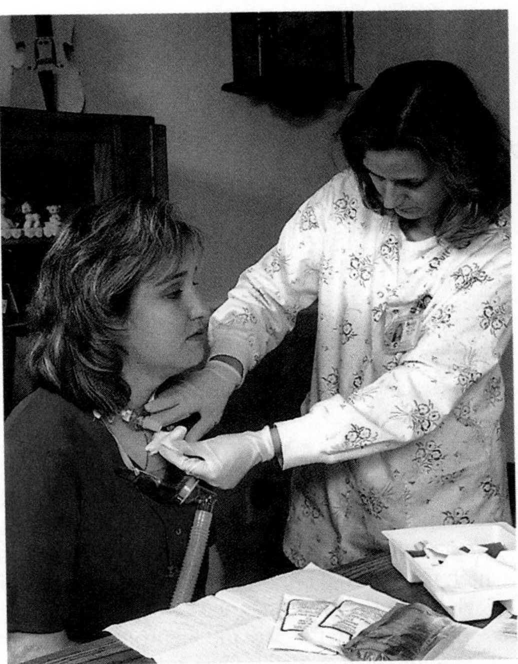

Figure 1-7 ● Nurses often care for clients in the home. (From Harkreader, H.C. (2000). *Fundamentals of nursing: Caring and clinical judgment.* W.B. Saunders: Philadelphia.)

standing today. Most are part of an integrated health care system (IHS) that typically comprises inpatient and ambulatory facilities and may include long-term care and home health components.

In the United States, most hospital care costs are paid for by third-party payers, either managed care organizations or traditional insurers. Medicare Part A (in-hospital coverage), a federal program, pays for most of the acute care given to people who are older than 65 years of age or who have been disabled for at least 2 years. State medical assistance programs, often managed care Medicaid, pay for some of the health care provided to clients of any age who are indigent.

In Canada, all people are entitled to free comprehensive health care for life. The Canadian government started this system in the 1960s with the belief that health care should be accessible to all Canadian citizens.

There are three general types of inpatient units in most hospital settings:

- Critical care units
- Intermediate or specialty care units
- Long-term care units (including subacute units)

Critical Care Units

Critical care units are areas for the intense care of critically ill clients. Examples are surgical or medical intensive care units, shock trauma and "step-down" units, and neurosurgical intensive care units. Emergency and operating departments are also considered critical care areas because of the acute and intense nature of the care provided in these parts of the hospital. Critical care areas require nurses who thrive in crisis situations and work effectively under high stress. Nurses in these areas must be highly skilled in making accurate observations of clients' conditions and in interpreting findings quickly and correctly. The nurse-to-client ratio in critical care units is typically 1:2 or 1:3 depending on the acuity of the clients.

Intermediate or Specialty Care Units

Intermediate care units have changed dramatically over the past decade. The clients on these units are much sicker today than in the past. Examples of specialty intermediate care areas are neuroscience (neurology) units, urology units, and orthopedic units. In hospitals that are too small to separate clients by specialty, intermediate care units provide treatment for a combination of medical and surgical health problems.

Nurses in intermediate care areas must be able to adapt to caring for various types of illness and must be competent in health teaching and discharge planning. As in critical care areas, nurses must also be highly skilled in critical thinking and psychomotor tasks.

Long-Term Care Units

Long-term care (LTC) units may be found within or adjacent to a hospital for clients with chronic illnesses or health problems that require a finite period of medical care or rehabilitation. These units may also be referred to as transitional care units, skilled nursing facilities (SNF), or subacute units. Most long-term care is provided in freestanding nursing homes. Chapter 2 describes long-term care in more detail.

OVERVIEW OF THE NURSING PROCESS

The nursing process is an organized, systematic approach used by medical-surgical nurses to meet the individualized health care needs of their clients, families, and communities. The term **nursing process** emerged in the mid-1960s. As nursing became more recognized and respected as a profession, there was a growing need to define more clearly what nurses do.

Comparison of the Nursing Process with the Scientific Method

The nursing process is a decision-making approach that enhances critical thinking. Many textbooks compare the nursing process with the scientific method of solving problems. The steps in these two approaches are similar—they both proceed from identification of the problem to evaluation of the solution. One difference is that the scientist identifies the problem first and then collects the data, whereas the nurse collects the data first and then determines the problem.

Intuitive Judgment in Nursing Practice

Over the past 20 years, research has shown that nurses sometimes use (and should use) intuitive judgment in clinical practice (Benner & Tanner, 1987). *Intuition* is the ability to understand immediately without using formal analysis; it is based on experience and knowledge. Intuition helps the nurse to act quickly if necessary, particularly in critical care settings or emergency situations in which he or she must assess the client and intervene at once.

The authors of this text use the nursing process as the organizing framework for its content. We do not believe that the nursing process is merely a technical skill with rules that apply in all situations but rather that nurses need to use intuition as well as a scientific basis for nursing care.

Steps of the Nursing Process

Most literature citations list five steps for the nursing process: assessment, analysis (nursing diagnosis), planning, implementation, and evaluation.

The steps are usually followed in sequence, from assessment to evaluation. However, once the nursing process begins, it is continuous or cyclic (Figure 1-8). For example, if the client's outcomes are not met on the basis of the initial evaluation, the nurse may need to reassess the client or implement new actions to help achieve the desired outcomes. To understand the nursing process as a whole, it is first necessary to briefly review each step and its associated activities. A more detailed discussion of the nursing process may be found in basic nursing textbooks.

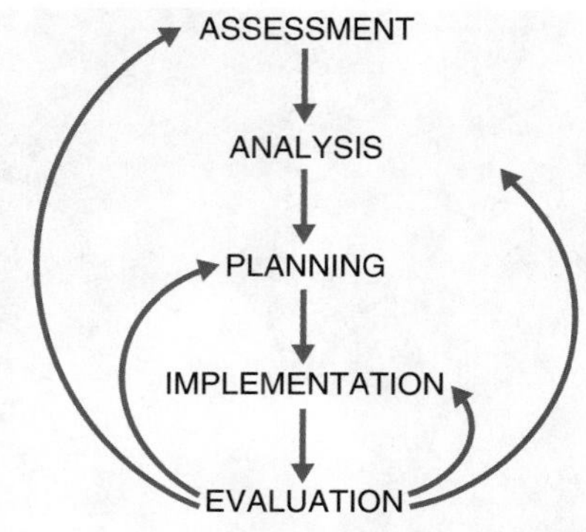

Figure 1-8 ● The nursing process cycle.

ASSESSMENT

Assessment, the first step of the nursing process, is a systematic method of collecting data about the client, family, or community for the purpose of identifying actual and potential health problems. The **database** is the organization of assessment data and often refers to the tool or chart form used to record the data.

Admission/First Visit Database

The complete database includes a thorough health history, physical assessment, and psychosocial assessment. In the acute care setting the admission database is usually completed during the first 8 hours after a client's admission to the hospital. Assessments are updated at least every shift throughout the client's stay. In the home or ambulatory care setting, the nurse completes the database during the first visit and updates it during subsequent visits.

In the skilled nursing unit or nursing home, the admission nursing assessment is documented within the first 24 hours. The federally mandated and standardized interdisciplinary Minimum Data Set (MDS) requires completion within 7 days of admission.

The information collected by the nurse is *not* a repetition of the medical history recorded by the health care provider. A *medical* history is obtained by the health care provider to determine the presence of a pathologic condition and to provide a basis for planning medical care. A *nursing* history is obtained by the nurse and focuses on the meaning of the illness and/or hospitalization to the client and family. It is used as a basis for planning nursing care. The nurse collects additional data regarding the client's response to health problems, functional ability, ability to perform activities of daily living, usual health behaviors, coping patterns, health goals, and support systems.

Episodic, or Problem-Centered, Database

An episodic database is collected for a limited or short-term problem. It focuses on one problem, and the data collected are associated with the problem. For example, an older hospitalized woman falls while trying to get out of bed and complains of hip pain. The nurse's history focuses on how the fall occurred, which parts of the client's body made contact with the floor, and what position she assumed after she fell. The physical assessment is centered on the neurologic and musculoskeletal systems, especially the head, hip, and knee. These data are usually recorded on a variance form according to agency policy.

In other situations, the nurse documents assessment findings on a flow sheet at frequent intervals during the day. For example, the client who is receiving epidural analgesia must be monitored continuously to determine whether the intervention is successful and whether adverse effects occur.

Sources of Data

The nurse obtains and documents data from several sources in the client's medical record according to the policies of the health care agency.

CLIENT

The client is the primary source of data. This information is direct and firsthand and is collected during an interview. Interviewing is a communication skill by which the nurse can explore the thoughts, feelings, and perceptions of the client. As in the teaching-learning process, the interview process is affected by many variables, including timing, environment, and demographic factors such as age. Chart 1-3 provides tips for interviewing an older adult.

FAMILY AND SIGNIFICANT OTHERS

The client's family members or significant others are secondary sources of data and can often supplement or verify information provided by the client. They may also be able to offer information about the client before the illness, provide a family history related to health and illness, and describe the client's home environment.

RECORDS

Previous medical histories, laboratory records, vital signs, and diagnostic reports provide pertinent data. These data can val-

CHART 1-3

NURSING FOCUS *on the* OLDER ADULT
Interviewing

- Review old records and the medical history, if available, before interviewing the client.
- Provide as much privacy as possible.
- Ask the client whether family or significant others should be present during the interview.
- Refer to the client by his or her last name (e.g., Mrs. Brown) unless he or she prefers another name.
- Make sure that eyeglasses, contact lenses, and hearing aids are available and working properly (if the client wears these devices).
- Conduct the interview when the client is not experiencing pain and after basic comfort needs have been met.
- Before conducting the interview, allow the client to adjust to a new environment.
- Sit at the client's eye level during the interview.
- Speak clearly, slowly, and in a low-pitched voice; do not shout.
- Be aware that the client may not be able to distinguish soft consonant blends such as "sh" or "ch."
- Interview in the morning, after breakfast, or in the early afternoon, after the client has rested.
- Whenever possible, use open-ended questions to gather more information; avoid questions that can be answered "yes" or "no."
- Consider the client's education, culture, and age when phrasing questions, especially about sensitive or controversial issues.
- Observe the client's nonverbal behavior as well as what he or she says.

idate information identified in the current history and physical examination or can serve as a comparison to indicate changes in the client's health condition. Records from previous hospital admissions supply additional pieces of information. The client's health care provider usually requests the old records from the agency's medical records department or other health care facility where the client has sought health care.

COLLABORATION

A nurse often gathers client information in collaboration with other members of the health care team. The physician or nurse practitioner is a key source of information. A social worker or home care nurse who has worked with the client can also contribute valuable information.

When a client is admitted to the hospital from another health care facility, such as a nursing home, the hospital nurse should contact the nurse who cared for the client in the previous facility for specific client information. Most nursing homes supply a transfer form that accompanies the client to the hospital or other facility. This form describes the client's abilities and limitations, drug therapy, diet therapy, and past and current health state. This information is particularly helpful when the client cannot communicate and when no family is available.

ANALYSIS

The second step of the nursing process is the analysis of data. In this phase, the nurse summarizes and analyzes the data and draws conclusions to determine what health problems the client may have or is at risk for. Client data are compared with "normal" findings and behaviors for the client's age, education, and cultural background. Abnormal data are reviewed to determine patterns of altered functioning. Client health problems are identified and categorized as potential problems requiring prevention or as actual problems being managed or requiring interventions.

In their classic book, Aspinall and Tanner (1981) state that nurses make two types of judgments or conclusions about the health state of a client: (1) those health problems that nurses, "by virtue of their education and experience, are licensed and able to treat" (nursing diagnoses), and (2) those problems that are diagnosed and treated by other members of the health care team but require continued nursing assessment and implementation of therapeutic interventions (collaborative problems) (p. 4). This textbook uses nursing diagnoses and collaborative problems that incorporate both types of client health problems.

Nursing Diagnosis

The nursing profession's acknowledgment and endorsement of the term *nursing diagnosis* began in 1973, when the American Nurses Association (ANA) published its first *Standards of Nursing Practice.* Since then, other countries have adopted nursing diagnoses as a way to describe client health problems.

Although many definitions of nursing diagnosis have been proposed by various nursing leaders, the authors of this text recognize the official definition approved by the North American Nursing Diagnosis Association (NANDA) at its Ninth Conference in 1990: "A nursing diagnosis is a clinical judgment about an individual, family, or community response to actual or potential health problems/life processes which provides the basis for definitive therapy toward achievement of outcomes for which the nurse is accountable" (Carpenito, 1995, p. 65).

Unlike medical diagnoses, which identify illness, nursing diagnoses identify the *responses* to health problems and life processes such as aging or death. A medical diagnosis is the basis for medical interventions; a nursing diagnosis is the basis for nursing interventions. Nursing diagnoses are not diagnostic tests, medical treatments, or problems experienced by the nurse while caring for the client. Table 1-3 differentiates between medical and nursing diagnoses.

Collaborative Problems

Collaborative problems, as identified in this text, are potential health problems for which the nurse monitors. If these problems occur, the nurse alerts the primary care provider. Measures that help to prevent the problem are implemented. Through keen assessment skills, the nurse detects the health problem as early as possible if it occurs. Then, in collaboration with members of the interdisciplinary care team, he or she carries out interventions to resolve the problem. An example of a collaborative problem is Potential for Hypoglycemia for a client with diabetes.

PLANNING

The planning step follows the analysis step of the nursing process. Throughout the planning process, the nurse performs

TABLE 1-3 • DIFFERENTIATION BETWEEN MEDICAL AND NURSING DIAGNOSES

Medical Diagnosis	Nursing Diagnosis
Identifies the pathologic basis for an illness	Identifies a response to illness
Focuses on the physical condition of the client	Focuses on the physical, psychosocial, and spiritual needs of the client
Addresses actual, existing problems	Addresses actual and potential problems
Is not validated with the client	Is validated with the client if possible
Uses standardized goals and treatments	Uses individualized outcomes and intervention
May not be resolvable	Is usually resolvable

several important functions: setting priorities and expected outcomes, selecting nursing interventions, and determining resources.

Setting Priorities and Outcomes

After analyzing the needs of the client to identify client health problems, the nurse decides on the urgency of these problems. This step is vital because some problems are more critical than others. Problems of higher priority require more immediate intervention than problems of lower priority. Setting priorities helps the nurse to organize and plan care to solve the most urgent problems first.

ESTABLISHING PRIORITIES

In determining the priority of the problems, the nurse must consider their impact on the client. Priorities may fluctuate as the client's level of wellness changes. The nurse should consider both actual and potential problems when establishing priorities. Actual problems are usually more important than potential problems; however, potential problems may at times be more important. For example, in a client who is asthmatic, the potential problem of Ineffective Airway Clearance is more life threatening than the actual problem of constipation.

ESTABLISHING OUTCOMES

After establishing priorities, the client and the nurse try to reach a mutual decision regarding expected outcomes on the basis of identified nursing diagnoses and collaborative problems. Outcomes serve as guides for selecting nursing interventions and for determining criteria for evaluating nursing interventions. The purpose of writing expected outcomes is to assist in evaluating the client's progress and in determining the resolution of the client's problem if possible.

Expected outcomes have the following characteristics:

- Client-centered
- Realistic in terms of the client's potential for achievement and the nurse's ability to help the client achieve them
- Specific and measurable to the extent possible (outcome criteria)

When writing outcomes, the nurse should state them in a clear, concise manner that can be understood and measured by all health care team members. Any health care professional caring for the client should be able to determine whether the outcomes have been achieved based on the specified measurable criteria. For example, "The client is expected to state that pain is reduced within 45 minutes after interdisciplinary intervention" is a specific outcome that can be measured easily. If after 45 minutes the client states that pain is reduced, the outcome has been met.

Johnson and Maas (2000) have published the Nursing Outcomes Classification (NOC) system, which lists outcomes based on nursing diagnoses. The expected outcomes for client care identified in this text are consistent with NOC but are not taken solely from this source. NOC continues to be developed and refined to ensure that outcomes are evidence based.

Selecting Nursing Interventions

After determining the outcomes, the nurse develops strategies to accomplish them. Nursing interventions, also known as nursing actions or measures, are designed to assist the client in achieving the desired outcomes. They are based on the client's health problems and define activities required to promote, maintain, or restore health.

McCloskey and Bulechek (2000) define an intervention as "any treatment, based upon clinical judgement and knowledge, that a nurse performs to enhance patient/client outcomes" (p. 3). In 1992 these authors published the results of the first phase of the Iowa Intervention Project. This research produced a Nursing Interventions Classification (NIC) system of 336 standardized nursing interventions. The newest update includes 486 evidence-based interventions that have been supported by a number of nursing specialty organizations. As with the development of nursing diagnoses and NOC, NIC is intended to help nurses standardize their terminology and practice. NIC interventions are included throughout the Interventions chapters of this text.

DEVELOPING THE COLLABORATIVE PLAN OF CARE

The collaborative plan of care (POC) is an interdisciplinary document that outlines the essential aspects of client care, often across a time sequence. The format commonly used is a clinical pathway, which is also called a critical path, care map, or coordinated POC.

The clinical pathway delineates what care must be provided, who will provide the care, and when the care will be provided. It is a guideline for care that can be individualized if needed. Most pathways also list expected outcomes for the client, which may be hourly, daily, or weekly depending on the nature of the health care setting. This text provides several samples of clinical pathways.

This text also includes Client Care Plans. Although these plans of care are not interdisciplinary, they are necessary for beginning students to learn the steps of the nursing process and to identify the rationale (scientific evidence) for selected nursing interventions. Interventions that the nurse can delegate to assistive nursing personnel are specified. This format is no longer used in many clinical practice settings because the accrediting agency for hospitals and other health care facilities, the Joint Commission on the Accreditation of Healthcare Organizations (JCAHO), does not require the use of columnar care plans. Instead JCAHO requires evidence that nurses plan and implement care on the basis of identified client health problems and in collaboration with the interdisciplinary team.

To save time and duplication, a number of computer programs and books have been developed to create standardized plans of care or clinical pathways that can be individualized as needed. As technology advances, these programs should be more widely available to nurses in all health care settings.

This text also provides examples of visual plans of care known as **concept maps.** Concept maps present assessment data, nursing diagnoses, and collaborative care for clients with complex health problems. They show the relationships among these components, thus enabling the reader to see the "big picture" regarding the client's interdisciplinary care. Concept maps are not used in the clinical practice setting, but they provide another learning tool for summarizing client care.

DETERMINING RESOURCES

When planning nursing interventions, the nurse determines what resources are necessary for implementation of these interventions. The client is a valuable source of information about health care resources that were successful in the past. For example, the client with an irritated stoma may mention that an enterostomal therapist was helpful with previous problems. Including the client and family in planning care often promotes their cooperation during the implementation phase.

Other nurses and health care team members are valuable resources. An interdisciplinary conference or "walking rounds" during which health care team members identify problems and the resources to solve them may be very helpful, especially in planning community-based care.

When the financial feasibility of the plan is explored, the nurse considers the availability of other resources for the client, such as equipment, time, personnel, and money. The client's value system is also considered. For instance, if the client requires dialysis in the home, the type of system implemented depends on the home water supply, electrical capability, space, available money, spiritual beliefs, and personal support system.

IMPLEMENTATION

Implementation involves the actual carrying out of a specific, individualized POC. This step of the nursing process is the action phase, in which the nurse assumes responsibility for implementing the POC based on the nursing diagnosis and collaborative problems. Best practice interventions are based on scientific evidence, identified standards of care and, at times, intuitive judgment. Best Practice for Nursing interventions are summarized in charts throughout this text.

Because planning and implementation are closely related, this text discusses them under one heading, Planning and Implementation, with expected outcomes and interventions clearly labeled.

EVALUATION

Evaluation, the fifth step of the nursing process, is a cognitive activity that completes the nursing process by indicating the degree to which the client's expected outcomes have been met.

Although evaluation is given as the final step of the nursing process, it is an ongoing and integral part of each step of the process (see Figure 1-8). The nurse reviews the data to determine whether sufficient information was collected and whether the appropriate behaviors were identified. Client health problems are evaluated for their accuracy and completeness. The nurse examines the expected outcomes, outcome criteria, and interventions to determine whether they were realistic, achievable, and effective.

The outcome of evaluation may be one or a combination of the following:

- The client responded as expected and the problem is resolved. No additional nursing actions are needed.
- Client behaviors indicate that the client's problem has not been resolved. Outcomes have been accomplished, but the overall long-term goal has not been achieved. Re-evaluation will continue.
- Client behaviors are similar to those present initially. Little or no evidence is available to show that the problem has been resolved. Reassessment and replanning are needed.
- Client behaviors indicate a new problem. Assessment, planning, and implementation of an additional plan of action are needed to resolve the problem.

In this text, outcomes are listed under the Planning and Implementation and Evaluation: Outcomes sections.

DOCUMENTATION

Documentation of each phase of the nursing process is essential and is accomplished by various means. Two general, traditional methods of documentation are still used in many health care settings: (1) source-oriented charting, which usually includes narrative notes that organize varied data and are entered into the medical record by health care professionals (e.g., nurses' notes, physicians' progress notes, dietary notes), and (2) the problem-oriented record (POR), in which a master health problem list is developed. Each problem is numbered, and all chart entries refer to one of the problems identified on the list.

All health care professionals may record their notes in a SOAP, SOAPIER, or PIE format (or one of its many variations) and on the same progress note form in the chart. The initials represent **S**ubjective data, **O**bjective data, **A**nalysis, **P**lan of action, **I**nterventions, **E**valuation, and **R**evision of the plan. This technique of documentation is systematic and limits data to only pertinent information related to the identified problem. Although this system assists the nurse in addressing each step of the nursing process, it is very time consuming and promotes duplication of record keeping. Many physicians, social workers, and dietitians still use the SOAP format, but new systems for nursing documentation have been and are being developed.

Documentation Systems

FOCUS CHARTING

A commonly used format in documentation is focus charting. Focus charting is not limited to specific client health problems but instead encourages nurses to document any significant changes in the client's condition, any client concern, or any significant client event. As seen in Figure 1-9, the record has

Date/Time	Focus/Problem	Notes
6/16/01 2:15 P.M.	Fever	D: T = 102.2° (R); face flushed; diaphoretic A: Give Tylenol 2 tab as ordered. Recheck temp. in 1 hr. R. Jones, RN
6/16/01 3:15 P.M.	Fever	R: T = 100.2° (R); face not flushed; not diaphoretic D. Ignas, LPN
6/17/01 3:30 A.M.	Impaired skin	D: 2-cm reddened area over coccyx; blanches A: Positioned on (L) side N. Smith, RNC

Figure 1-9 ● A sample of focus charting.

three columns. The actual notes are divided into **D**ata, **A**ction, and **R**esponse information. An **E** may be added for documenting client **E**ducation. This technique helps locate desired information but still uses the familiar narrative approach to recording pertinent data.

CHARTING BY EXCEPTION

Another system is charting by exception (CBE). CBE was started at St. Luke's Hospital in Milwaukee, Wisconsin, in an attempt to save nursing time. It incorporates three basic components (Burke & Murphy, 1988):

- Comprehensive flow sheets that list normal findings and require the nurse to initial them if they are present. If the findings are not present, the nurse writes an entry into the notes.
- References to preestablished nursing standards. The nurse initials the appropriate space when they are completed.
- Bedside accessibility of forms. All flow sheets are kept at the bedside, which prevents wasting the nurse's time in looking for a client's chart. Bedside charting also prevents transcription of data from one form to another, which can lead to errors and wasted time. The information is available for any health care professional to read.

COMPUTERIZED NURSING INFORMATION SYSTEMS (NIS)

One major advantage of documentation systems such as CBE is the ability to transfer the concept to computerization. Electronic charting, also known as point-of-care charting and online documentation, is common in hospitals, nursing homes, home care agencies, and ambulatory care settings. The literature suggests that the major advantages of point-of-care documentation are accuracy and time savings. Electronic charting at the bedside also increases the time that the nurse spends in the client's room. The goal of any system should be to streamline or diminish paperwork and save valuable nursing time, giving nurses more time for direct client care. Commonly used hospital systems are Meditech and HBOC.

CHART 1-4

BEST PRACTICE *for* Nursing Documentation

- Write clearly and legibly.
- Do not erase or "white-out" any part of the client's record.
- To correct an error, use one line to cross out the incorrect entry, then initial the change.
- Use only standard and facility-approved abbreviations and symbols.
- Document significant information as close as possible to the time it is collected instead of waiting until the end of a shift.
- Transcribe physicians' orders carefully and correctly.
- If using nurses' notes or progress notes, do not leave blank spaces between entries.
- Time and date each entry on the client's record.
- Use only blue or black ink (it visualizes best for copies or microfilm).
- Document like a reporter: State facts objectively and avoid judgment or criticism.
- Do not state that "an incident report has been completed" or refer to any unusual occurrence or special event as an "incident."
- Follow all facility policies for documentation.
- To add one or two words, use a caret (^) and insert the words, then initial the change; if agency policy does not allow this practice, write a late entry.
- To make a late entry, begin by stating that it is a "Late entry for (date and time);" if the entry is more than a day late, state the reason for the late entry (e.g., "on vacation for 3 days").
- If an order is discontinued on the record as indicated by a highlighter, be sure that the original can still be read, especially on copies.

Legal Aspects of Documentation

Regardless of the type of documentation system used, the nurse must remember that the client's chart is a legal document. Chart 1-4 lists basic charting guidelines that all nurses should follow.

ONLINE RESOURCES

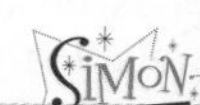

For suggested readings and Internet resources, go to http://www.wbsaunders.com/SIMON/Iggy/.

SELECTED BIBLIOGRAPHY

Asterisk indicates a classic or definitive work on this subject.

Alfaro-LeFevre, R. (1999). *Critical thinking in nursing: A practical approach* (2nd ed.). Philadelphia: W.B. Saunders.

Allen, K.M., & Phillips, J.M. (1997). *Women's health across the lifespan: A comprehensive perspective.* Philadelphia: Lippincott-Raven.

*Aspinall, M.J., & Tanner, C. (1981). *Decision-making for patient care.* Norwalk, CT: Appleton & Lange.

Barr, W.J., & Bush, H.A. (1998). Four factors of nurse caring in the ICU. *Dimensions of Critical Care Nursing, 17*(4), 214-223.

Beck, C.T. (1999). Quantitative measurement of caring. *Journal of Advanced Nursing, 30*(1), 24-32.

*Benner, P., & Tanner, C. (1987). How expert nurses use intuition. *American Journal of Nursing, 87,* 23-31.

*Bower, F. (1972). *The process of planning nursing care.* St. Louis: Mosby.

Bureau of the Census. (1997). *Resident population of the United States by race and origin.* Washington, DC: U.S. Department of Commerce.

*Burke, L.J., & Murphy, J. (1988). *Charting by exception: A cost-effective, quality approach.* New York: John Wiley & Sons.

*Carpenito, L.J. (1995). *Nursing care plans and documentation: Nursing diagnoses and collaborative problems.* Philadelphia: J.B. Lippincott.

*Cella, D.F. (1994). Quality of life: The concept and definition. *Journal of Pain and Symptom Management, 6,* 186-192.

Davis, C.M., & Curley, C.M. (1999). Disparities of health in African Americans. *Nursing Clinics of North America, 34*(2), 345-355.

*Dunn, H.L. (1980). *High level wellness.* Thorofare, NJ: Charles B. Slack.

*Eggland, E.T. (1995). Charting smarter: Using new mechanisms to organize your paperwork. *Nursing95, 25*(9), 34-41.

*Facione, N.C., & Facione, P.A. (1996). Externalizing the critical thinking in knowledge development and clinical judgment. *Nursing Outlook, 44*(3), 129-136.

*Ferrell, B.R. (1996). The quality of lives: 1,525 voices of cancer. *Oncology Nursing Forum, 23*(6), 907-916.

Ferrell, B.R. et al. (1998). Quality of life in breast cancer: Part 2. Psychological and spiritual well-being. *Cancer Nursing, 21*(1), 1-9.

Flaskerud, J.H., & Kim, S. (1999). Health problems of Asian and Latino immigrants. *Nursing Clinics of North America, 34*(2), 359-380.

Fonteyn, M.E. (1998). *Thinking strategies for nursing practice* (2nd ed.). Gaithersburg, MD: Aspen.

Hamer, S., & Collinson, G. (1999). *Achieving evidence-based practice: A handbook for practitioners.* Edinburgh: Bailliere Tindall.

Jarvis, C. (2000). *Physical examination and health assessment* (3rd ed.). Philadelphia: W.B. Saunders.

Johnson, M., & Maas, M. (2000). *Nursing outcomes classification (NOC)* (2nd ed.). Philadelphia: W.B. Saunders.

Lash, A.A. (1998). Quality of life in systemic lupus erythematosus. *Applied Nursing Research, 11*(3), 130-137.

McCance, T., McKenna, H., & Boone, J. (1997). Caring: Dealing with a difficult concept. *International Journal of Nursing Studies, 34*(4), 241-248.

McCloskey, J.C., & Bulechek, G.M. (2000). *Nursing interventions classification (NIC)* (3rd ed.). Philadelphia: W.B. Saunders.

*Pender, N.J. (1987). *Health promotion in nursing practice* (2nd ed.). Norwalk, CT: Appleton & Lange.

Schielke, C. (1997). Patient advocacy: The shield that empowers. *Continuing Care, 16*(3), 22-26.

Shinagawa, L.H., & Jang, M. (1998). *Atlas of American diversity.* Walnut Creek, CA: AltaMira Press.

*U.S. Department of Health and Human Services, Public Health Service. (1990). *Healthy People 2000: National health promotion and disease prevention objectives.* Washington, DC: U.S. Government Printing Office.

U.S. Department of Health and Human Services, Public Health Service. (2000). *Healthy People 2010: National health promotion and disease prevention objectives.* Washington, DC: U.S. Government Printing Office.

Wilkinson, J.M. (2000). *Nursing diagnosis handbook with NIC interventions and NOC outcomes* (7th ed.). Upper Saddle River, NJ: Prentice Hall Health.

*World Health Organization. (1947). *Constitution of the World Health Organization: Chronicle of the World Health Organization.* Geneva: Author.

CHAPTER 2

Community-Based Care

DEBORAH H. HEATHERLY • DONNA D. IGNATAVICIUS

Learning Objectives

After studying this chapter, you should be able to:

1. Explain the primary purpose of ambulatory care.
2. Discuss the growth of home care in the United States.
3. Describe the role of the nurse in home care.
4. Identify examples of interventions for which Medicare pays in home care.
5. Compare and contrast the common types of nursing homes.
6. Describe the term *subacute care.*

SIMON Go to http://www.wbsaunders.com/SIMON/Iggy/ for self-assessment questions related to these Learning Objectives.

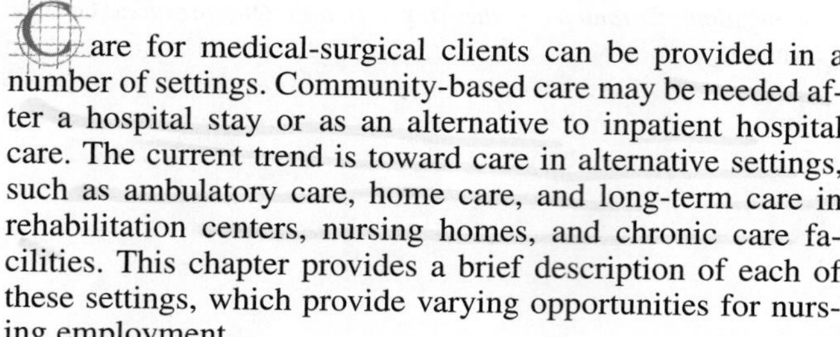

Care for medical-surgical clients can be provided in a number of settings. Community-based care may be needed after a hospital stay or as an alternative to inpatient hospital care. The current trend is toward care in alternative settings, such as ambulatory care, home care, and long-term care in rehabilitation centers, nursing homes, and chronic care facilities. This chapter provides a brief description of each of these settings, which provide varying opportunities for nursing employment.

This text covers care for clients in all settings in which medical-surgical nurses practice. The Community-Based Care sections that follow the discussions of major health problems highlight the most important aspects of care in nonhospital environments.

AMBULATORY CARE

Ambulatory health care is a general term for client care provided in myriad community settings, such as physician offices, hospital or freestanding outpatient clinics, freestanding surgicenters, and health maintenance organizations (a type of managed-care organization) (see Chapter 3). The purpose of ambulatory care is health promotion, health protection (illness prevention), short-term treatment (e.g., surgery), and follow-up for existing health problems.

Client visits to ambulatory care settings are episodic and based on need. For example, clients may visit their health care provider for annual physical examinations (health promotion). Alternatively, they may seek out providers for acute health care problems, chemotherapy, or selected surgeries such as cataract removal or laparoscopic cholecystectomy (removal of the gallbladder). Still others are monitored periodically for chronic health conditions such as diabetes mellitus and hypertension.

Clients discharged from the hospital are often followed in one or more ambulatory care settings. Many health care providers in these settings are nurse practitioners. The cost of ambulatory care is typically far less than that of a nursing home or home care agency.

Role of the Nurse in Ambulatory Care

One of the major roles of the nurse working in an ambulatory care setting is performing health promotion activities, including client education, health screening, and comprehensive assessment. In a surgicenter, for example, the nurse provides preoperative teaching to prepare clients for the surgical procedure and postoperative expectations. Their vital signs and general condition are assessed to ensure that they are ready for the surgery.

Many physicians employ nurses to assist in their practice. These nurses often triage clients who call; that is, they decide which clients need priority care and intervene accordingly. In some parts of the country large physician practices employ nurse case managers who monitor high-risk, high-cost, problem-prone clients throughout the continuum of health care in all settings. Case management is discussed in Chapter 3.

Nursing Community Centers

Nursing community centers are ambulatory care settings operated by nurses. Although the organizational structure and services provided vary among centers, most of them are affiliated with large university schools of nursing. The primary health care providers are typically nurse practitioners, nurse midwives, clinical nurse specialists, and students preparing to become one of these advanced-practice specialists. The funding for nursing community centers varies. Some monies come from city, state, and federal governments, whereas others come from grants obtained by university faculty.

HOME CARE

Home care in the United States is a diverse and rapidly growing industry. For many clients the home not only is the preferred health care setting but also is the lowest cost setting. There are a variety of definitions and models for home care, but the United States Public Health Service has put forth a definition that is both holistic and interdisciplinary. **Home health care** is part of a continuum of comprehensive health care in which health services are provided to individuals and families in their place of residence. The goal is to promote, maintain, or restore health or to maximize the level of independence while minimizing the effects of disability and illness, including terminal illness.

Historical Perspective and Trends of Home Care Nursing

Modern home care nursing has its roots in public health and community health nursing models. In the mid 1880s, visiting nurse associations (VNAs) evolved in Philadelphia, Boston, and Buffalo, New York. The traditions of Lillian Wald, who is regarded as the founder of public health nursing, began with the Henry Street Settlement in New York City in 1893. During the early twentieth century, most of the home health nursing care in the United States was provided by VNAs and the nursing divisions of governmental health agencies. Public health principles and practices, as well as components of family and community care, were integrated into home health nursing services. Nurses provided health promotion services to individuals, families, and communities while continuing to provide nursing care to the sick.

Home care, however, was a small entity until the passage of the Medicare Law in 1965. At that time Medicare required agencies to provide a minimum of nursing services plus one additional service, such as physical or occupational therapy, speech-language pathology, medical-social services, or home care aide services. The advent of Medicare began the trend toward and the basis for reimbursement of home care services. It has been estimated that only 1100 home care programs were in existence in 1963—3 years before Medicare became law. As of September 1998, the National Association for Home Care had identified more than 20,000 home care organizations that provide some type of service or product to clients in their homes, with more than 11,000 of those being Medicare-certified home care or hospice agencies that provide skilled nursing services (National Association for Home Care, 1999).

Many factors have contributed to the growth and acceptance of home care, including the following:

- A continued shift from inpatient-based care to community-based care and home care
- Increased acceptance by the medical community and the consumer community that home care is often a viable alternative to institutional care
- Baby boomers who, as they get older, are becoming more educated about health care alternatives and are becoming more involved in the decision-making process
- An aging population that has increased the need for health care for older adults
- Technology such as mobile x-ray machines, apnea monitors, and electrocardiographs, which allow clients to remain safely at home while having their health needs monitored; the introduction of telehealthcare services allows even more ways for clients to be monitored from their home (Kinsella, 1998)
- The generally lower cost of home care (compared to institutional care)
- The increase in managed care, which dictates a lower cost care environment

Although there has been significant growth in home care since the 1960s, the number of Medicare-certified agencies has decreased from more than 10,000 in 1997 to approximately 9655 in 1998; this number continues to decline. The National Association for Home Care (NAHC) believes this recent decline to be the direct result of changes in Medicare home care reimbursement, which were enacted as part of the Balanced Budget Act of 1997 (NAHC, 1999).

Types of Home Care

The term *home care* is used to describe a variety of products and services. There are different specialty areas within the home care industry, and nurses may work in any one of these areas (Figure 2-1). Some companies may provide all or just one of these home care services. There are generally four types of services provided by the home care industry:

1. *Skilled home care service.* This is the largest type of service, with these agencies employing most of the

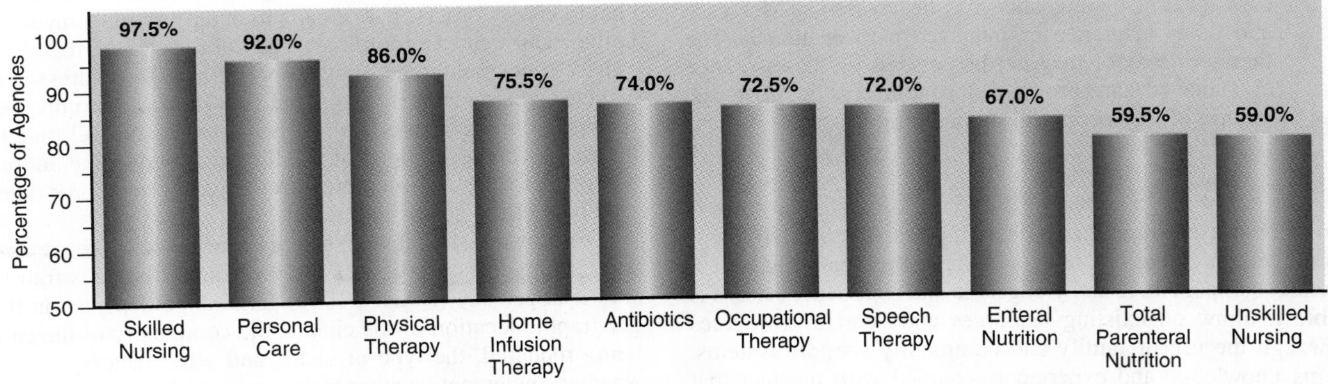

Figure 2-1 ● Ten most commonly offered home care services. (Courtesy Marion Merrell Dow, Inc., Managed Care Digest Series, *Institutional Digest,* 1995, and SMG Marketing Group, Inc.)

home care nurses and other health care professionals to provide care as needed. Skilled home care services are provided by home care organizations that are usually Medicare certified and provide two or more of the following services:

- Nursing (RN and LPN)
- Physical therapy (LPT, LPTA)
- Occupational therapy (OTR, COTA)
- Speech/language pathology
- Medical social services (MSW, BSW)
- Home care aides

The organization may also provide dietitian services, respiratory therapy, and other specialty services (e.g., enterostomal therapy, behavioral health nursing) depending on the specialty programs of the organization. In general, Medicare, Medicaid, and other insurance or managed care programs cover these skilled services when the qualifying criteria of the insurance program are met.

2. *Personal care or private duty service.* This type of service may provide "shifts" of nurses or home care aides to clients in their homes. It may also provide additional services such as homemaker services, transportation, respite for caregivers, meal preparation, and sitter services. Some insurance programs may pay for a limited amount of these services related to health care, but most of them are paid privately by the client or family.
3. *Home medical equipment (HME) service.* This service can also include durable medical equipment (DME). HME companies provide hospital beds, wheelchairs, bath benches, oxygen and related equipment and services, walkers, and other equipment. In general, Medicare and other insurance or managed care programs pay for HME when the qualifying criteria of the insurance program are met.
4. *Home infusion or intravenous (IV) service.* Companies providing this type of service have pharmacists that mix the infusion therapies. The company then delivers the infusion, sets it up in the home, trains the client/family on proper administration, and sometimes administers the infusion therapies. Therapies can be enteral or parenteral and can include tube feedings, antibiotics, hyperalimentation, blood and blood products, tocolytic therapy, antineoplastics, opioid analgesics, and catecholamines. Nursing services for activities such as observation and assessment, therapy administration, site care, and line maintenance may be covered by Medicare and other insurance or managed care programs. The therapies may or may not be covered by the insurance or managed care program depending on the coverage criteria of the specific insurance program.

Role of the Nurse in Home Care

In spite of everything that is changing in the home care environment, one thing has remained the same: nursing is an essential component. A knowledgeable and experienced nurse is able to draw on existing resources and "create" resources through the use of family and community support systems. This knowledge and experience, coupled with the fact that nursing is an essential component of home care, makes it possible for nurses to direct and manage home care effectively. Nurses can continue to support client advocacy by promoting nursing's unique contribution to the care of the client and caregivers.

In 1986 the American Nurses Association (ANA) published its *Standards of Home Health Nursing Practice,* identifying home care nursing as a component of community health nursing. These standards apply to nursing practice in any home care setting, including both health promotion and care of the sick, and they are targeted toward communities, families, and individuals. These standards apply to both nursing practice generalists and specialists and were written within the framework of the nursing process, with the associated criteria being divided into structure, process, and outcome. It is important to note that "outcomes" are becoming an integral part of the home care industry.

Home care has come to mean a variety of specialized and generalized nursing care provided to clients whose primary site for health care is their home. Adult health (medical-surgical) care, child (pediatric) care, perinatal care, older adult (geriatric) care, behavioral health care, and many other specialties are practiced routinely by home care nurses. Effective home care nursing incorporates the aspects of comprehensive assessment skills with current technology and the "hi-touch" care of skilled nurses. Home care *case management* uses the client care plan in conjunction with effective care coordination and ongoing communication to ensure that the client is receiving appropriate care. Collaborative communication among team members and active and ongoing client participation ensures that clients are truly equal partners in their health care. Table 2-1 compares nursing in the home care setting to nursing in the inpatient setting.

Home Visits

Home care provided by private duty or personal care companies is often rendered in "hours" or "shifts" of service delivery. In general, intermittent home care is provided in "visits" by Medicare-certified agencies. The actual visit time is the time spent in the client's home for the provision of the ordered care. The length of the visit depends on the complexity of the care being provided, the type of visit (e.g., the admission visit is typically longer because of the increased amount of data being collected and documented), how well the client tolerates the care, and how efficient the nurse is in providing the care. Although the actual visit time is the time spent in the client's home, several components go into effective visit provision: visit preparation, including phone calls to the physician to clarify orders; phone calls to other providers involved in the client's care to coordinate care delivery; gathering of required documentation and supplies (wound dressings, catheter, venipuncture); phone calls to insurance companies for visit authorization or care delivery updates; travel time to the client's home; completion of all necessary documentation; and further care coordination with the physician and/or other members of the health care team.

The number of visits nurses are expected to make per day varies from agency to agency. The national average is four to six visits per day (NAHC, 1999). The range depends on the geographic location of the clients, the complexity of the care being rendered, the type of visits, and other factors such as weather. Inclement weather poses another challenge to home care staff. Many staff use four-wheel drive vehicles, boats, and other alternate means of transportation. In areas of extremely heavy snowfall, nurses have even been known to use

TABLE 2-1 • MAJOR DIFFERENCES BETWEEN NURSING CARE IN THE HOME AND IN INPATIENT SETTINGS

Home Setting	Inpatient Setting
Nurse is more autonomous and is many times the "eyes and ears" of the physician.	Nurse relies heavily on physician directives.
Environment is controlled by the client/caregiver. Circumstances are often less than optimal for the provision of skilled care.	Environment is controlled by the facility and its staff.
Nurse must be knowledgeable about the care of all types and ages of clients.	Nurse is typically knowledgeable about the care of specific types of clients, often based on diagnosis.
Nurse must know and understand various reimbursement requirements and document accordingly.	Financial officer and accounting department usually handle reimbursement.
For older adults, only selected skilled and nonskilled services are reimbursed by Medicare.	For older adults, hospital care is largely reimbursed by Medicare.
There is limited direct supervision of assistive staff, such as home care aides.	There is continuous direct supervision of assistive staff. Nurse and staff work as a single unit.

skis, snowmobiles, or snowshoes to ensure that they can reach their clients. Staff assignments are generally based on the geographic location of the client, the client diagnosis, and/or the service to be delivered (e.g., infusion services, cardiac services, rehabilitative services).

Client Plan of Care

As with other care settings, a physician's order is needed for care interventions and care plan changes. Because home care nursing practice is more autonomous than many inpatient settings, it is imperative that orders be obtained from physicians for care and care changes. Sometimes the physician does not see the client for months and therefore relies on the nurse's assessments and reports to assist with development and revision of the care plan. Verbal and telephone orders are a large part of the home care practice and communication with physicians. For Medicare clients, agencies generally use the Form 485 from the Centers for Medicare and Medicaid Services (formerly the Health Care Financing Administration) as the client plan of care (Figure 2-2). This plan of care is developed with input from the client/caregiver, physician, and other members of the health care team. The plan of care must be signed by the physician before the agency bills for the services rendered under the plan of care.

Medicare will pay for home care services when the beneficiary meets one or more of certain qualifying conditions:

- The client is confined to the home
- Services are provided under a plan of care established and approved by a physician
- The client is under the care of a physician
- The client needs skilled nursing care on an intermittent basis or needs physical therapy or speech language pathology services
- The client has a continued need for occupational therapy services

Once client eligibility has been established, Medicare usually pays for any or all of the following skilled nursing services:

1. Observation and assessment of the client's condition when only the specialized skills of a medical professional can determine a client's status
2. Management and evaluation of a client care plan
3. Teaching and training activities
4. Administration of medications
5. Nasopharyngeal and tracheostomy aspiration
6. Urinary catheters
7. Wound care
8. Ostomy care
9. Rehabilitation nursing
10. Nursing student visits
11. Psychiatric evaluation, therapy, and teaching

Medicare principles governing reasonable and necessary skilled nursing services include the following (Health Care Financing Administration [HCFA], 1996):

1. A skilled nursing service is a service that must be provided by a registered nurse (or a licensed practical [vocational] nurse under the supervision of a registered nurse) to be safe and effective.
2. A service is not considered a skilled nursing service merely because it is performed by or under the direct supervision of a licensed nurse. A service is not considered a skilled nursing service if it can be performed safely and effectively by the average nonmedical person (or self-administered) without direct nursing supervision.
3. If a service requires the skills of a licensed nurse to be provided safely and effectively, it continues to be a skilled service even if it is taught to the client/caregiver.
4. The skilled nursing service must be reasonable and necessary to the diagnosis and treatment of the client's illness or injury within the context of the client's unique medical condition.

Documentation Systems

Reimbursement for home care relies heavily on the documentation of care. In many home care and other community-based settings, the Omaha Problem Classification System may be used instead of the nursing diagnoses from the North American Nursing Diagnosis Association. The Omaha system delineates four general areas that represent community and home care practice and provide organizational groupings for client problems: environmental, psychosocial, physiologic, and health-related behaviors. More than 40 nursing diagnoses with modifiers such as potential deficit, deficit, and health promotion are then listed within their appropriate domains (Martin & Scheet, 1992).

Computerization and Home Care

In an effort to facilitate the documentation and communication processes, many agencies have implemented some form of automation. At a minimum, most agencies have computerized Form 485 (Plan of Care) from the Centers for Medicare and Medicaid Services, and many agencies have implemented a clinical documentation system for their client care staff. Several software products are on the market and use a variety of hardware products, from the handheld to the personal computer. For agencies that have implemented an automated clinical documentation system, nurses carry a handheld, laptop, or other computer into the clients' homes to document their assessment findings and care delivery. This information is then transmitted to the main agency server.

One advantage of computerization is immediate access to the information by office personnel or other members of the health care team once the nurse has transmitted it to the agency. Another advantage is that the nurse can readily access client medical record information, day or night, without coming into the office. This allows the nurse more flexibility in scheduling his or her day. Many software programs also reduce the amount of times the information must be entered (or written if documentation is done by hand) because it flows to all appropriate locations within the documentation system. Computer literacy is becoming a requirement for nursing practice in many settings, and home care is no exception.

Outcomes and Home Care

In January 1999 new regulations were put into place that require Medicare-certified home care agencies to track and report client outcomes. The tool to be used by agencies is the **Out**come and **AS**sessment **I**nformation **S**et (OASIS), which was

Department of Health and Human Services
Health Care Financing Administration

Form Approved
OMB No. 0938-0357

HOME HEALTH CERTIFICATION AND PLAN OF CARE

1. Patient's HI Claim No. | 2. Start Of Care Date | 3. Certification Period From: To: | 4. Medical Record No. | 5. Provider No.

6. Patient's Name and Address

7. Provider's Name, Address and Telephone Number

8. Date of Birth

9. Sex ☐ M ☐ F

10. Medications: Dose/Frequency/Route (N)ew (C)hanged

11. ICD-9-CM | Principal Diagnosis | Date

12. ICD-9-CM | Surgical Procedure | Date

13. ICD-9-CM | Other Pertinent Diagnoses | Date

14. DME and Supplies

15. Safety Measures:

16. Nutritional Req.

17. Allergies:

18.A. Functional Limitations

1 ☐ Amputation
2 ☐ Bowel/Bladder (Incontinence)
3 ☐ Contracture
4 ☐ Hearing
5 ☐ Paralysis
6 ☐ Endurance
7 ☐ Ambulation
8 ☐ Speech
9 ☐ Legally Blind
A ☐ Dyspnea With Minimal Exertion
B ☐ Other (Specify)

18.B. Activities Permitted

1 ☐ Complete Bedrest
2 ☐ Bedrest BRP
3 ☐ Up As Tolerated
4 ☐ Transfer Bed/Chair
5 ☐ Exercises Prescribed
6 ☐ Partial Weight Bearing
7 ☐ Independent At Home
8 ☐ Crutches
9 ☐ Cane
A ☐ Wheelchair
B ☐ Walker
C ☐ No Restrictions
D ☐ Other (Specify)

19. Mental Status:

1 ☐ Oriented
2 ☐ Comatose
3 ☐ Forgetful
4 ☐ Depressed
5 ☐ Disoriented
6 ☐ Lethargic
7 ☐ Agitated
8 ☐ Other

20. Prognosis: 1 ☐ Poor 2 ☐ Guarded 3 ☐ Fair 4 ☐ Good 5 ☐ Excellent

21. Orders for Discipline and Treatments (Specify Amount/Frequency/Duration)

22. Goals/Rehabilitation Potential/Discharge Plans

23. Nurse's Signature and Date of Verbal SOC Where Applicable:

25. Date HHA Received Signed POT

24. Physician's Name and Address

26. I certify/recertify that this patient is confined to his/her home and needs intermittent skilled nursing care, physical therapy and/or speech therapy or continues to need occupational therapy. The patient is under my care, and I have authorized the services on this plan of care and will periodically review the plan.

27. Attending Physician's Signature and Date Signed

28. Anyone who misrepresents, falsifies, or conceals essential information required for payment of Federal funds may be subject to fine, imprisonment, or civil penalty under applicable Federal laws.

Figure 2-2 ● Centers for Medicare and Medicaid Services Form 485.

developed, extensively tested, and refined through the Center for Health Services and Policy Research at the University of Colorado. These outcome measures are the crux of Outcome Based Quality Improvement (OBQI), a systematic approach that home care agencies can implement and follow for continuous improvement of quality of care. With respect to OASIS and OBQI, the Health Care Financing Administration (now the Centers for Medicare and Medicaid Services) (1998) has defined *outcomes* as follows:

- A change in client health status between two or more points in time (Health status encompasses physiologic, functional, cognitive, emotional, and behavioral health. The definition of an outcome does not include a presumed direction; it is any deviation [or nondeviation] in health status between the initial time point and the follow-up time point.)
- Changes that are intrinsic to the client
- Positive, negative, or neutral changes in health status
- Changes that result from the care provided, the natural progression of disease and disability, or both

Before OASIS, there was no uniform data set that agencies could use to track their own outcomes and, perhaps more important, to compare themselves to similar agencies across the United States (HCFA, 1998).

NURSING HOME CARE

In clinical practice, long-term care (LTC) has become synonymous with nursing home care. LTC for adult clients with medical-surgical problems can occur either in the home or in facilities such as nursing homes, subacute units, chronic care facilities, or rehabilitation centers. In general, **long-term care** implies that clients receive care for a prolonged period of time, usually weeks or months. A small percentage of clients may remain in a facility indefinitely, perhaps a lifetime.

Nursing home care can be very expensive, with annual costs between $30,000 and $45,000 in the United States. As the proportion of older adults increases from 13% of the population in 2000 to 20% by 2030, the implication for increasing health care expenditures is profound. Older adults use health care services at a far greater rate than younger adults (see the Cost of Care box below).

Nursing homes in the United States provide care for clients with physical and cognitive impairments or chronic illness. Clients admitted to a nursing home are called **residents** because the facility is considered their home (see the Evidence-Based Practice for Nursing box below). The majority of residents are female and over 65 years of age. However, nursing homes are experiencing an increase in the number of younger residents as people live longer with debilitating chronic illnesses such as multiple sclerosis and muscular dystrophy.

Nursing homes are undergoing another major change. Most Medicare-certified facilities are increasingly admitting short-term (1 to 3 weeks) residents for rehabilitation or recovery from an illness or injury and then discharging them to home or another setting. Clients come from hospitals "quicker and sicker," and they often require complex or continuing care. Examples of common health problems that require short-term care in a nursing home include rehabilitation for total joint replacements, serious fractures, and strokes, and continued postoperative care following major surgeries such as a coronary artery bypass graft (CABG).

Types of Nursing Homes

Nursing homes can be divided into residential care homes, nursing facilities, skilled nursing facilities, and chronic care facilities. Some nursing homes are part of retirement communities, and others have specialty units, such as dementia, ventilator, or subacute units.

Residential facilities include domiciliary homes, care homes, rest homes, assisted-living facilities, and group homes. Some of these facilities are small and much like boarding homes before the advent of Medicare (Ignatavicius, 1998). Others are large communities managed by national

COST OF CARE IMPLICATIONS FOR NURSING

EFFECT OF AGING ON HEALTH CARE COSTS AND LONG-TERM CARE

Cost of Care

- Older adults use health care services for both acute and long-term care at a greater rate than younger adults.
- The longer a person lives, the greater the health care costs. For example, estimated health costs for an older adult who dies at age 65 is $32,000. This number increases to $200,000 for individuals who die at the age of 90.
- Health care costs during the last 2 years of life increase with longevity, but Medicare costs decline because the client needs more custodial care rather than skilled care.
- Health care spending is consistently higher for older women than for older men, even when adjusting for the increased longevity of women.

Implications for Nursing

Knowing the high costs of health care for older adults, nurses and other health care professionals need to focus their interventions on health promotion and illness prevention, especially in view of the aging 78 million "baby boomers," many of whom will be older adults by 2015. Nurses also need to conduct more research on quality of life and the use of complementary and alternative therapies, which can help reduce costs.

EVIDENCE-BASED PRACTICE FOR NURSING

Do older adults feel "at home" in life care or long-term care settings?

Hammer, R.M. (1999). The lived experience of being at home: A phenomenological investigation. *Journal of Gerontological Nursing, 25*(11), 10-18.

This qualitative research investigated the experience of 10 older adults who were relocated to either life care retirement centers or long-term care facilities. Data were gathered through interviews of the subjects.

The study identified 14 themes that clearly described feeling "at home" versus "not at home." Subjects who felt at home in their new settings had strong feelings of satisfaction with their lives, security, autonomy, and purpose. Older adults who did not feel at home were angry, anxious, depressed, and consumed by a desire to be elsewhere.

Critique. Although the researchers used a small convenience sample, the qualitative research design allowed them to collect a large amount of meaningful data in which the feelings of the subjects could be thoroughly explored. The findings cannot be generalized, but the study should be replicated to determine if other older adults have the same feelings as this study sample.

Implications for Nursing. Nurses need to be sensitive to the feelings of older adults who have been relocated. They can ask the clients what makes them feel at home and then try to provide, to the extent possible, an environment that helps in adjusting to the new setting.

TABLE 2-2 • CATEGORIES OF SUBACUTE CARE

Definition of Category	Examples of Services
TRANSITIONAL SUBACUTE CARE A substitute or alternative for continued hospital stays	Deep wound management Stroke rehabilitation Vascular or cardiac surgery Oncology surgery with chemotherapy Medically complex care Complicated orthopedic surgery
MEDICAL-SURGICAL SUBACUTE CARE A setting for stable residents who require a moderate level of care	Uncomplicated orthopedic surgery Individuals with human immunodeficiency virus Intravenous therapy Uncomplicated tracheostomy care Stroke rehabilitation
CHRONIC SUBACUTE CARE A setting for residents with little or no hope of recovery	Long-term comatose residents Ventilator-dependent residents Progressive neurologic diseases
LONG-TERM TRANSITIONAL SUBACUTE CARE A setting for residents with medically complex conditions	Acute ventilator support Medically complex residents requiring an extended stay

Data from Stahl, D.A. (1994). Subacute care: The future of health care. *Nursing Management,* 25(10), 34-40. Used with permission from Ignatavicius, D.D. (1998). *Introduction to long term care nursing: Principles and practice.* Philadelphia: F.A. Davis.

corporations. Many of the larger complexes are life care or continuing care retirement centers that offer a continuum of services, from independent living to skilled care. The typical resident in a residential facility is fairly independent and is able to perform most or all self-care activities. Employees in these facilities are usually unlicensed staff.

Formerly called intermediate care facilities, **nursing facilities (NFs)** provide a custodial, maintenance level of care. Certified, licensed NFs receive Medicaid funding for the care of residents who cannot perform activities of daily living independently. Each state has specific guidelines for reimbursement.

Skilled nursing facilities (SNFs, pronounced "snifs") provide care that requires licensed health care professionals, such as nurses and therapists. Only a small portion of most nursing home residents are categorized as skilled and therefore eligible for Medicare reimbursement. Examples of skilled care include new tube feedings, daily rehabilitative care for postoperative fractured hips, and care of stage 3 and stage 4 wounds.

Chronic care facilities provide care for long-term, chronically ill clients, such those with severe head injuries or those who need chronic ventilator support. These facilities are often managed by county or state governments.

Prospective Payment System

In the late 1990s the federally mandated Prospective Payment System (PPS) required that accurate assessment and documentation be directly linked to the amount of Medicare reimbursement for resident care. Although implementation of this system dramatically decreased financial reimbursement to skilled nursing facilities, the rates are usually better than those provided for residents who qualify for medical assistance funding. Medicaid and MediCal payments vary state to state.

Reimbursement issues can affect the quality of care for older adults. Limited reimbursement offers financial challenges for affording adequate resources to provide quality resident care (Boroughs, 1999).

Role of the Nurse in Nursing Home Care

Before 1965, nursing home care was not carefully monitored by external agencies. Poor sanitation, resident abuse, and inadequate care were common in the nursing home industry. Since 1965, nursing homes have been carefully scrutinized and highly regulated by both federal and state agencies. Nurses who work in these facilities must be aware of these laws, which are meant to protect both the residents and the staff.

In general, nurses employed by nursing homes are more autonomous than nurses working in hospitals. Health care providers are usually not present in the LTC facility on a continuous basis, because residents in these facilities are considered to be more medically "stable" than those in acute care. With early discharge from acute care, however, nursing home nurses are caring for sicker residents than in the past and therefore need increased skills and knowledge to manage them.

For the past decade, geriatric nursing research has helped validate best practice patterns for nurses who care for older adults in a variety of settings. Most notable is the work led by the John A. Hartford Institute for the Advancement of Geriatric Nursing Practice in New York City. Some of the areas studied include pain management, the use of physical restraints, fall prevention, and medication safety (Abraham et al., 1999).

Most nurses in nursing homes are placed "in charge" of a unit or shift because there are more unlicensed personnel (certified nursing assistants) than professional nurses. Therefore the nursing home or LTC nurse needs leadership, management, and clinical competencies to function in this interdisciplinary care environment. There may be only one nurse in charge of 30 to 40 residents and a number of certified nursing assistants.

Documentation in Long-Term Care

Documentation in nursing homes is highly regulated by both federal and state governments. The Minimum Data Set (MDS) is a federally mandated assessment form that is completed for all residents regardless of the level of care or reimbursement system. This document is an interdisciplinary tool completed by each member of the health care team.

The team develops an interdisciplinary care plan for all actual or potential resident problems. Depending on the resident's level of care, this plan is updated every 30 to 60 days, or more often as the resident's condition changes.

SUBACUTE CARE

Subacute care (SAC), one of the newest concepts in health care, is designed for clients who are too ill to be discharged from the hospital to a traditional nursing home or the client's own home. SAC "fills the gap" between the hospital and the long-term care (LTC) facility. Most SAC units are located in freestanding nursing home settings; a smaller percentage are located in hospital settings and provide a skilled level of care.

The American Health Care Association (AHCA), which represents the LTC industry, defines subacute care as a "comprehensive inpatient program designed for the individual who has an acute event as a result of an illness, injury or exacerbation (flare-up) of a disease process; has a determined course of treatment; and does not require intensive diagnostic and/or invasive procedures" (AHCA, 1994). Approximately one third of the health care provided by SAC units are rehabilitation services; the remainder are medical-surgical services (Stahl, 1994).

Types of Subacute Care

Most SAC units are part of traditional nursing homes. Some units are diagnostic specific, whereas others admit clients with a variety of health problems. Health problems for SAC units can be divided into four broad categories: transitional, general medical-surgical, chronic, and long-term transitional (Stahl, 1994). Table 2-2 lists examples of the services provided by each type.

Role of the Nurse in Subacute Care

Little has been published about the role of the nurse in SAC. Nurses who work in SAC must be knowledgeable about LTC and have medical-surgical, critical care, or rehabilitation skills depending on the type of unit in which they work. SAC nurses work closely with rehabilitation therapists to help residents meet functional outcomes. Restorative nursing aides assist the resident in returning to an optimal level of ADL functioning.

Few nurses have a background that encompasses all of the necessary SAC skills. Nursing homes and hospitals that employ nurses for their units are responsible for educating them to ensure that clients' needs are met.

REHABILITATIVE CARE

Rehabilitation is designed for clients who have experienced an acute injury or illness or for those who are coping with chronic conditions. Rehabilitation services may be provided in the home setting, nursing home, or rehabilitation unit or center. Chapter 10 discusses in detail the rehabilitation of individuals with chronic or disabling health problems.

ONLINE RESOURCES

For suggested readings and Internet resources, go to http://www.wbsaunders.com/SIMON/Iggy/.

SELECTED BIBLIOGRAPHY

Asterisk indicates a classic or definitive work on this subject.

Abraham, I., et al. (1999). *Geriatric nursing protocols for best practice.* New York: Springer.

*American Health Care Association. (1994). *Blueprint for the future vision.* Washington, DC: Author.

*American Nurses Association. (1986). *Standards of home health nursing practice.* Washington, DC: Author.

*Anderson, A. (1996). Nursing clinics in urban settings. *Home Healthcare Nurse, 14,* 542-546.

Bohny, B.J. (1997). A time for self-care: Role of the home healthcare nurse. *Home Healthcare Nurse, 15*(4), 281-286.

Boroughs, D.S. (1999). Documentation in the long-term care setting. *Journal of Nursing Administration, 29*(12), 46-49.

*Brown-Goebler, S. (1994). Subacute care: Nursing for the next century. *MEDSURG Nursing, 3,* 497-499.

Catanzaro, J., & Serembus, J.F. (1998). High-tech wound and ostomy care in the home setting. *Critical Care Nursing Clinics of North America, 10*(3), 327-338.

Congdon, J.G., & Magilvy, J.K. (1998). Rural nursing homes: A housing option for older adults. *Geriatric Nursing, 19*(3), 157-159.

Cox, R.A. (1998). Implementing nurse sensitive outcomes into care planning at a long-term care facility. *Journal of Nursing Care Quality, 12*(5), 41-51.

Hammer, R.M. (1999). The lived experience of being at home: A phenomenological investigation. *Journal of Gerontological Nursing, 25*(11), 10-18.

*Health Care Financing Administration. (1996). *Home health agency manual.* Baltimore: Author.

Health Care Financing Administration. (1998). *OASIS user's manual.* Baltimore: Author.

Ignatavicius, D.D. (1998). *Introduction to long term care nursing: Principles and practice.* Philadelphia: F.A. Davis.

Jones, A.M., & Foster, N. (1997). Transitional care: Bridging the gap. *MEDSURG Nursing, 6*(1), 32-38.

Kinsella, A. (1998). Home telehealthcare services: Their role on home care today. *Home Care Management, 2*(5), 17-22.

*Martin, K.S., & Scheet, N.J. (1992). *The Omaha system: Applications for community health nursing.* Philadelphia: W.B. Saunders.

McNeal, G.J. (1998). Care of the critically ill at home. *Critical Care Nursing Clinics of North America, 10*(3), 267-278.

National Association for Home Care. (1999). *Basic statistics about home care.* Washington, DC: Author.

Penrod, J., & Dellasega, C. (1998). Caregivers' experiences in making placement decisions. *Western Journal of Nursing Research, 20*(6), 723-732.

Spillman, B.C., & Lubitz, J. (2000). The effect of longevity on spending for acute and long-term care. *New England Journal of Medicine, 342*(19), 1409-1415.

*Stahl, D.A. (1994). Subacute care: The future of health care. *Nursing Management, 25*(10), 34-40.

Vaca, K.J., Vaca, B.L., & Daake, C.J. (1998). Review of nursing home regulations. *MEDSURG Nursing, 7*(3), 165-171.

*Walsh, G.G. (1995). How subacute care fills the gap. *Nursing95, 25*(3), 51.

CHAPTER

3

Introduction to Managed Care and Case Management

DONNA D. IGNATAVICIUS

Learning Objectives

After studying this chapter, you should be able to:

1. Explain the primary purpose of managed health care.
2. Contrast the fee-for-service and capitated reimbursement systems.
3. Describe the process of case management.
4. Identify at least three certifications for case managers.

SIMON

Go to http://www.wbsaunders.com/SIMON/Iggy/ for self-assessment questions related to these Learning Objectives.

The cost of health care in the United States has dramatically increased over the past 20 years and now accounts for nearly 15% of the gross national product (GNP). As a result, insurance companies and health care providers have reexamined how health care is paid and how client care is managed. Managed health care has evolved to consider both the quality and the cost of care.

Today managed care has grown to be the largest provider for health care in the United States. **Managed health care** is a system that attempts to control costs by using a select group of providers who have agreed to a predetermined payment before delivering care. In this system, client care is outcome driven and is managed by a utilization and/or a case management process. As participants in managed care, nurses have many roles in utilization management, case management, and outcomes management. They work in these roles as they focus on achieving client outcomes while maintaining costs.

MANAGED CARE

The managed care system is very different from the traditional way of paying for health care. Before the managed care movement, hospitals, physicians, and other health care providers were paid by health insurance companies on the basis of what the providers billed for their services. Under this **fee-for-service** arrangement, two physicians could perform identical services but could bill at their own rates. For example, one physician might bill $3000 for a surgical procedure, whereas another might bill $1800 for the same service. Under this fee-for-service system, the financial risk was largely taken by the insurance companies.

Purpose of Managed Care

Managed care organizations (MCOs) standardize and control costs. Under the managed care payment system, health care providers receive a uniform amount of money for each client; this is referred to as a **capitated reimbursement system** (Table 3-1). The MCO and the providers share the financial risks.

Balancing cost with quality is an important concept for managed care. Health care providers have been concerned that some MCOs may be too focused on saving money rather than on providing high-quality client care (Powell, 2000). The National Committee for Quality Assurance (NCQA) reviews and accredits MCOs that demonstrate high-quality care.

As discussed in Chapter 1, an important role for the nurse is to advocate for clients to ensure that they receive the necessary and appropriate care. As client advocates, care coordinators, and consumers, nurses need to know about managed care and the need for collaborative management of client care.

Role of Nurse Practitioners

Nurse practitioners (NPs) have become more predominant health care providers in the managed care environment because they can deliver more cost-effective health care. In addition, they work from a wellness model, with a focus on empowering clients to stay well and care for themselves. As a result of the increased demand for and success of this advanced practice role, many schools of nursing now offer graduate programs to prepare nurses to become NPs.

TABLE 3-1 • GLOSSARY OF TERMS RELATED TO MANAGED CARE

authorization The process used by managed health care organizations to grant services for a specified period for reimbursement of specific services

capitation A managed care reimbursement arrangement that prepays the physician or other health care provider a set dollar amount on a per-member, per-month basis for the delivery of services to a specified group of members

deductible The amount of money that an insured person must pay toward health care costs before the insurance company begins reimbursement for health care

fee-for-service A reimbursement arrangement in which health care services are paid for as billed by the provider

indemnity An arrangement in which benefits are paid in a predetermined amount in the event of a covered loss

integrated delivery system (IDS) A system created to manage or provide health care services ranging from primary to tertiary inpatient care and all other settings for care

risk sharing A mechanism that provides incentives to physicians and other health care providers to deliver cost-effective and efficient services

Types of Managed Care Organizations

Many businesses contract with a variety of MCOs to reduce health benefit costs. Government reimbursement systems have also entered into managed care arrangements to control escalating costs. For example, Medicare, a federal program for older adults and qualified disabled individuals, is expected to become a totally managed care system. Many state Medicaid programs, which pay for health services for the poor, have also entered managed care agreements.

The oldest and most common type of MCO is the health maintenance organization (HMO), which is sometimes referred to as a membership organization. Many models for HMOs are used, but all either employ health care professionals to serve subscribing members (enrollees) in an ambulatory setting or contract with physicians and other providers to treat clients in their private offices. The enrollee usually pays a small co-payment, typically $5 or $10, for each visit to their health care provider. Hospitalization or other inpatient services are provided by agencies that contract with the HMO.

Another popular type of MCO is the preferred provider organization (PPO). PPOs provide contractual arrangements with physicians, hospitals, and other providers who meet their criteria. In other words, they are the "preferred" providers who render care to a group of subscribers in the health plan.

COLLABORATIVE INTERDISCIPLINARY MANAGEMENT

As the United States moves forward with the managed care system, health care professionals have realized that they must work together as an **interdisciplinary team** to provide comprehensive, cost-effective care. Although this idea is not new in certain settings (e.g., rehabilitation, home care, and long-term care), health care professionals in hospitals have not always worked as a collaborative team. One of the constraints in acute care is the short-term stay. However, the Joint Commission on Accreditation of Healthcare Organizations (JCAHO) mandates that *all* JCAHO-accredited agencies must provide collaborative, interdisciplinary care for their clients.

This text has advocated collaborative management of care since the publication of its first edition in 1991. This edition continues to discuss client care under Collaborative Management headings. Nurses often take the lead role in the interdisciplinary team because they tend to be with clients for longer periods as they deliver and coordinate comprehensive, holistic care.

Focus on Outcomes

The primary focus of collaborative management is on the outcomes of care. The interdisciplinary team identifies expected outcomes for the client and provides interventions to help the client meet those outcomes. Both clinical and cost outcomes are established. This text identifies common clinical outcomes for clients with a number of diseases and illnesses. However, each client is an individual with unique problems and circumstances that may require modification of the commonly identified expected outcomes.

Cost of Care Implications boxes are also found throughout this text to increase awareness of costs and, in some cases, to show how nurses can help contain costs.

Development of Case Management

Although all clients need to have their care managed in a collaborative manner, not all clients need to be case managed. **Case management** is based on the assumption that certain clients with complex health problems need assistance in using the health care system and its resources effectively.

Case management is not a new concept. Since the turn of the twentieth century, social workers, psychologists, and others have "carried a caseload" of clients in the community for a variety of purposes. For instance, social workers and community health nurses have worked with at-risk older adults to keep them at home rather than admitting them to a nursing home.

In the mid-1980s Karen Zander and her colleagues at the New England Medical Center introduced a nursing case management (NCM) model. In this model, case managers followed up on high-risk, high-cost clients during their hospital stay to coordinate resources and ensure quality outcomes. Physician-nurse collaboration was a primary focus, which increased communication and coordination of care.

The Carondolet integrated health system in Arizona expanded on the NCM model by using case managers across the health care continuum. Sometimes referred to as "beyond the walls" case management, this model incorporated the ethnic values and culture of the community to ensure individualized, holistic care.

Definition and Process of Case Management

Many definitions for case management can be found in the literature. According to the Case Management Society of America (CMSA) (1995), case management is "a collaborative process which assesses, plans, implements, coordinates, monitors, and evaluates services and options to meet an individual's health needs through communications and available resources to promote quality, cost-effective outcomes" (p. 8). Sometimes case managers may meet the health needs of a population rather than a single individual (e.g., all diabetic clients or all asthmatic school-age children in a given community).

The case management process is reserved for clients who have complex health problems (high risk) and incur a high cost to the health care system. An example of a client who could benefit from case management is an older woman with pulmonary emphysema and congestive heart failure who has had repeated admissions to the hospital for pneumonia and lives alone at home. Where appropriate in this text, the role of the case manager is discussed under Community-Based Care sections.

Part of the definition of case management endorsed by CMSA is similar to the steps of the nursing process (Chart 3-1). Similarly, the American Nurses Association (ANA) states that nursing case management includes five components: assessment, planning, implementation, evaluation, and interaction.

The ANA also identifies the goals of case management:

- To provide quality health care along a continuum of care
- To decrease fragmentation [and duplication] of care across many health care settings
- To enhance the client's quality of life
- To increase cost containment (through appropriate use of resources)

In some agencies the case manager is referred to as the care coordinator or care manager. Most case managers are nurses, but some are social workers or mental health workers. Some case managers have little or no clinical health background.

In general, case managers can be considered as having either an internal or an external role. **Internal case managers** are employed by a health care agency and are usually nurses or social workers. Although these individuals manage resources, their primary focus is clinical care. **External case managers** are either employed by a managed care organization (MCO) or traditional insurance company or are self-employed and contract with the MCO or traditional insurance company. The primary focus of external case managers is the utilization of resources for insurance companies.

Standards for Case Management Practice

As the largest professional case management organization, CMSA (1995) published standards that specify the recommended preparation for a case manager. As listed in the criteria, the recommended educational preparation is a baccalaureate degree in a health or human service. Although most case managers today are approximately 40 years of age and are nurses prepared at the associate degree level, it is likely that new case managers in the twenty-first century will have at least a baccalaureate degree. Some nursing programs believe that case management is an advanced practice role and offer masters' preparation as a case manager.

According to CMSA (1995), the criteria for preparation as a case manager also includes working toward obtaining a certified case manager (CCM) credential. Since 1997, this certification process has required that the experienced case manager (with at least 2 years experience) successfully complete a national standardized examination. The CCM designation is a valued credential in the field of case management for any discipline.

A new certification is now available for nurses who want to be credentialed by their professional organization as a nursing case manager. In October 1997, the first nursing case management examination was given by the American Nurses Credentialing Center (ANCC).

Other certifications may also be acquired by case managers, such as the CRRN certification for case managers in rehabilitation nursing (Table 3-2). Information on certifying organizations can be found on the SIMON website at http://www.wbsaunders.com/SIMON/Iggy/.

CHART 3-1

BEST PRACTICE *for* The Process of Case Management

Needs Assessment
- Assesses/collects data
- Conducts case screening
- Identifies client's support systems and care providers
- Reviews history and determines current health care needs
- Obtains approvals for contracts

Plan Development
- Identifies services and funding options
- Reviews plan for consensus
- Advocates for client as needed
- Develops plan of care as indicated

Implementation and Coordination
- Communicates regularly with clients and support systems
- Coordinates treatment plan
- Promotes coordinated and efficient care
- Identifies needs for additional services

Outcomes Monitoring and Evaluation
- Assesses benefit value to cost and value to quality of life
- Reviews plan for continuity of care
- Evaluates client satisfaction and compliance with treatment plan

Documentation
- Records services and outcomes
- Submits reports and other documentation as needed

Roles of Case Managers

Although models for case management vary, all case managers assume a common set of roles and functions. The CMSA *Standards of Practice* outlines the major roles of the case manager, including assessment, planning, facilitation, and advocacy. For nurses, many of the skills needed to fulfill these roles are learned in basic nursing education programs.

As an assessor, the case manager gathers all relevant data from a variety of sources and evaluates this information to identify barriers, clarify or determine realistic outcomes, and seek potential alternatives. The case manager works with the client and family/significant other to develop a plan that ensures that outcomes will be met and costs will be contained. As a facilitator, the case manager uses expert communication skills with all parties involved, including the care providers, client, family, and managed care payer. The client's best interests are represented by the case manager's advocacy for necessary resources, including funding and the coordination of health care services.

From Case Management to Disease State Management

Case management models vary depending on the country's health care system or specific health care agency. For example, case managers in the United States practice disease state management, sometimes called disease management. Put simply, disease state management focuses on the care of clients with chronic disease or illness, such as asthma, diabetes, or congestive heart failure. The purpose of this approach is to keep clients with chronic conditions as healthy as possible in the community.

TABLE 3-2 • THE MOST COMMON TYPES OF CASE MANAGER CERTIFICATIONS

Type of Case Manager	Certification Designation
Case manager (generalist)	Certified Case Manager (CCM)
Disability manager	Certified Disability Management Specialist (CDMS), formerly the Certified Insurance Rehabilitation Specialist (CIRS)
Rehabilitation nurse	Certified Rehabilitation Registered Nurse (CRRN)
Occupational health nurse	Certified Occupational Health Nurse (COHN)
Continuity of care manager	Advanced Certification in Continuity of Care (A-CCC)
Vocational evaluator	Certified Vocational Evaluator (CVE)
Drug and alcohol counselor	Masters Addiction Counselor (MAC)
Life care planner	Certified Life Care Planner (CLCP)

Data taken in part from May, V.R. et al. (2000). The life care planning process and certification: Current trends in health care management. *The Journal of Care Management, 6*(1), 38-40, 45-49.

The Role of Clinical Pathways

As mentioned in Chapter 1, the clinical pathway (CP) is a commonly used format for delineating the client's plan of care. It is an interdisciplinary guideline for care that optimally sequences the interventions and expected outcomes for a client. Other names for the pathway include the collaborative plan of care (POC), multidisciplinary action plan (MAP), critical pathway, and care path.

The CP is developed by clinical experts for diagnoses, treatments, procedures, or symptoms that are costly, complex, and variable. The health care team follows the pathway in managing the client's care. If expected outcomes are not met, the case manager, nurse, or other health professional records these variances, or deviations, on a data collection tool. The variances are then analyzed to identify actual or potential problems. An action plan is implemented and followed up to determine if the problem was resolved or avoided. This entire sequence of data collection, problem identification, action plan, and follow-up is part of the continuous quality improvement (CQI) process that every health care agency uses to monitor and improve the care that it provides.

This text provides several examples of CPs with varying formats. Traditional client care plans are also included in this text to help students identify the difference between a nursing focused care plan and an interdisciplinary plan of care, the clinical pathway.

ONLINE RESOURCES

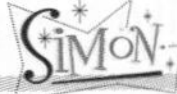

For suggested readings and Internet resources, go to http://www.wbsaunders.com/SIMON/Iggy/.

SELECTED BIBLIOGRAPHY

Asterisk indicates a classic or definitive work on this subject.

*Bower, K. (1992). *Case management by nurses.* Washington, DC: American Nurses Publishing.

*Case Management Society of America. (1995). *Standards of practice for case management.* Little Rock, AR: Author.

Cesta, T., Tahan, H., & Fink, L. (1998). *The case manager's survival guide.* St. Louis: Mosby.

Chan, F., et al. (1999). Foundational knowledge and major practice domains of case management. *The Journal of Care Management, 5*(1), 10-18, 26-30.

Cohen, E.L. (1997). *Nurse case management in the 21st century.* St. Louis: Mosby.

Conger, M. (1998). Integration of acute care CNS and case manager roles. *Critical Care Clinics of North America, 10*(1), 127-134.

Engen, C. (1998). Critical thinking in case management. *Inside Case Management, 5*(9), 11-12.

Fick, D.M., et al. (2000). Advance practice nursing care management model for elders in a managed care environment. *Journal of Care Management, 6*(1), 28-30, 33-37, 49.

Finkelman, A.W. (2001). *Managed care: A nursing perspective.* Upper Saddle River, NJ: Prentice Hall.

Forbes, M. (1999). The practice of professional nurse case management. *Nursing Case Management, 4*(1), 28-33.

Hogan, T.D. (1997). Case management in a wound care program. *Nursing Case Management, 2*(1), 2-15.

Howe, R. (1998). Population case management emerging as a significant approach to case management. *Inside Case Management, 5*(3), 3-5.

*Ignatavicius, D.D., & Hausman, K. (1995). *Clinical pathways for collaborative practice.* Philadelphia: W.B. Saunders.

May, V.R., et al. (2000). The life care planning process and certification: Current trends in health care management. *The Journal of Care Management, 6*(1), 38-40, 45-49.

McGregor, C. (1998). Building partnerships in managed care. *Inside Case Management, 4*(12), 2-5.

Mullahy, C.M. (1998). *Essential readings in case management.* Gaithersburg, MD: Aspen.

Mullahy, C.M. (1999). *The case manager's handbook.* (2nd ed.). Gaithersburg, MD: Aspen.

Owens, M. (1997). Hi, I'm your case manager. *Home Care Provider, 2*(6), 307-310.

Powell, S.K. (2000). *Nursing care management: A practical guide to success in managed care* (2nd ed.). Philadelphia: Lippincott-Raven.

Powell, S.K., & Ignatavicius, D. (2001). *CMSA core curriculum for case management.* Philadelphia: J.B. Lippincott.

Rognehaugh, R. (1998). *The managed care health care dictionary.* Gaithersburg, MD: Aspen.

Siefker, J.M., et al. (1998). *Fundamentals of case management: Guidelines for practicing case managers.* St. Louis: Mosby.

Taylor, P. (1999). Comprehensive nursing case management: An advanced practice model. *Nursing Case Management, 4*(1), 11-13.

Wrinn, P. (1998). A new frontier for case management outcomes. *Continuing Care, 17*(6), 16, 18, 20, 25, 35.

*Zander, K. (1996). *Handbook of nursing case management.* Gaithersburg, MD: Aspen.

CHAPTER 4

Introduction to Complementary and Alternative Therapies

DONNA D. IGNATAVICIUS

Learning Objectives

After studying this chapter, you should be able to:

1. Describe selected low-risk complementary and alternative therapies that nurses can use with their clients in a variety of health care settings.
2. Identify at least one purpose for each selected complementary and alternative therapy.
3. Discuss the implications of complementary and alternative therapies for health care professionals.

SIMON **Go to http://www.wbsaunders.com/SIMON/Iggy/ for self-assessment questions related to these Learning Objectives.**

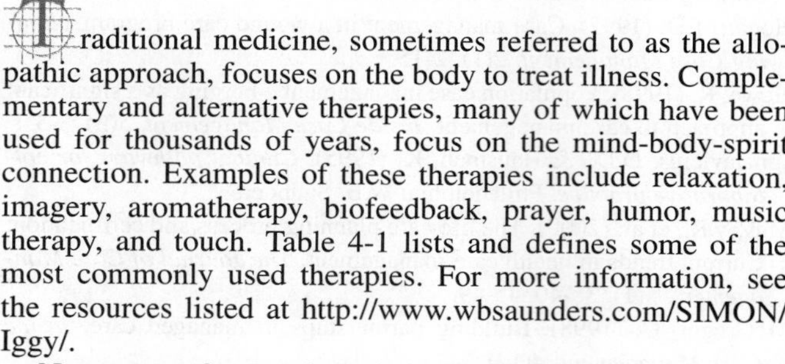

Traditional medicine, sometimes referred to as the allopathic approach, focuses on the body to treat illness. Complementary and alternative therapies, many of which have been used for thousands of years, focus on the mind-body-spirit connection. Examples of these therapies include relaxation, imagery, aromatherapy, biofeedback, prayer, humor, music therapy, and touch. Table 4-1 lists and defines some of the most commonly used therapies. For more information, see the resources listed at http://www.wbsaunders.com/SIMON/Iggy/.

Nurses are often not knowledgeable about the role of complementary and alternative therapies in the promotion of health or healing. Yet in 1997, more than 40% of adults in the United States visited practitioners for these therapies and spent more than $32 billion for treatment (Eisenberg et al., 1998). The majority of these dollars were out-of-pocket expenses because most insurance companies and managed care organizations (MCOs) do not cover complementary and alternative therapies (see the Cost of Care box on p. 31). Increasing consumer demand mandates that third-party payers include benefits for these therapies and that nurses be informed about these important interventions.

NATIONAL CENTER FOR COMPLEMENTARY AND ALTERNATIVE MEDICINE

Recognizing the growing trend toward CAM, the National Institutes of Health created the Office of Alternative Medicine (OAM) in 1992 to evaluate therapies that hold the most promise in treating illness and disease. OAM was recently changed to the National Center for Complementary and Alternative Medicine (NCCAM), and its budget has been significantly increased. The ultimate goal of the NCCAM is to integrate validated complementary therapies into current conventional medical practice. At this time, a number of studies are being conducted around the country by physicians, nurses, and others interested in CAM to determine which therapies are the most effective for which conditions. Many of these studies focus on mind-body control therapies (e.g., biofeedback and imagery), structural and energetic therapies (e.g., acupressure and therapeutic touch), and ethnomedicine (e.g., homeopathic medicine and herbal medicine). The safety, efficacy, mechanism of action, and cost-effectiveness of individual therapies are also being examined.

COMMONLY USED COMPLEMENTARY AND ALTERNATIVE THERAPIES

It is beyond the scope of this introductory chapter to list all of the many therapies used by consumers and health care professionals or to describe any one therapy in detail. The reader is referred to the books and articles included in the Bibliography. Some of the most common, low-risk therapies that nurses can use are briefly described here. In addition to this introduction, discussions of complementary and alternative therapies are found throughout the text, such as in the sections on pain (Chapter 7), arthritis (Chapter 21), acquired immunodeficiency syndrome (Chapter 22), cancer (Chapter 25), and burns (Chapter 68).

CULTURAL CONSIDERATIONS

Studies have shown that ethnicity and culture play a part in determining who seeks complementary and alternative medicine (CAM). Eisenberg et al. (1998) found that U.S. consumers of CAM tend to be educated, upper-income Caucasians in the 35- to 49-year age-group. Use is more common among women than men and less common among African Americans when compared with other minority racial groups. Arcury et al. (1996) found that less wealthy rural clients in North Carolina used a variety of conventional and alternative remedies, especially for arthritic pain. Prayer was the most common modality used (92% of the sample), and African Americans used prayer more often than did Caucasians.

Another study revealed that 44% of Mexican Americans in the Texas Rio Grande Valley visited an alternative practitioner one or more times during the study year (Keegan, 1996). The most commonly sought therapies were herbal medicine, spiritual healing and prayer, relaxation, and massage. Chapter 6 of this text describes additional information about the relationship of culture to healing, including the practice of folk medicine.

COST OF CARE IMPLICATIONS FOR NURSING

COMPLEMENTARY AND ALTERNATIVE THERAPIES

- The amount of money spent in the United States for treatments provided by practitioners of complementary and alternative therapies has been estimated at $32.6 billion—an increase of 45% between 1990 and 1997.
- The total out-of-pocket expense for complementary and alternative therapies in 1997 was approximately $27 billion.
- Estimated out-of-pocket expenses for vitamin supplements rose from $0.9 billion in 1990 to $3.3 billion in 1997.
- Expenditures for herbal products in 1997 were approximately $5.1 billion.
- Sales of herbal products are increasing at a rate of approximately 15% each year.

Data from Eisenberg, D.M., et al. (1998). Trends in alternative medicine use in the United States, 1990-1997: Results of a follow-up national survey. *Journal of the American Medical Association, 280*(18), 1569-1575.

Spirituality and Religion

Spirituality and religion are related concepts. **Spirituality** gives meaning to a person; that is, it is an aspect of humanity that helps a person find purpose in life. **Religion** refers to a belief system and the practices of worship related to that system. Religion usually includes a personal commitment or devotion to God or other higher power (Dossey, 1997; Nehring & Meraviglia, 2000).

Research has demonstrated that spirituality and religion can positively affect healing and minimize the demands of illness. For example, nursing researchers Fernsler, Klemm, and Miller (1999) found that clients with colorectal cancer who reported high levels of spiritual well-being had significantly fewer physical symptoms and treatment issues than those with lower levels of spiritual well-being. In another study, Ayele et al. (1999) determined that the religious perceptions and activities of physicians and older adults had a positive association with life satisfaction.

Because spirituality and religion take many forms, the nurse explores the way in which clients express their beliefs. For instance, the nurse can help clients reflect on the meaning of prayer and of other expressions of spirituality and religion, including inspirational readings and music, in their lives. Some of the questions that a nurse might ask to help clients to find and use meaning in spiritual or religious activities are listed in Table 4-2.

Relaxation

Relaxation is one of the simplest and easiest complementary and alternative therapies to use. The purpose of relaxation techniques is to reduce physical, mental, and emotional tension, resulting in changes opposite to those of the fight-or-flight mechanism (Dossey, 1997). The physiologic effects of relaxation involve the autonomic, immune, and endocrine systems (Table 4-3).

Commonly used relaxation techniques include progressive muscle relaxation (PMR), imagery, aromatherapy, and music. The nurse can easily use PMR, imagery, and music without special training. Aromatherapy usually requires special training.

TABLE 4-1 • DEFINITIONS OF COMMON COMPLEMENTARY AND ALTERNATIVE THERAPIES

acupressure Use of pressure from the fingers and hands to stimulate the energy points in the body, thereby removing energy blocks that are believed to produce health problems

acupuncture Use of needles to stimulate certain points on the body to treat pain, diseases, or dysfunctions of the body; the World Health Organization and National Institutes of Health currently list a number of medical conditions that may be effectively treated, including migraine, asthma, and arthritis (practitioners are usually licensed by the state)

aromatherapy Use of medicinal properties of essential oils extracted from plants and herbs; may be administered via inhalation, topically, or through ingestion

chiropractic Use of manipulation to realign the spine and nervous system so the body can heal (practitioners are usually licensed by the state)

imagery Use of a technique in which a client uses memories, dreams, and fantasies to relieve stress, decrease pain, and promote healing

homeopathy Use of dilute forms of biologic materials (plant, animal, and mineral) to produce symptoms similar to those caused by disease, causing the body to fight disease

hypnotherapy Use of hypnosis, posthypnotic suggestion, or any similar process that prepares the client to be susceptible to suggestion or direction

massage therapy Manipulation of skeletal muscle to relieve stress or muscle tension; includes stroking, kneading, or stretching of muscles

naturopathy A system of prevention, diagnosis, and management of health problems using natural medicines and therapies to stimulate the client's healing process

osteopathy Use of body positioning and manipulative techniques to detect faulty body structure and function

TABLE 4-2 • QUESTIONS THAT CAN BE USED AS PART OF A SPIRITUAL/RELIGIOUS ASSESSMENT

- What gives your life meaning?
- What brings you joy and peace in your life?
- What helps you cope when you are troubled or worried?
- How do you feel about yourself?
- Who are the significant people in your life?
- Are worship and religion important to you?
- Do you believe in God or a higher power?
- Is prayer helpful to you?
- Is faith important in your life?
- What is the most important or powerful thing in your life?
- To whom do you turn when you need help?
- What is your source of strength and hope?
- Can I contact someone for you now?

TABLE 4-3 • PHYSIOLOGIC EFFECTS OF RELAXATION

- Increased peripheral blood flow
- Decreased respiratory rate and volume
- Decreased heart rate
- Decreased blood pressure
- Decreased epinephrine level
- Decreased gastric acidity and motility
- Increased activity of killer cells
- Decreased oxygen consumption
- Decreased sweat gland activity

PROGRESSIVE MUSCLE RELAXATION

Progressive muscle relaxation (PMR) is based on the belief that stress increases skeletal muscle tension. Intentional tensing and releasing of successive muscle groups promotes relaxation and decreases anxiety. PMR has been used successfully for clients with hypertension, asthma, and panic attacks.

When caring for a client who is tense or anxious, the nurse assesses the client's perception of the need for relaxation, readiness and motivation to learn relaxation strategies, and past experience, if any, with relaxation techniques. The nurse also determines whether the client can remain still for a short time.

To begin PMR, the client closes his or her eyes and takes several deep breaths, in through the nose and out through the mouth. He or she tenses and releases each muscle group for several seconds, starting with the head and progressing to the toes. This entire procedure can be completed in a few minutes. The nurse evaluates the success of relaxation strategies by asking the client how he or she feels before and after the intervention and by assessing for the physiologic responses listed in Table 4-3.

IMAGERY

Imagery is a technique in which a person experiences memories, dreams, and visions as a bridge for making the body-mind-spirit connection. Images can occur spontaneously or be induced deliberately. All senses may be involved, but most images are visual; that is, people see positive "mental pictures" such as a beautiful sunset or a magnificent ocean. The inhalation or application of essential plant oils, sometimes referred to as aromatherapy, can enhance the formation of images and relaxation.

Imagery produces physiologic effects that affect healing. Images and thoughts are transmitted through the hypothalamus and limbic system of the brain by neurotransmitters, especially norepinephrine and acetylcholine. These substances affect both the peripheral and autonomic nervous systems to promote relaxation. Clients with terminal cancer or severe pain often use imagery as a complementary therapy.

A nursing study by Kolcaba and Fox (1999) explored the effects of guided imagery on the comfort of women with early breast cancer undergoing radiation therapy. Fifty-three women between 37 and 81 years of age were randomly assigned to an experimental group or a control group. The experimental group listened to a guided imagery audiotape once a day from the beginning of radiation therapy through 3 weeks after the completion of therapy. Results clearly demonstrated that guided imagery enhanced comfort and decreased anxiety, especially during the first 3 weeks. Audiotapes were cost-effective because they saved time for the staff.

EVIDENCE-BASED PRACTICE FOR NURSING

Music can help alleviate nausea and vomiting in clients receiving chemotherapy

Ezzone, S., et al. (1998). Music as an adjunct to antiemetic therapy. *Oncology Nursing Forum, 25*(9), 1551-1556.

To test whether the use of music during high-dose cyclophosphamide administration affects nausea and episodes of vomiting, the researchers randomly assigned 39 clients to either a treatment group or a control group. Both groups received the usual antiemetic medications. In addition, subjects in the treatment group listened to music during the 48 hours of chemotherapy administration. Subjects who listened to music had less perception of nausea and had fewer episodes of vomiting than subjects in the control group.

Critique. Although the sample size was small, the researchers used an experimental design and controlled for the type of chemotherapy administered. Further study using larger groups of subjects is needed for generalization, but it appears that music is helpful as a diversional adjunct intervention for clients receiving chemotherapy.

Implications for Nursing. Music is a cost-effective intervention that any nurse can use when giving chemotherapy. It can be individualized for each client and initiated independently by nurses to increase client comfort.

AROMATHERAPY

Aromatherapy is a branch of herbal medicine that uses scents from the essential oils of plants to cause physiologic and psychologic responses, including relaxation. Specific oils, such as chamomile, lavender, and tea tree, are believed to have relaxing effects. Others, such as eucalyptus and peppermint, act as stimulants. When absorbed by body tissues, they are thought to interact with enzymes and hormones and produce changes in vital signs and other body functions.

Although the demand for aromatherapy has dramatically increased in the United States during the past decade, it is most common in Europe. Aromatherapy can be self-administered or administered by a trained practitioner. The claims that aromatherapy can treat or cure disease have not yet been supported through research (Springhouse, 2000).

MUSIC

Soothing music can produce relaxation and a hypometabolic response in which the autonomic, immune, and endocrine systems are affected. Because music is nonverbal, it appeals to the right side of the brain; traditional verbalization appeals to the left side of the brain.

Music can complement conventional medical therapy by reducing pain, anxiety, nausea, and agitation. Music has been used for surgical clients in both the preoperative and postoperative phases of care. Preoperative clients who listened to music of their choice reported less anxiety than those who did not. Music can also lower the heart rates, blood pressures, and respiratory rates of preoperative clients (Augustin & Hains, 1996). Another nursing study showed that music in the immediate postoperative period functioned as a distractor and helped clients to relax (Heiser et al., 1997). Music can also reduce nausea and anxiety in clients who are receiving chemotherapy (see the Evidence-Based Practice for Nursing box on p. 32).

As with other relaxation methods, music therapy can be used in any health care setting or in the home. The nurse assesses the client's preferred types of music and how the music makes him or her feel. Recorded tapes can be played for several daily sessions, each lasting between 20 and 30 minutes. The nurse then evaluates the client's response to the therapy, including his or her vital signs and description of the experience (if possible) and its effects, such as decreased insomnia, pain relief, or decreased agitation.

CONSIDERATIONS FOR OLDER ADULTS

For older clients who are confused and restless, the calming effect of music may improve behavioral manifestations such as agitation and combativeness. Music causes a variety of experiences, including imagery, sensory stimulation, and relaxation. A nursing study of 18 older adults with Alzheimer's disease showed that audiotaped music played during bathing significantly decreased aggressive behaviors and promoted cooperation with the bathing activity (Clark, Lipe, & Bilbrey, 1998).

Touch

The use of touch for healing was documented more than 5000 years ago. All cultures have developed some form of touch therapy. Research has demonstrated that **touch therapy** slows heart rate, decreases diastolic blood pressure, and reduces anxiety (Sayre-Adams, 1996).

Many types of touch therapies are available, including massage, therapeutic touch, acupressure, and reflexology. A back rub is a therapeutic massage. Nurses have been administering back rubs for most of the twentieth century, but time constraints have limited this intervention in most settings. Back rubs and the massage of other parts of the body can promote relaxation and sleep and provide a distraction for clients with anxiety or pain (Richards, 1998).

Therapeutic touch (TT) is a commonly used healing modality for rebalancing or repatterning one's energy field to promote pain relief, relaxation, and healing. Dr. Dolores Kreiger, Professor of Nursing at New York University, is credited with naming and promoting this specialized therapy. Research on TT has demonstrated its effectiveness in healing, including improvement in headaches, insomnia, and hypertension. It also helps with wound healing, pain relief, anxiety reduction, and relaxation (Sayre-Adams, 1996).

Acupressure is based on the Oriental energy system of meridian lines and points. Applying the healer's finger and/or

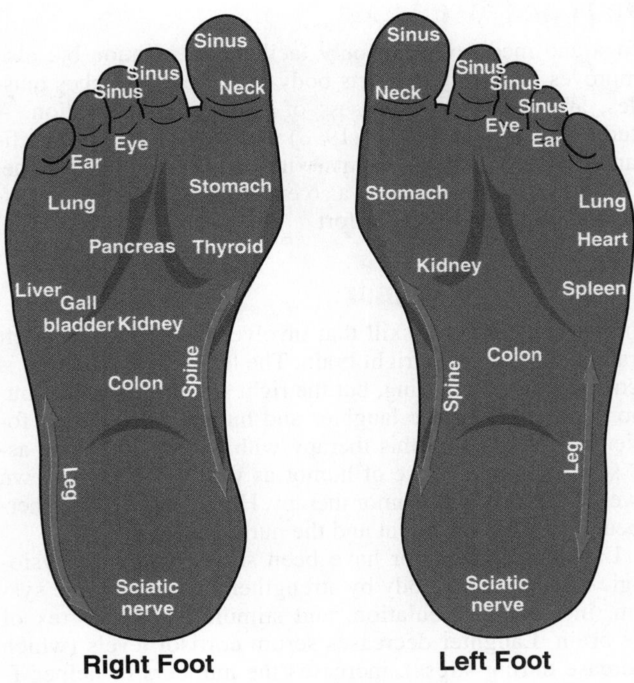

Figure 4-1 ● Reflexology chart of the foot. (From Dossey, B.M. [1995]. Using imagery to help your patient heal. *American Journal of Nursing, 95*[6], 41-46. Used with permission.)

thumb to one or more of 657 energy points that run along 12 pathways (meridian lines) releases congestion and promotes energy flow.

In the early 1900s Dr. William Fitzgerald noted that pressure applied to certain parts of the hands caused anesthesia in other parts of the body. His work was used by others to explore the field of **reflexology,** which is based on the theory that 10 equal, longitudinal zones run the length of the body. As with acupressure, applying pressure to certain points releases congestion and promotes energy flow. The other major goal of this therapy is relaxation. Figure 4-1 shows a foot reflexology chart and the location of some of the pressure points.

As with the previously described relaxation therapies, the nurse can use touch in any health care setting or in the client's home. Massage or simple touching is one of the most commonly used nursing interventions. Before using touch, however, the nurse assesses the client's feelings regarding touching, including cultural and age considerations. The nurse also evaluates the client's response to touch.

CONSIDERATIONS FOR OLDER ADULTS

Older clients are likely to receive the least amount of touch, but they need touch as much as or more than any other age-group. Older clients often have no family members or significant others. In addition, some clients cannot communicate and need touch as an effective communication tool.

Severely agitated older adults may not want to be touched; indeed, touch can cause an increase in aggressive behaviors. Some older adults may view touch as an invasion of their personal space.

Yoga and Meditation

Yoga and meditation not only facilitates relaxation but also improves flexibility, corrects body alignment, stretches muscles, and increases awareness of optimal joint position. A study by Garfinkel et al. (1998) showed that yoga significantly reduced pain in clients with carpal tunnel syndrome. Clients who practiced yoga also experienced fewer sleep disturbances related to discomfort.

Laughter and Humor

Humor is a cognitive skill that involves both the logical left brain and the creative right brain. The left side of the brain is active during joke telling, but the right side perceives the humor. Nurses often use laughter and humor when caring for clients. Before using this therapy with clients, the nurse assesses the client's sense of humor as well as his or her own level of comfort with humor therapy. Humor can be very therapeutic for both the client and the nurse.

Laughter and humor have been shown to have physiologic effects on the body by strengthening the immune system, increasing circulation, and stimulating the cortex of the brain. Laughter decreases serum cortisol levels (which increase during stress), increases the numbers of helper T-cells and natural killer cells (to destroy tumor cells), and increases salivary immunoglobulin A (to protect against upper respiratory and oral infections) (Berk & Tan, 1993). The physical activity of laughter dilates the peripheral blood vessels, which increases blood flow to the extremities (Dossey, 1997).

Laughter and humor also have psychologic effects that result in relaxation, stress reduction, and distraction. Individuals who have a strong sense of humor may deal better with stress than those who do not.

Herbalism

Many herbs, vitamins, minerals, and other natural supplements are available as over-the-counter compounds for a variety of preventive and curative purposes. However, clients need to be aware of their safety and efficacy. Some herbs have been researched, but others have not. Table 4-4 lists some of the most commonly used herbs, their purported benefits, and precautions.

Herbs are not classified as drugs in the United States, but they should be considered as drugs because they have pharmacologic effects on the body. In Germany and France, up to 40% of physicians use herbs and other botanicals in their practice and receive formal training in phytotherapy, the standardized use of herbal products (Glisson, Crawford, & Street, 1999a).

When caring for clients, the nurse should ask whether the client takes herbal products and for what purpose. In some cases, the herb may interact with prescription medications and cause toxic effects or other adverse reactions. Clients are reminded to inform all health care providers about their use of any supplement or herb. For more information, the nurse refers the client to an herbalist who is knowledgeable about high-quality herbs and where they can be purchased.

IMPLICATIONS FOR HEALTH CARE PROVIDERS

Physicians, nurses, and other health care professionals need to learn more about complementary and alternative therapies as more research becomes available. As discussed at the beginning of this chapter, healing requires a body-mind-spirit approach.

Eisenberg (1997) suggested that physicians incorporate the use of these therapies into their practices. He recommended that physicians discuss safety and efficacy issues with their

TABLE 4-4 • COMMONLY USED HERBS: PURPORTED BENEFITS AND PRECAUTIONS

Name of Herb	Purported Benefit	Precautions
Echinacea	Builds immunity, especially against upper respiratory infections; helps wound healing	Prolonged use may suppress immune system
Feverfew	Works with Echinacea to build immunity; preventive agent for migraines; antipyretic	May cause mouth ulcers and postfeverfew syndrome (aches, pains, stiffness)
Garlic	Helps to lower cholesterol level; antiplatelet agent	Can cause interaction with antiplatelet or anticoagulant drugs; chronic use can lower hemoglobin
Ginkgo biloba	Increases cerebral blood flow, resulting in improved memory; increases peripheral blood flow, resulting in improved tissue perfusion	Can cause interaction with antiplatelet or anticoagulant drugs; need to monitor for bruising and bleeding
Ginseng	Improves concentration, stamina, healing, and work efficiency; antistress agent	Should not be used for long-term therapy; can interact with caffeine to increase CNS effects
Green tea	Helps to prevent certain chronic conditions such as atherosclerosis, dental caries, and hypercholesterolemia; serves as a diuretic and stimulant	Should be used with caution in clients with asthma; avoid use with MAO inhibitors
Milk thistle	Protects the liver from disease, such as chronic hepatitis and cirrhosis	Clients with active liver disease should check with health care provider before taking this product
Saw palmetto	Decreases symptoms related to benign prostatic hypertrophy	Take with meals to reduce GI distress
St. John's wort	Improves mild to moderate depression	Take precautions against sun exposure; avoid use with other antidepressant agents

CNS, Central nervous system; *GI*, gastrointestinal; *MAO*, monoamine oxidase inhibitor.

clients and help them identify suitable licensed providers of alternative medicine. He further suggested that a follow-up visit after treatment by a practitioner of alternative therapies be made to review the response to treatment.

Medical and nursing education programs should incorporate low-risk therapies into their basic curricula. Practicing health care providers need continuing education to keep up with the public's demand for integrative therapies. More research is needed to better delineate the nurse's role in the use of these therapies.

ONLINE RESOURCES

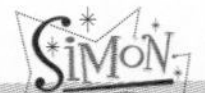

For suggested readings and Internet resources, go to http://www.wbsaunders.com/SIMON/Iggy/.

SELECTED BIBLIOGRAPHY

Asterisk indicates a classic or definitive work on this subject.

American Health Consultants. (1997). HMOs moving more toward alternative care coverage. *Case Management Advisor, 8*(1), 18-19.

*Arcury, T.A., et al. (1996). Gender and ethnic differences in alternative and conventional arthritis remedy use among community-dwelling rural adults with arthritis. *Arthritis Care Research, 9,* 384-390.

*Augustin, P., & Hains, A.A. (1996). Effect of music on ambulatory surgery patients' preoperative anxiety. *AORN Journal, 63,* 750, 753-758.

Ayele, H., et al. (1999). Religious activity improves life satisfaction for some physicians and older patients. *Journal of the American Geriatrics Society, 47*(4), 453-455.

*Berk, L.S., & Tan, S.A. (1993). Eustress of humor-associated laughter modulates specific immune system components. *Annals of Behavioral Medicine, 15,* S111.

Buselli, E.F., & Stuart, E.M. (1999). Influence of psychosocial factors and biopsychosocial interventions on outcomes after myocardial infarction. *Journal of Cardiovascular Nursing, 13*(3), 60-72.

Clark, M.E., Lipe, A.W., & Bilbrey, M. (1998). Use of music to decrease aggressive behaviors in people with dementia. *Journal of Gerontological Nursing, 24*(7), 10-17.

Collins, J.A., & Rice, V.H. (1997). Effects of relaxation intervention in phase II cardiac rehabilitation: Replication and extension. *Heart and Lung, 26,* 31-44.

*Dossey, B.M. (1995). Using imagery to help your patient heal. *American Journal of Nursing, 95*(6), 41-46.

Dossey, B.M. (1997). *Core curriculum for holistic nursing.* Gaithersburg, MD: Aspen.

Dossey, B.M., & Dossey, L. (1998). Body-mind-spirit: Attending to holistic care. *American Journal of Nursing, 98*(8), 35-38.

Dossey, B.M., Keegan, L., & Guzetta, C.E. (2000). *Holistic nursing: A handbook for practice* (3rd ed). Gaithersburg, MD: Aspen.

Eisenberg, D.M. (1997). Advising patients who seek alternative medical therapies. *Annals of Internal Medicine, 127,* 61-69.

Eisenberg, D.M., et al. (1998). Trends in alternative medicine use in the United States, 1990-1997: Results of a follow-up national survey. *Journal of the American Medical Association, 280*(18), 1569-1575.

Eliopoulos, C. (1999). *Integrating conventional alternative therapies: Holistic care for chronic conditions.* St. Louis: Mosby.

Ezzone, S., et al. (1998). Music as an adjunct to antiemetic therapy. *Oncology Nursing Forum, 25*(9), 1551-1556.

Fernsler, J.I., Klemm, P., & Miller, M.A. (1999). Spiritual well-being and demands of illness in people with colorectal cancer. *Cancer Nursing, 22*(2), 134-140.

Forbes, D.A. (1998). Strategies for managing behavioural symptomatology associated with dementia of the Alzheimer type: A systematic overview. *Canadian Journal of Nursing Research, 30*(2), 67-86.

Garfinkel, M.S., et al. (1998). Yoga-based intervention for carpal tunnel syndrome: A randomized trial. *Journal of the American Medical Association, 280,* 1601-1603.

Gimbel, M.A. (1998). Yoga, meditation, and imagery: Clinical applications. *Nurse Practitioner Forum, 9*(4), 243-255.

Glisson, J., Crawford, R., & Street, S. (1999a). Review, critique, and guidelines for the use of herbs and homeopathy. *The Nurse Practitioner, 24*(4), 44-46, 53, 60, 65-67.

Glisson, J., Crawford, R., & Street, S. (1999b). The clinical applications of ginkgo biloba, St. John's Wort, saw palmetto, and soy. *The Nurse Practitioner, 24*(6), 28-38, 43-47.

Hatler, C.W. (1998). Using guided imagery in the emergency department. *Journal of Emergency Nursing, 24*(6), 518-522.

Heiser, R.M., et al. (1997). The use of music during the immediate postoperative recovery period. *AORN Journal, 765,* 777-778, 781-785.

*Keegan, L. (1996). Use of alternative therapies among Mexican Americans in the Texas Rio Grande Valley. *Journal of Holistic Nursing, 14,* 277-294.

Keegan, L. (1998). Getting comfortable with alternative and complementary therapies. *Nursing98, 28*(4), 50-53.

Kendall, M.L. (1999). A holistic nursing model for spiritual care of the terminally ill. *American Journal of Hospice and Palliative Care, 16*(2), 473-476.

Kendig, S., & Sanford, D.G. (1998). Alternative aging: Using complementary therapies for midlife and menopause. *AWHONN Lifelines, 2*(3), 55-58.

Kolcaba, K., & Fox, C. (1999). The effects of guided imagery on comfort of women with early stage breast cancer undergoing radiation therapy. *Oncology Nursing Forum, 26*(1), 67-72.

Kwekkeboom, K., Huseby-Moore, K., & Ward, S. (1998). Imaging ability and the effective use of guided imagery. *Research in Nursing and Health, 21*(3), 189-198.

Marcus, C.L. (1999). Alternative medicine: The AMA reviews scientific evidence. *Clinician Reviews, 9*(2), 87-90.

Maxwell, J. (1997). The gentle power of acupressure. *RN, 60*(4), 53-56.

McDowell, B.J., et al. (1999). Effectiveness of behavioral therapy to treat incontinence in homebound older adults. *Journal of the American Geriatrics Society, 47*(3), 301-318.

Miller, T. (1998). The value of imagery in perioperative nursing. *Seminars in Perioperative Nursing, 7*(2), 108-113.

Nehring, V. & Meraviglia, M. (2000). Spirituality. In H. Harkreeder (Ed.), *Fundamentals of nursing* (pp. 1462-1486). Philadelphia: W.B. Saunders.

O'Neil, C., Avila, J.R., & Fetrow, C.W. (1999). Herbal medicines: Getting beyond the hype. *Nursing99, 29*(4), 58-61.

Papantonio, C. (1998). Alternative medicine and wound healing. *Ostomy and Wound Management, 44*(4), 44-46, 50.

Richards, K.C. (1998). Effect of a back massage and relaxation intervention on sleep in critically ill patients. *American Journal of Critical Care, 7*(4), 288-299.

Rimmer, L. (1998). The clinical use of aromatherapy in the reduction of stress. *Home Healthcare Nurse, 16*(2), 123-126.

*Sayre-Adams, J. (1996). Therapeutic touch. In V. Slater & V. Rankin-Box. *The nurses' handbook of complementary therapies* (pp. 163-169). New York: Churchill Livingstone.

Springhouse. (2000). *Nurse's handbook of alternative and complementary therapies.* Springhouse, PA: Author.

Toran, M.R. (1999). The magic of music. *The Case Manager, 10*(6), 41-43.

Wallace, K.G. (1997). Analysis of recent literature concerning relaxation and imagery interventions for cancer pain. *Cancer Nursing, 20*(2), 79-87.

CHAPTER

5

Health Care of Older Adults

DONNA D. IGNATAVICIUS

Learning Objectives

After studying this chapter, you should be able to:

1. Identify four subgroups of older adults.
2. Describe nursing interventions for relocation stress syndrome.
3. Discuss common health issues that may concern older adults.
4. Explain why older adults are often at high risk for falls.
5. State common interventions for older clients at high risk for falls.
6. Describe the nursing care required for clients who are restrained.
7. Explain the effects of drugs on the older adult.
8. Compare and contrast delirium and dementia.
9. Interpret the signs and symptoms of elder neglect or abuse.
10. Discuss potential economic issues for older adults.
11. Describe government and community resources that are available for older adults.

Go to http://www.wbsaunders.com/SIMON/Iggy/ for self-assessment questions related to these Learning Objectives.

In the United States, the percentage of people over 65 years of age is approximately 13%. This number is expected to grow as "baby boomers" approach late adulthood in the next 10 to 15 years. As many as 50% to 80% of hospitalized clients on medical-surgical units are over age 65. Health care professionals need to know about the special needs of older adults as they care for them in a variety of settings.

This chapter describes the major health issues associated with late adulthood. The care of older adults (sometimes referred to as elders or the elderly) with specific health problems, such as pain management, acute and chronic illnesses, and the need for surgical procedures, is discussed in appropriate chapters throughout this text. In addition, Nursing Focus on the Older Adult charts and Considerations for Older Adults headings highlight the most important information.

SUBGROUPS OF LATE ADULTHOOD

Late adulthood can be divided into four subgroups:

- 65 to 74 years of age: the young old
- 75 to 84 years of age: the middle old
- 85 to 99 years of age: the old old
- 100 years of age or more: the elite old

The fastest growing subgroup is the old old, sometimes referred to as the advanced older adult population. The needs and problems of this subgroup are generally different from those of adults between 65 and 74 years of age. The incidence of chronic disease increases markedly after age 80. At any age, however, the older adult has specific needs and problems.

DISTRIBUTION OF OLDER ADULTS IN THE HEALTH CARE SYSTEM

Approximately 80% to 85% of older adults are relatively healthy and live in the community at home, in assisted-living facilities, or in retirement complexes. Five percent reside in long-term care facilities (nursing homes), and another 10% to 15% are ill but are being cared for at home (Matteson, McConnell, & Linton, 1997). Older adults from any setting usually experience one or more hospitalizations in their lifetime. Approximately 40% of elders are admitted for short-term stays in a nursing home.

ADMISSION OF THE OLDER ADULT TO A HOSPITAL OR NURSING HOME

Being admitted to a hospital or nursing home is often a traumatic experience. Many older adults suffer from **relocation stress,** also known as relocation trauma or relocation syndrome. Most early studies of this syndrome examined the increased mortality rate associated with moving people from their own homes to a nursing home or hospital. Other studies have investigated the additional effects of relocation on behavior and health. Few studies have examined the negative impact of relocation on health status and function, although physical and mental changes have been noted (Matteson et al., 1997).

In some cases, an older adult who is admitted to the hospital or nursing home from the community can become disoriented, confused, agitated, or abusive. Risk factors thought to contribute to relocation syndrome are the lack of choice or

CHART 5-1

BEST PRACTICE *for*
Minimizing the Effects of Relocation Stress in Older Adults

- Provide opportunities for the client to assist in decision making.
- Carefully explain all procedures and routines to the client before they occur.
- Ask the family or significant others to provide familiar or special keepsakes to keep at the client's bedside (e.g., family picture, favorite hairbrush).
- Reorient the client frequently to his or her location.
- Ask the client about his or her expectations during hospitalization or nursing home placement.
- Encourage the client's family and friends to visit often.
- Establish a trusting relationship with the client as early as possible.
- Assess the client's usual lifestyle and daily activities, including food likes and dislikes and preferred time for bathing.
- Avoid unnecessary room changes.
- If possible, have a family member, significant other, staff member, or volunteer accompany the client when leaving the unit for special procedures or therapies.

preparation time and the major environmental change. Men older than age 75 who are physically and mentally impaired are at a very high risk for relocation syndrome. Chart 5-1 lists interventions that may help to minimize the effects of relocation.

HEALTH ISSUES FOR OLDER ADULTS

Common health issues and problems that can affect older adults in any setting include the following:

- Health promotion
- Self-management
- Nutritional awareness
- Physical fitness and mobility
- Stress management
- Accidents
- Drug use and misuse
- Mental health
- Elder neglect and abuse

Health Promotion

Health is a major concern of most older adults. Health status can affect the ability to perform basic activities of daily living and to participate in social roles. A failure to perform these activities may increase dependence on others and may have a negative effect on morale and life satisfaction. When older adults lose the ability to function independently, they often feel empty and worthless. Loss of autonomy is a painful event related to the physical and mental changes of aging, and it can be the result of physical illness (Davidhizar & Shearer, 2000).

Autonomy has been studied extensively in relation to ethical issues. Like any clients, older adults need to have control over decision making whenever possible. They should have the right to choose whether they access or forego health and social services.

For both middle-aged and older adults, heart disease and cancer are very common. Most fatalities among older adults are due to disorders resulting from diminished physiologic defenses, such as a severe infection related to cancer or cancer treatment.

CHART 5-2

CLIENT EDUCATION GUIDE
Lifestyles and Practices to Promote Wellness

Health-Protecting Behaviors

- Have yearly influenza vaccinations (after October 1).
- Obtain a pneumococcal vaccination. (A routine revaccination may be necessary.)
- Have a tetanus immunization, and get a booster every 10 years.
- Wear seat belts when you are in an automobile.
- Use alcohol in moderation or not at all.
- Avoid smoking.
- If you smoke at home, do not smoke in bed.
- Install and maintain working smoke detectors.
- Create a hazard-free environment to prevent falls; eliminate hazards such as scatter rugs and waxed floors.
- Use medications according to your physician's orders.
- Avoid over-the-counter medications unless your physician directs you to use them.
- Take one aspirin every day (any dose between 81 and 325 mg) to decrease the risk of myocardial infarction and colon cancer.

Health-Enhancing Behaviors

- Have a yearly physical examination; see your health care provider more often if health problems occur.
- Reduce dietary fat to not more than 30% of calories; saturated fat should provide less than 10% of your calories.
- Increase your dietary intake of complex carbohydrate and fiber-containing food to five or more servings of fruits and vegetables and six or more servings of grain products daily.
- Increase calcium intake to between 1000 and 1500 mg daily.
- Allow at least 10 to 15 minutes of sun exposure two to three times weekly for vitamin D intake; avoid prolonged sun exposure.
- Exercise regularly three to five times a week for 30 minutes per session.
- Manage stress through coping mechanisms that have been successful in the past.
- Get together with people in different settings.
- Reminisce about your life.

Based in part on data from Paist, S.S. (1999). Screening and preventive interventions in older patients: Which ones are useful? *Hospital Medicine, 35*(6), 16-21.

Like younger adults, older adults need to practice health promotion and illness prevention to maintain or achieve a high level of wellness. The nurse working with these clients in any setting needs to teach them the importance of promoting wellness and strategies for accomplishing this goal (Chart 5-2).

Self-Management

An older person's ability to maintain a positive self-concept and self-control may be hampered by the loss of resources in the late years of life. Older adults may also experience a number of losses that can affect their sense of control over their lives: the death of a spouse and significant others, the loss of social and work roles, and a decrease in physical mobility. The nurse can support older clients' self-esteem and feelings of competency by encouraging them to maintain as much control as possible over their lives, to participate in decision making, and to perform as many tasks as possible.

Regardless of the situation, it is important that older clients direct their lifestyle in a manner that encourages them to feel capable and valued. Most important, they need to find opportunities to be productive and take care of themselves as well as others.

A number of tools are available to the nurse in the community health or home health setting for assessing the self-care or self-management ability of older adults. (See Chapter 10 for examples of functional assessment tools.) When older adults are admitted to a hospital or nursing home, the nurse needs to assess self-management capabilities for discharge planning.

Nutritional Awareness

NUTRITIONAL NEEDS IN THE COMMUNITY

A person's need for adequate nutrition remains constant throughout the life span, yet many older people are at risk for malnutrition. Inflation, reduced income, and a lack of transportation are factors that may contribute to inadequate nutrition among older adults. Older adults whose diets consist of inappropriate or unbalanced foods (e.g., an excess of carbohydrates) may also be poorly nourished. Some clients reduce their intake of food to near-starvation levels, even with the availability of assistive programs such as food stamps, free food, and Meals on Wheels. The lack of transportation, the necessity of traveling to obtain such services, and the inability to carry large quantities of groceries prohibit some elders from taking advantage of food programs. Some older adults are too proud to accept free services.

Poor nutrition may also be related to loneliness. Older adults may respond to loneliness, depression, and boredom by not eating, which can lead to malnutrition. Many clients who live alone lose the incentive to prepare or eat balanced diets. Others respond to stress by overeating, which leads to obesity.

NUTRITIONAL REQUIREMENTS

The minimal nutritional requirements of the human body remain consistent from youth through old age, with a few exceptions. Older adults need an increased dietary intake of calcium, vitamin D, vitamin C, and vitamin A because alterations with age disrupt the ability to store, use, and absorb these substances. A sedentary lifestyle and reduced metabolic rate requires a reduction in total caloric intake to maintain an ideal body weight.

PHYSICAL CHANGES AFFECTING NUTRITION

Other physical aging changes influence nutritional status or the ability to consume needed nutrients. Diminished senses of taste and smell often result in a loss of appeal of food. Older adults experience a greater decline in the ability to taste sweet and salt than in the discrimination of bitter and sour. This physiologic change often results in an overuse of table sugar and salt to compensate. The nurse teaches the client to substitute herbs and spices to season food or to vary the textures of food substances to achieve satisfaction from food.

Tooth loss and poorly fitting dentures from inadequate dental care can also cause the older adult to avoid important foodstuffs. Older people with dentition problems often resort to eating soft, high-calorie foods such as ice cream and mashed potatoes, which lack roughage and fiber. Unless the person carefully chooses more nutritious soft foods, vitamin deficiencies, constipation, and other disorders can result. The extensive use of prescribed and over-the-counter (OTC) drugs may affect appetite, food tolerances, and food absorption and use.

Older adults sometimes respond to problems associated with mobility, prescribed diuretics, and limited bladder capacity by limiting fluid intake, especially in the evening. The nurse teaches older adults that fluid restrictions make them prone to dehydration and electrolyte imbalances that can cause serious illness or death.

NUTRITIONAL NEEDS IN THE HOSPITAL AND NURSING HOME

In addition to the nutritional needs described for older adults living in the community, those who are in the hospital or nursing home have special needs related to their illness and general health. For example, an older client with a pressure ulcer needs additional protein, vitamin C, and zinc to heal the open skin lesion. The health care provider, nurse, and dietitian collaborate to determine the best sources of these nutrients. The health care provider may prescribe a multivitamin tablet with zinc to be given every day. The dietitian may recommend that a high-calorie, high-protein supplement such as Ensure Plus be given several times a day. The nurse encourages the client to select and eat high-protein foods to promote healing and prevent undernutrition.

Anorexia and weight loss are the most common nutritional problems in both hospitals and long-term care settings. In nursing homes, the prevalence of undernutrition has been reported to range from 20% to 54% (Council for Nutritional Clinical Strategies in Long-Term Care, 1999). Common causes of undernutrition include drugs, chewing problems, immobility, infections, and Alzheimer's disease. Chapter 61 discusses nutrition in detail, including interdisciplinary interventions for the prevention and management of common problems.

Physical Fitness and Mobility

Exercise and activity are important for older adults as a means of promoting and maintaining health (Figure 5-1). Physical activity can help keep the body in shape and maintain an optimal level of functioning. In addition, regular and moderate exercise typically results in feelings of well-being. Numerous studies have shown that exercise can do the following (Christmas & Andersen, 2000):

- Decrease falls
- Increase strength
- Reduce arthritis pain
- Reduce depression
- Improve longevity
- Reduce risks for diabetes and coronary artery disease

Health care providers need to promote a less sedentary lifestyle for their clients and encourage physical activity. One of the best exercises for older adults is walking at least 30 minutes, three to five times a week. Swimming is also recommended but does not offer the weight-bearing advantage of walking. Elders who have been sedentary should start their exercise programs slowly and gradually increase the frequency and duration of activity over time.

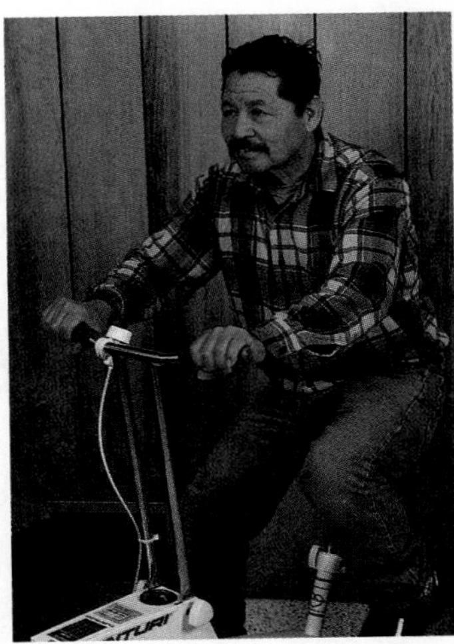

Figure 5-1 ● Exercise is important to older adults for health promotion and maintenance.

When older adults are hospitalized, the opportunity for continuing a program of physical fitness is interrupted, at least temporarily. During severe or prolonged illness, they are at high risk for complications of decreased physical mobility, such as pneumonia, skin impairment, contractures, muscle atrophy, constipation, and renal calculi. These problems are addressed elsewhere in this text.

Stress Management

FACTORS CONTRIBUTING TO STRESS IN OLDER ADULTS

According to many physiologic and psychologic theories of aging, stress and disease play significant roles. Stress can speed up the aging process over time, or it can lead to diseases that increase the rate of degeneration. Stress can impair the reserve capacity of older adults and lessen their ability to respond and adapt to changes in their environment.

Although no period of the life cycle is free from stress, the later years can be a time of especially high risk. Frequently observed sources of stress for the older population include rapid environmental changes that require immediate reaction, changes in lifestyle resulting from retirement or physical incapacity, acute or chronic illness, the loss of significant others, financial hardships, and relocation. How people react to these stresses depends on their personal coping skills and support networks. The loss of roles experienced by older adults often limits the availability of external support networks. For instance, losses leave many clients without friends to whom they can turn for support and help. As a result, many must rely solely on their personal resources to maintain their mental health. A combination of poor physical health and social problems leaves older adults susceptible to stress overload, which can result in illness and premature death.

COPING WITH STRESS

The ways in which people adapt to old age largely depend on the personality traits and coping strategies that have characterized them throughout their lives. Establishing and maintaining relationships with others throughout life is especially important to the older person's happiness. Even more important than having friends is the nature of the friendships. People who have close, intimate, stable relationships with others in whom they confide are more likely to maintain integrity in times of crisis.

ENVIRONMENTAL FACTORS

Most older adults live in and own their own homes. Physical incapacity or economic problems may force some to relocate to a retirement center or an assisted-living facility. Family members and facility staff need to be aware that older adults need personal space in their new surroundings. They need to participate in deciding how the space will be arranged and what they can keep in their new home. Such participation helps to offset the feelings of powerlessness and depersonalization that often accompany relocation to a group setting. The nurse suggests that the client or family bring in personal items, such as pictures of relatives and friends, favorite clothing, and valued knickknacks to assist in making the new setting seem more familiar and comfortable. This same intervention can be carried out in a hospital setting.

Changes in vision, touch, and motor ability can create difficulties for older adults in any environment. For example, decreased vision in old age, especially the poor perception of distance, may make walking more difficult; the person is less aware of the location of each step. A reduced sense of touch decreases the awareness of body orientation (e.g., whether the foot is squarely on the step). The decreased reaction time that commonly results from age-related changes in the neurologic system may also impair the ability to recognize or move from a dangerous setting.

Accidents

ACCIDENTS IN THE COMMUNITY

The nurse teaches older adults about the need to be aware of safety precautions to prevent accidents, such as falls. Incapacitating accidents are a primary cause of restricted physical fitness and decreased mobility in old age.

Safeguards such as handrails, slip-proof underpads for rugs, and adequate lighting are essential. To minimize sensory overload, the nurse advises the older adult to concentrate on one activity at a time. If needed, the nurse encourages the use of visual, hearing, or ambulatory assistive devices. High costs and a fear of appearing old sometimes prevent older adults from obtaining or using hearing aids, eyeglasses, walkers, or canes.

ACCIDENTS IN THE HOSPITAL AND NURSING HOME

The most common accident among older clients in a hospital or nursing home setting is falling. A **fall** is an event that results in the client's body coming to rest on the floor or another surface (Corrigan, et al., 1999). Many falls result in serious injuries such as fractures and head trauma. The nurse identifies clients at high risk for falls and takes action to prevent them.

Risk Assessment and Interventions for Preventing Falls

The nurse assesses the client for risk for falls. Many risk assessment tools have been developed to help the nurse focus on factors that increase an older person's risk of falling (Conley, Schultz, & Selvin, 1999). Chart 5-3 lists some of the common risk factors that the nurse should assess and the measures for preventing falls. A history of falling is the single most important predictor for falls.

Once an older client has been identified as being at high risk for falls, the nurse chooses interventions that help to prevent falls and possible serious injury. One of the most controversial issues in fall prevention is the use of siderails on the bed or of physical and chemical restraints, especially in the hospital setting.

CHART 5-3

BEST PRACTICE *for* Assessing Risk Factors and Preventing Falls in Older Adults

Assess for the presence of the following risk factors:

- History of falls
- Advanced age (>80 years)
- Multiple illnesses
- Generalized weakness or decreased mobility
- Disorientation or confusion
- The use of drugs that can cause increased confusion, mobility limitations, or orthostatic hypotension
- Urinary incontinence
- Communication impairments
- Major visual impairments or visual impairment without correction
- Substance abuse
- Location of client's room away from the nurses' station (in the hospital or nursing home)
- Change of shift or mealtime (in the hospital or nursing home)

Implement the following nursing interventions for all clients, regardless of risk:

- Monitor the client's activities and behavior as often as possible, preferably every 30 to 60 minutes.
- Remind the client to call for help before getting out of bed or a chair.
- Help the client to get out of bed or a chair.
- Provide, or remind the client to use, a walker or cane for ambulating.
- Remind the client to wear eyeglasses or a hearing aid if needed.
- Toilet the incontinent client every 1 to 2 hours.
- Clean up spills immediately.
- Arrange the furniture in the client's room or hallway to eliminate clutter or obstacles that could contribute to a fall.
- Provide adequate lighting at all times, especially at night.
- Observe for side effects and toxic effects of drug therapy.
- Orient the client to the environment.
- Keep the call light within reach, and ensure that the client can use it.
- Place the bed in the lowest position with the brakes locked.
- Place objects that the client needs within reach.
- Ensure that adequate handrails are present in the client's room, bathroom, and hall.
- Have the physical therapist assess the client for mobility and safety.

For clients at a high risk for falls:

- Implement all interventions listed above.
- Relocate the client for best visibility and supervision.
- Use bed and chair alarms.
- Encourage family members or significant others to stay with the client.

Use of Restraints

Older clients often have nocturia (urination at night) and get out of bed to go to the bathroom. They may forget to ask for assistance and may subsequently fall as a result of the darkness and disorientation in the unfamiliar environment. In some cases they may crawl over the siderail, which can make the fall more serious. Because of this, siderails are used less often in both hospitals and nursing homes.

Similar considerations have been given regarding the use of physical and chemical restraints. A **restraint** is any device or medication that prevents the client from moving freely. In 1990 the federal government enforced a law that gives nursing home residents the right to be restraint free. In nursing homes, siderails may be classified as restraints. Removing physical restraints from nursing home residents reduces serious injuries, although falls and minor injuries may increase.

Hospitals have also reduced the use of physical restraints, although the use of siderails has not been widely addressed. The Joint Commission on Accreditation of Healthcare Organizations (JCAHO) has specific standards that limit the use of physical restraints in hospitals and nursing homes. Chemical restraints or psychoactive drugs such as haloperidol (Haldol) have sometimes been used in place of physical restraints. JCAHO may also develop standards that limit the use of these drugs.

PHYSICAL RESTRAINTS

Experts agree that older adults should not be placed in a physical restraint or sedated just because they are old. Alternatives are used before applying any type of restraint (Chart 5-4). However, if all other interventions (e.g., reminding clients to call for assistance when needed or asking a family member to stay with clients) are ineffective in fall prevention, the nurse may need to use a physical restraint for a specified period. Applying a restraint is a serious intervention and should be analyzed for its risk versus its benefit. The nurse checks the client in a restraint every 30 to 60 minutes and releases the restraint at least every 2 hours for turning, repositioning, and toileting. Physical restraints such as vests have caused serious injury and even death. If restraint is needed, the least restrictive device should be used.

CHEMICAL RESTRAINTS

Chemical restraints, or psychoactive drugs, are often overused in hospital settings. Clients who are noisy, agitated, abusive, or combative may have an "as needed" order for a psychoactive drug. Such medications include the following:

- Antipsychotic drugs, such as haloperidol (Haldol, Peridol♣) and lorazepam (Ativan)
- Antianxiety drugs, such as alprazolam (Xanax)
- Antidepressant drugs, such as nortriptyline (Pamelor)
- Sedative-hypnotic drugs

These drugs produce serious side effects and toxic effects and therefore should be reserved for clients with a documented mental health disorder, such as anxiety or psychosis. Clients

CHART 5-4

BEST PRACTICE *for* Restraint Alternatives

- If the client is acutely confused, reorient him or her to reality as often as possible.
- If the client has dementia, use validation to reaffirm his or her feelings and concerns.
- Check the client often, at least every hour.
- If the client pulls tubes and lines, cover them with roller gauze or another protective device.
- Provide activities that keep the client busy, such as an activity pillow or apron, puzzle, or art activity.
- Provide soft, calming music.
- Place the client in an area where he or she can be supervised. (If the client is agitated, do not place him or her in a noisy area.)
- Turn off the television if the client is agitated.
- Ask a family member or friend to stay with the client at night.
- Toilet the client every 2 to 3 hours, including during the night.
- Be sure that the client's needs for food, fluids, and comfort are met.
- If agency policy allows, provide the client with a pet visit.
- Provide familiar objects or cherished items that the client can touch.
- Document the use of all alternative interventions.
- If a restraint is applied, use the least restrictive device (e.g., mitts rather than wrist restraints, a roller belt rather than a vest).

receiving these medications must be closely monitored for therapeutic and adverse effects.

The most potent group of psychoactive drugs is the antipsychotics. These drugs may be appropriate for the control of certain behavioral symptoms, such as hallucinations, delusions, and violent episodes. However, fewer than half of clients respond to these drugs.

If a psychoactive drug is used as a last resort to control behavior, the lowest dose should be given. Table 5-1 lists some of the drugs commonly used as chemical restraints.

TABLE 5-1 • DRUGS USED AS CHEMICAL RESTRAINTS

LOW POTENCY (HIGH SEDATION, HIGH ANTICHOLINERGIC EFFECTS)
Chlorpromazine (Thorazine)
Thioridazine (Mellaril)
Chlorprothixene (Taractan)
Mesoridazine (Serentil)
MEDIUM POTENCY (MEDIUM SEDATION, MEDIUM ANTICHOLINERGIC EFFECTS)
Triflupromazine (Vesprin)
Acetophenazine (Tindal)
Loxapine (Loxitane)
Molindone (Moban)
HIGH POTENCY (LOW SEDATION, LOW ANTICHOLINERGIC EFFECTS)
Trifluoperazine (Stelazine)
Thiothixene (Navane)
Fluphenazine (Prolixin)
Haloperidol (Haldol)
Pimozide (Orap)

From Ignatavicius, D.D. (1998). *Introduction to long term care: Principles and practice.* Philadelphia: F.A. Davis.

Drug Use and Misuse

Drug therapy for the older population in general is another major health issue. Because of the multiple chronic and acute illnesses that occur in this age-group, drugs for older adults account for approximately one third of all prescription drug costs. The term **polypharmacy** has been used to describe the use of multiple drugs by older adults.

Elders also commonly use nonprescription drugs, such as analgesics, antacids, cold and cough preparations, laxatives, and vitamins, often without consulting a physician. The occurrence of adverse drug reactions is directly related to the number of drugs taken and the frequency with which they are taken. Therefore older adults are at high risk for adverse drug reactions or interactions and are often admitted to the hospital for these problems.

PHYSIOLOGIC CHANGES AFFECTING DRUG USE

Older adults may not tolerate the standard dosage of medications traditionally prescribed for younger adults. The physiologic changes related to aging make drug therapy more complex and challenging. These changes affect the absorption, distribution, metabolism, and excretion of drugs from the body.

Age-related changes that can potentially affect drug absorption from an oral route include an increase in gastric pH, a decrease in gastric blood flow, and a decrease in gastrointestinal motility. Despite these changes, most clients do not have absorption difficulties because of age-related changes alone.

Age-related changes that affect drug distribution include smaller amounts of total body water, an increased ratio of adipose tissue to lean body mass, a decreased albumin level, and a decreased cardiac output. Increased adipose tissue in proportion to lean body mass can cause increased storage of lipid-soluble drugs. This leads to a decreased concentration of the drug in plasma but an increased concentration in tissue.

Drug metabolism most often occurs in the liver. Age-related changes affecting metabolism include a decrease in liver size, a decrease in liver blood flow, and a decrease in liver enzyme activity. These changes can result in increased plasma concentrations of a drug. Changes in the kidneys can also result in high plasma concentrations of drugs.

The excretion of drugs most often involves the renal system. Age-related changes of the renal system include decreased renal blood flow and reduced glomerular filtration rate. These changes result in a decreased creatinine clearance and thus a slower excretion time for medications (Matteson et al., 1997). Consequently, serum drug levels can become toxic, and the client can become extremely ill or die.

EFFECTS OF DRUGS ON OLDER ADULTS

Because of age-related physiologic changes, older adults are at a high risk for side effects and toxic effects from drugs. Elders have less reserve capacity in most organ systems. When chronic disease is added to the physiologic changes of aging, drug reactions have a more dramatic effect and take a longer time to correct. Often a lower dose of medication is necessary to prevent adverse effects. The policy of "start low, go slow" is appropriate when health care providers prescribe drugs for this group. The physiologic changes of aging are highly individual. Alterations in drug therapy should always be individualized according to the actual physiologic changes present and the occurrence and severity of chronic disease.

Common adverse drug reactions in older adults include edema, nausea, vomiting, anorexia, dry mouth, fatigue, weakness, dizziness, urinary retention, diarrhea, constipation, and confusion. Many of these signs and symptoms can be mistakenly attributed to a concurrent illness or assumed to be part of the aging process. The nurse assesses all older clients with such symptoms for possible adverse reactions to medications.

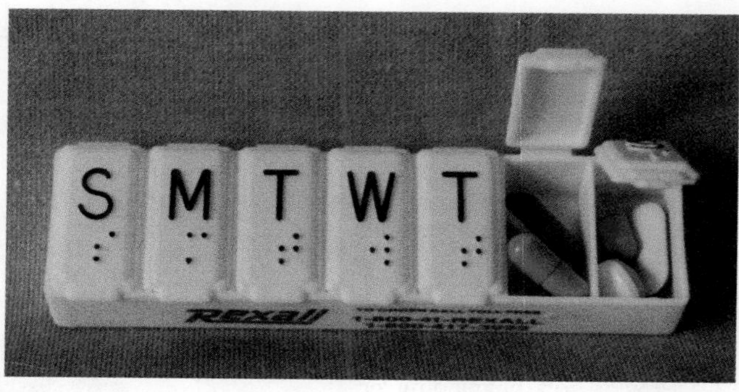

Figure 5-2 ● A medication system for safe self-administration.

SELF-ADMINISTRATION OF MEDICATION

Most people older than 65 years of age live at home and are responsible for taking their own medications. Because the risk of drug toxicity is considerably increased in the older population, the nurse should assist clients in assuming this task responsibly. He or she can help prevent problems by educating clients and their caregivers, providing clear and concise directions, and developing ways to assist them in overcoming handicaps or difficulties with self-administration.

Older adults make errors in self-administration for several reasons. First, they may simply forget. In the rush of daily activities, they may not take the drug at all or may take it too often because of an inability to remember when or whether their medications have been taken. It can be helpful for clients to associate pill taking with daily events (e.g., meals) or to keep a simple chart or calendar. Pill boxes have been devised so that a daily, weekly, or monthly supply of medicine can be placed in the appropriate compartments (Figure 5-2). Egg cartons can be very cost-effective pill boxes. Large print on the drug label assists clients who have poor visual acuity. Writing the drug regimen on the top of the bottle with large letters and numbers is also helpful.

A second reason that older adults often commit errors in taking medications is poor communication with health care professionals. These difficulties result from inadequate explanations or explanations that are not understood because of educational limitations or language barriers. Health care professionals often presume that their client has acquired the knowledge if they have told the client about the medications. The nurse or other health care provider needs to help older adults plan their medication schedules.

A third reason for medication errors is attitude and long-ingrained feelings about taking medicine. Some people add to their drug regimen by taking over-the-counter (OTC) drugs, which can interact with prescription drugs and cause serious problems. For example, a client receiving warfarin (Coumadin, Warfilone🍁) for anticoagulation may take aspirin (Ancasal🍁) regularly for arthritis. Because aspirin is also an anticoagulant, this combination can cause overt or occult bleeding. When obtaining a medication history, it is very important that the nurse ask clients about all OTC drugs, including herbal and food supplements.

Other older people avoid taking medication whenever they can. The fear of drug dependency or the cost of the drugs may cause many to discontinue their medications too soon. In addition, the actions or side effects of some drugs may not be desirable. For example, diuretics may cause incontinence when clients cannot get to the bathroom quickly enough. Others may think that two pills are twice as effective as one; some elders take medication that is leftover from a previous illness or take a drug that has been prescribed for someone else.

Health care providers can influence the attitudes of elders toward their medications and their health problems. One method being tried in some hospitals and nursing homes is supervised drug self-administration, in which clients are allowed to take their own medications under supervision. In this way, the nurse can be sure of a client's understanding and ability to self-administer medications at home or in another health care setting.

Mental Health

Most older adults are mentally sound and competent. A few changes in cognition have been identified as age related and are linked to specific cognitive functions rather than intellectual capacity. These changes include a decreased reaction time to stimuli and an impairment of memory for recent events. However, gross cognitive impairment, depression, hallucinations, and delusions are not part of the normal aging process.

Two forms of competence exist: legal competence and clinical competence. A person is **legally competent** if he or she is:

- 18 years of age or older
- Pregnant or a married minor
- A legally emancipated (free) minor who is self-supporting
- Not declared incompetent by a court of law

If a court determines that a person is not legally competent, a guardian is appointed to make financial and health care decisions.

A person is **clinically competent** if he or she is legally competent and has decisional capacity. Decisional capacity is determined by an individual's ability to identify problems, recognize options, make decisions, and provide the rationale supporting the decisions.

It is not surprising that mental illness does occur among the older population. Losses in income and physical health, a lack of comprehensive health care and social services, a loss of social roles, and the death of significant others may affect a person's emotional stability. Older adults are often unaware of early symptoms of emotional or mental impairments. Their symptoms may go unnoticed by family and friends and thus progress until crisis results. The three most common cognitive

TABLE 5-2 • MEDICATIONS COMMONLY USED FOR DEPRESSION IN OLDER ADULTS AND THEIR ADVERSE EFFECTS

Medication	Adverse Effects
TRICYCLIC ANTIDEPRESSANTS*	
Amitriptyline (Elavil, Endep) Clomipramine (Anafranil) Desipramine (Norpramin) Doxepin (Sinequan, Triadapin) Imipramine (Tofranil) Nortriptyline (Pamelor) Protriptyline (Vivactil) Trimipramine (Surmontil)	Cardiac dysrhythmias, orthostatic hypotension, weight gain, drowsiness, anticholinergic effects (dry mouth, constipation, urinary retention, visual disturbances); amitriptyline has the most anticholinergic effects of any medication in this group
HETEROCYCLIC ANTIDEPRESSANTS†	
Amoxapine (Asendin) Bupropion (Wellbutrin, Wellbutrin SR) Maprotiline (Ludiomil) Trazodone (Desyrel)	Drowsiness; maprotiline has the longest half-life in this group
SELECTIVE SEROTONIN REUPTAKE INHIBITORS (SSRIs)†	
Fluoxetine (Prozac) Paroxetine (Paxil) Sertraline (Zoloft) Citalopram (Celexa) Nefazodone (Serzone) Venlafaxine (Effexor, Effexor SR)	Insomnia, agitation, gastrointestinal distress, weight loss; fluoxetine has the longest half-life in this group
MONOAMINE OXIDASE INHIBITORS	
Isocarboxazid (Marplan) Phenelzine (Nardil) Tranylcypromine (Parnate)	Weight gain, insomnia, agitation Hypertensive crisis (avoid foods containing tyramine)

Data from Agency for Health Care Policy and Research. *Depression in Primary Care: Vol. 2: Treatment of major depression. Clinical Practice Guideline Number 5.* Rockville, MD: Agency for Health Care Policy and Research, Public Health Service, U.S. Department of Health and Human Services; and modified from Ignatavicius, D.D. (1998). *Introduction to long term care: Principles and practice.* Philadelphia: F.A. Davis.

*Do not give with antidysrhythmics or monoamine oxidase inhibitors.

†Do not give with monoamine oxidase inhibitors.

problems among older adults are depression, dementia, and delirium.

DEPRESSION

Depression, the most common mental health disorder among older adults, is a response to multiple life stresses, a single situation (situational depression), a primary disorder, or a problem associated with dementia. It can range from mild, transient feelings of sadness to a severe sense of helplessness and hopelessness. Depression is thought to result from a lack of the neurotransmitters norepinephrine and serotonin in the brain (Isaacs, 1998). It is often underdiagnosed by physicians and is therefore undertreated.

Without treatment, depression can result in the following:

- Worsening of medical conditions
- Risk of physical illness
- Alcoholism
- Increased pain and disability
- Delayed recovery from illness
- Suicide

Older adults have the highest suicide rate of any age-group (Uncapher & Arean, 2000). In their study, Uncapher and Arean (2000) sent two case studies of suicidal, depressed clients to primary care physicians to determine if any bias in treatment would be present. The two cases were the same except for age—one client was age 38, and the other was age 78. The 215 physician responses showed that all providers recognized the depression and suicide risk but were less willing to treat the older client. They believed that suicidal ideation was normal for the older client.

> **CULTURAL CONSIDERATIONS**
> Caucasian males older than 70 years of age, especially those living alone, are at the highest risk for suicide. Older adults contemplating suicide usually do not talk about their plans and choose a method that will ensure death (e.g., a gunshot).

Elders with depression may experience early morning insomnia, excessive daytime sleeping, poor appetite, a lack of energy, and an unwillingness to participate in social and recreational activities. The primary treatment for depression usually includes drug therapy and psychotherapy. In some parts of the country, electroconvulsive therapy (ECT) may be used either as a last resort or when drugs are not effective.

Table 5-2 lists the drugs commonly used for depression. Most of these drugs take 2 to 3 weeks to become effective. Selective serotonin reuptake inhibitors (SSRIs) are now the first choice for drug therapy. They act by increasing the amount of serotonin and norepinephrine at neuronal synapses in the brain (Isaacs, 1998). More information about depression is available in mental health nursing textbooks.

DEMENTIA

Dementia is a broad term used for a syndrome that is characterized by a slowly progressive cognitive decline. Formerly

TABLE 5-3 • THE CONFUSION ASSESSMENT METHOD (CAM)

1. Acute onset and fluctuating course (e.g., Is there evidence of an acute change in mental status from the client's baseline?)
2. Inattention (e.g., Does the client have difficulty focusing attention or keeping track of what is being said?)
3. Disorganized thinking (e.g., Is the client's thinking and conversation disorganized or incoherent?)
4. Altered level of consciousness (e.g., Is the client lethargic, hyperalert, or difficult to arouse?)

The diagnosis of delirium by the CAM is the presence of features 1 *and* 2 and either 3 *or* 4.

called organic brain syndrome (OBS) and chronic brain syndrome (CBS), dementia represents a global impairment of intellectual function and is generally chronic and progressive. There are many types of dementia, the most common being Alzheimer's disease (senile dementia, Alzheimer type). Multi-infarct dementia, the second most common dementia, is a vascular disorder and accounts for 20% to 25% of all dementias. Chapter 42 discusses dementias in detail, with a focus on Alzheimer's disease.

DELIRIUM

Whereas dementia is a chronic, progressive disorder, **delirium** is an acute state of confusion. Delirium also differs from dementia in that it is usually short-term and reversible within 3 weeks. It is often seen among older adults in a hospital setting or in a setting with which they are unfamiliar. Behavior typically fits into one of two categories: hyperactivity (most common) or hypoactivity (Ignatavicius, 1999). Hyperactive clients may try to climb out of bed or pull out invasive catheters (e.g., urinary catheters or intravenous cannulas), or they may become quite agitated and combative. Hypoactive clients are quiet, apathetic, and withdrawn.

Multiple factors can cause delirium, including the following:

- Medication (especially anticholinergic drugs)
- Metabolic disturbances
- Infections
- Surgical operations
- Circulatory, renal, and pulmonary disorders
- Nutritional deficiencies
- Major loss

Acutely confused clients who are discharged from the hospital are at an increased risk for functional dependence, falls, incontinence, infections, pressure ulcers, adverse drug reactions, and declining health status (Crawley & Miller, 1998). Therefore nurses should assess older clients for acute confusion. A number of assessment tools have been developed, including the Confusion Assessment Method (CAM), Delirium Rating Scale (DRS), and NEECHAM Confusion Scale. Although the CAM is easy to use (Table 5-3), Rapp et al. (2000) found that the most useful tool was the nurse-developed NEECHAM Confusion Scale (see the Evidence-Based Practice for Nursing box above).

To manage delirium, the nurse should use a calm voice in reorienting the client and try to divert attention away from devices or tubes. A number of innovative nursing interventions have been used with some success. For example, playing tapes of soothing music in the client's room may have a calming effect. Giving the client a doll or stuffed animal to "fidget" with may prevent the client from removing important medical instrumentation. Some nurses believe that providing dolls and stuffed animals is treating the adult like a child, but this intervention can sometimes be very effective when used for therapeutic purposes. If the client has a favorite item, such as an afghan or a picture, the nurse asks the family or significant others to provide it for the same purpose.

Table 5-4 briefly differentiates delirium and dementia and lists the major nursing considerations for each. The most difficult challenge is caring for a client who is experiencing both problems at the same time.

EVIDENCE-BASED PRACTICE FOR NURSING

Which tool is best for nurses to use when assessing clients who are acutely confused?

Rapp, C.G., et al. (2000). Acute confusion assessment instruments: Clinical versus research usability. *Applied Nursing Research,* 13(1), 37-45.

Acute confusion (AC), also known as delirium, is a common problem seen by nurses in a variety of health care settings. This study examined five AC assessment tools—Confusion Assessment Method (CAM), Delirium Rating Scale (DRS), Delirium Symptom Inventory (DSI), Mini-Mental State Examination (MMSE), and Neelon/Champagne (NEECHAM) Confusion Scale—to determine the most reliable indicator of acute confusion. The researchers also asked evaluators to identify which tool was the easiest to use. The NEECHAM tool was unanimously selected because it specifically assesses for AC and identifies both at-risk clients and those who actually have AC. They also liked the CAM because it was linked to the criteria for delirium as listed in the Diagnostic and Statistical Manual, fourth edition (DSM-IV). A protocol that includes both tools was written, and nurses from the authors' health care system have been trained in its use for screening clients.

Critique. The authors evaluated tools that had already been tested for reliability and validity and applied them for use in the practice setting. The NEECHAM tool, the only nurse-designed tool, was selected by the raters. Other authors have reported that this tool can be incorporated into daily practice.

Implications for Nursing. This study validated that nurses need to assess for AC using a standardized screening method, especially for older adults. Early identification of delirium alerts the health care team to the need for modifications in the client's plan of care.

Elder Neglect and Abuse

Another problem sometimes encountered by older adults is neglect and abuse, both verbal and physical. Some elders are very vulnerable to these problems, especially widowed women who may have difficulty being assertive. Older persons who are neglected or abused are often physically dependent. The abuser is often a family member who becomes frustrated or distraught over the burden of caring for the elder.

Prolonged caregiving by a family member is a new and unexpected role for adult children, most often women. This new role may result in role fatigue and role conflict. Caregiver Role Strain and Risk for Caregiver Role Strain were added to the list of nursing diagnoses approved by the North American Nursing Diagnosis Association (NANDA). From their research, McCloskey and Bulechek (2000) identified Caregiver Support as a major nursing intervention (Chart 5-5).

TABLE 5-4 • DIFFERENCES IN THE CHARACTERISTICS OF DELIRIUM AND DEMENTIA

Variable	Dementia	Delirium
Description	A chronic, progressive cognitive decline	An acute confusional state
Onset	Slow	Fast
Duration	Months to years	Hours to less than 1 month
Cause	Unknown, possibly familial, chemical	Multiple, such as surgery, infection, drugs
Reversibility	None	Usually
Management	Treat signs and symptoms	Remove or treat the cause
Nursing interventions	Reorientation not effective in the late stages; use validation therapy (acknowledge the client's feelings and do not argue); provide a safe environment; observe for associated behaviors, such as delusions and hallucinations	Reorient the client to reality; provide a safe environment

CHART 5-5

NIC INTERVENTION ACTIVITIES *for* Caregiver Support

Caregiver Support: *Provision of the necessary information, advocacy, and support to facilitate primary client care by someone other than a health care professional.*

- Determine caregiver's level of knowledge.
- Determine caregiver's acceptance of role.
- Teach caregiver stress management techniques.
- Monitor for indicators of stress.
- Identify sources of respite care.
- Teach the caregiver health care maintenance strategies to sustain own physical and mental health.
- Encourage caregiver participation in support groups.
- Educate caregiver about the grieving process.
- Teach caregiver strategies to access and maximize health care and community resources.
- Foster caregiver social networking.

NIC intervention activities selected from McCloskey, J.C., & Bulechek, G.M. (Eds.). (2000). *Nursing interventions classification (NIC)* (3rd ed.). St. Louis: Mosby. No part of this work is to be altered without prior written permission from the Publisher.

Gray-Vickery (2000) described four common types of abuse:

- **Neglect** occurs when a caregiver fails to provide for a client's basic needs, such as food, clothing, or assistance with activities of daily living (ADLs). Whether intentional or unintentional, neglect accounts for almost half of all cases of actual elder abuse.
- **Physical abuse** is the use of physical force that results in bodily injury, especially in the "bathing suit" zone (abdomen, buttocks, genital area, upper thighs). Examples of physical abuse include hitting, burning, pushing, and molesting the client. Approximately one fourth of all cases of actual elder abuse involve physical force.
- **Financial abuse** occurs when the client's property or resources are mismanaged or misused; this is more common than physical abuse.
- **Emotional abuse** is the intentional use of threats, humiliation, intimidation, and isolation toward older adults. It occurs in more than one third of all cases of actual elder abuse.

The nurse carefully assesses the client for signs of abuse, such as bruises in clusters or regular patterns; burns, commonly to the buttocks or the soles of the feet; unusual hair loss; or multiple injuries, especially fractures. If the older adult is too weak or has no other resources or support systems, he or she may not acknowledge that the abuse is occurring. Neglect may be manifested by pressure ulcers, contractures, dehydration or undernutrition, urine burns, excessive body odor, and listlessness (Gray-Vickrey, 1999). Dyer et al. (2000) found that depression and dementia were common in community elders who were abused or neglected.

If physical abuse or neglect is suspected, the nurse notifies the physician and social worker to investigate the situation. All states in the United States and other Western countries have laws requiring health care professionals to report suspected elder abuse.

ECONOMIC ISSUES FOR OLDER ADULTS

Income

Most adults hope to provide for their own needs throughout their life cycle. One of the greatest fears related to aging is becoming dependent on family, friends, or society. In many cases, older adults have not achieved economic self-sufficiency. One fifth of the total population of the United States is poor, and one fifth of the poor are older than age 65.

Most people expect their financial resources to decline in their retirement years compared with their working years. They also expect their level of expenses to decline, but this may not occur. In the United States, for example, the inflation that began in the 1970s has reduced the value of financial assets. Older adults have been especially hard hit because most rely on Social Security benefits or pension funds for the bulk of their income. Many elders are unable to adjust their income to changing economic circumstances and hence are powerless to combat declining real income. Health care purchases are paid for in large part by private insurance and federal health and social programs. However, the rising cost of these programs contributes substantially to rising government costs and may result in more out-of-pocket costs for the older health care consumer.

Housing

The popular belief that older adults are frail, dependent, senile people living out their last years in an institution has no factual basis. Many elders live in their own homes and have paid off their mortgages. However, living arrangements are a major problem for some people as they age. The nurse needs to be aware of this issue because it can increase the client's stress level and have an impact on health care planning.

In many countries the rising costs of energy and housing have joined the high costs of food and health care as factors that contribute to the economic hardship of older adults. In addition to financial difficulties, housing may be a problem because of a lack of environmental supports that would help older adults to continue residing and participating in the community.

Deterioration of property, escalation of property taxes, and maintenance service costs create many problems for older homeowners wishing to keep their homes. In some areas, older renters are extremely vulnerable to high rents, real estate speculation, and the loss of living quarters because of the removal of substandard, low-rent apartment or hotel buildings. Physical impairments and a lack of available and affordable support services (e.g., household help, transportation, home health care, and meal assistance) prevent some older adults from managing adequately in their own homes.

The need for special housing for older adults has long been recognized. Numbers of government and privately funded experiments in alternative housing have been tested. These projects incorporate variables such as personal care services, special health and safety remedies, and recreation and leisure plans. Although most of these projects provide security, improve life satisfaction, and prove to be cost-effective, many areas of the United States have no overall plan for alternative living arrangements for older adults.

RESOURCES FOR OLDER ADULTS

In the United States, Canada, and other countries, a broad range of government benefits and services is available to assist older adults with problems related to income, health insurance, housing, and social services. The nurse informs older adults and their families about the types of services available to help them achieve a higher quality of life.

Government Resources

INCOME

In the United States, the major portion of federal funds that support programs for elders is devoted to the Social Security program. The Social Security Act was passed in 1935, when many individuals were economically impoverished after the Depression. Since that time there has been a gradual shift from a program intended to provide a minimal supplement to retirees' sources of income to one that is the primary source of retirement income for many people. Other provisions of this act that are significant for people younger than 65 years of age are the disability and survivors' insurance provisions.

HEALTH INSURANCE

Medicare is a federal health insurance program that was enacted as part of the amendments to the Social Security Act of 1965. This program was created to help older adults meet the cost of health care. Despite its deficiencies, Medicare has provided a means for elders to obtain needed health care in times of escalating costs without decimating their total personal savings.

Medicare provides health insurance to people 65 years of age and older and to qualified disabled people of any age. Medicare A primarily pays for most in-hospital care and is paid for by the federal government. It covers only a very small portion of the care required in long-term care and only minimal home care services. Medicare B is an optional insurance and requires payment of a monthly premium. Medicare B pays most of the outpatient costs associated with health care provider visits, medication, and home care services.

Medical assistance (Medicaid) is a program designed to provide payment for medical services for the poor, including older adults who are poor. This program supplements the Medicare insurance program for eligible adults 65 years of age and older. Eligibility is related to determination of poverty level, and each state program determines its own criteria for eligibility. A number of states have completed the transition to managed care for their Medicaid recipients.

HOUSING PROGRAMS

The U.S. Congress has passed a number of legislative acts designed to alleviate housing problems for older citizens. Among these programs is rental assistance for low-income families, older adults, and the disabled. Direct low-interest loans are available to individuals to construct special rental housing facilities. For information related to these housing programs, nurses can contact the local public housing authority or the Housing and Urban Development area office in most communities.

SOCIAL SERVICES

The Older Americans Act of 1965 provided social services to older adults. Under this legislation, each state created an office to provide leadership in the coordination and development of services for older adults (Office on Aging). Some of the more significant programs and services carried out under this legislation are described in Chart 5-6.

RESEARCH AGENCIES

The National Institute on Aging was established in 1974. Its purpose is to conduct research on the biologic, population-

CHART 5-6

NURSING FOCUS *on the* OLDER ADULT
Social Services Provided by the Older Americans Act of 1965

- Senior centers to meet the need for a central place for older adults to congregate, develop new interests, and socialize
- Nutrition programs to provide nutritious meals in a centralized setting as well as to homebound older adults; recreation, education, and health activities are incorporated in many sites as a regular part of the program
- Transportation services to accommodate older adults via special fares on existing public transportation systems and the operation of specially equipped vehicles for frail and handicapped older adults
- Information and referral services to direct older adults to the appropriate agency that provides needed services
- In-home services such as household help, telephone reassurance, chore maintenance, and visitation by home care aides to enable impaired older adults to remain living in the community

related, and sociologic aspects of aging at its Gerontology Research Center in Baltimore. It also supports research by others at universities and laboratories across the United States.

One division within the National Institute for Mental Health—the Center for Studies of the Mental Health of the Aging—is devoted exclusively to problems of older adults. Its major role is to stimulate, coordinate, and support research training and to offer technical assistance related to aging and mental health. Although it provides no monies for programs of service delivery to older adults, it significantly affects the training of those working with older adults in community mental health centers and other service settings.

Community Resources

Over the years it has become evident that government programs cannot provide all of the services needed by older adults. In many areas, private efforts can supply the same services at lower costs and without the red tape involved with some government programs. Transportation is an area in which the private sector and local, state, and federal governments all have roles.

In many urban areas, governments have established Dial-A-Ride or similar services that provide free transportation. The federal government has subsidized the development and operation of transit systems, but the main focus of this aid has been on high-use systems and routes. For occasional travel, particularly in rural areas, the best solution may be for the older adult to rely on a friend or a neighbor. Churches and community groups often help organize this approach by using sign-up sheets and recruiting volunteers to drive each week.

Education, recreation, and cultural activities help to maintain a person's physical condition, mental alertness, and social contact. Education helps older people keep up with a rapidly changing world. Advances in the Internet and in cable and satellite television systems provide a broad range of new educational experiences at home. Nevertheless, the value of person-to-person discussion and the need to focus some educational activities on local issues means that community discussion groups and other informal education will remain important.

Churches and other religious institutions serve older adults in many ways. In addition to their primary role of providing organized worship, they sponsor many activities that bring people together with their peers as well as with younger people. Clergypersons and other spiritual leaders are often excellent counselors, and other members of the congregation or religious group are sometimes willing to help older members in time of trouble.

Many communities have access to community resource books (e.g., those published by the United Way). Area agencies on aging are excellent referral centers. Some of these agencies publish directories of services that are specifically geared toward the older adult. The nurse can help to inform older clients about the community resources they may need depending on their specific life situation.

THE FUTURE OF GERONTOLOGIC NURSING

Nurses in most adult health care settings encounter the challenges of caring for both healthy and ill older adults. In view of the rapidly increasing older population, especially the over-85 age-group, nurses in many settings are specializing in gerontological nursing or geriatric case management. Nurses can practice these specialties in acute care, long-term care, and community-based settings.

Just as nurses can achieve certification in medical-surgical nursing, they can become certified in gerontological nursing or case management. The American Nurses Credentialing Center (ANCC) provides three gerontology examinations for the certification of those who qualify: gerontological nurse, gerontological clinical specialist, and gerontological nurse practitioner. The ANCC also offers a nursing case management examination that is broad based and not specific for geriatric case management. Other professional organizations also certify case managers, including geriatric case managers.

ONLINE RESOURCES

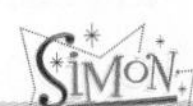

For suggested readings and Internet resources, go to http://www.wbsaunders.com/SIMON/Iggy/.

SELECTED BIBLIOGRAPHY

Asterisk indicates a classic or definitive work on this subject.

Burke, M.M., & Walsh, M.B. (1997). *Gerontologic nursing: Wholistic care of the older adult* (2nd ed.). St. Louis: Mosby.

Christmas, C., & Andersen, R.A. (2000). Exercise and older patients: Guidelines for the physician. *Journal of the American Geriatric Society, 48*(3), 318-324.

Conley, D., Schultz, A.A., & Selvin, R. (1999). The challenge of predicting patients at risk for falling: Development of the Conley Scale. *MEDSURG Nursing: The Journal of Adult Health, 8*(6), 348-354.

Corrigan, B., et al. (1999). Preventing falls in acute care. In I. Abraham et al. (Eds.), *Geriatric nursing protocols for best practice* (pp. 77-100). New York: Springer.

Council for Nutritional Clinical Strategies in Long-Term Care. (1999). *Anorexia in the elderly.* Plainsboro, NJ: MultiMedia Health Care/Freedom.

Crawley, E.J., & Miller, J. (1998). Acute confusion among hospitalized elders: Part 1. A rural hospital. *MEDSURG Nursing: The Journal of Adult Health, 7*(4), 199-206.

Davidhizar, R., & Shearer, R. (2000). Helping elders adjust to losing autonomy. *The Journal of Care Management, 6*(1), 53-54, 69-72.

Dyer, C.B., et al. (2000). The high prevalence of depression and dementia in elder abuse or neglect. *Journal of the American Geriatric Society, 48*(2), 205-208.

Eden, B.M., Foreman, M.D., & Sisk, R. (1998). Delirium: Comparison of four predictive models in hospitalized elderly patients. *Applied Nursing Research, 11*(1), 27-35.

Gray-Vickery, P. (1999). Recognizing elder abuse. *Nursing99, 29*(9), 52-63.

Gray-Vickery, P. (2000). Protecting the older adult. *Nursing2000, 30*(7), 34-37.

Hammond, M., & Levine, J.M. (1999). Bedrails: Choosing the best alternative. *Geriatric Nursing, 20*(6), 297-301.

Ignatavicius, D.D. (1998). *Introduction to long-term care: Principles and practice.* Philadelphia: F.A. Davis.

Ignatavicius, D.D. (1999). Resolving the delirium dilemma. *Nursing99, 29*(10), 41-47.

Isaacs, A. (1998). Depression and your patient. *American Journal of Nursing, 98*(7), 26-32.

Kessenich, C.R. (1998). Tai Chi as a method of fall prevention in the elderly. *Orthopaedic Nursing, 17*(4), 27-29.

Kurlowicz, L.W., & NICHE Faculty. (1999). Depression in elderly patients. In I. Abraham et al. (Eds.), *Geriatric nursing protocols for best practice* (pp. 77-100). New York: Springer.

Matteson, M.A., McConnell, E.S., & Linton, A.D. (1997). *Gerontological nursing: Concepts and practice* (2nd ed.). Philadelphia: W.B. Saunders.

McCloskey, J.C., & Bulechek, G.M. (2000). *Nursing interventions classification (NIC)* (3rd ed.). St. Louis: Mosby.

Musil, C.M., et al. (1998). Health problems and health actions among community-dwelling older adults: Results of a health diary study. *Applied Nursing Research, 11*(3), 130-137.

Paist, S.S. (1999). Screening and preventive interventions in older patients: Which ones are useful? *Hospital Medicine, 35*(6), 16-21.

Rapp, C.G., et al. (2000). Acute confusion assessment instruments: Clinical versus research usability. *Applied Nursing Research, 13*(1), 37-45.

Schiavento, M. (1997). The Hispanic elderly: Implications for nursing care. *Journal of Gerontological Nursing, 23*(6), 10-15.

Stevens, J.A. & Olson, S. (2000). Reducing falls and resulting hip fractures among older women. *Morbidity and Mortality Weekly Report, 49*(RR02), 1-12.

Uncapher, H., & Arean, P.A. (2000). Physicians are less willing to treat suicidal ideation in older patients. *Journal of the American Geriatric Society, 48*(2), 188-192.

Walton, J.C., & Miller, J.M. (1998). Evaluating physical and behavioral changes in older adults. *MEDSURG Nursing: The Journal of Adult Health, 7*(2), 85-90.

Wells, D.L., & Dawson, P. (2000). Description of retained abilities in older persons with dementia. *Research in Nursing and Health Care, 23*(2), 158-166.

UNIT

2

Biopsychosocial Concepts Related to Health Care

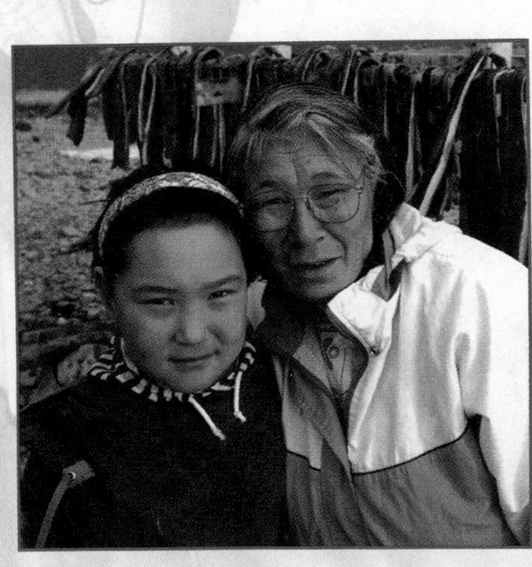

BIOPSYCHOSOCIAL CONCEPTS RELATED TO HEALTH CARE ■ Core Concepts Grid

Concepts	Assessment	Interventions	Pharmacology
• **Culture** Definition Cultural competence Assessment Cultural care plan Religion Folk medicine Pain Ethics • **Pain** Theories of pain Types of pain Addiction Dependence Tolerance Placebos • **Substance abuse** Stimulants Hallucinogens Depressants Narcotics Inhalants Steroids • **End-of life care** Goals Hospice care Death Postmortem care Euthanasia • **Rehabilitation** Settings Team	• **Pain** Site/location Intensity Quality/chronology Nonverbal indicators of pain Vital signs Anxiety Sweating Restlessness Confusion • **Substance abuse** Hallucinations Seizures Cardiac dysrhythmias Dilated pupils Vital sign changes Tremors Nausea/vomiting Abdominal cramps Mental health disorders Visual disturbances Euphoria Relaxation Sexual arousal Poor attention and memory • **End-of life care** Lethargy Decreased level of consciousness (LOC) Discomfort or pain Dyspnea Agitation Nausea/vomiting Dysphagia • **Rehabilitation** Body system assessment Functional assessment Psychosocial assessment Vocational assessment	• **Pain** Monitoring pain Cutaneous stimulation Distraction Acupuncture Imagery Transcutaneous electrical nerve stimulation (TENS) Heat/cold Touch • **Substance abuse** Health teaching Avoidance Rehabilitation Symptom management • **End-of life care** Oxygen Oral hygiene Alternative drug routes Positioning Rest Energy conservation Foley catheter Enema Physical support Presence Being realistic Promoting spirituality Referral to bereavement services Health teaching • **Rehabilitation** Transfers Gait training Prevention of complications of immobility Assistive/adaptive devices Energy conservation Skin care Bladder and bowel training Community-based care	• **Pain** Nonopioid drugs Opioid analgesics Tricyclic antidepressants Other adjunctive drugs • **End-of life care** Opioids in varying routes Diuretics Bronchodilators Corticosteroids Antibiotics Anticholinergics Sedatives Antianxiety drugs Barbiturates • **Rehabilitation** Cholinergics Rectal suppositories

CHAPTER 6

Cultural Aspects of Health

MARJORIE G. MORGAN

Learning Objectives

After studying this chapter, you should be able to:

1. Define cultural competence, culture, and subculture.
2. Explain the purpose of Healthy People 2010 as it relates to cultural groups.
3. Describe the three methods for assessing the culture of a client or group.
4. Identify two subcultures that have often been neglected.
5. Discuss specific cultural practices—religion, nutrition, and folk medicine—that the nurse should consider when assessing a client's culture.

SIMON Go to http://www.wbsaunders.com/SIMON/Iggy/ for self-assessment questions related to these Learning Objectives.

Population diversity—not only of the United States, but of the world—is increasing rapidly in this exciting century. As a result of the Internet, foreign travel, and global industrialization, there is more interaction between different peoples of the world. The citizens of each country have their own way of doing things, their own way of interacting with one another, and their own beliefs and practices. Although there are cultural similarities among many people in each country, there are also subgroups within each society—each with its own customs and beliefs.

THE NEED FOR CULTURAL CONSIDERATIONS OF HEALTH

Not only is the world population becoming more diverse, but people from other cultures continue to immigrate to the United States in large numbers, bringing different ideas with them. In addition, longtime citizens of the United States often have different cultural needs based on their ethnicity and background. According to the U.S. Census Bureau, the estimated figures for the U.S. population in 2000 showed the following percentages for different cultural groups:

- Caucasians: 71.5%
- African Americans: 12.2 %
- Hispanics: 12.6%
- Asian Americans/Pacific Islanders: 3.8%

In 2000 the number of minority populations in the United States accounted for 28% of the total population; the projection is that minorities will make up 43.8% of the population by 2050. The diversity in this population makes culturally sensitive health care imperative.

The U.S. government has an initiative for health care workers and organizations to become culturally competent. There are many definitions for cultural competence, and in 2000 the U.S. Department of Health and Human Services (DHHS) developed a widely recognized definition. **Cultural competence** is the ability of health care providers and organizations to understand and respond effectively to the cultural and linguistic needs that clients bring to the health care setting. Among other standards to achieve cultural competence, the DHHS made several suggestions for health care organizations. First, organizations are to ensure that staff members are trained to work respectfully and effectively with clients in culturally diverse health care environments. Second, organizations are to develop procedures to address cross-cultural ethical and legal conflicts in health care delivery, such as culturally insensitive or discriminatory treatment, difficulty in accessing service, or denial of services.

HEALTHY PEOPLE 2010

Another program created by the U.S. Department of Health and Human Services (2000) is **"Healthy People 2010."** Culture and language have a significant impact on how clients access and respond to health care services. The goal by 2010 is to eliminate the disparities in six areas of health status experienced by racial and ethnic minorities while trying to continue the overall health of all American people. These six target areas are infant mortality, cancer screening and management, cardiovascular disease, diabetes, human immunodeficiency virus (HIV) infection/acquired immunodeficiency syndrome (AIDS), and immunizations. Hopefully, this goal will be met through research, preventive programs, and consultation with members of minority groups. As a large force within the health care industry, nursing can play a vital role in helping to meet Healthy People 2010 objectives.

CULTURE AND NURSING

Among the diverse values, beliefs, and practices found in a cultural group are those relating to health, illness, professional health care, and folk health care. Nursing has a long history of

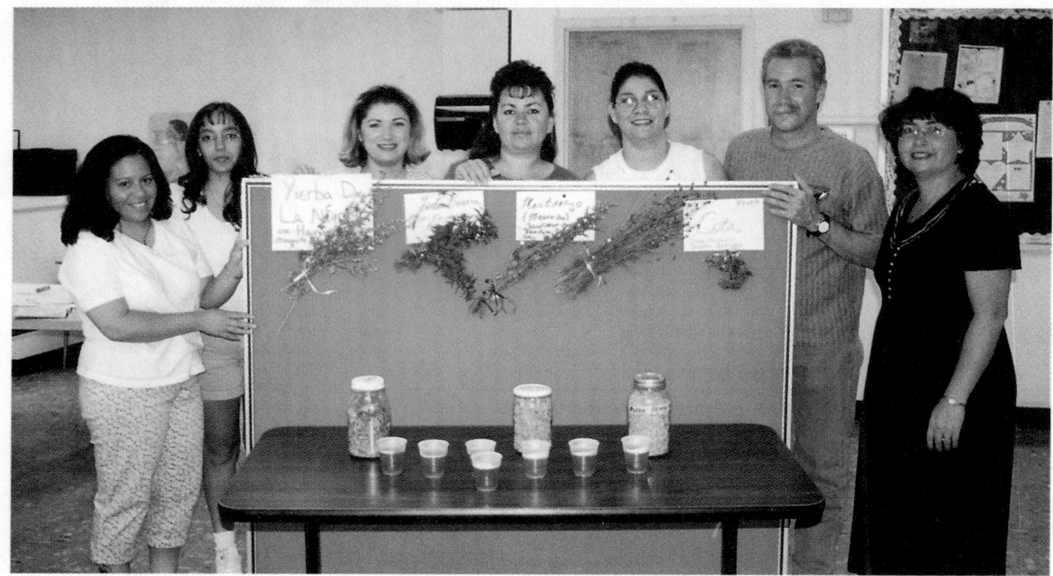

Figure 6-1 ● Nursing students in an associate degree program learning about the value of herbs for healing in the southwestern part of the United States. (Courtesy Luna Vocational Technical Institute, Las Vegas, NM.)

caring for people's physical and mental needs, and there is a newer emphasis on taking care of cultural needs. This focus is the basis for having nursing students learn about cultural considerations while in the academic setting (Figure 6-1).

A dictionary definition of **culture** suggests that it is an integrated pattern of human behavior that includes thought, speech, action, and artifacts and depends on a person's capacity for learning and transmitting knowledge to succeeding generations. Anthropologist Conrad P. Kottak states that "cultures are traditions and customs, transmitted learning that govern the beliefs and behaviors of the people exposed to them" (1991, p. 2). Madeline Leininger, a nurse anthropologist and theorist, defines culture as "the learned and shared beliefs, values and lifeways of a designated or particular group which are generally transmitted intergenerationally and influence one's thinking and action modes" (1995b, p. 8). A definition that includes all of the above is "a body of learned beliefs, traditions, and guides for behavior that are shared among members of a particular group" (Department of Health and Environmental Control of South Carolina, 1997, p. 3). Culture can include things such as language, art, morals, laws, customs, rituals, technology, economics, and kinship or family systems.

Culture also influences health and nursing care. It influences the way people think about health, the ways in which they express pain, what they consider to be symptoms, how they seek and accept help and care, and who they consider to be healers.

In the 1950s Leininger combined culture and nursing into a new field called **transcultural nursing.** She developed the theory of Culture Care Diversity and Universality. She specified that transcultural nursing is an area of study and practice that focuses on the care, health, and illness patterns of people with similarities and differences in their cultural beliefs, values, and practices. The practice of transcultural nurses is to provide care that considers the cultural aspects of the client (Leininger, 1995b). Over time, other nurses have become proficient in the field of cultural care, including Boyle, Andrews, Spector, Douglas, and Purnell.

Cultural considerations should certainly be given a role in the study and nursing care of people who move to the United States from other parts of the world. Many people within the same country have diverse needs in health care and fall into various categories. For example, cultural differences exist between residents of urban areas and rural areas and between residents of different geographic sections of a country. Differences are also found between young and old, male and female, and gay and straight people. Nurses and physicians also make up a culture within themselves according to their unique beliefs, values, and practices.

Culture can also be institutional or organizational. Hospitals, nursing homes, and health care offices in both the public and private sector have cultural beliefs, values, and practices, as do nursing programs in schools and universities. An example can be found in the culture of managed care organizations. Unlike a hospital environment, in which care is often for clients with emergent illness or surgery needs, a managed care organization focuses on lowering health care costs and is more likely to stress preventive and cost-effective screening tests (Ludwig-Beymer, 1999a). The organizational plan, beliefs, values, and practice of the managed care organization are different from those of a hospital.

ASSESSING AND MANAGING THE CULTURAL NEEDS OF CLIENTS

There are several ways to learn about the culture of clients. Cultural research in nursing relies on questioning clients, observing them, and participating in their cultural activities. Each of these methods can also be used in nursing practice.

The aspects of culture that need to be assessed depend on the situation. Several assessment guides created by expert cultural nurses are especially helpful. Leininger (1995a) bases her culturologic assessment on cultural social structure dimensions (Table 6-1). Purnell developed a second model for assessing the cultural aspects of a particular group (Table 6-2).

TABLE 6-1 • LEININGER'S FACTORS FOR ASSESSING CULTURAL GROUPS OR PERSONS

- Worldview of the group
- Technologic factors
- Kinship and social factors
- Economic factors
- Cultural values and lifeways
- Philosophic and religious factors
- Political and legal factors
- Educational factors

TABLE 6-2 • PURNELL'S FACTORS FOR ASSESSING CULTURAL GROUPS OR PERSONS

- Nutrition
- Communication
- Family roles
- Work issues
- Biocultural ecology
- High-risk behaviors
- Heritage
- Pregnancy and childbirth
- Death rituals
- Spirituality
- Health care practices
- Folk health practices

He points out that, although the model is given as a whole for assessment, the situation and culture studied may lead the health care provider to concentrate on one area before another. In a very religious community, for example, the provider may want to start the assessment with spirituality rather than with another domain.

Many of the same factors are found in both assessment models, with Purnell having added some extra dimensions. The nurse should use the parts of either model that are most appropriate for the person and the culture being considered.

Performing a Cultural Assessment

The three major methods for assessing the culture of a client are observation, interview, and participation. The health care setting often determines the order in which these methods are used.

OBSERVATION

A cultural assessment in the home probably starts with the observation phase. For example, the neighborhood and the geographic area in which the client and family live could be observed (Figure 6-2). Is the street in front of the house a busy one, or is it in a more rural area? Is public transportation available, or do residents have their own cars? Going into the client's house, the nurse observes for Bibles, other religious books, and religious symbols on the walls or tables. Evidence of technology, such as air-conditioning, televisions, telephones, kitchen appliances, and computers, is noted. The interactions among family members are also observed.

INTERVIEW

Following observation, the nurse could interview the client and possibly the family. Nurses often obtain health histories from their clients, and cultural interviewing is only slightly different. The best questions for cultural interviews are "semi-structured and open-ended" questions. The nurse usually has an interview guide or an outline for the questions. The following are a few of the questions used in one cultural study (Morgan, 1994):

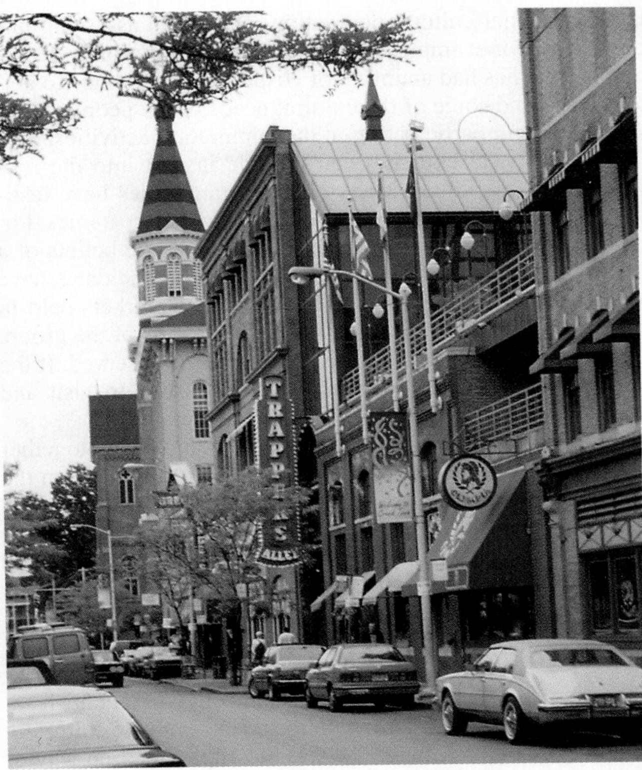

Figure 6-2 • Community assessment of Greektown in Detroit, Michigan.

1. I am interested in where you were born. Could you describe the community (or country)?
2. I would like to know where your parents were born. If they are living, where are they now?
3. Tell me about your household. Who lives in it? Are they related to you?
4. Describe how you usually spend your days. What do you like to do most?
5. Please describe your education for me.
6. I am also interested in the church and religion. What do they mean in your life?
7. Tell me about what you believe about health. What does it mean to "be healthy"? To whom do you look for health care?
8. Is there anything else you would like to tell me?

A good interviewer will often deviate from the form if the client shows interest in a particular question. Often more details are learned in such a circumstance. A large amount of information can usually be gleaned from actively listening to a client, whether during an interview or at any other time.

PARTICIPATION

Participation is the third method of collecting data for a cultural assessment. This process is very helpful for understanding a particular cultural population rather than assessing just one client. For example, a nurse may begin working in a community that has had an influx of Hispanic immigrants. To better understand some of the cultural needs of the people, he or she may begin participating in the community activities.

Trips to local churches can provide insight into the religious life of a culture. Many ethnic communities have festivals with handicrafts, special foods, music, and costumes. Political rallies are also a good place to observe the beliefs of a group. A number of local, state, and federal candidates have used these rallies to gather votes. Similarly, markets held in the community tell a lot about the buying habits of the group. Local foods, clothing, and other goods can be observed. If the nurse is fortunate, an invitation may be issued to visit and have a meal in the home of a community member.

In preparing a cultural assessment, the nurse puts together the information gathered from the cultural group or from the client about the lifestyles, general beliefs and practices and, specifically, health care beliefs. A cultural care plan can be developed from this information (see the Evidence-Based Practice for Nursing box below.

Developing the Cultural Care Plan

The nurse uses the data gathered about a client or clients from a particular culture to plan, implement, and evaluate culturally competent care. Leininger (1995a) has suggested one way of planning cultural care for a client, and this method is used by many nurses. She uses three modes for planning care (p. 106):

- *Culture care preservation or maintenance* is a way to help "people of a particular culture to retain or preserve relevant care values so they can maintain and/or preserve their well-being, recover from illness, or face handicaps and/or death."
- *Culture care accommodation or negotiation* refers to "professional actions and decisions that help people of a designated culture adapt to or negotiate with others for a beneficial or satisfying health outcome with professional care providers."
- *Culture care repatterning or restructuring* helps clients to "reorder, change or greatly modify their lifeways . . . providing a lifeway more beneficial or healthier than before the changes were co-established with the clients."

An example of applying these modes for planning care can be found in a study by Berry (1999). Berry outlined her decisions and actions according to what she had learned from assessing a group of Mexican-American women (Table 6-3).

RESEARCH APPLICATIONS

The same or similar methods of assessing a culture or a client have been used by many nurses interested in cultural care. Struthers and Littlejohn (1999) reported on research showing "the essence of Native American nursing," which was based on a summit held in Montana for Native American nurses. The thoughts and themes of the nurses during this 4-day gathering were analyzed using observation, participation, and interviews. The major themes arising from the data were caring, traditions, respect, connection,

EVIDENCE-BASED PRACTICE FOR NURSING

What is the relationship between culture and parish nursing?

Chase-Ziolek, M. (1999). The meaning and experience of health ministry within the culture of a congregation with a parish nurse. *Journal of Transcultural Nursing, 10*(1), 46-55.

The meaning and experience of a parish nurse with a health ministry for a United Methodist congregation was studied by the author, who used observation, participation, interviews, and a review of significant documents for her research. She found that the congregation understood that the parish nurse promoted health through nursing activities. The congregation also believed that the parish nurse was involved with church activities and experiences that were not specifically planned to promote health but led those involved to experience positive health benefits. The author concluded that it was important to be sensitive to the culture of a congregation in order to provide them with culturally competent care.

Critique. The use of observation, participation, interviews, and record review were appropriate methods to explore the effect of a parish ministry. In cultural studies, a lengthy period of time is required to immerse oneself in the culture before conclusions can be drawn. This researcher used a 14-month study period.

Implications for Nursing. All nurses need to understand the cultures of their clients. In parish nursing, the congregation as a whole is the client, and culturally competent care will enhance a health ministry. Religious beliefs are an important part of a client's or group's culture.

TABLE 6-3 • APPLICATION OF PLANNING CARE FOR HISPANIC WOMEN

CULTURE CARE PRESERVATION OR MAINTENANCE

A. Spiritual beliefs are a major source of strength.
  - Provide religious advisors and time for prayer.

B. Respect is an important pattern.
  - Address clients by last name.
  - Respect the generic care guidance provided by older females.
  - Understand the respect given to male authority as protective care in public and in family life.

CULTURE CARE ACCOMMODATION OR NEGOTIATION

A. Kin is important during illness.
  - Allow kin to be involved during treatment.
  - Consider female relatives at bedside rather than male because of the high value of modesty among women.

B. There is a belief that women should be quiet when in pain.
  - Explain and offer pain relief.
  - Provide assurance that vocalization is acceptable.

C. Generic (folk) beliefs involve hot/cold theories.
  - Provide blankets for warming.
  - Do not insist on iced water; give tepid water.

D. Communication and language are important.
  - Try to have a bilingual nurse available.
  - Have common phrases in Spanish and English illustrated with pictures for better communication.

CULTURE CARE REPATTERNING OR RESTRUCTURING

A. There can be a lack of understanding of ways to access health care.
  - Establish a communication hotline in Spanish.

B. Transportation can be a problem in getting care.
  - Work with public officials to initiate a van service.

C. The waiting time in clinics is long.
  - Consider adding late afternoon or evening appointments.

Data from Berry, A. (1999). Mexican American women's expressions of the meaning of culturally congruent prenatal care. *Journal of Transcultural Nursing, 10*(3), 203-212.

holism/holistic care, trust, and spirituality. The author points out that caring is universal to both Native American nursing and mainstream or Western nursing, whereas the other themes are more specific to the Native American nurses.

Another study examined the motivation, health beliefs, and access barriers experienced by older minority women in keeping mammography appointments (Bernstein, Mutschler, & Bernstein, 2000). Minority women have a high mortality rate for breast cancer and lower rates of routine mammography. The study sample contained mostly African-American women but also included Caucasian (Anglo-American), Hispanic, and Haitian participants. The method used was peer interaction with the participants concerning education about breast health, discussion of the pros and cons of mammography, assessment of the willingness to change behavior, and a no-cost, next-day appointment for a mammogram. Sixty percent of the study group kept their appointments or had a mammogram within 3 months.

According to Bernstein, Mutschler, and Bernstein (2000), the success of the program resulted from the following: (1) the interaction between the women and culturally-ompetent peers who offered education, (2) the use of interpreters for non–English speaking participants, and (3) the fact that the women in the study group were treated as experts in telling their own experiences and stories related to breast health.

In a study of health care for Anglo-American men in the Midwest, Sellers et al. (1999) point out that nurse researchers have generally neglected to study men. They used an ethnonursing method to find the specific needs for this group. Several cultural themes and corresponding nursing implications were identified from interviews with subjects:

- The importance for men to be individualists, independent, and self-reliant
- A delayed seeking of medical help, a preference for self-prescribed treatment, and a reluctance to discuss symptoms
- A definition of health as being able to work and meet responsibilities

Nursing implications regarding men's health in rural settings include the following:

- Providing information about health care at local community events, such as county fairs
- Scheduling health care services during less busy times of the year (e.g., avoiding the crop harvesting season)
- Reducing the wait time in clinics and physician's offices to prevent less time missed at work

SPECIAL CONSIDERATIONS FOR SELECTED SUBCULTURES

Subcultures are part of a larger culture of the client. For example, there are disabled people with Greek-American backgrounds whose cultural care plans would include both the major culture and the subculture. The same might be true of a lesbian client who is also African American. She would need special care for her sex orientation and for her overall culture. Two specific groups that make up subcultures in our society—disabled individuals and those with sexual orientations out of the mainstream—have often been neglected.

Disability

One subculture that should be considered by the health care professional is that of individuals with disabilities. There is not one disability subculture but rather several that are based on the variations of disabilities (see also Chapter 10). Some disabilities are acquired from various illnesses, conditions, and accidents, whereas others are a result of developmental problems. There are, however, some common themes that define the culture of all individuals with disabilities.

Individuals with disabilities make up the largest minority group in the United States. Approximately "15% to 20% of U.S. residents have a disabling condition that interferes with life activities" (National Organization on Disability, 1998). Disability activists express hostility to health care providers, arguing that they lack knowledge regarding the social nature of disability and have a reluctance to admit there is an environment that enhances the difficulties of those with disabilities. Cultural competence must be broadened to include this group (Lipson & Rogers, 2000).

Two other authors write about implications for health care providers in caring for disabled individuals. Treloar (1999) focused on clinical applications discovered from a qualitative research study. One of her subjects remarked that life becomes an "obstacle course with a way to get to the other end" (p. 363). This comment echoes the need for environmental considerations by nurses and others.

In "The Culture of the Deaf," Stebnicki and Coeling (1999) discuss modes of care specific to this group of individuals, again stressing the need for culturally competent care. The following are suggestions for cultural care for the deaf:

- Ensure that visiting arrangements in a hospital are made for the clients' support system.
- Have the hospital staff learn a few key phrases in American Sign Language (ASL).
- Recognize that facial expressions are another means of communication.

Sexual Orientation

Sexual orientation can influence the delivery of cultural care to a group of people. Spinks, Andrews, and Boyle (2000) discuss the provision of cultural care to lesbian clients, but many of their suggestions could include gay men. Unlike a group in which the language, dress, or country of residence give some clue to the culture, the identification of someone in the lesbian or gay community may be more difficult. The professional nurse may assume incorrectly that a client is heterosexual and thus not provide the unique health care that is needed. A lack of good communication, along with bias of the health care professional, is often involved.

A gay or lesbian client has the same physical health needs in screening and health promotion as any client but may also have specific issues that need to be addressed. For example, there is a higher risk of substance abuse among homosexuals, perhaps because of the stresses inherent in feeling the need to hide their sexual orientation. Other issues may involve help regarding whether to have children through adoption, artificial insemination, or intentional heterosexual contact. One group in a large city took a proactive role in providing culturally congruent care by forming a Feminist Women's Health Center to meet the needs of all women, including lesbian clients (Spinks, Andrews, & Boyle, 2000).

A note of caution regarding sexual orientation is that overt signs of affection between persons of the same sex may or may not be an indication of their sexual preference. As Andrews and Herberg (1999) emphasize, in some cultures such as the Nigerian population, women publicly hold hands or embrace other women as a sign of friendship. This author found a similar situation in her visits to Benin in West Africa. In that area, heterosexual men often held hands while casually walking down the street.

SELECTED CONCEPTS RELATED TO CULTURALLY SENSITIVE NURSING

Specific cultural practices involving religion, nutrition, and folk practices should be considered when assessing clients and planning their care.

Religion

The spiritual well-being of clients who practice a religion is an important consideration in nursing in that it has a bearing on many different aspects of health and illness. Some examples are the acceptance or nonacceptance of blood products, diet, the furnishing of religious support for the sick, and beliefs and practices related to death and dying.

In times of crisis, religion may well come to the forefront in caring for the client. As Andrews and Hanson (1999) state, "In the case of integration of health care and religious/spiritual beliefs, the focus of the nursing plan is to help the client maintain his/her own beliefs in the face of the health crisis and to use these beliefs to strengthen their individual coping patterns" (p. 382).

Under no circumstances should the nurse forget that many people are atheists (do not believe in a higher power) or agnostics (question whether there is a God or higher power). Although the majority of U.S. citizens are Christian, cultural diversity is bringing many varied religions that should be considered in planning care.

Generic or Folk Medicine

Although many Americans believe in using the professional medical and nursing system for health care, many more do not seek professional care for many reasons. Such reasons may include transportation difficulties, high cost of care, fear and distrust of health care workers, and poor communication between clients and professionals. Some cultural ways of healing might be considered unscientific and strange to many health care workers.

Where do folk health ideas come from? People within certain cultures look at their ideas as ways to preserve both their heritage and their health. Folk health beliefs, practices, and values are learned from experience and observations. They are passed down from generation to generation and have proved to be of value to the culture and the people.

Long before there were physicians and nurses, there were systems of caring for and curing people. For example, early ancestors found they could prevent or cure disease with plants. Digitalis (which comes from the foxglove plant) and belladonna have been used for many generations. Dr. Loudell Snow's book (1998) about folk health beliefs and practices is entitled *Walkin' Over Medicine.* As one of her subjects told her, "Why there's lotta weeds out there now, you're walkin' over medicine. . . . There's many vitamins out there right now that we're walkin' over" (p. vii).

Substances other than plants are also used. For example, in the South (and among Southerners who migrated to the North), the practice among African Americans and Euro Americans from the Appalachian mountains is to eat clay or dirt. This practice is called *geophagia.* Many Southern families have had their own clay banks for years. Some studies have shown this practice going back to Africa (Spector, 2000; Boyle & Mackey, 1999). Red clay is used for anemia, and white clay is preferred for indigestion. White clay consists of kaolin, the same ingredient found in some medications for indigestion today. The cost of these drugs far exceeds that of the natural clay.

There also are numerous hot/cold theories related to healing. It is important to remember that these theories are not necessarily based on temperature. Hot/cold theories of healing are found among Hispanic, Arab, Southeast Indian, African-American, and Southern Anglo-American cultures. If the nurse provides care to an adult who has some of these beliefs, he or she may find that the explanation for the present illness goes back to earlier life. For example, Hispanic women believe that partaking of "cold" foods and medicines after pregnancy will cause the bleeding to stop. They believe this blood is reabsorbed into the body to cause nervousness or insanity later in life. A similar belief is that cold can get into the open vagina after childbirth and stay in the body to cause arthritis in adult life. Health care providers who see these clients must realize that the etiology of the problem may be quite different from the scientific explanation.

The "evil eye" is a prominent belief in many cultures, including Hispanic and Arab cultures. The Spanish term for this belief is *mal de ojo.* One basis for this belief is envy or jealousy of the gods when there is excessive praise or admiration of a person. Another belief is that a person who is angry at another person can "put the evil eye on him or her." Various amulets are worn to reflect the evil eye back onto the person who caused it (Figure 6-3).

In addition to evil eye, there are "red eyes." To the health professional, "red eyes" are the same as conjunctivitis. A common folk cure for this ailment is the use of urine. A few drops of urine in the eye are believed to quickly remedy the condition. Health care professionals are often guilty of saying, "You put *what* in your eye?" A better approach is to suggest to the client that although it is fine to continue the home treatment, antibiotic ointment might help to speed the cure. These treatments have been used for years in some cultures and without a problem. However, the health care worker needs to stress that it is better to use the urine from someone who is healthy. Some cases of gonorrhea have occurred as a result of folk uses for urine.

Various methods are used to protect people from evil. Garlic or a substance such as asofoetida may be worn around the neck, often in a little red bag. Both of these substances are thought to protect against colds and flu. They both smell so bad that they may indeed work, because other people do not want to get close to the wearer.

A very important point to consider with folk medicine is the use of particular phrases to describe health problems.

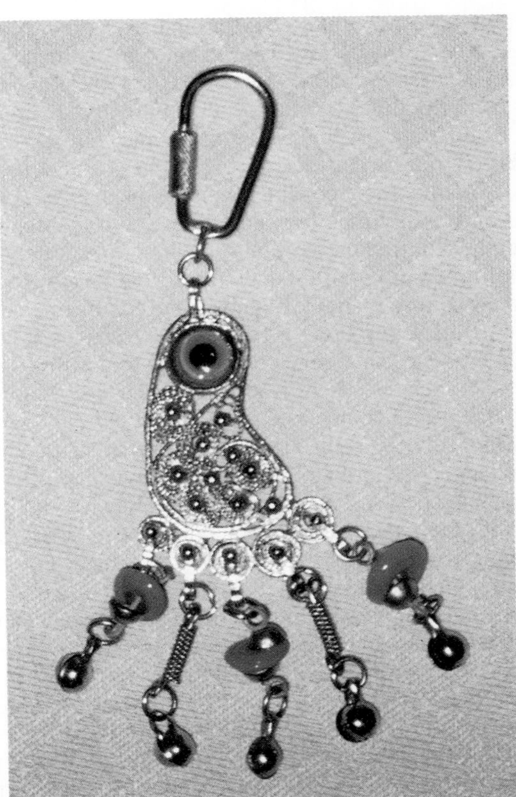

Figure 6-3 ● "Hand of God" amulet to protect the wearer from the "evil eye."

Many African Americans and some Appalachians refer to the blood in various ways that can have several meanings. For example, "high blood" can mean hypertension, or too much blood in the body, or it can mean the movement of blood to a higher part of the body such as the brain or head. The movement of blood into the head is commonly believed to cause strokes or nervousness or to make the person "fall out" (faint). A similar situation is "low blood," which can mean low blood pressure or anemia in the sense of not having enough blood. These different terms can cause clinical problems. For example, Snow (1998) refers to a man who was told his blood count was a little low. As a result, the man decided he should no longer take his medicine for hypertension. A similar use of language is the reference to "sweet blood" or "sugar in blood" (diabetes). When taking care of clients, the nurse must sometimes delve deeper into the meaning of certain phrases.

This section has described only a few examples of the generic or folk beliefs that are prevalent in almost any culture. What must nurses do to help people with these beliefs? Most folk practices are not hurtful, but when they are, nurses and physicians must deal with them. The worst thing a health care professional can do is make fun of or express dismay at folk beliefs and practices. People will often not return for care if they are treated as though they are ignorant for practicing folk health habits.

The subject of folk health is so broad that very few examples can be given in this chapter. Many books listed in the Selected Bibliography go into great detail. Readers who are interested in more information should consult these resources.

Pain

Pain is universal in all cultures, and yet the way in which people display and discuss pain varies greatly among and between cultures. Ludwig-Beymer (1999b) states that "pain is a highly personal experience, depending on cultural learning, the meaning of the situation, and other factors unique to the individual" (p. 284).

Douglas (1999) has suggested that pain be the fifth vital sign along with temperature, pulse, respiration, and blood pressure. However, she cautions that current pain assessment often depends on a numerical rating from 0 to 10. It is necessary that cultural definitions of pain be taken into consideration, because subjective rather than objective measurements are more culture specific.

Nurses often believe that silent suffering is a valued reaction to pain. Because of their socialization to the idea that stoicism and acceptance of pain is preferable, they often deny pain in themselves and use minimal analgesics when in pain. Thus they expect the same reactions from their clients (Ludwig-Beymer, 1999b). They prefer to see self-control in their clients rather than displays of strong feelings related to pain (Spector, 2000).

Ludwig-Beymer (1999b) reports an interesting study on the administration of analgesics by health care providers. The most vocal cultural groups received the most pain medication, whereas the more stoic groups received less. Therefore fewer pain medications were given to Japanese, Filipino, and Chinese clients, who were the least vocal.

Older adults were also included in this study. Older adults often believed that pain was just a normal part of the aging process and should be tolerated. They further thought that the health care staff was too busy to pay attention to their complaints and that further, more expensive tests would be ordered if they complained too much (Ludwig-Beymer, 1999b).

The alleviation of pain is also cultural. Techniques such as acupuncture, long used by the Chinese, have become more widespread in the United States. Similarly, herbal remedies have been used by many cultures through the ages (see also Chapters 4 and 7).

Religious practices also have a place in pain management. Catholics often use their rosaries to pray. Other denominations in the Christian faith have special healing services either in churches or in the sick room. Jewish clients may ask to speak to a rabbi. Native American clients have shamans who perform religious rituals for healing that involve the client, relatives, and other members of the cultural group. One role of the nurse is to provide privacy for religious practices.

Nutrition

Culture has a great impact on food and the way in which it is prepared and served. Technology, economics, and religion—all parts of the cultural assessment—influence the food that is eaten by different cultural groups.

Technology affects how food is produced. High-level technology is involved on large agricultural farms, but very few tools may be necessary to grow a backyard garden. Foods are much less seasonal now than they were before rapid transportation systems could move food from many countries with varying growing seasons.

Economics also affects the production and distribution of food. In Third World countries, food is produced on small farms. The food that is not needed by the family who produced it is brought to a central market area for sale. Custom also dictates how food is sold. In many European countries, people go to specialty stores or markets to buy fresh meat and produce each day. Many economically deprived countries experience famine and starvation.

Religion also dictates what different cultural groups eat and how the food is prepared. Many in the Hindu religion refrain from eating cows, and some are lacto-vegetarians, eating only milk products and vegetables. Jewish people do not eat pork or shellfish, and there are religious rituals for killing the meat to make it kosher. Many Jewish people believe that milk and meat should not be eaten at the same meal (Spector, 2000). Religion also influences whether specific things are eaten at different times. Many Christians who are Catholic or Episcopalian "give up" certain foods, commonly meat or desserts, during the Lenten season. Religious holidays also feature traditional meats, such as the Christmas turkey or the Easter ham.

Beliefs and practices related to the hot/cold theory often involve foods. Illness is often seen as an imbalance between elements, and food or herbs are used to therapeutically restore the body to its natural balance. Therefore curing a "hot" disease such as arthritis may require cold foods or medicines. Beliefs vary about what is hot and what is cold. When a nurse is faced with a client who has these beliefs, an assessment must be made by interviewing the client and family or by referring to books with details about these specific beliefs. A similar belief is the Chinese *yin* and *yang* balance of foods for health.

Foods are also important in planning care with certain cultural groups. For example, African Americans are often lactose intolerant and have problems with milk and milk products. They also have a tendency to have high blood pressure, which some health care providers and scientists attribute to high-salt diets and the intake of many fried foods.

Communication

One of the stumbling blocks to effective health care is communication. Not only do clients and nurses often speak different languages, there is also miscommunication when nurses use technical language, slang, or jargon. In addition, people in every culture have silent ways of expressing themselves through facial expressions, posture, and hand gestures; through the space between people; and through touch. Discomfort and a lack of understanding results if efforts are not made to overcome miscommunication or a lack of communication.

When nurses and clients speak an entirely different language, several interventions can be taken to try to effectively communicate with the client and the family. The first step is to assess the population for which care will be provided. If it is primarily a Hispanic group, then learning the language is the ideal answer. Although learning a complete language is often not possible, knowing and using a few words and phrases often go a long way in making a client comfortable and interested in the care provided.

Interpreters are often used in health care with different cultures. The best situation is to have someone on the health care team act as an interpreter. When this is not possible, arrangements can sometimes be made with people in the community. Some health care facilities have found that foreign language professors from nearby schools or colleges can act in this capacity. An important consideration is the use of a client's friends and family members and the need to maintain confidentiality. With friends and family in the room, the client may be less forthcoming with personal information—information that could be important to diagnosis and treatment.

One helpful resource is the AT&T Language Service (800-752-6096). This service contains translators in more than 150 languages. There is a fee for this service, but it can be very helpful in some cases.

Another solution is the use of pictures that contain both the foreign language word and the English equivalent. For example, Spanish-speaking clients would be shown a picture of a nurse with the words "enfermera" and "nurse" underneath it or a hypodermic syringe and needle with the words "inyección" and "shot" underneath it (Figure 6-4).

There can be confusion in communication even when English is the first language. The different meanings of health expressions such as high and low blood were discussed under Generic or Folk Medicine, p. 56. Clients can often get confused if they are told to "go to the bathroom and get a specimen." The client does not know whether he or she is expected to get a urine or a feces specimen when such vague terms are used. The nurse should be clear about the expectations or instructions for the clients.

Nonverbal communication can involve space, gestures, posture, and facial expressions, all of which vary with the culture of the person. When someone invades another's personal space, that person can get very uncomfortable and transmit feelings of discomfort. Andrews and Herberg (1999) point out that "Americans, Canadians, and British require the most personal space, whereas Latin American, Japanese, and Arabs need the least" (p. 33). Understanding that space is cultural can help in coping with feelings of being invaded.

Gestures are very much a cultural means of communication. They vary between cultures and can be seen as unacceptable or threatening depending on the ethnic group. In the American culture, the thumb and first finger make a circle and the other fingers are held upright to mean "everything's okay." In some Arab cultures, however, this same hand gesture means a woman's vagina. This example illustrates the concern that the use of certain gestures can cause.

Facial expressions and looking directly at someone can also cause discomfort in certain cultures. Some groups (e.g., Asian Americans) expect their health care providers to be serious and formal, whereas others (e.g., Hispanic clients) want a more intimate, personal reaction. American nurses value the use of eye-to-eye contact with clients, but some clients may avert their eyes because of cultural differences. Clients of Asian, Native American, Indochinese, Arab, and Appalachian descent fall into this last category (Andrews & Herberg, 1999).

ETHICS

According to Norton (1999), "Ethics is a systematic philosophical method of inquiry that assists people in understand-

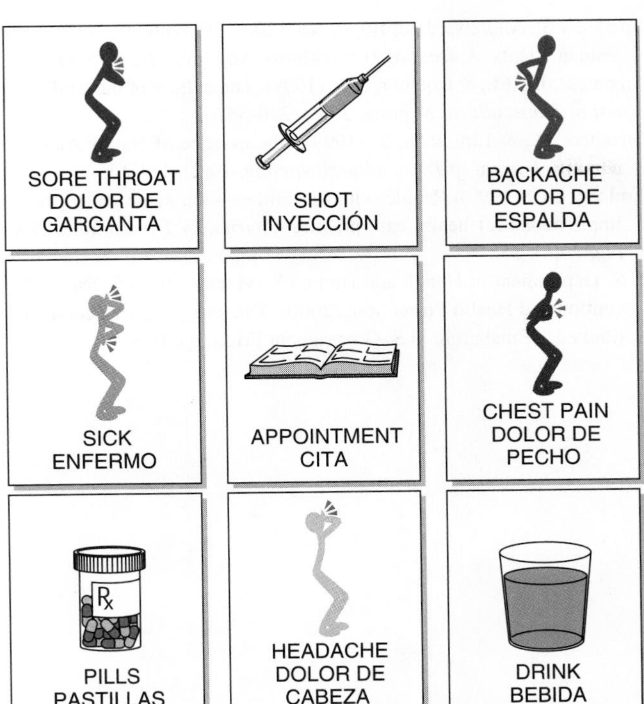

Figure 6-4 ● English/Spanish pictograph to assist with communication. (Courtesy Anne Grimmer, Xid Design, Tallahassee, FL.)

ing the morality (rightness or wrongness) of human behavior and social policies. Ethics also refers to the standards of behavior expected of members of a professional group" (p. 449). The ethics of nursing includes, but is not limited to, ensuring client confidentiality, getting informed consent for certain procedures and surgery, and respecting the right of clients to make autonomous decisions about their care. The ethics regarding the cultural care of clients goes further and considers the values of each individual client and his or her cultural beliefs and practices.

Some aspects of cultural care involve beliefs related to death and dying, the right to refuse medical care and blood transfusions, and cultural prerogatives in giving information to the client and family. The nurse must examine his or her own values and be ready to set them aside if faced with a conflict that involves the values, beliefs, and practices of the client. In some cases the nurse may not be able to provide care for the client.

Many conditions require the culturally competent nurse to make adjustments. For example, different cultures have different perspectives of time. In the United States, and particularly among Anglo-Americans, a high value is placed on punctuality and keeping appointments. Health care providers often refer to clients as being "noncompliant" when advice, appointments, or prescriptions are given and then ignored. The nurse needs to understand that not all cultures view the world in the same way as the majority of the population. Therefore the nurse or health organization must make culturally sound interventions or adjustments for the sake of good care. To help meet this goal, Cultural Considerations discussions are used throughout this text to describe how culture relates to various diseases and their management.

ONLINE RESOURCES

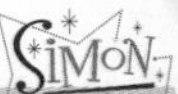

For suggested readings and Internet resources, go to http://www.wbsaunders.com/SIMON/Iggy/.

SELECTED BIBLIOGRAPHY

Asterisk indicates a classic or definitive work on this subject.

Andrews, M.M. (1999). Culture and nutrition. In M.M. Andrews & J.S. Boyle (Eds.), *Transcultural concepts in nursing care* (3rd ed., pp. 341-377). Philadelphia: J.B. Lippincott.

Andrews, M.M., & Hanson, P.A. (1999). Religion, culture, and nursing. In M.M. Andrews & J.A. Boyle (Eds.), *Transcultural concepts in nursing care* (3rd ed., pp. 378-443). Philadelphia: J.B. Lippincott.

Andrews, M.M., & Herberg, P. (1999). Transcultural nursing care. In M.M. Andrews & J.S. Boyle (Eds.), *Transcultural concepts in nursing care* (3rd ed., pp. 23-77). Philadelphia: J.B. Lippincott.

Bernstein, J., Mutschler, P., & Bernstein, E. (2000). Keeping mammography appointments: Motivation, health beliefs, and access barriers experienced by older minority women. *Journal of Midwifery and Women's Health, 45*(4), 308-313.

Berry, A. (1999). Mexican American women's expressions of the meaning of culturally congruent prenatal care. *Journal of Transcultural Nursing, 10*(3), 203-212.

Boyle, J.S., & Mackey, M.C. (1999). Pica: Sorting it out. *Journal of Transcultural Nursing, 10*(1), 65-68.

Chase-Ziolek, M. (1999). The meaning and experience of health ministry within the culture of a congregation with a parish nurse. *Journal of Transcultural Nursing, 10*(1), 46-55.

Department of Health and Environmental Control of South Carolina. (1997). *Basic cultural competence training manual: Office of Minority Health.* Columbia, SC: Author.

Douglas, M. (1999). Pain as the fifth vital sign: Will cultural variations be considered? *Journal of Transcultural Nursing, 10*(4),285.

*Kantrowitz, M.P., Mondragon, A., & Coleman, W.L. (1983). *Que paso? An English-Spanish guide for medical personnel.* Albuquerque: University of New Mexico Press.

*Kottak, C.P. (1991). *Anthropology: The examination of human diversity* (5th ed.). New York: McGraw-Hill.

*Leininger, M.M. (1995a). Overview of Leininger's culture care theory. In M.M. Leininger (Ed.), *Transcultural nursing: Concepts, theories, research, and practice* (2nd ed., pp. 93-114). New York: McGraw-Hill.

*Leininger, M.M. (1995b). Transcultural nursing: Development, focus, importance, and historical development. In M.M. Leininger (Ed.), *Transcultural nursing: Concepts, theories, research, and practice* (2nd ed., pp. 3-54). New York: McGraw-Hill.

Lipson, J.G., & Rogers, J.G. (2000). Cultural aspects of disability. *Journal of Transcultural Nursing, 11*(3), 212-219.

Ludwig-Beymer, P. (1999a). Transcultural aspects of pain. In M.M. Andrews & J.S. Boyle, (Eds.), *Transcultural concepts in nursing care* (3rd ed., pp. 283-307). Philadelphia: J.B. Lippincott.

Ludwig-Beymer, P. (1999b). Transcultural nursing's role in a managed care setting. *Journal of Transcultural Nursing, 10*(4), 286-287.

*Morgan, M.A. (1994). *Prenatal care of African American women in selected USA urban and rural cultural contexts conceptualized within Leininger's cultural care theory.* Unpublished doctoral dissertation, Wayne State University, Detroit, MI.

*Morgan, M.A. (1996). Prenatal care of African American women in selected USA urban and rural cultural contexts. *Journal of Transcultural Nursing, 7*(2), 3-9.

National Organization on Disability/Louis Harris Associates. (1998). *N.O.D./Harris 1998 Survey of Americans with Disabilities.*

Norton, M.E. (1999). Ethics and culture: Contemporary challenges. In M.M. Andrews & J.S. Boyle (Eds.), *Transcultural concepts in nursing care* (3rd ed., pp. 444-470). Philadelphia: J.B. Lippincott.

Purnell, L. (2000). A description of the Purnell model for cultural competence. *Journal of Transcultural Nursing, 11*(1), 40-46.

Sellers, S.C., et al. (1999). The healthcare meanings, values, and practices of Anglo-American males in the rural midwest. *Journal of Transcultural Nursing, 10*(4), 320-330.

Snow, L.F. (1998). *Walkin' over medicine* (2nd ed.). Detroit: Wayne State University.

Spector, R.E. (2000). *Cultural diversity in health and illness* (5th ed.). Upper Saddle River, NJ: Prentice-Hall Health.

Spinks, V.S., Andrews, J., & Boyle, J.S. (2000). Providing health care for lesbian clients. *Journal of Transcultural Nursing, 11*(2), 137-143.

Stebnicki, J.A.M., & Coeling, H.V. (1999). The culture of the deaf. *Journal of Transcultural Nursing, 10*(4), 350-357.

Struthers, R., & Littlejohn, S. (1999). The essence of Native American nursing. *Journal of Transcultural Nursing, 10*(2), 131-135.

Treloar, L.L. (1999). People with disabilities—the same, but different: Implications for health care practice. *Journal of Transcultural Nursing, 10*(4), 358-364.

U.S. Department of Health and Human Services, Office of Disease Prevention and Health Promotion. (2000). *Tracking Healthy People 2010* (2nd ed.). Pittsburgh: U.S. Government Printing Office.

CHAPTER 7

Pain: The Fifth Vital Sign

ANNE KEANE • ERIN M. McMENAMIN • ROSEMARY C. POLOMANO

Learning Objectives

After studying this chapter, you should be able to:

1. Define the concept of pain.
2. Describe briefly the gate control theory to explain the relationship between pain and emotion.
3. Explain the role of neuromodulators in the experience of pain.
4. Identify variables that influence a client's perception of pain.
5. Discuss the attitudes and knowledge of nurses, physicians, and clients regarding pain assessment and management.
6. Compare and contrast the characteristics of the major types of pain.
7. Describe the components of a comprehensive pain assessment.
8. Analyze assessment data to formulate nursing diagnoses for the client experiencing pain.
9. Plan nursing care for the client experiencing acute pain.
10. Differentiate commonly used drugs for acute pain and chronic pain.
11. Describe the nursing implications associated with drug therapy for clients with acute pain or chronic pain.
12. Identify special considerations for older adults related to pain assessment and management.
13. Discuss complementary and alternative therapies for clients experiencing pain.
14. Develop a teaching/learning plan for managing pain as part of community-based care for clients experiencing pain.

SIMON

Go to http://www.wbsaunders.com/SIMON/Iggy/ for self-assessment questions related to these Learning Objectives.

Pain is the number one symptom or complaint that causes people to seek health care. It alters or compromises quality of life more than any other single health-related problem. Despite more than 20 years of work by clinicians and professional organizations, there have been only slight improvements in pain management. Unrelieved and undertreated pain remains a major yet avoidable public health problem in the United States (Berry & Dahl, 2000).

In 1999, the Veteran's Health Administration endorsed a policy to add pain as the **fifth vital sign.** This means that nurses and other health care team members should assess and record pain just as they would for temperature, respirations, pulse, and blood pressure. The American Nurses Association and other national nursing organizations support this national movement for clients in all settings.

OVERVIEW

Everyone experiences pain at some point in life. Although this is likely a universal experience, it is also a complex and private one. Because pain is such a personal experience, it is very difficult to describe or explain to others. Many factors make it hard to understand and assess, including psychosocial, cultural, and developmental factors; the influence of gender and environment; and the subjectivity of the pain itself. The amount of pain and responses to it vary from person to person, and therefore interpreting pain solely on actions or behaviors can be misleading.

Definitions of Pain

Several attempts have been made to define **pain** in descriptive or measurable terms; no one definition is more accepted than another. Among the most popular definitions of pain are those of Sternbach (1968), McCaffery (1979), and the International Association on Pain (1979). Sternbach (1968) asserted that pain is "an abstract concept which refers to:

- A personal, private sensation of hurt
- A harmful stimulus which signals current or impending tissue damage
- A pattern of responses to protect the organism from harm" (p. 8)

This comprehensive definition serves to explain pain through a physiologic, psychologic, and social approach.

McCaffery (1979) offered a more personal explanation of pain when she stated that pain "is whatever the experiencing person says it is and exists whenever he says it does" (p. 11). This understanding of pain requires that the client be seen as the authority on the pain and the only one who can define the experience. Finally, the International Association on Pain

(1979) described pain as an unpleasant sensory and emotional experience associated with actual or potential tissue damage.

Regardless of the definition, most people agree that pain has both sensory and behavioral components and is strongly influenced by various physiologic, psychologic, and sociologic factors. A comprehensive understanding of pain requires knowing the descriptive definitions, theories, and physiology of pain. The nurse can use this knowledge in developing skill in pain intervention and in appreciating the different clinical pain situations. This understanding can also help the nurse develop a personal philosophy of pain management.

Theoretical Bases for Pain

Several theories have been proposed to explain the complex phenomenon of pain. Early theories emphasized the recognition of specific pathways of pain transmission. Later theories attempted to uncover the complexity of the central processing of pain in specific areas of the brain. The concept of a pain-modulating network was recently introduced. This concept describes the various links and connections in the spinal cord and brain, specifically the medulla and the midbrain.

Gate Control Theory

The **gate control theory** was proposed to explain the observed relationship between pain and emotion. Melzack and Wall (1982) first introduced this theory and concluded that pain is not just a physiologic response. Psychologic variables such as behavioral and emotional responses also influence the perception of pain.

According to this theory, a gating mechanism occurs in the spinal cord. Nerve fibers (A delta and C fibers) transmit pain impulses from the periphery of the body. These impulses travel to the dorsal horns of the spinal cord, specifically to the *substantia gelatinosa.* The cells of the substantia gelatinosa can inhibit or facilitate the pain impulses transmitted to the trigger cells (T-cells). When T-cell activity is inhibited, the gate is closed and impulses are less likely to be transmitted to the brain. When the gate is opened, pain impulses ascend to the brain (Figure 7-1).

Similar gating mechanisms exist in the nerve fibers descending from the thalamus and cerebral cortex. These areas of the brain regulate thoughts and emotions, including beliefs and values. When pain occurs, a person's thoughts and emotions can modify perceptual phenomena as they reach the level of conscious awareness.

The gate control theory has helped nurses and other health care professionals to recognize the *holistic* nature of pain. As a result, many complementary and alternative therapies (e.g., imagery and distraction [see p. 80]) are used to help relieve pain.

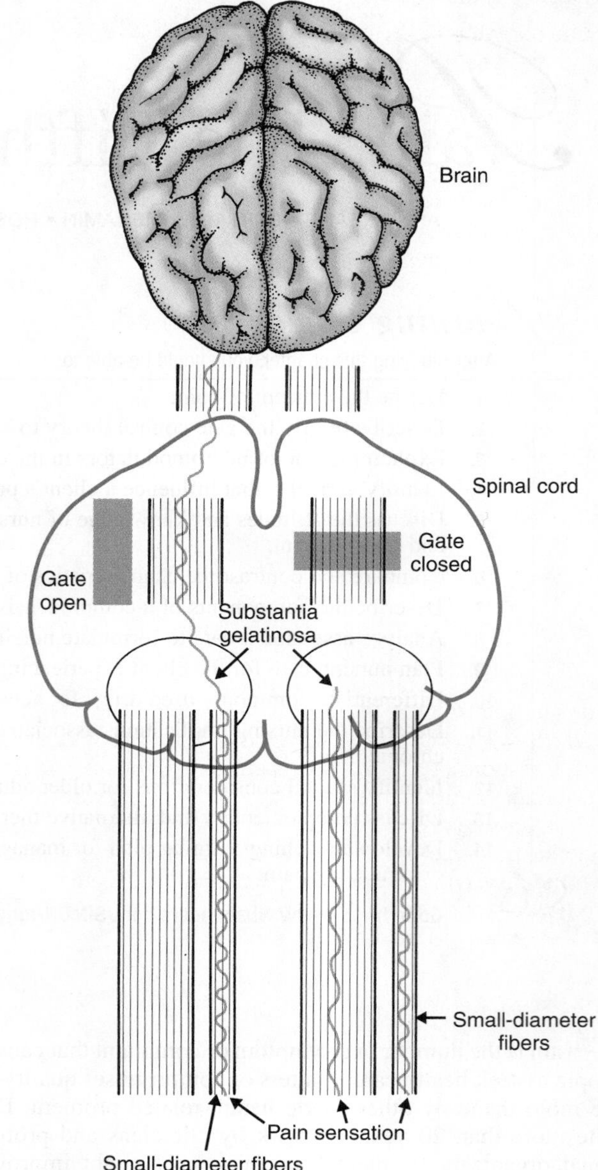

Figure 7-1 ● The gate control theory of pain.

Anatomic and Physiologic Bases for Pain

PAIN STIMULI

A wide range of sensory input is capable of producing pain. Tissue ischemia and muscle spasm also cause pain. Free nerve endings (receptors capable of responding to painful stimuli) are often referred to as nociceptors. Nociceptors are located in various body tissues and are activated by thermal, mechanical, and chemical stimuli. In addition to nociceptors, other receptors in the body respond to almost any type of intense stimulation, which sometimes results in pain.

In most circumstances painful stimuli cause actual tissue damage, which leads to the release of certain chemical substances (e.g., histamine, bradykinin, serotonin, norepinephrine) and certain acids that sensitize nociceptors, including leukotrienes, prostaglandins, and substance P. These chemicals are believed to activate pain receptors. For example, the accumulation of lactic acid leads to the pain associated with ischemic tissue damage. Muscle contraction or spasm can also produce ischemic-type pain. The oxygen demands of the muscle are increased, but the blood supply is limited because of compressed blood vessels.

PAIN FIBERS AND PATHWAYS

Painful stimuli often originate in the periphery (extremities) of the body. To be perceived, the stimuli must be transmitted first to the spinal cord and then to the central areas of the brain, as described by the gate control theory of pain (see Figure 7-1). In the periphery, two specific fibers can transmit stimuli: (1) A delta fibers, which are found primarily in the skin and muscle; and (2) C fibers, which are distributed in muscle, periosteum, and viscera. Both of these nerve fibers are first-order neurons capable of accepting nociceptive stimuli.

A delta fibers are myelinated fibers that carry rapid, sharp, pricking, or piercing sensations. A person feeling these sensations can generally localize them readily to a fairly well-defined area. Because these fibers respond predominantly to mechanical rather than chemical or thermal stimuli, they are called mechanical nociceptors.

C fibers are unmyelinated or poorly myelinated fibers that conduct thermal, chemical, and strong mechanical impulses. Pain conduction from C fibers is more diffuse and dull, burning, or achy—quite different from the sensations of A delta fibers. In contrast to the intermittent nature of A delta sensations, C fibers usually produce constant pain.

Second-order neurons, or pain pathways of the ascending pain tracts, are found in the dorsal horn of the spinal cord and terminate in the thalamus. The spinothalamic tract is divided into two spinal tracts: the lateral or neospinothalamic tract, and the medial or paleospinothalamic tract. The neospinothalamic tract is responsible for sensory pain discrimination. It transmits painful stimuli more directly to the sensory cortex, where pain is eventually perceived and interpreted. The paleospinothalamic tract synapses in other parts of the brain, such as the limbic system (emotional center) and the reticular formation (sleep-wake center). The painful stimuli is therefore subjected to emotional and behavioral influences.

CENTRAL NERVOUS SYSTEM PROCESSING

The central processing of pain occurs at three different levels of the brain: the thalamus, midbrain, and cortex. These areas cooperate to raise the awareness of pain, interpret painful stimuli, and produce a response to pain. The thalamus acts as the relay station for sensory input from the spinothalamic tract of the spinal cord. The midbrain signals the cortex to increase awareness of the stimuli. The cortex seems to be involved both in the discrimination of well-localized pain and in the interpretation of the pain experience.

INHIBITORY AND FACILITATORY MECHANISMS

Sensory input to the spinal cord may be influenced by chemical substances known as neuroregulators. Neuroregulators are classified as either neurotransmitters or neuromodulators.

NEUROTRANSMITTERS. **Neurotransmitters** are the chemicals that exert inhibitory (slowing down) or excitatory (speeding up) activity at postsynaptic nerve cell membranes. Acetylcholine, norepinephrine, epinephrine, and dopamine are documented neurotransmitters.

NEUROMODULATORS. **Neuromodulators,** also called endogenous opiates, are protein hormones in the brain. These substances are composed of large amino acid peptides called alpha-endorphins, beta-endorphins, and enkephalins. These natural opiate-like substances are responsible for pain relief.

Endorphins and enkephalins are similar to morphine-like substances, only more potent. They are believed to play a major role in the biologic response to pain. The larger peptides **(endorphins)** exert more prolonged analgesic (pain-relieving) effects than do the enkephalins. Endorphins are produced by the anterior pituitary gland and the hypothalamus. The smaller peptides **(enkephalins)** tend to be more widespread throughout the brain and the dorsal horn of the spinal cord. Several types of endorphins and enkephalins have been identified. Each acts on highly specific opiate receptors in the central nervous system.

Opioid receptors are binding sites not only for endogenous opiates but also for opioid analgesics taken to relieve pain. There are several types of opioid receptors: mu, kappa, delta, epsilon, and sigma. Mu receptors are found throughout the central nervous system, especially in the brainstem, limbic system, and dorsal horn of the spinal cord. Morphine and morphine agonists bind to mu receptors. Specific subtypes of the mu receptor are responsible for analgesia, bradycardia and sedation, and opioid agonist binding, which is associated with respiratory depression, euphoria, and physical dependence.

Various factors influence the production of neuromodulators. The activity of endorphins and enkephalins may be enhanced by prolonged strenuous activity, transcutaneous electrical nerve stimulators (see later discussions about interventions for acute pain [p. 74] and chronic pain [p. 80]), and antidepressant therapy, which often increases levels of serotonin in the body. Adequate amounts of serotonin, a neurotransmitter, have been shown to enhance analgesia through the activity of endorphins and enkephalins. Similarly, pain and stress are strong activators of the endogenous opiate system.

Sources of Pain

There are three major categories of pain: somatic, visceral, and neuropathic. Another classification for the physiologic sources of pain is pain that involves the activation of nociceptors and nonnociceptive pain or neuropathic pain. Table 7-1 provides a complete description of the physiologic sources of pain.

Pain Perception

The subjectivity of the pain experience limits the understanding of the perception of and response to pain. This situation is further complicated by the knowledge that the perception of pain may persist even when pain pathways are surgically interrupted. Even though the perception of pain is difficult to measure, it can be characterized as the actual awareness of a painful feeling or sensation.

The **pain threshold** is the amount or degree of noxious stimuli that leads a person to first interpret a sensation as painful. More specifically, this term refers to the point at which a person feels pain and reports it as such.

Even though all pain is real, it sometimes persists without any detectable physical cause. Such pain may be highly influenced by emotional and social factors. In such situations the lack of a physiologic or organic cause may lead health care professionals, families, and clients to doubt the validity of the pain.

TABLE 7-1 • PHYSIOLOGIC SOURCES OF PAIN

Physiologic Structures	Mechanism of Pain	Characteristics of Pain	Sources of Acute Postoperative Pain	Sources of Chronic Pain Syndromes
SOMATIC PAIN				
Cutaneous: skin and subcutaneous tissues Deep somatic: bone, muscle, blood vessels, connective tissues	Activation of nociceptors	Well localized Constant and achy	Incisional pain, pain at insertion sites of tubes and drains, wound complications, orthopaedic procedures, skeletal muscle spasms	Bony metastases, osteoarthritis and rheumatoid arthritis, low back pain, peripheral vascular disease
VISCERAL PAIN				
Organs and the linings of the body cavities	Activation of nociceptors	Poorly localized Diffuse, deep, cramping or splitting	Chest tubes, abdominal tubes and drains, bladder distention or spasms, intestinal distention	Pancreatitis, liver metastases, colitis
NEUROPATHIC PAIN				
Nerve fibers, spinal cord, and central nervous system	Nonnociceptive Injury to the nervous system structures	Poorly localized Shooting, burning, fiery, shocklike, sharp, painful numbness	Phantom limb pain, postmastectomy pain, pain from nerve compression	Diabetic, human immunodeficiency virus, chemotherapy-induced neuropathies, postherpetic neuralgia, cancer-related nerve injury

Pain tolerance refers to the ability to endure the intensity of pain. Pain tolerance is usually characterized by an overt expression of behavior. Unlike pain perception and pain threshold, the ability to tolerate pain is more a function of psychologic and social variables than of biologic characteristics.

The nurse should be aware that many variables affect the perception of and response to pain. Demographic factors (e.g., age, gender, sociocultural background), personality characteristics, and cognition may influence the client's ability to process and react to pain sensations.

AGE

Age can influence how pain is perceived and assessed.

CONSIDERATIONS FOR OLDER ADULTS

Some researchers believe that the perceptual acuity of pain diminishes as a result of aging, but this finding has not been validated (Acute Pain Management Guideline Panel, 1992). The perception of cutaneous pain may diminish because of age-related skin changes, but the perception of visceral (organ) pain may increase in older adults. Studies in older adults with cancer suggest that they experience similar levels of pain intensity but require lower levels of analgesia (Vigano, Bruera, & Suarez-Almazor, 1998).

Little attention has been given to assessing or managing pain in older adults who are cognitively impaired (confused) and unable to communicate. Feldt (2000) tested a Checklist of Nonverbal Pain Indicators (CNPI) to assess cognitively impaired older adults hospitalized for hip fracture. Feldt noted that older adults who were not cognitively impaired received significantly more pain medication in comparison to the impaired group.

Both malignant pain (resulting from cancer or other progressive disease) and nonmalignant pain are prevalent among older adults in nursing homes. However, Won and colleagues (1999) found that approximately 25% of residents with daily pain receive no analgesics. Even when nonmalignant pain was recognized, adults over 85 years of age, men, racial minorities, and cognitively impaired residents were less likely to be treated. Similar rates of undertreatment were identified in another analysis of older nursing home residents with cancer pain. Advanced age, racial minority status, low cognitive performance, and the number of other medications received increased the likelihood of undertreatment for pain (Bernabei et al., 1998).

In addition to receiving less analgesia, older adults tend to report pain less often than do younger adults. These findings may be related to beliefs and concerns about pain and the reporting of pain. Many older people hold the following beliefs and concerns about pain (Neeley, 1993):

- Pain is something that must be lived with.
- Expressing pain is unacceptable or is a sign of weakness.
- Complaining of pain will result in being labeled as a "bad" client.
- Nurses are too busy to listen to complaints of pain.
- Pain signifies a serious illness or impending death.

Nurses should be aware of the beliefs of older clients regarding pain management. Nurses and other caregivers often undermedicate these clients and are sometimes reluctant to administer the prescribed analgesics. Unfounded concerns about overmedication, addiction, and decreases in pain perception may contribute to undermedication (Berry & Dahl, 2000).

GENDER

Gender differences in the types of and responses to pain have been described by several researchers (Faucett, 1994; Vallerand, 1995). Physiologic, hormonal, and anatomic influences are unclear, but it is apparent that some painful conditions are more common in either men or women (Ruda,

1993). Women suffer more often from migraine headaches, arthritis, and facial pain, whereas cluster headaches, back pain, and chest pain are more common among men (Faucett, 1994; Vallerand, 1995).

The effects of gender on pain in clinical situations have been identified in some studies but not in others. Such studies must be interpreted with caution, because gender-oriented pain research is based largely on male responses. Women may be more likely to discuss their pain and distress and therefore are mistakenly labeled as less likely to deal effectively with pain. Some investigators have demonstrated that men are better than women in tolerating pain, whereas others have found no gender differences. It is widely believed that men exhibit greater stoicism than do women. Research has shown that nurses expect men to be stoic but accept more emotional responses from women in pain (Zatzick & Dimsdale, 1990).

WOMEN'S HEALTH CONSIDERATIONS

Whatever gender differences do exist in the perception of and response to pain, nurses must acknowledge the effects of gender bias. Studies investigating the attitudes of caregivers toward clients in pain suggest that women are treated less aggressively and that their complaints are viewed with suspicion (Vallerand, 1995). In one study of physicians' pain management practices for clients with cancer, being female was an important predictor of inadequate analgesia (Cleeland et al., 1994).

CULTURAL CONSIDERATIONS

Cultural sensitivity is critical to the understanding of factors that influence pain and expressions of pain. Certain sociocultural groups are still sometimes categorized according to their ability to tolerate pain. This leads to unfair stereotypes and expectations of certain ethnic groups, such as "Italian Americans are very dramatic when they are in pain" or "Mexican Americans have a low pain tolerance."

Many studies have shown a relationship between pain and culture, but the study methods and results have not been consistent (Zatzick & Dimsdale, 1990). Descriptions of the study sample must be carefully evaluated for similar and dissimilar characteristics compared with clients in clinical practice. Findings from ethnic groups studied in other countries may not apply to culturally diverse populations living in the United States and socialized in the American culture. Studies that lack evidence of acceptable psychometric or measurement properties for pain instruments must be interpreted with caution. Cross-cultural comparisons of pain measurement data substantially improve the ability to identify similarities and differences in the perceptions of and responses to pain across cultures.

Few nursing studies have examined the cultural aspects of pain, yet nurses assess pain and make decisions regarding pain management for individuals in various ethnic groups. For example, many Mexican-American clients, especially women, moan or cry when they are uncomfortable. As a result, they may be identified by nurses as complainers who cannot tolerate pain (Calvillo & Flaskerud, 1991). Nurses who value the stoic model or "norm" for pain response interpret behaviors such as moaning and crying as an inability to tolerate pain and as a request for intervention. In the Mexican culture, however, these behaviors might help to relieve pain rather than communicate a need for intervention (Calvillo & Flaskerud, 1991).

Nurses must also consider language when dealing with people from various cultures. If English is not a person's first language within an English-speaking culture, his or her ability to express pain may be limited or expressions of pain may be misinterpreted. The nurse may need to rely on nonverbal communication, which also can be misinterpreted. (See Chapter 6 on cultural aspects of health.)

PERSONALITY TRAITS

According to the gate control theory of pain, pain perception and pain tolerance can be influenced by personality and other psychosocial factors. For example, outgoing or extroverted people may be more likely to express their pain than individuals who are quiet and shy.

Anxiety is another personality factor that can influence pain perception and tolerance. Other associated characteristics are feelings of powerlessness and an inability to cope with anxiety and pain. Nursing interventions to reduce anxiety and increase coping ability may also help to relieve pain. The way in which pain is interpreted or appraised influences the coping strategies or methods selected by clients to deal with their pain.

In addition to personality and other factors that cannot be changed (e.g., age and gender), other factors may influence the experience of pain. Factors that tend to *decrease* the threshold for and tolerance of pain include discomfort, insomnia, fatigue, anxiety, fear, anger, sadness, depression, mental isolation, introversion, and past experience. Factors that tend to *increase* the threshold for and tolerance of pain include symptom relief, sleep, rest, sympathy, understanding, diversion, elevation of mood, analgesics, anxiolytic agents, and antidepressants. Many of these factors can be altered, and therefore nursing interventions often include minimizing factors that lower the pain threshold and tolerance and increasing or maximizing factors that increase the pain threshold and tolerance.

Attitudes and Practices Related to Pain

Negative and mistaken beliefs about pain and its treatment are common in the health care system. Studies have shown that many health care professionals do not have the knowledge and skills to manage pain adequately (Drayer, Henderson, & Reidenberg, 1999; Levin, Berry, & Leiter, 1998).

ATTITUDES AND KNOWLEDGE OF NURSES

Nurses' attitudes toward pain easily influence the way they perceive and interact with clients in pain. Without adequate assessment skills and a knowledge of pain and the principles of analgesic therapy, nurses may not be able to understand their clients' pain and confidently participate with physicians and other professionals in its treatment. Pain assessment skills are influenced by the nurse's cultural background, level of experience, and empathy for the client (Redmond, 1998).

Nurses who have little personal experience with pain may not appreciate the magnitude of painful conditions associated with diseases and medical and surgical interventions. They may expect clients with chronic pain to react similarly to those with acute pain. They may assume that reactions to pain, including complaints about pain, fall within a certain norm on the basis of their own cultural values. The more that a client's response varies from these expected norms, the more likely it is that a nurse's attitude toward the client will be positively or negatively biased.

Knowledge deficits are found even in groups of nurses who administer opioids (narcotics) on a frequent basis. Ferrell and McCaffery (1997) identified a lack of knowledge about equianalgesic dosing, dose escalation, the use of appropriate breakthrough doses, and the pharmacokinetics of transdermal opioids. Only two thirds of the nurses in their sample were able to correctly convert medications to an extended-release form.

ATTITUDES AND KNOWLEDGE OF CLIENTS

Many clients are reluctant to report pain. When they do, they may underestimate its severity (Berry & Dahl, 2000). Clients may not complain of pain because they want to be a "good" client or do not want to bother or distract their caregivers from other issues in their care. In clients with a history of cancer, pain can be an unwanted reminder of the disease and its progression.

Clients may also be reluctant to take pain medications, especially opioid analgesics, because they fear becoming addicted or used to the medication (Berry & Dahl, 2000). The complexity of the medication schedule or an experience with adverse effects (e.g., sedation or constipation) can also affect compliance.

ATTITUDES AND KNOWLEDGE OF PHYSICIANS

Undertreatment of pain, especially cancer pain, is a serious problem in the United States and elsewhere in the world. Between 50% and 80% of clients with cancer do not receive adequate pain control (Breitbart, Rosenfeld, & Passik, 1998).

Despite increased education about pain, there are several reasons why many physicians underprescribe medication for clients in pain, especially opioids such as morphine. First, cultural and societal attitudes exist regarding opioid use, especially in the United States. In some states, clients who use these drugs must register with state regulatory agencies in a manner similar to that required for people enrolled in methadone programs. Requiring such a procedure equates the client with a drug abuser. Some state regulations make it mandatory that triplicate prescriptions be used for schedule II controlled substances. This can deter physicians from prescribing some opioid analgesics.

Second, government regulatory agencies do not set practical guidelines for drug use for severe or chronic pain. A physician or other health care provider may be reprimanded by the governing state board for prescribing what the board considers an inappropriate amount or type of pain medication.

Third, there is still a lack of knowledge about the effects of analgesics. Even with knowledge about correct prescribing practices, physicians may fail to assess clients' complaints of pain. Levin, Berry, and Leiter (1998) found that 40% of primary care physicians caring for clients with cancer failed to prescribe medications for breakthrough pain (pain that occurs between doses of opioid medication). National efforts are underway to improve caregivers' knowledge and attitudes about pain management, such as the Network Project at Memorial Sloan-Kettering Cancer Center in New York.

Types of Pain

There are several ways to classify types of pain. In 1986 the National Institutes of Health Consensus Conference on Pain categorized pain according to its cause. Participants at the conference identified three types of pain: acute, chronic malignant, and chronic nonmalignant. This classification is still commonly used today.

Acute pain results from acute injury, disease, or surgery. **Chronic nonmalignant pain** is associated with tissue injury that has healed or is not progressive, such as the pain experienced by many clients with arthritis. Pain associated with cancer or another progressive disease is called **chronic malignant pain.**

ACUTE PAIN

CHARACTERISTICS OF ACUTE PAIN. Almost everyone experiences acute pain at some time. Certain characteristics distinguish this type of pain from the more chronic (long-term) pain often associated with chronic illness. A major distinction between acute and chronic pain is the effect on biologic responses. Acute pain serves a biologic purpose. It acts as a warning signal because it can activate the sympathetic nervous system, causing various physiologic responses. These responses are similar to those found in "fight-or-flight" reactions and include increased heart rate, blood pressure, and respiratory rate; dilated pupils; and sweating. Behavioral signs of acute pain may include restlessness, an inability to concentrate, apprehension, and overall distress (Table 7-2).

Acute pain is usually temporary, of sudden onset, and easily localized. The client can often describe the pain, which may subside with or without treatment. Acute pain often results from sudden, accidental trauma (e.g., fractures, burns, and lacerations) or from surgery, ischemia, and acute inflammation. Acute pain is often the result of trauma involving superficial or cutaneous structures. The pain is confined to the affected area. As this area heals, the quality or sensation of the pain changes. Although possibly severe, acute pain is limited

TABLE 7-2 • PHYSIOLOGIC AND BEHAVIORAL RESPONSES TO ACUTE AND CHRONIC PAIN

Physiologic Response	Behavioral Response
ACUTE PAIN	
Increased blood pressure initially	Restlessness
Increased pulse rate	Inability to concentrate
Increased respiratory rate	Apprehension
Dilated pupils	Distress
Perspiration	
CHRONIC PAIN	
Normal blood pressure	Immobility or physical inactivity
Normal pulse rate	Withdrawal
Normal respiratory rate	Despair
Normal pupils	
Dry skin	

over time and generally can be managed successfully. Both the caregiver and the client can see an end to the pain, which makes coping somewhat easier.

POSTOPERATIVE PAIN. Pain that accompanies surgery is one of the most common examples of acute pain, but it is poorly understood and not always well managed. Conservative estimates state that of all clients undergoing surgery, 20% experience mild pain, 20% to 40% experience moderate pain, and 40% to 70% experience severe pain. According to some authorities, the alarmingly high number of clients who experience pain after surgery can result from inadequate drug therapy (Acute Pain Management Guideline Panel, 1992). As discussed earlier, others believe that inadequate pain control stems from societal attitudes and beliefs that people in pain should "grin and bear it." Still others identify the fear of addiction as a major factor in practices such as administering less than optimal amounts of analgesics after surgery. Whatever the reason, some people undergoing surgery suffer needlessly.

The severity of postoperative pain may be a predictor of long-term pain. The use of **pre-emptive analgesia** is a fairly new technique designed to decrease pain in the postoperative period, decrease the requirements for a postoperative analgesic, improve morbidity, and decrease hospital stay (Siddall & Cousins, 1997). Pre-emptive analgesia includes administering local anesthetics, opioids, and NSAIDs in the preoperative, intraoperative, or postoperative period. This intervention may inhibit changes in the spinal cord—changes that can lead to a central sensitization that results in chronic pain.

According to several studies, the type and site of a surgery are some of the most important predictors in determining the incidence, severity, and duration of postoperative pain. Similarly, the extent of the operation, the degree of tissue trauma, and the positioning of the client during surgery contribute to the overall incidence and severity of postoperative pain.

In general, intrathoracic and upper intra-abdominal surgical approaches are associated with more severe, steady wound pain and with pain on movement in the postoperative period. Many clients who undergo superficial surgery of the head and neck, chest wall, or limbs report minimal or no postoperative pain. Muscle-splitting procedures are far more painful than muscle-stretching procedures. On the basis of this information, surgeons have changed their techniques over the years to reduce or minimize the components of this type of pain.

CRITICAL THINKING CHALLENGE

A 62-year-old woman has undergone an exploratory laparotomy and colon resection for a ruptured diverticulum. It is now 2 days after surgery, and she is receiving 50 mg of Demerol IM every 4 hours as needed for pain. She is not coughing because of her pain; a chest x-ray examination performed today reveals atelectasis.

- How would you assess the effectiveness of her pain management regimen?
- What changes would you recommend for her pain management regimen?
- How would you evaluate the success of these changes?

For suggested answer guidelines, go to SIMON http://www.wbsaunders.com/SIMON/Iggy/.

CHRONIC PAIN

CHARACTERISTICS OF CHRONIC PAIN. Chronic pain is a major health problem. In the United States alone it is estimated that 25% of people, many of them older than 65 years of age, are affected with a chronic illness and chronic pain. Unlike acute pain, chronic pain serves no biologic purpose. After the initial warning signal of pain, the body must learn to adapt to the persistent pain impulses by blocking or adjusting to activation of the sympathetic nervous system (which causes the fight-or-flight reaction in acute pain). Because of this adaptation, many of the obvious symptoms associated with acute pain are absent or less obvious with chronic pain.

Chronic pain is defined as pain that persists or recurs for indefinite periods, usually for more than 2 months. The onset is gradual, and the character and quality of the pain change over time. Because chronic pain often involves deep body structures, it is usually poorly localized and often difficult to describe. If the underlying cause cannot be treated medically, controlling the long-term effects of chronic pain may be a difficult clinical challenge.

Chronic pain is associated with a variety of health problems, such as cancer, connective tissue diseases, peripheral vascular diseases, and musculoskeletal disorders. It is also seen in post-traumatic problems, such as phantom limb pain and low back pain. The degree of chronic pain varies according to the type of problem and whether it is progressive, stable, or capable of resolution. Unless the disease process is treated or reversed, the severity of chronic pain may worsen to the point that the client is physically and emotionally debilitated. Even when physiologic pain stimuli are eliminated or tissue damage has resolved, the client's perception of pain may linger. This is sometimes called the "chronic pain syndrome." A client's response to chronic pain is influenced by his or her ability to cope, the availability of family support and social resources, and the severity of physiologic and emotional consequences (see Table 7-2).

Because chronic pain persists for extended periods, it can interfere with personal relationships and activities of daily living. It can also result in emotional and financial burdens. Thus the efforts of an interdisciplinary health care team are needed to manage the situation effectively. Inadequately managed pain is an overwhelming, frustrating experience for both the sufferer and the caregiver. Although many characteristics of chronic pain are similar in different clients, the nurse should be aware that each situation is unique and requires a highly specialized plan of care.

CHRONIC NONMALIGNANT PAIN. Chronic nonmalignant pain may be caused by chronic diseases such as rheumatoid arthritis, lupus, sickle cell anemia, diabetic neuropathy, and peripheral vascular disease. It may also be related to painful conditions such as fibromyalgia, low back pain, chronic headaches, osteoporosis, and facial pain. Whenever possible, the source(s) of the chronic nonmalignant pain should be targeted and managed with nonopioid analgesics and nondrug measures. Chronic opioid therapy has gained wide acceptance in selected populations when other therapies fail to provide optimal pain relief.

In the past, physicians were reluctant to consider opioid therapy for clients who did not have cancer. Clients experiencing nonmalignant pain were traditionally managed with nondrug measures and nonopioid analgesics or adjuvant drugs. Today some clients with chronic nonmalignant pain are managed with long-term opioid therapy. In general, this type of therapy is reserved for clients who have a documented physiologic source for the pain (more specifically, those with chronic diseases). Structured regimens using long-acting or extended-release opioids with occasional short-acting analgesics (if necessary) are preferred.

There is enough evidence to suggest that the benefits of alleviating pain and suffering with chronic opioid therapy far outweigh any risks. Several published reports in selected client populations have documented favorable clinical outcomes with the use of opioids, such as improved function, better quality of life, less psychologic distress, and less dependence on the health care system (Vallerand, 1991). Moreover, the risk of addiction remains exceedingly low. Drug-seeking behavior is seldom a significant problem, even when chronic opioids are given to clients who have nonmalignant pain and a known history of substance abuse (Dunbar & Katz, 1996).

CONSIDERATIONS FOR OLDER ADULTS

Only clients who have demonstrated measurable benefits from opioids should be considered for their long-term use for nonmalignant pain. The compassionate use of opioids may be considered for older adults with debilitating pain (e.g., compression fractures of the spine), both at home and in long-term care facilities. The nurse recognizes that the older client may be more prone to the side effects of opioids (i.e., sedation, constipation, mental status changes) and implements measures to reduce the risk of opioid-induced adverse effects.

CHRONIC PAIN SYNDROME. Clients sometimes have chronic pain associated with a physical problem. Eventually the physiologic changes resolve or become less obvious, and the cause of the pain is unclear. However, the perception or sensation of pain persists. These painful conditions are sometimes referred to as idiopathic pain, pain of unknown etiology, or chronic pain syndrome. The degree of pain appears to be out of proportion to the physical findings, yet the pain is real to the person experiencing it.

Clients in this situation often subject themselves to a variety of medical tests and frequent hospitalizations while searching for a cause or explanation for their pain. So-called doctor shopping is common in this group of clients. Some clients invest an incredible amount of time and energy in the health care system in the hope of uncovering a solution for their pain. Clients with chronic pain syndrome focus on what they cannot do rather than what they can do. Clients often demonstrate learned helplessness, powerlessness, dependency, and sick role behaviors. They may experience a loss of confidence, disuse of their bodies, risks of losing income, and difficulty in adapting to social and work situations. When pain persists for long periods, family members are often emotionally drained, frustrated, and in need of help in dealing with the client.

Interdisciplinary pain centers, such as pain clinics or programs, are best equipped to handle the complex psychosocial pain issues associated with chronic pain syndrome. Published data show that comprehensive pain centers have demonstrated modest success in eliminating the need for prescription analgesics, reducing dependence on the health care system, and reintegrating clients into social and occupational networks (Flor, Fydrich, & Turk, 1992). Behavioral and cognitive approaches, which focus on family-centered care, are useful strategies for these clients.

CHRONIC MALIGNANT (CANCER-RELATED) PAIN. Although many clients with advanced malignant disease experience severe pain, most of them can achieve adequate pain control. The complexity and progressive nature of this type of pain often limit the success of pain management efforts, even when the best pain management techniques are used.

Cancer-related pain arises from a variety of mechanisms. For example, chemicals known as prostaglandins are released as a malignant tumor invades bone. These substances sensitize nerve receptors in the bone and increase their sensitivity to painful stimuli. In part, this explains the extreme degree of pain associated with bony metastases. Other causes of cancer-related pain include arterial ischemia, venous engorgement, nerve compression, infection, inflammation, necrosis, and ulcerations. The sources of these problems are usually in deep somatic and visceral structures. These types of painful sensations and the diffuse nature of the pain hamper the client's ability to describe and localize cancer pain.

The psychologic impact of cancer can be devastating, especially if clients must contend with unrelieved pain (see the Evidence-Based Practice for Nursing box below. Investigators have documented marked psychologic distress among clients with higher pain intensities and poor relief of pain (Polomano, 1995; Zimmerman et al., 1996).

Most clients with advanced cancer have more than one location of and physiologic source for pain. Approximately one third of these clients experience a component of neuropathic pain or nerve injury pain (Polomano, 1995). Because the

EVIDENCE-BASED PRACTICE FOR NURSING

Are clients satisfied with their pain management?

McNeill, J.A., et al. (1998). Assessing clinical outcomes: Patient satisfaction with pain management. *Journal of Pain and Symptom Management, 16*(1), 29-40.

The purpose of this study was to determine the characteristics of the pain experience among hospitalized clients. In addition, the revised American Pain Society (APS) Patient Outcome Questionnaire was tested for reliability and validity. Data were collected on current pain intensity, worse pain, general level of pain, and interference with activity and sleep. Most subjects reported they were still in pain but did not wish to receive stronger pain medication. Subjects who requested more medication tended to be younger. Subjects requesting additional pain medication also reported more pain-related interference with activity and sleep. Measures of current pain intensity and general level of pain were inversely correlated with overall satisfaction with pain management. That is, if clients' current pain intensity and general level of pain were high, their satisfaction with pain management was low.

Critique. This study was an attempt to determine the correlation between client satisfaction and pain management in hospitalized clients using a revised version of the APS Patient Satisfaction Questionnaire. The results of this study differ from previous studies, because clients reporting more pain were less satisfied with their pain management.

Implications for Nursing. The data analysis does not explain the reason for the change in satisfaction compared with previous studies. Nurses need to realize that clients are more satisfied with their care if their pain is managed. Further efforts must be made to use the Agency for Health Care Policy and Research (AHCPR) pain guidelines to improve pain management in hospitalized clients.

pharmacologic approaches may vary depending on the source of pain, it is important that the nurse identify the cause(s) of the pain in each location. (See Chapter 25 for additional information on this type of pain, and consult Jacox et al. [1994], Management of Cancer Pain Clinical Practice Guidelines.)

CRITICAL THINKING CHALLENGE

A middle-aged man with advanced lung cancer was admitted to the emergency department with uncontrolled back pain. His disease has not responded to two chemotherapeutic regimens, and he was diagnosed last month with bony metastasis after complaining of left hip pain. He has been receiving 30 mg of MS Contin twice a day, with two tablets of Percocet every 4 hours as needed. The client reports only fair control of his pain. An x-ray examination of the lumbar spine performed today demonstrates new metastatic lesions of the spine.

- What changes do you think he needs in his opioid regimen?
- What factors lead practitioners to inadequately prescribe medications for pain?
- What factors lead clients and families to inadequately medicate pain?

For suggested answer guidelines, go to  http://www.wbsaunders.com/SIMON/Iggy/.

➤ COLLABORATIVE MANAGEMENT

Activity Link

Assessment

HISTORY

The nurse asks the client about the pain experience, including the sequence of events (precipitating and relieving factors); the nature of adjustments, if any, in life or in the family; and beliefs about the cause of the pain and what should be done about it (client's expectations). Personal characteristics (e.g., age and culture) influence attitudes about reporting a pain history. Families and significant others are included in this information-gathering process.

Clients may report pain in the absence of any observable or documented physiologic changes. The nurse keeps in mind that all pain is real and operates from the premise that pain is "whatever the person experiencing it says it is." The nurse respects the client's verbal and nonverbal expressions of pain without making judgments or inferences about the reality of the pain. If clients perceive that health care professionals doubt the existence of their pain, mistrust and other negative feelings can arise and interfere with a therapeutic nurse-client relationship.

The nurse also assesses the length of time the client has experienced pain. Clients may welcome an opportunity to discuss acute pain with the nurse because it is a relatively short-term experience and is easily described. However, clients with chronic pain can become frustrated when they are unable to adequately describe their vague, diffuse pain experience. Structured interviews using assessment aids (e.g., pain scales and descriptors) often help clients to express their pain.

CONSIDERATIONS FOR OLDER ADULTS

When obtaining a history from an older client, the nurse should consider that the client may be anxious or temporarily disoriented because of pain or being in an unusual environment. The nurse observes for nonverbal indicators of pain, such as grimacing, and checks for changes in behavior. If a client becomes restless, hostile, or combative, the nurse considers pain as a possible underlying reason. Too often a client behaving in this manner is labeled with a diagnosis of dementia or other cognitive impairment or is categorized by the nursing staff as "difficult." Chart 7-1 highlights key points for assessing an older adult in pain.

ESSENTIAL DATA FOR A COMPLETE PAIN HISTORY. Information about a client's pain can be helpful in understanding the factors associated with the present pain or previous episodes of pain. If the client is in pain when the nurse is obtaining the history, the session should be kept reasonably short or continued at a later time. Essential data include the following:

- *Precipitating factors.* Does the client associate any activities, food, or other environmental factors with the onset of pain? What does the client think causes the present pain? Was the onset of pain sudden or slow? Has the client done anything or taken anything to relieve the pain? What were the results of the intervention?

CHART 7-1

NURSING FOCUS *on the* OLDER ADULT
The Client Experiencing Pain

When taking a client history:

- Realize that the prevalence of pain is estimated to be double that of clients younger than 60 years and well over 70% among older adults in long-term care facilities.
- Consider the older adult at risk for the undertreatment of pain, especially cancer pain, because of inappropriate beliefs about pain sensitivity, tolerance, and ability to use opioids.
- Recognize that cognitive impairment in the older adult may pose barriers to pain assessment, but the client with mild to moderate cognitive impairment may be able to accurately report pain at the moment or when prompted.
- Cognitively impaired older adults may require more frequent assessments of pain than clients who are not impaired.
- Use visual representations of pain measures rather than mental images of pain rating scales. Be sure that the client is wearing glasses and hearing aid(s), if needed and available.
- Alter a written pain scale to include large lettering, adequate space between lines, nonglossy paper, and color for increased visualization.
- Provide adequate lighting and privacy to avoid distracting background noise.

If the client cannot verbally communicate:

- Assess for nonverbal indicators of pain, such as grimacing or crying.
- Observe for changes in the client's behavior, such as increased confusion or combativeness.
- Respond to complaints of pain promptly—they are typically not age-related complaints.
- Administer the prescribed amount of analgesics for postoperative pain in a timely manner. If pain is not relieved, evaluate the effectiveness of the analgesic regimen, and immediately notify the physician.
- Use nondrug pain relief measures.

Data from the Acute Pain Management Guideline Panel (1992). *Acute pain management: Operative or medical procedures and trauma. Clinical practice guidelines.* AHCPR Pub. No. 92-0032. Rockville, MD: Agency for Health Care Policy and Research, Public Health Service, U.S. Department of Health and Human Services.

- *Aggravating factors.* What factors make the pain worse? What influence has this pain had on the client's activity? What changes in life activity have been affected (e.g., diet, job, sleep)?
- *Localization of pain.* Can the client localize the pain or describe where it travels or radiates?
- *Character and quality of pain.* What words does the client use to describe the pain and its character, quality, or intensity?
- *Duration of pain.* How long has the client experienced this pain?

PHYSICAL ASSESSMENT/CLINICAL MANIFESTATIONS

The observable clinical manifestations of pain include physiologic responses, motor or body movements, and affective behaviors such as crying. Although physiologic changes occur in response to acute noxious stimuli, these changes are usually *not* reliable indicators of chronic pain. Acute pain, with its property of warning an individual about harm, causes several physiologic signs and symptoms, which are largely a function of sympathetic nervous system stimulation. Clients with acute pain often manifest major changes in vital body functions, such as tachycardia and blood pressure changes. Blood pressure is usually increased initially and then decreased. Clients with acute pain may also become diaphoretic, restless, and apprehensive.

Physiologic changes in response to chronic pain are usually masked as the body attempts to compensate for and adapt to noxious stimuli. The pain no longer serves as a necessary warning. Changes in vital signs related to chronic pain may be evident only when pre-existing pain occurs or as new sites of painful stimuli arise.

Certain motor or body movements may be associated with either acute or chronic pain. Some may be more exaggerated or obvious than others. Clients in pain may support or shield ("splint"), holding painful body parts while moving, or they may lie listlessly because they are afraid to move. The nurse assesses the functional status and degree of impairment in the client with pain.

LOCATION OF PAIN. The nurse assesses the pain from two dimensions: the level of pain (deep or superficial) and the position or location of pain. Most clients can usually describe the depth of acute pain or chronic pain. The actual area or location of the pain, however, may not be as easily identified. The nurse asks the client whether the pain is superficial or deep. In general, clients with pain involving superficial or cutaneous structures describe their pain as superficial and can often localize the pain to a specific area.

Pain may be described as belonging to one of four categories related to its location:

- **Localized pain** is pain confined to the site of origin.
- **Projected pain** is pain along a specific nerve or nerves.
- **Radiating pain** is diffuse pain around the site of origin that is not well localized.
- **Referred pain** is pain perceived in an area distant from the site of painful stimuli.

A client who has difficulty specifying the exact location of pain can be asked to point to the painful areas on his or her own body or on another person. It is sometimes helpful to have the client point to or shade in the painful areas on a diagram of the front and back of the human body (Figure 7-2). Clients who cannot identify the painful areas and state that they just "hurt all over" are encouraged to focus on parts of the body that are not painful. The nurse asks the client to con-

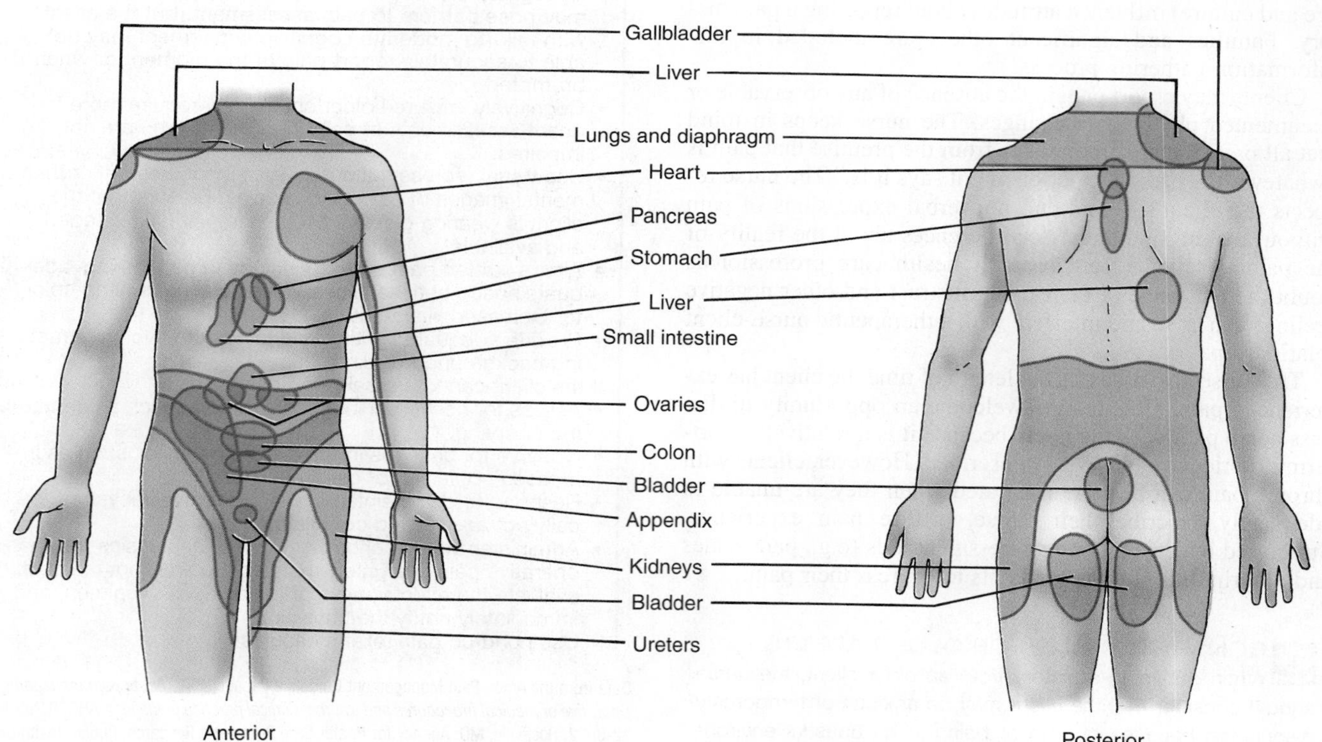

Figure 7-2 ● Anterior and posterior referred pain sites.

centrate on different body parts, beginning with the hand and fingers of one extremity, and identify the presence or absence of pain. As the nurse focuses attention on selected areas of the body, the client is assisted in localizing painful areas. Clients who state that they hurt everywhere often begin to realize that some parts of the body are not painful.

Clients may present with more than one discrete painful site. In fact, approximately one half of clients with advanced cancer report having pain in more than one location. As painful areas are identified, the nurse helps the client to understand the origin of the pain. This understanding is particularly important for clients with cancer, because every new pain often raises the suspicion of metastasis (spread of disease). The pain may be caused by other reasons, such as immobility or constipation.

CHARACTER AND QUALITY OF PAIN. After asking the client to locate the pain, the nurse asks him or her to describe it. Clients may use one word or a group of words to convey the sensations or feelings of the pain. The nurse avoids suggesting descriptive words for the pain. Some clients who are frustrated and are having difficulty describing their pain may benefit from using the McGill-Melzack Pain Questionnaire (Figure 7-3). Using this tool, the client circles descriptive terms in the appropriate categories to best describe the pain. This questionnaire may be too difficult for clients with poor reading or verbal skills.

Another useful strategy is to ask the client to describe the sensation by comparing it to a situation or event that may be comparable to the feeling of pain. For example, a man with excruciating diffuse abdominal pain from advanced cancer once said that his pain felt as if a soldier were walking around inside his abdomen, with no set path or destination, stepping on mines. For this man, the pain was unpredictable and never ending and produced "blowing-up" sensations.

PATTERN OF PAIN. Pain is rarely the same at all times. It is perceived differently over time and varies with factors such as physical activity and stress (see the earlier discussion under History, p. 69).

INTENSITY OF PAIN. Subjective measurements of pain intensity by the client are more reliable and accurate than observable qualities of pain. Only the client can determine the amount or severity of pain being experienced. Various visual analog scales (VAS), numeric rating scales (NRS), descriptive word scales, and other measures have been designed to help clients communicate the magnitude or severity of pain and to help nurses quantify the pain.

The nurse uses pain intensity scales to measure pain in the clinical or home setting and to assess and determine the effectiveness of pain relief interventions. The client is presented with an appropriate pain scale and asked to rate the amount of painful stimuli. Clients with more than one discrete painful site may wish to specify their pain levels by location. Some scales also assess the emotional aspects of pain.

Verbal descriptive scales typically group words such as "none," "moderate," or "severe" and permit an intensity rating of pain. However, the 0 to 10 NRS is most commonly used in clinical practice for adult clients who can communicate in English (Figure 7-4). For culturally diverse clients with language barriers, the Wong-Baker FACES pain rating scale (smile to frown) may be helpful. This scale is also used for children and developmentally disabled populations. For cognitively impaired clients, the nurse observes nonverbal behaviors such as restlessness, grimacing, and moaning.

ISSUES IN PAIN MANAGEMENT. It is critical that reliable and valid measures be used to evaluate dimensions of pain. Nurses should avoid using self-report scales that have not been adequately tested in clinical practice settings. Pain measures should be appropriate for the client's cognitive level and issues with pain.

> **CONSIDERATIONS FOR OLDER ADULTS**
> When using tools to measure pain in older clients, the nurse considers possible visual or hearing limitations. The client should wear glasses and hearing aids, if appropriate. Increased lighting with nonglare bulbs may improve visual perception. The tools may be altered to include large lettering, adequate spacing between lines, and color on a white background (Herr & Mobily, 1991).

PSYCHOSOCIAL ASSESSMENT

ACUTE PAIN. All pain holds significant meaning for the person experiencing it. Clients having acute pain from surgery may interpret their pain as necessary and expected. It may be viewed with relief as a sign that some greater problem has been resolved or alleviated by the surgery. Knowing that the duration of the pain is limited may allow the client to deal with unpleasant sensations without too much difficulty. In contrast, acute chest pain associated with angina may mark the beginning of a life of fear and uncertainty.

CHRONIC PAIN. Various psychosocial factors influence chronic pain. Some factors are similar to those found in the acute pain experience, such as anxiety or fear related to the meaning of the pain. Because chronic pain persists or is perhaps only partially relieved, the client may feel powerless, angry, hostile, or desperate. The client is also vulnerable to labels such as "chronic complainer" or "fake." Because many of the behavioral manifestations of acute pain (e.g., sweating, writhing, increased blood pressure) are absent in the client with chronic pain, the caregiver might doubt the existence of the pain. In some chronic pain conditions (e.g., myofacial pain disorders), there may be an absence of objective physical findings to corroborate the report of pain. This may produce problems of depression, socializing difficulties, and conflicts with others. Clients may need outside assistance to resolve their illness-specific controversies.

The status of family and other close relationships, along with the breadth of social resources available to the chronic pain client, must be assessed. The existence of a pain-specific conflict with a spouse or significant other may affect or limit pain coping strategies. Other people may react to chronic pain with depression, social withdrawal, and preoccupation with physical symptoms.

If the chronic pain is associated with a progressive disease such as cancer, rheumatoid arthritis, or peripheral vascular disease, the client may have worries and concerns about the consequences of the illness. Clients with cancer-related pain may fear death or body mutilation. Some may think they are being punished for some wrongdoing in life. Others may attach a religious or spiritual significance to lingering pain.

The nurse asks open-ended questions (e.g., "Tell me how your pain has affected your job or role as a mother") to allow

McGill-Melzack PAIN QUESTIONNAIRE

Patient's name ________ Age ________

File No. ________ Date ________

Clinical category (e.g., cardiac, neurologic)

Diagnosis: ________

____

____

Analgesic (if already administered):

1. Type ________
2. Dosage ________
3. Time given in relation to this test ________

Patient's intelligence: circle number that represents best estimate.

1 (low) 2 3 4 5 (high)

****

This questionnaire has been designed to tell us more about your pain. Four major questions we ask are

1. Where is your pain?
2. What does it feel like?
3. How does it change with time?
4. How strong is it?

It is important that you tell us how your pain feels now. Please follow the instructions at the beginning of each part.

Part 1. Where Is Your Pain?

Please mark, on the drawings below, the areas where you feel pain. Put E if external, or I if internal, near the areas you mark. Put EI if both external and internal.

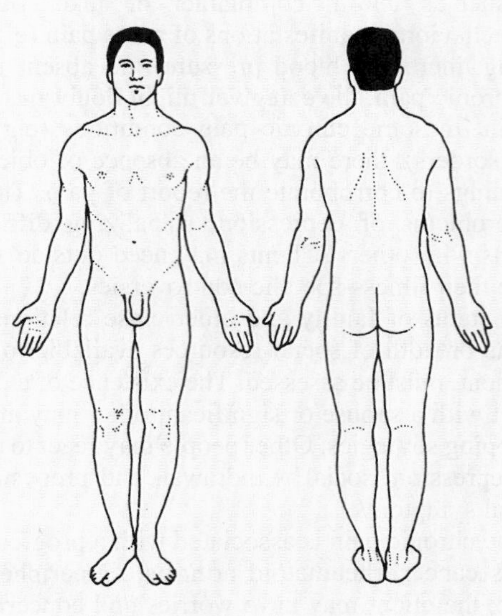

Part 2. What Does Your Pain Feel Like?

Some of the words below describe your *present* pain. Circle *ONLY* those words that best describe it. Leave out any category that is not suitable. Use only a single word in each appropriate category—the one that applies best.

1
Flickering
Quivering
Pulsing
Throbbing
Beating
Pounding

2
Jumping
Flashing
Shooting

3
Pricking
Boring
Drilling
Stabbing
Lancinating

4
Sharp
Cutting
Lacerating

5
Pinching
Pressing
Gnawing
Cramping
Crushing

6
Tugging
Pulling
Wrenching

7
Hot
Burning
Scalding
Searing

8
Tingling
Itchy
Smarting
Stinging

9
Dull
Sore
Hurting
Aching
Heavy

10
Tender
Taut
Rasping
Splitting

11
Tiring
Exhausting

12
Sickening
Suffocating

13
Fearful
Frightful
Terrifying

14
Punishing
Grueling
Cruel
Vicious
Killing

15
Wretched
Blinding

16
Annoying
Troublesome
Miserable
Intense
Unbearable

17
Spreading
Radiating
Penetrating
Piercing

18
Tight
Numb
Drawing
Squeezing
Tearing

19
Cool
Cold
Freezing

20
Nagging
Nauseating
Agonizing
Dreadful
Torturing

Part 3. How Does Your Pain Change With Time?

1. Which word or words would you use to describe the *pattern* of your pain?

1	2	3
Continuous	Rhythmic	Brief
Steady	Periodic	Momentary
Constant	Intermittent	Transient

2. What kind of things *relieve* your pain?

3. What kind of things *increase* your pain?

Part 4. How Strong Is Your Pain?

People agree that the following 5 words represent pain of increasing intensity. They are:

1	2	3	4	5
Mild	Discomforting	Distressing	Horrible	Excruciating

To answer each question below, write the number of the most appropriate word in the space beside the question.

1. Which word describes your pain right now? ___
2. Which word describes it at its worst? ___
3. Which word describes it when it is least? ___
4. Which word describes the worst toothache you ever had? ___
5. Which word describes the worst headache you ever had? ___
6. Which word describes the worst stomachache you ever had? ___

Figure 7-3 ● The McGill-Melzack Pain Questionnaire. (From Melzack, R. [1975]. The McGill Pain Questionnaire: Major properties and scoring methods. *Pain, 1,* 272-281.)

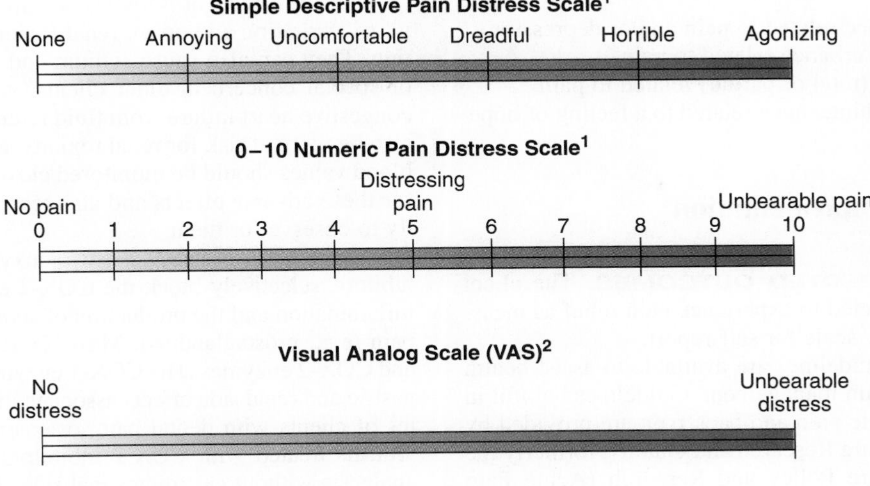

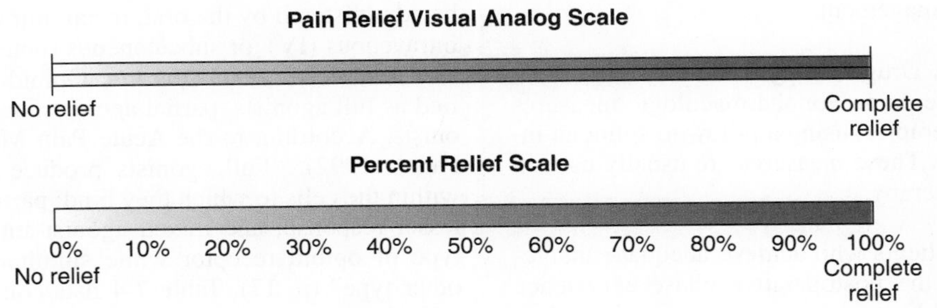

[1]If used as a graphic rating scale, a 10-cm baseline is recommended.

[2]A 10-cm baseline is recommended for VAS scales.

Figure 7-4 ● Pain rating scales and pain relief scales. (Simple Descriptive Pain Distress Scale, 0-10 Numeric Pain Distress Scale, and Visual Analog Scale redrawn from Acute Pain Management Guideline Panel. [1992]. *Acute pain management: Operative or medical procedures and trauma. Clinical practice guideline.* AHCPR Pub. No. 92-0032. Rockville, MD: Agency for Health Care Policy and Research, Public Health Service, U.S. Department of Health and Human Services; Pain Relief Visual Analog Scale redrawn from Fishman, B., et al. [1987]. The Memorial Pain Assessment Card: A valid instrument for the evaluation of cancer pain. *Cancer, 60*[5], 1151-1158; Percent Relief Scale redrawn from the Brief Pain Inventory. Pain Research Group, Department of Neurology, University of Wisconsin—Madison.)

the client to describe personal attitudes about pain and its influence on life. This opportunity can help a client whose life has been changed by pain. However, some clients choose not to share their private information or fears, and this decision should be respected by the nurse.

Analysis

COMMON NURSING DIAGNOSES AND COLLABORATIVE PROBLEMS

The actual diagnoses for a client with pain are divided into two main categories:

1. Acute Pain
2. Chronic Pain

Etiologic factors are not included here because they vary and depend on the cause of the pain and each client's response.

ADDITIONAL NURSING DIAGNOSES AND COLLABORATIVE PROBLEMS

In addition to the common nursing diagnoses, clients experiencing pain may have one or more of the following:

- Anxiety related to loss of control
- Fear related to pain
- Powerlessness related to the illness-related regimen
- Ineffective Role Performance related to a change in health status and impaired coping

- Altered Sexuality Patterns related to illness and pain
- Impaired Physical Mobility related to pain and discomfort
- Activity Intolerance related to pain and/or depression
- Sleep Pattern Disturbance related to pain
- Self-Care Deficit (total or partial) related to pain
- Altered Health Maintenance related to a feeling of hopelessness

Planning and Implementation

ACUTE PAIN

NOC **PLANNING: EXPECTED OUTCOMES.** The client with acute pain is expected to experience pain relief as measured by a pain intensity scale for self-report.

Several important guidelines are available to assist health care professionals in pain management. Guidelines helpful in the management of acute pain and back pain are provided by the Agency for Healthcare Research and Quality, formerly the Agency for Health Care Policy and Research (Acute Pain Management Guideline Panel, 1992; Bigos et al., 1994) and the American Pain Society (1999). These guidelines provide sound pain management principles arising from expert consensus and a careful review of the pain literature. In addition, clinical pathways or algorithms may be used in acute care settings to assist in pain management.

INTERVENTIONS. Drug therapy is the major intervention used to relieve acute pain. Nonpharmacologic measures (e.g., complementary therapies, using a pillow to splint an incision) are also effective. These measures are usually used in conjunction with drug therapy.

DRUG THERAPY. Clients who achieve adequate analgesia (pain relief) during the postoperative phase experience fewer complications and have shorter recovery periods than clients who have a significant degree of pain (Acute Pain Management Guideline Panel, 1992). Nurses must ensure that clients receive adequate interventions to manage their pain.

NONOPIOID ANALGESICS. Many people underestimate the effectiveness of nonopioid analgesics, also referred to as **peripheral-acting analgesics.** For mild pain, the nonopioids acetylsalicylic acid (ASA; aspirin, Ancasal♣) 650 mg and acetaminophen (Datril, Tylenol, Ace-Tabs♣) 650 mg produce pain relief comparable to that of the opioids codeine 32 mg PO and meperidine (Demerol) 50 mg PO. Aspirin has direct analgesic effects because it inhibits prostaglandin synthesis in the presence of inflammation.

Over-the-counter (OTC) medications are not given alone for the treatment of severe pain but are usually administered in conjunction with opioid analgesics. Aspirin or aspirin-containing compounds must be used with caution after surgery because they can irritate the gastrointestinal tract and interfere with blood clotting. The nurse monitors the client carefully for bleeding and bruising.

Nonsteroidal anti-inflammatory drugs (NSAIDs) are also popular nonopioids that possess anti-inflammatory properties, largely by inhibiting prostaglandins. These drugs are particularly useful in the management of acute inflammation caused by tissue destruction. Ketorolac (Toradol) is one of the most popular NSAIDs prescribed for short-term use in cases of acute pain. Unlike other NSAIDs, this drug is available in both oral and parenteral form. Table 7-3 outlines the NSAIDs most commonly prescribed for acute pain.

The side effects of NSAIDs are similar to those of aspirin: gastric irritation and upset, renal toxicity, and decreased clotting. They can also cause sodium and water retention; this is of special concern in older clients, who can easily develop congestive heart failure from fluid retention. Older adults may also be more at risk for renal toxicity, and their renal function blood values should be monitored closely. The nurse observes for these adverse effects and also teaches the client and family to observe for them.

A new class of NSAIDs, cyclooxygenase-2 (COX-2) inhibitors, selectively block the COX-2 enzyme responsible for inflammation and the production of substances associated with pain (e.g., prostaglandins). Most NSAIDs block both COX-1 and COX-2 enzymes. The COX-1 enzyme is responsible for the gastric and renal side effects associated with NSAID use. Studies of clients with dental pain, osteoarthritis, and rheumatoid arthritis treated with COX-2 inhibitors demonstrate effective analgesia without gastrointestinal side effects (Lane, 1997).

OPIOID ANALGESICS. **Opioid analgesics** (also called **opioids** or **narcotics**) are **central-acting analgesics.** These drugs work by binding with opioid receptors both within and outside of the central nervous system. For acute pain they may be administered by the oral, rectal, intramuscular, intraspinal, intravenous (IV), or subcutaneous route.

Classification of Opioids. Opioid analgesics are classified as full agonists, partial agonists, or mixed agonist-antagonists. According to the Acute Pain Management Guideline Panel (1992), "Full agonists produce a maximal response within the cells to which they bind; partial agonists produce a lesser response; and mixed agonist-antagonists activate one type of opioid receptor while simultaneously blocking another type" (p. 17). Table 7-4 lists common opioid agonists with dosing guidelines and additional information.

Meperidine (Demerol) used to be routinely prescribed by physicians after surgery because it was mistakenly thought to possess certain advantages over morphine and other opioids. An insufficient amount was often prescribed, resulting in less than optimal pain control. Meperidine is effective only for 2.5 to 3.5 hours, and a dose of 75 mg is equivalent to only 5 to 7.5 mg of morphine. Some health care providers continue this outdated practice of prescribing meperidine, especially for older adults.

CONSIDERATIONS FOR OLDER ADULTS

Older adults and those with renal disease should not take meperidine because of the prolonged half-life of its drug metabolite, normeperidine (Acute Pain Management Guideline Panel, 1992). Normeperidine, an excitotoxin, accumulates with repeated dosing and can lead to life-threatening seizures. Because of the physical changes associated with aging, older adults may excrete this metabolite more slowly. This puts them at greatest risk for cerebral irritation, which leads to seizures, memory loss, hallucinations, paranoia, and depression. Some health care agencies have established guidelines to restrict the use of meperidine, monitor the duration of therapy, and offer alternative choices for the use of other opioids.

The most important type of opioid receptor is the mu receptor. Mu opioids may cause urinary retention, constipation,

TABLE 7-3 • NONSTEROIDAL ANTI-INFLAMMATORY DRUGS FOR THE TREATMENT OF ACUTE PAIN

Drug	Usual Adult Dose	Comments
COX-2 INHIBITORS		
Celecoxib (Celebrex)	100-200 mg bid	Associated with fewer gastroduodenal ulcers than other NSAIDs
Rofecoxib (Vioxx)	25-50 mg q24h	Associated with fewer gastroduodenal ulcers than other NSAIDs
OTHER ORAL NSAIDs		
Acetaminophen	650-975 mg q4h	Lacks the peripheral anti-inflammatory activity of other NSAIDs
Aspirin	650-975 mg q4h	The standard against which other NSAIDs are compared; inhibits platelet aggregation; may cause postoperative bleeding
Choline magnesium trisalicylate (Trilisate)	1000-1500 mg bid	May have minimal antiplatelet activity; also available as oral liquid
Diflunisal (Dolobid)	1000 mg initial dose followed by 500 mg q12h	
Etodolac (Lodine)	200-400 mg q6-8h	
Fenoprofen calcium (Nalfon)	200 mg q4-6h	
Ibuprofen (Motrin, others)	400 mg q4-6h	Available as several brand names and as generic; also available as oral suspension
Ketoprofen (Orudis)	25-75 mg q6-8h	
Magnesium salicylate	650 mg q4h	Many brands and generic forms available
Meclofenamate sodium (Meclomen)	50 mg q4-6h	
Mefenamic acid (Ponstel)	250 mg q6h	
Naproxen (Naprosyn)	500 mg initial dose followed by 250 mg q6-8h	Also available as oral liquid
Naproxen sodium (Anaprox)	550 mg initial dose followed by 275 mg q6-8h	
Salsalate (Disalcid, others)	500 mg q4h	May have minimal antiplatelet activity
Sodium salicylate	325-650 mg q3-4h	Available in generic form from several distributors
PARENTERAL OR ORAL NSAID		
Ketorolac	30 or 60 mg IM initial dose followed by 15 or 30 mg q6h Oral dose following IM dosage: 10 mg q6-8h	Intramuscular dose not to exceed 5 days

From Acute Pain Management Guideline Panel. (1992). *Acute pain management: Operative or medical procedures and trauma. Clinical practice guideline.* AHCPR Pub. No. 92-0032. Rockville, MD: Agency for Health Care Policy and Research, Public Health Service, U.S. Department of Health and Human Services.

sedation, respiratory depression, and nausea and vomiting. Urinary retention and respiratory depression are less common among opioid-dependent clients or those who take opioids for extended periods. In general, the opioid-induced side effects correlate with the blood level of the medication. The nurse observes for these problems and reports them to the health care provider.

The pain, stress, and anxiety experienced by the client are potent respiratory *stimulants* that may override or negate the respiratory depression resulting from the drugs. The nurse also considers that the effect of all opioid analgesics may be greater in a client who is older, has reduced blood volume or renal disease, or has received anesthetic agents or other central nervous system depressants.

When respirations fall below 10, the nurse should rouse the client. If respirations do not increase, the health care provider typically orders naloxone (Narcan), an **opioid antagonist,** to reverse the respiratory depression. Naloxone can potentially reverse the effects of the opioid analgesic. Doses of more than 0.2 mg generally reverse analgesia and precipitate acute physiologic withdrawal in opioid-dependent clients. Smaller doses (<0.2 mg) can be given and titrated (adjusted) slowly to reduce the respiratory depressant effects of the opioid agonists. Naloxone is always given with caution to clients who are physically dependent on opioids and only in life-threatening situations. In the hospital or nursing home setting, this drug is kept in an emergency drug box or cabinet on each unit for use as necessary.

Opioid Analgesic Regimens. Immediately after surgery or traumatic injury, the health care provider typically prescribes oral or parenteral opioid analgesics on a continuous time schedule or an intermittent, as needed (prn) schedule. Around-the-clock dosing schedules should be used during the first 24 to 36 hours following surgery (Acute Pain Management Guideline Panel, 1992). Oral drugs are the most convenient and least expensive but should be prescribed in doses **equianalgesic** (equal in analgesic ability) to parenteral ones.

TABLE 7-4 • DOSING GUIDELINES FOR OPIOIDS IN THE TREATMENT OF ACUTE PAIN[a,b]

Drug	Approximate Equianalgesic Oral Dose	Approximate Equianalgesic Parenteral Dose	Recommended Starting Dose (Adults More Than 50 kg Body Weight)		Recommended Starting Dose (Children and Adults Less Than 50 kg Body Weight)[c]	
			ORAL	PARENTERAL	ORAL	PARENTERAL
OPIOID AGONIST						
Morphine[d]	30 mg q3-4h (around-the-clock dosing) 60 mg q3-4h (single dose or intermittent dosing)	10 mg q3-4h	30 mg q3-4h	10 mg q3-4h	0.3 mg/kg q3-4h	0.1 mg/kg q3-4h
Codeine[e]	130 mg q3-4h	75 mg q3-4h	60 mg q3-4h	60 mg q2h (IM/SC)	1 mg/kg q3-4h[f]	Not recommended
Hydromorphone[d] (Dilaudid)	7.5 mg q3-4h	1.5 mg q3-4h	6 mg q3-4h	1.5 mg q3-4h	0.06 mg/kg q3-4h	0.015 mg/kg q3-4h
Hydrocodone (in Lorcet, Lortab, Vicodin, others)	30 mg q3-4h	Not available	10 mg q3-4h	Not available	0.2 mg/kg q3-4h[f]	Not available
Levorphanol (Levo-Dromoran)	4 mg q6-8h	2 mg q6-8h	4 mg q6-8h	2 mg q6-8h	0.04 mg/kg q6-8h	0.02 mg/kg q6-8h
Meperidine (Demerol)	300 mg q2-3h	100 mg q3h	Not recommended	100 mg q3h	Not recommended	0.75 mg/kg q2-3h
Methadone (Dolophine, others)	20 mg q6-8h	10 mg q6-8h	20 mg q6-8h	10 mg q6-8h	0.2 mg/kg q6-8h	0.1 mg/kg q6-8h
Oxycodone (Roxicodone, also in Percocet, Percodan, Tylox, others)	30 mg q3-4h	Not available	10 mg q3-4h	Not available	0.2 mg/kg q3-4h[f]	Not available
Oxymorphone[d] (Numorphan)	Not available	1 mg q3-4h	Not available	1 mg q3-4h	Not recommended[f]	Not recommended
OPIOID AGONIST-ANTAGONIST AND PARTIAL AGONIST						
Buprenorphine (Buprenex)	Not available	0.3-0.4 mg q6-8h	Not available	0.4 mg q6-8h	Not available	0.004 mg/kg q6-8h
Butorphanol (Stadol)	Not available	2 mg q3-4h	Not available	2 mg q3-4h	Not available	Not recommended
Nalbuphine (Nubain)	Not available	10 mg q3-4h	Not available	10 mg q3-4h	Not available	0.1 mg/kg q3-4h
Pentazocine (Talwin, others)	150 mg q3-4h	60 mg q3-4h	50 mg q4-6h	Not recommended	Not recommended	Not recommended

From Acute Pain Management Guideline Panel. (1992). *Acute pain management: Operative or medical procedures and trauma. Clinical practice guideline.* AHCPR Pub. No. 92-0032. Rockville, MD: Agency for Health Care Policy and Research, Public Health Service, U.S. Department of Health and Human Services.

[a]NOTE: Published tables vary in the suggested doses that are equianalgesic to morphine. Clinical response is the criterion that must be applied for each client; titration to clinical response is necessary. Because there is not complete cross tolerance among these drugs, it is usually necessary to use a lower than equianalgesic dose when changing drugs and to retitrate to response.

[b]CAUTION: Recommended doses do not apply to clients with renal or hepatic insufficiency or other conditions affecting drug metabolism and kinetics.

[c]CAUTION: Doses listed for clients with body weight less than 50 kg cannot be used as initial starting doses in infants under 6 months of age. Consult the *Clinical Practice Guideline for Acute Pain Management: Operative or Medical Procedures and Trauma* section on management of pain in neonates for recommendations.

[d]For morphine, hydromorphone, and oxymorphone, rectal administration is an alternate route for clients unable to take oral medications, but equianalgesic doses may differ from oral and parenteral doses because of pharmacokinetic differences.

[e]CAUTION: Codeine doses above 65 mg often are not appropriate because of diminishing incremental analgesia with increasing doses but continually increasing constipation and other side effects.

[f]CAUTION: Doses of aspirin and acetaminophen in combination opioid/NSAID preparations must also be adjusted to the client's body weight.

When the health care provider orders an intermittent schedule, the client depends on the nurse to give the medication when requested. Not all clients will ask for medication. It is imperative for the nurse to offer the medication at the prescribed intervals and to anticipate the need for medication on the basis of behavioral and nonverbal cues.

Use of Opioids for Substance Abusers. Acute pain management for clients who are known or suspected substance abusers is a difficult but increasingly common problem. Some hospitals have pain management teams to assist with this type of problem. Team members usually represent several disciplines that include, but are not limited to, nurses, physicians, clinical pharmacists, and social workers.

Clients who are substance abusers often have traumatic injuries and other health problems that cause acute pain. Chart 7-2 lists some recommendations for the nurse when planning

CHART 7-2

BEST PRACTICE *for*
Pain Management for the Substance Abuser

- Define the exact source(s) of pain and treat them (e.g., heat for muscle spasms, antibiotics for infection).
- Follow the principles of opioid use, such as not giving agonist-antagonists to clients receiving opioid agonists.
- Use nonopioid therapies, including medication, cutaneous stimulation techniques, and cognitive and behavioral strategies.
- Monitor the client for substance abuse while in the health care agency to ensure that drugs are not being stolen or hoarded.
- Set limits and negotiate with the client about drug choices and dosing.
- Provide clear instructions about drug use and dosing schedules.
- Consult with other members of the health care team, such as physicians, psychiatrists, psychologists, pharmacists, and social workers.

Data from the Acute Pain Management Guideline Panel. (1992). *Acute pain management: Operative or medical procedures and trauma. Clinical practice guideline.* AHCPR Pub. No. 92-0032. Rockville, MD: Agency for Health Care Policy and Research, Public Health Service, U.S. Department of Health and Human Services.

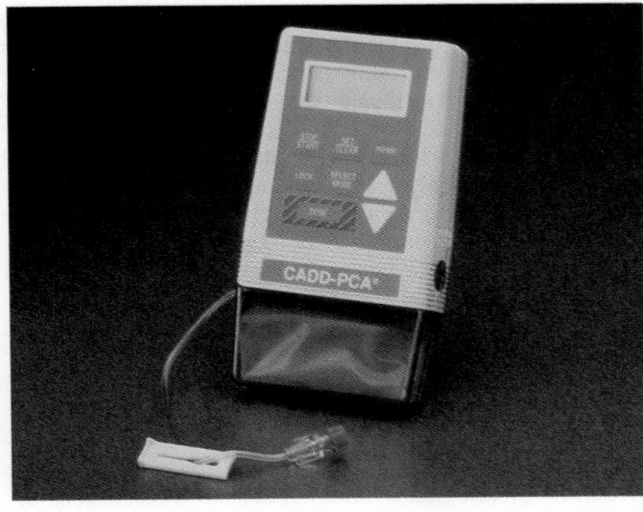

Figure 7-5 ● An ambulatory patient-controlled analgesia infusion pump. (CADD-PCA is a registered trademark of Pharmacia Deltec.)

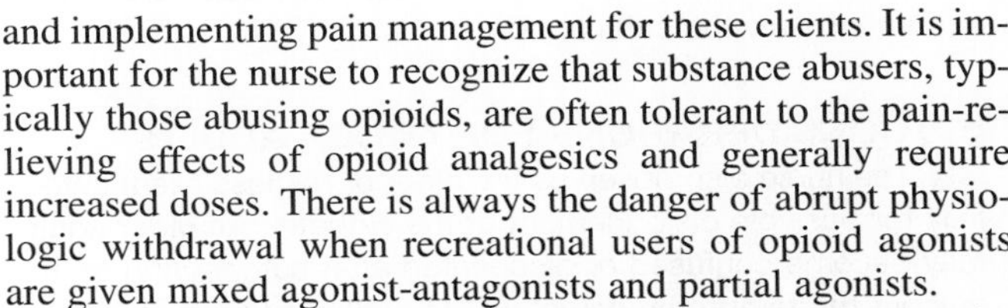

and implementing pain management for these clients. It is important for the nurse to recognize that substance abusers, typically those abusing opioids, are often tolerant to the pain-relieving effects of opioid analgesics and generally require increased doses. There is always the danger of abrupt physiologic withdrawal when recreational users of opioid agonists are given mixed agonist-antagonists and partial agonists.

Adjuvant Drugs for Acute Opioid Analgesia. A relatively common practice in the treatment of acute pain is the administration of adjuvant drugs that add to the action or effects of opioids. The most commonly used adjuvant drugs are hydroxyzine pamoate (Vistaril) and promethazine (Phenergan, Histantil✤). These drugs were once thought to potentiate the action of opioids, but evidence has shown that they enhance the sedating effects of the opioid and not the actual pain-relieving effects. They do help to relieve the anxiety and nausea that often follow general anesthesia and accompany acute pain. Some analgesic effects have been demonstrated with hydroxyzine alone in treating postoperative pain. The nurse observes for the side effect of sedation in clients receiving promethazine or hydroxyzine in addition to opioid analgesics.

Anxiolytic agents such as the benzodiazepines may be helpful in reducing the anxiety that accompanies acute pain. However, these agents cause sedation and should be cautiously administered along with opioids, especially in older adults.

Patient-Controlled Analgesia. **Patient-controlled analgesia (PCA)** is one way to combat the problem of inadequate analgesia in the management of acute and chronic pain. This method allows the client to control the dosage of opioid analgesia received. This approach to pain control can improve pain relief and increase client satisfaction. It can also decrease the amount of opioid consumption per day when compared with intermittent dosing methods.

Clients receiving medication on an as-needed basis for postoperative pain must sense the pain, report it to the nurse, and wait until the nurse is aware of the client's need and has the time to administer the analgesic. Considerable time may pass because the client may wait too long before asking for the medication. Alternatively, the nurse may not understand the need to respond promptly or may have other equally pressing responsibilities. Whatever the reasons, the client's pain may be more severe or out of control by the time he or she receives the analgesic. As a result, more medication is required to relieve the pain adequately.

Clients who have ready access to an analgesic are more likely to medicate themselves before the pain becomes severe, and thus they may require a reduced amount. Having such control over drug administration also reduces anxiety, which helps to relieve pain.

PCA is achieved through the use of a PCA infusion pump (Figure 7-5). Both stationary pole pumps (for hospital use) and ambulatory pumps (for nursing home or home use) are available. The infusion pump delivers the desired amount of medication through a conventional IV route for acute pain. Morphine is the most commonly used drug for PCA. However, the use of hydromorphone (Dilaudid) and fentanyl (Sublimaze) is gaining popularity. Meperidine (Demerol) is still reserved for short-term use (usually less than 48 to 72 hours) because its toxic metabolite, normeperidine, may accumulate in the blood and is capable of inducing confusion and seizures.

Drug security to avoid overdosing is achieved through a locked syringe pump system or locked drug reservoir system. The device is programmed to deliver a certain amount of drug within a specific interval known as a lockout interval. The physician specifies the amount of the demand dose. Morphine doses typically range from 1 to 2 mg; hydromorphone, 0.15 to 0.4 mg; fentanyl, 12.5 to 25.0 μg; and meperidine, 10 to 15 mg. Doses may vary according to the client's degree of pain and tolerance for opioids. The lockout interval is usually 5 to 15 minutes.

The nurse programs the dosing parameters into the PCA delivery device. When the client presses the button or pendant (on ambulatory pumps), the appropriate bolus or demand dose is delivered. No drug is administered if the client attempts to access the drug before the designated time interval between doses has elapsed. With this technique, there is little chance that clients will overmedicate themselves.

The PCA regimen may consist of a demand-dosing-only schedule or a continuous infusion or basal rate and demand dosing. With demand or self-administered dosing only, the client relies solely on a push of the pendant or bolus feature to seek pain relief. Continuous or basal infusions of the opioid in addition to demand dosing provide more consistent analgesia and allow the client to sleep without fear of missing any pain medication. The usual morphine dose prescribed by the health care provider for postoperative pain is 1 to 2 mg/hr; hydromorphone, 0.15 to 0.4 mg/hr; and fentanyl, 12.5 to 25.0 μg/hr. A continuous infusion of meperidine is not recommended. When a continuous infusion is added to the regimen, clients may be at greater risk for opioid-induced side effects (i.e., nausea and vomiting, sedation, respiratory depression), especially if the hourly dose is too much for the client.

The nurse's role in caring for clients using PCA is to teach them how to use the device and to report side effects, such as dizziness, nausea and vomiting, and inability to void. As with all opioids, the nurse monitors the client's vital signs frequently—at least every 4 hours. In some cases the nurse may need to anticipate the client's need for pain medication and administer doses of the drug if the client cannot. For example, a client who is confused or cannot move may need the nurse to push the pump button to administer the drug. The physician specifies the PCA demand doses, or bolus amounts, as well as the lockout interval.

Epidural Analgesia. **Epidural analgesia** (also known as peridural or extradural analgesia) refers to the instillation of a pain-blocking agent—usually an opioid analgesic alone or in combination with a local anesthetic—into the epidural space (the space between the dura mater and the vertebral column). Epidural analgesia is far more popular for the management of acute pain, such as postoperative pain. It has been used since the 1950s but has become more popular as newer and more innovative approaches to acute pain control are explored. Epidural analgesia is used with clients who are predisposed to respiratory complications (including those undergoing thoracic surgery), those with pre-existing respiratory disease, and those who are obese.

Morphine (preservative free), hydromorphone (Dilaudid), and fentanyl (Sublimaze) are the most commonly used opioids for epidural administration. A local anesthetic such as bupivacaine, which affects both sensory and motor nerves, may be given alone or in combination with an opioid. Low concentrations of local anesthetics are used to avoid the significant sensory and motor deficits that can accompany epidural anesthesia. The incidence of lower motor weakness is far less with the introduction of ropivacaine, a local anesthetic that is selective for sensory nerves (Cederholm, 1997).

A temporary, externalized epidural catheter is used for acute pain control. This device is not sutured to the skin and is easily dislodged. The nurse tapes the catheter in two places to anchor it properly. Some clinicians do not recommend transparent dressings because the catheter may be dislodged when the dressing is removed. The catheter is generally placed in either the lumbar or the thoracic region. Rarely is the catheter placed above the level of sixth thoracic vertebra, because the diaphragmatic muscle may be affected by the analgesic.

Complications of Epidural Analgesia. In caring for a client undergoing epidural analgesia, the nurse helps to prevent associated complications, monitors for them, and implements prescribed medical therapies for managing them. Complications that occur with epidural analgesia are directly related to catheter placement, catheter maintenance, and the type of analgesic.

Pruritus (itching) and nausea and vomiting are common side effects of epidural opioids. Pruritus is first treated with a small amount of naloxone (Narcan). Because epidural-induced pruritus does not appear to be mediated by histamine release, diphenhydramine (Benadryl, Allerdryl✦) may not be effective in relieving itching and may only work via its sedating effects. The physician usually prescribes an antiemetic for nausea and vomiting.

Infection results from a failure to maintain aseptic technique during catheter placement, direct drug instillation, and infusion solution and tubing changes. Infection also results from a failure to maintain aseptic conditions for indwelling catheters at the site of insertion or at the site of tube junctions. To prevent infections, the nurse ensures that all catheter line connections are secure and that an occlusive sterile dressing is maintained over the catheter site.

CONSIDERATIONS FOR OLDER ADULTS

The nurse also observes the older or restless client carefully for possible dislodgement of the catheter. An older adult may become confused or disoriented after surgery and try to pull out the temporary catheter. The catheter usually stays in place for approximately 48 to 72 hours, depending on the reason for the analgesia and the hospital policy.

Clients who receive epidural opioids are also at risk for respiratory depression resulting from high plasma and/or cerebrospinal fluid concentrations of the instilled drug. Clients receiving just epidural therapy with a local anesthetic are not at risk for respiratory depression. Because of its potential for greater spread up the spinal cord, morphine is more likely than fentanyl to cause respiratory depression. Morphine is preferred to fentanyl when a larger distribution of analgesia is required (e.g., pain relief from extensive abdominal wounds).

The nurse monitors the client's respirations at frequent intervals during and after the administration of epidural opioids and immediately reports to the physician respiratory rates below 10 per minute. Opioid-induced respiratory depression usually occurs within the first few hours of administering fentanyl but may not be seen for 12 hours or more when morphine is given. This complication is managed by administering low doses (0.2 mg) of naloxone (Narcan) either intravenously or intramuscularly.

Urinary retention is another common problem associated with epidural analgesia, but it occurs no more frequently than postoperative urinary retention in clients not receiving epidural analgesia. Although the cause is not clear, this problem usually occurs during the first or second day of analgesia administration and may be treated with bethanechol chloride (Urecholine) or intermittent urinary catheterization. The incidence of this complication is less than 25% and is more likely to occur in men than in women (Wild & Coyne, 1992).

Lower motor weakness is more common when an epidural local anesthetic is used. Clients who get out of bed for the first time should be assisted by the nurse to determine the degree of leg weakness.

Intrapleural Opioid Analgesia. Although not commonly used, local anesthetics may be administered via the intrapleural route to achieve pain control. This method is sometimes used postoperatively for clients who have undergone a videothoracoscopy and less commonly for an open thoracotomy (chest surgery).

PLACEBOS. The clinical use of placebos in non–research-based therapies has not been shown to have a sustained effect on pain relief. McCaffery's definition of a **placebo** is "any medical treatment (medication or procedure, including surgery) or nursing care that produces an effect in a client because of its implicit or explicit or nursing care therapeutic intent and not because of its specific nature (physical or chemical properties)" (1979, p. 160). Placebos are substances or actions that produce an effect regardless of their known intrinsic value. When a client responds favorably to a placebo, it is known as the placebo effect.

Placebos are sometimes used incorrectly and unethically. For example, placebos such as intramuscular saline may be administered and the client informed that the injection contains a pain medication. This practice deceives the client and perpetuates mistrust in caregivers and the health care system. Some health care providers are concerned that placebos may not be legal or ethical, and therefore they are not often used.

PHYSICAL MEASURES. Physical measures may be used instead of or in addition to drug therapy to relieve acute pain. Cutaneous (skin) stimulation strategies to relieve pain have been in use for many years. Various types of stimulation to the skin and subcutaneous tissue produce pain relief. Mobily, Herr, and Nicholson (1994) have identified areas of nursing practice that are critical to the successful implementation of cutaneous stimulation. Nurses play an important role in educating clients about these techniques. Methods of cutaneous stimulation include techniques such as the following:

- Transcutaneous electrical nerve stimulation (TENS)
- Application of heat, cold, and pressure
- Therapeutic touch
- Massage
- Vibration

Whichever method is used, several characteristics of cutaneous stimulation must be considered:

- The benefits of these techniques are highly unpredictable and may vary from application to application.
- Pain relief is generally sustained only as long as the stimulation continues.
- Multiple trials may be necessary to establish the desired effects.
- Stimulation itself may aggravate pre-existing pain or may produce new pain.

Despite the drawbacks to cutaneous stimulation, it is effective in the management of both acute pain and chronic pain. These techniques have both physiologic and psychologic effects on the client. Cutaneous stimulation techniques also give clients an opportunity to participate actively in the management of their pain.

PHYSICAL THERAPY. Physical therapy is used for clients experiencing pain to increase function, decrease pain, compensate for decreased function, and prevent further deterioration. Exercises and physical modalities such as heat, cold, massage, or TENS units may be used. Measures of client progress include an increase in the range of motion, strength, and function of the affected area (Nordin & Campello, 1999).

Transcutaneous Electrical Nerve Stimulation. **Transcutaneous electrical nerve stimulation (TENS)** involves the use of a battery-operated device capable of delivering small electrical currents to the skin and underlying tissues. The first-generation, or conventional, TENS unit is used most frequently. Electrodes connected to a small box are placed over the painful sites. The voltage or current is regulated by adjusting a dial to the point at which the client perceives a prickly, "pins-and-needles" sensation. The current is adjusted on the basis of the client's degree of pain relief and level of comfort.

The physician, nurse, or physical therapist (depending on the health care setting) assists the client in applying the electrodes either on the painful area or above or below it (Figure 7-6). A conducting substance (usually a gel) is placed between the electrode and the client's skin.

The advantages of TENS units are that the client can wear the unit and achieve a level of pain relief while participating in activities of daily living. The unit is easy to use and can be worn for several hours. However, the skin may become irritated at the site of the electrode placement. To prevent this, the nurse teaches the client to rotate electrode sites.

In general, clients use TENS units for the management of both acute pain and chronic pain. This type of therapy is indicated for localized pain, such as postoperative pain or local chronic pain, particularly low back pain (Fishbain et al., 1996).

Other Cutaneous Techniques. Additional cutaneous stimulation techniques, such as touch, pressure, massage, vi-

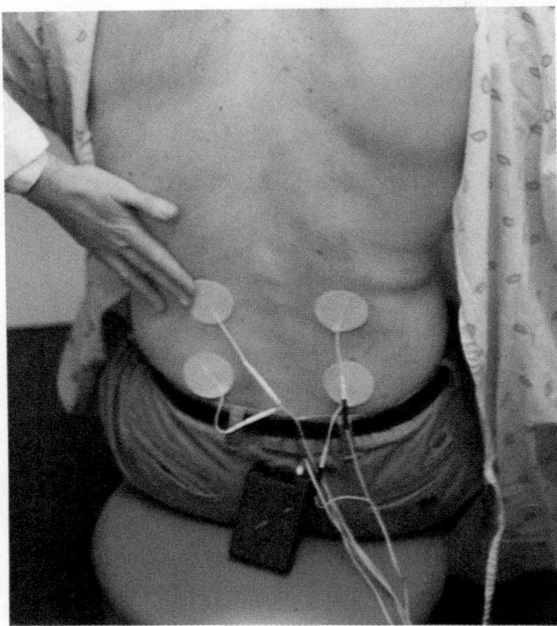

Figure 7-6 ● Application of a TENS unit.

bration, and heat and cold application, stimulate the skin and somehow interrupt the pain pathway. These interventions are relatively easy for the client to learn and are fairly economical. Table 7-5 summarizes these techniques.

COMPLEMENTARY AND ALTERNATIVE THERAPIES. Cognitive and behavioral strategies to relieve pain (e.g., distraction) have been popular for years either as adjuncts to drug therapy or as alternative interventions. Theoretical explanations for the effectiveness of these measures reflect the premises of the gate control theory.

Distraction can be an effective method of acute pain relief. Simple measures such as holding a client's hand, taking him or her for a walk, or encouraging deep breathing exercises can divert attention from the pain. Nurses often observe that clients request less pain medication when family members are present. After visiting hours are over, many clients request something for pain.

Instead of viewing distraction as a therapeutic pain relief measure, some nurses may question the presence or severity of the pain if a client is easily distracted from it. Distraction alters the perception of pain but does not influence the cause or peripheral mechanism of pain. It is a transient method of pain relief and is probably best used with other pain control measures.

Nurses can provide several methods of distraction. Visual distractors (e.g., pictures or television) can divert the client's attention to something pleasant or interesting. Auditory distractors, including music or relaxation tapes, can have a calming effect. Changing the environment can remove unpleasant stressors or reminders that may enhance pain. Physical distractions (e.g., deep breathing exercises) help the client concentrate on other physiologic sensations.

Distraction is used in the following situations:

- Exacerbations of pain
- Painful procedures (e.g., dressing changes or invasive procedures)
- Interrupting the client's constant perception of pain

The benefit of guided imagery in reducing preoperative and postoperative anxiety, pain, and opioid use was demonstrated by Tusek, Church, and Fazio (1997). Clients undergoing elective colorectal surgery were randomly assigned to a guided imagery group or to a control group. Both groups received standard care, including the use of patient-controlled analgesia (PCA). In the guided imagery group, total analgesia requirements were lower, and the first postoperative bowel movement was earlier.

CHRONIC PAIN

PLANNING: EXPECTED OUTCOMES. The client with chronic pain is expected to experience pain reduction or relief, pain modification, or prevention of recurring or worsening pain. Jacox et al. (1994) provide the nurse with information to suggest appropriate management of these conditions.

INTERVENTIONS. The goals for chronic pain management are accomplished by interrupting the relentless cycle of pain, anxiety and, sometimes, depression. Pain algorithms also assist the health care provider in delivering standardized measures to relieve chronic pain. In general, nonsurgical methods of pain reduction are used before surgical techniques

TABLE 7-5 • CUTANEOUS STIMULATION TECHNIQUES USED TO INTERRUPT THE PAIN PATHWAY

Method of Application	Comments
THERAPEUTIC TOUCH OR "LAYING ON OF HANDS" The hands of the caregiver are placed on or close to the client's body.	The caregiver's intent to help may contribute to the success of this technique. This technique may extend the nurse-client relationship.
PRESSURE A hand or other object is placed firmly over or around the painful area.	Pressure seems to relieve pain, decrease bleeding, and prevent swelling. Release of pressure is associated with increased blood flow and return of pain.
MASSAGE The hands or fingers are moved slowly or briskly over a body part. A lubricant or other substance is sometimes used.	Effects include muscle relaxation and sedation.
VIBRATION Electrical and battery-operated vibrators produce a massage effect.	Vibration may decrease the intensity of the noxious (pain) stimuli.
APPLICATION OF HEAT AND COLD Heat may be applied in a variety of ways, including short-wave diathermy, microwave diathermy, sonography, melted paraffin and Hubbard tank, hot water bottle or heating pad, heat cradle and lamp, moist pads or towels, hot tub or shower, or gel packs. Cold may be applied in a dry or moist way, similar to heat applications. Ice chips, cold towels and packs, and chilled gel packs are commonly used.	Both heat and cold may reduce muscle spasm and decrease pain. Cold probably slows the conduction velocity of nerves. Heat increases the tendency for bleeding and therefore should not be used after trauma. Heat may also increase edema and is not indicated if circulation is poor. Both heat and cold should be used cautiously if clients have impaired sensation or cannot communicate.

Data from McCaffery, M. (1979). *Nursing management of the patient with pain* (2nd ed.). Philadelphia: J.B. Lippincott.

are tried. The client may eventually need a combination of nonsurgical and surgical measures.

DRUG THERAPY. A pharmacologic approach to treating chronic pain is often the most effective and reliable method of pain management. Other measures may be used in combination with drug therapy. Although a number of drugs have been used to manage chronic pain, the health care provider most commonly prescribes nonopioid and opioid analgesics.

NONOPIOID ANALGESICS. Acetylsalicylic acid (aspirin, Ancasal✱), acetaminophen (Tylenol, Ace-Tabs✱), nonsteroidal anti-inflammatory drugs (NSAIDs) such as ibuprofen (Motrin, Amersol✱), and the newer COX-2 inhibitors celecoxib (Celebrex) and rofecoxib (Vioxx) may be effective in the management of mild chronic pain. They are also effective in combination with opioid analgesics. Aspirin and NSAIDs possess anti-inflammatory properties in that they peripherally inhibit prostaglandins. This property makes them particularly useful in treating the inflammation associated with arthritis and cancer. The use of aspirin and NSAIDs can reduce the need for opioid analgesics in the client with chronic pain.

However, both aspirin and NSAIDs can cause gastric disturbances and can have an effect on platelets, which results in a tendency toward bleeding. The nurse observes the client for gastric discomfort or vomiting and bleeding or bruising and reports these problems to the physician immediately. NSAIDs can cause renal toxicity; therefore renal function blood tests should be routinely monitored with long-term therapy, especially in the older adult. In addition, NSAIDs can cause sodium and water retention that may lead to congestive heart failure, more often in an older client.

Salicylates (choline magnesium trisalicylate [Trilisate]) also have anti-inflammatory effects, and this class of drugs has certain benefits. Compared with aspirin, salicylates cause less gastrointestinal upset, are less toxic to the kidneys, and have little effect on platelet aggregation. These advantages make salicylates a more favorable alternative to NSAIDs in clients undergoing cancer therapy, those at risk for bleeding, and older clients who may be more susceptible to the renal effects of NSAIDs (Table 7-6).

The health care provider also commonly prescribes acetaminophen for chronic pain. Acetaminophen exerts its analgesic action by blocking peripheral pain receptors, thus increasing the threshold of these receptors to painful stimuli. Reports of liver toxicity have been associated with higher doses of this drug (1000 mg) taken more frequently than every 4 hours for long-term use. Current recommendations restrict the total daily amount of acetaminophen to no more than 4000 mg (4 g). Therefore nurses must check all combination analgesic products for their acetaminophen content and caution the client regarding maximum dosing.

Capsaicin (Zostrix), an over-the-counter cream, can be applied to the skin in painful areas (Ellison et al., 1997). Its pain-relieving qualities lie in its ability to deplete the painful site of substance P, a pain mediator. This preparation is marketed for painful arthritis, diabetic neuropathy, and other chronic pain conditions. For the first few applications, the cream produces noticeable pain as the release of substance P is intensified; this reaction can be alleviated with the addition of a local anesthetic cream or ointment. Regular applications are recommended to sustain its pain-relieving properties.

ADJUVANT DRUGS. Other nonopioid drugs used to control the pain of certain neuralgias (pain along the distribution of nerves) or nerve injury include carbamazepine (Tegretol, Mazepine✱), phenytoin (Dilantin), and valproic acid (Depakene). The exact mechanism of action of these drugs is unknown, but it is believed that they inhibit or reduce the intermittent firing of nerve impulses. Both carbamazepine and phenytoin are associated with a wide variety of side effects (central nervous system toxicity and hematopoietic, hepatic, and pulmonary effects). These drugs are therefore used with extreme caution.

Gabapentin (Neurontin), a newer anticonvulsant, has proved to be effective in treating postherpetic neuralgia and the painful neuropathy associated with diabetes mellitus (Rowbotham, et al., 1998; Backonja et al., 1998). It has been associated with fewer and milder side effects than other anticonvulsants.

Tricyclic antidepressants such as amitriptyline (Elavil), nortriptyline (Pamelor), imipramine (Tofranil), and doxepin (Sinequan) may be beneficial in treating chronic neuropathic pain. Both tricyclic antidepressants and other antidepressants such as trazodone (Desyrel), paroxetine (Paxil), and sertraline (Zoloft) help treat the depression that can accompany chronic pain. They also stimulate the activity of endogenous opiates (endorphins and enkephalins) by increasing levels of the neurotransmitter serotonin. Perhaps the greatest advantage of this group of drugs, particularly the tricyclic antidepressants, is the sedative effect. This effect can be helpful in promoting sleep when administered at bedtime.

In some cases antianxiety agents help to relax the client and thus help to relieve pain. Many of these drugs cause confusion, drowsiness, and hypotension; the physician selects the drugs with the fewest side effects. Examples of antianxiety agents include alprazolam (Xanax), clorazepate (Tranxene, Novo-Clopate✱), lorazepam (Ativan), and oxazepam (Serax, Zapex✱). Clonazepam (Klonopin), also used for anxiety, has been shown to be particularly helpful for certain types of nerve injury pain.

Oral local anesthetics such as mexiletine (Mexitil) act by suppressing the electrical activity of both peripheral nerves and neurons in the central nervous system. They are useful for electric, shocklike pain and continuous pain. Mexiletine is contraindicated for clients who have cardiac conduction defects or dysrhythmias or are currently taking cardiac antiarrhythmic medications.

Other agents known to have some effect in relieving chronic pain include dextromethorphan (the active ingredient in many cough syrups) and ketamine. Both of these agents are *N*-methyl-D-aspartate (NMDA) antagonists. NMDA receptors are involved in the development of tolerance to opioids. The administration of NMDA antagonists is thought to potentiate the action of opioids and prevent the development of opioid tolerance (Siddall & Cousins, 1997).

OPIOID ANALGESICS. Opioid analgesics are capable of relieving pain by binding to various opiate receptors in the central nervous system (see the discussion under Interventions [Acute Pain], p. 74). For chronic pain, opioids are more commonly ad-

TABLE 7-6 • NONOPIOID ANALGESICS FOR CHRONIC PAIN

Drug	Usual Dose for Adults and Children ≥50 kg Body Weight	Usual Dose for Children[a] and Adults[b] ≤50 kg Body Weight
ACETAMINOPHEN AND OVER-THE-COUNTER NSAIDs		
Acetaminophen[c]	650 mg q4h 975 mg q6h	10-15 mg/kg q4h 15-20 mg/kg q4h (rectal)
Aspirin[d]	650 mg q4h 975 mg q6h	10-15 mg/kg q4h 15-20 mg/kg q4h (rectal)
Ibuprofen (Motrin, others)	400-600 mg q6h	10 mg/kg q6-8h[e]
PRESCRIPTION NSAIDs		
Celecoxib (Celebrex)	100-200 mg bid	
Choline magnesium trisalicylate (Trilisate)[f]	1000-1500 mg tid	25 mg/kg tid
Choline salicylate (Arthropan)[f]	870 mg q3-4h	
Diflunisal (Dolobid)[g]	500 mg q12h	
Etodolac (Lodine)	200-400 mg q6-8h	
Fenoprofen calcium (Nalfon)	300-600 mg q6h	
Ketoprofen (Orudis)	25-60 mg q6-8h	
Ketorolac tromethamine (Toradol)[h]	10 mg q4-6h to a maximum of 40 mg/day	
Magnesium salicylate (Doan's, Magan, Mobidin, others)	650 mg q4h	
Meclofenamate sodium (Meclomen)[i]	50-100 mg q6h	
Mefenamic acid (Ponstel)	250 mg q6h	
Naproxen (Naprosyn)	250-275 mg q6-8h	5 mg/kg q8h
Naproxen sodium (Anaprox)	275 mg q6-8h	
Refecoxib (Vioxx)	25-50 mg q24h	
Sodium salicylate (Generic)	325-650 mg q3-4h	
PARENTERAL AND ORAL NSAID		
Ketorolac tromethamine (Toradol)[h,j]	60 mg initially, then 30 mg q6h; IM dose not to exceed 5 days	

From Management of Cancer Pain Guideline Panel. (1994). *Management of cancer pain: Clinical practice guidelines* (pp. 48 and 49). AHCPR Pub. No. 94-0592. Rockville, MD: Agency for Health Care Policy and Research, Public Health Service, U.S. Department of Health and Human Services.

NOTE: Only the above NSAIDs have FDA approval for use as simple analgesics, but clinical experience has been gained with other drugs as well.

[a]Only drugs that are FDA approved as an analgesic for use in children are included.

[b]Acetaminophen and NSAID dosage for adults weighing less than 50 kg should be adjusted for weight.

[c]APAP lacks the peripheral anti-inflammatory and antiplatelet activities of the other NSAIDs.

[d]The standard against which other NSAIDs are compared. May inhibit platelet aggregation ≥1 week and may cause bleeding. Aspirin is contraindicated in children with fever or other viral disease because of its association with Reye's syndrome.

[e]Not FDA approved for use in children as an over-the-counter drug; has FDA approval for use in children as a prescription drug for fever. However, clinicians have experience in prescribing ibuprofen for pain in children.

[f]May have minimal antiplatelet activity.

[g]Administration with antacids may decrease absorption.

[h]For short-term use only.

[i]Coombs-positive autoimmune hemolytic anemia has been associated with prolonged use.

[j]Has the same gastrointestinal toxicities as oral NSAIDs.

ministered by the oral route; other acceptable routes include transdermal, rectal, sublingual, subcutaneous, IV, or intraspinal.

An equianalgesic guide can help determine the appropriate dose conversions when switching the type or route of a drug (Table 7-7). The term *equianalgesic* refers to the dose and route of administration of one drug that produces approximately the same degree of analgesia as the given dose and route of another drug. Most commonly, 10 mg of morphine is the standard dose against which other opioids are measured. Equianalgesic opioid drug guides provide only the comparative analgesic potencies among these drugs. Dose modifications may be necessary according to each client's response. When converting from one opioid to another in clients receiving higher than usual opioid amounts, the new opioid should be started at one-half the equianalgesic dose. This is necessary because incomplete cross-tolerance between opioids may occur.

Considerations with Long-Term Use of Opioids. The side effects of opioid analgesics are discussed under Interven-

TABLE 7-7 • DOSE EQUIVALENTS FOR OPIOID ANALGESICS IN OPIOID-NAIVE ADULTS[a]

Drug	Approximate Equianalgesic Dose		Usual Starting Dose for Moderate to Severe Pain	
	Oral	Parenteral	Oral	Parenteral
OPIOID AGONIST[b]				
Morphine[c]	30 mg q3-4h (repeat around-the-clock dosing) 60 mg q3-4h (single dose or intermittent dosing)	10 mg q3-4h	30 mg q3-4h	10 mg q3-4h
Morphine, controlled-release[b,d] (MS Contin, Oramorph)	90-120 mg q12h	N/A	90-120 mg q12h	N/A
Hydromorphone[c] (Dilaudid)	7.5 mg q3-4h	1.5 mg q3-4h	6 mg q3-4h	1.5 mg q3-4h
Levorphanol (Levo-Dromoran)	4 mg q6-8h	2 mg q6-8h	4 mg q6-8h	2 mg q6-8h
Meperidine (Demerol)	300 mg q2-3h	100 mg q3h	N/R	100 mg q3h
Methadone (Dolophine, other)	20 mg q6-8h	10 mg q6-8h	20 mg q6-8h	10 mg q6-8h
Oxymorphone[c] (Numorphan)	N/A	1 mg q3-4h	N/A	1 mg q3-4h
COMBINATION OPIOID/NSAID PREPARATIONS[e]				
Codeine[f] (with aspirin or acetaminophen)	18-200 mg q3-4h	130 mg q3-4h	60 mg q3-4h	60 mg q2h (IM/SC)
Hydrocodone (in Lorcet, Lortab, Vicodin, others)	30 mg q3-4h	N/A	10 mg q3-4h	N/A
Oxycodone (Roxicodone, also in Percocet, Percodan, Tylox, others)	30 mg q3-4h	N/A	10 mg q3-4h	N/A

From Management of Cancer Pain Guideline Panel. (1994). *Management of cancer pain: Clinical practice guidelines.* AHCPR Pub. No. 94-0592. Rockville, MD: Agency for Health Care Policy and Research, Public Health Service, U.S. Department of Health and Human Services.

N/A, not available; *N/R,* not recommended.

NOTE: Published tables vary in the suggested doses that are equianalgesic to morphine. Clinical response is the criterion that must be applied for each patient; titration to clinical responses is necessary. Because there is not complete cross tolerance among these drugs, it is usually necessary to use a lower-than-equianalgesic dose when changing drugs and to retitrate to response.

[a]CAUTION: Recommended doses do not apply for adult patients with body weight less than 50 kg. For recommended starting doses for children and adults <50 kg body weight, see Table 7-4.

[b]CAUTION: Recommended doses do not apply to patients with renal or hepatic insufficiency or other conditions affecting drug metabolism and kinetics.

[c]CAUTION: For morphine, hydromorphone, and oxymorphone, rectal administration is an alternate route for patients unable to take oral medications. Equianalgesic doses may differ from oral and parenteral doses because of pharmokinetic differences.

[d]Transdermal fentanyl (Duragesic) is an alternative option. Transdermal fentanyl dosage is not calculated as equianalgesic to a single morphine dosage. See the package insert for dosing calculations. Doses above 25 μg/hr should not be used in opioid-naive patients.

[e]CAUTION: Doses of aspirin and acetaminophen in combination opioid-NSAID preparations must also be adjusted to the patient's body weight. Aspirin is contraindicated in children in the presence of fever or other viral disease because of its association with Reye's syndrome.

[f]CAUTION: Codeine doses above 65 mg often are not appropriate because of diminishing incremental analgesia with increasing doses but increasing nausea, constipation, and other side effects.

tions (Acute Pain), p. 74. The long-term use of these agents is associated with some concerns.

Physical Dependency. Physical dependency is associated with the administration of opioids on a long-term basis. Physical dependency is *not* the same as addiction but is sometimes confused with addiction. **Physical dependency** is a physiologic adaptation of the body tissues so that continued administration of the drug is required for normal tissue function. So-called **withdrawal symptoms** result when a client who is physically dependent on opioids abruptly ceases using them. These symptoms result from autonomic nervous system responses and include nausea and vomiting, abdominal cramping, muscle twitching, profuse perspiration, delirium, and convulsions. When it is necessary to discontinue opioid analgesia for a client who is opioid dependent, a slow tapering (weaning) of the drug dosage lessens or alleviates the physical withdrawal symptoms.

Addiction. Addiction is a common fear of the health care professionals who administer or prescribe opioids and of the clients who receive them. **Addiction** is a term used to describe the persistent craving for and abuse of a drug for recreational purposes. It is a psychologic phenomenon, not a physical one. Physical dependence does not define the problem of addiction, but it does occur in many people who become addicted. Although addiction rarely occurs in clients who use opioids for medicinal pain relief, the fear of addiction is a major contributing factor in the inadequate prescription and administration of opioid analgesics.

Clients may worry about becoming addicted to analgesics. They may be concerned about the possibility of drug withdrawal symptoms, which are often associated with the "street addict." The nurse clarifies the term *addiction* with clients while stressing the concept of physical dependency.

Drug Tolerance. The client may also experience drug tolerance from opioid analgesic therapy. **Tolerance** is characterized by a gradual resistance of the body to the effects of an opioid, including its pain-relieving properties. When tolerance occurs, clients usually require more of the drug to achieve the same analgesic effects. Tolerance should be recognized and the appropriate analgesic plans designed to account for increased opioid requirements during acute episodes of chronic or procedure-related pain. Issues with sedation and analgesia for clients with cancer can be especially difficult (Polomano, Soulen, & McDaniel, 1997).

Tolerance to opioid analgesics is particularly a problem in clients who are substance abusers (see Chart 7-2). Tolerance is measured not only by the analgesic effects but also by the ability of the body to adjust to the adverse reactions.

Care management contracts can be effective tools when caring for substance abusers with pain. These contracts should be developed by both the client and the health care provider to keep the client as comfortable as possible. Essential components of the contract are pain relief without sedation and the avoidance of withdrawal symptoms (Vourakis, 1998). Contracts must clearly identify outcome expectations, including unacceptable client behaviors and their consequences.

Continuous Intravenous Opioid Analgesia. For chronic cancer pain management, hourly doses of continuous opioid infusions vary depending on the severity of the pain and the client's tolerance to the opioid. If the hourly dose needs to be increased, the physician usually increases it to no more than 10% to 20% of the hourly rate and to intervals no smaller than every 3 to 4 hours. The nurse may need to monitor the client's vital signs frequently (at least every hour) until an adequate and safe level of drug is achieved.

Patient-controlled analgesia (PCA) can provide effective relief of chronic pain. Although the principles of PCA are the same for both acute pain and chronic pain, the dosing guidelines and methods of administration do differ. PCA for chronic pain, typically cancer pain, can be administered either by IV or subcutaneous routes. The idea is to provide most of the analgesia at a continuous rate. The physician calculates demand doses based on the amount of continuous hourly opioid administration. Usually the PCA demand dose is a minimum of 33% of the basal or continuous rate, but sometimes it may be as high as 100% of the hourly rate. The lockout interval for chronic pain is usually longer than for acute pain. Longer lockout intervals with higher demand doses keep the client from needing to work hard to manage the pain.

Continuous Subcutaneous Opioid Analgesia. Continuous subcutaneous opioid analgesia is best for clients who have compromised venous access or have central venous lines that are being used for other fluids. Subcutaneous infusion is accomplished through the use of a small (25- or 27-gauge) butterfly-type catheter or a special subcutaneous needle device placed under the skin into the subcutaneous tissue.

The subclavicular tissue underneath the clavicle or the abdomen is typically used for continuous subcutaneous opioid analgesia. Placing the catheter in the extremities should be avoided if possible, especially in terminally ill clients, because peripheral circulation may be impaired or edema may be present, which could affect drug absorption. The nurse applies an occlusive dressing over the site and rotates the site every 3 to 7 days depending on the drug and the volume delivered. The physician usually orders no more than 3 to 6 mL/hr.

Morphine is the most common drug administered by this route. Hydromorphone (Dilaudid) is occasionally used, but it is more irritating to the tissues and requires more site changes. If the physician orders a PCA demand-dosing schedule in addition to the continuous infusion, the volume of the bolus dose does not usually exceed 1 mL. In addition, the lockout interval (the time during which the client cannot access more opioids) is usually no smaller than 30 to 60 minutes. Clients may require adjustments in their continuous rates if more than 6 to 12 PCA bolus doses are used each day. The nurse observes for and reports complications of subcutaneous infusion, including fluid leakage around the insertion site, inadequate pain relief, and edema around the site.

Neuraxial Delivery of Analgesia. Neuraxial drug delivery involves the epidural, subarachnoid or intrathecal, and intraventricular routes. Neuraxial administration is sometimes referred to as the intraspinal route. There are two major methods for administering intraspinal analgesia: epidural and intrathecal. Intraspinal therapy is particularly useful for **intractable pain** not relieved by systemic opioids (Rauck, 1997) or for clients who may not be able to tolerate the effects of systemic opioids. The administration of spinal opioids results from an understanding that opioid receptors are present not only in the brain but also in the spinal cord. It is therefore possible to give lower doses of opioids.

Long-term epidural analgesia, also known as peridural or extradural analgesia, refers to the instillation of a pain-blocking agent, usually an opioid analgesic alone or in combination with a local anesthetic. This agent is instilled into the epidural space (the space between the dura mater and the vertebral column) through an externalized catheter (see Figure 7-7), an implantable port, or an implantable drug delivery system. *Intrathecal* (subarachnoid) analgesia, in which a pain-blocking agent is introduced into the space between the arachnoid mater and pia mater of the spinal cord (where cerebrospinal fluid is located), is the route of choice for long-term management of intractable pain (more than 3 months).

Action of Intraspinal Analgesia. The goal of both types of intraspinal analgesia is to interrupt pain pathways where the sensory fibers exit the spinal cord. Morphine (preservative free) is the opioid of choice for long-term intraspinal administration, but fentanyl (Sublimaze) and hydromorphone (Dilaudid) may also be used. The addition of a local anesthetic (e.g., bupivacaine, ropivacaine) may provide an opioid-sparing effect and is often considered for many intractable neuropathic pain syndromes. Lower concentrations of local anesthetics are used to minimize the significant sensory and motor deficits that often accompany intraspinal anesthesia. As with opioids, tolerance to local anesthetics may develop, thus necessitating increasing doses over time.

Long-Term Intraspinal Analgesia. Long-term intraspinal opioid administration may be used for the management of chronic, intractable (uncontrollable or unyielding) pain. Such pain is usually the result of cancer or central sensitization. A permanent *epidural catheter* may be inserted, and several catheter devices are available for this purpose. The DuPen Silastic catheter (Davol) is the most commonly used *external* catheter. A portion of the catheter exits the skin. Drugs can be intermittently injected into this portion, or the catheter can be attached to an infusion device for continuous drug administration.

Implantable devices are also used. The epidural Port-A-Cath (SIMS Deltec, Inc.) is implanted under the skin, and the catheter portion is inserted into the epidural space. As with the

DuPen catheter, this device can be injected with drugs intermittently or can be connected to an infusion device for continuous opioid delivery. Injectable ports have been shown to reduce the incidence of catheter dislodgement and early infection. Systems consisting of either an externalized catheter or a drug delivery device are rarely used for intrathecal or subarachnoid drug administration. The SynchroMed pump (Medtronic, Inc.) is a totally implantable system that contains a drug reservoir. The drug reservoir is filled on a routine basis and is capable of continuously administering a certain volume of drug each day (Figure 7-7).

The side effects of intraspinal opioids are more common in clients who have had little exposure to opioids. Clients who receive intraspinal therapy are usually more tolerant of the effects of opioids and may not require the rigorous monitoring needed for postoperative analgesia. Male clients receiving long-term spinal opioids may complain of sexual dysfunction, decreased libido, and difficulty maintaining an erection; female clients may experience amenorrhea. Testosterone injections seem to help improve sexual function in male clients.

Transdermal Opioid Administration. Transdermal opioid administration is now possible with the transdermal fentanyl system (Duragesic). Duragesic is available in patch dose strengths of 25, 50, 75, and 100 μg/hr. It is reserved for clients with continuous and relatively stable pain who can take nothing by mouth, have difficulty taking pills, or cannot comply with their analgesic regimen. Because of the extended length of time needed to achieve optimal, steady-state serum concentrations of the opioid, the Duragesic patch is supplemented with intermittent administration of short-acting opioids. Intermittent "rescue" dosing should continue if the client has periods of episodic pain that lead to an increased need for opioid analgesia. Duragesic should be used for clients with a known opioid requirement for effective pain relief; it is difficult to titrate Duragesic quickly to pain relief.

The transdermal system is applied by removing the adhesive backing and placing it on the skin of the client's chest (front or back), preferably on an area without hair. The nurse clips any hair present on the chest. The patch delivers a specified amount of drug into the skin, and the drug absorbs over 72 hours. The physician calculates the appropriate dosage from the client's previous opioid requirement. If the client's need is known, the lowest patch strength is used initially. Transdermal administration should be used cautiously when the requirement is *not* known.

The nurse teaches the client and family how to apply the patch and to report side effects (e.g., dizziness, sedation, nausea, decreased respiratory rate) to the physician or nurse. The nurse also explains that it may take up to 24 hours after the unit is applied before pain relief is apparent. Supplemental analgesia with short-acting opioids is usually ordered until adequate blood levels of the transdermal drug are reached. The absorption of transdermal analgesics is affected by body temperature. The nurse teaches the client and family that a temperature of 102° F (38.9° C) or greater might accelerate drug absorption from the skin and increase side effects. Clients should be monitored closely for increased effects (e.g., sedation) when fever is present. The client is monitored for approximately 24 hours after the system is removed, because the drug may still be released into the bloodstream from the site of application.

Oral Transmucosal Administration. The oral transmucosal (OT) route of opioid delivery has been studied using fentanyl citrate. Fentanyl (Actiq) is delivered in a sucrose-based medium and fitted onto a radiopaque plastic handle. The medication is available with a raspberry flavor in six strengths: 200, 400, 600, 800, 1200, and 1600 μg. The client is instructed to swirl the unit onto the buccal mucosa until the medication dissolves. This takes 5 to 15 minutes. The benefit of the transmucosal route is that a portion of the medication is absorbed directly into the bloodstream, resulting in an onset effect equal to IV morphine (Chandler, 1999). The remaining portion of the drug is swallowed and absorbed through the gastrointestinal tract. The OT route of fentanyl administration produces a rapid peak effect and a short half-life. Oral trans-

A

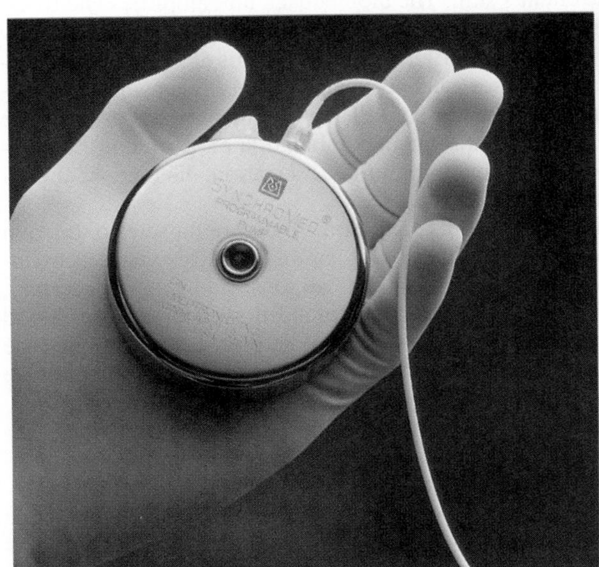

B

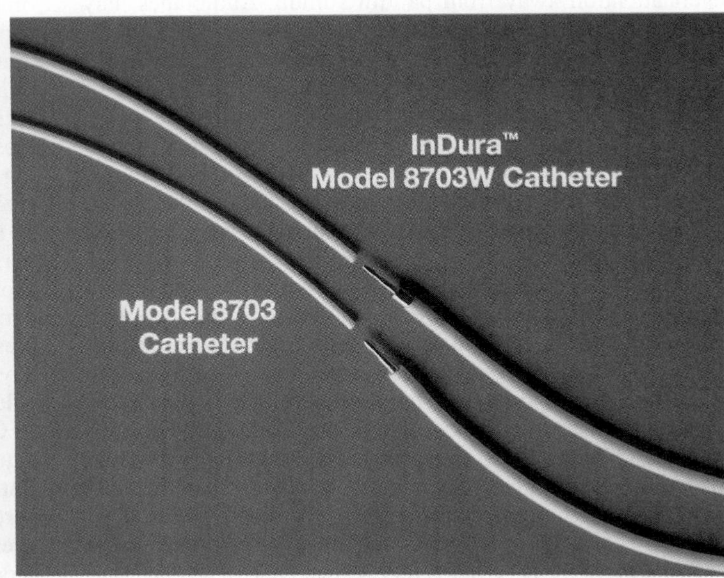

Figure 7-7 ● A SynchroMed implantable pump (*A*) and spinal catheters (*B*) for delivery of a precise volume of long-term intraspinal analgesia each day. (Courtesy of Medtronic, Inc., Columbia Heights, MN.)

mucosal fentanyl citrate (OTFC) has been approved by the Federal Drug Administration (FDA) for opioid-tolerant cancer clients who experience breakthrough pain.

COMPLEMENTARY AND ALTERNATIVE THERAPIES. Cognitive and behavioral strategies, including imagery, relaxation, hypnosis, biofeedback, and magnetic field therapy, may be effective in relieving chronic pain. Analgesic therapy is an essential component of pain management, but cognitive and behavioral strategies may be used effectively in addition to (and sometimes instead of) drug therapy.

IMAGERY. Imagery is a form of distraction in which the client is encouraged to visualize or think about some pleasant or desirable feeling, sensation, or event. Guided imagery occurs when a person, often a nurse, assists the client in sustaining a sequence of thoughts aimed at diverting attention away from the pain. Intense concentration is required to visualize images. Clients who are extremely anxious, agitated, or unable to concentrate may first benefit from mild distraction.

Imagery is particularly useful for chronic pain. Clients who practice this technique can mentally and vividly experience sights, sounds, smells, events, or other sensations. The nurse first assesses the client's level of concentration to determine if he or she can sustain a particular thought or thoughts for a desired time. The time interval for mental imagery can vary from 5 to 60 minutes. Behaviors that are helpful in assessing a client's capacity for imagery include the following:

- Reading and comprehending the newspaper
- Listening to music or other auditory stimuli
- Having the ability to follow and participate in sustained conversation
- Having an interest in environmental surroundings

When the client has demonstrated some ability to concentrate, the nurse assists in identifying a pleasant or favorable thought. The client is encouraged to focus on this thought to divert attention away from painful stimuli. Audiotapes may help in forming and maintaining images. The nurse, client, or family may wish to create audiotapes, or commercially available audiotapes may be used. The following is an example of guided imagery instructions: "Imagine yourself on the beach on some deserted island. You can hear the sound of waves rushing onto the shore, the cry of seagulls flying high above, and the rustling of trees as they are brushed gently by the wind. You can feel the warmth of the sun over your body and the cooling breeze."

Imagery works for some clients but not for others. It may even worsen symptoms in clients who become annoyed with imagery strategies (Kwekkeboom, Huseby-Moore, & Ward, 1998). The capacity to become engaged in the reality of the image may be important for the successful use of this complementary therapy. The work of Kwekkeboom, Huseby-Moore, and Ward (1998) suggests that the client's ability to be absorbed by the images may be more important than the ability to generate vivid mental images.

RELAXATION TECHNIQUES. Clients may use relaxation techniques to reduce anxiety, tension, and emotional stress, all of which may exacerbate pain. Techniques to help clients relax can be both physical and psychologic. Physical relaxation techniques include the following:

- Receiving a body massage, back rub, or warm or hot bath
- Modifying the environment to reduce distractions
- Moving into a comfortable position

Psychologic relaxation techniques include the following:

- Pleasant conversation
- Music
- Relaxation tapes

Some relaxation tapes assist the client with progressive relaxation of the muscles. Relaxation exercises can be effectively coupled with guided imagery, distraction, and hypnosis. Chapter 4 describes relaxation techniques in detail.

Many studies suggest the effectiveness of complementary therapies in pain relief. Wallace's analysis (1997) of studies of adults with cancer pain from 1982 to 1995 suggests that relaxation and imagery reduce the sensory experience of pain, have equivocal effects on affective measures of pain, and have no effect on functional status.

HYPNOSIS. **Hypnosis** is defined as an altered state of consciousness in which a person enters a trance and loses an overall sense of reality. Although the person is in a trance, he or she has some sense of awareness and contact with reality and has an understanding of what is actually happening. Hypnosis is used to treat a variety of pain syndromes, particularly chronic pain. It is used to help clients overcome the emotional consequences of pain and can promote a positive state of mind. Although nurses do not usually teach hypnosis, they are in a key position to help clarify misconceptions, instruct clients about relaxation and distraction, and encourage clients to practice self-hypnosis.

BIOFEEDBACK. Biofeedback is used to treat chronic pain, anxiety, and other stress conditions. Biofeedback involves monitoring various physiologic responses by an electric device capable of sensing bodily changes and reporting this information to the client. Certain physiologic signals are transmitted to the feedback unit by electrode sensors placed on the client's skin. The biofeedback unit amplifies and transforms this physiologic information into visual signals (usually meter readings or colored lights). Clients are alerted to stress-related responses, such as increased muscle tension or an elevation in blood pressure. They are then taught to regulate these responses through a combination of techniques, including deep breathing, progressive relaxation, distraction, and visual imagery.

Biofeedback units vary. Some measure muscle contraction via electromyography and brain activity via electroencephalography. Galvanic skin response and skin temperature, which can reflect changes in blood flow, heart rate, or blood pressure, are also measured. Whatever the technique, the physiologic responses that tend to worsen or prolong pain are voluntarily controlled.

Clients who are interested in learning biofeedback techniques to control pain are usually trained by a skilled therapist. They are taught to observe the feedback information, report sensations or feelings that become apparent, and practice stress-reducing or pain-reducing techniques. Clients may need several sessions before they can recognize and control these responses. Eventually they become aware of even the most subtle bodily changes that indicate the onset or worsening of pain, and they respond automatically without the help of the biofeedback unit.

Biofeedback training helps the client gain control over pain. Clients require training and self-discipline in order for biofeedback and all other cognitive therapy strategies to be effective.

MAGNETIC FIELD THERAPY. Magnetic field therapy, also called magnet therapy or biomagnetic therapy, involves the use of magnets to relieve acute and chronic pain. Practitioners claim they can also be used for basic first aid to treat sprains, strains, burns, headache, and insect bites. In the United States, most reports about magnetic therapy are based on anecdotal evidence rather than on research. However, clinical research is being conducted in various centers to investigate the use of magnets for fibromyalgia and phantom limb pain (Springhouse, 1999).

INVASIVE PAIN MANAGEMENT TECHNIQUES FOR CHRONIC PAIN. Invasive techniques are used to interrupt the pain pathways when pain is intractable (not able to be relieved) or severely debilitating. Depending on the technique, some degree of neurologic deficits and nerve destruction is expected. Various invasive techniques are used when chronic or persistent pain can no longer be adequately controlled with drugs or other pain-reducing methods.

NERVE BLOCKS. Nerve blocks can be used for both diagnostic and treatment purposes. These procedures are usually indicated for pain confined to a specific area or nerve distribution. This technique involves localizing a nerve root (or roots) and injecting it with either a local anesthetic for temporary relief or diagnostic evaluations or with a chemical agent (e.g., phenol or alcohol) to achieve permanent neurolysis or nerve destruction. Temporary blocks or permanent destruction (neuroablation) might be considered in areas such as the intercostal nerves, celiac plexus, superior hypogastric block, or craniofacial nerves.

The complications associated with nerve block vary. In general, injecting a local anesthetic or chemical agent into a peripheral nerve root leads to decreased sensation in the area; motor function is not affected. Injecting a local anesthetic into the lumbosacral area of the spinal cord area may cause transient motor and bowel and bladder dysfunction. Neurolysis of the lumbosacral nerves can damage motor nerve roots, resulting in lost or impaired bowel, bladder, or sexual function. This procedure is usually reserved for clients with intractable cancer-related pain.

Before permanent neurolysis is considered, a temporary nerve block may be given to determine the degree of relief obtained from disrupting the nerve impulses. Although the intent of neurolysis is to permanently destroy nerve transmission, clients may experience only short-term pain relief because of nerve cell regeneration or the development of alternative pathways capable of transmitting pain. Although relatively new, permanent ablation of nerve roots can be performed with thermal techniques such as radiofrequency ablation (uses heat) or cryoanalgesia (uses cold).

Because a nerve block is an invasive procedure performed by anesthesiologists, neurosurgeons, surgeons, and neurologists, the physician is responsible for informing the client about the procedure and its risks and alternative treatments. The nurse reinforces this information with the client and family.

Epidural steroids may also be used for pain, but their use in certain pain conditions is controversial. Some investigators have looked at the evidence for the use of epidural steroids for low back pain (Koes et al., 1995). Their review of 12 randomized clinical trials found this treatment to be effective in only half of the published studies. They concluded that the benefits of epidural injection, if any, are of short duration.

SPINAL CORD STIMULATION. Spinal cord stimulator therapy offers a more invasive method of nerve stimulation. This technique involves the use of electrodes implanted under the skin and into the area of nerve(s) responsible for the pain. At first, a trial of spinal cord stimulation is attempted through the use of temporary externalized electrodes that are implanted and connected to a stimulator device. The amount of electrical current is adjusted to provide pain relief without additional discomfort. If this trial is successful, the client undergoes surgery for placement of a permanent implantable stimulator. Forrest (1996) discusses the nursing implications associated with this technique.

SURGICAL TECHNIQUES. The surgical techniques aimed at surgically interrupting the transmission of pain include rhizotomy and cordotomy. These two procedures are not performed as commonly today because of the new, improved pain management measures currently available (Figure 7-8).

In **rhizotomy,** sensory nerve roots are destroyed where they enter the spinal cord. In a *closed* rhizotomy, a percutaneous catheter is inserted into the area, and the sensory nerve roots are destroyed by chemicals, coagulation, or cryodestruction (extreme cold). A laminectomy is necessary for an *open* rhizotomy. During this surgery, the physician isolates and destroys the nerve roots.

In a **cordotomy,** the surgeon cuts the pain pathways at the midline portion of the spinal cord—before nerve impulses ascend to the spinothalamic tract. As with the other surgical procedures, clients may experience impaired bowel, bladder, or sexual function. Because of the complexity of the pain experience, the interruption of nerve conduction and pain pathways may not completely interrupt the client's sensation of pain.

After surgical intervention, the nurse assesses the nature of the neurologic deficits, if any, and teaches the client how to adapt to them. If the client has lost sensation in a body area, he or she will need to learn how to protect that area from harm. The nurse also assesses expectations in relation to the surgery and helps the client to express realistic expectations.

STIMULATION TECHNIQUES. Acupuncture and dorsal column stimulation achieve pain control by stimulating certain parts of the nervous system.

ACUPUNCTURE. The practice of acupuncture originated in China. According to ancient beliefs, the body is divided into 10 sections by lines, or meridians. Specific acupuncture points are located within these meridians. The acupuncturist inserts tiny needles into the skin and subcutaneous tissues at these points, and manual vibration or electrical stimulation is delivered. This complementary technique is used to relieve pain and is thought to cure certain diseases.

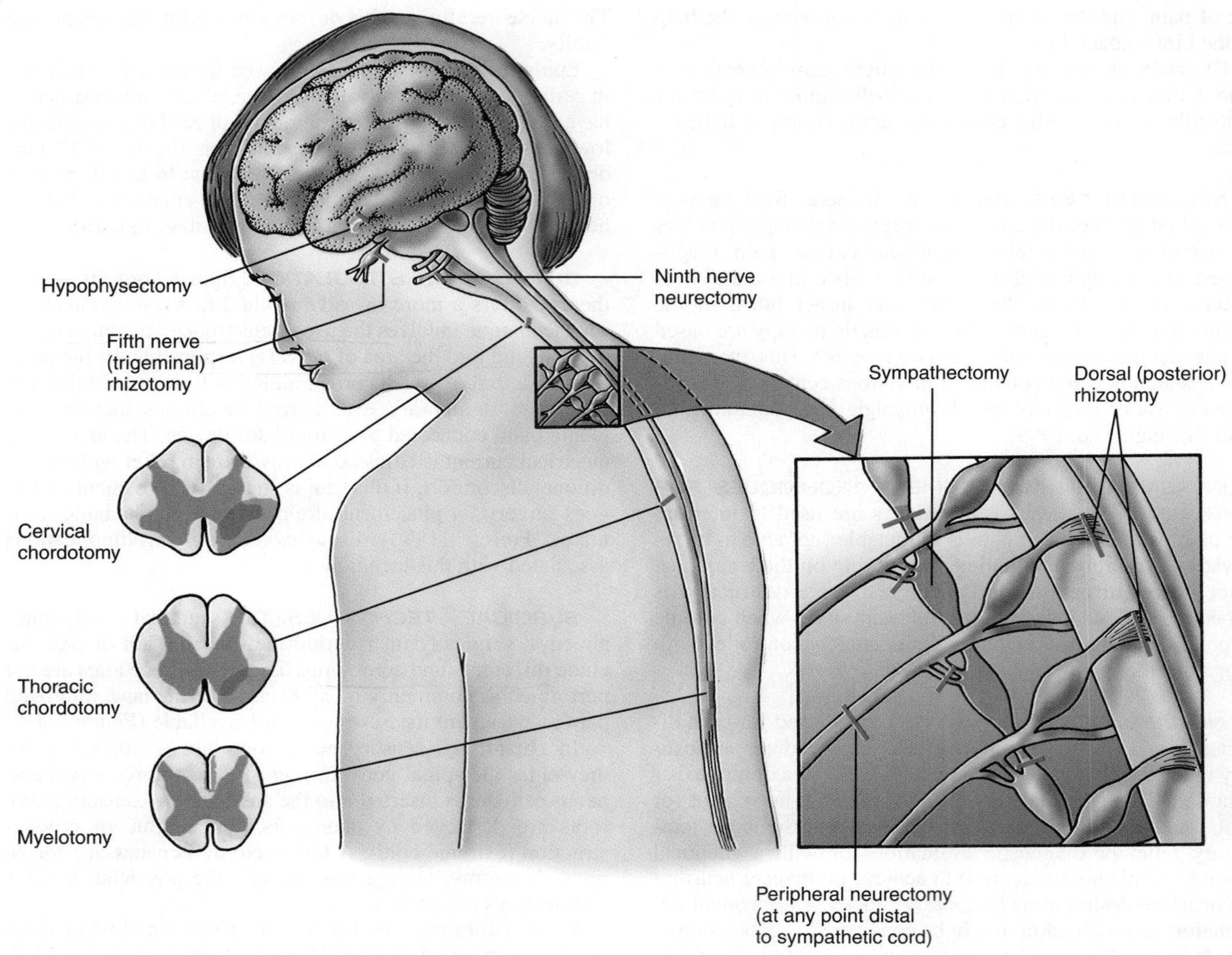

Figure 7-8 ● Surgical procedures designed to alleviate pain.

Acupuncture is still widely acclaimed in China but is less popular in the West. Because the physiologic basis for this technique is unclear, many Western health care professionals are skeptical about its usefulness. Nonetheless, acupuncture is practiced for the treatment of pain and for anesthetic purposes during diagnostic procedures, labor and delivery, and surgery. It is also used to help clients change their behavior (e.g., smoking cessation). More than 1000 acupuncture sites have been identified, and 14 "lines" exist as meridians (Figure 7-9).

DORSAL COLUMN STIMULATION. Dorsal column stimulation is a temporary or permanent way of stimulating nerve roots in the spinal cord to override painful stimuli. Good candidates for this procedure are usually those who derive some benefit from the application of transcutaneous electrical nerve stimulation (TENS). Percutaneous electrodes can be inserted into the epidural space in close proximity to nerve roots entering the dorsal horn of the spinal cord. The electrodes are connected to an external device capable of delivering an electrical current. Clients who respond to this technique may progress to permanent implantable stimulators.

Community-Based Care

For some clients, the pain experience extends beyond hospitalization. Effective analgesic regimens or pain-relieving strategies should be coordinated before discharge if clients are to leave the hospital with pain. The nurse ensures that the client, especially one who is opioid dependent, has enough pain medication to last at least until the first follow-up visit.

HOME CARE MANAGEMENT

Preparation for home care is carried out with the client and family. The nurse assesses the physical layout of the home and related environment. Together with the client and family, the nurse, discharge planner, or occupational therapist determines whether modifications are necessary for maintaining a

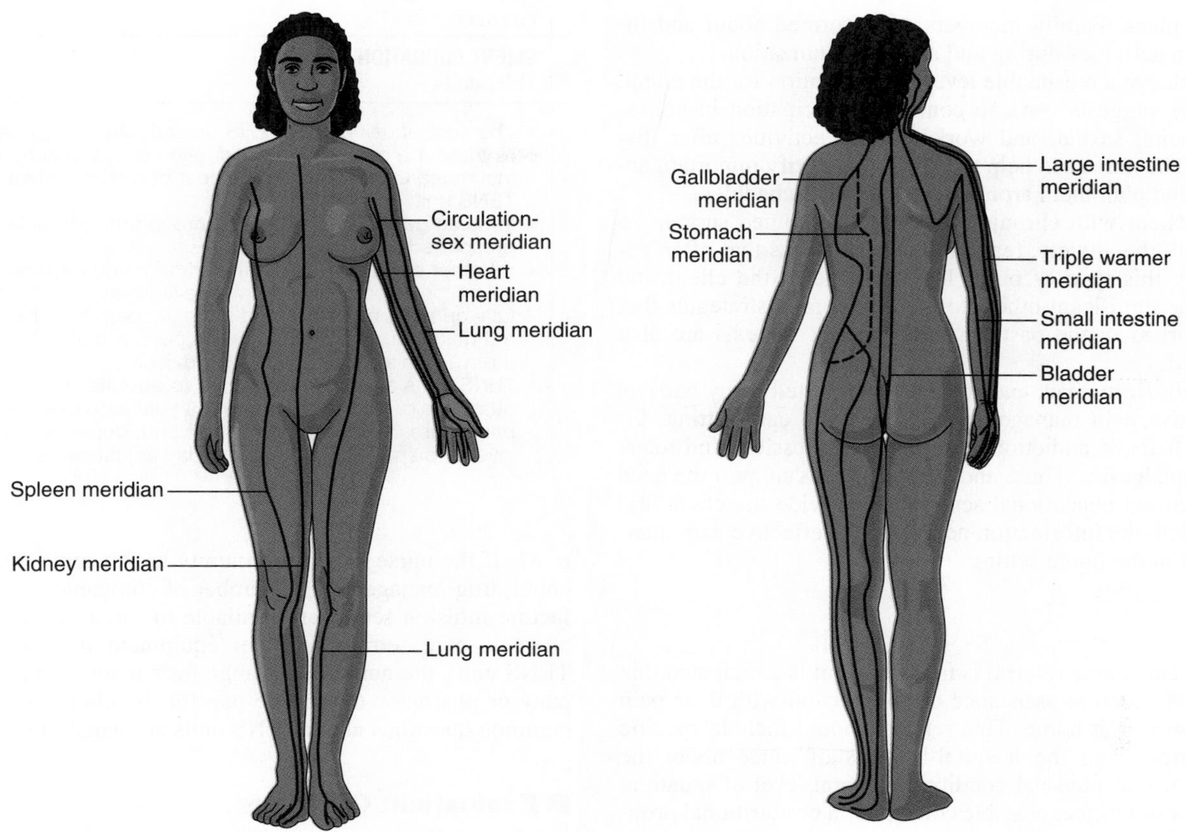

Figure 7-9 ● Acupuncture meridians.

reasonably pain-free regimen after discharge. Fatigue heightens the awareness of pain. If physical modifications (e.g., installing a downstairs bathroom) are unrealistic (too expensive or unacceptable to the client or family), the caregiver suggests schedule changes, role responsibilities, and daily routines to help avoid fatigue.

At home, clients may require a referral for physical therapy, especially to continue treatment with cutaneous stimulation, TENS, or heat or cold techniques. Clients may need a psychiatric clinical nurse specialist or social worker to assist them in developing coping strategies or maintaining adequate family dynamics. A hospice referral (hospital- or community-based) can help maintain continuity of care in the management of terminally ill clients. Clients with cancer may be at risk for developing uncontrolled pain that results in hospitalization if it cannot be managed at home (Plaisance, 1997). It is important that nurses be knowledgeable about palliative care and end-of-life issues so they are better able to manage pain crises.

The growing number of home infusion therapy programs provides a wide variety of services to clients who require technology-supported pain care at home. Many of these services depend on approval by the insurance carrier, usually before analgesic options are considered and placement of technology is performed. Well-defined home agency practices and professional support at home are key if clients are required to leave the hospital with infusional pain therapy.

HEALTH TEACHING

The nurse directs educational efforts toward involving clients and their families in continuing health care behaviors that relieve pain and improve psychologic well-being and overall functional status. The nurse teaches the client and family about analgesic regimens, including any technical skills needed to administer or deliver the analgesic, the purpose and action of medications, their side effects or adverse reactions, and the importance of dosage intervals. The nurse also teaches the client or family members how to prevent or treat the constipation commonly associated with taking opioid analgesics and other pain medications.

The nurse explains that, ideally, the analgesic regimen should not interfere with the client's sleep, rest, appetite, or level of physical mobility. If such interference occurs, the nurse encourages the family or significant other to consult with the physician or visiting nurse.

In clients with pain from advanced cancer, all efforts should be directed toward maximizing pain relief and symptom control at home to eliminate unnecessary readmissions. This may mean that the physician prescribes a flexible analgesic schedule that allows the client to adjust analgesics according to the amount of pain. The nurse teaches the client and family how to safely increase the medication within the prescribed dosing guidelines.

The nurse evaluates family support systems to assist the client in adhering to and continuing the proposed medical and nursing plans. Family members are informed about and included in activities during and after hospitalization.

To achieve a reasonable level of expectation for the client, the nurse suggests ways to continue participation in household, social, sexual, and work-oriented activities after discharge. The nurse can help the client to identify important activities and plan them around adequate rest schedules.

The client with chronic pain needs continued support to cope with the anxiety, fear, and powerlessness that often accompany this type of pain. The nurse helps the client and family or significant others to identify coping strategies that have worked in the past. Outside support systems are also identified.

Ferrell, Borneman, and Juarez (1998) noted many barriers to effective pain management in the home care setting, including fears of addiction, respiratory depression, and tolerance to analgesics. These and other concerns support the need for structured educational sessions to provide the client and family with the information necessary for effective pain management in the home setting.

HEALTH CARE RESOURCES

A home care nurse referral is made when it is anticipated that clients will require assistance or supervision with their pain relief regimen at home. This referral should include specific information from the hospital-based staff nurse about the client's overall physical condition, general level of sedation, weakness or fatigue, possible constipation or nutritional problems, and sleep patterns.

In addition to explaining the client's physical status to the home care nurse, the staff nurse also describes the client's levels of anxiety and depression and general expectations about pain status after discharge. The nurse describes family interactions and determines whether the client or family anticipates any altered role functions at home. The client's close relationships and available support network are important factors in providing ongoing support for effective pain intervention strategies.

Referrals to an advanced practice nurse pain specialist, social worker, or psychologist are appropriate ways to continue providing emotional support to the client and family, reinforce instructions for cognitive or behavioral strategies to deal with pain, and evaluate overall physical and emotional adaptation after discharge. These health care professionals can also direct the client and family to appropriate resources (e.g., pain clinics and support groups).

Clients with chronic pain often require treatment and support beyond that available in the traditional health care system. For this reason, pain clinics or programs have evolved over the past 25 years. The underlying premise of these clinics is to foster independence and self-care behaviors while promoting pain control and maximizing quality of life. These programs use analgesics, adjuvant drug therapy, physical measures, cognitive and behavioral strategies, surgical interventions, and individual and group counseling for clients and family. The emphasis on many of the measures differs according to the orientation of the program.

Some clients receive continuous or intermittent opioid administration at home or in a long-term care facility by any one of the methods described under Drug Therapy (Chronic Pain), p. 81. If the nurse in the community health setting is unsure about drug management, a number of companies that manufacture infusion setups are available to assist in the home or alternate care setting. If other equipment is needed (e.g., TENS unit), the nurse can arrange for a medical supply company or pharmacy to provide one for the client. Answers to common questions about TENS units are listed in Chart 7-3.

CHART 7-3

CLIENT EDUCATION GUIDE
TENS Units

- The cost of using your TENS unit should be comparable to that for a regimen of prescription drugs or surgery.
- Insurance usually covers the cost of buying or leasing a TENS unit.
- You can get a TENS unit only through the physician who prescribed it.
- Whether or not a TENS unit works for you depends on your type of pain. These units have been used successfully on back pain, arm and leg pain, pain from neuralgia, arthritis pain, and other types of pain. A trial period under a physician's care is generally advised.
- TENS units are relatively simple to operate. You simply attach color-coded electrodes to your skin over the painful area. You turn on the unit and, depending on your level of pain, you make day-to-day adjustments.

Evaluation: Outcomes

NOC Historically, inadequate attention has been given to evaluating the effects of pain interventions. Measures of evaluation in this area have focused on the impact of pain on the client's quality of life, the effect of pain on the client's functional status, and the role of family caregivers.

Many factors may interfere with adequate pain relief measures in the home setting. Caregivers may not assess the degree of pain relief and intensity accurately or often enough. Nurses may not establish pain relief goals that are consistent with the expectations of the client and family. Because of these and other factors, the client may be at risk for further pain, frustration, lack of control, feelings of abandonment, and social isolation.

The nurse evaluates care for the client with pain on the basis of the identified nursing diagnoses. The expected outcomes are that the client will:

- Report that acute pain is relieved or reduced
- Report that chronic pain is relieved or reduced or that the pain is not worsened
- Establish realistic goals given the limitations imposed by chronic pain
- Perform activities of daily living
- Participate in his or her usual daily lifestyle, with modifications as needed

PAIN AS A QUALITY IMPROVEMENT OUTCOME

Today many hospitals and other health care facilities rely on quality improvement (QI) programs to evaluate pain care and direct the implementation of pain care strategies. These programs focus on critical pain outcomes that serve as indicators

COST OF CARE
IMPLICATIONS FOR NURSING

CURRENT COSTS OF COMMON ANALGESIC AGENTS

	DOSE/FREQUENCY	COST/DAY (MANUFACTURER)
Opioids		
Roxanol (MSO_4)	30-mL bottle	$20.76
Morphine Liquid 20 mg/mL	120-mL bottle	$77.96
MSIR	15-mg tab/#100	$21.70
	30-mg tab/#100	$36.67
MS Contin	30-mg tab/#100	$189.34
	60-mg tab/#100	$369.44
Oramorph SR	30-mg tab/#100	$183.40
	60-mg tab/#100	$313.15
Kadian	20-mg caps/#60	$76.50
	50-mg caps/#60	$184.72
	100-mg caps/#60	$330.00
Dilaudid	2-mg tab/#100	$57.68
	4-mg tab/#100	$87.70
Oxycodone	5-mg tab/#100	$39.99 (Amide)
	5-mg tab/#10	$35.75 (Ethex)
	5-mg tab/#10	$41.99 (Global)
Oxyfast (Oxycodone HCL)	20 mg/mL/30 mL	$33.75
OxyContin	10-mg tab/#100	$117.10
	20-mg tab/#100	$224.11
	40-mg tab/#100	$397.66
Methadone	5-mg tab/#100	$32.53
	10-mg tab/#100	$37.01
Morphine	1 mg/mL/10 mL amp	$8.86-23.01
Dilaudid	1 mg/mL/1 mL amp	$12.19
	1 mg/mL 10 × 1 mL amp	$9.62 (generic cost)
NSAIDs		
Acetaminophen	650 mg q4h	OTC
Aspirin	650 mg q4h	OTC
Ibuprofen	400 mg q6h	$0.52
	600 mg q6h	$0.70
Choline Magnesium Trisalicylate	1000 mg tid	$1.73
Diflunisal	500 mg q12h	$1.80
Etodolac	400 mg q8h	$3.97
Fenoprofen	600 mg q6h	$1.92
Ketoprofen	50 mg q8h	$2.76
Ketorolac (Toradol)	10 mg q6h	$4.22
Meclofenamate sodium	50 mg q6h	$1.19
Mefenamic acid	250 mg q6h	$4.36
Naproxen	250 mg q6h	$2.80
Naproxen sodium	275 mg q6h	$2.75
Ketorolac (parenteral)	30 mg q6h	$18.58
Cyclooxygenase-2 Inhibitors		
Celecoxib (Celebrex)	200 mg/day	$2.42
Rofecoxib (Vioxx)	25 mg/day	$2.42

Data from *Drug Topics Red Book.* (1999). Montvale, NJ: Medical Economics Data Company.

of how well pain is managed. The indicators are assessed, documented, monitored over time, and evaluated against predetermined standards. The introduction of the Agency for Healthcare Research and Quality *Clinical Practice Guidelines* for acute pain (Acute Pain Management Guideline Panel, 1992) and cancer pain (Jacox et al., 1994) offers clinicians a useful framework for designing QI initiatives.

The American Pain Society Quality of Care Committee (1995) highlights five critical components of a QI program for pain. Programs should be based on the following tenets: (1) unrelieved pain should attract clinicians' attention, (2) information about analgesics should be accessible where orders are written, (3) clients should be assured of responsive analgesic care and urged to communicate pain, (4) policies and safeguards should be implemented for the use of technology-supported pain care, and (5) implementation of these measures should be assessed and coordinated. Many clients, however, report little use of the full range of approaches specified in the AHCPR Guidelines in the management of their pain (McNeill et al., 1998). Reports indicate that clients feel more satisfied with care when health care providers place a priority on pain management.

COSTS OF PAIN CARE

When caring for clients with pain, the nurse appreciates the financial aspects of pain care, especially in the current climate of managed care. Several factors are associated with medication costs. First, costs differ depending on the location of administration. Parenteral drug therapy may be more costly when administered in a hospital setting than at home. Second, the commercial success of the agent influences the price of a pharmaceutical product. Third, the type of manufacturer and the history of drug development and testing influences the market price of a drug. Drug innovations such as extended-release or controlled-release products may be more costly per tablet than short-acting agents. Although the cost of the overall therapy (dose per day) may be similar or only slightly more, many hospice-based care programs are reluctant to use sustained-release analgesics because of the increased cost. Despite the inflated costs of extended-release or controlled-release preparations, clients report better compliance and achieve better pain control. The approximate cost of common analgesics is found in the Cost of Care box at left. A cost-analysis framework for evaluating the economic implications for pain care is provided in Table 7-8.

Technology-supported pain care is always associated with increased costs, but the financial expenditures may be beneficial in terms of improved clinical outcomes. Epidural analgesia and patient-controlled analgesia in the immediate postoperative period have shown significant benefits in improving pain control and recovery compared with intermittent nurse-administered analgesics. The use of technology in delivering analgesia may also be cost-efficient for certain clients with intractable chronic nonmalignant and cancer-related pain.

The oral route is preferred for long-term pain management. The nurse considers the cost of both opioid and nonopioid analgesics to ensure that the cost of drug therapy is within the client's financial budget. Knowing the client's prescription plan aids the nurse in assessing "out-of-pocket" expenses.

TABLE 7-8 • ECONOMICS OF PAIN CARE: COST ANALYSIS FRAMEWORK

- Costs associated with oral alternative route medications
- Costs associated with parenteral/neuraxial administration
- Unreimbursed charges of medication therapy
- Costs of surgical interventions
- Costs of specialized pain care
- Costs of nondrug measures
- Expenditures to justify costs
- Reimbursement issues
- Expenditures by various health care settings and home costs associated with preventing and treating complications of pain/pain therapy

Modified from Agency for Health Care Policy and Research (1994). *Clinical Practice Guidelines for Cancer Pain;* from Ferrell, B.R., Griffith, H. (1994). Cost issues related to pain management: Report from the Cancer Pain Panel of the Agency for Health Care Policy and Research. *Journal of Pain and Symptom Management, 9*(4), 221-234.

The nurse must also factor in any other health care expenditures for the client or family. Some pharmaceutical companies, usually manufacturers of opioid analgesics, supply indigent clients with free medication if they meet certain eligibility criteria.

Significant health care costs are associated with hospitalizations for pain control. Many health insurance companies do not view a hospital admission for uncontrolled pain as necessary, especially in palliative care. Therefore reimbursement for hospital days is lower unless the client has another primary diagnosis. The nurse recognizes the importance of aggressive pain care to facilitate discharge and prevent subsequent hospitalizations for pain. The hospital-based case manager can assist in meeting this goal by coordinating communication with members of the health care team. Appropriate follow-up at home must be provided by knowledgeable home care nurses who can advocate for appropriate adjustments in analgesic regimens based on their clients' needs.

The cost of care must be understood in a broader way than just the money spent on pain medications or time lost from the job market. Pain, especially chronic pain, can disrupt the life of clients and families. Some of these costs are reimbursed by insurance, but many are not well understood or quantifiable.

ONLINE RESOURCES

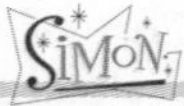

For suggested readings and Internet resources, go to http://www.wbsaunders.com/SIMON/Iggy/.

SELECTED BIBLIOGRAPHY

Asterisk indicates a classic or definitive work on this subject.

Acello, B. (2000). Meeting JCAHO standards for pain control. *Nursing2000, 30*(3), 52-54.

*Acute Pain Management Guideline Panel. (1992). *Acute pain management: Operative or medical procedures and trauma. Clinical practice guideline.* AHCPR Pub. No. 92-0032. Rockville, MD: Agency for Health Care Policy and Research, Public Health Service, U.S. Department of Health and Human Services.

American Pain Society. (1999). *Principles of analgesic use in the treatment of acute pain and cancer pain* (4th ed.). Glenview, IL: American Pain Society.

*American Pain Society Quality of Care Committee. (1995). Quality improvement guidelines for the treatment of acute pain and cancer pain. *Journal of American Medical Association, 274*(23), 1874-1880.

Backonja, M., et al. for the Gabapentin Diabetic Neuropathy Study Group. (1998). Gabapentin for the symptomatic treatment of painful neuropathy in patients with diabetes mellitus. A randomized controlled trial. *Journal of the American Medical Association, 280*(21), 1831-1836.

Bell, M.L., & Reeves, K.A. (1999). Postoperative pain management in the non-Hispanic white and Mexican American older adult. *Seminars in Perioperative Nursing, 8*(1), 7-11.

Bernabei, R., et al. for the SAGE Study Group.(1998). Management of pain in elderly patients with cancer. *Journal of the American Medical Association, 279*(23), 1877-1882.

Berry, P.H., & Dahl, J.L. (2000). The new JCAHO pain standards: Implications for pain management nurses. *Pain Management Nursing, 1*(1), 3-12.

*Bigos, S., et al. (1994). *Acute low back problems in adults. Clinical practice guideline: Quick reference guide number 14.* AHCPR Pub. No. 95-0643. Rockville, MD: Agency for Health Care Policy and Research, Public Health Service, U.S. Department of Health and Human Services.

Breitbart, W., Rosenfeld, B., & Passik, S.D. (1998). The Network Project: A multidisciplinary cancer education and training in pain management, rehabilitation, and psychosocial issues. *Journal of Pain and Symptom Management, 15(*1), 18-26.

*Calvillo, E.R., & Flaskerud, J.H. (1991). Review of literature on culture and pain of adults with focus of Mexican-Americans. *Journal of Transcultural Nursing, 2*(2), 16-23.

Cederholm, I. (1997). Preliminary risk-benefit analysis of ropivacaine in labour and following surgery. *Drug Safety, 16*(6), 391-402.

Chandler, S. (1999). Oral transmucosal fentanyl citrate: A new treatment for breakthrough pain. *American Journal of Hospice and Palliative Care, 16*(2), 489-491.

*Cleeland, C.S., et al. (1994). Pain and its treatment in outpatients with metastatic cancer. *The New England Journal of Medicine, 330*(9), 592-596.

*Cobb, S.C., & Mindel, S.A. (1996). Creating a cost-effective pain management task force in a community hospital. *MEDSURG Nursing, 5*(6), 445-448.

Drayer, R.A., Henderson, J., & Reidenberg, M. (1999). Barriers to better pain management control in hospitalized patients. *Journal of Pain and Symptom Management, 17,* 434-440.

*Dunbar, S.A., & Katz, N.P. (1996). Chronic opioid therapy for nonmalignant pain in clients with a history of substance abuse: Report of 20 cases. *Journal of Pain and Symptom Management, 11*(3), 163-171.

Eckes Peck, S.D. (1997). The effectiveness of therapeutic touch for decreasing pain in elders with degenerative arthritis. *Journal of Holistic Nursing, 15*(2), 176-198.

Ellison, N., et al. (1997). Phase III placebo-control trial of capsaicin cream in the management of surgical neuropathic pain in cancer patients. *Journal of Clinical Oncology, 15*(8), 2974-2980.

*Faucett, J.A. (1994). Depression in painful chronic disorders: The role of pain and conflict about pain. *Journal of Pain and Symptom Management, 9*(8), 520-526.

Feldt, K.S. (2000). The checklist of nonverbal pain indicators (CNPI). *Pain Management Nursing, 1*(1), 13-21.

*Ferrell, B.R., & Griffith, H. (1994). Cost issues related to pain management: Report from the Cancer Pain Panel of the Agency for Health Care Policy and Research. *Journal of Pain and Symptom Management, 9*(4), 221-234.

Ferrell, B.R., & McCaffery, M. (1997). Nurses' knowledge about equianalgesia and opioid dosing. *Cancer Nursing, 20*(3), 201-212.

Ferrell, B.R., Borneman, T., & Juarez, G. (1998). Integration of pain education in home care. *Journal of Palliative Care, 14(3)*, 62-68.

*Ferrell, B.A., Ferrell, B.R., & Osterweil, D. (1990). Pain in the nursing home. *Journal of the American Geriatrics Society, 38*, 409-414.

*Fishbain, D.A., et al. (1996). Transcutaneous electrical nerve stimulation (TENS) treatment outcome in long-term users. *Clinical Journal of Pain, 12*(3), 201-214.

*Flor, H., Fydrich, T., & Turk, D.C. (1992). Efficacy of multidisciplinary pain treatment centers: A meta-analytic review. *Pain, 49*(2), 221-230.

*Forrest, D.M. (1996). Spinal cord stimulator therapy. *Journal of Peri-Anesthesia Nursing, 11*(5), 349-352.

Furstenberg, C.T., et al. (1998). Knowledge and attitudes of health care providers toward cancer pain management: A comparison of physicians, nurses, and pharmacists in the state of New Hampshire. *Journal of Pain and Symptom Management, 15*(6), 335-349.

*Herr, KA., & Mobily, P.R. (1991). Complexities of pain assessment in the elderly. *Journal of Gerontological Nursing, 17*(4), 12-19.

*International Association on Pain, Subcommittee of Taxonomy. (1979). Pain terms: A list with definitions and notes on usage. *Pain, 6*, 249.

*Jacox, A.K., et al. (1994). *Management of cancer pain: Adults. Clinical practice guideline No. 9.* AHCPR Pub. No. 94-0593. Rockville, MD: Agency for Health Care Policy and Research, Public Health Service, U.S. Department of Health and Human Services.

Johnson, D.L. (1998). Pharmacologic pain management for the cancer patient at home. *Home Healthcare Nurse, 16*(3), 166-174.

*Keeney, S.A. (1993). Nursing care of the postoperative patient receiving epidural analgesia. *MEDSURG Nursing, 2*(3), 191-196.

*Keller, E., & Bzdek, V. (1986). Effects of therapeutic touch on tension headache pain. *Nursing Research, 35*, 101-105.

*Koes, B.W., et al. (1995). Efficacy of epidural steroid injections for low back pain and sciatica: A systematic review of randomized clinical trials. *Pain, 63*, 279-288.

*Kreiger, D. (1975). Therapeutic touch: The imprimatur of nursing. *American Journal of Nursing, 75*, 784-787.

Kwekkeboom, K.L. (1997). The placebo effect in symptom management. *Oncology Nursing Forum, 24*(8), 1393-1399.

Kwekkeboom, K., Huseby-Moore, K., Ward, S. (1998). Imaging ability and effective use of guided imagery. *Research in Nursing and Health, 21*, 189-198.

Lane, N.E. (1997). Pain management in osteoarthritis: The role of COX-2 inhibitors. *The Journal of Rheumatology, 24*(Suppl. 49), 20-24.

Levin, M.L., Berry, J.I., & Leiter, J. (1998). Management of pain in terminally ill patients: Physician report of knowledge, attitudes, and behavior. *Journal of Pain and symptom Management, 15*(1), 27-40.

Loeb, J.L. (1999). Pain management in long-term care. *American Journal of Nursing, 99*(2), 48-52.

*Malek, C.J., & Olivieri, R.J. (1996). Pain management: Documenting the decision making process. *Nursing Case Management, 1*(2), 64-74.

*McCaffery, M. (1979). *Nursing management of the patient with pain* (2nd ed.). Philadelphia: J.B. Lippincott.

McCaffery, M., & Ferrell, B.R. (1999). Opioids and pain management: What do nurses know? *Nursing99, 29*(3), 48-52.

*McGuire, L. (1994). The nurse's role in pain relief. *MEDSURG Nursing, 3*(2), 94-107.

McNeill, J.A., et al. (1998). Assessing clinical outcomes: Patient satisfaction with pain management. *Journal of Pain and Symptom Management, 16*(1), 29-40.

*Melzack, R. (1975). The McGill Pain Questionnaire: Major properties and scoring methods. *Pain, 1*, 277-299.

*Melzack, R., & Wall, P.D. (1982). *The challenge of pain.* New York: Basic Books.

*Miller, J., et al. (1996). The assessment of discomfort in elderly confused patients: A preliminary study. *Journal of Neuroscience Nursing, 28*(3), 175-182.

*Mobily, P.R., Herr, K.A., & Nicholson, A.C. (1994). Validation of cutaneous stimulation interventions for pain management. *International Journal of Nursing Studies, 31*(6), 533-544.

*Mulloney, S.S., & Wells-Federman, C. (1996). Therapeutic touch: A healing modality. *Journal of Cardiovascular Nursing, 10*(30), 27-49.

*Neeley, M.A. (1993). Pain management in elderly clients. *MEDSURG Nursing Quarterly, 1*(4), 32-51.

*Neill, K.M. (1993). Ethnic pain styles in acute myocardial infarction. *Western Journal of Nursing Research, 15*(5), 531-547.

Nordin, M., & Campello, M. (1999). Physical therapy exercises and the modalities: When, what, and why? *Neurologic Clinics of North America, 17*(1), 75-89.

*Pasero, C.L. (1994). Pain control. *American Journal of Nursing, 94*(2), 22-23.

Plaisance, L. (1997). Managing cancer pain crisis effectively in the home. *Home Healthcare Nurse, 15*(6), 411-413.

*Polomano, R.C. (1995). The relationship of pain characteristics, type of cancer, and opioid consumption to quality of life, psychological distress and pain outcomes. Unpublished doctoral dissertation, University of Maryland, Baltimore.

*Polomano, R.C., Blumenthal, N.P., & Riegler, F.X. (1993). Intrapleural analgesia for the management of postoperative pain. *MEDSURG Nursing, 2*(3), 185-190.

Polomano, R.C., Soulen, M., & McDaniel, C. (1997). Sedation and analgesia with interventional radiology for oncology patients. *Critical Care Nursing Clinics of North America, 9*(3), 335-353.

Ramer, L., et al. (1999). Multimeasure pain assessment in an ethnically diverse group of patients with cancer. *Journal of Transcultural Nursing, 10*(2), 94-101.

Rauck, R.L. (1997). Intraspinal therapy in the management of refractory cancer pain. *Techniques in Regional Anesthesia and Pain Management, 1*(1), 38-48.

Redmond, B. (1998). Barriers to the effective management of pain. *International Journal of Palliative Nursing, 4*(6), 276-283.

Rowbotham, M., et al. for the Gabapentin Post-Herpetic Neuralgia Study Group. (1998). Gabapentin for the treatment of postherpetic neuralgia: A randomized controlled trial. *Journal of the American Medical Association, 280*(21), 1837-1842.

*Ruda, M.A. (1993). Gender and pain. *Pain, 53*, 1-2.

Siddall, P.J., & Cousins, M.J. (1997). Spinal update: Spinal pain mechanisms. *Spine, 22*(1), 98-104.

*Sloman, R. (1995). Relaxation and the relief of cancer pain. *Nursing Clinics of North America, 30*(4), 697-709.

Springhouse. (1999). *Nurse's handbook of alternative and complementary therapies.* Springhouse, PA: Author.

*Sternbach, R.A. (1968). *Pain: A psychophysiological analysis.* New York: Academic Press.

Stuppy, D.J. (1998). The Faces Pain Scale: Reliability and validity with mature adults. *Applied Nursing Research, 11*(2), 84-89.

Tusek, D., Church, J.M., Fazio, V.W. (1997). Guided imagery as a coping strategy for perioperative patients. *AORN Journal, 66*(4), 644-649.

*Vallerand, A.H. (1991). The use of narcotic analgesics in chronic nonmalignant pain. *Holistic Nursing Practice, 6*(1), 17-23.

*Vallerand, A.H. (1994). Street addicts and patients with pain: Similarities and differences. *Clinical Nurse Specialist, 8*(1), 11-15.

*Vallerand, A.H. (1995). Gender differences in pain. *Image: Journal of Nursing Scholarship, 27*(3), 235-237.

Vigano, A., Bruera, E., & Suarez-Almazor, M. (1998). Age, pain intensity, and opioid dose in patients with advanced cancer. *Cancer, 83*(6), 1244-1250.

Vourakis, C. (1998). Substance abuse concerns in the treatment of pain. *Nursing Clinics of North America, 33*(1), 47-59.

Wallace, K.G. (1997). Analysis of recent literature concerning relaxation and imagery interventions for cancer pain. *Cancer Nursing, 20*(2), 79-87.

*Wild, L., & Coyne, C. (1992). The basics and beyond: Epidural analgesia. *American Journal of Nursing, 92*(4), 26-34.

Won, A. et al. (1999). Correlates and management of nonmalignant pain in the nursing home. SAGE Study Group: Systematic Assessment of Geriatric drug use via Epidemiology. *Journal of the American Geriatrics Society, 47*(8), 936-942.

*Zatzick, D.F., & Dimsdale, J.E. (1990). Cultural variations in response to painful stimuli. *Psychosomatic Medicine, 52*, 544-557.

*Zimmerman L., et al. (1996). Psychological variables and cancer pain. *Cancer Nursing, 19*(1), 44-53.

CHAPTER

8

Substance Abuse

TOMMIE WRIGHT PNIEWSKI • DONNA D. IGNATAVICIUS

Learning Objectives

After studying this chapter, you should be able to:

1. Discuss substance abuse as a major health problem in the United States.
2. Explain the effects of substance abuse on the mental and physical health of individuals and society.
3. Describe the relationship between stress and substance abuse.
4. Identify assessment findings associated with use of stimulants, hallucinogens, depressants, opioids, inhalants, and steroids.
5. Discuss priorities for care of clients who have or are experiencing substance abuse.
6. Identify signs and symptoms of alcohol withdrawal.

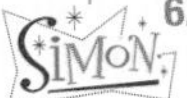

Go to http://www.wbsaunders.com/SIMON/Iggy/ for self-assessment questions related to these Learning Objectives.

OVERVIEW

Substance abuse is described as the overindulgence of a chemical substance and the resulting dependence that interferes with life's activities. Each year there are alarming increases in the abuse of mind- and mood-altering substances, such as alcohol, marijuana, methamphetamine, and nicotine products. The mental and physical health of the individual is affected by substance abuse, which can also significantly affect the lives of others. Productivity is drastically reduced, and the costs of abuse to society are enormous. In 1995 the economic cost of substance abuse was $276 billion—$166 billion due to alcohol abuse and $110 billion due to drug abuse (National Institute on Drug Abuse [NIDA], 2000).

Categories of substances commonly abused include stimulants, hallucinogens, depressants, opioids (narcotics), and other substances that alter the mind. Stimulants are abused by some clients because the need for "faster, better, and longer" exists as a mindset in society. Hallucinogens continue to be popular in various forms but are commonly encountered as mind-altering drugs such as phencyclidine (PCP) and lysergic acid (LSD). Depressants, such as the anxiolytic drugs, are becoming increasingly popular as a maladaptive alternative in responding to the ever-increasing demands of today's busy lifestyles. Opioids and morphine derivatives, although important for therapeutic uses for pain relief, continue to be abused and addictive in the drug community.

Prescription drugs can also easily become addictive because of the nature of their action in the brain and because of the tendency of the client to become comfortable with the effects of the drug long after the therapeutic need is satisfied. Improper use of therapeutic substances can result in addiction; such substances may also be used improperly for pleasure-seeking effects. Examples of therapeutic prescription drugs that can produce addiction or be used for maladaptive purposes are morphine, barbiturates, and benzodiazepines.

Challenges for the health care professional include preparedness to intervene in the risk behaviors created by substance use or abuse. This health problem is not limited to teenagers or to an impoverished population. All age-groups and socioeconomic groups are vulnerable to substance abuse. The professional who is knowledgeable about substance abuse will be able to identify and appropriately care for the client experiencing substance use or abuse problems. As the provision of health care moves further into the community at large, the nurse will need to have knowledge of commonly abused substances to adequately assess the needs of the public. Serving as a resource and provider of care to a diverse population of clients, the nurse will be able to influence them in improving their health status and productivity.

Approximately 1 out of 4 persons in the United States has a friend or family member with substance abuse problems or a history of drug abuse. Medical-surgical care is affected by substance abuse because of complications caused by the physical presence of or dependence on the substance. Management of clients with medical problems is more complex in the presence of an addiction.

Incidence and Extent of Substance Abuse

A chronic, long-standing problem, substance abuse continues to be prevalent in the United States. Studies conducted by and in conjunction with the National Institute on Drug Abuse (NIDA) are helpful in assessment of drug abuse. The data from three surveys are used throughout this chapter to describe the incidence and prevalence of drug use and abuse.

Monitoring the Future Study (MTF) is an annual survey on drug use and related attitudes of America's adolescents that began in 1975. The survey is conducted by the University of Michigan's Institute for Social Research and is funded by the NIDA. The *Community Epidemiology Work Group (CEWG)* is an NIDA-sponsored network of researchers from 20 major U.S. metropolitan areas and selected foreign countries who meet semiannually to discuss the current epidemiology of drug abuse. The *National Household Survey on Drug Abuse (NHSDA)* is an annual survey conducted by The Substance Abuse and Mental Health Services Administration. Reference to these surveys follows discussions of each major classification of drugs.

Cultural Competence Related to Substance Abuse

Culture influences every aspect of the client's life. The nurse needs to demonstrate competence in understanding the cultural influences that are related to drug abuse to plan care that will be amenable to the person with substance abuse problems. In addition, an understanding of the client's culture helps the nurse avoid making assumptions about substance abuse based on the client's body language. Some behaviors that are interpreted within the Western culture as negative responses are considered normal, even reverent, in some cultures, as in the case of avoiding eye contact.

The nurse adapts assessment and the subsequent planning of care within the norms of the client's culture. With the stigma associated with substance abuse, the nurse needs to be sensitive of those behaviors and norms that would alienate him or her. Often, substance abuse disorders are a result of interpersonal inadequacies wherein the user perceives the substance as helpful to reduce stress or assist him or her in coping. Success of drug treatment is often related to the use of external support, forcing the user to rely on other persons rather than the chemical.

The nurse must be open to the array of religious preferences to avoid conflicts between treatment modalities and the client's faith. In addition, the nurse must have a firm awareness of self to avoid reactive behaviors to the client's beliefs or absence of personal convictions. A posture of judgment is never appropriate and is particularly nontherapeutic when caring for the client with substance abuse. Chapter 6 describes cultural aspects of health in more detail, including how to perform a cultural assessment.

Substance Abuse, Stress, and Addiction

Many clients relate substance abuse to stress relief. However, external situational stress is not the only contributing factor resulting in substance abuse. The role that stress does play in substance abuse occurs more in a biologic response to stress, part of which is a normal response.

The introduction of stress in the brain, as perceived by the individual, results in stimulation of the hypothalamus. The hypothalamus, located beneath the thalamus, is the center for emotional responses and houses the limbic system (emotional part of the brain). In addition, the hypothalamus controls the involuntary nervous system and organ functions. Biologic rhythms and internal drives (e.g., sex drive) are directed by the nuclei of the hypothalamus. Perceptions of pleasure, fear, and rage are also found in the hypothalamus. Autonomic nervous system pathways act to initiate most physical expressions of these emotions, such as a pounding heart, increased blood pressure, pallor, increased perspiration, and a dry mouth.

Responses to external stress (situation or ingested chemicals) or internal stress (disease or withdrawal of drugs) trigger chemical and hormonal responses in the body arising from activity in the hypothalamus. Depending on the source of the stress, behavioral manifestations vary. The frequency of the stress has an influence on the quality of the body's response. Stress responses that are frequently triggered can result in a more sensitive response. Continued substance abuse creates a cycle of ever-increasing amounts of the drug to sustain the desired level of response to the drug. As with achieving the desired result, the body also responds with "withdrawal" responses (symptoms of withdrawal) when deprived of the substance. A cyclic ingestion-withdrawal response sets the stage for addiction.

Addiction can result in either physical or psychologic dependence or both, depending on the substance abused. Substance abuse is a documented nursing diagnosis when the following criteria are present:

- The client loses control of use of the drug.
- The client takes the drug even though the drug has caused adverse conditions in the body.
- The client demonstrates cognitive, behavioral, and physiologic disturbances with the abuse of drugs or inhalants.

Addiction is characterized as a condition that causes a habitual, compulsive, and uncontrollable urge to use a substance; and without the substance, the body experiences severe physiologic, psychologic, and emotional disturbances. Substance abuse in the presence of medical or surgical problems creates a very complicated situation in terms of helping clients to reach their highest level of function.

Substance Abuse and the Hospitalized Client

The client may be hospitalized when he or she can no longer be managed in an ambulatory care setting or when emergencies arise. As part of the comprehensive health assessment, the nurse carefully assesses for any signs, symptoms, or history of substance abuse.

In a comprehensive assessment, alcohol, tobacco, and prescription drug use is determined. The nurse should be adept in ascertaining substance abuse during the interview process. Failure to include a complete substance use history could have devastating effects on the client. The client who habitually uses substances will require closer observation for withdrawal than the occasional user, depending on the substance.

Caring for the client experiencing substance problems includes determining where he or she will be going at the time of discharge. If the client has focused on treatment and recovery from the substance, he or she may be discharged to a treatment center. If the client's plan includes continuation of the substance use, home may be the choice for discharge. Regardless of the best intentions of health care providers, the client may choose to handle his or her own substance abuse problem. The nurse is present to assist clients in reaching their optimal level of function as determined by both the client and the health care team.

Understanding the influence of abusive substances is an important educational aspect for the hospitalized client. Some chemicals have potentiating effects on therapeutic medications that can create a very dangerous situation. Room assignment, delegation to personnel, staffing assignments, and other nursing decisions are important with the substance-using client. The course of hospitalization may be altered as a result of substance abuse; treatment, care, and recovery are influenced by abuse of substances.

Referrals and community-based health resources are very important in assisting the client with substance abuse. Emotional support is necessary in coping with the reason for hospitalization, being in the hospital, and dealing with the adverse effects of the substance abuse.

WOMEN'S HEALTH CONSIDERATIONS

According to the NIDA (2000) report, 4 million women in the United States use drugs. Women of all races, ages, educational backgrounds, cultures, and community types are among the drug users in the United States. Drug use and abuse data among women are becoming increasingly available as the nursing profession seeks to improve the health of women. Usually women abuse more than one drug. Almost half of all women 15 to 44 years of age have used drugs at least once in their lifetime (includes the use of tobacco products and alcohol). Approximately 2 million women used cocaine and more than 6 million used marijuana in 1999 (NIDA, 2000).

Tobacco can have an adverse effect on women's health. Women who smoke experience the symptoms of menopause at an earlier age. Research concerning the combination of tobacco smoking and oral contraceptives has shown that women who smoke and take oral contraceptives have a greater risk for cardiovascular and cerebrovascular diseases than women who smoke and do not take oral contraceptives. Women over 30 years of age have an even greater risk for disease development with the combination of these drugs. Tobacco use increases the incidence of stillborn or premature infants. Babies born to smoking mothers usually have a lower birth weight. Maternal smoking also has been found to increase the tendency of the child to smoke.

Women are at risk for developing drug dependence as a result of biologic predisposition, stressors in the environment, and the availability of quality support services. These factors must be explored during the nursing assessment to be thorough in addressing the specific client's needs.

CONSIDERATIONS FOR OLDER ADULTS

Older women are at risk for substance abuse because of the body changes associated with the aging process. In the later years clients usually take prescription drugs for various conditions. These drugs, as well as over-the-counter medications, can become addictive.

STIMULANTS

Stimulants are drugs that excite the cerebral cortex of the brain, producing a variety of behavioral responses. Any substance that is introduced into the body that excites or stimulates an increase in body activity is referred to as a stimulant. Examples of stimulants are caffeine, nicotine, amphetamines, and methamphetamines. Although amphetamines and methamphetamines can be used for therapeutic purposes, their use is limited. Agents that are considered to be illicit and abused stimulants are crack (a potent form of cocaine), cocaine, and illegally produced methamphetamines. The incidence of stimulant use is varied among age-groups and chemicals (Table 8-1).

The therapeutic effects of stimulants are to:

- Increase mental alertness
- Improve one's sense of well-being
- Increase the capacity to work
- Improve the performance of motor skills and stimulate general metabolism by increasing respiratory and cardiac function

When a large amount of stimulant is introduced into the body, the effects can cause insomnia, tremor, and restlessness, with resulting loss of motor function. The prolonged and sustained use of a stimulant can result in toxicity; an overdose can cause hallucinations, seizures, and cardiac dysrhythmias.

Amphetamines

Amphetamines are stimulants that increase the body's activities. Prescribed therapeutically as a psychomotor stimulant, amphetamines and methamphetamines are effective for attention deficit hyperactivity disorder (ADHD), obesity, or narcolepsy. Use of stimulants results in energy, excitement, relief of fatigue, decreased appetite, insomnia, aggression, and a tendency toward menstrual problems in women. As a result of these effects, the nurse assesses the client for objective symptoms such as dilated pupils, weight loss, elevated vital signs, tremors, seizures, restlessness, and symptoms of emotional tension.

The purpose of amphetamine abuse is to obtain the euphoria and grandiosity achieved by use of the drug. Names for amphetamines (Biphetamine, Dexedrine) in the illicit drug community include "black beauties," "crosses," and "hearts." Knowledge of the "street" names for these drugs assists the nurse in assessment or identification of the abusive use of amphetamines. The routes for amphetamine use are varied, since they can be taken orally, injected, smoked, or sniffed. Amphetamines have a very high potential for addiction, both physically and psychologically.

Methamphetamine

Methamphetamine (Desoxyn) is a very powerful substance that is highly addictive. Therapeutically, methamphetamine is available as a Schedule II substance. It is available medically through a prescription for ADHD, narcolepsy, and obesity. Although it is similar to amphetamines, methamphetamine is more powerful and affects the brain more dramatically. High levels of the neurotransmitter dopamine are released as a result of ingestion of methamphetamine. There is evidence that this drug has neurotoxic effects on the brain, damaging cells that contain other transmitters such as serotonin. Symptoms of parkinsonism can be found in the long-term user. Even small amounts of methamphetamine can result in very dramatic results.

The object of drug use is to obtain a "rush" or "flash." Commonly known as "chalk," "speed," "crank," "crystal," "glass," and "ice," methamphetamines are manufactured illegally in "meth" labs across the United States. In addition to the results produced by amphetamines, methamphetamine can produce life-threatening conditions, such as hyperthermia and convulsions. Irreversible damage to the vessels in the brain can cause strokes, or brain attacks. Cardiovascular collapse, resulting in death, can be caused by methamphetamine use.

Cocaine

Cocaine is a stimulant that is commonly known as "coke," "crack," "flake," "rocks," and "snow." Cocaine, legally used as a Schedule II drug, is valuable as a topical anesthetic or a vasoconstrictor to stop bleeding. Its action is interference with the reabsorption process of dopamine. As a chemical messenger related to pleasure and movement, dopamine is released as part of the brain's reward system and is associated with the eupho-

TABLE 8-1 • INCIDENCE OF USE: STIMULANTS

METHAMPHETAMINE ("Speed," "Meth," "Chalk") AND METHAMPHETAMINE HYDROCHLORIDE ("Ice," "Crystal," "Glass," "Crank")

Monitoring the Future Study

In 1997, 4.4% of high school seniors had used crystal methamphetamine at least once in their lifetime—an increase from 2.7% in 1990. Data show that 2.3% of seniors reported past-year use of crystal methamphetamine in 1997—an increase from 1.3% in 1990.

Community Epidemiology Work Group

Methamphetamine is the dominant illicit drug used in San Diego. San Francisco and Honolulu also have substantial methamphetamine-using populations. Patterns of increasing use have been seen in Denver, Los Angeles, Minneapolis, Phoenix, Seattle, and Tucson. New trafficking patterns have increased availability of the drug in Missouri, Nebraska, and Iowa.

National Household Survey on Drug Abuse

According to the 1996 National Household Survey on Drug Abuse (NHSDA), 4.9 million people (age 12 and older) had tried methamphetamine at least once in their lifetime (2.3% of the population). This is not a statistically significant increase from the 4.7 million people (2.2%) who reported using methamphetamine at least once in their lifetime in the 1995 NHSDA.

COCAINE ("Crack," "Coke," "Flake," "Snow," "Rocks")

Monitoring the Future Study

The proportion of high school seniors who had used cocaine at least once in their lifetime increased from a low of 5.9% in 1994 to 9.8% in 1999. However, this is lower than the peak use of 17.3% in 1985. Current (past month) use of cocaine by seniors decreased from a high of 6.7% in 1985 to 2.6% in 1999. Also in 1999, 7.7% of tenth-graders had tried cocaine at least once, up from a low of 3.3% in 1992. The percentage of eighth-graders who had ever tried cocaine increased from a low of 2.3% in 1991 to 4.7% in 1999.

In 1995, 3.6% of college students 1 to 4 years beyond high school had used cocaine within the past year, and 0.7% had used cocaine within the past month.

Community Epidemiology Work Group

Although most demographic data continue to show most cocaine users to be older, inner-city crack addicts, isolated field reports indicate new groups of users: teenagers smoking crack with marijuana in some cities; Hispanic crack users in Texas; and in the Atlanta area, middle-class suburban users of cocaine hydrochloride and female crack users in their 30s with no prior drug history.

National Household Survey on Drug Abuse

In 1998 about 1.7 million Americans were current (at least once per month) cocaine users. This was about 0.8% of the population age 12 and older; about 437,000 of these used crack. The rate of current cocaine use in 1998 was highest among Americans ages 18 to 25 (2.0%). The rate of use for this age-group was significantly higher than in 1997, when it was 1.2%.

NICOTINE (Chew, Cigar, Cigarette, Snuff)

Monitoring the Future Study

Prevalence rates for smoking among young people remain high, in spite of the demonstrated health risk associated with smoking. Since 1975, cigarettes have consistently been the substance that the greatest number of high school students use daily.

Between 1998 and 1999, however, past-month smoking decreased significantly among eighth-graders, from 19.1% to 17.5%, and rates of use were stable or slightly decreased for tenth-graders (35.7%) and seniors (34.6%). Lifetime and daily use also leveled off in 1999 among all grades, as did use of smokeless tobacco.

National Household Survey on Drug Abuse

In 1998 an estimated 60 million Americans, or 28% of all Americans age 12 and older, were current smokers. Approximately 18% (4.1 million) of youths 12 to 17 years old were current smokers in 1998.

Data from National Institute on Drug Abuse, National Institute of Health, U.S. Department of Health and Human Services. (2000); http://www.nida.nih.gov: "Infofax: Methamphetamine; Methamphetamine: Abuse and addiction; Crack and cocaine; Cigarettes and other nicotine products."

ria achieved with cocaine use. Processing cocaine using ammonia or sodium bicarbonate transforms the cocaine into crack cocaine, a substance that can be smoked. This process is referred to as freebasing cocaine. Smoking cocaine is a more direct method of getting the drug to the brain. Cocaine use is severely addicting, and withdrawal can be a life-threatening situation. Adverse reactions include all of the reactions listed with stimulant use, including vertigo, nausea, vomiting, abdominal cramps, hypotension or hypertension, chills, fever, tachycardia, and tachypnea, progressing to collapse of the peripheral circulatory system, coma, and death.

When caring for the client using cocaine, the nurse must be able to differentiate symptoms that may be associated with crack/cocaine use. During the initial physical assessment, the nurse pays careful attention to the mucous membranes of the nose, since prolonged snorting can deteriorate the membranes and the nasal septum.

Cardiopulmonary arrest can occur with the first use of cocaine. Nursing care for clients using stimulants is determined by the exact chemical used and the current medical condition.

CRITICAL THINKING CHALLENGE

You are working in the emergency department when a group of people drop a young woman off at the door. She is approximately 22 years old and is about 5 feet 4 inches tall. Her body is emaciated; she is vomiting and holding her abdomen. You take her vital signs with the following findings: temperature, 101.4° F (38.6° C); pulse, 120; and blood pressure, 90/50.

- What other assessment data do you need?
- According to Maslow, what needs are present for this client?
- How would you triage this client, and what are your reasons for your decision?

For suggested answer guidelines, go to SIMON http://www.wbsaunders.com/SIMON/Iggy/.

Nicotine

Nicotine is one of the most addictive substances in the United States and is the addictive component of tobacco. Although the U.S. Surgeon General issued a report in 1989 about the health hazards of tobacco and cigarette smoking, tobacco products continue to be used. This report cited nicotine as a major contributing factor to strokes, or brain attacks, the third leading cause of death. According to the National Institute on Drug Abuse, there were 60 million smokers in the United States in 1989 (NIDA, 2000). Today, there is wide use of nicotine products in cigarettes, pipe tobacco, chewing tobacco, and spit tobacco.

Physiologically, nicotine has both stimulant and sedative properties that affect the central nervous system (CNS). First, nicotine stimulates the discharge of epinephrine from the adrenal cortex, causing a sudden release of glucose. Then, after recovery from the stimulant effect of the nicotine, depressant effects result in feelings of depression and fatigue. Daily ingestion of nicotine results in accumulation of nicotine in the body, lasting up to 24 hours. Because of the cyclic properties of nicotine, the body begins to require more nicotine usage to maintain the stimulant effects of the drug.

The addictive process begins with the cyclic use of nicotine for continuation of the stimulation experienced by the body. The addictive effects of nicotine have been compared to cocaine. With the cessation of nicotine, withdrawal symptoms are observed in the tobacco user. Lack of nicotine use in a 24-hour period can result in aggression, hostility, anger, and inappropriate social interactions. Research into the use of nicotine has resulted in data that show an increased level of dopamine, a neurotransmitter affecting brain pathways that control reward and pleasure. Tolerance for and dependence on additional nicotine increase as levels of stress rise. During periods of stress, there is a need for additional nicotine because the stress hormone corticosterone reduces the effects of nicotine. As stress and anxiety increase, the cycle of dependence grows stronger, leading the user to take in additional amounts of nicotine. Depriving the user of nicotine can result in a prolonged recovery period before emotional homeostasis is achieved after experiencing stress.

To help motivate the client to quit using nicotine, the nurse describes the negative effects of smoking, including chronic cardiovascular and respiratory diseases, as well as secondhand effects on other people. The nurse teaches the importance of smoking cessation. A number of community-based support groups and smoking cessation programs, using behavioral methods, hypnosis, acupressure, or other modalities, are available. Chapters 36 and 38 discuss smoking cessation in more detail.

HALLUCINOGENS AND RELATED COMPOUNDS

Chemical substances that possess mind-altering or mental perception–altering properties are known as **hallucinogens.** Examples of hallucinogenic substances are lysergic acid (LSD), phencyclidine (PCP), and marijuana. Of these three, the only therapeutic drug is PCP, which is used as a veterinary anesthetic agent. There are no therapeutic uses acceptable for medical treatment today, although marijuana has been used by some to treat cancer pain.

Hallucinogenic compounds are desirable to the drug user because of their thrill-seeking effects, caused by an alteration in perception. Action of these drugs produces changes in the neurotransmitters of the brain. Alterations in mood, sensory distortions, delusions, and depersonalization are some of the resulting behaviors. Physical changes experienced by the user are increased vital signs and pupillary dilation. A psychologic dependence may occur, or the client may experience suicidal or psychotic states. Flashbacks are a common phenomenon when psychedelic drugs are used and can occur at any time. The user is returned to the initial drug experience without warning, which can be very disturbing and can create a threat to safety. The nurse observes for objective signs of use, in addition to looking for paranoia and suspicious behavior. Addiction to hallucinogens is psychologic in nature rather than physical addiction (Table 8-2).

Lysergic Acid

Lysergic acid (LSD) is a major hallucinogenic drug, known as "acid" in the drug community. The drug is odorless and colorless with a slightly bitter taste. Usually taken orally, LSD is often distributed on absorbent, decorative paper, making it very attractive to adolescents and children. The health hazards of LSD are very unpredictable and are affected by the dose, personality and mood of the user, anticipated outcome, and environment at the time of use. Because the exact mechanism of action is not known, further studies in drug research are being conducted by the National Institute on Drug Abuse (NIDA), a component of the Institutes of Health in Washington D.C. LSD is known to influence neurotransmission in the CNS. The effects of the drug can last up to 12 hours and result in either pleasant or unpleasant experiences, also known as "good trips" or "bad trips." Thoughts and feelings can be bizarre and at times have resulted in suicide. LSD use can also result in psychiatric illness such as schizophrenia. Because LSD does not result in compulsive drug-seeking behaviors, it is not addictive. Tolerance can develop, so that an increased amount of the drug is needed to attain the same level of stimulation as earlier experiences.

3,4-Methylenedioxymethamphetamine

Amphetamine can be altered to become a hallucinogen, as in the case of 3,4-methylenedioxymethamphetamine (MDMA), an oral drug that is also called "Adam," "ecstasy," and the "date rape" drug. The desired effects are development of trust in others and easing of inhibitions between people. Other desired effects, as well as adverse effects, are the same as those of LSD. When the client uses MDMA, the nurse will observe psychologic difficulties, including confusion, depression, sleep disturbances, drug craving, severe anxiety, and paranoia. Physical symptoms of MDMA are muscle tension, involuntary teeth clenching, nausea, visual disturbances, faintness, and chills or sweating. Abnormal vital signs such as increased heart rate and blood pressure are also observed. Critical thinking and memory are affected by long-term use of MDMA. Demonstrating a structural relationship to methamphetamine, MDMA also causes a degeneration of

TABLE 8-2 • INCIDENCE OF USE: HALLUCINOGENS

LYSERGIC ACID (LSD; "Acid," "Microdot")

Monitoring the Future Study

From 1997 to 1999 the percentage of high school seniors who had used LSD remained relatively stable. Between 1975 and 1997 the lowest lifetime use of LSD was reported by the class of 1986, when 7.2% of seniors reported using LSD at least once in their lifetime. In 1997, 13.6% of seniors had experimented with LSD at least once in their lifetime. The percentage of seniors reporting use of LSD in the past year nearly doubled, from a low of 4.4% in 1985 to 8.4% in 1997.

In 1997, 34.7% of seniors perceived great risk in using LSD once or twice, and 76.6% said they saw great risk in using LSD regularly. More that 80% of seniors disapproved of people trying LSD once or twice, and almost 93% disapproved of people taking LSD regularly.

Almost 51% of seniors said it would have been fairly easy or very easy for them to get LSD if they had wanted it.

National Household Survey on Drug Abuse

In the 1996 National Household Survey on Drug Abuse (NHSDA) estimates, the percentage of the population age 12 and older who had ever used LSD (the lifetime prevalence rate) increased to 7.7% from 6.0% in 1988. Among youths 12 to 17 years old, the 1996 LSD lifetime prevalence rate was 4.3%, and for those ages 18 to 25, the rate was 13.9%. The rate for past-year use of LSD among the population age 12 and older was 1% in 1996. Past-year prevalence was highest among the age-groups 12 to 17 (2.8%) and 18 to 25 (4.6%). The rate of current LSD use in 1996 for those ages 18 to 25 was 0.9%, and it was 0.8% for 12- to 17-year-old youths.

PHENCYCLIDINE (PCP; "Angel Dust," "Boat," "Hog," "Love Boat")

Monitoring the Future Study

The 1997 Monitoring the Future Study (MTF) of the National Institute on Drug Abuse (NIDA) showed that use of PCP by high school seniors had declined steadily since 1979, when 7.0% of seniors had used PCP in the year preceding the survey. In 1997, however, 2.3% of seniors used PCP at least once in the past year, up from a low of 1.2% in 1990. Past-month use among seniors decreased from 1.3% in 1996 to 0.7% in 1997.

National Household Survey on Drug Abuse

According to the 1996 NHSDA, 3.2% of the population age 12 and older had used PCP at least once. Lifetime use of PCP was higher among those ages 26 through 34 (4.2%) than for those ages 18 through 25 (2.3%) and those ages 12 through 17 (1.2%).

3,4-METHYLENEDIOXYMETHAMPHETAMINE (MDMA; "Adam," "Ecstasy," "XTC")

Community Epidemiology Work Group

MDMA is used most often by young adults and adolescents at clubs, "raves" (large, all-night dance parties), and rock concerts.

Its abuse is increasingly reported in the 20 metropolitan areas included in the Community Epidemiology Work Group (CEWG).

In Kings County, Washington, a recently completed survey of young men who have sex with men showed that MDMA was among the frequently used drugs (20% of the sample).

A 1996 to 1997 survey of public schools in Boston found that about 14% of male and 7% of female twelfth-graders had used MDMA during their lifetime. Increased use of MDMA among youth was also reported in Seattle.

National Household Survey on Drug Abuse

According to NHSDA data on MDMA use among students, rates of use remained relatively stable from 1996 to 1999 for students in the eighth grade, whereas usage among tenth- and twelfth-graders increased.

The number of twelfth-graders who had used MDMA in their lifetime increased from 5.8% in 1998 to 8.0% in 1999. Use in the past year also increased from 3.6% in 1998 to 5.6% in 1999. In addition, twelfth-graders' use of MDMA in the past month also increased from 1.5% in 1998 to 2.5% in 1999.

On the other hand, the largest change for tenth-graders occurred in past-year use, which increased from 3.3% in 1998 to 4.4% in 1999.

MARIJUANA ("MJ," "Mary Jane," "Weed," "Pot," "Reefer," "Smoke," "Grass")

Monitoring the Future Study

After decreasing for over a decade, marijuana use among students began to increase in the early 1990s. From 1998 to 1999, use of marijuana at least once (lifetime use) increased among tenth- and twelfth-graders, continuing the trend seen in recent years. The seniors' rate of lifetime marijuana use was higher than in any year since 1987, but all rates remained well below those seen in the early 1970s and early 1980s. Past-year and past-month marijuana use did not change significantly from 1998 to 1999 in any of the three grades, suggesting that the sharp increases of recent years may be slowing. Daily marijuana use in the past month increased slightly among all three grades as well.

National Household Survey on Drug Abuse

Marijuana remains the most commonly used illicit drug in the United States. There were an estimated 2.1 million people who started using marijuana in 1998. According to data from the 1998 NHSDA, more than 72.0 million Americans (33%) 12 years of age and older have tried marijuana at least once in their lifetime, and almost 18.7 million (8.6%) have used marijuana in the past year. In 1985, 56.5 million Americans (29.4%) had tried marijuana at least once in their lifetime, and 26.1 million (13.6%) had used marijuana within the past year.

Data from National Institute on Drug Abuse, National Institute of Health, U.S. Department of Health and Human Services. (2000); http://www.nida.nih.gov: "Infofax: LSD; PCP; Ecstasy; Marijuana."

neurons containing dopamine, a neurotransmitter, resulting in parkinsonism.

Methylenedioxyamphetamine (MDA), the parent drug of MDMA, is an amphetamine-like drug that destroys serotonin-producing neurons in the brain. Serotonin plays a vital role in the regulation of aggression, mood, sexual activity, sleep, and pain sensitivity. Action of the serotonin interaction accounts for the report of heightened sexual experiences and tranquility.

Phencyclidine

Phencyclidine, commonly known as PCP, is an animal anesthetic that causes a feeling of detachment in humans. Clients using PCP ("angel dust") are unaware of their surroundings, which causes the detachment. Primarily affecting the CNS, the client exhibits flushing, increased perspiration, aggression, and incoherence. The user may experience feelings of superior strength and physical power. Some users state that their use is related to the numbing effects on the mind. However, the results may progress to a comatose state.

There is no evidence of physical addiction; however, psychologic addiction is common. There is evidence to suggest a decrease in the use of PCP, a commonly abused drug in the past. The nurse who suspects PCP abuse assesses for shallow respirations, generalized numbness of the extremities, and psychologic effects, including distinct changes in body awareness. High doses of PCP can produce vomiting, loss of balance, visual disturbances, and dizziness. Seizures, coma, and death have resulted from high doses of PCP. Lasting effects of PCP use can include memory loss, speech difficulties, and interference with thinking processes.

Marijuana

Another hallucinogen is marijuana. Widely used and distributed, this drug is illegal and does not have any accepted legal therapeutic uses. For some clients, it has been used experimentally for chronic pain control. Although there is a considerable and ongoing debate about the uses and need for legalization of marijuana, it remains a contraband substance in the United States. Commonly referred to as "weed," "smoke," "pot," "grass," "Mary Jane," and "herb," marijuana is a drug with a moderate potential for addiction. More common to marijuana is a psychologic dependence if it is used over long periods of time. Whether smoked or taken orally, the short-term effects of marijuana include problems with memory and learning, distorted perception, decreased critical thinking, and increased symptoms of anxiety.

The user enjoys marijuana because of the sensations of euphoria, sexual arousal, and relaxation. The "high" experience that users feel is a result of the action of tetrahydrocannabinol (THC), the main active substance in marijuana. THC changes the method by which sensory information gets to and is processed in the hippocampus. As a component of the brain's limbic system, the hippocampus is necessary for the integration of sensory experiences and emotion, as well as learning and memory. Frequent and long-term use of marijuana can create the same respiratory changes seen in long-term tobacco smokers. Studies of young adults who use marijuana demonstrate that learning and social behavior are affected by heavy marijuana use. Evidence suggests that marijuana use affects critical skills related to attention, memory, and learning. Heavy marijuana users make more mistakes in their work and have more difficulty maintaining attention.

CRITICAL THINKING CHALLENGE

When you are assessing a postoperative client, he suddenly jumps out of the bed and starts running around the room, talking about "getting rid of the bats." He makes karate gestures toward the sink. Then the client turns abruptly toward you, apologizes profusely, and returns to his bed.

- What is a clinical explanation of this behavior?
- What nursing diagnoses are appropriate for this client?
- How does the postoperative condition of the client affect your nursing care?

For suggested answer guidelines, go to SIMON http://www.wbsaunders.com/SIMON/Iggy/.

DEPRESSANTS

Drugs that reduce the activity of the central nervous system (CNS) are referred to as **depressants.** Benzodiazepines and barbiturates are discussed as depressants because of their activity in the ascending reticular activating system in the CNS. Both classes have valuable therapeutic properties in treating anxiety and emotional disorders. They are an adjunct to sleep and can be used as needed for situational tension. The route of ingestion is either oral or by injection. On the illicit drug market, barbiturates are called "barbs" and "ludes." The benzodiazepines are called "roofies" and "tranks." These are Schedule IV drugs because of the high potential for abuse.

Benzodiazepines

The desired results for the use of benzodiazepines include relaxation, sleep, seizure control, withdrawal from alcohol, and relief of anxiety. Abuse is present when the client continues to use the drug after the clinical signs have subsided. The street value of benzodiazepines and the drug effects make this drug popular. Physical and psychologic dependence on benzodiazepines is prevalent. The user can develop a high tolerance for the drug, causing increasing amounts to be needed to achieve the desired feeling. Benzodiazepines act to depress the CNS; therefore combination with other CNS substances has a potentiating effect.

Barbiturates

Barbiturates are depressant drugs that can depress the CNS through action in the cerebral cortex and the reticular formation. Effects of barbiturates include sedation, drowsiness, and a decrease in motor activity of the body. Dependence on barbiturates can occur in a very short time and can lead to withdrawal symptoms if the drug is discontinued abruptly. Street abuse of the drug often results in withdrawal, recognizable by CNS responses such as anxiety, restlessness, insomnia, irritability, and impaired attention. Physical illness may accompany the withdrawal of barbiturates. Because of the aging process, older adults can tolerate only small doses of the barbiturate group.

Alcohol

Alcohol in various mixed drinks, beer, wine, and liquor provides sedation, relaxation, and release of a person's inhibitions. A substantial number of people in the United States drink alcoholic beverages. For most people, alcohol is used for a pleasure experience. Alcohol acts as a depressant on the CNS and the respiratory system; therefore the signs and symptoms of the effects of alcohol use are primarily neurologic. One of every 13 adults in the United States abuses alcohol (Table 8-3).

Alcoholism (alcohol dependence syndrome) is a disease wherein the person has a strong need or compulsion to drink, is unable to quit once he or she begins drinking, experiences a physical dependence, and has a need to increase the amount of alcohol to get "high" (high tolerance). Physical dependence occurs when the person experiences withdrawal after alcohol use is stopped after a period of heavy drinking. When drinking alcohol relieves the symptoms of withdrawal, the person has an addiction to alcohol.

Alcohol abuse exists when a person does not have a strong craving for alcohol, loss of control, or physical dependence but has problems related to alcohol use. Failing to fulfill responsibilities at home, work, or school; drinking in unsafe situations; experiencing legal problems that are alcohol related, and/or continuing to drink when problems have been caused or worsened by use of alcohol are situations that help identify alcohol abuse. When one or more of these events occur within a 12-month period, the person is abusing alcohol.

The nurse in the medical-surgical setting must be knowledgeable about the signs, symptoms, and complications of alcohol use. The most threatening result of alcohol abuse or alcoholism is withdrawal from the substance. Symptoms of withdrawal range from mild to severe and can progress to death. Alcohol withdrawal can be evaluated by categories according to severity:

- *Minor*—restlessness, anxiety, sleeping difficulties, agitation and tremors, tachycardia, low-grade fever, diaphoresis, and elevated blood pressure
- *Major*—in addition to the signs and symptoms of mild withdrawal, visual or auditory hallucinations, tremors of the entire body (delirium tremens [DTs]), heart rate above 100 beats/min, diastolic pressure above 100 mm Hg, pronounced diaphoresis, and vomiting
- *Life threatening*—delirium tremens, disorientation ×3, global confusion, and inability to recognize familiar objects or people

The life-threatening stage of alcohol withdrawal has a 2% to 5% mortality rate, requiring emergency medical interventions. Alcohol seizures may occur 12 to 48 hours after the last drink.

When the client is experiencing withdrawal of alcohol—or another depressant—the nurse prevents the client from harming himself or herself or others and attempts to reorient him or her to reality. The health care provider often prescribes medications to calm or sedate the client according to agency protocol or physician preference. The nurse applies the nursing process in collaboration with the health care team (Table 8-4).

TABLE 8-3 • INCIDENCE OF USE: ALCOHOL

- Forty-four percent of adults age 18 years and older report having consumed 12 or more alcoholic drinks in the past year (more than 82 million).
- Forty-six percent of current drinkers report having been intoxicated at least once in the last year.
- Four percent of current drinkers report having been intoxicated weekly in the past year.
- Twenty percent of current drinkers report having consumed an average of more than two drinks per day in the past year.
- Ten percent of current drinkers meet the diagnostic criteria for alcohol dependence (approximately 8 million people).*
- Four percent of American women ages 18 and older can be classified as alcoholic or problem drinkers, one-third the number of men; of these women, 58% are between the ages of 18 and 29.†
- Men (21%) are twice as likely as women (10%) to be heavier drinkers who consume two or more drinks per day on the average.
- Prevalence of alcoholism is highest among people who have personal incomes of less than $10,000 (17%) and lowest among those whose incomes are $25,000 or more (6%).
- Beer is the most popular alcoholic beverage by far among men who express a preference; women prefer beer and wine in almost equal percentages.
- Fifty-nine percent of those who ever received treatment for an alcohol problem say they prefer drinking beer.‡

*http://www.health.gov/healthypeople: "Alcoholism: Getting the facts."
†http://www.nida.nih.gov. "Criteria for substance dependence diagnosis: How can we tell if someone is abusing or addicted to drugs."
‡http://www.ncadd.org.

CRITICAL THINKING CHALLENGE

You are admitting a 59-year-old man in the emergency department who is experiencing a "jumpy heart." He has slight tremors and is having difficulties giving the nurse details about his health history. He denies the use of alcohol. The client has a blood pressure of 182/110 with a pulse of 104. He has arrived alone and gives you some nitroglycerin tablets that he takes at home for angina.

- What problem might this client have? State the rationale for your answer.
- What are the appropriate nursing diagnoses for this client?
- What outcomes would be considered for the client's comfort and safety?

For suggested answer guidelines, go to SIMON http://www.wbsaunders.com/SIMON/Iggy/.

NARCOTICS: OPIOIDS AND MORPHINE DERIVATIVES

Narcotic is a broad term encompassing all drugs that are made from the Asian poppy or produced as a synthetic drug with the effects of opium. A general action of narcotics is to reduce the client's perception of pain. Drugs included in this category are codeine, morphine, heroin, methadone, hydromorphone (Dilaudid), and meperidine (Demerol). Common names for heroin and opium in the drug community are "horse" and "smack" for heroin and "Dover's powder" for opium (Table 8-5). The sites of action of these drugs are in the brain, binding in the receptor sites of the CNS (causing CNS depression) and in the gastrointestinal system (producing the antidiarrheal effects of opium).

Opioid and morphine derivatives are drugs of addiction because of their analgesic and euphoric effects. These drugs are therapeutically used for relief of severe pain, such as pain experienced in terminal cancer or postoperative pain. Sleep is an added feature of the drug when it is used for pain. The substance abuse user enjoys the therapeutic effects, as well as the escape effect in the mind. Aggression and sexual drives are usually minimized with use of the opioids and morphine drugs.

A high potential for addiction, tolerance, and dependence occurs with this class of drugs. The withdrawal effects can range from mild withdrawal symptoms to death. According to the National Institute on Drug Abuse, there are four categories of opiate withdrawal (NIDA, 2000):

- Grade 0 is characterized by drug craving, anxiety, and drug-seeking behaviors.
- Grade 1 is characterized by yawning, sweating, lacrimation, and rhinorrhea ("runny nose").
- Grade 2 is characterized by mydriasis (pupillary dilation), gooseflesh, muscle twitching, and anorexia.
- Grade 3, the most dangerous of the grades in opiate withdrawal, is characterized by increased pulse, respiratory rate, and blood pressure; abdominal cramps; diarrhea; vomiting; and weakness.

These drugs may be taken orally, injected, or inhaled. The nurse must have an understanding of the withdrawal symptoms to be aware of the severity of the medical condition created by withdrawal from opiates and their derivatives.

Heroin, a highly addictive drug, is an opiate derivative. Unlike the other opiate drugs noted earlier, heroin has no medical use. The health hazards of heroin are very serious and include fatal overdoses and spontaneous abortions. Intravenous use of heroin or other abused substances increases the risk of acquiring infectious diseases such as human immunodeficiency virus infection or acquired immunodeficiency syndrome (HIV/AIDS) and hepatitis. Short-term effects of heroin are felt immediately and continue for a few hours after a single dose. Users report an immediate feeling of extreme euphoria ("rush") when using. The person experiences a dry mouth, heavy extremities, and a warm, flushed feeling. Generally, there are alternate sensations of wakefulness and sleep. Common street names for heroin are "horse," "smack," "H," "skag," and "junk." Chronic use of heroin results in many physical problems, such as emaciation, frequent infections, cellulitis, and liver disease.

Care of the client with an opiate or heroin addiction becomes complex because of the physical condition, the addictive behaviors, and safety concerns both physically and psychologically. Other drugs with addictive properties in this class are used for therapeutic purposes and are part of the treatment regimen for conditions that the nurse frequently encounters. Implications for the nurse include the need for current information about addictions and the addictive drug cycle, both physically and mentally.

INHALANTS

Breathable chemical vapors that produce psychoactive effects are called **inhalants.** These substances are popular with young people because of their accessibility (in the home) and price (Table 8-6). Three categories of inhalants are common household items. **Solvents** produce a high when inhaled. Examples of solvents are paint thinners, gasoline, glues, paper correction fluid, felt-tip markers, and electronic contact cleaners. Gases are another source of inhalants and include products such as butane lighters, propane tanks, whipping cream aerosols, spray paints, hair or deodorant sprays, chloroform, ether, and nitrous oxide (laughing gas). **Nitrites** are the third

TABLE 8-4 • DEPRESSANT/SEDATIVE WITHDRAWAL AND THE NURSING PROCESS

ASSESSMENT

General head-to-toe physical assessment with the following as findings associated with depressant abuse:

- Positive findings of sedative and alcohol withdrawal, differentiating as to minor, major, or delirium tremens
- Presence of seizures within 12 to 24 hours after the last ingestion of alcohol
- Presence of seizures with barbiturate use within 72 hours after the last use

ANALYSIS

The following nursing diagnosis is applicable to these observations:

Injury (Physical and Psychologic)
Related to (cessation of alcohol or sedative use)
Manifested by (the symptoms identified in the nursing assessment)

If there are no signs or symptoms of withdrawal, the nursing diagnosis would be:

Risk for Injury
Related to (the abrupt withdrawal of alcohol or sedatives)
As evidenced by (not present; therefore there are no signs or symptoms to use in planning of care. Care would focus on early detection or observation.)

There are many other nursing diagnoses that would be applicable for this situation, depending on the actual client in the medical-surgical unit.

PLANNING AND IMPLEMENTATION

Planning: Expected Outcomes

The client will experience no physical injury. This is a simple yet profound outcome of the client with depressant abuse. What other outcomes would be applicable?

Interventions

The nurse will identify the client's stage of withdrawal (if the client is experiencing symptoms):

- Observe for the early signs of withdrawal (if the client does not have the signs or symptoms of withdrawal but does have the risk for development).
- Incorporate factors of the medical condition that was the primary purpose of admission (if not acute withdrawal).

This is a skeleton of a nursing care plan used to integrate substance abuse into the plan of care in a medical-surgical setting.

TABLE 8-5 • INCIDENCE OF USE: OPIOIDS AND MORPHINE DERIVATIVES

HEROIN ("Horse," "Smack")
Monitoring the Future Study
According to the 1997 Monitoring the Future Study (MTF), rates of heroin use remained relatively stable and low from the late 1970s to 1991. After 1991, however, use began to rise among tenth- and twelfth-graders, and after 1993, among eighth-graders. In 1997, prevalence of heroin use was comparable for all three grade levels. Although the annual prevalence rates for heroin use remained relatively low in 1997, these rates are approximately two to three times higher than those reported in 1991.

Community Epidemiology Work Group
In December 1996 the Community Epidemiology Work Group (CEWG) reported that the availability of low-priced, high-quality heroin has continued to increase, especially in the East and in some areas of the Midwest. This increase has also been reported in some cities that previously had escaped the influx of high-quality heroin.
Quantitative indicators and field reports continue to suggest an increasing incidence of new users (snorters) in the younger age-groups, often among women. One concern is that young heroin snorters may shift to needle injecting because of increasing tolerance, nasal soreness, or declining or unreliable purity. Injection use would place them at increased risk of contracting HIV/AIDS.
In some areas, such as Boston and San Francisco, the recent initiates increasingly include members of the middle class. In Newark, heroin users are usually found in suburban populations.

National Household Survey on Drug Abuse
The 1996 National Household Survey on Drug Abuse (NHSDA) shows a significant increase from 1993 in the estimated number of current (once in the past month) heroin users. The estimated number of users rose from 68,000 in 1993 to 216,000 in 1996.
Among individuals who had ever used heroin in their lives, the proportion who had ever smoked, sniffed, or snorted heroin increased from 55% in 1994 to 82% in 1996. During the same period, the proportion of users who injected remained about the same, at about 50%.

Data from National Institute on Drug Abuse, National Institute of Health, U.S. Department of Health and Human Services. (2000); http://www.nida.nih.gov: "Infofax: Heroin."

TABLE 8-6 • INCIDENCE OF USE: INHALANTS

HOUSEHOLD ITEMS: GASES—AEROSOLS; SOLVENTS—PAINT THINNER
Extent of Use
Initial use of inhalants often starts early. Some young people may use inhalants as a cheap, accessible substitute for alcohol. Research suggests that chronic or long-term inhalant abusers are among the most difficult to treat, and they may experience multiple psychologic and social problems.

Monitoring the Future Study
The National Institute on Drug Abuse's (NIDA's) national survey on drug abuse among high school students provides estimates of the percentage of seniors using inhalants since 1976. The annual rate of inhalant use among seniors steadily rose from 3.0% in 1976 to a peak of 8.0% in 1995. In 1997, 6.7% of seniors reported past-year inhalant use.
In 1997, 21.0% of eighth-graders and 18.3% of tenth-graders had used inhalants at least once in their lifetime; 11.8% of eighth-graders and 8.7% of tenth-graders had used inhalants in the past year.
The perceived harmfulness of inhalants varies among high school students. In 1997 almost 40.1% of eighth-graders and 47.5% of tenth-graders said there was great risk in trying inhalants once or twice; 68.7% of eighth-graders and 74.5% of tenth-graders saw great risk in using inhalants regularly.

National Household Survey on Drug Abuse
Data from the National Household Survey on Drug Abuse (NHSDA) show that in 1996, 5.9% of adolescents (1.3 million) reported use of inhalants at least once in their lifetime, and 4% (900,000) reported using inhalants in the past year.

Data from National Institute on Drug Abuse, National Institute of Health, U.S. Department of Health and Human Services. (2000); http://www.nida.nih/gov: "Infofax: Inhalants."

source of inhalants and include cyclohexyl nitrite, amyl nitrite, and butyl nitrite.

Inhalants produce anesthetic results, slowing the body functions. Users may feel intoxicated, less inhibited, and less in control with repeated use. The user may inhale enough chemical to become unconscious. Sniffing highly concentrated chemicals can result in death from cardiac failure. Suffocation can also occur because the inhalant takes the place of oxygen in the lungs and respirations cease. Irreversible effects, including hearing losses, limb spasms, brain damage, and/or bone marrow suppression, can occur from inhalants. Reversible effects that can occur with inhalants include liver and kidney damage and blood oxygen depletion. Pouring or dispensing the inhalant into a paper bag increases the concentration of the substance, inducing a quicker, more pronounced effect.

The nurse may come in contact with young adults who have had experience with inhalants. These clients may have been admitted to the hospital for complications of inhalant use or because of medical conditions. Once the client is stabilized, the nurse may try to determine with the client the reasons for his or her use of inhalants.

STEROIDS

Anabolic-androgenic steroids are growing in popularity among young athletes (Table 8-7). The term *anabolic* indicates muscle building, and the term *androgenic* refers to increased masculinity. Steroids are legally available through prescription use for people with hormonal difficulties such as delayed puberty or impotence. Athletes use steroids to increase strength and performance. Misuse of steroids can lead

TABLE 8-7 • INCIDENCE OF USE: STEROIDS

STEROIDS (ANABOLIC-ANDROGENIC)

Monitoring the Future Study

The Monitoring the Future Study (MTF) assesses drug abuse among eighth-, tenth-, and twelfth-graders nationwide and has been conducted annually since 1975. Because of growing professional and public concern over the abuse of anabolic steroids by adolescents and young adults, questions regarding anabolic steroid use were added to the MTF in 1989 to afford a better understanding of the extent of the problem. Between 1989 and 1999, lifetime prevalence of anabolic steroid use among twelfth-graders fluctuated between a 3% high in 1989 and a 1.9% low in 1996.

In 1991 the MTF was expanded to include assessment of eighth- and tenth-graders nationwide, in addition to twelfth-graders.

According to the 1999 survey, 2.7% of eighth-graders and tenth-graders reported that they had taken anabolic steroids at least once in their lifetime. These numbers are statistically significant increases from the 1991 data.

Additional statistically significant increases from 1989 to 1999 include the following:

- Among tenth-graders in 1999, 2.7% had used anabolic steroids at least once in their lifetime, up from 2.0% in 1998. The rates also increased for past-year use from 1.2% in 1998 to 1.7% in 1999 and increased for past-month use from 0.6% in 1998 to 0.9% in 1999.
- In 1999, 2.7% of eighth-graders had used anabolic steroids at least once in their lifetime. In addition, 1.7% of eighth-graders had used anabolic steroids in the past year, up from 1.2% in 1998. Use in the past month had also increased from 0.5% in 1998 to 0.7% in 1999.

In addition to data regarding use, the 1999 survey reported twelfth-graders' attitudes toward steroid use as follows:

- In 1999, 62.1% of twelfth-graders perceived a great risk in taking steroids—the lowest percentage reported since questions about steroids started appearing in 1989. This is a decrease from 68.1% in 1998.
- Of those surveyed, 88.9% said they disapproved of people who use steroids.

Data from National Institute on Drug Abuse, National Institute of Health, U.S. Department of Health and Human Services. (2000); http://www.nida.nih.gov: "Infofax: Steroids."

to serious medical problems, some of which are irreversible. Possible effects of steroids include the following:

- For men: shrinking testicles, reduced sperm count, infertility, baldness, development of breasts, and an increased risk for cancer
- For women: growth of facial hair, male pattern baldness, changes or cessation of menses, enlargement of the clitoris, and deepened voice
- For adolescents: premature skeletal maturation and accelerated puberty changes

Aggression is increased by the use of steroids. In addition, there may be a noted increase in mental illness as a result of mood disturbances. Discontinuation of steroids can result in depression.

CONSIDERATIONS FOR OLDER ADULTS

Substance abuse should not be overlooked in the older adult. The potential for nontherapeutic use or abuse is high because of the number of different types of medications taken. As part the aging process, older adults have more difficulty metabolizing and excreting drugs; therefore toxicity is a common situation. Self-medication is a problem in the older population, increasing the complexity of care. A thorough drug history is necessary for identifying patterns of drug use that are harmful to the client. Misuse of prescription medications can happen quite innocently as memory becomes altered. Regular drug administration times are difficult to remember, resulting in overdosing or underdosing.

The older adult also faces risks for alcohol-related problems. This group consumes low amounts of alcohol. However, when the older client uses alcohol in combination with other drugs, his or her health may be compromised.

ONLINE RESOURCES

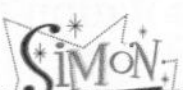

For suggested readings and Internet resources, go to http://www.wbsaunders.com/SIMON/Iggy/.

SELECTED BIBLIOGRAPHY

Acello, B. (2000). Controlling pain, facing fears about opioid addiction. *Nursing2000, 30*(5), 72.

Conrad, K.M., Furner, S.E., & Qian, Y. (1999). Occupational hazard exposure and at risk drinking. *AAOHN Journal, 47*(1), 9-16.

Gorman, M. (1998a). Substance abuse. *American Journal of Nursing, 98*(7), 16.

Gorman, M. (1998b). Substance abuse: What to do when your patient uses illicit drugs? *American Journal of Nursing, 98*(3), 54.

Keltner, N.L., Schwecke, L.H., & Bostrom, C.E. (1999). *Psychiatric nursing* (3rd ed.). St. Louis: Mosby.

Kuhn, M. (1998). *Pharmacotherapeutics: A nursing process approach* (4th ed.). Philadelphia: F.A. Davis.

Ludwick, R.E., et al. (2000). Alcohol use in elderly women: Nursing considerations in community settings. *Journal of Gerontological Nursing, 26*(2), 44-49.

Mason, M.G. (1999). The "crack belly": Newly recognized bowel sequelae after crack cocaine intoxication. *J Emergency Nursing 25*(5):373-376, 1999.

National Institute on Drug Abuse, National Institute of Health, U.S. Department of Health and Human Services. (2000). http://www.nida.nih.gov.

Powell, A.H. (1999). Alcohol withdrawal in critical care. *Dimensions in Critical Care Nursing, 18*(6), 24-28.

Ruppert, R.A. (1999). The last smoke: Your patients can quit smoking—for life. *American Journal of Nursing, 99*(11), 26-32.

Sachse, D. (2000). Emergency: Delirium tremens. *American Journal of Nursing, 100*(5), 41-42.

Segatore, M., Adams, D., & Lange, S. (1999). Managing alcohol withdrawal in the acutely ill hospitalized adult. *Journal of Neuroscience Nursing, 31*(1), 129-141.

Snow, D., & Gorman, M. (1999). Addiction, working with relapse. *American Journal of Nursing,* 99(7), 69.

Stewart, K.B., & Richards, A.B. (2000). Recognizing and managing your patient's alcohol abuse. *Nursing2000, 30*(2), 56-59.

CHAPTER 9

End-of-Life Care

MARY KAZANOWSKI

Learning Objectives

After studying this chapter, you should be able to:

1. Explain the goals of end-of-life care.
2. Describe the hospice concept.
3. Interpret the common physical and emotional signs of impending death.
4. Identify interventions for managing symptoms of distress at end of life.
5. Describe postmortem care.
6. Compare active euthanasia and passive euthanasia.

SIMON

Go to http://www.wbsaunders.com/SIMON/Iggy/ for self-assessment questions related to these Learning Objectives.

Nurses spend more time with clients and their families than do any other health care professionals. Therefore they are usually in the best and most immediate position to provide compassionate, palliative care when difficult decisions must be made at the end of life (EOL). **Palliative care** includes measures to promote comfort and support to both clients and their families.

OVERVIEW

Goals for End-of-Life Care

The goals for clients expected to recover from an illness may differ from the goals for clients near death. Efforts to discuss these goals are essential to the provision of quality care. In general, clients expected to recover from an illness or an exacerbation of symptoms are treated aggressively with medications and treatments intended to extend life—often at all costs. Clients who lack a reasonable chance for recovery often want to forgo aggressive treatments, which may cause discomfort, in favor of peace and comfort. Ignoring the possibility that a client is near death risks the implementation of interventions that could contribute to pain and suffering. It also risks inadequate preparation and interventions for the physical, emotional, spiritual, and/or developmental issues that occur near death.

The goals of care for a client near the end of life are to control symptoms, promote meaningful interactions between the client and significant others, and facilitate a peaceful death. Interventions that attend to the physical, psychologic, social, and spiritual needs of clients require an interdisciplinary approach to care that is accessible and committed to these goals. The interdisciplinary care of hospice is the most successful approach to end-of-life care to date. Although the perception of hospice is that it provides care for the dying, the emphasis of hospice care is on its provision of quality of life for clients with terminal disease. As a concept, **hospice** is an alternative approach to care for clients near the end of life. It has served as a catalyst for integrating palliative care into traditional health care services such as acute care, extended care, and home care facilities (American Association of Colleges of Nursing, 1998).

Hospice Care

Hospice care was developed in the United States during the 1970s in response to the unmet needs of terminally ill clients. As both a philosophy and a system of care, hospice care seeks to use an interdisciplinary approach to facilitate both quality of life and death with dignity for clients with terminal disease. Hospice programs are often affiliated with home care agencies, providing services to clients at home or in an extended care facility. Some communities also have hospice houses, which admit clients in the terminal phase of their illness and provide a safe haven where they can die.

Not all hospices restrict their services to the terminally ill. Some agencies have bridge programs that target clients who have advanced disease but do not meet the criteria for hospice (i.e., a prognosis limited to 6 months or less). The advantages of bridge programs are that they allow expert palliative care to be given to clients whose exact prognosis might not be known or to clients who are not ready to accept what they perceive as end-of-life care. Bridge programs also facilitate the delivery of palliative care to clients whose health care providers are reluctant to refer clients to hospice because of the negative connotation they may have.

Symptoms of Distress at End of Life

As death nears, clients often manifest physical symptoms of distress that require treatment to control them until death. Pain, dyspnea, agitation, nausea, and vomiting are common causes of distress at the end of life (Fainsinger et al., 1991; Kazanowski, 1996). Other symptoms of distress at the end of life include, but are not limited to, fatigue, weakness, constipation, anorexia, and delirium.

In general, the occurrence of symptoms such as pain, dyspnea, delirium, nausea, and vomiting requires the use of medications such as analgesics, sedatives, and/or antiemetics. Once these symptoms occur, medications are usually administered around-the-clock until death to prevent recurrence and attain control. With the appropriate knowledge and resources, the management of symptoms near death can usually be achieved with medication. In fact, studies show that symptoms of distress (e.g., pain near death) can be effectively controlled in more than 90% of cases when clients have access to palliative care providers (Management of Cancer Pain Guideline Panel, 1994)

COLLABORATIVE MANAGEMENT

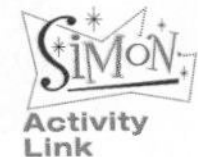

Assessment

HISTORY

The nurse obtains information about the client's diagnosis, past medical history, and recent state of health to identify possible risks for symptoms near death. For example, clients with lung cancer, cardiac failure, or chronic respiratory disease are at high risk for respiratory distress and dyspnea near death. Clients who have been experiencing pain often continue to have pain, and it may increase, decrease, or remain at the same level of intensity.

PHYSICAL ASSESSMENT/CLINICAL MANIFESTATIONS

Near the end of life, the client often grows weak and lethargic and sleeps for longer periods of time. This lethargy and sleep may progress to the point that the client has a decreased level of consciousness and rouses only to touch. In many cases, the ability of the client to communicate verbally diminishes and level of consciousness decreases, making it difficult to assess the client's perception of symptoms. When caring for clients who are unable to communicate their distress or needs, it is essential that health care providers identify alternative ways to assess symptoms of distress. Professional caregivers should teach family caregivers to watch closely for objective signs of discomfort (e.g., restlessness, grimacing, or moaning) and to identify when these symptoms occur in relation to positioning, movement, medication, or other external stimuli (Chart 9-1). For example, grimacing when turning from side to side in the bed is indicative of pain or discomfort with movement. When the head of the bed is flat, an increase in respiratory rate and effort indicates shortness of breath and is referred to as orthopnea.

Although the client's point of view is the most valid indicator of comfort or distress, the family's perception of symptoms is also important. The family's perceptions of symptoms should be obtained as part of each client's symptom assessment. Research has shown that family caregivers, health care providers, and clients may differ in their perceptions of symptoms in terms of intensity, significance, and meaning (McMillan, 1996; Weitzner, Moody, & McMillan, 1997). Whereas health care providers are often more adept at identifying symptoms of distress, families are often more knowledgeable about client habits and preferences. Health care providers need to incorporate all client-related information into the plan for symptom management and work with clients and families toward a common goal or outcome.

When first recognized, a symptom of distress is assessed in terms of intensity, frequency, duration, quality, exacerbating and relieving factors, and effect on the client's sleep and ability to participate in activities of daily living. A method for rating the intensity of that symptom should be used to facilitate

CHART 9-1

CLIENT EDUCATION GUIDE
Common Physical Signs and Symptoms of Approaching Death

Coolness of Extremities
Circulation to the extremities is decreased; the skin may become mottled or discolored.
- Cover the person with a blanket.
- Do not use an electric blanket, hot water bottle, electric heating pad, or hair dryer to warm the person.

Increased Sleeping
Metabolism is decreased.
- Spend time sitting quietly with the person.
- Do not force the person to stay awake.
- Talk to the person as you normally would, even if he or she does not respond.

Fluid and Food Decrease
Metabolic needs have decreased.
- Do not force the person to eat or drink.
- Offer ice chips or small sips of liquids at frequent intervals if the person is alert.
- Use glycerine swabs to keep the mouth moist and comfortable.
- Coat the lips with lip balm or petroleum jelly.

Incontinence
The perineal muscles relax.
- Keep the area clean and dry.
- If the person would be more comfortable, use urine catheters.

Congestion and Gurgling
The person is unable to cough up secretions effectively.
- Suctioning can be used to remove secretions, but this may cause discomfort.
- Medications can decrease the production of secretions.

Breathing Pattern Change
Slowed circulation to the brain may cause the breathing pattern to become irregular, with brief periods of no breathing or shallow breathing.
- Elevate the person's head.
- Position the person on his or her side.

Disorientation
Decreased metabolism and slowed circulation to the brain may occur.
- Identify yourself whenever you communicate with the person.
- Speak softly, clearly, and truthfully.

Restlessness
Decreased metabolism and slowed circulation to the brain may occur.
- Play soothing music.
- Do not restrain the person.
- Massage the person's forehead.
- Reduce the number of people in the room.

Modified from the Hospice of North Central Florida, Inc.

ongoing assessments and evaluate treatment response. A rating scale of 0 to 10 is commonly used, with 0 indicating no pain or dyspnea and 10 indicating the worst possible pain and dyspnea. The intensity of the symptom before and after an intervention (e.g., medication) is documented and is referred to daily to evaluate the client's overall comfort. (See Chapter 7 for a complete discussion of pain assessment.)

The nurse assesses the client for any sign or symptom that indicates pain, dyspnea, agitation, nausea, or vomiting. Pertinent information includes heart rate, respiratory rate and effort, breath sounds, bowel sounds, abdominal distention, last bowel movement, urine output, and temperature.

As death nears, peripheral circulation decreases and the client's skin often becomes cold, mottled, and cyanotic. If blood pressure has been monitored, the nurse will notice that it becomes lower and then disappears. The dying person's pulse may increase in rate, become irregular in rhythm, gradually decrease, and stop. Meanwhile, respirations become shallow until they, too, stop. Death has taken place when respirations and heartbeat cease.

> **CULTURAL CONSIDERATIONS**
>
> Mainstream values in the United States affect how middle class, upper middle class, and upper class people in the United States deal with "dying." These groups believe that an answer or solution is always possible and that choices should always be available. This is probably why the dying process in the United States is so often oriented to a "high-tech" hospital setting and why family demands for testing and treatment are common, even when the clients themselves prefer a palliative approach.
>
> Hispanic Americans tend to see dying as a family affair; one primary caregiver, usually a wife or daughter, tends to take responsibility for the majority of care. For Southeast Asians, discussing dying brings bad luck, and hospitals and treatments are alien. Some Southeast Asians, especially if uneducated, are likely to avoid visiting terminally ill family members for fear of contracting the disease.

Various other values, religious beliefs, healing practices (e.g., faith healing), and family structures can also affect dying in challenging ways. Nurses need to assess the cultural beliefs of both clients and their families to assess their potential effect on the process of dying and symptom control. (See Chapter 7 for cultural pain considerations.)

PSYCHOSOCIAL ASSESSMENT

Individuals facing death may have coping difficulties, fear, and anxiety with regard to their decline and/or their impending death. However, the existence of these manifestations is not universal and should not be assumed. Families of individuals near death are more likely to manifest fear, anxiety, and knowledge deficits regarding the process of death and their role in it.

The nurse assesses the client and individual family members for signs and symptoms of fear and anxiety and for their expectations regarding death. Families may have a preconceived notion about the dying process that may or may not be realistic. Chart 9-2 describes the common emotional signs of approaching death that the nurse should explain to the client, family, or significant others.

Analysis

COMMON NURSING DIAGNOSES AND COLLABORATIVE PROBLEMS

The major collaborative problem is Potential for Symptoms of Distress at End of Life.

The major nursing diagnosis is Risk for Ineffective Individual and/or Family Coping related to the loss of health and impending death.

ADDITIONAL NURSING DIAGNOSES AND COLLABORATIVE PROBLEMS

In addition to the major nursing diagnosis and collaborative problem, clients and their families may have one or more of the following:

- Anticipatory Grieving related to an actual loss
- Spiritual Distress related to a challenged belief and value system
- Hopelessness related to impending death

Planning and Implementation

POTENTIAL FOR SYMPTOMS OF DISTRESS AT END OF LIFE

PLANNING: EXPECTED OUTCOMES. The priority outcome for the client at the end of life is to achieve physical and psychologic comfort until the time of death. Client suffering at the end of life is unacceptable.

INTERVENTIONS. The most common symptoms of distress are dysphagia (impaired swallowing), pain, dyspnea, nausea and vomiting, and agitation. Interventions aim to promote comfort and manage these symptoms.

> **CHART 9-2**
>
> **CLIENT EDUCATION GUIDE**
> **Common Emotional Signs of Approaching Death**
>
> **Withdrawal**
> The person is preparing to "let go" from surroundings and relationships.
>
> **Vision-like Experiences**
> The person may talk to people you cannot see or hear and see objects and places not visible to you. These are not hallucinations or drug reactions.
> - Do not deny or argue with what the person claims.
> - Affirm the experience.
>
> **Letting Go**
> The person may become agitated or continue to perform repetitive tasks. Often this indicates that something is unresolved or is preventing the person from letting go. As difficult as it may be to do or say, the dying person takes on a more peaceful demeanor when loved ones are able to say things such as "It's okay to go. We'll be all right."
>
> **Saying Goodbye**
> When the person is ready to die and you are ready to let go, saying "Goodbye" is important for both of you. Touching, hugging, crying, and saying "I love you," "Thank you," "I'm sorry," or "I'll miss you so much" are all natural expressions of sadness and loss. Verbalizing these sentiments can bring comfort both to the dying person and to those left behind.

Modified from the Hospice of North Central Florida, Inc.

DYSPHAGIA MANAGEMENT. Clients near death often lose their ability to swallow because of changes in mental status and/or extreme weakness. Anorexia is also common. If the client is not awake, professional and family caregivers should avoid giving food or liquid orally because of the risk of aspiration. Nurses need to reassure the family that anorexia is often normal and that giving fluid or food can actually lead to discomfort. In general, families have great difficulty accepting that their loved ones are not being fed and may request that intravenous (IV) fluids be initiated. With great sensitivity, the nurse reinforces that the cessation of food and liquids is a natural process and that hydration can actually increase discomfort in a person with multisystem slowdown. Discomfort from fluid replacement could lead to respiratory secretions (and distress), increased gastrointestinal secretions, nausea, vomiting, edema, and ascites. Applying emollient to the lips and moistening the mouth and lips with applicators and saturated gauze can help prevent and/or relieve the dry mouth that may occur with a decreased oral intake.

Impaired swallowing near death also presents a problem for medication management. Clients often lose their ability to swallow their oral medications. Although some pills may be crushed, medications such as sustained-release capsules cannot be taken apart. Scheduled medications can often be discontinued, but medications for pain, dyspnea, agitation, nausea, and vomiting need to be continued to maintain symptom control until death. If faced with this situation, the nurse needs to identify alternatives such as sublingual, rectal, IV, or subcutaneous routes. A change in route of administration often requires a change in the dose of medication. The guiding principle for choice of route in clients near death is to choose the least invasive route with the most effective treatment (Coluzzi & Fairbairn, 1999). Identifying the appropriate routes and dosages often requires the input of a physician, nurse practitioner, nurse, or pharmacist who is knowledgeable in palliative care.

Although clients near death are often obtunded and/or withdrawn from the external environment, their sense of hearing remains intact until death. Conversation in the room and near the client should be conducted as if the client were alert. Caregivers are encouraged to talk softly to the client and to touch and gently stroke the skin. Although the dying person may not respond, these actions foster a sense of communication between the client and the caregiver.

PAIN MANAGEMENT. Pain is the symptom that dying clients fear the most. Although it is not universal, it is common and has many possible causes. Diseases such as cancer often cause tumor pain as a result of the infiltration of malignant cells into organs, nerves, and bones. Other causes of pain in dying clients include "disturbance" pain resulting from headaches, osteoarthritis, muscle spasms, and stiff joints caused by immobility.

Clients who have had their pain controlled with long-acting opioids must continue their scheduled doses of opioids to prevent any recurrence of pain. Depending on the brand of long-acting opioid, oral capsules may be given rectally (same dose and same capsule) when clients are no longer able to swallow. Increases in pain require immediate-relief analgesics (e.g., morphine sulfate immediate-release) and possibly an increase in long-acting opioids. Liquid morphine sulfate can be given sublingually, rectally, or via the buccal mucosa, and it is quick acting, effective, and safe to administer, even to comatose clients. Chapter 7 describes in detail the management of chronic malignant and nonmalignant pain, including complementary and alternative therapies.

DYSPNEA MANAGEMENT. Dyspnea is a subjective experience in which the client experiences an uncomfortable awareness of breathing, breathlessness, or severe shortness of breath (Hospice and Palliative Nurses Association, 1996). This condition can manifest itself as copious secretions, cough, chest pain, fatigue, or air hunger. It is a common symptom of distress near the end of life, occurring in 50% to 70% of dying clients. Many clients, families, and health care providers consider this to be the worst symptom of distress near death.

Dyspnea can be:

- Directly related to the client's primary diagnosis (e.g., lung cancer, breast cancer, or coronary artery disease)
- Secondary to the primary diagnosis (e.g., pleural effusion, metastasis to the lung or pleura)
- Related to treatment of the primary disease (e.g., congestive heart failure caused by chemotherapy, constrictive pericarditis due to radiation therapy, anemia related to chemotherapy)
- Related to an etiology unrelated to the primary disease (e.g., pneumonia)

Depending on the cause, the pathophysiology of dyspnea can involve the following:

- Obstructive, restrictive, or vascular disturbances in the airways with tumor or nodal involvement
- Pulmonary congestion secondary to fluid overload and or cardiac dysfunction
- Bronchoconstriction and bronchospasm as seen with respiratory infection, chronic obstructive pulmonary disease (COPD), or airway blockage by a tumor
- A decreased hemoglobin carrying capacity, as with anemia
- Hyperventilation secondary to neuromuscular disease, with limited movement of the diaphragm

The goal for the client with dyspnea near the end of life is to treat the primary cause and relieve the psychologic distress and autonomic response that accompany this symptom (Gavrin & Chapman, 1995). Because diagnostic testing to identify the cause of dyspnea at the end of life is usually inappropriate, the cause is determined by physical assessment and knowledge of the underlying condition. If the cause of dyspnea cannot be treated successfully, interventions are aimed at alleviating the distress.

OPIOIDS. Morphine sulfate is the standard treatment for dyspnea near death. Nurses need to understand that individuals who have not been taking daily opioids should initially receive low doses of morphine (e.g., 5 to 10 mg PO or sublingually), which can be repeated if necessary. Individuals who have been taking opioids for pain will need to have their breakthrough dose of morphine increased by 50% of their usual dose for effective treatment of dyspnea. If IV access is available, health care providers may order 1 to 2 mg of morphine to be given every 5 to 10 minutes until relief is obtained. However, health care providers should not initiate IV access in dying clients unless it is absolutely necessary.

Morphine via a facial nebulizer is another option for dyspnea near the end of life. Although some research suggests that the nebulized route is no more effective than the oral route, anecdotal reports indicate that nebulized morphine is effective, easy to administer, and has no side effects. The suggested dose for nebulized morphine is 4 mg morphine with 2.5 mL normal saline (Wrede-Seaman, 1996).

DIURETICS, BRONCHODILATORS, CORTICOSTEROIDS, AND ANTIBIOTICS. Individuals with signs of fluid volume excess as manifested by dyspnea, crackles on auscultation, peripheral edema, and other signs of heart failure should be given a diuretic such as furosemide (Lasix) to decrease blood volume, reduce vascular congestion, and reduce the workload of the heart. Furosemide can be administered by mouth, intravenously, subcutaneously, or intramuscularly. IV administration, which is effective in the pulmonary system within minutes, may be preferred for treating congestive heart failure and pulmonary edema.

Bronchodilators such as albuterol or ipratropium bromide via a metered dose inhaler (MDI) or nebulizer may be given for symptoms of bronchospasm (e.g., wheezes on auscultation of breath sounds). Corticosteroids may also be given for bronchospasm and inflammatory problems within and exterior to the lung. Superior vena cava syndrome and lymphangitis carcinomatosis can cause dyspnea and may respond to corticosteroids.

Antibiotics may be indicated in clients with dyspnea secondary to a respiratory infection. A thorough workup for a respiratory infection is not appropriate in clients in whom death is imminent. However, it is safe to assume they have an upper respiratory infection if they have developed dyspnea along with an elevated temperature, adventitious breath sounds, and a congested cough. A trial of an appropriate antibiotic should be considered if they are suffering from the infection.

ANTICHOLINERGICS. Secretions in the respiratory tract and oral cavity may contribute to a client's dyspnea near death. Loud, wet respirations (referred to as "death rattle") are disturbing to family and caregivers even when they do not seem to cause dyspnea or respiratory distress. Anticholinergics such as oral or sublingual hyoscyamine (Levsin) or transdermal scopolamine are used to reduce the production of secretions.

OXYGEN. The use of oxygen for clients with hypoxemia is recognized as an important part of treatment. However, oxygen for dyspnea near death has not been established as a standard of care for all individuals (Harwood, 1999). Some studies have shown significant improvement in dyspnea in the presence of hypoxia, but others have demonstrated no improvement in dyspnea despite the use of oxygen. Other studies have shown improvement in dyspnea in groups of clients who were not hypoxemic.

The need for oxygen for dyspnea at the end of life depends on the client's perception of the need and his or her perception of its effect. Many practitioners believe that oxygen is not necessary near the end of life and can actually cause discomfort; they believe comfort can be better achieved using morphine. Indeed, many clients with dyspnea near death often remove their oxygen and can be kept comfortable without it. It is imperative, however, that clients who do not respond promptly to morphine or other medications be given a trial dose of oxygen to assess its effect, whether or not they are hypoxemic.

SEDATIVES. Sedatives such as benzodiazepines are commonly used when morphine does not fully control the client's dyspnea. Lorazepam (Ativan) 0.5 mg is commonly administered orally or sublingually every 4 hours or around-the-clock to prevent or control dyspnea and anxiety.

NONPHARMACOLOGIC INTERVENTIONS. Pharmacologic interventions should be initiated early in the course of dyspnea near death. Nonpharmacologic interventions can be used in conjunction with, but not in place of, medications. Nonpharmacologic interventions include the following:

- Altering the environment to facilitate the circulation of cool air (e.g., via air-conditioner or fan)
- Cooling the body
- Positioning the client to facilitate chest expansion
- Encouraging imagery and deep breathing
- Intervening to conserve client energy
- Facilitating the client's rest

Positioning the body with the head of the bed elevated and the upper body supported to facilitate diaphragmatic excursion can be accomplished with a hospital bed or pillows or with the client out of bed and in a chair. Insertion of a Foley catheter to avoid the need for exertion with voiding may be considered if the client will benefit.

NAUSEA AND VOMITING MANAGEMENT. Although not as common a problem as pain or dyspnea, nausea and vomiting are thought to occur in approximately 40% of terminally ill individuals during the last week of life. Nausea and vomiting are particularly prevalent in individuals with acquired immunodeficiency syndrome (AIDS) or breast, stomach, or gynecologic cancers.

Common causes of nausea and vomiting at the end of life include the following:

- Initiation of opioid therapy (nausea usually lasts a few days)
- Uremia
- Hypercalcemia
- Increased intracranial pressure secondary to brain metastasis
- Vagal stimulation secondary to oral candida
- Stretching of the hepatic capsule
- Constipation or impaction
- Bowel obstruction

If constipation is identified as a problem, a biphosphate enema is administered in an attempt to release stool quickly. If stool in the rectum cannot be evacuated, a mineral oil enema followed by disimpaction may be required to relieve the client's distress.

Nausea and vomiting related to other causes can generally be controlled by one or more antiemetic agents. Combinations of antiemetics as rectal suppositories or oral troches can be tried and individualized for maximal relief and control (Chart 9-3).

AGITATION MANAGEMENT. Agitation at the end of life requires that the nurse assess for pain or urinary retention, constipation, or other reversible cause. If constipation is ruled out as the cause and if analgesia and catheterization do not re-

CHART 9-3

BEST PRACTICE *for* Symptom Relief

- For unrelieved pain: Morphine solution, 0.25 to 0.5 mL (PO/SL) (20 mg/1 mL solution) q2-3h prn
- For unrelieved dyspnea: Morphine solution, 0.25 to 0.5 mL (PO/SL) (20 mg/1 mL solution) q2h prn
- For nausea or vomiting: Prochlorperazine, 25-mg suppository, 1 PR q8h prn
- For unrelieved nausea or vomiting, or for agitation/restlessness: ABH* suppository, 1 PR q8h prn
- For severe agitation and restlessness:
  - Determine if client is in pain; treat accordingly.
  - Determine if client is constipated or experiencing urinary retention; take appropriate action.
  - If agitation persists and the safety of the client or caregiver is at risk, administer pentobarbitol suppository, 1 PR q4-6h prn.
- For loud, wet respirations or excessive secretions: Hyoscyamine (Levsin) SL tablets, 1 to 2 PO or SL q4-6h prn
- For unrelieved respiratory fluid accumulation: Furosemide (Lasix), 40 to 80 mg PO, SC, IM, or IV × 1

Printed with permission from VNA Hospice, Visiting Nurse Services, Manchester, NH.
SL, Sublingual; *PR,* per rectum.
*Many hospice and palliative care organizations use pharmacist-compounded suppositories for symptom relief. One such combination is ABH, which stands for Ativan (lorazepam), Benadryl (diphenhydramine), and Haldol (haloperidol). Reglan (metoclopramide) may be added to equate to ABHR Suppository.

lieve the restlessness, sedatives should be administered to provide some relief. Consultation with a spiritual and/or bereavement counselor should be considered to assess for unfinished business or spiritual distress as a possible cause of the agitation.

Benzodiazepines such as lorazepam (Ativan) or alprazolam (Xanax) are often given for anxiety, restlessness, or myoclonus near death. Lorazepam 1 to 2 mg is often crushed and given sublingually with a few drops of water; this is continued at 0.5 to 2 mg every 6 to 8 hours around-the-clock. If paradoxical agitation occurs, another benzodiazepine is substituted for lorazepam. Until recently, long-acting benzodiazepines such as diazepam (Valium) were not recommended for agitation near death. However, long-acting medications such as diazepam (Valium) and clonazepam (Klonopin) are now considered helpful in controlling anxiety near death.

Barbiturates such as phenobarbital or pentobarbital are given when benzodiazepines fail to control anxiety, delirium, or restlessness near death (March, 1998). The neuroleptic haloperidol (Haldol) may be administered when hallucinations or paranoia occur (Levy, 1999) (see Chart 9-3).

MANAGEMENT OF THE REFRACTORY SYMPTOMS OF DISTRESS. Studies show that the majority of clients with access to palliative care achieve control of symptoms such as pain, dyspnea, and agitation near death. However, a small percentage of clients (less than 5% to 10%) experience symptoms of distress that are refractory or resistant to treatment. They may require such high doses of analgesia that sedation occurs as a side effect, or they may actually need to be sedated to control symptoms of distress. Although sedation is not ideal, its occurrence as a side effect of treatment for symptoms of distress at the end of life may be acceptable if there is no alternative for comfort. It is important that both health care providers and the public understand that adequate symptom management may at times result in sedation. The sedation that occurs is a side effect of treatment—it is not a treatment goal or an effect meant to hasten death.

The administration of medications for symptoms of distress at the end of life is guided by protocols using doses of medications that are considered safe. These guidelines and protocols are used with the intention of alleviating suffering, not hastening death. The occurrence of an untoward effect of a medication is, however, a risk. According to the Guideline Panel for Management of Cancer Pain (1994), the increased risk of earlier death counts little against the benefit of pain relief and painless death in a client who faces imminent death from progression of a primary disease. The ethical duty of the nurse is to assist in relieving pain or other symptoms of distress in a client near death.

RISK FOR INEFFECTIVE INDIVIDUAL AND/OR FAMILY COPING

PLANNING: EXPECTED OUTCOMES. The client and family or significant others are expected to acknowledge the client's loss of health and independence and impending death.

INTERVENTIONS. Most research on loss, grieving, and coping with death has focused on Caucasian, English-speaking populations. The grieving responses and coping mechanisms of other cultural groups have not been widely studied except in reference to religious beliefs. Table 9-1 lists the specific beliefs and customs of various groups regarding death and dying. The nurse keeps these values in mind when planning and implementing interventions to assist with coping with the end of life.

Interventions are aimed at providing appropriate emotional support to allow clients and families to verbalize their fears and concerns. Nurses can also assist by keeping families informed of the client's level of comfort, keeping them involved in health care decisions, and reframing the situation to emphasize the goal of keeping the individual comfortable.

OFFERING PHYSICAL AND EMOTIONAL SUPPORT. The nurse intervenes with those grieving an impending death by "being with" as opposed to "being there." "Being with" implies that the nurse is physically and psychologically with the grieving client, empathizing to provide emotional support. Listening and somehow acknowledging the legitimacy of the client's pain are often more therapeutic than speaking; this concept is sometimes referred to as **presence.** Nurses facilitate the expression of grief by giving the person who is mourning permission to express herself or himself. The nurse's manner and words show that these expressions of grief are acceptable and expected. Nurses can say something such as, "This must be very difficult for you." or "I'm sorry this is happening."

BEING REALISTIC. The pain of loss cannot be, nor should it be, taken away no matter how committed the nurse may be to the client's comfort. The nurse avoids trite assurances such as, "Things will be fine. Don't cry" or "Don't be upset. She wouldn't want it that way" or "In a year you will have forgotten." Such comments can actually be barriers to demonstrating care and concern. The nurse accepts whatever the grieving person says about the situation and remains pres-

TABLE 9-1 • MAJOR RELIGIOUS GROUPS IN THE UNITED STATES: CONCEPTS AND PRACTICES RELATED TO DEATH

Afterlife	Rituals	Handling of the Body After Death	"Extraordinary" Life-Prolonging Measures
EASTERN ORTHODOXY (INCLUDING GREEK AND RUSSIAN ORTHODOXY)			
Yes, the soul blends into the spiritual cosmos.	The client's arms are crossed after death, with the fingers set in the shape of a cross. Special prayers are said for those who have been baptized to bless the sick and dying. Last Rites must be delivered while the person is still conscious. Holy Communion is obligatory.	Autopsy and embalming are discouraged. Organ and body donation are discouraged. Cremation is discouraged.	Encouraged
JUDAISM			
The dead will be resurrected with the coming of the Messiah. A person lives on in the memories of his or her survivors. For Reform Jews, there is no concept of eternal punishment.	The dying and dead are never left unattended before burial because the soul should depart in the presence of people. The body is ritually washed, sometimes by members of a ritual burial society. Burial is in a wooden casket within 24 hours or as soon as possible after death. Five stages of mourning extend over a year. Funerals are very simple, with no flowers (flowers are a symbol of life).	Orthodox Jews prohibit autopsy and do not allow removal of body parts. Conservative and Reform Jews permit autopsy. For Orthodox Jews, embalming is not allowed. Beliefs about organ and body donation vary. Orthodox Jews generally prohibit both but may agree with rabinical consent. Cremation is largely prohibited, but beliefs vary. Reform Jews allow cremation but recommend the burial of ashes in a Jewish cemetery.	Generally discouraged after irreversible brain damage is determined Orthodox Jews advocate life support without "heroic measures"
ROMAN CATHOLICISM			
The faithful go to Heaven, but those who reject God's grace go to Hell. The soul goes to Purgatory for a time and is released by prayers and Masses. Resurrection occurs at the second coming of Christ.	The family and priest choose the prayers. Holy Communion and rites for anointing the sick are mandatory. Confession may be desired but is not mandatory; however, repentance is recommended.	Autopsy is permitted, but all body parts must be buried appropriately. Organ and body donation are unrestricted provided that the donor is not harmed. Cremation is not restricted.	Discouraged
PROTESTANTISM			
Varies; Episcopalians, Presbyterians, and Lutherans strongly believe in an afterlife, Quakers strongly do not.	Varies, anointing rites, confession, and communion may be available but are not mandatory. Healing services may be available, but there are no official sacraments. The client and family may have a large role in planning services and prayer; services range from traditional funerals to memorial services. Clergy may minister through prayer, scripture reading, and counseling.	Beliefs about autopsy, organ and body donation, and cremation vary by group, from no restriction to individual choice to preferred.	Discouraged
NONAFFILIATED			
Varies.	Services are spontaneous and individualized, possibly including a reading of original or traditional prayers or songs such as Psalm 23. Traditional secular funeral or memorial services are used.	Autopsy, organ and body donation, and cremation are by individual preference.	Individual preference

ent, ready to listen attentively and guide gently. In this way, nurses help the bereaved prepare for the necessary reminiscence and integration of the loss.

ENCOURAGING REMINISCENCE. Storytelling through reminiscence and life review can be a very important activity for clients who are dying. **Life review** is a structured process of reflecting on one's life and is often facilitated by an interviewer. **Reminiscence** is the process of randomly reflecting on memories of events in one's life. The benefits of storytelling through either method include catharsis, the ability to attain perspective, and enhancement of meaning (Brady, 1999). The nurse suggests that the client and family tape autobiographical stories, record memories in a journal, or develop a scrapbook. If the client does not have enough energy for these activities, familiar objects such as photographs and favorite jewelry pieces can be used to spark ideas for stories that the client may want to tell.

PROMOTING SPIRITUALITY. **Spirituality,** a part of every human being, is the connection to self, others, the environment, and a Higher Power (e.g., God, Allah, Spirit). **Religiosity** describes the acts that are practiced alone or with others to preserve spiritual understanding (Cairns, 1999).

Spirituality and religiosity contribute to health but also have an impact on palliative care and the dying client. Studies have shown that religious acts (e.g., prayer, meditation, inspirational reading, recitation of mantras) help clients cope with death and the dying process (Cairns, 1999). The nurse encourages activities that promote spirituality and also supports family members as they help their loved ones to express their faith and beliefs.

FOSTERING HOPE. Hope involves picturing a reality that is not yet present and imagining what a situation might be like. This image sets the direction for clients and their families to give them purpose in life and to help them find the strength to go forward, even in the darkest times (Wang, 2000). Nurses can foster hope for clients and their families by listening and caring.

AVOIDING EXPLANATIONS OF THE LOSS. The nurse should not try to explain the loss in philosophic or religious terms. Statements such as "Everything happens for the best" or "God sends us only as much as we can bear" are not helpful when the bereaved person has yet to express feelings of anguish or anger. Telling someone too soon that they have other children to rely on or that there are other family members who need them does not diminish the intensity of the grief. In fact, doing so can create feelings of anger and resentment toward the nurse because it reflects an insensitivity to the acute initial pain.

"Being with" remains important as the weeks or months pass and the funeral crisis supports dissipate. The out-of-town relatives return home, and friends and local relatives resume their own lives. The nurse should consider contacting family members after the death to allow them the opportunity to voice their perceptions of the experience. In particular, family caregivers who assumed the role of symptom manager in the home often welcome the opportunity to discuss their experience.

PROVIDING REFERRALS TO BEREAVEMENT COUNSELORS. The nurse informs the family about bereavement counselors and support groups for persons who have loved ones with life-threatening diseases and/or loved ones who have died. Bereavement counselors are extremely knowledgeable about the grieving process and can be accessed through hospice agencies. Any nurse caring for clients experiencing loss through chronic or acute illness should know how to access this resource.

Participation in support groups by individuals who are grieving a person's pending or past death has been shown to facilitate the grieving process. Being a part of a support group (e.g., Alzheimer Caregiver support group) can help people to discover that others have suffered through an experience just as devastating as their own. This discovery makes them more likely to share their feelings with others and work toward some resolution of the experience.

TEACHING ABOUT THE PHYSICAL SIGNS OF DEATH. Although emotionally challenging, witnessing the death of a loved one may actually facilitate the family's acceptance of death. Witnessing how ill a person is makes the event real and enhances an understanding of how disease affects bodily function and decline. If death is anticipated, the nurse uses nontechnical language to give the client and family or significant others information about the signs of death. The physical signs are described in detail—realistic enough to be unmistakable yet not so graphic as to alarm the listeners. Chart 9-1 describes the common signs and symptoms of approaching death in lay terms. Such charts are often shared with family and friends who are anticipating the death of a loved one.

ENSURING PALLIATIVE CARE. Family and friends who are anticipating the death of a loved one often fear that the death will be characterized by pain and suffering. The nurse reassures families that clients will be monitored closely for any sign or symptom of distress and that appropriate medications and other measures will be administered as needed until pain is controlled. Families are reassured that significant advances have been made in pain and symptom control.

• Community-Based Care

Most people who choose hospice care prefer the home to other caregiving environments during the final episodes of illness. Although there are exceptions, being surrounded by familiar people and things, having ready access to friends and relatives, and having the freedom from institutional restriction often make the home setting more comfortable and give the client and family more control. Clients whose cases are being followed by home hospice agencies have access to nurses, social workers, spiritual and/or bereavement counselors, and volunteers to assist in dealing with multiple end-of-life issues. Interdisciplinary hospice team meetings are scheduled regularly to review client needs and solve problems.

Although home care is less costly than inpatient care, it generally requires that a friend or family member(s) take on the responsibility of providing most physical and emotional care. Some families may not be able to manage the physically and psychologically demanding schedule of 24-hour, 7-day-a-week care. Depending on insurance benefits, some families may be entitled to assistive nursing personnel for personal client care in the home. In general, health care aides are allowed to assist in the home for only 1 to 2 hours once each day, sometimes twice each day if clients are bedbound or incontinent. Families who require more assistance with personal (custodial) care are often referred to agencies that hire out private duty nursing assistants. However, the family must pay for these services, and many families cannot afford them. If families are exhausted from providing care, respite care of the client in a palliative care setting should be available to allow caregivers a few days of rest.

To ensure that client and family needs are promptly addressed as they arise, hospices generally provide 24-hour on-call services. It is not always possible to predict the final phase of the terminal process and or the development of symptoms of distress. To address this problem, some hospices have arranged for pharmacies to supply clients (by prescription) with "symptom relief kits." These kits provide a limited amount of commonly used medications that are effective in treating symptoms near death. Chart 9-3 describes the contents of and directions for a "hospice symptom relief kit" to facilitate safe passage in the home.

DEATH AND DYING

Death

Death is manifested as the cessation of respiration and heartbeat caused by physiologic dysfunction, generally related to an illness or trauma that overwhelms the compensatory mechanisms of the body. Direct causes of death include respiratory failure (PCO_2 accumulation and PO_2 deficit) and hypovolemic, septic, or cardiogenic shock manifested as inadequate blood flow to meet the demands of vital organs. Inadequate blood flow to the tissues deprives cells of their source of oxygen and biochemical exchange—the ultimate factor in their death.

Clinical death refers to the short interval after the cessation of heartbeat and breathing when no evidence of brain function is present. If this termination of function occurs suddenly, as in cardiac arrest or massive hemorrhage, a brief time remains before vital organs lose their viability, and cardiopulmonary resuscitation (CPR) may be successful.

People with healthy organs are most likely to survive resuscitation. CPR is likely to be futile and therefore inappropriate in those with terminal disease. However, legal and ethical standards of care must be followed. Most agencies require that CPR be initiated on clients whose breathing or heartbeat has ceased unless a physician's order of "do not resuscitate" (DNR) is obtained. CPR is meant to sustain a person's vital organs until a more definitive treatment is initiated. When clients with terminal disease are near death, CPR is usually inappropriate because it does nothing to reverse the progress of the terminal disease. CPR may be appropriate if it can reverse a life-threatening event.

Each and every individual has the right to decide if he or she wants CPR and aggressive treatment at the end of life. Clients with terminal disease should be educated about the goals of CPR and should be informed that it is usually ineffective in people with terminal disease. Nurses need to address the issue of CPR and advance directives with great sensitivity and as soon as possible when caring for a client who may be near death. Clients and or families often need time to process this information before deciding on their course of action.

CHART 9-4

FOCUSED ASSESSMENT *of* Physical Manifestations of Death

- No breathing
- No heartbeat
- Release of bowel and bladder contents
- No response to name, environmental sounds, touch, or pain
- Eyelids slightly open
- Pupils enlarged and not constricting in response to light
- Eyes fixed on a certain spot
- No blinking in response to air moving over the eyes or to a light touch on the eye
- Jaw relaxed and mouth slightly open

Dying

Death is the termination of life, whereas dying is a process. Individuals facing death may demonstrate emotional signs and symptoms of their response to the dying process through behaviors that equate to saying goodbye or through actual withdrawal. Families need to be educated that such behaviors are normal to the process of dying (see Chart 9-2).

Postmortem Care

The dying client may have such reduced physical activity that actual death can be difficult to ascertain. Chart 9-4 lists the physical manifestations of death.

After a client's death, the nurse or the physician (depending on the state) pronounces death. He or she then completes a death certificate, which must accompany the body to the funeral home. The nurse or other member of the nursing staff prepares the body for immediate postmortem viewing. All tubes and linens are removed or cut according to agency policy, the eyes are closed, dentures are replaced, and the body is straightened. The nurse removes all pillows except for one supporting the head, which is kept in place to delay blood pooling and face discoloration. Pads are placed under the client's hips and around the perineum to absorb fecal material and fluid. Each health care agency has its own policies and procedures for postmortem care. Chart 9-5 lists typical postmortem nursing interventions.

The family or significant others may then have privacy while they join the deceased in the room. They may perform religious or cultural customs as described in Table 9-1. If the family wishes to see a member of the clergy, the nurse notifies the hospital chaplain or appropriate community religious leader.

After the family or significant others view the body, the nurse follows agency procedure for preparing the client for transfer to either the morgue or a funeral home. The necessary materials, such as a shroud and identification tags, are usually supplied in a packet.

Euthanasia

Under some conditions, keeping someone alive through technologic life support rather than actively and arbitrarily ending

CHART 9-5

BEST PRACTICE *for* Postmortem Care

- Ensure that the nurse or physician has completed and signed the death certificate.
- Ask the family or significant others if they wish to wash or help wash the client.
- Remove or cut all tubes and lines according to health care agency policy.
- Close the client's eyes.
- Replace dentures or other dental appliances, if worn.
- Straighten the client and lower the bed to a flat position.
- Place a pillow under the client's head.
- Wash the client as needed; comb and arrange the client's hair.
- Place pads under the client's hips and around the perineum to absorb feces and urine.
- Clean up the client's room or unit.
- Allow the family or significant others to see the client in private and to perform any religious or cultural customs they wish.
- Notify the hospital chaplain or appropriate community religious leader if requested by the family or significant others.
- Prepare the client for transfer to either a morgue or funeral home; wrap the client in a shroud and attach identification tags per agency policy (if the client is to be transferred to the morgue).

his or her life can provide time to try an experimental new therapy or perhaps allow for remission. Unfortunately, an interval such as this does not always provide quality time for peace and growth. Instead this time may be fraught with pain, suffering, and confusion. The occurrence and fear of pain and suffering have stimulated movements that provide and support the controversial practice of euthanasia in society.

Euthanasia, derived from a Greek word meaning "easy or pleasant death," implies that under some circumstances death is preferable to life. **Active euthanasia** refers to an act of commission that directly and *intentionally* shortens a person's life. **Passive euthanasia** is an act of omission and usually refers to letting the person die by either withdrawing or withholding a treatment that might prolong life.

Although active euthanasia is condemned by many professional organizations (e.g., the American Nurses Association, the American Medical Association) and religious communities (e.g., the Catholic Church), the rights of clients or their surrogates to refuse or stop life-sustaining treatment (e.g., mechanical ventilation, tube feedings, antibiotics) are actually supported by these same communities. **Advance directives** (e.g., durable power of attorney for health care, living will) have allowed U.S. residents to make known their wishes about treatment at the end of life, which helps surrogate decision makers with their decisions when clients are unconscious or incompetent (Figure 9-1). The Patient Self-Determination Act (1990) requires that all clients admitted to health care agencies be asked if they have drafted advance directives. The intent of this Act was to facilitate end-of-life treatment decisions before a crisis situation occurs. Clients who have not drafted advance directives should be given information about the process and the implications of having (or not having) these in place and should be assisted in drafting them.

Much confusion exists regarding euthanasia and the treatment of dying clients. It is important that health care providers, clients, and families understand the distinction between active and passive euthanasia and assisted suicide versus the appropriate treatment of pain and symptoms of distress. Because nurses spend more time with clients than do other health care providers, they should be competent in and committed to initiating discussions of end-of-life issues when appropriate. Recent research indicates that many hospitalized clients die undergoing aggressive treatment and pain and without regard for their wishes. Better communication between clients and health care providers and more collaboration among physicians and nurses are needed if end-of-life decisions of clients in acute care are to be heeded (see the Evidence-Based Practice for Nursing box above.

EVIDENCE-BASED PRACTICE FOR NURSING

Painful deaths for seriously ill hospitalized clients continue despite a physician education intervention

Support Study Principal Investigators. (1995). A controlled trial to improve care for seriously ill hospitalized patients. *Journal of the American Medical Association, 274,* 1591-1598.

The objectives of this two-phase study were to improve end-of-life decision making and to reduce the frequency of mechanically supported, painful, prolonged dying in seriously ill hospitalized clients. The sample involved 9105 adults hospitalized with one or more of nine life-threatening diseases in one of five major teaching hospitals in the United States. Phase I, a 2-year prospective observational study, found that only 47% of physicians knew when their clients preferred to avoid cardiopulmonary resuscitation (CPR); 38% of clients who died spent at least 10 days in an intensive care unit. Family reports of moderate to severe pain occurred at least half the time in 50% of clients near death.

In phase II (intervention phase), physicians were provided with estimates of client 6-month survival (given their disease and condition), estimates of outcomes for CPR, and estimates on functional disability for clients at 2 months. This phase also included a specially trained nurse making multiple contacts with clients, families, physicians, and hospital staff to elicit preferences, improve understanding of outcomes, encourage attention to pain control, and facilitate advance directive planning and client-physician communication. The following were results of phase II: clients experienced no improvement in client-physician communication, no improvement occurred in physician's knowledge of client preferences not to be resuscitated, the number of days clients spent on mechanical ventilation or comatose in intensive care units did not decrease, and the level of pain reported by families of clients near death did not decrease.

Critique. This study was rigorous in its experimental design and large sample size. However, it does not explain why aggressive treatment was continued despite poor odds for recovery. For example, did clients change their minds? Did physicians simply ignore what clients and nurses communicated? Did they see the teaching hospital as one that assumes aggressive care, regardless of the odds? A qualitative component to the study might shed light on the findings.

Implications for Nursing. The role of the nurse in discussing end-of-life issues in acute care may not be deemed appropriate by providers making treatment decisions. Despite this perception, nurses are generally guided by state nurse practice acts to obtain comprehensive assessment data on all clients, and nurses are often the best equipped to initiate discussions on end-of-life issues. Nurses working with clients with serious illnesses should identify and fulfill their educational needs regarding end-of-life issues and effectively communicate their knowledge and concerns to physicians, clients, and families when appropriate.

DURABLE POWER OF ATTORNEY FOR HEALTH CARE

Power of Attorney made this ________ day of __________, 20 ____

1. I, the undersigned hereby appoint (insert name and address of agent)

____

as agent to act for me and in my name to make any and all decisions for me concerning my personal care, medical treatment, hospitalization and health care and to require, withhold or withdraw any type of medical treatment or procedure, even though my death may ensue. My agent shall have the same access to my medical records that I have, including the right to disclose the contents to others. My agent shall also have full power to make a disposition of any part or all of my body for medical purposes, authorize an autopsy and direct the disposition of my remains. (Neither the attending physician nor any other health care provider may act as your agent.)

2. The powers granted above shall be subject to the following rules or limitations (if none, leave blank):

____

____

(The subject of life-sustaining treatment is of particular importance. For your convenience in dealing with that subject some general statements concerning the withholding or removal of life-sustaining treatment are set forth below. If you agree with one of these statements, you may initial that statement; but do not initial more than one.)

(I do not want my life to be prolonged nor do I want life-sustaining treatment
(to be provided or continued if my agent believes the burdens of the treatment
(outweigh the expected benefits. I want my agent to consider the relief of
(suffering the expense involved and the quality as well as the possible extension
_____(of my life in making decisions concerning life-sustaining treatment.

(I want my life to be prolonged and I want life-sustaining treatment to be
(provided or continued unless I am in a coma which my attending physician
(believes to be irreversible, in accordance with reasonable medical standards at
(the time of reference. If and when I have suffered irreversible coma, I want
_____(life-sustaining treatment to be withheld or discontinued.

(I want my life to be prolonged to the greatest extent possible without regard to
_____(my condition, the chances I have for recovery or the cost of the procedures.

3. This power of attorney shall become effective on ______________________

____

4. This power of attorney shall terminate on ______________________

____

5. If any agent named by me shall die, become legally disabled, resign, refuse to act or be unavailable, I name the following (each to act alone and successively, in the order named) as successors to such agent:

____

____

6. If a guardian of my person is to be appointed, I nominate the following to serve as such guardian (if same as agent, leave blank):

____

Figure 9-1 ● An example of a durable power of attorney for health care.

7. **I am fully informed as to all the contents of this form and understand the full import of this grant of power to my agent.**

Signed ______________________
Principal

The principal has had an opportunity to read the above form and has signed the form or acknowledged his or her signature or mark on the form in my presence.

______________________ **Residing at** ______________________
Witness

(You may, but are not required to, request your agent and successor agents to provide specimen signature below. If you include specimen signature in this Power of Attorney, you must complete the certification opposite the signatures of the agents.)

Specimen signatures of agent (and successors)	**I certify that the signature of my agent (and successors) are correct.**
______________ **(agent)**	______________ **(principal)**
______________ **(successor agent)**	______________ **(principal)**
______________ **(successor agent)**	______________ **(principal)**

Figure 9-1, cont'd ● An example of a durable power of attorney for health care.

ONLINE RESOURCES

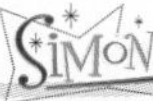

For suggested readings and Internet resources, go to http://www.wbsaunders.com/SIMON/Iggy/.

SELECTED BIBLIOGRAPHY

Asterisk indicates a classic or definitive work on this subject.

American Association of Colleges of Nursing. (1998). *Peaceful death: Recommended competencies and curricular guidelines for end-of-life nursing care.* Washington, DC: Author.

Bennett, J.A. (2000). Dehydration: Hazards and benefits. *Geriatric Nursing, 21*(2), 84-88.

Benzein, E., & Saveman, B. (1998). Nurses' perception of hope in patients with cancer: A palliative care perspective. *Cancer Nursing, 21*(1), 10-16.

Brady, E.M. (1999). Stories at the hour of our death. *Home Healthcare Nurse, 17*(3), 176-180.

Burke, A. (1997). Palliative care: An update in "terminal restlessness." *Medical Journal of Australia, 166*(1), 39-42.

Cairns, A.B. (1999). Spirituality and religiosity in palliative care. *Home Healthcare Nurse, 17*(7), 450-455.

Coluzzi, P.H. (1998). Sublingual morphine: Efficacy reviewed. *Journal of Pain and Symptom Management, 16,* 187-192.

Coluzzi, P.H., & Fairbairn, B.S. (1999). The management of pain in terminally ill cancer patients with difficulty swallowing. *American Journal of Hospice & Palliative Care, 16,* 731-737.

Committee on Care at the End of Life, Institute of Medicine. (1997). *Approaching death.* Washington, DC: National Academy Press.

Davis, A.J., & Konishi, E. (2000). End-of-life ethical issues in Japan. *Geriatric Nursing, 21*(2), 89-91.

*Escalante, C.P., et al. (1996). Dyspnea in cancer patients: Etiology, resource utilization, and survival implications in a managed care world. *Cancer, 78,* 1314-1319.

*Fainsinger, R., et al. (1991). Symptom control during the last week of life on a palliative care unit. *Journal of Palliative Care, 7*(1), 5-11.

*Gavrin, J., & Chapman, C. R. (1995). Clinical management of dying patients. *Caring for patients at the end of life [Special Issue]. Western Journal of Medicine, 163,* 268-277.

Harwood, K.V. (1999). Dyspnea. In C.H. Yarbro, M.H. Frogge, & M. Goodman (Eds.), *Cancer symptom management* (2nd ed., pp. 45-57). Boston: Jones & Bartlett.

*Hospice and Palliative Nurses Association. (1996). *Clinical practice protocol: Dyspnea.* Pittsburgh: Author.

Hospice and Palliative Nurses Association. (1997). *Clinical practice protocol: Terminal restlessness.* Pittsburgh, PA: Author.

International Council of Nurses. (1997). *Basic principles of nursing care.* Washington, DC: American Nurses Publishing.

James, K. (1998). In M. Snyder & R. Lindquist (Eds.). *Complementary/alternative therapies in nursing* (3rd ed., pp. 139-147). New York: Springer.

*Kazanowski, M. (June 1996). *Review of the literature on symptoms near death in patients with terminal cancer.* Paper presented at conference on research-based clinical practice, Dartmouth-Hitchcock Medical Center and Saint Anselm College, Nashua, NH.

Kazanowski, M. (1997). A commitment to palliative care: Could it impact assisted suicide? *Journal of Gerontological Nursing, 3*(3), 1-7.

Kazanowski, M. (1998). Commitment to the end: Family caregivers' medication management of symptoms in patients with cancer near death. (Doctoral dissertation, Boston College, Chestnut Hill, MA, 1998). *Dissertation Abstracts International.*

*Kubler-Ross, E. (1969). *On death and dying.* New York: Macmillan.

Levy, M. (1997). *Symptom control in advanced cancer.* Australia: Pharmacia & Upjohn.

Levy, M. (October 28, 1999). *Sedation in palliative care: Walking an ever-fine line.* 1999 Annual Conference, New Hampshire Cancer Pain Initiative and New Hampshire Hospice Organization, Portsmouth, NH.

*Management of Cancer Pain Guideline Panel. (1994). *Management of cancer pain. Clinical practice guidelines.* AHCPR Pub. No. 94-0592. Rockville, MD: Agency for Health Care Policy and Research, Public Health Service, U.S. Department of Health and Human Services.

March, P.A. (1998). Terminal restlessness. *The American Journal of Hospice and Palliative Care, 15*(1), 51-53.

Matzo, M. L., & Sherman, D.W. (2000). *Nursing education for quality care at end of life.* New York: Springer.

*McMillan, S.C. (1996). The quality of life of patients with cancer receiving hospice care. *Oncology Nursing Forum, 23,* 1221-1228.

Moritz, T., et al. (1999). Perceptions and decision-making on rehydration of terminally ill cancer patients and family members. *American Journal of Hospice and Palliative Care, 16,* 509-516.

*Musgrave C.F. (1990). Terminal dehydration: To give or not to give intravenous fluids. *Cancer Nursing, 13*(1), 62-66.

Norton, S.A., & Talerico, K.A. (2000). Facilitating end-of-life decision making: Strategies for communicating and assessing. *Journal of Gerontological Nursing, 26*(9), 6-13.

Paice, J. (1999). Pain. In C.H. Yarbro, M.H. Frogge, & M. Goodman (Eds.), *Cancer symptom management* (2nd ed., pp. 118-147). Boston: Jones & Bartlett.

Petrin, R. (1998). The symptom relief kit for hospice patients. *International Journal of Pharmaceutical Compounding,* 2(2), 116-117.

Robinson, C.B., et al. (2000). Development of a protocol to prevent opioid-induced constipation in patients with cancer: A research utilization project. *Clinical Journal of Oncology Nursing, 4,* 79-84.

*Support Study Principal Investigators. (1995). A controlled trial to improve care for seriously ill hospitalized patients. *Journal of the American Medical Association, 274,* 1591-1598.

Wang, C.H. (2000). Knowing and approaching hope as human experience: Implications for the medical-surgical nurse. *MEDSURG Nursing, 9*(4), 189-192.

Weitzner, M. A., Moody, L.N., & McMillan, S.C. (1997). Symptom management issues in hospice care. *The American Journal of Hospice and Palliative Care, 14,* 190-195.

*Wrede-Seaman, L. (1996). *Symptom management algorithms for palliative care.* Yakima, WA: Intellicard.

CHAPTER 10

Rehabilitation Concepts for Acute and Chronic Problems

DONNA D. IGNATAVICIUS

Learning Objectives

After studying this chapter, you should be able to:

1. Differentiate between impairment, disability, and handicap.
2. Identify the roles of each member of the interdisciplinary rehabilitation team.
3. Interpret physical assessment findings for the client in a rehabilitation program.
4. Describe the major components of a functional assessment.
5. Prioritize nursing care for the client in a rehabilitation program.
6. Develop a teaching plan for the rehabilitation client at risk for complications of impaired physical mobility.
7. Assess client outcomes of the interdisciplinary rehabilitation program. Explain the primary concerns for clients being discharged to home after rehabilitation.

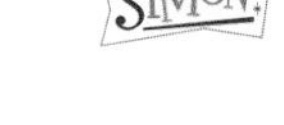

Go to http://www.wbsaunders.com/SIMON/Iggy/ for self-assessment questions related to these Learning Objectives.

A **chronic illness** or condition is one that has existed for at least 3 months. A **disabling condition** is any physical or mental health problem that can cause disability. This text focuses on physical health problems; mental health problems are discussed in textbooks on mental health nursing.

The rate of chronic and disabling illnesses will increase rapidly as baby boomers approach late adulthood. Medical-surgical nurses care for clients with chronic conditions in a variety of health care settings.

Clients with chronic and disabling conditions often participate in rehabilitation programs to prevent disability, maintain functional ability, and restore as much function as possible. The nurse is a vital member of the rehabilitation team.

OVERVIEW

Chronic illness is a major health problem in the United States, with approximately 50% of the population having one or more chronic illnesses. Approximately 35 million people (one in seven) experience activity limitations because of their chronic health problems. Many of these individuals are in residential settings, and others are managed at home.

In the United States, the annual cost of chronic and disabling conditions is more than $200 billion in medical care and lost productivity. Disability occurs slightly more often in men than in women and in families with lower incomes.

Stroke is the leading cause of disability, costing more than $30 billion each year in medical costs and loss of productivity (Collins, 1997). Coronary artery disease, cancer, chronic obstructive pulmonary disease (COPD), and arthritis are other common chronic conditions that may result in varying degrees of disability. Most of these conditions occur in people older than 65 years of age. These health problems are discussed throughout this text.

Chronic and disabling conditions are not always diseases such as cancer; they may also result from accidents. Accidents are the leading cause of death among young adults and the third leading cause of death in adults 45 to 54 years of age. Today increasing numbers of people survive accidents because of advances in medical technology. These survivors are often faced with chronic or disabling conditions, such as head and spinal cord injuries (SCIs), and they may need months to years of follow-up health care after returning to the community. As a result, the need for rehabilitation is on the rise.

CONCEPTS RELATED TO REHABILITATION

Rehabilitation is the process of learning to live with chronic and disabling conditions, often those resulting from trauma. The goal of rehabilitation is to return the client to the fullest possible physical, mental, social, vocational, and economic capacity. Rehabilitation is not limited to the return of function in post-traumatic situations. It also includes education and therapy for any chronic illness characterized by a change in a body system function or body structure. Rehabilitation programs related to respiratory, cardiac, musculoskeletal, and oncologic disorders are common examples that do not involve trauma.

In any discussion of rehabilitation, it is important to define and distinguish the terms *impairment, disability,* and *handicap.* These terms have been used interchangeably in some settings; for this chapter the terms are defined according to the classic, but still widely used, *International Classification of Impairments, Disabilities and Handicaps* (World Health Organization, 1980).

Impairment

Impairment is an abnormality of a body structure or structures or an alteration in a body system function resulting from any cause; it represents a disturbance at the organ level. Impairments can be temporary or permanent and may or may not be associated with an active pathologic condition.

Disability

Disability is the consequence of an impairment and is usually described in terms of a client's altered functional ability; it represents a disturbance at the personal level. A variety of diseases or traumas impair mobility and may result in a decreased ability to function.

Handicap

A **handicap** is the disadvantage experienced by a person as a result of impairments and disabilities; it represents a disturbance at the societal level. This disadvantage is based on interactions that the client experiences with the environment. Handicaps are associated with negative values that a person or society ascribes to the person's situation or experience. Although impairments and the disabilities that result from pathologic changes in a body organ are often unpreventable or irreversible, handicaps are both preventable and reversible.

REHABILITATION AS PART OF COMMUNITY-BASED CARE

After the acute condition or injury has been stabilized in a hospital, the client may be discharged to continue the healing process, generally under the follow-up care of a nonhospital health care provider (e.g., a family physician). The nurse provides home care preparation, health teaching, psychosocial preparation, and information about various health care resources to help the client resume his or her usual roles in society.

Some health problems require the intermediate step of rehabilitation, which can occur in a number of settings. Rehabilitation starts in the acute care hospital (sometimes called acute rehabilitation) and continues after discharge from the hospital. The nurse's coordination of care from acute care through community-based care is critical to the success of rehabilitation.

Settings for Rehabilitation

For continuing rehabilitation services, the most common settings are freestanding rehabilitation hospitals, rehabilitation units within hospitals, and skilled nursing home units to which the client is typically admitted for 1 to 4 weeks (Figure 10-1). Ambulatory care rehabilitation departments and home rehabilitation programs may be needed for continuing less intensive rehabilitative services after discharge from one of the inpatient settings or as an alternative to inpatient rehabilitation.

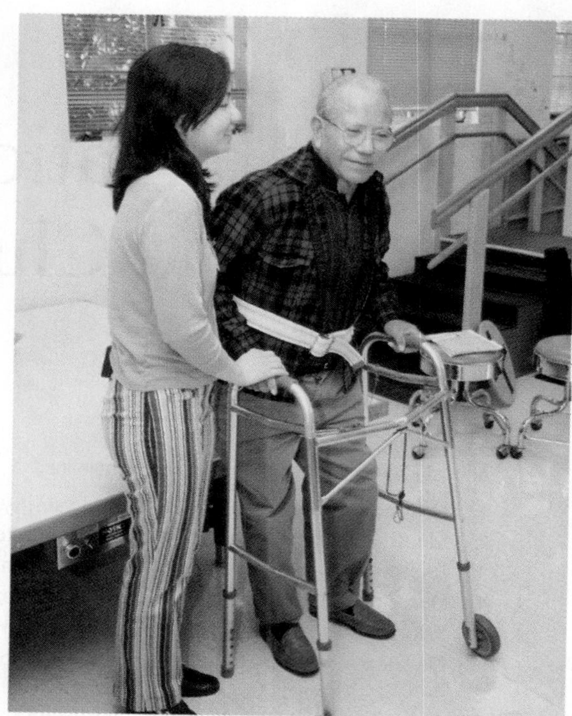

Figure 10-1 ● A physical therapist helping a client to ambulate.

Some hospitals and nursing homes have converted one or more inpatient units into subacute care units or transitional care units (TCUs). In this way, the client can stay in the same health care system for both acute and continuing rehabilitative care.

After disabled clients become more confident and independent in the inpatient setting, they may choose to live at home or in a group home. These group homes are facilities in which to live independently while together with other disabled adults. Each client or group of clients has a care provider, such as a personal care aide, to assist with the activities of daily living (ADLs) and decisions requiring accurate judgments. The clients may or may not be employed. The goal of these centers is to provide independent living arrangements outside an institution, especially for younger clients with head injury or spinal cord injury.

The Rehabilitation Team

Successful rehabilitation depends on the coordinated effort of a group of health care professionals, the interdisciplinary rehabilitation team, and the involvement of the client, family, and other support systems in planning and implementing care.

Goals of the Rehabilitation Team

The rehabilitation team has two basic goals: prevention of injury and restoration of function. The aim of prevention is to maintain the client's activity levels to avoid the deterioration of an unaffected organ or part and to eliminate possible hazards or factors that may contribute to further injury. Prevention is a continuous aspect of care for chronic illness or dis-

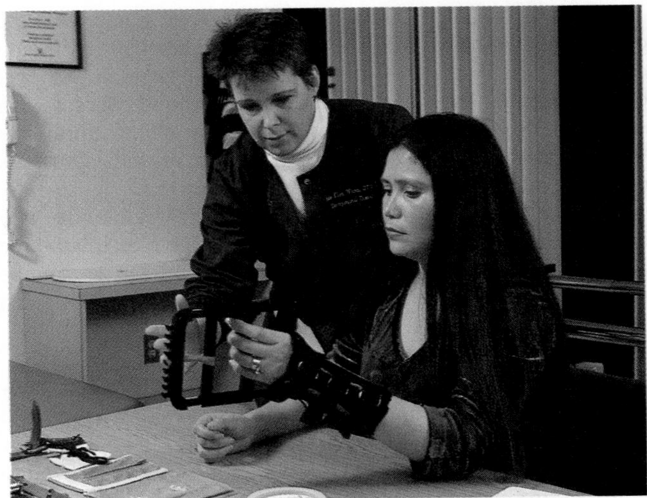

Figure 10-2 ● An occupational therapist working with a client.

ability. For example, meticulous skin care is necessary to prevent the formation of pressure ulcers. The other major goal of the rehabilitation team is to restore as much function as possible to the injured or diseased body part or system to facilitate the client's independence.

Members of the Rehabilitation Team

Members of the interdisciplinary health care team in the rehabilitation setting include physicians, nurses, physical therapists, occupational therapists, speech-language pathologists, recreational therapists, cognitive therapists, aides, social workers, psychologists, vocational counselors, clients, and family members or significant others. Not all settings that offer rehabilitation services have all of these members on their team.

PHYSIATRISTS

A physician who specializes in rehabilitative medicine is called a **physiatrist.** Except for most freestanding skilled nursing facilities, most inpatient rehabilitation settings employ physiatrists.

REHABILITATION NURSES

The rehabilitation nurse coordinates the efforts of the team members and therefore is usually designated as the client's case manager. In clients undergoing rehabilitation, health problems are characterized by an altered functional ability and a diminished quality of life. The goal of rehabilitation nursing is to assist in the restoration and maintenance of optimal health. The rehabilitation nurse must be innovative and patient in helping clients regain independence.

THERAPISTS

Physical therapists (PTs) intervene to help the client achieve mobility (e.g., by facilitating ambulation and teaching the client to use a walker). They may also teach techniques for performing certain ADLs, such as transferring (e.g., moving into and out of bed), ambulating, and toileting.

Occupational therapists (OTs) work to develop the client's fine motor skills used for ADLs, such as those required for eating, maintaining hygiene, dressing, and driving. OTs may also teach skills related to coordination (e.g., hand movements) and cognitive retraining (Figure 10-2).

Speech-language pathologists (SLPs) evaluate and retrain clients with speech, language, or swallowing problems. Speech is roughly defined as the ability to say words, and language is the ability to understand and put words together in a meaningful way. Some clients, especially those who have experienced a head injury or stroke, have difficulty with both speech and language. Clients who have experienced a stroke also typically have dysphagia (difficulty with swallowing). SLPs provide screening and testing for dysphagia. If the client has dysphagia, the SLP recommends appropriate foods and feeding techniques.

Recreational or **activity therapists** work to help clients continue or develop hobbies or interests. These therapists often coordinate their efforts with those of the OT.

Cognitive therapists, usually neuropsychologists, work primarily with clients who have experienced head injuries and have cognitive impairments. These therapists often use computers to assist with cognitive retraining.

Aides and health care assistants work in the nursing or therapy departments to assist in the care of clients. These members of the rehabilitation team are under the direct supervision of the nurse or therapist.

COUNSELORS

Various counselors are helpful in promoting community reintegration of the client and acceptance of the disability or chronic illness. Social workers help clients to identify support services and resources, including financial assistance, and they usually coordinate transfers to or discharges from the rehabilitation setting. Psychologists also counsel clients and families on their psychologic problems and on strategies to cope with disability.

Vocational counselors assist with job placement, training, or further education. Work-related skills are taught if the client needs to change careers because of the disability. If the client has not yet completed high school, educational tutors may help with completion of the requirements for graduation.

Interdisciplinary team conferences for the exchange of ideas are held on a regular basis with the client, family members and significant others, and health care providers. Chart documentation is shared and read by all team members.

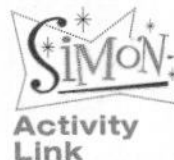

➤ COLLABORATIVE MANAGEMENT

● Assessment

HISTORY

The nurse collects the health history, including the history of the present condition, any current medications, and any treatment programs in progress.

GENERAL BACKGROUND DATA. General background data about the client and family are obtained. These data include financial status, occupations, educational levels, cultural background, and home situation. In collaboration with the occupational therapist, the nurse or case manager addresses the architectural features of the environment (e.g., the layout of the home). Together they determine whether the physical layout at home, such as the presence of stairs or the width of doorways, will present a problem to the client. Data are gathered on the client's neighborhood, such as the location of shopping centers and available transportation. The nurse or case manager determines who will do the client's shopping, cooking, and housework. This information is essential for discharge planning.

DAILY SCHEDULE AND HABITS. The nurse also assesses the client's usual daily schedule and habits of everyday living. These include hygiene practices, eating, elimination, sexual activity, and sleep. The nurse asks about the client's preferred method and time of bathing and hygiene activity. In assessing dietary patterns, food likes and dislikes are noted. Information about bowel and bladder function and the normal pattern of elimination is also obtained.

In assessing sexuality patterns, the nurse asks about changes in sexual function since the onset of the disability. The client's current and previous sleep habits, patterns, usual number of hours of sleep, and use of hypnotics are also assessed. The nurse should ask whether the client feels well rested after sleep. Sleep patterns have a significant impact on activity patterns. The assessment of activity patterns focuses on work, exercise, and recreational activities.

PHYSICAL ASSESSMENT/CLINICAL MANIFESTATIONS

The nurse collects the physical assessment data systematically according to major body systems (Chart 10-1). The focus of the assessment related to rehabilitation and chronic disease is on the functional abilities of the client.

CARDIOVASCULAR ASSESSMENT. An alteration in cardiac status may affect the client's cardiac output or cause activity intolerance. The nurse assesses the manifestations of decreased cardiac output (e.g., chest pain and fatigue) and determines when the client experiences these symptoms and what relieves them. The physician may order a change in medications or may prescribe a prophylactic dose of nitroglycerin to be taken before the client resumes activities. The nurse collaborates with the physician and appropriate therapists to determine whether activities can be modified to be accomplished without these symptoms.

For the client showing fatigue, the nurse and the client plan methods for using limited energy resources. For instance, frequent rest periods can be taken throughout the day, especially before performing activities. Major tasks could be performed in the morning because most people have the most energy at that time.

A great hindrance to rehabilitation for clients with cardiac disorders is fear. These clients may have survived a life-threatening experience (e.g., myocardial infarction) and are now so afraid of recurrence (and death) that they are unable or unwilling to resume any activity. They usually benefit from participation in a structured cardiac rehabilitation program. The nurse discusses available programs with the client and the family (see Chapter 35 for a complete description of cardiac rehabilitation).

RESPIRATORY ASSESSMENT. The nurse asks the client whether he or she is experiencing shortness of breath during or after activity. It is important to determine the level of activity that can be accomplished without experiencing shortness of breath. For example, can the client climb one flight of stairs without shortness of breath, or does shortness of breath occur after climbing only two steps?

The fear associated with any inability to breathe normally can render a person dependent in many facets of life. Some problems related to disorders of the respiratory system can be resolved or diminished, but some breathing difficulties must be endured (e.g., emphysema).

GASTROINTESTINAL AND NUTRITIONAL ASSESSMENT. The nurse monitors the client's oral intake and pattern of eating. He or she is also assessed for the presence of anorexia, dysphagia, nausea, vomiting, or discomfort related to or interfering with oral intake. In collaboration with the physician and the dietitian, the nurse reviews the client's height, weight, hemoglobin and hematocrit levels, and serum albumin, transferrin, and blood glucose concentrations (see Chapter 61 for a complete nutritional assessment). Weight loss or weight gain is particularly significant and may be related to an associated disease or to the illness that caused the disability.

Elimination habits vary from person to person; they are often related to daily job or activity schedules, dietary patterns, and family or cultural background. Elimination habits may be

CHART 10-1

FOCUSED ASSESSMENT *of* Clients Undergoing Rehabilitation

Body System	Relevant Data
Cardiovascular system	Chest pain Fatigue Fear of cardiac failure
Respiratory system	Shortness of breath or dyspnea Activity tolerance Fear of inability to breathe
Gastrointestinal system and nutrition	Oral intake, eating pattern Anorexia, nausea, and vomiting Dysphagia Laboratory data (e.g., serum albumin level) Weight loss or gain Bowel elimination pattern or habits Change in stool Ability to get to toilet
Renal-urinary system	Urinary pattern Fluid intake Urinary incontinence or retention Urine culture or urinalysis
Neurologic system	Motor function Sensation Cognitive abilities
Musculoskeletal system	Functional ability Range of motion Endurance Muscle strength
Integumentary system	Risk of skin breakdown Presence of skin lesions

difficult to assess, because many nurses are hesitant to request (and many clients are afraid to volunteer) information pertaining to elimination. When assessing elimination status, the nurse first asks about the client's usual elimination patterns before the injury or the illness.

The nurse is attuned to any changes in the client's bowel routine or stool consistency. If the client notices any change in elimination pattern, the nurse tries to determine whether this alteration can be attributed to a change in diet, activity pattern, or medication use that could cause increased or decreased motility of the gastrointestinal tract. Bowel habits are evaluated on the basis of what is normal for that person.

The nurse also determines whether the client can manage bowel functions independently. Independence in bowel elimination requires cognition, manual dexterity, sensation, muscle control, and mobility. If the client requires help, the nurse determines whether someone is available at home to provide the assistance. The client's (and family's) ability to cope with any dependency in bowel elimination must also be assessed.

RENAL AND URINARY ASSESSMENT. When assessing the urinary system, the nurse determines the client's baseline urinary patterns, asks about the number of times the client usually voids, and determines whether the client routinely awakens during the night to empty the bladder or has uninterrupted sleep. Fluid intake patterns and volume are recorded and include the type of fluids ingested and the timing of fluid consumption throughout the day.

The nurse determines whether the client has ever experienced any problems with urinary incontinence or retention. Laboratory reports, especially the results of the urinalysis, are also monitored.

NEUROLOGIC ASSESSMENT. In rehabilitation, the neurologic assessment identifies the functional aspects of motor ability, sensation, and cognition. The nurse assesses the client's pre-existing problems, general physical condition, and communication abilities.

MOTOR ABILITY. The movement of an extremity is compared with the function of the opposite extremity to identify **paresis** (weakness) or **paralysis** (absence of movement).

SENSATION. The identification of sensory-perceptual alterations is important in assessing the client's risk for injury. The nurse assesses the client's response to light touch, hot or cold temperature, and position change in each extremity and on the trunk. Levels of decreased sensation are identified. For a perceptual assessment, the nurse evaluates the client's ability to receive and understand what is heard and seen and the ability to express appropriate motor and verbal responses. During this portion of the assessment, the nurse can begin to assess short-term and long-term memory.

COGNITIVE ABILITIES. The nurse also assesses the client's cognitive abilities, especially if there is a head injury or stroke. Several tools are available to evaluate cognition. One of the most common is the Mini-Mental State Examination, which is described in detail in Chapter 42.

MUSCULOSKELETAL ASSESSMENT. As with other body systems, the rehabilitation nursing assessment of the musculoskeletal system focuses on function. The nurse assesses the client's musculoskeletal status, response to the impairment, and demands of the home, work, or school environment. The client's endurance level is determined, and both active and passive range of motion (ROM) of joints are measured. The nurse reviews the results of manual muscle testing by physical therapy, which identifies the client's ROM and resistance against gravity. In this procedure, the therapist determines the degree of muscle strength present in each body segment. The grading system usually ranges from 0 (no evidence of muscle contractility) to 5 (normal muscle contractility) (see Chapter 50).

SKIN ASSESSMENT. When assessing a client's skin, the nurse identifies actual or potential interruptions in its integrity.

RISK FOR SKIN BREAKDOWN. To maintain healthy skin, the body must have adequate food, water, and oxygen intake; intact waste removal mechanisms; sensation; and functional mobility. Changes in any of these variables can lead to rapid and extensive skin breakdown. If the client cannot protect or maintain the skin, the nurse must be able to assess and plan for his or her needs. The nurse monitors the client to determine the risk of skin breakdown before it occurs.

Some rehabilitation settings use special skin assessment tools to identify clients at risk for skin breakdown. For example, the classic Braden Scale for Predicting Pressure Sore Risk (see Chapter 67) assesses several areas: sensory perception, skin moisture, activity level, nutritional status, and potential for friction and shear.

Other skin risk assessment tools are available. Some tools also include additional indicators of nutritional status, such as the serum albumin or transferrin level. When either of these levels is low, the client is at high risk for pressure sores. Some tools include incontinence and altered mental state as risk factors. Regardless of which tool is used, Braden and Bergstrom (1992) have recommended the following schedule for skin assessment:

- For clients in critical care units: during every nursing shift when the client is unstable and at least daily when the client is stable
- For clients in medical-surgical units: every other day when the client's condition is stable and when the condition changes significantly (e.g., after surgery)
- For clients in nursing homes or rehabilitation units: weekly for 1 month and then monthly after the first month unless there is a significant change in the client's condition

ACTUAL SKIN BREAKDOWN. If a pressure ulcer or other change in skin integrity develops, the nurse accurately assesses the problem and its possible causes. The skin is inspected every 2 hours (more often if needed) until the client learns to inspect his or her own skin several times a day. The depth and diameter of the open skin area is measured in centimeters or inches, depending on the policy of the facility. The area around the open lesion must also be assessed to determine the presence of cellulitis or other tissue damage. Chapter 67 includes a widely used classification system for staging skin breakdown. The nurse also assesses the client's understanding of the cause and treatment of skin breakdown as well as his or her ability to inspect the skin and participate in maintaining skin integrity.

In many health care agencies, a skin assessment and documentation tool ("skin sheet") is used to keep track of each area of skin breakdown. A baseline assessment is conducted on admission to the agency, and the form is updated periodically depending on the agency's policy and the nurse's judgment. In some long-term care, acute care, or rehabilitation settings, and with the client's permission, photographs of the skin are taken on admission and at various intervals to document its condition.

FUNCTIONAL ASSESSMENT

Functional ability refers to the client's ability to perform **activities of daily living (ADLs),** such as bathing, dressing, feeding, and ambulating, as well as independent living skills such as using the telephone, shopping, preparing food, and housekeeping. **Functional assessment** tools are used to assess a client's abilities (see the Evidence-Based Practice for Nursing box below). Rehabilitation nurses, physiatrists, or therapists complete one or more of these assessment tools on the basis of the client's abilities and the policy of the health care setting. Some of the commonly used tools are described briefly in the following sections. For further information, consult the Bibliography at the end of this chapter.

PULSES PROFILE. One of the earliest tools used was the PULSES profile. It was developed in 1957 and adapted in 1975 to evaluate and classify functional capacity in the chronically ill and aging population. Six categories are included in the evaluation:

- Physical condition (basic health status)
- *U*pper limb function (self-care)
- *L*ower limb function (mobility)
- *S*ensory components (sight, communication)
- *E*xcretory function
- *S*upport factors

Scoring uses four numeric grades for each category. Scores increase as functional ability is diminished, and the maximum score is 24. High scores indicate greater levels of dependency. The adapted form of the PULSES profile has been a useful tool in many rehabilitation programs. It indicates the level of independence in life-functioning skills necessary for a person to make adaptations to community living.

KATZ INDEX OF ACTIVITIES OF DAILY LIVING. One of the best known and most widely used instruments was developed during the 1950s from observations of clients with fractured hips. The Katz Index of Activities of Daily Living addresses six functional tasks: bathing, dressing, toileting, achieving transfers, level of continence, and feeding (Katz et al., 1963). Each of the six areas is scored as either "dependent" or "independent" on the basis of the client's need for help in performing the task (Table 10-1). From the total scores, the overall functional status is assigned a grade from A (independent in feeding, continence, transferring, toileting, dressing, and bathing) through G (dependent in all six functions).

The Katz Index has been used for clients with many types of chronic illnesses. It is a valuable tool for evaluating care and developing data about the course of an illness over time.

BARTHEL INDEX. The Barthel Index was designed to measure functional levels and mobility in the physically impaired client. This tool consists of 10 variables, and clients are scored by their degree of independence in performance. Categories include feeding, bathing, and mobility. The scoring system consists of two descriptive areas: performing an activity with help and performing an activity independently. Scores range from 0, indicating total dependence, to 100, indicating complete independence. The Barthel Index was intended for use in both immediate and long-term care rehabilitation programs.

LEVEL OF REHABILITATION SCALE. The Level of Rehabilitation Scale (LORS) developed by Carey and Posavec (1978) provides a general assessment of the client's functioning for program evaluation rather than clinical assessment. The LORS provides an overview through measurement of function regarding ADLs, cognition, home activities, activities outside the home, and social interactions. The LORS was expanded to include 11 items related to activities of daily living, mobility, and communication (Posavec & Carey, 1982). These items receive a score of 0 to 4, which is determined through a coding manual that ascribes numeric values to behavioral terms.

FUNCTIONAL INDEPENDENCE MEASURES. Assessment tools have also been designed for use on a national level, which enables uniform outcome data to be obtained from numerous rehabilitation programs. An example of

EVIDENCE-BASED PRACTICE FOR NURSING

For older clients, which factors predict functional independence after hospital discharge?

Hansen, K., Mahoney, J., & Palta, M. (1999). Risk factors for lack of recovery of ADL independence after hospital discharge. *Journal of the American Geriatrics Society, 47*(3), 360-365.

The purpose of this descriptive study was to determine which risk factors contributed to the lack of activities of daily living (ADL) independence among older clients following hospital discharge. Evaluations for ADL ability were conducted at the time of discharge and 1 month later on 73 older clients who previously were ADL independent before hospitalization. The researchers used self-report and objective measures of function, mobility, and cognition. By 1 month after discharge, 59% had not returned to baseline. The likelihood of not returning to an independent level was 87% if the client had a Mini-Mental State Examination (MMSE) score (measuring cognition) of less than 24 at discharge. Among clients with adequate cognition (above a score of 24), 85% of those who used an ambulatory device before hospitalization did not return to baseline. The likelihood of recovering ADL independence was high if the client had no prehospital ambulatory device and received a good score on the MMSE.

Critique. Although this study was descriptive and used a relatively small number of subjects, it looked at an area that has not previously been studied. This research needs to be repeated using a larger number of clients followed over a longer period of time.

Implications for Nursing. As resources become more scarce and costs are highly considered, it would be very helpful to predict which clients are most likely to benefit from additional interventions after hospital discharge. With posthospital rehabilitative services, most older clients can return to their baseline level of functioning if they have good cognition and are able to ambulate with an assistive device.

TABLE 10-1 • KATZ INDEX OF ACTIVITIES OF DAILY LIVING

Independence means without supervision, direction, or active personal assistance, except as specifically noted below. This is based on actual status and not ability. A patient who refuses to perform a function is considered as not performing the function, even though he or she is deemed able.

BATHING (sponge, shower, or tub)
Independent: assistance only in bathing a single part (back or disabled extremity), or bathes self completely
Dependent: assistance in bathing more than one part of body; assistance in getting in or out of tub; does not bathe self

DRESSING
Independent: gets clothes from closets and drawers; puts on clothes, outer garments, braces; manages fasteners; act of tying shoes is excluded
Dependent: does not dress self, or remains partly undressed

GOING TO TOILET
Independent: gets to toilet; gets on and off toilet; arranges clothes; cleans organs of excretion (may manage own bedpan used at night only and may or may not be using mechanical supports)
Dependent: uses bedpan or commode or receives assistance in getting to and using toilet

TRANSFER
Independent: moves in and out of bed and in and out of chair independently (may or may not be using mechanical supports)
Dependent: assistance in moving in or out of bed and/or chair; does not perform one or more transfers

CONTINENCE
Independent: urination and defecation entirely self-controlled
Dependent: partial or total incontinence in urination or defecation; partial or total control by enemas, catheters, or regulated use of urinals and/or bedpans

FEEDING
Independent: gets food from plate or its equivalent into mouth (precutting of meat and preparation of food, such as buttering bread, are excluded from evaluation)
Dependent: assistance in act of feeding (see above); does not eat at all or requires parenteral feeding

EVALUATION FORM

Name ______________________ Date of Evaluation ______________________

For each area of functioning listed below, circle the description that applies (the word "assistance" means supervision, direction, or personal assistance).

BATHING—either sponge bath, tub bath, or shower

Receives no assistance (gets in and out of tub by self if tub is usual means of bathing)	Receives assistance in bathing only one part of body (such as back or a leg)	Receives assistance in bathing more than one part of body (or does not bathe self)

DRESSING—gets clothes from closets and drawers; puts on clothes, including underclothes, outer garments; manages fasteners (including braces, if worn)

Gets clothes and gets completely dressed without assistance	Gets clothes and gets dressed without assistance, except for tying shoes	Receives assistance in getting clothes or in getting dressed, or stays partly or completely undressed

TOILETING—going to the "toilet room" for bowel and urine elimination, cleaning self after elimination, and arranging clothes

Goes to "toilet room," cleans self, and arranges clothes without assistance (may use object for support, such as cane, walker, or wheelchair and may manage night bedpan or commode, emptying same in morning)	Receives assistance in going to "toilet room" or in cleansing self or in arranging clothes after elimination or in use of night bedpan or commode	Does not go to room termed "toilet" for the elimination process

TRANSFER

Moves in and out of bed and in and out of chair without assistance (may use object for support, such as cane or walker)	Moves in or out of bed or chair with assistance	Does not get out of bed

CONTINENCE

Controls urination and bowel movement completely by self	Has occasional "accidents"	Supervision helps keep urine or bowel control; uses catheter or is incontinent

FEEDING

Feeds self without assistance	Feeds self except for getting assistance in cutting meat or buttering bread	Receives assistance in feeding or is fed partly or completely by tubes or IV fluids

From Katz, S., et al. (1963). Studies of illness in the aged. The index of ADL: A standardized measure of biological and psychosocial function. *Journal of the American Medical Association, 185,* 914-919. Copyright 1963, American Medical Association.

this type of system—a uniform data system—is the Functional Independence Measure (FIM) developed by Granger and Gresham (1984). As a basic indicator of the severity of a disability, the FIM attempts to quantify what the person actually does, whatever the diagnosis or impairment. It does not measure what a person should do or how the person would perform under a different set of circumstances. To eliminate the bias of a particular discipline, the assessment may be performed by trained clinicians. The entire assessment may be performed by one person, or certain categories may be completed by representatives of various disciplines.

Categories for assessment are self-care, sphincter control, mobility and locomotion, communication, and cognition. Scoring is done with numbers that use predetermined criteria for measurement. The client is evaluated when he or she is admitted to and discharged from a rehabilitation institution and at a specified follow-up time. The FIM assessment system has also been adapted for use in other health care settings, including acute care and home care.

PSYCHOSOCIAL ASSESSMENT

The nurse must understand the theories of body image and self-esteem to assess the client's psychosocial needs adequately. These concepts serve as a basis for understanding psychologic responses to chronic illness and the resulting disability. The client's self-esteem and body image are assessed through verbal indicators and descriptions of self-care.

The nurse assesses the client's use of defense mechanisms and manifestations of anxiety, such as those noted in facial expressions and communication patterns. To assess the client's response to loss, the nurse asks the client to describe feelings concerning the loss of a body part or function. The presence of any stress-related physical problem is noted. The client may experience symptoms of depression, such as fatigue, a change in appetite, or feelings of powerlessness.

The nurse assesses the availability of support systems for the client. The major support system is typically the family or significant others. Family interactions and coping patterns are also assessed.

VOCATIONAL ASSESSMENT

The client is assisted in maximizing functional status to allow him or her to resume many usual activities. The nurse should be aware of the appropriate resources for each client in compiling a vocational database. Vocational counselors can help the client find meaningful training, education, or employment after discharge from the rehabilitation setting.

Clients in the United States are informed about the Americans with Disabilities Act, which was passed by Congress in 1991 to prevent employer discrimination against disabled people. The employer must offer reasonable assistance to a disabled employee to allow him or her to perform the job. For example, if an employee has a severe hearing loss, the employer may need to hire an interpreter for sign language.

The rehabilitation team assesses the cognitive and physical demands of the client's job and ascertains whether he or she can return to the former job or whether retraining in another field is necessary. The physical demands of jobs range from light in sedentary occupations (0 to 10 pounds often lifted) to heavy (more than 100 pounds often lifted). The nurse must also consider other aspects of the job, such as strength, mobility, or senses required (e.g., hearing).

Job analysis also involves assessing the work environment of the client's former job. The nurse works with the vocational counselor to determine whether the environment is conducive to the client's return. Union contracts must also be considered, and any job modifications must be noted. If an injured worker requires vocational rehabilitation, the nurse refers him or her to vocational rehabilitation personnel to evaluate present skills and learn new skills for employment if needed. In most states worker's compensation insurance helps to support vocational rehabilitation.

Analysis

COMMON NURSING DIAGNOSES AND COLLABORATIVE PROBLEMS

Regardless of the client's age or specific disability, the following nursing diagnoses are commonly applicable to the client with chronic illness or disability:

1. Impaired Physical Mobility related to neuromuscular impairment, sensory-perceptual impairment, pain, activity intolerance, fatigue, or the effects of trauma or surgery
2. Self-Care Deficit (Total or Partial) related to the effects of trauma or chronic illness, muscular weakness, pain, immobility, or perceptual or cognitive impairment
3. Risk for Impaired Skin Integrity related to altered sensation or immobility
4. Impaired Urinary Elimination related to sensorimotor impairment or immobility
5. Constipation related to neuromuscular or musculoskeletal impairment or immobility
6. Ineffective Coping related to the effects of chronic illness, the loss of control over a body part or a body function, or major changes in lifestyle

ADDITIONAL NURSING DIAGNOSES AND COLLABORATIVE PROBLEMS

Additional nursing diagnoses may apply depending on the client's specific disability. For example, a client with rheumatoid arthritis also experiences chronic pain. The client with a spinal cord injury may also have sexual dysfunction.

Planning and Implementation

IMPAIRED PHYSICAL MOBILITY

NOC **PLANNING: EXPECTED OUTCOMES.** The client with chronic illness or disability is expected to (1) achieve the maximal physical mobility possible with the least restriction of activity, and (2) not experience consequences resulting from immobility.

INTERVENTIONS. Most problems requiring rehabilitation relate to impaired physical mobility. Clients with neurologic disease or injury, amputations, arthritis, severe burns, and cardiopulmonary disease experience some degree of impaired mobility. Physical and occupational therapists are the key rehabilitation team members in helping clients meet their mobility goals. Depending on the setting, clients often spend several hours every day working in the physical therapy department to regain function and skills.

CONSIDERATIONS FOR OLDER ADULTS
Older clients may not be able to tolerate extensive therapy workouts and may need shorter sessions to prevent extreme fatigue or physical complications. The nurse reinforces the physical therapist's instructions and must be aware of the client's progress and abilities.

TRANSFER TECHNIQUES. Clients with decreased mobility may require assistance with transfers, such as from a bed to a chair, commode, or wheelchair. Because the degree of assistance required varies with the client and the specific disability, the nurse carefully assesses mobility status before attempting a transfer. The physical or occupational therapist usually specifies the type of transfer. For example, a quadriplegic client may use a sliding board for transfer, whereas a client with an above-knee amputation may need a wheelchair with removable arms. In any case, the nurse always plans the transfer technique before initiating it. The desired outcome is that the client will eventually be able to transfer independently and safely.

Basic techniques for the nurse to use when assisting in the transfer of the client from a bed to a chair or wheelchair (and vice versa) are identified in Chart 10-2. These techniques are also taught to the family member or other caregiver who will be caring for the client at home. Additional information about transfers can be found in basic nursing textbooks.

CHART 10-2

BEST PRACTICE *for* Transfer Techniques

Bed to Wheelchair or Chair

1. Place the chair at an angle to the bed on the client's strong side.
2. Lock the wheelchair brakes or secure the chair position.
3. Assist the client to stand, and move his or her strong hand to the armrest.
4. Keep the client's body weight forward and pivot.
5. When the client's legs touch the chair edge, assist the client in sitting.

Wheelchair or Chair to Bed

1. Place the chair with the client's strong side next to the bed.
2. Lock the wheelchair brakes or secure the chair position.
3. Assist the client to stand, and move his or her strong hand to the armrest.
4. Keep the client's body weight forward and pivot.
5. When the client's legs touch the bed edge, assist the client in sitting and then reclining.

Use of a Sliding Board

1. Place the chair or wheelchair as close to the bed as possible.
2. Remove the armrest from the chair or (if removable) wheelchair.
3. Powder the sliding board.
4. Place the sliding board under the client's buttocks.
5. Instruct the client to reach toward his or her side.
6. Assist the client in sliding gently to the bed.

ALTERNATIVE TRANSFER TECHNIQUES. Some clients cannot bear weight. For example, a spinal cord injury resulting in quadriplegia involves using either a **sliding board** (which requires balance skills) or, with the nurse or therapist, a "bear hug" technique. The sitting client places his or her arms around the nurse's neck while being lifted from the bed to the chair or vice versa. Another person assists with the transfer by stabilizing the wheelchair and holding onto the client's waist. Most physical therapists recommend that the client wear pants or a **gait belt** so the assistant can hold on to the belt during the transfer.

POTENTIAL PROBLEMS WITH TRANSFERS. Before any transfer, the nurse carefully observes for potential problems. Orthostatic, or postural, hypotension is a common problem in rehabilitation and contributes to falls, which are common in any client with impaired mobility. If the client moves from a lying to a sitting or standing position too quickly, his or her blood pressure drops; as a result, he or she becomes dizzy or faints. This problem is worsened by antihypertensive medications, especially in older adults. To prevent this, the nurse helps the client change positions slowly, with frequent rest periods to allow the blood pressure to stabilize. The nurse may measure blood pressure with the client in the lying, sitting, and standing positions to examine the differences. Orthostatic hypotension is indicated by a drop of more than 20 mm Hg in systolic pressure or 10 mm Hg in diastolic pressure between positions. The nurse notifies the physician about this change.

Weight gain is another potential problem. Because the client undergoing rehabilitation has impaired mobility, he or she tends to gain weight. Excessive weight hinders transfers both for the nurse or the therapist who is assisting and for the client who is learning to transfer independently. Weight is usually checked every week to monitor gains or losses.

GAIT TRAINING. The physical therapist works with clients for gait training if they are able to ambulate. While regaining the ability to ambulate, clients may need to use canes or walkers (Figure 10-3). When working with clients who are using such assistive devices, also known as **ambulatory aids,** the physical therapist ensures that there is a level surface on which to walk. The nurse reinforces the physical therapist's instructions and encourages practice, with the goal being to walk independently with or without an assistive device. Older clients typically use a walker for a broader base of support. Younger or minimally impaired clients often progress to the use of a hemi-cane or straight cane. Chart 10-3 outlines how to use assistive devices for ambulation.

Some clients never regain the ability to walk because of their impairment, such as multiple sclerosis or spinal cord injury. They may become wheelchair dependent and need to learn wheelchair mobility skills. With the help of physical and occupational therapy, most clients can learn to move anywhere in the wheelchair.

PREVENTION OF COMPLICATIONS. During the rehabilitation phase, clients are vulnerable to complications of immobility. Table 10-2 lists the common complications and the major strategies the nurse can use to help prevent each complication. Implementing range-of-motion (ROM) routines, adhering to schedules for turning and repositioning, and maintaining skin care are constant components of rehabilitation nursing care to prevent complications of immobility. The key is to increase mobility.

One way to increase mobility, even with clients who are bedridden, is through ROM exercises. ROM techniques are beneficial for any client with decreased mobility (Table 10-3). Although basic ROM techniques are presented in basic nursing textbooks, a few key principles are pertinent to rehabilitation nursing care:

- The human body contains more joints than simply the knees, hips, elbows, and shoulders. For ROM techniques to be effective in preventing musculoskeletal contractures, the client must exercise all joints, including each joint of the fingers, hands, toes, and so forth.
- In performing ROM activities, the nurse or client completes full-range movement of each joint at least five times and completes the entire process at least three times daily.
- The nurse does not move the joints beyond the point at which the client expresses pain or beyond the point at which the nurse perceives stiffness or difficulty.

Clients with decreased mobility who are able to follow directions are taught by the nurse and the physical therapist to perform active or active-assisted ROM exercises.

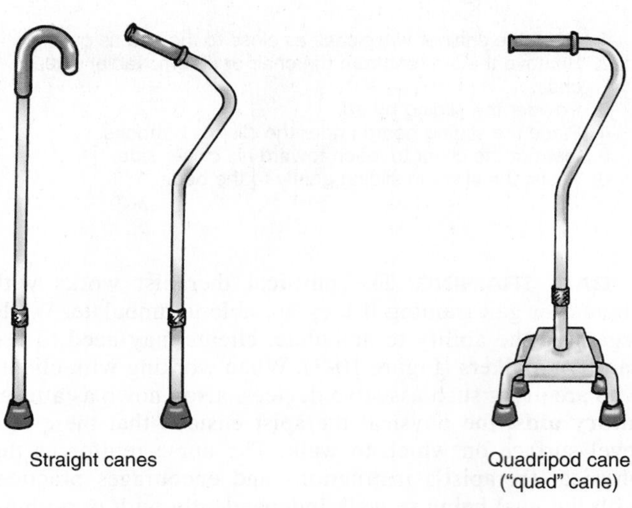

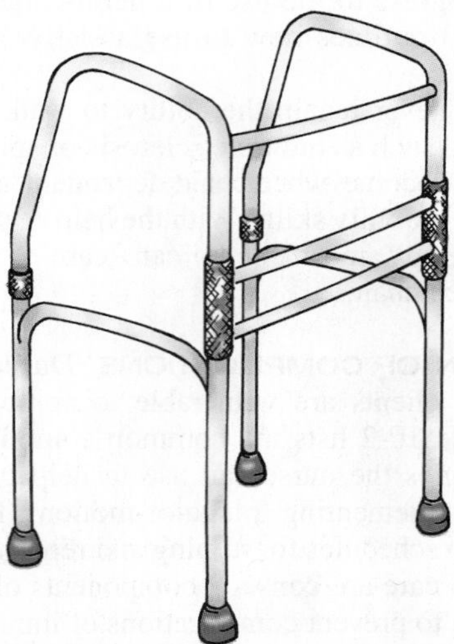

Figure 10-3 ● Assistive devices for ambulation. Assistive devices vary in the amount of support they provide. A straight cane provides less support than a quadripod cane or walker.

SELF-CARE DEFICIT

NOC PLANNING: EXPECTED OUTCOMES. The client with chronic illness or disability is expected to become independent in ADLs to the extent possible based on his or her disability.

INTERVENTIONS. Activities of daily living (ADLs), or self-care activities, include eating, bathing, dressing, grooming, and toileting. The nurse encourages the client to perform as much self-care as possible. The nurse and occupational therapist collaborate to identify ways in which self-care activities can be modified so the client can perform them independently. For example, the occupational therapist teaches a hemiplegic client to put on a shirt by first placing the affected arm in the sleeve and then putting the unaffected arm in the appropriate sleeve. The nurse reinforces this dressing technique and encourages the client to practice.

In long-term care settings (e.g., nursing homes), federal regulations require that residents not lose their functional skills. Therefore most facilities have developed **restorative nursing** programs and have coordinated these programs with rehabilitation therapy and activity therapy. The focus of this coordinated effort includes the following:

- Bed mobility
- Walking
- Transfers
- Dressing
- Grooming
- Active range of motion
- Communication

USE OF ASSISTIVE/ADAPTIVE DEVICES. A variety of **assistive/adaptive devices** are available for clients with chronic illness and disability. An assistive/adaptive device, or self-care support device, is any item that enables the client to perform all or part of an activity independently. Table 10-4 identifies common devices and describes their use.

CHART 10-3

BEST PRACTICE *for* Gait Training

Walker Assisted

1. Apply a gait belt around the client's waist.
2. Assist the client to a standing position.
3. Assist the client in placing both hands on the walker.
4. Ensure that the client is well balanced.
5. Assist the client repeatedly to perform the following sequence:
   a. Lift the walker.
   b. Move the walker 2 feet forward and set it down on all legs.
   c. While resting on the walker, take small steps.
   d. Check balance.

Cane Assisted

1. Apply a gait belt around the client's waist.
2. Assist the client to a standing position.
3. Assist the client in placing his or her strong hand on the cane.
4. Ensure that the client is well balanced.
5. Assist the client to perform the following sequence repeatedly:
   a. Move the cane forward.
   b. Move the weaker leg one step forward.
   c. Move the stronger leg one step forward.
   d. Check balance.

TABLE 10-2 • PREVENTION OF THE COMMON HAZARDS OF IMMOBILITY

Body System	Complication	Prevention
Musculoskeletal	Contractures	Range-of-motion exercises
	Foot drop	Foot support while in bed, range-of-motion exercises
	Osteoporosis	Range-of-motion exercises
	Susceptibility to fractures	Weight-bearing exercises
	Muscular atrophy	Passive or active range-of-motion exercises
Gastrointestinal	Constipation	Increased activity level Increased fluid intake
Cardiovascular	Decreased cardiac output	Range-of-motion exercises
	Increased venous stasis	Exercise, support hose, or antiembolism stockings
	Thrombus formation	Exercise, support hose, or antiembolism stockings
	Embolism	Avoidance of leg massage
Neurologic	Disorientation	Sleep-wake schedule in accord with light-dark pattern Reorientation (to person, place, and time) Control of sensory stimulation
	Postural hypotension	Avoidance of sudden position changes
Renal/urinary	Calculi	Decreased dietary calcium level Increased fluid intake Maintenance of acidic urine
Respiratory	Pneumonia	Frequent repositioning Respiratory exercises
Integumentary	Pressure ulcers	Frequent repositioning Pressure relief devices Skin care Adequate nutrition

Many department stores carry clothing and assistive/adaptive devices designed for clients with disabilities. The occupational therapist works with the client to determine specific needs with regard to such equipment. The nurse and the occupational therapist also help look for creative and inexpensive alternatives to meeting these needs. For example, barbecue tongs may be used as "reachers" for pulling up pants or obtaining items on high shelves. A foam curler with the plastic insert removed may be placed over a pencil or eating utensil to make a built-up device. The client might use an extended shoehorn to operate light switches from wheelchair height. Hook-and-loop fasteners (Velcro) sewn on clothes can prevent the frustrations caused by buttons and zippers.

ENERGY CONSERVATION. Fatigue is commonly associated with chronic and disabling conditions. Therefore nurses work with occupational therapists to assess the client's self-care abilities and to determine possible ways of conserving energy. The nurse and the therapist develop strategies for **energy conservation** after evaluating the client's self-care routines. Preparation for ADLs can be helpful in reducing effort and energy expenditure (e.g., gathering all necessary equipment before starting grooming routines). If a client has high energy levels in the morning, he or she can be taught to schedule energy-intensive activities in the morning rather than later in the day or evening. Spacing activities is also helpful for conserving energy. In addition, allowing time to rest before and after eating and toileting decreases the strain on the client's energy level.

RISK FOR IMPAIRED SKIN INTEGRITY

NOC **PLANNING: EXPECTED OUTCOMES.** The client with chronic illness or disability is expected to have intact skin.

INTERVENTIONS. An enormous variety of topical and mechanical remedies have been used with varying success to prevent and treat pressure ulcers. Pressure reduction is a nursing intervention that may be achieved when the nurse temporarily repositions the client or alters the physical properties of the mattress surface, such as adding a mattress overlay.

TURNING AND REPOSITIONING. The best intervention to prevent skin impairment is frequent position changes in combination with adequate skin care and sufficient nutritional intake. In general, the nurse turns and repositions the client every 2 hours; this may not be sufficient for people who are frail and have thin skin, especially older adults (Chart 10-4).

TABLE 10-3 • TYPES OF RANGE-OF-MOTION EXERCISES

Type	Description	Indications
Passive	Exercises are performed by the nurse for the client.	The client is too weak to participate actively.
Active	Exercises are performed by the client.	The client is able to complete range-of-motion movements.
Assisted, or active assisted	Exercises are performed by the client but are guided by the nurse or therapist.	The client is weak and needs assistance.
Resistive	The actions of the client are in opposition to those performed by the nurse or therapist.	The client has full range of motion, and an increase in strength is desired.

TABLE 10-4 • USES OF ASSISTIVE/ADAPTIVE DEVICES

Device	Use
Buttonhook	Threaded through the buttonhole to enable clients with weak finger mobility to button shirts Alternative uses include serving as pencil holder or cigarette holder
Extended shoe horn	Assists in the application of shoes for clients with decreased mobility Alternative uses include turning light switches off or on while client is in a wheelchair
Plate guard	Applied to a plate to assist clients with weak hand and arm mobility to feed themselves
Gel pad	Placed under a plate or a glass to prevent dishes from slipping and moving Alternative uses include placement under bathing and grooming items to prevent them from moving
Foam buildups	Applied to eating utensils to assist clients with weak hand grasps to feed themselves Alternative uses include application to pens and pencils to assist with writing or over a buttonhook to assist with grasping the device
Hook and loop fastener (Velcro) straps	Applied to utensils, a buttonhook, or a pencil to slip over the hand and provide a method of stabilizing the device when the client's hand grasp is weak
Long-handled reacher	Assists in obtaining items located on high shelves or at ground level for clients who are unable to change positions easily

CHART 10-4

NURSING FOCUS *on the* OLDER ADULT
Special Considerations in Rehabilitation

- When getting the client out of bed, move him or her (or instruct him or her to move or sit up) slowly to prevent orthostatic hypotension. This problem is most common in older adults who take antihypertensive medications.
- Turn the client more often than every 2 hours, even if it is just a minor position change. Skin becomes thinner and more fragile with age.
- Determine whether the client had any problem with urinary patterns before the illness or rehabilitation. A client with a previous problem may not have a successful bladder training program.
- Be aware that intestinal motility decreases with age, which leads to constipation.
- Assess the client's support system of family and significant others. Many older clients have no spouse or close friends, who would usually serve as a support network.

To determine the best turning schedule, the nurse assesses the client's skin condition during each turning and repositioning. For example, if the client has been sleeping for 2 hours and the nurse decides to postpone turning for 1 hour, reddened areas over the bony prominences may be present. If such reddened areas do not fade within 30 minutes after pressure relief or do not blanch, they may be classified as pre-ulcer areas, or stage I pressure areas (see Chapter 67).

Clients who sit for prolonged periods in a wheelchair are repositioned at least every 1 to 2 hours. Each client is evaluated by the physical or occupational therapist for the best seating pad that is comfortable yet reduces pressure on bony prominences. Clients who are able are taught to perform "wheelchair push-ups" by using their arms to lift their buttocks off the wheelchair seat for 10 seconds or longer every hour, or more often if needed. The physical therapist helps clients strengthen their arm muscles in preparation for performing wheelchair push-ups.

SKIN CARE. Adequate skin care is an essential component of prevention. The nurse performs or assists clients in completing skin care each time they are turned, repositioned, or bathed. Skin care includes cleaning soiled areas, drying carefully, and applying body lotion. If a client is incontinent, topical barrier creams or ointments can help to protect the skin from moisture, which facilitates skin breakdown. Reddened areas are not rubbed because doing so can cause extensive damage to the already fragile capillary system. Instead the nurse carefully observes the areas for further breakdown and relieves pressure on the areas as much as possible. Bed pillows are often good pressure-relieving devices. (See Chapter 67 for a complete discussion of skin care interventions.)

NUTRITION. Sufficient nutrition is needed both to repair wounds and to prevent pressure ulcers. The nurse collaborates with the dietitian to assess the client's food selection and ensure that it contains adequate protein and carbohydrates. Both the nurse and the dietitian closely monitor the client's weight and levels of serum albumin and transferrin. If either of these indexes decreases significantly, the client may be given high-protein, high-carbohydrate food supplements (e.g., milkshakes) or commercial preparations (e.g., Ensure Plus) (also see Chapter 61).

MECHANICAL DEVICES. Pressure-relieving devices include waterbeds, gel mattresses or pads, air mattresses, low–air loss overlays or beds, and air-fluidized beds. Mattress overlays, such as air and gel types, and replacement mattresses are often very effective in reducing pressure. The use of any mechanical device (except air-fluidized beds) does not eliminate the need for turning and repositioning.

Specialty beds are categorized as either "low air loss" or "air fluidized." Air-fluidized therapy (e.g., Clinitron or FluidAir bed) provides the most effective pressure relief; the client is maintained in a nearly pressure-free environment (Figure 10-4). In general, these beds are not used to prevent skin breakdown, because most insurers will not reimburse the agency for the use of the bed. Therefore special beds are usually reserved for severe skin problems that have not healed with the use of a conventional bed or other mechanical device. If optimal nutrition and healing conditions are maintained, skin breakdowns should heal with continued use of air-fluidized therapy. The primary disadvantage of

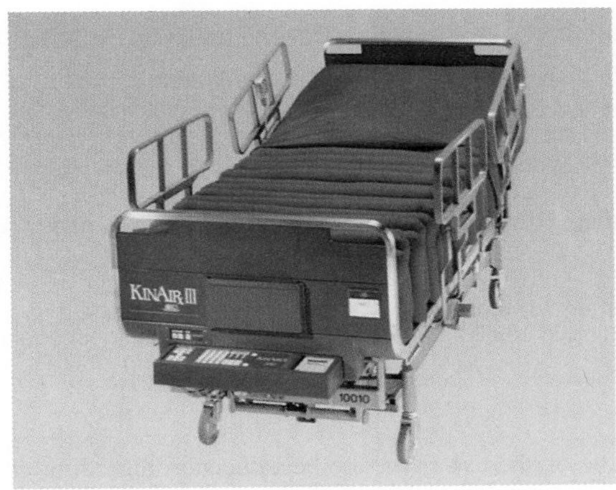

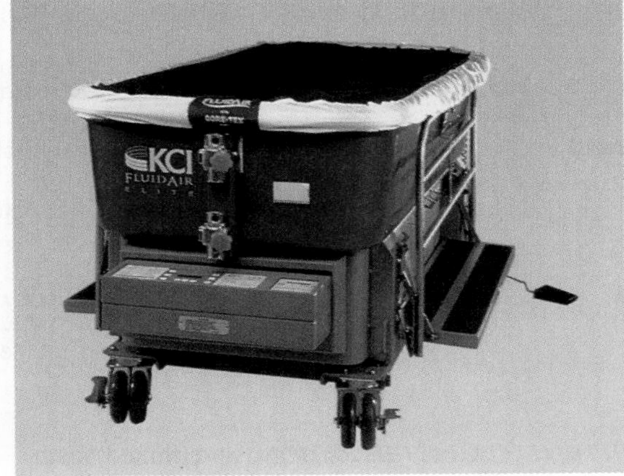

Figure 10-4 ● Pressure relief devices. *Left,* KinAirIII beds provide controlled air suspension to redistribute body weight away from bony prominences. *Right,* FluidAir Elite beds use airflow and bead fluidization. Both of these beds are covered with GORE-TEX fabric, which resists tearing. This fabric is also waterproof and acts as a barrier against bacteria. (Courtesy Kinetic Concepts, Inc., San Antonio, TX.)

this therapy is its expense, which may exceed several hundred dollars for each day of use. The cost of air-fluidized therapy may be reimbursed by some health insurance providers.

IMPAIRED URINARY ELIMINATION

PLANNING: EXPECTED OUTCOMES. The client with chronic illness or disability is expected to (1) achieve a personally acceptable form of urinary elimination, and (2) be free from urinary complications, such as infection.

INTERVENTIONS. Neurologic disabilities may interfere with successful bladder control in a client undergoing rehabilitation. These disabilities result in three basic functional types of neurogenic bladder: reflex (spastic) bladder, flaccid bladder, and uninhibited bladder.

A **reflex** or **spastic** (upper motor neuron) **bladder** causes incontinence that is characterized by sudden, gushing voids. The bladder does not usually empty completely. A reflex bladder is also sometimes referred to as a "spastic" bladder. Neurologic problems affecting the upper motor neuron typically occur with high-level or mid-level spinal cord injuries above the twelfth thoracic vertebra (T12). These injuries result in a failure of impulse transmission from the lower spinal cord areas to the cortex of the brain. When the bladder fills and transmits impulses to the spinal cord, the client is not conscious of the filling sensation. However, because there is no injury to the lower spinal cord and the voiding reflex arc is intact, the efferent (motor) impulse is relayed and the bladder contracts.

A **flaccid** (lower motor neuron) **bladder** results in urinary retention and overflow (dribbling). Injuries that cause damage to the lower motor neuron at the spinal cord level of S2-4 (e.g., multiple sclerosis and spinal cord injury below T12) may directly interfere with the reflex arc or may result in inappropriate interpretation of impulses to the brain. The bladder fills, and afferent (sensory) impulses conduct the message via the spinal cord to the cortical region of the brain. Because of the injury, the impulse is not interpreted correctly by the cortical bladder center in the brain, and there is a failure to respond with a message for the bladder to contract.

An **uninhibited bladder** may occur when the client has a neurologic problem that affects the cortical bladder center of the brain (frontal lobe), such as stroke or brain injury. When the bladder needs to empty, the client has little sensorimotor control and cannot wait until he or she is on the commode or bedpan before voiding. The client is incontinent, but the bladder may not completely empty.

BLADDER TRAINING. The nurse can teach three techniques to assist the client in "repatterning" voiding (bladder training):

- Facilitating, or triggering, techniques
- Intermittent catheterization
- Consistent scheduling of toileting routines

These techniques may not be as effective in clients with physiologic changes associated with aging.

FACILITATING OR TRIGGERING TECHNIQUES. Facilitating (triggering) techniques are used to stimulate voiding (Table 10-5). If there is an upper motor neuron problem but the reflex arc is intact (reflex bladder pattern), the voiding response can be initiated by any stimulus that sends the message to the spinal cord level S2-4 that the bladder might be full. Such techniques include stroking the medial aspect of the thigh, pinching the area above the groin, pulling pubic hair, massaging the penoscrotal area, pinching the posterior aspect of the glans penis, and providing digital anal stimulation.

When the client has a lower motor neuron problem, the voiding reflex arc is not intact (flaccid bladder pattern), and additional stimulation may be needed to initiate voiding. Two techniques used to facilitate voiding are the Valsalva maneuver and the Credé maneuver. In teaching the Valsalva maneuver, the nurse instructs the client to hold his or her breath and bear down as if trying to defecate. The nurse assists the client in performing the Credé maneuver by placing the client's hand in a cupped position directly over the bladder area and instructing the client to push inward and downward as if massaging the bladder to empty.

TABLE 10-5 • MANAGEMENT OF ALTERED URINARY ELIMINATION

Functional Type	Neurologic Disability	Clinical Manifestations	Reestablishing Voiding Patterns
Reflex (spastic)	Upper motor neuron spinal cord injury above T12	Urinary frequency, incontinence	Triggering or facilitating techniques Medications
Flaccid	Lower motor neuron spinal cord injury below T12 (affects S2-4 reflex arc)	Urinary retention, overflow	Valsalva and Credé maneuvers Medications
Uninhibited	Brain damage from injury or stroke	Frequency, urgency, incontinence, voiding in small amounts	Intermittent catheterization Consistent toileting schedule Regulation of fluid intake

INTERMITTENT CATHETERIZATION. Intermittent catheterization is often used for disorders that involve a flaccid bladder, which is generally caused by a lower motor neuron problem. In assisting the client with intermittent catheterization, the nurse initially inserts a urinary catheter every 2 to 3 hours—after the client has attempted voiding and has used the Valsalva and Credé maneuvers. If less than 150 mL of residual urine is obtained, the nurse typically increases the interval between catheterizations. This interval may be to 3 to 4 hours according to the health care provider's order or health care agency protocol. The interval may be gradually increased to 4 to 6 hours, but the client should not go beyond 8 hours between catheterizations. The exception occurs when the residual urine volume is less than 150 mL each time with an adequate intake of fluids. If the client will be performing intermittent self-catheterization at home after discharge from the rehabilitation facility, the nurse instructs the client about clean (not sterile) technique.

Intermittent catheterizations may also be performed to determine residual urine volumes for the client with a reflex (upper motor neuron) or uninhibited bladder. The client with this type of neurogenic bladder can void but often does not empty the bladder completely. The nurse catheterizes the client within 10 minutes of voiding to determine the residual amount of urine in the bladder. The desired amount is usually less than 100 mL.

TOILETING SCHEDULE. Consistent toileting routines may be the best way to reestablish voiding continence when the client displays an uninhibited bladder pattern (associated with brain damage or head injury). The nurse assesses the client's previous voiding pattern and determines his or her daily routine. At a minimum, the nurse assists the client with voiding after awakening in the morning, before and after meals, before and after physical activity, and at bedtime. The nurse considers the client's bladder capacity, which may range from 100 to 500 mL, as well as mobility limitations and restrictive clothing. Bladder capacity is determined by measuring urine output. The nurse ensures that the client is aware of nearby bathrooms at all times or has a call system to contact the nurse for assistance.

DRUG THERAPY. Medications that may be used for urinary elimination problems include cholinergics (to promote bladder emptying), antispasmodics (to prevent incontinence), and skeletal muscle relaxants (to decrease spasticity, which promotes self-care) (Chart 10-5). Medications are not usually prescribed by the health care provider in the initial management of bladder problems but may be used to assist with a bladder training program. The nurse reports the client's progress in bladder training to the health care provider so that he or she can make the best decision regarding drug therapy. In general, anticholinergics, antispasmodics, and skeletal muscle relaxants help to promote continence in clients with a reflex (upper motor neuron) bladder. Cholinergics, such as bethanechol chloride (Urecholine), may decrease urinary retention problems resulting from a flaccid bladder. They may also facilitate complete bladder emptying in a client with a large residual volume, which occurs with reflex bladder problems. An uninhibited bladder does not routinely require medications for bladder training programs unless urinary function is affected by additional pathologic changes.

FLUID INTAKE. The nurse instructs the client to maintain an adequate intake of fluids, at least 2000 to 2500 mL/day. An acidic urine usually minimizes the risk of urinary tract infection and calculus (stone) formation, although this belief is controversial. However, some microorganisms, such as *Escherichia coli,* do grow best in acidic environments. Therefore the nurse encourages the client to drink fluids that promote an acidic urine, including large amounts of cranberry juice, prune juice, bouillon, tomato juice, and water. Fluids that promote an alkaline urine are discouraged, including citrus juices, excessive amounts of milk and milk products, and carbonated beverages.

In addition, the nurse discourages high-calorie fluids for overweight clients. Disabled clients have more difficulty with mobility and self-care if their weight is not controlled.

CONSIDERATIONS FOR OLDER ADULTS

The nurse may decrease fluid intake to prevent complications in clients with congestive heart disease or renal problems, especially older clients. Some clients, especially those with flaccid bladder patterns, decrease fluid intake after 6 or 7 PM to avoid the need for catheterization during the night.

PREVENTION OF COMPLICATIONS. The client with altered urinary elimination is at risk for skin breakdown from incontinence, urinary tract infection from urinary retention, and urinary calculi from urinary retention and stasis. The nurse keeps the client clean and dry and provides skin care as described under Risk for Impaired Skin Integrity (p. 129). (See Chapter 70 for preventive measures for urinary tract infection and calculi.)

CONSTIPATION

PLANNING: EXPECTED OUTCOMES. The client with chronic illness or disability is expected to achieve a personally acceptable form of bowel elimination and be

CHART 10-5

DRUG THERAPY *for* Clients in Bladder Training Programs

Drug	Usual Dosage	Nursing Interventions	Rationale
CHOLINERGICS			
Bethanechol chloride (Urecholine)	10-50 mg bid-qid PO	Give 1 hr before or 2 hr after meals.	This agent may cause nausea and vomiting.
		Instruct clients to change positions slowly.	Orthostatic hypotension is a possible side effect.
		Give 1 hr before toileting or triggering or facilitating measure.	The drug is effective when using other measures for bladder training.
ANTISPASMODICS			
Oxybutynin chloride (Ditropan)	5 mg bid or tid PO	Instruct the client to avoid driving.	Vertigo, drowsiness, and blurred vision may occur.
		Instruct the client to avoid hot environmental temperatures.	Sweating is suppressed.
		Assess the client for urinary retention.	Retention may be a side effect of the drug.
Flavoxate hydrochloride (Urispas)	100-200 mg tid or qid PO	Instruct the client to avoid driving.	Drowsiness, mental confusion, and blurred vision may occur.
		Instruct the client to avoid hot environmental temperatures.	Sweating is suppressed.
		Assess the client for urinary retention.	Retention may be a side effect of the drug.
SKELETAL MUSCLE RELAXANTS			
Dantrolene (Dantrium)	25 mg once daily PO initially; increase to 25 mg bid-qid, then by 25-mg increments up to 100 mg	Instruct the client to avoid driving.	Fatigue, dizziness, and muscular weakness are side effects.
		Instruct the client to avoid prolonged sun exposure.	Photosensitivity may occur.
Baclofen (Lioresal)	5 mg tid PO; may increase by 5 mg daily until desired effect is attained to maximum of 80 mg	Instruct the client to avoid alcohol.	Alcohol potentiates the effects of this drug.
		Instruct the client to avoid driving.	Drowsiness and dizziness may occur.

free from bowel elimination complications, such as impaction or diarrhea.

INTERVENTIONS. Neurologic problems often affect the client's bowel pattern by causing a reflex (spastic) bowel, a flaccid bowel, or an uninhibited bowel.

Upper motor neuron diseases and injuries, such as a high-level or mid-level spinal cord injury, may result in a reflex (spastic) bowel pattern, with defecation occurring suddenly and without warning. With a reflex pattern, any facilitating or triggering mechanism may lead to defecation if the lower colon contains stool. Examples of facilitating or triggering techniques include providing anal stimulation (by inserting a finger, using either a finger cot or rubber glove and lubrication, to the first joint), gently pinching the anus, and pulling pubic hair. Digital stimulation should not be used for clients with cardiac disease because of the risk of inducing a vagal response (a rapid decrease in heart rate).

Lower motor neuron diseases and injuries interfere with transmission of the nervous impulse across the reflex arc and may result in a flaccid bowel pattern, with defecation occurring infrequently and in small amounts. The use of facilitating and triggering mechanisms in combination with a toileting schedule, suppository use, and disimpaction yields the best results. Clients may be able to self-administer the suppository or disimpact if necessary.

Neurologic injuries that affect the brain may cause an uninhibited bowel pattern, with frequent defecation, urgency, and complaints of hard stool. Clients may manage uninhibited bowel patterns through a consistent toileting schedule, a high-fiber diet, and the use of stool softeners.

BOWEL TRAINING. An overview of management techniques for bowel dysfunction is presented in Table 10-6. In many cases, clients are not able to regain control over their bowel function in the manner previously possible. The rehabilitation team assists in designing a bowel elimination program that accommodates the disability.

The nurse works with clients to schedule bowel elimination as close as possible to their previous routine. For example, a client who had stools at noon every other day before the illness or injury should have the bowel program scheduled in the same way. An exception is the client who prefers another time that best fits into his or her daily routine. If the client is employed during the day, a time-consuming bowel elimination program in the morning may not be reasonable. It may be preferable to change the bowel protocol to the evening, when there is more time.

DRUG THERAPY. Bowel training programs for clients with neurologic problems are often designed to include a combination of suppository use and a consistent toileting schedule.

TABLE 10-6 • MANAGEMENT OF BOWEL DYSFUNCTION

Functional Type	Neurologic Disability	Dysfunction	Reestablishing Defecation Patterns
Reflex (spastic)	Upper motor neuron spinal cord injury above T12	Defecation without warning	Triggering mechanisms Facilitation techniques High-fiber diet Suppository use Consistent toileting schedule
Flaccid	Lower motor neuron spinal cord injury below T12 (affects S2-4 reflex arc)	Infrequent, small stools	Triggering or facilitating techniques High-fiber diet Suppository use Consistent toileting schedule Manual disimpaction
Uninhibited	Brain damage from injury or stroke	Frequency, urgency, and constipation	Consistent toileting schedule High-fiber diet Stool softener use

Although medications should not be a first choice when formulating a bowel training program, the nurse routinely considers the need for a suppository if clients do not reestablish defecation habits through a consistent toileting schedule, dietary modification, anal stimulation, and disimpaction.

Bisacodyl (Dulcolax) and glycerin are common agents prescribed by physicians as suppositories in bowel training programs. Suppositories must be placed against the bowel wall to stimulate the sacral reflex arc and promote rectal emptying. Both agents are equivalent in effect, with results occurring in 15 to 30 minutes. The nurse administers the suppository when the client expects to defecate. For example, if a client had a previous bowel habit of defecating every other day after breakfast, the suppository is administered every other day after breakfast. Administering the suppository every second or third day is usually effective in reestablishing defecation patterns. Depending on each client's need, other medications (e.g., laxatives) may be indicated for bowel training programs.

NUTRITION. Bowel elimination is directly related to the type and quality of food and fluid ingested. A high-fiber diet is a mainstay of most bowel training programs and includes whole-grain foods, bran, and fresh and dried fruits. Increasing dietary fiber is effective in facilitating defecation only if the client reduces fat intake.

PREVENTION OF COMPLICATIONS. Constipation, diarrhea, and flatulence are common complications of any bowel training program. The nurse assesses for these complications and modifies the bowel training program accordingly in collaboration with the physician and the dietitian.

INEFFECTIVE COPING

PLANNING: EXPECTED OUTCOMES. The client with chronic illness or disability is expected to learn to cope with the chronic illness or disability and participate in the rehabilitation program.

INTERVENTIONS. The client with a disability often has a poor self-concept because of changes in body image from structural or functional changes. The use of an assistive device, such as a wheelchair, also differentiates the client from most other people, and the client may not want to accept the need for the device. The nurse encourages the client to discuss his or her feelings and asks questions to elicit specific information that can help in assessing his or her acceptance of and ability to cope with the disability.

A disability also affects a person's role in society. For instance, a young medical student may fall from a ladder and become a paraplegic; as a result, plans for a career as a surgeon are altered. A middle-aged farmer may be burned severely when his tractor catches on fire. He can no longer care for his farm, and his wife takes over during his rehabilitation process. An older adult who cares for her grandchildren is crippled with rheumatoid arthritis and can no longer provide child care. Disability requires role changes and always involves losses in the lives of those affected.

In addition to role changes, relationships with people change. Socializing with friends and family may be a strain when a person feels "different." Intimate relationships are affected because sexual dysfunction may result from disability. The nurse should be sensitive to these issues and should not avoid discussing them.

The nurse assesses the client's previous coping strategies and support systems so they can be used during rehabilitation if needed. The client is asked what strategies have been used to cope successfully with previous life crises, if any. Spiritual and religious beliefs are important for some people and should not be overlooked when helping to identify sources of support.

COMPLEMENTARY AND ALTERNATIVE THERAPIES. Some clients use complementary and alternative medicine (CAM) to cope with chronic disease and disability, especially if chronic pain is a problem. Examples of these therapies include acupuncture, acupressure, imagery, and music. Chapter 4 discusses CAM in detail.

Community-Based Care

Discharge planning begins during the client's admission. If the client is being transferred from a hospital to a rehabilitation unit or facility, the nurse orients him or her to the change in routine and emphasizes the importance of self-care. When the client is admitted to the rehabilitation unit or facility, the case manager assesses his or her current living situation at home. Together with the client and family members or significant others, the case manager determines the adequacy of the current situation and the potential needs after discharge to home. The client with chronic illness and disability may require home care, assistance with activities of daily living (ADLs), nursing care, or physical or occupational therapy after discharge. The case manager assesses these needs and plans with the client, family or significant other, social worker, physical or vocational therapist, and physician the best ways to meet identified needs.

Other health care professionals may be necessary to meet the unique needs of special populations. For example, clients with brain injury may benefit from life planning, a process that examines and plans to meet lifelong needs. Case managers specializing in life planning may be part of the interdisciplinary rehabilitation team.

HOME CARE MANAGEMENT

Before the client returns home, the nurse assesses his or her readiness for discharge from the rehabilitation facility or hospital. The home may be assessed in multiple ways.

PREDISCHARGE ASSESSMENT. Before discharge, the case manager or occupational therapist may visit the home to assess its layout and accessibility. These professionals may be employed by the health care agency or by a third-party payer, such as a health maintenance organization (see Chapter 3 for a discussion of third-party payers). Because of the stress of hospitalization, a client with a fractured hip who is ambulating well with a walker may neglect to explain to the nurse that the home has three steps at the entrance and that the bathroom is accessible by stairway only. The client may not consider it important to mention that throw rugs, which do not provide a completely level surface on which to use a cane, are scattered throughout the apartment.

During a predischarge visit to the home, the case manager assesses the accessibility of the home in general and of the bathrooms, bedrooms, and kitchen. If the client will be wheelchair dependent after discharge from the facility, ramps are needed to replace steps, and doorways should be checked for adequate width. A doorway width of 36 to 38 inches (slightly less than 1 m) is usually sufficient for a standard-sized wheelchair. Any room that the client needs to use is checked. The bedroom should have sufficient space for the client to maneuver transfers to and from the wheelchair and the bed.

Space requirements vary and depend on the client's need to use a wheelchair, walker, or cane. In the bathroom, grab bars may need to be installed before the client comes home. Bathtub benches can provide support for the client who has difficulty with mobility and, when used in combination with a handheld showerhead, can provide easily accessible bathing facilities. Assessment of the kitchen may or may not be critical depending on whether the client has help with cooking and preparing meals. If the client will be responsible for cooking after discharge, the kitchen is assessed for wheelchair or walker accessibility, appliance accessibility, and the need for adaptive equipment.

For hospitalized older clients returning home, cognitive assessment may help predict rehabilitation success. A study of 73 older clients being discharged with home care services showed that cognition correlated with the ability to return to ADL independence (see the Evidence-Based Practice for Nursing box on p. 124).

LEAVE-OF-ABSENCE VISIT. A second method of assessing the client's home is through a brief home visit, also called a leave-of-absence (LOA) visit, by the client before discharge. The nurse explains the need for the trial home visit and assesses the client's comfort level with this idea. The client who has been hospitalized for a lengthy period may feel intense anxiety about returning home. The nurse may allay such anxieties with careful preparation. Before the visit, the rehabilitation nurse meets with the client and family members or significant others to set goals for the visit and to identify specific tasks to be attempted while at home. After the home visit, the client is interviewed to determine the success of the visit and to assess additional education or training needs before final discharge.

Going home may not be an option for everyone. Some clients may not have a support network of family members or significant others. For example, many older adults have no spouse or close friends living nearby. Children may live far away, which can make home care difficult. If no caregiver is available, the family must decide whether care can be provided in the home by an outside resource or whether the client needs to be admitted to a 24-hour supervised health care setting, such as a nursing home. Rehabilitation services are available in most long-term care settings (skilled nursing facilities) at least 5 days a week.

HEALTH TEACHING

Education of the client and the family is the cornerstone of nursing care. The nurse assesses every component of care to determine how to teach the client to perform activities of daily living (ADLs) independently. The nurse assesses the client's learning potential and cognitive capacity and encourages him or her to perform or direct each skill or technique independently to verify understanding. Written material explaining the steps in the procedure is provided to the client and family members to reinforce learning and to provide support with the technique after discharge. Before distributing written material, the rehabilitation team assesses the reading level of the material and determines whether it is appropriate for the client's reading ability and language skills.

Any chronic illness or disability necessitates changes in lifestyle and body image. The nurse assists in dealing with such changes by encouraging the verbalization of feelings and emotions. A focus on existing capabilities instead of disabilities is emphasized.

The client may fail to relate psychologically to the disability during hospitalization. For example, he or she may display anger or frustration in attempting to perform self-care routines before discharge from the rehabilitation facility. The nurse encourages the client to be open about such feelings and to talk about ways to prevent worries from becoming realities after discharge.

The leave-of-absence home visit assists the client and family members or significant others in psychosocial preparation for discharge. It allows the experience of the home situation while being able to return to the hospital environment after a few hours. Often the client finds that his or her fears were not realized during the home visit but finds new problems in the home that must be addressed before discharge. The nurse reviews this information with the client in preparation for discharge to the home.

HEALTH CARE RESOURCES

After discharge to the home, various health care resources (e.g., physical therapy, home care nursing, and vocational counseling) are available to the client with chronic illness and disability. The nurse assesses the need for additional care and support throughout the hospitalization and works with the case manager and physician in arranging for home services.

• Evaluation: Outcomes

NOC The client and rehabilitation team evaluate the effectiveness of interdisciplinary interventions on the basis of the identified nursing diagnoses and collaborative problems. Expected outcomes may include that the client will:

- Ambulate independently, with or without assistive devices, or be independent in wheelchair mobility skills
- Perform ADLs independently with or without assistive/adaptive devices
- Have intact skin
- Demonstrate effective urinary elimination through an individualized bladder training program
- Demonstrate effective bowel elimination through an individualized bowel training program
- State acceptance of the disability and use coping strategies effectively

ONLINE RESOURCES

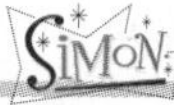

For suggested readings and Internet resources, go to http://www.wbsaunders.com/SIMON/Iggy/.

SELECTED BIBLIOGRAPHY

Asterisk indicates a classic or definitive work on this subject.

*Boss, B.J., et al. (1995). Self-care competence among persons with spinal cord injury. *SCI Nursing, 12*(2), 48-53.

*Braden, B.J., & Bergstrom, N. (1992). Pressure reduction. In G.M. Bulechek & J.C. McCloskey (Eds.), *Nursing interventions: Essential nursing treatments* (2nd ed., pp. 94-108). Philadelphia: W.B. Saunders.

*Carey, R.G., & Posavec, E.J. (1978). Program evaluation of a physical medicine and rehabilitation unit: A new approach. *Archives of Physical Medicine and Rehabilitation, 59,* 330-337.

Collins, R.C. (1997). *Neurology.* Philadelphia: W.B. Saunders.

Davis, F.N. (1999). Functional rehabilitation of employees with chronic musculoskeletal pain. *The Case Manager, 10*(3), 55-59.

Evans, R.W. (1997). The role of the neuropsychologist in life care planning for brain-injured populations. *The Journal of Care Management, 3*(5), 46-47, 49.

Gallagner, R.M. (2000). How long-term care is changing. *American Journal of Nursing, 100*(2), 65-67.

*Granger, C.V., & Gresham, G.E. (1984). *Functional assessment in rehabilitation medicine.* Baltimore: Williams & Wilkins.

*Granger, C.V., et al. (1993). Performance profiles of the Functional Independence Measure. *Journal of Physical Medicine and Rehabilitation, 72,* 84-89.

*Hamilton, L., & Lyon, P.S. (1995). A nursing-driven program to preserve and restore functional ability in hospitalized elderly patients. *Journal of Nursing Administration, 25*(4), 30-37.

Hansen, K., Mahoney, J., & Palta, M. (1999). Risk factors for lack of recovery of ADL independence after hospital discharge. *Journal of the American Geriatrics Society, 47*(3), 360-365.

Hickey, J.V. (1997). *The clinical practice of neurological and neurosurgical nursing* (4th ed.). Philadelphia: J.B. Lippincott.

Hosack, K. (1999). The model spinal cord injury system. *The Case Manager, 10*(2), 51-54.

Huntt, D.C., & Growick, B.S. (1997). Managed care for people with disabilities. *Journal of Rehabilitation,* July/August/September, pp. 10-14.

Ignatavicius, D.D. (1998). *Introduction to long term care nursing.* Philadelphia: F.A. Davis.

*Institute of Medicine. (1991). *Disability in America.* Washington, DC: National Academy Press.

*Katz, S., et al. (1963). Studies of illness in the aged. The index of ADL: A standardized measure of biological and psychosocial function. *Journal of the American Medical Association, 185,* 914-919.

*Miller, J.M. (1991). *Coping with chronic illness: Overcoming powerlessness* (2nd ed.). Philadelphia: F.A. Davis.

Monahan, K. (1999). A joint effort to save lives. The COPD Wellness Program. *Geriatric Nursing, 20*(4), 200-202.

Murphy, M.P., Pereira-Ogan, A., & Yody, B.B. (1998). Discharge planning for individuals with neurocognitive barriers. *The Journal of Care Management, 4*(4), 28-36.

Nazarko, L. (1999). Rehabilitation. *Nursing Management, 6*(5), 24-27.

*Neal, L.J. (1995). The rehabilitation nurse in the home care setting: Treating chronic wounds as a disability. *Rehabilitation Nursing, 20*(5), 261-264.

*Posavec, E.J., & Carey, R.G. (1982). Using a level of function scale (LORS-II) to evaluate the success of inpatient rehabilitation programs. *Rehabilitation Nursing, 7*(6), 17-19.

Somervill, B.A. (1997). Transitional and subacute care. *Case Review, 3*(3), 61-63.

Sorensen, B., & Luken, K. (1999). Improving functional outcomes with recreational therapy. *The Case Manager, 10*(5), 48-53.

Thrift, J. (1999). Case managers at the helm of return-to-productivity programs. *The Case Manager, 10*(4), 75-80.

Vierling, L. (1999). Four components for an improved return-to-work program. *The Case Manager, 10*(4), 52-54.

Wood, C., & Lui, J. (1999). The evolution of disability care and case management: Identifying core competencies. *The Case Manager, 10*(4), 41-46.

*World Health Organization. (1980). *International classification of impairments, disabilities and handicaps.* Geneva: Author.

UNIT

3

MANAGEMENT OF CLIENTS WITH FLUID, ELECTROLYTE, AND ACID-BASE IMBALANCES

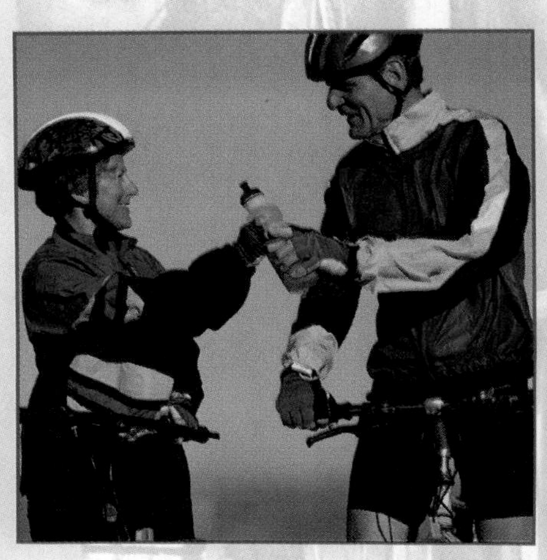

Management of Clients with Fluid, Electrolyte, and Acid-Base Imbalances

Core Concepts Grid

Anatomy	Physiology	Pathophysiology	History	Physical Exam	Diagnostic Tests	Interventions	Pharmacology
• **Body fluid** Intracellular Extracellular Intravascular Interstitial • **Lungs** • **Heart/vessels** • **Kidney**	• **Filtration** • **Osmosis** • **Diffusion** • **Active transport** • **Hydrostatic pressure** • **Tonicity** Isotonic Hypotonic Hypertonic • **Third-space fluids** • **Transport medium** • **Protection** • **Metabolism** • **Regulatory mechanisms for fluid-electrolyte balance** • **Regulatory mechanisms for acid-base balance**	• **Overhydration** • **Dehydration** Isotonic Hypertonic Hypotonic • **Solute excess** • **Solute deficit** • **Metabolic acidosis/ alkalosis** • **Respiratory acidosis/ alkalosis**	• **Client history** Anorexia Fatigue Headache Nausea/ vomiting Diarrhea Weakness Cramping Thirst Fever	• **Skin** Color/moisture Turgor • **Weight** • **Urine output** • **Vital signs** • **Breath sounds** • **Muscle weakness** • **Central nervous system** Mental status Hyperreflexia Tetany Chvostek's sign Trousseau's sign • **Cardiovascular system** Dysrhythmias Decreased cardiac output	• **Serum levels** Sodium Potassium Calcium Phosphorus Magnesium • **Urine tests** pH Specific gravity • **Blood urea nitrogen** • **Arterial blood gases** pH $Pa{O_2}$ $Pa{CO_2}$ HCO_3^- • **Anion gap** • **Hemoglobin/ hematocrit**	• **Oral rehydration** • **Therapeutic diets** • **Blood gas interpretation** • **Semi-Fowler's position** • **Respiratory** Oxygen Turn, cough, deep breathe Incentive spirometry • **Oral hygiene** • **Rest** • **Infusion therapy** Peripheral intravenous therapy Central intravenous therapy • **Health teaching**	• **Diuretics** • **Crystalloid/ colloid fluid replacement** • **Electrolyte replacement** • **Bronchodilators** • **Anti-inflammatory drugs** • **Antibiotics** • **Antidiarrheals** • **Kayexelate**

CHAPTER

11

Fluid and Electrolyte Balance

M. LINDA WORKMAN

Learning Objectives

After studying this chapter, you should be able to:

1. Explain why women and older adults have less total body water than do men and younger adults.
2. Interpret whether a client's serum electrolyte values are normal, elevated, or low.
3. Describe the expected blood volume and osmolarity responses when isotonic, hypertonic, or hypotonic intravenous fluids are infused.
4. Explain the relationships between antidiuretic hormone, urine output volume, and osmolarity.
5. Analyze a client's hydration status on the basis of physical assessment findings.
6. Evaluate a client's food choices for compliance with a low-sodium diet.

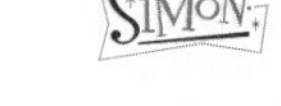

Go to http://www.wbsaunders.com/SIMON/Iggy/ for self-assessment questions related to these Learning Objectives.

HOMEOSTASIS

The human body functions best when certain conditions are kept within a narrow range of normal. Examples of such conditions include body temperature, specific serum electrolyte values (e.g., sodium, potassium, and calcium), blood pH, and blood volume. Nothing functions very well if the body gains or loses 2 liters of blood. To keep conditions as close to normal as possible (a situation called **homeostasis**), the body has many regulatory mechanisms **(homeostatic mechanisms)** to prevent unacceptable changes. For example, if a person is in a hot environment (e.g., 110° F) and does not have good homeostatic mechanisms, his or her body temperature could go as high as 110° F, resulting in death. The homeostatic mechanisms of sweating to cool by evaporation and dilating blood vessels to dissipate body heat help to prevent body temperature from going more than 1° F above the normal 98.6° F, thereby maintaining homeostasis of body temperature.

One area extremely important for homeostasis is maintenance of the body's normal fluid volume and composition. Water is the most common substance in the body. It is needed to deliver dissolved nutrients, electrolytes, and other substances to all organs, tissues, and cells. Changes in body fluid in terms of either the amount of water or the concentration of electrolytes can affect the functioning of all cells, tissues, and organs. For proper physiologic function, the volume of all body fluids and the types and amount of dissolved substances must be carefully regulated.

ANATOMY AND PHYSIOLOGY REVIEW

Physiologic Influences on Fluid and Electrolyte Balance

Many physical and biologic processes control the normal balance of body fluids and electrolytes. These processes work together to keep homeostatic balance so the internal environment remains stable even when the external environment undergoes dramatic changes.

Knowing the terminology related to solutions is necessary for understanding the processes involved in fluid and electrolyte balance (Table 11-1). Body fluids are composed of water and particles either dissolved or suspended in water. The **solvent** is the water portion of body fluids. **Solutes** are the particles dissolved in the water. Solutes vary in type and concentration from one body fluid compartment to another. Proper body function is dependent on keeping the correct balance of fluid and electrolytes within each body fluid compartment.

Important processes involved in fluid and electrolyte balance include filtration, diffusion, osmosis, and active transport. Capillary dynamics also affect fluid and electrolyte balance. All of these processes determine how, when, and where fluids and particles move across cell membranes.

FILTRATION

Definition

Filtration is the movement of fluid through a cell or blood vessel membrane because of hydrostatic pressure differences on both sides of the membrane. Basically, filtration depends on differences in water volume exerting pressure against confining walls.

All fluid has weight. The overall weight of a fluid is related to the amount of fluid present in the confined space. Water molecules in a confined space constantly press outward against the confining walls or boundaries. **Hydrostatic pressure** is the force exerted by water molecules against the confining walls of a space. This pressure is caused by the weight of fluid against the walls. Hydrostatic pressure may be thought of as "water-pushing" pressure, because it is a force that moves water outward from a confined space through a membrane (Figure 11-1).

Physiologic Activity

Water is the largest component of any body fluid. The amount of water in any body fluid compartment is a main factor in determining the hydrostatic pressure of that compartment. The proportion of water present in a fluid is inversely related to the **viscosity** (thickness) of that fluid. Thus more water and less solute results in decreased viscosity, and less water with more solute results in increased viscosity. Blood, a viscous fluid (more viscous than water), is confined within the blood vessels. Blood has hydrostatic pressure because of its weight and volume and also because the heart is pumping blood into the arterial circulation.

The hydrostatic pressures of two fluid compartments can be compared whenever a **permeable** (porous) membrane separates the two compartments. If the hydrostatic pressure is the same in both fluid compartments, a state of **equilibrium** exists for hydrostatic pressure. If the hydrostatic pressure is not the same in both compartments, a state of **disequilibrium** ex-

TABLE 11-1 • TERMINOLOGY ASSOCIATED WITH FLUID AND ELECTROLYTE BALANCE

active transport Assisted movement of a substance through a permeable membrane between two fluid compartments; occurs against a concentration, electrical, or pressure gradient; requires the expenditure of chemical energy

adenosine triphosphate (ATP) A substance that is generated by the metabolism of glucose or fat within cells and releases chemical energy for physiologic function when a high-energy phosphate bond (~P) is broken

aldosterone A hormone secreted by the adrenal cortex that stimulates the renal reabsorption of sodium and water and the renal excretion of potassium

anion A molecule (electrolyte) that carries an overall negative charge when dissolved in water

antidiuretic hormone (ADH) A hormone secreted from the posterior pituitary gland that increases the renal reabsorption of pure water and decreases urine output

atrial natriuretic peptide (ANP) A hormone secreted by cardiac atrial cells that increases the renal excretion of sodium and water

brownian motion Inherent molecular motion

capillary (plasma) hydrostatic pressure The force generated by fluid within a capillary that tends to move fluid out from the capillary and into the interstitial space

capillary (plasma) osmotic pressure The force generated by the concentration of plasma solutes (osmotic and oncotic pressures) that tends to retain fluid within the capillary or move fluid from the interstitial space into the capillary

cation A molecule (electrolyte) that carries an overall positive charge when dissolved in water

cofactor A substance required to enhance the activity of an enzyme or a physiologic reaction

colloidal oncotic pressure The osmotic pressure exerted by the concentration of colloids (proteins) within a solution

diffusion Unimpeded movement of a substance through a permeable membrane between two fluid compartments; occurs down a concentration gradient; does not require the expenditure of chemical energy

disequilibrium A state in which two fluid compartments are unequal in at least one characteristic

electrolytes Substances that carry an electrical charge when dissolved in water

electroneutrality A state in which a body fluid has an equal number of cations and anions so that the fluid does not express an electrical charge

equilibrium A state in which two fluid compartments are equal in one or more characteristics

extracellular fluid (ECF) Body fluid present outside of cells; includes plasma, interstitial fluid, and transcellular fluid

facilitated diffusion Assisted movement of a substance through a permeable membrane between two fluid compartments; occurs down a concentration gradient; does not require the expenditure of chemical energy

filtration The movement of fluid through a biologic membrane as a result of hydrostatic pressure differences on the two sides of the membrane

gradient A graded difference in some characteristic between two fluid compartments

hydrostatic pressure The force of pressure exerted by static water in a confined space—"water-pushing" pressure

hypertonic (hyperosmotic) Any solution with a solute concentration (osmolarity) greater than that of normal body fluids (>310 mOsm/L)

hypotonic (hyposmotic) Any solution with a solute concentration (osmolarity) less than that of normal body fluids (<270 mOsm/L)

impermeable membrane A membrane separating two fluid compartments that does not permit the movement of one or more substances through the membrane (by diffusion) from one compartment to the other

insensible fluid loss Unregulated fluid losses from the skin, gastrointestinal tract, wounds, and pulmonary epithelium

interstitial fluid Fluid present in tissues between cells

intracellular fluid (ICF) Fluid found inside cells

isotonic (isosmotic) Any solution with a solute concentration equal to the osmolarity of normal body fluids or normal saline (0.9% NaCl), ~300 mOsm/L

obligatory urine output The minimal amount of urine output necessary to ensure the excretion of metabolic wastes (~400 mL/day)

osmolality The concentration of solute within a solution as measured by the amount of solute osmoles per kilogram of solvent

osmolarity The concentration of solute within a solution as measured by the amount of solute osmoles per liter of solution

osmoreceptor Specialized sensory nerve cells in the thalamus or hypothalamus that are sensitive to changes in the osmolarity of extracellular fluid

osmosis Diffusion of water (no other substance) through a selectively permeable membrane from an area of lower osmotic pressure to an area of greater osmotic pressure

osmotic pressure The pressure exerted by a solution that contains a relatively high concentration of solute; this pressure draws water from areas or compartments with lower concentrations of solute into the areas or compartments with higher concentrations of solute—"water-pulling" pressure

permeable membrane A membrane separating two fluid compartments that permits the movement of one or more substances through the membrane (by diffusion) from one compartment to the other

solubility The degree to which any given solute completely dissolves (dissociates) in water

solute The solid particles dissolved in a solution

solvent The fluid (water) portion of a solution

tissue hydrostatic pressure (THP) The force generated by fluid within the interstitial spaces that tends to move fluid into the capillary from the interstitial space

tissue osmotic pressure (TOP) The force generated by the concentration of interstitial fluid solutes that tend to retain fluid in the interstitial space or move fluid from the capillary into the interstitial space

transcellular fluid Extracellular fluid confined to a specific area or region of the body (cerebrospinal fluid, pericardial fluid, visceral fluid, aqueous humor, peritoneal fluid, and pleural fluid)

viscosity Gumminess or thickness of the molecules in a solution, causing friction within that solution ists. This means that the two compartments have a **gradient,** or graded difference, of hydrostatic pressure: one compartment has a higher hydrostatic pressure than the other. Because the human body constantly seeks equilibrium, a gradient across a cell membrane causes forces to rearrange the distribution of substances on both sides of the membrane until an equilibrium is reached (Figure 11-2).

In most instances, substances move or are rearranged from the greater amount of pressure or concentration to the lesser amount. Thus when a hydrostatic pressure gradient exists between two fluid compartments, fluid from the compartment with the higher hydrostatic pressure moves through **(filters)** the membrane into the compartment with the lower hydrostatic pressure. This filtration continues only as long as the hydrostatic pressure gradient exists. An equilibrium is reached when enough fluid leaves one compartment and enters the other compartment to make the hydrostatic pressure in both compartments equal.

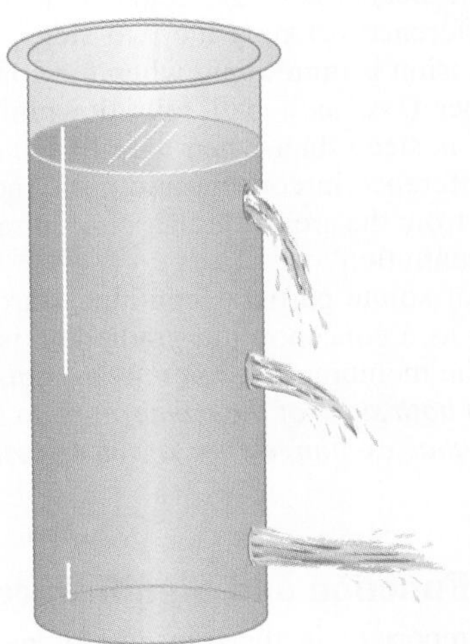

Figure 11-1 ● Hydrostatic pressure. The pressure that water molecules exert against the sides of the container is highest where the weight of the water is greatest. (From Nave, C., & Nave, B. [Eds.]. [1985]. *Physics for the health sciences* [3rd ed.]. Philadelphia, W.B. Saunders.)

When the two compartments are in equilibrium for hydrostatic pressure, a gradient no longer exists between them. Although water molecules may be exchanged evenly back and forth between two compartments in equilibrium, no net filtration of fluid occurs. In equilibrium, neither compartment gains or loses water molecules, and the hydrostatic pressure in both compartments remains the same.

Clinical Function and Significance

Blood pressure is a hydrostatic filtering force measured in millimeters of mercury (mm Hg). It moves whole blood from the heart to tissue areas where filtration can occur. Filtration is important for the exchange of water, nutrients, and waste products when blood arrives at the tissue capillaries. One factor that determines whether or not fluid leaves the blood vessels and enters the tissue spaces **(interstitial fluid)** is the difference between the hydrostatic pressure of the fluid in the capillaries and that of the fluid in the interstitial tissue spaces.

The lining of the capillaries is only one cell layer thick. Therefore the "wall" that holds blood in the capillaries is thin. Large spaces **(pores)** between the cells in the capillary membrane help water filter freely through capillary membranes in either direction if a hydrostatic pressure gradient is present

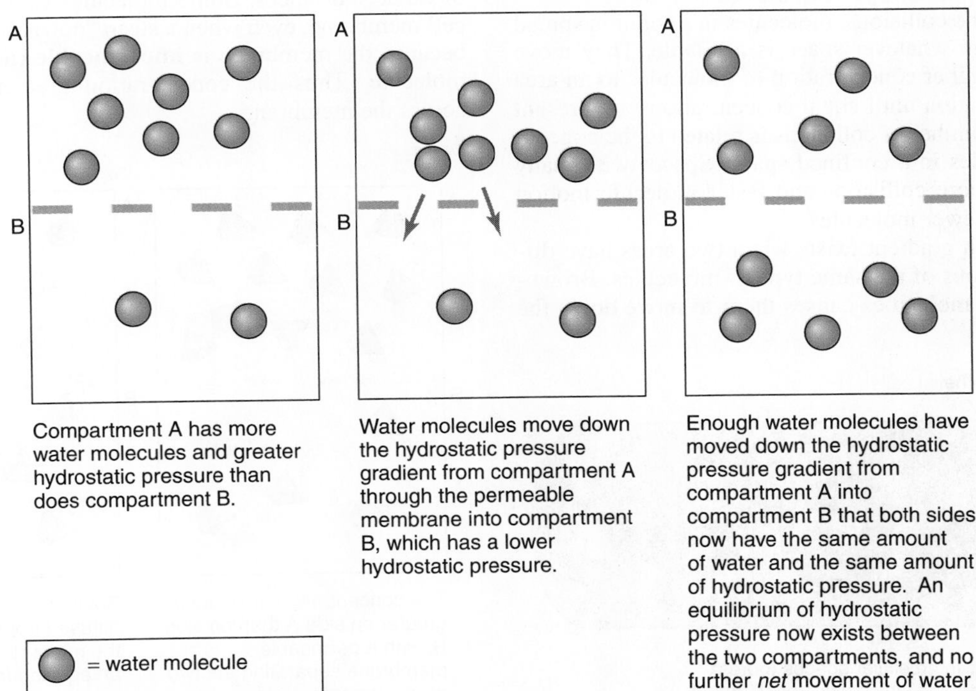

Figure 11-2 ● The process of filtration. (© 1992 M. Linda Workman. All rights reserved.)

(Figure 11-3). This concept is discussed later in this chapter under Capillary Dynamics, p. 145.

Edema (tissue swelling) can develop as a result of changes in normal hydrostatic pressure gradients, such as in clients with right-sided congestive heart failure. In this condition, the volume of blood in the right side of the heart increases greatly because the right ventricle is too weak to pump blood efficiently into the pulmonary blood vessels. As blood volume accumulates, blood backs up into the venous system, and venous hydrostatic pressure rises. The increased venous pressure causes capillary hydrostatic pressure to increase until it is higher than the hydrostatic pressure in the interstitial spaces. Excess filtration of fluid from the capillaries into the interstitial tissue spaces occurs, resulting in the formation of visible edema.

DIFFUSION

Definition

Diffusion is the free movement of particles (solute) across a permeable membrane down a **concentration gradient,** that is, from an area of higher concentration to an area of lower concentration. Diffusion controls the movement of particles in solution across various body membranes.

Physiologic Activity

The diffusion of particles into and out of cells and fluid compartments occurs via **brownian motion,** the kinetic energy of molecular motion. Brownian motion is the vibration of single molecules caused by electrons orbiting at the core of each molecule. Such motion produces totally random movement of molecules, which causes molecules to move and bump into each other within a confined space. These collisions cause a temporary increase in the speed of movement.

As a result of the collisions, molecules in a solution spread out evenly through whatever space is available. They move from an area of higher concentration of molecules to an area of lower concentration until equal concentrations are present in all areas. The number of collisions is related to the concentration of molecules in a confined space. Spaces with many molecules have more collisions and faster molecule motion than spaces with fewer molecules.

A concentration gradient exists when two areas have different concentrations of the same type of molecules. Brownian motion of the molecules causes them to move down the concentration gradient. As a result of brownian motion, any membrane that separates two areas is struck repeatedly by molecules. When the molecule strikes a pore in the membrane that is large enough for it to pass through, diffusion occurs (Figure 11-4). The likelihood of any single molecule colliding with the membrane and going through a pore is much greater on the side of the membrane with a higher molecule concentration.

The speed of diffusion is directly related to the degree of concentration difference between the two sides of the membrane. The degree of concentration difference is usually referred to as the *steepness* of the gradient: The larger the concentration difference between the two sides, the steeper the gradient. Diffusion is more rapid when the concentration gradient is steeper (just as a ball rolls downhill more rapidly when the hill is steep than when the hill is nearly flat). The greater the difference in concentration, the more rapidly diffusion occurs from the area of higher concentration to the area of lower concentration.

Diffusion of solute particles continues through the membrane as long as a concentration gradient exists between the two sides of the membrane. *When the concentration of solute is the same on both sides of the membrane, an equilibrium exists and an equal exchange (not a net movement) of solute continues.*

Clinical Function and Significance

Diffusion is important in the transport of gases and in the movement of most electrolytes, atoms, and molecules through cell membranes. Unlike capillary membranes, which permit the diffusion of most small-sized substances down a concentration gradient, cell membranes are *selective.* They permit the movement of some substances and inhibit the movement of other substances. Some molecules cannot move across a cell membrane, even when a steep "downhill" gradient exists, because the membrane is **impermeable** (not porous) to that molecule. Thus the concentration gradient is maintained across the membrane.

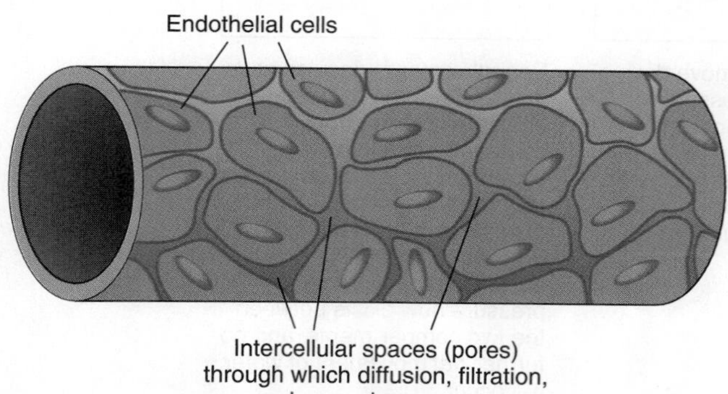

Figure 11-3 ● The basic structure of a capillary.

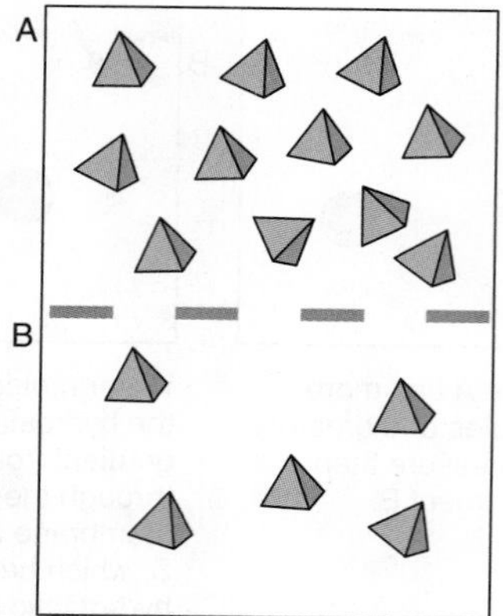

The concentration of solute is greater on side A than on side B, with a permeable membrane separating the two compartments.

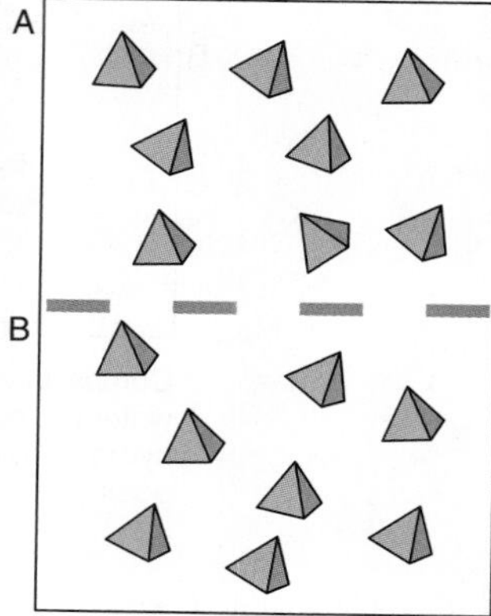

Solute molecules have diffused from side A through the membrane into side B until an equilibrium of solute exists and the concentration of solute is the same on both sides.

Figure 11-4 ● Diffusion of a solute.

Impermeability and special transport systems cause differences in the concentrations of specific substances from one fluid compartment to another. For example, under normal conditions the fluid outside of the cells, the **extracellular fluid (ECF),** contains almost ten times more sodium ions than the fluid inside the cell, the **intracellular fluid (ICF).** This extreme concentration difference results from the relative impermeability of the cell membrane to sodium and from a special "sodium pump" that moves any extra sodium out of the cell "uphill" against its concentration gradient and back into the ECF.

In some instances diffusion cannot occur without assistance, even down steep concentration gradients, because of membrane selectivity. A clinical example is the fact that even though the concentration of glucose is much higher in the ECF than in the ICF (creating a steep gradient for glucose), glucose cannot cross most cell membranes without the help of insulin. When insulin is present in the ECF, it binds to insulin receptor sites on cell membranes, which makes the membranes much more permeable to glucose. Glucose can then cross the cellular membrane down its concentration gradient until either an equilibrium of glucose concentration is created or insulin binding decreases.

Diffusion across a cell membrane that requires the assistance of a transport system or membrane-altering system (e.g., insulin) is called **facilitated diffusion** or **facilitated transport.** Because this type of transport occurs down a concentration gradient and requires no energy from the cell, it is a form of diffusion.

OSMOSIS

Definition

Osmosis is the process by which only water molecules (solvent) move through a selectively permeable membrane. For osmosis to occur, a membrane must separate two fluid compartments, at least one of which must contain a solute that cannot move through the membrane. (The membrane is therefore impermeable to this solute.) A concentration gradient of this solute must also exist. If the membrane were permeable to this solute, then the solute would diffuse through the membrane down its concentration gradient until the concentrations of solute were equal on both sides of the membrane. Because the membrane is impermeable to the solute, these particles cannot cross the membrane, but water molecules can.

Physiologic Activity

For the fluid compartments to have equal concentrations of solute, the water molecules must move down their concentration gradient from the side with the higher concentration of water molecules (and thus a lower concentration of solute molecules) to the side with the lower concentration of water molecules (and thus a higher concentration of solute molecules). This movement continues until both compartments contain the same proportions of solute to solvent. The more dilute (less concentrated) fluid contains proportionately fewer solute molecules and more water molecules than the more concentrated fluid. Thus water moves by osmosis down its concentration gradient from the area of more dilute solute to the area of more concentrated solute until a new equilibrium is achieved (Figure 11-5).

At this point, the concentrations of solute in the fluid compartments (the proportion of solute to solvent) on both sides of the membrane are equal, even though the total numbers of solute and volume of water may be different. This equilibrium is achieved by the movement of water molecules rather than the movement of solute molecules.

Factors that determine whether and how fast osmosis occurs include the overall concentration of particles (solute) in solution, how easily the solute dissolves in water **(solubility),** and the amount of membrane available for osmosis.

CONCENTRATION OF SOLUTE

The concentration of particles in body fluids is expressed in milliequivalents per liter (mEq/L), millimoles per liter (mmol/L), and milliosmoles per liter (mOsm/L). Osmoles and milliosmoles are used to describe the total concentration of solute particles (including electrolytes) contained in a solution. The number of milliosmoles present in body fluids can be expressed as either osmolarity or osmolality.

Osmolarity is the number of milliosmoles in a *liter* of solution; **osmolality** is the number of milliosmoles in a *kilogram* of solution. The normal osmolarity value for plasma and other body fluids ranges from 270 to 300 mOsm/L.

The body functions best when the osmolarity of the fluids in all compartments is approximately 300 mOsm/L. Many mechanisms work to keep the solute concentration close to optimum levels. When all body fluids have this solute concentration, the osmotic pressures (water-pulling) of the various fluid compartments are essentially equal, and no *net* water movement occurs. In such a situation, the body fluids are said to be **isosmotic** to each other. Another term with essentially the same meaning is **isotonic** (sometimes called **normotonic**). Examples of specific intravenous (IV) solutions with overall concentrations of specific substances equaling 270 to 300 mOsm/L include 0.9% sodium chloride in water and Ringer's lactate in water. Because these solutions are isotonic (or isosmotic) to plasma, their addition to plasma does not change the osmolarity or osmotic pressure of the plasma.

Fluids with osmolarities (solute concentrations) greater than 300 mOsm/L are **hyperosmotic,** or **hypertonic,** compared with isosmotic fluids. Hyperosmotic fluids have a greater osmotic pressure than do isosmotic fluids and tend to pull water from the isosmotic fluid compartment into the hyperosmotic fluid compartment until an osmotic balance is achieved.

Fluids with osmolarities of less than 270 mOsm/L are **hypo-osmotic,** or **hypotonic,** compared with isosmotic fluids. Hypo-osmolar fluids have a lower or smaller osmotic pressure than isosmotic fluids. As a result, water tends to be pulled from the hypo-osmotic fluid compartment into the isosmotic fluid compartment until an osmotic balance is achieved.

SOLUBILITY OF SOLUTE

Solubility refers to the degree to which a solute dissolves or dissociates completely in water. Solubility is directly related to osmotic pressure: The greater the solubility of the solutes in a fluid, the higher the osmotic pressure of that fluid.

AMOUNT OF AVAILABLE MEMBRANE

The greater the amount of membrane available for osmosis, the faster the rate of osmosis. More membrane increases the

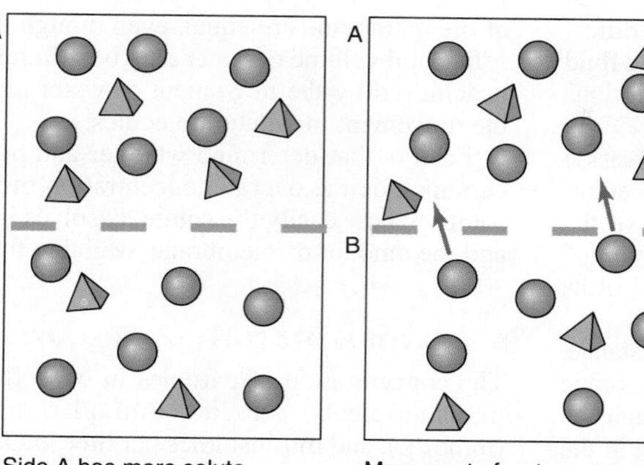

Side A has more solute molecules than does side B, even though the number of water molecules is the same on both sides. Thus side A has a greater osmotic (water pulling) pressure than does side B.

DISEQUILIBRIUM
Side A 1.5:1 ratio of water to solute
Side B 3:1 ratio of water to solute

Movement of water occurs by osmosis toward side A because it has greater osmotic pressure. The membrane is *not* permeable to the solute molecules, so the actual number of solute molecules on side A and side B does not change. *Only the water molecules move, because the membrane is not permeable to the solute molecules.*

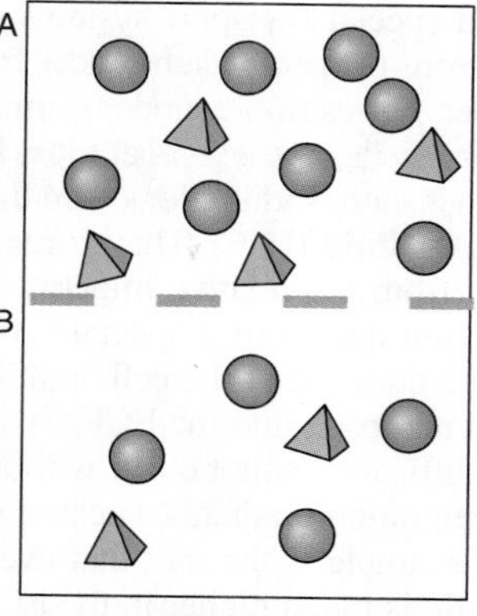

Enough water molecules have moved from side B into side A that the actual concentration of solute is now the same on both sides, with a ratio of water to solute of 2:1. An equilibrium of osmotic pressure now exists between the two compartments, and no further *net* movement of water molecules or solute molecules will occur.

EQUILIBRIUM
Side A 2:1 ratio of water to solute
Side B 2:1 ratio of water to solute

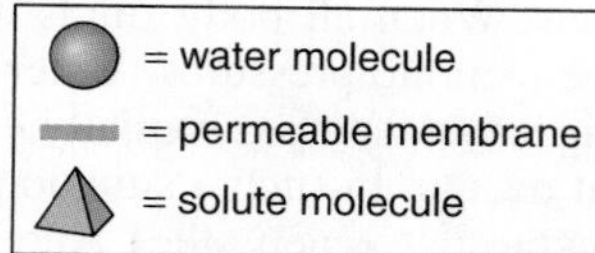

Figure 11-5 ● The process of osmosis.

chances that water molecules will strike the membrane at a point where penetration is possible.

Clinical Function and Significance

Osmosis and filtration act together in capillary fluid dynamics to regulate both extracellular and intracellular fluid volumes. The thirst mechanism is an excellent example of the importance of osmosis in maintaining homeostasis. Thirst results from the activation of cells in the hypothalamus of the brain that respond to changes in extracellular fluid (ECF) osmolarity. These cells are so sensitive to changes in ECF osmolarity that they are called *osmoreceptors.* When a person loses body water, such as through excessive sweating during prolonged heavy exercise, ECF volume is decreased and osmolarity is increased (hypertonic conditions exist). The cells in the thirst center shrink as water moves from the cells into the hypertonic ECF. The shrinking of these cells stimulates a person's awareness of thirst and increases the urge to drink. The person will usually drink enough fluid to replace the water lost through sweating and restore the ECF osmolarity to normal. After the ECF volume and osmolarity return to normal levels, the osmoreceptors return to their normal size and no longer send stimulatory messages.

ACTIVE TRANSPORT

Definition

A cell must use extra energy to move a substance across the cell membrane against a concentration gradient (uphill). This type of movement is called **active transport** because the cell must make active efforts for net movement to occur. Because of its energy demands and uphill movement, active transport is sometimes called "pumping," and the mechanisms are known as membrane pumps.

Physiologic Activity

Active transport systems, or pumps, are usually located in the cell membrane and act as "gatekeepers" to maintain special environments inside cells. Some active transport pumps can carry more than one substance across the membrane at the same time. The sodium-potassium pump is an example of a common active transport system that simultaneously moves two substances in opposite directions against concentration gradients.

Sodium tends to diffuse slightly down its concentration gradient into the intracellular fluid (ICF) because it has such a high extracellular fluid (ECF) concentration compared with its ICF concentration. Similarly, because potassium has such a high concentration inside the cells compared with its concentration in ECF, it tends to diffuse slightly down its concentration gradient into the ECF. The action of the sodium-potassium pump moves the extra sodium out of the cell and returns the lost potassium back into the cell. The sodium-potassium pump requires the use of cellular energy.

The energy for this process usually comes from breaking a high-energy bond (~P), which occurs when a phosphate group is split off from an adenosine triphosphate (ATP) molecule. The functioning of active transport pumps depends on the presence of adequate cellular ATP.

TABLE 11-2 • SUMMARY OF MEMBRANE-FLUID ACTIONS

Action	Definition	Specific Characteristics
Filtration	The movement of fluid through a biologic membrane as a result of hydrostatic pressure differences on both sides of the membrane	Does not require energy Is limited to solvent and low–molecular weight solute Usually occurs from capillaries to the interstitial fluid Depends on hydrostatic pressure differences Occurs more rapidly with steep gradients
Diffusion	The free movement of substances across a permeable membrane and down a concentration gradient	Does not require energy Is not pressure dependent Moves solute and solvent down their individual gradients Occurs more rapidly with steep gradients Is directly related in speed to the amount of membrane available Occurs in both directions across capillary and cell membranes Is responsible for maintaining tissue nutrition
Osmosis	The process by which only the *solvent* diffuses through a selectively permeable membrane	Does not require energy Involves movement of water only Depends on hydrostatic and osmotic pressures Occurs more rapidly with steep gradients
Active transport	The movement of a substance across a selectively permeable membrane and against a concentration, electrical, or pressure gradient	Requires energy Requires a transport system (pump) Helps to maintain a special intracellular environment

Clinical Function and Significance

Cells use active transport to regulate cell volume and to control the intracellular concentration of many substances. All cells function best when their internal environments are maintained separately from the changes occurring in the extracellular fluid (ECF) environment.

A clinical example of what occurs when active transport fails is what results from tissue **hypoxia** (decreased oxygen supply in the body). Without adequate oxygen, ATP cannot be produced in sufficient amounts. Without ATP, the sodium-potassium pump cannot remove the extra sodium ions that have diffused from the ECF into the cell. The increased sodium concentration inside the cell increases the osmolarity and the osmotic pressure of the fluid inside the cell. Water moves into the cell in response to the increased osmotic pressure, causing the cell to swell and perhaps to **lyse** (break open) and die if oxygen is not provided.

Table 11-2 summarizes the membrane processes involved in fluid and electrolyte balance.

CAPILLARY DYNAMICS

The circulatory system delivers nutrients and removes wastes at the tissue level. The important blood vessels for nutrient waste exchange are the thin-walled, porous capillaries. Nutrient delivery and waste removal depend on fluid movement in the capillary.

Fluid movement at the capillary level is dynamic not only because it is continuous but also because the homeostasis of plasma and interstitial fluid volumes must be maintained. Opposing processes must occur for nutrients to move into tissue spaces, for wastes to move into circulation, and for the fluid volumes of both the vascular and tissue spaces to be maintained.

During these processes, some fluid with nutrients must leave the capillary and enter the interstitial (tissue space) fluid compartment for a short period, which temporarily expands the interstitial fluid volume. The nutrients in the interstitial fluid are taken up by the cells through various membrane transport processes. Water may be exchanged between the intracellular compartment and the interstitial compartment, but under normal circumstances there is no net change in water volume. Metabolic wastes created in the cells are moved into the interstitial fluid. These waste products and any extra fluid in the interstitial space must be returned via the capillary to the systemic circulation. If there were no way to return the fluid originally lost into the interstitial compartment back to the blood, the blood volume would be depleted to the point of circulatory failure, and the interstitial fluid compartment would greatly expand.

Capillary Forces Influencing Fluid Movement

Forces at the capillary level permit capillary fluid loss to be followed by a return of fluid to the capillary so that a near-equilibrium of fluid distribution is maintained at the capillary tissue level. These forces, known as **Starling's forces,** are outlined in Figure 11-6. The near-equilibrium is based on the fact that the forces tending to move fluid out from the capillary at the arterial end are nearly equal to the forces tending to move fluid from the interstitial compartment back into the capillary at the venous end.

Blood flowing from the arterial end of the capillary to the venous end is controlled by the following:

- Hydrostatic pressure of the blood
- Dynamic ejection of the blood from the left ventricle of the heart
- **Patency** or openness of the capillaries

The blood entering the arterial end of the capillary has a blood pressure, or a capillary (plasma) hydrostatic pressure (PHP), of about 32 mm Hg. The capillary membrane is thin and permeable, and the usual tissue hydrostatic pressure is low. These factors create a natural tendency for filtration of fluid from the blood outward into the tissue spaces. The fluid portion of the blood, along with most of the smaller substances dissolved in the blood, filters through the capillary membrane into the tissue spaces. Through this process, nutrients and other essential substances can reach the cells.

If net filtration as a result of plasma hydrostatic pressure were the only force or factor involved at this level, blood volume would be progressively lost from circulation and would appear in the tissues. Fortunately, other mechanisms that favor the reabsorption of tissue fluid into the capillaries are also part of capillary dynamics. These mechanisms are plasma osmotic pressure and tissue hydrostatic pressure.

Osmosis (of water) through the capillary membrane (in either direction) occurs in response to differences in the concentrations of osmotically active substances in the capillary blood and tissue fluid. Tissue osmotic pressure (TOP) tends to draw fluid out of the capillary. Plasma osmotic pressure (POP) in the capillary tends to keep fluid in the capillary and draw fluid from the interstitial space into the capillary. Under normal conditions, osmotic pressure in capillary plasma is greater than osmotic pressure in tissue because there is a higher concentration of proteins in the blood than in the interstitial fluid.

Because the capillary membrane is highly impermeable to proteins, it does not allow blood proteins to pass freely through it into the tissue space. Therefore blood proteins remain in the capillary and add to the osmotic pressure. The specific type of osmotic pressure exerted by plasma proteins is called **colloidal** oncotic pressure because it is caused by the presence of proteins (colloidal substances) rather than by dissociated ions such as sodium (**crystalloid** substances). The average colloidal oncotic pressure in capillary blood is about 22 mm Hg.

Blood pressure (hydrostatic pressure) is greater than colloidal oncotic pressure at the arterial end of the capillary. Capillary hydrostatic pressure favors the filtration of fluid from

Capillary blood normally flows from the arterial end to the venous end:

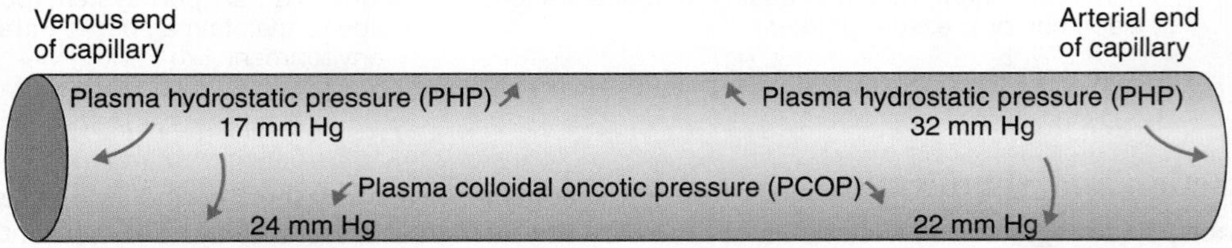

Venous end of capillary

Arterial end of capillary

Plasma hydrostatic pressure (PHP) 17 mm Hg

Plasma hydrostatic pressure (PHP) 32 mm Hg

Plasma colloidal oncotic pressure (PCOP)

24 mm Hg

22 mm Hg

Tissue hydrostatic pressure (THP) 8 mm Hg
Tissue osmotic pressure (TOP) 6 mm Hg

Tissue hydrostatic pressure (THP) 4 mm Hg
Tissue osmotic pressure (TOP) 10 mm Hg

At the arterial end, the forces that tend to move fluid from the capillary into the tissue space are

Plasma hydrostatic pressure 32 mm Hg
+
Tissue osmotic pressure 10 mm Hg

Total forces moving fluid out = 42 mm Hg

At the arterial end, the forces that tend to move fluid from the tissue spaces into the capillary are

Tissue hydrostatic pressure 4 mm Hg
+
Plasma colloidal oncotic pressure 22 mm Hg

Total forces moving fluid in = 26 mm Hg

The total forces tending to move fluid out at the arterial end are 16 mm Hg higher than the total forces tending to move fluid in at the arterial end (42 – 26 = 16). Thus, at the arterial end, fluid leaks out of the capillary into the tissue (interstitial) spaces.

At the venous end of the same capillary, the forces that tend to move fluid from the capillary into the tissue space are

Plasma hydrostatic pressure 17 mm Hg
+
Tissue osmotic pressure 6 mm Hg

Total forces moving fluid out = 23 mm Hg

At the venous end of the capillary, the forces that tend to move fluid from the tissue spaces back into the capillary are

Tissue hydrostatic pressure 8 mm Hg
+
Plasma colloidal oncotic pressure 24 mm Hg

Total forces moving fluid in = 32 mm Hg

The total forces tending to move fluid out at the venous end are 9 mm Hg lower than the total forces tending to move fluid into the capillary at the venous end (32 – 23 = 9). Thus, at the venous end, fluid moves from the tissue spaces back into the capillary.

Because the pressures tending to move fluid out of the capillary at the arterial end (16 mm Hg) are greater than the pressures that tend to move fluid back into the capillary at the venous end (9 mm Hg), more fluid is lost from the capillary than is returned to it. Lymph drainage eventually returns this extra lost fluid to the systemic circulation.

Figure 11-6 ● Capillary dynamics.

the capillary into the tissue spaces, and colloidal oncotic pressure favors the reabsorption of fluid from the interstitial space into the capillary. The difference between these two capillary pressures at the arterial end of the capillary indicates that the filtering force outward is greater than the reabsorbing force inward.

Tissue Forces Influencing Fluid Movement

Tissue forces also influence the movement of solutions at the capillary level. These forces are tissue hydrostatic pressure (THP) and tissue osmotic pressure (TOP), both of which are usually relatively small forces. In some diseases, however, these forces increase greatly and change capillary dynamics.

To determine the direction of fluid movement in any one area of the capillary, the forces that move fluid out from the capillary are compared with the forces that move fluid into the capillary. Two forces at the arterial end that move fluid out from the capillary are the plasma hydrostatic pressure (PHP) (normally about 32 mm Hg) and the TOP (normally about 10 mm Hg). The pressures at the arterial end that return fluid to the capillary are the plasma colloidal oncotic pressure (normally about 22 mm Hg) and the tissue hydrostatic pressure (THP) (normally about 4 mm Hg). Because the outward filtration force is 16 mm Hg higher than the inward reabsorbing force, the overall result at the arterial end of the capillary is the outward filtration of fluid and small solute particles into the tissue spaces.

Plasma hydrostatic pressure (PHP) decreases as blood flows through the length of the capillary. As filtration proceeds along the capillary, water is lost from the capillary, and the PHP gradually decreases. Therefore the pressures that create the outward filtration force (from the capillary into the interstitial fluid) decrease, whereas the pressures that create the inward reabsorption force (from the interstitial fluid into the capillary) remain the same. Eventually, the outward filtration pressures and the inward reabsorption pressures become equal.

Clinical Function and Significance

Finally, at the venous end of the capillary, the inward reabsorption forces exceed the outward filtration forces. The venous end of the capillary has a much lower hydrostatic pressure than does the arterial end. This decreased hydrostatic pressure has two causes:

- Because much of the water in the blood was filtered out of the capillary at the arterial end, the volume of water remaining in the blood at the venous end of the capillary is diminished.
- Because the venous portion of the capillary is farther away from the heart than the arterial end, blood pressure is lower in the venous end.

At the venous end of the capillary, the hydrostatic pressure is low and the interstitial fluid (tissue) hydrostatic pressure is high (because water has moved from the arterial end of the capillary into the interstitial space). The colloidal osmotic pressure at the venous end of the capillary exceeds that at the arterial end because water has been lost, which increases the concentration of proteins. The tissue osmotic pressure at the venous end of the capillary is lower than at the arterial end of the capillary because the water lost from the capillary has diluted the solute concentration of the tissue fluid. As a result, forces favoring the return of water from the tissues into the capillary are greater than the forces favoring filtration, and some water returns from the interstitial space back into the capillary at the venous end.

Lymph

In most cases, not all of the fluid that leaves the capillary at the arterial end and enters the interstitial space is returned to the capillary at the venous end. A small amount remains in the tissues. If this situation is not balanced by another mechanism to return the fluid to the systemic circulation, blood volume would become depleted and the interstitial areas would constantly be edematous. Instead, this extra fluid leaking out from the capillaries is returned to the systemic circulation as **lymph.**

Lymph fluid is similar to blood plasma (from which it is formed) but contains far less protein. It is returned to the circulation by lymph vessels, or **lymphatics.** Lymphatics begin as small, thin-walled, vein-like vessels that join to form larger lymphatic vessels. Two large groups of lymphatic vessels connect the entire lymph system with the general circulatory system. The left thoracic lymph duct drains lymph from the abdomen, gastrointestinal tract, pelvis, lower extremities, left side of the thorax, left arm, and left side of the head and neck into the left subclavian vein at the point where it joins the left internal jugular vein (Figure 11-7). Lymph from the right arm, right side of the thorax, and right side of the head and neck drains into the right subclavian vein through three lymph ducts. Lymph nodes are situated along the lymphatic paths and filter the lymph fluid.

Lymphatics carry lymph fluid in one direction: toward the heart. Lymph flow is slower than blood flow because lymph has no pump and no direct connection between the arterial blood circulation and the lymphatic system. Lymph flow is enhanced by skeletal muscle contractions, intrathoracic pressure changes during breathing, and a peristalsis-like motion in the lymph vessels.

Hormonal Regulation of Fluid and Electrolyte Balance

The endocrine system helps to control fluid and electrolyte balance. Three hormones that help control these critical balances are aldosterone, antidiuretic hormone (ADH), and atrial natriuretic peptide (ANP).

ALDOSTERONE

Aldosterone is a hormone secreted by the adrenal cortex. Aldosterone secretion is stimulated by either a decreased sodium level in the extracellular fluid (ECF) or an increased sodium level in urine. The secretion and function of aldosterone, angiotensinogen, and angiotensin are outlined in Figure 11-8. Aldosterone directly influences sodium balance by preventing sodium loss. Because sodium in body fluids exerts osmotic (water-pulling) pressure, water attempts to follow sodium in physiologically proportionate amounts (Guyton & Hall, 2000). As a result of this sodium-water relationship, aldosterone secretion also indirectly regulates water balance.

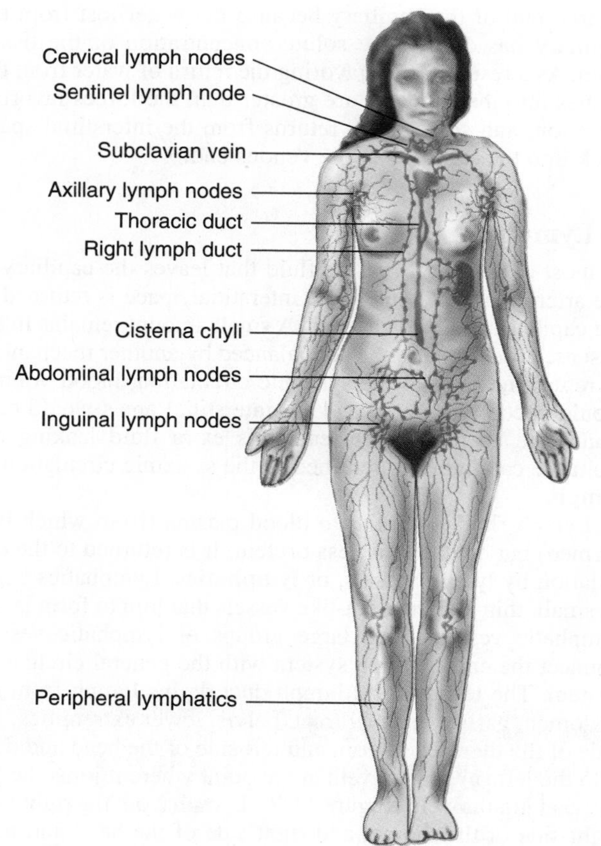

Figure 11-7 ● Patterns of lymph drainage. (From Guyton, A., & Hall, J. [1996]. *Textbook of medical physiology* [9th ed.]. Philadelphia, W.B. Saunders.)

In the kidney, blood is supplied to the nephrons via the afferent arteriole. Specialized cells **(juxtaglomerular cells)** inside the afferent arteriole near the nephron glomerulus are sensitive to changes in serum concentrations of sodium. This area of the afferent arteriole comes into direct contact with a specialized area of the distal convoluted tubule (the **macula densa**). Together, the juxtaglomerular cells and the macula densa form the **juxtaglomerular complex.** When this complex senses that actual serum sodium concentrations are lower than normal or that the total blood volume is low, the macula densa stimulates juxtaglomerular cells to secrete **renin.**

Renin acts on an inactive plasma protein called **angiotensinogen,** converting it to angiotensin I. Angiotensin I is immediately further degraded into angiotensin II by an enzyme called angiotensin-converting enzyme (ACE). **Angiotensin II** causes the constriction of many blood vessels and stimulates an increased secretion of aldosterone from the adrenal cortex.

Aldosterone acts on the distal convoluted tubules of the nephrons. When serum osmolarity is too low, aldosterone secretion stimulates these areas to reabsorb sodium from the urine back into the circulation (in exchange for potassium); this increases serum osmolarity. Aldosterone secretion increases when blood osmolarity or serum sodium levels are low, and its presence is normally required to prevent excessive renal excretion of sodium. Aldosterone secretion also helps to prevent serum potassium levels from becoming too high. The secretion of aldosterone is inhibited when blood osmolarity or serum sodium levels are greater than normal.

ANTIDIURETIC HORMONE

Antidiuretic hormone (ADH), also known as **vasopressin,** is produced in the brain and stored in the posterior pituitary gland. The release of ADH from the posterior pituitary gland is controlled by the hypothalamus in response to changes in blood osmolarity. The hypothalamus contains specialized cells **(osmoreceptors)** that are sensitive to changes in blood osmolarity. Increased blood osmolarity, especially an increase in the concentration of plasma sodium, results in a slight shrinkage of these cells and triggers the hypothalamus to stimulate the posterior pituitary to release ADH.

ADH acts directly on kidney tubules and collecting ducts, making them more permeable to water. As a result, more water is reabsorbed by these tubules and returned to the circulation, which in turn decreases the osmolarity of the blood by making it more dilute. When blood osmolarity decreases, especially when the plasma sodium concentration is below normal, the osmoreceptors swell slightly and inhibit the release of ADH. Less water is reabsorbed and more is lost from the body in the urine. As a result, the amount of water in the extracellular fluid (ECF) decreases, bringing osmolarity to normal.

ATRIAL NATRIURETIC PEPTIDE

Atrial natriuretic peptide (ANP) is secreted by special cells that line the atria of the heart. It is secreted in response to increased blood volume and blood pressure. ANP binds to receptor sites in the collecting ducts of the nephrons, creating effects opposite those of aldosterone. Kidney reabsorption of sodium is inhibited at the same time that glomerular filtration is increased (Briggs et al., 1996). The outcome is increased output of urine with a high sodium content, which results in decreased circulating blood volume and decreased blood osmolarity.

Body Fluids

Fluids, especially water, make up about 55% to 60% of total adult body weight and can be divided into the extracellular fluid (ECF) and intracellular fluid (ICF). The ECF compartment accounts for approximately 15 L (40%) of total body water and includes interstitial fluid, blood plasma, lymph, bone and connective tissue water, and the fluid within special spaces (transcellular fluid), such as cerebrospinal fluid, synovial fluid, peritoneal fluid, and pleural fluid. ICF accounts for the remaining 25 L (60%) of total body water. Figure 11-9 shows the normal distribution of total body water.

A person's age, gender, and ratio of lean mass to body fat influence the amount and distribution of body fluids. An older adult has less total body water than a younger adult. Because fat cells contain practically no water, an obese person has less total body water than a lean person of the same body weight.

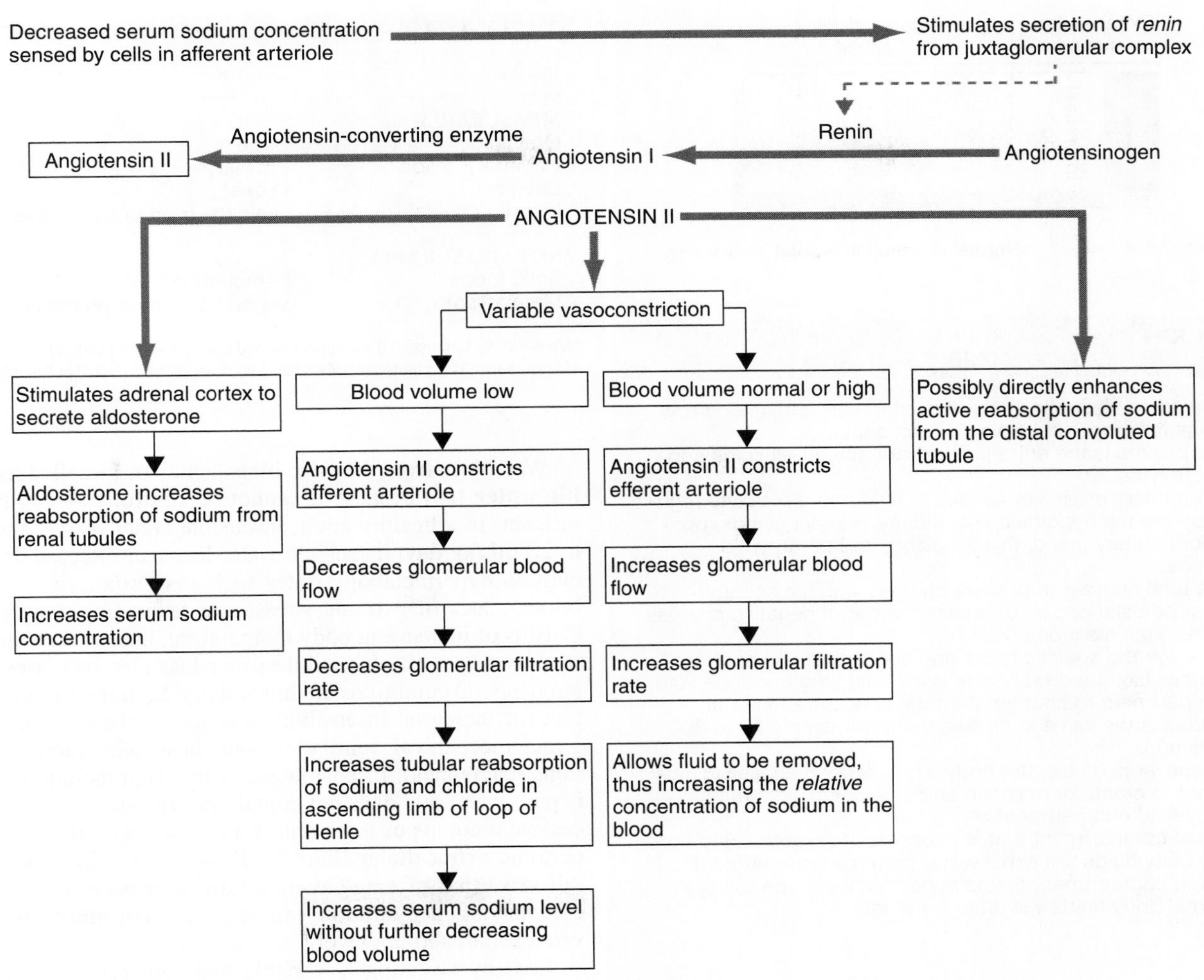

Figure 11-8 ● The role of aldosterone, angiotensinogen, angiotensin I, and angiotensin II in the renal regulation of water and sodium.

WOMEN'S HEALTH CONSIDERATIONS

A woman of any age usually has less total body water than does a man of similar size and age. This difference exists because men generally have more muscle mass than women and because women have a higher percentage of body fat. Differences in muscle mass and percentage of body fat are partly a result of the influence of sex hormones. These differences in fat to lean body weight may be responsible for some of the differences seen in women's and men's responses to drugs.

Body fluids allow cell nutrition and transport active molecules (e.g., hormones) that are important to the regulation of normal physiologic functions. Most physiologic processes occur only in a watery environment. Body fluids are constantly renewed, purified, and replaced as fluid balance is maintained through intake and output. The total amount of water within each fluid compartment is stable, but water moves continually among all compartments. Water is not static in any compartment but is exchanged constantly while maintaining a volume equilibrium. Table 11-3 summarizes the key points regarding fluid and electrolyte balance.

SOURCES OF FLUID INTAKE

Fluid intake is regulated through the thirst drive. Fluids enter the body primarily as liquids (Table 11-4). Because solid foods contain up to 85% water, some fluid also enters the body as ingested solid foods. In addition, water is a by-product of cellular metabolism. This metabolic water accounts for about 300 mL of the daily water requirement. A rising plasma osmolarity or a decreasing plasma volume stimulates the sensation of thirst. Sensations such as mouth dryness or the thought that a person has not had a drink recently can trigger the thirst drive. An adult drinks an average of 1500 mL of fluid per day and obtains an additional 800 mL of fluid from ingested foods.

ROUTES OF FLUID LOSS

The body has several ways to remove excess water and waste products (see Table 11-4). Of all the water loss pathways, the

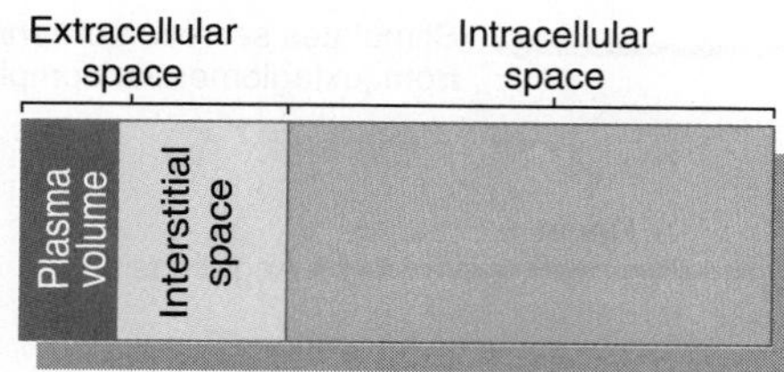

Figure 11-9 ● Normal distribution of total body water.

TABLE 11-3 • SUMMARY OF KEY POINTS REGARDING FLUID AND ELECTROLYTE BALANCE

- All plasma electrolyte values must remain within a narrow range for proper physiologic functioning.
- The plasma is the entrance and exit site for all fluids and electrolytes.
- The primary organs or tissues of fluid and electrolyte regulation are the hypothalamus, kidney, adrenal glands, posterior pituitary gland, thyroid gland, and parathyroid glands.
- The total number of positive charges within a solution must be balanced by an equal number of negative charges to maintain electroneutrality.
- Although the specific types and concentrations of substances (solute) dissolved in body fluid vary from one fluid compartment to another, the total concentration of all solutes is the same in all fluid compartments (270 to 300 mOsm/L).
- Whenever possible, the body's regulatory mechanisms attempt to create or maintain an osmolar equilibrium in all body fluid compartments.
- A fluid compartment that is hyposmolar (hypotonic) to normal body fluids will expel water from the compartment.
- A fluid compartment that is hyperosmolar (hypertonic) to normal body fluids will draw water into it.

TABLE 11-4 • ROUTES OF FLUID INGESTION AND EXCRETION

Intake	Output
MEASURABLE	
Oral fluids	Urine
Parenteral fluids	Emesis†
Enemas*	Feces†
Irrigation fluids*	Drainage from body cavities
NOT MEASURABLE	
Solid foods	Perspiration
Metabolism	Vaporization through the lungs

*Measured by subtracting the amount returned from the amount instilled.
†Measurement is accurate only when these substances are excreted in liquid form.

kidney is the most important and the most sensitive. Water loss via the kidney is closely regulated and is adjustable. The volume of urine excreted daily varies depending on the amount of fluid intake and the body's need to conserve fluids.

The minimum amount of urine per day needed to dissolve and excrete toxic waste products is 400 to 600 mL. This minimal volume is called the **obligatory urine output.** If the 24-hour urine output falls below the obligatory output amount, wastes are retained and can cause lethal electrolyte imbalances, acidosis, and a toxic build up of nitrogen. This urine is maximally concentrated, with a **specific gravity** (the weight of the liquid compared with the weight of pure water) of 1.032 or higher and an osmolarity of at least 1200 mOsm/L.

Urine can also become very dilute, with a specific gravity of 1.005 and an osmolarity of 200 mOsm/L. Dilution can result from a large fluid intake and is reflected in a large volume of urine output. The ability of the kidneys to make either concentrated or very dilute urine helps to maintain fluid and electrolyte balance. With the influence of aldosterone, antidiuretic hormone (ADH), and atrial natriuretic peptide (ANP), the kidney is able to respond when extracellular fluid concentrations, volumes, or pressures change.

Other normal water loss occurs through the skin, the lungs, and the gastrointestinal tract. Additional water losses can occur via salivation, drainage from fistulas and drains, and gastrointestinal suction.

Water loss from the skin, lungs, and stool—called **insensible water loss** because it cannot be controlled—can be significant. In a healthy adult, insensible water loss is about 15 to 20 mL/kg/day. Insensible water loss can increase dramatically in hypermetabolic states such as thyroid crisis, trauma, burns, states of extreme stress, and fever. For every degree Celsius of increase in body temperature, insensible water loss increases by 10%. Insensible water loss also increases when atmospheric conditions are hot and dry. Examples of clients at risk for increased insensible water loss include those undergoing mechanical ventilation and those with rapid respirations (tachypnea). Insensible water loss (not including sweat) is pure water and does not contain electrolytes. Therefore excessive amounts of insensible water loss result in a more hypertonic extracellular fluid (ECF) with a smaller volume. If this loss is not balanced by intake, the hypertonic ECF and accompanying dehydration can lead to **hypernatremia** (elevated serum sodium level).

Loss by sweating is variable and can reach a maximum rate of about 2 L/hr. Although it contains electrolytes, sweat is slightly hypotonic compared to plasma. The amount of sweating is regulated by the autonomic nervous system, body temperature, and blood flow in the skin.

Water loss through stool is normally minimal. However, this loss can increase significantly with severe diarrhea or excessive fistula drainage. Clients with ulcerative colitis can experience a diarrheal fluid loss of several liters per day. Diarrheal fluid contains water, potassium, sodium, bicarbonate, and chloride. Thus, with diarrhea, hypotonic fluid containing some electrolytes is lost.

Electrolytes

Electrolytes, or **ions,** are substances in body fluids that carry an electrical charge. **Cations** are positively charged ions; **anions** are negatively charged ions. Body fluids are electrochemically neutral, which means that the number of positive ions is balanced by an equal number of negative ions. However, the distribution of ions differs in the extracellular fluid (ECF) and the intracellular fluid (ICF) (Figure 11-10).

Most electrolytes have different concentrations in the ICF and ECF. This concentration difference helps maintain membrane excitability and transmit nerve impulses. The ranges of electrolyte concentration in these fluid compartments are extremely narrow. Thus even small changes in these concentrations can result in major pathologic alterations.

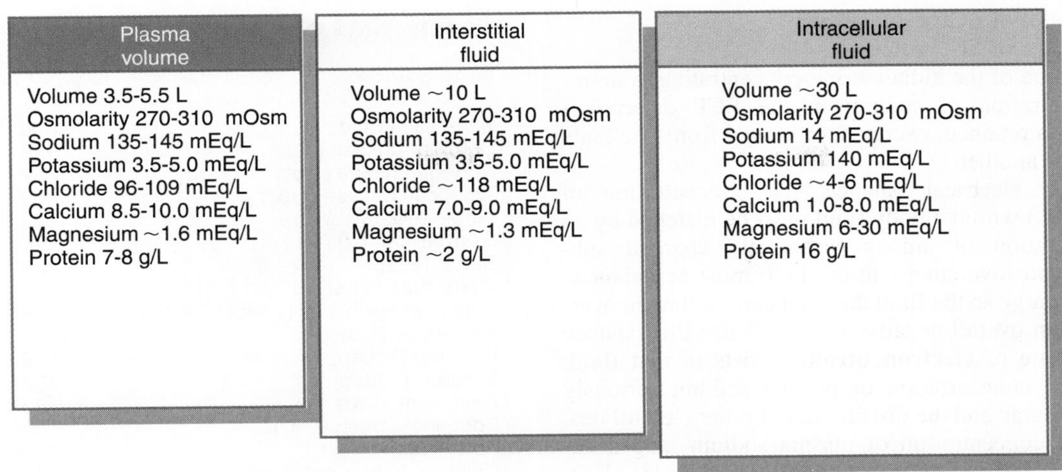

Figure 11-10 ● The composition of various body fluids.

TABLE 11-5 • MAJOR SERUM ELECTROLYTE CONCENTRATIONS AND FUNCTIONS

Electrolyte	Reference Range	International Recommended Units	Functions
Sodium (Na^+)	136-145 mEq/L	136-145 mmol/L	Maintenance of plasma and interstitial osmolarity Generation and transmission of action potentials Maintenance of acid-base balance Maintenance of electroneutrality
Potassium (K^+)	3.5-5.0 mEq/L	3.5-5.0 mmol/L	Regulation of intracellular osmolarity Maintenance of electrical membrane excitability Maintenance of plasma acid-base balance
Calcium (Ca^{2+})	9.0-10.5 mg/dL	2.25-2.75 mmol/L	Cofactor in blood-clotting cascade Excitable membrane stabilizer Adds strength/density to bones and teeth Essential element in cardiac, skeletal, and smooth muscle contraction
Chloride (Cl^-)	90-110 mEq/L	90-110 mmol/L	Maintenance of plasma acid-base balance Maintenance of plasma electroneutrality Formation of hydrochloric acid
Magnesium (Mg^{2+})	1.2-2.0 mg/dL	0.66-1.07 mmol/L	Excitable membrane stabilizer Essential element in cardiac, skeletal, and smooth muscle contraction Cofactor in blood-clotting cascade Cofactor in carbohydrate metabolism Cofactor in DNA and protein synthesis
Phosphorus (P_i)	3.0-4.5 mg/dL	0.97-1.45 mmol/L	Activation of B-complex vitamins Formation of adenosine triphosphate and other high-energy substances Cofactor in carbohydrate, protein, and lipid metabolism

Data from Pagana, K., & Pagana, T. (1999). *Diagnostic testing and nursing implications: A case study approach* (5th ed.). St. Louis: Mosby.

Table 11-5 lists the major body fluid electrolytes together with their normal serum concentrations and primary functions. Most electrolytes enter the body in the form of ingested food.

Electrolyte homeostasis is controlled by balancing the dietary intake of electrolytes with the renal excretion or reabsorption of electrolytes. For example, the concentration of plasma potassium is maintained between 3.5 and 5.0 mmol/L. In theory, the potassium in common foods could greatly increase the ECF potassium concentration and lead to major problems. Usually, however, the excretion of potassium by the kidney keeps pace with potassium intake and prevents major changes in the concentration of plasma potassium.

SODIUM

Sodium (Na^+) is the major cation in the extracellular fluid (ECF) and is the main factor responsible for maintaining ECF osmolarity. The activity of the sodium-potassium pump keeps the sodium concentration of the intracellular fluid (ICF) low (about 14 mmol/L) while maintaining high sodium concentrations in the plasma and other extracellular fluids. Maintaining this difference in sodium concentration is vital for the following physiologic functions:

- Initiation of skeletal muscle contraction
- Initiation of cardiac contractions
- Transmission of nerve impulses

- Maintenance of ECF osmolarity
- Maintenance of ECF volume
- Maintenance of the kidney urine-concentrating system

The concentration of sodium in the ECF determines whether water is retained, excreted, or moved from one body compartment to another.

To maintain electrical balance, the concentration of sodium (a cation) within a body fluid must be matched by an equal concentration of anions (negatively charged substances). Each positive charge in the ECF must be balanced by a negative charge so the fluid does not carry either an overall positive or an overall negative charge. When this balance is present, a state of **electroneutrality** exists in that fluid. Changes in the concentration of plasma sodium seriously change fluid volume and the distribution of other electrolytes.

The normal concentration of plasma sodium ranges between 136 and 145 mEq/L or mmol/L (see Table 11-5). Sodium enters the body through the ingestion of many foods and fluids (Table 11-6). The average dietary intake of sodium is about 6 to 12 g/day. Sodium is also stored deep within the kidney tissues and can be released to the ECF as needed. Despite great variations in sodium intake, the concentration of serum sodium usually remains within the normal range. Serum sodium balance is regulated by the kidney under the influences of aldosterone, antidiuretic hormone (ADH), and atrial natriuretic peptide (ANP).

Low serum sodium levels inhibit the secretion of ADH and ANP and stimulate aldosterone secretion. Together these actions increase serum sodium concentration by increasing kidney reabsorption of sodium and enhancing kidney loss of water.

High serum sodium levels inhibit aldosterone secretion and directly stimulate the secretion of ADH and ANP. Together these hormones cause an increase in kidney excretion of sodium and kidney reabsorption of water.

TABLE 11-6 • SODIUM VALUES OF COMMON FOODS*

Food Source	Amount (mg)
Table salt (1 tsp)	2000
Cheddar cheese (1 oz)	176
Cottage cheese (4 oz)	457
American cheese (1 oz)	439
Whole milk (8 oz)	120
Skim milk (8 oz)	126
Butter (1 tsp)	123
White bread (1 slice)	123
Whole-wheat bread (1 slice)	159
Soy sauce (1 tbsp)	1029
Ketchup (1 tbsp)	156
Mustard (1 tbsp)	188
Beef, lean (4 oz)	60
Pork, lean, fresh (4 oz)	60
Pork, cured (4 oz)	850
Chicken, light meat (4 oz)	70
Chicken, dark meat (4 oz)	70

Data from Pennington, J. (1998). *Bowe's and Church's food values of portions commonly used* (17th ed.). Philadelphia: J.B. Lippincott.
*U.S. Department of Agriculture recommended daily allowance for adults: 1100-3300 mg.

POTASSIUM

In contrast to sodium, potassium (K^+) is the major cation of the intracellular fluid (ICF). The normal plasma concentration of potassium ranges from 3.5 to 5.0 mEq/L or mmol/L (see Table 11-5). The normal ICF concentration of potassium is about 140 mEq/L (mmol/L). Because of its high concentration inside cells, potassium has some control over intracellular osmolarity and volume. Keeping this large difference in potassium concentration between the ICF and the extracellular fluid (ECF) is critical for excitable tissues to generate action potentials and transmit impulses. Functions of potassium include the following:

- Regulation of protein synthesis
- Regulation of glucose use and storage
- Maintenance of action potentials in excitable membranes

Because potassium levels in the plasma and interstitial fluid are so low, any change in concentration is poorly tolerated by the body and seriously affects physiologic activities. For example, a decrease in plasma potassium of only 1 mEq/L (from 4 mEq/L to 3 mEq/L) is a 25% difference in total ECF potassium concentration. In contrast, a decrease in plasma sodium of 1 mEq/L (from 140 mEq/L to 139 mEq/L) is, overall, a much smaller change (less than 1%) in total ECF sodium concentration.

Potassium drifts out of cells down its concentration gradient into the ECF. Almost all foods contain potassium (Table 11-7). Potassium intake averages approximately 2 to 20 g/day. Despite heavy potassium intake and the drifting of potassium from cellular storage sites into the ECF, the healthy body keeps plasma potassium levels within the narrow range of normal values required for physiologic function.

The primary controller of ECF potassium concentration is the sodium-potassium pump within the membranes of all body cells. This pump removes three sodium ions from the fluid inside the cell for every two potassium ions that it returns to the cell. In this way, the levels of both serum sodium and cellular potassium remain high.

Some potassium regulation also occurs through kidney function. The kidney is the excretory route for ridding the body of ECF potassium (80% of potassium removed from the body occurs via the kidney). Unlike sodium, no hormone has been identified that directly controls kidney reabsorption of potassium; thus the kidney does not conserve potassium directly.

CALCIUM

Calcium (Ca^{2+}) is a mineral whose presence and functions are closely related to those of phosphorus and magnesium. Calcium is a **divalent cation** (an ion having two positive charges) that exists in the body in two forms: bound and ionized (unbound or free).

Bound calcium is usually connected to specific serum proteins, especially albumin. Ionized calcium is present in the blood and other extracellular fluid (ECF) as free calcium. Free calcium is the active form and must be kept within a narrow range in the ECF. The body functions best when plasma calcium concentrations are maintained between 9.0 and 10.5 mg/dL, or between 2.25 and 2.75 mmol/L (see Table 11-5). Because the concentration of calcium in the intracellular fluid (ICF) is low, calcium has a steep gradient between ECF and ICF. Calcium functions in many ways and in many specialized body systems, including the following:

- Enhances the activity of enzymes or reactions
- Increases skeletal muscle contraction
- Increases cardiac muscle contraction
- Regulates nerve impulse transmission
- Assists in blood clotting
- Provides bone strength and density

TABLE 11-7 • POTASSIUM VALUES OF COMMON FOODS*

Food Source	Amount (mg)
Corn flakes (1¹/₄ c)	26
Cooked oatmeal (³/₄ c)	99
Egg (1 large)	66
Codfish, raw (4 oz)	400
Salmon, pink, raw (3¹/₂ oz)	306
Tuna fish (4 oz)	375
Apple, raw with skin (1 medium)	159
Banana (1 medium)	451
Cantaloupe (1 c pieces)	494
Grapefruit (¹/₂ medium)	175
Orange (1 medium)	250
Raisins (¹/₂ c)	700
Strawberries, raw (1 c)	247
Watermelon (1 c pieces)	186
White bread (1 slice)	27
Whole-wheat bread (1 slice)	44
Beef (4 oz)	480
Beef liver (3¹/₂ oz)	281
Pork, fresh (4 oz)	525
Pork, cured (4 oz)	325
Chicken (4 oz)	225
Veal cutlet (3¹/₂ oz)	448
Whole milk (8 oz)	370
Skim milk (8 oz)	406
Avocado (1 medium)	1097
Carrot (1 large)	341
Corn (4-inch ear)	196
Cauliflower (1 c pieces)	295
Celery (1 stalk)	170
Green beans (1 c)	189
Mushrooms (10 small)	410
Onion (1 medium)	157
Peas (³/₄ c)	316
Potato, white (1 medium)	407
Spinach, raw (3¹/₂ oz)	470
Tomato (1 medium)	366

Data from Pennington, J. (1998). *Bowe's and Church's food values of portions commonly used* (17th ed.). Philadelphia: J.B. Lippincott.
*U.S. Department of Agriculture recommended daily allowance for adults: 1875-5625 mg.

Calcium enters the body by dietary intake and absorption through the intestinal tract (Table 11-8). Absorption of dietary calcium requires the active form of vitamin D. Calcium is stored in the bones. When both plasma calcium levels and stored calcium levels are adequate, intestinal absorption of dietary calcium is inhibited and urine excretion of excess calcium increases. When more plasma calcium is needed, **parathyroid hormone (PTH)** is secreted and released from the parathyroid glands (Table 11-9). PTH causes serum calcium levels to increase in the following ways:

- Releasing free calcium from bone storage sites directly into the ECF **(resorption)**
- Stimulating vitamin D activation, thus increasing intestinal absorption of dietary calcium
- Inhibiting kidney excretion of calcium and stimulating kidney reabsorption of calcium

When excess calcium is present in plasma, secretion of PTH is inhibited and the secretion of **thyrocalcitonin (TCT),** a hormone secreted by the thyroid gland, is increased. TCT causes the plasma calcium level to decrease in the following ways:

- Inhibiting bone resorption of calcium
- Inhibiting activation of vitamin D, causing decreased gastrointestinal uptake of calcium
- Increasing kidney excretion of calcium in the urine

TABLE 11-8 • CALCIUM VALUES OF COMMON FOODS*

Food Source	Amount (mg)
Cheddar cheese (1 oz)	204
Cottage cheese (4 oz)	68
American cheese (1 oz)	174
Whole milk (8 oz)	288
Skim milk (8 oz)	302
Yogurt, low-fat (1 c)	415
Broccoli, raw (¹/₂ c)	75
Carrot (1 large)	37
Collard greens, raw (3 oz)	200
Green beans (1 c)	62
Rhubarb (1 c)	266
Spinach, raw (3¹/₂ oz)	93
Tofu (3 oz)	100

Data from Pennington, J. (1998). *Bowe's and Church's food values of portions commonly used* (17th ed.). Philadelphia: J.B. Lippincott.
*U.S. Department of Agriculture recommended daily allowance for adults: 800-1200 mg.

PHOSPHORUS

Phosphorus (P) is present in the body in both inorganic and organic forms. Normal serum levels of phosphorus range from 3.0 to 4.5 mg/dL, or 0.97 to 1.45 mmol/L (see Table 11-5). Most phosphorus (80%) can be found in the bones. Phosphorus is the major anion in the intracellular fluid (ICF), and its concentration inside cells is much higher than in extracellular fluid (ECF). Phosphorus is needed for the following cellular activities:

- Activating B-complex vitamins
- Forming and activating high-energy substances, including adenosine triphosphate (ATP)
- Assisting in cell division
- Cooperating in carbohydrate metabolism
- Cooperating in protein metabolism
- Cooperating in lipid (fat) metabolism

Other phosphorus functions include acid-base buffering and calcium homeostasis. Phosphorus is found in a variety of foods, such as nuts, legumes, dairy products, red meat, organ meat, bran, and whole grains (Table 11-10). The average North American diet is high in phosphorus (1 to 2 g/day).

Phosphorus balance and calcium balance are intertwined. Normally, plasma concentrations of calcium and phosphorus exist in a reciprocal relationship, which means that the product of the plasma concentrations remains constant. Therefore a change in the concentration of phosphorus results in an equal and opposite change in the concentration of calcium (and vice versa).

The regulation of ECF phosphorus occurs through the activity of parathyroid hormone (PTH). Increased PTH levels cause a net loss of phosphorus. Reduced PTH levels enhance kidney reabsorption of phosphorus, resulting in increased concentrations of ECF phosphorus.

MAGNESIUM

Magnesium (Mg^{2+}) is another mineral that forms a cation when dissolved in water. Adults have an average of 25 g of magnesium, most of which (60%) is stored in bones and cartilage. Little magnesium is present in the extracellular fluid (ECF). Serum levels of free magnesium range from 1.2 to 2.0 mg/dL, or 0.66 to 1.07 mmol/L (see Table 11-5). Much more magnesium is present in the intracellular fluid (ICF), and it

TABLE 11-9 • HORMONAL REGULATION OF CALCIUM

Hormone	Action
PARATHYROID HORMONE (PTH)	
Secreted in response to low or low-normal serum calcium levels Secretion results in a rise in serum calcium concentration	Increases bone resorption of calcium (leaching of stored calcium) Increases the absorption of ingested calcium from the gastrointestinal tract into the extracellular fluid Increases the renal reabsorption of calcium at the proximal convoluted tubule
THYROCALCITONIN (TCT)	
Secreted by the thyroid gland in response to high or high-normal serum calcium levels Secretion results in a reduction of the serum calcium concentration	Increases bone uptake of calcium Inhibits the absorption of calcium from the gastrointestinal tract so that ingested calcium is excreted from the body in the feces Inhibits the renal reabsorption of calcium at the proximal convoluted tubule so that more calcium is excreted in the urine

TABLE 11-10 • PHOSPHORUS VALUES OF COMMON FOODS*

Food Source	Amount (mg)
Rolled oats, cooked (3/4 c)	133
Egg (1 large)	90
Codfish (3 oz)	175
Tuna fish, white, canned (6 1/2 oz)	405
Raisins (1/2 c)	75
White bread (1 slice)	26
Whole-wheat bread (1 slice)	23
Cheddar cheese (1 oz)	145
American cheese (1 oz)	211
Whole milk (8 oz)	228
Skim milk (8 oz)	247
Yogurt, low-fat (8 oz)	326
Beef (4 oz)	215
Beef liver (4 oz)	375
Pork, fresh (4 oz)	325
Chicken (4 oz)	200
Almonds (1 oz)	141
Peanuts (1 oz)	110

Data from Pennington, J. (1998). *Bowe's and Church's food values of portions commonly used* (17th ed.). Philadelphia: J.B. Lippincott.
*U.S. Department of Agriculture recommended daily allowance for adults: 800 mg.

TABLE 11-11 • MAGNESIUM VALUES OF COMMON FOODS*

Food Source	Amount (mg)
Rolled oats, cooked (3/4 c)	42
Tuna fish, white, canned (6 1/2 oz)	59
Raisins (1/2 c)	25
Beef (4 oz)	24
Pork (4 oz)	30
Chicken (4 oz)	26
Whole milk (8 oz)	33
Skim milk (8 oz)	28
Yogurt, low-fat (8 oz)	40
Peanut butter (1 tbsp)	22
Avocado (1 medium)	70
Broccoli (1 stalk)	24
Cauliflower (1 c pieces)	24
Peas (3/4 c)	35
Potato (1 medium)	34
Spinach, raw (3 1/2 oz)	88

Data from Pennington, J. (1998). *Bowe's and Church's food values of portions commonly used* (17th ed.). Philadelphia: J.B. Lippincott.
*U.S. Department of Agriculture recommended daily allowance for adults: 300-350 mg.

has more functions inside the cells than in the plasma. Magnesium is critical for the following intracellular reactions or activities:

- Stimulating skeletal muscle contraction
- Participating in carbohydrate metabolism
- Activating adenosine triphosphate (ATP)
- Activating B-complex vitamins
- Enhancing deoxyribonucleic acid (DNA) synthesis
- Enhancing protein synthesis

Extracellular magnesium regulates blood coagulation and skeletal muscle contractility.

Magnesium is found in many foods, such as nuts, vegetables, fish, and whole grains (Table 11-11). The daily magnesium requirement for adults is approximately 300 mg.

Although magnesium is similar to calcium in many respects and its presence in serum must be kept within a narrow range of normal values, little is known about its regulation. Magnesium is absorbed from the intestinal tract at the same place as calcium. The absorption of phosphorus inhibits magnesium absorption. Parathyroid hormone (PTH) stimulates the release of magnesium from bone in much the same way that it stimulates the release of calcium.

CHLORIDE

Chloride (Cl^-) is the major anion of the extracellular fluid (ECF) and works with sodium in maintaining ECF osmotic pressure. Chloride is important in the formation of hydrochloric acid in the stomach. The normal plasma concentration of chloride ranges from 90 to 110 mEq/L or mmol/L (see Table 11-5).

Only a small amount of chloride is present inside the cells because negatively charged particles on the cell membrane repel chloride and prevent it from crossing the membrane. However, extracellular chloride can enter cells when exchanged for another anion that is leaving the cell. This situation, called a **chloride shift,** results in decreased concentrations of plasma chloride but no net body loss of chloride. Bicarbonate (HCO_3^-) is the anion most commonly exchanged for chloride. Chloride enters the body through dietary intake. Because chloride (along with sodium, potassium, and many other minerals) is a part of a salt, most diets contain enough chloride to meet the normal needs of the body.

Fluid and Electrolyte Changes Associated with Aging

Only 45% to 50% of the body weight of older adults is water, compared with 55% to 60% in younger adults. This decrease occurs because of a loss of muscle mass and a reduced ratio

CHART 11-1

NURSING FOCUS *on the* OLDER ADULT
Impact of Age-Related Changes on Fluid and Electrolyte Balance

System	Change	Result
Integumentary	Loss of elasticity Decreased turgor Decreased oil production	An unreliable indicator of fluid status Dry, easily damaged skin
Renal	Decreased glomerular filtration Decreased concentrating capacity	Poor excretion of waste products Increased water loss
Muscular	Decreased muscle mass	Decreased total body water Greater risk of dehydration
Neurologic	Diminished thirst reflex	Decreased fluid intake, increasing the risk of dehydration
Endocrine	Adrenal atrophy	Poor regulation of sodium and potassium, predisposing the client to hyponatremia and hyperkalemia

CHART 11-2

NURSING FOCUS *on the* OLDER ADULT
Normal Plasma Electrolyte Values for People Older Than 60 Years of Age

Electrolyte	Reference Range	International Recommended Units
Calcium (Ca^{2+})	8.8-10.2 mg/dL	2.2-2.55 mmol/L
>90 years	8.2-9.6 mg/dL	2.05-2.40 mmol/L
Chloride (Cl^-)	98-107 mEq/L	98-107 mmol/L
>90 years	98-111 mEq/L	98-111 mmol/L
Magnesium (Mg^{2+})	1.6-2.4 mg/dL	0.66-0.99 mmol/L
>90 years	1.7-2.3 mg/dL	0.70-0.95 mmol/L
Phosphorus (P_i)	2.3-3.7 mg/dL (male)	0.74-1.20 mmol/L
	2.8-4.1 mg/dL (female)	0.90-1.32 mmol/L
Potassium (K^+)	3.5-4.5 mEq/L (male)	3.5-4.5 mmol/L
	3.4-4.4 mEq/L (female)	3.4-4.4 mmol/L
Sodium (Na^+)	136-145 mEq/L	136-145 mmol/L
>90 years	132-146 mEq/L	132-146 mmol/L

Data from Tietz, N. (Ed.). (1995). *Clinical guide to laboratory tests* (3rd ed.). Philadelphia: W.B. Saunders.

of lean body weight to total body weight. This decrease in total body water places older adults at greater risk for dehydration. Multiple symptoms point to fluid volume deficit in the older adult.

Skin **turgor** (the normal resiliency of a pinched fold of skin) is not always an accurate assessment of extracellular fluid (ECF) volume deficit (dehydration) in the older adult because the natural aging process is associated with decreased turgor (Chart 11-1). Furthermore, the older adult may have a diminished thirst sensation and decreased kidney function, both of which contribute to the risk for dehydration and make assessment more difficult. When nurses work with older clients, it is extremely important that they accurately record intake and output and weight, because these measurements reflect hydration status more accurately than does skin turgor.

The normal concentration of serum electrolytes also changes with the aging process. Chart 11-2 lists the normal electrolyte values for people older than 60 years of age.

Electrolyte balance may be more difficult to maintain in older adults. In particular, small changes in the concentrations of potassium and calcium may produce unexpectedly serious results. Although the ranges of electrolytes in plasma and intracellular fluid (ICF) may remain normal, the balance is fragile and more easily disturbed in an older adult. Part of this fragility is related to decreased regulatory functions that occur with aging. Age-related kidney changes include decreased blood flow, decreased filtration, and decreased numbers of functional nephrons. Kidney and capillary changes associated with hypertension are more likely to be present in the older adult.

ASSESSMENT OF FLUID AND ELECTROLYTE BALANCE

History

One way of organizing history data to assess the client's fluid and electrolyte status is to use Gordon's Functional Health Patterns (Gordon, 2000). The patterns that most affect fluid and electrolyte status are the Nutritional-Metabolic Pattern and the Elimination Pattern (Chart 11-3).

The client's nutritional history can often reveal a problem that affects fluid and electrolyte balance. The nurse obtains this information directly because the client may not understand the connection between dietary intake and the onset of fluid and electrolyte imbalances.

The guidelines for obtaining a thorough fluid and electrolyte history do not differ from those for assessing any other system; however, the information collected is more specific. For example, exact intake and output volumes are important, as are serial daily weights. The nurse may need to guide the client in accurately reporting the amount of fluid ingested and changes in urine patterns. The nurse also assesses the types of fluids and foods ingested to determine amount and osmolarity. Many clients do not consider solid food to contain liquid. Solid foods such as ice cream, gelatin, and ices are liquids at body temperature, and the nurse includes them when calculating fluid intake.

Output fluids include losses not only through urine but also through perspiration, diarrhea, and insensible loss during fevers. The nurse asks specific questions about prescribed and over-the-counter medications and checks the dosage, the length of time taken, and the client's compliance with the medication regimen. A client who is taking diuretics can have

CHART 11-3

FLUID AND ELECTROLYTE ASSESSMENT
Using Gordon's Functional Health Patterns

Nutritional-Metabolic Pattern

What is your typical daily food intake? Describe a day's meals, snacks, and vitamins.
How much salt do you typically add to your food? Do you use salt substitutes?
How is your appetite?
Do you have any difficulty chewing or swallowing?
What is your typical daily fluid intake? What types of fluids (water, juices, soft drinks, coffee, tea)? How much?
Have you had any recent change in your weight? Weight gain? Weight loss? How much?
Have you noticed a change in tightness of your rings or shoes? Tighter? Looser?

Elimination Pattern

What is your usual bowel elimination pattern? Frequency? Character? Discomfort? Laxatives?
What is your usual urinary elimination pattern? Frequency? Amount? Color? Odor? Control?
Have you noticed a change in the amount of urine?
Do you have any problem with excessive perspiration?
Do you have any other type of drainage?

Based on Gordon, M. (2000). *Manual of nursing diagnosis* (9th ed.). St. Louis: Mosby.

an imbalance of fluid, potassium, sodium, or hydrogen ions if additional conditions of water loss, such as vomiting or excessive sweating, also occur.

Older adults often use laxatives, which can disturb fluid and electrolyte balance. Misuse and overuse of these drugs can lead to serious imbalances.

Other important areas of the client history include body weight changes, thirst or excessive drinking, exposure to hot environments, and the presence of other disorders, such as kidney or endocrine diseases (e.g., Cushing's disease, Addison's disease, diabetes mellitus, and diabetes insipidus). The nurse makes a general assessment of the client's level of consciousness and mental status, because changes in mental status may support findings of imbalance. In such cases, the nurse may need to check the accuracy of historical data with family members.

Physical Assessment

Hydration is the normal state of fluid balance. A normally hydrated adult is alert and has moist eyes and mucous membranes, a urine output nearly the same as the amount of fluid ingested (with a urine specific gravity of approximately 1.015), and good skin turgor.

The nurse assesses skin turgor by pinching a fold of skin. This pinched fold should return immediately to its original shape after release. Decreased turgor, a sign of dehydration, is present when the fold remains in a pinched shape after being released and rebounds slowly **(tenting)** (Figure 11-11). The nurse can best assess skin turgor in body areas that contain little fat tissue, such as over the sternum, on the forehead, or on the back of the hand. An older person may have poor skin turgor because of the loss of tissue elasticity related to the aging process; thus a true state of hydration may be more difficult to assess in an older adult than in a younger adult. The best areas for assessing turgor in the older adult are over the sternum and on the forehead.

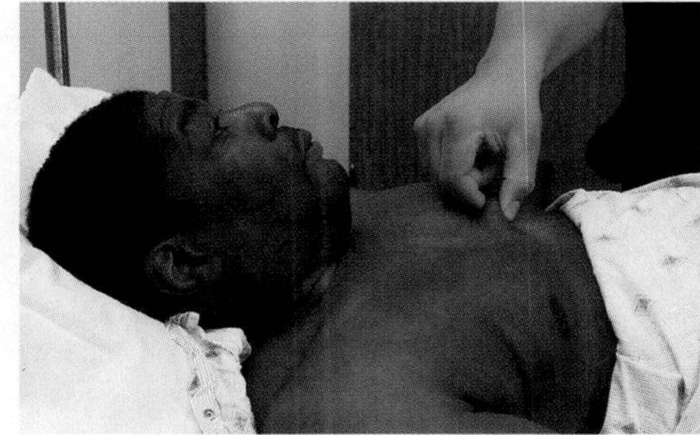

Figure 11-11 ● Examining the skin turgor of an older client.

Skin hydration assessment also includes an examination for dryness. The mucous membranes and the conjunctiva are normally moist. An assessment of fluid balance always includes an examination of the eyes, nose, and oral mucous membranes. A dry, sticky, "cottony" mouth; the absence of tearing; weight loss; and decreased urine output all indicate an actual fluid volume deficit.

A major criterion used in assessing fluid and electrolyte status is accurate measurement of fluid intake and output. Accurate assessment of actual fluid intake and output is the nurse's responsibility, and volumetric measuring devices must be used.

Behavioral and neurologic assessments are included in fluid assessment because changes in fluid balance can result in an alteration of neurologic function. In hypertonic states, neuronal cell shrinkage may induce serious nervous system excitability and hyperactivity, and convulsions may occur. Another variable to assess is the degree of thirst, but this may be difficult to gauge in a confused older client.

The nurse approximates insensible water loss (e.g., sweat) in every client. Special situations also require an assessment of fluid loss from other routes, including the following:

- Fluid losses from wounds
- Gastric or intestinal drainage
- Blood loss from hemorrhage
- Drainage of body secretions, such as bile and pancreatic juices, through fistulas

Electrolytes control the activity of excitable membranes, and electrolyte imbalances are associated with altered function of these membranes. Electrolyte assessment includes a complete neuromuscular assessment of muscle tone and strength, movement, coordination, and tremors. Assessment of other systems, including the cardiac system (heart rate, the strength of contractions, and the presence of dysrhythmias) and gastrointestinal system (peristalsis), may indicate changes of excitable membrane function.

Part of the nurse's assessment focuses on changes from previous findings (including mental status, physical examination data, and laboratory data). Fluid and electrolyte imbalances can occur quickly; therefore the nurse must be familiar with the client's baseline assessment data to detect any changes.

TABLE 11-12 • NORMAL URINE ELECTROLYTE VALUES

Electrolyte/Characteristics	Normal Value*	Significance of Abnormal Value†
Calcium	2.5-7.5 mmol/day	Increased: Malignancy, thyrotoxicosis, hyperparathyroidism, osteoporosis, vitamin D intoxication Decreased: Hypoparathyroidism, rickets, kidney disease, hypothyroidism
Chloride	100-250 mEq/day 110-250 mmol/day	Increased: Increased salt intake, drug-induced diuresis, adreno-cortical insufficiency Decreased: Reduced salt intake, water retention, vomiting, cerebral edema, adrenocortical hyperfunction
Magnesium	3.0-5.0 mmol/day	Increased: Alcohol intake, diuretics, corticosteroid therapy, cisplatin therapy Decreased: Dietary insufficiency
Phosphorus	12.9-42.0 mmol/day	Increased: Hyperparathyroidism, renal tubular damage, immobility, nonrenal acidosis Decreased: Hypoparathyroidism
Potassium	25-125 mmol/day (varies with diet)	Increased: Early starvation, hyperaldosteronism, metabolic acidosis Decreased: Addison's disease, renal disease
Sodium	40-220 mEq/day 40-220 mmol/day	Increased: Increased dietary intake, adrenal failure, diuretic therapy Decreased: Low sodium intake, sodium and water retention, adrenocortical hyperfunction, excessive diaphoresis, diarrhea
Osmolarity (osmolality)	300-900 mOsm/kg water	Increased: Dehydration, SIADH Decreased: Diabetes insipidus, primary polydipsia
Specific gravity	1.015-1.025	Increased: Dehydration, SIADH, diabetes mellitus, toxemia of pregnancy Decreased: Chronic renal insufficiency, diabetes insipidus, lithium toxicity, early renal disease

Data from Tietz, N. (Ed.). (1995). *Clinical guide to laboratory tests* (3rd ed.). Philadelphia: W.B. Saunders.
SIADH, Syndrome of inappropriate antidiuretic hormone.
*Based on a 24-hour total volume urine sample.
†Common conditions associated with abnormal values.

Psychosocial Assessment

Psychosocial assessment related to fluid and electrolyte status includes both psychologic and cultural factors that might influence balance. Depressed clients may refuse fluids or forget to drink adequate fluids. Clients with bulimia or anorexia nervosa (eating disorders) may use laxatives to excess or may induce vomiting, resulting in fluid and electrolyte imbalances. The nurse also assesses social practices. For example, excessive alcohol or drug use may lead to fluid or electrolyte imbalance.

Diagnostic Assessment

Laboratory results are important in identifying specific fluid and electrolyte imbalances or disorders that alter fluid and electrolyte status. Normal serum electrolyte values are presented in Table 11-5, and normal values for adults 60 years of age appear in Chart 11-2. Other laboratory values that are helpful in assessing fluid and electrolyte status include blood urea nitrogen level (BUN), glucose concentration, creatinine level, pH, bicarbonate level, osmolarity, hemoglobin, and hematocrit.

The urine test results may be helpful in assessing fluid status (Table 11-12). If a laboratory report is not available, the nurse can perform various tests using a dipstick to help determine fluid and electrolyte status, including detecting substances that should not be present in the urine, such as glucose, acetone, protein, and blood. Urine measurements such as pH and specific gravity also can be determined in this way.

ONLINE RESOURCES

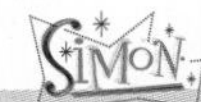

For suggested readings and Internet resources, go to http://www.wbsaunders.com/SIMON/Iggy/.

SELECTED BIBLIOGRAPHY

Asterisk indicates a classic or definitive work on this subject.

*Briggs, J., et al. (1996). Disorders of salt balance. In J. Kokko and R. Tannen (Eds.), *Fluids and electrolytes* (3rd ed., pp. 3-62). Philadelphia: W.B. Saunders.

Cook, L. (1999). The value of lab values. *American Journal of Nursing, 99*(5), 66-75.

Frizzell, J. (1998). Avoiding lab test pitfalls. *American Journal of Nursing, 98*(2), 34-38.

Gordon, M. (2000). *Manual of nursing diagnosis* (9th ed.). St. Louis: Mosby.

Guyton, A., & Hall, J. (2000). *Textbook of medical physiology* (10th ed.). Philadelphia: W.B. Saunders.

*Kokko, J., & Tannen, R. (1996). *Fluids and electrolytes* (3rd ed.). Philadelphia: W.B. Saunders.

McConnell, E. (1999). A bedside laboratory: Point-of-care blood analyzers. *Dimensions of Critical Care Nursing, 18*(5), 24-26.

*Metheny, N. (1996). *Fluid and electrolyte balance: Nursing considerations* (3rd ed.). Philadelphia: Lippincott-Raven.

*O'Donnell, M. (1995). Assessing fluid and electrolyte balance needs in elders. *American Journal of Nursing, 95*(1), 41-46.

Pagana, K., & Pagana, T. (1999). *Diagnostic testing and nursing implications: A case study approach.* St. Louis: Mosby.

Pennington, J. (1998). *Bowe's and Church's food values of portions commonly used* (17th ed.). Philadelphia: J.B. Lippincott.

Stark, J. (1998). A comprehensive analysis of the fluid and electrolytes system. *Critical Care Nursing Clinics of North America, 10*(4), 471-475.

Stark, J. (1998). Interpretation of BUN and serum creatinine. *Critical Care Nursing Clinics of North America, 10*(4), 491-496.

*Tietz, N.W. (Ed.). (1995). *Clinical guide to laboratory tests* (3rd ed.). Philadelphia: W.B. Saunders.

Toto, K. (1998). Fluid balance assessment: The total perspective. *Critical Care Nursing Clinics of North America, 10*(4), 383-400.

Trissel, L. (1998). *Handbook on injectable drugs* (10th ed.). Bethesda, MD: American Society of Health Systems.

CHAPTER 12

Interventions for Clients with Fluid Imbalances

M. LINDA WORKMAN

Learning Objectives

After studying this chapter, you should be able to:

1. Identify clients at risk for fluid imbalances.
2. Use laboratory data and clinical manifestations to determine the presence of fluid imbalance.
3. Apply appropriate nursing techniques to promote comfort and safety in the client with dehydration.
4. Prioritize nursing care for the client with fluid imbalance.
5. Develop a teaching plan to prevent dehydration in the older client at continuing risk for fluid loss.
6. Analyze changes in clinical manifestations to determine the effectiveness of therapy for the client with fluid imbalance.

SIMON

Go to http://www.wbsaunders.com/SIMON/Iggy/ for self-assessment questions related to these Learning Objectives.

Normal body functioning requires a proper balance of all body fluids. Many health problems can disrupt fluid intake or output, placing all clients at risk for some degree of fluid imbalance. Although most imbalances of fluid are accompanied by electrolyte imbalances, this chapter focuses only on client problems associated with fluid imbalances.

DEHYDRATION

OVERVIEW

In **dehydration,** the body's fluid intake is not sufficient to meet the body's fluid needs, resulting in a **fluid volume deficit.** Three basic types of dehydration are possible (Figure 12-1):

- **Isotonic dehydration,** in which water and dissolved electrolytes are lost in equal proportions
- **Hypertonic dehydration,** in which water loss is greater than electrolyte loss
- **Hypotonic dehydration,** in which electrolyte loss is greater than water loss

Dehydration is a clinical state rather than a disease and can be caused by many factors. Dehydration may be an *actual* decrease in total body water caused by either too little an intake of fluid or too great a loss of fluid. Dehydration also can occur without an actual decrease in total body water, such as when water shifts from the plasma into the interstitial space. This condition is called *relative* dehydration.

Pathophysiology

ISOTONIC DEHYDRATION

Isotonic dehydration is the most common type of fluid volume deficit. Problems caused by isotonic dehydration result from loss of plasma volume. Isotonic dehydration involves loss of isotonic fluids from the extracellular fluid (ECF) compartment, including both the plasma and the interstitial space. Because isotonic fluid is lost, plasma osmolarity remains normal. This type of dehydration does not cause a shift of fluids between compartments, so the intracellular fluid (ICF) volume remains normal. Isotonic dehydration decreases circulating blood volume **(hypovolemia)** and leads to inadequate tissue perfusion. Compensatory mechanisms attempt to maintain adequate tissue perfusion to vital organs in spite of decreased vascular volume (Figure 12-2).

Isotonic dehydration has many causes (Table 12-1). These include inadequate intake of fluids and solutes, fluid shifts between compartments, and excessive losses of isotonic body fluids.

HYPERTONIC DEHYDRATION

Hypertonic dehydration is the second most common type of fluid volume deficit. The problems caused by hypertonic dehydration result from changes in the concentrations of specific electrolytes.

Hypertonic dehydration occurs when water loss from the extracellular fluid (ECF) is greater than electrolyte loss. This water loss increases the osmolarity of the remaining plasma, making it *hypertonic* or *hyperosmolar* compared with normal ECF. The hyperosmolar plasma has an increased osmotic pressure that causes fluid to move from the intracellular fluid (ICF) into the plasma and interstitial fluid spaces. The fluid shift leads to cellular dehydration and shrinkage. The fluid shift also causes the plasma volume to increase to normal or greater than normal levels. *Thus the compensatory mechanisms and signs and symptoms of hy-*

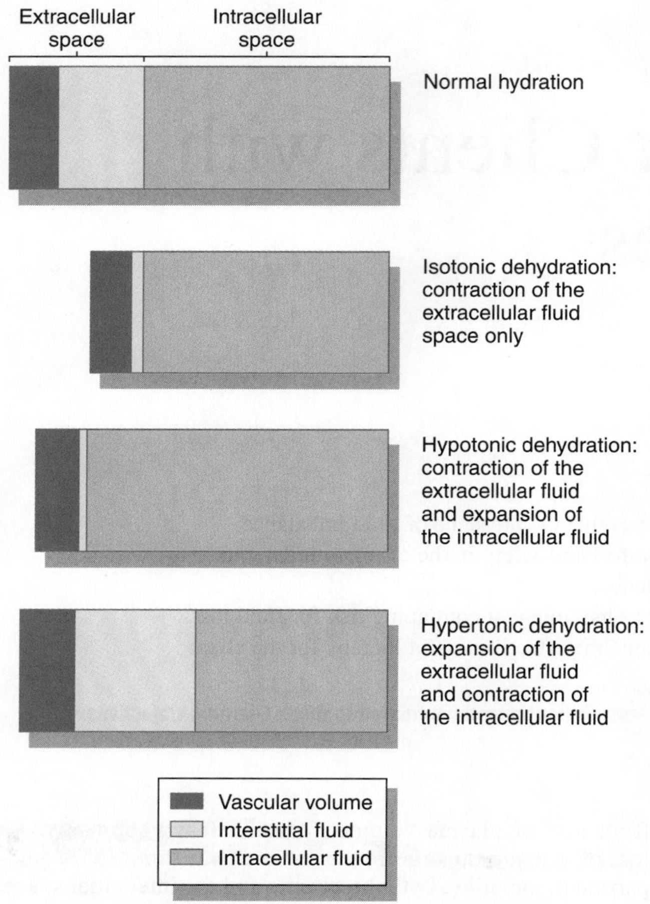

Figure 12-1 ● Three types of dehydration. (© 1992 M. Linda Workman. All rights reserved.)

TABLE 12-1 ● COMMON CAUSES OF DEHYDRATION

ISOTONIC DEHYDRATION
- Hemorrhage
- Vomiting
- Diarrhea
- Profuse salivation
- Fistulas
- Abscesses
- Ileostomy
- Cecostomy
- Frequent enemas
- Profuse diaphoresis
- Burns
- Severe wounds
- Long-term NPO (nothing by mouth)
- Diuretic therapy
- Gastrointestinal suction

HYPERTONIC DEHYDRATION
- Hyperventilation
- Watery diarrhea
- Renal failure
- Ketoacidosis
- Diabetes insipidus
- Excessive fluid replacement (hypertonic)
- Excessive sodium bicarbonate administration
- Tube feedings
- Dysphagia
- Impaired thirst
- Unconsciousness
- Fever
- Impaired motor function
- Systemic infection

HYPOTONIC DEHYDRATION
- Chronic illness
- Excessive fluid replacement (hypotonic)
- Renal failure
- Chronic or severe malnutrition

povolemic shock are not present. However, excitable membrane activity and cardiac contractility are affected by altered plasma levels of potassium and calcium. Compensatory mechanisms for hypertonic dehydration occur in response to the increased ECF osmolarity (Figure 12-3).

Hypertonic dehydration is caused by the loss of any body fluid that is hypotonic (low osmolarity, or decreased concentration of solute particles compared with isotonic body fluid) or occurs when water loss is greater than electrolyte loss. Common causes of hypertonic dehydration are conditions such as excessive perspiration, hyperventilation, ketoacidosis, prolonged fevers, diarrhea, early-stage renal failure, diabetes insipidus, and ketoacidosis in the diuretic phase (see Table 12-1).

HYPOTONIC DEHYDRATION

Hypotonic dehydration is the least common type of fluid volume deficit. The problems caused by hypotonic dehydration result from fluid shifts between compartments, causing a decrease in plasma volume.

Hypotonic dehydration involves excessive loss of sodium and potassium from the ECF. This loss leads to decreased osmolarity of the remaining ECF, making it hypotonic compared with normal ECF. The decreased ECF osmolarity lowers the osmotic pressure of plasma and interstitial fluids to below that of the fluid inside the cells, the ICF. As a result of this difference in osmotic pressure, water moves from the plasma and interstitial spaces into the cells, creating a plasma volume deficit and causing the cells to swell.

Cell swelling causes widespread problems and symptoms. Because brain cells are more sensitive to swelling than the cells of other tissues, neurologic problems usually occur with hypotonic dehydration. Hypotonic fluid also dilutes the normal electrolyte concentrations and causes sodium and potassium imbalances.

Hypotonic dehydration is usually associated with chronic illness. Chronic renal failure, in which the kidneys waste sodium, leads to hypotonic dehydration. Chronic malnutrition and taking in excessive amounts of hypotonic fluids also cause hypotonic dehydration.

Incidence/Prevalence

The actual incidence of dehydration is not known; however every ill client is at risk. Older clients are at high risk because they have less total body water than younger adults. Conditions contributing to inadequate fluid intake in the older adult include decreased thirst sensation and difficulty with ambulation or other motor skills necessary for ingesting fluids. Nurs-

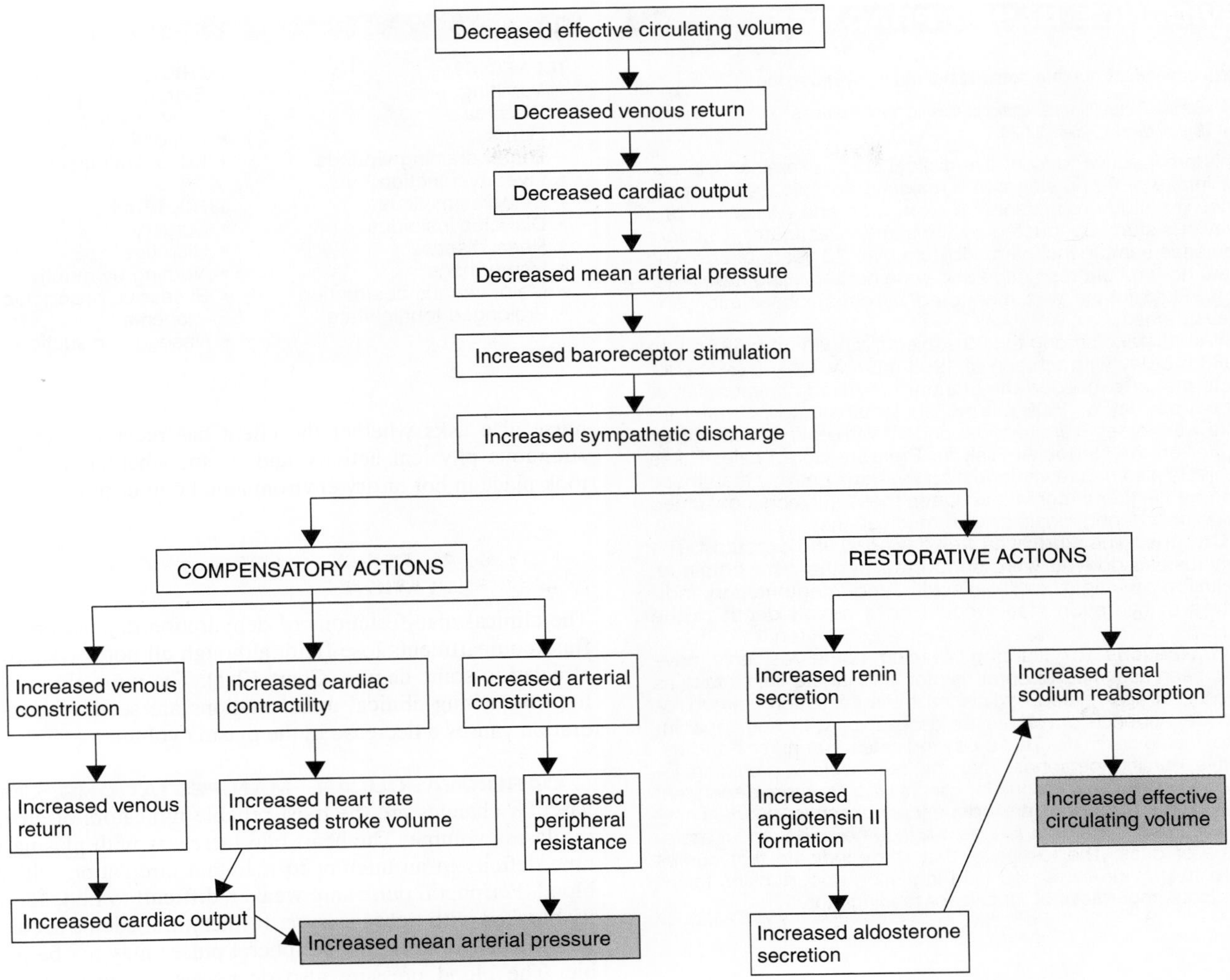

Decreased effective circulating volume
Decreased venous return
Decreased cardiac output
Decreased mean arterial pressure
Increased baroreceptor stimulation
Increased sympathetic discharge
COMPENSATORY ACTIONS
RESTORATIVE ACTIONS
Increased venous constriction
Increased cardiac contractility
Increased arterial constriction
Increased renin secretion
Increased renal sodium reabsorption
Increased venous return
Increased heart rate
Increased stroke volume
Increased peripheral resistance
Increased angiotensin II formation
Increased effective circulating volume
Increased cardiac output
Increased mean arterial pressure
Increased aldosterone secretion

Figure 12-2 ● Compensatory mechanisms associated with isotonic dehydration.

ing home residents older than 85 years of age who are semi-dependent with eating and are less dependent on others for function appear to be at greatest risk for dehydration (see the Evidence-Based Practice for Nursing box on p. 162).

➤ COLLABORATIVE MANAGEMENT

SIMON Activity Link

● Assessment

HISTORY

The nurse collects data on risk factors and factors causing dehydration (Table 12-2).

AGE. Age is an important consideration because dehydration in the older adult can develop quickly in response to relatively small fluid losses. In addition, older people are more likely to have chronic illnesses or to be taking medications, such as diuretics, that can lead to fluid and electrolyte imbalances.

HEIGHT AND WEIGHT. Measuring height and weight is important for calculating approximate fluid needs. If this

Solute-free water loss
Decreased ECF volume
Increased ECF osmolarity
Fluid shift (ICF to ECF)
Increased ADH secretion (posterior pituitary)
Stimulation of osmoreceptors (hypothalamus)
Cell shrinkage
Activation of thirst reflex
Increased renal reabsorption of water
Increased oral water intake
Decreased urine output
Increased ECF volume

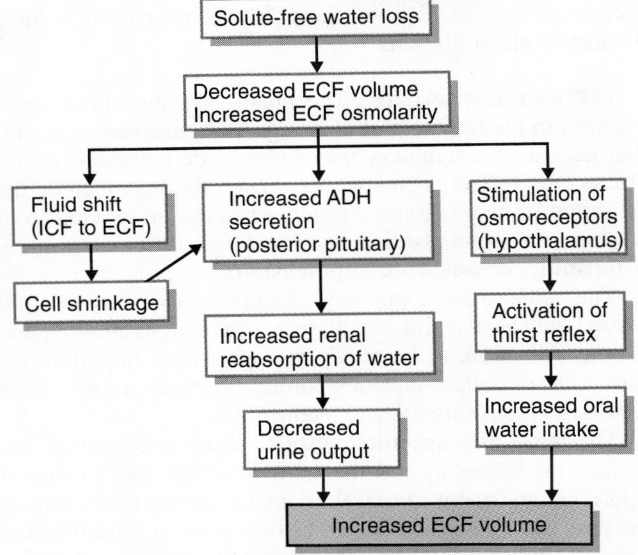

Figure 12-3 ● Compensatory mechanisms associated with hypertonic dehydration. (*ADH,* Antidiuretic hormone; *ECF,* extracellular fluid; *ICF,* intracellular fluid.)

EVIDENCE-BASED PRACTICE FOR NURSING

Less dependent nursing home residents need water, too

Gaspar, P. (1999). Water intake of nursing home residents. *Journal of Gerontological Nursing, 25*(4), 23-29.

This prospective, descriptive clinical study examined the water intake of 99 nursing home residents for two 24-hour periods. The study represents an expansion and replication of a previous study conducted by the same investigator. The convenience sample included subjects over 70 years of age who were not on fluid restriction and were not receiving tube feedings. Fluid intake was monitored by direct observation and measurement.

Water intake among the 99 subjects ranged from 597 mL to 2988 mL/day with a mean of 1968 mL/day. Only 8 (8%) subjects met or exceeded the standard required minimum water intake per day of 1600 mL/m². Subjects with lower water intake were older, were semidependent with eating, and scored higher on the Norton At-Risk for Pressure Sore Scale. These subjects also had fewer ingestion sessions per day than those who had higher water intake. Often these subjects consumed fluids only during meals or with medications.

Critique. The study was well designed and executed. The conclusions derived were supported by the data obtained. Inclusion of weight, cardiovascular, and integumentary indicators of hydration status could have added depth to the study.

Implications for Nursing. Nursing home residents have long been assumed to be at risk for inadequate fluid intake as a result of age-related diminished thirst sensation, immobility, and dependence on others for assistance with nutritional intake, including fluids. This study indicates that nurses and assistive nursing personnel may be purposefully providing increased ingestion sessions for clients who are more dependent with eating. Those who are independent or semidependent may be assumed to be able to ingest adequate fluid without assistance or cues. The results of this study indicate that nurses need to provide increased fluid ingestion opportunities for all residents, regardless of mobility or feeding status.

information is not known or if the client is confused, the nurse obtains these measurements directly. Because 1 L of water weighs about 2.2 pounds (1 kg), changes in daily weights are good indicators of fluid losses or excesses. A weight change of 1 pound corresponds to a fluid volume change of about 500 mL.

OTHER CHANGES. The nurse asks the client about changes in the tightness of clothing, rings, and shoes. A sudden decrease in tightness may indicate dehydration; an increase may reflect edema. Other related findings include the sensation of palpitations or lightheadedness on moving from a lying or a sitting position to a standing position (caused by **orthostatic, or postural, hypotension**).

The nurse asks about any abnormal or excessive fluid losses, such as perspiration, diarrhea, bleeding, vomiting, urination, salivation, and wound drainage. Other important information to collect includes chronic illnesses, recent acute illnesses, recent surgery, and medications.

The nurse asks specific questions about urine output, including the frequency and amount of voidings. The nurse also asks about the client's usual fluid intake and the intake during the previous 24 hours. It is just as important to determine the types of fluids ingested as it is to determine the amount of fluids ingested, because fluids vary widely in osmolarity. The

TABLE 12-2 • RISK FACTORS FOR DEHYDRATION

ILLNESSES	OTHER SITUATIONS
• Vomiting • Diarrhea • Burns • Large, draining wounds • Liver dysfunction • Diabetes mellitus • Diabetes insipidus • Renal disease • Hemorrhage • Major venous obstruction • Prolonged febrile state	• Extremes of age: older adults, infants • Unconsciousness • Motor limitations **THERAPIES** • Surgery • Diuretics • Nothing by mouth • Excessive hypertonic enemas • Nasogastric suction

nurse also asks whether the client has recently engaged in strenuous physical activity and, if so, whether the activity took place in hot or dry environmental conditions.

PHYSICAL ASSESSMENT/CLINICAL MANIFESTATIONS

The clinical manifestations of dehydration depend on which fluid compartments lose fluid, although all body systems are affected to some degree (Chart 12-1). The most obvious and life-threatening clinical manifestations are seen when dehydration causes a decrease in the plasma volume.

CARDIOVASCULAR MANIFESTATIONS. Cardiovascular changes are the most reliable indicators of changes in plasma volume. The heart rate increases with plasma volume deficits in an attempt to maintain circulation with less blood. Peripheral pulses are weaker, difficult to find, and easily blocked with light pressure. If interstitial edema accompanies the dehydration, the peripheral pulses may not be palpable. The blood pressure also decreases, as does the pulse pressure, with a greater decrease in the systolic blood pressure. Hypotension is more severe with the client in the standing position than with the client in the sitting or lying position. Because the blood pressure with the client standing may be much lower than in other positions, blood pressure is measured first with the client lying down, then sitting, and finally standing.

Another indicator of hydration status is the degree of neck and hand vein filling. Normally, hand veins fill and become engorged when the hands are lower than the level of the heart. As the hands are raised above the level of the heart, the veins flatten or collapse (Figure 12-4). Neck veins are normally distended when a client is in the supine position. These veins flatten when the client moves to a sitting position. When dehydration involves a plasma volume deficit, neck and hand veins are flat, even when the neck and hands are not raised above the level of the heart. These cardiovascular changes are not seen in hypertonic dehydration.

RESPIRATORY MANIFESTATIONS. The respiratory rate increases directly with the degree of fluid loss from plasma volume. The decreased blood volume is perceived by the body as decreased oxygen levels **(hypoxia),** and increased respiration is an attempt to maintain oxygen delivery.

CHART 12-1

KEY FEATURES *of* Dehydration

Manifestations of Dehydration in General*

Cardiovascular
- Increased pulse rate
- Thready pulse quality
- Decreased blood pressure
- Postural hypotension
- Flat neck and hand veins in dependent positions
- Diminished peripheral pulses

Respiratory
- Increased respiratory rate
- Increased depth of respirations

Neuromuscular
- Decreased central nervous system activity (lethargy to coma)
- Fever

Renal
- Decreased urine output
- Increased specific gravity

Integumentary
- Skin dry and scaly
- Turgor poor, tenting present
- Mouth dry and fissured, pastelike coating present

Gastrointestinal
- Decreased motility
- Diminished bowel sounds
- Constipation
- Thirst

Manifestations of Hypotonic Dehydration
- Skeletal muscle weakness

Manifestations of Hypertonic Dehydration
- Hyperactive deep tendon reflexes
- Increased sensation of thirst
- Pitting edema

*These manifestations are most severe with hypotonic dehydration.

INTEGUMENTARY MANIFESTATIONS. Changes in skin may be useful indicators of hydration. The nurse assesses for changes in the skin and mucous membranes that may indicate dehydration, including skin color, moisture, skin turgor, and edema. In older clients this information is less reliable because of poor skin turgor resulting from the loss of elastic tissue and the loss of tissue fluids with aging. The nurse assesses skin turgor by noting the following:

- How easily the skin over the back of the hand and arm can be gently pinched between the thumb and the forefinger to form a "tent"
- How soon the pinched skin resumes its normal position after release
- Whether depressions (pits) remain in the skin after a finger is pressed firmly but gently (over the shin, over the sternum, and over the sacrum)
- How deep the depression is (in millimeters)
- How long the depression remains

In generalized dehydration, skin turgor is poor, with the tenting remaining for minutes after pinching the skin, and no skin depressions occur with gentle pressure. The skin appears dry and scaly. The nurse assesses skin turgor in an

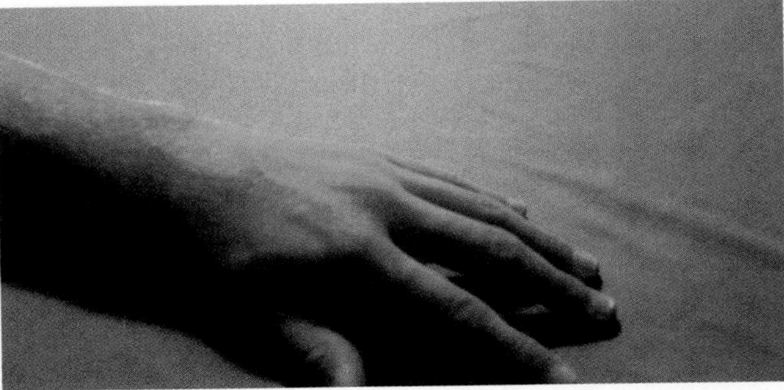

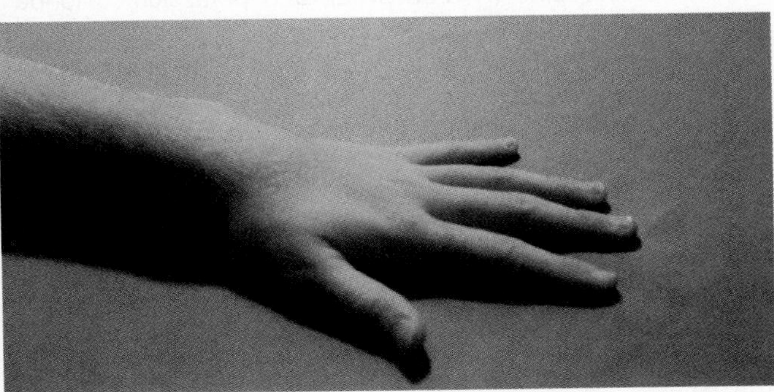

Figure 12-4 ● Hand veins full and bulging in the dependent position *(top)*. Hand veins collapsed *(bottom)*.

older adult by pinching the skin over the sternum, the forehead, or the abdomen because these areas more reliably indicate hydration (see Figure 11-11). As a person ages, the skin loses elasticity and tents on extremities even when the person is well hydrated.

In dehydration, oral mucous membranes are not moist. They may be covered with a thick, sticky, pastelike coating and may have cracks and fissures. The surface of the tongue may have deep furrows.

NEUROLOGIC MANIFESTATIONS. Dehydration may cause changes in body temperature and mental status as the brain is less perfused. The client with dehydration typically has a low-grade fever. One cause of the fever is the constriction of blood vessels that occurs as a compensation for hypovolemia. The blood vessel constriction makes heat dissipation more difficult.

Fever can also cause dehydration. A client with a temperature greater than 102° F (39° C) for longer than 6 hours is especially at risk. Older adults, who normally have a body temperature range of 96° to 98° F (35.4° to 36.6° C), are at greater risk for dehydration during episodes of fever. Mental status changes are also common with dehydration. Chart 12-2 outlines how to assess mental status quickly.

RENAL MANIFESTATIONS. The volume and the composition of urine output indicate the hydration status of the renal system. The nurse monitors urine output, comparing total output with total fluid intake and daily weights. Accurate intake and output measurement is a major nursing responsibility. Urine output below 500 mL/day for any client without renal disease is cause for concern. A client with fluid imbalance is weighed each day at the same time and on the same scale. When possible, the client wears the same amount and type of clothing for each weigh-in. Metabolic weight loss (even in starvation) usually accounts for only about ½ pound of weight loss per day. Any weight loss in excess of this amount is considered fluid loss.

CRITICAL THINKING CHALLENGE

You are making a home visit to a 75-year-old client who has long-standing mild congestive heart failure and hypertension. She lives alone and has been well managed with digoxin, hydrochlorothiazide (HydroDIURIL), and potassium chloride tablets. When she answers the door, you note that she is unsteady on her feet. She tells you she feels lightheaded.

- What vital sign would you assess first?
- What might you expect to find on physical assessment?
- What questions regarding her medication regimen should you ask?

For suggested answer guidelines, go to SIMON http://www.wbsaunders.com/SIMON/Iggy/.

PSYCHOSOCIAL ASSESSMENT

The nurse observes the client for behavioral changes that accompany dehydration. Initially, a dehydrated client may have a flat affect and may seem unconcerned about his or her state of health and possible treatment regimens. As dehydration worsens, psychosocial activities reflect abnormal functioning of the central nervous system. The client may become anxious, restless, lethargic, and confused. These behavioral changes are more obvious in hypertonic and hypotonic dehydration because of intracellular fluid (ICF) shifts in brain cells, resulting in shrinkage or swelling of the cells. If the conditions causing the dehydration continue, circulation to cerebral tissues becomes so impaired that delirium and coma can occur.

CHART 12-2

BEST PRACTICE *for* Brief Check of Mental Status

- Is the client awake?
- If the client is not awake, what type of stimulation is needed to waken the client?
  - Calling the client's name in a normal voice volume
  - Calling the client's name in a louder voice volume
  - Touching the client's arm or face while calling the client's name
  - Gently tapping or shaking an arm
  - Vigorously shaking a hand or arm
  - Applying a painful stimulus
- If the client is awake, ask questions that require more than a "yes" or "no" response to establish orientation to time and place.
- Avoid the use of nonsense questions (e.g., "Do helicopters eat their young?").
- Ask questions that are reasonable and likely to be known by the client, such as "When is your birthday?" Avoid questions such as "Who was vice president under Truman?"
- Is it necessary to repeat questions to obtain a response?
- Does the response answer the question asked?
- Does the client have difficulty with word choices in forming responses?
- Is the client irritated or upset by the questions?
- Can the client concentrate on a question long enough to provide an appropriate response, or is the attention span short?
- Can the client count by threes?
- Can the client count backward from 100 by threes?
- Does the client know the names of immediate family members?
- Does the client know who the questioner is (not necessarily the questioner's name but that person's role in the client's care, such as nurse, doctor, chaplain, therapist)?
- Does the client know his or her immediate location (e.g., home, hospital, clinic)?
- Does the client know the year?

LABORATORY ASSESSMENT

No single laboratory test result confirms or rules out dehydration. Instead, a diagnosis of dehydration is based on laboratory findings along with presenting signs and symptoms. Laboratory findings depend on the type of dehydration present (Chart 12-3). Isotonic and hypotonic dehydration states with accompanying plasma volume deficits show **hemoconcentration** (elevated levels of hemoglobin, hematocrit, serum osmolarity, glucose, protein, blood urea nitrogen, and various electrolytes) because only the water is lost and other substances remain. Hemoconcentration is not present when dehydration is caused by hemorrhage, because loss of all blood and plasma products occurs.

Specific urine laboratory values can help to confirm dehydration if the client does not have renal dysfunction. Usually the urine of the client with dehydration is concentrated, with a specific gravity greater than 1.030. Volume is decreased, and osmolarity is greatly increased. Usually the color is dark amber and a strong odor is evident.

Analysis

COMMON NURSING DIAGNOSES AND COLLABORATIVE PROBLEMS

The following are priority nursing diagnoses for clients with dehydration:

1. Deficient Fluid Volume related to excessive fluid loss or inadequate fluid intake
2. Decreased Cardiac Output related to decreased plasma volume
3. Impaired Oral Mucous Membrane related to inadequate oral secretions

The primary collaborative problem is Potential for Dysrhythmias.

ADDITIONAL NURSING DIAGNOSES AND COLLABORATIVE PROBLEMS

In addition to the common nursing diagnoses and collaborative problems, clients with dehydration may have one or more of the following:

- Constipation related to decreased body fluids
- Risk for Injury (fall) related to orthostatic (postural) hypotension
- Deficient Knowledge related to medication regimen and preventive measures
- Risk for Impaired Skin Integrity related to deficiencies of interstitial fluid and inadequate tissue perfusion
- Ineffective Airway Clearance related to thick, tenacious secretions
- Potential for Hypovolemic Shock
- Potential for Electrolyte Imbalances

CHART 12-3

LABORATORY PROFILE
Dehydration

Values*	Isotonic Dehydration	Hypotonic Dehydration	Hypertonic Dehydration
BLOOD VALUES			
BUN	Normal or increased	Increased	Increased
Creatinine	Normal or increased	Increased	Increased
Sodium	Normal	<120 mEq/L (mmol)	>150 mEq/L (mmol)
Osmolality	Normal	Decreased	Increased
Hematocrit	Increased	Increased	Normal or decreased
Hemoglobin	Increased	Increased	Normal or decreased
WBCs	Increased	Increased	Normal or decreased
Protein	Increased	Increased	Increased
URINE VALUES			
Specific gravity	>1.010	<1.010	>1.030
Osmolality	Increased	Increased	Increased
Volume	Decreased	Decreased	Decreased

BUN, Blood urea nitrogen; *WBC,* white blood cell.
*All values reflect dehydration states alone and not the underlying pathologic changes or disease states contributing to the dehydration.

CHART 12-4

NIC INTERVENTION ACTIVITIES *for* The Client with Fluid Volume Deficit

Fluid Monitoring: *Collection and analysis of client data to regulate fluid balance*
- Monitor serum and urine electrolyte values, as appropriate.
- Monitor BP, heart rate, and respiratory status.
- Monitor orthostatic blood pressure and change in cardiac rhythm, as appropriate.
- Monitor weight.
- Maintain intake and output.
- Note presence or absence of vertigo on rising.
- Monitor color, quantity, and specific gravity of urine.

Fluid Management: *Promotion of fluid balance and prevention of complications resulting from abnormal or undesired fluid levels*
- Administer IV therapy, as prescribed.
- Give fluids, as appropriate.
- Promote oral intake (e.g., provide a drinking straw, offer fluid between meals, change ice water routinely), as appropriate.
- Distribute the fluid intake over 24 hours, as appropriate.
- Encourage significant other to assist client with feedings, as appropriate.
- Offer snacks (e.g., frequent drinks and fresh fruit/fruit juice), as appropriate.

Oral Health Restoration: *Promotion of healing for a client who has an oral mucosa or dental lesion*
- Encourage frequent rinsing of mouth with any of the following: sodium bicarbonate solution, warm saline, or hydrogen peroxide solution.
- Monitor lips, tongue, mucous membranes, tonsillar fossae, and gums for moisture, color, texture, presence of debris, and infection, using good lighting and a tongue blade.
- Instruct client to avoid commercial mouthwashes.
- Monitor client every shift for dryness of the oral mucosa.
- Increase mouth care to every 2 hours and twice at night, if stomatitis is not controlled.
- Avoid use of lemon-glycerin swabs.
- Increase liquids on the meal tray.

NIC intervention activities selected from McCloskey, J.C., & Bulechek, G.M. (Eds.). (2000). *Nursing interventions classification (NIC)* (3rd ed.). St. Louis: Mosby.

Planning and Implementation

DEFICIENT FLUID VOLUME

PLANNING: EXPECTED OUTCOMES. The client with dehydration is expected to have body fluid levels restored to normal.

INTERVENTIONS. Management of dehydration aims to prevent further fluid losses and increase fluid compartment volumes to normal ranges.

NIC **FLUID MANAGEMENT.** Diet therapy, oral rehydration therapy, and drug therapy are the methods of choice to manage fluid volume deficit (Chart 12-4).

DIET THERAPY. Mild to moderate dehydration is corrected with oral fluid replacement if the client is alert enough to swallow and can tolerate oral fluids. The nurse or assistive nursing personnel encourages and measures fluid intake. The specific type of fluid needed for replacement varies with the type of dehydration.

The client's compliance in drinking oral replacement fluids can be enhanced by using fluids he or she enjoys and by carefully timing the intake schedule. Dividing the total amount of fluids needed by nursing shifts helps to meet fluid needs more evenly with less danger of overhydration. The conscious client is offered small volumes of fluids every hour to increase intake.

ORAL REHYDRATION THERAPY. Oral rehydration therapy (ORT) is the most cost-effective way to replace fluids for the client with dehydration. Specifically formulated solutions containing glucose and electrolytes cause water to be absorbed even when the client is vomiting or has diarrhea. Fluid losses from diarrhea are usually 2 to 3 L/day and should be replaced liter for liter, especially in older clients. A typical order might be "Resol 1 L every 8 hours." Table 12-3 lists commercially available ORT solutions.

DRUG THERAPY. Drug therapy for dehydration is directed at restoring fluid balance and controlling the causes

TABLE 12-3 • COMMERCIAL SOLUTIONS FOR ORAL REHYDRATION THERAPY

Brand Name	Na^+ (mEq/L)	K^+ (mEq/L)	Cl^- (mEq/L)	Citrate (mEq/L)	Sugar or Starch	Calories (kcal/L)
Ricelyte (Mead-Johnson)	50	25	45	34	Rice syrup (30 g)	126
Resol (Wyeth-Ayerst)	50	20	50	34	Dextrose (20 g)	84
Rehydralyte (Ross Labs)	75	20	65	30	Dextrose (25 g)	100
Pedialyte (Ross Labs)	45	20	35	30	Dextrose (25 g)	100
Gastrolyte (Rorer)	60	20	60	10	Dextrose (17.8 g)	75
Rapolyte (Richmond)	90	20	80	30	Dextrose (20 g)	84
Lytren (Mead-Johnson)	50	25	45	30	Dextrose (20 g)	84
Oralyte (Rugby)	45	20	25	48	Dextrose (25 g)	100
Kao Lectrolyte (Pharmacia & UpJohn)	50	20	—	30	Dextrose (20 g)	84

Data from *United States Pharmacopeia Dispensing Information (USP DI): Vol I. Drug information for the health care professional* (20th ed.). (2000). Englewood, CO: Micromedex.

TABLE 12-4 • CHARACTERISTICS OF COMMON INTRAVENOUS THERAPY SOLUTIONS

Solution	Osmolarity (mOsm/L)	pH	Calories* (kcal)	Tonicity
0.9% saline	308	5	0	Isotonic
0.45% saline	154	5	0	Hypotonic
5% dextrose in water (D_5W)	272	3.5-6.5	170	Isotonic†
10% dextrose in water ($D_{10}W$)	500	3.5-6.5	340	Hypertonic†
5% dextrose in 0.9% saline	560	3.5-6.5	170	Hypertonic†
5% dextrose in 0.45% saline	406	4	170	Hypertonic†
5% dextrose in 0.225% saline	321	4	170	Isotonic†
Ringer's lactate	273	6.5	9	Isotonic
5% dextrose in Ringer's lactate	525	4.0-6.5	179	Hypertonic†

Data from Trissel, L. (1998). *Handbook on injectable drugs* (10th ed.). Bethesda, MD: American Society of Hospital Pharmacists.
*Calories are calculated on the basis of a volume of 1000 mL.
†*Solution tonicity at the time of administration.* Within a short time after administration, the dextrose is metabolized, and the tonicity of the infused solution decreases in proportion to the osmolarity or tonicity of the nondextrose components (electrolytes) within the water.

of dehydration. Whenever possible, fluids are replaced by the oral route. When dehydration is severe or life threatening, intravenous (IV) fluid replacement may be necessary. Calculation of how much fluid to replace is based on the client's weight loss and clinical manifestations. The rate of fluid replacement depends on the degree of dehydration and the presence of pre-existing cardiac, pulmonary, or renal problems.

The type of fluid ordered by the health care provider varies with the type of dehydration and the client's cardiovascular status. The desired outcomes of therapy are appropriate fluid replacement and normal volumes in all body fluid compartments. Usually the client receives IV infusions of water with whatever solutes (especially electrolytes) are determined necessary on the basis of laboratory values. Table 12-4 lists the osmolarity, caloric content, and tonicity of common IV fluids. Generally, isotonic dehydration is treated with isotonic fluid solutions, hypertonic dehydration is treated with hypotonic fluid solutions, and hypotonic dehydration is treated with hypertonic fluid solutions.

Drug therapy includes the use of medications to correct the cause of the dehydration. Antidiarrheal medications are ordered when excessive diarrhea causes dehydration. Antimicrobial therapy may be used in clients with bacterial diarrhea. Antiemetics to control vomiting may be necessary when excessive vomiting produces dehydration. Antipyretics to reduce body temperature are helpful when fever contributes to dehydration.

CRITICAL THINKING CHALLENGE

The home care client with mild congestive heart failure tells you that she took two diuretics this morning (6 hours ago) because she ate salty ham the evening before.

- What type of dehydration is this client most likely to have?
- What types of fluids would you suggest for replacement?
- What criteria would you use to determine how much fluid to give this client?
- What criteria would you use to determine if the fluid replacement therapy was effective?

For suggested answer guidelines, go to SIMON http://www.wbsaunders.com/SIMON/Iggy/.

DECREASED CARDIAC OUTPUT

PLANNING: EXPECTED OUTCOMES. The client with dehydration is expected to have cardiac output restored to normal levels and to maintain adequate oxygenation to vital organs.

INTERVENTIONS. Interventions of drug and oxygen therapy aim to increase circulating fluid volume, support compensatory mechanisms, and prevent complications.

DRUG THERAPY. Drug therapy to increase body fluid volume and prevent excessive fluid loss is the same as that for the client with fluid volume deficit. Drugs to increase venous return or improve cardiac contractility are used only when a cardiac problem also is present.

OXYGEN THERAPY. Oxygen is usually delivered by mask or nasal cannula to the client with dehydration. The nurse administers water-nebulized oxygen at the rate or amount specified by the health care provider's order.

NIC ***FLUID MONITORING.*** Monitoring vital signs and level of consciousness is important when caring for clients with dehydration (see Chart 12-4). The nurse or assistive nursing personnel monitors the pulse, blood pressure, pulse pressure, central venous pressure, respiratory rate, skin and mucous membrane color, and urine output at least every hour until the fluid imbalance is resolved.

> **CRITICAL THINKING CHALLENGE**
>
> When you take the client's blood pressure in a sitting position and in a standing position, the systolic pressure is 24 mm Hg lower with the client standing compared with the pressure taken with the client sitting.
>
> - Is this finding supportive or nonsupportive of fluid volume deficit?
> - What would you teach this client to avoid complications associated with this problem?

For suggested answer guidelines, go to SIMON http://www.wbsaunders.com/SIMON/Iggy/.

IMPAIRED ORAL MUCOUS MEMBRANE

PLANNING: EXPECTED OUTCOMES. The client with dehydration is expected to have less discomfort and remain free of complications.

INTERVENTIONS

NIC **ORAL HEALTH RESTORATION.** Interventions include drug therapy, fluid replacement, and good oral hygiene, as well as the early diagnosis and prevention of complications (see Chart 12-4).

DRUG THERAPY. Drug therapy to increase fluid volume and prevent fluid loss is the same as that discussed earlier for deficient fluid volume (p. 165). Saliva substitutes, such as Salivart, can reduce the sensation of mouth dryness. To prevent aspiration, the nurse does not use such agents in an unconscious client.

ORAL HYGIENE. Nursing actions to promote oral hygiene can increase the client's comfort. The lips are kept clean and moist. The thick, sticky coating on the tongue and mouth during dehydration can be reduced with frequent mouth care.

Mouth care includes gentle toothbrushing several times a day and rinsing hourly. The nurse teaches the client to avoid mouthwashes and swabs that contain alcohol or glycerin because these products dry the oral mucosa further and may cause more discomfort by stinging or burning open areas of the mucosa. Rinsing the mouth with dilute solutions of hydrogen peroxide two or three times per day is a good form of oral hygiene; however, when used more frequently, this treatment increases oral dryness. Tap water and normal saline rinses can be used safely as often as the client wishes.

PREVENTION OF COMPLICATIONS. A dry mouth can lead to the development of sores and fissures in the mucosa, providing a portal of entry for many pathogens. The thick, sticky coating also is an excellent breeding ground for microorganisms. A major complication of mouth dryness is a wide variety of oral infections. Chart 12-4 summarizes nursing interventions for mouth care.

POTENTIAL FOR DYSRHYTHMIAS

PLANNING: EXPECTED OUTCOMES. The client with dehydration is expected to maintain his or her normal cardiac rhythm.

INTERVENTIONS. Interventions are aimed at correcting the dehydration and recognizing dysrhythmias so that appropriate drug therapy can be initiated.

DRUG THERAPY. Drug therapy to increase body fluid volume and prevent excessive fluid loss is the same as that discussed earlier for deficient fluid volume (p. 165).

Elevated potassium or calcium levels can cause life-threatening dysrhythmias. Drug therapy to reduce these electrolytes may be ordered. If potassium levels are elevated, a combination of 20 units of regular insulin in 100 mL of 20% dextrose may be administered to promote movement of potassium from the blood into the intracellular fluid (ICF). Drugs such as etidronate (Didronel) and plicamycin (Mithracin) may be administered to reduce an elevated serum calcium level.

MONITORING. The nurse monitors the client for signs and symptoms of cardiac dysrhythmias every 15 minutes until he or she is fully rehydrated. The rate, rhythm, and quality of the apical pulse are assessed and compared with the client's baseline measurements. The nurse further assesses for fatigue, chest discomfort or pain, and shortness of breath. Hand grasps and deep tendon reflexes are assessed, and changes from baseline are noted.

Clients at risk for dysrhythmias are monitored using electrocardiography (ECG). The pattern may show tall T waves or a shortened ST segment. Any change from the client's baseline ECG is reported to the physician immediately.

Community-Based Care

No extensive home care preparations are necessary for clients with mild dehydration or for those with dehydration of sudden onset. The imbalance is corrected before discharge from

CHART 12-5

FOCUSED ASSESSMENT *of* Home Care Clients at Risk for Dehydration

Assess cardiovascular status.
- Vital signs, including apical pulse, pulse pressure, presence or absence of orthostatic hypotension, and quality and rhythm of peripheral pulses
- Presence or absence of peripheral edema
- Hand vein filling in the dependent position
- Neck vein filling in the recumbent and sitting positions
- Weight gain or loss

Assess cognition and mental status.
- Level of consciousness
- Orientation to time, place, and person
- Can the client accurately read a seven-word sentence containing no words greater than three syllables?

Assess condition of skin and mucous membranes.
- Presence or absence of skin tenting over the sternum or the forehead
- Moistness of skin, most reliable on chest and back
- Presence or absence of coating on tongue or teeth
- Can the client spit?

Assess neutromuscular status.
- Reactivity of patellar and biceps reflexes
- Oral temperature
- Handgrip strength
- Steadiness of gait

Assess renal system.
- Observe urine specimen for color, odor, cloudiness, and amount

Ask about the following:
- 24-hour fluid intake and output
- 24-hour diet recall
- 24-hour activity recall
- Over-the-counter and prescribed medications the client has taken

Assess client's understanding of illness and compliance with treatment.
- Signs and symptoms to report to health care provider
- Medication plan (correct timing and dose)

the facility and, with minimal precautions, is unlikely to recur. Clients who are most likely to be discharged before the imbalance is completely corrected and who are susceptible to recurrent episodes are those with chronic pathologic conditions, such as renal insufficiency, diabetes, malignancy, adrenal insufficiency, and many endocrine disorders. These clients often require long-term diet and drug therapy.

The nurse performs a focused assessment (Chart 12-5) and a mental status check at every home visit to a client at risk for dehydration. Medications, signs and symptoms of dehydration, and health care resources are reviewed with the client and family.

Education is important in the prevention and early detection of dehydration. The nurse teaches the client at risk for dehydration about diet, drug regimens, and the signs and symptoms of dehydration, explaining the meaning of changes found on assessment.

The nurse stresses the importance of recording accurate daily weights in assessing hydration status. Clients are instructed to weigh themselves on the same scale daily, close to the same time each day, and with approximately the same amount of clothing on each time. Keeping a chart comparing the recorded weights from one day to the next can help the client recognize early-stage dehydration.

Clients are instructed to take medications as prescribed and not increase the use of diuretics. The nurse explains that if a diuretic is not taken one day, the next day's dose should not be doubled. Clients are taught how and where to assess skin turgor. The nurse teaches them how to measure their own peripheral pulse and obtains a return demonstration.

The nurse instructs the family to keep fluids for the client in places that he or she can access. Container modifications, such as opening zip-top cans and covering them with foil, can be made to ensure that the client can easily open container lids. "Sipper" containers not only provide easy access but also are unbreakable and reduce spillage.

CRITICAL THINKING CHALLENGE

Your client has had her fluid volume deficit corrected and will continue to live at home alone.
- What specific areas of teaching will you emphasize to her?

For suggested answer guidelines, go to SIMON http://www.wbsaunders.com/SIMON/Iggy/.

Evaluation: Outcomes

NOC The nurse evaluates the care of the client with dehydration on the basis of the identified nursing diagnoses and collaborative problems. The expected outcomes include that the client will:
- Ingest at least 1500 mL of hypotonic fluids each day
- Maintain a fluid output approximately equal to fluid intake
- State that oral mucosal discomfort is relieved
- Experience no oral mucosal complication

HEAT STROKE

OVERVIEW

Heat stroke, sometimes called **heat exhaustion,** is a combination of dehydration and **hyperthermia** (elevated body temperature) that can rapidly cause death. The excessive dehydration causes hypovolemic shock. The greatly increased core body temperature, sometimes in excess of 109° F (42.8° C) damages organs, particularly the heart and the brain.

The most common cause of heat stroke among younger adults is the performance of strenuous exercise under high environmental temperatures without adequate fluid replacement for the excessive fluid loss. In this condition, heavy muscle contractions generate heat faster than the body is able to dissipate it. Older adults are very prone to heat stroke in hot environments, even when physical activity is minimal, because they have proportionately less body water and heat dissipation mechanisms are not as effective. In addition, many older adults are less sensitive to high environmental temperatures than are younger adults and are less likely to increase fluid intake.

COLLABORATIVE MANAGEMENT

Assessment

The client with heat stroke initially sweats excessively and may complain of a headache and lightheadedness. As the condition worsens, he or she stops sweating and becomes unconscious. The skin is very warm and dry. Some clients will have a flushed appearance but, when dehydration is severe, no flush is evident. The heart rate is rapid and thready. The blood pressure, both systolic and diastolic, is low. Skin surface temperatures are elevated. Ear or rectal temperatures are very high, often exceeding 107° F (42° C). *This situation is a life-*

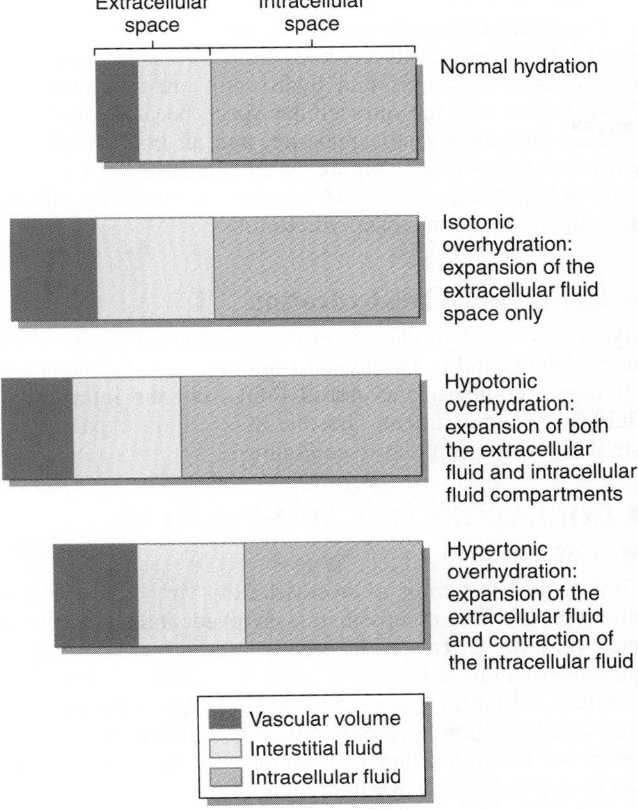

Figure 12-5 ● Three types of overhydration. (© 1992 M. Linda Workman. All rights reserved.)

threatening emergency. The client should be taken to the nearest emergency department or intensive care unit; however, interventions must be initiated at the scene.

Interventions

The focus of therapy is to reduce the client's body temperature and restore fluid volume. After determining a patent airway, the first priority is to cool the client. All clothing is removed. If possible, the client is taken immediately to an air-conditioned environment and placed in the position for shock with the legs elevated. If no air-conditioning is available, he or she is placed in the shade. Water is sprayed or poured on the client, and all surrounding personnel fan him or her. Ice packs are wrapped in cloth and positioned on the client's groin, head, and armpits.

Oxygen is administered by mask or nasal cannula. At least one IV line is started with a large-bore needle. When available, cooled normal saline (0.9% sodium chloride) is administered intravenously. Depending on how high the client's temperature is, cooled sterile saline may be administered by peritoneal lavage.

Vital signs, including rectal temperature, are monitored every 15 minutes until the client responds to therapy. An indwelling catheter is placed so that output can be monitored accurately. Depending on the severity of the client's condition, a pulmonary artery catheter may be needed to monitor hydration status.

CHART 12-6

KEY FEATURES *of* Overhydration

Manifestations of Overhydration in General

Cardiovascular
- Increased pulse rate
- Bounding pulse quality
- Peripheral pulses full
- Elevated blood pressure
- Decreased pulse pressure
- Elevated central venous pressure
- Distended neck and hand veins
- Engorged venous varicosities

Respiratory
- Respiratory rate increased
- Shallow respirations
- Dyspnea increases with exertion or in the supine position
- Moist crackles present on auscultation

Integumentary
- Pitting edema in dependent areas
- Skin pale and cool to touch

Neuromuscular
- Altered level of consciousness
- Headache
- Visual disturbances
- Skeletal muscle weakness
- Paresthesias

Gastrointestinal
- Increased motility

Manifestations of Isotonic Overhydration
- Liver enlargement
- Ascites formation

Manifestations of Hypotonic Overhydration
- Polyuria
- Diarrhea
- Nonpitting edema
- Cardiac dysrhythmias associated with electrolyte dilution
- Projectile vomiting

If interventions are started promptly, the client has a good chance for full recovery. Responses usually start to occur within half an hour. If vital signs remain poor in spite of intervention, extensive laboratory assessment may be needed to determine possible organ damage.

OVERHYDRATION

OVERVIEW

Overhydration, also called fluid overload, is an excess of body fluid. It is not an actual disease but rather a clinical sign of a physiologic problem in which fluid intake or retention is greater than the body's fluid needs. Overhydration may be either an actual excess of total body fluid or a relative fluid excess in one or more fluid compartments. The three basic types of fluid volume excess are isotonic overhydration, hypotonic overhydration, and hypertonic overhydration (Figure 12-5).

Most problems caused by overhydration are related to fluid volume excess in the vascular space or to dilution of specific electrolytes and blood components. Clinical manifestations vary with the type and degree of overhydration (Chart 12-6). The conditions leading to overhydration (fluid overload) are related to excessive intake or inadequate excretion of fluid. Table 12-5 lists common causes of overhydration.

Isotonic Overhydration

Isotonic overhydration is also called **hypervolemia** because the problems result from excessive fluid in the extracellular fluid (ECF) compartment. In isotonic overhydration, isotonic fluids are ingested or retained, so that osmolarity remains normal. Only the ECF compartment is expanded, and fluid does not shift between the extracellular and intracellular compartments. The problems caused by severe isotonic overhydration are circulatory overload and development of edema. Figure 12-6 outlines the compensatory mechanisms that occur in response to mild or moderate isotonic overhydration. When isotonic overhydration is severe, or when it occurs in a person with poor cardiac function, overhydration can lead to congestive heart failure and pulmonary edema.

TABLE 12-5 • COMMON CAUSES OF OVERHYDRATION

ISOTONIC OVERHYDRATION
- Poorly controlled IV therapy
- Renal failure
- Long-term corticosteroid therapy

HYPOTONIC OVERHYDRATION
- Early renal failure
- Congestive heart failure
- Syndrome of inappropriate antidiuretic hormone
- Poorly controlled IV therapy
- Replacement of isotonic fluid loss with hypotonic fluids
- Psychogenic polydipsia
- Irrigation of wounds and body cavities with hypotonic fluids

HYPERTONIC OVERHYDRATION
- Excessive sodium ingestion
- Rapid infusion of hypertonic saline
- Excessive sodium bicarbonate therapy

Hypotonic Overhydration

In hypotonic overhydration (water intoxication), the excess fluid is hypotonic to normal body fluids. Thus the osmolarity of the ECF decreases, and hydrostatic pressure increases. Fluid moves into the intracellular space because of the decreased vascular osmotic pressure, and all body fluid compartments expand (see Figure 12-5). Because the excessive fluid is hypotonic, electrolyte imbalances caused by dilution accompany hypotonic overhydration.

Hypertonic Overhydration

Hypertonic overhydration is rare and is caused by an excessive sodium intake. The hyperosmolarity of the plasma and interstitial compartments draws fluid from the intracellular fluid (ICF) compartment. Thus the ECF volume expands, and the ICF volume contracts (see Figure 12-5).

COLLABORATIVE MANAGEMENT

Assessment

Clinical manifestations of overhydration vary with the specific type, the fluid compartments involved, and the degree of overhydration. Clients with isotonic overhydration or hypertonic overhydration have signs and symptoms of circulatory overload and pitting edema (Figure 12-7). Clients with hypotonic overhydration have problems with cellular swelling and electrolyte dilution. Chart 12-6 summarizes the common clinical manifestations of overhydration.

A diagnosis of overhydration is based on assessment findings and the results of laboratory tests. In isotonic overhydration, serum electrolyte values are normal, but decreased hemoglobin, hematocrit, and serum protein levels may result from **hemodilution** (excessive water in the vascular compartment). Elevated levels of most electrolytes, along with increased blood urea nitrogen (BUN) and creatinine levels, accompany overhydration caused by kidney failure. Hypotonic

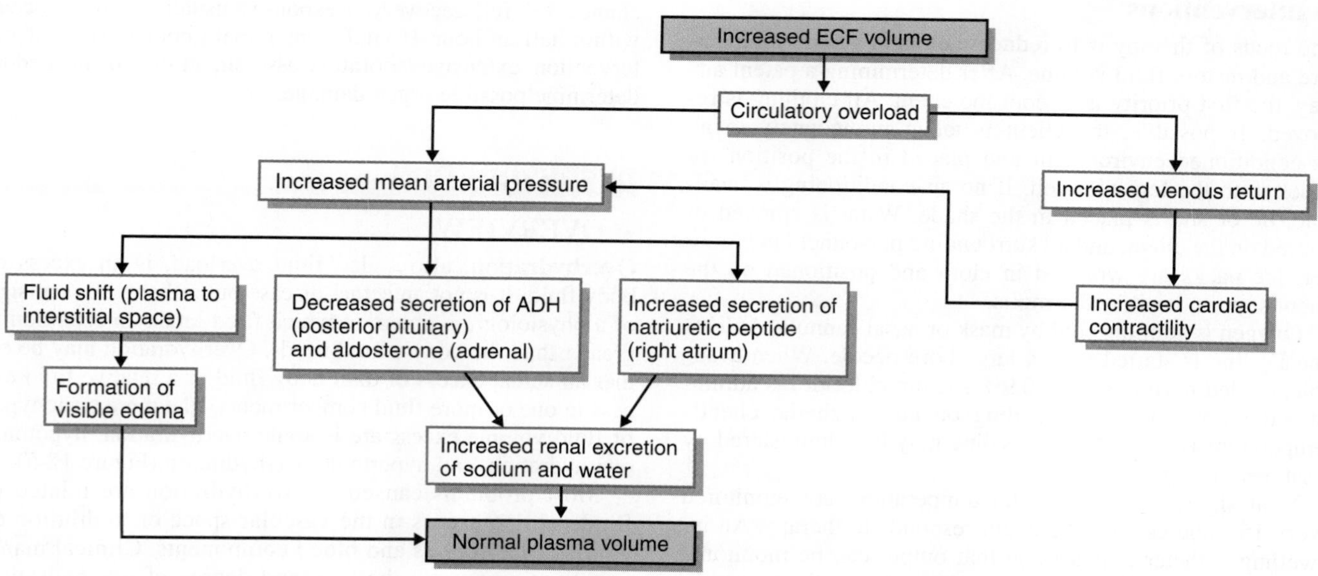

Figure 12-6 • Compensatory mechanisms associated with isotonic hypervolemia. (*ADH,* Antidiuretic hormone; *ECF,* extracellular fluid.)

overhydration is accompanied by a decreased complete blood count and decreased protein and electrolyte levels.

Interventions

Interventions for clients with fluid volume excess aim to restore normal fluid balance, provide supportive care until the imbalance is resolved, and prevent future fluid overload. Drug and diet therapies form the basis of intervention.

DRUG THERAPY. The health care provider may order diuretics for clients with overhydration if renal failure is not the cause. Diuretics work on the kidneys to increase the excretion of water or sodium from the body. Osmotic diuretics, such as mannitol (Osmitrol), are typically prescribed first to prevent severe electrolyte imbalances. If osmotic diuretics are not effective, high-ceiling (loop) diuretics, such as furosemide (Lasix, Furoside✤), may be prescribed.

The nurse monitors the client for response to medication, especially weight loss and increased urine output. The nurse also observes for signs and symptoms of electrolyte imbalance and assesses laboratory findings every 8 hours.

DIET THERAPY. For the client with mild or chronic overhydration, long-term diet therapy may be valuable in controlling fluid volume through restrictions of both fluid and sodium intake. The client's serum sodium concentration should be considered whenever overhydration is present.

MONITORING

Intake and Output. The nurse or assistive nursing personnel accurately measures fluid intake and output and explains the reason for any fluid restriction. In addition to regulating the total amount of fluid ingested in a 24-hour period, the nurse schedules fluid offerings throughout the 24 hours. Urine also is monitored for color, character, and specific gravity. If the client is receiving IV therapy, the nurse administers the exact amount ordered and monitors for increased fluid overload.

Weight. Fluid retention may not be visible. A sudden weight gain, however, indicates fluid retention. The nurse weighs the client at the same time every day (before breakfast), using the same scale. Whenever possible, the client wears the same type of clothing for each weigh-in.

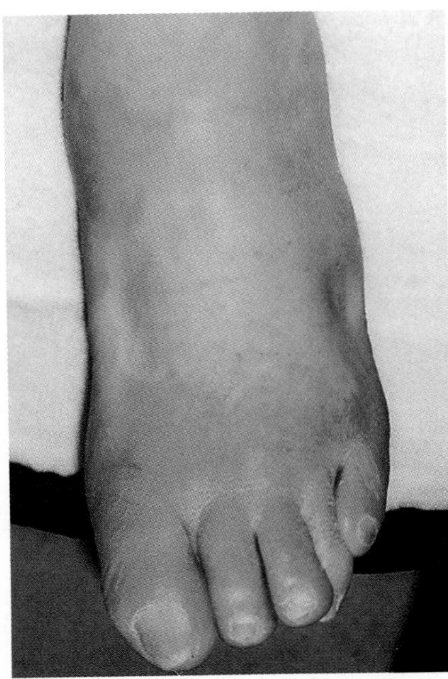

Figure 12-7 ● Pitting edema.

ONLINE RESOURCES

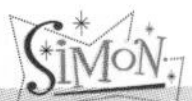

For suggested readings and Internet resources, go to http://www.wbsaunders.com/SIMON/Iggy/.

SELECTED BIBLIOGRAPHY

Asterisk indicates a classic or definitive work on this subject.

Armstrong, L., et al. (1998). Urinary indices during dehydration, exercise, and rehydration. *International Journal of Sports Nutrition, 8*(4), 345-355.

Cook, L. (1999). The value of lab values. *American Journal of Nursing, 99*(5), 66-75.

Day, M. (1997). Action stat: Heatstroke. *American Journal of Nursing, 97*(8), 33.

Edwards, S. (1998). Hypovolemia: Pathophysiology and management options. *Nursing in Critical Care, 3*(2), 73-82.

Epstein, Y., & Armstrong, L. (1999). Fluid-electrolyte balance during labor and exercise: Concepts and misconceptions. *International Journal of Sports Nutrition, 9*(1), 1-12.

Epstein, Y., et al.: (1999). Exertional heat stroke: A case series, *Medicine and Science in Sports and Exercise, 31*(2), 224-228.

Frizzell, J. (1998). Avoiding lab test pitfalls. *American Journal of Nursing, 98*(2), 34-38.

Gaspar, P. (1999). Water intake of nursing home residents. *Journal of Gerontological Nursing, 25*(4), 23-29.

Goldy, D. (1998). Emergency! Circulatory overload secondary to blood transfusion. *American Journal of Nursing, 98*(7), 33.

Gosling, P. (1999). Fluid balance in the critically ill: The sodium and water audit. *Care of the Critically Ill, 15*(1), 11-16.

Guyton, A., & Hall, J. (2000). *Textbook of medical physiology* (10th ed.). Philadelphia: W.B. Saunders.

Iggulden, H. (1999). Dehydration and electrolyte disturbance. *Nursing Standard, 13*(19), 48-56.

*Kokko, J., & Tannen, R. (1996). *Fluids and electrolytes* (3rd ed.). Philadelphia: W.B. Saunders.

Krau, S. (1998). Selecting and managing fluid therapy. *Critical Care Nursing Clinics of North America, 10*(4), 401-410.

Maughan, R. (1999). Dehydration, rehydration, and exercise in the heat. *Canadian Journal of Applied Physiology, 24*(2), 149-200.

McAlpine, L. (1998). CAVH: Principles and practical applications. *Critical Care Nursing Clinics of North America, 10*(2), 179-189.

McCloskey, J.C., & Bulechek, G.M. (2000). *Nursing interventions classification (NIC)* (3rd ed.). St. Louis: Mosby.

McConnell, E. (1999). A bedside laboratory: Point-of-care blood analyzers. *Dimensions of Critical Care Nursing, 18*(5), 24-26.

*Metheny, N. (1996). *Fluid and electrolyte balance: Nursing considerations* (3rd ed.) . Philadelphia: Lippincott-Raven.

Miekley, T.F. (1998). A patient-focused approach to managing diuretic therapy. *Critical Care Nursing Clinics of North America, 10*(4), 421-467.

*O'Donnell, M. (1995). Assessing fluid and electrolyte balance needs in elders. *American Journal of Nursing, 95*(1), 41-46.

Pagana, K.D., & Pagana, T.J. (1999). *Diagnostic testing and nursing implications: A case study approach* (5th ed.). St. Louis: Mosby.

Stark, J. (1998a). A comprehensive analysis of the fluid and electrolytes system. *Critical Care Nursing Clinics of North America, 10*(4), 471-475.

Stark, J. (1998b). Interpretation of BUN and serum creatinine. *Critical Care Nursing Clinics of North America, 10*(4), 491-496.

*Tietz, N.W. (Ed.). (1995). *Clinical guide to laboratory tests* (3rd ed.). Philadelphia: W.B. Saunders.

Toto, K. (1998). Fluid balance assessment: The total perspective. *Critical Care Nursing Clinics of North America, 10*(4), 383-400.

Trissel, L. (1998). *Handbook on injectable drugs* (10th ed.). Bethesda, MD: American Society of Health Systems.

Trotto, N. (1999). Keeping dehydrated patients out of the hospital. *Patient Care, 33,* 81-82, 84, 89-90.

CHAPTER 13

Interventions for Clients with Electrolyte Imbalances

M. LINDA WORKMAN

Learning Objectives

After studying this chapter, you should be able to:

1. Identify clients at risk for imbalances of potassium.
2. Use laboratory data and clinical manifestations to determine the presence of potassium imbalance.
3. Prioritize nursing care for the client with potassium imbalance.
4. Develop a teaching plan to prevent deficiencies or excesses of potassium in the older adult client at risk for potassium imbalance.
5. Analyze changes in clinical manifestations to determine the effectiveness of therapy for the client with potassium imbalance.
6. Identify clients at risk for imbalances of sodium.
7. Use laboratory data and clinical manifestations to determine the presence of sodium imbalance.
8. Prioritize nursing care for the client with sodium imbalance.
9. Develop a teaching plan to prevent deficiencies or excesses of sodium in the older adult client at risk for sodium imbalance.
10. Analyze changes in clinical manifestations to determine the effectiveness of therapy for the client with sodium imbalance.
11. Identify clients at risk for imbalances of calcium.
12. Use laboratory data and clinical manifestations to determine the presence of calcium imbalance.
13. Prioritize nursing care for the client with calcium imbalance.
14. Develop a teaching plan to prevent deficiencies or excesses of calcium in the older adult client at risk for calcium imbalance.
15. Analyze changes in clinical manifestations to determine the effectiveness of therapy for the client with calcium imbalance.

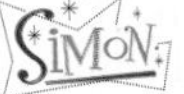

Go to http://www.wbsaunders.com/SIMON/Iggy/ for self-assessment questions related to these Learning Objectives.

All people are at some risk for electrolyte imbalances to some degree. Electrolyte imbalances can occur in healthy people as a result of variations in fluid intake and output. These imbalances are usually mild and are easily corrected without intervention from health care professionals. Severe electrolyte imbalances are life threatening and can occur in any setting. People at greatest risk for severe imbalances are older clients, clients with chronic renal or endocrine disorders, clients who are mentally impaired, and clients who are taking medications that alter fluid and electrolyte status.

POTASSIUM IMBALANCES

Hypokalemia

OVERVIEW

Because 98% of total body potassium (K^+) is intracellular, minor changes in extracellular potassium levels cause major changes in cell membrane excitability and in other cellular processes. **Hypokalemia** is a serum potassium level below 3.5 mEq/L (mmol/L). A relatively common electrolyte imbalance, hypokalemia is potentially life threatening because every body system can be affected.

Pathophysiology

Decreased serum potassium levels increase the difference in potassium concentration between the fluid inside the cells (**intracellular fluid [ICF]**), and the fluid outside the cells (**extracellular fluid (ECF]**). This increased difference reduces the excitability of cells. Consequently, the cell membranes of all excitable tissues, such as nerve and muscle, are less responsive to normal stimuli.

The severity of problems caused by hypokalemia is directly related to how rapidly the serum potassium level decreases. When the loss of extracellular potassium is gradual, cells adjust and intracellular potassium decreases in proportion to the ECF potassium level. In this situation, the potassium concentration difference between the two fluid compartments remains unchanged; symptoms of hypokalemia may

TABLE 13-1 • COMMON CAUSES OF HYPOKALEMIA

ACTUAL POTASSIUM DEFICITS

Excessive Potassium Loss
- Inappropriate or excessive use of drugs
  - Diuretics
  - Digitalis
  - Corticosteroids
- Increased secretion of aldosterone
  - Cushing's syndrome
- Diarrhea
- Vomiting
- Wound drainage (especially gastrointestinal)
- Prolonged nasogastric suction
- Heat-induced excessive diaphoresis
- Renal disease impairing reabsorption of potassium

Inadequate Potassium Intake
- Nothing by mouth

RELATIVE POTASSIUM DEFICITS

Movement of Potassium from Extracellular Fluid to Intracellular Fluid
- Alkalosis
- Hyperinsulinism
- Hyperalimentation
- Total parenteral nutrition

Dilution of Serum Potassium
- Water intoxication
- IV therapy with potassium-poor solutions

not appear until the potassium loss is extreme. Rapid changes in extracellular potassium levels (representing a more rapid loss of potassium) cannot be compensated for quickly and result in dramatic changes in body function.

Etiology

Hypokalemia may result either from an *actual* total body potassium loss or from the movement of potassium from the ECF to the ICF, causing a *relative* decrease in extracellular potassium level. Table 13-1 summarizes the common causes of hypokalemia.

Actual potassium depletion occurs when potassium loss is excessive or when potassium intake is not sufficient to match normal potassium loss. Relative hypokalemia occurs when total body potassium levels are normal but the potassium distribution between fluid compartments is abnormal. Conditions that increase the cellular uptake of potassium, leading to hypokalemia, include metabolic alkalosis and insulin administration.

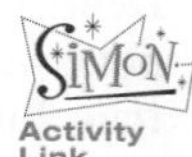

COLLABORATIVE MANAGEMENT

Assessment

HISTORY

The nurse collects data from clients at risk as well as from those with actual hypokalemia.

AGE. Age is an important consideration because renal capacity to concentrate urine decreases with aging, which increases potassium loss. Moreover, older adults are more likely to use medications that promote potassium loss.

CHART 13-1

KEY FEATURES *of* Hypokalemia

Cardiovascular Manifestations
- Variable pulse rate, more often rapid
- Pulse quality thready and weak
- Peripheral pulses difficult to palpate
- Orthostatic (postural) hypotension
- Electrocardiographic abnormalities
  - ST depression
  - Inverted T wave
  - Prominent U wave
  - Heart block

Respiratory Manifestations
- Shallow, ineffective respirations resulting from profound weakness of the skeletal muscles of respiration
- Diminished breath sounds

Neuromuscular Manifestations
- Anxiety, lethargy, confusion, coma
- Loss of tactile discrimination
- General skeletal muscle weakness
- Deep tendon hyporeflexia
- Eventual flaccid paralysis

Gastrointestinal Manifestations
- Decreased motility
- Hypoactive to absent bowel sounds
- Nausea
- Vomiting
- Abdominal distention
- Paralytic ileus
- Constipation

Renal Manifestations
- Decreased ability to concentrate urine
- Polyuria
- Decreased specific gravity

MEDICATION USE. The nurse asks the client about medication use, especially diuretics, corticosteroids, and beta-adrenergic agonists or antagonists. These drugs increase potassium loss through the kidneys. One of the most common causes of hypokalemia is the use and misuse of diuretics. In clients taking digoxin (Lanoxin, Novodigoxin♣), hypokalemia increases the sensitivity of the myocardium to the drug and may result in digoxin toxicity, even when the dosage is within the therapeutic range.

The nurse asks whether the client is taking a prescribed potassium supplement, such as potassium chloride (KCl). The client may not be taking the potassium chloride as prescribed because of its unpleasant taste.

OTHER FACTORS. Any acute or chronic disease state may lead to hypokalemia. The client is asked about recent illnesses and medical or surgical interventions. A thorough diet history, including a typical day's food and beverage intake, helps the nurse to identify clients at risk for hypokalemia.

PHYSICAL ASSESSMENT/CLINICAL MANIFESTATIONS

The clinical manifestations of hypokalemia are associated with the altered function of many systems (Chart 13-1).

MUSCULOSKELETAL MANIFESTATIONS. Skeletal muscles become weak in response to hypokalemia, and a stronger stimulus is needed to begin muscle contraction. A client may be so weak that he or she is unable to stand. Handgrasps are weak, and **hyporeflexia** (a decreased response to deep tendon reflex stimulation) may be noted. Severe hypokalemia can lead to flaccid paralysis. The nurse assesses the degree of muscle weakness and determines the client's ability to perform activities of daily living (ADLs).

RESPIRATORY MANIFESTATIONS. The respiratory system can be seriously affected by hypokalemia through the depression of the nerves and muscles needed for breathing. Weakness of the skeletal muscles of respiration results in shallow respirations. The nurse assesses the client's breath sounds, ease of respiratory effort, color of nail beds and mucous membranes, and rate and depth of respiration. Respiratory status is assessed at least every 2 hours because respiratory insufficiency often accompanies hypokalemia and is a major cause of death.

CARDIOVASCULAR MANIFESTATIONS. Cardiovascular changes often accompany hypokalemia. The nurse assesses the cardiovascular system by first palpating the peripheral pulses. In the client with hypokalemia, the pulse is usually thready and weak. Palpation is difficult, and the pulse is easily blocked with light pressure. The pulse rate ranges from excessively slow to excessively rapid, depending on whether a **dysrhythmia** (irregular heartbeat), especially premature ventricular contraction (PVC), is present. The nurse measures blood pressure with the client in the lying, sitting, and standing positions because orthostatic (postural) hypotension accompanies hypokalemia.

NEUROLOGIC MANIFESTATIONS. The neurologic manifestations of hypokalemia include changes in mental status. The client may experience short-term irritability and anxiety followed by lethargy that progresses to confusion and coma as hypokalemia worsens. Severe hypokalemia decreases sensory awareness. For example, the client may not be able to identify mild sensations of pain, touch, heat, and cold.

GASTROINTESTINAL MANIFESTATIONS. Hypokalemia decreases smooth muscle contractions within the gastrointestinal system, which leads to decreased peristalsis. The affected client has hypoactive bowel sounds and may experience nausea, vomiting, constipation, and abdominal distention. The nurse assesses distention by measuring abdominal girth. Bowel sounds are assessed in all four abdominal quadrants to determine the extent of decreased peristalsis. Severe hypokalemia can cause **paralytic ileus** (the absence of peristalsis).

CRITICAL THINKING CHALLENGE

Your client, an 86-year-old nursing home resident, states that she feels nauseated and constipated at breakfast. She has been taking digoxin and furosemide (Lasix) for 10 years for chronic congestive heart failure.

- Which vital sign would you assess first?
- What laboratory values would you examine to determine:
  The specific electrolyte imbalance?
  Whether the imbalance represents an electrolyte loss or electrolyte dilution?
- What other assessment data would you gather?

For suggested answer guidelines, go to SIMON http://www.wbsaunders.com/SIMON/Iggy/.

PSYCHOSOCIAL ASSESSMENT

Behavioral changes caused by hypokalemia usually occur within a short period. Information about the client's behavior may need to be obtained from close family members or friends, depending on the client's condition.

The nurse collects data about the onset and duration of behavioral changes as well as their association with any other physical signs and symptoms. The client may be lethargic and unable to perform simple problem-solving tasks that require concentration, such as counting backward from 100 by threes. As hypokalemia progresses, the client may become increasingly confused, especially to time and place. In severe hypokalemia, coma may develop.

LABORATORY ASSESSMENT

Hypokalemia is confirmed by a serum potassium value below 3.5 mEq/L (mmol/L). However, this value alone does not determine whether potassium loss has occurred or whether potassium has moved from the blood into the cells.

OTHER DIAGNOSTIC ASSESSMENTS

The health care provider may order a baseline electrocardiogram (ECG) and continuous cardiac monitoring for a client with severe hypokalemia. Hypokalemia causes electrical conduction abnormalities in the heart, including ST-segment depression, flat or inverted T waves, and increased U waves. Dysrhythmias can result in death, particularly in older adults who are taking digoxin.

Analysis

COMMON NURSING DIAGNOSES AND COLLABORATIVE PROBLEMS

The following are priority nursing diagnoses for clients with hypokalemia:

1. Risk for Injury related to skeletal muscle weakness
2. Constipation related to smooth muscle atony

The primary collaborative problem is High Risk for Ineffective Breathing Pattern related to neuromuscular impairment.

ADDITIONAL NURSING DIAGNOSES AND COLLABORATIVE PROBLEMS

In addition to the common nursing diagnoses and collaborative problems, clients with hypokalemia may have one or more of the following:

- Impaired Physical Mobility related to skeletal muscle weakness
- Total Self-Care Deficit related to skeletal muscle weakness
- Decreased Cardiac Output related to dysrhythmia

CHART 13-2

NIC INTERVENTION ACTIVITIES *for* The Client with Hypokalemia

Electrolyte Management: Hypokalemia: *Promotion of potassium balance and prevention of complications resulting from serum potassium levels lower than desired*

- Monitor lab values associated with hypokalemia (e.g., elevated glucose, metabolic alkalosis, reduced urine osmolality, urine potassium, hypochloremia, and hypocalcemia).
- Administer prescribed supplemental potassium (PO, NG, or IV), per policy.
- Prevent/reduce irritation from potassium supplement (e.g., administer PO or NG potassium supplements during or after meals to minimize GI irritation, dilute IV potassium adequately, administer IV supplement slowly, and apply topical anesthetic to IV site), as appropriate.
- Administer potassium-sparing diuretics (e.g., spironolactone [Aldactone] or triamterene [Dyrenium]), as appropriate.
- Avoid administration of alkaline substances (e.g., IV sodium bicarbonate and PO or NG antacids), as appropriate.
- Monitor neurologic manifestations of hypokalemia (e.g., muscle weakness, altered level of consciousness, drowsiness, apathy, lethargy, confusion, and depression).
- Monitor cardiac manifestations of hypokalemia (e.g., hypotension, broad T wave, U wave, ectopy, tachycardia, and weak pulse).
- Monitor renal manifestations of hypokalemia (e.g., acidic urine, reduced urine osmolality, nocturia, polyuria, and polydipsia).
- Monitor GI manifestations of hypokalemia (e.g., anorexia, nausea, cramps, constipation, distension, and paralytic ileus).
- Monitor pulmonary manifestations of hypokalemia (e.g., hypoventilation and respiratory muscle weakness).
- Monitor for symptoms of respiratory failure (e.g., low Pao_2 and elevated $Paco_2$ levels and respiratory muscle fatigue).
- Monitor for rebound hyperkalemia.
- Provide food rich in potassium (e.g., salt substitutes, dried fruits, bananas, green vegetables, tomatoes, yellow vegetables, chocolate, and dairy products), as appropriate.

NIC intervention activities selected from McCloskey, J.C., & Bulechek, G.M. (Eds.). (2000). *Nursing intervention classification (NIC)* (3rd ed.). St. Louis: Mosby. No part of this work is to be altered without prior written permission from the Publisher.

GI, Gastrointestinal; Pao_2, partial pressure of arterial oxygen; $Paco_2$, partial pressure of arterial carbon dioxide.

Planning and Implementation

RISK FOR INJURY

PLANNING: EXPECTED OUTCOMES. The client with hypokalemia is expected to avoid injury and have a return to a normal serum potassium level.

INTERVENTIONS

NIC ELECTROLYTE MANAGEMENT: HYPOKALEMIA. Interventions for hypokalemia aim to prevent potassium loss, increase serum potassium levels, and provide a safe environment for the client (Chart 13-2). Drug and diet therapies help to restore normal serum potassium levels.

DRUG THERAPY. Drug therapies for the treatment and prevention of hypokalemia include additional potassium and drugs to prevent potassium loss.

Potassium Supplements. Most potassium supplements are potassium chloride, potassium gluconate, potassium citrate, or a combination of these salts. The amount and the route of potassium replacement depend on the degree of potassium loss. A client with a serum potassium level of 3 mEq/L needs 100 to 200 mEq of potassium supplement; a client with a serum potassium level of 2.0 mEq/L needs 500 to 600 mEq (Tannen, 1996).

Potassium is given intravenously for severe hypokalemia. A dilution of no more than 1 mEq/10 mL of solution is recommended. *The maximum recommended infusion rate is 5 to 10 mEq/hr; this rate is never to exceed 20 mEq/hr under any circumstances.* Older clients may not be able to handle this rate. Because the rapid infusion of potassium can cause cardiac arrest, potassium is seldom given by intravenous (IV) push.

Potassium is a severe tissue irritant and is never administered as an intramuscular or subcutaneous injection. Tissues damaged by potassium can become necrotic and slough, leading to a loss of function and requiring reconstructive surgery. IV potassium solutions irritate veins and can cause phlebitis. The nurse checks the orders carefully to ensure that the client receives the correct amount of potassium. The IV site is assessed every 2 hours, and the client is asked whether he or she feels burning or pain at the site. The IV solution is stopped immediately if infiltration occurs.

Oral potassium preparations may be administered as liquids or solids. Potassium chloride has a strong, unpleasant taste that is difficult to mask. Because potassium chloride can cause nausea and vomiting, it should not be taken on an empty stomach.

Potassium-Sparing Diuretics. Diuretics that increase the renal excretion of potassium commonly cause hypokalemia. These classes of diuretics include high-ceiling (loop) diuretics (e.g., furosemide [Lasix, Furoside✦], bumetanide [Bumex], and ethacrynic acid [Edecrin]) and the thiazide diuretics (chlorothiazide [Diuril], hydrochlorothiazide [Esidrix, HydroDIURIL, Urozide✦], and quinethazone [Hydromox]). These drugs are avoided in clients with actual hypokalemia and in those who are at risk for hypokalemia. A potassium-sparing diuretic may be appropriate for clients with hypokalemia who require diuretic therapy. Potassium-sparing diuretics increase urine output without increasing potassium excretion. Potassium-sparing diuretics include spironolactone (Aldactone, Novospiroton✦), triamterene (Dyrenium), and amiloride (Midamor).

DIET THERAPY. The nurse consults with the dietitian in teaching the client how to increase dietary potassium intake. Eating foods that are naturally rich in potassium helps to restore normal potassium levels and prevent further loss. Table 11-7 lists the potassium content of common foods.

SAFETY MEASURES. For a client with muscle weakness from hypokalemia, the nurse uses safety measures, eliminates hazards, and assists with ambulation. Obstacles or slippery areas are removed from the ambulation path, and the client wears nonslip footgear. When ambulating with assistance, the client wears a gait belt around the waist.

CRITICAL THINKING CHALLENGE

Your client has been diagnosed as having actual hypokalemia. Her morning dose of Lasix has been withheld, and she has been prescribed to receive 20 mEq of potassium gluconate/potassium citrate (Twin K) suspension in 4 ounces of fruit juice four times daily. Two hours after her first dose of oral potassium, her vital signs are as follows: pulse, 64 (thready but regular); blood pressure (in the sitting position), 108/50; and respirations, 28 and shallow.

- What assessment data would you need to determine whether or not her electrolyte balance is improving?
- What activities might need to be modified until her serum potassium level is normal?

For suggested answer guidelines, go to SIMON http://www.wbsaunders.com/SIMON/Iggy/.

CONSTIPATION

NOC **PLANNING: EXPECTED OUTCOMES.** The client with hypokalemia is expected to experience a restoration of a normal bowel elimination pattern.

INTERVENTIONS. Interventions aim to restore normal serum potassium levels and induce gastric motility. Specific interventions include drug and diet therapies to restore serum potassium levels to normal values (discussed earlier under Drug Therapy and Diet Therapy [Risk for Injury], p. 176), stimulate intestinal peristalsis, and prevent constipation.

DRUG THERAPY. Laxatives that add bulk or fiber may be used to stimulate peristalsis. Other drugs that enhance gastric emptying and stimulate gastrointestinal motility, such as metoclopramide (Reglan, Maxeran♣), are used to treat constipation associated with hypokalemia.

DIET THERAPY. The nurse provides high-fiber foods and plenty of liquids for the client who is not on fluid restrictions. To ensure cooperation, the nurse prepares a list of foods that contain high concentrations of fiber and asks the client to select favorite items from that list.

COMFORT MEASURES. The nurse or assistive nursing personnel can help in maintaining normal bowel elimination patterns in several ways. Privacy is provided when the client uses the toilet or bedpan. The door is closed, privacy curtains are drawn, and visitors are asked to step out of the room. Because physical activity promotes gastric motility, the client is encouraged to ambulate whenever his or her condition permits. A bedridden client benefits from frequent position changes and mild bed exercises.

CRITICAL THINKING CHALLENGE

Your nursing home client with hypokalemia tells you that she does not eat the fruits on her meal trays because they are too hard to chew.

- What modifications would you make to increase her dietary intake of potassium?

For suggested answer guidelines, go to SIMON http://www.wbsaunders.com/SIMON/Iggy/.

INEFFECTIVE BREATHING PATTERN

NOC **PLANNING: EXPECTED OUTCOMES.** The client with hypokalemia is expected to have a breathing pattern adequate to maintain gas exchange.

INTERVENTIONS. The nurse monitors the client's respiratory rate and depth at least once per hour, noting in particular increased rate and decreased depth. The effectiveness of the respiratory muscles can also be determined by assessing the client's ability to cough. The face, oral mucosa, and nail beds are examined for pallor or cyanosis. The nurse evaluates arterial blood gas values for **hypoxemia** (decreased blood oxygen concentration) and **hypercapnia** (increased arterial carbon dioxide concentration). Chapters 27 and 28 discuss respiratory assessment and interventions in more detail.

Community-Based Care

No extensive home care preparations are necessary for clients with mild hypokalemia or sudden-onset hypokalemia. The imbalance is corrected before discharge and, with minimal precautions, is unlikely to recur. Clients with chronic pathologic conditions or diseases are most likely to be discharged before the imbalance is completely corrected and are susceptible to recurrent episodes of imbalance. These clients often require long-term diet and drug therapy. Health teaching for prevention and early detection is a major nursing responsibility.

The nurse instructs the at-risk client (especially one receiving diuretics or corticosteroids) regarding the proper use of medications, the signs and symptoms of hypokalemia, when to seek medical help, and foods rich in potassium. The client also is taught to assess the rate, rhythm, and quality of the peripheral pulses at least once each day and whenever any signs or symptoms of hypokalemia are present. For clients at chronic risk for hypokalemia, the nurse reinforces how often serum potassium levels should be checked.

A home care aide may be needed to assist with hygiene and ensure a safe environment. Weekly visits by a nurse may also be needed to assess changes and ensure compliance with the medication regimen. At every home visit to a client at risk for hypokalemia, the nurse performs a focused assessment (Chart 13-3). Medications, the signs and symptoms of hypokalemia, and health care resources are reviewed with the client and family.

Evaluation: Outcomes

NOC The nurse evaluates the care of the client with hypokalemia on the basis of the identified nursing diagnoses and collaborative problems. The expected outcomes are that the client will:

- Return to and maintain a normal serum potassium level (between 3.5 and 5.0 mEq/L)
- Comply with prescribed drug and diet therapies
- Identify the early signs and symptoms of hypokalemia
- Avoid injury
- Have normal bowel elimination patterns
- Maintain adequate gas exchange
- Maintain regular cardiac rate and rhythm

CHART 13-3

FOCUSED ASSESSMENT *of* Home Care Clients at Risk for Hypokalemia

Assess respiratory status.
- Rate, depth, rhythm of respiration
- Color of lips, tongue, nail beds
- Can the client complete a sentence without taking a breath?

Assess cardiovascular status.
- Vital signs, including apical pulse, pulse pressure, presence or absence of orthostatic hypotension, and quality and rhythm of peripheral pulses
- Presence or absence of peripheral edema
- Hand vein filling in the dependent position
- Neck vein filling in the recumbent and sitting positions
- Weight gain or loss

Assess cognition and mental status.
- Level of consciousness
- Orientation to time, place, and person
- Can the client accurately read a seven-word sentence containing no words greater than three syllables?

Assess condition of skin and mucous membranes.
- Presence or absence of skin tenting over the sternum or the forehead
- Moistness of skin, most reliable on chest and back
- Presence or absence of coating on tongue or teeth
- Can the client spit?

Assess neuromuscular status.
- Reactivity of patellar and biceps reflexes
- Oral temperature
- Handgrip strength
- Steadiness of gait

Assess renal system.
- Observe urine specimen for color, odor, cloudiness, and amount.

Ask about the following:
- 24-hour fluid intake and output
- 24-hour diet recall
- 24-hour activity recall
- What over-the-counter and prescribed medications has the client taken?
- Has the client experienced any dizziness or lightheadedness?
- Does the client have a headache (what time of day, associated with what activities)?
- Muscle twitches, cramps, pain, or spasms

Assess the client's understanding of illness and compliance with treatment.
- Signs and symptoms to report to health care provider
- Medication plan (correct timing and dose)

Hyperkalemia

OVERVIEW

Hyperkalemia is a serum potassium level greater than 5.0 mEq/L (mmol/L). Because the range of normal serum potassium values is narrow, even slight increases above normal values can have serious adverse effects on the physiologic function of excitable tissues, especially the heart.

Pathophysiology

An elevated serum potassium level decreases the potassium concentration difference between the intracellular fluid (ICF) and the extracellular fluid (ECF). This decreased difference increases cell excitability; as a result, excitable tissues respond to less intense stimuli and may even discharge spontaneously.

TABLE 13-2 • COMMON CAUSES OF HYPERKALEMIA

ACTUAL POTASSIUM EXCESSES

Excessive Potassium Intake
- Overingestion of potassium-containing foods or medications
  - Salt substitutes
  - Potassium chloride
- Rapid infusion of potassium-containing IV solution
- Bolus IV potassium injections

Decreased Potassium Excretion
- Adrenal insufficiency (Addison's disease, adrenalectomy)
- Renal failure
- Potassium-sparing diuretics

RELATIVE POTASSIUM EXCESSES

Movement of Potassium from Intracellular Fluid to Extracellular Fluid
- Tissue damage
- Acidosis
- Hyperuricemia
- Hypercatabolism
- Uncontrolled diabetes mellitus

Hyperkalemia alters the function of all excitable membranes to some degree. The excitable membrane in the heart is most sensitive to serum potassium increases, and therefore the more serious complications of hyperkalemia are associated with altered cardiac function.

The pathologic changes associated with hyperkalemia are directly related to how rapidly ECF potassium levels increase. Sudden increases in serum potassium levels cause severe functional changes at potassium levels between 6 and 7 mEq/L. When serum potassium levels increase slowly, problems with excitable membrane function may not be obvious until potassium levels reach 8 mEq/L or higher.

Hyperkalemia may result from an actual increase in the amount of total body potassium or from the movement of potassium from the cells into the blood. Table 13-2 summarizes the common causes of hyperkalemia.

Hyperkalemia is rare in people with normal kidney function. Most cases of hyperkalemia occur in hospitalized clients and in those undergoing medical treatment. Those at greatest risk for hyperkalemia are chronically ill clients, debilitated clients, and older adults.

➤ COLLABORATIVE MANAGEMENT

Assessment

The client's age is an important factor because renal function decreases with aging. The nurse asks about chronic illnesses (particularly renal disease and diabetes mellitus), recent medical or surgical interventions, and urine output, including frequency and amount of voidings. The nurse also inquires about medication use, particularly potassium-sparing diuretics. A diet history is obtained to determine the intake of potassium-rich foods or the use of salt substitutes, many of which contain potassium.

The nurse collects data regarding symptoms related to hyperkalemia. The client is asked if he or she has experienced palpitations, skipped heartbeats, other cardiac irregularities, muscle twitching, weakness in the leg muscles, and unusual tingling or numbness in the hands, feet, or face. The nurse in-

CHART 13-4

KEY FEATURES *of* Hyperkalemia

Cardiovascular Manifestations
- Irregular heart rate, usually slow
- Decreased blood pressure
- Electrocardiographic abnormalities
  - Tall T waves
  - Widened QRS complexes
  - Prolonged PR intervals
  - Flat P waves
- Ectopic beats
- Late: dysrhythmias, ventricular fibrillation, cardiac arrest in diastole

Respiratory Manifestations
- Unaffected until late, when profound weakness of the skeletal muscles causes respiratory failure

Neuromuscular Manifestations
- Early phase, or mild, hyperkalemia
  - Muscle twitches, cramps
  - Paresthesias
- Late phase, or severe, hyperkalemia
  - Profound weakness
  - Ascending flaccid paralysis in distal to proximal direction; involves the arms and legs

Gastrointestinal Manifestations
- Increased motility
- Hyperactive bowel sounds
- Diarrhea

quires about recent changes in bowel habits, especially diarrhea, colic, and explosive bowel movements.

PHYSICAL ASSESSMENT/CLINICAL MANIFESTATIONS

The clinical manifestations of hyperkalemia are summarized in Chart 13-4. Cardiovascular changes are the most severe results of hyperkalemia and are the most common cause of death in clients with hyperkalemia (Chmielewski, 1998). Cardiac manifestations of hyperkalemia include bradycardia, hypotension, and electrocardiographic (ECG) changes of tall, peaked T waves, prolonged PR intervals, flat or absent P waves, and wide QRS complexes (Figure 13-1). As serum potassium levels rise, **ectopic beats** (beats generated outside the normal conduction system in the ventricles) may appear. Complete heart block, ventricular standstill, and ventricular fibrillation are major life-threatening complications of severe hyperkalemia.

The neuromuscular response to hyperkalemia has two phases. Skeletal muscles twitch in the early stages of hyperkalemia, and the client may be aware of unusual nerve sensations (e.g., tingling and burning) that are followed by numbness in the hands and feet and around the mouth **(paresthesia).** As hyperkalemia progresses, muscle twitching changes to weakness followed by flaccid paralysis. The weakness ascends from the distal to the proximal areas and initially affects the muscles of the arms and legs. Trunk, head, and respiratory muscles are not affected until serum potassium levels reach lethal levels.

The smooth muscle of the gastrointestinal tract responds to hyperkalemia by increasing peristalsis. As a result, the client may experience diarrhea and spastic colonic activity.

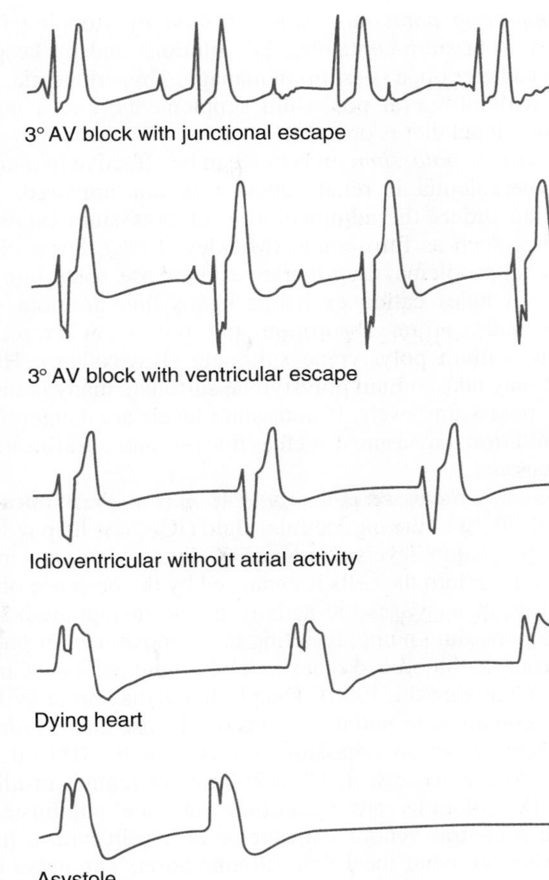

Figure 13-1 ● ECG changes associated with hyperkalemia. (Modified with permission from John M. Clochesy.)

The nurse listens to bowel sounds and observes stools. Bowel sounds are hyperactive, with frequent audible rushes and gurgles. Bowel movements may be frequent, watery, and explosive.

LABORATORY ASSESSMENT

A serum potassium value greater than 5.0 mEq/L confirms hyperkalemia. If hyperkalemia results from dehydration, levels of other serum electrolytes, hematocrit, and hemoglobin may be elevated. Hyperkalemia associated with renal failure is usually accompanied by elevated levels of serum creatinine and blood urea nitrogen, decreased blood pH, and normal or low hematocrit and hemoglobin levels.

Interventions

NIC **ELECTROLYTE MANAGEMENT: HYPERKALEMIA.** Interventions for hyperkalemia are aimed at immediately reducing the serum potassium level. Drug therapy is useful for restoring normal potassium balance by eliminating potassium administration, enhancing potassium excretion, and promoting the movement of potassium from the extracellular fluid (ECF) into the cells. Monitoring the client's response to intervention is another major nursing responsibility (Chart 13-5).

Eliminating potassium administration by stopping infusions of potassium-containing IV solutions and by keeping the IV catheter open is useful in managing hyperkalemia. The nurse withholds oral potassium supplements, and a potassium-restricted diet is ordered.

Increasing potassium excretion can be effective in managing hyperkalemia if renal function is not impaired. The physician orders the administration of potassium-excreting diuretics, such as furosemide (Miekley, 1998). For a client with renal problems, drug therapy to increase potassium excretion includes cation exchange resins that promote gastrointestinal sodium absorption and potassium excretion, such as sodium polystyrene sulfonate (Kayexalate). However, it may take sodium polystyrene sulfonate many hours to reduce potassium levels. If potassium levels are dangerously high, additional measures, such as dialysis and ultrafiltration, are necessary.

Promoting the movement of potassium from the extracellular fluid (ECF) to the intracellular fluid (ICF) can help reduce serum potassium levels temporarily. Potassium movement from the ECF into the cells is enhanced by the presence of insulin. Insulin increases the activity of the membrane-bound sodium-potassium pump, resulting in the movement of potassium from the blood and other ECFs into the cell (see Chapter 11) (Chmielewski, 1998). The physician may order IV fluids that contain substantial amounts of glucose and insulin to help decrease serum potassium levels (usually 100 mL of 10% to 20% glucose with 10 to 20 units of regular insulin). These IV solutions are hypertonic and are administered through a central venous catheter or in a vein with a high blood flow to avoid local vein inflammation. The nurse observes the client for signs and symptoms of hypokalemia and hypoglycemia during this therapy.

CHART 13-5

NIC INTERVENTION ACTIVITIES *for* The Client with Hyperkalemia

Electrolyte Management: Hyperkalemia: *Promotion of potassium balance and prevention of complications resulting from serum potassium levels higher than desired*

- Administer electrolyte-binding and electrolyte-excreting resins (e.g., Kayexalate) as prescribed, if appropriate.
- Monitor lab values for changes in oxygenation or acid-base balance, as appropriate.
- Administer prescribed medications to shift potassium into the cell (e.g., 50% dextrose and insulin, sodium bicarbonate, calcium chloride, and calcium gluconate), as appropriate.
- Avoid potassium-sparing medications (e.g., spironolactone [Aldactone] and triamterene [Dyrenium]), as appropriate.
- Maintain potassium restrictions.
- Administer prescribed diuretics, as appropriate.
- Monitor fluid status, including intake and output, as appropriate.
- Monitor potassium levels after diuresis.
- Monitor cardiac manifestations of hyperkalemia (e.g., decreased cardiac output, heart blocks, peaked T waves, fibrillation, or systole).
- Respond to cardiac arrest.

NIC intervention activities selected from McCloskey, J.C., & Bulechek, G.M. (Eds.). (2000). *Nursing interventions classification (NIC)* (3rd ed.). St. Louis: Mosby. No part of this work is to be altered without prior written permission from the Publisher.

Cardiac monitoring can help to prevent lethal dysrhythmias and allow for the early recognition of signs and symptoms of the adverse response of cardiac muscle. The nurse compares recent ECG tracings with the client's baseline tracings or with tracings obtained when the client's serum potassium level was close to normal.

Health teaching is a key factor in the prevention of hyperkalemia and in the early detection of its life-threatening complications. The teaching plan for the client at risk for hyperkalemia includes diet, medications, and recognition of the signs and symptoms of hyperkalemia. Diet education includes knowledge of foods to avoid (those high in potassium) and permissible foods containing little potassium (Chart 13-6). The nurse instructs the client to examine the labels on

CHART 13-6

CLIENT EDUCATION GUIDE
Dietary Management of Hyperkalemia

You Should Avoid

- Meats, especially organ meat and preserved meat
- Dairy products
- Dried fruit
- Fruits high in potassium
  - Bananas
  - Cantaloupe
  - Kiwi
  - Oranges
- Vegetables high in potassium
  - Avocados
  - Broccoli
  - Dried beans or peas
  - Lima beans
  - Mushrooms
  - Potatoes (white or sweet)
  - Seaweed
  - Soybeans
  - Spinach

You May Eat

- Eggs
- Breads
- Butter
- Cereals
- Sugar
- Fruits low in potassium (fresh, frozen, or canned)
  - Apples
  - Apricots
  - Berries
  - Cherries
  - Grapefruit
  - Peaches
  - Pineapple
  - Cranberries
- Vegetables low in potassium
  - Alfalfa sprouts
  - Cabbage
  - Carrots
  - Cauliflower
  - Celery
  - Eggplant
  - Green beans
  - Lettuce
  - Onions
  - Peas
  - Peppers
  - Squash

Data from Pennington, J. (1998). *Bowe's and Church's food values of portions commonly used* (17th ed.). Philadelphia: Lippincott-Raven.

medications and food packages to determine the potassium content and to avoid salt substitutes, which usually contain potassium.

SODIUM IMBALANCES

Hyponatremia

OVERVIEW

Hyponatremia is a serum sodium (Na^+) level below 135 mEq/L (mmol/L). Because sodium is the major cation of the blood and interstitial fluid and maintains the osmolarity of these fluids, sodium imbalances are often associated with fluid volume imbalances.

Pathophysiology

The pathologic changes caused by hyponatremia involve two mechanisms. The first mechanism is a change in cell excitability or activity. As the concentration of sodium in the blood and other extracellular fluid decreases, the difference in sodium concentration between the extracellular fluid (ECF) and the intracellular fluid (ICF) also decreases. Less sodium is available to move across the excitable membrane, causing delayed and slower membrane depolarization. The second mechanism is the movement of water from the ECF space into the ICF space. Cells swell, and their functions are impaired.

Etiology

Many conditions can lead to hyponatremia by causing either an actual or a relative decrease in sodium content (Table 13-3). Hyponatremia can result from the loss of total body sodium, the movement of sodium from the blood to other fluid spaces (such as in burns, extensive inflammatory responses, or severe crushing injuries), or the dilution of serum sodium as a result of excessive water in the plasma.

TABLE 13-3 • COMMON CAUSES OF HYPONATREMIA

ACTUAL SODIUM DEFICITS
Increased Sodium Excretion
- Excessive diaphoresis
- Diuretics (high-ceiling diuretics)
- Wound drainage (especially gastrointestinal)
- Decreased secretion of aldosterone
- Hyperlipidemia
- Renal disease (scarred distal convoluted tubule)

Inadequate Sodium Intake
- Nothing by mouth
- Low-salt diet

RELATIVE SODIUM DEFICITS
Dilution of Serum Sodium
- Excessive ingestion of hypotonic fluids
- Psychogenic polydipsia
- Freshwater drowning
- Renal failure (nephrotic syndrome)
- Irrigation with hypotonic fluids
- Syndrome of inappropriate antidiuretic hormone secretion
- Hyperglycemia
- Congestive heart failure

WOMEN'S HEALTH CONSIDERATIONS
Hyponatremia as a complication during early postoperative recovery has a relatively high occurrence in the United States, ranging from 1% to 5%. Although this complication occurs with equal frequency among men and women, more women develop brain damage and die from coma or seizure activity.

➤ COLLABORATIVE MANAGEMENT

Assessment

The clinical manifestations of hyponatremia are caused by its effects on excitable cellular activity. The cells especially affected are those involved in cerebral, neuromuscular, and gastric smooth muscle functions (Chart 13-7).

CEREBRAL MANIFESTATIONS

Changes in cerebral function are the most obvious signs and symptoms of hyponatremia. Because these changes may be seen as either depressed activity or excessive activity (and sometimes both), establishing the client's usual cerebral func-

CHART 13-7

KEY FEATURES *of* Hyponatremia

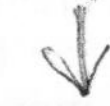

Cardiovascular Manifestations*
- Normovolemic
  - Rapid pulse rate
  - Normal blood pressure
- Hypovolemic
  - Rapid pulse rate
  - Pulse quality thready and weak
  - Hypotension
  - Central venous pressure normal or low
  - Flat neck veins
- Hypervolemic
  - Rapid, bounding pulse
  - Central venous pressure normal or elevated
  - Blood pressure normal or elevated

Respiratory Manifestations
- Late manifestations related to skeletal muscle weakness
  - Shallow, ineffective respiratory movements
- Hypervolemia
- Pulmonary edema
  - Rapid, shallow respiration
  - Moist crackles

Neuromuscular Manifestations
- Generalized skeletal muscle weakness
- Diminished deep tendon reflexes

Cerebral Manifestations
- Personality changes
- Headache

Renal Manifestations
- Increased urine output
- Decreased specific gravity

Gastrointestinal Manifestations
- Increased motility
- Nausea
- Hyperactive bowel sounds
- Diarrhea

*Symptoms vary with changes in vascular volume.

tion and behavioral patterns is essential to detecting the changes caused by hyponatremia. Behavioral changes result from cerebral edema and increased intracranial pressure. The nurse closely observes and documents the client's behavior and level of consciousness.

NEUROMUSCULAR MANIFESTATIONS

The client's neuromuscular status is assessed during each nursing shift for changes from baseline values. The neuromuscular response to hyponatremia is generalized muscle weakness. Muscle tone and deep tendon reflexes diminish.

Muscle weakness occurs bilaterally and is worse in the extremities. The nurse assesses deep tendon reflexes by lightly tapping the patellar (knee) tendons and Achilles (heel) tendons with a reflex hammer and documenting the degree of reflex movement. The technique for assessing motor strength and reflexes is described in depth in Chapter 41.

GASTROINTESTINAL MANIFESTATIONS

The smooth muscle of the gastrointestinal system responds to decreased serum sodium levels with increased motility, causing nausea, diarrhea, and abdominal cramping. The gastrointestinal system is assessed by listening to bowel sounds and observing stools. Bowel sounds are hyperactive, with frequent rushes and gurgles, especially over the splenic flexure and in the lower left quadrant. Bowel movements are frequent, watery, and explosive. Peristaltic movements may be palpated through the abdominal wall and may even be visible on the abdominal surface.

CARDIOVASCULAR MANIFESTATIONS

Hyponatremia has little direct effect on cardiac muscle contractility; however, alterations in cardiac output are associated with hyponatremia. When hyponatremia is accompanied by changes in blood volume, these fluid changes alter cardiac function. In general, the cardiac responses to hyponatremia with accompanying **hypovolemia** (decreased plasma volume, or fluid deficit) are a rapid, weak, thready pulse. Peripheral pulses are difficult to palpate and are easily blocked with light pressure. Neck veins may be flat when the client is in the supine position. Blood pressure, especially diastolic pressure, is decreased. The client may experience severe hypotension when moving from a lying or sitting position to a standing position. The central venous pressure is low.

When hyponatremia is accompanied by **hypervolemia** (increased plasma volume or fluid excess), cardiac manifestations include a rapid, full pulse. Blood pressure is normal or elevated. Central venous pressure is normal or elevated depending on how well the left ventricle handles the extra fluid. Peripheral pulses are full and difficult to block; however, the peripheral pulses may not be palpable if edema is present.

Interventions

NIC **ELECTROLYTE MANAGEMENT: HYPONATREMIA.** Interventions with drug therapy and diet therapy aim to restore serum sodium levels to normal values and prevent further decreases in serum sodium levels (Chart 13-8).

CHART 13-8

NIC INTERVENTION ACTIVITIES *for* The Client with Sodium Imbalances

Electrolyte Management: Hyponatremia: *Promotion of sodium balance and prevention of complications resulting from serum sodium levels lower than desired*

- Monitor for electrolyte imbalances associated with hyponatremia (e.g., hypokalemia, metabolic acidosis, and hypoglycemia), as appropriate.
- Monitor for renal loss of sodium (oliguria).
- Monitor intake and output.
- Weigh daily and monitor trends.
- Monitor for indications of fluid overload/retention (e.g., crackles, elevated CVP or pulmonary capillary wedge pressure, edema, neck vein distension, and ascites), as appropriate.
- Administer hypertonic (3% to 5%) saline at 3 mL/kg/hr or per policy for rapid correction of hyponatremia, as appropriate.
- Maintain fluid restriction, as appropriate.
- Monitor for neurologic and/or neuromuscular manifestations of hyponatremia (e.g., lethargy, ICP, confusion, headache, seizures, coma, fatigue, tremors, apprehension, muscle weakness, and hyperreflexia).
- Monitor for cardiac manifestations of hyponatremia (e.g., elevated blood pressure, cold and clammy skin, and hypo- or hypervolemia).

Electrolyte Management: Hypernatremia: *Promotion of sodium balance and prevention of complications resulting from serum sodium levels higher than desired*

- Monitor for indications of dehydration (e.g., decreased sweating, decreased urine, decreased skin turgor, and dry mucous membranes).
- Monitor vital signs, as appropriate.
- Weigh daily and monitor trends.
- Provide comfort measures to decrease thirst.
- Maintain patent IV access.
- Monitor intake and output.
- Provide frequent oral hygiene.
- Administer isotonic (0.9%) saline, hypotonic (0.45%) saline, hypotonic (5%) dextrose, or diuretics, as appropriate, based on fluid status and urine osmolality.
- Maintain sodium restrictions.

NIC intervention activities selected from McCloskey, J.C., & Bulechek, G.M. (Eds.). (2000). *Nursing interventions classification (NIC)* (3rd ed.). St. Louis: Mosby. No part of this work is to be altered without prior written permission from the Publisher.
CVP, Central venous pressure; *ICP,* intracranial pressure.

DRUG THERAPY. Drug therapy can restore serum sodium levels to normal. Drug therapy regimens vary depending on whether or not fluid imbalance accompanies hyponatremia and how fast the imbalance has developed. In chronic or asymptomatic hyponatremia, sodium is replaced slowly and carefully.

When hyponatremia occurs with a fluid deficit (hypovolemia), the physician orders IV saline infusions to restore both sodium content and fluid volume. Severe hyponatremia may be treated with small-volume infusions of hypertonic (2% to 3%) saline. The infusions are delivered through a controller to prevent accidental increases in infusion rate. The nurse monitors the infusion rate and the client's response.

When hyponatremia is accompanied by fluid excess, drug therapy includes the administration of osmotic diuretics that primarily promote the excretion of water rather than sodium, such as mannitol (Osmitrol). The nurse assesses the client hourly for signs of an excessive loss of fluids or potassium and for dramatic increases in sodium levels.

TABLE 13-4 • COMMON CAUSES OF HYPERNATREMIA

ACTUAL SODIUM EXCESSES

Decreased Sodium Excretion
- Hyperaldosteronism
- Renal failure
- Corticosteroids
- Cushing's syndrome

Increased Sodium Intake
- Excessive oral sodium ingestion
- Excessive administration of sodium-containing IV fluids

RELATIVE SODIUM EXCESSES

Decreased Water Intake
- Nothing by mouth

Increased Water Loss
- Increased rate of metabolism
- Fever
- Hyperventilation
- Infection
- Excessive diaphoresis
- Watery diarrhea
- Dehydration

Drug therapy for hyponatremia caused by inappropriate secretion of antidiuretic hormone (ADH) includes agents that antagonize ADH, such as lithium and demeclocycline (Declomycin).

DIET THERAPY. Diet therapy can help to restore normal sodium balance in mild hyponatremia. Table 11-6 lists the sodium content of common foods. The nurse collaborates with the dietitian in teaching the client about which foods to increase in the diet. Therapy consists of increasing oral sodium intake and restricting oral fluid intake. Fluid restriction may be a long-term regimen when overhydration with oral fluids is the cause of the hyponatremia or when renal fluid excretion is impaired. The nurse or assistive nursing personnel measures fluid intake and output and reinforces the purpose of the fluid restriction.

Hypernatremia

OVERVIEW

Hypernatremia is a serum sodium level greater than 145 mEq/L. Increased serum sodium levels can be caused by or can cause changes in fluid volumes. Table 13-4 lists the common causes of hypernatremia.

As the extracellular sodium level rises, a larger difference in sodium concentration occurs between the extracellular fluid (ECF) and the intracellular fluid (ICF). More sodium is available to move rapidly across cell membranes. With mild hypernatremia, almost all excitable tissues are excited more easily. This condition is called **irritability** and causes excitable tissues to overrespond to stimuli. In addition, the osmolarity of the ECF also increases as the concentration of extracellular sodium increases. This situation causes water to move from the cells into the ECF as a compensatory action to dilute the hyperosmolar ECF. Therefore when hypernatremia persists or worsens, the compensatory action causes severe cellular dehydration, and excitable tissues may no longer be able to respond to stimuli.

CHART 13-9

KEY FEATURES *of* Hypernatremia

Cardiovascular Manifestations
- Decreased myocardial contractility
- Diminished cardiac output
- Heart rate and blood pressure respond to vascular volume

Respiratory Manifestations
- Problems associated with pulmonary edema when hypernatremia is accompanied by hypervolemia

Central Nervous System Manifestations*
- Hypernatremia and normovolemia or hypovolemia
  - Increased neural activity
  - Agitation, confusion, seizures
- Hypernatremia and hypervolemia
  - Decreased neural activity
  - Lethargy, stupor, coma

Neuromuscular Manifestations
- Mild or early hypernatremia
  - Spontaneous muscle twitches
  - Irregular contractions
- Severe or late hypernatremia
  - Skeletal muscle weakness
  - Diminished or absent deep tendon reflexes

Renal Manifestations
- Decreased urine output
- Increased specific gravity

Integumentary Manifestations
- Dry, flaky skin
- Presence or absence of edema related to accompanying fluid volume changes

*Upper neural function changes are related to volume changes as well as sodium increases.

COLLABORATIVE MANAGEMENT

Assessment

The clinical manifestations of hypernatremia vary with the severity of imbalance and whether a fluid imbalance is also present. Rapid increases in serum sodium level generally cause more obvious and severe symptoms. Gradual increases in serum sodium levels may produce no observable physical changes, even when sodium levels increase to ranges that are well above normal. The clinical manifestations of hypernatremia involve changes in cell membrane activity, especially among excitable tissues involved in cerebral, neuromuscular, and cardiac functions (Chart 13-9).

CENTRAL NERVOUS SYSTEM MANIFESTATIONS

Altered cerebral function is the most common manifestation of hypernatremia. The nurse assesses the client's mental status in terms of attention span, recall of recent events, and ability to perform cognitive functions. In hypernatremia with normal or decreased fluid volumes, the client may have a short attention span and be agitated or confused about recent events. Manic episodes or seizures may occur if serum sodium concentration continues to increase. When hypernatremia is accompanied by a blood volume overload, the client may be lethargic, drowsy, stuporous, and even comatose.

NEUROMUSCULAR MANIFESTATIONS

Skeletal muscles respond differently to various degrees of hypernatremia. Mild hypernatremia causes muscle twitching and irregular muscle contractions. As hypernatremia worsens, the muscles and nerves are less able to respond to a stimulus. The muscles become progressively weaker and show rigid paralysis. Deep tendon reflexes are reduced or absent. Muscle weakness associated with hypernatremia occurs bilaterally and has no specific pattern. Neuromuscular status is assessed by observing for twitching in muscle groups. The nurse also assesses muscle strength by having the client perform handgrip and arm flexion against resistance. Peripheral nerve responses are assessed by lightly tapping the patellar (knee) tendons and Achilles (heel) tendons with a reflex hammer and measuring the degree of movement.

CARDIOVASCULAR MANIFESTATIONS

Increased serum sodium levels slow the movement of calcium into the heart cells, which decreases contractility. The nurse assesses cardiovascular status by measuring blood pressure and the rate and quality of the apical and peripheral pulses. Pulse rate and blood pressure may be normal, above normal, or below normal during hypernatremia, depending on the fluid volume and the speed with which the imbalance occurs.

Pulse rate is increased in clients with hypernatremia and hypovolemia. Peripheral pulses may be difficult to palpate and are easily blocked with light pressure. Hypotension and severe orthostatic (postural) hypotension are present, and pulse pressure is greatly diminished.

Clients with hypernatremia and hypervolemia have slow to normal bounding pulses. Peripheral pulses are full and difficult to block. Neck veins are distended, even with the client in the upright position. Blood pressure, especially diastolic blood pressure, is increased.

Interventions

NIC **ELECTROLYTE MANAGEMENT: HYPERNATREMIA.** Drug therapy and diet therapy aim to prevent further increases in serum sodium levels and decrease elevated serum sodium levels (see Chart 13-8). Other interventions used when hypernatremia becomes life threatening include hemodialysis, peritoneal dialysis, and blood ultrafiltration.

DRUG THERAPY. When hypernatremia is caused by fluid loss, drug therapy is used to restore fluid balance. The physician orders hypotonic IV infusions, usually 0.225% or 0.45% sodium chloride. Hypernatremia caused by fluid and sodium losses may necessitate fluid replacement with IV administration of isotonic sodium chloride (NaCl) solutions. Hypernatremia caused by inadequate renal excretion of sodium requires drug therapy with diuretics that promote sodium loss, such as furosemide (Lasix, Furoside♣), bumetanide (Bumex), and ethacrynic acid (Edecrin). The nurse assesses the client hourly for symptoms that indicate an excessive loss of fluids, sodium, or potassium.

DIET THERAPY. Mild hypernatremia can be prevented or corrected by ensuring adequate water intake among older adults or those who may not have self-access to water. Dietary sodium restriction may be needed to prevent hypernatremia when renal problems are present. In addition, fluids must often be restricted. The nurse collaborates with the dietitian in helping the client to understand how to determine the sodium content of foods, beverages, and medications, as well as the importance of complying with the diet.

CALCIUM IMBALANCES

Hypocalcemia

OVERVIEW

Hypocalcemia is a total serum calcium (Ca^{2+}) level below 9.0 mg/dL or 2.25 mmol/L. Calcium is stored in bone, with only a small fraction of total body calcium present in extracellular fluid (ECF). Because the normal serum level of calcium is so low, small changes in serum calcium levels have major effects on body function.

Pathophysiology

Calcium ions decrease the permeability of excitable membranes to sodium ions, thereby preventing spontaneous depolarization. Calcium is a membrane stabilizer, regulating depolarization and the generation of action potentials. Low serum calcium levels increase the permeability of excitable membranes to sodium, and as a result depolarization occurs more easily and at inappropriate times.

Excitable tissues vary in their sensitivity to low serum calcium levels. Peripheral nerves, skeletal muscles, cardiac muscle, and gastrointestinal smooth muscle are most sensitive to decreased serum calcium levels. The severity of the manifestations associated with hypocalcemia depends on the degree of calcium imbalance.

Hypocalcemia also has pathologic effects on bone. Bone is the primary storage site for calcium and can release calcium into the blood when needed. Excessive calcium loss from bone can weaken bone. Chronic hypocalcemia leads to progressive osteoporosis, which decreases bone density and makes the bones more susceptible to fracture or deformity. (See Chapter 51 for a discussion of osteoporosis.)

Etiology

Hypocalcemia can be caused by many chronic and acute pathologic states as well as specific medical or surgical treatments. Table 13-5 lists the common causes of hypocalcemia.

Actual calcium loss (a reduction in total body calcium) occurs when the absorption of calcium from the gastrointestinal tract is inhibited or when calcium is lost from the body. Relative calcium loss causes total body calcium concentration to remain normal while serum calcium levels are too low. This type of hypocalcemia occurs when the free or ionized (unbound) calcium in the body is reduced or when parathyroid gland function is decreased.

CULTURAL CONSIDERATIONS

Many African-American and Asian clients have a lactose intolerance caused by a deficiency of the enzyme lactase. These clients cannot use the nutrients present in milk and experience cramping, diarrhea, and abdominal pain after ingesting dairy products. Dairy products, especially milk, are a common and rich source of calcium and vitamin D. Therefore clients with lactose intolerance may experience difficulty in obtaining enough calcium and vitamin D from other sources to maintain normal calcium levels in the blood and bones.

WOMEN'S HEALTH CONSIDERATIONS

Postmenopausal women are susceptible to a loss of total body calcium. This occurrence appears to be related to reduced weight-bearing activities and a decrease in sex hormone (estrogen) levels. In general, women are smaller framed than men, and therefore the female skeleton does not experience as much weight bearing as the male skeleton. As they age, many women also decrease weight-bearing activities such as running and walking. Osteoporosis occurs when weight-bearing activity decreases or is limited. In addition, the estrogen secretion that protects against osteoporosis diminishes. All of these factors increase the risk for calcium loss in postmenopausal women.

CONSIDERATIONS FOR OLDER ADULTS

Older adults are at risk for most electrolyte imbalances. Major organs and body systems undergo changes with aging. For example, older adults have a smaller fluid volume per body weight than younger adults, and therefore any variation in fluid volumes or electrolyte levels leads to imbalances more quickly. They are also more likely to be taking prescription or over-the-counter medications that affect fluid or electrolyte balance. Some older adults have dietary calcium or vitamin D deficits because of economic conditions or general problems with obtaining, preparing, or eating food.

COLLABORATIVE MANAGEMENT

Assessment

The diet history is a critical factor in assessing for the risk of hypocalcemia. The nurse asks the client about his or her intake of calcium-containing foods and whether a calcium supplement is taken regularly (see Table 11-8).

One indicator of hypocalcemia is a report of frequent, painful muscle spasms ("charley horses") in the calf or foot during periods of inactivity or sleep. Other information that can alert the nurse to a possible risk of hypocalcemia is a history of recent orthopedic surgery or bone healing. Endocrine disturbances and treatments are risk factors for hypocalcemia. A history of thyroid surgery, therapeutic irradiation of the upper middle chest and neck area, or a recent anterior neck injury predisposes the client to hypocalcemia. The most common clinical manifestations of hypocalcemia are caused by overstimulation of the nerves and muscles (Chart 13-10).

NEUROMUSCULAR MANIFESTATIONS

The client usually notices symptoms first in the limbs, with distal to proximal movement from the hands and feet. Paresthesias may be noted initially, with sensations of tingling alternating with sensations of numbness. If hypocalcemia continues or worsens, these sensations may progress to actual muscle twitching or painful cramps and spasms. Paresthesias may also affect the lips, nose, and ears. These symptoms sig-

TABLE 13-5 • COMMON CAUSES OF HYPOCALCEMIA

ACTUAL CALCIUM DEFICITS

Inhibition of Calcium Absorption from the Gastrointestinal Tract
- Inadequate oral intake of calcium
- Lactose intolerance
- Malabsorption syndromes
  - Celiac sprue
  - Crohn's disease
- Inadequate intake of vitamin D
- End-stage renal disease

Increased Calcium Excretion
- Renal failure—polyuric phase
- Diarrhea
- Steatorrhea
- Wound drainage (especially gastrointestinal)

RELATIVE CALCIUM DEFICITS

Conditions That Decrease the Ionized Fraction of Calcium
- Hyperproteinemia
- Alkalosis
- Calcium chelators or binders
  - Citrate
  - Mithramycin
  - Penicillamine
  - Sodium cellulose phosphate (Calcibind)
  - Aredia
- Acute pancreatitis
- Hyperphosphatemia
- Immobility

Endocrine Disturbances
- Removal or destruction of parathyroid glands
  - Thyroidectomy
  - Irradiation of thyroid
  - Strangulation
  - Neck injuries

CHART 13-10

KEY FEATURES *of* Hypocalcemia

Cardiovascular Manifestations
- Decreased heart rate
- Decreased myocardial contractility
- Diminished peripheral pulses
- Hypotension
- Electrocardiographic abnormalities
  - Prolonged ST interval
  - Prolonged QT interval

Respiratory Manifestations
- Not directly affected
- Respiratory failure or arrest can result from decreased respiratory movement because of muscle tetany or seizure activity

Neuromuscular Manifestations*
- Anxiety, irritability, psychosis
- Paresthesias followed by numbness
- Irritable skeletal muscles—twitches, cramps, tetany, seizures
- Hyperactive deep tendon reflexes
- Positive Trousseau's sign
- Positive Chvostek's sign

Gastrointestinal Manifestations
- Increased gastric motility
- Hyperactive bowel sounds
- Abdominal cramping
- Diarrhea

*The neuromuscular system is most profoundly affected by hypocalcemia.

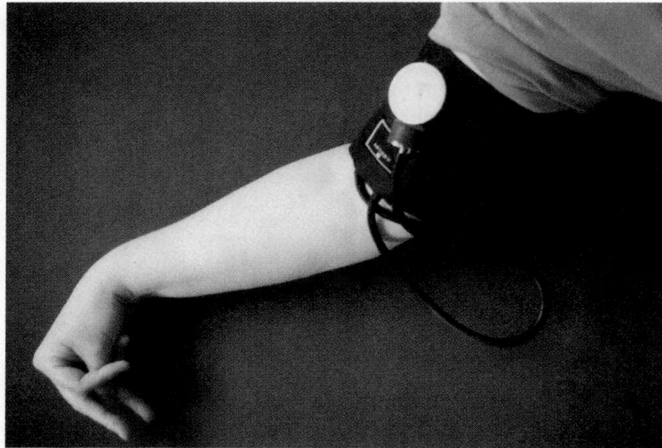

Figure 13-2 ● Palmar flexion—positive Trousseau's sign in hypocalcemia.

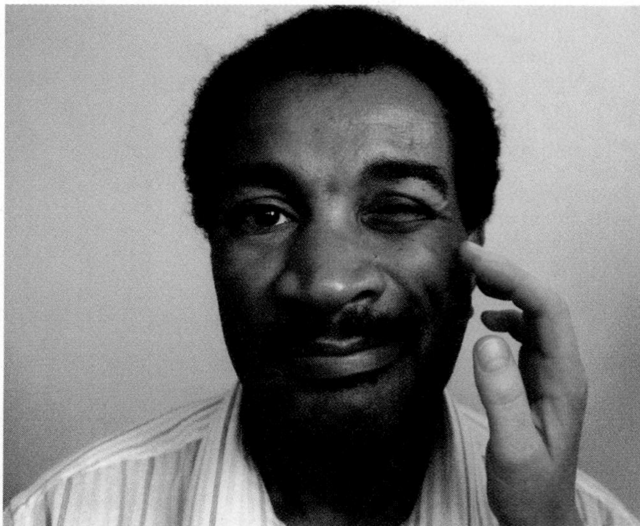

Figure 13-3 ● Facial muscle response—positive Chvostek's sign in hypocalcemia.

nal the approach of serious neuromuscular overstimulation and tetany.

The nurse assesses for hypocalcemia by testing for **Trousseau's** and **Chvostek's signs.** To test for Trousseau's sign, the nurse places a blood pressure cuff around the upper arm, inflates the cuff to greater than the client's systolic pressure, and keeps the cuff inflated for 1 to 4 minutes. Under these hypoxic conditions, a positive Trousseau's sign occurs if the hand and fingers go into spasm in palmar flexion (Figure 13-2). To test for Chvostek's sign, the nurse taps on the face just below and anterior to the ear (over the facial nerve) to trigger facial twitching of one side of the mouth, nose, and cheek (Figure 13-3).

CARDIOVASCULAR MANIFESTATIONS

With hypocalcemia, the heart rate may be slower or slightly faster than normal, with a weaker contraction and a decreased pulse quality. Severe hypocalcemia causes severe hypotension and electrocardiographic (ECG) changes, including a prolonged ST interval and a prolonged QT interval.

CHART 13-11

NIC INTERVENTION ACTIVITIES *for* The Client with Calcium Imbalances

Electrolyte Management: Hypocalcemia: *Promotion of calcium balance and prevention of complications resulting from serum calcium levels lower than desired*

- Monitor trends in serum levels of calcium (e.g., ionized calcium), as available.
- Monitor fluid status, including intake and output, as appropriate.
- Administer appropriate prescribed calcium salt (e.g., calcium carbonate, calcium chloride, and calcium gluconate), as indicated.
- Monitor for side effects of IV administration of ionized calcium (e.g., calcium chloride), such as thrombophlebitis, soft tissue damage with extravasation, clotting, and thrombus formation, as appropriate.
- Encourage intake of calcium (e.g., dairy products, seafood, nuts, broccoli, spinach, and supplements), as appropriate.
- Provide adequate intake of vitamin D (e.g., vitamin supplement and organ meats) to facilitate GI absorption of calcium, as appropriate.
- Monitor for neuromuscular manifestations of hypocalcemia (e.g., tetany, muscle twitching, cramping, grimacing, seizure, altered deep tendon reflexes, and spasm).
- Monitor for cardiovascular manifestations of hypocalcemia (e.g., decreased contractility, decreased cardiac output, hypotension, lengthened ST segment, and prolonged QT interval).
- Monitor for overcorrection and hypercalcemia.

Electrolyte Management: Hypercalcemia: *Promotion of calcium balance and prevention of complications resulting from serum calcium levels higher than desired*

- Monitor intake and output.
- Monitor trends in serum levels of calcium (e.g., ionized calcium), as available.
- Monitor for fluid overload resulting from hydration therapy (e.g., daily weight, urine output, jugular vein distention, lung sounds, and right atrial pressure), as appropriate.
- Monitor for neuromuscular manifestations of hypocalcemia (e.g., weakness, malaise, paresthesias, myalgia, hypotonia, decreased deep tendon reflexes, and poor coordination).
- Administer indomethacin (Indocin), calcitonin, or plicamycin (Mithracin), as appropriate.
- Encourage mobilization to prevent bone resorption.
- Monitor for recurring hypercalcemia 1 to 3 days after cessation of therapeutic measures.

NIC intervention activities selected from McCloskey, J.C., & Bulechek, G.M. (Eds.). (2000). *Nursing interventions classification (NIC)* (3rd ed.). St. Louis: Mosby.
GI, Gastrointestinal.

GASTROINTESTINAL MANIFESTATIONS

Hypocalcemia increases peristaltic activity. The nurse auscultates the abdomen for hyperactive bowel sounds. The client may report painful abdominal cramping and diarrhea.

Interventions

NIC **ELECTROLYTE MANAGEMENT: HYPOCALCEMIA.** Interventions aim to prevent further decreases in serum calcium levels, restore normal serum calcium levels, and prevent complications (Chart 13-11). Appropriate interventions in-

CHART 13-12

DRUG THERAPY *for* Hypocalcemia

Drug	Precautions
ORAL CALCIUM SUPPLEMENTS	
Calcium carbonate Calcium citrate Calcium gluconate Calcium lactate	Dose must be increased in older clients because of decreased intestinal absorption. Use with thiazide diuretics can increase the risk for hypercalcemia. Use with phenytoin decreases the bioavailability of both drugs; phenytoin should not be given within 3 hours of calcium administration.
INTRAVENOUS CALCIUM	
Calcium acetate Calcium chloride Calcium gluconate	All must be administered slowly, not to exceed 27 g/min. Clients should be monitored for electrocardiographic changes during administration. Observe the client for infiltration; calcium is a severe tissue irritant/vesicant. There is a potential for hypercalcemia and hypomagnesemia. The injection should be warmed to body temperature before administration.
AGENTS THAT INCREASE CALCIUM ABSORPTION	
Aluminum hydroxide	This agent reduces serum phosphorus levels, causing the countereffect of increasing calcium levels; there is a potential for hypophosphatemia. Signs and symptoms include bradycardia, decreased deep tendon reflexes, shortness of breath, and confusion.
Vitamin D Alfacalcidol♣ Calcifediol Calcitriol Dihydrotachysterol	This agent increases the intestinal absorption of calcium; there is a potential for hypercalcemia. This is a fat-soluble vitamin and is stored to some degree; there is a risk for vitamin D toxicity resulting in renal failure and/or cardiac failure.
AGENTS THAT REDUCE NERVE AND SKELETAL MUSCLE EXCITABILITY	
Magnesium sulfate	This agent is a tissue irritant; the preferred route of administration is intravenous. There is a potential for hypermagnesemia; signs and symptoms of toxicity include bradycardia, flushing, headache, nausea, vomiting, shortness of breath, hypotension.
Methocarbamol Robaxin Carbacot Metaxalone Skelaxin Orphenadrine Banflex Flexoject Myolin Diazepam Valium Vivol♣ E-pam♣ Carisoprodol Soma Vanadom	These agents act at the level of the central nervous system to decrease skeletal muscle activity. All have some sedative effect. All have some risk for psychologic dependency and abuse.

clude drug therapy, diet therapy, reduction of environmental stimuli, and prevention of injury.

DRUG THERAPY. Drug therapy for hypocalcemia consists of direct calcium supplements or replacements, drugs that enhance the absorption of calcium, and drugs that decrease the response of nerves and muscles to overstimulation. Chart 13-12 lists the different drug types used to manage hypocalcemia.

DIET THERAPY. A high-calcium diet is indicated for clients with mild hypocalcemia and for those with chronic conditions that cause them to be at continuous risk for hypocalcemia. The nurse and dietitian assist the client in selecting calcium-rich foods. The calcium content of common foods is listed in Table 11-8.

REDUCTION OF ENVIRONMENTAL STIMULI. The excitable membranes of both the nervous system and the skeletal system are overstimulated in hypocalcemia. Therefore the nurse provides an environment that reduces the stimulation of these systems.

PREVENTION OF INJURY. The nurse uses seizure precautions for the client with hypocalcemia. Such precautions include padding the siderails of the bed and keeping emergency equipment (e.g., oxygen and suction) at the bedside. An emergency cart equipped with emergency drugs and an

TABLE 13-6 • COMMON CAUSES OF HYPERCALCEMIA

ACTUAL CALCIUM EXCESSES

Increased Calcium Absorption
- Excessive oral intake of calcium
- Excessive oral intake of vitamin D

Decreased Calcium Excretion
- Renal failure
- Use of thiazide diuretics

RELATIVE CALCIUM EXCESSES

Increased Bone Resorption of Calcium
- Hyperparathyroidism
- Malignancy
  - Direct invasion (cancers of breast, lung, prostate, and osteoclastic bone and multiple myeloma)
  - Indirect resorption (liver cancer, small cell lung cancer, and cancer of the adrenal gland)
- Hyperthyroidism
- Immobility
- Use of glucocorticoids

Hemoconcentration
- Dehydration
- Use of lithium
- Adrenal insufficiency

endotracheal tray is positioned just outside the client's room.

The client with long-standing calcium loss may have brittle, fragile bones that fracture at only slight provocation and cause little pain. When lifting or moving a client with fragile bones, the nurse and assistive nursing personnel use a lift sheet rather than pull or grasp the client directly. The nurse also observes for normal range of joint motion and for any unusual surface projections or depressions over bony areas.

Hypercalcemia

OVERVIEW

Hypercalcemia occurs when the total serum calcium level exceeds 10.5 mg/dL or 2.75 mmol/L. Because the normal range for serum calcium is so narrow, even small increases can have severe effects on body function. Although the effects of hypercalcemia are most noticeable in body systems that depend on cell excitability, all body systems are affected to some degree.

Hypercalcemia indicates either that the amount of serum calcium is so great that the normal calcium-regulating mechanisms are overburdened or that at least one calcium-regulating mechanism is not functioning properly. Hypercalcemia causes excitable tissues to be less sensitive to normal stimuli and therefore require a stronger stimulus to function. The excitable tissues that respond most to hypercalcemia are cardiac muscle tissue, nerve tissue, skeletal muscle, and gastrointestinal smooth muscle.

Calcium is a cofactor for many of the enzymes involved in the blood-clotting process. Hypercalcemia usually causes faster clotting times. Clots may form at inappropriate times and in inappropriate places. Excessive clotting related to hypercalcemia is more likely in vessels in which blood flow is slow or blocked.

Causes of hypercalcemia include increased absorption of calcium, decreased excretion of calcium, and increased bone resorption of calcium (Table 13-6).

CHART 13-13

KEY FEATURES *of* Hypercalcemia

Cardiovascular Manifestations
- Increased heart rate (early phase)
- Increased blood pressure
- Bounding, full peripheral pulses
- Electrocardiographic abnormalities
  - Shortened ST segment
  - Widened T wave
- Potentiation of digoxin-associated toxicities
- Decreased clotting time
- Late phase
  - Bradycardia
  - Cardiac arrest, sinus arrest

Respiratory Manifestations
- Ineffective respiratory movement related to profound skeletal muscle weakness

Neuromuscular Manifestations
- Disorientation, lethargy, coma
- Profound muscle weakness
- Diminished or absent deep tendon reflexes

Renal Manifestations
- Increased urine output
- Dehydration
- Formation of renal calculi

Gastrointestinal Manifestations
- Decreased motility
- Hypoactive bowel sounds
- Anorexia, nausea
- Abdominal distention
- Constipation

COLLABORATIVE MANAGEMENT

Assessment

The clinical manifestations of hypercalcemia are related to both the severity of the imbalance and how quickly the imbalance occurred. The client with a mild but rapidly occurring excess of serum calcium usually experiences more severe signs and symptoms than the client whose hypercalcemia is severe but has developed slowly. The body systems most affected by hypercalcemia include the cardiovascular, neuromuscular, gastrointestinal, and renal urinary systems (Chart 13-13).

CARDIOVASCULAR MANIFESTATIONS

The most serious and life-threatening clinical manifestations of hypercalcemia are changes in cardiac function. Mild hypercalcemia initially causes increased heart rate and blood pressure. Severe or prolonged hypercalcemia affects electrical conduction.

The nurse assesses cardiac status by measuring pulse rate and blood pressure and observing for indications of poor tissue perfusion such as cyanosis and pallor. ECG tracings are observed for indications of dysrhythmias, especially a shortened QT interval.

Although hypercalcemia does not directly cause the formation of blood clots, they do form more easily whenever abnormal conditions are present. Thus the client with hypercalcemia may be at increased risk for clot formation in areas of blood vessel or tissue damage and in vessels in which blood flow is blocked. Blood clotting is more likely in the lower legs, the pelvic region, areas where blood flow is blocked by internal or external constrictions, and regions where internal blood vessel obstruction occurs.

The nurse assesses each client at risk for hypercalcemia for indications of slowed or impaired blood flow. Calf circumferences are measured with a soft tape measure and recorded. The client is asked to alternately dorsiflex and plantar flex the ankles and state whether calf pain occurs in either position **(Homan's sign).** The nurse assesses the lower legs for temperature, color, and capillary refill to determine the adequacy of blood flow to and from the area.

NEUROMUSCULAR MANIFESTATIONS

The neuromuscular manifestations of hypercalcemia include severe muscle weakness and decreased deep tendon reflexes without accompanying paresthesia. Central nervous system manifestations include an altered level of consciousness that can range from disorientation and lethargy to coma. Psychiatric disturbances can occur with hypercalcemia.

GASTROINTESTINAL MANIFESTATIONS

Decreased peristalsis is an early manifestation of hypercalcemia. The client may report constipation, anorexia, nausea, vomiting, and abdominal pain. Bowel sounds are hypoactive or absent. The nurse assesses the gastrointestinal tract by auscultating for bowel sounds in all four abdominal quadrants. The abdomen increases in size because the intestinal contents remain in the gastrointestinal tract instead of being propelled to the outside. The nurse assesses abdominal size by measuring abdominal girth with a soft tape measure in a line circling the abdomen at the umbilicus.

RENAL MANIFESTATIONS

Hypercalcemia causes increased urine output and leads to dehydration. Chronic hypercalcemia may result in the formation of renal **calculi** (stones) in the kidney, because the excess calcium precipitates out of solution in a solid form. The nurse or assistive nursing personnel measures intake and output, assesses voided urine for blood or cloudiness, and strains the urine for the presence of stones.

Interventions

NIC **ELECTROLYTE MANAGEMENT: HYPERCALCEMIA.** Interventions for hypercalcemia aim to prevent further increases in serum calcium levels and decrease excessive serum calcium levels through drug therapy and dialysis (see Chart 13-11).

DRUG THERAPY. Drug therapy for the treatment of hypercalcemia restores calcium balance by preventing additional calcium administration and promoting calcium excretion. IV infusions of solutions containing calcium are stopped. In addition, the administration of oral drugs containing calcium or vitamin D (e.g., calcium-based antacids) is discontinued.

Fluid volume replacement alone can help to restore normal serum calcium levels. The physician usually orders IV normal saline (isotonic sodium chloride) because sodium increases the excretion of calcium in the urine.

Thiazide diuretics are discontinued for clients with hypercalcemia and are replaced with diuretics that enhance the excretion of calcium, such as furosemide (Lasix, Furoside♣).

Agents that act as calcium chelators (calcium binders) can be useful in lowering serum calcium levels. Such drugs include plicamycin (Mithracin) and penicillamine (Cuprimine, Pendramine♣).

Other drugs that are often useful in treating hypercalcemia include agents that inhibit calcium resorption from bone, such as phosphorus, calcitonin (Calcimar), biphosphonates (etidronate), and prostaglandin synthesis inhibitors (aspirin, nonsteroidal anti-inflammatory drugs).

DIALYSIS. In severe hypercalcemia that causes life-threatening cardiac problems, drug therapy may not reduce serum calcium levels fast enough to prevent death. Dialysis (either hemodialysis or peritoneal dialysis) or blood ultrafiltration may be necessary.

CARDIAC MONITORING. Clients with hypercalcemia usually undergo continuous cardiac monitoring to identify dysrhythmias and decreased cardiac output. The nurse compares recently obtained electrocardiogram (ECG) tracings with the client's baseline tracings. The ECG is observed for changes in the T waves and the QT interval as well as changes in rate and rhythm.

PHOSPHOROUS IMBALANCES

Hypophosphatemia

OVERVIEW

Hypophosphatemia is a serum phosphorus level below 3.0 mg/dL. Even though the serum concentration of phosphorus has a narrow range of normal values (3.0 to 4.5 mg/dL), body functions are not significantly impaired as a result of rapid, wide changes in serum phosphorus levels. Alterations in function are more obvious with chronic hypophosphatemia.

Most of the pathologic effects of hypophosphatemia are related to decreased energy metabolism and altered levels of other electrolytes and body fluids. Because of the reciprocal relationship between phosphorus and calcium, decreases in serum phosphorus levels are accompanied by increases in serum calcium levels.

Three main processes cause decreased serum phosphorus levels: decreased absorption of phosphorus, increased excretion of phosphorus, and intracellular phosphorus shift (Table 13-7).

COLLABORATIVE MANAGEMENT

Assessment

The clinical manifestations of hypophosphatemia occur when the decrease in serum phosphorus levels is severe or prolonged. Acute manifestations of hypophosphatemia are related to the decreased availability of high-energy compounds (e.g., **adenosine triphosphate [ATP]**) necessary to perform normal metabolic functions. The clinical manifestations are apparent in the cardiac, musculoskeletal, hematologic, and central nervous systems (Chart 13-14).

CARDIOVASCULAR MANIFESTATIONS

Cardiac manifestations of hypophosphatemia are decreased stroke volume and decreased cardiac output. Peripheral pulses are slow, difficult to find, and easy to block. Myocardial depression is caused by low stores of intracellular energy. With-

TABLE 13-7 • COMMON CAUSES OF PHOSPHORUS IMBALANCE

HYPOPHOSPHATEMIA

Insufficient Phosphorus Intake
- Malnutrition
- Starvation
- Use of aluminum hydroxide–based antacids
- Use of magnesium-based antacids

Increased Phosphorus Excretion
- Hyperparathyroidism
- Hypercalcemia
- Renal failure
- Malignancy

Intracellular Shift
- Hyperglycemia
- Hyperalimentation
- Respiratory alkalosis
- Uncontrolled diabetes mellitus
- Alcohol abuse

HYPERPHOSPHATEMIA
- Decreased renal excretion resulting from renal insufficiency
- Tumor lysis syndrome
- Increased intake of phosphorus
- Hypoparathyroidism

out sufficient quantities of energy in myocardial cells, contractions are weak and ineffective. Prolonged hypophosphatemia can lead to progressive but reversible cardiac muscle damage.

MUSCULOSKELETAL MANIFESTATIONS

Hypophosphatemia weakens skeletal muscles and may cause acute muscle breakdown **(rhabdomyolysis).** The weakness is generalized, and paresthesias usually are not present. When skeletal muscle weakness becomes profound, respiratory movements are ineffective, which leads to respiratory failure. The nurse assesses for muscle strength and observes respiratory ability.

The clinical manifestations of chronic hypophosphatemia are most evident in the skeletal system. Bone density is decreased, which leads to fractures and changes in bone shape. These changes are caused by the calcium resorption that often accompanies hypophosphatemia. The nurse assesses the client for unusual lumps, projections, or depressions over bony areas that indicate bone fractures.

CENTRAL NERVOUS SYSTEM MANIFESTATIONS

Central nervous system manifestations are not apparent until hypophosphatemia is severe. These first appear as increased irritability and may progress to seizure activity followed by coma.

Interventions

The administration of drugs that contribute to the development of hypophosphatemia (e.g., antacids, osmotic diuretics, and calcium supplements) is discontinued. Oral replacement of phosphorus along with a vitamin D supplement, such as with milk or a commercial preparation, is often sufficient to correct moderate hypophosphatemia or to prevent hypophosphatemia in susceptible clients (see the Evidence-Based Practice for Nursing box above). The administration of IV phosphorus is initiated only when serum phosphorus levels fall below 1 mg/dL and the client has serious clinical manifestations. For cost-effectiveness and client tolerance, hypophosphatemia is prevented or corrected with the use of oral phosphorus replacement fluids rather than by the IV route whenever appropriate (see the Cost of Care box on p. 191). IV

CHART 13-14

KEY FEATURES *of* Hypophosphatemia

Cardiovascular Manifestations
- Decreased contractility
- Cardiomyopathy (reversible)

Respiratory Manifestations
- Shallow respirations

Musculoskeletal Manifestations
- Weakness
- Rhabdomyolysis
- Decreased deep tendon reflexes

Central Nervous System Manifestations
- Irritability
- Confusion
- Seizures

Hematologic Manifestations
- Increased bleeding
- Decreased platelet aggregation
- Immunosuppression

EVIDENCE-BASED PRACTICE FOR NURSING

Oral phosphate replacement reduces incidence and severity of hypophosphatemia

Mathews, J., Aleem, R., & Gamelli, R. (1999). Cost reduction strategies in burn nutrition services: Adjustments in dietary treatment of patients with hyponatremia and hypophosphatemia. *Journal of Burn Care and Rehabilitation, 20*(1), 80-84.

This study compared the incidence and severity of hypophosphatemia in severely burned clients with and without dietary phosphate adjustment. Eight clients with total body surface area burns of at least 20% were treated prophylactically from the first day of admission through day 10 with 16 to 24 mmol of oral phosphate supplementation (Neutra-Phos). Daily serum phosphorus levels were compared retrospectively to 45 clients with 20% or greater total body surface area burns who were treated intravenously for documented hypophosphatemia. Seven of the clients receiving prophylactic oral phosphate supplementation did become hypohosphatemic; however, the severity was far less than the group who did not receive oral phosphate supplementation. Only two clients receiving the prophylactic treatment experienced hypophosphatemia to the degree that IV phosphorus replacement was required.

Critique. The study compared a prospective protocol to retrospective documentation of postburn hypophosphatemia. Although the results are highly suggestive of an effective protocol, the study would have been strengthened by using a prospective approach with randomization of equal numbers of subjects to a prophylactic treatment versus a nonprophylactic treatment experimental design.

Implications for Nursing. IV electrolyte replacement is usually effective; however, the risks associated with IV therapy are greater than those of oral replacement. In addition, the cost of the product as well as nursing time for IV replacement may not be justified if oral replacement and prophylaxis prevent severe changes in electrolyte homeostasis.

COST OF CARE IMPLICATIONS FOR NURSING

ELECTROLYTE IMBALANCES

Cost of Care

- IV electrolyte replacement solutions cost two to five times as much as oral electrolyte replacement fluids.
- Clients tolerate the procedures and the solutions administered orally better than those administered parenterally.
- The risk of complications, especially too rapid an increase in serum electrolyte concentration, is greater with IV replacement than with oral replacement.
- Nursing care time, especially for registered nurses, is more costly with IV electrolyte replacement than with oral electrolyte replacement.
- Other members of the health care team can participate in administering oral electrolyte replacement.

Implications for Nursing

Because of the greater costs and risks associated with IV electrolyte fluid replacement therapy, nurses (especially those with prescriptive privileges) need to be more aware of "low-tech" modalities to treat mild or moderate electrolyte imbalances. Research has shown that oral electrolyte replacement fluids can be just as effective, more acceptable to clients, and less likely to cause other electrolyte imbalances than IV electrolyte replacement fluids. More staff education is needed to monitor client responses to oral electrolyte replacement therapy for the most effective titration.

Data from Mathews, J., Aleem, R., & Gamelli, R. (1999). Cost reduction strategies in burn nutrition services: Adjustments in dietary treatment of patients with hyponatremia and hypophosphatemia. *Journal of Burn Care and Rehabilitation, 20*(1), 80-84; and Trissel, L. (1998). *Handbook on injectable drugs* (10th ed.). Bethesda, MD: American Society of Health Systems.

phosphorus is administered slowly because the problems associated with hyperphosphatemia are equally serious.

Diet therapy for hypophosphatemia involves increasing the intake of phosphorus-rich foods while decreasing the intake of calcium-rich foods (Chart 13-15).

Hyperphosphatemia

OVERVIEW

Hyperphosphatemia occurs when the serum phosphorus level exceeds 4.5 mg/dL. Serum phosphorus levels above normal are well tolerated by most body systems.

The problems caused by hyperphosphatemia center on the hypocalcemia that results when serum phosphorus levels increase. These problems include increased sensitivity of excitable membranes to the extent that they may depolarize spontaneously and inappropriately.

Underlying causes of increased serum phosphorus levels include renal insufficiency, certain cancer treatments, increased phosphorus intake, and hypoparathyroidism. Table 13-7 lists the specific common causes of hyperphosphatemia.

COLLABORATIVE MANAGEMENT

Hyperphosphatemia causes few direct problems with body function. However, hypocalcemia is usually present because calcium and phosphorus ions exist in the blood in a balanced reciprocal relationship: when one increases, the other decreases. The accompanying hypocalcemia dramatically alters the physiologic functioning of many body systems and has the potential for causing serious and life-threatening side effects. Thus the management of hyperphosphatemia entails the management of hypocalcemia.

CHART 13-15

CLIENT EDUCATION GUIDE
Dietary Management of Hypophosphatemia

You Should Avoid	You May Eat
• Milk	• Fish
• Cheese	• Beef
• Yogurt	• Chicken
• Collard greens	• Pork
• Rhubarb	• Organ meats
	• Nuts
	• Whole-grain breads and cereals

MAGNESIUM IMBALANCES

Hypomagnesemia

OVERVIEW

Hypomagnesemia is a serum magnesium (Mg^{2+}) level below 1.2 mg/dL. Because most conditions resulting in hypomagnesemia are caused by decreased magnesium intake or increased magnesium loss, measurable hypomagnesemia reflects a decrease in the concentration of total body magnesium.

The direct pathophysiologic effects of hypomagnesemia are caused by changes in the function of excitable membranes and the accompanying imbalances of serum calcium and potassium. These problems include increased sensitivity of excitable membranes, especially nerve cell membranes, to the extent that they may depolarize spontaneously and inappropriately.

Hypomagnesemia results from conditions that decrease the absorption of dietary magnesium or increase the renal excretion of magnesium. Table 13-8 lists the specific causes of hypomagnesemia.

COLLABORATIVE MANAGEMENT

Assessment

Clinical manifestations of hypomagnesemia result from changes in the activity of excitable cell membranes. The most common manifestations are seen in the neuromuscular, central nervous, and gastrointestinal systems (Chart 13-16).

NEUROMUSCULAR MANIFESTATIONS

The neuromuscular manifestations of hypomagnesemia cause increased nerve impulse transmission. Normally, magnesium inhibits the release of the acetylcholine at nerve synapse areas. Decreased magnesium levels allow a greater release of acetylcholine, which increases the transmission of impulses from nerve to nerve or from nerve to skeletal muscle. The client with hypomagnesemia experiences hyperactive deep tendon reflexes (+4), painful paresthesia (numbness and tingling), and tetanic muscle contractions. Positive Chvostek's and Trousseau's signs may be present because hypomagnesemia may be accompanied by hypocalcemia (see the earlier discussion of these assessment signs under Neuromuscular Manifestations [Hypocalcemia], p. 185). Skeletal muscle weakness may be present if intracellular

TABLE 13-8 • COMMON CAUSES OF MAGNESIUM IMBALANCE

HYPOMAGNESEMIA

Insufficient Magnesium Intake
- Malnutrition
- Starvation
- Diarrhea
- Steatorrhea
- Celiac disease
- Crohn's disease

Increased Magnesium Excretion
- Drugs (diuretics, aminoglycoside antibiotics, cisplatin, amphotericin B, cyclosporine)
- Citrate (blood products)
- Ethanol ingestion

Intracellular Movement of Magnesium
- Hyperglycemia
- Insulin administration
- Sepsis
- Alkalosis

HYPERMAGNESEMIA
- Increased magnesium intake
  - Magnesium-containing antacids and laxatives
  - IV magnesium replacement
- Decreased renal excretion of magnesium resulting from renal insufficiency

CHART 13-16

KEY FEATURES *of* Hypomagnesemia

Cardiovascular Manifestations
- Electrocardiographic changes
  - Tall T waves
  - Depressed ST segments
- Dysrhythmias
  - Ectopic beats
  - Ventricular tachycardia
  - Ventricular fibrillation
- Hypertension

Gastrointestinal Manifestations
- Decreased motility
- Anorexia
- Nausea
- Abdominal distention
- Decreased bowel sounds

Respiratory Manifestations
- Shallow respirations

Neuromuscular Manifestations
- Fasciculations
- Twitches
- Paresthesias
- Positive Trousseau's sign
- Positive Chvostek's sign
- Hyperreflexia
- Tetany
- Seizures

Central Nervous System Manifestations
- Irritability
- Confusion
- Psychosis

magnesium levels are also decreased. The client may experience tetany and seizures as hypomagnesemia progresses.

CENTRAL NERVOUS SYSTEM MANIFESTATIONS

Central nervous system manifestations of hypomagnesemia are caused by a general increase in the transmission of nerve impulses. Increased central nervous system irritability may manifest as psychologic depression, psychosis, and confusion.

GASTROINTESTINAL MANIFESTATIONS

Gastrointestinal manifestations include decreased intestinal smooth muscle contraction. Clients have decreased gastric motility, anorexia, nausea, constipation, and abdominal distention. A paralytic ileus may occur when hypomagnesemia is severe.

Interventions

Interventions for hypomagnesemia aim to correct the electrolyte imbalance and manage the specific condition that caused the hypomagnesemia. In addition, because hypocalcemia often accompanies hypomagnesemia, some interventions also aim to restore normal serum calcium levels.

The administration of drugs that contribute to the development of hypomagnesemia, such as high-ceiling (loop) diuretics, osmotic diuretics, aminoglycosides, and drugs containing phosphorus, is discontinued. Magnesium is replaced intravenously in the form of magnesium sulfate ($MgSO_4$) when hypomagnesemia is severe. The IV route is used because $MgSO_4$ causes pain and tissue damage when injected intramuscularly. The nurse assesses deep tendon reflexes at least hourly in the client receiving IV magnesium to monitor effectiveness and prevent hypermagnesemia. Oral magnesium often causes diarrhea and can increase magnesium loss. If hypocalcemia is also present, the physician prescribes drug therapy to increase the concentration of serum calcium.

Diet therapy for hypomagnesemia consists of increasing the intake of foods that contain high concentrations of magnesium (see Table 11-11).

Hypermagnesemia

OVERVIEW

Hypermagnesemia occurs when the serum magnesium level exceeds 2.0 mg/dL. Magnesium is a membrane stabilizer. When excesses of magnesium occur, excitable membranes require a stronger-than-normal stimulus to respond and thus are less excitable. With severe hypermagnesemia, excitable membranes may not respond to any stimulus.

Hypermagnesemia results from an increased intake of magnesium coupled with a decreased renal excretion of magnesium. Table 13-8 lists the specific causes of hypermagnesemia.

COLLABORATIVE MANAGEMENT

Assessment

Most clinical manifestations of hypermagnesemia occur as a result of alterations in the activity of excitable cell membranes. These manifestations usually are not apparent until serum magnesium levels exceed 4 mg/dL. The most common manifestations are seen in the cardiac, central nervous, and neuromuscular systems.

The cardiac manifestations of hypermagnesemia are bradycardia, peripheral vasodilation, and hypotension. These problems become more severe as serum magnesium concentration increases. Electrocardiographic (ECG) changes include a prolonged PR interval with a widened QRS complex. Bradycardia can be severe, and cardiac arrest is possible. Hypotension with a wide pulse pressure is also severe; the diastolic pressure is much lower than normal. Clients with severe hypermagnesemia are in grave danger of cardiac arrest.

Central nervous system manifestations of hypermagnesemia are related to depressed transmission of nerve impulses at specific synaptic points. Clients may be drowsy to the point of lethargy. Coma may occur if the hypermagnesemia is prolonged or becomes severe.

Neuromuscular manifestations of hypermagnesemia are related to the decreased transmission of impulses from the nerves to the skeletal muscles. Deep tendon reflexes are greatly reduced or even absent. Voluntary skeletal muscle contractions become progressively weaker and finally stop.

Hypermagnesemia has no direct effect on the lungs; however, when the skeletal muscles of respiration are weak, respiratory insufficiency can lead to respiratory failure and death.

Interventions

Interventions for hypermagnesemia aim to reduce the serum magnesium level and correct the underlying problem that caused or contributed to the development of hypermagnesemia.

All oral and parenteral administration of magnesium is discontinued. When renal failure is not present, the administration of magnesium-free IV fluids can reduce serum magnesium levels. Administration of high-ceiling (loop) diuretics such as furosemide (Lasix, Furoside♣) can further reduce serum magnesium levels. When cardiac manifestations are severe, the administration of calcium may reverse the cardiac effects of hypermagnesemia.

Diet therapy is most effective in preventing hypermagnesemia when other chronic conditions predispose the client to the development of excess serum magnesium levels. Dietary restrictions involve limiting the ingestion of meat, nuts, legumes, fish, vegetables, and whole-grain cereal products. To prevent the recurrence of hypermagnesemia, the client is taught to avoid drugs or conditions that increase magnesium, such as magnesium-containing antacids, laxatives, or commercial enemas.

ONLINE RESOURCES

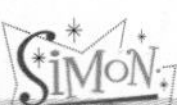

For suggested readings and Internet resources, go to http://www.wbsaunders.com/SIMON/Iggy/.

SELECTED BIBLIOGRAPHY

Asterisk indicates a classic or definitive work on this subject.

Ahern-Gould, K., & Stark, J. (1998). Quick resource for electrolyte imbalance. *Critical Care Nursing Clinics of North America, 10*(4), 477-490.

Barnett, M. (1999). Hypercalcemia. *Seminars in Oncology Nursing, 15*(3), 190-201.

Bass, M. (1998). Fluid and electrolyte management of ascites in patients with cirrhosis. *Critical Care Nursing Clinics of North America, 10*(4), 459-467.

Castiglione, K. (2000). Hyperkalemia. *American Journal of Nursing, 100*(1), 55.

Chmielewski, C. (1998). Hyperkalemic emergencies: Mechanisms, manifestations, and management. *Critical Care Clinics of North America, 10*(4), 449-457.

Clayton, K. (1997). Cancer-related hypercalcemia: How to spot it, how to manage it. *American Journal of Nursing, 97*(5), 42-48.

Cook, L. (1999). The value of lab values. *American Journal of Nursing, 99*(5), 66-75.

DeJong, M. (1998). Hyponatremia. *American Journal of Nursing, 98*(12), 36.

Edwards, R., Mitchell, M., & Twaddle, S. (1998). Hypophosphatemia in the critically ill patient: Aetiology and management. *Care of the Critically Ill, 14*(8), 267-270.

Epstein, Y., & Armstrong, L. (1999). Fluid-electrolyte balance during labor and exercise: Concepts and misconceptions. *International Journal of Sports Nutrition, 9*(1), 1-12.

Fabius, D. (1998). How to recognize electrolyte imbalances on an ECG. *Nursing98, 28*(2), 32hn1-32hn6.

Frizzell, J. (1998). Avoiding lab test pitfalls. *American Journal of Nursing, 98*(2), 34-38.

Fulop, M. (1998). Algorithms for diagnosing some electrolyte disorders. *American Journal of Emergency Medicine, 16*(1), 76-84.

Goldy, D. (1998). Circulatory overload secondary to blood transfusion. *American Journal of Nursing, 98*(7), 33.

Gosling, P. (1999). Fluid balance in the critically ill: The sodium and water audit. *Care of the Critically Ill, 15*(1), 11-16.

Guyton, A., & Hall, J. (2000). *Textbook of medical physiology* (10th ed.). Philadelphia: W.B. Saunders.

Heater, D. (1999). If ADH goes out of balance: SIADH. *RN, 62*(7), 47-50.

Iggulden, H. (1999). Dehydration and electrolyte disturbance. *Nursing Standard, 13*(19), 48-56.

Jordan, K. (2000). Fluid resuscitation in acutely injured patients. *Journal of Intravenous Nursing, 23*(2), 81-87.

Klotz, J. (1998). The effects of intravenous solutions on fluid and electrolyte balance. *Journal of Intravenous Nursing, 21*(1), 20-26.

*Kokko, J., & Tannen, R. (1996). *Fluids and electrolytes* (3rd ed.). Philadelphia: W.B. Saunders.

Krau, S. (1998). Selecting and managing fluid therapy. *Critical Care Nursing Clinics of North America, 10*(4), 401-410.

Mathews, J., Aleem, R., & Gamelli, R. (1999). Cost reduction strategies in burn nutrition services: Adjustments in dietary treatment of patients with hyponatremia and hypophosphatemia. *Journal of Burn Care and Rehabilitation, 20*(1), 80-84.

McAlpine, L. (1998). CAVH: Principles and practical applications. *Critical Care Nursing Clinics of North America, 10*(2), 179-189.

McCarty, M., Jagoda, A., & Fairweather, P. (1998). Hyperkalemic ascending paralysis. *Annals of Emergency Medicine, 32*(1), 104-107.

McCloskey, J.C., & Bulechek, G.M. (2000). *Nursing interventions classification (NIC)* (3rd ed.). St. Louis: Mosby.

*Metheny, N. (1996). *Fluid and electrolyte balance: Nursing considerations* (3rd ed.). Philadelphia: Lippincott-Raven.

Miekley, T.F. (1998). A patient-focused approach to managing diuretic therapy. *Critical Care Nursing Clinics of North America, 10*(4), 421-467.

Miller, M. (1998). Hyponatremia: Age-related risk factors and therapy decisions. *Geriatrics, 53*(7), 32-33, 37-38, & 41-42.

*O'Donnell, M. (1995). Assessing fluid and electrolyte balance needs in elders. *American Journal of Nursing, 95*(1), 41-46.

Pagana, K., & Pagana, T. (1999). *Diagnostic testing and nursing implications: A case study approach* (5th ed.). St. Louis: Mosby.

Rosenberg, K. (1998). Management of electrolyte abnormalities: Hypocalcemia, hypomagnesemia, and hypokalemia. *Journal of the American Academy of Nurse Practitioners, 10*(5), 209-217.

Santinelli, V., et al. (1999). Magnesium deficiency and dizziness: A case of electrolyte imbalance. *Geriatrics, 54*(3), 67-73.

Sobel, B., Rutecki, G., & Whittier, F. (1998). Life-threatening phosphate imbalance: When to suspect, how to treat. *Journal of Critical Illness, 13*(4), 217-218.

Stark, J. (1998). A comprehensive analysis of the fluid and electrolytes system. *Critical Care Nursing Clinics of North America, 10*(4), 471-475.

*Tannen, R. (1996). Potassium disorders. In J. Kokko & R. Tannen (Eds.), *Fluids and electrolytes* (3rd ed., pp. 111-119). Philadelphia: W.B. Saunders.

*Tietz, N.W. (Ed.). (1995). *Clinical guide to laboratory tests* (3rd ed.). Philadelphia: W.B. Saunders.

Trissel, L. (1998). *Handbook on injectable drugs* (10th ed.). Bethesda, MD: American Society of Health Systems.

United States Pharmacopeia. (1997). Intravenous potassium predicament. *Clinical Journal of Oncology Nursing, 1*(2), 45-49.

Young, J. (1998). A closer look at IV fluids. *Nursing98, 28*(10), 52-55.

CHAPTER 14

Infusion Therapy

ROBIN L. BARANOWSKI

Learning Objectives

After studying this chapter, you should be able to:

1. Explain the purpose of infusion filters.
2. Explain the primary advantage of needleless infusion systems.
3. Compare and contrast the use of controllers and pumps.
4. Identify important considerations when placing a venous access device (VAD).
5. Determine special needs of older adults who receive intravenous (IV) therapy.
6. Describe the major differences between nontunneled and tunneled central VADs.
7. Describe how a peripherally inserted central catheter differs from central lines.
8. Compare and contrast the major complications of peripheral and central IV therapy.
9. Identify the most common use for intra-arterial therapy.
10. Describe the nursing care of a client receiving hypodermoclysis.
11. Explain the indications for epidural and intrathecal therapy.

SIMON

Go to http://www.wbsaunders.com/SIMON/Iggy/ for self-assessment questions related to these Learning Objectives.

The term **infusion therapy** refers to a wide variety of techniques and procedures that health care professionals use to deliver parenteral medications and fluids to their clients. In intravenous (IV) therapy and arterial therapy, medications and fluids are infused into the vascular system. Intraperitoneal therapy is infusion of medications and fluids into the body cavity. Subcutaneous therapy, also known as hypodermoclysis, is infusion of medications and fluids into the subcutaneous tissue. Central nervous system therapy is infusion of medications and fluids into the epidural space or intrathecally. Intraosseous therapy is infusion of medications and fluids into the bones. This chapter focuses on access for and administration of infusion therapy. Various types of fluids for infusion are discussed throughout the text where appropriate.

INTRODUCTION TO INFUSION THERAPY

Approximately 90% of hospitalized clients receive some type of infusion therapy. Health care providers prescribe infusion therapy for a variety of reasons, including maintenance, replacement, treatment, palliation (promoting comfort), or a combination of these.

Not long ago, most clients received infusion therapy as inpatients in acute care facilities. With the advent of computerized ambulatory and implantable infusion control devices, as well as long-term infusion access devices, clients now receive infusion therapy in virtually any setting, including their homes.

Some agencies have specialized teams that focus on all of the procedures associated with infusion therapy. These infusion, or IV, teams:

- Develop infusion policies and procedures
- Start peripheral IV lines and place peripherally inserted central catheters
- Administer parenteral fluids and medications
- Administer parenteral nutrition and blood products
- Maintain infusion devices

They may also:

- Provide input to agency purchasing departments regarding infusion devices and equipment
- Monitor infusion-related complications
- Provide consultation to health care providers and clients regarding device selection and placement
- Engage in quality improvement activities

The continued use of IV teams in health care settings is a controversial issue. In this time of "downsizing," "right-sizing," and "re-engineering," most agencies have disbanded their IV teams, leaving these responsibilities to nurse generalists or unlicensed technicians. The impact of a dedicated IV team was recently tested by a large Veterans' Administration medical center. The medical center started a new IV team and subsequently found that the rate of primary nosocomial bloodstream infections decreased by 35%. There was a 51% decrease in bloodstream infections caused by *Staphylococcus aureus.* The excess costs per life saved and infection prevented were projected to be $53,000 and $14,000, respectively (Meier, 1998).

The Intravenous Nurses Society (INS), the professional nursing organization for infusion therapy nurses, publishes standards of care that provide the basis for the practice of infusion nursing. Its affiliate organization, the Intravenous Nurses Certification Corporation (INCC), offers a written certifying examination. Nurses who successfully complete this examination may use the initials *CRNI,* which stand for "certified registered nurse infusion." The INS is currently the only organization offering certification in infusion therapy. The Oncology Nurses Society (ONS) is another professional organization of registered nurses and other health care professionals that has developed access device guidelines for nursing practice (ONS, 1996). For more information on these organizations, see http://www.wbsaunders.com/SIMON/Iggy/.

INFUSION SYSTEMS

Nurses administering infusion therapies need to understand the way in which infusion systems work. This knowledge ensures that the nurse can benefit from a particular system's advantages while minimizing any potential complications.

Containers

Infusion containers are generally made of glass or plastic. Plastic containers are used most often. *Glass* infusion systems are of two types: the separate-airway system and the integral-airway system. The separate-airway system has a plastic tube or "straw" attached to the inside of the thick, hard cork-type stopper. This tube extends almost the entire length of the bottle to above the fluid level of a full bottle. Unfiltered air enters through the straw and exerts pressure on the surface of the fluid, allowing the fluid to pass through the administration set. The integral-airway system is also an "open" system. In this system, air enters through a side port filter on the administration set. This type of set is often referred to as "vented" tubing.

Plastic containers may be soft and totally collapsible or semirigid. Both of these types of containers are considered "closed" systems, since they do not rely on outside air to allow the fluid to infuse. Instead, atmospheric pressure pushes against the flexible sides of the container, allowing the fluid to flow by gravity. For this reason, plastic containers use "nonvented," or "unvented," tubing.

The totally collapsible plastic containers are usually made of polyvinyl chloride (PVC). Some PVC materials are incompatible with nitroglycerin, insulin, and fat emulsions. Nitroglycerin and insulin adhere to the walls of the PVC container, making it impossible to know exactly how much medication the client is receiving. Fat emulsions leach the plasticizer diethylhexylphthalate (DEHP), a component of some PVC containers, thereby making this substance an unintended part of the infusion.

Although they are plastic, semirigid containers do not have the same compatibility problems associated with containers made of PVC. These containers, as their name indicates, are less flexible than totally collapsible plastic containers.

Administration Sets

The administration set is the connection between the access device and the container with the infusion solution. Numerous administration sets are available in many different configurations. The type of administration set that the nurse chooses depends on the type and purpose of the infusion. Some sets are generic, meaning that they are appropriate for most infusions. Other sets are designed to be used for specific types of infusions. Still other sets are "dedicated," meaning that they must be used with a specific manufacturer's infusion control device. Information that describes their proper use is usually provided on the packaging of administration sets. Table 14-1 and Charts 14-1 and 14-2 describe some of the standard and miscellaneous components of administration sets and how to use them.

Filters remove particulate matter suspended in the infusion solution while allowing the fluid to pass through to the client. Filters may be membrane filters or depth filters. Both types of filters may be "in-line" (an integral part of the administration set) or "add-on" (a filter set that is separate and must be added to the administration set).

A membrane filter has tiny pores or holes sized to prevent the passage of particles into the filter. These pores capture any particles that may be in the solution and trap them on the surface of the filter. One problem associated with membrane filters is that they are prone to "loading." This means that the filter's surface becomes completely coated with particulate matter, so that the filter will no longer work as a filter. It is for this reason that membrane filters are best suited as final filters rather than as primary filters.

A depth filter has a mazelike configuration. Any particles suspended in the fluid pass through the surface and become trapped in the multitude of passages as they travel through the labyrinth. In addition, depth filters have adsorption properties that cause any particles to adhere to the filter material itself. The size of the particle does not influence the adsorption of the filter material.

Both membrane and depth filters are rated by the size of the smallest particles they hold back. A 0.22-micron filter retains any particles 0.22 micron or larger. These particles may be particulate matter or organisms, such as *Escherichia coli* and *Pseudomonas.*

Needleless Systems

In July 1992 the Occupational Safety and Health Administration (OSHA) published its guidelines entitled *Occupational Exposure to Bloodborne Pathogens, Final Rule.* This document requires health care organizations to initiate engineering controls "that isolate or remove the bloodborne pathogen hazard from the workplace." Currently there are a number of products available and more entering the market every day that are designed to minimize health care workers' exposure to contaminated needles. Some of these products include devices that use blunt metal cannulas or needles recessed into a plastic housing. Others use blunt plastic cannulas, and still others include valves. Figure 14-1 displays two common needleless systems currently available. Some companies have gone a step further to reduce the risk of needle sticks by manufacturing an IV catheter that, with the push of a button, retracts the needle (Figure 14-2).

Many studies have been conducted comparing various needleless systems with conventional venous access systems (see the Evidence-Based Practice for Nursing Box on p. 199). For example, Mendelson et al. (1998) concluded that the needleless system for peripheral infusions is effective in reducing percutaneous injuries to staff and is not associated with an increase in either insertion site complications or nosocomial bacteremia.

Infusion Regulation Devices

The ability to regulate the rate and volume of infusions is critical to the safe and accurate administration of medications and fluids to clients. Nurses have a choice of numerous devices designed to regulate infusions. Infusion devices can be mechanically or electronically regulated. Mechanically regulated systems, such as an elastomeric device, delivers medications and fluids by positive pressure and has no power source, such as a battery or alternating current. These small, portable devices administer small-volume, long-term, inter-

TABLE 14-1 • COMPONENTS OF ADMINISTRATION SETS

Component	Description or Characteristics	Purpose or Function
STANDARD COMPONENTS		
Spike	Hard plastic tube with a sharp point; plastic cover or sheath over the spike must be removed before use	Sharp point penetrates the solution container, sheath maintains sterility of the spike
Shield	Hard plastic disk below the spike	Prevents the nurse's hands from slipping onto the spike when inserting it into the fluid container
Drip chamber	Plastic tube between the shield and the tubing; the bottom of the spike extends into this chamber	Used to prime the administration set and to verify continued flow
Bottom of spike	Plastic or metal piece that extends into the drip chamber	Size controls the volume of fluid in each drop; may be macrodrip, minidrip, or microdrip; volume of a macrodrip varies among manufacturers from 10 to 20 drops/mL (gtt/mL); microdrip or minidrip is 60 gtt/mL
Tubing	May be of varying lengths and diameters	Connects the drip chamber to the connector device
Clamps	May be screw clamp or roller clamp	Controls the rate of fluid flow through the administration
Flashball	A piece of latex with small circles on the surface that highlight areas reinforced with self-sealing material	Connects the tubing to the connector; reinforced areas used for needle access to infusion to administer IV push medications
Connectors	At the end of the tubing, may be slip tip, Luer-Lok, or slip Luer-Lok	Connects the administration set to the client's access device
Y-site	Set may have one or more; may be called injection site or side-arm; hard plastic tube; upper end has either a self-sealing injection port or a valve; bottom of the Y-site is an integral part of the administration set tubing	Used for piggybacking intermittent medications into the client's primary infusion (see Chart 14-1)
MISCELLANEOUS COMPONENTS		
On-off clamps	May be slide or clip; not appropriate for regulating rate of flow	Used to open or close the administration set to flow
Burettes	Reservoir that is either incorporated into the administration set or an add-on device; the reservoir holds between 100 and 150 mL of fluid; the burette is calibrated on the side to assist with accurate measurement; at the top or bottom of the burette is a rubber cap that looks like the end of a Y-site; through this self-sealing cap, the nurse can add any medications or additives ordered for the client	The burette is useful for mixing IV medications for administration or for controlling the amount of fluid available for administration, a critical consideration in the care of the young child or the older client (see Chart 14-2)
Back-check valves	When present, a back-check valve is built into the administration set; the device is a hard plastic one-way valve	Back-check valves allow fluid to travel away from the solution container but prevents fluid from flowing upstream toward the container
Passive flow control devices	Usually an add-on device that looks like an extension set with a dial	Regulates the rate of infusion in mL/hr; all other clamps are left open, and the passive flow control device regulates administrations at the prescribed rate

CHART 14-1

BEST PRACTICE *for*
Piggybacking an Intermittent Medication

1. Verify the order from the health care provider.
2. Check the compatibility between the medication and the large-volume parenteral (LVP) infusion and its additives.
3. Spike the medication mini-bag with the secondary set.
4. Prime the secondary set, close the roller clamp, and hang the mini-bag on the other arm of the IV pole.
5. Place the hanger that comes with the secondary set on the IV pole with the LVP.
6. Cleanse the lowest Y-site injection port on the LVP administration set.
7. Attach the secondary set to the Y-site.
8. Lower the level of the LVP by hanging it from the hanger. Do not adjust the LVP roller clamp. (The rate will decrease and then stop when the secondary set is opened.)
9. Open the roller clamp on the secondary set and regulate the flow to the desired rate.
10. When the intermittent infusion completes, the LVP will automatically begin again. Hang the LVP from the IV pole and adjust the roller clamp to deliver the prescribed rate.

CHART 14-2

BEST PRACTICE *for*
Using a Burette

1. To fill the burette, close the main clamp below the burette.
2. Open the clamp between the solution container and the burette, allowing the fluid to flow into the burette.
3. When the burette contains the amount of fluid desired, close the clamp between the solution container and the burette.
4. If using the burette for administration of intermittent medications, add the prescribed medication now and gently swirl the burette.
5. Regulate the rate of the infusion from the burette with the lower clamp.

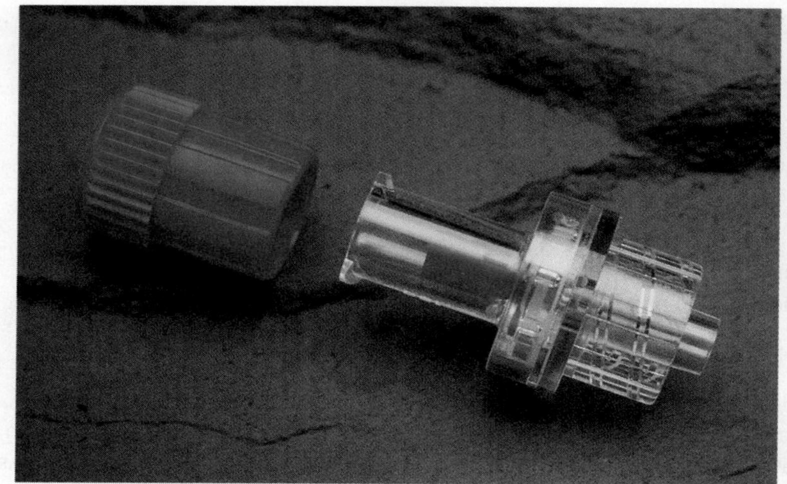

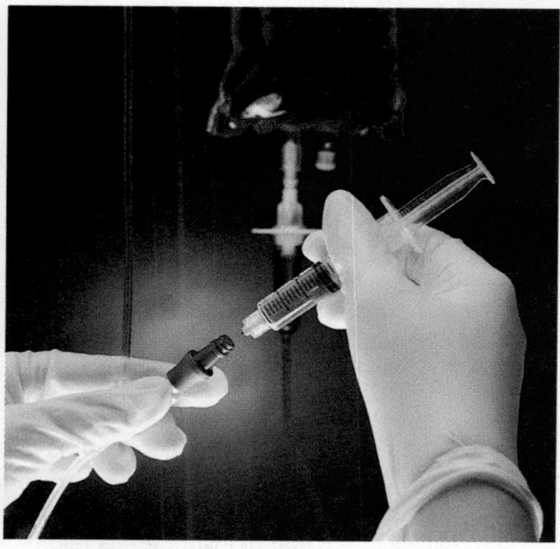

Figure 14-1 ● Needleless infusion systems. **A,** Burron Safesite IV System Valve and "deadhead." **B,** Clave system in use. (**A** courtesy B. Braun Medical, Inc., Bethlehem, PA; **B** courtesy ICU Medical, Inc., San Clemente, CA.)

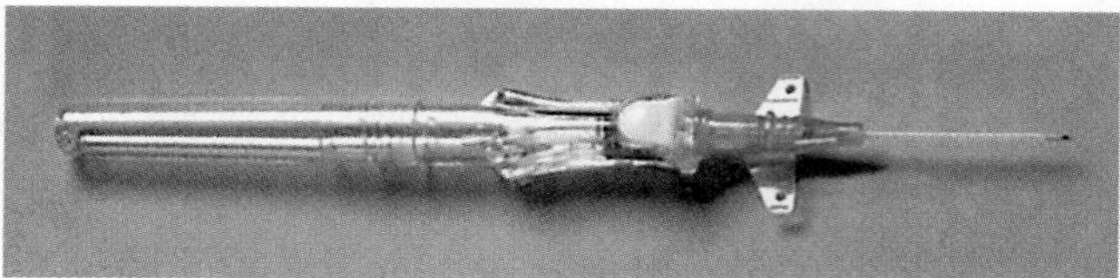

Figure 14-2 ● Insyte AutoGuard IV catheters. With the push of a button, the needle instantly retracts, reducing the risk of accidental needle stick injuries. (Courtesy Becton Dickinson Infusion Therapy Systems, Sandy, UT.)

mittent infusions, including chemotherapy, antivirals, and antibiotics (McConnell, 1999).

Electronic infusion devices fall into two categories: controllers and pumps, based on the principle of operation. Nurses and clients who use these electronic infusion devices reap the benefits of some of the latest computer technology. Infusion regulation devices can save nursing time, prevent clients from receiving too much infusion solution, reduce the incidence of infiltration, and keep infusion access devices patent. However, the nurse must remember that the use of these devices does not decrease the practitioner's responsibility to carefully monitor the client's infusion site and the infusion rate.

A **controller** is a stationary, pole-mounted electronic device that can be classified as either nonvolumetric or volumetric. Nonvolumetric controllers rely completely on gravity for flow. A drop sensor attached to the drip chamber of the administration set regulates flow. Volumetric controllers also count drops and electronically convert the drops to milliliters per hour. Because controllers rely on counting drops, which vary in size and therefore volume, controllers are not as accurate as pumps.

Pumps may be either stationary (pole mounted or tabletop), ambulatory (portable), or implantable (surgically implanted into the client). As their name indicates, these devices actually pump medications or solutions under pressure. Stationary pumps may be nonvolumetric or volumetric. Nonvolumetric pumps count drops and, as with controllers, are inherently inaccurate because of the variation in drop size.

Three types of volumetric pumps are available: syringe, cassette, and peristaltic. **Syringe pumps** use a mechanism that continuously closes the plunger at a selected milliliter-per-hour rate. The use of syringe pumps is limited to small-volume continuous infusions or intermittent infusions. Syringe pumps are generally not appropriate for continuous administration of larger volumes, since they require very frequent syringe changes. **Cassette pumps** use special sets (dedicated sets) that include a pumping chamber of exact volume. This volume is displaced by means of either a piston or a diaphragm at the selected milliliter-per-hour rate. Cassette pumps usually require special techniques to prime the administration set but are appropriate for use when delivering large-volume infusions. **Peristaltic pumps** are also appropriate for large-volume infusions. They control the rate of the infusion by squeezing the tubing with finger-like projections that intermittently "walk across" the administration set tubing.

Ambulatory pumps are generally used for home care clients and allow them to return to their usual activities while receiving infusion therapy.

Implantable pumps usually include a catheter as part of the pump. The physician places the catheter in a vessel that feeds the "target" organ or structure. Implantable pumps also have a chamber that holds the medication and at least one self-sealing septum. The clinician or trained layperson accesses the medication chamber through the septum to (re)fill or empty the chamber. Implantable pumps are placed in the client's trunk via a laparotomy. Usual implant sites are the lower abdomen, the subclavicular area, and the subscapular area. Common uses for these pumps include regional chemotherapy and continuous intraspinal pain management.

TYPES OF INFUSION THERAPY

Intravenous Therapy

Intravenous (IV) therapy involves infusing medications and/or solutions into the client's veins through a venous access device (VAD). The placement of the tip of the IV cannula

EVIDENCE-BASED PRACTICE FOR NURSING

Can a needleless system significantly benefit the staff, client, and health care agency?

Luebke, M.A. et al. (1998). Comparison of the microbial barrier properties of a needleless and a conventional needle-based intravenous access system. *American Journal of Infection Control, 26*(4), 437-441.

Nurses and clients have been exposed to risks since the institution of IV therapy. The greatest risks are needle stick injuries with possible exposure to bloodborne pathogens, as well as catheter-related infection or bacteremia. In 1992 the Occupational Safety and Health Administration (OSHA) published guidelines to decrease these risks. Since then, many different needleless systems have been developed and studied to determine the actual risks to staff and clients and the cost-effectiveness for the health care agency.

In a study conducted in a 1100-bed teaching medical center, a comparison was made between a needleless (NL) access system and a conventional heparin lock (CHL) system. A random selection of clients was assessed for local IV site complications, including the development of nosocomial bacteremia and device-related complications. Staff members were assessed for percutaneous injuries. During the study, 35 percutaneous injuries were reported. Eight were CHL related; no NL-related injuries were reported. Of 773 episodes of positive blood cultures on study and control units, 0.8% were device related, showing virtually no differences between an NL and a CHL system. The projected cost to the institution for hospital-wide implementation of an NL system for intermittent access for peripheral infusions was estimated at $82,845, or $230 per 1000 client days.

Critique. This study was performed on a large group of randomly selected clients. The data demonstrate that the needleless system performs as well as the conventional IV access system with respect to the risk of microbial contamination. The study examined only intermittent IV access systems for peripheral infusions and did not consider the effects of these systems when used on central venous access devices. However, since much of the data are based on technique and usage of these systems, similar outcomes could be concluded.

Implications for Nursing. The ability of the nurse to initiate and manage a client receiving IV therapy safely is of great concern to the nurse, the client, and the health care agency. A needleless IV access system provides a safer means of IV therapy for the nurse and virtually no greater risk to the client. Nurses must be meticulous in using the appropriate disinfection before accessing either system. Each health care agency should consider these data, their own available resources, and data regarding frequency and risk of intermittent access device–related injuries in its own staff when selecting any needleless system or safety device.

determines whether the therapy is considered peripheral or central venous therapy. In peripheral venous therapy, the tip of the cannula remains in the peripheral veins. Central venous therapy involves placing the tip of the cannula or catheter into the superior vena cava (SVC).

PERIPHERAL INTRAVENOUS THERAPY

Description

Peripheral IV therapy is the most common method of gaining access to the client's venous system. Nurses competent in venipuncture insert the needle or flexible cannula percutaneously (through the skin) into the vein. Under most circumstances the peripheral veins offer the quickest and easiest approach to establishing a route for administering IV solutions and medications. These solutions and medications may be administered for therapeutic or diagnostic purposes, including the following:

- Replacement of fluid, electrolyte, and nutrient losses
- Administration of anti-infectives
- Blood and blood product transfusions
- Administration of enhancing agents for diagnostic imaging

An order from a health care provider is necessary before the nurse initiates IV therapy. The order usually includes the following:

- Specific type of solution to be given
- Rate of administration written in milliliters per hour, milligrams per hour, grams per hour, or units per hour
- Total volume of the infusion
- Number of hours for infusion

If the health care provider orders medication for IV administration, the dose, volume, solution or diluent, rate, and frequency of administration are usually included in the order. In many agencies the infusion pharmacist determines the solution and volume for the medication admixture.

When determining which site to use to initiate peripheral IV therapy, the nurse considers the client's age, history, and diagnosis; the type and duration of the prescribed therapy; and whenever possible, the client's preference. Chart 14-3 lists some criteria for the placement of peripheral VADs.

CHART 14-3

BEST PRACTICE *for* Placement of Peripheral Venous Access Devices

- Obtain a health care provider's order for placing a peripheral IV cannula.
- For adults, place a peripheral IV catheter only in the upper extremities.
- Use the client's nondominant hand when possible.
- Do not use the arm on the side where the client has a mastectomy, a lymph node dissection, an arteriovenous shunt or fistula, or venous revision.
- Use the most distal area of the client's arm above the wrist for the initial insertion and work your way up the client's arm to more proximal sites for subsequent insertions.
- Avoid placing a peripheral IV catheter over a joint.
- Avoid placing a peripheral IV cannula in a vein that is bruised, has puncture wounds from other venipunctures, is streaked, is hard, has a palpable cord, or is tender to touch.

The veins considered the most appropriate for most types of peripheral IV therapy are in the upper extremities and include the metacarpal, basilic, cephalic, and median veins, as well as their branches (Figure 14-3). Veins that are resilient, long, and straight are the best choices for cannula placement. Veins that are hard, knotty, or sclerotic are difficult to cannulate and are likely to infiltrate. For short-term therapy it is recommended that the nurse place the initial IV catheter in the most distal site of the client's arm and use more proximal sites for subsequent IV cannula insertions.

When determining which vein and which type of peripheral access device to use, the nurse considers the product to be infused. The administration of an isotonic solution, such as 5% dextrose in water (D_5W), does not require any specific precautions related to the size of the vein or the type of catheter used for infusion. However, medications or solutions that are viscous or those with a high osmolality or a high or low pH can be harsh and cause vein irritation. For administration of medications or solutions with these properties, the nurse should consider using a larger vein to decrease the potential for complications.

Most veins may be used for IV administrations that are of short duration, such as a one-time dose of an IV push medication that does not have vein-irritating properties. An infusion of a medication or solution with vein-irritating properties requires a larger vessel to reduce the probability of complications.

Devices

The nurse considers the age and condition of the client; the size, location, and condition of the available veins; and the type and duration of the infusion. The shortest, smallest-gauge device that accommodates the vein, type of infusion, and duration of therapy is the nurse's best choice when selecting an IV catheter.

IV access devices, also known as venous access devices (VADs), may be categorized in a variety of ways. For the purpose of this discussion, peripheral IV catheters are categorized by dwell time (the amount of time the catheter may stay in the vein before being replaced)—either short-term dwell or long-term dwell.

SHORT-TERM DWELL CATHETERS

Winged metal sets and most over-the-needle catheters are short-term dwell catheters. Most **short-term dwell peripheral catheters** have a dwell time of 48 to 72 hours.

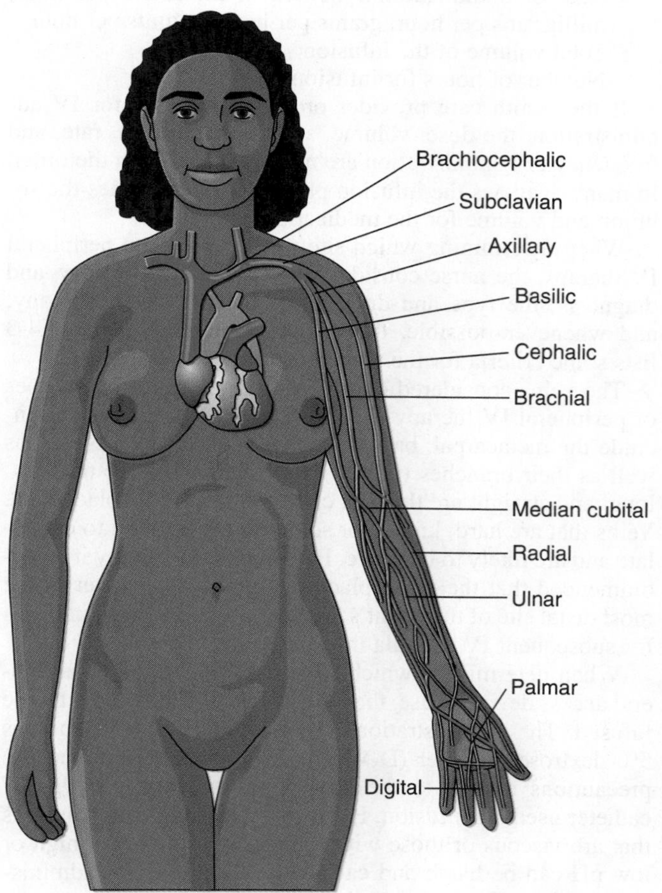

Figure 14-3 ● The superficial veins of the arm.

A metal winged IV set is commonly known as a butterfly. Many practitioners consider these catheters easy to insert, but they contribute to practitioner needle sticks. The practitioner holds the wings between the thumb and forefinger to insert the device. After insertion the wings lie flat against the client's skin.

The standard over-the-needle catheter is between $\frac{3}{4}$ and 3 inches long and ranges in size from 14 to 26 gauge. The over-the-needle catheter consists of a needle inside a polyethylene or plastic catheter. The practitioner removes the needle after making the venipuncture, and the plastic catheter remains inside the vessel.

LONG-TERM DWELL CATHETERS

Long-term dwell peripheral catheters, such as the midline or midclavicular catheters, are usually through-the-needle catheters. Through-the-needle catheters have either a break-away needle or a plastic peel-away sheath to encase the needle after the catheter is advanced through it. Some controversy exists over the amount of time these longer-dwell catheters may stay in place. Some believe that the midline and midclavicular catheters may remain in place for as long as the client exhibits no complications or until he or she no longer requires venous access. In a position paper, the Intravenous Nurses Society (INS) recommends that the maximum dwell time for midline catheters be limited to 2 to 4 weeks and that the maximum dwell time for midclavicular catheters be limited to 2 to 3 months (INS, 1997a). Blood specimens may be drawn from indwelling peripheral catheters, but consideration must be given to the guidelines set by the manufacturer. When a blood specimen is obtained from a venous access device, blood is withdrawn and discarded before sample collection. Table 14-2 describes the blood volume to be discarded before blood sample collection from each venous access device as recommended by the Oncology Nurses Society (ONS) standards of practice.

A midline catheter is a through-the-needle catheter that the nurse usually inserts at the antecubital fossa into the basilic, cephalic, or median cubital veins. The tip of the midline catheter rests in the vein about 6 to 8 inches above the insertion site.

A midclavicular catheter is a through-the-needle catheter that is longer than a midline catheter. The tip of the midclavicular catheter usually rests at the midclavicular line. This area is the approximate junction of the axillary and subclavian veins.

CONSIDERATIONS FOR OLDER ADULTS

Older adults receiving IV therapy have special needs. The normal aging process presents changes in the skin and vessels that require the nurse's attention.

The older person's skin is typically loose, thin, and transparent. As people age, they lose subcutaneous fat, the dermis thins, and the density and amount of collagen lessen. Elastin fibers just below the dermis become more abundant but less effectively organized. The fine elastin fibers in the dermis disappear. All of these changes account for the decreased elasticity found in the older client's skin.

The older adult's veins appear tortuous and large because of inadequate venous pressure. The veins are likely to roll, since there is little connective tissue to hold them, and the veins themselves become more fragile. These changes may require the nurse to alter the IV insertion technique. Chart 14-4 outlines special considerations for the older adult receiving peripheral IV therapy.

Fluid overload, electrolyte imbalances, and other problems can develop when administering fluids to the older client with compromised renal and cardiovascular function. The nurse can prevent complications of IV therapy through careful assessment and monitoring (Powers, 1999).

For older adults who are confused as a result of delirium or dementia, maintaining an intact IV system is often a challenge. The client tends to "pick" at the tubing or, in some cases, pull out the IV line. The nurse protects the site but ensures that it is visible at all times for assessment and maintenance (Figure 14-4).

CENTRAL INTRAVENOUS THERAPY

Description

Central venous therapy involves the placement of a flexible catheter into one of the client's central veins. The tip of the catheter is most commonly situated in the superior vena cava. Drugs, fluids, nutrients, enhancing diagnostic agents, and blood and blood products may be infused through a central IV line. At times, a central venous catheter (CVC) is placed because peripheral venous access is inadequate for the duration or type of IV therapy required. In some clients a CVC allows the nurse to measure and monitor central venous pressure (CVP). In other cases a CVC is inserted to ensure venous access when IV therapy is prescribed.

There are a number of criteria to consider when determining the type of CVC to use. The type and duration of therapy, the setting in which the therapy will be given, and the client's lifestyle, activity, and personal preference all play a role in determining the type of catheter the client will receive.

Each of the devices discussed here, with the exception of the peripherally inserted central catheter, requires a physician to insert the catheter.

Devices

NONTUNNELED CENTRAL VENOUS ACCESS DEVICES

Nontunneled catheters may be placed at the client's bedside. The physician inserts the catheter percutaneously (through the skin) in a manner similar to that for a through-the-needle peripheral IV catheter. The site of placement may

TABLE 14-2 • COMMON INTRAVENOUS MAINTENANCE PROCEDURES

VAD	Dressing	Flushing*	Cap Change†	Blood Withdrawal Discard
Nontunneled Peripheral	Transparent dressing every 5-7 days or gauze dressing qod or with catheter change	Normal saline 1-2 mL q8h, q12h, or q24h	Every week or with catheter change	0.5-1 mL
Central	Transparent dressing every 5-7 days or gauze dressing qod or with catheter change	Heparin 100 units/mL, 3 mL/day or 2 mL/day per each lumen	Every week	1-2 mL
PICC lines	24 hr postinsertion, then transparent dressing every 5-7 days or gauze dressing qod	Heparin 100 units/mL, 3 mL/day; or 10 units/mL, 3 mL 3 times a week	Every week	1-2 mL
Tunneled	Transparent dressing every 5-7 days or gauze dressing qod, then clean technique unless myelosuppressed	Heparin 100 units/mL, 3 mL/day or every other day	Every week	3-5 mL
Implanted port	For continuous access, change noncoring needle and transparent dressing every week or gauze dressing qod	Heparin 100 units/mL, 5 mL/month	Every week	5 mL
Groshong (*Bard Access Systems, Salt Lake City,* UT) VADs	Transparent dressing every 5-7 days or gauze dressing qod, then clean technique unless myelosuppressed	Normal saline 5-10 mL weekly	Every month	3-5 mL
Pheresis	Transparent dressing every 5-7 days or gauze dressing qod or with catheter change	Heparin 1000 units/mL-5000 units/mL 1-2 mL/day‡	Every week	5 mL
Hemodialysis	Transparent dressing every 5-7 days or gauze dressing qod or with catheter change	Heparin 1000 units/mL-5000 units/mL after each treatment‡	Every week	5 mL

From Oncology Nursing Society. (1996). *Access device guidelines: Recommendations for nursing and education.* Pittsburgh: Oncology Nursing Press.
VAD, Venous access device, *PICC,* peripherally inserted central catheter.
*Heparin solution may be 10 units/mL concentration.
†Change caps more frequently if damaged or used frequently.
‡Always aspirate heparin locked in device before using.

CHART 14-4

NURSING FOCUS *on the* OLDER ADULT

Considerations When Receiving Peripheral Intravenous Therapy

- If the client's veins appear large and tortuous, do not use a tourniquet. Having the client hold the arm in a dependent position may fill the veins sufficiently for venipuncture.
- Do not use hand veins for starting an IV line. These veins are too small and limit the older client's ability to perform activities of daily living.
- Use the smallest-gauge IV catheter possible, preferably 21 gauge or smaller. (Most 24-gauge catheters allow the delivery of 100 mL/hr.)
- Do not use a traditional tourniquet. A blood pressure cuff inflated to 80 to 90 mm Hg is easier on the older client's skin.
- Take time to find the most suitable vein.
- Use strict aseptic technique, because the older client is typically immunocompromised.
- Do not slap the arm to visualize the client's veins.
- Use a decreased angle for insertion—usually between 5 and 15 degrees.
- Set the flow rate of IV medications, especially antibiotics, to no more than 100 mL/hr; for clients with congestive heart failure or renal failure, set the rate at 50 mL/hr.
- Use a protective skin preparation before applying a transparent dressing over the IV insertion site; dry gauze pads may be best for clients with tissue-thin skin.
- Cover the IV dressing with flexible netting. If netting is unavailable, use minimal tape or an elastic bandage to secure the dressing and protect the site; keep the insertion site visible at all times.
- Do not use circumferential restraints on the extremity with the IV catheter.
- Do not use the client's lower extremities for IV insertion, because the circulation may be impaired in the client's legs and feet.
- Assess the client's mental status at least every 4 hours.
- Use pumps, controllers, or burettes to control infusion volume and rate.

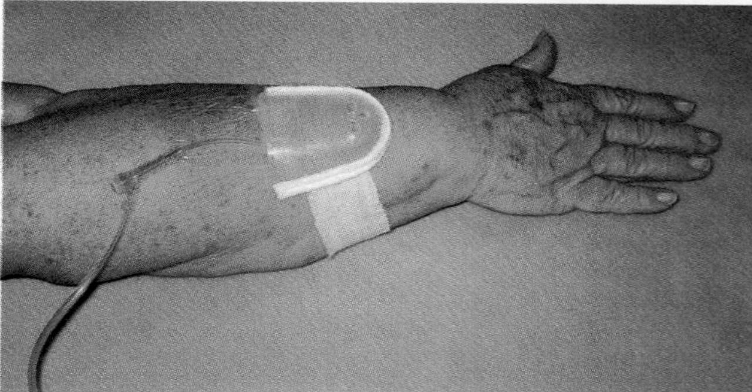

Figure 14-4 ● I.V. House, a commercially available safety device used for IV site protection, guards the integrity of the older adult's skin while helping to secure the site. (Courtesy I.V. House, Hazelwood, MO.)

be into the chest or neck veins (usually the subclavian, or internal or external jugular vein). The catheters are made of polyurethane or Silastic and may have a single lumen or multiple lumens. The chest and neck vein sites are generally used for short-term therapy. After placement and before it is used for infusions, the catheter's placement must be checked by x-ray examination.

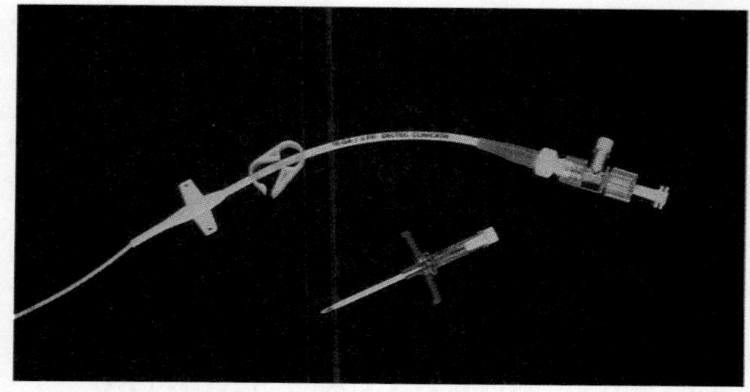

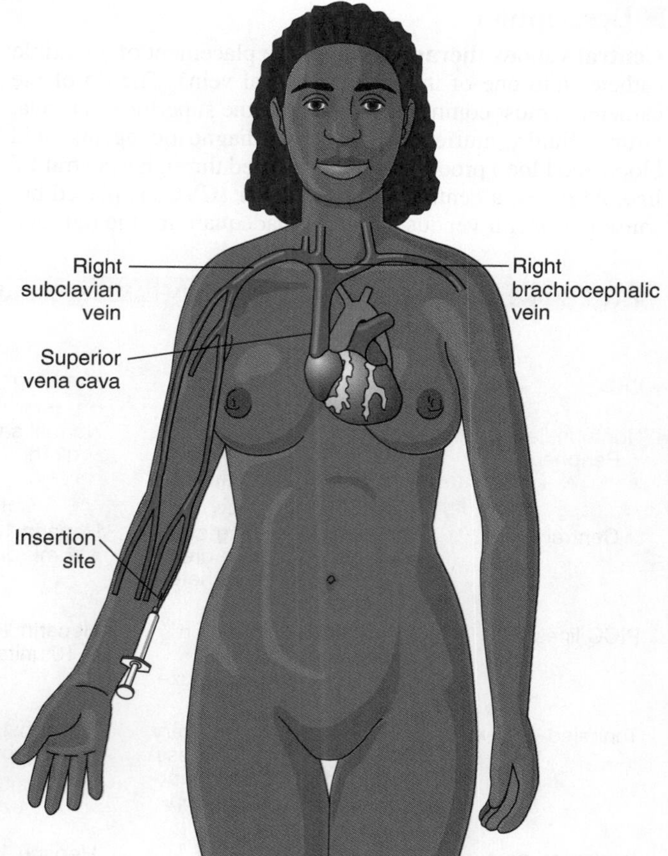

Figure 14-5 ● **A,** A ClinicCath peripherally inserted central venous catheter. **B,** Usual placement. (**A** courtesy SIMS Deltec, Inc., St. Paul, MN.)

PERIPHERALLY INSERTED CENTRAL CATHETER

The peripherally inserted central catheter (PICC) is a special type of nontunneled catheter (Figure 14-5). The PICC is currently the only type of central venous catheter for which placement falls within the realm of nursing practice. Boards of nursing in every state now recognize the specially trained nurse's ability to safely and efficiently access the client's central venous system with a PICC. Many agencies and regulating boards agree that before a nurse can be considered "PICC

COST OF CARE IMPLICATIONS FOR NURSING

VASCULAR ACCESS COST COMPARISON*

Peripheral Catheters		PICC Lines	
IV catheters	$10	IV catheter tray	$75
Start pack	$ 3	Dressing change kit	$ 8
External tubing with cap	$ 3	External tubing with cap	$ 3
Venipuncture charge (Routine change every 72 hr)	$12	Total per PICC insertion	$86
		Dressing kit and external tubing with cap ($8 + $3 × 7)	$77
TOTAL SUPPLY COST	$252	TOTAL SUPPLY COST	$163
Nursing visit at $85.00 per visit × 21 visits	$1785	Nursing visit at $85.00 per visit × 8 visits	$680
TOTAL COST	**$2037**	**TOTAL COST**	**$843**

Research courtesy Patte Strain, RN, BSN, CRNI, Med/EdCon, Ltd.
PICC, Peripherally inserted central catheter.
*Based on 6 weeks of IV antibiotic therapy: Tobramycin 1 g every 12 hours.

competent," he or she must complete a minimum of 8 hours of didactic (classroom) training and perform at least two or three successful PICC placements under the guidance of a preceptor or clinical trainer. Having a PICC placed by a qualified registered nurse (RN) instead of a CVC placed by a physician is less invasive to the client and avoids the surgical risk.

The PICC is appropriate for any setting and for administration of any IV therapy. PICC line placement is ideal for long-term antibiotic therapy in home care and may be more cost-effective than conventional peripheral catheters (see the Cost of Care box above). As with other direct-insertion catheters, PICCs are available as single- or multiple-lumen devices and require an x-ray study to verify placement before use. According to the INS position paper (1997b), a PICC that is functioning well may remain in place for up to 12 months.

TUNNELED CENTRAL VENOUS ACCESS DEVICES

Tunneled central venous catheters include the Broviac, Hickman, Leonard, and Groshong catheters. These central venous catheters (CVCs), named for their developers, are made of silicone or polyurethane. Some of the differences among these catheters relate to their inside diameter, or the gauge of the lumen, and the catheter tip. Before the nurse uses these catheters, the physician confirms the placement of the catheter tip by radiography.

The Broviac catheter is usually a smaller-bore catheter than the Hickman, Leonard, and Groshong catheters. Like the Hickman and Leonard catheters, the Broviac catheter is an open-ended catheter, meaning that it has a tip that is open, similar to that of peripheral venous catheters. The external portions of the Hickman and Broviac catheters have a reinforced area on each lumen. When the catheter is not being used for infusions, the lumens are clamped at the reinforced area to avoid air embolism.

The Groshong catheter is a closed-ended catheter. Toward the tip of the Groshong catheter on the side, there is a slit-valve that opens out and allows fluid to infuse if there is positive pressure in the catheter. It opens in and allows blood to be aspirated if there is negative pressure in the catheter. When the pressure in the catheter is neutral, the valve is closed. The Groshong catheter is not supplied with clamps, and the manufacturer's instructions state that to maintain the integrity of the valve, the catheter should not be clamped. The Groshong tip is available on PICC catheters, as well as on tunneled catheters.

The other features of the Broviac, Hickman, and Groshong catheters are similar in design. Each of these catheters is available with one to four lumens. The catheters are usually 19 to 41 inches (42 to 90 cm) long until the physician trims them during insertion. Each has a cuff positioned inside the subcutaneous tunnel. This cuff is designed to rest just inside the tunnel, under the skin. Fibrous tissue develops around the catheter after insertion to secure it in place and produce a physical barrier to the migration of organisms up the tunnel and into the client's bloodstream.

IMPLANTED PORTS

Implanted ports consist of a portal body, a central septum, a reservoir, and a catheter (Figure 14-6). The port is surgically placed in a subcutaneous pocket in the client's trunk. The surgeon threads the catheter into the central vascular system and positions the tip in the superior vena cava. The catheter is attached to the portal body. The distal tip of the catheter is either open ended or closed ended. The septum is made of self-sealing silicone and is located in either the center or on the side of the portal body. The nurse uses a noncoring needle device to access the system by piercing the skin over the portal body and puncturing the septum of the port.

Dialysis or pheresis catheters may be tunneled or nontunneled and are available in plastic for short-term needs and in silicone for long-term needs. Dialysis catheters have a much larger lumen than regular central lines and are shorter and less flexible. Being more rigid than other lines allows high blood volumes and rates. A catheter that becomes soft enough to collapse with the dynamics of a high flow rate would be disastrous to the dialysis process. Dialysis catheters can be used not only for dialysis but also for intermittent administration of medication. Because of their size, these catheters carry a greater risk for complications. Therefore the physician or an RN with specialized training in dialysis should be consulted before any access procedure.

Maintaining patency of these devices and preventing infection of the catheter/tunnel requires diligent care. Using aseptic technique when changing dressings and flushing the catheter on schedule with appropriate flush solution are very important.

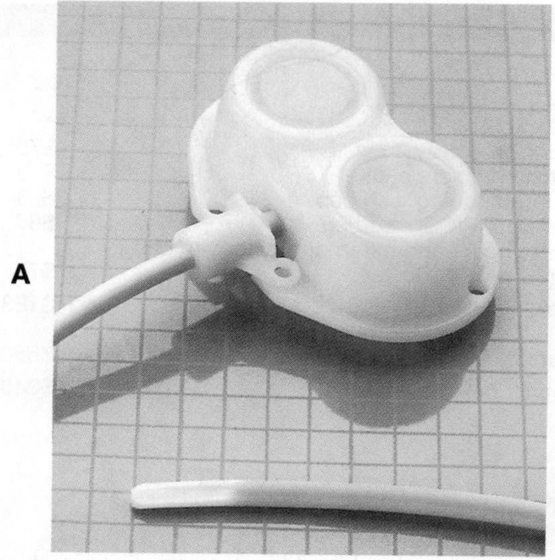

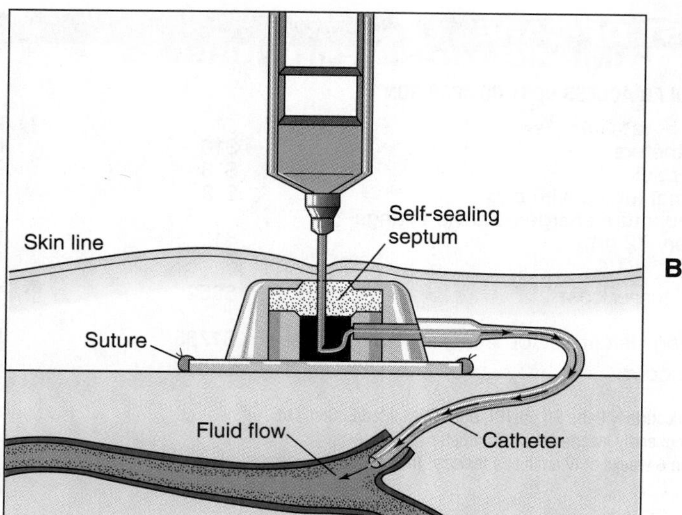

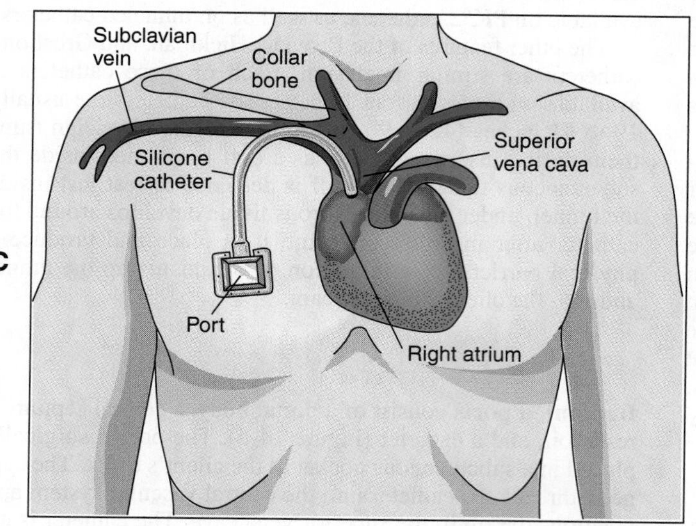

Figure 14-6 ● **A,** A dual-access implanted port for venous access. **B,** A needle puncture through the skin into the port allows drugs, fluids, and blood to be administered. **C,** For systemic drug and fluid delivery, the catheter is placed in the subclavian vein with the tip in the superior vena cava. (**A** courtesy HMP-Horizon Medical Products, Inc., Manchester, GA. **B** and **C** redrawn from Winters, B. [1984]. Implantable vascular devices. *Oncology Nursing Forum, 11*[6], 25-30.)

Complications

Table 14-3 describes local and systemic complications of peripheral IV therapy. When a CVC is used, insertion-related and postinsertion complications must be prevented or detected early (Table 14-4).

Nursing care is the key to decreasing the incidence of complications associated with all infusion therapy. A major nursing responsibility when caring for clients receiving infusion therapy is prevention, assessment, and management of complications.

Arterial Therapy

Description

Arteries are used for intra-arterial chemotherapy (IAC). Chemotherapy administered arterially allows a high concentration of drug to be administered to the tumor site before it is diluted in the circulatory system or metabolized by the liver or kidneys. A high drug concentration at the tumor site optimizes cell kill at the tumor site while minimizing systemic side effects. This action is important to clients who are receiving chemotherapy because debilitating systemic side effects often lead to discontinuation of some therapeutic regimens or alteration of others. In addition, enough drug is available systemically to treat undetected micrometastases.

The physician is responsible for placing the arterial catheter. This is usually done as a surgical procedure or as an interventional radiologic procedure. The nurse monitors and maintains the IAC.

The artery selected for **encannulation** (placement of a catheter) is specific to the diseased organ or structure to be treated. The physician usually prescribes IAC to treat a client's localized inoperable tumor in the liver, head, neck, or bones. Liver tumors are typically treated through the hepatic artery or branches of the celiac artery. The external carotid artery may be used in the treatment of head and neck tumors, and the internal carotid artery may be used in the treatment of brain tumors.

Generally, the duration of the therapy and the number of treatments to be given determine which type of catheter the client will receive. If the client is going to have intermittent therapy for a limited number of times, the physician will likely place a nonpermanent catheter using a radiologic pro-

TABLE 14-3 • COMPLICATIONS OF PERIPHERAL INTRAVENOUS THERAPY

Complication	Definition	Cause	Signs and Symptoms	Treatment	Prevention
LOCAL COMPLICATIONS					
Infiltration	Infusion or seepage of IV solution or medication into the extravascular tissue	Access device either partially or completely dislodges from the vein	IV rate slows down; increasing edema above the IV insertion site; client may complain of burning and tightness at the IV site.	If recent, ice may prevent any further seepage into the surrounding tissue; if older, warm moist compresses will assist with reabsorption of the fluid.	Stabilize IV catheter well; use smallest catheter that will accomplish the infusion; avoid placement over area of flexion; monitor site frequently.
Phlebitis	Inflammation of the vein	May be mechanical as a result of insertion technique or not stabilizing catheter well; may be chemical as a result of the pH or osmolality of the solution or medication	Client may complain of pain at the IV site; nurse may observe that vein appears red and inflamed along the length; client may spike temperature; vein may become hard and cordlike.	Remove catheter; use warm compresses to relieve pain; adjust infusion solution or admixture to prevent further injury.	Change short-term IV catheter every 72 hr, when infusing medications or solutions with high osmolality, choose large veins; anchor catheters well to avoid movement in vein.
Hemotoma	Leaking of blood into the surrounding tissue	May be caused by piercing the back of the vein during insertion of the catheter; client may have faulty coagulation ability or be taking anticoagulants	Discolored area of bruising around the IV site; client may complain of pain; area may be swollen.	Remove IV device and apply pressure; see treatment for infiltration.	Carefully advance catheter, staying parallel with the client's skin; select smallest catheter that will accomplish the task.
Local infection	Bacterial contamination at the IV site	Break in aseptic technique during insertion or the handling of sterile equipment	Site appears red, swollen, and warm; client may complain of tenderness at the site; may observe purulent or malodorous exudate.	Remove IV catheter, allow site to bleed for a few seconds, and use 2×2 gauze to express discharge; send catheter tip for culture; clean site with antibacterial solution and cover with dry sterile dressing; physician to evaluate for septic phlebitis and need for surgical intervention.	Use careful technique when inserting IV; change site every 72 hours.
Catheter embolism	A shaving or piece of catheter breaks off and floats freely in the vessel	May occur if the needle of an over-the-needle catheter is reinserted into the catheter or if the needle of a through-the-needle catheter is inadvertently pulled back through the catheter	Client will experience a decrease in blood pressure and complain of pain along the vein; pulse becomes weak, rapid, and thready, and nurse may note cyanosis of the nail beds and circumorally; client may lapse into unconsciousness.	Discontinue catheter and apply a tourniquet high on the limb of the catheter site; inspect catheter for any rough edges; an x-ray film is taken to determine the presence of any catheter piece; surgical intervention may be necessary.	When inserting over-the-needle catheters, never reinsert the needle into the catheter; avoid pulling a through-the-needle catheter back through the needle during insertion.

Continued

TABLE 14-3 • COMPLICATIONS OF PERIPHERAL INTRAVENOUS THERAPY—cont'd

Complication	Definition	Cause	Signs and Symptoms	Treatment	Prevention
SYSTEMIC COMPLICATIONS					
Bloodstream infection	Pathogenic organisms enter the client's circulation	Result of poor aseptic technique or contaminated infusion or if the catheter site is not changed regularly	Early symptoms include fever, chills, headache, and general malaise; if left untreated, client may experience severe infection, which may lead to vascular collapse and death.	Change the entire infusion system from solution to IV device; notify physician, obtain cultures, and administer antibiotics as ordered; if the infusate is the suspected cause, send a specimen to the laboratory for evaluation.	Same as for local infection above.
Circulatory overload	Disruption of fluid homeostasis with excess fluid in the circulatory system	Infusion of fluids at a rate greater than the client's system can accommodate	Client may complain of shortness of breath and cough; client's blood pressure is elevated, and there is puffiness around the eyes and edema in dependent areas; client's neck veins may be engorged, and nurse may hear moist breath sounds.	Slow the IV rate and notify physician; raise client to an upright position; monitor vital signs and administer oxygen as ordered; administer diuretics as ordered.	Monitor intake and output carefully and notify physician as soon as an imbalance is noticed between the client's intake and output.
Speed shock	Systemic reaction to the rapid infusion of a substance unfamiliar to the client's circulatory system	Rapid infusion of drugs or bolus infusion, which causes the drug to reach toxic levels quickly	Client may complain of lightheadedness or dizziness and chest tightness; nurse may note that client has a flushed face and an irregular pulse; without intervention, client may lose consciousness and go into shock and cardiac arrest.	Immediately discontinue the drug infusion and hang D_5W to keep the vein open; monitor vital signs carefully and notify physician for further treatment orders.	Nurse is aware of the appropriate infusion rate of medications and adheres to them; use of infusion control devices assists in prevention of speed shock.
Allergic reaction	Local or general response to an allergen	May be a response to tape, cleansing agent, drug, solution, or IV device	A client having a local reaction may exhibit a wheal, redness, or itching at the IV site; in the case of a general reaction, client may complain of itching, running nose, and tearing; nurse may note bronchospasm, wheezing, and a truncal rash; without treatment, client may experience anaphylaxis.		

TABLE 14-4 • CENTRAL LINE INSERTION-RELATED AND POSTINSERTION-RELATED COMPLICATIONS

Problem	Definition	Signs and Symptoms	Possible Causes	Treatment
INSERTION-RELATED COMPLICATIONS				
Pneumothorax	Collection of air in the pleural space (space between the lung and chest wall)	Chest pain Dyspnea Apprehension Cyanosis Decreased breath sounds on the affected side Abnormal chest x-ray findings	Puncture of the pleural covering of the lung by the introducer on insertion of a direct subclavian approach	Remove catheter or assist with removal Assess client by monitoring vital signs, and assess breath sounds Notify physician immediately if suspected after insertion Administer oxygen as ordered Assist with insertion of a chest tube
Hemothorax	Blood enters the pleural cavity	Similar to pneumothorax; usually see dyspnea first and then tachycardia Decreased hemoglobin because of blood pooling	Result of puncture or transection of the subclavian vein or artery	Same as for pneumothorax Apply pressure on insertion site after introducer needle and catheter are removed
Chylothorax	Lymph (chyle) enters the pleural cavity	Same as in hemothorax Usually noted on insertion with withdrawal of a milk-like substance	Transection of the thoracic duct on the left side	Same as for pneumothorax
Hydrothorax	Infusion of IV fluids directly into the thoracic cavity	Same as in pneumothorax with absence of vesicular breath sounds and a murmur with a flat sound over the location	Transection of the subclavian vein and placement of the catheter into the thoracic cavity	Same as for pneumothorax with removal of the catheter and aspiration of fluid
Air embolism	Air enters the central venous system	Loud churning heard over the pericardium on auscultation Chest pain, dyspnea, hypoxia Anxiety, tachycardia, hypotension	Air is introduced into the central venous system by insertion, tubing changes, or breaking of the catheter	Place client in lateral Trendelenburg position on left side Clamp catheter immediately Notify physician immediately
Arterial puncture	Cannulation of an artery	Pulsating of bright red blood from the introducer needle	Accessed the artery instead of the vein	Remove needle immediately and apply pressure to the site Secure a pressure dressing for 5-10 min
Difficult cannulation	Inability to access the vein	No blood return	Poor IV skills Lack of knowledge Small sclerotic veins Volume deficit Infiltration of local anesthetic	Good venous assessment before insertion Pull skin to side of vein to apply anesthetic
Nerve injury	Damage to one of the ulnar, median, or radial cords	Tingling to sensory motor deficit to complete paralysis	Ineffective cannulation of the vein	Careful cannulation without probing If resistance is met on catheter advancement, do not force catheter

Continued

Data from Robin M. McBeath, RN, BSN, Vascular Access Education Specialist; and Fern Zick, RN, Vascular Access Education Specialist. *Central line care and maintenance workbook.* Sinai Education Resource Center.
SVC, Superior vena cava; *PICC*, peripherally inserted central catheter.

TABLE 14-4 • CENTRAL LINE INSERTION-RELATED AND POSTINSERTION-RELATED COMPLICATIONS—cont'd

Problem	Definition	Signs and Symptoms	Possible Causes	Treatment
INSERTION-RELATED COMPLICATIONS—cont'd				
Difficult threading	Catheter will not advance in the vein	Resistance is met when trying to advance the catheter	Vasospasm Narrowed vessels Anatomic valve obstruction	Help client to relax Reposition extremity Inject saline to "float" catheter in Select another vein
POSTINSERTION COMPLICATIONS				
Malpositioned catheters	Catheter has moved from original placement to either the jugular vein or SVC above the right atrium	Ear or neck pain Water heard in the ear Palpitations or arrythmias Inability to irrigate	Changes in interthoracic pressure related to excessive vomiting or coughing	Place client in semi-Fowler's position Rapidly flush line Reposition line by guidewire exchange (physician) Partially withdraw catheter Reposition under fluoroscopy (physician)
Catheter rupture	Catheter is broken open and/or apart	Fluid leaking Pain or swelling during infusion Reflux of blood into the catheter extension	Using small syringes (<10 mL) Occluded catheter Forceful irrigation Pinch syndrome can cause catheter embolus	Guidewire exchange (physician) Repair damaged segment Remove catheter
Occlusion	Catheter lumen has become narrowed and/or closed as a result of precipitate, blood clot, or fibrin sheath	Infusion stops and/or pump alarm sounds Inability or difficulty administering fluids Inability or difficulty drawing blood Increased resistance to flushing of the catheter	Drug precipitate (calcium, diazepam, and phenytoin are common) Blood clots and fibrin sheath can form with ineffective flushing routine	For drug precipitate, use hydrochloric acid For blood clot, use thrombolytic enzymes such as urokinase (see procedure for declotting central lines)
Phlebitis	Inflammation of the vein wall	Pain, redness, slight swelling May progress to cellulitus and palpable cord or collateral circulation	Mechanical phlebitis is common with PICC lines and will appear within 7 days after insertion Chemical phlebitis may be seen with catheter rupture	Mechanical phlebitis: conservative measures, warm compresses applied for 20 min qid for approximately 48-72 hr Mild exercise Chemical: change catheter and/or medication
Thrombosis	Formation of a blood clot in a vessel within the neck, chest, or arms that occurs in the presence of a central venous catheter	Chest pain, earache, or jaw pain Edema of neck, supraclavicular area, or extremities Edema at puncture site Jugular distention Collateral circulation on the affected side	Statis, vessel wall injury, or hypercoagulability	Anticoagulant therapy Possible catheter removal
Infection	Infection may be localized at the insertion site or in the catheter, or may progress to systemic infection	Redness, warmth, tenderness, swelling at the insertion site Cellulitus Possible exudate of purulent material Local rash or pustules Fever, chills, malaise Leukocytosis Nausea and vomiting Elevated urine glucose level	Failure to maintain sterile technique during catheter insertion or care Wet or soiled dressing remaining on site Immunosuppression Contaminated catheter or solution	Monitor vital signs closely Monitor culture site Redress with sterile technique Treat systemically with antibiotics or antifungals, depending on culture results Blood cultures Remove catheter

Data from Robin M. McBeath, RN, BSN, Vascular Access Education Specialist; and Fern Zick, RN, Vascular Access Education Specialist. *Central line care and maintenance workbook.* Sinai Education Resource Center.
SVC, Superior vena cava; *PICC,* peripherally inserted central catheter.

cedure in the radiology department. If the client is prescribed continuous therapy over a period of weeks or months, the physician will likely place a permanent arterial catheter.

Devices

Catheters placed using a radiologic procedure are usually made of a polymer or Teflon. Catheters inserted surgically are usually ports. These ports are similar to those discussed under Central Intravenous Therapy (p. 201), but the lumen of the catheter is generally smaller.

Whether the physician is placing the catheter surgically or radiologically, the catheter is threaded into the main artery feeding the tumor site. Some clients may have several vessels supplying the tumor site, or it may not be possible to infuse the target vessel without infusing adjacent vessels. In either situation, the physician may elect to occlude vessels by injecting Gelfoam or metal coils through the catheter. Blocking the arteries in this way may cause the tumor to shrink without the chemotherapy. The body absorbs the Gelfoam within a few days, re-establishing circulation. Metal coils provide permanent vascular occlusion. Until the client's body establishes collateral circulation, he or she may complain of general malaise and pain in the area occluded.

Complications

Catheter displacement is the most common problem associated with temporary arterial catheters. Clients whose catheters become displaced may exhibit dyspepsia, excessive nausea and vomiting or diarrhea, gastric pain from peptic ulcers, or abdominal pain from pancreatitis. Management may include stopping the chemotherapy infusion temporarily until the client can be treated with antiemetics and antacids.

A subintimal tear is the separation of the intima and media of the arterial wall, resulting from manipulation during placement. The client may complain of pain near the target organ during the infusion. Subintimal tears can delay therapy for weeks until the tear heals.

Arterial occlusion may occur with either a radiologically placed catheter or a surgically placed catheter. The physician may order heparin to be added to the chemotherapy infusion or have the client take 650 mg of aspirin twice a day to avoid catheter occlusion. Even with this prophylactic therapy, the nurse may observe a transient or permanent loss or decrease in the pulse distal to the insertion site. The nurse must report this symptom immediately. If the physician diagnoses the client as having an embolism, the physician will either remove the catheter or use the fibrolytic agent urokinase (Abbokinase) in an attempt to lyse the clot.

Intraperitoneal Therapy

Description

Intraperitoneal (IP) therapy is the administration of therapeutic agents (cytotoxic drugs and biologic response modifiers [BRMs]) into the peritoneal cavity. IP therapy is usually prescribed for the treatment of tumors that are confined to the peritoneal cavity. Carcinomas of the ovaries and fallopian tubes generally meet this criterion.

Devices

There are three categories of IP catheters generally available: temporary indwelling catheters, semipermanent indwelling external catheters, and implantable IP ports. The placement of an IP catheter is a physician responsibility, but the administration and monitoring of the therapeutic agent is generally a nursing responsibility.

Administration of the IP therapy includes three phases: the instillation phase, the dwell phase, and the drain phase. The peritoneal cavity generally acts as a tumor refuge, separated from the bloodstream by a cellular enclosure similar to the blood-brain barrier. This enclosure protects IP tumors from systemically infused chemotherapeutic agents. IP therapy, like intra-arterial therapy, allows for the administration of antineoplastic agents directly to the tumor sites. This enhances the drug's penetration and cell kill while restricting systemic effects.

Temporary indwelling catheters include temporary peritoneal dialysis catheters, paracentesis catheters, and 16- or 18-gauge over-the-needle IV catheters. Semipermanent indwelling external catheters include the Tenckhoff, Gore-Tex, and column-disk catheters. IP implanted ports are similar to IV and arterial ports, but the portal body and the catheter diameter are larger.

Temporary indwelling catheters may be inserted and removed at the bedside. Clients receiving a temporary indwelling catheter benefit from having a new catheter inserted at the time of each therapy. Complications such as the development of fibrous sheaths and infection do not plague these clients.

Semipermanent indwelling external catheters and IP implanted ports are inserted in the operating room. Both of these catheters are appropriate for longer-term therapy.

Complications

Exit site infection, indicated by redness, tenderness, and warmth of the tissue around the catheter, is more often seen in clients who have a Tenckhoff catheter. Frequent dressing changes at the exit site using sterile technique can help prevent this complication.

Microbial peritonitis is inflammation of the peritoneal membranes from the invasion of microorganisms. The client may experience a fever and complain of abdominal pain. There may be abdominal rigidity and rebound tenderness. This condition is preventable with strict aseptic technique in the handling of all equipment and infusion supplies. Management includes antimicrobial therapy either intravenously or intraperitoneally.

Chemical peritonitis is irritation of the peritoneal membranes by the chemotherapeutic agent. The client may complain of symptoms similar to those experienced with microbial peritonitis. If chemical peritonitis is severe, it may delay further treatment.

Occlusion is the inability to administer fluids into the peritoneum or withdraw fluid from the peritoneum. **Occlusion** is caused by the formation of fibrous sheaths or fibrin clots or plugs inside the catheter or around the tip. It may also be caused by compartmentalization of fluid due to adhesions or to twisting, kinking, or displacement of the catheter. Management may include the infusion of a lysing agent such as urokinase. If the catheter is an indwelling external catheter, the physician may attempt to dislodge the clot by using a push-pull method with a syringe and 0.9% normal saline solution (NSS). Sometimes the physician may insert a sterile stylet through an external catheter to dislodge the catheter.

Subcutaneous Therapy

Description

Subcutaneous (SC) therapy involves the insertion of a small-gauge needle into the client's subcutaneous tissue and the continuous administration of isotonic fluids or medications at a slow rate of usually 1 mL/min. Continuous subcutaneous infusion (CSQI) has been used as an alternative to IV therapy, primarily for fluid replacement, and was referred to as **hypodermoclysis** or clysis in the 1950s and 1960s. Today, SC fluid replacement is again being referred to as hypodermoclysis in the health care literature.

SC infusion was virtually abandoned after the development of IV infusion. Recently it has been found to be beneficial primarily for older persons requiring short-term fluid administration to correct dehydration (Donnelly, 1999).

Other criteria for hypodermoclysis include that the client (Brown & Worobec, 2000):

- Needs less than 3000 mL of fluid per day
- Has no bleeding or coagulation problems
- Has intact skin sites available

To facilitate fluid absorption, an enzyme such as hyaluronidase (Wydase) may be mixed with the infusion fluid. Because this enzyme can cause an allergic reaction, a test dose is given intradermally. If the enzyme is not used, the infusion may not be well absorbed and redness at the insertion site is more likely (Brown & Worobec, 2000).

Devices

The nurse begins CSQI by cleansing any area on the client's body that has sufficient subcutaneous tissue. Such sites include the inner thigh and abdomen. The nurse primes the attached tubing and, gently pinching an area of approximately 2 inches (1 cm), inserts a small-gauge needle. Appropriate needle choices for CSQI include a 25- to 27-gauge butterfly needle or a Sub-Q-Set. A butterfly needle is inserted at a 35- to 45-degree angle, whereas a Sub-Q-Set is inserted at a 90-degree angle. After anchoring the needle, the nurse covers the site with a transparent dressing.

Clients who benefit from CSQI are those who:

- Are unable to take oral medications (e.g., have dysphagia, gastrointestinal obstruction, or malabsorption)
- Have intractable nausea and vomiting
- Require parenteral medication but have poor venous access
- Require subcutaneous injections for longer than 48 hours
- Have a need for prolonged use of parenteral medication
- Need a continuous level of medication to control pain
- Cannot cope with the expense of IV therapy

Complications

Insertion site irritation, evidenced by erythema, heat, or swelling, is a local complication of CSQI. Rotation of the SC site approximately every 5 to 7 days usually helps prevent this problem.

Other complications include pooling of the fluid at the insertion site and an uneven fluid drip rate. Both of these problems may be resolved by restarting the infusion in another location. An infusion pump may also be used.

Another possible complication is fluid overload. This problem can be prevented if the fluid rate is no more than 80 mL/hr. If signs of fluid overload occur, the infusion should be discontinued.

Central Nervous System Therapy

Central nervous system therapy involves the infusion of medications into the epidural space or intrathecally.

Epidural Therapy

In **epidural therapy,** the physician or specially trained nurse administers medication into the epidural space of the spinal column. Located between the wall of the vertebral canal and the dura mater, the epidural space consists of fat, connective tissue, and blood vessels that protect the spinal cord. The most common uses of epidural therapy are to relieve postoperative or chronic pain and the pain associated with labor and delivery. The physician, usually an anesthesiologist or neurosurgeon, initiates epidural therapy. There are four major categories of catheters used for epidural therapy. The choice of one over the other depends on the purpose and duration of the therapy. Table 14-5 describes each type and lists their indications.

Opioids administered epidurally slowly diffuse across the dura mater to the dorsal horn of the spinal cord. They lock onto receptors and block pain impulses from ascending to the brain. The client receives pain relief from the level of the injection caudally (toward the toes). Local anesthetics administered epidurally work on the sensory nerve roots in the epidural space to block pain impulses. The physician administers the first dose of medication; then, depending on state law, the type of medication, and facility policies, nurses trained in epidural therapy may administer subsequent doses. In all cases it is a nursing responsibility to monitor the client receiving epidural therapy for any signs of complications. In some states, specially trained nurses are permitted to remove the catheter when therapy is discontinued.

Complications associated with epidural therapy are usually caused by the medications administered. Table 14-6 outlines medication-related complications that may occur with the administration of epidural opiates and local anesthetics.

Intrathecal Therapy

Intrathecal therapy provides a means of administering chemotherapy, pain medication, or antibiotics directly into the ventricular cerebrospinal fluid (CSF) of clients who suffer from CSF malignancies or metastases, chronic cancer pain, or CSF infections. Some medications used to treat CSF neoplasms, such as methotrexate and cytarabine, cannot be administered intravenously because they cannot cross the blood-brain barrier. Others must be administered in very large doses to cross this natural protective mechanism. It may not be possible to administer large doses of chemotherapeutic agents intravenously because of the severe systemic side effects associated with them. Administration of medications via the intrathecal route

TABLE 14-5 • CATHETERS USED FOR EPIDURAL THERAPY

Type of Device	Description	Indications
Percutaneous catheter	Flexible nylon catheter threaded through a spinal needle into the epidural space. The external end has a standard female Luer-Lok hub, which accepts an intermittent injection cap.	Temporary pain relief postoperatively or during labor and delivery. For pain control in clients with end-stage cancer or a temporary measure to determine if the client with chronic pain will receive relief with epidural therapy.
Subcutaneous tunneled catheter	A Silastic catheter tunneled from the point where it exits the spine to a point on the client's trunk, usually on the side just above the waist. Like a tunneled central venous catheter, the catheter has a Dacron cuff that prevents the migration of microorganisms along the catheter into the epidural space.	A more permanent catheter indicated for clients in whom epidural therapy has proved to be effective and who have a life expectancy of weeks to months.
Totally implantable reservoir or port	Appears identical to a venous or arterial port. The surgeon places the portal body over a bony prominence, such as the spine itself, or one of the client's lower ribs.	Indicated for clients who respond to epidural therapy and have a life expectancy of months to years. Another indication is the client who is confused and repeatedly pulls out his or her subcutaneous tunneled catheter.
Totally implantable infusion pump	Consists of a catheter whose tip sits in the epidural space at the appropriate level. The catheter is tunneled subcutaneously and attached to the pump, which is usually implanted in a pocket in the abdominal region of the chest wall. As described earlier, the medication is in the pump's reservoir.	The most expensive method of administering epidural therapy. Indicated for clients who will require therapy for a long period (chronic pain) and who have a life expectancy of months to years.

TABLE 14-6 • MEDICATION-RELATED COMPLICATIONS OF EPIDURAL THERAPY

System	Epidural Opiates	Epidural Local Anesthetics
Cardiovascular	No postural hypotension Minor changes in heart rate	Postural hypotension Decrease in heart rate
Respiratory	If occurs, may be early at 1-2 hours due to systemic absorption or late after dose at 6-24 hours due to migration to brain	Usually unimpaired
Central nervous system	Sedation may be marked Convulsions absent	Sedation absent to mild Convulsions possible due to rapid vascular absorption Sensory losses Motor weakness
Genitourinary	Urinary retention	Urinary retention
Integumentary	Pruritus	Pruritus rarely occurs
Gastrointestinal	Nausea and vomiting	Nausea and vomiting rarely occurs

From Booker, M.F., & Ignatavicius, D.D. (1996). *Infusion therapy: Techniques and medications.* Philadelphia: W.B. Saunders.

eliminates this problem, since the medication is administered directly into the CSF.

The Ommaya reservoir is the catheter commonly used for intrathecal therapy. A neurosurgeon is usually responsible for the placement of the catheter in the operating room under strict asepsis. The Ommaya reservoir consists of two pieces: a mushroom-shaped self-sealing dome made of silicone and a catheter that attaches to the dome. The tip of the catheter is placed in one of the lateral ventricles. The reservoir is attached and placed beneath a flap in the client's scalp. Some models of the reservoir have a side outlet tube that can be used as a shunt to remove excess CSF in the client with increased intracranial pressure. The physician, or in some cases the chemotherapy nurse, administers the medication by inserting a needle through the skin into the Ommaya dome. After removing an amount of CSF equal to the volume of the medication to be administered, the physician slowly injects the medication. The physician removes the needle and pumps the dome of the reservoir to release the medication into the catheter for delivery to the CSF. The nurse is responsible for monitoring the client for any complications.

Complications

Infection in the client receiving either epidural or intrathecal therapy is the result of a lack of asepsis when handling the medication or during the administration. There may be local evidence of infection, such as redness or swelling at the catheter exit site or over the Ommaya reservoir. The client may also exhibit neurologic and systemic signs of infection, such as headache, stiff neck, or temperature higher than 101° F (38.3° C). The nurse may observe cloudy CSF, indicating a proliferation of white blood cells in clients undergoing intrathecal therapy.

Misplacement or migration of the catheter may occur at the time of placement, or the catheter may move or become kinked after placement. In clients with epidural catheters, when the nurse aspirates to check placement, he or she may observe clear, free-flowing fluid (CSF), indicating that the catheter has migrated into the subarachnoid space, or the nurse may withdraw blood, indicating that the catheter has migrated into a blood vessel. An inadvertent administration of local anesthetics directly into the subarachnoid space may lead to high or total spinal block and convulsions or cardiovascular depression. Clients who mistakenly receive local anesthetics intravenously may experience toxic reactions with convulsions. In the client receiving intrathecal therapy via an Ommaya reservoir, the physician may observe no or very slow filling when "pumping" the dome. The client may exhibit new neurologic symptoms if the catheter has migrated.

Intraosseous Therapy

Description

Intraosseous (IO) therapy is a previously used and reemerging method of gaining access to the vascular system. IO therapy is primarily used in critically injured clients with vascular collapse. However, a number of research studies have confirmed that it is a viable option for other clients requiring infusion therapy. In some states, prehospital providers such as emergency medical technicians (EMTs) and paramedics, as well as trained clinicians in trauma centers and emergency departments, initiate IO therapy.

IO therapy allows access to the rich vascular network located in the long bones. This vascular network is more prominent in children younger than 6 years of age. Victims of trauma, burns, cardiac arrest, and other life-threatening conditions benefit from IO therapy, because often clinicians are unable to access these clients' vascular systems using traditional methods such as IV therapy. Research indicates that absorption rates of large-volume parenteral (LVP) infusions and medications administered via the IO route are similar to those achieved with peripheral or central venous administration.

Devices

Theoretically, any needle may be used to provide IO therapy and access the medullary space. However, the following criteria make some needles superior to others for IO therapy:

- A needle with a removable stylet that screws into the cannula to keep the needle from retracting during insertion
- A short shaft to eliminate accidental dislodgment after placement
- An adjustable guard to stabilize the needle at skin level
- Graduations along the needle to guide the practitioner during insertion

Complications

Improper needle placement is the most common complication of IO therapy. An accumulation of fluid under the skin at either the insertion site or on the other side of the limb indicates that the needle is either not far enough in to penetrate the bone marrow or is too far into the limb and has protruded through the other side of the shaft.

Needle obstruction occurs when the puncture has been accomplished but there has been a delay in flushing. This delay may cause the needle to become clotted with bone marrow.

Osteomyelitis is a very serious complication of IO therapy. This infection in the bone tissue is unusual, but when it occurs, it is generally due to the cannula's being left in place too long or to the client's having had a source of infection before the needle's insertion.

An embolus is a complication of any orthopedic procedure, and IO therapy is no exception. An embolus occurs when a bone fragment or fat enters the peripheral circulation. The client exhibits classic symptoms of respiratory distress, tachycardia, hypertension, tachypnea, fever, and petechiae. Laboratory data indicate an increased sedimentation rate and decreased red blood cell and platelet counts.

Compartment syndrome is a condition in which increased tissue pressure in a confined anatomic space causes decreased blood flow to the area. The decreased circulation to the area leads to hypoxia and pain in the area. This is very rare in IO therapy, but the nurse should monitor the site of the IO therapy carefully and alert the physician promptly if the client exhibits any signs of decreased circulation to the limb, such as coolness, swelling, mottling, or discoloration. Without improvement in perfusion to the limb, the client may require amputation of the limb.

ONLINE RESOURCES

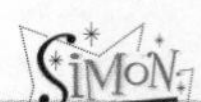

For suggested readings and Internet resources, go to http://www.wbsaunders.com/SIMON/Iggy/.

SELECTED BIBLIOGRAPHY

Asterisk indicates a classic or definitive work on this subject.

Andris, D.A., & Krzywda, E.A. (1997). Central venous access: Clinical practice issues. *Nursing Clinics of North America, 32*(4), 719-740.

Andris, D.A., & Krzywda, E.A. (1999). Central venous catheter occlusion: Successful management strategies. *MEDSURG Nursing, 8*(4), 229-237.

Bagnall-Reeb, H. (1998). Diagnosis of central venous access device occlusion: Implications for nursing practice. *Journal of Intravenous Nursing, 21*(5 Suppl.), S115-S121.

*Booker, M.F., & Ignatavicius, D.D. (1996). *Infusion therapy: techniques and medications.* Philadelphia: W.B. Saunders.

Donnelly, M. (1999). The benefits of hypodermoclysis. *Nursing Standard, 13*(52), 44-45.

Hadaway, L.C. (1999a). I.V. infiltration: Not just a peripheral problem. *Nursing99, 29*(9), 41-43.

Hadaway, L.C. (1999b). Vascular access devices: Meeting patients' needs. *MEDSURG Nursing, 8*(5), 296-302.

Herbst, S.L., Kaplan, L.K., & McKinnon, B.T. (1998). Vascular access devices: Managing occlusions and related complications in home infusion. *Infusion, 4*(8), 1-32.

Intravenous Nurses Society. (1997a). Position paper: Midline and midclavicular catheters. *Journal of Intravenous Nursing, 20*(4), 175-178.

Intravenous Nurses Society. (1997b). Position paper: Peripherally inserted central catheters. *Journal of Intravenous Nursing, 20*(4), 172-174.

Krzywda, E. (1998). Central venous access: Catheters, technology, and physiology. *MEDSURG Nursing, 7*(3), 132-140.

Laroure, E. (1999). The art of accessing an implanted port. *Nursing99, 29*(5), 56-58.

Luebke, M.A., et al. (1998). Comparison of the microbial barrier properties of a needleless and a conventional needle-based intravenous access system. *American Journal of Infection Control, 26*(4), 437-441.

Masoorli, S., Angeles, T., & Barbone, M. (1998). Danger points: How to prevent nerve injuries from venipuncture. *Nursing98, 28*(9), 35-39.

Mayo, D.J. (1998). Administering urokinase for catheter clearance. *Nursing98, 28*(12), 50-52.

McConnell, E.A. (1999). Pump primer: How to choose the right infusion device. *Nursing Management, 30*(8), 49-52.

Meier, P.A. (1998). Impact of a dedicated intravenous therapy team on nosocomial bloodstream infection rates. *American Journal of Infection Control, 26*(4), 388-392.

Mendelson, M.H., et al.(1998). Study of a needleless intermittent intravenous-access system for peripheral infusions: analysis of staff, patient, and institutional outcomes. *Infection Control and Hospital Epidemiology. 19*(6), 401-406.

*Oncology Nursing Society. (1996). *Access device guidelines: Recommendations for nursing practice and education.* Pittsburgh: Oncology Nursing Press.

*Pearson, M.L., et al. (1996). Guideline for prevention of intravascular device–related infections. *Infection Control and Hospital Epidemiology, 17*(7), 438-473.

Powers, F.A. (1999). Your elderly patient needs I.V. therapy . . . Can you keep her safe? *Nursing99, 29*(7), 54-55.

Treston-Aurand, J., et al. (1997). Impact of dressing materials on central venous catheter infection rates. *Journal of Intravenous Nursing, 20*(4), 201-206.

CHAPTER

15

Acid-Base Balance

M. LINDA WORKMAN

Learning Objectives

After studying this chapter, you should be able to:

1. Describe the relationship between hydrogen ion concentration and pH.
2. Explain the role of bicarbonate in the blood.
3. Explain the concept of compensation.
4. Compare the role of a buffer in conditions of acidosis and alkalosis.
5. Compare the roles of the respiratory system and the renal system in maintaining acid-base balance.
6. Describe the role of oxygen in maintaining acid-base balance.
7. Interpret whether the client's arterial blood gas values are normal, elevated, or low.

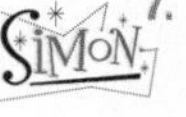

Go to http://www.wbsaunders.com/SIMON/Iggy/ for self-assessment questions related to these Learning Objectives.

Acid-base balance results from the regulation of hydrogen ion (H^+) production and elimination. Body fluid **pH** is a measure of the body fluid's hydrogen ion concentration. The hydrogen ion concentration, or pH, has the narrowest range of normal and the tightest control mechanisms of all electrolytes. The concentration of hydrogen ions, formed from acids, must be rigidly controlled for proper physiologic function. Even small changes in the hydrogen ion concentration, or pH, of body fluids can cause major problems in physiologic function. Keeping the pH within the normal range involves balancing acids and bases in body fluids.

The normal hydrogen ion concentration of blood and other body fluids is quite low (<0.0001 mEq/L) compared with the body fluid concentrations of other electrolytes (see Chapters 11 and 13). Because it is so low, hydrogen ion concentration is measured in pH units, calculated as the negative logarithm of the concentration in milliequivalents per liter (Figure 15-1). Normal pH ranges from 7.35 to 7.45 for arterial blood and from 7.31 to 7.41 for venous blood.

Because pH is calculated in negative logarithm units, the value of pH is inversely related (negatively related) to the concentration of hydrogen ions. In other words, the lower the pH value of a fluid, the higher the concentration of hydrogen ions in that fluid. The pH of a solution may range from 1 (as acidic as possible) to 14 (as alkaline as possible), with 7 being neutral. *A change of 1 pH unit actually represents a tenfold change in hydrogen ion concentration.* Therefore even a pH unit change of one tenth (e.g., a change from 7.4 to 7.3) represents a large increase in the hydrogen ion concentration. Table 15-1 lists terms used to describe acid-base balance.

Changes from normal blood pH (7.35 to 7.45) interfere with many normal physiologic functions by:

- Altering the shape of hormones and enzymes so that they may no longer perform their designated functions
- Changing the distribution of other electrolytes, causing fluid and electrolyte imbalances
- Altering the responses of excitable membranes so that the heart, nerves, skeletal muscles, and gastrointestinal tract are either less or more active than normal
- Decreasing the uptake, activity, distribution, and effectiveness of many hormones and drugs

Fortunately, the body has many well-regulated mechanisms to ensure minimal changes in hydrogen ion concentration. Table 15-2 lists the key concepts of acid-base balance.

INTRODUCTION TO ACID-BASE BALANCE

As discussed in Chapters 11 and 13, body fluids are electrically neutral even though they contain ions with an overall positive charge (**cations** or **protons**) and ions with an overall negative charge **(anions).** When fluids contain an equal number of positive and negative charges, the electrical charge of the fluid remains neutral. The body maintains a blood pH between 7.35 and 7.45 in a similar manner; however, this value is not strictly neutral (7.0 is neutral) but rather is slightly alkaline. Normal body fluid pH remains at a near-neutral value when the acid components and base components are in relative balance, limiting the total number of free hydrogen ions. Acid-base balance occurs by matching the rate of hydrogen ion production with the activities for hydrogen ion removal or uptake.

Acid-Base Chemistry

ACIDS

Acids are substances that release a hydrogen ion when the substance is dissolved in water (H_2O). An acid in solution *increases* the concentration of free hydrogen ions in that solution. The strength of an acid is determined by how easily it releases a hydrogen ion in solution. A strong acid, such as hydrochloric acid (HCl), **dissociates** (separates) completely

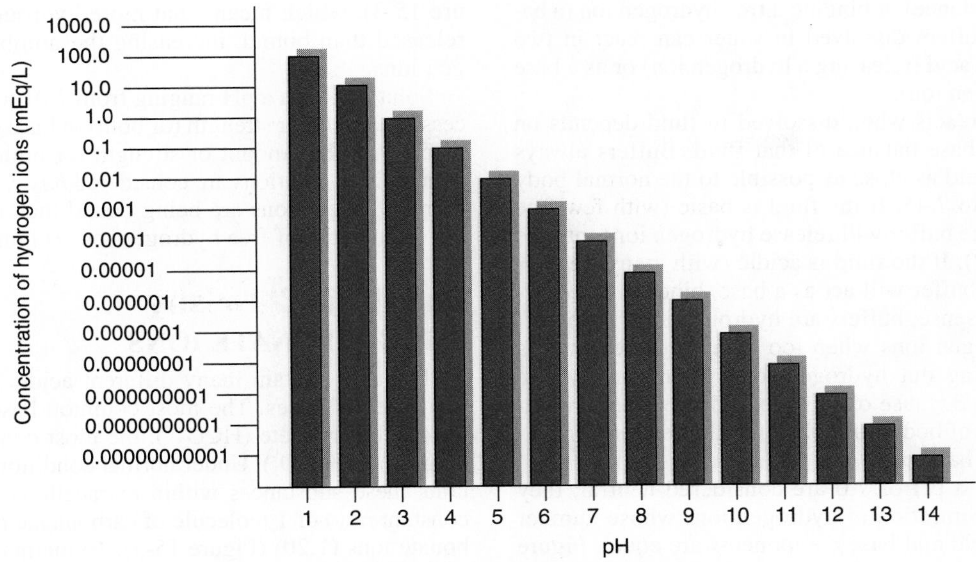

Figure 15-1 • Relationship between pH and concentration of hydrogen ions.

TABLE 15-1 • PERTINENT ACID-BASE BALANCE TERMINOLOGY

acid Any substance releasing a hydrogen ion when dissolved in water

anaerobic metabolism Cellular metabolism occurring without the presence of oxygen

base Any substance binding a hydrogen ion when dissolved in water

buffer A substance capable of binding a hydrogen ion from body fluids (acting as a base) or releasing a hydrogen ion into body fluids (acting as an acid)

chemoreceptors Special cells in the respiratory center of the brain sensitive to changes in the carbon dioxide concentration of extracellular fluid

pH The concentration of hydrogen ions in a solution, calculated as the negative logarithm of the milliequivalent concentration per liter

in water and readily releases all of its hydrogen ions:

$$\underset{\text{Hydrochloric acid}}{HCl} + \underset{\text{Water}}{H_2O} \Rightarrow \underset{\text{Hydrogen ion}}{H^+} + \underset{\text{Chloride ion}}{Cl^-} + \underset{\text{Water}}{H_2O}$$

A weak acid does not completely dissociate in water; it releases only some of its total hydrogen ions. In the following example, each molecule of acetic acid (CH_3COOH), a weak acid, contains a total of four hydrogen molecules. When acetic acid combines with water, it releases only one of its four hydrogen molecules. The other three hydrogen molecules remain bound to the acetic acid molecule:

$$CH_3COOH + H_2O \Rightarrow H^+ + CH_3COO + H_2O$$

BASES

A **base** is a substance that binds free hydrogen ions in solution. Thus bases are hydrogen acceptors and act to reduce the concentration of free hydrogen ions in solution. Strong bases bind hydrogen ions easily. Examples of strong bases include sodium hydroxide (NaOH) and ammonia (NH_3).

Weak bases bind hydrogen ions less readily. Examples of weak bases include aluminum hydroxide ($AlOH_3$) and bicarbonate (HCO_3^-). Although bicarbonate is a weak base, bicarbonate ions in the body are crucial in preventing major disturbances in body fluid pH.

TABLE 15-2 • KEY CONCEPTS OF ACID-BASE BALANCE

- The normal pH of the body's extracellular fluids (including blood) is 7.35 to 7.45.
- The pH in the body can be described as the relationship of bicarbonate to carbonic acid, or a 20:1 ratio.
- Carbon dioxide is the most changeable component of carbonic acid.
- The concentration of carbon dioxide is directly related to the concentration of hydrogen ions.
- An acid gives up hydrogen ions in solution; a base binds hydrogen ions in solution.
- Acids are formed in the body as a result of metabolism and incomplete oxidation of glucose and fats.
- Acid-base balance is regulated by chemical, respiratory, and renal mechanisms.
- Chemical buffers are the immediate way that acid-base imbalances are corrected.
- The lungs control the amount of carbon dioxide that is retained or exhaled.
- The kidneys regulate the amount of hydrogen and bicarbonate ions that are retained or excreted by the body.
- Compensation is the process in which the body uses its three regulatory mechanisms to correct for changes in the pH of body fluids.

BUFFERS

Buffers are substances that either release a hydrogen ion into a fluid or bind a hydrogen ion from a fluid. Most substances, when dissolved in water, react by either releasing a hydrogen ion (an acidic substance) or binding a free hydrogen ion (a basic substance). Buffers dissolved in water can react in two ways: either as an acid (releasing a hydrogen ion) or as a base (binding a hydrogen ion).

How a buffer reacts when dissolved in fluid depends on the existing acid-base balance of that fluid. Buffers always try to bring the fluid as close as possible to the normal body fluid pH of 7.35 to 7.45. If the fluid is basic (with few free hydrogen ions), the buffer will release hydrogen ions into the fluid (Figure 15-2). If the fluid is acidic (with many free hydrogen ions), the buffer will act as a base, binding some hydrogen ions. In a sense, buffers are hydrogen ion "sponges," soaking up hydrogen ions when too many are present in a fluid and squeezing out hydrogen ions when too few are present in a fluid. Because of this flexibility, buffers are important regulators of body fluid pH, or hydrogen ion concentration (acid-base balance).

Solutions with a pH of 7.0 are considered neutral; they contain a set concentration of hydrogen ions whose number and strength of acid and base components are equal. Figure 15-3 is an artificial yet concrete representation of the concept of neutral pH. This representation shows that the combined *strength* and *amount* of all acid components are equal to the combined *strength* and *amount* of all base components in a given solution. This is not the actual case in human physiology. However, in acid-base homeostasis, the relative amounts and strengths of acids and bases are approximately equal, so the overall hydrogen ion concentration remains constant.

Solutions with a pH ranging from 1.0 to 6.99 contain an excessive amount or strength (or both) of acid components compared with the amount or strength (or both) of base components. Such solutions are considered *acidic* (see Figure 15-3), which means that more hydrogen ions are being released than bound, increasing the number of free hydrogen ions.

Solutions with a pH ranging from 7.01 to 14.0 have an excessive amount or strength (or both) of base components compared with the amount or strength (or both) of acid components. These solutions are considered *basic,* which means that more hydrogen ions are being bound than released, decreasing the number of free hydrogen ions (Figure 15-4).

Body Fluid Chemistry

BICARBONATE IONS

Body fluids contain many different acidic substances and a few types of bases. The most common base in human body fluid is bicarbonate (HCO_3^-); the most common acid is carbonic acid (H_2CO_3). Under normal conditions the body maintains these substances within extracellular fluid (ECF) at a constant ratio of 1 molecule of carbonic acid to 20 free bicarbonate ions (1:20) (Figure 15-5). To maintain this ratio, both carbonic acid and bicarbonate must be carefully controlled. Both of these substances and their constant ratio are related to the production and elimination of carbon dioxide (CO_2) and hydrogen ions (H^+).

A key concept that aids in the understanding of acid-base balance is the *carbonic anhydrase equation.* This equation, driven by the enzyme carbonic anhydrase, demonstrates how hydrogen ion concentration and carbon dioxide concentration are directly related to one another, so that an increase in one causes a corresponding increase in the other:

$$\underset{\text{Carbon dioxide}}{CO_2} + \underset{\text{Water}}{H_2O} \Leftrightarrow \underset{\text{Carbonic acid}}{H_2CO_3} \Leftrightarrow \underset{\text{Hydrogen ion}}{H^+} + \underset{\text{Bicarbonate ion}}{HCO_3^-}$$

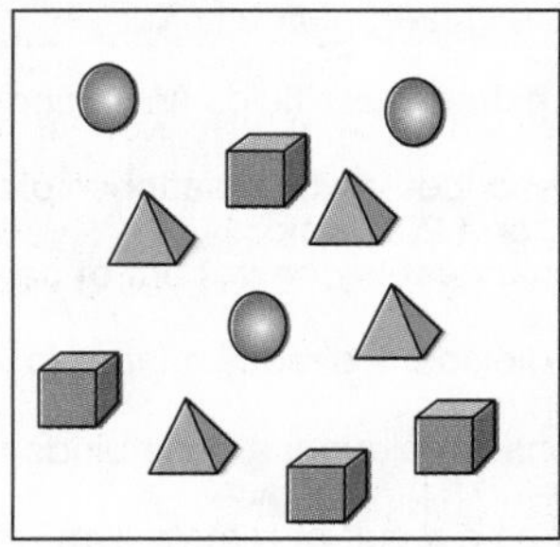

Fluid pH 7.38 (normal). The number and strength of acid components are equal to the number and strength of base components. Hydrogen ion concentration is limited and constant.

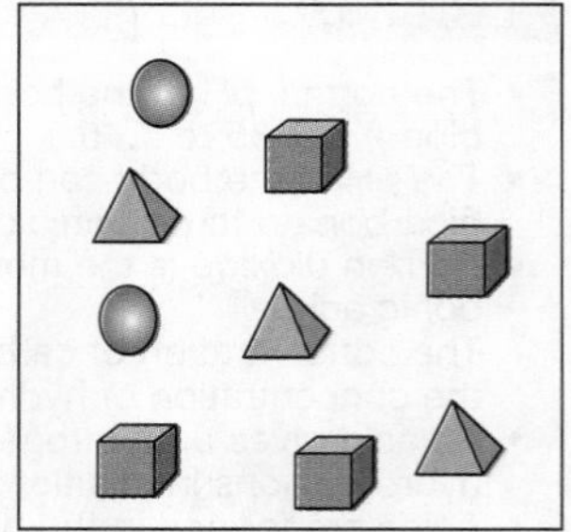

Fluid pH 7.51 (alkaline). The number and strength of base components are greater than the number and strength of acid components. Hydrogen ion concentration is below normal.

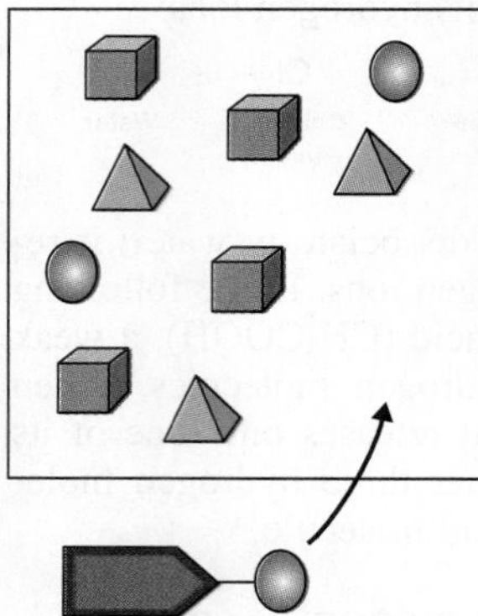

Buffer is added to the alkaline fluid.

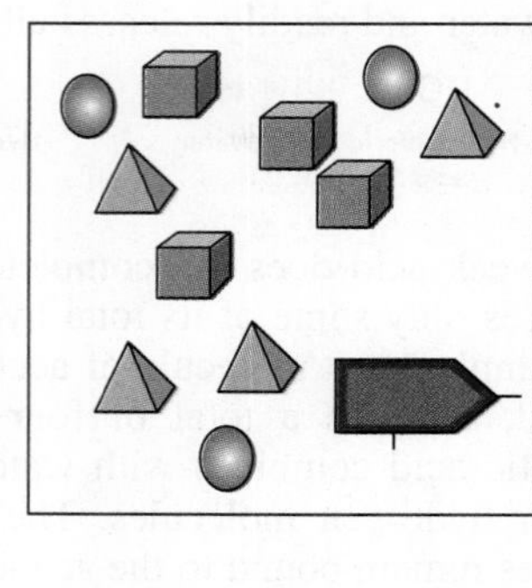

The buffer acts as an acid, releasing a hydrogen ion.

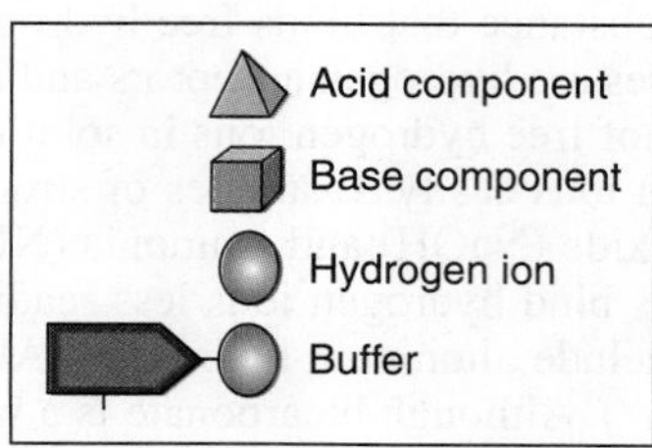

Figure 15-2 ● Action of buffer in solution.

Carbon dioxide is a gas that when combined with water, forms carbonic acid. Carbon dioxide is a changeable part of carbonic acid. Carbonic acid is not stable, and the body needs to maintain a 1:20 ratio of carbonic acid to bicarbonate. As soon as carbonic acid is formed from water and carbon dioxide, it immediately dissociates (separates) into free hydrogen ions and bicarbonate ions. *Therefore the carbon dioxide content of a fluid is directly related to the hydrogen ion concentration of that fluid. Whenever conditions cause carbon dioxide to increase, more hydrogen ions are created. Likewise, whenever hydrogen ion production increases, more carbon dioxide is produced.*

RELATIONSHIP BETWEEN CARBON DIOXIDE AND HYDROGEN IONS

When excess carbon dioxide is produced, the concentration of carbon dioxide increases and the carbonic anhydrase equation shifts to the right, causing an increase in the hydrogen ion concentration (and a decrease in pH):

$$CO_2 + H_2O \Leftrightarrow H_2CO_3 \Leftrightarrow H^+ + HCO_3^-$$

When very little carbon dioxide is produced, no hydrogen ions are generated by the carbonic anhydrase equation.

When excess hydrogen ions are produced or brought into the body, the carbonic anhydrase equation shifts to the left, causing the creation of more carbon dioxide:

$$CO_2 + H_2O \Leftrightarrow H_2CO_3 \Leftrightarrow H^+ + HCO_3^-$$

When the hydrogen ion concentration of body fluids is low, no extra carbon dioxide is produced.

CALCULATION OF HYDROGEN ION CONCENTRATION

The pH is a calculated measurement of hydrogen ion concentration in body fluids; the actual number or percentage of hydrogen ions in these fluids is not easily measured. The pH calculations come from a mathematical formula (the Henderson-Hasselbach equation) that shows how three factors are interrelated: the concentration of free hydrogen ions, the concentration of bases, and the concentration of acids in a solution. When temperature and pressure remain constant, if two of the three factors are known, the third factor can then be calculated.

Because the ratio of carbonic acid and bicarbonate concentration in ECF is 1:20, under normal conditions the only factor that changes is the carbon dioxide concentration. Whenever the carbon dioxide concentration changes, the pH changes correspondingly, in the opposite direction. Thus when the carbon dioxide concentration of a solution increases, the pH drops, indicating an increase in the hydrogen ion concentration (more acidic). Conversely, when the carbon dioxide concentration of a solution decreases, the pH rises, indicating a decrease in the hydrogen ion concentration (more alkaline).

An increase in the bicarbonate concentration causes the hydrogen ion concentration to decrease and the pH to increase, or become more alkaline (basic). Conversely, an increase in the carbon dioxide concentration causes the hydrogen ion concentration to increase and the pH to decrease, or become more acidic.

Because the kidneys control bicarbonate concentration and the lungs control carbon dioxide concentration in the body, pH can also be described as the function of the kidneys divided by the function of the lungs:

$$pH = \frac{\text{Kidneys (bicarbonate)}}{\text{Lungs (carbon dioxide)}}$$

SOURCES OF ACIDS

Acids are formed in the body as waste products of normal metabolism of carbohydrates, fats, and proteins. Metabolism of carbohydrates results in carbon dioxide formation, which can then be converted to hydrogen ions. Fat and protein metabolism directly create acids.

Glucose Metabolism (Production of Carbon Dioxide)

Carbon dioxide is a waste product of glucose breakdown and many other metabolic reactions. (The complete breakdown of 1 molecule of glucose results in the formation of 36 molecules of adenosine triphosphate, 6 molecules of water, and 6 mole-

AAABBB	AAAABBB	AAABB
AAABBB	AAAABBB	AAABB
AAABBB	AAAABBB	AAABB
Neutral	Acidic (acid excess)	Acidic (base deficit)

Figure 15-3 ● Concept of acidic versus normal pH. (*A*, Acid; *B*, base.)

AAABBB	AAABBBB	AABBB
AAABBB	AAABBBB	AABBB
AAABBB	AAABBBB	AABBB
Neutral	Alkaline (base excess)	Alkaline (acid deficit)

Figure 15-4 ● Concept of alkaline versus normal pH. (*A*, Acid; *B*, base.)

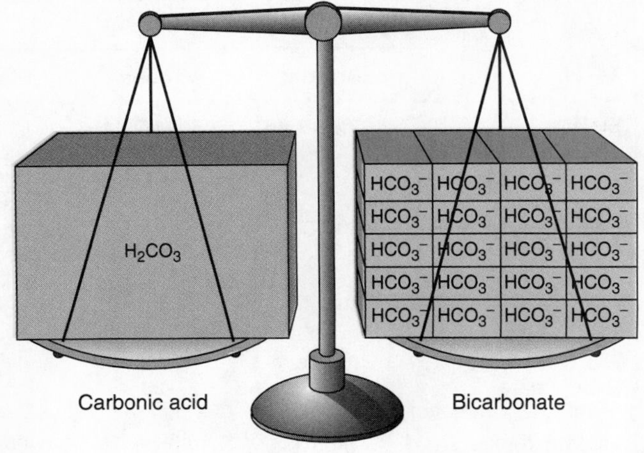

Figure 15-5 ● Normal ratio of carbonic acid to bicarbonate is 1:20.

cules of carbon dioxide.) Because of the relationship between carbon dioxide and hydrogen ions, any increase in carbon dioxide concentration in body fluids always leads to the formation of increased amounts of hydrogen ions in those fluids. The result is a decrease in pH.

Carbon dioxide is exhaled by the lungs during breathing. Therefore one determinant of blood pH is how much carbon dioxide is produced by body cells during metabolism versus how rapidly carbon dioxide is removed by respiration.

Metabolism of Fats and Proteins

The catabolism (breakdown) of food for energy results in the formation of *fixed acids.* Protein catabolism creates sulfuric acid. Fat catabolism creates fatty acids and ketoacids.

Anaerobic Metabolism of Glucose and Fats

Incomplete breakdown of glucose, which occurs whenever cells continue to metabolize substances under **anaerobic** (no oxygen) conditions, leads to the formation of lactic acid. Clinical conditions in which anaerobic metabolism can occur include hypoxia, sepsis, and shock. Incomplete breakdown of fatty acids, either because excessive amounts of fatty acids are being metabolized or because too little oxygen is present during any fatty acid breakdown, causes the formation of ketoacids (Guyton & Hall, 2000).

Destruction of Cells

Whenever cells are damaged or destroyed, plasma membranes are broken and cell contents are released. Some cell structures contain acids that are released into the extracellular fluid (ECF) when this occurs.

SOURCES OF BICARBONATE IONS

Bicarbonate is the primary buffer of the ECF. Sources of bicarbonate in the ECF include the breakdown of carbonic acid, intestinal absorption of ingested bicarbonate, pancreatic production of bicarbonate, movement of intracellular bicarbonate into the ECF, and kidney reabsorption of filtered bicarbonate. Once bicarbonate is in the ECF, it is maintained at a concentration 20 times greater than that of carbonic acid.

ACID-BASE HOMEOSTASIS

As long as body cells are capable of metabolism, the production of acids, carbon dioxide, and hydrogen ions is a normal and continuous process. Despite this production, homeostasis of body fluids (keeping hydrogen ion, bicarbonate, oxygen, and carbon dioxide concentrations within physiologic ranges) is maintained under normal conditions. Chart 15-1 lists normal values for these substances in arterial and venous blood. This homeostasis depends on three factors:

- Hydrogen ion production must be consistent, not excessive.
- Carbon dioxide loss from the body through breathing must keep pace with hydrogen ion production.
- The ratio between carbonic acid and bicarbonate must be maintained at 1:20.

Acid-Base Regulatory Mechanisms

To maintain the hydrogen ion concentration, or pH, of the ECF within the narrow ranges of normal, the body has three well-regulated mechanisms for acid-base balance: chemical, respiratory, and renal (Table 15-3).

CHEMICAL MECHANISMS

Buffers are the first line of defense against changes in hydrogen ion concentration. Because they are constantly present in body fluids, buffers can take immediate action to reduce or raise the hydrogen ion concentration to normal. By acting as hydrogen ion "sponges," buffers can bind hydrogen ions when the concentration is too high or release hydrogen ions when

CHART 15-1

LABORATORY PROFILE
Acid-Base Assessment

Test	Normal Range for Adults: Arterial	Venous	Significance of Abnormal Findings
pH >90 yr	7.35-7.45 7.25-7.45	7.31-7.41	Increased: metabolic alkalosis, loss of gastric fluids, decreased potassium intake, diuretic therapy, fever, salicylate toxicity Decreased: metabolic or respiratory acidosis, ketosis, renal failure, starvation, diarrhea, hyperthyroidism
Pao_2 (mm Hg) >90 yr	80-100 >50		Increased: increased ventilation, oxygen therapy, exercise Decreased: respiratory depression, high altitude, carbon monoxide poisoning, decreased cardiac output
$Paco_2$ (mm Hg)	35-45	40-50	Increased: respiratory acidosis, emphysema, pneumonia, cardiac failure, respiratory depression Decreased: respiratory alkalosis, excessive ventilation, diarrhea
Bicarbonate (mEq/L or mmol/L)	21-28	24-29	Increased: bicarbonate therapy, metabolic alkalosis Decreased: metabolic acidosis, diarrhea, pancreatitis
Lactate (mmol/L)	0.9-1.7	0.5-2.2	Increased: hypoxia, exercise, insulin infusion, alcoholism, pregnancy Decreased: fluid overload

Pao_2, Partial pressure of arterial oxygen; *$Paco_2$,* partial pressure of arterial carbon dioxide.

the concentration is too low. Fluid buffers are composed of chemicals or proteins.

Chemical Buffers

Chemical buffers are paired mixtures, usually consisting of a weak base and an acid salt. The two most common chemical buffer systems are bicarbonate buffers (which are active in both the extracellular fluid [ECF] and intracellular fluid [ICF]) and phosphate buffers (which are active in the ICF).

Protein Buffers

Proteins are the largest source of buffers. Proteins in body fluids can either bind or release hydrogen ions as needed. Both intracellular and extracellular proteins serve as buffers.

The major cellular protein buffer is hemoglobin. Hemoglobin buffers hydrogen ions directly and also buffers acids formed during the production of carbon dioxide. When the hydrogen ion concentration of the blood increases, some of the excess hydrogen ions cross the plasma membranes of red blood cells and bind to the large numbers of hemoglobin molecules in each red blood cell.

Extracellular buffering proteins include albumin and globulins. These proteins buffer carbonic acid and other acids present in the ECF as a result of catabolism.

TABLE 15-3 • ACID-BASE REGULATORY MECHANISMS

Mechanism	Characteristics
CHEMICAL MECHANISMS	
Protein buffers Extracellular Albumin Globulins Intracellular Hemoglobin Chemical buffers Extracellular Bicarbonate Intracellular Phosphate Bicarbonate	Very rapid Provide immediate response to changing conditions Can handle relatively small fluctuations in hydrogen ion production and elimination encountered under normal metabolic and health conditions
RESPIRATORY MECHANISMS	
Increased hydrogen ions Increased carbon dioxide Stimulates central respiratory neurons, leading to increased rate and depth of breathing, causing more carbon dioxide to be lost and decreasing the hydrogen ion concentration Decreased hydrogen ions Decreased carbon dioxide Inhibition of central respiratory neurons, leading to decreased rate and depth of breathing, causing normally produced carbon dioxide to be retained, increasing the hydrogen ion concentration	Primarily assist buffering systems when the fluctuation of hydrogen ion concentration is acute
RENAL MECHANISMS	
Mechanisms to decrease pH Increased renal excretion of bicarbonate Increased renal reabsorption of hydrogen ions Mechanisms to increase pH Decreased renal excretion of bicarbonate Decreased renal reabsorption of hydrogen ions	The most powerful regulator of acid-base balance Respond to large or chronic fluctuations in hydrogen ion production or elimination

RESPIRATORY MECHANISMS

When chemical buffers alone cannot prevent changes in body fluid pH, the respiratory system is the second line of defense against changes. Breathing controls hydrogen ion concentration by regulating the carbon dioxide concentration in arterial blood. Carbon dioxide is converted into hydrogen ions through the carbonic anhydrase reaction; therefore the carbon dioxide concentration is directly related to the hydrogen ion concentration. Breathing is a major mechanism for ridding the body of carbon dioxide, which is created as a by-product of metabolism.

The carbon dioxide concentration in venous blood increases during normal metabolism. This carbon dioxide is transported to the capillaries of the lungs. Because the partial pressure (concentration) of carbon dioxide is far higher in capillary blood than in the atmospheric air in the alveoli, carbon dioxide diffuses freely from the blood into the alveolar air. Once in the alveoli, carbon dioxide is exhaled during breathing and is lost from the body. Because the partial pressure (concentration) of carbon dioxide in atmospheric air is nearly zero, carbon dioxide usually continues to be exhaled at an appropriate rate even when breathing is impaired to some degree.

Hyperventilation

Respiratory regulation of acid-base balance is under the control of the nervous system (Figure 15-6). Special chemoreceptors in the areas of the brain that directly regulate the rate and depth of respiration are sensitive to changes in the carbon dioxide concentration in brain tissues. As the carbon dioxide concentration begins to rise in brain blood and tissues, these central chemoreceptors stimulate the neurons that control the rate and depth of respiration. Under this stimulation both the rate and the depth of respiration increase. As a result, more carbon dioxide is exhaled ("blown off") from the alveoli and the carbon dioxide concentration of the ECF decreases. When the arterial carbon dioxide concentration returns to normal, the rate and depth of respiration return to levels that are normal for the person.

Hypoventilation

If the ECF hydrogen ion concentration is too low, then the carbon dioxide concentration also is too low. Central chemoreceptors sense these low carbon dioxide levels and inhibit stimulation of neurons in the respiratory control centers, causing the rate and depth of respiration to dramatically decrease. As a result, less carbon dioxide is lost through the lungs and more carbon dioxide is retained in arterial blood. This retention of already-formed carbon dioxide, coupled with continuation of the normal generation of carbon dioxide from metabolic reactions, results in a rapid return of the arterial carbon dioxide concentration (and hydrogen ion concen-

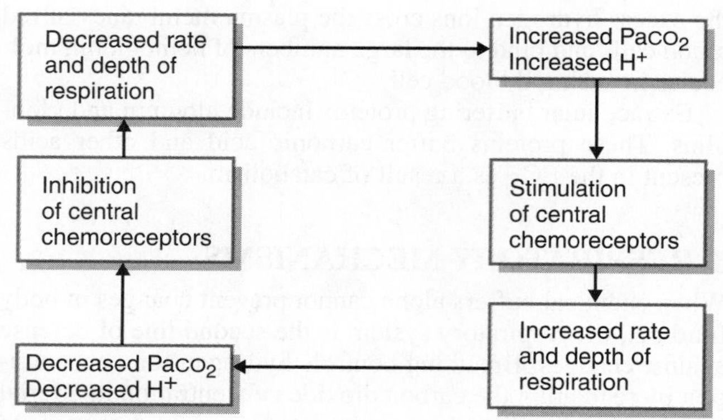

Figure 15-6 ● Neural regulation of respiration and hydrogen ion concentration. (*$PaCO_2$*, Partial pressure of arterial carbon dioxide; *H^+*, hydrogen ion.)

tration) to normal levels. When these levels are normal, the rate and depth of respiration also return to basal levels.

The respiratory system's response in regulating acid-base balance is rapid. Changes in the rate and depth of respiration occur within minutes after changes in the hydrogen ion concentration or carbon dioxide concentration of the ECF occur.

RENAL MECHANISMS

The kidneys are the third line of defense against fluctuations in body fluid pH. Renal mechanisms are the strongest mechanisms for regulating acid-base balance but take longer than chemical and respiratory mechanisms to completely respond. (They take 24 to 48 hours to respond.) When changes in body fluid pH are persistent, renal mechanisms that increase excretion and reabsorption rates of acids or bases (depending on the direction of the pH changes) begin to operate. These mechanisms are kidney movement of bicarbonate, formation of acids, and formation of ammonium.

Kidney Movement of Bicarbonate

This first renal mechanism occurs in the kidney tubules in two ways: (1) kidney movement of bicarbonate produced elsewhere in the body and (2) kidney movement of bicarbonate produced in the kidneys. Much of the bicarbonate made in other body areas is lost in the urine. When blood hydrogen ion levels are high, this bicarbonate is reabsorbed from the kidneys back into circulation, where it can help buffer excess hydrogen ions. When blood hydrogen ion levels are low, the bicarbonate remains in the urine and is excreted. When a hydrogen ion excess is evident, the kidney tubules can make additional bicarbonate that will be reabsorbed.

Formation of Acids

The second renal mechanism occurs through the phosphate-buffering system inside the cells of the kidney tubules. When the newly created bicarbonate made in the kidney cells is reabsorbed into circulation along with sodium, the urine has an excess of anions, including phosphate (HPO_4^{2-}). This negatively charged fluid draws hydrogen ions (which carry a positive charge) into the urine. Once the hydrogen ion is in the urine, it combines with the phosphate ion, forming an acid, H_2PO_4, which is then excreted in the urine.

Formation of Ammonium

In the third renal mechanism, ammonium (NH_4^+) is formed from ammonia (NH_3^+), which is normally made during protein breakdown (Guyton & Hall, 2000). Ammonia is secreted into the urine, where it can combine with free hydrogen ions to form ammonium, and then is excreted from the body. This trapping of free hydrogen ions in ammonium prevents the free hydrogen ion concentration in the urine from becoming so high that it inhibits movement of free hydrogen ions from the blood into the urine. The overall result of this process is a loss of hydrogen ions and an increase in blood pH.

COMPENSATION

In the process of *compensation,* the body attempts to correct for changes in body fluid (blood) pH. A pH below 6.9 or above 7.8 is usually fatal. The normal pH range for human extracellular fluid (ECF) is 7.35 to 7.45. Both the kidneys and the lungs can compensate for acid-base imbalances, but they are not equal in their compensatory actions and reactions. The respiratory system is much more sensitive to acid-base changes and can begin compensation efforts within seconds to minutes after a change in pH. However, these efforts are limited and can be overwhelmed easily. The renal compensatory mechanisms are much more powerful and result in dramatic changes in ECF composition. However, these more powerful mechanisms are not fully stimulated until the acid-base imbalance has been sustained for several hours to several days.

Respiratory Compensation

The lungs can usually compensate for acid-base imbalances of a metabolic origin. For example, when prolonged running causes excessive buildup of lactic acid, hydrogen ion concentration in the ECF increases and the pH drops. To bring the pH back to normal, the lungs are stimulated by the increased carbon dioxide concentration to increase both the rate and depth of respiration. These respiratory efforts cause the blood to lose carbon dioxide with each exhalation, so ECF levels of carbon dioxide and hydrogen ions gradually decrease. When the lungs can fully compensate, the pH returns to normal.

Renal Compensation

A healthy kidney can correct or compensate for changes in pH when the respiratory system is either overwhelmed or is actually a cause of the imbalance. For example, in a person with chronic obstructive pulmonary disease (COPD), the respiratory system cannot exchange gases adequately. Carbon dioxide is thus retained, and the pH of the ECF falls, or becomes more acidic. To counteract this process, the kidney increases its excretion of hydrogen ions and increases the reabsorption of bicarbonate back into the body. As a result, the pH of body fluids remains either within or closer to the normal range. When these backup mechanisms are completely effective, acid-base problems are fully compensated and the pH of the blood returns to normal, even though the concentration of other substances (such as oxygen and bicarbonate) may be abnormal.

CHART 15-2

NURSING FOCUS *on the* OLDER ADULT
Age-Related Risk Factors for Acid-Base Disturbances

Disturbance	Risk Factors
Increased hydrogen ion concentration	Pulmonary diseases Chronic obstructive pulmonary disease (COPD) Pneumonia Dehydration Infection Renal disease Vascular disease Atherosclerosis Arteriosclerosis Angiitis
Decreased hydrogen ion concentration	Overhydration Congestive heart failure Drugs Diuretics (loop and thiazide) Digoxin Insulin Antibiotics Chemotherapeutic agents

CHART 15-3

ACID-BASE ASSESSMENT
Using Gordon's Functional Health Patterns

Activity-Exercise Pattern

Have you had any shortness of breath or difficulty breathing at rest or during activity?
Have you noticed any changes in your breathing rate or depth?
Do you have a hard time "catching" your breath?
Do you have any difficulty clearing excretions?
Do you feel the need for additional energy to accomplish routine tasks?
Do you have any difficulty concentrating?
Have you noticed any changes in your interest in normal daily activities?
Have you noticed any changes in your leisure activities?

Elimination Pattern

What is your usual urinary elimination pattern? Frequency? Amount? Color? Odor? Control?
Have you noticed any changes in the amount of urine?
Has your urine changed color or odor?
What is your usual bowel elimination pattern? Frequency? Amount? Control?
Have you noticed any changes in the number or consistency of your stools?

Cognitive-Perceptual Pattern

Have you noticed any changes in memory lately?
Have you noticed an increase in anxiety or feelings of apprehension?
Are you sleeping more or sleeping less than usual for you?
Have you noticed any changes in your attention span?
Have your muscles seemed weak or "twitchy" lately?

Based on Gordon, M. (2000). *Manual of nursing diagnosis* (9th ed.). St. Louis: Mosby.

Sometimes, however, the respiratory factors contributing to the acid-base imbalance are so severe that kidney actions can only partially compensate, and the pH is not quite normal. Even partial compensation is very important to acid-base balance because it prevents the imbalance from becoming severe or life threatening.

Age-Related Changes in Acid-Base Balance

Older adults are more susceptible to pH disturbances than younger persons because their normal physiologic mechanisms are less able to respond to minor fluctuations in hydrogen ion production or elimination. In addition, an older adult may be taking medications that alter the activity of normal pH-compensating mechanisms (Chart 15-2).

Effective gas exchange during breathing is also reduced as a person ages. There is less alveolar membrane for gas exchange in older persons, and many also have some degree of blood vessel thickening, which further impairs gas diffusion through capillaries. These conditions can cause carbon dioxide retention, increasing the concentration of hydrogen ions.

Because kidney function decreases with age, older adults are less able to excrete hydrogen ions or produce bicarbonate ions. The kidneys may be able to handle ordinary changes resulting from normal metabolism but cannot compensate adequately when pathologic conditions (such as pneumonia, fever, or infection) interfere with acid-base balance.

Two medications often prescribed for older clients are diuretics and digoxin. Both agents increase kidney excretion of hydrogen ions, which can result in an increased blood pH.

All older clients are at risk for acid-base disturbances. This risk is even greater for clients with pulmonary, vascular, cardiac, or kidney impairments.

ASSESSMENT OF ACID-BASE BALANCE

Acid-base balance is a systemic process, and all cells and body systems are affected when acid-base balance is disturbed. Assessment of acid-base balance involves examining data that reflect the functioning of systems responsible for acid-base balance. Assessment also involves examining the data that reflect body responses to changes in the concentration of acids or bases. Behavioral and neurologic assessments also are included in assessment of acid-base balance because changes in pH can alter neurologic function.

History

One way of organizing history data to assess the client's fluid and electrolyte status is the use of Gordon's Functional Health Patterns (Gordon, 2000). The patterns that affect acid-base balance most are Activity-Exercise, Elimination, and Cognitive-Perceptual patterns (Chart 15-3), demonstrating the functional effectiveness of the lungs and kidneys.

Physical Assessment

Hydration status can indicate fluid balance. A normally hydrated adult is alert, has moist eyes and mucous membranes, has a urine output nearly the same as the amount of fluid ingested (with a urine specific gravity of approximately 1.015), and has good skin turgor (see Chapter 11). A dry, sticky, "cottony" mouth; the absence of tearing; weight loss; and decreased urine output all indicate either a problem with oral intake or excess fluid loss. Accurate assessment of fluid intake and output can assist in determining adequacy of kidney function and, indirectly, acid-base balance.

Hydrogen ions affect the activity of excitable membranes, and acid-base imbalances are associated with altered function of these membranes. Acid-base assessment includes a complete neuromuscular assessment of muscle tone and strength, movement, coordination, and tremors. Assessment of other systems, including the cardiac (heart rate, strength of contractions, and presence of dysrhythmias) and gastrointestinal (motility) systems, may indicate changes in excitable membrane function.

Part of the nurse's assessment focuses on changes from previous findings, including mental status, physical examination data, and laboratory data. Acid-base imbalances can occur quickly; therefore the nurse must be familiar with the client's baseline assessment data to detect any changes.

Diagnostic Assessment

Laboratory results, especially arterial blood gases (ABGs), are important in identifying specific acid-base imbalances and are discussed fully in Chapter 16 (see also Chart 15-1). Other laboratory values helpful in assessing acid-base balance include serum electrolyte concentration, blood urea nitrogen (BUN) level, glucose concentration, creatinine level, and osmolarity.

Urine test results may be helpful in determining whether a kidney or metabolic problem is affecting acid-base balance. Such tests include measurement of glomerular filtration and detection of substances that should not be present in the urine, such as glucose, acetone, protein, or blood.

ONLINE RESOURCES

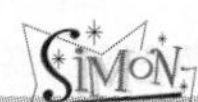

For suggested readings and Internet resources, go to http://www.wbsaunders.com/SIMON/Iggy/.

SELECTED BIBLIOGRAPHY

Asterisk indicates a classic or definitive work on this subject.

Coleman, N., & Houston, L. (1998). Demystifying acid-base regulation. *Australian Nurses Journal, 5*(8), 4-7.

Cook, L. (1999). The value of lab values. *American Journal of Nursing, 99*(5), 66-75.

Demers, B., & Morfei, J. (1999). Role of bicarbonate ion concentration in acid-base balance. *Respiratory Care, 44*(8), 963-964.

Faria, S. (1997). Interpretation of arterial blood gases by nurses. *Journal of Vascular Nursing, 15*(4), 128-130.

Frizzell, J. (1998). Avoiding lab test pitfalls. *American Journal of Nursing, 98*(2), 34-38.

Gordon, M. (2000). *Manual of nursing diagnosis* (9th ed.). St. Louis: Mosby.

Guyton, A., & Hall, J. (2000). *Textbook of medical physiology* (10th ed.). Philadelphia: W.B. Saunders.

Horne, C., & Derrico, D. (1999). Mastering ABGs. *American Journal of Nursing, 99*(8), 26-32.

*Metheny, N. (1996). *Fluid and electrolyte balance: Nursing considerations* (3rd ed.). Philadelphia: J.B. Lippincott.

Miekley, T.F. (1998). A patient-focused approach to managing diuretic therapy. *Critical Care Nursing Clinics of North America, 10*(4), 421-467.

Pagana, K.D., & Pagana, T.J. (1999). *Diagnostic testing and nursing implications: A case study approach* (5th ed.). St. Louis: Mosby.

Tasota, F., & Wesmiller, S. (1998). Balancing act: Keeping blood pH in equilibrium, *Nursing98, 28*(12), 35-40.

Wong, F. (1999). A new approach to ABG interpretation, *American Journal of Nursing, 99*(8), 34-35.

CHAPTER 16

Interventions for Clients with Acid-Base Imbalances

M. LINDA WORKMAN

Learning Objectives

After studying this chapter, you should be able to:

1. Identify clients at risk for acidosis.
2. Use laboratory data and clinical manifestations to determine the presence of acidosis.
3. Analyze arterial blood gases to determine whether acidosis is respiratory or metabolic in origin.
4. Analyze arterial blood gases to determine if respiratory acidosis is acute or chronic.
5. Prioritize nursing care for the client with acute acidosis.
6. Identify clients at risk for alkalosis.
7. Use laboratory data and clinical manifestations to determine the presence of alkalosis.
8. Analyze arterial blood gases to determine whether alkalosis is respiratory or metabolic in origin.
9. Prioritize nursing care for the client with alkalosis.

SIMON **Go to http://www.wbsaunders.com/SIMON/Iggy/ for self-assessment questions related to these Learning Objectives.**

Acid-base imbalances are changes in the hydrogen ion concentration or pH of the blood; these changes indicate either problems with the acid-base regulatory mechanisms of the body or exposure of the body to dangerous conditions. Imbalances in which the pH is below normal reflect **acidosis,** and imbalances in which the pH is above normal reflect **alkalosis.** Severe impairment of normal physiology may accompany acid-base imbalances and can be life threatening. Table 16-1 lists key points associated with acid-base imbalances.

ACIDOSIS

OVERVIEW

In acidosis, the acid-base balance of the blood and other extracellular fluid (ECF) is disturbed by an excess of hydrogen ions (H^+) and is reflected as an arterial blood pH below 7.35. The concentration or strength (or both) of acids is greater than normal compared with the concentration or strength of bases.

Acidosis is not a disease but rather a condition caused by a disease or pathologic process. Acidosis can be caused by metabolic problems, respiratory problems, or both. Clients at particular risk for acute acidosis are those with conditions that impair any aspect of respiratory function to any degree. The older adult with chronic health problems also is at greater risk for developing acidosis (Chart 16-1).

Pathophysiology

Acidosis can result from an actual or relative increase in the concentration or strength of acids. In an actual acid excess, acidosis results from processes that cause either an overproduction of acids (and release of hydrogen ions) or an underelimination of normally produced acids (retention of hydrogen ions). Examples of conditions that increase acid production include diabetic ketoacidosis and seizures. Examples of conditions that decrease acid elimination include respiratory or renal impairment.

In *relative* acidosis, the amount or strength of acids does not increase. Instead, the concentration or strength (or both) of the bases decreases (to create a *base deficit*), which makes the fluid relatively more acidic than basic. A relative acid-excess acidosis *(actual base deficit)* results from processes that cause either an overelimination of bases (bicarbonate ions [HCO_3^-]) or an underproduction of bases (Figure 16-1). Examples of conditions that cause an underproduction of bases include pancreatitis and dehydration. An example of a condition that causes an overelimination of bases is diarrhea.

Regardless of its origin, acidosis causes major changes in physiologic function. Its primary pathologic effects are related to the fact that hydrogen ions are cations (positively charged electrolytes). An increase in hydrogen ion concentration creates imbalances of other electrolytes, especially potassium, the principal cation in intracellular fluid. These induced electrolyte imbalances then disrupt the functions of excitable membranes, such as nerve and cardiac tissue. Many of the early signs and symptoms of acidosis first appear in the neuromuscular, cardiac, respiratory, and central nervous systems (Metheney, 1996). Even slight increases in hydrogen ion concentration cause many body hormones and enzymes, as well as medications, to become inactive; this may lead to death.

TABLE 16-1 • KEY POINTS RELATED TO ACID-BASE IMBALANCES

- Acidemia is defined as an increase in the hydrogen ion concentration (pH) of the blood and is reflected by an arterial blood pH below 7.35.
- Acidemia can result from an actual acid excess or a relative base deficit.
- Metabolic acidosis usually results from a lack of bicarbonate or from excess acid production in the body.
- Respiratory acidosis results from the retention of carbon dioxide in the body, causing increased carbonic acid production.
- Manifestations of acidemia are related to fluid and electrolyte imbalances that accompany acid-base imbalance, such as hyperkalemia.
- Chronic respiratory acidosis is common in the medical-surgical setting as a result of chronic obstructive pulmonary disease, such as emphysema.
- Alkalemia is defined as a decrease in the hydrogen ion concentration of the blood, which is reflected by an arterial blood pH above 7.45.
- Alkalemia can result from an actual base excess or an acid deficit.
- Metabolic alkalosis most often occurs when body acids are lost, such as in prolonged vomiting or nasogastric suctioning.
- Respiratory alkalosis most often occurs when hyperventilation causes excessive loss of carbon dioxide.
- Dehydration and hypokalemia are associated with metabolic alkalosis and account for most of the clinical manifestations seen in this type of acid-base imbalance.
- The goal of management for any type of acid-base imbalance is to restore fluid, electrolyte, and acid-base balance to normal or near-normal.

CHART 16-1

NURSING FOCUS *on the* OLDER ADULT
The Older Client Experiencing Acid-Base Imbalance

WHEN OBTAINING A CLIENT'S HISTORY

- Assess risk factors for acid-base imbalance, including medications, chronic health problems (especially renal disease, pulmonary disease), and acute health problems.
- Obtain the history when the client is awake and more familiar with his or her surroundings.
- Ask the client to list all prescribed and over-the-counter medications (especially diuretics and antacids). If the client cannot recall this information or seems confused, ask the significant other to bring medications from home to show the nurse.
- Ask the client to recall what liquids he or she has taken in the past 24 hours and whether he or she has urinated as much as usual.

WHEN ASSESSING THE CLIENT

- Compare the client's mental status with what the family, significant other, or health record states is the client's baseline.
- Observe the rate and depth of respiration.
  Can the client complete a sentence without stopping to take a breath?
  Examine the color of the client's nail beds and mucous membranes.
- Obtain a urine specimen and observe for color and character. Test for specific gravity and pH.
- Examine skin turgor for dehydration. Attempt to pinch the skin to form a tent over the sternum and on the forehead. If a tent forms, record how long it remains.
- Measure the rate and quality of the pulse.

Observe the client's clinical responses and laboratory values carefully while the acid-base imbalance is being corrected.
Administer IV therapy by pump or controller.

Etiology

Acidosis can be caused by metabolic disturbances, respiratory disturbances, or combined metabolic and respiratory disturbances. The causes of metabolic and respiratory acidosis are summarized in Table 16-2.

METABOLIC ACIDOSIS

Four processes can result in metabolic acidosis: overproduction of hydrogen ions, underelimination of hydrogen ions, underproduction of bicarbonate ions, and overelimination of bicarbonate ions.

OVERPRODUCTION OF HYDROGEN IONS. Three metabolic processes that can increase the concentration of hydrogen ions in body fluid are an excessive breakdown of fatty acids, hypermetabolism (anaerobic lactic acidosis), and an excessive ingestion of acidic substances.

An *excessive breakdown of fatty acids* is usually a result of diabetic ketoacidosis or starvation. When glucose is not readily available for fuel, the body metabolizes fats (lipids). The metabolites from excessive fatty acid breakdown form strong acids *(ketoacids),* which release large amounts of hydrogen ions.

Hypermetabolism (anaerobic lactic acidosis) occurs when cells are forced to use glucose without adequate oxygen (anaerobic metabolism); as a result, glucose is incompletely metabolized and forms lactic acid. Lactic acid molecules leave the cell, enter the extracellular fluid (ECF), and release hydrogen ions, causing acidosis. Anaerobic metabolism leading to lactic acidosis occurs whenever the body has insufficient oxygen. Conditions that cause lactic acidosis include strenuous exercise, seizure activity, fever, and the presence of tissue hypoxia.

AAABBB	AAAABBB	AAABB
AAABBB	AAAABBB	AAABB
AAABBB	AAAABBB	AAABB
Acid-base balance	Actual acidosis (acid excess)	Relative acidosis (base deficit)

Figure 16-1 • Concepts of actual and relative acidosis. (*A,* Acid; *B,* base.)

Excessive intake of acidic substances floods the body directly with hydrogen ions. Common substances that cause acidosis when ingested in excess include alcoholic beverages, methyl alcohol (a poison), and acetylsalicylic acid (aspirin).

UNDERELIMINATION OF HYDROGEN IONS. The major routes for hydrogen ion elimination are through the lungs and the kidneys. Kidney failure causes acidosis when the kidney tubules cannot secrete hydrogen ions into the urine. As a result, too many hydrogen ions are retained.

UNDERPRODUCTION OF BICARBONATE IONS. As discussed in Chapter 15, bicarbonate is the most common base in the fluid outside the cells and is responsible for buffering carbonic acid (H_2CO_3). A base-deficit state exists when body fluid levels of bicarbonate are too low. Base-deficit acidosis occurs when hydrogen ion production and elimination are normal but too few bicarbonate ions are present to balance the hydrogen ions. Such base deficits occur when bicarbonate ions are not produced at the normal rate. Because bicarbonate is made in the kidneys and in the pancreas, renal failure and reduced hepatic or pancreatic function can cause a base-deficit acidosis (Guyton & Hall, 2000).

OVERELIMINATION OF BICARBONATE IONS. Base-deficit acidosis can also occur when hydrogen ion production and elimination are normal but too many bicarbonate ions have been eliminated (overelimination). A common cause of overelimination is diarrhea.

RESPIRATORY ACIDOSIS

Respiratory acidosis results from an impairment in any area of respiratory function, causing an inadequate exchange of oxygen (O_2) and carbon dioxide (CO_2). This impairment causes carbon dioxide retention. Because any increase in carbon dioxide concentration causes a corresponding increase in hydrogen ion concentration, carbon dioxide retention leads to acidosis. This relationship is demonstrated in the following carbonic anhydrase equation:

$$CO_2 + H_2O \Leftrightarrow H_2CO_3 \Leftrightarrow H^+ + HCO_3$$

An excess of carbon dioxide forces the equation to the right, first increasing the production of carbonic acid. The carbonic acid then rapidly separates into hydrogen ions and bicarbonate ions. This increase in the concentration of free hydrogen ions in the blood is acidosis.

Unlike metabolic acidosis, respiratory acidosis results from only one mechanism: retention of carbon dioxide, which causes an underelimination of hydrogen ions. Virtually all causes of respiratory acidosis result in an acid-excess acidosis. Four types of respiratory problems can cause respiratory acidosis: respiratory depression, inadequate chest expansion, airway obstruction, and reduced alveolar-capillary diffusion.

RESPIRATORY DEPRESSION. Respiratory depression is a change in the function of the brainstem neurons that stimulate inhalation and exhalation. The overall result is a reduced rate and depth of respiration, which causes an inadequate gas exchange and a retention of carbon dioxide. Respiratory depression may be chemical or physical in origin.

Chemical depression of respiratory neurons in the brain can result from the action of anesthetic agents, drugs (especially opioids), and poisons such as methyl alcohol, pesticides, and botulinus toxin that cross the blood-brain barrier. Specific electrolyte imbalances also slow or inhibit respiratory neurons (see Chapter 13 for a discussion of hyponatremia, hypercalcemia, and hyperkalemia).

Physical depression of respiratory neurons can occur in response to many conditions. Respiratory neurons can be damaged or destroyed by trauma or when problems in other areas of the brain cause an increase in intracranial pressure. Such an increase causes edema of brain tissues, which leads to pressure on the respiratory centers located in the brainstem. Conditions causing cerebral edema with resultant respiratory depression include brain tumors, cerebral aneurysm, stroke, overhydration, and hyponatremia.

INADEQUATE CHEST EXPANSION. Any condition that restricts chest expansion can result in inadequate gas exchange. Inadequate chest expansion can result from skeletal trauma or deformities, respiratory muscle weakness, or nonrespiratory movement restrictions.

Skeletal problems restrict respiratory movement of the chest wall when broken or malformed bones distort the shape of the chest. Broken ribs restrict chest movement because they

TABLE 16-2 • COMMON CAUSES OF ACIDOSIS

Pathology	Condition
METABOLIC ACIDOSIS	
Overproduction of hydrogen ions	Excessive oxidation of fatty acids • Diabetic ketoacidosis • Starvation Hypermetabolism • Heavy exercise • Seizure activity • Fever • Hypoxia, ischemia Excessive ingestion of acids • Ethanol intoxication • Methanol ingestion • Salicylate intoxication
Underelimination of hydrogen ions	Renal failure
Underproduction of bicarbonate	Renal failure Pancreatitis Liver failure Dehydration
Overelimination of bicarbonate	Diarrhea Buffering of organic acids
RESPIRATORY ACIDOSIS	
Underelimination of hydrogen ions	Respiratory depression • Anesthetics • Drugs (especially opioids) • Poisons • Electrolyte imbalance • Trauma Cerebral edema Spinal cord injuries • Neurologic diseases Guillain-Barré Polio Myasthenia gravis Inadequate chest expansion • Skeletal deformities • Muscle weakness • Nonpulmonary restriction Obesity Fluid Tumor Body casts Chest eschar Airway obstruction • Asthma • Cancer • Bronchiolitis Alveolar-capillary block • Thrombus or embolus • Vascular occlusive disease • Pneumonia • Pulmonary edema • Tuberculosis • Cystic fibrosis • Atelectasis • Acute respiratory distress syndrome (ARDS) • Emphysema • Cancer

cannot provide the rigid structure needed for thoracic pressure changes (as in flail chest). Pain from broken ribs may also cause voluntary restriction of chest movement.

Respiratory muscle weakness makes chest expansion inadequate. This condition can be caused by electrolyte imbalances (especially hyperkalemia and hyponatremia), fatigue, muscular dystrophy, rhabdomyosarcoma, and inflammatory myositis.

Nonrespiratory conditions also can restrict the chest movement necessary for full lung expansion. Causes of restricted chest movement include body cast enclosure of the thoracic cavity, tight scar tissue formation around the chest, severe obesity, abdominal masses, ascites, and **hemothorax** (blood in the thoracic cavity).

AIRWAY OBSTRUCTION. Prevention of air movement into and out of the lungs through airway obstruction can lead to ineffective gas exchange, carbon dioxide retention, and acidosis. The upper airway can be obstructed externally by restrictive clothing, neck edema, and local lymph node enlargement. Internal obstruction of the upper airway can be caused by aspiration of foreign objects, constriction of bronchial smooth muscles, and edema. Internal obstruction of the lower airways is caused by constriction of smooth muscle, edema, and excessive mucus, conditions which occur in asthma, bronchiolitis, and emphysema.

REDUCED ALVEOLAR-CAPILLARY DIFFUSION. Most pulmonary gas exchange occurs by diffusion at the junction of the alveolar membrane and capillary membranes. Any condition that prevents or slows this diffusion process can cause retention of carbon dioxide and acidosis. Conditions or diseases that reduce alveolar-capillary diffusion include pneumonia, pulmonary edema, fluid aspiration, pneumonitis, tuberculosis, emphysema, acute respiratory distress syndrome, chest trauma, pulmonary emboli, and pulmonary edema.

COMBINED METABOLIC AND RESPIRATORY ACIDOSIS

Metabolic and respiratory acidosis can occur simultaneously. Uncorrected acute respiratory acidosis always leads to **anaerobic** (lacking adequate oxygen) metabolism and lactic acidosis (Metheney, 1996). The resulting acidosis is more profound than that caused by either metabolic acidosis or respiratory acidosis alone. Cardiac arrest is an example of a condition leading to combined metabolic and respiratory acidosis. Another example is the development of severe diarrhea in a client with chronic obstructive lung disease.

COLLABORATIVE MANAGEMENT

Assessment

HISTORY

When obtaining a history from any client, the nurse collects data about risk factors and causative factors related to the development of acidosis, specifically age, nutrition, and presenting symptoms.

Older adults are more prone to conditions that cause acid-base imbalance, including impairments of cardiac, renal, and pulmonary functions. In addition, older adults are more likely to be taking prescribed or over-the-counter medications that interfere with acid-base, fluid, and electrolyte balance, especially diuretics, aspirin, and products containing alcohol. The nurse asks about specific risk factors, such as any type of respiratory problem, kidney failure, diabetes mellitus, diarrhea, pancreatitis, and fever.

The nurse obtains a detailed diet history to determine total caloric intake and the proportions of carbohydrates, fats, and proteins ingested. The client is asked specifically whether he or she has fasted or followed a strict diet during the preceding week.

The nurse asks the client if he or she has experienced headaches, behavior changes, increased drowsiness, reduced alertness, reduced attention span, lethargy, anorexia, abdominal distention, nausea or vomiting, muscle weakness, or increased fatigue. Having the client relate his or her activities of the previous 24 hours may disclose additional information about activity intolerance, behavior changes, and unexplained fatigue. Because the central nervous system is often depressed in acidosis, the nurse may obtain this information from the client's significant other.

CHART 16-2

KEY FEATURES *of* Acidosis

Central Nervous System Manifestations
- Depressed activity (lethargy, confusion, stupor, and coma)

Neuromuscular Manifestations
- Hyporeflexia
- Skeletal muscle weakness
- Flaccid paralysis

Cardiovascular Manifestations
- Delayed electrical conduction
  - Ranges from bradycardia to heart block
  - Tall T waves
  - Widened QRS complex
  - Prolonged PR interval
- Hypotension
- Thready peripheral pulses

Respiratory Manifestations
- Kussmaul respirations (in metabolic acidosis with respiratory compensation)
- Variable respirations (generally ineffective in respiratory acidosis)

Integumentary Manifestations
- Warm, flushed, dry skin in metabolic acidosis
- Pale to cyanotic and dry skin in respiratory acidosis

PHYSICAL ASSESSMENT/CLINICAL MANIFESTATIONS

The key clinical manifestations of acidosis are similar whether the cause is metabolic or respiratory (Chart 16-2). Clinical manifestations appear primarily as changes in the activity of excitable membranes, including neurons, skeletal muscle, and gastric smooth muscle.

CENTRAL NERVOUS SYSTEM MANIFESTATIONS. Depression of central nervous system function is common in acidosis and may range from lethargy to confusion, especially in older clients. As acidosis worsens, the client may become stuporous and unresponsive. The nurse assesses the client's mental status (see Chapter 41).

CHART 16-3

LABORATORY PROFILE
Acid-Base Imbalances

Imbalance	Laboratory Value Changes						
	pH	HCO_3^-	Pao_2	$Paco_2$	K^+	Ca^{2+}	Cl^-
Metabolic acidosis	↓	↓	∅	∅	↑	∅	↑
Respiratory acidosis	↓	↑	↓	↑	↑	∅	↑↓
Combined acidosis	↓	↑	↓	↑	↑	∅	↑
Metabolic alkalosis	↑	↑	∅	↑	↓	↓	↓
Respiratory alkalosis	↑	↓	∅	↓	↓	↓	↑
Combined alkalosis	↑	↑	∅	↓	↓	↓	↓

↑, Above normal; ↓, below normal; ↑↓, value can increase or decrease depending on other factors; ∅, normal; HCO_3^-, bicarbonate ions; Pao_2, partial pressure of arterial oxygen; $Paco_2$, partial pressure of arterial carbon dioxide; K^+, potassium ions; Ca^{2+}, calcium ions; Cl^-, chloride ions.

NEUROMUSCULAR MANIFESTATIONS. An increase in serum hydrogen ion concentration, along with the accompanying hyperkalemia, causes a decrease in muscle tone and deep tendon reflexes. The nurse assesses muscle strength by having the client do the following:

- Squeeze the nurse's hand
- Keep arms flexed while the nurse pulls down on the lower arms
- Push both feet against a flat surface while the nurse applies resistance

Muscle weakness associated with acidosis is bilateral and can progress to flaccid paralysis. Respiratory efforts are reduced when skeletal muscles become weak.

CARDIOVASCULAR MANIFESTATIONS. The early cardiac manifestations of acidosis are increased heart rate and cardiac output. With worsening acidosis or with acidosis accompanied by hyperkalemia, electrical conduction through the heart is reduced and heart rate decreases. Peripheral pulses may be hard to find and are easily blocked with light pressure. The client may experience hypotension as a result of vasodilation.

RESPIRATORY MANIFESTATIONS. The nurse assesses the client's rate, depth, and ease of respirations. Pulse oximetry is performed to determine how well oxygen is delivered to the peripheral tissues.

If acidosis is metabolic in origin, the rate and depth of respiration increase in proportion to the increase in hydrogen ion concentration. Respirations are deep, rapid, and not under voluntary control. This pattern is called *Kussmaul respiration.*

If acidosis is respiratory in origin, the effectiveness of respiratory efforts is reduced. Respirations are usually shallow and rapid.

INTEGUMENTARY MANIFESTATIONS. With metabolic acidosis, respiration is unimpaired and respiratory rate is increased. This increased gas exchange coupled with a vasodilation makes the client's skin and mucous membranes warm, dry, and pink. With respiratory acidosis, respirations are ineffective; therefore skin and mucous membranes are pale to cyanotic.

PSYCHOSOCIAL ASSESSMENT

It is vital that the nurse complete a psychosocial assessment, because behavioral changes may be the first clinical manifestations of acidosis. The nurse observes and documents the client's presenting behavior by description (objectively) rather than by interpretation (subjectively). For example, the nurse may state that "the client is unable to recognize close family members" rather than "the client is confused" or may state that "the client spit out the oral medication" rather than "the client is uncooperative." The nurse questions significant others to determine whether the client's behavior and mental status are typical and to establish a baseline for comparison with later assessment findings.

LABORATORY ASSESSMENT

Arterial blood pH is the laboratory value used to confirm acidosis. Acidosis is present when arterial blood pH is less than 7.35. However, this test alone does not indicate the underlying pathologic condition or the origin of the acidosis. The clinical manifestations of metabolic acidosis and respiratory acidosis are similar, but their treatments are different. Therefore it is critical that the nurse obtain and interpret other laboratory data, such as arterial blood gas (ABG) values and the measurements of certain serum electrolytes (Chart 16-3).

METABOLIC ACIDOSIS. The following laboratory data indicate metabolic acidosis:

ABGs

Low pH (<7.35)
Low bicarbonate level (<21 mEq/L)
Normal partial pressure of arterial carbon dioxide ($Paco_2$)

Electrolytes

Elevated serum potassium level
Normal chloride levels (acid excess or high anion gap acidosis)
Elevated chloride levels (base deficit or normal anion gap acidosis)

The pH is low because buffering and respiratory compensation are not adequate to maintain the hydrogen ion concentration at a normal level. The bicarbonate level is below normal for any one (or all) of the following reasons: bicarbonate has been lost from the body, creating an actual base-deficit acidosis; bicarbonate has not been produced in sufficient quantities, creating an actual base-deficit acidosis; or bicarbonate may be bound to other substances. The carbon dioxide level is normal or even slightly decreased because gas exchange is adequate and carbon dioxide retention is not a factor. The oxygen level is normal because gas exchange is adequate.

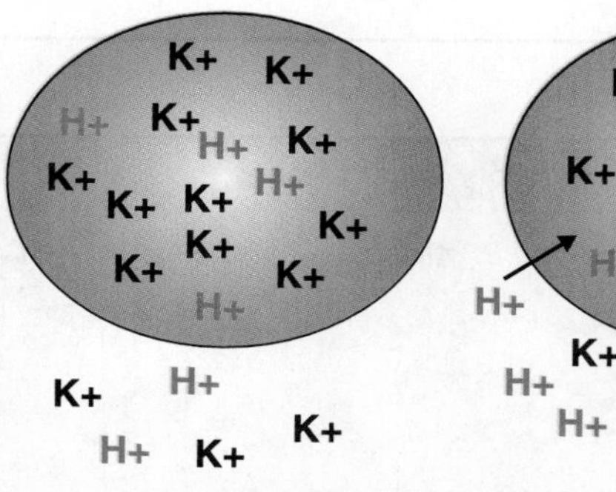

Under normal conditions, the intracellular potassium content is much greater than that of the extracellular fluid. The concentration of hydrogen ions is low in both compartments.

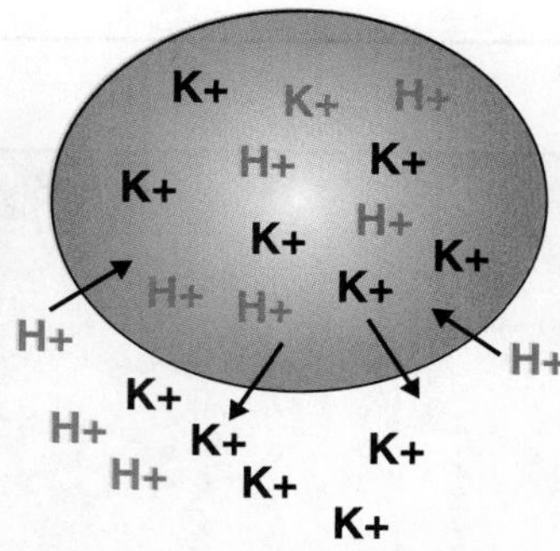

In acidemia, the extracellular hydrogen ion content increases, and the hydrogen ions move into the intracellular fluid. To keep the intracellular fluid electrically neutral, an equal number of potassium ions leave the cell, creating a relative hyperkalemia.

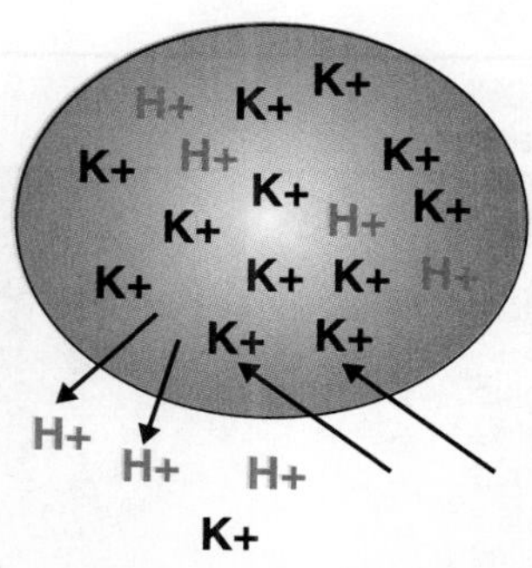

In alkalemia, more hydrogen ions are present in the intracellular fluid than in the extracellular fluid. Hydrogen ions move from the intracellular fluid into the extracellular fluid. To keep the intracellular fluid electrically neutral, potassium ions move from the extracellular fluid into the intracellular fluid, creating a relative hypokalemia.

Figure 16-2 ● Movement of potassium in response to changes in the extracellular fluid hydrogen ion concentration. (© 1992 M. Linda Workman. All rights reserved.)

The serum potassium level is often elevated in metabolic acidosis as a result of the body's attempt to maintain electroneutrality during buffering. Figure 16-2 shows the movement of potassium ions as serum pH changes. As the hydrogen ion concentration of the blood increases, some of the excess hydrogen ions enter cells (especially red blood cells) for intracellular buffering. The movement of hydrogen ions into the cells creates an intracellular excess of positive ions. To prevent imbalances of intracellular charge, an equal number of potassium ions move from the cells into the blood. This increases the extracellular potassium concentration, causing hyperkalemia.

RESPIRATORY ACIDOSIS. The following laboratory data indicate respiratory acidosis:

ABGs

Low pH (<7.35)
Elevated $Paco_2$
Low partial pressure of arterial oxygen (Pao_2)

Electrolytes

Elevated serum potassium levels
Variable serum bicarbonate levels

pH is lowered by the increase in the concentration of hydrogen ions in the extracellular fluid (ECF). If the kidneys partially compensate for this acidosis, pH is low but not as abnormal as could be expected, considering the degree of derangement in the retention of carbon dioxide. A rapid onset of respiratory acidosis is characterized by a normal bicarbonate level. When respiratory acidosis persists for 24 hours or longer, kidney compensation for the acidosis helps increase the generation and reabsorption of bicarbonate. Chronic respiratory acidosis is indicated by an elevated bicarbonate level and increased $Paco_2$.

$Paco_2$ is elevated and Pao_2 is decreased because the respiratory disorder impairs gas exchange, causing carbon dioxide retention and poor oxygenation. Carbon dioxide is approximately 20 times more diffusible than is oxygen across the alveolar membrane. Therefore a decreased Pao_2 usually occurs before an increased $Paco_2$ (Guyton & Hall, 2000).

Serum potassium levels are elevated in acute respiratory acidosis. They are normal or low in chronic respiratory acidosis when renal compensation is present.

● Interventions

Interventions for acidosis focus on correcting the underlying problem, supporting aerobic metabolism, and monitoring for changes (Chart 16-4). To ensure appropriate interventions, the specific type of acidosis must first be identified.

METABOLIC ACIDOSIS. Interventions for metabolic acidosis include hydration and drugs or treatments to control or eliminate the condition causing the acidosis. For example, if the acidosis is a result of diabetic ketoacidosis, insulin is given to correct the hyperglycemia and the production of ketone bodies. Rehydration and antidiarrheal drugs are administered if the acidosis is a result of prolonged diarrhea. *Bicarbonate is administered only if serum bicarbonate levels are low.*

RESPIRATORY ACIDOSIS. Interventions aim to maintain a patent airway and enhance gas exchange. Such interventions can include drug therapy, oxygen therapy, pulmonary hygiene (positioning and breathing techniques), ventilatory support, and prevention of complications. (See Chapter 30 for a complete discussion of interventions for common disorders causing respiratory acidosis.)

DRUG THERAPY. Drug therapy includes agents to increase the diameter of upper and lower airways and to thin

CHART 16-4

NIC INTERVENTION ACTIVITIES *for* The Client with Acidosis

Acid-Base Management: Metabolic Acidosis: *Promotion of acid-base balance and prevention of complications resulting from serum bicarbonate levels lower than desired*

- Monitor ABG levels for decreasing pH level, as appropriate.
- Maintain patent IV access.
- Monitor intake and output.
- Monitor determinants of oxygen delivery (e.g., Pao_2, Sao_2, and hemoglobin levels and cardiac output), if available.
- Monitor loss of bicarbonate through the GI tract (e.g., diarrhea, pancreatic fistula, small bowel fistula, and ileal conduit), as appropriate.
- Administer fluids as prescribed.
- Administer insulin and fluid hydration (isotonic and hypotonic) for diabetic ketoacidosis, causing metabolic acidosis, as appropriate.
- Prepare client for dialysis (e.g., assist with catheter placement for dialysis), as appropriate.
- Institute seizure precautions.

Acid-Base Management: Respiratory Acidosis: *Promotion of acid-base balance and prevention of complications resulting from serum pCO_2 levels higher than desired*

- Monitor ABG levels for decreasing pH level, as appropriate.
- Monitor determinants of tissue oxygen delivery (e.g., Pao_2, Sao_2, and hemoglobin levels and cardiac output), if available.
- Monitor for symptoms of respiratory failure (e.g., low Pao_2 and elevated $Paco_2$ levels and respiratory muscle fatigue).
- Monitor work of breathing (e.g., respiratory rate, heart rate, use of accessory muscles, and diaphoresis).
- Provide oxygen therapy, if necessary.
- Provide low-carbohydrate, high-fat diet (e.g., pulmocare feedings) to reduce CO_2 production, if indicated.
- Monitor neurologic status (e.g., level of consciousness and confusion).

NIC intervention activities selected from McCloskey, J.C., & Bulechek, G.M. (Eds.). (2000). *Nursing interventions classification (NIC)* (3rd ed.). St. Louis: Mosby. No part of this work is to be altered without prior written permission from the Publisher.
ABG, Arterial blood gas; *GI,* gastrointestinal; *Pao_2,* partial pressure of arterial oxygen; *Sao_2,* arterial oxygen saturation; *$Paco_2$,* partial pressure of arterial carbon dioxide.

pulmonary secretions. Drug therapy is not aimed directly at altering arterial pH.

Drugs to Increase Airway Diameter. Drugs that induce the relaxation of bronchial smooth muscle increase airway diameter. Many of these agents are adrenergic agonists, sympathomimetic agents, antimuscarinic drugs, and methylxanthines. Examples of these drugs include albuterol (Novo-Salmol✤, Proventil, Ventolin), ephedrine, fenoterol (Berotec✤), isoproterenol (Isuprel), metaproterenol (Alupent), pirbuterol (Maxair), terbutaline (Brethine, Bricanyl), ipratropium (Atrovent), atropine, aminophylline (Phyllocontin, Truphylline), and theophylline (Bronkodyl, Theo-Dur).

Clients may take agents that increase bronchodilation by reducing the inflammation of bronchial luminal tissues. These agents are primarily cortisol (steroid) based, such as beclomethasone (Vanceril, Beclovent), dexamethasone (Decadron Respihaler, Dexasone), flunisolide (AeroBid, Bronalide✤), and triamcinolone (Azmacort).

Drugs to Thin Bronchial Secretions. Some drugs can break up mucus when thick, tenacious pulmonary secretions contribute to airway obstruction. These agents are classified as mucolytic; one example is acetylcysteine (Mucomyst, Mucosil). (See Chapter 30 for a discussion of drugs used for clients with chronic obstructive pulmonary disease or chronic airflow limitation [CAL].)

OXYGEN THERAPY. Oxygen therapy can help promote gas exchange for clients with respiratory acidosis. However, the nurse must use caution when administering oxygen to clients with chronic obstructive pulmonary disease (COPD) and carbon dioxide retention as evidenced by a high $Paco_2$ level. The only respiratory trigger for these clients is a decreased arterial oxygen level. Administering too much oxygen to these clients decreases their respiratory efforts and may lead to respiratory arrest.

PULMONARY HYGIENE. To promote effective gas exchange, the nurse considers positioning, techniques to enhance the excretion of pulmonary secretions, and specific breathing techniques to change airway resistance and maintain inflated alveoli. The nurse helps clients assume a Fowler's or semi-Fowler's position to help increase lung expansion. Increasing fluid intake may reduce the thickness of pulmonary secretions and assist in excretion.

VENTILATORY SUPPORT. Mechanical ventilation may be needed for clients who are unable to maintain an oxygen saturation of at least 90% or are experiencing respiratory muscle fatigue. Chapter 28 discusses the criteria for initiating mechanical ventilation and the nursing care needs of clients who are being mechanically ventilated.

PREVENTION OF COMPLICATIONS. Monitoring clients' respiratory status is critical in preventing pulmonary complications. For clients experiencing chronic respiratory acidosis, the nurse assesses respiratory status at least every 2 hours. He or she also auscultates breath sounds and notes the ease with which air moves into and out of the lungs, including any muscle retractions, the use of accessory muscles, and whether respiratory effort produces a sound that can be heard without a stethoscope. The color of the nail beds and mucous membranes are assessed for cyanosis (a late finding).

CRITICAL THINKING CHALLENGE

The client is a 30-year-old male who received a head injury during a game of touch football. He is unconscious on arrival at the emergency department. Shortly after arrival, he has a generalized seizure that lasts approximately 2 minutes. After the seizure, his arterial blood gases (ABGs) are as follows: pH, 7.1; HCO_3^-, 22 mEq/L; $Paco_2$, 56 mm Hg; and Pao_2, 78 mm Hg.

- What type of acid-base imbalance is present?
- Is the origin of the imbalance metabolic or respiratory? Explain your answer.
- What should be the first intervention? Why?
- Should this client receive intravenous (IV) bicarbonate? Why or why not?

For suggested answer guidelines, go to SIMON http://www.wbsaunders.com/SIMON/Iggy/.

ALKALOSIS

OVERVIEW

In clients with alkalosis, the acid-base balance of the extracellular fluid (ECF) is disturbed and has an excess of bases, especially bicarbonate (HCO_3^-). The concentration or strength

TABLE 16-3 • COMMON CAUSES OF ALKALOSIS

Pathology	Condition
METABOLIC ALKALOSIS	
Increase of base components	Oral ingestion of bases • Antacids • Milk-alkali syndrome Parenteral base administration • Blood transfusion • Sodium bicarbonate • Total parenteral nutrition
Decrease of acid components	Prolonged vomiting Nasogastric suctioning Cushing's syndrome (hypercortisolism) Hyperaldosteronism Thiazide diuretics
RESPIRATORY ALKALOSIS	
Excessive loss of carbon dioxide	Hyperventilation • Fear • Anxiety • Mechanical ventilation • Central nervous system stimulation Salicylates Catecholamines Progesterone Hypoxemia • Asphyxiation • High altitudes • Shock • Early-stage pulmonary problems Pneumonia Asthma Pulmonary emboli

(or both) of the bases is greater than normal compared with the concentration or strength of the acids. Alkalosis is defined as a decrease in the hydrogen ion concentration of the blood and is reflected by an arterial blood pH above 7.45. Like acidosis, alkalosis is not a disease but rather a manifestation of a disease or pathologic process. Alkalosis can be caused by metabolic problems, respiratory problems, or both (Table 16-3).

Pathophysiology

Alkalosis can result from an actual or relative increase in the concentration or strength (or both) of bases. In an actual base excess, alkalosis occurs with processes that cause an overproduction of bases or an underelimination of normally produced bases (usually bicarbonate).

In *relative* alkalosis, the actual amount or strength of bases does not increase. Instead, the concentration or strength (or both) of the acids decreases, which creates an *acid deficit* and makes the fluid relatively more basic than acidic. A relative base-excess alkalosis (or *actual acid deficit*) results from an overelimination or underproduction of acids (Figure 16-3).

The physiologic consequences of alkalosis are serious and potentially life threatening. Treatment is aimed at correcting the cause of alkalosis. To provide the proper intervention, it is important to determine whether the alkalosis is respiratory or metabolic.

Whether its origin is metabolic, respiratory, or both, alkalosis greatly affects specific physiologic functions. Its pathologic effects are caused by accompanying electrolyte imbalances that occur in response to decreased blood cation

AAABBB AAABBB AAABBB	AAABBBB AAABBBB AAABBBB	AABBB AABBB AABBB
Acid-base balance	Actual alkalosis (base excess)	Relative alkalosis (acid deficit)

Figure 16-3 • Concepts of actual and relative alkalosis. (*A*, Acid; *B*, base.)

concentration. The most common problems of alkalosis are associated with increased stimulation of the central nervous, neuromuscular, and cardiovascular systems.

Etiology

METABOLIC ALKALOSIS

Most conditions that result in metabolic alkalosis create the acid-base imbalance through one of two mechanisms: an increase of bases (base excess) or a decrease of acids (acid deficit).

BASE EXCESS. Increases in bases are caused by the oral or parenteral ingestion of bicarbonates, carbonates, acetates, citrates, and lactates. Excessive use of oral antacids containing sodium bicarbonate or calcium carbonate can also cause a metabolic alkalosis. Other base excesses can occur during medical treatments, such as citrate excesses during rapid or massive blood transfusions, acetate and lactate excesses during hyperalimentation, and IV sodium bicarbonate administration to correct lactic acidosis or ketoacidosis.

ACID DEFICIT. Decreases in acids can be caused by disease processes or medical treatment. Contributing conditions include prolonged vomiting, Cushing's syndrome (hypercortisolism), and hyperaldosteronism. Medical treatments that promote acid loss and can cause metabolic alkalosis include the use of thiazide diuretics and prolonged nasogastric suctioning.

RESPIRATORY ALKALOSIS

The primary problem that causes respiratory alkalosis is the excessive loss of carbon dioxide through hyperventilation (rapid respirations). Clients may hyperventilate in response to anxiety, fear, or improper settings on mechanical ventilators. Hyperventilation can also result from direct stimulation of central respiratory centers because of fever, respiratory compensation for metabolic acidosis, central nervous system lesions, and drugs (e.g., salicylates, catecholamines, and progesterone).

➤ COLLABORATIVE MANAGEMENT

• Assessment

PHYSICAL ASSESSMENT/CLINICAL MANIFESTATIONS

Clinical manifestations are the same for metabolic or respiratory alkalosis. Many symptoms are the result of the hypocalcemia (low calcium levels) and hypokalemia (low potassium levels) that usually accompany alkalosis (see Figure 16-2). These problems cause changes in the functions of the central nervous, neuromuscular, and cardiovascular systems (Chart 16-5).

CHART 16-5

KEY FEATURES *of* Alkalosis

Central Nervous System Manifestations
- Increased activity
- Anxiety, irritability, tetany, seizures
- Positive Chvostek's sign
- Positive Trousseau's sign
- Paresthesias

Neuromuscular Manifestations
- Hyperreflexia
- Muscle cramping and twitching
- Skeletal muscle weakness

Cardiovascular Manifestations
- Increased heart rate
- Normal or low blood pressure
- Increased digitalis toxicity

Respiratory Manifestations
- Increased rate and depth of ventilation in respiratory alkalosis
- Decreased respiratory effort associated with skeletal muscle weakness in metabolic alkalosis

CENTRAL NERVOUS SYSTEM MANIFESTATIONS. Overexcitement of the central and peripheral nervous systems is the major cause of the symptoms associated with alkalosis. Clients experience lightheadedness, agitation, confusion, and hyperreflexia, which may progress to seizure activity. Tingling or numbness around the mouth and in the toes may be present. Other indicators of alkalosis with hypocalcemia are positive Chvostek's and Trousseau's signs (see Chapter 13).

NEUROMUSCULAR MANIFESTATIONS. Alkalosis is accompanied by hypocalcemia and hypokalemia, both of which alter neuromuscular function. Hypocalcemia increases nervous system activity, which in turn causes skeletal muscle cramps, twitches, and charley horses. Deep tendon reflexes are hyperactive. **Tetany** (continuous contractions) of muscle groups also may be present. Tetany is painful and indicates a rapidly worsening condition.

Skeletal muscles may contract as a result of nerve overstimulation, but they become weaker because of the hypokalemia. Handgrip strength decreases, and the client may be unable to walk or support his or her own weight. Respiratory efforts become less effective as the skeletal muscles of respiration weaken.

CARDIOVASCULAR MANIFESTATIONS. Alkalosis increases myocardial irritability, especially when accompanied by hypokalemia. Heart rate increases, and the pulse is thready. When hypovolemia (decreased blood volume) is also present, the client may have severe hypotension. The hypokalemia that accompanies alkalosis also increases myocardial sensitivity to digoxin, which increases the risk for digoxin toxicity.

RESPIRATORY MANIFESTATIONS. Increases in the rate and depth of respiration are the main causes of respiratory alkalosis. Tidal volume (the volume of air inhaled and exhaled with each breath) is nearly normal, but minute respiratory volume (the total volume of air inhaled and exhaled in 1 minute) rises in proportion to the increased respiratory rate. The increased minute volume may be caused by anxiety or other physiologic changes.

LABORATORY ASSESSMENT

Arterial blood pH greater than 7.45 confirms alkalosis, but this test alone does not identify the cause of the alkalosis. Because the clinical manifestations of metabolic alkalosis are similar to those of respiratory alkalosis, it is critical that the nurse obtain additional laboratory data, especially arterial blood gas (ABG) values and specific serum electrolytes levels (see Chart 16-3).

METABOLIC ALKALOSIS. The following laboratory data indicate metabolic alkalosis:

ABGs

High pH (>7.45)
Elevated bicarbonate level (>28 mEq/L)
Rising partial pressure of arterial carbon dioxide ($Paco_2$)
Normal partial pressure of arterial oxygen (Pao_2)

Electrolytes

Decreased serum potassium levels
Decreased serum calcium levels

The pH is high because buffering and respiratory compensation are not adequate to maintain the hydrogen ion concentration at a normal level. *The hallmark of metabolic alkalosis is an increased bicarbonate level with a rising $Paco_2$.* The rising $Paco_2$ compensates for the decreased hydrogen ion concentration. The serum potassium level decreases as the body attempts to maintain electroneutrality (see Figure 16-2). As the pH increases, calcium binding increases and serum calcium concentration decreases, which creates an accompanying state of hypocalcemia. Most of the serious clinical manifestations of alkalosis are caused by the accompanying hypocalcemia.

RESPIRATORY ALKALOSIS. The following laboratory data indicate respiratory alkalosis:

ABGs

High pH
Low bicarbonate level
Low $Paco_2$

Electrolytes

Low serum potassium level
Low serum calcium level

The pH is high because buffering and renal compensation cannot maintain the hydrogen ion concentration at a normal level.

The classic respiratory alkalosis profile is a reduced bicarbonate level (not usually <15 mEq/L) coupled with a very low $Paco_2$. The carbon dioxide level is so low because it is being exhaled more rapidly than it is being produced **(hyperventilation).** The bicarbonate level is low in response to the pH increase. Many blood and cellular buffers release hydrogen ions that immediately combine with the serum bicarbonate ions and form carbonic acid, thus reducing the serum concentration of bicarbonate.

CHART 16-6

NIC INTERVENTION ACTIVITIES *for* The Client with Alkalosis

Acid-Base Management: Metabolic Alkalosis: *Promotion of acid-base balance and prevention of complications resulting from serum HCO_3 levels higher than desired*

- Monitor ABG levels for increased pH level.
- Maintain patent IV access.
- Monitor intake and output.
- Monitor determinants of oxygen delivery (e.g., Pao_2, Sao_2, and hemoglobin levels and cardiac output), if available.
- Avoid administration of alkaline substances (e.g., IV sodium bicarbonate and PO or NG antacids) as appropriate.
- Monitor for electrolyte imbalances associated with metabolic alkalosis (e.g., hypokalemia, hypocalcemia, and hypochloremia), as appropriate.
- Monitor for renal loss of acid (e.g., diuretic therapy), as appropriate.
- Replace extracellular fluid deficit with IV saline, as appropriate.
- Administer antiemetics to reduce loss of HCl in emesis, as appropriate.

Acid-Base Management: Respiratory Alkalosis: *Promotion of acid-base balance and prevention of complications resulting from serum pCO_2 levels lower than desired*

- Monitor ABG levels for increased pH level.
- Monitor for indications of impending respiratory failure (e.g., low Pao_2 level, low Sao_2/Svo_2 level, respiratory muscle fatigue).
- Monitor for hyperventilation resulting in respiratory alkalosis (e.g., hypoxemia, CNS injury, hypermetabolic states, GI distension, pain, and stress).
- Monitor for cardiopulmonary manifestations of respiratory alkalosis (e.g., arrhythmias, decreased cardiac output, and hyperventilation).
- Provide oxygen therapy, if necessary.
- Reduce oxygen consumption to minimize hyperventilation (e.g., promote comfort, control fever, and reduce anxiety), as appropriate.
- Provide mechanical ventilatory support, if necessary.

NIC intervention activities selected from McCloskey, J.C., & Bulechek, G.M. (Eds.). (2000). *Nursing interventions classification (NIC)* (3rd ed.). St. Louis: Mosby. No part of this work is to be altered without prior written permission from the Publisher.

ABG, Arterial blood gas; *HCO_3,* bicarbonate; *Pao_2,* partial pressure of arterial oxygen; *Sao_2,* arterial oxygen saturation; *Svo_2,* venous oxygen saturation; *$Paco_2$,* partial pressure of arterial carbon dioxide; *GI,* gastrointestinal.

As in metabolic alkalosis, the serum potassium level is reduced as the body attempts to maintain electroneutrality. Again, as the pH increases, calcium binding increases and the concentration of serum calcium decreases, causing hypocalcemia.

Interventions

Interventions are planned to prevent further losses of hydrogen, potassium, calcium, and chloride ions; to restore fluid balance; and to monitor changes (Chart 16-6).

Drug therapy is the intervention of choice for alkalosis. Drugs are prescribed to resolve the causes of alkalosis and to restore normal fluid, electrolyte, and acid-base balance. For example, the client with metabolic alkalosis caused by diuretic therapy receives fluid and electrolyte replacement and is then re-evaluated by the physician for the need to resume a diuretic. The physician may prescribe a potassium-sparing diuretic to prevent potassium loss and also orders antiemetic medications if the client is vomiting. Fluids and electrolytes are replaced orally or parenterally. The nurse carefully monitors the client's progress and titrates fluid and electrolyte therapy. Serum electrolyte values are monitored daily until they return to normal or near-normal.

CRITICAL THINKING CHALLENGE

The client is an 82-year-old woman who lives alone. She has had diarrhea for 2 days as a result of mild food poisoning. Her vital signs are as follows: temperature, 101° F (38.3° C); pulse, 104; respirations, 32; and blood pressure, 100/78.

- What acid-base imbalance does this client most likely have?
- Which ABGs do you expect will be abnormal? How will they be abnormal? Why will they be abnormal?
- What electrolyte imbalance(s) may also be present?

For suggested answer guidelines, go to SIMON http://www.wbsaunders.com/SIMON/Iggy/.

ONLINE RESOURCES

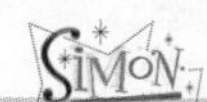

For suggested readings and Internet resources, go to http://www.wbsaunders.com/SIMON/Iggy/.

SELECTED BIBLIOGRAPHY

Asterisk indicates a classic or definitive work on this subject.

Adrogue, H., & Madias, N. (1998a). Management of life-threatening acid-base disorders (first of two parts). *New England Journal of Medicine, 338*(1), 26-34.

Adrogue, H., & Madias, N. (1998b). Management of life-threatening acid-base disorders (second of two parts). *New England Journal of Medicine, 338*(2), 107-111.

Chmielewski, C. (1998). Hyperkalemic emergencies: Mechanisms, manifestations, and management. *Critical Care Nursing Clinics of North America, 10*(4), 449-457.

Coleman, N., & Houston, L. (1998). Demystifying acid-base regulation. *Australian Nurses Journal, 5*(8), 4-7.

Cook, L. (1999). The value of lab values. *American Journal of Nursing, 99*(5), 66-75.

Demers, B., & Morfei, J. (1999). Role of bicarbonate ion concentration in acid-base balance. *Respiratory Care, 44*(8), 963-964.

Faria, S. (1997). Interpretation of arterial blood gases by nurses. *Journal of Vascular Nursing, 15*(4), 128-130.

Frizzell, J. (1998). Avoiding lab test pitfalls. *American Journal of Nursing, 98*(2), 34-38.

Guyton, A., & Hall, J. (2000). *Textbook of medical physiology* (10th ed.). Philadelphia: W.B. Saunders.

Horne, C., & Derrico, D. (1999). Mastering ABGs. *American Journal of Nursing, 99*(8), 26-32.

Markowitz, D., & Irwin, R. (1999). Evaluating acid-base disorders: Is venous blood gas testing sufficient? *Journal of Critical Illness, 14*(7), 403-406.

McCloskey, J., & Bulechek, G. (2000). *Nursing interventions classification (NIC)* (3rd ed.). St. Louis: Mosby.

*Metheney, N. (1996). *Fluid and electrolyte balance: Nursing considerations* (3rd ed.). Philadelphia: J.B. Lippincott.

Miekley, T.F. (1998). A patient-focused approach to managing diuretic therapy. *Critical Care Nursing Clinics of North America, 10*(4), 421-467.

Mizock, B., & Hathiwala, S. (1998). Using the sodium-chloride difference to diagnose acid-base disorders. *Journal of Critical Illness, 13*(11), 701-704.

Pagana, K., & Pagana, T. (1999). *Diagnostic testing and nursing implications: A case study approach.* St. Louis: Mosby.

Paulson, W. (1999). Quick take: Common causes of acid-base disorders. *Journal of Critical Illness, 14*(2), 110-111.

Szaflarski, N., & Hanson, C.W. (1997). Metabolic acidosis. *AACN Clinical Issues: Advanced Practice in Acute and Critical Care, 8*(3), 481-496.

Tasota, F., & Wesmiller, S. (1998). Balancing act: Keeping blood pH in equilibrium, *Nursing98, 28*(12), 35-40.

Wong, F. (1999). A new approach to ABG interpretation, *American Journal of Nursing, 99*(8), 34-35.

UNIT

4

MANAGEMENT OF PERIOPERATIVE CLIENTS

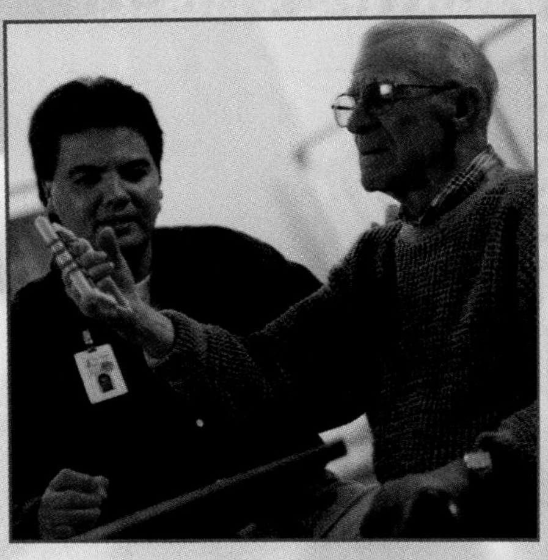

UNIT 4 MANAGEMENT OF PERIOPERATIVE CLIENTS ■ Core Concepts Grid

Anatomy	Physiology	Pathophysiology	History	Physical Exam	Diagnostic Tests	Interventions	Pharmacology
			• **Age** • **Previous medical history** • **Tobacco** • **Usual medications** • **Previous surgeries** • **Complications of surgeries** • **Autologous blood donation** • **Support** • **Advance directives**	• **Vital signs** • **Breath sounds** • **Nutritional status** • **Exposure to infection** • **Cardiovascular system** • **Renal/urinary system** • **Neurologic system** • **Musculoskeletal system**	• **Routine urinalysis** • **Complete blood count** • **Blood urea nitrogen** • **Creatinine** • **Coagulation studies** • **Electrolyte studies** • **Electrocardiogram**	• **Preoperative** Surgical consent Pulmonary toilet Exercises to facilitate venous return Pain management Tubes Drains Dressings Intravenous fluids Skin preparation • **Intraoperative** Surgical team Nursing roles Holding area Positioning Anesthesia Complications Skin closures • **Postoperative** PACU assessment Return to unit Assessment Wound care Complications Infection Pulmonary embolism Deep vein thrombosis Paralytic ileus Dehiscence/ Evisceration Fluid management Tubes/drains Dressings Respiratory care Pain management Health teaching	• **Anesthetic agents** Intravenous Inhaled Spinal Local or regional • **Adjunct drugs** Hypnotics Opioids Blocking agents

CHAPTER 17

Interventions for Preoperative Clients

REBECCA M. PATTON

Learning Objectives

After studying this chapter, you should be able to:

1. Assume the role of client advocate.
2. Describe the legal implications and proper procedures for obtaining informed consent.
3. Prioritize teaching needs for the client preparing for surgery.
4. Recognize client conditions or issues that need to be communicated to the surgical and postoperative teams.

Go to http://www.wbsaunders.com/SIMON/Iggy/ for self-assessment questions related to these Learning Objectives.

Today's trends in health care will be tomorrow's examples of how clients used to be treated. These constant changes reflect multiple advances and society's needs. The technology explosion is responsible for the development of new diagnostic and interventional devices that provide opportunities for the use and refinement of new surgical techniques. Examples of such technical advances include the GAMMA knife for brain tumor resections, as well as other minimally invasive surgery. Advances in anesthetic agents and techniques also have developed. These changes improve the ways that a surgical client is treated and has made anesthesia safer than ever before.

Cost reduction initiatives by third-party payers are also a driving force as to how the client is managed by the health care community. Shortened stays or outpatient treatment has become the expected. Ambulatory surgical services have rapidly been expanded, with more clients being admitted as inpatients *after* a procedure, rather than before. Some clients may only be observed after surgery and not admitted as an inpatient. In response to the ongoing health care delivery changes and the use of multiple settings, nurses have modified their interventions, remaining focused on client care before **(preoperative),** during **(intraoperative),** and after **(postoperative)** surgery.

OVERVIEW

The preoperative period begins when the client is scheduled for surgery and ends at the time of transfer to the surgical suite. The nurse acts as an educator, an advocate, and a promoter of health. Perioperative nursing places special emphasis on safety and client education.

Preoperative care consists of education and any intervention needed before surgery to reduce anxiety and postoperative complications and to promote cooperation in postoperative procedures. In preoperative teaching, the nurse uses adult teaching and learning principles, validating and clarifying information the physician has provided. In addition, during the preoperative assessment it is not uncommon for the nurse to identify situations that warrant further client assessment and/or intervention before surgery. In collaboration with the surgical team, appropriate action is taken to achieve the desired outcome.

Categories and Purposes of Surgery

Surgical procedures are usually categorized according to the following:

- The reason for the surgery
- The urgency of the procedure
- The degree of risk
- The anatomic location
- The extent of surgery required

The primary purposes, or reasons, for surgery can be divided into five general subcategories: diagnostic, curative, restorative, palliative, and cosmetic. **Palliative surgery** makes the client more comfortable, and **cosmetic surgery** reconstructs the skin and underlying structures. The urgency of the procedure can be divided into three subcategories: elective, urgent, and emergent. The degree of risk is classified as minor or major. Classification by location is based on the area of the body on which the surgery occurs (e.g., abdominal surgery, intracranial surgery, or heart surgery). The extent can be simple, modified, or radical. Table 17-1 explains the categories and gives examples of surgical procedures.

Surgical Settings

The term *inpatient* refers to a client who is admitted to a hospital. The client may be admitted the day before or, more of-

TABLE 17-1 • SELECTED CATEGORIES OF SURGICAL PROCEDURES

Category	Description	Condition or Surgical Procedure
REASONS FOR SURGERY		
Diagnostic	Performed to determine the origin and cause of a disorder or the cell type for cancer	Breast biopsy Exploratory laparotomy Arthroscopy
Curative	Performed to resolve a health problem by repairing or removing the cause	Laparoscopic cholecystectomy Mastectomy Hysterectomy
Restorative	Performed to improve a client's functional ability	Total knee replacement Finger reimplantation
Palliative	Performed to relieve symptoms of a disease process, but does not cure	Colostomy Nerve root resection Tumor debulking Ileostomy
Cosmetic	Performed primarily to alter or enhance personal appearance	Liposuction Revision of scars Rhinoplasty Blepharoplasty
URGENCY OF SURGERY		
Elective	Planned for correction of a nonacute problem	Cataract removal Hernia repair Hemorrhoidectomy Total joint replacement
Urgent	Requires prompt intervention; may be life threatening if treatment is delayed more than 24-48 hr	Intestinal obstruction Bladder obstruction Kidney or ureteral stones Bone fracture Eye injury Acute cholecystitis
Emergent	Requires immediate intervention because of life-threatening consequences	Gunshot or stab wound Severe bleeding Abdominal aortic aneurysm Compound fracture Appendectomy
DEGREE OF RISK OF SURGERY		
Minor	Procedure without significant risk; often done with local anesthesia	Incision and drainage (I&D) Implantation of a venous access device (VAD) Muscle biopsy
Major	Procedure of greater risk, usually longer and more extensive than a minor procedure	Mitral valve replacement Pancreas transplant Lymph node dissection
EXTENT OF SURGERY		
Simple	Only the most overtly affected areas involved in the surgery	Simple/partial mastectomy
Radical	Extensive surgery beyond the area obviously involved; is directed at finding a root cause	Radical prostatectomy Radical hysterectomy

ten, the day of surgery (often termed same-day admission [SDA]), or he or she may already be an inpatient when the need for surgical intervention is identified. In contrast, the terms *outpatient* and **ambulatory** refer to a client who goes to the surgical area the day of the surgery and returns home on the same day (i.e., same-day surgery [SDS]). Hospital-based ambulatory surgical centers, freestanding surgical centers, physicians' offices, and ambulatory care centers are becoming increasingly more common. It is estimated that 70% to 90% of all surgical procedures in the United States are performed in ambulatory centers (Poole, 1999).

One of the many advantages of outpatient surgery is that clients are not separated from the comfort and security of their home and family. With continuous improvements in surgical techniques and anesthesia, more procedures are performed safely on an outpatient basis. Changes in the surgical experience, however, present particular challenges for the client who does not have an adequate or available support system. An older spouse may be unable to assist in preoperative and postoperative care. Clients who are primarily responsible for others may be unable to perform their usual tasks within the family. They may try to continue their family role but jeopardize their own health by doing so. As a result, their stress, fears, and anxieties about the surgical experience and about returning home immediately after surgery may be increased.

➤ COLLABORATIVE MANAGEMENT

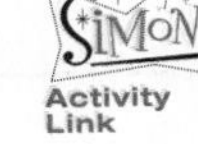

• Assessment

HISTORY

Collection of data about the client before surgery begins in various settings (e.g., the surgeon's office, the preadmission or admission office, the inpatient unit, and over the telephone). The nurse provides privacy to increase the client's comfort with the interview process. Anesthesia and surgery are both physical and emotional stressors. The nurse collects the following data:

- Age
- Use of tobacco, alcohol, or illicit substances, including marijuana
- Current medications
- Use of complementary or alternative medicines, such as herbal therapies, folk remedies, or acupuncture
- Medical history
- Prior surgical procedures and experiences
- Prior experience with anesthesia
- Autologous or directed blood donations
- Allergies, including sensitivity to latex products
- General health
- Family history
- Type of surgery planned
- Knowledge about and understanding of events during the perioperative period
- Adequacy and availability of the client's support system

When taking a history, the nurse screens the preoperative client for conditions that may increase the risk for complications during the perioperative period. Some conditions that could either increase the surgical risk or increase the possibility of postoperative complications are outlined in Table 17-2.

AGE. Older clients are at increased risk for perioperative complications. The normal aging process decreases immune system functioning and delays wound healing. The frequency of chronic illness increases in older clients. See Chart 17-1 for other physiologic changes in older adults that may have an impact on the perioperative experience.

MEDICATION AND SUBSTANCE USE. The use of tobacco products increases the risk of pulmonary complications because of changes they cause to the lungs and thoracic cavity. Excessive alcohol and illicit substance use can alter the effects of anesthesia and response to pain medication. Withdrawal of alcohol in preparation for surgery may precipitate delirium tremens. Prescription and over-the-counter medications may also affect how the client reacts to the perioperative experience. The potential effects of specific medications are listed in Table 17-3. Another area of concern is the potential for reaction or serious adverse effects with some herbs, such as those listed in Table 17-4.

MEDICAL HISTORY. The nurse asks the client about his or her medical history. The presence of many chronic illnesses increases perioperative risks and is considered when planning care. For example, a client with systemic lupus erythematosus may need additional medication to offset the physical and emotional stress of the surgery. A client with diabetes may need a more extensive preoperative bowel preparation because of decreased gastrointestinal motility. An infection may need to be treated before surgery.

TABLE 17-2 • SELECTED FACTORS THAT INCREASE SURGICAL RISK OR INCREASE THE RISK OF POSTOPERATIVE COMPLICATIONS

AGE
- Older than 65 years

MEDICATIONS
- Antihypertensives
- Tricyclic antidepressants
- Anticoagulants
- Nonsteroidal anti-inflammatory drugs (NSAIDs)

MEDICAL HISTORY
- Decreased immunity
- Diabetes
- Pulmonary disease
- Cardiac disease
- Hemodynamic instability
- Multisystem disease
- Coagulation defect or disorder
- Anemia
- Dehydration
- Infection
- Hypertension
- Hypotension
- Any chronic disease

PRIOR SURGICAL EXPERIENCES
- Less-than-optimal emotional reaction
- Anesthesia reactions or complications
- Postoperative complications

HEALTH HISTORY
- Malnutrition or obesity
- Medication, tobacco, alcohol, or illicit substance use or abuse
- Altered coping ability

FAMILY HISTORY
- Malignant hyperthermia
- Cancer
- Bleeding disorder

TYPE OF SURGICAL PROCEDURE PLANNED
- Neck, oral, or facial procedures (airway complications)
- Chest or high abdominal procedures (pulmonary complications)
- Abdominal surgery (paralytic ileus, deep vein thrombosis)

PRIOR CARDIAC HISTORY. The nurse obtains a history of cardiac disease because complications from anesthesia could occur in clients with cardiac problems. Cardiac disorders that increase risks associated with surgery include coronary artery disease, angina pectoris, myocardial infarction (MI) within 6 months before surgery, congestive heart failure, hypertension, and dysrhythmias. These disorders impair the ability to withstand and respond to both anesthesia and the hemodynamic changes associated with surgery. The risk of intraoperative MI is also higher in clients with pre-existing heart problems.

PULMONARY HISTORY. Adults with chronic respiratory problems, older persons, and smokers are at risk for pulmonary complications because of smoking-induced pul-

CHART 17-1

NURSING FOCUS *on the* OLDER ADULT

Changes of Aging as Surgical Risk Factors

Physiologic Change	Nursing Interventions	Rationale
CARDIOVASCULAR SYSTEM Decreased cardiac output Increased blood pressure Decreased peripheral circulation	Determine normal activity levels and note when the client tires. Monitor vital signs, peripheral pulses, and capillary refill.	Knowing limits helps prevent fatigue. Having baseline data helps detect deviations.
RESPIRATORY SYSTEM Reduced viral capacity Loss of lung elasticity Decreased oxygenation of blood	Teach coughing and deep breathing exercises. Monitor respirations and breathing effort.	Pulmonary exercises help prevent pulmonary complications. Having baseline data helps detect deviations.
RENAL/URINARY SYSTEM Decreased blood flow to kidneys Reduced ability to excrete waste products Decline in glomerular filtration rate Nocturia common	Monitor intake and output. Assess overall hydration. Monitor electrolyte status. Assist frequently with toileting needs, especially at night.	Ongoing assessment helps detect fluid and electrolyte imbalances and decreased renal function. Frequent toileting helps prevent incontinence and falls.
NEUROLOGIC SYSTEM Sensory deficits Slower reaction time Decreased ability to adjust to changes in the surroundings	Orient the client to the surroundings. Allow extra time for teaching the client. Provide for the client's safety.	An individualized preoperative teaching plan is developed on the basis of the client's orientation and any neurologic deficits. Safety measures help prevent falls and injury.
MUSCULOSKELETAL SYSTEM Increased incidence of deformities related to osteoporosis or arthritis	Assess the client's mobility. Teach turning and positioning. Encourage ambulation. Place on fall precautions, if indicated.	Interventions help prevent complications of immobility. Safety measures help prevent injury.

monary changes. Increased rigidity of the thoracic cavity and loss of lung elasticity reduce the efficiency of anesthesia excretion. Smoking increases the level of circulating **carboxyhemoglobin** (carbon monoxide in the oxygen-binding sites of the hemoglobin molecule), which in turn decreases oxygen delivery to organs. In addition, mucociliary transport decreases, which leads to increased secretions and predisposes the client to infection (pneumonia) and **atelectasis** (collapse of alveoli). Atelectasis prevents the exchange of oxygen and carbon dioxide and causes intolerance of anesthesia.

Chronic conditions such as asthma, emphysema, and chronic bronchitis also reduce the elasticity of the lungs, which causes an ineffective exchange of carbon dioxide and oxygen. As a result, clients with these conditions have decreased oxygen diffusion and decreased oxygenation of the tissues.

PREVIOUS SURGERY AND ANESTHESIA. The number and type of previous surgical procedures and previous surgical experiences affect the preoperative client's readiness for surgery. Previous perioperative experiences, particularly those with complications, may contribute to fears and concerns about the scheduled surgery. The nurse asks about the client's experience with anesthetic agents and all allergies. These data provide the nurse with information about tolerance of and possible fears about the use of anesthesia. A sensitivity or allergy to certain substances alerts the nurse to a possible reaction to anesthetic agents or to substances that are used for preoperative skin preparation. For example, povidone-iodine used for skin preparation contains some of the same components found in shellfish. Clients who are allergic to shellfish may have an adverse reaction to povidone-iodine. The family medical history and problems with anesthetics may indicate possible intraoperative needs and reactions to anesthesia, such as malignant hyperthermia (see Chapter 18).

AUTOLOGOUS OR DIRECTED BLOOD DONATIONS. Clients may donate their own blood (**autologous donations**) for a few weeks immediately before the scheduled surgery date. If they need blood during the perioperative period, an autologous blood transfusion can be given. This practice eliminates the possibility of transfusion reactions and the transmission of bloodborne disease.

Clients may be candidates for autologous blood donations up to 5 weeks preoperatively if they are afebrile, have a hemoglobin level greater than 11 g/dL (110 g/L), and have a physician's recommendation. Usually clients with a history of cardiovascular disease need additional clearance from their cardiologist. The physician may order supplemental iron beginning before the first donation. Autologous donations can be made as frequently as every 3 days if the other criteria are met. Usually a total of 2 to 4 units is donated. The last donation cannot be made within 72 hours before surgery.

A special tag is affixed to the transfusion bag when an autologous blood donation has been made. The blood donor center gives the client a matching tag that he or she brings to the surgical area preoperatively. This procedure helps to ensure that the client receives only his or her own blood. If the blood is not used, it goes to the blood bank to be used as would any other unit of donated blood.

TABLE 17-3 • EFFECTS OF ROUTINE MEDICATIONS TAKEN PREOPERATIVELY

Drug	Implications for the Perioperative Experience	Nursing Interventions	Rationale
ANTIARRHYTHMICS Quinidine gluconate (Quinate♣, Quinaglute Dura-Tabs) Procainamide hydrochloride (Pronestyl, Procan SR)	Antiarrhythmic medications affect the client's tolerance of anesthesia and potentiate anesthetics that are neuromuscular blockers. Antiarrhythmics depress cardiac function by decreasing cardiac output and slowing the pulse rate. Antiarrhythmics may cause peripheral vasodilation.	Communicate the use and type of antiarrhythmics to the anesthesia personnel. Monitor vital signs. Obtain a baseline electrocardiogram, as ordered. Assess the client's peripheral circulation.	Cardiac complications during surgery can be life threatening. Ongoing monitoring helps to detect deviations and potential complications.
ANTIHYPERTENSIVES Methyldopa (Aldomet, Novomedopa♣) Captopril (Capoten) Clonidine hydrochloride (Catapres)	Antihypertensive agents alter the client's response to muscle relaxants and opioid analgesics by inhibiting synthesis and storage of norepinephrine. Antihypertensives may cause a hypotensive crisis intraoperatively and postoperatively.	Monitor blood pressure and pulse frequently. Assess for hypotension during transfer and turning.	Ongoing monitoring helps to detect deviations and potential complications. Hypotensive crisis can occur and may be prevented through timely assessments.
CORTICOSTEROIDS Dexamethasone (Decadron, Dexasone) Hydrocortisone sodium (Solu-Cortef) Prednisone (Deltasone♣, Winpred)	Surgery increases the demand for corticosteroids in the client with no adrenal function. Steroids delay wound healing because of blockage of collagen formation. Steroids increase the serum glucose level and block fibroblast formation. Steroids increase the risk of hemorrhage. Steroids mask the signs and symptoms of infection.	Continue steroid therapy during surgery. Monitor vital signs. Assess for signs of hyperglycemia. Assess for subtle signs of infection and bleeding. Monitor wound healing, support the incision area with binders, and splint the wound when the client is turning, coughing, and deep breathing.	Continuation of steroid therapy avoids problems associated with abrupt withdrawal. Ongoing monitoring helps to detect deviations and potential complications. It is important to detect early signs and symptoms of infection. Specific wound and incision care helps to prevent complications.
ANTICOAGULANTS Wafarin sodium (Coumadin, Warfilone sodium♣) Heparin sodium (Leo-Heparin, Hepalean♣) Aspirin (acetylsalicylic acid, Ancasal♣, Astrin♣, Coryphen♣)	Anticoagulant therapy increases the risk of hemorrhage intraoperatively and postoperatively.	Monitor coagulation studies (aPTT, PT, INR). Monitor for signs of bleeding. Gradually discontinue anticoagulants 24-48 hr before surgery, as ordered. Have an antidote (protamine sulfate for heparin and vitamin K [Mephyton] for warfarin sodium) available to reverse the effects of the anticoagulant.	Coagulation studies help detect bleeding disorders. Anticoagulant administration is discontinued to avoid hemorrhage. An antidote needs to be available to prevent complications of bleeding in an emergency situation.
ANTISEIZURE MEDICATIONS Phenobarbital (Luminal, Gardenal♣)	Seizure activity can cause injury to the surgical wound. Antiseizure medications alter the metabolism of anesthetic agents.	Maintain use of the drug. Inform the anesthesiologist or anesthetist to allow for adjustment of the dosage of the anesthetic. Assess for seizure activity. Pad the siderails of the bed. Place suction equipment at the bedside.	Antiseizure medications prevent seizures. Safety measures prevent injury.

aPTT, Partial thromboplastin time, activated; *INR*, International Normalized Ratio; *NPO*, nothing by mouth; *PT*, prothrombin time.

Continued

TABLE 17-3 • EFFECTS OF ROUTINE MEDICATIONS TAKEN PREOPERATIVELY—cont'd

Drug	Implications for the Perioperative Experience	Nursing Interventions	Rationale
GLAUCOMA MEDICATIONS			
Demecarium bromide (Humorsol) Echothiophate (Phospholine iodide) Pilocarpine hydrochloride (Isopto Carpine, Pilocar, Miocarpine♣) Timolol maleate (Timoptic)	Glaucoma medications have cumulative systemic effects and can cause respiratory and cardiovascular collapse, especially during surgery.	Consult the physician about stopping Humorsol at least 2 weeks before surgery. Monitor respiratory status and cardiac output. Assess for increased intraocular pressure.	Collaboration with the physician helps prevent complications. Ongoing monitoring helps to detect complications.
ANTIDIABETIC AGENT			
Insulin	Insulin needs decrease preoperatively when the client is on NPO status. Postoperative insulin demands increase because of IV administration of dextrose. Insulin levels may fluctuate during healing because of dietary and activity restrictions and the physical stress of surgery.	Monitor serum glucose levels. Administer antibiotics and other intermittent medications in normal saline instead of dextrose when possible, as ordered, or as per facility policy.	Monitoring will detect an increased or a decreased need for insulin. The use of normal saline prevents complications.

aPTT, Partial thromboplastin time, activated; *INR,* International Normalized Ratio; *NPO,* nothing by mouth; *PT,* prothrombin time.

TABLE 17-4 • POTENTIAL EFFECTS OF HERBS

Herb	Potential Effect
Black cohosh	Bradycardia, hypotension, joint pains
Bloodroot	Bradycardia, dysrhythmia, dizziness, impaired vision, intense thirst
Boneset	Liver toxicity, mental changes, respiratory problems
Coltsfoot	Fever, liver toxicity
Dandelion	Interactions with diuretics, increased concentration of lithium or potassium
Ephedra	Headache, dizziness, insomnia, tachycardia, hypertension, anxiety, irritability, dry mouth
Feverfew	Interference with blood-clotting mechanisms
Garlic	Hypotension, blood-clotting inhibition, potentiation of diabetes drugs
Ginseng	Headache, anxiety, insomnia, hypertension, tachycardia, asthma attacks, postmenopausal bleeding
Goldenseal	Vasoconstriction
Hawthorn	Hypotension
Kava	Damage to the eyes, skin, liver, and spinal cord from long-term use
Licorice	Hypokalemia, hypernatremia
Lobelia	Hearing and vision problems
Motherwort	Increased anticoagulation
Nettle	Hypokalemia
Senna	Potentiation of digoxin
St. John's Wort	Antidepressant, photosensitivity
Valerian root	Mild sedative or tranquilizer effect, hepatotoxicity

Clients may wish to have family and friends donate blood exclusively for their use, if needed. This practice of **directed blood donation** is possible only if the blood types are compatible and the donor's blood is acceptable. Clients may fear disease transmission from unknown blood and feel more comfortable knowing who gave the blood. Increasingly, blood collection centers and other health care personnel are discouraging this practice. Some centers do not accept directed blood, stating that it gives a false sense of security. As with autologous blood donations, a special tag is affixed to the blood. This tag notes the names of the client and the donor and bears the client's signature.

The nurse asks whether autologous or directed blood donations have been made and documents this information in the chart. It may be important to know the specific blood collection center where the donation was made and whether the blood has arrived before the client goes into surgery.

PLANNING FOR BLOODLESS SURGERY. Increased use of "bloodless surgery," or minimally invasive surgery, programs is helping to provide another alternative for clients with religious or medical contraindications to blood transfusions. These programs reduce or eliminate the need for transfusion during and after surgery. Some techniques employed include limiting preoperative blood samples (the number of samples, as well as the volume of blood drawn per sample) and stimulating the client's own red blood cell production with epoetin alpha (Epogen, Procrit) before, during, and after surgery. The physician may prescribe supplemental iron, folic acid, vitamin B_{12}, and vitamin C preoperatively to further stimulate erythropoiesis. Special equipment and techniques used during the surgical procedure result in less blood loss than with older techniques. Such technologic advances include autotransfusion of suctioned blood during surgery to be recycled and immediately transfused back into the client. The nurse assesses, monitors, teaches, and supports the client during the bloodless surgery process (Vernon & Pfeifer, 1997).

DISCHARGE PLANNING. The nurse assesses the client's home environment, self-care capabilities, and support systems and anticipates postoperative needs during the preoperative period. All clients, regardless of how minor the procedure, should have discharge planning. Older persons and dependent adults may need referrals for transportation to and from the physician's office or the surgical setting. A home care nurse may be needed to monitor postoperative recovery and to provide instruction on wound care. All clients with inadequate support systems may need follow-up care at home. Some require a planned direct admission to a rehabilitation hospital or center for extensive physical therapy following surgery, as in the case of total hip arthroplasty. Shortened hospital stays necessitate adequate discharge planning to achieve the desired outcomes after surgery.

CHART 17-2

NURSING FOCUS *on the* OLDER ADULT

Specific Considerations When Planning Care for the Older Preoperative Client

- Greater incidence of chronic illness
- Greater incidence of malnutrition
- More allergies
- Increased incidence of impaired self-care abilities
- Inadequate support systems
- Decreased ability to withstand the stress of surgery and anesthesia
- Increased risk of postoperative cardiopulmonary complications
- Risk of a change in mental status when admitted (related to unfamiliar surroundings, change in routine, medications administered, and so forth)
- Increased risk of a fall and resultant injury

PHYSICAL ASSESSMENT/CLINICAL MANIFESTATIONS

The preoperative client may be of any age, with a health status that varies from well to debilitated. The nurse performs a complete preoperative physical assessment to obtain baseline data. During physical assessment the nurse also identifies current health problems, potential complications related to the administration of anesthesia, and potential postoperative complications.

When beginning the assessment, the nurse obtains a complete set of vital signs. The nurse may need to obtain vital signs several times for accurate baseline values. Abnormal vital signs may cause the postponement of surgery until the underlying problem is treated and the client's condition is stable. The nurse also assesses for anxiety, which could increase blood pressure, pulse, and respiratory rate. These findings are documented in the chart as part of the overall assessment.

Throughout the physical assessment, the nurse focuses on problem areas identified from the client's history and on all body systems affected directly or indirectly by the surgical procedure. The older adult (Chart 17-2; see also Chapter 5) or chronically ill client is at increased risk for intraoperative and postoperative complications. Perioperative morbidity and mortality are higher in older and chronically ill clients because of their preoperative physical condition.

The nurse reports any abnormalities found on physical assessment to the physician and anesthesiology personnel. In this manner, the nurse functions as a proactive client advocate and is exercising professional legal responsibility. Often, established protocols or care maps identify what interventions are to be performed in the preoperative period.

CARDIOVASCULAR SYSTEM. Alterations in cardiac status are responsible for as many as 30% of perioperative deaths. The nurse evaluates the client for hypertension, which is common, is often undiagnosed, and can affect the response to surgery. Cardiovascular assessment also includes auscultation of heart sounds for rate, regularity, and abnormalities. The nurse evaluates the client's extremities for temperature, color, peripheral pulses, capillary refill, and edema. Any physical alterations, such as absent peripheral pulses, pitting edema, or cardiac symptoms, such as chest pain, shortness of breath, and dyspnea, are reported to the physician for further assessment and evaluation. (Cardiovascular assessment is discussed further in Chapter 33.)

RESPIRATORY SYSTEM. In assessing the client's respiratory status, the nurse considers the client's age, smoking history, and the presence of any chronic illness. The nurse observes the client's posture; respiratory rate, rhythm, and depth; overall respiratory effort; and lung expansion. **Clubbing of the fingertips** (swelling at the base of the nail beds caused by a chronic lack of oxygen) or any cyanosis is noted. The nurse auscultates the lungs to determine the quality and presence of any adventitious (crackles, wheezes, rubs) or abnormal breath sounds. (More information on respiratory status assessment is found in Chapter 27.)

RENAL/URINARY SYSTEM. Renal and urinary function affects the filtration and eventual excretion of waste products, including anesthetic and analgesic agents. If renal and urinary function is less than optimal, fluid and electrolyte balance can be altered, especially in the older client. The nurse asks about the presence or absence of symptoms such as urinary frequency, **dysuria** (painful urination), **nocturia** (awakening during nighttime sleep because of a need to void), difficulty starting urine flow, and **oliguria** (scant amount of urine). The client is asked about the appearance and odor of the urine. Equally important is an assessment of usual fluid intake and degree of continence. If the client is suspected of having underlying renal or urinary problems, the nurse consults with the physician about further workup. (Renal/urinary assessment is discussed further in Chapter 69.)

Abnormal renal function can decrease the excretion rate of preoperative medications and anesthetic agents. As a result, the drug's effectiveness may be altered. Scopolamine (Buscopan♣), morphine, meperidine (Demerol), and barbiturates frequently cause confusion, disorientation, apprehension, and restlessness when administered to clients with decreased renal function.

NEUROLOGIC SYSTEM. The nurse assesses the client's overall mental status, including level of consciousness, orientation, and ability to follow commands, before planning preoperative teaching and postoperative care. A deficit in any of these areas affects the type of care required during the perioperative experience. The nurse determines the client's baseline neurologic status to be able to identify changes that may occur later. The nurse also assesses for any motor or sensory deficits. (See Chapter 41 for complete nervous system assessment.)

The usual neurologic status of a mentally impaired or older client may be difficult to assess. The client who has been independent and oriented while in the home environment may become disoriented in an unfamiliar hospital setting. Family members and significant others can often provide information about what the client was like at home.

Often, as part of the neurologic assessment, the nurse assesses the client's risk for falling, especially in older clients. Factors such as mental status, muscle strength, steadiness of gait, and sense of independence are evaluated to determine the client's risk. The client's ability to ambulate and his or her steadiness of gait are noted preoperatively as baseline data.

MUSCULOSKELETAL SYSTEM. Deformities of the musculoskeletal system may interfere with intraoperative and postoperative positioning. For example, clients with arthritis may be able to assume conventional intraoperative positions but have unnecessary discomfort postoperatively from prolonged immobilization of joints. Other anatomic characteristics, such as the shape and length of the neck and the shape of the thoracic cavity, may interfere with respiratory and cardiac function or require special positioning during surgery.

The nurse asks about a history of joint replacements and notes the exact location of any prostheses. During surgery the nurse ensures that electrocautery pads, which could cause an electrical burn, are not placed near the area of the prosthesis.

NUTRITIONAL STATUS. Malnutrition and obesity can increase surgical risk. Surgery usually increases the body's metabolic rate and consequently depletes potassium, ascorbic acid, and B vitamins, all of which are needed for wound healing and fibrin formation. In malnourished clients, hypoproteinemia slows postoperative recovery. Negative nitrogen balance may result from depleted protein stores. This situation increases the risk for perioperative morbidity and mortality from delayed wound healing, possible dehiscence or evisceration (see Chapter 19), fluid volume deficit, and sepsis.

Some older clients may have nutritional imbalances because of chronic illness, diuretic or laxative use, poor dietary planning or habits, anorexia, lack of motivation, or financial limitations. Clinical indications of poor fluid or nutritional status include brittle nails, muscle wasting, dry or flaky skin, hair alterations (e.g., dull, sparse, dry), decreased skin turgor, **orthostatic** (postural) hypotension, decreased serum albumin levels, and abnormal serum electrolyte values.

The obese client is often malnourished because of poor eating habits and an imbalanced diet. Obesity increases the risk for poor or incomplete wound healing because of excessive adipose tissue. Fatty tissue has poor vasculature, little collagen, and decreased nutrients, all of which are important for wound healing. Obesity causes increased stress on the heart and reduces the available lung volumes, which can affect the intraoperative experience and postoperative recovery. In addition, obese clients may require larger doses of medication and retain them longer in their systems postoperatively.

PSYCHOSOCIAL ASSESSMENT

The nurse performs a psychosocial assessment and preparation to determine the client's level of anxiety, coping ability, and support systems; provide information; and offer support.

Most clients scheduled for surgery experience some preoperative anxiety and fear. The extent and type of these reactions vary according to the type of surgery, the perceived effects of the surgery and its potential outcome, and the client's basic personality. Surgery may be seen as a threat to biologic integrity, body image, self-esteem, self-concept, or lifestyle. Clients may fear death, pain, helplessness, decreased socioeconomic status, a diagnosis of life-threatening conditions, possible disabling or crippling effects, or the unknown.

The client's anxiety and fear affect his or her ability to learn, cope, and cooperate with preoperative teaching and perioperative procedures. Anxiety and fear may also influence the amount and type of anesthesia needed and may retard postoperative recovery. The nurse is aware of potential fears and anxieties when interviewing the client and planning preoperative teaching.

The nurse assesses coping mechanisms used by the client under similar situations or in the past when confronted with a stressful situation. The nurse asks open-ended questions pertaining to the client's feelings about the entire perioperative experience. Factors to be assessed that influence coping include age; previous surgical or sick-role experiences; and emotional and physical signs of fear, anxiety, or discomfort. Signs of fear and anxiety include anger, crying, restlessness, **diaphoresis** (sweating, usually profusely), increased pulse rate, palpitations, sleeplessness, diarrhea, and urinary frequency.

LABORATORY ASSESSMENT

Preoperative laboratory tests provide baseline data about the client's health and help predict potential complications. The client scheduled for surgery in an ambulatory surgical center or admitted to the hospital on the morning of or day before surgery may have preadmission testing performed from 48 hours to 28 days before the scheduled surgery, depending on the facility's policy. The results of prior tests are usually valid unless there has been a change in the client's condition that warrants repeated testing or the client is taking medications that can alter laboratory values (such as warfarin [Coumadin], aspirin, or diuretics).

The choice of routine preoperative laboratory tests varies among facilities and depends on the client's age and medical history and the type of anesthesia planned. The most common tests are urinalysis, blood type and crossmatch, complete blood count or hemoglobin level and hematocrit, coagulation studies (prothrombin time [PT], International Normalized Ratio [INR], activated partial thromboplastin time [aPTT], and platelet count), electrolyte levels, and serum creatinine level. Depending on a female client's age and the nature of the planned procedure, a pregnancy test may also be ordered.

A preoperative urinalysis is performed to assess for the presence of protein, glucose, blood, and bacteria, all of which are abnormal constituents of the urine. If renal disease is suspected or the client is older, the physician may order other tests to determine the type and degree of disease present.

The nurse reports electrolyte imbalances or other abnormal results to the anesthesia team and the surgeon before surgery. **Hypokalemia** (decreased serum potassium level) increases the risk of digoxin toxicity (if the client is taking digoxin), slows recovery from anesthesia, and increases cardiac irritability. **Hyperkalemia** (increased serum potassium level) increases the risk for cardiac dysrhythmias, especially with the use of anesthesia. Both hypokalemia and hyperkalemia should be corrected before the surgery.

The physician may order other studies, depending on the client's medical history. For example, baseline arterial blood gas (ABG) values are assessed before surgery for clients with chronic pulmonary problems. Chart 17-3 presents abnormal laboratory findings and their possible causes.

CHART 17-3

LABORATORY PROFILE
Perioperative Assessment

Test	Normal Range for Adults	Significance of Abnormal Findings: Increased in	Significance of Abnormal Findings: Decreased in
Potassium (K^+) level	3.5-5.0 mEq/L, or 3.5-5.0 mmol/L	Dehydration Renal failure Acidosis Cellular/tissue damage Hemolysis of the specimen	NPO status when potassium replacement is inadequate Excessive use of non–potassium-sparing diuretics Vomiting Malnutrition Diarrhea Alkalosis
Sodium (Na^+)	Up to 90 yr: 136-145 mEq/L, or 136-145 mmol/L >90 yr: 132-146 mEq/L, or 132-146 mmol/L	Cardiac or renal failure Hypertension Excessive amounts of IV fluids containing normal saline Edema Dehydration (hemoconcentration)	Nasogastric drainage Vomiting or diarrhea Excessive use of laxatives or diuretics Excessive amounts of IV fluids containing water Syndrome of inappropriate antidiuretic hormone (SIADH)
Chloride (Cl^-)	Up to 90 yr: 90-110 mEq/L, or 98-106 mmol/L >90 yr: 98-111 mEq/L, or 98-111 mmol/L	Respiratory alkalosis Dehydration Renal failure Excessive amounts of IV fluids containing sodium chloride (NaCl)	Excessive nasogastric drainage Vomiting Excessive use of diuretics Diarrhea
Carbon dioxide (CO_2)	Up to 60 yr: 23-30 mEq/L, or 23-30 mmol/L 60-90 yr: 23-31 mEq/L, or 23-31 mmol/L >90 yr: 20-29 mEq/L, or 20-29 mmol/L	Chronic pulmonary disease Intestinal obstruction Vomiting or nasogastric suctioning Metabolic alkalosis	Hyperventilation Diabetic ketoacidosis Diarrhea Lactic acidosis Renal failure Salicylate toxicity
Glucose (fasting)	Up to 60 yr: 70-105 mg/dL, or 4.1-5.9 mmol/L 60-90 yr: 82-115 mg/dL, or 4.6-6.4 mmol/L >90 yr: 75-121 mg/dL, or 4.2-6.7 mmol/L	Hyperglycemia Excess amounts of IV fluids containing glucose Stress Steroid use Pancreatic or hepatic disease	Hypoglycemia Excess insulin
Creatinine	Females: Up to 60 yr: 0.5-1.1 mg/dL, or 53-97 μmol/L 60-90 yr: 0.6-1.2 mg/dL, or 53-106 μmol/L >90 yr: 0.6-1.3 mg/dL, or 53-115 μmol/L Males: Up to 60 yr: 0.6-1.2 mg/dL, or 80-115 μmol/L 60-90 yr: 0.8-1.3 mg/dL, or 71-115 μmol/L >90 yr: 1.0-1.7 mg/dL, or 88-150 μmol/L	Renal damage with destruction of large number of nephrons Renal insufficiency Acute renal failure Chronic renal failure End-stage renal disease (ESRD)	Atrophy of muscle tissue
Blood urea nitrogen (BUN)	Up to 60 yr: 10-20 mg/dL, or 2.1-7.1 mmol/L 60-90 yr: 8-23 mg/dL, or 2.9-8.2 mmol/L >90 yr: 10-31 mg/dL, or 3.6-11.1 mmol/L	Dehydration Renal failure Excessive protein in diet Liver failure	Overhydration Malnutrition

IRU, International recommended unit; *NPO,* nothing by mouth.

Continued

CHART 17-3

LABORATORY PROFILE
Perioperative Assessment—cont'd

Test	Normal Range for Adults	Significance of Abnormal Findings: Increased in	Significance of Abnormal Findings: Decreased in
Prothrombin time (Pro Time, PT) International Normalized Ratio (INR)	11-12.5 sec, 85%-100%, or 1-1.1 client-control ratio 0.7-1.8	Coagulation defect (bleeding disorder) Anticoagulant therapy (aspirin, warfarin)	Coagulation (clotting) disorder, such as thrombophlebitis or pulmonary embolus Extensive cancer
Partial thromboplastin time, activated (aPTT)	Less than 35 sec	Coagulation defect (bleeding disorder) Anticoagulant therapy (heparin) Liver disease	Coagulation (clotting) disorder, such as thrombophlebitis or pulmonary embolus Extensive cancer
White blood cell (WBC) count (leukocyte count)	Total: 5000-10,000/mm³, or 7.4 IRU	Infection Inflammation Stress Tissue necrosis	Immune disorder Immunosuppressant therapy
Hemoglobin, total	Females: 18-44 yr: 12-16 g/dL, or 117-155 g/L 45-64 yr: 11.7-16.0 g/dL, or 117-160 g/L 65-74 yr: 11.7-16.1 g/dL, or 117-161 g/L Males: 18-44 yr: 14-18 g/dL, or 132-173 g/L 45-64 yr: 13.1-17.2 g/dL, or 131-172 g/L 65-74 yr: 12.6-17.4 g/dL, or 126-174 g/L	Dehydration Polycythemia Chronic pulmonary disease Congestive heart failure	Blood loss Anemia Renal failure
Hematocrit	Females: 18-44 yr: 35%-45% 45-74 yr: 37%-47% Males: 18-44 yr: 42%-52% 45-64 yr: 39%-50% 65-74 yr: 37%-51%	Dehydration Polycythemia High altitude	Blood loss Anemia Renal failure

IRU, International recommended unit; *NPO,* nothing by mouth.

RADIOGRAPHIC ASSESSMENT

A chest x-ray film, ordered by the physician or anesthesiologist, is commonly obtained to determine the size and contour of the heart, lungs, and major vessels and to determine the presence of any infiltrates that could indicate pneumonia or tuberculosis. A chest x-ray study also provides baseline data in the event of postoperative complications. Abnormal x-ray findings alert the physician to potential cardiac or pulmonary complications. The presence of congestive heart failure, cardiomyopathy, pneumonia, or infiltrates may cause cancellation or delay of elective surgery. For emergency surgery, x-ray results assist the anesthesiologist in the selection of anesthesia. In many facilities, chest x-ray results are valid when done within 6 months before surgery, provided that there has not been a change in the client's condition.

Other radiographic studies are based on individual need, the medical history, and the nature of the surgical procedure. For example, a client with back pain may have computed tomography (CT) or magnetic resonance imaging (MRI) done before a **laminectomy** (spinal surgery) to identify the exact location of the abnormality.

OTHER DIAGNOSTIC ASSESSMENT

An electrocardiogram (ECG) may routinely be required for all clients older than a specific age who are to have general anesthesia. The age varies among facilities but is often 40 to 45 years. An ECG may also be ordered for clients with a history of cardiac disease or those at risk for cardiovascular complications. An ECG provides baseline information on new or pre-existing cardiac conditions, such as an old anterior wall myocardial infarction (MI). A client with a known cardiac condition may require a preoperative consultation with a cardiologist. Prophylactic medication, such as nitroglycerin and antibiotics, may be needed during the perioperative period to reduce or prevent stress on the cardiovascular system. Abnormal or potentially life-threatening ECG results may cause the cancellation of surgery until the client's cardiac status is stable.

CHART 17-4

FOCUSED ASSESSMENT *of*
The Preoperative Client

As part of the cardiopulmonary assessment, take and record vital signs; report the following:
- Hypotension or hypertension
- Heart rate of less than 60 or more than 120 beats/min
- Irregular heart rate
- Chest pain
- Shortness of breath or dyspnea
- Tachypnea
- Pulse oximetry reading of <94%

Assess for and report any signs or symptoms of infection, including the following:
- Fever
- Purulent sputum
- Dysuria or cloudy, foul-smelling urine
- Any red, swollen, draining IV or wound site
- Increased white blood cell count

Assess for and report signs or symptoms that could contraindicate surgery, including the following:
- Increased prothrombin time (PT), International Normalized Ratio (INR), or activated partial thromboplastin time (aPTT).
- Hypokalemia or hyperkalemia
- Client report of possible pregnancy or positive pregnancy test

Assess for and report other clinical conditions that may need to be evaluated by a physician or advanced nurse practitioner before proceeding with the surgical plans, including the following:
- Change in mental status
- Vomiting
- Rash
- Recent administration of an anticoagulant medication

A focused assessment of the preoperative client is shown in Chart 17-4.

Analysis

COMMON NURSING DIAGNOSES

The following are common nursing diagnoses for preoperative clients:

1. Deficient Knowledge related to a lack of education and lack of exposure to the specific perioperative experience
2. Anxiety related to the threat of a change in health status or fear of the unknown

ADDITIONAL NURSING DIAGNOSES

In addition to the common nursing diagnoses, preoperative clients may have one or more of the following:

- Disturbed Sleep Pattern related to internal sensory alterations (e.g., illness and anxiety)
- Ineffective Coping related to the impending surgery
- Anticipatory Grieving related to the effects of surgery
- Disturbed Body Image related to anticipated changes in the body's appearance or function
- Disabled Family Coping related to temporary family disorganization and role changes
- Powerlessness related to the health care environment, loss of independence, and loss of control of one's body
- Interrupted Family Processes related to situational crisis

CHART 17-5

NIC INTERVENTION ACTIVITIES *for*
The Preoperative Client

Preoperative Coordination: *Facilitating preadmission diagnostic testing and preparation of the surgical client*
- Review planned surgery.
- Obtain client history, as appropriate.
- Complete a physical assessment, as appropriate.
- Describe and explain preadmission treatments and diagnostic tests.
- Interpret diagnostic tests, as appropriate.
- Determine the client's expectations about the surgery.
- Provide time for the client and significant other to ask questions and voice concerns.
- Discuss postoperative discharge plans.
- Determine ability of caretakers.

NIC intervention activities selected from McCloskey, J.C., & Bulechek, G.M. (Eds.). (2000). *Nursing interventions classification (NIC)* (3rd ed.). St. Louis: Mosby.

Planning and Implementation

DEFICIENT KNOWLEDGE

NOC **PLANNING: EXPECTED OUTCOMES.** The preoperative client is expected to verbalize and comply with preoperative procedures and demonstrate techniques to prevent postoperative complications.

INTERVENTIONS. Interventions to increase the client's knowledge level are listed in Chart 17-5. Because the perioperative experience is foreign to many people, the nurse focuses on preoperative education of the client and family members. Preoperative teaching usually begins in the surgeon's office for planned or elective surgery. Pamphlets, written instructions, and videotapes may be given and sent to the client as well. More teaching may occur when the client has preadmission testing. Some facilities conduct preoperative classes for groups of clients or have videos for those who are having the same or similar surgical procedures. A tour of the operating suite and the postanesthesia care unit (PACU) may be included.

Information about informed consent, dietary restrictions, preoperative preparation (bowel and skin preparations), postoperative exercises, and plans for pain management promote clients' participation and help achieve the desired outcome in their health care (see the Evidence-Based Practice for Nursing box on p. 248). A sample preoperative educational checklist is shown in Table 17-5. Because education occurs in a variety of settings, coordination of client teaching efforts is particularly challenging. The nurse who cares for the client immediately before surgery (same-day, ambulatory surgery [outpatient] unit or inpatient hospital unit) assesses the client's and family member's knowledge and provides additional information as needed.

ENSURING INFORMED CONSENT. Surgery of any type involves invasion of the body and requires informed consent from the client or legal guardian (Figure 17-1). Clients deserve, and rightly demand, to be informed and involved in decisions affecting their health care. Consent implies that one has been provided with information necessary to understand the following:

- The nature of and reason for surgery
- All available options and the risks associated with each option

EVIDENCE-BASED PRACTICE FOR NURSING

Teach pain management strategies *before* clients hurt!

Knoerl, D., et al. (1999). Preoperative PCA teaching program to manage post-operative pain. *MEDSURG Nursing, 8*(1), 25-33.

The primary purpose of this prospective experimental nursing study was to determine if preoperative teaching about the correct use of a patient-controlled analgesia (PCA) pump system increased postoperative use of the system and increased clients' pain control. A total of 76 adult surgical clients were enrolled in this study and randomly assigned to an intervention group or a control group. All clients completed a preoperative questionnaire regarding PCAs and pain control strategies. Intervention group clients received an intervention in the form of an 11-minute instructional video and practice using a pump control button. The intervention took place in an ambulatory surgery unit waiting area before preoperative medications or surgical procedures were initiated. Clients in the control group received no structured preoperative information regarding PCA equipment or function. The two groups were homogeneous with regard to age, gender, ethnicity, and the types of surgical procedures.

After surgery, data were collected from both groups using a post-test with the PCA questionnaire and an 11-point scale to measure pain intensity. Pain intensity scores were obtained postoperatively at 4 hours, at 8 hours, and at the end of PCA therapy.

The pretest scores were not different between the two groups. The post-test scores were significantly different between the two groups, with the intervention group showing greater understanding of pain management strategies. However, clients in both groups scored poorly on the test item regarding the use of pain medication before pain becomes severe. The intervention group had lower mean and median pain scores at all points after surgery than did the control group, although the differences did not reach statistical significance.

Critique. The study was well designed and well controlled. The finding that even the clients who received the intervention were unsure about using medication before the pain becomes severe indicates the need for clarifying this issue in the videotape.

Implications for Nursing. Clients may be unfamiliar with the proper use of technical equipment designed to relieve postoperative pain. Timing the teaching about the equipment and providing time to practice using it before the client's focus is interrupted by pain or anesthesia increase the likelihood that the teaching will be effective.

- The risks of the surgical procedure and its potential outcomes
- The risks associated with the administration of anesthesia

Signed permission helps protect the client from any unwanted procedures and protects the physician and the facility from lawsuit claims related to unauthorized surgery or uninformed clients. As a competent adult, it is the client's right to refuse medical treatment for any reason, even when refusal might lead to death. For example, in the case of Jehovah's Witnesses, some clients will not accept blood transfusions because of their deep religious convictions.

The physician is responsible for having the consent form signed before preoperative sedation is given and before surgery is performed. The nurse is not responsible for providing detailed information about the surgical procedure. Rather, the nurse *clarifies* facts that have been presented by the physician and dispels myths that the client or family may have about the perioperative experience. The nurse ensures that the consent form is signed and serves as a witness to the signature, not to

TABLE 17-5 • PREOPERATIVE TEACHING CHECKLIST

Consider the following items when planning individualized preoperative teaching for clients and families:

- Fears and anxieties
- Surgical procedure
- Preoperative routines (e.g., NPO, enemas, blood samples, showering)
- Invasive procedures (e.g., lines, catheters)
- Coughing, turning, deep breathing
- Incentive spirometer
  - How to use
  - How to tell when used correctly
- Lower extremity exercises
- Stockings and pneumatic compression devices
- Early ambulation
- Splinting
- Pain management

NPO, Nothing by mouth.

the fact that the client is informed. The surgeon is contacted and requested to see the client for clarification of information if the nurse believes that the client has not been adequately informed. The nurse documents this action in the chart.

Clients who cannot write may sign with an *X,* which must be witnessed by two persons. In an emergency, telephone or telegram authorization is acceptable and should be followed with written consent as soon as possible. The number of witnesses (usually two) and the type of documentation vary according to the facility's policy. In a life-threatening situation in which every effort has been made to contact the person with medical power of attorney, consent is desired but not essential. In place of written or oral consent, written consultation by at least two physicians who are not associated with the case may be requested by the physician. This formal consultation legally supports the decision for surgery until the appropriate person can sign a consent form. If the client is not capable of giving consent and has no family, the court can appoint a legal guardian to represent the client's best interests.

A blind client is capable of signing his or her own consent form, which usually needs to be witnessed by two persons. Clients who speak a language other than the general language of the agency require a translator and a second witness. Some facilities have consent forms written in more than one language.

Some surgical procedures require a special permit in addition to the standard consent. National and local governing bodies and the individual surgical facility determine which procedures require a separate permit. Intraocular lens implants, sterilization, and experimental procedures are examples of procedures for which the extra form is usually required. Separate consents for anesthesia and the administration of blood products may be required as well.

CLIENT SELF-DETERMINATION ACT. All individuals receiving medical care have the right to have or initiate advance directives, such as living wills and durable power of attorney, as mandated by the Patient Self-Determination Act. Advance directives provide legal instructions to the health care providers about the client's wishes and are to be followed. Surgery does not provide an exception to a client's advance directives or living will.

IMPLEMENTING DIETARY RESTRICTIONS. Regardless of the type of surgery and anesthesia planned, the client is re-

Northwest Hospital Center

The hospital centered around its patients.

REQUEST AND AUTHORIZATION FOR MEDICAL AND/OR SURGICAL TREATMENT, BLOOD PRODUCTS ADMINISTRATION

1. I hereby request and authorize Dr.________________ and/or his/her associates and whomever they may designate as their assistants, to administer such treatment as is necessary and to perform the following operation________________________________ and such additional operations or procedures as are considered necessary on the basis of conditions that may be revealed during the course of said operation or treatment.
2. The reasons why the above named surgery and/or treatment is considered necessary, its advantages, probability of success, possible complications, and risks, as well as possible alternative modes of treatment were explained to me by Dr.________________.
3. I request and authorize the administration of such anesthetics and/or other medications as are necessary.
4. Final disposition of any tissues or parts surgically removed is to be handled in accordance with the customary practices of the hospital.
5. I am aware that the practice of medicine and surgery is not an exact science and I acknowledge that no guarantees have been made to me concerning the results of the operation or procedure.
6. I hereby acknowledge that I have read and fully understand the above request and authorization for medical and/or surgical treatment.
7. I consent to the admittance of permitted observers, the use of closed-circuit television, taking of photographs (including motion pictures), and the preparation of drawings and similar illustrative material, and I also consent to the use of such photographs and other material for scientific purposes, provided my identity is not revealed by the pictures or by the descriptive text accompanying them.
8. I consent to release of my social security number in accordance with the Safe Medical Device Act.

Date ________ Time ________ Signature of Patient or Patient Surrogate ________

Witness ________ Signature of Physician ________

CONSENT TO BLOOD/BLOOD PRODUCTS TRANSFUSION

After discussing the risks, benefits and alternatives to transfusion of blood (donor/autologous) (circle one or both) or blood products with my physician or his designee, I consent to the administration of these products.

Date ________ Time ________ Signature of Patient or Patient Surrogate ________

Witness ________ Signature of Physician ________

703/1019-3-R-8/97 (40-1331)

Figure 17-1 ● A surgical consent form. (Courtesy Northwest Hospital Center, Randallstown, MD.)

TABLE 17-6 • COMPLICATIONS OF COMMON BOWEL PREPARATIONS FOR THE SURGICAL CLIENT

Surgical Site	Preparation	Complications
Stomach, duodenum, and proximal jejunum	Oral laxative (e.g., castor oil preparation or bisacodyl [Dulcolax, Laxit♣]) Clear liquid diet the evening before surgery NPO after midnight	Abdominal cramping Dehydration Electrolyte imbalance Fatigue
Small intestine	Oral laxative (e.g., magnesium citrate) Clear liquid diet the evening before surgery Multiple-position enema the evening before surgery NPO after midnight	Abdominal cramping Dehydration Electrolyte imbalance Fatigue
Large intestine to rectum	Multiple or combination of oral laxatives 12-24 hr before surgery Multiple-position tap water or antibiotic (neomycin) enemas (three times or until the return flow is clear) the evening and morning before surgery Oral antibiotics to sterilize the bowel (e.g., neomycin and erythromycin) 24 hr before surgery Clear liquid diet the day before surgery NPO after midnight	Abdominal cramping Fatigue and weakness Fluid excess or deficit Potassium or sodium deficit Decreased cardiac output from vagal stimulation Irritation of bowel and rectal mucosa from enemas

NPO, Nothing by mouth.

stricted to **nothing by mouth (NPO)** for 6 to 8 hours before surgery. *NPO* means no eating, drinking (including water), or smoking (nicotine stimulates gastric secretions). It is common practice to begin NPO status for all preoperative clients at midnight on the night before surgery. This extra precaution ensures that the stomach contains a limited volume of gastric secretions, which helps decrease the possibility of aspiration. Outpatients and clients who are scheduled for admission to the hospital on the same day that surgery is performed must receive written and oral instructions about remaining NPO after midnight. The nurse emphasizes the importance of compliance; failure to comply can result in cancellation of surgery or an increased risk of intraoperative or postoperative aspiration.

ADMINISTERING REGULARLY SCHEDULED MEDICATIONS. On the day of surgery, the client's usual medication schedule may need to be altered. The nurse consults the medical physician and the anesthesiologist for instructions about administration of medications, such as those taken for diabetes mellitus, cardiac disease, or glaucoma, as well as regularly scheduled anticonvulsants, antihypertensives, anticoagulants, antidepressants, or corticosteroids. The physician may order some medications, including over-the-counter medications, such as aspirin, to be stopped until after surgery. The physician may order other medications to be administered by the intravenous (IV) route to maintain the level of the medication in the blood. Medications for cardiac disease and hypertension are commonly allowed with a sip of water if taken at least 2 hours before surgery. Some antihypertensive or antidepressant medications may be withheld on the day of surgery because of a possible adverse effect on the blood pressure intraoperatively.

The client with diabetes who is taking insulin may be given a reduced dose of intermediate- or long-acting insulin on the basis of the serum glucose level, or he or she may be given regular (fast-acting) insulin subcutaneously in divided doses on the day of surgery. An alternative method of diabetes management is an IV infusion of 5% dextrose in water given with the insulin to prevent hypoglycemia intraoperatively. Because of numerous treatment approaches to diabetes, the nurse clarifies medication and IV orders with the physician. (More information about the client with diabetes is found in Chapter 65.)

GASTROINTESTINAL PREPARATION. Bowel or gastrointestinal (GI) preparation procedures are performed to prevent injury to the colon and to reduce the number of intestinal bacteria. Evacuation of the GI tract is done when a client is having major abdominal, pelvic, perineal, or perianal surgery. The surgeon's preference and the type of surgical procedure determine the type of bowel preparation. Table 17-6 shows typical GI preparation regimens for common surgical procedures and complications of the regimens. An enema ordered to be given until return flow is clear is a physically stressful procedure for anyone, but especially for the older client. Repeated enemas can cause electrolyte imbalance (especially potassium depletion), fluid volume deficit, vagal stimulation, and postural (orthostatic) hypotension. Enemas also cause severe anorectal discomfort in clients with hemorrhoids. To prevent complications, some physicians prescribe potent laxatives (e.g., polyethylene glycol electrolyte solution [GoLYTELY]) instead of enemas, especially for older clients. Bowel preparation procedures can be exhausting, and the nurse takes safety precautions to prevent falls.

SKIN PREPARATION. The skin preparation may be embarrassing or uncomfortable for the client, especially if the surgical site is in a sensitive or generally private body area. The nurse provides a warm, comfortable, and private environment during the procedure.

The skin is the body's first line of defense against infection. A break in this protective mechanism increases the risk of infection, especially for older clients. Preoperative skin preparation is the initial step in the prevention of wound infection. One or two days before the scheduled surgery, the surgeon may require the client to shower using an antiseptic solution such as povidone-iodine (Betadine) or hexachlorophene. The physician may want the client to be especially attentive to cleaning around the proposed surgical site. If the client is hospitalized before surgery, the showering and cleaning is often repeated the night before surgery or in the morning before transfer to the surgical suite. This cleaning reduces contamination of the surgical field, as well as the number of microorganisms on the surgical field. After the final cleaning procedure, especially for an orthopedic surgical procedure, the area may be covered with sterile towels or drapes to prevent contamination.

A controversial step in preoperative skin preparation after the cleaning or showering is the shave. Many health care practitioners believe that the shaving procedure itself is a possible source of contamination of the surgical area and traumatizes the skin around the area where the incision will be made. Those factors believed to predispose the client to wound contamination include bacteria found in hair follicles, disruption of the normal protective mechanisms of the skin, and nicks in the skin (e.g., from shaving). Shaving of hair creates the potential for infection. Clipping of the hair with electrical surgical clippers is becoming increasingly popular to decrease the complications associated with traditional razors. In the United States the Centers for Disease Control and Prevention (CDC) recommend that if shaving is necessary, the hair should be removed using disposable sterile supplies and aseptic principles *immediately* before the start of the surgical procedure. Thus preparations for shaving are performed in the treatment room, the holding area of the operating suite, or the operating room (OR). Figure 17-2 shows areas shaved for various surgical procedures. Shaving of hair, especially from the head or genital area, can be emotionally upsetting to the client, and regrowth of this hair can be uncomfortable.

PREPARING THE CLIENT FOR TUBES, DRAINS, AND INTRAVENOUS ACCESS. The nurse prepares the client for possible insertion of tubes, drains, and IV access devices. Preparation reduces the client's postoperative anxiety and fear, and the family's negative reaction. The nurse is careful not to scare the client while providing information about the purpose of each tube.

TUBES. The client may require an indwelling urinary (Foley) catheter before, during, or after surgery to keep the bladder empty and to enable monitoring of renal function. The client having major abdominal or genitourinary surgery usually has a Foley catheter.

A nasogastric tube may be inserted before emergency surgery or major abdominal surgery for decompressing or emptying the stomach and the upper bowel. More often, however, the tube is inserted after the induction of anesthesia, when insertion is less disturbing to the client and is easier to perform.

DRAINS. Drains are frequently inserted during surgery to promote the evacuation of fluid from the surgical site. Some drains are under the dressing, whereas others are visible and require emptying. Drains come in various shapes and sizes (see Chapter 19). The nurse informs the client that drains are often used routinely and that generally they are not painful but may cause some discomfort. The nurse further discusses the reasons why they should not kink or pull on the drain.

INTRAVENOUS ACCESS. An IV access (line) is placed by the nurse or anesthesia personnel for all clients receiving general anesthesia and most clients receiving other types of anesthesia. An access is needed to administer medication and fluids before, during, and after surgery. Clients who are dehydrated or who are at risk for dehydration, such as older clients, may receive fluids before surgery.

> **CONSIDERATIONS FOR OLDER ADULTS**
> Older clients are more susceptible to dehydration because their fluid reserves are lower than those of young or middle-aged adults. Careful monitoring is required for older clients and for clients with cardiac disease who are receiving IV fluids. (See Chapter 14 for more information on IV therapy.)

The IV access is usually placed in the arm or the posterior aspect of the hand using a large, short catheter (e.g., 18-gauge, 1-inch catheter). This type of catheter provides the least resistance to fluid or blood infusion, especially in an emergency when rapid infusions may be necessary. Depending on the individual client's needs and the facility's policies and practices, the IV access can be placed before surgery when the client is in the hospital room, in the holding or admission area of the surgical suite, or in the OR.

TEACHING ABOUT POSTOPERATIVE PROCEDURES AND EXERCISES. The nurse instructs the client and family members about postoperative exercises and procedures (e.g., checking dressings and obtaining vital signs frequently). Preoperative teaching reduces apprehension and fear, increases cooperation and participation in postoperative care, and decreases the incidence and severity of postoperative complications. When the fear or anxiety level is high, however, the nurse explores the client's attitudes and feelings before discussing procedures (Cipperley, Butcher, & Hayes, 1995). Discussion, demonstration, and return demonstration and practice by the client aid in the ability to perform various breathing (Chart 17-6) and leg (Chart 17-7) exercises during postoperative recovery. The nurse emphasizes the need to begin exercises early in the recovery phase and to continue them, with five to ten repetitions each, every 1 to 2 hours after surgery for at least the first 48 hours. The nurse also explains that the client may need to be awakened for these activities.

BREATHING EXERCISES. In deep, or diaphragmatic, breathing, the diaphragm flattens during inspiration, enlarging the upper abdominal cavity. During expiration the abdominal muscles and diaphragm contract, which completely expands the lungs. After the nurse demonstrates and explains the technique, the client is encouraged to practice the five steps of deep breathing.

For clients with chronic pulmonary disease or limited upper chest expansion, as seen in older clients because of the aging process, expansion breathing exercises are useful. For the client having thoracic surgery, expansion breathing exercises strengthen accessory muscles and should be initiated preoperatively. Expansion breathing may be used postoperatively during chest physiotherapy (percussion, vibration, and postural drainage) to assist with loosening secretions and maintaining an adequate air exchange.

INCENTIVE SPIROMETRY. Incentive spirometry is another way to encourage the client to take deep breaths. Its purpose is to promote complete lung expansion and to prevent respiratory complications. Various types of incentive spirometers are available; some examples are shown in Figure 17-3.

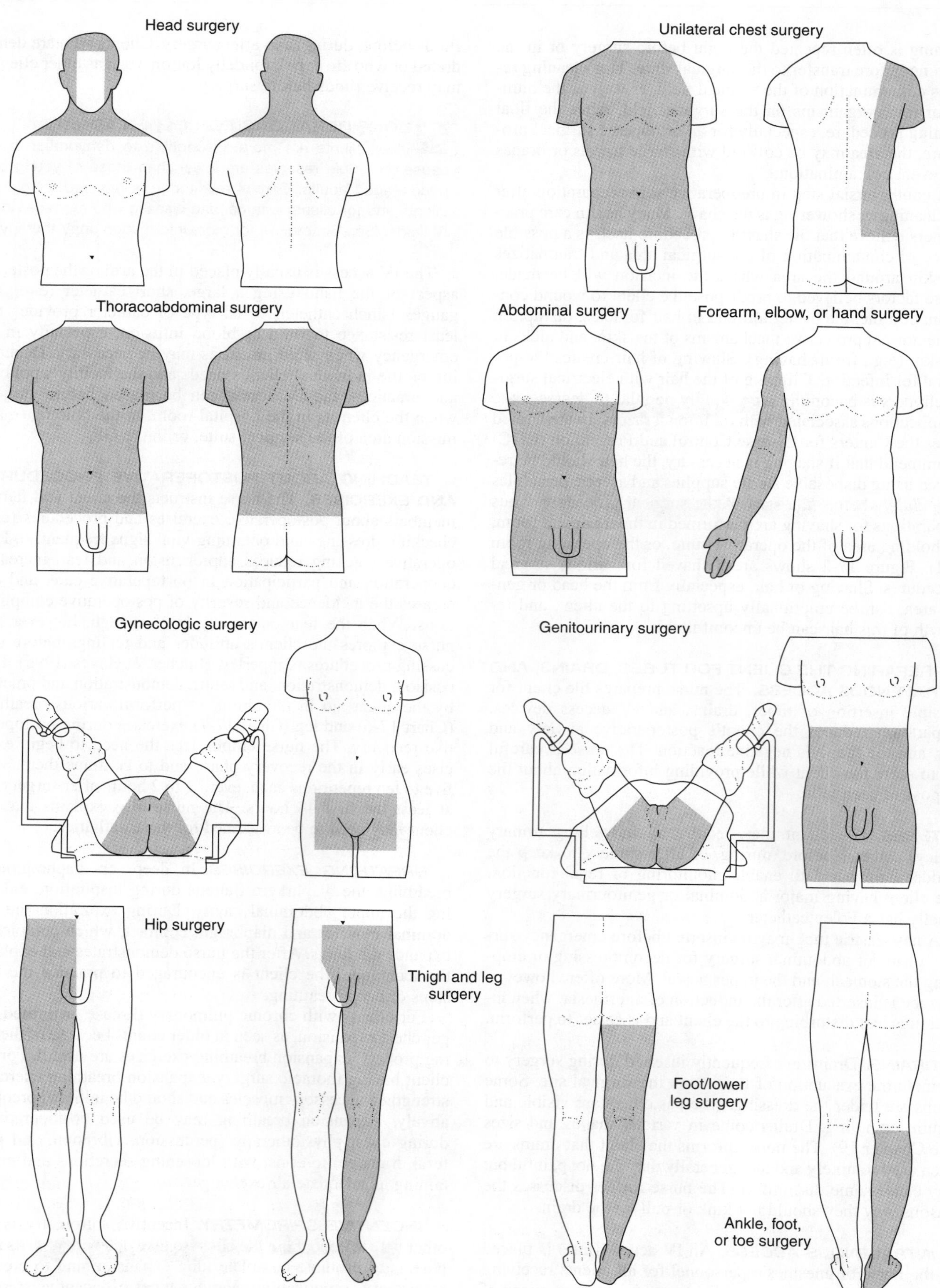

Figure 17-2 ● Skin preparation of common surgical sites. Shaded areas indicate areas of hair removal.

CHART 17-6

CLIENT EDUCATION GUIDE
Perioperative Respiratory Care

Deep (Diaphragmatic) Breathing

1. Sit upright on the edge of the bed or in a chair, being sure that your feet are placed firmly on the floor or a stool. [After surgery, deep breathing is done with the client in Fowler's position or in semi-Fowler's position.]
2. Take a gentle breath through your mouth.
3. Breathe out gently and completely.
4. Then take a deep breath through your nose and mouth, and hold this breath to the count of five.
5. Exhale through your nose and mouth.

Expansion Breathing

1. Find a comfortable upright position, with your knees slightly bent. [Bending the knees decreases tension on the abdominal muscles and decreases respiratory resistance and discomfort.]
2. Place your hands on each side of your lower rib cage, just above your waist.
3. Take a deep breath through your nose, using your shoulder muscles to expand your lower rib cage outward during inhalation.
4. Exhale, concentrating first on moving your chest, then on moving your lower ribs inward, while gently squeezing the rib cage and forcing air out of the base of your lungs.

Splinting of the Surgical Incision

1. Unless coughing is contraindicated, place a pillow, towel, or folded blanket over your surgical incision and hold the item firmly in place.
2. Take three slow, deep breaths to stimulate your cough reflex.
3. Inhale through your nose, then exhale through your mouth.
4. On your third deep breath, cough to clear secretions from your lungs while firmly holding the pillow, towel, or folded blanket against your incision.

With all types, the client must be able to seal his or her lips tightly around the mouthpiece, inhale spontaneously, and hold his or her breath for 3 to 5 seconds to achieve effective lung expansion. Goals (e.g., attaining specific volumes) can be set according to the client's ability and the type of incentive spirometer. Visualization through seeing a light move up a column or a bellows expanding often reinforces and motivates the client to continue performance.

COUGHING AND SPLINTING. Coughing may be performed in conjunction with deep breathing every 1 to 2 hours postoperatively. The purposes of coughing are to promote expectoration of secretions, keep the lungs clear, allow full aeration, and prevent pneumonia and atelectasis. Coughing may be uncomfortable for the client, but when performed correctly, it should not harm the surgical area. Splinting (e.g., holding) the incision area provides support, promotes a feeling of security, and reduces pain during coughing. The proper technique for splinting the incision site and coughing is described in Chart 17-6. A folded bath blanket is helpful to use as a splint.

Some practitioners think that coughing exercises should no longer be encouraged routinely. Their belief is that coughing has the potential to harm the surgical wound and that it would be better to emphasize other, safer measures for pulmonary hygiene, such as deep breathing and incentive spirometer exercises. When routine coughing exercises are contraindicated for a client, such as after a hernia repair, the physician usually writes a "do not cough" order.

LEG PROCEDURES AND EXERCISES. Antiembolism stockings (TED or Jobst stockings), elastic (Ace) wraps, or pneumatic compression devices (e.g., "sequentials" or "boots") may be used perioperatively in combination with leg exercises and early ambulation to promote venous return. Venous stasis can lead to deep vein thrombosis (DVT) or a pulmonary embolus (PE) if the blood clot breaks off and travels to the lungs. Interventions depend on the client's risk factors. Clients at greater risk for DVT:

- Are obese
- Are older than 40 years of age
- Have a concurrent diagnosis of cancer
- Have decreased mobility or immobility
- Have a fracture or leg trauma
- Have a history of DVT, PE, varicose veins, or edema
- Are taking estrogen or oral contraceptives
- Smoke
- Have decreased cardiac output
- Are undergoing pelvic surgery

Antiembolism Stockings and Elastic Wraps. Stockings and elastic wraps provide graduated compression of the lower extremities, starting distally at the foot and ankle. The nurse measures the client's leg length and circumference and orders the appropriate stocking size. Elastic wraps are used when the legs are too large or too small for the stockings. The nurse assists the client in applying the devices and ensures that they are neither too loose (are ineffective) nor too tight (inhibit blood flow). They also need to be worn as ordered to be effective and should be removed one to three times per day for 30 minutes for skin care and inspection.

Pneumatic Compression Devices. Pneumatic compression devices enhance venous blood flow by providing intermittent periods of compression on the lower extremities. The nurse measures the client's legs and orders the appropriate size. The nurse places the boots on the client's legs and sets and checks the prescribed or recommended compression pressures (often 35 to 55 mm Hg). Figure 17-4 shows various types of sequential devices. Antiembolism stockings may be worn in addition to the boots and may alleviate some of the uncomfortable sensations associated with the boots (e.g., itching, sweating, heat).

Leg Exercises. Leg exercises also promote venous return. The nurse teaches the postoperative leg exercises outlined in Chart 17-7 and then encourages the client to practice these exercises preoperatively. The exercises are important, even when the other devices are being used.

EARLY AMBULATION. Mobility soon after surgery (early ambulation) stimulates gastrointestinal motility, enhances lung expansion, mobilizes secretions, promotes venous return, prevents rigidity of joints, and relieves pressure. In general, the nurse instructs the client that he or she should turn at least every 2 hours after surgery while confined to bed. To aid clients, the nurse teaches them how to use the bed siderails safely for turning and how to protect the surgical wound (splinting) when turning. The nurse assures clients that assistance and pain medication will be given as needed to alleviate any anxiety and pain they may have in relation to this activity.

CHART 17-7

CLIENT EDUCATION GUIDE
Postoperative Leg Exercises

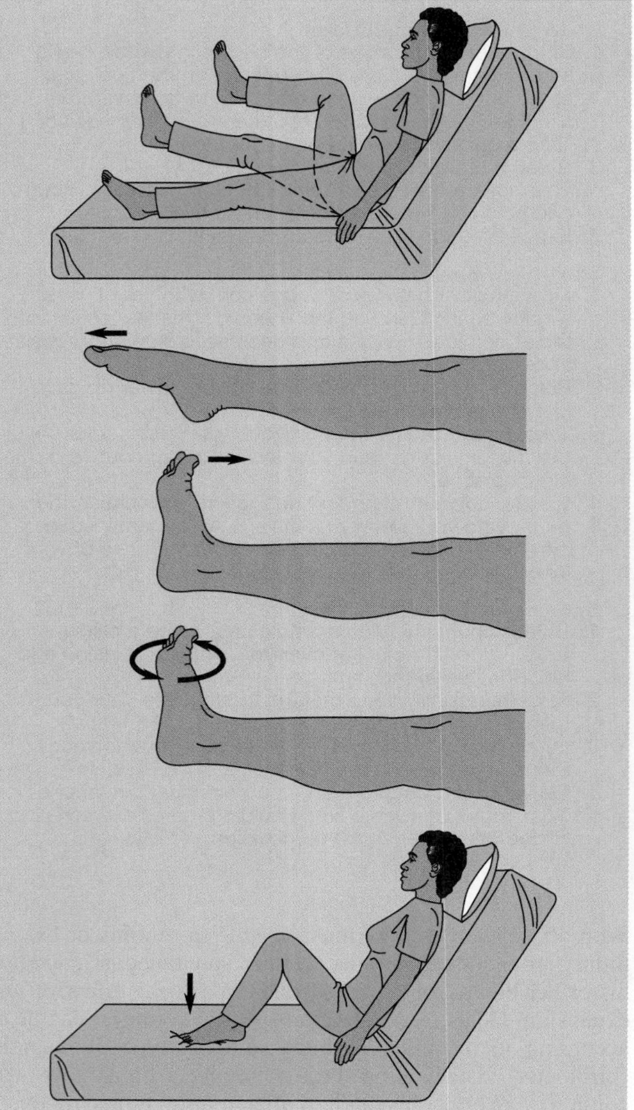

Exercise No. 1

1. Lie in bed with the head of your bed elevated to about 45 degrees. [Using semi-Fowler's position during postoperative leg exercises improves peripheral circulation, prevents thrombus formation, and strengthens muscles.]
2. Beginning with your right leg, bend your knee, raise your foot off the bed, and hold this position for a few seconds.
3. Extend your leg by unbending your knee, and lower the leg to the bed.
4. Repeat this sequence four more times with your right leg, then perform this same exercise five times with your left leg.

Exercise No. 2

1. Beginning with your right leg, point your toes toward the bottom of the bed.
2. With the same leg, point your toes up toward your face.
3. Repeat this exercise several times with your right leg, then perform this same exercise with your left leg.

Exercise No. 3

1. Beginning with your right leg, make circles with your ankles, first to the left, then to the right.
2. Repeat this exercise several times with your right leg, then perform this same exercise with your left leg.

Exercise No. 4

1. Beginning with your right leg, bend your knee and *push* the ball of your foot into the bed or floor until you feel your calf and thigh muscles contracting.
2. Repeat this exercise several times with your right leg, then perform this same exercise with your left leg.

For certain surgical procedures, such as some brain, spinal, and orthopedic procedures, the physician may order turning restrictions. The nurse discusses with the physician other interventions to prevent complications associated with immobility in clients with turning restrictions. The nurse informs the client of anticipated turning restrictions during preoperative teaching.

Many clients are allowed and encouraged to get out of bed the day of or the day after surgery. The nurse assists the client into a chair or with ambulation after the surgery or the next day, depending on the type and time of surgery and the physician's preference. If a client must remain in bed, he or she must turn, deep breathe, and perform leg exercises at least every 2 hours to prevent the complications of postoperative immobility.

RANGE-OF-MOTION EXERCISES. Passive or active range-of-motion (ROM) exercises help prevent joint rigidity and muscle contracture. The client should do these exercises three to five times each, three to four times a day while bedridden. The nurse instructs the client in these procedures and informs the client that he or she will receive assistance as needed postoperatively. (Guidelines for ROM exercises are found in Chapter 19.)

ANXIETY

NOC **PLANNING: EXPECTED OUTCOMES.** The preoperative client is expected to verbalize decreased or manageable preoperative anxiety and demonstrate evidence of relaxation when at rest.

INTERVENTIONS. Preoperative anxiety frequently causes physical symptoms such as restlessness and sleeplessness. The surgical client perceives the perioperative experience

A

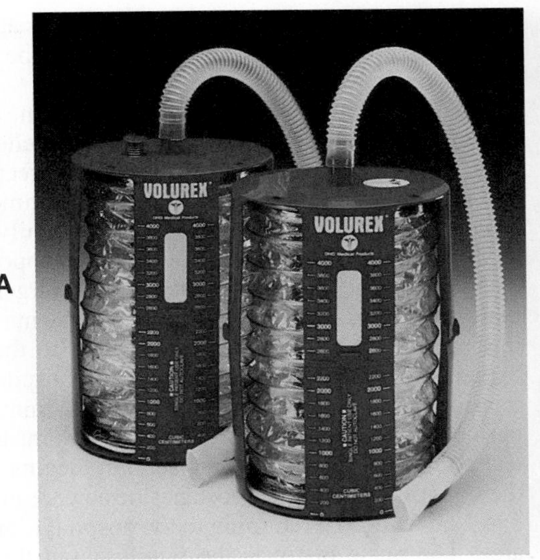

B

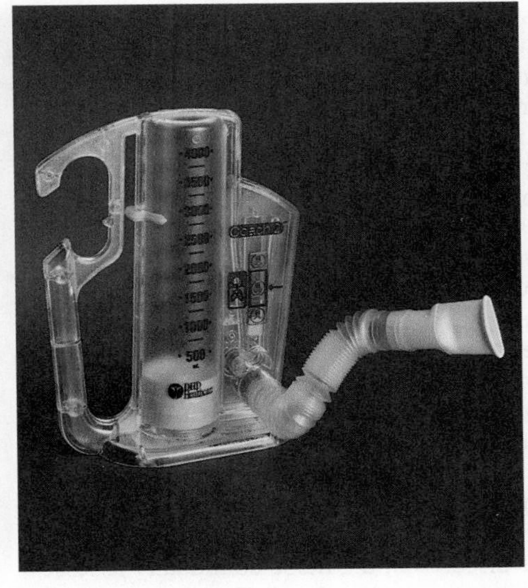

Figure 17-3 ● Examples of volume incentive spirometers for lung expansion. **A,** A volume displacement incentive spirometer. **B,** A volumetric incentive spirometer. (Courtesy DHD Healthcare, Canastota, NY.)

A

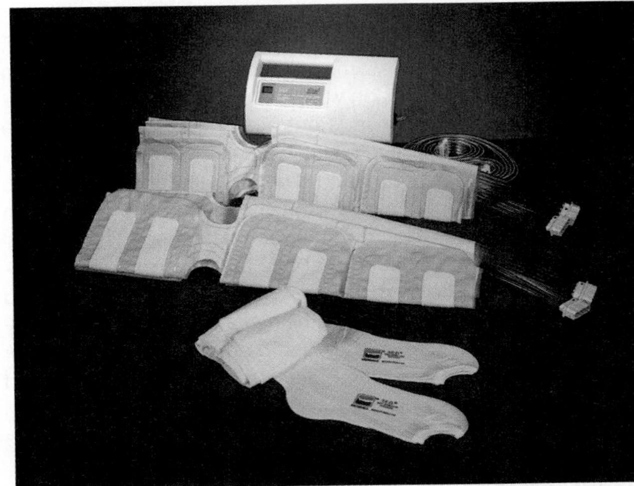

B

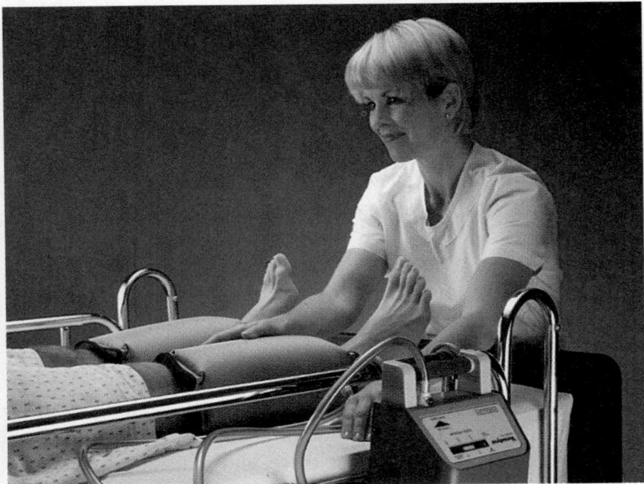

C

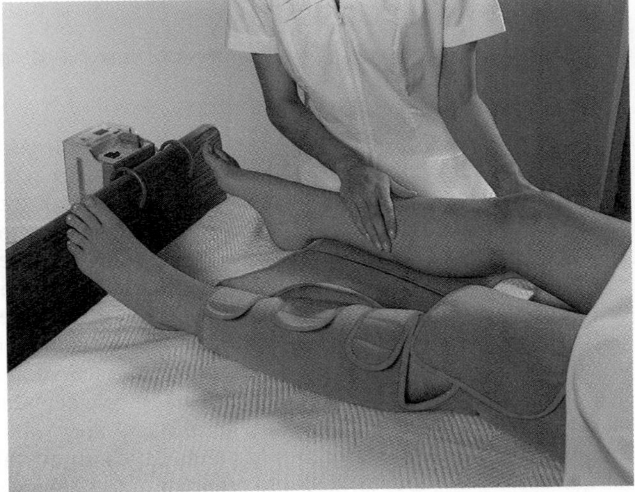

Figure 17-4 ● Examples of external pneumatic compression devices used to promote venous return and prevent deep vein thrombosis (DVT). **A,** Kendall SCD machine, sleeves, and TED stockings. **B,** Venodyne pneumatic compression system. **C,** Flowtron DVT calf garments. (**A** courtesy Kendall Healthcare Company; **B** courtesy Venodyne, Inc.; **C** courtesy Huntleigh Healthcare.)

as a threat to biopsychosocial integrity. The nurse first assesses the client's level of anxiety, as discussed earlier under Psychosocial Assessment, p. 244. Interventions such as teaching and communicating with the client preoperatively, enabling the client to use previously successful coping mechanisms, and administering antianxiety agents help to reduce the anxiety and subsequent complications. The nurse incorporates appropriate and available support systems into the plan of care.

PREOPERATIVE TEACHING. The nurse assesses the client's knowledge about the perioperative experience that he or she has acquired from prior surgical experiences and procedures and from other sources (see earlier discussion under Deficient Knowledge, p. 247). Factual information about the surgery and the perioperative experience is provided to promote the client's understanding. Ample time is allowed for questions. The nurse responds to the questions appropriately and accurately and refers unanswered questions to the proper person. During the discussion, the nurse continually assesses the client's responses and anxiety level. The nurse must be careful not to provide information that might increase anxiety. Clients have ranked psychosocial support as the most important component during preoperative teaching. The informed, educated client is better able to anticipate events and maintain self-control and is thus less anxious.

ENCOURAGING COMMUNICATION. Stating feelings, fears, and concerns is an appropriate way to reduce anxiety. The nurse develops a trusting relationship with the client so that he or she can express feelings freely without fear of ridicule or judgment. The nurse keeps the client informed, clarifies information, answers questions, and allays some apprehensions about the surgery.

PROMOTING REST. The stress and anxiety of impending surgery frequently interfere with the client's ability to sleep and rest the night before surgery. The preoperative experience is physically and emotionally stressful. To assist the client in relaxing, the nurse determines what the client usually does to relax and fall asleep. If permitted and able, the client is encouraged to continue these methods of relaxation. A back rub is a relaxing and therapeutic measure and can be performed by a nurse or family member. The physician may prescribe a sedative or short-acting hypnotic to ensure that the client is well rested for surgery.

USING DISTRACTION. The nurse may plan distraction as an intervention for anxiety. Especially in the 24 hours immediately before surgery, listening to music or audiotapes may decrease anxiety, as may watching television, reading, or visiting with family members.

TEACHING FAMILY AND SIGNIFICANT OTHERS. The nurse assesses the readiness and desire of the family or significant others to take an active part in the client's care. The involved family provides support and helps reduce anxiety. A positive sign of family interest is members' initiation of questions about the perioperative experience. After family readiness is determined, the nurse keeps family members informed and encourages their involvement in all aspects of preoperative education. The nurse emphasizes the important role of the family preoperatively but guides discussions and practice sessions so that family members do not dominate the sessions. Family members can encourage and help the client practice postoperative exercises.

The nurse informs the family of the time for surgery, if known, and of any schedule changes. If the client is an outpatient, he or she and the family need clear directions regarding any specific night-before procedures, what time and where to report, and what to bring with them. The family is encouraged to stay with the client preoperatively for support.

Most families are anxious about the surgery planned for their loved one. To reduce their anxiety, the nurse explains the intraoperative and postoperative routine to them. The nurse explains that after the client leaves the hospital room or admission area, there is usually a 30- to 60-minute preparation period in the operating area (holding room, treatment area, and so on) before the surgery actually begins. After surgery, the client is taken to the postanesthesia care unit (PACU) for 1 to 2 hours before returning to the hospital room or discharge area. The nurse instructs the family about the best place to wait for the client or surgeon according to the facility's policy and the physician's preference. Many hospitals and surgical centers have designated surgical waiting areas so that families can wait in comfortable surroundings and be easily located when the procedure is completed.

CRITICAL THINKING CHALLENGE

The client, a 49-year-old single retired military nurse, has been waiting for 45 minutes to go into surgery for an emergency open reduction with internal fixation of her left ankle. While visiting her friends out of town, she slipped on ice and fractured her ankle in multiple locations. The client is anxious about having surgery and her ability to get back home to her dog as scheduled before her fall. Her constant focus is on who will take care of her dog until she gets there. The medical record review documented that she minimized her preoperative teaching, since "I am a nurse" and appeared disinterested in the coughing and deep breathing exercises. During her preoperative assessment, she almost forgets to tell you about her sensitivity to latex but remembers as she is being measured for antiembolism stockings.

- As the preoperative nurse, how do you decrease this client's anxiety and assess her readiness for surgery?
- What nursing diagnoses should be anticipated in this client's care?

For suggested answer guidelines, go to SIMON http://www.wbsaunders.com/SIMON/Iggy/.

PREOPERATIVE CHART REVIEW

The nurse reviews the client's chart to ensure that all documentation, preoperative procedures, and orders are completed. The nurse checks the surgical informed consent form and, if indicated, any other special consent forms to see that they are signed and dated, and that they contain the witnesses' signatures. The nurse confirms that the scheduled procedure, including the identification of left versus right when necessary, is what is listed on the consent form. Allergies must be noted according to facility policy. Accurate documentation of height and weight is important for proper dosage calculation of the anesthetic agents. The results of all laboratory, radiographic, and diagnostic tests should be on the chart; any abnormal results are documented and reported to the physician and the anesthesiologist or anesthetist. If the client is an autologous blood donor or has had directed blood donations made, those special slips must be included in the chart. The nurse records a current set of vital signs (within 1 to 2 hours of the scheduled surgery time) and documents any significant physical or psychosocial observations. The nurse reports special needs, concerns, and instructions (advance directives) to the surgical team. For example, the nurse advises the surgical team whether the client is a member of Jehovah's Witnesses and does not accept blood products or whether the client is hard of hearing and does not have his or her hearing aid. This information assists the surgical team in providing continuity of care while the client is in the surgical area.

CRITICAL THINKING CHALLENGE

You are about to send the client, described in the earlier Critical Thinking Challenge (p. 256) to the surgical suite.

- How should you communicate this client's allergies?
- What interventions to prevent deep vein thrombosis (DVT) should be used with this client?

For suggested answer guidelines, go to SIMON http://www.wbsaunders.com/SIMON/Iggy/.

PREOPERATIVE CLIENT PREPARATION

Facilities generally require that the client remove most clothing and wear a hospital gown into the operating room (OR). Underwear may be permitted for surgery above the waist; socks may be worn, except for foot or leg surgery. If ordered by the surgeon, antiembolism stockings are applied preoperatively. In some ambulatory settings, such as for cataract surgery, minimal clothes are removed.

Clients are often advised to leave all valuables at home. If the client has valuables, including jewelry, money, and clothes, they are typically given to a family member or locked in a safe place, according to the facility's policy. The nurse tapes in place rings that cannot be removed. All pierced jewelry is removed. Religious emblems may be pinned or fastened securely to the client's gown; in some facilities, paper emblems are available from a religious leader.

The client wears an identification band that clearly gives his or her first and last name and hospital number. An optional bracelet, usually red, identifies any allergies. A bracelet designating that a blood sample for type and crossmatch has been drawn may be worn, depending on the facility's policy.

Dentures, including partial dental plates, are removed and placed in a labeled denture cup. The removal of dentures is a safety measure to prevent aspiration and obstruction of the airway. If a client has any capped teeth, the nurse documents this finding on the preoperative checklist.

All prosthetic devices, such as artificial eyes and limbs, are removed and given to a family member or safely stored, as are contact lenses, wigs, and toupees. The nurse checks for hairpins and clips, which, if not removed, can conduct electrical current used during surgery and cause scalp burns.

Some facilities allow hearing aids in the surgical suite to facilitate communication before and after surgery. If the client is sent to surgery with a hearing aid, the nurse communicates this to the surgical nurse to prevent accidental loss of or damage to the device. Some facilities allow items such as dentures, wigs, and glasses to be worn into the operating suite to prevent embarrassment to the client. These items can then be removed when absolutely necessary.

The removal of fingernail polish or artificial nails is controversial. Polish is flammable, and artificial nails may affect the accuracy of pulse oximetry readings. In some facilities at least one artificial nail must be removed for this reason.

After the client is prepared for surgery and the operating suite is ready to receive him or her, the nurse asks the client to empty his or her bladder to prevent incontinence or overdistention and to provide a starting point for intake and output measurement. An overly full bladder may hinder access to the surgical site. The nurse answers any final questions, offers reassurance as needed, and administers any ordered preoperative medication.

PREOPERATIVE MEDICATIONS

Preoperative medication may be ordered regardless of the type of planned anesthesia. Various preoperative medications reduce anxiety, promote relaxation, reduce pharyngeal secretions, prevent laryngospasm, inhibit gastric secretions, and decrease the amount of anesthetic required for the induction and maintenance of anesthesia. The selection of medication is based on the client's age, physical and psychologic condition, medical history, and height and weight; the medications that the client takes routinely; the results of preoperative tests; and the type and extensiveness of the surgical procedure. If more than one pharmacologic response is required, combination therapy may be ordered. A typical combination consists of a sedative or tranquilizer, an opioid analgesic, and an anticholinergic agent.

The preoperative medication is often ordered when the client is "on call" to the surgical suite. After the nurse positively identifies the client (using the arm band) and makes sure the operative permit is signed, the correct medication is administered. Then the nurse raises the siderails, places the call system within easy reach of the client while reminding him or her not to try to get out of bed, and places the bed in a low position. The nurse tells the client that he or she may become drowsy and have a dry mouth as a result of the medication.

An increasingly common practice is for the premedication to be given *after* the client is transferred to the operating area. This practice permits the surgical team and anesthesia personnel to make more accurate assessments and have last-minute discussions with a client not yet affected by medication. In addition, after the client is in the operating area, medications can be given via the IV route. The oral or intramuscular (IM) route is less desirable because of unpredictable absorption rates.

CLIENT TRANSFER TO THE SURGICAL SUITE

In the immediate preoperative preparation, the nurse reviews and updates the client's chart, reinforces preoperative teaching, ensures that the client is appropriately dressed for surgery, and administers preoperative medication if ordered. The nurse uses a preoperative checklist to assist in a smooth, efficient transfer to the surgical suite (Figure 17-5). The client, along with the signed consent form, the completed preoperative checklist, the chart, and the Addressograph plate, is transported to the surgical suite.

Most clients in the hospital setting are transferred to the surgical suite on a stretcher with the siderails up. In special circumstances (e.g., clients requiring traction, those having

NORTHWEST HOSPITAL CENTER
PRE-OPERATIVE CHECKLIST

Date of Surgery ______ Addressograph Plate

ALLERGIES

CLINICAL DATA:	YES	NO	COMMENTS
Authorization for Surgical Treatment Completed			
Height & Weight Charted			
History and Physical			
Chest X-Ray			
EKG Report			
Urine Report			
Blood Sugar Within Range of (75-250mg%)			
Hematocrit Within Range of (27-55%)			
Potassium Within Range of (3.2-5.5mEq/L)			
Results Out of Range Reported to Dept. of Anesthesia			
Anesthesiologist ______ Time:		By:	

PATIENT PREPARATION:	YES	NO	COMMENTS
Jewelry Removed			
Hair Piece, Wig, Hairpin, Barrettes, Beads, Rubberbands Removed			
Loose Teeth or Caps Noted			
Dentures Removed			
Artificial Eye, Contact Lenses, Glasses Removed			
Any Prosthetic Appliance Removed			
Voided or Catheterized - I&O Sheet on Chart			
Identification Bracelet in Place			
Parenteral Fluids Patent & Infusing at ______ cc/hr			
B/P, T.P.R. Charted			
Premedication Given As Ordered			
Side Rails Up-Pt. Care Data & Care Plan on Chart			
Is Patient on Isolation - If Yes, What Type			

COMMUNICATION ASSESSMENT:	Normal	Abnormal	COMMENTS
Vision			
Hearing			
Mental			
Speech			
Other			

Patient's Preferred Name:

Limb For Burial ☐ Yes ☐ No Funeral Home:

R.N. Completing Checklist

702/1091-3-R-4/95 (40-1471) pl/3133N

Figure 17-5 ● A preoperative checklist. (Courtesy Northwest Hospital Center, Randallstown, MD.)

orthopedic surgery, and those who should be moved as little as possible immediately after surgery) the client is transferred in his or her hospital bed. Other factors that influence the nurse's decision to transfer in a bed are the client's age, size, and physical condition. In ambulatory settings clients either walk or are transferred to the surgical suite on a stretcher or in a wheelchair.

Evaluation: Outcomes

NOC The nurse evaluates the care of the preoperative client on the basis of the identified nursing diagnoses. The expected outcomes include that the client:

- States that he or she understands informed consent as it applies to surgery
- Complies with the nothing-by-mouth (NPO) requirement before surgery
- Verbalizes an understanding of and the reason for a bowel preparation, if applicable
- States the purpose of the skin preparation
- Verbalizes an understanding of how tubes, drains, and IV lines and catheters may be used during and after surgery
- Demonstrates postoperative exercises: turning, deep breathing, splinting, coughing, and performing specific leg exercises
- Demonstrates the use of an incentive spirometer
- States that preoperative anxiety is lessened after preoperative teaching

ONLINE RESOURCES

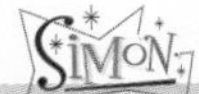

For suggested readings and Internet resources, go to http://www.wbsaunders.com/SIMON/Iggy/.

SELECTED BIBLIOGRAPHY

Asterisk indicates a classic or definitive work on this subject.

American Society of Anesthesiologists Task Force. (1999). Practice guidelines for preoperative fasting and the use of pharmacologic agents to reduce the risk of pulmonary aspiration: application to healthy patients undergoing elective procedures. *Anesthesiology, 90*(3), 896-905.

Association of Perioperative Registered Nurses. (1999a). ANA code for nurses with interpretive statements: Explications for perioperative nursing. In *Standards, recommended practices and guidelines* (pp. 39-56). Denver: Author.

Association of Perioperative Registered Nurses. (1999b). AORN clinical path template. In *Standards, recommended practices and guidelines* (pp. 109-117). Denver: Author.

Baker, B., et al. (1999). Ambulatory surgical clinical pathway. *Journal of PeriAnesthesia Nursing, 14*(1), 2-11.

Cipperley, J.A., Butcher, L.A., & Hayes, J.E. (1995). Research utilization: The development of a preoperative teaching protocol. *MEDSURG Nursing, 4*(3), 199-206.

DeFazio-Quinn, D.M. (1997). Ambulatory surgery. *Nursing Clinics of North America, 32*(2), 375-488.

Dunn, D. (1998). Preoperative assessment criteria and patient teaching for ambulatory surgery patients. *Journal of PeriAnesthesia Nursing, 13*(5), 274-291.

Fogg, D. (1999). Body piercing; perineal preps; insects in the OR; wound classification systems; recommended practices. *AORN Journal, 70*(1), 120, 122-124.

Geuder, D. (1999). Ambulatory surgery. In M.H. Meeker & J.C. Rothrock (Eds.), *Alexander's care of the patient in surgery* (11th ed., pp. 1189-1210). St. Louis: Mosby.

JCAHO's tips on wrong-site surgery risks. (1998). *OR Manager, 14*(12), 12.

Knoerl, D., et al. (1999). Preoperative PCA teaching program to manage postoperative pain. *MEDSURG Nursing, 8*(1), 25-33.

Lancaster, K. (1997). Patient teaching in ambulatory surgery. *Nursing Clinics of North America, 32*(2), 417-427.

Madsen, M., et al. (1999). American Society of Anesthesiologists news release. *Journal of PeriAnesthesia Nursing, 13*(4), 225-228.

McCloskey, J.C, & Bulechek, G.M. (2000). *Nursing interventions classification (NIC)* (3rd ed). St. Louis: Mosby.

Meckes, P.F. (1999). Geriatric surgery. In M.H. Meeker & J.C. Rothrock (Eds.), *Alexander's care of the patient in surgery* (11th ed., pp. 1283-1299). St. Louis: Mosby.

Meeker, M.H., & Rothrock, J.C. (Eds.). (1999). *Alexander's care of the patient in surgery* (11th ed.). St. Louis: Mosby.

Miller, C. (1998). How safe are herbs? *Geriatric Nursing, 19*(3), 163-164.

Murphy, J. (1999). Preoperative consideration with herbal medicines. *AORN Journal, 69*(1), 173-183.

Pagana, K.D, & Pagana, T.J. (1999). *Diagnostic testing and nursing implications: A case study approach* (5th ed.). St. Louis: Mosby.

Poole, E. (1999). Ambulatory surgery: the growth of an industry. *Journal of PeriAnesthesia Nursing, 14*(4), 201-206.

Tappen, R., Muzic, J., & Kennedy, P. (2001). Preoperative assessment and discharge planning for older adults undergoing ambulatory surgery. *AORN Journal, 73*(2), 464-474.

Thornton, L., & Gold, J. (1999). Integrating holism into health care for the new millennium. *Surgical Services Management, 5*(12), 41-44.

Vernon, S., & Pfeifer, G.M. (1997). Are you ready for bloodless surgery? *American Journal of Nursing, 97*(9), 40-47.

Walton, J. (2001). Helping high risk surgical patients beat the odds. *Nursing 2001, 31*(3), 54-59.

Williams, G. (1997). Preoperative assessment and health history interview. *Nursing Clinics of North America, 32*(2), 395-415.

Young, S. (1999). Practicing holism. *Surgical Services Management, 5*(8), 37-41.

CHAPTER 18

Interventions for Intraoperative Clients

REBECCA M. PATTON

Learning Objectives

After studying this chapter, you should be able to:

1. Discuss nursing interventions to reduce client and family anxiety.
2. Describe the roles and responsibilities of various intraoperative personnel.
3. Apply appropriate interventions to ensure the client's safety during an operative procedure.
4. Identify nursing responsibilities for management of clients receiving anesthesia.
5. Recognize the clinical manifestations of malignant hyperthermia.
6. Apply appropriate interventions for the client experiencing malignant hyperthermia.
7. Discuss the potential adverse reactions and complications of specific anesthetic agents.
8. Assess clients for specific problems related to positioning during surgical procedures.

SIMON

Go to http://www.wbsaunders.com/SIMON/Iggy/ for self-assessment questions related to these Learning Objectives.

Safety and advocacy for the client during surgical interventions are the primary concerns of perioperative nurses. Outcomes and numerous hazards can be managed, prevented, reduced, and controlled by deliberate actions and observations. The client entering the perioperative environment is at risk for infection, impaired skin integrity, increased anxiety, altered body temperature, and injury related to positioning and other hazards present. The intraoperative phase begins with unfamiliar experiences involving uncertain or nonguaranteed outcomes. Nursing care during the intraoperative period is critical, because all of the client's physical needs, comfort, safety, dignity, and psychologic status are dependent on the perioperative nurse. Specific procedures and policies may differ among agencies, but similarities are evident and reflect the standards and recommended practices for perioperative nursing, as published by AORN, the Association of periOperative Registered Nurses (formerly the Association of Operating Room Nurses).

OVERVIEW

Members of the Surgical Team

The surgical team consists of the surgeon, one or more surgical assistants, the anesthesiologist and/or nurse anesthetist, and perioperative staff.

Perioperative, or operating room (OR), nurses include the holding area nurse, circulating nurse, scrub nurse, and any specialty nurses. The number of assistants, circulating nurses, and scrub nurses depends on the complexity and projected length of the surgical procedure. For some minor diagnostic or outpatient procedures, only a scrub nurse or a circulating nurse may be required in addition to the surgeon. The more complex procedures may require additional nursing staff to either circulate or scrub.

SURGEON AND SURGICAL ASSISTANT

The **surgeon** is a physician who assumes responsibility for the surgical procedure and any surgical judgments about the client. The **surgical assistant** might be another surgeon (or physician, such as a resident or intern) or a physician's assistant, nurse, or surgical technologist. Under the direction of the surgeon and within the legal scope of practice within each state, the assistant may hold retractors, suction the wound (to allow visualization of the operative site), cut tissue, suture, and dress wounds. Regulating agencies determine who may qualify to be a surgical assistant and delineate the functions of the surgical assistant.

ANESTHESIOLOGIST AND NURSE ANESTHETIST

The **anesthesiologist** is a physician who specializes in the administration of anesthetic agents. A **certified registered nurse anesthetist (CRNA)** is a specially trained registered nurse with additional credentials who administers anesthetic agents under the supervision of an anesthesiologist, surgeon, dentist, or podiatrist. The anesthesiologist or CRNA administers anesthetic drugs to induce and maintain anesthesia and administers other medications as indicated to support the client's physical status during surgery.

The anesthesiologist or nurse anesthetist usually monitors the client intraoperatively by measuring, assessing, and monitoring the following:

- The level of anesthesia (i.e., by using a peripheral nerve stimulator or bispectral analysis)
- Cardiopulmonary function (using electrocardiographic [ECG] monitoring, pulse oximetry, end-tidal carbon dioxide monitoring, arterial blood gases, and hemodynamic monitoring via arterial lines and/or pulmonary artery catheters)
- Vital signs
- Intake and output

Depending on the client's needs, anesthesia personnel administer intravenous (IV) fluids, including blood and blood components, to maintain physiologic homeostasis.

PERIOPERATIVE STAFF

Perioperative, or OR, staff assume several roles within the operating suite, depending on their education, experience, skill, and job responsibilities.

HOLDING AREA NURSE. Some operating suites feature a presurgical holding area next to the main ORs. The client waits in this area until the OR is ready. The holding room nurse manages the client's care while he or she is in this area. This nurse greets the client on arrival, reviews the medical record and preoperative checklist, and ensures that the operative consent forms are signed. The nurse assesses the client's physical and emotional status, gives emotional support, answers questions, and provides additional education as needed. The nurse initiates documentation on a perioperative nursing record (Figure 18-1).

The holding area can be very busy, with many staff members performing a number of preoperative procedures (e.g., establishing IV lines or inserting epidural catheters). The holding area nurse maintains an atmosphere conducive to the client's overall well-being and intervenes on his or her behalf to maintain comfort, privacy, and confidentiality. Depending on the facility's policy, family members may be invited to wait with the client.

CIRCULATING NURSE. The **circulating nurse,** or **circulator** (who should be a registered nurse), coordinates, oversees, and participates in the client's nursing care while he or she is in the OR. The circulating nurse's actions are vital to the smooth flow of events before, during, and after the operation. This nurse is responsible for the activities within that particular OR. The circulator sets up the OR and ensures that necessary supplies, including blood products, are available as needed. All anticipated equipment is gathered and inspected by the circulator to make certain that all equipment is safe and functional before the surgery. Depending on the procedure and position required, the circulator makes up the operating bed (formerly called the OR table) with gel pads (to prevent pressure sores) and heating pads (to prevent hypothermia) under the sheets as indicated.

If there is no holding room nurse, the circulator assumes the responsibilities of that nursing role as well. Even when there is a holding room nurse, the circulator also greets the client and reviews findings with the holding area nurse, because the circulator is responsible for continuity of care.

Once the client is ready to move into the OR, the circulating nurse assists the OR team in the transfer to the operating bed. The nurse then positions the client, protecting bony prominences with extra padding as indicated while providing comfort and reassurance. While comforting and observing the client, the circulating nurse also assists the anesthesiologist or CRNA with the induction of anesthesia. The circulator then may "prep" (scrub) the surgical site before the client is draped with sterile drapes.

Throughout the surgery, the circulating nurse:

- Monitors traffic in the room
- Assesses the amount of urine and blood loss
- Reports findings to the surgeon and anesthesia personnel
- Ensures that the surgical team maintains sterile technique and a sterile field
- Anticipates the client's and surgical team's needs, providing supplies and equipment as needed
- Communicates information regarding the client's status with family members during long and unique procedures
- Documents care, events, interventions, and findings

Depending on facility policy, the circulating nurse may obtain and record medications, blood, and blood components. (This may be partially a function of anesthesia personnel.)

Before the surgical procedure is over, the circulating nurse completes documentation (Figure 18-2; see also Figure 18-1). The nurse notes drains or catheters in place, the length of the surgery, and a count of all sponges, "sharps" (needles, blades), and instruments. The nurse notifies the postanesthesia care unit (PACU) of the client's estimated time of arrival and any special needs.

SCRUB NURSE AND SURGICAL TECHNOLOGIST. The **scrub nurse** and/or the surgical technologist sets up the sterile field (Figure 18-3), assists with draping the client, and hands sterile supplies, sterile equipment, and instruments to the surgeon and the assistant. Knowledge of anatomy and physiology, as well as familiarity with the surgical procedure, allows the scrub nurse to anticipate the progression of the procedure and determine which instruments and types of sutures the surgeon will need. The nurse's ability to anticipate these needs reduces the duration of anesthesia for the client. Furthermore, the surgeon's anxiety and tension can be minimized with a scrub nurse who is familiar with the procedure and demonstrates the ability to anticipate and respond accordingly. Throughout the surgical procedure, the scrub nurse (with the circulating nurse) maintains an accurate account of the sponges, sharps, instruments, and amounts of irrigation fluid and medication used.

A specially trained person who is not a nurse may perform the scrub role. Such people are called **operating room technicians (ORTs)** or **surgical technologists.** Increasingly, certified surgical technologists (CSTs) are used in the perioperative environment.

SPECIALTY NURSE. The **specialty coordinator nurse** is educated in a particular type of surgery (e.g., orthopedic, cardiac, ophthalmologic) and is responsible for intraoperative nursing care specific to clients needing that type of surgery. The specialty coordinator nurse serves a critical role by assessing, maintaining, and recommending equipment, instruments, and supplies used in that specialty. They also typically are responsible for orienting and evaluating staff members to

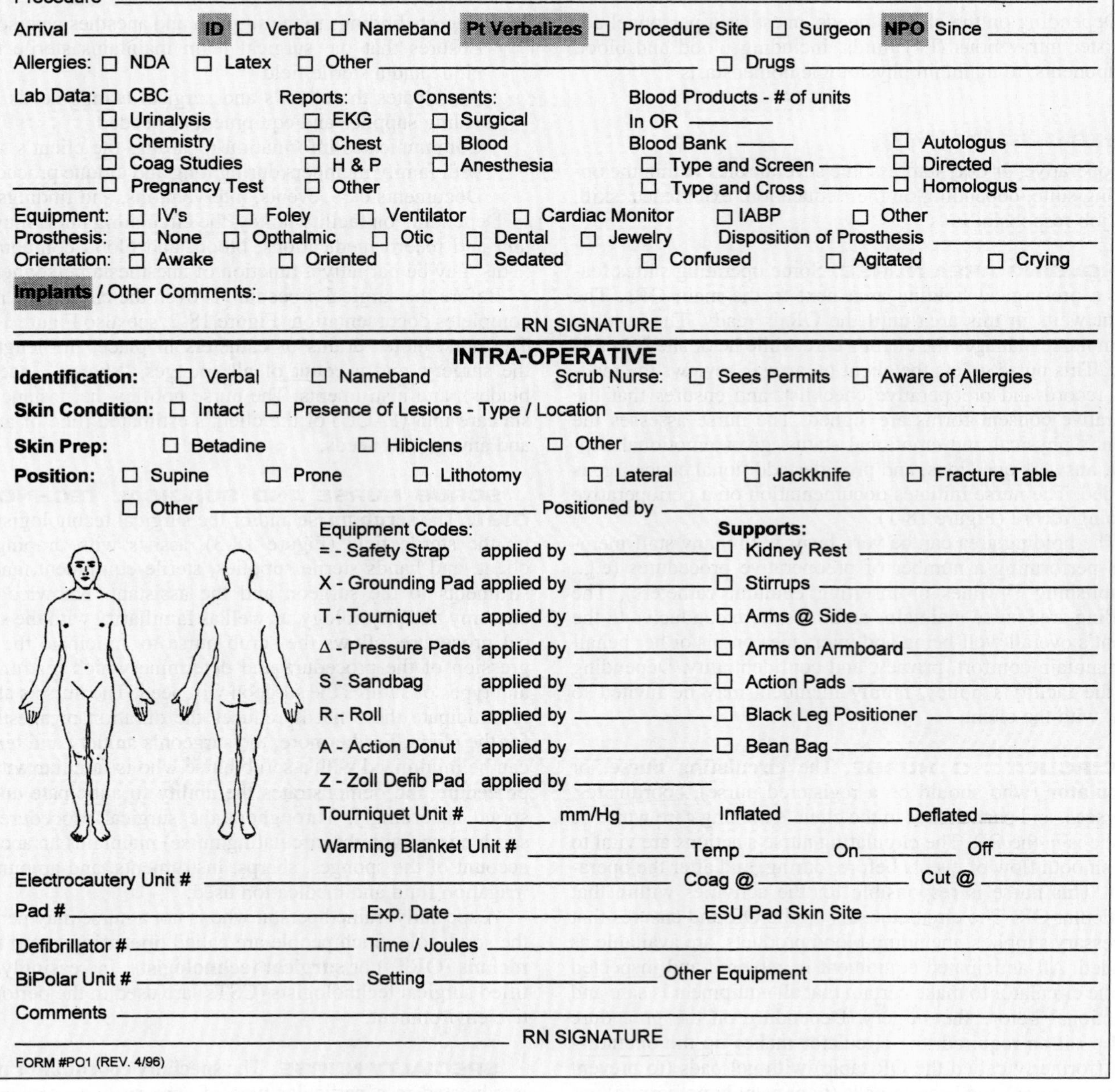

Our Lady of Lourdes Medical Center
1600 Haddon Avenue Camden, N.J. 08103

PRE-OPERATIVE RECORD

PRE-OPERATIVE

Patient Name ______ Surgeon ______ Date ______

Procedure ______

Arrival ______ ID ☐ Verbal ☐ Nameband Pt Verbalizes ☐ Procedure Site ☐ Surgeon NPO Since ______

Allergies: ☐ NDA ☐ Latex ☐ Other ______ ☐ Drugs ______

Lab Data: ☐ CBC ☐ Urinalysis ☐ Chemistry ☐ Coag Studies ☐ Pregnancy Test

Reports: ☐ EKG ☐ Chest ☐ H & P ☐ Other

Consents: ☐ Surgical ☐ Blood ☐ Anesthesia

Blood Products - # of units: In OR ______ Blood Bank ______ ☐ Type and Screen ______ ☐ Type and Cross ______ ☐ Autologus ______ ☐ Directed ______ ☐ Homologus ______

Equipment: ☐ IV's ☐ Foley ☐ Ventilator ☐ Cardiac Monitor ☐ IABP ☐ Other

Prosthesis: ☐ None ☐ Opthalmic ☐ Otic ☐ Dental ☐ Jewelry Disposition of Prosthesis ______

Orientation: ☐ Awake ☐ Oriented ☐ Sedated ☐ Confused ☐ Agitated ☐ Crying

Implants / Other Comments: ______

______ RN SIGNATURE ______

INTRA-OPERATIVE

Identification: ☐ Verbal ☐ Nameband Scrub Nurse: ☐ Sees Permits ☐ Aware of Allergies

Skin Condition: ☐ Intact ☐ Presence of Lesions - Type / Location ______

Skin Prep: ☐ Betadine ☐ Hibiclens ☐ Other ______

Position: ☐ Supine ☐ Prone ☐ Lithotomy ☐ Lateral ☐ Jackknife ☐ Fracture Table

☐ Other ______ Positioned by ______

Equipment Codes:
= - Safety Strap applied by ______
X - Grounding Pad applied by ______
T Tourniquet applied by ______
Δ Pressure Pads applied by ______
S - Sandbag applied by ______
R - Roll applied by ______
A - Action Donut applied by ______
Z - Zoll Defib Pad applied by ______

Supports:
☐ Kidney Rest ______
☐ Stirrups ______
☐ Arms @ Side ______
☐ Arms on Armboard ______
☐ Action Pads ______
☐ Black Leg Positioner ______
☐ Bean Bag ______

Tourniquet Unit # ______ mm/Hg ______ Inflated ______ Deflated ______

Warming Blanket Unit # ______ Temp ______ On ______ Off ______

Electrocautery Unit # ______ Coag @ ______ Cut @ ______

Pad # ______ Exp. Date ______ ESU Pad Skin Site ______

Defibrillator # ______ Time / Joules ______

BiPolar Unit # ______ Setting ______ Other Equipment ______

Comments ______

______ RN SIGNATURE ______

FORM #PO1 (REV. 4/96)

Figure 18-1 ● A perioperative nursing record with areas for charting preoperatively on the client's arrival in the operating suite and on initial preparation intraoperatively. (Courtesy Our Lady of Lourdes Medical Center, Camden, NJ.)

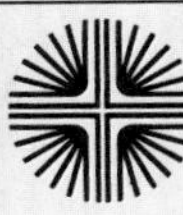

Our Lady of Lourdes Medical Center
1600 Haddon Avenue Camden, N.J. 08103

INTRA-OPERATIVE RECORD

Patient Name ______ Date ______ Suite ______

☐ Scheduled ☐ Emergency ☐ Add On In Room ______ Began ______ End ______ Out ______

Surgeon ______ Assistant ______

Anesthesia ______ Perfusion/Other ______

Type of Anesthesia: ☐ General ☐ Spinal ☐ Epidural ☐ Regional Block ☐ Local ASB ☐ Local

Scrub ______ Circulator ______

Relief ______ Relief ______

Preoperative Diagnosis ______

Postoperative Diagnosis ______

Procedure ______

Clamp/Bypass on ______ off ______ EBL ______

Specimens: Cultures ☐ **Aerobic** ☐ **Anaerobic**

Implant Log# ______

Irrigation: ______

Wound Classification:

Pre-Op I II III IV

Post-Op I II III IV

ASA Classification I II III IV

Medication Dispensed to OR Table (Include time, drug, amt used, site/route should be prepared by and given by)

Counts: ☐ Correct ______ ☐ Incorrect ______ Comments: ______

Intra-operative X-ray ☐ Yes ☐ No Type ______

Drains / Packing: ☐ None ☐ Foley Inserted by ______ ☐ Immediate urine output

☐ Jackson Pratt / Davol ______ ☐ Hemovac ______ ☐ Penrose ______ ☐ Packing Other

☐ Chest Tubes # and size ______ ☐ Pleuravac ☐ Auto transfusion pleuravac

Post Op Skin Condition: ______

ESU Pad Skin Site ______ Dressing Site ______

Receiving Unit ☐ PACU ☐ CVU ☐ ICU / CCU ☐ SDS ☐ Nursing Unit ______ Report given to ______

RN Signature ______ Surgeon Signature ______

FORM #PO2 (REV. 7/96) White - Original Copy Yellow - O.R. Copy Pink - Surgeon Copy Goldenrod - Pharmacy Copy

Figure 18-2 ● An interdisciplinary intraoperative record. Names of all personnel involved are listed, and both the circulating nurse's and surgeon's signatures are required for completion. (Courtesy Our Lady of Lourdes Medical Center, Camden, NJ.)

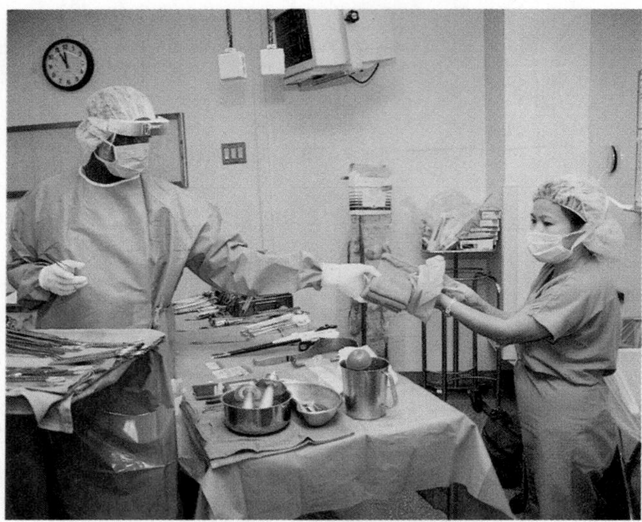

Figure 18-3 ● Setting up the sterile table.

this service. During surgery the specialty nurse may function as the scrub or circulating nurse.

If the facility has laser technology, nurses specially trained in the use, care, and maintenance of the laser should be on hand. Such a nurse may be called a laser specialty nurse or a laser nurse coordinator. **Laser** is an acronym for *l*ight *a*mplification by the *s*timulated *e*mission of *r*adiation. A laser emits a high-powered beam of light that cuts tissue cleaner than do scalpel blades. This process produces intense heat for rapid coagulation of blood vessels or tissue and can turn tissue (such as a tumor) into vapor. It is essential for all personnel to observe safety measures (e.g., eye shields, door signs) during laser procedures. Improper laser use and inadequate safety measures increase the risk for injury to both the client and staff.

Preparation of the Surgical Suite and Team Safety

During the intraoperative phase, when the client is unable to protect himself or herself, all members of the surgical team must provide protection. The operating room (OR) layout is designed to prevent infection by limiting the source of contaminants by air exchanges in the room and limiting the traffic and extraneous activities in the OR. Safety straps are used for the client, and the operating bed is locked in place. Heating pads are used to prevent hypothermia, and interventions are instituted to prevent skin breakdown.

The nurse ensures electrical safety through proper placement of grounding pads and use of electrical equipment that meets safety standards. All equipment that might be used during surgery must be functional and in proper working condition, checked per safety procedure of that facility, and appropriately cleaned and, when required, sterilized so that it can be used as a part of the procedure. The scrub and circulating nurses together ensure a correct count of surgical instruments, sharps, and sponges immediately before the beginning of the procedure, during the procedure, and immediately after the close of the surgical incision.

Fire prevention is of utmost concern to OR personnel, as is prevention of complications associated with the use of hazardous and potentially toxic substances. A cool room temperature (between 68° and 73° F [20° to 30° C]), with a low relative humidity of 30% to 60% is optimal, and staff and clients must be protected against thermal or chemical burns caused by fire or spills. The nurse is aware of appropriate emergency measures to take in the event of a fire or spill.

LAYOUT

The surgical suite should be located out of the mainstream of the hospital or facility and adjacent to the postanesthesia care unit (PACU) and support services (e.g., blood bank, pathology and laboratory departments). Traffic flow should be patterned to ensure minimal contamination from outside the suite. Within the suite, clean and contaminated areas must be separate. According to AORN, the Association of periOperative Registered Nurses, designation of the surgical area into three zones as unrestricted, semirestricted, and restricted facilitates appropriate movement of clients and personnel.

The size of a surgical suite depends on the size and surgical capabilities of the facility. The average suite contains staff changing rooms (staff locker rooms) and staff lounges, an admission or preoperative holding area, a scrub area for staff, a number of ORs, designated cabinets for sterile supplies, separate utility rooms for clean and soiled equipment, and a clean linen room.

Figure 18-4 shows a typical OR. The exact number of tables and specialized equipment used in the room is based on the needs of each client. A reliable communication system links the OR and the main desk of the surgical unit or suite to ensure safe client care. The system should include an intercom and the capability to differentiate between routine and emergency calls.

HEALTH AND HYGIENE OF THE SURGICAL TEAM

People are a major source of bacteria in the surgical setting. Everyone has a large number of potentially pathogenic bacteria on the skin and hair and in the respiratory tract. Because these pathogens can be transmitted to the client, special health standards and dress are required. Every surgical environment has written policies and procedures regarding personnel and acceptable attire. Health standards require that all members of the surgical team and other support personnel in the surgical suite be free from communicable diseases. Anyone who has an open wound, cold, or other infection should not participate in surgery.

Good personal hygiene aids in the prevention and control of infection, as does frequent and appropriate handwashing. Shedding of microorganisms and skin debris is greatest immediately after showering, so surgical staff should bathe a few hours before changing into OR attire. Jewelry, which can carry multiple microorganisms, should be minimal. In preparing for surgery, all personnel must wash their hands between procedures and more frequently when indicated. Microbial specimens from the hands of surgical personnel may be obtained for culture periodically to maintain an awareness of the potential for **nosocomial** (hospital-acquired) infections and to identify the source of pathogenic invasion. Further interventions or cultures are necessary if quality reports (e.g., through the facility's quality improvement program or quality reviews) indicate

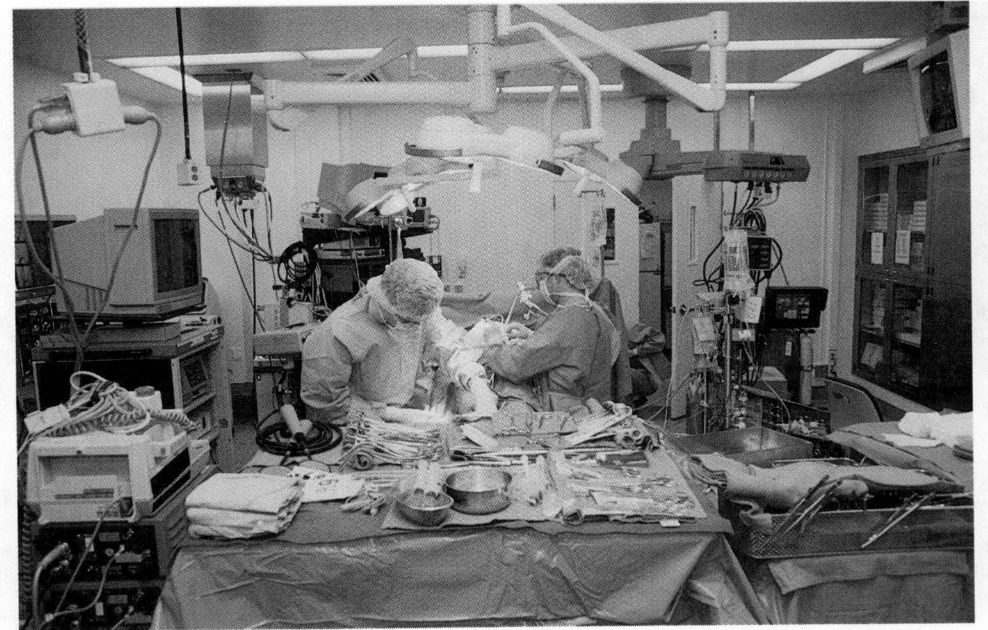

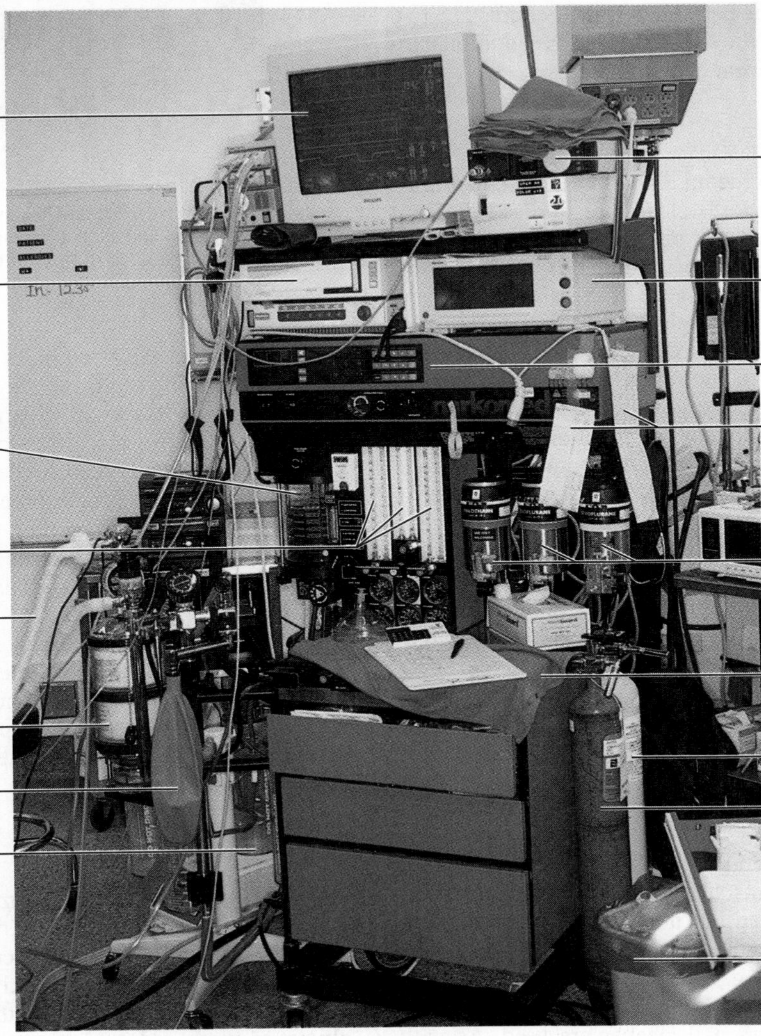

B

Monitor screen displaying client's heart rate and rhythm, blood pressure, and other hemodynamic parameters

Printer to accompany the monitor

Ventilator bellows

Nitrous oxide, air, and oxygen flow meters

Anesthesia circuit

Carbon dioxide absorber

Anesthesia breathing bag

Suction canister

Pulse oximeter

Blood pressure monitor

Ventilator

Laboratory results

Vaporizers

Airway equipment (under sterile towel)

Extra supply of air (yellow) and oxygen (green)

Hazardous waste ("red bag" trash)

Figure 18-4 ● **A,** A typical operating room. **B,** A typical anesthesia station with an anesthesia machine.

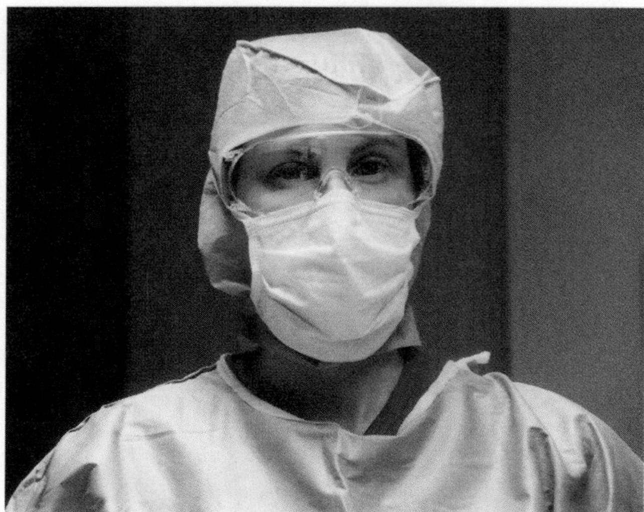

Figure 18-5 ● An example of a hood-type hair covering that adequately covers facial and scalp hair.

a problem. The average time between routine cultures is 3 to 6 months. Surgical attire and the surgical scrub are additional interventions that help to prevent contaminations.

SURGICAL ATTIRE

All members of the surgical team and all OR personnel must wear scrub attire. Scrub attire is clean, not sterile. It is worn to decrease contamination from microorganisms. The basic attire of personnel entering the operating *suite* consists of a shirt and pants, a cap or hood (Figure 18-5), and shoe coverings. Staff change into clean surgical attire in the operating suite locker rooms, not at home. All members of the surgical team must cover their hair, including facial hair when present.

In addition to basic attire, everyone must wear appropriate protective body attire depending on the situation. This includes a mask, eyewear, gloves, gown, and shoe covers. Everyone who enters an OR where a sterile field is present must wear a mask. Members of the surgical team who are scrubbed to be at the bedside of the client during the surgical procedure must also be in a sterile fluid-resistant gown, with sterile gloves and eye protectors (Figure 18-6). Members of the surgical team in the OR who are *not* scrubbed (e.g., anesthesiologist and circulating nurse) usually wear cover scrub jackets to prevent shedding of organisms from bare arms and eyewear, as warranted.

SURGICAL SCRUB

The surgeon, all assistants, and the scrub nurse perform a surgical scrub after putting on a mask and before putting on the sterile gown and gloves (Figure 18-7). The scrub does not make the hands and forearms sterile; however, when it is effectively carried out, it reduces the number of microorganisms from the hands, arms, and nails. Rings, watches, and bracelets are removed before scrubbing.

A disposable scrub brush or sponge, impregnated with an antimicrobial solution, and a nail cleaner are used. As with handwashing, the effectiveness of the scrub depends on the application of friction from the fingertips to the elbow. The surgical scrub usually continues for 3 to 5 minutes, followed by a rinse. During the rinse, surgical personnel position their hands and arms in such a way that water runs off, rather than up or down, their arms. After scrubbing, personnel enter the OR with their hands held higher than the elbows and thoroughly dry their hands and forearms with a sterile towel. The scrubbed staff member is then assisted into a sterile gown **("gowning")** and puts on sterile gloves **("gloving").**

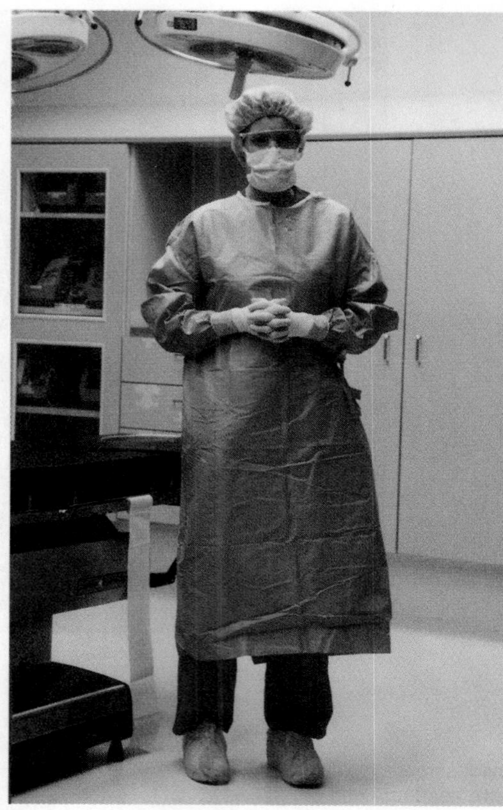

Figure 18-6 ● Typical attire for all scrubbed personnel. Note complete hair covering, eye shields, mask, sterile gloves over the sleeves of the sterile gown, and shoe coverings. Note that when not in use, the hands are typically folded in front of the body, never below the waist.

Gowns, gloves, and materials used at the operative field must be sterile and are changed between surgical procedures and as they become contaminated. The areas of the surgical gown considered sterile are the front of the gown from 2 inches below the neck to the waist area, and the elbow to the wrist area. Only when they are properly scrubbed and attired should members of the surgical team handle sterile drapes and other equipment.

Anesthesia

The word *anesthesia* comes from the Greek word *anesthesis,* meaning "negative sensation." Administration of anesthesia is an exact and sophisticated science. It requires the skill of a licensed anesthesiologist, a certified registered nurse anesthetist (CRNA) working under the direction of an anesthesiologist or another physician, or an anesthesiologist's assistant (AA)—which is similar to a physician's assistant—working under the direction of an anesthesiologist.

A

B

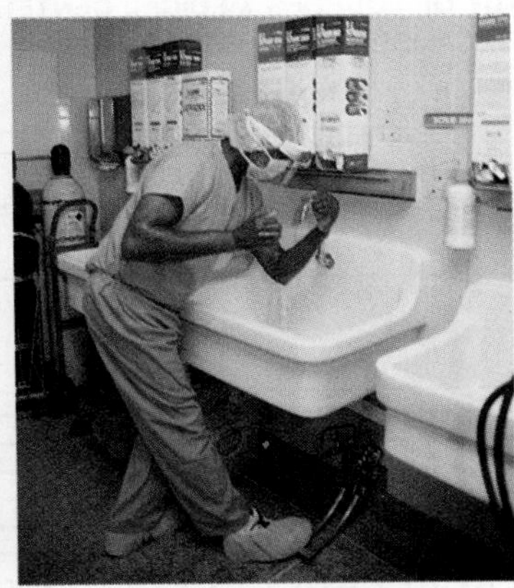

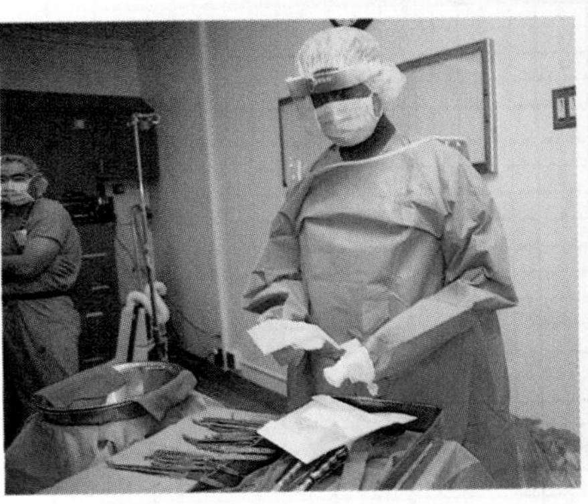

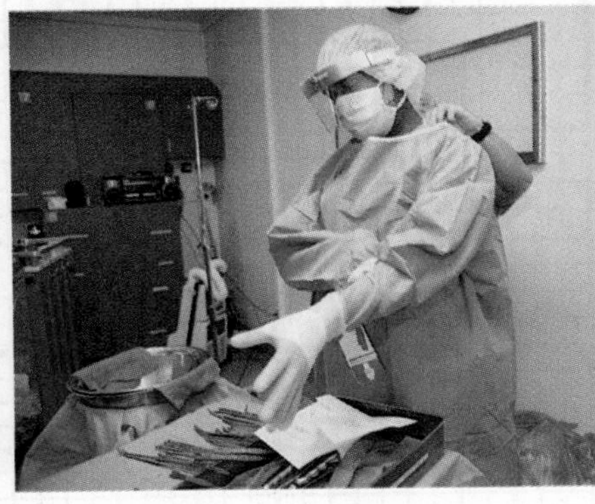

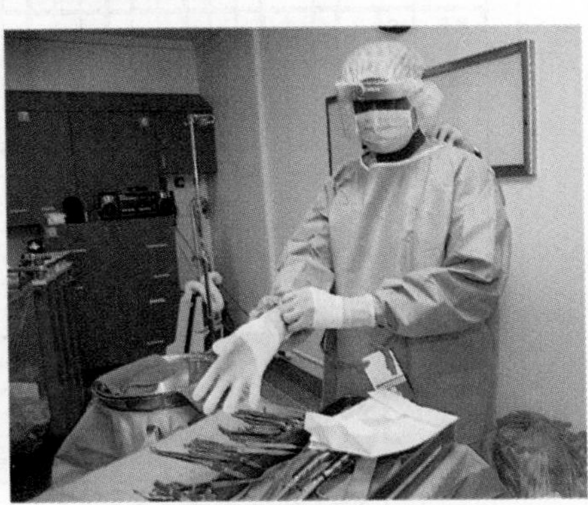

C D E

Figure 18-7 ● The scrubbing, gowning, and gloving process. **A,** The surgical scrub. **B,** Rinsing. Note the water falling off the hands and arms. Also note the foot-operated handle that controls the water flow. (After scrubbing and rinsing, the scrub nurse dries his hands and arms with a sterile towel inside the operating room and then is assisted into a sterile gown.) **C,** The scrub nurse prepares sterile gloves. Note that the scrub nurse's hands are *inside* the sleeves of the gown and that he is touching the sterile gloves only with the sterile sleeves. **D,** The scrub nurse puts on his first sterile glove while the sterile gown is being tied in the back. Note again that his hand never emerges from under the sterile sleeve. **E,** The scrub nurse puts on his second sterile glove.

Anesthesia is an artificially induced state of partial or total loss of sensation, occurring with or without loss of consciousness. The purpose of anesthesia is to block the transmission of nerve impulses, suppress reflexes, promote muscle relaxation, and in some cases, achieve a controlled level of unconsciousness. Anesthesia providers use a separate anesthesia record for documentation (Figure 18-8).

Usually the anesthesia provider determines the choice of anesthesia after consultation with the client and surgeon, and after consideration of specific client-related factors. The nurse or client or both communicate the preference and fears related to a particular type of anesthesia to the anesthesia provider. Specific problems noted in the client's history or preoperative physical examination are major factors in the selection and dosage of anesthesia. Selection is also influenced by the following:

- Type and duration of the procedure
- Area of the body being operated on
- Whether the procedure is an emergency
- Options for management of postoperative pain
- How long it has been since the client ate, had any liquids, or any medications
- Client position needed for the surgical procedure

The administration of anesthesia begins with the selection and administration of preoperative medication, if any (see Chapter 17). The nurse must know the pharmacologic characteristics of commonly used agents and their effects during and after surgery. Anesthesia produces multiple systemic effects, which can affect the client's care and can compound other coexisting problems. For example, most anesthetics are metabolized by the liver and excreted by the kidneys. Liver or kidney impairment can increase anesthetic effects and the risk for toxicity. In addition, drug interactions may occur between the anesthetic agents and other medications the client has been receiving.

The state of anesthesia may be produced in a number of ways (Table 18-1):

- General or balanced anesthesia
- Local or regional anesthesia
- Hypnosis or hypnoanesthesia
- Cryothermia
- Acupuncture

Hypnosis or **hypnoanesthesia** (which induces a passive, trancelike state), **cryothermia** (use of cold [e.g., ice] to lower the surface temperature of the surgical site), and

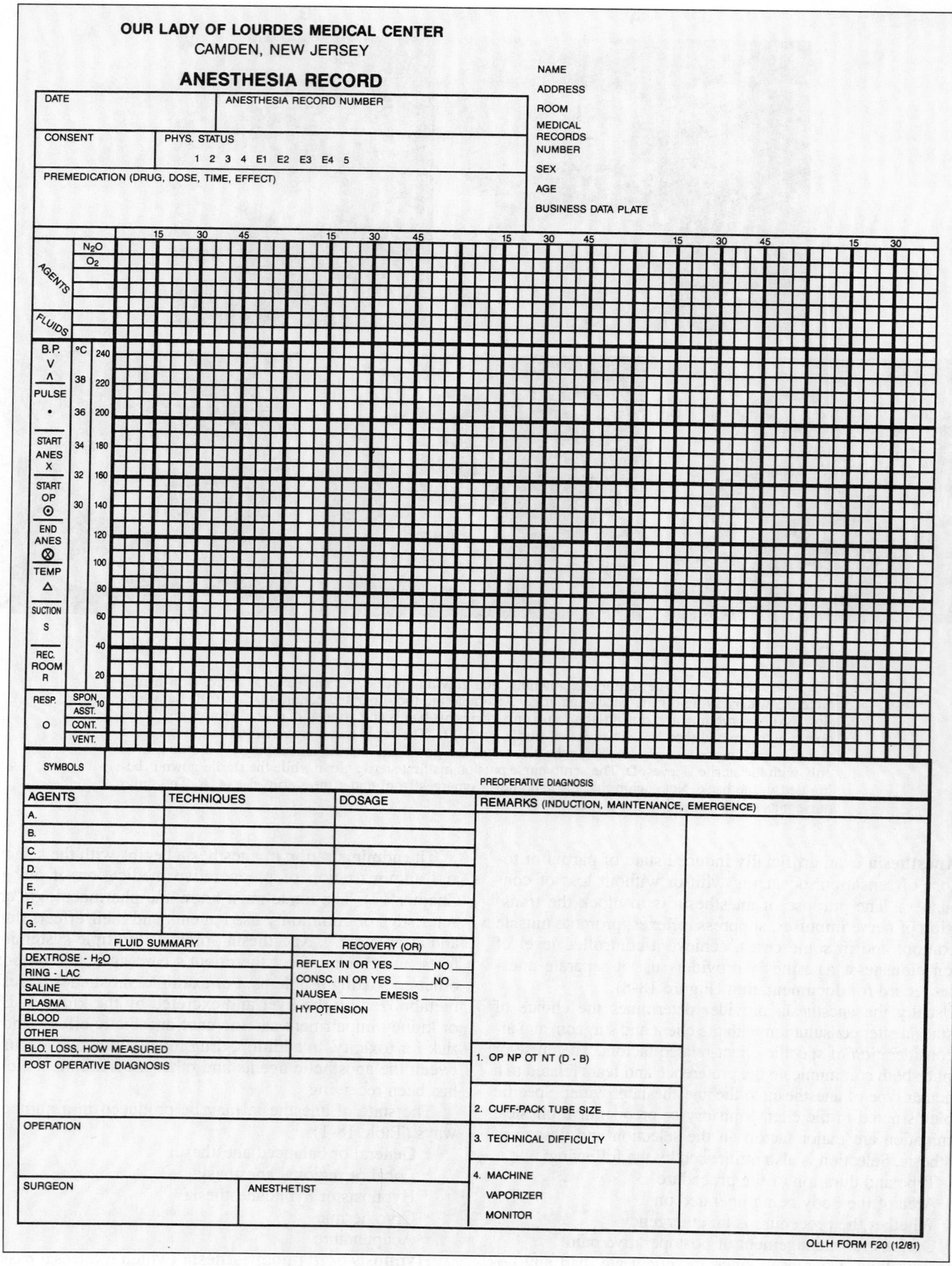

OUR LADY OF LOURDES MEDICAL CENTER
CAMDEN, NEW JERSEY

ANESTHESIA RECORD

DATE | ANESTHESIA RECORD NUMBER

CONSENT | PHYS. STATUS 1 2 3 4 E1 E2 E3 E4 5

PREMEDICATION (DRUG, DOSE, TIME, EFFECT)

NAME
ADDRESS
ROOM
MEDICAL RECORDS NUMBER
SEX
AGE
BUSINESS DATA PLATE

15 30 45 15 30 45 15 30 45 15 30 45 15 30

AGENTS: N_2O, O_2

FLUIDS

B.P. V Λ — PULSE • — START ANES X — START OP ⊙ — END ANES ⊗ — TEMP Δ — SUCTION S — REC. ROOM R

°C: 38, 36, 34, 32, 30

240, 220, 200, 180, 160, 140, 120, 100, 80, 60, 40, 20

RESP. O — SPON. 10 ASST. CONT. VENT.

SYMBOLS

PREOPERATIVE DIAGNOSIS

AGENTS	TECHNIQUES	DOSAGE
A.		
B.		
C.		
D.		
E.		
F.		
G.		

REMARKS (INDUCTION, MAINTENANCE, EMERGENCE)

FLUID SUMMARY
DEXTROSE - H_2O
RING - LAC
SALINE
PLASMA
BLOOD
OTHER
BLO. LOSS, HOW MEASURED

RECOVERY (OR)
REFLEX IN OR YES ______ NO ____
CONSC. IN OR YES ______ NO ____
NAUSEA ______ EMESIS ____
HYPOTENSION

POST OPERATIVE DIAGNOSIS

OPERATION

SURGEON | ANESTHETIST

1. OP NP OT NT (D - B)
2. CUFF-PACK TUBE SIZE
3. TECHNICAL DIFFICULTY
4. MACHINE
VAPORIZER
MONITOR

OLLH FORM F20 (12/81)

Figure 18-8 ● An anesthesia record. (Courtesy Our Lady of Lourdes Medical Center, Camden, NJ.)

TABLE 18-1 • ADVANTAGES AND DISADVANTAGES OF VARIOUS TYPES OF ANESTHESIA

Type	Advantages	Disadvantages
GENERAL		
Inhalation	Most controllable method Induction and reversal accomplished with pulmonary ventilation Few side effects	Must be used in combination with other agents for painful or prolonged procedures Limited muscle relaxant effects Postoperative nausea and shivering common Explosive
Intravenous	Rapid and pleasant induction Low incidence of postoperative nausea and vomiting Requires little equipment	Must be metabolized and excreted from the body for complete reversal Contraindicated in presence of hepatic or renal disease Increased cardiac and respiratory depression Retained by fat cells
Balanced	Minimal disturbance to physiologic function Minimal side effects Can be used with older and high-risk clients	Drug interactions can occur Pharmacologic effects on the body may be unpredictable
REGIONAL OR LOCAL	Gag and cough reflexes stay intact Allows participation and cooperation by the client Less disruption of physical and emotional body functions Decreased chance of sensitivity to the agent Decreased intraoperative stress	Difficult to administer to an uncooperative or upset client No way to control agent after administration Absorbs rapidly into the blood and causes cardiac depression (hypotension) or overdose Increased nervous system stimulation (overdose) Not practical for extensive procedures because of the amount of drug that would be required to maintain anesthesia

acupuncture are not commonly used in the United States or Canada. Interest in the use of these methods, however, is growing.

GENERAL ANESTHESIA

General anesthesia is a reversible state in which the client loses consciousness as a result of the inhibition of neuronal impulses in the several areas of the central nervous system (CNS). The administration of a single agent or a combination of chemical agents achieves this state. The anesthetic agents used induce CNS depression, characterized by **analgesia** (pain relief or pain suppression), **amnesia** (memory loss of the surgery), and unconsciousness, with loss of muscle tone and reflexes. The client is unconscious, unaware, and anesthetized. Indications for general anesthesia include surgery of the head, neck, and upper torso; extensive abdominal surgery; and situations in which clients are unable to cooperate.

STAGES OF GENERAL ANESTHESIA. Four stages of general anesthesia are classically described. Table 18-2 presents the client's physiologic responses and nursing interventions for each stage.

The speed of **emergence,** or recovery from the anesthesia, depends on the type of anesthetic agent, the length of time the client is anesthetized, and whether a reversal agent for the neuromuscular blocking agent has been administered. Although they are not as common as they once were (because of advances made in the pharmacology of anesthesia), retching, vomiting, and restlessness may occur during emergence. The nurse has suction equipment available to prevent aspiration. During recovery, shivering, rigidity, and slight cyanosis are not uncommon. These phenomena may reflect a temporary disturbance in the body's temperature control. The nurse provides the client with warm blankets, radiant light, and oxygen to decrease the undesirable effects of emergence.

ADMINISTRATION OF GENERAL ANESTHESIA. The two methods of administering general anesthesia are inhalation and IV injection.

INHALATION. **Inhalation** is the most controllable method of administering general anesthesia because intake and elimination of the anesthetic are accomplished primarily by respiration. The lungs act as a passageway for entrance and exit of the anesthetic agent. The client inhales the anesthetic vapor of a volatile liquid or the anesthetic gas via a mask. The anesthetic then passes across the alveolar membrane to the general circulation. The agent is transported through the bloodstream to the various tissues, where it is metabolized.

To improve ventilation and control the anesthesia, respiration may be assisted or controlled. With **assisted respiration,** an endotracheal (ET) tube is inserted. The ET tube is then connected to a reservoir (breathing) bag of the anesthesia machine (see Figure 18-4). The anesthesiologist overrides, or "assists," the client's own respiratory effort to initiate the respiratory cycle by manually compressing the reservoir bag.

Controlled respiration is accomplished with the use of a mechanical device, such as a mechanical ventilator, that automatically and rhythmically inflates the lungs with intermittent positive pressure; the client is not required to participate. Controlled ventilation is initiated after the anesthesiologist has produced **apnea** (absence of spontaneous respiratory effort) either through hyperventilation or by administering a respiratory depressant or neuromuscular blocking agent.

The anesthesiologist or certified registered nurse anesthetist (CRNA) inserts the ET tube with the assistance of the circulating nurse. A laryngoscope is used to visualize the vocal cords, and the tube is placed in the trachea (Figure 18-9).

TABLE 18-2 • THE FOUR STAGES OF GENERAL ANESTHESIA AND RELATED NURSING INTERVENTIONS

Stage	Description	Nursing Interventions	Rationale
Stage 1 (Analgesia and sedation, relaxation)	Begins with induction and ends with loss of consciousness. Client feels drowsy and dizzy, has a reduced sensation to pain, and is amnesic. Hearing is exaggerated.	Close operating room doors, dim the lights, and control traffic in the operating room. Position client securely with safety belts. Keep discussions about the client to a minimum.	Avoiding external stimuli in the environment promotes relaxation. Using safety measures in stage 1 prepares for stage 2. Being sensitive to the client maintains his or her dignity.
Stage 2 (Excitement, delirium)	Begins with loss of consciousness and ends with relaxation, regular breathing, and loss of the eyelid reflex. Client may have irregular breathing, increased muscle tone, and involuntary movement of the extremities during this stage. Laryngospasm or vomiting may occur. Client is susceptible to external stimuli.	Avoid auditory and physical stimuli. Protect the extremities. Assist the anesthesiologist or CRNA with suctioning as needed. Stay with client.	Sensory stimuli can contribute to the client's response. Safety measures help to prevent injury. Staying with the client is emotionally supportive.
Stage 3 (Operative anesthesia, surgical anesthesia)	Begins with generalized muscle relaxation and ends with loss of reflexes and depression of vital functions. The jaw is relaxed, and there is quiet, regular breathing. The client cannot hear. Sensations (i.e., to pain) are lost.	Assist the anesthesiologist or CRNA with intubation. Place client into operative position. Prep (scrub) the client's skin over the operative site as directed.	Providing assistance helps promote smooth intubation and prevent injury. Performing procedures as soon as possible promotes time management to minimize total anesthesia time for the client.
Stage 4 (Danger)	Begins with depression of vital functions and ends with respiratory failure, cardiac arrest, and possible death. Respiratory muscles are paralyzed; apnea occurs. Pupils are fixed and dilated.	Prepare for and assist in treatment of cardiac and/or pulmonary arrest. Document occurrence in the client's chart.	Teamwork and preparedness help decrease injuries and complications, and promote the possibility of a desired outcome for the client.

CRNA, Certified registered nurse anesthetist.

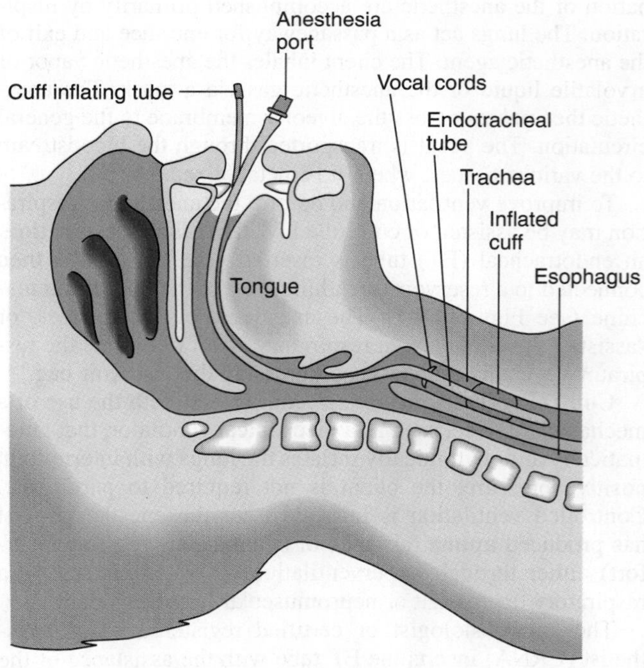

Figure 18-9 ● An oral endotracheal tube in position. The cuff of the tube was placed just below the vocal cords, then inflated to seal off the airway.

With the ET tube safely in place, the client has an open airway (through the tube) and an avenue for the safe administration of the inhaled anesthetic and oxygen.

Inhalation anesthetic agents are divided into two categories: gases and volatile agents. Table 18-3 lists the advantages, disadvantages, and related nursing implications of various inhalation anesthetic agents.

GASEOUS AGENTS. In the past, gaseous agents included ether and cyclopropane gas. *Nitrous oxide (N_2O)* is now the most commonly used gaseous anesthetic agent and is usually administered with oxygen. It is a colorless, odorless, nonirritating gas that provides analgesia equivalent to 10 mg of morphine sulfate.

VOLATILE AGENTS. Liquids vaporized for inhalation are considered volatile agents. Oxygen acts as a carrier, flowing over or bubbling through the liquid in the vaporizer system on the anesthesia machine. All volatile agents can produce postoperative shivering in the client because of their effect on the hypothalamus. Awakening is usually rapid, within 15 to 20 minutes.

Halothane (Fluothane). Halothane is a halogenated hydrocarbon that depresses the cardiovascular system. The intraoperative use of epinephrine to control bleeding may increase or precipitate a dysrhythmia when halothane is used.

TABLE 18-3 • ADVANTAGES, DISADVANTAGES, AND RELATED NURSING IMPLICATIONS OF VARIOUS GENERAL INHALATION ANESTHETIC AGENTS

Agent	Advantages	Disadvantages	Nursing Implications	Rationale
Nitrous oxide (N_2O)	Rapid induction and recovery Useful for short procedures When used with other agents, reduces the required concentration of the other agents Minimal cardiovascular and respiratory depression	Relatively weak anesthetic agent May produce hypoxia if the concentration is high Needs addition of other agents for longer procedures	Assess oxygenation via pulse oximetry, physical assessment.	Ongoing assessment leads to early detection and treatment of potential complications.
Halothane (Fluothane)	Rapid and smooth induction Low incidence of postoperative nausea and vomiting Less irritating to the respiratory tract than other inhalation agents Sweet smell makes it easy to use in children Tolerated well by children	Shivering common postoperatively Malignant hyperthermia is possible in susceptible clients Metabolized by the liver Hypotension and bradycardia may occur Can sensitize the myocardium to dysrhythmias	Monitor heart rate for bradycardia. Monitor blood pressure for hypotension. Provide warm blankets, radiant heat.	Ongoing assessment leads to early detection and treatment of potential complications. Warmth helps promote client comfort and decrease shivering.
Enflurane (Ethrane)	Rapid induction and recovery Does not alter heart rate or rhythm	Respiratory depression and hypotension may occur Malignant hyperthermia is possible in susceptible clients Lowers seizure threshold	Monitor respiratory rate and depth for hypoventilation. Assess oxygenation via pulse oximetry, physical assessment. Monitor blood pressure for hypotension.	Ongoing assessment leads to early detection and treatment of potential complications.
Isoflurane (Forane)	Rapid induction and recovery Has some muscle relaxant properties Stimulates the heart, which helps keep a stable heart rate Is not significantly metabolized; no renal or hepatic damage	Respiratory depression may occur Malignant hyperthermia is possible in susceptible clients	Monitor respiratory rate and depth for hypoventilation.	Ongoing assessment leads to early detection and treatment of potential complications.
Desflurane (Suprane)	Rapid induction, recovery, and awakening	May cause coughing and excitement during induction Deep levels of anesthesia may increase heart rate and blood pressure Malignant hyperthermia is possible in susceptible clients May cause changes in mental function	Monitor heart rate and blood pressure. Caution client and family that client should not drive or operate hazardous machinery until mental status has returned to preoperative baseline.	Ongoing assessment leads to early detection and treatment of potential complications. Specific instructions will help prevent other injuries or accidents.

Clients can have memory impairment for up to 24 hours after halothane is used.

Enflurane (Ethrane). Enflurane is an inhalation anesthetic agent that reduces ventilations and decreases blood pressure as the depth of anesthesia increases.

Isoflurane (Forane). Isoflurane is another halogenated compound and appears to be a preferred inhalation agent.

Desflurane (Suprane). Desflurane produces a rapid induction of anesthesia but can cause coughing and excitation during the process. The rapid elimination of desflurane produces awakening in 8 to 10 minutes. Cardiopulmonary depressant effects and malignant hyperthermia are the most common adverse effects.

Sevoflurane (Sevorane). Sevoflurane is like desflurane, except less coughing and laryngospasm occur with sevoflurane. Adverse effects are similar to those associated with desflurane.

INTRAVENOUS INJECTION. IV anesthetic agents are injected, usually through a peripheral IV line, into the circulation. A pleasant, rapid, and smooth dissipation of the agent occurs. The drug is diluted by the blood, but still travels in high concentration to the organs of high blood flow (brain, liver, and kidneys). The reversal and removal of the agent from circulation are not possible with IV injection, and the recovery from the agent is directly related to the client's metabolism. Table 18-4 lists advantages, disadvantages, and related nursing implications of various IV anesthetic agents.

BARBITURATES. Barbiturates are often used for IV induction of anesthesia. These drugs act directly on the central nervous system (CNS), producing a reaction ranging from mild sedation to unconsciousness. The principal barbiturate used is thiopental sodium (Pentothal), which can also be used for rectal induction. Intravenously, it acts rapidly, resulting in unconsciousness within 30 seconds of administration. Because thiopental is a potent respiratory and cardiovascular system depressant, the client's vital signs must be monitored continuously during administration.

KETAMINE (KETALAR). Ketamine is a **dissociative anesthetic agent** (one that promotes a feeling of dissociation from the environment). It acts by selectively interrupting various pathways in the brain. Rapid onset of a trancelike, analgesic state occurs. Ketamine is commonly used for diagnostic and short surgical procedures or to supplement weaker agents, such as nitrous oxide.

Emergence reactions are expected during recovery from ketamine. The operating room (OR) nurse reports the use of the drug to the postanesthesia nurse so that safety precautions can be implemented. If the client is combative or restless, the nurse pads the siderails of the bed to prevent injury. The nurse minimizes external stimuli until the client awakens naturally.

TABLE 18-4 • ADVANTAGES, DISADVANTAGES, AND RELATED NURSING IMPLICATIONS OF VARIOUS GENERAL INTRAVENOUS ANESTHETIC AGENTS

Agent	Advantages	Disadvantages	Nursing Implications	Rationale
BARBITURATES				
Thiopental sodium (Pentothal), methohexital sodium (Brevital)	Rapid, pleasant induction and recovery Acts directly on the central nervous system Short acting Low incidence of postoperative nausea and vomiting	Strong respiratory and cardiovascular depressant effect No antagonist medication available Mild to severe local tissue reaction with extravasation Poor analgesic, muscle relaxant effects	Monitor respiratory rate and depth for hypoventilation. Monitor heart rate for bradycardia. Monitor blood pressure for hypotension. Assess IV site.	Ongoing assessment leads to early detection and treatment of potential complications.
NONBARBITURATES				
Ketamine hydrochloride (Ketalar)	Rapid induction Short acting Can be given IM or IV No respiratory depression or loss of muscle tone (protects the airway) Protective reflexes remain intact Stimulates the cardiovascular system Can use for clients with respiratory or cardiac disorders Good amnesic effect Postoperative emergence reactions generally last only 24 hr	Emergence reactions—hallucinations, irrational behaviors, distorted images, unpleasant dreams, restlessness—are common Increased heart rate Increased blood pressure Increased cardiac output Poor muscle relaxant effect Nausea, vomiting, and aspiration can occur	Minimize external stimuli: noise, light, touch, movement. Speak in a calm, soothing voice. Reassure client and family that emergence reactions are common and temporary. Have suction equipment near. Monitor blood pressure for hypertension. Monitor heart rate for tachycardia.	Stimuli increase the severity of the emergence reaction. Quiet promotes comfort, decreases anxiety. Reassurance decreases anxiety. Suction may be needed in the event of vomiting to prevent aspiration. Ongoing assessment leads to early detection and treatment of potential complications.
Propofol (Diprivan)	Short acting Rapidly metabolized Client becomes responsive quickly postoperatively Minimal postoperative nausea, vomiting, or sedation	Allergic skin reactions have occurred Client becomes aware of postoperative pain and discomfort sooner than with other anesthetics	Be prepared to administer analgesic medications as ordered early in the postoperative period. Plan for nonpharmacologic pain interventions (see Chapter 7).	Awareness of pain very early in the postoperative period can be frightening. Pain can increase blood pressure and increase anxiety.
OPIOIDS (AS ADJUNCT)				
Fentanyl (Sublimaze)	Excellent postoperative analgesia Long-acting analgesia	Significant respiratory depression can occur several hours after administration Cardiovascular depression can occur	Monitor respiratory rate and depth for hypoventilation. Monitor blood pressure for hypotension. Have atropine, naloxone (Narcan), vasopressors, and resuscitative equipment nearby.	Ongoing assessment leads to early detection and treatment of potential complications. Having necessary supplies and equipment available provides for prompt response to an emergency.

For severe reactions during the recovery phase, small doses of diazepam (Valium, Vivol✱, Novo-Dipam✱) may be given as needed. The medical-surgical nurse continues interventions until the effects of the drug have worn off.

PROPOFOL (DIPRIVAN). Propofol is in a newer classification of IV anesthetic agents, the alkylphenols. Its short action makes it desirable as an anesthetic agent. Hypnosis occurs in less than 1 minute from the time of injection, and because the drug is so rapidly metabolized, it does not accumulate during maintenance of the anesthesia. The client becomes responsive quickly after the infusion is ended (within 8 minutes). Propofol is also used to supplement nitrous oxide during short procedures and is used as a hypnotic agent with regional anesthesia.

ADJUNCTS TO GENERAL ANESTHETIC AGENTS. Other drugs, such as hypnotics, opioid analgesics, and neuromuscular blocking agents, may be used as part of the anesthesia regimen.

HYPNOTICS. The benzodiazepines may be used for various effects. Common drugs in this classification include midazolam (Versed), lorazepam (Ativan, Novolorazem✱), and diazepam (Valium, Vivol✱, Novo-Dipam✱). All have hypnotic, sedative, antianxiety, muscle relaxant, and amnesic effects. Generally, lower doses are ordered for preoperative sedation. Each drug may be used as part of an IV conscious sedation regimen for diagnostic or endoscopic procedures. Higher doses of midazolam may be used to induce general anesthesia. The benzodiazepines may also be used intraoperatively in conjunction with regional or local anesthesia. Adverse reactions include respiratory depression, apnea, and oversedation.

OPIOID ANALGESICS. Common opioid analgesics used to supplement inhalation anesthesia include morphine sulfate (Statex✱), meperidine hydrochloride (Demerol), fentanyl citrate (Sublimaze), and sufentanil (Sufenta). The use of opioids during surgery contributes to postoperative analgesia. *All opioid analgesics are respiratory depressants and decrease alveolar ventilation.* The nurse monitors respirations and maintains an open airway. Reduced dosages are prescribed for older clients, clients with a circulatory problem (e.g., heart failure), and debilitated clients.

Fentanyl and sufentanil induce analgesia in lower doses, but at higher doses they can be used as the anesthetic agent. Fentanyl has a potency 75 to 125 times greater than that of morphine. Sufentanil has five to seven times the analgesic potency of fentanyl and produces a more rapid onset of CNS effects than does fentanyl. It is often used in open heart surgery when the sternum must be opened. The nurse monitors the client who has received sufentanil for bradycardia and decreased cardiac output.

NEUROMUSCULAR BLOCKING AGENTS. The neuromuscular blocking agents are used to relax the jaw and vocal cords immediately after induction so that the anesthesiologist or certified registered nurse anesthetist (CRNA) can place the endotracheal (ET) tube. These drugs are also used throughout the surgical procedure to provide continued overall muscle relaxation. Neuromuscular blocking agents act on the skeletal muscles of the body by interfering with impulse transmission at the neuromuscular junction. The drugs are administered intravenously in small amounts and may cause circulatory alterations, decreased respirations, or apnea from muscle paralysis. The nurse ensures the client's safety by securing him or her on the operating bed with safety straps and assists the anesthesiologist or CRNA with intubation. Throughout the surgery, the anesthesiologist or CRNA checks the effectiveness of the blocking agent by using a peripheral nerve stimulator. There are two types of neuromuscular blocking agents: nondepolarizing and depolarizing.

NONDEPOLARIZING BLOCKING AGENTS. The nondepolarizing blocking agents block acetylcholine at the neuromuscular junction. Only skeletal muscles are blocked, and the drug is easily reversed with an antidote of neostigmine and atropine. Examples of nondepolarizing blocking agents include pancuronium (Pavulon), atracurium (Tracrium), vecuronium (Norcuron), doxacurium (Nuromax), tubocurarine (Tubarine✱), and mivacurium (Mivacron). Pancuronium has a relatively long effect (45 to 60 minutes) compared with vecuronium (25 to 30 minutes) or mivacurium (6 to 16 minutes). The longer the duration of drug action, the longer it takes for the client to recover.

DEPOLARIZING BLOCKING AGENTS. The depolarizing blocking agents, also called "noncompetitive" blocking agents, depolarize the motor end plate at the neuromuscular junction. In the process, potassium is forced out of the muscle cells and into general circulation, which can cause hyperkalemia. Clients often experience transient intraoperative muscle twitching, which can result in generalized muscle aches after awakening. Other side effects include increased salivation (increasing the risk for aspiration) and increased intraocular pressure (thus the agents may be contraindicated with glaucoma). An example of a commonly used depolarizing blocking agent is succinylcholine (Anectine). There is no specific antidote for these agents.

BALANCED ANESTHESIA. In the past, the term **balanced anesthesia** was used when various combinations of IV medications were balanced to provide complete anesthesia. Today, the term is used to describe a combination of both IV medication and inhalation agents employed to obtain specific effects. Balanced anesthesia provides a safe and controlled anesthetic experience, especially for older and high-risk clients. A combination is used to provide hypnosis, amnesia, analgesia, muscle relaxation, and relaxation of reflexes with minimal disturbance of physiologic function. An example of balanced anesthesia is the use of a barbiturate (such as thiopental) administered intravenously for induction, nitrous oxide administered by inhalation for amnesia, morphine for analgesia, and a muscle relaxant (such as pancuronium) administered intravenously to provide additional muscle relaxation.

A second example of balanced anesthesia is the use of 70% nitrous oxide for induction and maintenance (to prevent awareness throughout the procedure and to prevent recall afterward), 30% oxygen to maintain oxygenation saturation at greater than 90%, an opioid, and a muscle relaxant. Many combinations are possible, and selection reflects assessment of the individual client and the specific surgical procedure.

COMPLICATIONS FROM GENERAL ANESTHESIA OR ANESTHESIA MANAGEMENT. Complications can range from minor and annoying (sore throat) to the most severe and irreversible—death. Despite surgical procedures being performed on increasingly sicker and higher-risk clients, however, there has been a significant decline in anesthesia-related deaths during the last 30 years (Voelker, 1995).

MALIGNANT HYPERTHERMIA. Malignant hyperthermia (MH) is an acute, life-threatening complication of general anesthesia that may be triggered by drugs commonly used in anesthesia. Inhalational anesthetics and succinylcholine are the most frequently implicated triggering agents. MH is a multifactorial disease and is genetically transmitted as an autosomal dominant trait. The client with a genetic predisposition for MH is at risk for this complication from agents such as halothane, enflurane, isoflurane, desflurane, sevoflurane, and succinylcholine. Stressors such as severe fatigue, strenuous exercise, trauma or muscle injury, and emotional stress may also trigger this crisis.

This rare but potentially deadly syndrome is most common in children and young adults. A biochemical reaction begins with a defect in skeletal muscle calcium regulation, and exposure to specific triggering stimuli results in intracellular hypercalcemia leading to increased metabolism. This hypermetabolic condition results in an increase in the circulating calcium level, an increase in the metabolic rate, hyperkalemia, metabolic and respiratory acidosis, cardiac dysrhythmias, and rapid elevation of the body temperature.

Onset of MH may occur immediately after induction of anesthesia, several hours into the procedure, or rarely, once the anesthetic has been terminated. Clinical features reflect the increased intracellular muscle calcium concentration and the greatly increased body metabolism. Common manifestations include tachycardia or other dysrhythmias; muscle rigidity (apparent in 75% of all MH cases), especially of the jaw and upper chest; hypotension; tachypnea; and skin mottling, cyanosis, and myoglobinuria (cola-colored urine). The most sensitive indication is an unexpected rise in the end-tidal carbon dioxide level with a decrease in oxygen saturation (Dunn, 1997). The second indication may be unexplained sinus tachycardia. *Extremely elevated temperature, perhaps as high as 111.2° F (44° C), is a late sign of MH.* Treatment and survival of the client depend on early diagnosis and the cooperation of the entire surgical team. Time is crucial when MH is diagnosed. Dantrolene sodium, a skeletal muscle relaxant, is the medication of choice along with other interventions.

Once a client or family history of MH is known, close family members can undergo a muscle biopsy to determine whether they are at risk. In the case of a known history or predetermination, the client can be treated preoperatively, intraoperatively, and postoperatively with dantrolene to prevent this complication. Chart 18-1 summarizes best practices for care of the client with malignant hyperthermia.

OVERDOSE. An anesthesia overdose can occur if the client's metabolism and drug elimination do not react or respond as expected. Drugs (e.g., antihypertensive medications) also alter anesthesia metabolism, and drug interactions can occur between the anesthetic agents and other regularly administered medications. Accurate, accessible information about the client, such as height, weight, and history, is vital in determining the anesthetic type and dosage. Intraoperative death, however, is more often related to pre-existing health problems than to overdose of anesthetics.

CHART 18-1

BEST PRACTICE *for* Care of the Client with Malignant Hyperthermia

- Stop all inhalation anesthetic agents and succinylcholine.
- If an endotracheal (ET) tube is not already in place, intubate immediately.
- Ventilate the client with 100% oxygen, using the highest possible flow rate.
- Administer dantrolene sodium (Dantrium) intravenously at a dose of 2 to 3 mg/kg.
- If possible, terminate surgery. If termination is not possible, continue surgery using anesthetic agents that do not trigger malignant hyperthermia (MH).
- Assess arterial blood gases (ABGs) and serum chemistries for metabolic acidosis and hyperkalemia.
  - If metabolic acidosis is evident by ABG analysis, administer sodium bicarbonate intravenously.
  - If hyperkalemia is present, administer 10 units of insulin in 50 mL of 20% dextrose intravenously.
- Use active cooling techniques.
  - Administer iced saline (0.9% NaCl) intravenously at a rate of 15 mL/kg every 15 minutes for three doses.
  - Apply a cooling blanket over the torso.
  - Wrap or rub extremities with cold, wet towels or ice wrapped in towels.
  - Lavage the stomach, bladder, rectum, and open body cavities (if appropriate) with sterile iced normal saline.
- Monitor core body temperature to assess effectiveness of interventions and avoid hypothermia.
- Monitor cardiac rhythm by electrocardiography (ECG) to assess for dysrhythmias.
- Insert a Foley catheter to monitor urine output.
- Treat any dysrhythmias that do not resolve on correction of hyperthermia and hyperkalemia with antidysrhythmic agents *other than calcium channel blockers.*
- Administer IV fluids at a rate and volume sufficient to maintain urine output above 2 mL/kg/hr.
- Monitor urine for presence of blood or myoglobin.
- If urine output falls below 2 mL/kg/hr, consider using osmotic or loop diuretics, depending on the client's cardiac and renal status.
- Contact the Malignant Hyperthermia Association of the United States (MHAUS) hotline for more information regarding treatment: (800) 644-9373.
- Transfer the client to the intensive care unit (ICU) when stable.
- Continue to monitor the client's temperature, ECG, ABGs, electrolytes, creatine kinase, coagulation studies, and serum and urine myoglobin levels until they have remained normal for 24 hours.
- Instruct the client and family about testing for MH risk.
- Refer the client and family to the Malignant Hyperthermia Association of the United States at (800) 986-4287 or http://www.mhaus.org.
- Report the incident to the North American Malignant Hyperthermia Registry at the University of Pittsburgh: (412) 692-5464.

Data from Malignant Hyperthermia Association of the United States; and Dunn, D. (1997). Malignant hyperthermia. *AORN Journal, 65*(4), 728-762.

UNRECOGNIZED HYPOVENTILATION. The respiratory system is most frequently involved when the client experiences an anesthesia-induced complication. Failure to ventilate adequately can lead to cardiac arrest, central nervous system (CNS) damage (e.g., permanent brain damage), and death. Monitoring standards include the use of an end-tidal carbon dioxide monitor to confirm carbon dioxide in the client's ex-

TABLE 18-5 • ADVANTAGES, DISADVANTAGES, AND RELATED NURSING IMPLICATIONS OF LOCAL OR REGIONAL ANESTHETIC AGENTS

Agent	Advantages	Disadvantages	Nursing Implications	Rationale
Procaine (Novocain) Tetracaine (Pontocaine) Lidocaine (Xylocaine) Mepivacaine (Carbocaine, Polocaine) Bupivacaine (Marcaine, Sensorcaine)	Easily administered Rapid onset (4-17 min) Can be administered topically or by injection Excellent muscle relaxant effects Protective reflexes (cough, gag) remain intact Client does not lose consciousness Many are available with epinephrine added	Absorbs into the bloodstream Can cause cardiac depression and dysrhythmias with absorption Difficult to control dosage Drug interactions with monoamine oxidase (MAO) inhibitors can cause hypertension Tremors, twitching shivering, respiratory arrest can occur with absorption	Assess for return of movement and sensation in the area anesthetized. Monitor blood pressure and pulse. Assess administration site for pallor, drainage. Protect area anesthetized until full sensation has returned.	Movement returns first, then sense of touch, pain, warmth, and cold, in that order. Ongoing assessment leads to early detection and treatment of potential complications. Protection prevents injury to the area. Duration of the anesthetic is 3-6 hr.

pired gas and a breathing system disconnect monitor to detect any break in the breathing circuit equipment.

COMPLICATIONS RELATED TO SPECIFIC ANESTHETIC AGENTS. Specific complications are discussed earlier in the chapter. The older or debilitated client may be more susceptible to complications of anesthesia because of intolerance to the agent, decreased metabolism, or his or her general physical condition. (For preoperative risk factors, see Chapter 17.)

COMPLICATIONS OF INTUBATION. Many complications can occur from intubation (e.g., broken or injured teeth and caps, swollen lip, or vocal cord trauma). Intubation may be difficult because of the individual anatomy or disease process (e.g., small oral cavity, tight mandibular joint, or presence of tumor). Improper extension of the neck during intubation also may cause injury. The surgeon should be in the operating room (OR) during the intubation process in case an emergency arises (e.g., a tracheostomy is needed) when the endotracheal (ET) tube is placed. Placement of the ET tube causes some degree of irritation and edema of the trachea and accounts for the client's sore throat postoperatively.

LOCAL OR REGIONAL ANESTHESIA

Local or regional anesthesia temporarily interrupts the transmission of sensory nerve impulses from a specific area or region. Motor function may or may not be affected, and the client does not lose consciousness. Thus the client is able to follow instructions throughout the procedure. Because the gag and cough reflexes remain intact, there is little risk of aspiration or complications from hypoventilation. Local or regional anesthesia is typically supplemented with sedatives, opioid analgesics, and/or hypnotics to reduce anxiety and increase comfort.

The OR nurse provides the client with information, directions, and emotional support before, during, and after the procedure. Table 18-5 describes various local and regional anesthetic agents and related nursing implications.

LOCAL ANESTHESIA. Techniques used to administer local anesthesia include topical anesthesia and local infiltration. Sometimes when the term *local* is used, it means *any* form of anesthesia that is not general anesthesia.

TOPICAL ANESTHESIA. **Topical anesthesia** involves use of an anesthetic agent applied *directly* to the surface of the area to be anesthetized. Often the anesthetic is an ointment or spray. This method is often used for respiratory intubation and for diagnostic procedures, such as laryngoscopy, bronchoscopy, or cystoscopy. The onset of action is 1 minute, and the duration is 20 to 30 minutes. Collapse or depression of the cardiovascular system is a potential complication of topical anesthetic agents applied to the respiratory tract.

LOCAL INFILTRATION. **Local infiltration** is the injection of an anesthetic agent intracutaneously and subcutaneously *into* the tissue surrounding an incision, wound, or lesion. The anesthetic agent blocks peripheral nerve stimulation at its origin. Local infiltration is commonly used during the suturing of superficial lacerations.

REGIONAL ANESTHESIA. Regional anesthesia, a type of local anesthesia, may be used as follows:

- When general anesthesia is contraindicated because of the presence of medical problems (e.g., dysrhythmias and respiratory disease)
- When the client has experienced previous adverse reactions to general anesthesia
- When the client has a preference and a choice is possible
- When pain management postoperatively is enhanced by regional anesthesia

If the client has eaten and the surgery is an emergency, it may be possible to perform the procedure with the client under regional anesthesia (depending on the procedure) to decrease the risks associated with gastric contents (e.g., aspiration). Types of regional anesthesia include field block, nerve block, spinal, and epidural.

FIELD BLOCK. A field block is produced by a series of injections *around* the operative field. Injecting around a specific nerve or group of nerves depresses the entire sensory nervous system of a localized area. This type of blocking is used for thoracic procedures, **herniorrhaphy** (hernia repair), dental procedures, and plastic surgery.

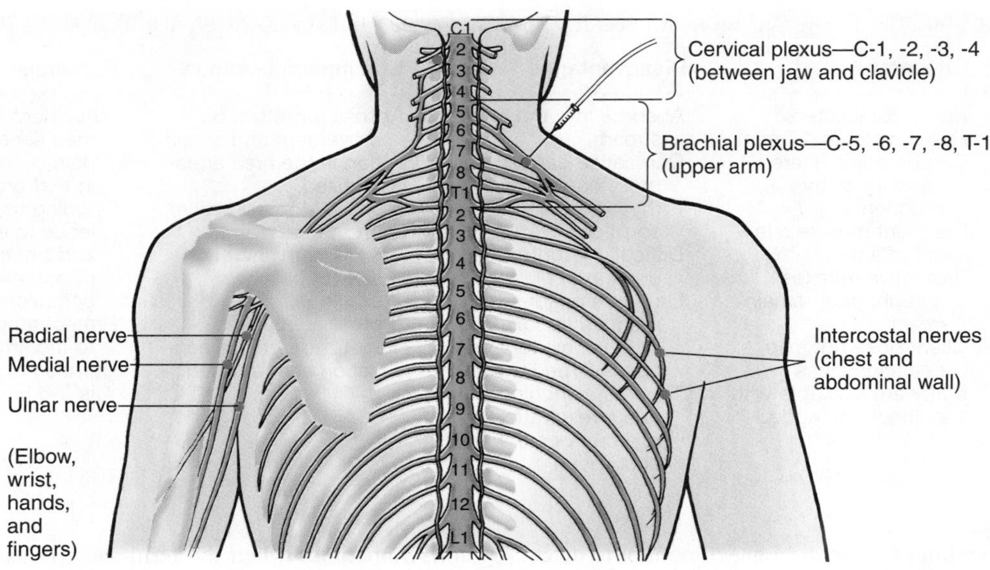

Figure 18-10 ● Nerve block sites.

NERVE BLOCK. A nerve block is achieved by injection of the local anesthetic agent *into or around* a nerve or group of nerves supplying the involved area. Nerve blocks interrupt sensory, motor, and sympathetic transmission. They are used surgically to prevent pain during a procedure, diagnostically to identify the cause of pain, and therapeutically to relieve chronic pain and increase circulation in some vascular diseases.

Figure 18-10 shows common nerve block sites. Lidocaine (Xylocaine) or bupivacaine (Marcaine) is frequently the agent used. A nerve block takes effect within minutes after the injection, and the anesthesia lasts longer than that achieved with local infiltration. Epinephrine added to the anesthetic agent potentates the drug, causing a prolonged effect. Seizures, cardiac depression, dysrhythmias, and/or respiratory depression may occur if the nerve-blocking agent is injected accidentally into the bloodstream. The nurse observes for signs of systemic absorption, sensitivity, or overdose.

SPINAL ANESTHESIA. Spinal anesthesia—intrathecal block—is achieved by injection of the anesthetic agent into the cerebrospinal fluid in the subarachnoid space (Figure 18-11). The drug acts on the nerves as they emerge from the spinal cord and before they leave the spinal canal, thereby inhibiting conduction in the autonomic, sensory, and motor systems. The drug is rapidly absorbed into the nerve fibers and produces analgesia with relaxation, which is effective for lower abdominal and pelvic surgical procedures.

EPIDURAL ANESTHESIA. The anesthetic agent is injected into the epidural space so that the protective coverings of the spinal cord (dura mater and arachnoid mater) are never entered. Because the anesthetic can diffuse or float up the vertebral column, the client can achieve anesthetic effects as high as the T4 level; however, potential respiratory complications may make injection at this high a level undesirable.

Epidural anesthesia is used for anorectal, vaginal, and perineal procedures, as well as for hip and lower extremity operations, such as total hip or knee replacements. Two important advantages are associated with this type of anesthesia:

- Decreased cardiopulmonary complications, which is particularly important for the older client
- Ability to retain the epidural catheter for postoperative analgesic administration (see Chapter 7)

COMPLICATIONS OF LOCAL OR REGIONAL ANESTHESIA. Major intraoperative complications of local or regional anesthesia are usually related to client sensitization to the anesthetic agent (anaphylaxis), incorrect administration technique, systemic absorption, or overdosage. The nurse observes for signs of a systemic toxic reaction, manifested by central nervous system (CNS) stimulation followed by CNS and cardiovascular depression. The nurse assesses for initial behaviors indicating a problem, such as restlessness, excitement, incoherent speech, headache, blurred vision, metallic taste, nausea, vomiting, tremors, seizures, and increased pulse, respirations, and blood pressure. Nursing interventions include establishing and maintaining an open airway, administering oxygen, and notifying the surgeon. Usually it is necessary to administer a fast-acting and short-acting barbiturate. If the client's toxic reaction remains untreated, unconsciousness, hypotension, apnea, cardiac arrest, and death may result.

A cardiac arrest may occur as a rare complication of spinal anesthesia, possibly related to unknown autonomic nervous system effects. Administration of epinephrine to a client who develops sudden, unexplained bradycardia may prevent cardiac arrest (Biddle, 1994).

Local complications include edema and inflammation, as early problems, with possible abscess, necrosis, and/or gangrene later. Inflammation and abscess usually result from a break in sterile technique occurring at the time of injection of the anesthetic agent. Necrosis and gangrene are rare but may occur as a result of prolonged vasoconstriction in the area of the injection.

The nurse's role in the administration of regional anesthesia consists of the following:

- Assisting the anesthesia provider
- Observing for breaks in sterile technique

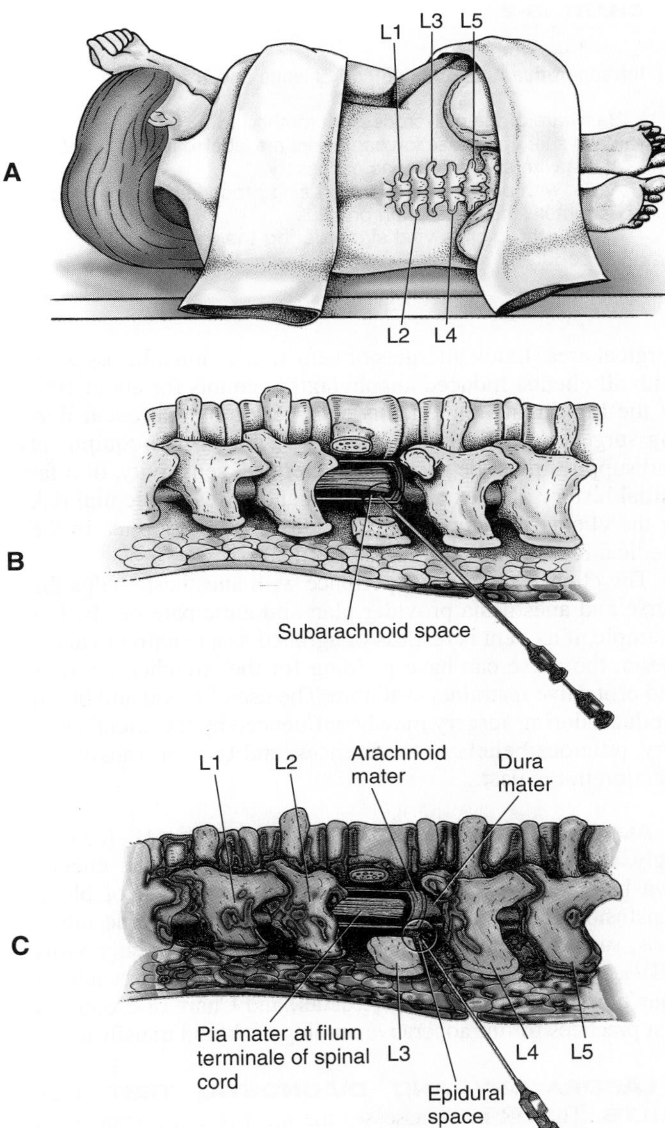

Figure 18-11 ● Administration of spinal and epidural anesthesia. **A,** Spinal or epidural anesthesia is administered by inserting a spinal needle between the second and third or the third and fourth lumbar vertebrae (L2-3 or L3-4). The client is placed in the flexed lateral (fetal) position (shown here) or seated on the edge of the operating bed with the back arched and the chin tucked to the chest. **B,** Spinal anesthesia (viewed from the side). A large needle is inserted to the surface of the dura mater, and a second, smaller needle is passed through the first to penetrate the dura mater and arachnoid mater. An anesthetic in injected, sometimes through an indwelling catheter, directly into the cerebrospinal fluid in the subarachnoid space. **C,** Epidural anesthesia (viewed from the side). The needle is inserted to the surface of the dura mater, and the anesthetic is injected, usually through an indwelling catheter, into the epidural space.

- Providing physical and emotional support for the client
- Staying with the client
- Offering information, encouragement, and reassurance
- Positioning the client comfortably and safely

CONSCIOUS SEDATION

Conscious sedation refers to the IV administration of sedative, hypnotic, and opioid medications to produce a condition in which the client has a depressed level of consciousness but retains the ability to independently maintain a patent airway and respond appropriately to verbal commands or physical stimulation. A rapid, safe return to activities of daily living is usually achieved with some degree of amnesia with conscious sedation. Diazepam (Valium, Vivol♣, Novo-Dipam♣), midazolam (Versed), meperidine (Demerol), fentanyl (Sublimaze), alfentanil (Alfenta), and morphine sulfate are the most commonly used drugs. Conscious sedation is typically used for procedures such as endoscopy, cardiac catheterization, closed fracture reduction, percutaneous transluminal cardiac angiography (PTCA), cardioversion, and other special but relatively short procedures.

Selection of clients for conscious sedation is based on established criteria developed by an interdisciplinary team. The physician determines whether the client is a candidate. In most states, a credentialed registered nurse may administer conscious sedation under physician supervision and within the state-defined scope of nursing practice (Bryan, 1997). Recommended credentialing includes advanced training in IV medication administration, airway management, and advanced cardiac life support (ACLS) (Landrum, 1997).

The nurse monitors the client during and after the procedure for his or her response to the procedure and drug administration. Specific responsibilities include careful monitoring of the client's airway, level of consciousness, oxygen saturation via pulse oximetry, electrocardiographic (ECG) status, and vital signs every 15 to 30 minutes until he or she is fully awake, alert, and oriented, and vital signs have returned to preprocedural levels.

The client receiving IV conscious sedation may be discharged to go home with a responsible adult. If the client returns to the general medical-surgical nursing unit, the unit staff nurses continue to monitor him or her. The client is expected to be sleepy but arousable for several hours after the procedure. The nurse usually does not permit oral intake until 30 minutes after the client has received medication or according to the physician's orders. When fluids are permitted, the nurse makes sure that the client is awake and positioned to avoid aspiration.

➤ COLLABORATIVE MANAGEMENT

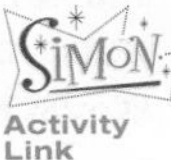

Activity Link

● Assessment

HISTORY

On arrival in the surgical suite, the client is taken to the holding area or directly into the operating suite. The holding area nurse and/or the circulating nurse greets the client on arrival. *Correct identification of the client is the responsibility of every member of the health care team.* The nurse verifies the client's identity with his or her identification bracelet and asks, "What is your name?" This practice prevents errors that may occur. For example, if a client is asked, "Are you Mr. James?" He may respond inappropriately if he is drowsy, anxious, or sedated. The nurse always validates the identification obtained using the medical record and the client's name and identification number.

After completing the identification process, the nurse validates that the surgical consent form has been signed and witnessed. The nurse asks the client, "What kind of operation are you having today?" to ascertain that his or her perception of the procedure, the operative permit, and the operative schedule coincide. This practice is especially important when the nurse is validating the side on which a procedure is to be performed (e.g., for amputation, cataract extraction, or hernia repair). Some facilities have the client and/or nurse initial the appropriate surgical site. Before proceeding, the nurse thoroughly investigates *any* discrepancy in information and notifies the surgeon and anesthesia provider.

The nurse asks the client about any allergies and determines if any autologous blood was donated. A red allergy bracelet on the client's wrist and the medical record must be verified with what has been communicated.

The nurse checks the client's attire to ensure compliance with facility policy. Dentures and dental prostheses (e.g., bridges and retainers), jewelry, eyeglasses, contact lenses, hearing aids, wigs, and other prostheses are removed for safety during surgery. The nurse pays special attention to the removal of dentures, because the denture plate could become loose and obstruct the airway during surgery. Occasionally the anesthesiology team may request that the dentures be left in place to ensure a snug fit of the anesthesia mask. In some facilities, clients may be permitted to retain their eyeglasses and hearing aids until after the induction phase of anesthesia.

MEDICAL RECORD REVIEW

The circulating nurse and anesthesia personnel review the client's medical record in the holding area (or in the operating room [OR] if there is no holding area). The medical record provides information needed to identify potential and actual needs of the client during the intraoperative period and allows the circulating nurse to assess and plan for his or her needs during and after surgery. The medical record is a primary source of information on the type and location of the planned surgical procedure. A check of the medical record ensures that all required data are present before the procedure is started.

ADVANCE DIRECTIVES AND DO-NOT-RESUSCITATE ORDERS. The perioperative nurse is subject to ethical dilemmas in the surgical environment. As a client advocate, the perioperative nurse may have to intervene on behalf of the client's rights and wishes. The perioperative nurse must be familiar with the advance directives and do-not-resuscitate (DNR) orders for each client.

The 1990 Patient Self-Determination Act requires health care providers to ask clients if they have advance directives. These directives are to be honored in the surgical environment regardless of the situation. It is difficult for some health care providers not to treat the client in the OR for an emergency situation, and they ignore advance directive or living will. In addition, it is a common practice to suspend DNR orders while a client is undergoing a surgical procedure. The position statement of AORN, the Association of periOperative Registered Nurses, regarding the perioperative care of clients with DNR orders states that automatically suspending a DNR order during surgery undermines a client's right to self-determination (AORN, 1999b). Many institutions are addressing this issue along with advance directives in a way that protects the client's rights in all environments.

ALLERGIES AND PREVIOUS REACTIONS TO ANESTHESIA OR TRANSFUSIONS. In reviewing the medical record, the nurse asks about allergies and previous reactions to anesthesia or blood transfusions. Allergies or sensitivity to iodine products or shellfish may indicate the potential for a reaction to the antimicrobial agents used to clean the surgical area. Latex allergies or sensitivities must be assessed with all clients. Induced anaphylaxis accounts for about 10% of the life-threatening anaphylactic reactions that occur during surgery (see Chapters 20 and 23). Latex-free equipment and supplies must be used when allergies, sensitivity, or a familial history of latex allergy exists and poses a potential risk to the client. The nurse clearly indicates the allergies in the medical record and notifies the OR team.

CHART 18-2

BEST PRACTICE *for* Intraoperative Autologous Blood Salvage and Transfusion

- Be aware of the cell-processing method to be used.
- Make sure that collection containers are labeled for the client.
- Assist with sterile setup as necessary.
- Assist with processing and reinfusing procedures as needed.
- Document the transfusion process.
- Monitor the client's vital signs during the transfusion procedure.

The client's previous experience with anesthesia helps the nurse and anesthesia provider plan and anticipate needs. For example, if a client is restless or agitated as a reaction to anesthesia, the nurse can have padding for the stretcher siderails and protective restraints available. The use of blood and blood products during surgery may be influenced by the client's history, religious beliefs or preferences, and type of transfusion reaction in the past.

AUTOLOGOUS BLOOD TRANSFUSION. Increasingly, **autologous blood transfusion** (reinfusing the client's own blood) is being used for surgery. This method of blood transfusion eliminates the risk of acquiring bloodborne infections, such as hepatitis B and human immunodeficiency virus (HIV), from another person. Chapters 17 and 40 discuss autologous blood transfusion in more detail, and Chart 18-2 outlines best practices for intraoperative autologous blood transfusion.

LABORATORY AND DIAGNOSTIC TEST RESULTS. The OR nurse assesses the most recent preoperative laboratory and diagnostic test results to inform the surgical team about the client's medical condition and to alert them to potential intraoperative and postoperative interventions. The most recent results are usually obtained within 24 to 28 hours before surgery for hospitalized clients and within 4 weeks for ambulatory surgery clients. The nurse reports all abnormalities to the surgeon and anesthesia provider. Laboratory values significantly greater than or less than the normal range are potentially life threatening for any client, but are especially so for the client undergoing surgery (see Chapter 17). For example, if the hemoglobin concentration is less than 10 g/dL, oxygen transport capacity is reduced, affecting the amount and type of anesthesia used as well as the potential impact of blood loss during surgery.

MEDICAL HISTORY AND PHYSICAL EXAMINATION FINDINGS. The OR nurse checks that the medical history and examination findings, including usual pulse and blood pressure, are recorded. This information provides the circulating nurse, surgeon, anesthesia provider, and postanesthesia care unit (PACU) nurse with baseline data to assess the client's reaction to the surgical procedure and anesthesia. Medications the client has routinely taken preoperatively may affect the reaction to surgery and wound healing. For exam-

CHART 18-3

NURSING FOCUS *on the* OLDER ADULT
Intraoperative Nursing Interventions

- Allow clients to retain eyeglasses and hearing aids until anesthesia has been administered.
- Use a small pillow under the client's head if his or her head and neck are normally bent slightly forward.
- Lift clients into position to prevent shearing forces on fragile skin.
- Position arthritic and artificial joints carefully to prevent postoperative pain and discomfort from strain on those joints.
- Pad bony prominences to prevent pressure sores.
- Provide extra padding for those clients with decreased peripheral circulation.
- Use head caps to prevent heat loss through the scalp.
- Place stockinette on extremities to conserve body heat.
- Warm prepping solutions and IV and irrigation fluids as indicated.
- Follow strict aseptic technique.
- Carefully monitor intake and output, including blood loss.

ple, aspirin has an anticoagulant effect and can cause increased clotting time and danger of hemorrhage.

Knowing the client's medical history and age (Chart 18-3) allows the nurse to take special precautions and plan appropriate interventions for the care and safety of high-risk clients. The nurse carefully monitors older clients and those with cardiac disease for potential fluid overload, which can be life threatening.

After completing the medical record review, the nurse may insert an IV catheter and perform a surgical shave. The circulating nurse provides additional emotional support and explains procedures to the client. *The client is never left unattended.* If the client is in the holding area, he or she is transferred to the OR after the preoperative routine is completed.

CRITICAL THINKING CHALLENGE

The client, a 69-year-old retired homemaker, has entered the surgical suite. The OR schedule lists that she is scheduled for a left total knee **arthroplasty** (total knee replacement). As the anesthesiologist is inserting the client's IV line, the client is questioned about which knee is being replaced. As the perioperative nurse, you overhear her answer, "I think it is my right knee, but both of them hurt and need to be replaced. I don't care which knee they do today."

- What should you do with the information?
- What steps do you take to ensure that the correct knee is operated on?
- Does it matter if the wrong knee is operated on first, since according to the client both knees need to be replaced?
- How do you prevent this situation from occurring again?

For suggested answer guidelines, go to SIMON http://www.wbsaunders.com/SIMON/Iggy/.

Analysis

COMMON NURSING DIAGNOSES AND COLLABORATIVE PROBLEMS

The following are common nursing diagnoses for intraoperative clients:

1. Risk for Perioperative Positioning Injury related to immobilization and effects of anesthesia
2. Impaired Skin Integrity and Impaired Tissue Integrity related to the surgical incision

A common collaborative problem for the intraoperative client is Potential for Hypoventilation.

ADDITIONAL NURSING DIAGNOSES AND COLLABORATIVE PROBLEMS

In addition to the common nursing diagnoses and collaborative problems, intraoperative clients may have one or more of the following:

- Risk for Infection related to a break in skin integrity (i.e., incision, invasive lines)
- Risk for Injury related to fire and electrical hazards within the operating environment
- Risk for Disuse Syndrome related to a decreased level of consciousness or to immobilization
- Hypothermia related to evaporation from skin and exposed tissue in a cool environment, body heat loss, alteration in the hypothalamus from anesthetic agents, inadequate body covering, or aging
- Ineffective Thermoregulation related to sedation, fluctuating environmental temperature, medications, or age extremes
- Fear related to the threat of death, actual or perceived, or to anticipation of events posing a threat to self-esteem
- Anxiety related to loss of control or the threat of death
- Deficient Fluid Volume related to decreased intake, evaporative fluid loss through the skin and exposed tissue, or blood loss
- Potential for Peripheral Neurovascular Dysfunction related to intraoperative positioning

Planning and Implementation

RISK FOR PERIOPERATIVE POSITIONING INJURY

PLANNING: EXPECTED OUTCOMES. The intraoperative client is expected to be free of injury.

INTERVENTIONS. Interventions are directed toward preventing injury resulting from intraoperative positioning. Because of preoperative medication, anesthetic agents, and the narrowness of the bed, the client's normal defense mechanisms cannot guard against nerve or joint damage and muscle stretch and strain. Proper positioning, therefore, is important. In addition, the incidence of pressure ulcer formation is greater in the postoperative client population than for those hospitalized clients who do not undergo surgery. The circulating nurse pads the operating bed with foam and/or silicone gel pads, properly places the grounding pads, coordinates the transfer to the operating bed, and helps the client obtain a comfortable position. The circulating nurse assesses the skin, especially of older clients, for bruising or injury, placing extra padding as indicated. A newer product designed to reduce pressure injury in the operating room (OR) is a mattress overlay made of urethane foam having a 25% indentation load deflection (ILD) of 30 pounds. The effectiveness of this device in preventing pressure ulcers during surgery is not consistent (see the Evidence-Based Practice for Nursing box on p. 280).

The client is usually in a **dorsal recumbent** (supine) position after transfer to the operating bed. Anesthesia may be administered with the client supine, and he or she may be repositioned for surgery. When general anesthesia is used, the nurse assists with repositioning (Figure 18-12).

EVIDENCE-BASED PRACTICE FOR NURSING

Is "newer" always "better?"

Schultz, A., et al. (1999). Etiology and incidence of pressure ulcers in surgical patients. *AORN Journal, 70*(3), 434-449.

This large, prospective, experimental study sought to determine whether an operating bed mattress overlay, made of foam with a 25% indentation load deflection (ILD) of 30 pounds and a density of 1.3, could reduce the incidence of pressure ulcer formation in surgical clients. A total of 413 surgical clients were randomized to a control (standard care) group or a treatment (mattress overlay) group during routine surgical procedures. The groups were highly homogeneous for *N* (control = 207; experimental = 206), mean age (~65 years), gender, surgical procedure, admission Braden Scale scores, body mass, operating room (OR) time, and the coexisting condition of diabetes. The time of first position change after surgery was recorded. All clients were examined for evidence of skin changes on postoperative days 1 through 6 by two research assistants blinded to the study groups. The research assistants received special training in use of the Braden Scale, and interrater reliability was set initially at 0.90 and re-established midway through the study.

The results showed that the incidence of early-stage pressure ulcers was not decreased by use of the mattress overlay. The incidence of pressure ulcers in the population studied was consistent with that found by other investigators; however, subjects in the study overall had less severe pressure ulcers than those in other studies of surgical clients. More severe pressure ulcers were correlated with greater age, the presence of diabetes, smaller body mass, and the use of the mattress overlay.

Critique. The study was well designed and implemented. Subjects were homogeneous and accrued from one setting, limiting the generalizability of the results. Pressure, as a variable, was not measured directly.

Implications for Nursing. Initially, it would seem that increased padding with the use of a mattress overlay would better protect clients from pressure ulcer development during surgical procedures when position cannot be changed. This study exemplifies the need to test all devices for effectiveness before changing standard procedures.

The circulating nurse coordinates repositioning of the client for surgery and modifies the position according to the client's safety and special needs. Factors influencing the *timing* of repositioning include the following:

- The surgical site
- The age and size of the client
- The anesthetic administration technique
- Pain experienced by the conscious client on movement

Factors influencing the actual *position* include the following:

- The specific procedure being performed
- The surgeon's request
- The client's age, size, and weight
- Any respiratory, skeletal, or neuromuscular limitations, such as rheumatoid arthritis, joint replacements, or emphysema

Table 18-6 presents possible complications related to prolonged surgical immobility and preventive nursing actions.

The dorsal recumbent, prone, lithotomy, and lateral positions are commonly used for surgery. Figure 18-12 illustrates common surgical positions and the use of protective padding. When general anesthesia is used, the nurse positions the client slowly to prevent blood vessel dilation that may produce hypotension. The nurse ensures proper positioning by assessing for the following:

- Physiologic alignment
- Minimal interference with circulation and respiration
- Protection of skeletal and neuromuscular structures
- Optimal exposure of the operative site and IV line
- Adequate access to the client for the anesthesia provider
- The client's comfort and safety
- Preservation of the client's dignity

The nurse must be aware of potential complications related to specific positions and modify care as indicated. For example, clients in the lithotomy position may develop leg swelling, pain in the legs or back, and diminished sensation or pulses. The nurse ensures proper padding and position changes at regular intervals. Throughout the intraoperative period, the nurse assists in preventing obstruction of circulation, respiratory efforts, or nerve impulse conduction caused by tight straps, improperly placed pads and pillows, or the position of the bed.

CRITICAL THINKING CHALLENGE

The 69-year-old client about to have knee replacement surgery is brought into the OR. She weighs 96 pounds and has type 2 diabetes.

- What areas on this client are most likely to be injured as a result of poor positioning or inadequate padding?
- In what position should you place this client for a left knee replacement?

For suggested answer guidelines, go to SIMON http://www.wbsaunders.com/SIMON/Iggy/.

IMPAIRED SKIN INTEGRITY AND IMPAIRED TISSUE INTEGRITY

PLANNING: EXPECTED OUTCOMES. The intraoperative client is expected to experience minimal skin and tissue impairment and contamination as a result of surgery.

INTERVENTIONS. Surgery is an invasive procedure that places the client at risk for complications related to the surgical wound (such as incisional tears and lacerations), bacterial contamination, and loss of body fluids from the wound during and after surgery. Sterile surgical technique and the use of protective drapes, skin closures, and dressings help to minimize complications and promote wound healing.

PLASTIC ADHESIVE DRAPE. If a sterile plastic adhesive drape is used, the scrub nurse helps the surgical assistant apply the drape after the surgical site has been cleaned and dried. The plastic drape is applied directly to the client's skin to prevent shifting and exposure of skin edges. *The surgeon makes the incision through the plastic drape.* The cut edge sticks to the skin and keeps the surgical incision sealed from the movement of bacteria into the wound. The scrub nurse and surgical assistant *gently* remove the drape after closure of the surgical incision. The nurse pays special attention to older clients and those with fragile skin to prevent skin tearing when the adhesive drape is removed.

SKIN CLOSURES. Skin and tissue closures, such as sutures and staples, are used to:

- Approximate wound edges until wound healing is complete
- Occlude blood vessels, preventing hemorrhage and fluid loss
- Prevent wound contamination

The quality of the wound edges and the type of closure material are two factors that determine the strength and integrity of

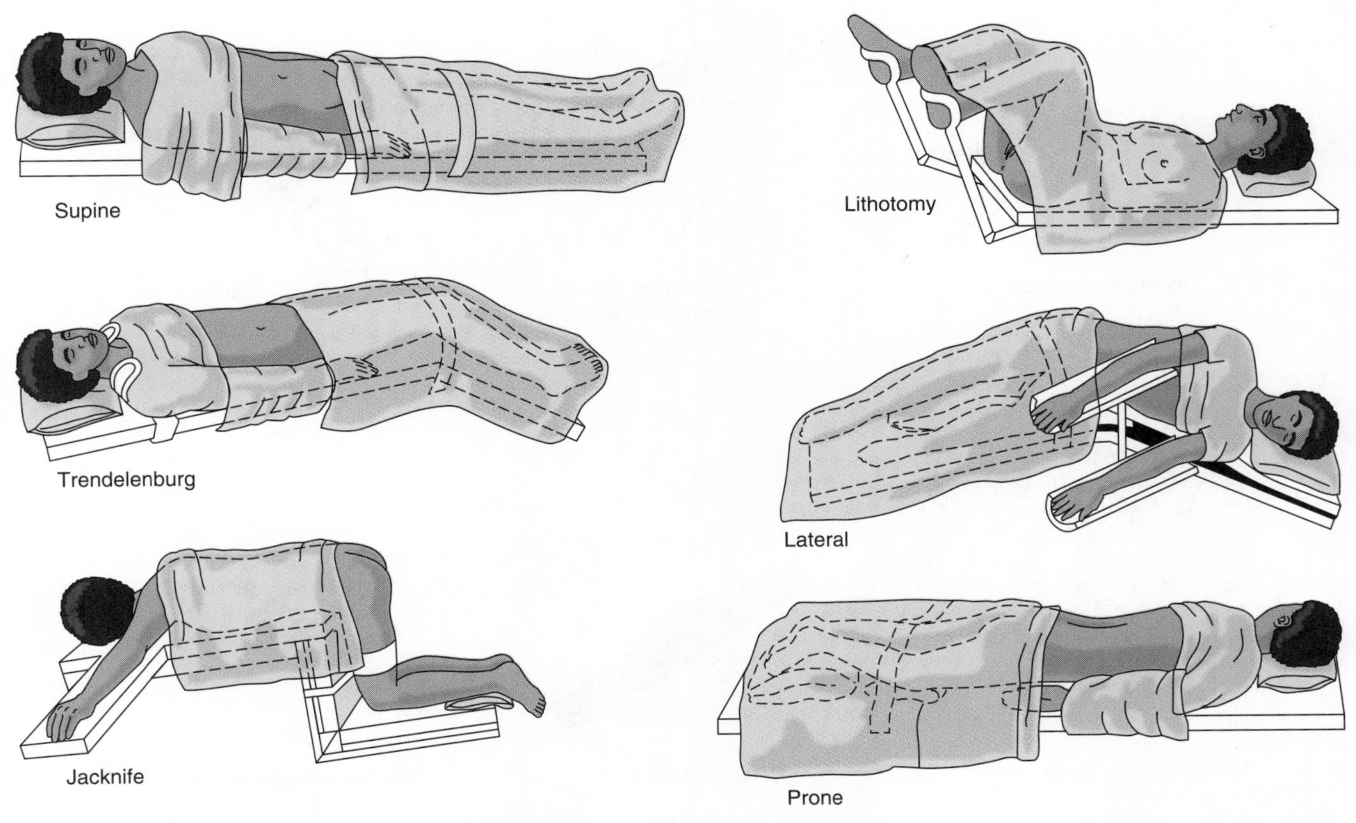

Figure 18-12 ● Common surgical positions.

TABLE 18-6 ● INTERVENTIONS TO PREVENT NEUROMUSCULAR COMPLICATIONS RELATED TO INTRAOPERATIVE POSITIONING

Anatomic Area	Complications	Interventions
Brachial plexus	Paralysis Loss of sensation in the arm and shoulder	Pad the elbow. Avoid excessive abduction. Secure the arm firmly on an arm board, positioned at shoulder level.
Radial nerve	Wrist drop	Support the wrist with padding. Do not overtighten wrist straps.
Medial or ulnar nerves	Hand deformities	Place a safety strap above or below the area.
Peroneal nerve	Foot drop	Place a pillow or padding under the knees. Support the lower extremities. Do not overtighten leg straps.
Tibial nerve	Loss of sensation on the plantar surface of the foot	Place a safety strap above the ankle. Do not place equipment on the lower extremities.
Joints	Stiffness Pain Inflammation	Place a pillow or foam padding under bony prominences. Maintain good body alignment. Slightly flex joints and support with pillows, trochanter rolls, or pads.

the closure. The wound is usually closed in layers to maintain tissue integrity and promote healing with minimal scarring. The surgeon selects the method and type of closures to be used on the basis of the surgical site, the tissue involved, the size and depth of the surgical wound, and the age and medical history of the client. A combination of sutures and clips is commonly used for closure of internal layers of the wound. Staples, retention (stay) sutures, and skin closure tapes (Steri-Strips) are used for closure of superficial wounds of the epidermis. Figure 18-13 illustrates commonly used wound closures.

A suture consists of one or more strands of material and is designated by its size, or gauge. The size designation sequence, from largest diameter to smallest, is 5, 4, 3, 2, 1, 0, 00 (2-0), 000 (3-0), 0000 (4-0), and so forth, to 11-0. Size 0

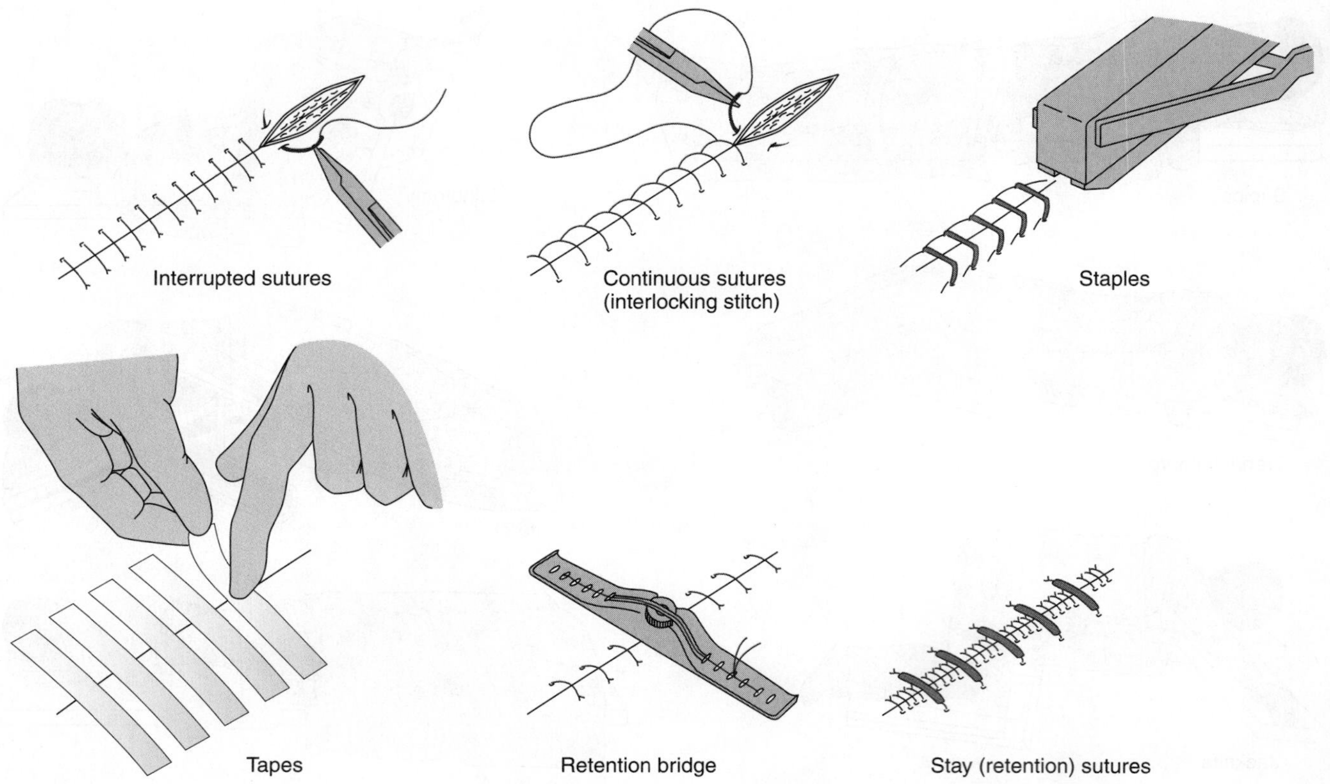

Figure 18-13 ● Common skin closures.

may be used to close the deep layers of an abdominal wound; 11-0 is the smallest-diameter suture and is used in plastic surgery and eye surgery. Other characteristics of the suture material, such as type (e.g., nylon, silk, Vicryl), color (e.g., green, blue, black, white, violet), and structure (e.g., twisted, braided), are listed on the package.

Suture material can be absorbable or nonabsorbable. **Absorbable sutures** are digested over time by body enzymes. These sutures first lose strength and then gradually disappear from the tissue. Catgut suture, such as "plain gut" and "chromic gut," is a type of natural absorbable suture material still in use today, although not as frequently as in the past. Other absorbable sutures are made of synthetic materials. The client's physical status, the presence of inflammation, and the type of suture used all influence the time for absorption, which is usually up to about 2 weeks.

Nonabsorbable sutures become encapsulated in the tissue during the healing process and remain embedded in the tissue unless they are removed. These sutures are made of silk, cotton, steel, nylon, polyester, or other synthetic material. *Body enzymes do not affect nonabsorbable sutures.* Nonabsorbable sutures are used for vascular anastomosis, "wiring" the sternum together after open heart surgery, and closing external wounds. The surgeon may use a double or interlocking stitch to increase the integrity of the closure. Retention (stay) sutures (see Figure 18-13) may be used in addition to standard suture material for clients at high risk for impaired wound healing (those having major abdominal surgery, obese clients, clients with diabetes, and clients taking steroids, which inhibit wound healing).

After the incision is closed, the physician may inject a local anesthetic or instill an antibiotic into the wound. A gauze or spray dressing may be applied to protect it from contamination. A variety of dressings may also be used to absorb drainage and provide support to the incision. A pressure dressing may be applied to prevent or stop a vascular area from bleeding postoperatively. One or more drains (see Chapter 19) may be inserted to prevent the accumulation of secretions and fluids within tissues around the surgical area. These secretions, if not drained, slow healing and promote bacterial growth, which could result in wound infection.

After the dressing is secure, the nurse coordinates the surgical team in repositioning and transfer. A roller board or a lift sheet is used for safe transfer from the operating bed to a stretcher or bed. Some clients are able to move themselves back over to the stretcher. The circulating nurse and anesthesia provider accompany the client to the postanesthesia care unit (PACU) and give a report of the client's intraoperative experience to the PACU nurse (see Chapter 19).

POTENTIAL FOR HYPOVENTILATION

PLANNING: EXPECTED OUTCOMES. The intraoperative client is expected to be free of damaging events related to hypoventilation.

INTERVENTIONS. Interventions are directed toward preventing injury resulting from anesthesia (see earlier discussion). The nurse, physician, and anesthesia provider monitor the client according to official standards. These standards, which have been adopted by both the American Society of Anesthesiologists and the American Association of Nurse Anesthetists, include continuous monitoring of ventilation, circulation, and cardiac rhythms; blood pressure and heart rate recordings every 5 minutes; and the continuous presence of an anesthesiology practitioner during the case (Biddle, 1994).

Evaluation: Outcomes

NOC The nurse evaluates the care of the intraoperative client on the basis of the identified nursing diagnoses and collaborative problems. The expected outcomes are that the client:

- Is safely anesthetized without complications
- Does not experience any injury related to intraoperative positioning or equipment
- Is free of skin or tissue contamination during surgery
- Is free of skin tears, bruises, redness, abrasion, or maceration over pressure points and elsewhere

ONLINE RESOURCES

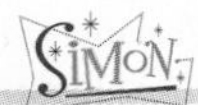

For suggested readings and Internet resources, go to http://www.wbsaunders.com/SIMON/Iggy/.

SELECTED BIBLIOGRAPHY

Asterisk indicates a classic or definitive work on this subject.

American Society of PeriAnesthesia Nurses. (1998). *Standards of perianesthesia nursing practice.* New Jersey: Author.

Arndt, K. (1999). Inadvertent hypothermia in the OR, *AORN Journal, 70*(2), 204-214.

Association of periOperative Registered Nurses. (1999a). Position statement: AORN official statement on RN first assistant. In *Standards, recommended practices and guidelines* (pp. 130-131). Denver: Author.

Association of periOperative Registered Nurses. (1999b). Position statement: Perioperative care of patients with do not resuscitate (DNR) orders. In *Standards, recommended practices and guidelines* (pp. 124-125). Denver: Author.

Association of periOperative Registered Nurses. (1999c). Recommended practices for the care and cleaning of surgical instruments and powered equipment. In *Standards, recommended practices and guidelines* (pp. 261-266). Denver: Author.

Association of periOperative Registered Nurses. (1999d). Recommended practices for disinfection. In *Standards, recommended practices and guidelines* (pp. 201-208). Denver: Author.

Association of periOperative Registered Nurses. (1999e). Recommended practices for documentation of perioperative nursing care. In *Standards, recommended practices and guidelines* (pp. 209-212). Denver: Author.

Association of periOperative Registered Nurses. (1999f). Recommended practices for environmental cleaning for the surgical practice setting. In *Standards, recommended practices and guidelines* (pp. 233-238). Denver: Author.

Association of periOperative Registered Nurses. (1999g). Recommended practices for hazards in the surgical environment. In *Standards, recommended practices and guidelines* (pp. 255-260). Denver: Author.

Association of periOperative Registered Nurses. (1999h). Recommended practices for laser safety in the practice setting. In *Standards, recommended practices and guidelines* (pp. 267-272). Denver: Author.

Association of periOperative Registered Nurses. (1999i). Recommended practices for managing the patient receiving conscious sedation/analgesia. In *Standards, recommended practices and guidelines* (pp. 189-194). Denver: Author.

Association of periOperative Registered Nurses. (1999j). Recommended practices for positioning the patient in the perioperative practice setting. In *Standards, recommended practices and guidelines* (pp. 289-292). Denver: Author.

Association of periOperative Registered Nurses. (1999k). Recommended practices for skin preparation. In *Standards, recommended practices and guidelines* (pp. 305-310). Denver: Author.

Association of periOperative Registered Nurses. (1999l). Recommended practices for sponge, sharp, and instrument counts. In *Standards, recommended practices and guidelines* (pp. 195-200). Denver: Author.

Association of periOperative Registered Nurses. (1999m). Recommended practices for sterile field-maintaining. In *Standards, recommended practices and guidelines* (pp. 317-322). Denver: Author.

Association of periOperative Registered Nurses. (1999n). Recommended practices for sterilization in the practice setting. In *Standards, recommended practices and guidelines* (pp. 323-334). Denver: Author.

Association of periOperative Registered Nurses. (1999o). Recommended practices for surgical attire. In *Standards, recommended practices and guidelines* (pp. 183-188). Denver: Author.

Association of periOperative Registered Nurses. (1999p). Recommended practices for surgical hand scrubs. In *Standards, recommended practices and guidelines* (pp. 249-254). Denver: Author.

Association of periOperative Registered Nurses. (1999q). Recommended practices for traffic patterns in the perioperative practice setting. In *Standards, recommended practices and guidelines* (pp. 341-345). Denver: Author.

Association of periOperative Registered Nurses. (1999r). Recommended practices for use and selection of barrier materials for surgical gowns and drapes. In *Standards, recommended practices and guidelines* (pp. 204-214). Denver: Author.

Association of periOperative Registered Nurses. (1999s). *Standards, recommended practices and guidelines.* Denver: Author.

Baker, B., et al. (1999). Ambulatory surgical clinical pathway. *Journal of PeriAnesthesia Nursing,* 14(1), 2-11.

*Ball, K.A. (1995). *Lasers: The perioperative challenge* (2nd ed.). St. Louis: Mosby.

*Ballantyne, G.H., Leahy, P.F., & Modlin, I.M. (1994). *Laparoscopic surgery.* Philadelphia: W.B. Saunders.

Belkin, N. (1997). APIC state of the art report: Use of scrubs and related apparel in health care facilities. *American Journal of Infection Control, 25*(5), 401-404.

Berg, M. (1998). An introduction to anesthesia-related medications. *Journal of PeriAnesthesia Nursing, 13*(4), 239-242.

Berkowitz, C.M. (1997). Conscious sedation: A primer. *RN, 60*(2), 32-36.

*Biddle, C. (1994). AANA journal course: Update for nurse anesthetists outcome measures in anesthesiology: Are we going in the right direction? *American Association of Nurse Anesthetists Journal, 62*(2), 117-124.

Bryan, R. (1997). Administering conscious sedation: Operational guidelines. *Critical Care Clinics of North America, 9*(3), 281-299.

Circulating by techs edges upward. (1998). *OR Manager, 14*(10), 23.

*Curry, M. (1994). Perioperative nursing care of the elderly patient: A case study. *ACORN Journal, 7*(2), 23-26.

Dunlap, K., & Wanzer, L. (1998). *AORN Journal, 68*(2), 265-272.

Dunn, D. (1997). Malignant hyperthermia. *AORN Journal, 65*(4), 728-762.

*Entrup, M.H. (1991). Perioperative complications of anesthesia. *Surgical Clinics of North America, 71*(6), 1151-1173.

Flower, J. (2000). Beyond surgery: Predictions for surgery in the next century. *Surgical Services Management, 6*(1), 29-32.

Folin, A., Nyberg, B., & Nordstrom, G. (2000). Reducing blood exposures during orthopedic surgical procedures. *AORN Journal, 71*(3), 573-582.

Friedman, C., et al. (1999). Special communication: requirements for infrastructure and essential activities of infection control and epidemiology in out-of-hospital settings: a consensus panel report. *American Journal of Infection Control, 27*(5), 418-430.

Gallo, S. (1999). Surgery in the twenty-first century. *Surgical Services Management, 5*(12), 18-21.

Geuder, D. (1999). Ambulatory surgery. In M.H. Meeker & J.C. Rothrock (Eds.), *Alexander's care of the patient in surgery* (11th ed., pp. 1189-1210). St. Louis: Mosby.

*Golanowski, M. (1995). Do not resuscitate: Informed consent in the operating room and postanesthesia care unit. *Journal of Post Anesthesia Nursing, 10*(1), 9-11.

*Green, S. (1996). Positioning the patient for surgery. *British Journal Theatre Nursing, 6*(5), 35-38.

Guidelines issued for infection control. (1998). *OR Manager, 14*(11), 26-28.

Homa, D., & Palfreyman, M. (2000). Infectious diseases in the O.R. *CRNA: The Clinical Forum for Nurse Anesthetists, 11*(1), 8-14.

Hussar, D.A. (1997). New drugs (ropivacaine HCl). *Nursing97, 27*(6), 38.

Jackson, S., & Van Norman, G. (1999) Goals and values–directed approach to informed consent in the "DNR" patient presenting for surgery. *Anesthesiology, 90*(1), 1-6.

Karlet, M. (1998). Ambulatory surgery: Malignant hyperthermia: Considerations for ambulatory surgery. *Journal of PeriAnesthesia Nursing, 13*(5), 304-312.

Kee, C., & Miller, V. (1999). Perioperative care of the older adult with auditory and visual changes. *AORN Journal, 70*(6), 1012-1019.

*Keffer, M.J. & Keffer, H.L. (1994). The do not resuscitate order: Moral responsibilities of the perioperative nurse. *AORN Journal, 59*(3), 641-650.

Kobs, A. (1997). Conscious sedation: Questions about the anesthesia continuum. *Nursing Management, 28*(4), 14, 17.

Kost, M. (1999). Conscious sedation: Guarding your patient against complications. *Nursing99, 29*(4), 34-39.

Landrum, L. (1997). A nursing guide to conscious sedation: Clarification of current practice issues. *Critical Care Clinics of North America, 9*(3), 411-422.

*Ley, S.J. (1996). Intraoperative and postoperative blood salvage. *AACN Clinical Issues: Advanced Practice in Acute and Critical Care, 7*(2), 238-248.

Mangram, A., et al. (1999). Guidelines for prevention of surgical site infection 1999. *Infection Control and Hospital Epidemiology, 20*(4), 250-278.

*McCraine, J. (1994). Fire safety in the operating room. *Today's OR Nurse, 16*(1), 33-37.

*McEwen, D.R. (1996). Intraoperative positioning of surgical patients. *AORN Journal, 63*(6), 1059-1063, 1066-1075, 1077-1082, 1084-1085.

Meckes, P.F. (1999). Geriatric surgery. In M.H. Meeker & J.C. Rothrock (Eds.), *Alexander's care of the patient in surgery* (11th ed., pp. 1283-1299). St. Louis: Mosby.

Meeker, M.H., & Rothrock, J.C. (1999). *Alexander's care of the patient in surgery* (11th ed.). St. Louis: Mosby.

O'Boyle, E.F. & Brochard, B. (1998). Latex allergy: Be prepared. *Surgical Services Management, 4*(3), 32-38.

*Omoigui, S. (1995). *The anesthesia drugs handbook* (2nd ed.). St. Louis: Mosby.

Ouellette, S., & Simpson, C. (1998). Monitoring for intraoperative awareness. *AORN Journal, 68*(6), 950-961.

Parker, L. (1999). Managing and maintaining a safe environment in the hospital setting. *British Journal of Nursing, 8*(16), 1053-1065.

Patient outcomes: Standards of perioperative care. (1997). *AORN Journal, 65*(2), 408-416.

Patty, C.M. (1999). Teaching affective competencies to surgical technologists. *AORN Journal, 70*(5), 776-781.

*Pearlman, R.C., et al. (1994). Intraoperative neural monitoring: An introduction for perioperative nurses . . . to determine whether nerve impulses are being conducted at normal levels. *AORN Journal, 60*(4), 648, 650-651.

Popolow, G. (1999). How robotics is transforming the OR. *Surgical Services Management, 5*(12), 35-39.

Regional, local blocks speed recovery. (1998). *OR Manager, 14*(11), 22-23.

*Rivelli, D. (1993). Local and regional anesthesia: Nursing implications. *Nursing Clinics of North America, 28*(3), 547-572.

*Roth, R.A. (1995). *Perioperative nursing core curriculum: Achieving competency in clinical practice.* Philadelphia: W.B. Saunders.

Schultz, A., et al. (1999). Etiology and incidence of pressure ulcers in surgical patients. *AORN Journal, 70*(3), 434-449.

*Stein, R.H. (1995). The perioperative nurse's role in anesthesia management. *AORN Journal, 62*(5), 794-795, 797-797, 801.

Vermett, E. (1998). Malignant hyperthermia. *American Journal of Nursing, 98*(4), 45.

*Voelker, R. (1995). Anesthesia-related risks have plummeted. *Journal of the American Medical Association, 273,* 445-446.

*Walsh, J. (1994). AANA journal course: Update for nurse anesthetists: Patient positioning. *American Association of Nurse Anesthetists Journal, 62*(3), 289-298.

Weighing cost savings with BIS. (1999). *OR Manager, 15*(11), 20-21.

Wheelock, S.M., & Lookinland, S. (1997). Effect of surgical hand scrub time on subsequent bacterial growth. *AORN Journal, 65*(6), 1087-1090, 1092, 1094-1098.

CHAPTER 19

Interventions for Postoperative Clients

REBECCA M. PATTON

Learning Objectives

After studying this chapter, you should be able to:

1. Describe the ongoing head-to-toe assessment of the postoperative client.
2. Recognize wound complications in the postoperative period.
3. Prioritize common nursing interventions for the client recovering from surgery and anesthesia during the first 24 hours.
4. Prioritize nursing care for the client experiencing postoperative respiratory depression.
5. Discuss the criteria for determining readiness of the postoperative client to be discharged from the postanesthesia care unit.
6. Discuss the teaching priorities for postoperative clients.

SIMON **Go to http://www.wbsaunders.com/SIMON/Iggy/ for self-assessment questions related to these Learning Objectives.**

The postoperative period begins with completion of the surgical procedure and transfer of the client to either the **postanesthesia care unit (PACU)** or, in the case of more critically ill clients, the intensive care unit. Discharge from these areas varies but is usually based on the stability of the client's condition and the meeting of specific discharge criteria. Many clients who have surgery are able to be discharged to home shortly after their procedure is completed. They are observed and monitored until discharge criteria are met and are then discharged. Some clients move from the specialized nursing care in the PACU to a hospital inpatient floor or critical care unit for additional nursing care during their postoperative period.

The actual postoperative period continues after the client's condition is stabilized, as well as after the client is discharged from the ambulatory surgery facility or hospital. The actual time spent away from home after surgery varies according to age, physical health, self-care ability, support systems, type and length of surgical procedure, anesthesia, complications (if any), and community resources.

OVERVIEW

The primary purpose of a PACU is the ongoing critical evaluation and stabilization of clients, with emphasis on anticipation, prevention, and treatment of complications after a surgical procedure. The PACU, or recovery room, is usually located close to the surgical suite or procedural rooms (e.g., endoscopy suite) for ease of access and client transfer. The unit is usually a large and open room to provide maximum visibility of clients, appropriate ventilation and lighting, and easy access to supplies and emergency equipment. Preferably, adults are separated from children. The client area in the unit is often divided into individual cubicles. Curtains or screens for privacy are available and are usually closed only during bedside procedures. Each cubicle is stocked with equipment and supplies commonly used by the nurse to monitor and care for the client, such as oxygen, suction equipment, cardiac monitors, airway equipment, and emergency medications.

After the surgical procedure is completed, the circulating nurse and the anesthesiologist, nurse anesthetist (certified registered nurse anesthetist [CRNA]), or anesthesia assistant (AA) accompany the client to the PACU. In some situations, such as when the client is in critical condition, he or she may go directly from the operating room (OR) to the intensive (critical) care unit. On arrival, the anesthesia provider and the circulating nurse give the postanesthesia nurse a verbal report (Table 19-1).

The postanesthesia nurse is skilled in the care of clients of all ages with multiple medical and surgical problems immediately after a surgical procedure. This nurse has in-depth knowledge of anesthetic agents, pharmacology, pain management, and surgical procedures; is skilled in physical and psychosocial assessment; and can make quick decisions if emergencies or complications occur. The postanesthesia nurse monitors the client closely and consults with the anesthesia provider and the surgeons as needed.

SIMON Activity Link

COLLABORATIVE MANAGEMENT

Assessment

HISTORY

The postanesthesia nurse uses the information from the surgical team's report in planning care. After receiving the report and assessing the client, the PACU nurse reviews the medical record for information about the client's history, presurgical physical

TABLE 19-1 • REPORT GUIDELINES ON ARRIVAL IN THE POSTANESTHESIA CARE UNIT

Anesthesiology personnel explain the following:
- Type and extent of the surgical procedure
- Type of anesthesia
- Client's tolerance of anesthesia and the surgical procedure
- Client's allergies
- Pathologic condition
- Status of vital signs
- Type and amount of IV fluids and medications administered
- Estimated blood loss (EBL)
- Any intraoperative complications, such as a traumatic intubation

The circulating nurse adds information related to the following:
- Client's primary language and any sensory impairments
- Client's anxiety level before receiving anesthesia
- Special requests that were verbalized by the client preoperatively
- Client's preoperative and intraoperative respiratory function and dysfunction
- Pertinent medical history
- Location and type of incisions, dressings, catheters, tubes, drains, or packing
- Intake and output, including current IV fluid administration and estimated blood loss
- Joint or limb immobility while in the operating room, especially in the older client
- Other intraoperative positioning that may be relevant in the postoperative phase
- Any other important intraoperative occurrences

condition, and emotional status. In ideal situations, the postanesthesia nurse reviews pertinent information before the client arrives in the unit. If the client is remaining as an inpatient, the nurse on the medical-surgical unit later incorporates all of the surgical and postanesthesia information into the postoperative plan of care. Chapter 17 identifies clinical situations that put a client at risk for the following postoperative complications:

- Allergic reactions
- Hypothermia
- Hyperthermia
- Hypertension
- Hypotension
- Hypovolemic shock
- Renal failure
- Electrolyte imbalances
- Dysrhythmias
- Congestive heart failure
- Paralytic ileus
- Acute urinary retention
- Deep vein thrombosis
- Pulmonary embolism
- Atelectasis or pneumonia
- Laryngeal edema
- Ventilator dependence
- Gastrointestinal (GI) bleeding
- Disseminated intravascular coagulation (DIC)
- Anemia
- Wound evisceration

PHYSICAL ASSESSMENT/CLINICAL MANIFESTATIONS

The postanesthesia nurse assesses the client and compiles data on a postanesthesia care unit (PACU) record form (Figure 19-1). Assessment data include level of consciousness, temperature, pulse, respiration, and blood pressure. The nurse examines the surgical area for bleeding. The postanesthesia nurse initiates assessments, and the intensive care or medical-surgical nurse continues assessments when the client is discharged to the inpatient unit. Vital signs are monitored with a frequency that is based on the facility's policy, the client's condition, and the surgeon's orders. Once the client is discharged from the PACU, vital signs are often recorded every 15 minutes for four times, every 30 minutes for four times, every 2 hours for four times, and then every 4 hours for 24 to 48 hours if the client's condition is stable. Thereafter, vital signs are assessed according to the facility's policy, the client's condition, and the nurse's judgment.

The health care team determines the client's readiness for discharge from the postanesthesia area by noting a postanesthesia recovery score on the postanesthesia recovery scale of at least 10 (see Figure 19-1). In addition, the facility may have specific criteria for discharge (e.g., stable vital signs; normothermia; no overt bleeding; return of gag, cough, and swallow reflexes; and the ability to take liquids). After the nurse determines that all criteria have been met, the client is discharged by the anesthesiologist to the hospital unit or to home. If an anesthesiologist has not been involved, which may be the case with local anesthesia or conscious sedation, the surgeon or nurse discharges the client once the discharge criteria have been met.

Physical assessment continues from the PACU to the intensive care or medical-surgical nursing unit. If the client is to be discharged from the PACU to home, physical assessment is continued by home care nurses or by the client or family members after adequate instruction.

RESPIRATORY SYSTEM

AIRWAY ASSESSMENT. When the client is admitted to the PACU, the nurse immediately assesses for a patent airway and adequate respiratory exchange. An artificial airway, such as an endotracheal (ET) tube, a nasal trumpet, or an oral airway, may be in place. If the client is receiving supplemental oxygen, the nurse notes the type of delivery device and the concentration or liter flow of the oxygen. The nurse usually maintains continuous pulse oximetry for monitoring oxygen saturation while the client is in the PACU.

The nurse assesses the rate, pattern, and depth of respirations to measure the adequacy of air exchange. A respiratory rate of fewer than 10 breaths per minute may indicate anesthetic or opioid analgesic depression. Rapid, shallow respirations signal cardiovascular compromise, increased metabolic rate, or pain.

BREATH SOUNDS. The nurse auscultates the lungs over all lung fields to determine the quality and adequacy of breath sounds. Symmetry of breath sounds also is assessed. If, for example, the client has an ET tube, it could move down into the right mainstem bronchus and prevent left lung expansion. In this case, lung sounds on the left would be absent or decreased and only the right chest wall would rise and fall with respirations.

OTHER RESPIRATORY ASSESSMENTS. Respiratory assessment by the postanesthesia nurse includes ongoing inspection of the chest wall for accessory muscle use, sternal retraction, and diaphragmatic breathing. These signs could indicate an excessive anesthetic effect, airway obstruction, or

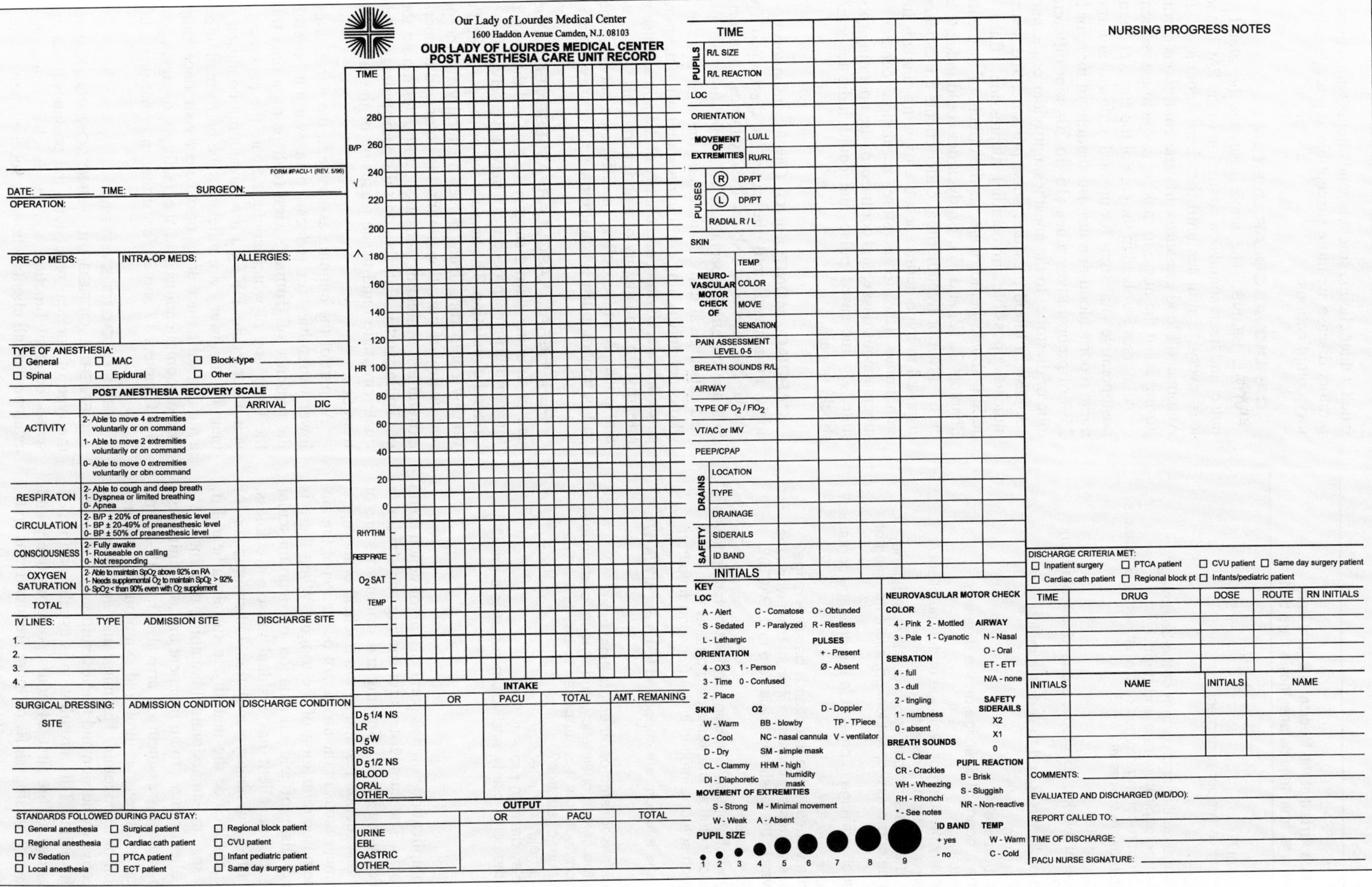

Our Lady of Lourdes Medical Center
1600 Haddon Avenue Camden, N.J. 08103

OUR LADY OF LOURDES MEDICAL CENTER
POST ANESTHESIA CARE UNIT RECORD

FORM #PACU-1 (REV. 5/96)

DATE: ______ TIME: ______ SURGEON: ______
OPERATION:

PRE-OP MEDS:	INTRA-OP MEDS:	ALLERGIES:

TYPE OF ANESTHESIA:
☐ General ☐ MAC ☐ Block-type ______
☐ Spinal ☐ Epidural ☐ Other ______

POST ANESTHESIA RECOVERY SCALE		ARRIVAL	DIC
ACTIVITY	2- Able to move 4 extremities voluntarily or on command 1- Able to move 2 extremities voluntarily or on command 0- Able to move 0 extremities voluntarily or obn command		
RESPIRATON	2- Able to cough and deep breath 1- Dyspnea or limited breathing 0- Apnea		
CIRCULATION	2- B/P ± 20% of preanesthesic level 1- BP ± 20-49% of preanesthesic level 0- BP ± 50% of preanesthesic level		
CONSCIOUSNESS	2- Fully awake 1- Rouseable on calling 0- Not responding		
OXYGEN SATURATION	2- Able to maintain SpO_2 above 92% on RA 1- Needs supplemental O_2 to maintain SpO_2 > 92% 0- SpO_2 < than 90% even with O_2 supplement		
TOTAL			

IV LINES:	TYPE	ADMISSION SITE	DISCHARGE SITE
1.			
2.			
3.			
4.			

SURGICAL DRESSING: SITE	ADMISSION CONDITION	DISCHARGE CONDITION

STANDARDS FOLLOWED DURING PACU STAY:
☐ General anesthesia ☐ Surgical patient ☐ Regional block patient
☐ Regional anesthesia ☐ Cardiac cath patient ☐ CVU patient
☐ IV Sedation ☐ PTCA patient ☐ Infant pediatric patient
☐ Local anesthesia ☐ ECT patient ☐ Same day surgery patient

TIME
B/P 280 260 240 √ 220 200 ^ 180 160 140 • 120 HR 100 80 60 40 20 0
RHYTHM
RESP RATE
O_2 SAT
TEMP

INTAKE	OR	PACU	TOTAL	AMT. REMANING
$D_5$1/4 NS LR D_5W PSS $D_5$1/2 NS BLOOD ORAL OTHER ____				

OUTPUT	OR	PACU	TOTAL
URINE EBL GASTRIC OTHER ____			

TIME						
PUPILS R/L SIZE						
PUPILS R/L REACTION						
LOC						
ORIENTATION						
MOVEMENT OF EXTREMITIES LU/LL						
MOVEMENT OF EXTREMITIES RU/RL						
PULSES (R) DP/PT						
PULSES (L) DP/PT						
PULSES RADIAL R / L						
SKIN						
NEURO-VASCULAR MOTOR CHECK OF TEMP						
COLOR						
MOVE						
SENSATION						
PAIN ASSESSMENT LEVEL 0-5						
BREATH SOUNDS R/L						
AIRWAY						
TYPE OF O_2 / FIO_2						
VT/AC or IMV						
PEEP/CPAP						
DRAINS LOCATION						
DRAINS TYPE						
DRAINS DRAINAGE						
SAFETY SIDERAILS						
SAFETY ID BAND						
INITIALS						

KEY
LOC
A - Alert C - Comatose O - Obtunded
S - Sedated P - Paralyzed R - Restless
L - Lethargic
ORIENTATION
4 - OX3 1 - Person
3 - Time 0 - Confused
2 - Place
PULSES
+ - Present
Ø - Absent
SKIN
W - Warm
C - Cool
D - Dry
CL - Clammy
DI - Diaphoretic
O2
BB - blowby
NC - nasal cannula
SM - simple mask
HHM - high humidity mask
D - Doppler
TP - TPiece
V - ventilator
MOVEMENT OF EXTREMITIES
S - Strong M - Minimal movement
W - Weak A - Absent
PUPIL SIZE
1 2 3 4 5 6 7 8 9

NEUROVASCULAR MOTOR CHECK
COLOR
4 - Pink 2 - Mottled
3 - Pale 1 - Cyanotic
SENSATION
4 - full
3 - dull
2 - tingling
1 - numbness
0 - absent
BREATH SOUNDS
CL - Clear
CR - Crackles
WH - Wheezing
RH - Rhonchi
* - See notes
AIRWAY
N - Nasal
O - Oral
ET - ETT
N/A - none
SAFETY SIDERAILS
X2
X1
0
PUPIL REACTION
B - Brisk
S - Sluggish
NR - Non-reactive
ID BAND
+ yes
- no
TEMP
W - Warm
C - Cold

NURSING PROGRESS NOTES

DISCHARGE CRITERIA MET:
☐ Inpatient surgery ☐ PTCA patient ☐ CVU patient ☐ Same day surgery patient
☐ Cardiac cath patient ☐ Regional block pt ☐ Infants/pediatric patient

TIME	DRUG	DOSE	ROUTE	RN INITIALS

INITIALS	NAME	INITIALS	NAME

COMMENTS: ______
EVALUATED AND DISCHARGED (MD/DO): ______
REPORT CALLED TO: ______
TIME OF DISCHARGE: ______
PACU NURSE SIGNATURE: ______

Figure 19-1 ● Example of a postanesthesia care unit record. (Courtesy Our Lady of Lourdes Medical Center, Camden, NJ.)

CHART 19-1

FOCUSED ASSESSMENT *of*
The Client on Arrival at the Medical-Surgical Unit After Discharge from the Postanesthesia Care Unit

Airway
- Is it patent?
- Is the neck in proper alignment?

Breathing
- What is the quality and pattern of the breathing?
- What is the respiratory rate and depth?
- Is the client receiving oxygen? At what setting? What is the pulse oximetry result?

Mental Status
- Is the client awake, able to be aroused, oriented, and aware?
- Does the client respond to verbal stimuli?

Surgical Incision Site
- How is it dressed?
- Mark the amount of drainage on the dressing immediately.
- Is there any bleeding or drainage under the client?
- Are there any drains present?
- Are the drains set properly (e.g., compressed if they should be compressed, not kinked, client not lying on them)?
- How much drainage is present in the drainage container?

Temperature, Pulse, and Blood Pressure
- Are these values within the client's baseline range?
- Are these values significantly different from when the client was in the postanesthesia care unit (PACU)?

Intravenous Fluids
- What type of solution is infusing and with what additives?
- How much solution was remaining on arrival?
- How much solution infused in the transport time from PACU?
- What is the infusion rate supposed to be set at? Is it?

Other Tubes
- Is there a nasogastric or other intestinal tube?
- What is the color, consistency, and amount of drainage?
- Is it set on suction if it is supposed to be? Is it on the right amount of suction?
- Is there a Foley catheter?
- Is the Foley draining properly?
- What is the color, clarity, and volume of urine output?

neurologic complications such as paralysis, all of which could result in hypoxia. The nurse listens for snoring and **stridor** (a high-pitched crowing sound). Snoring and stridor are signs of upper airway obstruction resulting from tracheal or laryngeal spasm or edema, mucus in the airway, or occlusion of the airway from edema or relaxation of the tongue. When there is delayed metabolism of and elimination of neuromuscular blocking agents, the client has residual muscle weakness, which could affect pulmonary ventilation. Other indicators of muscle weakness include the inability to sustain a head lift, weak handgrasps, and an abdominal breathing pattern.

When the client returns to an inpatient unit, the unit nurse completes an initial assessment on arrival (Chart 19-1) and then continues to assess for signs and symptoms of respiratory depression or hypoxemia. The nurse also auscultates the lungs for effective expansion and for adventitious or other abnormal breath sounds. This auscultation is usually performed every 4 hours during the first 24 hours postoperatively and then during every nursing shift, or more frequently, as indicated. Older clients, smokers, and clients with a history of respiratory disease are more susceptible to postoperative respiratory complications.

CARDIOVASCULAR SYSTEM

VITAL SIGNS. The nurse assesses the blood pressure, pulse, and heart sounds on admission to the PACU and then at least every 15 minutes until the client's condition stabilizes. Automated blood pressure cuffs and continuous cardiac monitoring assist the nurse in making frequent assessments.

All nurses involved in the care of the surgical client review postoperative vital signs for upward or downward trends. The nurse reports blood pressure fluctuations of more or less than 25% of preoperative values (15- to 20-point difference, systolic or diastolic) to the anesthesia provider or the surgeon. A decrease in blood pressure, pulse pressure, and heart sounds indicates possible myocardial depression, fluid volume deficit, shock, hemorrhage, or the effects of medication (see Chapters 7, 12, and 37). Bradycardia could indicate an anesthesia effect or hypothermia. Older clients are especially predisposed to hypothermia because of aging changes in the hypothalamus (the temperature regulation center), loss of subcutaneous tissue, and coolness of the operating room (OR) suite. An increased pulse rate could indicate hemorrhage, shock, or pain.

CARDIAC MONITORING. Cardiac monitoring is routinely maintained until the client is discharged from the PACU. For clients at risk for dysrhythmias, monitoring may continue on either specialized telemetry units or on general medical-surgical units. In assessing the vital signs of a client who is not undergoing continuous monitoring, the nurse compares the rate, rhythm, and quality of the apical pulse with the rate, rhythm, and quality of a peripheral pulse, such as the radial pulse. A **pulse deficit** (a difference between the apical and peripheral pulses) could indicate a dysrhythmia.

PERIPHERAL VASCULAR ASSESSMENT. Anesthesia and positioning during surgery (e.g., the lithotomy position for genitourinary procedures) may adversely affect the peripheral circulation. The nurse assesses the peripheral circulation by comparing distal pulses bilaterally for the presence and quality of pulsation, noting the color and temperature of extremities, evaluating sensation, and determining the speed of capillary refill. Palpable dorsalis pedis pulses indicate adequate circulation and tissue perfusion of the distal lower extremities.

As part of the ongoing assessment, the nurse assesses the lower extremities for redness, pain, warmth, swelling, and the presence of **Homan's sign** (calf pain on dorsiflexion of the foot), any of which could indicate the presence of deep vein thrombosis (DVT), a life-threatening condition. Assessment of the lower extremities may be performed once during a nursing shift, once daily, or once per visit, depending on the risk of complications and the facility's or agency's policy. (See Chapters 17 and 36 for further information on DVT.)

NEUROLOGIC SYSTEM

GENERAL CEREBRAL FUNCTIONING. Regardless of the type of surgical procedure, the postanesthesia nurse assesses cerebral function and the level of consciousness or awareness of all clients who have received general anesthesia

TABLE 19-2 • IMMEDIATE POSTOPERATIVE NEUROLOGIC ASSESSMENT: RETURN TO PREOPERATIVE LEVEL

ORDER OF RETURN TO CONSCIOUSNESS AFTER GENERAL ANESTHESIA
1. Muscular irritability
2. Restlessness and delirium
3. Recognition of pain
4. Ability to reason and control behavior

ORDER OF RETURN OF MOTOR AND SENSORY FUNCTIONING AFTER LOCAL OR REGIONAL ANESTHESIA
1. Sense of touch
2. Sense of pain
3. Sense of warmth
4. Sense of cold
5. Ability to move

(Table 19-2) or any type of sedation. To assess level of consciousness, the nurse observes for lethargy, restlessness, or irritability and tests coherence and orientation. The nurse determines awareness by observing responses to calling the client's name, touching the client, and giving simple commands such as "Open your eyes" and "Take a deep breath." Eye opening in response to a command indicates wakefulness or arousability but not necessarily awareness. The nurse determines the degree of orientation to person, place, and time by asking the conscious client to answer simple questions such as "What is your name?" (person), "Where are you?" (place), and "What day is it?" (time).

CONSIDERATIONS FOR OLDER ADULTS

For an older client, a rapid return to his or her prior level of orientation may not be realistic. Preoperative, intraoperative, and postoperative medications and anesthetic agents often affect the older client's reorientation ability (see Chapters 17 and 18).

The nurse compares the client's preoperative baseline neurologic status with the postoperative assessment findings. Clients with altered cerebral functioning preoperatively as a result of a pre-existing condition continue to have that alteration postoperatively. After the client has returned to a satisfactory level of consciousness (and all other criteria have been met), he or she is discharged from the postanesthesia care unit (PACU). Assessment of level of consciousness continues every 4 to 8 hours or as indicated by the client's condition and the facility's policy.

MOTOR/SENSORY ASSESSMENT. For all clients receiving general and regional anesthesia, motor and sensory function is assessed. General anesthesia renders clients unconscious and depresses voluntary motor function; regional anesthesia alters the motor and sensory function of only part of the body. (See Chapter 18 for more information on anesthesia.) Motor and sensory assessment is especially important after epidural or spinal anesthesia. The postanesthesia nurse evaluates motor function by instructing the client to move each extremity. The client who had epidural or spinal anesthesia remains in the PACU until sensory function (feeling) and voluntary motor movement of the lower extremities have returned (see Table 19-2). In addition, the nurse assesses the strength of each limb and compares the results bilaterally.

The postanesthesia nurse also tests for the return of sympathetic nervous system tone by gradually elevating the client's head and monitoring for hypotension. This evaluation begins after the client's sensation has returned to at least the spinal dermatome level of T10. (See Chapter 41 for further neurologic assessment.) After the client is transferred to the nursing unit, the medical-surgical nurse continues neurologic assessment as indicated.

FLUID AND ELECTROLYTE BALANCE. Fasting before and during surgery, the loss of fluid during the procedure, and the type and amount of blood or intravenous (IV) fluid administered affect the client's postoperative fluid and electrolyte balance. Fluid volume deficit or fluid volume overload may occur after surgery. Sodium, potassium, chloride, and calcium imbalances also may result, as may alterations in other electrolyte levels. Complications of fluid and electrolyte imbalances occur more often in older or debilitated clients and in clients with medical problems such as diabetes mellitus, Crohn's disease (especially after major intestinal surgery), or heart failure.

INTAKE AND OUTPUT. Intraoperative intake and output measurement is part of the operative record and part of the circulating nurse's report to the postanesthesia nurse. The postanesthesia nurse records any intake or output, including IV fluid intake, vomitus, urine, and nasogastric (NG) tube drainage. When receiving the report, the medical-surgical nurse needs to know the total intake and output from both the OR and the PACU to assess fluid balance accurately and to complete the 24-hour intake and output record.

HYDRATION ASSESSMENT. The medical-surgical nurse continues to assess the client's hydration. To determine hydration status, the nurse inspects the color and moist appearance of mucous membranes; the turgor, texture, and "tenting" of the skin (test over the sternum or forehead of an older client); the amount of drainage on dressings; and the presence of axillary sweat. Total output (e.g., NG tube drainage, urine output, and wound drainage) is measured and compared with total intake to identify a possible fluid imbalance. The nurse considers insensible fluid loss when reviewing total output. Intake and output continue to be assessed as long as the client is at risk for fluid imbalances. Some facilities have policies that require intake and output to be measured if the client receives IV fluids or has a catheter, drains, or an NG tube.

INTRAVENOUS FLUIDS. The nurse administers and closely monitors IV fluids to promote fluid and electrolyte balance. Standard isotonic solutions such as lactated Ringer's (LR) and 5% dextrose with lactated Ringer's (D_5/LR) are used for IV fluid replacement and maintenance in the PACU. After the client returns to the medical-surgical unit, the type and rate of administration of IV solutions are based on need. A typical IV solution for the client being admitted to the nursing unit is 5% dextrose with 0.45% normal saline (D_5 0.45% NSS). (See Chapters 12 and 14 for further discussion of IV fluid administration, electrolyte balance, and assessment of hydration.)

ACID-BASE BALANCE. Acid-base balance may be affected by preoperative, intraoperative, and postoperative respiratory status; intraoperative metabolic changes; and losses of acids or bases in drainage. For example, NG tube drainage or vomitus causes a loss of hydrochloric acid and contributes to alkalosis. The nurse assesses acid-base status through arterial blood gas measurement and other laboratory values. (See Chapter 16 for more detailed information on acid-base imbalances.)

RENAL/URINARY SYSTEM. Voluntary control of urinary system function may return immediately after surgery or may not return for 6 to 8 hours or longer after inhalation, IV, or epidural or spinal anesthesia. The effects of preoperative medications, anesthetic agents, or manipulation during surgery can cause urinary retention. The nurse assesses for this complication by inspection, palpation, and percussion of the lower abdomen for bladder distention. Assessment may be difficult to perform after lower abdominal surgery. Urinary retention is common in the early postoperative period and requires appropriate intervention, which is often one or more intermittent (straight) catheterizations to empty the bladder.

When the client has an indwelling urinary (Foley) catheter, the nurse assesses the urine for color, clarity, and amount. If the client is voiding, the nurse also assesses the urinary frequency, associated amount per void, and any symptoms. Urine output should correlate with total input for a 24-hour period, and other sources of output also need to be considered. The nurse reports a urine output of less than 30 mL/hr (240 mL per 8-hour nursing shift) to the physician. Decreased urine output may indicate hypovolemia or renal complications. (See Chapter 69 for complete information on the assessment of renal/urinary system function, including the interpretation of specific gravity, electrolyte values, and osmolality of urine.)

GASTROINTESTINAL SYSTEM

NAUSEA AND VOMITING. One of the most common postoperative reactions is nausea and vomiting. Approximately 30% of clients receiving general anesthesia have some form of gastrointestinal (GI) upset within the first 24 hours after surgery. Preventive therapy has been effective in reducing the incidence. A frequently used drug, especially in the ambulatory setting, is droperidol (Inapsine). Clients with a history of motion sickness are more likely to develop postoperative nausea and vomiting. Obese individuals may be at risk because many anesthetics are retained by fat cells and therefore have a lingering effect. Abdominal surgery and the use of opioid analgesics reduce intestinal peristalsis after surgery. These situations predispose the client to nausea and vomiting for longer than the first 24 hours after surgery.

Postoperative nausea and vomiting can cause stress and irritation of abdominal and GI wounds, increase intracranial pressure in clients who had head and neck surgery, elevate intraocular pressure in clients who had eye surgery, and increase the risk of aspiration and aspiration pneumonia. The nurse assesses for nausea and vomiting continuously. Often clients experience nausea as the head of the bed is raised in the early postoperative period. This symptom may occur with or without associated dizziness. By having the client in a side-lying position before raising his or her head slowly, the nurse can help reduce this distressing symptom.

GASTROINTESTINAL PERISTALSIS. The nurse in the postanesthesia care unit (PACU) and later on the medical-surgical unit assesses for the return of peristaltic function. Peristalsis may be delayed because of the length of time the client is under anesthesia, the amount of bowel handling intraoperatively, and opioid analgesic use. Clients who have abdominal surgery may have decreased peristalsis for at least 24 hours; this may persist for several days for those who have GI surgery.

ASSESSMENT. The nurse auscultates for bowel sounds in all four abdominal quadrants and at the umbilicus. If the client is undergoing NG suctioning, the suction must be turned off before auscultation of the abdomen to prevent mistaking the sound of the suction for bowel sounds. In addition, the nurse asks the client whether flatus has been passed. Both bowel sounds and flatus passage indicate peristalsis; abdominal cramping denotes trapped, nonmoving gas and not peristalsis.

COMPLICATIONS. Decreased peristalsis can occur in clients with paralytic ileus. The intestine wall is distended, and there is no movement of the intestinal wall **(aperistalsis).** The nurse assesses for the clinical manifestations of paralytic ileus. These include few or absent bowel sounds, a distended abdomen, diffuse abdominal discomfort (as a result of the distention), vomiting, lack of flatus, and no passage of stool.

The client may also experience constipation postoperatively as a result of anesthesia, analgesia (especially codeine and other opioid analgesics), decreased activity, and decreased oral intake. The nurse assesses the abdomen by inspection, palpation, percussion, and auscultation and records the elimination pattern to determine whether interventions are needed. Increased dietary fiber intake, the administration of mild laxatives or bulk-forming agents, or the use of enemas may be necessary.

NASOGASTRIC TUBE DRAINAGE. A nasogastric (NG) tube may be inserted intraoperatively to decompress and drain the stomach, to promote GI rest, to allow the lower GI tract to heal, and to provide an enteral feeding route. It may also be used to monitor the occurrence of bleeding and prevent intestinal obstruction. The Levin tube and the Salem sump tube are the two most common tubes used. The Salem tube is a double-lumen tube with an air vent to keep the tube from adhering to the gastric mucosa. This feature allows easy drainage of the stomach and prevents gastric mucosal damage. The Levin tube is a single-lumen tube with no air vent. To promote drainage, varying degrees of suction (high, medium, or low) are applied to the NG tube. Suction is either continuous (recommended for the Salem tube) or intermittent on the basis of the surgeon's preference and the tube type.

ASSESSMENT. The nurse records the color, consistency, and amount of the drained material every 8 hours (Table 19-3). In some instances, the results of an occult blood test (Gastroccult) may also be recorded. Normal NG drainage fluid is greenish yellow; red drainage fluid indicates active bleeding, and brown liquid or drainage with a coffee-ground appearance indicates the possibility of old bleeding.

COMPLICATIONS. The nurse assesses the client for possible complications related to NG tube use, including fluid and electrolyte imbalances, aspiration, and nares discomfort. To prevent aspiration, the nurse checks the tube placement every 4 to 8 hours and before the instillation of irrigation solution into the tube. (See Chapter 56 for information on tube place-

TABLE 19-3 • CALCULATING NASOGASTRIC TUBE DRAINAGE

FORMULA

Drainage in collection device − Amount of irrigant = True (actual) amount of drainage

EXAMPLE

A client's drainage container was marked at 150 mL at 7 AM. At 3 PM, there was 525 mL in the container. During the nursing shift, the nurse instilled 30 mL of saline as an irrigant into the tube four times, as ordered by the physician.

525 mL − 150 mL = 375 mL of drainage

30 mL × 4 = 120 mL of irrigant

375 mL − 120 mL = 255 mL of actual drainage

ment and care.) After gastric surgery, the tube should not be manipulated or irrigated without an order from the physician. Fluid and electrolyte imbalances can result from NG drainage and tube irrigation with water instead of saline. Imbalances include fluid volume deficit (see Chapter 12), hypokalemia and hyponatremia (see Chapter 13), hypochloremia, and metabolic alkalosis (see Chapter 16).

INTEGUMENTARY SYSTEM. The clean surgical wound heals itself at skin level in approximately 2 weeks in the absence of trauma, connective tissue disease, malnutrition, or the use of some medications, such as steroids. Smokers, older clients, obese clients, and those with diseases that decrease immunity have delayed wound healing. Complete healing of underlying tissue and return to presurgical integrity may take 6 months to 2 years. The physical condition and age of the client, size and location of the wound, and stress on the surgical wound also affect the length of time for wound healing. Because of the rich blood supply, wounds of the face and head heal more quickly than abdominal and leg wounds.

NORMAL WOUND HEALING. During the first few days of normal wound healing, the incised tissue regains blood supply and begins to bind together. Fibrin from the clotting process and a thin layer of epithelial cells seal the incision. After 1 to 4 days, epithelial cells continue to grow along the fibrin while growing strands of collagen begin to fill in the gaps in the wound (Strimike, Wojcik, & Stark, 1997). This process continues for 2 to 3 weeks, after which time the wound appears to be healed; however, healing is not complete for up to 2 years, until the scar is strengthened. (See Chapter 67 for discussion of wound healing and wound infection.)

When the client is an inpatient, the surgeon usually removes the original postoperative dressing on the first or second postoperative day. The nurse assesses the incision on a regular basis, usually every 8 hours, for redness, increased warmth, swelling, tenderness or pain, and the type and amount of drainage. Some drainage, changing from **sanguineous** (bloody) to serosanguineous to **serous** (serum-like, or yellow), is normal during the first few days. Serosanguineous drainage continuing beyond the fifth postoperative day should alert the nurse to the possibility of dehiscence, and the surgeon should be notified. Slight crusting on the incision line is normal, as is a pink color to the line itself, which is caused by inflammation from the surgical procedure. Slight swelling under the sutures or staples is also normal. Redness or swelling of or around the incision line, excessive tenderness or pain on palpation, and purulent or odorous drainage could indicate wound infection and is reported to the surgeon.

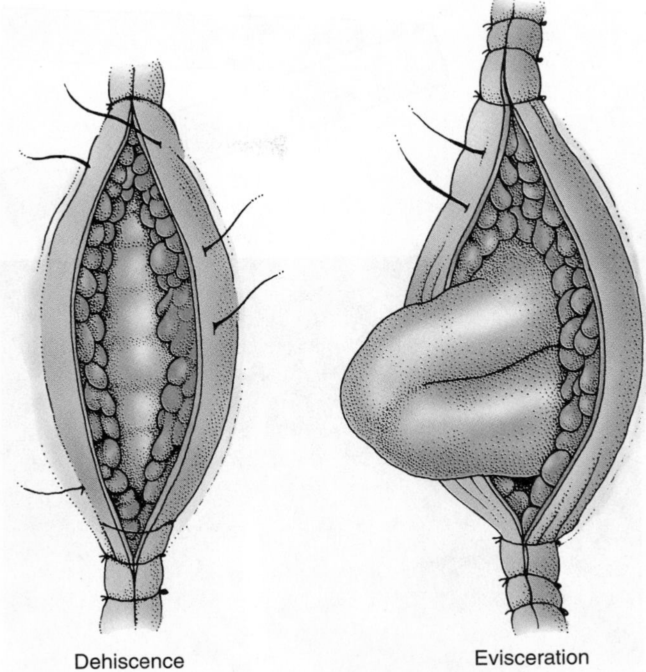

Figure 19-2 • Complications of wound healing.

INEFFECTIVE WOUND HEALING. Ineffective wound healing may be caused by wound infection, distention from edema or paralytic ileus, stress at the surgical site, and pre-existing conditions that cause delayed wound healing. Wound **dehiscence** is a partial or complete separation of the outer layers of the wound, sometimes described as a "splitting open of the wound." **Evisceration** is the total separation of the layers and extrusion of internal organs or viscera (usually abdominal) through the open wound (Figure 19-2). Both of these alterations in wound healing are more often seen between the fifth and tenth postoperative days and occur more frequently in obese clients or others predisposed to delayed wound healing. Wound dehiscence or evisceration may be preceded by excessive coughing, not splinting the surgical site during movement, vomiting, or straining. The client may state, "Something gave way" or "I feel as if I just split open."

DRESSINGS AND DRAINS. All dressings, including casts and elastic (Ace) bandages, are assessed for bleeding or other drainage on admission to the PACU and then frequently until the client is discharged to home or transferred to the inpatient unit. The nurse assesses the dressing each time vital signs are taken. When inspecting the dressing, the nurse checks for drainage and notes the amount, color, consistency, and odor of the drainage fluid. The area underneath the client is checked, because drainage (often blood from hemorrhage) may leak from the side of the dressing and yet not appear on the dressing itself. The dressing should not restrict circulation or sensation.

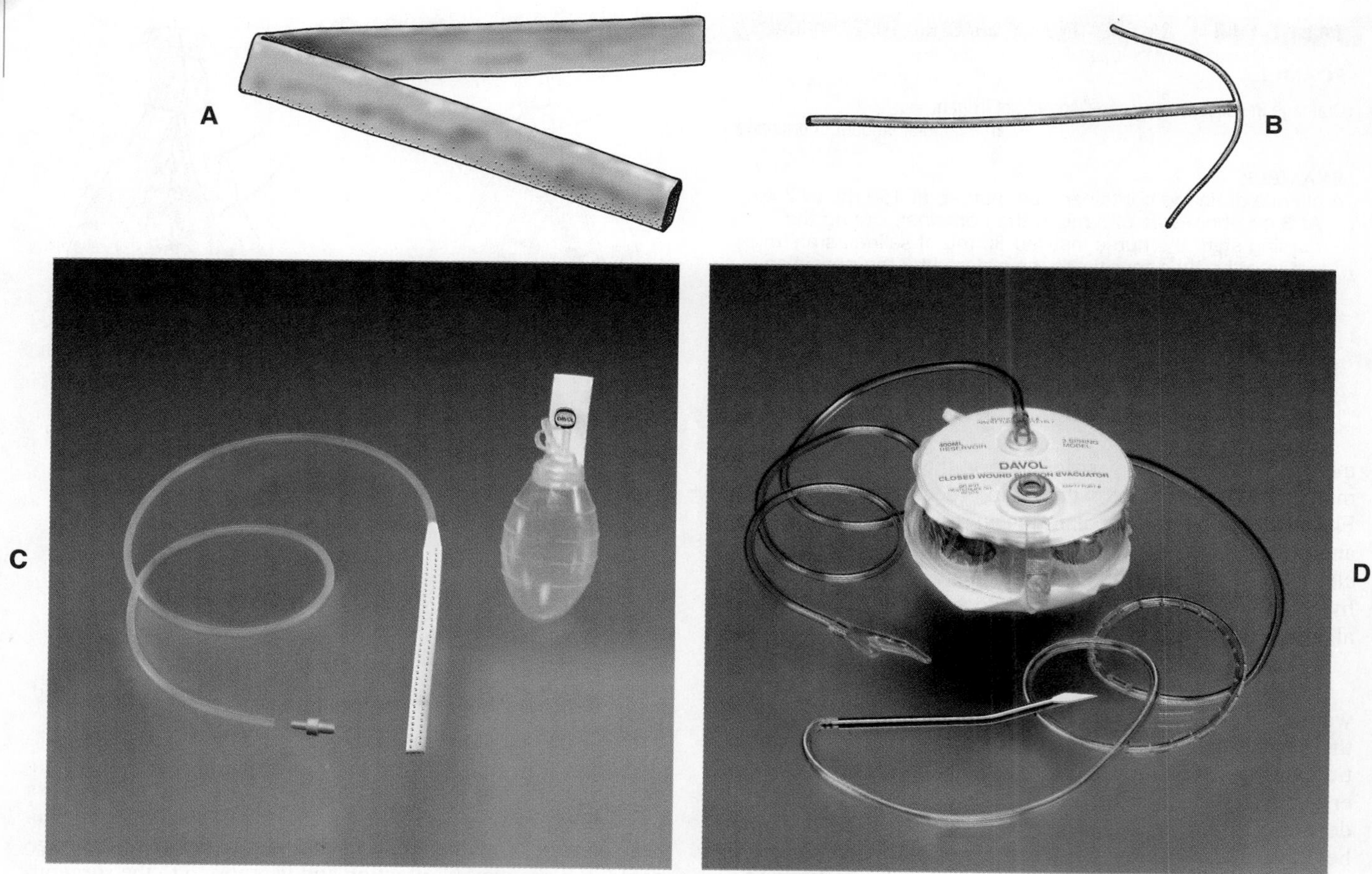

Figure 19-3 ● Types of surgical drains. Gravity drains, such as the Penrose (**A**) and the T-tube (**B**), drain directly through a tube from the surgical area. In closed wound drainage systems, such as the Jackson Pratt (**C**) and Hemovac (**D**), drainage collects in a collecting vessel by means of compression and re-expansion of the system. (**C** and **D** courtesy C.R. Bard, Inc., Covington, GA.)

To confine or contain drainage, the surgeon inserts a drain into or close to the wound if more than a minimal amount of drainage is expected. A Penrose drain (a single-lumen, soft latex tube) is a gravity-type drain under the dressing. The nurse assesses closed-suction drains such as Hemovac, VacuDrain, and Jackson-Pratt drains to ensure maintenance of compression and thus suction. The surgeon may place a T-tube after abdominal cholecystectomy to drain bile. Figure 19-3 shows commonly used drains.

The nurse assesses all drains for patency when the client is admitted to the PACU and every time vital signs are taken during the postoperative period. The nurse monitors the amount, color, and consistency of the drainage while the client is in the PACU and at least every 8 hours after the client is transferred to the medical-surgical nursing unit. For example, large amounts of sanguineous drainage may indicate internal bleeding.

DISCOMFORT/PAIN ASSESSMENT. The surgical client almost always reports pain or some level of discomfort. Pain is a subjective experience and may not be verbalized or appreciated by the providers to the extent that it is experienced by the client. Postoperative pain is related to the surgical wound, tissue manipulation, presence of drains, intraoperative positioning, and prolonged presence of an endotracheal (ET) tube. In assessing the client's discomfort or pain and need for medication, the nurse considers the type, extent, and length of the surgical procedure. The nurse assesses for physical and emotional signs of pain, such as increased pulse and blood pressure, increased respiratory rate or hyperventilation, diaphoresis (profuse perspiration), restlessness, increased confusion (in the older adult), wincing, moaning, and crying. When possible, the nurse asks the client to quantify or rate the discomfort or pain before and after medication is given (e.g., on a scale of 1 to 10, with 1 being least intense and 10 being extreme pain). The nurse plans the client's activities around the analgesia administration to improve mobility. In addition, the nurse observes for a return of normal (baseline) physical behaviors. (See Chapter 7 for further discussion of pain assessment.)

Discomfort or pain assessment is initiated by the postanesthesia nurse. After the client is transferred from the PACU, the medical-surgical nurse continues to assess his or her comfort level. Postoperative pain generally reaches its peak on the second postoperative day, when the client is more awake and the anesthetics and analgesics given intraoperatively have been metabolized and excreted.

PSYCHOSOCIAL ASSESSMENT

As the nurse completes the physical aspects of postoperative assessment, the psychologic, social, and cultural characteristics of the client are considered. This assessment may be delayed or difficult to perform in the postanesthesia care unit (PACU) when the client is drowsy or incoherent. The nurse considers the client's age and medical history, the surgical procedure, and the impact of the procedure on recovery, body image, roles, and lifestyle.

Physical signs indicating anxiety include restlessness; increased pulse, blood pressure, and respiratory rate; and crying. The client may be anxious and ask questions about the results or findings of the surgical procedure. The nurse reassures the client that the surgeon will speak with him or her after the client is fully awake. If the surgeon has already spoken with the client, the nurse reinforces what was said.

After the client returns to the medical-surgical unit, the medical-surgical nurse continues the psychosocial assessment and also assesses significant others.

LABORATORY ASSESSMENT

Postoperative laboratory tests are performed to monitor for complications. Tests are based on the surgical procedure and the client's medical history and postoperative clinical manifestations. Common postoperative serum tests include analysis of electrolytes and a complete blood count (see Chart 17-3). A change in laboratory test results (e.g., electrolyte levels, hematocrit, and hemoglobin levels) commonly occurs during the first 24 to 48 hours postoperatively because of blood and fluid loss and the body's reaction to the surgical process. Fluid loss without significant blood loss may result in hemoconcentrated laboratory values (decreased fluid in the blood with resultant increased concentration). The laboratory test result is reported as increased, but actually represents a concentrated normal value.

A subtle early indication of infection is an increase in the band cells (immature neutrophils) in the white blood cell differential count. This increase is termed a **left-shift.** The source of infection may be the respiratory system, urinary tract, wound, or IV site. The nurse obtains appropriate specimens for culture and sensitivity testing and monitors the culture results reported from the microbiology laboratory at 24, 48, and 72 hours. The nurse notifies the physician of positive culture results. (See Chapters 20 and 26 for more information on infection and assessment of immune function.)

Arterial blood gas (ABG) determinations may be indicated for clients with a history of respiratory or cardiac disease, those undergoing prolonged mechanical ventilation postoperatively, and those having had surgery involving the thoracic cavity. The nurse interprets ABG results and notifies the surgeon of any indication of acid-base imbalance or hypoxemia. (For more discussion on arterial blood gases and acidosis, see Chapters 15 and 16.)

Urine and renal laboratory studies are ordered as indicated (e.g., urinalysis, urine electrolyte levels, and serum creatinine levels). Other laboratory studies performed depend on the diagnosis, type of surgical procedure, and presence of additional disorders. Examples are a serum amylase level for a client who had pancreatic surgery and a blood glucose level for a client with diabetes.

> **CRITICAL THINKING CHALLENGE**
>
> The client is a 52-year-old man who experienced a compound fracture of the ankle 2 days ago when he fell from a bar stool. The surgery to place internal fixation devices in his ankle required 3 hours with the client under general anesthesia. His last vital signs before leaving the operating room (OR) were as follows: blood pressure, 150/110; pulse, 100; respirations, 12. He does not have a Foley catheter, and there is a vacuum-style drain from his wound.
>
> - What assessment data should you obtain first?
> - Where should you assess for hemorrhage?
> - In what position should you place this client?

For suggested answer guidelines, go to 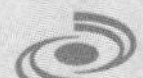 http://www.wbsaunders.com/SIMON/Iggy/.

Analysis

COMMON NURSING DIAGNOSES AND COLLABORATIVE PROBLEMS

The following are common nursing diagnoses for the postoperative client:

1. Impaired Gas Exchange related to the residual effects of anesthesia, pain, the use of opioid analgesics, and immobility
2. Impaired Skin Integrity related to surgical wounds, decreased mobility, inflammatory processes, drains and drainage, and tubes
3. Acute Pain related to the surgical incision, positioning during surgery, and endotracheal (ET) tube irritation

A common collaborative problem is Potential for Hypoxemia.

ADDITIONAL NURSING DIAGNOSES AND COLLABORATIVE PROBLEMS

In addition to the common nursing diagnoses and collaborative problems, postoperative clients may have one or more of the following depending on the type and extent of surgery, the family structure, and other presenting conditions:

- Risk for Aspiration related to decreased mobility, anesthesia, and opioid analgesic use
- Ineffective Airway Clearance related to ineffective or absent cough
- Potential for Hypovolemic Shock
- Potential for Deep Vein Thrombosis and Pulmonary Embolism
- Constipation related to decreased mobility, anesthesia, and opioid analgesic use
- Risk for Infection related to surgery and invasive lines, catheters, and tubes
- Urinary Retention related to anesthesia, surgical procedures, and decreased mobility
- Self-Care Deficit related to surgical procedures and decreased mobility
- Disturbed Body Image related to surgical procedures, loss of a body part or function, and pain

CHART 19-2

NIC INTERVENTION ACTIVITIES *for* The Postoperative Client

Postanesthesia Care: *Monitoring and management of the client who has recently undergone general or regional anesthesia*

- Administer oxygen, as appropriate.
- Monitor oxygenation.
- Ventilate, as appropriate.
- Monitor quality and number of respirations.
- Encourage client to cough and deep breathe.
- Monitor and record vital signs every 15 minutes or more often, as appropriate.
- Monitor urine output.
- Monitor return of sensorium and motor function.
- Monitor neurologic status.
- Monitor level of consciousness.
- Check surgical site, as appropriate.
- Administer narcotic antagonists, as appropriate, per agency protocol.
- Determine whether client meets discharge criteria.
- Report client information to postoperative nursing unit.
- Discharge client to next level of care.

- Interrupted Family Processes related to the impact of surgery and illness on the family system
- Ineffective Sexuality Patterns related to surgery, pain, and hospitalization

Planning and Implementation

IMPAIRED GAS EXCHANGE

PLANNING: EXPECTED OUTCOMES. The postoperative client is expected to attain or maintain optimal lung expansion and respiratory function with a partial pressure of arterial oxygen (Pa_{O_2}), partial pressure of arterial carbon dioxide (Pa_{CO_2}), and oxygen saturation values within baseline range.

INTERVENTIONS. NIC interventions for the postoperative client are listed in Chart 19-2.

AIRWAY MAINTENANCE. After assessing the airway, the postanesthesia nurse may need to insert an oral airway if the client does not already have one. The oral airway pulls the tongue forward and holds it down to prevent obstruction. If the client has clenched teeth, a large tongue, or upper airway obstruction, the nurse may insert a nasal airway (nasal trumpet) to keep the airway open. The manual resuscitation bag and emergency equipment for intubation or tracheostomy are kept nearby. For clients whose only airway is a tracheostomy or laryngectomy stoma, the nurse alerts other staff members by posting signs in the room and notes on the chart.

POSITIONING. Immediate care by the nurse in the postanesthesia care unit (PACU) includes positioning the client in a side-lying position or turning his or her head to the side to prevent aspiration of secretions (or vomitus) while he or she is still unreactive and vulnerable to aspiration. The nurse suctions the mouth, nose, and throat to keep the airway clear of mucus or vomitus as necessary.

The postanesthesia nurse keeps the client's head flat to prevent hypotension and possible shock, unless this position is contraindicated by the condition or surgical procedure. (For example, after intracranial surgery, the head of the bed or stretcher is elevated to promote respiratory function and prevent postoperative cerebral edema.) Oxygen is administered via a face tent, nasal cannula, or mask to facilitate the excretion of inhalation anesthetic agents, to increase arterial oxygen levels, and to raise the level of consciousness. After the client is fully reactive and stable, the postanesthesia nurse raises the head of the bed to promote respiratory function.

BREATHING EXERCISES. After the client regains the gag and cough reflex and meets the agency's criteria for extubation (if intubated), the airway or ET tube is removed. Examples of extubation criteria are the ability to raise and hold the head up and evidence of thoracic breathing. The nurse encourages the client to cough (with the incision splinted) and deep breathe to expand the lungs, promote gas exchange, and hasten the elimination of inhalation anesthetic agents. Chart 17-6 reviews the teaching of postoperative breathing exercises and splinting of the surgical wound area. As soon as the client is awake enough to follow commands, and throughout the postoperative period, the nurse encourages the client to cough, use the incentive spirometer, and take deep breaths. The client who is unable to expectorate mucus or sputum voluntarily may require oral or nasal suctioning. Meticulous mouth care is important after the removal of secretions.

MOBILIZATION. The client is out of bed and ambulating as soon as possible to help mobilize secretions and promote lung expansion. Even for the hospitalized client with extensive surgery, the goal may be to get out of bed the same day as or the first day after surgery. If this is not possible, depending on the situation, the nurse turns the client at least every 2 hours (side to side) and ensures that he or she performs his or her respiratory exercises and leg exercises (see Charts 17-6 and 17-7). Early ambulation reduces the risk of pulmonary complications, including a pulmonary embolism, which could arise from impaired venous circulation in the legs or pelvis. The client may report pain and resist getting up, but the nurse stresses the importance of activity to prevent postoperative complications. When indicated, the nurse offers pain medication 30 to 45 minutes before the client gets out of bed.

IMPAIRED SKIN INTEGRITY

PLANNING: EXPECTED OUTCOMES. The postoperative client is expected to have incision healing without postoperative wound complications.

INTERVENTIONS. Nursing assessment of the surgical area postoperatively is critical (see the discussion of integumentary system assessment on p. 291. Although most wound complications can be treated without additional surgical intervention, emergency surgical procedures may be necessary.

NONSURGICAL MANAGEMENT. Postoperative wound care usually includes changing and care of the dressing, assessment of the wound for signs of infection, and care of drains, including emptying, measuring, and documenting characteristics of the drainage. The nurse emphasizes the im-

CHART 19-3

NURSING FOCUS *on the* OLDER ADULT
Best Practices in Postoperative Skin Care

Improve perfusion to the wound to promote wound healing:
- Keep the client adequately hydrated to maintain cardiac output
- Keep the airway patent and provide adequate oxygenation.
- Keep the client's oxygen saturation on pulse oximetry at greater than 93%.

Conserve the client's energy:
- Allow the client to sleep in a darkened, quiet room.
- Administer medication to combat pain and sleeplessness, as ordered.
- Provide rest periods throughout the day.
- Control the client's room temperature.
- Assist in activities of daily living.

Place the client on a safety program to prevent falls, if indicated.

Maintain strict aseptic technique in caring for breaks in the integument (IV or other catheters, indwelling urethral catheter, wound).

Maintain the client's psychosocial health:
- Prevent unnecessary stressors.
- Allow the client liberal visitation of supportive others.
- Enable the client to use individual successful coping mechanisms.
- Keep the client well groomed and bathed.

Protect fragile skin:
- Minimize the use of tape on the skin.
- Use hypoallergenic tape or Montgomery straps.
- Change dressings as soon as they become wet.
- Lift the client during transfer or repositioning.

Data from Jones, P.L., & Millman, A. (1990). Wound healing and the aged patient. *Nursing Clinics of North America, 25*(1), 263-277.

portance of early deep breathing exercises to prevent respiratory complications that could cause forceful coughing. The nurse encourages hip flexion when the client is in the supine position to reduce tension on a chest or abdominal wound. The client is reminded to always splint the incision when coughing. The nurse promotes an atmosphere that is conducive to wound healing and protective of the skin in general, especially for the older client. Chart 19-3 lists best practices for skin care of the older postoperative client.

DRESSINGS. The surgeon usually performs the first dressing change to assess the wound, remove any packing, and advance (pull partially out) or remove drains as indicated. Before the first dressing change, the nurse reinforces the dressing if it becomes wet from drainage. The nurse documents the reinforcement, as well as the color, type, amount, and odor of drainage fluid and time of observation, in the client's chart. The nurse assesses the surgical area frequently and reports any unexpected findings to the surgeon.

After removal of the surgical dressing, the surgeon may wish to leave the suture or staple line open to the air, which allows easy assessment of the wound and early detection of poor approximation, drainage, swelling, or redness. Some surgeons believe that air-drying promotes healing. A draining wound, however, is always covered with a dressing.

Dressing changes are generally ordered by the surgeon; however, the facility or unit may have standards or policies that dictate specific protocols for postoperative dressing changes and incision care. An unchanged wet or damp dressing becomes a source of infection. The nurse performs dressing changes under aseptic conditions until the sutures or staples are removed.

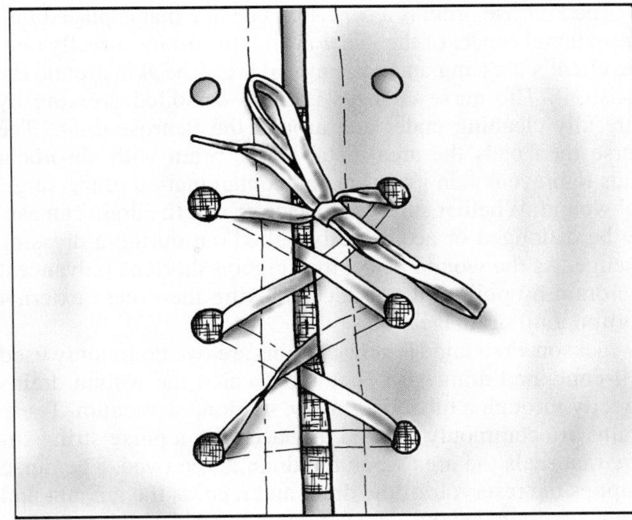

Figure 19-4 ● Montgomery straps may be used when frequent dressing changes are anticipated. They help to prevent skin irritation from frequent tape removal.

Dressings vary depending on the surgical procedure and the surgeon's preference. The standard postoperative dressing for a large incision consists of gauze or nonadherent pads covered with a larger absorbent pad held in place by tape or by Montgomery straps (Figure 19-4). In other cases, the incision may be covered with a transparent plastic surgical dressing (such as Op-Site) or a spray in the operating room (OR). This type of dressing stays intact for 3 to 6 days and allows direct visualization of the wound while preventing contamination and eliminating the need for dressing changes.

Wound or suture line care generally consists of changing gauze dressings at least once during a nursing shift or daily and may include cleaning the area with sterile saline or some other solution. Some suture lines are left open to air without any dressing to cover the incision. The hospital's policy, the unit's standards, and the surgeon's preference determine what solution, if any, is used on the wound and also the frequency of the dressing changes. For extensive dressing changes or drain removal, the nurse offers the client an ordered analgesic before the procedure.

Skin sutures or staples are usually removed 6 to 8 days postoperatively, and the incision is secured with Steri-Strips. Either the surgeon or the nurse removes the sutures or staples, depending on the agency's policy. Before removing sutures, the nurse notes the condition and healing stage of the wound. If the wound does not appear to be healing well, the nurse notifies the surgeon before proceeding with suture removal.

DRAINS. Drains (see Figure 19-3) may be inserted into the wound or through a separate small incision (known as a stab wound) close to the operative site during surgery. The drain provides an exit through which air and fluids, such as blood and bile, can be evacuated. Drains also help prevent deep infections and abscess formation within the wound during healing.

The Penrose drain is a superficial device that is placed into the external aspect of the incision and that drains directly onto the client's dressing and perisurgical area (the skin around the incision). The nurse changes a damp or soiled dressing by carefully cleaning under and around the Penrose drain. The nurse then pads the area distal to the drain with absorbent pads to prevent skin irritation and contamination of the surgical wound. Whether sutured in place or not, the drain can easily be dislodged or accidentally pulled out during a dressing change. As the wound heals, the surgeon shortens (advances) the drain by pulling it out and removing the excess external portion until drainage stops.

Jackson-Pratt and Hemovac drains are two commonly used self-contained drainage systems by which the wound drains directly through a tube via gravity, suction, or vacuum. These drains are commonly sutured in place with a purse-string suture that seals the area when the drain is removed. The nurse empties the reservoir of the drain and records the amount and color of drainage during every nursing shift or more frequently if ordered by the surgeon. After emptying and compressing the reservoir, the nurse secures the drain to the client's gown or pajamas (never to the sheet or mattress) to prevent pulling and stress on the surgical wound.

DRUG THERAPY. Wound infection is a major postoperative complication. It usually results from contamination during surgery, preoperative infection, debilitation, or immunosuppression. A client at risk for wound infection may receive prophylactic antibiotic therapy with a broad-spectrum antibiotic or one that is effective in fighting organisms common to the specific surgical site. These antibiotics are usually continued for 24 to 72 hours postoperatively to ensure that adequate antibiotic levels are reached in this critical time period. The first dose may be administered intravenously before or during the surgery.

Wounds that become infected and open (without intact sutures) are usually treated with specific dressing changes and prolonged systemic antibiotic administration. Depending on the physician's orders, the nurse irrigates the wound (e.g., with sterile saline, hydrogen peroxide, povidone-iodine, or acetic acid), loosely packs it with solution-soaked gauze (e.g., with neomycin, gentamicin, iodoform, povidone-iodine, saline, or acetic acid), and covers the wound with dry, sterile dressings. This procedure (wet-to-dry dressings) may be ordered to be done one to three times daily. The packing promotes healing from within the wound and **debridement** (removal) of the infected tissue as the wound heals.

SURGICAL MANAGEMENT

MANAGEMENT OF DEHISCENCE. If dehiscence (wound opening) occurs, the nurse applies a sterile nonadherent (such as Telfa) or saline dressing to the wound and notifies the surgeon. A wound that becomes infected dehisces by itself, or it may be opened by the surgeon through an **incision and drainage (I&D)** procedure. In either case, the wound is left open rather than re-sutured and is treated as described previously.

MANAGEMENT OF EVISCERATION. An evisceration (a wound opening with protrusion of internal organs or viscera) is a surgical emergency. One nurse tends to the client while another nurse immediately notifies the surgeon. Chart 19-4 outlines best practices for emergency care of the client with surgical wound evisceration. The nurse provides emotional support by explaining what happened and reassuring the client that the emergency will be handled by competent, capable individuals.

CHART 19-4

BEST PRACTICE *for*
The Client with Surgical Wound Evisceration

1. Call for help! Instruct the person who responds to notify the surgeon immediately and to bring any needed supplies into the client's room.
2. Stay with the client.
3. Cover the wound with a nonadherent dressing premoistened with warmed sterile normal saline. NOTE: The supplies needed for this emergency should be in the client's room, especially if the client is at high risk.
4. If premoistened dressings are not available, moisten sterile gauze or sterile towels in a sterile irrigation tray with sterile saline, then cover the wound.
5. If saline is not immediately available, cover the wound with gauze and then moisten with sterile saline using a sterile irrigation tray as soon as someone brings saline.
6. Do not attempt to reinsert the protruding organ or viscera.
7. While covering the wound, note the client's response and assess for signs and symptoms of shock.
8. Place the client in a supine position with the hips and knees bent.
9. Take and document vital signs. NOTE: If the person who answered the call for help is back in the room before this, instruct that individual to take vital signs while you focus on covering the wound and repositioning the client.
10. Provide support and reassurance to the client.
11. Continue assessing the client, including vital signs assessment, every 5 to 10 minutes until the surgeon arrives.
12. Keep dressings continuously moist by adding warmed sterile saline to the dressing as often as necessary. Do not let the dressing become dry.
13. When the surgeon arrives, report your finding and your interventions. Then follow the surgeon's directions.
14. Document the incident, the activity the client was engaged in at the time of the incident, your actions, and your assessments.

The surgeon may order a nasogastric (NG) tube to decompress the stomach and relieve some of the pressure internally or to remove the stomach's contents if the client has been eating and general anesthesia is planned. The nurse prepares the client for surgery (see Chapter 17) to close the wound. Regional or local anesthesia may be used, depending on the location of the wound and the surgeon's or the anesthesiologist's preference. Postoperative nausea and vomiting, which place undue stress on the already fragile incision, are minimized when regional or local anesthesia is used. To increase the incision's integrity, stay or retention sutures of wire or nylon are used over the standard suture or staple line (see Figure 18-13).

PREVENTION. In addition to impaired skin integrity from the surgical wound, clients are at risk for developing pressure ulcers from positioning during surgery, prolonged contact with damp surgical linens, and contact with unpadded surfaces. Pressure ulcers acquired during the perioperative period increase lengths of stay, health care costs, and the risk for complications (see the Cost of Care: Implications for Nursing

COST OF CARE IMPLICATIONS FOR NURSING

PERIOPERATIVE PRESSURE ULCERS

Cost of Care

- Approximately 1.5 to 1.6 million pressure ulcers develop among hospitalized clients in the United States each year (5.4% incidence rate).
- Over 900,000 of these ulcers are stage II and above.
- The number of intraoperative pressure ulcers is calculated to be 373,560 (23%) each year.
- Most occur in clients who were in surgery for 3 hours or longer.
- The estimated additional health care cost for intraoperative/perioperative pressure ulcer development ranges between $455 million and $725 million annually.
- Most ulcers are preventable.
- More ulcers develop in clients who are older, malnourished, or have diabetes.

Implications for Nursing

The monetary and personal cost of pressure ulcer management is enormous. Such ulcers can be prevented by implementing interventions to protect the skin, especially among high-risk clients. Diligent nursing assessment of the skin to prevent conversion of early-stage pressure ulcers to deeper ulcers is paramount in reducing costs and decreasing the length of stay. Nurses should consider continuing skin assessment during the postoperative period an essential nursing function.

Data from Beckrich, K., & Aronvitch, S. (1999). Hospital-acquired pressure ulcers: A comparison of costs in medical vs surgical patients. *Nursing Economics, 17*(5), 263-271.

box above). Addressing early-stage pressure ulcers can prevent progression and limit complications.

The PACU nurse examines the client's skin for areas of redness or lost integrity. Any abnormalities are documented and reported to the surgeon. Appropriate padding and positioning are used to relieve pressure. Any open areas are treated according to agency guidelines and the physician's orders. The PACU nurse ensures that information regarding skin condition is communicated to the medical-surgical nurse if the client remains as an inpatient.

ACUTE PAIN

PLANNING: EXPECTED OUTCOMES. The postoperative client is expected to attain or maintain optimal comfort levels throughout the postoperative phase. This outcome entails the alleviation or reduction of pain or discomfort associated with the surgical wound and positioning during surgery.

INTERVENTIONS. Postoperative pain management includes drug therapy and other methods of management, such as positioning, massage, relaxation techniques, and diversion. Often the client achieves greater benefit from a combination of approaches. The nurse assesses the client's comfort level and the effectiveness of the therapies. Chapter 7 provides a comprehensive discussion of pain assessment and management for the postoperative client. The client who has optimal pain control is better able to cooperate with the therapies and exercises designed to prevent postoperative complications and to promote the postoperative rehabilitation process.

DRUG THERAPY. The use of opioids or other analgesics for the management of pain may mask or increase the amount and severity of symptoms of an anesthesia reaction. Therefore these drugs must be administered with caution, especially in the postanesthesia care unit (PACU) when the client's condition is not stabilized. Pain medication, when administered in the PACU, is usually given intravenously in small doses. After the nurse administers medication for pain, the client remains in the PACU for a defined period (often 30 to 45 minutes). The postanesthesia nurse assesses for hypotension, respiratory depression, and other side effects. Approximately 5 to 10 minutes after an IV injection, the nurse assesses the effectiveness of the medication (i.e., on a rating scale) in relieving pain.

Opioid analgesics are routinely given during the first 24 to 48 hours after surgery to control acute pain. Around-the-clock administration is generally more effective than medicating on client demand because more constant blood levels can be obtained. Drugs commonly used include meperidine hydrochloride (Demerol), morphine sulfate (Statex✤), hydromorphone hydrochloride (Dilaudid), ketorolac (Toradol), codeine sulfate, butorphanol tartrate (Stadol), and oxycodone hydrochloride with aspirin (Percodan) or oxycodone hydrochloride with acetaminophen (Tylox, Percocet). The nurse assesses the type, location, and intensity of the pain before and after the administration of medication (see also Discomfort/Pain Assessment, p. 292). The nurse monitors the client's vital signs closely, especially for hypotension and hypoventilation, after the administration of opioid analgesics. Chart 19-5 contains further information on various analgesics used during the postoperative period.

Patient-controlled analgesia (PCA) via IV infusion or internal pump (the catheter is sutured into or near the surgical area) and epidural analgesia are becoming more common to achieve better pain control. In PCA, the client adjusts the rate or dosage of infusion of an opioid analgesic on the basis of the pain level and physical response to the drug. This method allows more consistent pain relief and more control by the client. The maximum dose per hour is "locked in" to the pump so that the client cannot accidentally overdose. Drugs commonly used by the PCA method include morphine, meperidine, and hydromorphone.

Epidural analgesia can be administered intermittently by the anesthesiologist or via continuous drip with or without PCA through an epidural catheter left in place after epidural anesthesia. Drugs commonly given by epidural catheter include the opioids fentanyl citrate (Sublimaze) and preservative-free morphine (Duramorph), and the local anesthetic bupivacaine (Marcaine).

The nurse takes care not to overmedicate or undermedicate, especially with older clients. In assessing for overmedication, the nurse monitors the vital signs, especially blood pressure and respiratory rate, and level of consciousness. Complications from the use of opioid analgesics include respiratory depression, hypotension, nausea, vomiting, and constipation. An opioid antagonist, such as naloxone hydrochloride (Narcan), may be administered to reverse the acute effects of opioid depression. Because of the short effect of the opioid antagonist, the nurse monitors the blood pressure and respirations closely (i.e., every 15 to 30 minutes) until the full effect of the opioid analgesic has passed. The nurse may need to give more doses of the opioid antagonist during this time. (See Chart 19-6 for more information on the opioid antagonists.) In addition, the

CHART 19-5

DRUG THERAPY *for* Management of Postoperative Pain

Drug	Usual Dosage	Nursing Interventions	Rationale
Meperidine hydrochloride (Demerol)	50-150 mg q3-4h PO or IM 12.5-25 mg IV Maximum 6-8 doses	Monitor blood pressure. Move and ambulate the client slowly. Monitor pulse rate.	Common side effects include decreased blood pressure, orthostatic (postural) hypotension, and bradycardia.
		Assess for decreased GI motility or GI upset.	Constipation, nausea, and vomiting can occur.
Morphine sulfate (Epimorph✤, Statex✤)	2-15 mg IM or IV incrementally 10-30 mg q4h PO Maximum 6 doses	Monitor respiratory status.	Respiratory depression can be severe and require medical intervention.
		Monitor blood pressure. Assess for GI motility and urine output.	Hypotension, constipation, and urinary retention can occur.
Hydromorphone hydrochloride (Dilaudid)	1-4 mg q3-4h IV or IM 2-4 mg q3-4h PO	Monitor respirations. Monitor blood pressure. Monitor for food intolerance. Monitor fluid and electrolyte balance. Assess GI motility.	Respiratory depression, hypotension, anorexia, nausea, vomiting, and constipation can occur.
Codeine sulfate, codeine phosphate (Paveral✤)	15-60 mg q4h IM or PO Maximum 6 doses	Monitor respiratory status. Monitor for food intolerance. Monitor fluid and electrolyte balance.	Respiratory depression, nausea, and vomiting can occur.
		Assess GI motility.	Constipation is common; prophylactic interventions may be indicated.
Butorphanol tartrate (Stadol)	1-4 mg q3-4h IM 0.5-2 mg IV Maximum 6-8 doses	Monitor neurologic status and changes in level of consciousness. Monitor respiratory status.	Butorphanol can cause increased intracranial pressure and respiratory depression.
Oxycodone hydrochloride and aspirin (Percodan, Endodan✤, Oxycodan✤)	1-2 tablets (5-10 mg) q3-4h PO Maximum 80 mg	Assess GI tolerance of medication. Assess for GI bleeding. Monitor GI motility.	The aspirin component can irritate the stomach and could cause GI bleeding.
		Monitor coagulation respiratory studies (PT, aPTT).	Bleeding times and other coagulation study results may be increased because of the aspirin component.
		Monitor respiratory status.	Respiratory depression and constipation can be caused by the oxycodone component.
Oxycodone hydrochloride and acetaminophen (Tylox, Percocet, Endocet✤, Oxycocet✤)	1-2 tablets q3-4h PO Maximum 12 tablets	Monitor blood pressure and respiratory status. Assess for GI motility.	Respiratory depression, hypotension, and constipation can occur.
Ketorolac tromethamine (Toradol)	15-60 mg IM or IV q6h Maximum 120 mg 5-day administration maximum	Monitor for GI bleeding.	GI bleeding, ulceration, and perforation can occur.
		Monitor for renal effects, especially in older adults.	Decreased urine output, increased serum creatinine, hematuria, and proteinuria can occur. Ketorolac is cleared more slowly in older adults. Older persons are more sensitive to the renal effects of NSAIDs.
Ibuprofen (Motrin, Amersol✤, Novoprofen✤)	300-800 mg q4-6h PO Maximum 2400 mg daily	Monitor upper GI tolerance of medication. Give with food or milk.	Food or milk helps decrease irritation of the stomach.
		Monitor coagulation studies (PT, aPTT).	Bleeding times and other coagulation study results may be increased.
		Assess for signs of bleeding or delayed clotting.	Monitoring leads to early detection of complications.

PT, Prothrombin time; *aPTT*, activated partial thromboplastin time; *NSAID*, nonsteroidal antiinflammatory drug; *GI*, gastrointestinal.

CHART 19-6

DRUG THERAPY *for* Management of Opioid Overdose

Drug	Usual Dosage	Nursing Interventions	Rationale
Naloxone hydrochloride (Narcan)	0.1-2 mg IV, SC, and IM; repeat every 2-3 min prn on the basis of the client's response up to 10 mg	Maintain an open airway.	A patent airway maximizes respiratory effort.
		Administer oxygen as ordered.	Oxygen helps to prevent hypoxemia.
		Have suction available.	Vomiting can occur with administration of naloxone; suction prevents aspiration.
		Closely monitor vital signs and pulse oximetry readings until the client responds.	The threat of hypoxemia and respiratory depression or arrest is a concern until the naloxone becomes effective.
		Do not leave the client unattended until he or she is fully responsive.	Staying with the client promotes safety.
		Observe for significant reversal of analgesia.	With reversal of the narcotic's respiratory-depressive effects, analgesic effects will also be reversed.
		Continue to monitor the client for effects of the naloxone for at least 1 hr.	Continued monitoring leads to early detection of hypertension, hypotension, tachycardia, and dysrhythmias, which can be effects of naloxone.

client has breakthrough pain after the opioid antagonist is administered, so the nurse initiates other interventions to promote comfort.

The nurse assesses for undermedication by questioning the client about the effects of the medication and observing for nonverbal cues that indicate pain or discomfort (e.g., restlessness, increased confusion, "picking" at bedcovers, and aggressive behaviors). The nurse offers pain medication after checking for hypotension and respiratory depression.

As recovery progresses, the nurse administers pain medications in reduced doses and frequency. The medications are changed from injectable or PCA to oral as soon as the client can tolerate oral administration. Nonopioid analgesics, such as acetaminophen (Tylenol, Atasol🍁), and nonsteroidal anti-inflammatory drugs (NSAIDs), such as ibuprofen (Motrin, Novo-Profen, Amersol🍁) and ketorolac (Toradol), are used during convalescence or can be given with an opioid analgesic as an adjunct. Antianxiety drugs, such as hydroxyzine (Vistaril, Novo-Hydroxyzin🍁), may be given in combination with an opioid analgesic. This combination decreases pain-related anxiety, alleviates muscle tension that could contribute to the client's pain or discomfort, and controls nausea.

COMPLEMENTARY AND ALTERNATIVE THERAPIES. The nurse provides comfort measures that may lower the amount of pain medication needed. These measures reduce anxiety and allow the client to relax and rest.

POSITIONING. In positioning the client, the nurse considers the position during surgery, the location of the surgical incision and drains, and medical problems such as arthritis and chronic pulmonary disease. The nurse assists the client in achieving a position of comfort while maintaining optimal function. The extremities are supported with pillows. No pillows are placed under the knees, and the knee gatch of the bed is not raised, because this position could restrict circulation and increase the risk for thrombophlebitis. The nurse turns or helps the client turn at least every 2 hours while he or she is bedridden to prevent pulmonary and other complications sometimes caused by immobility.

On the basis of the surgeon's orders and the nurse's assessment of the client's tolerance, the nurse encourages the client progressively to increase activity. Activity decreases stiffness, promotes lung expansion, and promotes venous circulation. When the client is initially allowed out of bed, the nurse assists him or her to the side of the bed and into a chair. The client splints the surgical wound for support and comfort during the transfer.

MASSAGE. The nurse uses gentle massage of stiff joints or a sore back to decrease postoperative discomfort. The client is positioned in a side-lying position, and lotion is applied with smooth, gentle strokes to increase blood flow to the area and promote general relaxation. The legs, especially the calves, are not massaged because of the increased risk of loosening a thrombus and causing a pulmonary embolus, which can be life threatening.

RELAXATION AND DIVERSION. Relaxation and diversion are also used to control acute episodes of pain, such as during painful procedures such as dressing changes and injections. Chapters 4 and 7 discuss how the nurse instructs and guides the client through these pain control methods. Music and noise reduction have been shown to decrease awareness of discomfort. Chart 19-7 lists examples of other interventions that may help to reduce pain and promote comfort.

CRITICAL THINKING CHALLENGE

The client (described earlier—a 52-year-old man postoperative from an internal fixation of a compound fracture of the ankle) has been in the PACU for 2 hours. He is irritable and has an increase in pulse rate and blood pressure. In addition, he is restless, diaphoretic, and has coarse hand tremors. Repeated repositioning and analgesic (IV morphine) medication failed to comfort the client.

- What historical data might be significant?
- What additional assessment data should you obtain?
- What nursing interventions could be implemented to manage this client's symptoms while in the PACU?
- What safety precautions should be planned?

For suggested answer guidelines, go to SIMON http://www.wbsaunders.com/SIMON/Iggy/.

CHART 19-7

BEST PRACTICE *for* Nonpharmacologic Interventions to Reduce Postoperative Pain and Promote Comfort

- Control or remove noxious stimuli.
- Cushion and elevate painful areas; avoid tension or pressure on those areas.
- Provide adequate rest to increase pain tolerance.
- Encourage the client's participation in diversional activities.
- Instruct the client in relaxation techniques; use audiotapes and breathing exercises.
- Provide opportunities for meditation.
- Help the client to stimulate sensory nerve endings near the painful areas to inhibit ascending pain impulses.
- Use ice to reduce and prevent swelling, as indicated.
- Find a general position of comfort for the client.
- Help the client to stimulate the area contralateral (opposite) to the painful area.

POTENTIAL FOR HYPOXEMIA

PLANNING: EXPECTED OUTCOMES. The postoperative client is expected to attain or maintain preoperative baseline partial pressure of arterial oxygen (Pao_2) values.

INTERVENTIONS. The key to preventing hypoxemia is to follow the interventions appropriate for the nursing diagnoses of Impaired Gas Exchange (p. 294), Ineffective Airway Clearance, and Ineffective Breathing Pattern. Postoperatively, the nurse and physician monitor the client's arterial blood gas (ABG) and pulse oximetry results. A client who received conscious sedation with midazolam (Versed) or lorazepam (Ativan, Nu-Loraz♣) may be overly sedated or have cardiopulmonary depression sufficient to require reversal with flumazenil (Romazicon) (Chart 19-8). Postoperative hypothermia and its associated shivering cause increased oxygen demands and can contribute to hypoxemia. Various rewarming methods are used in postanesthesia care units (PACUs), although prevention may be more important. The highest incidence of postoperative hypoxemia, however, is on the second postoperative day. Those clients who have a low normal Pao_2, such as those with underlying pulmonary disease or the older adult, are at higher risk for hypoxemia.

The physician treats the potential for hypoxemia with oxygen administration. Depending on the surgeon's preference and established guidelines, the physician may continue oxygen administration until after the second postoperative day. When hypoxemia occurs despite preventive care, the physician orders treatment to manage the cause of the hypoxemia and prescribes oxygen therapy, respiratory treatments, and mechanical ventilation as indicated.

Community-Based Care

Many clients are discharged after a brief hospital stay or directly from the PACU to home. Because of the shortened length of hospitalization, discharge planning, teaching, and referral begin preoperatively and continue postoperatively (see the Evidence-Based Practice for Nursing box on p. 301).

HEALTH TEACHING

The teaching plan for the postoperative client and appropriate others includes the following:

- Prevention of infection
- Care and assessment of the surgical wound
- Diet therapy
- Pain management
- Drug therapy
- Progressive increase in activity

If dressing changes are needed, the client and family members are instructed on the importance of proper handwashing to prevent infection. The nurse thoroughly explains and demonstrates wound care to the client and family, who then perform a return demonstration of that care. During teaching sessions, the nurse evaluates learning and promotes compliance after discharge. At the same time, the nurse teaches signs and symptoms of complications such as wound infection. The nurse also discusses with the client and family members appropriate measures to take if complications occur.

A diet high in protein, calories, and vitamin C promotes wound healing. A dietary consultation before the client is discharged helps him or her to select a balanced diet to promote healing. Supplemental vitamin C, iron, and multivitamins are often prescribed after surgery to aid in wound healing and in the formation of red blood cells. Often these supplements are prescribed for 10 to 14 days postoperatively. The nurse instructs the client with prior dietary restrictions about the importance of following the prescribed diet during convalescence. The older adult or debilitated client is encouraged to continue using dietary supplements, if ordered, between meals until the wound is completely healed and the energy levels are restored.

The nurse instructs the client about taking pain medication, with special attention to the proper dosage and frequency of administration. The client is instructed to notify the surgeon if the medication does not control the pain or if the pain suddenly increases. If antibiotics or other medications are prescribed, the client is instructed to finish the entire prescription as ordered by the surgeon.

Surgery places physical and emotional stress on the body, and time and rest are required for healing. The nurse instructs the client to increase his or her activity level slowly, balance rest with activity (e.g., plan rest periods), and avoid straining the surgical wound or the surrounding area. Depending on the type of surgery and the client's occupation and usual activities, the surgeon decides when the client may climb stairs, return to work, drive, and resume other usual activities, such as sexual intercourse. The amount of weight that can be lifted safely after discharge from the facility needs to be specifically defined by the surgeon (i.e., in pounds or kilograms, as ap-

CHART 19-8

DRUG THERAPY *for* Management of Benzodiazepine Overdose

Drug	Usual Dosage	Nursing Interventions	Rationale
Flumazenil (Romazicon)	0.2-1 mg IV at rate of 0.2 mg/min; repeat every 2-3 min prn up to 3 mg in any 1 hr	Maintain an open airway.	A patent airway maximizes respiratory effort.
		Administer oxygen as ordered.	Oxygen helps to prevent hypoxemia.
		Have suction available.	Vomiting can occur with administration of flumazenil; suction prevents aspiration.
		Closely monitor the client's level of sedation, vital signs, and pulse oximetry readings until the client responds.	Hypoventilation may not be fully reversed with flumazenil; sedation, amnesia, and psychomotor effects of the benzodiazepines should be reversed.
		Do not leave the client unattended until fully responsive.	Seizures have occurred with reversal.
		Observe for significant reversal of sedation.	With reversal of the benzodiazepine's sedative and amnesia effect, the client will become more aware of pain/discomfort.
		Observe for up to 2 hr for re-sedation and respiratory depression.	The duration of action of the benzodiazepines is longer than that of flumazenil.

EVIDENCE-BASED PRACTICE FOR NURSING

Clients identify areas of unmet postoperative teaching

Jacobs, V. (2000). Informational needs of surgical patients following discharge. *Applied Nursing Research, 13*(1), 12-18.

This prospective, descriptive study examined client reports of educational information received after surgery. A convenience sample included 45 clients who underwent common surgical procedures, usually requiring short hospital stays, and were surveyed for the type of information received and their satisfaction with the level of information provided.

Clients indicated that predischarge teaching did occur but that some of the areas of greatest concern to them were not sufficiently addressed before they were discharged. Overall, discharge instructions stressed medication regimens. Clients indicated that more information regarding self-monitoring of specific parameters, activity restrictions, wound care, potential complications, pain management, and elimination was needed for them to feel confident in their abilities to manage an early discharge after surgery.

Critique. The study methods were appropriate for the research question. The sample size was sufficient to allow generalizability of the results. The results were consistent with the findings of similar studies. The study could have been strengthened by including more subjects discharged within 24 hours after the surgical procedure.

Implications for Nursing. With shorter postoperative hospital stays, client teaching has become more challenging. Clients are discharged more quickly and must be adequately prepared to take responsibility for care and monitoring that previously had been an expected part of hospital care. Although instructions regarding medications are important, other issues are equally important for client safety. Nurses need to examine how and under what conditions discharge teaching is occurring. More emphasis should be placed on self-monitoring, activity restrictions, wound care, pain management, complications, and elimination. Nurses may want to consider multiple approaches and repetition when disseminating this information to ensure greater comprehension and retention.

propriate) and interpreted and reinforced as necessary by the nurse (e.g., grocery bags, laundry baskets, children, books).

The nurse also instructs the client in the use of proper body mechanics. A client whose work involves a moderate amount of physical labor may be allowed back to work 6 weeks after nonlaser abdominal surgery. However, he or she may be eager to return to work or to other activities and may not follow activity restrictions. The nurse emphasizes the importance of compliance to prevent complications or disability. It is imperative that the client receives written discharge instructions for reinforcement at home. A visiting nurse may be necessary for follow-up.

HOME CARE MANAGEMENT

If the client is discharged directly to home, the nurse reviews data to help assess the home environment for safety, cleanliness, and availability of caregivers. The database completed on admission to the hospital or ambulatory surgical unit is used to ascertain the client's needs. For example, if the client is unable or not allowed to climb stairs and lives in a two-story house with only one bathroom, the nurse advises the client to rent a bedside commode. The social worker or discharge planner, in collaboration with the nurse, helps in identifying needs related to postoperative care, including meal preparation, dressing changes, and personal hygiene. A referral to a home care nursing agency may be indicated.

The client is usually apprehensive about postoperative complications, pain, and changes in the usual activity level; thus the nurse must allay fears. The more extensive the surgical procedure is, the more fearful the client is of assuming self-care. The nurse supports the client and family members as they make discharge plans. The client whose surgical procedure has left visible scars may require more emotional support from and acceptance of his or her family. The client may express anger about the surgical outcome or about temporary or permanent role changes. The client may also express concern about financial matters and work. The surgical outcome may not have met the client's expectations, and further interventions may be necessary to assist in resolving his or her feelings. Referrals are made for additional counseling as indicated.

HEALTH CARE RESOURCES

After returning home, the client may need equipment and assistance with dressing changes, activities of daily living (ADLs), and meal preparation. Referral to a home care agency is made, if necessary; this may be paid for by third-party insurance payers, including Medicare, if the client is homebound and requires skilled care. The home care nurse provides skilled nursing assessments, dressing supplies, education in self-care, and referrals for services as needed. Such referrals include Meals on Wheels, support groups, and homemaker services (e.g., for housekeeping and food shopping).

Evaluation: Outcomes

NOC The nurse evaluates the care of the postoperative client on the basis of the identified nursing diagnoses and collaborative problems. The expected outcomes include that the client:

- Maintains a patent airway
- Maintains adequate lung expansion and respiratory function as evidenced by clear breath sounds
- Has stable vital signs and does not obtain an infection
- Returns to baseline arterial blood gas (ABG) values
- Returns to his or her preoperative mental state
- Has complete wound healing without complications
- States that postoperative pain is reduced or alleviated by interventions

ONLINE RESOURCES

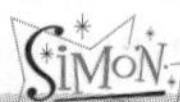

For suggested readings and Internet resources, go to http://www.wbsaunders.com/SIMON/Iggy/.

SELECTED BIBLIOGRAPHY

Asterisk indicates a classic or definitive work on this subject.

*Acute Pain Management Guideline Panel. (1992). *Acute pain management in adults: Operative procedures.* AHCPR Pub. No. 92-0019. Rockville, MD: Agency for Health Care Policy and Research, Public Health Service, U.S. Department of Health and Human Services.

American Society of PeriAnesthesia Nurses. (1998). *Standards of perianesthesia nursing practice.* New Jersey: Author.

Beckrich, K., & Aronvitch, S. (1999). Hospital-acquired pressure ulcers: A comparison of costs in medical vs surgical patients. *Nursing Economics, 17*(5), 263-271.

Brenner, Z. (1999). Preventing postoperative complications: What's old what's new, what's tried-and-true. *Nursing99, 29*(10), 34-40.

Cheever, K. (1999). Pain, analgesic use, and morbidity in appendectomy patients. *Clinical Nursing Research, 8*(3), 267-282.

Cole, L. (1999). Early enteral feeding after surgery. *Critical Care Clinics of North America, 11*(2), 227-231.

Dennison, R.D. (1997). Nurses' guide to common postoperative complications. *Nursing97,* 27 (11), 56-57.

Ennis, D. (1999). Reducing the risk of surgical site infection. *Nursing99, 29*(6), 32hn1-2, 32hn4-5.

Goldiner, P., & Rappaport, E. (1998). Postoperative respiratory dysfunction. *Current Reviews for Nurse Anesthetists, 21*(3), 21-28.

Greensmith, J., & Aker, J. (1998) Ventilatory management in the postanesthesia care unit. *Journal of PeriAnesthesia Nursing, 13*(6), 370-381.

Hershey, J., Valenciano, C., & Bookbinder, M. (1997). Comparison of three rewarming methods in a postanesthesia care unit. *AORN Journal, 65*(3), 597-601.

Hess, D. (2000). Detection and monitoring of hypoxemia and oxygen therapy. *Respiratory Care, 45*(1), 65-83.

Hulme, J., Waterman, J., & Hillier, V. (1999). The effect of foot massage on patients' perception of care following laparoscopic sterilization as day case patients. *Journal of Advanced Nursing, 30*(2), 460-468.

Jacobs, V. (2000). Informational needs of surgical patients following discharge. *Applied Nursing Research, 13*(1), 12-18.

Juran, N., et al. (1999). Nursing interventions to decrease bleeding at the femoral access site after percutaneous coronary intervention. *American Journal of Critical Care, 8*(5), 303-313.

Kirkland, K., et al. (1999). The impact of surgical-site infections in the 1990's: attributable mortality, excess length of hospitalization, and extra cost. *Infection Control and Hospital Epidemiology, 20*(11), 725-730.

Kuc, J., & Pietro, J. (1999). Safe discharge from the PACU and ambulatory care setting. *Journal of Nursing Law, 6*(2), 7-14.

Leininger, S. (1999). Helping your patient back on track after knee replacement surgery. *Nursing99, 29*(12), 32hn10-11.

Lezon, K. (1999). Teaching incentive spirometry. *Nursing 99, 29*(1), 60-61.

*Lusis, S.A. (1996). The challenges of nursing elderly surgical patients. *AORN Journal, 64*(6), 954-955, 957-962.

Managram, A., et al. (1999). Guideline for prevention of surgical site infection, 1999. *American Journal of Infection Control, 27*(2), 97-134.

Mann, E. (1999). Using acupuncture and acupressure to treat postoperative emesis. *Professional Nurse, 14*(10), 691-694.

McCloskey, J.C, & Bulechek, G.M. (2000). *Nursing interventions classification (NIC)* (3rd ed.). St. Louis: Mosby.

Mecca, R. (1998). Postoperative hypoxemia. *Current Reviews for PeriAnesthesia Nurses, 20*(21), 214-224.

Mecca, R. (1999). Postoperative hypercarbia. *Current Reviews for PeriAnesthesia Nurses, 21*(10), 90-100.

Mimnaugh, L., et al. (1999). Sensations experienced during removal of tubes in acute postoperative patients. *Applied Nursing Research, 12*(2), 78-85.

Nazarko, L. (1999). Paying the price of early discharge. *Nursing Times, 95*(12), 51-52.

Nebelkopf, H. (1999). Abdominal compartment syndrome. *American Journal of Nursing, 99*(11), 53-59.

Pandit, S. (1999). Ambulatory anesthesia and surgery in America: a historical background and recent innovations. *Journal of PeriAnesthesia Nursing 14*(5), 270-274.

*Pasero, C.L. (1996). Managing postoperative pain in the elderly. *American Journal of Nursing, 96*(10), 38-46.

Porter, N., Sidou, V., & Husson, J. (1999). Postoperative sore throat: incidence and severity after the use of lidocaine, saline, or air to inflate the endotracheal tube cuff. *Journal of the American Association of Nurse Anesthetists, 67*(1), 49-52.

Seymour, D. (1999). The aging surgical patient: An update. *Reviews in Clinical Gerontology, 9*(3), 221-233.

Sherman, D.W. (1997). Developing quality assurance programs in ambulatory surgery. *Nursing Management, 28*(9), 44-48.

Smith, L., Baker, F., & Stead, L. (1999). Practice procedures for nurses: Removal of staples. *Nursing Times, 95*(10), insert 2p.

Stays are shorter in Phase I PACU. (1998). *OR Manager, 14*(12), 13.

Strimike, C.L., Wojcik, J.M., & Stark, B.A. (1997). Incision care that really cuts it. *RN, 60*(7), 22-26.

Swan, B.A. (1998). Postoperative nursing care contributions to symptom distress and functional status after ambulatory surgery. *MedSurg Nursing, 7*(3), 148-158.

Tappen, R., Muzic, J., & Kennedy, P. (2001). Preoperative assessment and discharge planning for older adults undergoing ambulatory surgery. *AORN Journal, 73*(2), 464-474.

Taylor, L., et al. (1998). The effect of music in the postanesthesia care unit on pain levels in women who have had abdominal hysterectomies. *Journal of PeriAnesthesia Nursing, 13*(2), 88-94.

United States Pharmacopeia Dispensing Information (USP DI): Vol I. Drug information for the health care professional (20th ed.). (2000). Englewood, CO: Micromedix.

Walker, J. (1999). New glue, zipper for closing wounds. *OR Manager, 15*(1), 6.

Walton, J. (2001). Helping high-risk surgical patients beat the odds. *Nursing 2001, 31*(3), 54-59.

Wilson, M. (2000). Giving postanesthesia care in the critical care unit. *Dimensions of Critical Care Nursing, 19*(2), 38-43.

Zalon, M.L. (1997). Pain in frail, older adult women after surgery. *Image: Journal of Nursing Scholarship, 29*(1), 21-26.

UNIT

5

PROBLEMS OF PROTECTION

Management of Clients with Problems of the Immune System

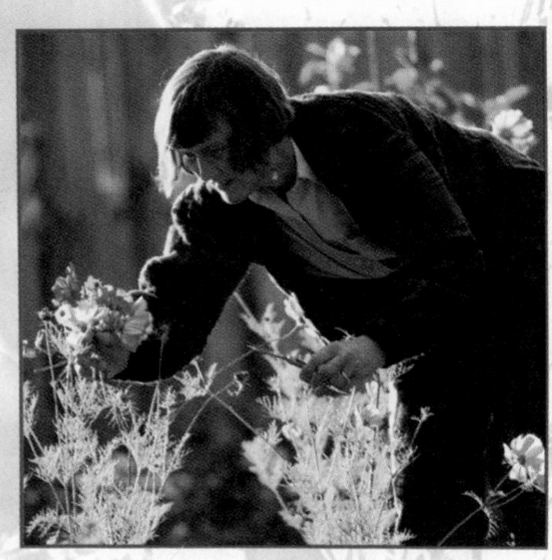

UNIT 5 PROBLEMS OF PROTECTION: IMMUNE SYSTEM ■ Core Concepts Grid

Anatomy	Physiology	Pathophysiology	History	Physical Exam	Diagnostic Tests	Interventions	Pharmacology
• **Lymph system** • **Mononuclear—phagocyte system** • **Cells** B-lymphocytes T-lymphocytes • **Antigens**	• **Phagocytosis** • **Specificity** • **Memory** • **Self-recognition** • **Human leukocyte antigen (HLA)** • **Inflammatory response** • **Immune response** Antibody-mediated Cell-mediated • **Types of immunity** Natural Acquired Active Passive	• **Hypersensitivity response** • **Autoimmune response** • **Immunodeficiency** • **Metastasis** • **Neoplasm** • **Inflammation** • **Infection** • **Transplant reaction** • **Tissue degeneration**	• **Past history of infections, allergies, malignancies, autoimmune disease** • **Immunization record** • **Family history** • **Social history** Occupation Nutrition	• **Liver size and location** • **Spleen** • **Thymus** • **Lymphatic system** Nodes • **Fever** • **Skin rashes** • **Urticaria** • **Itching** • **Fatigue** • **Malaise** • **Infection** • **Respiratory distress** • **Weight loss** • **Joint assessment** • **Cardiovascular system** • **Renal system**	• **Complete blood count** • **Carcinoembryonic antigen (CEA)** • **C-reactive protein** • **Immunoglobins IgA, IgG, IgM, IgD, IgE** • **Rheumatoid factor** • **Antinuclear antibody titer** • **Enzyme-linked immunosorbent assay (ELISA)** • **Western blot** • **Skin tests** • **Tumor staging**	• **Education** Avoidance of infection Avoidance of trigger substances • **Rest** • **Nutrition** • **Stress management** • **Lifestyle alterations** • **Radiation** • **Bone marrow transplantation** • **Therapeutic exercise** • **Energy conservation** • **Joint protection** • **Skin protection from the sun** • **Joint replacement** Total hip Total knee • **Abduction pillow** • **Continuous passive motion (CPM) machine** • **Postoperative complications** Infection Thromboembolitic complications Dislocation	• **Histamine blockers** • **Corticosteroids** • **Hyposensitization** • **Immunosuppressants** • **Chemotherapeutic agents** • **Biologic response modifiers (BRMs)** • **Antibiotics** • **Nonsteroidal anti-inflammatory drugs** • **Opioids**

CHAPTER 20

Concepts of Inflammation and the Immune Response

M. LINDA WORKMAN

Learning Objectives

After studying this chapter, you should be able to:

1. Describe the concept of self-tolerance.
2. Explain the difference between inflammation and infection.
3. Compare and contrast the cells, purposes, and features of inflammation and immunity.
4. Describe the basis for the five cardinal manifestations of inflammation.
5. Interpret a white blood cell count with differential to indicate no immune problems, an acute bacterial infection, a chronic bacterial infection, or an allergic reaction.
6. Explain how complement activation and fixation assists in protection from infection.
7. Compare the cells, function, and protective actions of antibody-mediated immunity and cell-mediated immunity.
8. Compare and contrast the types of antibody-mediated immunity.

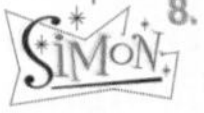

Go to http://www.wbsaunders.com/SIMON/Iggy/ for self-assessment questions related to these Learning Objectives.

Injury and infectious illnesses are common. Most people, however, are healthy more often than they are ill. Inflammation and immunity are the two major defense mechanisms protecting the immunocompetent person against diseases and other problems when the body is invaded by microorganisms. These same defenses also help the body to recover after injury or tissue damage. Therefore inflammation and immunity have critical roles in maintaining health and preventing disease.

Immune function is altered to some degree by many diseases, injuries, and medical therapies. These alterations in immune function may be temporary or permanent, but they always endanger the health of the client.

OVERVIEW

Immunity is composed of many cell functions that protect people against the effects of injury or microscopic invasion. People interact with many other living organisms in the environment. The size of these organisms varies from large (other humans and animals) to microscopic (bacteria, viruses, molds, spores, pollens, protozoa, and cells from other people or animals). As long as microorganisms do not enter the body's internal environment, they pose no threat to health. The body has some defenses to prevent microorganisms from gaining access to the internal environment. These defenses are not perfect, and invasion of the body's internal environment by microorganisms occurs often. Invasion occurs much more frequently than does an actual disease or illness because of proper immune functioning.

Purpose of Inflammation and Immunity

The purpose of inflammation and immunity is to neutralize, eliminate, or destroy microorganisms that invade the internal environment. To accomplish this purpose without harming the body, immune system cells use defensive actions only against non-self proteins and cells. Therefore immune system cells can distinguish between the body's own healthy self cells and other, non-self proteins and cells.

Self Versus Non-Self

Non-self proteins and cells include infected body cells, cancer cells, and all invading cells and microorganisms. This ability to recognize self versus non-self, which is necessary to prevent healthy body cells from being destroyed along with the invaders, is called **self-tolerance.** The immune system cells are the only body cells capable of distinguishing self from non-self. The process of self-tolerance is possible because of the different kinds of proteins present on cell membranes.

All organisms are made up of cells. Each cell is surrounded by a plasma membrane (Figure 20-1). With any cell, many different proteins protrude through the plasma membrane. For example, in liver cells, many different proteins are present on the cell surface (protruding through the membrane). The amino acid sequence of each protein type differs from that of all other protein types. Some of these proteins are found on the liver cells of all animals (including humans) that have livers, because these protein types are specific to the liver and actually serve as a marker for liver tissues.

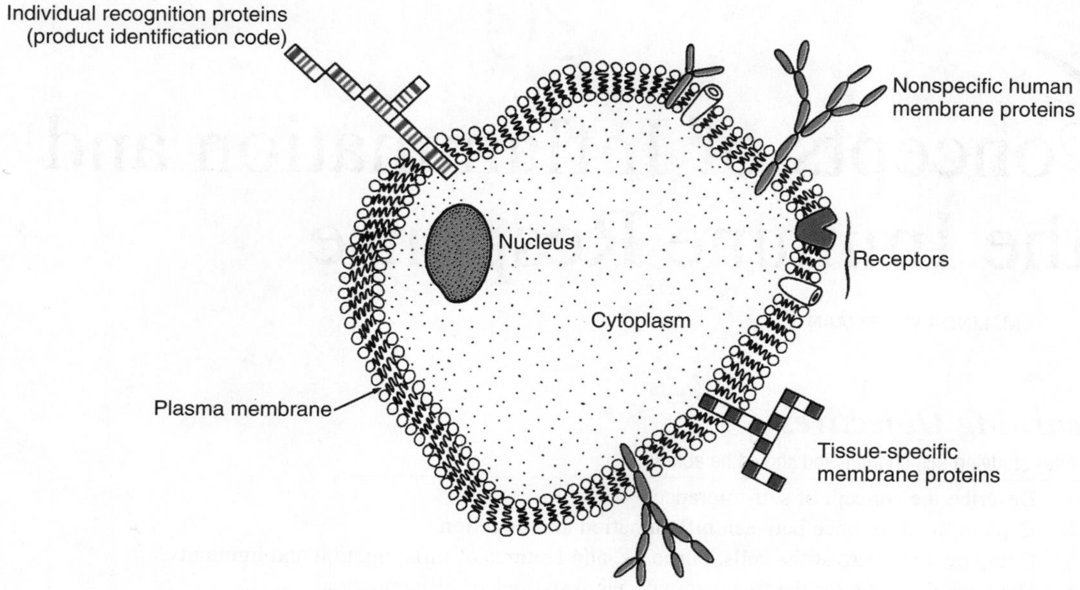

Figure 20-1 ● Properties of human cell membranes.

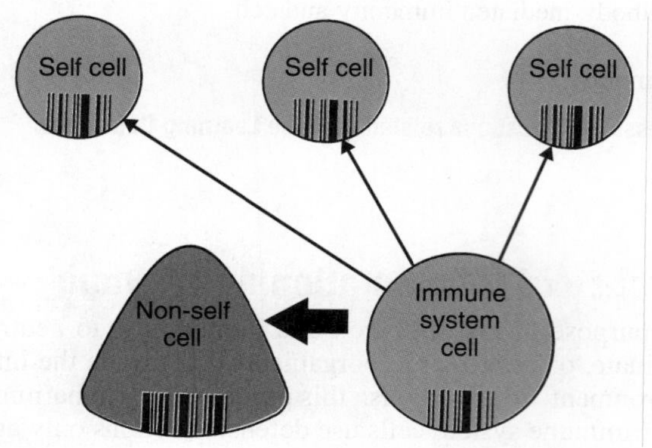

Figure 20-2 ● Determination of self versus non-self cells.

Other protein types are found only on the liver cells of humans, because these protein types are specific markers for humans. Still other protein types are found only on the liver cells of humans with a specific blood type. In addition, each person's liver cells have surface protein types that are specific to that individual. These proteins are unique to the person and would be identical only to the proteins of an identical twin. These unique proteins, found on the surface of all body cells of that individual, serve as a "universal product code" or a "cellular fingerprint" for that person (Workman, Ellerhorst-Ryan, & Koertge, 1993). The proteins that make up the universal product code for one person are recognized as "foreign," or non-self, by the immune system of another person. Because the cell-surface proteins are non-self to another person's immune system, they are **antigens,** proteins capable of stimulating an immune response.

This unique universal product code for each person is composed of the **human leukocyte antigens (HLAs).** "Leukocyte antigen" is actually an incorrect term, because these antigens are also present on the surfaces of nearly all body cells, not just on leukocytes. HLAs are a normal part of the person and act as antigens only if they enter another person's body. These antigens specify the **tissue type** of a person. Other names for these personal cellular fingerprints are *human transplantation antigens, human histocompatibility antigens,* and *class I antigens.*

Humans have about 40 major HLAs (known as *histocompatibility antigens*) that are determined by a series of genes collectively called the major histocompatibility complex (MHC). However, the exact number of minor HLAs that any person has is not known. The specific antigens that any person has (of a large number of possible antigens) are genetically determined by which MHC genes were inherited from his or her parents.

This universal product code (HLA) is a key feature for recognition and self-tolerance. The immune system cells constantly come into contact with other body cells and with any invader that happens to enter the body's internal environment. At each encounter, the immune system cells compare the surface protein universal product codes (HLAs) to determine whether or not the encountered cell belongs in the body's internal environment (Figure 20-2). If the encountered cell's universal product code (HLA) perfectly matches the HLA of the immune system cell, the encountered cell is considered self and is not attacked by the immune system cell. If the encountered cell's universal product code (HLA) does not perfectly match the HLA of the immune system cell, the encountered cell is considered non-self, or foreign. The immune system cell takes action to neutralize, destroy, or eliminate the foreign invader.

Immune function changes during a person's life, according to nutritional status, environmental conditions, medications, the presence of disease, and age. Immune function is most efficient when people are in their 20s and 30s and slowly declines with increasing age. The older adult has decreased immune function, causing greater susceptibility to a variety of pathologic conditions (Chart 20-1).

CHART 20-1

NURSING FOCUS *on the* OLDER ADULT
Changes in Immune Function Related to Aging

Immune Component	Functional Change	Nursing Implications
Inflammation	There is a probable defect in neutrophil function. Leukocytosis does not occur during episodes of acute infection. Older persons may not have a fever during inflammatory or infectious episodes.	Neutrophil counts may be normal, but activity is reduced or impaired. Clients may have an infection but not show standard changes in white blood cell counts. Not only is there potential loss of protection through inflammation, but minor infections may be overlooked until the client becomes severely infected or septic.
Antibody-mediated immunity	The total number of colony-forming B-lymphocytes and the ability of these cells to mature into antibody-secreting cells are diminished.	Older adults are less able to make new antibodies in response to the presence of new antigens. Thus they should receive immunizations, such as "flu shots" and the pneumococcal vaccination.
	There is a decline in natural antibodies, decreased response to antigens, and reduction in the amount of time the antibody response is maintained.	Older adults may not have sufficient antibodies present to provide protection when they are re-exposed to microorganisms against which they have already generated antibodies. Thus older clients need to avoid people with viral infections and to receive "booster" shots for old vaccinations and immunizations.
Cell-mediated immunity	Thymic activity decreases with aging, and the number of circulating T-lymphocytes decreases.	Skin tests for tuberculosis may be falsely negative. Older clients are more at risk for bacterial and fungal infections, especially on the skin and mucous membranes, in the respiratory tract, and in the genitourinary tract.

Organization of the Immune System

The immune system is not confined to any one organ or area of the body. The cells of the immune system originate in the bone marrow. Some of these cells mature in the bone marrow; others leave the bone marrow and mature in different specific body sites. After maturation, most immune system cells are released into the blood, where they circulate to most areas of the body and exert specific effects.

The bone marrow is the source of all blood cells, including immune system cells. The bone marrow produces an immature, undifferentiated cell called a **stem cell** (Guyton & Hall, 2000). This immature stem cell is also described as *pluripotent, multipotent,* and *totipotent.* These terms describe the potential future of the stem cell. When the stem cell is first created in the bone marrow, it is undifferentiated. The cell is not yet committed to maturing into a specific blood cell type. At this stage, the stem cell is flexible and has the potential to become any one of a variety of mature blood cells. Figure 20-3 presents a scheme showing the major possible maturational outcomes for the pluripotent stem cell. The type of mature blood cell the stem cell becomes depends on which maturational pathway it follows.

The maturational pathway of any stem cell depends on body needs at the time, as well as on the presence of specific hormones (cytokines, factors, or poietins) that direct commitment and induce maturation. For example, **erythropoietin** is made in the kidney. When immature stem cells are exposed to erythropoietin, the immature stem cells commit to following the erythrocyte maturational pathway and become mature red blood cells.

White blood cells **(leukocytes)** are cells that protect the body from the effects of invasion by foreign microorganisms. These cells are the immune system cells. Table 20-1 summarizes the functions of different immune system cells. The leukocytes can provide protection through a variety of defensive actions (Abbas, Lichtman, & Pober, 1997). These actions include the following:

- Recognition of self versus non-self
- Phagocytic destruction of foreign invaders, cellular debris, and unhealthy or abnormal self cells
- Lytic destruction of foreign invaders and unhealthy self cells
- Production of antibodies directed against invaders
- Activation of complement
- Production of hormones that stimulate increased formation of leukocytes in bone marrow
- Production of hormones that increase specific leukocyte growth and activity

The three processes necessary for immunity and the cell types involved in these responses can be categorized as inflammation; antibody-mediated immunity (AMI), also known as humoral immunity; and cell-mediated immunity (CMI). These three processes use different defensive actions, and each process influences or requires assistance from the other two processes (Figure 20-4). Therefore full immunity, or **immunocompetence,** requires the function and interaction of all three processes.

INFLAMMATION

Inflammation provides immediate protection against the effects of tissue injury and invading foreign proteins. The ability to produce an inflammatory response is critical to health and well-being. Inflammation differs from AMI and CMI in two important ways:

1. Inflammatory responses provide immediate but short-term protection against the effects of injury or foreign

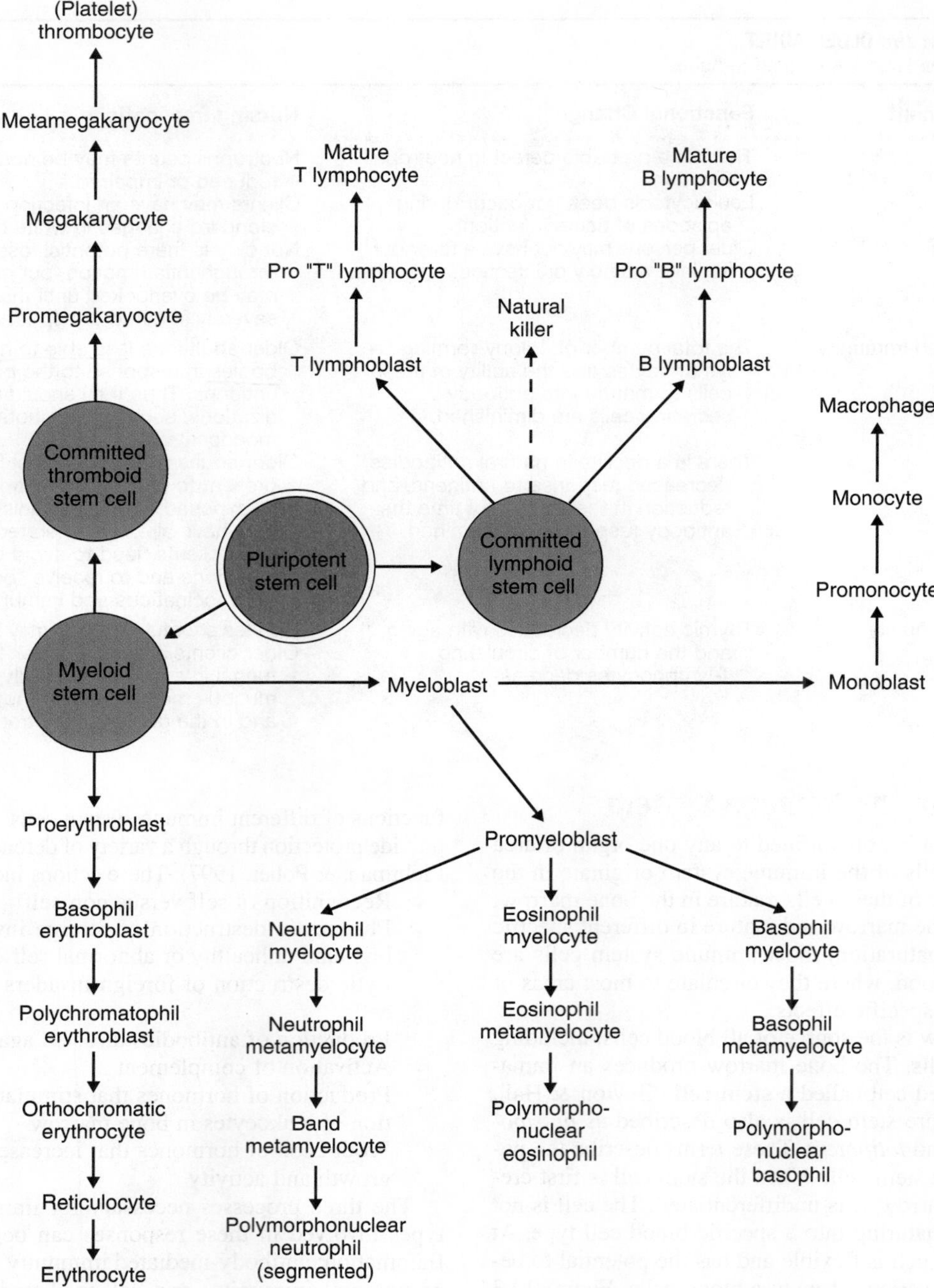

Figure 20-3 ● Stem cell differentiation and maturation.

invaders rather than sustained, long-term immunity on repeated exposure to the same foreign invaders.

2. Inflammation is a nonspecific body defense to invasion or injury and can be started quickly by almost any event.

Inflammation is nonspecific; the same tissue responses occur with any type of injury or invasion, regardless of the location on the body or the specific initiating agent. Therefore the inflammatory processes stimulated by a scald burn to the hand are the same as the inflammatory processes stimulated by excessive acid in the stomach or the presence of bacteria in the middle ear. How widespread the symptoms of inflammation are in the body depends on the intensity, severity, duration, and extent of exposure to the initiating injury or invasion. For example, a splinter in the finger triggers an inflammatory response only at the splinter site, whereas a burn injuring 60% of the skin surface results in an inflammatory response involving the entire body.

Purpose

Inflammatory responses start tissue actions that cause visible and uncomfortable symptoms. Despite the discomfort, these inflammatory actions are important in ridding the body of harmful microorganisms. However, if the inflammatory response is excessive, tissue damage may result. Inflammatory

TABLE 20-1 • IMMUNE FUNCTIONS OF SPECIFIC LEUKOCYTES

Variable	Leukocyte	Function
Inflammation	Neutrophil	Nonspecific ingestion and phagocytosis of microorganisms and foreign protein
	Macrophage	Nonspecific recognition of foreign proteins and microorganisms; ingestion and phagocytosis
	Monocyte	Destruction of bacteria and cellular debris; matures into macrophage
	Eosinophil	Weak phagocytic action; releases vasoactive amines during allergic reactions
	Basophil	Releases histamine and heparin in areas of tissue damage
Antibody-mediated immunity	B-lymphocyte	Becomes sensitized to foreign cells and proteins
	Plasma cell	Secretes immunoglobulins in response to the presence of a specific antigen
	Memory cell	Remains sensitized to a specific antigen and can secrete increased amounts of immunoglobulins specific to the antigen
Cell-mediated immunity	T-lymphocyte helper/inducer T-cell	Enhances immune activity through secretion of various factors, cytokines, and lymphokines
	Cytotoxic/cytolytic T-cell	Selectively attacks and destroys non-self cells, including virally infected cells, grafts, and transplanted organs
	Natural killer cell	Nonselectively attacks non-self cells, especially body cells that have undergone mutation and become malignant; also attacks grafts and transplanted organs

responses also help stimulate both antibody-mediated and cell-mediated actions to activate a full immune response.

Infection

A confusing issue regarding inflammation is that this process occurs in response to tissue injury, as well as to invasion by microorganisms or other foreign proteins. Infection is usually accompanied by inflammation; however, *inflammation can occur without invasion by microorganisms.* For example, inflammatory responses not associated with infection occur with sprain injuries to joints, myocardial infarction, sterile surgical incisions, thrombophlebitis, and blister formation. Examples of inflammatory responses caused by noninfectious invasion by foreign proteins include allergic rhinitis, contact dermatitis, and other allergic reactions. Inflammatory responses caused by infection with microorganisms include otitis media, appendicitis, bacterial peritonitis, viral hepatitis, and bacterial myocarditis, among others. Thus inflammation does not always mean that an infection is present.

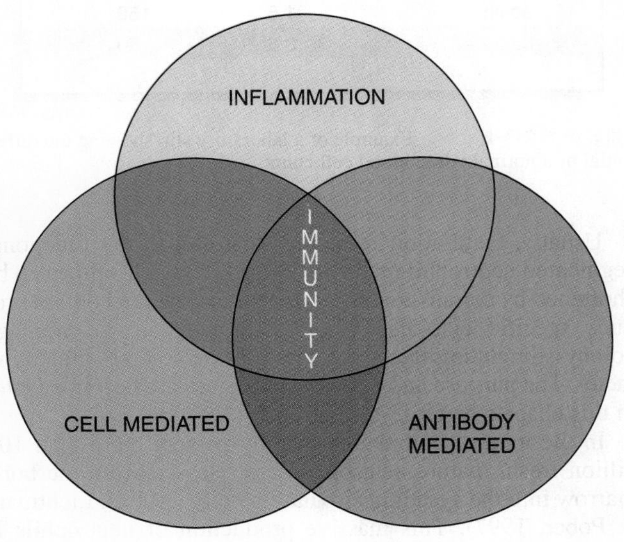

Figure 20-4 ● The three divisions of immunity. Each division (inflammation, antibody-mediated immunity, and cell-mediated immunity) has an important independent function. In addition, the function of each division of immunity is profoundly influenced by the other two divisions. Most important, optimal function of all three divisions is necessary for complete immunity.

Cell Types Involved in Inflammation

The leukocytes associated with inflammatory responses are neutrophils, macrophages, eosinophils, and basophils. Neutrophils and macrophages participate in phagocytosis, destroying and eliminating foreign invaders. Basophils and eosinophils act on blood vessels to cause tissue-level responses.

NEUTROPHILS

Description and Origin

Mature neutrophils normally make up between 55% and 70% of the total white blood cell count. **Neutrophils** arise from the stem cells and complete the maturation process in the bone marrow (Figure 20-5). They belong to the class of leukocytes known as **granulocytes** because of the large number of granules present inside each cell. Other names for neutrophils are based on their physical appearance and degree of maturation. Mature neutrophils are also called *segmented neutrophils* ("segs") or *polymorphonuclear cells* ("polys," PNMs,) because of their segmented nucleus. Less mature neutrophils are called *band neutrophils* ("bands" or "stabs") because of their nuclear appearance.

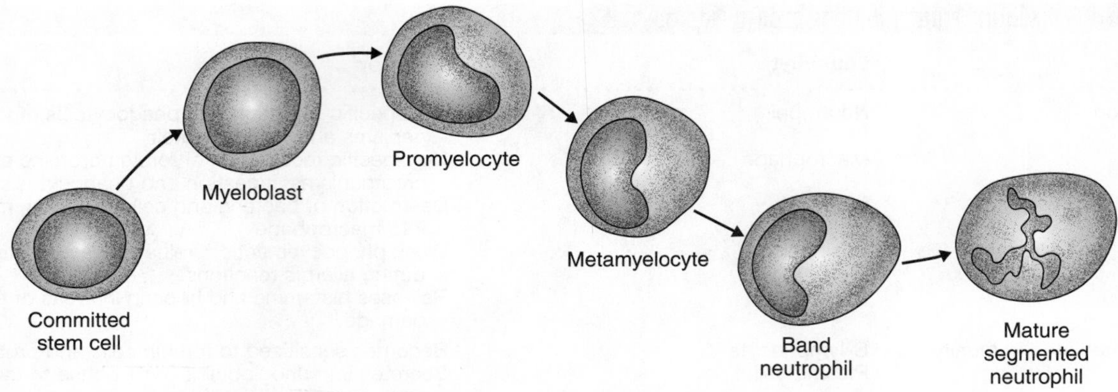

Figure 20-5 ● Neutrophil maturation.

Differential	%	/mm³
Total WBC	100	10,000
segs	62	6200
bands	5	500
monos	3	300
lymphs	28	2800
eosin	1.5	150
baso	0.5	50

Figure 20-6 ● Example of a laboratory slip showing the differential of a normal white blood cell count.

Usually, maturation from the stem cell to the functional segmented neutrophil requires 12 to 14 days. This time can be shortened by certain conditions that stimulate the body to produce specific cytokines, such as granulocyte-macrophage colony-stimulating factor and granulocyte colony-stimulating factor. The purpose and action of cytokines are described later in this chapter under Cytokines, p. 322.

In the immunocompetent, healthy person, more than 100 billion fresh, mature neutrophils are released from the bone marrow into the systemic circulation daily (Abbas, Lichtman, & Pober, 1997). This massive production of neutrophils is necessary because the life span of a circulating neutrophil is extremely short, averaging only about 12 to 18 hours.

Function

Although the neutrophils are the largest group of circulating leukocytes, each individual cell is small. This army of powerful small cells provides the first internal line of defense, via phagocytosis, against foreign invaders (especially bacteria) in blood and extracellular fluid. It is the granules inside the neutrophils that cause the phagocytic destruction of foreign invaders. The mature neutrophil has many granules containing different enzymes that can degrade invaders.

Neutrophils have a small energy supply and no way of replenishing either that energy supply or the enzymes used in degradation. Thus each neutrophil can take part in only one episode of phagocytic destruction before supplies are exhausted.

The mature, segmented neutrophil is the only neutrophil stage capable of effective phagocytosis. Because this cell type is responsible for continuous, instant, nonspecific protection against microorganisms, the percentage and actual number of circulating white blood cells that are mature neutrophils reliably measure a client's susceptibility to infection: the higher the numbers, the greater the resistance to infection. This measurement is the **absolute neutrophil count** (sometimes called the absolute granulocyte count or total granulocyte count).

The differential of a normal white blood cell count shows the number and percent of all the different types of circulating leukocytes (Figure 20-6). This test indicates that most of the neutrophils released into the blood from the bone marrow are segmented neutrophils; only a small percentage are band neutrophils. The less mature neutrophil forms should not be present in the blood. Some conditions cause the population of neutrophils in the blood to change from mostly segmented neutrophils to less mature forms. This situation is termed a **left shift** because the segmented neutrophil, which is seen at the far right of the neutrophil maturational pathway (see Figure 20-5), no longer represents the greatest number of circulating neutrophils. Instead, the population is made up primarily of one of the cell types found farther left on the neutrophil maturational pathway.

A left shift is a clinical sign indicating that the client's bone marrow cannot produce enough mature neutrophils to keep pace with the continuing presence of microorganisms and is releasing immature neutrophils into the blood. Unfortunately, most of these immature neutrophils are of no benefit, because they are not capable of phagocytosis.

MACROPHAGES

Description and Origin

Macrophages arise from the committed myeloid stem cells in the bone marrow and form the **mononuclear-phagocyte system.** The stem cells first form monocytes and are released into the blood at this stage. Until they mature, monocytes have only limited activity. Most monocytes move from the blood into various tissues, where they complete

TABLE 20-2 • TISSUE MACROPHAGES

Tissue	Macrophage
Lung	Alveolar macrophage
Connective tissue	Histiocyte
Brain	Microglial cell
Liver	Kupffer cell
Peritoneum	Peritoneal macrophage
Bone	Osteoclast
Joints	Synovial type A cell
Kidney	Mesangial cell

the maturation process into macrophages. Some macrophages become "fixed" in position within the tissues, whereas others remain mobile in the tissue's interstitial fluid. Macrophages in various tissues have slightly different appearances and different names. Table 20-2 lists the names of the different tissue macrophages. Figure 20-7 shows the distribution of tissue macrophages throughout the body. The liver and spleen contain the greatest concentration of these cells.

Tissue macrophages have relatively long life spans, lasting from months to years. Macrophages are the largest of all the leukocytes and contain many lytic enzymes.

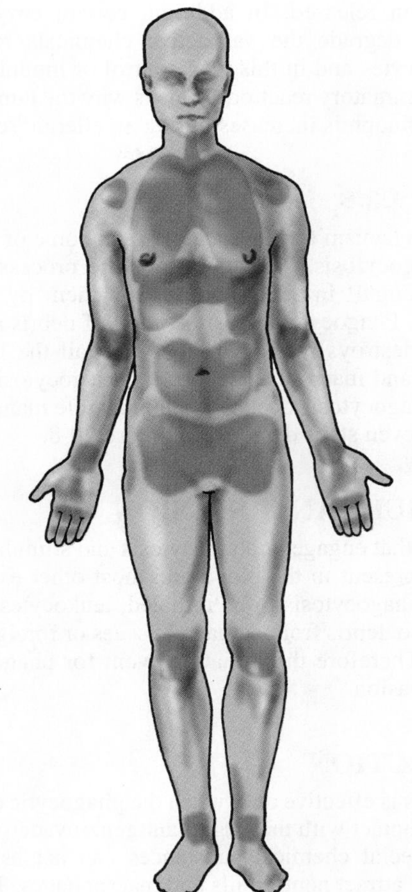

Figure 20-7 ● Areas of highest concentration of tissue macrophages.

Function

Macrophages play more than one role in protecting against invasion and tissue injury. These cells are important in immediate inflammatory responses and can also stimulate the longer-lasting immune responses associated with antibody-mediated immunity (AMI) and cell-mediated immunity (CMI). Specific macrophage functions include phagocytosis, repair of injured tissues, antigen presenting/processing, and secretion of cytokines that help control the immune system.

The inflammation-associated macrophage function is phagocytosis. Macrophages are efficient at distinguishing between self and non-self and are especially effective at trapping invading cells. Unlike neutrophils, macrophages are able to regenerate the energy supplies and enzymes needed to degrade foreign protein. Therefore each macrophage can take part in many phagocytic events during its life span.

BASOPHILS

Description and Origin

The rarest leukocytes, **basophils,** arise from myeloid stem cells and are released from the bone marrow after a short maturation period. Basophils cause the obvious signs and symptoms accompanying inflammation, as described in the following section (Function) and under Sequence of Inflammatory Responses, p. 315.

Function

Basophils have granules containing many chemicals (vasoactive amines) that act on blood vessels, including heparin, histamine, serotonin, kinins, and leukotrienes. When released into the blood, most of these chemicals act on smooth muscle and blood vessel walls. **Heparin** inhibits coagulation of blood and other protein-containing fluids. **Histamine** constricts the smooth muscles of the respiratory system and small veins. Constriction of respiratory smooth muscle narrows the lumen of airways and restricts breathing. Constriction of veins inhibits blood flow through small veins and decreases venous return. This effect causes blood to collect in capillaries and small arterioles. **Kinins** cause vasodilation of arterioles and, together with serotonin, increased capillary permeability. These actions permit the plasma portion of the blood to leak into the interstitial space. This chemical-induced process is called **vascular leak syndrome.**

EOSINOPHILS

Description and Origin

Eosinophils arise from the myeloid line and contain more vasoactive chemicals. Usually, only 1% to 2% of the total white blood cell count is composed of eosinophils.

Function

Eosinophils are not efficient phagocytes, although they can act against infestations of parasitic larvae. Eosinophil granules contain many substances with vastly different actions. Some substances are chemicals that produce inflammatory reactions when released. In addition, certain enzymes from eosinophils degrade the vasoactive chemicals released by other leukocytes and in this way control or modulate the extent of inflammatory reactions. This is why the number of circulating eosinophils increases during an allergic response.

Phagocytosis

The key mechanism for the successful outcome of inflammation is **phagocytosis.** Phagocytosis is the process by which leukocytes engulf invaders and destroy them by enzymatic degradation. Phagocytosis rids the body of debris after tissue injury and destroys foreign invaders. Of all the leukocytes, neutrophils and macrophages perform phagocytosis most efficiently. Phagocytosis occurs in a predictable manner and involves the seven steps depicted in Figure 20-8.

EXPOSURE AND INVASION

Leukocytes that engage in phagocytosis and stimulate inflammation are present in the blood and most other extracellular fluids. For phagocytosis to be initiated, leukocytes must first be exposed to debris from damaged tissues or foreign proteins (antigens). Therefore the initiating event for phagocytosis is injury or invasion.

ATTRACTION

Phagocytosis is effective only when the phagocytic cell comes into direct contact with the target (antigen, invader, or foreign protein). Special chemical substances can act as chemical magnets that attract neutrophils and macrophages. These substances are called **chemotaxins** or **leukotaxins.** Damaged tissues and blood vessels secrete chemotaxins. In addition, substances that combine with the surface of invading foreign proteins serve as chemotaxins. This combining (and attracting) mechanism is described next.

ADHERENCE

Because phagocytosis requires direct contact of the leukocyte with its intended target, the phagocytic cell must first bind to the surface of the target. A special process called **opsonization** helps provide direct contact of the phagocyte with its target.

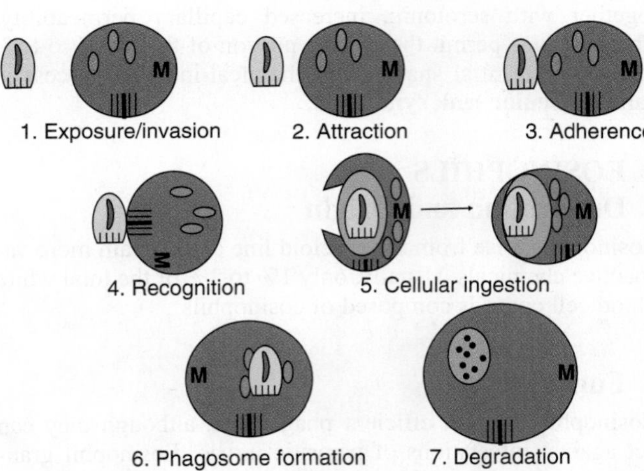

Figure 20-8 ● Steps of phagocytosis.

Opsonization

The word *opsonin* is Greek and literally means "to cover food with a sauce in preparation for eating." In inflammation, opsonins coat a target cell (antigen or foreign protein); this changes the target cell's surface charge and makes it easier for phagocytic cells to stick to it. Many substances can act as opsonins. Some of these substances are particles from dead neutrophils, antibodies, and activated (fixated) complement components.

Complement Activation and Fixation

One mechanism of opsonization and phagocytic adherence to target cells is **complement activation and fixation.** Twenty different inactive protein components of the complement system are present in the blood. These components are made by the liver. With proper stimulation, individual complement proteins become activated, join together, surround an antigen, and cause dramatic actions as a result of fixation (adherence) to the antigen. Complement fixation must occur quickly, but consequences can be devastating if its effects are exerted at the wrong time or in the wrong place. Therefore the complement system works as a cascade reaction (chain reaction), with many sites of activation and control.

RECOGNITION

When the phagocytic cell sticks to the surface of the target cell, recognition of non-self occurs. The body's phagocytic cells examine the universal product codes (human leukocyte antigens [HLAs]) of whatever they encounter. Recognition of non-self is enhanced by opsonins on the surface of the target cell. Phagocytic cells proceed with phagocytosis only if the target cell is recognized either as foreign or as debris from damaged self cells.

CELLULAR INGESTION

Because phagocytic destruction occurs inside the cell, the target cell or foreign protein must be brought inside the phagocytic cell. The phagocytic cell changes its shape and bends its membrane around to enclose (engulf) the target cell. Once the target is enclosed in the phagocytic cells, a vacuole is formed.

PHAGOSOME FORMATION

When the phagocyte's granules are inside the vacuole, the structure is called a **phagosome** (or **phagolysosome**). These granules break open and release enzymes into the fluid of the phagosome and destroy the ingested target.

DEGRADATION

The enzymes within the phagosome exert their specific effects on different parts of the ingested target. The target is broken down into smaller pieces until only minute particles remain to be removed from the body as debris.

Sequence of Inflammatory Responses

Inflammatory responses that protect the body against the effects of tissue injury or invasion by foreign proteins occur in a predictable sequence. The sequence is the same regardless of the initiating stimulus. Responses at the tissue level cause the **five cardinal manifestations of inflammation:** warmth, redness, swelling, pain, and decreased function. These inflammatory responses occur in three distinct stages, although the timing of the stages may overlap (Table 20-3).

STAGE I (VASCULAR)

In stage I of the inflammatory response, the early effects involve changes at the blood vessel level. When inflammation results from tissue injury, this stage has two phases.

Phase I

The first phase is an immediate, short-term constriction of arterioles and venules as a direct result of physical trauma to vascular smooth muscle. This phase lasts only seconds to minutes and may be so short that the person undergoing the response is unaware of the vasoconstriction.

Phase II

The second phase is characterized by increased blood flow to the area **(hyperemia)** and swelling **(edema formation)** at the site of injury or invasion. Injured tissues and the leukocytes in this area secrete vasoactive chemicals (histamine, serotonin, and kinins) that cause constriction of the small veins and dilation of the arterioles in the immediate area. These changes in blood vessel dilation lead to redness and increased warmth of the tissues. This response increases the supply of nutrients at the tissue level by increasing blood flow.

Some of these chemicals increase capillary permeability, allowing blood plasma to leak into the interstitial space. This response causes swelling and pain. Pain, although uncomfortable, increases the person's awareness that a problem exists and encourages action to avoid further injury or inflammation. Edema formation at the site of injury or invasion is also a helpful event. This swelling protects the area from further injury by creating a cushion of fluid. The extra fluid can dilute the concentration of any toxins or microorganisms that have entered the area. The duration of these responses depends on the severity of the initiating event.

The major leukocyte involved in stage I of the inflammatory response is the tissue macrophage. The response of tissue macrophages is immediate, because they are already in place at the site of injury or invasion. This response, however, is limited, because the number of macrophages is so small. In addition to functioning in phagocytosis, the tissue macrophages secrete several cytokines to enhance the inflammatory response. One cytokine is colony-stimulating factor, which stimulates the bone marrow to reduce the time of leukocyte production from 14 days to a matter of hours. Tissue macrophages also secrete substances that increase the release of neutrophils from the bone marrow and attract them to the site of injury or invasion, which leads to the next stage of inflammation.

STAGE II (CELLULAR EXUDATE)

Stage II of inflammation is characterized by **neutrophilia** (increased number of circulating neutrophils), secretion of many

TABLE 20-3 • STAGES OF INFLAMMATION

Onset	Cells Involved	Actions
STAGE I: VASCULAR		
Minutes after injury or invasion	Tissue macrophages	Limited phagocytosis of invading microorganisms or cell debris from injured tissues Secretion of vasoactive amines (histamine, bradykinin, serotonin) to dilate blood vessels and increase capillary leak; this action results in redness, warmth, swelling, and pain at the site but also increases bloodflow to the area; more nutrients are available to the tissues; plasma proteins move into the tissues, clot, and "wall off" microorganisms, limiting their spread Secretion of chemotaxins to draw more leukocytes into the area to sustain the inflammatory response Secretion of cytokines to increase bone marrow production of granulocytes
STAGE II: CELLULAR EXUDATE		
Hours after injury or invasion	Granular myeloid cells • Neutrophils • Basophils • Eosinophils	Increased phagocytosis Secretion of slow-acting vasoactive amines to ensure a sustained inflammatory response Secretion of substances to increase the rate of neutrophil maturation and macrophage maturation
STAGE III: TISSUE REPAIR AND REPLACEMENT		
Begins at initial injury and continues until new tissues are formed and mature or are functional	Neutrophils Macrophages	Stimulation of mitotically active cells to divide; stimulation of fibroblasts in blood vessels to grow and release collagen to form scaffold on which to build scar tissue

factors into the interstitial fluid, and the formation of exudate, commonly called **pus.**

The most active leukocyte in this stage is the neutrophil. Under the influence of chemotactic agents and cytokines, the neutrophil count can increase up to five times within 12 hours after the onset of inflammation. At the site of inflammation, neutrophils attack and destroy foreign materials and remove dead tissue through phagocytosis.

During acute inflammatory responses, the healthy person can produce enough mature neutrophils to keep pace with the effects of injury or invasion and to prevent the invaders from multiplying. At the same time, the leukocytes secrete cytokines, which increase reproduction of tissue macrophages and bone marrow production of monocytes. Although this reaction begins slowly, its effects are long lasting.

When infectious processes stimulating inflammation are longer or chronic, the bone marrow cannot produce and release enough mature neutrophils into the blood to keep pace with the ability of microorganisms to multiply. In this situation, the bone marrow begins to release only immature neutrophils. Such a reduction in the number of functional phagocytic neutrophils limits the effectiveness of the inflammatory response and increases the susceptibility to microbial infections.

STAGE III (TISSUE REPAIR AND REPLACEMENT)

Although stage III is completed last, it begins at the time of injury and is critical to the ultimate function of the inflamed area.

Some of the leukocytes involved in inflammation start the replacement of lost tissues or repair of damaged tissues by inducing the remaining healthy tissue to divide. In tissues that are unable to divide, leukocytes stimulate new blood vessel growth and scar tissue formation. Because scar tissue does not behave like normal tissue, loss of function occurs where damaged tissues are replaced with scar tissue. The extent of the functional loss is determined by the percentage of tissue replaced by scar tissue.

Inflammation alone cannot confer immunity; however, the interaction of inflammatory cells with lymphocytes helps provide long-lasting immunity against re-exposure to the same microorganisms. Long-lasting immune actions are generated by antibody-mediated immunity (AMI) and cell-mediated immunity (CMI).

ANTIBODY-MEDIATED IMMUNITY

Antibody-mediated immunity (AMI), also known as humoral immunity, involves antigen-antibody interactions to neutralize, eliminate, or destroy foreign proteins. Antibodies for these actions are produced by populations of B-lymphocytes.

Purpose

The primary functions of B-lymphocytes are to become sensitized to a specific foreign protein (antigen) and to produce antibodies directed specifically against that protein. The antibody (rather than the actual B-lymphocyte) then takes part in one of several actions to neutralize, eliminate, or destroy that antigen.

Cell Types Involved in Antibody-Mediated Immunity

The leukocytes with the most direct role in AMI are the B-lymphocytes. Macrophages and T-lymphocytes (discussed later under Cell-Mediated Immunity, p. 321) cooperate with B-lymphocytes to start and complete antigen-antibody interactions. Therefore for optimal AMI, the entire immune system must function adequately.

B-lymphocytes start life as pluripotent stem cells in the bone marrow, the primary lymphoid tissue. The pluripotent stem cells destined to become B-lymphocytes commit early to following the lymphocyte maturational pathway (see Figure 20-3). At the point of commitment these stem cells are no longer pluripotent but are limited to differentiation into lymphocytes. The committed lymphocyte stem cells are released from the bone marrow into the blood. They then migrate into various secondary lymphoid tissues, where maturation is completed.

In humans the secondary lymphoid tissues for B-lymphocyte maturation are the spleen, germinal centers of lymph nodes, tonsils, and Peyer's patches of the intestinal tract.

Antigen-Antibody Interactions

The body learns to make enough of any specific antibody to provide long-lasting immunity against specific microorganisms or toxins. Seven steps in a series of special interactions are required for the production of a unique and specific antibody directed against a unique and specific antigen whenever the person is exposed to that antigen. These steps are exposure and invasion, antigen recognition, lymphocyte sensitization, antibody production and release, antigen-antibody binding, antibody-binding reactions, and sustained immunity memory (Figure 20-9).

EXPOSURE AND INVASION

Antigen-antibody interactions occur in the body's internal environment. For the body to make an antibody that can exert its effects on a specific antigen, the antigen must first enter the body. Not all exposures result in antibody production, even when exposure includes penetration. Invasion by the antigen must occur in such large numbers that some of the antigen evades detection by the normal nonspecific defenses or overwhelms the ability of the inflammatory response to get rid of the invader.

Take, for example, a person who has never contracted or even been exposed to the childhood viral disease chickenpox. This person baby-sits for three children who develop chickenpox lesions within the next 10 hours. These children, in the pre-eruption stage, shed many millions of live chickenpox virus particles via droplets from the upper respiratory tract. Because small children are often unconcerned about the finer points of infection control, they drink out of the baby-sitter's cup, kiss the baby-sitter directly (and wetly) on the lips, and sneeze and cough directly into the sitter's face. During the 5 hours spent with the children at close range, the baby-sitter is overwhelmingly invaded by the chickenpox virus (varicella-zoster) and will become sick with this disease within 14 to 21 days. While the virus is incubating and the disease is developing, the sitter's leukocytes are taking part in the next steps in the series of antibody-antigen interactions to prevent the development of chickenpox more than once.

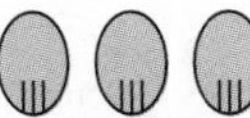
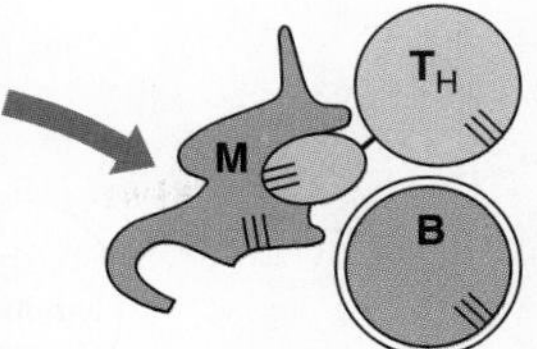
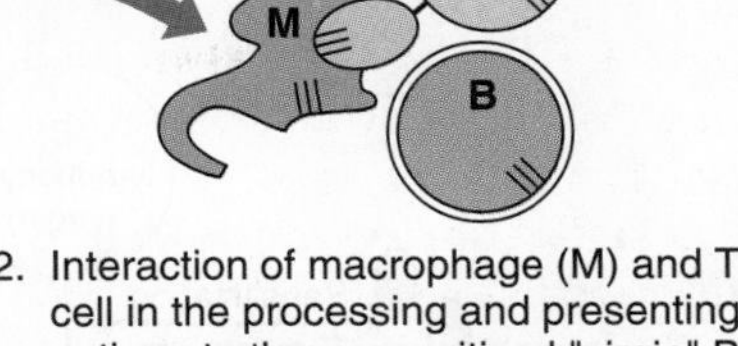
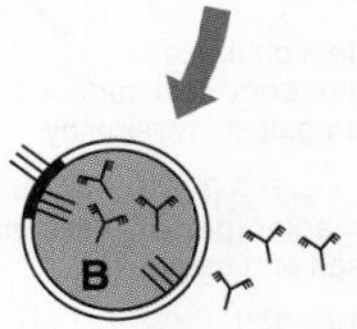
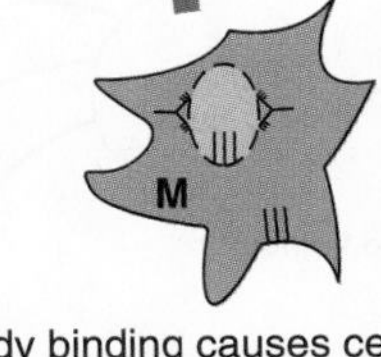
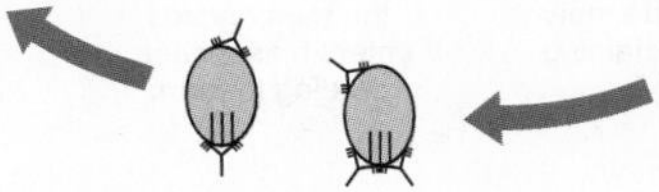

Figure 20-9 ● Sequence of events stimulating antibody-mediated immunity.

ANTIGEN RECOGNITION

To begin to make antibodies against an antigen, the "virgin" or previously unsensitized B-lymphocyte must first recognize the antigen as non-self. B-lymphocytes cannot carry out this important function alone; they require the actions of macrophages and helper/inducer T-cells.

This cooperative effort is started by the macrophages. After the membrane of the antigen has been altered somewhat by opsonization (previously discussed under Adherence, p. 314), the macrophage recognizes the invading foreign protein (antigen) as non-self and physically attaches itself to the antigen. This attachment to the antigen does not result in phagocytosis or in immediate destruction of the antigen. Instead, the macrophage presents the attached antigen to the helper/inducer T-cell. At this time, the helper/inducer T-cell and the macrophage process the antigen in such a way as to expose the antigen's recognition sites (universal product code). After processing the antigen, the helper/inducer T-cell brings the antigen into contact with the B-lymphocyte so that the B-lymphocyte can recognize the antigen as non-self.

LYMPHOCYTE SENSITIZATION

Once the B-lymphocyte recognizes the antigen as non-self, the B-lymphocyte becomes sensitized to this antigen. A single virgin B-lymphocyte can undergo sensitization only once. Therefore each B-lymphocyte can be sensitized to only one antigen.

As a result of sensitization, this B-lymphocyte can respond to any substance that carries the same antigens (codes) as the original antigen. Once it is sensitized to a specific antigen, the B-lymphocyte always remains sensitized to that specific antigen. In addition, all daughter cells of that sensitized B-lymphocyte are sensitized to that same specific antigen.

Immediately after it is sensitized, the B-lymphocyte (or B-blast) divides and forms two different types of lymphocytes, each one remaining sensitized to that specific antigen (Figure 20-10). One new cell becomes a **plasma cell** and immediately starts to produce antibody directed specifically against the antigen that originally sensitized the B-lymphocyte. The other new cell becomes a **memory cell.** The plasma cell functions immediately and has a short life span. The memory cell remains sensitized but functionally dormant until the next exposure to the same antigen (discussed later under Sustained Immunity: Memory, p. 319).

ANTIBODY PRODUCTION AND RELEASE

Antibodies are produced by the plasma cell. When fully stimulated, each plasma cell can produce as much as 300 mole-

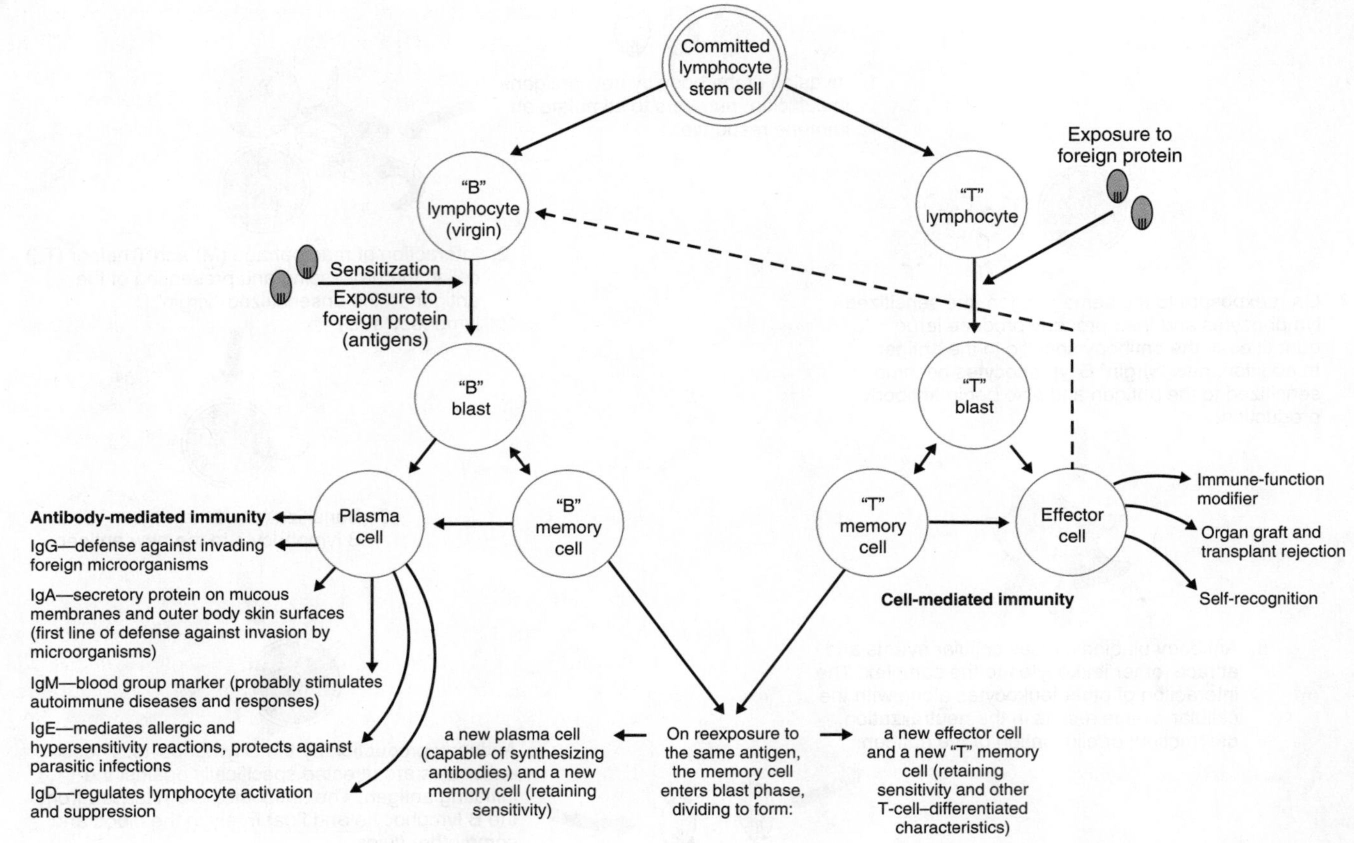

Committed lymphocyte stem cell
"B" lymphocyte (virgin)
"T" lymphocyte
Exposure to foreign protein
Sensitization
Exposure to foreign protein (antigens)
"B" blast
"T" blast
Plasma cell
"B" memory cell
"T" memory cell
Effector cell
Antibody-mediated immunity
IgG—defense against invading foreign microorganisms
IgA—secretory protein on mucous membranes and outer body skin surfaces (first line of defense against invasion by microorganisms)
IgM—blood group marker (probably stimulates autoimmune diseases and responses)
IgE—mediates allergic and hypersensitivity reactions, protects against parasitic infections
IgD—regulates lymphocyte activation and suppression
Immune-function modifier
Organ graft and transplant rejection
Self-recognition
Cell-mediated immunity
a new plasma cell (capable of synthesizing antibodies) and a new memory cell (retaining sensitivity)
On reexposure to the same antigen, the memory cell enters blast phase, dividing to form:
a new effector cell and a new "T" memory cell (retaining sensitivity and other T-cell–differentiated characteristics)

Figure 20-10 ● Differentiated functions of lymphocytes.

Antigen recognition and binding sites
Heavy chain
Hinge region
Fab fragment
Light chain
S–S
Disulfide bonds
Fc fragment

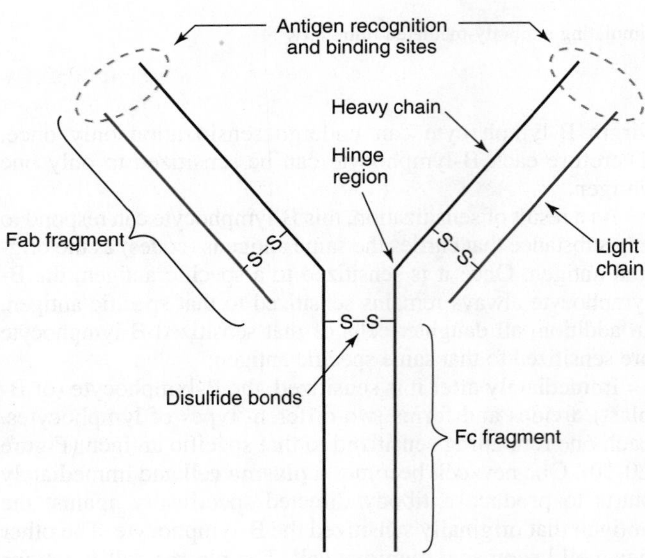

Figure 20-11 ● Basic antibody structure.

cules of antibody per second. Each plasma cell produces antibody specific only to the antigen that originally sensitized the parent B-lymphocyte. For example, in the case of the baby-sitter who was exposed to and invaded by the chickenpox virus, the plasma cells that are derived from the B-lymphocytes sensitized to the chickenpox virus can produce only antichickenpox antibodies. The exact antibody type (e.g., immunoglobulin G [IgG] or immunoglobulin M [IgM]) that the plasma cell can produce may vary, but the specificity of that antibody remains forever directed against the chickenpox virus.

Antibody molecules produced by the plasma cells are secreted into the blood and other extracellular fluids as free antibody. Individual molecules of free antibody remain in the blood for 3 to 30 days. Because the antibody circulates in body fluids (or body "humors") and is separate from the B-lymphocytes, the immunity provided is sometimes called **humoral immunity.** Circulating antibodies can be transferred from one person to another to provide the receiving person with immediate immunity of short duration.

ANTIGEN-ANTIBODY BINDING

An antibody is a Y-shaped molecule (Figure 20-11). The tips of the short arms of the Y are the areas that recognize the specific antigen and bind to it. Because each antibody molecule has two tips (Fab fragments, or arms), antibody molecules can bind either to two separate antigen molecules or to two areas of the same antigen molecule.

The stem of the Y forms what is called the Fc fragment. This area of the antibody molecule can bind to Fc receptor sites on leukocytes. The leukocyte then has not only its own mechanisms of attacking antigens but also the added power of having antibodies on its surface that stick to antigens (Figure 20-12).

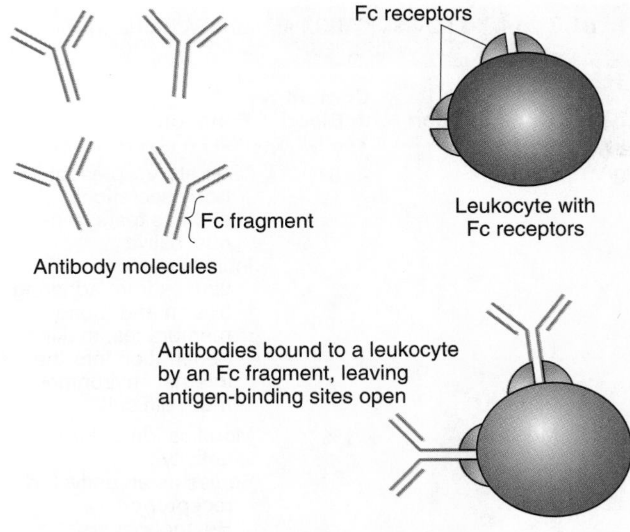

Figure 20-12 ● Antibody Fc receptors on leukocytes.

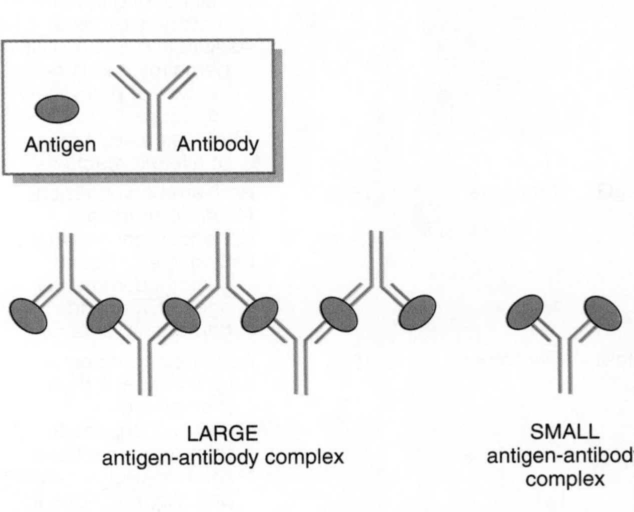

Figure 20-13 ● Antibody-antigen complexes.

The actual binding of antibody to antigen is usually not lethal to the antigen. Instead, the physical binding of the antibody to the antigen starts other actions that neutralize, eliminate, or destroy the antigen.

ANTIBODY-BINDING REACTIONS

The action of binding antibody to antigen allows or triggers specific reactions to cause the neutralization, elimination, or destruction of the antigen. These reactions include agglutination, lysis, complement fixation, precipitation, and inactivation or neutralization.

Agglutination

Agglutination is a clumping-like antibody action that results from an antibody molecule's having at least two antigen-binding sites. This clumping links antigens together, forming large and small immune complexes (Figure 20-13). The binding of more than one antigen molecule to each antibody does not directly destroy the antigen. Agglutination starts defensive effects in at least two ways. First, it slows the movement of the antigen through the extracellular fluids. Second, the irregular shape of the antigen-antibody complex (see Figure 20-13) increases the chances of the complex being attacked by other leukocytes (e.g., macrophages, neutrophils, and cytotoxic/cytolytic T-cells [discussed later under Cell-Mediated Immunity, p. 321]).

Lysis

Lysis, cell membrane destruction, occurs because of antibody binding to membrane-bound antigens of some invaders. The actual binding creates holes in the invader's membrane, changing the intracellular environment. This response usually requires that complement be involved in the antigen-antibody interaction. Bacteria and viruses are the non-self cells most susceptible to damage through lysis caused by the binding of antibody to membrane-surface antigens.

Complement Fixation

Specific classes of antibodies can remove or destroy the non-self antigen through activation of the complement cascade and complement fixation. (The mechanism by which complement assists in immunity is discussed earlier under Adherence, p. 314.) The two classes of antibody capable of stimulating the complement system are IgG and IgM. Binding of antibody from either of these classes to an appropriate antigen provides a binding site for the first component of complement (C1q). Once C1q is activated, other components of the complement system are activated in a cascade.

Precipitation

Precipitation is similar to agglutination. However, in precipitation, antibody molecules bind so much antigen that large, insoluble antigen-antibody complexes are formed. These complexes cannot stay in suspension in the blood. Instead, they form a large precipitate, which can be acted on and removed by neutrophils and macrophages.

Inactivation-Neutralization

Inactivation-neutralization does not result in the immediate destruction of the antigen. Usually, only a small area of the antigen, the **active site,** is actually responsible for causing harmful effects. The rest of the antigen is not harmful to the host. Inactivation-neutralization, through binding of antibody to an antigen, covers up the active site or changes its shape. Either mechanism inhibits the activity of the antigen and makes it harmless without destroying or eliminating it.

SUSTAINED IMMUNITY: MEMORY

The sustained immunity, or memory, function of antibody-mediated immunity (AMI) provides humans with long-lasting immunity to a specific antigen. Sustained immunity occurs through the action of the B-lymphocyte memory cells made during the lymphocyte sensitization stage. These memory cells remain sensitized to the specific antigen to which they were originally exposed. On re-exposure to the same antigen, the memory cells rapidly respond. First, the cells divide and form new sensitized blast cells and new sensitized plasma cells. The blast cells continue to divide to produce even more sensitized plasma cells. The sensitized plasma cells rapidly begin to make and secrete large amounts of the antibody specific for the sensitizing antigen.

This ability of the sensitized memory cells to initiate events on re-exposure to the same antigen that originally sensitized the B-lymphocyte allows a rapid and widespread immune **(anamnestic)** response to the antigen. This response usually removes the invading antigen completely, so that the person does not become ill. Because of this process, most people do not become ill with chickenpox or other viral diseases more than once, even though they are exposed many times to the causative organism. Without the process or action of memory, people would remain susceptible to specific diseases on subsequent exposure to the antigen, and no sustained immunity would be generated.

General Antibody Classification

All antibodies are **immunoglobulins,** also called **gamma globulins.** These names are based on the structure and function of antibodies. A globulin is a type of protein structure that is globular rather than straight. Because antibodies are composed of this type of protein, they are globulins. The term *immunoglobulin* is appropriate for antibodies because they are globular proteins that provide immunity. Antibodies are called gamma globulins because all free antibodies in the plasma separate out in the gamma fraction of plasma proteins during electrophoresis (based on size and electrical charge). The five antibody types are classified by differences in antibody structure, molecular weight, and association (Table 20-4).

TABLE 20-4 • CLASSIFICATION AND CHARACTERIZATION OF ANTIBODIES

Type	Configuration	Content in Blood	Function
IgA	Dimer	<15%	"Secretory"; present in body secretions, such as tears, mucus, saliva Inhibits bacteria and viruses from adhering to skin and mucous membranes, making penetration into the internal environment more difficult
IgD	Monomer	<1%	Modification of IgM activity Serves as an activated receptor on B-lymphocytes
IgE	Monomer	<1%	Degranulation of basophils and mast cells during inflammatory responses Assists in clearance of parasites and prevention of pulmonary infections Mediates many types of allergic reactions
IgG	Monomer	75%	Activates complement Neutralizes toxins Enhances phagocytosis Provides significant sustained immunity against viral and bacterial infections
IgM	Pentomer	10%	Activates complement Clears antigens through precipitation Possibly mediates autoimmune reactions Mediates ABO incompatibility reactions in blood transfusions

Ig, Immunoglobulin.

Acquiring Antibody-Mediated Immunity

Two broad categories of immunity are innate-native immunity and acquired immunity.

INNATE-NATIVE IMMUNITY

Innate-native immunity (sometimes called "natural immunity") is a genetically determined characteristic of an individual, group, or species. A person either has or does not have innate immunity. For example, humans have many innate immunities to viruses and other microorganisms that cause specific diseases in animals. As a result, humans are not susceptible to such diseases as mange, distemper, hog cholera, or any of a variety of animal afflictions. This type of immunity cannot be developed or transferred from one person to another and is not an adaptive response to exposure or invasion by foreign proteins.

Innate-native immunity is nonspecific and encompasses the inflammatory responses. Other components of innate-native immunity include skin, mucosa, antimicrobial chemicals, complement, and natural killer cells (Abbas, Lichtman, & Pober, 1997).

ACQUIRED IMMUNITY

Acquired immunity is the immunity that every person's body makes (or can receive) as an adaptive response to invasion by foreign proteins. AMI is an acquired immunity. Acquired immunity occurs either naturally or artificially and can be either active or passive.

Active Immunity

Active immunity occurs when antigens enter the body and the body responds by making specific antibodies against the antigen. This type of immunity is active because the body takes an active part in making the antibodies. Active immunity can occur under natural or artificial conditions.

NATURAL ACTIVE IMMUNITY

Natural active immunity occurs when an antigen enters the body without human assistance and the body responds by actively making antibodies against that antigen (e.g., chickenpox virus). Most of the time, the first invasion of the body by the antigen results in development of disease. However, processes occurring in the body at the same time confer immunity to that antigen. Thus the person will not become ill after a second exposure to the same antigen. *This type of immunity is the most effective and the longest lasting.*

ARTIFICIAL ACTIVE IMMUNITY

Artificial active immunity is a type of protection developed against serious illnesses for which total avoidance is most desirable. Examples of diseases for which artificially acquired active immunity can be obtained include tetanus, diphtheria, measles, smallpox, mumps, and rubella. Small amounts of specific antigens are deliberately placed (as a vaccination) in the body, so that the body responds by actively making antibodies against the antigen. Because antigens used for this procedure have been specially processed **(attenuated)** to make them less likely to proliferate within the body, this exposure does not cause the disease. Artificial active immunity lasts many years, although repeated but smaller doses of the original antigen are required as a "booster" for maintaining complete protection against the antigen.

Passive Immunity

Passive immunity occurs when antibodies against a specific antigen are in a person's body but were not created there. Rather, these antibodies are transferred to the person's body after being made in the body of another person or animal. Because these antibodies are foreign to the individual, the body recognizes the antibodies as non-self and takes steps to eliminate them relatively quickly. For this reason, passive immunity can provide only immediate, short-term protection against a specific antigen.

Natural passive immunity occurs when antibodies are passed from the mother to the fetus via the placenta or to the infant through colostrum and breast milk.

Artificial passive immunity involves deliberately injecting a person with antibodies that were produced in another person or animal. This type of immunity is used when a person is exposed to a serious disease or illness for which he or she has little or no known actively acquired immunity. Instead, the injected antibodies are expected to inactivate the antigen. This type of immunity provides only temporary protection lasting for days to a few weeks. Some of the conditions or diseases for which artificial passive immunity may be used include exposure to rabies, tetanus, and poisonous snake bites.

AMI works with the inflammatory responses to provide protection against infection. However, AMI can provide the most effective, long-lasting immunity only when its actions are combined with those of cell-mediated immunity (CMI).

CELL-MEDIATED IMMUNITY

Cell-mediated immunity (CMI), or cellular immunity, involves many leukocyte actions, reactions, and interactions ranging from simple to complex. This type of immunity is provided by committed lymphocyte stem cells that mature in the secondary lymphoid tissues of the thymus and pericortical areas of lymph nodes. Certain CMI responses influence and regulate the activities of antibody-mediated immunity (AMI) and inflammation by producing and releasing cytokines. Therefore for total immunocompetence, CMI must function optimally.

Cell Types Involved in Cell-Mediated Immunity

The leukocytes playing the most important roles in CMI include several specific T-lymphocyte subsets along with a special population of cells known as natural killer (NK) cells. T-lymphocytes further differentiate into a variety of subsets, each of which has a specific function.

One way of identifying different T-lymphocyte subsets is to determine the presence or absence of certain "marker proteins" (antigens) on the cell membrane's surface. More than 50 different T-lymphocyte proteins have been identified on the cell membrane, and 11 of these (named T1 through T11) are commonly used clinically to identify specific cells. Antibodies have been made against each of these 11 proteins. Thus each T-lymphocyte subset can be identified by how the T-lymphocyte reacts to the commercial antibodies. Most T-lymphocytes have more than one antigen on their cell membrane. For example, all mature T-lymphocytes contain T1, T3, T10, and T11 proteins. Certain subsets of T-lymphocytes also contain other specific T-lymphocyte membrane antigens.

The names used to identify specific T-lymphocyte subsets include the specific membrane antigen and the overall functional activities of the cells in a subset. The three T-lymphocyte subsets that are critically important for the development and continuation of CMI are helper/inducer T-cells, suppressor T-cells, and cytotoxic/cytolytic T-cells.

HELPER/INDUCER T-CELLS

Description

The cell membranes of helper/inducer T-cells contain the T4 protein. These cells are usually called T4+-cells or T_H-cells. A newer name for helper/inducer T-cells is CD4+ (cluster of differentiation 4). Several antibodies to the T4-cell membrane protein have been made commercially. These antibodies include OKT4 and Leu-3; thus the helper/inducer T-cells may also be referred to as cells that are OKT4 positive or Leu-3 positive.

Function

Helper/inducer T-cells are efficient in recognizing self versus non-self. These cells participate in CMI by stimulating the activity of many other leukocytes. In response to the recognition of non-self (antigen), helper/inducer T-cells secrete lymphokines that can regulate the activity of other leukocytes.

Most lymphokines secreted by the helper/inducer T-cells have overall stimulating effects on immune function. These lymphokines increase bone marrow production of stem cells and speed up the maturation of cells of myeloid and lymphoid origin. Thus helper/inducer T-cells act as organizers in "calling to arms" various squads of leukocytes involved in inflammatory, antibody, and cellular defensive actions to destroy, eliminate, or neutralize antigens.

SUPPRESSOR T-CELLS

Description

The cell membranes of suppressor T-cells contain the T8-lymphocyte antigen, and these cells are commonly called T8-cells or T_S-cells. Suppressor T-cells help regulate CMI.

Function

Suppressor T-cells prevent continuous overreactions **(hypersensitivity reactions)** to exposure to non-self cells or proteins. This function is important in preventing the formation of autoantibodies directed against normal, healthy self cells, which is the basis for many autoimmune diseases.

The suppressor T-cells secrete lymphokines that have an overall *inhibitory* action on most cells of the immune system. These lymphokines inhibit both the growth and activation of immune system cells.

Suppressor T-cells have the opposite action of helper/inducer T-cells. Therefore for optimal function of CMI, a balance between helper/inducer T-cell activity and suppressor T-cell activity must be maintained. This balance occurs when the helper/inducer T-cells outnumber the suppressor T-cells by a ratio of 2:1. When this ratio increases, overreactions can occur, some of which are tissue damaging, as well as unpleasant. When the helper-suppressor ratio decreases, immune function is suppressed, and the body is more vulnerable to invasion by non-self cells and to infections of all types.

CYTOTOXIC/CYTOLYTIC T-CELLS

Description

Cytotoxic/cytolytic T-cells are also called T_C-cells. Because they have the T8 protein present on their surfaces, they are a subset of suppressor cells. Cytotoxic/cytolytic T-cells function in CMI by destroying cells that contain a processed antigen major histocompatibility complex (MHC). This activity is most effective against self cells infected by parasitic organisms, such as viruses or protozoa.

Function

Parasite-infected self cells have both self MHC proteins (universal product code) and the parasite's antigens on the cell surface. This allows the person's immune system cells to recognize the infected self cell as abnormal, and the cytotoxic/cytolytic T-cell can bind to it.

The binding of the cytotoxic/cytolytic T-cell to the infected cell's antigen MHC complex stimulates activities that result in the death of the infected cell. The cytotoxic/cytolytic T-cell makes holes in the membrane of the infected cell and delivers a "lethal hit" of enzymes to the infected cell, causing it to lyse and die. Once the lethal hit has been administered to the infected cell, the cytotoxic/cytolytic T-cell releases the dying infected cell and can attack and destroy other infected cells that carry the same antigen MHC complex.

NATURAL KILLER CELLS

Description

Natural killer (NK) cells are extremely important in providing CMI. The actual site of differentiation and maturation of NK cells is unknown. Although this cell population has some T-cell characteristics, it is not considered a true T-cell subset (Abbas, Lichtman, & Pober, 1997).

Function

NK cells direct cytotoxic effects on target non-self cells. Unlike cytotoxic/cytolytic T-cells, NK cells can exert these cytotoxic effects without first undergoing a period of sensitization to non-self cell membrane antigens. Moreover, NK cells do not need to share any of the MHC proteins in common with the non-self cell to initiate defensive actions against the non-self cell. The defensive actions of NK cells appear to be totally unrelated to either antigen sensitivity or the interactions of other leukocytes. NK cells conduct "seek and destroy" missions in the body to eliminate invaders and unhealthy self cells.

NK cells are most effective in destroying unhealthy or abnormal self cells. The non-self cells most susceptible to defensive actions of NK cells are those body cells that are virally infected and cancer cells.

Cytokines

The inducing and regulatory aspects of CMI are controlled through the selected production and activity of cytokines. **Cytokines** are small protein hormones produced by the various leukocytes. Cytokines made by the mononuclear phagocytes (macrophages, neutrophils, eosinophils, and monocytes) are termed **monokines;** cytokines produced by T-lymphocytes are termed **lymphokines.**

Cytokine activity is similar to the action of any other kind of hormone: one cell produces and secretes a cytokine, which in turn exerts its effects on other cells of the immune system. The cells responding to the cytokine may be located close to or remote from the cytokine-secreting cell. The cells that change their activity in response to the cytokine are known as "responder" cells. For a responder cell to respond to the presence of a cytokine, the membrane of the responder cell must have a specific receptor for the cytokine to bind to and initiate changes in the responder cell's activity (Figure 20-14).

Cytokines regulate a variety of inflammatory and immune responses. Most cytokines are produced as needed, rather than stored. The actions of some cytokines are **pleiotropic** in that the effects are widespread within the immune system, setting into motion various immunomodulating actions. Other cytokines have specific actions limited to only one type of cell. Table 20-5 summarizes the activities of the currently known cytokines.

Protection Provided by Cell-Mediated Immunity

Cell-mediated immunity (CMI) helps provide protection to the body through its highly developed ability to differentiate self from non-self. The non-self cells most easily recognized by CMI are those self cells infected by organisms that live within host cells and cancer cells. CMI provides a surveillance system for ridding the body of self cells that might potentially harm the body. *CMI is important in preventing the development of cancer and metastasis after exposure to carcinogens.*

Transplant Rejection

Natural killer (NK) cells and cytotoxic/cytolytic T-cells also destroy cells from other people or animals. Although this action is generally helpful, it is also responsible for rejection of grafts and transplanted organs. Because the solid organ transplanted into the host is seldom a perfectly identical match of universal product codes (human leukocyte antigens [HLAs]) between the donated organ and the recipient host, the client's immune system cells recognize a newly transplanted organ as non-self. Without intervention, the host's immune system initiates standard inflammatory and immunologic actions to destroy or eliminate these non-self cells. This activity causes rejection of the transplanted organ. Graft rejection is a result of a complex series of responses that change over time and involve different components of the immune system. Graft rejection can be hyperacute, acute, or chronic.

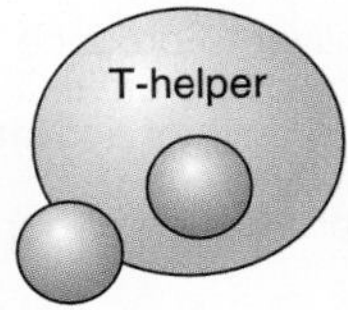

T-helper cell making and releasing a cytokine (MAF—macrophage activating factor)

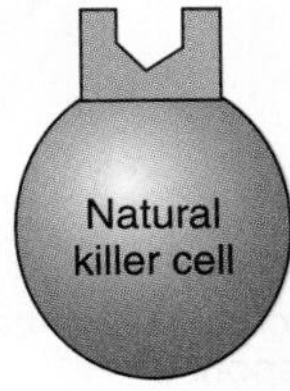

Leukocyte with one type of surface receptor

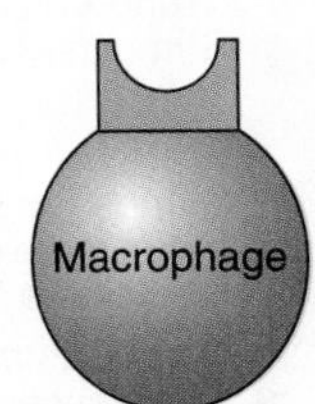

Leukocyte with a surface receptor specific for the cytokine released by the T-helper cell

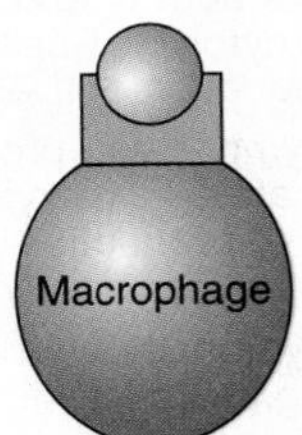

Cytokine binding to a cytokine-specific receptor on the leukocyte (macrophage)

Figure 20-14 ● Cytokine receptors on leukocytes.

HYPERACUTE REJECTION

Hyperacute graft rejection begins immediately on transplantation and is an antibody-mediated response. Antigen-antibody complexes form in the blood vessels of the transplanted organ (Cotran, Kumar, & Collins, 1999). The host's blood has pre-existing antibodies to one or more of the antigens (including blood group antigens) present in the donated organ. The antigen-antibody complexes adhere to the lining of blood vessels and activate complement. The activated-fixated complement in the blood vessel linings initiates the blood clotting cascade; microcoagulation occurs throughout the organ vasculature. Widespread coagulation and occlusion lead to ischemic necrosis, inflammation with phagocytosis of the necrotic blood vessels, and release of lytic enzymes into the transplanted organ. These enzymes cause massive cellular destruction and graft loss.

Hyperacute rejection occurs primarily in transplanted kidneys. The following persons are at greatest risk for hyperacute rejection:

1. Those who have received donated organs of an ABO blood type different from their own
2. Those who have received multiple blood transfusions at any time in life before transplantation
3. Those who have a history of multiple pregnancies
4. Those who have received a previous transplant

The manifestations of hyperacute rejection become apparent within minutes of attachment of the donated organ to the host's blood supply. The process cannot be stopped once it has started, and the rejected organ must be removed as soon as hyperacute rejection is diagnosed.

TABLE 20-5 • SUMMARY OF CYTOKINE ACTIVITY

Cytokine	Cellular Origin	Inducing Event	Cytokine Action
IL-1	Macrophages Monocytes NK cells	Contact with gram-negative bacterial products Contact with CD4+ cell Presence of TNF	Stimulates increased production of prostaglandins Induces fever Increases proliferation of CD4+ cells Stimulates growth and differentiation of B-lymphocytes Induces further secretion of IL-1 and IL-6
IL-2	Helper T-cells (CD4+ T-cells) CD8+ T-cells	T-cell activation by antigens	Increases growth and differentiation of T-lymphocytes Stimulates increased production of IL-2 from activated lymphocytes Enhances NK activity and activity of tumor-infiltrating lymphocytes
IL-3 (multilineage colony-stimulating factor)	Helper T-cells (CD4+ T-cells)	Infection or antigen invasion	Pluripotent (pleiotropic) stimulation of bone marrow stem cells

IL, Interleukin; *TNF*, tumor necrosis factor, *NK*, natural killer; *Ig*, immunoglobulin; *INF*, interferon; *G*, granulocyte, *M*, macrophage, *CSF*, colony-stimulating factor.

Continued

TABLE 20-5 • SUMMARY OF CYTOKINE ACTIVITY—cont'd

Cytokine	Cellular Origin	Inducing Event	Cytokine Action
IL-4 (B-cell stimulatory factor)	Helper T-cells (CD4+ T-cells) Activated mast cells	Presence of anti-Ig antibody	Stimulates growth and differentiation of B-lymphocytes Stimulates increased production of IgG and IgE Induces further secretion of IL-4, IL-5, and IL-6 Suppresses inflammation
IL-5 (B-cell growth factor)	Helper T-cells (CD4+ T-cells) Activated mast cells	Helminth infection Pulmonary infection	Stimulates growth and differentiation of eosinophils Stimulates increased production of IgA and IgE
IL-6	Activated T-cells Fibroblasts Vascular endothelial cells Macrophages Monocytes	Infection or inflammation Presence of IL-1 TNF	Stimulates liver to produce fibrinogen, macroglobulin, protein C Stimulates growth of activated B-lymphocytes Increases production of bone marrow stem cells
IL-7 (B-cell growth factor)	Bone marrow stromal cells	Presence of antigens	Stimulates growth and differentiation of committed B-lymphocyte stem cells Stimulates T-cell production of IL-2
IL-8 (monocyte chemotactic factor)	Activated T-cells Macrophages Platelets Fibroblasts Endothelial cells	Infection or inflammation	Chemotactic factor for neutrophils, basophils, and eosinophils Stimulates neutrophil activation
IL-9	Helper T-cells (CD4+ T-cells)	Infection or inflammation	Stimulates mast cell growth Induces IL-4 production Stimulates lymphocyte activation
IL-10	Mature lymphocytes Macrophages Monocytes	Infection or inflammation	Enhances activity of cytotoxic/cytolytic T-cells Suppresses inflammatory response
IL-11	Bone marrow stromal cells	Viral infection or inflammation	Enhances B-lymphocyte activity Stimulates platelet proliferation and maturation
IL-12	Macrophages Activated B-cells	Infection or inflammation	Induces production of interferon Enhances NK activity and activity of cytotoxic/cytolytic T-cells Induces production of IL-2 and IL-4
IL-13	Activated T-cells (CD4+ T-cells and CD8+ T-cells)	Infection	Induces B-lymphocyte proliferation Increases platelet and erythrocyte production Increases IL-6 production Decreases neutrophil activity
IL-14	Activated T-cells	Infection, plasma cell malignancies	Induces B-lymphocyte proliferation Decreases Ig secretion Enhances B-cell differentiation
INF-α	Macrophages	Viral infection	Decreases viral proliferation
INF-β	Fibroblasts	Viral infection	Decreases viral proliferation
INF-γ	Helper T-cells (CD4+ T-cells) Suppressor T-cells (CD8+ T-cells) NK cells	Viral infection	Decreases viral proliferation Activates macrophages Induces differentiation of committed lymphoid stem cells Activates neutrophils Activates NK cells
TNF	Activated macrophages Activated mast cells Activated NK cells Activated T-cells	Infection or inflammation (especially infection with gram-negative microorganisms)	Increases leukocyte adhesion Induces fever Stimulates production of CSF Induces cytolysis of virally infected cells Induces secretion of IL-1 and IL-6
GM-CSF	Activated T-cells Macrophages Fibroblasts Vascular endothelial cells	Infection or inflammation	Increases growth and differentiation of committed myeloid stem cells Slightly activates macrophages
M-CSF	Fibroblasts Vascular endothelial cells	Infection or inflammation	Increases growth and differentiation of committed monocyte-macrophage progenitor cells
G-CSF	Macrophages Vascular endothelial cells Fibroblasts	Infection or inflammation	Increases proliferation and maturation of neutrophils

IL, Interleukin; *TNF*, tumor necrosis factor; *NK*, natural killer; *Ig*, immunoglobulin; *INF*, interferon; *G*, granulocyte; *M*, macrophage; *GM*, granulocyte-macrophage; *CSF*, colony-stimulating factor.

ACUTE REJECTION

Acute graft rejection occurs within 1 week to 3 months after transplantation. Two mechanisms are responsible. The first mechanism is antibody mediated and results in vasculitis within the transplanted organ. This reaction differs from that of hyperacute rejection in that blood vessel necrosis (rather than thrombotic occlusion) leads to the organ's destruction.

The second mechanism is cellular. Host cytotoxic/cytolytic T-cells and NK cells enter the transplanted organ through the blood, infiltrate the organ cells (rather than the blood vessel cells), and cause lysis of the organ cells (Bush, 1999).

Diagnosis of acute rejection is made by laboratory tests indicating impaired function of the specific organ, along with biopsy of the grafted organ. Symptoms of acute rejection vary with the individual and with the specific organ transplanted. For example, when acute rejection occurs in a transplanted kidney, the client usually experiences some tenderness in the kidney area and may experience other general symptoms of inflammation.

An episode of acute rejection after solid organ transplantation does not automatically mean that the client will lose the transplant. Pharmacologic manipulation of host immune responses at this time may limit the damage to the organ and allow the graft to be maintained (Bush, 1999).

CHRONIC REJECTION

The origin of **chronic rejection** is not clear, but it resembles the aftermath of chronic inflammation and scarring. Functional tissue of the transplanted organ is replaced with fibrotic, scarlike tissue. Because this fibrotic tissue does not resemble the organ tissue in either structure or function, the ability of the transplanted organ to perform differentiated tasks diminishes in proportion to the percentage of normal tissue replaced by fibrotic tissue. This type of reaction is longstanding and occurs continuously as a response to chronic ischemia caused by blood vessel injury. In transplanted hearts this process is called **accelerated graft atherosclerosis (AGA)** and is the major cause of death in clients who have survived 1 or more years after heart transplantation (Augustine, 2000).

Although good control over host immune function can delay the manifestations of this type of rejection, the process probably occurs to some degree with all solid organ transplants. Because the fibrotic changes are permanent, there is no cure for chronic graft rejection. When the fibrosis increases to the extent that it significantly interferes with the functional capacity of the transplanted organ, the only recourse is retransplantation.

TREATMENT OF TRANSPLANT REJECTION

Rejection of transplanted solid organs involves all three components of immunity, although cell-mediated immune responses are most significant in the rejection process.

Maintenance Therapy

The drugs generally used for routine immunosuppressive therapy after solid organ transplantation are combinations of very specific immunosuppressants (cyclosporine [Sandimmune]), less specific immunosuppressants (azathioprine [Imuran] or mycophenolate mofetil [CellCept]), and one of the corticosteroids, such as prednisone (Apo-Prednisone✤, Deltasone✤) or prednisolone (Delta-Cortef) (Table 20-6). Cyclosporine induces the most specific and the most effective suppression of rejection. This drug, however, induces significant long-term adverse actions and is very expensive (see the Cost of Care box on p. 327). The dosage of all immunosuppressive agents is adjusted to the immune response of each client. Treatment with these agents increases the risk for bacterial and fungal infections.

A newer approach to prevention of transplant rejection for clients undergoing kidney transplantation is the use of monoclonal antibodies directed against the interleukin-2 receptor site on activated T-lymphocytes (especially helper/inducer T-cells). These antibodies, basiliximab (Simulect) or daclizumab (Zenapax), are administered intravenously within 2 hours before the transplant surgery and within the first few days after the surgery. By binding the antibodies to the interleukin-2 receptor site, T-lymphocyte proliferation and activation are reduced for several months.

Rescue Therapy

Certain agents are used not to maintain the graft within the host but rather to reduce the host's immunologic responses during rejection episodes, especially acute rejection. These agents may be used in addition to or in place of any of the maintenance drugs in the host's post-transplantation treatment regimen.

ANTILYMPHOCYTE GLOBULIN

Antilymphocyte globulin (ALG) is an antibody (or group of antibodies) produced in an animal after the animal has been exposed to human lymphocytes. The globulin can be made more specific by exposing the animal to human T-cells instead of mixed lymphocytes. When these antihuman lymphocyte antibodies are administered to humans, the antibodies selectively attack and clear lymphocytes from the blood, extracellular fluids, and tissues into which they have infiltrated (such as the transplanted organ). This agent is given only for a short time to combat the acute rejection episode.

Most clients receiving ALG have some immunologic side effects, ranging from low-grade fever and malaise to serum sickness and anaphylaxis. The response usually increases in intensity on repeated exposure to ALG.

MUROMONAB-CD3 (ORTHOCLONE OKT3)

Muromonab-CD3 is an antibody directed specifically against the human T-cell cell-surface antigen, CD3. This antibody is generated with a murine (mouse) model rather than an equine (horse) model. Because the agent is generated in mice, the humans receiving it rapidly develop antimouse antibodies. These antimouse antibodies attack the CD3 and prevent its anti–T-cell activities. Thus this antibody is most effective against rejection during the first episode for which it is used. Its utility in combating graft rejection decreases with each subsequent use.

TABLE 20-6 • DRUGS USED TO PREVENT OR TREAT TRANSPLANT REJECTION

Drug	Action	Problems/Precautions
MAINTENANCE		
Cyclosporine (Sandimmune, Neoral)	Reduces T-lymphocyte production of cytokines, which are important in stimulating T-lymphocyte proliferation and activation (especially interleukin-2)	Has nephrotoxic, neurotoxic, and hepatoxic properties Stimulates hyperglycemia—may cause diabetes mellitus Increases body and facial hair Causes gingival hyperplasia Blood levels are sensitive to the presence of other drugs Must be mixed following strict manufacturer guidelines Do not administer to clients receiving tacrolimus
Azathioprine (Immuran)	Converts to an antimetabolite that inhibits DNA synthesis and cell division in T- and B-lymphocytes and myeloid cells	Has hepatotoxic properties Has high incidence of nausea and vomiting Suppresses hematologic functions Use is less frequent compared with mycophenolate mofetil
Mycophenolate mofetil (CellCept)	Selectively inhibits T- and B-lymphocyte proliferation by interfering with purine synthesis and cell division	Has fewer side effects than azathioprine Has been demonstrated to be more effective as part of triple therapy in clients after kidney transplantation Is less selective than cyclosporine
Tacrolimus/FK 506 (Prograf)	Similar to cyclosporine	Used primarily after liver transplantation Do not administer with cyclosporine Has nephrotoxic and neurotoxic properties Induces hyperglycemia Has a frequent incidence of nausea, vomiting, and weight loss May be used as a rescue agent in kidney rejection
Corticosteroids (prednisone, prednisilone, dexamethasone [Decadron], many others)	Directly cytotoxic to circulating lymphocytes Suppresses bone marrow stem cell proliferation	Induces general immunosuppression Immunosuppression more profound than with other agents Suppresses adrenal cortical activity Numerous metabolic and endocrine side effects
Interleukin-2 receptor antagonists: Basiliximab (Simulect) Daclizumab (Zenapax)	Binds to interleukin-2 receptors on activated lymphocytes, especially helper/inducer T-cells, preventing proliferation and limiting activation	Used as initial induction therapy—not as continuing therapy IV administration only Approved as prophylaxis for kidney transplant only Synthesized through recombinant DNA technology and contains both human (90%) and mouse (10%) DNA sequences May induce anaphylaxis High incidence of flu-like symptoms
RESCUE		
Antithymocyte globulin (Atgam)	Depletes existing T-lymphocytes through antigen-antibody binding actions	Is a polyclonal antibody raised in horses May induce anaphylaxis or other immune side effects Side effects increase on re-exposure Has limited duration of action
Muromonab-CD3 (Orthoclone OKT3)	Binds to the OKT3 receptor on lymphocytes, down-regulating the receptor action Depletes circulating T-lymphocytes through antigen-antibody binding actions May induce programmed cell death (apoptosis of bound T-lymphocytes)	Is a monoclonal antibody raised in a mouse model May induce anaphylaxis or other immune side effects Has limited duration of action May be inactivated by human antimouse antibodies Induction of capillary leak syndrome is common May require premedication with corticosteroids

Tacrolimus/FK 506 (Prograf)

Tacrolimus is used in maintenance therapy and rescue therapy, primarily after liver transplantation. It is similar in chemical composition to erythromycin and specifically suppresses T-cell actions, including production of interleukin-2 (IL-2). These effects are achieved through various mechanisms. In the presence of tacrolimus/FK 506, receptor sites for IL-2 are inhibited on helper/inducer T-cells and cytotoxic/cytolytic T-cells. Without continuous stimulation by IL-2, these lymphocytes are slow to reproduce and do not perform their usual functions. In addition, tacrolimus/FK 506 is able to prevent activation of immature or unsensitized cytotoxic/cytolytic T-cells. Because cytotoxic/cytolytic T-cells are responsible for immunologic destruction of transplanted cells and tissues, and because helper/inducer T-cells boost the activity of cytotoxic/cytolytic T-cells, selective suppression of the activity of

COST OF CARE IMPLICATIONS FOR NURSING

TRANSPLANT REJECTION PROPHYLAXIS

Cost of Care

- The most useful agent in preventing rejection of transplanted solid organs is cyclosporine.
- The cost of maintaining therapeutic levels of this drug for an average-size adult ranges between $1100 and $1500 per month.
- Clients must take this drug daily for the life of the transplanted organ.
- The effectiveness of this drug is highly dependent on following the manufacturer's directions for mixing and administering.
- An antifungal agent, ketoconazole, when taken orally, has been demonstrated to slow metabolism of cyclosporine and maintain therapeutic blood levels at lower doses (approximately 40% to 50% of cyclosporine dose needed when taken without ketoconazole).
- The cost of ketoconazole daily maintenance therapy is approximately $100 per month.

Implications for Nursing

Because of the high cost of medications for preventing transplant rejection, nurses need to incorporate proper medication administration into their client teaching plans and reinforce this information frequently. Nurses can assist in cost reductions by observing for sustained therapeutic blood levels of cyclosporine in clients and exploring what factors may be contributing to this effect.

Data from Augustine, S. (2000). Heart transplantation: Long-term management related to immunosuppression, complications, and psychosocial adjustments. *Critical Care Clinics of North America, 12*(1), 69-77; *United States Pharmacopeia Dispensing Information (USP DI): Vol. I. Drug information for the health care professional* (20th ed.). (2000). Englewood, CO: Micromedix; and CVS Pharmacies. (March 2000). Personal communication.

these two cell populations allows the transplanted organ to remain free from immunologic destruction. It does this without resulting in so profound an immunosuppressive state as to put the host at great risk for infection.

ONLINE RESOURCES

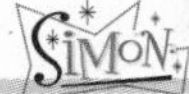

For suggested readings and Internet resources, go to http://www.wbsaunders.com/SIMON/Iggy/.

SELECTED BIBLIOGRAPHY

Asterisk indicates a classic or definitive work on this subject.

Abbas, A., Lichtman, A., & Pober, J. (1997). *Cellular and molecular immunology* (3rd ed.). Philadelphia: W.B. Saunders.

Alam, R. (1998). A brief review of the immune system. *Primary Care: Clinics in Office Practice, 25*(4), 727-738.

Augustine, S. (2000). Heart transplantation: Long-term management related to immunosuppression, complications, and psychosocial adjustments. *Critical Care Clinics of North America, 12*(1), 69-77.

Bush, W. (1999). Overview of transplantation and the pharmacotherapy of adult solid organ transplant recipients: Focus on immunosuppression. *AACN Clinical Issues: Advanced Practice in Acute and Critical Care, 10*(2), 253-269.

Coleman, C. (1998). Overview of biotherapy and nursing considerations. *Journal of Intravenous Nursing, 21*(6), 367-373.

Cotran, R., Kumar, V., & Collins, T. (1999). *Robbins pathologic basis of disease* (6th ed.). Philadelphia: W.B. Saunders.

Guyton, A., & Hall, J. (2000). *Textbook of medical physiology* (10th ed.). Philadelphia: W.B. Saunders.

Nieman, D. (1999). Nutrition, exercise, and immune system function. *Clinics in Sports Medicine, 18*(3), 537-548.

United States Pharmacopeia Dispensing Information (USP DI): Vol. I. Drug information for the health care professional (20th ed.). (2000). Englewood, CO: Micromedix.

Vasquez, E., & Westin, E. (1999). Transplant immunopharmacology: You CAN fool with mother nature! *Nursing Case Management, 4*(1), 37-48.

Workman, M. (1998). The lymphoid system and its role in maintaining immunocompetence. *Seminars in Oncology Nursing, 14*(4), 248-255.

*Workman, M., Ellerhorst-Ryan, J., & Koertge, V. (1993). *Nursing care of the immunocompromised patient.* Philadelphia: W.B. Saunders.

CHAPTER 21

Interventions for Clients with Connective Tissue Disease

DONNA D. IGNATAVICIUS

Learning Objectives

After studying this chapter, you should be able to:

1. Compare and contrast the pathophysiology and clinical manifestations of degenerative joint disease (DJD) and rheumatoid disease (RA).
2. Discuss the priority collaborative interventions for clients with DJD and RA.
3. Determine common nursing diagnoses for postoperative clients having total joint replacement surgery.
4. Evaluate the expected outcomes for clients having total joint replacement surgery.
5. Interpret laboratory findings for clients with rheumatoid disease.
6. Discuss the differences between anti-inflammatory and disease-modifying drugs for clients with rheumatoid arthritis.
7. Identify educational needs for clients with arthritis.
8. Differentiate between discoid lupus erythematosus and systemic lupus erythematosus.
9. Describe the priority nursing interventions for clients who have progressive systemic sclerosis.
10. Identify the pathophysiology and etiology of gout.
11. Explain the differences between polymyositis, systemic necrotizing vasculitis, polymyalgia rheumatica, ankylosing spondylitis, Reiter's syndrome, and Sjögren's syndrome.
12. Describe interventions that clients can use to prevent Lyme disease.
13. Identify the primary concern in care for clients with Marfan syndrome.
14. Describe the common clinical manifestations of fibromyalgia.

Go to http://www.wbsaunders.com/SIMON/Iggy/ for self-assessment questions related to these Learning Objectives.

Connective tissue disease (CTD) is the major focus of *rheumatology,* the study of rheumatic disease. A **rheumatic disease** is any disease or condition involving the musculoskeletal system. In this text, CTDs are discussed separately from other musculoskeletal conditions because most CTDs are classified as probably autoimmune.

More than 38 million people in the United States (1 in 7) have at least one of more than 100 CTDs. The primary clinical manifestation of many of these diseases is **arthritis,** the inflammation of one or more joints. In clinical practice, however, arthritis usually refers to either degenerative arthritis or rheumatoid arthritis.

Most common CTDs are characterized by chronic pain and progressive joint deterioration, which results in decreased function. Some of these disorders have additional localized clinical manifestations, whereas others are systemic. The economic and social costs of these diseases are staggering and will increase steadily as "baby boomers" continue to age. Client management requires an interdisciplinary approach, including medicine, surgery, nursing, and physical and occupational therapy.

DEGENERATIVE JOINT DISEASE (OSTEOARTHRITIS)

OVERVIEW

Several terms describe degenerative joint disease (DJD), the most common connective tissue disease and the second most common cause of disability among adults in the United States. It is the eighth most common cause of disability worldwide (Kee, 2000). **Osteoarthritis (OA)** is used interchangeably with DJD; however, this condition is not a primary inflammatory disease, and thus osteoarthritis may not be the most accurate term.

Pathophysiology

DJD is characterized by the progressive deterioration of and loss of cartilage in the joints. Weight-bearing joints (hips and knees), the vertebral column, and the hands are primarily affected because they are used most often and, except for the hands, bear the mechanical stress of body weight. Therefore DJD is sometimes called the "wear and tear disease." Most

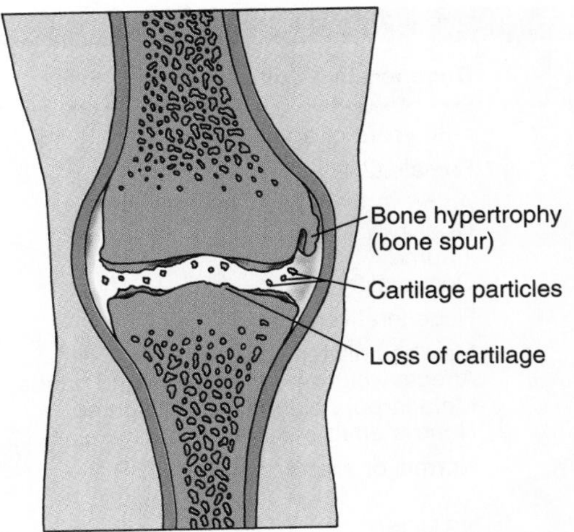

Figure 21-1 ● Joint changes in degenerative joint disease.

clients have the primary (idiopathic) form of the disease; secondary DJD can result from other musculoskeletal conditions or from trauma. DJD can also be classified as *nodal* (with hand involvement) or *non-nodal* (without hand involvement) (Kee, 2000).

In affected joints, the normal bluish-white, translucent cartilage becomes soft, opaque, and yellow. Fissures, pitting, and ulcerations develop, and the cartilage thins. As cartilage and the bone beneath the cartilage begin to erode, the joint space narrows and osteophytes (bone spurs) form (Figure 21-1). Inflammatory enzymes enhance tissue deterioration as a result of altered cartilage metabolism. As a result, the repair process is unable to overcome the rapid process of degeneration. Bone cysts and secondary synovitis are common in advanced disease. Subluxation and joint deformities eventually cause marked immobility, pain, muscle spasm and, possibly, inflammation.

Etiology

Although the causative mechanisms of *primary* DJD at the cellular level have not been well identified, the disease may be initiated by developmental, genetic, metabolic, and traumatic factors. Age is the strongest risk factor, but research does not support that aging is the only cause of DJD (Mankin & Brandt, 1997). Some clients report a family history of DJD, which supports a possible genetic cause, especially for women who have the nodal type. Obesity also contributes to the likelihood of degeneration, particularly in the knees. Recent research has found that postmenopausal women who are not on hormone replacement therapy (HRT) are prone to nodal DJD. This finding suggests that estrogen reduction may be a contributing factor to the disease (Kee, 2000).

Trauma to the joints from excessive use or abuse predisposes a person to DJD. Certain heavy manual occupations (e.g., carpet installation, construction, and farming) cause high intensity or repetitive stress to the joints. The risk of hip and knee DJD is significantly increased in professional athletes, especially football and soccer players, runners, and gymnasts.

Lack of exercise can also contribute to DJD, causing **sarcopenia** (muscle loss). Muscle tissue helps to support joints, particularly those that bear weight (e.g., hips and knees).

In a small percentage of people, congenital anomalies, trauma, and joint sepsis can result in *secondary* DJD. For example, injuries from motor vehicle accidents can cause DJD in later years. Certain metabolic diseases (e.g., diabetes mellitus, Paget's disease) and blood disorders (e.g., hemophilia, sickle cell disease) can also cause joint degeneration. Inflammatory joint diseases, such as rheumatoid arthritis, often lead to secondary DJD.

Incidence/Prevalence

The prevalence of DJD varies among different populations but is a universal problem. Approximately 70% to 85% of people over 55 years of age have x-ray changes associated with the disease.

CONSIDERATIONS FOR OLDER ADULTS

The prevalence of DJD increases with age; almost everyone older than 60 years of age has some degree of symptomatic joint degeneration. DJD of the hands is especially common among older adults, affecting more than 70% of individuals older than 70 years of age (Solomon, 1997).

WOMEN'S HEALTH CONSIDERATIONS

Before 50 years of age, more men than women have DJD. The disease is much more common in women, especially African-American women, after 50 years of age. Women are more prone to hand involvement, especially in the distal and proximal interphalangeal joints of the fingers, which often produces painful, bony nodes. Women also have a greater number of affected joints when compared with men, but men have more hip involvement.

CULTURAL CONSIDERATIONS

Native Americans, especially Pima and Blackfoot Indians, African Americans, and South African blacks, are affected more often than Caucasians in the United States. Alaskan Eskimos have a lower prevalence of DJD when compared with Caucasians.

DJD of the hip occurs less often in Asians when compared with other ethnic groups. African Americans have more knee involvement but less hand involvement than other groups (Kee, 2000).

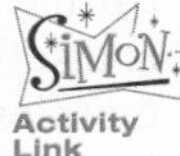

➤ COLLABORATIVE MANAGEMENT

● Assessment

HISTORY

At the initial interview, the nurse collects information specifically related to degenerative joint disease (DJD). Because this disease is observed more often in older women, age, gender, and ethnicity are important factors for the nursing history. Women should also be asked whether they are currently taking or have taken estrogen or hormone replacement therapy (ERT or HRT).

The nurse asks all clients about their occupation, nature of work, history of trauma, weight history, exercise, and current or previous involvement in sports. A history of obesity is significant, even for clients currently within the ideal range for body weight. A family history of arthritis is also noted.

TABLE 21-1 • DIFFERENTIAL FEATURES OF RHEUMATOID ARTHRITIS AND DEGENERATIVE JOINT DISEASE

Characteristic	Rheumatoid Arthritis	Degenerative Joint Disease
Typical onset	35-45 years of age	>60 years of age
Sex affected	Female (3:1)	Female (2:1)
Risk factors or cause	Probably autoimmune Emotional stress	Aging Obesity Trauma Occupation
Disease process	Inflammatory	Degenerative
Disease pattern	Bilateral, symmetric, multiple joints Usually affects upper extremities first Distal interphalangeal joints of hands spared Systemic	May be unilateral, single joint Affects weight-bearing joints and hands, spine Metacarpophalangeal joints spared Nonsystemic
Laboratory findings	Elevated rheumatoid factor, antinuclear antibody, ESR	Normal or slightly elevated ESR
Drug therapy	Salicylates NSAIDs Methotrexate Gold or penicillamine Corticosteroids Other immunosuppressive agents Other analgesics	NSAIDs Acetaminophen Other analgesics

ESR, Erythrocyte sedimentation rate; *NSAIDs*, nonsteroidal anti-inflammatory drugs.

Finally, the nurse determines whether the client has a current or previous medical condition that may cause joint manifestations. As with all musculoskeletal disorders, the nurse asks questions about the course of the disease.

PHYSICAL ASSESSMENT/CLINICAL MANIFESTATIONS

In the early stage of the disease, the clinical manifestations of DJD may appear similar to those of rheumatoid arthritis (RA). The distinction between DJD and RA becomes more evident as the disease progresses. Table 21-1 differentiates the major characteristics of both diseases and their treatments.

JOINT PAIN. The typical client with DJD is a middle-aged or older woman who complains of joint pain and stiffness. Early in the course of the disease, the pain diminishes after rest and intensifies after activity. Later the pain occurs with slight motion or even when the client is at rest. Because cartilage has no nerve supply, the pain is probably due to joint and soft-tissue involvement and to spasms of the surrounding muscles. During examination of the joints, the nurse can often elicit pain or tenderness by palpation or by putting the joint through range of motion. **Crepitus,** a continuous grating sensation caused by irregular cartilage, may be felt or heard as the joint is put through passive range of motion. One or more joints are affected. The client may also complain of joint stiffness that usually lasts less than 30 minutes after a period of inactivity.

JOINT CHANGES. On inspection, the nurse notes that the joint is often enlarged because of bony hypertrophy; rarely does a joint appear to be hot and inflamed. The presence of inflammation in clients with DJD usually indicates a secondary synovitis. Approximately 50% of clients with hand involvement display the characteristic **Heberden's nodes** (at the distal interphalangeal joints) and **Bouchard's nodes** (at the proximal interphalangeal joints). Although DJD is not a bilateral, symmetric disease, these large bony nodes appear in that pattern, especially in women. The nodes may be painful and red, but some clients do not experience discomfort from their presence. They have a familial tendency and are usually a cosmetic concern to clients. The nodes feel hard when the nurse palpates them, and clients may complain of tenderness on palpation.

OTHER CLINICAL MANIFESTATIONS. Joint effusions are common when the knees are involved. When trying to differentiate the presence of fluid from subcutaneous tissue, the nurse may be able to move fluid from the infrapatellar notch (the area directly below the knee) into the suprapatellar notch (the area directly above the knee). Subcutaneous tissue cannot be relocated.

The nurse may also observe atrophy of skeletal muscle from disuse. The vicious pain cycle of the disease discourages the movement of painful joints, which then results in contractures, muscle atrophy, and further pain. Loss of function may result depending on which joints are involved. Hip or knee pain may cause the client to limp and restrict walking distance.

DJD can often affect the spine, especially the lumbar region at the L3-4 level or the cervical region at C4-6. Compression of spinal nerve roots may occur as a result of vertebral facet bone spurs. The client typically complains of radiating pain, stiffness, and muscle spasms in one or both extremities. Spinal and vertebral arteries may also become compressed.

Severe pain and deformity interfere with ambulation and self-care. In addition to performing a musculoskeletal assessment, the nurse performs a functional assessment of the client with DJD to determine mobility and the ability to perform activities of daily living (ADLs). Chapter 10 describes ADLs and functional assessment in depth.

CRITICAL THINKING CHALLENGE

You are assigned to care for an older adult in an assisted-living facility. She has long-standing DJD of both the hips and knees and a history of diabetes mellitus, congestive heart failure, and hypertension. She is able to care for herself but uses a walker for ambulation because of chronic joint pain and deterioration.

- How would you perform a physical assessment of this client?
- What might you expect to find during the physical assessment?
- How might her other medical diagnoses affect the findings of the physical assessment?

For suggested answer guidelines, go to SIMON http://www.wbsaunders.com/SIMON/Iggy/.

PSYCHOSOCIAL ASSESSMENT

DJD is a chronic condition that may cause permanent changes in lifestyle. An inability to care for oneself in advanced disease prevents socialization and results in role changes and other losses. Therefore the client may exhibit a variety of behaviors indicative of the grieving process, such as anger and depression.

The client may experience a role change in the family, workplace, or both. To identify changes that have been or need to be made, the nurse asks the client about his or her roles before the disease developed. Coping strategies to help in living with the disease are also identified. Kee (1998) found four themes that help people cope with DJD (see the Evidence-Based Practice for Nursing box at right):

- Refusal to give up
- Pragmatism toward treatment strategies
- Staying in charge
- Tangible caring by others

In addition to role changes, joint deformities and bony nodules often cause an alteration in body image and self-esteem. The nurse observes the client's response to body changes. Does the client ignore them or seem overly occupied with them? How does he or she refer to the changes—with anger, degradation, or humor? These clues help the nurse assess the client's acceptance of body alterations.

LABORATORY ASSESSMENT

The health care provider uses the history and physical examination to make the diagnosis of DJD. The results of routine laboratory tests are usually normal but can be helpful in screening for associated conditions. The erythrocyte sedimentation rate (ESR) may be slightly elevated when secondary synovitis (synovial inflammation) occurs. ESR also tends to rise with age and infection.

RADIOGRAPHIC ASSESSMENT

Routine x-ray examinations are useful in determining structural joint changes. Specialized views are obtained when the disease cannot be visualized on standard x-ray film but is suspected. A computed tomography (CT) scan may be used to determine vertebral involvement.

EVIDENCE-BASED PRACTICE FOR NURSING

How do older people cope with osteoarthritis?

Kee, C.C. (1998). Living with osteoarthritis: Insiders' views. *Applied Nursing Research, 11*(1), 19-26.

The purpose of this qualitative study was to explore the daily experiences of older adults with symptomatic osteoarthritis (OA), or degenerative joint disease, and to determine if older adults with varying socioeconomic status have different coping strategies. A semistructured interview was used for all 20 subjects.

Some differences in understanding the cause and treatment of OA were found. For example, less advantaged subjects used rubbing alcohol on their joints, whereas the more advantaged group used more expensive creams and ointments. Overall coping strategies were similar for both groups. Four themes emerged regarding living with OA: (1) refusing to give up, (2) pragmatism toward treatment strategies, (3) staying in charge, and (4) tangible caring by others.

Critique. Although the sample size was small, this study is important in beginning to understand the ways in which people live with a chronic disease such as OA on a day-to-day basis. Open-ended questions on the interview allowed subjects to express their real experiences.

Implications for Nursing. Support and caring for the person with OA was a valuable asset for all subjects. Nurses can help to identify support systems or organizations that provide interaction for clients with OA. In addition, they can be encouraged to view their illness as something they can live with and control.

OTHER DIAGNOSTIC ASSESSMENT

The health care provider may order magnetic resonance imaging (MRI) studies of the vertebral column to detect degenerative bony changes in the spine. A bone scan using technetium (Tc^{99m}) can often show early DJD—years before typical changes appear on x-ray film.

Analysis

COMMON NURSING DIAGNOSES AND COLLABORATIVE PROBLEMS

The following are priority nursing diagnoses for clients with degenerative joint disease (DJD):

1. Chronic Pain related to muscle spasm, cartilage deterioration, or joint inflammation
2. Impaired Physical Mobility related to pain and muscle atrophy

ADDITIONAL NURSING DIAGNOSES AND COLLABORATIVE PROBLEMS

In addition to the common nursing diagnoses, clients may have secondary problems caused by the pain and immobility common in DJD, including one or more of the following:

- Activity Intolerance related to pain and fatigue
- Self-Care Deficit (Partial) related to pain, fatigue, and immobility
- Disturbed Body Image related to the effects of loss of body function
- Impaired Walking related to joint pain
- Ineffective Coping related to chronic pain and decreased function
- Imbalanced Nutrition: More than Body Requirements related to decreased activity and mobility

Planning and Implementation

CHRONIC PAIN

NOC **PLANNING: EXPECTED OUTCOMES.** The major concern of the client with DJD is pain control. Therefore the client is expected to state that chronic pain is reduced or relieved.

INTERVENTIONS. Pain control may be accomplished at home with drug and nondrug measures. If these measures become ineffective, surgery may be performed to reduce pain. The nurse performs a comprehensive pain assessment before and after implementing interventions (Chart 21-1).

NONSURGICAL MANAGEMENT. Management of chronic joint pain is difficult for both the client and the health care professional. A combination of modalities is often used, including analgesics, rest, positioning, thermal modalities, weight control, and integrative therapies. Chapter 7 elaborates on pain assessment and methods of pain control for chronic, nonmalignant pain.

CHART 21-1

NIC INTERVENTION ACTIVITIES *for* The Client with Degenerative Joint Disease

Analgesic Administration: *Use of pharmacologic agents to reduce or eliminate pain*
- Determine pain location, characteristics, quality, and severity before medicating client.
- Check medical order for drug, dose, and frequency of analgesic prescribed.
- Attend to comfort needs and other activities that assist relaxation to facilitate response to analgesia.
- Administer analgesics around-the-clock to prevent the peaks and troughs of analgesia, especially with severe pain.
- Set positive expectations regarding the effectiveness of analgesics to optimize client response.
- Document response to analgesic and any untoward effects.

Pain Management: *Alleviation of pain or a reduction in pain to a level of comfort that is acceptable to the client*
- Observe for nonverbal cues of discomfort, especially in clients who are unable to communicate effectively.
- Consider cultural influences on pain response.
- Determine the impact of the pain experience on quality of life (e.g., sleep, appetite, activity, cognition, mood, relationships, performance of job, and role responsibilities).
- Evaluate, with the client and the health care team, the effectiveness of past pain control measures that have been used.
- Consider the client's willingness to participate, ability to participate, preference, support of significant others for method, and contraindications when selecting a pain relief strategy.
- Teach the use of nonpharmacologic techniques (e.g., biofeedback, TENS, hypnosis, relaxation, guided imagery, music therapy, distraction, activity therapy, hot/cold application, and massage) before, after and, if possible, during painful activities; before pain occurs or increases; and along with other pain relief measures.
- Promote adequate rest/sleep to facilitate pain relief.
- Utilize a multidisciplinary approach to pain management, when appropriate.
- Consider referrals for client, family, and significant others to support groups and other resources, as appropriate.
- Monitor client satisfaction with pain management at specified intervals.

NIC intervention activities selected from McCloskey, J.C., & Bulechek, G.M. (Eds.). (2000). *Nursing interventions classification (NIC)* (3rd ed.). St. Louis: Mosby. No part of this work is to be altered without prior written permission from the Publisher.
TENS, Transcutaneous electrical nerve stimulation.

NIC ***ANALGESIC ADMINISTRATION.*** The purpose of drug therapy is to reduce pain and secondary joint inflammation if present. Acetaminophen (Tylenol, Atasol✱) is the primary drug of choice for pain relief. Clients are at risk for liver damage if they take more than 4000 mg/day, have concurrent alcoholism, or have pre-existing liver disease.

Topical salicylates, such as over-the-counter (OTC) Aspercreme, are useful for some clients as a temporary pain reliever. The Food and Drug Administration (FDA) has recently approved topical capsaicin products for DJD. This expensive OTC drug works by blocking substance P, a neurotransmitter for pain (Kee, 2000). The nurse teaches the client to expect a burning sensation for a short time after applying capsaicin.

If acetaminophen or topical agents are not successful in relieving pain, the analgesic drug class of choice is usually **nonsteroidal anti-inflammatory drugs (NSAIDs)** (Chart 21-2). Most NSAIDs work by inhibiting both forms of the enzyme cyclooxygenase, COX-1 and COX-2. COX-1 produces prostaglandins that help regulate normal cell activity, including protecting the lining of the gastrointestinal (GI) tract. COX-2 produces prostaglandins mainly at the sites of inflammation. A subgroup of NSAIDs has been developed to inhibit only the COX-2 enzyme. These new COX-2–inhibiting medications, such as celecoxib (Celebrex) and rofecoxib (Vioxx), appear to manage pain and inflammation without the adverse side effects of GI distress or bleeding.

For temporary relief of pain in a single joint, the health care provider may inject an individual joint with cortisone. Frequently injected joints include the knee, base of the thumb, shoulder, and hip.

Newer agents, such as hyaluronate (Hyalgan) and hylan GF 20 (Synvisc), are used for DJD of the knee. These synthetic joint fluid implants replace or supplement the body's natural hyaluronic acid, which is broken down by inflammation. Muscle relaxants, such as cyclobenzaprine hydrochloride (Flexeril), are sometimes given for painful muscle spasms, especially those occurring in the back. Potent analgesics are not usually appropriate for the client with DJD because of the chronic nature of the pain.

NIC ***PAIN MANAGEMENT.*** In addition to analgesics, many nondrug measures can be used for clients with DJD.

Rest. Several types of rest are used to treat clients with DJD:
- *Local* rest involves immobilizing a joint with a splint or brace. If a joint becomes acutely inflamed, the joint is rested until inflammation subsides. The nurse consults with the occupational therapist (OT), who fits the client for the appropriate device and explains its use.
- *Systemic* rest refers to immobilizing the entire body, such as during a nap. The nurse teaches the client about the importance of sleeping approximately 10 hours and, if possible, resting an additional 1 to 2 hours each day.
- *Psychologic* rest is equally important because it allows relief from the daily stresses that can enhance pain.

Positioning. Joints should be placed in their functional position, which may not be the position of comfort. When the client is in a supine position (recumbent), he or she should use a small pillow under the head or neck but avoid the use of other pillows. The use of large pillows under the knees or head may quickly result in flexion contractures. If needed, the legs may be elevated 8 to 12 inches (20.3 to 30.5 cm) to reduce back discomfort. Lying in the prone position twice a day is recommended if tolerated. The nurse also reminds the client to use proper posture when standing and sitting to reduce undue strain on the vertebral column.

Thermal Modalities. In general, the client with DJD uses heat instead of cold to reduce pain. The application of cold is usually reserved for acutely inflamed joints. In collaboration with the physical therapist, the nurse suggests hot showers and baths, hot packs or compresses, and moist heating pads. Regardless of treatment, the nurse teaches the client to check that the heat source is not too heavy or so hot that it causes

CHART 21-2

DRUG THERAPY *for* Connective Tissue Disease

Drug	Usual Dosage	Nursing Interventions	Rationale
Salicylates (e.g., aspirin, buffered aspirin) (Ecotrin, Ascriptin, Ancasal✤)	12-18 tablets/day (4-6 g) are given in divided doses to achieve therapeutic effect.	Give with meals or snacks.	Aspirin products can cause gastrointestinal problems, including bleeding and ulcers, because of increased stomach acid production. Drugs can damage eighth cranial nerve and prevent platelet aggregation, which causes clotting.
		Instruct client to observe for and report tinnitus, bleeding, or bruising (especially seen in older clients). Teach client to use a toothbrush.	Gums may bleed easily because of decreased clotting.
NSAIDs, e.g., naproxen (Naprosyn, Apo-Naproxen✤), sulindac (Clinoril), indomethacin (Indocin, Apo-Indomethacin✤), ibuprofen (Motrin, Advil, Amersol✤), mefenamic acid (Ponstel, Ponstan✤), phenylbutazone (Butazolidin, Novobutazone✤), piroxicam (Feldene, Apo-Piroxicam✤), diclofenac sodium (Voltaren), flurbiprofen (Ansaid)	Dosage varies depending on which drug is used. Piroxicam and naproxen are given in fewer doses because of their longer half-life. Indomethacin and phenylbutazone are not as commonly used because of their tendencies to cause peptic ulcers and CNS changes.	Same as for salicylates (above).	Same as for salicylates above.
		In addition, observe for fluid retention, increased blood pressure, and changes in renal function.	Most NSAIDs cause sodium retention, which can lead to edema, hypertension, renal damage, and/or congestive heart failure. Drugs should be used with caution in older adults.
		Monitor electrolyte and complete blood count values.	Most NSAIDs cause increased sodium levels and can cause bone marrow suppression.
		Observe for CNS changes (e.g., dizziness or confusion).	Most NSAIDs can cause CNS effects, especially in older adults.
		If a client is taking aspirin and an NSAID or is taking two NSAIDs, observe carefully for side effects or toxic effects.	Drugs are often used in combination, especially in clients with rheumatoid arthritis. Additive effects can cause serious complications.
Gold Auranofin (Ridaura)	Dosage is 3 mg bid PO.	Observe for and instruct client to report gastrointestinal problems such as diarrhea, nausea/vomiting, and abdominal cramping.	This side effect causes discomfort and can lead to electrolyte imbalance.
Gold sodium thiomalate (water-based gold) (Myochrysine)	After a 10-mg test dose, 25 mg and then 50 mg is given every week until monthly maintenance of 50 mg IM is reached.	Observe for rash or other skin changes and for mouth ulceration (stomatitis).	Drug may be discontinued for a short period and then restarted.

NSAIDs, Nonsteroidal anti-inflammatory drugs; *CNS,* central nervous system; *CBC,* complete blood count; *CTDs,* connective tissue diseases.

Continued

CHART 21-2

DRUG THERAPY *for* Connective Tissue Disease—cont'd

Drug	Usual Dosage	Nursing Interventions	Rationale
Aurothioglucose (oil-based gold) (Solganal)	Same as for gold sodium thiomalate. If total of 1000 mg is used and no clinical change is seen, gold is discontinued.	Instruct client to expect metallic taste in mouth; teach importance of proper mouth care.	Proper, frequent mouth care reduces risk of stomatitis and metallic taste.
		Monitor urine for protein and serum for CBC. If CBC is markedly decreased or if proteinuria is present, discontinue drug.	These changes indicate serious toxic effects, and the drug needs to be discontinued.
		Give *deep* IM administration, preferably by Z-track technique.	Drug is locally irritating to soft tissue.
		After IM administration, observe for nitroid crisis, a form of anaphylactic reaction.	Flushing, dyspnea, and anxiety may occur shortly after drug administration.
Hydroxychloroquine sulfate (Plaquenil)	Dosage is 200 mg PO each day.	Instruct client to have frequent (every 3-6 mo) ophthalmologic examination.	Drug can cause retinal damage.
Penicillamine (Cuprimine)	Dosage is 125-250 mg PO each day (may be given in two divided doses).	Same as for IM gold, except no nitroid crisis occurs.	Same as for IM gold.
Immunosuppressive agents, e.g., azathioprine (Imuran), cyclophosphamide (Cytoxan, Procytox✤), methotrexate (Mexate)	Dosage varies depending on disease activity and route of drug administration.	Observe for side effects and toxic effects, including but not limited to nausea/vomiting, bone marrow suppression, alopecia, and increased liver enzymes.	The side effects and toxic effects of these drugs can be devastating. Drugs are reserved for severe forms of CTDs in which organ involvement is potentially life threatening.
		Take medications with meals.	
		Instruct client to avoid crowds and people with infections such as influenza.	Bone marrow suppression or immune suppression increases the risk of infection.
Prednisone (Deltasone, Apo-Prednisone✤)	Dosage is 10-150 mg PO each day. For maintenance, attempt to give dose every other day (to allow client's adrenal glands to function).	Observe for cushiongoid changes, such as moonface, buffalo hump, striae, acne, thin skin, bruising, fluid retention, and increased blood pressure.	These changes are expected and tend to be dose related. Changes diminish as dose decreases.
		Monitor electrolyte and glucose levels.	Chronic steroid therapy can cause sodium or fluid retention, potassium depletion, and elevated glucose level.
		Observe for long-term effects of chronic steroid therapy, such as osteoporosis, cataracts, hypertension, diabetes, and impaired healing.	These complications may need to be treated with other drugs or modalities.
		Instruct client to avoid crowds and individuals with infections such as influenza.	Drug suppresses immune system (lymphocytes) and increases risk of infection or decreased healing.

NSAIDs, Nonsteroidal anti-inflammatory drugs; *CNS,* central nervous system; *CBC,* complete blood count; *CTDs,* connective tissue diseases.

burns. A temperature just above body temperature is adequate to promote comfort.

A physical therapist may provide special heat treatments, such as paraffin dips, diathermy (electrical current), and ultrasonography (sound waves). A 15- to 20-minute heat application usually is sufficient to temporarily reduce pain, spasm, and stiffness.

Weight Control. Contrary to what has been proposed by the media and uninformed authors, there is no "arthritis diet." In collaboration with the dietitian, the nurse explains which foods are high in protein and vitamin C to promote tissue healing. People who consume adequate amounts of antioxidants, such as vitamins C and D, have a lower incidence of DJD (Kee, 2000). In addition, the nurse encourages clients who are obese to lose weight to lessen the stress on weight-bearing joints. Less weight reduces pain and slows the disease process in affected joints. If needed, the nurse collaborates with the dietitian to provide more in-depth teaching about nutrition and meal planning.

Complementary and Alternative Therapies. Additional measures may be used for pain reduction. Transcutaneous electrical nerve stimulation (TENS) may be particularly helpful for vertebral involvement. The health care provider collaborates with the nurse and physical therapist to determine whether this pain management modality would be beneficial. The client must be able to control the TENS unit for pain relief.

Clients may also use acupuncture, acupressure, tai chi, therapeutic touch, hypnosis, magnets, music therapy, and imagery for pain relief (see Chapters 4 and 7). In a study by Berman et al. (1999), acupuncture was found to be an effective and safe adjunct to conventional pain management for clients with DJD of the knee. After using therapeutic touch, Gordon et al. (1998) and Evanoff et al. (1999) observed decreased pain and improved function in clients with DJD in one or both knees.

Cayenne pepper (the source of capsaicin products) and other dietary supplements, gamma linolenic acid (GLA), glucosamine, and chondroitin are the most recent additions to complement traditional therapies. GLA can be found in evening primrose oil, borage seed oil, and currant seed oil. Many clients have reported positive results from these dietary supplements and topical analgesics, especially decreased pain and inflammation. However, scientific data are lacking (Kee, 2000).

CRITICAL THINKING CHALLENGE

Your hospitalized client with DJD tells you that she receives Tylenol for pain only when she requests it. She gets very little relief from the drug and sometimes is unable to sleep because of severe pain. The client also states that she uses glucosamine at home.

- What should you include in her comprehensive pain assessment?
- What options does she have for pain control?
- What actions should you take based on her pain assessment?

For suggested answer guidelines, go to SIMON http://www.wbsaunders.com/SIMON/Iggy/.

SURGICAL MANAGEMENT. Surgery may be indicated when all other measures are inadequate to provide pain control for clients with degenerative joint disease (DJD). The most common surgical procedure performed for these clients is total joint replacement (TJR). A surgical arthroscopy may be used to remove damaged cartilage (see Chapter 50). An osteotomy may be performed to correct joint deformity, but this procedure is less common because of the success rate of TJR.

Almost any synovial joint of the body can be replaced with a prosthetic system that consists of at least two parts, one for each joint surface. A TJR is the major type of arthroplasty (surgical creation of a joint) performed.

INDICATIONS. TJR is a procedure of last resort for pain management; it is used when all other methods of pain relief have been unsuccessful. The hips and knees are the joints most commonly replaced, but replacements of finger and wrist joints, elbows, shoulders, toe joints, and ankles have become more popular in the past 20 years.

Although TJRs are performed most often for clients with DJD, other conditions causing joint damage may also require surgery. These disorders include rheumatoid arthritis (RA), congenital anomalies, trauma, and avascular necrosis (bony necrosis secondary to lack of blood flow, usually from trauma or chronic steroid therapy).

CONTRAINDICATIONS. The primary contraindications for TJR are infection anywhere in the body, advanced osteoporosis, and severe inflammation. An infection elsewhere in the body or from the joint being replaced can result in an infected TJR and subsequent prosthetic failure. Therefore if a client has a urinary tract infection, for example, the physician treats the infection before surgery. Advanced osteoporosis can cause bone shattering during insertion of the prosthetic device. Acute joint inflammation is treated before surgery because the mechanical stress of the procedure may promote further inflammation and prosthetic failure.

As a group, TJRs are quite successful. Many clients who have lived with chronic, unbearable pain for years and could not function independently at home or in the workplace no longer experience pain in the diseased joint. The pain relief and psychologic benefit may outweigh the perioperative risks and costs, but the surgeon and client must make that decision with the case manager. When the client is of advanced age, this decision may become an ethical issue in addition to a physical risk and cost-versus-benefit decision (see the Legal/Ethical Issues in Health Care box on p. 336).

TOTAL HIP REPLACEMENT. The most commonly replaced joint is the hip. Although clients of any age can undergo total hip replacement (THR), the procedure is performed most often in clients over 60 years of age. The special needs and normal physiologic changes of older clients often complicate the perioperative period and may result in additional postoperative complications. (See Chapters 17 to 19 for routine perioperative care and the special considerations needed for care of the older client.)

PREOPERATIVE CARE. Most managed care companies assign TJR candidates to case managers (CMs) before surgery. During the assessment process, the CM determines whether the client will have postoperative support and care-giving services. If none are available, the client's surgery may

LEGAL/ETHICAL ISSUES IN HEALTH CARE

QUALITY OF LIFE FOR CLIENTS HAVING TOTAL JOINT REPLACEMENT

Quality of life (QOL) or quality of well-being (QWB) is a difficult concept to define. In general, it is determined by the client's opinion about the importance of certain elements of his or her life and satisfaction with those elements. Few studies have compared the high cost of surgery with QOL following total joint replacement. This *utilitarian* ethical approach is based on the belief that a person deserves resources based on the real or potential productivity that he or she offers to society.

Health economists consider a resource or intervention a bargain for society if it costs less than $30,000 per quality of well year. Lavernia, Guzman, and Gachupin-Garcia (1999) calculated the cost per quality of well year for 100 clients undergoing a total knee replacement. The clients completed the QWB Index before surgery and at 3 months, 6 months, 1 year, and 2 years after surgery. The differences in the scores before and after surgery were multiplied by the client's life expectancy to obtain the cost per quality of well year. The calculated costs were about $30,700 at 3 months but steadily decreased to about $6,600 by 2 years postsurgery. Based on this study, total knee replacement meets the utilitarian approach to ethical decision making and should be considered an appropriate investment by society.

From Lavernia, C.J., Guzman, J.F., & Gachupin-Garcia, A. (1999). Cost effectiveness and quality of life in knee arthroplasty. *Clinical Orthopaedics, 345*, 134-139.

not be approved until arrangements can be made for care in a nursing home or alternative setting.

As with any surgical procedure, preoperative care begins with assessing the client's level of understanding about the impending replacement. The surgeon explains the procedure and realistic postoperative care expectations during the office visit, but this education may have occurred weeks or months before the scheduled surgery. Older clients in particular may forget some of the information or may not know what questions to ask. Many orthopedic surgeons employ nurses who follow up and address client concerns. An interdisciplinary clinical pathway that outlines expectations during preadmission, hospitalization, and posthospitalization phases of care should be reviewed with the client and family or significant other.

In addition, nurse educators or orthopedic nurses may lead formal classes in the hospital or clinic several weeks before surgery to answer questions and clarify information. Preadmission sessions are an excellent way for nurses to provide education and support and to improve customer satisfaction. During the class, the client sees the prosthesis or a picture of the device and receives written instructions or a teaching booklet to reinforce the information.

In some hospitals or orthopedic office practices, the physical therapist may meet the client before surgery to explain transfers, precautions, ambulation, and postoperative exercises. An occupational therapist may be available to demonstrate assistive/adaptive devices that facilitate independent activities of daily living (ADLs).

Preadmission programs are beginning to include outcomes measurement using a quality-of-life assessment tool, such as the Health Status Profile (SF-36). (See Chapter 1 for discussion of quality-of-life assessments.) This widely used form is typically completed by the client during preadmission, 6 months after surgery, and every year thereafter to compare measurable outcomes such as ability to perform ADLs and mobility skills.

Clients are admitted to the hospital on the morning of surgery and are transferred to the orthopedic, surgical, or medical-surgical unit after surgery.

OPERATIVE PROCEDURES. Before the start of the procedure, the operating room may be specially cleaned to reduce the risk of infection. Laminar airflow surgical suites and body exhaust systems ("spacesuits") may be used. The surgery is usually scheduled early in the morning, if possible, and movement into and out of the room is kept to a minimum. The client is given a dose of intravenous (IV) antibiotics, usually a cephalosporin such as cefazolin (Ancef), at least 1 hour before the initial surgical incision is made. Vancomycin (Vancocin) or clindamycin (Cleocin) may be used for clients who are allergic to cephalosporins.

The anesthesiologist or nurse anesthetist places the client under general or epidural anesthesia. Epidural induction reduces blood loss and the incidence of deep vein thrombosis. Intraoperative blood loss with hypotensive epidural anesthesia is usually less than 300 mL, which decreases the need for postoperative blood transfusions (Ranawat et al., 1997).

The 8- to 10-inch (20.3 to 24.5 cm) incision is usually longitudinal on the anterolateral thigh. A posterior incision may be used instead to preserve muscle, depending on the surgeon's preference.

If the prosthesis is cemented, polymethyl methacrylate (an acrylic fixating substance) is used. During the surgical procedure, the operative area is irrigated with a cool solution. To help prevent infection, the surgeon may mix an antibiotic with the cement or may plant antibiotic-impregnated beads deep into the wound. The surgeon also inserts one or two wound drains to remove exudate from the tissues, which might serve as a medium for pathogenic growth and cause wound infection.

A major advance in joint replacement surgery is the increased use of noncemented prostheses, especially for hip replacements. Although polymethyl methacrylate is an excellent initial fixator, it has a finite life span and deteriorates over time, which loosens the implant and causes pain. The average life span of a cemented hip is 10 years. When a prosthesis eventually loosens and causes pain, it is replaced in a procedure called a *revision arthroplasty.* To prevent repeated replacements, several devices that do not require a fixating substance have been designed. Clients who are older than 75 years or age or who do not have sufficient bone mass are often not candidates for a noncemented hip.

The most common mechanism used to avoid polymethyl methacrylate is a porous metal coating on the shaft of the femoral component and the back of the acetabular cap. By using a tight fit, known as a "press fit," the surgeon places the implant (prosthesis) snugly against the client's bone tissue. Most of the prostheses used today are custom designed by computers to match the size of the prosthesis with the size of the joint. Figure 21-2 illustrates a typical noncemented hip replacement system.

New bone tissue grows between the pores of the prosthesis and "grafts" to the device within 6 to 12 weeks. The older the client, the longer the bone grafting may take. This bony ingrowth serves as the fixating mechanism and, ideally, lasts a lifetime. The earliest noncemented total joint systems, which were inserted in the 1970s and 1980s, have needed revisions, primarily because of undersizing of the prosthesis. These

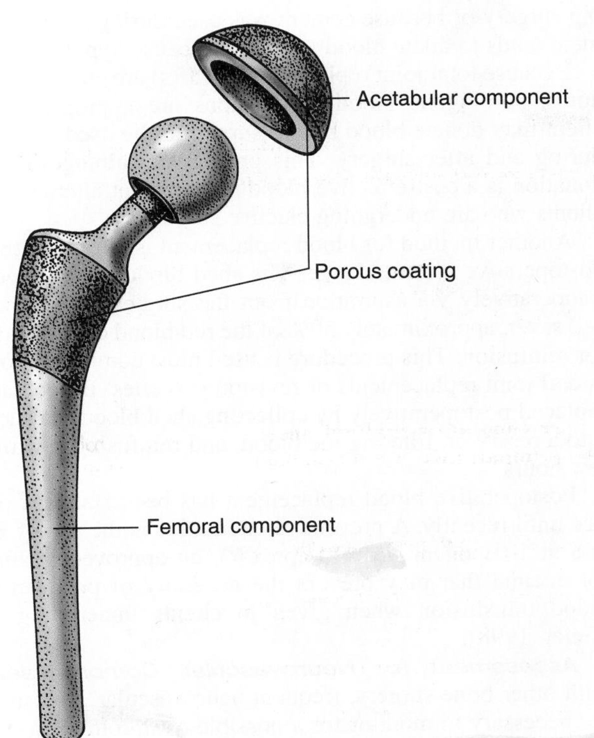

Figure 21-2 ● Noncemented, porous-coated hip replacement system.

older devices have loosened and have been replaced with a new noncemented device. Freeze-dried bone grafts *(allografts)* are used to fill in the bony defects that result from removing the old prosthesis. During the healing process, the essentially dead bone revascularizes and grafts with the client's own bone.

POSTOPERATIVE CARE. In addition to providing the routine postoperative care discussed in Chapter 19, the nurse assesses for and assists in the prevention of possible postoperative complications following a joint replacement. Table 21-2 summarizes common postoperative complications of total hip replacement surgery, including nursing measures for prevention, assessment, and intervention. Chart 21-3 highlights special concerns for the care of older adults in the postoperative period.

Prevention of Dislocation. A common complication of total hip replacement is subluxation (partial dislocation) or total dislocation. Therefore correct positioning is maintained at all times. When the client returns from the postanesthesia care unit (PACU), the nurse places him or her in a supine position with the head slightly elevated. The nurse may place a trapezoid-shaped abduction pillow, wedge, sling, or splint (with or without straps) between the client's legs to prevent adduction beyond the midline of the body. In some hospitals this device is no longer used because it is uncomfortable and unnecessary in most cases. Abduction devices are usually reserved for clients who are very restless or are unable to follow instructions, especially older adults. One or two regular bed pillows are used in most cases.

TABLE 21-2 ● NURSING INTERVENTIONS TO PREVENT COMPLICATIONS OF TOTAL JOINT REPLACEMENT SURGERY

Complication	Prevention/Intervention
Dislocation	Position correctly. For hip, keep legs slightly abducted. For hip, prevent hip flexion beyond 90 degrees. Assess for pain, rotation, and/or extremity shortening. Keep client in bed. Report immediately to physician.
Infection	Use aseptic technique for wound care and emptying of drains. Wash hands thoroughly when caring for client. Culture drainage fluid. Monitor temperature. Report excessive inflammation and/or drainage to physician.
Deep vein thrombosis/pulmonary embolism	Have client wear elastic stockings and/or sequential compression stockings. Teach leg exercises to client. Encourage fluid intake. Observe for signs of thrombosis (redness, swelling, or pain). Observe client for changes in mental status. Keep client in bed. Do not massage legs. Do not use knee gatch on bed.
Hypotension, bleeding, or infection	Take vital signs at least every 4 hours. Observe client for bleeding. Report excessively low blood pressure or bleeding to physician.

The nurse may place and support the affected leg in neutral rotation by using a device such as the cradle boot. The cradle boot not only prevents rotation but also elevates the leg to the desired functional position and keeps the heel off the bed linen to prevent the breakdown of heel tissue. Keeping the heels off the bed is particularly important for an older client, who is at high risk for pressure ulcers.

The nurse turns the client toward either side as long as the abduction device or other pillow is in place. Some surgeons only allow turning directly onto one side or the other. This policy varies according to the surgeon's preference and the policy of the hospital unit.

The nurse observes for possible signs of hip dislocation, which include increased hip pain, shortening of the affected leg, and leg rotation. If any of these clinical manifestations occur, the nurse keeps the client in bed and notifies the surgeon immediately. The surgeon manipulates and relocates the affected hip after the client receives an analgesic or is anesthetized. The hip is then immobilized by an abduction splint or other device until healing occurs, usually in approximately 6 weeks.

Prevention of Infection. Another common potential complication of hip replacement is infection. As soon as the client's bowel sounds return and he or she is voiding in sufficient quantity, the nurse discontinues IV therapy unless otherwise contraindicated.

CHART 21-3

NURSING FOCUS *on the* OLDER ADULT
Total Hip Replacement

- Use an abduction pillow or splint to prevent adduction after surgery if the client is very restless or has an altered mental state.
- Keep the client's heels off the bed to prevent pressure sores.
- Do not rely on fever as a sign of infection; older clients often have infection without fever. Decreasing mental status typically occurs when the client has an infection.
- When assisting the client out of bed, move him or her slowly to prevent orthostatic (postural) hypotension.
- Encourage the client to deep breathe and cough, and use the incentive spirometer every 2 hours to prevent atelectasis and pneumonia.
- As soon as permitted, get the client out of bed to prevent complications of immobility.
- Anticipate the client's need for pain medication, especially if he or she is unable to verbalize the need for pain control.
- Expect a temporary change in mental state immediately after surgery as a result of the anesthetic and unfamiliar sensory stimuli. Reorient the client frequently.

The nurse also monitors the surgical incision and vital signs carefully—every 4 hours for the first several days and every 8 hours thereafter. The nurse observes for signs of infection, such as an elevated temperature and excessive or foul-smelling drainage from the incision. An older client may not have a fever with infection but instead may experience an altered mental state. The nurse obtains a sample of the drainage for culture and sensitivity to determine the offending organisms and the antibiotics that may be needed for treatment.

An infection that occurs within 1 year of surgery is referred to as an early infection. It is most often due to contamination during surgery. In addition to antibiotics, laminar airflow operating rooms, body exhaust systems, ultraviolet light, and double gloving help reduce the incidence of infection. If an early infection occurs, the surgeon usually prescribes IV antibiotic therapy. Late infection can occur anytime after 1 year following surgery. If the late infection does not resolve with treatment, the surgeon may replace the prosthesis.

The clinical manifestations of infection are variable. The erythrocyte sedimentation rate (ESR) is elevated, and the client typically complains of incisional pain, swelling, erythema, and wound drainage.

Assessment of Bleeding and Prevention of Anemia. The nurse observes the surgical hip dressing for bleeding or other type of drainage at least every 4 hours or when vital signs are taken. The nurse or assistive nursing personnel empties and measures the bloody fluid in the drain every shift. The total amount of drainage is usually less than 50 mL every 8 hours (possibly more if the client has received a plasma expander such as dextran). The surgeon removes the drains and operative dressing 48 to 72 hours after surgery. Care must be taken to prevent tape burns when the surgical dressing is removed, especially in older adults.

The surgeon also orders periodic hemoglobin and hematocrit assessments to determine whether the client is anemic and requires blood transfusions. Although some clients receive several units of blood during surgery, the hematocrit and hemoglobin may fall below the normal level, in which case additional blood is needed 2 or 3 days after surgery. Blood pressure may be lower than usual because of blood loss during surgery or because cement was used during surgery. (Cement tends to dilate blood vessels and cause hypotension.)

Because total joint replacements (TJRs) are elective procedures, autologous blood transfusions are appropriate. The client may donate blood before surgery to be used as needed during and after surgery. This predeposit autologous blood donation is a cost-effective blood replacement alternative for clients who are undergoing elective surgeries.

Another method for blood replacement is intraoperative or postoperative blood salvage. The shed blood is collected intraoperatively via aspiration from the surgical site. Using a cell saver, approximately 50% of the red blood cells are saved for reinfusion. This procedure is used most commonly for bilateral joint replacements or revision surgeries. Blood can be replaced postoperatively by collecting shed blood via suction into a reservoir, filtering the blood, and reinfusing it within a few hours.

Postoperative blood replacement has been standard practice until recently. A preventive alternative is the use of Epoetin alfa (Epogen, Procrit, Eprex🍁), an approved treatment for anemia that may prevent the necessity of postoperative blood transfusion when given to clients undergoing TJR (Geier, 1998).

Assessment for Neurovascular Compromise. As with other bone surgery, frequent neurovascular assessments are necessary to monitor for a possible compromise in circulation to the distal extremity. Such assessments are performed at the same time the vital signs are checked.

Management of Incisional Pain. Although hip replacement is performed to relieve joint pain, the client does experience pain related to the surgical procedure. Many clients state that they have pain after surgery but that it is of a different type and is less excruciating than the pain before surgery. Pain control may be achieved by epidural analgesia, patient-controlled analgesia (PCA), intramuscular opioid analgesia, or a combination of techniques. Chapter 7 contains a chart of commonly used opioid analgesics and related nursing interventions.

A new device for pain control after TJR (hip or knee) is a small pump called the PainBuster. This pump continuously infuses a local anesthetic, such as bupivacaine, directly into the surgical site. The local infusion decreases the amount of opioids that the client needs (e.g., morphine), thus reducing the risk of adverse drug reactions. The device is also ideal for ambulatory surgical clients, who may go home with the device (Kettelman, 2000). After the catheter is removed in 48 to 72 hours, the entire device is discarded and the site is covered with a sterile dressing.

The nurse anticipates the older client's need for pain medication if he or she cannot verbalize the need. Many older adults experience several days of increased disorientation or delirium as a result of surgery and anesthesia.

Regardless of the pain management method used, most clients do not require parenteral analgesia after the first 2 days. Oral opioids, such as oxycodone (Supeudol🍁) or oxycodone plus acetaminophen (Percocet, Tylox), are then commonly prescribed until the pain can be controlled by NSAIDs such as ketorolac (Toradol, Acular) or ibuprofen (Motrin, Apo–Ibuprofen🍁).

Progression of Activity. The client with a total hip replacement is usually allowed to get out of bed the day after

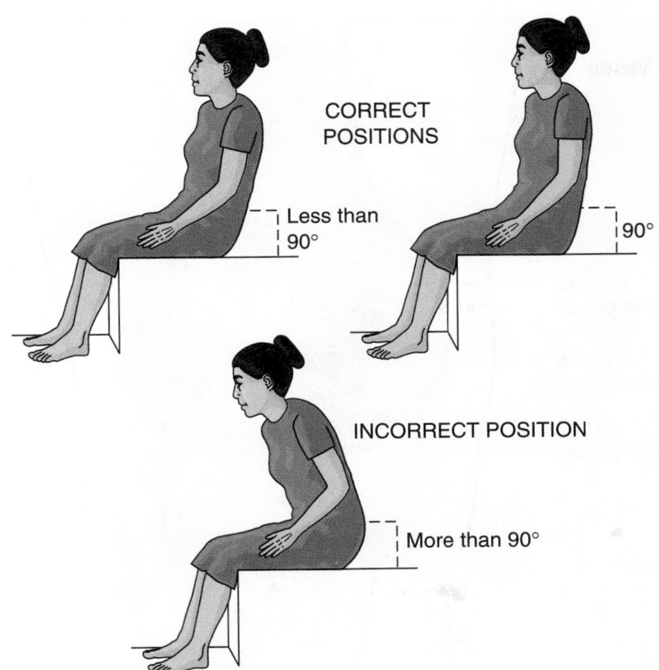

Figure 21-3 ● Correct and incorrect hip flexion after a total hip replacement.

surgery, and physical therapy is initiated. Permitted activities differ among surgeons and hospitals, but prolonged bedrest can cause numerous complications (e.g., atelectasis and pneumonia), especially in the older adults. When getting the client out of bed, the nurse stands on the same side of the bed as the affected leg. After achieving a sitting position, the client stands on the unaffected leg and pivots to the chair with assistance. To prevent hip dislocation, the nurse at all times ensures that the client does not flex the hips beyond 90 degrees (Figure 21-3). Raised toilet seats, straight-back chairs, and reclining wheelchairs help prevent hyperflexion.

The surgeon, the type of prosthesis, and the surgical approach determine the resumption of weight bearing on the affected leg. A client with a cemented implant is usually allowed immediate partial weight bearing (PWB) or full weight bearing (FWB) to tolerance. A client with an uncemented prosthesis cannot tolerate FWB until bony ingrowth occurs. Typically, only PWB is permitted for the first 6 weeks or until there is x-ray evidence of bony ingrowth.

The physical therapist (PT) teaches the client how to follow these weight-bearing restrictions and helps the client progress to FWB status, if possible. Most clients use a walker, but young clients may use crutches. Clients are usually advanced to a single cane or crutch if they can walk without a severe limp 1 month after surgery. When the limp disappears, they no longer need an ambulatory/assistive device and are permitted to sit in chairs of normal height, use regular toilets, and drive a car.

Prevention of Thromboembolic Complications. The risk of developing deep venous thrombosis (DVT) postoperatively is high. Fatal pulmonary embolism syndrome occurs in 0.5% to 2% of cases (Ranawat et al., 1997). Older clients are especially at increased risk for thrombi because of age and compromised circulation before surgery. Obese clients and those with a history of DVT are also at high risk for thrombi. In clients with total hip replacement, thrombi usually develop in the thigh; these thrombi become life-threatening emboli more readily than thrombi in the calf and other areas. For this reason, thigh-high stockings, elastic bandages, and sequential compression devices (SCDs) are used during the hospital stay (see Chapter 17).

Anticoagulants, such as aspirin (Ecotrin, buffered aspirin), warfarin (Coumadin, Warfilone✱), or a subcutaneous low-molecular-weight (LMW) heparin (Lovenox), are prescribed. Studies indicate that LMW heparins are superior and decrease the risk of DVT in clients undergoing total hip and knee replacement (Morris et al., 1998). If the client takes warfarin, the dosage is usually adjusted to maintain an International Normalized Ratio (INR) of 2.0 to 3.0.

The PT teaches leg exercises, which are begun in the immediate postoperative period and continue until the client is fully ambulatory. These exercises include plantar flexion and dorsiflexion (heel pumping), circumduction (circles) of the feet, gluteal and quadriceps muscle setting, and straight-leg raises (SLRs). The client performs gluteal exercises by pushing the heels into the bed and achieves quadriceps-setting exercises ("quad sets") by straightening the legs and pushing the back of the knees into the bed. In addition to preventing clots, these exercises improve muscle tone, which aids restoring the function of the extremity.

Promotion of Self-Care. The hospital's occupational therapy department often supplies assistive/adaptive devices to help with activities of daily living (ADLs). Particularly important for clients are devices designed for reaching to prevent them from bending or stooping and flexing at the hips more than 90 degrees. Extended handles on shoehorns and dressing sticks are particularly useful for helping clients achieve independence in ADLs.

The length of stay in the acute care hospital is typically 3 days, but older clients or those experiencing postoperative complications may stay longer. Discharge may be to the home, a rehabilitation unit, transitional care unit (subacute unit), or long-term care facility for rehabilitation or custodial care. The interdisciplinary team provides written instructions for posthospital care and reviews them with clients and their family members (Chart 21-4). A copy of the posthospital instructions is sent with clients who are transferred to a facility.

CRITICAL THINKING CHALLENGE

Your client is unable to obtain pain control for degenerative joint disease (DJD) of the hip and knee and therefore undergoes a left cemented total hip replacement. She returns to the assisted living facility for rehabilitation following a 3-day hospital stay. She is able to ambulate with a walker in her room and wears thigh-high elastic stockings. Her medication orders include Coumadin and Tylox for pain.

- What teaching should you reinforce with her related to Coumadin?
- What weight-bearing allowance will she most likely have?
- What surgical complications is she still at risk for, and how can you help prevent them?

For suggested answer guidelines, go to SIMON http://www.wbsaunders.com/SIMON/Iggy/.

TOTAL KNEE REPLACEMENT. After total hip replacement, the second most common total joint replacement (TJR)

CHART 21-4

CLIENT EDUCATION GUIDE
Total Hip Replacement

Hip Precautions
- Do not sit or stand for prolonged periods.
- Do not cross your legs beyond the midline of your body.
- Do not bend your hips more than 90 degrees.
- Use an ambulatory aid, such as a walker, when walking.
- Use assistive/adaptive devices for dressing, such as for putting on shoes and socks.
- You can resume sexual intercourse as usual, but use the hip precautions learned in the hospital.

Pain Management
- Report increased hip pain to the physician immediately.
- Take oral analgesics as prescribed and only as needed.
- Do not overexert yourself; take frequent rests.

Incisional Care
- Inspect your hip incision every day for redness, heat, or drainage; if any of these are present, call your physician immediately.
- Cleanse your hip incision with a mild soap and water every day; be sure to dry it thoroughly.

Other Care
- Continue walking and performing the leg exercises as you learned in the hospital.
- Report pain, redness, or swelling in your legs to your physician immediately.
- Report chest pain and/or shortness of breath to your physician immediately.
- If you are taking an anticoagulant for 4 to 6 weeks, follow the precautions learned in the hospital to prevent bleeding: avoid using a straight razor, avoid injuries, and report bleeding or excessive bruising to your physician immediately.

procedure involves the knee, or total knee replacement (TKR). Before 1980, attempts at knee replacement were not successful, and most of the prostheses inserted before then have been removed. The knee is not a simple, hinged joint; it is a condylar joint that rotates slightly when flexed and extended. As seen in Figure 21-4, the typical total knee prosthesis is a three-part system: a femoral component, a tibial plate, and a patellar button. With some clients, only one surface is replaced.

PREOPERATIVE CARE. Only severe symptoms and disability justify TKR in clients with DJD. TKRs are typically avoided in people younger than 60 years of age (Windsor & Insall, 1997). The preoperative care for clients undergoing a TKR is similar to that for total hip replacement. The major difference is the teaching, which depends on the postoperative protocol used by the orthopedic surgeon.

OPERATIVE PROCEDURES. As with the hip, the knee can be replaced with the client under general or epidural anesthesia. The surgeon typically makes a central longitudinal incision approximately 8 inches (20.3 cm) long. Osteotomies of the femoral and tibial condyles and of the posterior patella are performed, and the surfaces are prepared for the prosthesis. Noncemented implants, once popular in the 1980s, are used less for the knee than they are for the hip. The surgeon inserts one or two surgical drains and applies a pressure dressing to prevent bleeding. Some clients have bilateral knee replacements as part of one surgery.

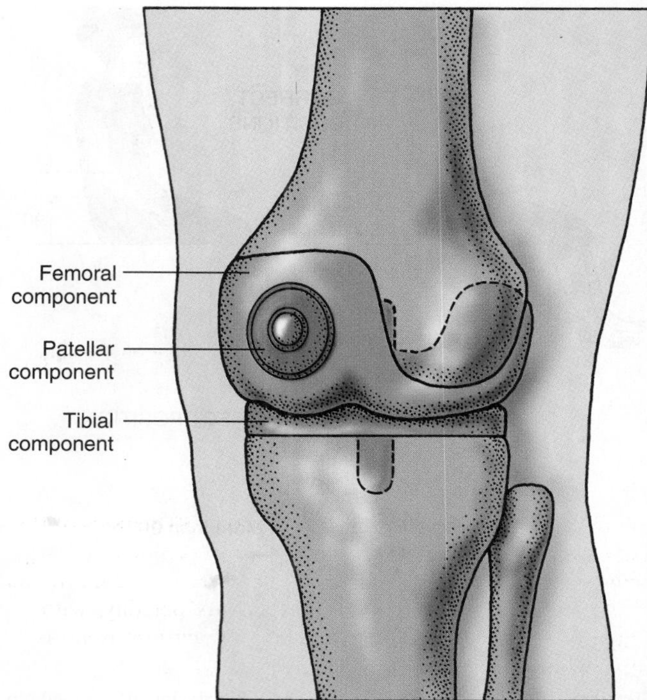

Figure 21-4 ● Typical three-part condylar knee replacement system.

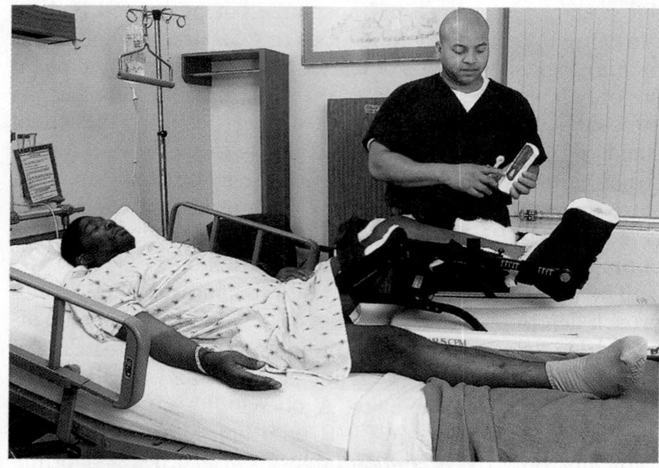

Figure 21-5 ● A continuous passive motion machine in use.

POSTOPERATIVE CARE. Postoperative nursing care of the client with a TKR is similar to that for the client with a total hip replacement; however, maintaining abduction is not necessary. The surgeon usually orders the use of a continuous passive motion (CPM) machine, which can be applied in the postanesthesia care unit (PACU) or not used until 1 to 2 days after surgery (Figure 21-5). The CPM keeps the prosthetic knee in motion and prevents the formation of scar tissue, which could impede mobility of the knee and exacerbate postoperative pain. In the immediate postoperative period, the surgeon may also order ice packs or a Hot/Ice Machine to decrease swelling at the surgical site.

CHART 21-5

BEST PRACTICE *for*
The Client Using a Continuous Passive Motion (CPM) Machine

- Ensure that the machine is well padded with sheepskin or other similar material.
- Check the cycle and range-of-motion settings at least once per shift (every 8 hours).
- Ensure that the joint being moved is properly positioned on the machine.
- If the client is confused, place the controls to the machine out of his or her reach.
- Assess the client's response to the machine.
- Turn off the machine while the client is having a meal in bed.
- When the machine is not in use, do not store it on the floor.

The surgeon, physical therapist, or technician presets the CPM machine for the appropriate range of motion and cycles per minute. A typical initial setting is 20 to 30 degrees of flexion and full extension (0 degrees) at 2 cycles/min, but this setting varies according to surgeon preference. The CPM machine is generally used for 8 to 12 hours per day, with the range of motion increased gradually. The current trend is intermittent use for several hours at a time. Each day the nurse notes the client's response to the device.

Some machines do not allow the leg to achieve full extension, thus promoting flexion contractures. One solution is for the client to use the CPM machine during the day and sleep in a knee immobilizer at night to achieve the desired extension. Chart 21-5 outlines the nurse's responsibility when caring for a client using the CPM machine.

In general, pain control measures for clients with TKR are similar to clients with total hip replacement. Ritter et al. (1999) found that intra-articular morphine for the first 24 hours after surgery is a safe and effective alternative for pain management.

Because dislocation is a rare problem for a client with TKR, special positioning is not required. Other complications that affect clients with total hip replacement may also affect clients with TKR. The preventive measures described earlier for total hip replacement are used for TKR.

The goal for discharge from the hospital is that the client should walk independently with a cane or walker and have 90 degrees of flexion in the operative knee. The use of a stationary bicycle can help gain flexion. After discharge from the hospital, the client should not hyperflex the knee or kneel for prolonged periods.

TOTAL SHOULDER REPLACEMENT. Shoulder replacements have not been performed as often as other types of replacement techniques. Because the joint is complex and has many articulations, subluxation (or dislocation) is a major complication. A Neer-type prosthesis is commonly used, with or without cement.

The client's affected arm is typically placed in a CPM machine shortly after surgery (see Chart 21-5). During the first few postoperative days, frequent neurovascular assessments are important. The hospital stay is shorter than for a total hip replacement or total knee replacement.

TOTAL ELBOW REPLACEMENT. Total elbow replacement is performed most commonly for clients with rheumatoid arthritis. It is usually successful in increasing range of motion, but infection is fairly common because of extensive tissue cutting during surgery. A Mayo prosthesis is commonly inserted, and the CPM device is often used postoperatively. In general, elbow motion is allowed as tolerated. Physical therapy is not usually necessary. Generalized swelling usually resolves in 3 to 6 months.

FINGER AND WRIST REPLACEMENTS. Any joint of the hand can be replaced, often for clients with rheumatoid arthritis. Flexible, silicone prostheses are implanted without the use of polymethyl methacrylate because no weight bearing is required.

A bulky dressing is used temporarily after surgery and is then replaced with a dynamic splint, brace, cast, or very small CPM machine. Edema formation is controlled if the client elevates the arm as much as possible. The rehabilitation program for finger arthroplasties may last for weeks, until normal function and strength return. These procedures are typically performed in specialized hand centers.

Any bone of the wrist can be replaced, including the heads of the radius and ulna. The postoperative pressure dressing is removed in 2 to 3 days, and a splint or short arm cast is applied. The client usually regains full function within 6 to 12 weeks, but lifting may be restricted for a longer period. Occupational therapists are usually involved with upper extremity rehabilitation.

ANKLE AND TOE REPLACEMENTS. Because the ankles support approximately 25% of the body's weight, developing an implant that is both small enough and strong enough has been difficult. When the ankle is replaced, an arthrodesis (bone fusion) is usually performed for added stability. Replacing the ankle is not a common procedure because of implant failures. The long-term results of newer-designed prostheses are not yet known.

Metatarsal implants are made of silicone and cannot bear excessive weight. Typically the client has one or more osteotomies and fusions, which are immobilized by wires and a cast while healing occurs. Chapter 51 discusses foot osteotomies and their associated nursing care.

IMPAIRED PHYSICAL MOBILITY

NOC **PLANNING: EXPECTED OUTCOMES.** The client with degenerative joint disease (DJD) is expected to function independently in performing activities of daily living (ADLs) and ambulation.

INTERVENTIONS. Management of the client with DJD is an interdisciplinary effort. The nurse collaborates with physical and occupational therapists to meet the goal of independent function. Major interventions include therapeutic exercise and the promotion of ADLs and ambulation by teaching about health and the use of assistive/adaptive devices.

EXERCISE. Two types of exercise are recommended for the client with DJD: recreational and therapeutic. Recreational exercise includes hobbies and sports, with no planned purpose other than relaxation. Therapeutic exercise includes carefully planned activities that are designed to improve muscle strength, muscle tone, and joint range of motion. Thera-

CHART 21-6

CLIENT EDUCATION GUIDE
Exercises for Clients with Degenerative Joint Disease or Rheumatoid Arthritis

- Follow the exercise instructions that have been specifically prescribed for you. There are no universal exercises; your exercises have been specifically tailored to your own needs.
- Do your exercises on both "good" and "bad" days. Consistency is important.
- Respect pain. If pain increases as you exercise, stop and report this to your physician.
- Use active rather than active-assist or passive exercise whenever possible.
- Reduce the number of repetitions when the inflammation is severe and you have more pain.
- Do not substitute your normal activities or household tasks for the prescribed exercises.
- Avoid resistive exercises when your joints are severely inflamed.

peutic exercise can also reduce pain and improve the client's psychologic health.

Certain recreational activities may also be therapeutic, such as doing the breaststroke during swimming to enhance chest and arm muscles. Aerobic exercises (e.g., walking, biking, swimming, and aerobic dance) are recommended. Usually the physical therapist prescribes exercises for the client with DJD, but the nurse reinforces their techniques and principles. The ideal time for exercise is immediately after the application of heat. To prevent further joint damage, clients should rigorously follow the instructions for exercise outlined in Chart 21-6.

USE OF ASSISTIVE/ADAPTIVE DEVICES. The physical therapist evaluates the client's need for ambulatory aids such as canes, walkers, or platform crutches. Although many clients do not like to use these aids or may forget how to use them, they do help prevent further joint deterioration and pain. An occupational therapist evaluates the client's ability to perform ADLs and can provide ideas and devices for assistance.

Community-Based Care

The client with DJD is not usually hospitalized for the disease itself but for surgical management. The cost of medical and surgical care for clients with DJD has been evaluated (see the Cost of Care box above).

HOME CARE MANAGEMENT

If weight-bearing joints are markedly involved, the client may have difficulty going up or down stairs. Making arrangements to live on one floor with accessibility to all rooms is often the best solution. A home care nurse, physical therapist, or occupational therapist assesses the need for structural alterations to the home to accommodate ambulatory aids and enable the client to perform activities. For example, a kitchen counter may need to be lowered, or a seat and handrails may need to be installed in the shower. If the client has undergone a total hip replacement, an elevated toilet seat is necessary for several weeks postoperatively to prevent excessive hip flexion.

COST OF CARE IMPLICATIONS FOR NURSING

DEGENERATIVE JOINT DISEASE

Cost of Care

- The cost of medical care for older clients with degenerative joint disease (DJD) is approximately twice that of older clients with no symptomatic DJD.
- The average individual cost of arthritis-related care for clients with rheumatoid arthritis (RA) is approximately $2200 per year. Medications account for almost two thirds of the cost, and hospital care accounts for 16%. By contrast, the average individual cost for clients with DJD is approximately $550 per year. Medications account for approximately one third of the cost, and hospital care accounts for close to one half of the cost (most due to total joint replacement).
- Although the individual cost of care for clients with DJD is approximately one fourth of that for clients with RA, the total cost for DJD is about seven times greater because the higher prevalence of DJD.
- One half of the costs for DJD is due to sick days from work—$15.5 billion in the United States.
- Clinical pathways for total hip replacement reduce the length of stay and hospital costs.

Implications for Nursing

Because of the high cost of medications for DJD and RA, nurses need to become more familiar with the use of integrative therapies for pain management. Research has shown that some modalities are as effective as analgesics, and others serve as excellent adjuncts for pain control. For clients undergoing total joint replacement, extensive staff and client education is needed to follow clinical pathways and ensure positive clinical and cost outcomes.

Data from Lanes, S.F. (1997). Resource utilization and cost of care for rheumatoid arthritis and osteoarthritis in a managed care setting: The importance of drug and surgery costs. *Arthritis and Rheumatism, 40*(8), 1475-1481; and MacLean, C.H. (1998). Costs attributable to osteoarthritis. *Journal of Rheumatology, 25*(11), 2213-2218.

HEALTH TEACHING

Learning how to protect the joint is the most important feature of client education. Preventing further damage to joints slows the progression of DJD and minimizes pain. The nurse explains the general rules of joint protection and cites examples (Chart 21-7).

As with other diseases in which drugs and diet therapy are used, the nurse teaches the drug protocol, side effects, and toxic effects to the client and family. The nurse also emphasizes the importance of reducing weight and eating a well-balanced diet to promote tissue healing.

Many clients with "arthritis" look for a cure after becoming frustrated and desperate about the course of the disease and treatment. Unfortunately, there is no cure for these joint diseases, even though tabloids, books, and the media often cite "curative" remedies. People spend billions of dollars each year on quackery, including liniments, special diets, and copper bracelets. More hazardous substances, such as snake venom and industrial cleaners, are also advertised as remedies. The nurse instructs the client always to check with The Arthritis Foundation about new "cures." For example, if a client believes it is helpful to wear a copper bracelet or to eat more

CHART 21-7

CLIENT EDUCATION GUIDE
Evidence-Based Instructions for Joint Protection

- Use large joints instead of small ones; for example, place your purse strap over your shoulder instead of grasping the purse with your hand.
- Do not turn a doorknob clockwise. Turn it counterclockwise to avoid twisting your arm and promoting ulnar deviation.
- Use two hands instead of one to hold objects.
- Sit in a chair that has a high, straight back.
- When getting out of bed, do not push off with your fingers; use the entire palm of both hands.
- Do not bend at your waist; instead bend your knees while keeping your back straight.
- Use long-handled devices, such as a hairbrush with an extended handle.
- Use assistive/adaptive devices, such as Velcro closures and built-up utensil handles, to protect your joints.
- Do not use pillows in bed, except a small one under your head.
- Avoid twisting or wringing your hands.

foods with a high vitamin C content, the nurse may encourage continuation of the practice as long as it is not harmful. If there is a potential for harm, the nurse instructs the client to avoid the modality and provides the rationale for doing so.

With most types of connective tissue disease (CTD), clients must live with a chronic, unpredictable, and painful disorder. Their roles, self-esteem, and body image may be affected by these diseases. Body image is often not as devastating in DJD as in the inflammatory arthritic diseases, such as rheumatoid arthritis. This psychosocial component is discussed in more detail under Psychosocial Assessment (Rheumatoid Arthritis), p. 346.

HEALTH CARE RESOURCES

The client who has undergone surgery is most likely to need help from community resources. After a joint replacement, he or she needs extensive assistance with mobility. He or she may be discharged to home, a long-term care facility, a subacute unit (transitional care unit), or a rehabilitation unit. The nurse collaborates with the case manager and physician to find the best placement. If the client is discharged to home, home care nurses may be approved for several visits, depending on the concurrent systemic diseases. A nursing assistant may visit the home to help with hygiene-related needs, and a physical therapist may work with ambulatory and mobility skills. A client who has undergone a total hip or knee replacement should not be discharged to home alone. A family member or significant other must be in the home at all times for at least the first 4 to 6 weeks—when the client needs the most assistance.

The nurse provides written instructions about the required care, regardless of whether the client goes home or to another inpatient facility. Communication with the new care provider is essential for seamless continuity of care. Arrangements are made for the client to return to the same acute care hospital if needed.

The Arthritis Foundation is an important community resource for all clients with CTD. This organization provides information to lay people and health care professionals and refers clients and their families to other resources as needed. Local support groups can help clients and their families cope with these diseases.

Evaluation: Outcomes

NOC The nurse evaluates the care of the client with DJD on the basis of the identified nursing diagnoses. The expected outcomes are that the client:

- States that chronic pain is reduced as a result of interdisciplinary interventions for pain control
- Ambulates without personal assistance (although a mechanical aid such as a walker may be used)
- Is independent in ADLs (may use assistive/adaptive devices)

RHEUMATOID ARTHRITIS

OVERVIEW

Rheumatoid arthritis (RA) is the second most common connective tissue disease and is the most destructive to the joints. It is a chronic, progressive, systemic inflammatory process that primarily affects the synovial joints.

The onset of RA is characterized by synovitis, or inflammation of the synovial tissue in joints. Inflammatory mediators, such as cytokines, chemokines, and proteases, attract and activate neutrophils and other cells. (See Chapter 20 for a complete discussion of the inflammatory response.) The synovium thickens and becomes hyperemic, fluid accumulates in the joint space, and a pannus forms. The pannus is vascular granulation tissue composed of inflammatory cells; it erodes articular cartilage and eventually destroys bone. As a result, fibrous adhesions, bony ankylosis, and calcifications occur; bone loses density and secondary osteoporosis occurs.

Permanent joint changes may be avoided if RA is diagnosed early. Early, aggressive treatment to suppress synovitis may cause a remission; approximately 25% of clients experience a remission, which may last as long as 20 years. Some clients experience spontaneous remissions and exacerbations without treatment.

RA is a systemic disease; that is, areas of the body besides the synovial joints can be affected. Inflammatory responses similar to those occurring in synovial tissue may be seen in any organ or body system in which connective tissue is prevalent. If blood vessel involvement **(vasculitis)** occurs, the organ supplied by that vessel can be affected. The result is malfunction and eventual failure of the organ or system. These pathologic changes occur late in the disease process and cause life-threatening problems.

The etiology of RA remains a mystery, but research suggests a combination of environmental and genetic factors. The most popular theory to date—the immune complex hypothesis—states that unusual antibodies of the immunoglobulin G (IgG) or immunoglobulin M (IgM) type (rheumatoid factor) develop against IgG antigenic determinants to form complexes that lodge in synovium and other connective tissues. Local and systemic inflammatory responses result. RA has been found to be strongly associated with the human leukocyte antigen (HLA) DRw4. Other antigens have been identified but are observed less frequently. (See Chapter 20 on inflammation and the immune response.)

Although RA is probably an autoimmune disease, the origin of rheumatoid factor is unclear. A genetic predisposition to RA is most likely because the disease affects people with a family history of RA two to three times more often than the rest of the population.

Some researchers suspect that female reproductive hormones influence the development of RA because it affects women more often than men. Others suspect that a virus, such as the Epstein-Barr virus, may trigger the autoimmune process. Physical and emotional stresses have been linked to exacerbations of the disorder and may be contributing factors in its development. Most recently, smoking and coffee drinking have been found to increase the incidence of RA (Wolfe, 2000; Heliovaara et al., 2000).

WOMEN'S HEALTH CONSIDERATIONS

RA affects 1% of the world's population, with women being affected three times more often than men. Women who are taking or have taken oral contraceptives are less likely to have RA. The onset of the disease is typically between 35 and 45 years of age, but it can occur at any age.

CULTURAL CONSIDERATIONS

Despite the common lay belief that warm, dry climates can be beneficial to people with RA, there are no significant differences in its prevalence among geographic locations. The incidence of RA in China is somewhat lower than elsewhere in the world (approximately 0.3%) and substantially higher among the Pima Indians in North America (approximately 5%) (Harris, 1997).

COLLABORATIVE MANAGEMENT

Assessment

The onset of rheumatoid arthritis (RA) may be acute and severe or slow and insidious; clients may have vague complaints that last for several months before diagnosis. The onset of the disease is more common in the winter months than in the warmer months. The manifestations of RA can be categorized as early or late disease and as articular or extra-articular (Chart 21-8).

PHYSICAL ASSESSMENT/CLINICAL MANIFESTATIONS

EARLY DISEASE MANIFESTATIONS. The client with RA typically complains of fatigue, generalized weakness, stiffness, anorexia, and a weight loss of approximately 2 or 3 pounds (1 kg) early in the disease process. Persistent low-grade fever may accompany these complaints because RA is an inflammatory disease. In clients with early disease, the nurse notes that the upper extremity joints are involved initially, typically the proximal interphalangeal (PIP) and metacarpophalangeal (MCP) joints of the hands. These joints may be slightly reddened, warm, stiff, swollen, and tender or painful, particularly on palpation **(synovitis).** The typical pattern of joint involvement in RA is bilateral and symmetric (e.g., both wrists), and the number of joints involved usually increases as the disease progresses.

CONSIDERATIONS FOR OLDER ADULTS

RA that develops in older adults affects men more often than women. The client typically complains of stiffness; swelling of the hands, wrists, and forearms; and limb girdle (shoulder and hip) pain (Harris, 1997).

LATE DISEASE MANIFESTATIONS. As the disease worsens, the joints become progressively inflamed and quite painful. The client complains of morning stiffness (also called the gel phenomenon), which lasts between 30 minutes and several hours after awakening. On palpation, the nurse notes that the joints feel soft because of synovitis and effusions. The fingers often appear spindle-like. The nurse may observe muscle atrophy (which can result from disuse secondary to joint pain) and a decreased range of motion in the affected joints.

Most or all synovial joints are eventually affected. The temporomandibular joint (TMJ) may be involved in severe disease, but such involvement is uncommon. When the TMJ is affected, the client typically complains of pain when chewing or opening the mouth.

When the spinal column is involved, the cervical joints are most likely to be affected. The nurse palpates the posterior cervical spine to elicit pain or tenderness. Cervical disease may result in subluxation, especially with the first and second vertebrae. This is a life-threatening complication because branches of the phrenic nerve that supply the diaphragm can be compressed, and respiratory function may be subsequently compromised. The client is also in danger of becoming quadriparetic or quadriplegic (also called tetraplegic).

JOINT MANIFESTATIONS. Joint deformity occurs as a late, articular manifestation, and secondary osteoporosis can

CHART 21-8

KEY FEATURES *of* The Client with Rheumatoid Arthritis

Early Manifestations

Joint

- Inflammation

Systemic

- Low-grade fever
- Fatigue
- Weakness
- Anorexia
- Paresthesias

Late Manifestations

Joint

- Deformities (e.g., swan neck or ulnar deviation)
- Moderate to severe pain and morning stiffness

Systemic

- Osteoporosis
- Severe fatigue
- Anemia
- Weight loss
- Subcutaneous nodules
- Peripheral neuropathy
- Vasculitis
- Pericarditis
- Fibrotic lung disease
- Sjögren's syndrome
- Renal disease

cause bone fractures. The nurse observes common deformities, especially in the hands and feet (Figure 21-6). Extensive wrist involvement can result in carpal tunnel syndrome (see Chapter 51 for assessment and management of carpal tunnel syndrome).

The nurse palpates the tissues around the joints to elicit pain or tenderness associated with other rheumatoid complications. For example, Baker's cysts (enlarged popliteal bursae) may occur and cause tissue compression and pain. Tendon rupture is also common, particularly rupture of the Achilles tendon.

A

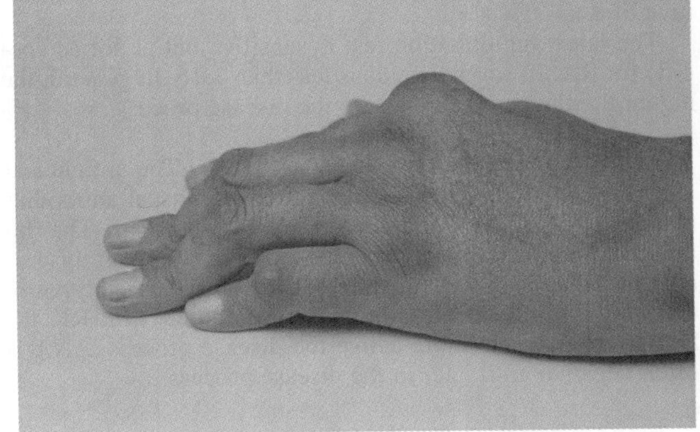

B

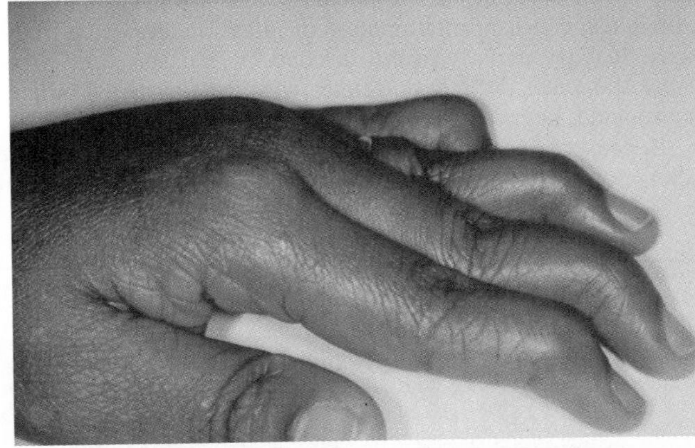

C

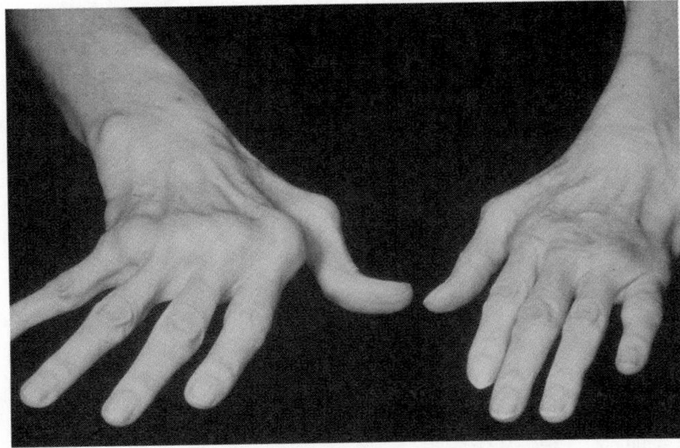

Figure 21-6 ● Common joint deformities seen in rheumatoid arthritis. **A,** Boutonniere, or buttonhole. **B,** Swan neck. **C,** Ulnar deviation *(on left).* (From the Arthritis Teaching Slide Collection, copyright 1980. Used by permission of the Arthritis Foundation.)

SYSTEMIC MANIFESTATIONS. Numerous extra-articular clinical manifestations are associated with advanced disease. Consequently, the nurse assesses other body systems to ascertain systemic involvement. Moderate to severe weight loss, fever, and extreme fatigue are common in late disease exacerbations, often called "flares." Approximately 25% of clients have the characteristic round, movable, nontender subcutaneous nodules, which most often appear on the ulnar surface of the arm. These nodules can disappear and reappear at any time and are associated with severe, destructive disease. They occasionally open and become infected, but otherwise they do not usually cause a problem.

Inflammation of the blood vessels results in vasculitis, particularly of small- to medium-sized vessels. When arterial involvement (RA) occurs, major organs and body systems become ischemic and malfunction. Ischemic skin lesions appear in groups as small, brownish spots, most commonly around the nail bed (periungual lesions). The nurse and health care provider monitor the number of lesions and note their location each day. An increased number of lesions indicates increased vasculitis, and a decreased number indicates decreased vasculitis. The nurse also carefully assesses any larger lesions that appear on the lower extremities; such lesions often lead to ulcerations, which heal slowly as a result of decreased circulation. Peripheral neuropathy associated with decreased circulation can cause foot drop and paresthesias (burning and tingling sensations), most often in older adults.

Respiratory complications manifest as pleurisy, pneumonitis, diffuse interstitial fibrosis, and pulmonary hypertension. Cardiac complications include pericarditis and myocarditis. The nurse also assesses for ocular involvement, which typically manifests as iritis and scleritis. If either of these complications is present, the nurse notes that the sclera of one or both eyes is reddened and that the pupils have an irregular shape.

ASSOCIATED SYNDROMES. Several syndromes are seen in clients with advanced RA. The most common is Sjögren's syndrome, which includes a triad of the following:

- Dry eyes (keratoconjunctivitis sicca [KCS], or the sicca syndrome)
- Dry mouth **(xerostomia)**
- Dry vagina (in some cases)

In **Sjögren's syndrome,** immune complexes and inflammatory cells are thought to obstruct secretory glands and ducts. The syndrome is usually associated with connective tissue diseases such as RA but may occur alone. The nurse notes the client's complaint of dry mouth or dry eyes. Some clients state that their eyes feel "gritty," as if sand is in their eyes. The nurse also inspects the mouth for dry, sticky membranes and the eyes for redness and lack of tearing.

Less commonly observed is Felty's syndrome, which is characterized by RA, hepatosplenomegaly (enlarged liver and spleen), and leukopenia.

Caplan's syndrome is characterized by the presence of rheumatoid nodules in the lungs and pneumoconiosis, which is noted primarily in coal miners and asbestos workers. The health care provider diagnoses these syndromes by physical examination and diagnostic testing.

PSYCHOSOCIAL ASSESSMENT

Rheumatoid arthritis (RA) can be a crippling disease. After having the disease for 10 to 15 years, fewer than 50% of clients are totally independent in activities of daily living (ADLs). These physical limitations result in role changes in the family and society. For example, the person may not be able to cook for the family or be an active sexual partner. In addition, extreme fatigue often causes clients to desire an early bedtime and may result in a reluctance to socialize.

Body changes may also cause poor self-esteem and body image. Because many societies value people with physically fit, attractive bodies, the client with RA may be embarrassed to be seen in public places. The client may grieve, experience depression, or attempt suicide. The client may experience a feeling of helplessness accompanied by a loss of control over a disease that can "consume" the body.

Living with a chronic disease and the pain that results is difficult for the client, family, and significant others. The client experiences a loss of control and independence. Chronic suffering affects quality of life. The nurse assesses the client's emotional and mental status in relation to the disease and its problems and evaluates the client's support systems and resources.

LABORATORY ASSESSMENT

Laboratory tests help to support a diagnosis of RA, but no single test or group of tests can confirm it. Chart 21-9 summarizes the common laboratory tests that the health care provider uses for diagnosing connective tissue disease.

RHEUMATOID FACTOR. The test for **rheumatoid factor (RF)** measures the presence of unusual antibodies of the IgG and IgM type that develop in a number of connective tissue diseases. Two methods may be used to ascertain the degree to which these antibodies are present in the body: Rose-Waaler and latex agglutination. In both procedures, values are reported as titers.

The Rose-Waaler test is more specific for a diagnosis of RA than the latex agglutination test, but it is not as sensitive. A client with a positive Rose-Waaler result probably has RA and is seropositive; a client with a negative test result may or may not have the disease and is seronegative. Approximately 60% of individuals with RA are seropositive and have a positive titer.

The latex agglutination test is sensitive but is not as specific for RA. Its normal value is less than 1:16. In general, the higher the titer, the more active the disease process.

ANTINUCLEAR ANTIBODY TITER. The antinuclear antibody (ANA) test measures the titer of unusual antibodies that destroy the nuclei of cells and cause tissue death. The fluorescent method is sometimes referred to as FANA. If this test result is positive (a value higher than 1:8), various subtypes of this antibody are identified and measured. As with RF, the higher the titer, the more active the disease process. ANA is often negative until later in the disease process.

ERYTHROCYTE SEDIMENTATION RATE. The "sed rate," as the erythrocyte sedimentation rate (ESR) is sometimes called, can confirm inflammation or infection anywhere in the body. It is particularly useful in connective tissue disease because the value directly correlates with the degree of inflammation and, later, with the severity of the disease.

Because several laboratory procedures are used to measure ESR, normal values will vary; women have higher normal

CHART 21-9

LABORATORY PROFILE
Connective Tissue Disease

Test	Normal Range for Adults	Significance of Abnormal Findings
Rheumatoid factor		
Rose-Waaler	Negative	Elevations of either titer (increase in number at right of colon) indicative of possible CTD Increased Rose's titer indicative of RA (seropositive); not a sensitive test
Latex agglutination	<1:16	Latex titer not as specific to one disease, but quite a sensitive test
ANA (total)	Negative (if positive, types of ANA identified [e.g., anti-DNA, anti-DNP, anti-RNA] to indicate what part of cells are involved)	Elevations common in SLE, PSS, RA, and other inflammatory CTDs (5% of healthy adults have positive ANA results)
Serum complement (C′ or CH_{50})	Varies greatly among laboratories	Decreased value indicative of active autoimmune disease such as SLE
LE preparation	Negative	A type of ANA (anti-DNP); not reliable because negative result does not rule out SLE; can be used as screening test
SPEP		
Albumin	3.5-5.0 g/dL	Increased levels of gamma globulins indicative of CTD (inflammatory type)
Globulin		Increased level of alpha globulins possible in RA
$Alpha_1$ globulin	0.1-0.3 g/dL	
$Alpha_2$ globulin	0.6-1.0 g/dL	
Beta globulin	0.7-1.1 g/dL	
Gamma globulin	0.8-1.6 g/dL	
HLA testing (HLA-B27)	None	Presence of HLA-B27 indicative of Reiter's syndrome or ankylosing spondylitis

ANA, Antinuclear antibody; *CTD*, connective tissue disease; *DNP*, dinitrophenol; *SLE*, systemic lupus erythematosus; *PSS*, progressive systemic sclerosis; *LE*, lupus erythematosus; *SPEP*, serum protein electrophoresis; *RA*, rheumatoid arthritis; *HLA*, human leukocyte antigen; *ESR*, erythrocyte sedimentation rate.

values than men. In general, a value of 20 to 40 mm/hr indicates mild inflammation; 40 to 70 mm/hr, moderate inflammation; and 70 to 150 mm/hr, severe inflammation.

The ESR is also used to monitor a client's response to anti-inflammatory drug therapy. This value should decrease if the drug dosage is effective.

SERUM COMPLEMENT. Complement (C') attaches to immune complexes in an attempt to destroy them. If a large amount of complement is used in this lytic process, the concentration of free-floating complement in the blood diminishes. Normal values vary considerably depending on the laboratory technique used. An abnormal finding is indicated by a decrease in serum complement and is seen primarily in clients with vasculitis.

SERUM PROTEIN ELECTROPHORESIS. In **serum protein electrophoresis,** the protein fractions of the plasma are measured, and an electrical current is used to separate them. The level of alpha globulin is raised in acute inflammation; in chronic inflammatory conditions such as RA, the level of gamma globulin is increased because of the increase in immunoglobulins.

IMMUNOGLOBULINS. The serum immunoglobulins can be separated into subtypes. In chronic inflammation, immunoglobulin G (IgG) is needed to combine with RF. Thus in RA the IgG value is typically elevated.

OTHER LABORATORY TESTS. The presence of most chronic diseases usually causes mild to moderate anemia, which contributes to the client's fatigue. Therefore the client's complete blood count (CBC) is monitored for a low hemoglobin, hematocrit, and red blood cell (RBC) count. An increase in white blood cell (WBC) count is consistent with an inflammatory response. A decrease in the WBC count may indicate Felty's syndrome. Thrombocytosis (increased platelets) is common in clients with RA. Additional laboratory tests may be performed depending on the body systems and organs that may be affected by the disease. For example, if heart involvement is suspected, the health care provider may order cardiac enzymes.

RADIOGRAPHIC ASSESSMENT

A standard x-ray study is used to visualize the joint changes and deformities typical of RA. A computed tomography (CT) scan may help to determine the presence and degree of cervical spine involvement.

OTHER DIAGNOSTIC ASSESSMENT

An **arthrocentesis** is a diagnostic procedure that may be used for clients with joint involvement. It may be performed at the bedside or in a physician's office or clinic. After administering a local anesthetic, the physician inserts a large-gauge needle into the joint (usually the knee) to aspirate a sample of synovial fluid; this procedure may also relieve pressure. The fluid is analyzed for inflammatory cells and immune complexes, including RF. Fluid from clients with RA shows increased WBCs, turbidity, and volume. After the procedure, the nurse monitors the insertion site for bleeding or leakage of synovial fluid. The nurse notifies the physician if either of these problems occur.

A bone scan or joint scan can also assess the extent of joint involvement. Magnetic resonance imaging (MRI) may be performed to assess spinal column disease.

Because RA can affect multiple body systems, tests to diagnose specific systemic manifestations are performed as necessary. For example, electromyography helps to confirm peripheral neuropathy. Pulmonary function tests help to determine the presence of lung involvement.

Interventions

As in other types of arthritis, the health care team manages pain by using a combination of drug and nondrug measures. Surgery may be indicated when these measures are no longer effective. The accompanying Client Care Plan on p. 348 highlights the most important nursing interventions for the client with rheumatoid arthritis (RA).

DRUG THERAPY. Although numerous pain relief modalities are available, the client with RA often needs a variety of medications to relieve pain or slow the progression of the disease. As with degenerative arthritis, clients with RA often have cortisone injections in single joints to relieve local pain.

The medications prescribed for RA have analgesic, antipyretic, and/or anti-inflammatory actions. Some drugs are disease modifying and often cause a remission of the illness.

SALICYLATES. Salicylates are a type of nonsteroidal anti-inflammatory drug (NSAID) and are a common drug of choice for pain and inflammation. However, the selection of drugs varies by health care provider and geographic area. As seen in Chart 21-2, any one of several agents may be used. Large doses of aspirin (ASA, Ancasal✱) may be prescribed unless the client is experiencing or has a history of gastrointestinal distress (nausea, vomiting, or ulcers).

The initial dosage of aspirin is typically 12 to 18 tablets each day in divided doses (usually four times a day) until a therapeutic serum salicylate level of 20 to 25 mg/100 mL (25 mg/dL) is achieved—usually in 3 to 6 weeks. The health care provider regulates the dosage so that side effects are minimized and the serum level is less than 30 mg/100 mL. Higher serum levels often result in signs of toxicity, such as tinnitus. The nurse asks the client if he or she has experienced this symptom. If so, the health care provider usually reduces the daily dosage of the drug. Once pain and other clinical manifestations are alleviated or reduced, the dosage can be adjusted to a maintenance level, which usually falls between 15 and 20 mg/100 mL (not >1.45 mmol/L).

NONSTEROIDAL ANTI-INFLAMMATORY DRUGS. NSAIDs are often the drug of choice for inflammatory arthritis to relieve pain and inflammation. The choice of which one to administer depends on the client's needs and the physician's preference. To minimize gastrointestinal problems, the NSAID may be given with misoprostol (Cytotec), 100 to 200 μg/day. If there is no clinical change after 6 to 8 weeks, the health care provider may discontinue the current NSAID and try another one. This process may be repeated until an effective drug is found for that client. Celecoxib (Celebrex) and rofecoxib (Vioxx) are two of the newest NSAIDs and are COX-2 in-

Client Care Plan • THE CLIENT WITH RHEUMATOID ARTHRITIS

NURSING DIAGNOSIS NO. 1 • Chronic Pain related to joint inflammation

Expected Outcomes	Nursing Interventions	Rationale
The client will experience a reduction in joint pain.	Give prescribed drugs, as ordered, on time.	Giving drugs on time ensures a consistent blood level (e.g., salicylates).
	Give analgesic drugs as needed, if ordered, and periods of rest, especially after periods of increased activity (e.g., physical therapy).	Supplemental analgesics may be needed to control chronic pain; rest is necessary to prevent overuse of joints and help decreased inflammation.
	Provide a warm shower, tub bath, and/or hot compresses after periods of decreased activity or rest. [D]	Heat application increases blood flow to the joints to decrease pain and increase joint mobility.
	Provide nonpharmacologic pain relief measures, such as imagery, massage, and music therapy. (Determine which of these measures are effective for each client.) [D]	Independent nursing interventions help reduce pain and decrease the amount of analgesics needed for pain relief.
	Evaluate the effectiveness of all pain relief interventions and document/communicate the outcome to the physician and other involved health care team members. (Also see Chapter 7 for additional interventions and pain assessment tools.)	Evaluation of the effectiveness of pain relief interventions helps the health care team plan care for the client. Changes may be necessary if the plan is not effective in meeting the expected outcome.

NURSING DIAGNOSIS NO. 2 • Impaired Physical Mobility related to fatigue, inflammation, and pain

Expected Outcomes	Nursing Interventions	Rationale
The client will ambulate independently, with or without ambulatory aids.	Reinforce the importance of and techniques for therapeutic joint and muscle exercises as taught by the physical therapist.	Therapeutic joint and muscle exercises increase joint mobility, decrease pain, and increase muscle strength.
	Teach the importance of recreational exercises, such as walking and swimming.	Walking and swimming increase muscle tone and enhance psychologic well-being.
	Reinforce the importance of and techniques for use of ambulatory aids, such as a cane or walker; allow rest periods during ambulation. [D]	Ambulatory aids help to reduce stress on affected joints and, therefore, reduce pain and inflammation.
	Emphasize the client's abilities and strengths in mobility skills. [D]	Focusing on the client's abilities rather than deficits builds the client's self-esteem and confidence.

NURSING DIAGNOSIS NO. 3 • Self-Care Deficit (Partial) related to fatigue, pain, stiffness, and joint deformity

Expected Outcomes	Nursing Interventions	Rationale
The client will independently perform activities of daily living (ADLs) with or without the use of assistive/adaptive devices.	In collaboration with the occupational therapist, assess the client's ability to perform ADLs.	The nurse allows the client to perform all ADLs independently. If the client needs assistance, the nurse plans ways to promote independence in these areas.
	Set up the client's tray, if needed, by opening packages and cartons and cutting food; assess the need for assistive/adaptive devices. [D]	The client may be able to self-feed if the tray is set up and/or if assistive devices (e.g., a plate guard) are obtained.
	For dressing activities, assess the need for long-handled assistive/adaptive devices and other mechanical aids.	The client may be able to dress independently if assistive/adaptive devices are available.
	Encourage the client to use large muscle groups and joints instead of smaller ones, if possible. [D]	Using larger joints helps to prevent stress and pain in small joints (joint protection).
	Emphasize the client's abilities in performing ADLs. [D]	Focusing on the client's abilities builds self-esteem and confidence.
	Teach the client to allow rest periods during ADLs. [D]	Rest reduces the fatigue that contributes to a decreased ability to perform ADLs.
	Assess the client's pain level and intervene appropriately (see Nursing Diagnosis 1).	Pain and stiffness contribute to a decreased ability to perform ADLs.

[D] Indicates tasks that can be delegated to assistive nursing personnel.

hibitors. These drugs do not cause the major side effects associated with older NSAIDs (for further information, see Analgesic Administration [Degenerative Joint Disease], p. 332).

CONSIDERATIONS FOR OLDER ADULTS

The adverse effects of older NSAIDs include gastrointestinal distress and central nervous system changes, especially in older adults. Many of these agents also cause sodium and water retention, which poses a life-threatening risk to clients with hypertension, renal disease, or congestive heart failure. Older clients are especially vulnerable to these problems. The nurse carefully monitors these clients and reports problems as early as possible to the health care provider.

DISEASE-MODIFYING AGENTS. Other agents may be prescribed to slow the disease or produce disease remission, such as the antimalarial drug hydroxychloroquine (Plaquenil) or penicillamine (Cuprimine, Depen). Some health care providers may use Plaquenil as one of the initial treatments for mild disease. The health care provider recommends that clients receiving Plaquenil have an eye examination every 3 to 6 months to detect changes in vision, because retinal toxicity may occur and result in decreased visual acuity. If this complication occurs, the health care provider discontinues the drug. The side and toxic effects of penicillamine are similar to those of gold, which is described later.

CYTOTOXIC DRUGS. Methotrexate (Mexate, Rheumatrex) in a low, once-a-week dosage has become the mainstay of therapy for advancing and sustaining RA because it is inexpensive, less toxic than other cytotoxic drugs, and effective. Because any cytotoxic drug can cause *Pneumocystis carinii* pneumonia, some rheumatologists advocate giving pentamidine to clients who are receiving methotrexate (Harris, 1997).

The nurse observes for the side and toxic effects of methotrexate, which include mouth sores, acute dyspnea from pneumonitis, chronic liver inflammation, and bone marrow suppression.

Other cytotoxic agents that may be used are azathioprine (Imuran) and cyclophosphamide (Cytoxan, Procytox✱). In addition to these adverse drug effects, lymphoma and bone marrow suppression may occur with azathioprine administration. Cyclophosphamide is sometimes given to control RA vasculitis, but it may cause leukemia or other types of malignancy.

GOLD SALTS. When pain and inflammation are not reduced by NSAIDs and cytotoxic drugs do not produce disease remission, gold therapy may be added to the drug regimen. Gold therapy may modify the disease and reduce pain and inflammation. The most commonly used parenteral preparation is gold sodium thiomalate (Myochrysine). A small test dose of 10 mg is given intramuscularly to detect an allergy to the drug, and weekly gold injections are given thereafter. The dosage increases from 25 to 50 mg/week until improvement is evident or a cumulative total of 1000 mg is administered.

If the client responds to gold without having toxic effects (e.g., rash, blood dyscrasias, renal involvement), the injections are slowly tapered to every 2 weeks, then every 3 weeks, and then once a month. Before each administration, the client's urine is tested for protein level and a complete blood count is taken. If remission does not occur after a total of 1000 mg has been given, the drug is usually discontinued.

Because intramuscular administration of gold preparations is painful, the oral gold product auranofin (Ridaura) is used more commonly. The client must take this drug daily to achieve a therapeutic serum level. Its major side effect is gastrointestinal symptoms, especially diarrhea, nausea, and vomiting. The nurse teaches the client to report any gastrointestinal problems to the health care provider.

MINOCYCLINE. In recent years, minocycline (a form of the antibiotic tetracycline) has gained recognition as a treatment for RA. Although its mechanism of action is not known, it has both antimicrobial and anti-inflammatory effects. It is also an immune modifier, inhibiting certain chemicals that cause bone and cartilage damage.

Minocycline differs from other agents used for RA in that it has a low incidence of adverse effects. In addition, the client does not develop a resistance to the drug after prolonged use (Sears & Ganger, 2000).

CHRONIC STEROID THERAPY. If clients do not experience relief of symptoms from the commonly administered medications, steroids—usually prednisone (Deltasone, Winpred✱, Apo-Prednisone✱)—are given for their anti-inflammatory and immunosuppressive effects. Prednisone may also be used as a short-term bridge therapy when NSAIDs are insufficient and other disease-modifying agents have not yet had an effect.

Unfortunately, chronic steroid therapy can result in devastating complications, such as diabetes mellitus, infection, fluid and electrolyte imbalances, hypertension, osteoporosis, and glaucoma. As shown in Chart 21-2, some drug effects are dose related, whereas others are not. The nurse observes the client for complications associated with chronic steroid therapy and reports them to the health care provider. For example, if blood pressure becomes elevated or significant laboratory values change, the nurse notifies the physician.

ETANERCEPT. One of the newest drugs for RA is etanercept (Enbrel), which is given subcutaneously by injection twice a week. This antiarthritic medication binds to tumor necrosis factor (TNF) to block the interaction of TNF with TNF receptors. TNF is involved in inflammatory and immune responses. Elevated levels of TNF are found in the synovial fluid of most clients who have RA.

Etanercept is a very expensive drug, and the client or family member must be taught how to self-administer the injections. Injection site reactions, infections (especially respiratory), and headache are common side effects.

INFLIXIMAB. Infliximab (Remicade), first approved to treat Crohn's disease, is now also classified as an antiarthritic agent that neutralizes the biologic activity of TNF by inhibiting its binding with TNF receptors. Unlike etanercept, infliximab is given in a single IV infusion over several hours. The dose is repeated usually 2, 6, and 8 weeks after the first infusion. The nurse teaches the client that chest pain, tachycardia, and anemia are common adverse effects.

ANALGESIC DRUGS. Other analgesic drugs may be prescribed to supplement the anti-inflammatory drugs specific for

RA. Some analgesics include acetaminophen (Tylenol, Exdol✤), propoxyphene (Darvon, Novopropoxyn✤), and propoxyphene napsylate (Darvocet-N). Propoxyphene and its associated products can cause headache, dizziness, and drowsiness. In clients with decreased metabolic rates, this slowly excreted drug may accumulate in the body over a long period and may cause death. The nurse teaches the client about the side effects and toxic effects of these drugs and advises the client to report any unusual symptoms or complaints to the physician.

REST, POSITIONING, ICE, AND HEAT. Adequate rest, proper positioning, and ice and heat application are important in pain management (see Pain Management [Degenerative Joint Disease], p. 332). If acute inflammation is present, the physical therapist (PT) or assistive nursing personnel applies ice to the "hot" joints for pain relief until the inflammation lessens. The ice pack should not be too heavy. Heated paraffin wax dips for painful hands often provides pain relief and increased mobility.

To relieve morning stiffness or the pain of late-stage disease, the nurse recommends a hot shower rather than a sponge bath or a tub bath. It is often difficult for the client with RA to get into and out of a bathtub, although special hydraulic lifts and tub chairs may be available. Hot packs applied directly to involved joints are also beneficial. Most physical therapy departments have hydrocollators that keep hot packs ready any time they are needed (Figure 21-7).

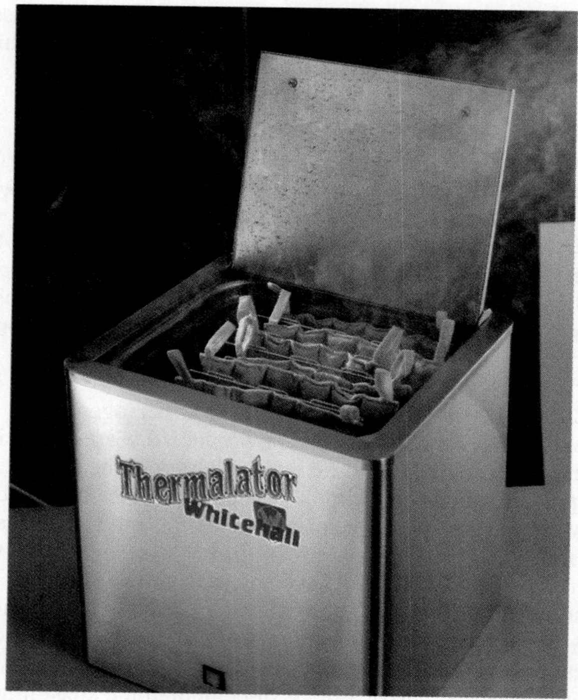

Figure 21-7 ● Heating units used to keep hot packs warm. (Courtesy Whitehall Manufacturing, City of Industry, CA.)

COMPLEMENTARY AND ALTERNATIVE THERAPIES. As for any client with arthritis, other nonpharmacologic pain relief techniques are available for rheumatoid arthritis (RA). Some clients may achieve relief with transcutaneous electrical nerve stimulation (TENS), hypnosis, acupuncture, magnet therapy, imagery, or music therapy. Stress management is also becoming more popular as a pain relief intervention. Chapters 4 and 7 discuss these therapies in detail.

Good nutrition is an important part of the management of RA, and special attention is given to certain types of foods (Yen, 1999):

- Omega 3 fatty acids (found in coldwater fish such as salmon and tuna) to decrease inflammation; Eskimos eat whale blubber and have a low incidence of RA
- Fish oil capsules at 2.5 to 5.0 g/day (should not be taken if the client is taking anticoagulant therapy)
- Antioxidant vitamins A, C, and E

EXPERIMENTAL THERAPIES. In addition to the drug regimens described earlier, two techniques—pulse therapy and plasmapheresis—have been tried and evaluated in the treatment of severe RA. In pulse therapy, the client receives rapid infusions of high-dose steroids or chemotherapeutic agents, usually over a period of several days. Plasmapheresis (sometimes called plasma exchange) is a procedure in which the client's plasma is treated to remove the antibodies causing the disease. This procedure may be combined with pulse therapy for clients with severe, life-threatening disease.

PROMOTION OF SELF-CARE. Although the physical appearance of a client with severe RA may lead the nurse to believe that independence in activities of daily living (ADLs) is not possible, a number of alternative methods can be used to perform these activities. The nurse should not automatically perform these activities; clients with RA do not want to be dependent. For example, hand deformities often prevent a client from opening packages of food, such as a box of crackers. However, he or she may prefer to use his or her teeth to open the crackers rather than depend on someone else.

In the hospital or long-term care facility, a client may not eat because of the barriers of heavy plate covers, milk cartons, small packages of condiments, and heavy containers. Styrofoam or paper cups may bend and collapse as the client attempts to hold them. A china or heavy plastic cup with handles may be easier to manipulate. The nurse and client collaborate with the dietitian to allow access to food and total independence in eating.

When fine motor activities (e.g., squeezing a tube of toothpaste) become impossible, larger joints or body surfaces can substitute for smaller ones. For example, the nurse teaches the client to use the palm of the hand to press the paste onto the brush. Devices such as long-handled brushes can allow clients to brush their hair; dressing sticks can facilitate putting on pants. These examples illustrate the need for the nurse to assess the problem area, suggest alternative methods, and refer the client to an occupational or physical therapist for special assistive and adaptive devices if necessary.

MANAGEMENT OF FATIGUE. Nursing interventions depend in part on identifying the factors contributing to fatigue. For example, increases in pain, sleep disturbances, and weakness are positively associated with increased fatigue. Anemia may also be a contributing factor and may be treated with iron (if an iron deficiency anemia is present), folic acid, or vitamin supplements prescribed by the health care provider. Chronic normochromic or chronic hypochromic anemia often occurs in most chronic, systemic diseases. The nurse also assesses for drug-related blood loss, such as that caused by salicylate therapy or other NSAIDs, by checking the stool for gross or occult blood. Older Caucasian women are the most likely clients to experience gastrointestinal bleeding as a result of taking these medications.

When fatigue results from muscle atrophy, the physician prescribes an aggressive physical therapy program to strengthen muscles and prevent further atrophy. Clients experience increased fatigue when pain prevents them from getting adequate rest and sleep. Measures to facilitate sleep include promoting a quiet environment, giving warm beverages, and administering hypnotics or relaxants as prescribed, if necessary. Pain relief measures were discussed earlier in this chapter under Chronic Pain (Degenerative Joint Disease), p. 332.

In addition to identifying and managing specific reasons for fatigue, the nurse assesses the client's daily activities and teaches principles of energy conservation, including:

- Pacing activities
- Allowing rest periods
- Setting priorities
- Obtaining assistance when needed

Chart 21-10 lists specific suggestions for conserving energy and thus increasing activity tolerance.

ENHANCEMENT OF BODY IMAGE. Body image may be affected by both the disease process and drug therapy. Steroids can cause a moon-faced appearance, acne, striae, "buffalo humps," and weight gain. The nurse determines the client's perception of these changes and the impact of the reactions of family and significant others. The most important intervention for the nurse is communicating acceptance of the client. When a trusting relationship is established, the nurse encourages the client to express his or her feelings.

Another way to improve body image while in the hospital or nursing home is to use personal items. A hospital gown reinforces the sick role. The nurse encourages clients to wear their own clothes, to brush their hair, and to use makeup if desired. The nurse assists in making the client as presentable as possible. The use of colored hair bows, nail polish, and perfume may improve a female client's image and self-concept.

As a reaction to body image disturbance and the presence of a chronic, painful disease, clients may display behaviors indicative of loss. They may use coping strategies that range from denial or fear to anger or depression. In an attempt to regain control over the effects of the disease process, they may appear to be manipulative and demanding and may sometimes be referred to as having an "arthritis personality." This personality, which has negative connotations, is a myth. Clients are trying to cope with the effects of their illness and should be treated with patience and understanding. The nurse continually assesses and accepts these behaviors but remains realistic in discussing goals to improve self-esteem. Clients' strengths are emphasized, and previously successful coping strategies are identified.

Nurses need to assess and intervene appropriately if clients are in pain and are suffering. A qualitative nursing study by Dildy (1996) found that clients with RA benefit from nurses who are empathetic, gentle, caring, and cheerful. In addition, clients want nurses to decrease their suffering and provide comfort.

CHART 21-10

CLIENT EDUCATION GUIDE
Energy Conservation for the Client with Arthritis

- Balance activity with rest. Take one or two naps each day.
- Pace yourself; do not plan too much for one day.
- Set priorities. Determine which activities are most important, and do them first.
- Delegate responsibility and tasks to your family and friends.
- Plan ahead to prevent last-minute rushing and stress.
- Learn your own activity tolerance and do not exceed it.

Community-Based Care

Clients with rheumatoid arthritis (RA) are usually managed at home but may be institutionalized in a long-term care setting if they become restricted to bed or a wheelchair. Some clients may be discharged to a rehabilitation facility for several weeks to aid in developing strategies, techniques, and skills for independent living at home.

HOME CARE MANAGEMENT

The amount of home care preparation depends on the severity of the disease. Structural changes may be necessary if there are deficits in activities of daily living (ADLs) or mobility. Doors must be wide enough to accommodate a wheelchair or walker if one is used. Ramps are needed to prevent the client in a wheelchair from being homebound. If the client cannot negotiate stairs, he or she must have access to facilities for all ADLs on one floor. Handrails should be available in the bathroom and halls.

To promote continued homemaking functions, countertops and appliances may require structural changes. The client may also require handrails and elevated chairs and toilet seats, which facilitate transfers (Figure 21-8).

CRITICAL THINKING CHALLENGE

A 70-year-old woman has had RA for nearly 10 years. Although she is independent in her activities of daily living (ADLs), she complains of constant pain. She is taking Rheumatrex, Plaquenil, Celebrex, and prednisone, but her disease continues to progress slowly. Because of diabetes mellitus, she receives only a low dose of prednisone. Her husband died 3 years ago, but she has several children who live close by. Lately, her children have tended to ignore her because she is very moody, negative, and often tearful.

- What are this client's priority nursing diagnoses?
- What factors are contributing to her emotional state?
- What outcomes are desired for this client?

For suggested answer guidelines, go to SIMON http://www.wbsaunders.com/SIMON/Iggy/.

HEALTH TEACHING

Health teaching is a vital role for nurses in the diagnosis and management of arthritis. Many people have signs and symptoms of joint inflammation but do not seek medical attention.

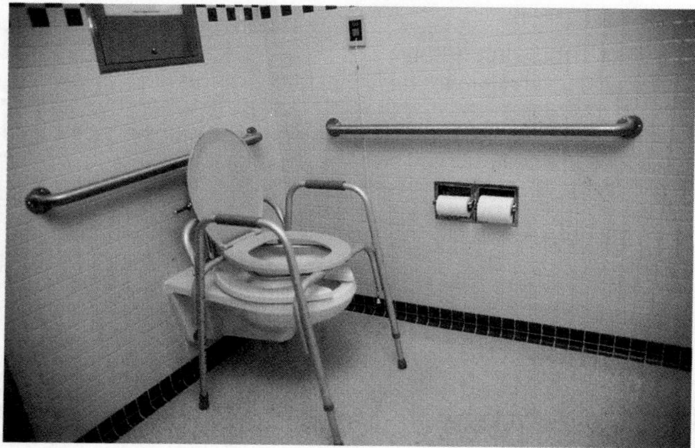

Figure 21-8 ● Handrails and an elevated toilet seat make transfers easier for the client.

The nurse teaches about the need to seek professional health care to reduce pain and disability (see the Meeting Healthy People 2010 Objectives box at right).

Health teaching is also important for promoting compliance with a treatment plan. The nurse should take precautions regarding myths and quackery to protect the client from harm. Information about drug therapy, joint protection, energy conservation, rest, and exercise is reviewed with the client, family, and significant others. This information is summarized in Charts 21-2, 21-6, 21-7, and 21-10.

The client with RA often complains of being on an "emotional roller coaster" from coping with a chronic illness every day. Control over one's life is an important human need. The client with an unpredictable chronic disease may lose this control, and this lowers self-esteem. Health care providers must allow the client to make decisions about care. Families and significant others must also include the client in decision making. Although the client's behavior may be perceived as demanding or manipulative, his or her self-esteem cannot be improved without this important aspect of interpersonal relationships.

Increased dependency also affects a sense of control and self-esteem. Some clients ignore their health needs and portray a tough image for others by insisting that they need no assistance. The nurse emphasizes to the client and family that asking for help may be the best decision at times to prevent further joint damage and disease progression.

Social and work roles are dramatically affected by RA. The client may find new friends among others who have the same problem; such friends provide a support system in coping with these changes. Becoming an active member of and volunteering for The Arthritis Foundation can help the client to meet his or her social and work needs. Loss of income from an inability to be gainfully employed can also be a major source of stress. The client may qualify for disability benefits through the federal Social Security program. If possible, he or she can learn new skills for a less stressful career.

In addition to the interventions just described for self-esteem disturbance, the nurse may need to refer the client to a counselor or religious or spiritual leader for emotional support and guidance during times of crisis. The nurse should identify and recommend other support systems within the family and community when necessary.

MEETING HEALTHY PEOPLE 2010 OBJECTIVES

ARTHRITIS AND OTHER RHEUMATIC CONDITIONS

Objective 2.7: Increase the proportion of adults who have seen a health care provider for their chronic joint symptoms

- Teach clients with suspected arthritis the importance of seeing a health care provider for initial evaluation and follow-up care.
- Educate clients that maintaining functional ability and managing pain can reduce arthritis pain and disability.
- Remind older adults that arthritis is not a normal part of the aging process.
- Assist the client in locating local health care providers who specialize in arthritis management (e.g., rheumatologists, internists).
- Teach clients about the availability of community support groups for people with arthritis.

Objective 2.8: Increase the proportion of persons with arthritis who have had effective evidence-based arthritis education as an integral part of the management of their condition

- Teach clients about community education programs at local hospitals or through the Arthritis Foundation, such as the Arthritis Self-Help course.
- Educate clients about the value of evidence-based education programs (reduces pain and visits to the health care provider).
- Provide client and family education about arthritis and its management, as needed.

HEALTH CARE RESOURCES

The need for health care resources for the client with RA is similar to that for the client with degenerative joint disease. A home care nurse or aide, physical therapist, or occupational therapist may be indicated. In collaboration with the discharge planner, the nurse in the hospital or nursing home identifies these resources and makes sure they are available before discharge.

LUPUS ERYTHEMATOSUS

OVERVIEW

The word *lupus* is the Latin term for "wolf." In the mid-nineteenth century, the facial rash accompanying this disease was thought to look like bites caused by a wolf. The rash was usually red, and thus the term *erythematosus,* a Latin word meaning "reddened," was added to describe the disease.

There are two main classifications of lupus: **discoid lupus erythematosus (DLE)** and **systemic lupus erythematosus (SLE).** A small percentage of clients with lupus have the DLE type, which affects only the skin.

SLE is a chronic, progressive, inflammatory connective tissue disorder that can cause major body organs and systems to fail. It is characterized by spontaneous remissions and exacerbations, and the onset may be acute or insidious. The condition is potentially fatal, but the survival rate has improved dramatically over the past 20 years. Today more than 85% of clients with SLE are alive 5 years after diagnosis (Hahn, 1997). Improvements in determining the cause, diagnosis, and treatment of lupus account for the prolonged survival of these clients.

Lupus is thought to be an autoimmune process; that is, abnormal antibodies are produced and react with the client's tissues. These antinuclear antibodies (ANAs) primarily affect the deoxyribonucleic acid (DNA) within the cell nuclei. As a result, immune complexes form in the serum and organ tissues, which causes inflammation and damage. These complexes invade organs directly or cause vasculitis (vessel inflammation), which deprives the organs of arterial blood and oxygen.

Many clients with SLE have some degree of kidney involvement—the leading cause of death. Other causes of death from SLE are cardiac and central nervous system involvement.

In kidney disease, renal biopsies show the following progressive changes within the glomeruli:

- In minimal lupus nephritis, the glomeruli are slightly irregular; immunoglobulins and complement are seen by electron microscopy.
- Focal, or mild, lupus nephritis is characterized by further glomerular changes, and immune complex deposits are common. In this type of lupus, the client begins to show clinical signs of renal impairment.
- In diffuse, severe proliferative nephritis, more than 50% of the glomeruli are affected, and the client is in renal failure.

Lupus affects women between the ages of 15 and 40 years at a rate 8 to 10 times more often than men. The onset of the disease occurs most often during the childbearing years, but it has been reported in young children and older adults.

CHART 21-11

KEY FEATURES *of* Systemic Lupus Erythematosus and Progressive Systemic Sclerosis

Systemic Lupus Erythematosus	Progressive Systemic Sclerosis
Skin Manifestations	
• Inflamed, red rash • Discoid lesions	• Inflamed • Fibrotic • Sclerotic • Edematous
Renal Manifestations	
• Nephritis	• Renal failure
Cardiovascular Manifestations	
• Pericarditis • Raynaud's phenomenon	• Myocardial fibrosis • Raynaud's phenomenon
Pulmonary Manifestations	
• Pleural effusions	• Interstitial fibrosis
Neurologic Manifestations	
• CNS lupus	• Not common
Gastrointestinal Manifestations	
• Abdominal pain	• Esophagitis • Ulcers
Musculoskeletal Manifestations	
• Joint inflammation • Myositis	• Joint inflammation • Myositis
Other Manifestations	
• Fever • Fatigue • Anorexia • Vasculitis	• Fever • Fatigue • Anorexia • Vasculitis

CNS, Central nervous system.

CULTURAL CONSIDERATIONS

Although incidence and prevalence data vary, approximately 1 in 700 women between 15 and 64 years of age are affected with lupus; 1 in 250 African-American women of this age-group are affected.

➤ COLLABORATIVE MANAGEMENT

• Assessment

It is impossible to describe a typical textbook picture of a client with lupus because of the extreme variability of symptoms. When the disease is in remission, the client may appear healthy and have no activity limitations. When the disease flares, the client may be so ill that admission to a critical care unit is required. Chart 21-11 highlights the clinical manifestations that occur with systemic lupus.

PHYSICAL ASSESSMENT/CLINICAL MANIFESTATIONS

SKIN INVOLVEMENT. The major and usually only manifestation of DLE is a dry, scaly, raised rash on the face ("butterfly" rash) or upper body or individual round lesions that are sometimes referred to as **discoid** (coinlike) **lesions** (Figure 21-9). The lesions are especially evident when the client is exposed to sunlight or ultraviolet light. Alopecia is also common. The nurse observes all skin changes and monitors them daily while the client is in an acute care setting.

MUSCULOSKELETAL CHANGES. In addition to skin changes, **polyarthritis** occurs in 90% of clients with SLE. The initial joint changes are similar to those seen in rheumatoid arthritis (RA), but severe deformities are not common. Small joints and the knees are most commonly involved. **Avascular necrosis** (bone necrosis from lack of oxygen) is often seen in clients with SLE who have been treated for at least 5 years, usually with steroids. Chronic steroid therapy may cause the constriction of small blood vessels supplying the joint, which causes the tissue to die. The hip is most commonly affected, and complaints of pain and decreased mobility result.

The nurse observes for muscle atrophy, which can result from disuse or from skeletal muscle invasion by the immune complexes **(myositis).** Myalgia (muscle pain) may also occur. The nurse inspects and palpates the major muscles, especially those in the extremities.

SYSTEMIC MANIFESTATIONS. Because SLE is an inflammatory condition, fever and fatigue are common findings. Fever is the classic sign of a flare, or exacerbation. Various degrees of generalized weakness, fatigue, anorexia, and weight loss occur. These signs may be the only evidence of impending disease, which makes diagnosis by the health care

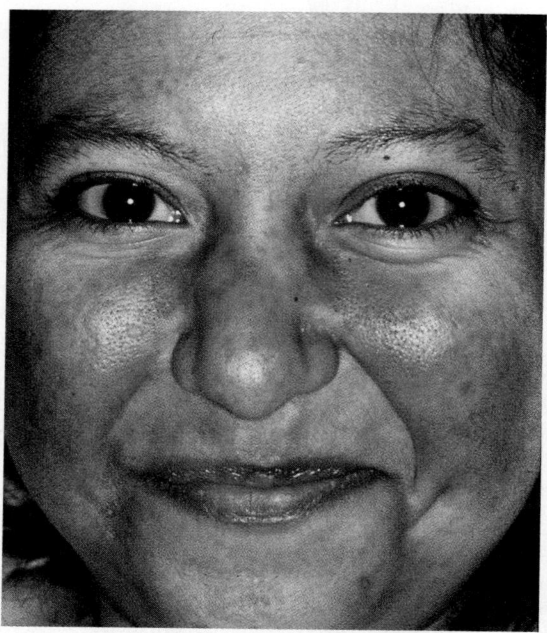

Figure 21-9 ● The characteristic "butterfly" rash of systemic lupus erythematosus.

provider difficult. Consequently, some clients have a diagnosis of "probable SLE."

Any or all body systems may be affected by SLE. Because lupus nephritis is the leading cause of death, the nurse carefully assesses for signs of renal involvement (e.g., changes in urinary output, proteinuria, hematuria, and fluid retention). Approximately 50% of clients with SLE have some type of nephritis.

Pleural effusions or pneumonia are found in almost half of all cases of SLE, but this complication is usually not life threatening. Pulmonary restrictive or obstructive changes may not result in overt clinical signs. However, progressive involvement can lead to dyspnea and arterial blood gas abnormalities. The nurse performs a complete respiratory assessment to determine any abnormalities in respiratory pattern or breath sounds.

Pericarditis is the most common cardiovascular manifestation and causes tachycardia, chest pain, and myocardial ischemia. The nurse monitors the vital signs at least every 4 hours while the client is in the hospital and reports chest pain immediately to the physician.

Raynaud's phenomenon is noted in 15% of cases of lupus. On exposure to cold or extreme stress, the client with Raynaud's phenomenon complains of the characteristic red, white, and blue color changes and severe pain in the digits; these changes are caused by arteriolar vasospasm. The nurse may not observe these episodes but should ask clients whether color changes occur when their hands or feet are exposed to cold or when they are extremely stressed.

Neurologic manifestations are varied. Central nervous system effects include psychoses, paresis, seizures, migraine headaches, and cranial nerve palsies. Peripheral neuropathies are also common. The nurse performs a neurologic assessment as described in Chapter 41.

The nurse monitors for reports of abdominal pain, which most often result from serositis (peritoneal involvement). Mesenteric arteritis, pancreatitis from arteritis of the pancreatic artery, and colonic ulcers also can cause abdominal pain with lupus. The nurse may note liver enlargement on assessment of the abdomen, but jaundice is rare. More than 50% of clients have lymph enlargement, and 10% have splenomegaly. The nurse palpates the lymph nodes and documents the findings. Vasculitis affecting any major or small vessels can lead to organ failure.

PSYCHOSOCIAL ASSESSMENT

The psychosocial results of lupus can be devastating. With either DLE or SLE, the rash can be disfiguring and embarrassing. Young adult women who never had a blemish are confronted with a rash that cannot be completely covered with makeup. If chronic steroid therapy is used, side effects such as acne, striae, fat pads, and weight gain intensify the problem of an already altered body image.

Chronic fatigue and generalized weakness may prevent the client from being as active as in the past. He or she may avoid social gatherings and may withdraw from family activities. The unpredictability and chronicity of SLE can cause fear and anxiety. Fear may increase if the client knows another person with the disease, particularly if the other person has more advanced, severe disease. The myth that lupus is always fatal is still common.

The nurse assesses the client's feelings about the illness to identify areas requiring intervention. The nurse should assess the usual coping mechanisms and support systems before developing a plan of care. See Psychosocial Assessment (Rheumatoid Arthritis), p. 346, for additional information about the psychosocial assessment of clients with chronic illness.

LABORATORY ASSESSMENT

Because DLE is not a systemic condition, the only significant test is a skin biopsy. The physician gently scrapes skin cells from the rash for microscopic evaluation. The characteristic lupus cell and a number of inflammatory cells confirm the diagnosis.

Some of the immunologic-based laboratory tests used to diagnose SLE are the same as those performed for rheumatoid arthritis (RA): positive rheumatoid factor, antinuclear antibody, erythrocyte sedimentation rate, serum protein electrophoresis, serum complement (especially C_3 and C_4), and immunoglobulins (see Chart 21-9). The lupus cell preparation (LE cell prep) may also be performed, but this assay is a poor indicator of disease; it is best used for screening. A false-positive VDRL (syphilis) test is common with lupus. Newer and more specific immunologic tests, such as anti-Rho (SSA), anti-La (SSB), anti-RNP, anti-Smith (anti-Sm), Anti-DNA, and antiphospholipid antibodies (AP) are also performed. High titers of these antibodies are associated with lupus (Kuper & Failla, 2000).

In addition to immunologic testing, several tests are performed to evaluate the possible involvement of major organs and body systems. A complete blood count (CBC) commonly shows pancytopenia (a decrease of all cell types), probably caused by direct attack of the blood cells or bone marrow by immune complexes. Serum electrolyte levels, renal function, cardiac and liver enzymes, and clotting factors are also routinely assessed to determine other body system functioning. APs prolong the partial thromboplastin time, causing clots.

Interventions

The health care provider often prescribes potent drugs that are used topically and systemically. In addition, precautions are taken to prevent further skin impairment and exacerbations (flare-ups). Many of the skin lesions do not disappear, even with treatment, but they usually fade when the disease is in remission.

DRUG THERAPY. With discoid lupus erythematosus (DLE), the client's major concern is the rash or discoid lesions. Clients with systemic lupus erythematosus (SLE) may also be concerned about skin changes. Topical cortisone preparations help to reduce inflammation and promote fading of the skin lesions. In addition, the health care provider may prescribe the antimalarial hydroxychloroquine (Plaquenil) for some clients to decrease the inflammatory response; other systemic medications are usually not used (see Chart 21-2).

The aim of management of SLE is to treat the disease aggressively until remission. In addition to medications for skin lesions, the health care provider often prescribes chronic steroid therapy to treat the systemic disease process. For renal or central nervous system lupus, the health care provider may also order immunosuppressive agents (e.g., azathioprine [Imuran]), which are sometimes used for clients with RA (see Chart 21-2). Although clinical manifestations improve during remission, maintenance doses of these drugs are usually continued to prevent further exacerbations of the disease. The nurse observes for side effects and toxic effects of these medications and reports their occurrence to the physician.

For severe renal involvement, azathioprine or cyclophosphamide (Cytoxan) may be given in combination with steroids. For clients who do not respond to this regimen, IV pulse (high dose) cyclophosphamide and plasmapheresis may be tried (see Experimental Therapies [Rheumatoid Arthritis], p. 350). Renal transplantation has been successful for some clients. Recent advances in allogenic stem cell transplantation have improved symptoms in clients who respond poorly to steroids or immunosuppressive drugs (Kuper & Failla, 2000).

SKIN PROTECTION. Clients with lupus should avoid prolonged exposure to sunlight and other forms of ultraviolet lighting, including certain types of fluorescent light. The nurse instructs clients that they may need to wear long sleeves and a large-brimmed hat when outdoors. They should use sunblocking agents with an SPF (sun protection factor) of 30 or higher on exposed skin surfaces.

In addition, the nurse teaches the client to clean the skin with mild soap (e.g., Ivory) and to avoid harsh, perfumed substances. The skin is rinsed and dried well, and lotion is applied. Excess powder and other drying substances are avoided. Cosmetics are carefully selected and should include moisturizers and sun protectors. The nurse may refer the client to a medical cosmetologist who specializes in applying makeup for skin lesions of all types.

The hair should receive special attention because alopecia (hair loss) is common. The nurse recommends the use of mild protein shampoos and the avoidance of harsh treatments (e.g., permanents or frostings) until the hair regrows during remission.

CHART 21-12

CLIENT EDUCATION GUIDE
Evidence-Based Practice for Skin Protection in Clients with Lupus Erythematosus

- Cleanse your skin with a mild soap, such as Ivory.
- Dry your skin thoroughly by patting rather than rubbing.
- Apply lotion liberally to dry skin areas.
- Avoid powder and other drying agents, such as rubbing alcohol.
- Use cosmetics that contain moisturizers.
- Avoid direct sunlight and any other type of ultraviolet lighting, including tanning beds.
- Wear a large-brimmed hat, long sleeves, and long pants when in the sun.
- Use a sun-blocking agent with a sun protection factor (SPF) of at least 30.
- Inspect your skin daily for open areas and rashes.

CRITICAL THINKING CHALLENGE

A 32-year-old Caucasian female visits her physician's office (where you are a nurse) with complaints of a facial rash. On further questioning, you find that she has been more fatigued than usual and has an achy left ankle. Her infant son is 4 months old, and she has just stopped bleeding from her traumatic vaginal delivery (the infant weighed 10 pounds, and she was in labor for 18 hours).

- When obtaining a complete history, what other questions should you ask the client?
- What risk factors does she have for SLE?
- What laboratory tests will the health care provider most likely order?
- If the client is diagnosed with SLE, what type of health teaching will she need?

For suggested answer guidelines, go to SIMON http://www.wbsaunders.com/SIMON/Iggy/.

Community-Based Care

Community-based care for the client with lupus is similar to that for rheumatoid arthritis. In general, the client is managed at home but may need repeated hospitalizations during exacerbations of disease. The client usually does not need rehabilitation or a long-term care facility, because severe joint deformity and prolonged immobility are not common.

Two major differences exist between SLE and rheumatoid arthritis in terms of education of the client and family or significant others. First, the nurse teaches the client with SLE how to protect the skin (Chart 21-12). Second, body temperature is monitored carefully with SLE. Fever is the major sign of an exacerbation, during which the client can become seriously ill. The nurse teaches the client to report any other unusual or new clinical manifestations to the health care provider immediately.

Many clients become frustrated that family members, significant others, and laypeople do not have a good understanding of lupus. When lupus is in complete remission, the client appears to be healthy. However, an exacerbation can necessitate rapid admission to a critical care unit. This unpredictability disrupts the client's life and can cause fear and anxiety. The nurse helps the client identify coping strategies and support systems that can help with functioning in the community.

The nurse teaches about possible effects of the disease on lifestyle, including fatigue. Women of childbearing age need to know that pregnancy can be a stressor and cause an exacerbation of the disease, either during pregnancy or after delivery. The pregnant client also has an increased risk of miscarriage, stillbirth, or premature birth. Pregnancy is not recommended for those with cardiac, renal, or central nervous system involvement. Sexual counseling regarding contraception options may be necessary.

Although The Arthritis Foundation is a general resource for all clients with connective tissue disease, the Lupus Foundation is a national organization and has chapters in every state to provide information and assistance for clients with lupus. Local support groups and services are offered free of charge.

PROGRESSIVE SYSTEMIC SCLEROSIS

OVERVIEW

Progressive systemic sclerosis (PSS), one of a family of diseases, is often referred to as **systemic scleroderma.** "Scleroderma" means hardening of the skin, which is only one clinical manifestation of PSS. As the name implies, PSS is a systemic disease. It is less common than systemic lupus erythematosus (SLE) but is associated with a higher mortality rate. Chart 21-11 shows a comparison of the clinical manifestations of these two diseases.

PSS is a chronic connective tissue disease characterized by inflammation, fibrosis, and sclerosis of the skin and vital organs. The inflammatory process is so similar to that of lupus that clients are often diagnosed as having probable SLE until the disease progresses. The inflamed tissue undergoes fibrotic and then sclerotic changes. The tissue most obviously affected is the skin, but renal involvement is the leading cause of death. Unfortunately, clients with PSS do not respond well to the steroids and immunosuppressants used for lupus, and therefore the mortality rate is higher.

The prognosis seems to be worse when the client presents with a group of manifestations that occur at the same time (the CREST syndrome):

- Calcinosis (calcium deposits)
- *R*aynaud's phenomenon
- *E*sophageal dysmotility
- *S*clerodactyly (scleroderma of the digits)
- *T*elangiectasia (spiderlike hemangiomas)

The disease tends to progress rapidly, but spontaneous remissions and exacerbations can occur.

Little is known about the cause of PSS, but autoimmunity is suspected. The occurrence of more than one case per family is uncommon, but other connective tissue diseases may be noted in the family history.

PSS has been described in people of all races and in all geographic areas. Women are affected three to four times more often than men. The onset of the disease is usually between 30 and 50 years of age. The incidence is higher in coal miners, who have a high incidence of silicosis, a possible predisposing or contributing factor to PSS. Prolonged exposure to other toxins, such as vinyl chloride and epoxy resins, may also predispose an individual to PSS.

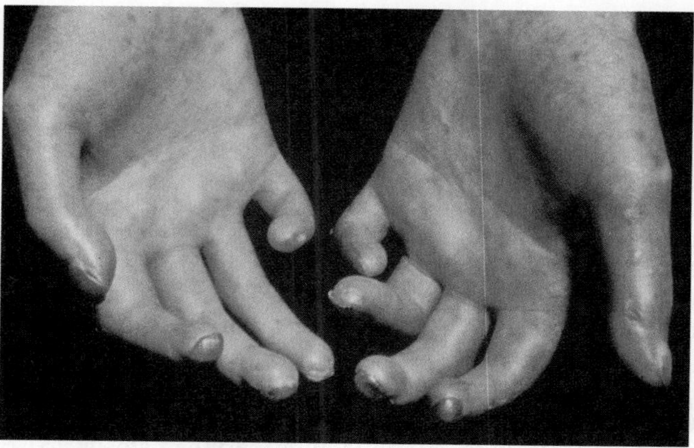

Figure 21-10 • Late-stage skin changes seen in clients with progressive systemic sclerosis. (From the Arthritis Teaching Slide Collection, copyright 1980. Used by permission of the Arthritis Foundation.)

COLLABORATIVE MANAGEMENT

Assessment

PHYSICAL ASSESSMENT/CLINICAL MANIFESTATIONS

Arthralgia (joint pain) and stiffness are common manifestations that the nurse can elicit during the musculoskeletal examination. The acute inflammation that occurs with rheumatoid arthritis (RA) is not common, and deformities are rare.

Findings on inspection of the skin depend on the stage of the scleroderma. Typically there is a painless, symmetric, pitting edema of the hands and fingers; this edema may progress to include the entire upper and lower extremities and face. In this edematous phase, the fingers are described as sausage-like. The skin is taut, shiny, and free of wrinkles. If diffuse scleroderma occurs, swelling is replaced by tightening, hardening, and thickening of skin tissue; this phase is sometimes called the *indurative phase* (Figure 21-10). The skin loses its elasticity, and range of motion is markedly decreased; ulcerations may occur. Joint contractures may develop, and the client may be unable to perform activities of daily living (ADLs) independently.

Major organ damage is likely to develop with diffuse scleroderma, and it specifically affects the following areas:

- Gastrointestinal tract
- Cardiovascular system
- Pulmonary system
- Renal system

Involvement of the gastrointestinal tract, particularly the esophagus, is common. The esophagus loses its motility, resulting in dysphagia and esophageal reflux. A small, sliding hiatal hernia may be present, and swallowing may be difficult. Reflux of the gastric contents can cause esophagitis and subsequent ulceration, particularly in the lower two thirds of the esophagus. Intestinal changes are similar to those of the esophagus. Peristalsis is diminished, which causes clinical manifestations similar to a partial bowel obstruction. Malabsorption is a common complication, causing malodorous diarrheal stools.

In addition to assessing problems of the digestive tract, the nurse observes for cardiovascular manifestations. Raynaud's phenomenon occurs in various degrees in most clients with PSS. On exposure to cold or emotional stress, the small arterioles in the digits of both hands and feet rapidly constrict, which causes decreased blood flow. In severe cases, the client experiences digit necrosis, excruciating pain, and autoamputation of the distal digits (the tips of the digits fall off spontaneously). (See Chapter 36 for a complete discussion of this disorder.) In many clients the nurse notes vasculitic lesions, often around the nail beds **(periungual lesions).** Myocardial fibrosis, another common problem, is evidenced by electrocardiographic (ECG) changes, cardiac dysrhythmias, and chest pain.

Lung involvement in the client with PSS may go undetected until autopsy. Fibrosis of the alveoli and interstitial tissues is present in almost all cases of the disease, but clinical manifestations may not be present.

Renal involvement is an important aspect of the overall disease process and often causes malignant hypertension and death. The nurse assesses for signs of impending organ failure, such as changes in urinary output.

LABORATORY ASSESSMENT

The laboratory findings for PSS are similar to those for SLE. Clinical findings and the client's response to drug therapy help the health care provider differentiate between the two diseases. Additional tests depend on which organs seem to be affected. Upper and lower gastrointestinal series are commonly performed because of the frequency of gastrointestinal clinical manifestations.

Interventions

The medical management of progressive systemic sclerosis (PSS) aims to force the disease into remission and thus slow disease progression. The health care provider uses drug therapy primarily for this purpose, but it is often unsuccessful. Systemic steroids and immunosuppressants are used in large doses and often in combination.

Local skin protective measures can help to maintain skin integrity. The nurse teaches the client to use mild soap and lotions and gentle cleaning techniques. The skin should be inspected daily for further changes or open lesions. Skin ulcers are treated according to their type and location.

In addition to drug therapy to control the overall disease process, specific measures can provide comfort. The client with PSS not only experiences chronic joint pain but also has severe, acute pain during episodes of Raynaud's phenomenon. A bed cradle and footboard keep bed covers away from the skin in severe cases. The nurse adjusts the room temperature to prevent chilling, which can precipitate digit vasospasm. The client who can tolerate touching of the affected areas can wear gloves and socks to increase warmth. Because cigarette smoking and extreme emotional stress can also cause symptoms to recur, the client should try to avoid or minimize these factors as much as possible. Chapter 36 describes the management of clients with Raynaud's phenomenon in more detail.

The client with esophageal involvement may need small, frequent meals rather than the traditional three meals daily. He or she should minimize the intake of foods and liquids that stimulate gastric secretion (e.g., spicy foods, caffeine, and alcohol). The nurse instructs the client to keep his or her head elevated for 1 to 2 hours after meals. The client may need to be in this position continuously. Histamine antagonists and antacids help to reduce and neutralize gastric acid. To help prevent choking, the nurse collaborates with the dietitian for dietary changes (Chart 21-13).

CHART 21-13

BEST PRACTICE *for*
The Client with Progressive Systemic Sclerosis and Esophagitis

- Keep the client's head elevated at least 60 degrees during meals and for at least 1 hour after each meal.
- Provide small, frequent meals rather than three large meals each day.
- Give the client small amounts of food for each bite, and explain the importance of chewing each bite carefully before swallowing.
- Provide semisoft foods, such as mashed potatoes and pudding or custard; liquids are most likely to cause choking.
- Collaborate with the dietitian about the client's diet.
- Teach the client to avoid foods that increase gastric secretion, such as caffeine, pepper, and other spices.
- Give antacids if the health care provider prescribes them.

Nursing care for the client with joint pain and decreased mobility is very similar to that for the client with rheumatoid arthritis (see Interventions [Rheumatoid Arthritis], p. 347).

Community-Based Care

Community-based care for the client with PSS is similar to that for the client with lupus. The client is treated at home but may need frequent hospitalizations if major organ involvement occurs during exacerbations.

GOUT

OVERVIEW

Gout, or gouty arthritis, is a systemic disease in which urate crystals deposit in the joints and other body tissues, causing inflammation. The cause and treatment of gout have been firmly established. The classic case of well-advanced disease is seldom seen today unless the client does not comply with the therapeutic regimen. There are two major types of gout: primary and secondary.

Primary gout is the most common type and results from one of several inborn errors of purine metabolism. An end product of purine metabolism is uric acid, which is usually excreted by the kidneys. In primary gout, the production of uric acid exceeds the excretion capability of the kidneys; sodium urate is deposited in synovium and other tissues, resulting in inflammation. Primary gout is inherited as an X-linked trait; males are affected through female carriers. Approximately 25% of clients have a family history of gout. Primary gout affects middle-aged and older men (85% to 90% of clients with gout) and postmenopausal women. The peak time of onset is during a person's 30s and 40s.

Secondary gout involves hyperuricemia (excessive uric acid in the blood) caused by another disease. Secondary gout affects people of all ages. Renal insufficiency, diuretic therapy, and certain chemotherapeutic agents decrease the normal excretion of uric acid and other waste products. Disorders such as multiple myeloma and certain carcinomas result in increased production of uric acid because of a greater turnover of cellular nucleic acids. Treatment involves management of the underlying disorder.

There are four phases of the primary disease process: asymptomatic hyperuricemic, acute, intercritical (intercurrent), and chronic. The client is usually unaware of the asymptomatic hyperuricemic phase unless he or she has had a serum uric acid level determination. The serum level is elevated, but no overt signs of the disease are present.

The first "attack" of gouty arthritis begins the acute phase. The client experiences excruciating pain and inflammation in one or more small joints, usually the metatarsophalangeal joint of the great toe. Of all clients with gout, 75% experience inflammation of this joint **(podagra)** as the initial manifestation. The erythrocyte sedimentation rate (ESR) and white blood cell count are increased as a result of the inflammatory process.

Months or perhaps years can pass before additional attacks occur; this is the intercritical, or intercurrent, phase of the disease. The client is asymptomatic, and no abnormalities are found during examination of the joints.

After repeated episodes of acute gout, deposits of urate crystals develop under the skin and within the major organs, particularly in the renal system. The client is then classified as having chronic tophaceous gout. In chronic gout, urate kidney stone formation is more common than renal insufficiency.

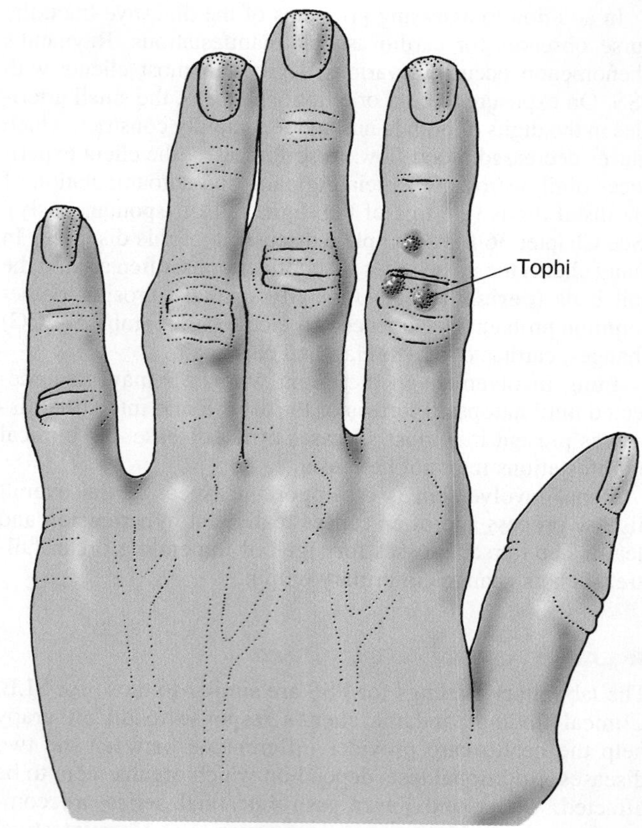

Figure 21-11 ● Typical appearance of tophi, which may occur in chronic gout, on an index finger.

COLLABORATIVE MANAGEMENT

Assessment

The nurse collects historical data, including age, sex, and a family history of gout. Gout affects more men than women, particularly men who have relatives with gout. A complete medical history is needed to determine whether gout has been caused by another problem. There is a tendency to overuse diuretics, especially among women, which can lead to secondary gout.

ACUTE GOUT

Overt manifestations are present in the acute and chronic phases of gout. The nurse most often encounters a client with acute gout; chronic gout is not common in the United States today. Joint inflammation is the most common finding and is usually so painful that the client seeks medical care. The nurse uses inspection skills only; the inflamed area is usually too painful and swollen to be touched or moved.

CHRONIC GOUT

With chronic gout, the nurse inspects the skin for tophi, or deposits of sodium urate crystals (Figure 21-11). Although tophi may occur anywhere, they commonly appear on the outer ear. Other common sites for tophi are the arms and fingers near the joints. The tophi are hard on palpation and are irregular in shape. When the skin over the tophi is irritated, it may break open, and a yellow, gritty substance is discharged. Infection may result.

Other manifestations of chronic gout include signs of renal calculi (stones) or renal dysfunction. Stones develop in approximately 20% of clients with gout. In some cases, urate kidney stones occur before the arthritis is present.

The health care provider orders determinations of serum uric acid levels to validate hyperuricemia. Because the serum uric acid level can be altered by food intake, serial measurements are usually obtained. A consistent level of more than 8 mg/100 mL is generally considered abnormal. Urinary uric acid levels are also measured; an overproduction of uric acid is confirmed by an excretion of more than 600 mg/24 hr after a 5-day restriction of purine intake.

The health care provider may order renal function tests, such as blood urea nitrogen (BUN) and serum creatinine level, to monitor possible kidney involvement. A definitive diagnostic test for the disease is synovial fluid aspiration (arthrocentesis) to detect the needle-like crystals that are characteristic of the disorder (see Other Diagnostic Assessment [Rheumatoid Arthritis], p. 347).

Interventions

Gout is one of the easiest diseases for the health care provider to diagnose and treat in its early phases. If the client receives treatment and complies with drug therapy, he or she should experience no further symptoms and no change in body image or lifestyle. The client with gout is usually treated on an outpatient basis.

DRUG THERAPY. Drug therapy is the primary component of management for clients with gout. In acute gouty "attacks," the inflammation subsides spontaneously within 3 to 5 days; however, most clients cannot tolerate the pain for that long. The drugs used for acute gout are different from those used for chronic gout. The health care provider typically prescribes a combination of colchicine (Colsalide, Novocolchicine✤) and a nonsteroidal anti-inflammatory drug such as indomethacin (Indocin, Novomethacin✤) or ibuprofen (Motrin, Amersol✤), for acute gout. IV colchicine works within 12 hours. The client takes oral medications until the inflammation subsides, usually for 4 to 7 days.

For clients with chronic gout, the health care provider prescribes drugs to promote uric acid excretion or to reduce its production on a continuous, maintenance basis. Allopurinol (Zyloprim) is the drug of choice. As a xanthine oxidase inhibitor, it prevents the conversion of xanthine to uric acid. Probenecid (Benemid, Benuryl✤) is also effective as a uricosuric drug in gout because it promotes the excretion of excess uric acid. Combination drugs that contain probenecid and colchicine (e.g., ColBenemid) are also available. The health care provider and nurse monitor serum uric acid levels to determine the effectiveness of these medications. Aspirin should be avoided because it inactivates the effects of the drug.

DIET THERAPY. Whether or not to recommend special dietary restrictions for clients with gout is controversial. Some physicians advocate a strict low-purine diet and advise clients to avoid foods such as organ meats, shellfish, and oily fish with bones (e.g., sardines). Some health care providers and dietitians believe that limiting protein foods, especially red and organ meats, is sufficient. Still others do not believe that diet restrictions affect treatment. It is well known, however, that excessive alcohol intake and fad "starvation" diets can cause a gouty attack. The nurse helps clients determine which foods may precipitate such an attack.

In addition to food and beverage restrictions, clients with gout should avoid all forms of aspirin and diuretics because they may precipitate an attack. Likewise, excessive physical or emotional stress can exacerbate the disease. The nurse may need to teach stress management techniques.

Having the client drink more fluids is one of the best measures to prevent the formation of urinary stones. Such a measure helps to dilute urine and prevent sediment formation. Uric acid is more soluble in urine with a high pH and therefore is less likely to form urinary stones in that environment. The client's urinary pH can be increased with an intake of alkaline ash foods, such as citrus fruits and juices, milk, and certain dairy products. However, the value of adhering to a strict diet rich in these foods is questionable.

The client with a diagnosis of gout is seldom hospitalized unless renal complications develop. If the client follows the prescribed interventions, chronic tophaceous gout should not develop.

OTHER CONNECTIVE TISSUE DISEASES

The care of clients with connective tissue diseases (CTDs) is often similar regardless of the specific diagnosis. This section describes other fairly common diseases that are classified as CTDs.

Polymyositis/Dermatomyositis

Polymyositis is a diffuse, inflammatory disease of striated muscle that causes symmetric weakness and atrophy. When a rash accompanies polymyositis, the disease is called **dermatomyositis.** Both diseases vary in their mode of onset and progression and are characterized by spontaneous remissions and exacerbations. Women are affected twice as often as men, and men and women between 30 and 60 years of age are most susceptible to either disease.

In addition to proximal muscle and possible skin involvement, clients typically have polyarthritis, **polyarthralgia** (pain around multiple joints), and Raynaud's phenomenon (see Chapter 36). Clients with dermatomyositis have the characteristic heliotrope (lilac) rash and periorbital edema. Malignant neoplasms are more common in these clients than in the rest of the population; as many as 30% of clients older than 55 have internal malignancies. Many clients have difficulty swallowing or talking because of severe muscle weakness.

This condition is treated with high-dose steroids, immunosuppressive agents, and supportive care, and particular attention is given to nutrition.

Systemic Necrotizing Vasculitis

Necrotizing vasculitis is a term for a group of diseases whose primary manifestation is arteritis (inflammation of arterial walls), which causes ischemia in the tissues usually supplied by the involved vessels. The drug of choice for most types of vasculitis is chronic steroid therapy.

Polyarteritis nodosa affects middle-aged men and involves every body system. Treatment is similar to that for systemic lupus, but the prognosis is not as promising. Renal disorders and cardiac involvement are the most common causes of death. Hypersensitivity vasculitis is the most common form of vasculitis and primarily causes skin lesions as an allergic response to drugs, infections, or tumors. Takayasu's arteritis, or the aortic arch syndrome, is also called the "pulseless" disease. Women in their 20s, particularly those of Japanese descent, are affected most often. Cerebral ischemia is manifested by visual changes, syncope, and vertigo.

Polymyalgia Rheumatica and Temporal Arteritis

Polymyalgia rheumatica (PMR) is a clinical syndrome characterized by stiffness, weakness, and aching of the proximal musculature (i.e., the shoulder and pelvic girdles).

> **CULTURAL CONSIDERATIONS**
> The incidence of PMR is greater among people in the northern regions of the United States and Europe. It is very uncommon in the African-American population.

Systemic manifestations such as low-grade fever, arthralgias (pain around joints), and weight loss occur in the majority of cases. Most clients have an increased erythrocyte sedimentation rate (ESR) and a normochromic, normocytic anemia (see Chart 21-9). The disease commonly occurs in women over 50 years of age and typically responds to low-dose steroid therapy in 1 to 3 days (Mikanowicz & Leslie, 2000).

Giant cell, or temporal arteritis (TA) occurs in as many as 20% of people with PMR. TA is a systemic vasculitis that affects large and midsized arteries. Clinical manifestations may be classified as systemic, myalgic, and arteritic (Chart 21-14).

CHART 21-14

KEY FEATURES *of* Temporal Arteritis

Systemic Manifestations
- Fatigue, malaise
- Fever
- Weight loss
- Night sweats

Myalgic Manifestations (if client has polymyalgia rheumatica [PMR])
- Proximal, symmetrical muscle pain
- Stiffness

Arteritic Manifestations
- Erythema
- Pain (especially localized temporal headache)
- Swelling
- Tenderness (especially scalp)
- Amaurosis fugax (temporary vision loss in one eye)
- Diplopia

The cause of both PMR and TA is unknown, but a genetic predisposition related to HLA-DRB1 is likely. The disorder is easy to miss because most clients are older women who complain of declining vision (also an age-related change). TA is treated with high doses of corticosteroids, often as high as 40 to 80 mg/day (Mikanowicz & Leslie, 2000).

Ankylosing Spondylitis

Ankylosing spondylitis is also known as Marie-Strümpell disease and, more recently, as rheumatoid spondylitis. As shown in Figure 21-12, the disease affects the vertebral column and causes spinal deformities. Although this disorder is present in both sexes at any age in adulthood, young Caucasian males under age 40 are most commonly affected. Other features include iritis (inflammation of the iris), arthritis or arthralgia, and nonspecific systemic manifestations such as malaise and weight loss.

Although the exact cause is unknown, ankylosing spondylitis is associated with the HLA-B27 antigen. Compromised respiratory function caused by a rigid chest wall is the major threat to health. Most clients function normally but live with chronic discomfort. Anti-inflammatory drugs and physical therapy are the key components of management.

Reiter's Syndrome

As with ankylosing spondylitis, **Reiter's syndrome** is associated with the HLA-B27 antigen. This disease most often affects young Caucasian males. The complete syndrome is a triad of arthritis, conjunctivitis, and urethritis (inflammation of the urethra) resulting from exposure to sexually transmitted disease or dysentery (infectious diarrhea). Urethritis is often the first clinical manifestation.

Although the disease is characterized by this triad of manifestations, other conditions such as balanitis circinata (ringlike inflammation of the glans penis) and skin lesions are equally significant for confirmation of the diagnosis.

Management is symptomatic and may be complex if there is organ involvement. Nonsteroidal anti-inflammatory drugs and physical therapy are generally prescribed.

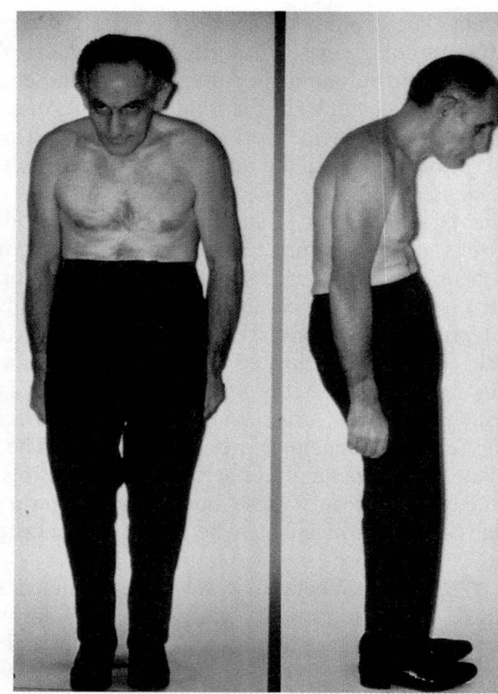

Figure 21-12 ● Spinal deformity and posture often seen in clients with advanced spondylitis. (From the Arthritis Teaching Slide Collection, copyright 1980. Used by permission of the Arthritis Foundation.)

Sjögren's Syndrome

With **Sjögren's syndrome,** inflammatory cells and immune complexes obstruct secretory ducts and glands. As a result, the client has dry eyes (sicca syndrome), a dry mouth (xerostomia), and a dry vagina. Severe cases involve swelling of the parotid and lacrimal areas and systemic manifestations (e.g., fever, fatigue). Of clients with the syndrome, 50% have an associated disease, such as rheumatoid arthritis (RA).

Local management includes meticulous care of the mouth, eyes, and perineal areas and the use of artificial tears and saliva. Systemic steroids may also be administered. Without treatment, the client can lose vision, and oral ulcerations, dental caries, and difficulty in swallowing or talking may ensue.

Marfan Syndrome

Marfan syndrome is inherited as an autosomal, dominant trait with equal prevalence in males and females. Clients with this syndrome have abnormalities of the skeletal, ocular, cardiopulmonary, and central nervous systems as a result of a basic defect in extracellular microfibrils. Microfibrils are very small fibers within cells.

Clients with the classic form of Marfan syndrome tend to be excessively tall and have elongated hands and feet. The diagnosis of milder forms of Marfan syndrome is often missed in young men, especially athletes involved in sports such as basketball.

Other skeletal abnormalities include scoliosis, a funnel-shaped chest, loss of the normal cervical curve, and hyperextensibility of the joints. Subluxation of the lens is usually bilateral and occurs by age 5, causing decreased visual acuity or glaucoma.

Cardiovascular problems are responsible for most deaths resulting from Marfan syndrome. The average life span is 32 years. Mitral valve prolapse with regurgitation, as well as aortic aneurysm with regurgitation and aortic rupture, are common. The client is closely monitored by echocardiography (Holcomb, 2000).

Management is both palliative and preventive and includes careful monitoring, cardiovascular medications, and orthopedic surgery if needed. Genetic counseling should also be part of the treatment plan, especially for women of childbearing age. Many pregnant women with Marfan-related cardiovascular complications die just before, during, or after birth (Eaton & Meiner, 1999).

Infectious Arthritis

Any infectious agent can invade the joint space and cause inflammation and tissue destruction. Certain pathogens, such as *Staphylococcus aureus,* destroy tissue rapidly; others, especially viruses, do not cause irreversible damage. The cornerstone of management is local or systemic antibiotic therapy.

Lyme Disease

Lyme disease has been added to the list of connective tissue diseases (CTDs). Unlike with many CTDs, however, the cause has been identified. The infected deer tick (*Ixodes* genus) transmits a bacterium (spirochete) that usually starts with a circular rash, malaise, fever, headache, and muscle or joint aches. The disease is common in the New England, Mid-Atlantic, and Great Lakes regions of the United States, especially during the summer months. Lyme disease has also been reported in Europe, Asia, and Australia (Meyers, 1998).

In the early and localized Stage I, the client appears with flu-like symptoms, rash (erythema migrans, the "bull's eye" rash), and pain and stiffness in the muscles and joints. Symptoms begin within 3 to 32 days of the tick bite. Doxycycline, amoxicillin, or cefuroxime is prescribed for 10 to 21 days.

Stage II (early disseminated stage) occurs 2 to 12 weeks after the tick bite. The client experiences carditis with dysrhythmias, dyspnea, dizziness, or palpitations, as well as central nervous system disorders such as meningitis, facial paralysis (often misdiagnosed as Bell's palsy), and peripheral neuritis. For severe disease, IV antibiotics (e.g., ceftriaxone or cefotaxime) are given.

If Lyme disease is not diagnosed and treated in the earlier stages, later chronic complications (e.g., arthritis, enlarged lymph nodes, and neurologic problems) can result. This late Stage III (chronic persistent stage) occurs 6 weeks to 2 years after the tick bite. For some clients, the first and only sign of Lyme disease is arthritis. In other cases the disease may not respond to antibiotics, and the client develops permanent damage to joints and the nervous system (Meyers, 1998).

A new vaccine to prevent Lyme disease, Lymrex, is now available for use in people between 15 and 60 years of age. Prevention is the best strategy for Lyme disease (Chart 21-15).

CHART 21-15

CLIENT EDUCATION GUIDE
Prevention and Early Detection of Lyme Disease

- Avoid heavily wooded areas or areas with thick underbrush.
- Walk in the center of the trail.
- Avoid dark clothing. Lighter colored clothing makes spotting ticks easier.
- Use an insect repellent on your skin and clothes when in an area where ticks are likely to be found.
- Wear long-sleeved tops and long pants.
- Wear closed shoes and a hat or cap.
- Bathe immediately after being in an infested area, and inspect your body for ticks (about the size of a pinhead); pay special attention to your arms, legs, and hairline.
- Gently remove with tweezers or fingers any tick that you find. Dispose of the tick by flushing it down the toilet (burning a tick could spread infection).
- Wait 4 to 6 weeks after being bitten by a tick before being tested for Lyme disease (testing before this time is not reliable).
- Report symptoms, such as a rash or influenza-like illness, to your physician.
- Obtain a vaccine to prevent disease if you live in a high-risk area.

Pseudogout

Pseudogout is a disease that mimics the clinical manifestations of gout. In this disease, however, the crystals deposited in the joints are calcium pyrophosphate, not sodium urate. These crystals usually migrate to cartilage, but they can also deposit in tendons, ligaments, and synovium.

The client most susceptible to pseudogout is an older, hospitalized male. Although the cause is not certain, the incidence is highest in men with metastatic cancer or endocrine imbalances such as hypothyroidism. Nonsteroidal anti-inflammatory drugs usually control manifestations of the disease.

Disease-Associated Arthritis

A number of diseases can cause secondary arthritis. Tuberculosis, Crohn's disease, ulcerative colitis, hemophilia, psoriasis, and sickle-cell anemia are typical examples. To manage joint involvement, the primary disease is treated. For example, when a client with Crohn's disease is in remission, joint manifestations also subside. Conditions in which joint involvement can occur are presented in Table 21-3.

Fibromyalgia

The term **fibromyalgia,** also called fibrositis, describes a syndrome characterized by trunk, extremity, and facial pain and tenderness without other objective findings. The primary manifestations are pain, muscle stiffness and spasm, sensory changes, and exhaustion, which may be attributable to severe sleep disturbances. Tender areas, known as trigger points, typically can be palpated to elicit pain in a predictable, reproducible pattern. Physical therapy, nonsteroidal anti-inflammatory drugs, and muscle relaxants usually provide temporary relief.

In most clients, fibrositis is the result of deep-sleep deprivation. Clients may need hypnotics and other sleep-inducing

TABLE 21-3 • COMMON DISORDERS ASSOCIATED WITH ARTHRITIS

• Crohn's disease	• Hyperparathyroidism
• Ulcerative colitis	• Hyperthyroidism
• Tuberculosis	• Diabetes mellitus
• Hemophilia	• Sickle-cell anemia crisis
• Whipple's disease	• Psoriasis
• Intestinal bypass surgery	• Infection

methods to overcome this sleep disturbance. Antidepressive agents such as amitriptyline (Elavil, Apo-Amitriptyline♣) or nortriptyline (Pamelor) may promote sleep and reduce muscle spasm. These drugs should be used with caution in older adults because they can cause confusion and orthostatic hypotension. Trazodone (Desyrel) may be preferred for this population because of its minimal side effects. The nurse observes for side effects and monitors for postural blood pressure changes.

Secondary fibrosis syndromes can accompany any connective tissue disease (CTD), particularly lupus and rheumatoid disease, and may not necessarily be related to sleep patterns.

Local Inflammatory Disorders

Two of the most common inflammatory conditions, bursitis and tendinitis, are localized to specific connective tissues. Both problems are caused by repetitive motion and overuse related to aging, sports, or work injuries. Bursitis is an irritation of subcutaneous tissues and inflammation of the underlying bursae. Tendinitis is inflammation of one or more tendon sheaths.

Tight shoes often irritate the heel and cause bursitis. Aerobic exercise and diseases such as rheumatoid arthritis (RA) and gout can lead to bursitis and tendinitis.

The conservative management for both inflammatory conditions includes rest, ice, and nonsteroidal anti-inflammatory agents to relieve pain. More aggressive treatment may include corticosteroid injections or surgery to remove the inflamed tissue.

Mixed Connective Tissue Disease

A diagnosis of mixed CTD is made when a client presents with clinical manifestations that are not typical of any one CTD. Approximately 10% of clients with CTDs are classified as having mixed disease. Some of these are overlap syndromes, in which two or more diseases occur at the same time. Common examples are systemic lupus erythematosus (SLE) plus progressive systemic sclerosis (PSS), and rheumatoid arthritis (RA) plus SLE. Management depends of the clinical manifestations, but often the client is treated as having SLE.

ONLINE RESOURCES

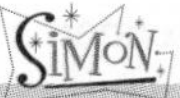

For suggested readings and Internet resources, go to http://www.wbsaunders.com/SIMON/Iggy/.

SELECTED BIBLIOGRAPHY

Asterisk indicates a classic or definitive work on this subject.

Berman, B.M, et al. (1999). A randomized trial of acupuncture as an adjunctive therapy in osteoarthritis of the knee. *Rheumatology, 38*(4), 346-354.

*Dildy, S.P. (1996). Suffering in people with rheumatoid arthritis. *Applied Nursing Research, 9,* 177-183.

Eaton, L. & Meiner, S.E. (1999). Marfan syndrome: Identification and management. *MEDSURG Nursing, 8*(2), 113-117.

Evanoff, A., et al. (1999). Therapeutic touch and osteoarthritis of the knee. *Journal of Family Practice, 48*(1), 11-12.

Geier, K. (1998). Perioperative blood management. *Orthopaedic Nursing, 17*(Suppl. 1), 6-36.

Gordon, A., et al. (1998). The effects of therapeutic touch on patients with osteoarthritis of the knee. *Journal of Family Practice, 47*(4), 271-277.

Hahn, B. H. (1997). Management of systemic lupus erythematosus. In W.N. Kelley et al. (Eds.), *Textbook of rheumatology* (5th ed., pp. 1040-1056). Philadelphia: W.B. Saunders.

Harris, E.D. (1997). Treatment of rheumatoid arthritis. In W.N. Kelley et al. (Eds.), *Textbook of rheumatology* (5th ed., pp. 933-950). Philadelphia: W.B. Saunders.

Heliovaara, M., et al. (2000). Coffee consumption, rheumatoid factor, and the risk of rheumatoid arthritis. *Annals of Rheumatic Diseases, 59*(8), 631-635.

Holcomb, S.S. (2000). Reviewing Marfan syndrome. *Nursing2000, 30*(5), 32cc10-32cc12.

Ignatavicius, D.D. (2001). Rheumatoid arthritis and the older adult. *Geriatric Nursing, 22*(3), 139-142.

Kee, C.C. (1998). Living with osteoarthritis: Insiders' views. *Applied Nursing Research, 11*(1), 19-26.

Kee, C.C. (2000). Osteoarthritis: Manageable scourge of aging. *Nursing Clinics of North America, 35*(1), 199-208.

Kettelman, K. (2000). Soothing the ache of joint surgery. *Nursing 2000, 30*(7), 14.

Klippel, J.H. (1997). *Primer on the rheumatic diseases* (11th ed.). Atlanta: The Arthritis Foundation.

Kuper, B.C., & Failla, S. (2000). Systemic lupus erythematosus: A multisystem autoimmune disorder. *Nursing Clinics of North America, 35*(1), 253-266.

Lash, A.A. (1998). Quality of life in systemic lupus erythematosus. *Applied Nursing Research, 11*(3), 130-137.

Lavernia C.J., Guzman, J.F., & Gachupin-Garcia, A. (1999). Cost effectiveness and quality of life in knee arthroplasty. *Clinical Orthopaedics, 345,* 134-139.

Maher, A.B., Salmond, S.W., & Pellino, T.A. (1999). *Orthopedic nursing* (2nd ed.). Philadelphia: W.B. Saunders.

Mankin, H.J., & Brandt, K.D. (1997). Pathogenesis of osteo-arthritis. In W.N. Kelley et al. (Eds.), *Textbook of rheumatology* (5th ed., pp. 1369-1382). Philadelphia: W.B. Saunders.

Matula, P.A., & Shollenberger, D. (1999). Total joint project: Acute care to home care. *MEDSURG Nursing, 8*(2), 92-98.

McGrath, A. (1997). Clinical snapshot: Raynaud's syndrome. *American Journal of Nursing, 97*(1), 34-35.

Meyers, J. (1998). Lyme disease: A challenge and an opportunity for nurse practitioners. *Journal of the American Academy of Nurse Practitioners, 10*(7), 315-319.

Mikanowicz, C.K., & Leslie, M. (2000). Polymyalgia rheumatica and temporal arteritis: A case presentation. *Nursing Clinics of North America, 35*(1), 245-252.

Morris, B.A., Colwell, C.W., & Hardwick, M.E. (1998). The use of low molecular weight heparins in the prevention of venous thromboembolic disease. *Orthopaedic Nursing, 17*(6), 23-29.

Pepper, G.A. (2000). Nonsteroidal anti-inflammatory drugs: New perspectives on a familiar class. *Nursing Clinics of North America, 35*(1), 223-244.

Ranawat, C.S., et al. (1997). The hip. In W.N. Kelley et al. (Eds.), *Textbook of rheumatology* (5th ed., pp. 1723-1738). Philadelphia: W.B. Saunders.

Ritter, M.A., et al. (1999). Intra-articular morphine and/or bupivacaine after total knee replacement. *Journal of Bone and Joint Surgery, 81*(2), 301-303.

Sears, J.R., & Ganger, P.M. (2000). Antibiotics to treat RA. *RN, 63*(1), 41-42.

Sharkey, N.A., Williams, N.I., & Guerin, J.B. (2000). The role of exercise in the prevention and treatment of osteoporosis and osteoarthritis. *Nursing Clinics of North America, 35*(1), 209-222.

Solomon, L. (1997). Clinical features of osteoarthritis. In W.N. Kelley et al. (Eds.), *Textbook of rheumatology* (5th ed., pp. 1383-1393). Philadelphia: W.B. Saunders.

Windsor, R.E.M., & Insall, J.N. (1997). The knee. In W.N. Kelley et al. (Eds.), *Textbook of rheumatology* (5th ed., pp. 1739-1758). Philadelphia: W.B. Saunders.

Wolfe, F. (2000). The effect of smoking on clinical, laboratory, and radiographic status in rheumatoid arthritis. *Journal of Rheumatology, 27*(3), 630-637.

Yen, P.K. (1999). Diet, complementary therapy, and arthritis. *Geriatric Nursing, 20*(6), 337-338.

CHAPTER 22

Interventions for Clients with HIV/AIDS and Other Immunodeficiencies

LUCILLE SANZERO ELLER

Learning Objectives

After studying this chapter, you should be able to:

1. Compare and contrast primary versus secondary immunodeficiencies for causes and onset of problems.
2. Explain the differences in nursing care required for a client with a pathogenic infection versus a client with an opportunistic infection.
3. Distinguish between the conditions of human immunodeficiency virus (HIV) infection and acquired immunodeficiency syndrome (AIDS) for clinical manifestations and risks for complications.
4. Describe the ways in which HIV is transmitted.
5. Identify techniques to reduce the risk for infection in an immunocompromised client.
6. Develop a teaching plan for condom use among sexually active, non–English-speaking adults.
7. Prioritize nursing care for the client with AIDS who has impaired gas exchange.
8. Identify teaching priorities for the HIV-positive client receiving highly active antiretroviral therapy.
9. Plan a week of meals for the client who has protein-calorie malnutrition.
10. Describe the nursing actions and responsibilities for administration of IV immunoglobulin.

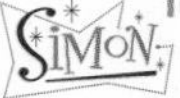

Go to http://www.wbsaunders.com/SIMON/Iggy/ for self-assessment questions related to these Learning Objectives.

Immune function protects the body from infectious disease and development of cancer. Any decrease in immune function increases the client's risk for infection and cancer. Malfunction of the immune system can be either the cause of disease or the result of other disease processes.

A deficient response of the immune system resulting from a missing or damaged immune component is an **immunodeficiency.** An immunodeficient person's immune system cannot recognize infectious agents or other antigens and eliminate them. Thus the immunodeficient person cannot defend adequately against potentially harmful substances that an immunocompetent person can.

A **primary** or **congenital** immunodeficiency is one in which the immune malfunction is present from birth. An **acquired** or **secondary** immunodeficiency is one that occurs in a person who has a normally functioning immune system at birth but later becomes immunodeficient as a consequence of disease, injury, exposure to toxins, medical therapy, or unknown cause. These people are referred to as **immunocompromised** because their immune systems have been compromised, resulting in an impaired ability to neutralize, destroy, or eliminate antigens (see Chapter 20).

The immunodeficient client has clinical symptoms that vary in severity and occur in multiple body systems. For many immunodeficiencies, the cause is unknown or uncontrollable, the pathophysiology is not well understood, and effective treatment may not be available. *The complications of immunodeficiencies, not the actual immune defect, can be treated.* Most immunodeficiencies are chronic conditions, and periods of wellness are interspersed with clinical problems.

Regardless of the cause, the immunodeficient person constantly faces the possibility that the next infection might be fatal. Normal environmental exposures to people, objects, and microorganisms may pose significant danger. The nurse is instrumental in teaching the immunodeficient person how to avoid infection and the signs and symptoms of infection.

ACQUIRED (SECONDARY) IMMUNODEFICIENCIES

ACQUIRED IMMUNODEFICIENCY SYNDROME

OVERVIEW

Acquired immunodeficiency syndrome (AIDS) is the late stage of a continuum of symptoms that result from infection with the human immunodeficiency virus (HIV). AIDS is not the same as HIV infection, and not everyone infected with

HIV has AIDS. People with AIDS are profoundly immunosuppressed and have usually lived with HIV infection for several years before AIDS develops. The nurse provides education, physical care, and psychologic support for the person living with HIV **(PLWH).**

AIDS is a serious, debilitating, and eventually fatal disease that can occur in any age-group. To date, 86% of those with AIDS have been between the ages of 25 and 49 years (Table 22-1). To be diagnosed as having AIDS, a person must be infected with HIV and have a clinical disease that indicates cellular immunodeficiency, a CD4+ T-lymphocyte (T4) count below 200/mm^3, or a CD4+ T-lymphocyte total percentage below 14 (Table 22-2).

TABLE 22-1 • AIDS CASES AMONG ADULTS AND ADOLESCENTS IN THE UNITED STATES, JUNE 1981 TO JUNE 2000

Age (years)	No. Cases
<13	8,704
13-19	3,865
20-24	26,518
25-29	99,587
30-34	168,273
35-39	168,778
40-44	124,398
45-49	72,128
50-54	38,118
55-59	20,971
60-64	11,636
65+	10,378
TOTAL	753,907 (438,795 DEATHS)

Data from Centers for Disease Control and Prevention. (2000). *HIV/AIDS Surveillance Report, 12*(1), Atlanta: Author.

Providing care to the person with AIDS can evoke complex personal issues for nurses. Nurses must acknowledge their own fear of acquiring HIV and any negative attitudes regarding possible lifestyles contributing to HIV infection, such as injection drug use or homosexual behaviors. Knowledge and practice of appropriate infection control techniques can reduce nurses' fears about becoming infected. To provide competent, compassionate nursing care to the person with AIDS, nurses must suspend judgment.

Pathophysiology

The Centers for Disease Control and Prevention (CDC) classification scheme for HIV infection combines clinical conditions associated with HIV infection and three ranges of CD4+ T-lymphocyte counts (see Table 22-2). The clinical classification begins with acute HIV infection (A) and spans a continuum that ends with AIDS (clinical category C). The clinical classifications are subdivided into 1, 2, and 3 on the basis of the client's CD4 T-lymphocyte cell count. *The person*

TABLE 22-2 • CENTERS FOR DISEASE CONTROL AND PREVENTION CLASSIFICATION SYSTEM FOR HIV INFECTION AND AIDS CASE DEFINITION

CD4 Cell Categories	Clinical Categories A	B	C*
	HIV positive, asymptomatic *or* Persistent generalized lymphadenopathy *or* Acute (primary) HIV infection with accompanying illness or history of acute infection as the only manifestations	Bacterial endocarditis, meningitis, pneumonia, or sepsis Vulvovaginal candidiasis that is persistent for more than 1 month or poorly responsive to therapy Oropharyngeal candidiasis (thrush) Severe cervical dysplasia or carcinoma Constitutional symptoms, such as fever or diarrhea lasting longer than 1 month Oral hairy leukoplakia Herpes zoster (shingles), involving at least two distinct episodes or more than 1 dermatome Idiopathic thrombocytopenic purpura Listeriosis Pulmonary *Mycobacterium tuberculosis* Nocardiosis Pelvic inflammatory disease Peripheral neuropathy	Bronchial, tracheal, pulmonary, or esophageal candidiasis Invasive cervical cancer Disseminated or extrapulmonary coccidioidomycosis Chronic intestinal cryptosporidiosis Cytomegalovirus disease of other than the liver, spleen, or lymph nodes Cytomegalovirus retinitis with vision loss HIV-related encephalopathy Herpes simplex (chronic, or bronchitis, pneumonitis, or esophagitis) Disseminated or extrapulmonary histoplasmosis Chronic intestinal isosporiasis Kaposi's sarcoma Lymphoma (Burkitt's, immunoblastic, or primary brain) Disseminated or extrapulmonary *Mycobacterium avium-intracellulare* complex or *M. kansasii* Extrapulmonary *Mycobacterium tuberculosis* *Pneumocystis carinii* pneumonia Recurrent infectious pneumonia Progressive multifocal leukoencephalopathy Salmonella septicemia Toxoplasmosis (brain) Wasting syndrome
1 ≥500/μL	A1	B1	C1
2 200-499/μL	A2	B2	C2
3 <200/μL*	A3	B3	C3

Data from Centers for Disease Control and Prevention, 1992.
*AIDS indicator conditions or counts.

with HIV infection can transmit the virus to others at all stages of disease.

CLINICAL CATEGORY A

A person in clinical category A is HIV positive and is either asymptomatic, has persistent lymphadenopathy, or has acute (primary) HIV infection with accompanying illness or a history of acute infection as the only manifestations. Clients with the above criteria have disease classifications of A1, A2, or A3 depending on their CD4+ T-lymphocyte cell count. When the count is equal to or greater than 500/μL, the disease is classified as A1. When the count is between 200 and 499/μL, the disease is classified as A2. When the count is less than 200/μL, the disease is classified as A3.

CLINICAL CATEGORY B

The client with HIV infection is considered to be in clinical category B if one or more of the following conditions are present and are (1) attributed to HIV infection or are indicative of a deficiency in cell-mediated immunity, or (2) are complicated by HIV infection:

- Bacterial endocarditis, meningitis, pneumonia, or sepsis
- Vulvovaginal candidiasis that is persistent for more than 1 month or poorly responsive to therapy
- Oropharyngeal candidiasis **(thrush)**
- Severe cervical dysplasia or carcinoma
- Constitutional symptoms, such as fever or diarrhea, lasting longer than 1 month
- Oral hairy leukoplakia
- Herpes zoster **(shingles)** involving at least two distinct episodes or more than one dermatome
- Idiopathic thrombocytopenic purpura
- Listeriosis
- Pulmonary *Mycobacterium tuberculosis*
- Nocardiosis
- Pelvic inflammatory disease
- Peripheral neuropathy

This list provides examples of category B clinical conditions but is not comprehensive. Clients with the above criteria have disease classifications of B1, B2, or B3 depending on their CD4+ T-lymphocyte cell count. When the count is equal to or greater than 500/μL, the disease is classified as B1. When the count is between 200 and 499/μL, the disease is classified as B2. When the count is less than 200/μL, the disease is classified as B3.

CLINICAL CATEGORY C

The HIV-positive client in clinical category C is considered to have AIDS if any one of the following conditions that meet the CDC surveillance case definition for AIDS is present:

- Bronchial, tracheal, pulmonary, or esophageal candidiasis
- Invasive cervical cancer
- Disseminated or extrapulmonary coccidioidomycosis
- Chronic intestinal cryptosporidiosis
- Cytomegalovirus disease of other than the liver, spleen, or lymph nodes
- Cytomegalovirus retinitis with vision loss
- HIV-related encephalopathy
- Herpes simplex (chronic, or bronchitis, pneumonitis, or esophagitis)
- Disseminated or extrapulmonary histoplasmosis
- Chronic intestinal isosporiasis
- Kaposi's sarcoma
- Lymphoma (Burkitt's, immunoblastic, or primary brain)
- Disseminated or extrapulmonary *Mycobacterium avium-intracellulare* complex or *M. kansasii*
- Extrapulmonary *Mycobacterium tuberculosis*
- *Pneumocystis carinii* pneumonia
- Recurrent infectious pneumonia
- Progressive multifocal leukoencephalopathy
- Salmonella septicemia
- Toxoplasmosis (brain)
- Wasting syndrome

Clients with the above criteria have disease classifications of C1, C2, or C3 depending on their CD4+ T-lymphocyte count. When the count is equal to or greater than 500/μL, the disease is classified as C1. When the count is between 200 and 499/μL, the disease is classified as C2. When the count is less than 200/μL, the disease is classified as C3.

PROGRESSION

The time from initial HIV infection to development of AIDS ranges from months to years. The range depends on how HIV was acquired, a variety of personal factors, and therapeutic intervention. For people who have been transfused with HIV-contaminated blood, for instance, AIDS develops more quickly; for those who become HIV positive as a result of a single sexual encounter, there is a longer latency period before the condition progresses to AIDS. Other personal factors that may influence progression to AIDS include frequency of re-exposure to HIV, presence of other sexually transmitted diseases (STDs), nutritional status, pregnancy, and stress.

Etiology

AIDS is caused by the profound suppression of immune responses resulting from infection with HIV. Two subtypes of the virus have been identified: type 1 (HIV-1) and type 2 (HIV-2). Type 1 is the form most frequently isolated from infected persons in the Western Hemisphere, Europe, and Asia. Type 2 is endemic to West Africa. Although they differ in viral markers, both subtypes can cause AIDS. More recently, variants within each subtype have been identified. Although these variations are thought to be related to differences in virulence or efficiency of infection, the exact significance of the variants has yet to be determined.

HIV belongs to a special class of viruses known as **retroviruses,** which differ from other viruses in their efficiency of cellular infection. Retroviruses have only ribonucleic acid (RNA) as their genetic material. The most important difference between retroviruses and other viruses is a special complex of enzymes within the retrovirus called **reverse transcriptase (RT).** This enzyme complex increases the efficiency of viral replication once the retrovirus enters a human cell.

Once a retrovirus gains entry into the body and infects a human cell, the RT enzymes force the human cell's deoxyribonucleic acid (DNA) synthesis machinery to use the viral RNA as a pattern and make a piece of human DNA complementary to the viral RNA. This new piece of DNA is then incorporated successfully into the person's cellular DNA, where it acts as a template for viral production. HIV then spreads quickly throughout the lymphoid system, hiding in macrophages and in the centers of lymph nodes (Sande & Volberding, 1999). Throughout the course of infection, HIV is actively replicated by infected T-lymphocytes, synthesizing up to 2 billion viral particles daily (Figure 22-1). After many rounds of replication, these numerous viral particles exhaust the immune system.

The HIV retrovirus attaches to, infects, and finally causes the destruction of those immune system cells with a CD4 surface receptor. These cells include CD4+ lymphocytes and macrophages. The CD4+ lymphocyte (also called the T4-lymphocyte or helper/inducer T-lymphocyte) regulates the activity of all immune system cells (see Chapter 20). When infected by HIV, the CD4 cell does not function normally, causing general malfunction and suppression of the whole immune system. The results of HIV infection are as follows:

- **Lymphocytopenia** (decreased numbers of lymphocytes) with selective CD4 cell depletion
- Abnormal T-cell function
- Increased production of incomplete and nonfunctional antibodies
- Abnormally functioning macrophages

As a result of these immune dysfunctions, the client with HIV infection is susceptible to opportunistic infections and cancer. Macrophages infected by HIV are not destroyed by infection; they act as a reservoir for the virus.

Incidence/Prevalence

The incidence of AIDS in the United States has grown exponentially from the early 1980s. In 1981, 291 new cases of AIDS were reported; in 1995, 74,180 new cases were reported. From June 1981 through June 2000, there have been 753,907 reported cases and 458,795 AIDS-related deaths in the United States (Centers for Disease Control and Prevention [CDC], 2000). The CDC estimates that 1 million persons in the United States are infected with HIV. This includes those living with AIDS, those who have tested positive for HIV, and those who are HIV positive but have not been tested.

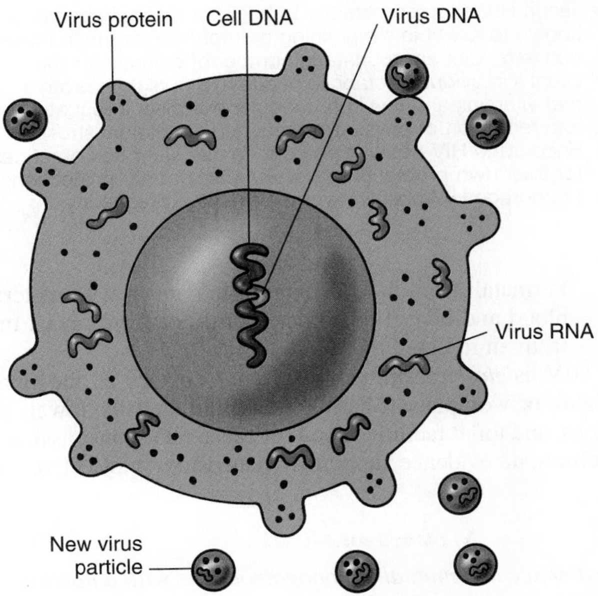

Figure 22-1 ● A T-lymphocyte infected with human immunodeficiency virus. The virus can be seen budding from the infected T-cell.

Epidemiologic and demographic data have shown that most people with AIDS in the United States are (1) men who have had sex with other men **(MSM)** (47%) or (2) persons of either gender who have used injection drugs (22%) (Table 22-3). The fastest-growing infected groups are women and minorities, with a disproportionate number of cases reported in racial and ethnic minority groups. Approximately 52% of all AIDS cases in North America have occurred in African Americans and Hispanics, who constitute only 18.5% of the population. Between 1985 and 1995, the demographics of the disease changed dramatically. The rates for women increased 8.2%, and the incidence of AIDS in minority groups increased 41.7% (Table 22-4).

AIDS is a disease with high mortality. The overall fatality rate is about 60% for adults (CDC, 1999a) and to date there have been no reports of a cure. Therefore a major focus for health care in North America and worldwide is prevention of HIV infection. The United States has highlighted several goals related to HIV and AIDS prevention, as shown in the Meeting Healthy People 2010 Objectives box on p. 368.

Currently, there are over 30 persons with HIV infection who have been identified as **nonprogressors,** individuals infected with HIV for at least 10 years who remain asymptomatic and have maintained CD4+ T-lymphocyte counts within a normal range. Researchers are studying nonprogressors to determine whether they resist disease because of differences in viral factors, such as infection with a weak HIV strain, or because they have an unusually strong immune response (Barnes, 1995; Cohen et al., 1997).

TABLE 22-3 ● AIDS CASES AMONG ADULTS AND ADOLESCENTS IN THE UNITED STATES BY EXPOSURE CATEGORY, JUNE 1981 TO JUNE 1999

Category	No. Cases	%
Men who have sex with men	348,657	47
Injecting drug users (female and male heterosexual)	189,242	25
Men who have sex with men and inject drugs	47,820	6
Hemophilia	5,121	1
Heterosexual contact	78,210	10
Recipients of blood transfusion, blood components, or tissue	8,666	1
Other and unidentified risk	67,368	9
TOTAL	753,907	100

Data from Centers for Disease Control and Prevention. (2000). *HIV/AIDS Surveillance Report, 12*(1), Atlanta: Author.

TABLE 22-4 ● DISTRIBUTION OF ADULT/ADOLESCENT AIDS CASES IN THE UNITED STATES BY RACE AND ETHNIC GROUP, JUNE 1981 TO JUNE 1999

Race/Ethnicity	No. Cases
Caucasian, not Hispanic	324,822
African American, not Hispanic	282,720
Hispanic	137,575
Asian/Pacific Islander	5,546
Native American	2,234
Unknown	1,010
TOTAL	753,907

Data from Centers for Disease Control and Prevention. (2000). *HIV/AIDS Surveillance Report, 12* (1), Atlanta: Author.

CULTURAL CONSIDERATIONS

More than 56% of HIV/AIDS cases reported in the United States occur in minorities, particularly among African Americans and Hispanics (CDC, 1999a). These two groups show an increasing trend in HIV infection compared with a leveling off among Caucasians. Some of the factors that appear to increase the incidence of HIV infection and progression to AIDS among people of color include the following:

- Limited access to health care
- Cost of highly active antiretroviral therapy
- Insufficient or inadequate culturally sensitive information about risk and prevention
- Ethnic and cultural differences in health beliefs, values, sexual practices, roles of women, and reproductive importance

WOMEN'S HEALTH CONSIDERATIONS

Women make up the fastest-growing group with HIV infection and AIDS (CDC, 1999a). Women with HIV infection appear to have a poorer outcome with shorter survival than men. This outcome may be a result of late diagnosis and social and economic factors that reduce access to medical care rather than any viral pathology.

Gynecologic symptoms, particularly persistent or recurrent vaginal candidiasis, may be the first signs of HIV infection in women. Additional symptoms include genital herpes, pelvic inflammatory disease, and cervical neoplasia (Ungvarski & Flaskerud, 1999).

Most women with HIV infection are of childbearing age. The effect of pregnancy on the course of HIV infection is not known. There is conflicting evidence that it may or may not speed up the progression of disease.

CONSIDERATIONS FOR OLDER ADULTS

Infection with HIV can occur at any age. The nurse or assistive nursing personnel should assess the older client for risk behaviors, including a sexual and drug use history. Decline in immune function may increase susceptibility to HIV infection in this population. In the older woman, changes in vaginal tissue as a result of aging may increase susceptibility to sexually transmitted HIV infection.

Prevention

The most important aspect for prevention of HIV transmission is education. All people, regardless of age, gender, ethnicity, or sexual orientation, are susceptible to HIV infection. HIV infection is preventable because of the modes of viral transmission and the fragile nature of the virus.

HIV has been isolated from multiple body secretions and tissues, including blood, semen, vaginal secretions, breast milk, amniotic fluid, urine, feces, saliva, tears, cerebrospinal fluid, lymph nodes, cervical cells, Langerhans' cells, corneal tissue, and brain tissue. HIV is primarily transmitted in three ways:

- Sexual: genital, anal, or oral sexual contact with exposure of mucous membranes to infected semen or vaginal secretions
- Parenteral: sharing needles or equipment contaminated with infected blood or receiving contaminated blood products
- Perinatal: from the placenta, from contact with maternal blood and body fluids during birth, or from breast milk from an infected mother to child

HIV is *not* transmitted by casual contact in the home, school, or workplace. Sharing household utensils, towels and linens, and toilet facilities does not cause HIV transmission. In addition, no evidence supports transmission by insect vectors.

SEXUAL TRANSMISSION

Abstinence and mutually monogamous sex with a noninfected partner are the only absolutely safe methods of preventing HIV infection through sexual contact. These practices may

Meeting HEALTHY PEOPLE 2010 OBJECTIVES

HIV/AIDS

Objective 21.1a: Confine annual incidence of diagnosed AIDS cases among adolescents and adults to no more than 12 per 100,000 population

- Include questions regarding sexual activity and use of safer sex practices whenever obtaining a health history from a client of any age, gender, occupation, socioeconomic status, religion, or educational background.
- Assess all clients for current and past exposures to blood-borne or sexually transmitted diseases.
- Encourage clients to know their own and their partners' HIV status.
- Teach clients safer sex practices.
- Direct clients who are IV drug users to drug rehabilitation programs and support groups.
- Direct clients who abuse alcohol to alcohol rehabilitation programs and support groups.
- Develop culturally sensitive and age-appropriate education materials of various literacy levels for HIV prevention.
- Enlist the assistance of educational, religious, and civic groups and institutions in the dissemination of information regarding prevention of HIV infection.
- Encourage people who are HIV positive to:
  - Avoid sharing toothbrushes, razors, or other items that could become contaminated with blood
  - Not donate sperm, blood, plasma, body organs, or other body tissues
  - Inform their partner, physician, dentist, and eye doctor about their HIV status
  - Clean blood or other body fluid spills on household or other surfaces with freshly diluted household bleach: 1 part bleach to 10 parts water. (Do not use bleach on wounds.)

Objective 21.11: Increase years of healthy life of an individual infected with HIV by extending the interval of time between an initial diagnosis of HIV infection and AIDS diagnosis and between AIDS diagnosis and death

- Teach HIV-positive persons who have no signs or symptoms of immunodeficiency to seek regular medical evaluation and follow-up.
- Encourage HIV-positive persons to adhere to drug regimen, especially highly active antiretroviral therapy (HAART).
- Teach HIV-infected persons to begin or maintain behaviors known to assist in maintaining or improving immune function (e.g., diet appropriate in number of calories for the client's individual metabolic needs that is high in protein and vitamins and low in fat; regular exercise; adequate rest; and reduction of physical, emotional, or spiritual stress).
- Encourage HIV-positive persons to use safer sex practices for their own protection, as well as for partner protection.
- Encourage HIV-positive women to avoid pregnancy.

not be feasible, however, because of personal, cultural, or economic factors.

Many forms of physical sexual expression can spread HIV infection if one partner is infected. The risk of acquiring the infection with a partner who is HIV positive is always present, although some sexual practices are more risky than others. The virus tends to concentrate most heavily in blood and seminal fluid, although it is also present in vaginal secretions. Thus risk differs by gender, specific sexual act, and the degree of viral load of the infected partner.

GENDER. HIV is most easily transmitted when infected body fluids come into contact with mucous membranes or nonintact skin. The vagina has considerably more mucous membrane than does the penis. Thus HIV, like all other sexually transmitted diseases (STDs), is more easily transmitted from infected male to uninfected female than vice versa.

SPECIFIC SEXUAL ACTS. Sexual acts or practices that permit infected seminal fluid to come into contact with mucous membranes or nonintact skin are the most risky for sexual transmission of HIV. Such practices include oral sex, in which the penis and seminal fluid of an infected individual come into contact with the mucous membranes of the mouth and throat **(fellatio),** and anal intercourse, in which the penis and seminal fluid of an infected individual come into contact with the mucous membranes of the uninfected partner's rectum. Anal intercourse wherein the semen depositor is infected is one of the most risky sexual practices regardless of whether the semen receiver is male or female. Anal intercourse not only allows seminal fluid contact with the mucous membranes of the rectum, but also usually causes some degree of tearing or fissuring of the mucous membranes, making infection more likely.

Oral sex in which the uninfected partner's oral mucous membranes and tongue come into contact with infected vaginal secretions **(cunnilingus)** also places the uninfected person at risk. This risk is increased if sores or other open areas are present in the mouth.

DEGREE OF VIRAL LOAD. The higher the blood concentration of HIV **(viremia),** the greater the risk for sexual transmission. Current highly active antiretroviral therapy (HAART) has caused the viral load of some infected individuals to drop below detectable levels. Although it is assumed that such individuals would have far less virus in seminal or vaginal fluids, the risk of disease transmission is presumed to still exist.

Safer sex practices are those that reduce the risk of nonintact skin or mucous membranes coming in contact with potentially infected body fluids and blood. Such practices include using the following:

- A latex condom for genital and anal intercourse (Chart 22-1)
- A condom or latex barrier (dental dam) over the genitals or anus during oral-genital or oral-anal sexual contact
- Latex gloves for finger or hand contact with the vagina or rectum

PARENTERAL TRANSMISSION

Preventive practices to reduce parenteral transmission among injection drug users include the use of proper cleaning of "works" (needles, syringes, and other drug paraphernalia).

CHART 22-1

CLIENT EDUCATION GUIDE

Condom Use to Prevent Sexually Transmitted Diseases

- Use latex condoms rather than natural membrane condoms.
- Store condoms in a cool, dry place.
- Do not use condoms that were in damaged packages or those that show signs of age, such as those that are brittle, sticky, or discolored.
- Handle condoms carefully to avoid puncturing them.
- Put a condom on before making any genital contact. Hold the tip of the condom and unroll it onto the erect penis, making sure that no air is trapped in the tip. Leave space at the tip to collect semen.
- Use adequate lubrication. Use water-based lubricants only. Petroleum or oil-based lubricants such as petroleum jelly, cooking oil, shortening, and lotions can damage the condom.
- Replace a broken condom immediately. If ejaculation occurs after the condom breaks, there may be some protection in the immediate use of a spermicide.
- After ejaculation, the condom must remain on until the penis is withdrawn. While the penis is still erect, hold the condom against the base of the penis while withdrawing.
- Never reuse condoms.

From Centers for Disease Control. (1988). Condoms for prevention of sexually transmitted diseases. *Morbidity and Mortality Weekly Report, 37*(9), 133-137.

Clients are instructed to clean a used needle and syringe by first filling and flushing with clear water. Next, the syringe should be filled with ordinary household bleach. The bleach-filled syringe should be shaken for 30 to 60 seconds. Drug users are advised to carry a small container with this solution whenever sharing needles. Some communities have a needle exchange program in which needles and syringes are used only once and exchanged for clean ones.

The risk of AIDS transmission through blood and blood products has been reduced to a national average of 0.02%. Several measures have been implemented to protect the nation's blood supply. All donated blood in North America is screened for the HIV antibody, and blood that reacts positively is discarded. However, current tests detect the antibody, not the virus itself. Because of the time lag in antibody production **(seroconversion)** after exposure to HIV, infected blood can test negative for HIV antibodies. False-negative results also can occur. The small but real possibility of HIV transmission through blood and blood products has resulted in more stringent indications for transfusion and an increase in autologous transfusion.

PERINATAL TRANSMISSION

The risk of perinatal transmission in pregnant clients with AIDS has been reported at 14% to 45% for each pregnancy. Studies have shown that pregnant women who received zidovudine had an 8.3% perinatal transmission rate compared with 25.5% in women who received a placebo (National Institute of Allergy and Infectious Disease, 1994). HIV transmission is thought to occur transplacentally in utero, intrapartally during exposure to blood and vaginal secretions during birth, or postpartally through breast milk. Women of childbearing age with HIV infection should be fully informed of the risks of perinatal transmission. Consult a maternal-child textbook for more information about reducing perinatal transmission of HIV.

CHART 22-2

BEST PRACTICE *for*
Postexposure Prophylaxis for Occupational HIV Exposure

Source client is HIV negative.
and/or
Health care worker had exposure confined to intact skin.

- No HIV prophylaxis is needed.

Source client is HIV positive, asymptomatic, has a low viral load, and has a high CD4+ count
and/or
Health care worker had exposure to blood; or the contaminating substance (small amount) had contact with mucous membranes or nonintact skin for a short duration.

- Basic prophylaxis regimen
  Zidovudine (Retrovir) 600 mg in divided doses (300 mg twice daily, 200 mg three times daily, or 100 mg every 4 hours)
  Lamivudine (Epivir) 150 mg twice daily
  Continue both medications for 4 weeks

Source client is HIV positive with any of the following conditions: high or increasing viral load, AIDS, low CD4+ count, primary HIV infection. Health care worker exposure to contaminating substance (large amount) had deeper than superficial skin contact or had prolonged contact.

- Expanded prophylaxis regimen
  Zidovudine (Retrovir) 600 mg in divided doses (300 mg twice daily, 200 mg three times daily, or 100 mg every 4 hours)
  Lamivudine (Epivir) 150 mg twice daily
  Indinavir (Crixivan) 800 mg every 8 hours or nelfinavir (Viracept) 750 mg twice daily
  Continue regimen for 4 weeks

HIV status of source client is unknown—consider basic prophylaxis regimen unless health care worker exposure is consistent with the need for the expanded regimen.

Data from Centers for Disease Control and Prevention. (1998). Public Health Service guidelines for the management of health-care worker exposure to HIV and recommendations for postexposure prophylaxis. *Morbidity and Mortality Weekly Report, 47*(RR-7), 1-32.

TRANSMISSION AND HEALTH CARE WORKERS

Needle stick injuries are the primary means of HIV infection for health care workers. In addition, health care workers can be infected through exposure of nonintact skin and mucous membranes to blood and body fluids. Because there is a time lag between the time of infection with HIV and the production of serum antibodies (seroconversion), infected people can test negative for HIV and still transmit the virus. Therefore the best prevention for health care providers is the scrupulous and consistent application of standard precautions for all clients as recommended by the Centers for Disease Control and Prevention (CDC) (see Chapter 26). Chart 22-2 outlines recommended actions for prevention of HIV infection after a needle stick or other occupational exposure.

The public may be alarmed about HIV transmission by health care workers. It is recommended that HIV-infected health care workers wear gloves when in contact with clients' mucous membranes or nonintact skin. Infected workers with weeping dermatitis or exudative lesions should not perform direct care activities. The CDC (1991) has issued recommendations for preventing HIV transmission by health care workers during exposure-prone invasive procedures. These include any procedure in which there is a risk of percutaneous injury to the health care worker and the worker's blood is likely to make contact with the client's body cavity, subcutaneous tissues, or mucous membranes. These recommendations aim to reduce the risk of HIV transmission to clients (Table 22-5).

TABLE 22-5 • RECOMMENDATIONS FOR PREVENTING HUMAN IMMUNODEFICIENCY VIRUS TRANSMISSION BY HEALTH CARE WORKERS

- Workers should adhere to standard precautions.
- Workers with exudative lesions or weeping dermatitis should not perform direct patient care or handle patient care equipment and devices used in invasive procedures.
- Workers must follow guidelines for disinfection and sterilization of reusable equipment used in invasive procedures.
- Workers infected with HIV are not restricted from practice of non–exposure-prone procedures, provided that they comply with standard precautions and sterilization/disinfection recommendations.
- Workers should identify exposure-prone procedures by institutions where they are performed.
- Workers who perform exposure-prone procedures should know their HIV antibody status.
- Workers who are infected with HIV should seek advice from an expert review panel before performing exposure-prone procedures to determine under what circumstances they may continue to practice these procedures. These circumstances would include notification of prospective clients of HIV positivity.

Modified from Centers for Disease Control. (1991). Recommendations for preventing transmission of human immunodeficiency virus and hepatitis B virus to patients during exposure-prone invasive procedures. *Morbidity and Mortality Weekly Report, 40*(RR-8), 1-9.

TESTING

Testing plays a role in prevention, because those who test positive can be educated and encouraged to modify their behaviors to prevent transmission to others. The CDC has issued recommendations describing who should be advised to seek HIV antibody testing (Chart 22-3). Pre-test and post-test counseling must be performed by appropriately trained personnel. Counseling helps the client make an informed decision about testing and provides an opportunity to teach risk reduction behaviors. Post-test counseling is needed to interpret the results, discuss risk reduction, and provide psychologic support and health promotion information for the client with a positive test result.

Recommendations for people who have had positive test results for antibody to HIV are presented in the Meeting Healthy People 2010 Objectives box on p. 368. People who test positive should also be counseled on how to inform sexual partners and those with whom they have shared needles.

➤ COLLABORATIVE MANAGEMENT

SIMON Activity Link

The care of the client with HIV disease or AIDS is complex, affecting all body systems. The concept map on p. 372 addresses assessment and nursing care issues related to clients who have HIV disease or AIDS.

CHART 22-3

CLIENT EDUCATION GUIDE

Centers for Disease Control and Prevention Recommendations for HIV Testing

You should be tested for AIDS if you fall within one or more of the following groups:

- People with sexually transmitted disease
- Injection drug abusers
- People who consider themselves at risk
- Women of childbearing age with identifiable risks, including the following:
  - Having used injection drugs
  - Having engaged in prostitution
  - Having had sexual partners who were infected or at risk
  - Having had contact with men from countries with high HIV prevalence
  - Having received a transfusion between 1978 and 1985
- People planning to get married
- People undergoing medical evaluation or treatment for signs and symptoms that may be HIV related
- People admitted to hospitals
- People in correctional institutions such as jails and prisons
- Prostitutes and their customers

Modified from Centers for Disease Control. (1987). Public Health Service guidelines for counseling and antibody testing to prevent HIV infection and AIDS. *Morbidity and Mortality Weekly Report, 36*(31), 509-515.

Assessment

The person who has HIV disease should be monitored on a regular basis for changes in immune function or health status that indicate disease progression and warrant prophylaxis or therapeutic intervention. Continuous, careful, comprehensive assessment of the client with AIDS is crucial, because he or she may have signs and symptoms related to disease in multiple organ systems. Subtle changes must be assessed so that infections and other clinical problems can be found early and treated effectively.

HISTORY

Information relevant to HIV infection and AIDS from the general history includes age, gender, occupation, and residence. The nurse thoroughly assesses the current complaint or current illness, including its nature, when it started, the severity of symptoms, associated problems, and any interventions to date. The client is asked about when AIDS was diagnosed and what clinical symptoms led to that diagnosis. The client is asked to give a chronology of infections and clinical problems since the diagnosis. The nurse assesses the client's health history, including whether he or she received a blood transfusion between 1978 and 1985. (Since 1985, donated blood in the United States has been routinely tested for HIV contamination.)

The client is also questioned about sexual practices, any history of sexually transmitted diseases (STDs), and any history of major infectious diseases, including tuberculosis and hepatitis. If the client has hemophilia, the nurse asks about treatment with clotting factors. The client is asked about past or present drug use, including needle exposure and sharing. The nurse assesses the client's level of knowledge regarding the diagnosis, symptom management, diagnostic tests, treatments, community resources, and modes of transmission of the virus. The client's understanding and use of safer sex practices is also assessed.

PHYSICAL ASSESSMENT/CLINICAL MANIFESTATIONS

HIV disease and AIDS represent a progression continuum. The client with HIV disease, as defined in Table 22-2, may either have few clinical manifestations or problems or may have problems that are acute in duration rather than chronically present. The client with AIDS, however, usually experiences more problems of longer duration and greater severity. The nurse or assistive nursing personnel looks for many possible signs and symptoms. These include shortness of breath or cough, fever, night sweats, fatigue, nausea and vomiting, weight loss, lymphadenopathy, diarrhea, visual changes, headache, memory loss, confusion, seizures, personality changes, dry skin, rashes, skin lesions, pain, and discomfort (Chart 22-4).

OPPORTUNISTIC INFECTIONS. The client with HIV/AIDS can develop pathogenic infections and opportunistic infections. **Pathogenic infections** are caused by virulent microorganisms and occur even among people whose immune systems are functioning at an optimal level. **Opportunistic infections** are those caused by microorganisms that are continually present as part of the normal environment and are kept in check by normal immune function. Only when immune function is depressed or compromised are such organisms capable of causing infection.

Opportunistic infections occur because of the profound immune suppression of the person with AIDS (see Chart 22-4). They may result from primary infection or reactivation of a latent infection. Opportunistic infections account for many of the clinical manifestations observed in AIDS and can be protozoan, fungal, bacterial, or viral. More than one infection may be present in a client with AIDS.

Opportunistic infections do not pose a threat to the immunocompetent health care worker caring for a client with HIV infection or AIDS. When the client with HIV infection or AIDS has a pathogenic infection, however, such as tuberculosis at a transmissible stage, health care personnel must use appropriate precautions to prevent disease spread.

PROTOZOAL INFECTIONS. *Pneumocystis carinii pneumonia (PCP)* is the most common opportunistic infection in persons infected with HIV; its incidence ranges from 75% to 80%. The nurse notes dyspnea on exertion, tachypnea, a persistent dry cough, and fever. The client with PCP complains of fatigue and weight loss. On auscultation of the lungs, crackles are present.

Toxoplasmosis encephalitis, caused by *Toxoplasma gondii,* is acquired through contact with contaminated cat feces or by ingesting infected, undercooked meat. The client may experience subtle changes in mental status, neurologic deficits, headaches, and fever. Other symptoms include difficulties with speech, gait, and vision; seizures; lethargy; and confusion. The nurse performs a comprehensive baseline mental status examination and monitors the client to detect subtle changes.

Cryptosporidiosis is a gastroenteritis caused by *Cryptosporidium* organisms. In AIDS, this illness ranges from a mild diarrhea to a cholera-like syndrome with wasting and electrolyte imbalance. The nurse notes voluminous diarrhea, with a volume loss of up to 15 to 20 L/day.

FUNGAL INFECTIONS. *Candida albicans* is part of the natural flora of the gastrointestinal tract. In the person with

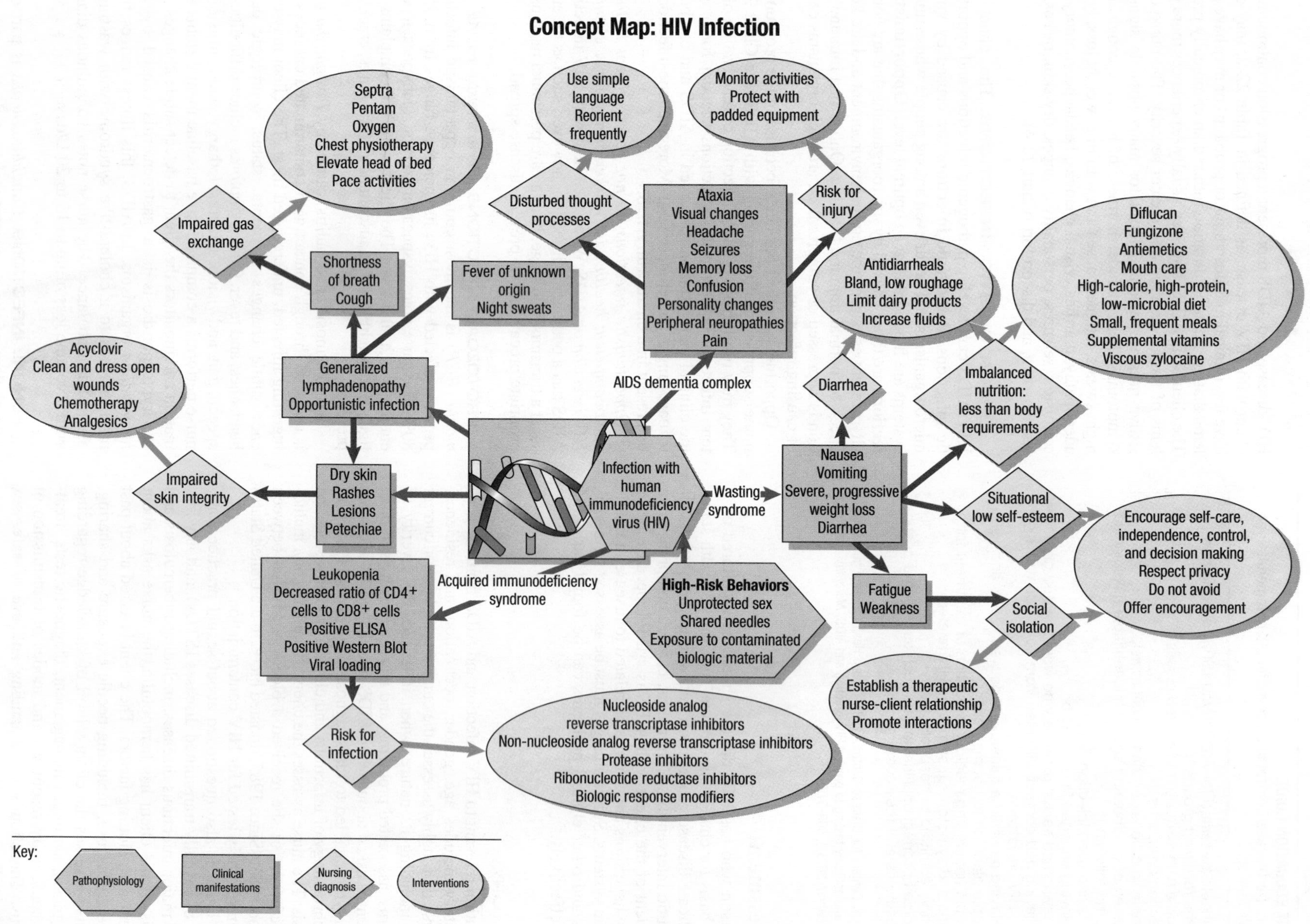
Concept Map: HIV Infection
Septra
Pentam
Oxygen
Chest physiotherapy
Elevate head of bed
Pace activities
Use simple language
Reorient frequently
Monitor activities
Protect with padded equipment
Impaired gas exchange
Disturbed thought processes
Ataxia
Visual changes
Headache
Seizures
Memory loss
Confusion
Personality changes
Peripheral neuropathies
Pain
Risk for injury
Diflucan
Fungizone
Antiemetics
Mouth care
High-calorie, high-protein, low-microbial diet
Small, frequent meals
Supplemental vitamins
Viscous zylocaine
Shortness of breath
Cough
Fever of unknown origin
Night sweats
Antidiarrheals
Bland, low roughage
Limit dairy products
Increase fluids
Acyclovir
Clean and dress open wounds
Chemotherapy
Analgesics
Generalized lymphadenopathy
Opportunistic infection
AIDS dementia complex
Diarrhea
Imbalanced nutrition: less than body requirements
Infection with human immunodeficiency virus (HIV)
Wasting syndrome
Nausea
Vomiting
Severe, progressive weight loss
Diarrhea
Impaired skin integrity
Dry skin
Rashes
Lesions
Petechiae
Situational low self-esteem
Encourage self-care, independence, control, and decision making
Respect privacy
Do not avoid
Offer encouragement
Leukopenia
Decreased ratio of CD4+ cells to CD8+ cells
Positive ELISA
Positive Western Blot
Viral loading
Acquired immunodeficiency syndrome
High-Risk Behaviors
Unprotected sex
Shared needles
Exposure to contaminated biologic material
Fatigue
Weakness
Social isolation
Establish a therapeutic nurse-client relationship
Promote interactions
Risk for infection
Nucleoside analog reverse transcriptase inhibitors
Non-nucleoside analog reverse transcriptase inhibitors
Protease inhibitors
Ribonucleotide reductase inhibitors
Biologic response modifiers
Key:
Pathophysiology
Clinical manifestations
Nursing diagnosis
Interventions

CHART 22-4

KEY FEATURES *of* AIDS

Immunologic Manifestations
- Low white blood cell counts:
  - CD4+/CD8+ ratio <2
  - CD4+ count <200/mm^3
- Hypergammaglobulinemia
- Opportunistic infections
- Lymphadenopathy
- Fatigue

Integumentary Manifestations
- Dry skin
- Poor wound healing
- Skin lesions
- Night sweats

Respiratory Manifestations
- Cough
- Shortness of breath

Gastrointestinal Manifestations
- Diarrhea
- Weight loss
- Nausea and vomiting

Central Nervous System Manifestations
- Confusion
- Dementia
- Headache
- Fever
- Visual changes
- Memory loss
- Personality changes
- Pain
- Seizures

Opportunistic Infections
- Protozoal infections
  - *Pneumocystis carinii* pneumonia
  - Toxoplasmosis
  - Cryptosporidiosis
  - Isosporiasis
  - Microsporidiosis
  - Strongyloidiasis
  - Giardiasis
- Fungal infections
  - Candidiasis
  - Cryptococcosis
  - Histoplasmosis
  - Coccidioidomycosis
- Bacterial infections
  - *Mycobacterium avium-intracellulare* complex infection
  - Tuberculosis
  - Nocardiosis
- Viral infections
  - Cytomegalovirus infection
  - Herpes simplex virus infection
  - Varicella-zoster virus infection

Malignancies
- Kaposi's sarcoma
- Non-Hodgkin's lymphoma
- Hodgkin's lymphoma
- Invasive cervical carcinoma

AIDS, candidiasis occurs because the regulatory mechanisms of the immune system can no longer control fungal overgrowth. *Candida* stomatitis or esophagitis is a frequent finding in AIDS; clients complain of food tasting "funny," mouth pain, difficulty in swallowing, and **retrosternal pain** (pain behind the ribs). On examination of the mouth and the back of the throat, the nurse sees the characteristic cottage cheese–like, yellow-white plaques and inflammation. Esophagitis is diagnosed by endoscopic biopsy and culture. Women with HIV disease or AIDS may have persistent vaginal candidiasis, characterized by severe **pruritus** (itching), perineal irritation, and a thick, white vaginal discharge.

Cryptococcosis is a severe, debilitating meningitis and occasionally a disseminated disease in AIDS. It is caused by *Cryptococcus neoformans.* Clinical manifestations of meningitis include fever, headache, blurred vision, nausea and vomiting, **nuchal rigidity** (stiff neck), mild confusion, and other mental status changes. Some clients experience seizures and other focal neurologic abnormalities or may have mild symptoms and complain only of malaise and fever with or without headaches.

Histoplasmosis, caused by *Histoplasma capsulatum,* begins as a respiratory infection and progresses to widespread infection in the person with AIDS. The nurse may note dyspnea, fever, cough, and weight loss. The spleen, liver, and lymph nodes may be enlarged.

BACTERIAL INFECTIONS. ***Mycobacterium avium-intracellulare* complex (MAC)** is the most common bacterial infection associated with AIDS. This complex is caused by *Mycobacterium intracellulare* or *Mycobacterium avium,* which infects the respiratory or gastrointestinal tract. MAC is a systemic infection. Positive cultures may be obtained from lymph nodes, bone marrow, and blood. Clinical manifestations include fever, debility, weight loss, malaise, and sometimes lymphadenopathy or organ disease.

Tuberculosis, caused by *Mycobacterium tuberculosis,* occurs in 2% to 10% of persons with AIDS. People with HIV disease are at increased risk for active tuberculosis. More than 50% of all clients who have AIDS and tuberculosis have extrapulmonary disease sites, including the central nervous system, bones, liver, spleen, skin, and gastrointestinal tract. Systemic symptoms include fever, chills, night sweats, weight loss, and anorexia. Pulmonary involvement causes cough, dyspnea, and chest pain. Symptoms of extrapulmonary infection vary with the site. The person with tuberculosis and a CD4+ count below 200/mm^3 may not have a positive purified protein derivative (PPD) skin test because of an inability to mount an immune response to the antigen, a condition known as **anergy.** Other diagnostic tests include a chest x-ray film, acid-fast sputum smear, and sputum culture.

The nurse or respiratory therapist giving aerosol treatments, such as pentamidine isethionate prophylaxis, that induce coughing to clients with AIDS should be screened with a PPD skin test every 6 months.

Recurrent pneumonia from bacterial infections occurs frequently among immunocompromised clients. In the current CDC classification system for AIDS, two or more episodes of pneumonia in a 12-month period is an AIDS case definition. Symptoms include chest pain, productive cough, fever, and dyspnea.

VIRAL INFECTIONS. **Cytomegalovirus (CMV)** can infect multiple sites in persons with AIDS, including the eye (CMV retinitis), respiratory and gastrointestinal tracts, and central nervous system. CMV infection can also result in many nonspecific symptoms associated with AIDS, such as fever, malaise, weight loss, fatigue, and lymphadenopathy.

CMV retinitis causes visual impairment ranging from slight to total bilateral blindness.

CMV infection also causes colitis, with diarrhea, abdominal bloating and discomfort, and weight loss. In addition, CMV can cause encephalitis, pneumonitis, adrenalitis, hepatitis, and disseminated infection.

Herpes simplex virus (HSV) infections in people with HIV disease or AIDS occur in the perirectal, oral, and genital areas. The manifestations tend to be more widespread and of longer duration among clients with HIV/AIDS than among those who are immunocompetent. Clients describe numbness or tingling at the site of infection up to 24 hours before **vesicle** (blister) formation. Vesicular lesions are painful, with chronic ulcerative lesions after vesicle rupture. The nurse notes fever, pain, bleeding, and lymph node enlargement in the affected area. Systemic symptoms include headache, myalgia, and malaise.

Varicella-zoster virus (VZV) infection is usually not a new infection for people with AIDS. This virus, present in the nerve ganglia of many people, causes chickenpox. When people who have had the chickenpox in childhood are immunocompromised, VZV leaves the nerve ganglia and enters body fluids and other tissue areas, causing shingles. Symptoms begin with pain and burning along dermatome nerve tracts. Large fluid-filled vesicles form and eventually crust over. Systemic symptoms include headache and low-grade fever.

MALIGNANCIES. The altered immunocompetence of AIDS increases the risk for cancer in this group. Cancers associated with AIDS include Kaposi's sarcoma, Hodgkin's lymphoma, non-Hodgkin's lymphoma, invasive cervical cancer, seminoma, plasmocytoma, and squamous carcinoma conjunctivitis (CDC, 1999a).

KAPOSI'S SARCOMA. Kaposi's sarcoma (KS) is the most common malignancy associated with AIDS, occurring in 1% to 21% of clients with AIDS. The risk for KS appears to vary with the way in which HIV was acquired. Clients with hemophilia who have HIV have the lowest incidence of KS, and men infected through homosexual contact have the highest incidence.

KS develops as small, purplish brown, raised lesions that are usually not painful or pruritic. The lesions can occur anywhere on the body. Most clients with KS have **mucocutaneous** (skin or mucous membrane) lesions. In some clients, lesions develop in the lymph nodes, gastrointestinal tract, or lungs. The nurse assesses KS lesions for number, size, and location and monitors their progression. KS is diagnosed by biopsy and histologic examination of the lesion.

MALIGNANT LYMPHOMAS. Malignant lymphomas associated with AIDS are primarily non-Hodgkin's B-cell lymphomas, such as Burkitt's lymphoma, immunoblastic lymphoma, and primary brain lymphoma. Systemic symptoms include weight loss, fever, and night sweats. (See Chapter 40 on the clinical course and care relevant to malignant lymphomas.)

OTHER CLINICAL MANIFESTATIONS. All body systems are affected to some degree in AIDS; however, manifestations most consistently appear as changes in cognitive function, weight, and the skin.

CHART 22-5

KEY FEATURES *of* AIDS Dementia Complex

Cognitive Impairment
- Slowed thinking
- Slowed reaction time to external stimuli
- Loss of concentration while thinking or speaking
- Memory loss
- Forgetfulness
- Wandering attention

Motor Impairment
- Loss of coordination
- Loss of balance
- Increased minor accidents such as tripping, bumping into things, or dropping things
- Slowed motor performance
- Leg weakness

Behavioral Impairment
- Apathy
- Withdrawal

or
- Irritability
- Hyperactivity

AIDS DEMENTIA COMPLEX AND OTHER NEUROLOGIC COMPLICATIONS. HIV-associated dementia complex, or **AIDS dementia complex (ADC),** refers to the signs and symptoms of central nervous system involvement. ADC occurs in up to 70% of persons with AIDS. It is probably a result of direct infection of cells within the central nervous system by HIV. ADC causes cognitive, motor, and behavioral impairments (Chart 22-5). Symptoms range from barely noticeable to severe dementia.

Other neurologic complications may be due to HIV infection or drug side effects, including peripheral neuropathies and myopathies. Symptoms of peripheral neuropathies include paresthesias and burning sensations, pain, and gait changes. Myopathies are accompanied by leg weakness, ataxia, and muscle pain.

WASTING SYNDROME. AIDS wasting syndrome is not due to any single factor. It may be a result of altered metabolism from malignancy or opportunistic infection. Diarrhea, malabsorption, anorexia, and oral and esophageal lesions can all contribute to persistent and sometimes extreme weight loss, and the client may appear quite emaciated.

INTEGUMENTARY CHANGES. Many clients complain of dry, itchy, irritated skin and many types of skin rashes. Folliculitis, eczema, or psoriasis may also be present. When the platelet count is low, petechiae or bleeding gums may be present.

PSYCHOSOCIAL ASSESSMENT

Psychosocial data collection for a client with AIDS is extremely important. The nurse asks about the client's social support system, including family, significant others, and friends. To protect confidentiality, the nurse assesses who in this support system is aware of the client's diagnosis so that it is not inadvertently mentioned. Some clients, because of real or threatened discrimination, are quite selective about whom they tell. Health care providers must respect the client's choices as much as possible without compromising care. The nurse can offer resources to help with disclosure to sexual partners or significant others.

The client may be closest to a lover or a friend who is not legally recognized as next of kin. The nurse obtains the name and telephone number of that person and learns whether a health care proxy or durable power-of-attorney document has been executed.

The nurse obtains information about the client's activities of daily living, as well as any changes that may have occurred since the diagnosis. Employment status and occupation, social activities and hobbies, living arrangements, and financial resources, including health insurance, are assessed.

To plan care and monitor changes, the nurse assesses the client's anxiety level, mood, and cognitive ability. The client is also asked about any experiences with discrimination and how they were handled. After the nurse assesses the client's level of self-esteem and changes in body image, together the nurse and client identify strengths and coping strategies. Information is gathered about any suicidal ideation, depression, or other psychologic problems. In addition, information about the client's involvement with support groups or other community resources is obtained.

LABORATORY ASSESSMENT

LYMPHOCYTE COUNTS. A lymphocyte count is performed as part of a complete blood count (CBC) with differential (see Chapter 20). The normal white blood cell (WBC) count is between 4500 and 11,000 cells/mm^3, with a differential of approximately 30% to 40% lymphocytes (an absolute number of 1500 to 4500). Clients with AIDS are often **leukopenic,** with a WBC count of less than 3500 cells/mm^3, and usually **lymphopenic** (less than 1500 lymphocytes/mm^3).

CD4/CD8 COUNTS. The percentage and number of CD4+ (T4) and CD8+ (T8) cells are an important part of an immune profile. People with HIV disease usually have a lower than normal number of CD4+ cells. Some clients with AIDS have fewer than 100 cells/mm^3 (normal: between 500 and 1600 cells/mm^3), whereas the number of CD8+ cells remains normal. The normal ratio of CD4+ to CD8+ cells is approximately 2:1. In HIV disease and AIDS, because of a low number of CD4+ cells, this ratio is low. Low CD4+ cell counts and a low CD4+/CD8+ ratio are associated with increased clinical manifestations of disease.

ANTIBODY TESTS. Antibody tests measure the client's response to the presence of the virus (the antigen) rather than measuring parts of the virus or the virus itself. HIV antibody can be measured by enzyme-linked immunosorbent assay (ELISA) and Western blot analysis. After infection with the virus, it usually takes from 3 weeks to 3 months for a person to test positive for HIV antibodies. In some infected people, however, it can take up to 36 months for antibodies to be detectable (Imagawa et al., 1989). False-negative results (incorrectly indicating the absence of HIV infection) have been reported early in the infection, in people with cancer, and in people receiving long-term immunosuppressive therapy.

ENZYME-LINKED IMMUNOSORBENT ASSAY. The client's serum is mixed with HIV grown in culture. If the client has antibodies to HIV, they will bind to the HIV antigens and can be detected (a positive test). False-positive test results (incorrectly indicating HIV infection) occur in approximately 0.1% of those tested with the enzyme-linked immunosorbent assay (ELISA). False-positive results have been reported in multiparous or pregnant women, injection drug users, people with a history of malaria, clients with lymphomas, and those with reactivity to the HLA-DR4 leukocyte antigen.

WESTERN BLOT. If the results of an ELISA are positive, they are confirmed by Western blot analysis. This test is not as widely available as ELISA because of its cost and complexity. The Western blot analysis is a more specific test to detect serum antibodies to four specific major HIV antigens. A positive Western blot result is based on the presence of antibodies to at least two of the major HIV antigens.

The result is considered indeterminate if two of the major antibodies are not detected but other antibodies to HIV are. The person should then be retested. In people whose tests are positive, conversion from an indeterminate to a positive Western blot usually occurs within 6 months. *If a person has a positive test result for HIV antibodies, it does not mean that he or she has AIDS, only that he or she has been infected with the virus.*

VIRAL CULTURE. Virus culture techniques also can determine the presence of HIV. One method involves placing the infected client's blood cells in a culture medium and measuring the amount of reverse transcriptase (RT) activity over a 28-day period. The more RT present, the more actively the virus is thought to be replicating.

VIRAL LOAD TESTING. **Viral load testing** (also called viral burden testing) measures the presence of HIV viral genetic material (ribonucleic acid [RNA]) or another actual viral protein in the client's blood rather than the body's response to the presence of the virus. These test types are quantitative and more directly indicate the level of viral burden or viral load. Such tests are very useful in monitoring disease progression and treatment effectiveness.

QUANTITATIVE RNA ASSAYS. Currently, three quantitative assays are available in some areas for viral load testing: the RT-polymerase chain reaction (RT-PCR), the branched deoxyribonucleic acid (DNA) method (bDNA), and the nucleic acid sequence-based assay (NASBA). All three assays use gene amplification processes to determine the amount of HIV RNA present in a client's serum, and all have a specificity of 100%. Even if only a few infected cells are present in a serum sample, tiny amounts of the HIV RNA are amplified by these methods in sufficient quantities to be detected. Such tests are useful in the clinical management of disease and in diagnosing HIV infection in people who have no other indication of infection. These tests are used to determine therapy effectiveness and as indicators of the need to change the drug regimen.

p24 ANTIGEN ASSAY. The p24 antigen assay quantifies the amount of **p24** (HIV viral core protein) in the client's serum. Antibodies to p24 are mixed with the serum and can detect even low levels of viral antigen present in serum. However, the assay is not as sensitive as antibody tests or assays of viral genetic material. This test is seldom used and has been largely replaced by the more quantitative tests of HIV RNA.

OTHER LABORATORY TESTS. Other laboratory tests monitor the overall condition of the client and detect or diagnose any infections or secondary clinical processes. Standard tests include blood chemistries, a complete blood count (CBC) with differential and platelets, prothrombin time and partial thromboplastin time, a serologic test for syphilis (STS), hepatitis B antigens, and immunoglobulin levels. Tests to further evaluate the immune profile of a client may include bone marrow aspiration with biopsy and cultures.

OTHER DIAGNOSTIC ASSESSMENT

On the basis of the clinical symptoms, other diagnostic tests are chosen, including stool for ova and parasites; biopsies of the skin, lymph nodes, lungs, liver, gastrointestinal tract, or brain; a chest x-ray film; gallium scans; bronchoscopy, endoscopy, or colonoscopy; liver and spleen scans; computed tomography scans; pulmonary function tests; and arterial blood gas analysis.

CRITICAL THINKING CHALLENGE

The client is a 28-year-old Hispanic woman admitted for multiple fractures, lacerations, and abrasions sustained in a car accident. She tells you she has symptoms of a vaginal yeast infection and complains that this is her sixth yeast infection in 7 months, even though she has treated herself each time with an over-the-counter antifungal product.

- What additional assessment data should you obtain?
- What questions should you ask about this client's sexual activity?
- What laboratory data already obtained should you examine more closely?
- How should you approach this client about her HIV status?

For suggested answer guidelines, go to SIMON http://www.wbsaunders.com/SIMON/Iggy/.

Analysis

COMMON NURSING DIAGNOSES AND COLLABORATIVE PROBLEMS

The following are the most common nursing diagnoses for clients with AIDS:

1. Risk for Infection related to immunodeficiency
2. Impaired Gas Exchange related to anemia, respiratory infection or malignancy (*Pneumocystis carinii* pneumonia [PCP], cytomegalovirus [CMV] pneumonitis, pulmonary Kaposi's sarcoma [KS], and/or *Mycobacterium* infection), anemia, fatigue, or pain
3. Acute Pain or Chronic Pain related to neuropathy, myelopathy, malignancy, or infection
4. Imbalanced Nutrition: Less Than Body Requirements related to high metabolic need, nausea and vomiting, diarrhea, difficulty chewing or swallowing, or anorexia
5. Diarrhea related to infection, food intolerance, or medications
6. Impaired Skin Integrity related to KS, infection, altered nutritional state, incontinence, immobility, hyperthermia, or malignancy
7. Disturbed Thought Processes related to AIDS dementia complex (ADC), central nervous system infection, or malignancy
8. Situational Low Self-Esteem or Chronic Low Self-Esteem related to changes in body image, decreased self-esteem, or helplessness
9. Social Isolation related to stigma, virus transmissibility, infection control practices, or fear

The primary collaborative problem is Potential for Infection (processed under Risk for Infection, below).

ADDITIONAL NURSING DIAGNOSES AND COLLABORATIVE PROBLEMS

In addition to the common nursing diagnoses and collaborative problems, clients with AIDS may have one or more of the following:

- Activity Intolerance related to fatigue, discomfort, central nervous system defect, weakness, or anemia
- Risk for Injury related to central nervous system defect, mental status changes, depression, or thrombocytopenia
- Disturbed Sensory Perception (Visual) related to CMV retinitis or blindness
- Disturbed Sleep Pattern related to pain, discomfort, anxiety, or depression
- Ineffective Coping related to the diagnosis of AIDS
- Disabled Family Coping related to the diagnosis of AIDS
- Anticipatory Grieving related to potential loss of role and function or impending death

Planning and Implementation

RISK FOR INFECTION

The client with AIDS is susceptible to opportunistic infections because of immunodeficiency secondary to HIV infection.

PLANNING: EXPECTED OUTCOMES. The client is expected to remain free of opportunistic diseases.

INTERVENTIONS. NIC interventions that can help the client minimize the chances of acquiring an infection are provided in Chart 22-6. Chart 22-7 outlines best practices for prevention of infection in a hospitalized immunocompromised client. Some strategies are investigational, including drug therapy and immune function enhancement.

DRUG THERAPY. Chart 22-8 lists treatments for opportunistic infections. Some medications have demonstrated antiretroviral effects; however, *it is important to remember that antiretroviral therapy only inhibits viral replication and does not kill the virus* (Chart 22-9). Treatment with only one antiretroviral agent, known as **monotherapy,** does not significantly improve the duration or quality of life for the client with HIV/AIDS. Instead, multiple drugs are used together in regimens called "cocktails." These regimens consist of combinations of different types of antiretroviral agents. Such a therapeutic approach is termed **highly active antiretroviral therapy (HAART)** and is showing good results as measured by reduced viral load and improved CD4+ lymphocyte counts. Major drawbacks to HIV/AIDS drug therapy include the expense of the drugs (see the Cost of Care box on p. 381),

CHART 22-6

NIC INTERVENTION ACTIVITIES *for* The Client at Risk for Infection

Infection Protection: *Prevention and early detection of infection in a client at risk*

- Monitor for systemic and localized signs and symptoms of infection.
- Monitor vulnerability to infection.
- Monitor absolute granulocyte count, WBC, and differential results.
- Follow neutropenic precautions, as appropriate.
- Screen all visitors for communicable disease.
- Maintain asepsis for client at risk.
- Inspect skin and mucous membranes for redness, extreme warmth, or drainage.
- Obtain cultures, as needed.
- Promote sufficient nutritional intake.
- Monitor for change in energy level/malaise.
- Instruct client to take medications as prescribed.
- Teach client and family members how to avoid infections.

NIC intervention activities selected from McCloskey, J.C., & Bulechek, G.M. (Eds.). (2000). *Nursing interventions classification (NIC)* (3rd ed.). St. Louis: Mosby. No part of this work is to be altered without prior written permission from the Publisher.
WBC, white blood cell.

the numerous side effects, and the sheer volume of daily medications. The main actions of each drug category are explained below. The specific drugs, dosages, and nursing implications are presented in Chart 22-9.

NUCLEOSIDE ANALOG REVERSE TRANSCRIPTASE INHIBITORS. Nucleoside analogs are structurally similar to various nucleotides (nucleosides) that are important in making DNA. These drugs are converted in the virally infected cell into a "counterfeit" form of a nucleoside and compete with the actual nucleoside for incorporation into reverse transcriptase–dependent DNA chains. Thus they suppress production of reverse transcriptase and inhibit viral DNA synthesis and genetic replication. This class of antiretroviral agents includes zidovudine (Retrovir), didanosine (ddI, Videx), zalcitabine (ddC, HIVID), lamivudine (Epivir, 3TC✤), stavudine (d4T, Zerit), and abacavir (Ziagen).

NON-NUCLEOSIDE ANALOG REVERSE TRANSCRIPTASE INHIBITORS. Non-nucleoside analog reverse transcriptase inhibitors, through an unknown mechanism, inhibit synthesis of the enzyme reverse transcriptase. Like nucleoside analogs, these drugs protect uninfected cells and suppress viral replication but do not kill the virus. These drugs include nevirapine (Viramune), delavirdine (Rescriptor), and efavirenz (Sustiva) (see Chart 22-9).

PROTEASE INHIBITORS. Protease inhibitors block the HIV protease enzyme, preventing viral replication and release of viral particles. The HIV initially produces all of its proteins, including the ones necessary to move viral particles out of a cell, in one long strand. For the proteins to be active, the large initial protein must be broken down into individual smaller proteins through the action of the viral enzyme protease. The protease inhibitor drugs, when taken into an HIV-infected cell, make the protease work on the drug rather than on the initial large protein. As a result, active proteins are not

CHART 22-7

BEST PRACTICE *for* Prevention of Infection in an Immunocompromised Client

- Place the client in a private room whenever possible.
- Use good handwashing technique before touching the client or any of his or her belongings.
- Ensure that the client's room and bathroom are cleaned at least once each day.
- Do not use supplies from common areas for immunosuppressed clients. For example, keep a sleeve or box of paper cups in the client's room, and do not share this box with any other client. Other articles include drinking straws, plastic knives and forks, dressing materials, gloves, and bandages.
- Limit the number of health care personnel entering the client's room.
- Monitor vital signs every 4 hours; note minor temperature elevation, which may suggest early sepsis.
- Inspect the client's mouth at least every 8 hours.
- Inspect the client's skin and mucous membranes (especially the anal area) for the presence of fissures and abscesses at least every 8 hours.
- Inspect open areas, such as IV sites, every 4 hours for manifestations of infection.
- Change wound dressings daily.
- Obtain specimens of all suspicious areas for culture, and promptly notify physician.
- Assist the client in performing coughing and deep-breathing exercises.
- Encourage activity at appropriate level for the client's current health status.
- Change IV tubing daily.
- Keep frequently used equipment in the room for use by the client only (e.g., blood pressure cuff, stethoscope, thermometer).
- Limit visitors to healthy adults.
- Use strict aseptic technique for all invasive procedures.
- Monitor the white blood cell count, especially the absolute neutrophil count (ANC), daily.
- Avoid the use of indwelling urinary catheters.
- Keep fresh flowers and potted plants out of the client's room.

produced and the newly made viral particles cannot leave the cell to infect other cells. Drugs in this class include ritonavir (Norvir), indinavir (Crixivan), saquinavir (Invirase), nelfinavir (Viracept), amprenavir (Agenerase), and lopinavir (ABT-378r, Kaletra). All protease inhibitors have fewer side effects than the nucleoside analogs but have shown rapid resistance (see Chart 22-9).

RIBONUCLEOTIDE REDUCTASE INHIBITORS. Ribonucleotide reductase inhibitors actually represent a new use for other cytotoxic therapies. The drug hydroxyurea (Hydrea) has been successfully used for cancer chemotherapy as an antimetabolite. The drug is structurally similar to the DNA base thymidine. When it is taken up by the cell, this drug interferes with DNA synthesis, stopping viral replication.

IMMUNE ENHANCEMENT. Research is also being conducted to evaluate treatments that may enhance or reconstitute the immune system of clients who are made immunodeficient by HIV infection. Some of these methods include bone marrow transplantation, lymphocyte transfusion, and administration of lymphokines, particularly interleukin-2, and other biologic response modifiers (Ungvarski, 1997).

CHART 22-8

DRUG THERAPY *for* AIDS-Related Opportunistic Infections

Drug	Indication	Usual Dosage	Nursing Interventions	Rationale
Trimethoprim (TMP)/ sulfamethoxazole (SMX) (Apo-Sulfatrim🍁, Bactrim🍁, Cotrim, Septra)	*Pneumocystis carinii* pneumonia	PO 160 mg TMP and 800 mg SMX q12h	Monitor I&O. Encourage fluids. Monitor CBC, urinalysis, bilirubin, creatinine, alkaline phosphatase. Assess for sore throat, pallor, purpura, jaundice, weakness.	I&O are monitored because TMP/SMX is nephrotoxic. These values are monitored because TMP/SMX suppresses the immune system. These signs are assessed for because TMP/SMX is hepatotoxic.
Pentamidine isethionate (Pentam)	*P. carinii* pneumonia	IM or IV 4 mg/kg once daily for 14-21 days	Monitor blood pressure, heart rate, and rhythm. Administer with client lying down. Monitor for hypoglycemia. Administer IV over 1 hr. Monitor liver function, CBC.	BP and heart rate are monitored because pentamidine causes hypotension when administered rapidly. Monitoring is necessary because pentamidine causes severe hypoglycemia that may be fatal. Liver function and CBC are monitored because pentamidine is heptotoxic and immunosuppressive.
Pentamidine isethionate (Pentam, Pentarcarinat🍁)	*P. carinii* pneumonia	Inhalant 300 mg every 4 wk via nebulizer	See above.	See above.
Pyrimethamine (with sulfadiazine) (Daraprim)	Toxoplasmosis	PO 50-75 mg/day for 1-3 wk, then 25 mg/day for 4-5 wk	Administer with food or milk. Monitor CBC and platelets.	Pyrimethamine irritates the GI tract. The CBC and platelets are monitored because pyrimethamine suppresses bone marrow activity.
Sulfadiazine	Toxoplasmosis Nocardiasis	PO 500-2000 mg daily q6h for 3-4 wk	Monitor urine output, CBC. Encourage fluids. Advise client to avoid sun. Assess for sore throat, pallor, purpura, jaundice, weakness.	Urine output and the CBC are monitored because sulfadiazine causes renal toxicity. Fluids are necessary because sulfadiazine suppresses bone marrow activity. Clients should avoid the sun because sulfadiazine increases photosensitivity.
Dapsone (Avlosulfon🍁, DDS)	Toxoplasmosis	PO 50-100 mg daily	Monitor CBC. Assess for fever, sore throat, purpura, jaundice.	The CBC is monitored because dapsone suppresses bone marrow activity.
Metronidazole (Flagyl, Novonidazole🍁)	Cryptosporidiosis Giardiasis	PO 7.5 mg/kg q6h, IV 15 mg/kg initial dose, then 7.5 mg/kg q6h	Administer with food or milk. Teach client to avoid alcohol during treatment. Assess for dry mouth, dizziness, fungal infection.	Food or milk is recommended because metronidazole irritates the GI tract. Alcohol causes formation of acetaldehyde and headache, nausea, vomiting, and diarrhea.
Ketoconazole (Nizoral)	Candidiasis Coccidioidomycosis Histoplasmosis	PO 200-400 mg/day, single dose	Administer with food or milk. Avoid antacids for 2 hr. Teach client to avoid sun and alcohol during treatment. Monitor hepatic function.	Ketoconazole irritates the GI tract. Gastric acid is needed to activate drug. Ketoconazole increases photosensitivity. Hepatic function is monitored because ketoconazole is hepatotoxic.
Fluconazole (Diflucan)	Candidiasis Cryptococcal meningitis	PO, IV 200-400 mg initially, then 100-200 mg daily for 2-4 wk	Monitor hepatic function. Assess for abdominal pain, fever, diarrhea.	Hepatic function is monitored because fluconazole is hepatotoxic.

Rifampin (Rifadin, Rofact🍁)	*Mycobacterium avium* complex Tuberculosis	PO 10 mg/kg/day	Assess breath sounds, sputum. Monitor hepatic function, CBC. May turn body secretions orange.	Assessment of breath sounds and sputum determines treatment effectiveness. Rifampin is hepatotoxic.
Ethambutol (Myambutol, Etibi🍁)	*Mycobacterium avium-intracellulare* complex Tuberculosis	PO 25-30 mg/kg 2-3 times/wk	Assess vision changes. Assess hepatic and renal function, CBC, urinalysis.	Vision changes are assessed because ethambutol causes retrobulbar neuritis and decreased visual acuity (reversible). This assessment is necessary because ethambutol increases uric acid concentrations. Ethambutol suppresses bone marrow activity.
Amphotericin B (Fungizone)	Candidiasis Other fungal infections	IV 0.3-1 mg/kg/day, maximum 50 mg/day	Assess renal function. Assess infusion site. Assess CBC.	Renal function is assessed because amphotericin B is nephrotoxic. Amphotericin B causes thrombophlebitis. The CBC is checked because amphotericin B suppresses bone marrow activity. Amphotericin B is *very* toxic.
Ciprofloxacin (Cipro)	*Mycobacterium avium-intracellulare* complex Urinary tract infections	PO 250-750 mg q12h, IV 200-400 mg q12h	Monitor I&O. Encourage fluids. Administer on empty stomach (1 hr before or 2 hr after meals) if tolerated. Teach client to avoid sun. Assess for dizziness, fungal infection. Infuse over 1 hr.	An empty stomach is recommended for best absorption. Client should avoid the sun because ciprofloxacin increases photosensitivity.
Clofazimine (Lamprene)	*Mycobacterium avium-intracellulare* complex	PO 50-300 mg every day	Assess vision changes, dizziness, drowsiness. Instruct client to avoid sun. Use lotions for dry skin. Monitor hepatic and renal function.	Vision changes and dizziness are assessed because clofazimine increases sedation. Clofazimine increases photosensitivity (especially of eyes). Clients should use lotions because clofazimine causes dry, scaly skin.
Pyrazinamide (Tebrazid🍁)	Tuberculosis	PO 20-30 mg/kg/day	Monitor hepatic function, uric acid. Assess temperature q4h.	Pyrazinamide is hepatotoxic and increases uric acid concentration. The client's temperature is assessed because pyrazinamide stimulates fever.
Isoniazid (Laniazid, Isotamine)	Tuberculosis	PO, IM 5-10 mg/kg/day or 15 mg/kg 2-3 times/wk	Administer on empty stomach. Monitor hepatic function. Assess for vision changes. Instruct client to avoid alcohol and tyramine-containing foods.	Taking isoniazid on an empty stomach enhances absorption. Isoniazid is hepatotoxic. Vision changes are assessed because isoniazid is neurotoxic. Isoniazid is an MAO inhibitor.
Ganciclovir (Cytovene)	Cytomegalovirus retinitis	IV 5 mg/kg q12h for 14-21 days PO 1000 mg q8h	Monitor neutrophil and platelet count. Infuse over 1 hr. Give with food.	Neutrophil and platelet counts are monitored because ganciclovir suppresses bone marrow activity.
Acyclovir (Zovirax)	Herpes simplex Herpes zoster Varicella zoster	PO 200-800 mg 5 times/day, IV 5-10 mg/kg q8h for 7-10 days	Monitor renal function. Encourage fluids. Rotate infusion site.	Acyclovir is nephrotoxic. Various infusion sites are used because acyclovir is a blood vessel irritant.

I&O, Intake and output; *CBC*, complete blood count; *GI*, gastrointestinal; *MAO*, monoamine oxidase.

CHART 22-9

DRUG THERAPY *for* HIV Infection

Drug	Usual Dosage	Nursing Interventions	Rationale
NUCLEOSIDE ANALOG REVERSE TRANSCRIPTASE INHIBITORS			
Zidovudine (Retrovir)	300 mg q12h	Assess for dizziness.	Drug crosses the blood-brain barrier, causing dizziness.
		Monitor CBC, hepatic and renal function.	Zidovudine induces bone marrow suppression, hepatotoxicities, and nephrotoxicities.
Didanosine (ddl, Videx)	125-300 mg q12h	Administer on an empty stomach.	Food decreases drug absorption.
		Assess vision, hearing, touch, and balance.	Drug induces peripheral neuropathy.
		Monitor CBC.	Drug induces bone marrow suppression.
Zalcitabine (ddC, HIVID)	0.75 mg q8h	Assess vision, hearing, touch, and balance.	Drug induces peripheral neuropathy.
		Tell client to avoid alcoholic beverages.	Drug elevates liver enzymes.
Lamivudine (Epivir, 3TC✱)	150 mg q8h	Teach client to avoid fatty foods.	Drug can cause severe pancreatitis.
		Assess vision, hearing, touch, and balance.	Drug induces peripheral neuropathy.
Stavudine (d4T, Zerit)	40 mg q12h	Assess vision, hearing, touch, and balance.	Drug induces peripheral neuropathy.
		Assess for generalized pain.	Drug induces arthralgias.
Abacavir (Ziagen)	300 mg q12h	Assess for flu-like symptoms.	Drug can cause manifestations of a hypersensitivity reaction.
		If flu-like symptoms are present, stop drug permanently.	Hypersensitivity can progress to life-threatening emergency.
NON-NUCLEOSIDE ANALOG REVERSE TRANSCRIPTASE INHIBITORS			
Nevirapine (Viramune)	200 mg q12h	Give 1 hr before or after antacids.	Absorption is inhibited by antacids.
		Assess for headache.	Headache is most common side effect.
		Assess for generalized pain.	Drug induces arthralgias.
Efavirenz (Sustiva)	600 mg once per day	Assess for headaches, dysphoria, and nightmares.	Drug crosses blood-brain barrier and induces headaches, dysphoria, and nightmares.
		Avoid contact with medication during pregnancy.	Drug is mutagenic and can induce birth defects.
Delavirdine (Rescriptor)	200 mg tid × 14 days 400 mg tid	Store at room temperature.	Room temperature is recommended storage.
		Assess for headache or rash.	Headache and rash are common side effects.
PROTEASE INHIBITORS			
Saquinavir (Invirase)	600 mg q8h	Tell client to take with or just after a high-fat, high-calorie meal.	Drug is best absorbed with a fatty meal.
		Instruct client to wear sunscreen.	Drug increases photosensitivity.
Indinavir (Crixivan)	800 mg q8h	Administer on an empty stomach.	An empty stomach enhances drug absorption.
		Assess for jaundice.	Drug induces hyperbilirubinemia.
		Assess for flank pain or hematuria.	Drug induces nephrolithiasis.
Ritonavir (Norvir)	600 mg q12h	Administer on an empty stomach.	An empty stomach enhances drug absorption.
		Monitor triglyceride levels.	Drug can elevate triglyceride synthesis.
Nelfinavir (Viracept)	750 mg q8h	Administer with food.	Drug causes diarrhea, which is lessened when drug is taken with food.
		Monitor blood glucose levels.	Drug can induce hyperglycemia.
Amprenavir (Agenerase)	200 mg q12h	Monitor blood glucose levels.	Drug can induce hyperglycemia.
Lopinavir (Kaletra; ABT-378/r)	400 mg q12h	Administer with food.	Food enhances drug absorption.
		Administer with 100 mg ritonavir.	Ritonavir synergizes drug activity.
		Avoid giving to clients with known sulfonamide allergy.	Cross-reactivity is possible.
RIBONUCLEOTIDE REDUCTASE INHIBITORS			
Hydroxyurea (Hydrea)	500-1000 mg daily	Monitor CBC.	Drug induces bone marrow suppression.

Data from *United States Pharmacopeia Dispensing Information (USP DI): Vol. I. Drug information for the health care professional* (20th ed.). (2000). Englewood, CO: Micromedix.
CBC, Complete blood count.

COST OF CARE IMPLICATIONS FOR NURSING

ANTIRETROVIRAL DISEASE

Cost of Care

- The most useful agents in suppressing retroviral replication are combinations of nucleoside analog reverse transcriptase inhibitors, non-nucleoside analog reverse transcriptase inhibitors, and protease inhibitors.
- The cost of maintaining therapeutic levels of these drug combinations ranges between $1100 and $2000 per month.
- These drug combinations cause many unpleasant and severe side effects.
- Without these drugs, clients progress in HIV disease and opportunistic infections.
- Inpatient care costs are high in terms of length of stay and intensive therapies.
- Compliance with drug regimens is difficult, and most drugs are ineffective unless taken regularly as prescribed.

Implications for Nursing

Because of the high cost of antiretrovirals and adherence issues, nurses need to develop individualized plans in conjunction with clients to increase adherence with the drug regimen. Helping clients to take medications as prescribed can reduce hospitalizations for opportunistic infections and contribute to health maintenance.

Data from Bechtel-Boenning, C. (1996). State of the art: Antiviral treatment of HIV infection. *Nursing Clinics of North America, 31*(1), 1-13; Williams, A. (1999). Adherence to highly active antiretroviral therapy. *Nursing Clinics of North America, 34*(1), 113-129; *United States Pharmacopeia Dispensing Information USP DI: Vol. I. Drug information for the health care professional* (20th ed.). (2000). Englewood, CO: Micromedex; and CVS Pharmacies. (March 2000). Personal communication.

TABLE 22-6 • COMPLEMENTARY AND ALTERNATIVE THERAPIES FOR HIV/AIDS

AGENTS WITH ANTIVIRAL EFFECTS	IMMUNE-ENHANCING AGENTS
• Shark cartilage	• Astragalus
• Curcumin	• Echinacea
• Hypercin	• Ascorbic acid
• Compound Q	
• SPV-30	
• Aloe vera	

COMPLEMENTARY AND ALTERNATIVE THERAPIES. Complementary therapies to increase immune function are frequently used by people with HIV/AIDS. Such therapies include vitamins, shark cartilage, and botanical products available at health food stores. The clinical usefulness of these products has yet to be established through well-controlled clinical trials. In addition, some botanicals alter the effects of prescription drugs. The nurse asks the client which botanicals are being used and checks with the pharmacist to determine known drug interactions. Table 22-6 lists the botanical agents used to enhance immune function or slow viral replication.

HEALTH PROMOTION. HIV can remain latent inside a cell for long periods and cause active infection when the cell is stimulated. The specific signals for the cell to become activated are not known, but concurrent viral or parasitic infections are suspected. The nurse teaches the client to avoid exposure to infection (Chart 22-10).

CHART 22-10

CLIENT EDUCATION GUIDE
Prevention of Infection

- Avoid crowds and other large gatherings of people who might be ill.
- Do not share personal toilet articles, such as toothbrushes, toothpaste, washcloths, or deodorant sticks, with others.
- If possible, bathe daily.
- Wash the armpits, groin, genitals, and anal area at least twice a day with an antimicrobial soap.
- Clean your toothbrush daily by either running it through the dishwasher or rinsing it in liquid laundry bleach.
- Wash your hands thoroughly with an antimicrobial soap before you eat or drink, after touching a pet, after shaking hands with anyone, as soon as you come home from any outing, and after using the toilet.
- Eat a low-bacteria diet, and avoid salads, raw fruit and vegetables, undercooked meat, pepper, and paprika.
- Wash dishes between use with hot, sudsy water or use a dishwasher.
- Do not drink water that has been standing for longer than 15 minutes.
- Do not reuse cups and glasses without washing.
- Avoid changing pet litter boxes. If unavoidable, use gloves or wash hands immediately.
- Avoid turtles and reptiles as pets.
- Do not feed pets raw or undercooked meat.
- Take your temperature at least once a day.
- Report any of the following signs or symptoms of infection to your physician immediately:
  - Temperature greater than 100° F (38° C)
  - Persistent cough (with or without sputum)
  - Pus or foul-smelling drainage from any open skin area or normal body opening
  - Presence of a boil or abscess
  - Urine that is cloudy or foul smelling or that causes burning on urination
- Take all prescribed medications as ordered.
- Do not dig in the garden or work with houseplants.
- Avoid travel to areas of the world with poor sanitation or less-than-adequate health care facilities.

IMPAIRED GAS EXCHANGE

PLANNING: EXPECTED OUTCOMES. The client is expected to maintain adequate oxygenation and perfusion, and experience minimal dyspnea and discomfort.

INTERVENTIONS. The nurse, respiratory therapist, or assistive nursing personnel provides interventions, including drug therapy, respiratory support and maintenance, comfort, and rest.

DRUG THERAPY. Appropriate drug therapy is initiated after identification of an infectious or neoplastic cause for respiratory difficulty (see Chart 22-8). A common respiratory infection among people with HIV disease or AIDS is ***Pneumocystis carinii pneumonia (PCP).*** The treatment of choice for PCP is trimethoprim/sulfamethoxazole (Apo-Sulfatrim✤, Bactrim, Cotrim, Septra), given intravenously or orally, depending on the severity of infection. A high percentage of clients with AIDS experience adverse reactions to this medication, including nausea, vomiting, hyponatremia, rashes, fever, leukopenia, thrombocytopenia, and hepatitis.

Pentamidine isethionate (Pentacarinat✤, Pentam), usually given intravenously or intramuscularly, is also used to treat

PCP. Aerosolized pentamidine isethionate is used prophylactically in those with CD4+ counts below 200 and in those who have already had PCP.

Other drug therapies include dapsone (Avlosulfon) and atovaquone (Mepron), which can be used as therapy for existing PCP or as prophylaxis. For moderate to severe PCP, steroids may be added to the regimen to reduce the inflammation.

RESPIRATORY SUPPORT AND MAINTENANCE. The client also needs appropriate care to maintain respiratory function and avoid complications. The nurse, respiratory therapist, or assistive nursing personnel assesses the respiratory rate, rhythm, and depth; breath sounds; and vital signs and monitors for cyanosis at least every 8 hours. Oxygen therapy and room humidification are applied as ordered. In addition, the nurse monitors mechanical ventilation, performs suctioning and chest physical therapy as needed, and evaluates blood gas results.

COMFORT. The nurse or assistive nursing personnel assesses the client's comfort. The client with respiratory difficulties often is more comfortable with the head of the bed elevated. Activities are paced to minimize shortness of breath and exhaustion. The nurse provides psychologic support during periods of respiratory distress.

REST AND ACTIVITY. Most clients with HIV/AIDS experience some degree of fatigue, especially when respiratory problems also are present. Fatigue can be made worse by certain therapies (see the Evidence-Based Practice for Nursing box at right). The nurse consults with the client to pace activities to conserve energy. The client is guided in active and passive range-of-motion (ROM) exercises. Non–time-critical activities, such as bathing, are scheduled so that the client is not fatigued at mealtime.

EVIDENCE-BASED PRACTICE FOR NURSING

HIV-related fatigue may worsen with biologic response modifier therapy

Grady, C., Anderson, R., & Chase, G. (1998). Fatigue in HIV-infected men receiving investigational interleukin-2. *Nursing Research, 47*(4), 227-234.

This purpose of this prospective, descriptive study was to quantify and characterize fatigue experienced by men living with HIV/AIDS. The study was an adjunct to a randomized clinical trial of the biologic response modifier (BRM) interleukin-2 (IL-2). Fifty subjects diagnosed with HIV/AIDS were randomized to an IL-2 treatment group (28 subjects) or a control group (22 subjects). In addition, 20 control subjects who later crossed over to IL-2 treatment also were studied. Data regarding fatigue were collected for all subjects using self-reports of fatigue and subscales of the Piper Fatigue Scale ([PFS], an established measure of fatigue with strong internal consistency, content validity, and concurrent criterion validity), as well as the Global Fatigue Index (GFI). All subjects completed fatigue measures at baseline and at designated intervals for 6 months.

All subjects experienced fatigue as indicated by fatigue scores and self-reports. Subjects in the IL-2 treatment and crossover groups experienced significantly higher scores than did controls within the week following IL-2 treatment, although these scores returned to baseline and were comparable with those of the control group 1 month after initiation of IL-2 therapy.

Critique. This clinical study was well designed and implemented. The number of subjects was appropriate for the measurements used. Results are generalizable within the population studied.

Implications for Nursing. Nurses can validate the fatigue experience in clients with HIV/AIDS. Together, the client and nurse can adjust health care, work-related, and social schedules to allow the client to maintain as near normal an activity level as possible during periods of fatigue.

PAIN

The client with more severe HIV disease or AIDS frequently has pain from a variety of causes. Pain can result from enlarged organs stretching the viscera or compressing nerves. Tumor invasion of bone and other tissues can cause pain. Many clients with AIDS experience peripheral neuropathy-induced pain from the disease or drug therapies. Many suffer from generalized joint and muscle pain.

NOC **PLANNING: EXPECTED OUTCOMES.** The client is expected to achieve an acceptable level of comfort and pain reduction from appropriate interventions.

INTERVENTIONS. Pharmacologic and nonpharmacologic approaches are used to manage pain in the client with HIV/AIDS, depending on the cause of the pain.

COMFORT MEASURES. The use of pressure-relieving mattress pads, warm baths, or other forms of hydrotherapy, massage, and the application of heat or cold to painful areas may reduce pain levels, with or without drug therapy. Care is taken when moving or otherwise physically assisting the client in order to avoid pulling or grasping the client with joint pain. Lift sheets are used whenever possible. The client may be thin and have poor circulation, contributing to pain and discomfort. The nurse helps him or her to change positions frequently.

DRUG THERAPY. The type of drugs used depends on what is thought to be causing the pain. For general arthralgia and myalgia, nonsteroidal anti-inflammatory drugs (NSAIDs) may be helpful in reducing inflammation and increasing comfort without inducing drowsiness.

The neuropathic pain associated with peripheral neuropathy may respond best to tricyclic antidepressants such as amitriptyline (Elavil) or to anticonvulsant medication such as phenytoin (Dilantin) or carbamazepine (Tegretol). Drugs for neuropathic pain may take from several days to weeks before a full effect is seen. During this time, opioids may be needed to temporarily control pain.

When opioids are needed to control pain, the client is evaluated for pain intensity. Mild to moderate pain is treated with weak opioids such as oxycodone or codeine. More intense pain is treated with stronger opioids such as morphine, hydromorphone (Dilaudid), or fentanyl transdermal (Duragesic). Individualized combinations of weak and strong opioids along with nonopioid medications may be used to provide the best sustained pain relief and allow the client to participate in activities to the extent that he or she wishes.

COMPLEMENTARY AND ALTERNATIVE THERAPY. Many clients with pain from HIV/AIDS use therapies such as guided imagery, distraction, progressive relaxation, and biofeedback to help control pain. Such therapies can be used with more traditional and pharmacologic measures to promote maximal comfort.

IMBALANCED NUTRITION: LESS THAN BODY REQUIREMENTS

Many clients with AIDS have difficulty maintaining their weight and nutritional status. This problem may be associated with fatigue, anorexia, nausea and vomiting, difficult or painful swallowing, diarrhea, or wasting syndrome.

NOC **PLANNING: EXPECTED OUTCOMES.** The client is expected to maintain optimal weight through adequate nutrition and hydration.

INTERVENTIONS. Because there are multiple factors for alterations in nutrition in AIDS, diagnostic procedures are undertaken to determine the cause. Once the cause is determined, appropriate therapy is initiated. For example, in the client who has candidal esophagitis, nutrition is affected because of swallowing difficulties.

DRUG THERAPY. Therapy can include ketoconazole (Nizoral) or fluconazole (Diflucan) orally, or intravenous (IV) amphotericin B (Fungizone). The nurse administers the medication as ordered and monitors for side effects such as nausea and vomiting, which further compromise nutritional status. The nurse provides mouth care and ice chips and keeps unpleasant odors out of the client's environment. Antiemetics are used as ordered.

DIET THERAPY. The client's weight, intake and output, and calorie count are monitored. The nurse assesses food preferences and any dietary cultural or religious practices. The client is instructed about a high-calorie, high-protein, low-microbial, nutritionally sound diet. In most cases, he or she is encouraged to avoid dietary fat, since fat intolerance often occurs as a result of the disease and as a side effect of some antiretroviral medications. In collaboration with the dietitian, the nurse provides an appropriate diet, including small, frequent meals (better tolerated than large meals). Supplemental vitamins and fluids are indicated in some cases. For the client who cannot achieve adequate nutrition through food, tube feedings or total parenteral nutrition may be needed.

MOUTH CARE. For clients susceptible to oral ulceration or infection, the nurse or nursing staff member provides meticulous mouth care. Rinses of sodium bicarbonate with normal saline every 2 hours or several times a day are helpful. The client is given a soft toothbrush and advised to drink plenty of fluids. For oral pain that interferes with eating ability, analgesics or viscous lidocaine may be necessary.

DIARRHEA

Clients with AIDS frequently suffer from diarrhea. Sometimes an infectious cause (e.g., *Giardia* or *Amoeba*) can be determined and treated, or the cause is determined but no effective therapy is available, as in cryptosporidiosis or cytomegalovirus (CMV) colitis. Many clients, especially non-Caucasians, are lactose intolerant, and HIV disease may aggravate this pre-existing condition. Diarrhea may occur as a side effect of therapy with protease inhibitors. In some cases, clients with AIDS have diarrhea and no cause can be identified.

PLANNING: EXPECTED OUTCOMES. The client is expected to experience decreased diarrhea; maintain fluid, electrolyte, and nutritional status; and minimize incontinence.

INTERVENTIONS. For most clients with AIDS and diarrhea, symptomatic management is all that is available. Antidiarrheals, such as diphenoxylate hydrochloride (Diarsed✤, Lomotil), given on a regular schedule, provide some degree of relief. In collaboration with the dietitian, the nurse offers dietary counseling and appropriate foods. Recommended dietary changes include less roughage; less fatty, spicy, and sweet food; and no alcohol or caffeine. Some clients experience symptomatic relief if they eliminate dairy products from the diet or eat smaller amounts of food more often and drink plenty of fluids, especially between meals.

The nurse or assistive nursing personnel provides the client a bedside commode or a bedpan if needed. Some clients cannot reach the bathroom in time because of immobility or anal sphincter weakness, others because of the urgency to defecate. The nurse provides privacy, support, and understanding.

IMPAIRED SKIN INTEGRITY

The most common skin lesion in AIDS is Kaposi's sarcoma (KS). Skin involvement may be localized or widespread. Large lesions can cause pain and restrict movement or ambulation. They can impede circulation, causing open, weeping, painful lesions. Another cause of impaired skin integrity is herpes simplex virus (HSV) infection.

PLANNING: EXPECTED OUTCOMES. The client is expected to have healing of any existing lesions and avoid increased skin breakdown or secondary infection.

INTERVENTIONS. KS can be treated locally with radiotherapy, intralesional chemotherapy, or cryotherapy. KS responds to local radiation therapy but only transiently.

Systemic therapy is used in clients with rapidly progressive disease or with significant involvement of the gastrointestinal tract, lungs, or other organs. These therapies include chemotherapy (single agent or combination), interferon-alpha, and interferon-alpha plus zidovudine.

Treatment of painful KS lesions includes the use of analgesics and comfort measures. Open, weeping KS lesions must be kept clean and dressed to minimize the risk of secondary infection. Many clients with cutaneous KS are concerned about their appearance and the risk of being identified as HIV positive. Makeup (if open lesions are not present), long-sleeved shirts, and hats may help in maintaining a normal appearance.

For the client with an HSV abscess, the nurse provides meticulous skin care. Abscesses are cleaned regularly with a diluted solution of povidone-iodine (Betadine) and left to air-dry or dry with a heat lamp. This infection can be painful and requires analgesics, assistance with position, and other comfort measures. Modified Burow's solution (Domeboro) soaks help to promote healing for some clients. HSV infection is treated with acyclovir (Zovirax) given intravenously, orally, or in some cases, topically, depending on the severity of the infection.

DISTURBED THOUGHT PROCESSES

Neurologic changes and alterations in thought processes are major areas of concern for clients with HIV disease or AIDS. These changes may be due to psychologic stressors accompanying the disease or to organic disorders caused by opportunistic infections, cancer, or HIV encephalitis.

PLANNING: EXPECTED OUTCOMES. The client is expected to demonstrate improved mental status and sustain no injury.

INTERVENTIONS. Clients with AIDS suffer from enormous loss and psychologic stress, which complicates the assessment of any changes in behavior or affect. The nurse or assistive nursing personnel establishes baseline neurologic and mental status by using neurologic assessment tools (see Chapter 41) to compare any changes. Subtle changes in memory, ability to concentrate, affect, and behavior are evaluated. Differential diagnosis is important to determine whether the cause of the neurologic changes is treatable.

ORIENTATION. The nurse reorients the confused client to person, time, and place as needed, reminding the client of the nurse's identity and explaining what is to be done at any given time. Using calendars, clocks, and radios and putting the bed close to a window also may help keep the client oriented. The nurse gives simple directions; uses short, uncomplicated sentences; explains activities in simple language; and involves the client in planning the daily schedule. Relatives or significant others are asked to bring in familiar items from home, and all items in the client's environment are arranged in the same location as at home.

DRUG THERAPY. Charts 22-8 and 22-9 list agents appropriate for different conditions contributing to altered thought processes in the person with AIDS. In addition, psychotropic medications can be used to treat ongoing behavioral problems or emotional disorders. Antidepressants and anxiolytics are commonly used to help this population.

SAFETY MEASURES. Attention to safety is crucial to the well-being of the neurologically impaired client with AIDS. He or she may not be aware of activities or surroundings and may need assistance with bathing, dressing, eating, ambulating, and other activities of daily living. The environment, whether a hospital room, long-term care facility, or home, is made safe and comfortable. Some clients are prone to seizures. The nurse or assistive nursing personnel institutes seizure precautions, including using padded siderails and having an artificial oral airway available. Anticonvulsants may be added to the medications.

The nurse assesses the client with neurologic disease for signs and symptoms of increased intracranial pressure. Any changes in level of consciousness, vital signs, pupil size or reactivity, or limb strength are reported immediately to the physician for appropriate intervention. Some clients are given corticosteroids to reduce intracranial pressure.

SUPPORT. The nurse and assistive nursing personnel work closely with the family and significant others of the neurologically impaired client. There is great trauma in seeing a loved one unable to care for himself or herself or demonstrating unusual or childlike behavior. The nurse answers questions honestly and sensitively and teaches the family and significant others how to reorient the client. They are encouraged to continue to provide the client with news of family happenings or current events. The nurse, in collaboration with the social worker, identifies community resources for the client and family.

SITUATIONAL LOW SELF-ESTEEM

The client with AIDS is susceptible to changes in self-esteem and self-concept. Contributing to this are real and often dramatic changes in appearance that alter the person's body image. Many clients also experience abrupt, significant changes in their relationships with others and in day-to-day activities, including a job or other productive activities. All changes can disrupt the self-concept.

NOC **PLANNING: EXPECTED OUTCOMES.** The client is expected to identify positive aspects of himself or herself and accept himself or herself.

INTERVENTIONS. The entire health care team provides a climate of acceptance for clients with AIDS by promoting a trusting relationship and helping clients express feelings and identify positive aspects of themselves. The nurse allows for privacy but does not avoid or isolate the client. Self-care, independence, control, and decision making are encouraged by helping the client formulate short-term, attainable goals and offering encouragement and praise when these are achieved.

COMPLEMENTARY AND ALTERNATIVE THERAPIES. Complementary therapy in the form of guided imagery is used by many clients to increase their sense of control and enhance self-esteem. Imagery can focus on helping clients cope with distressing side effects or painful procedures. Other uses of imagery include picturing battle scenes in which the virus is killed by immune system cells.

SOCIAL ISOLATION

Many clients with AIDS face discrimination, rejection, and isolation. Friends or health care workers sometimes avoid or refuse to have anything to do with them. Misunderstanding and fear lead to misuse of proper infection control procedures, and clients are inappropriately isolated.

PLANNING: EXPECTED OUTCOMES. The client is expected to identify behaviors that cause social isolation and demonstrate behaviors that reduce social isolation.

INTERVENTIONS. Interventions for social isolation focus on promoting interactions and on education to reduce fear of AIDS transmission.

PROMOTION OF INTERACTION. The nurse does not isolate the client but establishes a therapeutic nurse-client relationship. Showing understanding and concern while helping the client find ways to minimize feelings of rejection and isolation is important. The nurse reduces barriers to social contact. Social support resources are assessed. Family and significant others are taught about HIV transmission and the use of standard precautions to reduce anxiety and increase contact with the client (see Chapter 26).

The client is encouraged to verbalize feelings about self, coping skills, and a sense of ability to control the situation. The nurse helps in identifying support systems, including those already in place and those that need to be arranged.

EDUCATION. The most important aspect for prevention of HIV transmission is education. All people, regardless of age, gender, ethnicity, or sexual orientation, are susceptible to HIV infection. HIV infection is preventable because of the mode of viral transmission and the fragile nature of the virus. (See earlier discussion under Prevention, pp. 368-370).

CRITICAL THINKING CHALLENGE

Your client, a 28-year-old sexually active woman, has been diagnosed with HIV/AIDS at CDC classification B2. In addition, she tells you she is about 11 weeks pregnant and does not want to take medications that might harm the baby. She does not want her husband to know she has AIDS, because she is certain that she acquired the disease from another sexual contact in the past.

- How will your care of this client be different to protect yourself and others from exposure to HIV?
- What should you tell her about antiretroviral medications?
- How should you handle her request not to tell her husband about her HIV status?

For suggested answer guidelines, go to SIMON http://www.wbsaunders.com/SIMON/Iggy/.

CHART 22-11

BEST PRACTICE *for* Infection Control for Home Care of the Person with AIDS

Direct Care
- Follow standard precautions and good handwashing techniques.
- Do not share razors or toothbrushes.

Housekeeping
- Wipe up feces, vomitus, sputum, urine, or blood or other body fluids and the area with soap and water. Dispose of solid wastes and solutions used for cleaning by flushing them down the toilet. Disinfect the area by wiping with a 1:10 solution of household bleach (1 part bleach to 10 parts water). Wear gloves during cleaning.
- Soak rags, mops, and sponges used for cleaning in a 1:10 bleach solution for 5 minutes to disinfect them.
- Wash dishes and eating utensils in hot water and dishwashing soap or detergent.
- Clean bathroom surfaces with regular household cleaners, then disinfect them with a 1:10 solution of household bleach.

Laundry
- Rinse clothes, towels, or bedclothes if they become soiled with feces, vomitus, sputum, urine, or blood. Then dispose of the soiled water by flushing it down the toilet. Launder these clothes with hot water and detergent with 1 cup of bleach added per load of laundry.
- Keep soiled clothes in a plastic bag.

Waste Disposal
- Dispose of needles and other "sharps" in a labeled puncture-proof container such as a coffee can with a lid, using standard precautions to avoid needle stick injuries. Decontaminate full containers by adding a 1:10 bleach solution. Then seal the container with tape and place it in a paper bag. Dispose of the container in the regular trash.
- Remove solid waste from contaminated trash such as paper towels or tissues, dressings, disposable incontinence pads, and disposable gloves, then flush the waste down the toilet. Place these items in tied plastic bags and dispose of them in the regular trash.

Community-Based Care

The usual course of illness is one of intermittent acute infections interspersed with periods of relative wellness over months or years and, ultimately, a chronic, progressive debilitation. Because of the fluctuating nature of HIV infection, the client often spends long periods at home between hospital admissions or clinic visits. In some instances, especially as the illness becomes more severe, he or she may need referral to a long-term care facility, home care agency, or hospice.

The nurse, in collaboration with the social worker, dietitian, and other available resources, works with clients to plan what will be needed and how they will manage at home with self-care and activities of daily living.

HEALTH TEACHING

Educating the client, family, and significant others is a high priority, especially when preparing the client for discharge. The nurse instructs about modes of transmission and preventive behaviors (guidelines for safer sex; not sharing toothbrushes, razors, and other potentially blood-contaminated articles). Caregivers also need instruction about best practices for infection control precautions to prevent transmission while caring for the client in the home (Chart 22-11), nursing techniques to use in the home, and coping and support strategies.

The nurse teaches the client, family, and significant others how to protect the client from infection, how to identify signs and symptoms of potential infections, and what to do if these appear. The nurse instructs about the importance of self-care strategies, such as good hygiene, balanced rest and exercise, skin care, mouth care, and safe administration of any ordered medications (including potential side effects). Dietary teaching stresses the following:

- Good nutrition
- Avoidance of raw or rare fish, fowl, or meat
- Thorough washing of fruits and vegetables
- Proper food handling
- Refrigeration practices

The nurse also teaches the client about preventing infections by avoiding large crowds, especially in enclosed areas, not traveling to countries with poor sanitation, and not cleaning pet litter boxes.

HOME CARE MANAGEMENT

When the client is discharged to home, the nurse carefully assesses the client's status, ability to function, and actual or potential needs for care. Some clients do not need home care but do need to maintain a link with the physician or primary care providers. Home care can range from assistance with activities of daily living for clients with weakness, debility, or limited function to around-the-clock nursing care, medications, and nutritional support for severely or terminally ill clients. The nurse assesses available resources, including family members and significant others willing and able to be caregivers. The nurse helps to make arrangements for outside caregivers or respite care, if needed. Clients may need referrals or help in planning housing, finances, insurance, legal services, funeral arrangements, and spiritual counseling.

Home care aides may be involved in daily or weekly care of the client with AIDS in the home. Usually a home care nurse makes routine visits for assessment purposes, especially as he or she becomes increasingly debilitated. Chart 22-12 lists focused assessment areas for the client with AIDS at home.

CHART 22-12

FOCUSED ASSESSMENT *of* The Home Care Client with AIDS

Assess cardiovascular and respiratory status.
- Vital signs
- Presence of acute chest pain or dyspnea
- Presence of cough
- Presence of fever
- Activity tolerance

Assess nutritional status.
- Food intake
- Weight loss or gain
- General condition of skin
- Financial resources

Assess neurologic status.
- Cognitive changes
- Motor changes
- Sensory disturbances

Assess gastrointestinal status.
- Mouth and oropharynx
- Presence of dysphagia
- Presence of abdominal pain
- Presence of nausea, vomiting, diarrhea

Assess psychologic status.
- Presence of anxiety
- Presence of depression

Assess activity and rest.
- Activities of daily living
- Mobility and ambulation
- Fatigue
- Sleep pattern
- Presence of pain

Assess home environment.
- Safety hazards
- Structural barriers affecting functional ability

Assess client's and caregiver's adherence and understanding of illness and treatment, including the following:
- Signs and symptoms to report to nurse
- Medication schedule and side or toxic effects

Assess client's and caregiver's coping skills.

PSYCHOSOCIAL PREPARATION

Clients with AIDS are often concerned about the possible social stigma and rejection that they may experience. The nurse is aware that this fear is realistic and helps identify ways to avoid problems, as well as coping strategies for difficult situations. Family and significant others are supported in efforts to help the client and provide protection from discrimination.

The nurse encourages clients to continue as many usual activities as possible. Except when too ill or too weak, they can continue to work and participate in most social activities. Because of potential stigma and discrimination, clients are supported in their selection of friends and relatives with whom to discuss the diagnosis. Sexual partners and care providers should be informed; beyond that, it is up to the client. Some clients experience severe depression or anxiety about the future. Almost all feel the burden of having a fatal disease widely considered unacceptable and feel compelled to maintain some secrecy about the illness. Referrals to community resources, mental health professionals, and support groups can help the client verbalize fears and frustrations and cope with the illness.

HEALTH CARE RESOURCES

In many cities, community organizations have been set up to assist people with AIDS. Often composed of volunteers, they offer excellent services to the community. The types and number of services vary by agency and city, but many include HIV testing and counseling, clinic services, buddy systems, support groups, respite care, education and outreach, referral services, and even housing. Clients may also need referrals to other local resources, such as home care agencies, companies that provide home IV therapy, community mental health agencies, Meals on Wheels, and others. In addition, educational materials and support groups are available through Internet access.

CRITICAL THINKING CHALLENGE

The 28-year-old pregnant client with CDC category B2 HIV disease is at home on a drug regimen that includes zidovudine therapy. During a home visit, she tells the visiting nurse that she is short of breath and has pains in her chest.

- What physical assessment techniques should you perform?
- What questions regarding this new problem should you ask?
- On further assessment, you find her oral temperature to be 102.2° F (39° C), and there are crackles in both lower lobes of the lungs.
- What should you do first?

For suggested answer guidelines, go to SIMON http://www.wbsaunders.com/SIMON/Iggy/.

Evaluation: Outcomes

NOC The overall goals for care of clients with AIDS are to maintain the maximum possible level of function for as long as possible, minimize infections, and maintain quality of life and dignity during the course of progressive illness. The nurse evaluates the care of the client with AIDS on the basis of the identified nursing diagnoses and collaborative problems. Expected outcomes include that the client will:

- Not develop opportunistic infections
- Demonstrate adequate respiratory function
- Achieve an acceptable level of physical comfort
- Attain adequate weight, nutritional, and fluid status
- Maintain skin integrity
- Remain oriented and/or in a safe environment
- Maintain self-esteem
- Maintain a support system and involvement with others
- Comply with the appropriate and available therapy

NUTRITION-RELATED DEFICIENCIES

Adequate and balanced nutrition is necessary for the proper functioning of the immune system. For example, lymphocytes are highly active metabolic cells that constantly shed surface components (such as immunoglobulin and marker antigens) and need nutrients to resynthesize these components. Immunodeficiency related to nutrition is an acquired abnormality and results from multiple factors: biologic, political, economic, and cultural. Acquired immunodeficiencies from inadequate or inappropriate nutrition are preventable and treatable.

Malnutrition is a major cause of global immunodeficiency, seen with the greatest frequency in developing countries, in the urban and rural poor of developed countries, and in the chronically ill. Hospitalized adult medical-surgical clients also are at high risk for malnutrition. Four points should be kept in mind:

- Anorexia associated with chronic disease, acute infection, or treatment often leads to reduced oral intake.
- Absorption, assimilation, or utilization of nutrients is sometimes impaired because of gastrointestinal diseases or absorption problems.
- Host defense mechanisms mobilized in infection result in increased demand for nutrients, which is met at the expense of the body's stores.
- Hospitalized clients often receive a semistarvation regimen with many hours of nothing by mouth because of procedures that will be performed or because of IV fluid administration lacking essential nutrients.

Malnutrition can impair any or all aspects of the immune system; the degree of impairment is related to the severity of the malnutrition. An excess of nutrients, especially fats and certain carbohydrates, can also have a detrimental effect on immune function. Nutritional problems are almost never simple, but a complex of deficiency or excess of one or more nutrients.

Protein-Calorie Malnutrition

OVERVIEW

Protein-calorie malnutrition (PCM) affects all aspects of the immune system. The greatest impairment is noted in cell-mediated immunity, with a decreased number of T-lymphocytes, reduced delayed hypersensitivity, and thymic changes. The result is anergy and an increased incidence of infection. The incidence of PCM is unknown, but estimates range from 25% to 50% of hospitalized adult medical-surgical clients. PCM causes a deficiency in energy and protein synthesis, requiring that other body stores (if available) be used.

The following are the usual manifestations of PCM in adults:

- Leanness and cachexia
- Decreased effort tolerance
- Lethargy
- Intolerance to cold
- Ankle edema
- Dry, flaking skin and various types of dermatitis
- Poor wound healing
- A higher than usual incidence of postoperative infection

COLLABORATIVE MANAGEMENT

The management strategy for clients with PCM is to treat the precipitating event and supply protein and calories, sometimes with nutrient supplements. In clients with severe PCM, any infection is treated first and then fluid and electrolyte imbalances are corrected. Then a gradual but steady repletion of protein and energy is undertaken. Often this refeeding begins parenterally, because a severely malnourished gut undergoes atrophy of the mucosa and depletion of gastric enzymes, resulting in an inability to tolerate food. Replenishment of protein and calories is accompanied by vitamin supplementation as appropriate, nutrition education, psychosocial stimulation, and a progressive increase in physical activity.

PCM is easier to prevent than to treat. The nurse is aware of hospitalized clients at risk for PCM. Chart 22-13 outlines best practices to reduce the risk for PCM in hospitalized clients.

CHART 22-13

BEST PRACTICE *for* Reducing the Risk for Protein-Calorie Malnutrition in the Hospitalized Client

- Measure height and weight when the client is admitted to the agency, reweighing at least weekly.
- Monitor the client's ability to eat the ordered diet and the amounts eaten.
- Obtain dietary consultation when needed.
- Evaluate whether nutrients consumed are sufficient to meet basal and stress-related energy needs.
- Avoid prolonged use of standard IV fluids that provide less than 200 calories/L.
- Assess and monitor laboratory values for serum albumin, prealbumin, and leukocyte counts.
- Schedule tests and procedures so that the client spends minimal time fasting.

Obesity

OVERVIEW

The incidence and severity of infectious disease increase among obese people. Impaired cell-mediated immunity and decreased intracellular killing by neutrophils are associated with obesity, making obese people more susceptible to infection. Excess dietary fats have a generalized suppressive action on all aspects of immune function. In addition, the obese client may have a coexisting PCM.

Often the obese client is not recognized as malnourished because of the excessive weight. For these clients, nutritional status must be assessed by laboratory measurements and diet history.

COLLABORATIVE MANAGEMENT

Although more research is needed regarding the interaction between obesity and specific immune functions, appropriate nutrition is an important factor in maintaining and improving host immunologic defenses. The nurse, in consultation with the physician and dietitian, provides a diet that has sufficient calories and protein but is low in fat.

Because the obese client is somewhat immunodeficient, the nurse protects him or her by maintaining a safe environment. Good handwashing is practiced before all contact with the client. All invasive procedures are conducted using strict aseptic technique. The nurse assesses the client every shift for signs and symptoms of local or systemic infection and notifies the physician of any suspected infection.

THERAPY-INDUCED IMMUNODEFICIENCIES

OVERVIEW

Some secondary immunodeficiencies may be related to other conditions that cause the loss of immunoglobulins or destruction of lymphocytes (T- and B-cells). The most common cause of secondary immunodeficiency is iatrogenesis, drugs, and other treatment modalities used for various diseases. Sometimes this is a desired effect, as in organ transplantation or the treatment of certain autoimmune disorders. At other times, immunosuppression is an undesirable, complicating side effect of therapy that is used for another intent, such as cancer chemotherapy, and may even necessitate altering the therapeutic regimen. Various therapies cause different types and degrees of immunosuppression. The challenge is to derive maximal therapeutic effect without leaving the client overly immunosuppressed and susceptible to potentially serious complications.

Drug-Induced Immunodeficiencies

Several classes of drugs have powerful and significant immunosuppressive effects. Some induce general immunosuppression; others are more specific and target one part of the immune system more than another.

CYTOTOXIC DRUGS

Cytotoxic drugs are usually not selective but interfere with all rapidly proliferating cells. White blood cells, including immunocompetent lymphocytes and phagocytes, rapidly proliferate and are therefore susceptible to this type of destruction (see Chapters 20 and 25). The result is a decrease in the number of lymphocytes and phagocytic cells. Cytotoxic agents also interfere with the ability of lymphocytes to synthesize and release products such as lymphokines and antibodies, thereby causing a general immunosuppression. Most cytotoxic drugs are used to treat cancer (see Chapter 25) and autoimmune disorders.

CORTICOSTEROIDS

Corticosteroids are adrenocortical hormones used to treat many immunologically mediated diseases, neoplasms, and several neurologic and endocrine disorders. Corticosteroids have both anti-inflammatory and immunosuppressive effects. They inhibit inflammation by stabilizing the vascular membrane and decreasing permeability, thereby blocking the migration and mobilization of neutrophils and monocytes. Corticosteroids disrupt the synthesis of arachidonic acid, the main precursor for a variety of vasoactive amines.

Corticosteroids sequester T-cells in the bone marrow, reducing the number of circulating T-cells and resulting in lymphopenia and suppressed cell-mediated immunity.

Corticosteroids appear to interfere with immunoglobulin G (IgG) synthesis and immunoglobulin binding to antigen. These drugs have many physiologic and immunologic effects, which can alter disease activity, and numerous side effects, including the following:

- Central nervous system changes, such as euphoria, insomnia, or psychosis
- Cardiovascular changes, such as hypertension or edema
- Gastrointestinal tract effects, such as gastric irritation, ulcers, or increased appetite (with weight gain)
- Other changes, such as cataracts, hyperglycemia and glucose intolerance, muscle weakness, osteoporosis, delayed wound healing, or redistribution of body fat

CYCLOSPORINE

Cyclosporine (Sandimmune) is a specific immunosuppressant that selectively suppresses the helper subset of T-lymphocytes by blocking proliferation and development (see Chapter 20). Cyclosporine is most commonly used to prevent organ transplant rejection and graft-versus-host disease (see Chapter 40). The drug is undergoing clinical trials for use in other disorders, such as uveitis, rheumatoid arthritis, and other autoimmune diseases.

Radiation-Induced Immunodeficiencies

Radiation is cytotoxic to proliferating and resting cells. Because most lymphocytes are sensitive to radiation, exposure can induce profound lymphopenia in lymphoid organs and in the circulation, causing general immunosuppression. Whether or not immunodeficiency occurs after radiation therapy depends on the location and dose of radiation. Exposure to the iliac and femur in adults can cause generalized immunosuppression because these medullary areas are the primary blood cell–producing sites. Total nodal irradiation is used in certain diseases, such as Hodgkin's disease, to induce immunosuppression, causing lymphopenia and decreased T-cell function.

➤ COLLABORATIVE MANAGEMENT

Management of the client with treatment-induced immunodeficiency aims to improve immune function and protect him or her from infection. The most severe immunosuppression occurs while he or she is receiving the immunosuppressive drugs or during radiation treatment. The severity and duration of the immunosuppression are related directly to the dosage of specific drugs. Although this impairment is usually temporary, with good recovery of immune and inflammatory responses evident within weeks or months of therapy completion, the seriousness of the potential infection complications makes this problem a major treatment concern. The infectious processes most commonly observed during this period include those of fungal origin, yeast, some residual viral breakthrough, and a wide variety of bacteria.

The nurse works closely with clients and other health care professionals to provide safe care to those at risk for infection. Chart 22-7 lists specific nursing care actions to prevent infection among clients with drug-induced or any type of immunosuppression. Good handwashing by all health care professionals and assistive nursing personnel before contact with the client is the cornerstone for prevention of infection. Health care professionals must practice asepsis (prevention of contact with microorganisms) when any invasive technique or procedure must be done.

In some instances, drug-induced immunosuppression can be reduced or avoided by the administration of biologic response modifiers (BRMs) to stimulate bone marrow production of immune system cells. Although not appropriate for all types of disorders, this supportive treatment can reduce the client's risk for infection during drug therapy. BRMs are expensive, however, and not consistently covered by insurance. (See Chapters 25 and 40 for further discussion of this treatment.)

Many clients remain at home during periods of immunosuppression. The nurse teaches the client and family best practices to reduce the client's chances of developing an infection (see Chart 22-11).

For clients receiving chronic therapy with immunosuppressive drugs, drug dosages are regulated according to their responses. The aim is to give the lowest dose that will achieve the desired effect.

CONGENITAL (PRIMARY) IMMUNODEFICIENCIES

Congenital, or primary, immunodeficiencies are disorders in which the immunodeficient person is born with a defect in the development or function of one or more of the immune components. As a result, the immune response does not adequately protect the client from infection, cancer, or other disease. Fortunately, most congenital immunodeficiencies are rare.

Some congenital immunodeficiencies are inherited as an X-linked trait (such as Bruton's agammaglobulinemia or Wiskott-Aldrich syndrome), and some are autosomal recessive (such as immunodeficiency with ataxia-telangiectasia). For many congenital immunodeficiencies, however, the genetic defect and inheritance pattern have not been clearly identified. Examples of congenital immunodeficiencies are listed in Table 22-7.

Congenital immunodeficiencies are classified according to the type of immune function that is impaired: antibody mediated, cell mediated, or combined. Because cell-mediated and combined immunodeficiencies are so severe that the affected person usually does not survive infancy or childhood, only antibody-mediated immunodeficiencies (seen in adults) are discussed in this chapter.

TABLE 22-7 • CONGENITAL IMMUNODEFICIENCIES

ANTIBODY-MEDIATED IMMUNODEFICIENCIES
- X-linked agammaglobulinemia (Bruton's)
- Acquired hypogammaglobulinemia (common variable immunodeficiency)
- Selective IgA deficiency

CELL-MEDIATED IMMUNODEFICIENCIES
- Congenital thymic aplasia (DiGeorge syndrome)
- Chronic mucocutaneous candidiasis

COMBINED IMMUNODEFICIENCIES
- Severe combined immunodeficiencies
- Wiskott-Aldrich syndrome
- Immunodeficiency with ataxia-telangiectasia
- Nezelof syndrome

BRUTON'S AGAMMAGLOBULINEMIA

OVERVIEW

A classic congenital antibody-mediated immunodeficiency is Bruton's, or X-linked, agammaglobulinemia. Boys born with this disease usually start to have problems at about 6 months of age, after maternal antibodies, transferred through the placenta, have been lost. The first signs and symptoms are recurrent sinusitis, pneumonia, otitis, furunculosis, meningitis, and septicemia with organisms such as *Pneumococcus, Streptococcus,* and *Haemophilus.* Laboratory evaluation of the client with Bruton's agammaglobulinemia shows an absence of circulating immunoglobulin.

COLLABORATIVE MANAGEMENT

Except for clients with poliomyelitis, chronic echovirus infection, or a lymphoreticular malignancy, the overall prognosis for Bruton's agammaglobulinemia is fairly good if antibody replacement is started early. IV or intramuscular (IM) immune serum globulin is regularly given to these clients, usually about 100 to 400 mg/kg every 3 to 4 weeks (Table 22-8). The dosage and schedule are individualized. Intermittent courses of antibiotics are used for specific infections. Long-term prophylactic antibiotic therapy may also be used. Despite therapy, severe sinopulmonary disease later develops in some clients.

COMMON VARIABLE IMMUNODEFICIENCY

OVERVIEW

The client with common variable immunodeficiency, or acquired hypogammaglobulinemia, has recurrent bacterial infections similar to those seen with Bruton's agammaglobulinemia. The client has low levels of circulating antibodies (immunoglobulins) of all classes.

Acquired hypogammaglobulinemia differs from Bruton's agammaglobulinemia in that it usually first appears later (in adolescence or young adulthood), occurs almost equally in males and females, and is associated with a less severe susceptibility to infection. Frequent complications include **giardiasis** (intestinal infection with the protozoon *Giardia lamblia*), bronchiectasis, gastric carcinoma, lymphoreticular malignancy, and **cholelithiasis** (gallbladder stones).

COLLABORATIVE MANAGEMENT

Treatment is similar to that for Bruton's agammaglobulinemia. Regular administration of IV or IM immune serum globulin and regular or intermittent use of antibiotics protect the affected person against infection.

SELECTIVE IMMUNOGLOBULIN A DEFICIENCY

OVERVIEW

Selective immunoglobulin A (IgA) deficiency is the most common congenital immunodeficiency, occurring in 1 per 600 to 800 individuals (Cotran, Kumar, & Collins, 1999). The client may be asymptomatic or have chronic recurrent upper respiratory tract infections, skin infections, urinary tract infections, vaginal infections, and diarrhea. Usually clients with selective IgA deficiency have a normal life span. Because IgA is the major antibody in secretions, bacterial infections are seen primarily in the respiratory, gastrointestinal, and urogenital tracts. Some adults with IgA deficiency also have malabsorption syndrome.

COLLABORATIVE MANAGEMENT

Therapy for selective IgA deficiency is limited to appropriate and vigorous treatment of infections. Unlike other immunoglobulin deficiencies, *selective IgA deficiency should never be treated with exogenous immune globulin* for two reasons. First, exogenous immune globulin contains very little IgA, and administration would not help boost IgA levels. Second, because clients with selective IgA deficiency make normal amounts of all other antibodies, they are at high risk for severe allergic reactions to exogenous immune globulin. If malabsorption syndrome accompanies the selective IgA deficiency, the client will need nutritional supplementation (such as partial or total enteral or parenteral nutrition).

TABLE 22-8 • ADMINISTRATION OF INTRAVENOUS IMMUNE SERUM GLOBULIN

Indications	Dosage	Interventions	Rationale
B cell or humoral immunodeficiencies • Bruton's hypogammaglobulinemia • Common variable immunodeficiency • Combined immunodeficiencies: severe combined immunodeficiencies Pediatric AIDS	Gamimmune 100-200 mg/kg or 2-4 mL/kg IV once monthly *or* Sandoglobulin 0.2-0.3 g/kg IV once monthly Gammagard 200-400 mg/kg IV once monthly Iveegam 200-800 mg/kg IV once monthly	Observe client closely and monitor vital signs during infusion and for 30-60 min thereafter.	Monitoring detects signs of anaphylaxis and routine side effects. Side effects occur in 10% of clients and include skeletal pain, back pain, nausea, chills, headache, chest tightness, and abdominal cramps.
		Slow the rate of infusion or stop it temporarily if side effects occur.	Side effects appear to be related to the rate of infusion.

ONLINE RESOURCES

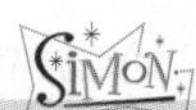

For suggested readings and Internet resources, go to http://www.wbsaunders.com/SIMON/Iggy/.

SELECTED BIBLIOGRAPHY

Asterisk indicates a classic or definitive work on this subject.

Abbas, A., Lichtman, A., & Pober, J. (1997). *Cellular and molecular immunology* (3rd ed.). Philadelphia: W.B. Saunders.

*Barnes, D. (1995). HIV-1-infected long-term non-progressors: A distinct group or part of a continuum? *Journal of NIH Research, 7*(2), 19-21.

*Bechtel-Boenning, C. (1996). State of the art: Antiviral treatment of HIV infection. *Nursing Clinics of North America, 31*(1), 1-13.

Bjorgen, S. (1998). Clinical snapshot: Herpes zoster. *American Journal of Nursing, 98*(2), 46-47.

Bursaw, M., Keenan, K., & Ehrhart, M. (2001). HIV update. *Nursing 2001, 31*(2), 62-63.

*Centers for Disease Control. (1987). Public Health Service guidelines for counseling and antibody testing to prevent HIV infection and AIDS. *Morbidity and Mortality Weekly Report, 36*(31), 509-515.

*Centers for Disease Control. (1991). Recommendations for preventing transmission of human immunodeficiency virus and hepatitis B virus to patients during exposure-prone invasive procedures. *Morbidity and Mortality Weekly Report, 40*(RR-8), 1-9.

Centers for Disease Control and Prevention. (1998a). Public Health Service guidelines for the management of health-care worker exposure to HIV and recommendations for postexposure prophylaxis. *Morbidity and Mortality Weekly Report, 47*(RR-7), 1-32.

Centers for Disease Control and Prevention. (1998b). Public Health Service taskforce recommendations for the use of anti-retroviral drugs in pregnant women infected with HIV-1 for maternal health and reducing perinatal HIV-1 transmission in the U.S. *Morbidity and Mortality Weekly Report, 47*(RR-2), 1-30.

Centers for Disease Control and Prevention. (1999a). *HIV/AIDS Surveillance Report, 11*(1), Atlanta: Author.

Centers for Disease Control and Prevention. (1999b). 1999 USPHS/IDSA guidelines for the prevention of opportunistic infections in persons infected with human immunodeficiency virus. *Morbidity and Mortality Weekly Report, 48*(RR-10), 1-66.

Centers for Disease Control and Prevention. (2000). *HIV/AIDS Surveillance Report, 12*(1), Atlanta: Author.

Cochran, A., & Wilson, B.A. (1999). Current management of AIDS and related opportunistic infections. *MEDSURG Nursing, 8*(4), 257-266.

Cohen, O., et al. (1997). Heterozygosity for a defective gene for CC chemokine receptor 5 is not the sole determinant for the immunologic and virologic phenotype of HIV-infected long-term nonprogressors. *Journal of Clinical Investigation, 100*(7), 1581-1589.

Cotran, R., Kumar, V., & Collins, T. (1999). *Robbins' pathologic basis of disease* (6th ed.). Philadelphia: W.B. Saunders.

Dube, M., & Sattler, F. (1998). Metabolic complications of antiretroviral therapy. *AIDS Clinical Care, 10*(6), 41-44.

Emlet, C. (1997). HIV/AIDS in the elderly. *Home Care Provider, 2*(2), 69-75.

Evans, B. (1999). Complementary therapies and HIV infection. *American Journal of Nursing, 99*(2), 42-45.

Freeman, E., & MacIntyre, R. (1999). Evaluating alternative treatments for HIV infection. *Nursing Clinics of North America, 34*(1), 147-162.

Gallagher, D. (1999). The era of managed care: The struggle of cost containment and compassionate, effective care of persons with HIV/AIDS. *Nursing Clinics of North America, 34*(1), 227-235.

Grady, C., Anderson, R., & Chase, G. (1998). Fatigue in HIV-infected men receiving investigational interleukin-2. *Nursing Research, 47*(4), 227-234.

Greene, K., et al. (1999). Most frequently used alternative and complementary therapies and activities by participants in the AMCOA study. *Journal of the Association of Nurses in AIDS Care, 10*(3), 60-73.

*Imagawa, D.T., et al. (1989). Human immunodeficiency virus type 1 infection in homosexual men who remain seronegative for prolonged periods. *New England Journal of Medicine, 320*(22), 1458-1489.

Jagger, J., & Perry, J. (1999). Power in numbers: Reducing your risk of bloodborne exposures. *Nursing99, 29*(1), 51-52.

Keithley, J., & Swanson, B. (1998). Minimizing HIV/AIDS malnutrition. *MEDSURG Nursing, 7*(5), 256-267.

Kemppainen, J.K. (2001). Prediction of quality of life in AIDS patients. *Journal of the Association of Nurses in AIDS Care, 12*(1), 61-70.

Konkle-Parker, D. (1998). Early HIV detection and treatment. *ADVANCE for Nurse Practitioners, 6*(9), 63-66.

Lisanti, P., & Zwolski, K. (1997). Understanding the devastation of AIDS. *American Journal of Nursing, 97*(1), 26-35.

McClinsey, S. (1999). Occupational exposure to HIV: Considerations for postexposure prophylaxis and prevention. *Nursing Clinics of North America, 34*(1), 213-225.

McCloskey, J.C, & Bulechek, G.M (2000). *Nursing interventions classification (NIC)* (3rd ed.). St. Louis: Mosby.

Mitsuyasu, R. (1999). Immune reconstitution in HIV disease. *Disease Management Digest, 3*(3), 2-3.

*National Institute of Allergy and Infectious Disease. (February 21, 1994). AZT reduces rate of maternal transmission of HIV. *NIAID News.*

O'Neill, D., & Elaine, K. (1998). Spirituality and chronic illness. *Image: The Journal of Nursing Scholarship, 30*(3), 275-280.

Porche, D. (1999). State of the art: Antiviral and prophylactic treatments in HIV/AIDS. *Nursing Clinics of North America, 34*(1), 95-112.

Sande, M.A., & Volberding, P.A. (1999). *The medical management of AIDS* (6th ed.). Philadelphia: W.B. Saunders.

Sowell, R., Moneyham, L., & Aradno-Naranjo, A. (1999). The care of women with AIDS: Special needs and considerations. *Nursing Clinics of North America, 34*(1), 179-197.

Tetreault, D. (1998). Managing and treating AIDS-related diarrhea. *ADVANCE for Nurse Practitioners, 6*(7), 55-60.

Ungvarski, P. (1997). Update on HIV infection. *American Journal of Nursing, 97(*1), 44-52.

Ungvarski, P., & Flaskerud, J. (1999). *HIV/AIDS: A guide to primary care management* (4th ed.). Philadelphia: W.B. Saunders.

United States Pharmacopeia Dispensing Information (USP DI): Vol. I. Drug information for the health care professional (20th ed.). (2000). Englewood, CO: Micromedix.

Williams, A. (1999a). Adherence to highly active antiretroviral therapy. *Nursing Clinics of North America, 34*(1), 113-129.

Williams, A. (1999b). Bridging the gap: Bringing new antiretroviral medications into the clinic. *ADVANCE for Nurse Practitioners, 7*(1), 24-32.

Wolfe, G. (1999). Anemia-related fatigue in patients with HIV/AIDS. *Journal of Care Management, 5*(3), 86, 88, 93-94, 96, 98.

Yeargin, P. (1998). An important risk group: Managing occupational HIV exposure. *ADVANCE for Nurse Practitioners, 6*(11), 55-60, 93.

CHAPTER 23

Interventions for Clients with Immune Function Excess: Hypersensitivity (Allergy) and Autoimmunity

M. LINDA WORKMAN

Learning Objectives

After studying this chapter, you should be able to:

1. Compare and contrast the bases for and manifestations of allergy and autoimmunity.
2. Discuss the nursing responsibility for a client experiencing anaphylaxis.
3. Describe allergy testing techniques.
4. List the defining characteristics of type I, type II, type III, type IV, and type V hypersensitivity reactions.
5. Explain the differences in mechanisms of action between antihistamines and mast cell stabilizers.

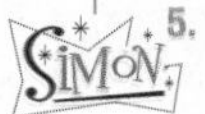

Go to http://www.wbsaunders.com/SIMON/Iggy/ for self-assessment questions related to these Learning Objectives.

The inflammatory and immune responses are normally beneficial. They not only protect the body against microorganism invasion and cancer development, but they also stimulate tissue growth and repair after injury. However, when inflammation or immune responses are prolonged, excessive, or occur at an inappropriate time, normal tissues can be damaged instead of protected. These responses are considered "overreactions" to invaders and foreign antigens and are known as **hypersensitivity** or **allergic** responses. In addition, inflammatory and immune responses can fail to recognize self-cells and literally attack normal body tissues. This type of reaction is known as an **autoimmune** response. Both hypersensitivity and autoimmune responses can damage cells, tissues, or organs and have serious consequences.

HYPERSENSITIVITY/ALLERGY

A hypersensitivity or allergy is a state of increased or excessive response to the presence of an **antigen** (foreign protein or **allergen**) to which the client has been previously exposed. These responses cause symptoms that range from uncomfortable (e.g., itchy, watery eyes or sneezing) to life threatening (e.g., allergic asthma, anaphylaxis, bronchoconstriction, or circulatory collapse). The terms *hypersensitivity* and *allergy* are synonymous and are used interchangeably. Hypersensitivity or allergy reactions are classified into five basic types, which are determined by differences in timing, mechanism, pathophysiology, and clinical manifestations (Table 23-1). Each type may occur alone or in combination with one or more other types.

TYPE I: RAPID HYPERSENSITIVITY REACTIONS

Type I (rapid) hypersensitivity, sometimes called **atopic** allergy, is the most common type of hypersensitivity. This type results from increased production of the immunoglobulin E (IgE) antibody class. An acute inflammatory reaction occurs when IgE responds to an otherwise harmless antigen (e.g., pollen) and causes the release of histamine and other vasoactive amines from basophils, eosinophils and mast cells. Clinical examples of type I reactions include systemic anaphylaxis, allergic asthma (discussed extensively in Chapter 30), and atopic (genetic tendency) allergies such as hay fever, allergic rhinitis, and allergies to specific allergens such as latex, bee venom, peanuts, iodine, shellfish, drugs, and thousands of other environmental antigens. Allergens can be encountered in the following ways:

- Inhaled (plant pollens, fungal spores, animal dander, house dust, grass, ragweed)
- Ingested (foods, food additives, drugs)
- Injected (bee venom, drugs, biologic substances such as contrast dyes and adrenocorticotropic hormone)
- Contacted (pollens, foods, environmental proteins)

Some reactions are confined to the areas exposed to the antigen, such as the mucous membranes of the nose and eyes,

TABLE 23-1 • MECHANISMS AND EXAMPLES OF TYPES OF HYPERSENSITIVITIES

Mechanism	Clinical Examples
TYPE 1: IMMEDIATE	
Reaction of IgE antibody on mast cells with antigen, which results in release of mediators	Hay fever Allergic asthma Anaphylaxis
TYPE II: CYTOTOXIC	
Reaction of IgG with host cell membrane or antigen adsorbed by host cell membrane	Autoimmune hemolytic anemia Goodpasture's syndrome Myasthenia gravis
TYPE III: IMMUNE COMPLEX–MEDIATED	
Formation of immune complex of antigen and antibody, which deposits in walls of blood vessels and results in complement release and inflammation	Serum sickness Vasculitis Systemic lupus erythematosus Rheumatoid arthritis
TYPE IV: DELAYED	
Reaction of sensitized T-cells with antigen and release of lymphokines, which activate macrophages and induce inflammation	Poison ivy Graft rejection Tuberculosis Sarcoidosis
TYPE V: STIMULATED	
Reaction of autoantibodies with normal cell-surface receptors, which stimulates a continual overreaction of the target cell	Graves' disease B-cell gammopathies

IgE, Immunoglobulin E; *IgG*, immunoglobulin G.

causing symptoms of rhinorrhea, sneezing, and itchy, red, and watery eyes. Other reactions may involve all blood vessels and bronchiolar smooth muscle, causing widespread vasodilation, decreased cardiac output, and severe bronchoconstriction; this condition is known as **anaphylaxis.**

Allergic Rhinitis

OVERVIEW

Allergic rhinitis, often called "hay fever," is triggered by hypersensitivity reactions to airborne allergens, especially plant pollens, molds, dust, animal dander, wool, food, and industrial pollutants. Some acute episodes are "seasonal" in that they tend to recur at the same time each year; they coincide with the timing of large environmental exposure and last only a few weeks. Chronic rhinitis, or perennial rhinitis, tends to occur intermittently (with no predictable seasonal pattern) or continuously on exposure to certain allergens. In "nonallergic rhinitis," the same clinical manifestations are present although no allergic cause is identified and the immune system does not appear to be involved.

Pathophysiology

On first exposure to an allergen (an antigen that provokes allergic sensitization with IgE), the person responds by making antigen-specific IgE. This antigen-specific IgE binds to the surface of basophils and mast cells (Figure 23-1). These cells have large numbers of granules containing vasoactive amines (including histamine) that are released when stimulated. Once the antigen-specific IgE has formed, the person is sensitized to that allergen.

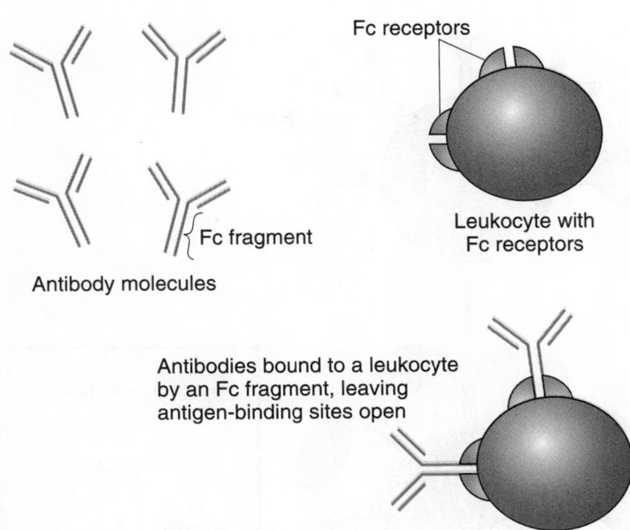

Figure 23-1 • Antibody Fc (fragment, crystalline) receptors on basophils and mast cells.

In a type I hypersensitivity reaction, the previously sensitized person is re-exposed to the provoking allergen. The resulting response has a primary phase and a secondary phase. In the primary phase, the allergen binds to two adjacent IgE molecules on the surface of a basophil or mast cell, which breaks or distorts the cell membrane. These membrane changes cause the cell to **degranulate** and release the vasoactive amines within the granules into the tissue fluids (Figure 23-2).

The most abundant vasoactive amine is *histamine,* a short-acting biochemical. Histamine causes increased capillary permeability, nasal and conjunctival mucous secretion, and itching **(pruritus),** sometimes accompanied by **erythema** (redness). These symptoms last for approximately 10 minutes after the histamine is released. When the allergen is continuously present, mast cells continuously release histamine and other vasoactive amines, thus prolonging the response.

The secondary phase results from the secretion of other vasoactive amines during the primary phase. These other vasoactive amines draw more white blood cells to the area and stimulate a more general inflammatory reaction through the action of the biochemicals leukotriene and prostaglandins. This reaction occurs in addition to the allergic reaction stimulated in the primary phase. The resulting inflammation increases the clinical manifestations and is probably responsible for continuing the response.

Etiology

The tendency to produce IgE in response to antigen exposure is based on genetic inheritance, but no single gene has been found to be responsible. Specific allergies are *not* inherited. Approximately 50% of clients with allergic rhinitis have one parent with type I hypersensitivities/allergies.

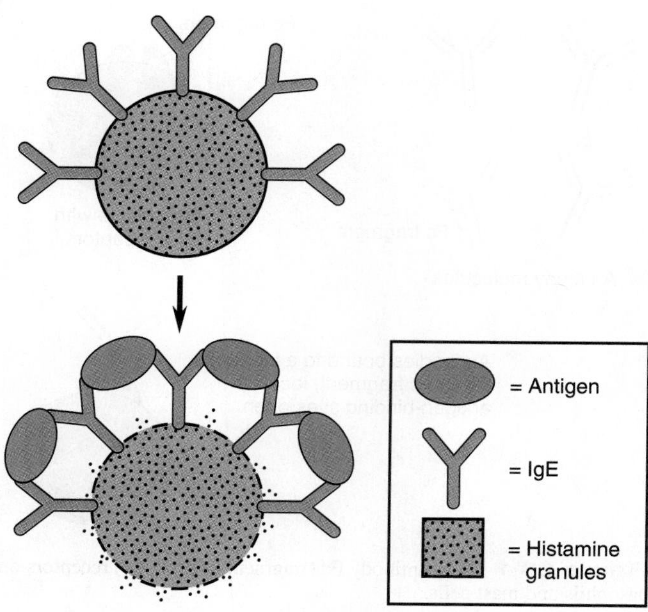

Figure 23-2 ● Degranulation and histamine release. *Top,* Mast cell with immunoglobulin E (IgE). *Bottom,* Mast cell degranulation and histamine release when allergen binds to IgE.

Incidence/Prevalence

Atopic allergies, including allergic rhinitis, affect approximately 10% of the population in North America (Cotran, Kumar, & Collins, 1999). Males and females are affected equally. Racial differences have not been documented.

COLLABORATIVE MANAGEMENT

Assessment

HISTORY

An accurate and detailed history may provide insight into the possibility of allergic rhinitis. The client is asked to describe the onset and duration of symptoms in relation to possible allergen exposure. The nurse asks about work, school, home environments, and possible exposures through hobbies, leisure time, or sports activities. Because a tendency toward type I hypersensitivities can be inherited, the client is asked about the presence of allergies among close relatives.

PHYSICAL ASSESSMENT/CLINICAL MANIFESTATIONS

The client with allergic rhinitis usually has **rhinorrhea** (a "runny" nose), a "stuffy" nose sensation, and itchy, watery eyes. Mouth breathing may be evident, and the voice can have a nasal sound. Drainage from the nose is usually clear or white. The nasal mucosa appears swollen and pink on inspection. The client may have a headache or feel pressure over the frontal and maxillary sinuses. Transillumination of the sinuses may be decreased. If nasal secretions drip posteriorly, the client may have a dry, scratchy throat and the appearance of pharyngitis. The client often feels as though he or she has a cold that has lasted longer than a week. Fever is not usually present unless an infection accompanies the rhinitis.

LABORATORY ASSESSMENT

A complete blood count and differential may be ordered. An increase in the percentage of eosinophils is consistent with allergic rhinitis. A client with severe seasonal allergic rhinitis may have an eosinophil count as high as 12% (with normal being 1% to 2%). Some clients have an increased total white blood cell count, but the percentage of neutrophils remains normal (55% to 70%). If an acute infection accompanies allergic rhinitis, both the total white blood cell count and the number of neutrophils may increase.

Other laboratory tests that indicate the presence of a hypersensitivity reaction include serum immunoglobulin E (IgE) levels and the **Radioallergosorbent Test (RAST).** Normal levels of IgE for nonallergic adults is approximately 39 IU/mL (or less than 100 IU/mL). This level can increase many times in the presence of allergies. The usual IgE test does not indicate the specific allergen—only the tendency to have allergic responses. The RAST can determine the blood concentration of IgE directed against a specific antigen and thus can determine specific allergies. However, the expense of this study limits its use in allergy testing.

ALLERGY TESTING

SKIN TESTING. With most type I hypersensitivities, skin testing can reveal which specific allergens are causing the reaction. Skin testing can be performed as scratch testing and intradermal testing. Patch testing is generally reserved for contact dermatitis and other manifestations of type IV hypersensitivities.

SCRATCH TESTING. A scratch or prick test results in an *immediate* hypersensitivity reaction to an allergen. Scratch tests are used in routine allergy testing to determine the possible cause of allergic rhinitis, asthma, **urticaria** (hives), or any other type I hypersensitivity/allergic reactions. Allergens introduced through a superficial scratch or prick cause a localized reaction (wheal) when the test result is positive. Results are usually determined after 15 to 20 minutes.

CLIENT PREPARATION. For best results, systemic corticosteroids or antihistamines are discontinued for 5 days before the test; this prevents suppression of the inflammatory response to an allergen. Nasal sprays to reduce mucous membrane swelling are permitted, except for antihistamine sprays such as azelastine (Astelin). Some allergists recommend that aspirin and other nonsteroidal anti-inflammatory agents be withheld before allergy testing.

PROCEDURE. The preferred site for scratch testing is the inside of the arm or the back. Alternate sites may be used if a rash or other skin problem is present in these areas. The skin is gently cleaned with soap and water, and surface oils are removed with alcohol.

Small drops of sera containing different known allergens are placed on the skin approximately 20 mm apart. Using a bifurcated skin testing needle, the skin is scratched or pricked through the drop. Skin areas are then examined for the presence and size of a reaction. Areas showing erythema and wheal formation are considered positive for that antigen. The degree of sensitivity is grossly estimated by the size of the response.

Control drops are also applied during the scratch test. Normal saline drops are negative controls, and histamine drops are positive controls. A variation from the expected response to the controls can invalidate the skin test results. If a positive reaction to the saline control occurs, the client may have very sensitive skin or a condition called **dermographism.** In such cases, the reddened test areas may be skin reactions to the scratch or prick rather than an allergic response to the sera. If the histamine control produces a negative reaction, the client may have used an antihistamine recently.

Serious reactions in response to scratch testing are rare. However, the nurse ensures that emergency equipment is readily available during a scratch test.

FOLLOW-UP CARE. After testing is completed, the nurse washes the solution from the skin. Topical steroids and oral antihistamines may be administered to reduce itching and increase client comfort. If the administered antihistamine can cause sedation, the client will need to have another person drive him or her home.

INTRADERMAL TESTING. Intradermal testing is reserved for substances that are strongly suspected of causing allergy but did not test positive during scratch testing. Intradermal testing increases the risk for a greater adverse reaction, including anaphylaxis, but it is a relatively safe procedure. The nurse ensures that emergency equipment is in the room with the client. Small amounts of testing sera (0.1 mL) are injected intradermally on the client's upper arm, and the area is observed for erythema and wheal formation. The degree of hypersensitivity is grossly estimated by the size of the response. Client preparation and follow-up care are the same as for scratch testing.

ORAL FOOD CHALLENGE. Some clients experience allergic rhinitis (and other hypersensitivity manifestations) when the allergen does not come into direct contact with the nasal mucosa but is ingested orally. The oral food challenge has been effective for some individuals in identifying specific allergens when skin testing has been inconclusive and keeping a food diary has failed to determine the offending food items. This test requires the client to eliminate suspected foods for 7 to 14 days before testing. After this time, the client is directed to eat a defined food for at least one day and to monitor for clinical manifestations. When many food allergies are present, the client may need to eat only one food type per day of testing.

IN VITRO TESTING. Hypersensitivity to specific allergens can be tested using an *in vitro* method. One method, the ALCAT, is available in some areas of the United States and is more widely used in Europe. This method involves drawing blood from a client and exposing it to different panels containing food and mold allergens. After incubation, the red blood cells are eliminated, and a Coulter Counter is used to examine the remaining cells (white blood cells and platelets) for size increases and other changes. Positive reactions are those in which the white blood cell size increases by at least 12% and platelets increase aggregation.

CHART 23-1

NIC INTERVENTION ACTIVITIES *for* The Client with Hypersensitivity/Allergy or Anaphylaxis

Allergy Management: *Identification, treatment, and prevention of allergic responses to food, medications, insect bites, contrast material, blood, or other substances*

- Identify known allergies and usual reaction (e.g., medication, food, insect, environmental).
- Notify caregivers and health care providers of known allergies.
- Document all allergies in clinical record, according to protocol.
- Place an allergy band on client, as appropriate.
- Monitor client for allergic reactions to new medications, formulas, foods, and/or test dyes.
- Encourage client to wear a medical alert tab, as appropriate.
- Provide medication to reduce or minimize an allergic response.
- Assist with allergy testing, as appropriate.
- Administer allergy injections, as needed.
- Instruct client to avoid allergic substances, as appropriate.
- Instruct client to avoid further use of substances causing allergic responses.
- Discuss methods to control environmental allergens (e.g., dust, mold, and pollen).
- Instruct client and caregiver(s) on how to avoid situations that put them at risk and how to respond if an anaphylactic reaction should occur.
- Instruct client and caregiver on use of epinephrine pen.

Anaphylaxis Management: *Promotion of adequate ventilation and tissue perfusion for a client with a severe allergic (antigen-antibody) reaction*

- Place client in Fowler's or high Fowler's position.
- Apply tourniquet immediately proximal to the allergen point of entry (e.g., injection site, IV site, insect bite, etc.), when possible.
- Administer aqueous epinephrine 1:1000 (0.3-0.5 mL) subcutaneously at the contact site, if applicable, and proximal to the tourniquet and repeat every 3 minutes, as needed.
- Establish and maintain a patent airway.
- Administer oxygen by mask.
- Start an IV infusion of normal saline, lactated Ringer's, or a plasma volume expander, as appropriate.
- Reassure the client and family members.
- Monitor for signs of shock, airway obstruction, cardiac arrhythmia, aspiration of gastric contents, and seizures.
- Administer spasmolytics, antihistamines, or corticosteroids as indicated if urticaria, angioedema, or bronchospasm present.
- Monitor for recurrence of anaphylaxis within 24 hours.

NIC intervention activities selected from McCloskey, J.C., & Bulechek, G.M. (Eds.). (2000). *Nursing interventions classification (NIC)* (3rd ed.). St. Louis: Mosby.

Interventions

Chart 23-1 lists NIC interventions for allergy management. Common interventions include avoidance therapy, desensitization therapy, and symptomatic therapy. Many clients use a combination of all three interventions for the effective management of allergic rhinitis and other manifestations of type I hypersensitivity.

AVOIDANCE THERAPY. When specific environmental allergens have been identified, the client is encouraged to avoid direct or close contact with these agents. Some allergens, such as

CHART 23-2

DRUG THERAPY *for* Allergic Rhinitis

Drug	Usual Dosage	Nursing Interventions	Rationale
ANTIHISTAMINES			
Diphenhydramine (Benadryl, Allerdryl♣ Hyrexin)	25-50 mg q4-6h	Instruct client not to drive or operate heavy machinery. Do not give during an acute asthma attack.	Drug can cause significant sedation. Sedation decreases the voluntary muscle contractions needed for breathing.
Chlorpheniramine (Chlor-Trimeton, Telachlor, Teldrin, Phenetron)	2-8 mg 1-3 times/day	Avoid alcoholic beverages. Same as for diphenhydramine.	Drug potentiates the effects of alcohol.
Loratadine (Claritin)	10 mg qd	Give every other day to clients with renal or hepatic dysfunction.	Renal or hepatic dysfunction reduces drug clearance.
Cetirizine (Zyrtec)	5-10 mg qd	Reduce dose for clients with renal or hepatic dysfunction.	Same as for loratadine.
Fexofenadine (Allegra)	60 mg bid or 180 mg qd	Same as for loratadine.	Same as for loratadine
CORTICOSTEROIDS (ORAL) *(may be given as a "taper" or "short-term burst")*			
Prednisilone (Cotolone, Delta-Cortef)	5-40 mg/day	Not recommended unless symptoms are severe or debilitating.	Systemic side effects are common and serious: • GI ulceration • Poor wound healing • Decreased immune function • Increased risk for infections • Weight gain • Hyperglycemia • Personality changes • Fluid retention
Prednisone (Deltasone, Prednicot, Orasone, Pred-Pak)	5-60 mg/day	Same as for prednisilone.	Same as for prednisilone.

Data from *United States Pharmacopeia Dispensing Information (USP DI): Vol. I. Drug information for the health care professional* (20th ed.). (2000). Englewood, CO: Micromedix.
GI, Gastrointestinal.

specific foods or drugs, may be easy to avoid. Other substances that are more common in the environment, such as pollen, mold, or dust mites, may require environmental changes.

Many airborne allergens can be minimized by the use of air-conditioning/air-cleaning units. Removing cloth drapes, upholstered furniture, and carpeting reduces airborne allergens. Covering mattresses and pillows with plastic or ultra-fine mesh hypoallergenic covers also reduces exposure to dust mites and mold.

Pet-induced allergies pose special challenges. Sometimes even simple interventions (e.g., keeping pets out of the bedroom, thoroughly cleaning the room to remove animal hair/dander) may help reduce symptoms. Bathing the pet frequently or keeping the pet outdoors can decrease allergen exposure. Depending on the severity of the allergy and how well other methods provide relief, pets with feathers or dander may need to be removed from the household.

SYMPTOMATIC THERAPY. When avoidance therapy is impractical, symptomatic therapy can be very effective in reducing the intensity of the allergic response and making the client more comfortable.

DRUG THERAPY. Drug therapy involves the use of steroidal and nonsteroidal agents (to reduce inflammation), vasoconstrictors, antihistamines, mast cell stabilizers, and new agents that inhibit the release or action of leukotrienes. Some drugs reduce the response, and others actually prevent the response. Chart 23-2 lists common agents used for symptomatic therapy of allergic rhinitis.

Decongestants. Decongestants are available in systemic oral medications or nasal sprays. These agents do not clear the allergen or prevent the release of histamine or leukotrienes. They often have actions similar to those of adrenergic drugs and generally work by causing vasoconstriction in the inflamed tissue, thereby reducing the edema. Common vasoconstrictors used in decongestant preparations are ephedrine, phenylephrine, phenylpropanolamine, and pseudoephedrine. Secretions are inhibited when the vasoconstrictor is combined with an anticholinergic agent such as scopolamine or atropine. Numerous combination decongestants are available by prescription and as over-the-counter cold and allergy medications. Common side effects include dry mouth, increased blood pressure, and sleep alterations. Because the effects are systemic, clients with hypertension, glaucoma, and urinary

CHART 23-2

DRUG THERAPY *for* Allergic Rhinitis—cont'd

Drug	Usual Dosage	Nursing Interventions	Rationale
LEUKOTRIENE ANTAGONISTS			
Zafirlukast (Accolate)	20 mg bid	Take 1 hr before or 2 hr after eating.	Drug absorption is slowed by the presence of food.
		There is an increased incidence of upper respiratory infections when coadministered with inhaled corticosteroids.	Drugs reduce local inflammatory and immune responses.
		Reduce dose in clients who are also taking aspirin.	Aspirin increases plasma concentration of drug.
Zileuton (Zyflo)	600 mg qid	Do not take with terfenadine or theophylline.	Drug increases plasma concentrations of terfenadine and theophylline.
CORTICOSTEROIDS (NASAL)*			
Beclomethasone (Beconase)	1-2 metered sprays per nostril, 1-2 times/day (approximately 50 μg/metered spray)	Use daily as directed.	Effectiveness depends on regular use.
		Symptoms may persist for 2-3 days after initial administration.	Maximum effectiveness requires continued use for 48-72 hr.
Fluticasone (Flonase)	2 metered sprays per nostril qd (approximately 50 μg/metered spray)	Same as for beclomethasone.	Same as for beclomethasone.
MAST CELL STABILIZERS (NASAL)			
Cromolyn sodium (Nasalcrom)	1 spray/nostril 4-6 times/day	Use daily as directed.	Effectiveness depends on regular use.
		Start therapy 3-4 wk before expected allergy season.	Requires regular use for prophylactic effect.
DECONGESTANTS (NASAL)			
Phenylephrine (Neo-Synephrine, dozens of others)	1 spray/nostril 4-6 times/day	Caution client not to use more frequently than directed or for longer than 4 days.	Overuse or continued use causes a rebound nasal congestion and worsens symptoms.
Oxymetazoline (Afrin, many others)	1 spray/nostril bid	Same as for phenylephrine.	Same as for phenylephrine.

*Additional drugs include Nasacort, Nasonex, and many others.

retention should consult with a health care professional before taking any decongestant.

Antihistamines. Antihistamines compete with histamine at the histamine receptor site and essentially block it from binding to its receptor. This action prevents vasodilation and capillary leak. Many antihistamines also have some anticholinergic effects, which assists in relief by decreasing secretions. First-generation antihistamines, which include diphenhydramine (Allerdryl♣, Benadryl) and chlorpheniramine (Chlor-Trimeton, Chlor-Tripolon♣) often induce sedation. Second-generation antihistamines, which include loratadine (Claritin), cetirizine (Zyrtec), and fexofenadine (Allegra), are less sedating.

Corticosteroids. Corticosteroids decrease inflammatory and immune responses in many ways, one of which is preventing the synthesis of mediators. Local corticosteroids in the form of nasal sprays can be helpful in preventing the symptoms of rhinitis. Systemic corticosteroids can produce severe side effects. Therefore they are avoided for rhinitis and are used only on a short-term basis for other problems associated with type I hypersensitivities.

Mast Cell Stabilizers. Nasal sprays containing mast cell stabilizers, such as cromolyn sodium (Nasalcrom), prevent mast cell membranes from opening when an allergen binds to IgE. Thus these agents are helpful in preventing the symptoms of allergic rhinitis but are not useful during an acute episode.

Leukotriene Antagonists. Two leukotriene antagonists are currently available to treat allergic rhinitis. Zileuton (Zyflo) prevents leukotriene synthesis. Zafirlukast (Accolate) blocks the leukotriene receptor. Both are oral agents and work best in the prevention of allergic rhinitis.

COMPLEMENTARY AND ALTERNATIVE THERAPY. Some clients with allergic rhinitis have found relief through the use of aromatherapy. Possible mechanisms of action include competition and desensitization. Some clients with pollen-induced allergic rhinitis report decreased sensitivity after ingesting unprocessed honey.

DESENSITIZATION THERAPY. Desensitization therapy, commonly called "allergy shots," may be needed when allergens have been identified but cannot be avoided consistently. The most common form of desensitization involves subcutaneous injections of small amounts of the allergen. After the allergen has been identified, a very dilute injection solution

(1:100,000 or 1:1,000,000) of the allergen is compounded. A 0.05-mL dose of the initial solution is injected subcutaneously. An increasing dose is usually given weekly (or more frequently) until the client is receiving a 0.5-mL dose. The client is then started on the lowest dose of the next higher concentration of allergen solution. This process is repeated with increasing concentrations of allergen solutions until the client is receiving the maximum dose of the greatest concentration determined to be needed (usually 1:100), depending on his or her response. In general, injections are given at weekly intervals during the first year, every other week for the second year, and every 3 to 4 weeks for the third year. The recommended course of treatment is approximately 5 years.

The mechanism of action to reduce allergic responses by desensitization is thought to be competition. In theory, the very small amounts of allergen initially injected are too low to bind to the immunoglobulin E (IgE) already present but are enough to induce the immune system to make immunoglobulin G (IgG) against that allergen. Because IgG is not associated with either mast cells or basal cells, allergens that bind to IgG do not trigger degranulation and are removed from the body by precipitation (see Chapter 20). By gradually increasing the amount and concentration of the allergen injection, large amounts of IgG are generated specifically against the allergen. When the client is exposed to the allergen, IgG will bind to it and clear it from the body before IgE can bind to it and trigger a hypersensitivity reaction. Because so much more IgG can be produced compared with IgE, IgG is successful in the competition to bind the allergen.

Desensitization can also be accomplished orally. Oral desensitization (sometimes called oral immunotherapy) is more common in Europe and is not yet widely available in the United States. Instead of injections, the allergen is introduced either by swallowing a gelatin capsule (to prevent the allergen from being destroyed by gastric enzymes and acid) or by allowing sublingual absorption. The encapsulated allergen is absorbed in the small intestine, whereas the sublingual allergen is absorbed directly into the circulatory system through the blood vessels under the tongue. Two major drawbacks of the oral desensitization method are expense and the difficulty of dose control. Both methods require higher concentrations of the allergen (compared to subcutaneous injections), and this increases the cost.

TABLE 23-2 • COMMON AGENTS THAT CAUSE ANAPHYLAXIS

DRUGS/FOREIGN PROTEINS
Antibiotics (penicillin, cephalosporins, tetracycline, sulfonamides, streptomycin, vancomycin, chloramphenicol, amphotericin B, others)
Adrenocorticotropic hormone, insulin, vasopressin, protamine*
Allergen extracts, muscle relaxants, hydrocortisone, vaccines, local anesthetics (lidocaine, procaine)*
Whole blood, cryoprecipitate, immune serum globulin*
Radiocontrast media*
Opiates

FOODS	OTHER AGENTS
Shellfish	Pollens
Eggs	Exercise
Legumes, nuts	Heat/cold
Grains	Other
Berries	
Preservatives	

INSECTS/ANIMALS
Hymenoptera: bees, wasps, hornets
Fire ants
Snake venom

*Anaphylaxis caused by these substances is probably a result of direct mast cell degranulation rather than an IgE-mediated hypersensitivity event.

Anaphylaxis

OVERVIEW

Anaphylaxis, the most dramatic and life-threatening example of a type I hypersensitivity reaction, occurs rapidly and systemically. It affects multiple organs within seconds to minutes of exposure to an allergen. Anaphylaxis is not common, and the episodes can vary in severity and symptom. It can be fatal. Many substances can trigger anaphylaxis in a susceptible person (Table 23-2).

COLLABORATIVE MANAGEMENT

Assessment

Typically, a client experiencing an anaphylactic reaction first complains of feelings of uneasiness, apprehension, weakness, and impending doom. The nurse notes that the client is anxious and frightened. These feelings are followed, often quickly, by a generalized pruritus and urticaria (hives). The nurse sees erythema and sometimes **angioedema** (diffuse swelling) of the eyes, lips, or tongue. Intensely pruritic skin wheals or hives commonly appear, and these sometimes merge together in a large, red blotch.

Histamine and other biochemicals cause bronchoconstriction, mucosal edema, and excess mucus production. On respiratory assessment, the nurse notes congestion, rhinorrhea, dyspnea, and increasing respiratory distress with audible wheezing.

On auscultation the nurse detects crackles, wheezing, and diminished breath sounds. Clients may experience laryngeal edema as a "lump in the throat," hoarseness, and **stridor** (a crowing sound). Distress increases as the tongue and larynx become more edematous and excess mucous secretion continues. The nurse may note increasing stridor and anxiety as the airway begins to close. Respiratory failure may follow quickly as a complication of laryngeal edema, suffocation, or lower airway bronchoconstriction causing **hypoxemia** (insufficient oxygenation of blood) and **hypercapnia** (increased carbon dioxide in the blood).

The client is usually hypotensive and has a rapid, weak, and irregular pulse. These findings are due to vasodilation and increased capillary permeability with a resultant leakage of intravascular fluids. The nurse notes faintness and diaphoresis, increasing anxiety, confusion and, if the client is not treated immediately, loss of consciousness. Dysrhythmias, shock, and cardiac arrest may occur within minutes as intravascular volume is lost. Abdominal cramping, diarrhea, or vomiting is less common. Respiratory failure or shock and cardiac dysrhythmias account for 70% of deaths from anaphylaxis.

Interventions

NIC interventions for clients with anaphylaxis are listed in Chart 23-1.

EMERGENCY RESPIRATORY MANAGEMENT. Emergency respiratory management is critical for clients experiencing an anaphylactic reaction, because the severity of the

CHART 23-3

DRUG THERAPY *for* Anaphylaxis

Drug	Mechanism	Side Effects
SYMPATHOMIMETICS		
Epinephrine (Adrenalin)	Rapidly stimulates alpha- and beta-adrenergic receptors of autonomic nervous system (alpha: vasoconstriction; beta: bronchodilation)	Pallor, tachycardia and palpitations, nervousness, muscle twitching, sweating, anxiety, insomnia, hypertension, headache, hyperglycemia
Isoproterenol (Isuprel)	Stimulated beta-adrenergic receptors, relaxing bronchial muscle and dilating vessels	Same as for epinephrine
Ephedrine sulfate (Vatronol)	Similar to isoproterenol, but with longer duration of action	Same as for epinephrine
ANTIHISTAMINES		
Diphenhydramine HCl (Allerdryl✤, Benadryl)	Competes with histamine for H_1 receptors on effector cells, thus blocking effects of histamine on bronchioles, gastrointestinal tract, and blood vessels	Drowsiness, confusion, insomnia, headache, vertigo, photosensitivity, diplopia, nausea, vomiting, dry mouth
CORTICOSTEROIDS		
Prednisone (PO) Hydrocortisone sodium succinate (Solu-Cortef) (IV/IM) Methylprednisolone sodium succinate (Solu-Medrol) (IV/IM) Beclomethasone (inhalant)	Anti-inflammatory; inhibits mast cell degranulation	Fluid and sodium retention, hypertension, cushingoid state, gastric distress, adrenal suppression, psychosis, osteoporosis, susceptibility to infection
METHYLXANTHINES		
Aminophylline (Truphylline)	Relaxes bronchial smooth muscle	Restlessness, dizziness, palpitations, tachycardia, nausea, vomiting, epigastric distress, headache, convulsions
VASOPRESSORS		
Norepinephrine (Levophed)	Raises blood pressure and cardiac output in severely decompensated states	Headache, tachycardia, fibrillation, decreased urine output, hypertension, metabolic acidosis
Dopamine (Intropin)		Dysrhythmias, tachycardia, hypertension, dyspnea, nausea and vomiting, azotemia, headache
INHALED BETA-ADRENERGIC AGONISTS		
Metaproterenol (Alupent, Metaprel)	Rapidly stimulates $beta_2$-receptor sites in pulmonary smooth muscle, causing bronchodilation	Palpitations, tachycardia, dysrhythmias, hypokalemia
Albuterol (Proventil, Ventolin)	Same as for metaproterenol	Same as for metaproterenol, plus painful urination, flushing of the face

reaction and consequences increases with time. An airway must be established or stabilized immediately. The nurse may need to initiate cardiopulmonary resuscitation. Epinephrine (1:1000) 0.3 to 0.5 mL should be given subcutaneously as soon as possible after the appearance of symptoms of systemic anaphylaxis. This drug constricts the blood vessels, increases myocardial contraction, and dilates the bronchioles. The same dose may be repeated every 15 to 20 minutes if needed. Other commonly administered drugs are listed in Chart 23-3.

Antihistamines such as diphenhydramine (Allerdryl✤, Benadryl) 25 to 100 mg are usually given intravenously, intramuscularly, or orally to treat angioedema and urticaria. This agent blocks the histamine receptor site (H_1) in vascular and bronchiolar smooth muscle. If necessitated by the extent of upper airway narrowing, the physician may insert a small endotracheal tube or perform an emergency tracheostomy.

If the client can breathe independently, the nurse administers oxygen to minimize hypoxemia. Oxygen is started via nasal cannula at 2 to 6 L/min or via face mask at 40% to 60% before arterial blood gas results are obtained. The nurse monitors pulse oximetry to determine oxygenation adequacy, with the goal of maintaining an oxygen saturation greater than 90%. If pulse oximetry readings are not satisfactory, arterial blood gases may be tested to determine the effectiveness of therapy. Suction is used to remove excess mucous secretions if indicated. The client's rate, rhythm, and depth of respirations, as well as the presence of bronchospasm and abnormal breath sounds, are assessed continually. The nurse or other assistive nursing personnel elevates the client's bed to 45 degrees unless contraindicated because of hypotension.

For severe bronchospasm, the client is given aminophylline 6 mg/kg IV over 20 to 30 minutes. If the client is tak-

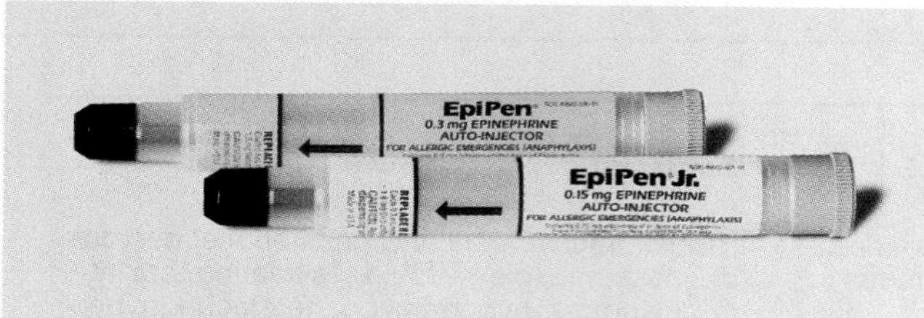

Figure 23-3 ● EpiPen and EpiPen Jr. self-injectors for epinephrine. (Courtesy Dey Pharmaceuticals, Napa, CA.)

ing aminophylline regularly, no more than 3 mg/kg is given. Maintenance aminophylline (0.3 to 0.5 mg/kg/hr) is initiated. The client may be given an inhaled beta-adrenergic agonist such as metaproterenol (Alupent) or albuterol (Proventil) via high flow nebulizer every 2 to 4 hours. Corticosteroids are added to emergency interventions, but they are not effective immediately. To prevent the late recurrence of symptoms, tapered doses of oral steroids are started after the anaphylaxis is under control.

The nurse's primary role in caring for the client with anaphylaxis is to assess for changes in any body system or for adverse effects of drug therapy. For severe anaphylaxis, the client is admitted to a critical care unit for cardiac, pulmonary arterial, and capillary wedge pressure monitoring. The nurse carefully observes for fluid overload from the rapid administration of medications and IV fluids and reports changes to the physician immediately. The client may be discharged from the hospital when respiratory and cardiovascular systems have returned to baseline.

PREVENTION. Because of the rapid onset of life-threatening symptoms and the potentially fatal outcome of this condition, sometimes even with appropriate medical intervention, preventing anaphylaxis is critical. The nurse teaches the client with a history of allergic reactions to avoid allergens whenever possible, wear a medical alert bracelet, and alert health care personnel about specific allergies. Some clients must carry an emergency anaphylaxis kit (e.g., a bee sting kit with injectable epinephrine) or an epinephrine injector such as the EpiPen automatic injector (Dey Laboratories, Napa, CA). The EpiPen device is an easy-to-use, spring-loaded injector that delivers 0.3 mg of epinephrine per a 2-mL dose (Figure 23-3).

The medical record of clients with a history of anaphylactic symptoms should prominently display the list of allergens to which they are sensitive. A careful history is obtained before administering any drug or therapeutic agent. Skin tests should be performed before administering any substance with a highly associated incidence of anaphylactic reactions, such as iodine-containing dyes. Physicians and nurses must be aware of common cross-reacting agents. For example, a client with a history of penicillin sensitivity is also likely to react to cephalosporins because both have a similar chemical structure. Clients with an allergy to bananas are also likely to have a latex sensitivity.

Precautionary measures must be taken if an agent must be used despite a history of allergenic reactions. An IV solution is started, and intubation equipment and a tracheostomy set are placed at the bedside. The client is often premedicated with diphenhydramine (Allerdryl✱, Benadryl). The substance is given first intradermally, then subcutaneously, and then intramuscularly in increasing doses at 20- to 30-minute intervals so the initial dose by the next route does not exceed the final dose by the previous route. When carefully performed, this procedure is fairly safe.

CRITICAL THINKING CHALLENGE

The client is a 52-year-old woman with type 1 diabetes who comes to an urgent care center. She fell 1 day ago and scraped her left shin. She now has a large, red, and indurated area around the abrasion. She is diagnosed with cellulitis and is to begin her first dose of penicillin intravenously because of her diabetes. The client explains that she is allergic to penicillin. When asked what type of reaction she has to penicillin, the client says she gets a severe rash over most of her body. The physician changes the order to cephalothin (Keflin) to be given intravenously for the first dose, followed by oral cephalexin (Keflex).

With the client in an examination room, you start an IV with normal saline and hang a 50-mL piggyback containing 1 g cephalothin and normal saline. The piggyback line is placed in the port closest to the IV needle.

Approximately 5 minutes after the infusion begins, the client says she is having a hard time catching her breath. She feels dizzy and scared. You find her pulse to be thready and too rapid to count. Her lips are dusky, and she begins to wheeze.

- What should you do with the IV?
- What is your next response?
- Why should you or should you not start oxygen on this client?
- Would epinephrine be helpful in this situation? Why or why not? Where, how much, and by what route would you administer it?
- Would diphenhydramine (Benadryl) be helpful in this situation? Why or why not?
- What is the explanation for this reaction to cephalothin?

For suggested answer guidelines, go to SIMON http://www.wbsaunders.com/SIMON/Iggy/.

Latex Allergy

OVERVIEW

Latex allergy or hypersensitivity is a type I hypersensitivity reaction in which the specific allergen is a protein found in processed natural latex rubber products. When the allergen enters the body through inhalation or direct contact with blood vessels (such as might occur during surgery), interaction with immunoglobulin E (IgE) occurs and causes clinical manifestations of type I hypersensitivity reactions, including anaphylaxis. For some people, contact with the latex allergen is limited to the skin or mucous membranes. This causes contact dermatitis, a type IV delayed hypersensitivity reaction (see p. 402). Others may have a "mixed" hypersensitivity response to the latex allergen and experience symptoms of both type I and type IV hypersensitivities. Others may express only one or the other type of reaction.

The incidence of latex hypersensitivity is increasing (Becker, 2000; Floyd, 2000). The individuals most at risk are those with a high exposure to natural latex products, such as

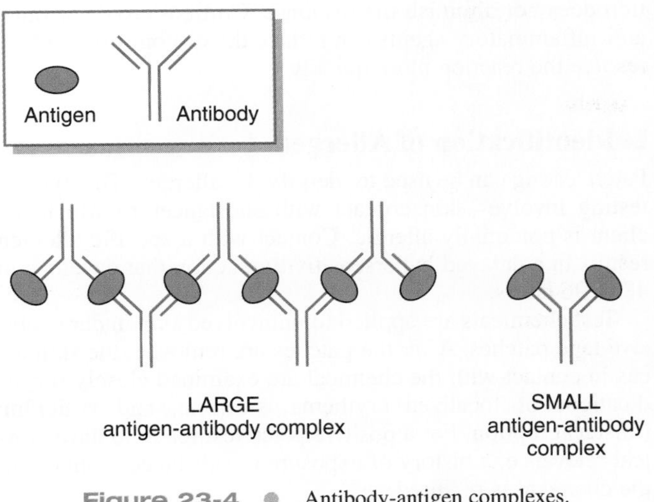

Figure 23-4 ● Antibody-antigen complexes.

health care workers (Karvonen, 1999), clients with spina bifida, and people who routinely use latex condoms.

COLLABORATIVE MANAGEMENT

The nurse questions all clients regarding the use of and known reactions to natural latex products. In addition, the nurse and other health care workers need to consider their own exposure and risk for hypersensitivities to natural latex products.

Avoiding products containing natural latex proteins can prevent reactions and initial sensitivity. More elastomeric products such as surgical gloves, tubing, and vial closures are now being made from synthetic substances containing no latex proteins. One such product is the thermoplastic elastomer glove, ElastyLite. It is essential that latex-free products be used in the care of a client with a known latex allergy. Interventions for the client experiencing a type I or type IV hypersensitivity reaction to latex are the same as for hypersensitivities caused by other allergens.

TYPE II: CYTOTOXIC REACTIONS

OVERVIEW

In a type II (cytotoxic) reaction, the body makes special autoantibodies directed against self-cells or tissues that have some form of foreign protein attached to them. The autoantibody binds to the self-cell and forms an antigen-antibody complex, or immune complex (Figure 23-4). The self-cell is then destroyed by phagocytosis or complement-mediated lysis (see Chapter 20). Clinical examples of type II reactions include Coombs'-positive hemolytic anemias, thrombocytopenic purpura, hemolytic transfusion reactions (when an individual receives the wrong blood type during a transfusion), hemolytic disease of the newborn, Goodpasture's syndrome, and drug-induced hemolytic anemia.

COLLABORATIVE MANAGEMENT

Treatment of type II cytotoxic reactions begins with discontinuing the offending drug or blood product. **Plasmapheresis** (filtration of the plasma to remove specific substances) to remove autoantibodies may be beneficial. Otherwise, treatment is symptomatic. Complications such as hemolytic crisis and renal failure can be life threatening.

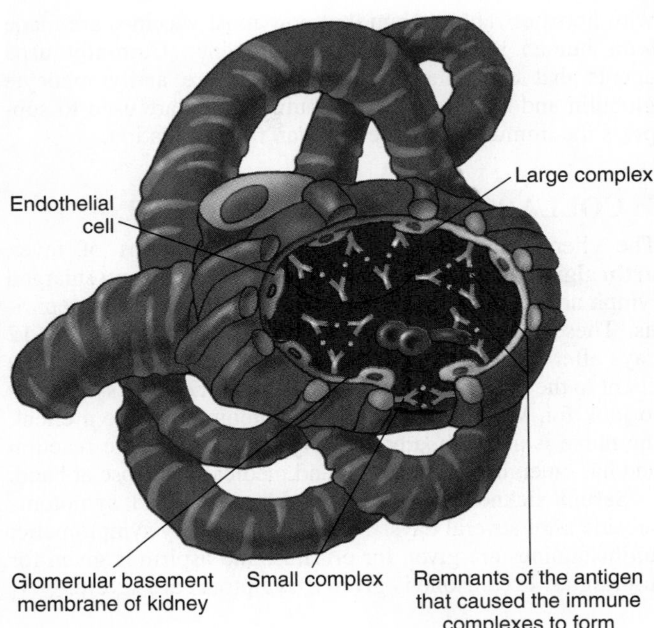

Figure 23-5 ● An immune complex in a type III hypersensitivity reaction.

TYPE III: IMMUNE COMPLEX REACTIONS

OVERVIEW

In a type III reaction, soluble immune complexes are formed, usually with antigen excess (Figure 23-5). These circulating immune complexes are usually deposited in the walls of small blood vessels. Common sites include the kidneys, skin, joints, and other small blood vessels. The deposited immune complex activates complement, resulting in tissue or vessel damage.

There are many immune complex disorders (mostly connective tissue disorders) in which the type III reaction is the major mechanism of disease. For example, the clinical manifestations of rheumatoid arthritis are caused by immune complexes that lodge in joint spaces; this is followed by tissue destruction and, later, scarring and fibrous changes. Similarly, the clinical manifestations of systemic lupus erythematosus result from the deposition of immune complex in the vessels (vasculitis), glomeruli (nephritis), joints (arthralgia, arthritis), and other organs and tissues. In this disorder, the immune complex is composed of cellular deoxyribonucleic acid (DNA) and anti-DNA antibodies. (See Chapter 21 for a detailed discussion of these and other connective tissue disorders.)

Serum sickness is a complex of symptoms that occurs after the administration of a foreign serum or certain drugs. It is caused by the collection of immune complexes deposited in the walls of blood vessels in the skin, joints, and kidney. The most common causes of serum sickness today are penicillin and related drugs and some animal serum antitoxins. Serum sickness used to be quite common when vaccines were made with horse or rabbit serum, but now most vaccines are made with human serum or antigen fragments. Currently used agents that can cause serum sickness are antilymphocyte globulin and antithymocyte globulin, which are used to suppress the immune response in organ transplantation.

COLLABORATIVE MANAGEMENT

The client with serum sickness has symptoms of fever, **arthralgia** (achy joints), rash, **lymphadenopathy** (enlarged lymph nodes), malaise, and possibly polyarthritis and nephritis. These symptoms usually appear approximately 7 to 12 days after receiving the causative agent. The nurse alerts the client to the possibility of serum sickness and what symptoms to look for. When administering a foreign serum to a client, the nurse is also prepared for a type I anaphylactic reaction and has emergency equipment and medications close at hand.

Serum sickness is usually self-limiting, and symptoms subside after several days. Treatment is usually symptomatic; antihistamines are given for pruritus, and aspirin is given for arthralgias. Prednisone is given if symptoms are severe.

TYPE IV: DELAYED HYPERSENSITIVITY REACTIONS

OVERVIEW

In a type IV reaction, the reactive cell is the T-lymphocyte. Antibodies and complement are not involved. Sensitized T-lymphocytes (from a previous exposure) respond to an antigen by producing and releasing certain lymphokines (chemical mediators), and they recruit, retain, and activate macrophages to destroy the antigen. Unlike with a type I hypersensitivity reaction, which occurs immediately, a type IV response typically occurs hours to days after exposure. A type IV reaction is characterized by an accumulation of lymphocytes and macrophages, which causes edema, ischemia, and tissue destruction at the site.

An example of a small type IV reaction is a positive purified protein derivative (PPD) test for tuberculosis. In a client previously exposed to tuberculosis, an intradermal injection of this agent causes sensitized T-cells to accumulate at the injection site, release lymphokines, and recruit and activate macrophages. Induration and erythema at the site of the injection appear after approximately 24 to 48 hours.

Other clinical examples of type IV hypersensitivity reactions include contact dermatitis, poison ivy skin rashes, a local response to insect stings, allograft (tissue transplant) rejections, and granulomatous diseases in which the antigen is unknown (e.g., sarcoidosis).

COLLABORATIVE MANAGEMENT

Intervention

Removal of the offending antigen is the major focus of management. The reaction is self-limiting in 5 to 7 days, and the client is treated symptomatically. Nursing responsibilities include monitoring the reaction site and sites distal to the reaction for circulation adequacy. Diphenhydramine (Benadryl) is of minimal benefit for type IV reactions because histamine is not the main mediator. In addition, IgE does not appear to play a role in this type of reaction, and therefore desensitization does not diminish the response. Corticosteroids or other anti-inflammatory agents can reduce the discomfort and help resolve the reaction more quickly.

Identification of Allergen

Patch testing can be used to identify the allergen. This type of testing involves skin contact with substances to which the client is potentially allergic. Contact with a specific allergen results in a delayed hypersensitivity reaction that develops in 48 to 96 hours.

Test chemicals are applied to uninvolved skin under occlusive tape patches. After the patches are removed, the skin areas in contact with the chemical are examined closely for indications of localized erythema, swelling, and **vesicular** (blister) eruption. For a positive patch test result to have clinical relevance, a history of exposure to substances containing the chemical is required.

CLIENT PREPARATION. To prevent suppression of the inflammatory response to an allergen, systemic corticosteroids or antihistamines are discontinued for at least 48 hours before the test. Topical steroid therapy may be continued as long as the agent is not applied on the area to be tested. To allay the client's anxiety, the nurse explains that patch testing does not involve pricking the skin with needles. The client is informed that testing will involve three separate visits to the allergist or dermatologist: one to apply the test patches, a second for an initial reading, and a third for detection of any delayed hypersensitivity reactions.

PROCEDURE. The upper back is the preferred site for the application of test patches. After the client has disrobed, the back is inspected for evidence of rash and the presence of hair. If a rash is present, alternative test sites are the flanks, the lower back, and the upper arms. Any hair in the area is shaved to prevent poor contact and subsequent false-negative results. Removing skin oils with alcohol allows better adhesion of the patches.

Small quantities of chemicals and solutions in standardized concentrations are placed in separate metal chambers that are backed with hypoallergenic adhesive tape. The tape is carefully applied to the skin so each chemical is held in contact with the skin surface. Each chamber is marked for later identification. As many as 60 or more chemicals may be tested simultaneously.

The nurse instructs the client to keep the test sites dry at all times. Baths are substituted for showers until testing is complete. The client is instructed to use caution when washing the hair to avoid getting the patches wet. Excessive physical activity that results in sweating is discouraged. Reapplying patches that come loose can interfere with an accurate interpretation of true allergic reactions. Thus the nurse reinforces the necessity of removing loose or nonadherent test patches for later reapplication by the allergist or nurse.

The initial reading is performed 2 days after application. The tape containing the chemical-filled chambers is peeled away from the skin, and each area of contact is marked with indelible ink for future reading. The nurse documents any initial allergic or irritant reactions in the client's medical record. The final reading occurs in 2 to 5 days.

FOLLOW-UP CARE. If a potential allergen is identified, the client is given a list of items containing that chemical. These items are to be avoided.

CRITICAL THINKING CHALLENGE

The client is a 25-year-old man who was stung by a wasp on the right hand yesterday while hiking. He experienced no problem except for pain at the site. When he woke up today, however, his right hand was twice the size of his left hand, and it was red, nontender, and very warm. He wonders if he has an infection.

- What additional assessment data should you obtain?
- Why should you or should you not start oxygen on this client?
- Would epinephrine be helpful in this situation? Why or why not? Where, how much, and by what route would you administer it?
- Would diphenhydramine (Benadryl) be helpful in this situation? Why or why not?

For suggested answer guidelines, go to SIMON http://www.wbsaunders.com/SIMON/Iggy/.

TYPE V: STIMULATORY REACTIONS

OVERVIEW

This relatively new category of hypersensitivity reactions involves inappropriate stimulation of a normal cell surface receptor by an autoantibody, resulting in a continuous "turned-on" state for the cell. The classic example of a stimulatory reaction is Graves' disease, a form of hyperthyroidism. In Graves' disease an autoantibody binds to thyroid-stimulating hormone (TSH) receptor sites on the thyroid gland. This binding continually stimulates the thyroid cells to produce thyroid hormones, causing the client to have symptoms of severe hyperthyroidism (see Chapter 64). These symptoms occur even though the thyroid gland itself is completely normal. In a sense, the tissue responding to the autoantibody is "out of control" from the body's normal feedback system of checks and balances.

COLLABORATIVE MANAGEMENT

For type V reactions involving only one organ, management focuses on removing enough of the responding (stimulated) tissue to return the function to normal. With Graves' disease, thyroid tissue is usually either surgically removed or destroyed with radiation. If more than one tissue is being stimulated by the autoantibodies or if the tissue is widespread, the focus of treatment is on reducing the production of autoantibodies through immunosuppression.

TABLE 23-3 • KNOWN OR PROBABLE AUTOIMMUNE DISORDERS

Disorder	Autoantigen
SYSTEMIC OR NON–ORGAN SPECIFIC	
Systemic lupus erythematosus	DNA, DNA proteins
Rheumatoid arthritis	IgG, possibly cartilage
Progressive systemic sclerosis	DNA proteins
Mixed connective tissue disorder	DNA proteins
ORGAN SPECIFIC	
Autoimmune hemolytic anemia	Erythrocytes
Autoimmune thrombocytopenic purpura	Platelets
Diabetes mellitus, Type I	Islet cells, insulin, insulin receptor
Dermatomyositis	Unknown
Glomerulonephritis	Glomerular basement membranes
Goodpasture's syndrome	Glomerular basement membranes, pulmonary basement membranes
Graves' disease	Thyroid-stimulating hormone receptor
Hashimoto's thyroiditis	Thyroid cell surface
Idiopathic Addison's disease	Adrenal cell
Myasthenia gravis	Acetylcholine receptor, acetylcholine
Pernicious anemia	Intrinsic factor, parietal cell, B_{12} complexes
Psoriasis	Stratum corneum
Reiter's syndrome	Possibly collagen, conjunctival cells
Sjögren's syndrome	Salivary gland cells, vaginal mucous cells, lacrimal gland cells
Uveitis	Uveal tract cells (eye)
Vasculitis	Unknown, possibly collagen or endothelial cells

IgG, Immunoglobulin G.

AUTOIMMUNITY

Autoimmunity is a process whereby a person develops and expresses an inappropriate immune response. In this response, antibodies and/or lymphocytes are directed against healthy normal cells and tissues. For unknown reasons, certain cells or tissues of the body are recognized as non–self-cells or are no longer tolerated as self-cells, and immune reactions occur. The resulting antibody-mediated and cell-mediated responses are similar to normal immune responses against non–self-cells, but they are inappropriate and sometimes excessive. The causes of alterations in self-tolerance are not known, but there are multiple theories.

Autoimmunity research is ongoing, and there are few confirmed, established data. Not only is the cause of autoimmunity uncertain, but there is also a lack of consensus regarding which diseases are truly autoimmune. Examples of diseases generally believed to be autoimmune include systemic lupus erythematosus, polyarteritis nodosa, rheumatoid arthritis, autoimmune hemolytic anemia, rheumatic fever, and Hashimoto's thyroiditis (Table 23-3). Other diseases, such as type I diabetes mellitus, may have multiple causes, one of which is autoimmune.

Connective tissue disorders, sometimes referred to as collagen disorders or rheumatic disorders, are characterized by changes in connective tissue. Many of these diseases are considered autoimmune; autoantibodies have been detected for most of these disorders. Connective tissue disorders include systemic lupus erythematosus, rheumatoid arthritis, scleroderma, and polyarteritis nodosa. Most of these tissue disorders are characterized as **organ-nonspecific autoimmunities,** which means that the autoantibodies and the tissue damage are not limited to a specific organ. In organ-specific autoimmunities, tissue damage occurs in a specific organ (see Chapter 21).

COST OF CARE IMPLICATIONS FOR NURSING

NSAID THERAPY

Cost of Care

- Drug therapy with nonsteroidal anti-inflammatory drugs (NSAIDs) remains a standard for autoimmune disorders that are associated with chronic inflammation or chronic pain (e.g., fibromyalgia, rheumatoid arthritis, and systemic lupus erythematosus).
- Aspirin is the oldest and most widely used NSAID.
- Side effects of chronic aspirin therapy include gastrointestinal ulceration and bleeding, increased bleeding tendency, and liver toxicities.
- Newer NSAIDs, especially the COX-2 selective inhibitors, have main effects similar to aspirin and were thought to have fewer side effects.
- The cost for 50 tablets of newer NSAIDs, especially the COX-2 selective inhibitors, ranges from 10 to 30 times more than the cost of aspirin.
- Recent studies using large sample sizes indicate that all NSAIDs, including COX-2 selective drugs, have serious side effects when taken chronically.
- The major side effect for which hospitalization and intervention may be required is gastrointestinal ulceration. In addition, some NSAIDs are known to significantly reduce kidney function to the point that intervention is necessary.
- The major benefit to the use of NSAIDs other than aspirin may be solely in the convenience of once- or twice-per-day dosing.

Implications for Nursing

There may be little advantage to using the newer, more expensive NSAIDs for inflammation and pain. The nurse must caution any client using NSAIDs for more than just a couple of days that these drugs are not harmless. Teaching priorities include administration of the drugs with meals, prophylactic use of antacids or H_2 histamine blockers, and the clinical manifestations of gastrointestinal, liver, or kidney function changes.

Data from Crain, A., DiGioia-Ross, L., & Pham-Vo, T. (1998). The changing face of NSAID therapy. *ADVANCE for Nurse Practitioners, 6*(10), 51-54, 91; *United States Pharmacopeia Dispensing Information (USP DI): Vol. I. Drug information for the health care professional* (20th ed.). (2000). Englewood, CO: Micromedix; and CVS Pharmacies. (March 2000). Personal communication.

Management of autoimmunities depends on the organ or organs affected. Anti-inflammatory drugs and immunosuppressive drugs are commonly used along with symptomatic treatment. (See the Cost of Care box above.)

WOMEN'S HEALTH CONSIDERATIONS

Virtually all autoimmune disorders, especially rheumatic disorders, occur much more commonly among women than men (Cotran, Kumar, & Collins, 1999; Workman, 2000). The risk for autoimmune disease among women compared to men ranges from 5:1 to 20:1. In addition, most autoimmune disorders are more common among Caucasian women than among women of any other race.

SJÖGREN'S SYNDROME

OVERVIEW

Sjögren's syndrome (SS) is a group of problems that often appear in association with other autoimmune disorders. Problems include dry eyes **(keratoconjunctivitis sicca),** dry mucous membranes of the nose and mouth **(xerostomia),** and vaginal dryness. These problems are thought to be caused by autoimmune destruction of the lacrimal, salivary, and vaginal mucus-producing glands. Most commonly, the client with Sjögren's syndrome also has rheumatoid arthritis. Fibromyalgia also is associated with SS.

Ninety percent of clients with Sjögren's syndrome are women between 35 and 45 years of age. SS is more common among clients with certain tissue types, specifically HLA-DRW52, HLA-DR3, and HLA-B8. Although an exact triggering agent has yet to be identified, viral infection is strongly suspected. The three viruses thought to be possible triggers for the autoimmune changes leading to Sjögren's syndrome are human immunodeficiency virus type 1 (HIV-1), human T-cell lymphotrophic virus type 1 (HTLV-1), and Epstein-Barr Virus (EBV).

Insufficient tears cause inflammation and ulceration of the cornea. Insufficient saliva decreases the digestion of carbohydrates, promotes tooth decay, and increases the incidence of oral/nasal infections. Vaginal dryness increases the incidence of infection and may cause pain during sexual intercourse **(dyspareunia).**

COLLABORATIVE MANAGEMENT

Assessment

The client with SS usually has blurred vision, burning and itching of the eyes, and thick mattering in the conjunctiva. Difficulty swallowing food is common, and the client often experiences changes in taste sensation. The nurse asks the client about the presence of nosebleeds **(epistaxis)** and frequent upper respiratory infections.

Physical examination reveals enlarged lymph nodes. If rheumatoid arthritis (RA) accompanies SS, the client has swollen, painful joints and limited joint mobility (see Chapter 21 for a complete discussion of RA). Laboratory assessment may show an increased presence of general antinuclear antibodies, anti-SS-A or anti-SS-B antibodies, and elevated levels of IgM rheumatoid factor.

Interventions

IMMUNOMODULATION. Currently, there is no cure for SS. The intensity and progression of the disorder can be slowed by suppressing immune and inflammatory responses. The agents often used to modulate the immune system in clients with SS include low-dose chemotherapy with methotrexate (Rheumatrex) or cyclophosphamide (Cytoxan). Both agents can have serious long-term detrimental effects, especially on liver and bone marrow function. Other immunosuppressive agents that have shown benefit in managing SS are corticosteroids, cyclosporine (Neoral, Sandimmune), and hydroxychloroquine (Plaquenil).

SYMPTOMATIC THERAPY. A variety of artificial tears and artificial saliva can help reduce symptoms of dry eye and dry mouth. Clients are instructed to use humidifiers in the home to increase the environmental moisture content. The use of water-soluble vaginal lubricants and moisturizers can increase comfort and reduce the incidence of vaginitis. Some clients have obtained significant relief from dry mouth with the use of systemic pilocarpine (Salagen). This agent is a cholinergic agonist that mimics the effects of the parasympathetic nervous system, including increased salivation.

A nonpharmacologic intervention for dry eyes is to block the tear outflow channel (nasal punctum). The punctum can be blocked temporarily with small plugs or closed surgically. Either method allows the scant amount of tears produced to have longer contact with the eye.

Pain control is an issue for clients who have both SS and either rheumatoid arthritis or fibromyalgia. Nonsteroidal anti-inflammatory drugs (NSAIDs), rather than pure analgesics, are most commonly used to decrease inflammation and reduce the associated pain. Many different types and strengths of NSAIDs are available by prescription and over-the-counter. The mechanism of action and side effects are similar for all NSAIDs, although the duration of action and cost can vary considerably (see the Cost of Care box on p. 404).

GOODPASTURE'S SYNDROME

OVERVIEW

Goodpasture's syndrome is an autoimmune disorder in which autoantibodies are made against the glomerular basement membrane and neutrophils. The two organs sustaining the most damage are the lungs and the kidney. Lung damage is manifested as pulmonary hemorrhage. Kidney damage manifests as glomerulonephritis, which may rapidly progress to complete renal failure (see Chapters 71 and 72). Unlike other autoimmune disorders, Goodpasture's syndrome is more common among males and generally occurs in adolescents or young adults (Cotran, Kumar, & Collins, 1999). The exact cause or triggering agent(s) is unknown.

COLLABORATIVE MANAGEMENT

The client with Goodpasture's syndrome usually is not diagnosed until significant pulmonary and/or kidney problems are evident. Clinical manifestations include shortness of breath, **hemoptysis** (bloody sputum), decreased urine output, weight gain, generalized nondependent edema, hypertension, and tachycardia. A chest x-ray study reveals multiple areas of consolidation. The most common cause of death is uremia as a result of renal failure.

Spontaneous resolution of Goodpasture's syndrome has been known to occur but is rare. Interventions focus on reducing immune-mediated damage and in performing some type of renal supportive therapy.

Immunomodulation

DRUG THERAPY. The mainstay of drug therapy for Goodpasture's syndrome is high-dose corticosteroids. Additional drug therapy to suppress the autoimmune response is the same as that for Sjögren's syndrome.

OTHER THERAPY. Additional therapy to modulate the immune responses with this autoimmune disorder involves plasmapheresis (filtration of the plasma to remove some proteins) to remove the autoantibodies. If the lungs and kidneys have not sustained permanent damage, clients undergoing plasmapheresis have shown clinical improvement. Some clients using plasmapheresis need supplemental administration of IV immunoglobulin (IVIG) to maintain antibody protection against infection.

Renal Support Therapy

Depending on the level of remaining renal function, the client may need ongoing dialysis. Therapy usually begins with hemodialysis. For chronic therapy, peritoneal or hemodialysis may be instituted depending on the client's health status, ability to self-manage the infusion and drainage systems, and lifestyle (see Chapter 72).

Renal transplantation is an option for some clients with Goodpasture's syndrome. After transplantation, renal function is normal. In rare instances, clients are disease free after transplantation. In others, the renal problems are improved but pulmonary destruction continues. Some of the drugs required for immunomodulation for the transplanted kidney also suppress the autoimmune response.

ONLINE RESOURCES

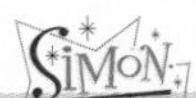

For suggested readings and Internet resources, go to http://www.wbsaunders.com/SIMON/Iggy/.

SELECTED BIBLIOGRAPHY

Abbas, A., Lichtman, A., & Pober, J. (1997). *Cellular and molecular immunology* (3rd ed.). Philadelphia: W.B. Saunders.

Alfonso, L., & Hogan, D. (1999). Contact dermatitis for primary care providers. *Nurse Practitioner Forum, 10*(2), 67-73.

Avella, P., & Walker, M. (2000). Goodpasture's syndrome: A nursing challenge. *Nursing2000, 30*(3), 32cc1-2, 32cc4, 32cc6.

Barrow, S., & Higgins, B. (1998). Self-administered epinephrine: A guide. *ADVANCE for Nurse Practitioners, 6*(4), 55-57.

Becker, H. (2000). An analysis of the epidemiology of latex allergy: Implications for primary prevention. *MEDSURG Nursing, 9*(3), 135-143.

Brewin, A. (1998). Allergy avoidance. *Nursing Standard, 12*(32), 49-56.

Bunn, B. (1999). Itch, scratch, sweat and wheeze: Managing allergic reactions. *Emergency Medical Services, 28*(7), 75-77.

Burt, S. (1999). What you need to know about latex allergy. *Nursing Management, 30*(8), 18, 20-26.

Cohen, S. (2001). About latex allergy. *Nursing 2001, 31*(2), 76.

Cotran, R., Kumar, V., & Collins, T. (1999). *Robbins' pathologic basis of disease* (6th ed). Philadelphia: W.B. Saunders.

Crain, A., DiGioia-Ross, L., & Pham-Vo, T. (1998). The changing face of NSAID therapy. *ADVANCE for Nurse Practitioners, 6*(10), 51-54, 91.

Cunning, S. (2000). When the diagnosis is myasthenia gravis. *RN, 63*(4), 26-31.

D'Epiro, N. (2000). Deciphering autoimmune disease in women. *Patient Care, 34*(7), 49-52, 54, 59, 63-66.

Dowling, M. (1997). Multiple myeloma. *Professional Nurse, 12*(5), 354-357.

Fisher, D., & Sawin, K. (1998). Latex allergy in the primary care setting. *Journal of the American Academy of Nurse Practitioners, 10*(5), 203-208.

Floyd, P. (2000). Latex allergy update. *Journal of Perianesthesia Nursing, 15*(1), 26-30.

Gritter, M. (1998). The latex threat. *American Journal of Nursing, 98*(9), 26-32.

Handley, D., & Graff, F. (1998). A look ahead: Third-generation antihistamines. *ADVANCE for Nurse Practitioners, 6*(4), 53-54, 72.

Henderson, N. (1998). Anaphylaxis. *Nursing Standard, 12*(47), 49-55.

Karvonen, C. (1999). Latex allergy in health care workers: What are the risks? *AAOHN Journal, 47*(11), 519-525.

Ledford, D., & Lockey, R. (1998). Allergic rhinitis. *Journal of Respiratory Diseases, 19*(7), 576-578, 581-584.

McCloskey, J., & Bulechek, G. (2000). *Nursing interventions classification (NIC)* (3rd ed.). St. Louis: Mosby.

Myers, J. (2000). Emergency: Chemotherapy-induced hypersensitivity reaction. *American Journal of Nursing, 100*(4), 53-54.

Pepper, G. (2000). Nonsteroidal anti-inflammatory drugs: New perspectives on a familiar drug class. *Nursing Clinics of North America, 35*(1), 223-244.

United States Pharmacopeia Dispensing Information (USP DI): Vol. I. Drug information for the health care professional (20th ed.). (2000). Englewood, CO: Micromedex.

Vale, D. (2000). Recognition and management of Sjögren's syndrome: Strategies for the advanced practice nurse. *Nursing Clinics of North America, 35*(1), 267-278.

Van Deusen, M., et al. (1997). Efficacy and safety of oral immunotherapy with short ragweed extract. *Annals of Allergy, Asthma, and Immunology, 78*(6), 573-580.

Walpert, N. (1998). The highs and lows of autoimmune thyroid disease. *Nursing98, 28*(12), 58-60.

Workman, M.L. (2000). Immune mechanisms in rheumatic disease. *Nursing Clinics of North America, 35*(1), 175-188.

CHAPTER 24

Altered Cell Growth and Cancer Development

M. LINDA WORKMAN

Learning Objectives

After studying this chapter, you should be able to:

1. Explain why causes of cancer can be hard to establish.
2. Compare and contrast the characteristics of benign and malignant tumors.
3. List three cancer types associated with exposure to tobacco.
4. Identify cancer types for which primary prevention is possible.
5. Compare and contrast the cancer development processes of initiation and promotion.
6. Describe the TNM system for cancer staging.
7. Explain the differences between a "low-grade" cancer and a "high-grade" cancer.
8. Discuss the roles of oncogenes and suppressor genes in cancer development.
9. Identify four common sites of distant metastasis for cancer.
10. Discuss the role of immunity in protection against cancer.
11. Identify which cancer types arise from connective tissues and which types arise from glandular tissues.
12. Describe how genetic predisposition can increase a person's risk for cancer development.
13. Identify behaviors that reduce the risk for cancer development and cancer death.

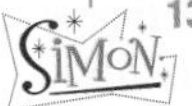

Go to http://www.wbsaunders.com/SIMON/Iggy/ for self-assessment questions related to these Learning Objectives.

Most people experience some form of altered cell growth. The most common types of altered cell growth are harmless (benign) and do not require intervention. Malignant cell growth or cancer, however, is serious and, without intervention, leads to death. Cancer is a common health problem in the United States and Canada, and approximately 1.5 million people are newly diagnosed with cancer each year (American Cancer Society, 2001). Some types of cancer can be prevented, and others have better cure rates if diagnosed early. The nurse can have a vital impact in educating the public about cancer prevention and early detection methods.

HISTORICAL PERSPECTIVE

Although cancer is very prevalent today, it is not a new disorder. Research has determined that even prehistoric humans experienced cancer. Some types of cancer are more prevalent today, especially among industrialized societies, than in centuries past. Two reasons for this increase are the longevity of people in industrialized countries and increased environmental exposure to substances that stimulate cancer development.

Cancer will occur in approximately 1 out of every 3 persons currently living in North America (American Cancer Society, 2001), although cancer risk differs for each person. Cancer prevention is a major health focus for the United States (see the Meeting Healthy People 2010 Objectives box on p. 408). More than 10 million Americans with a history of cancer are alive today, nearly 5 million of whom can be considered cured (American Cancer Society, 2001). Terms used to describe abnormal cell growth and cancer are presented in Table 24-1.

OVERVIEW

The continuous growth of cells and tissues is expected during infancy and childhood, and many human body cells continue to "grow" by cell division (mitosis) long after development and maturation are complete. Such cells are located in tissues where constant damage or wear is likely and where continued cell growth is necessary to replace dead tissues. Cells of the skin, hair, mucous membranes, bone marrow, and linings of glandular organs (lungs, stomach, intestines, bladder, uterus), as well as support cells of the brain (glial cells), among others, maintain the ability to divide throughout a person's life span. The growth of these cells is well controlled, ensuring that only the right number of cells is always present in any tissue or organ.

Some tissues and organs stop growing by cell division after development is complete. For example, heart muscle cells

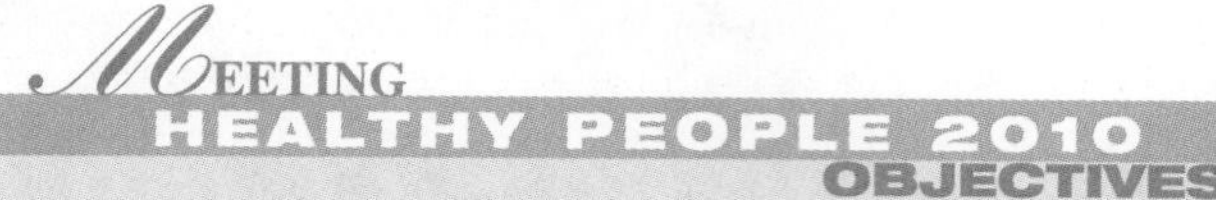

CANCER

Objective 17.1: Reduce cancer deaths to a rate of no more than 103 per 100,000 people

- Assess all clients for current and past exposures to carcinogens.
- Help clients to identify personal cancer risks.
- Help clients to avoid known environmental carcinogens.
- Assess all clients for a family history of cancer to identify clients at a genetic high risk for cancer.
- Refer identified clients at a genetic high risk for cancer to an appropriate-level counselor.
- Teach clients to avoid excessive sun exposure and to use protective clothing, hats, and sun-screening agents when sun exposure is not avoidable.
- Teach clients about tobacco-related cancers.
- Help clients who smoke to reduce or quit smoking.
- Teach clients about alcohol-related cancers.
- Teach clients about the importance of limiting dietary fat, smoked meats, and red meats.
- Teach clients about the importance of increasing dietary fiber.
- Encourage clients to see a health care provider at least once per year for cancer screening.
- Teach clients the correct technique for breast self-examination or testicular self-examination.
- Encourage clients to engage in self-screening measures, such as whole-body skin examination, breast self-examination, or testicular self-examination, on a monthly basis.
- Instruct clients who have any of the seven warning signs of cancer to follow up with their primary care provider as soon as possible.
- Encourage female clients to follow American Cancer Society guidelines for cervical, breast, and colorectal cancer screening appropriate for age and risk categories.
- Encourage male clients to follow American Cancer Society guidelines for prostate and colorectal cancer screening appropriate for age and risk categories.

no longer divide after fetal life; the number of heart muscle cells is fixed at birth. The size of the heart increases as the person grows because each of the cells gets larger, but the number of muscle cells in the heart does not increase. Growth that causes tissue to increase in size by enlarging individual cells is called **hypertrophy.** Growth that causes tissue to increase in size by increasing the number of cells is called **hyperplasia** (Figure 24-1).

Any new or continued cell growth not needed for normal development or replacement of dead and damaged tissues is called **neoplasia** and is always considered abnormal even if it causes no harm. Whether the new cells are benign or malignant, neoplastic cells develop from normal cells (parent tissues or cells). Thus cancer or any neoplastic cells were once normal cells but changed to no longer look, grow, or function normally. The strict processes controlling normal growth and function have been lost or suppressed. To understand how cancer cells grow, it is first necessary to understand the regulation and function of normal cells.

Biology of Normal Cells

Different types of normal cells work together to make the whole person function at an optimal level. To achieve optimal function, each individual cell must perform in a predictable manner.

CHARACTERISTICS OF NORMAL CELLS

- **Have limited cell division.** Normal cells divide (undergo mitosis) for one of two reasons: (1) to develop normal tissue or (2) to replace lost or damaged normal tissue. Even when they are capable of mitosis, normal cells divide only when all internal body conditions and nutrition are just right to promote cell division.

TABLE 24-1 • TERMINOLOGY COMMONLY ASSOCIATED WITH ABNORMAL CELL GROWTH

anaplastic Without shape or differentiation, small and round
benign New, nonmalignant cell growth not needed for normal growth or replacement
carcinogenesis The transformation of a normal cell into a cancer cell
doubling time The amount of time it takes for a tumor to double in size by mitotic cell divisions
fibronectin A large, extracellular, transformation-sensitive cell-surface protein present on normal cells that allows normal cells to adhere tightly together
gene expression The activation, or "turning on," of a specific gene to the extent that it synthesizes a specific protein that influences the activity of a cell or group of cells
gene repression The deactivation, or "turning off," of a specific gene so that it is silent and does not synthesize a protein
generation time The period of time necessary for one cell to enter and complete one round of cell division by mitosis
initiation The damage of a normal cell's DNA by a carcinogen
latency The period of time between when a carcinogenic agent or substance damaged the DNA of a normal cell (initiated it) and when an overt cancer is present
malignant Cancerous, new growth of cells by invasion that is not needed for normal development or tissue replacement
metastasis Invasive growth of cancer cells from the original tumor into distant areas
mitosis Cell division by exact duplication
morphology Appearance or shape
multipotent An undifferentiated cell that has multiple potentials for maturation and differentiation (also called totipotent and pluripotent)
neoplasia New cell growth not needed for normal body growth or replacement of dead or missing tissue
oncogene A developmental gene (proto-oncogene) expressed at an inappropriate time, capable of transforming a normal cell into a cancer cell
ploidy The chromosome content of a cell
  aneuploid ploidy The chromosome content of a cell that is greater or lesser than the normal chromosome number for the species
  diploid (euploid) ploidy The normal chromosome content of a cell for the species (e.g., human cells have 46 chromosomes [23 pairs] per cell)
primary tumor A tumor formed in a specific tissue as a result of a carcinogenic agent or event
promotion Enhancement of cell division in a cell initiated by a carcinogen
proto-oncogene A developmental gene expressed during early embryonic development
secondary tumor A tumor formed as a result of breaking off from a primary tumor and spreading to distant sites (metastasis)
transformation The changing of a normal cell into a cancer cell by a carcinogenic agent or event

- **Show specific morphology.** Each normal cell type has a distinct and recognizable appearance, size, and shape, as shown in Figure 24-2.
- **Have a small nuclear-cytoplasmic ratio.** As shown in Figure 24-2, the space that the nucleus occupies inside a normal cell is small compared with the size of the cell. The nuclear space is small in proportion to the cytoplasmic space.
- **Perform specific differentiated functions.** Every normal cell must perform at least one special function to contribute to whole-body homeostasis. For example, skin cells make keratin, liver cells make bile, cardiac muscle cells contract rhythmically, nerve cells generate and conduct impulses, and red blood cells make hemoglobin to carry oxygen.
- **Adhere tightly together.** Normal cells make and secrete proteins that protrude from the cell surface, allowing cells to bind closely and tightly together. In the presence of a protein called fibronectin, normal cells composing most normal tissues are bound tightly to each other. Exceptions are blood cells. Erythrocytes and leukocytes produce no fibronectin and do not adhere to one another under normal circumstances.
- **Are nonmigratory.** Because normal cells are tightly bound together, they do not wander from one tissue to the next (with the exception of erythrocytes and leukocytes).
- **Grow in an orderly and well-regulated manner.** Normal cells capable of mitosis do not divide unless all internal body conditions are optimal for cell division. These conditions include the need for more cells, adequate space, and sufficient nutrients and other resources. Cell division, occurring in a well-recognized pattern, is described by the cell cycle. Figure 24-3 shows the phases of the cell cycle.

Living cells not actively reproducing are not in the cell cycle but in a reproductive resting state termed G_0. During the G_0 period, cells actively carry out specific functions but do not divide. Most normal cells spend most of their existence in the G_0 state, just like most humans spend the majority of their lives in a nonpregnant state.

Mitotic cell division makes a cell divide into two cells. These two cells are identical to each other and to the original cell that started the mitotic cell division. The processes of entering and completing the cell cycle are rigidly controlled. Figure 24-4 shows the activities occurring during the phases of the cell cycle:

G_1. The cell is preparing for division by taking on extra nutrients, generating more energy, and making extra membrane. The amount of cell fluid (cytoplasm) also increases.

S. Because making one cell into two cells requires twice as much of everything, including deoxyribonucleic acid (DNA), the cell doubles its DNA content through DNA synthesis.

G_2. The cell makes important proteins that will be used in actual cell division and in normal physiologic function after cell division is complete.

M. The single cell splits apart into two cells (actual mitosis).

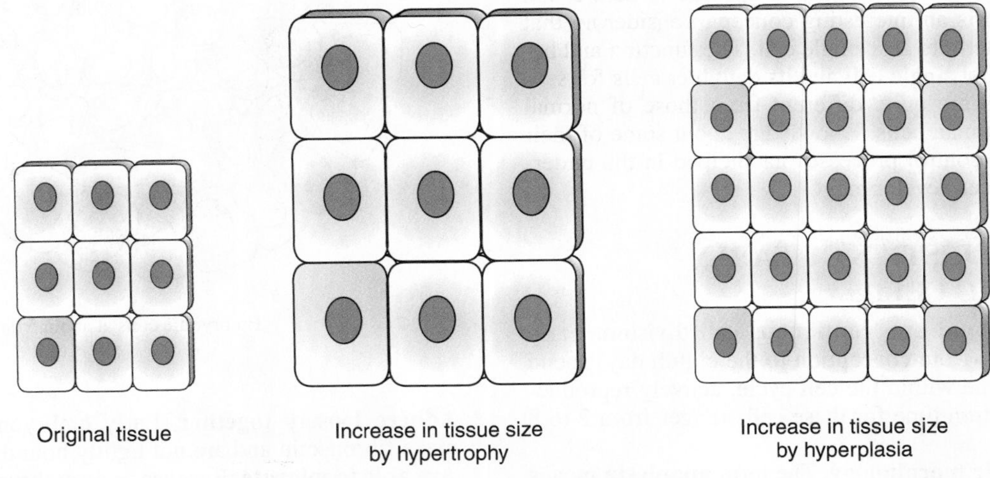

Figure 24-1 ● Tissue growth by hypertrophy and hyperplasia.

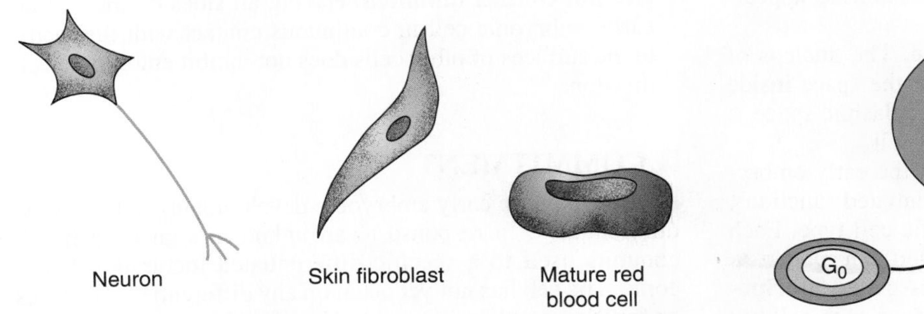

Figure 24-2 ● Distinctive morphology of some normal cells.

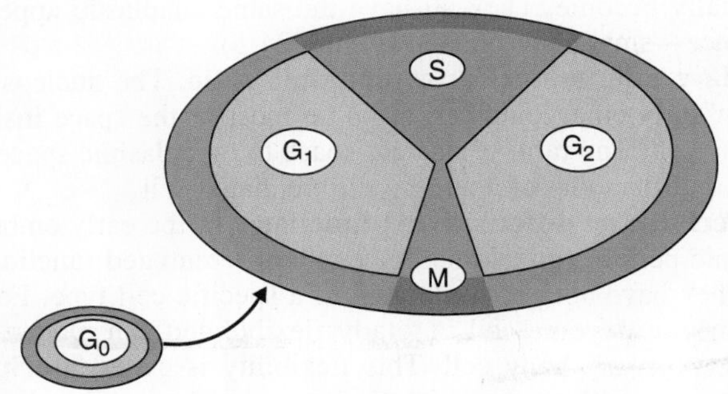

Figure 24-3 ● The cell cycle.

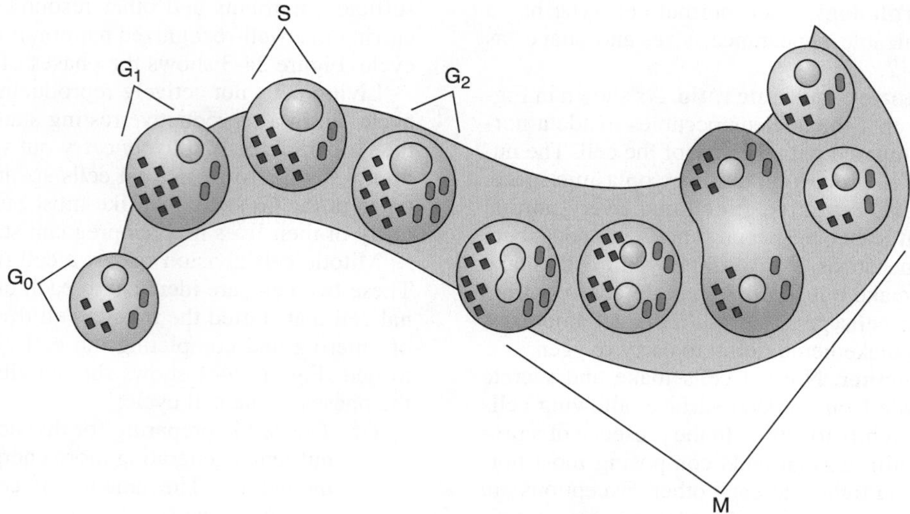

Figure 24-4 ● Cellular events during mitotic cell division.

- **Are contact inhibited.** Among normal cells capable of cell division, each individual cell will divide only as long as it has some surface not in direct contact with another cell. Once a normal cell is in direct contact on all surface areas with other cell membranes, it no longer undergoes mitosis. Thus normal cell division is **contact inhibited.** Contact inhibition is also called **density-dependent inhibition of cell growth.**

Each normal, mature cell has a specific structure and function, which is an interesting concept, considering that all humans started life as a single cell. The function and behavior of that first single cell and its daughter cells for several generations are quite different from those of normal differentiated human cells. Knowledge about some of their differences and control processes has helped in the understanding of cancer development.

CHARACTERISTICS OF EARLY EMBRYONIC CELLS

- **Demonstrate rapid and continuous cell division.** Early embryonic cells (from conception to the eighth day) spend most of their time within the cell cycle, actively reproducing. The generation time for these cells ranges from 2 to 8 hours.
- **Show anaplastic morphology.** The term **anaplasia** means "without structural shape or differentiation." Early embryonic cells do not look like the mature cells they will eventually become. They all have the same anaplastic appearance—small and rounded (Figure 24-5).
- **Have a large nuclear-cytoplasmic ratio.** The nucleus of an early embryonic cell takes up most of the space inside the cell. The ratio of nuclear space to cytoplasmic space is larger than that of a normal differentiated cell.
- **Perform no differentiated functions.** In the early embryonic period, cells do not have any differentiated functions. They have not yet committed to a specific cell type. Each early embryonic cell is totally flexible and can mature to become any body cell. This flexibility is called **pluripotency, multipotency,** or **totipotency** because each cell has an unlimited potential for maturation.

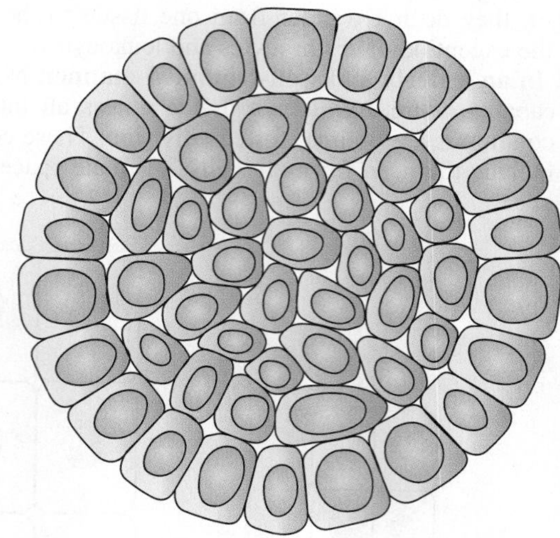

Figure 24-5 ● Embryonic cells at about 5 days after conception.

- **Adhere loosely together.** Early embryonic cells do not make fibronectin and are not tightly bound together.
- **Are able to migrate.** Because early embryonic cells are not tightly bound together, they do not remain in one place within the embryo but migrate throughout the early embryo.
- **Are not contact inhibited.** Having all sides or areas of an early embryonic cell in continuous contact with the membrane surfaces of other cells does not inhibit embryonic cell division.

COMMITMENT

At some point in early embryonic development, cells become differentiated. In response to an unknown signal, each cell commits itself to a specific differentiated maturational outcome. The cell has not yet taken on any differentiated features or functions; rather, it positions itself within a group of cells that will eventually become only one specific organ or tissue.

TABLE 24-2 • CHARACTERISTICS OF NORMAL AND ABNORMAL CELLS

Characteristic	Normal Cell	Embryonic Cell	Benign Tumor Cell	Malignant Cell
Cell division	None or slow	Rapid, continuous	Continuous or inappropriate	Rapid or continuous
Appearance	Specific morphologic features	Anaplastic	Specific morphologic features	Anaplastic
Nuclear-cytoplasmic ratio	Small	Large	Small	Large
Differentiated functions	Many	None	Many	Some or none
Adherence	Tight	Loose	Tight	Loose
Migratory	No	Yes	No	Yes
Growth	Well regulated	Well regulated	Expansion	Invasion
Chromosomes	Diploid (euploid)	Diploid (euploid)	Diploid (euploid)	Aneuploid*
Mitotic index	Low	High	Low	High*

*Depends on the degree of malignant transformation.

Commitment involves turning off specific early embryonic genes that controlled or regulated early rapid growth. These genes, called **proto-oncogenes,** have no apparent normal function at any other point in life.

After the early embryonic regulatory genes are "turned off" (**repressed** or **suppressed**), other specific genes that control the expression of specific differentiated functions must be "turned on" **(expressed)** selectively in different cell types. For example, the gene for insulin is actively expressed only in fetal pancreatic beta cells and is repressed in all other cells. This selective gene expression directs the normal growth and differentiation of specific body cells.

Biology of Abnormal Cells

Body cells do not exist in isolation but are exposed to personal and environmental changes, which can alter how the cells grow or function. When either cell growth or cell function is changed, the cells are considered abnormal. Table 24-2 compares characteristics of normal, embryonic, benign tumor, and cancer cells.

CHARACTERISTICS OF BENIGN CELLS

Benign tumor cells are normal cells growing in the wrong place, at the wrong time, or at the wrong rate. Examples include moles, uterine fibroid tumors, skin tags, endometriosis, and nasal polyps. Benign cells:

- **Demonstrate continuous or inappropriate cell growth.** Benign tumors are tissues unnecessary for normal function, growing too much or in the wrong place.
- **Show specific morphology.** Benign tumors strongly resemble their parent tissues, retaining the specific morphologic features of parent tissue.
- **Have a small nuclear-cytoplasmic ratio.** Just like completely normal cells, benign tumor cells have a small nucleus compared with the rest of the cell.
- **Perform differentiated functions.** Not only do benign tumors look like their parent tissues, but they also perform the same differentiated functions. For example, in endometriosis, one type of benign tumor, the normal lining of the uterus (endometrium) grows in an abnormal place (such as on an ovary, on the peritoneum, or in the chest cavity). This displaced endometrium acts just like normal endometrium by increasing vascularity and tissue thickness each month under the influence of estrogen and progesterone. When these hormone levels drop and the normal endometrium sheds from the uterus, the displaced endometrium, wherever it is, also sheds.
- **Adhere tightly together.** Benign tumor cells make and secrete fibronectin, and benign tumor cells bind tightly to one another. In addition, many benign tissues are "encapsulated," or surrounded with fibrous connective tissue, helping to hold the benign tissue together.
- **Are nonmigratory.** Benign tissues do not wander but remain tightly bound and do not invade other body tissues.
- **Grow in an orderly manner.** Benign tumor cells follow normal cell growth patterns even though their growth is not needed. Growth may continue beyond an appropriate time, but the rate of growth is normal for the parent tissue. The benign tumor grows by hyperplastic expansion.

CHARACTERISTICS OF MALIGNANT CELLS

Cancer (malignant) cells are abnormal, serve no useful function, and are harmful to normal body tissues. Malignant tumors commonly:

- **Demonstrate rapid or continuous cell division.** Some cancer cells have a short generation time (2 to 4 hours); others have a generation time even longer than that of normal cells. Most cancer cells have a generation time similar to that of the parent tissue.

  A major distinction between normal and cancer cells is that cancer cells divide nearly continuously. Almost as soon as one round of mitosis is complete, the daughter cells begin a new round.
- **Show anaplastic morphology.** Cancer cells lose the specific appearance of their parent cells, becoming **anaplastic.** As a cancer cell becomes even more malignant, it becomes smaller and rounder. This loss of specific appearance can make diagnosis of cancer type difficult, because many types of cancer cells look alike.
- **Have a large nuclear-cytoplasmic ratio.** The nucleus of a cancer cell is larger than that of a normal cell, and the cancer cell is small. The nucleus occupies much of

the space within the cancer cell, creating a large nuclear-cytoplasmic ratio.

- **Lose some or all differentiated functions.** Along with losing the appearance of the parent cell, cancer cells lose some differentiated functions the parent tissue performed. Cancer cells serve no useful purpose.
- **Adhere loosely together.** Cancer cells make little, if any, fibronectin. As a result, they adhere poorly to each other, and little pressure is needed to allow some cancer cells to break off from the primary tumor.
- **Are able to migrate.** Because cancer cells do not bind tightly together and have many enzymes on their cell surfaces, they are able to slip through blood vessels and tissues and spread from the original tumor site to many other body sites. This ability to spread **(metastasize)** is a key characteristic of cancer cells and a frequent cause of death among people with cancer.
- **Grow by invasion.** Cancer cells expand and extend into other tissues, both close by and more remote from the original tumor, by invasion or metastasis. Together with persistent growth, metastasis makes untreated cancer deadly.
- **Are not contact inhibited.** Cancer cells continue to divide even when contacted on all surface areas by other cells; thus their growth is not contact inhibited. The persistence of cancer cell division, even under adverse conditions, is one factor making the disease so difficult to control.

CANCER DEVELOPMENT

Carcinogenesis/Oncogenesis

Carcinogenesis and **oncogenesis** are synonyms for cancer development. Table 24-3 summarizes key concepts about cancer development. The process of changing a cell with a normal appearance and function into a cell with malignant characteristics is called **malignant transformation.** Malignant transformation occurs through the steps of *initiation, promotion, progression,* and *metastasis.*

INITIATION

The first step in carcinogenesis is **initiation.** Normal cells can become cancer cells if their proto-oncogenes are turned back on at any time after early embryonic development is complete. Anything that can penetrate a cell, get into the nucleus, and damage the DNA can damage the genes, turning on genes that should remain suppressed and turning off normal genes (Cooper, 1995). Substances that can change the activity of a cell's genes so that the cell has malignant characteristics are called **carcinogens.** Carcinogens may be chemicals, physical agents, or viruses. Table 24-4 lists common carcinogens and the types of cancer they are known to cause. Chapters presenting the care of clients with specific cancers discuss specific carcinogens (when known) within the Etiology sections.

Pure carcinogens initiate mutational changes in a cell's genes and are thus called *initiators.* Initiation is an irreversible event that can lead to cancer development if it does not interfere with the cell's ability to divide.

Once a cell has been initiated, it can become a cancer cell if the cellular changes that occurred during initiation are enhanced by **promotion.** One cancer cell is not significant, however, unless it can divide. If it cannot divide, it cannot form a tumor. *If growth conditions are right, however, widespread metastatic disease can develop from just one cancer cell.*

TABLE 24-3 • KEY CONCEPTS RELATED TO CANCER DEVELOPMENT

- Neoplastic cells originate from normal body cells.
- Transformation of a normal cell into a cancer cell involves mutation of the genes (DNA) of the normal cell.
- Early embryonic genes activated at an inappropriate time can cause a cell to develop into a tumor.
- Only one cell has to undergo malignant transformation for cancer to begin.
- Benign tumors grow by expansion, whereas malignant tumors grow by invasion.
- Most tumors arise from cells that are capable of cell division.
- Primary prevention of cancer involves avoiding exposure to known causes of cancer.
- Secondary prevention of cancer involves screening for early detection.
- Tobacco use is a causative or permissive factor in 30% of all malignant neoplasms.
- Tumors that metastasize from the primary site into another organ are still designated as tumors of the originating tissue.

TABLE 24-4 • KNOWN ENVIRONMENTAL CARCINOGENS

Carcinogen	Associated Cancer Site or Neoplasm
Alcoholic beverages	Liver, esophagus, mouth, pharynx, breast, colon, and rectum
Anabolic steroids	Liver
Arsenic	Lung, skin
Asbestos	Lung, pleura, peritoneum, pericardium
Benzene	Myelogenous leukemia
Chemotherapy drugs Alkylating agents Anthracycline antibiotics Antimetabolites	Acute leukemia, lymphoma
Cyclosporine	Non-Hodgkin's lymphoma
Diesel exhaust	Lung
Formaldehyde	Nasopharynx
Hair dyes	Bladder
Ionizing radiation	Bone marrow, thyroid, many organs
Mineral oils	Skin
Pesticides	Lung
Polycyclic hydrocarbons	Lung, skin, scrotum
Polychlorinated biphenyls	Liver, skin
Sunlight	Skin, eyes
Tobacco	Lung, esophagus, mouth, pharynx, larynx, pancreas, bladder, kidney, liver, stomach, colon, rectum, leukemia

PROMOTION

Once a normal cell has been initiated by a carcinogen and has cancer cell characteristics, it can become a tumor if its growth is enhanced. The time between a cell's initiation and development of an overt tumor is called the **latency period,** which can range from months to years and depends on the type of cell initiated and the presence of promoters.

Promoters are substances that promote or enhance initiated cell growth (Weinberg, 1996). They can also shorten the latency period. Promoters may be hormones, drugs, or a wide variety of industrial chemicals.

PROGRESSION

After cancer cells have grown to the point that a detectable tumor is formed (a 1-cm tumor has at least 1 billion cells in it), other events must occur for this tumor to become a health problem. First, the tumor must establish its own blood supply. In the early stages, the center cells of the tumor receive nutrition only by diffusion from the surrounding fluids. After the tumor reaches 1 cm, however, diffusion is not efficient, and cells in the center of the tumor become hypoxic and start to die. To continue to grow and survive, the tumor makes **tumor angiogenesis factor (TAF).** TAF stimulates capillaries and other blood vessels in the area to grow new branches into the tumor (Pitot, 1986). These blood vessels ensure the tumor's continued nourishment.

As tumor cells continue to divide, some of the new cells experience more changes from the original, initiated cancer cell. Actual colonies or subpopulations within the tumor begin to appear. These subpopulations differ from the original cancer cell. Some of the differences provide these subpopulations with advantages that allow them to live and divide no matter how the environmental conditions around them change; these differences are thus called "selection advantages." Changes that a tumor undergoes at this time allow it to become more malignant. Over time, the tumor cells come to have fewer and fewer normal cell characteristics.

The original tumor formed from transformed normal cells is called the **primary tumor.** It is usually identified by the tissue from which it arose (parent tissue), such as in breast cancer or lung cancer. When primary tumors are located in vital organs, such as the brain or lungs, they can grow to such an extent that they either lethally damage the vital organ or "crowd out" healthy organ tissue and interfere with that organ's ability to perform its vital function. At other times, the primary tumor is located in soft tissue that can expand without damage as the tumor grows. One such site is the breast. The breast is not a vital organ, and even if it had a large tumor in it, the primary tumor would not cause the client's death. When the tumor spreads from the original site into vital areas, life functions can be disrupted.

METASTASIS

In metastasis, cancer cells move from their original location by breaking off from the original group and establishing remote colonies. These additional tumors are called **metastatic** or *secondary tumors.* Even though the tumor is now in another organ, it is still a cancer from the original altered tissue. For example, when breast cancer spreads to the lung and the bone, it is breast cancer in the lung and bone, not lung cancer and not bone cancer. Metastasis occurs through several progressive steps, as shown in Figure 24-6 (Liotta, 1992).

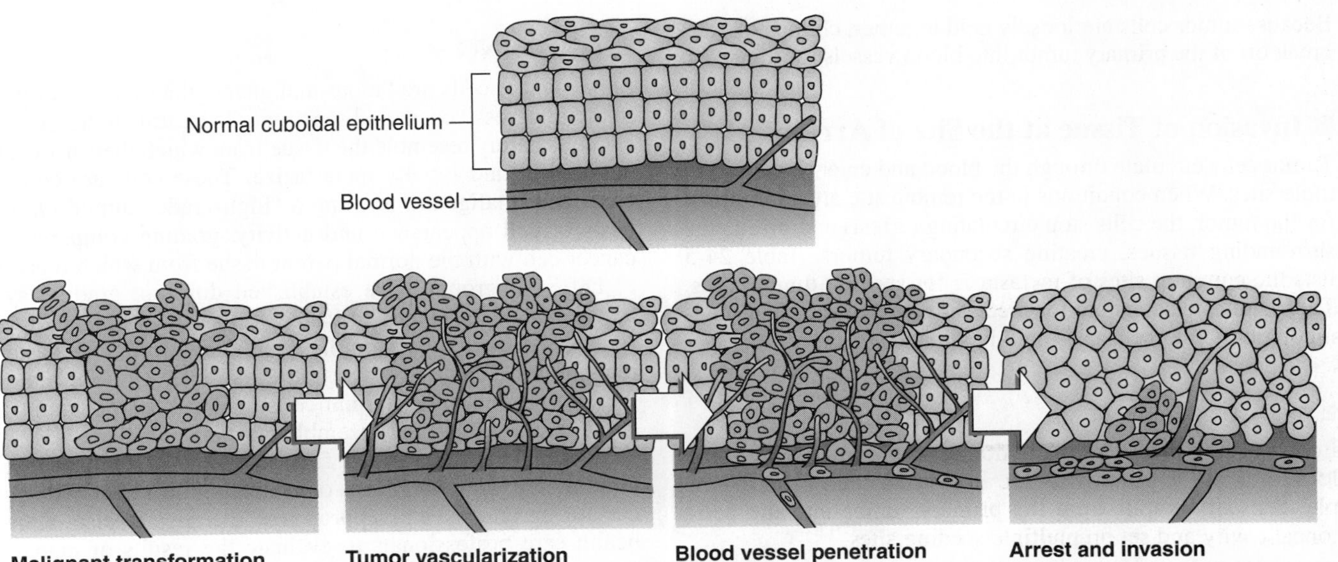

Figure 24-6 • The steps of metastasis.

TABLE 24-5 • COMMON SITES OF METASTASIS FOR DIFFERENT CANCER TYPES

BREAST CANCER Bone* Lung* Liver Brain	**PROSTATE CANCER** Bone (especially spine and legs)* Pelvic nodes
LUNG CANCER Brain* Bone Liver Lymph nodes Pancreas	**MELANOMA** Gastrointestinal tract Lymph nodes Lung Brain
COLORECTAL CANCER Liver* Lymph nodes Adjacent structures	**PRIMARY BRAIN CANCER** Central nervous system

*Most common site of metastasis for the specific malignant neoplasm.

Extension into Surrounding Tissues

Tumors secrete enzymes that open up areas of surrounding tissue. Mechanical pressure, created as the tumor increases in size, forces tumor cells to invade new territory.

Penetration into Blood Vessels

The same enzymes that open up areas of surrounding tissue make large pores in the client's blood vessels, allowing tumor cells to enter the blood and circulate throughout the body.

Release of Tumor Cells

Because tumor cells are loosely held together, clumps of cells break off of the primary tumor into blood vessels for transport.

Invasion of Tissue at the Site of Arrest

Tumor cells circulate through the blood and enter tissues at remote sites. When conditions in the remote site are appropriate for the tumor, the cells stop circulating (arrest) and invade the surrounding tissues, creating secondary tumors. Table 24-5 lists the common sites of metastasis for specific tumor types. Three routes responsible for metastatic spread are local seeding, bloodborne metastasis, and lymphatic spread.

LOCAL SEEDING

Local seeding involves distribution of shed cancer cells in the local area of the primary tumor. In ovarian cancer, for example, cells often spill from the primary tumor into the peritoneal cavity and set up multiple seeding sites.

BLOODBORNE METASTASIS

Bloodborne metastasis (tumor cell release into the blood) is the most common cause of cancer spread. Combined with seeding, distribution via the bloodstream determines the area of metastases.

Many circulating tumor cells are destroyed by factors in the circulation, immune responses, or unsuitable environments in the organs in which the cells stop. Clumps of tumor cells can become trapped in capillaries. These clumps damage the capillary wall and allow tumor cells to enter the surrounding tissue.

LYMPHATIC SPREAD

Lymphatic spread is related to the number, structure, and location of lymph nodes and vessels. Primary sites that are rich in lymphatics are more susceptible to early metastatic spread than are areas with few lymphatics.

Cancer Classification

Terms that describe neoplasia by tissue origin and classify the tumor as benign or malignant are listed in Table 24-6. Other terms describe the tumor's biologic behavior, anatomic site, and degree of differentiation.

Approximately 100 different types of cancer arise from various tissues or organs. Figure 24-7 compares cancer distribution by site and gender. Cancers are divided into two major categories: solid and hematologic.

Solid tumors are associated with the organs from which they develop (e.g., breast cancer and lung cancer). Hematologic cancers (e.g., leukemias and lymphomas) originate from blood cell–forming tissues, which communicate with all organs.

Cancer Grade and Stage

To help standardize cancer diagnosis, prognosis, and treatment, classification systems of grading and staging were developed. Grading of a tumor classifies cellular aspects of the cancer. Staging of the client classifies clinical aspects of the cancer.

GRADING

Some cancer cells are "more malignant" than others, varying in their aggressiveness and sensitivity to treatment. Some cancer cells barely resemble the tissue from which they arose, are aggressive, and rapidly metastasize. These cells are considered more malignant, forming a "high-grade" tumor. On the basis of cell appearance and activity, grading compares the cancer cell with the normal parent tissue from which it arose.

Different groups have established different grading systems for different types of cancer cells, but overall they resemble the standard system listed in Table 24-7. This system rates tumor cells; the lowest rating is given to those tumors that closely resemble normal cells, and the highest rating is given to those that little resemble normal cells.

Grading the cells is the first step in confirming cancer. Grading provides one means of evaluating the client with cancer for prognosis and appropriate therapy. It also allows health care professionals to evaluate the results of management and compare local, regional, national, and international statistics.

PLOIDY

Another biologic feature describing cancer cells is chromosome number and appearance, or **ploidy.** Normal human cells have 46 chromosomes (23 pairs), the normal diploid number. When malignant transformation occurs, changes in the genes and chromosomes also occur. Some tumor cells gain or lose

TABLE 24-6 • CLASSIFICATION OF TUMORS BY TISSUE OF ORIGIN

Prefix	Tissue of Origin	Benign Tumor	Malignant Tumor*
Adeno	Epithelial glands	Adenoma	Adenocarcinoma
Chondro	Cartilage	Chrondroma	Chondrosarcoma
Fibro	Fibrous connective	Fibroma	Fibrosarcoma
Glio	Glial cells (brain)	Glioma	Glioblastoma
Hemangio	Blood vessel	Hemangioma	Hemangiosarcoma
Hepato	Liver	Hepatoma	Hepatocarcinoma Hepatoblastoma
Leiomyo	Smooth muscle	Leiomyoma	Leiomyosarcoma
Lipo	Fat/adipose	Lipoma	Liposarcoma
Lympho	Lymphoid tissues		Malignant lymphomas Hodgkin's lymphoma Non-Hodgkin's lymphoma Burkitt's lymphoma Cutaneous T-cell
Melano	Pigment-producing skin		Melanoma
Meningio	Meninges	Meningioma	Malignant meningioma Meningioblastoma
Neuro	Nerve tissue	Neuroma Neurofibroma	Neurosarcoma Neuroblastoma
Osteo	Bone	Osteoma	Osteosarcoma
Renal	Kidney		Renal cell carcinoma
Rhabdo	Skeletal muscle	Rhabdomyoma	Rhabdomyosarcoma
Squamous	Epithelial layer of skin, mucous membranes, and organ linings	Papilloma	Squamous cell carcinoma of skin, bladder, lungs, cervix

*Carcinomas are tumors of glandular tissue; sarcomas are tumors of connective tissue; blastomas are tumors of less differentiated, embryonal tissues.

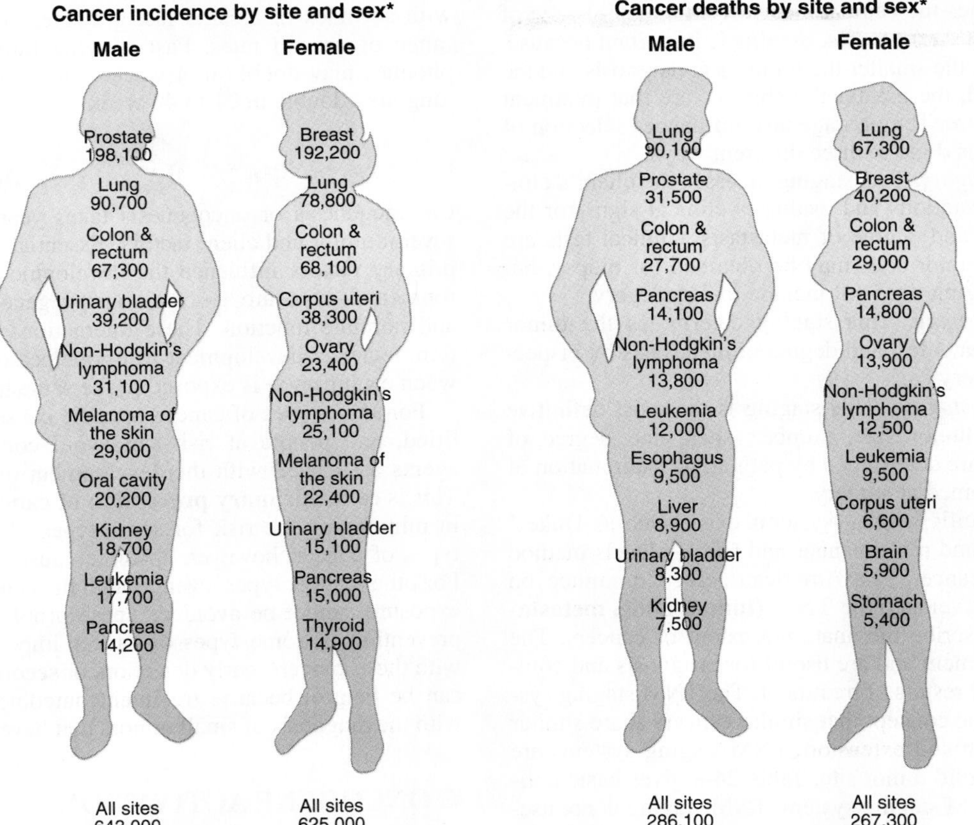

Figure 24-7 ● Cancer incidence and death by site and sex. (From American Cancer Society. [2001]. *Cancer facts and figures—2001.* Report No. 01-300M-No. 5008.01. Atlanta: Author.)

TABLE 24-7 • GRADING OF MALIGNANT TUMORS

Grade	Cellular Characteristics
G_X	Grade cannot be determined.
G_1	Tumor cells are well differentiated and closely resemble the normal cells from which they arose. This grade is considered a low grade of malignant change. These tumors are malignant but are relatively slow growing.
G_2	Tumor cells are moderately differentiated; they still retain some of the characteristics of normal cells but also have more malignant characteristics than do G_1 tumor cells.
G_3	Tumor cells are poorly differentiated, but the tissue of origin can usually be established. The cells have few normal cell characteristics.
G_4	Tumor cells are poorly differentiated and retain no normal cell characteristics. Determination of the tissue of origin is difficult and perhaps impossible.

TABLE 24-8 • STAGING OF CANCER: TNM CLASSIFICATION

	Primary Tumor (T)
T_X	Primary tumor cannot be assessed
T_0	No evidence of primary tumor
T_{is}	Carcinoma in situ
T_1, T_2, T_3, T_4	Increasing size and/or local extent of the primary tumor
	Regional Lymph Nodes (N)
N_X	Regional lymph nodes cannot be assessed
N_0	No regional lymph node metastasis
N_1, N_2, N_3	Increasing involvement of regional lymph nodes
	Distant Metastasis (M)
M_X	Presence of distant metastasis cannot be assessed
M_0	No distant metastasis
M_1	Distant metastasis

Modified from American Joint Committee on Cancer. (1988). In O.H. Beahrs et al. (Eds.), *Manual for staging of cancer* (3rd ed., p. 7). Philadelphia: J.B. Lippincott.

whole chromosomes and may have structural abnormalities of the remaining chromosomes. When a tumor cell has more or less than the normal diploid number, it is said to be **aneuploid.** The degree of aneuploidy generally increases with the degree of malignant transformation.

STAGING

Staging determines the cancer's exact location and degree of metastasis present at diagnosis. Staging is important because, for most cancers, the smaller the tumor is at diagnosis and the less it has spread, the greater the chances are that treatment will result in a cure. Tumor stage also influences selection of therapy. Staging is done in three different ways:

1. *Clinical staging.* This staging assesses the client's clinical manifestations and evaluates clinical signs for the tumor size and degree of metastasis. Clinical tests are used, and tumor cells may be obtained for biopsy, but clinical staging does not include major surgery.
2. *Surgical staging.* This staging determines the tumor size, number, sites, and degree of metastasis by inspection at surgery.
3. *Pathologic staging.* This staging is the most definitive type. The tumor size, number, sites, and degree of metastasis are determined by pathologic examination of tissues obtained at surgery.

Some site-specific staging systems exist, such as Dukes' staging of colon and rectal cancer and Clark's levels method of staging skin cancer. The American Joint Committee on Cancer (AJCC) developed the **TNM (tumor, node, metastasis)** system to describe the anatomic extent of cancers. The stages guide treatment and are useful for prognosis and comparison of the end results of treatment. The TNM staging system is based on the concept that similar cancers share similar patterns of growth and extension. TNM staging systems are specific to each solid tumor site. Table 24-8 gives basic definitions for the TNM staging system. TNM staging is not useful for cancers that arise in the bone marrow or lymphoid tissues. Staging for these cancers is discussed in Chapter 40.

Tumor growth is discussed in terms of doubling time (the amount of time it takes for a tumor to double in size) and mitotic index (the percentage of actively dividing cells within a tumor). The smallest tumor likely to be detected by a physical examination or diagnostic test is about 1 cm in diameter and contains 1 billion cells. To reach this size, a tumor will have undergone at least 30 doublings. A tumor with a mitotic index of less than 10% is a relatively slow growing tumor; a tumor with an index of 85% is fast growing. Tumors have a wide range of growth rates. Fast-growing tumors, such as lymphomas, may double in 4 weeks; an adenocarcinoma of the lung may double in 21 to 40 weeks.

Causes of Cancer Development

Carcinogenesis or oncogenesis takes years and depends on several tumor and client factors. Essentially, three interacting primary factors influence the development of cancer: environmental exposure to carcinogens, genetic predisposition, and immune function. These interactions account for variation in cancer development from one person to another, even when each person is exposed to the same hazards.

For some types of cancer, specific causes have been identified, and people at risk can avoid contact with specific agents associated with the development of that cancer type. This is called **primary prevention of cancer** and is effective in minimizing the risk for some types of cancer. For many types of cancer, however, absolute causes remain unknown. For other cancer types, even though the cause may be known, exposure cannot be avoided. These problems make primary prevention of some types of cancer impossible. For people with these cancers, early detection, or **secondary prevention,** can be helpful because treatment outcome is usually better with the diagnosis of small tumors that have not metastasized.

ONCOGENE ACTIVATION

Regardless of specific cause, the mechanism of carcinogenesis appears to be the same: the activation of proto-oncogenes into **oncogenes.** When a normal cell is exposed to any carcinogen (initiator), the normal cell's DNA can be damaged or

TABLE 24-9 • MALIGNANCIES ASSOCIATED WITH ALTERED ONCOGENE ACTIVITY

Oncogene	Malignancies
abl	Chronic myelogenous leukemia, other leukemias
bcl-2	Breast, colorectal, testicular, and laryngeal carcinomas
c-myc	Burkitt's lymphoma; T-cell and B-cell neoplasms; non-Hodgkin's lymphoma; breast, stomach, and lung carcinomas
erb B	Glioblastoma, squamous cell carcinomas
erb B-2	Breast, salivary gland, ovarian, gastric, and endometrial carcinomas
ets	Lymphomas
HER-2/neu	Breast carcinoma
hst-1	Breast and testicular carcinomas, squamous cell carcinomas
int-2	Breast carcinoma, squamous cell carcinomas
jun-B	Breast carcinoma
L-*myc*	Lung carcinoma
met	Osteosarcoma
myb	Colorectal carcinoma, leukemia
PRAD-1	Breast carcinoma, squamous cell carcinomas
ras H *ras* K *ras* N	Carcinomas, sarcomas, neuroblastoma, leukemias, lymphomas
ret	Thyroid carcinoma
Tpl-2/cot	Breast carcinoma
trk	Colorectal and thyroid carcinomas

mutated. The mutations can cause the early embryonic genes (proto-oncogenes), which should be suppressed forever, to be turned on or activated again. These genes are then oncogenes and can cause the cell to change from normal to malignant (Cooper, 1995).

About 50 different proto-oncogenes that can be activated into oncogenes have been identified so far, and scientists estimate that at least 50 more exist. *These oncogenes are not abnormal genes* but are part of every cell's normal makeup and were critically important in early development. Oncogenes become a problem only if they are activated (derepressed) after development is complete, as a result of exposure to carcinogenic agents or events. Activation of some specific oncogenes causes specific cancers. Table 24-9 lists known oncogenes and the malignancies they have been found to cause. Extrinsic and intrinsic factors are associated with oncogene activation.

EXTRINSIC FACTORS INFLUENCING CANCER DEVELOPMENT

Up to 80% of cancer in North America may be the result of environmental, or extrinsic, factors (Trichopoulos, Li, & Hunter, 1996). Environmental carcinogens are chemical, physical, or viral agents that cause cancer. Table 24-4 lists known environmental causes of human cancer.

Chemical Carcinogenesis

Many chemicals capable of causing malignant transformation appear to have similar chemical structures. More than 20 organic and inorganic industrial chemicals, drugs, and other products used in everyday life are known to be carcinogenic, and hundreds more are suspected of being carcinogenic.

TABLE 24-10 • MALIGNANCIES ASSOCIATED WITH TOBACCO USE

• Lung	• Oral cavity
• Pharyngeal	• Laryngeal
• Esophagus	• Pancreatic
• Cervical	• Kidney
• Bladder	

Data from American Cancer Society. (2001). *Cancer facts and figures—2001*. Report No. 00-300M-No. 5008.01. Atlanta: Author.

Some chemicals are complete carcinogens that can both initiate and promote cancer. Others are pure initiating agents, or incomplete carcinogens. Still others are only promoting agents. Some substances, such as tobacco and alcohol, appear to be only mildly carcinogenic; it takes chronic exposure to large amounts before a cancer develops. However, these two substances can act as co-carcinogens; when taken together, they enhance the carcinogenic activity of each other and of other carcinogens.

Cells are not equally susceptible to chemically induced malignant transformation. Normal cells that retain the capacity for cell division are at greater risk for cancer development than are normal cells that are not capable of cell division. Cancers commonly arise in bone marrow, skin, lining of the gastrointestinal tract, ductal cells of the breast, and lining of the lungs. All of these cells normally undergo mitotic cell division. Cancers of nerve tissue, cardiac muscle, and skeletal muscle are rare. These cells do not normally undergo mitotic cell division.

Approximately 30% of cancers diagnosed in North America are related to tobacco use (American Cancer Society, 2001). Tobacco is the single most important source of preventable chemical carcinogenesis. It contains many different chemical compounds, including complete carcinogens and co-carcinogens. Tobacco use or ingestion can initiate and promote cancer. The risk of cancer development for a person who uses tobacco depends on his or her immune function; amount, depth, and mode of exposure; and tobacco tar content. The type of cancer that develops depends on the susceptibility of specific sites to various concentrations of tobacco and its metabolites.

Tissues associated with the greatest risk for cancer are those with direct contact with tobacco smoke. Cigarette smoking and tobacco use are also implicated in the development of cancers remote from tissues with direct contact with tobacco. Table 24-10 summarizes the association of tobacco and development of specific cancers.

Physical Carcinogenesis

Physical agents or events may cause cancer by the same mechanism as for chemical carcinogens (i.e., by induction of DNA damage). Two types of physical agents suspected of causing cancer are radiation and chronic irritation (Pitot, 1986).

RADIATION

Radiation is a physical agent capable of carcinogenesis. Even small doses of radiation affect cells. Some effects are temporary and reparable; others are irreversible and may be lethal to the

TABLE 24-11 • MALIGNANCIES ASSOCIATED WITH A KNOWN VIRAL ORIGIN

Virus	Malignancies
Epstein-Barr virus	Burkitt's lymphoma, B-cell lymphoma, nasopharyngeal carcinoma
Hepatitis B virus	Primary liver carcinoma
Human papillomavirus	Cervical carcinoma, vulvar carcinoma, and other anogenital carcinomas
Human lymphotrophic virus type I	Adult T-cell leukemia
Human lymphotrophic virus type II	Hairy cell leukemia

Data from Cooper, G. (1995). *Oncogenes* (2nd ed.). Boston: Jones & Bartlett.

damaged cell. The two types of radiation associated with carcinogenesis are ionizing and ultraviolet (UV). Ionizing radiation occurs naturally in such minerals as radon, uranium, and radium. Most rocks and soil contain various concentrations of uranium and radium. Other sources of ionizing radiation include diagnostic and therapeutic radiation, as well as cosmic radiation. UV radiation is the most common type of solar radiation. Other sources of UV radiation include tanning beds and germicidal lights. UV rays do not penetrate deeply, and the most common type of cancer associated with UV exposure is skin cancer.

Both ionizing and UV radiation produce gene mutations and chromosomal damage. Although radiation exposure induces cancers more frequently among cells that can divide, it can cause cancer among nondividing cells as well.

CHRONIC IRRITATION

Chronic irritation and tissue trauma have been suspected as predisposing physical agents to cancer development, but this theory has not yet been supported directly. The incidence of skin cancer is higher in people with burn scars and other tissues that have sustained severe injury. Chronically irritated tissues may undergo frequent mitosis and thus are at an increased risk for spontaneous DNA mutation (Pitot, 1986).

Viral Carcinogenesis

Relatively few viruses have yet been proved to be carcinogenic to humans, although some are suspected to play major roles in cancer development. When viruses infect body cells, they break the DNA chain and insert their own genetic material into the human DNA chain. Breaking the DNA, along with viral gene insertion, mutates the normal cell's DNA and can either activate an oncogene or repress a suppressor gene. Viruses capable of causing cancer are known as oncoviruses. Table 24-11 lists specific cancers of known viral origin.

Dietary Factors Related to Carcinogenesis

Epidemiologic data relate cancer development to many dietary practices or combinations of dietary practices and environmental exposures. However, the relationship of diet to carcinogenesis is poorly understood. Because dietary considerations are rarely independent of other possible carcinogenic agents, evidence of dietary contributions to cancer development is clouded. Suspected dietary factors include low crude fiber intake, high intake of red meat, and high animal fat intake. Preservatives, contaminants, preparation methods, and additives (dyes, flavorings, and sweeteners) are being assessed for possible carcinogenic effects. Chart 24-1 identifies foods considered to have high carcinogenic potential.

CHART 24-1

CLIENT EDUCATION GUIDE
Dietary Habits to Reduce Cancer Risk

- Avoid excessive intake of animal fat.
- Avoid nitrites (prepared lunch meats, sausage, bacon).
- Minimize your intake of red meat.
- Keep your alcohol consumption to no more than one or two drinks per day.
- Eat more bran.
- Eat more cruciferous vegetables, such as broccoli, cauliflower, Brussels sprouts, and cabbage.
- Eat foods high in vitamin A (such as apricots, carrots, and leafy green and yellow vegetables) and vitamin C (such as fresh fruits and vegetables, especially citrus fruits).

INTRINSIC FACTORS INFLUENCING CANCER DEVELOPMENT

Intrinsic factors, including immune function, age, and genetic predisposition, also affect whether a person is likely to develop cancer.

Immune Function

The immune system protects the body from foreign invaders and non-self cells (see Chapter 20). Non-self cells include cells made in the body that are no longer normal, such as cancer cells. The part of the immune system responsible for cancer protection is cell-mediated immunity. Natural killer (NK) and helper T-cells are most important to immune surveillance.

The instrumental role of the immune system in protecting the body from cancer is supported by cancer incidence statistics in immunosuppressed people. Children younger than 2 years of age and adults older than 60 years of age have immune systems that function at less than optimal levels, and both groups have a higher incidence of cancer compared with that of the general population. Organ transplant recipients taking immunosuppressive drugs to reduce the risk of organ rejection also have a higher incidence of cancer. In clients with AIDS, incidence may be as high as 70%.

Age

Advancing age is the single most significant risk factor related to the development of cancer (American Cancer Society, 1991). Of all cancers, 50% occur in people older than 65 years of age (American Cancer Society, 2001). The higher cancer incidence in this age-group may reflect lifelong accumulation of DNA mutations that result in cell transformation and cancer. The body may no longer be able to repair these mutations as it once did. The effectiveness of the immune system, especially cell-mediated immunity, is also reduced in the older adult, resulting in a limited ability to recognize and

CHART 24-2

NURSING FOCUS *on the* OLDER ADULT
Cancer Assessment Considerations

Cancer Type	Assessment Consideration
Colorectal cancer	Ask the client whether bowel habits have changed over the past year (e.g., in consistency, frequency, or color). Is there any obvious blood in the stool? Test at least one stool specimen for occult blood during the client's hospitalization. Encourage the client to have a baseline colonoscopy. Encourage the client to reduce dietary intake of animal fats, red meat, and smoked meats. Encourage the client to increase dietary intake of bran, vegetables, and fruit.
Bladder cancer	Ask the client about the presence of: Pain on urination Blood in the urine Cloudy urine Increased frequency or urgency
Prostate cancer	Ask the client about: Hesitancy Change in the size of the urine stream Pain in the back or legs History of urinary tract infections
Skin cancer	Examine skin areas for moles or warts. Ask the client about changes in moles (e.g., color, edges, or sensation).
Leukemia	Observe the skin for color, petechiae, or ecchymosis. Ask the client about: Fatigue Bruising Bleeding tendency History of infections and illnesses Night sweats Unexplained fevers
Lung cancer	Observe the skin and mucous membranes for color. How many words can the client say between breaths? Ask the client about: Cough Hoarseness Smoking history Exposure to inhalation irritants Shortness of breath Activity tolerance Frothy or bloody sputum Pain in the arms or chest Difficulty swallowing

TABLE 24-12 • THE SEVEN WARNING SIGNS OF CANCER

C	Changes in bowel or bladder habits
A	A sore that does not heal
U	Unusual bleeding or discharge
T	Thickening or lump in the breast or elsewhere
I	Indigestion or difficulty swallowing
O	Obvious change in a wart or mole
N	Nagging cough or hoarseness

eliminate altered self cells. Cancer assessment considerations for the older adult are given in Chart 24-2.

Manifestations of cancer in older clients may be overlooked and attributed to changes that coincide with normal aging. Older adults must be aware of and report symptoms such as the seven warning signs of cancer (Table 24-12) to health care providers. Health care providers must treat these reports with respect and thoroughly investigate all manifestations suggestive of disease.

Genetic Predisposition

As previously discussed, oncogenes are primarily intrinsic factors related to carcinogenesis. Proto-oncogenes, precursors of oncogenes, are passed on from generation to generation. The development of cancer, however, depends on more than these genes. The proto-oncogene needs to be altered to allow expression of the oncogene. In some people, the location of specific proto-oncogenes is different, which may allow them to be activated more easily (Cooper, 1995). In other people, the position of the oncogene may be normal, but the gene controlling the oncogene's activity, the **suppressor gene,** may be abnormal or out of place. These variations in gene location are inheritable. Table 24-9 lists specific malignancies associated with altered oncogene activity; Table 24-13 lists specific malignancies associated with altered suppressor gene activity.

TABLE 24-13 • MALIGNANCIES ASSOCIATED WITH ALTERED SUPPRESSOR GENE ACTIVITY

Suppressor Gene	Malignancies
APC	Colorectal, stomach, and pancreatic carcinomas
DCC	Colorectal carcinoma
MTS1	Melanoma; brain tumors; leukemias; sarcomas; breast, bladder, ovarian, lung, and kidney carcinomas
NF1	Neurofibroma, colon carcinoma, astrocytoma
NF2	Neurofibroma, meningioma, schwannoma
p53	Breast, bladder, colorectal, esophageal, liver, lung and ovarian carcinomas; brain tumors; sarcomas; leukemias and lymphomas
Rb	Retinoblastoma; sarcomas; breast, bladder, esophageal, and lung carcinomas
pVHL	Renal cell carcinoma, pheochromocytoma, hemangioblastoma

TABLE 24-14 • CONDITIONS ASSOCIATED WITH A GENETIC PREDISPOSITION FOR CANCER

Condition	Specific Cancer Type
Inherited cancers*	Breast cancer Prostate cancer Ovarian cancer
Familial clustering	Breast cancer Melanoma
Bloom's syndrome	Leukemia
Familial polyposis	Colorectal cancer
Chromosomal aberrations	
Down syndrome (47 chromosomes)	Leukemia
Klinefelter's syndrome (47, XXY)	Breast cancer
Turner's syndrome (45, XO)	Leukemia Gonadal carcinoma Meningioma Colorectal cancer

*Not all breast, prostate, or ovarian cancers are inherited.

Patterns of genetic predisposition for cancer other than oncogenes have also been identified, including the following:

- Inherited predisposition for specific cancers
- Inherited conditions associated with cancer
- Familial clustering
- Chromosomal aberrations

Table 24-14 lists different conditions associated with a genetic predisposition for cancer development.

CULTURAL CONSIDERATIONS

The incidence of cancer varies among races. American Cancer Society data (2001) show that African Americans have a higher incidence of cancer than Caucasians do, and the death rate is higher for African Americans. Since 1960 the overall incidence among African Americans has increased 27%, whereas for Caucasians it has increased 12%. Cancer sites and cancer-related mortality vary along racial lines as well. Table 24-15 summarizes common cancers among Caucasian, African-American, Asian, and Hispanic populations.

When risks for cancer development are assessed, however, race and genetic predisposition cannot be considered alone. Behavior related to a cultural or ethnic group, geographic location, diet, and socioeconomic factors must also be assessed. The American Cancer Society (2001) has reported that cancer incidence and survival are often related to socioeconomic factors, such as the availability of health care services or the belief that seeking early health care has a positive effect on the outcome of cancer diagnosis (see the Evidence-Based Practice for Nursing box at right).

CANCER PREVENTION

Avoidance of Known or Potential Carcinogens

A very effective means of preventing cancer development is avoidance of known or potential carcinogens. This method of prevention is appropriate when the cause of a specific cancer

TABLE 24-15 • RACIAL DIFFERENCES IN CANCER DEVELOPMENT

CAUCASIAN
Common Cancer Types
1. Lung
2. Breast
3. Colorectal
4. Prostate

AFRICAN AMERICAN
Common Cancer Types
1. Lung
2. Prostate
3. Breast
4. Colorectal
5. Uterine

ASIAN
Common Cancer Types
1. Breast
2. Colorectal
3. Prostate
4. Lung
5. Stomach

HISPANIC
Common Cancer Types
1. Prostate
2. Breast
3. Colorectal
4. Lung

Data from American Cancer Society. (2001). *Cancer facts and figures—2001.* Report No. 00-300M-No. 5008.01. Atlanta: Author.

EVIDENCE-BASED PRACTICE FOR NURSING

African-American women's attitudes toward breast cancer

Phillips, J., Cohen, M., & Moses, G. (1999). Breast cancer screening and African-American women: Fear, fatalism, and silence. *Oncology Nursing Forum, 26*(3), 561-571.

The investigators of this prospective qualitative study explored the beliefs of 26 African-American women from different educational, employment, and socioeconomic strata. The women were between the ages of 40 and 66; groups consisted of women employed as teachers (middle income), women employed as service workers (low income), and women who were unemployed (low income). Data were collected through three 90-minute focus group discussions regarding breast cancer beliefs, experiences, attitudes, and screening practices. All focus group sessions were audiotaped, transcribed verbatim, reviewed for completeness, and reviewed line by line for similar themes.

The results indicated that all participants related a cancer diagnosis with panic and fear of death. In addition, the participants viewed breast cancer as largely a "white disease." The most significant differences noted among the participants was in the area of breast health and breast screening. The women with more education and higher incomes expressed greater reliance on breast examinations and mammography. In addition, these women expressed concern about the lack of access to these screening methods for African-American women with low incomes.

The investigators suggest that culturally sensitive educational interventions targeted to African Americans could dispel myths, reduce fatalism, and contribute to greater compliance with recommended cancer screening regimens.

Critique. This study was well designed and well implemented for the purpose of examining the influence of education and socioeconomic factors separate from race for breast health and breast cancer screening. The study supports the literature demonstrating differences among groups of African-American women regarding the stage at diagnosis and death rates from breast cancer, with low-income women being diagnosed at later stages and having poorer outcomes compared with African-American women with more education and higher incomes.

Implications for Nursing. Many African-American women with fatalistic beliefs either have had negative experiences with cancer, are basing their opinions on out-of-date cancer statistics, or view breast cancer as a "white disease." Socioeconomic factors, as well as race and cultural factors, must be taken into consideration when determining each client's beliefs regarding cancer prognosis. Development of culturally appropriate breast health and cancer educational materials using African-American women as models or informants could increase compliance with recommended screening guidelines.

is known or strongly implicated and avoidance is easily accomplished. Examples of effective avoidance are using skin protection during sun exposure, avoiding tobacco, and eliminating environmental asbestos. As more causes of cancer are identified, the prevention method of avoidance will likely become even more effective.

Avoidance or Modification of Associated Factors

Absolute causes are not known for many cancers, but specific conditions or exposures appear to have an associated risk. Some examples are the increased incidence of some cancer types among people who consume alcohol; the association of a diet high in fat and low in fiber with colon cancer, breast cancer, and ovarian cancer; and the greater incidence of cervical cancer among women with many sexual partners. It is thought that avoidance or reduction of exposure to the associated condition or factor might result in decreased risks for cancer development.

Chemoprevention

A new form of cancer prevention, **chemoprevention,** is currently under study to determine its effectiveness. This strategy uses exogenous chemicals, such as synthetic chemicals, natural nutrients, or other substances found in plant food sources, to disrupt one or more steps important to cancer development. Such agents may be able to reverse existing damage or halt the progression of the transformation process. Chemopreventive agents have a variety of actions, including the following, that disrupt at least one important step in the process of cancer:

- Blocking an inactive compound from becoming an active carcinogen
- Blocking the direct action of a carcinogen on DNA
- Enhancing the rate of elimination of a carcinogen from the body
- Suppressing the activity of a carcinogen
- Suppressing the promoting activity of a carcinogen
- Suppressing the progression of a premalignant or early-stage malignancy into a more malignant state

Table 24-16 lists agents under current investigation for effectiveness in chemoprevention.

The ultimate goal of chemopreventive strategies is prevention of cancer development. Target populations for whom chemoprevention might be effective include the following:

- Healthy people with no known specific cancer risk
- People at greater than normal risk because of increased environmental exposure or decreased immune function
- People with precancerous lesions
- People with a history of cancer

TABLE 24-16 • AGENTS UNDER INVESTIGATION FOR CHEMOPREVENTION OF CANCER

Category of Prevention	Specific Agents
Prevention of carcinogen formation	Ascorbic acid (vitamin C) Tocopherol (type of vitamin E) Selenium Caffeic acid
Blocking the action of a carcinogen on DNA ("antimutagens")	Carotenoids (vitamin A derivative) Retinoids (vitamin A derivative) Ellagic acid Flavones Oltipraz Butylated hydroxyanisole
Enhancing the elimination of a carcinogen	Isothiocyanate Indole-3-carbinol
Suppression of carcinogenic action	Aspirin Retinoids Indomethacin Selenium Steroidal anti-inflammatory agents Protease inhibitors
Antipromotion activity	Carotenoids Retinoids Selenium Coumarin Piroxicam Indomethacin Calciferol (vitamin D) Hormone antagonists Tamoxifen Fenasteride
Suppression of progression	Danazol Interferon Cysteamine Vorozole

Gene Alteration as a Potential Form of Cancer Prevention

Because cancer development clearly involves gene changes (either congenital genetic abnormalities or acquired gene damage), researchers have suggested that altering damaged genes could prevent cancer development. At the present stage of scientific development, people can be screened for some gene alterations that will eventually lead to cancer. Such screening can help a genetically susceptible person either alter lifestyle factors or participate in early detection methods to identify a malignancy when cure is more likely. Although it is not yet possible to "fix" or remove an abnormal gene in humans, gene therapy in the future is not out of the realm of possibility.

ONLINE RESOURCES

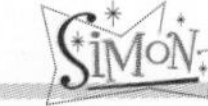

For suggested readings and Internet resources, go to http://www.wbsaunders.com/SIMON/Iggy/.

SELECTED BIBLIOGRAPHY

Asterisk indicates a classic or definitive work on this subject.

*American Cancer Society. (1991). *Proceedings of the National Workshop on Cancer Control and the Older Person.* Report No. 91-3M-No. 3043. Atlanta: Author.

American Cancer Society. (2001). *Cancer facts and figures—2001.* Report No. 00-300M-No. 5008.01. Atlanta: Author.

*Ames, B., Gold, L., & Willett, W. (1995). The causes and prevention of cancer. *Proceedings of the National Academy of Sciences, 92*(12), 5258-5265.

Baron, R., & Borgen, P. (1997). Genetic susceptibility for breast cancer: Testing and primary prevention options. *Oncology Nursing Forum, 24*(3), 461-468.

*Bishop, J. (1982). Oncogenes. *Scientific American, 246*(3), 80-92.

Brown, P. (1999). Nutrition and cancer. *MEDSURG Nursing, 8*(6), 333-345.

Byers, T., et al. (1999). Cancer genetics counseling. *Cancer Practice, 7*(2), 93-95.

Calzone, K. (1997). Genetic predisposition testing: Clinical implications for oncology nurses. *Oncology Nursing Forum, 24*(4), 712-718.

Clark, P., & Gomez, E. (2001). Details on demand: Consumers, cancer information, and the internet. *Clinical Journal of Oncology Nursing, 5*(1), 19-24.

*Cooper, G. (1995). *Oncogenes* (2nd ed.). Boston: Jones & Bartlett.

Daley, E. (1998). Clinical update on the role of HPV and cervical cancer. *Cancer Nursing, 21*(1), 31-35.

Dimond, E., et al. (1998). Programmed instruction: The role of the nurse in cancer genetics. *Cancer Nursing, 21*(1), 57-74.

*Frank-Stromborg, M., & Olsen, S. (2001). *Cancer prevention in diverse populations: Cultural implications for health care professionals.* Pittsburgh: Oncology Nursing Society.

*Glaser, E. (1990). Inherited predisposition to colon cancer. *Cancer Nursing, 21*(6), 377-383.

Greenlee, R., et al. (2001). Cancer statistics 2001.*CA: A Cancer Journal for Clinicians, 51*(1), 15-37.

Haylock, P. (1998). Cancer metastasis: An update. *Seminars in Oncology Nursing, 14*(3), 172-177.

Khuri, F. (1999). Chemoprevention of cancer. *Highlights in Oncology Practice, 16*(4), 100-109.

*Liotta, L. (1992). Cancer cell invasion and metastasis. *Scientific American, 266*(2), 54-62.

Loescher, L. (1998). DNA testing for cancer predisposition. *Oncology Nursing Forum, 25*(8), 1317-1326.

Machia, J. (2001). Breast cancer: Risk, prevention, and tamoxifen. *American Journal of Nursing, 101*(4), 26-35.

Mahan, S. (1998). Cancer risk assessment: Conceptual considerations for clinical practice. *Oncology Nursing Forum, 25*(9), 1535-1547.

Miaskowski, C., & Buchsel, P. (1999). *Oncology nursing: Assessment and clinical care.* St. Louis: Mosby.

*Nicolson, G. (1979). Cancer metastasis. *Scientific American, 240,* 66-79.

*Olsen, S., & Frank-Stromborg, M. (1994). Cancer prevention and screening activities reported by African-American nurses. *Oncology Nursing Forum, 21*(3), 487-494.

Phillips, J., Cohen, M., & Moses, G. (1999). Breast cancer screening and African-American women: Fear, fatalism, and silence. *Oncology Nursing Forum, 26*(3), 561-571.

*Pitot, H. (1986). *Fundamentals of oncology* (2nd ed.). New York: Marcel Dekker.

*Ruoslahti, E. (1996). How cancer spreads. *Scientific American, 275*(3), 72-77.

Sarna, L. (1999). Prevention: Tobacco control and cancer nursing. *Cancer Nursing, 21*(1), 21-28.

Singh, D., & Lippman, S. (1998). Cancer chemoprevention: Part 1. Retinoids, carotenoids and other classic antioxidants. *Oncology, 12*(11), 1643-1658.

Swan, D., & Ford, B. (1997). Chemoprevention of cancer: Review of the literature. *Oncology Nursing Forum, 24*(4), 719-727.

*Trichopoulos, D., Li, F., & Hunter, D. (1996). What causes cancer? *Scientific American, 275*(3), 80-87.

*Weinberg, R. (1996). How cancer arises. *Scientific American, 275*(3), 62-70.

Weinrich, S., et al. (1998). The impact of prostate cancer knowledge on cancer screening. *Oncology Nursing Forum, 25*(3), 527-534.

CHAPTER 25

Interventions for Clients with Cancer

M. LINDA WORKMAN

Learning Objectives

After studying this chapter, you should be able to:

1. Identify the goals of cancer therapy.
2. Differentiate between cancer surgery for cure and cancer surgery for palliation.
3. Discuss how the nursing care needs for the client undergoing cancer surgery compare to those for the client undergoing any other type of surgery.
4. Compare and contrast the purposes and side effects of radiation therapy and chemotherapy for cancer.
5. Prioritize nursing care for the client with radiation-induced skin problems.
6. Prioritize educational needs for the client receiving external beam radiation.
7. Compare the personnel safety issues for working with clients receiving teletherapy radiation versus those receiving brachytherapy radiation.
8. Identify nursing interventions to promote safety for the client experiencing chemotherapy-induced anemia or thrombocytopenia.
9. Prioritize nursing care for the client with chemotherapy-induced neutropenia.
10. Prioritize nursing care for the client with mucositis.
11. Explain the rationale for hormonal manipulation therapy.
12. Discuss the uses of biologic response modifiers as supportive therapy in the treatment of cancer.
13. Identify clients at risk for oncologic emergencies.

SIMON

Go to http://www.wbsaunders.com/SIMON/Iggy/ for self-assessment questions related to these Learning Objectives.

Most people fear a diagnosis of cancer, equating the disease with suffering and death. However, more than 50% of people in North America diagnosed with cancer are cured, and thousands of others live 5 years or longer after the diagnosis (American Cancer Society, 2001). Regardless of treatment type, the experience of cancer always alters a person's physical and psychologic functioning to some degree.

Providing care to clients and families experiencing cancer is complex and challenging. This chapter describes the general interventions for and the consequences of cancer and its treatment. For individualized treatment requirements and client problems associated with specific cancer types, consult the interventions chapters in which the cancer is described. Table 25-1 lists common cancer types and the specific locations within this text where the interventions are presented. Table 25-2 lists key concepts about cancer treatment.

GENERAL DISEASE-RELATED CONSEQUENCES OF CANCER

Cancer can develop in any organ or tissue but tends to occur more commonly in some tissues than in others. Cancer destroys normal tissue, resulting in decreased function in that tissue or organ. Even when cancers occur in nonvital tissues or organs, they can cause death by **metastasizing** (spreading) into vital organs and disrupting critical physiologic processes (see Chapter 24). Cancers that are left untreated produce serious health problems, such as the following:

- Impaired immune and hematopoietic (blood-producing) function
- Altered gastrointestinal (GI) tract structure and function
- Motor and sensory deficits
- Decreased respiratory function

These impairments cause great physical and emotional distress. Without intervention, persistent cancer invasion of normal tissues leads to death.

Impaired Immune and Hematopoietic Function

Impaired immune and hematopoietic function occurs most often in clients with leukemia and lymphoma, but such impairment can occur with any cancer that invades the bone marrow. Tumor cells enter the bone marrow and cause decreased production of healthy white blood cells **(leukopenia),** which are needed for normal immune function (see Chapter 20). Thus clients who have cancer, especially leukemia, are at an increased risk for infection.

When cancer invades the bone marrow, it also decreases the number of red blood cells **(anemia)** and platelets **(throm-**

TABLE 25-1 • TEXT LOCATION OF SPECIFIC CANCER CONTENT

Cancer Type	Chapter	Patho/ Etiol	Treatment and Nursing Intervention
Breast	74	1736-1738	1738-1749
Lung	30	559-561	562-565
Prostate	76	1789-1790	1791-1793
Colorectal	57	1245-1246	1248-1253
Skin	67	1545-1546	1546-1548
Leukemia	40	846-847	849-858
Lymphoma	40	858-859	859-860
Ovarian	75	1776	1776-1778
Head and neck	54	1182-1183	1184-1190
Cervical	75	1772-1773	1774-1776
Bladder	70	1637	1638-1639
Stomach	56	1235	1236-1238
Esophageal	55	1205	1206-1212
Kidney	71	1658	1658-1659

TABLE 25-2 • KEY POINTS ABOUT CANCER TREATMENT

- With a multiapproach to cancer treatment, 50% of clients with cancer can be cured.
- Surgery is most effective for cancer therapy when tumors are small and well localized.
- Radiation therapy is effective only on the tissues directly within the radiation path.
- Side effects of radiation therapy are confined to the tissues within the radiation path.
- The most common side effects of radiation therapy are skin irritation, fatigue, and altered taste sensation.
- Chemotherapy is systemic therapy for cancer and affects all body tissues.
- The most common side effects of chemotherapy are alopecia, nausea and vomiting, mucositis, skin changes, and bone marrow suppression.
- The most life-threatening side effect of chemotherapy is bone marrow suppression.

bocytopenia). These changes may be caused by the cancer itself, such as in leukemia, or by the cancer treatment. In either case, the client becomes anemic and has an increased tendency to bleed.

Altered Gastrointestinal Structure and Function

Cancer can alter GI function and disturb nutritional status. For example, tumors may cause obstruction or compression anywhere along the GI tract and interfere with the client's ability to obtain adequate nutrients and eliminate waste products. Tumors also can affect basal metabolic rate and increase a client's requirements for protein, carbohydrates, and fat at the same time he or she has less energy available to prepare and eat meals.

Many tumors spread to the liver, causing profound damage to this organ. The liver has many important metabolic functions and helps digest and use proteins and fats. Altered liver function contributes to malnutrition and death among clients with cancer.

The anorexia experienced by clients with cancer often interferes with their ability to meet energy requirements. **Cachexia** (extreme body wasting and malnutrition) develops from an imbalance between food intake and energy use. This condition may occur in spite of what appears to be adequate nutritional intake. Changes in a client's taste can result from the cancer or the treatment and cause a decrease in appetite. A complete list of cancer-related factors that can contribute to malnutrition is presented in Table 25-3.

Nutritional support for the client with cancer, especially one undergoing cancer therapy, is complex and controversial. A diet high in protein and carbohydrates is often ordered to help the client maintain weight and to provide the necessary nutrients for energy and cellular repair. However, some scientists believe that an excessive intake of protein, carbohydrates, and vitamins increases the nutrition of the cancer cells and contributes to cancer progression. Clients often believe their cancer can be cured more easily by eating more food, especially a diet low in fat and high in fiber, grains, fruit, and vegetables. Currently no one nutritional plan meets the needs of all clients with cancer (Brown, 1999; Wilson, 2000).

Motor and Sensory Deficits

Motor (movement) and sensory deficits can occur when cancers invade bone or the brain or compress nerves. In adult clients with bone metastases, the primary cancer started in another organ (e.g., the prostate, breast, or lung). The bone sites most affected include the vertebrae, ribs, pelvis, and femur. The humerus, scapula, sternum, skull, and clavicle are also common metastatic sites. Bone metastases can cause fractures, spinal cord compression, and hypercalcemia, each of which results in decreased mobility for the client.

The client may also experience sensory changes if the spinal cord is damaged by tumor compression or if nerve ganglia are compressed. Sensory, motor, and cognitive functions are severely disrupted when tumors metastasize to the brain.

The client with cancer may also experience pain. Pain does not always accompany cancer, but it can be a significant problem for clients with terminal cancer. Chapter 7 provides an in-depth discussion of the causes and management of cancer pain.

Decreased Respiratory Function

Cancer can disrupt a client's respiratory function in several ways and often results in death. For example, tumors involving the airways can cause airway obstruction. If lung tissue is involved, lung capacity is decreased. Tumor growth can also press on vascular and lymphatic structures in the chest, blocking blood flow through the chest and lungs and resulting in pulmonary edema and dyspnea. In addition, tumors can thicken the alveolar membrane and damage pulmonary blood vessels, reducing gas exchange.

TREATMENT-RELATED CONSEQUENCES OF CANCER

The purpose of any cancer treatment is to prolong survival time or improve quality of life (see the Meeting Healthy People 2010 Objectives box on p. 425). Although a few spontaneous regressions of malignant tumors have been reported, most clients would die within months of diagnosis without appropriate cancer therapy. Therapies for cancer include surgery, radiation, chemotherapy, hormonal manipulation, im-

TABLE 25-3 • CAUSES OF MALNUTRITION IN CLIENTS WITH CANCER

ANOREXIA

Local causes
- Pelvic or abdominal tumors
- Hepatic metastases
- Intestinal compression or obstruction
- Others

Remote causes
- Food aversions
- Early satiety

Treatment-related causes
- Postsurgical small stomach or stasis
- Drugs, including chemotherapy
- Radiation—local and systemic effects

Systemic illness
- Infection
- Hepatitis or pancreatitis
- Endocrinopathies

Taste disorders
- Drugs (e.g., metronidazole)
- Remote effects of neoplasm and its treatment
- Local disease and its treatment (e.g., stomatitis, nasopharyngeal tumor, radiation, and surgery)
- Nausea and vomiting

Psychogenic causes
- Depression
- Anxiety
- Conditioned aversions

Intolerance of institutional food

DIFFICULTY IN EATING

Head and neck tumors and their treatment
Xerostomia
Stomatitis
Loss of teeth and dental problems
Dysphagia and odynophagia

MALDIGESTION OR MALABSORPTION

Pancreatic insufficiency
Bile salt deficiency
Hypersecretory syndrome
- Zollinger-Ellison syndrome
- Pancreatic cholera
- Bowel infiltration
- Diffuse invasion (e.g., lymphoma)
- Local blockage
- Fistula

Postsurgical causes
- Esophageal surgery (with vagotomy, gastric statis, diarrhea, and steatorrhea)
- Gastrectomy—dumping, achlorhydria, or afferent loop syndrome
- Small intestine resections

Postirradiation causes
- Enteritis (may occur as late sequelae)
- Fistula
- Stenosis
- Obstruction

PROTEIN-LOSING ENTEROPATHY MALUTILIZATION

Cancer cachexia
Steroids
- Nitrogen wasting
- Hyperglycemia
- Calcium loss

munotherapy, and gene therapy. These therapies may be used individually or in combination to kill tumor cells. The type and amount of therapy depends on the specific type of cancer, the extent of the disease, and the overall health of the client. One or more regimens **(protocols)** have been established for most types of cancer. These regimens are based on experiments with cancer cells and animals and on experience with other clients with cancer.

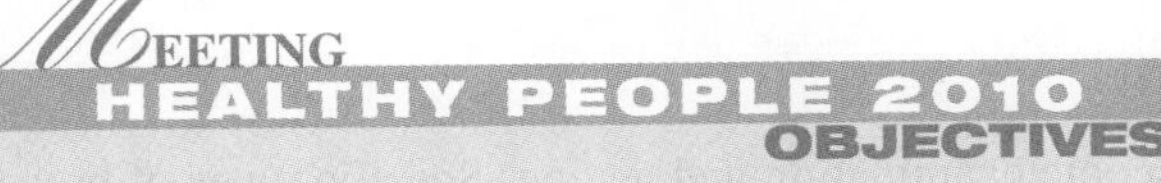

CANCER

Objective 17.16: Increase the number of cancer survivors who are living 5 years or longer after diagnosis.

- Encourage clients to seek early health care advice whenever one of the seven warning signs of cancer are present.
- Teach clients being treated for cancer the importance of compliance with the scheduled treatment regimen.
- Teach the client to follow up with health care visits after cancer treatment is completed.
- Teach the client with cancer to continue with recommended screening practices.
- Encourage the client who has been treated for cancer to avoid known environmental carcinogens.
- Assist clients who smoke to reduce or quit smoking.
- Teach clients about the importance of limiting dietary fat, smoked meats, and red meats.

Surgery

RATIONALE FOR CANCER TREATMENT

Surgery for cancer involves the removal of diseased tissue. If cancer is confined to the removed tissue, surgery alone can result in a "cure" for that cancer. Although many cancers have spread too far at the time of diagnosis for surgery alone to be curative, it may still be a useful part of diagnosis, treatment, follow-up, and rehabilitation.

MECHANISM OF ACTION

Surgery is the oldest form of cancer treatment and is the first method to cure cancer. Cancer surgery may be prescribed for any of the following purposes: prophylaxis, diagnosis, cure, control, palliation, determination of therapy effectiveness, and reconstruction.

Prophylaxis

Prophylactic surgery is performed when a client has either an existing "premalignant" condition or a known family history that strongly predisposes the person to the development of cancer. An attempt is made to remove the "at-risk" tissue or organ to prevent the development of cancer. An example of prophylactic surgery for a premalignant condition is removing a benign mole from a location where it would receive continuous irritation or exposure to sunlight.

Diagnosis (Biopsy)

Diagnostic surgery provides histologic proof of malignancy. All or part of a suspected lesion is usually removed for mi-

TABLE 25-4 • DIAGNOSTIC/BIOPSY SURGERIES FOR CANCER

Biopsy Type	Description	Problem/Limitations
Needle	Aspirating cells in a fluid or in very soft tissue Boring a "core" of solid tissue by using a long needle or making a punch, scrape, or bite	Sample error—may biopsy only noncancerous cells in a tissue or organ Sample size may not be adequate for accurate testing Procedure may spread cancer by seeding it into surrounding tissues Procedure may damage healthy tissue
Incisional	Removing a wedge of suspected tissue from a larger tissue mass, leaving some tumor cells in the tissue	Sample error Tumor seeding Damage to healthy tissue
Excisional	Completely removing an entire lesion without removing any adjacent normal tissues	Tumor seeding Leaving micrometastasis Damage to healthy tissue
Staging	Performing multiple needle or incisional biopsies in tissues where metastasis is suspected or likely	Tumor seeding Sample error Damage to healthy tissue

TABLE 25-5 • CURATIVE SURGERIES FOR CANCER

Surgery Type	Description	Purpose/Use
Local excision	Removal of all identifiable tumor along with a small margin of normal tissues	Small, localized tumors
Wide local excision (radical)	Removal of identifiable tumor plus immediate tissue or adjacent tissue	Small tumors with only local tissue invasion
Wide excision	Removal of tumor, surrounding tissue, adjacent structures, and usual lymph channels draining the area	Small to moderate-size tumors with known local invasion
Extended radical excision	Removal of tumor, lymphatics, adjacent organs, and all tissues in the region	Tumor infiltrate in a wide area but with no known distant metastasis

croscopic examination and testing. Specific types of biopsies are summarized in Table 25-4.

Cure

Without additional therapy, surgery for cure can result in a cure rate of 25% to 30%. All gross and microscopic tumor is either removed or destroyed. Types of curative surgeries are described in Table 25-5.

Control (Cytoreductive Surgery)

Cancer control, or cytoreductive surgery, is a "debulking" procedure that consists of removing part of the tumor and leaving a known amount of gross tumor. This type of surgery alone cannot result in a cure, but it does decrease the number of cancer cells and increases the chances that other therapies can be successful.

Palliation

Palliative surgery aims not to cure (or even increase survival time in many instances) but to improve quality of life during the survival time. The surgeon removes the tumor tissue that is causing pain, intestinal obstruction, or difficulty swallowing. The specific procedure used during palliative surgery depends on the client's specific problem.

Determination of Therapy Effectiveness ("Second Look")

Second-look surgery is essentially a "rediagnosis" after treatment. This procedure is performed to assess the disease status in clients who have been treated and have no symptoms of remaining or recurrent tumor. The results of this surgery serve as a basis for discontinuing or continuing specific therapy.

Reconstructive or Rehabilitative Surgery

Reconstructive-rehabilitative surgery is relatively new. People with cancer are surviving long enough to need reconstruction. This type of surgery increases function, enhances cosmetic appearance, or both. Examples include breast reconstruction after mastectomy, replacement of the esophagus after radiation damage, bowel reconstruction, revision of scars, release of contractures, and placement of penile implants.

SIDE EFFECTS OF SURGICAL THERAPY

Unlike surgery performed for many other reasons, cancer surgery often involves the loss of a specific body part or its function. Sometimes whole organs are removed, such as the kidney, lung, breast, testes, arm, or tongue. Any organ loss results in reduced function. The amount of function that is lost and how much the loss physically affects clients depends on the location and extent of the surgery. Some surgical procedures for cancer may result in significant scarring or disfigurement. In addition to actual body part loss and anxiety about the chances of surviving, clients may be grieving about a loss of body image or a change in lifestyle imposed by the cancer or its treatment.

NURSING CARE OF CLIENTS UNDERGOING SURGICAL THERAPY

The nursing care associated with cancer surgery is not vastly different from that related to surgery for other reasons (see Chapters 17 to 19). The nurse considers all the physical and psychosocial factors related to the client's ability (and the ability of family and significant others) to cope with the uncertainty of cancer and its treatment and with the changes in body image and role. For example, surgery involving the genitals, urinary tract, colon, and rectum may permanently damage these organs. Surgical procedures that create a urinary or fecal diversion (e.g., a colostomy) may disturb innervation, causing erectile impotence or ejaculatory dysfunction in men and painful intercourse **(dyspareunia)** in women.

Radiation

RATIONALE FOR CANCER TREATMENT

The purpose of all types of radiation therapy for cancer is to destroy cancer cells with minimal exposure of the normal cells to the damaging actions of radiation. The effects of radiation are seen only in the tissues in the path of the radiation beam. Some effects are apparent within days or weeks, whereas other effects may not be apparent for months to years after the completion of radiation therapy.

MECHANISM OF ACTION

Most of the radiation used to treat malignant tumors is **ionizing radiation.** When cells are exposed to this type of radiation, atoms within the cell are "kicked out" of orbit, resulting in a tremendous release of intracellular energy. Ionizing radiation is given off naturally by some substances, such as radium and cobalt, and can also be generated by machines called linear accelerators. Naturally occurring radiation is called **gamma radiation;** radiation that is generated by machine is called **roentgen radiation.** Their effect on cells is exactly the same.

Cells damaged by radiation either die outright or become unable to divide. Radiation damage can occur any time a cell is exposed to radiation; it is not confined to cells actively in the cell cycle. However, cells in the cell cycle do experience more damage when exposed to radiation than do nondividing cells.

Three different types of energy, or rays, are produced by gamma radiation: **gamma, beta,** and **alpha rays.** These rays vary in their ability to penetrate tissues and damage cells. Table 25-6 summarizes the features of these three types of gamma radiation, and Figure 25-1 shows the penetrating ability of each.

The amount of radiation aimed at or delivered to a tissue is called **exposure,** and the amount of radiation absorbed by the recipient tissue is called the **dose.** The dose is always somewhat less than the exposure. Three major factors determine the absorbed dose: intensity of exposure, duration of exposure, and proximity of the radiation source to the cells.

TABLE 25-6 • CHARACTERISTICS OF DIFFERENT TYPES OF GAMMA RADIATION

GAMMA RAY

Gamma rays are very light and have a low energy-transfer potential. They travel at the speed of light, allowing them to be concentrated and penetrate deeply into tissues.

This is the most common type of radiation used for the treatment of cancer.

This type of radiation can also cause serious, irreversible harm to tissues.

Exposure to this type of radiation must be avoided or severely limited.

BETA RAY

Beta rays are heavier and travel at a moderate to high speed. They have a high linear energy-transfer potential and do not penetrate tissues or other substances well.

Some beta rays are used inside the body for specific radiation therapy.

Beta rays are used in some diagnostic tests.

Beta rays pose health hazards to humans exposed to them, but exposure must be considerable for damage to occur.

ALPHA RAY

Alpha rays are very heavy and slow. They easily transfer energy to their surroundings and quickly lose their ability to penetrate tissues (0.04 mm into tissue).

Currently, alpha rays are used in laboratory tests rather than as treatment for cancer.

This type of radiation is harmful to humans only if it is ingested chronically.

The intensity of the radiation emitted decreases with the distance from the radiation source (Figure 25-2). This phenomenon is known as the **inverse square law.** For example, the radiation dose received at a distance of 2 feet from the radiation source is only one fourth of the dose received at a distance of 1 foot from the radiation source; the dose of radiation received at 3 feet is only one ninth of the dose received at 1 foot (Hassey, 1987).

Killing Effects of Radiation

If the dose of radiation is high enough, all cells are killed immediately. This does not usually happen. Radiation damage to the deoxyribonucleic acid (DNA) of the cell is not usually apparent until the cell attempts to divide. In a tumor treated with a single exposure of radiation, all cells within the tumor absorb the radiation slightly differently. Therefore their overall response to the radiation is slightly different. A few cells die immediately, and more die within the next 24 hours as they attempt to divide. Some cells become sterile as a result of this single treatment, whereas others repair the radiation-induced damage and continue to reproduce for many cell generations.

Because of the varying responses of all cancer cells within a given tumor, radiation is administered as a series of divided doses. Small doses of radiation are delivered on a daily basis for a set period of time. Giving radiation treatments sequentially rather than as a single dose allows multiple opportunities to catch and destroy cancer cells that survived the initial hit of radiation while minimizing the damage to normal tissues. This

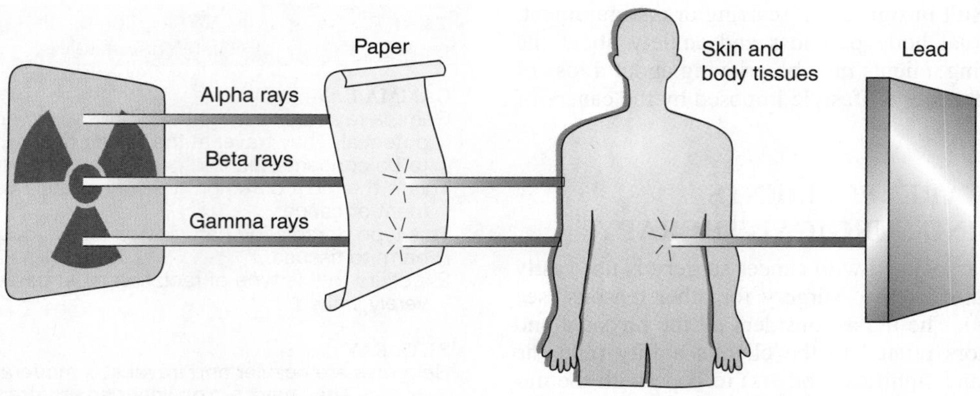

Figure 25-1 ● Penetrating capacity of different types of radiation.

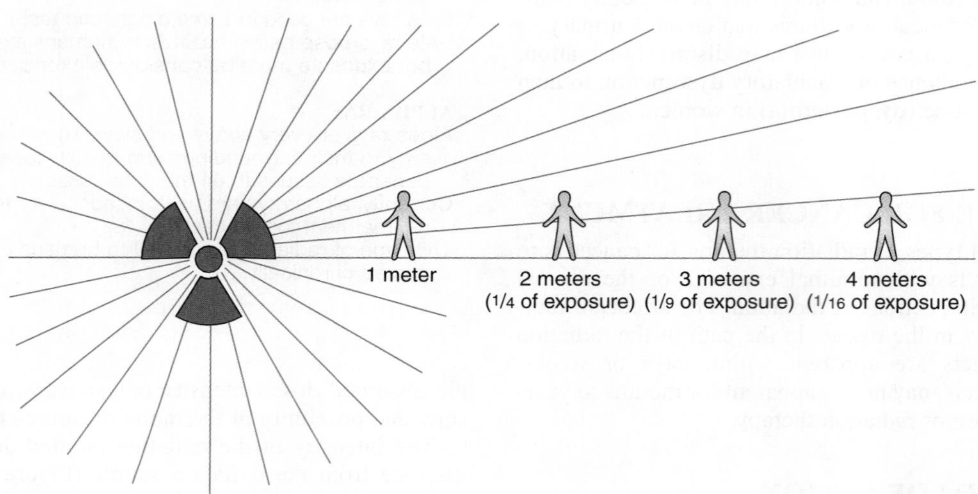

Figure 25-2 ● The inverse square law of radiation exposure.

dose division is called **fractionation.** Standard radiotherapy is usually fractionated between 180 and 250 rad/day, multiplied by as many days as needed to achieve the total prescribed dose. (Rad is an acronym meaning "radiation absorbed dose.")

The total therapeutic dose of radiation to a tumor depends on the size and location of the tumor and on the radiation sensitivity of the tumor and surrounding normal tissues. Some normal tissues are more sensitive than others to radiation. For example, a total dose of 1200 rad might be prescribed for a primary liver tumor, but a total dose of 5000 to 6000 rad might be necessary for a breast carcinoma (delivered over 25 to 30 separate days). A 6000-rad dose delivered to the liver would lead to such extensive damage of liver tissue that the client would experience liver failure and die, even if the tumor were destroyed. Healthy breast tissue can tolerate much higher doses of radiation.

Two types of radiation delivery are most commonly used for cancer therapy: teletherapy and brachytherapy. The type used depends on the client's general condition and state of health and on the site, stage (including size and depth of the lesion), and radiosensitivity of the tumor. Regardless of how it is administered, the optimum dose of radiation is one that can kill the cancer cells with an acceptable level of damage to normal tissues (some damage to normal tissues cannot be avoided).

Teletherapy

Teletherapy is derived from the Greek prefix *"tele,"* meaning distant. In teletherapy, the actual radiation source is external to the client and remote from the tumor site. Because the source is external, the client never emits radiation and poses no hazard to anyone else. This type of therapy is also called **beam radiation.**

To increase the accuracy of radiation delivery to cancer cells, the exact location of the tumor is determined. Once the pattern of radiation delivery is established, the client must always be in exactly the same position for all treatments. The nurse ensures that the client can get into and maintain this position with relative ease. Position-fixing devices and markings, either on the client's body or on the devices, ensure the proper position each day of treatment.

Brachytherapy

Brachytherapy is derived from the Greek word *"brach,"* meaning short. With brachytherapy, the radiation source must come into direct, continuous contact with the tumor tissues for a specific period of time. The rationale is to provide a high absorbed dose of radiation in tumor tissues and a very limited absorbed low dose in surrounding normal tissues. The radiation delivered by brachytherapy has the same tissue effects as ionizing radiation delivered by external sources.

Brachytherapy involves the use of radioactive isotopes either in solid form or within body fluids. Isotopes can be delivered to the tumor tissues in several ways. With all types of brachytherapy, the radiation source is within the client. Therefore the client emits radiation for a period of time and can pose a hazard to others.

UNSEALED RADIATION SOURCES

Soluble isotopes are unsealed radioactive sources administered via the oral or intravenous (IV) routes or as an instillation into body cavities, such as the peritoneal cavity and the spinal fluid space. Because the isotopes are unsealed, they are not completely confined to any one body area. However, they may concentrate more in some body tissues than in others. These soluble isotopes enter body fluids and eventually are eliminated from the body in various excreta (waste products), which are radioactive and can be harmful to other people.

An example of brachytherapy with soluble isotopes is the ingestion or injection of the radionuclide iodine^{131} (an iodine base with a half-life of 8.05 days) to treat hyperthyroidism and some thyroid malignancies. The radioactive iodine concentrates in the thyroid gland and destroys the thyroid cancer cells. Most of this isotope is eliminated from the body within 48 hours. Once eliminated, neither the client nor the excreta are radioactive.

SEALED RADIATION SOURCES

The solid forms of brachytherapy involve sealed radiation sources implanted within the tumor target tissues. These radiation sources can be temporary or permanent. Most of the implants emit continuous, low-energy radiation to tumor tissues. Some devices (e.g., seeds or needles) can be placed into the tissues and stay in place by themselves. Other solid radiation sources must be held in place within the tissue or cavity by special applicators. Needles and seeds are preloaded with the radioactive isotope and are radioactive at the time of insertion ("hot implantation"). Some of these devices are so small and the half-life of the isotope so short that the device is permanently left in place (most often for clients with prostate cancer). Other devices are removed and reused in other clients.

In afterloading, the implant is placed within the cavity without the radioactive isotope. Special applicators hold the implant in position. When placement has been ascertained and the client is in the proper environment, the implant is loaded with the radioisotope. After the prescribed dose has been delivered, the implant, radioisotopes, and position-holding applicators are removed. *With solid implants, the client emits radiation while the implant is in place, but the excreta are not radioactive.* Chart 25-1 lists the best practices for the client with sealed implant radiation sources.

SIDE EFFECTS OF RADIATION THERAPY

The immediate and long-term side effects of all types of radiation are limited to the tissues exposed to the radiation. Therefore the side effects vary according to the site. Skin changes and hair loss are local but are likely to be permanent depending on the total absorbed dose.

CHART 25-1

BEST PRACTICE *for*
Care of the Client with Sealed Implants of Radioactive Sources

- Assign the client to a private room with a private bath.
- Place a "Caution: Radioactive Material" sign on the door of the client's room.
- Wear a dosimeter film badge at all times while caring for clients with radioactive implants. The badge offers no protection but measures an individual's exposure to radiation and should be used by only one individual.
- Pregnant nurses should not care for these clients; do not allow pregnant women or children younger than 16 to visit.
- Limit each visitor to one-half hour per day. Be sure visitors are at least 6 feet from the source.
- Never touch the radioactive source with bare hands. In the rare instance that it is dislodged, use a long-handled forceps to retrieve it. Deposit the radioactive source in the lead container kept in the client's room.
- Save all dressings and bed linens until after the radioactive source is removed. After the source is removed, dispose of dressings and linens in the usual manner. Other equipment can be removed from the room at any time.

Depending on the dose, altered taste sensations and fatigue are two systemic side effects often noted by clients receiving external beam radiation—regardless of the radiation site. Taste changes are thought to be caused by metabolites released from dead and dying cells. In particular, many clients experience an aversion to the taste of red meats. Fatigue may be related to the increased energy demands needed to repair radiation-damaged cells. Regardless of the physiologic cause, radiation-induced fatigue can be debilitating and may last for weeks to months (see the Evidence-Based Practice for Nursing box on p. 430). Many clients are unprepared for the degree of fatigue experienced and require lifestyle adjustments to manage this symptom.

Radiation damage to normal tissues during cancer therapy can initiate the inflammatory responses that cause tissue fibrosis and scarring. Their effects may not be apparent for many years after radiation treatment. For example, women who receive high-dose radiation therapy for uterine cancer may experience radiation-induced changes in the colon years later, resulting in constipation and obstruction.

NURSING CARE OF CLIENTS UNDERGOING RADIATION THERAPY

Most clients are anxious about radiation. The nurse must be knowledgeable about its nature and be able to explain its purpose and side effects to clients and families. When clients receive concrete, objective information regarding radiation therapy, they are better able to cope with the treatment and continue to participate in normal activities.

Chart 25-2 summarizes skin care and other precautions during external radiation therapy. The nurse instructs clients not to remove the markings when cleaning the skin until the entire course of radiation therapy is completed. Skin in the path of radiation becomes very dry and may break down. The nurse instructs clients not to use lotions or ointments in these areas unless the radiologist prescribes them. Because skin in the radiation path is more sensitive to sun damage, the nurse advises against direct skin exposure to the sun during treatment and for at least 1 year after completing radiation therapy.

EVIDENCE-BASED PRACTICE FOR NURSING

Radiation-induced fatigue is real and common

Irvine, D., et al. (1998). Fatigue in women with breast cancer receiving radiation therapy. *Cancer Nursing, 21*(2), 127-135.

This prospective, longitudinal, descriptive study examined the experience of radiation-induced fatigue among 76 women receiving radiation therapy (alone) for breast cancer. Measures of fatigue (Pearson Byars Fatigue Feeling Checklist [PBFFC]), psychologic distress (Linear Analogue Self-Assessment Scale [LASA]), symptom distress (Piper Fatigue Scale), and functional ability (Sickness Impact Profile [SIP]) were obtained at six time points throughout the treatment period. Time points for data collection consisted of before treatment, 1 week after onset of radiation, 2 weeks after onset of radiation, final week of radiation, 3 months after completion of radiation, and 6 months after completion of radiation.

Subjects experienced little fatigue before treatment and 1 week into treatment. In contrast, significant differences in the report of fatigue occurred at time points 3 and 4 (2 weeks after initiation of treatment and during the final week of treatment). The level of fatigue reported 3 months and 6 months after completion of treatment did not differ significantly from the pretreatment level. The pattern of decreased functional status closely paralleled fatigue in timing, whereas the patients of psychologic distress and symptom distress did not parallel the experience of fatigue in timing.

Critique. The study approached a pervasive yet subjective problem using quantitative measures. In addition, the PBFFC is a unidimensional rather than multidimensional measure of fatigue. The sample size was relatively large but not randomized.

Implications for Nursing. Clients and families are unprepared for the experience of fatigue with radiation therapy for cancer. In fact, because radiation therapy results in relatively few overt changes in clinical manifestations, both clients and families have indicated disbelief at the existence and severity of radiation-induced fatigue. Families have become impatient and clients have felt guilty for not participating in work-related or family activities to the degree expected. The nurse can help the client and family accept and prepare for fatigue as an expected and reversible side effect of radiation therapy for cancer.

CHART 25-2

CLIENT EDUCATION GUIDE
Radiation Therapy for Cancer

- Wash the irradiated area gently each day with either water alone or with a mild soap and water.
- Use your hand rather than a washcloth to be more gentle.
- Rinse soap thoroughly from your skin.
- Take care not to remove the markings that indicate exactly where the beam of radiation is to be focused.
- Dry the irradiated area with patting motions rather than rubbing motions; use a clean, soft towel or cloth.
- Use no powders, ointments, lotions, or creams on your skin at the radiation site unless they are prescribed by your *radiologist.*
- Wear soft clothing over the skin at the radiation site.
- Avoid wearing belts, buckles, straps, or any type of clothing that binds or rubs the skin at the radiation site.
- Avoid exposure of the irradiated area to the sun.
- Avoid heat exposure.

The normal tissues most sensitive to external radiation are hematopoietic (blood-producing), epithelial (including skin, mucous membranes, and hair follicles), and gonadal (reproductive) tissues. Some changes caused by radiation are permanent. The long-term problems experienced by clients vary with the location and dose of radiation administered. For example, radiation to the throat and upper chest can cause difficulty in swallowing. Head and neck radiation may damage the salivary glands and cause dry mouth **(xerostomia).** Bone exposed to radiation therapy may be less dense and break more easily. The nurse teaches about the types of symptoms that might be expected from the location and dose of radiation delivered.

CRITICAL THINKING CHALLENGE

The client is a 28-year-old woman diagnosed with breast cancer who is going to receive radiation therapy to the left breast and axillary area after a lumpectomy. She is a professional golfer and wonders how radiation therapy will affect her game and her appearance.

- How long will her radiation therapy last?
- Are there contraindications to playing golf while receiving radiation therapy?
- What modifications for time of day or dress will you suggest to this client? Why?
- What will you tell this client about hair loss?

For suggested answer guidelines, go to SIMON http://www.wbsaunders.com/SIMON/Iggy/.

Chemotherapy

Chemotherapy, the treatment of disease through chemical agents, has assumed a major role in managing clients with cancer. Chemotherapy as a cancer treatment is used to cure, increase mean survival time, and decrease the risk for specific life-threatening complications.

RATIONALE FOR CANCER TREATMENT

As described in Chapter 24, one characteristic of cancer growth is the ability of cancer cells to separate from the original tumor, spread to new areas, and establish new cancers at distant sites **(metastasize).** Clients with metastatic disease will die unless treatment focuses on eliminating the metastatic cancer cells and the original cancer cells. Chemotherapy is useful in treating cancer because its effects are systemic and thus provide the opportunity to kill metastatic cancer cells that may have escaped local treatment.

MECHANISM OF ACTION

Chemotherapy can be successful in treating cancer because it has some demonstrated selectivity for killing cancer cells over normal cells. This killing effect on cancer cells appears to be related to the ability of chemotherapy to damage DNA and interfere with cell division. Thus the tumors most sensitive to chemotherapy are those that have rapid growth.

Unfortunately, chemotherapeutic agents usually are administered systemically and exert their cell-damaging **(cytotoxic)** effects against both healthy cells and cancerous cells. The normal cells most profoundly affected by systemic chemotherapy are those that undergo frequent cell division, including skin, hair, epithelial lining of the gastrointestinal (GI) tract, spermatocytes, and hematopoietic cells.

Chemotherapy includes many drugs or chemical compounds that are effective in killing cancer cells. They are classified by the specific types of biologic action they exert in the cancer cell and by the period in the life of a cell during which the agent is most likely to succeed in disrupting vital processes. Table 25-7 lists categories and specific chemotherapeutic agents.

TABLE 25-7 • CATEGORIES OF CHEMOTHERAPEUTIC AGENTS

Generic Name	Usual Dose	Nadir
ANTIMETABOLITES		
Methotrexate (Mexate, Folex)	3.3 mg/m²	10-14 days
6-Mercaptopurine (Purinethol)	80-100 mg/m²	5-40 days
6-Thioguanine (Lanvis)	2-3 mg/kg	1-4 wk
5-Fluorouracil (Adrucil, Efudex, Fluoroplex)	300-750 mg/m²	9-14 days
Fludarabine (Fludara)	25 mg/m²	3-25 days
Floxuridine (FUDR)	0.1-0.6 mg/kg	4-7 days
Cytarabine (Cytosar, Ara-C)	100-300 mg/m²	4-7 days
Pentostatin (Nipent)	4 mg/m²	3-10 days
Capecitabine (Xeloda)	2500 mg/m²	Not reported
Trimetrexate (Neutrexin)	45 mg/m²	10-14 days
Gemcitabine (Gemzar)	1000-1250 mg/m²	7-12 days
ANTIBIOTICS		
Bleomycin (Blenoxane)	10-20 units/m²	7-14 days
Dactinomycin (Cosmegen)	0.4-0.6 mg/m²	14-21 days
Doxorubicin (Adriamycin, Rubex)	50-80 mg/m²	10-15 days
Daunorubicin (Cerubidine)	30-60 mg/m²	10-14 days
Epirubicin (Ellence)	100-120 mg/m²	10-14 days
Idarubicin (Idamycin)	12-25 mg/m²	10-14 days
Plicamycin (Mithracin)	0.025-0.030 mg/m²	10-12 days
Mitomycin C (Mutamycin)	10-20 mg/m²	21-50 days
Mitoxantrone (Novantrone)	12-14 mg/m²	7-10 days
ALKYLATING AGENTS		
Cyclophosphamide (Cytoxan, Procytox♣)	50-500 mg/m²	7-14 days
Altretamine (Hexalen)	260 mg/m²	3-4 wk
Cisplatin (Platinol)	25-120 mg/m²	10-20 days
Carboplatin (Paraplatin)	360 mg/m²	21-28 days
Ifosfamide (IFEX)	1.2 g/m²	10 days
ALKYLATING AGENTS—CONT'D		
Mechlorethamine (Mustargen)	0.2-0.3 mg/kg	10-14 days
Busulfan (Myleran)	1-8 mg	14-21 days
Chlorambucil (Leukeran)	1-4 mg/m²	28 days
Melphalan (Alkeran)	1-6 mg/m²	14-21 days
Carmustine (BiCNU)	200-250 mg/m²	4-6 wk
Lomustine (CCNU, CeeNU)	130 mg/m²	4-6 wk
Temozolomide (Temodar)	150-200 mg/m²	20-22 days
Thiotepa (Thioplex)	0.3-0.8 mg/kg	15-30 days
Streptozocin (Zanosar)	500-1500 mg/m²	14 days
ANTIMITOTICS		
Vincristine (Oncovin, Leurocristine, VCR)	0.5-2.0 mg/m²	7 days
Vinblastine (Velban, Velbe♣, Velsar)	5-10 mg/m²	5-11 days
Vindesine (DAVA, Eldisine♣)	2 mg/m²	2-7 days
Vinorelbine (Navelbine)	30 mg/m²	7-10 days
Paclitaxel (Taxol)	100-250 mg/m²	8-11 days
Docetaxel (Taxotere)	60-100 mg/m²	8-10 days
TOPOISOMERASE INHIBITORS		
Irinotecan (Camptosar)	125-150 mg/m²	18-25 days
Topotecan (Hycamtin)	1.5 mg/m²	7-14 days
Etoposide (VP-16, VePesid)	50-100 mg/m²	8-10 days
Teniposide (Vumon, VM-26)	100-180 mg/m²	8-10 days
Estramustine (Emcyt)	600 mg/m²	Rare
OTHER AGENTS		
Procarbazine (Matulane, Natulan♣)	100-300 mg	14-28 days
Dacarbazine (DTIC♣)	75-250 mg/m²	10-14 days
Hydroxyurea (Hydrea)	25 mg/kg	4-7 days
Asparaginase (Elspar)	200-1000 IU/kg	4-10 days

Data from *United States Pharmacopeia Dispensing Information (USP DI): Vol I. Drug information for the health care professional.* (20th ed). (2000). Englewood, CO: Micromedex.

Antimetabolites

Antimetabolites are chemicals similar to normal metabolites (cofactors, vitamins, and nucleotides [purines and pyrimidines]) that play critical roles in essential cell processes. Most cellular reactions require metabolites in order to begin or continue the reaction. Antimetabolites closely resemble normal metabolites and can be considered "counterfeit" metabolites that literally fool cancer cells into using the antimetabolites in cellular reactions. Because antimetabolites cannot function as proper metabolites, their presence impairs or prevents cell division.

Antitumor Antibiotics

Antitumor antibiotics are a class of anticancer drugs initially developed to combat bacterial infections by causing major damage to the cell's DNA and interrupting DNA or ribonucleic acid (RNA) synthesis. Exactly how the interruptions occur varies with each antibiotic.

Alkylating Agents

All alkylating agents cross-link DNA by various means. Whatever the mechanism, the double strands of DNA become more tightly bound together. This tight binding prevents proper DNA and RNA synthesis, resulting in an inhibition of cell division.

Antimitotic Agents

Antimitotic agents are substances made from plant sources. Their primary mechanism of action is to interfere with the proper formation of microtubules so cells cannot complete mitosis during cell division. As a result, the cell either does not divide at all or divides only once, resulting in two daughter cells with unequal amounts of DNA that cannot continue to divide.

Topoisomerase Inhibitors

Topoisomerase is an enzyme needed for DNA synthesis and cell division. It nicks and straightens the DNA helix, allowing the DNA to be copied, and then reattaches the DNA together. Topoisomerase inhibitors prevent these processes, causing DNA breakage and cell death.

Miscellaneous Chemotherapeutic Agents

The actions of other chemotherapeutic agents do not fit any of the broad categories of chemotherapeutic agents and include the following:

- Inhibition of important enzyme systems
- Competition for important substances in metabolic pathways

Combination Chemotherapy

Chemotherapy for cancer usually involves the timed administration of more than one specific anticancer drug. This technique is called **combination chemotherapy.** Using more than one drug is much more effective in killing cancer cells than using a single agent. Unfortunately, the damage caused to normal tissues also increases with combination chemotherapy.

The selection of drugs is based on known tumor sensitivity to the drugs and the degree of side effects expected. For example, most chemotherapeutic drugs suppress bone marrow activity and immune function to some degree, but some agents are more profoundly immunosuppressive than others. Such agents include busulfan, cyclophosphamide, etoposide, dactinomycin, doxorubicin, and mechlorethamine. There is also variation in the timing of drug-induced immunosuppression.

The time during which bone marrow activity and peripheral white blood cell counts are at their lowest levels after chemotherapy is the **nadir.** The nadir occurs at different times for different chemotherapeutic agents (see Table 25-7). For instance, the expected nadir after cytosine arabinoside administration is 5 to 7 days; after methotrexate, 10 to 14 days; and after mitomycin C, approximately 4 weeks. To minimize immunosuppression, combination chemotherapy is planned to avoid prescribing different drugs with nadirs that occur at or near the same time.

TABLE 25-8 • ROUTES OF CHEMOTHERAPY ADMINISTRATION

Route	Typical Cancer
Oral	Hodgkin's lymphoma Leukemia (maintenance phase) Small cell lung cancer
Intravenous	Most solid tumors, leukemias Lymphomas
Intra-arterial	Hepatic tumors (primary and metastatic) Head and neck cancers
Isolated limb perfusion	Cancers confined to a limb • Osteogenic sarcoma • Ewing's sarcoma • Rhabdomyosarcoma • Regional melanoma
Intracavitary	
• Intraperitoneal	Ovarian cancer
• Intraventricular	Brain tumors
• Intrathecal	Brain tumors Prophylaxis for acute lymphocytic leukemia
• Intravesical	Bladder tumors

Drug Dosage

The doses of most chemotherapeutic agents are calculated according to the type of cancer and the client's size. A few drug dosages are calculated in terms of milligrams per kilogram of body weight. More commonly, calculations are based on milligrams per square meter of total body surface area (TBSA). This parameter also considers the client's height and weight and is calculated as follows: the height of the client (in centimeters) is multiplied by his or her weight (in kilograms), and the result is divided by 10,000 (moving the decimal point four spaces to the left). For example, a woman who is 68 inches tall (173 cm) and weighs 143 pounds (65 kg) has a TBSA of 11,245 cm^2, or 1.12 m^2.

Drug Schedule

Chemotherapeutic agents are administered on a regular basis and are timed to maximize cancer cell kill and minimize damage to normal cells. The schedule may vary somewhat to accommodate a client's response to therapy, but chemotherapy is usually scheduled every 3 to 4 weeks for a specified number of times (on average, 6 to 12 times). The entire planned schedule is the *course* of chemotherapy; the individual days of administration are the *rounds.*

Drug Administration

Most chemotherapeutic drugs are administered intravenously, although other routes may be used for specific cancers (Table 25-8). The techniques and nursing care considerations for different routes are described with the specific cancer type most commonly associated with the specific administration route. Chapter 14 describes various types of venous access devices, many of which are used to administer chemotherapy.

TABLE 25-9 • CHEMOTHERAPY TISSUE VESICANTS AND IRRITANTS

VESICANTS	IRRITANTS
Amsacrine	Bleomycin
Dactinomycin	Carmustine
Daunorubicin	Cisplatin
Doxorubicin	Dacarbazine
Epirubicin	Etoposide
Esorubicin	Fluorouracil
Idarubicin	Mitoxantrone
Mechlorethamine	Paclitaxel
Menogaril	Plicamycin
Mitomycin C	Streptozocin
Pyrazofurin	Teniposide
Vinblastine	
Vincristine	
Vindesine	
Vinorelbine	

The IV route is the most preferred route for chemotherapy because the therapeutic effects of the drugs are rapid and because many of these agents are irritating or damaging to tissues. A major complication of IV administration is **extravasation,** or the movement of the IV needle so the drug leaks into the surrounding skin and subcutaneous tissues. When the administered agents are vesicants (chemicals that cause tissue damage on direct contact), the results of extravasation can include pain, infection, and tissue loss. Surgical intervention is sometimes necessary. Table 25-9 lists known vesicant or irritant chemotherapeutic agents.

The most important nursing intervention for extravasation is prevention (Wood & Gullo, 1993). Most extravasations resolve without extensive treatment if less than 0.5 mL of the irritating drug has infiltrated into the tissues. If a larger amount has leaked, extensive tissue damage occurs and surgical intervention may be necessary. Immediate treatment depends on the specific agent extravasated. With some agents, cold compresses to the area are appropriate; for other agents, warm compresses are used. Antidotes may be injected into the site of extravasation. The nurse consults with the oncologist and pharmacist to determine the specific antidote needed for the extravasated agent. Chart 25-3 outlines the best practices for documenting an extravasation event.

Most chemotherapeutic agents are readily absorbed through the skin and mucous membranes. As a result, the health care workers who prepare or administer these chemotherapeutic agents (especially nurses and pharmacists) are at risk for absorbing them (DelGaudio & Menonna-Quinn, 1998). Even at low doses, chronic exposure to chemotherapeutic agents can seriously affect health. Nurses and other health care professionals must use extreme caution and wear protective clothing whenever preparing, administering, or disposing of chemotherapeutic agents. The Occupational Safety and Health Administration (OSHA) and the Oncology Nursing Society have established practice guidelines and protective standards.

SIDE EFFECTS OF CHEMOTHERAPY

Serious side effects are associated with aggressive chemotherapy, including alopecia (hair loss), nausea and vomiting, open sores on mucous membranes (mucositis), and various skin changes.

CHART 25-3

BEST PRACTICE *for* Documentation of Extravasation

- Document the date and time when extravasation was suspected or identified.
- Note the date and time when the infusion was started.
- Record the time when the infusion was stopped.
- Note the exact contents of the infusion fluid and the volume of fluid infused.
- Document the estimated amount of fluid extravasated.
- Note the needle type and size.
- Diagram the exact insertion site.
- Indicate on the diagram the location and number of venipuncture attempts.
- Record the time between the extravasation and the last full blood return.
- Identify all agents administered in the previous 24 hours through this site (list agent administered, dosage and volume, and order of administration).
- Note the client's vital signs.
- Take a photograph of the site.
- Document the administration of neutralizing or antidote agents.
- Note the application of compresses.
- Note other nursing interventions.
- Record the client's responses to nursing interventions.
- Document the physician notification (including the time).
- Document the written and oral instructions given to the client about follow-up care.
- Note any consultation request.
- Sign the documentation.

TABLE 25-10 • AGENTS USED FOR CHEMOPROTECTION

Agent	Cytotoxic Problem Prevented
Amifostine (Ethyol)	Xerostomia
Dexrazoxane (Zinecard)	Cardiomyopathy
Mesna (MESNEX)	Hemorrhagic cystitis
Pamidronate (Aredia)	Skeletal complications

The common side effects on the hematopoietic (blood-producing) system can be life threatening and are the most common reason for altering the dosage or schedule. The chemotoxic effects on the blood-forming cells of the bone marrow also produce specific side effects, including immunosuppression, anemia, and thrombocytopenia (decreased numbers of platelets).

A newer approach to decrease the impact of chemotherapeutic agents on normal tissues is to administer the agents with drugs that exert a protective influence on specific healthy cells. These drugs, called **cytoprotectants,** have little if any effect on cancer cells but do offer some protection to normal cells (Table 25-10).

NURSING CARE OF CLIENTS UNDERGOING CHEMOTHERAPY

The major nursing care issue during chemotherapy is managing the distressing symptoms associated with therapy. For some clients, the symptoms are so disagreeable that they discontinue treatment. Chart 25-4 presents NIC interventions appropriate for the client undergoing chemotherapy.

CHART 25-4

NIC INTERVENTION ACTIVITIES *for* **The Client with Cancer**

Chemotherapy Management: *Assisting the client and family to understand the action and minimize side effects of antineoplastic agents*

- Monitor for side effects and toxic effects of chemotherapeutic agents.
- Provide information to client and family on how antineoplastic drugs work on cancer cells.
- Instruct client and family on ways to prevent infection, such as avoiding crowds and using good hygiene and handwashing techniques.
- Instruct client to promptly report fever, chills, nosebleeds, excessive bruising, and tarry stools.
- Instruct client to avoid the use of aspirin products.
- Administer antiemetic drugs for nausea and vomiting.
- Teach the client relaxation and imagery techniques to use before, during, and after treatments, as appropriate.
- Ensure adequate fluid intake to prevent dehydration and electrolyte imbalance.
- Monitor the effectiveness of measures to control nausea and vomiting.
- Teach client and family to monitor for signs and symptoms of stomatitis.
- Instruct client on proper oral hygiene techniques.
- Inform client that hair loss is expected, as determined by type of chemotherapeutic agent used.
- Assist client in obtaining a wig or other head-covering device, as appropriate.
- Provide nutritious, appetizing foods of client's choice.
- Monitor nutritional status and weight.
- Discuss with client the possibility of sterility and other reproductive system impairments, as appropriate.
- Instruct long-term survivors and their families of the possibility of second malignancies and the importance of reporting increased susceptibility to infection, fatigue, or bleeding.

Alopecia

Clients receiving chemotherapy for cancer often experience whole-body hair loss. Some drugs (e.g., methotrexate) may cause only thinning of the scalp hair. Others (e.g., doxorubicin, vincristine, and cisplatin) cause a more complete hair loss.

The nurse reassures clients that hair loss is temporary. Hair regrowth usually begins approximately 1 month after completion of chemotherapy. The nurse cautions that the new hair may differ from the original hair in color, texture, and thickness.

No known treatment completely prevents alopecia. However, techniques to reduce the amount of chemotherapeutic agent that reaches the hair follicles during treatment have been somewhat effective in reducing hair loss. These techniques include applying ice packs and caps to the scalp or applying a scalp tourniquet during chemotherapy administration and for a few hours immediately afterward. These techniques are not endorsed by oncologists or oncology nurses because it is believed that some circulating cancer cells may escape chemotherapy, resulting in a less favorable treatment outcome.

Nurses can assist clients in selecting a type of head covering that suits their financial means and lifestyle. High-quality wigs are expensive but can look very much like the client's own hair. Many local units of the American Cancer Society offer wigs that other clients have used temporarily and have donated to be lent to other clients with cancer. Clients can disguise hair loss relatively inexpensively with caps or by the creative use of scarves and turbans, which are available in many fabrics, styles, and prices.

Nausea and Vomiting

Chemotherapy-induced nausea and vomiting arises from a variety of local and central nervous system mechanisms. Most chemotherapeutic agents are *emetogenic* (vomiting inducing) to some degree, depending on the dose. The agents producing the most severe nausea and vomiting include cisplatin, doxorubicin, mithramycin, nitrogen mustard, vinblastine, and etoposide. Most of these agents induce nausea and vomiting during drug administration and for 1 to 2 days afterward. Some agents, such as cisplatin, induce delayed nausea and vomiting that can continue as long as 5 to 7 days after administration. Clients who experienced chemotherapy-related nausea and vomiting during one round of chemotherapy may begin experiencing the same symptoms before the next round as a result of sheer anticipation.

CONSIDERATIONS FOR OLDER ADULTS

At times older clients have received lower doses of chemotherapy agents in anticipation of a reduced capacity to tolerate the side effects of nausea and vomiting. More recent research indicates that older clients do not experience greater nausea and vomiting than do younger clients. Therefore their chemotherapy regimens should not be altered on this basis alone.

DRUG THERAPY

Many oral and parenteral antiemetics (agents that alleviate nausea and vomiting) are available. These agents vary in their production of side effects and in their effectiveness in controlling chemotherapy-induced nausea and vomiting. One or more antiemetics are usually administered before and after chemotherapy. The drugs commonly used to control chemotherapy-induced nausea and vomiting are presented in Chart 25-5. Client response to antiemetic therapy is highly variable, and the drug combinations must be individualized for best effect. In addition, different antiemetic agents vary considerably in cost (see the Cost of Care box on p. 435).

COMPLIMENTARY AND ALTERNATIVE THERAPIES

The nurse also assists the client with chemotherapy-induced nausea and vomiting to achieve comfort through nonpharmacologic means, either alone or in conjunction with antiemetics. Progressive muscle relaxation, guided imagery, music, acupressure, or distraction may help to reduce anxiety and relieve some nausea and vomiting (see the Evidence-Based Practice for Nursing box on p. 436). The nurse also assesses the client for complications associated with excessive vomiting, such as dehydration and electrolyte imbalances.

Mucositis

Clients undergoing chemotherapy for cancer often experience *mucositis* (sores in mucous membranes) of the entire gastrointestinal (GI) tract, especially in the mouth (stomatitis). Normally, the mucous membrane of the GI tract undergoes rapid

CHART 25-5

DRUG THERAPY *for* Chemotherapy-Induced Nausea and Vomiting

Drug	Usual Dosage	Side Effects
SEROTONIN ANTAGONISTS		
Ondansetron (Zofran)	8 mg q8h	Constipation, diarrhea, fever, lightheadedness, drowsiness
Granisetron (Kytril)	1 mg q12h	Fever, dysrhythmias, chest pain, fainting
Dolasetron (Anzemet)	1.8 mg/kg	
CNS DEPRESSANTS		
Trimethobenzamide (Tigan, Benzacot, Arrestin, T-Gen)	200 mg tid or qid	Drowsiness, blurred vision, dizziness, diarrhea, headache, mental depression, tremors
BENZODIAZEPINES		
Lorazepam (Ativan)	1-3 mg bid or tid	Amnesia, bradycardia, hypotension, muscle weakness, anemia
PHENOTHIAZINES		
Prochlorperazine (Compazine, Stemetil✱)	10-20 mg qid	Hypotension, CNS depression, extrapyramidal reactions, dry mouth, blurred vision
Chlorpromazine (Thorazine, Ormazine)	25-50 mg qid	Hypotension, CNS depression, extrapyramidal reactions, dry mouth, blurred vision
ANTIHISTAMINES		
Diphenhydramine (Benadryl)	25-50 mg qid	Drowsiness, dry mouth, hypotension
CORTICOSTEROIDS		
Dexamethasone (Decadron)	5-10 mg qd	Fluid and electrolyte imbalances, immunosuppression, GI bleeding, bruising, cushingoid symptoms

CNS, Central nervous system; *GI,* gastrointestinal.

COST OF CARE IMPLICATIONS FOR NURSING

ANTIEMETIC THERAPY FOR CHEMOTHERAPY-INDUCED NAUSEA AND VOMITING

Cost of Care

- Prolonged nausea and vomiting is a common and distressful side effect of cancer chemotherapy.
- Chemotherapy-induced nausea and vomiting reduces a client's productivity and has contributed to increased length of stay and costs of care.
- Antiemetic agents vary in cost from less than $1 per dose to more than $130 per dose.
- In general, the newer and more expensive antiemetic agents are more clinically effective in reducing the severity of chemotherapy-induced nausea and vomiting than older, less expensive agents.
- Medicare and managed care organizations have reduced the reimbursement for these agents.
- Not all clients experience relief from chemotherapy-induced nausea and vomiting when using the more expensive agents.

Implications for Nursing

Because of the higher costs associated with the administration of serotonin antagonists, nurses need to explore the use of complementary and integrative therapies to assist in the reduction of chemotherapy-induced nausea and vomiting. Working collaboratively with pharmacists and physicians, nurses can suggest reducing the dosage of the more expensive antiemetic agents and using them in combination with less expensive agents. In addition, nurses can reduce costs to the institution and reduce out-of-pocket expenses for the client by helping clients take advantage of drug company–sponsored "medications for the indigent" programs.

Data from Doherty, K. (1999). Closing the gap in prophylactic antiemetic therapy: Patient factors in calculating the emetogenic potential of chemotherapy. *Clinical Journal of Oncology Nursing, 3*(3), 113-119; Engstrom, C., et al. (1999). The efficacy and cost-effectiveness of new antiemetic guidelines. *Oncology Nursing Forum, 26*(9), 1453-1458; and Goldsmith, M., & Wodinsky, H. (1999). Controlling costs using evidenced-based guidelines: 5-HT3 antagonists as a model. *Managed Care and Cancer, 1*(3), 20-24.

cell division and quickly replaces dead or damaged cells. In chemotherapy, mucous membrane cells are killed more rapidly than they are replaced, resulting in sore formation. Mouth sores are painful and interfere with the desire and ability to eat. Chart 25-6 lists the best practices for clients with mucositis.

Frequent mouth assessment and appropriate hygiene are key in managing stomatitis and mucositis. A major component in managing oral mucositis is oral hygiene. The nurse stresses the importance of good and frequent oral hygiene, including tooth cleaning and mouth rinsing. Because most clients with chemotherapy-induced mucositis also have bone marrow suppression, they must take care to avoid traumatizing the oral mucosa. They are instructed to use a soft-bristled toothbrush or disposable mouth sponges and to avoid using dental floss and water pressure gum cleaners (e.g., a Water Pik). The nurse encourages clients to rinse the mouth with plain water or saline every hour while awake. Commercial mouthwashes that contain alcohol or other drying agents that may further irritate the mucosa are avoided.

Oral hygiene equipment must be kept clean. The nurse reminds clients not to share toothbrushes with anyone. Toothbrushes can be cleaned daily by running them through a home dishwasher or by rinsing them with a concentrated solution of liquid bleach or hydrogen peroxide.

Many compounds are available for pain relief from stomatitis or mucositis. Many hospitals offer their own special "swish and spit" mixtures, which usually contain a local anesthetic combined with anti-inflammatory agents. The nurse stresses that these mixtures are not to be swallowed.

Bone Marrow Suppression

Bone marrow suppression results in decreased numbers of circulating leukocytes, erythrocytes, and platelets. Decreased leukocyte numbers cause immunosuppression. Decreased

EVIDENCE-BASED PRACTICE FOR NURSING

Complementary therapy for chemotherapy-induced nausea

Dibble, S. et al. (2000). Acupressure for nausea: Results of a pilot study. *Oncology Nursing Forum, 27*(1), 41-47.

This prospective, single-cycle, randomized study measured the effectiveness of acupressure in combination with standard pharmacologic antiemetic therapy among women receiving chemotherapy for breast cancer. Seventeen women who previously experienced nausea as a side effect of breast cancer chemotherapy were enrolled in the study. These women were randomized to either a treatment group (receiving self-applied acupressure and the usual antiemetic therapy) or a control group (receiving only the usual antiemetic therapy). The women using acupressure were taught the technique using the P6 and ST36 meridians as the acupressure points for nausea. All subjects kept a daily log of nausea episodes (from the Rhodes Index of Nausea, Vomiting and Retching [INVR]), medication regimen, and (for the experimental subjects) timing of the intervention. In addition, all subjects completed the Chemotherapy Problem Checklist (CPC) at the end of the study. The investigators examined the daily logs from all subjects to compare the incidence and severity of nausea experienced.

During the first 10 days after chemotherapy, subjects who received the acupressure intervention experienced fewer incidences of nausea and less severe nausea than did the subjects who received only the usual pharmacologic intervention. The difference was statistically significant to the $p = 0.01$ level for incidence and to the $p = 0.04$ level for intensity.

Critique. The study represented pilot work in the area of complementary and alternative therapies for chemotherapy-induced nausea and vomiting. The subject populations were largely homogenous and the sample size was small, which limits the generalizability of the results.

Implications for Nursing. Acupressure has been found to reduce nausea and vomiting in morning sickness and motion sickness. It is inexpensive, easy to learn, noninvasive, and requires client engagement. These preliminary results are promising. Nurses could teach clients how to use acupressure and perhaps reduce costs related to antiemetic therapy by reducing the amount of drug needed to achieve adequate control over nausea and vomiting.

erythrocytes and platelets cause hypoxia, fatigue, and an increased tendency to bleed.

Immunosuppression, which places the client at extreme risk for infection, is the major dose-limiting side effect of cancer chemotherapy. Most chemotherapeutic agents suppress bone marrow function to some degree. The agents associated with severe bone marrow suppression include busulfan, cyclophosphamide, cytosine arabinoside, dactinomycin, doxorubicin, daunorubicin, etoposide, mitomycin-C, nitrogen mustard, and triethylenethiophosphoramide. Suppression of immune function is the most life-threatening side effect and presents the nurse with the serious challenge of providing the client with the understanding, environment, and support to withstand this potentially devastating complication.

The clinical problems associated with immunosuppression are related primarily to a temporary reduction of circulating neutrophils and tissue macrophages, which decreases the body's protective inflammatory responses to microorganism invasion. The severity and duration of the impairment are related directly to the dosage of specific chemo-therapeutic agents. This impairment is usually temporary, with good recovery of inflammatory responses evident within weeks or months of therapy completion. However, the seriousness of potential infection complications makes this problem a major treatment concern. The infectious processes most commonly observed include those of fungal origin, yeast, some residual viral breakthrough, and a wide variety of bacteria.

Decreased numbers of circulating erythrocytes (anemia) and platelets (thrombocytopenia) result from the generalized bone marrow suppression caused by some chemotherapeutic agents. Anemia causes clients to feel fatigued, and some tissues must operate under hypoxic conditions. The cardiac and respiratory systems may be overtaxed in their effort to maintain adequate oxygenation. Thrombocytopenia increases the risk for uncontrolled bleeding. When the concentration of platelets is less than 50,000/mm^3, any small trauma can lead to episodes of prolonged bleeding. Clients with a concentration less than 20,000/mm^3 may experience spontaneous and uncontrollable bleeding, which requires extensive transfusion therapy and other interventions.

CHART 25-6

BEST PRACTICE *for* Mouth Care for Clients with Mucositis

- Examine the client's mouth (including the roof, under the tongue, and between the teeth and cheek) every 4 hours.
- Document the location, size, and character of fissures, blisters, sores, or drainage.
- Get an order to obtain specimens of sores or drainage for culture.
- Brush the teeth and tongue with a soft-bristled brush or sponges every 8 hours.
- Rinse the mouth with a solution of $^1/_2$ peroxide and $^1/_2$ normal saline every 12 hours.
- Avoid the use of alcohol or glycerin-based mouthwashes.
- Administer antimicrobial medications as prescribed.
- Administer topical analgesic medications as prescribed or as needed.
- Help the conscious client to "swish and spit" room-temperature tap water or normal saline as needed.
- Apply petrolatum jelly to the client's lips after each episode of mouth care and as needed.
- Assist the client in using "artificial saliva" as needed, if ordered.
- Assist the client in menu choices to avoid spicy or hard food.
- Offer complete mouth care before and after every meal.

DRUG THERAPY

In some instances immunosuppression can be managed medically by the administration of biologic response modifiers (BRMs) to stimulate the production of immune system cells in the bone marrow. Although not appropriate for all types of cancer, this supportive treatment can reduce the risk for infection during chemotherapy. However, BRMs are expensive and not consistently covered by insurance. Further discussion of this treatment is presented under Immunotherapy, pp. 439-440.

COMPLEMENTARY AND ALTERNATIVE THERAPIES

Many clients experiencing treatment-induced immunosuppression use complementary and alternative therapies to boost immune function and prevent infection. Common therapies include shark cartilage, Echinacea, and megadoses of vitamin C. Although the benefit of such therapies has not yet been deter-

CHART 25-7

BEST PRACTICE *for*
Care of the Client with Immunosuppression

- Place the client in a private room whenever possible.
- Use good handwashing technique before touching the client or any of the client's belongings.
- Ensure that the client's room and bathroom are cleaned at least once each day.
- Do not use supplies from common areas for immunosuppressed clients. For example, keep a sleeve or box of paper cups in the client's room, and do not share this box with any other client. Other articles include drinking straws, plastic knives and forks, dressing materials, gloves, and bandages.
- Limit the number of health care personnel entering the client's room.
- Monitor vital signs every 4 hours; note minor temperature elevation, which may suggest early sepsis.
- Inspect the client's mouth at least every 8 hours.
- Inspect the client's skin and mucous membranes (especially the anal area) for the presence of fissures and abscesses at least every 8 hours.
- Inspect open areas, such as IV sites, every 4 hours for manifestations of infection.
- Change wound dressings daily.
- Obtain specimens of all suspicious areas for culture, and promptly notify the physician.
- Assist the client in performing coughing and deep-breathing exercises.
- Encourage activity at a level appropriate for the client's current health status.
- Change IV tubing daily.
- Keep frequently used equipment in the room for use with this client only (e.g., blood pressure cuff, stethoscope, thermometer).
- Limit visitors to healthy adults.
- Use strict aseptic technique for all invasive procedures.
- Monitor the white blood cell count, especially the absolute neutrophil count (ANC), daily.
- Avoid the use of indwelling urinary catheters.
- Keep fresh flowers and potted plants out of the client's room.
- Teach the client to eat a low-bacteria diet.

mined in organized clinical trials, there appear to be few harmful effects associated with their use.

PROTECTION FROM INFECTION

The nurse works closely with clients and other health care professionals to provide safe care to clients at risk for infection. Chart 25-7 lists the best practices to prevent infection among immunosuppressed clients. Good handwashing by all health care professionals and assistive nursing personnel before contact is the cornerstone for prevention of infection. Health care professionals must practice asepsis (prevention of contact with microorganisms) when performing any invasive technique or procedure.

Many clients remain at home during periods of immunosuppression. The nurse teaches clients and family members precautions to take to reduce the chances of developing an infection (Chart 25-8).

The nurse provides a safe hospital environment for clients with thrombocytopenia and teaches them how to avoid excessive bleeding when they are discharged before the platelet count has returned to normal. Chart 25-9 lists the best practices for reducing the risk for bleeding during hospitalization. The nurse teaches how to prevent bleeding and what to do if bleeding should occur after discharge (Chart 25-10).

CHART 25-8

CLIENT EDUCATION GUIDE
Prevention of Infection

- Avoid crowds and other large gatherings of people who might be ill.
- Do not share personal toilet articles, such as toothbrushes, toothpaste, washcloths, or deodorant sticks, with others.
- If possible, bathe daily.
- Wash the armpits, groin, genitals, and anal area at least twice a day with an antimicrobial soap.
- Clean your toothbrush daily by either running it through the dishwasher or rinsing it in liquid laundry bleach.
- Wash your hands thoroughly with an antimicrobial soap before you eat or drink, after touching a pet, after shaking hands with anyone, as soon as you come home from any outing, and after using the toilet.
- Eat a low-bacteria diet, and avoid salads, raw fruit and vegetables, undercooked meat, pepper, and paprika.
- Wash dishes between use with hot, sudsy water, or use a dishwasher.
- Do not drink water that has been standing for longer than 15 minutes.
- Do not reuse cups and glasses without washing.
- Do not change pet litter boxes.
- Take your temperature at least once a day.
- Report any of the following signs or symptoms of infection to your physician immediately:
  - Temperature greater than 100° F (38° C)
  - Persistent cough (with or without sputum)
  - Pus or foul-smelling drainage from any open skin area or normal body opening
  - Presence of a boil or abscess
  - Urine that is cloudy or foul smelling or that causes burning on urination
- Take all prescribed medications as ordered.
- Do not dig in the garden or work with houseplants.

CHART 25-9

BEST PRACTICE *for*
Care of the Client with Thrombocytopenia

- Handle the client gently.
- Use a lift sheet when moving and positioning the client in bed.
- Avoid intramuscular injections and venipunctures.
- When injections or venipunctures are necessary, use the smallest-gauge needle for the task.
- Apply firm pressure to the needle stick site for 10 minutes or until the site no longer oozes blood.
- Apply ice to areas of trauma.
- Test all urine and stool for the presence of occult blood.
- Observe IV sites every 2 hours for bleeding
- Avoid trauma to rectal tissues:
  - Do not take temperatures rectally.
  - Do not administer enemas.
  - Administer well-lubricated suppositories and with caution.
  - Advise the client not to have anal intercourse.
- Measure the client's abdominal girth daily.
- Use an electric razor.
- Teach the client to avoid mouth trauma by:
  - Using soft-bristled toothbrush or tooth sponges
  - Not flossing
  - Avoiding dental work, especially extractions
  - Avoiding hard foods
  - Making certain that dentures fit and do not rub
- Encourage the client not to blow the nose or insert objects into the nose.
- Instruct the client to avoid contact sports.
- Advise the client to wear shoes with firm soles whenever he or she is ambulating.

CHART 25-10

CLIENT EDUCATION GUIDE
The Client at Risk for Bleeding

- Use an electric razor.
- Use a soft-bristled toothbrush, and do not floss.
- Do not have dental work performed without consulting your doctor.
- Do not take aspirin or any aspirin-containing products. Read the label to be sure that the product does not contain aspirin or salicylates.
- Do not participate in contact sports or any activity likely to result in your being bumped, scratched, or scraped.
- If you are bumped, apply ice to the site for at least 1 hour.
- Notify your doctor if you:
  - Experience an injury and persistent bleeding results
  - Have excessive menstrual bleeding
  - See blood in your urine or bowel movement
- Avoid anal intercourse.
- Take a stool softener to prevent straining during a bowel movement.
- Do not use enemas or rectal suppositories.
- Avoid bending over at the waist.
- Do not wear clothing or shoes that are tight or that rub.
- Avoid blowing your nose or placing objects in your nose. If you must blow your nose, do so gently without blocking either nasal passage.

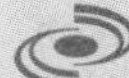

CRITICAL THINKING CHALLENGE

Your client with cancer is receiving IV doxorubicin. She tells you that her arm is burning and hurts around the IV site. You lower the infusion set and get a brisk blood return.

- Should you continue or discontinue the infusion?
- What other questions should you ask the client about her discomfort?
- What should you look for at the site?
- How will you document this complaint?

For suggested answer guidelines, go to SIMON http://www.wbsaunders.com/SIMON/Iggy/.

Hormonal Manipulation

RATIONALE FOR CANCER TREATMENT

Hormones are naturally occurring chemicals secreted by endocrine (ductless) glands and picked up by capillaries. Once in the bloodstream, hormones circulate to all body areas but exert their effects only on their specific target tissues. Some hormones make hormone-sensitive tumors grow more rapidly. Some tumors actually require specific hormones to divide. Therefore altering the availability of these hormones to hormone-sensitive tumors can directly alter the rate of tumor growth.

MECHANISM OF ACTION

Hormones

Hormonal manipulation can help to control some types of cancer for many years. However, this therapy does not lead to a cure. The endocrine system usually keeps hormones within narrow ranges and maintains a balance. When a large amount of one hormone is administered, it upsets the balance and disturbs the uptake of other hormones. If a tumor depends on hormone A for growth and a large quantity of hormone B (structurally but not functionally related to A) is given to the client, hormone B will interfere with the tumor's uptake of hormone A or will limit the amount of hormone A produced (through competition or feedback inhibition). As a result, tumor growth is slowed. Thus hormonal therapy may increase survival time. Table 25-11 lists the drugs commonly used in hormonal manipulation for cancer therapy.

TABLE 25-11 • COMMON AGENTS USED FOR HORMONAL MANIPULATION OF CANCER

Type of Agent	Example
HORMONE AGONISTS	
Androgen	Calusterone Danocrine Fluoxymesterone Testosterone Testolactone
Estrogen	Conjugated estrogens Diethylstilbestrol Ethinyl estradiol
Progestin	Medroxyprogesterone Megestrol
Luteinizing-hormone releasing hormone (LHRH)	Leuprolide Goserelin
HORMONE ANTAGONISTS	
Antiandrogens	Flutamide Cyproterone acetate
Antiprogestins	Mifepristone
Antiestrogens	Droloxifen Idoxifene Tamoxifen Toremifene Trioxifene mesylate Zindoxifene
Gonadotropin-releasing hormone (GnRH)	Abarelix

Hormone Antagonists

Hormone antagonists, competitors for the hormones at the receptor sites, may be antibodies specific to the receptor. When hormone antagonists are administered, they bind to the specific hormone receptor of the tumor cell and prevent the needed hormone from binding to the receptor. If a tumor requires a certain hormone to grow and the hormone can enter or activate the cell only through a receptor, hormone antagonists can slow down tumor growth.

SIDE EFFECTS OF HORMONAL MANIPULATION

Androgens and the antiestrogen receptor drugs cause masculinizing manifestations in women. Chest and facial hair may develop, menstrual periods stop, and breast tissue shrinks. Women usually experience some fluid retention. For men and women receiving androgens, acne may develop, hypercalcemia is common, and liver dysfunction may occur with prolonged therapy. Women receiving estrogens or progestins have irregular but heavy menses, fluid retention, and breast tenderness. Male and female clients who take estrogen or progestins are at an increased risk for thrombus formation.

Certain feminine clinical manifestations usually develop in men who take estrogens, progestins, or antiandrogen receptor drugs. Facial hair thins or disappears, facial skin becomes smoother, body fat is redistributed, and **gynecomastia** (breast development in men) can occur. In addition, testicular and penile atrophy occurs to some degree. Although sexual function may continue, achieving and maintaining an erection are much more difficult.

Immunotherapy: Biologic Response Modifiers

Biologic response modifiers (BRMs) are agents or approaches that modify the client's biologic responses to tumor cells to produce a beneficial result (Clark & Longo, 1986). The BRMs in current use or under investigation for use as cancer therapy are cytokines, small protein hormones synthesized by the various leukocytes. Cytokines synthesized by mononuclear phagocytes (macrophages, neutrophils, eosinophils, and monocytes) are monokines; cytokines produced by lymphocytes (especially the T-lymphocytes) are lymphokines. Cytokines essentially make the immune system work better (see Chapter 20, especially Table 20-5).

RATIONALE FOR CANCER TREATMENT

Cytokines enhance the effectiveness of the immune system. Immune function plays an important role in cancer prevention (see Chapters 20 and 24). Cytokines and other BRMs are potentially therapeutic as a cancer treatment by stimulating the immune system to recognize cancer cells and take actions to eliminate or destroy them. Some BRMs may also be useful in a supporting role. Other BRMs (colony-stimulating factors) stimulate faster recovery of bone marrow function after treatment-induced suppression.

MECHANISM OF ACTION

The activity of cytokines is similar to that of any other type of peptide hormone in that one cell produces and secretes a cytokine, which then exerts its effects on other cells of the immune system. The cells responding to the cytokine may be right next to the cytokine-secreting cell or quite remote from it. Cells that change their activity in response to the cytokine are *responder* cells. For a responder cell to be able to respond to a cytokine, the membrane of the responder cell must have a specific receptor for the cytokine. The cytokine binds to this receptor and initiates changes in the activity of the responder cell.

Biologic Response Modifiers for Cancer Therapy

Three categories of BRMs are being used as cytotoxic therapy for cancer: interleukins, interferons, and monoclonal antibodies. Some agents can stimulate specific immune system cells to attack and destroy cancer cells; other agents block access of the cancer cell to some essential function or nutrient.

INTERLEUKINS

Sixteen interleukins (ILs) have been identified (see Table 20-5). Many of these are now synthetically produced through recombinant DNA technology. Interleukins help different immune system cells recognize and destroy abnormal body cells. In particular, IL-1, -2, and -6 appear to "charge up" the immune system and enhance attacks on cancer cells by macrophages, natural killer (NK) cells, lymphokine-activated killer (LAK) cells, and tumor-infiltrating lymphocytes. Cancer treatment with interleukins is currently experimental, but good responses have occurred for renal cell carcinoma, colorectal cancer, and melanoma.

INTERFERONS

Interferons are cell-produced substances that can protect noninfected cells from viral infection and replication. There are many types of interferons. Although all of them have similar functions, each type has unique properties and functions. The most completely characterized interferon is interferon alfa-2b.

Different body cells can produce interferon, with leukocytes producing the most. Today interferons are synthetically mass produced by recombinant DNA technology. Cancer-related functions of interferon include the ability to do the following:

- Slow down tumor cell division
- Stimulate the proliferation and activation of NK cells
- Help cancer cells resume a more normal appearance and revert to their previous characteristics
- Inhibit the expression of oncogenes

Although interferons are approved for limited use as a cancer treatment, they have been effective to some degree in the treatment of hairy cell leukemia, renal cell carcinoma, ovarian cancer, and cutaneous T-cell lymphoma.

MONOCLONAL ANTIBODIES

Antibodies to one or more parts of cancer cells have been used experimentally and in cancer diagnosis for many years. Two monoclonal antibodies for cancer treatment have recently been approved and are currently in use. Trastuzumab (Herceptin) binds to a protein made by some breast cancer cells. Binding this protein prevents the division of cancer cells and makes them more easily killed by immune system cells. Another monoclonal antibody, rituximab (Rituxan) performs a similar function in some types of non-Hodgkin's lymphoma.

Biologic Response Modifiers for Cancer Support

BRMs approved for use as supportive therapy during cancer treatment are the colony-stimulating factors (Table 25-12). Essentially, these factors induce more rapid recovery of the bone marrow after suppression by chemotherapy.

This effect may have two benefits. First, when bone marrow suppression is less severe or of shorter duration, clients are less at risk for life-threatening infections and anemia. Second, because the colony-stimulating factors allow more rapid bone marrow recovery, clients can receive their chemotherapy on time and may even be able to tolerate higher doses, potentially improving the curative outcome of chemotherapy. These agents must be used cautiously for malignancies in which the cancer cells may also have a BRM receptor, such as leukemias and lymphomas.

TABLE 25-12 • COLONY-STIMULATING FACTORS

Agent	Cell Type Affected	Indications
Sargramostim (Leukine, Prokine)	All granulocytes • Neutrophils • Eosinophils Monocytes Macrophages	Chemotherapy-induced leukopenia
Filgrastim (Neupogen)	Neutrophils	Chemotherapy-induced neutropenia
Epoetin alfa (Epogen Procrit)	Erythrocytes	Chemotherapy-induced anemia Chemotherapy-induced fatigue Anemia induced by renal failure
Oprelvekin (Neumega)	Platelets	Chemotherapy-induced thrombocytopenia

SIDE EFFECTS OF BIOLOGIC RESPONSE MODIFIER THERAPY

Clients receiving interleukins at therapeutic doses experience generalized and sometimes severe inflammatory reactions. Fluid shifts and capillary leak are widespread. Tissue swelling affects the function of all major organs and can be life threatening. Clients receiving high-dose BRM therapy should receive care in an intensive care or monitoring unit. The effects of BRM therapy are limited to the period of acute drug administration and resolve spontaneously when treatment is completed.

Many BRMs induce general symptoms of mild inflammatory reactions during and immediately after administration, including fever, chills, rigors, and flu-like general malaise. Symptoms are worse when higher doses are given, and they seem to become less severe over time. Fever is treated with acetaminophen. Clients with severe rigors are managed with meperidine (Demerol).

Allergic reactions are an issue in clients receiving monoclonal antibodies. Most of these antibodies were raised in other animal species and may express some of those animal proteins. Clients receiving monoclonal antibodies over time may develop their own antibodies to the drugs, making them less effective and possibly causing severe inflammatory or allergic reactions.

Gene Therapy

Gene therapy as a primary or adjunct cancer treatment modality currently has only investigational status. Although response rates have been limited, experimental successes indicate the potential for gene therapy as a form of cancer treatment.

INCREASED TUMOR CELL SUSCEPTIBILITY

One method of using gene therapy for cancer is to render the tumor cells more susceptible to damage or death by other treatments. Inserting a viral enzyme gene into brain tumor cells makes them more susceptible to being killed by antiviral agents. Other techniques involve inserting human leukocyte antigen (HLA) genes different from the client's own HLAs into the tumor cells. This technique makes the client's immune system cells better able to recognize the cancer cells as foreign and take steps to eliminate or destroy them. Both methods of gene therapy for cancer have shown some success in early-phase clinical trials.

INCREASED IMMUNE SYSTEM CELL ACTIVITY

Some immune system cells are capable of attacking and killing cancer cells (see Chapter 20). This ability is increased when more of certain cytokines, such as IL-2, are present. Some gene therapy involves inserting additional genes for cytokines into the client's own immune system cells. These "charged-up" cancer-fighting immune system cells remain active for up to 6 months and can participate in cancer cell–killing episodes.

POTENTIAL USES OF GENE THERAPY FOR CANCER

Because cancer is caused by one or more changes in the genes of a normal cell, it is not unreasonable to think that gene alterations could influence a cancer cell to become normal. Areas under current research for gene therapy against cancer include the following:

- Inserting additional or healthy suppressor genes into cancer cells
- Inserting chemotherapy resistance genes into normal cells so higher doses of chemotherapy can be given without affecting normal cells
- Removing damaged, mutated, or activated oncogenes
- Inserting multiple genes into cancer cells to make them more easily recognized by immune system cells and more susceptible to other treatment modalities

ONCOLOGIC EMERGENCIES

Cancer is considered a chronic disease. However, a number of acute conditions associated with cancer and its treatment can occur. These conditions, or complications, often require immediate medical intervention and are thus considered *oncologic emergencies.* Early diagnosis of such conditions is essential to avoid life-threatening situations.

Sepsis and Disseminated Intravascular Coagulation

OVERVIEW

Sepsis, or septicemia, is a condition in which microorganisms enter the bloodstream. Septic shock is a life-threatening result of sepsis and a common cause of death in clients with cancer. Clients with cancer are at increased risk for infection and sepsis because their white blood cell counts are often low and their immune function is usually impaired. Chapter 37 describes the pathophysiology of sepsis and septic shock.

Disseminated intravascular coagulation (DIC) is a condition that indicates a problem with the blood-clotting process. DIC is triggered by many severe illnesses, including cancer. In clients with cancer, DIC is caused by sepsis (usually a gram-negative infection), by the release of thrombin or thromboplastin (clotting factors) from cancer cells, or by blood transfusions. DIC is most often associated with leukemia and with adenocarcinomas of the lung, pancreas, stomach, and prostate.

Extensive, abnormal clot formation occurs throughout the small blood vessels of clients with DIC. This widespread clotting consumes all circulating clotting factors and platelets. This process is followed by extensive bleeding. Bleeding from many sites is the most common problem and ranges from minimal to fatal hemorrhage. The blockage of blood vessels from clots decreases blood flow to major body organs and results in pain, stroke-like signs and symptoms, dyspnea, tachycardia, oliguria (decreased urine output), and bowel necrosis (tissue death). Chapter 37 describes the pathophysiology and collaborative management of sepsis-induced DIC.

➤ COLLABORATIVE MANAGEMENT

DIC is a life-threatening problem and has a mortality rate greater than 70% even when appropriate therapies are instituted. Therefore the best treatment plan for sepsis and DIC is prevention. The nurse identifies those clients at greatest risk for the development of sepsis and DIC. Strict adherence to aseptic technique is practiced during invasive procedures and during the manipulation of nonintact skin and mucous membranes in immunocompromised clients. The nurse teaches clients and family members the early clinical manifestations of infection and sepsis and when to seek medical assistance.

When sepsis is present and DIC is likely, treatment focuses on reducing the infection and halting the DIC process. Appropriate IV antibiotic therapy is initiated. During the early phase of DIC, anticoagulants (especially heparin) are administered to limit unnecessary clotting and prevent the rapid consumption of circulating clotting factors. Cryoprecipitated clotting factors are administered when DIC has progressed to the later phase and hemorrhage is the primary problem.

Syndrome of Inappropriate Antidiuretic Hormone

OVERVIEW

In healthy people, antidiuretic hormone (ADH) is secreted by the posterior pituitary gland only when more fluid (water) is needed in the body, such as when plasma volume is decreased (see Chapter 11). In people with certain health problems, ADH is secreted inappropriately or when not needed by the body.

Cancer is the most common cause of the syndrome of inappropriate antidiuretic hormone (SIADH). The type of cancer most commonly associated with SIADH is carcinoma of the lung (especially small cell lung cancer), but SIADH may occur in other types of cancer, especially when tumors are present in the brain. Some tumors actually make and secrete ADH, whereas others stimulate the brain to synthesize and secrete ADH. In addition, certain drugs commonly used in clients with cancer can cause the problem (most notably morphine sulfate and cyclophosphamide).

In SIADH, excessive amounts of water are reabsorbed by the kidney and put into systemic circulation. The increased water causes hyponatremia (decreased serum sodium levels) and some degree of fluid retention. Mild symptoms occur and include weakness, muscle cramps, loss of appetite, and fatigue. Serum sodium levels range from 115 to 120 mEq/L (normal range is 135 to 145 mEq/L). More serious signs and symptoms are related to water intoxication, including weight gain, nervous system changes (especially personality changes), confusion, and extreme muscle weakness. As the sodium level approaches 110 mEq/L, seizures, coma and, eventually, death may follow unless the condition is rapidly treated.

➤ COLLABORATIVE MANAGEMENT

SIADH is managed by treating the condition and the cause. Treatment regimens for SIADH usually include fluid restriction (sometimes total fluid intake is reduced to 1 L/day), increased sodium intake, and drug therapy. A commonly used drug for this condition is demeclocycline, a form of tetracycline antibiotic, which is taken orally. The mechanism of action appears to be antagonistic to ADH. Serum sodium levels must be monitored closely, because hypernatremia can develop suddenly as a result of this treatment.

A second method for managing SIADH is to reduce or eliminate the underlying cause. The immediate institution of appropriate cancer therapy, usually either radiation or chemotherapy, can cause such tumor regression that ADH synthesis and release processes return to normal.

Spinal Cord Compression

OVERVIEW

Spinal cord compression and damage occur when a tumor directly enters the spinal cord or when the vertebral column collapses from tumor entry. Tumors may begin in the spinal cord but more commonly spread from other areas of the body, such as the lung, prostate, breast, and colon. Spinal cord compression causes back pain, usually before neurologic deficits occur. Neurologic deficits are related to the spinal level of compression and include numbness; tingling; loss of urethral, vaginal, and rectal sensation; and muscle weakness. If paralysis occurs, it is usually permanent.

➤ COLLABORATIVE MANAGEMENT

Nurses caring for clients with spinal cord compression must recognize the condition early. The nurse assesses the client for neurologic changes consistent with spinal cord compression. The nurse also teaches clients and families to recognize the symptoms of early spinal cord compression and to seek medical assistance as soon as symptoms are apparent.

Treatment is largely palliative. High-dose radiation is usually administered to reduce the size of the tumor in the area and relieve compression. Radiation may be given in conjunction with chemotherapy to treat the total disease. Surgery is occasionally performed to remove the tumor from the area and rearrange the bony tissue so less pressure is placed on the spinal cord. External back or neck braces may be prescribed to reduce the weight borne by the spinal column and to reduce pressure on the spinal cord or spinal nerves.

Hypercalcemia

OVERVIEW

Hypercalcemia (increased serum calcium level), a late manifestation of extensive malignancy, occurs most often in clients with bone metastasis. Cancer in bone causes the bone to release calcium into the bloodstream. In clients with cancer in other parts of the body—especially the lung, head and neck, kidney, or lymph nodes—the tumor secretes parathyroid hormone (parathormone), causing bone to release calcium. Decreased physical mobility also contributes to or worsens hypercalcemia.

Early signs and symptoms of hypercalcemia include fatigue, loss of appetite, nausea, vomiting, constipation, and polyuria (increased urine output). More serious signs and symptoms include severe muscle weakness, diminished deep tendon reflexes, paralytic ileus, dehydration, and electrocardiographic (ECG) changes. The severity of signs and symptoms depends on how high the serum calcium level is and how quickly it developed (see also Chapter 13).

▶ COLLABORATIVE MANAGEMENT

Hypercalcemia as a consequence of cancer develops very slowly for many clients, which allows the body time to adapt to this electrolyte change. As a result, symptoms of hypercalcemia may not be evident until the serum calcium level is greatly elevated. Because adaptation does occur, hypercalcemia associated with cancer is treated only when clinical manifestations are present.

Conservative management, such as oral hydration alone, may be enough to reduce the serum calcium to an acceptable level. Normal saline is the fluid of choice when parenteral hydration is needed.

Many drugs lower serum calcium levels. Some agents, such oral glucocorticoids, calcitonin, diphosphonate, gallium nitrate, and mithramycin, lower levels quite dramatically. These agents do not cure hypercalcemia but instead reduce serum calcium levels temporarily. When cancer-induced hypercalcemia is life threatening or accompanied by renal impairment, dialysis can temporarily reduce serum calcium levels.

Superior Vena Cava Syndrome

OVERVIEW

Superior vena cava (SVC) syndrome occurs when the SVC is compressed or obstructed by tumor growth (Figure 25-3). SVC compression can lead to a painful and life-threatening emergency, most often in clients with lymphomas and bronchogenic carcinoma. Clients with cancer of the breast, esophagus, colon, and testes may also be affected.

The signs and symptoms associated with SVC syndrome result from the blockage of blood flow in the venous system of the head, neck, and upper trunk. In general, early signs and symptoms occur in the early morning and include edema of the face, especially around the eyes (periorbital edema), and tightness of the shirt or blouse collar (Stokes' sign). As the compression worsens, the client typically experiences edema in the arms and hands, dyspnea, erythema of the upper body, and epistaxis (nosebleeds). Late life-threatening signs and symptoms include hemorrhage, cyanosis, mental status changes from lack of blood to the brain, decreased cardiac output, and hypotension (low blood pressure). Death can result if compression is not relieved.

▶ COLLABORATIVE MANAGEMENT

SVC syndrome is a late-stage manifestation; the tumor is usually widespread. High-dose radiation therapy to the mediastinal area is the most common treatment of choice and can provide temporary relief in approximately 70% of clients. Surgery is not performed for this condition because the tumor may have increased intrathoracic pressure to such a level that it may be impossible to close the chest after the procedure.

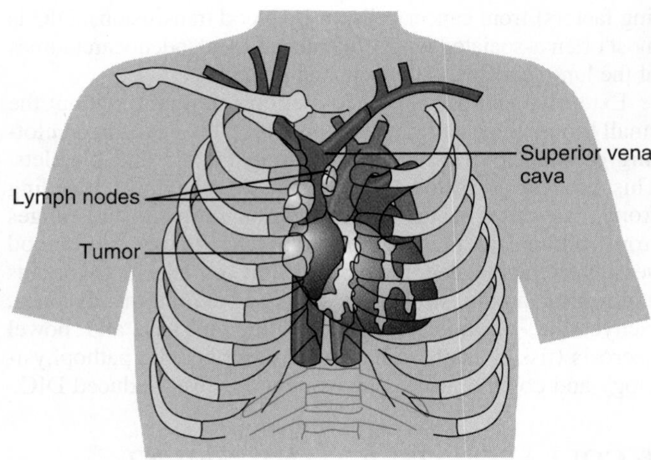

Figure 25-3 ● Compression of the superior vena cava in superior vena cava syndrome.

The best therapeutic and palliative results occur when SVC syndrome is in the early stages. The nurse assesses each client for signs and symptoms of SVC syndrome and notifies the physician.

Tumor Lysis Syndrome

OVERVIEW

In tumor lysis syndrome (TLS), large quantities of tumor cells are destroyed rapidly. Their intracellular contents, including potassium and purines (DNA components), are released into the bloodstream faster than the body's homeostatic mechanisms can handle them (Figure 25-4). Unlike other oncologic emergencies, TLS is a positive sign that cancer treatment is effective.

Severe or untreated TLS can cause severe tissue damage and death. Serum potassium levels can increase to the point of hyperkalemia, causing severe cardiac dysfunction (see Chapter 13). In addition, the large quantities of released purines are converted in the liver to uric acid and released into the systemic circulation, causing hyperuricemia. These uric acid molecules precipitate in the kidney, forming a sludge in the kidney tubules; this effect blocks them and leads to acute renal failure.

TLS is most commonly seen in clients receiving radiation or drug therapy for cancers initially very sensitive to these therapies, including leukemia, lymphoma, small cell lung cancer, and multiple myeloma.

▶ COLLABORATIVE MANAGEMENT

Prevention through hydration is the best management for TLS. Hydration alone can dilute the serum potassium level and increases the glomerular filtration rate. As a result, urine flows through the kidney at a greatly increased rate. This action prevents the precipitation of uric acid crystals, increases

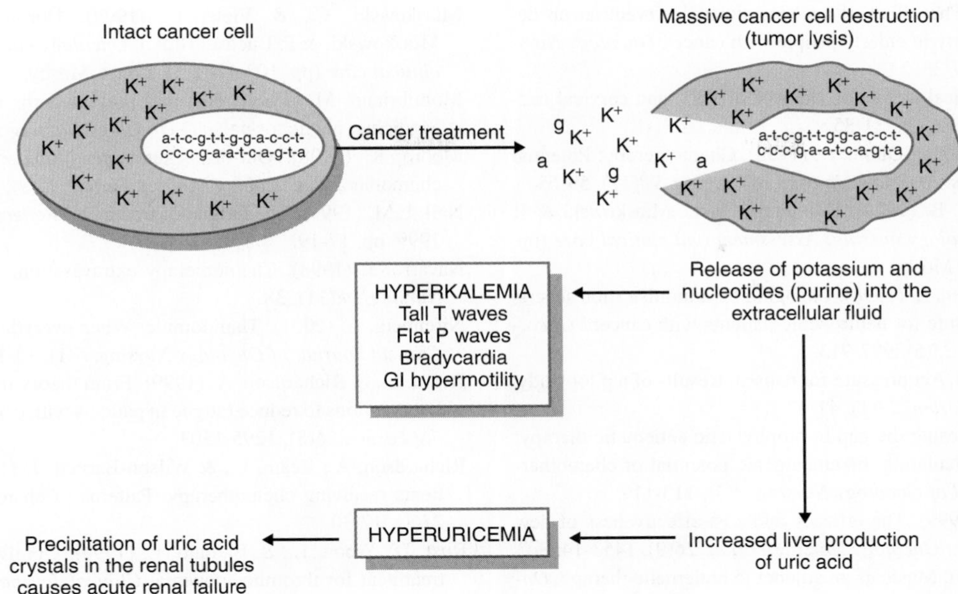

Figure 25-4 ● Pathology of tumor lysis syndrome.

the renal excretion of potassium, and mechanically flushes any renal tubular sludge.

With tumors known to be very sensitive to cancer therapy, the nurse instructs clients to drink at least 3000 mL (5000 mL is more desirable) of fluid the day before, the day of, and for 3 days after treatment. Some fluids should be alkaline to help prevent the crystallization of uric acid. The nurse stresses the importance of keeping fluid intake relatively consistent throughout the 24-hour day and helps clients draw up a schedule of fluid intake.

Because some clients experience nausea and vomiting after cancer therapy and may not feel like ingesting oral fluids, the nurse stresses the importance of following the antiemetic regimen. The nurse also instructs clients to contact their health care provider or cancer clinic immediately if nausea and vomiting prevent adequate fluid intake so they can be started on parenteral fluids.

Treatment becomes more aggressive for clients who become hyperkalemic or hyperuricemic. In addition to increased fluid intake (oral or parenteral), diuretics (especially osmotic types) are given to increase urine flow through the kidney. These agents are administered with caution because clients must not become dehydrated. Drugs that increase the excretion of purines, such as allopurinol (Alloprin, Zyloprim), are administered. To reduce serum potassium levels, IV infusions containing glucose and insulin may be administered. Clients who experience more severe and persistent hyperkalemia and hyperuricemia may require dialysis.

CANCER TREATMENT FAILURE

More than 50% of people diagnosed with cancer in North America this year will be cured of their disease, and many others will live 2 years or longer. However, some will experience cancer treatment failure and die. With cancer, the process of dying is usually long, lasting weeks or months. Clients and families require special support and assistance during this time. Chapter 9 addresses hospice care and other important physical, emotional, social, and spiritual needs of clients and families during and after the dying process.

ONLINE RESOURCES

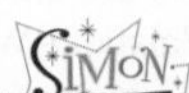

For suggested readings and Internet resources, go to http://www.wbsaunders.com/SIMON/Iggy/.

SELECTED BIBLIOGRAPHY

Asterisk indicates a classic or definitive work on this subject.

*American Cancer Society. (1991). *Proceedings of the National Workshop on Cancer Control and the Older Person.* Atlanta: Author.

American Cancer Society. (2001). *Cancer facts and figures 2001.* Report No. 00-300M-No. 5008.01. Atlanta: Author.

Anastasia, P. (2001). Nursing considerations for managing topotecan-related hematologic side effects. *Clinical Journal of Oncology Nursing, 5*(1), 9-13.

Barsevick, A. (2001). Assessment and management of cancer fatigue. *Clinical Journal of Oncology Nursing, 5*(1), 39-40.

Bennett, M., & Lengacher, C. (1999). Use of complementary therapies in a rural cancer population. *Oncology Nursing Forum, 26*(8), 1287-1294.

Berkowitz, N., et al. (1999). Comparing the cost-effectiveness of chemo in the treatment of metastatic breast cancer. *Managed Care & Cancer, 1*(5), 18-25.

Brown, D., et al. (1999). Economic evaluation of breast cancer screening. *Cancer Practice, 7*(1), 28-33.

Brown, P. (1999). Nutrition and cancer. *MEDSURG Nursing, 8*(6), 333-345.

Burke, C. (1999). Surgical treatment. In C. Miaskowski & P. Buchsel (Eds.), *Oncology nursing: Assessment and clinical care* (pp. 29-58). St. Louis: Mosby.

*Clark, J., & Longo, D. (1986). Biologic response modifiers. *Mediguide to Oncology, 6,* 1-10.

Clayton, K. (1997). Cancer-related hypercalcemia: How to spot it, how to manage it. *American Journal of Nursing, 97*(5), 42-49.

Clofelter, C. (1999). The effect of an educational intervention on decreasing pain intensity in elderly people with cancer. *Oncology Nursing Forum, 26*(1), 27-33.

Daley, E. (1998). Clinical update on the role of HPV and cervical cancer. *Cancer Nursing, 21*(1), 31-35.

DelGaudio, D., & Menonna-Quinn, D. (1998). Chemotherapy: Potential occupational hazards. *American Journal of Nursing, 98*(11), 59-65.

DeMeyer, E., & Stein, B. (1999). Biotherapy. In C. Miaskowski & P. Buchsel (Eds.), *Oncology nursing: Assessment and clinical care* (pp. 119-141). St. Louis: Mosby.

deMoissac, D., & Jensen, L. (1998). Changing IV administration sets: Is 48 versus 24 hours safe for neutropenic patients with cancer? *Oncology Nursing Forum, 25*(5), 907-913.

Dibble, S., et al. (2000). Acupressure for nausea: Results of a pilot study. *Oncology Nursing Forum, 27*(1), 41-47.

Doherty, K. (1999). Closing the gap in prophylactic antiemetic therapy: Patient factors in calculating the emetogenic potential of chemotherapy. *Clinical Journal of Oncology Nursing, 3*(3), 113-119.

Engstrom, C., et al. (1999). The efficacy and cost-effectiveness of new antiemetic guidelines. *Oncology Nursing Forum, 26*(9), 1453-1458.

Ezzone, S., et al. (1998). Music as an adjunct to antiemetic therapy. *Oncology Nursing Forum, 25*(9), 1551-1556.

*Folkman, J. (1996). Fighting cancer by attacking its blood supply. *Scientific American, 275*(3), 150-154.

Garner, C. (1999). Cancer-related spinal cord compression. *American Journal of Nursing, 99*(7), 34-35.

Goldsmith, M., & Wodinsky, H. (1999). Controlling costs using evidenced-based guidelines: 5-HT3 antagonists as a model. *Managed Care and Cancer, 1*(3), 20-24.

Haisfield-Wolfe, M., & Rund, C. (2000). A nursing protocol for the management of perineal-rectal skin alterations. *Clinical Journal of Oncology Nursing, 4*(1), 15-21.

*Hassey, K. (1987). Principles of radiation therapy and protection. *Seminars in Oncology Nursing, 3,* 23-29.

Houston, D. (1997). Supportive therapies for cancer chemotherapy patients and the role of the oncology nurse. *Cancer Nursing, 20*(6), 409-413.

Irvine, D., et al. (1998). Fatigue in women with breast cancer receiving radiation therapy. *Cancer Nursing, 21*(2), 127-135.

Johnson, M., Moroney, C., & Gay, C. (1997). Relieving nausea and vomiting in patients with cancer: A treatment algorithm. *Oncology Nursing Forum, 24*(1), 51-57.

Karius, D., & Marriott, M. (1997). Immunologic advances in monoclonal antibody therapy: Implications for oncology nursing. *Oncology Nursing Forum, 24*(3), 483-494.

Larson, P., et al. (1998). The PRO-SELF mouth aware program: An effective approach for reducing chemotherapy-induced mucositis. *Cancer Nursing, 21*(4), 263-268.

Loney, M., & Chernecky, C. (2000). Anemia. *Oncology Nursing Forum, 27*(6), 951-962.

*Maddock, P. (1987). Brachytherapy sources and applicators. *Seminars in Oncology Nursing, 3*(1), 15.

Miaskowski, C., & Buchsel, P. (1999). *Oncology nursing: Assessment and clinical care.* St. Louis: Mosby.

Miaskowski, C., & Viele, C. (1999). Cancer chemotherapy. In C. Miaskowski, & P. Buchsel (Eds.), *Oncology nursing: Assessment and clinical care* (pp. 83-106). St. Louis: Mosby.

Miaskowski, C., & Viele, C. (1999). Hormonal therapy. In C. Miaskowski, & P. Buchsel (Eds.), *Oncology nursing: Assessment and clinical care* (pp. 107-118). St. Louis: Mosby.

Montibriand, M. (1999). Past and present herbs used to treat cancer: Medicine, magic, or poison? *Oncology Nursing Forum, 26*(1), 49-60.

Moore, K. (1998). Out-of-pocket expenditures of patients receiving chemotherapy. *Oncology Nursing Forum, 25*(9), 1615-1622.

Nail, L.M. (1999). The fatigue of treatment. *Reflections,* Fourth Quarter 1999, pp. 17-19.

Navarro, T. (1998). Chemotherapy extravasation. *American Journal of Nursing, 98*(11), 38.

Nirenberg, A. (2001). Thalidomide: When everything old is new again. *Clinical Journal of Oncology Nursing, 5*(1), 15-18.

Ream, E., & Richardson, A. (1999). From theory to practice: Designing interventions to reduce fatigue in patients with cancer. *Oncology Nursing Forum, 26*(8), 1295-1303.

Richardson, A., Ream, E., & Wilson-Barnett, J. (1998). Fatigue in patients receiving chemotherapy: Patterns of change. *Cancer Nursing, 21*(1), 17-30.

Rust, D., Wood, L., & Battiato, L. (1999). Oprelvekin: An alternative treatment for thrombocytopenia. *Clinical Journal of Oncology Nursing, 3*(2), 57-61.

Schulmeister, L. (1999). Discrimination in the workplace. *Clinical Journal of Oncology Nursing, 3*(3), 123-124.

Shelton, B. (2000). Preventing crises in the patient with cancer. *Oncology Nursing Forum, 27*(6), 905-913.

Strohl, R. (1999). Radiation therapy. In C. Miaskowski, & P. Buchsel (Eds.), *Oncology nursing: Assessment and clinical care* (pp. 59-81). St. Louis: Mosby.

United States Pharmacopeia Dispensing Information (USP DI): Vol. I. Drug information for the health care professional (20th ed.). (2000). Englewood, CO: Micromedix.

Vanegas, G., et al. (1998). Side effects of morphine administration in cancer patients. *Cancer Nursing, 21*(4), 289-297.

Viele, C., & Holmes, B. (1998). Amifostine: Drug profile and nursing implications of the first pancytoprotectant. *Oncology Nursing Forum, 25*(3), 515-523.

Webster, A. (1999). Mind/body medicine: Self-care skills for persons with cancer. *Cancer Practice, 7*(1), 43-45.

Wells, N. (2000). Pain intensity and pain interference in hospitalized clients with cancer. *Oncology Nursing Forum, 27*(6), 985-991.

Williams, J., Wood, C., & Cunningham-Warburton, P. (1999). A narrative study of chemotherapy-induced alopecia. *Oncology Nursing Forum, 26*(9), 1463-1468.

Wilson, R. (2000). Optimizing nutrition for patients with cancer. *Clinical Journal of Oncology Nursing, 4*(1), 23-28.

Witt, M. (1998). Radiation and chemotherapy as combined treatment for advanced head and neck cancer. *MEDSURG Nursing, 7*(3), 159-164.

*Wood, L., & Gullo, S. (1993). IV vesicants: How to avoid extravasation. *American Journal of Nursing, 93*(4), 42-46.

Wyatt, G., et al. (1999). Complementary therapy use among older cancer patients. *Cancer Practice, 7*(3), 136-144.

CHAPTER 26

Interventions for Clients with Infection

JUDITH P. STURGIS

Learning Objectives

After studying this chapter, you should be able to:

1. Explain the chain of infection.
2. Describe the principles of infection control in inpatient and community-based settings.
3. Discuss the risk of gloves and other products made with latex.
4. Interpret the four types of transmission-based precautions.
5. Identify the major complications of infection.
6. Describe the common clinical manifestations of infection for which the nurse should assess.
7. Interpret laboratory test findings related to infections and infectious diseases.
8. Evaluate nursing interventions for fever management.

SIMON

Go to http://www.wbsaunders.com/SIMON/Iggy/ for self-assessment questions related to these Learning Objectives.

Infectious diseases have been the major cause of death worldwide for centuries. Today, there are threats of drug-resistant and re-emerging infections with the added possibility of bioterrorism. Appropriately used, antibiotics and vaccines prevent many types of infection, but their utility is limited by misuse, cost, and distribution issues. World marketing and people traveling and interacting with each other and their diversified environments cause exposure to a wider variety of infectious agents than in the past. Advancing technology and invasive procedures introduce previously harmless microorganisms into the body with resulting infection. Understanding of these issues, the infectious process, and transmission prevention will help prevent or minimize the effects of infection.

OVERVIEW

Definitions

The infection process requires a pathogen (cause agent), a susceptible host (infection recipient), and a means of transmission. A pathogen is any microorganism capable of producing disease. Infections can be communicable (e.g., influenza) or not communicable (e.g., pancreatitis). Microorganisms with differing levels of **pathogenicity** (ability to cause disease) surround everyone. **Virulence** is a term often used as a synonym for *pathogenicity.* However, virulence is related more to the frequency with which a pathogen causes disease (degree of communicability) and its ability to invade and damage a host. Virulence can also indicate the severity of the disease. Another important characteristic is **invasiveness** (ability of pathogens to spread and grow in the tissues of a host after entrance).

Most microorganisms commonly live in or on the human host without causing disease. Some microbes are beneficial. Each body location harbors its own characteristic bacteria, or **normal flora.** Normal flora often function to compete with and prevent infection from unfamiliar microorganisms attempting to invade a body site. In some instances, microorganisms that are often pathogenic may be present in the tissues of the host and yet not cause symptomatic disease; this process is called **colonization.**

Microorganisms often behave as parasites; that is, they live at the expense of their human hosts. Through this relationship, microbes gain some advantage and infection occurs. Infection is the establishment of a host-parasite interaction.

Subclinical infection causes no apparent reaction in the host and thus elicits no detectable symptoms. Most often, subclinical infection can be identified only by the host immune response. This is demonstrated by a rise in the antibody titer directed against the infecting agent. Clinically apparent infection in which the host-parasite interaction causes obvious injury is accompanied by one or more clinical manifestations and is known as infectious disease. Disease caused by an infectious agent may range from mild to fatal.

The Centers for Disease Control and Prevention (CDC) collects epidemiologic information about the occurrence and nature of infectious diseases. The CDC then makes recommendations to health care agencies for infection control and prevention. Certain diseases must be reported to health departments and the CDC (Table 26-1).

TABLE 26-1 • INFECTIOUS DISEASES THAT MUST BE REPORTED TO THE CENTERS FOR DISEASE CONTROL AND PREVENTION

- Acquired immunodeficiency syndrome (AIDS)
- Anthrax
- Botulism*
- Brucellosis
- Chancroid
- *Chlamydia trachomatis:* genital infection
- Cholera
- Coccidioidomycosis*
- Congenital rubella syndrome
- Congenital syphilis
- Cryptosporidiosis
- Diphtheria
- Encephalitis: California, eastern equine, St. Louis, western equine
- *Escherichia coli* 0157:H7
- Gonorrhea
- *Haemophilus influenzae:* invasive disease
- Hansen's disease (leprosy)
- Hantavirus: pulmonary syndrome
- Hemolytic-uremic syndrome following diarrhea*
- Hepatitis A
- Hepatitis B
- Hepatitis C
- Human immunodeficiency virus (HIV) infection, pediatric (<13 years)
- Legionellosis
- Lyme disease
- Malaria
- Measles (rubeola)
- Meningococcal disease
- Mumps
- Pertussis
- Plague
- Poliomyelitis, paralytic
- Psittacosis
- Rabies, animal
- Rabies, human
- Rocky Mountain spotted fever
- Rubella
- Salmonellosis*
- Shigellosis*
- Streptococcal disease, invasive, group A*
- Streptococcal toxic shock syndrome*
- *Streptococcus pneumoniae,* drug-resistant*
- Syphilis
- Tetanus
- Toxic shock syndrome
- Trichinosis
- Tuberculosis
- Typhoid fever
- Yellow fever*
- Varicella (chickenpox)†

Data from Centers for Disease Control and Prevention. (1999). *Summary of notifiable diseases, United States, 1998. Morbidity and Mortality Weekly Report, 47*(53), ii-92.
*Not currently published in the weekly tables.
†Although varicella is not a nationally notifiable disease, the Council of State and Territorial Epidemiologists recommends reporting cases of this disease to the Centers for Disease Control and Prevention (CDC).

Chain of Infection

Infectious disease development depends on a series of factors noted as the chain of infection (Figure 26-1).

To prevent the spread of infection, break the chain of infection at any point. Eliminating microorganisms, establishing host immunity, or interrupting transmission breaks the chain of infection. Nurses interrupt pathogen transmission by scrupulous handwashing, the use of standard precautions, and cleansing with antimicrobial agents.

RESERVOIR

Reservoirs (sources of infectious agents) are numerous. Animate reservoirs include people, animals, and insects. Inanimate reservoirs include soil, water, other environmental sources, or medical equipment (e.g., intravenous [IV] solutions and urine collection devices). The host's body can be a reservoir; pathogens can colonize in skin and body substances (e.g., feces, sputum, saliva, or wound drainage). A person with an active infection or an asymptomatic carrier (one who harbors an infectious agent without active disease) is a reservoir. A carrier can be incubating the pathogen before signs and symptoms develop, have a subclinical infection, be convalescing from an infection, or be a chronic carrier of the pathogen. Examples of community reservoirs include sewage, stagnant or contaminated water, and certain improperly handled foods.

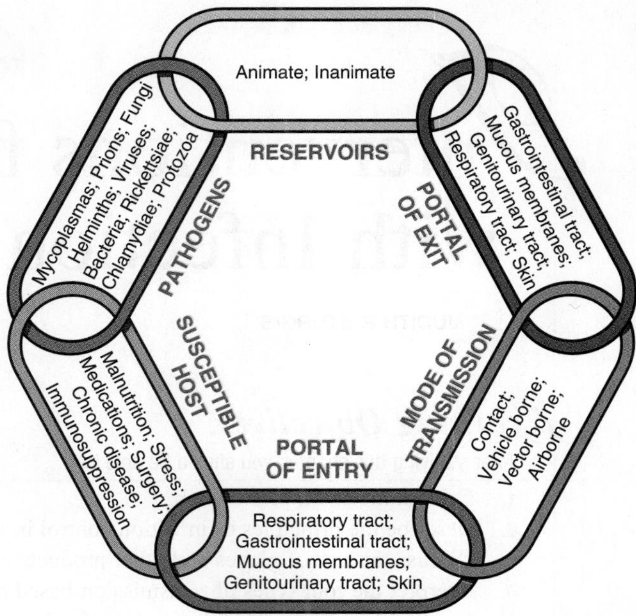

Figure 26-1 ● The chain of infection: the process by which pathogens are transmitted from the environment to a host, invade the host, and cause infection.

PATHOGEN

Several classes of microorganisms produce infection (Table 26-2). Continued multiplication of a pathogen is often accompanied by toxin production. **Toxins** are protein molecules released by bacteria to affect host cells at a distant site. **Exotoxins** are produced and released by certain bacteria into the surrounding environment. Botulism, tetanus, diphtheria, and *Escherichia coli* 0157:H7–related systemic disease are attributed to exotoxins. **Endotoxins** are produced in the cell walls of certain bacteria and released only with cell lysis. Typhoid and meningococcal diseases are caused by endotoxins.

HOST

Host factors influence the development of infection (Table 26-3). Host defenses provide the body with an efficient system for protection against pathogens. Breakdown of these defense mechanisms may increase the susceptibility of the host to infection.

The client's immune status plays the largest role in determining risk for infection. Congenital abnormalities, as well as acquired health problems (e.g., renal failure, steroid dependence, cancer, acquired immunodeficiency syndrome [AIDS]), can result in numerous immunologic deficiencies. Such depression of the immune system may render the host more susceptible to infection or cripple the host's ability to combat organisms that have gained entry.

IMMUNITY. Immunity is resistance to infection; it is usually associated with the presence of antibodies or cells that

TABLE 26-2 • INFECTIOUS ORGANISMS*

Organism Class	Common Examples	Common Disease Manifestations
Prions		Bovine spongiform encephalitis (BSE),‡ Creutzfeldt-Jakob disease, Kuru‡ Possible role in Alzheimer's disease, Parkinson's disease, and amyotrophic lateral sclerosis (ALS)†
Viruses	Poliovirus Hepatitis A virus Rhinovirus Influenza A virus Mumps virus	Poliomyelitis Hepatitis Common cold Influenza Mumps
Chlamydiae	*Chlamydia trachomatis* *Chlamydia psittaci*	Trachoma, lymphogranuloma venereum, conjunctivitis Psittacosis (parrot fever)
Mycoplasmas	*Mycoplasma pneumoniae* *Ureaplasma urealyticum* *Mycoplasma hominis*	Pneumonia Urethritis Pyelonephritis, pelvic inflammatory disease
Rickettsiae	*Rickettsia rickettsii* *Rickettsia prowazekii* *Coxiella burnetii*	Rocky Mountain spotted fever Typhus Q fever
Bacteria	*Staphylococcus* sp. *Streptococcus* sp. *Neisseria meningitidis* *Escherichia coli* *Pseudomonas aeruginosa*	Superficial skin infections, osteomyelitis, pneumonia, bacteremia Pharyngitis, skin infections, pneumonia Meningitis Urinary tract infection Skin infection, otitis, urinary tract infection
Fungi	*Candida albicans* *Aspergillus* sp. *Cryptococcus neoformans* *Histoplasma capsulatum* *Coccidioides immitis*	Thrush, vaginitis Sinusitis, brain abscess Meningitis, pneumonia Pneumonia Pneumonia
Protozoa	*Entamoeba histolytica* *Plasmodium* sp. *Leishmania* sp. *Toxoplasma gondii* *Pneumocystis carinii*	Diarrhea, colitis Malaria Fever, weight loss, cutaneous lesions Chorioretinitis, encephalitis Pneumonia
Helminths	*Ancylostoma duodenale* (hookworm) *Ascaris lumbricoides* (roundworm) *Enterobius vermicularis* (pinworm) *Schistosoma* sp. (blood flukes) *Taenia solium* (pork tapeworm)	Anemia Intestinal obstruction Anal pruritus Hydronephrosis Epilepsy from cysticercosis

*Organisms are presented in order of increasing complexity.

†Prusiner, S. Nobelist believes prions may be at root of Alzheimer's, Parkinson's, ALS. *Reuter's Health,* October 20, 1999; http://www.reutershealth.com. (Dr. Stanley Prusiner is a 1997 Nobel Prize winner for the discovery of prions.)

‡Mastrianni, J.A., & Roos, R.P. (2000). The prion diseases. *Seminars in Neurology, 20*(3), 337-352.

TABLE 26-3 • HOST FACTORS THAT INFLUENCE THE DEVELOPMENT OF INFECTION

Host Factor	Increased Risk of Infection
Natural immunity	Congenital or acquired immunodeficiencies
Normal flora	Alteration of normal flora by antibiotic therapy
Age	Infants and older clients
Hormonal factors	Pregnancy, diabetes, corticosteroid therapy, and adrenal insufficiency
Phagocytosis	Defective phagocytic function, circulatory disturbances, and neutropenia
Skin/mucous membranes/ normal excretory secretions	Break in skin or mucous membrane integrity; interference with flow of urine, tears, or saliva; interference with cough reflex or ciliary action; changes in gastric secretions
Nutrition	Malnutrition or dehydration
Environmental factors	Smoking, alcohol consumption, and inhalation of toxic chemicals
Medical interventions	Invasive therapy, chemotherapy, radiation therapy, and steroid therapy; surgery

CHART 26-1

NURSING FOCUS *on the* OLDER ADULT

Prevention of Infection

- Assess for atypical clinical manifestations of infection, such as confusion and unusual behavior. Typical manifestations (e.g., fever and pain) may not be present.
- Monitor renal function carefully when the client receives antibiotic therapy, especially aminoglycosides.
- Observe for and report adverse effects of antibiotic therapy because they may cause serious complications or death in older adults.
- Monitor for diarrhea from *Clostridium difficile* infection; obtain a specimen for culture if diarrhea occurs.
- Keep the client well hydrated, because older clients are at high risk for dehydration.

act on specific microorganisms. **Passive immunity** is of short duration (days or months) and either natural by transplacental transfer from the mother or artificial by injection of antibodies (e.g., immune globulin). **Active immunity** lasts for years and is natural by infection or artificial by injection of the agent itself (e.g., vaccine).

CONSIDERATIONS FOR OLDER ADULTS

Host factors such as age may influence immunity. Because of their decreased ability to produce an adequate immune response, older clients are at increased risk for infection. Immunity declines as people age, as evidenced by decreasing T-cell and primary antibody responses (see Chapter 20). Pneumonia following respiratory infection is more likely in older people. Vaccine for pneumococcal pneumonia, vaccine for influenza (annually), and/or antiviral medications are critical preventives for older adults (Chart 26-1).

OTHER FACTORS. Hormonal factors play a role in the incidence and mortality rate of many infectious diseases. People with diabetes mellitus and adrenal insufficiency experience increased numbers of acute and chronic bacterial infections.

Environmental factors may influence clients' immune status and thus their susceptibility to or ability to fight infection. Examples include alcohol consumption, nicotine use, inhalation of bone marrow–suppressing toxic chemicals, and certain vitamin deficiencies. Malnutrition, especially protein-calorie malnutrition, places clients at increased risk for infection.

Finally, some medical interventions may impair normal immune response. Steroid therapy, chemotherapy for malignant neoplasms, and cytotoxic therapy intended to suppress the immune response (e.g., cyclophosphamide [Cytoxan] for lupus nephritis and cyclosporine in organ transplant recipients) increase the risk of infection. Medical devices (e.g., intravascular or urethral catheters, endotracheal tubes) also may violate normal host defense mechanisms.

PORTAL OF ENTRY

Microorganisms may enter the body in a variety of ways (Table 26-4), and some specific sites of infection have key features (Chart 26-2).

TABLE 26-4 • PORTALS OF ENTRY OF SELECTED DISEASE-PRODUCING ORGANISMS

Infecting Organisms	Resultant Diseases
RESPIRATORY TRACT	
Neisseria meningitidis	Meningococcal pneumonia, meningocccal meningitis, meningococcemia
Cryptococcus neoformans	Cryptococcal meningitis, cryptococcal pneumonia
Mycobacterium tuberculosis	Tuberculosis
Influenza A virus	Influenza
Streptococcus pneumoniae	Pneumococcal pneumonia
Measles virus (rubeola)	Measles
Legionella pneumophila	Legionnaires' disease
Varicella-zoster virus	Chickenpox
GASTROINTESTINAL TRACT	
Salmonella enteritidis	Gastroenteritis
Salmonella typhi	Typhoid fever
Clostridium botulinum	Botulism
Poliovirus	Poliomyelitis
Hepatitis A virus	Hepatitis A
Escherichia coli 0157:H7	Possibly, hemolytic uremic syndrome
GENITOURINARY TRACT	
Neisseria gonorrhoeae	Gonorrhea
Chlamydia trachomatis	Lymphogranuloma venereum, cervicitis, urethritis, endometritis
Enterobacteriaceae (*E. coli, Klebsiella* sp., *Serratia* sp., *Proteus* sp.)	Urinary tract infections
INTACT SKIN OR MUCOUS MEMBRANES	
Rhinovirus	Common cold
Respiratory syncytial virus	Pneumonia, bronchiolitis, tracheobronchitis
Schistosoma sp.	Schistosome dermatitis (swimmer's disease)
Herpes simplex virus	Oral or genital herpes
BLOODSTREAM	
Hepatitis B or C viruses	Hepatitis B or C
Plasmodium sp.	Malaria
Clostridium tetani	Tetanus
Human immunodeficiency virus	Acquired immunodeficiency syndrome

RESPIRATORY TRACT. Pathogens may enter the body through the respiratory tract. Microbes in droplets are sprayed into the air when people with infected oral or nasal tissue talk, cough, or sneeze. A susceptible host then inhales droplets, and pathogens localize in the lungs or are distributed via the lymphatic system or bloodstream to other areas of the body. Microorganisms that enter the body by the respiratory tract and produce distant infection include influenza virus, *Mycobacterium tuberculosis,* and *Neisseria meningitidis* (often responsible for epidemic meningitis).

WOMEN'S HEALTH CONSIDERATIONS

A recent study tested for gender differences in outcome after treatment of infection in hospitalized clients. Hospital-acquired pneumonia mortality risk was noted as 18% for men and 34% for women (Crabtree et al., 1999).

CHART 26-2

KEY FEATURES *of* Infection of Specific Sites

Gastrointestinal Infections
- Fever
- Nausea and vomiting
- Diarrhea
- Abdominal distention and/or tenderness

Genitourinary Infections
- Dysuria
- Frequency
- Urgency
- Hematuria
- Fever
- Purulent discharge
- Pelvic or flank pain

Respiratory Infections
- Cough
- Congestion
- Rhinitis
- Sore throat
- Sputum
- Fever
- Chest pain

Skin Infections
- Redness
- Warmth
- Swelling
- Drainage
- Pain
- Pruritus

Generalized Infections
- Fever
- Malaise
- Fatigue
- Muscle aches
- Joint pain

GASTROINTESTINAL TRACT. Some pathogens enter the body by ingestion through the gastrointestinal (GI) tract. Some of these stay in the GI tract and produce disease (e.g., enteroviruses and organisms causing self-limited food poisoning). Others invade the GI tract to produce local and distant infection (e.g., *Salmonella enteritidis*). Some produce limited GI symptoms, causing systemic infection (e.g., *Salmonella typhi*) or profound involvement of organs (e.g., hepatitis A virus). Reported foodborne disease outbreaks affected 86,058 persons, causing 29 deaths in the United States from 1993 to 1999; however, actual numbers of individuals with foodborne illness are much higher (Centers for Disease Control and Prevention [CDC], 2000).

CONSIDERATIONS FOR OLDER ADULTS
Clostridium difficile can cause diarrhea, especially in older adults. Illness most often occurs after antibiotic therapy that destroys normal bowel flora. *C. difficile* multiplies opportunistically, and illness-causing toxin increases. Stool cultures may still be positive for *C. difficile* after diarrhea subsides.

GENITOURINARY TRACT. Microorganisms also enter through the genitourinary tract. Urinary tract infection (UTI) is one of the most common infectious diseases. Up to 25% of hospitalized clients have bladder catheterization, and about 5% per catheter day develop UTI. The use of urinary catheters coated with silver alloy may reduce the risk of UTI (Saint & Lipsky, 1999).

WOMEN'S HEALTH CONSIDERATIONS
Microorganisms (often colonic flora) colonize the perineal area, the urethral meatus, and the bladder, especially in women. The older woman is at even greater risk because of decreased resistance to infection, stress incontinence, or possibly, inability to practice proper hygiene.

SKIN/MUCOUS MEMBRANES. Some pathogens, such as *Treponema pallidum,* can enter the body through intact skin or mucous membranes. Most enter through breaks in these normally effective surface barriers. Sometimes a medical procedure creates a break in cutaneous or mucocutaneous barriers, as in catheter-acquired bacteremia (bacteria in the bloodstream) and surgical wound infections. Fragile skin of older clients and of those receiving prolonged steroid therapy increases infection risk.

BLOODSTREAM. Microorganisms can gain direct access to the bloodstream. The National Nosocomial Infection Surveillance (NNIS) reported that normal skin bacteria caused 40.9% of hospital-acquired (nosocomial) bloodstream infections in medical/surgical and intensive care unit (ICU) clients, which were probably introduced by intravascular devices (NNIS, 1999). In the community setting, biting insects can inject organisms into the bloodstream, causing infection (e.g., malaria, Lyme disease, or West Nile viral encephalitis).

MODE OF TRANSMISSION

For infection to be transmitted from an infected source to a susceptible host, a transport mechanism is required. Microorganisms are transmitted by several routes. The following are four common routes:

- Contact transmission
- Airborne transmission
- Vehicle transmission
- Vectorborne transmission

CONTACT TRANSMISSION. Contact transmission is the usual mode of transmission causing nosocomial infections. Of particular concern are the antibiotic-resistant infections that are difficult to treat. The NNIS (1999) reported a 37% increase in methicillin-resistant *Staphylococcus aureus* (MRSA) (52.3% of nosocomial *S. aureus* isolates) and a 43% increase in vancomycin-resistant enterococcus (VRE) (25.2% of enterococcus isolates) in ICU clients with nosocomial infections compared with the previous 4 years. Community-acquired MRSA has been seen in some persons who were not previously hospitalized (CDC, 1999).

Many infections are spread by direct or indirect contact. With **direct contact,** the source and host have physical contact; microorganisms are transferred directly from skin to skin or from mucous membrane to mucous membrane. Often called person-to-person transmission, direct contact is best illustrated by the spread of sexually transmitted diseases.

Indirect contact transmission involves transfer of microorganisms from a source to a host by passive transfer from an inanimate object (a fomite). Contaminated articles may serve as sources of infection (e.g., the transfer of hepatitis B virus to a susceptible host by a contaminated needle stick).

Indirect contact transmission may involve contact with infected secretions or *droplet spread.* Droplets are relatively large, usually greater than 5 μm in size. Produced when a person talks or sneezes, these droplets travel short distances (less than 1 m). Susceptible hosts may acquire infection by contact with droplets deposited on the nasal, oral, or conjunctival membranes. A common example of droplet-spread infection is influenza.

Oral-fecal transmission is another route of indirect contact infection. Ingestion of enteric pathogens (e.g., eating food prepared by a hepatitis A–infected person with unwashed hands) can cause disease transmission.

AIRBORNE TRANSMISSION. Airborne transmission occurs when small, airborne, infected particles leave the infected source, travel 3 feet, or are suspended in the air for a prolonged time. These particles are usually contained in droplet nuclei or dust; they are most often propelled from the respiratory tract by coughing or sneezing. A susceptible person then inhales the particles directly into the respiratory tract.

VEHICLE TRANSMISSION. Vehicle transmission occurs when infectious agents are transmitted through a common source, such as contaminated food, water, or IV fluid. Salmonellosis is an example of a disease that is frequently vehicle transmitted.

VECTORBORNE TRANSMISSION. Vectorborne transmission of infection involves insects and animals as intermediaries between two or more hosts (e.g., ticks transmit Rocky Mountain spotted fever and Lyme disease; mosquitoes spread malaria).

PORTAL OF EXIT

The portal of exit completes the chain of infection. An infecting organism exits from the once-susceptible person who has become a reservoir for infection. Exit from the host often occurs through the portal of entry. An organism, such as *Mycobacterium tuberculosis,* enters the respiratory tract and then exits the respiratory tract as the infected host coughs. Some organisms may exit from the infected host by several routes. For example, varicella-zoster virus can spread through direct contact with infective fluid in vesicles and by droplet contact.

Defense Against Infection

Strong and intact host defenses can prevent microbes from entering the body or destroy a pathogen that has entered. Conversely, impaired host defenses may be unable to defend against microbial invasion, allowing entry of microbes that can destroy cells and cause infection. Host defense mechanisms may be classified as nonspecific or specific.

NONSPECIFIC DEFENSES

Nonspecific mechanisms, usually representing the first encounter an invading pathogen has with its human host, include invasion of body tissues, such as skin and mucous membranes; phagocytosis; and inflammation (Table 26-5).

TABLE 26-5 • NONSPECIFIC DEFENSES AGAINST INFECTION

Body Tissue	Type of Action	Defense Action
Intact skin	Physical	Barrier action
	Chemical	Action of normal flora and acid pH (creates a hostile environment)
Mucous membranes	Mechanical	Mucociliary action (clears bacteria)
	Chemical	Lysosome action (dissolves bacterial wall)
Respiratory tract	Mechanical	Mucociliary action, cough
	Chemical	Lysosome action, humidification
Gastrointestinal tract	Mechanical	Peristalsis
	Chemical	Action of enzymes, acid pH, normal bowel flora
Genitourinary tract	Mechanical	Flushing action of urine
	Chemical	Action of acid pH

BODY TISSUES. Intact skin forms the first and most important physical barrier to the entry of microorganisms. In addition to providing a mechanical barrier, the skin's slightly acidic pH (resulting from breakdown of lipids into fatty acids), together with normal skin flora, creates an unfriendly environment for pathogenic bacteria.

Mucous membranes' mucociliary action provides some mechanical protection against pathogenic invasion. More important, however, mucous membranes are bathed in secretions that inactivate many microorganisms. Lysozymes, which dissolve the cell walls of some bacteria, are present in large quantities in many body secretions, particularly in nasal mucus and tears.

Other body systems provide natural barriers to infection. The healthy respiratory tract clears about 90% of all inhaled material by upper airway filtration, humidification, mucociliary transport, and expulsion by coughing. Peristaltic action mechanically empties the gastrointestinal (GI) tract of pathogenic organisms. Stomach acid, intestinal secretions, pancreatic enzymes, and bile, together with the competition from normal bowel flora, provide an environment that protects the GI tract from invasion by harmful organisms. In the genitourinary tract the flushing action of urine eliminates pathogenic organisms. The low pH of urine also maintains a sterile environment, although some microorganisms, such as *Escherichia coli,* thrive in an acid medium.

PHAGOCYTOSIS. Phagocytosis occurs when a foreign substance evades the first-line mechanical barriers and enters the body. Various leukocyte types function differently in the immune reaction, but neutrophils bear primary responsibility for phagocytosis. This process of engulfing, ingesting, killing, and disposing of an invading organism is an essential mechanism in host defense. Phagocytic dysfunction dramatically increases a client's risk for infection.

INFLAMMATION. Inflammation is another important nonspecific defense mechanism in preventing the spread of infection. Inflammation occurs when tissue becomes damaged. Damaged cells release enzymes, and polymorphonuclear leukocytes are attracted to the infected site from the bloodstream. One important enzyme, histamine, increases the permeability of the capillaries in inflamed tissues, thus allowing fluid, proteins, and white blood cells to enter an inflamed area. Other enzymes activate fibrinogen, which causes leaked fluid to clot and prevents its flow away from the damaged site into unaffected tissue, essentially "walling off" the inflamed tissue. The process of phagocytosis disposes of the invading microorganism and, often, dead tissue. If inflammation is caused by infection, the end products of inflammation form pus, which is subsequently absorbed or exits the body through a break in the skin.

SPECIFIC DEFENSES

Specific defense responses to specific microorganisms are provided by the antibody- and cell-mediated immune systems. The **antibody-mediated immune system** produces antibodies directed against certain pathogens. These antibodies inactivate or destroy invading microorganisms, as well as protect against future infection from that microorganism. Resistance to other microorganisms is mediated by the action of specifically sensitized T-lymphocytes and is called **cell-mediated immunity.** The components of the immune system work both independently and together to protect against infection.

INFECTION CONTROL IN INPATIENT HEALTH CARE AGENCIES

Infection acquired in the inpatient health care setting (not present or incubating at admission) is termed *nosocomial.* Nosocomial infection can be endogenous (from a client's flora) or exogenous (from outside the client, often from the hands of health care personnel). Nosocomial infections are acquired by about 2 million inpatients yearly, with a cost of approximately $3.5 billion annually (CDC, 2001). Clients who develop nosocomial surgical site infection (SSI) have longer and costlier hospitalizations, are 60% more likely to spend time in an intensive care unit (ICU), and are twice as likely to die as those who do not have an SSI (Kirkland et al., 1999).

Infection control within a health care facility is designed to reduce the risk of nosocomial infection and thus reduce morbidity and mortality. Infection control and prevention programs include facility- and department-specific infection control policies and procedures, surveillance and analysis, client and staff education, community and multidisciplinary networking, and product evaluation with an emphasis on quality and cost savings. Monitoring hospital-acquired (nosocomial) infections promotes client safety, as evidenced by the decreased nosocomial rate in intensive care units (ICUs) during 1990 and 1999 (CDC, 2000). The program is usually coordinated and implemented by a person certified in infection control (CIC) who has varied clinical and administrative experience.

INFECTION CONTROL IN THE COMMUNITY

Community-based caregivers follow epidemiologically sound infection control guidelines when caring for clients with infection. The Association for Professionals in Infection Control and Epidemiology (APIC) and the Society for Healthcare Epidemiology of America (SHEA) consensus panel have published requirements for activities of infection control and epidemiology in community-based settings (Friedman et al., 1999). Three primary goals were noted:

- Protect the client.
- Protect health care providers, visitors, and others in the health care environment.
- Accomplish these goals in a timely, efficient, and cost-effective manner.

Of special note are the CDC guidelines for pregnant health care personnel (Table 26-6).

The goals for infection control and epidemiology are the same for all health care settings. Functions of infection control and epidemiolgy, including the following principal functions, were summarized by the APIC and SHEA consensus report:

- Obtain and manage critical data, including infection surveillance.
- Develop and recommend policies and procedures.
- Intervene directly to prevent infections.
- Educate and train health care workers, clients, and nonmedical caregivers.

Methods of Infection Control

All health care facility employees who come in contact with clients or care areas are involved in some aspect of the infection control program of the agency. Infections can be prevented or controlled in at least five ways:

- Handwashing
- Hygiene
- Sanitation
- Disinfection/sterilization
- Barriers (e.g., gloves; see transmission precautions)

HANDWASHING

Handwashing is the most effective mechanism to prevent the spread of infection. Effective handwashing takes 15 seconds and includes wetting, soaping, lathering, applying friction under running water, rinsing, and adequate drying. Friction is essential to emulsify skin oils and to disperse transient bacteria and soil from hand surfaces (see the Evidence-Based Practice for Nursing box on p. 453).

The Centers for Disease Control and Prevention (CDC) recommend the use of antiseptic solutions, such as chlorhexidine, povidone-iodine, or PCMX, for handwashing in the care of clients who are at high risk (e.g., immunocompromised clients). The use of these solutions is also recommended after caring for clients who are infected with multiply resistant or other virulent organisms.

FALSE FINGERNAILS. Many health care workers have false fingernails, such as tips or sculptured nails. In a comparative study done by Virginia Medical Center and the University of Michigan, health care workers with false fingernails were compared with those without them. After proper handwashing, multiple bacteria, including pathogens, were found on 68% of those with false fingernails and 26% of those without false nails. The study concluded that false fingernails harbor bacteria that can be transmitted to clients.

GLOVES. Health care personnel must always wash their hands before and after direct contact with a client and immediately after contact with blood, secretions, and excretions,

TABLE 26-6 • PREGNANT HEALTH CARE PERSONNEL: PERTINENT FACTS TO GUIDE MANAGEMENT OF OCCUPATIONAL EXPOSURES TO INFECTIOUS AGENTS

Agent	Potential Effect on Fetus	Rate of Perinatal Transmission	Maternal Screening	Prevention
CMV	Hearing loss; congenital syndrome*	15% post–maternal infection; 5% with symptoms	Antibody gives some, but not complete, protection against clinical disease; routine screening not recommended	**Standard precautions**
Influenza virus	Inconsistent	Rare	None	Vaccine (safe during pregnancy); **droplet precautions**
HBV	Hepatitis; development of chronic infection in infant	HBeAg positive: 90%; HBeAg negative: 0-25%	HBsAg routine screening recommended	Vaccine and hepatitis B immune globulin to infant; **standard precautions**
HCV	Hepatitis	2%-5%	Routine screening not recommended Anti-HCV; HCV RNA	**Standard precautions**
HSV	Mucocutaneous lesions, sepsis, encephalitis, rare congenital malformations	Unlikely from nosocomial exposure primary: 33%-50%; recurrent: 4%	Antibody testing not useful; inspect for lesions at delivery	**Standard precautions**
HIV	AIDS by 2-3 yr	8%-30%	HIV and Western blot	Avoid high-risk behaviors; consider postexposure prophylaxis after high-risk exposure; intrapartum and postnatal zidovudine (AZT) for HIV-positive mothers and their infants; **standard precautions**
Measles	Prematurity, abortion	Rare	History, antibody	Vaccine†; **airborne precautions**
Parvovirus (B19)	Hydrops, stillbirth	Rare; 3%-9% maximum for adverse outcome	IgM and IgG antibody before pregnancy; antibody protective	**Droplet precautions**
Rubella virus	Congenital syndrome*	45%-50% overall; 90% in first 12 wk	Antibody	Vaccine†; **droplet precautions** for acute infection; **contact precautions** if congenital rubella
Mycobacterium tuberculosis	Hepatomegaly, pulmonary, CNS	Rare	Skin test	Isoniazid (INH) ± ethambutol for disease; **airborne isolation‡**
Varicella-zoster virus	Malformations (skin, limb, CNS, eye), chickenpox	Total: 25%; congenital syndrome: 0%-4%	Antibody	Vaccine†; VZIG within 96 hr of exposure if susceptible; **airborne plus contact isolation**

Data from Centers for Disease Control and Prevention. (1998). Guidelines for infection control in health care personnel, 1998. *American Journal of Infection Control, 26,* 322.
CMV, Cytomegalovirus; *HBV,* hepatitis B virus; *HCV,* hepatitis C virus, *HbeAg,* hepatitis B e antigen; *HbsAg,* hepatitis B surface antigen; *RNA,* ribonucleic acid; *HSV,* herpes simplex virus; *HIV,* human immunodeficiency virus; *AIDS,* acquired immunodeficiency syndrome; *Ig,* immunoglobulin; *TB,* tuberculosis; *CNS,* central nervous system; *VZIG,* varicella-zoster immune globulin.
*Congenital syndrome: varying combinations of jaundice, hepatosplenomegaly, microcephaly, CNS abnormalities, thrombocytopenia, anemia, retinopathy, and skin and bone lesions.
†Live-virus vaccines are given routinely before pregnancy.
‡Airborne isolation: apply guidelines related to TB transmission prevention.

and after glove removal. The use of gloves does not eliminate the need for handwashing. Studies have shown that up to 34% of gloves allow bacterial penetration, and as many as 53% leak or allow bacterial penetration during use (Beaumont, 1997).

The National Institute of Occupational Safety and Health (NIOSH) issued a public warning about potential allergic reactions to those exposed to latex in gloves and other medical products. Reactions include rashes, nasal or eye symptoms, asthma, and (rarely) shock (NIOSH, 1998). People with **latex allergy** are also more likely to develop an allergy to foods such as bananas, kiwis, and avocados. Types of reactions to latex include the following:

- *Irritant contact dermatitis*—dry, itchy, irritated skin, usually on the hands, which can result from frequent and/or inappropriate handwashing or cleansers. This dermatitis is not a true allergy.

EVIDENCE-BASED PRACTICE FOR NURSING

What is the effect of client education on staff compliance with handwashing?

McGuckin, M., et al. (1999). Patient education model for increasing hand washing compliance. *American Journal of Infection Control, 27*(4), 309-314.

The purpose of this prospective, controlled, 6-week study was to determine whether educated clients affected staff handwashing compliance. Four community hospitals in South New Jersey participated. Clients were educated within 24 hours of admission about the importance of asking health care providers to wash their hands. Phone follow-up was conducted 2 weeks after discharge. Soap use was measured based on bed-days.

Soap use increased an average of 34% for all hospitals, regardless of initial use rates. Of clients interviewed, 81% reported having read educational materials, and 57% asked health care providers if they washed their hands, 81% of those who asked received positive answers.

Critique. Current handwashing programs are directed toward health care providers with inconsistent results. This "partners in care" program furnished continuous handwashing education by using clients as prompters. Infections could be decreased by 32% with the use of this education model. A 300-bed hospital would save $57,600 annually. The study needs to be replicated using a larger sample and more hospitals in various geographic areas.

Implications for Nursing. Although this was only a 6-week study, positive outcomes could be projected for the future. Clients should be provided needed education to be involved in a partnership with health care providers in their care. Risk of infection is reduced and client outcomes improve with client education.

- *Chemical sensitivity dermatitis*—(delayed hypersensitivity) results from exposure to chemicals added to latex during harvesting or manufacturing.
- *Latex allergy*—(immediate sensitivity) true allergy in which certain proteins in latex may cause sensitization (positive blood test, with or without symptoms). Exposure to even low levels may trigger allergic reactions in some sensitized persons.

The following are recommendations by NIOSH for latex-allergy prevention:

- Use nonlatex gloves when there is no blood exposure risk (e.g., dietary functions).
- Avoid oil-based hand lotions while using latex gloves.
- Wash hands appropriately after removal of latex gloves.
- Seek medical evaluation for suspected latex allergy and inform employer.
- If allergic, avoid contact with latex-containing gloves and other products.

Latex-alternative product lists are readily available (Baumann, 1999).

OTHER INFECTION CONTROL MEASURES

Potentially harmful microbes are eliminated or greatly reduced through various methods. Good hygienic practices help prevent infection for clients and health care personnel. Strict sanitation and infectious waste disposal practices must be followed according to state, local, or federal regulations. Sterilization and disinfection procedures keep equipment and the environment clean. Housekeeping personnel use appropriate disinfectants to eliminate or minimize microbes.

TABLE 26-7 • STANDARD PRECAUTIONS

These precautions are to be used with all clients to protect health care providers from contracting or transmitting communicable disease.

- *Gloves* should be worn for contact with all body fluids, moist body tissues and mucous membranes, and nonintact skin of all clients; for handling other potentially infectious materials (OPIM), items, or surfaces; and for performing venipuncture and other vascular access procedures. Gloves should be changed after each client contact.
- *Masks and/or protective eyewear* should be worn during procedures that are likely to cause splashes of body fluids.
- *Gowns or aprons* should be worn during procedures likely to result in splashes of blood or body fluids.
- *Handwashing* should be done immediately on contact with body fluids or OPIM. Hands should be washed as soon as gloves are removed.
- *Needles and sharp instruments* should be placed in puncture-resistant containers for disposal to prevent injuries from needles or other sharp items. Needles should not be recapped, bent, or removed from syringe.
- *Mouth-to-mouth resuscitation* should be performed with use of mouthpieces or other ventilation devices.

Modified from Garner, J.S., & Hospital Infection Control Practices Advisory Committee (HICPAC). (1996). Guidelines for isolation precautions in hospitals. *American Journal of Infection Control, 24,* 24-52.

TABLE 26-8 • TRANSMISSION OF BLOODBORNE DISEASE BY VARIOUS BODY FLUIDS

BODY FLUIDS LIKELY TO TRANSMIT BLOODBORNE DISEASE

- Blood and other body fluids containing visible blood
- Semen and vaginal/cervical secretions
- Tissues
- Cerebrospinal fluid
- Amniotic fluid
- Synovial fluid
- Pleural fluid
- Peritoneal fluid
- Pericardial fluid
- Breast milk—from mother to child

BODY FLUIDS NOT LIKELY TO TRANSMIT BLOODBORNE DISEASE UNLESS BLOOD IS VISIBLE

- Feces
- Nasal secretions
- Sputum
- Vomitus
- Sweat
- Tears
- Urine
- Saliva, except in oral surgery or dentistry

Clients with immunocompromise or recent surgery are more susceptible to infections. Nurses must try to keep infectious clients apart from those who are highly susceptible to help prevent client-to-client infection transmission.

CENTERS FOR DISEASE CONTROL AND PREVENTION TRANSMISSION-BASED GUIDELINES

The newest isolation guidelines from the Centers for Disease Control and Prevention (CDC) focus on transmission mechanisms and combine the best aspects of previous guidelines. Included in these guidelines are standard, airborne, droplet, and contact precautions.

TABLE 26-9 • TRANSMISSION-BASED INFECTION CONTROL PRECAUTIONS*

Precautions (In Addition to Standard Precautions)	Examples of Diseases in Category
AIRBORNE PRECAUTIONS	
1. Private room with monitored negative airflow (with appropriate number of air exchanges and air discharge to outside or through HEPA); keep door(s) closed 2. Special respiratory protection: N-95† or HEPA† respirator for known or suspected TB Susceptible persons not to enter room of client with known or suspected measles or varicella unless immune caregivers are not available Susceptible persons who must enter room must wear N-95 or HEPA 3. Transport: client to leave room only for essential clinical reasons, wearing surgical mask	Diseases that are known or suspected to be transmitted by air: Measles (rubeola) *M. tuberculosis,* including multidrug–resistant TB (MDRTB) Varicella (chickenpox)‡; disseminated zoster (shingles)‡
DROPLET PRECAUTIONS	
1. Private room: if not available, may cohort with client with same active infection with same microorganisms if no other infection present; maintain distance of at least 3 feet from other clients if private room not available 2. Mask: required when working within 3 feet of client 3. Transport: as above	Diseases that are known or suspected to be transmitted by droplets: Diphtheria (pharyngeal) Streptococcal pharyngitis Pneumonia Scarlet fever (in infants or young children) Influenza Rubella Invasive disease (meningitis, pneumonia, sepsis) caused by *Haemophilus influenzae* type B or *Neisseria meningitidis* Mumps Pertussis
CONTACT PRECAUTIONS	
1. Private room: if not available, may cohort with client with same active infection with same microorganisms if no other infection present 2. Wear gloves when entering room 3. Wash hands with antimicrobial soap before leaving client's room 4. Wear gown to prevent contact with client or client-contaminated items or if client has uncontrolled body fluids; remove gown before leaving room 5. Transport: client to leave room only for essential clinical reasons; during transport, use needed precautions to prevent disease transmission 6. Dedicated equipment for this client only (or disinfect after use before taking from room)	Diseases that are known or suspected to be transmitted by direct contact: *Clostridium difficile* Colonization or infection caused by multidrug–resistant organisms (e.g., MRSA, VRE) Pediculosis Respiratory syncytial virus Scabies Viral hemorrhagic infections (Ebola, Lassa, or Marburg)

Modified from Garner, J.S., & Hospital Infection Control Practices Advisory Committee (HICPAC). (1996). Guidelines for isolation precautions in hospitals. *American Journal of Infection Control, 24,* 24-52.
HEPA, High-efficiency particulate air filter; *TB,* tuberculosis; *MRSA,* methicillin-resistant *Staphylococcus aureus; VRE,* vancomycin-resistant *Enterococcus.*
*Modification by facilities: The Centers for Disease Control and Prevention encourages facilities to adapt these guidelines, still following sound epidemiologic principles (e.g., some have removed TB transmission prevention guidelines from the airborne precautions category and added a separate category).
†Before use: training and fit testing required for personnel.
‡Add contact precautions for draining lesions.

Standard precautions acknowledge that all body excretions, secretions, and moist membranes and tissues, excluding perspiration, are potentially infectious. The protective measures from universal precautions and body substance isolation are combined. Table 26-7 outlines the guidelines for standard precautions, and Table 26-8 notes which body fluids have the highest risk for transmission of bloodborne disease and which do not.

Airborne precautions are used for clients known or suspected to have infections transmitted by the airborne transmission route; such infections are caused by organisms that can be suspended in air for prolonged periods. Negative airflow rooms are required to prevent airborne spread of microbes through ventilation ducts. Enclosed booths with high-efficiency particulate air (HEPA) filtration and/or ultraviolet light may be used for sputum induction procedures. Tuberculosis, measles (rubeola), and chickenpox (varicella) are examples of airborne diseases (Table 26-9).

Droplet precautions are used for clients known or suspected to have infections transmitted by the droplet transmission route. Such infections are caused by organisms in droplets that may travel 3 feet but are not suspended for long time periods. Examples of infectious conditions requiring droplet precautions include influenza, mumps, pertussis, and meningitis caused by either *Neisseria meningitidis* or *Haemophilus influenzae* type B (see Table 26-9).

Contact precautions are used for clients known or suspected to have infections transmitted by direct contact or contact with items in the client's environment. Clients with significant multidrug-resistant organism infection or colonization (e.g., methicillin-resistant *Staphylococcus aureus* [MRSA] or

CHART 26-3

BEST PRACTICE *for* Drug-Resistant Infections

Prevalent Resistant Organisms

- Aminoglycoside-resistant *Pseudomonas* (gentamicin, tobramycin, amikacin)
- Methicillin-resistant *Staphylococcus aureus* (MRSA)
- Vancomycin-resistant *Enterococcus* (VRE)

Enabling and Contributing Factors

- Long-term antibiotic use and misuse (health care provider and client's roles)
- Fewer new antibiotics being developed
- Invasive devices or procedures, especially the following:
  - Gastric/endotracheal tubes
  - Catheters
- Surgical drains or wounds
- Vascular devices
- Increased exposure risk through prolonged or repeated hospital stays
- Compromised or weakened defenses
- Inadequate health care handwashing facilities or practices
- Inconsistent cleaning of health care equipment or environment
- Food preparation or handling inconsistencies
- Delayed identification and institution of infection control precautions

Centers for Disease Control and Prevention

- Rapid national and international detection and response
- Applied research in disease diagnosis and prevention
- Better communication and implementation of prevention strategies
- Stronger connections among local, state, and federal public health providers to support tracking, prevention, and control programs

Implications for Nursing

- Early identification is important. Look for the following:
  - Signs of new or spreading infection
  - Culture and sensitivity (C&S) result that shows resistance (e.g., MRSA, VRE)
  - C&S result that matches another client's drug sensitivity pattern (possibly indicating a cluster of infections from the same source)
- Implement infection control measures in a timely manner:
  - Use standard precautions consistently.
  - Implement special additional precautions promptly (contact precautions).
  - Post signs and labels to notify others as per hospital policy.
  - Educate the client and family about infection control measures.
  - Notify the physician and infection control practitioner about infection.
- Appropriately administer antibiotics and teach discharged client and family about appropriate antibiotic use.

vancomycin-resistant *Enterococcus* [VRE]) are placed on contact precautions. Other infections requiring contact precautions include pediculosis, scabies, respiratory syncytial virus (RSV), and *Clostridium difficile* (see Table 26-9). Information about drug-resistant infections is found in Chart 26-3.

CRITICAL THINKING CHALLENGE

You have received surgical site culture and sensitivity (C&S) reports for two clients in the same hospital room. Both post–orthopedic surgery clients have *Staphylococcus aureus* resistant to methicillin, penicillin, and erythromycin, labeled by the laboratory as MRSA.

- Who should be informed of these matching MRSA C&S reports?
- What transmission route(s) may have caused the matching MRSA C&S results?
- Why is it important to identify the probable nosocomial transmission route?
- What are the implications for the clients' postdischarge care?

For suggested answer guidelines, go to SIMON http://www.wbsaunders.com/SIMON/Iggy/.

Occupational Exposure to Sources of Infection

The Occupational Safety and Health Administration (OSHA) is a federal agency that protects workers from injury or illness at their place of employment. Unlike the voluntary guidelines developed by the CDC, OSHA regulations are law. Employers can be fined or disciplined for noncompliance with OSHA regulations. The regulation for prevention of exposure to bloodborne pathogens, such as hepatitis B and C or the human immunodeficiency virus (HIV), is one example of an OSHA regulation (Table 26-10).

BLOODBORNE PATHOGENS

Reduction of percutaneous injuries (e.g., needle sticks) is of utmost importance to reduce bloodborne pathogen transmission to health care personnel. OSHA mandates that sharp objects ("sharps") and needles be handled with care. Availability and consistency in the use of protective devices are vital. Almost half of contaminated sharp-object exposures involve nurses. Many exposures go unreported.

In a case control study among health care workers occupationally exposed to HIV, the CDC (1998b) reported a 79% decrease in the risk for HIV seroconversion for those who took zidovudine (ZDV) after exposure, compared with exposed health care workers who did *not* take ZDV. In 1998 the CDC issued revised guidelines for postexposure prophylaxis (PEP) following HIV exposure, increasing PEP from ZDV alone to ZDV plus lamivudine as the basic regimen and adding a third drug (e.g., nelfinavir) for higher-risk HIV exposures (CDC, 1998b). The revised PEP regimens are expected to further reduce HIV work-related transmission to health care providers.

TUBERCULOSIS

Tuberculosis (TB) continues to be a problem worldwide. Although numbers of cases have decreased in the United States, 44% of 1998 TB cases were linked to foreign-born persons. Incomplete TB treatment in some parts of the world has resulted in increased numbers of TB and drug-resistant TB cases.

In addition to standards protecting workers from bloodborne diseases, OSHA has issued draft regulations that address protection from tuberculosis and drug-resistant strains of tuberculosis. To prevent occupational exposure, agencies will be required to provide employee education, tuberculosis screening at the appropriate frequency, specially designed client isolation rooms, and special respirators (N-95 or HEPA) with fit testing to protect the health care provider.

Complications of Infection

Most complications of infection relate to inadequate treatment. This may range from an incorrect choice of antibiotics to poor

TABLE 26-10 • OCCUPATIONAL SAFETY AND HEALTH ADMINISTRATION BLOODBORNE PATHOGENS STANDARD

- Employers whose workers are at risk of "occupational exposure" must establish a written exposure control plan that is updated annually.
- Employers must implement and enforce procedures to reduce the risk of occupational exposure, including, but not limited to, standard precautions, handwashing, and providing supplies for avoidance of blood or other potentially infectious materials.
- Employers must provide and launder protective garments and other equipment, such as gloves, gowns, masks, eye shields, goggles, and ventilation devices. For those with allergies, special gloves must be provided.
- Employers must provide hepatitis B vaccine to all employees at risk for work exposure at no cost to the employee within 10 days of employment. The employee must sign a refusal statement if vaccine is declined.
- Employers must provide postexposure evaluation for all employees who are exposed to blood or other infectious material.
- Employers must annually train employees about the hazards of blood and other infectious materials and the bloodborne pathogens standard.

Modified from Occupational Safety and Health Administration (OSHA), U.S. Department of Labor (1991). Occupational exposure to bloodborne pathogens: Final rule. *Federal Register,* 29CFR.1910.1030.

compliance. Some infections relapse in a subtle fashion when a client thinks he or she is slowly getting better. Drug regimen noncompliance (e.g., taking medicines when the client feels like it) prevents contact of harmful microorganisms with sufficient concentrations of antibiotics and contributes to resistant organism development. In addition, the cost of care for clients with infections is high (see the Cost of Care box above).

LOCAL COMPLICATIONS

Serious complications of infection may result from incomplete antibiotic therapy. Local infections that could be cured without complications, such as cellulitis and pneumonia, may progress to abscess formation if appropriate drug therapy is not continued. Although adequate antibiotic therapy does not always prevent abscess, early therapy may prevent or limit the size of an abscess.

SYSTEMIC COMPLICATIONS

In addition to abscess formation, inadequate therapy may promote systemic complications. If the infection is not resolved, or if it is treated with drugs that are ineffective for the offending microorganism, the pathogen may enter the bloodstream. Systemic sepsis or septicemia results. Inadequately treated small local infections may also spread to produce significant complications, such as leukocytosis (increased white blood cell count) or leukopenia (decreased white blood cell count) and disseminated intravascular coagulation (DIC). After pathogens invade the bloodstream, no site is protected from invasion.

Sepsis may progress to septic shock. In septic shock, insufficient cardiac output is compounded by hypovolemia; inadequate blood supply to vital organs leads to hypoxia (lack of oxygen) and metabolic failure.

COST OF CARE — IMPLICATIONS FOR NURSING

INFECTIOUS DISEASES IN THE UNITED STATES

Costs of infectious diseases are high. The following are examples of costs for several infectious diseases:

- Additional treatment cost averages $2100 (1992 dollars) for a hospitalized client who acquires an infection. Bloodstream infection causes an average of 7 additional hospital days and $3517 increased cost per infected client.
- The lifetime cost of treating a client with HIV is $96,000 (multidrug therapy not included).
- Recent outbreaks of cryptosporidiosis in several U.S. cities cost an average of $330 per case. Cases that required hospital care cost up to 10 times more.
- Lyme disease diagnosed in the early stages costs about $74 for medical treatment. Resulting complications from delayed treatment cost $2228 to $6724 per patient in the first year.

Modified from Binder, S., & Levitt, A. Centers for Disease Control and Prevention. (1998). *Preventing emerging infectious diseases: A strategy for the 21st century.* Atlanta: Centers for Disease Control and Prevention.

COLLABORATIVE MANAGEMENT

SIMON Activity Link

Assessment

HISTORY

Careful attention to the history of a client with a possible infectious disease helps the nurse determine risk factors for infection. The age of the client, a history of cigarette smoking or alcohol use, current illness or disease (such as diabetes), past and current medication use (such as steroids), familial predisposition, and poor nutritional status may place him or her at increased risk for a number of infectious diseases.

The nurse determines whether the client has been exposed to infectious agents. A history of recent exposure to someone with similar clinical symptoms (does a family member have the same symptoms?) or to contaminated food or water, as well as the time of exposure, assists in identifying a possible source for infection. This information will be helpful for determining the incubation period for the disease and thus for providing a clue to its cause.

Contact with animals, including pets, may facilitate exposure to infection. The nurse asks the client about recent animal contact at home or work, or in leisure activities (e.g., hunting). Insect bites should be documented.

A travel history should be obtained. Travel to areas both within and outside the client's home country may expose a susceptible client to infectious organisms not encountered in the local community.

A thorough sexual history may reveal sexual behavior associated with increased risk of sexually transmitted diseases. The nurse should obtain a history of IV drug use and a transfusion history to assess the client's risk for hepatitis B, hepatitis C, and HIV infections.

Identifying the type and location of symptoms may point to affected organ systems. The onset order of symptoms gives clues to the specific problem.

PHYSICAL ASSESSMENT/CLINICAL MANIFESTATIONS

Disorders caused by pathogens vary, depending on the infection cause and site. Common clinical manifestations are associated with specific sites of infection (see Chart 26-2). The nurse carefully inspects the skin for symptoms of local infection at any site (pain, swelling, heat, redness, and/or pus).

Fever (generally a temperature above 101° F [38° C]), chills, and malaise are primary indicators of a systemic infection. Fever may accompany other, noninfectious disorders, and infection can be present without fever. The older adult, whose normal temperature may be 1° to 2° lower than the normal temperature in younger adults, may manifest fever at 99° F (37° C). The nurse assesses the client for these symptoms and carefully asks about the history and patterns of symptoms.

Lymphadenopathy, photophobia, pharyngitis, and gastrointestinal (GI) disturbance (usually diarrhea or vomiting) are often associated with infection. To detect enlargement, the nurse should palpate the cervical, axillary, and other lymph nodes. The throat is examined for redness.

CONSIDERATIONS FOR OLDER ADULTS

In the older adult a change in mental status may be the first, possibly the only, presenting symptom. The client's baseline mental status should be determined for comparison. The infected older client typically becomes increasingly confused and disoriented (Table 26-11; see also Chart 26-1).

TABLE 26-11 • FACTORS THAT MAY PROMOTE INFECTION IN THE OLDER CLIENT

Factor	Aging-Associated Changes or Conditions
Immune system	Decreased antibody production, lymphocytes, and fever response
Integumentary system	Thinning skin, decreased subcutaneous tissue, decreased vascularity, slower wound healing
Respiratory system	Decreased cough and gag reflexes
Gastrointestinal system	Decreased gastric acid and intestinal motility
Chronic illness	Diabetes mellitus, chronic airflow limitation, neurologic impairments
Functional/cognitive impairments	Immobility, incontinence, dementia
Invasive devices	Urinary catheters, feeding tubes, IV devices, tracheostomies
Institutionalization	Increased person-to-person contact and transmission

PSYCHOSOCIAL ASSESSMENT

The client with an infectious disease often has psychosocial concerns. Delay in diagnosis due to the need to await clinical test results produces anxiety. The nurse should assess the client's level of understanding about various diagnostic procedures and the time required to obtain test results.

Feelings of malaise and fatigue often accompany infection. The client's current level of activity and the impact of these symptoms on family, occupational, and recreational activities should be assessed by the nurse.

The potential spread of infection to others is an additional stress associated with the diagnosis of infection. The client may curtail family and social interactions for fear of spreading the illness. The nurse assesses the client and family's levels of understanding of the infection, the mode of transmission, and mechanisms that may limit or prevent transmission.

Finally, a number of transmissible infectious diseases, especially those associated with socially unacceptable lifestyles (such as IV drug abuse), are associated with some degree of social labeling. The client may feel socially isolated and may experience guilt related to behavior that increases the risk for infection. The nurse observes carefully for signs a client's reaction to social labels and how these feelings further affect socialization.

CRITICAL THINKING CHALLENGE

In admitting a client to your nursing home, you identify a painful vesicular rash on her trunk.

- What other physical assessment should be documented for this client?
- What history needs to be obtained about this client?
- What transmission prevention precautions should be implemented?

For suggested answer guidelines, go to SIMON http://www.wbsaunders.com/SIMON/Iggy/.

LABORATORY ASSESSMENT

The definitive diagnosis of an infectious disease requires identification of a microorganism in the tissues of an infected client. Direct examination of blood, body fluids, and tissues under a microscope in the laboratory may not yield positive identification. However, laboratory assessment usually provides helpful information about microorganisms, such as shape, motility, and reaction to staining agents. Even when direct microscopy does not prove diagnostic, enough information is often gathered for initiating appropriate antibiotic therapy.

CULTURE AND SENSITIVITY. The most definitive procedure for identification of a microorganism is **culture,** or isolation of the pathogen by cultivation in tissue cultures or artificial media. Specimens for culture may be obtained from almost any body fluid or tissue. The health care provider usually decides when and where the specimen for culture is taken.

Proper collection and handling of specimens for culture, following standard precautions, is essential for obtaining accurate results. Specimens collected must be appropriate for the suspected infection. Material must be of adequate quantity, freshly obtained and placed in a sterile container to preserve the specimen and microorganism, and properly labeled.

After isolation of a microorganism in culture, antibiotic sensitivity testing is usually performed to determine the effects of various antibiotics on that particular microorganism. A microorganism that is killed by acceptable levels of an antibiotic is considered sensitive to that drug. An organism that is not killed by tolerable levels of an antibiotic is considered resistant to that drug. Preliminary results are usually available in 24 to 48 hours, but the final results generally take 72 hours. Antibiotic therapy should not begin until the culture specimen is obtained.

COMPLETE BLOOD COUNT. A complete blood count (CBC) is nearly always performed on the client with a suspected infectious disease. Five types of leukocytes (white blood cells) have been identified: neutrophils, lymphocytes, monocytes, eosinophils, and basophils. In most active infections, especially those caused by bacteria, the total leukocyte count is elevated. Various diseases are characterized by changes in the percentages of the different types of leukocytes. The differential count most often shows an increased number of immature neutrophils, or a shift to the left. A few infectious diseases, however, such as malaria and infectious mononucleosis, are associated with neutropenia (decreased neutrophils).

ERYTHROCYTE SEDIMENTATION RATE. The erythrocyte sedimentation rate (ESR) measures the rate at which red blood cells fall through plasma. This rate is most significantly affected by an increased number of acute-phase reactants, which occurs with inflammation. Thus an elevated ESR (>20 mm/hr) indicates inflammation or infection somewhere in the body. Chronic infection, most notably osteomyelitis, and chronic abscesses are commonly associated with an elevated ESR. The ESR is chronically elevated with arthritis, as well. The effectiveness of therapy is often monitored by a fall in this value.

RADIOGRAPHIC ASSESSMENT

X-ray films are often obtained to determine activity or destruction by an infectious microorganism. Radiologic studies (such as chest films, sinus films, joint films, GI studies, and renal films) are typically done for diagnosis of infection in a specific body site.

More sophisticated techniques for infection diagnosis include computed tomography (CT) scans and magnetic resonance imaging (MRI). Tomography is helpful in assessing for abscesses. CT scans help identify suspected osteomyelitis and fluid collections that point to possible infection. MRI scans provide a cross-sectional assessment for infection.

OTHER DIAGNOSTIC ASSESSMENT

Another diagnostic tool for the evaluation of a client with an infectious disease is *ultrasonography.* This noninvasive procedure is particularly helpful in detecting infection involving the heart valves.

Scanning techniques using radioactive substances, such as gallium, can determine the presence of inflammation. Inflammatory tissue is identified by its increased uptake of the injected radioactive material.

Biopsy of the infected site may be needed for tissue culture. Biopsy sites may include the liver, bone marrow, skin, pleura, lymph nodes, kidney, bone, or even the brain. To obtain specimens, invasive procedures (e.g., bronchoscopy or endoscopy) or surgery (e.g., open lung biopsy or laparotomy) may be necessary.

Analysis

COMMON NURSING DIAGNOSES AND COLLABORATIVE PROBLEMS

The following are the most common nursing diagnoses for clients with an infection or infectious disease:

1. Hyperthermia related to an increased metabolic state
2. Social Isolation related to effects of illness

The inclusion of other nursing diagnoses depends on the type and extent of the infection. For example, a client with pneumonia might experience Ineffective Airway Clearance and Fatigue; a client with a sexually transmitted disease may have Altered Sexuality Patterns. Altered Protection (suprainfection) is another potential diagnosis.

CHART 26-4

NIC INTERVENTION ACTIVITIES *for* The Client with Infection

Fever Treatment: *Management of a client with hyperpyrexia caused by nonenvironmental factors*

- Monitor temperature as frequently as is appropriate.
- Monitor blood pressure, pulse, and respiration as appropriate.
- Monitor skin color and temperature.
- Monitor for decreasing levels of consciousness.
- Monitor for intake and output.
- Monitor for seizure activity.
- Monitor WBC, Hgb, and Hct values.
- Administer antipyretic medication, as appropriate.
- Cover the client with a sheet, only as appropriate.
- Administer a tepid sponge bath, as appropriate.
- Encourage increased intake of oral fluids, as appropriate.
- Administer IV fluids, as appropriate.
- Encourage or administer oral hygiene, as appropriate.
- Place client on hypothermia blanket, as appropriate.
- Monitor temperature closely to prevent treatment-induced hypothermia.

NIC intervention activities selected from McCloskey, J.C., & Bulechek, G.M. (Eds.). (2000). *Nursing interventions classification (NIC)* (3rd ed.). St. Louis: Mosby. No part of this work is to be altered without prior written permission from the Publisher.
WBC, White blood cell; *Hgb,* hemoglobin; *Hct,* hematocrit.

ADDITIONAL NURSING DIAGNOSES AND COLLABORATIVE PROBLEMS

The primary collaborative problem is Risk for Sepsis, Septic Shock, and Disseminated Intravascular Coagulation (DIC).

Planning and Implementation

HYPERTHERMIA

NOC **PLANNING: EXPECTED OUTCOMES.** The body temperature of the client with an infection or infectious disease is expected to return to baseline, or within normal limits (WNL).

INTERVENTIONS. The primary concern is to provide measures to eliminate the underlying cause of hyperthermia and to destroy the causative microorganism.

NIC **FEVER TREATMENT.** Interventions to reduce fever may include antipyretic therapy, external cooling, fluid administration, and antimicrobial therapy. The nurse performs a thorough assessment before and after interventions are implemented.

ANTIPYRETIC THERAPY. In collaboration with the health care team, the nurse uses a variety of methods to manage fever (Chart 26-4). One method is the use of antipyretic drugs, such as aspirin (Ancasal♣) and acetaminophen (Tylenol, Ace-Tabs♣), to reduce hyperthermia. However, because antipyretics mask fever, monitoring the course of the disease may be difficult. Therefore unless the client is extremely uncomfortable or if hyperthermia presents a significant risk (e.g., in the client with heart failure, febrile seizures, or head injury), antipyretics are not always ordered.

The nurse must be alert for waves of sweating after each dose. Sweating may be accompanied by a fall in blood pressure followed by return of fever. These unpleasant side effects of antipyretic therapy can often be alleviated by liberal administration of fluids and by regular scheduling of drug administration.

EXTERNAL COOLING. Cooling or hypothermia blankets, or ice bags and packs, are highly effective external mechanisms for reducing fever. For convenience, cooling blankets are used extensively in the hospital setting, yet there are no universal guidelines for their use.

Alternative cooling methods may be used, particularly in settings other than hospitals. The nurse or assistive nursing personnel may sponge the client's body with tepid water or saline solution or apply cool compresses to the skin and pulse points to reduce body temperature. The client is observed for shivering during any form of external cooling. Shivering may indicate that he or she is being cooled too quickly.

FLUID ADMINISTRATION. In clients with fever, fluid volume loss is increased from rapid evaporation of body fluids and increased perspiration. As body temperature increases, fluid volume loss increases. The nurse monitors carefully for signs of dehydration, such as increased thirst, decreased skin turgor, dry mucous membranes, and disorientation, especially in older adults. Increased oral fluid intake and IV fluids are administered as prescribed.

ANTIMICROBIAL THERAPY. The cornerstone of therapy for infectious diseases is antimicrobial drug therapy, also called anti-infective therapy. Antibiotics, antiviral agents, and antifungals are types of antimicrobials. The sulfonamides, the first antibiotic group, were used in the mid-1930s. Shortly thereafter, in the 1940s, penicillin became the primary antibiotic used systemically. Since then, a wide variety of antimicrobial drugs have been developed for treatment, as well as prevention, of infection associated with virtually every class of microorganism. Effective antibiotics are available to treat nearly all bacterial infections, but misuse of antibiotics has contributed to the development of antibiotic-resistant bacteria (see Chart 26-3). A few effective antifungal agents have been developed, but these drugs generally exhibit more toxicity than do antibacterial agents. Effective agents are currently available for the treatment of influenza type A virus infection and HIV, but viruses mutate rapidly; thus these agents have a limited duration of effectiveness.

Effective antimicrobial therapy requires delivery of an appropriate agent, sufficient dosage, proper administration route, and sufficient therapy duration. These four requirements ensure delivery of a concentration of drug sufficient to inhibit or kill infecting microorganisms. Health care providers, often in consultation with a pharmacist, decide about the requirements. Nurses must know drug actions, side effects, and toxic effects and teach them to clients. Antimicrobials act on susceptible pathogens by:

- Inhibiting cell wall synthesis (penicillins and cephalosporins)
- Injuring the cytoplasmic membrane (antifungal agents)
- Inhibiting biosynthesis, or reproduction (erythromycin, tetracycline, and gentamicin)
- Inhibiting nucleic acid synthesis (actinomycin)

The nurse observes and reports side effects and toxic effects, which vary according to the specific classification of the drug. Most antibiotics can cause nausea, vomiting, and rashes, along with a long list of other problems. The nurse ensures that the prescribed drug is not one to which the client is allergic. An accurate allergy history before drug therapy begins is essential (Table 26-12).

TABLE 26-12 • ALLERGIC REACTIONS TO ANTIBIOTIC THERAPY

- Flushing
- Wheezing
- Sneezing
- Pruritus
- Urticaria
- Rashes
- Maculopapular to exfoliative dermatitis
- Vascular eruptions
- Erythema multiforme (Stevens-Johnson syndrome)
- Angioneurotic edema
- Serum sickness (headache, fever, chills, hives, malaise, and conjunctivitis)
- Anaphylaxis (laryngeal edema, bronchospasm, hypotension, vascular collapse, and cardiac arrest)
- Death

SOCIAL ISOLATION

NOC **PLANNING: EXPECTED OUTCOMES.** The client with an infection or infectious disease is expected to be free of feelings of social isolation and interact with others.

INTERVENTIONS. Education is the major intervention for meeting this goal. The nurse develops an educational program to instruct the client and the family about the mode of transmission of infection and mechanisms that prevent spread to others.

The nurse ensures that the client and family understand the disease process and its cause. The mode of transmission of the infecting microorganism, risk for transmission to others, and mechanisms that may prevent transmission are explained. If necessary, the nurse ensures that the client and family can state specific ways in which precautions will be instituted in the home after discharge from the hospital.

Because the client requiring precautions may feel secluded, health care personnel, as well as family members and friends, are encouraged to maintain contact with the client. Personnel caring for the client are reminded as needed that the disease, not the client, requires isolation. Family members and friends are encouraged to visit and to use appropriate infection control when necessary. Communication by telephone is often effective for continuing contact with loved ones. Television and radio help bring the outside world into the life of the client confined to the room.

In the nursing home setting, an outbreak of respiratory or gastrointestinal (GI) infection usually requires limiting visitors, activities, and admissions to the facility. The nurse working in a nursing home needs to be familiar with state regulations regarding handling infections in nursing homes.

Community-Based Care

Clients with infections may be cared for in the home, hospital, nursing home, or an ambulatory setting, depending on the type and severity of the infection. Infections among older adults in nursing homes are very common (see Table 26-11).

HEALTH TEACHING

INFECTION CONTROL. The nurse explains the disease and makes certain that the client understands what is causing the illness. Whether the pathogen causing the infection can be spread to family members, social contacts, or other community contacts is discussed.

If the client has an infectious disease that is potentially transmissible, the nurse teaches the client, family, or home caregivers transmission prevention precautions. General household cleaning measures are often sufficient (e.g., a dishwasher for dishes, and a washer and dryer for laundry). If a dishwasher is not available, dishes can be sanitized with a weak bleach solution (100 parts per million [ppm] available chlorine), attained by adding 1 ounce (30 mL) of bleach to 4 gallons of water. Clothing soiled with blood or other body fluids can be washed with bleach or disinfectant (e.g., Lysol). Recommended cleaning measures should be based on actual available equipment or facilities.

DRUG THERAPY. For the client who is discharged to the home setting to complete a course of antibiotic therapy, the importance of compliance with the planned drug regimen is stressed. The importance of both the timing of doses and the completion of the planned number of days of therapy is explained. The client (and family as appropriate) is also taught how the agents should be taken (e.g., before meals, with meals, and without other agents) and the possible side effects. Side effects include those that are expected (such as gastric distress after oral administration of erythromycin), as well as more severe adverse reactions (such as rash, fever, or other systemic signs and symptoms of an acute adverse drug reaction). Emphasis is placed on teaching about allergic manifestations and the need for notifying the health care provider if adverse reactions occur (see Table 26-12).

In the past, many clients with severe infection were hospitalized for several weeks or more, simply to receive IV antibiotic therapy. Since the implementation of managed care, many clients have been discharged with an IV device in place and continue to receive IV antibiotics at home or in the nursing home. Clients, a family member, or a nurse administers the drugs. When clients are discharged with an indwelling intravascular device in place, the nurse teaches them or their assisting family members how to care for it. They are also instructed to be alert for malfunction of the device, as well as for signs of inflammation resulting from infection at the catheter insertion site (e.g., redness, heat, pain, swelling, and purulent discharge).

PSYCHOSOCIAL SUPPORT

The client with an infection is often anxious and fearful that the infection will be transmitted to family members or friends. These fears are allayed by teaching the client and the family ways of preventing the spread of disease. Careful attention is paid to the client's concerns. The nurse also makes concrete suggestions (e.g., "Your wife can wear gloves when changing your dressing") to address specific concerns.

The client with an infectious disease associated with lifestyle behaviors, such as sexual activity or IV drug abuse, may experience guilt related to the disease. The nurse encourages verbalization of feelings associated with the illness and assists in locating support systems that may help alleviate these problems.

HOME CARE MANAGEMENT

The client with an infectious disease, such as osteomyelitis, who is discharged from the hospital to home may require continued, long-term antibiotic therapy. The nurse emphasizes the importance of a clean home environment, especially for the client who continues to be immunocompromised or who is uniquely susceptible to superinfection (i.e., reinfection or a second infection of the same kind) because of antimicrobial drug therapy. Medications often need to be refrigerated. The nurse ensures that the client has access to proper storage facilities and instructs him or her to check for signs of improper storage, such as discoloration of the medication.

The client is questioned to be sure that handwashing facilities are available in the home and that supplies and instructions are provided as needed.

HEALTH CARE RESOURCES

In unusual instances, a client who has been hospitalized for an infectious disease may not be able to return to the home setting immediately. In such circumstances, temporary placement in a long-term care facility may be advantageous. Care requirements, medication schedules, and personal needs and preferences are carefully noted on transfer documents. When possible, person-to-person communication is done verbally between the two facilities to facilitate a smooth transition from the hospital to the intermediate care setting.

Because of the early discharge trend from hospitals, the client with severe or chronic infections may be discharged to home before completing long-term antibiotic therapy. Implanted ports may be used for convenience and to decrease the chance of infection at the skin site for the client who receives IV therapy at home. The nurse communicates with the outpatient facility to effect a smooth transition from the hospital to the outpatient setting.

Home care services are often used to ensure appropriate administration of antibiotics in the client's home. These services have proved efficient, effective, psychologically supportive, and less expensive than hospitalization or intermediate care facilities. Occasional visits and phone calls from a home care nurse may also facilitate detection of early antimicrobial failures, toxic reactions, or other side effects of therapy.

Evaluation: Outcomes

NOC The nurse evaluates the care of the client with an infection or infectious disease on the basis of the identified nursing diagnoses and collaborative problems. The expected outcomes include that the client:

- Describes and complies with the antimicrobial regimen as ordered
- Maintains baseline body temperature
- Returns to his or her usual level of activity
- Describes and implements precautions to prevent infection transmission
- Exhibits no clinical manifestations of recurrence, relapse, or reinfection
- Interacts with others

CRITICAL ISSUES FOR THE NEXT DECADE

Plans are being made to address certain critical issues internationally, nationally, and locally in some cases. These issues include bioterrorism (Table 26-13), pandemic influenza, gene

TABLE 26-13 • SAMPLE BIOTERRORISM AGENTS AND CLINICAL MANAGEMENT

Pathogen or Agent and Disease Information	Clinical Management*
ANTHRAX (*BACILLUS ANTHRACIS*) **Cutaneous:** 1-7 days after contact, exposed skin itching progressing to papular and vesicular lesions, eschar, edema, ulceration and sloughing. If untreated, may spread to lymph nodes and bloodstream. Fatality 5%-20%. **Inhalation:** 48 hr after organism or spore inhalation, flu-like illness with possible brief improvement. 2-4 days from initial symptoms, abrupt onset of severe cardiopulmonary illness (dyspnea, tachycardia, fever, diaphoresis, thoracic edema, shock, and respiratory failure). If antibiotics delayed until onset of cardiopulmonary symptoms, mortality high. **Other forms:** Gastrointestinal, meningeal, and sepsis.	**For cutaneous and inhaled anthrax:** No person-to-person spread. Contact precautions until decontamination is complete: • Avoid contact with organism while handling contaminated clothes; wear protective attire (gloves, gown, respiratory protection). • Bag client's clothes (do not agitate or shake clothes). • Have client shower and shampoo hair thoroughly with soap and water. • Disinfect contaminated surfaces with sporicidal or bleach solution (1 part household bleach in 9 parts water). Standard precautions for: • Prescribed wound cleansing and management of lesions • Ventilator support for respiratory failure • Postmortem care
BOTULISM (*CLOSTRIDIUM BOTULINUM* AND NEUROTOXIN) Toxin ingestion results in dysphasia, dry mouth, drooping eyelids, and blurred or double vision. Vomiting and constipation or diarrhea may be present initially, extending to symmetric flaccid paralysis in an alert person. Acute bilateral cranial nerve impairment and descending weakness or paralysis follow. Neurologic symptoms after 12-36 hr for foodborne botulism and in 24-72 hr after aerosol exposure. Case fatality up to 10%. Recovery may take months.	Standard precautions—decontamination of client is not required. No person-to-person spread. Consider outbreak with suspicion of a single case. Consult with Centers for Disease Control and Prevention (CDC) and health departments. Advise careful cleanup and disposal of suspected contaminated food source—*after* consultation with health department about any needed laboratory sampling. Interdisciplinary planning for nutrition and rehabilitation support during lengthy neuromuscular and respiratory recovery.
PLAGUE (*YERSINIA PESTIS*) **Lymphatic infection:** 2-8 days after bites from fleas of an infected rodent (rarely after infected tissue or body fluid contact), onset of fever and chills, painful lymphadenopathy (or bubo—usually inquinal, axillary, or cervical lymph nodes), headache, gastrointestinal (GI) symptoms, and rapidly progressive weakness. 50%-60% fatality if untreated. **Pneumonic:** 1-3 days after aerosolized organism inhalation, fever and chills, productive cough, hemoptysis, rapidly progressive weakness, GI symptoms and bronchopneumonia. Survival unlikely if not treated within 18 hr of symptom onset. **Other forms:** Sepsis with coagulopathy, rarely meningitis.	Droplet precautions—required for pneumonic plague (until 72 hr of antibiotic therapy). Contact precautions until decontamination is complete: • For any suspected gross contamination. See documentation information listed under Anthrax—above. Standard precautions: • For prescribed management of bubo(s) if incised to drain. Community and other environmental modifications: • Apply insecticide to infested environment and pets (to kill fleas). • Reduce food and water supply for rodents. • Avoid sick or dead animals.
SMALLPOX (VARIOLA VIRUS) (VARIOLA MAJOR AND MINOR) 10-17 days after droplet or airborne virus inhalation or contact with bleeding lesions, onset of severe myalgias, headache, and high fever. 2-3 days later, a papular rash appears on face and spreads to extremities (and palms and soles). The rash quickly (simultaneously) becomes vesicular, then painful and pustular (contrasted to varicella rash that crops and concentrates more on trunk with various stages of macules to vesicles seen at one time). Clients are infectious at onset of rash until scabs separate (3 weeks). Historically, variola major kills 20%.	Standard, contact, and airborne precautions for clients with vesicular rash pending diagnosis. Same for varicella and variola. • Also, avoid contact with organism while handling contaminated clothes and bedding. Wear protective attire (gloves, gown, and N-95 respirator). One case is a public health emergency—highly communicable. Consult CDC and health departments at earliest suspicion. Vaccine does not give reliable lifelong immunity. Previously vaccinated persons are considered susceptible. *Following exposure*: Initiate airborne precautions and observe for unprotected contacts (from days 10-17). Vaccinate within 2-3 days of exposure.

OTHER KEY POINTS

Other agents besides the above may be used (e.g., salmonella, shigella, tuleremia, brucellosis, and various bacterial toxins).

Assessment: Include account of symptoms, client's incident (what, where, when, how, others exposed or ill, and officials aware).

Treatment: Antibiotic-resistance possible. Vaccine and postexposure prophylaxis are subject to change. If any of the above diseases are suspected, consult infection control practitioner for coordination with community health officials and CDC about current recommendations and specimen collection). *If terrorism suspected*, Federal Bureau of Investigation (FBI) will coordinate evidence collection and delivery.

Multiple exposures planning: Emergency and critical care managers must address availability and acquisition of stocks of medications, vaccines, equipment (e.g., ventilators), and communications with officials, as well as public information needs.

Data from *CDC Emerging Infectious Diseases Journal, 5*(4), July-August 1999, http://www.cdc.gov/ncidod/eid/; and English, J., et al. (1999). *Bioterrorism readiness plan: A template for healthcare facilities* (pp. 11-26). APIC Bioterrorism Task Force and CDC Hospital Infections Program Bioterrorism Working Group (http://www.apic.org/bioterror/).

*See CDC transmission precautions.

therapy, and emerging and re-emerging infectious diseases. Ongoing surveillance; availability, control, and distribution of supplies; communication systems; a network of diagnostic laboratories; and emergency preparedness are all parts of these plans (Kahn et al., 2000). An expanded focus on critical national and international public health infrastructures is needed to respond to these complex infectious disease issues (Osterholm, 2000). More information can be obtained on these subjects from the *Emerging Infectious Diseases Journal* (see http://www.cdc.gov/ncidod/eid/). The impact and costs of bioterrorism and pandemic influenza are predicted as follows (Meltzer, Cox, & Fukuda, 1999; Kaufmann, Meltzer, & Schmid, 1997):

- Bioterrorism
  Projected impact: Depends on the type
  Estimated cost: $4541 to $7582 per day per person for those hospitalized (average 7 to 10 days) and $422 to $1418 per day per nonhospitalized exposed person
- Pandemic influenza
  Projected impact (United States): 20 to 47 million people ill, 314,000 to 734,000 hospitalizations, and 89,000 to 207,000 deaths
  Estimated economic impact (United States): $71.3 to $166.5 billion, excluding disruptions to commerce and society

ONLINE RESOURCES

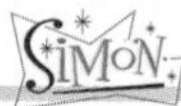

For suggested readings and Internet resources, go to http://www.wbsaunders.com/SIMON/Iggy/.

SELECTED BIBLIOGRAPHY

Asterisk indicates a classic or definitive work on this subject.

Baumann, N.H. (1999). Latex allergy: An orthopaedic case presentation and considerations in patient care. *Orthopaedic Nursing,* 18(3), 15-20.

Beaumont, E. (1997). Technology scorecard: Focus on infection control. *American Journal of Nursing, 97*(12), 51-54.

Binder, S., & Levitt, A. Centers for Disease Control and Prevention. (1998). *Preventing emerging infectious diseases: A strategy for the 21st century.* Atlanta: Centers for Disease Control and Prevention.

Boden, M. (1999). Infection control in moving and handling. *Professional Nurse, 14* (6), 387-389.

*Centers for Disease Control and Prevention. (1994). Guidelines for preventing the transmission of *Mycobacterium tuberculosis* in health-care facilities, 1994. *Morbidity and Mortality Weekly Report, 43*(RR-13), 1-132.

Centers for Disease Control and Prevention. (1998a). Guidelines for infection control in health care personnel, 1998. *American Journal of Infection Control, 26,* 322.

Centers for Disease Control and Prevention. (1998b). Public Health Service guidelines for the management of health-care worker exposure to HIV and recommendations for postexposure prophylaxis. *Morbidity and Mortality Weekly Report, 47*(RR-7), 1-33.

Centers for Disease Control and Prevention. (1999). Summary of notifiable diseases, United States, 1998. *Morbidity and Mortality Weekly Report, 47*(53), ii-92.

Centers for Disease Control and Prevention & Hospital Infection Control Practices Advisory Committee (HICPAC). (1999). Guidelines for prevention of surgical site infection. *Infection Control and Hospital Epidemiology, 20*(4), 254-255, 257.

Centers for Disease Control and Prevention. (2000). Monitoring hospital-acquired infections to promote patient safety, 1990-1999. *Morbidity and Mortality Weekly Report, 49*(8), 149-153.

Centers for Disease Control and Prevention. National Center for Infectious Diseases Hospital Infections Program. (2001). *Hospital infections program download brochure,* p. 1; http://www.cdc.gov/ncidod/publications/brochures/hip.htm.

Chin, J. (Ed.) (2000). *Control of communicable diseases manual* (17th ed., pp. 20-25, 70-75, 381-387, 455-457). Washington, DC: American Public Health Association.

Crabtree, T.D., et al. (1999). Gender-dependent differences in outcome after the treatment of infection in hospitalized patients. *Journal of the American Medical Association, 282*(22), 2143-2148.

English, J., et al. (1999). *Bioterrorism readiness plan: A template for healthcare facilities* (pp. 11-26). APIC Bioterrorism Task Force and CDC Hospital Infections Program Bioterrorism Working Group; download from http://www.apic.org/bioterror/.

Friedman, C., et al. (1999). Requirements for infrastructure and essential activities of infection control and epidemiology in out-of-hospital settings: A Consensus Panel report. *American Journal of Infection Control, 27*(5), 418-430.

Friedman, M.M., & Rhinehart, E. (1999). Putting infection control principles into practice in home care. *Nursing Clinics of North America, 34*(2), 463-482.

*Garner, J.S., & Hospital Infection Control Practices Advisory Committee (HICPAC). (1996). Guidelines for isolation precautions in hospitals. *American Journal of Infection Control, 24,* 24-52.

Gehring, L.L., & Ring, P. (1999). Latex allergy: Creating a safe environment. *MEDSURG Nursing, 8*(6), 358-362.

Henderson, D.A. (1999). Consensus statement of smallpox: Clinical and epidemiologic features. *Emerging Infectious Diseases Journal, 5*(4).

Henderson, D.A., et al. (1999). Smallpox as a biological weapon: Medical and public health management. *Journal of the American Medical Association, 281*(22), 2127-2137.

Herwaldt, L.A., Smith, S.D., & Carter, C.D. (1998). Infection control in the outpatient setting. *Infection Control and Hospital Epidemiology, 19*(1), 41-73.

Jagger, J., et al. (Ed.). (1999). Uniform needlestick and sharp-object injury report: U.S. EPINet Network, 1998, 52 hospitals. *Advances in Exposure Prevention, 4*(5), 54.

Kahn, A.S., et al. (2000). Biological and chemical terrorism: Strategic plan for preparedness and response: Recommendations of the CDC Strategic Planning Workgroup. *Morbidity and Mortality Weekly Report, 49*(RR-4), 1-14.

Kaufmann, A.F., Meltzer, M.I., & Schmid, G.P. (1997). The economic impact of a bioterrorism attack: Are prevention and postattack intervention programs justifiable? *Emerging Infectious Diseases Journal, 3*(2), 4.

Kirkland, K.B., et al. (1999). The impact of surgical site infections in the 1990's: Attributable mortality, excess length of hospitalization, and extra costs. *Infection Control and Hospital Epidemiology, 20*(11), 725-730.

McGuckin, M., et al. (1999). Patient education model for increasing hand washing compliance. *American Journal of Infection Control, 27*(4), 309-314.

Meltzer, M.I., Cox, N.J., & Fukuda, K. (1999). The economic impact of pandemic influenza in the United States: Priorities for intervention. *Emerging Infectious Diseases Journal, 5*(5), 659-670.

National Institute for Occupational Safety and Health. (1998). *NISOH alert: Preventing allergic reactions to natural rubber latex in the workplace* (updated September 1998, pp. 1, 3, 5-7). U.S. Government Printing Office. No. 97-135; http://www.cdc.gov/niosh/latexalt.html.

National Nosocomial Infections Surveillance System. (1999). *NNIS antimicrobial resistance report of selected antimicrobial resistant pathogens associated with nosocomial infections in intensive care unit patients.* Atlanta: Hospital Infection Program, National Center for Infectious Diseases, Centers for Disease Control and Prevention; http://www.cdc.gov/ncidod/hip/surveill/nnis.htm.

National Nosocomial Infections Surveillance System. (2000). *NNIS report, data summary from January 1990-December 1999, issued March 2000.* Atlanta: Hospital Infection Program, National Center for Infectious Diseases, Centers for Disease Control and Prevention.

Olsen, S.J., et al. (2000). Surveillance for foodborne disease outbreaks—United States, 1993-1997. *Morbidity and Mortality Weekly Report, 49*(SS01), 1-62.

Osterholm, M.T. (2000). Emerging infections—Another warning. *New England Journal of Medicine,* 342(17), 1280-1281.

Parini, S. (2000). Combating infection: How to collect specimens. *Nursing2000, 30*(5), 66-67.

Saint, S., & Lipsky, B.A. (1999). Preventing catheter-related bacteriuria. *Archives of Internal Medicine, 159*(8), 800-808.

Sarver-Steffensen, J.A. (1999). When MRSA reaches into long-term care. *RN, 62*(3), 39-41.

Sheff, B. (1998). VRE & MRSA: Putting bad bugs out of business. *Nursing98,* 28(3), 40-44.

Smith, P.W., & Rusnak, P.G. (1997). Infection prevention and control in the long-term-care facility. *American Journal of Infection Control, 25*(6), 488-512.

Steed, C.J. (1999). Common infections in the hospital: The nurse's role in prevention. *Nursing Clinics of North America, 34*(2), 443-461.

Williamson, J. (Ed.). (1999). Summary of APIC bioterrorism readiness plan. *ICP Report,* 4(5), 51-52.

UNIT

6

PROBLEMS OF OXYGENATION

Management of Clients with Problems of the Respiratory Tract

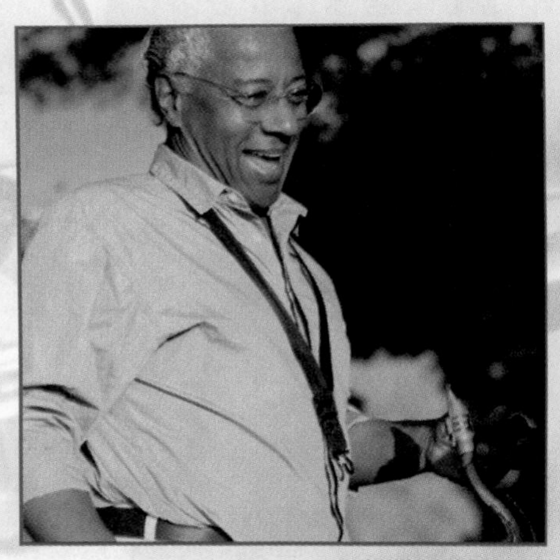

PROBLEMS OF OXYGENATION: RESPIRATORY TRACT ■ Core Concepts Grid

Anatomy	Physiology	Pathophysiology	History	Physical Exam	Diagnostic Tests	Interventions	Pharmacology
• **Upper respiratory tract** • **Lower respiratory tract** • **Alveolar level** • **Thoracic structure**	• **Ventilation** • **Thoracic pressure**	• **Obstruction** • **Inflammation** • **Trauma** • **Hypoxia** • **Infection** • **Fibrosis** • **Tumor** • **Respiratory failure**	• **Risk factors** Smoking Age Occupation Previous health Socioeconomic status • **Cardinal symptoms** Fatigue Cough Sputum Chest pain • **Growth and development**	• **Respiratory rate, rhythm, depth** • **Breath sounds** • **Dyspnea** • **Cyanosis/pallor** • **Restlessness** • **Irritability** • **Confusion** • **Hoarseness** • **Dysrhythmias**	• **Chest x-ray** • **Arterial blood gas (ABG)** • **Pulse oximetry** • **Lung volumes** • **Sputum cultures** • **Acid-fast bacillus** • **Bronchoscopy** • **Thoracentesis** • **Complete blood count** • **$\dot{V}/\dot{Q}$ lung scan**	• **Positioning** • **Oxygen** • **Incentive spirometry** • **Chest physiotherapy** • **Postural drainage** • **Breathing techniques** • **Intubation** Endotracheal Tracheotomy Tracheostomy • **Suction** • **Chest tubes** • **Mechanical ventilation** • **Lung transplantation** • **Health teaching**	• **Antitussives** • **Anti-infectives** Antibiotics Antituberculars • **Bronchodilators** • **Mucolytics** • **Anti-inflammatory drugs** • **Corticosteroids** • **Chemotherapeutic agents** • **Anticoagulants**

CHAPTER 27

Assessment of the Respiratory System

M. LINDA WORKMAN

Learning Objectives

After studying this chapter, you should be able to:

1. Compare and contrast the structures and functions of the upper airways to those of the lower airways.
2. Distinguish between normal and abnormal (adventitious) breath sounds.
3. Describe the respiratory changes associated with aging.
4. Calculate the pack-year smoking history for the client who smokes or who has ever smoked cigarettes.
5. Demonstrate proper technique when using observation and auscultation to assess the respiratory system.
6. Demonstrate proper technique when using palpation and percussion to assess the respiratory system.
7. Interpret arterial blood gas values to assess the client's respiratory status.
8. Prioritize educational needs for the client undergoing pulmonary function tests.
9. Prioritize nursing care needs for the client after bronchoscopy or open lung biopsy.

SIMON

Go to http://www.wbsaunders.com/SIMON/Iggy/ for self-assessment questions related to these Learning Objectives.

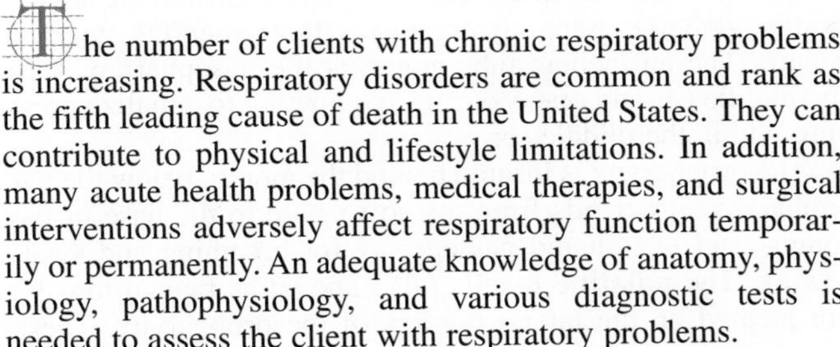

The number of clients with chronic respiratory problems is increasing. Respiratory disorders are common and rank as the fifth leading cause of death in the United States. They can contribute to physical and lifestyle limitations. In addition, many acute health problems, medical therapies, and surgical interventions adversely affect respiratory function temporarily or permanently. An adequate knowledge of anatomy, physiology, pathophysiology, and various diagnostic tests is needed to assess the client with respiratory problems.

ANATOMY AND PHYSIOLOGY REVIEW

The two purposes of the respiratory system are to provide a source of oxygen for tissue metabolism and to remove carbon dioxide, the major waste product of metabolism. The respiratory system also influences the following functions:

- Acid-base balance
- Speech
- Sense of smell
- Fluid balance
- Thermoregulation

Upper Respiratory Tract

The upper airways consist of the nose, the sinuses, the **pharynx** (throat), and the **larynx** ("voice box") (Figure 27-1).

NOSE AND SINUSES

The nose is the organ of smell, with receptors from cranial nerve I (olfactory) located in the upper areas. This organ is a rigid structure that contains two passages separated in the middle by the **septum.** The upper one third of the nose is composed of bone; the lower two thirds is composed of cartilage, which allows limited movement. The septum and interior walls of the nasal cavity are lined with mucous membranes that have a rich blood supply. The **anterior nares** (nostrils or external openings into the nasal cavities) are lined with skin and hair follicles, which help keep foreign particles or organisms from entering the lungs. The posterior nares are openings from the nasal cavity into the nasopharynx.

Three bony projections **(turbinates)** protrude into the nasal cavities from the walls of the internal portion of the nose (see Figure 27-1). Turbinates increase the total surface area for filtering, heating, and humidifying inspired air before it passes into the nasopharynx. Inspired air entering the nose is first filtered by vibrissae in the nares. Particles not filtered out in the nares are trapped in the mucous layer of the turbinates. These particles are moved by cilia (hairlike projections) to the oropharynx, where they are either swallowed or expectorated. Inspired air is humidified by contact with the mucous membrane and is warmed by exposure to heat from the vascular network.

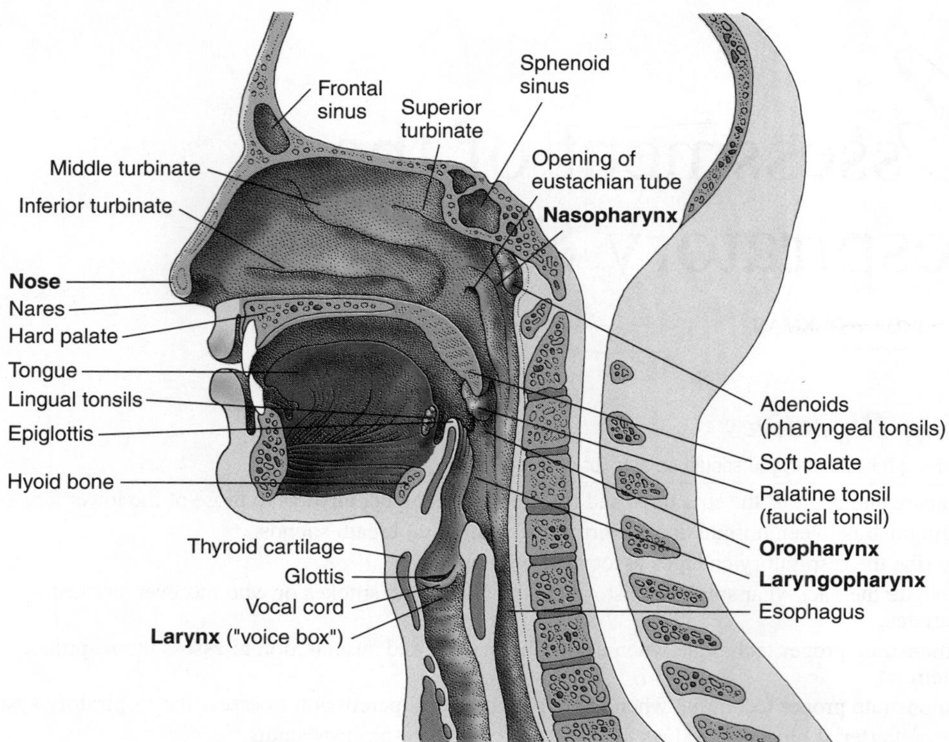

Figure 27-1 ● Structures of the upper respiratory tract.

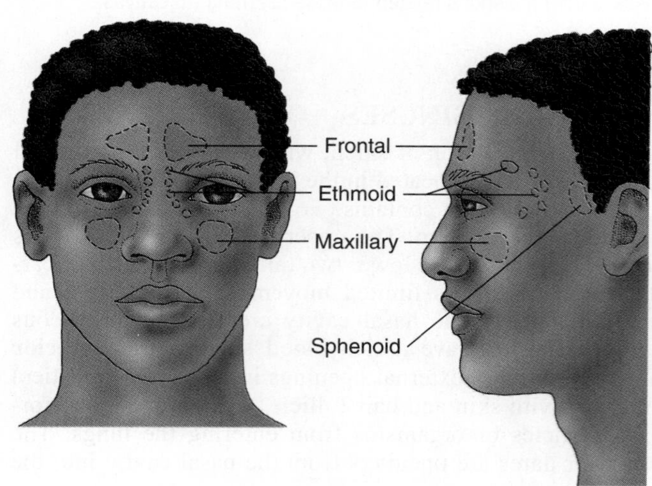

Figure 27-2 ● The paranasal sinuses.

The **paranasal sinuses** are air-filled cavities within the bones that surround the nasal passages (Figure 27-2). Lined with ciliated epithelium, the purposes of the sinuses are to provide resonance during speech and to decrease the weight of the skull.

PHARYNX

The pharynx, or throat, serves as a passageway for both the respiratory and digestive tracts and is located behind the oral and nasal cavities. It is divided into the nasopharynx, the oropharynx, and the laryngopharynx (see Figure 27-1).

The nasopharynx is located behind the nose, above the soft palate. It contains the adenoids and the distal opening of the eustachian tube. The **adenoids** (pharyngeal tonsils) are an important defense, trapping organisms that enter the nose or mouth. The eustachian tube connects the nasopharynx with the middle ear and opens during swallowing to equalize pressure within the middle ear.

The oropharynx is located behind the mouth, below the nasopharynx. It extends from the soft palate to the base of the tongue and is a shared passageway for breathing and swallowing. The **palatine tonsils** (also known as faucial tonsils) are located on the lateral borders of the oropharynx. These tonsils also guard the body against invading organisms.

The laryngopharynx is located behind the larynx and extends from the base of the tongue to the esophagus. The **laryngopharynx** is the critical dividing point where solid foods and fluids are separated from air. At this point, the passageway divides into the larynx and the esophagus.

LARYNX

The larynx is located above the trachea, just below the pharynx at the base of the tongue. It is innervated by the recurrent laryngeal nerves. The larynx is composed of several cartilages (Figure 27-3). The thyroid cartilage is the largest and is commonly referred to as the Adam's apple. The cricoid cartilage, which contains the vocal cords, lies below the thyroid cartilage. The cricothyroid membrane is located below the level of the vocal cords and joins the thyroid and cricoid cartilages. This site is used in an emergency for access to the lower airways. In this procedure, called a **cricothyroidotomy** (or cricothyrotomy), an opening is made between the thyroid and

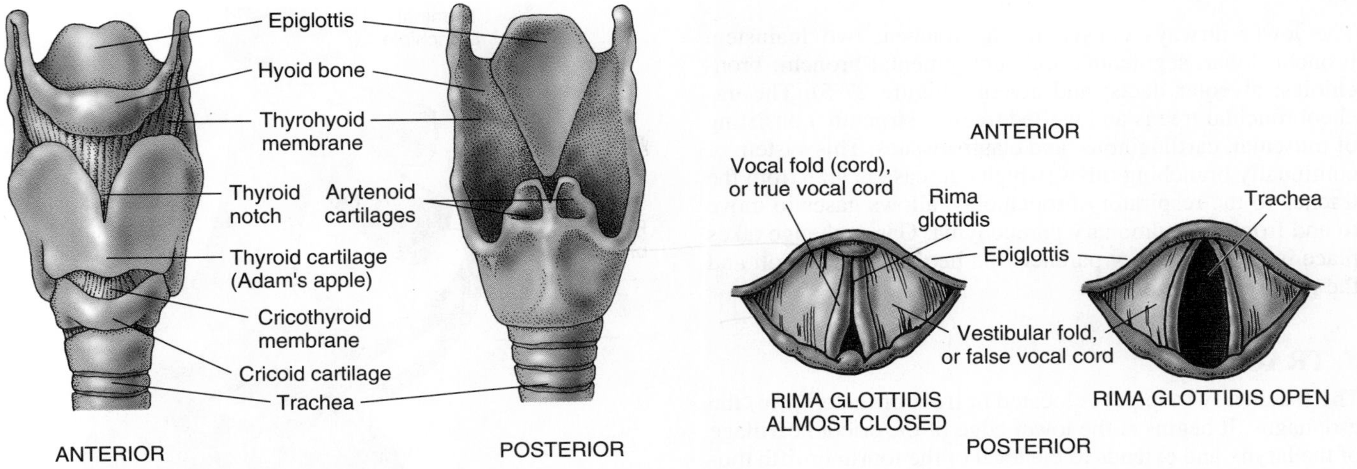

Figure 27-3 ● Structures of the larynx.

Figure 27-4 ● Detail of the glottis (two vocal folds and the intervening space, the rima glottidis).

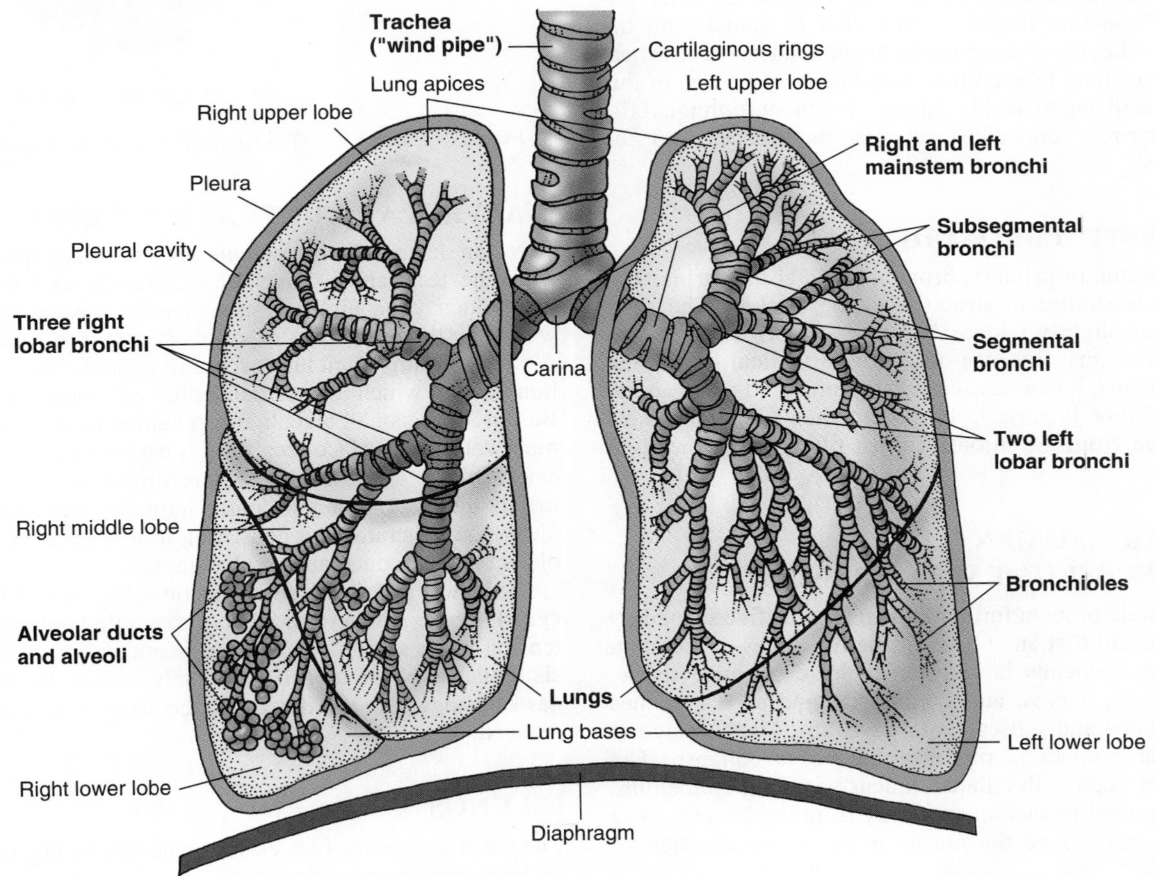

Figure 27-5 ● Structures of the lower respiratory tract (structural size and proportions not drawn to scale).

cricoid cartilage and results in a tracheostomy. The two arytenoid cartilages, which attach at the posterior ends of the vocal cords, are used together with the thyroid cartilage in vocal cord movement.

Inside the larynx are two pairs of vocal cords: the false vocal cords and the true vocal cords. The opening between the true vocal cords is the **glottis** (Figure 27-4). The **epiglottis** is a leaf-shaped, elastic structure that is attached along one edge to the top of the larynx. Its hinge-like action prevents food from entering the tracheobronchial tree **(aspiration)** by closing over the glottis during swallowing. The epiglottis opens during breathing and coughing.

Lower Respiratory Tract

The lower airways consist of the trachea; two mainstem bronchi; lobar, segmental, and subsegmental bronchi; bronchioles; alveolar ducts; and alveoli (Figure 27-5). The tracheobronchial tree is an inverted treelike structure consisting of muscular, cartilaginous, and elastic tissues. This system of continually branching tubes, which decrease in size from the trachea to the respiratory bronchioles, allows gases to move to and from the pulmonary parenchyma. Gas exchange takes place in the pulmonary parenchyma between the alveoli and the pulmonary capillaries.

TRACHEA

The **trachea** (windpipe) is located in front of (anterior to) the esophagus. It begins at the lower edge of the cricoid cartilage of the larynx and extends to the level of the fourth or fifth thoracic vertebra. The trachea branches into the right and left mainstem bronchi at the **carina.**

The trachea is composed of 6 to 10 C-shaped cartilaginous rings. The open portion of the C is the back portion of the trachea and contains smooth muscle that is shared with the esophagus. Low pressure must be maintained in endotracheal and tracheostomy tube cuffs to avoid causing erosion of this posterior wall and to avoid creating a **tracheoesophageal** fistula (abnormal connection between the trachea and the esophagus).

MAINSTEM BRONCHI

The mainstem, or primary, bronchi begin at the carina. The bronchus is similar in structure to the trachea. The right bronchus is slightly wider, shorter, and more vertical than the left bronchus. Because of the more vertical line of the right bronchus, it can be accidentally intubated when an endotracheal tube is passed. Similarly, when a foreign object is aspirated from the throat, it most often enters the right bronchus.

LOBAR, SEGMENTAL, AND SUBSEGMENTAL BRONCHI

The mainstem bronchi further branch into the five secondary (lobar) bronchi that enter each of the five lobes of the lung. Each lobar bronchus is surrounded by connective tissue, blood vessels, nerves, and lymphatics, and each branches into segmental and subsegmental divisions. The cartilage of these lobar bronchi is ringlike and resists collapse. The bronchi are lined with ciliated, mucus-secreting epithelium. The cilia propel mucus up and away from the lower airway to the trachea, where the mucus is either expectorated or swallowed.

BRONCHIOLES

The bronchioles branch from the secondary bronchi and subdivide into smaller and smaller tubes: the terminal and respiratory bronchioles (Figure 27-6). These terminal and respiratory tubes are less than 1 mm in diameter. They have no cartilage and therefore depend entirely on the elastic recoil of the lung to remain open **(patent).** The terminal bronchioles do not participate in gas exchange.

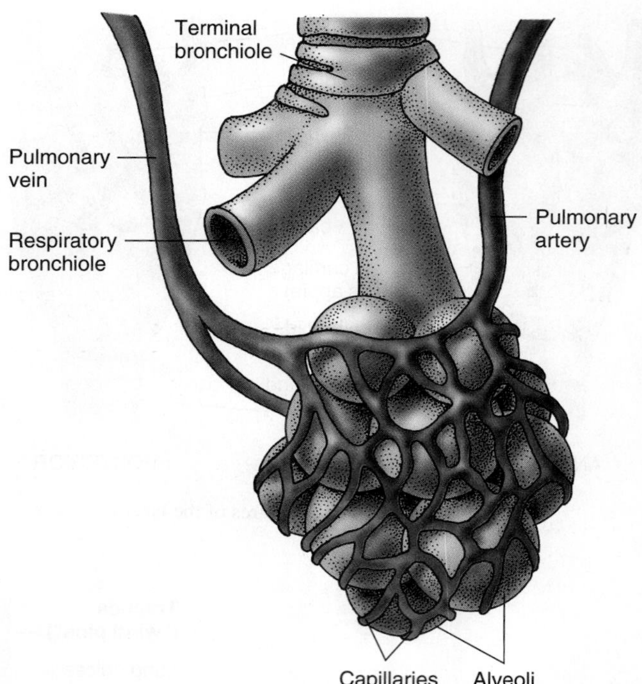

Figure 27-6 ● The terminal bronchioles and the acinus.

ALVEOLAR DUCTS AND ALVEOLI

Alveolar ducts, which resemble a bunch of grapes, branch from the respiratory bronchioles. Alveolar sacs arise from these ducts. The alveolar sacs contain clusters of alveoli, which are the basic units of gas exchange (see Figure 27-6). A pair of healthy adult lungs contains approximately 300 million alveoli, which are surrounded by pulmonary capillaries. Because these small alveoli are so numerous and share common walls, the surface area for gas exchange in the lungs is extensive. In a healthy adult, this surface area is approximately the size of a tennis court. **Acinus** is a term used to indicate the structural unit consisting of a respiratory bronchiole, an alveolar duct, and an alveolar sac.

In the walls of the alveoli, specific cells **(type II pneumocytes)** secrete **surfactant,** a fatty protein that reduces surface tension in the alveoli. Without sufficient surfactant, **atelectasis** (collapse of the alveoli) ultimately occurs. In atelectasis, gas exchange is reduced because the alveolar surface area is reduced.

LUNGS

The lungs are sponge-like, elastic, cone-shaped organs located in the pleural cavity in the thorax. The apex (top) of each lung extends above the clavicle; the base (bottom) of each lung lies just above the **diaphragm** (the major muscle of inspiration). The lungs are composed of millions of alveoli and their related ducts, bronchioles, and bronchi. The right lung, which is larger than the left, is divided into three lobes: upper, middle, and lower. The left lung, which is somewhat narrower than the right lung to make room for the heart, is divided into two lobes.

The hilum is the point at which the primary bronchus, pulmonary blood vessels, nerves, and lymphatics enter each lung. Innervation of the chest wall is via the phrenic (pleura) and intercostal (diaphragm, ribs, and muscles) nerves. Innervation of the bronchi is via the vagus nerve.

The **pleura** is a continuous smooth membrane composed of two surfaces that totally enclose the lung. The **parietal pleura** lines the inside of the thoracic cavity and the upper surface of the diaphragm. The **visceral pleura** covers the lung surfaces, including the major fissures between the lobes. These two surfaces are lubricated by a thin fluid that is produced by the cells lining the pleura. This lubrication allows the surfaces to glide smoothly and painlessly during respirations.

Blood flow through the lungs occurs via two separate systems: bronchial and pulmonary. The bronchial system carries the blood necessary to meet the metabolic demands of the lungs. The bronchial arteries, which arise from the thoracic aorta, are part of the systemic circulation and do not participate in gas exchange.

The pulmonary circulation is composed of a highly vascular capillary network. Oxygen-depleted blood travels from the right ventricle of the heart into the pulmonary artery, which eventually branches into arterioles that form the capillary networks. The capillaries are enmeshed around and through the alveoli, the site of gas exchange (see Figure 27-6). Freshly oxygenated blood travels from the capillaries and through the venules to the pulmonary veins and then to the left atrium. From the left atrium, oxygenated blood flows into the left ventricle, where it is pumped throughout the systemic circulation.

Accessory Muscles of Respiration

Breathing occurs through changes in the size of and pressure within the thoracic cavity. Contraction and relaxation of specific skeletal muscles (and the diaphragm) cause changes in the size and pressure of the thoracic cavity. Accessory muscles of respiration include the scalene muscles, which elevate the first two ribs; the sternocleidomastoid muscles, which raise the sternum; and the trapezius and pectoralis muscles, which fix the shoulders. In addition, various back and abdominal muscles are used when the work of breathing is increased.

Respiratory Changes Associated with Aging

The respiratory changes that occur with aging are described in Chart 27-1 (Ebersole & Hess, 1998). Many changes associated with older clients result from heredity and a lifetime of exposure to environmental stimuli (e.g., cigarette smoke, bacteria, air pollutants, and industrial fumes and irritants). Table 27-1 shows the age-related changes in the partial pressure of arterial oxygen (Pa_{O_2}).

Respiratory disease is a major cause of acute illness and chronic disability in older clients. Although respiratory function normally declines with age, there is usually little difficulty with the demands of ordinary activity. However, the sedentary older adult often reports feeling breathless during exercise.

It is difficult to determine which respiratory changes in older adults are related to normal aging and which changes are pathologic and associated with respiratory disease or exposure to pollutants. In addition, age-related disorders of the neuromuscular and cardiovascular systems may cause abnormal respiration, even if the lungs are normal.

ASSESSMENT TECHNIQUES

History

Obtaining accurate information from the client is important in determining the type and severity of pulmonary problems. Chart 27-2 lists questions to ask clients (based on Gordon's Functional Health Patterns) to determine the impact of pulmonary function.

DEMOGRAPHIC DATA

Age, gender, and race can affect the physical and diagnostic findings related to respiratory function. Many of the diagnostic studies relevant to respiratory disorders (e.g., pulmonary function tests) use these demographic data for determining predicted normal values.

WOMEN'S HEALTH CONSIDERATIONS

Women, especially smokers, have greater bronchial responsiveness (i.e., bronchial hyperreactivity) and larger airways than men. Increased bronchial responsiveness is a risk factor for a more rapid decline in lung function as an older adult, particularly in former and current smokers.

CULTURAL CONSIDERATIONS

The largest chest volumes are found in Caucasians; the smallest volumes are found in Native Americans. The chest volumes of African Americans are significantly larger than those of Asian Americans but not as large as those of Caucasians (Jarvis, 2000). Compared to Caucasians, African Americans and other people with dark skin usually show a lower oxygen saturation (3% to 5% lower) as measured by pulse oximeter; this results from deeper coloration of the nail bed.

PERSONAL AND FAMILY HISTORY

Medical History

The nurse asks clients about their own respiratory history and that of their family members (Table 27-2). The family history is obtained to consider respiratory disorders with a genetic component, such as cystic fibrosis, some lung cancers, and alpha$_1$-antitrypsin deficiency (one risk factor for emphysema). Clients with asthma often have a family history of allergic symptoms and reactive airways. The nurse assesses for a history of infectious disease, such as tuberculosis, and considers that family members may have similar environmental or occupational exposures.

Smoking History

The nurse questions the client about the use of cigarettes, cigars, pipe tobacco, marijuana, and other controlled substances, and he or she notes whether the client has passive exposure to smoke in the home or workplace. If the client smokes, the nurse asks for how long, how many packs a day, and whether the client has quit smoking (and how long ago). The smoking history is documented in **pack-years** (number of packs smoked per day multiplied by number of years). Because the client may have guilt or denial about this habit, the nurse assumes a nonjudgmental attitude during the interview.

CHART 27-1

Nursing Focus *on the* Older Adult
Changes in the Respiratory System Related to Aging

Physiologic Change	Nursing Interventions	Rationale
ALVEOLI		
Alveolar surface area decreases. Diffusion capacity decreases. Elastic recoil decreases. Bronchioles and alveolar ducts dilate. Ability to cough decreases. Airways close early.	Encourage vigorous pulmonary hygiene (i.e., encourage the client to turn, cough, and deep breathe), especially if he or she is confined to bed or has had surgery.	There is increased potential for mechanical or infectious respiratory complications in these situations.
	Encourage upright position.	The upright position minimizes ventilation-perfusion mismatching.
LUNGS		
Residual volume increases. Vital capacity decreases. Efficiency of oxygen and carbon dioxide exchange decreases. Elasticity decreases.	Include inspection, palpation, percussion, and auscultation in lung assessments.	Inspection, palpation, percussion, and auscultation are needed to detect normal age-related changes.
	Help client in actively maintaining health and fitness.	Health and fitness helps to keep losses in respiratory functioning to a minimum.
	Assess the client's respirations for abnormal breathing patterns.	Periodic breathing patterns (e.g., Cheyne-Stokes) can occur.
	Encourage frequent oral hygiene.	Oral hygiene aids in the removal of secretions.
PHARYNX AND LARYNX		
Muscles atrophy. Vocal cords become slack. Laryngeal muscles lose elasticity and cartilage.	Have face-to-face conversations with client when possible.	Client's voice may be soft and difficult to understand.
PULMONARY VASCULATURE		
Increased vascular resistance to blood flow through pulmonary vascular system occurs. Pulmonary capillary blood volume decreases. Risk of hypoxia increases.	Assess the client's level of consciousness.	Client can become confused during acute respiratory conditions.
EXERCISE TOLERANCE		
Body's response to hypoxia and hypercarbia decreases.	Assess for subtle signs and symptoms of hypoxia.	Early assessment helps to prevent complications.
MUSCLE STRENGTH		
Respiratory muscle strength, especially the diaphragm and the intercostals, decreases.	Encourage pulmonary hygiene and help the client in actively maintaining health and fitness.	Regular pulmonary hygiene and overall fitness help maintain maximal functioning of the respiratory system and prevent illness.
SUSCEPTIBILITY TO INFECTION		
Effectiveness of the cilia decreases. Immunoglobulin A decreases. Alveolar macrophages are altered.	Encourage pulmonary hygiene and help the client in actively maintaining health and fitness.	Regular pulmonary hygiene and overall fitness help maintain maximal functioning of the respiratory system and prevent illness.
CHEST WALL		
Anteroposterior diameter increases. Thorax becomes shorter. Progressive kyphoscoliosis occurs. Chest wall compliance (elasticity) decreases. Mobility may decrease. Osteoporosis is possible.	Discuss the normal changes of aging.	Clients may be anxious because they must work harder to breathe.
	Discuss the need for increased rest periods during exercise.	Older clients have less tolerance for exercise.
	Encourage adequate calcium intake (especially during a woman's premenopause phase).	Calcium intake helps prevent osteoporosis by building bone in younger clients.

Smoking induces anatomic changes in the large and peripheral airways, and these changes lead to varying degrees of airway obstruction. Men who continue to smoke experience a more rapid decline in their pulmonary function than do nonsmokers. The pulmonary function of clients who have quit smoking for 2 or more years appears to decline less rapidly than in clients who continue to smoke.

Medication Use

The nurse asks about medications taken for breathing problems and about drugs taken for other conditions. For example, a cough can be a side effect of the angiotensin-converting enzyme (ACE) inhibitors. The nurse determines which over-the-counter medications (e.g., cough syrups, antihistamines, decongestants, inhalants, and nasal sprays) the client is using.

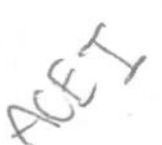

TABLE 27-1 • AGE DISTRIBUTIONS AND PARTIAL PRESSURE OF ARTERIAL OXYGEN (Pa_{O_2}) VALUES (MEAN)

Age (years)	Pa_{O_2}
40-44	95
45-49	88.6
50-54	87.1
55-59	85.1
60-64	84.8
65-69	82.3
70-74	79.1
75-79	82.9
80-84	83.4
85-90	83.2

Modified with permission from Cerveri, I., et al. (1995). Reference values of arterial oxygen tension in the middle-aged and elderly. *American Journal of Respiratory and Critical Care Medicine, 152,* 934-941.

CHART 27-2

Respiratory Assessment Using Gordon's Functional Health Patterns

Health Perception–Health Management Pattern

How has your general health been?
Have you had any colds this past year?
Have you missed work or school because of illness this past year?
Do you use cigarettes? For how many years? How many packs per day?

Activity-Exercise Pattern

Do you feel you have sufficient energy to perform tasks or routines that are required of you?
Do you feel you have sufficient energy to do what you would like to do?
Do you exercise? How often? For how long each time? What type(s) of exercise do you perform?
What activities do you perform in your spare time?
What is your ability to perform the following tasks?

Feeding ______	Grooming ______
Bathing ______	General Mobility ______
Toileting ______	Cooking ______
Bed Mobility ______	Home Maintenance ______
Dressing ______	Shopping ______

Functional Levels Code

Level 0: Full self-care
Level I: Requires use of equipment or device
Level II: Requires assistance or supervision of another person
Level III: Requires assistance or supervision of another person and the use of equipment or devices
Level IV: Is dependent and does not participate

Based on Gordon, M. (2000). *Manual of nursing diagnosis* (9th ed.). St. Louis: Mosby.

The use of home remedies also is assessed. The client is asked about past medication use and the reason for its discontinuation. For example, he or she may have used numerous bronchodilator metered dose inhalers but may prefer one particular drug for relieving breathlessness. In addition, some medications for other conditions can cause permanent changes in pulmonary function. For example, clients may have residual pulmonary fibrosis if they received bleomycin (Blenoxane) as chemotherapy for cancer or amiodarone (Cordarone) for cardiac problems.

TABLE 27-2 • IMPORTANT ASPECTS TO ASSESS IN A RESPIRATORY SYSTEM HISTORY

Smoking history
Childhood illnesses
- Asthma
- Pneumonia
- Communicable diseases
- Hay fever
- Allergies
- Eczema
- Frequent colds
- Croup
- Cystic fibrosis

Adult illnesses
- Pneumonia
- Sinusitis
- Tuberculosis
- HIV and AIDS
- Lung disease such as emphysema and sarcoidosis
- Diabetes
- Hypertension
- Heart disease

Influenza, pneumococcal (Pneumovax) and BCG vaccinations
Surgeries of the upper or lower respiratory system
Injuries to the upper or lower respiratory system
Hospitalizations
Date of last chest x-ray examination, pulmonary function test, tuberculin test, or other diagnostic tests and results
Recent weight loss
Night sweats
Sleep disturbances
Lung disease and condition of family members

BCG, Bacille Calmette-Guérin.

Allergies

Information about allergies is important to the respiratory history. The nurse determines whether the client has any known allergies to environmental substances such as foods, dust, molds, pollen, bee stings, trees, grass, animal dander and saliva, or medications. The client is asked to explain a specific allergic response. For example, does he or she wheeze, have trouble breathing, cough, sneeze, or experience rhinitis after exposure to the allergen? Has he or she ever been treated for an allergic response? If the client has received treatment for allergies, the nurse asks about the circumstances leading up to the need for treatment, the type of treatment, and the response to treatment.

Travel and Area of Residence

Travel and area of residence may be relevant for a history of exposure to certain diseases. For example, *histoplasmosis,* a fungal disease caused by inhalation of contaminated dust, is found in the central United States, the Mississippi and Missouri river valleys, and Central America. *Coccidioidomycosis,* another fungal disease, is found predominantly in the western and southwestern United States, Mexico, and portions of Central America.

DIET HISTORY

An evaluation of the client's diet history may reveal allergic reactions to certain foods or preservatives. Signs and symptoms range from rhinitis, chest tightness, weakness, shortness of breath, urticaria, and severe wheezing to loss of consciousness. The nurse documents in a prominent location of the client's record any known allergies and the specific type of allergic response experienced. The client is asked about his or her usual food intake and whether any symptoms occur with eating. Malnutrition may occur if he or she has difficulty breathing during eating or the food preparation process.

OCCUPATIONAL HISTORY AND SOCIOECONOMIC STATUS

The nurse considers the home, community, and workplace for environmental factors that could cause or contribute to lung disease. Occupational pulmonary diseases include pneumoconiosis, which results from the inhalation of dust (e.g., coal dust, stone dust, silicone dust); toxic lung injury; and hypersensitivity disease (e.g., hypersensitivity to latex). The occupational history includes the exact dates of employment and a brief job description. Exposure to industrial dusts of any type or to the noxious chemicals found in smoke and fumes may cause respiratory disease. Coal miners, stone masons, cotton handlers, welders, potters, plastic and rubber manufacturers, printers, farm workers, and steel foundry workers are among the most susceptible.

The nurse obtains information about the home and living conditions, such as the type of heat used (e.g., gas heater, wood-burning stove, fireplace, and kerosene heater) and exposure to environmental irritants (e.g., noxious fumes, chemicals, animals, birds, and air pollutants). The client is asked about hobbies and leisure activities. Pastimes such as painting, working with ceramics, model airplane building, furniture refinishing, or woodworking may have exposed the client to harmful chemical irritants.

CURRENT HEALTH PROBLEMS

Whether the pulmonary problem is acute or chronic, the chief complaint is likely to include cough, sputum production, chest pain, and shortness of breath at rest or on exertion. During the interview, the nurse explores the history of the present illness, preferably in chronologic order. This analysis of the problem(s) includes the following:

- Onset
- Duration
- Location
- Frequency
- Progressing and radiating patterns
- Quality and number of symptoms
- Aggravating and relieving factors
- Associated signs and symptoms
- Treatments

Cough

Cough is the cardinal sign of respiratory disease. The nurse asks the client how long the cough has persisted (e.g., 1 week, 3 months) and whether it occurs at a specific time of day (e.g., on awakening in the morning, which is common in smokers) or in relation to any physical activity. The nurse determines whether the cough is productive or nonproductive, congested, dry, tickling, or hacking.

Sputum Production

Sputum production is an important symptom associated with coughing. The nurse notes the duration, color, consistency, odor, and amount of sputum. Sputum may be clear, white, tan, gray or, if infection is present, yellow or green.

The nurse describes the consistency of sputum as thin, thick, watery, or frothy. Smokers with chronic bronchitis have mucoid sputum because of chronic stimulation and hypertrophy of the bronchial glands. Voluminous, pink, frothy sputum is characteristic of pulmonary edema. Pneumococcal pneumonia is often associated with rust-colored sputum, and foul-smelling sputum is often found in anaerobic infections such as a lung abscess. Blood in the sputum (hemoptysis) is most commonly noted in clients with chronic bronchitis or bronchogenic carcinoma. Clients with tuberculosis, pulmonary infarction, bronchial adenoma, or lung abscess may expectorate grossly bloody sputum.

Sputum can be quantified by describing its production in terms of measurements such as teaspoon, tablespoon, and cups or fractions of cups. Normally, the tracheobronchial tree can produce up to 3 ounces (90 mL) of sputum per day. The nurse determines whether sputum production is increasing, possibly from external stimuli (e.g., an irritant in the work setting) or an internal cause (e.g., chronic bronchitis or a pulmonary abscess).

Chest Pain

A detailed description of chest pain helps the nurse differentiate pleural, musculoskeletal, cardiac, and gastrointestinal pain. Because the perception of pain is subjective, pain is analyzed in relation to the characteristics described in the history of the present illness. Coughing, deep breathing, or swallowing usually worsens chest wall pain.

Dyspnea

The perception of **dyspnea** (difficulty in breathing or breathlessness) is subjective and varies among clients. A client's perception may not be consistent with the severity of the presenting problem. Therefore the nurse determines the type of onset (slow or abrupt), the duration (number of hours, time of day), relieving factors (changes of position, medication use, activity cessation), and evidence of audible sounds (wheezing, crackles, stridor).

The nurse tries to quantify dyspnea by asking whether this symptom interferes with **activities of daily living (ADLs)** and, if so, how severely. For example, is the client breathless while dressing, showering, shaving, or eating? Does dyspnea on exertion occur after walking one block or climbing one flight of stairs? Table 27-3 classifies dyspnea with changes in ADL performance. A dyspnea assessment scale may be used to assess dyspnea (see Chapter 30).

The nurse asks about **paroxysmal nocturnal dyspnea (PND),** which involves intermittent dyspnea during sleep, and about **orthopnea,** which is demonstrated by a shortness of breath that occurs when lying down but is relieved by sitting up. These two conditions are commonly associated with chronic pulmonary disease and left ventricular failure. In PND, the client has a sudden onset of breathing difficulty that is severe enough to awaken the client from sleep.

TABLE 27-3 • CORRELATION OF DYSPNEA CLASSIFICATION WITH PERFORMANCE OF ACTIVITIES OF DAILY LIVING

Classification	Activities of Daily Living Key
Class I: No significant restrictions in normal activity. Employable. Dyspnea occurs only on more than normal or strenuous exertion.	*4:* No breathlessness, normal.
Class II: Independent in essential ADLs but restricted in some other activities. Dyspneic on climbing stairs or on walking on an incline but not on level walking. Employable for only sedentary job or under special circumstances.	*3:* Satisfactory, mild breathlessness. Complete performance is possible without pause or assistance but not entirely normal.
Class III: Dyspnea commonly occurs during usual activities, such as showering or dressing, but the client can manage without assistance from others. Not dyspneic at rest; can walk for more than a city block at own pace but cannot keep up with others of own age. May stop to catch breath partway up a flight of stairs. Is probably not employable in any occupation.	*2:* Fair, moderate breathlessness. Must stop during activity. Complete performance is possible without assistance, but performance may be too debilitating or time consuming.
Class IV: Dyspnea produces dependence on help in some essential ADLs such as dressing and bathing. Not usually dyspneic at rest. Dyspneic on minimal exertion; must pause on climbing one flight, walking more than 100 yards, or dressing. Often restricted to home if lives alone. Has minimal or no activities outside of home..	*1:* Poor, marked breathlessness. Incomplete performance; assistance is necessary.
Class V: Entirely restricted to home and often limited to bed or chair. Dyspneic at rest. Dependent on help for most needs.	*0:* Performance not indicated or recommended; too difficult.

ADLs, Activities of daily living.

Physical Assessment

ASSESSMENT OF THE NOSE AND SINUSES

The nurse inspects the client's external nose for deformities or tumors and inspects the nostrils for symmetry of size and shape. Nasal flaring may indicate an increased respiratory effort. To observe the interior nose, the nurse asks the client to tilt the head back for a penlight examination. The nurse may use a nasal speculum and nasopharyngeal mirror for a more thorough examination of the nasal cavity.

The nurse inspects for color, swelling, drainage, and bleeding. The mucous membrane of the nose normally appears redder than the oral mucosa, but it may appear pale, engorged, and bluish gray in clients with allergic rhinitis. The nasal septum is checked for evidence of bleeding, perforation, or deviation. Some degree of septal deviation is common in most adults and appears as an S shape, inclining toward one side or the other. A perforated septum is noted if the light shines through the perforation into the opposite nostril; this condition is often found in cocaine users. Nasal polyps, a common cause of obstruction, appear as pale, shiny, gelatinous structures attached to the turbinates.

The nurse occludes one nare at a time to check whether air moves through the nonoccluded side easily. The nose and paranasal sinuses are palpated to detect tenderness or swelling. Only the frontal and maxillary sinuses are readily accessible to clinical examination because the ethmoid and sphenoid sinuses lie deep within the skull (see Figure 27-2). Using the thumbs, the nurse checks for sinus tenderness by pressing upward on the frontal and maxillary areas; both sides are assessed simultaneously. Tenderness in these areas suggests inflammation or acute sinusitis. Tenderness in response to tapping a finger over these areas also indicates inflammation.

Transillumination of the sinuses may be used to detect sinusitis. In a darkened room, the nurse places the bulb of a penlight on the client's cheek (just under the corner of the eye) and observes for light penetration through the roof of the mouth. Normally, a faint glow of light through the bone outlines the sinus. Transillumination is absent or decreased in sinusitis. However, this test is not conclusive for sinusitis.

ASSESSMENT OF THE PHARYNX, TRACHEA, AND LARYNX

Examination of the pharynx begins with inspection of the external structures of the mouth. To examine the structures of the posterior pharynx, the nurse uses a tongue depressor to press down one side of the tongue at a time (to avoid stimulating the gag reflex). As the client says "ah," the nurse notes the rise and fall of the soft palate and uvula and observes for color and symmetry, evidence of discharge (postnasal drainage), edema or ulceration, and tonsillar enlargement or inflammation.

The neck is inspected for symmetry, alignment, masses, swelling, bruises, and the use of accessory neck muscles in breathing. Lymph nodes are palpated for size, shape, mobility, consistency, and tenderness. Tender nodes are usually movable and suggest inflammation. Malignant nodes are often hard and are fixed to the surrounding tissue.

The nurse gently palpates the trachea for deviation, mobility, tenderness, and masses. Firm palpation may elicit coughing or gagging. The space on either side of the trachea should be equal. Many pulmonary disorders cause the trachea to deviate from the midline. Tension pneumothorax, large pleural effusion, mediastinal mass, and neck tumors push the trachea away from the affected area, whereas pneumonectomy, fibrosis, and atelectasis cause a pull toward the affected area. Decreased tracheal mobility may occur with carcinoma or fibrosis of the mediastinum.

The larynx is usually examined by a specialist with a laryngoscope. The nurse may observe an abnormal voice, especially hoarseness, when there are abnormalities of the larynx.

ASSESSMENT OF THE LUNGS AND THORAX

Inspection

Inspection of the chest begins with an assessment of the anterior and posterior thorax. Normal landmarks of the chest and thorax are shown in Figure 27-7. If possible, the client is in a sitting position during the assessment. He or she should be undressed to the waist and draped for privacy and warmth. The chest is observed by comparing one side with the other. The nurse works from the top (apex) and moves downward toward the base while inspecting for discoloration, scars, lesions, masses, and spinal deformities such as kyphosis, scoliosis, and lordosis.

The nurse observes the rate, rhythm, and depth of inspirations as well as the symmetry of chest movement. An impaired movement or unequal expansion may indicate an underlying disease of the lung or the pleura. The nurse observes the type of breathing (e.g., pursed-lip or diaphragmatic breathing) and the use of accessory muscles. In observing respiration, the nurse documents the duration of the inspiratory (I) and expiratory (E) phases. The ratio of these phases (the I/E ratio) is normally 1:2. A prolonged expiratory phase indicates an obstruction of air outflow and is often seen in clients with asthma or chronic obstructive pulmonary disease (COPD).

The nurse examines the shape of the client's chest and compares the anteroposterior (AP) diameter with the lateral diameter. This ratio normally ranges from 1:2 to approximately 5:7, depending on body build. The ratio increases to 1:1 in clients with emphysema, which results in the typical barrel chest appearance.

Normally, the ribs slope downward. However, clients with air trapping in the lungs caused by chronic asthma or emphysema have little or no slope to the ribs (i.e., the ribs are more horizontal).

The nurse also checks for abnormal retractions of the intercostal spaces during inspiration, which indicate airflow obstruction. These retractions may be due to fibrosis of the underlying lung, severe acute asthma, emphysema, or tracheal or laryngeal obstruction.

Palpation

Palpation of the chest occurs after inspection. Palpation allows the nurse to assess respiratory movement symmetry and observable abnormalities, to identify areas of tenderness, and to elicit vocal or tactile **fremitus** (vibration).

The nurse assesses thoracic expansion by placing the thumbs posteriorly on the spine at the level of the ninth ribs and extending the fingers laterally around the rib cage. As the client inhales, both sides of the chest should move upward and outward together in one symmetric movement, and the nurse's thumbs move apart. On exhalation, the thumbs should come back together as they return to the midline. Decreased movement on one side (unilateral or unequal expansion) may be a result of pain, trauma, or **pneumothorax** (air in the pleural cavity). Respiratory lag or slowed movement on one side may indicate the presence of a pulmonary mass, pleural fibrosis, atelectasis, pneumonia, or a lung abscess.

The nurse palpates any abnormalities found on inspection (e.g., masses, lesions, bruises, and swelling). The nurse also palpates for tenderness, particularly if the client has reported pain. **Crepitus** (subcutaneous emphysema) is felt as a crackling sensation beneath the fingertips and should be documented, especially if it occurs around a wound site or if a pneumothorax is suspected. Crepitus indicates that air is trapped within the tissues.

Tactile (vocal) fremitus is a vibration of the chest wall produced when the client speaks. This vibration can be palpated on the chest wall. To elicit tactile fremitus, the nurse

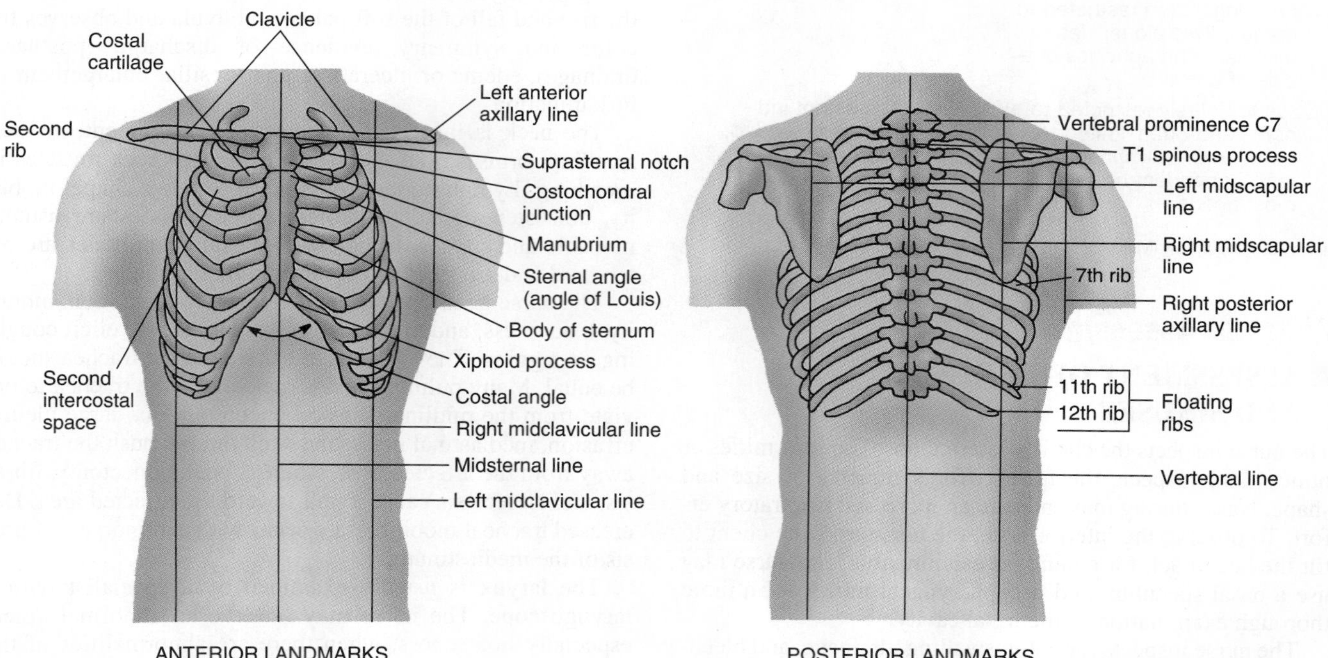

Figure 27-7 ● Anterior and posterior thoracic landmarks.

places the palm or the base of the fingers against the client's chest wall and instructs him or her to say the number *99*. Using the same hand and moving from the apices to the bases, the nurse compares vibrations from one side of the chest with those from the other side. Palpable vibrations are transmitted from the tracheobronchial tree, along the solid surface of chest wall, and to the nurse's hand.

The nurse notes the symmetry of the vibrations and areas of enhanced, diminished, or absent fremitus. Fremitus is decreased if the transmission of sound waves from the larynx to the chest wall is slowed. This situation can occur when the pleural space is filled with air (pneumothorax) or fluid **(pleural effusion)** or when the bronchus is obstructed. Fremitus is increased over large bronchi because of their proximity to the chest wall. Disease processes such as pneumonia and abscesses increase the density of the thorax and enhance transmission of the vibrations.

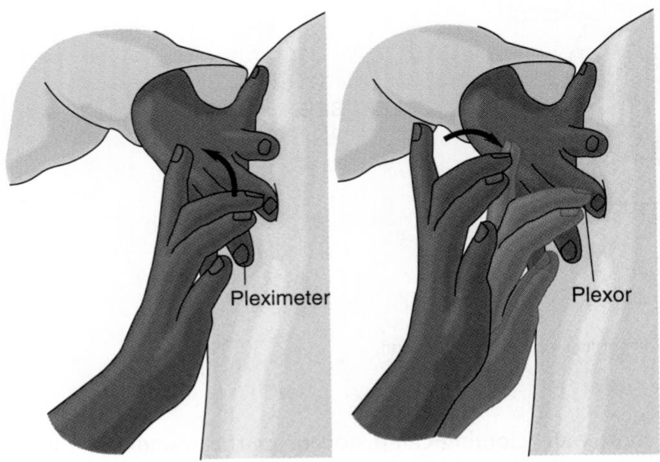

Figure 27-8 ● Percussion technique.

Percussion

The nurse uses percussion to assess for pulmonary resonance, the boundaries of organs, and diaphragmatic excursion. Percussion involves tapping the chest wall, which sets the underlying tissues into motion and produces audible sounds. The nurse places the distal joint of the middle finger of the less dominant hand firmly over the intercostal space to be percussed. No other part of the nurse's hand touches the client's chest wall because doing so absorbs the vibrations. The middle finger of the dominant hand then delivers quick, sharp strikes to the distal joint of the positioned finger (Figure 27-8). The nurse maintains a loose, relaxed wrist while delivering the taps with the tip of the finger, not the finger pad. This technique is repeated two or three times to determine the intensity, pitch, quality, and duration of the sound produced. Long fingernails limit the ability to percuss.

Percussion produces five distinguishable notes (Table 27-4). These sounds assist the nurse in determining the density of the underlying structures (i.e., whether the lung tissue contains air or fluid or is solid). Percussion of the thorax is performed over the intercostal spaces because percussing the sternum, ribs, or scapulae yields sound indicating solid bone. Percussion penetrates only 2 to 3 inches (5 to 7 cm), and therefore deeper lesions are not detected with this technique.

Percussion begins with the client sitting in an upright position. The nurse assesses the posterior thorax first and proceeds systematically, beginning at the apex and working toward the base. The apex of the lung extends anteriorly approximately ¾ to 1½ inches (2 to 4 cm) above the clavicle. Posteriorly, there is approximately a 2-inch (5-cm) width of lung tissue at the apex.

TABLE 27-4 • CHARACTERISTIC FEATURES OF THE FIVE PERCUSSION NOTES

Note	Pitch	Intensity	Quality	Duration	Findings
Resonance	Low	Moderate to loud	Hollow	Long	Resonance is characteristic of normal lung tissue.
Hyperresonance	Higher than resonance	Very loud	Booming	Longer than resonance	Hyperresonance indicates the presence of trapped air, so it is commonly heard over an emphysematous or asthmatic lung and occasionally over a pneumothorax.
Flatness	High	Soft	Extreme dullness	Short	An example location is the sternum. Flatness percussed over the lung fields may indicate a massive pleural effusion.
Dullness	Medium	Medium	Thudlike	Medium	An example location is over the liver and the kidneys. Dullness can be percussed over an atelectatic lung or a consolidated lung.
Tympany	High	Loud	Musical, drumlike	Short	Examples are the cheek filled with air and the abdomen distended with air. Over the lung, a tympanic note usually indicates a large pneumothorax.

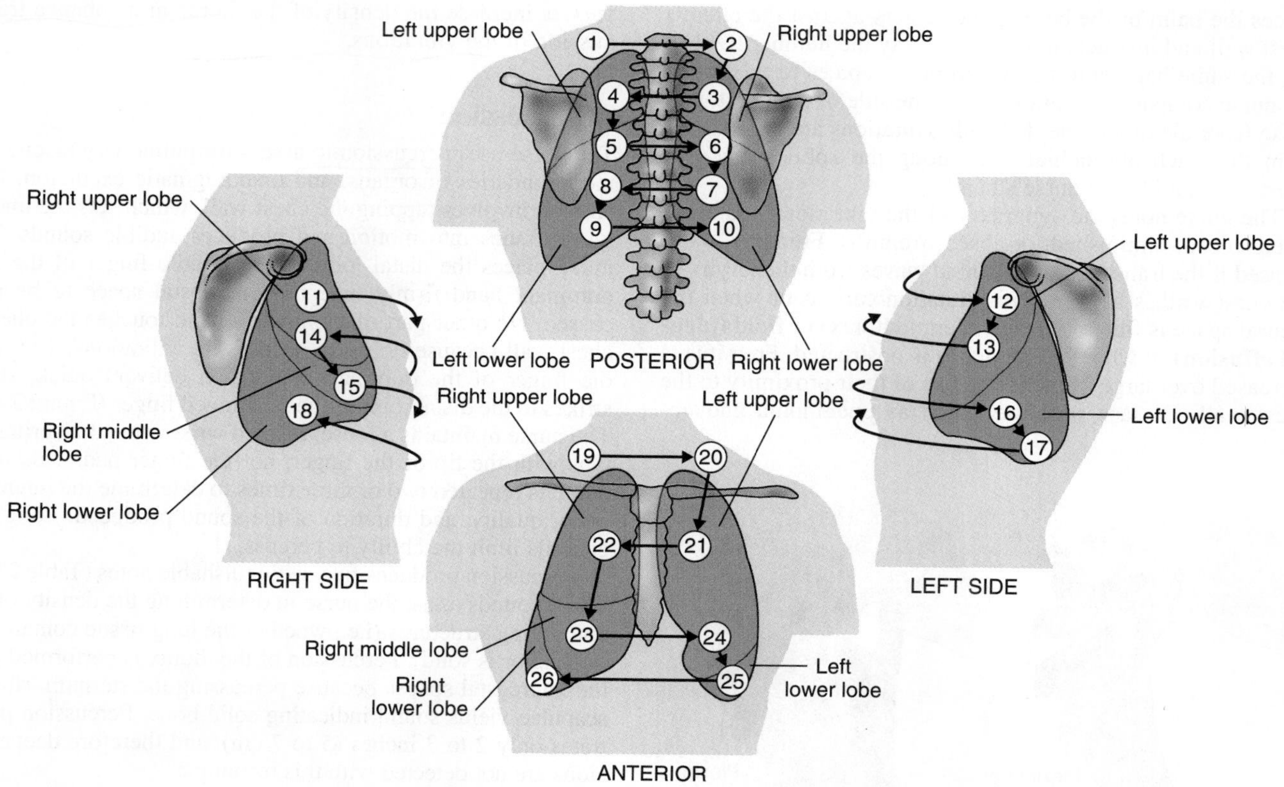

Figure 27-9 ● Sequence for percussion and auscultation.

The nurse assesses diaphragmatic excursion by instructing the client to "take a deep breath and hold it" while percussing downward until dullness is noted at the lower border of the lung. Normal resonance of the lung stops at the diaphragm, where the sound becomes dull; this site is marked. The nurse repeats the process after instructing the client to "let out all your breath and hold." The difference between the two markings or sounds is the diaphragmatic excursion, which may range from 1 to 2 inches (3 to 5 cm). The diaphragm is normally higher on the right because of the location of the liver. Diaphragmatic excursion may be decreased or absent in clients with pleurisy, diaphragm paralysis, or emphysema.

The nurse continues to assess the thorax with percussion of the anterior and lateral chest. The percussion note changes from resonance of the normal lung to dullness at the borders of the heart and liver. The presence of fluid or solid material is indicated by a dull percussion note over lung tissue (as occurs with pneumonia, pleural effusion, fibrosis, atelectasis, and tumors).

Auscultation

Auscultation includes listening for normal breath sounds, adventitious sounds, and voice sounds. Auscultation provides information about the flow of air through the tracheobronchial tree and helps the listener to identify fluid, mucus, or obstruction in the respiratory system. The diaphragm of the stethoscope is designed to detect high-pitched sounds.

Auscultation begins with the client sitting in an upright position. With the stethoscope pressed firmly against the client's chest wall (clothing can distort or muffle sounds), the nurse instructs him or her to breathe slowly and deeply through an open mouth. (Breathing through the nose would set up turbulent sounds that are transmitted to the lungs.) A systematic approach is used, beginning at the apices and moving down through the intercostal spaces to the bases (Figure 27-9). Listening over bony structures is avoided while auscultating the thorax posteriorly, laterally, and anteriorly. The nurse listens to a full respiratory cycle, noting the quality and intensity of the breath sounds. The client is observed for signs of lightheadedness or dizziness caused by hyperventilation during auscultation. If these symptoms occur, the client is told to breathe normally for a few minutes.

NORMAL BREATH SOUNDS

Normal breath sounds are produced as air vibrates while passing through the respiratory passages from the larynx to the alveoli. Breath sounds are identified by their location, intensity, pitch, and duration within the respiratory cycle (e.g., early or late inspiration and expiration). Normal breath sounds are known as **bronchial** or tubular (harsh hollow sounds heard over the trachea and mainstem bronchi), **bronchovesicular** (heard over the branching bronchi), and **vesicular** (a soft rustling sound heard in the periphery over small bronchioles) (Table 27-5). The nurse describes these sounds as normal, increased, decreased (diminished), or absent.

When bronchial breath sounds are heard peripherally, they are abnormal. This increased sound occurs when centrally

TABLE 27-5 • CHARACTERISTICS OF NORMAL BREATH SOUNDS

	Pitch	Amplitude	Duration	Quality	Normal Location
Bronchial (tubular, tracheal)	High	Loud	Inspiration < Expiration	Harsh, hollow, tubular, blowing	Trachea and larynx
Bronchovesicular	Moderate	Moderate	Inspiration = Expiration	Mixed	Over major bronchi where fewer alveoli are located: posterior, between scapulae (especially on right); anterior, around upper sternum in first and second intercostal spaces
Vesicular	Low	Soft	Inspiration > Expiration	Rustling, like the sound of the wind in the trees	Over peripheral lung fields where air flows through smaller bronchioles and alveoli

From Jarvis, C. (2000). *Physical examination and health assessment* (3rd ed.). Philadelphia: W.B. Saunders. Used with permission.

TABLE 27-6 • CHARACTERISTIC FEATURES OF ADVENTITIOUS BREATH SOUNDS

Adventitious Sound	Occurrence in the Respiratory Cycle	Character	Association
DISCONTINUOUS			
Fine crackles Fine rales High-pitched rales	Either early or late inspiration	Popping, discontinuous sounds caused by air moving into previously deflated airways; sounds like hair being rolled between fingers near the ear "Velcro" sounds late in inspiration usually associated with restrictive disorders	Asbestosis Atelectasis Interstitial fibrosis Bronchitis Pneumonia Chronic pulmonary diseases
Coarse crackles Low-pitched crackles	More common on expiration but may be present early in inspiration	Lower pitched, coarse, discontinuous rattling sounds caused by fluid or secretions in large airways; likely to change with coughing or suctioning	Bronchitis Pneumonia Tumors Pulmonary edema
CONTINUOUS			
Wheeze	Audible during either inspiration, expiration, or both	Squeaky, musical, continuous sounds associated with air rushing through narrowed airways; may be heard without a stethoscope Arise from the small airways Usually do not clear with coughing	Inflammation Bronchospasm Edema Secretions Pulmonary vessel engorgement (as in cardiac "asthma")
Rhonchus (rhonchi)	Audible during both inspiration and expiration, but commonly more prominent on expiration	Lower-pitched, coarse, continuous snoring sounds Arise from the large airways	Thick, tenacious secretions Sputum production Obstruction by foreign body Tumors
PLEURAL FRICTION RUB	Heard during both inspiration and expiration, generally at the end of inspiration and the beginning of expiration	Loud, rough, grating, scratching sounds caused by the inflamed surfaces of the pleura rubbing together; often associated with pain on deep inspirations Heard in lateral lung fields	Pleurisy Tuberculosis Pulmonary infarction Pneumonia Lung cancer

generated bronchial sounds are transmitted to an area of increased density, such as in clients with atelectasis, tumor, or pneumonia. When audible in an abnormal location, bronchovesicular breath sounds may indicate normal aging or an abnormality such as pulmonary consolidation and chronic airway disease.

ADVENTITIOUS BREATH SOUNDS

Adventitious sounds are additional breath sounds superimposed on normal sounds, and they indicate pathologic changes in the tracheobronchial tree. Table 27-6 classifies and describes adventitious sounds: crackle, wheeze, rhonchus, and pleural friction rub. Adventitious sounds vary in pitch, intensity, duration, and the phase of the respiratory cycle in which they occur. The nurse documents exactly what is heard on auscultation.

VOICE SOUNDS

If the nurse discovers abnormalities during the physical assessment of the lungs and thorax, the client is assessed for vocal resonance. Auscultation of voice sounds through the normally air-filled lung produces a muffled, unclear sound because sound vibrations travel poorly through air. Vocal resonance is increased when the sound must travel through a solid or liquid medium, as it does in clients with a consolidated area of the lung, pneumonia, atelectasis, pleural effusion, tumor, or abscess.

BRONCHOPHONY. Bronchophony is the abnormally loud and clear transmission of voice sounds through an area of increased density. For assessment of bronchophony, the client repeats the number *99* while the nurse systematically auscultates the thorax.

WHISPERED PECTORILOQUY. Whispered pectoriloquy is the enhanced voice heard through the chest wall. It is much more sensitive than bronchophony and is perceived by having the client whisper the number sequence *one, two, three.* Whispered words normally sound faint and indistinct. If they are heard loudly and distinctly, the nurse suspects consolidation of lung tissue.

EGOPHONY. Egophony is another form of abnormally enhanced vocal resonance and has a high-pitched, bleating, nasal quality. The nurse auscultates the thorax while the client repeats the letter *E.* Egophony exists when this letter is heard as a flat, nasal sound of *A* through the stethoscope. This abnormal sound indicates an area of consolidation, pleural effusion, or abscess.

OTHER INDICATORS OF RESPIRATORY ADEQUACY

The nurse evaluates additional indicators of respiratory adequacy because gas exchange affects all body systems. Some indicators (e.g., cyanosis) indicate immediate oxygenation problems. Other changes (e.g., clubbing, weight loss, unevenly developed muscles) reflect a more long-standing oxygenation problem.

Skin and Mucous Membranes

The skin and mucous membranes are assessed for the presence of pallor or cyanosis, which could indicate inadequate ventilation. Areas to assess include the nail beds and the mucous membranes of the oral cavity. The fingers are examined for clubbing (see Figure 30-8), which would indicate hypoxia of long duration.

General Appearance

The nurse observes the client for muscle development and general body build. Long-term respiratory problems are often associated with an inability to maintain body weight and a loss of general muscle mass. Arms and legs may appear thin or poorly muscled. The muscles of the neck and chest may be hypertrophied, especially in the client with chronic obstructive pulmonary disease (COPD).

Endurance

The nurse observes how easily the client moves and whether he or she is short of breath while resting or becomes short of breath when walking 10 to 20 steps. As the client speaks, the nurse observes how often he or she pauses for breath between words.

Psychosocial Assessment

The nurse assesses aspects of the client's lifestyle that may significantly affect respiratory function. Some respiratory conditions may be worsened by stress. The nurse asks about present life stresses and usual coping mechanisms.

Chronic respiratory illnesses may cause changes in family roles and relationships, social isolation, financial problems, and unemployment or disability. By discussing coping mechanisms, the nurse assesses the client's reaction to these psychosocial stressors and discovers strengths and ineffective behaviors. For example, the client may react to stress with dependence on family members, withdrawal, or noncompliance with interventions. After completing the psychosocial assessment, the nurse assists the client in determining the support systems available to help cope with respiratory impairment.

CRITICAL THINKING CHALLENGE

The client is a 38-year-old male bank employee who says that he is a little short of breath and has noticed a reduced level of energy and endurance over the past year. He is quite anxious because his mother died of emphysema at age 62. He tells you that he smoked for 10 years when he was in college and first working but has been a nonsmoker for the last 11 years.

- What specific family information should you obtain?
- Is the client's occupational or socioeconomic status relevant to this problem? Why or why not?
- What other assessment questions should you ask?

For suggested answer guidelines, go to SIMON http://www.wbsaunders.com/SIMON/Iggy/.

Diagnostic Assessment

LABORATORY TESTS

Blood Tests

Several laboratory tests (Chart 27-3) are relevant to the care of clients with respiratory disorders. A red blood cell count provides data regarding the transport of oxygen from the lungs. A hemoglobin deficiency directly affects tissue oxygenation because hemoglobin transports oxygen to the cells and could cause hypoxemia.

Arterial blood gas (ABG) analysis assesses oxygenation (partial pressure of arterial oxygen [Pa_{O_2}]), alveolar ventilation (partial pressure of arterial carbon dioxide [Pa_{CO_2}]), and acid-base balance. Blood gas studies provide valuable information for monitoring treatment results, adjusting oxygen therapy, and evaluating the client's responses to treatment and therapy, such as during weaning from mechanical ventilation.

CHART 27-3

LABORATORY PROFILE

Respiratory Assessment

Test	Normal Range for Adults	Significance of Abnormal Findings
BLOOD STUDIES		
Complete Blood Count		
Red blood cells	*Females:* 18-44 yr: 3.8-5.1 million/mm^3 45-64 yr: 3.8-5.3 million/mm^3 65-74 yr: 3.8-5.2 million/mm^3 *Males:* 18-44 yr: 4.3-5.7 million/mm^3 45-64 yr: 4.2-5.6 million/mm^3 65-74 yr: 3.8-5.8 million/mm^3	*Elevated levels* (polycythemia) may be due to the excessive production of erythropoietin, which occurs in response to a hypoxic stimulus, as in COPD, and from living at a high altitude. *Decreased levels* indicate possible anemia, hemorrhage, or hemolysis.
Hemoglobin, total	*Females:* 18-44 yr: 11.7-15.5 g/dL, or 117-155 g/L 45-64 yr: 11.7-16 g/dL, or 117-160 g/L 65-74 yr: 11.7-16.1 g/dL, or 117-161 g/L *Males:* 18-44 yr: 13.2-17.3 g/dL, or 132-173 g/L 45-64 yr: 13.1-17.2 g/dL, or 131-172 g/L	Same as for red blood cells.
Hematocrit	*Females:* 18-44 yr: 35%-45% 45-74 yr: 35%-47% *Males:* 18-44 yr: 39%-49% 45-64 yr: 39%-50% 65-74 yr: 37%-51%	Same as for red blood cells.
White blood cell count (leukocyte count, WBC count)	Total: 4.5-11.0 × 10^3 cells/μL, or 7.4 IRU African Americans: 3.6-10.2 × 10^3 cells/μL	*Elevations* indicate possible acute infections or inflammations, pneumonia, meningitis, tonsillitis, or emphysema. *Decreased levels* may indicate an overwhelming infection, an autoimmune disorder, or immunosuppressant therapy.
Differential White Blood Cell (Leukocyte) Count		
Neutrophils	1.8-7.7 × 10^3 cells/μL; 18%-77% of total African Americans: slightly lower	*Elevations* indicate possible acute bacterial infection (pneumonia), COPD, or inflammatory conditions (smoking). *Decreased levels* indicate possible viral disease (influenza).
Eosinophils	0-0.7 × 10^3 cells/μL; 0%-7% of total	*Elevations* indicate possible COPD, asthma, or allergies. *Decreased levels* indicate pyogenic infections.
Basophils	0-0.15 × 10^3 cells/μL; 0%-1.5% of total	*Elevations* indicate possible inflammation; seen in chronic sinusitis, hypersensitivity reactions. *Decreased levels* may be seen in an acute infection.
Lymphocytes	1.5-4.0 × 10^3 cells/μL; 15%-40% of total	*Elevations* indicate possible viral infection, pertussis, and infectious mononucleosis. *Decreased levels* may be seen during corticosteroid therapy.
Monocytes	0-0.8 × 10^3 cells/μL; 0%-8% of total	*Elevations:* see Lymphocytes; also may indicate active tuberculosis. *Decreased levels:* see Lymphocytes.
Arterial Blood Gases		
Pao_2	83-100 mm Hg *Older adults:* values may be lower	*Elevations* indicate possible excessive oxygen administration. *Decreased levels* indicate possible COPD, asthma, chronic bronchitis, cancer of the bronchi and lungs, cystic fibrosis, respiratory distress syndrome, anemias, atelectasis, or any other cause of hypoxia.

COPD, Chronic obstructive pulmonary disease; *IRU,* international recommended unit; Pao_2, partial pressure of arterial oxygen; $Paco_2$, partial pressure of arterial carbon dioxide; HCO_3^-, bicarbonate ion; Sao_2, arterial oxygen saturation.

Continued

CHART 27-3

LABORATORY PROFILE
Respiratory Assessment—cont'd

Test	Normal Range for Adults	Significance of Abnormal Findings
Arterial Blood Gases—cont'd		
$Paco_2$	*Females:* 32-45 mm Hg *Males:* 35-48 mm Hg	*Elevations* indicate possible COPD, asthma, pneumonia, anesthesia effects, or use of opioids (respiratory acidosis). *Decreased levels* indicate hyperventilation/respiratory alkalosis.
pH	Up to 60 yr: 7.35-7.45 60-90 yr: 7.31-7.42 >90 yr: 7.26-7.43	*Elevations* indicate metabolic or respiratory alkalosis. *Decreased levels* indicate metabolic or respiratory acidosis.
HCO_3^-	22-26 mEq/L	*Elevations* indicate possible respiratory acidosis as compensation for a primary metabolic alkalosis. *Decreased levels* indicate possible respiratory alkalosis as compensation for a primary metabolic acidosis.
Sao_2	94%-98% *Older adults:* values may be slightly lower	*Decreased levels* indicate possible impaired ability of hemoglobin to release oxygen to tissues.
SPUTUM STUDIES		
Gram stain	Negative	Presence of gram-positive or gram-negative bacteria indicates the type of microorganism causing the respiratory infection.
Culture and sensitivity	Negative	Presence of microorganisms indicates possible respiratory infections (e.g., pneumonia or bronchitis).
Acid-fast stain	No acid-fast bacilli	Presence of bacilli indicates possible tuberculosis.
Cytologic tests	Negative	Presence of abnormal cells indicates possible malignancy.

COPD, Chronic obstructive pulmonary disease; *IRU,* international recommended unit; *Pao_2,* partial pressure of arterial oxygen; *$Paco_2$,* partial pressure of arterial carbon dioxide; *HCO_3^-,* bicarbonate ion; *Sao_2,* arterial oxygen saturation.

Sputum Tests

Sputum specimens obtained by expectoration or tracheal suctioning assist in the identification of pathogenic organisms or abnormal cells, such as in a malignancy or a hypersensitivity state. Sputum culture and sensitivity analyses identify bacterial infection with either gram-negative or gram-positive organisms and determine the vulnerability to specific antibiotics. Cytologic examination is performed on sputum to help diagnose malignant lesions by identifying cancer cells. Benign conditions, such as a hypersensitivity state, may also be identified by cytologic testing. Eosinophils and Curschmann's spirals (a mucous form) are often found by cytologic study in clients with allergic asthma.

RADIOGRAPHIC EXAMINATIONS

Standard Radiography

Chest x-ray examinations are performed for clients with respiratory tract disorders to evaluate the present status of the chest and to provide a baseline for comparison with future changes. Standard chest x-ray examinations are performed from **posteroanterior** (PA; back to front) and left lateral (LL) projections. Portable chest x-ray studies (taken anteroposterior [AP], front to back) cost more, and the films produced are of lower quality and are more difficult for the radiologist to interpret.

Chest x-ray studies can be used to assess pathologic changes in the lung, such as with pneumonia, atelectasis, pneumothorax, and tumor. Chest x-ray studies can also be used to detect the presence of pleural fluid and the position and placement of an endotracheal tube or other invasive catheters. However, these films have limitations and may appear normal, even in a severe form of certain diseases such as chronic bronchitis, asthma, and emphysema.

Sinus and facial x-ray studies are used to assess fluid levels in the sinus cavities to assist in the diagnosis of acute or chronic sinusitis.

Digital Chest Radiography

By using a computer, bone images can be eliminated from the chest x-ray film, thereby creating better views of nonbone images. This type of test is useful in detecting lung lesions.

Tomography

Tomography is valuable in assessing clients with respiratory disorders because pulmonary soft tissue densities, tumors, and lesions can be seen. **Positron emission tomography (PET)** is useful for studying ventilation-perfusion ($\dot{V}/\dot{Q}$) relationships in the lung. Computed tomography (CT) provides consecutive, 10-mm cross-sectional views of the thorax and produces a three-dimensional assessment of the lungs and thorax.

Fat, cystic, and solid tissue can be distinguished with CT. By adding an intravenously injected contrast agent, vessels and other soft tissue structures can be identified. CT is especially valuable in studying the mediastinum, hilar region, and pleural space. The newer high-resolution CT (HRCT) uses 1.5- to 2-mm "slices" to assist in assessing bronchial abnormalities, interstitial disease, and emphysema. Nursing interventions for the client undergoing CT include education about the procedure and determination of the client's sensitivity to the contrast medium (very important for anaphylaxis prevention).

Ventilation and Perfusion Scanning

A ventilation and perfusion scan ($\dot{V}/\dot{Q}$ scan) identifies the areas of the lung being ventilated and the distribution of pulmonary blood. It is used primarily to support or rule out a diagnosis of pulmonary embolism.

To perform the study, the physician first injects a radionuclide with the client in a supine position and then takes six perfusion views: anterior, posterior, right and left lateral, and two obliques. If the perfusion scan is normal, there is no reason to continue with the ventilation scan. Otherwise, the client inhales a radioactive gas or radioaerosol, and the lung is scanned continuously—as the gas makes its way into the lungs (the "wash-in" phase), once the gas has reached equilibrium within the lungs, and then while the gas is leaving the lungs (the "wash-out" phase).

The nurse teaches the client about the procedure and explains that the radioactive substance clears from the body in approximately 8 hours.

OTHER NONINVASIVE DIAGNOSTIC TESTS

Pulse Oximetry

Pulse oximetry identifies hemoglobin saturation. Usually hemoglobin is almost 100% saturated with oxygen. The pulse oximeter uses a wave of infrared light and a sensor placed on the client's finger, toe, nose, earlobe, or forehead. Ideal normal pulse oximetry values are 95% to 100%; values may be a little lower in older clients and in clients with dark skin. To avoid confusion with the Pao_2 values from arterial blood gases, pulse oximetry readings are recorded as the Sao_2 (arterial oxygen saturation), or Spo_2.

A pulse oximetry reading can alert the nurse to desaturation before clinical signs occur (e.g., dusky skin, pale mucosa, and nail beds). The nurse considers client movement, hypothermia, decreased peripheral blood flow, ambient light (sunlight, infrared lamps), decreased hemoglobin, edema, and fingernail polish as possible causes for low readings. Covering the sensor or changing its positioning could yield better accuracy if too much ambient light is present.

Results lower than 91% (and certainly below 86%) constitute an emergency and necessitate immediate treatment. When the Sao_2 is below 85%, the tissues of the body have a difficult time becoming oxygenated. An Sao_2 of less than 70% is usually life threatening, but in some cases values below 80% may be life threatening. *Pulse oximetry is less accurate at lower values.*

Pulmonary Function Tests

Pulmonary function tests (PFTs) evaluate lung function and dysfunction and include studies such as lung volumes and capacities, flow rates, diffusion capacity, gas exchange, airway resistance, and distribution of ventilation. The physician interprets the results by comparing the client's data with normal findings predicted according to age, gender, race, height, weight, and smoking status.

PFTs are useful in screening clients for pulmonary disease even before the onset of signs or symptoms. Serial testing provides objective data that may be used as a guide to treatment (e.g., changes in pulmonary function can support a decision to continue, change, or discontinue a specific therapy). Preoperative evaluation with PFTs may identify the client at risk for postoperative pulmonary complications. One of the most common reasons for performing such tests is to determine the cause of dyspnea. When performed while the client exercises, PFTs help to determine whether dyspnea is caused by pulmonary or cardiac dysfunction or by muscle deconditioning. These tests are also useful for determining the effect of the client's occupation on pulmonary function and for evaluating any related disability for legal purposes.

CLIENT PREPARATION. The nurse prepares the client for PFTs by explaining the purpose of the tests for planning care. He or she is advised not to smoke for 6 to 8 hours before testing. According to institutional policy and procedure, bronchodilator medication is withheld for 4 to 6 hours before the test. The client with respiratory impairment often fears further breathlessness and is usually anxious before these "breathing" tests. The nurse helps to reduce apprehension by describing what will be experienced during and after the testing.

PROCEDURE. PFTs can be performed at the bedside or in the respiratory laboratory. The client is asked to breathe through the mouth only. A nose clip may be used to prevent air from escaping. The client performs different breathing maneuvers while measurements are obtained (Figure 27-10). Table 27-7 describes the most commonly used PFTs and their purpose.

FOLLOW-UP CARE. Because numerous breathing maneuvers are performed during PFTs, the nurse observes for increased dyspnea or bronchospasm after such studies. The nurse documents whether bronchodilator medication was administered during testing and alters the client's medication schedule as indicated.

Exercise Testing

Exercise, or activity in general, increases metabolism and gas transport as energy is generated. Five reasons for exercise testing are listed in Table 27-8. These tests are performed on a treadmill or bicycle or by a self-paced 12-minute walking test. The normal client's exercise is limited by hemodynamic factors, whereas the pulmonary client is limited by ventilatory capacity, pulmonary gas exchange compromise, or both. The nurse explains exercise testing and assures the client of close monitoring by trained professionals throughout the test.

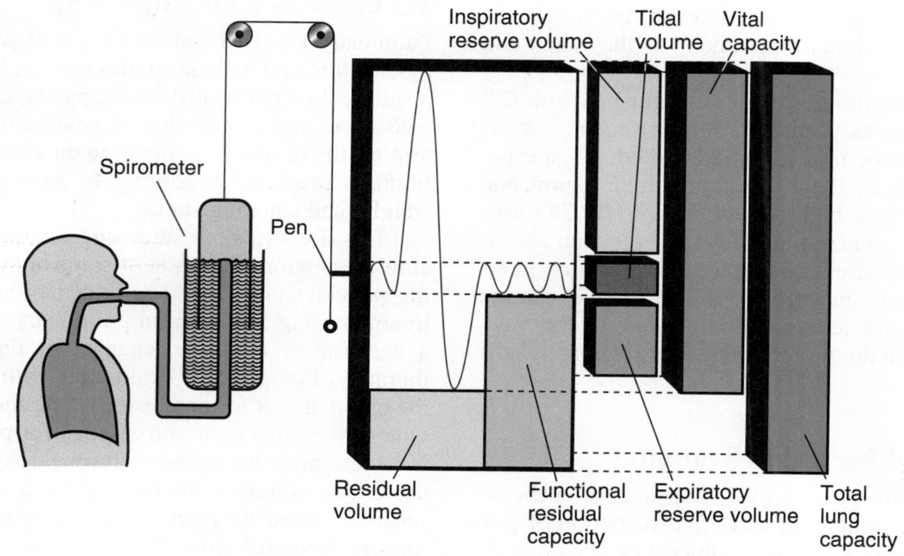

Figure 27-10 ● Common measurements in pulmonary function testing. (Modified from Luce, J.M., Pierson, D.J., & Tyler, M.L. [1993]. *Intensive respiratory care* [2nd ed.]. Philadelphia: W.B. Saunders.)

TABLE 27-7 • CHARACTERISTICS AND PURPOSES OF PULMONARY FUNCTION TESTS

Test	Purpose
FVC (forced vital capacity) records the maximum amount of air that can be exhaled as quickly as possible after maximum inspiration.	*FVC* gives an indication of respiratory muscle strength and ventilatory reserve. FVC is often reduced in obstructive disease (because of air trapping) and in restrictive disease.
FEV_1 (forced expiratory volume in 1 second) records the maximal amount of air that can be exhaled in the first second of expiration.	*FEV_1* is effort dependent and declines normally with age. It is reduced in certain obstructive and restrictive disorders.
FEV_1/FVC is the ratio of expiratory volume in 1 second to FVC.	This ratio provides a much more sensitive indication of obstruction to airflow. This ratio is the hallmark of obstructive pulmonary disease. It is normal or increased in restrictive disease.
$FEF_{25\%-75\%}$ records the forced expiratory flow over the 25%-75% volume (middle half) of the FVC.	This measure provides a more sensitive index of obstruction in the smaller airways.
FRC (functional residual capacity) is the amount of air remaining in the lungs after normal expiration. FRC test requires use of the helium dilution technique.	Increased FRC indicates hyperinflation or air trapping, which may result from obstructive pulmonary disease. FRC is normal or decreased in restrictive pulmonary diseases.
TLC (total lung capacity) is the amount of air in the lungs at the end of maximum inhalation.	Increased TLC indicates air trapping associated with obstructive pulmonary disease. Decreased TLC indicates restrictive disease.
RV (residual volume) is the amount of air remaining in the lungs at the end of a full, forced exhalation.	RV is increased in obstructive pulmonary disease such as emphysema.
DLCO (diffusion capacity of carbon monoxide) reflects the surface area of the alveolocapillary membrane. The client inhales a small amount of CO, holds for 10 seconds, and then exhales. The amount inhaled is compared with the amount exhaled.	DLCO is reduced whenever the alveolocapillary membrane is diminished, such as occurs in emphysema, pulmonary hypertension, and pulmonary fibrosis. It is increased with exercise and in conditions such as polycythemia and congestive heart disease.

Skin Tests

Skin tests are used in combination with other diagnostic data to identify various infectious diseases (e.g., tuberculosis), viral diseases (e.g., mononucleosis and mumps), and fungal diseases (e.g., coccidioidomycosis and histoplasmosis). The presence of allergic hypersensitivity and the status of the immune system can be demonstrated through skin testing. Exposure to the allergen or organism used in testing produces a specific reaction (delayed hypersensitivity reaction) of the client's immune system. (See Chapters 20 and 23 for further discussion of these tests.)

Magnetic Resonance Imaging

Magnetic resonance imaging (MRI) is used in the diagnosis of respiratory system disorders to provide information about

TABLE 27-8 • FIVE INDICATIONS FOR EXERCISE TESTING

- To assess a client's functional capacity (ability to work and perform activities of daily living)
- To determine the reason for exercise limitation: cardiac, pulmonary, or poor conditioning
- To evaluate changes in exercise capacity related to disease or treatment
- To determine the basis for the development of a pulmonary rehabilitation program
- To determine whether supplemental oxygen is required during exercise

the type and condition of the tissues being imaged along any plane inside the body: vertically, horizontally, and diagonally. This costly procedure requires little client preparation other than the removal of all metal objects. Because of the powerful magnets used in MRI, clients with pacemakers, aneurysm clips, inner-ear implants, cardiac valves, or any other metallic foreign objects in the body are not candidates for MRI.

The nurse informs the client of possible claustrophobia and discomfort from lying on a hard, cool table inside the magnet's small cylinder. The nurse instructs the client in the use of relaxation techniques and imagery to help decrease these sensations. Sedation may be necessary in some cases. The nurse explains that the noises heard during the examination are the natural, rhythmic sounds of radiofrequency pulses. These noises may range from barely audible to noticeable.

CRITICAL THINKING CHALLENGE

The 38-year-old male bank employee has a history of shortness of breath and decreased exercise tolerance. He has a respiratory rate of 16 breaths per minute, with bilateral chest movement, no retractions, no visible pallor or cyanosis, and no clubbing of the fingers. His pulse oximetry shows an oxygen saturation of 97%.

- Is it safe to assume this client does not have serious pulmonary problems? Why or why not?
- What additional physical assessment data (noninvasive) should you obtain?
- How could you ascertain whether the data you have already obtained (respiratory rate, respiratory effort, skin and mucous membrane color, pulse oximetry) accurately reflect this client's respiratory status?

For suggested answer guidelines, go to SIMON http://www.wbsaunders.com/SIMON/Iggy/.

OTHER INVASIVE DIAGNOSTIC TESTS

Endoscopic Examinations

Endoscopic diagnostic studies to assess respiratory disorders include bronchoscopy, laryngoscopy, and mediastinoscopy. These procedures are summarized in Table 27-9. The most common complications are those related to the medications and bleeding.

Thoracentesis

Thoracentesis is used for diagnosis or treatment and involves the aspiration of pleural fluid or air from the pleural space. Microscopic examination of the pleural fluid helps in making a diagnosis. Pleural fluid may be drained to relieve pulmonary compression and the resultant respiratory distress caused by cancer, empyema, pleurisy, or tuberculosis. Thoracentesis is often followed by pleural biopsy to assist in further assessment of the parietal pleura. Thoracentesis also allows the instillation of medications into the pleural space.

CLIENT PREPARATION. Adequate client preparation is essential before thoracentesis to ensure cooperation during the procedure and to prevent complications. The nurse tells the client to expect a stinging sensation from the local anesthetic agent and a feeling of pressure when the needle is inserted. The nurse reinforces the importance of not moving during the procedure (avoiding coughing, deep breathing, or sudden movement) to avoid puncture of the visceral pleura or lung.

Figure 27-11 shows the appropriate positions for thoracentesis. These positions widen the intercostal spaces and permit easy access to the pleural fluid. The nurse properly positions and physically supports the client. Pillows are used to make the client comfortable and to provide physical support.

Before the procedure, the nurse checks the client's history for hypersensitivity to local anesthetic agents and checks to make sure the client has signed an informed consent. The entire chest or back is exposed, and the aspiration site is shaved if necessary. The actual site depends on the volume and location of the effusion, which are determined by radiography and physical examination procedures such as percussion.

PROCEDURE. Thoracentesis is usually performed at the bedside, although ultrasonography or computed tomography may be used to guide it. After draping the client and cleaning the skin with a germicidal solution, the physician uses aseptic technique and injects a local anesthetic agent into the selected intercostal space. The nurse keeps the client informed of the procedure while observing for shock, pain, nausea, pallor, diaphoresis, cyanosis, tachypnea, and dyspnea.

The physician advances the short 18- to 25-gauge thoracentesis needle (with an attached syringe) into the pleural space. Gentle suction is applied as the fluid in the pleural space is slowly aspirated. A vacuum collection bottle is sometimes necessary to remove larger volumes of fluid. To prevent re-expansion pulmonary edema, usually no more than 1000 mL of fluid is removed at one time. If a pleural biopsy is to be performed, a second, larger needle with a cutting edge and collection chamber is used. After the physician withdraws the needle, pressure is applied to the puncture site, and a small sterile dressing is applied.

FOLLOW-UP CARE. After thoracentesis, the physician orders a chest x-ray study to rule out possible pneumothorax and subsequent **mediastinal shift** (shift of center thoracic structure toward one side). The nurse monitors the client's vital signs and auscultates breath sounds while noting absent or diminished sounds on the affected side. The puncture site and dressing are observed for leakage or bleeding. The nurse also assesses for other complications, such as reaccumulation of fluid in the pleural space, subcutaneous emphysema, pyrogenic infection, and tension pneumothorax. The client is encouraged to breathe deeply to promote reexpansion of the lung. The nurse documents the procedure, including the client's tolerance, the volume and char-

TABLE 27-9 • CARE OF THE CLIENT UNDERGOING ENDOSCOPIC TESTS FOR RESPIRATORY DISORDERS

Purpose and Description	Nursing Interventions	Rationale
BRONCHOSCOPY		
To assess airway anatomy for tumors, obstruction, and atelectasis.	Allow the client nothing by mouth for several hours before the test.	The client may aspirate gastric contents if vomiting occurs.
To assist in the diagnosis of infection or cancer by biopsy of lesions; biopsy techniques include the brush biopsy and needle aspiration.	Assess for allergies to iodine, local anesthetics, or pretest medications.	A knowledge of allergies helps prevent allergic reactions.
To remove thick secretions, mucus plugs, or foreign bodies.	Place pulse oximeter.	Pulse oximetry allows continuous monitoring throughout the procedure.
A flexible fiberoptic bronchoscope is inserted through the mouth, nose, endotracheal tube, or tracheostomy tube. The procedure may be performed in the operating room or radiology department. Oxygen administration and blood pressure monitoring are standard procedures.	Administer pretest medications (atropine, diazepam) as ordered.	Pretest medications help decrease secretions and reduce anxiety.
	Prepare the client for topical anesthetic administration into the oropharynx.	Explanations about the effects of the anesthetic agent (numbness and gagging) help to decrease anxiety.
	Remove the client's dentures if present.	Injury may occur if dentures are left in place.
	After the procedure, monitor the client's vital signs for 15 min until stable, and monitor for hemoptysis.	Assessment helps the nurse detect respiratory distress and signs of complications related to the procedure.
	After the procedure, allow the client nothing by mouth until the gag reflex returns.	Allowing the client nothing by mouth reduces the possibility of aspiration.
	Discourage smoking, talking, and coughing for several hours.	Throat irritation is decreased by avoiding these activities.
LARYNGOSCOPY		
Direct: To detect or remove lesions or foreign bodies in the larynx or to diagnose cancer by removing tissue for biopsy or samples for culture. A fiberoptic laryngoscope is used.	Allow the client nothing by mouth for several hours before the test.	Aspiration is possible if vomiting occurs.
Indirect: To assess the function of the vocal cords or to obtain tissue for biopsy. Observations are made during rest and phonation by using a laryngeal mirror, head mirror, and light source.	Assess the client for allergies to iodine, contrast media, or local anesthetics.	A knowledge of allergies helps prevent allergic reactions.
	Administer pretest medications (atropine, diazepam) as ordered.	Pretest medications help decrease secretions and reduce anxiety.
	Assess the client for fears concerning the procedure. Assure the client that he or she will be monitored for any respiratory problems.	Reassurance helps decrease fears about not being able to breathe during the procedure.
	For indirect laryngoscopy, assist the client to sit in an upright position, and encourage normal breathing.	An upright sitting position facilitates the passage of the laryngeal mirror into the mouth.
	After the procedure, allow the client nothing by mouth until the gag reflex returns.	The client may aspirate gastric contents if vomiting occurs.
	Encourage coughing and fluid intake.	Hydration and coughing promote the expectoration of secretions.
	Assess vital signs frequently for 24 hr. Assess the client for bleeding.	Frequent monitoring of vital signs enables the nurse to detect changes such as dyspnea.
	After the procedure, administer lozenges or gargles as ordered.	Lozenges and gargles help to relieve a sore throat.
MEDIASTINOSCOPY		
To inspect and remove samples for biopsy of lymph nodes that drain the lung.	Explain preoperative measures and the procedure to the client.	Explanations about the anticipated procedure help to decrease anxiety.
To detect metastasis of lung cancer.	Assess the client postoperatively for bleeding, pneumothorax, and vocal cord paralysis.	Ongoing assessment for complications helps to ensure prompt treatment.
To obtain tissue for biopsy for diagnosis of tuberculosis or sarcoidosis.	Assess the client for pain, and administer analgesics as ordered.	Medication decreases the discomfort associated with the procedure.
The procedure is performed in the operating room with the client under local or general anesthesia; a suprasternal incision is used.		

acter of the fluid removed, any specimens sent to the laboratory, the location of the puncture site, and respiratory assessment findings before, during, and after the procedure.

Lung Biopsy

A lung biopsy is performed to obtain tissue for histologic analysis, culture, or cytologic examination. The physician uses tissue samples to make a definite diagnosis regarding the type of malignancy, infection, inflammation, or lung disease. Biopsy procedures include transbronchial biopsy (TBB) and transbronchial needle aspiration (TBNA), both of which are performed during bronchoscopy; transthoracic needle aspiration (percutaneous approach for areas not accessible by bronchoscopy); and open lung biopsy (in the operating room).

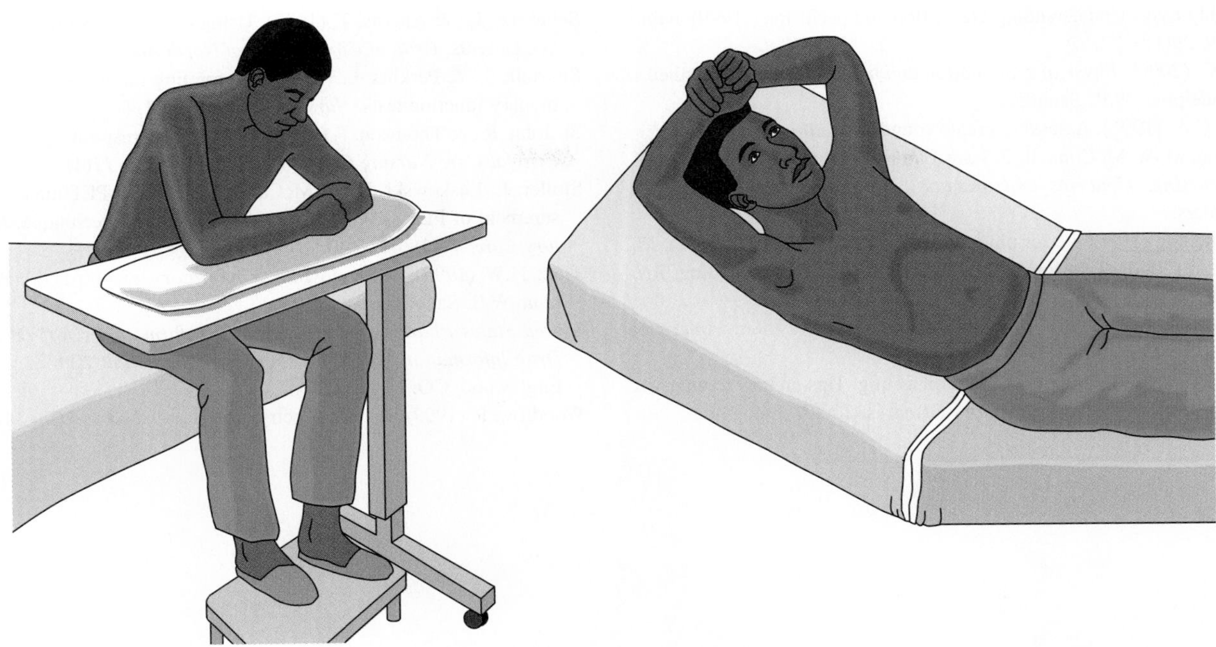

Figure 27-11 ● Positions for thoracentesis.

CLIENT PREPARATION. The client may have predetermined ideas about the outcome of the biopsy and may closely associate the terms *biopsy* and *cancer.* Therefore the nurse explains what to expect before and after the procedure and explores the client's feelings and fears. To reduce discomfort and anxiety, the physician may prescribe an analgesic or sedative before the procedure. The nurse informs the client undergoing percutaneous biopsy that discomfort is minimized with a local anesthetic agent but that a sensation of pressure may be experienced during needle insertion and tissue aspiration. Open lung biopsy is usually performed in the operating room with the client under general anesthesia, and the usual preoperative preparations apply.

PROCEDURE. Percutaneous lung biopsy may be performed in the client's room or in the radiology department after an informed consent has been obtained. Fluoroscopy, CT, or ultrasonography is often used to better visualize the area undergoing biopsy and to guide the procedure. Positioning of the client is similar to that for thoracentesis. The physician cleans the skin with an antibacterial agent and administers a local anesthetic agent. Under sterile conditions, the physician inserts a spinal-type 18- to 22-gauge needle through the skin into the desired area (e.g., tissue, nodule, or lymph node) and obtains the tissue needed for microscopic examination. The nurse applies a dressing after the procedure.

An open lung biopsy is performed in the operating room. The client undergoes a thoracotomy where lung tissue is exposed. At least two tissue specimens are taken (usually from an upper lobe and a lower lobe site). The surgeon places a chest tube to remove air and fluid so the lung can reinflate and then closes the chest.

FOLLOW-UP CARE. The nurse monitors the client's vital signs and breath sounds every 4 hours for 24 hours and assesses for signs of respiratory distress (e.g., dyspnea, pallor, diaphoresis, and tachypnea). Pneumothorax is a serious complication of needle biopsy and open lung biopsy, and therefore it is important for the nurse to report untoward signs and symptoms promptly. The nurse also monitors for hemoptysis (which may be scant and transient) or, in rare cases, for frank bleeding from vascular or lung trauma.

ONLINE RESOURCES

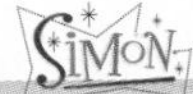

For suggested readings and Internet resources, go to http://www.wbsaunders.com/SIMON/Iggy/.

SELECTED BIBLIOGRAPHY

Asterisk indicates a classic or definitive work on this subject.

Aherns, T., & Tucker, K. (1999). Pulse oximetry. *Critical Care Nursing Clinics of North America, 11*(1), 87-98.

Aherns, T., Wijeweera, H., & Ray, S. (1999). Capnography: A key underutilized technology. *Critical Care Nursing Clinics of North America, 11*(1), 49-62.

Carroll, P. (1997). Pulse oximetry at your fingertips. *RN, 60*(2), 22-27.

Carroll, P. (1999). Evolutions: Capnography. *RN, 62*(5), 69-71.

Carroll, P. (1999). Revolutions: Continuous spirometry. *RN, 62*(5), 72-74, 77-78.

Ebersole, P., & Hess, P. (1998). *Toward healthy aging: Human needs and nursing response* (5th ed.). St. Louis: Mosby.

Finesilver, C. (2001). Perfecting your skills: Respiratory assessment. *RN,* April suppl., pp. 16-28.

Gordon, M. (2000). *Manual of nursing diagnosis* (9th ed.). St. Louis: Mosby.

Guyton, A., & Hall, J. (2000). *Textbook of medical physiology* (10th ed.). Philadelphia: W.B. Saunders.

Hess, D. (2000). Detection and monitoring of hypoxemia and oxygen therapy. *Respiratory Care, 45*(1), 65-83.

Incredibly easy! Understanding ventilation and perfusion. (1999). *Nursing99, 29*(10), 22.

Jarvis, C. (2000). *Physical examination and health assessment* (3rd ed.). Philadelphia: W.B. Saunders.

*Kirton, C.A. (1996). Assessing breath sounds. *Nursing, 26*(6), 50-51.

Matteson, M.A., McConnell, E.S., & Linton, A.D. (1997). *Gerontological nursing: Concepts and practice* (2nd ed.). Philadelphia: W.B. Saunders.

McConnell, E. (1999). Performing pulse oximetry. *Nursing99, 29*(11), 17.

Moore, A. (2000). Tips for getting a more reliable O_2 sat reading. *RN, 63*(2), 73.

O'Hanlon-Nichols, T. (1998). The adult respiratory system. *American Journal of Nursing, 98*(2), 39-45.

Salzman, S. (1999). Pulmonary function testing: Tips on how to interpret the results. *Journal of Respiratory Diseases, 20*(12), 809-812.

Schallom, L., & Aherns, T. (1999). Using oxygenation profiles to manage patients. *Critical Care Clinics of North America, 11*(4), 437-446.

Shortall, S., & Perkins, L. (1999). Interpreting the ins and outs of pulmonary function tests. *Nursing 99, 29*(12), 41-47.

St. John, R., & Thomson, P. (1999). Noninvasive respiratory monitoring. *Critical Care Nursing Clinics of North America, 11*(4), 423-435.

Stoller, J., Laskowski, D., & McCarthy, K. (1999). PFT nuggets: Measurement of FEV_1 using the modified spirometry technique. *Respiratory Care, 44*(4), 441-442.

*Tietz, N.W. (1995). *Clinical guide to laboratory tests* (3rd ed.). Philadelphia: W.B. Saunders.

United States Pharmacopeia Dispensing Information (USP DI): Vol. I. Drug information for the health care professional (20th ed.). (2000). Englewood, CO: Micromedix.

Woodrow, P. (1999). Pulse oximetry. *Emergency Nurse, 7*(5), 34-39.

CHAPTER 28

Interventions for Clients Requiring Oxygen Therapy or Tracheostomy

M. LINDA WORKMAN

Learning Objectives

After studying this chapter, you should be able to:

1. Compare and contrast the uses and nursing care issues of oxygen delivery by nasal cannula with oxygen delivery by mask.
2. Explain the problems associated with oxygen therapy for those clients whose respiratory efforts are controlled by the hypoxic drive.
3. Analyze changes in clinical manifestations to determine the effectiveness of therapy for the client receiving oxygen.
4. Use laboratory data and clinical manifestations to determine the presence of hypoxemia or hypercarbia.
5. Prioritize educational needs for the client receiving supportive oxygen therapy at home.
6. Prioritize nursing care needs for the client with a new tracheostomy.
7. Identify techniques to minimize the risk for aspiration when helping the client with a tracheostomy to eat.

SIMON

Go to http://www.wbsaunders.com/SIMON/Iggy/ for self-assessment questions related to these Learning Objectives.

OXYGEN THERAPY

OVERVIEW

Oxygen (O_2) is a gas that is essential for life, as well as a potent drug prescribed by the physician for relief of symptoms of **hypoxemia** (low levels of oxygen in the blood) and the resulting **hypoxia** (decreased tissue oxygenation). The oxygen content of atmospheric air is about 21%. Therapeutic oxygen is prescribed when the oxygen needs of the body cannot be met by atmospheric or "room air" alone. Therapeutic oxygen is used for both acute and chronic respiratory conditions associated with decreased blood and tissue oxygen levels as indicated by decreased partial pressure of arterial oxygen (Pa_{O_2}) levels or by decreased arterial oxygen saturation (Sa_{O_2}). Conditions outside the respiratory system that increase oxygen demand, decrease oxygen-carrying capability of the blood, or decrease cardiac output also are indications for oxygen therapy. Such conditions include sepsis, fever, and decreased hemoglobin levels or poor hemoglobin quality.

The goal of oxygen therapy is to use the lowest **fraction of inspired oxygen (F_{IO_2})** to obtain the most acceptable oxygenation without causing the development of harmful side effects. Although oxygen improves the Pa_{O_2} level, it does not cure the condition or stop the disease process. The average client requires an oxygen flow of 2 to 4 L/min via nasal cannula or up to 40% via Venturi mask. The client who is hypoxemic and also has chronic **hypercarbia** (increased partial pressure of arterial carbon dioxide [Pa_{CO_2}] levels) requires lower levels of oxygen delivery, usually 1 to 2 L/min via nasal cannula, to prevent decreased respiratory effort. (A low Pa_{O_2} level is this client's primary drive for breathing.)

COLLABORATIVE MANAGEMENT

Arterial blood gas (ABG) analysis is the best measure for determining the need for oxygen therapy and for evaluating its effects. Oxygen need can also be determined by noninvasive monitoring, such as pulse oximetry.

The nurse administers prescribed oxygen therapy. Before initiating oxygen therapy and while caring for a client receiving oxygen therapy, the nurse is knowledgeable about associated hazards and complications. The nurse also knows the rationale and the expected outcome related to oxygen therapy for each client receiving oxygen. Chart 28-1 lists NIC interventions for clients requiring oxygen therapy.

Hazards and Complications of Oxygen Therapy

COMBUSTION

Oxygen itself does not burn, but its presence supports and enhances combustion. Therefore a fire burns more readily in the presence of oxygen. The nurse takes special precautions dur-

CHART 28-1

NIC INTERVENTION ACTIVITIES *for* The Client with Respiratory Problems

Oxygen Therapy: *Administration of oxygen and monitoring of its effectiveness*
- Clear oral, nasal, and tracheal secretions, as appropriate.
- Maintain airway patency.
- Set up oxygen equipment and administer through a heated, humidified system.
- Monitor the oxygen liter flow.
- Monitor position of oxygen delivery device.
- Periodically check oxygen delivery device to ensure that the prescribed concentration is being delivered.
- Monitor the effectiveness of oxygen therapy (e.g., pulse oximetry, ABGs), as appropriate.
- Ensure replacement of oxygen mask/cannula whenever the device is removed.
- Observe for signs of oxygen-induced hypoventilation.
- Monitor for signs of oxygen toxicity and absorption atelectasis.
- Monitor oxygen equipment to ensure that it is not interfering with the client's attempts to breathe.
- Monitor client's anxiety related to need for oxygen therapy.
- Monitor for skin breakdown from friction of oxygen device.
- Provide for oxygen when client is transported.
- Instruct client and family about use of oxygen at home.
- Arrange for use of oxygen devices that facilitate mobility and teach client accordingly.

Artificial Airway Management: *Maintenance of endotracheal and tracheostomy tubes and preventing complications associated with their use*
- Provide 100% humidification of inspired gas/air.
- Provide adequate systemic hydration via oral or intravenous fluid administration.
- Inflate endotracheal/tracheostomy cuff using minimal occlusive volume technique or minimal leak technique.
- Suction the oropharynx and secretions from the top of the tube cuff before deflating cuff.
- Monitor cuff pressures every 4 to 8 hours during expiration using a three-way stopcock, calibrated syringe, and mercury manometer.
- Change endotracheal tapes/ties every 24 hours, inspect the skin and oral mucosa, and move endotracheal tube to the other side of the mouth.
- Monitor for presence of crackles and rhonchi over large airways.
- Institute measures to prevent spontaneous decannulation: secure artificial airway with tape/ties; administer sedation and muscle paralyzing agent, as appropriate, and use arm restraints, as appropriate.
- Provide additional intubation equipment and ambu bag in a readily available location.
- Provide trachea care every 4 to 8 hours as appropriate: clean the inner cannula, clean and dry the area around the stoma, and change tracheostomy ties.
- Inspect skin around tracheal stoma for drainage, redness, and irritation.
- Maintain sterile technique when suctioning and providing tracheostomy care.
- Shield the tracheostomy from water.
- Tape the tracheostomy obturator to head of bed.
- Tape a second tracheostomy tube and obturator (same type and size) and forceps to the head of the bed.
- Institute chest physiotherapy, as appropriate.
- Elevate head of the bed or assist client to a sitting position in a chair during feedings, as appropriate.
- Add food coloring to enteral feedings as appropriate.

NIC intervention activities selected from McCloskey, J.C., & Bulechek, G.M. (Eds.). (2000). *Nursing interventions classification (NIC)* (3rd ed.). St. Louis: Mosby.
ABG, Arterial blood gas.

ing oxygen administration, including posting a sign on the door of the client's room. Smoking is prohibited in the client's room, including at home, when he or she is receiving oxygen. All electrical equipment must be grounded (i.e., with three prongs having a green or red dot on the plate). Frayed cords must be repaired because they can cause a spark that can ignite a flame. Any type of flammable solution containing alcohol or oil is prohibited from the room when oxygen is in use.

OXYGEN-INDUCED HYPOVENTILATION

The nurse assesses for oxygen-induced hypoventilation in the client whose principal respiratory drive is hypoxia (hypoxic drive), such as in the client with chronic lung disease who also has hypercarbia. The partial pressure of arterial carbon dioxide ($Paco_2$) level for these clients gradually rises over time. The central chemoreceptors in the brain (medulla) are normally sensitive to increased $Paco_2$ levels, which stimulate breathing and cause an increased respiratory rate. When the $Paco_2$ increases over time to above 60 to 65 mm Hg, this normal mechanism shuts off. The central chemoreceptors lose their sensitivity to increased levels of $Paco_2$ and no longer respond by increasing the rate and depth of respiration, a condition called **CO_2 narcosis.** For these clients, the stimulus to breathe is a decreased arterial oxygen concentration as sensed by peripheral chemoreceptors found in the carotid sinus areas and aortic arch. When partial pressure of arterial oxygen (Pao_2) levels drop (hypoxemia), these receptors signal the brain to increase the respiratory rate and depth—the **hypoxic drive** to breathe.

The hypoxic drive occurs only in the presence of severely elevated $Paco_2$ levels (i.e., in the client who has hypoxemia and hypercarbia). When the client with low Pao_2 levels and high $Paco_2$ levels receives oxygen therapy, the Pao_2 level increases, removing the stimulation for breathing, and the client experiences respiratory depression. (The client being ventilated mechanically is not at risk for this complication.)

The health care provider prescribes oxygen therapy at the lowest liter flow (usually 1, 2 or 3 L/min) necessary to treat the hypoxemia without raising the $Paco_2$. A system that delivers precise oxygen concentrations (e.g., a Venturi mask) is preferred for this client. However, a client with chronic obstructive pulmonary disease may not tolerate a face mask.

The nurse closely monitors the respiratory rate and depth while the client is receiving oxygen. This monitoring is especially important when it is the first time he or she has received oxygen or when the $Paco_2$ levels are not known. Signs and symptoms of hypoventilation are seen during the first 30 minutes of oxygen administration; the client's color improves (from ashen or gray to pink) because of an increase in the Pao_2 level before the apnea or respiratory arrest occurs from loss of the hypoxic drive. The nurse therefore carefully monitors the level of consciousness, respiratory pattern and rate, and pulse oximetry for clients at risk for oxygen-induced hypoventilation, apnea, and respiratory arrest. *Although oxygen-induced hypoventilation is a serious concern, untreated or inadequately treated hypoxemia is a greater threat to life.*

OXYGEN TOXICITY

Oxygen toxicity is related to the concentration of oxygen delivered, duration of oxygen therapy, and degree of lung disease present before oxygen therapy is started. In general, an oxygen concentration greater than 50% administered continuously for more than 24 to 48 hours may damage the lungs. *It is important to remember that although oxygen toxicity is a serious concern, untreated or inadequately treated hypoxemia is a greater threat to life.*

The pathophysiologic mechanism and clinical manifestations of lung injury associated with oxygen toxicity are the same as those for acute respiratory distress syndrome (ARDS) (see Chapter 32). The nurse observes for initial symptoms, which include nonproductive cough, substernal chest pain, gastrointestinal (GI) upset, and dyspnea. As exposure to high concentrations of oxygen continues, the symptoms become more severe and are accompanied by decreased vital capacity, decreased compliance (which results in more dyspnea), crackles, and hypoxemia. Prolonged exposure to high concentrations of oxygen causes structural damage to the lungs. Atelectasis, pulmonary edema, pulmonary hemorrhages, and hyaline membrane formation result. Surviving this life-threatening condition depends on the ability of the health care team to correct the underlying disease process and to decrease the oxygen amount delivered.

The toxic effects of oxygen are difficult to treat, making prevention a priority. The physician orders the lowest concentration of oxygen required to prevent oxygen toxicity. The nurse closely monitors arterial blood gases during oxygen administration and notifies the physician of Pao_2 levels greater than 90 mm Hg. The nurse also monitors the prescribed oxygen concentration and length of time of administration to identify the client at higher risk. High concentrations of oxygen are avoided unless absolutely necessary. The addition of **continuous positive airway pressure (CPAP)** with an oxygen mask, **bilevel positive airway pressure (BiPAP),** or **positive end-expiratory pressure (PEEP)** on the mechanical ventilator (see Chapter 32) may reduce the amount of oxygen needed. As soon as the client's clinical condition allows, the physician decreases the prescribed amount of oxygen.

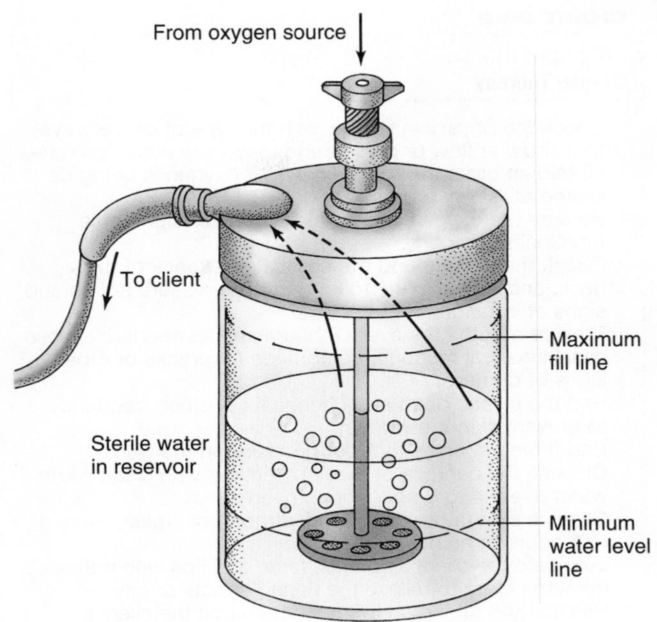

Figure 28-1 ● A bubble humidifier bottle used with oxygen therapy.

ABSORPTION ATELECTASIS

Nitrogen normally plays a large role in the maintenance of patent airways and alveoli. Making up 79% of room air, nitrogen prevents alveolar collapse. When high concentrations of oxygen are delivered, nitrogen is diluted, oxygen diffuses from the alveoli into the pulmonary circulation, and the alveoli collapse. Collapsed alveoli cause atelectasis (called **absorption atelectasis**), which is detected by auscultation. The nurse monitors the client closely for crackles and decreased breath sounds every 1 to 2 hours when oxygen therapy is initiated and as frequently as needed thereafter.

DRYING OF THE MUCOUS MEMBRANES

When an oxygen flow rate higher than 4 L/min is needed, humidification is added to the delivery system (Figure 28-1). The nurse ensures that oxygen can be seen bubbling through the water in the humidifier.

Oxygen can also be humidified via a nebulizer in mist form (aerosol). A heated nebulizer raises the humidity even more and is used when oxygen is administered via an artificial airway. Usually the upper airway passages have sufficient warming ability, but these passages are bypassed when an artificial airway is in use.

A sufficient amount of sterile water must be in the humidification container, and an adequate flow rate must be maintained so that proper humidification is delivered to the client. Condensation often forms in the tubing and is removed as needed by disconnecting the tubing and emptying the water appropriately. Some manufacturers place a water trap that hangs from the tubing so that the condensation can be drained without disconnecting. *For prevention of bacterial contamination, the fluid is never drained back into the humidification container.* The nurse checks the water level and changes the humidifier as needed.

CHART 28-2

BEST PRACTICE *for* Oxygen Therapy

- Check the physician's order with the type of delivery system and liter flow or percentage of oxygen actually in use.
- Obtain an order for humidification if oxygen is being delivered at 4 L/min or more.
- Be sure the oxygen and humidification equipment is functioning properly.
- Check the skin around the client's ears, back of the neck, and face every 4 to 8 hours for pressure points and signs of irritation.
- Provide mouth care every 8 hours and as needed; assess nasal and oral mucous membranes for cracks or other signs of dryness.
- Pad the elastic band and change its position frequently to prevent skin breakdown.
- Pad tubing in areas that put pressure on the skin.
- Cleanse the cannula or mask by rinsing with clear, warm water every 4 to 8 hours or as needed.
- Cleanse skin under the tubing, straps, and mask every 4 to 8 hours or as needed.
- Lubricate the client's nostrils, face, and lips with nonpetroleum cream to relieve the drying effects of oxygen.
- Position the tubing so it does not pull on the client's face, nose, or artificial airway.
- Ensure that there is no smoking and that no candles or matches are lit in the immediate area.
- Assess and document the client's response to oxygen therapy.
- Provide the client with ongoing teaching and reassurance to enhance the client's compliance with oxygen therapy.

INFECTION

The humidification system may be a source of bacteria. *Pseudomonas aeruginosa* is frequently the organism involved. Oxygen delivery equipment such as cannulas and masks can also harbor organisms. The nurse changes equipment as per policy or protocol, which can range from every 24 hours for humidification systems to every 7 days or whenever necessary for cannulas and masks.

Oxygen Delivery Systems

Oxygen can be delivered by many systems. Regardless of the type of delivery system used, the nurse needs to understand its indications, advantages, and disadvantages. The nurse uses the equipment properly and ensures appropriate equipment maintenance. A respiratory therapist is consulted whenever there is a question or concern about an oxygen delivery system.

The type of delivery system selected depends on the following:

- Oxygen concentration required by the client
- Oxygen concentration achieved by a delivery system
- Importance of accuracy and control of the oxygen concentration
- Client comfort
- Expense to the client
- Importance of humidity
- Client mobility

Oxygen delivery systems are classified according to the rate at which oxygen is delivered. There are two systems: low-flow systems and high-flow systems. Low-flow systems do not provide enough flow of oxygen to meet the total inspiratory effort of the client. Part of the tidal volume is supplied by inspiring room air. The total concentration of oxygen received depends on the respiratory rate and tidal volume. In contrast, high-flow systems provide a flow rate that is adequate to meet the entire inspiratory effort and tidal volume of the client regardless of the respiratory pattern. High-flow systems are used for critically ill clients and when it is particularly important to know the precise concentration of oxygen being delivered.

If the client requires a mask but is able to eat, the nurse requests an order for a nasal cannula at an appropriate liter flow for mealtimes only. The mask is replaced after the meal is completed. To increase mobility, up to 50 feet of connecting tubing can be used with proper connecting pieces. Best nursing practices for clients receiving oxygen therapy are listed in Chart 28-2.

LOW-FLOW OXYGEN DELIVERY SYSTEMS

Low-flow delivery systems include the nasal cannula, simple face mask, partial rebreather mask, and non-rebreather mask (Table 28-1). These systems are inexpensive, easy to use, and fairly comfortable. A major disadvantage is that the actual amount of oxygen obtained per liter is variable and depends on the client's breathing pattern. The oxygen delivered by the system is diluted with room air (21%), which lowers the amount of oxygen actually received.

NASAL CANNULA. The nasal cannula, or nasal prongs (Figure 28-2), is used at flow rates of 1 to 6 L/min. Approximate oxygen concentrations of 24% (at 1 L/min) to 44% (at 6 L/min) can be achieved. Flow rates greater than 6 L/min do not significantly increase oxygenation because the **anatomic dead space** (places where air flows but the structures are too thick for gas exchange; includes the oral and nasal cavities, pharynx, trachea, mainstem bronchi, secondary bronchi, and smaller airways down to the alveolar ducts) is full. In addition, high flow rates increase mucosal irritation. With the use of a nasal cannula, an effective oxygen concentration can be delivered to both nose breathers and mouth breathers.

The nasal cannula is frequently used for chronic lung disease and for long-term maintenance of clients with other illnesses. The client who retains carbon dioxide rarely receives oxygen at a rate higher than 2 to 3 L/min because of the concern for losing the drive to breathe, increasing the risk for apnea or respiratory arrest. The nurse places the nasal prongs in the nostrils, with the openings facing the client.

SIMPLE FACE MASK. A simple face mask is used to deliver oxygen concentrations of 40% to 60% for short-term oxygen therapy or in an emergency (Figure 28-3). A minimum flow rate of 5 L/min is needed to prevent the rebreathing of exhaled air. The nurse gives special attention to skin care and to the proper fitting of the mask so that inspired oxygen concentration is maintained.

PARTIAL REBREATHER MASK. A partial rebreather mask provides oxygen concentrations of 60% to 75%, with flow rates of 6 to 11 L/min. It consists of a mask with a reservoir bag but no flaps (Figure 28-4). The client first rebreathes one third of the exhaled tidal volume, which is high in oxygen, thus providing a high fraction of inspired oxygen (FIO_2). The nurse ensures that the bag remains slightly inflated at the end of inspiration; otherwise, the client will not be getting the desired oxygen prescription. If needed, the nurse calls the respiratory therapist for assistance.

TABLE 28-1 • COMPARISON OF LOW-FLOW OXYGEN DELIVERY SYSTEMS

FIO_2 Delivered	Nursing Interventions	Rationale
NASAL CANNULA 24%-40% FIO_2 at 1-6 L/min ≈24% at 1 L/min ≈28% at 2 L/min ≈32% at 3 L/min ≈36% at 4 L/min ≈40% at 5 L/min ≈44% at 6 L/min	Ensure that prongs are in the nares properly.	A poorly fitting nasal cannula leads to hypoxemia and skin breakdown.
	Provide water-soluble jelly to nares prn.	This substance prevents mucosal irritation related to the drying effect of oxygen; promotes comfort.
	Assess the patency of the nostrils.	Congestion or a deviated septum prevents effective delivery of oxygen through the nares.
	Assess the client for changes in respiratory rate or depth.	The respiratory pattern affects the amount of oxygen delivered. A different delivery system may be needed.
SIMPLE FACE MASK 40%-60% FIO_2 at 5-8 L/min; flow rate must be set at at least 5 L/min to flush mask of carbon dioxide ≈40% at 5 L/min ≈45%-50% at 6 L/min ≈55%-60% at 8 L/min	Be sure mask fits securely over nose and mouth.	A poorly fitting mask reduces the FIO_2 delivered.
	Assess skin and provide skin care to the area covered by the mask.	Pressure and moisture under the mask may cause skin breakdown.
	Monitor the client closely for risk of aspiration.	The mask limits the client's ability to clear the mouth, especially if vomiting occurs.
	Provide emotional support to the client who feels claustrophobic.	Emotional support decreases anxiety, which contributes to a claustrophobic feeling.
	Suggest to the physician to switch the client from a mask to the nasal cannula during eating.	Use of the cannula prevents hypoxemia during eating.
PARTIAL REBREATHER MASK 60%-75% at 6-11 L/min, a liter flow rate high enough to maintain reservoir bag two-thirds full during inspiration and expiration	Make sure that the reservoir does not twist or kink, which results in a deflated bag.	Deflation results in decreased oxygen delivered and rebreathing of exhaled air.
	Adjust the flow rate to keep the reservoir bag inflated.	The flow rate is adjusted to meet the pattern of the client.
NON-REBREATHER MASK 80%-95% FIO_2 at liter flow to maintain reservoir bag two-thirds full	Interventions as for partial rebreather mask; this client requires close monitoring.	Rationales as for partial rebreather mask. Monitoring ensures proper functioning and prevents harm.
	Make sure that valves and rubber flaps are patent, functional, and not stuck. Remove mucus or saliva.	Valves should open during expiration and close during inhalation to prevent dramatic decrease in FIO_2. Suffocation can occur if the reservoir bag kinks or if the oxygen source disconnects.
	Closely assess the client on increased FIO_2 via non-rebreather mask. Intubation is the only way to provide more precise FIO_2.	The client may require intubation.

FIO_2, Fraction of inspired oxygen.

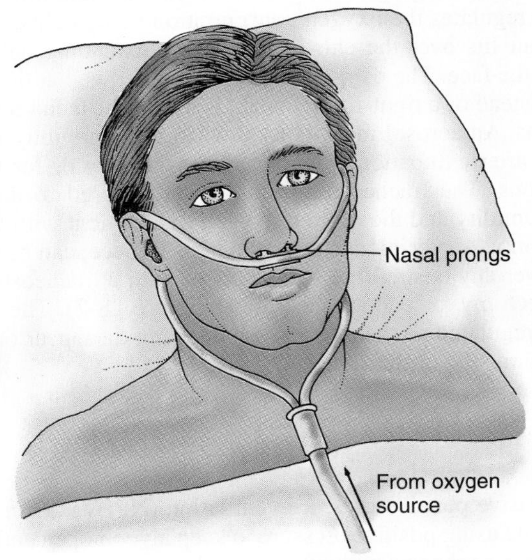

Figure 28-2 • A nasal cannula (prongs).

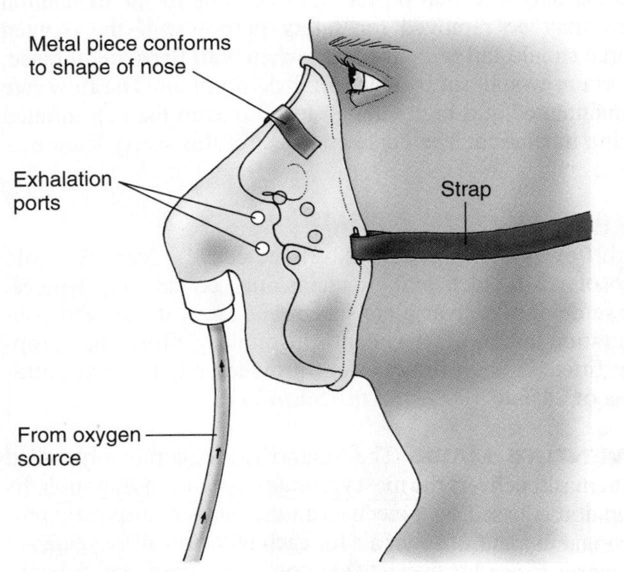

Figure 28-3 • A simple face mask used to deliver oxygen.

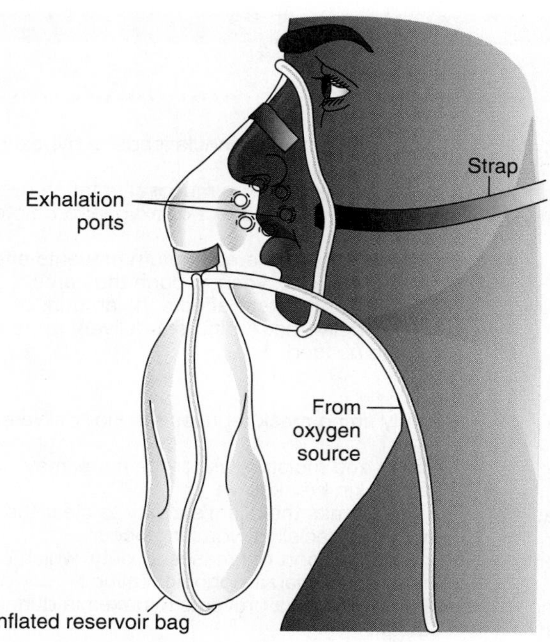

Figure 28-4 ● A partial rebreather mask.

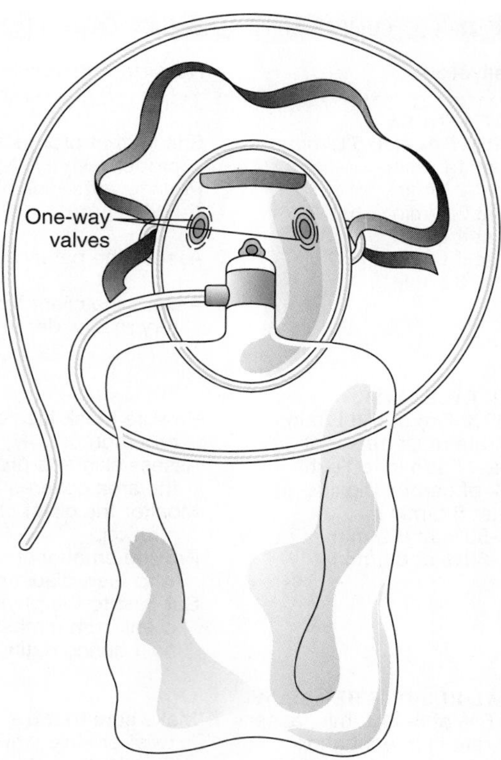

Figure 28-5 ● A non-rebreather mask.

NON-REBREATHER MASK. A non-rebreather mask provides the highest concentration of the low-flow systems and can deliver an FIO_2 greater than 90%, depending on the client's breathing pattern. The non-rebreather mask is used most often with deteriorating respiratory status who might soon require intubation.

The non-rebreather mask has a one-way valve between the mask and the reservoir and two flaps over the exhalation ports (Figure 28-5). The valve allows the client to draw all needed oxygen from the reservoir bag, and the flaps prevent room air from entering through the exhalation ports. During exhalation, air leaves through these exhalation ports while the one-way valve prevents exhaled air from re-entering the reservoir bag. It is crucial for the nurse to ensure that the valve and flaps are intact and functional during each breath. Some manufacturers include only one flap on the mask, or one of the exhalation flaps may be removed for safety purposes. If the oxygen source should fail or be depleted when both flaps are in place, the client would not be able to inhale room air. The flow rate is maintained at a high-enough level to keep the bag inflated during inhalation. The nurse assesses for this safety feature.

HIGH-FLOW OXYGEN DELIVERY SYSTEMS

High-flow systems (Table 28-2) include the Venturi mask, aerosol mask, face tent, tracheostomy collar, and T-piece. These devices deliver a consistent and accurate oxygen concentration that meets the client's inspiratory effort when properly fitted. A high-flow system provides oxygen concentrations of 24% to 100% at 8 to 15 L/min.

VENTURI MASK. The Venturi mask (commonly called Venti mask) delivers the most accurate oxygen concentration. Its operation is based on a mechanism that pulls in a specific proportional amount of room air for each liter flow of oxygen. An adaptor is located between the bottom of the mask and the oxygen source (Figure 28-6). Adaptors with holes of different sizes allow only specific amounts of air to mix with the oxygen. Precise delivery of oxygen results. Each adaptor also specifies the flow rate to be used; for example, to deliver 24% of oxygen, the flow rate must be 4 L/min. Another type of Venturi mask has one adaptor with a dial that the nurse uses to select the amount of oxygen desired. Humidification is not necessary with the Venturi mask. The Venturi system is best for the client with chronic lung disease because it delivers a precise oxygen concentration.

OTHER HIGH-FLOW SYSTEMS. The face tent, aerosol mask, tracheostomy collar, and T-piece are often used to administer high humidity. A dial on the humidification source regulates the oxygen concentration being delivered. A face tent fits over the chin, with the top extending halfway across the face. The oxygen concentration varies, but the face tent, instead of a tight-fitting mask, is useful for facial trauma or burns. An aerosol mask is used when high humidity is required after extubation or upper airway surgery or for thick secretions. The tracheostomy collar can be used to deliver high humidity and the desired oxygen to the client with a tracheostomy. A special adaptor, called the **T-piece,** can be used to deliver any desired FIO_2 to the client with a tracheostomy, laryngectomy, or endotracheal tube (Figure 28-7). The flow rate is regulated so that the aerosol does not disappear on the exhalation side of the T-piece.

NONINVASIVE POSITIVE-PRESSURE VENTILATION

Noninvasive positive-pressure ventilation (NPPV) is a newer technique using positive pressure to keep alveoli open and improve gas exchange without the need for airway intubation (Perkins & Shortall, 2000). This type of ventilation can de-

TABLE 28-2 • COMPARISON OF HIGH-FLOW OXYGEN DELIVERY SYSTEMS

FIO_2 Delivered	Nursing Interventions	Rationale
VENTURI MASK (VENTI MASK)		
24%-55% FIO_2 with flow rates as recommended by the manufacturer, usually 4-10 L/min; provides high humidity	Perform constant surveillance to ensure an accurate flow rate for the specific FIO_2.	An accurate flow rate ensures FIO_2 delivery.
	Keep the orifice for the Venturi adaptor open and uncovered.	If the Venturi orifice is covered, the adaptor does not function and oxygen delivery varies.
	Provide a mask that fits snugly and tubing that is free of kinks.	FIO_2 is altered if kinking occurs or if the mask fits poorly.
	Assess the client for dry mucous membranes.	Comfort measures may be indicated.
	Change to a nasal cannula during mealtimes.	Oxygen is a drug that needs to be given continuously.
AEROSOL MASK, FACE TENT, TRACHEOSTOMY COLLAR		
24%-100% FIO_2 with flow rates of at least 10 L/min; provides high humidity	Assess that aerosol mist escapes from the vents of the delivery system during inspiration and expiration.	Humidification should be delivered to the client.
	Empty condensation from the tubing.	Emptying prevents the client from being lavaged with water and promotes an adequate flow rate.
	Change the aerosol water container as needed.	Adequate humidification is ensured only when there is sufficient water in the canister.
T-PIECE		
24%-100% FIO_2 with flow rates of at least 10 L/min; provides high humidity	Empty condensation from the tubing.	Condensation interferes with flow rate and may drain into the tracheostomy if not emptied.
	Keep the exhalation port open and uncovered.	If the port is occluded, the client can suffocate.
	Position the T-piece so that it does not pull on the tracheostomy or endotracheal tube.	The weight of the T-piece pulls on the tracheostomy and causes pain or erosion of skin at the insertion site.
	Make sure the humidifier creates enough mist. A mist should be seen during inspiration and expiration.	An adequate flow rate is needed to meet the inspiration effort of the client. If not, FIO_2 is decreased.

FIO_2, Fraction of inspired oxygen.

liver oxygen or may just use room air. Essentially, a nasal mask or full-face mask delivery system allows mechanical delivery of either bi-level positive airway pressure (BiPAP) or continuous nasal positive airway pressure.

For BiPAP, a cycling machine delivers a set inspiratory positive airway pressure each time the client begins to inspire. As the client begins to exhale, the machine delivers a lower set end expiratory pressure. Together, these two pressures improve tidal volume.

Nasal continuous positive airway pressure delivers a set positive airway pressure continually throughout each cycle of inhalation and exhalation. The effect is to open collapsed alveoli. Clients who might benefit from this form of oxygen or air delivery include those with postoperative atelectasis or cardiac-induced pulmonary edema. This technique is also used for sleep apnea. The effect of this use is to hold open the upper airways.

TRANSTRACHEAL OXYGEN THERAPY

Transtracheal oxygen (TTO) is a long-term method of delivering oxygen directly into the lungs. The physician passes a small, flexible catheter into the trachea via a small incision (Figure 28-8) with the use of local anesthesia. TTO allows better compliance and avoids the irritation that nasal prongs cause. Clients also report it to be more cosmetically acceptable. A TTO team provides formal client education, including the purpose of TTO and care of the catheter. The physician prescribes a TTO flow rate for rest and for activity and a flow rate for the nasal cannula, to be used when the TTO catheter is being cleaned. The average client will have a 55% reduction in required oxygen flow at rest and a 30% decrease with activity.

Community-Based Care

HOME CARE MANAGEMENT

CRITERIA FOR HOME OXYGEN THERAPY. The client must be clinically stable and optimally treated before the need for home oxygen is considered. For Medicare to cover the cost of continuous oxygen therapy, the client must have severe hypoxemia. For reimbursement purposes, severe hypoxemia is generally defined as a partial pressure of arterial oxygen (PaO_2) level of less than 55 mm Hg or an arterial oxygen saturation (SaO_2) of less than 88% on room air and at rest. The criteria are variable when hypoxemia is caused by cardiac rather than pulmonary problems, or when oxygen is needed only at night or with exercise.

CLIENT EDUCATION. After the need for home oxygen therapy is verified, the nurse begins a teaching plan about oxygen therapy. The client, with the nurse's assistance, selects a durable medical equipment (DME) company to deliver oxygen equipment and a community health nursing agency for follow-up care in the home. The physician re-evaluates the

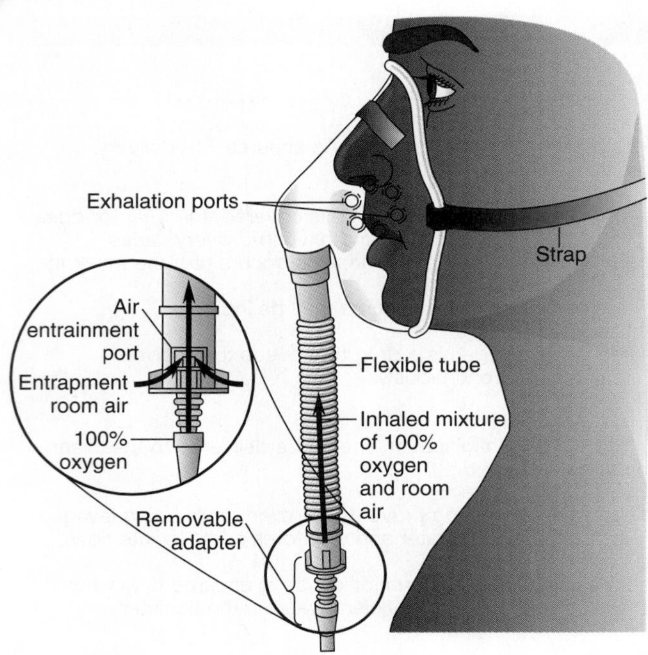

Figure 28-6 ● A Venturi mask for precise oxygen delivery.

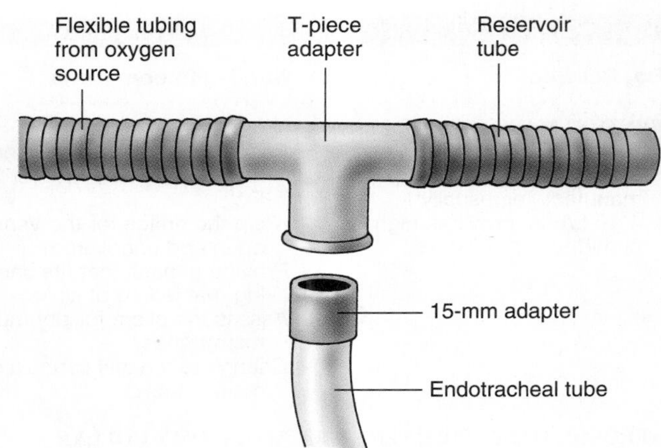

Figure 28-7 ● A T-piece apparatus for attachment to an endotracheal or tracheostomy tube.

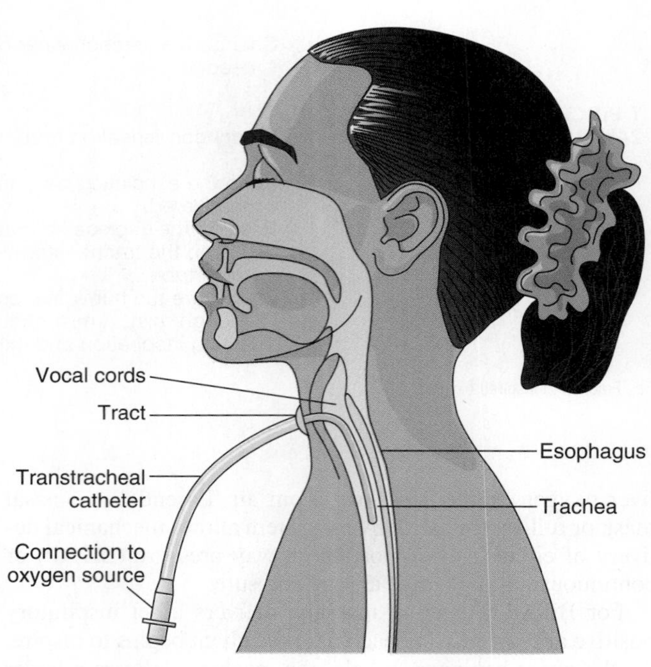

Figure 28-8 ● Example of transtracheal oxygen delivery.

need for oxygen therapy approximately 6 months after discharge from the health care facility and yearly thereafter.

While providing discharge planning and teaching, the nurse is sensitive to the client's psychologic adjustment to oxygen therapy. The nurse encourages the client to share feelings and concerns. The client may be concerned about social acceptance and misconceptions of friends. The nurse helps him or her realize that compliance with oxygen therapy is important so that normal activities of daily living (ADLs) and events that bring enjoyment can be continued.

HOME CARE PREPARATION

EQUIPMENT FOR HOME OXYGEN THERAPY. The nurse or respiratory therapist teaches the client about the equipment needed for home oxygen therapy:

- Oxygen source
- Oxygen delivery device
- Humidification source
- Safety aspects of using and maintaining the equipment

Home oxygen therapy is provided in one of three ways: compressed gas in a tank or a cylinder, liquid oxygen in a reservoir, or an oxygen concentrator. Compressed gas in an oxygen tank (green) is the most common oxygen source. An oxygen tank is economical, and pure oxygen can be delivered at a wide range of flow rates. The large H cylinder may be used as a stationary source; the small E tank is available for transporting the client (Figure 28-9). As a safety precaution, the tanks must always be in a stand or rack. A tank that is accidentally knocked over could suddenly decompress and move around in an uncontrolled manner. Even smaller (and lighter) D or C cylinders are available for the client to carry.

The second type of home oxygen, **liquid oxygen,** is oxygen gas that has been liquefied by cooling to −300° F (−147° C); thus a concentrated amount of oxygen is available in a lightweight and easy-to-carry container similar to a Thermos bottle (Figure 28-10). The client is able to fill the portable tank from the large stationary liquid vessel. This type of oxygen lasts longer than oxygen in a conventional tank of the same size; however, it is expensive, and the oxygen evaporates if it is not used continuously.

The last type of home oxygen source is the **oxygen concentrator,** which is a machine that removes nitrogen, water vapor, and hydrocarbons from room air. It is sometimes referred to as an **oxygen extractor.** Oxygen is concentrated from room air and is delivered at more than 90%. The concentrator, although noisy and not portable, is the most common stationary oxygen delivery system used in the home. Portable tanks are used when the client leaves home. The major advantages of the concentrator are that it is the least expensive of the systems and does not need to be filled.

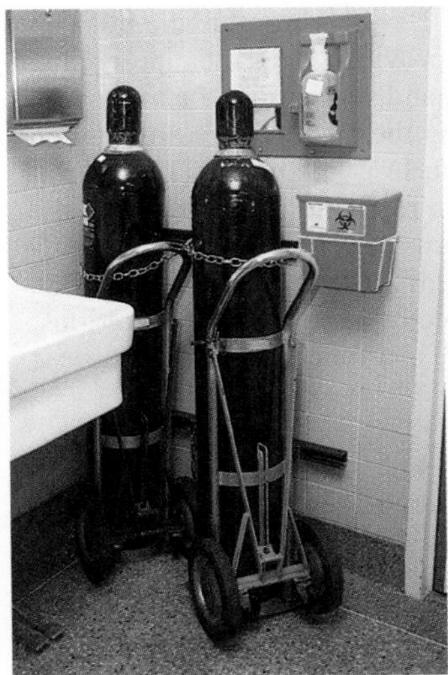

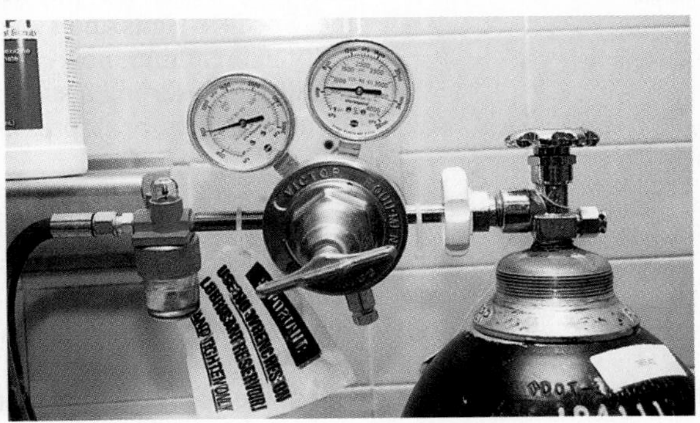

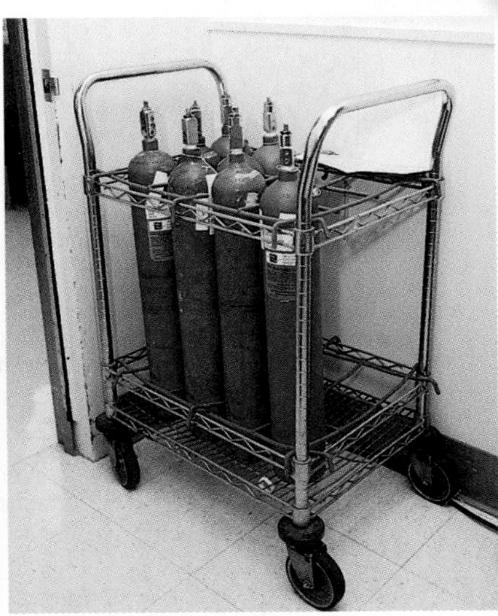

Figure 28-9 ● Comparison of a large H oxygen cylinder, with a stand *(left)*, regulator, and flowmeter *(middle)*, and several small E cylinders *(right)*.

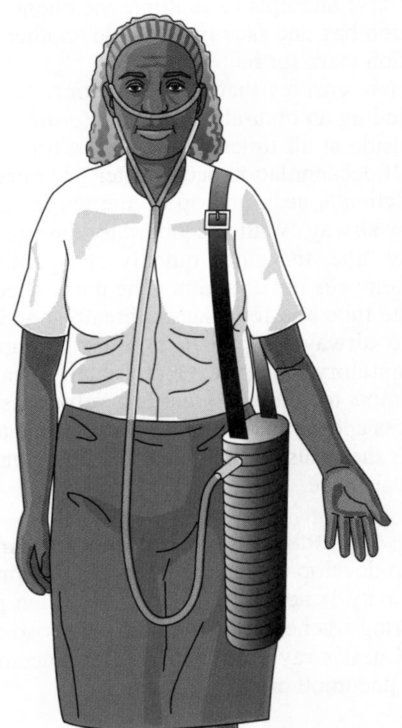

Figure 28-10 ● Liquid oxygen.

Humidification is rarely needed for any of these oxygen systems. Humidification may be helpful, however, when the prescribed flow rate is higher than 4 L/min.

In any of the three home oxygen systems, an oxygen-conserving reservoir-type nasal cannula can be used to reduce oxygen flow requirements by approximately 50%. Two types currently available are the mustache type and the pendant type. Attached to the tubing is a reservoir where exhaled oxygen is stored and then redelivered back to the client on the next inhalation. The reservoir sits on top of the upper lip (mustache type) or hangs around the neck (pendant type).

TABLE 28-3 • INDICATIONS FOR TRACHEOSTOMY

- Acute airway obstruction when oral or nasal intubation is not feasible
- Airway protection (e.g., after head and neck cancer surgery)
- Prolonged intubation or need for mechanical ventilation
- Decreased airway dead space in combination with other indicators
- Control of pulmonary secretions refractory to conventional methods
- Airway reconstruction after laryngeal trauma or laryngeal cancer surgery
- Obstructive sleep apnea refractory to conventional therapy

TRACHEOSTOMY

OVERVIEW

Tracheotomy is the surgical incision into the trachea for the purpose of establishing an airway. **Tracheostomy** is the (tracheal) stoma, or opening, that results from the tracheotomy. A tracheostomy can be performed as an emergency procedure or as a scheduled surgical procedure and can be temporary or permanent. Indications for tracheostomy are listed in Table 28-3. Tracheostomy as an emergency procedure for upper airway obstruction is covered in Chapter 29.

COLLABORATIVE MANAGEMENT

Once the determination of need for a tracheostomy has been established, the nurse prepares the client for surgery.

Preoperative Care

The preoperative care for the client undergoing a tracheostomy is similar to that for a laryngectomy (see Chapter 29). The nurse focuses on the client's knowledge deficits

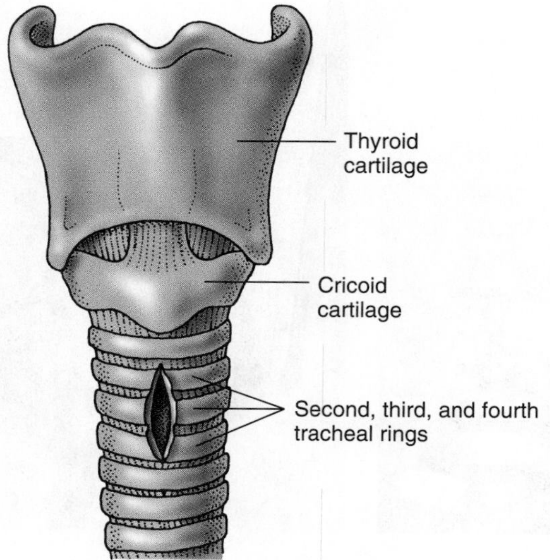

Figure 28-11 ● A vertical tracheal incision for a tracheostomy.

through teaching and discusses tracheostomy care, communication, and speech.

Operative Procedures

Initially, the anesthesiologist or nurse anesthetist extends the neck and places an endotracheal (ET) tube to maintain the airway. The surgeon then makes an incision through the anterior skin of the neck, dissects the subcutaneous tissue for exposure, separates the thyroid, and identifies the thyroid artery and tracheal rings. Another incision is made through the second and third or third and fourth tracheal rings to enter the trachea (Figure 28-11). The types of incisions and specific techniques vary, depending on the surgeon's preference and the reason for the surgery.

After the surgeon enters the trachea, the ET tube is carefully removed while the tracheostomy tube is inserted. The surgeon secures the tracheostomy tube in place with sutures and tracheostomy ties (or Velcro tube holders) and orders a chest x-ray study to ensure proper placement of the tube. If intubation is not possible, a tracheostomy can be done with the client awake under local anesthesia.

Postoperative Care

Immediate postoperative nursing care focuses on ensuring a patent airway, confirming the presence of bilateral breath sounds, recovering the client from anesthesia, and assessing for complications from the procedure.

COMPLICATIONS

Six major complications may arise in the postoperative period: tube obstruction with secretions, tube dislodgment or accidental decannulation, pneumothorax, subcutaneous emphysema, bleeding, and infection. Table 28-4 summarizes signs and symptoms, management, and prevention of other serious complications of tracheostomy.

TUBE OBSTRUCTION. By helping the client with coughing and deep breathing, providing inner cannula care, humidifying the oxygen source, and suctioning, the nurse prevents secretions from obstructing the tube. If tube obstruction occurs as a result of cuff prolapse over the end of the tracheostomy tube, the physician repositions or replaces the tube. Specific signs and symptoms of obstruction include difficulty in breathing; noisy respirations from the tracheostomy; difficulty in inserting a suction catheter; thick, dry secretions; and unexplained peak pressures if a mechanical ventilator is in use.

TUBE DISLODGMENT OR ACCIDENTAL DECANNULATION. The nurse prevents tube dislodgment and decannulation by securing the tube in place, thus minimizing manipulation and traction on the tube from oxygen or ventilator tubing or accidental pulling by the client. Tube dislodgment in the first 72 hours after surgery is a medical emergency because the tracheostomy tract has not matured and tissue planes are not well defined. Attempts at replacement of a fresh tracheostomy tube can lead to cannulation of subcutaneous tissue planes instead of the trachea itself. In this situation, the nurse attempts to ventilate the client using a manual resuscitation bag and face mask while another nurse calls the resuscitation team for help.

The nurse ensures that a tracheostomy tube of the same type (including an obturator) and size (or one size smaller) is at the bedside at all times, along with a tracheostomy insertion tray. If decannulation occurs after 72 hours, the nurse extends the client's neck and opens the tissues of the stoma to secure the airway. With the obturator inserted into the tracheostomy tube, the nurse quickly and gently replaces the tube and removes the obturator. The nurse checks for airflow through the tube and for bilateral breath sounds. If unable to secure the airway, the nurse notifies a more experienced nurse, respiratory therapist, or physician for assistance. The nurse attempts to ventilate via a bag-valve mask. If the client is in distress and further attempts to secure the airway fail, the nurse calls the resuscitation team, including an anesthesiologist, for assistance.

PNEUMOTHORAX. **Pneumothorax** (air in the chest cavity) can develop during the tracheostomy procedure if the thoracic cavity is accidentally entered. When pneumothorax occurs during tracheotomy, it usually does so at the apex of the lung. Chest x-ray examination after placement is used to assess for pneumothorax.

SUBCUTANEOUS EMPHYSEMA. When there is an opening (rent) in the trachea, air escapes into fresh tissue planes of the neck, causing subcutaneous emphysema. Air can also progress throughout the chest and axillary tissues into the face. The nurse inspects and palpates for air under the skin of a client with a new tracheostomy.

BLEEDING. A small amount of bleeding from the tracheostomy incision can be expected for the first few days, but constant oozing warrants surgical intervention, cauterization, or ligation of vessels. The nurse wraps gauze around the tube and packs it gently into the wound to apply pressure to the bleeding sites.

TABLE 28-4 • COMPLICATIONS OF TRACHEOSTOMY

Complications and Description	Signs and Symptoms	Management	Prevention
Tracheomalacia: constant pressure exerted by the cuff causes tracheal dilation and erosion of cartilage.	An increased amount of air is required in the cuff to maintain the seal. A larger tracheostomy tube is required to prevent an air leak at the stoma. Food particles are seen in tracheal secretions. The client does not receive the set tidal volume on the ventilator.	No special management is needed unless bleeding occurs.	Use an uncuffed tube as soon as possible. Monitor cuff pressure and air volumes closely and detect changes.
Tracheal stenosis: narrowed tracheal lumen is due to scar formation from irritation of tracheal mucosa by the cuff.	Stenosis usually seen after the cuff is deflated or the tracheostomy tube is removed. The client has increased coughing, inability to expectorate secretions, or difficulty in breathing or talking.	Tracheal dilation or surgical intervention is used.	Prevent pulling of and traction on the tracheostomy tube. Properly secure the tube in the midline position. Maintain proper cuff pressure. Minimize oronasal intubation time.
Tracheoesophageal fistula (TEF): excessive cuff pressure causes erosion of the posterior wall of the trachea. A hole is created between the trachea and the anterior esophagus. The client at highest risk also has a nasogastric tube present.	Similar to tracheomalacia: • Food particles are seen in tracheal secretions. • Increased air in cuff is needed to achieve a seal. • The client has increased coughing and choking while eating. • The client does not receive the set tidal volume on the ventilator.	Manually administer oxygen by mask to prevent hypoxemia. A small soft feeding tube is used instead of a nasogastric tube for tube feedings. A gastrostomy or jejunostomy may be performed. Monitor the client with a nasogastric tube closely; assess for TEF and aspiration.	Maintain cuff pressure. Monitor the amount of air needed for inflation and detect changes. Progress to a deflated cuff or cuffless tube as soon as possible.
Trachea-innominate artery fistula: a malpositioned tube causes its distal tip to push against the lateral wall of the tracheostomy. Continued pressure causes necrosis and erosion of the innominate artery. ***This is a medical emergency.***	The tracheostomy tube pulsates in synchrony with the heartbeat. There is heavy bleeding from the stoma. This is a life-threatening complication.	Remove the tracheostomy tube immediately. Apply direct pressure to the innominate artery at the stoma site. Prepare the client for immediate repair surgery.	Correct the tube size, length, and midline position. Prevent pulling or tugging on the tracheostomy tube. Immediately notify the physician of the pulsating tube.

INFECTION. While in the hospital, the nurse uses sterile technique to prevent infection during suctioning and tracheostomy care and assesses the stoma site for purulent drainage, redness, pain, swelling, or cellulitis. Tracheostomy dressings may be used to keep the stoma clean and dry; moist dressings provide an excellent medium for bacterial growth. Prevention and early detection of a local infection are therefore important. Diligent wound care prevents most local infections.

TRACHEOSTOMY TUBES

A variety of tracheostomy tubes are available (Table 28-5 and Figure 28-12). The one chosen depends on the specific needs of the client. Tracheostomy tubes are available in numerous sizes and are made of various types of materials, such as plastic or metal. The tubes may be disposable or reusable. A tracheostomy tube may or may not have a cuff. It also may have an inner cannula that can be either disposable or reusable. For clients receiving mechanical ventilation, a cuffed tube is used in acute care settings. A noncuffed tube is used for airway maintenance when mechanical ventilation is not required.

For tubes with an inner cannula, the nurse inspects, suctions, and cleans the inner cannula. During the immediate postoperative period, the nurse may provide cannula care frequently as needed, perhaps every 30 to 60 minutes. Thereafter care is usually determined by the client's needs and agency policy. In planning for self-care, the nurse teaches the client to remove the inner cannula and check for cleanliness. As teaching progresses, the nurse also instructs about suctioning and tracheostomy cleaning.

Because movement of breathing and swallowing moves the tube, a cuffed tube is not protective against aspiration. Having a cuffed tube inflated may give the nurse or other caregiver a false sense of security that aspiration cannot occur during activities such as feeding or mouth care (St. John, 1999). In addition, the pilot balloon does not reflect whether the correct amount of air is present in the cuff.

A fenestrated tube can function in many different ways. When the inner cannula is in place, the fenestration is covered over (closed), and the tube functions as a double-lumen tube. With the inner cannula removed and the plug or red decannulation stopper locked in place, air can pass through the

TABLE 28-5 • TYPES OF TRACHEOSTOMY TUBES

DOUBLE-LUMEN TUBE

The double-lumen tube has three major parts:

- Outer cannula—fits into the stoma and keeps the airway open. The faceplate indicates the size and type of tube and has small holes on both sides for securing the tube with tracheostomy ties.
- Inner cannula—fits snugly into the outer cannula and locks into place. Provides the universal adaptor for use with the ventilator and other respiratory therapy equipment. Some may be removed, cleaned, and reused; others are disposable.
- Obturator—is a stylet with a blunt end used to facilitate the direction of the tube when inserting or changing a tracheostomy tube. It is removed immediately after tube placement and is always kept with the client and at the bedside in case of accidental decannulation.

SINGLE-LUMEN TUBE

The single-lumen tube is a long tube used for clients with long or extra-thick necks. Often called a "bull neck trach" because of the long distance from the skin to the trachea or the longer length of the trachea in large people. More intensive nursing care is required with this tube because there is no inner cannula to ensure a patent lumen.

CUFFED TUBE

A cuff, when inflated, seals the airway. Used with mechanical ventilation, in preventing aspiration of oral or gastric secretions, or for tube feeding. A pilot balloon attached to the outside of the tube indicates the presence or absence of air in the cuff.

CUFFLESS TUBE

The cuffless tube is a plastic, silicone-like (Silastic), or metal tube, usually double lumen. Used for long-term airway management in those clients who require a tracheostomy, who can protect themselves from aspiration, and who do not require mechanical ventilation. Many people can speak with this tube in place.

FENESTRATED TUBE

The fenestrated tube has a precut opening (fenestration) in the upper posterior wall of the outer cannula. It is used to wean the client from a tracheostomy by ensuring that the client can tolerate breathing through his or her natural airway before the entire tube is removed. This tube allows the client to speak.

CUFFED FENESTRATED TUBE

The cuffed fenestrated tube facilitates mechanical ventilation and speech. It is often used for clients with spinal cord paralysis or neuromuscular disease who do not require ventilation all the time. When not on the ventilator, the client can have the cuff deflated and the tube capped for speech. A cuffed fenestrated tube is never used in weaning from a tracheostomy because the cuff, even fully deflated, may partially obstruct the airway.

METAL TRACHEOSTOMY TUBE

The metal tracheostomy tube is used for permanent tracheostomy. It is a cuffless double-lumen tube and can be cleaned and reused indefinitely. A special adaptor attaches a manual resuscitation bag. Popular types are the Jackson and Holinger tubes.

TALKING TRACHEOSTOMY TUBE

The talking tracheostomy tube provides a means of communication for the client who is using a ventilator on a long-term basis. An extra air channel allows air to flow up through the vocal cords so that the client can speak with the cuff inflated. The air can cause drying of the vocal cords from constant dry airflow. Examples are the Pitt Trach Speaking Tube (National Catheter Corporation) and Communitrach (Implant Technologies, Inc.).

fenestration, as well as around the tube and up through the natural airway. The client can cough and speak, becoming reaccustomed to breathing through the upper air passages. If the client has trouble with any of these maneuvers, the nurse, respiratory therapist, and physician evaluate him or her for proper tube placement, patency, size, and fenestration. The nurse does not cap the tube until the problem is identified and corrected. A fenestrated tube may or may not have a cuff.

With a cuffed fenestrated tube, some air flows through the natural airway when the client is not depending on mechanical ventilation. *The nurse always deflates the cuff before capping the tube with the decannulation cap; otherwise, the client has no airway* (Figure 28-13).

Care Issues for the Client with a Tracheostomy

PREVENTION OF TISSUE DAMAGE

Tissue damage can occur at the point where the inflated cuff presses against the tracheal mucosa. Mucosal ischemia occurs when the pressure of the cuff exerted on the mucosa exceeds the capillary perfusion pressure. To reduce the incidence of tracheal damage, the nurse ensures a cuff pressure between 14 and 20 mm Hg.

Most cuffs are designed to use a high volume of air while maintaining a low pressure on the tracheal mucosa. The nurse inflates the cuff to provide an adequate seal between the trachea and the cuff while creating the least amount of pressure. If the cuff cannot be inflated to seal well enough, a larger-diameter tube may be needed. There are two methods of cuff inflation: the **minimal leak technique** (for cuffs without pressure relief valves) and the **occlusive technique** (for cuffs with pressure relief valves).

The nurse checks the cuff pressure during each shift, especially with the minimal leak technique, and maintains the pressure at 14 to 20 mm Hg. In rare situations, the cuff pressure is increased to maintain ventilator volumes when peak pressures are greater than 50 mm Hg and positive end-expiratory pressure (PEEP) is greater than 10 mm Hg. Manufacturers provide guidelines for the approximate recommended volumes allowed for each tracheostomy cuff size. Most cuffs are sufficiently inflated with less than 10 mL of air.

Although a high cuff pressure causes tracheal damage, other factors contribute to the severity of the damage. The client's condition determines, to a degree, susceptibility to tissue damage. The client who is malnourished, hypotensive, dehydrated, hypoxic, an older adult, or receiving corticosteroids is unable to promote adequate tissue healing and is vulnerable to further tissue damage. The duration of intubation, extent and technique of suctioning, and stabilization of the tube against friction and

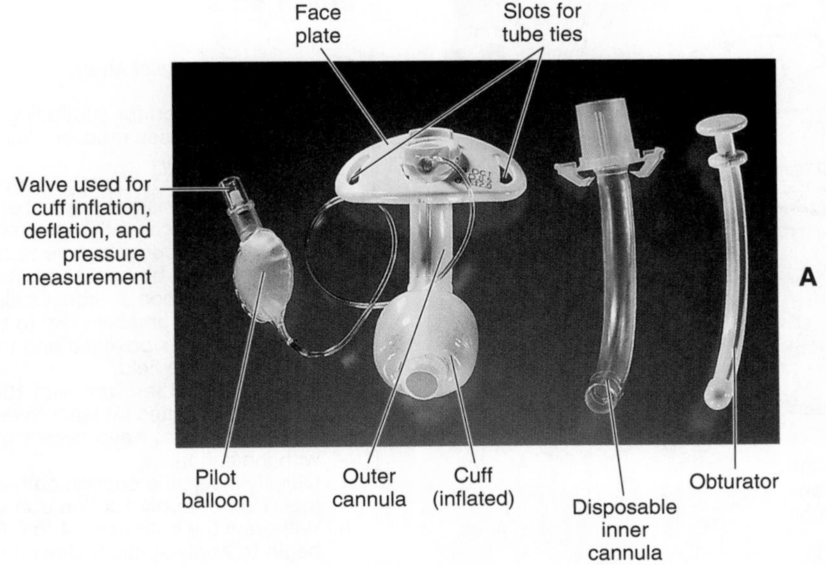

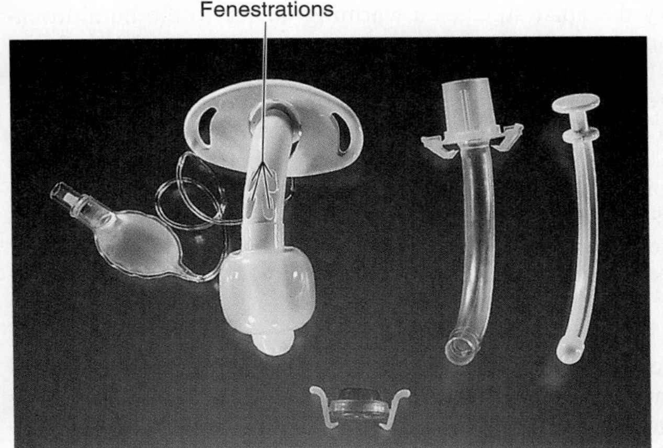

Figure 28-12 ● Tracheostomy tubes. **A,** Dual-lumen cuffed tracheostomy tube with disposable inner cannula. **B,** Single-lumen cannula cuffed tracheostomy tube. **C,** Dual-lumen cannula cuffed fenestrated tracheostomy tube. (Courtesy Mallinckrodt, Inc., Shiley Tracheostomy Products, St. Louis, MO.)

movement are important factors that determine the extent of tracheal mucosa damage. The nurse minimizes local airway damage by maintaining proper cuff pressures, stabilizing the tube, suctioning judiciously, and preventing and treating malnutrition, hemodynamic instability, or hypoxia.

A newer experimental tube design uses a series of 8 to 20 thin, pliable sheets, or "gills," in place of a cuff. These gills are soft enough to conform to the shape of the trachea and form a no-pressure seal with minimal leakage. Although more testing needs to be done regarding the long-term effects of this system, this alternative shows promise of additional comfort and safety (St. John, 1999).

HUMIDIFICATION AND WARMING OF AIR

The tracheostomy tube bypasses the upper air passages of the nose and mouth, which normally humidify, warm, and filter the air before it reaches the lower part of the respiratory tract. If humidification and warming are not adequate, tracheal damage can result from extremes in humidity and air temperature. In addition, thick, dried secretions can occlude the airways.

To prevent these complications, the nurse provides humidification, as ordered. The nurse then assesses, on an ongoing basis, for a fine mist emerging from the tracheostomy collar or T-piece during inspiration and expiration. To increase the amount of humidification delivered, the respira-

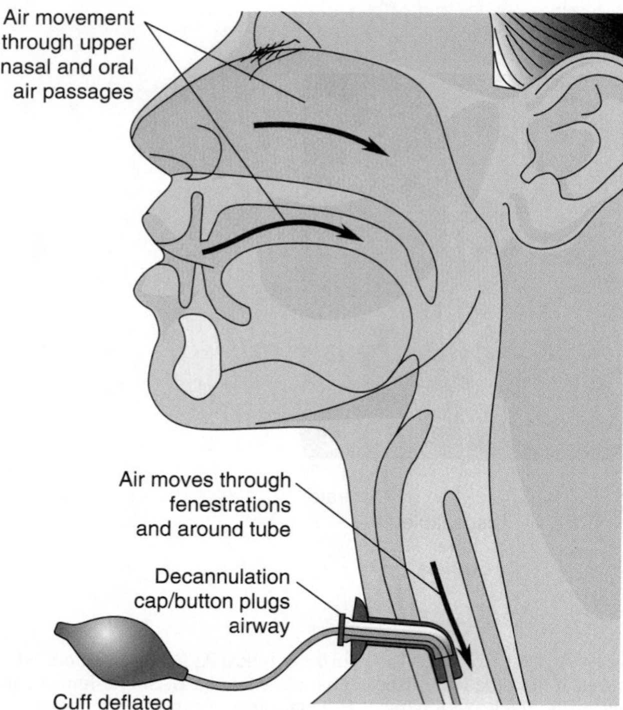

Figure 28-13 ● Breathing through a fenestrated tracheostomy tube with a cap in place and the cuff deflated.

CHART 28-3

BEST PRACTICE *for* Suctioning the Artificial Airway

1. Assess the need for suctioning (routine unnecessary suctioning causes mucosal damage, bleeding, and bronchospasm).
2. Wash hands. Don protective eyewear. Maintain standard precautions or body substance precautions.
3. Explain to the client that sensations such as shortness of breath and coughing are to be expected but that any discomfort will be very short in duration.
4. Check the suction source. Occlude the suction source, and adjust the pressure dial to between 80 and 120 mm Hg to prevent hypoxemia and trauma to the mucosa.
5. Set up a sterile field.
6. Preoxygenate the client with 100% oxygen for 30 seconds to 3 minutes (at least three hyperinflations) to prevent hypoxemia. Keep hyperinflations synchronized with inhalation.
7. Quickly insert the suction catheter until resistance is met. Do not apply suction during insertion.
8. Withdraw the catheter 0.4 to 0.8 inch (1 to 2 cm), and begin to apply suction. Use intermittent suction and a twirling motion of the catheter during withdrawal. *Never suction longer than 10 to 15 seconds.*
9. Hyperoxygenate for 1 to 5 minutes or until the client's baseline heart rate and oxygen saturation are within normal limits.
10. Repeat as needed for up to three total suction passes.
11. Suction mouth as needed, and provide mouth care.
12. Describe secretions, and document client's responses.

tory therapist attaches a warming device to the humidification source. At the same time, a temperature probe is placed in the tubing circuit. The temperature is constantly monitored and is generally maintained between 98.6° and 100.4° F (37° and 38° C); it is not allowed to exceed 104° F (40° C). The nurse monitors the circuit temperature by feeling the tubing and by checking the temperature probe. In addition, the nurse ensures adequate hydration, which also helps to liquefy secretions.

SUCTIONING

Suctioning maintains a patent airway and promotes gas exchange by removing secretions from the client who cannot cough adequately. Chart 28-3 lists best practices for suctioning. The nurse assesses the client's need for suction, which is indicated by audible or noisy secretions, crackles or rhonchi on auscultation, restlessness, increased pulse or respiratory rates, presence of mucus in the artificial airway, client requests for suctioning, or an increase in the peak airway pressure on the ventilator.

Suctioning is performed most often through an artificial airway but can be accomplished either through the nose or the mouth. Suctioning of both routes is considered routine for the client with retained secretions.

The technique of suctioning through the nose is associated with similar complications as suctioning through an artificial airway. Entry through the nasal vault into the nasopharynx can be painful. Slow, careful placement of the catheter, with a good understanding of the nasopharyngeal anatomy, can make the procedure less traumatic. The nurse may place a nasopharyngeal airway through which to suction to prevent trauma to the nasal mucosa. The catheter is advanced through the nasopharynx and into the laryngopharynx while the client receives oxygen by mask or nasal cannula. Once the catheter enters the larynx, the client may cough. On inhalation, the nurse inserts the catheter through the vocal cords and into the trachea. Occasionally, the catheter can be disconnected from suction and attached to an oxygen source, with the client receiving oxygen via the catheter.

Suctioning is associated with several complications, including hypoxia, tissue (mucosal) trauma, infection, vagal stimulation, and bronchospasm.

HYPOXIA. The following are causes of hypoxia in the client with a tracheostomy:

- Ineffective oxygenation before, during, and after suctioning
- Use of a catheter that is too large for the artificial airway
- Prolonged suctioning time
- Excessive suction pressure
- Too frequent suctioning

The nurse prevents hypoxia by hyperoxygenating the client with 100% oxygen from an oxygen delivery device (manual resuscitation bag attached to an oxygen source). If the client is able to take deep breaths, the nurse instructs him or her to do so three or four times with the existing oxygen delivery system before suctioning. If possible, simultaneous monitoring of the heart rate or use of a pulse oximeter is helpful in assessing tolerance of the suctioning procedure. The nurse assesses for signs and symptoms of hypoxia (e.g., increased heart rate and blood pressure, oxygen desaturation, cyanosis, restlessness, anxiety, and cardiac dysrhythmias). Oxygen desaturation below 90% as determined by pulse oximetry indicates hypoxemia. If hypoxia occurs, the nurse terminates the suctioning procedure. Using the 100% oxygen delivery system, the client is reoxygenated until baseline parameters are achieved.

The nurse also prevents hypoxia by using a catheter of the correct size. The size should not exceed half of the size of the tracheal lumen. In adults the standard catheter size is 12 or 14 Fr. Adequate catheter size facilitates efficient removal of secretions without causing hypoxemia.

TISSUE TRAUMA. The mucosa of the respiratory tract is extremely fragile, and frequent suctioning, prolonged suctioning time, excessive suction pressure, and nonrotation of the catheter cause damage. The nurse prevents tissue trauma by suctioning only when indicated. The catheter is lubricated with sterile water or saline before insertion, and suction is applied only during the withdrawal of the catheter. Use of a twirling motion during withdrawal prevents excessive grabbing of the mucosa.

In addition, the nurse applies suction intermittently for only 10 to 15 seconds. The nurse can estimate this time frame by holding his or her own breath and counting to 10 or 15 during suctioning. At the end of the 15 seconds the suctioning procedure is finished. Fifteen seconds does not seem long to a healthy person, but most clients requiring suctioning have respiratory compromise and cannot tolerate more than 15 seconds of suctioning.

INFECTION. Each catheter pass introduces bacteria into the trachea. In the hospital the nurse uses sterile technique for suctioning and for all suctioning equipment, including suction catheters, gloves, and saline or water. After suctioning the artificial airway, the nurse then suctions the mouth. *Oral suction equipment is never used for suctioning an artificial airway, because the mouth is contaminated with bacteria, which could be introduced into the lungs.* Home suctioning procedures emphasize clean technique, because the number of virulent organisms in the home environment is lower than in the hospital.

VAGAL STIMULATION AND BRONCHOSPASM. Vagal stimulation results in severe bradycardia, hypotension, heart block, ventricular tachycardia, or asystole. *If vagal stimulation occurs, the nurse stops suctioning immediately and oxygenates the client manually with 100% oxygen.* Bronchospasm sometimes occurs when the catheter passes into the airway. The client may need a bronchodilator to relieve bronchospasm and respiratory distress.

TRACHEOSTOMY CARE

Tracheostomy care keeps the tracheostomy tube free of obstructing secretions, maintains a patent airway, and provides wound care. This procedure is performed whether or not the client is able to clear secretions. The nurse performs tracheostomy care according to agency policy, usually every shift and as needed. Chart 28-4 outlines best practices for tracheostomy care.

Before proceeding with tracheostomy care, the nurse assesses the client as shown in Chart 28-5. The extent of both suctioning and tracheostomy care depends entirely on the needs of the client. The need for suctioning and tracheostomy care is determined by the amount and consistency of secretions, medical diagnosis (specifically pulmonary diseases), ability of the client to cough and deep breathe, need for mechanical ventilation, and wound care required. The nurse inspects the inner lumen of a single-lumen tube with a flashlight or penlight to assess for the presence of secretions.

Tracheostomy tubes are secured in place using either twill tape ties or Velcro tracheostomy tube holders. Both devices re-

CHART 28-4

BEST PRACTICE *for* Tracheostomy Care

1. Assemble the necessary equipment.
2. Wash hands. Maintain standard precautions or body substance precautions.
3. Suction the tracheostomy tube if necessary.
4. Remove old dressings and excess secretions.
5. Set up a sterile field.
6. Remove and clean the inner cannula. Use half-strength hydrogen peroxide to clean the cannula and sterile saline to rinse it. If the inner cannula is disposable, remove the cannula and replace it with a new one.
7. Clean the stoma site and then the tracheostomy plate with half-strength hydrogen peroxide followed by sterile saline. Ensure that none of the solutions enters the tracheostomy.
8. Change tracheostomy ties if they are soiled. Secure new ties in place before removing soiled ones to prevent accidental decannulation. If a knot is needed, tie a square knot that is visible on the side of the neck. One or two fingers should be able to be placed between the tie tape and the neck.
9. Document the type and amount of secretions and the general condition of the stoma and surrounding skin. Document the client's response to the procedure and any teaching or learning that occurred.

CHART 28-5

FOCUSED ASSESSMENT *of* The Client with a Tracheostomy

Note the quality, pattern, and rate of breathing:
- Within client's baseline?
  - Tachypnea can indicate hypoxia.
  - Dyspnea can indicate secretions in the airway.

Assess for any cyanosis, especially around the lips, which could indicate hypoxia.
Check the client's pulse oximetry reading.
If oxygen is ordered, is the client receiving the correct amount, with the correct equipment and humidification?
Assess the tracheostomy site:
- Note the color, consistency, and amount of secretions in the tube or externally.
- If the tracheostomy is sutured in place, is there any redness, swelling, or drainage from suture sites?
- If the tracheostomy is secured with ties, what is the condition of the ties? Are they moist with secretions or perspiration? Are the secretions dried on the ties? Is the tie secure?
- Assess the condition of the skin around the tracheostomy and neck. Be sure to check underneath the neck for secretions that may have drained to the back. Check for any breakdown related to pressure from the ties or from excess secretions.
- Assess behind the faceplate for the size of the space between the outer cannula and the client's tissue. Are any secretions collected in this area?

If the tube is cuffed, check cuff pressure.
Auscultate the lungs.
Is a second (emergency) tracheostomy tube and obturator available?

EVIDENCE-BASED PRACTICE FOR NURSING

Are we being "penny-wise and pound foolish"?

Dixon, L., & Wasson, D. (1998). Comparing use and cost effectiveness of tracheostomy tube securing devices. *MEDSURG Nursing, 7*(5), 270-274.

This prospective and descriptive study compared the time spent by experienced clinical nurses in changing two types of tracheostomy tube securing devices. The first type was the traditional twill tape ties that are inexpensive, costing less than $0.10 per change, and the second type was a commercially available Velcro tracheostomy tube holder, costing $2 per change. The convenience sample of nurses who participated in the study were selected on the basis of self-reports that they performed the procedure frequently, on a routine basis. A simulation clinical laboratory was used for this study. A total of 65 nurses performed the procedure using the two methods of securing the tracheostomy tubes. The procedures were time-tested at two stations. Timing was performed at each station by a nurse anesthetist and a designated quality control officer.

Consistently, almost twice as much time (mean of 146.2 seconds) was required to change the traditional twill tape ties compared with the time required to change the Velcro tracheostomy tube holders (73.6 seconds). The participants reported that the Velcro tracheostomy tube holders were easier to use and did not require the assistance of an additional nurse to safely complete the procedure.

Critique. Although all participants self-reported skill in this procedure, no standard skill test was established to determine participant eligibility and quantitative skill level. The controlled environment, although contributing to testing homogeneity, may not have accurately reflected clinical practice settings.

Implications for Nursing. Nurses are not used to costing out their time as part of procedural costs and tend to consider only the cost of equipment or products. It is clear that labor costs associated with any task or procedure can be significant and must be taken into consideration when calculating procedural costs. In the case of a complex or labor-intensive procedure, using a more expensive product or piece of equipment that results in less time is indeed contributing to a decreased procedural cost. Nurses need to examine their general and specialty practices where being "penny-wise" has become "pound foolish."

quire changing at least once a day to keep them clean and to avoid having them act as a medium for infection. Velcro holders cost significantly more than traditional twill tape ties; however, less nursing time is required to change Velcro holders and may cost less overall (see the Evidence-Based Practice for Nursing box above and the Cost of Care box above). A properly secured tie or holder allows space for only one or two fingers to be placed between the tie or holder and the neck. Tube movement causes irritation and coughing, which in turn may cause decannulation. Keeping the tube secure while changing the ties or holder to prevent accidental decannulation is imperative. One way to accomplish this safely is to keep the old ties or holder on the tube while changing tubes, but a secure hand on the tube is the most reliable method of tube stabilization. The nurse includes the client in this process as a step toward self-care. Figure 28-14 demonstrates a correct technique for applying a tracheostomy dressing. Figure 28-15 shows the use of Velcro tracheostomy tube holders.

BRONCHIAL AND ORAL HYGIENE

Bronchial hygiene promotes a patent airway, prevents pulmonary infections, and stimulates the pulmonary system. The

COST OF CARE IMPLICATIONS FOR NURSING

SECURING TRACHEOSTOMY TUBES

Cost of Care

- Tracheostomy tubes must be secured to prevent complications.
- Standard twill tape ties are changed at least daily and cost approximately $5/100 yards (less than 1 yard required per tie change).
- Changing these tapes requires considerable time and dexterity.
- Many nurses use the assistance of an additional nurse during changes with standard twill tape ties.
- Commercially available Velcro tracheostomy tube holders cost approximately $2 each.
- The Velcro tracheostomy tube holders are easier and faster to change than standard twill tape ties and do not require assistance from another nurse.
- When both labor costs and product or equipment costs are taken into consideration, the more expensive product results in a reduced procedure cost.

Implications for Nursing

Nurses are not used to costing out their time as part of procedural costs and tend to consider only the cost of equipment or products. It is clear that labor costs associated with any task or procedure can be significant and must be taken into consideration when calculating procedural costs. In the case of a complex or labor-intensive procedure, using a more expensive product or piece of equipment that results in less time is indeed contributing to a decreased procedural cost. Nurses need to examine their general and specialty practices where being "penny-wise" has become "pound foolish."

Data from Dixon, L., & Wasson, D. (1998). Comparing use and cost effectiveness of tracheostomy tube securing devices. *MEDSURG Nursing, 7*(5), 270-274.

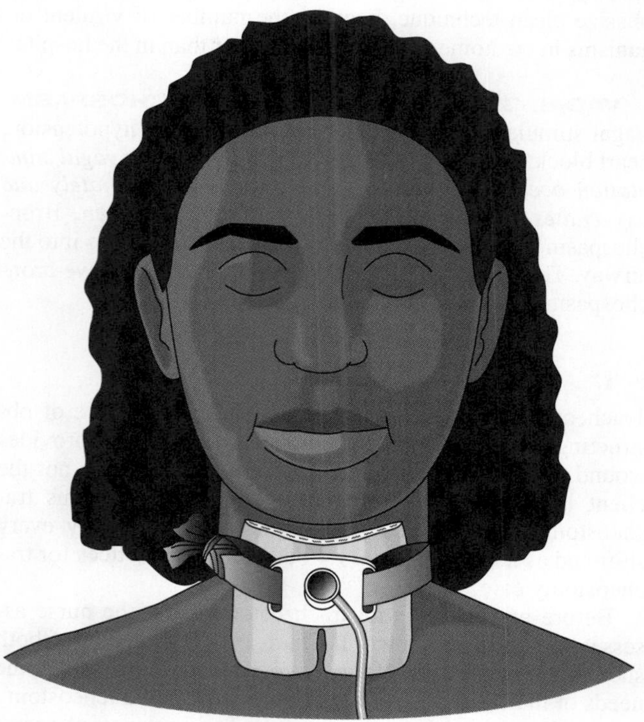

Figure 28-14 ● Placement of precut gauze and tie around a tracheostomy tube.

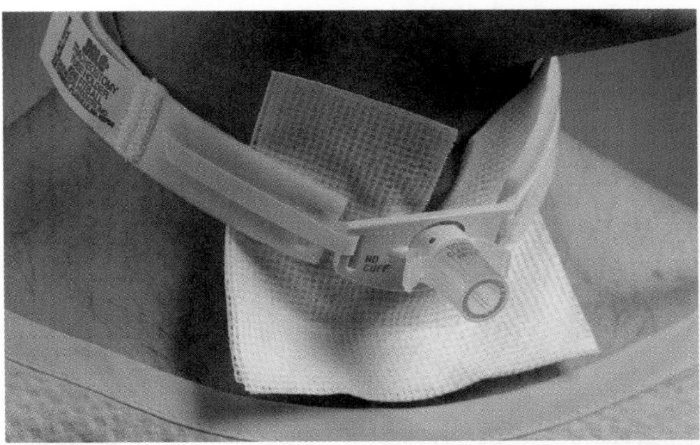

Figure 28-15 ● Velcro tracheostomy tube holder. (Courtesy Dale Medical Products, Inc., Plainville, MA.)

nurse turns and repositions the client every 1 to 2 hours, supports out-of-bed activities, and encourages ambulation. These interventions promote lung expansion and gas exchange, and facilitate the mobilization of secretions. Coughing and deep breathing, combined with the chest physical therapy techniques of percussion, vibration, and postural drainage, are powerful measures in promoting pulmonary care (see Chapter 30).

Frequent oral hygiene is important not only to ensure a patent airway but also to prevent bacterial overgrowth and dental caries and to promote comfort. The nurse maintains standard or body substance precautions during the procedure. Cleansing the mouth with glycerin swabs or mouthwash, which contains significant amounts of alcohol, is contraindicated because these products dry the oral mucosa, change its pH, and promote bacterial growth. Instead, a toothette or soft-bristled toothbrush moistened in water is used for mouth care. Hydrogen peroxide solutions can help to remove crusted materials but may break down granulating tissue and are used only with a physician's order.

During oral care, the nurse examines the mouth for any alterations in mucosal integrity, dental abnormalities, or alterations in tissue integrity. Ulcers (aphthous or herpes simplex), bacterial or fungal *(Candida)* growth, and other infections are treated medically. Application of lip balms or water-soluble jelly can prevent cracked lips and further skin breakdown and can help keep the client comfortable. Providing mouth care is a simple but very effective method of promoting oral health, comfort, and aesthetic appearance. Offering an opportunity for the client or family member to perform mouth care encourages participation in care and increases self-esteem.

Oral secretions can move down the trachea and collect above the inflated cuff of the endotracheal tube. When the cuff is deflated, the secretions can move into the lungs. A new endotracheal tube, the Hi-Lo Evac, has an additional lumen open to the area above the cuff and can help prevent aspiration of oral secretions (Figure 28-16). The additional lumen allows the nurse to suction the airway above the cuff before deflating, thus preventing movement of oral secretions deeper into the airway.

NUTRITION

Swallowing can be a major problem for the client with a tracheostomy tube in place. In a normal swallow, the larynx ele-

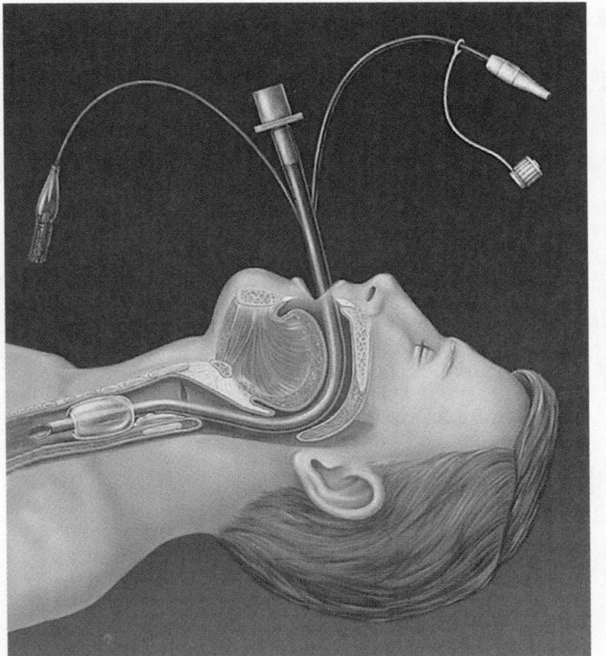

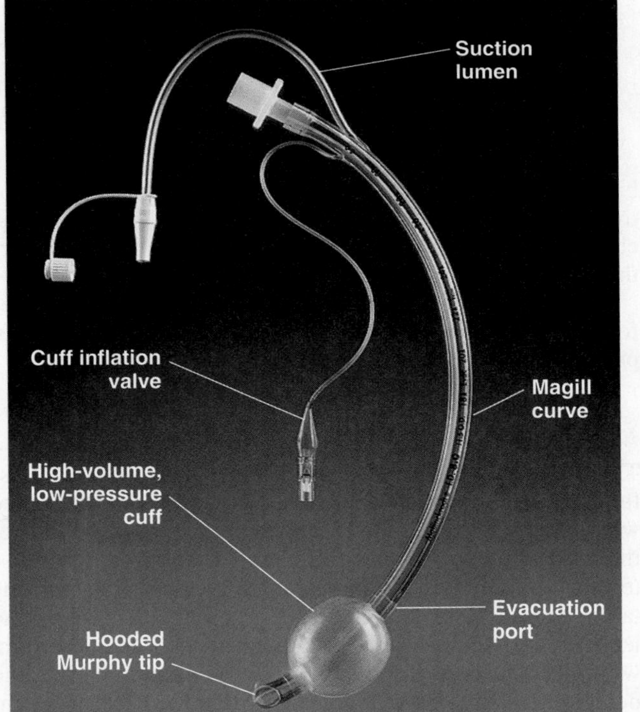

Figure 28-16 ● The Hi-Lo Evac endotracheal tube system. **A,** The system positioned within a client. **B,** The Hi-Lo Evac tube. (Courtesy Malinckrodt, Inc., Shiley Tracheostomy Products, St. Louis, MO.)

vates and moves forward to protect itself from the passing stream of food and saliva. Laryngeal elevation also assists in the opening of the cricopharyngeal muscle, the upper esophageal sphincter. The tracheostomy tube sometimes tethers the larynx in place, making it unable to execute this motion efficiently. The result is difficulty in swallowing. Likewise, when the tracheostomy tube cuff is inflated, it can

CHART 28-6

BEST PRACTICE *for*
Preventing Aspiration During Swallowing

- Avoid having meals when the client is fatigued.
- Provide smaller and more frequent meals.
- Provide adequate time; do not "hurry" the client.
- Provide close supervision if the client is self-feeding.
- Keep emergency suctioning equipment close at hand.
- Avoid water and other "thin" liquids.
- Thicken liquids.
- Avoid foods that generate thin liquids during the chewing process, such as fruit.
- Position the client in the most upright position possible.
- When possible, completely (or at least partially) deflate the tube cuff during meals.
- Suction after initial cuff deflation to clear the airway and allow maximal comfort during the meal.
- Feed each bite or encourage the client to take each bite slowly.
- Encourage the client to "dry swallow" after each bite to clear residue from the throat.
- Avoid consecutive swallows by cup or straw.
- Provide controlled small volumes of liquids, using a spoon.
- Encourage the client to "tuck" his or her chin down and forward while swallowing.
- Allow the client to indicate when he or she is ready for the next bite.
- If the client coughs, stop the feeding until the client indicates that the airway has been cleared.
- Continuously monitor tolerance to oral food intake by assessing respiratory rate, ease, pulse oximetry, and heart rate.

balloon posteriorly and interfere with the passage of food through the esophagus. The common wall of the posterior trachea (trachealis muscle) and the anterior esophagus is very thin, allowing this pushing phenomenon.

The client is instructed to keep the head of the bed elevated for at least 30 minutes after feeding. Chart 28-6 outlines best practices to prevent aspiration during swallowing.

SPEECH AND COMMUNICATION

The client will be able to speak when there is a cuffless tube, when a fenestrated tracheostomy tube is in place, and when the fenestrated tube is capped or covered. Until one of the methods for natural vocalization is feasible, the nurse teaches alternative communication methods. A writing tablet, Magic Slate, communication board with pictures and letters, hand signals, or a computer, as well as a call light within reach, is essential to promote communication and decrease frustration from not being able to speak or be understood. Questions phrased for "yes" or "no" answers help the client respond efficiently. The nurse moves the client closer to the nurses' station and marks the central call light system with indicators to communicate that the client cannot speak.

The inability to talk is a major stressor for the client. Every effort to facilitate communication and speech is important. When the client can tolerate cuff deflation, he or she places a finger over the tracheostomy tube on exhalation. This forces air up through the larynx, vocal cords, and mouth and allows speech. During the process of decannulation, when the fenestrated tube is "capped," the client experiences a very positive but secondary benefit of speech without the need to cover the tube.

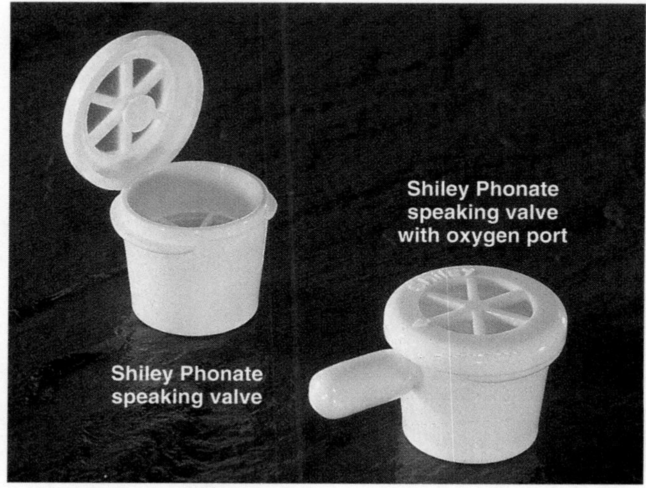

Figure 28-17 ● The Shiley Phonate Speaking Valve. (Courtesy Malinckrodt, Inc., Shiley Tracheostomy Products, St. Louis, MO.)

A device to increase speech for the client with a tracheostomy is a special one-way valve that fits over the tube and replaces the need for finger occlusion (Figure 28-17). The valve allows him or her to breathe in through the tracheostomy tube. On exhalation, the valve closes so that air is forced through the vocal cords and upper airways, allowing speech in the same manner that finger occlusion does. For this valve to effectively assist in speech, the client must not be connected to a ventilator, must have the cuff deflated, and must be able to breathe around the tube. Some valves have an extra port for administration of supplemental oxygen without impairing the ability to speak.

EMOTIONAL CARE

Addressing psychologic concerns is an important aspect of nursing care of clients recovering from a tracheostomy. While providing physical care, the nurse keeps in mind the emotional impact of an artificial airway. Acknowledging the client's frustration in communication and allowing sufficient time for communication are critically important. When speaking to the client, the nurse uses a normal tone of voice. The tracheostomy tube has not altered the ability to hear or understand.

BODY IMAGE

The client experiences a change in body image because of deformity, the presence of a stoma or artificial airway, speech changes, a change in the method of eating, and possibly difficulty with speech. The nurse helps the client to set realistic goals, starting with involvement in self-care.

The nurse and family must make all attempts to ease the client into a more normal social environment. The nurse provides encouragement and positive reinforcement while demonstrating acceptance and caring behaviors. The family may benefit from counseling sessions that the nurse initiates in the hospital.

After surgery, the client may feel shy and socially isolated. To cover the tracheostomy tube, he or she can wear loose-fitting shirts, decorative collars, or scarves.

WEANING

Weaning the client from a tracheostomy tube entails a gradual decrease in the tube size and ultimate removal of the tube. The nurse carefully monitors this process, especially after each change. The physician, nurse practitioner, or respiratory advanced-practice nurse performs the steps in the process.

First, the cuff is deflated as soon as the client can manage secretions and does not require mechanical ventilation. This change allows him or her to breathe through the tube and also through the upper airway. Next, the tube is changed to an uncuffed tube; then the size of the tube is gradually decreased. When a small fenestrated tube is placed (No. 4 or 6, depending on the size of the airway), the tube is capped so that all air passes through the upper airway and the fenestra, with none passing through the tube. The client is assessed to be certain there is adequate airflow around the tube when it is capped. The tube may be removed after he or she tolerates more than 24 hours of capping. The nurse places a dry dressing over the stoma, which then gradually heals on its own. A small scar remains.

Another device used for the transition from tracheostomy to natural breathing is a **tracheostomy button.** The button maintains patency of the stoma and facilitates spontaneous breathing. The Kistner tracheostomy tube and Olympic tracheostomy button are examples of this type of device. To function, they must fit properly. A disadvantage of these buttons is the possibility of decannulation: the tube dislodges from the trachea but remains in the anterior subcutaneous tissues of the neck.

Community-Based Care

By the time of discharge from the hospital, the client should be able to provide self-care, which may include tracheostomy care, nutritional care, suctioning, and methods of communication. Although education begins during preoperative teaching sessions, most self-care is taught in the hospital. The nurse teaches the client and family how to care for the tracheostomy tube. Airway care is reviewed, including cleaning and inspecting for signs of infection. The nurse teaches clean suction technique and reviews the plan of care.

The client is instructed to use a shower shield over the tracheostomy tube when bathing to prevent water from entering the airway. To shield the airway during the day, he or she may wear a protective cover. Covering the permanent opening has several benefits: filtering the air entering the stoma, keeping humidity in the airway, and enhancing aesthetic appearance. To protect the airway and increase humidity, the nurse instructs the client to cover the airway with cotton or foam. Attractive coverings are available in the form of cotton scarves, decorative collars, crocheted bibs, and jewelry. Using colored seam binding for tracheostomy ties after the stoma has matured may enhance overall body image. Shirt or dress color can be matched or coordinated with seam bindings of various colors. The nurse also teaches the client to increase humidity in the home.

The nurse may teach the client to instill normal saline into the artificial airway 10 to 15 times a day, as ordered. The client continues the selected method of alternative communication that began in the hospital and wears a medical alert bracelet.

The client should feel safe and secure with the extended plan of care. The multidisciplinary care team assesses specific discharge needs and makes appropriate referrals to home care agencies and durable medical equipment (DME) companies (for suction equipment and tracheostomy supplies). Clinic or physician follow-up visits occur early after discharge, but the home care nurse also becomes a very important resource for the client and family. The home care nurse initiates (with a physician's order) and coordinates the services of professionals such as nutritionists, nurses, speech pathologists, and social workers. The home care or hospital nurse informs the client and family of community organizations that can offer support and friendships. When the client has problems paying for health care services, equipment supply, and prescriptions, the visiting nurse agency may be helpful in directing him or her to available resources.

ONLINE RESOURCES

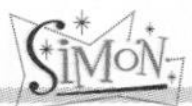

For suggested readings and Internet resources, go to http://www.wbsaunders.com/SIMON/Iggy/.

SELECTED BIBLIOGRAPHY

Asterisk indicates a classic or definitive work on this subject.

Ahrens, T., Wijeweera, H., & Ray, S. (1999). Capnopraphy: A key underutilized technology. *Critical Care Clinics of North America, 11*(1), 49-62.

*Albarren, J.W. (1991). A review of communication with intubated patients and those with tracheostomies within an intensive care environment. *Intensive Care Nursing, 7*(3), 179-186.

Carlson-Catalano, J., et al. (1998). Clinical validation of Ineffective Breathing Pattern, Ineffective Airway Clearance, and Impaired Gas Exchange. *Image: The Journal of Nursing Scholarship, 30*(3), 243-248.

Corbett, N. (1998). Homecare, technology, and the management of respiratory disease. *Critical Care Clinics of North America, 10*(3), 305-313.

Dixon, L., & Wasson, D. (1998). Comparing use and cost effectiveness of tracheostomy tube securing devices. *MEDSURG Nursing, 7*(5), 270-274.

Hatfield, B.O. (1997). Cost effective trach teaching. *RN, 60*(3), 48-49.

McCarley, C. (1999). A model of chronic dyspnea. *Image: The Journal of Nursing Scholarship, 31*(3), 231-236.

McCloskey, J.C, & Bulechek, G.M. (2000). *Nursing interventions classification (NIC)* (3rd ed.). St. Louis: Mosby.

McConnell, E.A. (1997). Administering oxygen by mask. *Nursing97, 21*(9), 26.

Murray, K., & Brzozowski, L. (1998). Swallowing in patients with tracheostomies. *AACN Clinical Issues: Advanced Practice in Acute and Critical Care, 9*(3), 416-426.

Nield, M. (2000). Dyspnea self-management in African Americans with chronic lung disease. *Heart and Lung, 29*(1), 50-55.

Paul-Allen, J., & Ostrow, L. (2000). Survey of nursing practices with closed-system suctioning. *American Journal of Critical Care, 9*(1), 9-19.

Perkins, L., & Shortall, S. (2000). Ventilation without intubation. *RN, 63*(1), 34-38.

Peterson, A., & Hall, T. (1999). Nursing challenge: Caring for a patient with complex, multiple complications. *Heart and Lung, 28*(5), 373-376.

St. John, R. (1999). Advances in artificial airway management. *Critical Care Clinics of North America, 11*(1), 7-17.

Schallom, L., & Aherns, T. (1999). Using oxygenation profiles to manage patients. *Critical Care Clinics of North America, 11*(4), 437-446.

CHAPTER 29

Interventions for Clients with Noninfectious Upper Respiratory Problems

M. LINDA WORKMAN

Learning Objectives

After studying this chapter, you should be able to:

1. Compare the clinical manifestations and care needs of a client with an anterior nosebleed to those of a client with a posterior nosebleed.
2. Prioritize nursing care needs for a client with facial trauma.
3. Identify the potential complications of sleep apnea.
4. Develop a plan of communication for a client who has a disruption of speech and cannot read.
5. Use clinical manifestations and laboratory data to determine airway adequacy in a client with laryngeal or neck injury.
6. Identify the risk factors that predispose a client to the development of head and neck cancer.
7. Develop a teaching plan for the client who is getting ready to go home after undergoing a complete laryngectomy.

Go to http://www.wbsaunders.com/SIMON/Iggy/ for self-assessment questions related to these Learning Objectives.

The upper airway structures include the nose, sinuses, oropharynx, larynx, and trachea. These structures are vulnerable to specific problems and also may be affected by other common acute and chronic disorders. Clients with upper respiratory problems are found across the health care continuum. The major nursing priority with disorders of the upper respiratory tract is maintaining a patent airway.

NONINFECTIOUS DISORDERS OF THE NOSE AND SINUSES

Fracture of the Nose

OVERVIEW

Nasal fractures commonly result from injuries received during falls, sports activities, motor vehicle accidents, or physical assaults. If the bone or cartilage is not displaced, serious complications usually do not result from the fracture, and treatment may not be necessary. However, displacement of either the bone or cartilage can cause airway obstruction or cosmetic deformity and is a potential source of infection.

COLLABORATIVE MANAGEMENT

Assessment

The nurse documents any nasal problem, including deviation, malaligned nasal bridge, change in nasal breathing, crepitus on palpation, midface bruising, and pain. Blood or clear (cerebrospinal) fluid rarely drains from one or both nares. The presence of drainage could indicate a skull fracture. Although important in evaluating general facial fractures, radiographic examination is not always useful in the diagnosis of nasal fractures.

Interventions

The physician performs a simple closed reduction of the nasal fracture (using local or general anesthesia) within the first 24 hours after injury. After 24 hours the fracture is more difficult to reduce because of edema and scar formation. Simple closed fractures need not be surgically treated. Treatment focuses on pain relief and local cold compresses to decrease swelling.

RHINOPLASTY. A reduction and surgery may be required for severe fractures or for those that do not heal properly. **Rhinoplasty** is a surgical reconstruction of the nose for cosmetic purposes and for functional improvement of airflow. The client returns from surgery with packing in both nostrils; this packing prevents bleeding and provides a **stent** (object that provides support and structure) for the reconstructed nose. The gauze packing is typically treated with an antibiotic ointment, such as bacitracin (Bacitin♣) to reduce the risk of infection. A "moustache" dressing (or drip pad), usually a folded 2 × 2 gauze pad, is usually placed under the nose (Figure 29-1). A splint or cast may cover the nose for additional

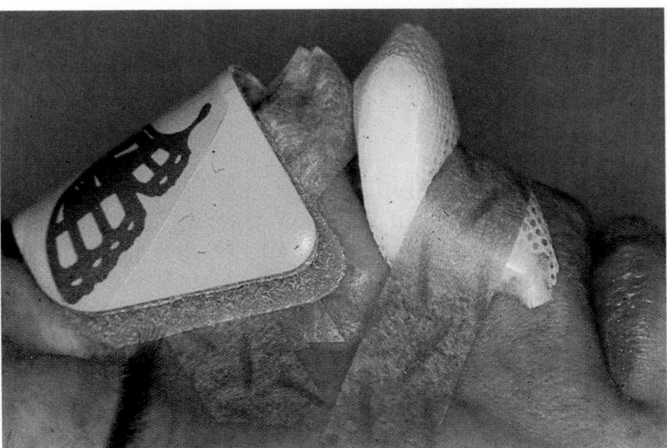

Figure 29-1 ● Immediate postoperative appearance of a client who has undergone rhinoplasty. Note the splint and gauze drip pad (moustache dressing). (From Tardy, M.E. [1997]. *Rhinoplasty: The art and science.* Philadelphia: W.B. Saunders. Used with permission.)

alignment and protection. The nurse or client changes the drip pad as necessary.

Postoperatively, the client is observed for edema and bleeding, and vital signs are obtained every 4 hours until discharge. Assessing how often the client swallows is a priority. Repeated swallowing may indicate posterior nasal bleeding. Using a penlight, the nurse examines the pharynx for bleeding and notifies the surgeon if bleeding is present. The client with uncomplicated rhinoplasty with or without related surgical procedures (browlifts, blepharoplasties, face lifts) is usually discharged the day of surgery. The client and family or significant other are instructed in routine care.

The nurse and/or family places the client in a semi-Fowler's position and instructs him or her to move slowly and to rest as much as possible. Cool compresses are applied to the nose, eyes, or face to reduce swelling and prevent excessive discoloration. If a general anesthetic was used, the client may eat soft foods once the effects of anesthesia have been eliminated (e.g., the client is alert and the gag reflex has returned) and the surgeon has so ordered. An oral fluid intake of at least 2500 mL/day is encouraged.

To prevent bleeding, the client is instructed to limit Valsalva maneuvers (e.g., forceful coughing or straining during a bowel movement) for the first few days after removing the nasal packing. Laxatives or stool softeners may be prescribed to facilitate bowel movement. Aspirin and nonsteroidal anti-inflammatory drugs are avoided during this time to prevent the possibility of bleeding. The surgeon may order prophylactic antibiotics to prevent postoperative infection and pain medication to relieve discomfort. The nurse explains that edema and discoloration usually last for several weeks, with the final surgical result evident in 6 to 12 months.

NASOSEPTOPLASTY. Nasoseptoplasty, or **submucous resection (SMR),** may be necessary to straighten a deviated septum when chronic symptoms (e.g., a "stuffy" nose) or discomfort occur. A slight deviation of the nasal septum is present in most adults and causes no symptoms. Major deviations, however, may obstruct the nasal passages or interfere with airflow and sinus drainage. The surgeon removes the deviated

CHART 29-1

BEST PRACTICE *for*
Emergency Care of a Nosebleed

- Position the client upright and leaning forward to prevent blood from entering the stomach and possible aspiration.
- Reassure the client and attempt to keep him or her quiet to reduce anxiety and blood pressure.
- Apply direct lateral pressure to the nose for 5 minutes, and apply ice or cool compresses to the nose and face if possible.
- Maintain standard or body substance precautions.
- If nasal packing is necessary, loosely pack both nares with gauze or nasal tampons.
- To prevent rebleeding from dislodging clots, instruct the client not to blow the nose for several hours after the bleeding stops.
- Seek medical assistance if these measures are ineffective or if the bleeding occurs frequently.

section of the cartilage and bone. The amount resected depends on the type and degree of deformity.

Nursing care is similar to that for a rhinoplasty. Nasoseptoplasty is usually an outpatient procedure.

Epistaxis

OVERVIEW

Epistaxis (nosebleed) is a common problem because of the rich capillary network within the nose. Nosebleeds may occur as a result of trauma, hypertension, blood dyscrasia (e.g., leukemias), inflammation, tumor, decreased humidity, excessive nose blowing, nose picking, chronic cocaine use, and selected nursing procedures such as nasogastric suctioning. Men are usually affected more often than women, and older adults tend to bleed most often from the posterior portion of the nose.

COLLABORATIVE MANAGEMENT

Assessment

The client will usually report that the bleeding started after sneezing or blowing the nose. The nurse documents the amount and color of the blood and takes the vital signs. The client is asked about the number, duration, and causes of previous bleeding episodes. This information is documented in the client's medical record.

Interventions

Chart 29-1 summarizes best practices for emergency care of the client with a nosebleed. Medical attention is needed if the nosebleed does not respond to these interventions. In such cases the physician cauterizes the affected capillaries with silver nitrate or electrocautery and follows with anterior packing. Anterior packing is very effective in controlling bleeding from the anterior nasal cavity.

The physician uses a posterior pack to stop bleeding that originates in the posterior nasal region. A string is attached to a large gauze pack and then threaded through the nose and out the mouth. The physician positions the pack in the posterior nasal cavity above the pharynx and then tapes the string to the client's cheek to prevent movement of the pack. This procedure is uncomfortable, and the airway may be obstructed if the pack slips. Most clients who require posterior packing are hospitalized.

The nurse observes the client for respiratory distress and for tolerance of the packing. The physician may prescribe humidification, oxygen, bed rest, and antibiotics. To maintain gag and cough reflexes and an optimal level of consciousness, the client should not receive any sedatives and only limited pain medication. The nurse provides oral care and ensures adequate hydration, which is important because of mouth breathing. Pulse oximetry is used to monitor for hypoxemia. The physician removes the packing after 2 to 5 days.

Petroleum jelly can be applied to the nares for lubrication and comfort. Nasal saline solution and humidification may be helpful to add moisture and prevent crusting and rebleeding. To prevent further crusting and subsequent rebleeding, the client is taught to continue gentle saline irrigations and lubrication to the nasal cavity after discharge. Other instructions include the avoidance of vigorous nose blowing, the use of aspirin or other nonsteroidal anti-inflammatory agents (NSAIDs), and strenuous activities such as lifting.

Nasal Polyps

OVERVIEW

Nasal polyps are benign, grapelike clusters of mucous membrane and loose connective tissue. Polyps usually occur bilaterally and are often caused by irritation to the nasal mucosa or sinuses, allergies, or infection (chronic sinusitis). If polyps become too large, airway obstruction may result.

COLLABORATIVE MANAGEMENT

Assessment

Clinical manifestations of nasal polyps include obstructed nasal breathing, the presence of or a change in the character of nasal discharge, and a change in speech quality. Clients who have had polyps are at risk for recurrence.

Interventions

Surgery is the treatment of choice for nasal polyps. The extent of the surgery required depends on the type of polyp present.

Benign nasal polyps are treated medically with nasally inhaled steroids and surgical removal **(polypectomy).** A polypectomy can be performed using either local or general anesthesia. The nurse observes the client for postoperative bleeding. After surgery, the nostrils are usually packed with gauze for 24 hours. Nasal polyps tend to recur if not completely resected.

Inverting papilloma is a rare, benign, space-occupying lesion that erodes nasal and maxillary skeletal structures. Often initially diagnosed as benign polyps, inverting papillomas grow by pressure into adjacent structures. Extensive sinus and nasal surgery is necessary for complete removal. If these papillomas are completely resected, they do not recur.

Juvenile angiofibromas are similar in growth pattern but cellularly different from other polyps. These tumors usually occur in adolescent males and may undergo resolution when the client reaches adulthood. These lesions may be removed by traditional nasal surgery or may require skull base resections for more invasive tumors.

Cancer of the Nose and Sinuses

OVERVIEW

Tumors of the nasal cavities and sinuses are relatively uncommon and may be either benign or malignant. Malignant lesions of these areas can occur at all ages, but the peak incidence is 40 to 45 years of age in males and 60 to 65 years of age in females. Asian Americans have a higher incidence of nasopharyngeal cancer.

COLLABORATIVE MANAGEMENT

Assessment

The onset of sinus cancer is slow, with symptoms resembling sinusitis. Therefore the client may have relatively advanced disease at diagnosis. Nasal or sinus malignancy is suggested by persistent nasal obstruction, drainage, bloody discharge, and pain that does not improve after treatment of sinusitis. Local lymph node enlargement usually occurs on the side with greater tumor mass.

Interventions

Radiation therapy is the primary treatment for nasopharyngeal cancers. Chart 29-2 lists some NIC interventions for clients undergoing radiation therapy. Surgical resection may be indicated if radiation therapy is not successful. Chemotherapy has not proved to be effective.

The specific surgical procedure depends on the amount of tumor, its anatomic location, and the degree of tissue invasion. The primary deficit is a change in body image or speech and an alteration in nutrition, especially when the maxilla and floor of the nose are involved in the resection. These procedures often cause the client to experience changes in taste and smell.

The nurse provides general postoperative care (see Chapter 19), including maintaining a patent airway, monitoring for hemorrhage, providing wound care, giving strict attention to nutrition, and providing tracheostomy care (if necessary). (See Chapter 28 for tracheostomy care.) Meticulous mouth and maxillary cavity care is carried out with saline irrigations using a water pick (e.g., Water Pik) or a syringe. The client is assessed for alterations in comfort and for infection. Optimal nutrition is essential during the perioperative period for adequate healing to occur.

Facial Trauma

OVERVIEW

Facial trauma is defined by the specific bones (e.g., mandibular, maxillary, zygomatic, orbital, or nasal fractures) and the side of the face involved. Mandibular (lower jaw) fractures can occur at any location on the mandible and account for the majority of facial fractures. **Le Fort I** is a nasoethmoid complex fracture. **Le Fort II** is a transverse maxillary *and* nasoethmoid complex fracture. **Le Fort III** is a combination of I and II plus an orbital-zygoma fracture, often called "craniofacial disjunction" because it leaves the midface with no con-

CHART 29-2

NIC INTERVENTION ACTIVITIES *for* The Client with Noninfectious Disorders of the Nose and Sinus

Radiation Therapy Management: *Assisting the client to understand and minimize the side effects of radiation treatments*
- Monitor for alterations in skin integrity and treat appropriately.
- Avoid use of adhesive tapes and other skin-irritating substances.
- Avoid application of deodorants and aftershave lotion to treated area.
- Discuss the need for skin care, such as maintenance of dye markings, avoidance of soap and other ointments, and protection during sunbathing or heat application.
- Monitor for indications of infection of oral mucous membranes.
- Encourage good oral hygiene with use of dental floss or Water Pik, as appropriate.
- Initiate oral health restoration activities, such as use of artificial saliva, mouth sprays, and sugarless mints, as appropriate.
- Monitor client for anorexia, nausea, vomiting, changes in taste, esophagitis, and diarrhea, as appropriate.
- Promote adequate fluid and nutritional intake.
- Assist client in managing fatigue by planning frequent rest periods, spacing activities, and limiting daily demands, as appropriate.
- Encourage rest immediately after radiation treatment.
- Facilitate expression of fears about prognosis or success of radiation treatments.

Communication Enhancement: Speech Deficit: *Assistance in accepting and learning alternate methods for living with impaired speech*
- Provide verbal prompts/reminders.
- Listen attentively.
- Refrain from shouting at the client with communication disorders.
- Use picture board, if appropriate.
- Use hand gestures, as appropriate.
- Perform prescriptive speech-language therapies during informal interactions with client.
- Teach esophageal speech, as appropriate.
- Instruct client and family on use of speech aids (e.g., tracheal-esophageal prosthesis and artificial larynx).
- Encourage client to repeat words.
- Provide positive reinforcement and praise, as appropriate.
- Carry on one-way conversations, as appropriate.
- Reinforce need for follow-up with speech pathologist after discharge.

NIC intervention activities selected from McCloskey, J.C., & Bulechek, G.M. (Eds.). (2000). *Nursing interventions classification (NIC)* (3rd ed.). St. Louis: Mosby.

nection to the skull. There is often much bleeding with facial trauma because the face is very vascular.

COLLABORATIVE MANAGEMENT

Assessment

The priority in the management of facial trauma is assessment for a patent airway. Signs and symptoms of an upper airway obstruction include stridor, shortness of breath, dyspnea, anxiety, restlessness, hypoxia, hypercarbia, decreased oxygen saturation, cyanosis, and loss of consciousness. After establishing the airway, the nurse assesses the amount and site of soft-tissue trauma, bleeding, and palpable fractures. Additional findings on assessment include edema of soft tissue, asymmetry, pain, or leakage of cerebrospinal fluid through the ears and/or nose, indicating a temporal bone or basilar skull fracture. Because orbital and maxillary fractures can entrap the eye, the nurse assesses vision and extraocular movement (EOM) and also observes for neurologic changes (see Chapter 41). Because spinal cord trauma and skull fractures often occur in conjunction with facial trauma, cranial computed tomography, facial series, and cervical spine films also are obtained.

Interventions

The priority action is to establish and maintain a patent airway. The nurse must anticipate the need for emergency intubation, tracheotomy, or cricothyroidotomy. When the client arrives at a trauma center, care focuses on establishing an airway, controlling hemorrhage, and assessing for the extent of injury. If signs and symptoms of shock are present, fluid resuscitation and identification of bleeding sites must be initiated immediately.

In head and neck trauma, the nurse must be astute in trauma and critical care nursing. Time is critical in stabilizing the client. Early treatment and response of the appropriate services, including the trauma team, maxillofacial surgeon, general surgeon, otolaryngologist, plastic surgeon, and dentist, optimize the client's post-trauma recovery.

Stabilization of the fractured segment of a *mandibular fracture* allows the teeth to heal in proper alignment or occlusion. The client remains in fixed centric occlusion for 6 to 10 weeks. Antibiotic therapy may be prescribed because of oral wound contamination. Delay in treatment, infection of the adjacent tooth, or poor oral care may result in infection in the mandibular bone segment. The client may then require surgical debridement, intravenous (IV) antibiotic therapy, and an extended period in fixation.

Facial fractures often are repaired with microplating surgical systems. These shaping plates fix the bone fragments in place until **osteoneogenesis** (new bone growth) occurs. Large areas of skull can be replaced with BoneSource. Bone cells grow into the BoneSource and rematrix into a stabilized bone support. In the United States the plates remain in place permanently; in Europe the plates are removed after healing has occurred.

If the mandibular fracture is repaired with titanium plates, the nurse teaches the client oral care, soft-diet restrictions, and follow-up care with a dentist. The plates are permanent and do not interfere with magnetic resonance imaging (MRI) studies.

A newer method of fixation is the use of resorbable devices (plates and screws) to hold tissues in alignment. These devices are made from a nonmetallic copolymer that retains its integrity for approximately 8 weeks and then undergoes water-mediated biodegradation. Total degradation of the product requires approximately 15 months (Abernathy et al., 2000). Contraindications for this type of fixation include prior irradiation of the area, smoking, drug or alcohol dependence, uncontrolled diabetes mellitus, immunosuppression, and impaired cardiovascular function.

Inner maxillary fixation (IMF) is another common method of securing a mandibular fracture. The bones are realigned and then wired in place with the bite closed. The physician can repair nondisplaced aligned fractures in a clinic or office using local dental anesthesia. General anesthesia is used to repair displaced or complex fractures or fractures that occur with other facial bone fractures.

Postoperatively, the client is taught about oral care with an irrigating device, such as a Water Pik. If the client is in inner maxillary fixation, the nurse teaches self-care with wires in place, including a dental liquid diet. There is a risk for aspiration if vomiting should occur because of the inability to open the jaws to allow ejection of the emesis. The client is taught the proper method of cutting the wires if emesis occurs. *Wire cutters are kept with the client at all times in preparation for this emergency.* If the wires are cut, the client is instructed to return to the physician for rewiring as soon as possible to reinstitute fixation.

Nutrition is important for any client with fractures. Because of oral fixation, pain, and surgery, nutritional needs may be ignored. Dietary consultations are important for teaching and support.

CRITICAL THINKING CHALLENGE

The client is a 22-year-old male who sustained facial trauma while playing touch football with his friends. His jaws have been wired together. His nose is also broken but is not displaced. He is to be discharged 6 hours after the intermaxillary fixation. He tells you that he is a little sick to his stomach from swallowing blood. He is also wondering if he could eat pizza if the pieces are cut up.

- What is the teaching priority for this client?
- What should you do for his subjective symptom of nausea?
- Design a diet appropriate for his size (height 6'2", weight 195 pounds).

For suggested answer guidelines, go to SIMON http://www.wbsaunders.com/SIMON/Iggy/.

NONINFECTIOUS DISORDERS OF THE ORAL PHARYNX AND TONSILS

Obstructive Sleep Apnea

OVERVIEW

Sleep apnea is a breathing disruption during sleep that lasts at least 10 seconds and occurs a minimum of 5 times in an hour. Although sleep apnea can have a neurologic or central origin, the most common form occurs as a result of upper airway obstruction by the soft palate or tongue. Factors that contribute to sleep apnea include obesity, a large uvula, a short neck, smoking, enlarged tonsils or adenoids, and oropharyngeal edema. Men are more commonly affected than women, and the incidence increases with age.

During sleep, the skeletal muscles relax and the tongue and neck structures are displaced. As a result, the upper airway is obstructed even though chest wall movement is unimpaired. The apnea increases the arterial carbon dioxide level and decreases the pH. These blood gas changes stimulate neural activity. The sleeper is aroused spontaneously after 10 or more seconds of apnea and corrects the obstruction, and respiration resumes. The cycle begins again, sometimes as often as every 5 minutes.

This cyclic pattern of disrupted sleep prevents reaching the prolonged state of deep sleep necessary for maximum rest. As a result, the person may experience excessive daytime sleepiness, an inability to concentrate, and irritability.

COLLABORATIVE MANAGEMENT

Assessment

Clients may have sleep apnea if they experience excessive daytime sleepiness or complain of "waking up tired," particularly if they snore heavily. Other clinical manifestations include irritability and personality changes. In some cases sleep apnea can be diagnosed through the observation of family members while the client sleeps in a supine position. A complete health assessment should be performed when excessive daytime sleepiness is a problem.

The most definitive test for diagnosing sleep apnea is polysomnography (PSG) performed during an overnight sleep study. Overnight sleep studies are preferred because the client is more likely to experience all phases of sleep, including rapid eye movement (REM) sleep and deep sleep. The client is directly observed while wearing a variety of monitoring equipment, including an electroencephalograph (EEG), an electrocardiograph (ECG), a pulse oximeter, and an electromyograph (EMG). Such equipment determines the depth of sleep, type of sleep, respiratory effort, oxygen saturation adequacy, and muscle movement.

Interventions

A change in sleeping position or weight loss may be all that is required to reduce or correct mild sleep apnea. Simple position-fixing devices that prevent subluxation of the tongue and neck structures also may be effective in preventing obstruction. For more severe sleep apnea, nonsurgical or surgical methods to prevent obstruction may be necessary.

A common nonsurgical method to prevent airway collapse is the use of noninvasive positive-pressure ventilation (NPPV) to hold open the upper airways. Essentially, a nasal mask or full-face mask delivery system allows mechanical delivery of either Bi-level positive airway pressure (BiPAP) or nasal continuous positive airway pressure. With BiPAP, a cycling machine delivers a set inspiratory positive airway pressure at the beginning of each inspiration. As the client begins to exhale, the machine delivers a lower set end expiratory pressure. Together these two pressures improve tidal volume and hold open the upper airways.

Nasal continuous positive airway pressure (CPAP) delivers a set positive airway pressure continually throughout each cycle of inhalation and exhalation. For CPAP ventilation through a face mask during sleep, a small electric compressor delivers positive pressure at an individually determined setting. Proper fit of the mask over the nose and mouth is key to successful treatment. Although intrusive, these methods are well accepted by clients after an initial adjustment period.

Surgical intervention for sleep apnea may involve a simple adenoidectomy or uvulectomy or may require remodeling of the entire posterior oropharynx **(uvulopalatopharyngoplasty).** Both conventional and laser surgeries are used for this purpose. A tracheostomy may be needed for very severe sleep apnea that is not relieved by more moderate interventions.

Oropharyngeal Cancer

Clients with cancer of the mouth, tongue, tonsils, and pharynx present special nursing needs related to airway maintenance, communication, nutrition, and self-image. Chapter 54 provides an in-depth discussion of the collaborative management of clients with oropharyngeal cancer.

NONINFECTIOUS DISORDERS OF THE LARYNX

Vocal Cord Paralysis

OVERVIEW

Vocal fold (cord) paralysis may result from injury, trauma, or disease that affects the larynx, laryngeal nerves, or vagus nerve. Prolonged intubation with an endotracheal (ET) tube may cause temporary or, rarely, permanent paralysis. Laryngeal paralysis may occur in clients with neurologic disorders. Damage to the vagus nerve (by chest injury) or brainstem may lead to nerve dysfunction. The superior and recurrent laryngeal nerves may be damaged as a result of trauma or disorders that involve the chest, esophagus, or thyroid. Paralysis of both vocal cords may result from direct traumatic injury or bilateral stroke, especially involving the brainstem or following total thyroidectomy.

COLLABORATIVE MANAGEMENT

Assessment

Vocal fold paralysis may be unilateral or bilateral. When only one vocal cord is involved, as is commonly the case, the airway usually remains patent but voice use may be affected. Symptoms of **abducted** (open) bilateral vocal cord paralysis include hoarseness; a breathy, weak voice; and aspiration of food. Bilateral **adducted** (closed) vocal cord paralysis causes airway obstruction and dyspnea and is a medical emergency if the symptoms are severe and the client is unable to compensate. Stridor is the major presenting symptom. The client with vocal cord dysfunction is at risk for aspiration because of an inability to protect the airway by normal vocal cord closure.

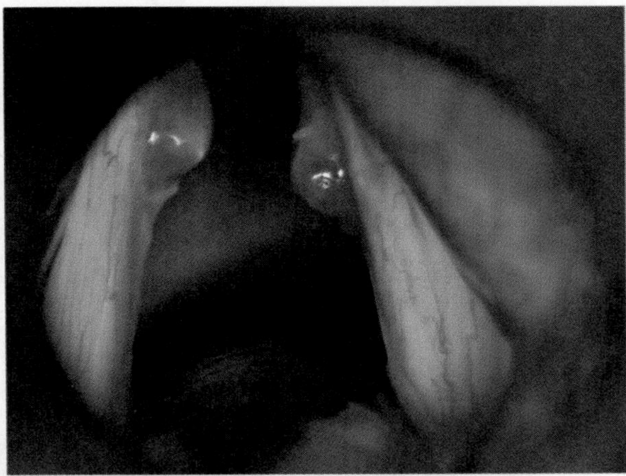

Figure 29-2 ● Bilateral vocal cord nodules caused by contact and voice abuse, often seen after viral illnesses. The differential diagnosis includes cancer and trauma. The origin of the nodules may be scar tissue, bacteria, or viruses. (From Damjanov, I., & Linder, J. [2000]. *Pathology: A color atlas.* St. Louis: Mosby.)

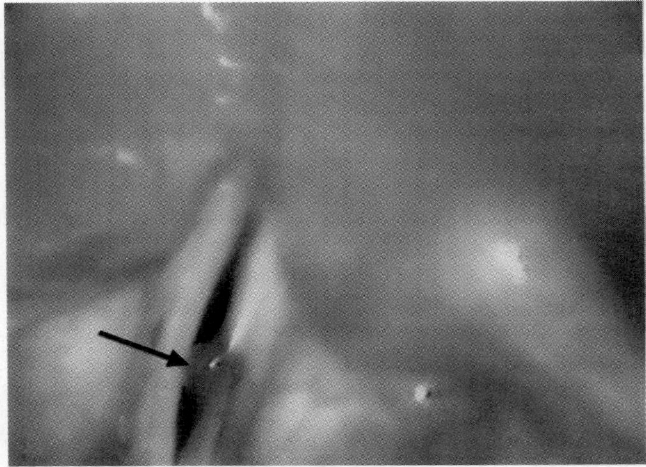

Figure 29-3 ● A hemorrhagic vocal cord polyp.

Interventions

The nurse assesses for symptoms of upper airway obstruction. Securing a patent airway is the primary intervention. The client is placed in a high Fowler's position to aid in breathing and proper alignment of airway structures. Dyspnea with stridor indicates an inadequate airway, and the nurse immediately notifies the physician. Emergency endotracheal intubation, cricothyroidotomy, or tracheostomy may be necessary.

Many surgical procedures have been used to improve the voice. One procedure for abducted vocal cord paresis involves injecting polytef (Teflon) into the affected cord so it enlarges toward the unaffected cord. This technique improves closure during speaking and eating.

Additional nursing interventions include teaching clients to hold their breath during swallowing. This intervention allows the larynx to elevate, close, and divert the food stream back into the esophagus during swallowing. Another protective technique involves the client tucking his or her chin down and forward during swallowing. The nurse evaluates the client for aspiration of liquids and saliva related to vocal cord dysfunction. Signs and symptoms include immediate coughing on swallowing of liquids or solids, a "wet"-sounding voice, and "tearing up" or watery eyes on swallowing. Chest x-ray studies and laryngeal and chest auscultation are also useful to diagnose the signs and symptoms of aspiration pneumonia.

Nodules and Polyps of the Vocal Cords

OVERVIEW

Nodules often appear at the point at which the vocal cords touch during speech. **Nodules** are hypertrophied fibrous tissue (Figure 29-2) that result from an infectious process or overuse of the voice. The populations most affected are teachers, coaches, sports fans, singers, and people who use their voices in noisy environments.

Vocal cord polyps (Figure 29-3) are chronic, edematous masses. They occur most commonly in adults who smoke, have many allergies, or live in dry climates. Vocal cysts also may occur.

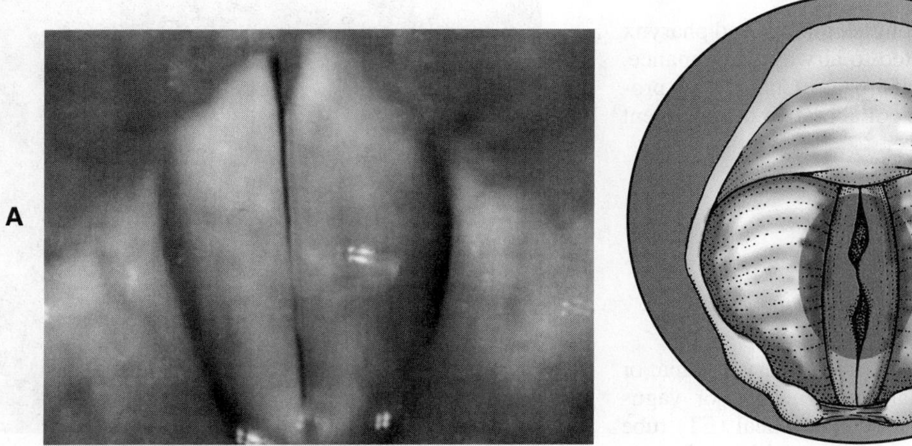

Figure 29-4 ● **A,** Close-up view of normal vocal cords in phonation. Saying the letter E in a high pitch allows the examiner to evaluate the total movement of the cords in all pitch ranges and to evaluate membrane contact. **B,** Vocal cord nodules and polyps prevent approximation of the vocal cords. Hoarseness results.

➤ COLLABORATIVE MANAGEMENT

Both nodules and polyps are painless, but they produce hoarseness because of the loss of coordinated closure of the vocal cords and vocal wave (Figure 29-4).

Nursing management with vocal cord nodules or polyps is aimed at educating the client and family. The client is instructed about the tobacco use hazards, smoking cessation programs, and the importance of voice rest. Conservative treatment includes not whispering and avoiding heavy lifting. Stool softeners are used to avoid bearing down during elimination **(Valsalva maneuvers),** which would cause the glottis to close. Humidification of inspired air may soothe the vocal cords and prevent overdrying.

Speech therapy is a primary treatment for behavioral voice changes and helps to reduce the intensity of speech. A conservative approach using speech therapy may make surgery unnecessary.

If hoarseness or another voice disturbance is not relieved by voice rest or speech therapy, the physician may remove the nodules or polyps under direct laryngoscopy. Laser and surgical resection are used to remove the mucous membrane of the affected cord. If both cords are involved, one cord is usually allowed to heal before surgery is performed on the other cord.

After surgery, the client must maintain complete voice rest for approximately 14 days to promote healing. Chart 29-2 lists NIC interventions for communication enhancement. Alternative methods of communication such as a slate board, pen and paper, "magic slate," or alphabet board are used. A sign is placed on the client's door, over the bed, and on the intercom system to help implement this important nursing intervention. Education is imperative *before* the operation and before the client returns home, because these procedures are often performed in an outpatient setting.

Laryngeal Trauma

OVERVIEW

Laryngeal trauma is a result of a crushing or direct blow injury, fracture, or intrinsic injury such as that induced by prolonged endotracheal intubation.

➤ COLLABORATIVE MANAGEMENT

Symptoms of laryngeal trauma include **dyspnea** (difficulty breathing), **aphonia** (inability to produce sound), hoarseness, and **subcutaneous emphysema** (air present in the subcutaneous tissue). Bleeding from the airway **(hemoptysis)** may occur depending on the location of the trauma. The physician performs a direct visual examination by laryngoscopy or fiberoptic laryngoscopy of the larynx to determine the nature and extent of the injury.

The management of clients with laryngeal injuries consists of assessing and frequently monitoring vital signs (every 15 to 30 minutes), including respiratory status and pulse oximetry. The nursing priority is to maintain a patent airway. Oxygen and humidification are administered as ordered to maintain adequate oxygen saturation. If the client is experiencing respiratory difficulty, the nurse stays with him or her and instructs other trauma team members to prepare for an emergency cricothyroidotomy (cricothyrotomy) or tracheostomy. Respiratory difficulty is evidenced by signs such as increasing tachypnea, anxiety, sternal retraction, shortness of breath, dyspnea, restlessness, decreased oxygen saturation, decreased level of consciousness, nasal flaring, and **stridor** (high-pitched, harsh blowing sound heard during breathing).

Surgical intervention is necessary for lacerations of the mucous membranes, cartilage exposure, and paralysis of the cords. Laryngeal repair is performed as soon as possible to prevent laryngeal stenosis and to cover any exposed cartilage. An artificial airway may be indicated. Maintenance of a patent airway is the utmost priority.

OTHER UPPER AIRWAY DISORDERS

Upper Airway Obstruction

OVERVIEW

Upper airway obstruction is a life-threatening emergency. It is defined as any significant interruption in airflow through the nose, mouth, pharynx, or larynx. Early recognition is essential to prevent further complications, including respiratory ar-

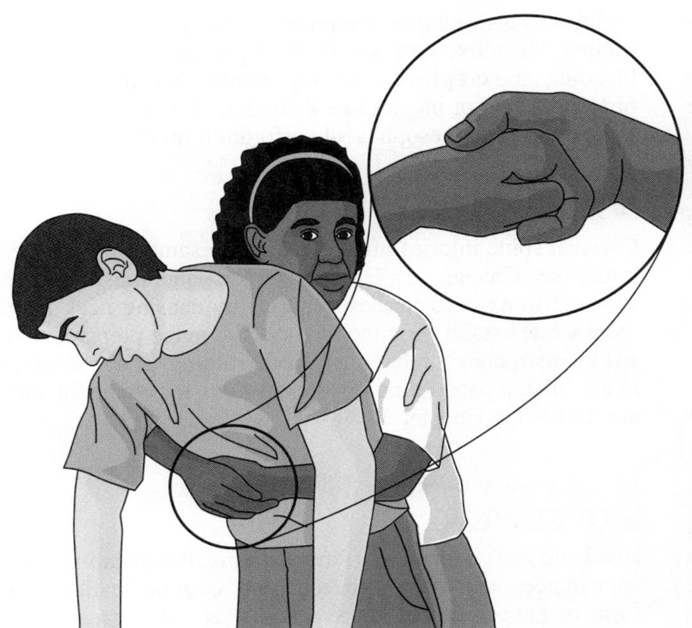

With the conscious victim standing or sitting, place your fist between the victim's lower rib cage and navel. Wrap the palm of your hand around your fist. A quick inward, upward thrust expels the air remaining in the victim's lungs, and with it the foreign body. If the first thrust is unsuccessful, repeat several thrusts in rapid succession until the foreign body is expelled or until the victim loses consciousness.

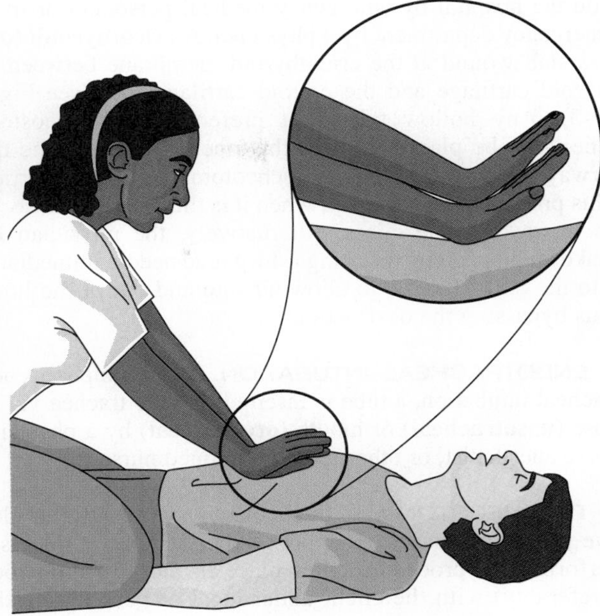

With the unconscious victim lying supine, straddle the victim's thighs. Place one hand on top of the other as shown, with the heel of the bottom hand just above the victim's navel. Quickly thrust inward and upward, toward the victim's head.

Figure 29-5 ● The abdominal thrust maneuver (formerly know as the Heimlich maneuver) for relief of upper airway obstruction caused by a foreign body.

rest. The following are some potential causes of upper airway obstruction:

- Tongue edema (surgery, trauma)
- Occlusion by the tongue (e.g., with loss of protective reflexes, loss of pharyngeal muscle tone, unconsciousness, and coma)
- Laryngeal edema
- Peritonsillar and pharyngeal abscess
- Head and neck carcinoma
- Thick secretions in the airway
- Cerebral disorders (i.e., stroke)
- Smoke inhalation edema
- Facial, tracheal, and/or laryngeal trauma
- Foreign body aspiration
- Burns of the head and/or neck area
- Anaphylaxis

COLLABORATIVE MANAGEMENT

Assessment

Upper airway obstruction can be a frightening experience for the client and family. Prompt nursing and medical care are essential to prevent a partial airway obstruction from progressing to a complete obstruction. A client with a partial obstruction (e.g., caused by limited edema or a small foreign body) may have few symptoms or only subtle and general symptoms such as diaphoresis, tachycardia, and elevated blood pressure. Unexplained or persistent recurrent symptoms warrant evaluation even though the symptoms are vague. To rule out any potentially life-threatening condition (e.g., tumor, foreign body, or infection), the physician orders diagnostic procedures, such as a chest x-ray study, lateral neck films, direct laryngoscopic examination, and computed tomography.

The nurse observes for signs of hypoxia and hypercapnia, restlessness, increasing anxiety, sternal retractions, a "seesawing" chest, abdominal movements, or a feeling of impending doom related to actual air hunger. Pulse oximetry is used for the ongoing monitoring of oxygen saturation. The client is continually assessed for stridor, cyanosis, and changes in level of consciousness.

Interventions

The nurse assesses for the cause of the obstruction. When the obstruction is due to the tongue falling back or the accumulation of secretions, the client's head and neck are placed in a slightly extended position, an oral airway is inserted, and suction may be used to remove obstructing secretions. If the airway obstruction results from a foreign body, abdominal thrusts are performed (Figure 29-5).

Upper airway obstruction may require emergency procedures such as a cricothyroidotomy, an endotracheal intubation, or a tracheostomy. These procedures are often preceded or followed by direct laryngoscopy to evaluate the cause of obstruction. The physician uses direct laryngoscopy in a controlled situation as the treatment of choice for the removal of foreign bodies.

CRICOTHYROIDOTOMY. Cricothyroidotomy is a lifesaving emergency procedure and is usually performed outside the hospital by emergency medical personnel or in the emergency department by a physician. A **cricothyroidotomy** is a stab wound at the cricothyroid membrane between the thyroid cartilage and the cricoid cartilage ring (see Figure 27-3). Any hollow tube—but preferably a tracheostomy tube—can be placed through this opening to keep the new airway open until a formal tracheotomy can be performed. This procedure is warranted when it is the *only* way to secure an airway for the client. Alternatively, the physician can make an incision by inserting a 14-gauge needle immediately into the cricoid space to allow air into and out of the lungs, thus bypassing the obstruction.

ENDOTRACHEAL INTUBATION. To accomplish endotracheal intubation, a tube is inserted into the trachea via the nose **(nasotracheal)** or mouth **(orotracheal)** by a physician, nurse anesthetist, or other specially trained nurse.

TRACHEOSTOMY. A tracheostomy is usually an elective procedure that takes approximately 5 to 10 minutes to perform. The procedure takes place in the operating room (preferably) with the client under local or general anesthesia, or it can be performed at the bedside. Infrequently, an awake tracheostomy with local anesthesia is performed if there is concern that the airway will be lost during the induction of anesthesia. An emergency tracheostomy is reserved for the client who cannot be immediately intubated with an oral or nasal endotracheal tube. The airway can be established in less than 2 minutes in an emergency situation. Care of the client with a tracheostomy is discussed in detail in Chapter 28.

Clients receiving mechanical ventilation as part of the treatment for upper airway obstruction or respiratory failure may require an elective tracheostomy after 7 or more days of continuous oral or nasal intubation. In such cases the procedure is performed to prevent laryngeal injury by the endotracheal tube.

Neck Trauma

OVERVIEW

Neck injuries are most often caused by a knife, gunshot, or traumatic accident. The client with neck trauma may have multiple injuries, including cardiovascular, respiratory, gastrointestinal, and neurologic damage. The final outcome of this type of injury depends on the initial assessment and management. Consult a critical care or emergency textbook and see Chapter 45 for more in-depth information.

➤ COLLABORATIVE MANAGEMENT

• Assessment

The priority in the management of neck trauma is assessment for a patent airway. The cardiovascular system is then assessed for signs of internal or external bleeding or impending shock.

The nurse performs a baseline neurologic assessment for mental status, sensory level, and motor function. Injury to the carotid artery may result in death, stroke, or paralysis related to the interruption of blood to the brain. The physician may order a carotid angiogram (see Chapter 33) to rule out vascular injuries.

Injuries involving the esophagus may also occur with neck trauma. The nurse assesses for chest pain and tenderness, oral bleeding, and **crepitus** (crackling sounds). The physician may order a barium or meglumine diatrizoate (Gastrografin) swallow to rule out an esophageal perforation injury.

• Interventions

Cervical spine injuries often occur at the same time as a neck injury (see Chapter 43). Health care personnel must take great care not to exacerbate these injuries by causing neck movement while establishing the airway. The nurse prepares to assist in emergency intubation, cricothyrotomy, or tracheostomy to establish a patent airway. Interventions for clients in shock are detailed in Chapter 37.

Head and Neck Cancer

OVERVIEW

Head and neck cancer interferes with breathing, eating, facial appearance, self-image, speech, and communication. This form of cancer can be devastating, even when treated successfully. The nurse is challenged in caring for clients with these complex problems. The client can receive appropriate care only through accurate identification of the location and size of the original tumor. An interdisciplinary approach by the health care team is essential to addressing the entire spectrum of needs for these clients.

Head and neck cancer can be curable when treated early. The prognosis for those who have more advanced disease at diagnosis depends on the extent and location of the tumor. Untreated cancer of the head and neck is a fatal disease, with untreated clients usually dying within 2 years of diagnosis.

Pathophysiology

Most head and neck cancers (80%) are squamous cell (mucosal epithelial) carcinomas that usually require several years to develop (Figure 29-6). Many head and neck tumors first present as malignant ulcerations with underlying infiltration.

Initially, the mucosa is subjected to an irritating substance and transforms itself into a tougher mucosa **(squamous metaplasia)** by increasing the mucosal thickness (**acanthosis** or hyperplasia) or by developing a keratin layer **(keratosis).** At the same time, cellular gene changes lead to the growth of abnormal epithelial cells that eventually become malignant. These lesions may then take the form of white, patchy lesions or red, velvety patches. Head and neck carcinoma is often diagnosed on the basis of white, patchy mucosal lesions **(leukoplakia)** or red patches **(erythroplasia).**

The growth and spread **(metastasis)** of head and neck cancer depends on the site of the primary tumor. Spread usually occurs in adjacent anatomic areas such as mucosa, muscle, and bone. Systemic spread through the blood and lymphatic systems may also occur. When metastasis occurs, it is most commonly to the lungs or liver.

The histologic description of squamous cell cancers includes carcinoma in situ, well-differentiated carcinoma, moderately differentiated carcinoma, or poorly differentiated carcinoma. Most head and neck cancers are of squamous origin, but they also can be of salivary gland or thyroid origin. Less commonly, tumors can be epidermoid, adenoid cystic, malig-

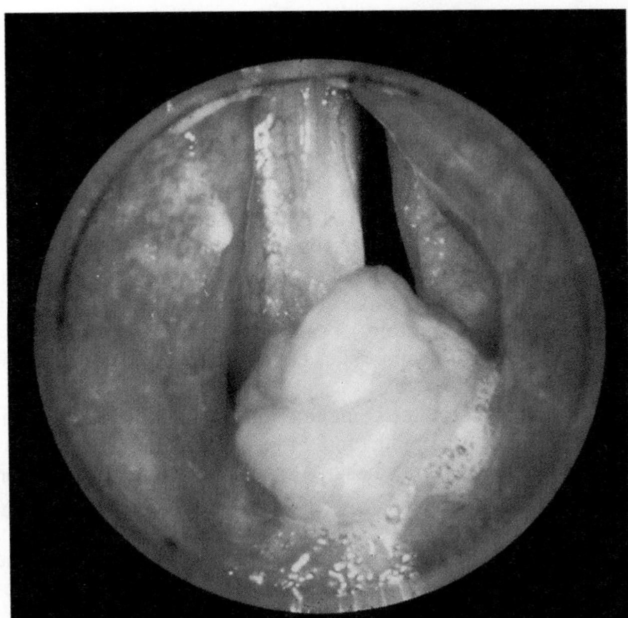

Figure 29-6 ● Laryngeal cancer is often caused by the combination of alcohol and tobacco. This laryngoscopic photograph shows a large granular cell tumor of the true vocal cord. (From Wenig, B.M. [1993]. *Atlas of head and neck pathology.* Philadelphia: W.B. Saunders. Used with permission.)

nant melanoma, or adenocarcinoma. These tumors are treated by various methods depending on the type of tumor and its known response to therapies.

Etiology

Numerous risk factors have been identified as contributing to the development of head and neck cancer, but the actual cause is unknown. The two most important risk factors are tobacco and alcohol use, especially in combination. Other risk factors include chewing tobacco, pipe smoking, marijuana, voice abuse, chronic laryngitis, exposure to industrial chemicals or hardwood dust, and complete neglect of oral hygiene.

Incidence/Prevalence

The frequency of occurrence of head and neck carcinoma is increasing. The American Cancer Society (ACS) estimates 43,000 newly diagnosed cases of *oral* and *laryngeal* cancers per year, which accounts for more than 4% of all carcinomas and more than 11,000 deaths per year (ACS, 2000). Approximately three times more males than females are affected, and most head and neck cancers occur in people over 60 years of age.

CULTURAL CONSIDERATIONS

The rate of death from laryngeal cancer for men of all races has not shown any changes over three decades. However, there has been a 110% increase in the non-Caucasian population—up from 2.3 to 4.9 cases per 100,000. Death rates for women with oral or laryngeal cancers have increased for all races over the past three decades.

TABLE 29-1 • WARNING SIGNS OF HEAD AND NECK CANCER

- Pain
- Lump in the mouth, throat, or neck
- Difficulty in swallowing
- Color changes in the mouth or tongue to red, white, gray, dark brown, or black
- Oral lesion or sore that does not heal in 2 weeks
- Persistent or unexplained oral bleeding
- Numbness of the mouth, lips, or face
- Change in the fit of dentures
- Burning sensation when drinking citrus juices or hot liquids
- Persistent, unilateral ear pain
- Hoarseness or change in voice quality
- Persistent or recurrent sore throat
- Shortness of breath
- Anorexia and weight loss

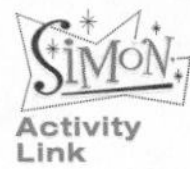

COLLABORATIVE MANAGEMENT

Assessment

HISTORY

The client with head and neck cancer may have difficulty speaking because of hoarseness, shortness of breath, tumor bulk, and pain. The nurse is sensitive to these difficulties during the interview.

The client is asked about tobacco and alcohol use, history of recurrent acute or chronic laryngitis or pharyngitis, oral sores, and lumps in the neck. The client's smoking history is calculated in **pack-years** (the number of packs smoked per day times the number of years the client has smoked). The nurse asks about alcohol intake (how many drinks per day and for how many years). Questions of this nature may be uncomfortable for both the client and the nurse but are an important part of the history. The nurse also asks about exposure to any environmental or occupational pollutants.

Problems related to risk factors are assessed. For example, nutrition may be poor because of alcohol intake and impaired liver function. The nurse assesses dietary habits and any reported weight loss. A history of chronic lung disease, which has an impact on the client's breathing pattern, is an important operative risk factor.

PHYSICAL ASSESSMENT/CLINICAL MANIFESTATIONS

Table 29-1 summarizes the warning signs of head and neck cancer. With *laryngeal* cancer, hoarseness may occur because of tumor bulk and a lack of ability to approximate the vocal cords in a normal fashion during phonation. Figure 29-7 illustrates the common sites of laryngeal cancer. Lesions of the true vocal cords are the earliest form of laryngeal cancer. A careful evaluation is important for anyone who has a history of hoarseness, mouth sores, or a lump in the neck for 3 to 4 weeks or longer.

Inspection and palpation of the head and neck are important parts of the physical examination. A specially trained nurse may perform a laryngeal examination, which includes the use of the laryngeal mirror or fiberoptic laryngoscope. Lesions may be visible on direct inspection, and the nurse palpates the neck for tumor nodal involvement.

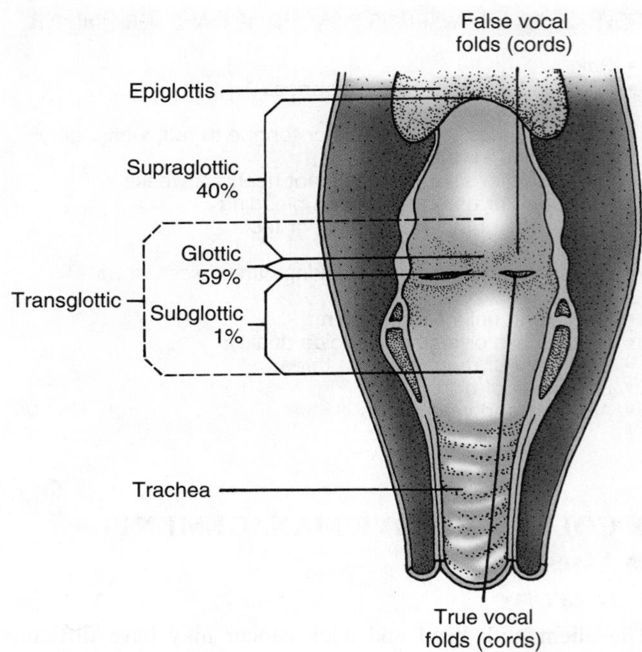

Figure 29-7 ● Sites and incidence of primary laryngeal tumors.

PSYCHOSOCIAL ASSESSMENT

The typical client with head and neck carcinoma has a long-standing history of cigarette and/or alcohol use. The client or family may experience denial, guilt, blame, or shame once the diagnosis is suspected. The nurse assesses the availability and adequacy of support systems and coping mechanisms. Because the client often requires extensive assistance at home following treatment, assessment and documentation of social and family support are essential. The social worker is consulted for assistance as needed. Because of the importance of preoperative and postoperative teaching, cognitive functioning (see Chapter 41) and the level of education and literacy of the client and family are evaluated.

The nurse notes any family history of cancer as well as the client's age, gender, occupation, interests, and ability to perform the activities of daily living. The client is asked whether his or her occupation requires continual oral communication. Retraining in other vocational areas may be needed if speech has been affected.

LABORATORY ASSESSMENT

Routine diagnostic laboratory tests include a complete blood count, bleeding times, urinalysis, and SMA-20. Decreased protein and albumin levels indicate a loss of protein stores and define the nutritional risks often seen in clients with alcoholism. Renal and liver function tests are performed to rule out metastatic disease and to evaluate the client's ability to metabolize medications and chemotherapeutic agents.

RADIOGRAPHIC ASSESSMENT

Many types of radiographic studies, including x-ray studies of the skull, sinuses, neck, and chest, are useful in diagnosing metastases, second primary tumors, and the extent of tumor invasion. Computed tomography (CT) of the head and neck, with or without contrast media, helps to evaluate the tumor's exact location.

OTHER DIAGNOSTIC ASSESSMENT

Magnetic resonance imaging (MRI) can differentiate normal from diseased tissue. An MRI is more sensitive than a CT in defining the extent of soft-tissue invasion.

The brain, bone, and liver may also be evaluated with nuclear imaging, bone scans, SPECT (single photon emission computerized tomography) scans, and PET (positron emission tomography) scans. These tests help in locating additional tumor sites.

Other diagnostic tests include direct and indirect laryngoscopy, tumor mapping, and biopsy. Panendoscopy is performed with general anesthesia to define the extent of the tumor. This procedure includes laryngoscopy, nasopharyngoscopy, esophagoscopy, and bronchoscopy. Anatomic tumor mapping uses biopsy to outline and identify tumor location. At the time of the panendoscopy, the biopsy confirms the diagnosis and determines the tumor type, cellular characteristics, and location. Tumor staging by the TNM (tumor, nodes, metastasis) classification (see Chapter 24) is performed at this time.

● Analysis

COMMON NURSING DIAGNOSES AND COLLABORATIVE PROBLEMS

The primary collaborative problem for clients with head and neck carcinomas is Risk for Ineffective Breathing Pattern related to impaired airway from the disease process (i.e., tumor invasion or obstruction, edema, and chronic lung disease).

The following are priority nursing diagnoses for these clients:

1. Risk for Aspiration related to edema, anatomic changes, or alteration of protective oropharyngeal reflexes
2. Anxiety related to fear of the unknown
3. Disturbed Body Image related to tumor and treatment modalities

ADDITIONAL NURSING DIAGNOSES AND COLLABORATIVE PROBLEMS

In addition to the common nursing diagnoses and collaborative problems, clients with head and neck carcinomas may have one or more of the following:

- Acute Pain or Chronic Pain related to tumor invasion of tissues and nerves and surgical intervention
- Imbalanced Nutrition: Less Than Body Requirements related to dysphagia, anxiety, tumor process, surgical resection, or chronic alcohol intake
- Impaired Verbal Communication related to tumor invasion, associated aphonia, hoarseness, pain, and/or surgical resection
- Impaired Tissue Integrity related to altered circulation, nutritional deficit, tumor invasion, radiation, chemical factors (body secretions or substances), or surgical wound
- Impaired Skin Integrity related to altered circulation, nutritional deficit, tumor invasion, radiation, chemical factors (body secretions or substances), or surgical wound

- Ineffective Coping related to altered body image, communication method, and/or ineffective social support
- Impaired Social Interaction related to body image disturbance and lifestyle practices
- Impaired Adjustment related to self-care of the tracheostomy and nasogastric tubes, alternative communication methods, and body image disturbance
- Deficient Knowledge related to treatment regimen and unfamiliarity with information resources

CRITICAL THINKING CHALLENGE

The client is a 58-year-old woman who has just been diagnosed with head and neck cancer. She has smoked two and a half packs of cigarettes per day for 33 years and says she drinks only a glass of wine before dinner each day. She is upset, telling you she has heard that cancer is "genetic." She worries that her three grown children may "inherit" this type of cancer.

- What is her pack-year smoking history?
- What will you tell her regarding her grown children's risk for head and neck cancer?
- What other information should you obtain from this client in order to plan appropriate preoperative teaching?

For suggested answer guidelines, go to SIMON http://www.wbsaunders.com/SIMON/Iggy/.

Planning and Implementation

INEFFECTIVE BREATHING PATTERN

NOC **PLANNING: EXPECTED OUTCOMES.** The client with head and neck carcinomas is expected to attain and/or maintain adequate ventilation and oxygenation as evidenced by the partial pressure of arterial oxygen ($Pa{O_2}$), partial pressure of arterial carbon dioxide ($Pa{CO_2}$), and $Sp{O_2}$ all being within normal limits (WNL).

INTERVENTIONS. The goal of treatment is to remove or eradicate the cancer while preserving as much normal function as possible. The physician presents the available treatment options. Modalities of surgery, radiation, or chemotherapy may be used alone or in combination. When planning treatment options, the physician considers the client's general physical condition, nutritional status, and age; the effects of the tumor on body function; and most important, the client's personal choice. Before recommending extensive surgery, the physician considers the client's ability to manage his or her own care postoperatively.

Treatment for laryngeal cancer may range from radiation therapy (for a small specific area or tumor) to total laryngopharyngectomy, with bilateral neck dissections followed by radiation therapy. The specific treatment depends on the extent and location of the lesion. Voice conservation procedures are elected only if they can be accomplished without risking incomplete removal of the tumor. The nurse focuses on the client's total needs, including preoperative preparation, competent in-hospital care, discharge planning and teaching, and extensive outpatient rehabilitation.

NONSURGICAL MANAGEMENT. The nurse monitors the respiratory system by assessing respiratory rate, breath sounds, pulse oximetry, arterial blood gas values, and the results of pulmonary function tests. Signs of respiratory distress may indicate narrowing of the airway related to tumor growth, edema, or both. The client is positioned for optimal air exchange. The nurse educates the client and family about the use of Fowler's and semi-Fowler's positions. Sitting upright in a reclining chair may promote more comfortable breathing. Chapters 7 and 9 provide additional information on palliation and pain control for clients who elect not to have therapy and for those whose therapy has not been effective.

RADIATION THERAPY. Radiation treatment of small cancers in specific locations offers a cure rate of at least 80%. The cure rate for larger cancers is lower when radiation is used as a single-modality therapy. Standard therapy uses 5000 to 7500 rad (radiation absorbed dose), usually over 6 weeks and in daily or twice-daily doses. The physician may recommend radiation alone or in combination with surgery. Because radiation therapy causes alterations in tissue healing, it might *not* be recommended preoperatively. Radiation therapy is commonly an outpatient procedure (see Chapter 25). Most clients experience uncomfortable side effects during and for a few weeks following radiation therapy (see Chart 29-2).

Hoarseness may become worse. The nurse reassures the client and family that vocalization will improve to at least pretreatment levels within 4 to 6 weeks after completion of radiation therapy. The client is encouraged to use voice rest and alternative means of communication until the effects of radiation therapy have subsided.

Most clients have a sore throat and difficulty swallowing while undergoing radiation therapy. Gargling with saline or sucking ice may decrease discomfort. Mouthwashes and throat sprays containing a local anesthetic agent such as diphenhydramine or lidocaine can provide temporary relief. Pain medication is ordered as needed.

The skin at the site of irradiation becomes red and tender and may peel during therapy. The client must avoid exposing this area to sun, heat, cold, and abrasive treatments such as shaving. The nurse instructs the client to wear protective clothing made of soft cotton and to wash this area gently with a mild soap, such as Dove. Only the lotions or powders prescribed by the radiologist should be used until the area has healed.

If the salivary glands are in the path of irradiation, the client will have a dry mouth. This side effect is long term and may be permanent. Heavy fluid intake, particularly water, and a humidified atmosphere can help relieve the discomfort. Some clients benefit from the use of artificial saliva, such as Salivart. Additional interventions for dry mouth include chewing gum and sucking hard candy.

CHEMOTHERAPY. Chemotherapy is not usually used alone for cancers of the head and neck. At times, it is **adjuvant** (additional) to surgery or radiation. Chapter 25 discusses the general care needs of clients receiving chemotherapy.

SURGICAL MANAGEMENT. Tumor size and location (TNM classification) defines the extent of surgical intervention for cancer of the head and neck. The method of reconstruction is also determined by the tumor size and amount of tissue to be resected and reconstructed. Surgical procedures for head and neck cancers include laryngectomy (total and partial), tracheostomy, and oropharyngeal cancer resections.

LARYNGECTOMY AND RELATED SURGICAL PROCEDURES. The major types of resections for laryngeal cancer include cordal stripping, **cordectomy** (excision of a vocal cord), partial laryngectomy, and total laryngectomy. If lymph nodes in the neck are involved or if it is known that the tumor has a high rate of nodal spread, the surgeon performs a nodal neck dissection in conjunction with removal of the primary tumor. A pathologist evaluates the resected lymph nodes for tumor invasion.

Preoperative Care. As the client advocate, the nurse teaches the client and family about the tumor. The physician explains the surgical procedure and obtains informed consent. The nurse discusses and interprets the implications of such consent.

The nurse explains about self-care of the airway, compensatory methods of communication, suctioning, pain control methods, the critical care environment (including ventilators and critical care routines), nutritional support, feeding tubes, and goals for discharge. The client will need to learn new methods of speech. He or she is prepared for this change through preoperative teaching and the establishment of an alternative form of communication (e.g., pen and pencil, "magic slate," picture or alphabet board) before surgery.

The explanations of routines and outcomes of care are very important because these discussions are used to plan the hospitalization and rehabilitation. Multidisciplinary teams of nurses, physicians, speech pathologists, social workers, dietitians, and occupational and physical therapists are vitally important in the preoperative evaluation and preparation of clients with cancer. Chapter 17 describes general preoperative assessment and education in detail.

CRITICAL THINKING CHALLENGE

The client is a 58-year-old woman with laryngeal cancer. She has been scheduled for a total laryngectomy and is in the preoperative holding area. You check her chart and find that she has signed the informed consent and has received a preoperative sedative intramuscularly. She tells you that she does not understand why she needs to be put to sleep just to have this small tumor removed. In talking further with her, you discover that she does not understand what a total laryngectomy is and thinks her outcome will be similar to dental surgery.

- What should you do with this information?
- How do you verify what type of surgery is about to take place?
- What will you tell this client?

For suggested answer guidelines, go to SIMON http://www.wbsaunders.com/SIMON/Iggy/.

Operative Procedures. Hemilaryngectomy (vertical or horizontal) and supraglottic laryngectomy are types of partial voice conservation laryngectomies. Table 29-2 presents more specific information about the various surgical procedures for laryngeal cancer.

To protect the airway, a temporary or permanent tracheostomy is usually performed with a partial laryngectomy. With a total laryngectomy, the upper airway is separated from the pharynx and esophagus, and the trachea is brought out through the skin in the neck and sutured in place, creating a stoma. This airway opening is *always* permanent and is referred to as a laryngectomy stoma.

Neck dissection includes the removal of tumor-involved lymph nodes, the sternocleidomastoid muscle, the jugular vein, the eleventh cranial nerve, and surrounding involved soft tissue. Because the eleventh cranial nerve (spinal accessory nerve) is resected during the nodal dissection, shoulder drop will be present after surgery. Physical therapy exercises are imperative and help the client ease the shoulder drop by increasing the use of other muscle groups.

TABLE 29-2 • SURGICAL PROCEDURES FOR LARYNGEAL CANCER AND THEIR EFFECT ON VOICE QUALITY

Procedure	Description	Resulting Voice Quality
Laser surgery	Tumor reduced or destroyed by laser beam through laryngoscope	Normal/hoarse
Transoral cordectomy	Tumor (early lesion) resected through laryngoscope	Normal/hoarse (high cure rate)
Laryngo-fissure	No cord removed (early lesion)	Normal (high cure rate)
Supraglottic partial laryngectomy	Hyoid bone, false cords, and epiglottis removed Neck dissection on affected side performed if nodes involved	Normal/hoarse
Hemilaryngectomy or vertical laryngectomy	One true cord, one false cord, and one half of thyroid cartilage removed	Hoarse voice
Total laryngectomy	Entire larynx, hyoid bone, strap muscles, one or two tracheal rings removed Nodal neck dissection if nodes involved	No natural voice

Postoperative Care. Head and neck surgical procedures often last 8 hours or longer. Because of the duration of anesthesia and the amount of resection and reconstruction, the client may spend the immediate postoperative period in the surgical intensive care unit. The nurse monitors the client's airway patency, vital signs, hemodynamic status, and comfort level. Manifestations of postoperative hemorrhage and other general complications of anesthesia and surgery are closely monitored (see Chapter 19). Vital signs are monitored every hour for the first 24 hours and then every 2 hours until the client is stable. After the client is transferred from the critical care unit, the vital signs can be monitored every 4 hours or according to agency policy. The client is generally out of bed by the second postoperative day.

Complications after a head and neck cancer resection include airway obstruction, hemorrhage, wound breakdown, and tumor recurrence. The priorities in postoperative head and neck cancer care include airway maintenance and ventilation; wound, flap, and reconstructive tissue care; pain management; nutrition; and psychologic adjustment, including speech therapy.

Airway Maintenance and Ventilation. In the immediate postoperative period, the client may need ventilatory assistance because of a long-term smoking history, chronic lung

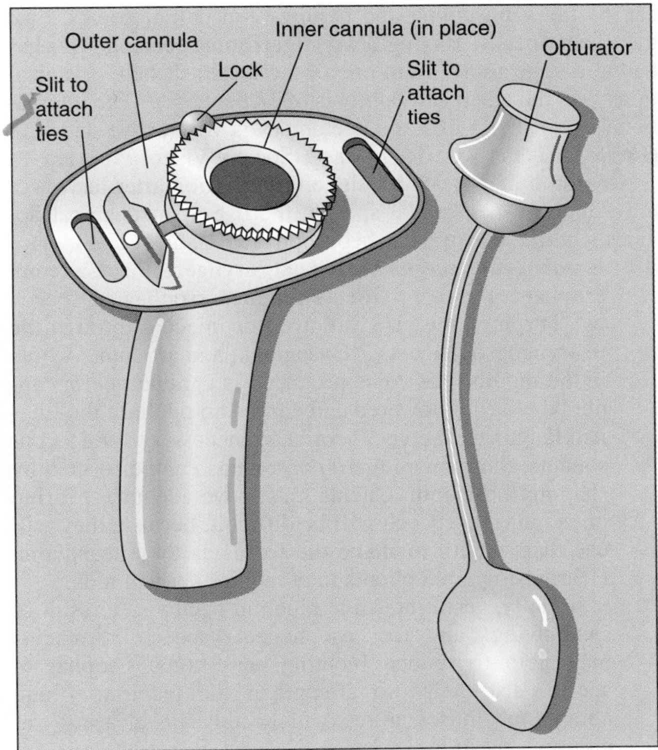

Figure 29-8 ● Laryngectomy tube. Note that the outer cannula is shorter and has a diameter wider than that of a tracheostomy tube.

disease, and a long duration of anesthesia. Although many clients also have chronic lung disease, weaning is usually not difficult because the thoracic and abdominal cavities are not entered during the surgical procedure and because the cough mechanism is intact. When weaned from the ventilator, the client usually uses a tracheostomy collar (over the artificial airway or open stoma) with oxygen and humidification to help mobilize mucus secretions. Secretions may remain blood tinged for 1 to 2 days. The nurse maintains body substance precautions and reports any increase in bleeding to the physician. Humidification helps to remove crusts and prevent obstruction of the tube with secretions. A sterile saline instillation of 5 to 10 mL every 2 hours or as needed may also be ordered; however, this practice is controversial.

A laryngectomy tube is used for clients who have undergone a *total laryngectomy* and need an appliance to prevent scar tissue contracture at the skin-tracheal border. This tube is similar to a conventional tracheostomy tube but is shorter and fatter and has a larger lumen and more acute angle (Figure 29-8). Laryngectomy tube care is similar to tracheostomy tube care (see Chapter 28), except that the client can change the laryngectomy tube daily or as needed. A laryngectomy button is similar to a laryngectomy tube but is made of a silicone-like substance (Silastic), has a single lumen, and is very short. A button is very comfortable for the laryngectomy client, is easily removed for cleaning, and is available in various sizes and lengths for a custom fit. The nurse provides a "magic slate" or paper and pencil for communication because the client has no immediate oral communication capabilities other than mouthing words.

Coughing, deep breathing, and saline instillation are often totally effective in clearing secretions. The lack of surgical interruption in the thoracic cavity or abdomen improves the ability to cough. The nurse instructs the client in the proper techniques for coughing and deep breathing to clear secretions (see Chapter 17).

Oral secretions can be suctioned with a Yankauer or tonsillar suction or with a soft red latex catheter. The nurse teaches clients to suction away from the side of an oral cavity cancer resection to prevent wound opening immediately after surgery. Clients can participate in their own care by using a table mirror for visibility. The nurse provides a clean environment for the catheter.

Stoma care following a total laryngectomy is a combination of wound care and airway care. Careful inspection of the stoma with a flashlight is routine. The suture line is cleaned with half-strength hydrogen peroxide to prevent secretions from forming crusts and obstructing the airway. Suture line care is performed every 1 to 2 hours initially, advancing to every 4 hours by the fifth postoperative day. The mucosa of the stoma and trachea should be bright and shiny and without crusts, similar to the appearance of the oral mucosa.

Wound, Flap, and Reconstructive Tissue Care. Tissue "flaps" may be used to close the wound and provide a cosmetically acceptable appearance. Commonly used reconstructive flaps are pectoralis major myocutaneous flaps, island flaps, rotation flaps, trapezius flaps, split-thickness skin grafts (STSGs), and free flaps with microvascular anastomosis (scapula, fibula, or radial forearm free flaps). These flaps may be used for reconstruction after any type of head and neck resection. After neck dissection, the surgeon places an STSG over the exposed carotid artery before covering it with skin flaps or reconstructive flaps.

The first 24 hours are critical. The nurse evaluates all flaps every hour for the first 72 hours and monitors capillary refill, color, and Doppler activity of the major feeding vessel. Any changes are reported to the surgeon immediately because surgical intervention may be indicated. The client is positioned to protect the blood supply of the reconstructed flaps.

Hemorrhage. Hemorrhage is a possible postoperative complication for all clients undergoing surgery, but it is uncommon with laryngectomy. The physician often places a closed surgical drain (see Chapter 19) in the neck area to collect blood and drainage for approximately 72 hours postoperatively. The drain also helps to maintain the position of the reconstructed skin flaps. Any drain obstruction or equipment malfunction may cause a buildup of blood or serum under the flaps. This accumulation jeopardizes the blood supply of the flaps by interfering with both arterial supply and venous drainage. Malfunctioning drains may require surgery to remove accumulated clots. Nursing responsibilities for drain management include monitoring and reporting the amount and character of drainage; emptying the drainage container; and milking the drainage tube as directed by the physician.

Wound Breakdown. Wound breakdown is a common complication because of poor nutrition in these clients, wound contamination from the oral cavity, and previous radiation therapy. A history of alcohol use further complicates the nutritional status.

The nurse treats such wound breakdown with packing and local care as ordered to keep the wound clean and to stimulate the growth of healthy granulation tissue. Wounds may be extensive, and the carotid artery may be exposed. At the initial surgical resection, split-thickness skin grafts are placed over the carotid artery for protection in the event of wound dehiscence. As the wound heals, granulation tissue covers the artery and prevents rupture. If granulation is slow and the carotid artery is at risk, another surgical flap may be made to cover the carotid artery and close the wound.

If the carotid artery ruptures because of drying or infection, the nurse places *immediate constant pressure* over the site and secures the airway. With direct manual pressure maintained on the carotid artery, the client is *immediately* transported to the operating room for carotid resection. *Carotid artery rupture has a high risk of stroke and death.* An immediate nursing response can save the client's life.

Pain Management. After cancer surgery, pain should be controlled and the client should still be able to participate in care. Morphine (Statex✤) often is given by IV bolus and continuously for the first days after surgery. As the client progresses, acetaminophen with codeine, then acetaminophen alone, can be given by feeding tube. Oral medications for pain and discomfort are started only after the client can tolerate oral nutrition. After discharge, the client still requires pain medication, especially if he or she is receiving radiation therapy. An adjunct to the pain regimen may be liquid nonsteroidal anti-inflammatory drugs (NSAIDs). These drugs provide excellent pain relief and can be used in conjunction with opioid analgesics (see also Chapter 7). Amitriptyline (Elavil) or other tricyclic antidepressants may also be used as an adjunct to pain medication for the lancinating pain of nerve root involvement.

Nutrition. A nasogastric, gastrostomy, or jejunostomy tube is placed intraoperatively for nutritional support while the aerodigestive tract heals. Initially the client receives IV fluids or parenteral nutrition until the gastrointestinal tract has recovered from the effects of anesthesia. After that, nutrients may be administered via the feeding tube. The nutritional support team or dietitian assesses the client preoperatively and is available for consultations after surgery. A standard postoperative therapeutic goal is 35 to 40 kcal/kg of body weight. Replacement of protein and insensible water loss must also be calculated very carefully.

The nasogastric tube (the most commonly used type of tube) usually remains in place for approximately 10 days after surgery. Before removing the tube, the nurse assesses the client's ability to swallow if nutrition is to be given by mouth. Aspiration *cannot* occur following an uncomplicated total laryngectomy because the airway and esophagus have been completely separated. The nurse reassures the client that aspiration will not occur and stays with him or her during the first few swallowing attempts. Swallowing may be uncomfortable at first, and analgesics are administered as ordered.

Speech Rehabilitation. Because the voice and speech can be expected to be altered after surgery, the speech pathologist and nurse discuss the principles of speech therapy with the client and family early in the course of the treatment plan (see Chart 29-2). Voice and speech differences depend on the type of surgical resection (see Table 29-2). Speech production varies with client practice, amount of resection, and radiation effects, but the speech can be very understandable.

The speech rehabilitation plan for clients undergoing a total laryngectomy consists initially of writing, then using an artificial larynx, then learning esophageal speech. The client needs support and encouragement from the speech pathologist, hospital team, and family while relearning to speak. This process can be time-consuming and requires concentration each time the client speaks. Having a **laryngectomee** (person who has had a laryngectomy) from one of the local self-help organizations visit the client and family is often beneficial. The International Association of Laryngectomees is very active and supportive, as is the American Cancer Society Visitor Program.

Common means of speech communication after laryngectomy include esophageal speech, the use of mechanical devices, and the use of a tracheoesophageal fistula (TEF).

- *Esophageal speech.* Most total laryngectomees attempt esophageal speech. Clients produce esophageal speech by "burping" the air swallowed or injected through the pharyngoesophageal (P-E) segment and articulate words in the mouth. The voice produced is a monotone; it cannot be raised or lowered and carries no pitch. In the English language, the vocal cords are necessary for 15 consonants; the remaining 10 consonants can be formed by shaping the mouth. Clients must have adequate hearing or esophageal speech will be difficult, because they will use their mouth to shape the words as they hear them. Hearing-impaired clients may require hearing aids.

  Initially, gastrointestinal bloating occurs as a result of swallowing air for esophageal speech. Antacids may help to reduce bloating sensations. Esophageal speech also helps to strengthen the respiratory and abdominal musculature, which aids in clearing secretions and in breathing.
- *Mechanical devices.* The client who cannot attain esophageal speech can use mechanical devices called **electro-larynges.** Most are battery-powered devices placed against the side of the neck or cheek. The air inside the mouth and pharynx is vibrated, and the client moves his or her lips and tongue as usual. Another external device (Cooper-Rand), also battery powered, consists of a plastic tube that is placed within the client's mouth and vibrates during speech. The quality of speech generated with these devices is robot-like and does not sound natural.
- *Tracheoesophageal fistula.* A tracheoesophageal fistula (TEF) may be used if esophageal speech is insufficient for communication and if the client meets strict criteria. A surgical fistula is created between the trachea and the esophagus either at the time of the laryngectomy or in the postoperative period (Figure 29-9). The surgeon places a catheter into the laryngectomy stoma and surgically creates a fistula into the esophagus. The catheter is usually sutured to the neck to prevent accidental dislodgment. After the fistula heals, a silicone prosthesis (e.g., the Blom-Singer prosthesis) is inserted in place of the catheter (Figure 29-10). The client covers the stoma and the opening of the prosthesis with a finger or opens and closes the opening with a special valve to divert air from the lungs, through the trachea, into the esophagus, and out of the mouth. Lip and tongue movement, not the prosthesis itself, produces speech.

SURGICAL PROCEDURES FOR OTHER HEAD AND NECK CANCERS. The major types of resections, defined by the tumor location of the *oropharyngeal cancer,* are called composite resections. **Composite resections** are a combination of surgical procedures that include partial or total glossectomies, partial mandibulectomies and, if required, nodal neck dissections. Tracheostomy may be planned to provide an adequate airway. (See Chapter 54 for more information about oral cancer.)

TRACHEOSTOMY. A **tracheostomy** is the (tracheal) stoma, or opening, that results from a tracheotomy. A **tracheotomy** is a surgical incision into the trachea for the purpose of establishing an airway. It can be performed as an emergency procedure or as a scheduled surgical procedure. A tracheostomy can be temporary or permanent. Chapter 28 presents in detail the nursing care requirements of a client with a tracheostomy.

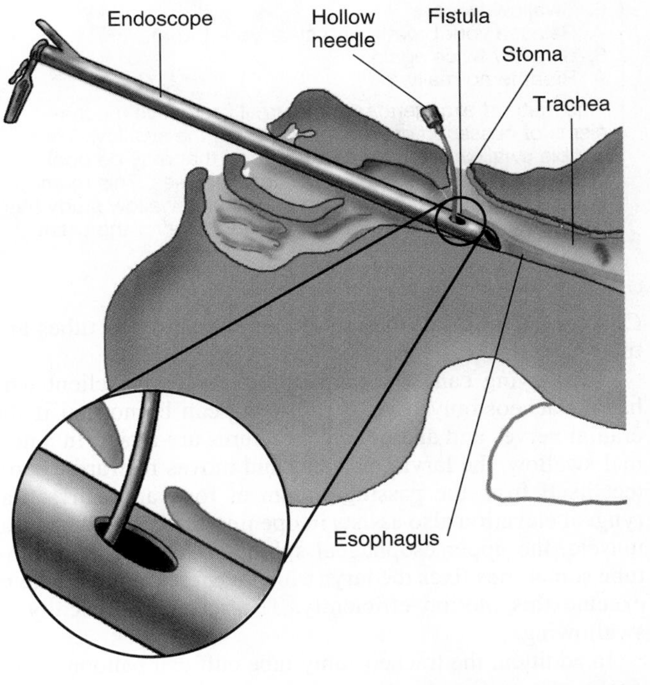

Figure 29-9 ● One method of creating a tracheoesophageal fistula.

RISK FOR ASPIRATION

NOC PLANNING: EXPECTED OUTCOMES. The client with head and neck carcinomas is expected not to aspirate food, gastrointestinal contents, or oral secretions into the lungs.

INTERVENTIONS. Depending on tumor size and location or type of tumor resection, the client may aspirate during eating. This incident can result in life-threatening pneumonia, weight loss, further hospitalization, and increased costs. Chart 29-3 lists NIC interventions for aspiration prevention.

Because of anatomic or surgical changes in the upper respiratory tract and altered swallowing mechanisms, the client with head and neck cancer is at risk for aspiration. The presence of a nasogastric (NG) feeding tube may further increase the potential for aspiration because of the incompetent lower esophageal sphincter (LES). The one exception is the client who has undergone a total laryngectomy. In these cases the airway is separated from the esophagus, making aspiration impossible; such a client is *not* at risk.

A dynamic swallow study, such as a barium swallow under fluoroscopy, evaluates a client's ability to protect the airway from aspiration and helps to determine the appropriate method of swallow rehabilitation. Bedside clinical assessment of swallowing is important but has a high rate of inaccuracy. In many cases the physician must institute enteral feedings either because of the client's inability to swallow or because of continued aspiration potential.

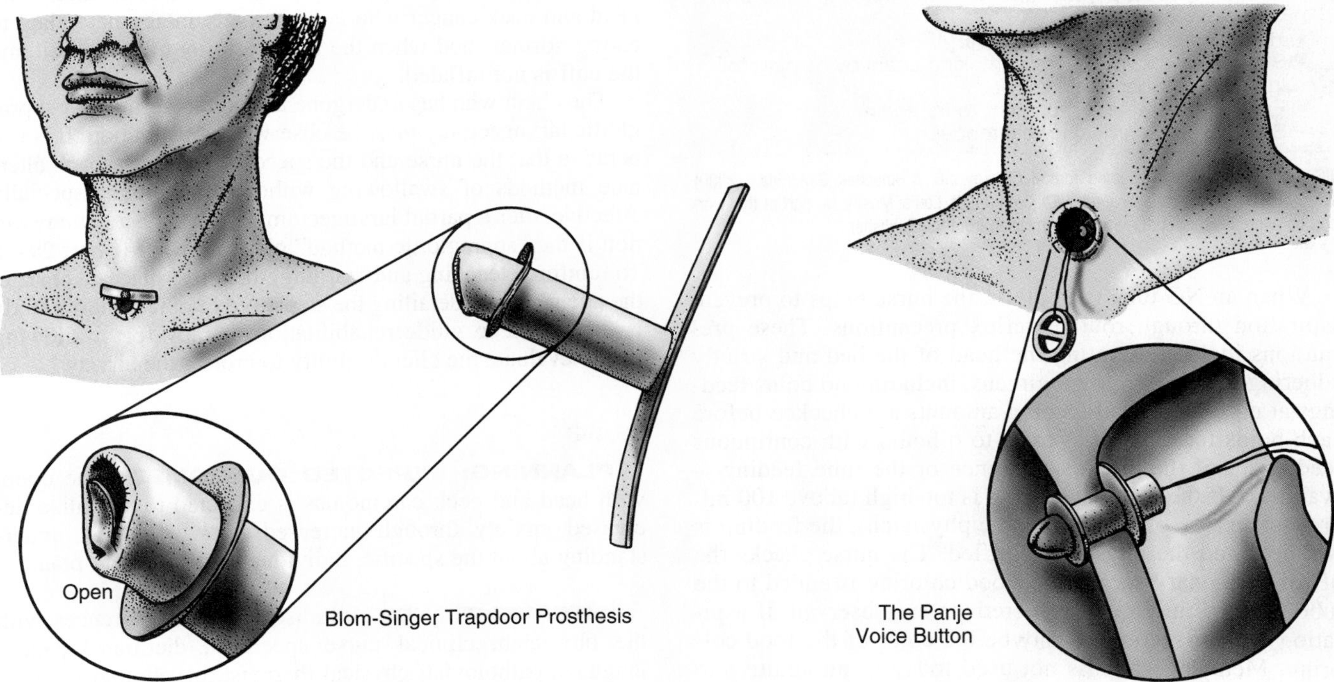

Figure 29-10 ● Examples of tracheoesophageal prostheses.

CHART 29-3

NIC INTERVENTION ACTIVITIES *for* The Client with Head and Neck Cancer

Aspiration Precautions: *Prevention or minimization of risk factors in the client at risk for aspiration*

- Monitor level of consciousness, cough reflex, gag reflex, and swallowing ability.
- Monitor pulmonary status.
- Maintain an airway.
- Position upright 90 degrees or as far as possible.
- Keep suction setup available.
- Feed in small amounts.
- Check NG or gastrostomy placement before feeding.
- Check NG or gastrostomy residual before feeding.
- Avoid liquids or use thickening agent.
- Offer foods or liquids that can be formed into a bolus before swallowing.
- Cut food into small pieces.
- Request medication in elixir form.
- Break or crush pills before administration.
- Keep head of bed elevated 30 to 45 minutes after feeding.

Smoking Cessation Assistance: *Helping another to stop smoking*

- Give smoker clear, consistent advice to quit smoking.
- Help choose best method for giving up cigarettes, when client is ready to quit.
- Refer to group programs or individual therapists, as appropriate.
- Assist client with any self-help methods.
- Help client plan specific coping strategies and resolve problems that result from quitting.
- Inform client that dry mouth, cough, scratchy throat, and feeling on edge are symptoms that may occur after quitting; the patch or gum may help with cravings.
- Advise client to keep a list of "slips" or near-slips, what causes them, and what client learned from them.
- Advise client to avoid smokeless tobacco, dipping, and chewing.
- Manage nicotine replacement therapy.
- Contact national and local resource organizations for resource materials.
- Follow client for 2 years after quitting, if possible, to provide encouragement.
- Help client deal with any lapses.
- Support client who begins smoking again by helping to identify what has been learned.
- Encourage the relapsed client to try again.
- Serve as a nonsmoking role model.

NIC intervention activities selected from McCloskey, J.C., & Bulechek, G.M. (Eds.). (2000). *Nursing interventions classification (NIC)* (3rd ed.). St. Louis: Mosby. No part of this work is to be altered without prior written permission from the Publisher.

When an NG tube is in place, the nurse helps to prevent aspiration through routine reflux precautions. These precautions include elevating the head of the bed and strictly adhering to tube feeding regimens, including no bolus feedings at night. Residual feeding amounts are checked before each bolus feeding (or every 4 to 6 hours with continuous feeding), and the client's tolerance of the tube feeding is evaluated. If the residual volume is too high (above 100 mL or as otherwise prescribed by the physician), the feeding is withheld and the physician notified. The nurse checks the pH of pulmonary secretions. Food coloring is added to the tube feeding, and tracheal secretions are observed. If aspiration occurs, secretions may be the color of the food coloring. Methylene blue is not used today as an additive to tube feedings because it is systemically excreted through the lungs and can appear in pulmonary secretions. (See Chapter 61 for other interventions related to NG tubes and tube feedings.)

CHART 29-4

CLIENT EDUCATION GUIDE The Supraglottic Method of Swallowing

1. Place yourself in an upright, preferably out-of-bed, position.
2. Clear your throat.
3. Take a deep breath.
4. Place 1/2 to 1 teaspoon of food into your mouth.
5. Hold your breath or "bear down" (Valsalva maneuver).
6. Swallow twice.
7. Release your breath, and clear your throat.
8. Swallow twice again.
9. Breathe normally.

This method exaggerates the normal protective mechanisms of cessation of respiration during the swallow. The double swallow attempts to clear food that may be pooling in the pharynx, vallecula, and piriform sinuses. This method is used only after a dynamic radiographic swallow study has demonstrated that it is appropriate and safe for the client.

Swallowing can be a major problem for the client who has a tracheostomy tube. Swallowing can be normal if the cranial nerves and anatomical structures are intact. In a normal swallow, the larynx elevates and moves forward to protect itself from the passing stream of food and saliva. Laryngeal elevation also assists in opening the cricopharyngeal muscle, the upper esophageal sphincter. The tracheostomy tube sometimes fixes the larynx in place, making it unable to execute this motion efficiently. The result is difficulty in swallowing.

In addition, the tracheostomy tube cuff can balloon posteriorly when inflated and interfere with the passage of food through the esophagus. The common wall of the posterior trachea (trachealis muscle) and the anterior esophagus is very thin, which allows this pushing phenomenon. The client with head and neck cancer who is cognitively intact may adapt to eating normal food when the tracheostomy tube is small and the cuff is not inflated.

The client who has undergone a subtotal, vertical, or supraglottic laryngectomy *must* be observed for aspiration. It is imperative that the nurse and the speech pathologist teach alternate methods of swallowing without aspirating. Especially effective after a partial laryngectomy or base-of-tongue resection is the "supraglottic method" of swallowing (Chart 29-4). To reinforce teaching and learning, the nurse places a chart in the client's room detailing the steps. A dynamic swallow study is performed to guide rehabilitation therapy for swallowing and to evaluate the client's ability to protect the airway.

ANXIETY

PLANNING: EXPECTED OUTCOMES. The client with head and neck carcinomas is expected to verbalize decreased anxiety through increased knowledge and understanding about the specific, individualized treatment plan.

INTERVENTIONS. Multidisciplinary conferences with the physician, clinical nurse specialist, dietitian, speech-language pathologist, physical therapist, psychologist, social worker, discharge-planning nurse, and general nursing staff may be beneficial. The nurse explores the reason for anxiety (e.g., fear of the unknown, lack of preoperative teaching, fear of pain, fear of airway compromise, fear of hospitalization, and loss of control). The client and family often benefit from further information. Before the client is scheduled for surgery (and while still at home), home care nurses or community-sponsored associations (e.g., American Cancer Society) may be able to decrease fears about the disease process and surgical interventions.

The nurse administers antianxiety agents, such as diazepam (Valium, Meval♣), with caution because of the possibility of hypercarbia and hypoxia in an already compromised client. The location of the tumor and the presence of any other lung disease may cause some degree of airway obstruction. For anxiety in these clients, the physician prescribes drug therapy judiciously and may choose lorazepam (Ativan, Novo-Lorazem♣) rather than a solely sedating agent.

DISTURBED BODY IMAGE

PLANNING: EXPECTED OUTCOMES. The client with head and neck carcinomas is expected to state an understanding and, in time, an acceptance of body image changes and return to the previous lifestyle within the limits of the disease.

INTERVENTIONS. The client with head and neck cancer experiences a permanent change in body image because of deformity, the presence of a stoma or artificial airway, speech changes, and a change in the method of eating. The client may be aphonic or have permanent hoarseness or speech deficits. The nurse helps in setting realistic goals, starting with involvement in self-care. Alternative communication methods are taught so the client can functionally communicate in the hospital and after discharge.

The nurse and family must make all attempts to ease the client into a more normal social environment. The nurse provides encouragement and positive reinforcement while demonstrating acceptance and caring behaviors. The family also may benefit from counseling sessions initiated while the client is still in the hospital.

After surgery, the client may feel reserved and socially isolated because of the change in voice and facial appearance. Loose-fitting, high-collar shirts or sweaters (e.g., turtleneck), scarves, and jewelry can be worn to cover the laryngectomy stoma, tracheostomy tube, and postoperative changes related to surgery. Cosmetics may aid in covering any disfigurement. Most surgeons try to place the surgical incisions in the natural skin fold lines if doing so does not pose a risk for cancer recurrence.

CRITICAL THINKING CHALLENGE

The client, a 68-year-old man 5 days postoperative after a supraglottic partial laryngectomy, is being discharged to home. After hearing the discharge order, his wife becomes agitated and says that "home isn't ready for him yet." She asks if he can remain in the hospital for another week.

- Should you try to get this client's discharge orders changed?
- What question(s) should you ask the wife?
- What might be causing the wife's anxiety?
- What teaching priorities are needed?

For suggested answer guidelines, go to SIMON http://www.wbsaunders.com/SIMON/Iggy/.

CHART 29-5

CLIENT EDUCATION GUIDE
Home Laryngectomy Care

- Avoid swimming, and use care when showering or shaving.
- Lean slightly forward and cover the stoma when coughing or sneezing.
- Wear a stoma guard or loose clothing to cover the stoma.
- Clean the stoma with mild soap and water. Lubricate the stoma with a non-oil–based ointment as needed.
- Increase humidity by using saline in the stoma as instructed, a bedside humidifier, pans of water, and houseplants.
- Obtain and wear a MedicAlert bracelet and emergency care card for life-threatening situations.

Community-Based Care

If no complications occur, the client is usually ready to be discharged home or to an extended care facility within 2 weeks. At the time of discharge, he or she should be able to provide self-care, which may include tracheostomy or stoma care, nutrition, wound care, and methods of communication.

The client and family may feel more secure about discharge if they receive a referral to selected support groups or a community health agency familiar with the care of clients recovering from head and neck cancer. The multidisciplinary team assesses the specific discharge needs and makes the appropriate referrals to home care agencies, including professionals such as nutritionists, nurses, physical therapists, speech pathologists, and social workers. The nurse coordinates the scheduling for chemotherapy or radiation therapy with the client and family.

HEALTH TEACHING

Although education begins during preoperative teaching sessions, most self-care is taught in the hospital. The nurse teaches the client and family how to care for the stoma or tracheostomy or laryngectomy tube, depending on the type of surgery performed. Incision and airway care are reviewed, including cleaning and inspecting for signs of infection.

Chart 29-5 summarizes the highlights of self-care for the client who is discharged after laryngeal cancer surgery. Many of these highlights are also applicable to any resection for head and neck cancer.

STOMA CARE. To prevent water from entering the airway, the client is instructed to use a shower shield over the tracheostomy tube or laryngectomy stoma when bathing. To shield the airway during the day, the client may wear a protective cover or stoma guard.

For clients with permanent stomas following laryngectomy or for those with permanent tracheostomies, covering the permanent opening has a double benefit: (1) filtering the air entering the stoma while keeping humidity in the airway, and (2) enhancing esthetic appearance. To protect the airway and increase humidity, the nurse instructs the client to cover the airway with cotton or foam. Attractive coverings are available in the form of cotton scarves, crocheted bibs, and jewelry. Using colored seam binding for tracheostomy ties after the stoma has matured may enhance overall body image. Shirt or

TOTAL NECK BREATHER
(Front of Card)

EMERGENCY!

I am a Total Neck Breather
(Laryngectomee—No Vocal Cords)

I breathe ONLY through an opening in my neck, NOT through my nose or mouth.

If I have stopped breathing:

1. Expose my entire neck.
2. Give me **mouth to neck breathing only.**
3. Keep my head straight—chin up.
4. Keep neck opening clear with clean CLOTH (not tissue).
5. Use oxygen supply to neck opening, ONLY, when I start to breathe again.

BE PROMPT—SECONDS COUNT
I NEED AIR NOW!

(Back of All Cards)

Medical Problems
☐ Epilepsy ☐ Glaucoma
☐ Diabetes ☐ Peptic Ulcer
Other ______

Medicines Taken Regularly
☐ Anticoagulants ☐ Cortisone or ACTH
☐ Heart Drugs (Name and Dose)
Other ______

Dangerous Allergies
☐ Drugs (Name)
☐ Penicillin
Other ______

Other Information
☐ Hard of Hearing
☐ Speaks No English (Other)
☐ Wearing Contact Lenses
Other ______

NAME ______
ADDRESS ______

PLEASE NOTIFY:

NAME ______
PHONE ______
ADDRESS ______
CITY ______

OR

NAME ______
PHONE ______
ADDRESS ______

INTERNATIONAL ASSOCIATION OF LARYNGECTOMEES

Figure 29-11 ● Emergency wallet card for identification of laryngectomy.

dress color can be matched or coordinated with seam bindings of various colors. The client is instructed how to increase humidity in the home. The nurse may teach him or her to instill normal saline into the artificial airway 10 to 15 times a day as ordered.

COMMUNICATION. The client continues the selected method of alternative communication that began in the hospital. He or she wears a medical alert (MedicAlert) bracelet and carries a special identification card (Figure 29-11). For clients who have undergone a laryngectomy, this card is available from the local chapters of the International Association of Laryngectomees. The card instructs the reader in providing an emergency airway or resuscitating someone who has a stoma.

SMOKING CESSATION. A difficult but important issue after head and neck cancer surgery is smoking cessation. Smoking plays a major role in the development of head and neck cancer. The nurse stresses that smoking cessation can reduce the risk for developing additional malignancies and can increase the rate of healing from surgery.

Smoking cessation is not an easy task, and most clients require continuing support and reinforcement to sustain this action (see the Evidence-Based Practice for Nursing box above). Chemical and psychologic assistance are available for smoking cessation (see Chart 29-3).

PSYCHOSOCIAL PREPARATION

The many physical changes resulting from a laryngectomy influence physical, social, and emotional functioning. Many clients perceive changes in their quality of life. The nurse begins to prepare the client and family for these changes, but another individual who has adjusted to these changes is usually more effective.

The client who is discharged to home with a permanent stoma, tracheostomy tube, nasogastric tube, and wounds experiences an alteration in body image. The nurse stresses the importance of returning to as normal a lifestyle as possible. Approximately half of the clients return to full-time employment, and the rest work part time or apply for disability income. Most clients can resume many of their usual activities within 4 to 6 weeks after surgery or longer after a combination of radiation therapy and surgery. The client may be frustrated at times while trying to adjust to changes in smell, taste, and communication.

The client with a total laryngectomy cannot produce sounds during laughing and crying, and mucous secretions may appear unexpectedly when these emotions or coughing or sneezing occur. The mucus can be embarrassing, and the client needs to be prepared to cover the stoma with a handkerchief or gauze. The client who has undergone composite resections will have difficulty with speech *and* swallowing.

EVIDENCE-BASED PRACTICE FOR NURSING

Smoking cessation is hard!

Griebel, B., Wewers, M., & Baker, C. (1998). The effectiveness of a nurse-managed minimal smoking cessation intervention among hospitalized patients with cancer. *Oncology Nursing Forum, 25*(5), 897-902.

This prospective study sought to determine the effectiveness of a nurse-managed minimal smoking-cessation intervention provided to hospitalized clients with cancer. Two groups of subjects, 14 in each, were enrolled in the study. All subjects had undergone cancer surgery for a type of cancer known to be influenced by cigarette smoking, and all expressed interest in smoking cessation. The intervention group received a 20-minute visit from an advanced practice nurse certified as an American Cancer Society "Fresh Start" facilitator. During the visit, this nurse discussed the benefits of quitting, approaches to quitting, and management of withdrawal symptoms. Intervention group subjects also received the names and numbers of community resources along with a booklet guide to smoking cessation. In addition to the one-time in-person discussion, the facilitator also provided each intervention subject with a weekly 10-minute phone call to encourage cessation maintenance. Subjects in the control group received routine care. Although smoking cessation materials were available to this group, there was no concerted effort to provide information.

Smoking status by self-report and biochemical analysis of salivary cotinine levels was examined in all subjects 6 weeks after surgery. The number of subjects in the intervention group who were successful in smoking cessation was not significantly different from the number of successful subjects in the control group. However, the intervention group did appear to have a greater reduction in the number of cigarettes smoked each day compared to the control group. It was determined that the intervention was not effective in helping people achieve success in smoking cessation.

Critique. The sample, although homogeneous, was small in size. Timing for delivery of the intervention was not addressed and could have been a factor in the subjects' readiness for the intervention. None of the subjects used a nicotine replacement therapy.

Implications for Nursing. Cigarette smoking is an addiction with emotional and physiologic components. Successful smoking cessation requires addressing both of these components. Nurses who begin discussions with clients regarding smoking cessation need to present honest, comprehensive information and demonstrate a commitment to assist the client in achieving an appropriate level of support/positive reinforcement of the cessation behavior.

CHART 29-6

FOCUSED ASSESSMENT *of*
Home Care Clients After Laryngectomy

Assess respiratory status.
- Observe rate and depth of respiration.
- Auscultate lungs.
- Check patency of airway.
- Examine the tracheostomy exudate for amount, color, and character.
- Examine nail beds and mucous membranes for evidence of cyanosis.
- Obtain a pulse oximetry reading.

Assess condition of wound.
- Remove dressings (noting condition of dressings).
- Cleanse the wound.
- Compare with previous notations of wound condition:
  - Presence, amount, and nature of exudate
  - Presence/absence of cellulitis
  - Presence/absence of odor

Assess client's psychosocial functioning.
- Ask the client about passing the time, visitors, and trips outside the house.
- Observe whether the client communicates responses directly or whether a family member speaks for the client.
- Observe client and family member interactions.
- Determine what method of communication the client has selected, and observe the client's skill with it.
- Is the client wearing pajamas, or is the client dressed?

Take the client's temperature.

Assess the client's understanding of illness and compliance with treatment.
- Signs and symptoms to report to the health care provider
- Medication plan (correct timing and dose)
- Ambulation or positioning schedule
- Dressing changes/skin care
- Diet modifications (24-hour diet recall)
- Skill in tracheostomy or dressing care

Assess client's nutritional status.
- Change in muscle mass
- Lackluster nails/sparse hair
- Recent weight loss >10% of usual weight
- Impaired oral intake
- Difficulty swallowing
- Generalized edema

He or she may need to deal with tracheostomy and feeding tubes in public places.

HOME CARE MANAGEMENT

Extensive home care preparation is required after a laryngectomy for cancer. The convalescent period is long, and airway management is complicated. The client or family must be able to take an active role in care.

General cleanliness of the home is assessed. If the client has severe or long-standing respiratory problems, adjustments in the home to allow for one-floor living may be necessary. Increased humidification is needed. A humidifier add-on to a forced-air furnace can be obtained. If the cost of this add-on is not manageable or if the home is heated by radiators, a room humidifier or vaporizer may be appropriate.

A home care nurse is involved with care after discharge and is a very important resource for the client and family. The home care nurse assesses the client and home situation for problems in self-care, complications, adjustment, and adherence to the medical regimen. Chart 29-6 lists assessment areas for the client in the home following a laryngectomy. The nurse reinforces health care teaching, self-care teaching, and smoking cessation regimens.

HEALTH CARE RESOURCES

The home care or hospital nurse informs the client and family of community organizations (e.g., American Cancer Society) and local laryngectomee clubs, which can offer support, accurate information, and friendships. When the client has problems paying for health care services, equipment, and prescriptions, a visiting nurse agency may be helpful in directing him or her to available resources.

In many areas the local unit of the American Cancer Society or Canadian Cancer Society can help provide dressing materials and nutritional supplements to clients in need. This organization may also provide transportation to and from follow-up visits or radiation therapy.

Evaluation: Outcomes

NOC The nurse evaluates the care of the client with head and neck carcinomas on the basis of the identified nursing diagnoses and collaborative problems. The expected outcomes are that the client:

- Maintains a patent airway
- Attains or maintains clear lung sounds in all lung fields
- Demonstrates an understanding of head and neck cancer and its treatment
- Performs self-care of the artificial airway and wound
- Performs activities of daily living (ADLs) independently or with minimal assistance
- States that levels of anxiety are reduced
- Resumes as normal a lifestyle as possible through rehabilitation
- States an understanding of and adjusts to changes in physical appearance and body function
- Attains or maintains adequate nutrition
- Does not aspirate gastric contents or food
- Complies with smoking and alcohol cessation

ONLINE RESOURCES

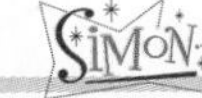

For suggested readings and Internet resources, go to http://www.wbsaunders.com/SIMON/Iggy/.

SELECTED BIBLIOGRAPHY

Abernathy, W., et al. (2000). Nonmetallic fixation in elective maxillofacial surgery. *AORN Journal, 71*(1), 193-198.

American Cancer Society. (2001). *Cancer facts and figures, 2001.* 01-300M-No.5008.01. Atlanta: Author.

Biddle, C. (1999). Sleep apnea and other disordered-breathing syndromes. *Current Reviews for Nurse Anesthetists, 22*(1), 3-8.

Bird, D. (1999). Epistaxis. *Emergency Nurse, 7*(3), 10-13.

Carr, M., et al. (2000). Communication after laryngectomy: An assessment of quality of life. *Otolaryngology—Head and Neck Surgery, 122*(1), 39-43.

Centers for Disease Control and Prevention. (1998). Preventing and controlling oral and pharyngeal cancer: Recommendations from a national strategic planning conference. *Oncology, 12*(11), 1629-1630, 1633, 1637-1638, 1640.

Crum, R. (1998). Pre and post laryngectomee: One patient's point of view. *ORL—Head and Neck Nursing, 16*(4), 23, 30-31.

Davidson, P. (1998). Voice restoration prostheses: The options. *Nursing Times, 94*(12), 56-58.

Dempsey, H., et al. (1998). Cold facts about epistaxis. *American Journal of Nursing, 98*(7), 21.

Dropkin, M.L. (1997). Coping with disfigurement/dysfunction and length of hospital stay after head and neck cancer surgery. *ORL—Head and Neck Nursing, 15*(1), 22-26.

Edwards, S., & Metheny, N. (2000). Measurement of gastric residual volume: State of the science. *MEDSURG Nursing, 9*(3), 125-128.

Griebel, B., Wewers, M., & Baker, C. (1998). The effectiveness of a nurse-managed minimal smoking cessation intervention among hospitalized patients with cancer. *Oncology Nursing Forum, 25*(5), 897-902.

Jarrell, L. (1999). The preoperative diagnosis and postoperative management of adult patients with obstructive sleep apnea syndrome: A review of the literature. *Journal of PeriAnesthesia Nursing, 14*(4), 193-200.

Krouse, J. (1999). Introduction to sinus disease: Part 1. Anatomy and physiology. *ORL—Head and Neck Nursing, 17*(2), 7-12.

Krouse, J., & Krouse, H. (1999). Introduction to sinus disease: Part 2. Diagnosis and treatment. *ORL—Head and Neck Nursing, 17*(3), 6-17.

Krug, P. (1999). Snoring and obstructive sleep apnea. *AORN Journal, 69*(4), 792-801.

Leccese, C. (1998). To each his own: Tailored approach works best for smoking cessation. *ADVANCE for Nursing Practitioners, 6*(4), 67-69.

Logemann, J., et al. (1997). Speech and swallowing rehabilitation for head and neck cancer patients. *Oncology, 11*(5), 651-659.

Martinelli, A. (1999). Testing a model of avoiding environmental tobacco smoke in young adults. *Image: Journal of Nursing Scholarship, 31*(3), 237-241.

McCloskey, J., & Bulechek, G. (2000). *Nursing interventions classification (NIC)* (3rd ed.). St. Louis: Mosby.

McConnell, E. (1998). Myths & facts about epistaxis. *Nursing98, 28*(3), 67.

McHale, J., et al. (1998). Expert nursing knowledge in the care of patients at risk of impaired swallowing. *Image: Journal of Nursing Scholarship, 30*(2), 137-142.

Metheny, N., et al. (1998). pH, color, and feeding tubes. *RN, 61*(1), 25-27.

Multidisciplinary rounds: Meeting nutritional needs after head and neck surgery. (1999). *Cancer Practice, 7*(1), 5-9.

Murray, K., & Brzozowski, L. (1998). Swallowing in patients with tracheostomies. *AACN Clinical Issues: Advanced Practice in Acute and Critical Care, 9*(3), 416-426.

Olsen, M. (1999). Oral cavity cancer. In C. Miaskowski & P. Buchsel (Eds.), *Oncology nursing: Assessment and clinical care* (pp. 1177-1201). St. Louis: Mosby.

Perkins, L., & Shortall, S. (2000). Ventilation without intubation. *RN, 63*(1), 34-38.

Philip, G., & Togias, A. (1999). Allergic rhinitis: Up-to-date strategies for management. *Journal of Respiratory Diseases, 20*(9), 580-582, 585-588.

Phillips, S. (1997). Obstructive sleep apnea: Diagnosis and management. *Nursing Standard, 11*(17), 43-46.

Sarna, L. (1999). Prevention: Tobacco control and cancer nursing. *Cancer Nursing, 22*(1), 21-28.

Schoem, S. (2000). Oral appliances for the treatment of snoring and obstructive sleep apnea. *Otolaryngology—Head and Neck Surgery, 122*(2), 259-262.

Shellenbarger, T. (2000). Nosebleeds: Not just kids' stuff. *RN, 63*(2), 50-54, 56.

Shiba, G. (1999). Nasopharyngeal cancer. In C. Miaskowski & P. Buchsel (Eds.), *Oncology nursing: Assessment and clinical care* (pp. 1145-1168). St. Louis: Mosby.

Wellen, D. (1999). Laryngeal cancer. In C. Miaskowski & P. Buchsel (Eds.), *Oncology nursing: Assessment and clinical care* (pp. 1121-1143). St. Louis: Mosby.

Yantis, M. (1999). Sleep apnea. *American Journal of Nursing, 99*(9), 24AA-BB.

CHAPTER

30

Interventions for Clients with Noninfectious Lower Respiratory Problems

M. LINDA WORKMAN

Learning Objectives

After studying this chapter, you should be able to:

1. Explain the differences in pathophysiology between asthma and bronchoconstriction, and between asthma and inflammation.
2. Prioritize educational needs for the client at step III of stepped therapy for asthma.
3. Interpret peak expiratory flow readings for the need for intervention.
4. Discuss the complications of chronic oral steroid therapy for treatment of chronic airflow limitation (CAL).
5. Compare and contrast the pathophysiology and clinical manifestations of asthma, bronchitis, and emphysema.
6. Identify risk factors for the development of chronic obstructive pulmonary disease (COPD).
7. Prioritize educational needs for the client with COPD who is receiving oxygen therapy at home.
8. Describe interventions for energy conservation for the client with COPD.
9. Prioritize nursing care needs for the client immediately following lung volume reduction surgery.
10. Explain the nutritional requirements for the client with severe COPD.
11. Use laboratory data and clinical manifestations to determine the effectiveness of therapy for impaired gas exchange in a client with CAL.
12. Identify the risk factors that predispose to the development of lung cancer.
13. Compare and contrast the side effects of radiation treatment for lung cancer with those of chemotherapy for lung cancer.
14. Explain how to troubleshoot the chest tube drainage system in a client 1 day after a thoracotomy.
15. Develop a teaching plan for a client getting ready to go home after a pneumonectomy.

SIMON

Go to http://www.wbsaunders.com/SIMON/Iggy/ for self-assessment questions related to these Learning Objectives.

Lower airway disorders directly affect gas exchange and have serious consequences. Many of these noninfectious disorders are chronic and progressive, requiring major changes in a person's lifestyle. The older client with a lower airway problem may require special considerations or assistance even before the disorder becomes severe. Chart 30-1 lists some general nursing considerations for the older client with a respiratory disorder.

CHRONIC AIRFLOW LIMITATION

Chronic airflow limitation (CAL) is a category of chronic lung diseases that includes asthma, chronic bronchitis, and pulmonary emphysema. Emphysema and chronic bronchitis, often termed **chronic obstructive pulmonary disease (COPD),** are characterized by bronchoconstriction and dyspnea (Figure 30-1). The tissue damage associated with these conditions is not reversible and tends to increase in severity over time, eventually leading to respiratory failure. Asthma, unlike emphysema and chronic bronchitis, is an intermittent process that involves *reversible* airflow obstruction and wheezing.

More than 40 million Americans suffer from some form of CAL, and 1 million people between the ages of 40 and 65 have moderate to severe disability from CAL. Although some problems are not reversible, newer management strategies can help maintain optimal functioning and improve overall health (see the Meeting Healthy People 2010 Objectives box on p. 532).

Asthma

OVERVIEW

Bronchial asthma is a condition of intermittent, reversible airflow obstruction affecting only the airways, not the alveoli (see Figure 30-1). Airway obstruction can occur in two ways: inflammation and airway hyperresponsiveness, sometimes called "twitchy airways." Inflammation obstructs the lumen, or the inside, of airways. Airway hyperresponsiveness results in airway obstruction by constriction of bronchial smooth muscle causing a narrowing of the airway from the outside. Airway inflammation can trigger bronchiolar hyperresponsiveness, and many people with asthma have both problems at the same time. Severe airway obstruction can be fatal, and more than 5000 deaths from acute asthma occur in the United States each year (Centers for Disease Control and Prevention, 1998).

Pathophysiology/Etiology

Asthma has been categorized in the past into different types based on the events known to trigger the attacks; however, the pathophysiologic events appear similar for all types of asthma. Inflammation of the mucous membranes lining the airways is a key event in precipitating an asthma attack. Inflammation can be stimulated by the presence of specific allergens; nonallergenic general irritants such as cold air, dry air, or fine airborne particles; microorganisms; and aspirin. Airway hyperresponsiveness can occur with exercise, in association with upper respiratory illnesses, and for unknown reasons. Susceptibility to airway inflammation and/or to hyperresponsive airways may have a genetic component.

When asthma is well controlled, the pathologic changes are temporary and reversible. When asthma is not well controlled, the presence of chronic inflammation can lead to damage and hyperplasia of the bronchial epithelial cells and of the bronchial smooth muscle. In addition, when asthma attacks are more frequent, even exposure to reduced levels of the triggering agent or event is sufficient to stimulate an attack. In rare instances severe, chronic asthma can result in such bronchial tissue damage that blood flow through the lungs is difficult and right-sided heart failure results **(cor pulmonale).**

INFLAMMATION

For some people, allergens bind to specific immunoglobulin molecules (especially immunoglobulin E [IgE]). These molecules are attached to tissue cells called mast cells and white blood cells called basophils. These cells are filled with granules containing biochemical substances that initiate local inflammatory responses (see Chapters 20 and 23). Some of these biochemicals, such as histamine, start an immediate inflammatory response. Other biochemicals, such as leukotriene, interleukin-4, and eotaxin, are slower and are responsible for later, prolonged inflammatory responses. These substances also attract more white blood cells (eosinophils, macrophages, and basophils) to the area, which release even more inflammatory-stimulating biochemicals **(mediators).** When allergens bind to the IgE molecules on mast cells, biochemicals are released that start inflammatory responses in the airway mucous membranes (see Figure 23-2). Responses include blood vessel dilation and capillary leakage, resulting in swollen tissue with increased secretions and mucus production. This is the most common cause of asthma and is often termed **atopic asthma** (Cotran, Kumar, & Collins, 1999).

Inflammation can also occur through processes that do not involve IgE and are considered general irritation rather than true allergic responses. Although some of the same cells and biochemicals play a role in this response, allergy desensitization therapy is not useful for general irritation-induced asthma.

BRONCHOCONSTRICTION

Hyperresponsive or hyperactive airways result in **bronchoconstriction,** narrowing of the bronchial tubes through constriction of the smooth muscle surrounding and within the bronchial walls. In some individuals, small amounts of pollutants or the presence of respiratory viruses stimulate vagal nerve fibers, causing constriction of bronchial smooth muscle. If these same substances stimulate an inflammatory response at the same time, the biochemicals released during inflammation bind to smooth muscle receptors and cause constriction. Severe bronchoconstriction alone, especially in smaller bronchioles, can profoundly limit airflow to the alveoli.

ASPIRIN AND OTHER NONSTEROIDAL ANTI-INFLAMMATORY DRUGS

Some clients may experience asthma after taking aspirin and other nonsteroidal anti-inflammatory drugs (NSAIDs). This response is not a true allergy. Rather, it results from an increased production of leukotriene when other inflammatory pathways are suppressed. One substance, arachidonic acid, can be converted into different substances when it is acted on by different enzymes. Aspirin and other NSAIDs inhibit one enzyme pathway, cyclooxygenase. When the cyclooxygenase pathway is inhibited, more arachidonic acid is available to be acted on by another enzyme, lipoxygenase, and converted into leukotriene (Figure 30-2).

CHART 30-1

NURSING FOCUS *on the* OLDER ADULT
Respiratory Disorders

- Provide rest periods between such activities as bathing, meals, and ambulation.
- Place the client in an upright position for meals to prevent aspiration.
- Encourage nutritional fluid intake after the meal to promote increased calorie intake.
- Schedule medications around routine activities to increase medication compliance.
- Arrange chairs in strategic locations to allow the client with dyspnea to walk and rest as needed.
- Encourage prompt access to a health care facility for any sign or symptom of infection.
- Ensure that the client has received the pneumococcal vaccine.
- Encourage the client to have an annual flu vaccination.

Incidence/Prevalence

Asthma can begin at any age, but in approximately half of those with asthma, the disease developed before age 10 years. About half of children with asthma have remission as adults. Asthma is more common in urban settings than in rural settings and is more prevalent in minority populations.

CONSIDERATIONS FOR OLDER ADULTS

Asthma occurs as a new disorder in about 3% of people over 55 years of age (Jablonski, 2000). In addition, another 3% of people over 60 years of age have asthma as a continuing chronic disorder. Lung and airway changes as a part of aging make any pulmonary problem more serious in the older adult. One problem thought to be related to aging is a change in the sensitivity of beta-adrenergic receptors. When stimulated, these receptors relax bronchial smooth muscle and cause bronchodilation. As these receptors become less sensitive, they no longer respond as quickly or as strongly to naturally occurring agonists (epinephrine, dopamine) and beta-adrenergic medications.

COLLABORATIVE MANAGEMENT

Assessment

Asthma is diagnosed and categorized on the basis of the frequency and severity of the symptoms, as well as the client's response to asthma medications. This categorization forms the basis for current asthma therapy (Chart 30-2).

HISTORY

The client with asthma usually has a pattern of episodes of shortness of breath **(dyspnea),** chest tightness, coughing, wheezing, and excessive mucus production. The nurse questions the client to determine if these symptoms occur continuously, seasonally, in association with specific activities or exposures, or more frequently at night. Some clients have a history of such symptoms lasting 4 to 8 weeks following a chest cold or other upper respiratory tract infection. The client with atopic or allergic asthma may also have other allergic symptoms such as rhinitis, skin rash, or pruritus. The nurse

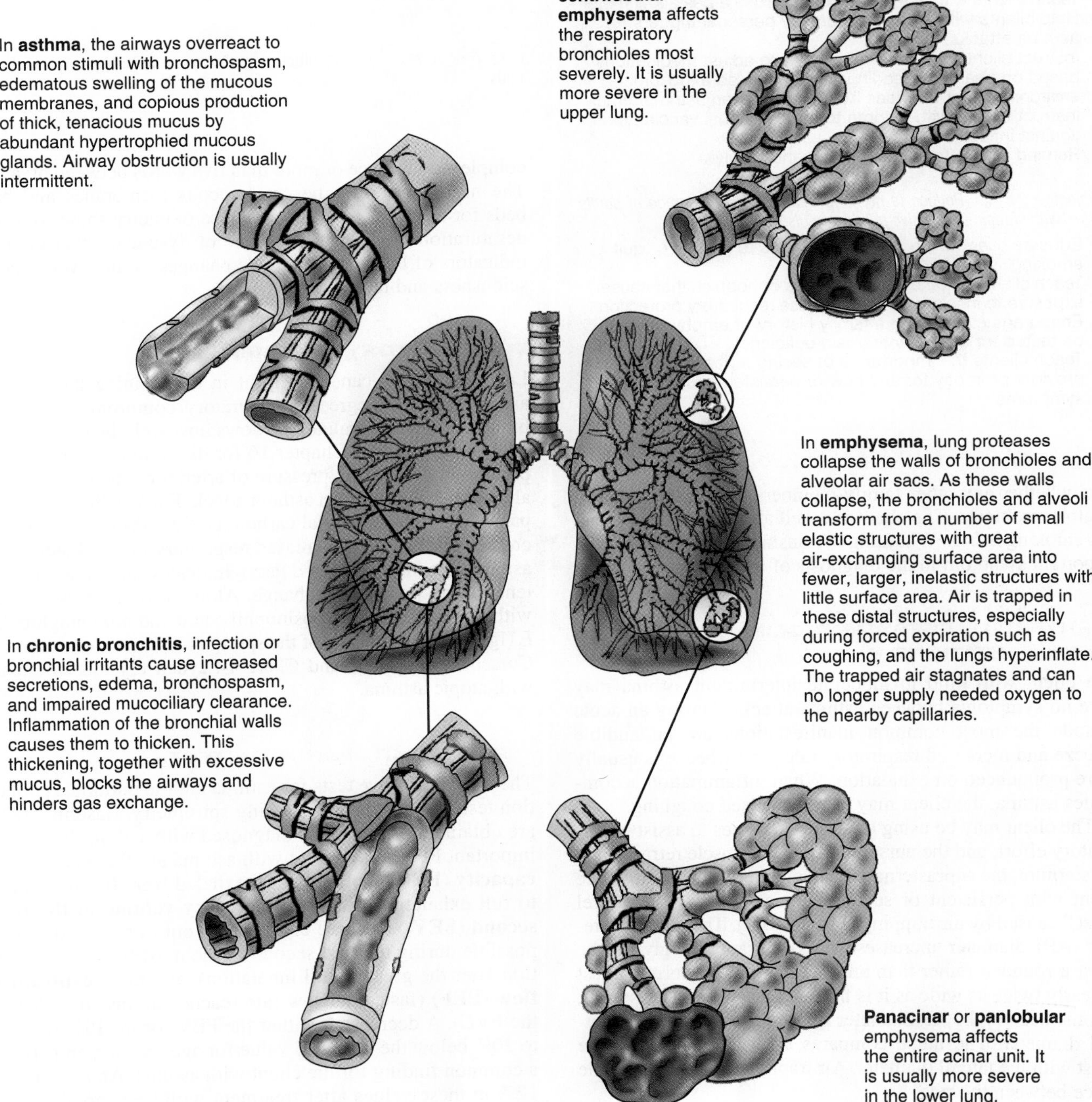

Figure 30-1 ● The pathophysiology of chronic airflow limitation.

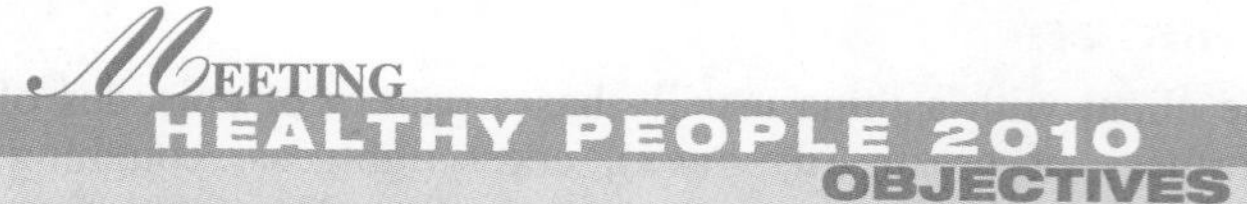

RESPIRATORY DISEASES

Objective 24.2: Reduce the overall asthma morbidity, as measured by a reduction in asthma hospitalization rates to 10 per 10,000 people.

- Teach clients with asthma to develop an asthma action plan in conjunction with their primary health care provider.
- Help clients with asthma who smoke to reduce or quit smoking.
- Instruct clients with asthma regarding the correct technique for use of an inhaler.
- Educate clients with asthma that taking asthma medications as prescribed can reduce asthma exacerbations and morbidity.
- Teach clients with asthma to correctly use a peak flow meter.
- Help clients with asthma to identify personal triggers for asthma attacks.
- Instruct clients with asthma on how to adjust medications based on peak flow readings and expected exposures to environments or activities likely to trigger an asthma attack.
- Instruct clients with asthma to obtain annual vaccinations against influenza.
- Remind clients to avoid secondhand smoke.

Objective 24.14: Reduce to no more than 3% the proportion of adults 45+ with chronic obstructive pulmonary disease.

- Educate clients who smoke cigarettes to reduce or quit smoking.
- Teach clients who have occupations or hobbies that cause exposure to inhalation irritants to use respiratory protection.
- Encourage clients with a family history of emphysema to be tested for alpha$_1$-antitrypsin deficiency.
- Teach clients the importance of seeing a health care provider promptly for any new or persistent respiratory symptoms.

asks whether any other family members have asthma or respiratory problems. The client is asked about current or previous smoking habits. Wheezing in nonsmokers is a particularly important symptom in the diagnosis of asthma.

PHYSICAL ASSESSMENT/CLINICAL MANIFESTATIONS

The client with mild to moderate intermittent asthma may have no symptoms between asthma attacks. During an acute episode the most common manifestations are an audible wheeze and increased respiratory rate. The wheeze is usually more pronounced on exhalation. When inflammation accompanies asthma, the client may have increased coughing.

The client may be using accessory muscles to assist in respiratory effort, and the nurse observes for muscle retraction at the sternum, the suprasternal notch, and between the ribs. The client with persistent or severe asthma may have a "barrel chest," caused by air trapping (Figure 30-3). The anteroposterior (AP) diameter increases with air trapping, giving the chest a rounded rather than an oval shape. The normal chest is nearly twice as wide as it is thick. In the client with severe, chronic asthma the AP diameter may equal or exceed the lateral diameter. The nurse compares the AP diameter of the chest with the lateral diameter. Air trapping also increases the space between the ribs.

In addition to an audible wheeze, the respiratory cycle is longer and requires greater effort. The client may be unable to

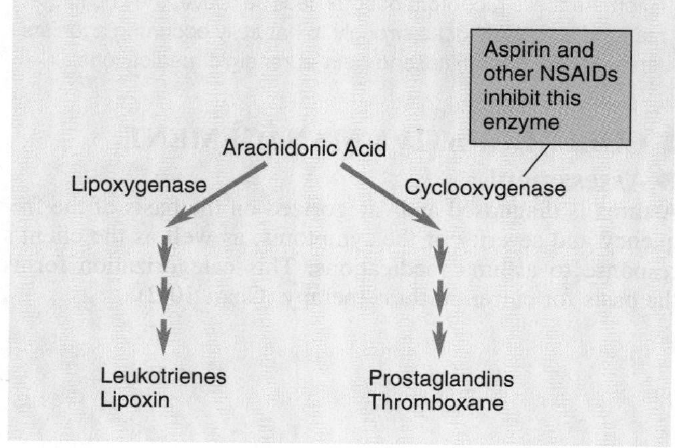

Figure 30-2 ● Production pathways of inflammatory biochemicals.

complete a sentence of more than five words between breaths. The nurse examines the oral mucous membranes and nail beds for evidence of cyanosis. Pulse oximetry shows oxygen desaturation related to the degree of dyspnea. Other clinical indicators of hypoxemia include changes in the level of consciousness and tachycardia.

LABORATORY ASSESSMENT

Laboratory tests can be helpful in determining the type of asthma and the degree of respiratory compromise. Arterial blood gas (ABG) evaluation shows how well the client is obtaining oxygen (see Chapter 16 for discussion of ABG interpretation). The partial pressure of arterial oxygen (Pao_2) usually decreases during an asthma attack. Early in the attack, the partial pressure of arterial carbon dioxide ($Paco_2$) may be decreased as the client increases respiratory effort. Later in an asthma episode an elevated $Paco_2$ indicates carbon dioxide retention and poor gas exchange. Atopic asthma is associated with an elevated serum eosinophil count and immunoglobulin E (IgE) levels. Analysis of the sputum may reveal eosinophils, Curschmann spirals, and Charcot-Leyden crystals in clients with atopic asthma.

PULMONARY FUNCTION TESTS

The most definitive tests for asthma are the pulmonary function tests (PFTs) measured using spirometry. Baseline PFTs are obtained for all clients diagnosed with asthma. The most important PFTs for a client with asthma are the **forced vital capacity (FVC)** (volume of air exhaled from full inhalation to full exhalation), **forced expiratory volume in the first second (FEV$_1$)** (volume of air blown out as hard and fast as possible during the first second of the most forceful exhalation after the greatest full inhalation), and **peak expiratory flow (PEF)** (fastest airflow rate reached at any time during the FVC). A decrease in either the FEV$_1$ or the PEF of 15% to 20% below the expected value for age, gender, and size is a common finding for the client with asthma. An increase of 12% in these values after treatment with bronchodilators is diagnostic for asthma. Airway hyperresponsiveness is tested by measuring the PEF and FEV$_1$ before and after the client

CHART 30-2

KEY FEATURES *of* Asthma: The Step System

Clinical Manifestations	Treatment Recommendations
I. Mild intermittent Symptoms or episodes occur twice per week or less. Client is symptom free between episodes/exacerbations. Episodes/exacerbations are short, lasting only a few hours. Symptoms are present at night no more frequently than twice per month. PFTs are normal between episodes. During episodes/exacerbations, FEV_1 or PEF is at least 80% of normal. PEF variability is less than 20%.	No daily medication needed Use of short-acting inhaled beta agonist during episodes (rescue inhaler) Increased use of rescue inhaler indicates the need to start long-term therapy
II. Mild persistent Symptoms or episodes occur more than twice per week but not daily. Symptoms are present at night more than twice per month. During episodes/exacerbations, FEV_1 or PEF is at least 80% of normal. PEF variability is 20%-30%. Activity is affected during episodes/exacerbations.	Use of a daily anti-inflammatory: Inhaled corticosteroid (CSC) Inhaled cromolyn Leukotriene antagonist Use of a rescue inhaler for relief during episodes
III. Moderate persistent Symptoms occur daily. Symptoms or episodes occur more than twice per week and may persist for days. Client uses short-acting inhaled bronchodilator daily. Symptoms are present at night at least once per week. PEF variability is greater than 30%.	Daily use of inhaled CSC (low to moderate dose) Use of long-acting inhaled beta agonist (bronchodilator) Use of a rescue inhaler for relief during episodes (daily use means the client should be evaluated for progression to step IV)
IV. Severe persistent Symptoms are continuously present. Episodes/exacerbations are frequent. During episodes/exacerbations, FEV_1 or PEF is less than 60% of normal. Physical activity is limited. Symptoms are frequently present at night. PEF variability is greater than 30%.	Daily use of inhaled CSC (high dose) Daily use of long-acting inhaled bronchodilator Frequent courses of systemic corticosteroids May include systemic methylxanthines

Modified from National Institutes of Health. (1997). *Guidelines for the diagnosis and management of asthma.* Expert panel report 2(97 4051). Bethesda, MD: U.S. Department of Health and Human Services.

PFTs, Pulmonary function tests; *PEF,* peak expiratory flow; FEV_1, volume of air blown out as hard and fast as possible during the first second of the most forceful exhalation after the greatest full inhalation.

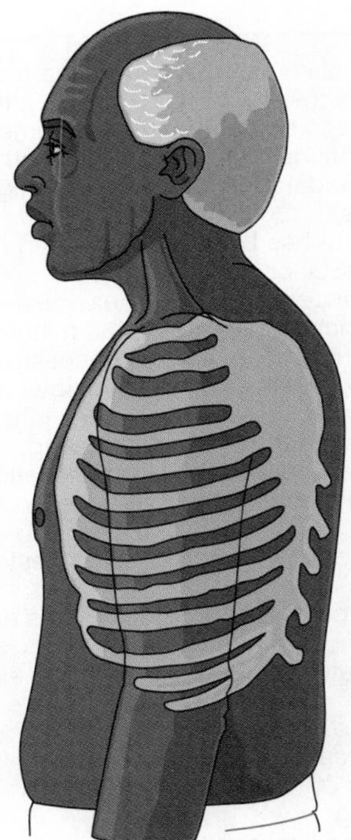

Figure 30-3 ● Typical barrel chest in a client with chronic obstructive pulmonary disease.

inhales an agent called methacholine, which induces bronchoconstriction in susceptible individuals.

OTHER DIAGNOSTIC ASSESSMENT

Chest x-ray films may be obtained to rule out other causes of dyspnea or to demonstrate changes in chest structure over time. For the client taking a drug such as theophylline, blood levels are obtained to determine whether a therapeutic level is being maintained.

Interventions

The treatment of adults with asthma has changed dramatically in recent years. The current goals of therapy are to improve airflow, relieve symptoms, and prevent episodes. The most effective management of adult asthma occurs when the client is included as a key partner in the management plan by active participation in self-care (see the Evidence-Based Practice for Nursing box on p. 534). The successful and cost-effective intervention plan incorporates client education, drug therapy, and lifestyle management, including exercise.

CLIENT EDUCATION. Asthma is largely an intermittent disease process. Through the technique of health care provider–guided self-care, clients can co-manage this disease, increasing symptom-free periods, decreasing the number and severity of attacks/exacerbations, decreasing the number of hospital admissions, and increasing participation in client-chosen pleasure, work, and family activities. Overall improved management through guided self-care has been shown to decrease health care costs (see the Cost of Care box at right).

Self-care requires extensive education for the client to be able to self-treat (including adjusting the frequency and dosage of prescribed medications) and determine when to consult the health care provider. Essentially, the client is taught how to assess symptom severity at least twice daily with a peak flow meter and adjust medications to manage inflammation and bronchoconstriction to prevent or relieve symptoms. Education in this area involves a specified drug therapy plan that is tailored to meet the personal pattern of asthma expression. The client keeps a symptom and intervention diary to learn his or her triggers of asthma symptoms, early cues for impending attacks, and personal response to medications. Proper use of an asthma action plan can be beneficial for any severity of asthma. Chart 30-3 lists areas to emphasize when providing instructions to the client with asthma.

DRUG THERAPY. Pharmacologic management of adult clients with asthma is based on the step category for severity

EVIDENCE-BASED PRACTICE FOR NURSING

Self-care can reduce emergency room visits by clients with asthma

Schott-Baer, D., & Christensen, M. (1999). A pilot program to increase self-care of adult asthma patients. *MEDSURG Nursing, 8*(3), 178-183.

This experimental pilot project sought to determine whether a focused intervention in the form of an asthma client education program stressing self-monitoring would increase self-efficacy and improve self-care behaviors. A convenience sample of 36 adult clients with asthma were randomly assigned to the intervention group (n = 17) or a control group (n = 19). Subjects for both groups were similar in age, gender, race, time since diagnosis, and education. Subjects in the intervention group had higher mean incomes and greater percentages of employment than those in the control group. Subjects in both groups received information about asthma, the prescribed medications, and how to record daily peak flow measurements. The intervention group also received a 3-hour instruction program with more information about asthma, daily self-monitoring, self-management techniques, and daily log/diary instruction. In addition, the subjects in the control group were contacted by telephone for information reinforcement.

Data were collected from subjects in both groups at three time points. The KASE-AQ, a 60-item multiple-choice tool, was used to collect data regarding knowledge, attitude, and self-efficacy regarding asthma. In addition, diaries were analyzed by the investigators, and the number of emergency department and clinic visits was tallied.

There were minimal differences between the groups in terms of knowledge and self-efficacy scores. The major difference between the two groups was that the intervention group reduced their emergency department visit rate by more than 50% and the control group increased their emergency department visit rate by nearly 50%.

Critique. This study represents important work in helping clients with asthma to be empowered to accept more control and responsibility for disease and symptom management. A larger sample size with more homogeneity between the groups with regard to mean income and employment may strengthen the study. In addition, only 2 out of 19 members of the control group returned diaries, limiting the incoming data. The investigators suggest that at least one face-to-face follow-up with the intervention group might have been beneficial.

Implications for Nursing. Sustaining self-care behaviors can be important to reduction of costs and improvement of function in clients with asthma. Self-care behaviors may take time and considerable positive reinforcement for clients to incorporate them into their lifestyle. Nurses as client educators and coaches can be the most important factor in helping clients to change self-care behaviors.

COST OF CARE IMPLICATIONS FOR NURSING

ASTHMA ACTION PLAN

Cost of Care

- Billions of dollars are spent on inpatient management of acute asthma exacerbations.
- Many millions of additional health care dollars are spent on emergency department management of acute asthma exacerbations.
- Any disorder affecting ventilation can cause the client to panic and seek emergency intervention before or in place of any type of self-management.
- Appropriate self-management has been demonstrated to reduce costs and increase quality of life for the client with asthma.

Implications for Nursing

Self-care strategies are successful only when the client completely understands all aspects of care and has confidence in his or her own ability to correctly assess and intervene. Empowering the client with asthma to increase participation and take responsibility for self-management is a critical task for nurses.

Data from Reinke, L., & Hoffman, L. (2000). Asthma education: Creating a partnership. *Heart and Lung, 29*(3), 225-236; and Steinhauser, K. (1999). Making "cents" of asthma. *Continuing Care, 18*(6), 22, 24-29.

CHART 30-3

CLIENT EDUCATION GUIDE
Asthma

- Avoid potential environmental asthma triggers, such as smoke, fireplaces, dust, mold, and weather changes (especially warm to cold, or sudden barometric changes).
- Avoid medications that could trigger asthma (e.g., aspirin, nonsteroidal anti-inflammatory drugs [NSAIDs], and beta blockers).
- Avoid food that has been prepared with monosodium glutamate (MSG) or metabisulfite.
- If you experience symptoms of exercise-induced asthma, use your bronchodilator inhaler 30 minutes before exercise to prevent or reduce bronchospasm.
- Be sure you know the proper technique and correct sequence when you use metered dose inhalers.
- Be sure to get adequate rest and sleep.
- Reduce stress and anxiety; learn relaxation techniques; adopt coping mechanisms that have worked for you in the past.
- Wash all bedding with hot water to destroy the dust mite.
- Monitor your peak expiratory flow rates as you were instructed.
- Seek immediate emergency care if you experience any of the following:
  - Gray or blue fingertips or lips
  - Difficulty breathing, walking, or talking
  - Retractions of the neck, chest, or ribs
  - Nasal flaring
  - Failure of medications to control worsening symptoms
  - Peak expiratory flow rates declining steadily after treatment, or a flow rate 50% below your usual flow rate

and treatment (see Chart 30-2). Some may require drug therapy only during an asthma episode. For others, daily medication regimens are needed to keep asthma episodic rather than a more frequent problem. This therapy involves the use of bronchodilators, steroidal and nonsteroidal agents to reduce inflammation, mast cell stabilizers, and new agents that inhibit the release or action of leukotrienes. Thus some drugs reduce the response, and other drugs actually prevent the response. Chart 30-4 lists common agents used for preventive and symptomatic therapy of asthma.

CHART 30-4

DRUG THERAPY *for* Asthma

Drug	Usual Dosage	Nursing Interventions	Rationale
BRONCHODILATORS			
Short-Acting Beta₂ Agonists			
Albuterol (Proventil, Ventolin)	1-2 inhalations q4-6h (90 μg per inhaled dose)	Teach client to monitor heart rate.	Excessive use causes systemic symptoms, especially tachycardia.
		Increase water/fluid intake.	Chronic use increases mouth and throat dryness.
		Instruct client to use bronchodilator at least 5 min before other inhaled drugs.	Bronchodilation allows better penetration of other inhaled drugs.
		Teach client the correct technique for using the inhaler and obtain a return demonstration.	Correct technique is essential in getting the medication to the site of action. If the client does not inhale during medication delivery, drug exits the nose or is swallowed.
Bitolterol (Tornalate)	2 inhalations q8h (370 μg per inhalation)	Same as for albuterol.	Same as for albuterol.
Pirbuterol (Maxair)	1-2 inhalations q4-6h (200 μg per inhalation)	Same as for albuterol.	Same as for albuterol.
Terbutaline (Brethaire)	2 inhalations q4-6h (200 μg per inhalation)	Same as for albuterol.	Same as for albuterol.
Long-Acting Beta₂ Agonists			
Salmeterol (Serevent)	2 inhalations q12h (25 μg per inhalation)	Do not use to relieve acute symptoms.	Drug has slow onset of action.
		Shake inhaler well before using.	Drug separates easily.
Methylxanthines			
Theophylline (Theo-Dur)	10-12 mg/kg/day PO (loading dose)	Monitor drug levels.	Drug has a narrow therapeutic range and many toxicities.
	Maintenance dose is usually 200-800 mg/day	Space doses equally throughout the 24-hour day.	Client maintains more even blood drug levels.
		Observe client for nausea, vomiting, diarrhea, tachycardia, dysrhythmias, and restlessness.	These are symptoms of toxicity.
		Teach client to avoid caffeine intake while taking this drug.	Caffeine potentiates side effects.
		Encourage client to take as prescribed daily.	Efficacy is related to continued correct use.
		Teach client to take oral dose with meals.	Food reduces gastrointestinal irritation.
		Administer IV doses using a pump or controller.	A pump or controller prevents accidental overdose.
Aminophylline (Truphylline)	5-7 mg/kg IV (loading dose) Maintenance dose is 0.5-1.2 mg/kg/hr	Observe for skin rash or sloughing.	A drug component, ethylenediamine, can cause severe skin reactions.
		Same as for theophylline.	Drug is 80% theophylline.
Oxtriphylline (Apo-Oxtriphylline✤, Choledyl✤)	75-150 mg qid PO	Same as for theophylline.	Drug contains significant amounts of theophylline.
Cholinergic Antagonists			
Ipratropium (Atrovent, Apo-Ipravent✤)	2-4 inhalations 4-6 times/day 18 μg per inhalation	Shake container well.	Drug separates on standing.
		Increase water/fluid intake.	Drug causes mouth dryness.
		Teach client to observe for blurred vision, eye pain, headache, nausea, nervousness, and palpitations.	These are systemic symptoms of overdose.

Data from *United States Pharmacopeia Dispensing Information (USP DI): Vol. I. Drug information for the health care professional* (20th ed.). (2000). Englewood, CO: Micromedex.

Continued

CHART 30-4

DRUG THERAPY *for* Asthma—cont'd

Drug	Usual Dosage	Nursing Interventions	Rationale
ANTI-INFLAMMATORIES			
Corticosteroids—Oral			
Prednisolone (Cotolone, Delta-Cortef)	5-40 mg/day	Not recommended unless symptoms are severe or debilitating.	The following systemic side effects are common and serious: • GI ulceration • Poor wound healing • Decreased immune function • Increased risk for infections • Weight gain • Hyperglycemia • Personality changes • Fluid retention
Prednisone (Deltasone♣, Prednicot, Orasone, Pred-Pak)	5-60 mg/day	Same as for prednisolone.	Same as for prednisolone.
Corticosteroids—Inhaler			
Budesonide (Pulmicort)	1-2 metered sprays qd (50 μg per metered spray)	Use daily as directed. Symptoms may persist for 2-3 days after initial administration. Observe mouth and throat for lesions.	Effectiveness depends on regular use. Maximum effectiveness requires continued use for 48-72 hr. Excessive use decreases local immune response and increases susceptibility to oral infections, especially candidiasis.
Fluticasone (Flovent)	2 metered sprays qd (50 μg per metered spray)	Same as for budesonide.	Same as for budesonide.
Beclomethasone (Vanceril, Beclovent, Becloforte♣)	2-4 inhalations tid-qid (42 μg per inhalation)	Same as for budesonide.	Same as for budesonide.
Triamcinolone (Azmacort)	2 inhalations tid-qid (100 μg per inhalation)	Same as for budesonide.	Same as for budesonide.
Flunisolide (AeroBid, Bronalide♣)	2 inhalations bid (250 μg per inhalation)	Same as for budesonide.	Same as for budesonide.
Leukotriene Antagonists			
Zafirlukast (Accolate)	20 mg bid	Take 1 hr before or 2 hr after eating. Increased incidence of upper respiratory tract infections when administered with inhaled corticosteroids. Reduce dose in clients also taking aspirin.	Drug absorption is slowed by presence of food. Drugs reduce local inflammatory and immune responses. Aspirin increases plasma concentration of drug.
Zileuton (Zyflo)	600 mg qid	Do not take with terfenadine or theophylline.	Drug increases plasma concentrations of terfenadine and theophylline.
Montelukast (Singulair)	10 mg qd (evenings)	Do not abruptly substitute for oral or inhaled steroids. Reduce dose in clients with hepatic impairment.	Drug requires time to reach peak action. Hepatic impairment prolongs blood levels of the drug.
Inhaled Anti-inflammatory			
Nedocromil (Tilade)	2 inhalations q6h (2 mg per inhalation)	Not for use during acute attack. Instruct client to use daily even when no symptoms are present. Discontinue use if symptoms worsen with drug.	Drug has slow onset to peak action. Efficacy is related to continued correct use. Client may be sensitive to propellents.
MAST CELL STABILIZERS			
Cromolyn sodium (Intal)	1-2 inhalations qid	Use daily as directed. Start therapy 3-4 wk before expected allergy season.	Effectiveness depends on regular use. Drug requires regular use for prophylactic effect.

Data from *United States Pharmacopeia Dispensing Information (USP DI): Vol. I. Drug information for the health care professional* (20th ed.). (2000). Englewood, CO: Micromedex.

BRONCHODILATORS. Bronchodilators increase bronchiolar smooth muscle relaxation. They have no effect on the inflammatory processes. Thus when a client with asthma experiences airflow obstruction by both bronchoconstriction and inflammation, at least two categories of drug therapy are required. Most bronchodilators exert their effects by stimulating the $beta_2$-adrenergic receptors on respiratory smooth muscle in much the same way that the sympathetic nervous system transmitters epinephrine and norepinephrine, do. These drugs include $beta_2$ agonists, cholinergic antagonists, and methylxanthines

$Beta_2$ Agonists. $Beta_2$ agonists bind to the $beta_2$-adrenergic receptors and cause a series of events to occur that result in an increase in the intracellular level of a substance called cyclic adenosine monophosphate (cAMP). This substance triggers smooth muscle relaxation.

Short-Acting $Beta_2$ Agonists. Short-acting $beta_2$ agents provide rapid but short-term relief. These inhaled agents are most useful when an attack begins or as premedication when the client is about to enter an environment or begin an activity that is likely to induce an asthma attack. Such agents include albuterol (Proventil, Ventolin), bitolterol (Tornalate), pirbuterol (Maxair), and terbutaline (Brethaire). When inhaled as either a metered dose inhaler (MDI) or a dry powder inhaler (DPI), the drug is delivered directly to the site of action and systemic effects are minimal (unless the agent is overused or abused). The nurse must teach the client the correct technique to use during administration of an inhaled drug to achieve the greatest benefit from the drug. Chart 30-5 describes proper inhaler use.

Long-Acting $Beta_2$ Agonists. Long-acting $beta_2$ agonists are also delivered by MDI directly to the site of action: the bronchioles. Unlike short-acting agonists, long-acting agonists require time to build up an effect, but the effects are longer lasting. Thus these drugs, such as salmeterol (Serevent), are useful in preventing an asthma attack but have no value during an acute attack. Appropriate use of the long-acting agonists is thought to decrease reliance on and abuse of short-acting agonists.

Cholinergic Antagonists. Cholinergic antagonists, sometimes called anticholinergic agents, are similar to atropine and block the parasympathetic nervous system. This block allows the sympathetic nervous system to act more prominently, allowing increased bronchodilation and decreased pulmonary secretions. The most common drug in this category is ipratropium (Atrovent), which is used as an inhalant.

Methylxanthines. Methylxanthines, once considered the mainstay of asthma therapy, are used only rarely when other types of management are ineffective. The classic agent in this category is theophylline (Theo-Dur). Other agents include aminophylline (Truphylline), oxtriphylline (Choledyl✱), and dyphylline (Dilor, Lufyllin). These agents are administered systemically, have fairly narrow therapeutic ranges, and have many side effects. Blood levels of these agents need to be monitored closely. The most dangerous side effects result from cardiac and central nervous system overstimulation.

ANTI-INFLAMMATORY AGENTS. Anti-inflammatory agents decrease the general and allergic inflammatory responses in the airways. Some are administered systemically and have more side effects. Others are administered as inhalants and have few, if any, systemic side effects.

CHART 30-5

CLIENT EDUCATION GUIDE

How to Use an Inhaler Correctly*

Without a Spacer (Preferred Technique)

1. Before each use, remove the cap and shake the inhaler according to the instructions in the package insert.
2. Tilt your head back slightly and breathe out fully.
3. Open your mouth and place the mouthpiece 1 to 2 inches away.
4. As you begin to breathe in deeply through your mouth, press down firmly on the canister of the inhaler to release one dose of medication.
5. Continue to breathe in slowly and deeply (usually over 3 to 5 seconds).
6. Hold your breath for at least 10 seconds to allow the medication to reach deep into the lungs, then breathe out slowly.
7. Wait at least 1 minute between puffs.
8. Replace the cap on the inhaler.
9. At least once a day, remove the canister and clean the plastic case and cap of the inhaler by thoroughly rinsing in warm, running tap water.

Without a Spacer (Alternative Method)

1. Follow steps 1 and 2 above.
2. Place the mouthpiece into your mouth, over your tongue, and seal your lips tightly around it.
3. Follow steps 4 to 9 above.

With a Spacer

1. Before each use, remove the caps from the inhaler and the spacer.
2. Insert the mouthpiece of the inhaler into the nonmouthpiece end of the spacer.
3. Shake the whole unit vigorously three or four times.
4. Place the mouthpiece into your mouth, over your tongue, and seal your lips tightly around it.
5. Press down firmly on the canister of the inhaler to release one dose of medication into the spacer.
6. Breathe in slowly and deeply. If the spacer makes a whistling sound, you are breathing in too rapidly.
7. Remove the mouthpiece from your mouth and, keeping your lips closed, hold your breath for at least 10 seconds, then breathe out slowly.
8. Wait at least 1 minute between puffs.
9. Replace the caps on the inhaler and the spacer.
10. At least once a day, clean the plastic case and cap of the inhaler by thoroughly rinsing in warm, running tap water; at least once a week, clean the spacer in the same manner.

*Avoid spraying in the direction of the eyes.

Corticosteroids. Corticosteroids decrease inflammatory and immune responses in many ways, including by preventing the synthesis of mediators. Local corticosteroids in the form of inhaled sprays can be helpful in preventing the symptoms of asthma. Newer high-potency steroid inhalers, such as fluticasone (Flovent) and budesonide (Pulmicort), may be used once per day for maintenance. Systemic corticosteroids, because of severe side effects, are avoided for mild to moderate asthma and are generally used on a short-term basis for moderate asthma. For some clients with severe asthma, daily systemic corticosteroids are required.

Inhaled Anti-inflammatory Agents. A newer category of nonsteroidal inhaled anti-inflammatory agent is nedocromil (Tilade). This agent appears to inhibit the release of inflammatory mediators from respiratory epithelial and white blood cells. In addition, it is thought to reduce sensory nerve stimulation in the lung. These actions are most helpful in preventing an asthma episode rather than in reversing an episode.

Mast Cell Stabilizers. Inhaled sprays containing mast cell stabilizers, such as cromolyn sodium (Intal), prevent mast cell membranes from opening when an allergen binds to IgE. Thus these agents are helpful in preventing the symptoms of atopic asthma but are not useful during an acute episode.

Leukotriene Antagonists. Currently three leukotriene antagonists are available to treat persistent asthma. Zileuton (Zyflo) prevents leukotriene synthesis. Zafirlukast (Accolate) and montelukast (Singulair) block the leukotriene receptor. All are oral agents and have good client compliance. Their efficacy at preventing episodes is considered moderate, and they are expensive.

EXERCISE/ACTIVITY. Regular exercise, including aerobic exercise, once thought to be impossible for anyone with moderate to severe asthma, is now a recommended part of asthma therapy. Aerobic exercise assists in maintaining cardiovascular health, enhancing skeletal muscle strength, and promoting ventilation and perfusion. Clients with asthma need to examine the conditions that trigger an attack and adjust the exercise routine appropriately. Some may need to premedicate with inhaled beta agonists before beginning activity. For others, adjusting the environment may be necessary. For example, outdoor ice-skating in cold, dry air can precipitate an attack; indoor ice-skating may be less of a problem. Sports that involve more "rest" action, such as baseball, seem to cause fewer severe symptoms than "nonrest" action sports, such as basketball (Reinke & Hoffman, 2000).

STATUS ASTHMATICUS. Status asthmaticus is a major complication associated with bronchial asthma. It is a severe, potentially life-threatening acute episode of airway obstruction that tends to intensify once it begins and often does not respond to common therapy. The client arrives in the emergency department of the hospital with extremely labored breathing and wheezing. Use of accessory muscles for breathing and distention of neck veins are commonly noted. If the condition is not reversed, the client may experience cor pulmonale, pneumothorax, and eventual cardiac or respiratory arrest. The physician immediately orders intravenous (IV) fluids, potent systemic bronchodilators, steroids (to decrease inflammation), epinephrine, and oxygen in an attempt to reverse the acute condition. The nurse prepares for emergency intubation. When wheezing diminishes, management is similar to that for any client with asthma.

CRITICAL THINKING CHALLENGE

The client is a 50-year-old man recently diagnosed with asthma. He comes to the emergency department with audible wheezes on inhalation and exhalation. His peak flow reading is 40% below the expected value for his age and size. His respiratory rate is 34 breaths per minute; pulse is 122 beats/min. He has suprasternal and intercostal retractions. He indicates that his medications include the following: salmeterol (Serevent) 2 puffs every 12 hours, terbutaline (Brethaire) 2 puffs prn, fluticasone (Flovent) 2 puffs once a day, and cromolyn sodium (Intal) 1 to 2 puffs four times a day.

His wife tells you that he has not used any of his inhalers for the past week because he has felt well and the medications leave a bad taste in his mouth.

- Should you start oxygen with this client? Why or why not?
- What additional assessment data should you obtain?
- Which of the client's current medications should be administered immediately? Why?
- What is your interpretation of this client's immediate condition based on his peak flow reading?
- What teaching priorities are needed for this client?

For suggested answer guidelines, go to SIMON http://www.wbsaunders.com/SIMON/Iggy/.

Chronic Obstructive Pulmonary Disease

OVERVIEW

Most clients with emphysema usually have chronic bronchitis simultaneously, but each condition has its own pathophysiologic process (Figure 30-4).

Pathophysiology

EMPHYSEMA

ANATOMIC AND FUNCTIONAL CHANGES. Two primary pathologic changes occurring in the client with pulmonary emphysema are loss of lung elasticity and hyperinflation of the lung (see Figure 30-1). These changes result in dyspnea and the need for an increased respiratory rate.

Enzymes that degrade protein (**proteases**) alter or destroy the alveoli and the small airways by breaking down elastin. As a result, the alveolar sacs lose their elasticity, and the small airways collapse or narrow. Some alveoli are destroyed, and others become large and flabby, with decreased surface area for gas exchange.

An increased amount of air becomes trapped in the lungs. Causes of air trapping are loss of elastic recoil in the alveolar walls, overstretching and enlargement of alveoli into air-filled spaces called **bullae**, and collapse of small airways (**bronchioles**). These changes greatly increase the work of breathing. The hyperinflated lung flattens the diaphragm (Figure 30-5), weakening the effect of this major muscle of respiration. As a result, the client with emphysema needs to use additional muscles (**accessory muscles**) in the neck, chest wall, and abdomen to inhale and exhale. This increased effort increases the need for oxygen and metabolic nutrients, making the

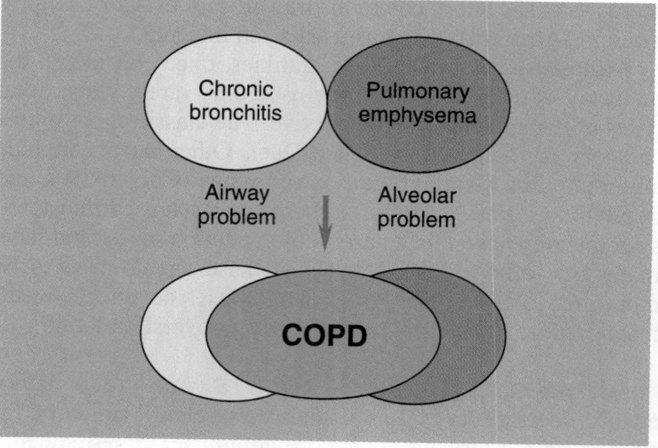

Figure 30-4 ● The interaction of chronic bronchitis and emphysema in chronic obstructive pulmonary disease.

client work harder and experience an "air hunger" sensation. He or she usually starts inhalation before exhalation is completed, resulting in dyspnea with an uncoordinated pattern of breathing.

Gas exchange is affected by the increased work of breathing and the loss of alveolar tissue. Although some alveoli enlarge, the curves of alveolar walls decrease and there is less surface area available for gas exchange. Usually the client adjusts by increasing the respiratory rate, so arterial blood gas (ABG) values may not show gas exchange problems until the client has advanced disease. Then carbon dioxide may be produced faster than the body can eliminate it, resulting in carbon dioxide retention and chronic respiratory acidosis (see Chapter 16). The client with late-stage emphysema has a low partial pressure of arterial oxygen (Pao_2) as well, because it is difficult for oxygen to move from diseased lung tissue into the bloodstream.

CLASSIFICATION OF EMPHYSEMA. Emphysema is classified as panlobular, centrilobular, or paraseptal emphysema according to the pattern of destruction and dilation of the gas-exchanging units **(acini)** of the lung (see Figure 30-1). Each type can occur alone or in combination in the same lung.

Panlobular (panacinar) emphysema (PLE) involves destruction of the entire alveolus uniformly. This type is diffuse and more severe in the lower lung areas.

In centrilobular (centriacinar) emphysema (CLE), openings occur in the bronchioles and allow spaces to develop as tissue walls disintegrate. Although this is a diffuse disease, the upper lung sections are most severely affected. This type of emphysema is often seen in long-standing cigarette smokers.

In paraseptal or distal acinar emphysema, the disease is confined to the distal portion of the acinus; only alveolar ducts and alveoli are involved. This disease type is associated with bullae formation and more commonly affects the upper half of the lungs.

CHRONIC BRONCHITIS

Bronchitis is an inflammation of the bronchi and bronchioles caused by continuous exposure to infectious or noninfectious irritants, especially tobacco smoke. The irritant produces an inflammatory response, which causes vasodilation, congestion, mucosal edema, and bronchospasm. Unlike emphysema, bronchitis affects only the small and large airways rather than the alveoli.

Chronic inflammation results in mucous gland hypertrophy and hyperplasia, which produce large amounts of thick mucus. The bronchial walls thicken (often to twice the normal thickness) and impair airflow. This thickening, together with production of excessive mucus, blocks some of the smaller airways and narrows larger ones. Small airways are affected before the large airways become involved.

Chronic bronchitis hinders airflow and gas exchange because of mucous plugs and secondary infections. As a result, the Pao_2 decreases **(hypoxemia)** and the arterial blood carbon dioxide concentration ($Paco_2$) increases (respiratory acidosis).

Etiology

CIGARETTE SMOKING

Smoking is the most important risk factor for chronic obstructive pulmonary disease (COPD). The client with an 8–pack-year history usually has obstructive lung changes but no signs and symptoms of disease. The client with a 20–pack-year history or longer typically has COPD with identified changes in pulmonary function tests (PFTs).

The harmful effects of tobacco result in part because inhaled smoke stimulates release of excessive amounts of the enzyme elastase protease from cells normally found in the lungs. The elastase protease breaks down elastin, the major component in alveoli. By impairing the action of cilia, smoking also inhibits the cilia from clearing the tracheobronchial tree of mucus, cellular debris, and fluid.

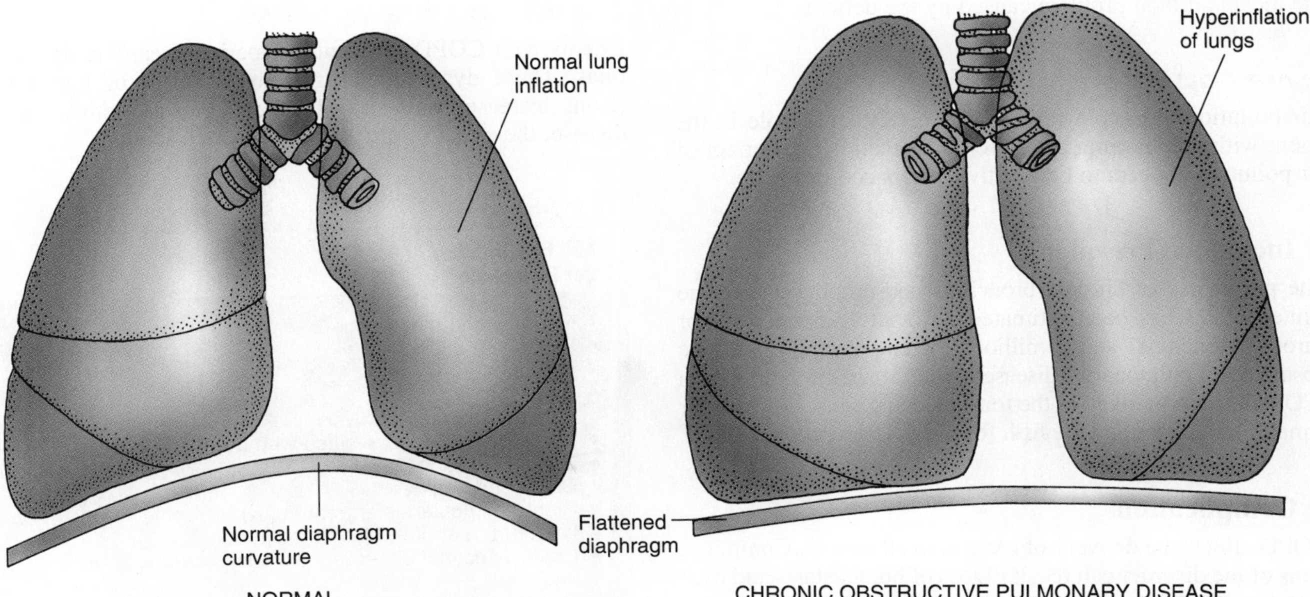

Figure 30-5 ● Diaphragm shape and lung inflation in the normal client and in the client with chronic obstructive pulmonary disease.

In addition to the increased risk of COPD from active smoking, passive smoking (or secondhand smoke) is also thought to contribute to the development of upper and lower respiratory tract problems. The risk appears greater when exposure occurs in small, confined spaces.

CULTURAL CONSIDERATIONS

The prevalence of smoking remains higher among African Americans, blue-collar workers, and less educated people than in the overall population of the United States. Smoking prevalence is highest among Northern Plains Native Americans and Alaskan Natives. The overall prevalence of smoking for both men and women has decreased over the past two decades, but the decrease for women has been proportionately less than for men (American Cancer Society, 2001; Sarna, 1999).

ALPHA$_1$-ANTITRYPSIN DEFICIENCY

A special enzyme, alpha$_1$-antitrypsin (AAT), is made by the liver and is normally present in the lungs. One purpose of ATT is to regulate the other enzymes (proteases) that are present to break down inhaled pollutants and microorganisms. AAT prevents the proteases from working on lung structures.

The production of sufficient quantities of AAT is dependent on the inheritance of a pair of normal genes. The AAT gene is co-dominant. Thus if one of the pair of genes is missing or faulty and the other gene is normal, the person makes enough AAT to prevent COPD unless there is significant exposure to cigarette smoke and other precipitating factors. This person, however, is a carrier for AAT deficiency. If both pairs of the gene are missing or faulty, COPD develops at a fairly young age even when the person is not exposed to cigarette smoke or other irritants.

Approximately 100,000 Americans have severe AAT deficiency, and many more have mild to moderate deficiencies (Stoller, 1997). Although an AAT deficiency causes problems in other organs, such as the skin and liver, lung diseases are the most common problem caused by the deficiency.

AIR POLLUTION

Air pollution alone plays only a relatively small role in the client with emphysema and chronic bronchitis. The effect of air pollution appears to be additive to tobacco exposure.

Incidence/Prevalence

The prevalence of chronic bronchitis and emphysema in the United States has been estimated at about 13.5 million (for chronic bronchitis) and 2 million (for emphysema). Chronic obstructive pulmonary disease/chronic airflow limitation (COPD/CAL) is ranked as the fourth leading cause of death for females of all ages and the fifth for males (Parker et al., 1997).

Complications

COPD affects the delivery of oxygen to all tissues. Complications of the disorder can result in loss of homeostasis and dysfunction of major organs. Major problems occur as hypoxemia, acidosis, respiratory tract infection, cardiac failure, and dysrhythmias.

HYPOXEMIA AND ACIDOSIS

As the client with COPD is less able to exchange gas, oxygenation decreases and carbon dioxide levels increase, leading to hypoxemia and acidosis. As a result, most tissues experience decreased function.

RESPIRATORY TRACT INFECTIONS

The client with COPD is susceptible to respiratory tract infections from the presence of increased mucus and poor oxygenation. The organisms frequently associated with bacterial infections include *Streptococcus pneumoniae, Haemophilus influenzae,* and *Moraxella catarrhalis.* Acute respiratory tract infections make symptoms of COPD worse by increasing inflammation and mucus production, and inducing more bronchoconstriction. Airflow becomes even more limited, the work of breathing increases, and dyspnea results.

CARDIAC FAILURE

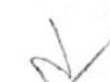

Cardiac failure, especially **cor pulmonale** (right-sided ventricular heart failure caused by pulmonary disease), can result from bronchitis or emphysema. Air trapping, airway collapse, and inelastic alveolar walls increase the pressure in the lungs, making blood flow through lung vessels more difficult. The increased lung pressure places a heavy workload on the right side of the heart, which is responsible for pumping blood into the lungs. As the disease progresses, the amount of oxygen in the blood decreases, causing major blood vessels in the lung to constrict. To pump blood through these narrowed vessels, the right side of the heart must generate high pressures. In response to this heavy workload, the right chambers of the heart enlarge and thicken, causing right-sided heart failure. Chart 30-6 lists key features of cor pulmonale.

CARDIAC DYSRHYTHMIAS

Clients with COPD frequently experience cardiac dysrhythmias. These dysrhythmias may be a result of hypoxemia (from decreased oxygen to the heart muscle), other cardiac disease, the effect of drugs, or respiratory acidosis.

CHART 30-6

KEY FEATURES *of* Cor Pulmonale

- Hypoxia and hypoxemia
- Increasing dyspnea
- Fatigue
- Weakness
- Enlarged and tender liver
- Warm, cyanotic extremities with bounding pulses
- Cyanotic lips
- Distended neck veins
- Right ventricular enlargement (hypertrophy)
- Lower sternal or epigastric pulsations
- Gastrointestinal disturbances, such as nausea or anorexia
- Dependent edema
- Metabolic and respiratory acidosis
- Pulmonary hypertension

COLLABORATIVE MANAGEMENT

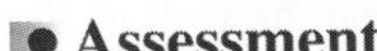

SIMON Activity Link

Assessment

HISTORY

RISK FACTORS. The nurse considers age, gender, occupational history, and ethnic-cultural background when taking a history from a client who has, or is suspected of having, chronic obstructive pulmonary disease (COPD). COPD is seen more often in older men. Certain types of diseases resulting in chronic airflow limitation (CAL), especially panlobular emphysema, occur in families, especially those with alpha$_1$-antitrypsin (AAT) deficiency.

Obtaining a thorough smoking history is critical, because tobacco use is a major risk factor. The information needed includes the length of time the client has smoked, the number of packs smoked daily, and the tar and nicotine content of the tobacco used. The nurse uses this information to determine the pack-year smoking history.

CURRENT PROBLEM. The client is asked to describe his or her breathing problems. The nurse notes whether the client has any difficulty breathing while talking. Can he or she speak in complete sentences, or does he or she take a breath between every one or two words? The client is asked about the presence, duration, or worsening of wheezing, coughing, and shortness of breath. The nurse determines when these symptoms are present and assesses the client's cough pattern. If the cough is productive, the nurse asks whether sputum is clear or colored and how much is expectorated each day. The client is asked to recall the time of day when the most sputum is expectorated. Smokers typically have a productive cough when they get up in the morning; nonsmokers generally do not. The nurse asks whether sputum production has increased or changed during the past year.

The nurse asks about the relationship between activity tolerance and dyspnea. The client is asked to compare his or her activity level and shortness of breath with those of a month ago and a year ago. Likewise, the nurse asks about any difficulty with eating and sleeping. Many clients sleep in a semi-sitting position because breathlessness is worse when lying down **(orthopnea).** In addition, information is obtained about usual daily activities and any difficulty with sleeping, bathing, dressing, or sexual activity.

WEIGHT AND DIET. The client is weighed, and this weight is compared with previous weights. Unplanned weight loss is associated with an increase in COPD severity. The client with COPD has increased metabolic requirements associated with the increased work of breathing. The increased metabolism plus dyspnea and mucus production often result in poor food intake and inadequate nutrition. The client is asked to recall a typical day's meals and fluid intake.

PHYSICAL ASSESSMENT/CLINICAL MANIFESTATIONS

GENERAL APPEARANCE. The nurse observes the client's general appearance, including weight in proportion to height, posture, mobility, muscle mass, and overall hygiene. The client with increasingly severe COPD is thin, with loss of muscle mass in the extremities, although the neck muscles may be enlarged. The client is typically slow moving and slightly stooped. Usually he or she will sit with a forward-bending posture, sometimes with the arms held forward (Figure 30-6). When dyspnea becomes severe, the client may have activity intolerance to the degree that bathing and general grooming are neglected.

RESPIRATORY MANIFESTATIONS. The chest is inspected to determine the breathing rate and pattern. The client with respiratory muscle fatigue typically breathes with rapid, shallow respirations and may have paradoxical respirations or use accessory muscles in the abdomen or neck. The respira-

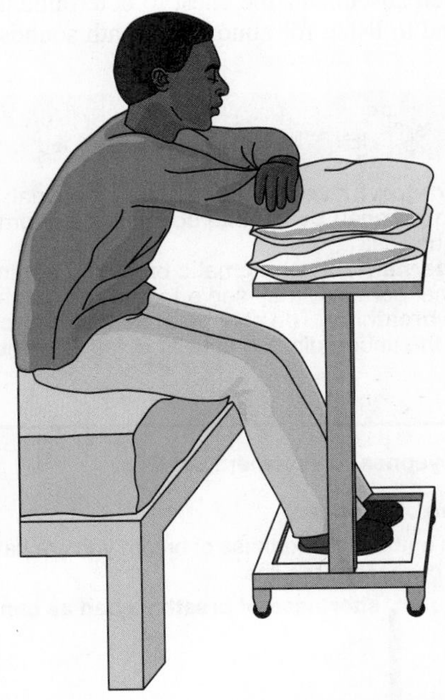

Sitting on the edge of a bed with the arms folded and placed on two or three pillows positioned over a nightstand.

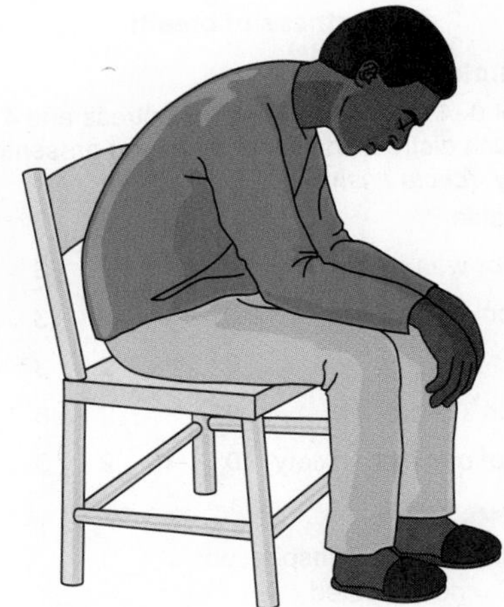

Sitting in a chair with the feet spread a shoulder-width apart and leaning forward with the elbows on the knees. Arms and hands are relaxed.

Figure 30-6 ● Orthopnea positions that clients with chronic obstructive pulmonary disease can assume to ease the work of breathing.

tory rate could be as high as 40 to 50 breaths per minute. Three breathing patterns commonly seen with respiratory muscle fatigue are abdominal paradox, respiratory alternans, and asynchronous breathing (Table 30-1).

The nurse systematically palpates the client's anterior chest for areas of tenderness and abnormal retractions and for symmetric chest expansion. The client with emphysema has limited diaphragmatic movement **(excursion)** because the diaphragm is flattened and below its usual resting state. Decreased vibration **(fremitus)** is noted when the client says "ninety-nine" because vibrations are not transmitted through obstructed airways. On percussion the chest is hyperresonant because of the presence of trapped air.

The nurse then auscultates the chest to determine the depth of inspiration and to listen for abnormal breath sounds. Crackles are associated with emphysema and chronic bronchitis. The nurse notes the pitch and location of the sound, as well as the point in the respiratory cycle at which the sound is heard. A silent chest may indicate airflow obstruction or pneumothorax.

TABLE 30-1 • THREE BREATHING PATTERNS COMMONLY SEEN IN CLIENTS WITH RESPIRATORY MUSCLE FATIGUE

Abdominal paradox. The diaphragm is nonfunctional; inspiration is accomplished by the intercostal and abdominal accessory muscles.
Respiratory alternans. Diaphragmatic breathing alternates with abdominal paradox; may serve to rest the diaphragm.
Asynchronous breathing. The chest wall motion is unorganized; reflects the uncoordinated activity of fatigued muscles.

Dyspnea Assessment Guide

Direct Measure of Dyspnea

Indicate the amount of shortness of breath you are having at this time by marking the line.

shortness of breath as bad as can be

no shortness of breath

Subjective Symptoms

On a scale of 0–4 with 0 indicating no distress and 4 indicating much distress, how much are you presently distressed by: *(circle answer).*

poor appetite	0	1	2	3	4
worn out or weak	0	1	2	3	4
suffocation	0	1	2	3	4
tightness	0	1	2	3	4
congestion	0	1	2	3	4
a feeling of panic or anxiety	0	1	2	3	4

Objective Sign

Rise of the clavicle during inspiration:
ABSENT = not detected
MILD = seen but not pronounced
SEVERE = pronounced

Figure 30-7 • A dyspnea assessment tool. (Redrawn from Gift, A. [1989]. A dyspnea assessment guide. *Critical Care Nurse, 9*[8], 79.)

The degree of dyspnea is assessed by questioning the client and using an assessment tool called a Visual Analog Dyspnea Scale (VADS). The VADS is a straight line with verbal anchors at the beginning and end of a 100-mm line. The client is asked to place a mark on the line to indicate breathing difficulty. The Modified Borg Scale, a 10-point scale that rates breathlessness from nothing at all to maximal, also may be used to rate perceived breathlessness. Figure 30-7 illustrates an assessment guide that combines subjective and objective assessments. These scales are used to assess dyspnea, determine the effectiveness of therapy, and pace the client's activities.

The nurse examines the client's chest, which usually has an altered shape known as a barrel chest (see Figure 30-3). With a barrel chest, the ratio between the anteroposterior (AP) diameter of the chest and its lateral diameter is 2:2 rather than the normal ratio of 1:2. This change in shape results from hyperinflation of alveoli and flattening of the diaphragm, which are typical of emphysema.

The client with chronic bronchitis often has a cyanotic, or blue-tinged, dusky appearance and has excessive sputum production. The nurse observes the client for cyanosis, delayed capillary refill, and clubbing of the fingers (Figure 30-8), which indicate chronically decreased arterial oxygen levels.

CARDIAC MANIFESTATIONS. The nurse determines the client's heart rate and rhythm and assesses for swelling of the feet and ankles (dependent edema) or other signs and symptoms of right-sided heart failure. Nail beds and oral mucous membranes are examined for color. The client with later-stage emphysema may have pallor or frank cyanosis.

PSYCHOSOCIAL ASSESSMENT

COPD affects all aspects of a person's life: social, economic, and psychologic. Socialization of the client with COPD may be reduced when friends avoid him or her because of annoying coughs, excessive sputum, or dyspnea. In addition, the client may choose to be isolated because dyspnea causes fatigue or because of embarrassment from coughing and exces-

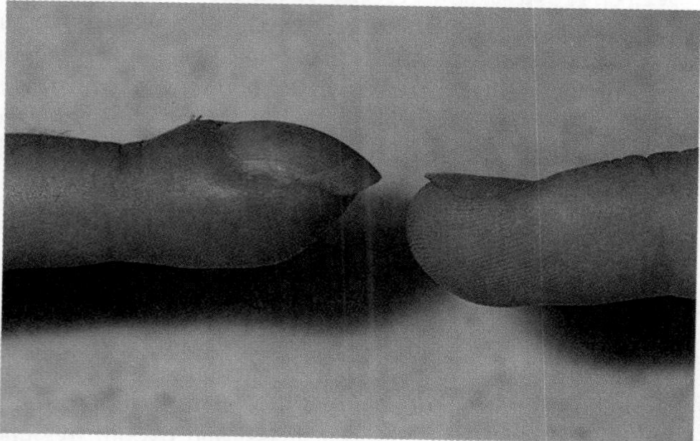

Figure 30-8 • Late digital clubbing *(left)* compared with a normal digit *(right).* (From Swartz, M.H. [1998]. *Textbook of physical diagnosis: History and examination.* Philadelphia: W.B. Saunders.)

sive sputum production. The nurse asks the client about interests and hobbies to determine if socialization has decreased or if hobbies cause exposure to chemicals, smoke, aerosols, or fine particles. He or she is asked about home conditions for exposure to inhalation irritants or crowded living conditions that promote transmission of respiratory tract infections.

The client's economic status may be affected by the disease through changes in income and health insurance coverage. If the client is the head of the household, severe COPD may require role reversal with the partner. Such a change may have a negative impact on self-image. Medications, especially the metered dose inhalers (MDIs), are expensive, and many clients with limited incomes may use these medications only during exacerbations of the disease and not as prescribed on a scheduled basis.

Anxiety and fear related to episodes of dyspnea and feelings of breathlessness may directly influence the client's ability to participate in a full life. Work, family, social, and sexual roles can be affected. The nurse determines the client's awareness and use of support groups and services.

LABORATORY ASSESSMENT

Arterial blood gas (ABG) values identify abnormalities of oxygenation, ventilation, and acid-base status. Serial or repeated ABG values are compared to assess changes in the client's respiratory status over time. Once baseline ABG values are obtained, pulse oximetry can gauge the response to treatment. In general, as COPD progresses, the amount of oxygen in the blood decreases (hypoxemia) and the amount of carbon dioxide in the blood increases **(hypercarbia).** Chronic respiratory acidosis (increased partial pressure of arterial carbon dioxide [$Paco_2$]) then results; metabolic alkalosis (increased arterial bicarbonate) occurs as compensation. Not all clients with COPD are carbon dioxide retainers, even when hypoxemia is present. Carbon dioxide is more easily diffused across the alveolar membrane than is oxygen. Hypercarbia is mostly a problem in advanced or exacerbated emphysema (because the alveoli are affected) rather than in bronchitis (wherein the airways are affected).

Sputum samples are collected for culture from hospitalized clients who exhibit signs of an acute respiratory tract infection. In the ambulatory care setting, sputum cultures are rarely obtained; the client is treated on the basis of signs and symptoms and the usual cause of bacterial organisms. A white blood cell count may confirm the presence of infection.

Other blood tests that may be indicated in clients with COPD include hemoglobin and hematocrit to determine **polycythemia** (a compensatory increase in red blood cells in the chronically hypoxic client). Serum electrolyte levels are examined because hypophosphatemia, hyperkalemia, hypocalcemia, and hypomagnesemia reduce muscle strength. In clients suspected of alpha$_1$-antitrypsin (AAT) deficiency, serum AAT levels are drawn.

RADIOGRAPHIC ASSESSMENT

Chest x-ray studies are done to rule out other chest diseases and to determine the progress of clients with respiratory tract infections and chronic disease. With advanced emphysema, chest x-ray films may show marked hyperinflation and a flattened diaphragm. Chest x-rays studies, however, may not be helpful in the diagnosis of early or moderate disease.

OTHER DIAGNOSTIC ASSESSMENT

COPD is classified from mild to severe on the basis of results of pulmonary function tests (PFTs) (Table 30-2). Airflow rates and lung volume measurements help distinguish airway disease from restrictive patterns typical of interstitial lung disease. The three major components of PFTs are measurements that determine lung volumes, flow volume curves, and diffusion capacity. Each test is performed before and after the client inhales a bronchodilator agent.

The usual lung volumes measured for COPD are vital capacity (VC), residual volume (RV), and total lung capacity (TLC). RV is usually most profoundly affected, although all volumes and capacities change to some degree in COPD. The RV increase reflects the trapped, stagnant air remaining in the lungs.

Flow volume curves measure the client's ability to move air into and out of the lung. The rate of airflow out of the lungs during a rapid, forceful, and complete exhalation from TLC to RV (forced expiratory volume [FEV]) indirectly measures the flow resistance of the lung. A diagnosis of

TABLE 30-2 • PULMONARY FUNCTION FINDINGS IN CHRONIC AIRFLOW LIMITATION

Test	Findings
Residual volume (RV)—the volume of gas remaining in the lungs after a maximal expiration	Loss of elastic recoil causes RV to be increased in emphysema and chronic bronchitis because of the narrowing and obstruction of airways.
Total lung capacity (TLC)—the total amount of gas in the lungs at the end of a maximal inspiration	TLC is increased in emphysematous clients because of loss of elastic recoil. TLC is normal in clients with chronic bronchitis.
Vital capacity (VC)—the maximum amount of gas that can be expired after a maximal inspiration	VC may be normal or decreased in the client with chronic obstructive pulmonary disease (COPD).
Forced vital capacity (FVC)—VC that is produced from a maximal forced expiratory effort	FVC is often increased in clients with emphysema secondary to air trapping.
Forced expiratory volume (FEV_1, FEV_2)—volume of air that is exhaled during a specified time (in seconds) while measuring FVC	FEV mainly reflects resistance in large airways and is usually reduced in the client with asthma (during an attack) and bronchitis.
Functional residual capacity (FRC)—the amount of gas remaining in the lungs at the end of a tidal expiration	FRC is increased in clients with chronic bronchitis if obstruction is severe.
Diffusion—measure of carbon monoxide uptake across the alveolar-capillary membrane	The diffusion value is decreased in severe emphysema. Chronic bronchitis has little effect on diffusion.

COPD is based primarily on the FEV_1 (the FEV in the first second of exhalation). FEV_1 can also be expressed as a percentage of the forced vital capacity (FVC). As the disease progresses, the ratio of FEV_1 to FVC becomes smaller.

The diffusion test measures how well a test gas (carbon monoxide) diffuses across the alveolar-capillary membrane and combines with the hemoglobin of red blood cells. In emphysema, destruction of alveolar walls causes a large decrease in surface area for diffusion of gas into the blood, leading to a decreased diffusion capacity. In bronchitis, even though lung volumes are increased, the diffusion capacity is usually normal.

The client with COPD may have a decreased oxygen saturation, often as low as 91%. Pulse oximetry results lower than 90% (and certainly below 86%) are considered an emergency necessitating immediate treatment.

Peak expiratory flow meters are monitors used by the client and health care professionals to determine the effectiveness of the prescribed treatment to alleviate obstruction. Peak flow rates increase as obstruction resolves. The client is taught to continue to self-monitor the peak expiratory flow rates at home and adjust medications accordingly.

CRITICAL THINKING CHALLENGE

The client is a 66-year-old African-American man who is a resident of the nursing home because of severe dyspnea related to long-standing COPD. He is receiving continuous oxygen by nasal cannula at 2 L/min. When you assess him today, he seems disoriented. His vital signs are as follows: pulse, 112, thready and irregular; respirations, 38 breaths per minute through pursed lips; and blood pressure, 140/110.

- What additional assessment data should you obtain?
- Should you increase the client's oxygen flow rate? Why or why not?

When you weigh the client today, his weight has increased by 7 pounds in 2 days. His fingers are clubbed, he has a "barrel" chest, he has pitting edema of his lower extremities, and his neck veins are flat in the upright position.

- Which of these assessment findings is important? Why?

For suggested answer guidelines, go to SIMON http://www.wbsaunders.com/SIMON/Iggy/.

Analysis

COMMON NURSING DIAGNOSES AND COLLABORATIVE PROBLEMS

The following are the most common nursing diagnoses for clients with chronic obstructive pulmonary disease (COPD):

1. Impaired Gas Exchange related to alveolar membrane changes, diminished airway size, airflow limitation, respiratory muscle fatigue, and excessive mucus production
2. Ineffective Breathing Pattern related to airway obstruction, flattening of the diaphragm, fatigue, and decreased energy
3. Ineffective Airway Clearance related to excessive secretions, fatigue, decreased energy, and ineffective cough
4. Imbalanced Nutrition: Less Than Body Requirements related to dyspnea, excessive secretions, anorexia, and fatigue
5. Anxiety related to loss of control during dyspneic episodes, dyspnea, a change in health status, and situational crisis
6. Activity Intolerance related to fatigue, dyspnea, and an imbalance between oxygen supply and demand

A common collaborative problem for clients with chronic obstructive pulmonary disease/chronic airflow limitation (COPD/CAL) is Potential for Pneumonia or Other Respiratory Infections.

ADDITIONAL NURSING DIAGNOSES AND COLLABORATIVE PROBLEMS

In addition to the common nursing diagnoses and collaborative problems, clients with COPD may have one or more of the following:

- Fatigue related to a change in metabolic energy or hypoxemia
- Knowledge Deficit (disease process, prescribed treatments, activity limitations) related to unfamiliarity with information resources
- Altered Sexuality Patterns related to extreme fatigue
- Inability to Sustain Spontaneous Ventilation related to respiratory muscle fatigue
- Sleep Pattern Disturbance related to dyspnea or an unfamiliar environment (hospitalization)
- Altered Thought Processes related to hypoxemia or sleep deprivation
- Ineffective Individual Coping related to the effects of chronic illness, loss of control over body function, major changes in lifestyle, situational crisis, or knowledge deficit
- Altered Role Performance related to a change in health status or role loss

Other collaborative problems for clients with COPD include Potential for Respiratory Failure and Potential for Right-Sided Heart Failure.

Planning and Implementation

IMPAIRED GAS EXCHANGE

NOC **PLANNING: EXPECTED OUTCOMES.** The client with COPD is expected to attain and maintain partial pressure of arterial oxygen (Pao_2) and arterial carbon dioxide ($Paco_2$) levels within normal ranges or within his or her chronic baseline values. The client is also expected to have a decrease in tachypnea, dyspnea, and confusion; state that fatigue is reduced; and use breathing techniques to improve oxygenation.

INTERVENTIONS. NIC interventions for the client with COPD are listed in Chart 30-7. Most clients with COPD use nonsurgical management to improve or maintain oxygenation. Surgical management is newer and requires that the client meet strict criteria.

NONSURGICAL MANAGEMENT. The mainstays of COPD management include airway maintenance, monitoring, drug therapy, and oxygen therapy.

AIRWAY MAINTENANCE. *The first intervention to improve gas exchange is to maintain a patent airway.* The nurse maintains the client's head, neck, and chest in alignment; assists him or her in liquefying secretions; and clears the airway of secretions.

MONITORING. The nurse assesses the hospitalized client with COPD at frequent intervals (every 2 hours), even when

CHART 30-7

NIC INTERVENTION ACTIVITIES *for* The Client with Chronic Obstructive Pulmonary Disease

Airway Management: *Facilitation of patency of air passages*
- Position client to maximize ventilation potential.
- Perform chest physiotherapy, as appropriate.
- Remove secretions by encouraging coughing or suctioning.
- Instruct how to cough effectively.
- Assist with incentive spirometer, as appropriate.
- Auscultate breath sounds, noting areas of decreased or absent ventilation and presence of adventitious sounds.
- Administer bronchodilators, as appropriate.
- Teach client how to use prescribed inhalers, as appropriate.
- Administer aerosol treatments, as appropriate.
- Administer ultrasonic nebulizer treatments, as appropriate.
- Administer humidified air or oxygen, as appropriate.
- Regulate fluid intake to optimize fluid balance.
- Position to alleviate dyspnea.
- Monitor respiratory and oxygenation status, as appropriate.

Cough Enhancement: *Promotion of deep inhalation by the client with subsequent generation of high intrathoracic pressures and compression of underlying lung parenchyma for the forceful expulsion of air*
- Monitor results of pulmonary function tests, particularly vital capacity, maximal inspiratory force, forced expiratory volume in 1 second (FEV_1), and FEV_1/FVC, as appropriate.
- Assist client to a sitting position with neck slightly flexed, shoulders relaxed, and knees flexed.
- Encourage client to take several deep breaths.
- Encourage client to take a deep breath, hold it for 2 seconds, and cough two or three times in succession.
- Instruct client to inhale deeply several times, to exhale slowly, and to cough at the end of exhalation.

Oxygen Therapy: *Administration of oxygen and monitoring of its effectiveness.*
- Clear oral, nasal, and tracheal secretions, as appropriate.
- Maintain airway patency.
- Set up oxygen equipment and administer through a heated, humidified system.
- Monitor the oxygen liter flow.
- Monitor position of oxygen delivery device.
- Periodically check oxygen delivery device to ensure that the prescribed concentration is being delivered.
- Monitor the effectiveness of oxygen therapy (e.g., pulse oximetry, ABGs), as appropriate.
- Ensure replacement of oxygen mask/cannula whenever the device is removed.
- Monitor client's ability to tolerate removal of oxygen while eating.
- Observe for signs of oxygen-induced hypoventilation.
- Monitor for signs of oxygen toxicity and absorption atelectasis.
- Monitor oxygen equipment to ensure that it is not interfering with the client's attempt to breathe.
- Monitor client's anxiety related to need for oxygen therapy.
- Monitor for skin breakdown from friction of oxygen device.
- Provide for oxygen when client is transported.
- Instruct client and family about use of oxygen at home.
- Arrange for use of oxygen devices that facilitate mobility and teach client accordingly.

Energy Management: *Regulating energy use to treat or prevent fatigue and optimize function.*
- Determine client's physical limitations.
- Encourage verbalization of feelings about limitations.
- Monitor nutritional intake to ensure adequate energy resources.
- Consult with dietitian about ways to increase intake of high-energy foods.
- Monitor cardiorespiratory response to activity (e.g., tachycardia, other dysrhythmias, dyspnea, diaphoresis, pallor, hemodynamic pressures, and respiratory rate).
- Limit environmental stimuli (e.g., light and noise) to facilitate relaxation.
- Promote bedrest/activity limitation (e.g., increase number of rest periods).
- Arrange physical activities to reduce competition for oxygen supply to vital body functions (e.g., avoid activity immediately after meals).
- Assist client to schedule rest periods.
- Avoid care activities during scheduled rest periods.
- Plan activities for periods when the client has the most energy.
- Assist with regular physical activities (e.g., ambulation, transfers, turning, and personal care), as needed.
- Monitor client's oxygen response (e.g., pulse rate, cardiac rhythm, and respiratory rate) to self-care or nursing activities.
- Teach client and significant other techniques of self-care that will minimize oxygen consumption (e.g., self-monitoring and pacing techniques for performance of activities of daily living).
- Assist the client to identify tasks that family and friends can perform in the home to prevent/relieve fatigue.
- Assist the client in assigning priority to activities to accommodate energy levels.
- Assist client to identify preferences for activity.
- Evaluate programmed increases in levels of activities.

NIC intervention activities selected from McCloskey, J.C., & Bulechek, G.M. (Eds.). (2000). *Nursing interventions classification (NIC)* (3rd ed.). St. Louis: Mosby.

ABG, Arterial blood gas.

the purpose of hospitalization is not COPD management. The nurse provides the prescribed oxygen, assesses the response to treatment, and intervenes to prevent complications.

If the client's condition continues to deteriorate despite treatment, more aggressive therapy is required. Intubation and mechanical ventilation may be necessary for clients in respiratory failure, including those who are unable to sustain spontaneous breathing patterns.

OXYGEN THERAPY. Oxygen is prescribed for relief of symptoms of hypoxemia (decreased blood oxygen levels) and **hypoxia** (decreased tissue oxygenation). Arterial blood gas (ABG) analysis is the best tool for determining the need for oxygen therapy and for evaluating its effects. Oxygen need can also be determined by pulse oximetry.

The average client requires an oxygen flow of 2 to 4 L/min via nasal cannula or up to 40% via Venturi mask. The client who is hypoxemic and also has chronic hypercarbia requires lower levels of oxygen delivery, usually 1 to 2 L/min via nasal cannula. *A low arterial oxygen level is this client's primary drive for breathing.* More information on oxygen therapy is found in Chapter 28.

DRUG THERAPY. Drug therapy for COPD involves many of the same inhaled and systemic drugs as for asthma, including beta-adrenergic agents, cholinergic antagonists, methylxanthines, corticosteroids, cromolyn sodium/nedocromil, and leukotriene modifiers (see Chart 30-4). The client with COPD is more likely to be taking systemic agents (in addition to inhaled drugs) than is the client with asthma. An additional drug class for COPD is the mucolytics, which are thought to thin secretions, making them easier to expectorate.

Mucolytic agents are prescribed for the client with thick, tenacious (sticky) mucous secretions. Nebulizer treatments with normal saline or with a mucolytic agent such as acetylcysteine (Mucomyst✤, Airbron✤) or dornase alfa (Pulmozyme) and normal saline help to thin secretions and facilitate expectoration. Guaifenesin (Organidin, Naldecon Senior EX) is a systemic mucolytic that is taken orally.

Stepped therapy is recommended for clients with chronic bronchitis or emphysema (Table 30-3). The key elements of stepped therapy include pharmacologic therapy, monitoring, and control of environmental irritants and allergens. The expected outcomes of stepped therapy are for the client to have more awareness of the disease and to increase participation symptom management.

TABLE 30-3 • PHARMACOLOGIC STEPPED APPROACH TO TREATING CHRONIC BRONCHITIS AND EMPHYSEMA

STEP 1. MILD SYMPTOMS
$Beta_2$ agonist 1-2 puffs q2-6h prn (not to exceed 8-12 puffs in 24 hr)

STEP 2. MILD TO MODERATE SYMPTOMS DAILY
Ipratropium bromide 2-6 puffs q6-8h
$Beta_2$ agonist 1-4 puffs for rescue treatment or as regular supplement

STEP 3. UNSATISFACTORY RESPONSE TO STEP 2
Add theophylline 200-400 mg bid or 400-800 mg hs (nocturnal bronchospasms) or albuterol SR 4-8 mg bid or hs only

STEP 4. UNSATISFACTORY RESPONSE TO STEP 3
Add prednisone 40 mg/day for 10-14 days
- Wean when improvement noted to low daily or qod dose
- Place on steroid metered dose inhaler if client has bronchial hyperreactivity
- Stop steroids if no improvement noted

STEP 5. SEVERE EXACERBATION
$Beta_2$ agonist with spacer, 6-8 puffs q½-2 h
Ipratropium bromide with spacer, 6-8 puffs q3-4h
Theophylline IV
Methylprednisolone 50-100 mg IV STAT, then q6-8h; wean as soon as possible.
Antibiotics if indicated
Mucokinetic agents if sputum tenacious

SURGICAL MANAGEMENT. At one time, single-lung transplantation offered some improved oxygenation for clients with end-stage COPD. This surgery is considered an impractical intervention because of limited donor lung availability and the problem of comorbidities. A newer intervention is lung reduction surgery. The goal of this surgery is improvement of gas exchange through removal of hyperinflated lung tissue. The hyperinflated areas of the lungs are filled with stagnant air that is not renewed with some atmospheric air (containing oxygen) during each respiratory cycle. Instead, this stagnant air continues to receive carbon dioxide until the level of carbon dioxide in the hyperinflated alveolus is the same as that in the capillary. Essentially, these hyperinflated lung areas are useless for gas exchange. Most clients having successful lung reduction surgery have at least a 75% improvement in the forced expiratory volume in the first second of exhalation (FEV_1), decreased total lung capacity (TLC) and residual volume (RV), and increased activity tolerance, and they may not need to use supplemental oxygen therapy.

PREOPERATIVE CARE. Clients are selected for this procedure on the basis of having end-stage emphysema, minimal chronic bronchitis, and stable cardiac function; being ambulatory and not dependent on a ventilator; not having pulmonary fibrosis, asthma, or late-stage cancer; and having been nonsmokers for at least 6 months (Schedel & Connolly, 1999). The client must undergo pulmonary rehabilitation before surgery to maximize lung and muscle function. The client must reach a state in which he or she is able to walk, without stopping, for 30 minutes at 1 mile/hr and maintain a 90% or better oxygen saturation level.

In addition to standard preoperative testing, the client having lung reduction surgery has tests to determine the location of greatest hyperinflation and poorest perfusion. These tests include pulmonary plethysmography, gas dilution, and perfusion scans.

OPERATIVE PROCEDURE. Usually, lung reduction is performed bilaterally through either a large midline incision or a transverse anterior thoracotomy. Each lung is deflated separately and examined for color and texture differences. Normal lung tissue darkens to purple or gray when deflated and becomes more dense or rubbery in texture. Hyperinflated areas do not deflate, and they remain pink with a spongy texture. After the hyperinflated areas have been identified, the surgeon removes as much of this tissue as possible, sealing off and reinforcing the remaining normal lung tissue.

POSTOPERATIVE CARE. The client having lung reduction surgery requires close monitoring for continuing respiratory problems, as well as usual postoperative complications. In addition to the usual care required after thoracotomy (see Surgical Management [Lung Cancer], p. 563), the client initially maintains bronchodilator and mucolytic therapy. Pulmonary hygiene includes incentive spirometry 10 times per hour while awake, chest physiotherapy starting on the first postoperative day, and hourly pulmonary assessment.

Pain is usually managed by epidural administration of opioids during the early postoperative period. This type of analgesic administration reduces pain, limits sedation and cognitive dysfunction, and allows the client to remain reasonably alert and more fully participate in pulmonary hygiene measures.

INEFFECTIVE BREATHING PATTERN

PLANNING: EXPECTED OUTCOMES. The client with COPD is expected to achieve an effective breathing pattern that decreases the work of breathing as evidenced by a respiratory rhythm within normal limits for the client's age, synchronous thoracoabdominal movement, use of accessory muscles appropriate to his or her activity level, and increased activity tolerance.

INTERVENTIONS. Before any interventions can be implemented, the client is assessed to determine the breathing pattern, especially the rate, rhythm, depth, and use of accessory muscles. The client with COPD relies more on accessory muscles than on the diaphragm for breathing. These muscles, however, are less efficient than the diaphragm; as a result, the work of breathing increases. The nurse determines whether there are any contributing factors to the increased work of breathing, such as respiratory tract infection. Interventions are aimed at improving the client's breathing efforts and decreasing the work of breathing through the use of specific breathing techniques, positioning, exercise conditioning, and energy conservation.

BREATHING TECHNIQUES. Diaphragmatic or abdominal and pursed-lip breathing maneuvers may be beneficial interventions for managing dyspneic episodes. The client uses these techniques, shown in Chart 30-8, during all activities. The amount of stagnant air in the lungs is minimized, and the client gains confidence and control in managing dyspnea. The nurse teaches these techniques when the client is free from dyspnea.

DIAPHRAGMATIC OR ABDOMINAL BREATHING. In diaphragmatic breathing, the client consciously increases diaphragmatic movement. Lying on the back allows the abdomen to relax.

PURSED-LIP BREATHING. The technique of breathing through pursed lips uses the mild resistance of partially opposed lips to prolong exhalation and to increase airway pressure, thereby delaying airway compression and reducing air trapping. Pursed-lip breathing can be used during diaphragmatic or abdominal breathing.

POSITIONING. The client is assisted to an upright position, with the head of the bed elevated. Various positions can be used to assist in alleviating dyspnea (see Figure 30-6) by increasing chest expansion, relaxing the chest muscles, and placing the diaphragm in the proper position to contract. These positions conserve energy by supporting the client's arms and upper body.

The client uses the standing position when there is no place to sit (Figure 30-9). Clients with COPD use a greater proportion of their accessory muscles for breathing. Supporting the thorax allows these muscles to work better.

EXERCISE CONDITIONING. Clients who experience exercise-induced shortness of breath respond to dyspnea by limiting their activity, even basic **activities of daily living (ADLs).** Over time, the muscles of respiration and other large muscle groups weaken and are less efficient in the use of oxygen. The result is increased dyspnea with lower activity levels.

Exercise conditioning of the large muscle groups (indirect) or retraining of the respiratory muscles (direct) can be done as part of a pulmonary rehabilitation program. Two direct techniques are isocapneic hyperventilation and resistive breathing. Isocapneic hyperventilation increases endurance. The client hyperventilates into a machine that controls the concentrations of oxygen and carbon dioxide. In resistive breathing, the client breathes against a set resistance. Resistive breathing increases respiratory muscle strength and endurance.

CHART 30-8

CLIENT EDUCATION GUIDE
Breathing Exercises

Diaphragmatic or Abdominal Breathing

- Lie on your back with your knees bent.
- Place your hands or a book on your abdomen to create resistance.
- Begin breathing from your abdomen while keeping your chest still. You can tell if you are breathing correctly if your hands or the book rises and falls accordingly.

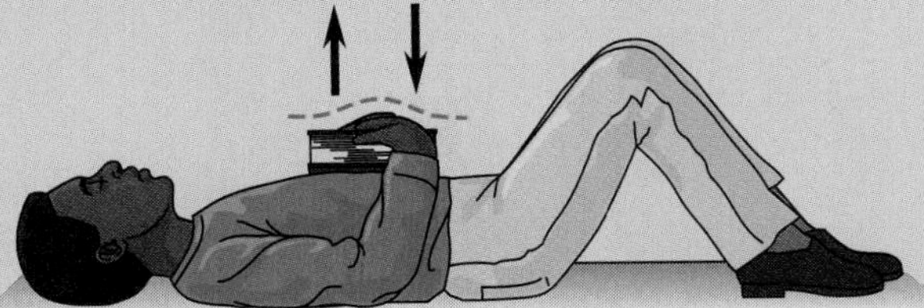

Pursed-Lip Breathing

- Close your mouth and breathe in through your nose.
- Purse your lips as you would to whistle. Breathe out slowly through your mouth, without puffing your cheeks. Spend at least twice the amount of time it took you to breathe in. Use your abdominal muscles to squeeze out every bit of air you can.
- Remember to use pursed-lip breathing during any physical activity. Always inhale before beginning the activity and exhale while performing the activity. Never hold your breath.

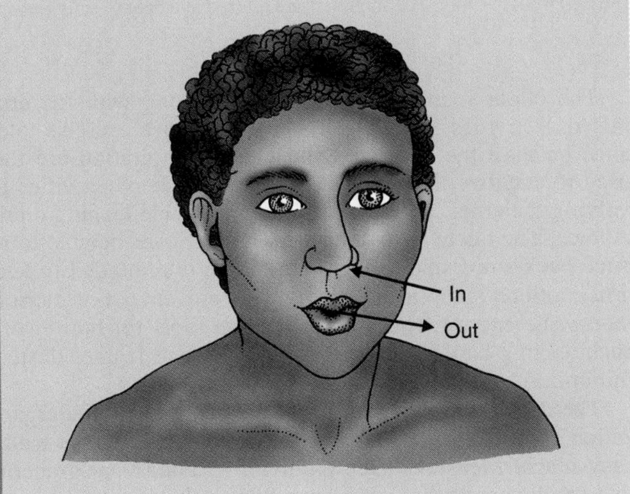

ENERGY CONSERVATION. Energy conservation is the planning and pacing of activities for maximal tolerance and minimal discomfort. Once the FEV_1 falls below 50% predicted, the client's ability to perform ADLs is limited. The nurse or therapist (physical or occupational) asks the client to describe a typical daily schedule. Each activity is divided into its smaller parts to determine whether that task can be performed in a different way or at a different time of the day. The nurse assists in planning and pacing activities for the day. Rest periods are paced between activities. Development of a personal chart outlining the day's activities and planned rest periods is helpful.

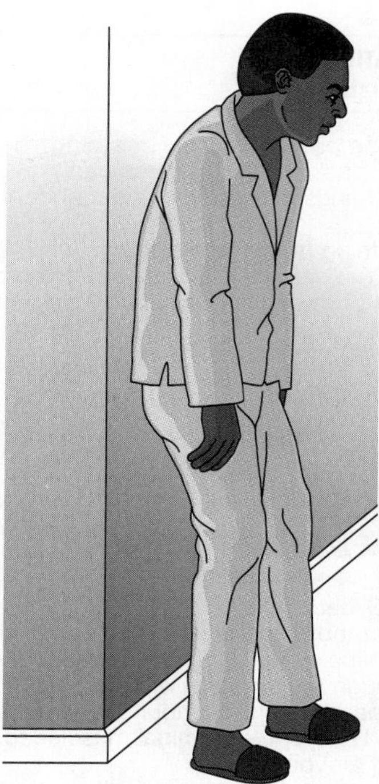

Figure 30-9 ● The standing position that is used to help clients with chronic obstructive pulmonary disease to breathe. The client stands with the back and hips against a wall and with the feet about 12 inches (30 cm) from the wall. The shoulders are relaxed and bent slightly forward.

The client is instructed to avoid working with the arms raised. Activities involving the arms decrease exercise tolerance because the accessory muscles of respiration are then used to stabilize the arms and shoulders. Many activities involving the arms can be done sitting at a table leaning on the elbows. The client is instructed to adjust work heights to reduce back strain and fatigue. He or she is reminded to keep arm motions smooth and flowing to prevent jerky motions that waste energy. The use of adaptive tools for housework, such as long-handled dustpans, sponges, and feather dusters, minimizes bending and reaching.

The nurse gives suggestions to the client about the organization of work spaces so that items used most often are within easy reach. Measures such as dividing laundry or groceries into small parcels that can be handled easily, using disposable plates to save washing time, and letting dishes dry in the rack also conserve energy. Talking requires energy and use of the lungs; therefore the client is instructed not to talk when engaged in other activities that require energy, such as walking. In addition, he or she is instructed to avoid holding his or her breath while performing any activity.

INEFFECTIVE AIRWAY CLEARANCE

PLANNING: EXPECTED OUTCOMES. The client with COPD is expected to maintain a patent airway, cough effectively, remain free from aspiration, and use the stepped therapy approach to control symptoms.

INTERVENTIONS. The client with chronic bronchitis and advanced emphysema often has difficulty with removal of secretions, which results in compromised breathing and inadequate oxygenation. Excessive mucus also predisposes the client to respiratory tract infections. The nurse assesses breath sounds routinely as part of physical assessment and before and after interventions. Careful use of drugs combined with controlled coughing, hydration, and postural drainage may help in airway clearance. If these measures fail, a tracheostomy may be required on a temporary or permanent basis.

CONTROLLED COUGHING. Because the client with COPD produces excessive mucus, specific coughing at certain times of the day is beneficial. The nurse teaches the client to cough on arising in the morning to eliminate mucus that collected during the night. Coughing to expectorate mucus before mealtimes may facilitate a more pleasant meal, and coughing before bedtime may ensure clear lungs for an uninterrupted night's sleep.

To cough effectively, the client sits in a chair or on the side of a bed with feet placed firmly on the floor. He or she is instructed to turn the shoulders inward and to bend the head slightly downward, hugging a pillow against the stomach. The client then takes a few diaphragmatic breaths. After the third to fifth deep breath (in through the nose, out through pursed lips), the nurse instructs the client to bend forward slowly while producing two or three strong coughs from the same breath. The color, consistency, odor, and amount of secretions are noted. On return to a sitting position, the client takes a comfortable deep breath. The entire coughing procedure is repeated at least twice. After coughing exercises, the nurse allows the client to rest and then assists in providing mouth care.

CHEST PHYSIOTHERAPY AND POSTURAL DRAINAGE. Chest physiotherapy (PT) with postural drainage (Figure 30-10) assists in moving secretions from peripheral to central airways, in re-expanding lung tissue, and in promoting efficient use of the respiratory muscles. Chest PT combines chest percussion with vibration to loosen secretions. Postural drainage uses specific positions and gravity to assist in removing bronchial secretions. Postural drainage with chest PT may be helpful for clients with excessive secretions and airway clearance problems but should not be used routinely on all clients with COPD.

SUCTIONING. Suctioning is performed only when abnormal breath sounds are present, not on a routine schedule. For the client with a weak cough, weak pulmonary muscles, and inability to expectorate effectively, the nurse or respiratory therapist performs nasotracheal suctioning. The client is assessed for dyspnea and tachycardia or other dysrhythmias during the suctioning procedure and for improved breath sounds afterward. Suctioning is discussed in detail in Chapter 28.

POSITIONING. The client who can tolerate sitting in a chair is assisted out of bed for 1-hour periods two to three times a day. This intervention helps mobilize secretions and keeps the diaphragm in a position to ventilate the lungs better.

HYDRATION. Unless hydration is contraindicated for other health problems, the client with COPD is instructed to drink 2 to 3 L/day to maintain adequate hydration, which helps liquefy secretions. Humidifiers may be useful for clients living in a dry climate or who use dry heat during the winter.

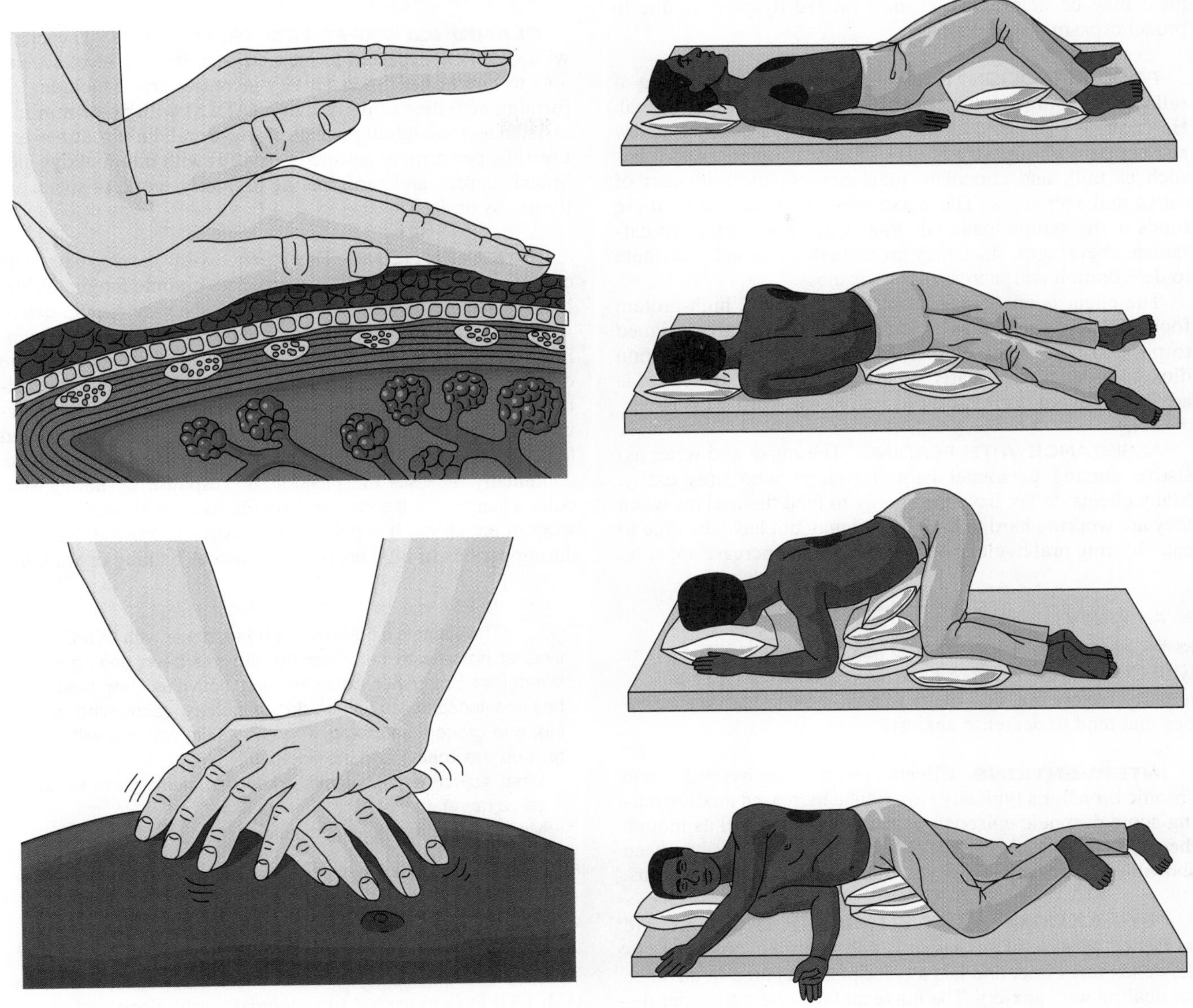

Figure 30-10 ● Chest physiotherapy and postural drainage. *Left,* Percussion and vibration techniques. The nurse may use one or two hands with vibration, which is performed when the client exhales or coughs. *Right,* Positions for postural drainage of respiratory secretions.

The client is instructed to clean the humidifier daily to prevent the growth of mold spores.

IMBALANCED NUTRITION: LESS THAN BODY REQUIREMENTS

NOC **PLANNING: EXPECTED OUTCOMES.** The client with COPD is expected to achieve and maintain a body weight within 10% of ideal.

INTERVENTIONS. The client with COPD often has food intolerance, nausea, early satiety, loss of appetite, and meal-related dyspnea. In addition, the increased work of breathing raises calorie and protein requirements. These situations lead to protein-calorie malnutrition for many clients. Malnourished clients lose total body mass, respiratory muscle mass, respiratory muscle strength, lung elasticity, and alveolar-capillary surface area, which contributes to an ineffective breathing pattern.

The nurse identifies the client who is at risk for or who is experiencing this complication and initiates dietary consultation. The client's weight and other indicators of nutrition, such as skin condition and serum prealbumin levels, are monitored.

DYSPNEA MANAGEMENT. Shortness of breath (dyspnea) is the most common problem related to eating. Dyspnea during mealtimes can be minimized by resting before meals. The biggest meal of the day is planned for the time when the client is most hungry and well rested. Four to six small meals a day may be preferred to three larger ones. The client is instructed to use pursed-lip and abdominal breathing to alleviate dyspnea. A bronchodilator used 30 minutes before the meal may be helpful if the meal-related dyspnea is due to bronchospasm or secretions.

FOOD SELECTION. Abdominal bloating and a feeling of fullness often prevent the client from eating a complete meal. He or she is instructed to choose foods that are easy to chew and not gas forming. Dry foods stimulate coughing, and foods such as milk and chocolate may increase the thickness of saliva and secretions. The nurse advises avoidance of these foods in the symptomatic client, as well as avoidance of caffeinated beverages, since they promote diuresis and contribute to dehydration and increased nervousness.

The client is encouraged to eat high-calorie, high-protein foods. Dietary supplements, such as Pulmocare, are designed to provide nutritional supplementation with reduced carbon dioxide production. If early satiety is a problem, the client is advised to avoid drinking fluids before and during the meal.

ASSISTANCE WITH FEEDING. The nurse and other assistive nursing personnel help the client who tires easily. Many clients do not have the energy to feed themselves when they are working hard to breathe and may not have the urge to eat. Offering oral hygiene before meals may increase appetite.

ANXIETY

NOC **PLANNING: EXPECTED OUTCOMES.** The client with COPD is expected to have decreased anxiety, be able to identify factors that contribute to anxiety, and identify activities that tend to decrease anxiety.

INTERVENTIONS. Clients with emphysema and chronic bronchitis typically experience increased anxiety during acute dyspneic episodes, especially if they feel as though they are choking on excessive secretions. Anxiety has been shown to cause dyspnea, which then affects functional status.

PSYCHOLOGIC INTERVENTIONS. If symptoms are worsened because of anxiety, it is important that he or she understands this effect and has a clear plan prepared in advance for dealing with anxiety. The nurse and the client together develop a written plan that states exactly what the client should do if symptoms flare. Having a plan provides confidence and control in knowing exactly what to do, which often helps reduce anxiety. The nurse stresses the importance of using pursed-lip and diaphragmatic breathing techniques during periods of anxiety or panic.

Family, friends, and support groups can be quite helpful. Professional counseling, if needed, is recommended as a positive suggestion and in no way suggests that this need represents a failure of the client to cope. The nurse reinforces that talking with a professional counselor can help identify techniques to maintain control over the dyspnea and feelings of panic.

COMPLEMENTARY AND ALTERNATIVE THERAPY. The nurse explores other approaches to help the client control dyspneic episodes and panic attacks. Examples include relaxation techniques, hypnosis therapy, and biofeedback. Biofeedback helps the client determine the impact of various stimuli on symptoms. Ultimately the client learns to relax and control these stimuli to avoid the aggravating symptoms.

ACTIVITY INTOLERANCE

PLANNING: EXPECTED OUTCOMES. The client with COPD is expected to increase activity to a level acceptable to him or her. Such activity increases could include performing activities of daily living (ADLs) with no or minimal assistance, maintaining usual or near-usual daily routines and lifestyle, performing selected activities with minimal dyspnea or tachycardia, and participating in family, work, or social activities as desired.

INTERVENTIONS. The client with emphysema and chronic bronchitis typically experiences chronic fatigue. While in the acute phases of the illness, he or she may require extensive assistance with the ADLs of eating, bathing, and grooming. As the acute episode resolves, the nurse encourages the client to pace activities and provide as much self-care as possible. The client is instructed not to rush through morning activities, because rushing is likely to increase dyspnea, fatigue, and hypoxemia. As the client gradually increases activity, the nurse continually assesses the physiologic response by noting skin color changes, pulse rate and regularity, blood pressure, and work of breathing. If supplemental oxygen is ordered, it is used during periods of high energy use, such as bathing or walking.

CRITICAL THINKING CHALLENGE

The client is a 58-year-old homemaker with COPD. She lives at home with her husband and has been getting more breathless doing her housekeeping activities. Her husband has convinced her to let him do the laundry, vacuuming, dusting, and grocery shopping. The client tells you she will never give up the ironing and the cooking.

- What adjustments in tasks could this client make to conserve her energy?
- Make a sample activity/rest plan for this client.

For suggested answer guidelines, go to SIMON http://www.wbsaunders.com/SIMON/Iggy/.

POTENTIAL FOR PNEUMONIA OR OTHER RESPIRATORY INFECTION

PLANNING: EXPECTED OUTCOMES. The client with COPD is expected to recognize early signs and symptoms of infection and seek treatment promptly.

INTERVENTIONS. Pneumonia is one of the most common complications of COPD. Clients who have excessive secretions or who have artificial airways are at increased risk for respiratory tract infections. The risk is greatly increased in the older client. He or she is taught to avoid large crowds of people, such as at a shopping center. The nurse stresses the importance of receiving a pneumonia vaccination and an annual influenza vaccine ("flu shot").

Community-Based Care

HEALTH TEACHING

The client with a chronic, disabling disease like chronic obstructive pulmonary disease (COPD) needs to know as much about the disease as possible so that he or she can better manage it and themselves. The client and significant others should be able to discuss medications, signs and symptoms of infection, avoidance of respiratory irritants, the diet therapy regimen, and activity progression. The client is instructed to identify and avoid stressors that can exacerbate the disease.

The nurse instructs the client in techniques of breathing, including pursed-lip breathing, diaphragmatic breathing, positioning, relaxation therapy, energy conservation, and coughing and deep breathing. Figure 30-11 is a sample client education checklist used for discharge teaching of the client with COPD. Two factors may interfere with teaching hospitalized clients: the shortened length of stay coupled with a multitude of topics to discuss and the level of tolerance and dyspnea. It may be unrealistic to cover all of the topics in the education checklist during a single hospitalization. The primary nurse or case manager must coordinate teaching with the home care or clinic staff.

Hypoxemic clients can benefit from long-term use of oxygen at home. Home oxygen may be needed only during periods of exercise or sleep if hypoxemia occurs only during these times. Continuous, long-term administration of oxygen can reverse tissue hypoxia and decrease pulmonary vascular resistance; it can also improve cognitive ability and well-being. More information on oxygen therapy is found in Chapter 28.

HOME CARE MANAGEMENT

Most clients with COPD are treated in the ambulatory care setting and cared for at home. When pneumonia or a severe exacerbation of the disease develops, the client is usually treated and discharged from the hospital to a previous home setting. For clients with advanced disease, however, 24-hour care may be needed for ADLs and for monitoring for acute episodes or progression of the illness. They may not be able to enjoy work or recreational activities because of severe dyspnea and fatigue. If arrangements for home care are not possible, placement in a long-term care setting may be necessary.

Most clients can benefit from a structured pulmonary rehabilitation program. Pulmonary rehabilitation programs vary, but the overall goal of these multidisciplinary programs is to increase a person's ability to compensate for and live with COPD. The client with COPD is referred to a pulmonary rehabilitation program before illness becomes severe. Clients with the least severe functional abnormality benefit the most.

The nurse works with the hospital nursing case manager to obtain the necessary equipment for care at home. Often the case manager coordinates the necessary resources to facilitate a smooth transition back to the community and ensures appropriate follow-up in the community. Client needs may include oxygen therapy, a hospital-type bed, a nebulizer, a tub transfer bench, and arrangements for a home care nurse to continue monitoring the health status, review medication compliance, and evaluate home care needs.

The client with COPD faces a lifelong disease with remissions and exacerbations. The nurse explains to the client and family that the client may experience periods of anxiety, depression, and ineffective coping. The client who was a smoker may also have self-directed anger, particularly if he or she recognizes that smoking contributed to the disease.

Financial concerns often increase the client's and family's anxiety and interfere with disease management. The condition may worsen to the point that he or she cannot work. Disability benefits through Social Security or private disability insurance plans can help ease the financial burden. Medicare or other health insurers may assist with payment for home oxygen therapy and nebulizer treatments. The nurse collaborates with the social worker or case manager to help the client make the necessary arrangements.

HEALTH CARE RESOURCES

The nurse provides appropriate referrals as necessary. Home care visits may be warranted, particularly if the client must use home oxygen therapy for the first time. Chart 30-9 lists assessment areas for the client with COPD at home. Referral to assistance programs, such as Meals on Wheels, can be extremely helpful. The nurse provides a list of various support groups, as well as Better Breathing groups sponsored by the American Lung Association. If the client is having difficulty with smoking cessation and indicates the desire for assistance, the nurse makes the appropriate referrals.

Evaluation: Outcomes

NOC The nurse evaluates the care of the client with chronic obstructive pulmonary disease (COPD) on the basis of the identified nursing diagnoses and collaborative problems. The expected outcomes are that the client:

- Attains and maintains ventilation parameters (partial pressure of arterial oxygen [Pa_{O_2}], partial pressure of arterial carbon dioxide [Pa_{CO_2}]) within the normal range for the client
- Adheres to the prescribed pharmacologic therapy
- Uses techniques of pursed-lip breathing and abdominal or diaphragmatic breathing
- Uses correct positioning techniques during dyspneic episodes
- Performs work simplification techniques
- Uses energy conservation techniques
- Adapts lifestyle to energy level
- Maintains a patent airway by removing excessive secretions
- Uses controlled coughing
- Increases or maintains fluid intake
- Attains and maintains body weight within 10% of ideal
- Identifies multiple coping strategies
- Identifies personal strengths
- Performs self-care independently or with minimal assistance for as long as possible
- States the need to avoid irritants and sources of infection
- Participates in social and family activities as desired
- Maintains employment or the same level of activity
- Decreases exacerbations of symptoms
- Reduces emergency department use and hospitalizations

CYSTIC FIBROSIS

OVERVIEW

Cystic fibrosis (CF) is a genetic disease that affects many organs and lethally impairs pulmonary function. Although this disorder is present from birth and is usually manifested in early childhood, advances in management have resulted in many affected clients living into adulthood.

Many clients with CF require frequent hospitalizations. Some acute care environments have specialized units for these clients because interventions are specific to the disease.

Checklist for COPD Client Education

The Client Has Received the Following Education:	Date	Signature
A. Basic anatomy and physiology of the respiratory system 1. Structures composing the respiratory system 2. Functions of the respiratory passageways		
B. Pathophysiology related to condition 1. Name of lung disease 2. Generalized physiologic effects 3. Generalized psychosocial effects		
C. Medications 1. Medication safety 2. Name of each medication 3. Action of each medication 4. Dosage 5. How to take each medication 6. How to use a metered dose inhaler with or without a "spacer" 7. Recognition of side effects 8. Importance of carrying a medication list and a medical alert (Medic Alert) bracelet or card		
D. Respiratory therapy interventions and bronchial hygiene 1. Proper care and cleaning of home equipment (i.e., oxygen, cannulas, nebulizers) 2. Sequence of treatments 3. Adequate hydration 4. Postural drainage and chest physiotherapy (optional and only with excessive secretions) 5. Prevention of respiratory tract infection: a. Avoid exposure to crowds and people with respiratory tract infections b. Signs and symptoms of respiratory tract infection c. Use of prescribed antibiotics with as-needed (prn) schedule d. Influenza immunization; pneumococcal immunization e. Use of measures to promote oronasal hygiene		
E. Management of dyspnea 1. Controlled cough maneuver 2. Pursed-lip breathing 3. Diaphragmatic breathing 4. Positioning techniques 5. Stress management and relaxation techniques		
F. Adaptation of a daily routine 1. Daily schedule of graded exercises 2. Walking exercise on level ground 3. Stair climbing 4. Activities of daily living: adjust activities according to individual fatigue patterns		
G. Nutrition 1. Type of diet prescribed 2. Balanced diet: meat, dairy, grain, fruit and vegetables (2:2:4:4 ratio) 3. Low salt intake		
H. Control of environment 1. Environmental problems related to pulmonary disease 2. Ways to make the environment conducive to living with pulmonary disease a. Avoid irritants and use air purification system b. Use mask when exposed to dusts and cold air c. Stay indoors with air-conditioning operating when air quality is poor d. Check air quality telephone recording		
I. Smoking 1. Rationale for smoking cessation 2. Suggest ways to stop smoking		
J. Body image and human sexuality 1. Alterations in self-esteem and body image related to pulmonary disease 2. Communication in human relationships 3. Alterations in sexual relationships related to pulmonary disease		
K. Available community resources 1. Discharge planning; referral to home care professionals 2. Available community services: Meals on Wheels, American Lung Association, American Heart Association, American Cancer Society		

Figure 30-11 ● A checklist for education of the client with chronic obstructive pulmonary disease (COPD).

CHART 30-9

FOCUSED ASSESSMENT *of*
The Home Care Client with Chronic Obstructive Pulmonary Disease

Assess respiratory status and adequacy of ventilation.
- Measure rate, depth, and rhythm of respirations.
- Examine mucous membranes and nail beds for evidence of hypoxia.
- Determine use of accessory muscles.
- Examine chest and abdomen for paradoxic breathing.
- Count number of words client can speak between breaths.
- Determine need and use of supplemental oxygen. (How many liters per minute is the client using?)
- Determine level of consciousness and presence/absence of confusion.
- Auscultate lungs for abnormal breath sounds.
- Measure oxygen saturation by pulse oximetry.
- Determine sputum production, color, and amount.
- Ask about activity level.
- Observe general hygiene.
- Measure body temperature.

Assess cardiac status.
- Measure rate, quality, and rhythm of pulse.
- Check dependent areas for edema.
- Check neck veins for distention with the client in a sitting position.
- Measure capillary refill.

Assess nutritional status.
- Weight maintenance, loss, or gain
- Food and fluid intake
- Use of nutritional supplements
- General condition of the skin

Assess client's and caregiver's compliance and understanding of illness and treatment, including the following:
- Correct use of supplemental oxygen
- Correct use of inhalers
- Medication schedule and side effects
- Signs and symptoms to report to the health care provider
- Use of pursed-lip and diaphragmatic breathing techniques
- Scheduling of rest periods and priority activities
- Participation in rehabilitation activities

Clients are often encouraged to continue to self-medicate using their customary medications during hospitalizations.

Pathophysiology

CF is a genetic disorder that results in blocked chloride transport in the cell membranes. The error in chloride transport causes the formation of mucus that has little water content. The thick, sticky mucus causes problems in the lungs, pancreas, liver, salivary glands, and testes. Essentially, the mucus plugs up glands in these organs, causing glandular atrophy and organ dysfunction. Nonpulmonary problems include pancreatic insufficiency with malnutrition and gastrointestinal obstruction, poor growth, male sterility, and cirrhosis of the liver. These primary problems cause a multitude of secondary problems. The primary cause of death in the client with CF is respiratory failure.

The pulmonary problems of CF result from the constant presence of thick, sticky mucus and are the most serious complications of the disease. The mucus narrows airways, reducing airflow. The constant presence of mucus results in chronic lower respiratory tract bacterial infections with chronic bronchitis and chronic dilation of the bronchioles **(bronchiectasis).** Lung abscesses are common. Changes occur in the bronchioles over time, including bronchiole distention, increased numbers **(hyperplasia)** of mucus-producing cells, and increased mucus-producing cell size **(hypertrophy).** Complications of CF are common and include pneumothorax, arterial erosion and hemorrhage, and respiratory failure.

Etiology

CF is an autosomal recessive disorder in which both genes of the pair must be defective for the disease to be expressed. The CF pair of genes is located on chromosome 7 and produces a protein that regulates chloride movement across cell membranes. There is great variation in the severity of CF; however, life expectancy is always considerably reduced, with a median life expectancy of 30 years. Those people with one abnormal gene of the pair are **carriers** and do not have any symptoms of CF but can pass the abnormal gene on to their children.

Incidence/Prevalence

The disorder is most common among Caucasians, and approximately 4% are carriers. CF is very rare among African Americans or Asians. Males and females are affected equally.

COLLABORATIVE MANAGEMENT

Assessment

Usually cystic fibrosis (CF) is diagnosed in childhood. The major diagnostic test is sweat chloride analysis. The defect in chloride movement prevents absorption of sodium chloride in the sweat glands; thus more chloride than normal is present in the sweat. The quantitative test shows levels of chloride in the sweat from 60 to 200 mEq/L (mmol/L), compared with the normal value of 5 to 35 mEq/L.

NONPULMONARY MANIFESTATIONS

The adult client with CF is usually smaller and thinner than average. Other nonpulmonary manifestations include abdominal distention, gastroesophageal reflux, rectal prolapse, foul-smelling stools, and **steatorrhea** (excessive fat in stools). The client may be malnourished and have many vitamin deficiencies. As pancreatic function decreases, the client has symptoms of diabetes mellitus from loss of insulin production.

PULMONARY MANIFESTATIONS

The pulmonary problems caused by CF are progressive in nature. The respiratory tract infections are frequent or chronic with periods of exacerbations. Adult clients usually have chest congestion, limited exercise tolerance, cough, sputum production, use of accessory muscles, and decreased pulmonary function (especially forced vital capacity [FVC] and forced expiratory volume in 1 second [FEV_1]). Chest x-ray studies show persistent infiltrate and an increased anteroposterior (AP) diameter.

During an acute exacerbation or when the disease progresses to end-stage, the client has increased chest congestion, reduced activity tolerance, increased crackles, increased cough, increased sputum production (often with hemoptysis), and increased dyspnea. Fatigue increases in proportion with the dyspnea. Arterial blood gas (ABG) studies show acidosis with greatly reduced partial pressure of arterial oxygen (Pao_2), increased partial pressure of arterial carbon dioxide ($Paco_2$), increased bicarbonate levels, and low pH.

When infection is present, the client has fever, an elevated white blood cell count, and decreased arterial oxygen saturation (Sao_2). Other manifestations of infection include tachypnea, tachycardia, intercostal retractions, weight loss, and increased fatigue.

Interventions

The client with CF requires continuing daily therapy to slow the progress of the disease and enhance gas exchange. At the present time, there is no cure for CF, although gene therapy is being tried experimentally.

NONSURGICAL MANAGEMENT. The nonsurgical management of the client with CF is complex, lifelong, and changing with technical advances. Nutritional management focuses on weight maintenance, vitamin supplementation, and diabetes management. Pulmonary management is focused on preventive maintenance and management of pulmonary exacerbation.

PREVENTIVE/MAINTENANCE THERAPY. The client with CF is maintained on a regimen of chest physiotherapy, positive expiratory pressure, active cycle breathing technique, and an individualized regular exercise program. Pulmonary function tests (PFTs), especially FEV_1, are monitored regularly.

Maintenance pulmonary medications include bronchodilators, anti-inflammatory agents, mucolytics, and antibiotics. At some centers, clients with CF also may be receiving a recombinant secretory leukocyte protease inhibitor or gene therapy.

PULMONARY EXACERBATION THERAPY. Pulmonary exacerbation therapy is needed when the client with CF experiences a change in signs and symptoms from baseline. Such changes include increased chest congestion, decreased activity tolerance, increased or new-onset crackles, and at least a 10% decrease in FEV_1. Other symptoms associated with exacerbation include increased sputum production with bloody or purulent sputum, increased frequency and duration of coughing, decreased appetite, weight loss, fatigue, decreased Sao_2, and respiratory muscle retractions. Often infection is present and the client also has fever, increased lung infiltrate on x-ray examination, and an elevated white blood count.

Every attempt is made to avoid having the client with CF mechanically ventilated. Treatment focuses on airway clearance, increased oxygenation, and antibiotic therapy. Supplemental oxygen is prescribed on the basis of Sao_2 levels. The respiratory therapist initiates airway clearance techniques (ACTs) four times a day. Bronchodilator and mucolytic therapies are intensified (higher doses given more frequently than for maintenance). Steroidal anti-inflammatory agents are started or increased.

Depending on the severity of the exacerbation, a 10- to 14-day course of oral antibiotics may be prescribed. If the exacerbation is more severe, aerosolized tobramycin is prescribed. If oral/inhaled antibiotics are not effective, or if the exacerbation is very severe, IV antibiotics are ordered. At least two antipseudomonal antibiotics are used, one of which is an aminoglycoside. Other antibiotics in the regimen may include colistin and meropenem (Merrem).

SURGICAL MANAGEMENT. The surgical management of the client with CF involves lung and/or pancreatic transplantation. *These procedures do not result in cure of the disease, because the genetic defect in chloride transport and production of thick, sticky mucus remains.* Rather, the client experiences a reduction of symptoms initially and gradual progression of the disease. Transplantation offers a 10- to 20-year extension of life, depending on other factors.

Fewer lung transplants are performed in the United States compared with transplantation of other solid organs. The problem is related to the scarcity of available lungs rather than to technical difficulty. In addition, many of the people who could benefit from lung transplantation have serious problems in other organs that may make them poor candidates for extended surgical procedures.

The scarcity of transplantable lungs has resulted in development of transplant procedures for a lobe or a single lung, as well as double-lung transplantation. The type of procedure done is determined by the client's age and overall condition, the cause of the lung problem, and the life expectancy after transplantation. The most common procedure for the client with CF is a bilateral lobe transplant from a living, related donor.

PREOPERATIVE CARE. Many factors are taken into consideration before lung transplantation is undertaken. Recipient and donor criteria may vary slightly from one program to another, but some criteria are universal.

Recipient Criteria. The person who will receive the transplant, the recipient, must have severe, irreversible lung problems. It is important, however, that the client be well enough to be expected to survive the surgery. Usually clients must be younger than 55 years of age, although transplantation is considered on an individual basis. The following are exclusion criteria:

- Severe psychiatric disorders
- Tendency toward self-destruction
- Proven history of noncompliance or poor compliance with medical regimens
- Current cancer or cancer within the last 5 years
- Systemic infection
- Irreversible kidney or liver damage/disease
- Chronic, progressive right-sided heart failure
- Presence of any problem that would be made worse by immunosuppression

Donor Criteria. The following are donor criteria, regardless of whether the lung tissue is obtained from a cadaver or from a living-related donor:

- Donor is free from infection.
- Donor is free from cancer.
- Lung tissue is healthy.
- Donor is a close tissue match with the recipient.
- Donor has the same blood type as the recipient.

When the donor is living-related, the following are additional criteria:

- Donor is under 55 years of age.
- Donor has normal cardiac function.
- Donor's pulmonary function will remain sufficiently adequate after removal of the tissue.

- Donor has had no previous chest surgery on the donor side.
- Donor is psychologically stable.
- Donor has not been coerced into this situation.

Teaching. Regardless of the disease process that led to the need for lung transplantation, two particular activities are important in the preoperative period. These activities are teaching the client the expected regimen of pulmonary hygiene to be used in the immediate postoperative period and assisting the client in a pulmonary muscle strengthening/conditioning regimen.

OPERATIVE PROCEDURE. The client may or may not need to be placed on cardiopulmonary bypass, depending on the exact procedure. The client having single-lung or lobe transplantation usually does not need bypass. The client having double-lung transplantation needs cardiopulmonary bypass.

The most common incision used for lung transplantation is a transverse thoracotomy "clamshell" approach for best access, even to the more posterior structures. The diseased lung or lungs are removed. The new lobes, lung, or lungs are placed in the chest cavity with anastomoses (connections) made to the proper airways (trachea, mainstem bronchus, or secondary bronchus) and blood vessel structures. Some procedures involve wrapping a section of the omentum (from the peritoneal cavity) around the newly transplanted lung to increase oxygenation of the new tissue. In general, surgery for lung transplantation is usually completed within 4 to 6 hours.

POSTOPERATIVE CARE. The client is intubated for at least 48 hours. In addition, chest tubes and arterial lines are in place. Much of the care needed is the same as that for any thoracic surgery.

Major problem areas following lung transplantation are bleeding, infection, and transplant rejection. Bleeding is most common in those clients who had cardiopulmonary bypass, since this procedure requires anticoagulation. Usually the client remains in the intensive care unit for several days following transplantation.

Immunosuppressive drug regimens must be started in the immediate postoperative period, which increases the risk for infection. The pharmacologic agents generally used for routine long-term immunosuppressive therapy after organ transplantation are combinations of very specific immunosuppressants (cyclosporine [Sandimmune]), less specific immunosuppressants (azathioprine [Imuran] or mycophenolate mofetil [CellCept]), and one of the corticosteroids, such as prednisone (Apo-Prednisone♣, Deltasone♣) or prednisolone (Delta-Cortef). In the immediate postoperative period, however, corticosteroids are avoided in the first 10 to 14 days after surgery because of their negative impact on the healing process. (See Chapter 20 for more information on antirejection therapy.)

PRIMARY PULMONARY HYPERTENSION

OVERVIEW

Pulmonary hypertension can occur as a complication of other lung disorders. Primary or idiopathic pulmonary hypertension occurs in the absence of other lung disorders, and its cause is unknown, although autoimmunity may play a role. This disorder is rare and occurs mostly in women between the ages of 20 and 40.

The pathophysiologic process in primary pulmonary hypertension involves vasoconstriction and increasing vascular resistance of pulmonary blood vessels. Pulmonary blood pressure rises and blood flow decreases, leading to poor perfusion and hypoxemia. Eventually, the right side of the heart fails (cor pulmonale) from the continuous workload of pumping against the high pulmonary pressures. Without treatment, death usually occurs within 2 years after diagnosis. Newer treatments have extended the survival time for many clients to over 5 years.

COLLABORATIVE MANAGEMENT

Assessment

The most common symptoms are dyspnea and fatigue in an otherwise healthy adult. Some clients also experience an angina-like chest pain.

Diagnosis is made from the results of right-sided heart catheterization showing elevated pulmonary pressures. Other test results suggesting pulmonary hypertension include abnormal ventilation-perfusion scans and pulmonary function tests (PFTs) showing some reduction in functional pulmonary volumes with reduced diffusion capacity.

Interventions

Nonsurgical interventions that reduce pulmonary pressures and slow the development of cor pulmonale involve drugs that dilate pulmonary vessels and prevent clot formation. Warfarin (Coumadin) therapy is taken daily. A current experimental therapy involves continuous infusion of a prostacyclin analog, epoprostenol (Flolan), through a small IV pump. When the heart has undergone some hypertrophy and cardiac output has fallen, the client may be started on a regimen of digoxin (Lanoxin) and diuretics. Oxygen therapy is used when dyspnea is continuous or uncomfortable. These therapies do not cure the disorder; they just temporarily improve function and reduce symptoms.

Surgical management of primary pulmonary hypertension involves whole-lung transplantation. When cor pulmonale also is present, the client may need a combined heart-lung transplantation. It is not known whether the process of pulmonary vasoconstriction can begin again in the transplanted lungs or if the transplant is a "cure."

INTERSTITIAL PULMONARY DISEASES

The category of interstitial pulmonary diseases contains a wide variety of lung disorders, also called **fibrotic lung** diseases, that have some characteristics in common. All affect the interstitium of the lungs (alveoli, blood vessels, and surrounding support tissue) rather than the airways. Therefore these disorders are **restrictive** (preventing good expansion and recoil of the gas exchange unit) in nature rather than obstructive. With restrictive pulmonary disease, the lung tissues generally thicken, causing reduced gas exchange and "stiff" lungs that do not expand well. Unlike obstructive disorders, air trapping does not occur and the client does not develop a "barrel chest." Often the onset of these disorders is slow and insidious, with dyspnea as the most common symptom.

Sarcoidosis

OVERVIEW

Sarcoidosis is a multisystem granulomatous disorder of unknown cause that can affect virtually any organ; however, the lung is involved most frequently. Pulmonary sarcoidosis develops over time in a step-by-step manner. Growths called **granulomas** characterize the disease. Granulomas are composed of lymphocytes, macrophages, epithelioid cells, and giant cells.

The development of pulmonary sarcoidosis involves autoimmune responses in which the normally helpful and protective T-lymphocytes increase and initiate damaging actions against normal lung tissue. Alveolar cells are the primary targets of the damaging actions. No single cause for T-lymphocyte activation has yet been identified; however, infection and genetic predisposition appear to play a role. **Alveolitis** occurs as a result of accumulation of inflammatory immune cells in the alveoli. The presence of chronic inflammation causes **fibrosis** (scar tissue formation in the lungs). The fibrosis results in a loss of **lung compliance** (elasticity) and a loss of ability to exchange gases. **Cor pulmonale** (right-sided cardiac failure) is often present, because the heart can no longer pump effectively against the stiff, fibrotic lung.

The disease usually affects young adults, peaking between ages 20 and 30 years and again between ages 45 and 65 years. Clinical manifestations include enlarged lymph nodes in the hilar area of the lungs, lung infiltrate on x-ray examination, skin lesions, and eye lesions. The first indication of disease may be an abnormal chest x-ray finding in an otherwise healthy client. The most common symptoms include cough, dyspnea, hemoptysis, and chest discomfort. In many clients the illness resolves permanently. Others may experience progressive pulmonary fibrosis and severe systemic disease.

> **CULTURAL CONSIDERATIONS**
>
> In the United States, sarcoidosis affects African Americans 10 times more frequently than Caucasians (Cotran, Kumar, & Collins, 1999). The incidence, as in many autoimmune disorders, is higher among women than among men and is twice as common in women of childbearing age as in women of other ages.

COLLABORATIVE MANAGEMENT

Assessment

Sarcoidosis is suspected in the client who has symptoms of cough, dyspnea, and abnormal chest x-ray findings but is otherwise asymptomatic. Other conditions to rule out before diagnosing sarcoidosis are pulmonary infections and malignancies. Fiberoptic bronchoscopy may also be used in the diagnosis of this disorder (see Chapter 27).

Sarcoidosis is staged on the basis of x-ray findings. Higher stages are associated with greater damage and more widespread disease. Pulmonary function studies often show a restrictive pattern of decreased lung volumes and impaired diffusing capacity. Irreversible lung changes develop in 10% to 15% of clients. Those clients who develop severe restrictive disease may also develop secondary pulmonary hypertension.

Interventions

The goal of therapy is to lessen symptoms and prevent fibrosis. Indications for treatment vary. If the client is asymptomatic and has normal pulmonary function, no treatment is given. Indications for treatment include clinical symptoms; decreased total lung capacity (TLC), diffusing capacity, or forced vital capacity (FVC); extrapulmonary involvement; and hypercalcemia.

Corticosteroids are the cornerstone of therapy. Protocols may vary from 40 to 60 mg/day with tapering doses over 6 to 8 weeks, to a maintenance dose of 10 to 15 mg for 6 months. Further therapy may occur over 12 months. Follow-up and monitoring includes a review of symptoms, pulmonary function studies, chest x-ray studies, a complete blood count, serum creatinine, serum calcium, and urinalysis. The nurse and pharmacist teach the client and family about side effects of steroid therapy and other aspects of physical care as indicated.

Idiopathic Pulmonary Fibrosis

OVERVIEW

Idiopathic pulmonary fibrosis is a common form of interstitial pulmonary disease. The typical client is an older adult with a history of cigarette smoking or chronic exposure to inhalation irritants such as metal particles, dust, organic chemicals, and wood fires. Unlike sarcoidosis, pulmonary fibrosis is highly lethal, since most clients have progressive disease with few remission periods. Even with appropriate treatment, clients usually survive less than 5 years after diagnosis.

Pulmonary fibrosis has been described as a model of excessive wound healing. Once lung injury occurs, an inflammatory process begins to initiate tissue repair. Unfortunately, the inflammation continues beyond normal healing time and causes extensive fibrosis and scarring. These changes thicken alveolar tissues, making gas exchange difficult.

COLLABORATIVE MANAGEMENT

Assessment

The onset of disease is slow, with early symptoms of mild dyspnea on exertion. Pulmonary function studies show decreased FVC. As the fibrosis progresses, the client becomes more dyspneic and hypoxemia becomes severe. Eventually, the client requires high levels of oxygen and often is still hypoxemic. Respirations are rapid and shallow.

Interventions

The goal of therapy is to slow the progressive fibrotic process and manage symptoms. Systemic corticosteroids and other immunosuppressants are the mainstays of therapy. Immunosuppressant drugs include cytotoxic drugs such as cyclophosphamide (Cytoxan, Neosar, Procytox♣), azathioprine, chlorambucil (Leukeran), or methotrexate (Folex). These agents have many side effects and toxicities, including immunosuppression, nausea, and lung and liver damage. Early initiation of therapy is critical, even though not all clients respond to therapy. Even among those who have a response to therapy, the disease continues to progress and leads to death by respiratory failure.

Lung transplantation is a curative therapy; however, the selection criteria, cost, and availability of organs make this option unlikely for most candidates.

The client and family require support and assistance with community resources once the diagnosis is made. The health care team assists the client and family in understanding the disease process and maintaining hope for control of the fibrosis. It is important to prevent further lung insult from respiratory tract infections. The client and family are educated regarding the signs and symptoms of infection and encouraged to avoid respiratory irritants, crowds, and those with known infections.

Home oxygen is usually required by the time the client becomes symptomatic because significant fibrosis has already occurred. He or she is instructed about oxygen use as a continuous therapy. As in most severe lung disorders, fatigue is a major concern, and the nurse instructs the client and family about energy conservation measures (see Energy Conservation [Chronic Obstructive Pulmonary Disease], p. 547). Activity limitations and rest help reduce the work of breathing and oxygen consumption.

The nurse supports the client's need to be as independent as possible and yet encourages him or her to pace activities and accept assistance as needed. The disease can be economically devastating, because the client is often unable to continue work and may need home care.

In the later stages of the disease, the focus is to minimize the sensation of shortness of breath, which is often accomplished with the use of oral or parenteral morphine. The nurse provides information regarding hospice, which supports and coordinates resources to meet the needs of the client and family when the prognosis for survival is less than 6 months.

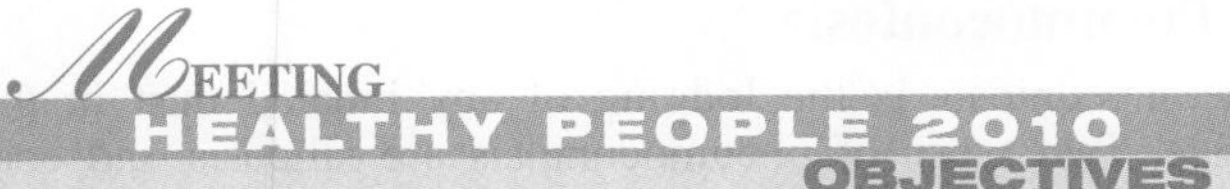

TOBACCO USE

Objective 3.1: Reduce to 13% the proportion of adults (18 and older) who use tobacco.

Teach the client who smokes cigarettes the following techniques to quit smoking:

- Make a list of the reasons you want to stop smoking (e.g., your health and the health of those around you, saving money, social reasons).
- Set a date to stop smoking and keep it. Decide whether you are going to begin to cut down on the amount you smoke or are going to stop "cold turkey." Whatever way you decide to do it, keep this important date!
- Ask for help from those around you. Find someone who wants to quit smoking and "buddy up" for support. Look for assistance in your community, such as formal smoking cessation programs, counselors, and certified acupuncture specialists or hypnotists.
- Consult your health care provider about nicotine replacement therapy (i.e., patch or gum).
- Remove ashtrays and lighters from your view.
- Talk to yourself! Remind yourself of all the reasons you want to quit.
- Think of a way to reward yourself with the money you save from not smoking for a year.
- Avoid places that might tempt you to smoke. If you are used to having a cigarette after meals, get up from the table as soon as you are finished eating. Think of new things to do at times when you used to smoke.
- Find activities that keep your hands busy: needlework, painting, gardening, even holding a pencil.
- Take five deep breaths of clean, fresh air through your nose and out your mouth if you feel the urge to smoke.
- Keep plenty of healthy, low-calorie snacks, such as fruits and vegetables, on hand to nibble on. Try sugarless gum or mints as a substitute for tobacco.
- Drink at least eight glasses of water each day.
- Begin an exercise program with the approval of your health care provider. Be aware of the positive, healthy changes in your body since you stopped smoking.
- List the many reasons why you are glad that you quit. Keep the list handy as a reminder of the positive things you are doing for yourself.
- Think of each day without tobacco as a major accomplishment. It is!

OCCUPATIONAL PULMONARY DISEASE

OVERVIEW

Exposure to occupational or environmental fumes, dust, vapors, gases, bacterial or fungal antigens, and allergens can result in a variety of obstructive and/or restrictive respiratory disorders. Depending on the degree, frequency, and intensity of exposure, and on underlying pulmonary disease, clients may experience acute reversible effects or chronic pulmonary disease. All occupational pulmonary diseases are worsened by the cofactor of cigarette smoking. Therefore smoking cessation efforts are critically important (see the Meeting Healthy People 2010 Objectives box at right).

Many occupational diseases have an onset of symptoms long after the initial exposure to the offending agent. Through skilled history taking, the nurse investigates respiratory symptoms associated with the work environment over a lifetime.

Occupational Asthma

Occupational asthma (OA) is the most common form of occupational lung disease in the United States. OA differs from other forms of asthma in that it is associated with variable airway narrowing related to an exposure in the working environment and not to stimuli outside the workplace. Symptoms may develop after several years of exposure. Exposure to virtually any industrial agent can trigger OA.

OA is divided into two types, which are differentiated by onset of symptoms and whether or not immunoglobulin E (IgE) serves as a mediator. The most common type is OA with a latency period. The disease develops after a period of exposure, which can vary from a few weeks to several years. This type of OA is associated with IgE mediation, similar to atopic asthma (discussed earlier under Pathophysiology [Asthma], p. 530).

Clients diagnosed with latency OA related to a specific allergen have a permanent impairment or disability, which is observed when performing pulmonary function testing using a bronchial provocation test to stimulate hyperresponsiveness. These clients demonstrate airflow limitation.

The second type of OA does not have a latency period and is frequently referred to as *irritant-induced asthma.* Onset of symptoms usually occurs within 24 hours of exposure. The most commonly occurring precipitating agents include chlorine, ammonia, and phosgene. Exposure to massive concentrations of the chemical can result in pulmonary edema, adult respiratory distress syndrome (ARDS), and death.

Pathologic changes associated with irritant-induced OA include sloughing of the epithelial layer, thickening of the basement membrane, and inflammation of cells of the bronchial mucosa. Symptoms often persist for 3 months but can occur for years or even permanently after the exposure. These symptoms frequently include cough, wheeze, and dyspnea. Some clients report a burning sensation in the throat and nose and chest discomfort.

Pneumoconiosis

Pneumoconiosis is the lodging of any inhaled dust in the lungs. Two types of pneumoconiosis are silicosis and coal miners' pneumoconiosis.

SILICOSIS

Silicosis is a chronic fibrosing disease of the lungs caused by long-term inhalation of free crystalline silica dust. Mining and quarrying are associated with a high incidence of silicosis. Hazardous exposure to silica dust also occurs in foundry work, tunneling, sandblasting, pottery making, stone masonry, and manufacture of glass, tile, and bricks. The finely ground silica used in soaps, polishes, and filters is especially dangerous.

In addition to progressive fibrosis, nodules form in the pulmonary parenchyma. Uncomplicated, or simple, silicosis is often entirely asymptomatic and causes only mild restriction with evidence of fibrosis on an x-ray film. Clients with chronic complicated silicosis have severe dyspnea on exertion with reduction in lung volume and massive fibrosis of the upper lobes. Malaise, anorexia, and weight loss may be present, and death from respiratory failure is common.

COAL MINERS' PNEUMOCONIOSIS

Chronic pneumoconiosis of coal miners, also known as **black lung disease,** is massive pulmonary fibrosis as a result of deposits of coal dust in the lung. The problem develops earlier in coal miners who also smoke cigarettes. Initial symptoms are similar to bronchitis, with eventual development of emphysema.

Diffuse Interstitial Fibrosis

Diffuse interstitial fibrosis caused by occupational exposure to inhalation irritants damages the lungs in a manner similar to that of other types of fibrotic lungs disorders. The most common agents to cause diffuse interstitial fibrosis are asbestos, talc dust, and beryllium. Usually exposures of at least 10 years are required for disease development. All result in a restrictive problem interfering with alveolar gas exchange. The chances of arresting the disease are best in its early stages. Clients with diffuse interstitial fibrosis of any origin are at high risk for respiratory tract infections.

ASBESTOSIS

Asbestosis is most common among asbestos miners, millers, and those employed in the building trades and shipyards. Asbestos causes a diffuse pleural thickening with diaphragmatic calcification. Calcified plaques are seen on chest x-ray examination. Malignant asbestosis includes lung cancers and malignant mesotheliomas of the pleura and peritoneum.

TALCOSIS

Talcosis occurs after years of exposure to high concentrations of talc dust. Significant exposures can occur during the manufacture of paints, ceramics, asphalt, roofing materials, cosmetics, and rubber goods.

BERYLLIOSIS

Berylliosis is a chronic granulomatous disorder of the lungs caused by inhalation of beryllium. Clients most likely to be exposed to beryllium are those involved in occupations in which metals are heated, creating fumes (e.g., welding, burning, or casting) or are machined, creating dust.

Although fibrosis is present, this disorder closely resembles sarcoidosis, and the client is more likely to have advanced irreversible disease. Genetic susceptibility appears to play a role in the development of berylliosis, because only about 2% of people heavily exposed to beryllium eventually develop the disease (Cotran, Kumar, & Collins, 1999).

Extrinsic Allergic Alveolitis

Extrinsic allergic alveolitis is a hypersensitivity pneumonitis caused by an immunologic response to inhaled organic dust or chemicals containing bacteria or fungal antigens. The immunologic response causes an inflammatory reaction that leads to the formation of granulomas. Three of the most common forms of this disease include *farmer's lung, bird fancier's lung,* and *machine operator's lung.* The degree of impairment is related to the extent of pulmonary exposure and the intensity of the inflammatory response.

➤ COLLABORATIVE MANAGEMENT

● Assessment

An occupational cause is considered for all clients with new-onset asthma or dyspnea. A thorough history regarding occupational exposure and onset of symptoms is obtained because there may or may not be a latency period between exposure and onset of symptoms. The nurse ascertains whether the symptoms are acute or chronic. The client is questioned about the use of inhalation protection and about cigarette smoking.

● Interventions

Prevention is extremely important in avoiding pulmonary disability caused by occupationally related disease. The health care professional stresses the importance of using special respirators and ensuring adequate ventilation when working in potentially harmful environments.

The client with occupational asthma with a latency period should be removed from the site of exposure, transferred to a job without exposure, and treated with medications for asthma. Nursing care is similar to the care for asthma not caused by the workplace environment. The nurse refers the client to a social worker, who provides information regarding compensation and pensions.

Nursing interventions for clients experiencing occupational pulmonary restrictive disease are the same as for those with emphysema. Hypoxemic clients require supplemental oxygen. In addition, respiratory therapies to promote sputum clearance are essential.

LUNG CANCER

OVERVIEW

Lung cancer is a leading cause of cancer-related deaths worldwide. In the United States, more deaths from lung cancer occur each year than from prostate cancer, breast cancer, and

TABLE 30-4 • DIFFERENTIAL FEATURES OF THE MAJOR TYPES OF LUNG CANCER

Approximate Incidence	Characteristics	Treatment
SMALL CELL (OAT CELL)		
20%	Centrally located tumors, rapidly growing, most malignant type High rate of metastasis via the lymph and circulatory systems with early extrathoracic involvement Associated with paraneoplastic syndromes Prognosis poor; survival usually not more than 2 yr with treatment	Combination chemotherapy is the initial treatment of choice Surgical resectability poor Palliative endobronchial laser therapy to relieve obstruction Radiation not recommended for metastatic disease
NON–SMALL CELL EPIDERMOID (SQUAMOUS CELL)		
30%	Frequently originates in a central or hilar location and at the bifurcation points of segmental bronchi In a peripheral location, cavities may form in lung tissue Strong association with cigarette smoking Slower growing, less invasive, metastasis often limited to the thorax, including regional nodes, pleura, and chest wall Commonly associated with obstructive symptoms and pneumonias; client presents with chest pain, cough, dyspnea, and hemoptysis	Surgical resectability good if stage I or stage II Chemotherapy and radiation therapy may be used to palliate symptoms
ADENOCARCINOMA		
30%-35%	Tumors are located peripherally Slow growing Hematogenous spread occurs frequently and usually early in the course of the disease High frequency of metastasis to brain; other sites include adrenals, liver, bone, and kidneys Predominant type in nonsmokers; most frequent type of lung cancer found in women Often arises in previously scarred or fibrotic lungs	Surgical resectability good if stage I or stage II Moderately good response to chemotherapy Radiation therapy used to palliate pulmonary and metastatic disease
LARGE CELL		
11%	Peripheral, subpleural lesions with necrotic surfaces or cavities Often form larger tumor masses than adenocarcinoma Slow growing Metastasis is similar to that for adenocarcinoma with addition of gastrointestinal tract Prognosis poor	Surgical resectability good if stage I or stage II Chemotherapy has limited benefit Palliative radiation therapy

colon cancer combined. The American Cancer Society predicted that 164,100 new cases of lung cancer would be diagnosed in the year 2000 and that 156,900 people with lung cancer would die (Greenlee et al., 2000). The overall 5-year survival rate for all clients with lung cancer is only 14%. This poor long-term survival rate is due to the fact that most lung cancers are diagnosed at a late stage, when metastasis is present. Only 15% of clients have small tumors and localized disease at the time of diagnosis (American Cancer Society, 2001).

In spite of many advances in cancer treatment, the prognosis for lung cancer remains poor unless the tumor can be removed completely by surgery. Treatment of lung cancer is often aimed toward relieving symptoms **(palliation)** rather than cure, because of the presence of metastasis.

A major focus for control of lung cancer is prevention. It has been estimated that 85% of lung cancers might be prevented through the elimination of cigarette smoking. The nurse plays a major role in public education to prevent the initiation of smoking.

Pathophysiology

More than 90% of all primary lung cancers arise from the bronchial epithelium. These cancers are collectively called bronchogenic carcinomas. Lung cancers can be classified according to their histologic cell type as small cell lung cancer (SCLC), epidermoid (squamous cell) cancer, adenocarcinoma, and large cell cancer. Most recently, the last three types have been referred to as non–small cell lung cancer (NSCLC). Major types of lung cancer are summarized in Table 30-4. Chapter 24 discusses the general mechanisms and processes of cancer development.

METASTASIS

Lung cancers **metastasize** (spread) by direct extension, through the blood, and by lymphatic invasion. Tumors in the bronchial tubes can grow and obstruct the bronchus partially or completely. Tumors in other areas of lung tissue can grow so large that they can cause airway obstruction by encircling

TABLE 30-5 • ENDOCRINE PARANEOPLASTIC SYNDROMES ASSOCIATED WITH LUNG CANCER

Ectopic Hormone	Manifestation
Adrenocorticotropic hormone (ACTH)	Cushing's syndrome
Antidiuretic hormone	Syndrome of inappropriate antidiuretic hormone (SIADH) • Weight gain • General edema • Dilution of serum electrolytes
Follicle-stimulating hormone (FSH)	Gynecomastia
Parathyroid hormone	Hypercalcemia
Ectopic insulin	Hypoglycemia

TABLE 30-6 • NONENDOCRINE PARANEOPLASTIC SYNDROMES ASSOCIATED WITH LUNG CANCER

Tissue/System	Manifestation
Connective tissue	Arthralgia Digital clubbing
Hematologic system	Anemia Leukocytosis Thrombocytopenia purpura Polycythemia Thrombocytosis
Neuromuscular system	Peripheral neuropathy Carcinomatous myopathy Cortical cerebellar degeneration Seizure Polymyositis Myasthenia-like syndrome
Integumentary system	Dermatomyositis Scleroderma Acanthosis nigricans
Vascular system	Thrombophlebitis Nonbacterial endocarditis
Renal system	Arterial thrombosis Nephrotic syndrome Proteinuria

the airway. Tumors in the edges of the lungs spread and can compress lung structures other than the airway, including the alveoli, nerves, blood vessels, and lymph vessels.

The patterns of metastasis depend on the type of tumor cell and the anatomic location of the tumor. Lung lymph nodes (especially mediastinal, paratracheal, and central hilar lymph nodes), as well as more distant lymph nodes, can be invaded.

Hematogenous (bloodborne) metastasis of lung cancer is due to invasion of the pulmonary blood vessels. Tumor pieces **(emboli)** spread to distant body areas. Distant sites of metastasis include the bone, liver, brain, adrenal glands, and abdominal lymph nodes.

Additional pathophysiologic manifestations, known as **paraneoplastic syndromes,** complicate certain lung cancers. The paraneoplastic syndromes are caused by various hormones, antigens, or enzymes secreted by tumor cells. SCLC is most commonly associated with paraneoplastic syndromes. Tables 30-5 and 30-6 list the endocrine and nonendocrine paraneoplastic syndromes, respectively, that may be associated with lung cancer.

TABLE 30-7 • TMN STAGE GROUPING FOR LUNG CANCER

Stage	Tumors	Nodes	Distant Metastasis
Occult carcinoma	T_X	N_0	M_0
Stage 0	T_{IS}	Carcinoma in situ	
Stage I	T_1	N_0	M_0
	T_2	N_0	M_0
Stage II	T_1	N_1	M_0
	T_2	N_1	M_0
Stage IIIa	T_3	N_0	M_0
	T_3	N_1	M_0
	T_{1-3}	N_2	M_0
Stage IIIb	Any T	N_3	M_0
	T_4	Any N	M_0
Stage IV	Any T	Any N	M_1

From Mountain, C.F., Greenberg, M.D., & Fraire, A.E. (1991). Tumor stages in non–small cell carcinoma of the lung. *Chest, 99*(5), 1258-1260.

STAGING

Lung cancer is staged to determine the size and extent of the disease. The stage of the cancer is correlated to survival rate. The staging of lung cancer is based on the TNM system (T, primary *t*umor; N, regional lymph *n*odes; M, distant *m*etastasis). Table 30-7 demonstrates the TNM system for lung cancer staging.

Higher numbers represent later stages and less chance for cure or long-term survival.

Etiology

Lung cancers have been associated with repeated exposure to inhaled substances that cause chronic tissue irritation or inflammation. Cigarette smoking is the major risk factor and is responsible for 85% of all lung cancer deaths (Parker et al., 1997). The risk for lung cancer is directly related to the total exposure to cigarette smoke as determined by the number of years of smoking, number of cigarettes smoked per day, depth of inhalation, and the tar and nicotine content of the cigarettes. Pipe and cigar smoking also increase risk. The incidence of lung cancer decreases when smoking stops, and after 15 years of smoking cessation, it approaches that of those who have never smoked. Approximately 48,000 ex-smokers, however, develop lung cancer in the United States each year.

Nonsmokers exposed to "passive" smoke (also referred to as sidestream smoke and environmental tobacco smoke) appear to have a greater risk for lung cancer than do nonsmokers who are minimally exposed to cigarette smoke. Passive smoke contains many of the carcinogens found in actively inhaled, or "mainstream," tobacco smoke.

Other risk factors for lung cancer include occupational exposure to asbestos, beryllium, chromium, coal distillates, cobalt, iron oxide, mustard gas, petroleum distillates, radiation, tar, nickel, and uranium. Atmospheric and industrial pollution that contains benzopyrenes and hydrocarbons have also been associated with an increased incidence of lung cancer.

Some hereditary conditions predispose to cancer, although they are not strongly linked to bronchogenic carcinoma. This predisposition does not seem to be related to smoking and is found in families with other tumors, acquired immunodeficiency syndrome (AIDS), or inheritable disorders of the lung.

Such predisposition supports a genetic basis for susceptibility to lung cancer development. Clients with chronic respiratory diseases are also at higher risk for lung cancer.

Incidence/Prevalence

Lung cancer is a major health problem throughout the world. Lung cancer represents 13% of new cancers in both men and women.

CULTURAL CONSIDERATIONS

Lung cancer occurs more frequently and with higher mortality in non-Caucasians. Lung cancer is the most common newly diagnosed cancer in African Americans (Greenlee et al., 2000), occurring at a rate of 73.9 per 100,000, compared with the rate of 55.9 per 100,000 in Caucasians.

WOMEN'S HEALTH CONSIDERATIONS

Demographic data have indicated that female smokers are at higher risk for lung cancer than male smokers. Possible explanations for this difference included that women have smaller lung volumes, resulting in the amount of carcinogens per cigarette smoked being spread over a smaller area, concentrating the dose. Recent studies indicate that a gene missing in some women (the glutathione S-transferase M1 gene [GSTM1]) correlates strongly with lung cancer development when women missing this gene also smoke (Tang et al., 1998). This missing gene has not been correlated with an increased risk for lung cancer among men who smoke.

Prevention

Primary prevention for lung cancer is directed at reducing the number of new and existing cases of tobacco smoking. Extensive educational strategies start with elementary school children to discourage them from beginning to smoke. Nurses are actively involved in encouraging nonsmokers not to begin to smoke, in promoting smoking cessation programs, and in establishing a smoke-free environment. For example, nurses from the Canadian Cancer Society's Industrial Education Program visit places of employment to educate workers about the dangers of smoking. Such educational strategies have also been successfully used in the United States (see the Meeting Healthy People 2010 Objectives box on p. 557). The nurse also encourages nonsmokers to avoid passive, or sidestream, smoking by avoiding environmental exposure.

Workers in industrial settings are educated about safety precautions, such as wearing specialized masks and protective clothing, to reduce occupational hazards. The nurse encourages people who are at high risk for lung cancer development to seek frequent health examinations.

COLLABORATIVE MANAGEMENT

Assessment

HISTORY

The nurse extensively questions the client about risk factors, including smoking and occupational hazards in the workplace, and warning signals (Table 30-8). The client is asked to describe how many pack of cigarettes have been smoked for how many years to determine the pack-year smoking history.

TABLE 30-8 • WARNING SIGNALS ASSOCIATED WITH LUNG CANCER

- Hoarseness
- Change in respiratory pattern
- Persistent cough or change in cough
- Blood-streaked sputum
- Rust-colored or purulent sputum
- Frank hemoptysis
- Chest pain or chest tightness
- Shoulder, arm, or chest wall pain
- Recurring episodes of pleural effusion, pneumonia, or bronchitis
- Dyspnea
- Fever associated with one or two other signs
- Wheezing
- Weight loss
- Clubbing

The nurse asks about the presence of symptoms associated with lung cancer, such as hoarseness, cough, sputum production, hemoptysis, shortness of breath, or change in endurance. Many of the symptoms of lung cancer are common and may have been present for years. The client is asked to describe any recent changes in symptoms or if position affects symptoms.

The nurse assesses for chest pain or discomfort, which can occur at any stage of tumor development. Chest pain may be localized or unilateral and can range from mild to severe. The nurse assesses for any vague sensation of fullness, tightness, or pressure in the chest, which may suggest obstruction. A piercing chest pain or pleuritic pain may accompany inspiration. Subscapular pain radiating to the arm commonly results from tumor invasion of nerve plexuses in advanced disease.

PHYSICAL ASSESSMENT/CLINICAL MANIFESTATIONS

PULMONARY

OBSERVATION. Clinical manifestations associated with lung cancer are often nonspecific and appear late in the disease process. Clinical signs and symptoms depend on the type of primary tumor. Persistent chills, fever, and cough may be related to pneumonitis or bronchitis and are associated with obstruction of the bronchi.

Sputum quantity and quality are assessed. Blood-tinged sputum may be associated with bleeding from a malignant tumor. Hemoptysis is a later finding in the course of the disease. If infection or necrosis is present, sputum may be purulent and copious.

Breathing patterns may be labored or painful. An obstructive breathing pattern may be evident as prolonged exhalation alternating with periods of shallow breathing. Rapid, shallow breathing is associated with pleuritic chest pain and an elevated diaphragm. Inspiratory efforts may be diminished in advanced disease. The nurse assesses for abnormal retractions, the use of accessory muscles, flared nares, stridor, and asymmetric diaphragmatic movement on inspiration. Dyspnea and wheezing may be present with airway obstruction. The client's level of dyspnea at rest, with activity, and in the supine position (orthopnea) is assessed.

PALPATION. On palpation of the chest wall, the nurse may find areas of tenderness or masses. Increased vibrations felt on the chest wall **(fremitus)** indicate areas of the lung in which airspaces are replaced with other material, such as tumor or fluid. Fremitus is decreased or absent when the bronchus is obstructed. The position of the trachea may be displaced from midline if a mass is present in the area.

PERCUSSION. Lung areas with masses sound dull or flat rather than hollow or resonant on chest percussion.

AUSCULTATION. Breath sounds may change as a result of the presence of a tumor. Wheezes indicate partial obstruction of airflow in passages narrowed by tumors. Decreased or absent breath sounds indicate impairment of air passages from obstruction by a tumor or replacement of lung tissue with a solid tumor or fluid. Increased loudness or sound intensity of the voice while listening to breath sounds indicates consolidation or compression of the pleural tissue by tumor. A pleural friction rub is heard when inflammation also is present.

NONPULMONARY. Many other systems can be affected by lung cancer and demonstrate changes at the time of diagnosis.

Heart sounds may be muffled by a tumor or the presence of tumor-induced cardiac tamponade. Dysrhythmias may be present as a result of hypoxemia or direct pressure of the tumor on the heart. Cyanosis of the lips and fingertips or clubbing of the fingers may be present (see Figure 30-8).

Bones become thin with tumor invasion and break easily. The client may have bone pain or experience pathologic fractures.

Late manifestations of lung cancer may include nonspecific systemic symptoms, such as fatigue, recent weight loss, anorexia, dysphagia, and nausea and vomiting. Superior vena cava syndrome may result from intrathoracic spread of the malignant tumor; this syndrome is an emergency (see Chapter 25). Lethargy and somnolence may develop, and the client may experience confusion or personality changes as a result of brain metastasis. Bowel and bladder tone or function may be affected by tumor spread to the spine and spinal cord.

PSYCHOSOCIAL ASSESSMENT

The poor prognosis for lung cancer has made it a much-feared disease. Symptoms associated with lung cancer, especially dyspnea, often add to the client's fear and anxiety. The client with a history of cigarette smoking may experience guilt and shame. The nurse conveys acceptance and interacts in a nonjudgmental way.

Few clients with lung cancer are candidates for curative therapy. Many are given palliative treatment limited to relief of symptoms. Fear of pain, abandonment, and death is common in the client with lung cancer.

DIAGNOSTIC ASSESSMENT

The diagnosis of lung cancer is made by direct examination of cancer cells. Cytologic examination of early morning sputum specimens may identify tumor cells; however, cancer cells may not be present in the sputum. With pleural effusion, fluid can be obtained for cytologic examination by thoracentesis.

Pulmonary lesions are frequently seen on chest x-ray examination; however, tomograms and computed tomography (CT) are used to identify the lesions clearly. CT scans identify and localize the extent of masses in the chest, including mediastinal and lymph node involvement. New, low-dose spiral CT scans are thought to detect lung cancers at earlier stages; however, the cost of this technique currently limits its use to diagnosis rather than screening.

Fiberoptic bronchoscopy provides direct visibility of the tracheobronchial tree. Specimens and bronchial brushings can be obtained with this technique, especially when lesions are located within or close to an airway. Needle biopsy during bronchoscopy also may be used to obtain malignant cells.

A thoracoscopy may be performed through a video-assisted thoracoscope entering the chest cavity via small incisions through the chest wall. This procedure allows direct visualization of the lung tissue. To identify metastasis in mediastinal lymph nodes, the physician may perform mediastinoscopy, inserting a scope through a small chest incision.

Other diagnostic studies may be needed to determine how widely the cancer has spread. Such tests include percutaneous needle biopsy, direct surgical biopsy, and thoracentesis with pleural biopsy. Studies (e.g., magnetic resonance imaging [MRI]; radionuclide scans of the liver, spleen, brain, and bone; and pulmonary function studies and arterial blood gas [ABG] analysis) are done to determine the overall respiratory status.

Interventions for Cure

Interventions for the client with lung cancer can be aimed at curing the disease, increasing the client's survival time, and enhancing the client's quality of life through palliation. Both nonsurgical and surgical interventions are used to achieve these aims. Some clients with lung cancer may undergo interventions for all three aims at different stages in the disease process.

NONSURGICAL MANAGEMENT

CHEMOTHERAPY. Chemotherapy is frequently the treatment of choice for lung cancers, especially small cell lung cancer (SCLC), and as adjuvant therapy in combination with surgery or in the presence of metastasis for non–small cell lung cancer (NSCLC). Table 30-9 lists common chemotherapeutic agents used in combination for treatment of lung cancer. The exact combination of drugs used may vary depending on the response of the tumor and the overall health of the client.

Serious side effects are associated with aggressive chemotherapy for lung cancer, including **alopecia** (hair loss), nausea and vomiting, open sores on mucous membranes **(mucositis),** immunosuppression, anemia, and **thrombocytopenia** (decreased numbers of platelets).

The nurse reassures clients that hair loss is temporary. Usually hair regrowth begins about 1 month after chemotherapy is completed. The client can disguise hair loss by the use of wigs, scarves, turbans, and caps.

The chemotherapy agents used for lung cancer treatment are moderately to highly **emetogenic** (inducing nausea and vomiting). Many oral and parenteral antiemetics are available. Usually one or more antiemetics are administered before and after chemotherapy. Drugs commonly used to control chemotherapy-induced nausea and vomiting are presented in Chart 25-5. Client response to antiemetic therapy is highly

TABLE 30-9 • COMMON CHEMOTHERAPEUTIC AGENTS USED IN THE TREATMENT OF LUNG CANCER

	Side Effects				
Drug	**Alopecia**	**Nausea and Vomiting**	**Bone Marrow Suppression**	**Diarrhea**	**Specific Toxic Effects**
Cisplatin (Platinol)	+	++++	+++	−	Constipation Nephrotoxic effects Ototoxic effects Hypophosphatemia
Cyclophosphamide (Cytoxan, Procytox♣)	++	++	++	+	Hemorrhagic cystitis Syndrome of inappropriate antidiuretic hormone (SIADH) Hyperpigmentation
Doxorubicin (Adriamycin)	+++	++	+++	+	Tissue vesicant Cardiotoxic effects Mucositis Hyperpigmentation
Etoposide (VP-16, VePesid)	+++	+++	++++	−	Constipation Postural hypotension
Ifosfamide (IFEX)	++	++	++	+	Hemorrhagic cystitis Cardiotoxic
Methotrexate (MTX)	+	++	+++	+	Mucositis
Mitomycin-C (Mutamycin)	+++	++	+++	+	Tissue vesicant Pulmonary injury
Procarbazine (Matulane)	+	+++	+++	+++	Postural hypotension Myalgia Arthralgia
Vinblastine (VLB, Velban)	+	+++	+	−	Tissue vesicant Pain at tumor site Jaw pain Neurotoxic effects Loss of deep tendon reflexes
Vinorelbine (Navelbine)	++	++	+++	+	Tissue vesicant Numbness in fingers and toes Mucositis Asthenia Jaw pain

+, Positive; ++, moderately positive; +++, strongly positive; −, negative.

variable, and the drug combinations must be individualized for best effect.

Frequent mouth assessment and appropriate hygiene are key in managing mucositis. The nurse stresses the importance of good, frequent oral hygiene, including tooth cleaning and mouth rinsing. Clients are instructed to use a soft-bristled toothbrush or disposable mouth sponges and to avoid using dental floss and water-pressure gum cleaners (such as a Water Pik).

Immunosuppression, which places the client at extreme risk for infection, is the major dose-limiting side effect of chemotherapy for lung cancer. Immunosuppression can be managed medically by the administration of biologic response modifiers (BRMs) to stimulate bone marrow production of immune system cells. In addition, the client and family are taught precautions to take to reduce the client's chances of developing an infection (see Chart 25-8). (See Chapter 25 for further discussion of chemotherapeutic agents and associated nursing care.)

RADIATION THERAPY. Radiation therapy can be an effective primary treatment for locally advanced, intrathoracic lung tumors. Best results are seen when radiation is used in addition to surgery or chemotherapy. In some clients radiation is performed before surgery to shrink the tumor and make resection easier.

Usually radiation therapy for lung cancer is performed daily for a 5- to 6-week period. Only the areas thought to have cancer are in the radiation path. The major immediate side effects of this treatment are skin irritation and peeling, fatigue, nausea, and taste changes. Some clients experience esophagitis during therapy. Narrowing of the esophagus can occur as a late response to radiation therapy for lung cancer.

Skin care in the radiation-treated area can be difficult. If the area has been marked with a dye to outline the areas for radiation, the client is instructed not to wash off the markings. Few treatment centers continue to use ink or dye markings, preferring instead to use small permanent tattoos. The nurse instructs clients not to use lotions or ointments on the skin of the chest unless the radiologist prescribes them. Because skin in the radiation path is more sensitive to sun damage, the nurse advises clients to avoid direct skin exposure to the sun during treatment and for at least 1 year after radiation is completed.

SURGICAL MANAGEMENT. Surgery is the treatment of choice for stage I and stage II NSCLC. Total resection of a non–small cell primary lung cancer is undertaken in hope of achieving a cure. If complete resection is not possible, the surgeon removes the bulk of the tumor. The choice of surgical procedure depends on the findings of the staging process and the

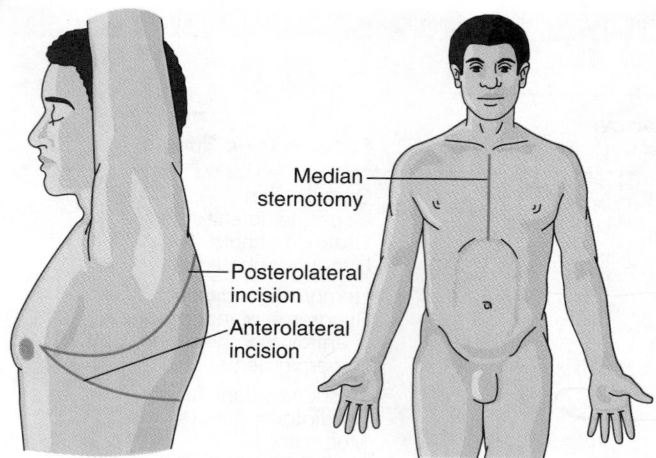

Figure 30-12 ● Common incision locations for partial or total pneumonectomy.

client's overall health and functional status. The procedure may involve only a thoracotomy with tumor removal. More frequently, thoracotomy for lung cancer involves removal of a lung segment, lobe **(lobectomy),** or entire lung **(pneumonectomy).**

PREOPERATIVE CARE. The goals of preoperative care are to relieve anxiety and promote the client's participation (see Chapter 17 for routine preoperative care). The nurse encourages the client to express fears and concerns, reinforces the surgeon's explanation of the surgical procedure, and provides education related to the postoperative course. The nurse teaches the anticipated location of the surgical incision, shoulder exercises, and about the chest tube and drainage system (except after pneumonectomy).

OPERATIVE PROCEDURES. Three types of thoracotomy incisions can be made depending on the location of the tissue to be removed: posterolateral, anterolateral, and median sternotomy (Figure 30-12). The incisions are large and are held open with retractors during surgery, contributing to postoperative discomfort.

A limited pulmonary resection is any surgical resection of the lung that does not involve a complete lobectomy. A segmental resection **(segmentectomy)** is a pulmonary resection that includes the bronchus, pulmonary artery and vein, and lung parenchyma of the involved lung segment or segments, which are divisions of lobes. A **wedge resection** is removal of the peripheral portion of small localized areas of disease.

When a pneumonectomy is performed, the mainstem bronchus is severed and sutured at its bifurcation. The pulmonary artery and veins are also ligated. The resection of a single pulmonary lobe is extended to the mainstem bronchus and is followed by a bronchial anastomosis.

POSTOPERATIVE CARE. General care of the client after thoracotomy is reviewed in the Client Care Plan on pp. 565 and 566. Postoperative management of clients who have undergone thoracotomy (except for pneumonectomy) requires closed-chest drainage to drain air and blood that may accumulate in the pleural space. A chest tube, a drain placed in the pleural space to restore intrapleural pressure, allows re-expansion of the lung (Figure 30-13). The chest tube also prevents air and fluid from returning to the chest. The drainage system consists of one or more chest tubes or drains, a collection container placed below the chest level, and a water seal to keep air from entering the chest. The drainage system may use actual bottles (Figure 30-14) or a commercially available self-contained system (Figure 30-15). The basic principles of gravity and pressure are the same with both systems.

Chest Tube Placement. The tip of the tube used to drain air is usually placed anteriorly near the lung apex (see Figure 30-13). The tube that drains liquid is placed laterally near the base of the lung. After lung resection, two tubes, anterior and posterior, are used. The puncture wounds are covered with airtight dressings.

The chest tube is connected to approximately 6 feet of tubing that leads to a collection bottle or device placed several feet below the chest. The tubing allows the client to turn and move easily. Positioning the collection device below the chest allows gravity to drain the pleural space. When two chest tubes are inserted, they are usually joined by a Y-connector near the client's body; the 6 feet of tubing are attached to the Y-connector.

Drainage System. The chest drainage system has a separate water seal mechanism that acts as a one-way valve to prevent air or liquid from moving back into the chest cavity. Earlier chest drainage consisted of one-, two-, and three-bottle systems. Technology has greatly improved these bulky glass bottle systems through the availability of one-piece disposable chest drainage devices. The Pleur-Evac system, one of the most widely distributed, uses a one-piece disposable, molded plastic unit with three chambers. This system duplicates the older three-bottle system.

The three-bottle system (see Figure 30-14) is used to explain the principles and actions of water-seal chest drainage. The three bottles are connected to one another. The tube(s) from the client are connected to the first bottle in the series of three, which serves as a collection container. The second bottle in the series serves as the water seal to prevent air from moving back up the tubing system and into the chest. The third bottle, when suction is applied, serves as a suction regulator.

Bottle One. In setting up the system, bottle one (nearest to the client) does not initially have fluid in it. The tubing from the client penetrates shallowly into the bottle, as does the tube connecting with bottle two. *It is critically important that the stopper remain tightly connected to the bottle to maintain a closed system. If the stopper loosens and the chest tube is unclamped, the negative pressure in the pleural space will pull air into the space and cause a pneumothorax.*

Bottle one collects the fluid draining from the client. This fluid is measured hourly during the first 24 hours. The fluid must never come into direct contact with either the tube draining from the client or the tube connecting this bottle to bottle two. If the tubing from the client enters the fluid, drainage stops.

Bottle Two. Bottle two serves as a water seal to prevent air from entering the client's pleural space. Air from the pleural space also enters bottle one but is immediately transported to bottle two through the connecting tube. This tube must always be under the water level in bottle two to prevent air from returning to the client. The bubbling of the water in bottle two indicates air drainage from the client and is usually seen when intrathoracic pressure is greater than atmospheric pressure,

CLIENT CARE PLAN • THE CLIENT WHO HAS HAD A THORACOTOMY FOR LUNG CANCER

NURSING DIAGNOSIS NO. 1 • Impaired Gas Exchange related to ventilation-perfusion imbalance secondary to removal of all or part of a lung and ineffective airway clearance

Expected Outcomes	Nursing Interventions	Rationale
The client is expected to have adequate lung expansion and mobilization of secretions.	Perform complete respiratory assessment every 2 hr. Assess breath sounds; rate, depth, and pattern of respirations; signs and symptoms of hypoxia, including restlessness and irritability; and position of mediastinum.	Ongoing astute assessments alert the nurse to subtle and early signs and symptoms of changes in respiratory status.
The client's blood gases and pulse oximetry are expected to be within normal range.	Monitor vital signs, pulse oximetry, and arterial blood gases as ordered. Report abnormalities to the physician.	Prompt reporting of abnormalities enable the physician to institute early treatment and prevent further complications.
	Administer oxygen therapy as ordered. D	Supplemental oxygen will help correct hypoxemia.
	Maintain patency and integrity of the chest tube and drainage system, if present.	A properly functioning chest drainage system promotes adequate drainage of blood and air that may accumulate in the pleural space, allowing reexpansion of the lung.
	Assess for and report signs and symptoms of air leak from the chest tube or hemorrhage.	Prompt reporting of abnormalities helps prevent further complications.
	Perform pain assessment and administer analgesics as ordered. (Observe for signs and symptoms of respiratory depression related to opioids.) D	Effective pain management promotes the client's participation in deep breathing and mobility, thus fostering optimal respiratory effort.
	Reposition the client every 2 hr. Check order for positioning carefully and seek clarification if necessary. (Do not place the client on the operative side after pneumonectomy.) D	Repositioning promotes lung expansion.
	Encourage the client to perform deep breathing exercises every 2 hr and to use incentive spirometry devices as soon as he or she is physically able. D	Breathing exercises promote lung expansion and help prevent atelectasis and pneumonia.
	Coach in effective coughing technique if secretions are present. Assist to high-Fowler's position with knees bent and feet flat on bed. Instruct the client to obtain maximal inspiration and to hold the breath for 2 sec; follow by having the client cough twice with the mouth open, pause, and then inhale through the nose and rest. D	Effective coughing improves airway clearance and prevents stasis of secretions.
	Assist the client in removing and properly disposing of secretions. D	Proper disposal of secretions is required for infection control purposes.
	Help the client to sit in a chair, when ordered, and monitor tolerance. D	Lung expansion is enhanced when the client is able to be out of bed.

NURSING DIAGNOSIS NO. 2 • Acute Pain related to tissue trauma as a result of surgery, inflammation of incised muscles, and presence of chest tubes

Expected Outcomes	Nursing Interventions	Rationale
The client is expected to reach an acceptable level of comfort.	Perform a complete pain assessment using designed pain level scale (i.e., 0 = no pain; 5 = severe pain).	Obtain the baseline pain assessment rating and use it for comparison with the routine pain assessment score to determine the effectiveness of pain management interventions.
	Assist with incisional splinting during deep breathing exercises, with turning, and in anticipation of cough stimulation. D	Splinting promotes the client's comfort and participation in measures that promote respiratory function.
	Secure the chest tube to prevent excessive discomfort resulting from movement of the tube. Promote optimal comfort through proper positioning, hygiene, gentle massage, and relaxation techniques. D	Nonpharmacologic nursing interventions are instrumental in helping the client to achieve optimal comfort.
	Administer analgesics as ordered. Plan activities to coincide with peak of analgesic effectiveness. Observe for signs and symptoms of respiratory depression associated with opioids. Use diversional activities as appropriate. D	The client's participation in respiratory excursion activities will be increased with effective pain management.
	Document the client's response to the pain control regimen and seek adjustment as needed.	Ongoing assessment and evaluation of the effectiveness of the pain control regimen are essential to the client's optimal comfort.

D indicates tasks that can be delegated to assistive nursing personnel.

Continued

NURSING DIAGNOSIS NO. 3 • Activity Intolerance related to restricted arm and shoulder movement

Expected Outcomes	Nursing Interventions	Rationale
The client is expected to maintain normal arm and shoulder movement and function as evidenced by the ability to perform range-of-motion exercises on the operative side.	Educate the client about the possible complication and prevention of "frozen shoulder syndrome."	The client is more likely to actively participate in preventive measures when he or she is knowledgeable about this potential postoperative complication.
	Monitor and report restricted arm and shoulder movement postoperatively. D	Ongoing assessments help detect early signs of complications.
	Perform passive range-of-motion exercises to the affected arm and shoulder 2 times every 4 hr during the first 24 hr postoperatively and then 10 times every 2 hr. D	Exercising maintains strength, facilitates mobility, and prevents fixation.
	Instruct the client in active range-of-motion exercises beginning the second day after surgery. Encourage the client to use the affected arm for activities of daily living and place frequently used items on the same side of the bed as the operative side to facilitate reaching and gentle stretching. D	Active participation by the client promotes well-being, autonomy, and independence.
	Administer analgesic as needed to promote active participation in exercises.	Effective levels of analgesia allow the client to perform prescribed exercises and prevent complications.
	Offer encouragement and support for the client's progress. D	Positive reinforcement enables the client to continue the rehabilitation process.

NURSING DIAGNOSIS NO. 4 • Disturbed Body Image related to actual change in body structure and function

Expected Outcomes	Nursing Interventions	Rationale
The client is expected to verbalize feelings about the loss of all or part of a lung and identify ways in which to compensate for altered lung capacity.	Establish a therapeutic nurse-client relationship by building trust and confidence.	Sincere behaviors that display concern and caring enable the client to feel comfortable and at ease with the nurse.
	Encourage expression of feelings and concerns related to lung cancer diagnosis, grief about loss of lung, and effects on lifestyle. D	Ventilation of feelings and concerns can serve as an effective coping strategy and help the client to express needs.
	Support a realistic hope of regaining aspects of usual activities. D	Hope is a universal coping mechanism and can enable the client to attain activity potential within the present physical limitations.
	Assist the client in identifying activities that can be performed with present lung capacity.	Identification of activities that can be performed by the client encourages independence and increased self-esteem.
	Identify measures to promote increased endurance and participation in activities (i.e., carefully schedule activities; ensure rest periods and proper nutrition).	Energy conservation and health promotion activities help the client to achieve optimal physical activity.
	Provide support for accomplishments and encourage the concept of slow progression without compromising respiratory status. D	Positive reinforcement of achievements enhances body image and self-esteem.

NURSING DIAGNOSIS NO. 5 • Knowledge Deficit related to care after hospitalization

Expected Outcomes	Nursing Interventions	Rationale
The client is expected to verbalize follow-up care and signs and symptoms to report to the primary care provider.	Review the discharge instructions with the client, including follow-up visit, medications, permitted activities, and arm and shoulder exercises.	Ensuring that the client understands required information before discharge promotes the client's participation in the treatment plan and minimizes anxiety after discharge.
	Instruct the client to report signs and symptoms of fever, cough and sputum production, increased discomfort, or dyspnea to the primary care provider (physician or nurse).	Early detection and treatment of possible respiratory infection or other respiratory complications can reduce the extent of the complication.
	Encourage the client to pace tolerable activities and rest periods. Reinforce that heavy lifting is to be avoided for 6 months and to stop any activity that provokes excessive dyspnea or discomfort.	When the client understands how to balance and limit activities, complications can be prevented.
	Review and educate the client about additional proposed treatment as indicated (chemotherapy, radiation therapy).	Education related to further treatment modalities fosters the client's understanding of and compliance with the treatment plan and can reduce anxiety and possible misconceptions.
	Refer the client to appropriate community resources, if indicated (e.g., home health agency, American Cancer Society, American Lung Association).	Community resources are an additional avenue for information and support.

D indicates tasks that can be delegated to assistive nursing personnel.

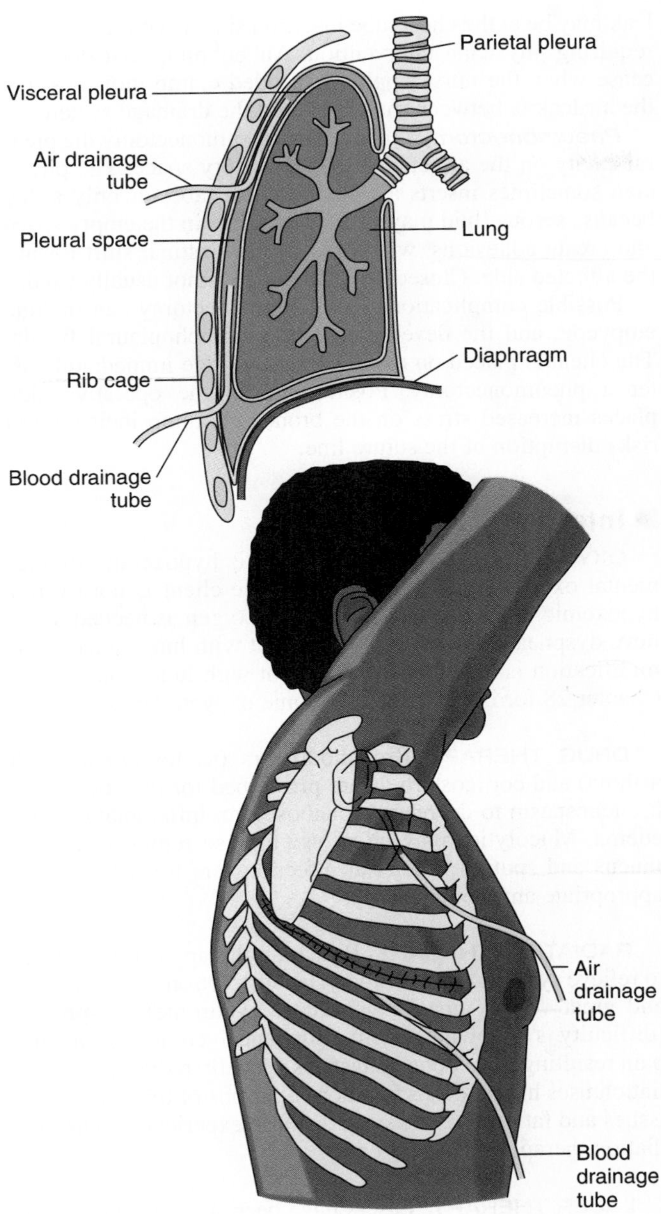

Figure 30-13 ● Chest tube placement.

such as during exhalation, coughing, or sneezing. When the air in the pleural space has been sufficiently removed, bubbling stops. Other causes of loss of bubbling include a blocked or kinked chest tube. Excessive bubbling in the second bottle may indicate an air leak. In addition, the water in the long tube of the second bottle rises and falls slightly with the client's respiratory cycle. A rise of 2 to 4 inches during inhalation and a corresponding fall during exhalation are normal. An absence of fluctuation may mean that the chest tube is obstructed, the expanded lung has blocked the eyelets of the chest tube, or no more air is leaking into the pleural space.

If the system consisted only of two bottles, drainage could occur only by gravity. In that situation the second tube in the second bottle would be open to the air to prevent a buildup of pressure sufficient to hinder air drainage.

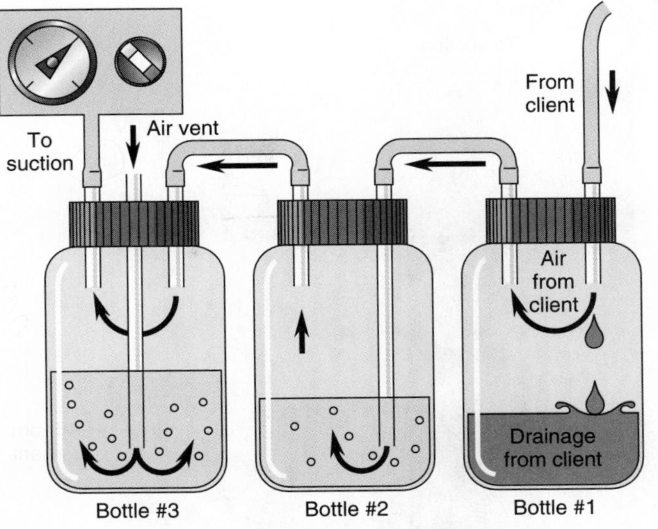

Figure 30-14 ● Three-bottle chest drainage system.

Bottle Three. The third bottle is the suction control bottle of the system. This stopper has three tubing connections: a short tube from the second bottle, a long open tube dipped into the water, and a short tube connecting to the suction unit. Suction can be added to the system on the physician's order. Suction enhances the pressure difference between the pleural space and the drainage system, causing the pressure to drop inside the system by 15 to 20 cm. Although the amount of suction generated by the suction unit can be increased, the amount of suction in the system is determined not by the suction unit but by the depth of the open tube in the water. While suction is applied, the nurse notes gentle bubbling in the chamber.

Commercial Chest Drainage Units. Chest drainage units are self-contained units that work in exactly the same way that the bulky three-bottle system does. From right to left, the system contains chambers for drainage, a water seal, and suction control (see Figure 30-15). The plastic devices reduce the risk of breakage or contamination of the drainage system and allow the client increased mobility.

The nurse routinely checks to ensure the sterility and patency of any chest drainage system. Tubing junctions are taped to prevent accidental disconnections, and an occlusive dressing is maintained at the chest tube insertion site. Sterile gauze is kept at the bedside to cover the insertion site immediately if the chest tube becomes dislodged. Padded clamps are also kept at the bedside for use if the drainage system is interrupted. The nurse positions the drainage tubing to prevent kinks and large loops of tubing, which can block drainage and prevent lung re-expansion. Vigorous stripping of the chest tube is avoided. Gentle milking of the tube, however, may prevent obstruction by moving any blood clots.

The nurse assesses the client's respiratory status and notes the amount and type of drainage. Usually the drainage in bottle one or chamber one is not emptied unless the container is so full that the fluid is in danger of coming into contact with the chest drainage tube. For the bottle system the nurse places a tape marking for volume on the side of the bottle. When volume is checked, the nurse marks the fluid level and the time on the tape. The self-contained systems have calibrations

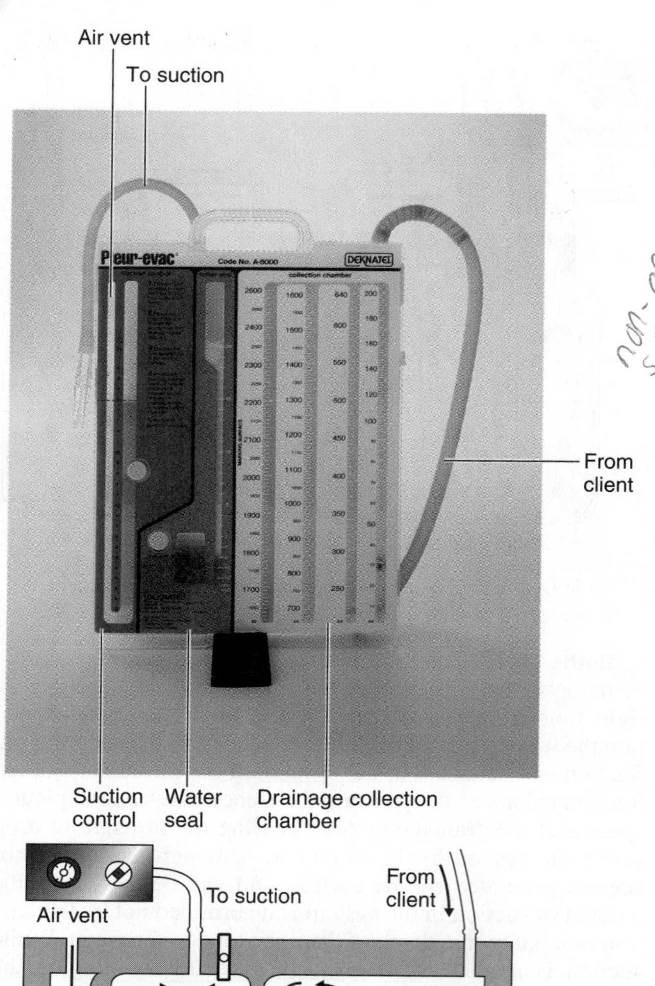

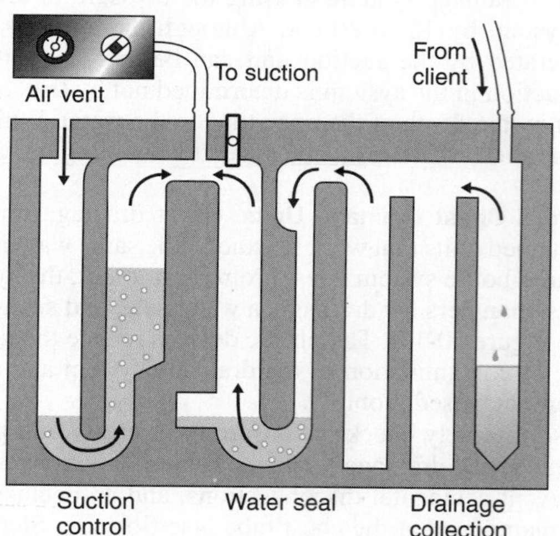

Figure 30-15 ● *Top,* The Pleur-Evac drainage system, a commercial three-bottle chest drainage device. *Bottom,* Schematic of the drainage device.

marked on the collection chamber. The amount of hourly drainage is recorded. Drainage of more than 100 mL/hr is considered excessive, and the physician is notified. After the first 24 hours, drainage is assessed at least every 8 hours.

The nurse checks the water seal chamber for unexpected bubbling created by an air leak in the system. Bubbling is normal during forceful expiration or coughing because air in the chest is being expelled. Continuous bubbling indicates an air leak that must be identified. On the physician's order, the nurse gently applies a padded clamp on the drainage tubing close to the occlusive dressing. If the bubbling stops, the air leak may be at the chest tube insertion site or within the chest, requiring physician intervention. Air bubbling that does not cease when the nurse applies a padded clamp indicates that the air leak is between the clamp and the drainage system.

Pneumonectomy Care. After pneumonectomy the pleural cavity on the affected side is an empty space. The physician sometimes inserts a clamped chest tube for only a day because serous fluid may then accumulate in the empty space and create adhesions, which reduce mediastinal shift toward the affected side. Closed-chest drainage is not usually used.

Possible complications of a pneumonectomy can include empyema and the development of a bronchopleural fistula. The client is placed on the nonoperative side immediately after a pneumonectomy. Positioning on the operative side places increased stress on the bronchial stump incision and risks disruption of the suture line.

Interventions for Palliation

OXYGEN THERAPY. If the client is hypoxemic, supplemental oxygen is provided. Even if the client is not overtly hypoxemic, the physician may order oxygen as needed to relieve dyspnea and anxiety in the client with lung cancer. Humidification is essential for the client with lung cancer. (See Chapter 28 for issues related to home oxygen therapy.)

DRUG THERAPY. Bronchodilators (as for clients with asthma) and corticosteroids are prescribed for the client with bronchospasm to decrease bronchospasm, inflammation, and edema. Mucolytics may be of use to ease removal of thick mucus and sputum. Bacterial infections are treated with the appropriate antibiotic therapy.

RADIATION THERAPY. Radiation therapy can be helpful to relieve symptoms of hemoptysis, obstruction of the bronchi and great veins (superior vena cava syndrome), **dysphagia** (difficulty swallowing) from esophageal compression, and pain resulting from bone metastasis. Usually radiation for palliation uses higher doses for shorter periods of time. Skin care issues and fatigue are the same as those experienced when radiation therapy is used for cure.

LASER THERAPY. Lasers have been used to remove endobronchial obstruction in clients with tumors that are accessible by bronchoscopy. The obstructive portion of the tumor is debulked, and the airway is reopened. Laser therapy does not produce systemic or toxic effects and is well tolerated by most clients.

THORACENTESIS AND PLEURODESIS. Malignant pleural effusions can be a problem for the client with lung cancer. The accumulation of fluid increases dyspnea, discomfort, and the risk for infection. The goal of treatment is to remove pleural fluid and prevent its reaccumulation. Fluid can be removed rapidly through the placement of a large needle or catheter into the intrapleural space and application of suction **(thoracentesis).** Fluid removal relieves immediate signs and symptoms of hypoxia; however, the fluid can rapidly reaccumulate in the pleural space.

As an alternative to repeated thoracentesis, the physician inserts a chest tube to drain the fluid and instills a **sclerosing** agent, an irritant that causes inflammation. Common scleros-

CHART 30-10

BEST PRACTICE *for* The Client Undergoing Pleurodesis

- Reinforce explanation of the pleurodesis and inform the client that medication will be provided to promote comfort before the procedure. (The physician may administer IV analgesia/sedation immediately before the procedure.)
- Ensure that the client tube is clamped after instillation of the sclerosing agent.
- Monitor vital signs and respiratory status at the completion of the procedure and then at least every 30 minutes until the effects of the IV medication have dissipated.
- Thereafter, monitor vital signs every 4 hours for 24 hours. (The client may experience a low-grade fever. Pleurodesis creates pleuritis between the visceral and parietal layers, thus preventing reaccumulation of fluid.)
- If a rotation schedule is ordered, assist the client to the correct position for appropriate time frames and provide reassurance.
- Unclamp the chest tube after completion of the rotation schedule or at the specified time ordered by the physician.
- Assess chest tube drainage and document the amount and character of the drainage.
- Perform a complete respiratory assessment every 2 hours and observe for signs and symptoms of distress, including those of pneumothorax.
- Analgesics may be administered as needed to promote the client's comfort.
- When drainage has decreased (<150 mL in 12 to 24 hours), the physician may remove the chest tube. Maintain an occlusive dressing at the insertion site for a minimum of 48 hours.

ing agents include doxycycline, thiotepa, bleomycin, minocycline, nitrogen mustard, 5-fluorouracil, and talc. The aim of thoracentesis and sclerosis is to create a **pleurodesis,** an inflammatory response that causes adherence of the pleura to the chest wall, preventing reaccumulation of effusion fluid.

The procedure can be done in a procedure room or at the bedside with the client under local anesthesia. Usually the client is also given an analgesic or sedative. Once the sclerosing agent is instilled, the chest tube is clamped to prevent drainage of the agent. Chart 30-10 reviews best practices for care of the client undergoing pleurodesis.

DYSPNEA MANAGEMENT. The client with lung cancer fatigues easily and is often most comfortable resting in a semi-Fowler's position. Dyspnea can be reduced with supplemental oxygen, use of a morphine drip, and positioning for comfort and to facilitate drainage of secretions. The severely dyspneic client may be most comfortable sitting in a lounge chair or reclining chair.

PAIN MANAGEMENT. The client with lung cancer may experience chest pain and subscapular pain radiating to the arm. With bone metastasis the client may also experience bone pain. The nurse performs a complete pain assessment with attention to onset, intensity, quality, duration, and the client's description of the pain. The goal of therapy is to help the client to be as pain free and as comfortable as possible.

The primary intervention for this type of pain is pharmacologic management with opioid medications as oral, parenteral, or transdermal preparations. Nonpharmacologic measures, such as positioning, hot or cold compresses, distractions, and guided imagery, may also be helpful. Prescribed analgesic medications are most effective when administered around the clock. Ongoing assessment and evaluation of the effectiveness of the pain control regimen is a primary nursing responsibility.

HOSPICE AND END-OF-LIFE ISSUES. For the client in the terminal phase of lung cancer, a referral to a hospice program can be beneficial. The nurse, case manager, or social worker can assist in making these arrangements. Hospice programs provide support to the terminally ill client and the family by meeting physical and psychosocial needs, adjusting the palliative care regimen as needed, making home visits, and providing volunteers for errands and respite care. (See Chapter 9 for a more complete discussion of end-of-life issues.) The American Cancer Society may also be able to provide assistance through support groups for clients and families or through the use of equipment, such as a hospital bed.

ONLINE RESOURCES

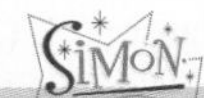

For suggested readings and Internet resources, go to http://www.wbsaunders.com/SIMON/Iggy/.

SELECTED BIBLIOGRAPHY

Asterisk indicates a classic or definitive work on this subject.

American Cancer Society. (2001). *Cancer facts and figures—2000.* Report No. 01-300M-No. 5008.01. Atlanta: Author.

*American Thoracic Society. (1995). Standards for the diagnosis and care of patients with chronic obstructive pulmonary disease. *American Journal of Respiratory and Critical Care Medicine, 152*(5), S78-S121.

Archer-Chicko, C. (2000). Continuous intravenous prostacyclin for advanced primary pulmonary hypertension. *Dimensions of Critical Care Nursing, 19*(2), 14-21.

Baldini, E.H. (1997). Palliative radiation therapy for non small cell lung cancer. *Hematology/Oncology Clinics of North America, 11*(20), 303-319.

Berg, D.T. (1997). New chemotherapy treatment options and implications for nursing care. *Oncology Nursing Forum, 24*(Suppl. 1), 5-12.

Bressler, T. (1999). Small cell lung cancer. In C. Miaskowski & P. Buchsel (Eds.), *Oncology nursing: Assessment and clinical care* (pp. 1301-1329). St. Louis: Mosby.

Brown, J., & Radke, K. (1998). Nutritional assessment, intervention, and evaluation of weight loss in patients with non–small cell lung cancer. *Oncology Nursing Forum, 25*(4), 547-553.

Centers for Disease Control and Prevention. (1998). Forecasted state-specific estimates of self-reported asthma prevalence—United States, 1998. *Morbidity and Mortality Weekly Report, 47*(47), 1022-1025.

Chain, L., et al. (1998). Promoting adherence to an electronic home spirometry research program after lung transplantation. *Applied Nursing Research, 11*(1), 36-40.

Chiocca, E., & Russo, L. (1997). Action stat: Acute asthma attack. *Nursing97, 27*(7), 43.

Corbett, N. (1998). Homecare, technology, and the management of respiratory disease. *Critical Care Clinics of North America, 10*(3), 305-313.

Cotran, R., Kumar, V., & Collins, T. (1999). *Robbins' pathologic basis of disease* (6th ed.). Philadelphia: W.B. Saunders.

Davidson, J.E., & Colt, H.G. (1997). Thoracoscopy: Nursing implications for optimal patient outcomes. *Dimensions of Critical Care Nursing, 16*(1), 20-28.

Dow, J.S., & Mest, C.G. (1997). Psychosocial interventions for patients with chronic obstructive pulmonary disease. *Home Healthcare Nurse, 15*(6), 414-420.

Dunn, N. (2001). Keeping COPD patients out of the ED. *RN, 64*(2), 33-37.

Duquette, S., LaLonde, L.C., & Traiger, G. (2000). Living-donor lobar lung transplantation: A case study. *Critical Care Nurse, 20*(1), 69-80.

Fiel, S. (1998). Aerosolized antibiotic treatment of cystic fibrosis. *RT: The Journal for Respiratory Care Practitioners, 11*(6), 79-81.

Fiocco, M., & Krasna, M.J. (1997). The management of pleural and pericardial effusions. *Hematology/Oncology Clinics of North America, 11*(20), 253-265.

Gazarian, P.K. (1997). Teaching your patient to use a metered-dose inhaler: The direct route for asthma therapy. *Nursing97, 27*(10), 52-54.

Greenlee, R., et al. (2000). Cancer statistics, 2000. *CA: A Cancer Journal for Clinicians, 50*(1), 7-33.

Imbruce, R.P., & Selevan, J. (1997). Pharmacoeconomics and the quality of life in the diagnosis and management of asthma: What is your FEEVY? *Journal of Care Management, 3*(Suppl. 3), 1-10.

Jablonski, R. (2000). Discovering asthma in the older adult. *Nurse Practitioner, 25*(3), 14, 24-25, 29-39.

Janson, S. (2000). Biologic markers of airway inflammation in asthma. *AACN Clinical Issues: Advanced Practice in Acute and Critical Care, 11*(2), 232-240.

Jones, A., & Rowe, B. (2000). Bronchopulmonary hygiene physical therapy and chronic obstructive pulmonary disease: A systematic review. *Heart and Lung, 29*(2), 125-135.

Judson, M. (2000). Clinical aspects of pulmonary sarcoidosis. *Journal of the South Carolina Medical Association, 96*(1), 9-17.

Lanuza, D., Lefaiver, C., & Farcas, G. (2000). Research on the quality of life of lung transplant candidates and recipients: An integrative review. *Heart and Lung, 29*(3), 180-195.

Lindsey, L., & Thielvoldt, D. (1999). Non–small cell lung cancer. In C. Miaskowski & P. Buchsel (Eds.), *Oncology nursing: Assessment and clinical care* (pp. 1331-1351). St. Louis: Mosby.

Mathews, P.J. (1997). Using a peak flowmeter. *Nursing97, 27*(6), 57-59.

McCarley, C. (1999). A model of chronic dyspnea. *Image: The Journal of Nursing Scholarship, 31*(3), 231-235.

McCloskey, J.C, & Bulechek, G.M. (2000). *Nursing interventions classification (NIC)* (3rd ed.). St. Louis: Mosby.

McHale, J., & Barth, M. (2000). Nursing care after pneumonectomy in patients with invasive pulmonary aspergillosis. *Critical Care Nurse, 20*(1), 37-44.

Meek, P. (2000). Influence of attention and judgment on perception of breathlessness in healthy individuals and patients with chronic obstructive pulmonary disease. *Nursing Research, 49*(1), 11-19.

Middleton, A.D. (1997). Managing asthma: It takes team work. *American Journal of Nursing, 97*(1), 39-43.

Mimnaugh, L., et al. (1999). Sensations experienced during removal of tubes in acute postoperative patients. *Applied Nursing Research, 12*(2), 78-85.

Miracle, V. (2001). Taking the wind out of asthma. *Dimensions in Critical Care Nursing, 20*(1), 2-9.

Miracle, V., & Miller, D. (1997). Lung volume reduction surgery: Making room for easier breathing. *Nursing97, 27*(6), 65-68.

Monahan, K. (1999). A joint effort to affect lives: The COPD wellness program. *Geriatric Nursing, 20*(4), 200-202.

National Institutes of Health. (1997). *Guidelines for the diagnosis and management of asthma.* Expert panel report 2(97 4051). Bethesda, MD: U.S. Department of Health and Human Services.

Nield, M. (2000). Dyspnea self-management in African-Americans with chronic lung disease. *Heart and Lung, 29*(1), 50-55.

Ochoa, L., & Richardson, G. (1999). The current status of lung transplantation: A nursing perspective. *AACN Clinical Issues: Advanced Practice in Acute and Critical Care, 10*(2), 229-239.

Parker, S., et al. (1997). Cancer statistics, 1997. *CA: A Cancer Journal for Clinicians, 47*(1), 5-27.

Phillip, M. (2000). Primary pulmonary hypertension. *MEDSURG Nursing, 9*(1), 17-20.

Ramsey, B., et al. (1999). Intermittent administration of inhaled tobramycin in patients with cystic fibrosis. *New England Journal of Medicine, 340*(1), 23-30.

Reinke, L., & Hoffman, L. (2000). Asthma education: Creating a partnership. *Heart and Lung, 29*(3), 225-236.

Sabo, J., & Nord, P. (2000). Intravenous epoprostenol: A new therapy for primary pulmonary hypertension. *Critical Care Nurse, 20*(6), 31-40.

*Sahn, S. (1996). Chemical pleurodesis for malignant effusions: What is the best agent? *Pulmonary Perspectives, 13*(1), 1-3.

Sarna, L. (1998). Effectiveness of structured nursing assessment of symptom distress in advanced lung cancer. *Oncology Nursing Forum, 25*(6), 1041-1048.

Sarna, L. (1999). Prevention: Tobacco control and cancer nursing. *Cancer Nursing, 22*(1), 21-28.

Schedel, E., & Connolly, M. (1999). Lung volume reduction surgery: New hope for emphysema patients. *Dimensions of Critical Care Nursing, 18*(1), 28-34.

Schmeltz, J., et al. (1999). Effects of position of chest drainage tube on volume drained and pressure. *American Journal of Critical Care, 8*(5), 319-323.

Schott-Baer, D., & Christensen, M. (1999). A pilot program to increase self-care of adult asthma patients. *MEDSURG Nursing, 8*(3), 178-183.

Small, S., & Lamb, M. (1999). Fatigue in chronic illness: The experience of individuals with chronic obstructive pulmonary disease and with asthma. *Journal of Advanced Nursing, 30*(2), 469-478.

Steinhauser, K. (1999). Making "cents" of asthma. *Continuing Care, 18*(6), 22, 24-29.

Stoller, J. (1997). Clinical features and natural history of severe α_1-antitrypsin deficiency. *Chest, 111*(1), 123S-128S.

Sweed, M. (1999). Shedding light on sarcoidosis. *Office Nursing, 12*(7), 22-24.

Tang, D., et al. (1998). Association between both genetic and environmental biomarkers and lung cancer: Evidence of a greater risk of lung cancer in women smokers. *Carcinogenesis, 19*(11), 1949-1953.

Tishelman, C., Degner, L., & Mueller, B. (2000). Measuring symptom distress in patients with lung cancer. *Cancer Nursing, 23*(2), 82-90.

United States Pharmacopeia Dispensing Information (USP DI): Vol. I. Drug information for the health care professional (20th ed.). (2000). Englewood, CO: Micromedix.

Weaver, T.E., Richmond, T.S., & Narsavage, G.L. (1997). An explanatory model of functional status in chronic obstructive pulmonary disease. *Nursing Research, 46*(1), 26-31.

Wilson, D. (1997). Pulmonary rehabilitation exercise program for high-risk thoracic surgical patients. *Chest Surgery Clinics of North America, 7*(4), 697-706.

Witta, K. (1997). COPD in the elderly. *ADVANCE for Nurse Practitioners, 5*(7), 18-20, 22-23, 27, 72.

CHAPTER 31

Interventions for Clients with Infectious Respiratory Problems

M. LINDA WORKMAN

Learning Objectives

After studying this chapter, you should be able to:

1. Explain the consequences of an untreated streptococcal infection of the upper respiratory tract.
2. Identify adult populations at highest risk for contracting influenza.
3. Develop a teaching plan to prevent influenza in the older adult.
4. Identify clients at risk for developing community-acquired or hospital-acquired pneumonia.
5. Compare the clinical manifestations of pneumonia in the younger client to those exhibited by the older client with pneumonia.
6. Identify adult populations at risk for tuberculosis.
7. Interpret correctly the purified protein derivative test results for an person with normal immune function and a person with human immunodeficiency virus/acquired immunodeficiency syndrome.
8. Prioritize educational needs for the client undergoing treatment at home for active tuberculosis.

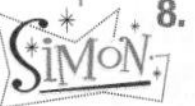

Go to http://www.wbsaunders.com/SIMON/Iggy/ for self-assessment questions related to these Learning Objectives.

Infections of the respiratory system range from minor "colds" to life-threatening pneumonias and abscesses. When a respiratory infection occurs at the same time as other respiratory problems, the client's risk for ineffective breathing and need for intervention increases.

DISORDERS OF THE NOSE AND SINUSES

Rhinitis

OVERVIEW

Rhinitis, an inflammation of the nasal mucosa, is the most common problem to affect the nose and sinuses of adults. The cause of the inflammation can be infectious (viral or bacterial) or can result from contact with allergens. Often an allergic rhinitis will make the mucous membranes more susceptible to invasion, and an infection will accompany the allergy.

Allergic rhinitis, often called "hay fever" or "allergies," is triggered by hypersensitivity reactions to airborne allergens, especially plant pollens or molds (see Chapter 23). Some acute episodes are "seasonal" in that they tend to recur at the same time each year; they coincide with the timing of a large environmental exposure and last only a few weeks. Chronic rhinitis, or perennial rhinitis, tends to occur intermittently (with no predictable seasonal pattern) or continuously with exposure to certain allergens such as dust, animal dander, wool, and foods (e.g., seafood). Rhinitis also can occur after excessive use of nose drops or sprays **(rhinitis medicamentosa)** as a rebound effect causing nasal congestion or after nasal inhalation of cocaine.

Acute viral rhinitis (**coryza,** or the common cold) is caused by any one of at least 200 viruses. It usually spreads from one person to another by droplets from sneezing or coughing and is most contagious in the first 2 to 3 days after symptoms begin to appear. The condition is self-limiting unless complicated by a bacterial infection such as otitis media, sinusitis, bronchitis, or pneumonia. Complications are most often seen in older adults or immunosuppressed people, especially if they live or work in crowded conditions or in group settings such as a long-term care facility.

COLLABORATIVE MANAGEMENT

Assessment

In both acute and chronic allergic rhinitis, the presence of the offending substance causes a release of natural biochemicals from basophils and mast cells in the nasal mucosa; this release causes changes in blood vessels. The released biochemicals include histamine, serotonin, bradykinin, and prostaglandins. When these substances bind to blood vessels they induce dilation and increase capillary permeability, causing edema and swelling of the nasal mucosa. The resulting symptoms include headache, nasal irritation, sneezing, nasal congestion, **rhinorrhea** (watery drainage from the nose), and itchy, watery eyes.

Viral or bacterial invasion of the nasal passages causes the same local tissue responses as allergic rhinitis. In addition, the client also may have more systemic manifestations, including a sore, dry throat and, at times, a low-grade fever with chills.

Interventions

Management of the client with any type of rhinitis includes symptomatic relief and client education. The health care provider prescribes appropriate drug therapy, and the nurse instructs the client as indicated.

DRUG THERAPY. Drugs, including antihistamines and decongestants, are commonly given but must be used with caution in the older adult because of side effects such as vertigo, hypertension, urinary retention, and insomnia. Antihistamines prevent the reactive biochemicals released from the mast cells and basophils from binding to sites on blood vessels and tissue receptors. Thus antihistamines prevent local edema and itching. Decongestants work by causing vasoconstriction and, subsequently, by decreasing edema. Antipyretics are administered if fever is present. Antibiotics are not usually prescribed for viral rhinitis because these agents do not kill the offending virus. Rhinitis medicamentosa is treated by decreasing or discontinuing the offending drug.

COMPLEMENTARY AND ALTERNATIVE THERAPY. Some people are able to decrease the severity of acute viral rhinitis by using complementary and alternative therapy early in the course of the problem. Agents commonly used are Echinacea, large doses of vitamin C, and oral ionic zinc preparations such as Cold-Eeze. It is not clear how these agents reduce symptom severity or duration of illness, but it is believed they may help increase nonspecific immune function.

SUPPORTIVE THERAPY. The nurse instructs the client about the importance of rest (8 to 10 hours a day) and fluid intake of at least 2000 mL/day (approximately eight glasses) unless other conditions (e.g., congestive heart failure, chronic renal failure) cannot tolerate this amount. Humidification of air helps to relieve congestion; the nurse suggests inhaling steam from a pan of boiled water after removing it from the heat. Hot shower water produces the same effect. The client is instructed to avoid people who are susceptible to infection for 2 to 3 days after symptoms begin. Thorough handwashing is another important precaution, especially after the client blows the nose or sneezes. An uncomplicated cold typically subsides within 7 to 10 days.

The client with recurrent allergic rhinitis can undergo allergy testing to determine the cause. The client may be able to avoid the offending substance to prevent further episodes or undergo desensitization for allergy relief (see Chapter 23).

Sinusitis

OVERVIEW

Sinusitis is an inflammation of the mucous membranes of one or more of the sinuses. Swelling can obstruct the flow of secretions from the sinuses, which may subsequently become infected. The disorder often accompanies or follows acute or chronic allergic rhinitis. Other conditions contributing to sinusitis include a deviated nasal septum, polyps, tumors, chronically inhaled air pollutants or cocaine, facial trauma, nasotracheal intubation, dental infection, or cystic fibrosis. In chronic sinusitis, the mucous membrane becomes permanently thickened from prolonged or repeated inflammation or infection.

The causative organism in sinus infection is usually *Streptococcus pneumoniae, Haemophilus influenzae, Diplococcus,* or *Bacteroides.* Anaerobic infections also can cause sinusitis. Sinusitis most often develops in the maxillary and frontal sinuses. Complications include cellulitis, abscess, and meningitis.

Diagnosis is made on the basis of the client's history, signs, and symptoms. Transillumination of the affected sinus is decreased. Other diagnostic tests for sinusitis include sinus x-ray studies, endoscopic examination, and computed tomography (CT) of the sinuses.

COLLABORATIVE MANAGEMENT

Assessment

The clinical manifestations of sinusitis include nasal swelling and congestion, headache, facial pressure, pain (usually made worse by movement of the head to a dependent position), tenderness on percussion over the involved area, low-grade fever, cough, and purulent or bloody nasal drainage.

Interventions

NONSURGICAL MANAGEMENT. Treatment for sinusitis includes the use of broad-spectrum antibiotics (e.g., amoxicillin), analgesics for pain and fever (e.g., acetaminophen [Tylenol, Atasol✱]), decongestants (e.g., phenylephrine [Neo-Synephrine]), steam humidification, hot and wet packs over the sinus area, and nasal saline irrigations. The nurse instructs the client to increase free water intake to more than 10 glasses of water or juice per day unless medically contraindicated. When this treatment plan is not successful, the physician orders an additional evaluation with sinus x-ray films and a CT scan. Surgical intervention may be necessary.

SURGICAL MANAGEMENT

ANTRAL IRRIGATION. **Antral irrigation,** also known as maxillary antral puncture and lavage, is an outpatient surgical procedure. With the client under local anesthesia, a large-gauge needle is inserted under the inferior turbinate of the nose and into the maxillary sinus on the affected side. Fluid or purulent material from the sinus is withdrawn. The sinus is then irrigated with saline solution, an antibiotic solution, or both.

OTHER SURGICAL PROCEDURES. If antral irrigation is not successful, other surgical procedures may be used to open the sinus cavities in clients with chronic sinusitis. In the Caldwell-Luc procedure, the surgeon makes an incision in the anterior wall of the maxillary sinus (under the upper lip). The infected mucosa in the maxillary sinus is then removed. With the nasal antral window procedure, the surgeon creates an opening in the anterior portion of the inferior turbinate to allow unobstructed drainage through the nares. After either procedure, the client may have difficulty eating for a few

CHART 31-1

BEST PRACTICE *for*
Postoperative Care for Clients with Sinus Surgery

- Place the client in the semi-Fowler's position to promote drainage and prevent swelling.
- Perform gentle oral hygiene to promote healing and prevent injury to the surgical incision.
- Use ice compresses as ordered for 24 hours.
- Change the "mustache" dressing under the nose as needed, and record the type and amount of drainage.
- Instruct the client to eat soft foods and increase fluid intake.
- Instruct the client to limit the Valsalva maneuver (no coughing, blowing the nose, or straining at stool) for at least 2 weeks postoperatively to prevent bleeding and tissue damage.

days because of pain and swelling. Chart 31-1 describes best practices for postoperative care for clients undergoing these procedures.

When the ethmoid sinuses need to be opened, the surgeon uses an external approach for better visibility and preservation of structures. The surgical incision is made along the side of the nose from the middle of the eyebrow (Weber-Ferguson incision).

ENDOSCOPIC SINUS SURGERY. Endoscopic sinus surgery has become a revolutionary method of diagnosing and treating sinus disorders. Direct inspection of the sinuses through a sinus endoscope is an improved surgical procedure for refractory sinus disorders. Completed with the client under general anesthesia in an outpatient surgical center, the procedure takes only minutes. The client goes home the same day and can return to work in 4 to 5 days. The nasal mucosa may take up to 4 to 6 weeks to heal. The nurse instructs the client in the frequent use of saline nasal sprays to prevent intranasal and sinus crusting and to promote healing.

DISORDERS OF THE ORAL PHARYNX AND TONSILS

Pharyngitis

OVERVIEW

Pharyngitis or "sore throat," is a common inflammation of the mucous membranes of the pharynx, and it accounts for more than 15 million office visits each year in the United States (Abaza, Spiegel, & Sataloff, 1999). This condition may precede acute rhinitis or sinusitis, or these conditions may occur simultaneously.

Acute pharyngitis has multiple causes (Table 31-1). The most common bacterial organism causing pharyngitis is group A beta-hemolytic *Streptococcus,* but most adult cases are caused by a virus. The incidence of streptococcal infection rises between late fall and spring, especially in colder climates.

TABLE 31-1 • CAUSES OF PHARYNGITIS

BACTERIAL CAUSES	OTHER CAUSES
• *Streptococcus*	• *Chlamydia*
• *Staphylococcus*	• *Mycoplasma pneumoniae*
• *Haemophilus influenzae*	• *Candida*
• Pneumococcus	• Physical and chemical causes
• *Corynebacterium diphtheriae*	Alcohol
• *Neisseria gonorrhoeae*	Tobacco
	Heat
VIRAL CAUSES	Irritants
• Adenovirus	Dehydration
• Rhinovirus	Trauma
• Epstein-Barr virus	
• Cytomegalovirus (CMV)	
• Influenza virus	
• Parainfluenza virus	
• Herpesvirus	
• Coxsackievirus A	
• Echovirus	

COLLABORATIVE MANAGEMENT

Assessment

The client with pharyngitis experiences soreness and dryness in the throat, pain, pain on swallowing **(odynophagia),** difficulty in swallowing **(dysphagia),** and fever. Viral and bacterial pharyngitis are often difficult to differentiate on physical assessment. When inspecting the mucous membranes of a throat infected with virus or bacteria, the nurse may note a mild to severe hyperemia (redness) with or without enlarged erythematous tonsils and with or without exudate. The client is asked about nasal discharge, which can vary from thin and watery to thick and purulent. Enlarged cervical lymph nodes may be present in either viral or bacterial pharyngitis. With a parapharyngeal (or tonsillar) abscess, the client may have a characteristic "hot potato" voice, a thickened voice of poor quality.

Clinical studies indicate that streptococcal or other bacterial infections are more often associated with enlarged erythematous tonsils, exudate, purulent nasal discharge, and cervical lymph node enlargement. Chart 31-2 compares the clinical manifestations of viral and bacterial pharyngitis. Viral pharyngitis is communicable for 2 to 3 days; symptoms usually subside within 3 to 10 days after onset. The disease is usually self-limiting.

Bacterial pharyngitis, such as group A streptococcal infection, can lead to dangerous medical complications (Table 31-2). The two most serious complications, acute glomerulonephritis (see Chapter 71) and rheumatic fever carditis (see Chapter 35), occur in 1% to 3% of cases. Acute glomerulonephritis generally occurs 7 to 10 days after the acute infection, and rheumatic fever may develop 3 to 5 weeks after an acute streptococcal infection.

Throat cultures are important in distinguishing a viral infection from a group A beta-hemolytic streptococcal infection. However, the results are not entirely accurate. False-negative cultures can occur, some of which are due to incorrect throat culture technique. In such cases the microorganisms are not uniformly distributed throughout the pharynx. To obtain a specimen, the nurse rubs a cotton swab first over the right tonsillar area, across the right arch to the uvula, and then across left arch to the left tonsillar area. The cotton swab is streaked on a blood agar plate, which is then incubated for 24 to 48 hours.

There are many types of rapid tests and screens for group A beta-hemolytic streptococcal antigen. These tests vary in specificity and sensitivity and cost about the same as a culture and sensitivity, but the results are available more quickly than

CHART 31-2

KEY FEATURES *of* Acute Viral and Bacterial Pharyngitis

Feature	Viral Pharyngitis	Bacterial Pharyngitis
Temperature	Low-grade fever or no fever	High temperature (above 101° F [38° C], and usually 102°-104° F [38.5°-40° C])*
Ear manifestations	Retracted and/or dull tympanic membrane	Retracted and/or dull tympanic membrane
Throat manifestations	Scant or no tonsillar exudate	Severe hyperemia of pharyngeal mucosa, tonsils, and uvula
	Slight erythema of pharynx and tonsils	Erythema of tonsils with yellow exudate
Neck manifestations	Possible lymphadenopathy	Anterior cervical lymphadenopathy and tenderness
Skin manifestations	No rash	Possible scarlatiniform rash Possible petechiae on chest and/or abdomen
Dysphagia, odynophagia	Present	Present
Other symptoms	No cough Rhinitis	No cough
	Mild hoarseness	Voice characterized by pain on voicing and slurred speech
	Headache	Headache Arthralgia Myalgia
Laboratory data	Complete blood count usually normal White blood cell count usually lower than 10,000/mm^3 Negative throat culture results	Complete blood count abnormal White blood cell count usually higher than 12,000/mm^3* Throat culture results positive for beta-hemolytic streptococcus
Onset	Gradual	Abrupt

*May not be present in adults over 65 years of age.

TABLE 31-2 • COMPLICATIONS OF GROUP A STREPTOCOCCAL INFECTION

- Rheumatic fever
- Acute glomerulonephritis
- Peritonsillar abscess
- Retropharyngeal abscess
- Otitis media
- Sinusitis
- Mastoiditis
- Bronchitis
- Pneumonia
- Scarlet fever

with standard cultures. Two of the most efficient tests are the Gen-Probe and the OIA (Optical Immunoassay). See the Cost of Care box on p. 575 for a discussion of cost issues related to detecting and treating pharyngitis.

A complete blood count is performed when the client's condition is severe or does not improve. The client may exhibit extremely high temperatures, lethargy, or signs and symptoms of complications. A complete blood count may indicate other causes of pharyngitis.

When obtaining a history, the nurse inquires about the client's recent contacts (within the last 10 days) with people who have been ill. Of particular importance is whether the client has recently been ill with symptoms of a cold or upper respiratory tract infection. Documenting previous streptococcal infections is essential. The nurse also documents a history of rheumatic fever, valvular heart disease, streptococcal infections, or penicillin allergy. Because diphtheria (*Corynebacterium diphtheriae*) can cause pharyngitis, the nurse asks about and documents whether the client has had a diphtheria immunization.

Interventions

Most sore throats in adults are viral and do not require antibiotic therapy. The treatment plan includes rest, increased fluid intake, humidification of the air, analgesics for pain, warm saline throat gargles, and throat lozenges containing mild anesthetics.

The management of bacterial pharyngitis involves the use of antibiotics and the same supportive care provided for viral pharyngitis. For a streptococcal infection, an oral penicillin or cephalosporin is prescribed. Erythromycin is the alternative if the client is allergic to penicillin. The nurse counsels the client on the importance of completing the entire antibiotic prescription, even if symptoms subside. If the client cannot tolerate the medication, the nurse notifies the physician so the antibiotic regimen can be changed. If compliance is a concern or the client cannot swallow pills, 1.2 million units of long-acting benzathine penicillin can be administered intramuscularly in a single dose to eradicate the organism.

The client should be re-evaluated if there is no improvement in 3 days or if symptoms are still present after the antibiotic course is completed. One cause of persistent bacterial pharyngitis is a positive human immunodeficiency virus (HIV) status with immunosuppression. Any client who fails to respond to the appropriate therapy should be considered for HIV testing (Leiner, 2000).

A rare complication of pharyngitis in adults is infection of the epiglottis and supraglottic structures **(epiglottitis).** The epiglottis is a flaplike structure that closes over the trachea during swallowing to prevent aspiration. An inflamed epiglottis can partially or completely obstruct the airway and is considered a medical emergency. The client with pharyngitis who

COST OF CARE IMPLICATIONS FOR NURSING

THE CLIENT WITH PHARYNGITIS

Cost of Care

- Most cases of pharyngitis in adults are viral rather than bacterial in origin.
- Antibiotics (especially antibacterial agents) are not effective against viral pharyngitis and contribute to the environmental development of antibiotic-resistant microorganisms.
- Viral pharyngitis can have the same clinical manifestations as bacterial (streptococcal) pharyngitis.
- Streptococcal pharyngitis may have long-term systemic complications such as renal failure and valvular heart disease.
- Standard antibiotic therapy for streptococcal pharyngitis is relatively inexpensive ($7 to $15 for a 10-day course of therapy).
- The average retail cost for a throat culture and sensitivity at a commercial laboratory ranges between $90 and $150.
- No laboratory test for streptococcal pharyngitis is 100% sensitive and 100% specific. All will have some false-positives and false-negatives.

Implications for Nursing

Although overtreating a viral pharyngitis may not have as many long-term consequences as under treating a streptococcal pharyngitis, it is not without personal and environmental risk. Nurses need to reinforce to their clients the knowledge that antibiotic therapy is not appropriate for viral pharyngitis or the common cold.

Data from DiMatteo, L. (1999). Managing streptococcal pharyngitis: A review of clinical decision-managing strategies, diagnostic evaluation, and treatment. *Journal of the American Academy of Nurse Practitioners, 11(2),* 57-62; *United States Pharmacopeia Dispensing Information (USP DI): Vol I. Drug information for the health care professional* (20th ed.). (2000). Englewood, CO: Micromedix, and Laboratory Corporation of America (personal communication), June 2000.

begins to have stridor or other symptoms of airway obstruction should be evaluated immediately by a health care provider in a setting in which intubation or a tracheostomy can be performed quickly and safely.

The nurse teaches the proper procedure for obtaining an oral temperature reading. This reading should be taken in the morning and in the evening until the infection resolves. The client is not contagious after 24 hours of antibiotic therapy. Family members or significant others who experience a sore throat should be evaluated, and a throat culture may be indicated.

Tonsillitis

OVERVIEW

Tonsillitis is an inflammation and infection of the tonsils and lymphatic tissue, which are located on each side of the oropharynx (where the palatine, or faucial, tonsils are located). The tonsils are lymphatic tissue shaped like a small almond. Each tonsil is covered by a mucous membrane and has small valleys **(crypts)** across the surface. Tonsils filter microorganisms, thus protecting the respiratory and gastrointestinal tracts.

Tonsillitis is a contagious airborne infection. Acute or chronic tonsillitis can occur in any age-group, but children are affected most often. The infection is usually more severe when it occurs in adolescents or adults.

The acute form of tonsillitis usually lasts 7 to 10 days and is usually caused by a bacterial organism. The most common organism is *Streptococcus.* Other bacterial pathogens include *Staphylococcus aureus, Haemophilus influenzae,* and *Pneumococcus.* Viruses may also cause tonsillitis. Chronic tonsillitis usually results from either an unresolved acute infection or recurrent infections.

CHART 31-3

KEY FEATURES *of* Acute Tonsillitis

- Sudden onset of a mild to severe sore throat
- Fever
- Muscle aches
- Chills
- Dysphagia, odynophagia (painful swallowing of food)
- Pain in the ears
- Headache
- Anorexia
- Malaise
- "Hot potato" voice (thickened voice of poor quality)
- Tonsils visually swollen and red with pus
- Tonsils may be covered with a white or yellow exudate
- Purulent drainage may be expressed upon pressing a tonsil
- Uvula visually edematous or inflamed
- Cervical lymph nodes usually tender and enlarged

COLLABORATIVE MANAGEMENT

Assessment

Chart 31-3 summarizes the signs and symptoms of acute tonsillitis. Diagnostic studies are performed to rule out other causes of the sore throat and fever (e.g., acute pharyngitis). A complete blood count, throat culture and sensitivity (C&S) studies, monospot test and, if respiratory symptoms are present, chest x-ray studies may be ordered for a client with suspected tonsillitis. The white blood cell count is elevated in bacterial infections. Throat C&S studies identify the causative bacterial organism and direct the choice of drug therapy.

Interventions

The health care provider orders systemic antibiotics (usually penicillin or erythromycin) for 7 to 10 days. Warm saline throat gargles, analgesics, antipyretics, and lozenges with topical anesthetic ingredients may provide symptomatic relief.

Indications for surgical intervention include recurrent acute infections or chronic infections that have not responded to antibiotic therapy, a peritonsillar abscess, and infected hypertrophy of the tonsils or adenoids that obstructs the airway. The indication for surgery becomes stronger with repeated group A beta-hemolytic streptococcal infections. In general, surgery is not indicated if the client is experiencing an acute tonsillar infection (except with an acute peritonsillar abscess) or has a blood dyscrasia such as aplastic anemia, hemophilia, or leukemia.

The most common surgical procedure to remove the tonsils is dissection and snare. The adenoids are removed with an adenoid curette or adenotome. Recently, laser tonsillectomy has been showing good success with decreased postoperative discomfort compared to standard surgery. A tonsillectomy and adenoidectomy (T&A) is usually performed with the client under general anesthesia. Postoperatively, the nurse focuses care on assessing for airway clearance, providing pain relief, and monitoring for excessive bleeding.

Peritonsillar Abscess

OVERVIEW

Peritonsillar abscess (PTA), or *quinsy,* is a complication of acute tonsillitis. The acute infection spreads from the tonsil to the surrounding peritonsillar tissue, which forms an abscess. PTA is one of the most common abscesses of the head and neck area. The common cause is group A beta-hemolytic streptococcus. Anaerobic organisms also may be the cause.

COLLABORATIVE MANAGEMENT

Signs of infection are pronounced at the physical examination. Pus forms behind the tonsil and causes a marked asymmetric swelling and deviation of the uvula. The client may experience drooling, severe throat pain that may radiate to the ear, a voice change, and difficulty swallowing because of the swelling. He or she may also have a tonic contraction of the muscles of chewing **(trismus)** and complain of breathing difficulties.

The nurse instructs about comfort measures (e.g., warm saline gargles or irrigations, ice collar, analgesics) and the importance of completing the antibiotic regimen. The client should improve in 24 to 48 hours. Outpatient management using percutaneous needle aspiration and antibiotic therapy may be needed. Hospitalization is required when the airway is in jeopardy or when the infection does not respond to antibiotic therapy. **Incision and drainage (I&D)** of the abscess and additional antibiotic therapy may be indicated. A tonsillectomy may be performed to prevent recurrence.

DISORDERS OF THE LARYNX AND LUNGS

Laryngitis

OVERVIEW

Laryngitis is an inflammation of the mucous membranes lining the larynx and may or may not include edema of the vocal cords. It is commonly associated with upper respiratory tract infections, and it can be a solitary problem or a symptom of a related disease process. Causes include exposure to irritating inhalants and pollutants (chemical agents, tobacco, alcohol, and smoke), overuse of the voice, inhalation of volatile gases (e.g., glue, paint thinner, and butane), or intubation.

COLLABORATIVE MANAGEMENT

The nurse assesses the client for acute hoarseness, dry cough, and dysphagia. Complete but temporary voice loss **(aphonia)** also may occur. A laryngeal examination is performed to assist in the diagnosis. A laryngeal mirror is used to examine the larynx and to differentiate inflammation, polyps, edema, or tumor. The physician may order an x-ray study, computed tomography (CT) scan, or fiberoptic laryngoscopic examination. Most clients are referred to an ear, nose, and throat (ENT) specialist for any suspected disorder other than acute laryngitis.

Nursing management is aimed toward symptom relief and prevention. Treatment consists of voice rest, steam inhalations, increased fluid intake, and topical throat lozenges. The physician may order antibiotic therapy and bronchodilators when sinusitis, bronchitis, or a bacterial upper respiratory tract infection is also present. The nurse informs the client and family about immediate acute care therapies, infection prevention, and the avoidance of alcohol, tobacco, and pollutants.

Preventive therapy is aimed toward increasing the client's and family's awareness of the hazards of tobacco and alcohol use. The nurse also emphasizes the activities that place an added strain on the larynx, such as singing, cheering, public speaking, heavy lifting, and whispering. Speech therapy is often the treatment of choice for vocal cord injuries and should be implemented for any voice disorder. For recurrent bouts of laryngitis, further medical and speech therapy evaluation are necessary.

Influenza

OVERVIEW

Influenza, or the "flu," is a highly contagious, acute viral respiratory infection that can occur in adults of all ages. Epidemics are common and lead to complications of pneumonia or death, especially in older adults or debilitated or immunocompromised clients. Hospitalization may be required. Influenza may be caused by one of several viruses, which are usually referred to as A, B, and C.

The client with influenza usually has a severe headache, muscle aches, fever, chills, fatigue, weakness, and anorexia. Clinical manifestations associated with the respiratory system, such as a sore throat, cough, and rhinorrhea (watery discharge from the nose), generally follow the initial symptoms for a week or more. Most clients continue to experience general malaise for 1 to 2 weeks after the acute episode has resolved.

COLLABORATIVE MANAGEMENT

Traditional antibiotic therapy is ineffective against viral infections. Antiviral agents may be effective for the prevention and treatment of some types of influenza. Amantadine (Symmetrel) and rimantadine (Flumadine) have been effective in the prevention and treatment of influenza A. Ribavirin (Virazole) has been used for severe influenza B. Newer antivirals include zanamivir (Relenza), which is administered as a nasal spray, and oseltamivir (Tamiflu), which is taken orally. Both of these antivirals inhibit the enzyme neuraminidase and are effective in shortening the duration of influenza if taken within 24 to 48 hours after the onset of symptoms. Both agents are approved for preventive use.

The nurse recommends that the client remain in bed for several days and drink large amounts of fluids unless contraindicated by some other physical condition such as chronic renal failure or congestive heart failure. Saline gargles may ease sore throat pain. Antihistamines may be ordered to reduce the rhinorrhea. Other supportive and comfort measures are the same as those for acute rhinitis.

During the past two decades vaccinations for the prevention of influenza have been developed and widely administered. With advanced refinement of the vaccine, allergic reaction is rare. The vaccine is altered every year on the basis of specific viral strains that are likely to pose a problem during the influenza season (i.e., late fall and winter). It is highly recommended that persons older than 50 years of age, those with chronic illness or immune compromise, those living in institutions, and health care personnel providing direct care to clients receive the vaccine each year, typically during October or November (Centers for Disease Control and Prevention [CDC], 2000).

Pneumonia

OVERVIEW

Pneumonia is an inflammatory process that results in edema of lung tissue and movement of fluid into the alveoli, causing hypoxemia. It can be caused by infectious or noninfectious irritating agents, such as inhaled fumes or aspirated food or fluids. Pneumonias are classified as **community acquired** or **hospital acquired (nosocomial).** In the past, antibiotics could reduce the mortality from pneumonia. However, the recent emergence of new or resistant organisms has made pneumonia a more serious problem.

Pathophysiology

The inflammation in pneumonia occurs in the interstitial spaces, the alveoli, and often the bronchioles. The process begins when pathogens successfully penetrate the airway mucus and multiply in the alveolar spaces. To do this, they must survive the lung's many defenses against microbial invasion. Fluid and exudate forms as the organisms multiply, and other evidence of inflammation becomes apparent. White blood cells migrate into the alveoli and cause thickening of the alveolar wall. Red blood cells and fibrin move into the alveoli. Fluid fills the alveoli, which protects the organisms from phagocytosis and facilitates the movement of organisms to other alveoli. As a result, the infection spreads. If the invading organisms obtain access to the bloodstream, **septicemia** results; if the infection extends into the pleural cavity, **empyema** results.

The fibrin and edema of inflammation stiffen the lung, causing decreased lung compliance and a decline in the vital capacity (VC) of the lung. Decreased production of surfactant further reduces compliance and leads to **atelectasis** (alveolar collapse). Some of the venous blood coming into the lungs passes through the underventilated area. This unoxygenated blood then travels to the left side of the heart. As a result, arterial oxygen tension falls, causing **hypoxemia** (insufficient oxygen in the blood).

Systemically, fever results from the infection. The client may develop shaking chills. Hypoxemia and an increase in metabolic demand cause tachypnea with tachycardia. Blood pressure may fall as a result of peripheral vasodilation and dehydration. Cardiac function may be compromised by hypoxemia and enhanced metabolism. Congestive heart failure or shock may result, and cardiac irritability may be enhanced because of inadequate tissue oxygenation, thus causing dysrhythmias.

Pneumonia may occur as either lobar pneumonia, with **consolidation** (solidification, lack of air spaces) in a segment or an entire lobe of the lung, or as bronchopneumonia, with diffusely scattered patches around the bronchi. The extent of lung involvement after microbial invasion depends on the defenses of the host. Bacteria can multiply quickly in a person whose immune system is compromised. Tissue necrosis results when multiplying organisms form an abscess that perforates the bronchial wall.

Etiology

In general, individuals develop pneumonia when their defense mechanisms are unable to combat the virulence of the invading organisms. Organisms from the environment, invasive devices, equipment and supplies, staff, or other people can invade the body. Risk factors are listed in Table 31-3. Pneumonia can be caused by bacteria, viruses, mycoplasmas, fungi, rickettsiae, protozoa, or helminths (worms) (Table 31-4). Noninfectious causes of pneumonia include inhalation of toxic gases, chemicals, or smoke or the aspiration of water, food, fluid, and vomitus.

Prevention is aimed at immunizing against the causative agent when possible and reducing the other risks for infection or exposure.

There are different types of the pneumoniae organism, the most common being 6B, 23F, 14, 9V, 19A, and 19F. All of these types are included in the 23-valent pneumococcal vaccine that has been available since 1983. Client education is an important factor in the prevention of pneumonia (Chart 31-4), as is making the vaccines readily available to those most at risk.

The nurse follows strict handwashing and aseptic techniques to avoid the spread of organisms. Respiratory therapy equipment is well maintained and is decontaminated or

TABLE 31-3 • RISK FACTORS ASSOCIATED WITH PNEUMONIA

COMMUNITY-ACQUIRED PNEUMONIAS
- Older adult
- No history of pneumococcal vaccination
- No history of having received the influenza vaccine in the previous year
- Chronic or other coexisting condition
- Recent history of or exposure to viral or influenza infections
- History of tobacco or alcohol use

NOSOCOMIAL PNEUMONIAS
- Older adult
- Chronic lung disease
- Gram-negative colonization of the oropharynx and stomach
- Altered level of consciousness
- Aspiration
- Endotracheal, tracheostomy, or nasogastric tube
- Poor nutritional status
- Immunocompromised status (from disease, medications)
- Medications that increase gastric pH (H_2 blockers, antacids) or alkaline tube feedings
- Mechanical ventilation

TABLE 31-4 • COMMON ORGANISMS CAUSING PNEUMONIA*

COMMUNITY-ACQUIRED PNEUMONIAS
- *Streptococcus pneumoniae* (Gram positive)
- *Staphylococcus aureus* (Gram positive)
- *Haemophilus influenzae* (Gram negative)
- *Legionella pneumophila* (Gram negative)
- *Mycoplasma pneumoniae* (smallest free-living organism)
- *Chlamydia pneumoniae* (parasite)

NOSOCOMIAL PNEUMONIAS
- *Staphylococcus aureus* (Gram positive)
- *Pseudomonas aeruginosa* (Gram negative)
- *Enterobacter* (Gram negative)
- *Klebsiella* (Gram negative)
- *Haemophilus influenzae* (Gram negative)
- *Acinetobacter* (Gram negative)
- *Candida albicans* (fungus)

*Because of various factors influencing the incidence of the pathogenic causes of pneumonia, these organisms are listed loosely in order of incidence.

CHART 31-4

CLIENT EDUCATION GUIDE
Preventing Pneumonia

- Know whether you are at risk for pneumonia.
- Have the annual influenza vaccine after discussing appropriate timing of the vaccination with your primary health care provider.
- Discuss the pneumococcal vaccine with your primary health care provider, and have the vaccination as recommended.
- Avoid crowded public areas during flu and holiday seasons.
- Cough, turn, move about, and perform deep-breathing exercises as directed by your nurse or other health care professional.
- If you are using respiration equipment at home, clean the equipment as you have been taught.
- Avoid indoor pollutants, such as dust, secondhand (passive) smoke, and aerosols.
- If you don't smoke, don't start.
- If you smoke, seek professional help on how to stop (or at least decrease) your habit.
- Be sure to get enough rest and sleep on a daily basis.
- Eat a healthy, balanced diet and take in a sufficient amount of nonalcoholic fluids each day.

changed as recommended. Sterile water rather than tap water is used in gastrointestinal tubes, and aspiration precautions are initiated as indicated. Specific interventions to prevent aspiration are discussed in Chapters 28 and 29.

CULTURAL CONSIDERATIONS

Differences in vaccination rates among different races may contribute to a greater morbidity and mortality from respiratory infections. Among adults older than 64 years of age, the highest levels of vaccination were found in women and Caucasians (CDC, 1997a).

Incidence/Prevalence

In the United States, 2 to 4 million cases of pneumonia occur each year. Among adults, the highest incidence occurs in older adults, nursing home residents, hospitalized clients, and those being mechanically ventilated (CDC, 2000). During late fall and winter, a higher incidence of community-acquired pneumonia is likely because it often follows viral or influenza infection. Community-acquired pneumonia, although more responsive to antibiotic therapy, is more common than hospital-acquired pneumonia and is the sixth leading cause of death in the United States (Vergis et al., 2000). Hospital-acquired pneumonia is a common nosocomial infection. Nosocomial pneumonia has a 20% to 50% mortality; the highest incidence is in those with *Pseudomonas aeruginosa, Acinetobacter,* other "high-risk" organisms, or secondary bacteremia. Mortality also is higher in clients who experience complications (Table 31-5).

CONSIDERATIONS FOR OLDER ADULTS

Pneumonia and influenza constitute the third leading cause of death for clients older than 85 years of age. Between 1979 and 1998, the death rate increased by one third for clients older than 64 years of age (CDC, 2000).

TABLE 31-5 • COMMON COMPLICATIONS OF PNEUMONIA

Complication	Description
Hypoxemia	Arterial oxygen <80 mm Hg
Ventilatory failure	Lungs unable to move gas in and out of lungs mechanically, resulting in hypoxemia and hypercapnia
Atelectasis	Collapse of the affected alveoli and associated lobes of the lungs
Pleural effusion	Collection of fluid in the pleural space (usually sterile fluid that resolves)
Pleurisy	Pain caused by friction between layers of pleura

SIMON Activity Link

➤ COLLABORATIVE MANAGEMENT

The concept map on p. 579 addresses assessment and nursing care issues related to clients who have pneumonia.

Assessment

HISTORY

In preparing to obtain a history from the client who may have pneumonia, the nurse considers risk factors consistent with infection (see Table 31-3). Information may be obtained from a family member or significant other if the client is too dyspneic.

The nurse documents data regarding age; living, work, or school environment; diet, exercise, and sleep routines; swallowing problems; nasogastrointestional tube; tobacco and alcohol use; past and current use of medications; and history of drug addiction or intravenous (IV) drug use. The client is asked about past illnesses, particularly those with a respiratory origin, and whether the client has been exposed to influenza or pneumonia or has experienced a recent viral episode. In addition, the nurse notes a history of any rashes, insect bites, or exposure to animals.

If the client has chronic respiratory problems, the nurse asks whether respiratory equipment is used in the home. It is essential to determine whether the client's housecleaning is adequate to prevent infection. The client is asked about inoculations with influenza or pneumococcal vaccine.

PHYSICAL ASSESSMENT/CLINICAL MANIFESTATIONS

The nurse first observes the general appearance of the client, who may present with flushed cheeks, bright eyes, and an anxious expression. He or she may have chest or pleuritic pain or discomfort, myalgia, headache, chills, fever, cough, tachycardia, dyspnea, tachypnea, and sputum production. Severe chest muscle weakness also may be present from sustained coughing.

The client's breathing pattern, position, and use of accessory muscles are observed. The acutely compromised client is uncomfortable in a lying position and sits upright, balancing with the hands. The nurse assesses the client's cough and the amount, color, consistency, and odor of sputum produced for diagnostic clues about the offending pathogen.

Crackles are heard on auscultation when there is fluid in interstitial and alveolar areas. Wheezing may be heard as a result of inflammation and exudate in the airways. Bronchial breath sounds are heard over areas of density or consolida-

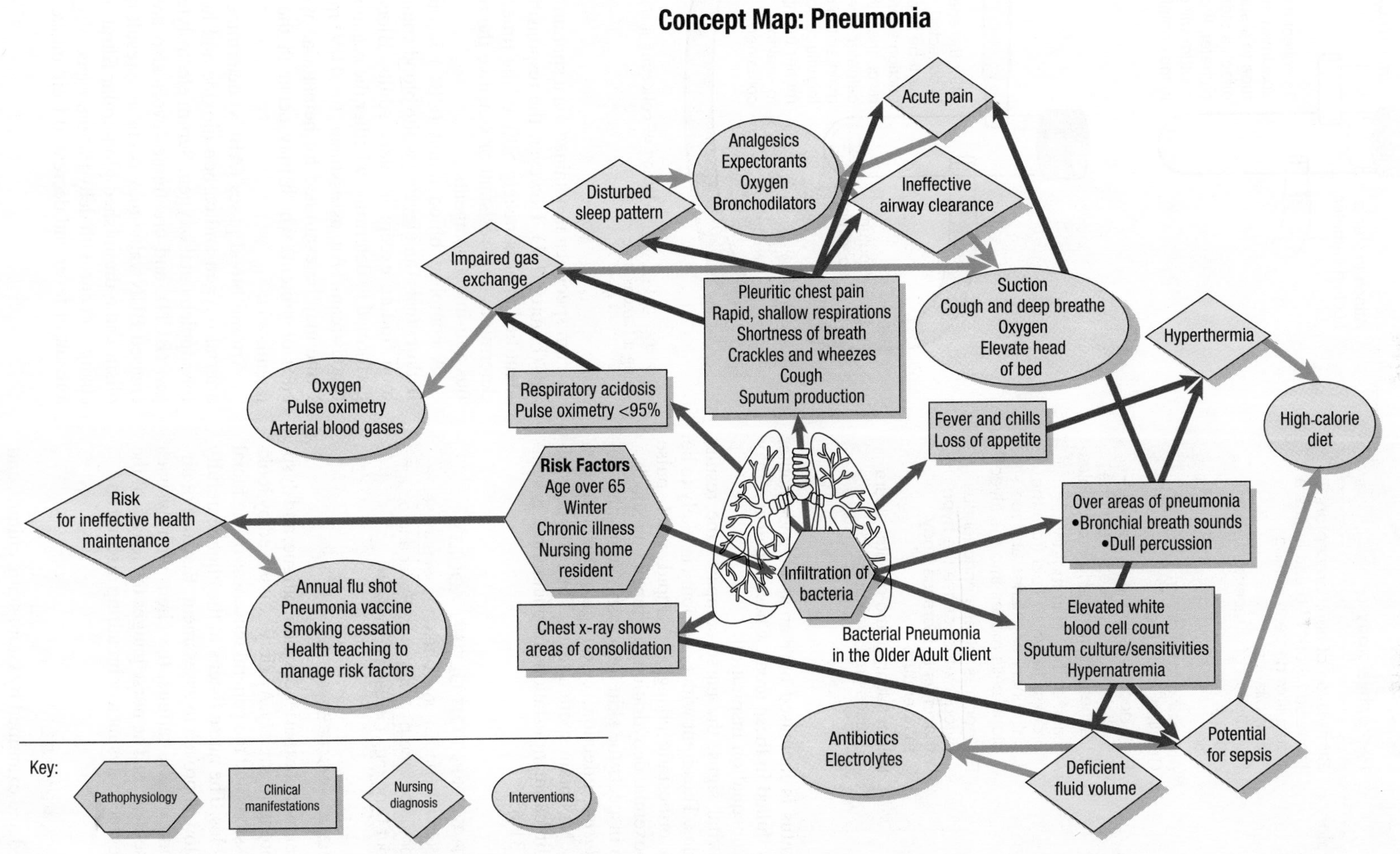
Concept Map: Pneumonia
Acute pain
Analgesics
Expectorants
Oxygen
Bronchodilators
Ineffective
airway clearance
Disturbed
sleep pattern
Impaired gas
exchange
Pleuritic chest pain
Rapid, shallow respirations
Shortness of breath
Crackles and wheezes
Cough
Sputum production
Suction
Cough and deep breathe
Oxygen
Elevate head
of bed
Hyperthermia
High-calorie
diet
Oxygen
Pulse oximetry
Arterial blood gases
Respiratory acidosis
Pulse oximetry <95%
Fever and chills
Loss of appetite
Risk Factors
Age over 65
Winter
Chronic illness
Nursing home
resident
Risk
for ineffective health
maintenance
Over areas of pneumonia
•Bronchial breath sounds
•Dull percussion
Infiltration of
bacteria
Annual flu shot
Pneumonia vaccine
Smoking cessation
Health teaching to
manage risk factors
Chest x-ray shows
areas of consolidation
Bacterial Pneumonia
in the Older Adult Client
Elevated white
blood cell count
Sputum culture/sensitivities
Hypernatremia
Antibiotics
Electrolytes
Potential
for sepsis
Deficient
fluid volume
Key:
Pathophysiology
Clinical
manifestations
Nursing
diagnosis
Interventions

TABLE 31-6 • PATHOPHYSIOLOGY OF SELECTED CLINICAL MANIFESTATIONS OF PNEUMONIA

Clinical Manifestation	Pathophysiology
Increased respiratory rate/dyspnea	Stimulation of chemoreceptors Increased work of breathing as a result of decreased lung compliance Stimulation of J receptors Anxiety Pain
Hypoxemia	Alveolar consolidation Capillary shunting
Cough	Fluid accumulation in the subepithelial mechanoreceptors in the trachea, bronchi, and bronchioles
Purulent, blood-tinged, or rust-colored sputum	A result of the inflammatory process in which fluid from the pulmonary capillaries and red blood cells moves into the alveoli
Fever	Phagocytes release endogenous pyrogens that cause the hypothalamus to increase body temperature
Pleuritic chest discomfort	Inflammation of the parietal pleura causes pain on inspiration

tion. Tactile fremitus is increased over areas of pneumonia, and percussion is dulled in these areas. Chest expansion may be diminished or unequal on inspiration.

In evaluating vital signs, the nurse compares the results with baseline values. The client with pneumonia is likely to be hypotensive with orthostatic changes. A rapid, weak pulse may indicate hypoxemia, dehydration, or impending shock.

The nurse also inspects the skin for a rash, which may occur with *Mycoplasma* infection, cytomegalovirus infection (CMV), or Rocky Mountain spotted fever. The pathophysiology of selected clinical manifestations of pneumonia is summarized in Table 31-6.

CONSIDERATIONS FOR OLDER ADULTS

The older adult with pneumonia often has weakness, fatigue, lethargy, confusion, and poor appetite. Fever and cough may be absent, but hypoxemia is usually present.

PSYCHOSOCIAL ASSESSMENT

The client with pneumonia experiences pain, fatigue, and dyspnea, all of which promote anxiety. Anxiety is assessed by looking at facial expressions and the general tenseness of the facial and shoulder muscles. The nurse listens to the client carefully and uses a calm, slow approach to assessment. Because of airway obstruction and muscle fatigue, the client with dyspnea speaks in broken sentences. The nurse gauges the length of the interview on the degree of dyspnea or breathing discomfort.

LABORATORY ASSESSMENT

Sputum is obtained and examined by Gram stain, culture, and sensitivity testing. A sputum sample is easily obtained from a client who can cough into a specimen container. Extremely ill clients may require nasotracheal suctioning or suctioning via a tracheostomy or endotracheal tube. In these situations, a sputum specimen is obtained via a sputum trap while suctioning (Figure 31-1). However, the responsible organism is not identified approximately 50% of the time. Sensitivity testing determines how resistant or sensitive the organism is to various anti-infective agents.

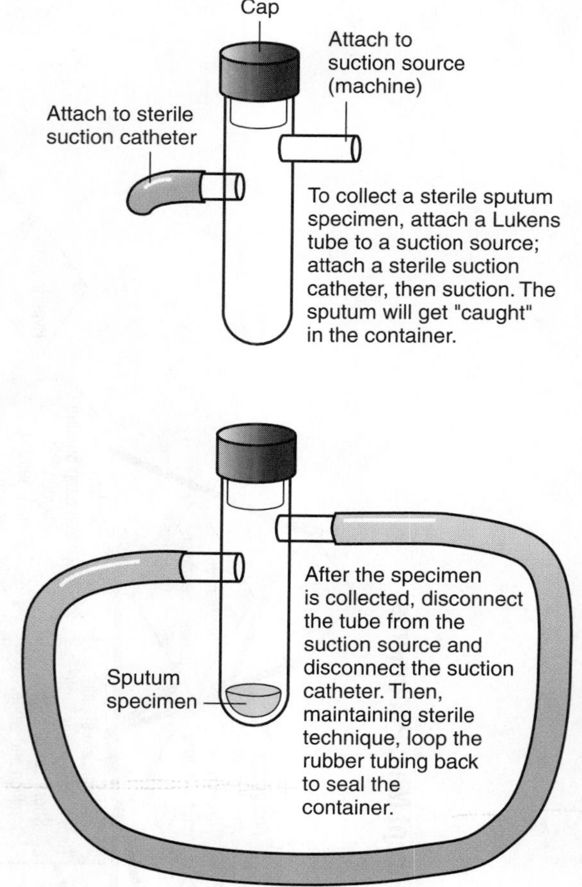

Figure 31-1 • Method of collecting a sterile sputum specimen using a Lukens tube.

A complete blood count (CBC) is obtained to identify **leukocytosis** (an elevated white blood count), which is a common finding except in older adults. Blood cultures may be performed to determine whether the organism has invaded the bloodstream. An assessment for HIV may be performed. Urine may be examined for hematuria, pyuria, and the presence of protein, which may occur in the septic client with pneumonia.

Arterial blood gases (ABGs) determine baseline levels of arterial oxygen and carbon dioxide and help identify a need for supplemental oxygen. Serum electrolyte, blood urea nitrogen (BUN), and creatinine levels also are assessed. An increased BUN value may occur as a result of increased catabolism and a diminished glomerular filtration rate. Electrolyte changes occur with dehydration, especially hypernatremia, as a result of fever and decreased fluid intake.

RADIOGRAPHIC ASSESSMENT

In general, pneumonia appears on chest x-ray films as an area of increased density. It may involve a lung segment, a lobe, one lung, or both lungs. In the older adult, the chest x-ray film is essential for early diagnosis of pneumonia because symptoms are often vague.

OTHER DIAGNOSTIC ASSESSMENT

The nurse uses pulse oximetry to assess for hypoxemia. The physician may order invasive tests such as transtracheal aspiration, bronchoscopy, or direct needle aspiration of the lung to obtain lower airway specimens in selected clients. Thoracentesis is most often used in clients who have an accompanying pleural effusion.

CRITICAL THINKING CHALLENGE

The client, a 93-year-old woman, is brought to the urgent care center by her son, who tells you he found his mother confused and on lying the floor of the bathroom. He also tells you that his father is hospitalized for pain control for advanced prostate cancer and that his mother has been spending long hours at her husband's bedside. The client's vital signs are as follows: temperature, 97° F (36.5° C); pulse, 112; respirations, 32 and shallow; and blood pressure, 94/50. On auscultation you find diminished breath sounds over the right lower and middle lobes. She is pale with some cyanosis around her mouth and at her nail beds. The son tells you that his mother had a cold 3 days ago and has been taking an over-the-counter cough suppressant for the symptoms.

- Which assessment technique should you perform next?
- What additional information should you obtain from the son?
- What intervention should you initiate first?

For suggested answer guidelines, go to SIMON http://www.wbsaunders.com/SIMON/Iggy/.

Analysis

COMMON NURSING DIAGNOSES AND COLLABORATIVE PROBLEMS

The following are common nursing diagnoses for clients with pneumonia:

1. Impaired Gas Exchange related to the effects of alveolar-capillary membrane changes
2. Ineffective Airway Clearance related to the effects of infection, excessive tracheobronchial secretions, fatigue and decreased energy, chest discomfort, and muscle weakness

A common collaborative problem for the client with pneumonia is Potential for Sepsis related to an infectious organism.

ADDITIONAL NURSING DIAGNOSES AND COLLABORATIVE PROBLEMS

In addition to the common nursing diagnoses and collaborative problem, clients with pneumonia may have one or more of the following:

- Acute Pain related to the effects of inflammation of parietal pleura, coughing
- Hyperthermia related to an increased metabolic rate, dehydration
- Deficient Fluid Volume related to fever, infection, and increased metabolic rate
- Disturbed Sleep Pattern related to pain, dyspnea, and unfamiliar environment (hospitalization)
- Potential for Pleural Effusion related to spread of the infection

Planning and Implementation

IMPAIRED GAS EXCHANGE

NOC **PLANNING: EXPECTED OUTCOMES.** The client with pneumonia is expected to attain or maintain the partial pressure of arterial oxygen and carbon dioxide (Pa_{O_2} and Pa_{CO_2}, respectively) and oxygen saturation values within baseline ranges.

INTERVENTIONS. NIC interventions for the client with pneumonia are listed in Chart 31-5. Interventions to treat and manage impaired gas exchange are similar to those for the client with chronic obstructive pulmonary disease (COPD) or asthma (see Chapter 30). In pneumonia, oxygen is the gas exchange most affected; therefore hypoxemia is the primary problem. Carbon dioxide retention is not as common in pneumonia as it is, for example, in chronic emphysema.

Incentive spirometry, also referred to as **sustained maximal inspiration,** is a type of bronchial hygiene used in pneumonia. The objective is to improve inspiratory muscle performance and prevent or reverse atelectasis (alveolar collapse). The nurse instructs the client to exhale fully, place the mouthpiece in the mouth, and take a long, slow, deep breath for 3 to 5 seconds. The nurse evaluates the client's technique and records the volume of air inspired. The client performs 5 to 10 breaths per session every hour while awake.

INEFFECTIVE AIRWAY CLEARANCE

NOC **PLANNING: EXPECTED OUTCOMES.** The client with pneumonia is expected to have auscultated breath sounds in the expected range.

INTERVENTIONS. For the client with pneumonia, interventions for the treatment and management of ineffective airway clearance are similar to those for COPD or asthma. Because of fatigue, muscle weakness, chest discomfort, and excessive secretions, the client with pneumonia often has difficulty clearing secretions. The nurse helps the client to cough and deep breathe at least every 2 hours. The alert client may use an incentive spirometer to facilitate deep breathing and stimulate coughing. Chest physiotherapy (CPT or chest PT), which was once thought to be useful for clearing secretions in pneumonia, is no longer recommended for uncomplicated pneumonia. Dehydration should be avoided, but there is no evidence that hydration helps to clear secretions. Adequate hydration may help to thin secretions and make them easier to remove. To ensure adequate hydration when fever and tachypnea are present, the nurse monitors intake and output.

The physician prescribes bronchodilators, especially beta-2 agonists (see Chart 30-4), when bronchospasm is part of the disease process. These are usually administered initially by aerosol nebulizer and then by metered dose inhaler (see Chart 30-4). In general, inhaled steroid preparations are not used with acute pneumonia except when the client also has bronchial asthma or respiratory failure.

POTENTIAL FOR SEPSIS

PLANNING: EXPECTED OUTCOMES. The client with pneumonia is expected to be free of the invading organism and return to a prepneumonia health status.

CHART 31-5

NIC INTERVENTION ACTIVITIES *for* The Client with Pneumonia

Cough Enhancement: *Promotion of deep inhalation by the client with subsequent generation of high intrathoracic pressures and compression of the underlying lung parenchyma for the forceful expulsion of air*

- Assist client to a sitting position with neck slightly flexed, shoulders relaxed, and knees flexed.
- Encourage client to take several deep breaths.
- Encourage client to take a deep breath, hold it for 2 seconds, and cough two or three times in succession.
- Instruct client to inhale deeply, bend forward slightly, and perform three or four huffs (against an open glottis).
- Instruct client to inhale deeply several times, to exhale slowly, and to cough at the end of exhalation.
- Initiate lateral chest wall rib spring techniques during the expiration phase of the cough maneuver, as appropriate.
- Instruct client to follow coughing with several maximal inhalation breaths.
- Encourage use of incentive spirometry, as appropriate.
- Promote systemic fluid hydration, as appropriate.

Oxygen Therapy: *Administration of oxygen and monitoring of its effectiveness*

- Clear oral, nasal, and tracheal secretions, as appropriate.
- Restrict smoking.
- Maintain airway patency.
- Set up oxygen equipment and administer through a heated, humidified system.
- Administer supplemental oxygen as ordered.
- Monitor the oxygen liter flow.
- Monitor position of oxygen delivery device.
- Instruct client about importance of leaving oxygen delivery device on.
- Periodically check oxygen delivery device to ensure that the prescribed concentration is being delivered.
- Monitor the effectiveness of oxygen therapy (e.g., pulse oximetry, ABGs), as appropriate.
- Ensure replacement of oxygen mask/cannula whenever the device is removed.
- Monitor client's ability to tolerate removal of oxygen while eating.
- Change oxygen delivery device from mask to nasal prongs during meals, as tolerated.
- Observe for signs of oxygen-induced hypoventilation.
- Monitor for signs of oxygen toxicity and absorption atelectasis.
- Monitor client's anxiety related to need for oxygen therapy.
- Monitor for skin breakdown from friction of oxygen device.
- Provide for oxygen when client is transported.

Respiratory Monitoring: *Collection and analysis of client data to ensure airway patency and adequate gas exchange*

- Monitor rate, rhythm, depth, and effort of respirations.
- Note chest movement, watching for symmetry, use of accessory muscles, and supraclavicular and intercostal muscle retractions.
- Monitor for breathing patterns: bradypnea, tachypnea, hyperventilation, Kussmaul respirations, Cheyne-Stokes respirations, apneustic, Biot, and ataxic patterns.
- Palpate for equal lung expansion.
- Monitor for diaphragmatic muscle fatigue (paradoxical motion).
- Auscultate breath sounds, noting areas of decreased/absent ventilation and presence of adventitious sounds.
- Determine the need for suctioning by auscultating for crackles and rhonchi over major airways.
- Auscultate lung sounds after treatments to note results.
- Monitor for increased restlessness, anxiety, and air hunger.
- Note changes in Sa_{O_2}, Sv_{O_2}, end tidal CO_2, and changes in ABG values, as appropriate.
- Monitor client's ability to cough effectively.
- Note onset, characteristics, and duration of cough.
- Monitor client's respiratory secretions.
- Monitor for dyspnea and events that improve and worsen it.
- Monitor chest x-ray reports.
- Place the client on side, as indicated, to prevent aspiration.
- Institute respiratory therapy treatments (e.g., nebulizer), as needed.

NIC intervention activities selected from McCloskey, J.C., & Bulechek, G.M. (Eds.). (2000). *Nursing interventions classification (NIC)* (3rd ed.). St. Louis: Mosby. No part of this work is to be altered without prior written permission from the Publisher.

ABG, Arterial blood gas; Sa_{O_a}, arterial oxygen saturation; Sv_{O_2}, venous oxygen saturation; CO_2, carbon dioxide.

INTERVENTIONS. The key to the effective treatment of pneumonia is identification and eradication of the organism causing the infection. Anti-infectives are given for all types of pneumonias except those caused by viruses. The physician prescribes anti-infective therapy depending on the organism suspected or identified, whether the pneumonia is community acquired or hospital acquired, and whether there are other contributing factors (Table 31-7). Treatment is often initiated based on presenting clinical manifestations and prior experience, and it may be continued if the specific organism is not identified.

The client may be able to switch from IV to oral therapy in 2 or 3 days depending on the response (e.g., stable clinical condition, afebrile). The course of anti-infective therapy varies with the characteristics of the drug and the organism(s) involved and generally ranges from a low of 5 days for a client with uncomplicated community-acquired pneumonia to up to 21 days for an immunocompromised client.

For pneumonia resulting from aspiration of food or stomach contents, interventions are focused on preventing lung damage and treating the infection. Aspiration of acidic substances (e.g., vomitus or stomach contents) can cause widespread inflammation and lead to complications such as acute respiratory distress syndrome (ARDS) and permanent lung damage. Thus steroids and nonsteroidal anti-inflammatory agents are used in conjunction with antibiotics to reduce the inflammatory response.

Community-Based Care

The client needs to continue the anti-infective medications as prescribed by the physician or primary care provider. The nurse reinforces, clarifies, and provides additional information to the client and family as indicated. Completion of the entire medication regimen is stressed.

HEALTH TEACHING

The most important aspect of education for the client and family is the avoidance of upper respiratory tract infections

TABLE 31-7 • RECOMMENDED DRUG CATEGORIES FOR THE TREATMENT OF PNEUMONIA

Pneumonia Type	Recommended Drug Categories with Alternatives
COMMUNITY-ACQUIRED PNEUMONIAS	
Age <60 with no comorbidity	Cefuroxime (add erythromycin if concern for *Mycoplasma, Chlamydia,* or *Legionella* is high) Azithromycin (alternative if client is allergic to penicillin/cephalosporin or is erythromycin intolerant) Levofloxacin (if client is macrolide* intolerant or pneumonia fails to resolve)
Age >60 or <60 with comorbidity	Ceftriaxone and azithromycin (or erythromycin) Levofloxacin (alternative if macrolide intolerant or pneumonia fails to resolve) Trovafloxacin
Aspiration pneumonia	Ampicillin/sulbactam and clindamycin Trovafloxacin (alternative if penicillin/cephalosporin allergy) Ceftriaxone and clindamycin
HOSPITAL-ACQUIRED (NOSOCOMIAL) PNEUMONIAS	
Gram-positive infections	Ticarcillin/clavulanate Vancomycin Imipenem/cilastatin Piperacillin/tazobactam Cefepime and metronidazole
Gram-negative infections	Ciprofloxaxin Aminoglycoside (amikacin, gentamicin) if renal function is stable Ceftazidime Aztreonam Ticarcillin

*Macrolides include erythromycin, azithromycin, clarithromycin, and dirithromycin.

and viruses. The client is instructed to avoid crowds (especially in the fall and winter, when viruses are prevalent), persons who have a cold or flu, and exposure to irritants such as smoke. An annual influenza vaccine is recommended, and the pneumococcal vaccine is currently recommended once every 5 years (possibly more often in some high-risk cases). A balanced diet and adequate fluid intake are essential.

The nurse reviews all medication with the client and family and emphasizes completing anti-infective therapy. The client is instructed to notify the physician if chills, fever, persistent cough, dyspnea, wheezing, hemoptysis, increased sputum production, chest discomfort, or increasing fatigue recurs or if symptoms fail to resolve. The nurse emphasizes the importance of getting plenty of rest and gradually increasing exercise.

HOME CARE MANAGEMENT

No special structural changes are needed in the home. If the home consists of more than one story, the client may prefer to stay on the first floor for a few weeks, because stair climbing may increase fatigue and dyspnea. Bath and hygiene needs may be met by using a bedside commode if a bathroom is not located on the first level. Home care needs depend on level of fatigue, dyspnea, and family and social support.

The prolonged convalescent phase of the disease process, particularly in the older client, can be frustrating and perhaps depressing. Fatigue, weakness, and a residual cough can last for weeks. Some clients fear they will never return to a "normal" level of functioning. It is important that the nurse prepare the client for the course of disease and offer reassurance so that complete recovery will occur. Initially after discharge, a home care nursing assessment may be beneficial (Chart 31-6).

CHART 31-6

FOCUSED ASSESSMENT *of* The Client Recovering from Pneumonia

Ascertain whether the client has had any of the following:
- Chills
- Fever
- Persistent cough
- Dyspnea
- Wheezing
- Hemoptysis
- Increased sputum production
- Chest discomfort
- Increasing fatigue
- Any other symptoms that have failed to resolve

Assess the client for the following:
- Fever
- Diaphoresis
- Cyanosis, especially around the mouth or conjunctiva
- Dyspnea, tachypnea, or tachycardia
- Adventitious or abnormal breath sounds
- Weakness

HEALTH CARE RESOURCES

Clients who smoke are taught that smoking is a risk factor for pneumonia. The nurse provides information on smoking cessation classes through the American Lung Association (ALA) and American Cancer Society. The physician or nurse practitioner may prescribe nicotine patches. The client is warned of the danger of myocardial infarction if smoking is continued while using the patches. The client should be enrolled in a smoking cessation program to assist in the nicotine withdrawal process in conjunction with nicotine patches. The nurse also can give the client information booklets on pneumonia provided by the ALA. A client who has not already been vaccinated against influenza or pneumococcal pneumonia is encouraged to take this preventive measure when the pneumonia has resolved.

Evaluation: Outcomes

NOC The nurse evaluates the care of the client with pneumonia on the basis of the identified nursing diagnoses and collaborative problems. The expected outcomes are that the client:

- Attains and/or maintains a $Pa{O_2}$, $Pa{CO_2}$, and oxygen saturation values within expected ranges
- Has optimal breath sounds, either clear lungs in all lobes on auscultation or, minimally, improved breath sounds
- Is free of the invading organism
- Returns to his or her prepneumonia health status

Pulmonary Tuberculosis

OVERVIEW

In 1900 tuberculosis (TB) was the leading cause of death in the United States and Europe. After a significant reduction in its incidence, TB has been on the rise, especially in clients with HIV and acquired immunodeficiency syndrome (AIDS). Continuous assessment and intervention to prevent and treat the disease must continue. Increasing poverty, numbers of homeless people, people with AIDS, and resistant strains of the TB organism (multidrug-resistant TB [MDR-TB]) present new challenges to the control and prevention of TB.

Pathophysiology

TB is a highly communicable disease caused by *Mycobacterium tuberculosis.* The tubercle bacillus is transmitted via **aerosolization** (i.e., an airborne route). When an infected person coughs, laughs, sneezes, whistles, or sings, droplet nuclei are produced, become airborne, and may be inhaled by others. The tubercle bacillus multiplies freely when it reaches a susceptible site (bronchi or alveoli). An exudative response occurs, causing a nonspecific pneumonitis. With the development of acquired immunity, further multiplication of bacilli is controlled in most initial lesions. The lesions typically resolve and leave little or no residual. However, a small percentage of individuals who are initially infected will acquire the disease (5% to 15%). The greatest risk for acquiring the disease for the non–HIV-infected person is during the first 2 years after infection.

Cell-mediated immunity develops 2 to 10 weeks after infection and is manifested by a significant reaction to a tuberculin test. A primary infection may be microscopic in size and may never appear on an x-ray film. The process of infection occurs in the following order:

- The granulomatous inflammation created by the tubercle bacillus in the lung becomes surrounded by collagen, fibroblasts, and lymphocytes.
- **Caseation necrosis** (necrotic tissue being turned into a granular mass) occurs in the center of the lesion. If this area becomes evident on x-ray, it is called a **Ghon tubercle,** or the primary lesion.

Areas of caseation then undergo resorption, hyaline degeneration, and fibrosis. These necrotic areas may calcify **(calcification)** or liquefy **(liquefaction).** If liquefaction occurs, the liquid material empties into a bronchus, and the evacuated area becomes a cavity **(cavitation).** Bacilli continue to grow in the necrotic cavity wall and spread via the tracheobronchial lymph nodes into new areas of the lung.

A lesion also may progress by direct extension if bacilli multiply rapidly with marked exudative response to the inflammation. These lesions may extend through the pleura, which results in tuberculous pleural effusion with a small number of organisms. Pericardial effusions also may occur.

Miliary or **hematogenous TB** occurs when a large number of organisms enter the bloodstream and the disease spreads throughout the body. Many tiny, discrete nodules scattered throughout the lung are seen on the chest x-ray film. The brain, meninges, liver, kidney, or bone marrow are commonly involved as a result of spread through the blood.

Initial infection is seen more often in the middle or lower lobes of the lung. The regional lymph nodes, particularly the hilar and paratracheal nodes, are commonly involved. There is usually an asymptomatic interval after the primary infection that lasts for years or decades—before clinical symptoms develop. An infected individual is not infectious to others until symptoms of disease occur.

Secondary TB occurs in a previously infected person and is a reactivation (sometimes inaccurately termed a reinfection) of the primary disease. Reactivation is more likely whenever defenses are lowered, which may be part of the reason why older adults are susceptible to the development of TB. The upper lobes are the most common site of reactivation and are referred to as **Simon's foci.** The TB classification adopted and revised by the ALA is shown in Table 31-8.

TABLE 31-8 • AMERICAN LUNG ASSOCIATION CLASSIFICATION OF TUBERCULOSIS

0	No TB exposure, not infected
1	TB exposure, no evidence of infection
2	TB infection, no disease
3	TB clinically active (clients with completed diagnostic evidence of TB—both a significant reaction to TB skin test and clinical or x-ray evidence of TB)
4	TB: not clinically active (clients with history of TB or abnormal chest x-ray film but no significant TB skin test reaction or clinical evidence)
5	TB: suspect (diagnosis pending); used during diagnostic testing of suspect clients for no longer than a 3-month period

Etiology

The organism *M. tuberculosis* is a nonmoving, slow-growing, nonsporulating, acid-fast rod. The bacillus is transmitted via aerosolization.

The people most commonly infected are those having repeated close contact with an infectious person who has not yet been diagnosed with TB. The risk of transmission is greatly reduced after the infectious person has received the proper medication for 2 to 3 weeks and after clinical signs of improvement are seen (including the reduction of acid-fast bacilli [AFB] in the sputum).

Incidence/Prevalence

Figures for 1981 reveal that TB accounted for only 0.8% of deaths in the United States and that its incidence was declining steadily. From 1985 through 1992, the number of new TB cases increased to more than 20,000 annually. This increase is largely related to the onset of HIV infection. For the past 6 years, the incidence of TB in the United States has continually decreased among all segments of the population except among foreign-born individuals (CDC, 1999). The highest at-risk populations currently include those persons:

- In constant, frequent contact with an untreated individual
- With immune dysfunction or HIV
- Living in crowded areas such as long-term care facilities, prisons, and mental health facilities
- Who are older, homeless, and minorities
- Who abuse IV drugs or alcohol
- From a lower socioeconomic group
- Who are foreign immigrants (especially from Mexico, the Philippines, and Vietnam)

COLLABORATIVE MANAGEMENT

Assessment

Early detection of tuberculosis (TB) depends on subjective findings rather than the presentation of symptoms. TB has an insidious onset, and many clients are not aware of symptoms until the disease is well advanced. A diagnosis of TB should be considered for a persistent cough or other symptoms compatible with TB, such as weight loss, anorexia, night sweats, hemoptysis, shortness of breath, fever, or chills.

HISTORY

A thorough history includes an assessment of past exposure to TB. The nurse inquires about the client's country of origin and travel to foreign countries in which there is a high incidence of TB. It is important to note the results of any previous tests for TB. In addition, the client is asked whether he or she has had a bacille Calmette-Guérin (BCG) vaccine. The BCG vaccine contains attenuated tubercle bacilli and is given routinely in many foreign countries to produce increased resistance to TB. *Anyone who has received a BCG vaccine within the previous 10 years will have a somewhat positive skin test that can complicate interpretation.* The size of the skin response usually decreases each year after vaccination. These clients should be evaluated for TB with a chest x-ray film. The effectiveness of the BCG vaccine in preventing TB is controversial and not recommended by the Centers for Disease Control and Prevention (CDC).

PHYSICAL ASSESSMENT/CLINICAL MANIFESTATIONS

The client with TB usually has progressive fatigue, lethargy, nausea, anorexia, weight loss, irregular menses, and a low-grade fever, which may have been present for weeks or months. Fever also may be accompanied by night sweats. The client finally notices a cough and the production of mucoid and mucopurulent sputum, which is occasionally streaked with blood. Chest tightness and a dull, aching chest pain may accompany the cough.

Physical examination of the chest does not provide conclusive evidence of TB. The nurse may hear dullness with percussion over involved parenchymal areas, bronchial breath sounds, crackles, and increased transmission of spoken or whispered sounds. Partial obstruction of a bronchus because of endobronchial disease or compression by lymph nodes may produce localized wheezing.

DIAGNOSTIC ASSESSMENT

A diagnosis of TB is suggested by the clinical manifestations and a positive smear for acid-fast bacillus. Sputum is obtained, smeared on a slide, and stained with a dye (usually fuchsin). After the slide has dried, it is treated with an acid alcohol to remove the stain. The TB bacillus does not destain with this procedure and remains red. The acid-fast bacillus test is not specific for TB (other mycobacterium are also acid-fast) but is used as a quick method to determine whether TB treatment and precautions should be started until more definitive testing can be completed.

Sputum culture of *Mycobacterium tuberculosis* confirms the diagnosis. Traditionally, these cultures are slow-growing, with weeks required to determine a positive or negative result. Some newer techniques (BACTEC) promote faster culture growth in a liquid rather than a solid culture environment and allow the microorganism to be identified in 1 to 3 weeks instead of 4 to 6 weeks. Three samples are usually obtained for an acid-fast smear. After medications are started, sputum samples are obtained again to determine the effectiveness of therapy. Most clients have negative cultures after 3 months of treatment.

The polymerase chain reaction (PCR) assay is performed for rapid identification of mycobacteria in selected situations. This process allows amplification of mycobacterial genetic material (deoxyribonucleic acid [DNA]) and identification of mycobacteria within hours instead of days to weeks. This test allows for earlier diagnosis of TB. Although highly accurate, the high cost and limited availability of PCR currently prohibit its widespread use as a screening or diagnostic tool for TB.

The tuberculin test (Mantoux test) is the most reliable determinant of TB infection. A small amount (0.1 mL) of intermediate-strength purified protein derivative (PPD) containing 5 tuberculin units is given intradermally in the forearm. An area of induration (not redness) measuring 10 mm or more in diameter 48 to 72 hours after injection indicates exposure to and infection with TB. A positive reaction does not mean that active disease is present but indicates exposure to TB or the presence of inactive (dormant) disease. A reaction of 5 mm or greater is considered positive in persons with HIV infection. A reduced skin reaction or a negative skin test does not rule out TB disease or infection, especially among the very old or anyone who is severely immunocompromised.

Yearly screening is recommended for anyone at greater risk of coming into contact with persons infected with TB. Screening is particularly important for foreign-born persons and migrant workers. Participation in screening programs can be enhanced when such programs are delivered in a culturally sensitive and nonthreatening manner (see the Evidence-Based Practice for Nursing box on p. 586).

Once a person's skin test is positive, a chest x-ray study is essential to rule out clinically active TB or to detect old, healed lesions. Caseation and inflammation may be seen on the x-ray film if the disease is active. Routine, repeat skin tests and chest x-ray studies are no longer recommended. Clients are instructed to seek medical attention if they experience symptoms suggestive of TB.

EVIDENCE-BASED PRACTICE FOR NURSING

Intention and perceived susceptibility positively influence tuberculosis screening behaviors

Poss, J. (2000). Factors associated with participation by Mexican migrant farmworkers in a tuberculosis screening program. *Nursing Research, 49*(1), 20-28.

This prospective and descriptive study integrated components of the Health Belief Model (HBM) and the Theory of Reasoned Action (TRA) into a new reduced model to explain the level of participation in a TB screening program for Mexican migrant farmworkers. A total of 206 Mexican migrant farmworkers agreed to be interviewed and initially participate in a comprehensive TB education and screening program. The program consisted of an evening class that provided information about TB education, detection, and treatment. The program was presented in Spanish by Mexican migrant workers who had received on-the-job training regarding the disease and adult education principles. All participants completed (with assistance) a 66-item Spanish-language TB interview instrument developed for the study. Educational techniques included skits, presentations, demonstrations, and audience participation. The next day, participants were screened for TB using intradermal positive protein derivative (PPD) PPD skin testing. The skin tests were read 48 to 72 hours later.

Of the 206 participants who attended the education sessions, 152 (73.4%) received the skin test. Ninety-eight percent (149) of those subjects tested returned to have the skin test read. Forty-four subjects had positive skin tests for TB and were further screened by chest x-ray examination. Analysis of the data obtained using the interview instrument indicated that the two most significant factors that determined complete participation in all aspects of the training program were the intention to participate and the perceived personal level of susceptibility to the disease or its consequences.

Critique. The study was well controlled for the elimination of confounding variables such as language and cultural differences as well as geographic barriers to access. Major strengths included the level of cultural sensitivity demonstrated by the investigators and the location of the screening at the migrant camps. No details were provided regarding the immigration status of the subjects or what consequences would follow a diagnosis of TB. Although the overall purpose of the study was to test the reduced model, a secondary purpose was to determine what factors increase complete participation in a TB screening program. Approximately 25% of the subjects did not participate in screening. Examining the responses of those who did not participate could provide direction for interventions to improve screening behaviors in this vulnerable population.

Implications for Nursing. Providing accurate information at an appropriate literacy level and a culturally sensitive manner can increase a person's belief of personal susceptibility to a disease or negative health outcome. Increasing such beliefs has the potential to increase individual health screening behaviors, which may identify the presence of the disease earlier and allow more timely treatment.

The radiographic presentation in HIV-infected clients may be unusual. In such cases the chest x-ray may be normal or may show infiltrates in any lung zone, which are often associated with hilar lymph node enlargement.

CRITICAL THINKING CHALLENGE

The client is a 72-year-old man from Mexico who is visiting his daughter. He speaks no English and was found to have a positive TB skin test at a church-run screening program. His daughter, who speaks a little English, tells you he has been coughing and has lost at least 25 pounds since his visit 1 year ago.

- What additional information about the client should you obtain?
- What information about the daughter should you obtain?

You are to prepare the client for a chest x-ray study and obtain a sputum specimen from him.

- How will you prepare this client for his diagnostic testing?
- Describe three approaches you might use to teach this

For suggested answer guidelines, go to SIMON http://www.wbsaunders.com/SIMON/Iggy/.

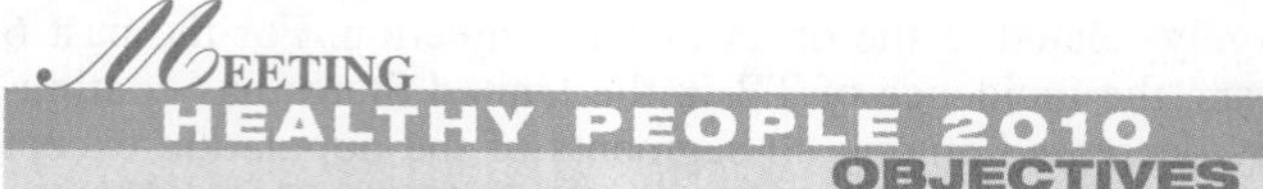

MEETING HEALTHY PEOPLE 2010 OBJECTIVES

TUBERCULOSIS

Objective 22.25 Increase to at least 90% the proportion of all tuberculosis patients who complete curative therapy within 12 months

- Teach all clients to have yearly tuberculosis (TB) skin tests.
- Assist clients who have a positive TB skin test to have a follow-up screening for a definitive diagnosis.
- Develop culturally appropriate education materials.
- Ensure that education materials are written or presented at no greater than a fourth-grade literacy level.
- Educate those clients who are diagnosed with TB to:
  - Take all medication as ordered
  - Keep all follow-up appointments
  - Identify contacts
- Implement a direction observation therapy (DOT) program for clients who have not consistently taken their medication as prescribed.
- Refer clients who do not have money for medications to the appropriate resource for obtaining low-cost or no-cost TB drugs.

Interventions

Combination drug therapy is the most effective method of treating tuberculosis (TB) and preventing transmission. Increasing the number of clients with TB who complete curative therapy is a major focus for Healthy People 2010 (see the Meeting Healthy People 2010 Objectives box above). Active TB is treated with a combination of drugs to which the organism is susceptible. Therapy is continued until the disease is under control. The use of multiple-drug regimens destroys organisms as quickly as possible and minimizes the emergence of drug-resistant organisms. Current therapy uses isoniazid (INH) and rifampin throughout the therapy; pyrazinamide is added for the first 2 months (Chart 31-7). This protocol shortens the therapy for most clients from 6 to 12 months to 6 months. Ethambutol and streptomycin are often added to the treatment regimen as the fourth drug. Additional therapies under investigation for treatment of TB include aerosolized interferon-gamma and thalidomide (Synovir, Thalomid♣).

Strict adherence to the prescribed drug regimen is crucial to suppressing the disease. Thus the nurse's major role is teaching the client about drug therapy. Accurate information provided in multiple formats (e.g., pamphlets, videos, drug schedule worksheets) can be valuable in client education. The nurse recognizes that the anxious client may not absorb information well. The nurse repeats the information and obtains the assistance of available family members. The client is asked to describe the treatment regimen and major

CHART 31-7

DRUG THERAPY *for* Tuberculosis*

Drug	Usual Dosage	Nursing Interventions	Drug Action/Rationale for Use
Isoniazid (INH)	5 mg/kg PO, IM (maximum 300 mg) daily; 15 mg/kg (maximum 900 mg) biweekly	Observe for drug interactions. It may inhibit drug metabolism of phenytoin, carbamazepine, primidone, and warfarin. Instruct the client to take on empty stomach and avoid antacids. Monitor for signs of hepatitis and neurotoxicity effects.	Isoniazid inhibits the synthesis of mycolic acids and acts to kill actively growing organisms in the extracellular environment and inhibits the growth of dormant organisms in the macrophages and caseating granulomas.
Rifampin (RIF)	10 mg/kg PO (maximum 600 mg) daily or biweekly	Instruct the client that secretions, including urine, will be orange in color and that the drug will permanently discolor soft contact lenses. Observe for drug interactions. It may enhance elimination of theophylline, steroids, opioids, oral hypoglycemics, warfarin, and occasionally vitamin D. Observe for hepatotoxic effects. RIF decreases effectiveness of oral contraceptives.	Rifampin has the unique ability to kill slower growing organisms that reside in the caseating granuloma and macrophage.
Pyrazinamide (PZA)	15-30 mg/kg PO (maximum 2000 mg) daily; 50 mg/kg biweekly	Observe for hepatotoxic effects.	Pyrazinamide is the most active drug at killing mycobacteria present in macrophages. The acidic environment in the macrophage inhibits most agents.
Ethambutol (EMB)	15 mg/kg daily PO; 50 mg/kg biweekly	Obtain baseline visual acuity and color discrimination, especially to the color green. Repeat testing every 1-2 mo.	Ethambutol inhibits bacterial ribonucleic acid (RNA) synthesis. It is slow acting and must be used in combination with other bactericidal agents.
Streptomycin (SM)	1000 mg IM, IV over 1 hr, daily for 2 mo followed by biweekly injections until treatment is completed	Obtain baseline audiometric test every 1-2 mo. It can impair the eighth cranial nerve. Older clients are especially susceptible.	Streptomycin is an aminoglycoside antibiotic that is active against extracellular organisms only.
Amikacin	15 mg/kg daily IM, IV (usual dose 1 g)	Ensure adequate hydration, monitor renal function and hearing. Amikacin can lead to renal toxicity and ototoxicity.	Amikacin is an aminoglycoside antibiotic that can be used if streptomycin is not available.
Rifapentine (Priftin)	600 mg twice weekly	Doses must be separated by at least 72 hr. Instruct the client that metabolism of other drugs may be faster, causing lower blood concentrations and a need for higher doses (especially for antidiabetic drugs, barbiturates, and antibiotics). Instruct female clients to use additional forms of birth control, because this drug decreases the effectiveness of oral contraceptives. Observe for hepatotoxic effects.	Rifapentine has high bacteriostatic and bactericidal action against slow-growing intracellular bacteria.

*Newer drugs contain combinations of rifampin and isoniazid (Rifamate) or of rifampin, isoniazid, and pyrazinamide (Rifater).

side effects for which to call the health care agency and physician.

TB is often treated outside the acute care setting, with the client convalescing in the home setting. Airborne precautions are not necessary in this setting because family members have already been exposed; however, all members of the household need to undergo TB testing. The nurse instructs the client to cover the mouth and nose when coughing or sneezing, to confine used tissues to plastic bags, and to wear a mask when in contact with crowds until the medication is effective in suppressing the infection.

The client is informed that sputum needs to be examined every 2 to 4 weeks once drug therapy is initiated. When the results of three sputum cultures are negative, the client is considered to be no longer infectious and can usually return to former employment. The nurse reminds the client to avoid ex-

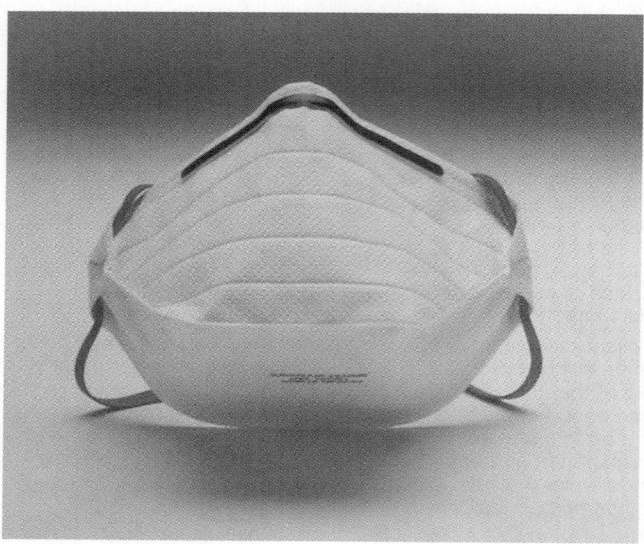

Figure 31-2 ● A HEPA respirator used in the care of clients with active or "rule-out" tuberculosis. (Courtesy Uvex Safety, Smithfield, RI.)

cessive exposure to silicone or dust because these substances can cause further lung damage.

The hospitalized client with active TB is placed under airborne precautions (see Chapter 26) in a well-ventilated room. The room should have at least six exchanges of fresh air per minute and should be ventilated to the outside if possible. All health care workers wear a N95 or high-efficiency particulate air (HEPA) respirator when caring for the client (Figure 31-2). When there is risk of hand and clothing contamination, standard precautions are implemented by using appropriate barrier protection (i.e., gowns and gloves). Thorough handwashing is performed before and after client care. Precautions are discontinued when the client is no longer considered infectious.

Nausea related to the medications may be prevented by taking the daily dose at bedtime. Antiemetics may also prevent this symptom. The client with TB is instructed about the need for adequate nutrition and a well-balanced diet to promote healing. An increased intake of foods that are rich in iron, protein, and vitamin C is recommended. The nurse consults the nutritionist for specialized needs.

The client with TB may be frightened by changes in physical stamina and also faces concerns about the prognosis of the disease. The nurse is realistic in offering a positive outlook for the client who complies with the medication regimen and suggests that fatigue will diminish as the treatment progresses. With current resistant strains of TB, the nurse must emphasize that noncompliance with the medication regimen could lead to an infection that is difficult to treat or has total drug resistance.

Community-Based Care

HEALTH TEACHING

The client is instructed to follow the drug regimen exactly as prescribed and always to have a supply of medication on hand. The nurse stresses the side effects and ways of minimizing them to ensure compliance. The client is reminded that the disease is usually no longer communicable after the medication has been taken for 2 to 3 consecutive weeks and clinical improvement is seen. However, the prescribed medication must be continued for 6 months or longer as ordered. Directly observed therapy (DOT), in which the nurse watches the client swallow the medications, may be indicated in some situations. This practice contributes to more treatment successes, fewer relapses, and less drug resistance.

The client who has experienced weight loss and severe lethargy should gradually resume his or her usual activities. Proper nutrition must be maintained to prevent a recurrence of infection.

To help with concerns about the contagious aspect of the infection, the nurse provides information about TB. A key to preventing transmission is identifying those in close contact with the infected person so they can be tested and treated as necessary. Public health professionals have an important role in this aspect of care. Identified contacts are assessed with a TB test and possibly a chest x-ray examination to determine infection. Multiple-drug therapy may be indicated. In addition, certain high-risk contacts receive prophylactic therapy, usually with isoniazid (INH).

HOME CARE MANAGEMENT

Most clients with TB are managed outside the hospital. However, clients may be diagnosed with TB while in the hospital if pneumonia is suspected or other possible complications exist. Discharge may be delayed if the living situation is considered high risk or if noncompliance is likely. The nurse consults with the social service worker in the hospital or the community health nursing agency to ensure that the client is discharged to the appropriate environment with continued supervision.

HEALTH CARE RESOURCES

The nurse instructs the client to receive follow-up care by a physician for at least 1 year during active treatment. The American Lung Association (ALA), an organization that uses volunteers, can provide free information about the disease and its treatment. In addition, Alcoholics Anonymous and other health care resources for clients with alcoholism are available if needed. The nurse assists the client who uses drugs to locate an appropriate drug treatment program.

CRITICAL THINKING CHALLENGE

The client, a 72-year-old man from Mexico who speaks no English, is diagnosed with active TB. He is prescribed to take rifampin 150 mg, INH 75 mg, and pyrazinamide 400 mg daily. He is to be discharged to the care of his daughter. You discover that the daughter has 5 children (ages 8 to 17) and lives in a 5-room apartment.

- What are the teaching priorities for this client?
- What modifications should the daughter make in her home environment (assuming that she cannot move and that all 5 children must remain in the home)?
- What types of community services should you assist this client and family in obtaining?
- How often should the daughter and children have skin testing for TB?

For suggested answer guidelines, go to SIMON http://www.wbsaunders.com/SIMON/Iggy/.

Lung Abscess

OVERVIEW

A lung abscess is a localized area of lung destruction caused by liquefaction necrosis, which is usually related to pyogenic bacteria. Clients with this problem often have a history of pneumonia, possibly complicated by the aspiration of oropharyngeal contents or proximal obstruction as a result of a tumor or foreign body. Other causes of aspiration leading to abscess include alcoholism that causes loss of consciousness, seizure disorders or other neurologic deficits, and swallowing disorders. An obstruction of a bronchus may cause a necrotizing process in the lung that eventually becomes an abscess.

Multiple abscesses and cavities commonly form in clients with tuberculosis (TB) or fungal infections of the lung. Immunosuppressed clients, such as those receiving chemotherapy or those with a disease such as leukemia or AIDS, are particularly susceptible to fungal infections. The most common organisms are anaerobic bacteria, *Staphylococcus* or other gram-positive organism, or gram-negative or opportunistic infections such as fungi.

COLLABORATIVE MANAGEMENT

Assessment

The nurse notes any recent history of influenza, pneumonia, febrile illness, cough, and foul-smelling sputum production. The client is asked about the color and odor of the sputum and about any pleuritic chest pain (a stabbing pain, especially when taking a deep breath). The client is often febrile, pale, fatigued, and cachectic. Decreased breath sounds may be noted on auscultation, and there is dullness on percussion in the involved area. Bronchial breath sounds and crackles are often heard over the site of the lesion. The health care professional orders a chest x-ray examination and sputum samples to assist in the diagnosis.

Interventions

The nursing diagnoses and interventions identified for the client with pneumonia also apply to the client with a lung abscess. Medical treatment is directed toward antibiotics and drainage of the abscess. The physician may prescribe more than one antibiotic. The nurse provides frequent mouth care and observes for oral overgrowth of *Candida albicans*.

Pulmonary Empyema

OVERVIEW

Empyema is a collection of pus in the pleural space. The most common cause of empyema is a pulmonary infection, lung abscess, or infected pleural effusion. Pneumonia or a lung abscess can spread across the pleura, or obstruction of the lymph nodes can cause a retrograde flood of infected lymph into the pleural space. In addition, a liver abscess or abscess under the diaphragm can spread through the diaphragm's lymphatic system into the lung area. Thoracic surgery and chest trauma are common predisposing conditions in which bacteria are introduced directly into the pleural space. Blood from trauma may accumulate in the pleural space, and incomplete drainage of this blood promotes bacterial growth.

COLLABORATIVE MANAGEMENT

Assessment

Important history findings include recent febrile illness (including pneumonia), chest pain, dyspnea, cough, and trauma. The nurse documents the character of the sputum. Chest wall motion may be reduced on physical assessment. If a pleural effusion is present, fremitus may be decreased or absent on palpation, percussion may sound flat, and breath sounds are decreased on auscultation. With compression of lung tissue near or next to the effusion, auscultation abnormalities include bronchial breath sounds, egophony, and whispered pectoriloquy (see Chapter 27).

Some clients experience fever, chills, night sweats, and weight loss. If there is cardiorespiratory compromise, the client may be hypotensive because of a mediastinal deviation. The PMI (point of maximal impulse) may be displaced on cardiac palpation.

The health care provider orders a chest x-ray examination and obtains a sample of the pleural fluid via thoracentesis for help in making the diagnosis (see Chapter 27). Empyema fluid is thick, opaque, exudative, and intensely foul smelling. The pleural fluid is sent to the laboratory and is analyzed for color, red blood cell count, white blood cell count and differential, glucose and protein levels, lactate dehydrogenase (LDH), and pH. Gram stains, acid-fast stains, and cytology studies are also performed. A protein concentration higher than 3 g/100 mL indicates an exudative process.

Interventions

Therapy for empyema is focused on emptying the empyema cavity, reexpanding the lung, and controlling the infection. The physician usually treats the client with antibiotics appropriate for the isolated pathogen. In addition, closed-chest drainage (see Chapter 30) is used to promote lung expansion. The physician places one or more chest tubes in the lower parts of the empyema sac. Underwater seal drainage is used without suction initially, but suction may be added if the lung fails to expand with gravity drainage alone. The physician removes the tube when the lung is fully expanded and the infectious process is under control. Open thoracotomy and removal of a portion of the pleura may be needed for thick pus or marked pleural thickening. Nursing considerations are the same as those for clients with a pleural effusion, pneumothorax, or infection.

ONLINE RESOURCES

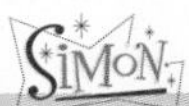

For suggested readings and Internet resources, go to http://www.wbsaunders.com/SIMON/Iggy/.

SELECTED BIBLIOGRAPHY

Asterisk indicates a classic or definitive work on this subject.

Abaza, M., Spiegel, J., & Sataloff, R. (1999). Managing uncommon causes of pharyngitis. *Hospital Medicine, 35*(1), 12-19.

Baek, C., et al. (2000). Polymerase chain reaction detection of Mycobacterium tuberculosis from fine-needle aspirate for the diagnosis of cervical tuberculosis lymphadenitis. *Laryngoscope, 110*(1), 30-34.

Brooks, J. (2001). Postoperative nosocomial pneumonia: Nurse-sensitive interventions. *AACN Clinical Issues: Advanced Practice in Acute and Critical Care, 12*(2), 305-323.

Centers for Disease Control and Prevention. (1997a). Pneumococcal and influenza vaccination among adults aged >65 years—United States, 1995. *Morbidity and Mortality Weekly Report, 46*(39), 913-919.

Centers for Disease Control and Prevention. (1997b). Recommendations of the Advisory Committee on immunization practices: Prevention of pneumococcal disease. *Morbidity and Mortality Weekly Report, 46*(RR 8), 1-24.

Centers for Disease Control and Prevention. (1999). Progress toward the elimination of tuberculosis—United States, 1998. *Morbidity and Mortality Weekly Report, 48*(33), 732-736.

Centers for Disease Control and Prevention. (2000). Update: Influenza activity—United States and worldwide, 1999-2000 season, and composition of the 2000-2001 influenza vaccine. *Morbidity and Mortality Weekly Report, 49*(17), 375-381.

Condos, R., Rom, W.N., & Schluger, N.W. (1997). Treatment of multidrug-resistant pulmonary tuberculosis with interferon-gamma via aerosol. *Lancet, 349,* 1513-1515.

Cotran, R., Kumar, V., & Collins, T. (1999). *Robbins' pathologic basis of disease* (6th ed.). Philadelphia: W.B. Saunders.

DiMatteo, L. (1999). Managing streptococcal pharyngitis: A review of clinical decision-managing strategies, diagnostic evaluation, and treatment. *Journal of the American Academy of Nurse Practitioners, 11*(2), 57-62.

*Finklestein, L., & Petrec, C.A. (1996). Sputum testing for TB: Getting good specimens. *American Journal of Nursing, 96*(2), 14.

Goolsby, M. (2001). Viral upper respiratory infections. *Journal of the American Academy of Nurse Practitioners, 13*(2), 50-54.

Hanchett, M. (1999). Clinical practice: New weapons in the struggle against TB. *Home Health Focus, 5*(11), 81, 83.

Harris, R. (1998). The integration of a tuberculosis control plan into a standard of care for tuberculosis. *MEDSURG Nursing, 7*(1), 19-27.

Harris, J., & Miller, T. (2000). Preventing nosocomial pneumonia: Evidence-based practice. *Critical Care Nurse, 20*(1), 51-67.

Harris, J., et al. (2000). Risk factors for nosocomial pneumonia in critically ill trauma patients. *AACN Clinical Issues: Advanced Practice in Acute and Critical Care, 11*(2), 198-231.

Johnson, J.M., & Force, R.W. (2000). Oseltamivir for flu prevention. *Journal of Family Practice, 49*(2), 183-184.

King, D.E., & Pippin, H.J. (1997). Community-acquired pneumonia in adults: Initial antibiotic therapy. *American Family Physician, 56*(2), 544-550.

Klein, L. (2001). Sinusitis: When to treat and how. *RN, 64*(1), 42-48.

Krouse, J. (1999). Introduction to sinus disease: I. Anatomy and physiology. *ORL—Head and Neck Nursing, 17*(2), 7-12.

Krouse, J., & Krouse, H. (1999). Introduction to sinus disease: II. Diagnosis and treatment. *ORL—Head and Neck Nursing, 17*(3), 6-17.

Leiner, S. (2000). Acute pharyngitis with lifelong implications. *The Nurse Practitioner,* 25(4), 119-122.

Lezon, K. (1999). Teaching incentive spirometry. *Nursing99, 29*(2), 61-62.

Loud, B. (2001). A WaterPik to clear sinuses? *RN, 64*(1), 48-49.

McCloskey, J., & Bulechek, G. (2000). *Nursing interventions classification (NIC)* (3rd ed.). St. Louis: Mosby.

McGrath, P. (2000). Address the rising levels of seasonal allergy. *Practice Nurse, 19*(6), 262-264, 268-269.

Phillips, G., & Togias, A. (1999). Allergic rhinitis: Up-to-date strategies for management. *Journal of Respiratory Diseases, 20*(9), 580-582, 585-588.

Poss, J. (2000). Factors associated with participation by Mexican migrant farmworkers in a tuberculosis screening program. *Nursing Research, 49*(1), 20-28.

United States Pharmacopeia Dispensing Information (USP DI): Vol. I. Drug information for the health care professional (20th ed.). (2000). Englewood, CO: Micromedix.

Vergis, E., et al. (2000). Azithromycin vs cefuroxime plus erythromycin for empirical treatment of community-acquired pneumonia in hospitalized patients. *Archives of Internal Medicine, 160*(9), 1294-1300.

CHAPTER 32

Interventions for Critically Ill Clients with Respiratory Problems

KATHLEEN ELLSTROM

Learning Objectives

After studying this chapter, you should be able to:

1. Identify clients at risk for development of pulmonary embolism.
2. Describe the clinical manifestations of pulmonary embolism.
3. Use laboratory data and clinical manifestations to determine the presence of acidosis.
4. Compare and contrast the ventilation-perfusion ratios for respiratory failure of ventilatory origin and respiratory failure of oxygenation origin.
5. Distinguish between normal and abnormal pulmonary capillary wedge pressure readings.
6. Use laboratory data and clinical manifestations to determine the adequacy of ventilatory interventions.
7. Describe the indications for intubation.
8. Prioritize nursing care for the conscious client being mechanically ventilated.
9. Identify clients at risk for development of pneumothorax.

Go to http://www.wbsaunders.com/SIMON/Iggy/ for self-assessment questions related to these Learning Objectives.

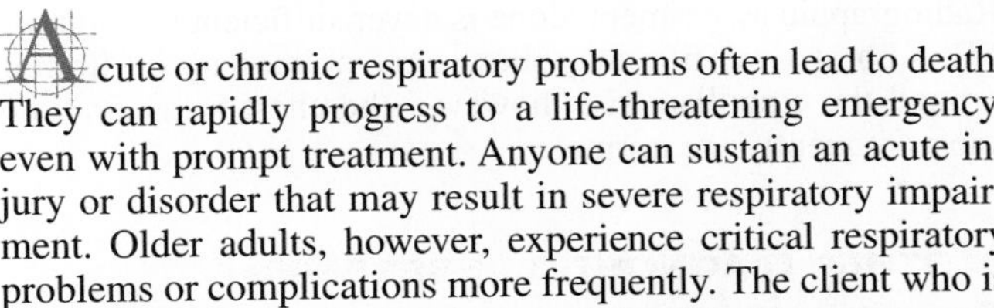

Acute or chronic respiratory problems often lead to death. They can rapidly progress to a life-threatening emergency, even with prompt treatment. Anyone can sustain an acute injury or disorder that may result in severe respiratory impairment. Older adults, however, experience critical respiratory problems or complications more frequently. The client who is short of breath is also anxious and fearful. The nurse must therefore be prepared to manage both the physical and emotional needs of the client during the respiratory emergency.

PULMONARY EMBOLISM

OVERVIEW

A **pulmonary embolism (PE)** is a collection of particulate matter (solids, liquids, or gaseous substances) that enters systemic venous circulation and lodges in the pulmonary vessels. Large emboli obstruct pulmonary circulation, leading to decreased systemic oxygenation, pulmonary tissue hypoxia, and potential death. Any substance can cause an embolism, but a blood clot is the most common.

Pathophysiology

PE is the most common acute pulmonary disease (90%) among hospitalized clients. In most people with PE, a blood clot from a deep vein thrombosis (DVT) breaks loose from one of the veins in the legs or the pelvis. The thrombus breaks off, travels through the vena cava and right side of the heart, and then lodges in a smaller blood vessel off of the pulmonary artery. Platelets collect behind the embolus, triggering the release of serotonin and thromboxane A_2, which causes vasoconstriction. Widespread pulmonary vasoconstriction and pulmonary hypertension impair ventilation and perfusion. Deoxygenated blood shunts into the arterial circulation to produce hypoxemia. Approximately 12% of clients with PE do *not,* however, have hypoxemia.

Etiology

The following are major risk factors for DVT leading to PE:

- Prolonged immobilization
- Surgery
- Obesity
- Advancing age
- Hypercoagulability
- History of thromboembolism

In addition, smoking, pregnancy, estrogen therapy, congestive heart failure, stroke, malignant neoplasms (particularly of the lung or prostate), Trousseau's syndrome, and major trauma increase the risk for DVT and PE.

Fat, oil, air, tumor cells, amniotic fluid, foreign objects (e.g., broken intravenous [IV] catheters), injected particles, and infected fibrin clots or pus can enter the venous system and cause

PE. Fat emboli from fracture of a long bone and oil emboli from lymphangiography do not impede blood flow; rather, they result in vascular injury and **acute respiratory distress syndrome (ARDS).** Amniotic fluid embolus is associated with a mortality rate of 80% to 90%; it occurs in 1 per 20,000 to 30,000 deliveries and can be a complication of abortion or amniocentesis. Septic emboli commonly arise from a pelvic abscess, an infected IV catheter, and nonsterile injections of illegal drugs. The problem with septic emboli lies in the toxic effects of the infection more than in the vascular occlusion.

CHART 32-1

KEY FEATURES *of* Pulmonary Embolism

Symptoms
- Dyspnea, sudden onset
- Pleuritic chest pain
- Apprehension, restlessness
- Feeling of impending doom
- Cough
- Hemoptysis

Signs
- Tachypnea
- Crackles
- Pleural friction rub
- Tachycardia
- S_3 or S_4 heart sound
- Diaphoresis
- Fever, low grade
- Petechiae over chest and axillae
- Decreased arterial oxygen saturation (Sa_{O_2})

Incidence/Prevalence

PE affects at least 500,000 people a year in the United States, approximately 10% of whom die. Many die within 1 hour of the onset of symptoms or before the diagnosis has even been suspected.

COLLABORATIVE MANAGEMENT

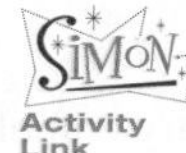

Assessment

HISTORY

The nurse questions any client with sudden onset of respiratory difficulty about the risk factors for PE, especially a history of DVT, recent surgery, or prolonged immobilization.

PHYSICAL ASSESSMENT/CLINICAL MANIFESTATIONS

RESPIRATORY MANIFESTATIONS. Chart 32-1 outlines the key features of PE. The nurse assesses the client for dyspnea accompanied by tachypnea, tachycardia, and pleuritic chest pain (sharp, stabbing-type pain on inspiration). These symptoms are found in 80% of clients diagnosed with PE. Other symptoms vary considerably depending on the severity and the type of embolism. Breath sounds may be normal, but crackles occur in 50% of clients with PE. The nurse typically notes a dry cough. **Hemoptysis** (blood sputum) may result from pulmonary infarction.

CARDIOVASCULAR MANIFESTATIONS. The nurse assesses for distended neck veins, **syncope** (fainting or loss of consciousness), cyanosis, and hypotension. Hypotension associated with massive emboli indicates acute pulmonary hypertension. Auscultation of heart sounds may reveal an S_3 or S_4 sound with an altered pulmonic component of S_2.

Electrocardiogram findings are abnormal, nonspecific, and transient. T-wave changes and ST-segment abnormalities develop in 50% of clients, but left- and right-axis deviations occur with equal frequency.

MISCELLANEOUS MANIFESTATIONS. A low-grade fever may be present. Petechiae may be present on the skin over the chest and in the axillae. Some clients have more vague symptoms resembling the flu, such as nausea, vomiting, and general malaise.

LABORATORY ASSESSMENT

The hyperventilation from hypoxia and pain initially leads to respiratory alkalosis, which the nurse confirms with low partial pressure of arterial carbon dioxide (Pa_{CO_2}) values on arterial blood gas (ABG) analysis. The alveolar-arterial (A-a) gradient is increased. As blood continues to be shunted without picking up oxygen from the lungs, the Pa_{CO_2} level starts to rise, leading to respiratory acidosis. Later, metabolic acidosis results from tissue hypoxia.

ABG studies and pulse oximetry may reveal hypoxemia, but these results alone are not sufficient for the diagnosis of PE. A client with a small embolus may not be hypoxemic, and PE is not the only cause of hypoxemia.

RADIOGRAPHIC ASSESSMENT

Radiographic assessment alone is never sufficient to diagnose PE. A chest x-ray film may show some pulmonary infiltration around the embolism site; however, the chest x-ray findings most frequently are normal.

OTHER DIAGNOSTIC ASSESSMENT

One of the most important studies to determine PE is the ventilation-perfusion ($\dot{V}/\dot{Q}$) lung scan. A negative perfusion scan rules out PE. If the $\dot{V}/\dot{Q}$ scan is inconclusive, pulmonary angiography, the most definitive and specific test for PE, may be done. Spiral computed tomography (CT) scans are increasingly being used to noninvasively diagnose PE.

In a few clients the physician performs thoracentesis (see Chapter 27) or transesophageal echocardiography (TEE) (see Chapter 33) for help in detecting PE. The physician often orders Doppler ultrasound studies or impedance plethysmography (IPG) to document the presence of DVT and to support a diagnosis of PE.

PSYCHOSOCIAL ASSESSMENT

Because the onset of symptoms is usually abrupt, the client with PE generally is extremely anxious and fearful. Hypoxemia may cause the client to have a sense of impending doom and increased restlessness. The emergency nature of the disorder and admission to an intensive care unit (ICU) may increase the client's anxiety and fear of death.

CHART 32-2

BEST PRACTICE *for* Prevention of Pulmonary Embolism

- Initiate passive and active range-of-motion exercises for the extremities of immobilized and postoperative clients.
- Ambulate postoperative clients soon after surgery.
- Use antiembolism and pneumatic compression stockings and devices postoperatively.
- Avoid the use of tight garters, girdles, and constricting clothing.
- Prevent pressure under the popliteal space (such as with a pillow).
- Perform a comprehensive appraisal of peripheral circulation.
- Elevate the affected limb 20 degrees or greater, above the level of the heart, to improve venous return, as appropriate.
- Change client position every 2 hours or ambulating as tolerated.
- Prevent injury to the vessel lumen by preventing local pressure, trauma, infection, or sepsis.
- Refrain from massaging or compressing leg muscles.
- Instruct client not to cross legs.
- Administer prophylactic low-dose anticoagulant and/or antiplatelet medication.
- Instruct the client to avoid activities that result in the Valsalva maneuver.
- Administer medications that will prevent episodes of the Valsalva maneuver, as appropriate.
- Instruct the client and/or family on appropriate precautions.
- Encourage smoking cessation.

Analysis

PREVENTION

Although pulmonary embolism (PE) can occur in apparently healthy people and may have no warning, it occurs more frequently in some situations. Thus prevention of conditions contributing to PE is a major nursing concern. Preventive actions for PE are those that also prevent venous stasis and DVT. Best practices for PE prevention are outlined in Chart 32-2.

The physician may order small doses of prophylactic heparin administered subcutaneously every 8 to 12 hours. Heparin prevents hypercoagulation in clients immobilized for a prolonged period, after trauma or surgery, or restricted to bedrest. Adequate fluid intake and avoidance of oral contraceptives are also preventive. Further information on the prevention of DVT is found in Chapter 17.

When a client complains of the acute onset of dyspnea with associated pleuritic chest pain, the physician is notified immediately. The client is given reassurance and assisted to a position of comfort with the head of the bed elevated. The nurse prepares for oxygen administration and blood gas analysis while continuing to monitor and assess for additional signs and symptoms.

COMMON NURSING DIAGNOSES AND COLLABORATIVE PROBLEMS

The primary collaborative problem for clients with PE is Hypoxemia related to an imbalanced $\dot{V}/\dot{Q}$ ratio.

The following are priority nursing diagnoses for clients with PE:

1. Decreased Cardiac Output related to acute pulmonary hypertension
2. Anxiety related to hypoxemia and life-threatening illness
3. Risk for Injury (Bleeding) related to anticoagulation thrombolytic therapy

ADDITIONAL NURSING DIAGNOSES AND COLLABORATIVE PROBLEMS

In addition to the common nursing diagnoses and collaborative problems, clients with PE may have one or more of the following:

- Activity Intolerance related to hypoxemia
- Impaired Gas Exchange related to disrupted pulmonary perfusion
- Fatigue related to ineffective gas exchange
- Impaired Oral Mucous Membrane related to oxygen therapy
- Acute Confusion related to hypoxemia
- Disturbed Sleep Pattern related to the ICU environment

Planning and Implementation

HYPOXEMIA

NOC **PLANNING: EXPECTED OUTCOMES.** The client with PE is expected to have adequate tissue perfusion in all major organs as evidenced by ABGs within normal limits (WNL) and $\dot{V}/\dot{Q}$ scan WNL.

INTERVENTIONS. Nonsurgical approaches to management of PE are most common. In some cases, surgical approaches may be needed in addition to drug therapy. NIC interventions for the client with PE are listed in Chart 32-3.

NONSURGICAL MANAGEMENT. Goals of management for PE are to increase alveolar gas exchange, improve pulmonary perfusion, eliminate the embolism, and prevent complications. Interventions include oxygen therapy, monitoring, and anticoagulation/antithrombolytic therapy.

OXYGEN THERAPY. Oxygen therapy is important for the client with PE (see Chapter 28). The severely hypoxemic client may require mechanical ventilation and close monitoring with arterial blood gas (ABG) studies. In less severe cases, oxygen may be administered by nasal cannula or mask. Pulse oximetry is useful in monitoring arterial oxygen saturation, which reflects the degree of hypoxemia.

MONITORING. The nurse assesses the client continually for any changes in status. Vital signs, lung sounds, and cardiac and respiratory status are assessed at least every 1 to 2 hours. Increasing dyspnea, dysrhythmias, distended neck veins, and pedal or sacral edema are documented. The nurse also notes the presence of crackles and adventitious sounds on auscultation of the lungs along with cyanosis of the lips, conjunctiva, oral mucous membranes, and nail beds.

ANTICOAGULATION/THROMBOLYTIC THERAPY. The physician usually orders anticoagulation to keep the embolus from enlarging and to prevent the formation of new clots. Active bleeding, stroke, and recent trauma are some contraindications to the use of anticoagulants. Before proceeding, the physician evaluates each client for risks and determines the risk versus the benefit of therapy.

CHART 32-3

NIC INTERVENTION ACTIVITIES *for* The Client with Pulmonary Embolism

Embolus Care: Pulmonary: *Limitation of complications for a client experiencing, or at risk for, occlusion of pulmonary circulation*

- Evaluate chest pain (e.g., intensity, location, radiation, duration, and precipitating and alleviating factors).
- Auscultate lung sounds for crackles or other adventitious sounds.
- Monitor respiratory pattern for symptoms of respiratory difficulty (e.g., dyspnea, tachypnea, and shortness of breath).
- Monitor determinants of tissue oxygen delivery (e.g., $Pa{O_2}$, $Sa{O_2}$, and hemoglobin levels and cardiac output), if available.
- Monitor for symptoms of inadequate tissue oxygenation (e.g., pallor, cyanosis, and sluggish capillary refill).
- Monitor for symptoms of respiratory failure (e.g., low $Pa{O_2}$ and elevated $Pa{CO_2}$ levels and respiratory muscle fatigue).
- Encourage good ventilation (e.g., incentive spirometry and cough and deep breathe every 2 hours).
- Monitor lab values for changes in oxygenation or acid-base balance, as appropriate.
- Instruct the client and/or family regarding diagnostic procedures (e.g., $\dot{V}/\dot{Q}$ scan), as appropriate.
- Encourage the client to relax.
- Monitor side effects of anticoagulant medications, if appropriate.

NIC intervention activities selected from McCloskey, J.C., & Bulechek, G.M. (Eds.). (2000). *Nursing interventions classification (NIC)* (3rd ed.). St. Louis: Mosby. No part of this work is to be altered without prior written permission from the Publisher.

$\dot{V}/\dot{Q}$, Ventilation-perfusion; *$Pa{O_2}$*, partial pressure of arterial oxygen; $Sa{O_2}$, arterial oxygen saturation; *$Pa{CO_2}$*, partial pressure of arterial carbon dioxide.

Heparin is commonly used unless the PE is massive or is accompanied by hemodynamic instability. A thrombolytic enzyme agent may then be used to break up the existing clot. The physician and nurse review the client's partial thromboplastin time (PTT)—also called activated partial thromboplastin time (aPTT)—before therapy is initiated, every 4 hours when therapy is initiated, and then usually daily thereafter. Therapeutic PTT values usually range between 1.5 and 2.5 times the control value.

Heparin therapy usually continues for 5 to 10 days. The physician starts most clients on a regimen of oral anticoagulants, such as warfarin (Coumadin, Warfilone✱), on the third day of heparin use. Therapy with both heparin and warfarin continues until the client has an International Normalized Ratio (INR) of 2.0 to 3.0. Heparin is then discontinued. The nurse and physician monitor the INR daily. The physician usually continues warfarin for 3 to 6 weeks, but some clients at high risk may take warfarin indefinitely. Charts 32-4 and 32-5 present the drugs used and laboratory tests monitored. Anticoagulants and associated nursing care are also discussed in Chapters 36 and 39.

SURGICAL MANAGEMENT. Two surgical procedures for the management of PE are embolectomy and inferior vena caval interruption.

EMBOLECTOMY. When thrombolytic enzyme therapy is contraindicated in a client with massive or multiple large pulmonary emboli with shock, surgical embolectomy may be necessary. **Embolectomy** is the removal of the embolus or emboli from the pulmonary arteries.

INFERIOR VENA CAVAL INTERRUPTION. The physician considers placing a vena caval filter as a lifesaving measure and to prevent further embolus formation for some clients. Candidates for this procedure include clients with an absolute contraindication to anticoagulation, recurrent or major bleeding while receiving anticoagulants, or septic PE, and those undergoing pulmonary embolectomy. The physician orders a pulmonary angiogram before placing the filter. Placement of a vena caval filter is detailed in Chapter 36.

DECREASED CARDIAC OUTPUT

PLANNING: EXPECTED OUTCOMES. The client with PE is expected to have adequate circulation.

INTERVENTIONS. In addition to the interventions used for hypoxemia induced by PE, IV fluid therapy and drug therapy are used to increase cardiac output.

INTRAVENOUS FLUID THERAPY. IV access is initiated and maintained for fluid and drug therapy. Fluid therapy involves administration of crystalloid solutions to restore plasma volume and prevent shock (see Chapter 37). The client with PE receiving IV fluids undergoes continuous cardiac monitoring and monitoring of pulmonary artery and central venous/right atrial pressures because the increased fluids can worsen pulmonary hypertension and contribute to right-sided heart failure.

DRUG THERAPY. When IV therapy alone is not effective in improving cardiac output, drug therapy with agents that increase myocardial contractility **(positive inotropic agents)** may be prescribed. Such agents include amrinone (Inocor) and dobutamine (Dobutrex). The nurse assesses the client's cardiac status hourly during therapy with inotropic agents. Vasodilators, such as nitroprusside (Nipride, Nitropress), may be used to decrease pulmonary artery pressure if it is impeding cardiac contractility.

ANXIETY

NOC **PLANNING: EXPECTED OUTCOMES.** The client with PE is expected to express a reduction in the level of anxiety and use effective coping strategies.

INTERVENTIONS. The client with PE is anxious and fearful for a variety of physiologic and psychologic reasons. Interventions for reducing anxiety in clients with PE include oxygen therapy (see the interventions for hypoxemia, p. 593), communication, and drug therapy.

COMMUNICATION. The nurse acknowledges the anxiety and the client's perception of a life-threatening situation. Speaking calmly and clearly, the nurse assures the client that appropriate measures are being taken. When administering a drug, changing position, taking vital signs, or obtaining assessment data, the nurse explains the rationale to the client and shares information appropriately.

DRUG THERAPY. If the client's anxiety increases or prevents adequate rest, an antianxiety drug may be prescribed. Unless the client is intubated and mechanically ventilated, agents that have a sedating effect are avoided.

CHART 32-4

DRUG THERAPY *for* Pulmonary Embolism

Drug	Usual Dosage	Nursing Interventions	Rationale
Heparin sodium (Hepalean✤)	5000-10,000 units IVP initially; then dose adjustment is based on PTT, 1300 units/hr on continuous drip or, less preferably, intermittent infusion	Monitor PTT. Know expected therapeutic PTT range for each client. Report PTT results. Monitor client for bleeding or bruising. Rebolus every time infusion is increased.	Ongoing assessment helps detect side effects and prevent complications. Reporting enables the physician to begin early treatment of a prolonged PTT.
		Do not use with salicylates.	An increased anticoagulation effect can occur with salicylates.
		Monitor platelets daily for thrombocytopenia.	White clot syndrome, a type of arterial thrombosis, can occur.
		Have the antidote, protamine sulfate, available.	Being prepared for an emergency helps prevent further complications.
		Avoid puncture sites and apply pressure to venipuncture and IM injection sites.	Pressure at puncture sites helps promote clotting.
		Avoid use of firm toothbrushes, straight razors, and rectal thermometers.	Safety measures help prevent bleeding.
Warfarin sodium (Coumadin, Warfilone sodium✤)	10-15 mg PO for 3 days initially; then dose adjustment is based on INR, usually 5-10 mg PO daily	Monitor INR. Know expected therapeutic INR range for each client. Report INR results. Monitor the client for bleeding or bruising.	Ongoing assessment helps detect side effects and prevent complications. Reporting enables the physician to begin early treatment of a prolonged INR.
		Monitor for fever and skin rash.	Adverse drug reaction can occur.
		Consult the pharmacist about potential drug interactions.	There are many drug interactions with warfarin.
		Have the antidote, vitamin K, available.	Being prepared for an emergency helps prevent further complications.
		Apply pressure to venipuncture and IM injection sites.	Pressure at puncture sites helps promote clotting.
		Avoid use of firm toothbrushes, straight razors, and rectal thermometers.	Safety measures help prevent bleeding.
		Teach the client which foods are high in vitamin K.	Food sources of vitamin K will alter INR.
Alteplase (tissue plasminogen activator, recombinant; tPA; Activase)	100 mg IV infusion over 2 hr	Assess for internal and external bleeding.	Bleeding is the most common adverse effect.
		Reconstitute with sterile water without preservative immediately before use.	Recommended preparation ensures drug stability.
		Administer with caution to clients who have been receiving aspirin, dipyridamole, heparin, or other anticoagulants.	Other drugs with anticoagulation effects increase the risk of bleeding.
Streptokinase	250,000-1,500,000 IU by IV infusion over 30 min as loading dose, then 100,000 IU/hr over 24-72 hr via continuous IV infusion pump	Draw blood samples for PTT and INR before starting infusion.	The rate of infusion depends on blood studies.
		Reconstitute and further dilute with sterile normal saline; roll to mix—do not shake.	Recommended preparation ensures drug stability.
		Monitor the client for internal and external bleeding.	Bleeding is a common adverse effect.
		Avoid IM injections, venipunctures, other invasive procedures, or excessive handling of the client during therapy.	Safety measures help prevent bleeding. Bruising is common.

IVP, Intravenous push, or bolus; *PTT,* partial thromboplastin time; *IU,* international units; *INR,* International Normalized Ratio.

CHART 32-5

LABORATORY PROFILE
Blood Tests Used to Monitor Anticoagulation Therapy

Test	Normal Range for Adults	Significance of Abnormal Findings
Partial thromboplastin time (PTT, aPTT [APTT])	Normal values for each local laboratory may vary. When activator reagents are used by the laboratory, the normal clotting time is shortened. Common normal ranges are 20-30 sec in some laboratories and 30-40 sec in others. Therapeutic range for PE is 1.5-2.5 times the normal value (e.g., if normal is 20-30 sec, then therapeutic range is 40-75 sec).	*Subtherapeutic times* may signify that the client is not receiving enough heparin to prevent extension of the blood clot. An increase in the dosage or rate of infusion is usually indicated. *Therapeutic times* mean that the clotting time is increased from normal, but this increase is indicated in the case of PE. *Prolonged times* in clients with PE (i.e., >75 sec) indicate that the client is at risk of serious spontaneous bleeding. Heparin is usually held or decreased unit the PTT drops back into the therapeutic range.
Prothrombin time (protime, PT)	11-12.5 sec Therapeutic range for anticoagulant therapy in PE is 1.5-2 times the normal or control value in seconds. Control values can vary day to day because reagents used may vary. If INR values are reported with the PT, therapeutic range for PE is 2.5-3.0, or 3.0-4.5 for recurrent PE.	*Subtherapeutic values* may signify that the client is not receiving enough warfarin. An increase in the dosage is usually indicated. *Therapeutic values* mean that the protime is increased from normal, but this increase is indicated in the case of PE. *Prolonged values* in the treatment of PE indicate that the client is at risk for bleeding. The warfarin dose is usually decreased or held, the client is instructed to eat foods high in vitamin K, or an injection of vitamin K may be given.

PE, Pulmonary embolism; *INR,* international normalized ratio; *aPTT* or *APTT,* activated partial thromboplastin time.

RISK FOR INJURY (BLEEDING)

PLANNING: EXPECTED OUTCOMES. The client with PE is expected to remain free from bleeding.

INTERVENTIONS. As a result of anticoagulation or thrombolytic therapy, the client's ability to initiate and continue the blood-clotting cascade when injured is seriously impaired, and he or she is at great risk for bleeding. The nurse's major objectives are to protect the client from situations that could lead to bleeding and to monitor closely the amount of bleeding that is occurring.

The nurse assesses frequently for evidence of bleeding in the form of oozing, confluent ecchymoses, petechiae, or purpura. All stools, urine, nasogastric drainage, and vomitus are examined visually for the appearance of blood and are tested for occult blood. The nurse measures any blood loss as accurately as possible. The client's abdominal girth is measured every 8 hours. Increases in abdominal girth can indicate internal hemorrhage. Best practices to prevent bleeding are outlined in Chart 32-6.

The nurse monitors laboratory values daily. The complete blood count (CBC) results are reviewed to determine the client's risk for bleeding, as well as to determine whether actual blood loss has occurred. If the client sustains a severe blood loss, packed red blood cells may be ordered (see the discussion of transfusion therapy in Chapter 40).

CHART 32-6

BEST PRACTICE *for*
Bleeding Precautions

- Handle the client gently.
- Use a lift sheet when moving or positioning the client in bed.
- Avoid IM injections and venipunctures.
- When injections are necessary, use the smallest gauge needle appropriate for the task.
- Apply firm pressure to the needle stick site for 10 minutes or until the site no longer oozes blood.
- Apply ice to areas of trauma.
- Test all urine and stool for the presence of occult blood.
- Check IV sites every 2 hours for bleeding.
- Avoid trauma to rectal tissue:
  - Do not take temperatures rectally.
  - Do not give enemas.
  - Administer well-lubricated suppositories with caution.
- Measure abdominal girth daily.
- If the client is to be shaved, use an electric razor.
- Use a soft-bristled toothbrush or tooth sponge for oral care.
- Inspect the mouth and gums for bleeding every 4 hours.
- Pad the siderails of the bed.
- Encourage the client not to blow the nose or insert objects into the nose.
- If the client is to ambulate, ensure that the footwear has a firm sole.

Community-Based Care

The client with pulmonary embolism (PE) is usually discharged after the embolism has been resolved but may continue anticoagulation therapy.

HEALTH TEACHING

The client with PE may continue anticoagulation therapy for weeks, months, or years after discharge, depending on the contributing factors. The nurse teaches the client and family about bleeding precautions, activities to reduce the risk for deep vein thrombosis (DVT) and recurrence of PE, signs and

CHART 32-7

CLIENT EDUCATION GUIDE
The Client After Pulmonary Embolism

- Use an electric razor.
- Use a soft-bristled toothbrush, and do not floss.
- Do not have dental work done without consulting your health care provider.
- Do not take aspirin or aspirin-containing products. Read the labels of all over-the-counter medications to be sure that the product does not contain aspirin or salicylates.
- Do not participate in contact sports or in any activity in which you might be bumped, scraped, or scratched.
- Apply ice immediately to any site of injury.
- Avoid anal intercourse.
- Take a stool softener to prevent straining during a bowel movement.
- Do not use enemas or rectal suppositories.
- Do not wear clothing that is tight or rubs.
- Avoid bending over at the waist.
- Avoid positions in which your knees are bent for any length of time.
- Wear elastic stockings as prescribed.
- Avoid prolonged sitting or standing.
- Avoid blowing your nose or placing objects in your nose. If you must blow your nose, do so gently without blocking either nasal passage.
- Take the prescribed dosage of medication at the precise time it was ordered to be given.
- Do not stop taking the medication abruptly or without a physician's order.
- Notify your doctor if you:
  Have an injury and persistent bleeding results.
  Have excessive menstrual bleeding.
  See blood in your urine or bowel movement.
  Notice large bruises or areas of small red or purple marks over the skin.

symptoms of complications, and the importance of follow-up care (Chart 32-7).

HOME CARE MANAGEMENT

Some clients will be discharged to home with minimal risk for recurrence and no permanent physiologic changes. Others may have extensive lung damage and require lifestyle modifications.

Clients with extensive lung damage may have activity intolerance and become fatigued easily. The living arrangements may need to be modified so that clients can spend all or most of the time on one floor and avoid stair climbing. Depending on the degree of impairment, clients may require some or much assistance with activities of daily living.

HEALTH CARE RESOURCES

For clients continuing with anticoagulation therapy, a home care nurse usually visits at least once per week to draw blood and perform an assessment (see Chart 32-8 for a focused assessment guide). Clients with severe dyspnea may require intermittent or continual home oxygen therapy. Respiratory therapy treatments can be performed in the home. The nurse or case manager coordinates arrangements for oxygen and other respiratory therapy to be available if needed at home.

CHART 32-8

FOCUSED ASSESSMENT *of*
Home Care Clients After Pulmonary Embolism

Assess respiratory status.
- Observe rate and depth of respiration.
- Auscultate lungs.
- Examine nail beds and mucous membranes for evidence of cyanosis.
- Take a pulse oximetry reading.
- Ask the client if chest pain or shortness of breath is experienced in any position.
- Ask the client about the presence of sputum and its color and character.

Assess cardiovascular status.
- Take vital signs, including apical pulse, pulse pressure; assess for presence or absence of orthostatic hypotension and quality and rhythm of peripheral pulses.
- Take blood pressure in both arms.
- Note presence or absence of peripheral edema.
- Examine hand vein filling in the dependent position.
- Examine neck vein filling in the recumbent and sitting positions.

Assess lower extremities for deep vein thrombosis.
- Examine lower legs and compare with each other for the following:
  General edema
  Calf swelling
  Surface temperature
  Presence of red streaks or cordlike palpable structure
- Measure calf circumference.
- Ask the client to dorsiflex and plantarflex each foot. Note the ease with which the client can do this, and ask whether pain is experienced in either position.
- Gently squeeze the calf of each leg laterally and from front to back. Ask the client whether pain or tenderness is experienced with either maneuver.

Assess for evidence of bleeding.
- Examine the mouth and gums for oozing or frank bleeding.
- Examine all skin areas for bruising or petechiae.
- If the client voids during the visit, test the urine for occult blood.

Assess cognition and mental status.
- Level of consciousness
- Orientation to time, place, and person
- Can the client accurately read a seven-word sentence containing no words greater than three syllables?

Assess the client's understanding of illness and compliance with treatment.
- Signs and symptoms to report to health care provider
- Medication plan (correct timing and dose)
- Bleeding precautions
- Prevention of deep vein thrombosis

Evaluation: Outcomes

NOC The nurse evaluates the care of the client with PE on the basis of the identified nursing diagnoses and collaborative problems. The expected outcomes are that the client:

- Attains and maintains adequate gas exchange and oxygenation as evidenced by arterial blood gases (ABGs) within normal limits (WNL) and ventilation-perfusion $\dot{V}/\dot{Q}$ scan WNL.
- Does not experience hypovolemia and shock
- Remains free from bleeding episodes
- States that levels of anxiety are reduced
- Uses effective coping strategies

CRITICAL THINKING CHALLENGE

The client is a 38-year-old woman admitted following a bicycle–motor vehicle accident. She has multiple pelvic fractures and multiple fractured ribs on the right side. On day three, during her bath, you notice petechiae over her axillae and chest. She has been requiring slowly increasing levels of oxygen to maintain good saturation.

- What is the most likely diagnosis for this client?
- For what other clinical manifestations should you assess?
- What additional information regarding her medical history should you obtain?

For suggested answer guidelines, go to SIMON http://www.wbsaunders.com/SIMON/Iggy/.

ACUTE RESPIRATORY FAILURE

OVERVIEW

Pathophysiology

Acute respiratory failure is categorized according to abnormal blood gases. The critical values are partial pressure of arterial oxygen (Pa_{O_2}) less than 60 mm Hg, arterial oxygen saturation (Sa_{O_2}) less than 90%, or partial pressure of arterial carbon dioxide (Pa_{CO_2}) greater than 50 mm Hg with accompanying acidemia (pH <7.30). Acute respiratory failure is further classified as *ventilatory failure, oxygenation failure,* or a *combination of both ventilatory and oxygenation failure.* Whatever the underlying disorder, the client in acute respiratory failure is always hypoxemic.

VENTILATORY FAILURE

Ventilatory failure is the type of ventilation-perfusion ($\dot{V}/\dot{Q}$) mismatching in which perfusion is normal but ventilation is inadequate. Ventilatory failure occurs when the thoracic pressure cannot be changed sufficiently to permit appropriate air movement into and out of the lungs. As a result, insufficient oxygen reaches the alveoli and carbon dioxide is retained. Both problems lead to hypoxemia.

Ventilatory failure is usually the result of one or more of the following three mechanisms: a mechanical abnormality of the lungs or chest wall, a defect in the respiratory control center in the brain, or an impairment in the function of the respiratory muscles. Ventilatory failure is usually defined by a Pa_{CO_2} level above 45 mm Hg in clients who have otherwise healthy lungs.

OXYGENATION FAILURE

In oxygenation failure, thoracic pressure changes are normal, and the lungs can move air sufficiently but cannot oxygenate the pulmonary blood properly. Oxygenation failure can result from the type of $\dot{V}/\dot{Q}$ mismatch in which ventilation is normal but perfusion is decreased.

COMBINED VENTILATORY AND OXYGENATION FAILURE

Combined ventilatory and oxygenation failure involves insufficient respiratory movements **(hypoventilation).** Gas exchange at the alveolar-capillary membrane is inadequate, so that too little oxygen reaches the blood and carbon dioxide is retained. The condition may or may not include poor pulmonary circulation. When pulmonary circulation is not adequate, $\dot{V}/\dot{Q}$ mismatching occurs and both ventilation and perfusion are inadequate. This type of respiratory failure results in a more profound hypoxemia than either ventilatory failure or oxygenation failure alone.

TABLE 32-1 • COMMON CAUSES OF VENTILATORY FAILURE

EXTRAPULMONARY CAUSES

Neuromuscular disorders
- Multiple sclerosis
- Myasthenia gravis
- Guillain-Barré syndrome
- Poliomyelitis

Spinal cord injuries affecting nerves to intercostal muscles

Central nervous system dysfunction
- Stroke
- Cerebral edema
- Increased intracranial pressure
- Meningitis

Chemical depression
- Opioid analgesics
- Sedatives
- Anesthetic agents

Kyphoscoliosis

Massive obesity

Sleep apnea

External obstruction/constriction

INTRAPULMONARY CAUSES

Airway disease
- Chronic obstructive pulmonary disease
- Asthma

Ventilation-perfusion ($\dot{V}/\dot{Q}$) mismatching
- Pulmonary embolism
- Pneumothorax
- Acute respiratory distress syndrome (ARDS)
- Amyloidosis
- Pulmonary edema
- Interstitial fibrosis

Etiology

VENTILATORY FAILURE

Numerous diseases and conditions can result in ventilatory failure. Causes of ventilatory failure are categorized as either **extrapulmonary** (involving nonpulmonary tissues but affecting respiratory function) or **intrapulmonary** (disorders of the respiratory tract). Table 32-1 lists common extrapulmonary and intrapulmonary causes of ventilatory failure.

OXYGENATION FAILURE

Many diseases and disorders of the lung can cause oxygenation failure. Mechanisms include impaired diffusion of oxygen at the alveolar level, right-to-left shunting of blood in the pulmonary vessels, $\dot{V}/\dot{Q}$ mismatching, breathing air with a low partial pressure of oxygen (a rare problem), and abnormal hemoglobin that fails to absorb the oxygen. In one type of $\dot{V}/\dot{Q}$ mismatching, areas of the lungs are still being perfused but gas exchange is not able to occur, which leads to hypoxemia. An extreme example of $\dot{V}/\dot{Q}$ mismatching is a right-to-left shunt. A normal shunt is less than 5% of cardiac output. With a right-to-left shunt, increased amounts of venous blood are not oxygenated, and 100% oxygen does not correct the defi-

TABLE 32-2 • COMMON CAUSES OF OXYGENATION FAILURE

- Low atmospheric oxygen concentration
  - High altitudes
  - Smoke inhalation
  - Carbon monoxide poisoning
- Pneumonia
- Abnormal hemoglobin
- Pulmonary embolism
- Pulmonary edema
- Interstitial pneumonitis-fibrosis
- Acute respiratory distress syndrome (ARDS)
- Mechanical obstruction
- Congestive heart failure
- Hypovolemic shock
- Hypoventilation

ciency. A classic cause of such a $\dot{V}/\dot{Q}$ mismatch is acute respiratory distress syndrome (ARDS). Table 32-2 lists specific causes of oxygenation failure.

COMBINED VENTILATORY AND OXYGENATION FAILURE

A combination of ventilatory failure and oxygenation failure occurs in clients who have abnormal lungs, such as those who have any form of **chronic airflow limitation (CAL),** such as chronic bronchitis, emphysema, or asthma). The bronchioles and alveoli are diseased (causing oxygenation failure), and the work of breathing increases until the respiratory muscles are unable to continue (causing ventilatory failure). Acute respiratory failure results. This process can also occur in clients who have cardiac failure, as well as respiratory failure. This is a very dangerous situation because the cardiac system cannot compensate for the decreased oxygen by increasing the cardiac output.

COLLABORATIVE MANAGEMENT

Assessment

The nurse assesses for **dyspnea** (difficulty breathing), the hallmark of respiratory failure. With use of a dyspnea assessment guide (Figure 32-1), if one is available, the nurse objectively evaluates the dyspnea. Depending on the process, nature, and course of the underlying condition, the client may or may not be aware of dyspnea. In addition, the client needs to be alert enough to perceive the sensation of difficult breathing.

Dyspnea tends to be more intense when it develops rapidly. Slowly progressive respiratory failure may first manifest as dyspnea on exertion (DOE) or when lying down. The client notes **orthopnea,** finding it is easier to breathe in an upright position. In the client with chronic respiratory problems, a minor increase in dyspnea from the baseline condition may represent severe gas exchange abnormalities.

The nurse assesses for a change in the client's respiratory rate or pattern, a change in lung sounds, and the signs and symptoms of hypoxemia and hypercapnia (see Chapter 31). Pulse oximetry may indicate decreased oxygen saturation, but an arterial blood gas (ABG) analysis is needed for adequate assessment of oxygenation status. The health care provider reviews the ABG studies to identify the degree of hypercapnia and hypoxemia.

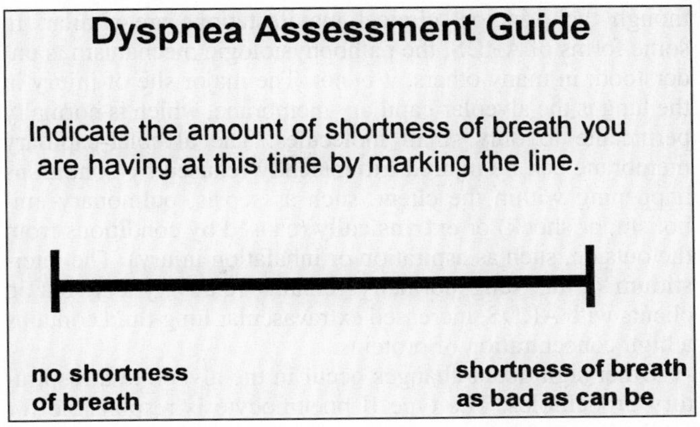

Dyspnea Assessment Guide

Indicate the amount of shortness of breath you are having at this time by marking the line.

no shortness of breath | shortness of breath as bad as can be

Figure 32-1 ● A dyspnea assessment tool. (Modified from Gift, A. [1989]. A dyspnea assessment guide. *Critical Care Nurse, 9*[8], 79, 82-88.)

Interventions

The physician orders oxygen therapy for the client with acute respiratory failure to keep the partial pressure of arterial oxygen ($Pa O_2$) level above 60 mm Hg while treating the underlying cause of the respiratory failure. Oxygen therapy is discussed in detail in Chapter 28. If supplemental oxygen cannot maintain acceptable $Pa O_2$ levels, the physician may order mechanical ventilation.

The nurse or assistive nursing personnel helps the client find a position of comfort that allows easier breathing. To decrease the anxiety commonly associated with dyspnea, the nurse assists with interventions such as relaxation, guided imagery, and diversion. Energy-conserving measures, such as minimal self-care and no unnecessary procedures, are instituted. The physician may order pulmonary medications administered systemically or by metered dose inhaler (MDI) to open the bronchioles and promote gas exchange. The client is instructed about the use of the inhaler and about the medications. Deep breathing and other breathing exercises are encouraged. (See Chapter 31 for further discussion of interventions for dyspnea and hypoxemia.)

ACUTE RESPIRATORY DISTRESS SYNDROME

OVERVIEW

Acute respiratory distress syndrome (ARDS) is a form of acute respiratory failure characterized by the following:

- Refractory hypoxemia
- Decreased pulmonary compliance
- Dyspnea
- Noncardiogenic bilateral pulmonary edema
- Dense pulmonary infiltrates (ground-glass appearance)

ARDS usually occurs after an acute catastrophic event in people with no previous pulmonary disease. The mortality rate remains at 50% to 60% despite continuing research. Terminology for ARDS includes the current term **noncardiogenic pulmonary edema** and the former term **shock lung.**

Pathophysiology

Despite diverse causes leading to injury of the lung in ARDS, no common pathway has been found in its development, although the principal clinical manifestations are similar. In some forms of ARDS, the pathophysiologic mechanism is understood; in many others, it is not. The major site of injury in the lung is the alveolar-capillary membrane, which is normally permeable to only small molecules. The alveolar-capillary membrane can be injured **intrinsically** (caused by conditions happening within the client, such as sepsis, pulmonary embolism, or shock) or **extrinsically** (caused by conditions from the outside, such as aspiration or inhalation injury). The interstitium of the lung normally remains relatively dry, but in clients with ARDS, increased extravascular lung fluid contains a high concentration of proteins.

Other significant changes occur in the alveoli and respiratory bronchioles. The type II pneumocyte is responsible for producing surfactant, a substance that maintains the elasticity of lung tissue and prevents alveolar collapse on expiration. Surfactant activity is reduced in ARDS either because of destruction of the type II pneumocyte or inactivation or dilution of surfactant. Consequently, the alveoli become unstable and tend to collapse unless they are filled with fluid from the interstitial space. These alveoli can no longer participate in gas exchange. As a result, interstitial edema forms around terminal airways, which are compressed and obliterated. Lung volume is further reduced, and there is even less **compliance** (elasticity). As the leak expands, fluid, protein, and blood cells collect in the interstitium and alveoli. Lymph channels are compressed and ineffective. Poorly ventilated alveoli receive blood. Thus the shunt fraction increases, and hypoxemia and ventilation-perfusion ($\dot{V}/\dot{Q}$) mismatching result.

Etiology

ARDS is associated with a number of causative factors (Table 32-3). Some causes involve direct injury to lung tissue; others do not directly involve the respiratory system. Serious nervous system injury, such as trauma, strokes, tumors, and sudden increases in cerebrospinal fluid pressure, may cause massive sympathetic discharge. Systemic vasoconstriction results, with redistribution of large volumes of blood into the pulmonary circuit. The marked elevation of hydrostatic pressure, then, probably causes lung injury. Processes that produce cerebral hypoxia, such as shock and ascent to high altitudes, may operate by a similar mechanism.

Some factors produce ARDS by direct injury to the lung. For example, aspiration of gastric contents leads to mechanical obstruction or produces an acid burn to the airway when the pH of the gastric contents is less than 2.5. In such a direct injury, rapid necrosis of the alveolar type I pneumocyte occurs. The injured capillary endothelium allows protein and cellular elements to escape from the intravascular space. Radiation, near-drowning, and inhalation of toxic gases similarly injure the alveolar and capillary endothelium. In addition, trauma, sepsis, drowning, and burns cause the release of thromboplastins, which form fibrin clots in the peripheral blood. The clots, together with platelets and leukocytes, are filtered out in the lung. In many cases of ARDS, especially after trauma, production of plasminogen activation inhibitors by the liver is enhanced. **Fibrinolysis** (clot breakdown) is prevented, and small emboli remain in the lung. Disseminated intravascular coagulation (DIC) plays a role in some clients.

TABLE 32-3 • COMMON CAUSES OF ACUTE RESPIRATORY DISTRESS SYNDROME

- Shock
- Trauma
- Serious nervous system injury
- Pancreatitis
- Fat and amniotic fluid emboli
- Pulmonary infections
- Sepsis
- Inhalation of toxic gases (smoke, oxygen)
- Pulmonary aspiration
- Drug ingestion (e.g., heroin, opioids, aspirin)
- Hemolytic disorders
- Multiple blood transfusions
- Cardiopulmonary bypass
- Near-drowning (especially in fresh water)

Incidence/Prevalence

Because of varying definitions, the incidence of ARDS is unknown, although a 1995 estimate suggested that 150,000 to 250,000 cases of ARDS occur yearly in the United States. Its high rank on the list of common diseases may be a result of the improved treatment of other catastrophic illnesses.

A major goal in the prevention of ARDS is early recognition of clients at high risk for the syndrome. Because clients with aspiration of gastric contents are at great risk, the nurse closely assesses and monitors older clients receiving tube feeding and those with neurologic deficits and altered swallowing and gag reflexes. All personnel meticulously follow all infection control guidelines, including handwashing, invasive catheter and wound care, and body substance precautions. In addition, the nurse carefully observes clients who are being treated for any of the diseases or disorders associated with ARDS.

COLLABORATIVE MANAGEMENT

Assessment

The nurse assesses the client's respirations and notes whether increased work of breathing is evident, as indicated by hyperpnea, grunting respiration, cyanosis, pallor, and retraction **intercostally** (between the ribs) or **suprasternally** (above the ribs). The presence of diaphoresis and any change in mental status is documented. No abnormal lung sounds are present on auscultation because the edema of acute respiratory distress syndrome (ARDS) occurs first in the interstitial spaces and not in the airways. Vital signs are monitored at least hourly to assess for hypotension, tachycardia, and dysrhythmias.

The primary laboratory study for establishing the diagnosis of ARDS is a lowered partial pressure of arterial oxygen (Pa_{O_2}) value, determined by arterial blood gas (ABG) measurements. Because a widening alveolar oxygen gradient (increased fraction of inspired oxygen [F_{IO_2}] does not yield corresponding increased Pa_{O_2} levels) develops with increased shunting of blood, the client has a progressive need for higher concentrations of oxygen. However, the client with ARDS is poorly responsive to high concentrations of oxygen **(refractory hypoxemia)** and invariably requires intubation and mechanical ventilation. A large difference between the predicted and actual alveolar oxygen tension indicates shunting. The physician orders sputum cultures to isolate any organisms causing an infection that must be treated. Because decreased mortality depends on aggressive therapy, sputum may be obtained through bronchoscopy with protective brushings and by transtracheal aspiration.

The chest x-ray film shows the diagnostic diffuse haziness or "whited-out" (ground-glass) appearance of the lung. An electrocardiogram rules out cardiac abnormalities and usually reveals no specific changes. The placement of a Swan-Ganz hemodynamic monitoring catheter is a diagnostic tool: in the client with ARDS, the pulmonary capillary wedge pressure (PCWP) is usually low to normal. This pressure differs from that in the client with cardiogenic pulmonary edema, in whom the PCWP is higher than 15 mm Hg.

Interventions

The client with ARDS usually requires endotracheal intubation and mechanical ventilation with positive end-expiratory pressure (PEEP) or continuous positive airway pressure (CPAP). Sedation and paralysis may be necessary for adequate ventilation and for reducing oxygen requirements. Because one of the side effects of PEEP is tension pneumothorax, the nurse assesses lung sounds frequently and maintains a patent airway with suctioning. Positioning may be important in promoting gas exchange.

DRUG AND FLUID THERAPY. Corticosteroids are seldom used in the treatment of ARDS, although they may help decrease neutrophil mobilization and stabilize the capillary membrane. Their effectiveness, however, has not been determined. Antibiotics are used to treat infections with organisms identified by culture.

Many interventions are under investigation, but none has been shown to be effective in decreasing mortality. Some of these interventions include mediators (vitamins C and E, interleukin, prostacyclin, aspirin), nitric oxide, surfactant replacement, and prone positioning.

The optimal type of fluid therapy for the client with ARDS remains unknown. A colloidal solution may be effective for intravascular volume expansion. Fluid volume should be titrated to maintain adequate cardiac output and tissue perfusion. Induced diuresis may help decrease lung edema, but care should be taken to prevent overall dehydration and hypotension.

NUTRITION THERAPY. The client with ARDS is at risk for malnutrition, which further compromises the respiratory system. An altered immune response, as well as an altered ventilatory response to hypoxemia, may occur with undernourished clients. Diaphragm function is also altered. Therefore enteral nutrition in the form of tube feeding or parenteral nutrition in the form of hyperalimentation is instituted as soon as possible.

CASE MANAGEMENT. Case management of the client with ARDS focuses on the phases of ARDS rather than day-to-day care. The course of ARDS and its management are divided into four phases:

Phase 1. This phase includes early changes with the client exhibiting dyspnea and tachypnea. Early interventions focus on supporting the client and providing oxygen.

Phase 2. Patchy infiltrates form from increasing pulmonary edema. Interventions include mechanical ventilation and prevention of complications.

Phase 3. This phase occurs over days 2 to 10, and the client exhibits progressive refractory hypoxemia. Interventions focus on maintaining adequate oxygen transport, preventing complications, and supporting the failing lung until it has had time to heal.

Phase 4. Pulmonary fibrosis pneumonia with progression occurs after 10 days. This phase is irreversible and is frequently referred to as "late" or "chronic" ARDS. Interventions focus on preventing sepsis, pneumonia, and multiple organ dysfunction syndrome (MODS), as well as weaning the client from the ventilator. The client in this phase may be ventilator dependent for weeks to months. He or she may be cared for in specialized units or facilities that focus on rehabilitation and long-term weaning. Some clients may not be weanable and go home ventilator dependent (see the Clinical Pathway on pp. 1855 and 1856).

THE CLIENT REQUIRING INTUBATION AND VENTILATION

OVERVIEW

Through the use of mechanical ventilation, the client who has severe problems of gas exchange may be supported until the underlying process has resolved or has been adequately treated. Thus mechanical ventilation is nearly always a temporary life support technique. The need for ventilatory support may, however, be lifelong, especially for those clients with chronic, progressive neuromuscular diseases that preclude effective spontaneous ventilation.

Mechanical ventilation is most commonly used for clients with hypoxemia and progressive alveolar hypoventilation with respiratory acidosis. The hypoxemia is usually due to intrapulmonary shunting of blood when external devices cannot provide a sufficiently high fraction of inspired oxygen (FIO_2). Mechanical ventilation is also indicated for clients who need respiratory support after surgery, who are barely maintaining adequate gas exchange at the cost of expending energy with the high work of breathing, or who require general anesthesia or heavy sedation to allow diagnostic or therapeutic interventions.

COLLABORATIVE MANAGEMENT

Assessment

The nurse assesses the client about to undergo intubation in the same way as for other respiratory problems. Once mechanical ventilation has been initiated, the respiratory system is assessed on an ongoing basis. The nurse monitors and assesses for complications related to the artificial airway or ventilator, as well as for those related to mechanical ventilation.

Interventions

ENDOTRACHEAL INTUBATION. The client who needs mechanical ventilation requires an artificial airway. The most common type of artificial airway for establishing and maintaining the airway on a short-term basis is the endotracheal

(ET) tube. If the client requires an artificial airway for longer than a specified period, usually longer than 10 to 14 days, the physician considers a tracheostomy (see Chapter 28) to avoid mucosal and vocal cord damage.

The goals of intubation include maintaining a patent airway, reducing the work of breathing, providing a means to remove secretions, and providing ventilation and oxygen. Major indications for intubation are listed in Table 32-4.

ENDOTRACHEAL TUBE. An ET tube is a long polyvinyl chloride tube that is passed through the mouth or nose and into the trachea (Figure 32-2). When properly positioned, the tip of the ET tube rests approximately 0.8 to 1.2 inches (2 to 3 cm) above the carina (where the trachea divides into the right and left mainstem bronchi). Oral intubation is the easiest and quickest method of establishing an airway; therefore it is also performed as an emergency procedure. The nasal route is reserved for elective intubation, for some facial or oral traumas and surgeries, and when oral intubation is not possible. This route is contraindicated if the client has a blood dyscrasia. An experienced, specially trained professional, such as an anesthesiologist, nurse anesthetist, or pulmonologist (physician), performs the intubation.

An ET tube has several parts (see Figure 32-2). The shaft of the tube contains a radiopaque vertical line for the length of the tube, which permits demonstration of correct placement by chest x-ray examination. Short horizontal lines (depth markings) are used to designate correct placement of the tube at the nares or mouth (at the incisor tooth) and to identify how far the tube has been inserted.

The cuff at the distal end of the tube, with proper inflation, produces a seal between the trachea and the cuff. The seal ensures delivery of a set tidal volume when mechanical ventilation is used. When the cuff is inflated to an adequate sealing volume, no air can pass through the cuff to the vocal cords, nose, or mouth; therefore the client is not able to talk when the cuff is inflated. The cuff should be inflated to a pressure of 20 to 25 cm H_2O using minimal-leak or no-leak techniques.

The pilot balloon with a one-way valve permits air to be inserted into the cuff and yet prevents air from escaping. This balloon is used as a general guideline for determining the absence or presence of air in the cuff, although it will not show how much or how little air is present.

The universal adaptor, which is 15 mm in diameter, enables attachment to ventilator tubing or other types of oxygen delivery systems. The tubing size is indicated on the adaptor or the shaft of the tube. Adult tube sizes range from 5 to 10 mm. Sizes used are 8.0 to 9.0 for large adults, 7.0 to 8.0 for medium-size adults, and 6.0 to 7.0 for small adults.

TABLE 32-4 • MAJOR INDICATIONS FOR INTUBATION

- Airway protection when the client loses reflexes because of anesthesia, medications, disease, or decreased level of consciousness
- To provide positive pressure or high oxygen concentration
- To bypass airway obstruction
- Facilitating pulmonary hygiene and suctioning of secretions when the client cannot handle secretions (as in diseases of chronic airflow limitation)

PREPARING FOR INTUBATION. The nurse and assistive nursing personnel know the proper procedure for summoning intubation personnel to the bedside in an emergency situation. The nurse explains the procedure to the client as clearly as possible under the circumstances. Basic life support measures, such as the establishment of a patent airway and the administration of 100% oxygen via a resuscitation (Ambu) bag with a face mask, are crucial to the client's survival until help arrives. The coordination for resuscitation with a bag and mask device can be cumbersome; therefore practice is necessary.

In an emergency the nurse or assistive personnel brings the code (or "crash") cart, respiratory equipment box, and suction equipment (which is often already on the code cart) to the bedside. The nurse maintains a patent airway through positioning and the insertion of an oral airway until the client is intubated. During intubation the nurse continuously monitors for changes in vital signs, signs of hypoxia or hypoxemia, dysrhythmias, and aspiration. The nurse also ensures that each intubation attempt lasts no longer than 30 seconds, preferably less than 15 seconds. After 30 seconds, oxygen is provided by means of a mask and manual resuscitation bag to prevent hypoxia and potential cardiac arrest. Suctioning is performed as necessary.

VERIFYING TUBE PLACEMENT. Immediately after an ET tube is inserted, its placement must be verified. The most

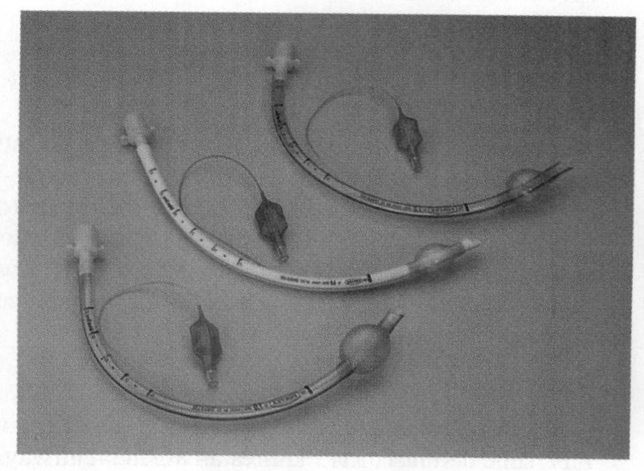

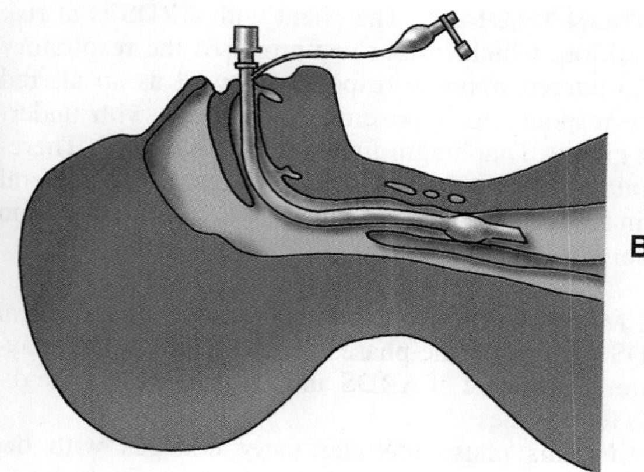

Figure 32-2 • **A,** Endotracheal tubes. **B,** Correct placement of an oral endotracheal tube. (**A** Courtesy Sims Porter, Inc.)

accurate way of verifying placement is by checking end-tidal carbon dioxide concentration, if available. The nurse assesses for bilateral equal breath sounds, bilateral equal chest excursion, and air emerging from the ET tube. If breath sounds and chest wall movement are absent on the left side, the tube may be in the right mainstem bronchus. The person intubating the client should be able to reposition the tube without repeating the entire intubation procedure.

The nurse auscultates over the stomach to rule out esophageal intubation. If the tube is in the stomach, louder breath sounds are heard over the stomach than over the chest and abdominal distention may be present. Chest wall movement and breath sounds are continuously monitored until tube placement is verified by chest x-ray examination.

STABILIZING THE TUBE. The nurse, respiratory therapist, or anesthesia personnel stabilize the ET tube at the mouth or nose. The tube is marked at the level at which it touches the incisor tooth or naris. Two persons working together use a head halter technique to secure the tube. Chart 32-9 outlines best practices for securing an oral or nasal ET tube.

An oral airway may also need to be inserted to keep the client from biting an oral tube. One person stabilizes the tube at the correct position and prevents head movement while a second person applies the tape. After the procedure is completed, the nurse verifies the presence of bilateral and equal breath sounds and the level of the tube.

NURSING CARE. The nurse assesses tube placement, cuff pressure, breath sounds, and chest wall movement regularly. The nurse prevents pulling or tugging on the tube by the client to prevent dislodgment or "slipping" of the tube and checks the pilot balloon to ensure that the cuff is inflated. Suctioning, coughing, and speaking attempts place extra stress on the tube and also can cause dislodgment (see the Cost of Care box on p. 605). Neck flexion moves the tube away from the carina; neck extension moves the tube closer to the carina. Rotation of the head also causes the tube to move. Mouth secretions and tongue movement can loosen the tape and allow malposition of the tube. When other measures fail, the nurse applies soft wrist restraints, as ordered, for the client who is voluntarily or involuntarily pulling on the tube. This intervention is a last resort to prevent accidental extubation. Adequate sedation (chemical restraint) may be necessary to decrease agitation or prevent extubation. The nurse obtains permission for restraints from the client or family after explaining the rationale. More information on management of the artificial airway is found in Chapter 28.

Complications of an ET or nasotracheal tube can occur at each stage of the process: during placement, while in place, during extubation, or after extubation (either early or late). Trauma and complications can occur to the face; eye; nasal and paranasal areas; oral, pharyngeal, bronchial, tracheal, and pulmonary areas; esophageal and gastric areas; and cardiovascular, musculoskeletal, and neurologic systems.

MECHANICAL VENTILATION. Mechanical ventilation to support and maintain respiratory function is widely used on medical-surgical units, in nursing homes, and in the home setting, as well as in critical care units. The nurse plays a pivotal role in the coordination of care and the prevention of complications. Chart 32-10 reviews best practices for care of the client during mechanical ventilation.

The goals of mechanical ventilation are to improve oxygenation and ventilation and decrease the amount of oxygen and work needed to accomplish an effective breathing pattern. Mechanical ventilation is used to support the client until lung function is adequate or until the acute episode has passed. A ventilator does not cure diseased lungs; it provides ventilation until the lungs are able to resume the process of breathing. Therefore the nurse must remember why the client is using the ventilator so that aggressive attempts to correct the underlying cause of the respiratory failure are always at the forefront of the management plan. If normal oxygenation, ventilation, and respiratory muscle strength are achieved, mechanical ventilation can be discontinued.

TYPES OF VENTILATORS. A wide variety of ventilators are available. The ventilator selected depends on the severity of the disease process and the length of time that ventilator support is required. Two major types of ventilators are negative-pressure and positive-pressure ventilators.

Negative-Pressure Ventilators. The negative-pressure ventilator is noninvasive (Figure 32-3). The iron lung, widely used during the poliomyelitis epidemic in the 1940s, is the prototype for the negative-pressure ventilator. The client is placed in an airtight apparatus that surrounds either the chest area or the entire body and leaves the head exposed. During inspiration, with the expansion of the chest wall, negative pressure is generated in the chest cavity. Because of the pressure gradient, air rushes from the atmosphere (high pressure) into the thoracic cavity (low pressure). At a preset time, negative pressure ceases and expiration occurs. Thus negative-pressure ventilators create pressure gradients that mimic normal physiologic ventilation.

Newer negative-pressure ventilators include the cuirass, poncho, and body wrap. These ventilators are used for clients with neuromuscular disease, central nervous system disorders, spinal cord injuries, and chronic obstructive pulmonary disease (COPD). Clients may use negative-pressure ventilation for home nighttime ventilatory support so that their muscles can rest. Advantages are that an artificial airway is not required and the newer models are lightweight and easy to use. The enclosing ventilator makes some direct nursing care more difficult. The client must be able to clear oral secretions and must have compliant (elastic) lungs to benefit from this mode of ventilation.

Positive-Pressure Ventilators. The positive-pressure ventilator is the most widely used type of ventilator in the acute care setting. During inspiration, pressure is generated that pushes air into the lungs and expands the chest. In most instances an endotracheal (ET) tube or tracheostomy is needed. Positive-pressure ventilators are classified according to the mechanism that ends inspiration and starts expiration. Inspiration is terminated or cycled in three major ways: pressure cycled, time cycled, or volume cycled.

Pressure-Cycled Ventilators. Pressure-cycled ventilators (which are infrequently used) push air into the lungs until a preset airway pressure is reached. Tidal volumes and inspiratory time are variable. Pressure-cycled ventilators may be used for short periods, such as in the postanesthesia care unit and for respiratory therapy.

CHART 32-9

BEST PRACTICE *for*
Securing an Oral and Nasal Endotracheal Tube

Little evidence is available to provide clinical direction on the best method to secure endotracheal (ET) and nasotracheal tubes. However, adhesive tape is the easiest, cheapest, and most frequently used.

Adhesive tape may be irritating to the skin, and frequent tape changes may disrupt the skin integrity. An additional reported complication is nosocomial cutaneous mucormycosis occurring around the surgical tape securing the ET tube. Protecting the skin, especially on the face, is a high priority for patients and nurses. This must be balanced against making sure the ET tube is not dislodged. A simple yet effective method of securing the oral and nasotracheal tube is demonstrated here:

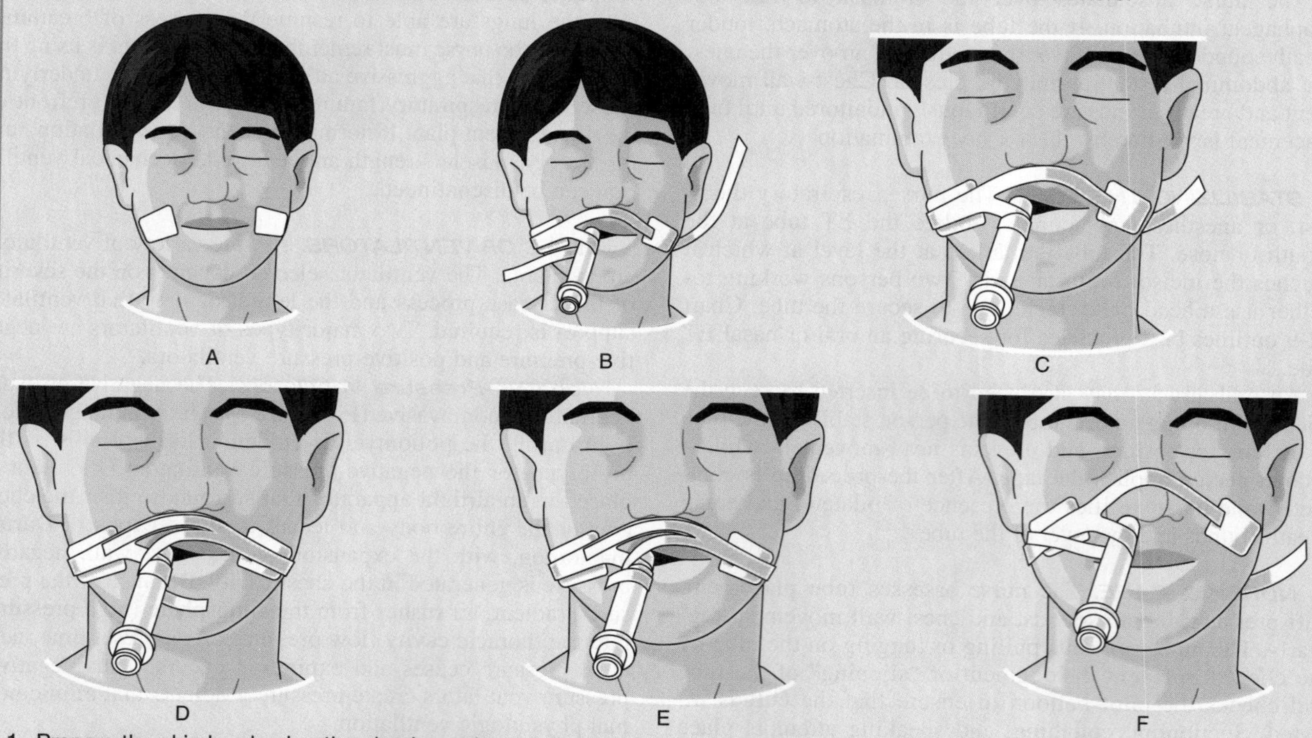

1. Prepare the skin by shaving the cheeks and upper lip, if possible.
2. Protect the skin by applying tincture of benzoin to the skin and ET tube and allow to dry (Mastisol may also be used, but Detachol **must** be used before removing the tape); then apply a 1 × 3 inch piece of thin DuoDerm or other protective or hydrocolloid membrane to the skin on the cheeks *(A)*.
3. Take a 30-inch (about 2½-foot) piece of adhesive tape and lay it on a flat surface, sticky side up. Take another piece of tape (about 10 inches) and cover the middle portion of the tape (sticky side to sticky side) to protect the back of the patient's neck. A tongue blade on each end folded over can keep it from getting tangled or sticking prematurely.
4. Place the tape behind the patient's neck. Remove the tongue blades and place the tape on the protective membrane up to the end of the mouth on each side. Trim the tape as needed and split each end of the tape.
5. Take the upper part of one end of the tape and place it on the upper lip. Take the lower part of the tape and wrap it securely around the tube *(B, C)*. Take the upper part of the other end of the tape, place it on the upper lip, and wrap the lower part securely around the tube *(D, E)*. Do not have the tube too far to either side of the mouth, or it can cause skin breakdown in the corner of the mouth or lips.
6. The same method can be used for nasal tubes, but do not tape the tube too tightly to the nose or skin breakdown will occur on the nares *(F)*.
7. Always tape the tube to the upper lip, never the lower. The lower jaw moves too much with attempts to speak or oral care, which will move the tube and cause irritation and discomfort for the patient. The tape should be inspected at least every shift for signs of loosening or skin irritation or breakdown, especially with increased oral secretions. Tightness of the tape should also be checked each shift if swelling in the face and neck occurs or if there is an increase in fluid retention (as in anasarca, sepsis, or acute respiratory distress syndrome).

An additional technique for securing tubing that can decrease ET tube movement and provide a fulcrum for pulling on ventilator tubing is to attach a 6-inch (50-mL) piece of flexible ventilator tubing between the ET tube adaptor and the Y-connector of the ventilator tubing. The procedure for this technique is as follows:

1. Shave the chest or clean with alcohol a portion of the chest at right angles to the angle of Louis. Apply tincture of benzoin and allow to dry.
2. Prepare Montgomery straps by taking two 6-inch pieces of 2-inch wide adhesive tape. Double-back one end of each piece of tape, and cut a small hole in the ends that are doubled over.
3. Apply the tape to the prepared chest with the ends with the hole over each other. Take a 12-inch piece of twill (trach) tape and thread through both holes. Position the tubing with the Y-connector over the holes and tie into place. This procedure allows all pulling on the tubing to place strain on the tape (straps) and not on the face or the tube. Caution should be taken if patients have increased partial pressure of arterial carbon dioxide retention, and end-tidal carbon dioxide monitoring may be useful when weaning.

COST OF CARE IMPLICATIONS FOR NURSING

THE CLIENT BEING MECHANICALLY VENTILATED

Cost of Care

Studies evaluating cost examine long-term ventilation costs rather than short-term costs. Inferences can be made, however, by considering length of stay as correlated with costs. Rosen and Bone (1990) discussed the financial implications of ventilator costs. Nonphysician charges for hospital care in clients intubated at least 48 hours averaged about $12,000 to $15,000. This was 8 to 10 times the charge of the average client. Costs for clients on mechanical ventilation can be four times the cost for a similarly ill client in the intensive care unit (ICU).

In a study examining outcomes of unplanned extubation (Ellstrom, 2000), preventing an unplanned extubation would have saved 3.4 hospital days. The average hospital cost per day was $790. Multiplying the hospital days saved by the average hospital cost per day gave a $2686 cost saving per patient. In this study, if the 112 unplanned extubations had been prevented, a cost savings of $300,847 would have been realized.

Implications for Nursing

Nurses who know their clients well are in a position to notice subtle changes in the client's cognition, psychologic affect, and immediate environment. Such observations can be critical in the prevention of unplanned or premature extubations, thereby saving the costs related to the need for reintubation.

Data from Rosen, RL, & Bone, RC. (1990). Financial implications of ventilator care. *Critical Care Clinics, 6*(3), 797-805; and Ellstrom, K. (2000). Relationship of psychoneurological, physiological, and environmental constructs to risk of unplanned extubation and outcomes in medical ICU patients. Doctoral dissertation, University of California—Los Angeles.

Time-Cycled Ventilators. Time-cycled ventilators push air into the lungs until a preset time has elapsed. Tidal volume and pressure are variable, depending on the characteristics of the client and the ventilator. The time-cycled ventilator is used primarily in pediatric and neonatal populations.

Volume-Cycled Ventilators. Volume-cycled ventilators push gas into the lungs until a preset volume is delivered. A constant tidal volume is delivered regardless of the pressure needed to deliver the tidal volume. However, a pressure limit is set to prevent excessive pressure from being exerted on the lungs. The advantage of the volume-cycled ventilator is that a constant tidal volume is delivered regardless of the changing compliance of the lungs and chest wall or the airway resistance found in the client or ventilator.

Microprocessor Ventilators. Microprocessor ventilators are the most sophisticated of the positive-pressure ventilators. A computer or microprocessor is built into the ventilator to allow ongoing monitoring of ventilatory functions, alarms, and client parameters. The ventilator often has components of volume-, time-, and pressure-cycled ventilators. The microprocessor ventilator is more responsive to clients who have severe lung disease, who require prolonged weaning trials, and who may not be able to be ventilated on older, volume-cycled ventilators. Examples include the Bear IV and V, Puritan-Bennett 7200, Erisa, and Siemens Servo C and Servo D.

MODES OF VENTILATION. The mode of ventilation describes the way in which the client receives breaths from the ventilator.

CHART 32-10

BEST PRACTICE *for*
Care of the Client on Mechanical Ventilation

- At least once every shift check to be sure the ventilator settings are set as ordered.
- Check to be sure alarms are set (especially low pressure and low exhaled volume).
- Observe the exhaled volume digital display to be sure the client is receiving the prescribed tidal volume.
- Empty ventilator tubings when moisture collects. Never empty fluid in the tubing back into the cascade.
- Ensure adequate humidity by keeping delivered air temperature maintained at body temperature.
- If the client is on PEEP, observe the peak airway pressure dial to determine the proper level of PEEP.
- Assess the client's respiratory status each shift and as needed:
  - Observe the client's color (especially lips and nail beds).
  - Observe the client's chest for bilateral expansion.
  - Auscultate the lungs for rales, rhonchi, wheezes, equal breath sounds, and decreased or absent breath sounds.
  - Obtain pulse oximetry reading.
  - Evaluate ABGs as ordered.
- Take vital signs at least every 4 hours.
- Be sure the tracheostomy cuff (or the endotracheal cuff) is adequately inflated to ensure tidal volume.
- Administer mouth care every 2 to 4 hours.
- Observe the client's need for tracheal/oral/nasal suctioning every 2 hours. Provide adequate suctioning as needed.
- Provide tracheostomy care every shift.
- Change tracheostomy tape or endotracheal tube tape as needed. Observe the client's mouth around the endotracheal tube for pressure sores.
- Move the oral endotracheal tube to the opposite side of the mouth once every 24 hours to prevent ulcers.
- Maintain accurate intake and output records to monitor fluid balance.
- Turn the client at least every 2 hours and get the client out of bed as ordered to promote pulmonary hygiene and prevent complications of immobility.
- Schedule treatments and nursing care at intervals to provide rest.
- Explain all procedures and treatments; provide access to a call bell; visit the client frequently.
- Include the client and his or her family in care whenever possible (especially suctioning and tracheostomy care).
- Provide a letter board or pencil and paper for communication. Request consultation with a speech therapist for assistance, if necessary.
- Observe ventilated clients for gastrointestinal distress (diarrhea, constipation, tarry stools).
- Document pertinent observations in the client's medical record (chart).
- Administer muscle-paralyzing agents, sedatives, and narcotic analgesics, as appropriate.
- Monitor the effectiveness of mechanical ventilation in terms of the client's physiologic and psychologic status.
- Initiate relaxation techniques, as appropriate.
- Monitor the client's progress on current ventilator settings and make appropriate changes as ordered.
- Monitor for adverse effects of mechanical ventilation: infection, barotrauma, reduced cardiac output.
- Position to facilitate ventilation/perfusion matching ("good lung down"), as appropriate.
- Monitor effects of ventilator changes on oxygenation and the client's subjective response.
- Monitor readiness to wean.

Courtesy Our Lady of Lourdes Medical Center, Camden, NJ.
PEEP, Positive end-expiratory pressure; *ABGs,* arterial blood gases.

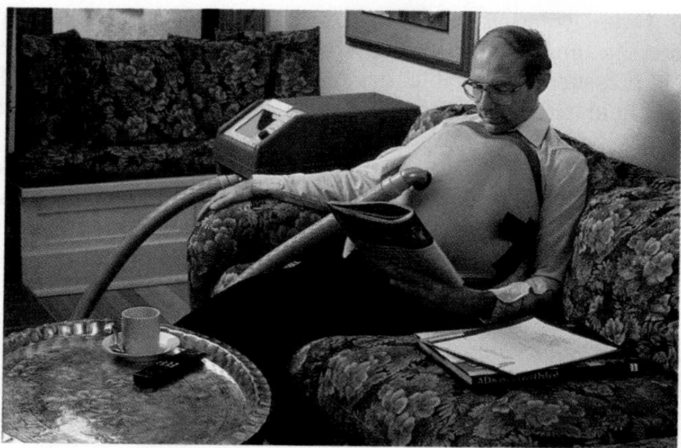

Figure 32-3 ● A portable negative-pressure ventilator. (Courtesy Repironics, Pittsburgh, PA.)

Controlled Ventilation. Controlled ventilation is the least-used mode. The client receives a set tidal volume at a set rate. This mode may be used for clients who cannot initiate respiratory effort (e.g., those with polio or Guillain-Barré syndrome). It may also be used for clients who are "paralyzed" as part of their medical management, such as those in status epilepticus or those with severely elevated intracranial pressure. With controlled ventilation, if the client attempts to initiate a breath, the efforts are blocked by the ventilator. This maneuver may result in the client's "fighting" the ventilator.

Assist-Control Ventilation. Assist-control (AC) ventilation is the most commonly used mode. It is used mainly as a resting mode. The ventilator takes over the work of breathing for the client. The tidal volume and ventilatory rate are preset on the ventilator. If the client does not trigger spontaneous breaths, a minimal ventilatory pattern is established. The ventilator is also programmed to respond to the client's inspiratory effort if he or she does initiate a breath. In this case, the ventilator delivers the preset tidal volume while allowing the client to control the rate of breathing.

One disadvantage of the AC mode is that if the client's spontaneous ventilatory rate increases, the ventilator continues to deliver a preset tidal volume with each breath. He or she may then hyperventilate, and respiratory alkalosis occurs. Causes of hyperventilation, such as pain, anxiety, or acid-base imbalances, must be corrected.

Synchronized Intermittent Mandatory Ventilation. Synchronized intermittent mandatory ventilation (SIMV) is similar to AC ventilation in that tidal volume and ventilatory rate are preset on the ventilator. Therefore if the client does not breathe, a minimal ventilatory pattern is established. In contrast to the AC mode, SIMV allows breathing spontaneously at the client's own rate and tidal volume between the ventilator breaths. SIMV can be used as a primary ventilatory mode or as a weaning modality. When SIMV is used as a weaning mode, the number of mechanical breaths (SIMV breaths) is gradually decreased (e.g., from 12 to 2), and the client gradually resumes spontaneous breathing. The mandatory ventilator breaths are delivered when the client is ready to inspire, promoting synchrony between the ventilator and the client.

Other Modes of Ventilation. Newer modes of ventilation, such as pressure support and continuous flow (flow-by), are available only in microprocessor ventilators. Both modalities decrease the work of breathing and are often used for weaning clients from mechanical ventilation. Other modes are maximum mandatory ventilation (MMV), inverse inspiration-expiration (I/E) ratio, permissive hypercapnia, airway pressure release ventilation, proportional assist ventilation, high-frequency ventilation, jet ventilation, and high-frequency oscillation. Many of these modes need specialized ventilators, tubing, or airways.

EVIDENCE-BASED PRACTICE FOR NURSING

Less is better for tidal volumes

The Acute Respiratory Distress Syndrome Network. (2000). Ventilation with lower tidal volumes as compared with traditional tidal volumes for acute lung injury. *New England Journal of Medicine, 342*(18), 1301-1308.

Traditionally, tidal volumes of 10 to 15 mg/kg of body weight are used in mechanical ventilation. However, these volumes may cause stretch-induced lung injury in clients with acute lung injury and acute respiratory distress syndrome (ARDS) (so-called volutrauma). The purpose of this study was to compare these volumes with a lower tidal volume and evaluate clinical outcomes.

Clients were enrolled in a multicenter, randomized trial. The trial compared traditional treatment (tidal volume of 12 ml/kg and plateau pressure of 50 cm of water or less) with management in the treatment group (tidal volume of 6 ml/kg and plateau pressure of 30 cm of water or less). The outcomes were death before discharge or breathing without assistance and the number of days without ventilator use from day 1 through day 28. The trial was stopped prematurely because mortality was lower in the treatment group; also, there was a greater number of days without ventilator use during the first 28 days.

Critique. This study has major implications for decreasing complications related to the use of mechanical ventilation. Lessening the effect of volutrauma can impact costs and length of stay, as well as functional status after hospitalization. The study has limitations, however, in that the volume-assist-control mode was used until the client was weaned. This is not consistently used in clinical practice; synchronized intermittent mandatory ventilation (SIMV) is more commonly used.

Implications for Nursing. Decreasing complications is a major role for nurses in critical care. Clients on mechanical ventilation are vulnerable to numerous insults, and diligent care is required to assess and intervene when an untoward event occurs. This treatment change is simple yet may impact the survival of clients with acute lung injury and ARDS.

VENTILATOR CONTROLS AND SETTINGS. The volume-cycled ventilator is the most widely used ventilator in the acute care setting. Regardless of the type of volume-cycled ventilator used, the controls and types of settings are universal (Figure 32-4). The physician prescribes the ventilator settings, and usually the ventilator is readied or set up by the respiratory department. The nurse assists in connecting the client to the ventilator. Monitoring of the ventilator settings is part of the nursing care.

Tidal Volume. Tidal volume (V_T) is the volume of air that the client receives with each breath; it can be measured on either inspiration or expiration. The average prescribed V_T ranges between 7 and 10 mL/kg of body weight (see the Evidence-Based Practice for Nursing box above). Adding a zero to the weight of clients in kilograms gives an estimate of tidal volume.

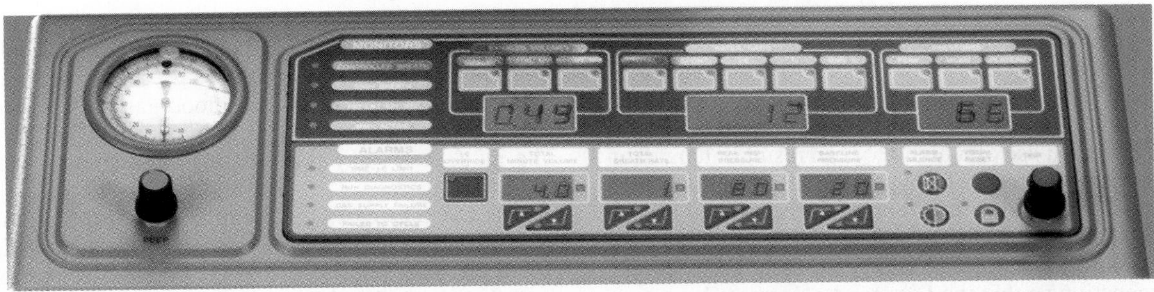

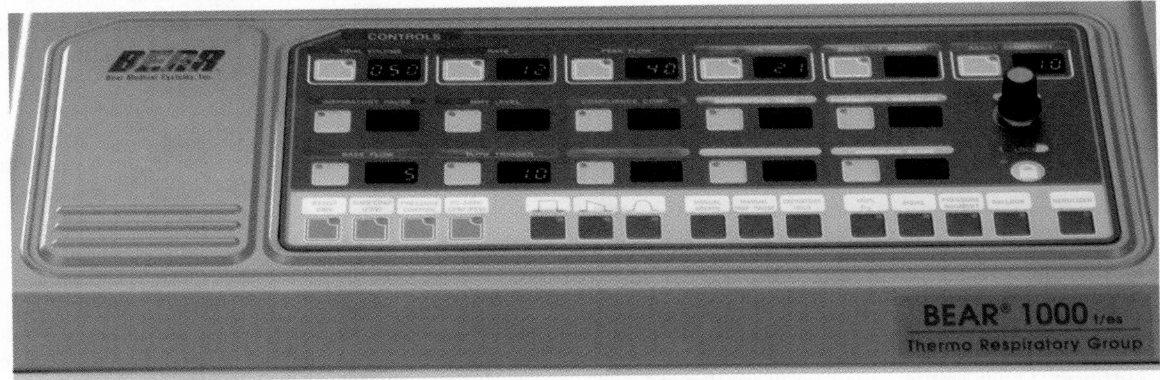

Figure 32-4 ● Display signals and alarms *(top)* and control panel *(bottom)* of a typical volume-cycled ventilator. (Bear 1000t/es Adult Volume Ventilator. Courtesy Bear Medical Systems, Thermo Respiratory Group, Palm Springs, CA.)

Rate, or Breaths per Minute. Rate, or breaths per minute, is the number of ventilator breaths delivered per minute. The rate is usually set between 10 and 14 breaths per minute.

Fraction of Inspired Oxygen. The **fraction of inspired oxygen (FIO_2)** is the oxygen concentration delivered to the client. The prescribed FIO_2 is determined by the arterial blood gas (ABG) value and the condition. Ventilators can provide 21% to 100% oxygen, depending on need.

The oxygen delivered to the client is warmed to body temperature (98.6° F [37° C]) and humidified to 100%. Humidification and warming are necessary because upper air passages of the respiratory tree, which normally warm, humidify, and filter air, are bypassed by the endotracheal (ET) tube or tracheostomy tube. Humidification and warming prevent mucosal damage and facilitate clearance of secretions.

Sighs. **Sighs** are volumes of air that are 1.5 to 2 times the set tidal volume, delivered 6 to 10 times per hour. These may be used to prevent atelectasis in special circumstances. Sighs are rarely used, however, because they can cause **barotrauma** (lung damage from excessive pressure) and have not been shown to be useful.

Peak Airway (Inspiratory) Pressure. Peak airway (inspiratory) pressure (PIP) indicates the pressure needed by the ventilator to deliver a set tidal volume at a given dynamic compliance. The PIP measurement appears on the digital readout or display on the front or top of the ventilator. Peak pressure is the highest pressure indicated during inspiration. Monitoring trends in PIP reflect changes in resistance of the lungs and resistance in the ventilator. An increased PIP reading means increased airway resistance (bronchospasm, or pinched tubing), increased amount of secretions, pulmonary edema, or decreased pulmonary compliance (the lungs or chest wall are "stiffer" or harder to inflate). An upper pressure limit is set on the ventilator to prevent barotrauma. When the limit is reached, the high-pressure alarm sounds, and the remaining volume is not given.

Continuous Positive Airway Pressure. Continuous positive airway pressure (CPAP) is the application of positive airway pressure throughout the entire respiratory cycle for spontaneously breathing clients. Sedating medications should be given cautiously or not at all when receiving CPAP so that respiratory effort is not suppressed. CPAP keeps the alveoli open during inspiration and prevents alveolar collapse during expiration. This process results in increased functional residual capacity (FRC), improved gas exchange, and improved oxygenation.

CPAP is used primarily to help in the weaning process. During CPAP, no ventilator breaths are delivered; the ventilator delivers oxygen and provides monitoring and an alarm system. The respiratory pattern is determined by the client's efforts. Normal levels of CPAP are 5 to 15 cm H_2O, adjusted to promote adequate oxygenation. If no pressure is set on the ventilator, the client receives no positive pressure. The client is essentially using the ventilator as a T-piece with alarms.

Newer modifications of CPAP include nasal CPAP and bilevel positive airway pressure (BiPAP). The physician uses these modifications for select indications.

Positive End-Expiratory Pressure. Positive end-expiratory pressure (PEEP) is positive pressure exerted during the expiratory phase of ventilation. PEEP improves oxygenation by enhancing gas exchange and preventing atelectasis. It is indicated for the treatment of persistent hypoxemia that does not improve with an acceptable oxygen concentration. PEEP is often added when the partial pressure of arterial oxygen ($Pa{O_2}$) value remains low with an $F{IO_2}$ of 50% to 70% or greater.

The need for PEEP indicates a severe gas exchange disturbance. It is important to lower the $F{IO_2}$ delivered whenever possible. Prolonged use of a high $F{IO_2}$ can result in lung damage from the toxic effects of oxygen. PEEP prevents alveoli from collapsing; the lungs are kept partially inflated so that alveolar-capillary gas exchange is facilitated throughout the ventilatory cycle. The effect should be an increase in arterial blood oxygenation so that the $F{IO_2}$ can be decreased.

PEEP is "dialed in" with the PEEP dial on the control panel. The amount of PEEP is often 5 to 15 cm H_2O and is read (monitored) on the peak airway pressure dial, the same dial used to read the PIP. When PEEP is added, the dial does not return to zero at the end of exhalation; rather, it returns to a baseline that has been increased from zero by the amount of PEEP applied.

Flow. **Flow** is how fast the ventilator delivers each breath. It is usually set at 40 L/min. If a client is agitated, is restless, has a widely fluctuating pressure reading on inspiration, or has other signs of air hunger, the flow may be set too low. Increasing the flow should be tried before using chemical restraints.

Other Settings. Other settings may be used, depending on the type of ventilator and mode of ventilation. Examples of additional settings include inspiratory and expiratory cycle, waveform, expiratory resistance, and plateau.

NURSING MANAGEMENT. The institution of mechanical ventilation involves a complex decision-making process for both the client/family and the health care professionals. Both physical and psychologic concerns of the client and family must be addressed. The mechanical ventilator frequently causes anxiety for the client and family. Therefore the nurse carefully explains the purpose of the ventilator and notes that the client might feel some different sensations. The client and family are encouraged to express their concerns. The nurse acts as the coach who both physically and psychologically helps and supports the client and family through this experience. In emergencies these explanations may not be accomplished until the emergency has been controlled. Clients undergoing mechanical ventilation in intensive care units (ICUs) often experience delirium, or "ICU psychosis." These persons require frequent, repetitive explanations and reassurance.

When caring for a ventilated client, the nurse is concerned with the client first and the ventilator second. It is vital that the nurse understand why the mechanical ventilation is required. Causes such as excessive amounts of secretions, sepsis, and trauma require different interventions to facilitate ventilator independence. In addition, an appreciation of the client's chronic health problems, particularly chronic obstructive pulmonary disease (COPD), left-sided heart failure, anemia, and malnutrition, is essential. These problems may impede weaning from mechanical ventilation and therefore warrant close monitoring and intervention.

Three nursing goals in caring for the client with mechanical ventilation are to monitor and evaluate the response to the ventilator, manage the ventilator system safely, and prevent complications.

Monitoring the Client's Response. A major nursing responsibility is to monitor and evaluate the client's response to the ventilator. The nurse assesses vital signs and listens to breath sounds every 30 to 60 minutes initially, monitors noninvasive respiratory parameters (e.g., capnography and pulse oximetry), and checks arterial blood gas (ABG) values. Vital signs change during episodes of hypercapnia and hypoxemia. The nurse notes any precipitating causes and corrects them promptly.

The nurse assesses the breathing pattern in relation to the ventilatory cycle to determine whether the client is fighting or tolerating the ventilator. Breath sounds are assessed and recorded, including bilateral equal breath sounds to ensure proper endotracheal (ET) tube placement. To determine the frequency of suctioning needed, the nurse observes secretions for type, color, and amount.

The area around the ET tube or tracheostomy site is assessed at least every 4 hours for color, tenderness, skin irritation, and drainage. Continuous noninvasive monitoring provides information to guide the client's activities, such as weaning, physical or occupational therapy, and self-care. These activities can be paced so that oxygenation and ventilation are adequate. The nurse interprets ABG values to evaluate ventilation and suggests ventilator settings that help the client.

Because the nurse spends the most time with the client, he or she is most likely to be the first person to recognize slight changes in vital signs or ABG values and fatigue or distress. The nurse promptly confers with the physician and implements the appropriate interventions.

While monitoring and evaluating the client's clinical status, the nurse also serves as a resource for addressing the psychologic needs of the client and family. Anxiety can play a major role in the tolerance of mechanical ventilation. Therefore skilled and sensitive nursing care promotes psychologic well-being and facilitates synchrony with the ventilator. Because the client cannot speak, communication can be frustrating and anxiety producing. The client and family may panic because they believe that the voice has been lost. They must be reassured that although the ET tube prevents speech, it is temporary.

Alternative, creative methods of communication must be individualized to meet the client's needs. Magic Slates, writing paper, computers, and tracheostomy tubes that permit talking are potential means of facilitating communication. Finding a successful means for communication is important because the client often feels isolated as a result of the inability to speak. Anticipation of the client's needs; easy access to frequently used belongings; visits from family, friends, and pets; and a nursing call light within reach are effective ways of giving a sense of control over the environment. In addition, the client can participate in self-care.

Managing the Ventilator System. Ventilator settings are ordered by the physician and include tidal volume, respiratory rate, fraction of inspired oxygen ($F{IO_2}$), mode of ventilation (assist-control [AC] ventilation, synchronized intermittent mandatory ventilation [SIMV]), and any adjunctive modes, such as positive end-expiratory pressure (PEEP), pressure support, or continuous flow.

The nurse performs and documents ventilator checks according to the standards of the unit or facility and responds promptly to emergencies as indicated by alarms. During a ventilator check, the ventilator settings ordered by the physician are compared with the actual settings. The level of water

TABLE 32-5 • NURSING INTERVENTIONS FOR VARIOUS CAUSES OF VENTILATOR ALARMS

Cause	Nursing Interventions
High-Pressure Alarm (sounds when peak inspiratory pressure reaches the set alarm limit [usually set 10–20 mm Hg above the client's baseline PIP])	
There is an increased amount of secretions in the airways or a mucous plug.	Suction as needed.
The client coughs, gags, or bites on the oral ET tube.	Insert oral airway to prevent biting on the ET tube.
The client is anxious or fights the ventilator.	Provide emotional support to decrease anxiety. Increase the flow rate. Explain all procedures to the client. Provide sedation or paralyzing agent per the physician's order.
Airway size decreases related to wheezing or bronchospasm.	Auscultate breath sounds. Consult with the physician for management of bronchospasm.
Pneumothorax occurs.	Auscultate breath sounds. Consult with the physician about a new onset of decreased breath sounds or unequal chest excursion, which may be due to pneumothorax.
The artificial airway is displaced; the ET tube may have slipped into the right mainstem bronchus.	Assess the chest for unequal breath sounds and chest excursion. Obtain a chest x-ray film as ordered to evaluate the position of the ET tube. After the proper position is verified, tape the tube securely in place.
Obstruction in tubing occurs because the client is lying on the tubing or there is water or a kink in the tubing.	Assess the system, moving from the artificial airway toward the ventilator. Empty water from the ventilator tubing and remove any kinks.
There is increased PIP associated with deliverance of a sigh.	Consult with respiratory therapist or physician to adjust the pressure alarm.
Decreased compliance of the lung is noted; a trend of gradually increasing PIP is noted over several hours or a day.	Evaluate the reasons for the decreased compliance of the lungs. Increased PIP occurs in ARDS, pneumonia, or any worsening of pulmonary disease.
Low Exhaled Volume (or Low-Pressure) Alarm (sounds when there is a disconnection or leak in the ventilator circuit or a leak in the client's artificial airway cuff)	
A leak in the ventilator circuit prevents breath from being delivered.	Assess all connections and all ventilator tubings for disconnection.
The client stops spontaneous breathing in the SIMV or CPAP mode or on pressure support ventilation.	Evaluate the client's tolerance of the mode.
A cuff leak occurs in the ET or tracheostomy tube.	Evaluate the client for a cuff leak. A cuff leak is suspected when the client is able to talk (air escapes from the mouth) or when the pilot balloon on the artificial airway is flat (see section on tracheostomy tubes in Chapter 28).
The exhalation valve on Bear I or II is wet.	Keep exhalation valve and flow tube vertical. Unsnap and check the membrane for dampness. If the sensor is wet, gently dab dry and resnap.

PIP, Peak inspiratory pressure; *ET,* endotracheal; *ARDS,* acute respiratory distress syndrome; *CPAP,* continuous positive airway pressure; *SIMV,* synchronized intermittent mandatory ventilation.

in the humidifier and the temperature of the humidification system are checked to ensure that they are within normal limits. Extremes in temperature cause damage to the mucosa of the airways. Any condensation in the ventilator tubing is removed by draining water into drainage collection receptacles, which should be emptied frequently. For prevention of bacterial contamination, moisture and water from the tubing are never allowed to enter the humidifier.

Mechanical ventilators have alarm systems that warn the nurse of a problem with either the client or the ventilator. Alarm systems must be activated and functional at all times. The nurse must recognize an emergency and intervene promptly so that complications are prevented. If the cause of the alarm cannot be determined, the nurse ventilates the client manually with a resuscitation bag until the problem is corrected by a second nurse, the respiratory therapist, or a physician. The two major alarms on a ventilator indicate either a high pressure or a low exhaled volume. Table 32-5 presents nursing interventions for various causes of ventilator alarms.

Ensuring proper functioning of the ventilator also includes care of the ET or tracheostomy tube. A patent airway is maintained through suctioning only as needed. The following are indications for suctioning in the ventilated client:

- Presence of secretions
- Increased peak airway (inspiratory) pressure (PIP)
- Presence of rhonchi (wheezes)
- Decreased breath sounds

Careful maintenance of the ET or tracheostomy tube also ensures a patent airway. The nurse frequently assesses the tube's position, especially for the client whose airway is attached to heavy ventilator tubing that may pull on the tracheostomy or ET tube. The ventilator tubing is positioned in such a way that the client can move without pulling on the ET or tracheostomy tube. The ET tube can move and slip into the right mainstem bronchus. To detect minimal changes in the tube's position, the level at which the tube touches the client's teeth or nose is marked. The nurse gives mouth care frequently to promote adequate oral hygiene and to prevent loosening of the tape that holds the tube.

Preventing Complications. Most complications are due to the positive pressure from the ventilator. Nearly every body system is affected.

Cardiac Complications. Cardiac complications of mechanical ventilation include hypotension and fluid retention. Hypotension is caused by the application of positive pressure, which increases intrathoracic pressure and inhibits blood return to the heart. The decreased venous return to the right side of the heart decreases cardiac output and is clinically reflected as hypotension. Hypotension is most frequently seen in the client who is dehydrated or requires a high PIP to be ventilated. The nurse instructs the client to avoid a Valsalva maneuver and plans care to prevent constipation, which could result in a Valsalva maneuver.

Fluid is retained because of decreased cardiac output. The kidneys receive less blood flow and stimulate the renin-angiotensin-aldosterone system to retain fluid. In addition, humidified air via the ventilator system can contribute to fluid retention. If humidification is not adequate, the airways become dehydrated and the secretions solidify. The nurse monitors the client's fluid intake and output, weight, hydration, and signs of hypovolemia.

Lung Complications. The lungs experience barotrauma (damage to the lungs by positive pressure), **volutrauma** (damage to the lung by excess volume delivered to one lung over the other), and acid-base abnormalities. Barotrauma includes pneumothorax, subcutaneous emphysema, and pneumomediastinum. Clients at risk for barotrauma have diseases of chronic airflow limitation (CAL), have blebs, are on PEEP, have dynamic hyperinflation, or require high pressures to ventilate the lungs (because of decreased compliance or "stiff" lungs, as seen in acute respiratory distress syndrome [ARDS]). Blood gas abnormalities, another pulmonary complication of mechanical ventilation, can be corrected by appropriate ventilator changes and adjustment of fluid and electrolyte imbalances.

Gastrointestinal and Nutritional Complications. Gastrointestinal (GI) alterations result from the stress of mechanical ventilation. Stress ulcers occur in approximately 25% of clients receiving mechanical ventilation. Prophylactic antacids, sucralfate (Carafate, Sulcrate🍁), and the histamine blockers cimetidine (Tagamet) and ranitidine (Zantac) are often instituted as soon as the client is intubated. Changes in the pressure relationship between the thoracic and abdominal cavities can also produce or induce a paralytic ileus. This problem may affect absorption of nutrients through the GI system, requiring short-term parenteral nutritional support.

Malnutrition is a prevalent problem in clients receiving mechanical ventilation. Because many other acute or life-threatening events are occurring simultaneously, nutrition is often neglected. Malnutrition is an extreme problem for these clients and is a major reason why they cannot be weaned from the ventilator. In malnourished clients the respiratory muscles lose their mass and strength. The diaphragm, which is the major muscle of inspiration, is affected early in this process. When the diaphragm and other muscles of respiration are weakened, an ineffective breathing pattern emerges, fatigue occurs, and the client cannot be weaned from the ventilator.

A balanced diet via the parenteral or enteral route is essential whenever a ventilator is used. Furthermore, nutrition for the client with chronic obstructive pulmonary disease (COPD) requires that special attention be given to the percentage of carbohydrates in the diet. During metabolism, carbohydrates are broken down to glucose to produce energy (adenosine triphosphate), carbon dioxide, and water. Excessive carbohydrate loads increase carbon dioxide production, which the client with chronic obstructive pulmonary disease (COPD) may be unable to exhale. Hypercapnic respiratory failure results. Enteral and parenteral formulas with a higher fat content (e.g., Pulmocare, NutriVent, intralipids) can be an alternative source of calories to combat this problem.

Another important aspect of nutritional support is electrolyte replacement. Electrolytes also have a major impact on the efficiency of respiratory muscle function. Specifically, the nurse and physician closely monitor potassium, calcium, magnesium, and phosphate levels, and the nurse replenishes deficiencies as ordered. All four electrolytes are important in respiratory muscle contraction and function and can easily be added to the nutritional regimen.

Infection. Infections are always a potential threat for the client requiring a ventilator. The ET or tracheostomy tube bypasses the body's normal process of filtering and warming air and provides bacteria with direct access to the lower parts of the respiratory system. Within 48 hours, the artificial airway is usually colonized with bacteria, and an environment is established in which pneumonia can develop. In addition, aspiration of colonized fluid from the mouth or the stomach can occur and be a source of pathogens. Pneumonia is associated with prolonged hospitalization and increased morbidity. Therefore the focus must be on prevention of infections through strict adherence to infection control, especially handwashing, during suctioning and care of the tracheostomy or ET tube. To prevent pneumonia, the nurse implements ongoing oral care and pulmonary hygiene, including chest physiotherapy, postural drainage, and turning and positioning. Further information on pneumonia can be found in Chapter 31.

Muscular Complications. Overall muscle deconditioning can occur because of immobility. Getting out of bed, ambulating with assistance, and performing exercises with the nurse, physical therapist, and occupational therapist not only improve muscle tone and strength but also boost morale, facilitate gas exchange, and promote oxygen delivery to all muscles.

Ventilator Dependence. The final complication of mechanical ventilation is ventilator dependence, or inability to wean. Ventilator dependence can be psychologic or physiologic but more often has a physiologic basis. The longer a client uses a ventilator, the more difficult is the weaning process because the respiratory muscles fatigue and cannot assume breathing. The health care team attempts to optimize all major body systems and to exhaust every method of weaning before a client is declared unweanable.

The physician and nurse, often with a social worker or psychologist and a member of the clergy, discuss with the family and the client, as able, the client's quality of life, goals,

TABLE 32-6 • WEANING METHODS

SYNCHRONOUS INTERMITTENT MANDATORY VENTILATION
- The client breathes between the machine's preset breaths-per-minute rate.
- The machine is initially set on an SIMV rate of 12, meaning the client receives a minimum of 12 breaths per minute by the ventilator.
- The client's respiratory rate will be a combination of ventilator breaths and spontaneous breaths.
- As the weaning process ensues, the physician orders gradual decreases in the SIMV rate, usually at a decrease of 1 to 2 breaths per minute.

T-PIECE TECHNIQUE
- The client is taken off the ventilator for short periods (initially 5 to 10 minutes) and allowed to breathe spontaneously.
- The ventilator is replaced with a T-piece (see Chapter 28) or CPAP, which delivers humidified oxygen.
- The ordered FIO_2 may be higher for the client on the T-piece than on the ventilator.
- Weaning progresses as the client is able to tolerate progressively longer periods off the ventilator.
- Nighttime weaning is not usually attempted until the client is able to maintain spontaneous respirations most of the day.

PRESSURE SUPPORT VENTILATION
- PSV allows the client's respiratory effort to be augmented by a predetermined pressure assist from the ventilator.
- As the weaning process ensues, the amount of pressure applied to inspiration is gradually decreased.
- Another method of weaning with PSV is to maintain the pressure but gradually decrease the ventilator's preset breaths-per-minute rate.

SIMV, Synchronized intermittent mandatory ventilation; *CPAP,* continuous positive airway pressure; *FIO_2,* fraction of inspired oxygen; *PSV,* pressure support ventilation.

and values. In accordance with this discussion, arrangements are made for home ventilation, nursing home placement, or withdrawal of life support (in terminal cases). Special units and facilities are available to maximize the rehabilitation and weaning of ventilator-dependent clients.

WEANING. Weaning is the process of going from ventilatory dependence to spontaneous breathing. The weaning process can be prolonged if complications develop. Many of these complications can be avoided by skillful nursing care. For example, turning and positioning the client not only promote comfort and prevent skin breakdown but also facilitate gas exchange and prevent pulmonary complications, such as pneumonia and atelectasis. Table 32-6 summarizes various weaning techniques.

CONSIDERATIONS FOR OLDER ADULTS

The older client, especially one who has smoked or who has an underlying lung dysfunction such as COPD, is at risk for ventilator dependence and failure to wean. Age-related changes that decrease the likelihood of weaning result in ventilatory failure and include increased chest wall stiffness, reduced respiratory muscle strength, and decreased lung elasticity. Because the usual manifestations of ventilatory failure—hypoxemia and hypercapnia—may be blunted in the older adult, the nurse must use other clinical measures of oxygenation, such as a change in mental status.

EXTUBATION. Removal of the endotracheal (ET) tube is termed **extubation.** The tube is removed when the indication for intubation has been resolved. Before removal, the nurse explains the procedure. The nurse or respiratory therapist sets up the prescribed oxygen delivery system at the bedside and brings in the equipment for emergency reintubation. The client is hyperoxygenated and the ET tube thoroughly suctioned, as is the oral cavity. The cuff of the ET tube is then rapidly deflated, and the tube is removed at peak inspiration. The nurse instructs the client to take deep breaths and to cough. It is normal for large amounts of oral secretions to have accumulated in the back of the throat. Oxygen is administered by face mask or nasal cannula. The fraction of inspired oxygen (FIO_2) is usually ordered at 10% higher than the level that was maintained while the ET tube was in place.

Monitoring after extubation is essential. The nurse monitors the vital signs every hour initially, assesses the ventilatory pattern, and assesses for any signs or symptoms of respiratory distress. It is common to experience hoarseness and a sore throat for a few days after extubation. The client is instructed to sit in a semi-Fowler's position, take deep breaths every ½ hour, use an incentive spirometer (see Chapters 17 and 27) every 2 hours, and limit speaking in the immediate period after extubation. These measures facilitate gas exchange and decrease laryngeal edema and vocal cord irritation. The client is observed closely for signs or symptoms of upper airway obstruction (see Chapter 29). Early signs are mild dyspnea, coughing, and the inability to expectorate secretions. With the onset of these signs, the nurse notifies the physician, who evaluates the need for reintubation. The nurse is especially concerned if the client develops stridor, a late sign of a narrowed airway. **Stridor** is a high-pitched, crowing noise during inspiration caused by laryngospasm or edema above or below the glottis. Racemic epinephrine, a topical aerosol vasoconstrictor, is given, and reintubation may be performed.

CRITICAL THINKING CHALLENGE

The client, a 38-year-old woman with pulmonary embolism following multiple fractures and pelvic trauma, is started on a regimen of low-dose IV heparin, keeping her partial thromboplastin time (PTT) 2.5 to 3 times the normal range. That night she develops severe hypoxemia requiring that she be intubated and mechanically ventilated. The postintubation chest x-ray film shows bilateral fluffy infiltrates.

- What is the most likely cause of the client's acute respiratory decompensation?
- Her partial pressure of arterial oxygen (PaO_2) value remains low despite receiving 100% oxygen.
- What therapy should be instituted to correct her continuing hypoxemia?

For suggested answer guidelines, go to SIMON http://www.wbsaunders.com/SIMON/Iggy/.

CHEST TRAUMA

Chest injuries are directly responsible for approximately 25% of all civilian traumatic deaths; 50% of the injured succumb before arriving at health care facilities. Only 5% to 15% of all chest injuries require thoracotomy. The remainder can be treated with basic resuscitation, intubation, or chest tube placement. The emergency initial approach to all chest injuries is ABC (*a*irway, *b*reathing, *c*irculation) followed by rapid assessment and treatment of potentially life-threatening conditions.

Pulmonary Contusion

OVERVIEW

Pulmonary contusion, a potentially lethal injury, is the most common chest injury seen in the United States. After a contusion, respiratory failure can develop over time rather than instantaneously. This condition most frequently follows injuries caused by rapid deceleration during vehicular accidents. Interstitial hemorrhage, which is almost invariably associated with intra-alveolar hemorrhage, accompanies pulmonary contusion. The resultant interstitial edema causes a decrease in pulmonary compliance and a decreased area for gas exchange. The client usually becomes hypoxemic and dyspneic. The bronchial mucosa becomes irritated, and the client has increased bronchial secretions.

COLLABORATIVE MANAGEMENT

Assessment

Clients with pulmonary contusion who may initially be asymptomatic can develop respiratory failure. These clients present with hemoptysis, decreased breath sounds, crackles, and wheezes. The chest x-ray film of the client with pulmonary contusion may show a hazy opacity in the lobes or parenchyma. If there is no disruption of the parenchyma, resorption of the lesion often occurs without treatment.

Interventions

Treatment includes maintenance of ventilation and oxygenation. Central venous pressure (CVP) is monitored closely, and fluid intake is restricted accordingly. The client in obvious respiratory distress may require mechanical ventilation with positive end-expiratory pressure (PEEP) to inflate the lungs and provide positive-pressure ventilation.

A vicious circle occurs in which more muscle effort is required for ventilation, and the client becomes progressively hypoxemic. Attempting to compensate causes the client to tire easily, become less efficient in breathing, and become more fatigued and hypoxemic. Flail chest may also be associated with a pulmonary contusion accompanied by parenchymal damage. The sequela to this situation is the probable development of acute respiratory distress syndrome (ARDS).

Rib Fracture

OVERVIEW

After chest wall contusion, rib fractures are the next most common injury to the chest wall. Rib fractures most frequently result from direct blunt trauma to the chest, usually with involvement of the fifth through ninth ribs. Direct force applied to the ribs tends to fracture them and drive the bone ends into the thorax. Thus there is a potential for intrathoracic injury, such as pneumothorax or pulmonary contusion. Pneumothorax is almost invariably present if ribs one through four are fractured.

COLLABORATIVE MANAGEMENT

The client usually experiences pain with movement and splints the chest defensively. Thoracic splinting results in impaired ventilation and inadequate clearance of tracheobronchial secretions. If the client has pre-existing pulmonary disease, the likelihood of atelectasis and pneumonia related to the rib fracture is increased. Clients with injuries to the first or second ribs, flail chest, seven or more fractured ribs, or expired volumes less than 15 mL/kg have a poor prognosis; intrathoracic injury occurs in 50% of these cases.

Treatment for uncomplicated rib fractures is nonspecific because the fractured ribs unite spontaneously. The chest is usually not splinted by tape or other materials. The primary consideration for the client is to decrease pain so that adequate ventilatory status is maintained. An intercostal nerve block may be used if pain is severe. Potent analgesia that causes respiratory depression is avoided.

Flail Chest

OVERVIEW

Flail chest (paradoxical respiration) is the inward movement of the thorax during inspiration, with outward movement during expiration. It usually involves one hemithorax (one side of the chest) and results from multiple rib fractures caused by blunt chest trauma. Flail chest is frequently associated with high-speed vehicular accidents. It is more common in older clients. It is associated with a high mortality rate (40%) and is one of the most critical chest injuries.

Flail chest occurs when a loose segment of chest wall is left because of a fracture of two or more adjacent ribs. The movement of this segment becomes paradoxic to the expansion and contraction of the rest of the chest wall. Flail chest can also occur from bilateral fracture of multiple costochondral junctions (without rib fracture) anteriorly, such as might occur during cardiopulmonary resuscitation on an older adult. There may be associated injury to the lung tissue under the flail segment. Gas exchange is significantly impaired, as is the ability to cough and clear secretions. Defensive splinting because of the rib fracture further reduces the client's ability to exert the extra effort required for breathing, which may contribute later to failure to wean.

COLLABORATIVE MANAGEMENT

Assessment

The nurse assesses the client with a flail chest for paradoxic chest movement, dyspnea, cyanosis, tachycardia, and hypotension. Anxiety is often associated with pain and dyspnea.

Interventions

Interventions for flail chest include administration of humidified oxygen, pain management, promotion of lung expansion through deep breathing and positioning, and secretion clearance by coughing and tracheal aspiration.

The client with a flail chest may be treated conservatively with vigilant respiratory care. The physician may prescribe mechanical ventilation if such complications as respiratory failure or shock ensue. The physician and the nurse monitor arterial blood gas (ABG) values closely, along with vital capacity. With severe hypoxemia and hypercapnia, the client is intubated and mechanically ventilated with PEEP. With pulmonary contusion or an underlying pulmonary disease, the potential for respiratory failure increases. Flail chest is best stabilized by positive-pressure ventilation rather than surgical intervention. Operative stabilization is reserved for extreme cases of flail chest.

The nurse monitors the client's vital signs and fluid and electrolyte balance closely so that hypovolemia or shock can be treated immediately. If the client has a pulmonary contusion, the nurse monitors central venous pressure (CVP) and administers fluids as ordered. The nurse assesses for pain and intervenes to relieve the pain. The physician may order analgesic medication by the IV, epidural, or nerve block route.

The nurse gives psychosocial support to the extremely anxious client by explaining all procedures, talking slowly, and allowing time to verbalize feelings and concerns.

Pneumothorax

OVERVIEW

Any thoracic injury that allows accumulation of atmospheric air in the pleural space results in a rise in intrathoracic pressure and a reduction in vital capacity, depending on the amount of pulmonary collapse produced. Pneumothorax is often caused by blunt chest trauma and is associated with some degree of hemothorax. The pneumothorax can be open (when the pleural cavity has become exposed to the outside air, as through an open wound in the chest wall) or closed.

COLLABORATIVE MANAGEMENT

Assessment findings commonly include the following:

- Diminished breath sounds on auscultation
- Hyperresonance on percussion
- Prominence of the involved side of the chest, which moves poorly with respirations
- Deviation of the trachea away from (closed) or toward (open) the affected side

In addition, the client may have pleuritic pain, tachypnea, and **subcutaneous emphysema** (air under the skin in the subcutaneous tissues).

A chest x-ray study is used for diagnosis. Chest tubes may be indicated to allow the air to escape and the lung segment to reinflate.

Tension Pneumothorax

OVERVIEW

Tension pneumothorax, one of the most rapidly developing and life-threatening complications of blunt chest trauma, results from an air leak in the lung or chest wall. Air forced into the thoracic cavity causes complete collapse of the affected lung. Air that enters the pleural space during expiration does not exit during inspiration. As a result, air progressively accumulates under pressure, compresses the mediastinal vessels, and interferes with venous return. Because this process leads to decreased diastolic filling of the heart, cardiac output is compromised. If not promptly detected and treated, tension pneumothorax is quickly fatal. Typical causes of tension pneumothorax are blunt chest trauma, mechanical ventilation with positive end-expiratory pressure (PEEP), closed-chest drainage (chest tubes), and insertion of central venous access catheters.

COLLABORATIVE MANAGEMENT

Assessment

Assessment findings with tension pneumothorax include the following:

- Asymmetry of the thorax
- Tracheal deviation to the unaffected side
- Respiratory distress
- Absence of breath sounds on one side
- Distended neck veins
- Cyanosis
- Hypertympanic sound on percussion over the affected side

Pneumothorax is detectable on a chest x-ray film. ABG assays demonstrate hypoxia and respiratory alkalosis.

Interventions

The physician inserts a large-bore needle into the second intercostal space in the midclavicular line of the affected side as initial treatment for tension pneumothorax. After this lifesaving measure is completed, the physician places a chest tube into the fourth intercostal space of the midaxillary line and attaches the tube to a water seal drainage system until the lung reinflates.

CRITICAL THINKING CHALLENGE

The 38-year-old female client with pulmonary embolism who is now being mechanically ventilated suddenly becomes agitated and starts "bucking" the ventilator. You notice that her blood pressure is starting to fall, she is using accessory muscles, and she has no breath sounds on the right side of her chest.

- What is the most likely cause of these symptoms?
- What should you do first?

Two days later, this client is switched from assist-control (AC) ventilation of 12 to synchronized intermittent mandatory ventilation (SIMV) of 10, to start weaning. You notice that she is grimacing and holding her breath.

- What is the most likely cause of her pain?
- What is the best way of relieving her pain?

For suggested answer guidelines, go to SIMON http://www.wbsaunders.com/SIMON/Iggy/.

Hemothorax

OVERVIEW

Hemothorax is one of the most common problems encountered after blunt chest trauma or penetrating injuries. A *simple* hemothorax is a blood loss of less than 1500 mL into the thoracic cavity; a *massive* hemothorax is a blood loss of more than 1500 mL.

Bleeding is frequently caused by injuries to the lung parenchyma, such as pulmonary contusions or lacerations, which are often associated with rib and sternal fractures. Massive intrathoracic bleeding in blunt chest trauma generally stems from the heart, great vessels, or major systemic arteries, such as the intercostal arteries.

COLLABORATIVE MANAGEMENT

Assessment

Physical assessment findings vary with the size of the hemothorax. If the hemothorax is small, the client may be asymptomatic. If the hemothorax is larger, the client experiences respiratory distress. In addition, breath sounds are diminished on auscultation. The percussion note on the involved side is dull. Blood in the pleural space is visible on a chest x-ray film and confirmed by diagnostic thoracentesis.

Interventions

Interventions are aimed at evacuating the blood in the pleural space to normalize pulmonary function and to prevent infection related to blood accumulation. The physician inserts anterior and posterolateral chest tubes to evacuate the pleural space and to reduce the rush of clotted blood. The physician and the nurse carefully monitor the chest tube drainage, and chest x-ray films are evaluated serially.

The physician considers open thoracotomy when there is initial evacuation of 1500 to 2000 mL of blood or persistent bleeding at the rate of 200 mL/hr over 3 hours. The nurse monitors the vital signs, blood loss, and overall intake and output; assesses the client's response to the chest tubes; and administers IV fluids and blood as ordered. Autotransfusion of the blood lost through chest drainage should be considered.

Tracheobronchial Trauma

OVERVIEW

Most tears of the tracheobronchial tree result from severe blunt trauma primarily involving the mainstem bronchi. Injuries to the cervical trachea usually occur at the junction of the trachea and cricoid cartilage. These injuries are frequently caused by striking the anterior neck against the dashboard or steering wheel during a vehicular accident. Clients with lacerations of the trachea develop massive air leaks, which produce pneumomediastinum (air in the mediastinum) and extensive subcutaneous emphysema. Upper airway obstruction may also occur and produce severe respiratory distress and inspiratory stridor. Major cervical tears are managed by cricothyroidotomy or tracheostomy below the level of injury.

COLLABORATIVE MANAGEMENT

The nurse assesses the client for hypoxemia by ABG assays. The nurse administers oxygen appropriately. Depending on the degree of injury, the client may require mechanical ventilation or surgical repair. Frequent assessment of vital signs is essential because the client is likely to be hypotensive and in shock. The nurse continues to assess for subcutaneous emphysema and auscultates the lungs to assess for further complications every 1 to 2 hours initially. Decreased breath sounds or wheezing may indicate further obstruction, atelectasis, or pneumothorax. Care of the client with a tracheostomy is discussed in Chapter 28.

ONLINE RESOURCES

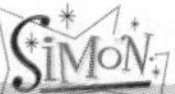

For suggested readings and Internet resources, go to http://www.wbsaunders.com/SIMON/Iggy/.

SELECTED BIBLIOGRAPHY

Asterisk indicates a classic or definitive work on this subject.

The Acute Respiratory Distress Syndrome Network. (2000). Ventilation with lower tidal volumes as compared with traditional tidal volumes for acute lung injury. *New England Journal of Medicine, 342*(18), 1301-1308.

Anderson, R. (1998). Another way to open an airway. *RN, 61*(3), 42-44.

Arcasoy, S.M., Kreit, J.W. (1999). Thrombolytic therapy of pulmonary embolism: A comprehensive review of current evidence. *Chest, 115*(6), 1695-1707.

Balas, M. (2000). Prone positioning of patients with acute respiratory distress syndrome: Applying research to practice. *Critical Care Nurse, 20*(1), 24-36.

*Baldwin-Myers, A., et al. (1994). *Standards of care for the ventilator-assisted individual: A comprehensive management plan from hospital to home.* Loma Linda, CA: Loma Linda University/Respiratory Nursing Society.

Brandstetter, R., et al. (1997). Adult respiratory distress syndrome: A disorder in need of improved outcome. *Heart and Lung, 26*(1), 3-14.

Burns, S. (1998). Making weaning easier: Pathways and protocols that work. *Critical Care Nursing Clinics of North America, 11*(4), 465-479.

Burns, S. (1999). The long-term mechanically ventilated patient: An outcomes management approach. *Critical Care Nursing Clinics of North America, 10*(1), 87-97.

Burns, S.M. (1999). Weaning from long-term mechanical ventilation. In C.M. Chulay & S.M. Burns (Eds.), *Care of the mechanically ventilated patient series.* Aliso Viejo, CA: American Association of Critical Care Nurses.

Carroll, P. (1997). When you WANT humidity. *RN, 60*(5), 30-35.

Cheever, K.H. (1999). Reducing the effects of acute pain in critically ill patients. *Dimensions of Critical Care Nursing 18*(3), 14-23.

Christie, F. (1998). Pulmonary embolism. *American Journal of Nursing, 98*(11), 36-37.

*Clochesy, J., Daly, B., & Montenegro, H. (1995). Weaning chronically critically ill adults from mechanical ventilatory support: A descriptive study. *American Journal of Critical Care, 4*(2), 93-99.

*Connolly, M.A., & Shekleton, M.E. (1991). Communicating with ventilator dependent patients. *Dimensions of Critical Care Nursing, 10*(2), 115-121.

Curley, M.A.Q. (1999). Prone positioning of patients with acute respiratory distress syndrome: A systematic review. *American Journal of Critical Care, 8*(6), 397-405.

Cushinotto, N. (1997). Pharmacology update: Clinical considerations of heparinization. *Journal of the American Academy of Nurse Practitioners, 9*(6), 273-276.

Dalen, J., & Hirsh, J. (Eds.). (1998). Fifth ACCP Consensus Conference on Antithrombotic Therapy. *Chest, 114*(Suppl.), 439S-769S.

*Dellenger, R. (Ed). (1993). Adult respiratory distress syndrome: Current considerations in future directions. *New Horizons, 1*(4), 463.

*Demling, R. (1993). Acute respiratory failure. *New Horizons, 1*(3), 361.

*Demling, R. (1993). Adult respiratory distress syndrome: Current concepts. *New Horizons, 1*(3), 388-401.

Ecklund, M. (1999). Successful outcomes for the ventilator-dependent patient. *Critical Care Nursing Clinics of North America, 11*(2), 249-260.

Ellstrom, K. (1997). Procedure for taping oral and nasal endotracheal tubes. *Perspectives in Respiratory Nursing, 8*(1), 7-8.

Ellstrom, K. (1999). Breathing easier in the intensive care unit: Pneumonia. *Critical Care Nursing Clinics of North America. 11*(4), 409-422.

Ellstrom, K. (2000). Relationship of psychoneurological, physiological, and environmental constructs to risk of unplanned extubation and outcomes in medical ICU patients. Doctoral Disseration, University of California–Los Angeles.

Fetzer, S. (1998). Laryngeal mask airway: Indications and management for critical care. *Critical Care Nurse, 18*(1), 83-87.

Frawley, P., & Habashi, N. (2001). Airway pressure release ventilation: Theory and practice. *AACN Clinical Issues: Advanced Practice in Acute and Critical Care, 12*(2), 234-246.

*Frederick, C. (1994). Noninvasive mechanical ventilation with the iron lung. *Critical Care Nursing Clinics of North America, 6*(4), 831-840.

Glass, C., Grap, M., & Battle, G. (1999). Preparing the patient and family for home mechanical ventilation. *MEDSURG Nursing, 8*(2), 99-107.

Hanneman, S.K. (1999). Weaning from short-term mechanical ventilation. In C.M. Chulay & S.M. Burns (Eds.), *Care of the mechanically ventilated patient series.* Aliso Viejo, CA: American Association of Critical Care Nurses.

Happ, M.B. (2000). Preventing treatment interference: The nurse's role in maintaining technological devices. *Heart and Lung,* 29(1), 60-69.

Happ, M.B. (2001). Communicating with mechanically ventilated patients: State of the science. *AACN Clinical Issues: Advanced Practice in Acute and Critical Care, 12*(2), 247-258.

*Henneman, E. (1996). Patients with acute respiratory failure. In J. Clochesy et al. (Eds.), *Critical care nursing* (2nd ed., pp. 630-655). Philadelphia: W.B. Saunders.

Henneman, E., Ellstrom, K., & St. John, R.E. (1999). Airway management. In C.M. Chulay & S.M. Burns (Eds.), *Care of the mechanically ventilated patient series.* Aliso Viejo, CA: American Association of Critical Care Nurses.

Johnson, R., Beneda, H. (1999). Reducing patient restraint use. *Dimensions of Critical Care Nursing, 18*(3), 34-37.

Klein, D.G. (1999). Prone positioning in patients with acute respiratory distress syndrome: The Vollman prone positioner. *Critical Care Nurse, 19*(4), 66-71.

*Knebel, A., Strider, V., & Wood, C. (1994). The art and science of caring for ventilator-assisted patients: Learning from our clinical practice. *Critical Care Nursing Clinics of North America, 6*(4), 819-830.

Marion, B. (2001). A turn for the better: "Prone positioning" of patients with ARDS. *American Journal of Nursing, 101*(5), 26-35.

McCloskey, J.C., & Bulechek, G.M. (2000). *Nursing interventions classification (NIC)* (3rd ed.). St. Louis: Mosby.

Metheny, N., et al. (1998). pH, color, and tube feedings. *RN, 61*(1), 25-27.

*Misasi, R., & Keyes, J. (1996). Matching and mismatching ventilation and perfusion in the lung. *Critical Care Nurse, 16*(3), 23-38.

O'Keefe, G. et al. (2001). Indicators of fatigue and of prolonged weaning from mechanical ventilation in surgical patients. *World Journal of Surgery,* 25(1), 98-103.

*Pierce, J.D., et al. (1993). Pressure support ventilation: Reducing the work of breathing during weaning. *Dimensions of Critical Care Nursing, 12*(6), 282-290.

Pierce, L. (2000). Traditional and nontraditional modes of mechanical ventilation. *Critical Care Nurse, 20*(1), 81-84.

Powers, J. (1999). A sedation protocol for preventing patient self-extubation. *Dimensions of Critical Care Nursing, 18*(2), 30-34.

Reid, E. (1999). Adult/elderly care nursing: Pulmonary embolism: An overview of treatment and nursing issue. *British Journal of Nursing, 8*(20), 1373-1378.

*Rosen, R.L., & Bone, R.C. (1990). Financial implications of ventilator care. *Critical Care Clinics, 6*(3), 797-805.

*Saul, L. (Ed.). (1991). *Activase therapy in acute myocardial infarction and acute massive pulmonary embolism.* Califon, NJ: Gardiner-Caldwell SynerMed.

Severson, A., Baldwin, L., & DeLoughery, T. (1997). International normalized ratio in anticoagulation therapy: Understanding the issues. *American Journal of Critical Care, 6*(2), 88-92.

*Thompson, L.F. (1996). Failure to wean: Exploration of the influence of age-related pulmonary changes. *Critical Care Nursing Clinics of North America, 8*(1), 7-16.

*Tobin, M.J. (Ed). (1994). *Principles and practice of mechanical ventilation.* New York: McGraw-Hill.

West, J.B. (1998). *Pulmonary pathophysiology: The essentials* (5th ed.). Baltimore, MD: Williams & Wilkins.

Wunderlish, R.J., et al. (1999). Patients' perceptions of uncertainty and stress during weaning from mechanical ventilation. *Dimensions of Critical Care Nursing, 18*(1), 2-8.

Yagan, M., White, D., & Staab, J. (2000). Sedation of the mechanically ventilated patient. *Critical Care Nursing Quarterly, 22*(4), 90-100.

UNIT

7

PROBLEMS OF CARDIAC OUTPUT AND TISSUE PERFUSION

Management of Clients with Problems of the Cardiovascular System

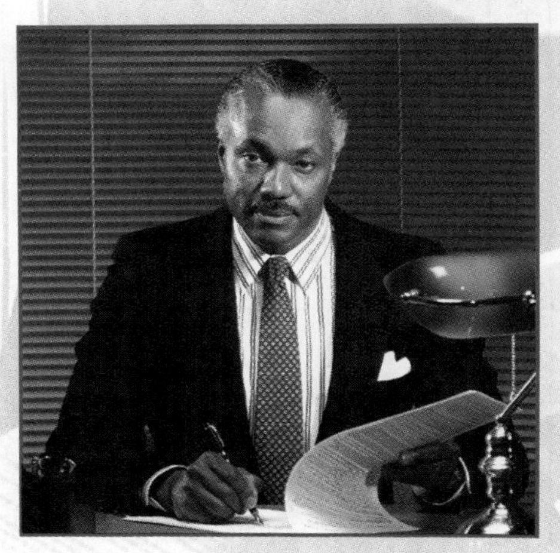

Problems of Cardiac Output and Tissue Perfusion: Cardiovascular System

■ Core Concepts Grid

Anatomy	Physiology	Pathophysiology	History	Physical Exam	Diagnostic Tests	Interventions	Pharmacology
• **Heart chambers** • **Heart valves** • **Major vessels** • **Blood flow through the heart** • **Conduction system** SA node AV node His Bundle Purkinje fibers • **Peripheral vascular system** Arteries Arterioles Capillaries Venules Veins	• **Heart rate** • **Stroke volume** • **Cardiac output** • **Cardiac cycle** • **Blood pressure**	• **Hypertension** • **Infarction** • **Atherosclerosis** • **Pump failure** • **Inflammation** • **Hypertrophy** • **Infection/ sepsis** • **Hypovolemia**	• **History of cardiac symptoms** • **Dyspnea** • **Fatigue** • **Paroxysmal nocturnal dyspnea** • **Orthopnea** • **Chest pain** • **Palpitations** • **Syncope** • **Cough** • **Past health history** • **Medications** • **Risk factors** Age Diet Activity Smoking	• **Cyanosis** • **Petechiae** • **Edema** • **Pulses** • **Heart sounds** S1-S4 • **Murmurs** • **Bruits** • **Blood pressure** • **Neck vein distention** • **Skin color** • **Hair distribution on extremities** • **Lesions** • **Clubbing** • **Dysrhythmias**	• **Chest x-ray** • **Electrocardiogram** • **Cardiac catheterization** • **Arteriography** • **Thallium scan** • **Exercise stress test** • **CK-MB** • **Lactate dehydrogenase** • **Cholesterol** • **Triglycerides** • **Lipoproteins** • **Myoglobin** • **Troponins** • **C-reactive protein**	• **Risk factor modification** • **Oxygen** • **Positioning** • **Pain control** • **Dysrhythmia monitoring** • **Diet modification** • **Heart transplantation** • **Coronary artery bypass graft (CABG)** • **MIDCAB** • **Percutaneous cardiac interventions (e.g., PTCA)** • **Fluid replacement** • **Hemodynamic monitoring** • **Mechanical ventilation** • **Cardiac rehabilitation** • **Health teaching**	• **Inotropic agent** • **Diuretics** • **Antidysrhythmics** • **Beta blockers** • **Vasodilators** • **Angiotensin-converting enzyme inhibitors** • **Calcium channel blockers** • **Nitrates** • **Anticoagulants** • **Antiplatelet agents** • **Morphine** • **Antibiotics** • **Antilipidemic agents**

CHAPTER 33

Assessment of the Cardiovascular System

KATHLEEN OUIMET PERRIN

Learning Objectives

After studying this chapter, you should be able to:

1. Review the anatomy and physiology of the cardiovascular system.
2. Describe cardiovascular changes associated with aging.
3. Identify factors that place clients at risk for cardiovascular problems.
4. Perform appropriate assessments for clients with cardiovascular problems.
5. Interpret diagnostic test findings for clients with suspected or actual cardiovascular disease.
6. Explain the purpose of hemodynamic monitoring.

SIMON

Go to http://www.wbsaunders.com/SIMON/Iggy/ for self-assessment questions related to these Learning Objectives.

In every year since 1900 (except 1918), cardiovascular disease has been the number one cause of death in the United States. It remains the major cause of mortality in the twenty-first century, resulting in 42% of all deaths, or nearly 1 million deaths, each year in the United States. In addition, the American Heart Association (AHA) estimates that approximately one in five people has experienced, and is living with, some form of cardiovascular disease (AHA, 1998).

ANATOMY AND PHYSIOLOGY REVIEW

Heart

Structure

The human heart is a cone-shaped, hollow, muscular organ located in the mediastinum between the lungs (Figure 33-1). It is approximately the size of an adult fist. The heart rests on the diaphragm, tilting forward and to the left in the client's chest. This small organ must pump continuously. Each beat of the heart pumps approximately 60 mL of blood, or approximately 5 L/min. During strenuous physical activity, the heart can double the amount of blood pumped to meet the increased oxygen needs of the peripheral tissues.

The heart is encapsulated by a protective covering called the pericardium (Figure 33-2). Cardiac muscle tissue is composed of three layers: epicardium, myocardium, and endocardium. The epicardium, the outer surface, is a thin, transparent tissue. The myocardium, the middle layer, is composed of striated muscle fibers interlaced into bundles. This layer is responsible for the contractile force of the heart. The innermost layer, the endocardium, is composed of endothelial tissue. This tissue lines the inside of the chambers of the heart and covers the four heart valves.

CHAMBERS OF THE HEART

A muscular wall (septum), separates the heart into two halves: right and left. Each half has an upper chamber (atrium) and a lower chamber (ventricle) (Figure 33-3).

RIGHT SIDE. The right atrium is a thin-walled structure that receives deoxygenated venous blood (venous return) from all peripheral tissues by way of the superior and inferior venae cavae and from the heart muscle by way of the coronary sinus. Most of this venous return flows passively from the right atrium, through the opened tricuspid valve, and to the right ventricle during ventricular diastole, or filling. The remaining venous return is actively propelled by the right atrium into the right ventricle during atrial systole, or contraction.

The right ventricle is a flat muscular pump located behind the sternum. The right ventricle generates enough pressure (approximately 25 mm Hg) to close the tricuspid valve, open the pulmonic valve, and propel blood into the pulmonary artery and the lungs. The workload of the right ventricle is light compared with that of the left ventricle because the pulmonary system is a low-pressure system, which imposes less resistance to flow.

LEFT SIDE. After blood is reoxygenated in the lungs, it flows freely from the four pulmonary veins into the left atrium. Blood then flows through an opened mitral valve into the left ventricle during ventricular diastole. When the left ventricle is almost full, the left atrium contracts, pumping the remaining blood volume into the left ventricle. With systolic contraction, the left ventricle generates enough pressure (approximately 120 mm Hg) to close the mitral valve and open the aortic valve. Blood is propelled into the aorta and into the

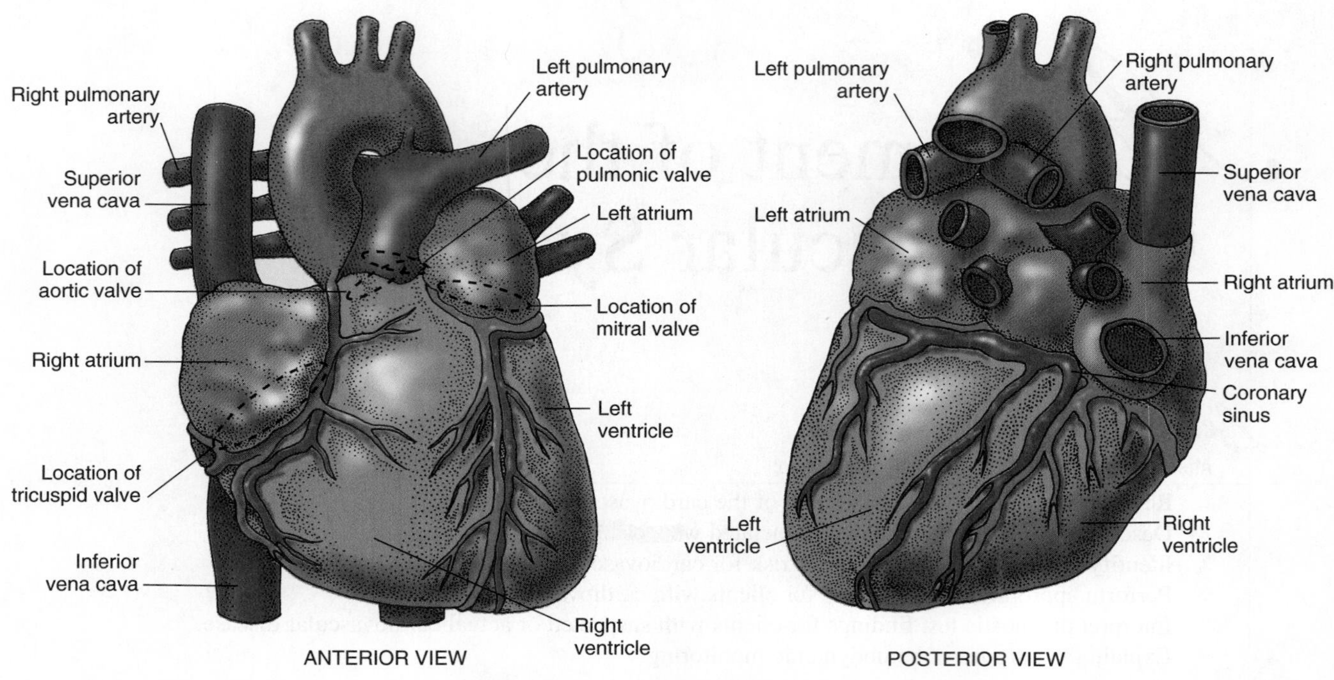

Figure 33-1 ● Surface anatomy of the heart.

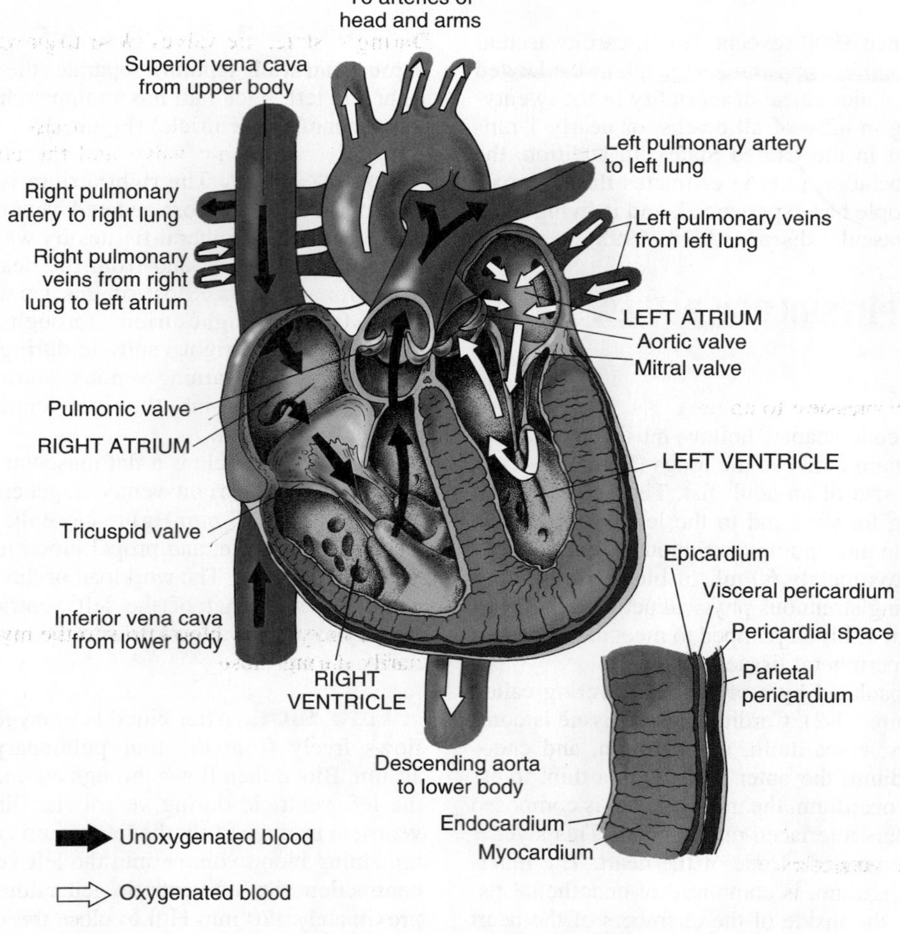

Figure 33-2 ● Blood flow through the heart.

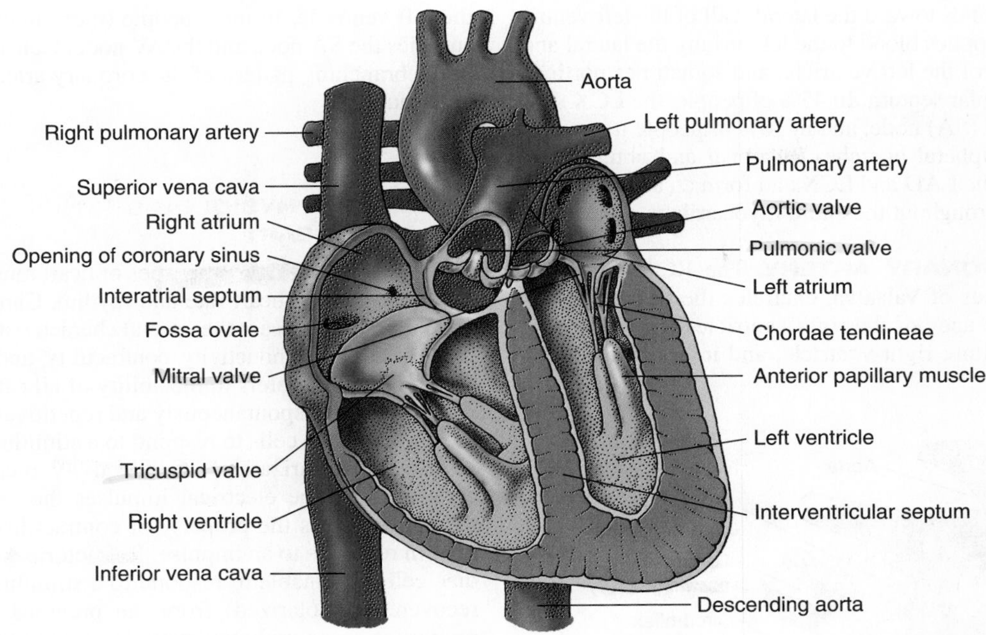

Figure 33-3 ● Cross section of the heart.

systemic arterial circulation. Blood flow through the heart is shown in Figure 33-2.

The left ventricle is ellipsoid in shape and is the largest and most muscular chamber of the heart. Its wall is two to three times the thickness of the right ventricular wall. The left ventricle must generate a higher pressure than the right ventricle because it must contract against a high–pressure systemic circulation, which imposes a greater resistance to flow.

Blood is propelled from the aorta throughout the systemic circulation to the various tissues of the body; blood returns to the right atrium because of pressure differences. The pressure of blood in the aorta of a young adult averages approximately 100 to 120 mm Hg, whereas the pressure of blood in the right atrium averages about 0 to 5 mm Hg. These differences in pressure produce a pressure gradient, with blood flowing from an area of higher pressure to an area of lower pressure. The heart and vascular structures are responsible for maintaining these pressures.

HEART VALVES

The four cardiac valves are responsible for maintaining the forward flow of blood through the chambers of the heart (see Figure 33-2). These valves open and close passively in response to pressure and volume changes within the cardiac chambers. The cardiac valves are classified into two types: atrioventricular (AV) valves and semilunar valves. Both AV valves are supported by chordae tendineae, which keep them from everting into the atria during systole.

ATRIOVENTRICULAR VALVES. The AV valves separate the atria from the ventricles. The tricuspid valve is composed of three leaflets and separates the right atrium from the right ventricle. The mitral (bicuspid) valve is composed of two leaflets and separates the left atrium from the left ventricle.

During ventricular diastole, the valves act as funnels and facilitate the flow of blood from the atria to the ventricles. During systole, the valves close to prevent the backflow (regurgitation) of blood into the atria.

SEMILUNAR VALVES. There are two semilunar valves: the pulmonic valve and the aortic valve. The pulmonic valve separates the right ventricle from the pulmonary artery. The aortic valve separates the left ventricle from the aorta. Each semilunar valve consists of three cuplike cusps, or pockets, around the inside wall of the artery. These cusps prevent blood from flowing back into the ventricles during ventricular diastole. During ventricular systole, these valves are open to permit blood flow into the pulmonary artery and the aorta.

CORONARY ARTERIES

The heart muscle receives blood to meet its metabolic needs through the coronary arterial system (Figure 33-4). The coronary arteries originate from an area on the aorta just beyond the aortic valve. There are two main coronary arteries: the left coronary artery (LCA) and the right coronary artery (RCA).

Coronary artery blood flow to the myocardium occurs primarily during diastole, when coronary vascular resistance is minimized. To maintain adequate blood flow through the coronary arteries, diastolic blood pressure must be at least 60 mm Hg.

LEFT CORONARY ARTERY. The LCA divides into two branches: the left anterior descending (LAD) and the circumflex coronary artery (LCX). The LAD branch descends toward the anterior wall and the apex of the left ventricle. It supplies blood to portions of the left ventricle, ventricular septum, chordae tendineae, papillary muscle, and right ventricle.

The LCX descends toward the lateral wall of the left ventricle and apex. It supplies blood to the left atrium, the lateral and posterior surfaces of the left ventricle, and sometimes portions of the interventricular septum. In 45% of people, the LCX supplies the sinoatrial (SA) node, and in 10% of people it supplies the AV node. Peripheral branches (diagonal and obtuse marginal) arise from the LAD and LCX and form an abundant network of vessels throughout the entire myocardium.

RIGHT CORONARY ARTERY. The RCA originates from the right sinus of Valsalva, encircles the heart, and descends toward the apex of the right ventricle. The RCA supplies the right atrium, right ventricle, and inferior portion of the left ventricle. In most people (more than 50%), the RCA supplies the SA node and the AV node. Considerable variation in the branching pattern of the coronary arteries exists among individuals.

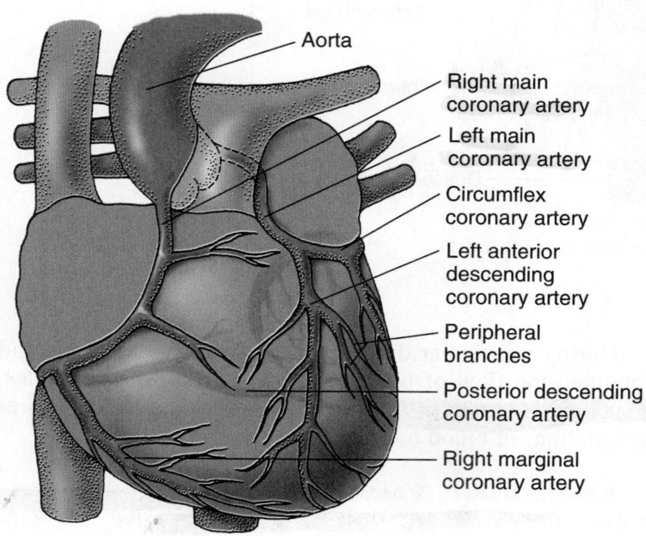

Figure 33-4 ● Coronary arterial system.

Function

ELECTROPHYSIOLOGIC PROPERTIES OF THE HEART

The electrophysiologic properties of heart muscle are responsible for regulating heart rate and rhythm. Cardiac muscle cells are unique and possess the special characteristics of automaticity, excitability, conductivity, contractility, and refractoriness.

Automaticity refers to the ability of all cardiac cells to initiate an impulse spontaneously and repetitively. Excitability is the ability of the cells to respond to a stimulus by initiating an impulse (depolarization). Conductivity means that cardiac cells transmit the electrical impulses they receive. Because the cells possess the property of contractility, they also contract in response to an impulse. Refractoriness means that cardiac cells are unable to respond to a stimulus until they have recovered (repolarized) from the previous stimulus. These properties are more completely described in Chapter 34.

CONDUCTION SYSTEM OF THE HEART

The cardiac conduction system is composed of specialized tissue capable of rhythmic electrical impulse formation (Figure 33-5). It can conduct impulses much more rapidly than other cells located in the myocardium. The SA node, located at the junction of the right atrium and the superior vena cava, is considered the main regulator of heart rate. The SA node is composed of pacemaker cells, which spontaneously initiate impulses at a rate of 60 to 100 times per minute and myocardial working cells, which transmit the impulses to the surrounding atrial muscle.

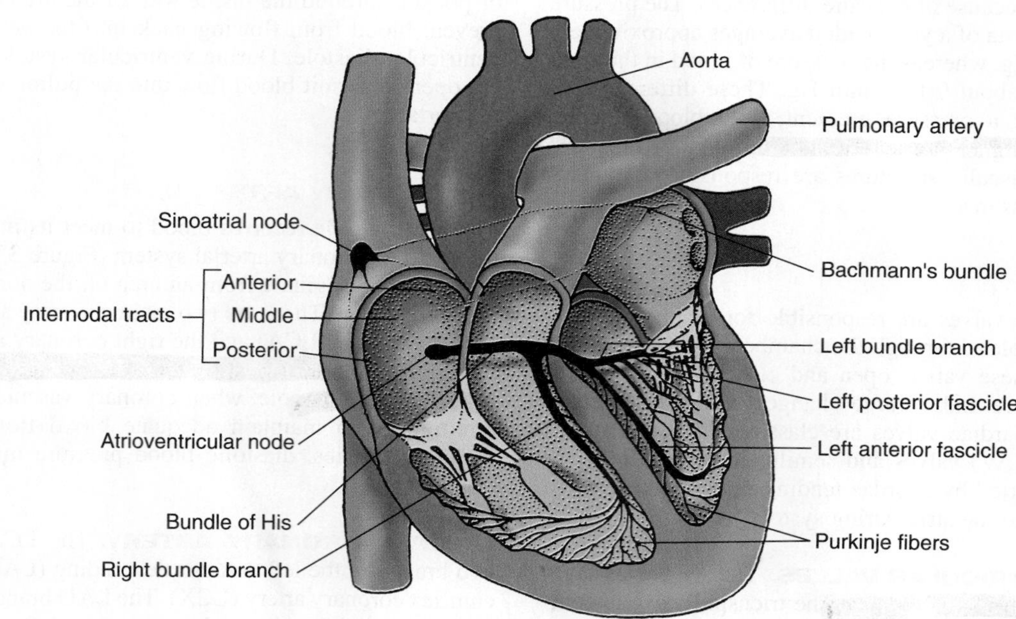

Figure 33-5 ● Conduction system of the heart.

An impulse from the SA node initiates the process of depolarization and hence the activation of all myocardial cells. The impulse travels through both atria to the atrioventricular (AV) node located in the junctional area. After the impulse reaches the AV node, conduction of the impulse is delayed briefly. This delay allows the atria to contract completely before the ventricles are stimulated to contract. The intrinsic rate of the AV node is 40 to 60 beats/min.

The Bundle of His is a continuation of the AV node and is located in the interventricular septum. It divides into the right and left bundle branches. The bundle branches extend downward through the ventricular septum and fuse with the Purkinje fiber system. The Purkinje fibers are the terminal branches of the conduction system and are responsible for carrying the wave of depolarization to both ventricular walls. Purkinje fibers can act as an intrinsic pacemaker, but their discharge rate is only 20 to 40 beats/min. Thus these intrinsic pacemakers seldom initiate an electrical impulse.

SEQUENCE OF EVENTS DURING THE CARDIAC CYCLE

The phases of the cardiac cycle are generally described in relation to changes in pressure and volume in the left ventricle during filling (diastole) and ventricular contraction (systole) (Figure 33-6). **Diastole,** normally about two thirds of the cardiac cycle, consists of relaxation and filling of the atria and ventricles, whereas **systole** consists of the contraction and emptying of the atria and ventricles.

Cardiac muscle contraction results from the release of large numbers of calcium ions from the sarcoplasmic reticulum. These ions diffuse into the myofibril sarcomere (the basic con-

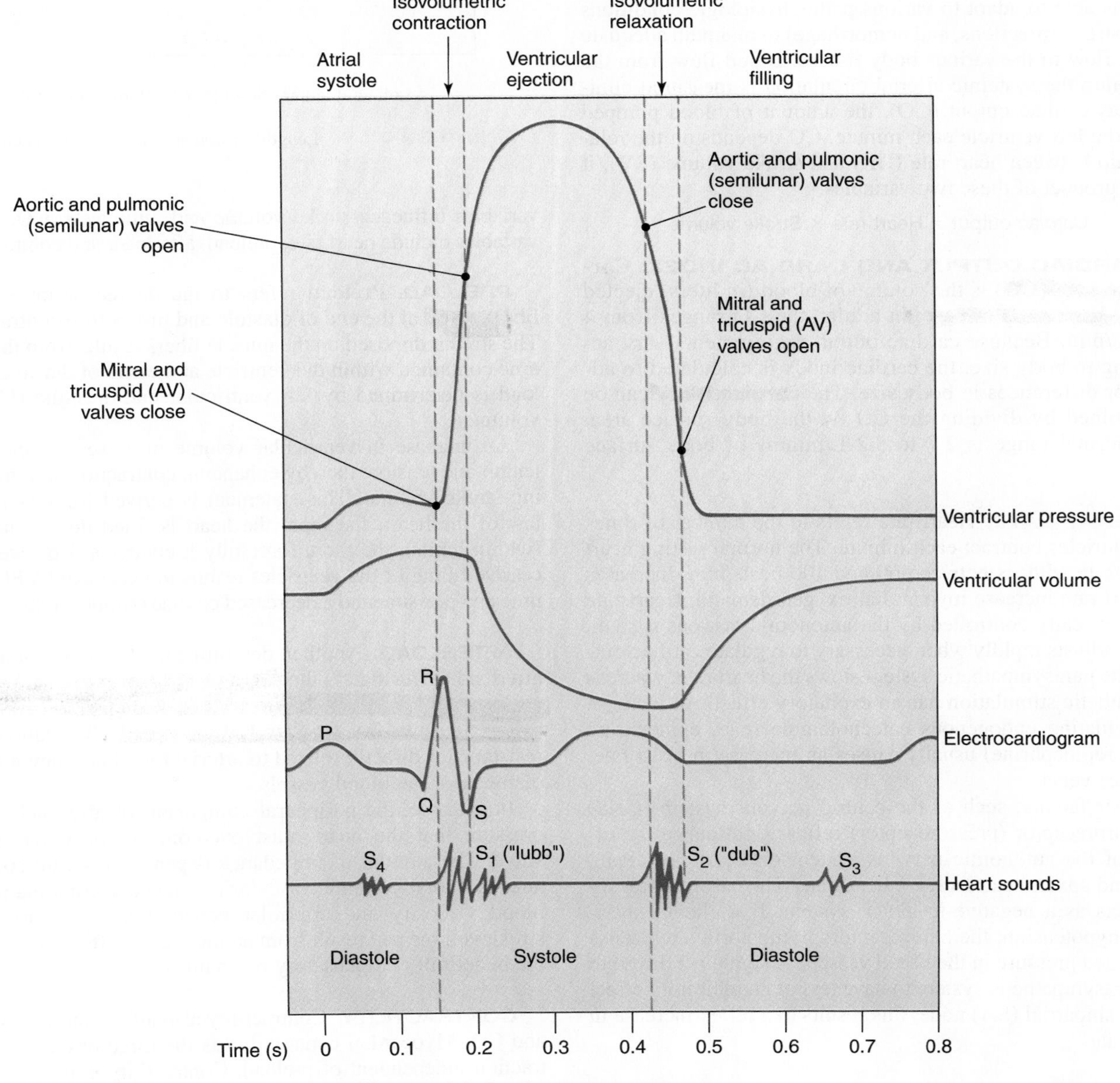

Figure 33-6 ● Events of the cardiac cycle.

tractile unit of the myocardial cell). Calcium ions promote the interaction of actin and myosin protein filaments, causing these filaments to link and overlap. Cross-bridges, or linkages, are formed as the protein filaments slide over or overlap each other. These cross-bridges act as force-generating sites. The sliding of these protein filaments of multiple myofibril sarcomeres shortens the sarcomeres, producing myocardial contraction.

Cardiac muscle relaxes when calcium ions are pumped back into the sarcoplasmic reticulum, causing a decrease in the number of calcium ions around the myofibrils. This reduced number of ions causes the protein filaments to disengage or dissociate, the sarcomere to lengthen, and the muscle to relax.

MECHANICAL PROPERTIES OF THE HEART

The electrical and mechanical properties of cardiac muscle determine the function of the cardiovascular system. The heart is able to adapt to various pathophysiologic conditions (e.g., stress, infections, and hemorrhage) to maintain adequate blood flow to the various body tissues. Blood flow from the heart into the systemic arterial circulation is measured clinically as cardiac output (CO), the amount of blood pumped from the left ventricle each minute. CO depends on the relationship between heart rate (HR) and stroke volume (SV); it is the product of these two variables:

Cardiac output = Heart rate × Stroke volume

CARDIAC OUTPUT AND CARDIAC INDEX. Cardiac output (CO) is the volume of blood (in liters) ejected by the heart each minute. In adults, the CO ranges from 4 to 7 L/min. Because cardiac output requirements vary according to body size, the cardiac index is calculated to adjust for differences in body size. The **cardiac index** can be determined by dividing the CO by the body surface area. The normal range is 2.7 to 3.2 L/min/m² of body surface area.

HEART RATE. Heart rate refers to the number of times the ventricles contract each minute. The normal resting heart rate for an adult is between 60 and 100 beats/min. Increases in heart rate increase myocardial oxygen demand. Heart rate is extrinsically controlled by the autonomic nervous system, which adjusts rapidly when necessary to regulate cardiac output. The parasympathetic system slows the heart rate, whereas sympathetic stimulation has an excitatory effect. An increase in circulating endogenous catecholamine (e.g., epinephrine and norepinephrine) usually causes an increase in heart rate, and vice versa.

Other factors, such as the central nervous system (CNS) and baroreceptor (pressoreceptor) reflexes, influence the effects of the autonomic nervous system on heart rate. Pain, fear, and anxiety can increase heart rate. The baroreceptor reflex acts as a negative-feedback system. If a client experiences hypotension, the baroreceptors in the aortic arch sense a lessened pressure in the blood vessels. A signal is relayed to the parasympathetic system to have less of an inhibitory effect on the sinoatrial (SA) node; this results in a reflex increase in heart rate.

STROKE VOLUME. Stroke volume is the amount of blood ejected by the left ventricle during each systole. Several variables influence stroke volume and, ultimately, CO. These variables include heart rate, preload, afterload, and contractility.

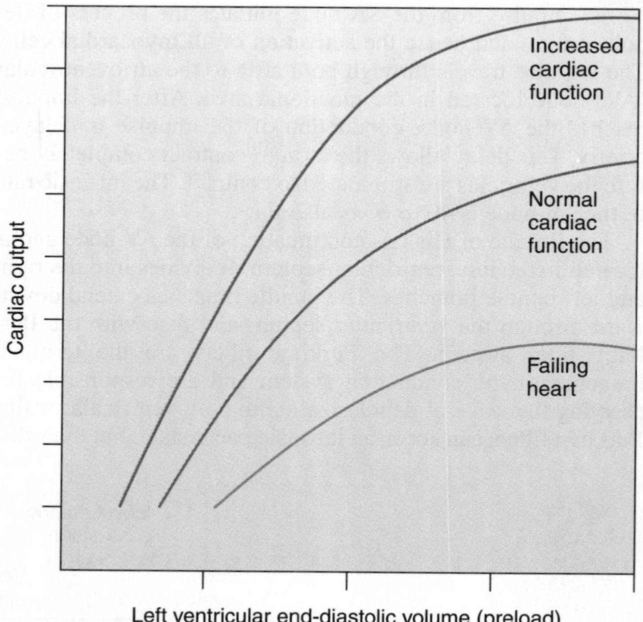

Figure 33-7 ● Length-tension ventricular function curves.

PRELOAD. Preload refers to the degree of myocardial fiber stretch at the end of diastole and just before contraction. The stretch imposed on the muscle fibers results from the volume contained within the ventricle at the end of diastole. Preload is determined by left ventricular end-diastolic (LVED) volume.

An increase in ventricular volume increases muscle fiber length and tension, thereby enhancing contraction and improving stroke volume. This statement is derived from Starling's law of the heart: the more the heart is filled during diastole (within limits), the more forcefully it contracts. However, excessive filling of the ventricles results in excessive LVED volume and pressure and a decreased cardiac output (Figure 33-7).

AFTERLOAD. Another determinant of stroke volume is afterload. **Afterload** is the pressure or resistance that the ventricles must overcome to eject blood through the semilunar valves and into the peripheral blood vessels. The amount of resistance is directly related to arterial blood pressure and the diameter of the blood vessels.

Impedance, the peripheral component of afterload, is the pressure that the heart must overcome to open the aortic valve. The amount of impedance depends on aortic compliance and total systemic vascular resistance, a combination of blood viscosity and arteriolar constriction. A decrease in stroke volume can result from an increase in afterload without the benefit of compensatory mechanisms.

CONTRACTILITY. Contractility also affects stroke volume and CO. Myocardial contractility is the force of cardiac contraction independent of preload. Contractility is increased by factors such as sympathetic stimulation and calcium release. Factors such as hypoxia and acidemia decrease contractility.

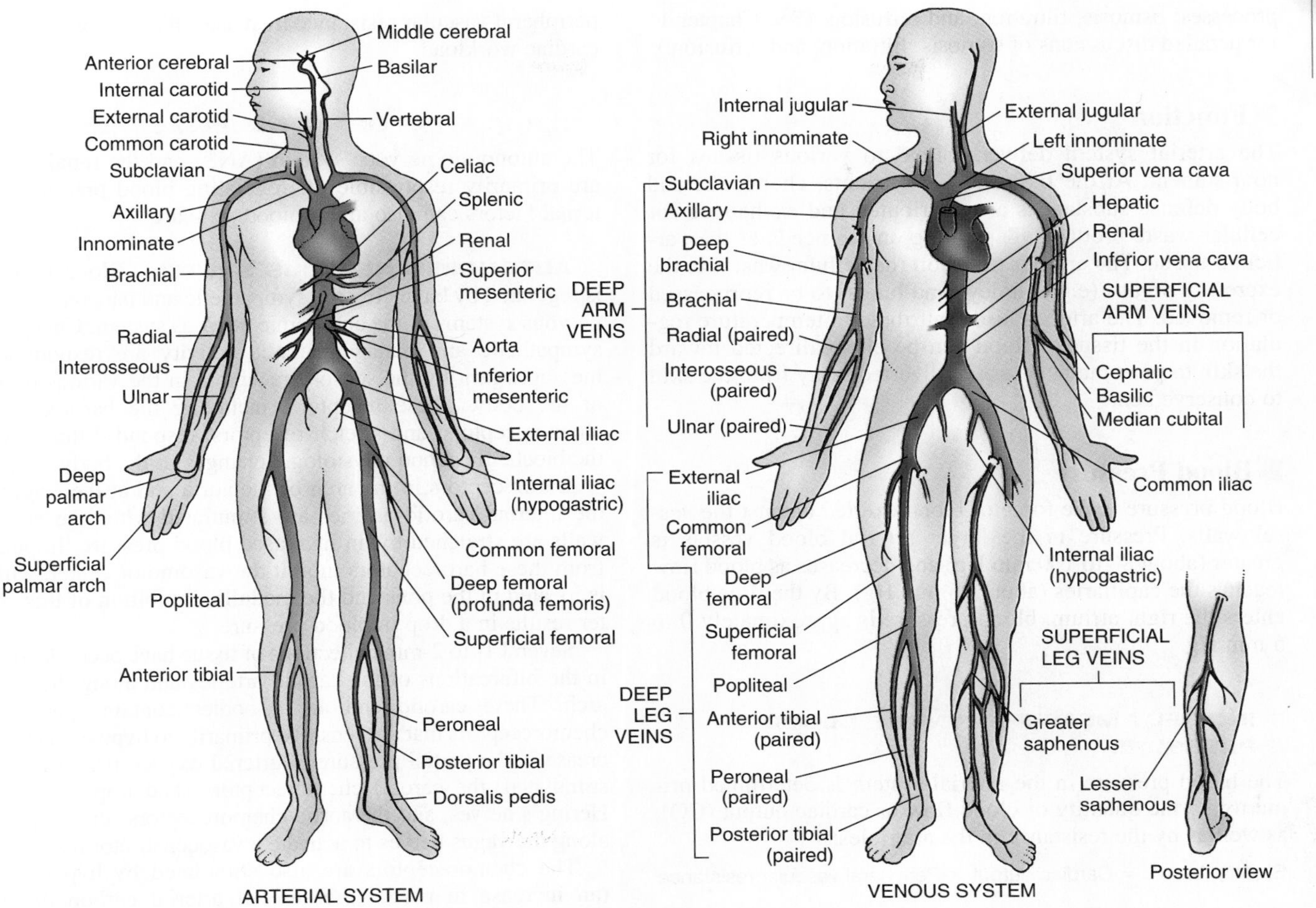

Figure 33-8 ● Anatomy of the arterial and venous systems.

Vascular System

The vascular system serves several purposes:

- To provide conduits for blood to travel from the heart to nourish the various tissues of the body
- To carry cellular wastes to the excretory organs
- To allow lymphatic flow to drain tissue fluid back into the circulation
- To return blood to the heart for recirculation

This system of conduits depends on an efficient heart and patent blood vessels to regulate and maintain systemic and regional blood flow and temperature.

The vascular system is divided into the arterial system and the venous system (Figure 33-8). In the arterial system, blood moves from the larger conduits to a network of smaller blood vessels. In the venous system, blood travels from the capillaries to the venules and to the larger system of veins, eventually returning in the venae cavae to the heart for recirculation.

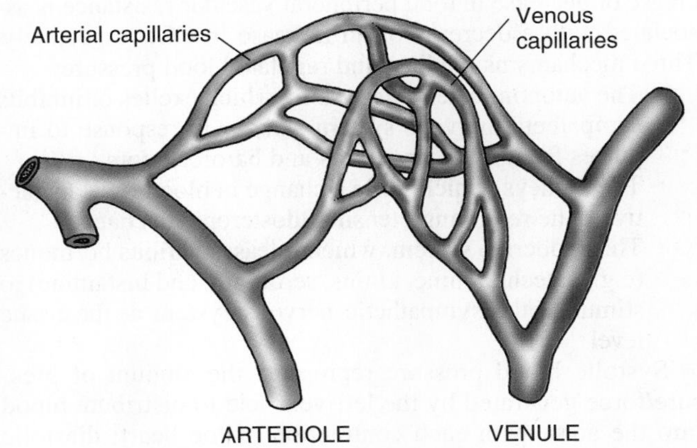

Figure 33-9 ● Structure of the capillary bed.

ARTERIAL SYSTEM

Structure

The high-pressure blood vessels of the arterial vascular system may be classified according to their size and wall structure. The large arteries, such as the aorta and femoral arteries, follow relatively straight routes and have few branches. Smaller arteries, such as the internal iliac and mesenteric arteries, divide from larger ones and have multiple branches.

Arteries may branch into arterioles or anastomose with other arteries. The arterioles branch into terminal arterioles, which join with capillaries and ultimately with venules to form the capillary network (Figure 33-9). The exchange of nutrients across the capillary membrane occurs primarily by three processes: osmosis, filtration, and diffusion. (See Chapter 11 for detailed discussions of osmosis, filtration, and diffusion.)

Function

The arterial system delivers blood to various tissues for nourishment. At the tissue level, nutrients, chemicals, and body defense substances are distributed and exchanged for cellular waste products, depending on the needs of the particular tissue. The arteries transport the cellular wastes to the excretory organs (e.g., kidneys and lungs) to be reprocessed or removed. The arteries also contribute to temperature regulation in the tissues. Blood can be either directed toward the skin to promote heat loss or diverted away from the skin to conserve heat.

Blood Pressure

Blood pressure is the force of blood exerted against the vessel walls. Pressure in the larger arterial blood vessels is greater (about 80 to 100 mm Hg) and decreases as blood flow reaches the capillaries (about 25 mm Hg). By the time blood enters the right atrium, blood pressure is approximately 0 to 5 mm Hg.

INDIRECT MEASUREMENT OF BLOOD PRESSURE

The blood pressure in the arterial system is determined primarily by the quantity of blood flow or cardiac output (CO), as well as by the resistance in the arterioles:

Blood pressure = Cardiac output × Peripheral vascular resistance

Any factor that increases CO or total peripheral vascular resistance increases blood pressure. In general, blood pressure is maintained at a relatively constant level; therefore an increase or decrease in total peripheral vascular resistance is associated with a decrease or an increase in CO, respectively. Three mechanisms mediate and regulate blood pressure:

- The autonomic nervous system, which excites or inhibits sympathetic nervous system activity in response to impulses from chemoreceptors and baroreceptors
- The kidneys, which sense a change in blood flow and activate the renin-angiotensin-aldosterone mechanism
- The endocrine system, which releases various hormones (e.g., catecholamine, kinins, serotonin, and histamine) to stimulate the sympathetic nervous system at the tissue level

Systolic blood pressure represents the amount of pressure/force generated by the left ventricle to distribute blood into the aorta with each contraction of the heart; diastolic blood pressure represents the amount of pressure/force sustained by the arteries during the relaxation phase of the heart. In the adult, systolic pressure is normally 90 to 135 mm Hg, and diastolic pressure is normally 60 to 85 mm Hg. Blood pressure is expressed as systolic pressure/diastolic pressure.

Systolic pressure is affected by a number of factors, including CO. When CO decreases, systolic pressure also decreases. Diastolic pressure is primarily determined by the amount of vasoconstriction in the periphery. An increase in peripheral vascular resistance increases diastolic pressure and cardiac workload.

REGULATION OF BLOOD PRESSURE

The autonomic nervous system (ANS) and the renal system are primarily responsible for regulating blood pressure. External factors can also affect blood pressure.

AUTONOMIC NERVOUS SYSTEM. Blood pressure is regulated by balancing the sympathetic and parasympathetic nervous systems of the autonomic nervous system. Changes in sympathetic and parasympathetic activity are responses to messages sent by the sensory receptors in the various tissues of the body. These receptors, including the baroreceptors, chemoreceptors, and stretch receptors, respond differently to the biochemical and physiologic changes of the body.

Baroreceptors in the arch of the aorta and at the origin of the internal carotid arteries are stimulated when the arterial walls are stretched by an increased blood pressure. Impulses from these baroreceptors inhibit the vasomotor center, which is located in the pons and the medulla. Inhibition of this center results in a drop in blood pressure.

Several 1- to 2-mm collections of tissue have been identified in the bifurcations of the carotid arteries and along the aortic arch. These carotid and aortic bodies contain specialized chemoreceptors that are sensitive primarily to hypoxemia (a decrease in the partial pressure of arterial oxygen [$Pa{O_2}$]). When stimulated, the carotid chemoreceptors send impulses along Hering's nerves, and the aortic chemoreceptors send impulses along the vagus nerves to activate a vasoconstrictor response.

The chemoreceptors are also stimulated by hypercapnia (an increase in partial pressure of arterial carbon dioxide [$Pa{CO_2}$]) and acidosis. However, the direct effect of carbon dioxide on the central nervous system is 10 times stronger than the effect it produces by stimulating the chemoreceptors.

Stretch receptors found in the venae cavae and the right atrium are sensitive to pressure or volume changes. When a client is hypovolemic, the stretch receptors in the blood vessels sense a reduced volume or pressure and send fewer impulses to the central nervous system. This reaction stimulates the sympathetic nervous system to increase heart rate and constrict the peripheral blood vessels.

RENAL SYSTEM. The renal system also helps to regulate cardiovascular activity. When renal blood flow or pressure decreases, the kidneys retain sodium and water. Blood pressure tends to rise because of fluid retention and because of activation of the renin-angiotensin-aldosterone mechanism. Vascular volume is also regulated by the release of antidiuretic hormone (vasopressin) from the posterior pituitary gland (see Chapter 11).

EXTERNAL FACTORS. Other factors can influence the activity of the cardiovascular system. Emotional behaviors (e.g., excitement, pain, anger) stimulate the sympathetic nervous system to increase blood pressure and heart rate. Increased physical activity such as exercise increases blood pressure and pulse rate. Body temperature can affect the metabolic needs of the tissues, thereby influencing the delivery of blood. In hypothermia, tissues require fewer nutrients and blood pressure falls. In hyperthermia, the metabolic requirement of the tissues is greater, and blood pressure and pulse rate rise.

VENOUS SYSTEM

Structure

The venous system is composed of a series of veins that are located adjacent to the arterial system. A second superficial venous circulation runs parallel to the subcutaneous tissue of the extremity. These two venous systems are connected by communicating veins that provide a means for blood to travel from the superficial veins to the deep veins. Blood flow is directed toward the deep venous circulation.

The venules collect blood from the capillaries and the terminal arterioles. White blood cells also enter and exit the body tissues at the venules.

Venules branch into veins, which are low-pressure blood vessels. Veins have the ability to accommodate large shifts in volume with minimal changes in venous pressure. This flexibility allows the venous system to accommodate the administration of intravenous (IV) fluids and blood transfusions, blood loss, and dehydration. All veins in the superficial and deep venous systems in the legs (except the smallest and the largest veins) have valves that direct blood flow back to the heart; this prevents retrograde flow (backflow).

Function

The primary function of the venous system is to complete the circulation of blood by returning blood from the capillaries to the right side of the heart. The venous system also acts as a reservoir for a large portion of the blood volume. In contrast to the arterial system, which consists of a high-pressure, continuous flow system through relatively rigid conduits, the venous system consists of a low-pressure, intermittent flow system through collapsible tubes that work against the effects of gravity.

Gravity exerts an increase in hydrostatic pressure (capillary blood pressure) when the client is in an upright position, which delays venous return. Hydrostatic pressure is lessened when the client is lying down, and thus there is less hindrance of venous return to the heart.

Cardiovascular Changes Associated with Aging

A number of physiologic changes in the cardiovascular system occur with advancing age (Chart 33-1). Many of these changes result in a loss of cardiac reserve. Thus these changes are usually not evident when the older adult is resting. They become apparent only when the person is physically or emotionally stressed and the heart cannot meet the increased metabolic demands of the body.

ASSESSMENT TECHNIQUES

History

The nurse obtains a thorough history, which includes demographic data, personal and family history, diet, socioeconomic status, and a functional assessment. The focus of the history is on obtaining information relative to client's risk factors and symptoms of cardiovascular disease (Chart 33-2).

DEMOGRAPHIC DATA

Demographic data include the client's age, sex, and ethnic origin. The incidence of conditions such as coronary artery disease (CAD) and valvular disease increases with age (AHA, 1998). The incidence of CAD also varies with the client's sex. Women who are premenopausal have a lower incidence of CAD than do men.

CULTURAL CONSIDERATIONS

Information about the client's ethnic or cultural background is important because some disease conditions may be more prevalent in specific ethnic groups. For example, African Americans and Mexican Americans have a higher incidence of hypertension than do Caucasians (AHA, 1998). The nurse should be aware that some clients may refer to their hypertension as "high blood."

Age, sex, ethnic background, and family history of cardiovascular disease are considered nonmodifiable or uncontrollable risk factors for cardiovascular disease. Modifiable risk factors (e.g., high blood pressure and excessive blood cholesterol), if controlled, can reduce the risk of heart disease. These factors are discussed under Modifiable Risk Factors, p. 629.

PERSONAL AND FAMILY HISTORY

The nurse reviews the client's history, noting any major illnesses such as diabetes mellitus, renal disease, anemia, high blood pressure, stroke, bleeding disorders, connective tissue diseases, chronic pulmonary diseases, heart disease, and thrombophlebitis. These conditions can influence the client's cardiovascular status.

The nurse asks about previous treatment for cardiovascular disease, identifies previous diagnostic procedures (e.g., electrocardiography and cardiac catheterization), and requests information about any medical or invasive treatment of cardiovascular disease. It is important for the nurse to ask specifically about recurrent tonsillitis, streptococcal infections, and rheumatic fever, because these conditions may lead to valvular abnormalities of the heart. In addition, the nurse inquires about any known congenital heart defects. Many clients with congenital heart problems are living into adulthood because of improved treatment and surgical modalities.

Clients are asked in detail about their medication history, beginning with any current or recent use of prescription or over-the-counter (OTC) medications or herbal/natural products (e.g., ginseng). The nurse inquires about known sensitivities to any drug and the nature of the reaction (e.g., nausea, rash). Clients should be asked whether they have recently used cocaine or any IV "street" drugs, because they may be associated with chest pain or endocarditis.

The nurse also asks female clients whether they are taking oral contraceptives or an estrogen replacement. There is an increased incidence of myocardial infarction (MI) and stroke in women over the age of 35 who take oral contraceptives, but only if they smoke, have diabetes, or have hypertension.

CHART 33-1

NURSING FOCUS *on the* OLDER ADULT

Changes in the Cardiovascular System Related to Aging

Change	Nursing Implications	Rationale
CARDIAC VALVES		
Calcification and mucoid degeneration occur, especially in mitral and aortic valves	Assess heart rate and rhythm and heart sounds for murmurs. Question clients about dyspnea.	Murmurs may be detected before other symptoms. Valvular abnormalities may result in rhythm changes.
CONDUCTION SYSTEM		
Pacemaker cells decrease in number. Fibrous tissue and fat in the sinoatrial node increase. Few muscle fibers remain in the atrial myocardium and bundle of His. Conduction time increases.	Assess the electrocardiogram (ECG) and heart rhythm for dysrhythmias or a heart rate less than 60 beats/min.	The sinoatrial (SA) node may lose its inherent rhythm. Atrial dysrhythmias occur in 50%-90% of elders; 80% of elders experience premature ventricular contractions (PVCs).
LEFT VENTRICLE		
The size of the left ventricle increases. The left ventricle becomes stiff and less distensible. Fibrotic changes in the left ventricle decrease the speed of early diastolic filling by about 50%.	Assess the ECG for a widening QRS complex and a longer QT interval. Assess for activity intolerance. Assess the heart rate at rest and with activity. Assess for activity intolerance.	Ventricular changes result in decreased stroke volume, ejection fraction, and cardiac output during exercise; the heart is less able to meet increased oxygen demands. Maximum heart rate with exercise is decreased. The heart is less able to meet increased oxygen demands.
AORTA AND OTHER LARGE ARTERIES		
The aorta and other large arteries thicken and become stiffer and less distensible. Systolic blood pressure increases to compensate for the stiff arteries. Systemic vascular resistance increases as a result of less distensible arteries; therefore the left ventricle pumps against greater resistance, contributing to left ventricular hypertrophy.	Assess blood pressure. Note increases in systolic, diastolic, and pulse pressures. Assess for activity intolerance and shortness of breath. Assess the peripheral pulses.	Hypertension may occur and must be treated to avoid target organ damage.
BARORECEPTORS		
Baroreceptors become less sensitive.	Assess the client's blood pressure with the client lying and then sitting or standing. Assess for dizziness when the client changes from a lying to a sitting or standing position. Teach the client to change positions slowly.	Orthostatic (postural) and postprandial changes occur because of ineffective baroreceptors. Changes may include blood pressure decreases of 10 mm Hg or more, dizziness, and fainting.

The nurse reviews the family history and obtains information about the age, health status, and cause of death of immediate family members. A family history of hypertension, obesity, diabetes, or sudden cardiac death is especially significant.

DIET HISTORY

A diet history includes the client's recall of food and fluid intake during a 24-hour period, self-imposed or medically prescribed dietary restrictions or supplementations, and the amount and type of alcohol consumption. The dietitian reviews the type of foods selected by the client for the amount of sodium, sugar, cholesterol, fiber, and fat. The nurse or dietitian also explores the client's attitude toward food, knowledge level of essential and nonessential dietary elements, and willingness to make changes in the diet. Cultural beliefs and economic status can influence the choice of food items and therefore must be reviewed. Family members or significant others who are responsible for shopping and cooking are included in this discussion.

SOCIOECONOMIC STATUS

The social history includes information about the client's domestic situation, such as marital status, number of children, household members, living environment, and occupation. The nurse also identifies support systems. It is especially important to explore the possibility that the client might have difficulty paying for medications or treatment.

The nurse asks about the client's occupation, including the type of work performed and the requirements of the specific job. For instance, does the job involve lifting of heavy objects? Is the job emotionally stressful? What does a day's work entail? Does the client's job require him or her to be outside in extreme weather conditions?

CHART 33-2

CARDIOVASCULAR ASSESSMENT
Using Gordon's Functional Health Patterns

Health Perception-Health Management
What advice has your health care provider offered you about exercise, diet, or smoking?
Are you able to follow that advice?
What medications (both over-the-counter and prescription) are you supposed to be taking?
Are you taking them as suggested or prescribed?
What problems have you had with the medications?

Nutrition-Metabolic
What is your usual daily diet? (Analyze the diet for saturated fat, cholesterol, total calorie, and sodium content.)
How much fluid do you drink daily? Are you thirsty?
What do you weigh? When did you last weigh yourself? How often do you weigh yourself?
What is your height?
Do you know your cholesterol level? What is it?
How often do you feel nauseated or not interested in eating?
Do your feet/ankles swell during the day? At night, too?

Elimination
How often do you urinate in the daytime?
How often do you wake up at night to urinate?

Activity-Exercise
What is the most strenuous exercise that you did last week?
How active are you compared with 6 months ago? 1 year ago?
How often do you feel fatigued or tired?
Can you climb a flight of stairs and walk a block without feeling short of breath or experiencing chest pain?
Do you experience leg cramps when you walk or climb stairs?

Sleep-Rest
Where do you sleep? (In bed? In a lounge chair?)
How many pillows do you sleep on?
Do you ever wake up at night short of breath?
What happens when you wake up short of breath?
Do you ever wake up at night with pain or cramps in your legs? How do you relieve that sensation?

Cognitive-Perceptual
How is your memory? What does your family say about your memory?
How often do you feel dizzy, disoriented, or faint?
Do you ever have chest discomfort? How often? What precipitates it? What is it like? How do you relieve it? What is its level on a scale of 0 to 10?
Do you ever have leg or buttock pain? What are its characteristics?
How do you learn best?

Role-Relationship
What is your job?
What does a day's work entail?
What are your family responsibilities?
Whom do you live with?
Who is available to help you?

Sexuality-Reproductive
Has your ability to engage in sexual activity changed in the past year?
If so, how?
Do you take any medications that affect your sexual response? If so, what?

Coping-Stress Tolerance
What do you think has been happening to you?
How do you respond to being caught in a traffic jam or meeting a deadline?
What do you do to relax?
What do you do when you feel stressed?

Based on Gordon, M. (2000). *Manual of nursing diagnosis* (9th ed.). St. Louis: Mosby.

MODIFIABLE RISK FACTORS

Personal habits that are risk factors for heart disease include cigarette smoking, physical inactivity, obesity, and type A behavior. These factors are considered modifiable or controllable risk factors. The nurse inquires about each of the following modifiable risk factors.

Cigarette Smoking

Cigarette smoking is a major risk factor for cardiovascular disease, specifically CAD and peripheral vascular disease (PVD) (AHA, 1998). According to the U.S. Department of Health and Human Services (DHHS), cigarette smoking is directly responsible for 21% of all deaths from CAD. Three compounds in cigarette smoke have been implicated in the development of CAD: tar, nicotine, and carbon monoxide.

The risks to the cardiovascular system from cigarette smoking appear to be dose related, noncumulative, and transient. The smoking history should include the number of cigarettes smoked daily, the duration of the smoking habit, and the age of the client when smoking started. A person who smokes fewer than 4 cigarettes per day has twice the risk of cardiovascular disease of a person who does not smoke; a person who smokes more than 20 cigarettes per day has four times the risk. Typically, the nurse records the smoking history in pack-years, which is the number of packs per day multiplied by the number of years the client has smoked.

The nurse should inquire about the client's desire to quit, past attempts to quit, and the methods used. The nurse may ascertain nicotine dependence by asking questions such as the following:

- How soon after you wake up in the morning do you smoke?
- Do you find it difficult not to smoke in places where smoking is prohibited?
- Do you smoke when you are ill?

Three to four years after a client has stopped smoking, his or her cardiovascular risk appears to be similar to that of a person who has never smoked. The nurse asks clients who do not currently smoke whether they have ever smoked and when they quit.

Physical Inactivity

A sedentary lifestyle is also considered a significant risk factor in the development of heart disease. Regular physical activity promotes cardiovascular fitness and produces beneficial changes in blood pressure and levels of blood lipids and clotting factors. Unfortunately, few people in the United States engage in the recommended exercise guidelines: 30 minutes daily of light to moderate exercise, which is equivalent to a 30-minute brisk walk. According to the American Heart Association, only 22% of Americans engage in this much exercise five times a week, and only 15% engage in vigorous physical activity (enough to promote cardiopulmonary fitness) three times a week (AHA, 1998). Therefore more people are at risk for CAD from physical inactivity than from any other factor. The nurse questions clients concerning the type of exercise in which they engage, the period for which they have participated in the exercise, and the frequency and intensity of the exercise.

Obesity

Approximately 104 million Americans adults are overweight when defined as a body mass index (BMI) of 25 to 30. Another 42 million Americans are obese, which is defined as a BMI greater than 30 (AHA, 1998). Obesity in the American population has increased 36% in the last 30 years; it is particularly a problem for African-American females, Mexican Americans, and native Hawaiians (AHA, 1998). Obesity is associated with hypertension, hyperlipidemia, and diabetes; all are known contributors to cardiovascular disease.

The nurse weighs the client, calculates the BMI, and examines the pattern of obesity, also known as the waist-hip ratio. Chapter 61 describes these assessments in detail.

> **WOMEN'S HEALTH CONSIDERATIONS**
>
> Caucasian women with abdominal obesity (greater waist circumference than hip circumference) are more likely to experience cardiovascular disease than are Caucasian women with fat distributed in their buttocks, hips, and thighs (greater hip circumference than waist circumference). Clients with an early onset of obesity (during adolescence) and an elevated waist-hip ratio appear to be at especially high risk for cardiovascular disease.

Type A Personality

Researchers have identified that people with type A personalities are more vulnerable to the development of heart disease. Type A personalities are highly competitive, overly concerned about meeting deadlines, and are often hostile or angry. The nurse might ask the client: "Have you ever experienced road rage?" or "How do you respond when you have to wait for an appointment?" The chronic anger and hostility displayed by type A people appear to be most closely associated with cardiovascular disease. The constant arousal of the sympathetic nervous system as a result of anger may influence blood pressure, serum fatty acids and lipids, and clotting mechanisms. The nurse observes the client and determines his or her response to stressful situations.

CURRENT HEALTH PROBLEMS

Inquiring about major concerns helps the nurse to establish priorities in nursing care and management. The client is asked to describe his or her health concerns. The nurse expands on the description of these concerns by obtaining information about their onset, duration, chronology, frequency, location, quality, intensity, associated symptoms, and precipitating, aggravating, and relieving factors. Major symptoms identified by clients with cardiovascular disease include chest pain or discomfort, dyspnea, fatigue, palpitations, weight gain, syncope, and extremity pain.

Chest Pain

Chest pain or discomfort, a cardinal symptom of heart disease, can result from ischemic heart disease, pericarditis, and aortic dissection. Chest pain can also be due to noncardiac conditions such as pleurisy, pulmonary embolus, hiatal hernia, and anxiety. Nurses must thoroughly evaluate the nature and characteristics of the chest pain. Because chest pain resulting from myocardial ischemia is life threatening and can lead to serious complications, its cause should be considered ischemic (reduced or obstructed blood flow to the myocardium) until proven otherwise.

When assessing for chest pain, the nurse uses alternative terms such as "discomfort," "heaviness," and "indigestion." Clients often do not experience pain in the chest but instead feel discomfort or indigestion. The client may also describe the sensation as aching, choking, strangling, tingling, squeezing, constricting, or vise-like.

The nurse asks the client to identify when the pain was first noticed (onset). Did the pain begin suddenly or develop gradually (manner of onset)? How long did it last (duration)? If the client has repeated chest pain episodes, the nurse assesses how often the pain occurs (frequency). The nurse asks whether this pain is different from any other episodes of pain. The nurse asks the client to describe what activities he or she was doing when it first occurred, such as sleeping, arguing, or running (precipitating factors). The client can be asked to point to the area where the chest pain occurred (location) and to describe how the pain spread (radiation).

In addition, the client describes how the pain feels and whether it is sharp or dull (quality). To understand the severity of the pain, the nurse asks the client to grade it from 0 to 10, with 0 indicating an absence of pain and 10 indicating severe pain (intensity). The client may also report other signs and symptoms that occur at the same time (associated symptoms), such as dyspnea, diaphoresis, nausea, and vomiting. Other factors that need to be addressed are those that may have made the chest pain worse (aggravating factors) or less intense (relieving factors). Chest pain may arise from a variety of sources (Table 33-1). By obtaining the appropriate information, the nurse may assist in identifying the source of the chest discomfort.

Dyspnea

Dyspnea can occur as a result of both cardiac and pulmonary disease. Dyspnea is objectively described as difficult or labored breathing and is subjectively experienced as uncomfortable breathing or shortness of breath. When obtaining the client's history, the nurse ascertains what factors precipitate and relieve dyspnea, what level of activity produces dyspnea, and the client's body position when dyspnea occurred.

There are several types of dyspnea. Dyspnea that is associated with activity, such as climbing stairs, is referred to as dyspnea on exertion (DOE). This is usually an early symptom of heart failure.

The client with advanced heart disease may experience orthopnea, or dyspnea that appears when the client lies flat. The client may use several pillows at night to elevate the head and chest or may sleep in a recliner to prevent nighttime breathlessness. The severity of orthopnea is measured by the number of pillows or the amount of head elevation needed to provide restful sleep. Orthopnea is usually relieved within a matter of minutes by sitting up or standing.

Paroxysmal nocturnal dyspnea develops after the client has been lying down for several hours. In this position, blood from the lower extremities is redistributed to the venous system, which increases venous return to the heart. A diseased heart is unable to compensate for the increased volume and is ineffective in pumping the additional fluid into the circulatory system. Pulmonary congestion results. The client awakens

TABLE 33-1 • ASSESSMENT OF CHEST DISCOMFORT: HOW VARIOUS TYPES OF CHEST PAIN DIFFER

Onset	Quality and Severity	Location and Radiation	Duration and Relieving Factors
ANGINA			
Sudden, usually in response to exertion, emotion, or extremes in temperature	Squeezing, vise-like pain	Substernal; may spread across the chest and the back and/or down the arms	Usually lasts less than 15 min; relieved with rest, nitrate administration, or oxygen therapy
MYOCARDIAL INFARCTION			
Sudden, without precipitating factors, often in early morning	Intense stabbing, vise-like pain or pressure, severe	Substernal; may spread throughout the anterior chest and to the arms, jaw, back, or neck	Usually lasts 30 min or longer or is relieved with opioids
PERICARDITIS			
Sudden	Sharp stabbing, moderate to severe	Substernal; usually spreads to the left side or the back	Intermittent; relieved with sitting upright, analgesia, or administration of anti-inflammatory agents
PLEUROPULMONARY			
Variable	Moderate ache, worse on inspiration	Lung fields	Continuous until the underlying condition is treated or the client has rested
ESOPHAGEAL-GASTRIC			
Variable	Squeezing, heartburn, variable severity	Substernal; may spread to the shoulders or the abdomen	Variable; may be relieved with antacid administration or food intake
ANXIETY			
Variable, may be in response to stress or fatigue	Dull ache to sharp stabbing; may be associated with numbness in fingers	Usually the left side of chest without radiation	Usually lasts a few minutes

abruptly, often with a feeling of suffocation and panic. The client usually sits upright with the legs dangled over the bedside to relieve the dyspnea. This sensation may last for 20 minutes before disappearing.

Fatigue

Fatigue may be described as a feeling of tiredness or weariness resulting from activity. The client may complain that a certain activity takes longer to complete or that he or she tires easily after activity. Although fatigue in itself is not diagnostic of heart disease, many people with heart failure are limited by leg fatigue during exercise. Fatigue that occurs after mild activity and exertion usually indicates inadequate cardiac output (low stroke volume) and anaerobic metabolism in skeletal muscle.

The nurse questions the client to determine the time of day he or she experiences fatigue as well as the activities that he or she can perform. Fatigue resulting from decreased cardiac output is often worse in the evening. The nurse asks whether the client can perform the same activities as a year ago or the same activities as others of the same age. Often the client limits activities in response to fatigue and unless questioned is unaware how much less active he or she has become.

Palpitations

A feeling of fluttering in the chest or an unpleasant awareness of the heartbeat is referred to as **palpitations.** Palpitations may result from a change in heart rate or rhythm or from an increase in the force of heart contractions. Rhythm disturbances that may cause palpitations include paroxysmal supraventricular tachycardia, premature contractions, and sinus tachycardia. Those that occur during or after strenuous physical activity, such as running and swimming, may indicate overexertion or possibly heart disease. Noncardiac factors that may precipitate palpitations include anxiety, stress, fatigue, insomnia, hyperthyroidism, and the ingestion of caffeine, nicotine, or alcohol.

Weight Gain

A sudden weight increase of 2.2 pounds (1 kg) can result from an accumulation of excessive fluid (1 L) in the interstitial spaces. This condition is commonly known as **edema.** It is possible for weight gains of up to 10 to 15 pounds (4.5 to 6.8 kg, or 4 to 7 L of fluid) to occur before edema is apparent. The nurse should inquire whether the client has noticed a tightness of shoes, indentations from socks, or tightness of rings.

Syncope

Syncope refers to a transient loss of consciousness. The most common cause is decreased perfusion to the brain. Any condition that suddenly reduces cardiac output, resulting in decreased cerebral blood flow, can potentiate a syncopal episode. Conditions such as cardiac rhythm disturbances (ventricular dysrhythmia or Stokes-Adams attack) and valvular disorders (aortic stenosis) may potentiate this symptom.

Near-syncope refers to dizziness with an inability to remain in an upright position. The nurse explores the circumstances that lead to dizziness or syncope.

CONSIDERATIONS FOR OLDER ADULTS
Syncope in an aging client may result from hypersensitivity of the carotid sinus bodies, which are located in the neck arteries. Pressure applied to the carotid arteries (e.g., while turning the head, shrugging the shoulders, shaving, or buttoning a shirt) stimulates a vagal response. A decrease in blood pressure and heart rate usually results, but an exaggerated response may produce syncope. The problem may also result from orthostatic (postural) or postprandial hypotension as a result of an age-affected baroreceptor response.

Extremity Pain

Extremity pain may be caused by two conditions: ischemia from atherosclerosis and venous insufficiency of the peripheral blood vessels. Clients who report a moderate to severe cramping sensation in their legs or buttocks associated with an activity such as walking have intermittent claudication related to reduced arterial tissue perfusion. Claudication pain is usually relieved by resting or lowering the affected extremity to decrease tissue demands or to enhance arterial blood flow. Leg pain that results from prolonged standing or sitting is related to venous insufficiency from either incompetent valves or venous obstruction. This pain may be relieved by elevating the extremity.

FUNCTIONAL HISTORY

After the history of the client's cardiovascular status is obtained, he or she may be classified according to the New York Heart Association's Functional Classification (Table 33-2). The four classifications (I, II, III, and IV) depend on the degree to which ordinary physical activities (routine activities of daily living [ADLs]) are affected by heart disease.

CRITICAL THINKING CHALLENGE
Your client, an older adult, has a history of multiple myocardial infarctions ("heart attacks"), heart failure, atrial fibrillation, two total hip replacements, and difficulty hearing. His medications include digoxin, Demadex, Coumadin, and Prinivil. He states that he does not take his prescribed Demadex in the morning when he is going to be leaving home. He no longer smokes cigarettes but continues to consume two or three alcoholic drinks every day.

- What additional information should you collect as part of his health history?
- What factors can you identify that place this client at risk for further cardiovascular problems?

For suggested answer guidelines, go to SIMON http://www.wbsaunders.com/SIMON/Iggy/.

Physical Assessment

A thorough physical assessment is the foundation for the nursing database and the formation of nursing diagnoses and collaborative problems. Any changes noted during the course of illness can be compared with this initial database. The nurse evaluates the client's vital signs on admission to the hospital or during the initial visit to the clinic or health care provider's office.

TABLE 33-2 • NEW YORK HEART ASSOCIATION FUNCTIONAL CLASSIFICATION OF CARDIOVASCULAR DISABILITY

CLASS I
- Clients with cardiac disease but without resulting limitations of physical activity
- Ordinary physical activity does not cause undue fatigue, palpitation, dyspnea, or anginal pain

CLASS II
- Clients with cardiac disease resulting in slight limitation of physical activity
- They are comfortable at rest
- Ordinary physical activity results in fatigue, palpitation, dyspnea, or anginal pain

CLASS III
- Clients with cardiac disease resulting in marked limitation of physical activity
- They are comfortable at rest
- Less than ordinary physical activity causes fatigue, palpitation, dyspnea, or anginal pain

CLASS IV
- Clients with cardiac disease resulting in inability to carry on any physical activity without discomfort
- Symptoms of cardiac insufficiency or of the anginal syndrome may be present, even at rest
- If any physical activity is undertaken, discomfort is increased

Excerpted from *Diseases of the heart and blood vessels–nomenclature and criteria for diagnosis* (6th ed.). Boston: Little, Brown; copyright 1964 by the New York Heart Association.

GENERAL APPEARANCE

Physical assessment begins with the client's general appearance. The nurse assesses the following areas: general build and appearance, skin color, distress level, level of consciousness, shortness of breath, position, and verbal responses.

Clients with chronic heart failure may appear malnourished, thin, and cachectic. Latent signs of severe heart failure are ascites, jaundice, and anasarca (generalized edema) as a result of prolonged congestion of the liver. Heart failure may cause fluid retention, and clients may have engorged neck veins and generalized dependent edema.

Coronary artery disease is suspected in clients with yellow, lipid-filled plaques on the upper eyelids (xanthelasma) or earlobe creases. Clients with poor cardiac output and decreased cerebral perfusion may experience mental confusion, memory loss, and slowed verbal responses.

INTEGUMENTARY SYSTEM

Assessment and evaluation of the integumentary system are determined primarily by the color and temperature of the skin. The best areas in which to assess circulation include the nail beds, mucous membranes, and conjunctival mucosa because small blood vessels are located near the surface of the skin.

Skin Color

If there is normal blood flow or adequate perfusion to a given area in light-colored skin, it appears pink, perhaps rosy in

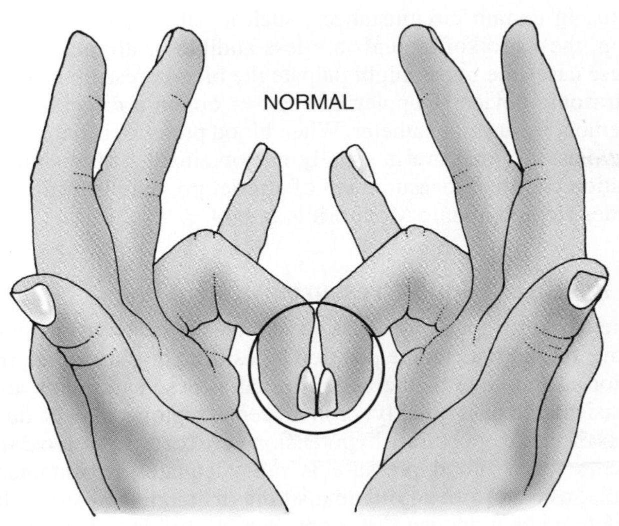

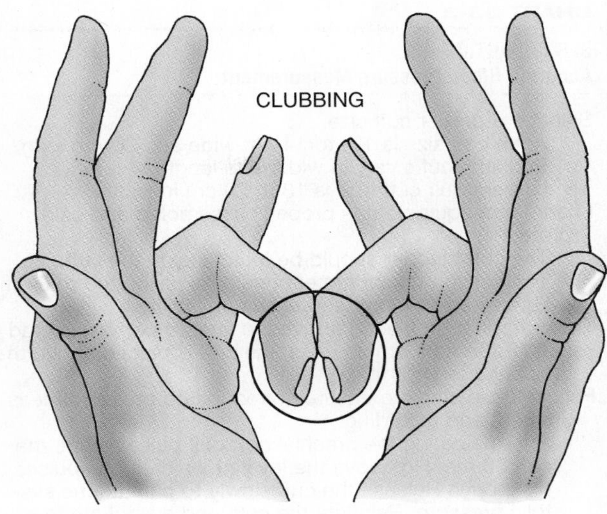

Figure 33-10 ● Assessment of clubbing by the Schamroth method. The client places the fingernails of the ring fingers together and holds them up to a light. If the examiner can see a diamond shape between the nails, there is no clubbing. Clubbing is identified by the absence of the diamond shape.

color, and it is warm to the touch. Decreased flow is depicted as cool, pale, and moist skin. Pallor is characteristic of anemia and can be seen in areas such as the nail beds, palms, and conjunctival mucous membranes.

A bluish or darkened discoloration of the skin and mucous membranes in Caucasians is referred to as **cyanosis.** This condition results from an increased amount of deoxygenated hemoglobin. Dark-skinned individuals may express cyanosis as a graying of the same tissues.

Central cyanosis involves decreased oxygenation of the arterial blood in the lungs and appears as a bluish tinge of the conjunctivae and the mucous membranes of the mouth and tongue. Central cyanosis may indicate impaired lung function or a right-to-left shunt found in congenital heart conditions. Because of impaired circulation, there is a marked desaturation of hemoglobin in the peripheral tissues, which produces a bluish or darkened discoloration of the nail beds, earlobes, lips, and toes.

Peripheral cyanosis occurs when blood flow to the peripheral vessels is decreased by peripheral vasoconstriction. The clamping down of the peripheral blood vessels results from a low cardiac output or an increased extraction of oxygen from the peripheral tissues. Peripheral cyanosis localized in an extremity is usually a result of arterial or venous obstruction.

Skin Temperature

Skin temperature can be assessed for symmetry by touching different areas of the client's body (e.g., arms, hands, legs, and feet) with the dorsal surface of the hand or fingers. Decreased blood flow results in decreased skin temperature. Skin temperature is lowered in several clinical conditions, including heart failure, peripheral vascular disease, and shock.

EXTREMITIES

The nurse assesses the client's hands, arms, feet, and legs for skin changes, vascular changes, clubbing, capillary filling, and edema. Skin mobility and turgor are affected by the fluid status of the client. Dehydration and aging reduce skin turgor, and edema decreases skin mobility. Vascular changes in an affected extremity may include paresthesia, muscle fatigue and discomfort, numbness, pain, coolness, and loss of hair distribution from a reduced blood supply.

Clubbing of the fingers and toes results from chronic oxygen deprivation in these tissue beds. Clubbing is characteristic in clients with advanced chronic pulmonary disease, congenital heart defects, and cor pulmonale. Clubbing can be identified by assessing the angle of the nail bed. The angle of the normal nail bed is 160 degrees. With **clubbing,** this angle increases to greater than 180 degrees, and the base of the nail becomes spongy. Figure 33-10 describes the assessment of clubbing using the Schamroth method.

Capillary filling of the fingers and the toes is an indicator of peripheral circulation. Pressing or blanching the nail bed of a finger or a toe produces a whitening effect; when pressure is released, a brisk return of color should occur. If color returns within 3 seconds, peripheral circulation is considered intact. If the capillary refill time exceeds 3 seconds, the lack of circulation may be due to arterial insufficiency from atherosclerosis or spasm. Older adults typically have a prolonged capillary refill. Rubor (dusky redness) that replaces pallor in a dependent foot suggests arterial insufficiency.

Peripheral edema is a common finding in clients with cardiovascular problems. The location of edema helps the nurse to determine its potential cause. Bilateral edema of the legs may be seen in clients with heart failure or chronic venous insufficiency. Abdominal and leg edema can be seen in clients with heart disease and cirrhosis of the liver. Localized edema in one extremity may be the result of venous obstruction (thrombosis) or lymphatic blockage of the extremity (lymphedema). Edema may also be noted in dependent areas, such as the sacrum, when a client is confined to bed.

The nurse documents the location of edema as precisely as possible (e.g., midtibial or sacral) and the number of centimeters from an anatomic landmark. Although some health care

CHART 33-3

BEST PRACTICE *for*
Accurate Blood Pressure Measurement

Select the proper cuff size.
- Adult cuff size is 12- to 14-cm wide and 30-cm long.
- Pediatric cuffs vary in width and length.
- Larger adult cuff size is 18 to 20 cm in width.

Ensure that equipment is properly assembled and calibrated.
- The cuff bladder should be intact inside the cuff.
- The sphygmomanometer should be calibrated to 0 mm Hg every few months to ensure reliability.

The cuff must be placed above the area to be auscultated (e.g., if the right arm is used, the cuff is placed above the brachial artery).

Follow these steps to ensure correct blood pressure measurement and recording:
- After palpating the brachial or radial pulse, inflate the cuff 30 mm Hg above the level at which those pulses disappear. Release the cuff slowly to palpate the systolic pressure. Reinflate the cuff, and auscultate the systolic and diastolic pressures. The auscultated pulses are referred to as the Korotkoff sounds.
- Record measurements on both arms to rule out dissecting aortic aneurysm, coarctation of the aorta, vascular obstruction, and possibly errors in measurement. Perform subsequent readings on the extremity with the highest pressure.
- If the client's arms are inaccessible (after amputation or mastectomy), you can obtain readings using the client's thigh or calf. Auscultate the popliteal artery or the posterior tibial artery, respectively.
- Obtain and record the client's blood pressure with the client in different positions, including supine, sitting, and standing positions.
- Record the position of the client and the site used to obtain the blood pressure.

practitioners attempt to grade edema as mild, moderate, and severe (or 1+, 2+, 3+, or 4+), there is no universal scale. In addition, these values are not precise and are subjective. Instead of using a grading scale, the nurse determines whether the edema is pitting (the skin can be indented) or nonpitting, the depth of the pit (in millimeters), and the amount of time the pit lasts (in seconds).

BLOOD PRESSURE

Arterial blood pressure is measured indirectly by sphygmomanometry (Chart 33-3). This technique of measurement is described in greater detail in nursing skills textbooks.

Normal blood pressure in adults older than 45 years of age ranges from 90 to 140 mm Hg for systolic pressure and from 60 to 90 mm Hg for diastolic pressure (AHA, 1998). A blood pressure that exceeds 135/85 mm Hg increases the workload of the left ventricle and oxygen consumption. Approximately 50 million Americans (one out of every 5 Americans) have hypertension, which is defined as a blood pressure greater than 140/90 mm Hg. Although the cause of hypertension is not known in 90% of people, it can be effectively controlled with lifestyle modification and/or medication. Hypertension is a cause of approximately 5 million deaths each year on its own and is a major contributor to the development of coronary artery disease and heart failure.

A blood pressure less than 90/60 mm Hg may be inadequate for providing proper and sufficient nutrition to body cells. In certain circumstances, such as shock and hypotension, the Korotkoff sounds are less audible or are absent. In these cases the nurse might palpate the blood pressure, use an ultrasonic device (Doppler device), or obtain a direct measurement by arterial catheter. When blood pressure is palpated, the diastolic pressure is usually not obtainable. More information on direct measurement of arterial pressure is available under Hemodynamic Monitoring, p. 649.

Postural Blood Pressure

Clients may report dizziness or lightheadedness when they move from a flat, supine position to a sitting or a standing position at the edge of the bed. Normally these symptoms are transient and pass quickly; pronounced symptoms may be due to orthostatic (postural) hypotension. **Postural hypotension** occurs when blood pressure is not adequately maintained while moving from a lying to a sitting or standing position. It is defined as a decrease of more than 20 mm Hg of the systolic pressure or more than 10 mm Hg of the diastolic pressure, as well as a 10% to 20% increase in heart rate. The causes of postural hypotension include medications, depletion of blood volume, prolonged bedrest, and age-related changes or disorders of the autonomic nervous system.

To detect orthostatic changes in blood pressure, the nurse first measures the blood pressure when the client is supine. After remaining supine for at least 3 minutes, the client changes position to sitting or standing. Normally systolic pressure drops slightly or remains unchanged as the client rises, whereas diastolic pressure rises slightly. After the position change, a time delay of 1 to 5 minutes should be permitted before auscultating blood pressure and palpating the radial pulse. The cuff should remain in the proper position on the client's arm. The nurse observes and records any signs or symptoms of distress. If the client is unable to tolerate the position change, he or she is returned to the previous position of comfort.

CONSIDERATIONS FOR OLDER ADULTS

As a person ages, the autonomic nervous system may lose the ability to compensate rapidly for the gravitational effects of position change and may therefore cause postural hypotension. With autonomic insufficiency, there is no increase in heart rate when moving to an upright position. Autonomic insufficiency can also result from the effects of some cardiac drugs that inhibit increases in heart rate, including digoxin, calcium channel blockers, and beta-adrenergic blockers. Antiparkinsonian drugs, such as carbidopa/levodopa (Sinemet), can cause severe postural hypotension. Some older adults experience a similar phenomenon after a heavy meal (postprandial hypotension).

Paradoxical Blood Pressure

Paradoxical blood pressure is defined as an exaggerated decrease in systolic pressure by more than 10 mm Hg during the inspiratory phase of the respiratory cycle (normal is 3 to 10 mm Hg). Certain clinical conditions that potentially alter the filling pressures in the right and left ventricles may produce a paradoxical blood pressure. Such conditions include pericardial tamponade, constrictive pericarditis, and pulmonary hypertension. During inspiration, the filling pressures normally decrease slightly. However, the decreased fluid volume in the ventricles resulting from these pathologic conditions produces an exaggerated or marked reduction in cardiac output. The procedure for assessing a paradoxical blood pressure is found in Chart 35-12.

Pulse Pressure

The difference between the systolic and diastolic values is referred to as pulse pressure. A normal pulse pressure for an adult is 30 to 40 mm Hg. This value can be used as an indirect measure of cardiac output. A more precise measurement, proportional pulse pressure, is calculated as follows:

$$\text{Proportional pulse pressure} = \frac{\text{Systolic blood pressure} - \text{Diastolic blood pressure}}{\text{Systolic blood pressure}}$$

A proportional pulse pressure less than 25% usually indicates a cardiac index of less than 2.2, as well as a critically low cardiac output (Stevenson & Braunwald, 1998). Narrowed pulse pressure is rarely normal and results from increased peripheral vascular resistance or decreased stroke volume in clients with heart failure, hypovolemia, or shock. Narrowed pulse pressure can also be seen in clients who have mitral stenosis or regurgitation. An increased pulse pressure may be seen in clients with slow heart rates, aortic regurgitation, atherosclerosis, hypertension, and aging.

Ankle Brachial Index

The **ankle brachial index (ABI)** can be used to assess the vascular status of the lower extremities. The nurse applies a blood pressure cuff to the lower extremities just above the malleoli and measures the systolic pressure by Doppler ultrasound at both the dorsalis pedis and posterior tibial pulses. The higher of these two pressures is then divided by the higher of the two brachial pulses to obtain the ankle brachial index:

$$\text{Ankle brachial index} = \frac{\text{Higher systolic ankle pressure}}{\text{Higher systolic brachial pressure}}$$

Normal values for ABI are 1 or higher, because blood pressure in the legs is usually higher than blood pressure in the arms. ABI values less than 0.80 usually indicate moderate vascular disease, whereas values less than 0.50 indicate severe vascular compromise. (See Chapter 36 for more information on ABI.)

VENOUS AND ARTERIAL PULSATIONS

Venous Pulsations

The nurse observes the venous pulsations in the neck to assess the adequacy of blood volume and central venous pressure (CVP). The nurse can assess **jugular venous pressure (JVP)** to estimate the filling volume and pressure on the right side of the heart (Chart 33-4). The right internal jugular vein is usually used to estimate JVP.

JVP is normally 3 to 10 cm H_2O. Increases in JVP are usually caused by right ventricular failure. Other causes include tricuspid regurgitation or stenosis, pulmonary hypertension, cardiac tamponade, constrictive pericarditis, hypervolemia, and superior vena cava obstruction.

Hepatojugular reflux is determined by locating the internal jugular vein after positioning the client with the head of the bed elevated to 45 degrees. The nurse compresses the right upper abdomen for 30 to 40 seconds. Sudden distention of the neck veins after abdominal compression is usually indicative of right-sided heart failure.

Arterial Pulsations

Assessment of arterial pulsations gives the nurse information about vascular integrity and circulation. For clients with suspected or actual vascular disease, all major peripheral pulses, including the temporal, carotid, brachial, radial, ulnar, femoral, popliteal, posterior tibial, and dorsalis pedis pulses, need to be assessed for presence or absence, amplitude, contour, rhythm, rate, and equality. The nurse examines the peripheral arteries in a head-to-toe approach with a side-to-side comparison (Figure 33-11).

A hypokinetic pulse is a weak pulsation indicative of a narrow pulse pressure. It is seen in clients with hypovolemia, aortic stenosis, and decreased cardiac output.

A hyperkinetic pulse is a large, "bounding" pulse caused by an increased ejection of blood. It is seen in clients with a high cardiac output (with exercise or thyrotoxicosis) and in those with increased sympathetic system activity (with pain, fever, or anxiety).

In **pulsus alternans,** a weak pulse alternates with a strong pulse despite a regular heart rhythm. It is seen in clients with severely depressed cardiac function. Clients may be asked to hold their breath to exclude any false readings. The nurse may palpate the brachial or radial arteries to assess this condition, but it is more accurately assessed by auscultation of blood pressure.

Auscultation of the major arteries (e.g., carotid and aorta) is necessary to assess for bruits. **Bruits** are swishing sounds that may develop in narrowed arteries and are usually associated with atherosclerotic disease. The nurse can assess for the absence or presence of bruits by placing the bell of the stethoscope over the skin of the carotid artery while the client holds his or her breath. Normally there are no sounds if the artery has uninterrupted blood flow. A bruit may develop when the internal diameter of the vessel is narrowed by 50% or more, but this does not indicate the severity of disease in the arteries. Severity is determined by Doppler flow studies and arteriography.

PRECORDIUM

Assessment of the precordium (the area over the heart) involves inspection, palpation, percussion, and auscultation. In most settings the medical-surgical nurse seldom performs precordial palpation and percussion. However, the critical care nurse should perform a complete assessment (McGrath & Cox, 1998). The nurse places the client in a supine position, with the head of the bed slightly elevated for comfort. Some clients may require elevation of the head of the bed to 45 degrees for ease and comfort in breathing.

Inspection

A cardiac examination is usually performed in a systematic order, beginning with inspection. The nurse inspects the chest from the side, at a right angle, and downward over areas of the precordium where vibrations are visible. Cardiac motion is of low amplitude, and sometimes the inward movements are more easily detected by the naked eye.

The nurse examines the entire precordium, focusing on the seven precordial areas (Figure 33-12) and noting any prominent precordial pulsations. Movement over the aortic, pulmonic, and tricuspid areas is abnormal. Pulsations in the mitral area (the apex of the heart) are considered normal and are referred to as the apical impulse, or the **point of maximal impulse (PMI).** The PMI should be located at the left fifth intercostal space (ICS) in the midclavicular line. If the apical impulse appears in more than one intercostal space and has shifted lateral to the midclavicular line, it may indicate left ventricular hypertrophy.

Palpation

The nurse palpates with the fingers and the most sensitive part of the palm of the hand to detect precordial motion and thrills, respectively. The nurse palpates by inching his or her hand in a Z pattern along the chest, starting with the aortic area and passing through all seven areas. Turning the client on his or her left side brings the heart closer to the surface of the chest. This may be helpful in achieving maximum tactile sensitivity.

An abnormal forceful thrust accompanied by a sustaining outward movement over the left anterior side of the chest usually indicates left ventricular enlargement. An outward systolic lift along the left sternal border that extends from the fourth to the fifth intercostal space represents right ventricular enlargement.

Heaves and *lifts* are terms found with pulsations associated with valvular diseases or pulmonary hypertension. Thrills are vibrations associated with abnormal heart valve function (mitral regurgitation, tricuspid regurgitation, and pulmonic stenosis). When palpating for heaves or thrills, the nurse should consider several factors, including location, amplitude, duration, distribution, and timing in relation to the cardiac cycle.

Percussion

Cardiac size is determined most accurately by chest x-ray examination; percussion is now rarely used to determine the size of the heart. However, the size of the left ventricle can be estimated by locating the apical impulse by inspection and palpation.

CHART 33-4

BEST PRACTICE *for*
Assessment of Jugular Venous Pressure and Central Venous Pressure

1. Place the client in a supine position.
2. Raise the head of the bed to approximately 30 to 45 degrees.
3. Shine a light across the client's neck (tangential lighting) to highlight the pulsations of the internal jugular vein.
4. To differentiate the internal jugular vein from the carotid artery, occlude the internal jugular vein with a fingertip at its base, then release. This maneuver easily eliminates the pulse wave in the internal jugular vein.

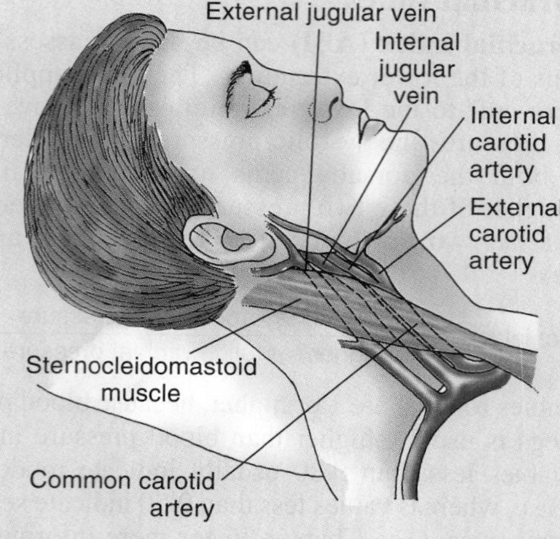

5. Locate the meniscus (the highest point at which pulsations of the internal jugular vein can be seen).
6. Locate the sternal angle (angle of Louis), which can be felt as a notch at the top of the sternum. It is roughly 4 cm above the right atrium.
7. With a centimeter rule, measure the vertical distance from the sternal angle to the meniscus of the internal jugular vein. The reading in centimeters equals the jugular venous pressure (JVP), which generally does not exceed 4 cm.
8. To calculate central venous pressure (CVP), add 4 cm to the JVP.

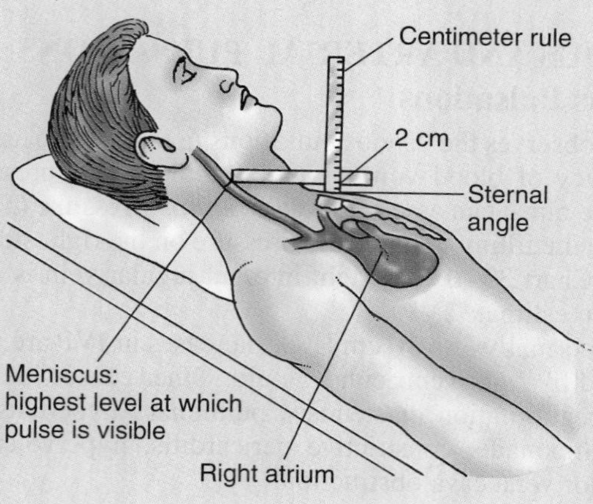

Auscultation

Auscultation evaluates heart rate and rhythm, cardiac cycle (systole and diastole), and valvular function. The technique of auscultation requires a good-quality stethoscope and extensive clinical practice. The medical-surgical nurse needs to be familiar with normal heart sounds. The critical care nurse, telemetry nurse, and advance practice nurse should be able to identify common abnormal heart sounds.

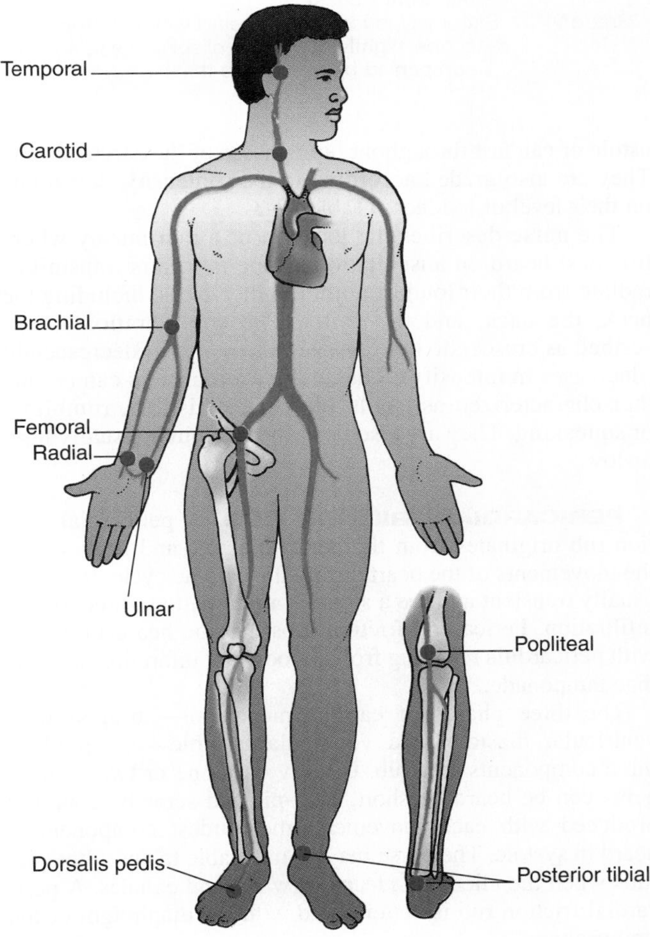

Figure 33-11 ● Pulse points for assessment of arterial pulses.

The nurse evaluates heart sounds in a systematic order. Examination usually begins at the aortic outflow tract area and progresses slowly to the apex of the heart. The diaphragm of the stethoscope is pressed tightly against the chest to listen for high-frequency sounds and is useful in listening to the first and second heart sounds and high-frequency murmurs. The nurse then repeats the progression from the base to the apex of the heart using the bell of the stethoscope, which is held lightly against the chest. The bell is able to screen out high-frequency sounds and is useful in listening for low-frequency gallops (diastolic filling sounds) and murmurs.

The nurse auscultates by inching a stethoscope in a Zpattern across the base of the heart, down the left sternal border, then over to the apex. Attention is given to the areas in Figure 33-12 (except the epigastric area). Auscultation checks for heart rate and rhythm, murmurs, extrasystolic sounds, and rubs in the presence of a current or suspected cardiac problem.

NORMAL HEART SOUNDS

The first heart sound (S_1) is created by the closure of the mitral and tricuspid valves (atrioventricular valves) (see Figure 33-6). When auscultated, the first heart sound is softer and longer; it is of a low pitch and is best heard at the lower left sternal border or the apex of the heart. It may be identified by palpating the carotid pulse while listening. S_1 marks the beginning of ventricular systole and occurs right after the QRS complex on the electrocardiogram (ECG).

The first heart sound can be accentuated or intensified in conditions such as exercise, hyperthyroidism, and mitral stenosis. A decrease in sound intensity occurs in clients with mitral regurgitation and heart failure.

The second heart sound (S_2) is caused mainly by the closing of the aortic and pulmonic valves (semilunar valves) (see Figure 33-6). S_2 is characteristically shorter. It is higher pitched and is heard best at the base of the heart at the end of ventricular systole.

The splitting of heart sounds is often difficult to differentiate from diastolic filling sounds (gallops). A splitting of S_1 (closure of the mitral valve followed by closure of the tricus-

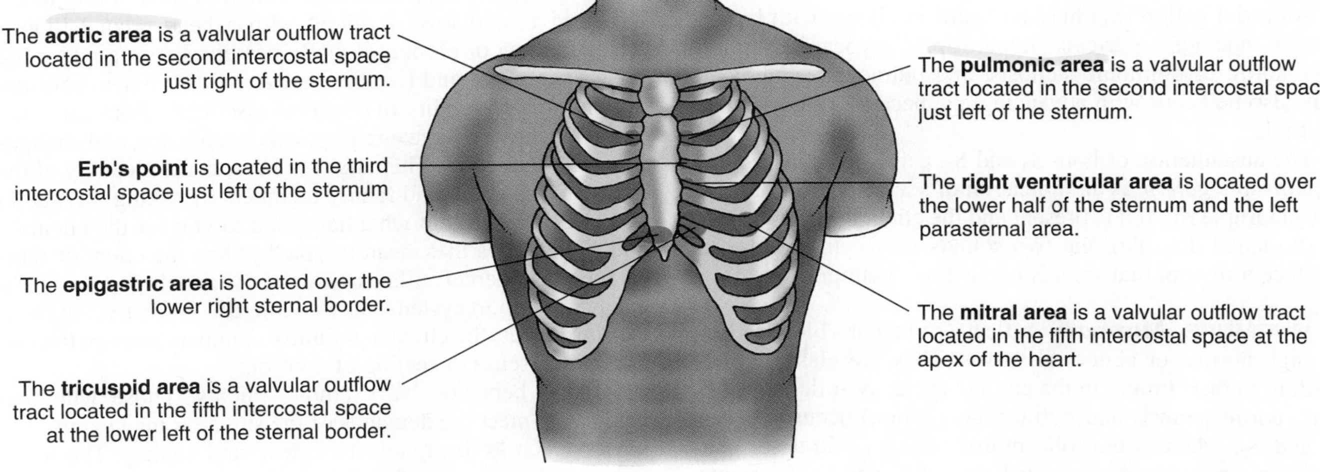

Figure 33-12 ● Areas for myocardial inspection, palpation, and auscultation.

pid valve) occurs physiologically because left ventricular contraction occurs slightly before right ventricular contraction. However, closure of the mitral valve is louder than closure of the tricuspid valve, so splitting is often not heard. Normal splitting of S_2 occurs because of the longer systolic phase of the right ventricle. Splitting of S_1 and S_2 can be accentuated by inspiration (increased venous return), and it narrows during expiration.

ABNORMAL HEART SOUNDS

PARADOXICAL SPLITTING. Abnormal splitting of S_2 is referred to as paradoxical splitting and is characteristic of a wider split heard on expiration. Paradoxical splitting of S_2 is heard in clients with severe myocardial depression that causes early closure of the pulmonic valve or a delay in aortic valve closure. Such conditions include myocardial infarction, left bundle branch block, aortic stenosis, aortic regurgitation, and right ventricular pacing.

GALLOPS AND MURMURS. Gallops and murmurs are common abnormal heart sounds that may occur with heart disease.

GALLOPS. Diastolic filling sounds (S_3) and (S_4) are produced when blood enters a noncompliant chamber during rapid ventricular filling. The third heart sound (S_3) is produced during the rapid passive filling phase of ventricular diastole when blood flows from the atrium to a noncompliant ventricle. The sound arises from vibrations of the valves and supporting structures. The fourth heart sound (S_4) occurs as blood enters the ventricles during the active filling phase at the end of ventricular diastole.

S_3 is termed **ventricular gallop,** and S_4 is referred to as **atrial gallop.** These sounds can be caused by decreased compliance of either or both ventricles. The nurse can best hear left ventricular diastolic filling sounds with the client on his or her left side. The bell of the stethoscope is placed at the apex and at the left lower sternal border during expiration.

An S_3 heart sound is probably a normal finding in children or young adults up to 30 years of age. An S_3 gallop in clients older than 40 years of age is considered abnormal and represents a decrease in left ventricular compliance. S_3 can be detected as an early sign of heart failure or as a ventricular septal defect.

An atrial gallop (S_4) may be heard in clients with hypertension, anemia, ventricular hypertrophy, myocardial infarction, aortic or pulmonic stenosis, and pulmonary emboli. It may also be heard with advancing age because of a stiffened ventricle.

The auscultation of both S_3 and S_4, called a *summation* or a *quadruple gallop,* is an indication of severe heart failure. If the quadruple rhythm is present and the client has tachycardia (a shortened diastole), the two sounds may actually fuse to produce a rhythm that sounds like a horse galloping.

MURMURS. Murmurs reflect turbulent blood flow through normal or abnormal valves. They are classified according to their timing in the cardiac cycle: systolic murmurs (e.g., aortic stenosis and mitral regurgitation) occur between S_1 and S_2, whereas diastolic murmurs (e.g., mitral stenosis and aortic regurgitation) occur between S_2 and S_1. Murmurs can occur during presystole, midsystole, or late systole or diastole or can last throughout both phases of the cardiac cycle. They are also graded according to their intensity, depending on their level of loudness (Table 33-3).

TABLE 33-3 • GRADING OF HEART MURMURS

Grade	Description
Grade I	Very faint
Grade II	Faint, but recognizable
Grade III	Loud, but moderate in intensity
Grade IV	Loud and accompanied by a palpable thrill
Grade V	Very loud, accompanied by a palpable thrill, and audible with the stethoscope partially off the client's chest
Grade VI	Extremely loud, may be heard with the stethoscope slightly above the client's chest, accompanied by a palpable thrill

The nurse describes the location of a murmur by where it is best heard on auscultation. Some murmurs transmit or radiate from their loudest point to other areas, including the neck, the back, and the axilla. The configuration is described as crescendo (increases in intensity) or decrescendo (decreases in intensity). The quality of murmurs can be further characterized as harsh, blowing, whistling, rumbling, or squeaking. They are also described by pitch, usually high or low.

PERICARDIAL FRICTION RUB. A pericardial friction rub originates from the pericardial sac and occurs with the movements of the heart during the cardiac cycle. Rubs are usually transient and are a sign of inflammation, infection, or infiltration. Pericardial friction rubs may be heard in clients with pericarditis resulting from myocardial infarction and cardiac tamponade.

The three phases of cardiac movement—atrial systole, ventricular diastole, and ventricular systole—can produce three components of a rub. Usually only one or two components can be heard. A short, high-pitched scratchy sound is produced with each movement; the loudest component is heard in systole. The nurse may be most able to auscultate the rubs when the client sits, leans forward, and exhales. A pericardial friction rub is better heard with the diaphragm of the stethoscope.

Psychosocial Assessment

To many people, their heart is a symbol of their ability to exist, survive, and love. A client with a heart-related illness, whether acute or chronic, usually perceives it as a major life crisis. The client and families and significant others confront not only the possibility of death but also fears about pain, disability, lack of self-esteem, physical dependence, and changes in family dynamics. The nurse may assess the meaning of the illness to the client and family members by asking, "What do you understand about what happened to you (or the client)?" and "What does that mean to you?" When the client or family members perceive the stressor as overwhelming, formerly adequate support systems may no longer be effective. In these circumstances, the client and family members attempt to cope to regain a sense or feeling of control.

Coping behaviors vary among clients. Those who feel helpless to meet the demands of the situation may exhibit behaviors such as disorganization, fear, and anxiety. The nurse may ask the client or family members, "Have you ever encountered such a situation before?", "How did you manage

CHART 33-5

LABORATORY PROFILE
Cardiovascular Assessment

Normal Range	Significance of Abnormal Findings
SERUM CARDIAC ENZYMES	
Creatine kinase (CK) *Females:* 10-55 units/mL, or 26-140 units/L *Males:* 12-70 units/mL, or 38-174 units/L Values higher after exercise	Elevations indicate possible brain, myocardial, and skeletal muscle necrosis or injury.
CK-MM (CK_3) 95%-100% of total CK	Elevations occur with muscle injury.
CK-MB (CK_2) 0%-5% of total CK	Elevations occur with myocardial injury or after percutaneous transluminal angioplasty and intracoronary streptokinase infusion.
CK-BB (CK_1) 0%	Elevations occur with brain tissue injury.
SERUM LIPIDS	
Total lipids 400-1000 mg/dL	Elevation indicates increased risk of CAD.
Cholesterol 122-200 mg/dL, or 3.16-6.5 mmol/L *Older adult (>70 yr):* 144-280 mg/dL, or 3.73-7.25 mmol/L	Elevation indicates increased risk of CAD.
Triglycerides *Females:* 39-262 mg/dL, or 0.44-2.96 mmol/L *Males:* 37-286 mg/dL, or 0.42-3.23 mmol/L *Older adult (>65 yr):* 55-260 mg/dL, or 0.62-2.94 mmol/L	Elevation indicates increased risk of CAD.
Plasma high-density lipoproteins (HDLs) *Females:* mean 55-60 mg/dL *Males:* mean, 45-50 mg/dL Older adult range increases with age	Elevations protect against CAD.
Plasma low-density lipoproteins (LDLs) 57-197 mg/dL, or 1.48-5.10 mmol/L *Older adult (>65 yr):* 92-221 mg/dL, or 2.38-5.72 mmol/L	Elevation indicates increased risk of CAD.
HDL:LDL ratio 3:1	Elevated ratios may protect against CAD.

CAD, Coronary artery disease.

that situation?", and "To whom can you turn for help?" The answers to these questions often reassure the client that he or she has encountered difficult situations in the past and has the ability and resources to cope with them.

A common and normal response is *denial,* which is a defense mechanism that enables the client to cope with threatening circumstances. The client may deny that he or she has the current cardiovascular condition, may state that it was present but is now absent, or may be excessively cheerful. Denying the seriousness of the illness while following the treatment regimen is a protective response. Denial becomes maladaptive when the client is noncompliant with significant portions of medical and nursing care.

Family members and significant others may be more anxious than the client. Often they recall all events of the illness, are unprotected by denial, and are afraid of recurrence. Disagreements often occur between the client and family members over compliance with appropriate follow-up care.

Diagnostic Assessment

LABORATORY TESTS

Assessment of the client with cardiac dysfunction includes examination of the blood for abnormalities. The examination is performed to establish a diagnosis, detect concurrent disease, assess risk factors, and monitor response to treatment. Normal values for serum cardiac enzymes and serum lipids are listed in Chart 33-5.

Serum Markers of Myocardial Damage

Events leading to cellular injury cause a release of enzymes from intracellular storage, and circulating levels of these enzymes are dramatically elevated. Acute myocardial infarction (MI) ("heart attack") can be confirmed by abnormally high levels of enzymes, isoenzymes, or markers in the serum.

CREATINE KINASE

Creatine kinase (CK) is an enzyme specific to cells of the brain, myocardium, and skeletal muscle. The appearance of CK in the blood indicates tissue necrosis or injury, with CK levels following a predictable rise and fall during a specified period. Cardiac specificity must be determined by measuring isoenzyme activity. There are three isoenzymes of CK: CK-MM is the predominant isoenzyme of skeletal muscle; CK-MB is found in myocardial muscle; and CK-BB occurs in the brain. CK-MB activity is most specific for MI and shows a predictable rise and fall during 3 days; a peak level occurs approximately 24 hours after the onset of chest pain.

EARLY MARKERS OF MYOCARDIAL DAMAGE

Newer treatment modalities for early intervention after acute MI and acute ischemia require more rapid diagnosis of MI. An assay using monoclonal anti–CK-MB antibodies (stat CK) can detect myocardial necrosis accurately 3 hours after emergency department admission when examined with an electrocardiogram (ECG). Two subforms of CK-MB (CK-MB_1, CK-MB_2) have also been identified. Abnormal elevations of these CK subforms may occur as early as 2 hours after MI. These subforms remain elevated for up to 12 hours after MI and appear to be very sensitive and specific early diagnostic markers of MI.

Other early markers of MI are myoglobin and troponin. Myoglobin, a low–molecular weight protein found in skeletal muscle, is an early and sensitive but nonspecific marker for myocardial injury. It can be detected as early as 2 hours after an MI but is relatively nonspecific. Troponin T and I are specific markers of myocardial injury and have a wide diagnostic time frame, making them useful for clients who present several hours after the onset of chest pain. Table 33-4 describes the characteristics of these new serum assays for myocardial damage.

LACTATE DEHYDROGENASE

Lactate dehydrogenase (LDH) is widely distributed in the body and is found in the heart, liver, kidney, brain, and erythrocytes. LDH elevation starts within 12 to 24 hours after an MI, peaks between 48 and 72 hours, and falls to normal in 7 days. Because LDH is not specific to the myocardial cell, an assessment of isoenzymes and patterns of elevation is necessary for confirmation of MI. There are five isoenzymes for LDH; LDH_1 and LDH_2 are found in the heart. If the serum level of LDH_1 is higher than the concentration of LDH_2, the pattern is said to have flipped, which signifies myocardial damage. LDH is being used less frequently now that the newer serum markers of myocardial damage, myoglobin and troponin, have been identified.

Serum Lipids

Elevated lipid levels are considered a risk factor for coronary artery disease (CAD). Cholesterol, triglycerides, and the protein components of high-density lipoproteins (HDL) and low-density lipoproteins (LDL) are evaluated to assess a client's degree of risk for CAD. The risk for CAD is three times greater in clients with a serum cholesterol level greater than 260 mg/dL than in clients with a serum level less than 200 mg/dL.

Each of the lipoproteins contains varying proportions of cholesterol, triglyceride, protein, and phospholipid. HDL contains mainly protein and 20% cholesterol, whereas LDL is predominantly cholesterol. Elevated LDL levels are positively correlated with CAD, whereas elevated HDL levels are negatively correlated and appear to be a protective factor.

A nonfasting blood sample for the measurement of serum cholesterol levels is acceptable. If triglycerides are to be evaluated, the physician requests the specimen after a 12-hour fast.

> **WOMEN'S HEALTH CONSIDERATIONS**
> Early studies have demonstrated that high blood levels of C-reactive protein are better predictors of cardiovascular disease (CVD) in women than are elevated levels of LDL (the current gold standard). Both tests are similar in cost, averaging approximately $20.

Homocysteine

Homocysteine, an amino acid, may be an independent risk factor for the development of CVD. Although the relationship between homocysteine and CVD remains controversial, some studies suggest that elevated levels of homocysteine increase the risk of CVD as much as smoking and hyperlipemia. Clients usually fast for 10 to 12 hours before the test, and the blood must be separated and frozen within 1 hour of collection. A level less than 12 mmol/dL is considered optimal. Most insurance policies do not cover this laboratory test, which costs from $50 to $110. Eating foods rich in B vitamins and folic acid appears to lower homocysteine levels and may decrease the risk for CVD (AHA, 1998).

Blood Coagulation Tests

Blood coagulation tests evaluate the ability of the blood to clot and are important in clients with a greater tendency to form thrombi (e.g., clients with atrial fibrillation, prosthetic valves, or infective endocarditis). They are also important for clients receiving anticoagulant therapy (e.g., during cardiac surgery, after thrombolytic therapy, and during treatment of an established thrombus).

PROTHROMBIN TIME AND INTERNATIONAL NORMALIZED RATIO

Prothrombin time (PT) and International Normalized Ratio (INR) are used when initiating and maintaining therapy with oral anticoagulants, such as sodium warfarin (Coumadin, Warfilone♣). They measure the activity of prothrombin, fibrinogen, and factors V, VII, and X. INR is the most reliable way to monitor anticoagulant status in warfarin therapy. The therapeutic ranges for standard anticoagulant therapy are 2.0 to 3.0 (INR).

TABLE 33-4 • CHARACTERISTICS OF NEW SERUM ASSAYS FOR MYOCARDIAL DAMAGE

Test	Time to Elevation (hr)	Time to Peak (hr)	Time to Normal	Assay Time (min)
Stat CK-MB	3-8	12-24	2-3 days	8-34
CK-MB subforms	1-3	5-7	24 hr	25
Myoglobin	2-3	6-9	24 hr	10-20
Troponin T&I	4-6	10-24	10-14 days	10-90

PARTIAL THROMBOPLASTIN TIME

Partial thromboplastin time (PTT) is assessed in clients who are receiving heparin (Hepalean♣). It measures deficiencies in all coagulation factors except VII and XIII.

Arterial Blood Gases

Arterial blood gas (ABG) determinations are often obtained in clients with cardiovascular disease. Determination of tissue oxygenation, carbon dioxide removal, and acid-base status is essential to appropriate intervention and treatment. (See Chapter 15 for a complete discussion of ABGs.)

Serum Electrolytes

Fluid and electrolyte balance is essential for normal cardiovascular performance. Cardiac manifestations often occur when there is an imbalance in either fluids or electrolytes in the body. For example, the cardiac effects of hypokalemia (low serum potassium level) include increased electrical instability, ventricular dysrhythmias, the appearance of U waves on the electrocardiogram, and an increased risk of digitalis toxicity. The effects of hyperkalemia on the myocardium include slowed ventricular conduction and contraction followed by asystole (cardiac standstill).

Cardiac manifestations of hypocalcemia are ventricular dysrhythmias, a prolonged QT interval, and cardiac arrest. Hypercalcemia shortens the QT interval and causes AV block, digitalis hypersensitivity, and cardiac arrest.

Serum sodium values reflect fluid balance and may be decreased, indicating a fluid excess in clients with heart failure (dilutional hyponatremia).

Because magnesium regulates some aspects of myocardial electrical activity, hypomagnesemia has been implicated in some forms of rapid ventricular dysrhythmias. Another manifestation of hypomagnesemia is hypokalemia that is unresponsive to potassium replacement.

Complete Blood Count

The erythrocyte (red blood cell) count is usually decreased in rheumatic fever and infective endocarditis. It is increased in heart diseases characterized by inadequate tissue oxygenation.

Decreased hematocrit and hemoglobin levels (e.g., caused by hemorrhage or hemolysis from prosthetic valves) indicate anemia and can lead to angina or aggravate heart failure. Vascular volume depletion with hemoconcentration (e.g., hypovolemic shock and excessive diuresis) results in an elevated hematocrit.

The leukocyte (white blood cell) count is typically elevated after a myocardial infarction and in various infectious and inflammatory diseases of the heart (e.g., infective endocarditis and pericarditis). Chapter 39 discusses the complete blood count in detail.

CRITICAL THINKING CHALLENGE

During a physical assessment, you discover that an older client's heart rate is 54 and irregular. His blood pressure is 110/84, and he has pitting edema in both his legs below mid-calf. His lungs are clear and his respirations are 32 per minute and regular. The client has a history of congestive heart failure and multiple "heart attacks."

- What additional physical assessment should you perform at this time?
- What is his highest priority nursing diagnosis?
- What diagnostic tests might the health care provider order for this client?

For suggested answer guidelines, go to SIMON http://www.wbsaunders.com/SIMON/Iggy/.

RADIOGRAPHIC EXAMINATIONS

Chest Radiography

Posteroanterior and left lateral x-ray views of the chest are routinely obtained to determine the size, silhouette, and position of the heart. In acutely ill clients, a simple anteroposterior view is obtained at the bedside. Cardiac enlargement, pulmonary congestion, cardiac calcifications, and placement of central venous catheters, endotracheal tubes, and hemodynamic monitoring devices are assessed by x-ray examination.

Cardiac Fluoroscopy

Fluoroscopy is a simple x-ray examination that reveals the action of the heart. Continuous visual observation of the heart, lungs, and vessel movement on a luminescent x-ray screen in a darkened room is provided. Fluoroscopy is used to place and position intracardiac catheters and IV pacemaker wires and can be helpful in identifying abnormal structures, calcifications, and tumors of the heart. In critically ill clients, fluoroscopy can be performed at the bedside for the placement of intracardiac catheters or IV pacemaker wires. Client preparation and follow-up depend on the procedure. Fluoroscopy is commonly used in conjunction with cardiac catheterization, and the client is taken to a special cardiac catheterization room (see the discussion under Cardiac Catheterization, p. 642).

Angiography

Angiography of the arterial vessels, or **arteriography,** is an invasive diagnostic procedure that involves fluoroscopy and the use of contrast media. This procedure is performed when an arterial obstruction, narrowing, or aneurysm is suspected. The radiologist performs selective arteriography to evaluate specific areas of the arterial system. For example, a coronary arteriography, which is performed during left-sided cardiac catheterization, assesses arterial circulation within the heart (see Left-Sided Heart Catheterization, p. 643). Angiography can also be performed on arteries in the extremities, mesentery, and cerebrum.

CLIENT PREPARATION. The radiologist explains the procedure and the risks before the client or designated responsible party signs a consent form. Because this procedure involves an injection of contrast medium (sometimes called a dye) into the arterial system, the risks are serious. Risks include allergic reaction, hemorrhage, thrombosis, embolism, renal failure, and death. The client is told to expect a warm sensation when the dye is injected.

The nurse assesses the client for any allergies to contrast medium, iodine-containing substances such as seafood, or local anesthetics. The femoral area is prepared according to the policy and procedure of the health care agency. The nurse

TABLE 33-5 • INDICATIONS FOR CARDIAC CATHETERIZATION

- To confirm suspected heart disease, including coronary artery disease, myocardial disease, valvular disease, and valvular dysfunction
- To determine the location and extent of the disease process
- To assess the following:
  - Stable, severe angina unresponsive to medical management
  - Unstable angina pectoris
  - Uncontrolled heart failure, ventricular dysrhythmias, or cardiogenic shock associated with acute myocardial infarction, papillary muscle dysfunction, ventricular aneurysm, or septal perforation
- To determine best therapeutic option (percutaneous transluminal coronary angioplasty, stents, coronary artery bypass graft, valvulotomy versus valve replacement)
- To evaluate effects of medical or invasive treatment on cardiovascular function, percutaneous transluminal coronary angioplasty, or coronary artery bypass graft patency

TABLE 33-6 • COMPLICATIONS OF CARDIAC CATHETERIZATION

RIGHT-SIDED HEART CATHETERIZATION
- Thrombophlebitis
- Pulmonary embolism
- Vagal response

LEFT-SIDED HEART CATHETERIZATION AND CORONARY ARTERIOGRAPHY
- Myocardial infarction
- Stroke
- Arterial bleeding or thromboembolism
- Dysrhythmias

RIGHT- OR LEFT-SIDED HEART CATHETERIZATION*
- Cardiac tamponade
- Hypovolemia
- Pulmonary edema
- Hematoma or blood less at insertion site
- Reaction to contrast medium

*In addition to those cited for each procedure.

documents vital signs and marks and describes pulses distal to the puncture site in the client's medical record.

PROCEDURE. The radiologist or technician places the client in a supine position on an x-ray table in the radiology department. A radiologist usually performs this procedure and begins by injecting a local anesthetic into the tissue surrounding the artery being catheterized. Contrast medium is injected via this catheter, and fluoroscopy and x-ray studies are performed.

FOLLOW-UP CARE. After the procedure, the client is typically restricted to bedrest in the supine position for 4 to 6 hours. The nurse ensures that the extremity that was catheterized is not flexed during this time. A pressure dressing or bandage is kept in place over the injection site; a sandbag may be placed over the dressing.

The nurse assesses the insertion site for bloody drainage or hematoma formation, assesses the distal pulses, and compares skin temperature in the affected extremity with that in the opposite extremity. Vital signs are assessed at every dressing, pulse, and temperature check; the first measurement is obtained immediately after the client is transferred from the radiology department. These assessments usually continue every 15 minutes for 1 hour, then every 30 minutes for 2 hours, and then every 4 hours or as necessary per the health care agency's protocol. The nurse notifies the radiologist immediately if bleeding, loss of pulses, or changes in vital signs occur. The nurse carefully administers the prescribed IV or oral fluids after the procedure, because the contrast medium may damage the kidneys.

Cardiac Catheterization

The most definitive, but most invasive, test in the diagnosis of heart disease is cardiac catheterization. Cardiac catheterization may include studies of the right or left side of the heart and the coronary arteries. Some of the most common indications for cardiac catheterization are listed in Table 33-5.

CLIENT PREPARATION. Many clients express anxiety and fear regarding cardiac catheterization. The nurse assesses their physical and psychosocial readiness and knowledge level.

The nurse reviews the purpose of the procedure, informs the client how long it usually takes, states who will be present, and describes the appearance of the catheterization laboratory. The client is also informed about the sensations that may be experienced during the procedure, such as palpitations (as the catheter is passed up to the left ventricle), a feeling of heat or a hot flash (as the dye is injected into either side of the heart), and a desire to cough (as the dye is injected into the right side of the heart). The nurse may use written or illustrated materials or videotapes, if available, to assist in the client's understanding.

The risks of cardiac catheterization are usually explained by the cardiologist. The risks vary with the procedures to be performed and the client's physical status (Table 33-6). Right-sided heart catheterization is less risky than left-sided catheterization. Several complications may follow coronary arteriography, such as the following:

- Myocardial infarction (MI)
- Stroke
- Arterial bleeding
- Thromboembolism
- Lethal dysrhythmias
- Death

The cardiologist or radiologist obtains a written informed consent from the client or responsible party.

The client may be admitted to the hospital on the day of the catheterization procedure. Standard preoperative tests are performed, which usually include a chest x-ray examination, complete blood count, coagulation studies, urinalysis, and 12-lead electrocardiogram. The client receives nothing by mouth after midnight or has only a liquid breakfast if the catheterization is to take place in the afternoon. The catheterization site is shaved and antiseptically prepared according to policy.

Nursing assessment before the procedure includes measuring the client's vital signs, auscultating the heart and the lungs, and evaluating the peripheral pulses. The nurse questions the client about any history of allergy to iodine-containing substances (e.g., seafood and contrast agents). An antihistamine may be given to a client with a positive history. A mild sedative is administered before the procedure. If the client normally takes a digitalis preparation or diuretic, it is usually withheld before the catheterization.

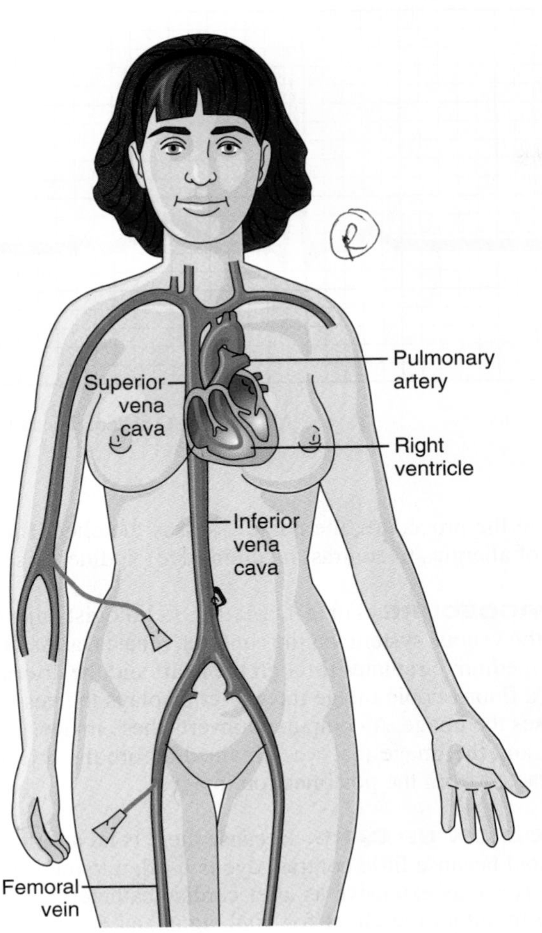

Figure 33-13 ● Right-sided heart catheterization. The catheter is inserted into the femoral vein and advanced through the inferior vena cava (or, if into an antecubital or basilic vein, through the superior vena cava), right atrium, and right ventricle and into the pulmonary artery.

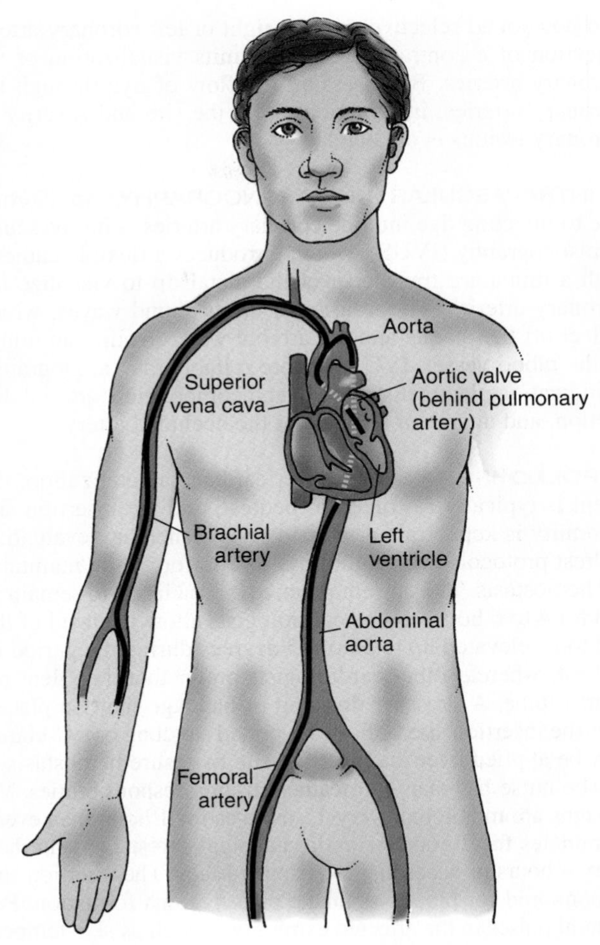

Figure 33-14 ● Left-sided heart catheterization. The catheter is inserted into the femoral artery or antecubital artery. The catheter is passed through the ascending aorta, through the aortic valve, and into the left ventricle.

PROCEDURE. The client is taken to the cardiac catheterization laboratory (sometimes referred to as the "cath lab"), placed in the supine position on the x-ray table, and securely strapped to the table. The nurse informs the client that this precaution is necessary because the table turns like a cradle during the procedure. The physician injects a local anesthetic at the insertion site. The nurse in the catheterization laboratory instructs the client to report any chest pain or other symptoms to the staff.

RIGHT-SIDED HEART CATHETERIZATION. The right side of the heart is catheterized first and may be the only side examined. The cardiologist inserts a catheter through the femoral vein to the inferior vena cava or through the basilic vein to the superior vena cava. The catheter is advanced through either the inferior or the superior vena cava and, guided by fluoroscopy, is advanced through the right atrium, through the right ventricle and, at times, into the pulmonary artery (Figure 33-13). Intracardiac pressures (right atrial, right ventricular, pulmonary artery, and pulmonary artery wedge pressures) and blood samples are obtained. A contrast dye or medium is usually injected to detect any cardiac shunts or regurgitation from the pulmonic or tricuspid valves.

LEFT-SIDED HEART CATHETERIZATION. Left-sided heart catheterization is more risky than right-sided heart catheterization. The cardiologist advances the catheter retrogradely from the femoral or brachial artery up the aorta, across the aortic valve, and into the left ventricle (Figure 33-14). Alternatively, the cardiologist may pass the catheter from the right side of the heart through the atrial septum, using a special needle to puncture the septum. Intracardiac pressures and blood samples are obtained. The pressures of the left atrium, left ventricle, and aorta, as well as mitral and aortic valve status, are evaluated. The cardiologist injects contrast dye into the ventricle; cineangiograms (rapidly changing films) evaluate left ventricular motion. Calculations are made regarding end-systolic volume, end-diastolic volume, stroke volume, and ejection fraction.

CORONARY ARTERIOGRAPHY. The technique for coronary arteriography is the same as for left-sided heart catheterization. The catheter is advanced into the aortic arch and positioned selectively in the right or left coronary artery. Injection of a contrast medium permits visualization of the coronary arteries. By assessing the flow of dye through the coronary arteries, information about the site and severity of coronary lesions is obtained.

INTRAVASCULAR ULTRASONOGRAPHY. An alternative to injecting dye into the coronary arteries is intravascular ultrasonography (IVUS), which introduces a flexible catheter with a miniature transducer at the distal tip to visualize the coronary arteries. The transducer emits sound waves, which reflect off the plaque and the arterial wall, creating an image of the blood vessel. IVUS is more reliable than angiography in indicating plaque distribution and composition, arterial dissection, and degree of stenosis of the occluded artery.

FOLLOW-UP CARE. After cardiac catheterization, the client is typically restricted to bedrest, and the insertion site extremity is kept straight. Nursing researchers are evaluating bedrest protocols that might limit discomfort while maintaining hemostasis. The current practice is for clients to remain in bed for 4 to 6 hours. Some cardiologists allow the head of the bed to be elevated up to 30 or 45 degrees during the period of bedrest, whereas other cardiologists prefer that the client remain supine. A pressure dressing or bandage may be placed over the insertion site. A 5- or 10-pound sandbag or a C-clamp may be applied over the insertion site to ensure hemostasis.

The nurse has many postcatheterization responsibilities. Vital signs are monitored every 15 minutes for 1 hour, then every 30 minutes for 2 hours or until vital signs are stable, and then every 4 hours or according to hospital policy. The insertion site is monitored for bloody drainage or hematoma formation. Peripheral pulses in the affected extremity, as well as skin temperature and color, are monitored with every vital sign check.

The nurse must observe for complications of cardiac catheterization (see Table 33-5). Complaints of pain and discomfort at the insertion site, chest pain, nausea, or feelings of lightheadedness should be reported. The client is often attached to a cardiac monitor. If not, the nurse auscultates the heart sounds, noting rhythm and rate to detect dysrhythmias. Because the contrast medium acts as an osmotic diuretic, the nurse monitors urinary output and ensures that the client receives sufficient oral and IV fluids for adequate excretion of the dye. Pain medication for insertion site or back discomfort may be given, as ordered.

If the client experiences chest pain, dysrhythmias, bleeding, hematoma formation, or a dramatic change in peripheral pulses in the affected extremity, the nurse contacts the physician immediately and provides prompt intervention. Neurologic changes, such as visual disturbances, slurred speech, swallowing difficulties, and extremity weakness, should also be reported.

Digital Subtraction Angiography

Digital subtraction angiography (DSA) combines x-ray detection methods and a computerized subtraction technique with fluoroscopy for visualization of the cardiovascular system. There is no interference from adjacent structures, such as bone and soft tissue.

CLIENT PREPARATION. Digital subtraction angiography involves the injection of dye into the venous system.

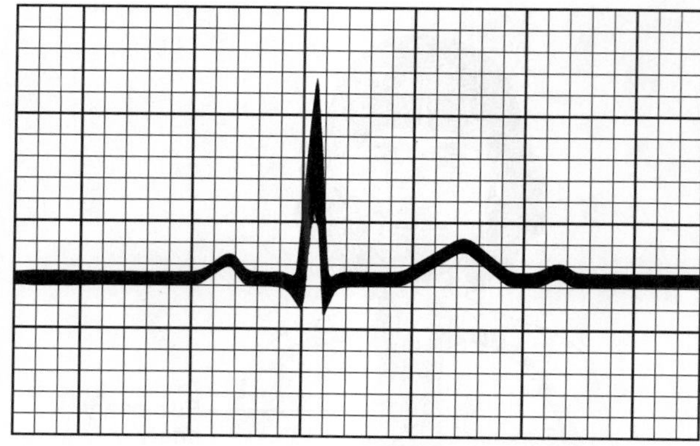

Figure 33-15 ● A normal ECG pattern in lead II.

Before the procedure, the nurse assesses the client for a history of allergies to contrast medium (dye), iodine, or seafood.

PROCEDURE. For a DSA, the radiologist injects dye into the venous system via the superior vena cava. As the contrast medium circulates through the heart and the arterial system, a fluoroscopic image intensifier displays the vessels and focuses the image. A computer converts these images to numbers, and the image that was obtained before the injection is subtracted from the postinjection images.

FOLLOW-UP CARE. Because there is no arterial puncture and because little contrast dye is used, nursing care after DSA is not as extensive as after cardiac catheterization. The nurse monitors the client for vital signs and assesses the injection site for bleeding or discomfort.

OTHER DIAGNOSTIC TESTS

Electrocardiography

The electrocardiogram (ECG) is a routine part of every cardiovascular evaluation and is one of the most valuable diagnostic tests. Various forms are available: resting ECG, continuous ambulatory ECG (Holter monitoring), exercise ECG (stress test), and signal-averaged ECG. The resting ECG provides information about cardiac dysrhythmias, myocardial ischemia, the site and extent of myocardial infarction, cardiac hypertrophy, electrolyte imbalances, and the effectiveness of cardiac drugs. The normal ECG pattern of one cardiac cycle is illustrated in Figure 33-15. Further discussion of the interpretation and evaluation of normal and abnormal patterns is found in Chapter 34.

RESTING ELECTROCARDIOGRAPHY

The ECG graphically records the electrical current generated by the heart. This current is measured by electrodes that are placed on the skin and connected to an amplifier and strip chart recorder (Figure 33-16). In the standard 12-lead ECG, five electrodes attached to the arms, legs, and chest measure current from 12 different views or leads: three bipolar limb leads (Figure 33-17), three unipolar augmented leads (Figure 33-18), and six unipolar precordial leads (Figure 33-19). Placement of the leads allows the health care provider to view myocardial electrical conduction from different axes or posi-

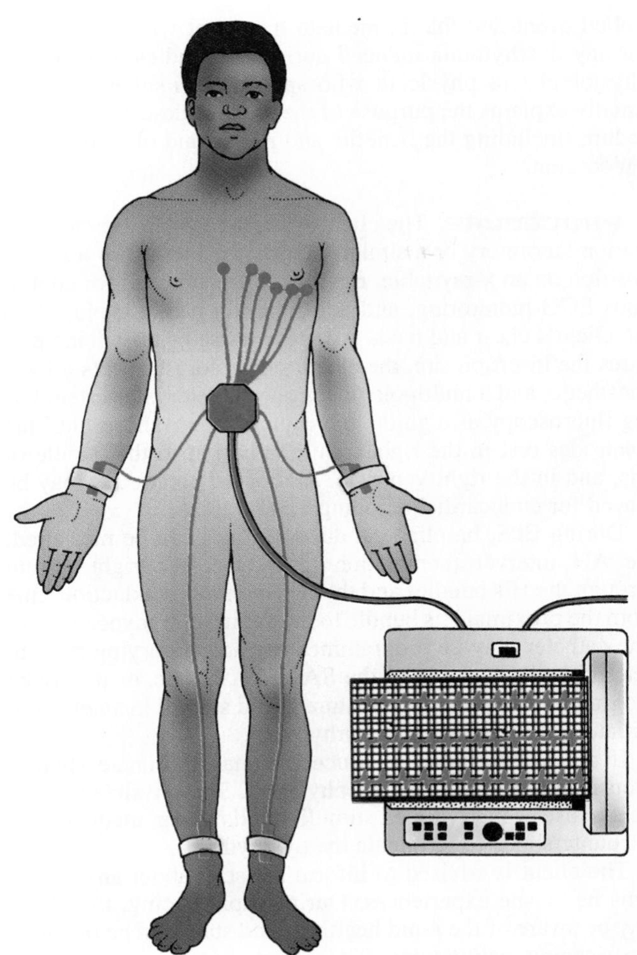

Figure 33-16 ● Electrode placement for a 12-lead ECG.

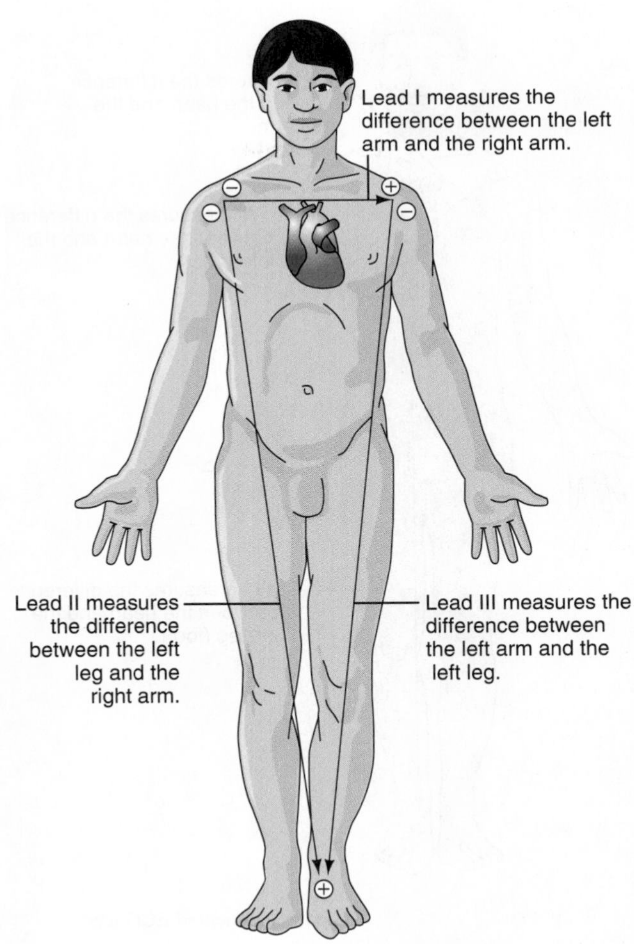

Figure 33-17 ● Standard ECG limb leads.

tions, identifying sections of the heart in which electrical conduction is abnormal.

CLIENT PREPARATION. The nurse explains the purpose and procedure of the resting ECG, informs the client that the test is safe and painless, and reminds him or her to lie as still as possible during the test.

PROCEDURE. The ECG is performed with the client in a supine position with the chest exposed. Before applying the electrodes, the nurse or the technician washes the skin to reduce skin oils and improve electrode contact. To ensure good contact between the skin and the electrodes for the limb leads, the electrodes should be placed on a flat surface above the wrists and the ankles. A total of 10 electrodes are used for a standard ECG and are attached to lead wires that connect to the ECG machine. The 12-lead ECG reading is obtained by selecting the indicators on the machine.

FOLLOW-UP CARE. No specific follow-up care is warranted.

AMBULATORY ELECTROCARDIOGRAPHY

Ambulatory ECG (also called Holter monitoring) allows continuous recording of cardiac activity during an extended period (usually 24 hours) while the client is performing his or her usual activities of daily living (ADLs). The ambulatory ECG allows the assessment and correlation of dyspnea, chest pain, central nervous system symptoms (e.g., lightheadedness and syncope), and palpitations with actual cardiac events and the client's activities.

CLIENT PREPARATION. The nurse encourages the client to maintain a normal day's schedule. He or she is instructed to keep a diary, or log. In this diary the client notes the time of activities (e.g., eating, sleeping, walking, and working) and records any symptoms such as chest pain, lightheadedness, fainting, and palpitations. The nurse instructs the client to avoid operating heavy machinery, using electric shavers and hair dryers, and bathing or showering, because these activities may interfere with the ECG recorder. If the client is hospitalized, the nurse may need to make the diary entries.

PROCEDURE. The ECG technician places the electrodes on the client's chest and attaches them to the Holter monitor. The monitor is a small portable ECG tape recorder about the size of a transistor radio. It is worn in a sling or holder around the client's chest or waist. After the prescribed monitoring period, the technician removes the electrodes and the monitor system. The ECG tape is analyzed by a micro-

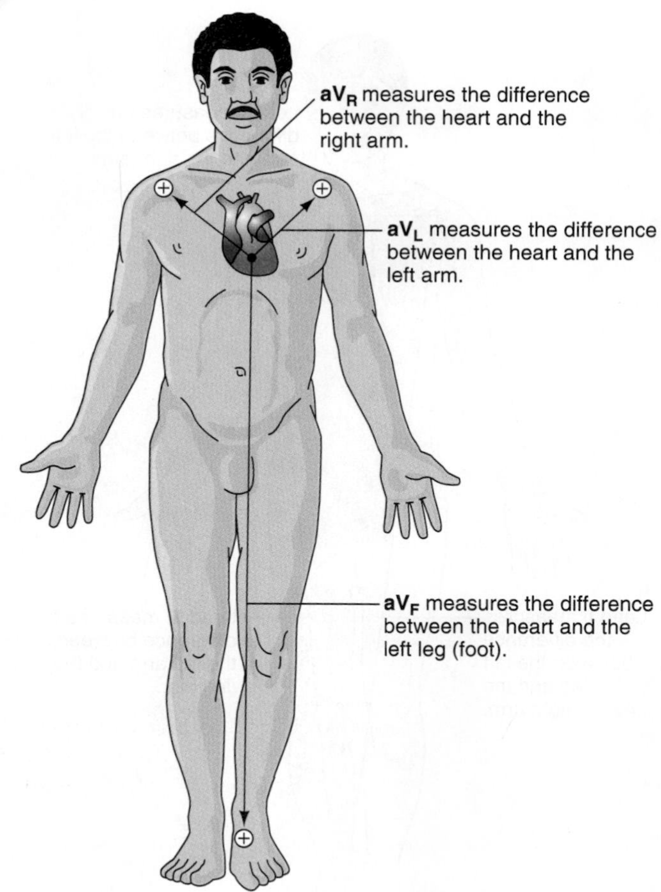

Figure 33-18 ● Unipolar augmented ECG leads.

computer to allow correlation of the ECG findings with the activities noted in the client's diary.

FOLLOW-UP CARE. No specific follow-up care is needed for a client who has undergone an ambulatory ECG.

ELECTROPHYSIOLOGIC STUDIES

An electrophysiologic study (EPS) is an invasive procedure during which programmed electrical stimulation of the heart is used to induce and evaluate lethal dysrhythmias and conduction abnormalities. Clients who have survived cardiac arrest, have recurrent tachydysrhythmias, or experience unexplained syncopal episodes may be referred for EPS. Induction of the dysrhythmia during EPS permits accurate diagnosis of the dysrhythmia and aids in the search for an effective treatment. These procedures have risks similar to those for cardiac catheterization and are performed in a special catheterization laboratory, where conditions are strictly controlled and immediate treatment is available for any adverse effects.

CLIENT PREPARATION. The preparation for EPS parallels that for cardiac catheterization (see Cardiac Catheterization, p. 642). Clients may express fear or anxiety, because attempts are made to induce lethal dysrhythmias similar to those that led to the initial hospitalization or resuscitation. The nurse reassures clients that EPS is a planned, controlled event and that immediate treatment will be available for any dysrhythmia induced during the studies. An electrophysiologist (a physician who specializes in these studies) usually explains the purpose of the studies, describes the procedure (including the benefits and risks), and obtains a written consent.

PROCEDURE. The client is taken to a cardiac catheterization laboratory or a similar laboratory and lies in a supine position on an x-ray table. Electrodes are attached for continuous ECG monitoring, and defibrillation pads are placed on the client's chest and back. After the nurse or technician prepares the insertion site, the electrophysiologist injects a local anesthetic, and a multipolar electrode catheter is inserted. Using fluoroscopy as a guide, the catheter is advanced until the electrodes rest in the right atrium, adjacent to the bundle of His, and in the right ventricle. Additional electrodes may be placed for endocardial mapping.

During EPS, baseline conduction times can be measured: the AH interval (conduction time from the right atrium through the His bundle) and the HV interval (conduction time from the proximal His bundle to the ventricular myocardium). The catheter may be programmed to pace at varying rates to determine the function of the SA and AV node, or it may be programmed to deliver premature paced stimuli in an effort to initiate and evaluate tachydysrhythmia.

If the dysrhythmia is induced, it may terminate spontaneously or be treated by the physician. The physician might elect to use properly timed stimuli, rapid pacing, medications, or countershock to terminate the dysrhythmia.

The client is advised to inform the staff about any symptoms he or she experiences. During rapid pacing, the client may be aware of the rapid heartbeat and state that he or she is experiencing palpitations. The client may also experience chest pain or loss of consciousness if he or she becomes hypotensive. The client often experiences back discomfort during the procedure, because he or she must remain supine for 2 to 6 hours. Pain may develop at the insertion site as the anesthetic wears off.

FOLLOW-UP CARE. Follow-up care for EPS is the same as for cardiac catheterization. The nurse may provide comfort measures to alleviate back discomfort, including massage and position changes. If the client lost consciousness during the procedure and received electrical cardioversion or defibrillation, he or she may complain of chest discomfort over the area where the electrical current was applied. The nurse assesses the skin for any signs of redness, swelling, or burns. In addition, there may be memory loss for the events during the procedure, and the nurse needs to provide reassurance and calmly explain the events of the procedure.

EXERCISE ELECTROCARDIOGRAPHY (STRESS TEST)

The exercise electrocardiography test (also known as exercise tolerance, or stress, test) assesses cardiovascular response to an increased workload. The stress test helps to determine the functional capacity of the heart and screens for asymptomatic coronary artery disease. Dysrhythmias that develop during exercise may be identified, and the effectiveness of antidysrhythmic drugs can be evaluated.

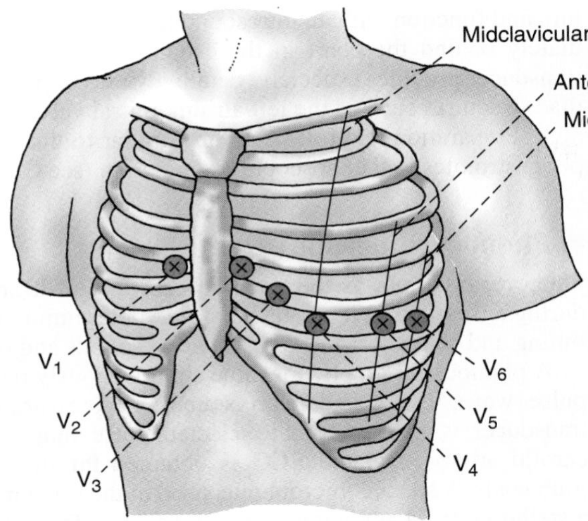

V_1 measures horizontally at the fourth intercostal space at the right sternal border.
V_2 measures horizontally at the fourth intercostal space at the left sternal border.
V_3 measures horizontally midway between V_2 and V_4.
V_4 measures horizontally at the fifth intercostal space at the midclavicular line.
V_5 measures horizontally at the fifth intercostal space at the anterior axillary line.
V_6 measures horizontally at the fifth intercostal space at the midaxillary line.

Figure 33-19 ● Unipolar precordial ECG leads.

CLIENT PREPARATION. Because there are risks associated with exercising, the client must be adequately informed about the purpose of the test, the procedure, and the risks involved. A written consent must be obtained. Anxiety and fear are common before stress testing. The nurse assures the client that the procedure is performed in a controlled environment where prompt nursing and medical attention is available.

The client is instructed to get plenty of rest the night before the procedure. The client may have a light meal 2 hours before the test but should avoid smoking or drinking alcohol or caffeine-containing beverages on the day of the test. The cardiologist decides whether the client should stop taking any cardiac medications. He or she is advised to wear comfortable, loose clothing and rubber-soled, supportive shoes. The nurse instructs the client to tell the physician if symptoms such as chest pain, dizziness, shortness of breath, and an irregular heartbeat are experienced during the test.

Before the stress test, a resting 12-lead ECG, cardiovascular history, and physical examination are performed to check for any ECG abnormalities or medical factors that might contraindicate the test.

Emergency supplies such as cardiac drugs, a defibrillator, and other necessary resuscitation equipment are available in the room in which the stress test is performed. The nurse assisting the physician should be proficient in the use of resuscitation equipment, because chest pain, dysrhythmias, and other ECG changes may occur during this test.

PROCEDURE. The technician places electrodes on the client's chest and attaches them to a multilead monitoring system. The nurse notes baseline blood pressure, heart rate, and respiratory rate. The two major modes of exercise available for stress testing are pedaling a bicycle ergometer and walking on a treadmill. A bicycle ergometer has a wheel operated by pedals that can be adjusted to increase the resistance to pedaling. The treadmill is a motorized device with an adjustable conveyor belt; it can reach speeds of 1 to 10 miles/hr and can also be adjusted from a flat position to a 22-degree gradient.

After the nurse shows the client how to use the bicycle or to walk on the treadmill, he or she begins to exercise. During the test, the blood pressure and electrocardiogram (ECG) are closely monitored as the speed and incline of the treadmill or the resistance to cycling are increased. The client exercises until one of the following occurs:

- A predetermined heart rate is reached and maintained.
- Signs and symptoms such as chest pain, fatigue, extreme dyspnea, vertigo, hypotension, and ventricular dysrhythmias appear.
- Significant ST-segment depression occurs.

FOLLOW-UP CARE. After the test, the nurse continues to monitor the ECG and blood pressure until the client has completely recovered. After the client has recovered, he or she can return home if the test was performed on an outpatient basis. The nurse advises avoiding a hot shower for 1 to 2 hours after the test, because this may precipitate hypotension. If the client does not recover but continues to have chest pain or ventricular dysrhythmias or appears medically unstable, he or she is admitted to a coronary care unit for observation.

For clients who are unable to exercise because of conditions such as peripheral vascular disease or arthritis, pharmacologic stress testing with agents such as dobutamine may be indicated. The nursing considerations are similar to those for the client who has undergone an exercise electrocardiography.

Echocardiography

As a noninvasive, risk-free test, echocardiography is easily performed at the bedside or on an ambulatory care basis. Echocardiography uses ultrasound waves to assess cardiac structure and mobility, particularly of the valves. ECGs help to assess and diagnose cardiomyopathy, valvular disorders, pericardial effusion, left ventricular function, ventricular aneurysms, and cardiac tumors.

CLIENT PREPARATION. There is no special preparation for echocardiography. The nurse informs the client that the test is painless and takes 30 to 60 minutes to complete. The client is instructed to lie quietly during the test and on his or her left side with the head elevated 15 to 20 degrees.

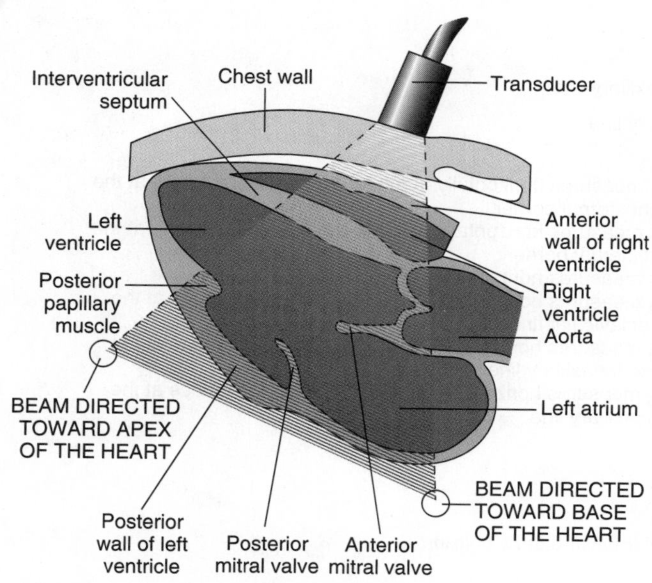

Figure 33-20 ● Echocardiographic imaging of the heart.

PROCEDURE. During an echocardiogram, a small transducer lubricated with gel to facilitate movement and conduction is placed on the client's chest at the level of the third or fourth intercostal space near the left sternal border. The transducer transmits high-frequency sound waves and receives them as they are reflected from different structures. These echoes are usually videotaped simultaneously with the echocardiogram and can be recorded on graph paper for a permanent record.

Figure 33-20 is a representation of how echocardiograms examine the heart. After the images are taped, cardiac measurements that require several images can be obtained. Routine measurements include chamber size, ejection fraction, and flow gradient across the valves.

FOLLOW-UP CARE. There is no specific follow-up care for a client who has undergone an echocardiogram.

Dobutamine Stress Echocardiogram

A slightly more aggressive form of echocardiogram is a dobutamine stress echocardiogram (DSE), which is used to provoke physiologic stress and identify patterns of cardiac response to the stress (e.g., chamber size, wall motion, and ejection fraction). Clients are required to have nothing by mouth (NPO status) for 3 to 6 hours before the test, except for sips of water with medications. The nurse or technician ensures that IV access is present before the procedure and monitors blood pressure and pulse continuously throughout the procedure. The nurse also monitors for the development of such severe responses as angina, life-threatening dysrhythmias, and syncope, although such reactions are uncommon. After the procedure, the nurse or technician continues to monitor the blood pressure until it returns to baseline and monitors the pulse rate until it slows to less than 100.

Transesophageal Echocardiography

Echocardiograms may also be performed transesophageally. Transesophageal echocardiography examines cardiac structure and function with an ultrasound transducer placed immediately behind the heart in the esophagus or stomach. The transducer provides especially detailed views of posterior cardiac structures such as the left atrium, mitral valve, and aortic arch. Preparation and follow-up are similar to that for an upper gastrointestinal endoscopic examination (see Chapter 53).

Phonocardiography

Phonocardiography is the graphic recording of heart sounds during auscultation. It can be helpful in determining the exact timing and characteristics of extra heart sounds and murmurs.

A phonocardiography machine simultaneously records the pulse wave, ECG, and heart sounds. A pressure-sensitive transducer is applied to the selected pulse (e.g., apical or carotid artery), and the ECG is obtained through standard limb leads. A special microphone, used in the same manner as a stethoscope, is applied to the various areas for auscultation on the client's chest. Client preparation and follow-up care are similar to those for echocardiography (see p. 647).

Myocardial Nuclear Perfusion Imaging

The use of radionuclide techniques in cardiovascular assessment is called myocardial nuclear perfusion imaging (MNPI). Cardiovascular abnormalities can be viewed, recorded, and evaluated using radioactive tracer substances. These studies are useful for detecting myocardial infarction (MI) and decreased myocardial blood flow and for evaluating left ventricular ejection. Conducting myocardial nuclear imaging tests in conjunction with exercise or the administration of vasodilating agents such as dipyridamole and adenosine allows clearer identification of how the heart responds to stress and involves only a slight increase in risk.

CLIENT PREPARATION. The nurse informs the client that the tests are relatively noninvasive and that the radiation exposure and risks are minimal. The client is informed that the test involves the IV injection of small amounts of radioisotope. If a dilating agent is to be used, the client is advised to abstain from cigarettes and caffeinated food or drinks for 4 hours before administration of the vasodilator. The client or responsible party must give written consent.

PROCEDURE. The most common tests in nuclear cardiology include technetium (^{99m}Tc) pyrophosphate scanning, thallium imaging, sestamibi exercise testing and scan, and multigated cardiac blood pool imaging.

TECHNETIUM PYROPHOSPHATE SCANNING. For technetium pyrophosphate scanning, a small dose of ^{99m}Tc pyrophosphate is injected into the antecubital vein. The client waits at least 2 hours while the renal system clears the unbound technetium. A gamma-scintillation camera scans the heart to identify the areas of increased uptake of the radioisotope. The radioisotope accumulates in damaged myocardial tissue and is referred to as a "hot spot." This test helps to detect an acute MI and define its location and size, but it does not show an old infarction.

THALLIUM IMAGING. For thallium imaging, a small dose of ^{201}Tl is injected into the client's antecubital vein. A nuclear camera takes images of the heart 10 minutes later to detect areas of normal blood flow and intact cells, which rapidly take up the thallium. Necrotic or ischemic tissue does not take up the radioisotope and appears as "cold spots" on the scan. Scanning is repeated in 2 to 4 hours to evaluate thallium clearance.

Thallium imaging may be performed with the client at rest or during an exercise test. Dipyridamole (Persantine, Apo-Dipyridamole✤) is administered before the Persantine thallium test. Dobutamine hydrochloride (Dobutrex) or Adenosine (Adenocard) may be given instead. By causing vasodilation, these drugs simulate the effects of exercise and are used for clients who are unable to exercise on a bike or treadmill. These medications may cause flushing, headache, dyspnea, and chest tightness for a few moments after injection.

Thallium imaging performed during an exercise test may demonstrate perfusion deficits not apparent at rest. First, the stress test procedure is performed (see Exercise Electrocardiography [Stress Test], p. 646). After the client reaches maximum activity level, a small dose of ^{201}Tl is injected intravenously. The client continues to exercise for approximately 1 to 2 minutes, after which the scanning is performed. Nuclear cardiologists often compare the resting and stress images to differentiate between fixed and reversible defects in the myocardium.

Thallium imaging is used to assess myocardial scarring and perfusion, detect the location and extent of an acute or chronic MI, evaluate graft patency after coronary bypass surgery, and evaluate antianginal therapy, thrombolytic therapy, or balloon angioplasty.

WOMEN'S HEALTH CONSIDERATIONS

Sestamibi (technetium–99m pertechnetate) may be used rather than thallium for exercise testing with scanning. Sestamibi more accurately identifies ischemic areas in women, and high-quality images may be obtained on the first scan.

CARDIAC BLOOD POOL IMAGING. Cardiac blood pool imaging is a noninvasive test for evaluating cardiac motion and calculating ejection fraction. It uses a computer to synchronize the client's electrocardiogram (ECG) with pictures taken by a gamma-scintillation camera. The technician attaches the client to an ECG and injects a small amount of ^{99m}Tc intravenously. The radioisotope is not taken up by tissue but remains "tagged" to red blood cells in the circulation. The camera may take pictures of the radioactive material as it makes its first pass through the heart.

During **multigated blood pool scanning,** the computer breaks the time between R waves on the ECG into fractions of a second, called "gates." The camera records blood flow through the heart during each of these gates. By analyzing the information from multiple gates, the computer can evaluate the ventricular wall motion and calculate ejection fraction (percentage of the left ventricular volume that is ejected with each contraction) and ejection velocity. Areas of decreased, absent, or paradoxical movement of the left ventricle may also be identified.

POSITRON EMISSION TOMOGRAPHY. Positron emission scans are used to compare cardiac perfusion and metabolic function and differentiate normal from diseased myocardium. The technician administers the first radioisotope (nitrogen-13-ammonia) and then begins a 20-minute scan to detect myocardial perfusion. Next, the technician administers a second radioisotope (fluoro-18-deoxyglucose). After a pause, a second scan is performed to detect the metabolically active myocardium, which is using glucose.

The two scans are compared. In a normal heart, performance and metabolic function will match. In an ischemic heart, there will be a mismatch: a reduction in perfusion and increased glucose uptake by the ischemic myocardium. The scanning procedure takes 2 to 3 hours, and the client may be asked to use a treadmill or exercise bicycle in conjunction with the scan.

FOLLOW-UP CARE. Depending on which test is performed, the client may complain of fatigue or discomfort at the antecubital injection site. If a stress test was paired with the study, the nurse needs to be aware of the same follow-up care as for the stress test.

Magnetic Resonance Imaging

Magnetic resonance imaging (MRI) is a noninvasive diagnostic option. An image of the heart or great vessels is produced through the interaction of magnetic fields, radio waves, and atomic nuclei showing hydrogen density. Simply put, the radio waves "bounce off" the body tissue being examined. Because each tissue has its own density, the computer image clearly differentiates between different types of tissues. MRI permits determination of cardiac wall thickness, chamber dilation, valve and ventricular function, and blood movement in the great vessels. Improved MRI techniques allow coronary artery blood flow to be mapped with nearly the accuracy of a cardiac catheterization.

Before an MRI, the nurse ensures that the client has removed all metallic objects, including watches, jewelry, clothing with metal fasteners, and hair clips. Clients with pacemakers should not undergo an MRI because the magnetic fields can deactivate the pacemaker. Approximately 5% of clients experience claustrophobia during the 15 to 60 minutes required to complete the scan.

Hemodynamic Monitoring

Hemodynamic monitoring is an invasive system used in critical care areas to provide quantitative information about vascular capacity, blood volume, pump effectiveness, and tissue perfusion. Hemodynamic monitoring is often referred to as direct monitoring because it involves procedures that directly measure pressures in the heart and great vessels. This procedure is usually performed for more seriously ill clients and can provide more accurate measurements of blood pressure, heart function, and volume status.

Hemodynamic monitoring does involve significant risks, although complications are uncommon. Therefore informed consent is required. After obtaining consent, the nurse prepares a pressure-monitoring system. The components of this system are a catheter with an infusion system, a transducer, and a monitor (Figure 33-21). The catheter receives the pressure waves (mechanical energy) from the heart or the great vessels. The transducer converts the mechanical energy into electrical energy, which is displayed as waveforms or numbers on the monitor. The nurse prepares a heparinized solution to maintain the patency of the catheter. This solution is usually infused at 3 to 4 mL/hr under pres-

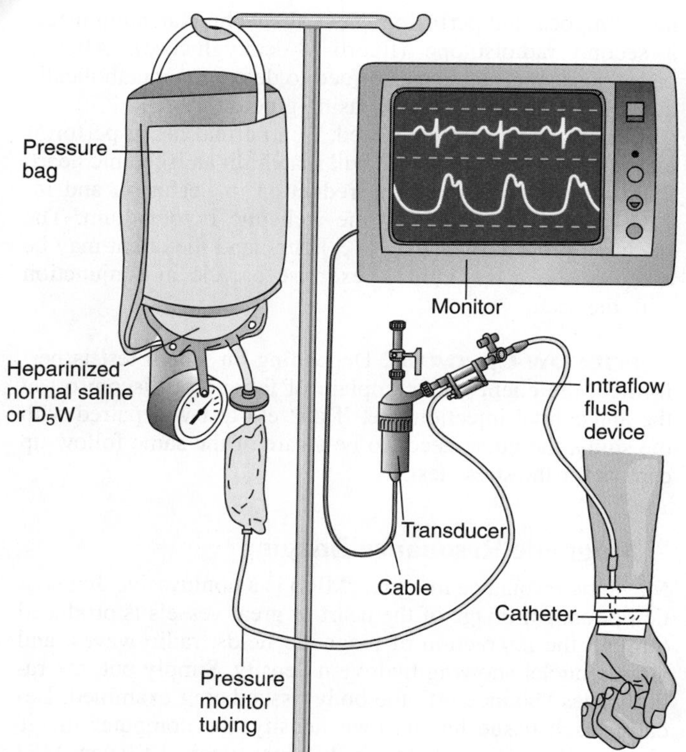

Figure 33-21 ● Components of a hemodynamic monitoring system.

CHART 33-6

BEST PRACTICE *for* Identification of the Phlebostatic Axis

1. Position the client supine.
2. Palpate the fourth intercostal space at the sternum.

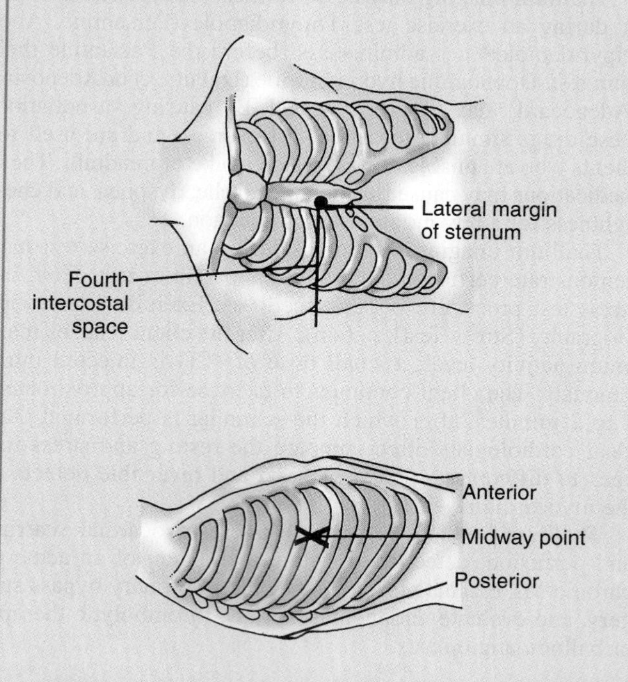

3. Follow the fourth intercostal space to the side of the client's chest.
4. Determine the midway point between anterior and posterior.
5. Find the intersection between the midway point and the line from the fourth intercostal space, and mark it with an X in indelible ink. This is the phlebostatic axis.

sure to prevent the back up of blood and occlusion of the catheter.

To prepare the transducer, the nurse must balance and calibrate it according to hospital policy and the manufacturer's specifications. Finally, the nurse must identify the phlebostatic axis (Chart 33-6) and level the transducer to it. When the monitoring system is prepared, the physician inserts the catheter.

RIGHT ATRIAL, PULMONARY ARTERY, AND PULMONARY WEDGE PRESSURES

A pulmonary artery catheter is a triple– or quadruple–lumen catheter with the capacity to measure right atrial and indirect left atrial pressures or pulmonary artery wedge pressure (PAWP), also known as the **pulmonary artery occlusive pressure (PAOP).** A cardiac output measurement may also be obtained.

CLIENT PREPARATION. The physician explains the procedure and advises the client and family members or significant others of the risks. The physician then obtains a written consent for the procedure. The client and family should understand that the hemodynamic monitoring system represents an assessment tool. Although it is used to guide therapy, it is not itself a treatment. The nurse asks the client to remain still and in the supine position for insertion of the catheter.

PROCEDURE. The physician inserts a balloon-tipped catheter percutaneously through a large vein and directs it to the right atrium (RA). When the catheter tip reaches the RA, the physician inflates the balloon. The catheter advances with the flow of blood through the tricuspid valve, into the right ventricle, past the pulmonic valve, and into a branch of the pulmonary artery. The balloon is deflated after the catheter tip reaches the pulmonary artery. Waveforms are visualized on the oscilloscope as the pulmonary artery catheter is advanced (Figure 33-22); fluoroscopy is used to monitor the location of the catheter.

Right atrial pressure is measured by a pressure sensor on the catheter inside the RA. Normal RA pressure ranges from 1 to 8 mm Hg. Increased RA pressures may occur with right ventricular failure, whereas low RA pressures are usually indicative of hypovolemia.

Normal pulmonary artery pressure (PAP) ranges from 15 to 28 mm Hg/5 to 16 mm Hg (a mean of 15) and may be constantly visible on the monitor. When the balloon at the catheter tip is inflated, the catheter advances and wedges in a branch of the pulmonary artery. The tip of the catheter is able to sense pressures transmitted from the left atrium, which reflect left ventricular end-diastolic pressure (LVEDP). The pressure measured during balloon inflation is called the **pulmonary artery wedge pressure (PAWP).** PAWP closely approximates left atrial pressure and LVEDP in clients with normal left ventricular function, normal heart rates, and no mitral valve disease. The PAWP is a mean pressure and normally ranges between 4 and 12 mm Hg.

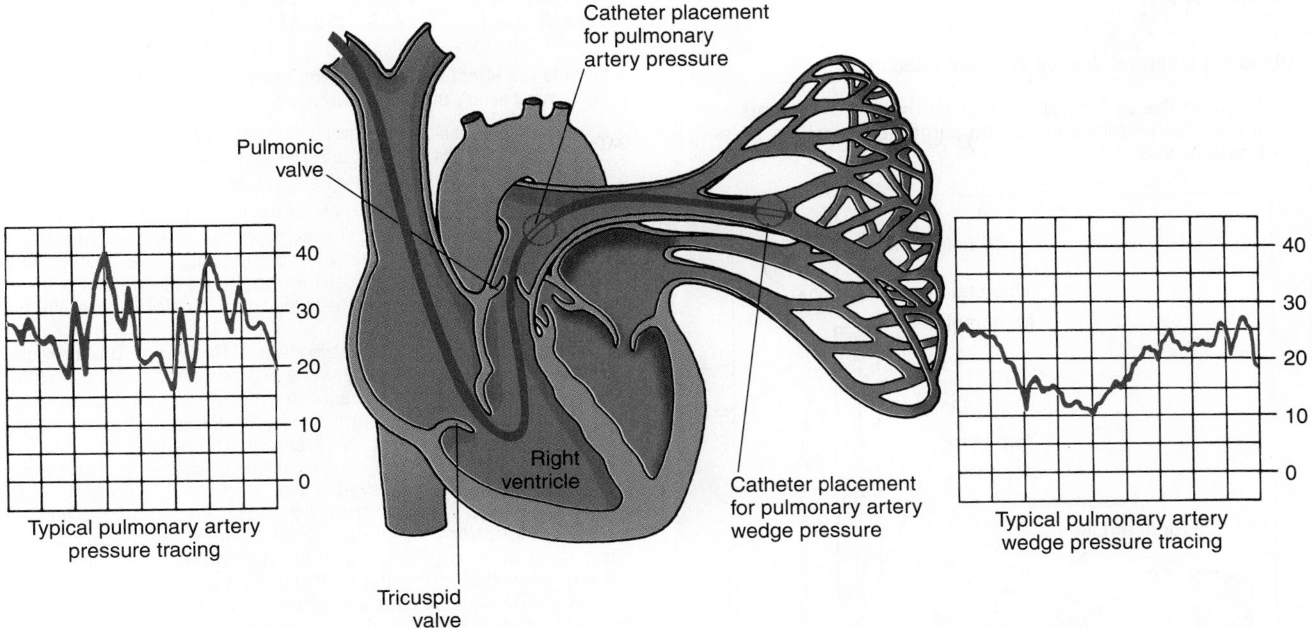

Figure 33-22 ● Cardiac pressure waveforms can be visualized on the oscilloscope.

Elevated PAWP measurements may indicate left ventricular failure, hypervolemia, mitral regurgitation, or intracardiac shunt. A decreased PAWP is seen with hypovolemia or afterload reduction. Individual values may be less important than the trend in values.

FOLLOW-UP CARE. The patency of the catheter is maintained with infusion of a heparinized solution under pressure. The nurse obtains and records RA pressure, PAP, and PAWP at appropriate intervals (usually every 1 to 4 hours). The trend of these pressures helps to guide medical therapy. During pressure recording, it is important that the transducer be at the level of the phlebostatic axis and that the client's position be appropriate. The client is usually supine with the head elevated up to 45 degrees or turned slightly to the side while PAWPs are obtained (see the Evidence-Based Practice for Nursing box on p. 652). If the balloon remains in the wedge position after PAWP measurement, the nurse attempts to change the catheter's position by asking the client to cough or by changing the client's position. If these methods are not successful, the nurse notifies the physician immediately.

The nurse changes the occlusive dressing over the catheter aseptically according to hospital policy. The insertion site is inspected for redness, heat, swelling, drainage, and intactness of the sutures. Detailed discussion of the management and care of clients with pulmonary artery catheters can be found in textbooks on critical care nursing.

The nurse assesses for a number of complications associated with pulmonary artery catheters. For example, pulmonary infarction or pulmonary rupture may occur if the catheter remains in the wedge position. Air embolism is possible if the balloon has ruptured and repeated attempts are made to inflate it. Ventricular dysrhythmias may occur if the catheter tip slips back into the right ventricle and irritates the myocardium. Thrombus and embolus formation may occur at the catheter site. Infection may result and bleeding may be pronounced if the infusion system becomes disconnected.

CARDIAC OUTPUT

Cardiac output can be measured using the thermodilution method when the client has a pulmonary artery catheter with a thermistor. The nurse injects a specified amount (5 or 10 mL) of iced or room-temperature IV solution (normal saline or dextrose in water) into the proximal port of the catheter. The solution mixes with the blood in the right atrium and travels with the flow of blood through the heart. A temperature-sensitive device located on the tip of the catheter in the pulmonary artery registers and senses the change in blood temperature. This information is transmitted to a cardiac output computer, which displays a digital value.

MIXED VENOUS OXYGEN SATURATION MONITORING

Mixed venous oxygen saturation (SvO_2) reflects the balance between the client's oxygen supply and demand. SvO_2 may be measured with a pulmonary artery catheter with fiberoptics. Light travels down one optical fiber, is reflected by the red blood cells according to the oxygen saturation of the hemoglobin, and returns to an optical module for interpretation and continuous display. The normal range for SvO_2 is 60% to 80%. Using SvO_2 monitoring, the nurse can individualize the plan of care so the SvO_2 remains in the normal range and the client's oxygen supply and demand are in balance.

CENTRAL VENOUS PRESSURE MONITORING

If the health care provider wants to measure pressures from the right atrium or central veins but a pulmonary artery catheter and pressure-monitoring system are not appropriate,

CHART 33-7

BEST PRACTICE *for*
Obtaining a Central Venous Pressure Reading

1. Position the water manometer so that the zero mark or the air-fluid interface is at the same height as the phlebostatic axis.

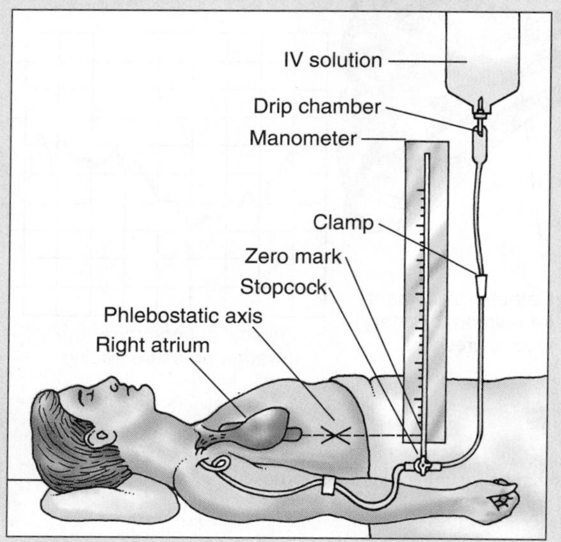

2. Turn the stopcock as shown to fill the manometer with IV fluid.
3. Turn the stopcock as shown to record the central venous pressure. With each respiration, the fluid level in the manometer should fluctuate. When the level has stabilized, read the highest level of the fluid column.
4. Return the stopcock to the position shown to resume the flow of IV fluid to the client.

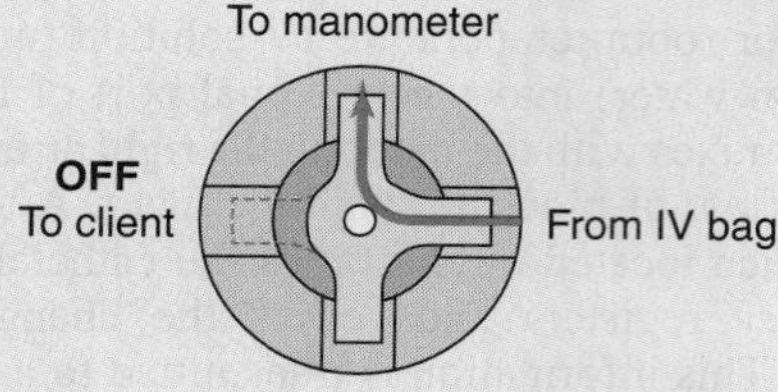

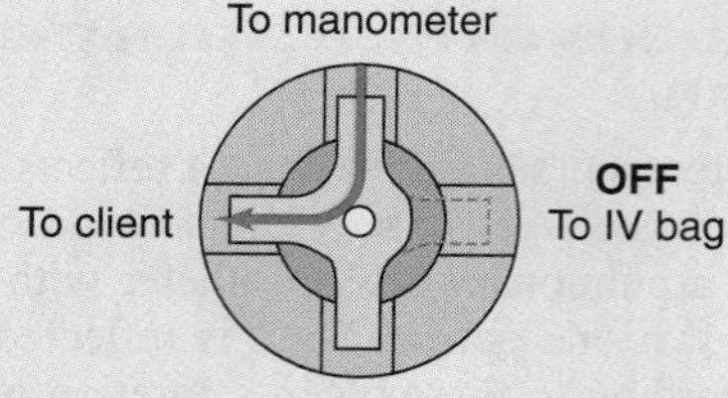

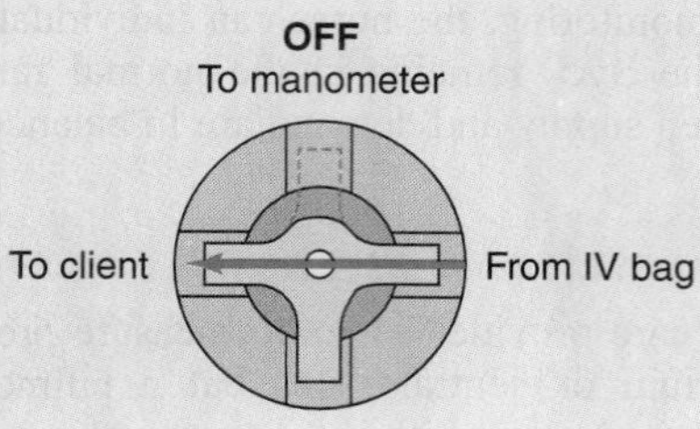

EVIDENCE-BASED PRACTICE FOR NURSING

What is the effect of the side-lying position on the accuracy of pulmonary artery pressure readings?

Bridges, E.J., et al. (2000). Effect of the 30° lateral recumbent position in pulmonary artery and pulmonary artery wedge pressures in critically ill adult cardiac surgery patients. *American Journal of Critical Care, 9*(4), 262-275.

The purpose of this study was to determine if pulmonary artery (PA) pressures and PA wedge pressures could be accurately determined in a side-lying position. This would allow critically ill clients to be therapeutically positioned in a lateral position without frequent repositioning to determine PA and wedge pressures.

Thirty-five clients with stable PA and PA wedge pressures after coronary artery surgery were studied. Although the differences between the PA measurements taken in the supine and lateral positions were statistically significant, they were not clinically significant. Clinically significant position-related differences occurred in only 2.1% of the position/pressure pairs.

Critique. This study was conducted by well-known, highly qualified nurse researchers. They used an experimental two-group, repeated-measures design, which is appropriate for this type of study. They carefully described their sample and adequately described the well-planned procedure. A two-way analysis of variance for repeated measures and a post hoc paired t test (to detect significant group differences) were the statistical tests used. The results were clearly described and the study limitations clearly explained.

Implications for Nursing. After coronary artery surgery, it may be possible to therapeutically position stable clients in the lateral position and obtain accurate PA and PA wedge readings. The ability to use pressures obtained with clients in the lateral position would prevent them from needing to remain supine for long periods following coronary artery surgery or from needing repeated turning from the lateral to the supine position to obtain accurate readings.

pressures may be obtained with a water manometer attached to a conventional IV system. Central venous pressures (CVPs) are similar to right atrial pressures, but CVPs are measured in centimeters of water rather than in millimeters of mercury. A normal CVP is 3 to 8 mm Hg, or 7 to 12 cm H_2O.

The physician inserts a catheter through the venous system into the right atrium. A chest x-ray film is obtained to assess placement. The nurse levels the manometer with the phlebostatic axis to ensure accurate pressure measurement (Chart 33-7).

Elevated CVPs may indicate right ventricular failure. Low CVPs may indicate hypovolemia. Caution must be used in predicting the function of the left side of the heart from a CVP reading.

Care of the site is similar to that for the pulmonary artery catheter site. Complications include pneumothorax during insertion, hemorrhage, infection, and catheter occlusion.

SYSTEMIC INTRA-ARTERIAL MONITORING

Direct measurement of arterial blood pressure is by invasive arterial catheter in critically ill clients. The physician usually inserts an intra-arterial catheter into the radial artery, but the femoral, brachial, or dorsalis pedis arteries may also be used. After the physician has inserted the catheter, it is attached to pressure tubing. A heparinized solution is infused constantly under pressure to maintain the integrity of the system. A transducer attached to the tubing allows continuous direct monitoring of the arterial blood pressure. Direct measurements of blood pressure are usually 10 to 15 mm Hg greater than indirect (cuff) measurements. The arterial catheter may also be used to obtain blood samples for arterial blood gas values and other blood tests.

Because the arterial vasculature is a high-pressure system, frequent assessment of the arterial site and infusion system is essential. The nurse notes any bleeding around the intra-arterial catheter or any loose connections and corrects the situation immediately. Collateral circulation is assessed by Doppler or Allen's tests before and while the arterial catheter is in place. Color, pulse, and temperature at the insertion site should be scrupulously monitored for any early signs of circulatory compromise. Complications of systemic intra-arterial monitoring may include pain, infection, arteriospasm, or obstruction at the site with the potential for distal infarction, air embolism, and hemorrhage.

IMPEDANCE CARDIOGRAPHY

Unlike conventional hemodynamic monitoring, **impedance cardiography (ICG)** is a noninvasive monitoring system that consists of four ICG electrodes, four electrocardiogram (ECG) electrodes, and a portable ICG monitor. Simply stated, it measures the total impedance (resistance) to the flow of electricity in the heart. ICG can be used in any setting, including the home. It provides measures of thoracic fluid, left ventricular function (cardiac output and cardiac index), preload, afterload, and contractility of the heart (Turner, 2000).

ONLINE RESOURCES

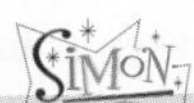

For suggested readings and Internet resources, go to http://www.wbsaunders.com/SIMON/Iggy/.

SELECTED BIBLIOGRAPHY

Asterisk indicates a classic or definitive work on this subject.

American Heart Association. (1998). *1999 heart and stroke statistical update.* Dallas: American Heart Association.

Beattie, S., & Stapleton, A. (1997). Noninvasive evaluation of coronary artery disease and myocardial viability through stress echocardiography and myocardial perfusion imaging. *The Nurse Practitioner, 22*(8), 39-40.

Beresford, A.A., et al. (1997). A dietary intervention in primary care practice: The eating patterns study. *American Journal of Public Health, 87*(4), 610-616.

Braunwald, E. (1998). The clinical examination. In L. Goldman & E. Braunwald (Eds.), *Primary cardiology* (pp. 27-43). Philadelphia: W.B. Saunders.

Bridges, E.J., et al. (2000). Effect of the 30° lateral recumbent position in pulmonary artery and pulmonary artery wedge pressures in critically ill adult cardiac surgery patients. *American Journal of Critical Care, 9*(4), 262-275.

Burke, M.M., & Walsh, M.B. (1997). *Gerontologic nursing: Wholistic care of the older adult* (2nd ed.). St. Louis: Mosby.

Chernecky, C.C., & Berger, B.J. (1997). *Laboratory tests and diagnostic procedures* (2nd ed.). Philadelphia: W.B. Saunders.

Coyne, K.S., & Allen, J.K. (1998). Assessment of functional status in patients with cardiac disease. *Heart and Lung, 27*(4), 263-273.

Cupples, S.A., Paige-Dobson, B., & Armstrong, D. (1998). Psychological manifestations of anxiety in patients undergoing electrophysiology studies. *Heart and Lung, 27*(6), 374-385.

Diez-Roux, A.V., et al. (1999). Prevalence and social correlates of cardiovascular disease risk factors in Harlem. *American Journal of Public Health, 89*(3), 302-307.

Garrett, A.P. (1997). Assessing cardiovascular status in the older adult with cognitive impairments. *Journal of Cardiovascular Nursing, 11*(4), 1-11.

Goldman, L. (1998). Clinical decision making. In L. Goldman & E. Braunwald (Eds.), *Primary cardiology* (pp. 13-26). Philadelphia: W.B. Saunders.

Goldman, L. (1998). Evidence-based medicine. In L. Goldman & E. Braunwald (Eds.), *Primary cardiology* (pp. 2-12). Philadelphia: W.B. Saunders.

Haapanen, N.N., Vuori, I., & Pasanan, M. (1999). Public health burden of coronary artery disease risk factors among middle-aged men and elderly men. *Preventive Medicine, 28*(4), 343-348.

Handley, R.T. (1999). Standard cardiovascular exercise stress testing: Indications, contraindications, and alternative testing modalities. *Physician Assistant, 23*(4), 37-50.

Hill, B., & Geraci, S.A. (1998). A diagnostic approach to chest pain based on history and ancillary evaluation. *The Nurse Practitioner, 23*(4), 22-24, 29-30.

Hogsten, P. (1997). Hemodynamic monitoring. In P.S. Kidd (Ed.), *High acuity nursing* (pp. 227-256). Stamford, CT: Appleton & Lange.

LaRosa, J.C. (1998). Cholesterol and atherosclerosis: A controversy resolved. *ADVANCE for Nurse Practitioners, 6*(5), 36-41.

Lee, T.H. (1998). Cardiac Non-Invasive Testing. In L. Goldman & E. Braunwald (Eds.), *Primary cardiology* (pp. 44-56). Philadelphia: W.B. Saunders.

Ludwig, L.M. (1998). Cardiovascular assessment for home health care nurses: Part 1. Initial cardiovascular assessment. *Home Healthcare Nurse, 16*(7), 450-456.

Ludwig, L.M. (1998). Cardiovascular assessment for home health care nurses: Part 2. Assessing blood pressure and cardiac functioning. *Home Healthcare Nurse, 16*(8), 547-554.

McGrath, A. & Cox, C.L. (1998). Cardiac and circulatory assessment in intensive care units. *Intensive and Critical Care Nursing, 14,* 283-287.

Meininger, J.C., et al. (1998). Genetic and environmental influences on cardiovascular disease risk factors in adolescence. *Nursing Research, 47*(1), 11-18.

Milligan, N.P., Havey, J.,& Dossa, A. (1997). Using a six minute walk to predict outcomes in patients with left ventricular dysfunction. *Rehabilitation Nursing, 22*(4), 177-181.

Murphy, M.J., & Berdiag, C.S. (1999). Use of measurements of myoglobin and cardiac troponins in the diagnosis of acute myocardial infarction. *Critical Care Nurse, 19*(1), 58-66.

*New York Heart Association Criteria Committee. (1964). *Diseases of the heart and blood vessels: Nomenclature and criteria for diagnosis* (6th ed.). Boston: Little, Brown.

Siomko, A.J. (2000). Demystifying cardiac markers. *American Journal of Nursing, 100*(1), 36-41.

Sox, H.C. (1998). Screening for coronary artery disease and its risk factors. In L. Goldman & E. Braunwald (Eds.), *Primary cardiology* (pp. 57-69). Philadelphia: W.B. Saunders.

Stevenson, L.W., & Braunwald, E. (1998). Recognition and management of patients with heart failure. In L. Goldman & E. Braunwald (Eds.), *Primary cardiology* (pp. 310-329). Philadelphia: W.B. Saunders.

Tobin, L.J. (1999). Evaluating mild to moderate hypertension. *The Nurse Practitioner, 24*(5), 22-41.

Turner, M.A. (2000). Monitoring hemodynamics noninvasively. *Nursing2000, 30*(5), 32cc1-32cc8.

Wenger, N.K. (1998). Cardiovascular disease in the elderly and in women. In L. Goldman & E. Braunwald (Eds.), *Primary cardiology* (pp. 70-82). Philadelphia: W.B. Saunders.

Wilbur, J. et al. (1999). Women's occupations, energy expenditure, and cardiovascular risk factors. *Journal of Women's Health, 8*(3), 377-387.

CHAPTER 34

Interventions for Clients with Dysrhythmias

MARCIA CHORBA

Learning Objectives

After studying this chapter, you should be able to:

1. Correlate the components of the electrocardiogram with the cardiac conduction system.
2. Interpret common cardiac dysrhythmias.
3. Identify typical physical assessment findings associated with common dysrhythmias.
4. Identify priority nursing diagnoses for clients experiencing dysrhythmias.
5. Plan care for clients experiencing common dysrhythmias.
6. Develop a teaching plan for clients experiencing common dysrhythmias.
7. Compare and contrast classes of antidysrhythmic drugs.
8. Compare and contrast types of atrioventricular blocks.
9. Explain the purpose and types of pacing used as interventions for clients with dysrhythmias.
10. Outline the procedure and precautions associated with defibrillation.
11. Plan community-based care for a client after pacemaker or implantable cardioverter/defibrillator insertion.

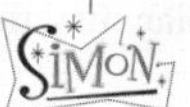

Go to http://www.wbsaunders.com/SIMON/Iggy/ for self-assessment questions related to these Learning Objectives.

Cardiac dysrhythmias are disturbances of cardiac electrical impulse formation, conduction, or both. Many diseases can affect the electrical activity of the heart, causing dysrhythmias. Although more common in older adults, dysrhythmias may occur in people of any age. Many dysrhythmias are benign; however, some cause cardiac dysfunction, and a few result in cardiac arrest. To understand dysrhythmias and to interpret these disturbances correctly, an understanding of cardiac electrophysiology, the conduction system of the heart, and the principles of electrocardiography is needed.

REVIEW OF CARDIAC ELECTROPHYSIOLOGY

Electrophysiologic Properties

The electrophysiologic properties of cardiac cells regulate heart rate and rhythm. Specialized cardiac muscle cells possess unique properties: automaticity, excitability, conductivity, and contractility.

AUTOMATICITY

Automaticity (spontaneous depolarization) is the ability of cardiac cells to generate an electrical impulse spontaneously and repetitively. Normally, only primary pacemaker cells possess this property. Under certain conditions, such as myocardial ischemia (decreased blood flow) and infarction (cell death), any cardiac cell may exhibit this property, generating electrical impulses independently and creating dysrhythmias.

EXCITABILITY

Excitability is the ability of nonpacemaker cardiac cells to respond to an electrical impulse generated from pacemaker cells and to depolarize. Depolarization occurs when the normally negatively charged cells develop a positive charge.

CONDUCTIVITY

Conductivity is the ability to transmit an electrical stimulus from cell membrane to cell membrane. Consequently, excitable cells depolarize in rapid succession from cell to cell until all cells have depolarized. This wave of depolarization gives rise to the deflections of the electrocardiogram (ECG) waveforms that are recognized as the P wave and the QRS complex.

CONTRACTILITY

Contractility is the ability of atrial and ventricular muscle cells to shorten their fiber length in response to electrical stimulation, generating sufficient pressure to propel blood forward. This is the mechanical activity of the heart.

Action Potential

The cardiac cell membrane (sarcolemma) exhibits selective permeability to ions. An ion is an electrically charged particle. This creates an electrical imbalance, known as an *action potential,* across the cell membrane.

The cardiac cell at rest has an internal negative charge, whereas the charge outside the cell is positive. This state of electrical imbalance of the resting cell is called *resting membrane potential.*

CARDIAC CONDUCTION SYSTEM

The cardiac conduction system consists of specialized cells (Figure 34-1). It is responsible for the generation and conduction of electrical impulses that cause atrial and ventricular depolarization. The conduction system consists of the sinoatrial node, atrioventricular junctional area, and bundle branch system.

Sinoatrial Node

The conduction system begins with the sinoatrial (SA) node (also called the sinus node), located close to the epicardial surface of the right atrium near its junction with the superior vena cava. The SA node is the heart's primary pacemaker. It can spontaneously and rhythmically generate electrical impulses at a rate of 60 to 100 beats/min, possessing the greatest degree of automaticity.

The SA node is richly supplied by the sympathetic and parasympathetic nervous systems, which accelerate and decelerate the rate of discharge of the sinus node, respectively. This process results in changes in the heart rate.

Impulses from the sinus node move directly through atrial muscle without specialized pathways. The impulses lead to atrial depolarization and are reflected by a P wave on the ECG. Atrial muscle contraction should follow. Within the atrial muscle are slow and fast conduction pathways, leading to the atrioventricular node.

Atrioventricular Junctional Area

The atrioventricular (AV) junctional area consists of a transitional cell zone, the AV node itself, and the His bundle. The AV node lies just beneath the right atrial endocardium, between the tricuspid valve and the ostium of the coronary sinus. Here, T-cells (transitional cells) cause impulses to slow down or be delayed in the AV node before proceeding to the ventricles. This delay is reflected by the PR segment on the ECG. This slow conduction provides a short delay, allowing the atria to contract. Blood can then fill the ventricle completely before ventricular contraction. This is known as the "atrial kick" and contributes 15% to 30% of additional blood volume for a greater cardiac output. The AV node is also controlled by both the sympathetic and the parasympathetic nervous systems. The His bundle connects with the distal portion of the AV node and continues on to perforate the interventricular septum.

Bundle Branch System

The His bundle extends as a right bundle branch down the right side of the interventricular septum to the apex of the right ventricle. On the left side it extends as a left bundle branch, which further divides into two fascicles.

At the ends of both right and left bundle branch systems are the Purkinje fibers. These fibers are an interweaving network located on the endocardial surface of both ventricles, from apex to base. The fibers then partially penetrate into the myocardium.

Purkinje cells make up the His bundle, bundle branches, and terminal Purkinje fibers. These cells are responsible for the rapid conduction of electrical impulses throughout the ventricles, leading to ventricular depolarization and the subsequent ventricular muscle contraction. A few nodal cells in

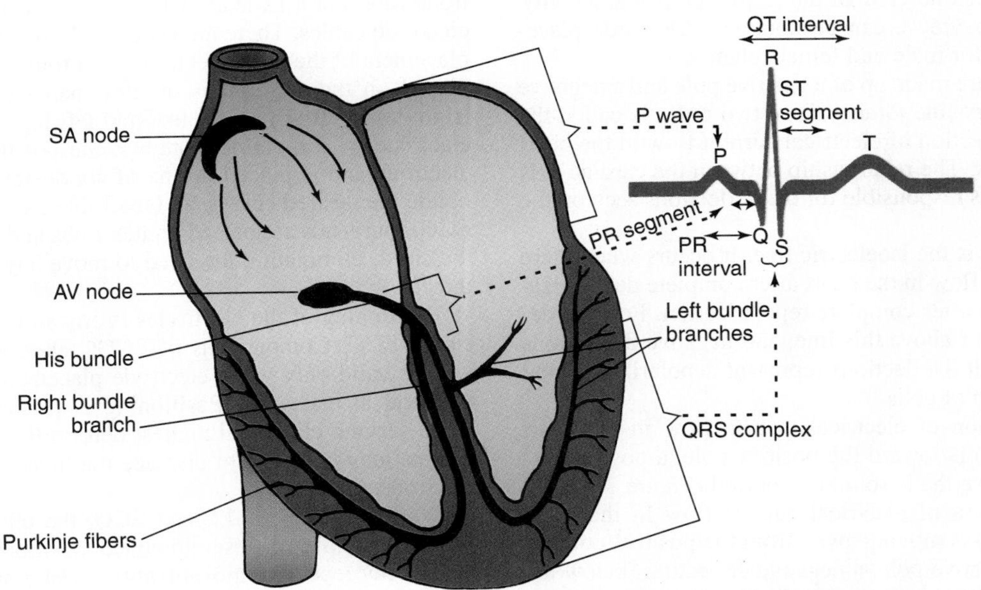

Figure 34-1 ● The cardiac conduction system.

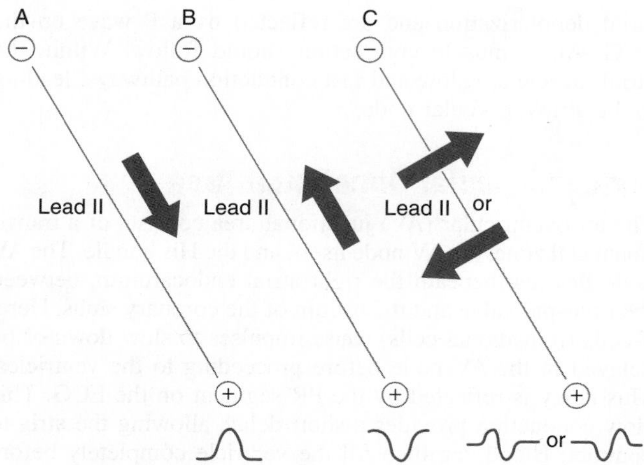

Figure 34-2 ● **A,** The cardiac axis (*bold arrow*) is parallel to the lead axis (the line between the negative and the positive electrodes), going toward the positive electrode; a positive deflection is inscribed. **B,** The cardiac axis is parallel to the lead axis, going toward the negative electrode; a negative deflection is inscribed. **C,** The cardiac axis is perpendicular to the lead axis, going neither toward the positive electrode nor toward the negative electrode; a biphasic deflection is inscribed.

the ventricles may also occasionally demonstrate automaticity, giving rise to ventricular beats or rhythms.

ELECTROCARDIOGRAPHY

The **electrocardiogram (ECG)** provides a graphic representation, or picture, of cardiac activity. The weak cardiac electrical currents are transmitted to the body surface. Electrodes, consisting of a conductive gel on an adhesive pad, are placed on specific sites on the body and attached to cables connected to an ECG machine or to a monitor. The cardiac electrical current is transmitted via the electrodes and through the lead wires to the machine or monitor, which displays the cardiac electrical activity.

A **lead** provides one view of the heart's electrical activity. Multiple leads, or views, can be obtained. Electrode placement is the same for male and female clients.

Lead systems are made up of a positive pole and a negative pole. An imaginary line joining these two poles is called the *lead axis.* The direction of electrical current flow in the heart is the *cardiac axis.* The relationship between the cardiac axis and the lead axis is responsible for the deflections seen on the ECG pattern:

- The baseline is the isoelectric line. It occurs when there is no current flow in the heart after complete depolarization and also after complete repolarization. Positive deflections occur above this line, and negative deflections occur below it. Deflections represent depolarization and repolarization of cells.
- If the direction of electrical current flow in the heart (cardiac axis) is toward the positive pole, a positive deflection (above the baseline) is viewed (Figure 34-2, *A*).
- If the direction of electrical current flow in the heart (cardiac axis) is moving away from the positive pole toward the negative pole, a negative deflection (below the baseline) is viewed (Figure 34-2, *B*).
- If the cardiac axis is moving neither toward nor away from the positive pole, a biphasic complex (both above and below baseline) will result (Figure 34-2, *C*).

Lead Systems

The standard 12-lead ECG consists of 12 leads (or views) of the heart's electrical activity. Six of the leads are called limb leads because the electrodes are placed on the four limbs in the frontal plane. The remaining six leads are called chest (precordial) leads because the electrodes are placed on the chest in the horizontal plane (see Chapter 33).

LIMB LEADS

Standard bipolar limb leads consist of three leads that each measure the electrical activity between two points, and a fourth lead (right leg) that acts solely as a ground electrode. Of the three measuring leads, the right arm is always negative, the left leg is always positive, and the left arm can be either positive or negative. Bipolar leads can be obtained by using a monitor with either three or five electrode cables or a 12-lead ECG machine. Leads I, II, and III are bipolar leads (Table 34-1; see also Chapter 33).

Unipolar limb leads consist of a positive electrode only. These leads can be obtained only by using a monitor with four or five electrode cables or a 12-lead ECG machine. The unipolar limb leads are aVR, aVL, and aVF, with *a* meaning augmented. *V* is a designation for a unipolar lead. The third letter denotes the positive electrode placement: *R* for right arm, *L* for left arm, and *F* for foot (left leg). The positive electrode is at one end of the lead axis. The other end is the center of the electrical field, at approximately the center of the heart (see Table 34-1).

CHEST LEADS

Chest (precordial) leads are also unipolar, or V, leads and therefore can be obtained only from a monitor with five electrode cables or a 12-lead ECG machine, which usually has 10 electrode cables. There are six chest leads, determined by the placement of the chest electrode. The four limb electrodes are placed on the extremities, as designated on each electrode (right arm, left arm, right leg, and left leg). The fifth (chest) electrode on a monitor system is the positive, or exploring, electrode and is placed in one of six designated positions to obtain the desired chest lead (see Table 34-1). With a 12-lead ECG, four leads are placed on the limbs and six are placed on the chest, eliminating the need to move any electrodes about the chest.

Positioning of the electrodes is crucial in obtaining an accurate ECG. Comparisons of ECGs taken at different times will be valid only when electrode placement is accurate and identical at each test. Positioning is particularly important when serving clients with chest deformities or large breasts. Clients may be asked to displace the breast to ensure proper electrode placement.

While obtaining a 12-lead ECG, the client should be as still as possible in a semireclined position, breathing normally. Any repetitive movement will cause artifact and could lead to inaccurate interpretation of the ECG.

TABLE 34-1 • ELECTRODE PLACEMENT FOR 12 LEADS

Lead	Negative Electrode	Positive Electrode	Ground Electrode
I	Right arm, or under the right clavicle	Left arm, or under the left clavicle	Right leg, or lowest rib, left midclavicular line
II	Right arm, or under the right clavicle	Left leg, or lowest rib, left midclavicular line	Right leg, or under the left clavicle
III	Left arm, or under the left clavicle	Left leg, or lowest rib, left midclavicular line	Right leg, or under the right clavicle
aVR	Average potential of left arm (or under the left clavicle) and left leg (or lowest rib, left midclavicular line)	Right arm, or under the right clavicle	Right leg, or lowest rib, right midclavicular line
aVL	Average potential of right arm (or under the right clavicle) and left leg (or lowest rib, left midclavicular line)	Left arm, or under the left clavicle	Same as for aVR
aVF	Average potential of right arm (or under the right clavicle) and left arm (or under the left clavicle)	Left leg, or lowest rib, left midclavicular line	Same as for aVR
V_1	Average potential of right arm, left arm, and left leg	Fourth intercostal space (ICS), right sternal border	Same as for aVR
V_2	Same as for V_1	Fourth ICS, left sternal border	Same as for aVR
V_3	Same as for V_1	Midway between V_2 and V_4	Same as for aVR
V_4	Same as for V_1	Fifth ICS, left midclavicular line	Same as for aVR
V_5	Same as for V_1	Horizontal to V_4, left anterior axillary line	Same as for aVR
V_6	Same as for V_1	Horizontal to V_4, left midaxillary line	Same as for aVR

Often, nurses are responsible for obtaining 12-lead ECGs, but technicians are more commonly trained to take 12-lead ECGs in various health care settings. It is imperative that the technician bring any suspected abnormality to the attention of a nurse or physician. A nurse may direct a technician to take a 12-lead ECG on a client experiencing chest pain to observe for diagnostic changes, but it is ultimately the physician's responsibility to interpret the ECG.

Continuous Electrocardiographic Monitoring

For continuous electrocardiographic (ECG) monitoring, the electrodes are not placed on the limbs, because movement of the extremities causes "noise," or motion artifact, on the ECG signal. The nurse places the electrodes on the trunk, a more stable area, to minimize such artifacts and to obtain a clearer signal. If the monitoring system provides five electrode cables, the nurse places the electrodes as follows:

- Right arm electrode just below the right clavicle
- Left arm electrode just below the left clavicle
- Right leg electrode on the lowest palpable rib, on the right midclavicular line
- Left leg electrode on the lowest palpable rib, on the left midclavicular line
- Fifth electrode placed to obtain one of the six chest leads

With this placement, the monitor lead select control may be changed to provide lead I, II, III, aVR, aVL, or aVF or one chest lead. The monitor automatically alters the polarity of the electrodes to provide the lead selected.

If the monitoring system provides only three electrode cables, the nurse places the right arm, the left arm, and the left leg electrodes as described. In this case, the lead selected provides only lead I, II, or III.

The popular MCL_1 lead is a modified *(M)* bipolar chest *(C)* lead. It approximates the V_1 lead without requiring a five-electrode cable monitoring system because it is a bipolar lead system. To obtain MCL_1, the nurse places the negative electrode just below the left *(L)* midclavicle and the positive electrode in the V_1 position. The ground electrode may be placed anywhere but is usually placed under the right clavicle. The nurse uses this lead for bedside or telemetry monitoring to differentiate left from right electrical activity, such as left from right bundle branch block or left from right premature ventricular complexes, and to differentiate certain supraventricular beats from ventricular ectopic beats. The MCL_1 lead provides a right-sided view of cardiac electrical activity.

Another bipolar lead, MCL_6, is frequently used. It can be achieved by placing the negative and ground electrodes as for MCL_1 and moving the positive electrode to the V_6 position. This approximates the V_6 lead and provides a left-sided view of cardiac electrical activity. It is used for the same reasons as MCL_1.

The clarity of continuous ECG monitor recordings is affected by skin preparation and electrode quality. To ensure the best signal transmission, the nurse or assistive nursing personnel decreases skin impedance by cleaning the skin with soap and water. The area is shaved if needed, and the electrode sites are wiped with an alcohol or other skin preparation pad and dried. The gel on each electrode must be moist and fresh. The nurse or assistive nursing personnel attaches the electrode to the lead cable, rubs the skin briskly with a gauze square or a washcloth until the skin is slightly reddened, and then applies the electrode onto the site for proper contact. This action rubs off surface cells and increases capillary blood flow to the area to improve transmission of electrical activity. The contact site should not have any lotion, tincture, or other substance on it that increases skin impedance. Electrodes cannot be placed on irritated skin or over scar tissue. The application of electrodes may be done by an assistive nursing personnel, but the nurse must determine which lead to select. The nurse assesses the quality of the ECG rhythm transmission to the monitoring system and is responsible for assessment and management of the client.

ECG cables may be attached directly to a wall-mounted monitor (a hard-wired system) if the client's activity is restricted to bedrest and sitting in a chair, as in a critical care unit. For an ambulatory client, the ECG cable is attached to a battery-operated transmitter (a **telemetry** system) held in a pouch worn by the client. The ECG is transmitted via antennae located in strategic places, usually in the ceiling, to a remote monitor. This device allows freedom of movement within a certain radius without losing transmission of the ECG.

Some acute care facilities employ monitor technicians who are educated in ECG rhythm interpretation and are responsible for the following:

- Watching a bank of monitors on a unit
- Printing ECG rhythm strips routinely and as needed
- Interpreting rhythms
- Communicating with the nurse to report the client's rhythm and significant changes

This technical support is particularly helpful on a telemetry unit that does not have monitors at the bedside. The nurse is reasonably assured that the ECG rhythm is being monitored "continuously," although some rhythms will not be observed by technicians. The nurse remains ultimately responsible for accurate ECG rhythm interpretation, as well as client assessment and management.

Some units have full-disclosure monitors, which continuously store ECG rhythms in memory up to a maximum amount of time, allowing nurses and physicians to access and print them for more thorough assessment and management of clients with dysrhythmias. Routine strips, as well as any changes in rhythm, are printed and documented in the client's record.

The physician is responsible for determining when monitoring can be suspended, such as when the client is showering. The health care provider also determines whether monitoring is needed during transportation and off-unit testing procedures. The nurse collaborates with the physician in making these determinations.

Prehospital personnel, such as paramedics and EMTs with advanced training, frequently monitor a client's ECG rhythm at the scene and en route to a health care facility. They function under medical direction and protocols but may also be in communication with a nurse.

Electrocardiographic Paper

The electrocardiogram (ECG) strip is printed on graph paper (Figure 34-3), with each small block measuring 1 mm in height and width. ECG recorders and monitors are standardized at a speed of 25 mm/sec. Time is measured on the horizontal axis. At this speed, each small block represents 0.04 second. Five small blocks make up one large block, defined by darker bold lines and representing 0.20 second. Five large blocks represent 1 second, whereas 30 large blocks represent 6 seconds. Vertical lines in the top margin of the graph paper are usually 15 large blocks apart, representing 3-second segments.

Electrocardiographic Complexes, Segments, and Intervals

Complexes that make up a normal ECG consist of a P wave, a QRS complex, a T wave, and possibly a U wave. Segments include the PR segment, the ST segment, and the TP segment. Intervals include the PR interval, the QRS duration, and the QT interval (Figure 34-4).

P WAVE

The P wave is a deflection representing atrial depolarization. The shape of the P wave may be a positive, negative, or biphasic deflection, depending on the lead selected. When the electrical impulse is consistently generated from the sinoatrial (SA) node, the P waves have a consistent shape in a given lead. If an impulse is then generated from a different (ectopic) focus, such as atrial tissue, the shape of the P wave changes in that lead, indicating that an ectopic focus has fired.

PR SEGMENT

The PR segment is the isoelectric line from the end of the P wave to the beginning of the QRS complex, when the electri-

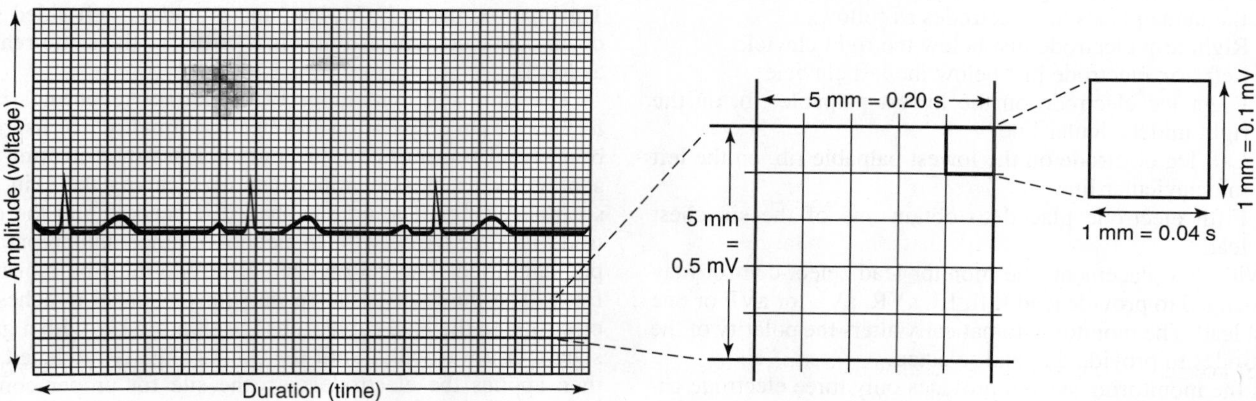

Figure 34-3 ● ECG waveforms are measured in amplitude (voltage) and duration (time).

cal impulse is traveling through the atrioventricular (AV) node, where it is delayed. It then travels through the ventricular conduction system to the Purkinje fibers.

PR INTERVAL

The PR interval is measured from the beginning of the P wave to the end of the PR segment. It represents the time required for atrial depolarization, as well as the impulse delay in the AV node and the travel time to the Purkinje fibers. It normally measures from 0.12 to 0.20 second.

QRS COMPLEX

The QRS complex represents ventricular depolarization. The shape of the QRS complex depends on the lead selected. The

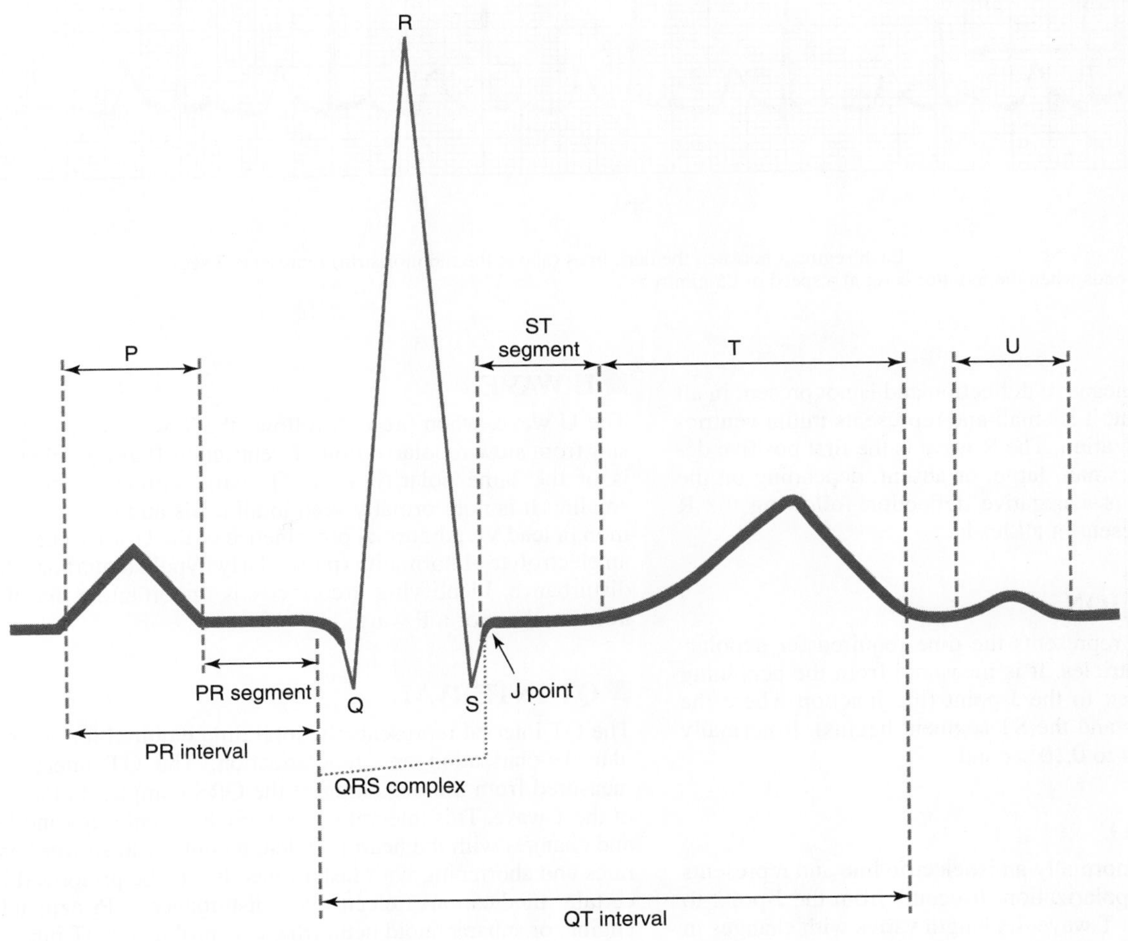

P wave:	Represents atrial depolarization.
PR segment:	Represents the time required for the impulse to travel through the AV node, where it is delayed, and through the His bundle, bundle branches, and Purkinje fiber network, just before ventricular depolarization.
PR interval:	Represents the time required for atrial depolarization as well as impulse travel through the conduction system and Purkinje fiber network, inclusive of the P wave and PR segment. It is measured from the beginning of the P wave to the end of the PR segment.
QRS complex:	Represents ventricular depolarization and is measured from the beginning of the Q (or R) wave to the end of the S wave.
J point:	Represents the junction where the QRS complex ends and the ST segment begins.
ST segment:	Represents early ventricular repolarization.
T wave:	Represents ventricular repolarization.
U wave:	Represents late ventricular repolarization.
QT interval:	Represents the total time required for ventricular depolarization and repolarization and is measured from the beginning of the QRS complex to the end of the T wave.

Figure 34-4 ● The components of a normal electrocardiogram.

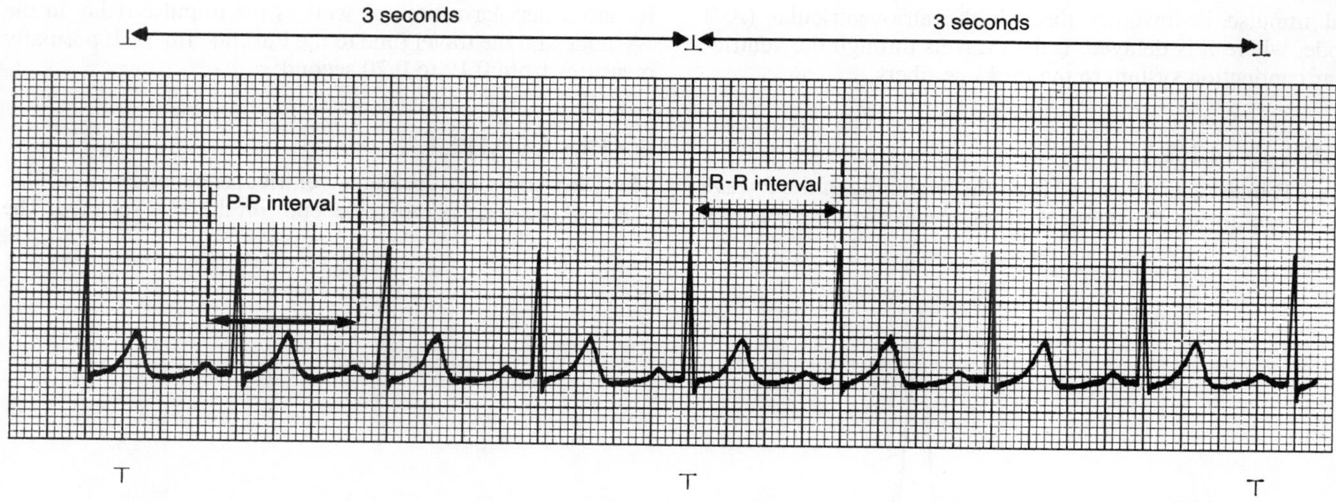

Figure 34-5 ● Each segment between the dark lines (above the monitor strip) represents 3 seconds when the monitor is set at a speed of 25 mm/sec.

Q wave is the first negative deflection and is not present in all leads. When present, it is small and represents initial ventricular septal depolarization. The R wave is the first positive deflection. It may be small, large, or absent, depending on the lead. The S wave is a negative deflection following the R wave and is not present in all leads.

QRS DURATION

The QRS duration represents the time required for depolarization of both ventricles. It is measured from the beginning of the QRS complex to the J-point (the junction where the QRS complex ends and the ST segment begins). It normally measures from 0.04 to 0.10 second.

ST SEGMENT

The ST segment is normally an isoelectric line and represents early ventricular repolarization. It occurs from the J-point to the beginning of the T wave. Its length varies with changes in the heart rate, the administration of medications, and electrolyte disturbances. It is normally not elevated more than 1 mm or depressed more than 0.5 mm from the isoelectric line. Its amplitude is measured at a point 1.5 to 2 mm after the J-point. ST elevation or depression can be caused by myocardial ischemia or infarction, conduction abnormalities, or the administration of medications.

T WAVE

The T wave follows the ST segment and represents ventricular repolarization. It is usually positive, rounded, and slightly asymmetric. If an ectopic stimulus excites the ventricles during this time, it may cause ventricular irritability and possible cardiac arrest in the vulnerable heart. This is known as the *R-on-T phenomenon.* T waves may become tall and peaked, inverted (negative), or flat as a result of myocardial ischemia, potassium or calcium imbalances, medications, or autonomic nervous system effects.

U WAVE

The U wave, when present, follows the T wave and may result from slow repolarization of ventricular Purkinje fibers. It is of the same polarity as the T wave, although generally smaller. It is not normally seen in all leads and is more common in lead V_3. Abnormal prominence of the U wave suggests an electrolyte abnormality (particularly hypokalemia) or other disturbance. Identifying it correctly is important so that it is not mistaken for a P wave.

QT INTERVAL

The QT interval represents the total time required for ventricular depolarization and repolarization. The QT interval is measured from the beginning of the QRS complex to the end of the T wave. This interval varies with the client's age and sex and changes with the heart rate, lengthening with slower heart rates and shortening with faster rates. It may be prolonged by certain medications, electrolyte disturbances, Prinzmetal's angina, or subarachnoid hemorrhage. A prolonged QT interval may lead to a unique type of ventricular tachycardia called Torsades de Pointes.

Determination of Heart Rate

The heart rate may be estimated by counting the number of P-P intervals (atrial rate) or R-R intervals (ventricular rate) in 6 seconds and multiplying that number by 10 to calculate the rate for a full minute (Figures 34-5 and 34-6). For accuracy, timing should begin with the P wave or the QRS complex and end exactly 30 large blocks (150 small blocks) later. The initial complex is the reference point and counts as zero. Subsequent complexes are counted until the end of 6 seconds, to include a fraction of the last interval; for example, if there are exactly seven R-R intervals, the heart rate is 70 beats/min; if there are 9½ intervals, the heart rate is 95 beats/min. This method may be used for both regular and irregular rhythms. It is called the 6-second strip method.

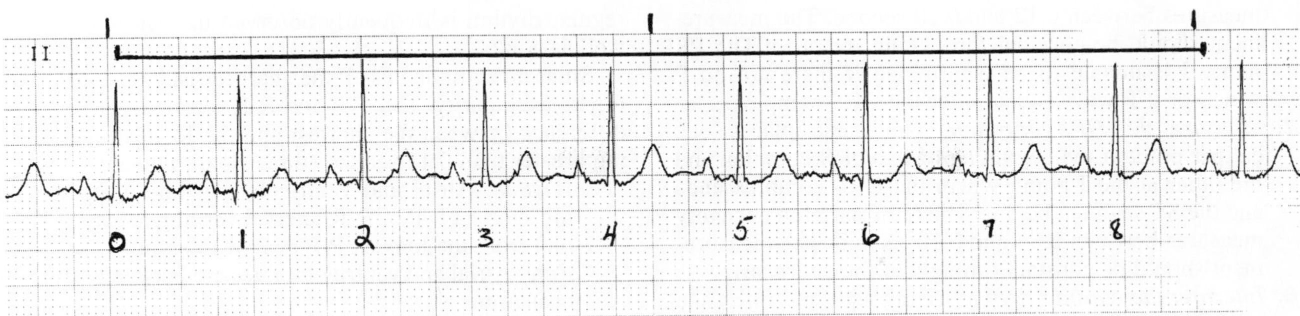

Figure 34-6 ● To estimate the ventricular rate, the 6-second timing is adjusted to begin on the R wave and end exactly 150 small blocks later. The R-R intervals are counted in the 6-second strip, and that number is multiplied by 10 to estimate the rate for a full minute. In this example there are approximately 8¾ R-R intervals in 6 seconds. Therefore the heart rate can be estimated to be 87 or 88 beats/min.

Another method, which may be used *only* if the rhythm is regular, relies on either of the following mathematic calculations:

- Count the number of small blocks in a P-P or R-R interval and divide into 1500 (the number of small blocks in 1 minute). For example, 20 small blocks equals a heart rate of 75 beats/min (1500/20 = 75).
- Count the number of large blocks in an interval and divide into 300 (the number of large blocks in 1 minute). For example, three large blocks equals a heart rate of 100 beats/min (300/3 = 100).

Commercially prepared electrocardiogram (ECG) rate rulers are based on these calculations and may be used for regular rhythms. Current monitoring systems will display a continuous heart rate and print the heart rate on the ECG strip. The nurse must, however, use caution and confirm that the rate is correct by assessing the client's heart rate directly. Many factors can incorrectly alter the rate displayed by the monitor.

Electrocardiographic Rhythm Analysis

Analysis of an ECG rhythm strip requires a systematic approach and is facilitated by the use of an **ECG caliper** (Chart 34-1):

1. *Analyze the P waves.* The nurse checks that the P-wave shape is consistent throughout the strip, indicating that atrial depolarization is occurring from impulses originating from one focus, normally the SA node. The nurse determines whether there is one P wave occurring before each QRS complex, establishing that a relationship exists between the P wave and the QRS complex. This relationship indicates that impulses from one focus are responsible for both atrial and ventricular depolarization. The nurse may observe more than one P wave shape, more P waves than QRS complexes, absent P waves, or P waves coming after the QRS, each indicating that a dysrhythmia exists.
2. *Analyze the QRS complexes.* The nurse checks that the QRS complexes are consistent throughout the strip. More than one QRS complex pattern or occasionally missing QRS complexes may be observed, indicating a dysrhythmia.
3. *Determine the atrial rhythm or regularity.* The nurse checks the regularity of the atrial rhythm by assessing the P-P intervals, placing one caliper point on a P wave and the other point on the precise spot on the next P wave. Then the caliper is moved from P wave to P wave along the entire strip ("walking out" the P waves) to determine the regularity of the rhythm. P waves of a different shape (ectopic waves), if present, create an irregularity and do not walk out with the other P waves. A slight irregularity in the P-P intervals, varying no more than three small blocks, is considered essentially regular if the P waves are all of the same shape.
4. *Determine the ventricular rhythm or regularity.* The nurse checks the regularity of the ventricular rhythm by assessing the R-R intervals, placing one caliper point on a portion of the QRS complex (usually the most prominent portion of the deflection) and the other point on the precise spot of the next QRS complex. The caliper is then moved from QRS complex to QRS complex along the entire strip (walking out the QRS complexes) to determine the regularity of the rhythm. QRS complexes of a different shape (ectopic QRS complexes), if present, create an irregularity and do not walk out with the other QRS complexes. A slight irregularity of no more than three small blocks between intervals is considered essentially regular if the QRS complexes are all of the same shape.
5. *Determine the heart rate.* If the atrial and ventricular rhythms are regular, the nurse may use any of the methods previously described to calculate the heart rate. If the rhythms are irregular, the nurse must use the 6-second strip method for accuracy.
6. *Measure the PR interval.* The nurse places one caliper point at the beginning of the P wave and the other point at the end of the PR segment. The PR interval normally

CHART 34-1

BEST PRACTICE *for* Electrocardiographic Rhythm Analysis

1. Analyze the P waves.
2. Analyze the QRS complexes.
3. Determine the atrial rhythm or regularity.
4. Determine the ventricular rhythm or regularity.
5. Determine the heart rate.
6. Measure the PR interval.
7. Measure the QRS duration.
8. Interpret the rhythm.

measures between 0.12 and 0.20 second. The measurement should be constant throughout the strip. The PR interval is unable to be determined if there are no P waves or if P waves occur after the QRS complex.

7. *Measure the QRS duration.* The nurse places one caliper point at the beginning of the QRS complex and the other at the J-point, where the QRS complex ends and the ST segment begins. The QRS duration normally measures between 0.04 and 0.10 second. The measurement should be constant throughout the entire strip.
8. *Interpret the cardiac rhythm.* Using accepted rules, the nurse can now interpret the cardiac rhythm.

These steps can be reorganized and formatted as the basis for rules or criteria to differentiate normal and abnormal cardiac rhythms. The following format is used to describe ECG criteria:

- *Rhythm:* Atrial and ventricular rhythms (regular or irregular)
- *Rate:* Atrial and ventricular rates
- *P waves:* Presence, shape, and relationship to QRS complexes
- *PR interval:* Measurement and constancy
- *QRS duration:* Measurement and constancy

NORMAL RHYTHMS

Normal Sinus Rhythm

Normal sinus rhythm (NSR) is the rhythm originating from the sinoatrial (SA) node (dominant pacemaker) that meets the following electrocardiographic (ECG) criteria (Figure 34-7):

- *Rhythm:* Atrial and ventricular rhythms regular
- *Rate:* Atrial and ventricular rates of 60 to 100 beats/min
- *P waves:* Present, consistent configuration, one P wave before each QRS complex
- *PR interval:* 0.12 to 0.20 second and constant
- *QRS duration:* 0.04 to 0.10 second and constant

Sinus Arrhythmia

Sinus arrhythmia is a variant of NSR. It results from changes in intrathoracic pressure during breathing. In this context the term *arrhythmia* does not denote an absence of rhythm, as the term suggests. Instead, the heart rate increases slightly during inspiration and decreases slightly during exhalation. This irregular rhythm is frequently observed in healthy children, as well as adults.

Sinus arrhythmia has all the characteristics of NSR, except for its irregularity. The P-P and R-R intervals vary, with the difference between the shortest and the longest intervals being greater than 0.12 second (three small blocks):

- *Rhythm:* Atrial and ventricular rhythms irregular, with the shortest P-P or R-R interval varying at least 0.12 second from the longest P-P or R-R interval
- *Rate:* Atrial and ventricular rates are between 60 and 100 beats/min
- *P waves:* One P wave before each QRS complex; consistent configuration
- *PR interval:* Normal, constant
- *QRS duration:* Normal, constant

Sinus arrhythmias may occasionally be due to nonrespiratory causes, such as the administration of digitalis or morphine. These drugs enhance vagal tone and cause decreased heart rate and irregularity unrelated to the respiratory cycle.

DYSRHYTHMIAS

OVERVIEW

Any disorder of the heartbeat is termed dysrhythmia. Historically, the term **arrhythmia** has been used in the literature; however, it means an absence of cardiac rhythm. Although the terms are often used interchangeably, **dysrhythmia,** which means a disturbance in cardiac rhythm, is more accurate.

Dysrhythmias result from a disturbance in impulse formation (either from an abnormal rate or from an ectopic focus), from a disturbance in impulse conduction (delays and blocks), or from both mechanisms. Although many dysrhythmias have no clinical manifestations, many others have serious consequences. A summary of key features is provided in Chart 34-2.

Dysrhythmia Terminology

TACHYDYSRHYTHMIAS

Tachydysrhythmias are heart rates greater than 100 beats/min. These rhythms may have serious hemodynamic consequences in the adult client with coronary artery disease (CAD). Coronary artery blood flow occurs predominantly during diastole, when the aortic valve is closed, and is deter-

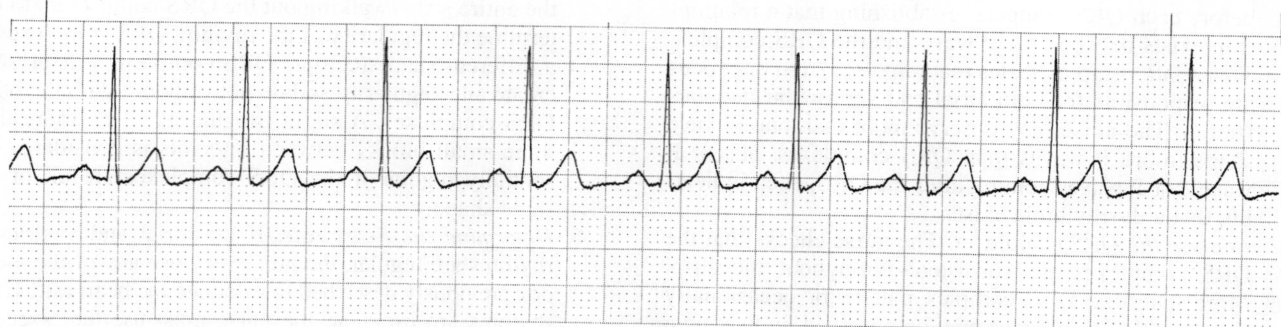

Figure 34-7 ● Normal sinus rhythm. Both atrial and ventricular rhythms are essentially regular (a slight variation in rhythm is normal). Atrial and ventricular rates are both 83 beats/min. There is one P wave before each QRS complex, and all of the P waves are of a consistent morphology, or shape. The PR interval measures 0.18 second and is constant; the QRS complex measures 0.06 second and is constant.

mined by diastolic time and blood pressure in the root of the aorta. The nurse must understand three important points to appreciate the seriousness of tachydysrhythmias:

- Tachydysrhythmias shorten the diastolic time and therefore the coronary perfusion time (the amount of time available for blood to flow through the coronary arteries to the myocardium).
- Tachydysrhythmias initially increase cardiac output and blood pressure. However, a continued rise in heart rate decreases the ventricular filling time because of a shortened diastole, decreasing the stroke volume. Consequently, cardiac output and blood pressure will begin to decrease, reducing aortic pressure and therefore coronary perfusion pressure.
- Tachydysrhythmias increase the work of the heart, increasing myocardial oxygen demand.

The client with a tachydysrhythmia may have palpitations; chest discomfort; pressure or pain from myocardial ischemia or infarction; restlessness; anxiety; pale, cool skin; and syncope from hypotension. Tachydysrhythmias may also lead to heart failure. Presenting symptoms may include dyspnea, orthopnea, pulmonary crackles, distended neck veins, fatigue, and weakness (see Chapter 35).

BRADYDYSRHYTHMIAS

Bradydysrhythmias are characterized by a heart rate less than 60 beats/min. These rhythms can also have serious hemodynamic consequences. The nurse considers the following three points:

- Myocardial oxygen demand is reduced from the slow heart rate, which is beneficial.
- Coronary perfusion time is adequate because of a prolonged diastole, which is desirable.
- Coronary perfusion pressure may decrease if the heart rate is too slow to provide adequate cardiac output and blood pressure; this is a serious consequence.

Therefore the client may tolerate the bradydysrhythmia well if the blood pressure is adequate. If the blood pressure is not adequate, symptomatic bradydysrhythmias may lead to myocardial ischemia or infarction, dysrhythmias, hypotension, and heart failure.

CHART 34-2

KEY FEATURES *of* Sustained Tachydysrhythmias and Bradydysrhythmias

- Chest discomfort, pressure, or pain, which may radiate to the jaw, the back, or the arm
- Restlessness, anxiety, nervousness, confusion
- Dizziness, syncope
- Palpitations (in tachydysrhythmias)
- Change in pulse strength, rate, and rhythm
- Pulse deficit
- Shortness of breath, dyspnea
- Tachypnea
- Pulmonary crackles
- Orthopnea
- S_3 or S_4 heart sounds
- Jugular venous distention
- Weakness, fatigue
- Pale, cool skin; diaphoresis
- Nausea, vomiting
- Decreased urine output
- Delayed capillary refill
- Hypotension

PREMATURE COMPLEXES

Premature complexes are early complexes. They occur when a cardiac cell or cell group, other than the sinoatrial (SA) node, becomes irritable and fires an impulse before the next sinus impulse is generated. This abnormal focus is called an *ectopic focus* and may be generated by atrial, junctional, or ventricular tissue. Following the premature complex, there is a pause before the next normal complex, creating an irregularity in the rhythm. The client with premature complexes may be unaware of them or may feel palpitations or a "skipping" of the heartbeat. If premature complexes, especially those that are ventricular in nature, become more frequent, the client may experience symptoms of decreased cardiac output.

REPETITIVE RHYTHMS

Premature complexes may occur repetitively in a rhythmic fashion:

- **Bigeminy** exists when normal complexes and premature complexes occur alternately in a repetitive two-beat pattern, with a pause occurring after each premature complex so that complexes occur in pairs.
- **Trigeminy** is a repetitive three-beat pattern, usually occurring as two sequential normal complexes followed by a premature complex and a pause, with the same pattern repeating itself in triplets.
- **Quadrigeminy** is a repetitive four-beat pattern, usually occurring as three sequential normal complexes followed by a premature complex and a pause, with the same pattern repeating itself in a four-beat pattern.

Such patterns may occur with atrial, junctional, or ventricular premature complexes. Clients may be unaware of the premature beats or may feel palpitations.

ESCAPE COMPLEXES AND RHYTHMS

Escape complexes or escape rhythms may occur when the SA node fails to discharge or is blocked or when a sinus impulse fails to depolarize the ventricles because of an atrioventricular (AV) nodal block. Escape complexes or rhythms serve as a secondary or escape pacemaker and are seen after a pause. Such impulses may originate from AV junctional or ventricular tissue. They cease when the SA node or the AV node regains the ability to function normally. If there are pauses followed by escape beats or rhythms, clients may feel lightheaded, dizzy, or faint during the pause.

Classification of Dysrhythmias

Dysrhythmias are classified according to their site of origin. The sites include the SA node, atrial tissue, AV node, junctional tissue, and ventricular tissue. Dysrhythmias may be caused by a disturbance in impulse formation or by conduction delays or blocks. The incidence and the prevalence of dysrhythmias are not precisely known, because they usually result from an underlying condition, such as heart disease. The incidence of dysrhythmias increases with age. A summary of the common dysrhythmias and their treatment is provided in Table 34-2.

TABLE 34-2 • COMMON DYSRHYTHMIAS AND THEIR TREATMENT

Dysrhythmia	Treatment
Sinus tachycardia	Correction of the underlying problem (e.g., fever, hypovolemia, pain, anxiety, or CHF) Beta-adrenergic blockade if increased catecholamine secretion is the underlying problem
Sinus bradycardia	Treatment necessary only if the client is symptomatic (has hypotension, diaphoresis, chest discomfort or pain, pulmonary congestion, or altered level of consciousness) • Atropine • Pacemaker • Avoidance of parasympathetic stimulation, such as prolonged suctioning or stimulation of the gag reflex
PREMATURE BEATS AND ECTOPIC RHYTHMS	
Supraventricular beats (PACs, PJCs)	Correction of any underlying problem (e.g., anxiety, stress, caffeine or nicotine intake, CHF, effects of drugs, COPD, or asthma) Medication administration • Quinidine • Procainamide • Digitalis • Propranolol • Sedatives
Supraventricular rhythms	Correction of any underlying problem (e.g., CHF, COPD, asthma, stress, or drugs) Medication administration • Verapamil • Diltiazem • Adenosine • Digitalis • Propranolol • Esmolol • Quinidine • Procainamide • Amiodarone Vagal stimulation with carotid massage Valsalva maneuvers Overdrive atrial pacing Synchronized cardioversion if the above measures are unsuccessful
Premature ventricular complexes and ventricular tachycardia (not sustained)	Correction of any underlying problem (e.g., infection, electrolyte imbalance, effects of drugs, myocardial infarction, CHF, stress, fatigue, or nicotine) Medication administration • Lidocaine bolus and infusion • Procainamide bolus and infusion • Bretylium tosylate bolus and infusion • Magnesium sulfate infusion • Class I and II antidysrhythmics • Amiodarone Restoration of electrolyte balance
Atrial flutter	Medication administration • Diltiazem • Verapamil
PREMATURE BEATS AND ECTOPIC RHYTHMS—cont'd	
Atrial flutter—cont'd	• Digitalis • Propranolol • Esmolol • Quinidine • Procainamide Atrial overdrive pacing Cardioversion Catheter or surgical ablation
Atrial fibrillation	Medication administration • Digitalis • Diltiazem • Verapamil • Quinidine • Procainamide Anticoagulation Atrial overdrive pacing Cardioversion Surgery
Escape beats and rhythms	Correction of the underlying cause if the client is symptomatic Atropine administration Pacemaker Isoproterenol administration if pacemaker unavailable
CONDUCTION DELAYS	
First-degree AV block	Treatment necessary only if the client is symptomatic Withhold digitalis (if the cause) Atropine administration if block is associated with symptomatic bradycardia
Second-degree AV block type I	Same as for first-degree AV block
Second-degree AV block type II	Pacemaker Isoproterenol administration if pacemaker unavailable
Third-degree AV block	Pacemaker Isoproterenol administration if pacemaker unavailable
LIFE-THREATENING DYSRHYTHMIAS	
Sustained ventricular tachycardia	Medication administration • Lidocaine bolus and infusion • Procainamide bolus and infusion • Bretylium tosylate bolus and infusion • Magnesium sulfate infusion If unstable: synchronized cardioversion If pulseless: defibrillation, CPR
Ventricular fibrillation	Defibrillation CPR Medication administration • Epinephrine • Lidocaine • Bretylium tosylate • Procainamide • Magnesium sulfate
Ventricular asystole	CPR Medication administration • Epinephrine • Atropine • Pacemaker

CHF, Congestive heart failure; *PACs*, premature atrial complexes; *PJCs*, premature junctional complexes; *COPD*, chronic obstructive pulmonary disease; *AV*; atrioventricular; *CPR*, cardiopulmonary resuscitation.

SINUS DYSRHYTHMIAS

The sinus node is the **pacemaker** in all sinus dysrhythmias. Sympathetic and parasympathetic nerve fibers are distributed to the SA node. Innervation from these two systems is normally in balance to ensure a normal sinus rhythm (NSR). An imbalance increases or decreases the rate of SA node discharge either as a normal response to activity or physiologic changes or as a pathologic response to disease.

SINUS TACHYCARDIA

PATHOPHYSIOLOGY. Dominant sympathetic nervous system stimulation of the heart or vagal inhibition results in an increased rate of SA node discharge, which increases the heart rate (positive chronotropic effect).

When the rate of SA node discharge exceeds 100 beats/min, the rhythm is called **sinus tachycardia** (Figure 34-8, *A*). Sinus tachycardia, with heart rates of 200 to 220 beats/min, is normal in infants and children. The rate gradually decreases until age 10 years. From age 10 years to adulthood, the heart rate normally does not exceed 100 beats/min except in response to activity and then usually does not exceed 160 beats/min. Rarely, the heart rate may reach 180 beats/min. Sinus tachycardia initially enhances cardiac output and blood pressure. However, sustained increases in heart rate decrease coronary perfusion time and coronary perfusion pressure, while increasing myocardial oxygen demand.

ETIOLOGY. Increased sympathetic stimulation is a normal response to physical activity but may also be caused by anxiety, pain, stress, fear, fever, anemia, hypoxemia, hyperthyroidism, and pulmonary embolism. Drugs such as catecholamines, atropine, caffeine, alcohol, nicotine, aminophylline, and thyroid medications may also increase the heart rate. In some cases, sinus tachycardia is a compensatory response to decreased cardiac output or blood pressure, as occurs in hypovolemia, shock, myocardial infarction, and heart failure.

PHYSICAL ASSESSMENT/CLINICAL MANIFESTATIONS. The client may be asymptomatic except for the increased pulse rate. However, if the rhythm is not well tolerated, he or she may become symptomatic. The client is assessed for fatigue, weakness, shortness of breath, orthopnea, neck vein distention, decreased oxygen saturation, and decreased blood pressure. The nurse also assesses for restlessness and anxiety from decreased cerebral perfusion and for decreased urine output from decreased renal perfusion. The adult client may experience anginal pain. The electrocardiographic (ECG) pattern may show T-wave inversion or ST-segment elevation or depression in response to myocardial ischemia.

INTERVENTIONS. The nurse and health care provider collaborate to identify the cause of sinus tachycardia and select the appropriate treatment. The goal is to decrease the heart rate to normal levels by treating the underlying cause. For example, if the client has angina, the nurse administers oxygen, helps the client to rest, and administers nitroglycerin or morphine as prescribed. Diuretics and inotropic agents

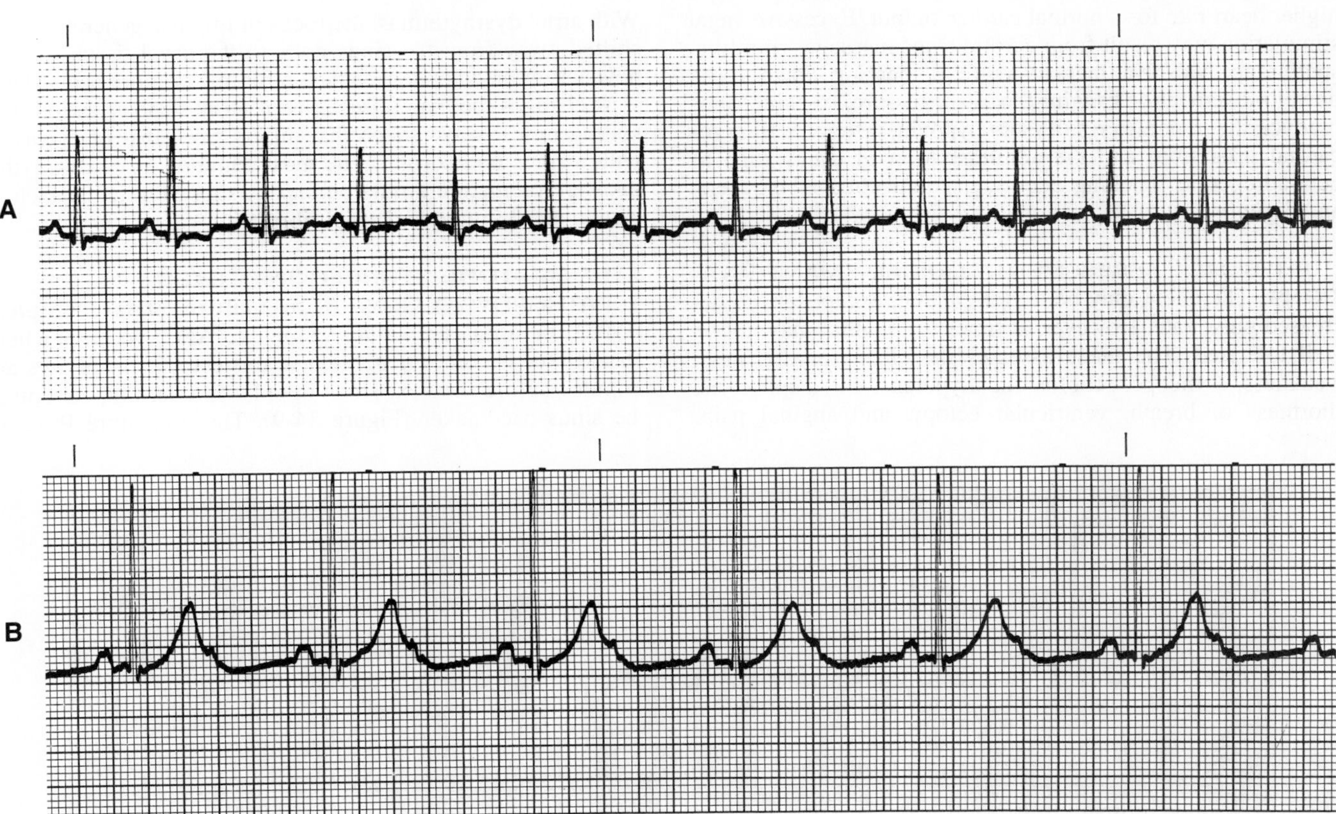

Figure 34-8 ● Sinus rhythms. **A,** Sinus tachycardia (heart rate, 110 beats/min; PR interval, 0.12 second; QRS complex, 0.08 second). **B,** Sinus bradycardia (heart rate, 52 beats/min; PR interval, 0.18 second; QRS complex, 0.08 second).

may be given for heart failure. The nurse initiates intravascular volume replacement for hypovolemia, administers antipyretics and antibiotics to the client with fever and infection, or provides comfort measures and administers analgesics or opioids to the client with noncardiac pain, as ordered.

The nurse collaborates with the respiratory therapist when indicated to oxygenate and suction the client with hypoxemia from excessive airway secretions. Beta-adrenergic blocking agents may be prescribed for the client with inappropriate sympathetic nervous system stimulation. Emotional support and relevant teaching are important for the client and family.

SINUS BRADYCARDIA

PATHOPHYSIOLOGY. Dominance of the parasympathetic nervous system, with excessive vagal stimulation to the heart, causes a decreased rate of sinus node discharge. This slows the heart rate and decreases the speed of conduction through the AV node and conduction system. When the rate of sinus node discharge is less than 60 beats/min in adults or below the normal range in infants and children, the rhythm is called **sinus bradycardia** (Figure 34-8, *B*). Sinus bradycardia increases coronary perfusion time but may decrease coronary perfusion pressure. However, myocardial oxygen demand is decreased.

ETIOLOGY. Increased parasympathetic stimulation of the heart by the vagus nerve is a normal response to decreased physical activity. It also often occurs in well-conditioned athletes because the strong heart muscle is extremely efficient in providing an adequate stroke volume while not requiring a higher heart rate for a normal cardiac output. Excessive vagal stimulation may result from carotid sinus massage, vomiting, suctioning, Valsalva maneuvers (e.g., bearing down for a bowel movement or gagging), ocular pressure, or pain. Sinus bradycardia may also result from hypoxia, inferior wall myocardial infarction, and the administration of drugs such as beta-adrenergic blocking agents, calcium channel blockers, and digitalis.

PHYSICAL ASSESSMENT/CLINICAL MANIFESTATIONS. The client may be asymptomatic, except for the decreased pulse rate. However, at times the rhythm may not be well tolerated. The nurse assesses the client for dizziness, weakness, syncope, confusion, hypotension, diaphoresis, shortness of breath, ventricular ectopy, and anginal pain. T-wave inversion or ST-segment elevation or depression may occur in response to myocardial ischemia.

INTERVENTIONS. If the client is symptomatic and the underlying cause cannot be determined, the treatment of choice is atropine administration, given as prescribed to increase the heart rate to approximately 60 beats/min. Oxygen should be applied. If the heart rate does not increase sufficiently, the nurse may apply an external pacemaker to increase the heart rate and notify the physician. However, if atropine administration succeeds in achieving an adequate heart rate but the client remains hypotensive, the nurse initiates intravascular volume replacement, as ordered, rather than administering another dose of atropine. Excessive atropine may induce tachycardia. If a medication is determined to be the cause, the nurse withholds the drug and notifies the physician for an order to discontinue the drug temporarily or permanently.

CRITICAL THINKING CHALLENGE

A 21-year-old male student, who is the captain of the college's ice hockey team, comes into the college health clinic where you are working. While taking his vital signs, you discover that his apical pulse is 46 beats/min and regular. He has no other symptoms.

- What other assessment data are needed?
- Does this dysrhythmia need treatment? Why or why not?

For suggested answer guidelines, go to SIMON http://www.wbsaunders.com/SIMON/Iggy/.

ATRIAL DYSRHYTHMIAS

With atrial dysrhythmias, the focus of impulse generation has shifted away from the sinus node to the atrial tissue, which now acts as an ectopic pacemaker, for one or more beats. This shift changes the axis (direction) of atrial depolarization, resulting in a P-wave shape that differs from that of P waves with a sinus node origin. The most common atrial dysrhythmias are premature atrial complexes, supraventricular tachycardia, atrial flutter, and atrial fibrillation.

PREMATURE ATRIAL COMPLEXES

PATHOPHYSIOLOGY. A **premature atrial complex (PAC),** or atrial premature complex (APC), occurs when atrial tissue becomes irritable, and this ectopic focus fires an impulse before the next sinus impulse is due, thus usurping the sinus pacemaker (Figure 34-9). The premature P wave

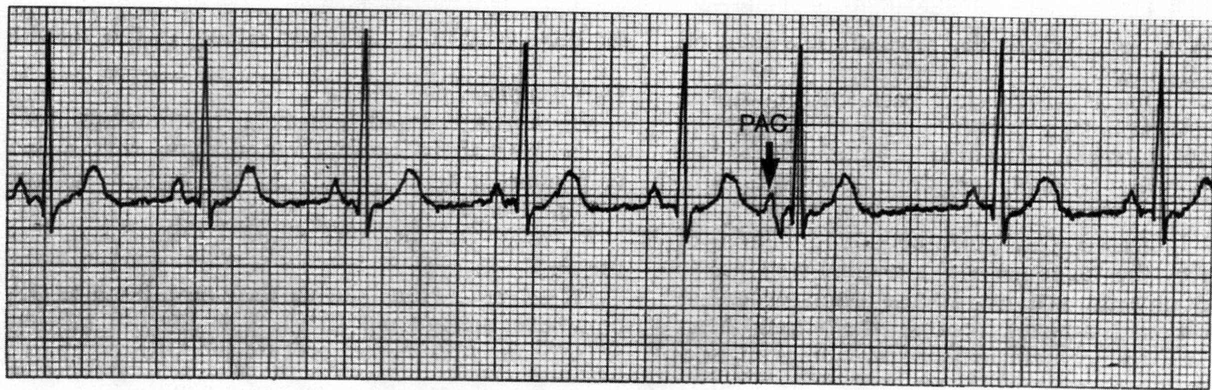

Figure 34-9 ● Normal sinus rhythm with a premature atrial complex (PAC) at arrow.

from the atrial focus is early and has a shape different from that of the P wave generated from the sinus node. The premature P wave may not always be clearly visible, since it can be hidden in the preceding T wave. The T wave must be closely examined for any change in shape and compared with other T waves to reveal a hidden P wave. A PAC is usually followed by a pause.

ETIOLOGY. The causes of atrial irritability include stress; fatigue; anxiety; inflammation; infection; intake of caffeine, nicotine, or alcohol; and the administration of drugs such as catecholamines, sympathomimetics, amphetamines, digitalis, or anesthetic agents. PACs may also result from myocardial ischemia, hypermetabolic states, electrolyte imbalance, or atrial stretch, as may occur with congestive heart failure, valvular disease, and pulmonary hypertension with cor pulmonale.

PHYSICAL ASSESSMENT/CLINICAL MANIFESTATIONS. The client is usually asymptomatic, except for possible heart palpitations, because PACs usually have no hemodynamic consequences.

INTERVENTIONS. No intervention is usually needed except to treat the cause, such as heart failure or valvular disease. If PACs occur frequently, they may signal the onset of more serious atrial tachydysrhythmias and therefore may warrant treatment. The nurse administers prescribed type IA antidysrhythmics, such as quinidine and procainamide (Pronestyl), or other drugs such as digitalis and propranolol (Inderal, Apo-Propranolol✱). Measures to reduce stress are also initiated, and the client is taught to avoid substances known to increase atrial irritability.

SUPRAVENTRICULAR TACHYCARDIA

PATHOPHYSIOLOGY. **Supraventricular tachycardia (SVT)** involves the rapid stimulation of atrial tissue at a rate of 100 to 280 beats/min, with a mean of 170 beats/min in adults (Figure 34-10) and 200 to 300 beats/min in children. SVT is most often due to a re-entry mechanism in which one impulse circulates repeatedly throughout the atrial pathway, restimulating the atrial tissue at a rapid rate. The term *paroxysmal supraventricular tachycardia (PSVT)* is used when the rhythm is intermittent, initiated suddenly by a premature complex such as a PAC, and terminated suddenly with or without intervention.

During SVT the P waves have a shape different from that of sinus P waves. The P waves may not be visible, especially if there is a 1:1 conduction with rapid rates, because the P waves are obscured in the preceding T wave.

ETIOLOGY. The causes of SVT are the same as those for PACs. SVT may occur in healthy young people without evidence of heart disease, usually women under 40 years of age. The condition commonly occurs in clients with a pre-excitation syndrome, such as Wolff-Parkinson-White (WPW) syndrome.

PHYSICAL ASSESSMENT/CLINICAL MANIFESTATIONS. The clinical manifestations depend on the duration of the SVT and the rate of the ventricular response. In clients with a sustained rapid ventricular response, the nurse assesses for palpitations, weakness, fatigue, shortness of breath, nervousness, anxiety, hypotension, and syncope. Hemodynamic deterioration may occur in the client with cardiac disease, causing angina, heart failure, and shock. With a nonsustained or slower ventricular response, the client may be asymptomatic except for transient palpitations.

INTERVENTIONS. If SVT occurs in a healthy person and terminates spontaneously, no intervention is necessary other than eliminating identified causative factors. If it is recurrent, the client should be studied in the electrophysiology laboratory. The preferred treatment for recurrent SVT is radiofrequency catheter ablation. In sustained SVT with a rapid ventricular response, the goals of treatment are to decrease the ventricular response, convert the dysrhythmia to a sinus rhythm, and treat the cause. Vagal stimulation (e.g., carotid massage) may be successful, but often only transiently, and must be performed only by a physician.

The nurse administers oxygen and prescribed antidysrhythmic drugs, which slow the ventricular rate by increasing the AV block (Chart 34-3). Some may also succeed in converting the dysrhythmia.

In the severely compromised client, the nurse may assist the physician in attempting atrial overdrive pacing or in delivering a synchronized electrical shock (cardioversion) to re-establish an organized rhythm and regain cardiac stability.

Text continued on page 672

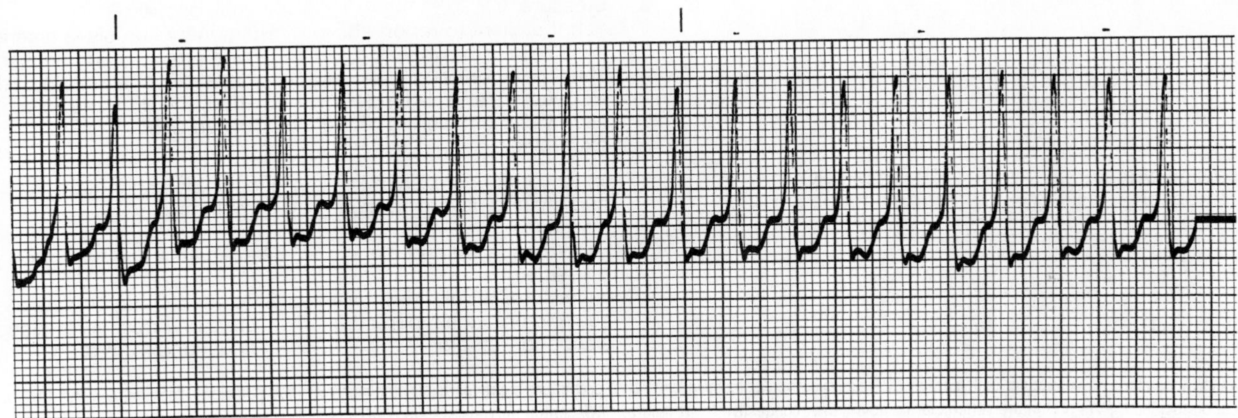

Figure 34-10 ● Sustained supraventricular tachycardia in a client with Wolff-Parkinson-White syndrome. Heart rate is 200 beats/min.

CHART 34-3

DRUG THERAPY *for* Dysrhythmias

Drug	Usual Dosage	Nursing Interventions	Rationale
CLASS I DRUGS			
Type IA			
Quinidine sulfate (quinidine, Apo-Quinidine✤)	300-600 mg q8-12h PO 6-10 mg/kg IV slowly; may be given IM	Monitor blood pressure.	Hypotension is a common side effect.
		Watch for diarrhea, nausea, or vomiting and administer with food if these occur.	Diarrhea is common during early therapy. Diarrhea and other gastrointestinal symptoms often decrease when quinidine is administered with food.
		Monitor for widening QRS complex, prolonged QT interval, heart block, and onset or increase in number of PVCs.	Toxic side effects necessitate stopping quinidine administration.
Procainamide hydrochloride (Pronestyl)	50 mg/kg/day PO in 4 divided doses 20-30 mg IV, not to exceed 17 mg/kg, followed by infusion of 1-4 mg/min	Monitor blood pressure.	Hypotension warrants drug discontinuation.
		Monitor for widening QRS complex, prolonged QT or PR interval, or heart block.	Toxic side effects necessitate stopping procainamide administration.
Disopyramide phosphate (Norpace)	100-200 mg q6h PO	Monitor blood pressure.	Hypotension is a common side effect.
		Watch for shortness of breath and weight gain.	Disopyramide can cause heart failure in a client with CAD.
		Monitor for widening QRS complex, prolonged QT or PR interval, or heart block	Toxic side effects necessitate stopping disopyramide administration.
Type IB			
Lidocaine (Xylocaine)	1-1.5 mg/kg IV bolus, then 0.5-0.75 mg/kg IV boluses q5-10min to a loading dose of 3 mg/kg, followed by 2-4 mg/min infusion For VF or pulseless VT: 1-1.5 mg/kg IV bolus q3-5min to a loading dose of 3 mg/kg, followed by 2-4 mg/min infusion	Watch for confusion, paresthesias, slurring of speech, drowsiness, or seizure activity.	CNS adverse effects predominate; they may require a decrease in dosage or discontinuation of the infusion.
Mexiletine hydrochloride (Mexitil)	200-300 mg q8h PO with food 125-250 mg IV bolus for 5-10 min 0.5-1.5 mg/min infusion	Monitor blood pressure and heart rate.	Hypotension and bradycardia may occur.
		Assess for tremors, blurred vision, dizziness, ataxia, or confusion.	CNS adverse reactions predominate.
Tocainide hydrochloride (Tonocard)	400 mg q8h PO initially 400-800 mg q8h PO Maximum of 2.4 g/day Take with food	Watch for tremors.	Tremors indicate that the maximum dose is being approached.
		Monitor heart rate and blood pressure.	Bradycardia and hypotension may occur.
		Teach the client to report shortness of breath, wheezing, chest pain, or cough, as well as dyspnea and distended neck veins or swelling of the extremities.	Pulmonary fibrosis is a serious side effect, which necessitates discontinuation of the drug; the drug may also cause CHF.
Type IC			
Flecainide acetate (Tambocor)	100 mg bid PO Maximum dose of 400 mg/day	Monitor for an increase in frequency and severity of dysrhythmias.	Flecainide can induce dysrhythmias.
		Monitor heart rate and blood pressure.	Bradycardia and hypotension may occur.
		Monitor for CHF dizziness, visual disturbances, paresthesias, and tremors.	Side effects may require a decrease in dosage or discontinuation of the drug.

VF, Ventricular fibrillation; *VT,* ventricular tachycardia; *SVT,* supraventricular tachycardia; *PSVT,* premature supraventricular tachycardia; *PEA,* pulseless electrical activity; *EMD,* electromechanical dissociation; *PVC,* premature ventricular complex; *CHF,* congestive heart failure; *CNS,* central nervous system; *CAD,* coronary artery disease; *AV,* atrioventricular; D_5W, 5% dextrose in water.

CHART 34-3

DRUG THERAPY *for* Dysrhythmias—cont'd

Drug	Usual Dosage	Nursing Interventions	Rationale
CLASS I DRUGS—cont'd			
Type IC—cont'd			
Propafenone hydrochloride (Rythmol)	150-300 mg q8h PO	Monitor for an increase in dysrhythmias.	Propafenone can induce dysrhythmias.
		Monitor heart rate and blood pressure.	Bradycardia and hypotension may occur.
		Monitor for CNS effects, dizziness, anxiety, ataxia, insomnia, confusion, and seizures, as well as CHF and gastrointestinal distress.	Side effects may require a decrease in dosage or discontinuation of the drug.
Moricizine hydrochloride (Ethmozine)	200-300 mg q8h PO	Monitor for an increase in dysrhythmias.	Drug can induce dysrhythmias.
		Monitor heart rate and blood pressure.	Bradycardia and hypotension may occur.
		Monitor for dizziness, hyperesthesias, anxiety, ataxia, insomnia, confusion, and seizures.	Side effects may require a decrease in dosage or discontinuation of the drug.
CLASS II DRUGS			
Propranolol hydrochloride (Inderal, Apo-Propranolol✱)	10-80 mg qid PO before meals 0.1 mg/kg slow IV bolus divided into 3 equal doses given at intervals of 2-3 min at rate of 1 mg/min	Monitor heart rate and blood pressure.	Bradycardia and decreased blood pressure are expected effects.
		Assess for shortness of breath or wheezing.	$Beta_2$-blocking effects on the lungs can cause bronchospasm.
		Assess for insomnia, fatigue, and dizziness.	Side effects may require decrease in dosage or discontinuation of the drug.
Acebutolol hydrochloride (Sectral)	600-1200 mg daily PO	Monitor heart rate and blood pressure.	Bradycardia and decreased blood pressure are expected effects.
		Assess for shortness of breath or wheezing.	$Beta_2$-blocking effects on the lungs can cause bronchospasm.
		Assess for insomnia, fatigue, and dizziness.	Side effects may require a decrease in dosage or discontinuation of the drug.
Esmolol hydrochloride (Brevibloc)	Initially, 500 μg/kg/min for 1 min, then 50 μg/kg/min for 4 min IV Titrate up if necessary	Monitor heart rate and blood pressure.	Bradycardia and decreased blood pressure are expected effects.
		Assess for shortness of breath or wheezing.	$Beta_2$-blocking effects on the lungs can cause bronchospasm.
		Assess for insomnia, fatigue, and seizures.	Side effects may require a decrease in dosage or discontinuation of the drug.
Sotalol hydrochloride (Betapace)	Initial dose of 80 mg bid PO Dosage may be increased every 2-3 days, if necessary, to 240-320 mg/day in 2-3 divided doses	Assess ECG rhythm for torsades de pointes and other serious new ventricular dysrhythmias.	Sotalol may have proarrhythmic effects.
		Assess for fatigue, bradycardia, dyspnea, CHF, chest pain, hypotension, dizziness, hypoglycemia, nausea, and vomiting.	Adverse reactions may warrant drug discontinuation.
		Sotalol should not be administered to clients with hypokalemia or hypomagnesemia before correction of these imbalances.	Hypokalemia or hypomagnesemia may prolong the QT interval and cause torsades de pointes.
		Sotalol is contraindicated in clients with bronchial asthma, sinus bradycardia, or second- and third-degree AV block (unless a functioning pacemaker is present), prolonged QT syndrome, cardiogenic shock, or CHF.	Sotalol has beta-blocking (class II) effects and class III effects.

Continued

CHART 34-3

DRUG THERAPY *for* Dysrhythmias—cont'd

Drug	Usual Dosage	Nursing Interventions	Rationale
CLASS III DRUGS			
Bretylium tosylate (Bretylol, Bretylate✤)	5-10 mg/kg, diluted in 50 mL IV, for 8-10 min, may repeat in 1-2 hr; maximum of 30-35 mg/kg 1-2 mg/min infusion For VF or pulseless VT: 5 mg/kg IV undiluted (IV bolus), followed by defibrillation; may give 10 mg/kg IV bolus, followed by defibrillation, and repeat q5min to maximum of 30-35 mg/kg	Observe cardiac monitor for PVCs, increased heart rate, and other dysrhythmias.	PVCs and increased heart rate commonly occur within 30 min.
		Monitor blood pressure.	Hypertension may occur in the first hour, followed by significant hypotension.
		Maintain the client in a supine position for up to 8 hr.	Orthostatic hypotension is a significant problem until tolerance to the drug develops.
		When the client begins to sit up or get out of bed, raise the head of the bed slowly and advise the client to make position changes slowly.	The client could become dizzy and faint.
		Anticipate vomiting during drug administration. Except in cardiac arrest, the drug must be diluted and given slowly.	Vomiting is a common side effect.
Amiodarone hydrochloride (Cordarone)	800-1600 mg qd PO in divided doses for 1-3 wk, then 600-800 mg qd for 1 mo, then 200-600 mg qd (average of 400 mg qd)	Administer IV dose diluted in D_5W in glass bottle; use volumetric infusion pump and PVC tubing with in-line filter and infuse via central line.	Drug is irritating to peripheral vasculature; drug is more stable in glass bottle.
	Rapid loading dose: 150 mg IV over first 10 min (15 mg/min); slow loading dose: 360 mg IV over next 6 hr (1 mg/min); maintenance infusion: 540 mg IV over next 18 hr (0.5 mg/min), then 720 mg/24 hr (0.5 mg/min)	Rapid-loading IV dose must not be administered faster than 10 min. Must stay with client and monitor heart rate and BP.	Hypotension may occur. It should be treated by slowing the infusion and other standard therapy. Cordarone should not be discontinued unless necessary.
		Continually monitor ECG rhythm during IV infusion; measure QT and QT_c.	Bradycardia and AV block may occur and are treated by slowing the infusion rate and providing pacemaker therapy, if necessary. May cause a worsening of ventricular dysrhythmias.
		Assess the client's knowledge of the treatment regimen and side effects.	Drug has major side effects, which make noncompliance a problem; clients may take the drug for 1½-3 mo before full clinical effects are apparent.
		Monitor heart rate, blood pressure, and cardiac rhythm when initiating therapy.	Bradycardia, hypotension, and worsening dysrhythmia can occur.
		Teach clients to report any muscle weakness, tremors, or difficulty with ambulation.	Muscle-related side effects usually develop during the first week of treatment.
		Teach clients to report shortness of breath, cough, pleuritic pain, or fever.	Pulmonary side effects may indicate drug induced pulmonary toxicity.
		Teach clients to report any visual disturbances and to wear sunglasses outdoors in the daytime if they have photophobia.	Corneal pigmentation occurs in most clients but generally does not interfere with vision; if it does, the dosage is decreased.
		Teach clients to use barrier sunscreens.	Photosensitivity reactions may occur.
		Teach clients to report any signs of thyroid problems or hepatotoxicity.	Thyroid problems or hepatotoxicity may occur, necessitating a decrease in dosage or discontinuation of the drug.

VF, Ventricular fibrillation; *VT,* ventricular tachycardia; *SVT,* supraventricular tachycardia; *PSVT,* premature supraventricular tachycardia; *PEA,* pulseless electrical activity; *EMD,* electromechanical dissociation; *PVC,* premature ventricular complex; *CHF,* congestive heart failure; *CNS,* central nervous system; *CAD,* coronary artery disease; *AV,* atrioventricular; D_5W, 5% dextrose in water.

CHART 34-3

DRUG THERAPY *for* Dysrhythmias—cont'd

Drug	Usual Dosage	Nursing Interventions	Rationale
CLASS III DRUGS—cont'd			
Ibutilide fumarate (Covert)	1 mg IV over 10 min for clients >60 kg; 0.01 mg/kg over 10 min for clients <60 kg May repeat dose 10 min after completion of first infusion if necessary	Stop infusion as soon as dysrhythmia is terminated, or in event of sustained or non-sustained VT, or marked prolongation of QT or QT_c.	Drug may cause potentially fatal dysrhythmias.
		Observe clients with continuous ECG monitoring and measure QT or QT_c for at least 4 hr following infusion or until QT_c has returned to baseline.	Acute ventricular dysrhythmias must be promptly identified and treated. Client may develop heart blocks.
		Clients with atrial fibrillation of >2-3 days' duration must be adequately anticoagulated for at least 2 wk.	Atrial fibrillation is associated with formation of thrombi in atrial chambers.
		Hypokalemia and hypomagnesemia must be corrected before Covert infusion.	This is important to reduce potential for proarrhythmia effects.
CLASS IV DRUGS			
Verapamil hydrochloride (Calan, Isoptin✱)	2.5-5 mg IV for 1-2 min for narrow-complex SVT or PSVT; after 15-30 min may give 5-10 mg IV for 1-2 min, if necessary, and repeat to a maximum of 20 mg 80-120 mg q6-8h PO	Monitor heart rate and blood pressure.	Bradycardia and hypotension are common side effects.
		Teach clients to remain recumbent for at least 1 hr after IV administration.	Hypotension may occur; may be reversed with calcium chloride ($CaCl_2$), 0.5-1 g slow IV.
		Teach clients to change positions slowly when receiving oral therapy.	Dizziness and orthostatic hypotension often occur until tolerance develops.
		Teach clients to report dyspnea, orthopnea, distended neck veins, or swelling of the extremities.	Heart failure may occur, necessitating a decrease in dosage or discontinuation of the drug.
Diltiazem hydrochloride (Cardizem)	0.25 mg/kg IV for 2 min After 15 min, give 0.35 mg/kg IV for 2 min 5-15 mg/hr IV infusion	Monitor heart rate and blood pressure.	Bradycardia and hypotension are common side effects.
		Teach clients to remain recumbent for at least 1 hr after IV administration.	Hypotension may occur.
		Teach clients to report dyspnea, orthopnea, distended neck veins, or swelling of the extremities.	Heart failure may occur, necessitating a decrease in dosage or discontinuation of the drug.
OTHER DRUGS			
Digoxin (Lanoxin, Novodigoxin✱)	Rapid digitalization: 0.5-1 mg PO or IV initially; 0.125-0.5 mg q6h PO or IV until a total of 1-1.5 mg is reached Maintenance: 0.125-0.25 mg qd or qod PO or IV (may be less for older adults)	Assess apical heart rate for 1 min before each dose; withhold the dose if the heart rate is less than 60 beats per min.	Decreased heart rate is an expected response, but bradycardia may indicate toxicity.
		Assess for sudden increase in heart rate and change of rhythm from regular to irregular, or irregular to regular.	Changes in heart rate or rhythm may indicate toxicity.
		Teach clients to report anorexia, nausea, vomiting, diarrhea, paresthesias, confusion, or visual disturbances.	Side effect can indicate toxicity.
		Monitor serum potassium levels.	Hypokalemia increases the risk of toxicity and ventricular dysrhythmias.
		Monitor serum creatinine levels.	Impaired renal function can cause toxicity; the dosage is altered if this occurs.

Continued

CHART 34-3

DRUG THERAPY *for* Dysrhythmias—cont'd

Drug	Usual Dosage	Nursing Interventions	Rationale
OTHER DRUGS—cont'd			
Atropine sulfate	0.5-1 mg IV bolus may be repeated q3-5min, if necessary, to a maximum of 0.04 mg/kg For asystole, PEA, or EMD: 1 mg IV bolus q3-5min, if necessary, to a total of 0.04 mg/kg	Monitor heart rate and rhythm after administration. Assess for chest pain after administration. Assess for urinary retention and dry mouth after administration. Avoid using in clients with angle-closure glaucoma	Increased heart rate is expected. Increased heart rate may cause ischemia in clients with CAD. Atropine is an anticholinergic agent. Atropine increases intraocular pressure.
Adenosine (Adenocard)	6 mg IV for 1-3 sec followed by 20-mL saline flush; may repeat in 1-2 min, if necessary, at 12 mg IV for 1-3 sec with 20-mL flush; may repeat 12 mg IV after 1-2 min if necessary	Monitor heart rate and rhythm after administration. Assess clients for facial flushing, shortness of breath, dyspnea, and chest pain. Assess clients for recurrence of PSVT or ventricular ectopy.	A short period of asystole is common after administration; bradycardia and hypotension may occur. These side effects commonly occur. Recurrence of PSVT is common; PVCs may occur.
Magnesium sulfate	1-2 g diluted in 100 mL of D_5W administered for 1-2 min for VF or VT 1-2 g in 50-100 mL of D_5W for 5-60 min for loading dose; 0.5-1 g/hr for 24 hr for supplementation	Assess ECG rhythm for conversion to sinus rhythm. Assess clients for facial flushing, hypotension, and respiratory and CNS depression.	Hypomagnesemia may precipitate refractory VF. Magnesium sulfate causes vasodilation and respiratory and CNS depression.

VF, Ventricular fibrillation; *VT,* ventricular tachycardia; *SVT,* supraventricular tachycardia; *PSVT,* premature supraventricular tachycardia; *PEA,* pulseless electrical activity; *EMD,* electromechanical dissociation; *PVC,* premature ventricular complex; *CHF,* congestive heart failure; *CNS,* central nervous system; *CAD,* coronary artery disease; *AV,* atrioventricular; D_5W, 5% dextrose in water.

CRITICAL THINKING CHALLENGE

A 29-year-old woman enters the emergency department with sudden onset of palpitations, shortness of breath, and syncope. Her past medical history includes anemia and mitral valve disease. She smokes approximately 2 packs of cigarettes a day, and she states that she has been recently divorced and is the sole caretaker of her two young children. Her vital signs are as follows: heart rate, 162; respirations, 32; and blood pressure, 92/50. She is pale, diaphoretic, and very anxious.

- What other assessment data do you need to obtain?
- What dysrhythmias should you assess for and why?
- What treatments might you anticipate that the physician will order?
- What health teaching could you provide?

For suggested answer guidelines, go to SIMON http://www.wbsaunders.com/SIMON/Iggy/.

ATRIAL FLUTTER

PATHOPHYSIOLOGY. **Atrial flutter** is rapid atrial depolarization occurring at a rate of 250 to 350 times per minute. The most common rate is approximately 300 times per minute. An atrioventricular (AV) node blocks the number of impulses that reach the ventricles as a protective mechanism (Figure 34-11, *A*). When untreated, atrial flutter results in a 2:1 block (Figure 34-11, *B*). In general, when the ventricular rate is 150 beats/min, the nurse should suspect atrial flutter with 2:1 block and carefully scrutinize the electrocardiographic (ECG) baseline for evidence of atrial flutter waves.

ETIOLOGY. Atrial flutter may be caused by rheumatic or ischemic heart disease, congestive heart failure, AV valve disease, pre-excitation syndromes, septal defects, pulmonary emboli, thyrotoxicosis, alcoholism, or pericarditis. The dysrhythmia commonly occurs after cardiac surgery.

PHYSICAL ASSESSMENT/CLINICAL MANIFESTATIONS. The clinical manifestations depend on the rate of ventricular response. The nurse assesses the client for palpitations, weakness, fatigue, shortness of breath, nervousness, anxiety, syncope, angina, and evidence of heart failure and shock. Carotid sinus massage transiently decreases the ventricular rate to facilitate rhythm interpretation but can be performed only by the physician. The client with a normal ventricular rate is usually asymptomatic.

INTERVENTIONS. The treatment goals are the same as those for supraventricular tachycardia (SVT). The nurse administers oxygen and prescribed drugs such as ibutilide (Covert), amiodarone (Cordarone), diltiazem (Cardizem), and verapamil (Calan, Isoptin) to slow the rapid ventricular response. Quinidine or procainamide (Pronestyl) must not be administered unless one of the above agents has slowed the ventricular response. Both drugs slow the atrial rate and may increase AV conduction, which could cause a 1:1 conduction with an increase in ventricular rate and hemodynamic deterioration.

The nurse helps the physician to attempt rapid atrial overdrive pacing or to achieve cardioversion if the client is hemodynamically compromised. If he or she fails to respond to these therapies, radiofrequency catheter ablation may be necessary.

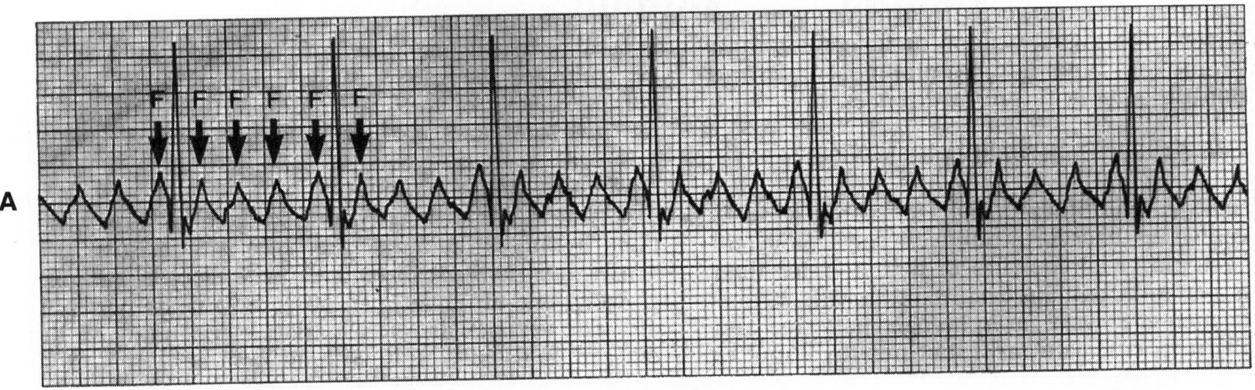

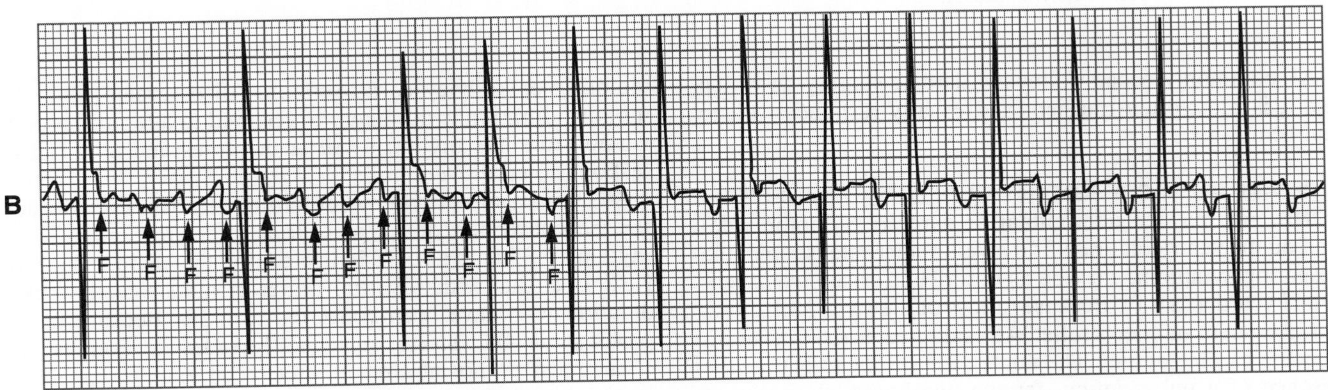

Figure 34-11 ● Atrial dysrhythmias. **A,** Atrial flutter *(F)* with 4:1 block. The atrial rate is 280 beats/min; the ventricular rate is 70 beats/min. **B,** Atrial flutter with 4:1 conduction, then an 11-beat run with 2:1 conduction.

ATRIAL FIBRILLATION

PATHOPHYSIOLOGY. **Atrial fibrillation (AF)** is the most common dysrhythmia in the United States. Long-range epidemiologic studies, such as the Framingham Heart Study, show a dramatic incidence of AF in the aging population. In fact, the incidence of AF increases more than 20 times between middle age (55 to 64 years of age) and older adulthood (85 to 94 years of age). It is estimated that millions of cases of intermittent or sustained AF occur each year in the United States (see the Cost of Care box at right). AF causes increased morbidity and mortality among those who experience it (Resnick, 1999).

Multiple, rapid impulses from many atrial foci, at a rate of 350 to 600 times per minute, depolarize the atria in a totally disorganized manner. The result is chaos, with no P waves, no atrial contractions, loss of the atrial kick, and an irregular ventricular response (Figure 34-12). The atria merely quiver in fibrillation (commonly called "A fib"), which may lead to the formation of mural thrombi (within the cardiac chambers) and potential embolic events.

ETIOLOGY. AF occurs most commonly in clients with systemic hypertension and is frequently seen in older adults (Resnick, 1999). It may also occur in clients with the following conditions:

- Myocardial infarction
- Rheumatic heart disease with mitral stenosis
- Atrial septal defect
- Congestive heart failure
- Cardiomyopathy
- Hyperthyroidism
- Pulmonary emboli
- Wolff-Parkinson-White (WPW) syndrome
- Congenital heart disease
- Chronic constrictive pericarditis

COST OF CARE IMPLICATIONS FOR NURSING

ATRIAL FIBRILLATION

Cost of Care

- The costs associated with the treatment of atrial fibrillation (AF) are enormous. Clients with AF make up the largest group of those hospitalized with *any* dysrhythmia, including all of the life-threatening ventricular dysrhythmias combined.
- Hospital stays for AF are the longest of any hospitalizations wherein the principal diagnosis is a dysrhythmia.
- Economists estimate the annual cost of treating AF at a staggering 1 billion dollars.

Implications for Nursing

- Prevention of AF must be a priority; health promotion, especially for the older adult, is essential, and health teaching must target the components of treatment in a clear and concise manner that is accessible to all.
- Evaluations of any older adult should include assessment for AF.
- Once AF is identified, restoration of normal sinus rhythm is crucial to prevent strokes and improve quality of life.

Data from Resnick, B. (1999). Atrial fibrillation in the older adult: Presentation and management issues. *Geriatric Nursing, 20* (4), 188-194.

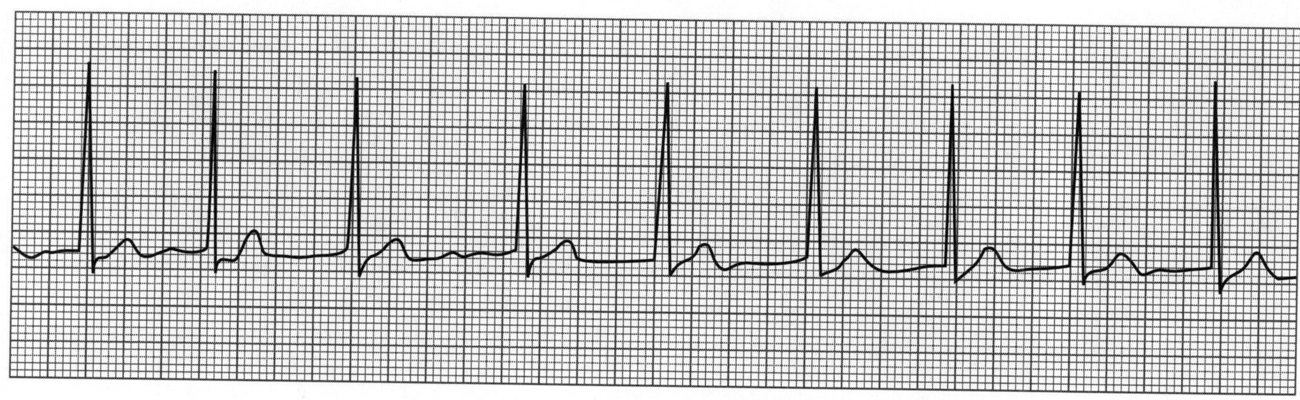

Figure 34-12 ● Atrial dysrhythmias. Atrial fibrillation, controlled, with a ventricular rate of approximately 80 beats/min.

AF commonly occurs following cardiac surgery, in which case it is most often transient and usually responds well to treatment.

PHYSICAL ASSESSMENT/CLINICAL MANIFESTATIONS. AF may be intermittent or chronic. Symptoms depend on the ventricular rate. If the ventricular rate is rapid, the presenting symptoms may be as described for supraventricular tachycardia (SVT). Because of loss of the atrial kick, however, the client in uncontrolled AF is at greater risk for an inadequate cardiac output. The nurse assesses the client for the presence of a pulse deficit, fatigue, weakness, shortness of breath, distended neck veins, dizziness, decreased exercise tolerance, anxiety, syncope, palpitations, chest discomfort or pain, and hypotension.

The client is also at risk for pulmonary embolism. Thrombi may accumulate within the right atrium and be transported through the right ventricle to the lungs. The nurse should assess for shortness of breath, chest pain, hemoptysis, and a feeling of impending doom.

In addition, the client is at risk for systemic emboli, particularly an embolic stroke, which may cause severe neurologic impairment or death. Because approximately one third of clients with AF have thromboemboli, the nurse must be astute in assessing the client for evidence of embolic events. Changes in mentation, speech, sensory function, and motor function are particularly noted. The nurse also assesses pulses, urine output, back pain, and complaints of gastrointestinal (GI) disturbances. Any of these symptoms should be reported to the health care provider immediately. Clients with AF who have valvular disease are particularly at risk for thromboemboli.

INTERVENTIONS. Treatment is the same as for atrial flutter. In addition, the nurse may administer anticoagulants, such as heparin, enoxaparin (Lovenox), and sodium warfarin, as prescribed by the physician for clients considered to be at high risk for emboli. Before elective cardioversion, the nurse must initiate anticoagulation therapy for 4 to 5 weeks as prescribed to prevent a thromboembolic event if the rhythm is successfully converted. To assess for the presence of atrial clots, a contraindication for cardioversion in the compromised client, the physician may order a transesophageal echocardiogram (TEE) before attempting emergency cardioversion. AF of greater than 12 months' duration is not likely to respond to attempts at conversion to sinus rhythm by drug therapies and may fail to respond to cardioversion.

A class III antiarrhythmic, dofetilide (Tikosyn) is indicated for the conversion of AF and atrial flutter to normal sinus rhythm (NSR). It also is indicated for the maintenance of NSR in clients with AF/atrial flutter of more than 1 weeks' duration who have been converted to NSR. Because it can prolong the QT interval, causing Torsades de Pointes, the client must be hospitalized for telemetry monitoring for at least 3 days during the initiation of therapy. In addition to cardiac rhythm and QT interval monitoring, the dose of Tikosyn must be adjusted to creatine clearance levels.

Clients with recurring, symptomatic AF resistant to medical therapies may be treated with radiofrequency catheter ablation to the His bundle to interrupt all conduction between the atria and the ventricles. However, this requires implantation of a permanent ventricular pacemaker and does not stop the atria from fibrillating. The atrial kick is not restored, and clients remain at risk for embolic events.

Clients may benefit from the "maze" procedure, an open heart surgical technique. In this procedure the nurse first prepares the client for electrophysiologic mapping studies for confirmation of the diagnosis of AF. The nurse then prepares him or her for surgery. The surgeon places a maze of sutures in strategic places in the atrial myocardium to prevent electrical circuits from developing and perpetuating AF. Sinus impulses can then depolarize the atria before reaching the AV node and preserve the atrial kick. Postoperative care is similar to that after other open heart surgical procedures (see Chapter 38).

JUNCTIONAL DYSRHYTHMIAS

Nodal cells in the atrioventricular (AV) junctional area can generate electrical impulses and are therefore secondary or latent pacemaker cells. They have a slower rate of discharge, usually 40 to 60 beats/min, and are usually suppressed. Occasionally, these cells do generate impulses as an escape pacemaker when the sinus node is excessively slow, or the cells may do so inappropriately as irritable rhythms. These rhythms are most commonly transient, and clients usually remain hemodynamically stable.

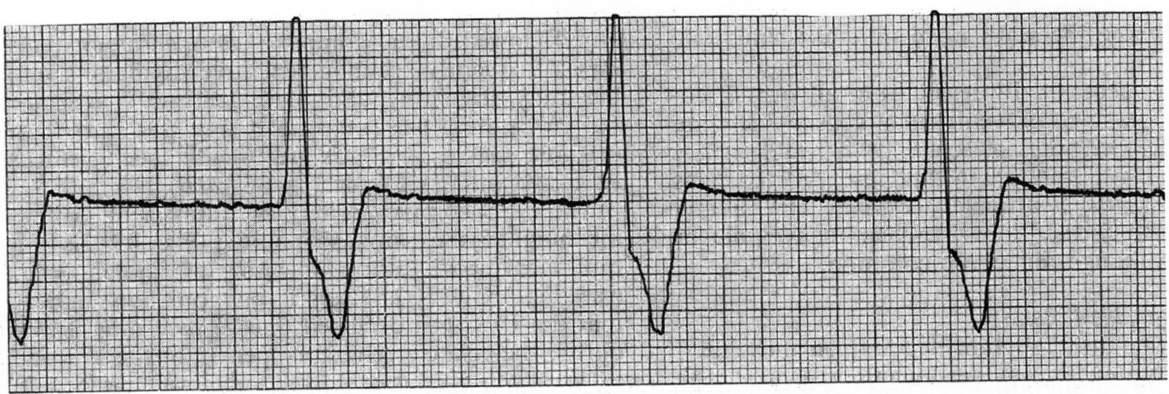

Figure 34-13 ● Idioventricular rhythm with a rate of 35 beats/min.

VENTRICULAR DYSRHYTHMIAS

The ventricles have the fewest number of nodal cells and are the slowest secondary pacemaker, generally being usurped by faster, higher pacemakers. However, irritable ventricular cells may generate electrical impulses and fire prematurely. Because the impulse originates in and depolarizes one ventricle first, then spreads to depolarize the other, the resultant QRS complex is wide, usually measuring greater than 0.12 second. The QRS complex is bizarre or odd in shape, looking different from the normal QRS complexes. The repolarization sequence is also different, so that the T wave is large and occurs in a direction opposite to the largest deflection of the QRS complex. The impulse most commonly is blocked in the AV node and cannot proceed further with retrograde conduction, so that the atria and the sinoatrial (SA) node are usually not affected by the ventricular impulse. The atrial rhythm typically remains regular, unless the underlying rhythm is sinus arrhythmia.

IDIOVENTRICULAR RHYTHM (VENTRICULAR ESCAPE RHYTHM)

PATHOPHYSIOLOGY. During idioventricular rhythm (ventricular escape rhythm), the ventricular nodal cells pace the ventricles. Because their inherent rate of firing is slow, the rate is usually less than 40 beats/min (Figure 34-13). If P waves are seen, they are independent of the QRS complexes and not related (AV dissociation).

ETIOLOGY. Idioventricular rhythm is seen as a rhythm in the dying heart, where downward displacement of the pacemaker has occurred. It is sometimes referred to as an "agonal" rhythm. Pulseless electrical activity (PEA) is characterized by no palpable pulse and therefore no perfusion, although electrical activity is displayed on the monitor. The most common causes of PEA are hypovolemia, hypoxia, and cardiac tamponade.

PHYSICAL ASSESSMENT/CLINICAL MANIFESTATIONS. Because idioventricular pacemakers are unstable, unreliable, and slow, the client is hypotensive and in shock or, most typically, is pulseless and therefore in cardiac arrest. The nurse assesses the client's airway, breathing, circulation, level of consciousness, and pupillary response.

INTERVENTIONS. Usually, idioventricular rhythms require immediate resuscitation measures, unless there is a do-not-resuscitate (DNR) order. The nurse initiates cardiopulmonary resuscitation (CPR) and summons assistance. The team may initiate advanced cardiac life support (ACLS) measures, including epinephrine administration, intravascular volume replacement, and other measures. The physician may attempt pacemaker therapy or discontinue resuscitation efforts.

PREMATURE VENTRICULAR COMPLEXES

PATHOPHYSIOLOGY. Premature ventricular complexes (PVCs), also called ventricular premature beats (VPBs), result from increased irritability of ventricular cells. PVCs are early ventricular complexes, followed by a pause. When multiple PVCs are present, the QRS complexes may be unifocal or uniform, meaning that they are of the same shape (Figure 34-14, *A*), or multifocal or multiform, meaning that they are of different shapes (Figure 34-14, *B*). PVCs frequently occur in repetitive rhythms, such as bigeminy, trigeminy, and quadrigeminy. Two sequential PVCs are a pair, or couplet. Three or more successive PVCs are usually called nonsustained ventricular tachycardia (NSVT) (Figure 34-14, *C*).

ETIOLOGY. PVCs are common, and their frequency increases with age. PVCs may be insignificant or may occur with myocardial ischemia or infarction, ccngestive heart failure, chronic hypoxemia, chronic airway limitation (CAL), anemia, hypokalemia, or hypomagnesemia. The administration of catecholamines, sympathomimetic drugs, and digitalis, as well as acidosis, anesthesia, stress, nicotine intake, ingestion of caffeine and alcohol, infection, trauma, or surgery, can also cause PVCs.

PHYSICAL ASSESSMENT/CLINICAL MANIFESTATIONS. The client may be asymptomatic or may experience palpitations or chest discomfort caused by increased stroke volume of the normal beat after the pause. Peripheral pulses may be diminished or absent with the PVCs themselves because the decreased stroke volume of the premature beats may decrease peripheral perfusion. Since other rhythms also cause widened QRS complexes, it is essential that the nurse assess whether the premature complexes perfuse. This is done by palpating the carotid, brachial, or femoral arteries while observing the monitor for widened complexes, or auscultating for the apical heart sounds. With acute myocardial infarction, PVCs may be considered warning dysrhythmias, possibly heralding the onset of ventricular tachycardia (VT) or ven-

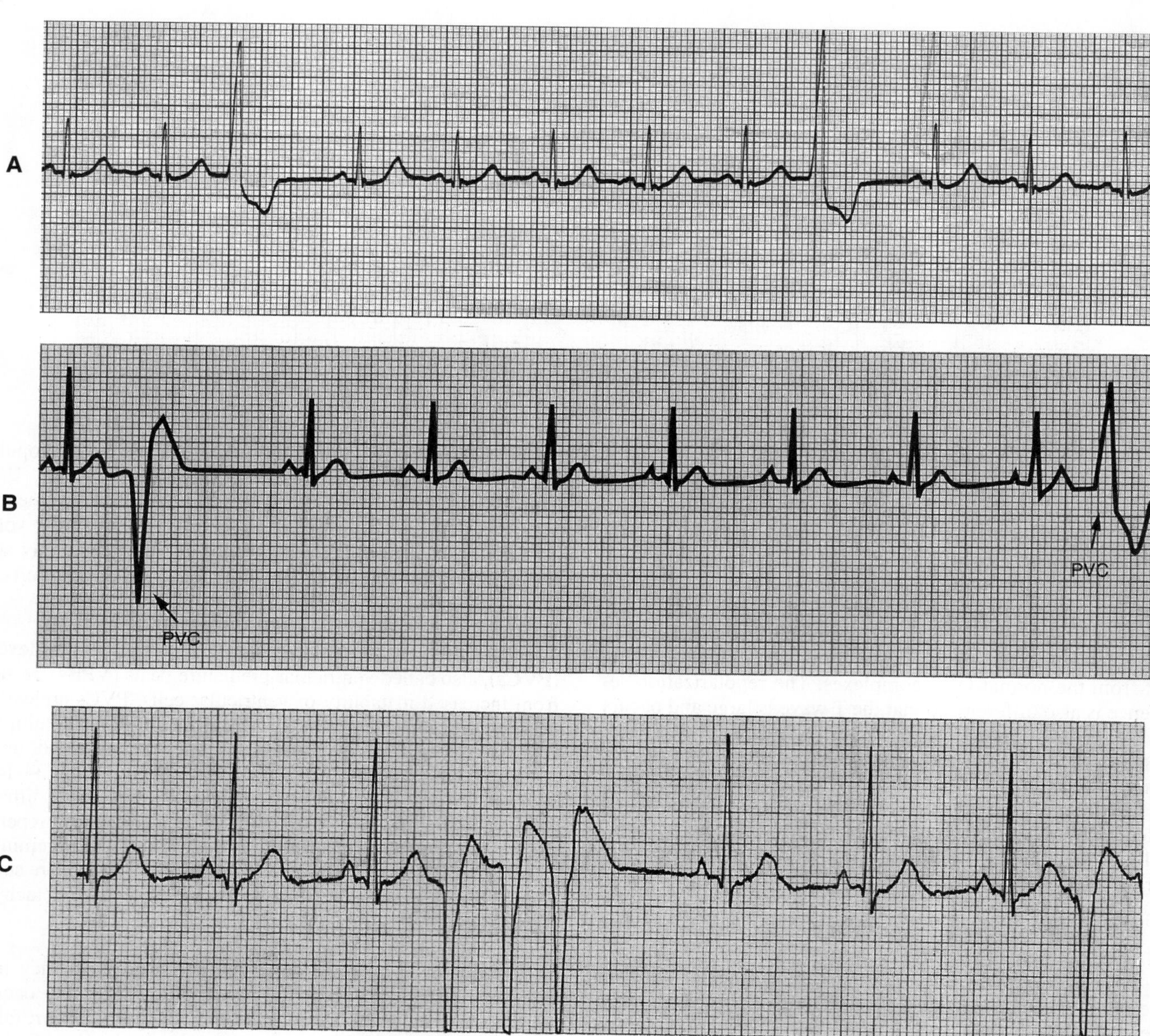

Figure 34-14 ● Ventricular dysrhythmias. **A,** Normal sinus rhythm with unifocal premature ventricular complexes (PVCs). **B,** Normal sinus rhythm with multifocal PVCs (one negative and the other positive). **C,** Normal sinus rhythm with three consecutive PVCs (nonsustained ventricular tachycardia) and another unifocal PVC.

tricular fibrillation (VF). For a client with chest discomfort or pain, the nurse reports to the physician whether PVCs increase in frequency, are multiform, are R-on-T phenomena, or occur in runs of VT.

INTERVENTIONS. If there is no underlying heart disease, PVCs are not usually treated other than by eliminating any contributing cause (e.g., caffeine, stress). With acute myocardial ischemia or infarction, the nurse treats significant PVCs by administering oxygen and lidocaine as prescribed. The nurse may administer other drugs as ordered, including procainamide (Pronestyl), bretylium (Bretylol, Bretylate✦), magnesium sulfate, propranolol (Inderal, Apo-Propranolol✦), quinidine, and mexiletine (Mexitil) (see Chart 34-3). Potassium is administered as ordered for replacement therapy if hypokalemia is the cause.

CRITICAL THINKING CHALLENGE

Your 77-year-old client has been recovering without complications from an acute anterior wall myocardial infarction, which occurred 3 days ago. He was transferred from the coronary care unit (CCU) today and has been walking in the hall, has been visiting with family, and has just returned from the cardiac rehabilitation center. The ECG monitor technician notifies you that the client has an increase in PVCs. You assess him as follows: heart rate, 92 and irregular; respirations, 24; and blood pressure, 112/60. He has no complaints of chest pain or shortness of breath.

- What are the possible causes of his increase in PVCs?
- Should you notify his physician?
- What are your treatment priorities?

For suggested answer guidelines, go to SIMON http://www.wbsaunders.com/SIMON/Iggy/.

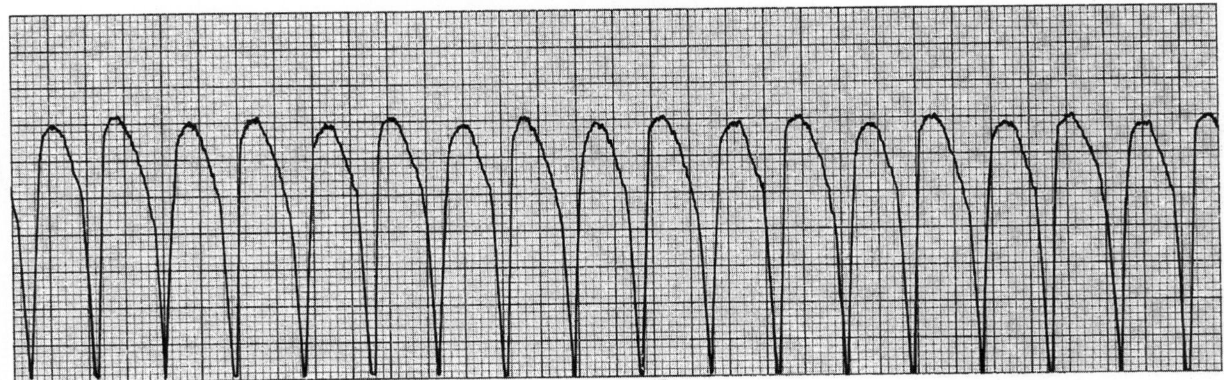

Figure 34-15 ● Ventricular dysrhythmias. Sustained ventricular tachycardia at a rate of 166 beats/min.

VENTRICULAR TACHYCARDIA

PATHOPHYSIOLOGY. Ventricular tachycardia (VT), sometimes referred to as "V tach," occurs with repetitive firing of an irritable ventricular ectopic focus, usually at a rate of 140 to 180 beats/min or more (Figure 34-15). VT may result from increased automaticity or a re-entry mechanism. VT may be intermittent, as in three or more self-limiting beats (nonsustained VT), or sustained, lasting longer than 15 to 30 seconds. The sinus node continues to discharge independently, depolarizing the atria but not the ventricles (atrioventricular [AV] dissociation), although P waves are seldom seen in sustained VT.

ETIOLOGY. VT may occur in clients with ischemic heart disease, myocardial infarction, cardiomyopathy, hypokalemia, hypomagnesemia, valvular heart disease, heart failure, drug toxicity, hypotension, or ventricular aneurysm. In clients who go into cardiac arrest, VT is commonly the initial rhythm before deterioration into ventricular fibrillation (VF) as the terminal rhythm. VT is not common in infants and children unless they have cardiac disease.

PHYSICAL ASSESSMENT/CLINICAL MANIFESTATIONS. Clinical manifestations of sustained VT partially depend on the ventricular rate. Slower rates are better tolerated. Clients may be hemodynamically compromised if the cardiac output decreases because of the shortened ventricular filling time and loss of the atrial kick. In some clients, VT causes cardiac arrest. The nurse assesses the client's airway, breathing, circulation, level of consciousness, and pupillary response.

INTERVENTIONS. For the stable client with sustained VT, the nurse administers oxygen and confirms the rhythm via a 12-lead electrocardiogram (ECG). Amiodarone, procainamide, or magnesium sulfate may be given. Lidocaine, a long-established antidysrhythmic, has not been recommended for prophylaxis of ventricular dysrhythmias in acute myocardial infarction. Current advanced cardiac life support (ACLS) guidelines state that elective cardioversion is highly recommended for stable VT. Bretylium has been dropped from ACLS algorithms because of a severe shortage of the world's natural sources of bretylium.

The physician may prescribe an oral antidysrhythmic agent, such as procainamide (Procan SR), mexiletine (Mexitil), or sotalol (Betapace, Sotacor🍁).

CHART 34-4

BEST PRACTICE *for*
Care of Unstable Ventricular Tachycardia

- Assist the physician with cardioversion.
- Provide oxygen and antidysrhythmic drugs as ordered.
- Teach the client how to perform cough cardiopulmonary resuscitation (CPR), if ordered.
- Assist with or provide defibrillation (if you are certified in advanced cardiac life support [ACLS]).
- Initiate CPR if the client does not respond to the above measures.
- Maintain a patent airway at all times. Administer oxygen.
- Monitor the client for premature ventricular complexes (PVCs) and the recurrence of ventricular tachycardia (VT).
- Assess for signs and symptoms of myocardial infarction, hypokalemia, or hypomagnesemia.

For the client with unstable VT, the nurse assists the physician in attempting emergency cardioversion followed by oxygen and antidysrhythmic therapy (Chart 34-4). The nurse may instruct the client to perform cough cardiopulmonary resuscitation (CPR) if prescribed, telling him or her to inhale deeply and cough hard every 1 to 3 seconds. Cough CPR is sometimes successful in either terminating the VT or at least briefly sustaining cerebral and coronary perfusion until other measures can be initiated. The physician may attempt rapid atrial or ventricular overdrive pacing if the VT is related to a significant bradydysrhythmia.

A precordial thump is sometimes successful in terminating VT, at least transiently. The physician or the ACLS-qualified nurse may administer a precordial thump to a client with unstable VT only if a defibrillator and pacemaker are immediately available.

With pulseless VT, the physician or ACLS-qualified nurse or other health care provider must *immediately* defibrillate the client or initiate CPR and defibrillate as soon as possible. A precordial thump may be administered initially, although it is frequently not successful in terminating VT. If the client remains pulseless, the nurse or other health care provider must resume CPR and full resuscitative measures following defibrillation. This includes airway management and administration of oxygen, epinephrine, and antidysrhythmic therapy with amiodarone, magnesium sulfate, and procainamide.

If the rhythm has been successfully converted, attention is given to treating reversible causes of VT, such as myocardial

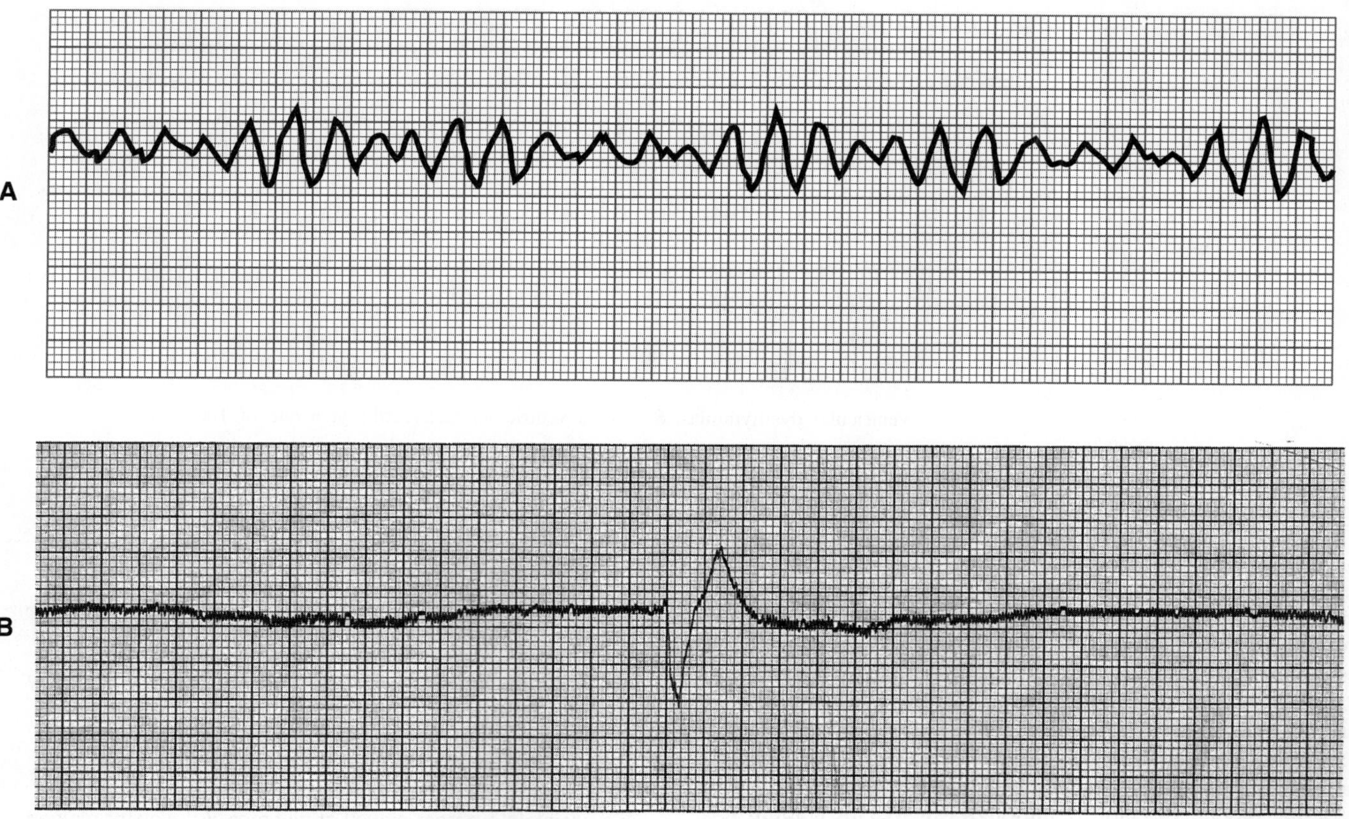

Figure 34-16 ● Ventricular dysrhythmias. **A,** Coarse ventricular fibrillation. **B,** Ventricular asystole with one idioventricular complex.

ischemia, hypokalemia, and hypomagnesemia. The nurse ensures that oxygen therapy and antidysrhythmic agent administration are continued, and the client is closely monitored for premature ventricular complexes (PVCs) and the recurrence of VT. The client with recurrent, medically refractory VT should be studied in the electrophysiology laboratory and may benefit from radiofrequency catheter ablation. Some forms of VT may require surgical intervention, such as coronary artery bypass graft (CABG) surgery, implantation of a cardioverter/defibrillator, aneurysmectomy, encircling endocardial ventriculotomy, cryosurgery, or endocardial resection (see Chapter 38).

VENTRICULAR FIBRILLATION

PATHOPHYSIOLOGY. Ventricular fibrillation (VF), sometimes called "V fib," is the result of electrical chaos in the ventricles. Impulses from many irritable foci fire in a totally disorganized manner so that ventricular contraction cannot occur. There are no recognizable deflections. Instead, there are irregular undulations of varying amplitudes, from coarse to fine (Figure 34-16, *A*). The ventricles merely quiver, consuming a tremendous amount of oxygen. There is no cardiac output and therefore no cerebral, myocardial, or systemic perfusion. This rhythm is *rapidly fatal* if not successfully terminated within 3 to 5 minutes.

ETIOLOGY. VF may be the first manifestation of coronary artery disease (CAD). Clients with myocardial infarction are at great risk for VF. VF may also occur in clients with myocardial ischemia, hypokalemia, hypomagnesemia, hemorrhage, antidysrhythmic therapy, rapid supraventricular tachydysrhythmias, shock, asynchronous pacing with competition, or severe metabolic disease. VF also occurs following surgery or trauma.

PHYSICAL ASSESSMENT/CLINICAL MANIFESTATIONS. On initiation of VF, the client becomes faint, immediately loses consciousness, and becomes pulseless and apneic. There is no blood pressure, and heart sounds are absent. Respiratory and metabolic acidosis develop. Seizures may occur. Within minutes, the pupils become fixed and dilated, and the skin becomes cold and mottled. Death ensues without prompt restoration of an organized rhythm and cardiac output.

INTERVENTIONS. The goals of treatment are to terminate VF promptly and convert it to an organized rhythm. The physician or the ACLS nurse or other health care provider must immediately defibrillate the client to accomplish this goal. This is the management priority, and the ACLS algorithm for VF must be followed. If a defibrillator is not readily available, a precordial thump may be delivered. CPR must be continued until the defibrillator arrives.

If the VF does not terminate after three rapid successive shocks of increasing energy, the nurse and resuscitation team resume CPR and provide airway management. They also administer oxygen and antidysrhythmic therapy with epinephrine, amiodarone, procainamide (Pronestyl), lidocaine, and magnesium sulfate, along with attempting defibrillation frequently. If VF is successfully converted to an organized rhythm, the nurse continues supportive therapy and assists the physician in treating potential causes of VF and preventing its recurrence.

CRITICAL THINKING CHALLENGE

You find a middle-aged client pulseless and without respiration on the floor of the bathroom.

- What should you do first?
- What actions will the cardiac arrest team take?
- What are the steps for safe defibrillation?

For suggested answer guidelines, go to SIMON http://www.wbsaunders.com/SIMON/Iggy/.

VENTRICULAR ASYSTOLE

PATHOPHYSIOLOGY. Ventricular asystole, sometimes called *ventricular standstill,* is the complete absence of any ventricular rhythm (Figure 34-16, *B*). There are no electrical impulses in the ventricles and therefore *no* ventricular depolarization, no QRS complex, no contraction, no cardiac output, and no pulse, respirations, or blood pressure. The client is in full cardiac arrest. The sinoatrial (SA) node, in some cases, may continue to fire and depolarize the atria, with only P waves seen on the electrocardiogram (ECG), but the sinus impulses do not conduct to the ventricles, and QRS complexes remain absent. In most cases, the entire conduction system is electrically silent, with no P waves seen on the ECG. There is only a mildly undulating line on the ECG. Fine ventricular fibrillation (VF) may resemble asystole in some leads. Because treatment of these two rhythms differs significantly, the nurse must assess two ECG leads for an accurate rhythm interpretation.

ETIOLOGY. Ventricular asystole usually results from myocardial hypoxia, which may be a consequence of advanced heart failure. It may also be caused by severe hyperkalemia and acidosis. If P waves are seen, asystole is likely because of severe ventricular conduction blocks. Rarely, excessive vagal stimulation may cause asystole.

PHYSICAL ASSESSMENT/CLINICAL MANIFESTATIONS. Clients are in full cardiac arrest with loss of consciousness and absence of pulse, respirations, and blood pressure. Ventricular asystole is often unresponsive to resuscitation measures and fatal.

INTERVENTIONS. The goal of treatment is to restore cardiac electrical activity. The nurse or other health care provider initiates CPR immediately and summons assistance. Another ECG lead is assessed to ensure that the rhythm is asystole and not fine VF, which warrants immediate defibrillation. When in doubt, the client should be defibrillated. The nurse and resuscitation team manage the airway and administer oxygen, epinephrine, and atropine. The nurse assists the physician with the initiation of noninvasive pacing or invasive transvenous or epicardial pacing, although pacemaker therapy is generally not effective. An isoproterenol infusion may also be tried. The prognosis for clients with asystole is poor.

ATRIOVENTRICULAR BLOCKS

Atrioventricular (AV) blocks exist when supraventricular impulses are excessively delayed or totally blocked in the AV node or intraventricular conduction system. Conduction may be transiently or permanently abnormal for a number of reasons. The SA node continues to function normally, and atrial depolarizations and P waves occur regularly. Because of the conduction dysfunction, ventricular depolarizations and QRS complexes are either delayed or blocked.

There are different degrees of heart blocks, as follows:

- In *first-degree* AV block, all sinus impulses eventually reach the ventricles.
- In *second-degree* heart block, some sinus impulses reach the ventricles, but others do not because they are blocked.
- In *third-degree* heart block (complete heart block), none of the sinus impulses reach the ventricles. The ventricles, therefore, are depolarized by a second, independent pacemaker.

AV blocks are differentiated by their PR intervals.

FIRST-DEGREE ATRIOVENTRICULAR BLOCK

PATHOPHYSIOLOGY. First-degree AV block is actually a conduction delay rather than a block. AV node conduction is slow, prolonging the PR interval to greater than 0.20 second. However, all sinus impulses eventually reach the ventricles. The underlying rhythm must still be identified (e.g., sinus rhythm with first-degree AV block) (Figure 34-17, *A*).

ETIOLOGY. First-degree AV block may be due to AV nodal ischemia from occlusion of the right coronary artery, as with an inferior or posterior myocardial infarction. It may also result from hypokalemia or hyperkalemia; the administration of digitalis, beta-adrenergic blockers, calcium channel blockers, or narcotics; excessive vagal stimulation; or degenerative AV nodal disease. It may also occur following cardiac surgery as a result of edema in the AV nodal area and usually resolves without treatment.

PHYSICAL ASSESSMENT/CLINICAL MANIFESTATIONS. First-degree AV block has no hemodynamic consequences and produces no symptoms. Any symptoms are the result of the underlying rhythm (e.g., sinus bradycardia). First-degree AV block may be insignificant and transient or may progress to more severe AV blocks.

INTERVENTIONS. In the stable client, no treatment is needed. If the PR interval is particularly long or is getting progressively longer, the nurse must notify the physician. If the first-degree AV block is due to drug therapy, the nurse must withhold the offending drug and notify the physician. When first-degree AV block is associated with symptomatic bradycardia, oxygen and atropine are administered as prescribed to accelerate AV conduction.

SECOND-DEGREE ATRIOVENTRICULAR BLOCK TYPE I (ATRIOVENTRICULAR WENCKEBACH OR MOBITZ TYPE I)

PATHOPHYSIOLOGY. In second-degree AV block type I, each successive sinus impulse takes a little longer to conduct through the impaired AV node, until one impulse is completely blocked and fails to depolarize the ventricles. This block results in a nonconducted or dropped beat (missing QRS complex). There is progressive prolongation of the PR interval, followed by a dropped beat and a pause (a character-

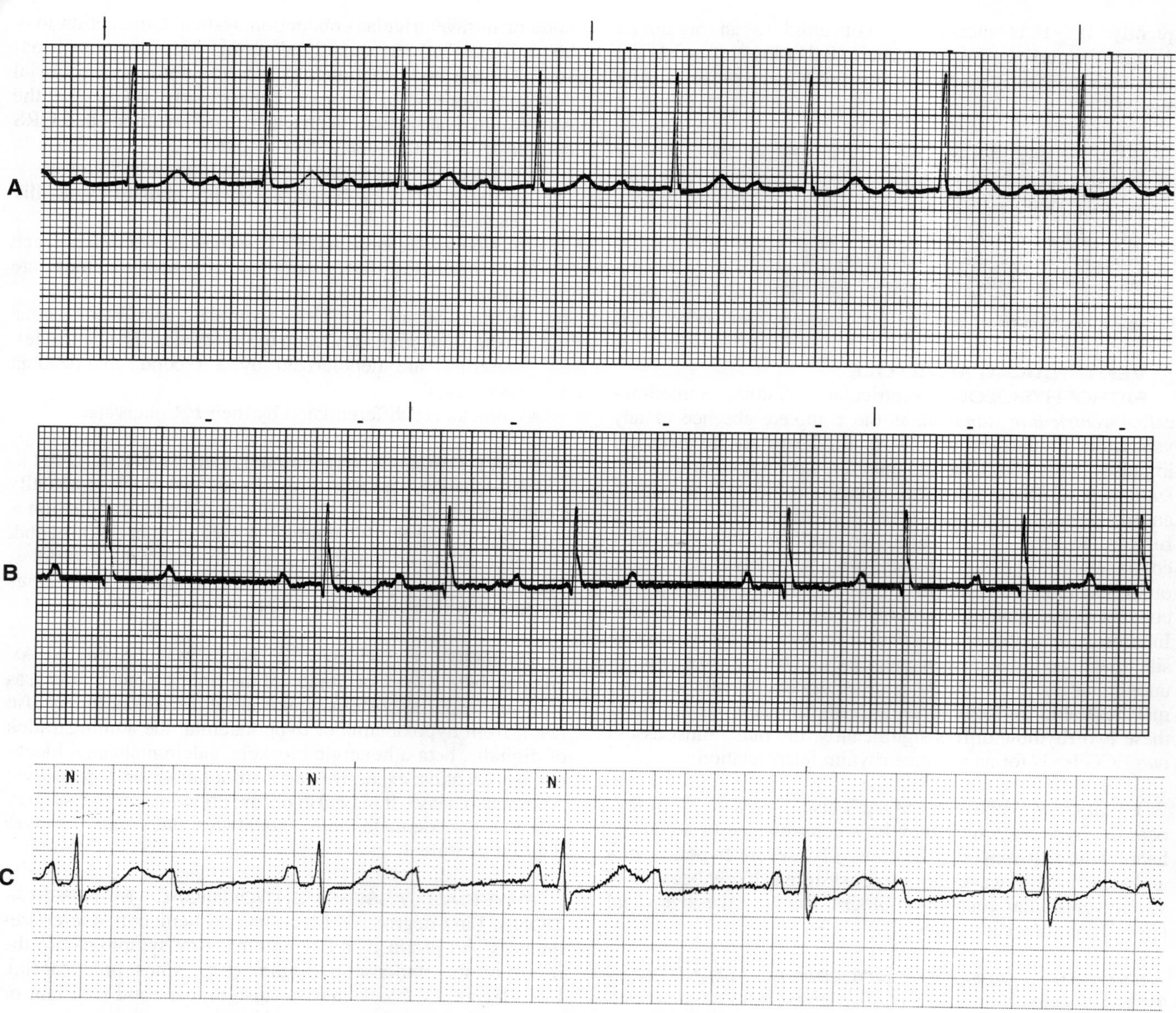

Figure 34-17 ● Atrioventricular (AV) blocks. **A,** Normal sinus rhythm with first-degree AV block (PR interval, 0.36 second). **B,** Second-degree AV block type I (Wenckebach AV) with an irregular rhythm, grouped beating, and progressive prolongation of the PR interval until a P wave is completely blocked and not followed by a QRS complex. **C,** Second-degree AV block type II (Mobitz II) with 2:1 conduction, a constant PR interval, and wide QRS complex.

istic feature of this rhythm). The pause allows sufficient time for the AV node to recover so that the next beat is conducted with a shorter PR interval and the Wenckebach sequence is repeated. Although the atrial rhythm is usually regular, the ventricular rhythm is irregular, with an appearance of grouped beats separated by pauses. Group size (conduction ratios) may be constant or may vary. Because of the dropped QRS complex, each group normally has one more P wave than QRS complexes (Figure 34-17, *B*).

ETIOLOGY. The causes of AV Wenckebach block are the same as for first-degree AV block. It is often a transient rhythm and may revert to first-degree AV block or even a normal sinus rhythm (NSR). However, Mobitz I may progress to third-degree or complete heart block. Second-degree AV block type I is also seen with rheumatic fever and digitalis administration.

PHYSICAL ASSESSMENT/CLINICAL MANIFESTATIONS. The client is usually asymptomatic if the frequency of dropped beats and the overall ventricular rate do not decrease the cardiac output. If the ventricular rate is too slow, decreasing the cardiac output, the client will have symptoms of a symptomatic bradydysrhythmia. This rhythm is usually transient and terminates spontaneously.

INTERVENTIONS. No intervention is required in the stable client, because this rhythm rarely progresses to a more severe block. In the symptomatic client, the nurse administers oxygen and atropine as prescribed. If atropine is not successful in speeding AV nodal conduction time and increasing the heart rate, the nurse initiates pacemaker therapy as ordered and notifies the physician.

SECOND-DEGREE HEART BLOCK TYPE II (MOBITZ TYPE II)

PATHOPHYSIOLOGY. In Mobitz type II block, the block is actually infranodal, occurring below the His bundle. It involves a constant block in one of the bundle branches, resulting in a wide QRS complex in conducted beats and an intermittent block in the other bundle branch, resulting in dropped beats because both bundles are blocked (P waves are not followed by a QRS complex). Because the block is not in the AV node, sinus impulses that conduct to the ventricles always do so with a constant PR interval. Impulses may be blocked randomly, making the ventricular rhythm irregular. Alternatively, the impulses may be blocked at regular intervals, such as in 2:1 block, in which case the ventricular rhythm is regular (Figure 34-17, *C*).

ETIOLOGY. Second-degree AV block type II is less common than type I. It may occur in the adult with an anterior wall myocardial infarction because of severe ischemic damage to the conduction system. It may also be caused by rheumatic heart disease or degenerative disease of the conduction system. It is a serious block that may progress suddenly to a third-degree AV block (complete heart block) and an ominous prognosis.

PHYSICAL ASSESSMENT/CLINICAL MANIFESTATIONS. Symptoms depend on the frequency of dropped beats and the overall ventricular rate. If the cardiac output is inadequate, the client presents with a symptomatic brady-dysrhythmia.

INTERVENTIONS. In the asymptomatic client, the nurse may assist the physician in initiating prophylactic pacing to avert the threat of sudden third-degree AV block. If slow ventricular rates are present, the nurse administers oxygen and atropine as prescribed. Atropine is usually ineffective because it does not reverse the infranodal block. An isoproterenol (Isuprel) infusion may be administered with caution but may be dangerous in adults with ischemic heart disease. Noninvasive (external) or invasive pacing is preferred. A permanent pacemaker may be required with recurrent Mobitz type II block.

THIRD-DEGREE HEART BLOCK (COMPLETE HEART BLOCK)

PATHOPHYSIOLOGY. In third-degree heart block, none of the sinus impulses conduct to the ventricles. The sinoatrial (SA) node is usually the pacemaker for the atria, producing P waves at a normal or even accelerated rate. A separate, independent pacemaker paces the ventricles. Thus AV dissociation exists. If the block is in the AV node, a junctional escape focus paces the ventricles, producing normal QRS complexes at a rate of 40 to 60 beats/min (Figure 34-18, *A*). If the block is below the His bundle (infranodal), a ventricular escape focus paces the ventricles, producing wide QRS complexes at a rate usually less than 40 beats/min (Figure 34-18, *B*). In either case, the atrial and ventricular rhythms are usually regular but independent of each other, with more P waves than QRS complexes.

Because the P waves and the QRS complexes are totally independent and bear no relationship to each other, the PR interval is not constant, which is the most characteristic feature of this rhythm. The ventricular escape pacemaker is the least dependable pacemaker. It may abruptly fail, causing ventricular asystole, or it may predispose to irritability in the form of premature ventricular complexes (PVCs), ventricular tachycardia (VT), or ventricular fibrillation (VF).

ETIOLOGY. Third-degree heart block in the adult may occur from ischemic injury with coronary artery disease (CAD) or myocardial infarction, degenerative disease of the conduction system, hypoxia, or calcific aortic stenosis. Third-degree heart block may occur with congenital heart disease, the effects of drugs or electrolyte disturbances, or cardiac surgery.

PHYSICAL ASSESSMENT/CLINICAL MANIFESTATIONS. Clinical manifestations depend on the overall ventricular rate and cardiac output. Transient third-degree heart block may be well tolerated, particularly when the block is in the AV node. If the block is infranodal, it may have serious hemodynamic consequences. If cerebral perfusion is inadequate, clients may be confused and lightheaded or may experience episodes of syncope with or without seizures (Stokes-Adams attacks). Inadequate cardiac output may cause myocardial ischemia or infarction, heart failure, or hypotension. Third-degree heart block may predispose to cardiac arrest, causing VT, VF, or asystole. Therefore it is regarded as a dangerous rhythm.

INTERVENTIONS. Third-degree AV block with a junctional escape pacemaker is often transient and well tolerated. If the client is symptomatic, the nurse administers oxygen and atropine as prescribed. Clients with third-degree heart block with a ventricular escape pacemaker are frequently symptomatic. The nurse administers oxygen and assists the physician in initiating pacing to avert the threat of cardiac arrest. Atropine is usually not successful in infranodal blocks with wide QRS complexes. Cautious use of isoproterenol (Isuprel) infusions may be necessary as a temporary measure while awaiting pacemaker therapy but is dangerous in clients with acute myocardial infarction. Implantation of a permanent pacemaker may be required for clients with recurrent third-degree infranodal block.

BUNDLE BRANCH BLOCKS

PATHOPHYSIOLOGY. Bundle branch block is a conduction delay or block within one of the two main bundle branches below the bifurcation of the His bundle. When one bundle branch is blocked, the supraventricular impulse is able to descend only down the unblocked bundle branch and to depolarize that ventricle. The other ventricle is depolarized afterward, as the wave of depolarization from the first ventricle proceeds from cell to cell to the other ventricle. Such slow depolarization prolongs the QRS duration to 0.12 second or longer. The underlying rhythm is usually sinus in origin (e.g., sinus rhythm with bundle branch block) (Figure 34-18, *C*).

ETIOLOGY. Bundle branch block may be a temporary or permanent conduction disorder. Right or left bundle branch blocks may occasionally be seen in clients with normal hearts. More commonly, they are seen in clients with cardiovascular disease, such as congenital heart disease, rheumatic heart disease, ventricular hypertrophy, cardiomyopathy, severe aortic stenosis, chronic degenerative disease of the conduction system, or fibrotic scarring of the conduction system. Transient bundle branch block may be seen with acute conditions such

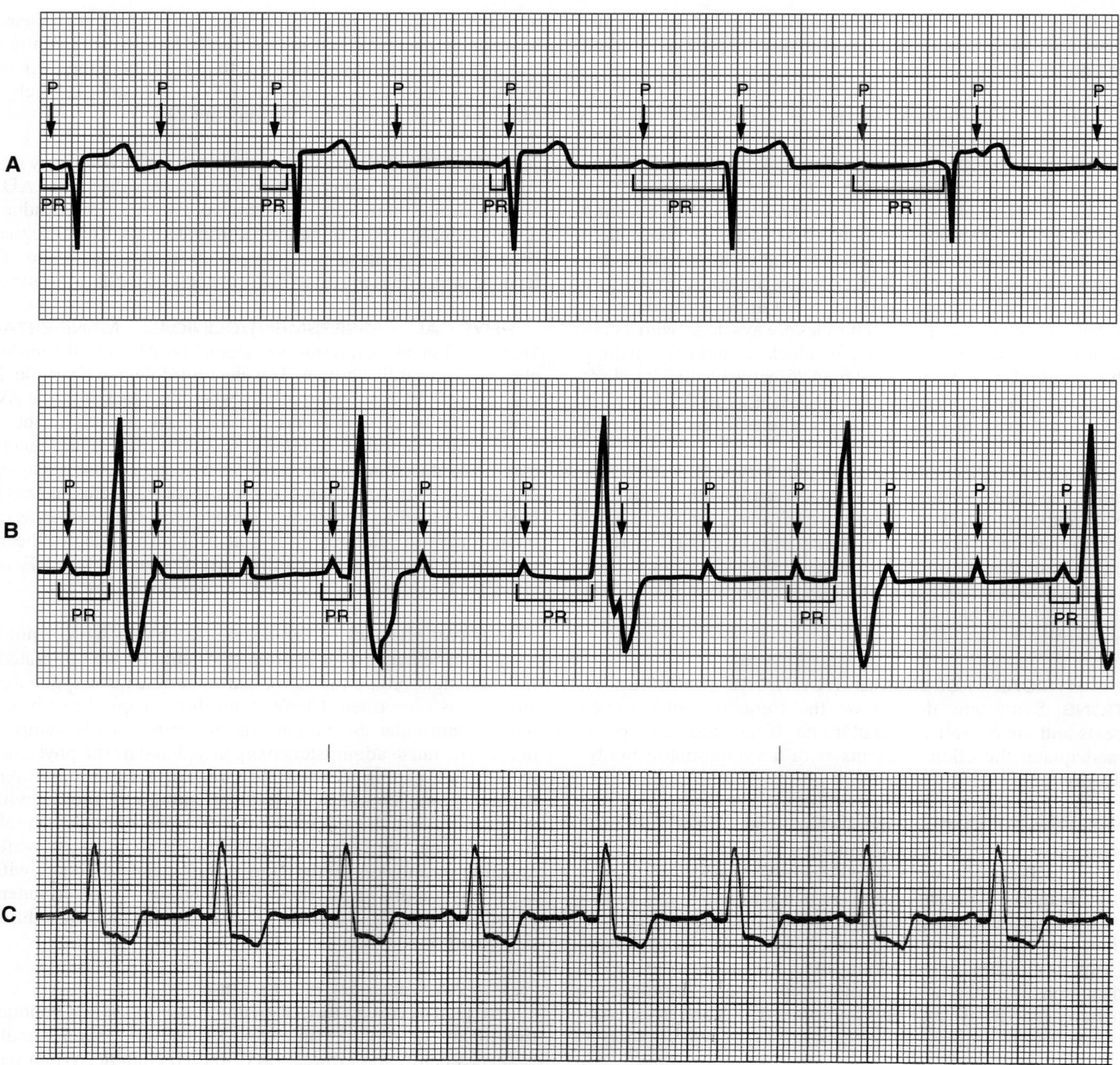

Figure 34-18 ● Atrioventricular (AV) blocks. **A,** Third-degree AV block (complete heart block) with regular atrial and ventricular rhythms, inconstant PR intervals (AV dissociation), and a junctional escape focus (normal QRS complexes) pacing the ventricles at a rate of 44 beats/min. **B,** Third-degree AV block with regular atrial and ventricular rhythms, inconstant PR intervals (AV dissociation), and a ventricular escape focus pacing the ventricles at a rate of 38 beats/min, with wide QRS complexes. **C,** Normal sinus rhythm with bundle branch block (wide QRS complexes measuring 0.12 second).

as coronary insufficiency, myocardial infarction, or heart failure; during right-sided heart catheterization; or with rapid supraventricular rates.

PHYSICAL ASSESSMENT/CLINICAL MANIFESTATIONS. There are no clinical manifestations specifically related to bundle branch block. The nurse must notify the physician when a new bundle branch block develops, especially in the client with an acute myocardial infarction. The conduction disorder may deteriorate to a more significant block requiring pacemaker therapy.

INTERVENTIONS. No interventions are specifically related to bundle branch block. The client is assessed during alterations in heart rate for symptoms of hemodynamic compromise, which are reported to the physician. The nurse ensures that the client is resting and has adequate ventilation and oxygenation.

COLLABORATIVE MANAGEMENT

Analysis

COMMON NURSING DIAGNOSES AND COLLABORATIVE PROBLEMS

The following are the most common nursing diagnoses for clients with dysrhythmias:

1. Decreased Cardiac Output related to electrical and mechanical dysfunction
2. Ineffective Tissue Perfusion related to decreased cardiac output

ADDITIONAL NURSING DIAGNOSES AND COLLABORATIVE PROBLEMS

In addition to the common nursing diagnoses, clients with dysrhythmias may have one or more of the following:

- Impaired Gas Exchange related to altered oxygen supply
- Ineffective Coping related to fear of death
- Activity Intolerance related to fatigue from decreased oxygen supply
- Self-Care Deficit related to activity intolerance

An additional collaborative problem is Potential for Pulmonary Edema.

Planning and Implementation

DECREASED CARDIAC OUTPUT AND INEFFECTIVE TISSUE PERFUSION

NOC **PLANNING: EXPECTED OUTCOMES.** The client with dysrhythmias is expected to demonstrate satisfactory cardiac output as evidenced by the following:

- Normal, regular heart rate
- No adventitious breath sounds
- Cognitive status in expected range (IER)
- Baseline skin color and temperature
- Blood pressure IER

In addition, the client is expected to perform activities of daily living without dyspnea or excessive fatigue.

INTERVENTIONS. The nurse's major role is to assess for complications and monitor the client for response to treatment (Chart 34-5). Interventions are specific to the type of dysrhythmia, the cause, the effect it has on cardiac output, and the risk it presents to the client. Interventions for specific dysrhythmias are summarized in Table 34-2.

NIC **CARDIAC CARE.** The nurse or assistive nursing personnel monitors the client's electrocardiographic (ECG) rhythm and/or assesses the client for signs and symptoms associated with dysrhythmias, such as abnormal pulse rate and rhythm, palpitations, chest pain, syncope, decreased blood pressure, and dyspnea.

The nurse may assess the client's apical and radial pulses for a full minute for any irregularity, which may occur with premature beats, escape beats, atrial fibrillation (AF), or second-degree heart blocks. If the apical pulse rate differs from the radial pulse rate, a pulse deficit exists and suggests that not all beats are perfusing. Clinical manifestations of sustained tachydysrhythmias and bradydysrhythmias are summarized in Chart 34-2.

In a critical care setting, if the client has a pulmonary artery catheter and an arterial line, his or her hemodynamic profile is reviewed to determine the physiologic effects of the dysrhythmia. The nurse must also assess the psychosocial impact of dysrhythmias on clients and families and the effectiveness of their coping mechanisms.

CHART 34-5

NIC INTERVENTION ACTIVITIES *for* The Client with Dysrhythmias

Cardiac Care: *Limitation of complications resulting from an imbalance between myocardial oxygen supply and demand for a client with symptoms of impaired cardiac function*

- Evaluate chest pain (e.g., intensity, location, radiation, duration, and precipitating and alleviating factors).
- Perform a comprehensive appraisal of peripheral circulation (e.g., check peripheral pulses, edema, capillary refill, color, and temperature of extremity).
- Monitor cardiovascular status.
- Document cardiac dysrhythmias.
- Monitor vital signs frequently.
- Evaluate the client's response to ectopy or dysrhythmias.
- Monitor appropriate laboratory values (e.g., cardiac enzymes, electrolyte levels).
- Provide antiarrhythmic therapy according to unit policy (e.g., antiarrhythmic medication, cardioversion, or defibrillation), as appropriate.
- Monitor client's response to antiarrhythmic medications.
- Arrange exercise and rest periods to avoid fatigue.
- Monitor the client's activity tolerance.
- Monitor for dyspnea, fatigue, tachypnea, and orthopnea.
- Promote stress reduction.
- Instruct the client on the importance of immediately reporting any chest discomfort.
- Offer spiritual support to the client and/or family (e.g., contact clergy), as appropriate.

NIC intervention activities selected from McCloskey J.C., & Bulechek, G.M. (2000). *Nursing interventions classification (NIC)* (3rd ed.). St. Louis: Mosby. No part of this work is to be altered without prior written permission from the Publisher.

Assessment of the client's past and current history is essential because dysrhythmias are associated with both acute and chronic disorders and also with medical and surgical therapies. The nurse should also review the interpretation of the client's 12-lead ECG and other ECG diagnostic tests, such as the Holter monitor, event monitor, or signal-averaged ECG.

NONSURGICAL MANAGEMENT. Nonsurgical management of dysrhythmias includes drug therapy, vagal maneuvers, temporary pacing, cardioversion, cardiopulmonary resuscitation (CPR), defibrillation, and catheter ablation.

DRUG THERAPY. Pharmacologic therapy administered for the control of dysrhythmias often includes drugs from one or more classes of antidysrhythmic agents (see Chart 34-3). The Vaughn-Williams classification is commonly used to classify drugs according to their effects on the action potential of cardiac cells. Other drugs also have antidysrhythmic effects but do not fit the Vaughn-Williams classification.

Vaughn-Williams Classification. Class I antidysrhythmics are membrane-stabilizing agents, stabilizing phase 4 to decrease automaticity. There are three subclassifications in this group. Type IA drugs moderately slow conduction and prolong repolarization, prolonging the QT interval. These drugs are used to treat or to prevent supraventricular and ventricular premature beats and tachydysrhythmias. Examples include quinidine sulfate and procainamide hydrochloride

(Pronestyl). Type IB drugs shorten repolarization. These drugs are used to treat or prevent ventricular premature beats, ventricular tachycardia (VT), and ventricular fibrillation (VF). Examples include lidocaine and mexiletine hydrochloride (Mexitil). Type IC drugs markedly slow conduction and widen the QRS complex. These drugs are used primarily to treat or to prevent recurrent, life-threatening ventricular premature beats, VT, and VF. Examples include flecainide acetate (Tambocor) and propafenone hydrochloride (Rythmol).

Class II antidysrhythmics control dysrhythmias associated with excessive beta-adrenergic stimulation by competing for receptor sites and thereby decreasing heart rate and conduction velocity. Beta-adrenergic blocking agents, such as propranolol (Inderal, Apo-Propranolol🍁) and esmolol hydrochloride (Brevibloc), are class II drugs. They are used to treat or to prevent supraventricular and ventricular premature beats and tachydysrhythmias. Sotalol hydrochloride (Betapace, Sotacor🍁) is an antidysrhythmic agent with both noncardioselective beta-adrenergic blocking effects (class II) and action potential duration prolongation properties (class III). It is an oral agent recommended for the treatment of documented ventricular dysrhythmias, such as VT, that are life threatening.

Class III antidysrhythmics lengthen the absolute refractory period and prolong repolarization and the action potential duration of ischemic cells. They decrease the disparity with normal cells to prevent a re-entry response. Class III drugs include bretylium (Bretylol, Bretylate🍁), amiodarone (Cordarone), and ibutilide (Covert) and are used to treat or prevent ventricular premature beats, VT, and VF.

Class IV antidysrhythmics impede the flow of calcium into the cell during depolarization, thereby depressing automaticity of the sinoatrial (SA) and atrioventricular (AV) nodes, decreasing the heart rate, and prolonging the AV nodal refractory period and conduction. Calcium channel blockers, such as verapamil hydrochloride (Calan, Isoptin🍁) and diltiazem hydrochloride (Cardizem), are class IV drugs. They are used to treat supraventricular tachycardia (SVT), atrial flutter, and atrial fibrillation (AF) to slow down the ventricular response.

Other Antidysrhythmic Drugs. Other drugs, such as digoxin, atropine, adenosine, and magnesium sulfate, are frequently used to treat dysrhythmias. Digoxin (Lanoxin, Novodigoxin🍁) increases vagal tone, slowing AV nodal conduction. It is useful in treating supraventricular tachydysrhythmias, particularly chronic AF, by controlling the rate of ventricular response. Atropine is a parasympatholytic or vagolytic agent. It is used to treat vagally induced symptomatic bradydysrhythmias. Adenosine is an endogenous nucleoside that slows AV nodal conduction to interrupt re-entry pathways. It is effective in terminating paroxysmal SVT, a reentrant tachydysrhythmia. Magnesium sulfate is an electrolyte administered to treat refractory VT or VF because these clients may be hypomagnesemic, with increased ventricular irritability.

Emergency Cardiac Drugs. In addition to antidysrhythmics, several other drugs are used during cardiac arrest (Chart 34-6). Epinephrine (Adrenalin) is a first-line agent in all cardiac arrests. It is given predominantly for its alpha-adrenergic effects to increase vasomotor tone for myocardial and cerebral perfusion. Its beta-adrenergic effects may stimulate the heart and increase myocardial contractility to improve cardiac output. Dopamine hydrochloride (Intropin) is generally used for its beta-adrenergic effects after cardiac arrest but may be used for its alpha-adrenergic effects during resuscitation. Dobutamine hydrochloride (Dobutrex) is a beta-adrenergic agent used to improve myocardial contractility and increase cardiac output.

Norepinephrine (Levophed) or phenylephrine hydrochloride (Neo-Synephrine) may be used for its alpha-adrenergic effects to increase vasomotor tone and increase perfusion pressure. Sodium bicarbonate is administered during cardiac arrest for clients who are hyperkalemic. It may also be used, if necessary, to treat a bicarbonate metabolic acidosis, as occurs in diabetic ketoacidosis or tricyclic antidepressant overdose. Isoproterenol (Isuprel) is indicated to increase the heart rate in heart transplant clients, but pacing is preferred. Calcium chloride, which increases myocardial contractility, is also rarely indicated. It is reserved for clients with hyperkalemia, hypocalcemia, or calcium channel blocker toxicity because it may cause cell damage and cerebrovascular vasospasm.

VAGAL MANEUVERS. Vagal maneuvers induce vagal stimulation of the cardiac conduction system, specifically the SA and AV nodes. Vagal maneuvers are used to terminate supraventricular tachydysrhythmias. They include carotid sinus massage and Valsalva maneuvers.

Carotid Sinus Massage. The physician massages over one carotid artery for a few seconds, observing for a change in cardiac rhythm. Massaging the carotid sinus causes vagal stimulation, slowing SA nodal and AV nodal conduction. The nurse prepares the client for this procedure, instructs him or her to turn the head slightly away from the side to be massaged, and observes the cardiac monitor for a change in rhythm. An electrocardiographic (ECG) rhythm strip is recorded before, during, and after the procedure. The nurse then assesses vital signs and the level of consciousness. Complications include bradydysrhythmias, asystole, VF, and cerebral damage. Because of these risks, carotid massage is not commonly performed. A defibrillator and resuscitative equipment must be immediately available during the procedure.

Valsalva Maneuvers. To stimulate a vagal reflex, the health care provider instructs the client to bear down as if straining to have a bowel movement or induces the gag reflex. The nurse prepares the client for the procedure; assesses the heart rate, heart rhythm, and blood pressure; observes the cardiac monitor; and records an ECG rhythm strip before, during, and after the procedure to determine the effect of therapy. If gagging is induced and the client vomits, the nurse provides an emesis basin and oral hygiene and takes measures to prevent aspiration.

Unintended vagal stimulation may sometimes occur, and the nurse must be cautious when performing procedures that may inadvertently cause vagal stimulation. For example, tracheal suctioning, enema administration, and rectal temperature checks can stimulate the vagus nerve and decrease the heart rate inappropriately. The nurse administers stool softeners as prescribed. The client is instructed not to strain during bowel movements and to avoid constipation through proper diet and exercise. He or she is also told to avoid inducing gagging during oral hygiene, which triggers a vagal response. The heart rate and rhythm of a client who is vomiting is monitored because a vagal reflex can result. Some clients experience a vagal response when raising their arms above their head and must be instructed to avoid this movement.

CHART 34-6

DRUG THERAPY *for* Cardiac Arrest

Drug	Usual Dosage	Nursing Interventions	Rationale
Epinephrine (Adrenalin)	1-mg IV bolus followed by 20-mL saline flush q3-5min If this fails, may consider 2-5 mg IV bolus q3-5min; 1-mg, 3-mg, and 5-mg IV boluses (3 min apart); or 0.1 mg/kg IV bolus q3-5min If necessary, may give endotracheally with dose at least 2-2½ times IV dose	Monitor for return of rhythm and pulse when used for asystole or VF.	Return of rhythm and pulse is the expected response.
		Assess for tachycardia, dysrhythmias, or hypertension.	Adverse reactions can occur with a dramatic response.
		Assess for the development of coarse VF when given during the VF.	This may improve the response to defibrillation.
Amiodarone hydrochloride (Cordarone)	150 mg IVP over 10 min (15 mg/min), followed by 360 mg IV over next 6 hr (1 mg/min), followed by 540 mg IV over next 18 hr (0.5 mg/min) After first 24 hr, continue maintenance infusion of 720 mg/24 hr (0.5 mg/min)	Monitor for return of rhythm and pulse when used for recurrent unstable VT or VF.	Return of rhythm and pulse is the expected response.
		Use with extreme caution in patients receiving other antiarrhythmias.	Amiodarone reduces the hepatic and renal clearance of certain antiarrhythmics, specifically procainamide, quinidine, and flecainide.
		Use caution in patients with pulmonary, hepatic, or thyroid disease.	Amiodarone can cause fatal toxicity, especially in patients receiving more than 600 mg/day.
		Perform continuous cardiac monitoring while the patient is receiving the loading dose.	There is a slow onset of antiarrhythmic effect and a high risk of life-threatening arrhythmias.
Dopamine hydrochloride (Intropin)	2.5-5 μg/kg/min IV infusion; titrate to desired clinical response 1-2 μg/kg/min for renal and mesenteric vasodilation 2-10 μg/kg/min for beta-adrenergic effects 10-20 μg/kg/min for alpha-adrenergic effects	Assess clients for increased blood pressure.	Increased blood pressure is the expected response.
		Monitor for tachycardia, dysrhythmias, or hypertension.	Adverse reactions may occur.
		Monitor for IV site for infiltration.	Extravasation of drug can occur, causing necrosis.
		Assess for urine output <30 mL/hr, or pallor, cyanosis, pain, or numbness in the extremities.	Dosages >10 μg/kg/min cause vasoconstriction of renal and peripheral blood vessels; dosages of 2-5 μg/kg/min may improve urine output by causing renal vasodilation and improving renal blood flow.
Dobutamine hydrochloride (Dobutrex)	2-20 μg/kg/min IV infusion	Assess for increased blood pressure.	Increased blood pressure is the expected response.
		Assess for hypertension and dysrhythmias.	Adverse reactions may occur.
Norepinephrine (Levophed)	0.5-1 μg/min IV infusion, titrate to desired effect, up to 8-30 μg/min	Assess for increased blood pressure.	Increased blood pressure is the expected response.
		Monitor for bradycardia.	Reflex bradycardia may occur with a rise in blood pressure.
		Monitor for hypertension and dysrhythmias.	Adverse reactions may occur with a dramatic response.
		Monitor the IV site for infiltration.	Extravasation can occur, which necessitates immediate treatment with phentolamine injected at the site.
		Assess for urine output <30 mL/hr or pallor, cyanosis, pain, or numbness in the extremities.	Norepinephrine is a powerful vasoconstrictor.
		Assess for chest pain after resuscitation.	Norepinephrine increases myocardial oxygen demand.
Sodium bicarbonate	1 mEq/kg IV bolus given after the first 10 min of cardiac arrest if necessary 0.5 mEq/kg IV bolus q10min thereafter if necessary	Assess arterial blood gas values for metabolic acidosis.	Administration without evidence of metabolic acidosis can result in alkalosis, which can hinder resuscitation efforts.

VF, Ventricular fibrillation; *VT,* ventricular tachycardia.

Continued

CHART 34-6

DRUG THERAPY *for* Cardiac Arrest—cont'd

Drug	Usual Dosage	Nursing Interventions	Rationale
Isoproterenol (Isuprel)	2-10 μg/min IV infusion; titrate to desired clinical response	Assess for increased heart rate.	Increased heart rate is the expected response.
		Assess for tachycardia, hypotension, or hypertension.	Adverse reactions may occur with a dramatic response.
		Assess for chest pain after resuscitation.	Isoproterenol increases myocardial oxygen demand.
		Monitor for ventricular dysrhythmias.	Isoproterenol increases ventricular irritability, especially in clients who are hypokalemic or who are receiving digitalis.
Calcium chloride ($CaCl_2$)	2-4 mg/kg IV slowly; may repeat q10min if necessary	Calcium chloride is indicated only for cardiac arrest associated with hyperkalemia, hypocalcemia, or calcium channel blocker toxicity.	Calcium chloride may cause cellular damage and cerebrovascular spasm.

VF, Ventricular fibrillation; *VT,* ventricular tachycardia.

TEMPORARY PACING. Temporary pacing is a nonsurgical intervention that provides a timed electrical stimulus to the heart when either the impulse initiation or the intrinsic conduction system of the heart is defective. The electrical stimulus then spreads throughout the heart to depolarize the cells, which should be followed by contraction and cardiac output. Electrical stimuli may be delivered to the right atrium or right ventricle (single-chamber pacemakers) or to both (dual-chamber pacemakers).

When a pacing stimulus is delivered to the heart, a spike (or pacemaker artifact) is seen on the monitor or ECG strip. The spike should be followed by evidence of depolarization (i.e., a P wave, indicating atrial depolarization, or a QRS complex, indicating ventricular depolarization). This pattern is referred to as *capture,* indicating that the pacemaker successfully depolarized, or captured, the chamber.

Temporary pacing is generally initiated in clients with symptomatic, atropine-refractory bradydysrhythmias, particularly second-degree heart block type II and third-degree heart block, or in clients with asystole. Temporary pacing may also be initiated prophylactically in hemodynamically stable clients with left bundle branch block in certain situations, such as insertion of a pulmonary artery catheter.

A different type of pacing may be used to terminate symptomatic tachydysrhythmias. Occasionally, atrial overdrive pacing is attempted to terminate atrial tachydysrhythmias, such as atrial flutter or atrial fibrillation (AF). Overdrive pacing is accomplished by rapidly pacing the atrium to capture the heart and control depolarization, followed by no pacing, in the hope that the sinus node will regain control of the heart. Ventricular overdrive pacing may be done to terminate ventricular tachydysrhythmias in much the same way. Overdrive pacing is usually performed by the physician or the physician's assistant. The nurse must have emergency equipment available in case the client becomes more unstable or goes into cardiac arrest.

Modes of Pacing. There are two basic modes of pacing: synchronous (demand) pacing and asynchronous (fixed-rate) pacing.

Synchronous (Demand) Pacing. Temporary pacing is most commonly done in the demand mode. The pacemaker's sensitivity is set to sense the client's own beats. When the client's intrinsic rate is above the rate set on the pulse generator, the pacemaker is inhibited from firing. When the client's rate is below that set on the generator, the pacemaker fires electrical impulses to stimulate depolarization (Figure 34-19, *A*).

Asynchronous (Fixed-Rate) Pacing. The asynchronous mode is used when the client is asystolic or profoundly bradycardic, as may occur after open heart surgery. When the pulse generator is set in an asynchronous mode, it does not sense any intrinsic beats of the client. The pacemaker continues to fire at a fixed rate as set on the generator, regardless of the intrinsic rhythm. This continued firing is not a problem as long as the client remains asystolic or has a rate slower than the pacemaker rate, because all beats come from the pacemaker and there is no competition from the client's beats (Figure 34-19, *B*). However, if the client's rate increases and equals or exceeds the pacemaker rate, competition (undersensing) is noted. The danger is that a pacemaker stimulus may reach the heart during the vulnerable period of repolarization (R-on-T phenomenon, with the pacer spike falling on the T wave) and possibly induce ventricular fibrillation (VF). The nurse must observe for pacemaker competition and set the pacemaker to a synchronous mode to avert potential problems.

Universal Pacemaker Code. In 1974 the Intersociety Commission for Heart Disease established a three-position pacemaker code (ICHD code) to standardize the description of pacemaker systems.

This code is used universally and makes it easier to quickly identify the primary functions of the pacemaker. AAI denotes an atrial demand pacemaker. AOO denotes an asynchronous atrial pacemaker. VVI denotes a ventricular demand pacemaker. VOO refers to an asynchronous ventricular pacemaker. DVI denotes a demand AV sequential pacemaker that can pace both chambers but senses only the ventricular chamber. DOO indicates an asynchronous dual-chamber pacemaker. DDD denotes a demand dual-chamber pacemaker that paces and senses both chambers and has a dual mode of response.

The code was expanded to five positions for standardization of multiprogrammable pacemakers and tachydysrhythmia functions, incorporating the original three-position code. This

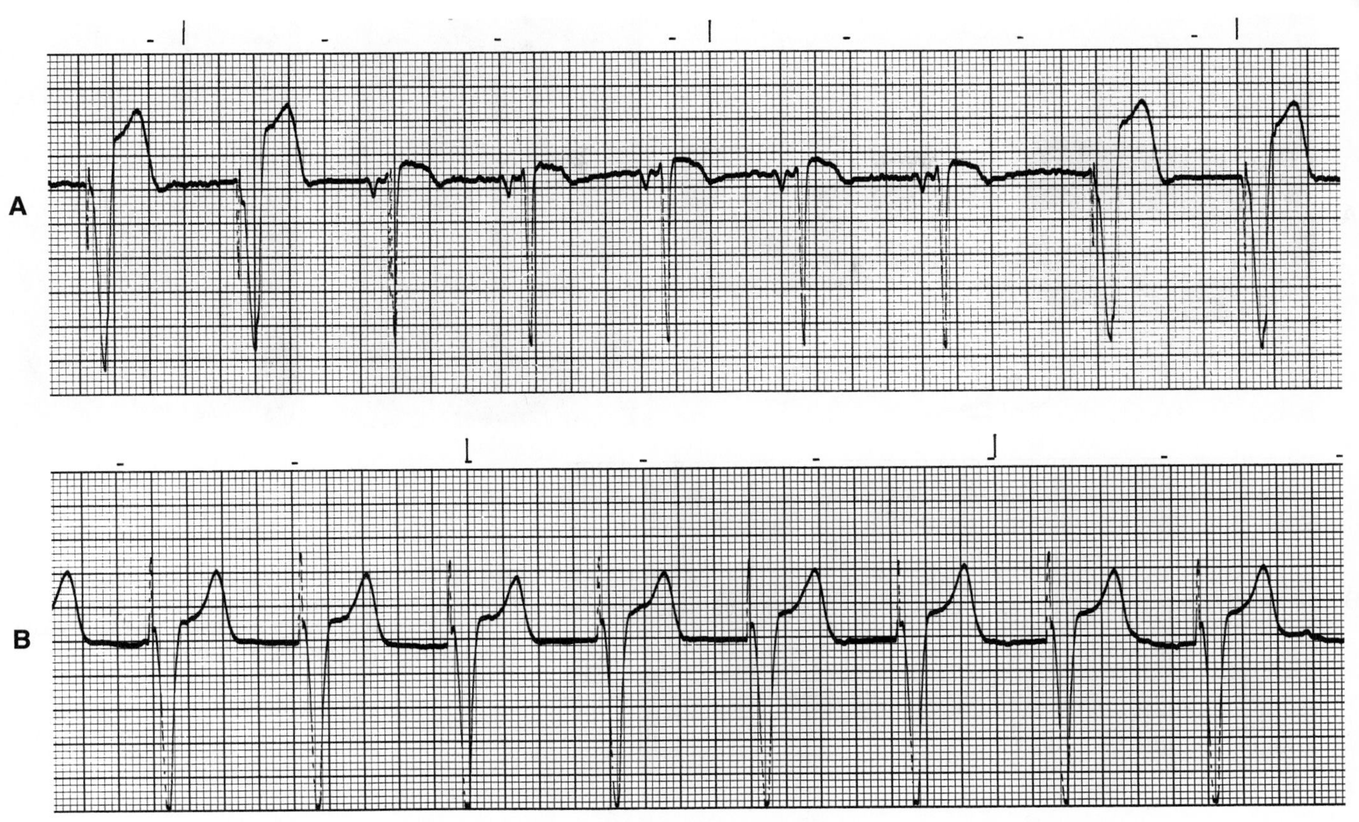

Figure 34-19 ● Modes of pacing. **A,** Synchronous (demand) ventricular pacing (VVI). **B,** Asynchronous (fixed-rate) ventricular pacing at a rate of 70 beats/min (VOO). (See Table 34-3.)

TABLE 34-3 • THE FIVE-POSITION PACEMAKER CODE*

I Chamber(s) Paced	II Chamber(s) Sensed	III Mode of Response	IV Programmability, Rate Modulation	V Antitachycardia Function(s)
A = Atrium V = Ventricle D = Dual (atrium and ventricle) O = None	A = Atrium V = Ventricle D = Dual (atrium and ventricle) O = None	I = Inhibited T = Triggered D = Atrial triggered and ventricular inhibited O = None	P = Simple programmable M = Multiprogrammable C = Communicating R = Rate modulation O = None	P = Pacing S = Shock D = Dual (pacing and shock) O = None

From Bernstein, A.D., et al. (1987). The NASPE/BPEG pacemaker code. *PACE, 10*(4), 794.
*The North American Society for Pacing and Electrophysiology (NASPE) and the British Pacing and Electrophysiology Group (BPEG) code (the NASE/BPEG generic [NBG] code).

code was designed by the North American Society for Pacing and Electrophysiology (NASPE) and the British Pacing and Electrophysiology Group (BPEG). The code is referred to as the NASPE/BPEG generic (or NBG) code (Table 34-3).

There are two basic types of temporary pacing: noninvasive (external) temporary pacing and invasive temporary pacing.

Noninvasive Temporary Pacing. Noninvasive temporary pacing (NTP) is accomplished through the application of two large patch electrodes. The electrodes are attached to an external pulse generator, which can operate on alternating current (AC) or battery power (Figure 34-20). The generator emits electrical pulses, which are transmitted through the cutaneous patches and then transcutaneously to stimulate ventricular depolarization when the client's heart rate is slower than the rate set on the pacemaker. Electrical currents of 60 milliamperes (mA) or more are usually required to achieve ventricular depolarization. The current is applied for 20 to 40 milliseconds (msec), producing a pacing stimulus, or spike, that occupies 0.02 to 0.04 second on the electrocardiographic (ECG) paper.

NTP is used as an emergency measure to provide demand ventricular pacing in a profoundly bradycardic or asystolic client until invasive pacing can be instituted or the client's intrinsic rate returns to normal. It may be used prophylactically when performing procedures or transporting clients at risk for bradydysrhythmias. Prophylactic use of NTP may be costly because of the high cost of the external electrodes, and its use should therefore be carefully considered.

Procedure. The nurse explains NTP to the client and prepares the equipment. The skin is washed with soap and water.

A

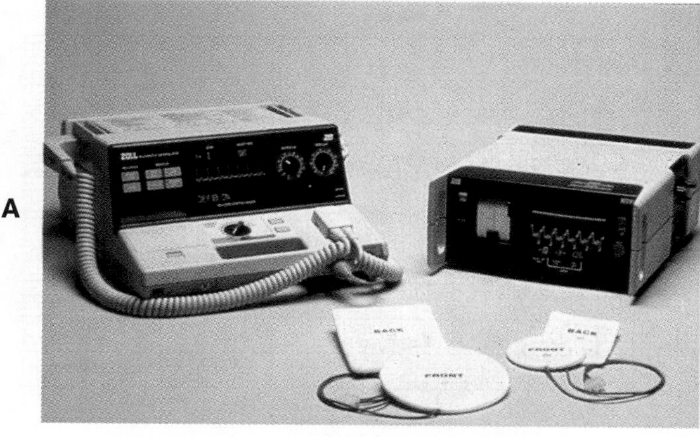

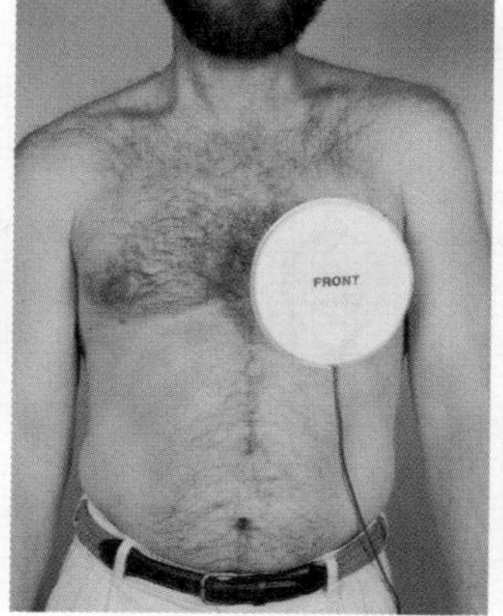

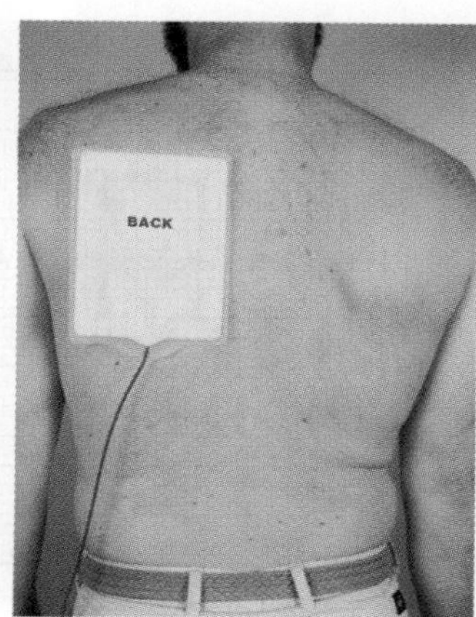

B

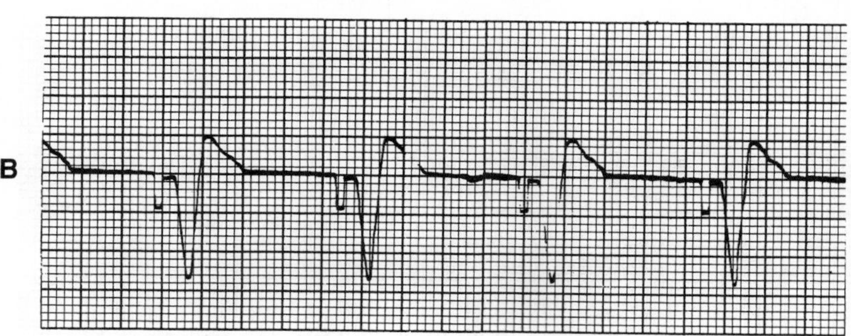

Figure 34-20 ● **A,** Equipment and electrode placement for transcutaneous external pacing. **B,** ECG rhythm strip showing wide pacing spikes. (**A** courtesy Zoll Medical Corporation, Burlington, MA.)

To prevent skin abrasion, the skin must not be shaved. The nurse or assistive nursing personnel should not rub the skin or apply alcohol or tinctures on the skin, because electrical current flows from the patches through the skin and causes discomfort. The nurse then applies the large posterior electrode on the client's back, between the spine and the left scapula, behind the heart. The electrode should not be placed higher over bone because bone is a poor conductor of electrical current. The anterior electrode is then applied on the chest, between the V_2 and the V_5 positions, over the heart. The electrode cannot be placed over female breast tissue. The breast tissue is displaced to position the electrode underneath the breast.

The nurse sets the pacing rate as ordered and establishes the stimulation threshold, the lowest current that achieves capture with each pacing spike followed by a QRS complex. The QRS complex is wide because one ventricle depolarizes first, followed by the other. The electrical current is then set 10% above threshold levels.

The nurse palpates the right radial or carotid pulse and assesses the blood pressure using the client's right arm, ensuring that each paced beat is perfused. Vital signs are not taken on the left side of the body because they may not be accurate, particularly if a high milliamperage is used.

Complications. Three complications may arise with NTP. The first is discomfort from cutaneous and muscle stimulation and skin irritation, as well as diaphoresis from the patch electrodes. The nurse ensures that the electrodes are in good contact with the skin and in the best location to achieve the lowest threshold for consistent capture. Analgesics or sedatives are given as prescribed to provide comfort.

The second problem is loss of capture, which occurs when the pacing spike is not followed by a QRS complex. The nurse ensures that the electrodes are in good contact with the skin and, if necessary, increases the current until capture is regained; however, higher currents cause more discomfort.

The third problem is inappropriate pacing, which occurs when the pacemaker does not sense the client's intrinsic QRS complex and therefore fires impulses at its preset rate, competing with the client's rhythm. The nurse must assess electrode contact and the effect of the client's position on pacemaker function. The client may need to avoid lying on the left side. If diaphoresis has caused poor contact and the electrodes must be replaced, the nurse must first turn the pacing function off to avoid receiving electrical shocks when touching the gel side of the electrodes.

Invasive Temporary Pacing. An invasive temporary pacemaker system consists of an external, battery-operated pulse generator and pacing electrodes, or lead wires. These wires attach to the generator on one end and are in contact with the heart on the other end. Electrical pulses, or stimuli, are emitted from the negative terminal of the generator, flow through a lead wire, and stimulate the cardiac cells to depolarize. The current seeks ground by returning through the other lead wire to the positive terminal of the generator, thus completing a circuitous route. The intensity of electrical current is set by selecting the appropriate current output, measured in milliamperes.

The client does not usually feel invasive pacemaker stimuli; however, clients occasionally feel an uncomfortable sensation from the stimuli if strong electrical currents (high milliamperage) are delivered by the pacemaker. The discomfort may be alleviated by decreasing the current if possible.

The two types of invasive temporary pacing are transvenous pacing and epicardial pacing.

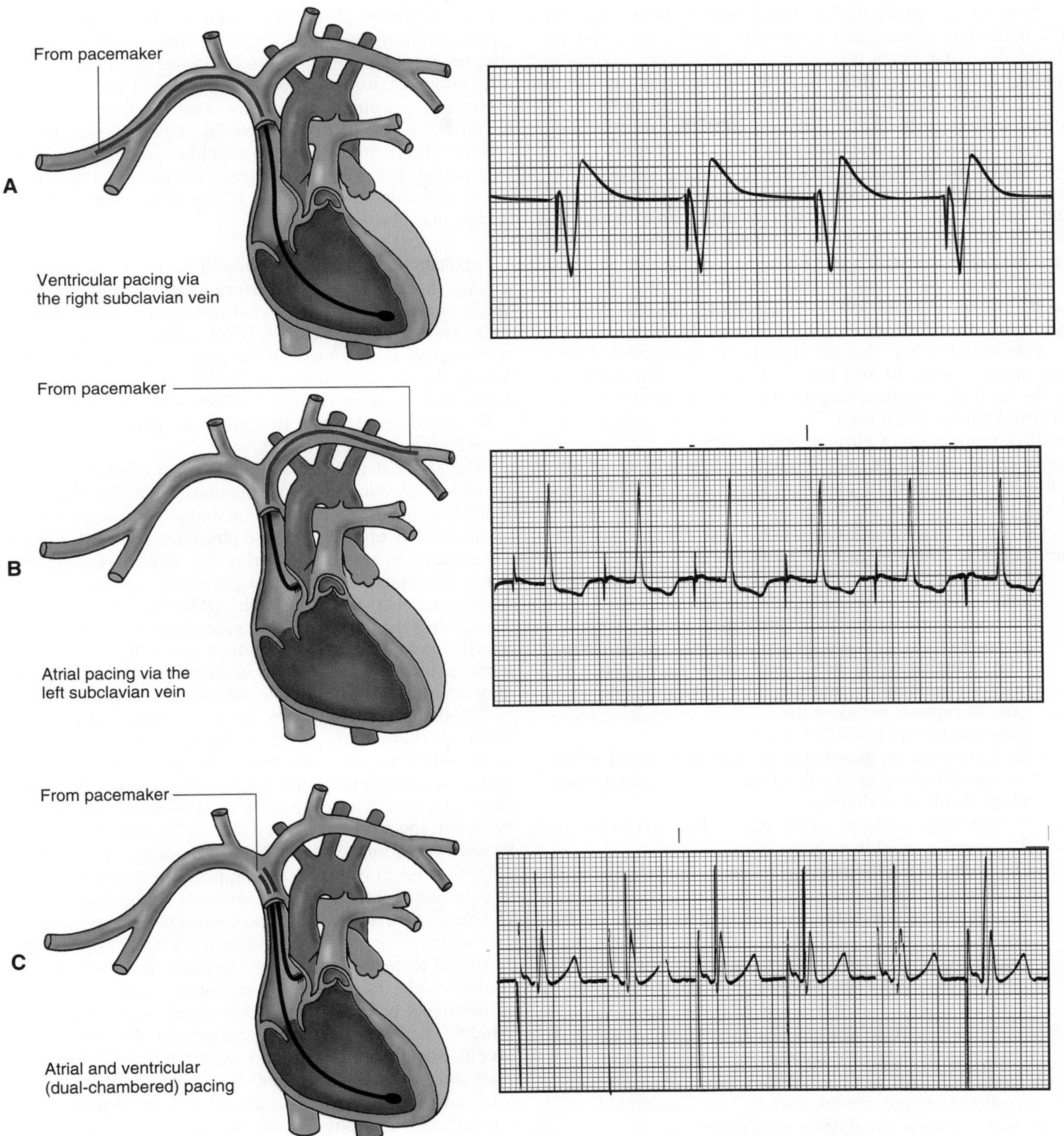

Figure 34-21 ● Pacemaker catheter electrode placement and corresponding ECG patterns in temporary transvenous pacing. **A,** Ventricular pacing at a rate of 72 beats/min. **B,** Atrial pacing at a rate of 88 beats/min, with intrinsic QRS complexes. **C,** AV pacing at a rate of 80 beats/min.

Transvenous Pacing. Transvenous ventricular pacing involves the use of fluoroscopy to thread a sterile catheter, containing two lead wires, percutaneously through a vein to the right ventricle for temporary pacing. The catheter electrode tip (negative electrode) is in contact with the endocardial surface of the ventricle, where it fixates for stability (Figure 34-21, *A*). The positive electrode is located just proximal to the tip of the catheter. The bifurcated external end of the catheter is attached to the negative and positive terminals of a battery-operated pulse generator. The generator provides the electrical current needed to stimulate the myocardial cells to depolarize.

Some clients with a dysfunctional sinus node but an intact AV node may require only temporary atrial pacing (Figure 34-21, *B*). If the client needs the atrial kick from atrial contractions, a temporary dual-chamber pacemaker is used, with one catheter tip in the right atrium and the other in the right ventricle (Figure 34-21, *C*). This preserves the normal timing of atrial contraction preceding ventricular contraction.

Nursing management of the client after temporary transvenous pacemaker insertion includes continuous ECG monitoring, frequent assessment of vital signs and the pacemaker insertion site, restriction of the client's movement to prevent lead wire displacement, and documentation of pacemaker settings. The qualified nurse or other health care provider must assess stimulation and sensitivity thresholds according to institutional protocols.

Epicardial Pacing. Epicardial pacing is accomplished with separate lead wires loosely threaded on the epicardial surface of the heart after cardiac surgery. The other ends of the wires exit through the chest wall. They attach to the negative and positive terminals of a pulse generator. The electrical current flows from epicardium to endocardium, from right to left. Nursing management of the client following cardiac surgery is detailed in Chapter 38.

Complications. Complications of invasive temporary pacing may be serious and include the following:

- Infection or hematoma at the pacemaker wire insertion site
- Ectopic complexes (usually premature ventricular complexes [PVCs]), caused by irritability from the pacing wire in the ventricle, use of high current, or undersensing with pacemaker competition
- Loss of capture, noted by the presence of a pacing stimulus or spike but no QRS complex
- Undersensing or pacemaker competition, noted when pacing stimuli occur at a fixed rate in the presence of an adequate intrinsic rhythm
- Oversensing, noted when the pacemaker fails to fire in the presence of an inadequate intrinsic rhythm
- Electromagnetic interference, noted by altered generator variables
- Stimulation of the chest wall or diaphragm, noted by rhythmic contraction of the chest wall muscles or hiccups with use of high current or from lead wire perforation, which could cause cardiac tamponade

CRITICAL THINKING CHALLENGE

Your client suddenly develops symptomatic third-degree heart block. The physician orders external cardiac pacing.

- How should you prepare the client for this procedure?
- How should the external pacer pads be applied?
- External pacemaking fails, and the physician tells you to prepare for insertion of a temporary pacemaker.
- What is the difference between a temporary pacemaker and external cardiac pacing?
- What health teaching should you do in preparation for this treatment modality?

For suggested answer guidelines, go to SIMON http://www.wbsaunders.com/SIMON/Iggy/.

Prevention of Microshock. When the metal external ends of lead wires are not attached to a pulse generator, the nurse must insulate the wire ends to prevent microshock. The fingertips of rubber gloves work well for this purpose, and the wire ends may then be looped and covered with nonconductive tape. All electrical equipment in the room must be properly grounded, using a three-pronged plug. The nurse must report faulty electrical equipment, such as frayed or broken electrical wires, to the biomedical engineering department. Neither the client nor the bed should be in contact with such equipment. The risk is that ungrounded electrical current may conduct through the lead wire, stimulate the heart, and induce ventricular fibrillation (VF).

CARDIOVERSION. Cardioversion is a synchronized countershock that may be performed in emergencies for hemodynamically unstable ventricular or supraventricular tachydysrhythmias or electively for stable tachydysrhythmias that are resistant to medical therapies. If the client has been taking digitalis, the nurse withholds the drug for up to 48 hours preceding an elective cardioversion, as ordered. Digitalis increases ventricular irritability and puts the client at risk for VF after the countershock.

The shock depolarizes a critical mass of myocardium simultaneously during intrinsic depolarization. The shock is intended to stop the re-entry circuit and allow the sinus node to regain control of the heart. The physician and skilled personnel must be in attendance during this procedure, with emergency equipment at hand. The physician explains the procedure to the client and assists him or her in signing a consent form unless the procedure is an emergency for a life-threatening dysrhythmia. Because the client is usually conscious, the nurse administers IV sedation as ordered. An anesthesiologist may administer a short-acting anesthetic agent.

The defibrillator should be in the synchronized mode. This avoids discharging the shock during the vulnerable period (T wave), which may increase ventricular irritability, causing VF. The nurse charges the defibrillator to the energy ordered by the physician, usually starting at 50 to 100 Joules. The nurse ensures that the oxygen delivery device has been removed and turned away from the client. Oxygen supports combustion, and a fire may result if there is arcing from the paddles. Arcing is usually due to improper paddle contact on the chest. At least 25 pounds of pressure should be applied to each paddle to prevent arcing. The nurse then loudly and clearly commands all personnel to clear contact with the client and the bed, as required for electrical safety. The nurse ensures compliance of all personnel before delivering the shock. While the client is exhaling, both paddles are discharged simultaneously to deliver the shock at end-expiration, when the heart is closer to the chest wall, so that more current flow can reach the heart for a better chance of success. This procedure may be performed by a qualified nurse, physician's assistant, paramedic, or other qualified health care provider following medical protocols.

After cardioversion, the nurse assesses the client's response and heart rhythm. Therapy is repeated as ordered, if necessary, until the desired result is obtained or alternative therapies are considered. If the client goes into VF after cardioversion, the nurse must ensure that the synchronizer is turned off and then immediately defibrillate the client.

Nursing care after cardioversion includes the following:

- Maintaining a patent airway
- Administering oxygen
- Assessing vital signs and the level of consciousness
- Administering antidysrhythmic drug therapy

- Monitoring for dysrhythmias
- Assessing for chest burns from paddle edges that may not have been on the conductive pad
- Providing emotional support
- Documenting the results of cardioversion

CARDIOPULMONARY RESUSCITATION. Management of the client in cardiac arrest depends on prompt recognition and therapeutic interventions for successful reversal of a potentially fatal event.

When cardiac arrest occurs, cardiac output ceases. The underlying rhythm is usually ventricular tachycardia (VT), ventricular fibrillation (VF), or asystole. In rare instances, cardiac arrest occurs in the presence of an organized electrocardiographic (ECG) rhythm, but with no effectual mechanical response, a condition referred to as pulseless electrical activity (PEA). Without cardiac output, the client is pulseless and becomes unconscious because of inadequate cerebral perfusion. Shortly after cardiac arrest, respiratory arrest occurs.

Cardiopulmonary resuscitation (CPR) must be initiated immediately to help prevent brain damage and death. The nurse, finding an unresponsive client, calls 911 or notifies the emergency response team before initiating CPR. The initial priorities are as follows:

- Maintenance of a patent airway
- Ventilation with a mouth-to-mask device
- Chest compressions

As soon as help arrives, a board is placed under the client who is not on a firm surface. To make room for the resuscitation team and the crash cart, the nurse commands that the area be cleared of movable items and unnecessary personnel.

Complications of CPR include rib fractures, fracture of the sternum, costochondral separation, lacerations of the liver and spleen, pneumothorax, hemothorax, cardiac tamponade, lung contusions, and fat emboli. The goal of resuscitation is the rapid return of a pulse, blood pressure, and consciousness. This is rarely achieved by CPR and basic measures alone. More definitive therapy must be initiated as soon as possible with advanced cardiac life support (ACLS) measures, including defibrillation, if warranted.

The goal is to be able to give a defibrillatory shock within 5 minutes of collapse outside of a hospital, and within 3 minutes in a hospital. To help meet this goal, automated external defibrillators (AEDs) should be placed where there is a probability of at least one sudden cardiac arrest every 5 years, such as on airplanes.

ADVANCED CARDIAC LIFE SUPPORT. When the crash cart arrives, the nurse applies ECG electrodes to the client's chest and turns on the monitor, directing the team to continue CPR. If the client is found to be in VF or pulseless VT, the immediate priority is to defibrillate. Following defibrillation, CPR is resumed. An oropharyngeal airway is inserted to facilitate proper ventilation. A manual resuscitation bag (MRB) with mask is attached to an oxygen flowmeter set at 10 to 15 L/min. The nurse directs that the person managing the airway now ventilate the lungs with the MRB, maintaining the proper head-tilt, chin-lift position of the client. Nurses initiate two large-bore IV lines if the client does not have any, infusing normal saline. These lines provide access for emergency drug administration. Suction equipment is also set up, with a tonsillar suction tube for suctioning vomitus and a suction catheter for endotracheal suctioning. Carotid or femoral pulse checks during chest compressions and without chest compressions, blood pressure measurements, and pupil assessments are done at frequent intervals. A nurse documents all assessments and findings, therapeutic measures, and the client's responses throughout the resuscitation.

Additional measures include endotracheal intubation with ventilation and oxygenation, IV administration of emergency cardiac drugs, and occasionally, external pacing. Chest compressions are continued as long as the client remains pulseless or until a physician decides to terminate resuscitation attempts.

DEFIBRILLATION. Defibrillation, an asynchronous countershock, depolarizes a critical mass of myocardium simultaneously to stop the re-entry circuit and to allow the sinus node to regain control of the heart. Early defibrillation is critical to terminate pulseless VT or VF. It must not be delayed for any reason after the equipment and skilled personnel are present. The earlier defibrillation is performed, the greater the chance of survival.

If a defibrillator is not immediately available, an ACLS-qualified nurse may deliver a precordial thump to a pulseless client in VF. There is a slight chance that it may succeed in terminating the VF. A precordial thump is performed by striking the lower half of the sternum with a closed fist from a height of 8 to 12 inches (12 to 30 cm) above the sternum. If the client remains in VF, CPR is resumed and the nurse prepares the client's chest for defibrillation. The nurse loudly and clearly commands all personnel to clear contact with the client and the bed and ensures their compliance before delivering the shock.

AUTOMATIC EXTERNAL DEFIBRILLATION. The American Heart Association promotes the use of automatic external defibrillators (AEDs) for use by laypersons and health care providers responding to cardiac arrest emergencies. The client in cardiac arrest must be on a firm, dry surface. The rescuer places two large adhesive patch electrodes on the client's chest in the same positions as for defibrillator paddles. The rescuer stops CPR and commands anyone present to move away, ensuring that no one is touching the client. This measure eliminates motion artifact when the machine analyzes the rhythm. The rescuer presses the "analyze" button on the machine. After rhythm analysis, which may take up to 30 seconds, the machine either advises that a shock is necessary or advises that a shock is not indicated. Shocks are recommended for pulseless VF or VT only.

After issuing a command to clear all contact with the client, the rescuer charges the defibrillator and presses both discharge buttons on the machine simultaneously, delivering the first shock at 200 Joules. The shock is delivered through the patches, so it is hands-off defibrillation, which is safer for the rescuer. The rescuer then presses the analyze button again, repeating the sequence. With sustained VF or VT, two more shocks may be delivered, with the third at 360 Joules. If the client remains in cardiac arrest, CPR is performed for 1 minute, and then another series of three shocks may be delivered, each at 360 Joules. It is imperative that ACLS be provided as soon as possible. Use of automatic external defibrillators (AEDs) results in earlier defibrillation of clients and therefore a greater chance of successful rhythm conversion and survival.

A

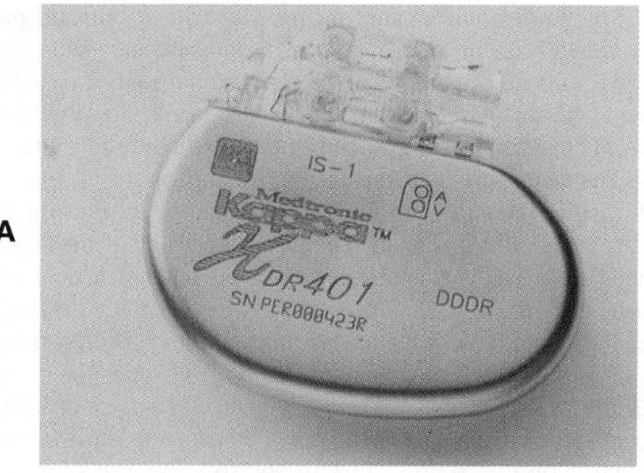

B

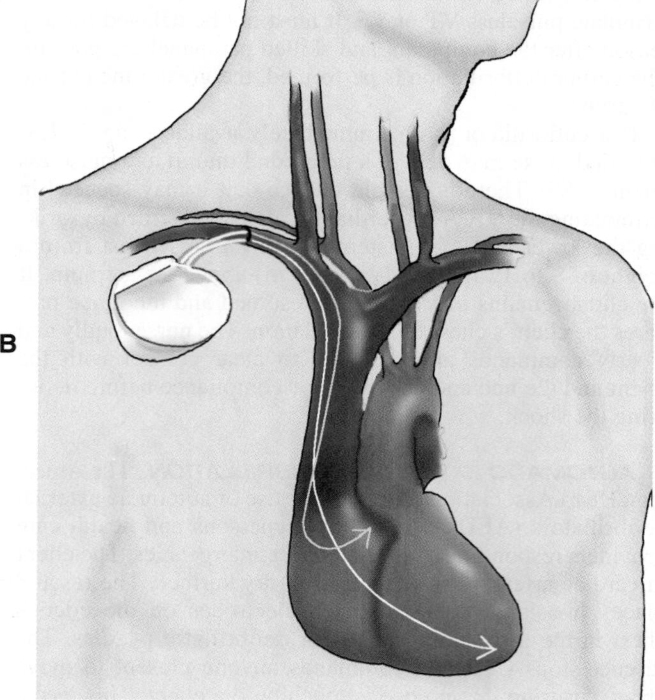

Figure 34-22 ● **A,** Permanent dual-chamber pacemaker. **B,** Implanted permanent dual-chamber pacemaker with endocardial leads introduced via the right subclavian vein into the right atrium and right ventricle. (A Courtesy Medtronic, Inc., Minneapolis, MN.)

RADIOFREQUENCY CATHETER ABLATION. Radiofrequency catheter ablation is an invasive procedure that may be used to abolish an irritable focus causing a supraventricular or ventricular tachydysrhythmia. The client must undergo electrophysiologic studies and mapping procedures to locate the focus. Then radiofrequency waves are delivered to abolish the irritable focus. When ablation is performed in the AV nodal or His bundle area, damage may also occur to the normal conduction system, causing heart blocks and requiring implantation of a permanent pacemaker.

SURGICAL MANAGEMENT. Clients who experience life-threatening dysrhythmias may require surgical treatment for long-term management. The type of treatment depends on the nature of the dysrhythmia. Procedures include permanent pacing, coronary artery bypass grafting, aneurysmectomy, insertion of an implantable cardioverter/defibrillator, and open-chest cardiac massage.

PERMANENT PACING. Permanent pacemaker insertion is performed for the resolution of conduction disorders that are not temporary, including complete heart block and sick sinus syndrome. Permanent pacemakers are usually powered by a lithium battery and have an average life span of 10 years. After the battery power is depleted, the generator must be replaced, a procedure done with the client under local anesthesia. Some pacemakers are nuclear powered and have a life span of 20 years or longer. Other pacemakers can be recharged externally.

Types of Pacemakers. Pacemakers may have a single chamber or dual chambers. With single-chamber pacemakers, a lead wire is positioned in the chamber to be paced, most commonly the right ventricle. Occasionally it is positioned in the right atrium for bradydysrhythmias originating from sinoatrial (SA) node disease with an intact atrioventricular (AV) conduction system (Figure 34-22, *A*).

Dual-chamber pacemakers have lead wires placed in the right atrium and the right ventricle for a more physiologic effect, preserving the atrial kick. A programmed AV interval, which closely relates to the PR interval, ensures a ventricular response shortly after atrial depolarization (Figure 34-22, *B*). The DDD pacemaker is commonly implanted. It is able to sense both atrial and ventricular intrinsic activity and pace both the atrium and the ventricle. It allows sinus control of the ventricular rate to meet increased metabolic demands when the sinus node is functioning well. If the client's sinus rate drops below the lower rate set, the generator paces both the atrium and the ventricle.

Another feature of many pacemakers is rate responsiveness. To allow faster pacing rates to meet increased body demands, the generator changes the pacing rate in response to a detected change in a physiologic variable, such as muscle movement within the client with impaired sinus or atrial function. Hysteresis, on the other hand, is a feature that allows the client's rate to slow to 10 to 20 beats lower than the generator's preset rate before the generator paces the client. The slower pace allows for a more normal physiologic slowing response during rest or sleep.

Surgical Procedures. For both single-chamber and dual-chamber pacemakers, the surgeon most commonly implants the pulse generator in a surgically made subcutaneous pocket at the shoulder in the right or left subclavicular area. The leads are introduced transvenously via the cephalic or the subclavian vein to the endocardium on the right side of the heart. After the procedure, the nurse monitors the client's electrocardiographic (ECG) rhythm to ensure that the pacemaker is functioning correctly. The implantation site is assessed for evidence of bleeding, swelling, redness, tenderness, or infection. The dressing over the site should remain clean and dry, and the client should be afebrile and have stable vital signs. The physician orders activity restrictions to enhance lead fixation. After 24 hours, activity is gradually increased. Complications of permanent pacemakers are similar to those for temporary invasive pacing.

Pacemaker checks are done on an ambulatory care basis at regular intervals. Reprogramming may be warranted if there are pacemaker problems. The pulse generator is interrogated using an electronic device to determine the pacemaker settings and battery life.

For clients who live far from the pacemaker clinic or physician's office, pacemaker information can be sent via transtelephonic transmission of data. The client attaches ECG electrodes to the wrists and places the telephone receiver in a transmitting unit. The sound signals are relayed via telephone lines to the clinic or office, where they are converted and recorded as the client's ECG rhythm strip and information about the pacemaker variables. The nurse stresses the need to keep clinic appointments for more detailed pacemaker checks and reprogramming, if necessary, as well as assessment.

CORONARY ARTERY BYPASS GRAFTING. Coronary artery bypass grafting (CABG) is performed if the cause of the dysrhythmia is coronary artery insufficiency that is unresponsive to medical therapy. This procedure is described in Chapter 38.

ANEURYSMECTOMY. Ventricular aneurysms are a complication of myocardial infarction and may be the source of intractable ventricular tachydysrhythmias. The surgeon resects the aneurysm, a dyskinetic or ballooning portion of the ventricular wall. Resection of the area eliminates the dangerous irritable focus and thus the cause of the dysrhythmias. Care of the client is similar to that for CABG, described in Chapter 38.

INSERTION OF IMPLANTABLE CARDIOVERTER/DEFIBRILLATOR. The implantable cardioverter/defibrillator (ICD) is indicated for clients who have experienced one or more episodes of spontaneous sustained ventricular tachycardia (VT) or ventricular fibrillation (VF) unrelated to a myocardial infarction or other causes amenable to correction.

Clients undergo electrophysiologic studies to assess the inducibility of VTs and their response to medication. If the dysrhythmias can be induced despite medical therapy, the client is considered a candidate for ICD implantation. The nurse collaborates with the physician and the electrophysiology nurse to prepare the client for an ICD. A psychologic profile is done to determine whether the client will be able to cope with the discomfort and fear associated with internal defibrillation from the ICD.

The leads are introduced percutaneously, and the generator is implanted in the left pectoral area, similar to a permanent pacemaker insertion procedure. This procedure is performed in the electrophysiology laboratory.

The electronic pulse generator is designed to monitor and to defibrillate for VT or VF. The generator is powered by a lithium battery and is connected to a transvenous endocardial lead. The ends of the lead are tunneled under the skin to attach to the generator. The sensing lead transmits electrical signals from the heart to the generator, which continuously monitors the heart rhythm. If the client's heart rate exceeds the generator's programmed rate, such as with VT, the generator takes a few seconds to sense the cardiac electrical activity and then delivers a burst of antitachycardial pacing (ATP) to overdrive pace the rhythm. A programmed number of ATP therapies may be delivered. If the client's rate continues to exceed the rate cutoff, the device can deliver a programmed number of low-energy and high-energy cardioversion shocks. In response to VF, the device delivers defibrillation shocks. Following such therapy, the client may develop a transient bradycardia. Many ICD devices are capable of delivering bradycardial pacing (VVI or ventricular demand pacing). This technology is rapidly changing.

If the ICD therapies are not successful and the client remains in VF or pulseless VT, the qualified nurse or health care provider must promptly externally defibrillate the client.

The generator may be activated or deactivated by the physician's placing a magnet over the implantation site for a few moments. The client requires close monitoring in the postimplantation period for the occurrence of dysrhythmias and complications such as bleeding and cardiac tamponade. The nurse must know if the ICD is activated or deactivated. Care of the client is similar to that following implantation of a permanent pacemaker.

OPEN-CHEST CARDIAC MASSAGE. When external chest compressions and advanced cardiac life support measures are unsuccessful in resuscitating a client in cardiac arrest, the physician may decide to perform open-chest cardiac massage through a thoracotomy approach or through the median sternotomy incision in post–cardiac surgery clients. Internal defibrillation may also be performed. Open-chest cardiac massage is usually reserved for the client who goes into cardiac arrest during cardiac surgery, often because of cardiac tamponade. It may also be beneficial but is rarely indicated for hypothermia, crushing or penetrating chest injuries, penetrating abdominal trauma, or chest deformities prohibiting external chest compressions.

Community-Based Care

For many clients, dysrhythmias are a chronic disorder resulting from chronic cardiac and pulmonary diseases. Clients may be cared for in a variety of settings, including the acute care hospital, subacute unit, traditional nursing home, or their own home. They are admitted to the hospital when they experience life-threatening or potentially life-threatening dysrhythmias, often associated with an acute disorder. Others can be managed with office or clinic visits or in other settings.

Clients discharged from the hospital may have considerable needs, often more related to their underlying chronic diseases than to their dysrhythmias, which should be essentially controlled by drug or device therapy. A case manager or care coordinator can assess the need for health care resources and coordinate access to services.

HEALTH TEACHING

PREVENTION OF RECURRENCE. Clients who have experienced a dysrhythmia associated with an acute disorder, such as electrolyte imbalance or ischemia related to a myocardial infarction, are instructed in the prevention, early recognition, and management of that disorder. The nurse teaches the client and family about lifestyle modifications designed to prevent, decrease, or control the occurrence of dysrhythmias, as outlined in Chart 34-7. This teaching may be provided in the acute care setting, physician's office, health care clinic, or home setting.

DRUG THERAPY. Clients and designated caregivers must have a thorough understanding of the prescribed medications, including antidysrhythmic agents. Pharmacies provide written instructions with filled prescriptions. The nurse

CHART 34-7

CLIENT EDUCATION GUIDE
How to Prevent or Decrease Dysrhythmias

For Clients at Risk for Vasovagal Attacks Causing Bradydysrhythmias
- Avoid doing things that stimulate the vagus nerve, such as raising your arms above your head, applying pressure over your carotid artery, applying pressure on your eyes, bearing down or straining during a bowel movement, and stimulating a gag reflex when brushing your teeth or putting objects in your mouth.

For Clients with Premature Beats and Ectopic Rhythms
- Take the medications that have been prescribed for you, and report any adverse effects to your physician.
- Stop smoking, avoid caffeinated beverages as much as possible, and drink alcohol only in moderation.
- Learn ways to manage stress and avoid getting too tired.

For Clients with Ischemic Heart Disease
- If you have an angina attack, treat it promptly with rest and nitroglycerin administration as prescribed by your physician. This decreases your chances of experiencing a dysrhythmia.
- If chest pain is not relieved after taking the amount of nitroglycerin that has been prescribed for you, seek medical attention promptly. Also, seek prompt medical attention if the pain becomes more severe or you experience other symptoms, such as sweating, nausea, weakness, and palpitations.

For Clients at Risk for Potassium Imbalance
- Know the symptoms of decreased potassium levels, such as muscle weakness and cardiac irregularity.
- Eat foods high in potassium, such as tomatoes, beans, prunes, avocados, bananas, strawberries, and lettuce.
- Take the potassium supplements that have been prescribed for you.

teaches clients and families the generic and trade names of their drugs, as well as the drugs' purposes, using basic terms that are easily understood. Clear instructions regarding dosage schedules and common side effects are important (see Chart 34-3). The nurse emphasizes the importance of reporting these side effects and any dizziness, nausea, vomiting, chest discomfort, or shortness of breath to the health care provider. Chart 34-8 highlights special considerations for older adults receiving antidysrhythmic therapy.

PULSE CHECK. The nurse teaches all clients and their significant others or family members how to take a pulse. The nurse instructs them to report any signs of a change in heart rhythm, such as a significant decrease in pulse rate, a rate greater than 100 beats/min, or increased rhythm irregularity.

PACEMAKER. Clients who have a permanent pacemaker are given written and verbal information about the type and settings of their pacemaker. They are taught to report any pulse rate lower than that set on the pacemaker or lower than the hysteresis rate. The nurse also reviews the proper care of the pacemaker insertion site and the importance of reporting any fever or any redness, swelling, or drainage at the pacemaker insertion site. If the surgical incision is near either shoulder, the nurse teaches and demonstrates range-of-motion exercises to perform to prevent shoulder stiffness.

Clients with pacemakers are also instructed to keep handheld cellular phones at least 6 inches away from the generator, with the handset on the ear opposite the side of the generator. The nurse also teaches them to avoid sources of strong electromagnetic fields, such as magnets and telecommunications transmitters. These may cause interference and could change the pacemaker settings, causing a malfunction. Magnetic resonance imaging is contraindicated. The nurse instructs clients to carry a pacemaker identification card and to wear a medical alert bracelet. Chart 34-9 outlines the major points for client and family teaching after the insertion of a permanent pacemaker.

IMPLANTABLE CARDIOVERTER/DEFIBRILLATOR. Clients with an implantable cardioverter/defibrillator (ICD) usually continue to receive antidysrhythmic drugs after discharge from the hospital. The nurse provides clear instructions about the purposes of the medications, the dosage schedules, special instructions for taking the medications, and side effects to report. If clients experience an internal defibrillator shock, they must sit or lie down immediately and notify the physician. Some clients describe the experience of a shock as a quick thud or kick in the chest, whereas others relate severe pain similar to that of external defibrillation. The nurse informs family members that they may feel an electrical shock if they are touching the client during delivery of the shock but that it is not harmful. Information on how to access the emergency medical services (EMS) system in the community is provided. The nurse also recommends resources for the family to learn how to perform cardiopulmonary resuscitation (CPR).

The nurse teaches clients with an ICD to avoid sources of strong electromagnetic fields, such as large electrical generators and radio or television transmitters. These may inhibit tachydysrhythmia detection and therapy or may cause inadvertent antitachycardial pacing or shocks. Magnetic resonance imaging is contraindicated for clients with ICDs. Handheld cellular phones must be at least 6 inches away from the generator, with the handset held to the ear opposite the side of the ICD. If the pulse generator emits a beeping sound or provides some other indicator, the client must move away from the area as quickly as possible to prevent deactivation of the device. The client with an ICD should carry an ICD identification card and wear a medical alert bracelet. Chart 34-10 highlights the important points for teaching clients and family members and significant others.

HOME CARE MANAGEMENT

The focus of the home care nurse's interventions is assessment and health teaching. Clients and families often fear recurrence of a life-threatening dysrhythmia. Clients with an ICD may dread or fear the activation of the ICD. The community-based nurse provides the client and family members with an opportunity to verbalize their concerns and fears. The nurse provides emotional support, as well as information about support groups in the community, and makes appropriate referrals. The client is assessed for possible side effects of antidysrhythmic agents or complications from a pacemaker or ICD.

HEALTH CARE RESOURCES

The cardiac rehabilitation nurse typically provides written and oral information about dysrhythmias, antidysrhythmic drugs, pacemakers, and ICDs, as well as information about cardiac exercise programs, educational programs, and support groups. The office or clinic nurse may also provide informa-

CHART 34-8

NURSING FOCUS *on the* OLDER ADULT
Dysrhythmias

Older adults are at increased risk for dysrhythmias because of changes in their cardiac conduction system. The sinoatrial node has fewer pacemaker cells. There is a loss of fibers in the bundle branch system. Therefore older adults are at risk for sinus node dysfunction and may require pacemaker therapy. The most common dysrhythmias are premature atrial contractions, premature ventricular contractions, and atrial fibrillation. Dysrhythmias tend to be more serious in older clients because of underlying heart disease, causing cardiac decompensation. Consequently, blood flow to organs, which may already be decreased because of the aging process, is further compromised, leading to multisystem organ dysfunction. The following are special nursing considerations for the older client with dysrhythmias:

- Evaluate the client with dysrhythmias immediately for the presence of a life-threatening dysrhythmia or hemodynamic deterioration.
- Assess the client with a dysrhythmia for angina, hypotension, heart failure, and decreased cerebral and renal perfusion.
- Consider the following causes of dysrhythmias when taking the client's history: hypoxia, drug toxicity, electrolyte imbalances, heart failure, and myocardial ischemia or infarction.
- Assess the client's level of education, hearing, learning style, and ability to understand and recall instructions to determine the best approaches for teaching.
- Assess the client's ability to read written instructions.
- Teach the client the generic and trade names of prescribed antidysrhythmic drugs, as well as their purposes, dosage, side effects, and special instructions for their use.
- Provide clear, written instructions in basic language and easy-to-read print.
- Provide a written drug dosage schedule for the client, taking into account all of the medications the client is taking and possible drug interactions.
- Assess the client for possible side effects or adverse reactions to drugs, considering the client's age and health status.
- Teach the client to take his or her pulse and to report significant changes in heart rate or rhythm to the physician.
- Inform the client of available resources for blood pressure and pulse checks, such as blood pressure clinics, home health agencies, and cardiac rehabilitation programs.
- Instruct the client on the importance of keeping follow-up appointments with the physician and of reporting symptoms promptly.
- Include the client's family members or significant other in all teaching whenever possible.
- Instruct the client to avoid drinking caffeinated beverages, to stop smoking, to drink alcohol only in moderation, and to follow his or her prescribed diet.

CHART 34-9

CLIENT EDUCATION GUIDE
Permanent Pacemakers

- Follow the instructions for pacemaker site skin care that have been specifically prepared for you. Report any fever or redness, swelling, or drainage from the incision site to your physician.
- Keep your pacemaker identification card in your wallet and wear a medical alert bracelet.
- Take your pulse for 1 full minute at the same time each day and record the rate in your pacemaker diary. Take your pulse any time you feel symptoms of a possible pacemaker failure, and report your heart rate and symptoms to your physician.
- Know the rate at which your pacemaker is set and the basic functioning of your pacemaker. Know what rate changes to report to your physician.
- Do not apply pressure over your generator. Avoid tight clothing or belts.
- You may take baths or showers without concern for your pacemaker.
- Inform other physicians and dentists that you have a pacemaker. Certain tests they may wish to perform (such as magnetic resonance imaging) could affect or damage your pacemaker.
- Know the indications of battery failure for your pacemaker as you were instructed, and report these findings to your physician if they occur.
- Do not operate electrical appliances directly over your pacemaker site, because this may cause your pacemaker to malfunction.
- Do not lean over electrical or gasoline engines or motors. Be sure that electrical appliances or motors are properly grounded.
- Avoid all transmitter towers for radio, television, and radar. Radio, television, other home appliances, and antennas do not pose a hazard.
- Be aware that antitheft devices in stores may cause temporary pacemaker malfunction. If symptoms develop, move away from the device.
- Inform airport personnel of your pacemaker before passing through a metal detector and show them your pacemaker identification card. The metal in your pacemaker will trigger the alarm in the metal detector device.
- Stay away from any arc welding equipment.
- Be aware that it is safe to operate a microwave oven unless it does not have proper shielding (old microwave ovens) or is defective.
- Report any of the following symptoms to your physician if you experience them: difficulty breathing, dizziness, fainting, chest pain, weight gain, and prolonged hiccupping. If you have any of these symptoms, check your pulse rate and call your physician.
- If you feel symptoms when near any device, move 5 to 10 feet away from it and then check your pulse. Your pulse rate should return to normal.
- Keep all of your physician and pacemaker clinic appointments.
- Take all medications prescribed for you as instructed.
- Follow your prescribed diet.
- Follow instructions on restrictions on physical activity, such as no sudden, jerky movement for 8 weeks to allow the pacemaker to settle in place.

tion about resources. The nurse instructs the client on how to contact the local affiliate of the American Heart Association or the provincial affiliate of the Heart and Stroke Foundation in Canada for information about dysrhythmias, pacemakers, and CPR training.

Manufacturers of pacemakers and ICDs provide helpful booklets and videotapes to give clients and their families a better understanding of these therapies. Clients with pacemakers may have transtelephonic systems for transmission of their rhythms to a clinic or health care provider's office. The

CHART 34-10

CLIENT EDUCATION GUIDE
Implantable Cardioverter/Defibrillator

- Follow the instructions for implantable cardioverter defibrillator (ICD) site skin care that have been specifically prepared for you.
- Report to your physician any fever or redness, swelling, soreness, or drainage from your incision site.
- Do not wear tight clothing or belts that could cause irritation over the ICD generator.
- Avoid activities that involve rough contact with the ICD implantation site.
- Keep your ICD identification card in your wallet and consider wearing a medical alert bracelet.
- Know the basic functioning of your ICD device and its rate cutoff, as well as the number of consecutive shocks it can deliver.
- Avoid magnets directly over your ICD because they can inactivate the device. If beeping tones are coming from the ICD, move away from the electromagnetic field immediately (within 30 seconds) before the inactivation sequence is completed, and notify your physician.
- Inform all physicians and dentists caring for you that you have an ICD implanted, because certain diagnostic tests and procedures must be avoided to prevent ICD malfunction. These include diathermy, electrocautery, and nuclear magnetic resonance tests.
- Avoid other sources of electromagnetic interference, such as devices emitting microwaves (not microwave ovens); transformers; radio, television, and radar transmitters; large electrical generators; metal detectors, including handheld security devices at airports; antitheft devices; arc welding equipment; and sources of 60-cycle (Hz) interference. Also avoid leaning directly over the alternator of a running motor of a car or boat.
- Report to your physician symptoms such as fainting, nausea, weakness, blackout, and rapid pulse rates.
- Take all medications prescribed for you as instructed.
- Follow instructions on restrictions on physical activity, such as not swimming, driving motor vehicles, or operating dangerous equipment.
- Follow your prescribed diet.
- Keep all physician and ICD clinic appointments.
- Sit or lie down immediately if you feel dizzy or faint to avoid falling if the ICD discharges.
- Post emergency telephone numbers.
- Know how to contact the local emergency medical services (EMS) systems in your community. Inform them in advance that you have an ICD so that they can be prepared if they need to respond to an emergency call for you.
- Know how to perform cough cardiopulmonary resuscitation (CPR) as instructed.
- Encourage family members to learn how to perform CPR. Family members should know that if they are touching you when the device discharges, they may feel a slight shock, but that this is not harmful to them.
- Follow instructions on what to do if the ICD successfully discharges, after which you feel well. This may include maintaining a diary of the date, the time, activity preceding the shock, symptoms, the number of shocks delivered, and how you feel after the shock. The physician may wish to be notified each time the device discharges.
- Avoid strenuous activities that may cause your heart rate to meet or exceed the rate cutoff of your ICD, because this causes the device to discharge inappropriately.
- Notify your physician if you are leaving town or are relocating for information regarding access to health care.

nurse teaches clients how to use these systems. The importance of keeping scheduled appointments for office visits with the cardiologist and pacemaker or ICD clinic is stressed. The nurse instructs clients with an ICD to contact the local ambulance or paramedic services and emergency facilities to inform them that they have these devices implanted. The client and family are encouraged to attend pacemaker or ICD support groups.

Evaluation: Outcomes

NOC The nurse evaluates the care of the client with dysrhythmias on the basis of the identified nursing diagnoses and collaborative problems. The expected outcomes are that the client will:

- Have vital signs in the expected range (IER)
- Have cognitive status IER
- Perform activities of daily living without dyspnea or fatigue
- Be free of pulmonary edema

ONLINE RESOURCES

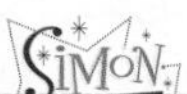

For suggested readings and Internet resources, go to http://www.wbsaunders.com/SIMON/Iggy/.

SELECTED BIBLIOGRAPHY

Asterisk indicates a classic or definitive work on this subject.

Alspach, J. (1998). *Core curriculum for critical care nursing* (5th ed.). Philadelphia: W.B. Saunders.

American Heart Association. (2000). Guidelines 2000 for cardiopulmonary resuscitation and emergency cardiovascular care. *Circulation, 102*(8), 112-124.

Ballew, C.C., & Reigle, J. (1998). Mechanisms and management of ventricular dysrhythmias in heart failure. *AACN Clinical Issues: Advanced Practice in Acute and Critical Care, 9*(2), 208-224.

Benner, P.E., et al. (1998). *Clinical wisdom and interventions in critical care: A thinking-in-action approach.* Philadelphia: W.B. Saunders.

*Conover, M.B. (1996). *Understanding electrocardiography: Arrhythmias and the 12-lead ECG* (7th ed.). St. Louis: Mosby.

Crowley, A. (1997). Emergency! Paroxysmal supraventricular tachycardia. *American Journal of Nursing, 97*(1), 53.

Davenport, J., & Morton, P.G. (1997). Identifying nonischemic causes of life-threatening arrhythmias. *American Journal of Nursing, 97*(11), 50-56.

Dubin, D. (1998). *Rapid interpretation of EKGs* (5th ed.). Tampa, FL: Cover Publishing.

Ellis, M.F. (1998). Atrial fibrillation following cardiac surgery. *Dimensions of Critical Care Nursing, 17*(5), 241-242.

Hartshorn, J., et al: (1997). *Introduction to critical care nursing* (7th ed.). Philadelphia: W.B. Saunders.

Hayes, D.D. (1997). Bradycardia: Keeping the current flowing. *Nursing97, 27*(6), 50-56.

Hellstedt, L.F. (1998). Treating ventricular tachyarrhythmias correctly. *Nursing98, 28*(9), 32cc1-32cc5.

Hiller, G.A. (1999). Atrial fibrillation: Soothing the savage beat. *Nursing99, 29*(2), 26-31.

Jung, F., & DiMarco, J.P. (1998). Treatment strategies for atrial fibrillation. *American Journal of Medicine, 104,* 272-286.

Kern, L.S. (1998). Management of post-operative atrial fibrillation. *Journal of Cardiovascular Nursing, 12*(3), 57-77.

Kinney, M.R., et al. (1998). *AACN clinical reference for critical care nursing* (4th ed.). St. Louis: Mosby.

Kruse, L., et al. (1998). Keeping pace with implanted defibrillators. *RN, 61*(8), 30-35.

Lazzara, D. (1999). Shocking facts about semiautomatic defibrillation. *Nursing99, 29*(4), 55-57.

Lezon, K. (1998). Code blue: Defibrillate. *Nursing98, 28*(4), 56-57.

Mancini, M.E., Richards, N., & Kaye, W. (1997). Saving lives with automated external defibrillators. *Nursing97, 27*(10), 42-43.

Marriott, H.J.L., & Conover, M.B. (1998). *Advanced concepts in arrhythmias* (3rd ed.). St. Louis: Mosby.

McCauley, K.M., Beauchamp, K., & Haber, H. (1998). Dysrhythmia update . . . the effects of intermittent heart block on the central venous pressure trace. *Cardiovascular Nursing, 12*(3), 78-81.

McCloskey, J.C., & Bulechek, G.M. (2000). *Nursing interventions classification (NIC)* (3rd ed.). St. Louis: Mosby.

Miracle, V., & Sims, J.M. (1998). Atrioventricular blocks. *Nursing98, 28*(6), 56-57.

Miracle, V., & Sims, J.M. (1999). Easy ECG series: Part 1. Making sense of the 12-lead ECG. *Nursing99, 29*(7), 34-40.

Moccia, M.M. (1998). When an arrhythmia hides a myocardial infarction . . . left bundle-branch block. *Nursing98, 28*(4), 32cc1-32cc3.

Newton, J.L. (2000). Action stat: Amiodarone overdose. *Nursing2000, 30*(2), 33.

Paul, S., et al. (1998). *The nurse's guide to cardiac rhythm interpretation: Implications for patient care.* Philadelphia: W.B. Saunders.

Resnick, B. (1999). Atrial fibrillation in the older adult: Presentation and management issues. *Geriatric Nursing, 20*(4), 188-194.

Riley, M. (1997). Elective cardioversion: Who, when, and how. *RN, 60*(5), 27-29.

Sargent, D.A. (1999). Using Ibutilide to convert atrial fibrillation and flutter. *Dimensions of Critical Care Nursing, 18*(4), 2-12.

Schull, P. (1997). *ECG interpretation made incredibly easy.* Springhouse, PA: Springhouse Publishing.

Shaffer, R.B. (1999). Keeping pace with permanent pacemakers: Part 1. *Nursing99, 18*(6), 2-8.

Sims, J.M., & Miracle, V. (1999). Easy ECG series: Part 2. Using the ECG to detect myocardial infarction. *Nursing99, 29*(8), 41-47.

Squires, A. (2000). Critical care: Teaching patients about telemetry. *Nursing2000, 30*(7), 32cc1-32cc4.

Thaler, M.S. (1999). *The only EKG book you'll ever need* (3rd ed.). Philadelphia: Lippincott, Williams & Wilkins.

Thelan, L.A., et al. (1998). *Critical care nursing: Diagnosis and management* (3rd ed.). St. Louis: Mosby.

Valenti, L.M., et al. (1998). *Critical care nursing.* Philadelphia: Lippincott, Williams & Wilkins.

Van Orden Wallace, C.J. (1998). Dual-chamber pacemakers in the management of severe heart failure. *Critical Care Nurse, 18*(2), 57-67.

Walraven, G. (1999). *Basic arrhythmias* (5th ed.). Upper Saddle River, NJ: Brady/Prentice-Hall.

CHAPTER 35

Interventions for Clients with Cardiac Problems

KATHLEEN OUIMET PERRIN

Learning Objectives

After studying this chapter, you should be able to:

1. Explain the pathophysiology of heart failure.
2. Compare and contrast left-sided and right-sided heart failure.
3. Perform a comprehensive assessment of clients experiencing heart failure.
4. Identify common nursing diagnoses and collaborative problems for clients with heart failure.
5. Evaluate the effects of interventions for reducing preload and afterload.
6. Describe special considerations for older adults with heart failure.
7. Discuss the prevention of complications for clients with heart failure.
8. Prioritize nursing care for clients experiencing heart failure.
9. Identify essential focused assessments used by the home care nurse for clients with heart failure.
10. Compare and contrast common valvular disorders.
11. Discuss surgical management for clients with valvular disease.
12. Develop a teaching/learning plan for clients with valvular disease.
13. Differentiate between common cardiac inflammations and infections—endocarditis, pericarditis, and rheumatic carditis.
14. Discuss the legal/ethical aspects related to heart transplantation, including cost of care.

SIMON

Go to http://www.wbsaunders.com/SIMON/Iggy/ for self-assessment questions related to these Learning Objectives.

Primary cardiac dysfunction may have a number of causes, including impaired cardiac muscle function, structural cardiac defects, infections within the heart, and inflammatory conditions of the heart. Although most Americans do not consider heart disease an incurable illness, more people die from heart disease than from the next seven leading causes of death combined. "More than 2600 Americans die of cardiovascular disease (CVD) every day, an average of one death every 33 seconds" (American Heart Association [AHA], 1998, p. 3). Survival following the onset of heart failure is poor, with a median survival rate of 1.7 years for men and 3.2 years for women.

Long-term survival of clients with heart disease depends on a coordinated interdisciplinary approach to ensure the best management of the illness and the highest possible quality of life. Therefore, as described in Chapter 3, high-risk clients are often targeted for case management to coordinate their care through the health care continuum.

HEART FAILURE

OVERVIEW

Heart failure, also called *cardiac failure* or *pump failure,* is the inability of the heart to pump sufficient blood to meet the demands of the body. Because fluid excess is not always present, the term **congestive heart failure** may not be applicable. Heart failure may be due to either increased cellular demands or, more commonly, to impaired pumping of the heart. When the heart fails, cardiac output is diminished and peripheral tissue is not adequately perfused. Congestion of the lungs and periphery may also develop.

Pathophysiology

COMPENSATORY MECHANISMS

When cardiac output is insufficient to meet the demands of the body, compensatory mechanisms operate to improve cardiac output. Although these compensatory mechanisms may initially increase cardiac output, they eventually have a damaging effect on pump function. Compensatory mechanisms include the following:

- Increased heart rate
- Improved stroke volume
- Arterial vasoconstriction
- Sodium and water retention
- Myocardial hypertrophy

In heart failure, stimulation of the sympathetic nervous system represents the most immediate compensatory mechanism. Stimulation of the adrenergic receptors causes an increase in heart rate (beta adrenergic) and vasoconstriction (alpha adrenergic).

INCREASED HEART RATE. Because cardiac output is the product of heart rate and stroke volume, an increase in heart rate results in an immediate increase in cardiac output. An increase in heart rate is limited in its ability to compensate for decreased cardiac output. If heart rate becomes too rapid, diastolic filling time is limited and cardiac output may start to fall. An increase in heart rate also significantly increases oxygen demand by the myocardium. If the heart is poorly perfused because of arteriosclerosis, heart failure may worsen.

IMPROVED STROKE VOLUME. Stroke volume is also improved by sympathetic stimulation. Sympathetic stimulation increases venous return to the heart, which further stretches the myocardial fibers. This increased stretch is referred to as **preload.** In accordance with Starling's law of the heart, increased myocardial stretch results in more forceful contraction, which increases stroke volume and cardiac output. After a critical point is reached, further volume and stretch reduce the force of contraction and cardiac output.

ARTERIAL VASOCONSTRICTION. Sympathetic stimulation also results in arterial vasoconstriction. Constriction of the arteries has the benefit of maintaining blood pressure and improving tissue perfusion in low-output states. However, constriction of the arteries increases **afterload,** the resistance against which the heart must pump. Afterload is the major determinant of myocardial oxygen requirements. As afterload increases, the left ventricle requires more energy to eject its contents, and stroke volume may decline.

SODIUM AND WATER RETENTION. Reduced blood flow to the kidneys, a common occurrence in low-output states, results in the activation of the renin-angiotensin-aldosterone mechanism. Vasoconstriction becomes more pronounced in response to angiotensin, and aldosterone secretion causes sodium and water retention. The volume of blood returning to the left ventricle is further increased by activation of this mechanism.

MYOCARDIAL HYPERTROPHY. Myocardial hypertrophy, with or without chamber dilation, is the final compensatory mechanism. The walls of the heart thicken to provide more muscle mass. This results in more forceful contractions, further increasing cardiac output. However, cardiac muscle may hypertrophy more rapidly than collateral circulation can provide adequate blood supply to the muscle. Often, a hypertrophied heart is slightly oxygen deprived.

• • •

These mechanisms of compensation act primarily to restore cardiac output to near-normal levels. However, when these cardiac and peripheral circulatory adjustments become excessive, they may actually decrease pump function. All of them contribute to an increase in the consumption of myocardial oxygen. When this occurs and the myocardial reserve has been exhausted, clinical manifestations of heart failure develop.

CLASSIFICATION OF HEART FAILURE

Heart failure can be classified in many ways. Several important categories are discussed in the following sections.

SYSTOLIC VERSUS DIASTOLIC DYSFUNCTION. **Systolic dysfunction** results when the ventricle is unable to contract forcefully enough during systole to eject adequate amounts of blood into the circulation. The ejection fraction (the percentage of blood ejected from the heart during systole) drops from a normal of 50% to 70% to below 40%. As the ejection fraction decreases, tissue perfusion diminishes and blood accumulates in the pulmonary vasculature. Symptoms of systolic dysfunction may be symptoms of inadequate tissue perfusion or pulmonary and systemic congestion.

In contrast, **diastolic failure** occurs when the left ventricle is unable to relax adequately during diastole. Inadequate relaxation prevents the ventricle from filling with sufficient blood to ensure an adequate cardiac output. Diastolic failure may represent 20% to 40% of all heart failure, primarily in older adults and in women following a myocardial infarction. Symptoms of diastolic failure are similar to those of systolic dysfunction. However, treatment is not clearly established and is not discussed in this text.

LEFT VERSUS RIGHT VENTRICULAR FAILURE. Because the two ventricles of the heart represent two separate pumping systems, it is possible for one to fail by itself for a short period. Most heart failure begins with failure of the left ventricle and progresses to failure of both ventricles. Typical causes of **left ventricular failure** include hypertensive disease, coronary artery disease, and valvular disease involving the mitral or aortic valve. Decreased tissue perfusion from poor cardiac output and pulmonary congestion from increased pressure in the pulmonary vessels indicate left ventricular failure.

Right ventricular failure may be caused by left ventricular failure, right ventricular myocardial infarction, or pulmonary hypertension. In right ventricular failure, the right ventricle is unable to empty completely. Increased volume and pressure develop in the systemic veins, and systemic venous congestion and peripheral edema develop. Figure 35-1 illustrates the pathophysiology of heart failure.

LOW-OUTPUT VERSUS HIGH-OUTPUT SYNDROME. **Low-output syndrome,** the more common type of heart failure, occurs when the heart fails as a pump, resulting in impaired peripheral circulation and peripheral vasoconstriction. **High-output syndrome** is present when

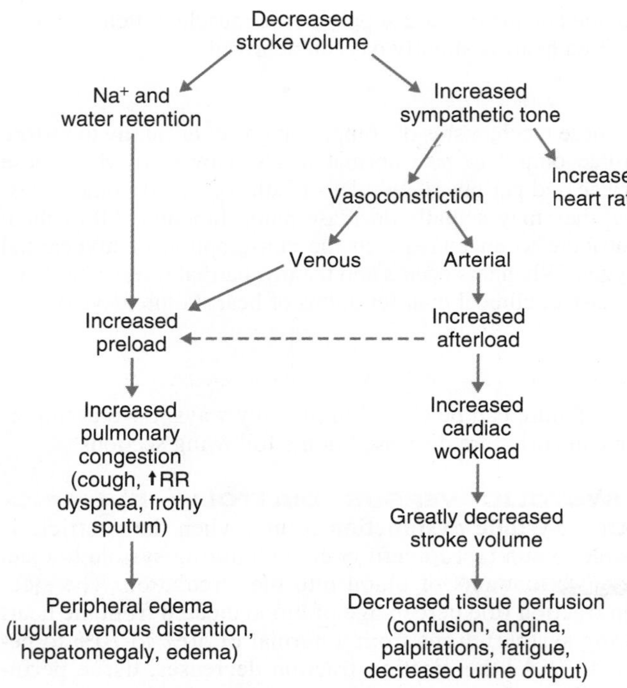

Figure 35-1 ● Pathophysiology of heart failure. (↑*RR*, Increased respiratory rate.)

TABLE 35-1 • COMMON PREDISPOSING FACTORS TO SYSTOLIC HEART FAILURE
• Hypertension (see Chapter 36) • Coronary artery disease (see Chapter 38) • Cardiomyopathy • Substance abuse (alcohol and illicit/prescribed drugs) (see Chapter 8) • Valvular disease • Congenital defects

cardiac output remains normal or above normal but the metabolic needs of the body are not met. It may be caused by increased metabolic needs (hyperthyroidism, fever, pregnancy) or hyperkinetic conditions (arteriovenous fistulas, Paget's disease).

FUNCTIONAL STATUS. Heart failure may also be categorized by its effect on the client's functional status. Table 33-2 in Chapter 33 summarizes the New York Heart Association (NYHA) categories.

Etiology

The most common cause of heart failure is myocardial infarction. The next most common causes are conditions such as systemic hypertension and pulmonary or aortic stenosis, which cause pressure or volume overload on the heart. Other direct causes of heart failure are myocardial dysfunction, filling disorders, and increased metabolic demand. Some of the conditions capable of causing heart failure are listed in Table 35-1.

COST OF CARE IMPLICATIONS FOR NURSING

HEART FAILURE

Cost of Care

Heart failure is the most common cause of hospitalization for clients 65 years of age and older. According to the American Heart Association, hospitalizations for heart failure cost $3.4 billion in 1995, or $5,153 per hospital discharge. Estimated additional costs for heart failure include the following (AHA, 1998):

- $11.4 billion in additional hospital and nursing home charges
- $1.4 billion in health care provider charges
- $1 billion for medications
- $2.1 billion for home health care and medical durables

In 1997, 2290 heart transplants were performed in the United States at 158 different transplant centers. The estimated cost for the first year of care following a heart transplant is $253,200, and the estimated cost for subsequent yearly follow-up is $21,200 (AHA, 1998).

Implications for Nursing

Because of the high cost of hospitalization and nursing home care for clients with heart failure, nurses must be attuned to enhancing client education, promoting client self-management of heart failure, and developing ways to deliver effective nursing care in the home to clients with heart failure.

Incidence/Prevalence

More than 4.5 million people in the United States are living with heart failure (AHA, 1998), with approximately 400,000 new cases occurring each year. Heart failure is more common in men than in women. The cost of providing care for this number of people with heart failure is detailed in the Cost of Care box above.

CONSIDERATIONS FOR OLDER ADULTS

Heart failure occurs most commonly in older adults; 50% of clients with heart failure are older than 70 years of age. The prevalence of heart failure steadily increases with aging; heart failure occurs in 3% of people 45 to 64 years of age, 6% of people 65 years and older, and 10% of people older than 80 years (Albert, 1999).

One of the Healthy People 2010 objectives for the United States is to reduce by 50% the number of hospitalizations of older adults with heart failure as the principal diagnosis. Interventions aimed at client and family education can help meet this objective (see the Meeting Healthy People 2010 Objectives box on p. 701).

➤ COLLABORATIVE MANAGEMENT

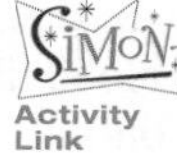

● Assessment

Manifestations of heart failure depend on the type of failure, the ventricle involved, and the underlying cause. Impaired tissue perfusion, pulmonary congestion, and edema dominate the picture of left ventricular failure (Chart 35-1). Systemic venous congestion and peripheral edema are associated with right ventricular failure (Chart 35-2).

HISTORY

When obtaining a history, the nurse should keep in mind the many conditions that can lead to heart failure. The client is

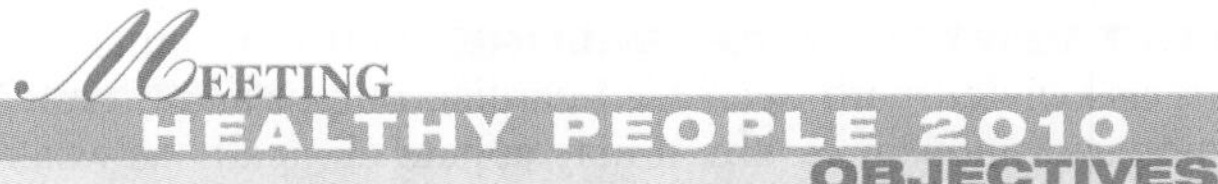

CARDIAC DISEASE

Objective 12.6: Reduce hospitalizations of older adults with heart failure as the principal diagnosis.

- For clients hospitalized for heart failure, collaborate with the case manager for discharge planning, including adequate support in the community.
- Provide a continuing plan of care for clients and their families or other caregivers when the client is discharged from the hospital.
- If the client is discharged to home, call the client to check that he or she has no impending signs and symptoms of heart failure (the case manager may make calls).
- Teach the client and family or other caregiver about when to call the health care provider for health changes so the client can be treated at home.
- Ensure that the interdisciplinary team provides the client with follow-up care in the home or nursing home.

CHART 35-1

KEY FEATURES *of* Left-Sided Heart Failure

Decreased Cardiac Output
- Fatigue
- Weakness
- Oliguria during the day
- Angina
- Confusion, restlessness
- Dizziness
- Tachycardia, palpitations
- Pallor
- Weak peripheral pulses
- Cool extremities

Pulmonary Congestion
- Hacking cough, worse at night
- Dyspnea/breathlessness
- Crackles or wheezes in lungs
- Frothy, pink-tinged sputum
- Tachypnea
- S_3/S_4 summation gallop

CHART 35-2

KEY FEATURES *of* Right-Sided Heart Failure

Systemic Congestion
- Jugular (neck vein) distention
- Enlarged liver and spleen
- Anorexia and nausea
- Dependent edema (legs and sacrum)
- Distended abdomen
- Swollen hands and fingers
- Polyuria at night
- Weight gain
- Increased blood pressure (from excess volume) or decreased blood pressure (from failure)

EVIDENCE-BASED PRACTICE FOR NURSING

What do hospitalized clients think they need to know about heart failure?

Wehby, D., & Brenner, P.S. (1999). Perceived learning needs of patients with heart failure. *Heart and Lung, 28*(1), 31-40.

The purpose of this quantitative research study was to compare the perceived learning needs identified by hospitalized clients experiencing heart failure with the learning needs identified by registered nurses (RNs) employed on the hospital units.

The primary differences between nurses and clients were that clients perceived knowledge of signs and symptoms of worsening heart failure and instruction about diet to be less important than did nurses. Clients also perceived it to be more realistic to include all the components of heart failure teaching during hospitalization than did nurses.

Critique. The study used purposeful sampling to ensure a heterogeneous population. The sample (83 clients and 83 nurses) was adequate to achieve a power of 0.80 and an effect size of 0.30. A reliable questionnaire based on the suggestions of the Agency for Healthcare Research and Quality for education of heart failure clients was used to identify client learning needs. One limitation was that the study did not address the client's baseline knowledge of heart failure.

Implications for Nursing. Other studies have demonstrated that increased sodium intake may trigger readmission for heart failure. Thus it is interesting that nurses perceive dietary teaching to be more important than do clients. The authors of the study suggest that clients may believe their dietary habits to be deeply ingrained and unchangeable. Nurses must be able to explain how sodium intake affects fluid retention so that clients can understand why diet, especially sodium restriction, is an important component of self-management.

carefully questioned about his or her medical history, including high blood pressure, angina, myocardial infarction, rheumatic heart disease, valvular disorders, endocarditis, and pericarditis. The nurse also asks about the client's perception of his or her activity tolerance, breathing pattern, urinary pattern, and fluid volume status, as well as his or her knowledge about heart failure (see the Evidence-Based Practice for Nursing box at right).

LEFT VENTRICULAR FAILURE. With left ventricular systolic dysfunction, cardiac output is diminished, impaired tissue perfusion results, anaerobic metabolism occurs, and the client often reports unusual fatigue. The nurse assesses activity tolerance by asking if the client can perform normal activities of daily living (ADLs) or climb flights of stairs without fatigue or dyspnea. Many clients with heart failure experience weakness or fatigue with activity or have a feeling of heaviness in their arms or legs. They should be asked about their ability to perform simultaneous arm and leg work (e.g., walking while carrying a bag of groceries). Such activity may place an unacceptable demand on the failing heart. The nurse asks clients to name their most strenuous activity in the past week. Many unconsciously limit their activities in response to fatigue or dyspnea and may not realize how limited they have become.

Perfusion to the myocardium is often impaired with left ventricular failure, especially if cardiac muscle has hypertrophied. The client may report chest discomfort or may describe palpitations, skipped beats, or a fast heartbeat.

As the amount of blood ejected from the left ventricle diminishes, pressure builds in the pulmonary venous system and results in fluid-filled alveoli and pulmonary congestion. Thus cough is often an early manifestation of heart failure. The client in early heart failure describes the cough as irritating, nocturnal, and usually nonproductive. As heart failure becomes very severe, the client may begin expectorating frothy, pink-tinged sputum—a sign of pulmonary edema.

Dyspnea also results from rising pulmonary venous pressure and pulmonary congestion. The nurse carefully questions the client about the presence of dyspnea and when and how it developed. The client may refer to dyspnea as "trouble in catching my breath," "breathlessness," or "difficulty in breathing."

As exertional dyspnea develops, the client often discontinues previously tolerated levels of activity because of shortness of breath. Dyspnea at rest in the recumbent position is known as **orthopnea.** The nurse asks the client how many pillows he or she usually uses to sleep or if he or she sleeps in an upright position in a bed or a chair.

Clients who describe sudden awakening with a feeling of breathlessness 2 to 5 hours after falling asleep have **paroxysmal nocturnal dyspnea (PND).** Sitting upright, dangling the feet, or walking usually relieves this condition.

CONSIDERATIONS FOR OLDER ADULTS

Decreased cerebral perfusion resulting from low cardiac output leads to changes in mental status. Confusion may occur with even mild or moderate heart failure in a very old client. The nurse asks the client and his or her family members if any memory lapses or periods of disorientation have occurred.

RIGHT VENTRICULAR FAILURE. Signs of systemic congestion occur as the right ventricle fails, fluid is retained, and pressure builds in the venous system. Edema develops in the lower legs and ascends to the thighs and abdominal wall. Clients may note that their shoes fit more tightly, or their shoes or socks may leave indentations on their swollen feet. They have removed their rings because of swelling in their fingers and hands. The nurse asks about weight gain. An adult may retain 4 to 7 L of fluid (10 to 15 pounds [4.5 to 6.8 kg]) before pitting edema occurs.

Gastrointestinal complaints of nausea and anorexia may be a direct consequence of liver engorgement resulting from fluid retention. In advanced heart failure, ascites and an increased abdominal girth may develop from the pronounced liver congestion. Another finding related to fluid retention is diuresis at rest. At rest, fluid in the peripheral tissue is mobilized and excreted, and the client describes frequent awakening at night to urinate.

The nurse or dietitian obtains a careful nutritional history, questioning the client about the use of salt and the types of food consumed. The nurse also asks about daily fluid intake. Clients with heart failure may experience increased thirst and take in excessive fluid (4000 to 5000 mL) because of aldosterone secretion.

PHYSICAL ASSESSMENT/CLINICAL MANIFESTATIONS

The signs and symptoms of heart failure can be considered in the context of these components of the syndrome:

- Failure of the left ventricle as a pump with decreased tissue perfusion and pulmonary venous congestion
- Failure of the right ventricle as a pump with systemic venous congestion

LEFT VENTRICULAR FAILURE. Left ventricular failure is associated with decreased cardiac output and elevated pulmonary venous pressure. It may appear clinically as weakness, fatigue, dizziness, confusion, pulmonary congestion, breathlessness, oliguria, or death (see Chart 35-1). Decreased blood flow to the major body organs can cause organ failure, especially renal failure.

The nurse or a nursing staff member obtains the client's vital signs. When obtaining blood pressure, the nurse should note if an auscultatory gap or orthostatic (postural) hypotension is present. The proportional pulse pressure ([systolic pressure − diastolic pressure] ÷ systolic pressure) is calculated. A proportional pulse pressure less than 25% indicates severely compromised cardiac output. The pulse may be tachycardiac (fast) or may alternate in strength (pulsus alternans). The nurse takes the apical pulse for a full minute, noting any irregularity in heart rhythm. An irregular heart rhythm resulting from premature atrial contractions (PACs), premature ventricular contractions (PVCs), and/or atrial fibrillation is common in heart failure. The sudden development of an irregular rhythm may further compromise cardiac output. The client's respiratory rate, rhythm, and character are carefully monitored. The respiratory rate typically exceeds 20 breaths/min.

The nurse also determines whether the client is oriented to person, place, and time. A short mental status examination may be used if there are concerns about orientation. Objective data are important because many people are skillful at covering up memory losses in daily conversation.

The cardiac nurse palpates the precordium. Increased heart size is common, with a displacement of the apical impulse to the left. On auscultation, the nurse may hear a third heart sound (S_3) gallop, an early diastolic filling sound indicating an increase in left ventricular pressure. A fourth heart sound (S_4) can also occur; it is not a sign of failure but is a reflection of decreased ventricular compliance.

Crackles and wheezes may be present on auscultation of the lungs. Late inspiratory crackles and fine profuse crackles that repeat themselves from breath to breath and do not diminish with coughing indicate heart failure. Crackles are produced by intra-alveolar fluid and are often noted first in the dependent areas of the lungs. Crackles usually develop in the bases and spread upward as the condition worsens. The nurse identifies the precise location of the crackles. Wheezes indicate a narrowing of the bronchial lumen caused by engorged pulmonary vessels.

RIGHT VENTRICULAR FAILURE. Right ventricular failure is associated with increased systemic venous pressures and congestion. Signs and symptoms are listed in Chart 35-2.

On inspection, the nurse may assess the neck veins for distention (see Chapter 33). The nurse may also measure abdominal girth and assess for hepatomegaly (liver engorgement), hepatojugular reflux (see Chapter 33), and ascites. Abdominal fluid can reach volumes of more than 10 L.

The nurse also examines for dependent edema. In ambulatory clients, edema is normally located in the ankles and legs. When the client is restricted to bedrest, the sacrum is dependent and edema accumulates there. Edema is an extremely unreliable sign of heart failure, and therefore accurate daily weights are needed to document fluid retention. *Weight is the most reliable indicator of fluid gain or loss.*

PSYCHOSOCIAL ASSESSMENT

Many clients with heart failure have symptoms that are not well controlled. These clients may have anxiety and frustrations or be depressed about dealing with a chronic illness. The nurse assesses clients and their families for fears, anxieties, and frustrations and also assesses their usual methods of coping.

Acute episodes of heart failure may be precipitated in susceptible people by stressful life situations. Acute exacerbations of heart failure may result from feelings of rejection, insecurity, frustration, or rage. The nurse needs to question clients sensitively about any recent stressors in their lives. The nurse asks them to rate their current level of stress and to describe any significant recent life changes.

Hope is a major determinant of well-being for clients in heart failure. Clients who are hopeful tend to feel better and are more socially involved. The nurse might ask clients about their activities and the significant people in their life and how often they are able to interact with them.

LABORATORY ASSESSMENT

Electrolyte imbalance may occur from complications of heart failure or as side effects of drug therapy, especially diuretic therapy. Regular evaluations of a client's serum electrolytes, including sodium, potassium, magnesium, calcium, and chloride, are essential. Any impairment of renal function may be reflected by elevated blood urea nitrogen, serum creatinine, and creatinine clearance levels. Urinalysis may reveal proteinuria and high specific gravity. Hemoglobin and hematocrit tests should be performed to identify heart failure resulting from anemia.

Arterial blood gas values often reveal hypoxia (low oxygen level) because oxygen does not diffuse easily through fluid-filled alveoli. Respiratory alkalosis may occur because of hyperventilation, and respiratory acidosis may occur because of carbon dioxide retention. Metabolic acidosis may indicate an accumulation of lactic acid.

> **CONSIDERATIONS FOR OLDER ADULTS**
> Thyroxine (T_4) and thyroid-stimulating hormone (TSH) levels should be determined in clients who are over 65 years of age, have atrial fibrillation, or have evidence of thyroid disease. Heart failure may be caused or aggravated by hypothyroidism or hyperthyroidism.

RADIOGRAPHIC ASSESSMENT

Chest x-ray studies can be helpful in diagnosing left ventricular failure. Typically, the heart is enlarged (cardiomegaly), representing hypertrophy or dilation. Pleural effusions develop less often and generally reflect biventricular failure.

OTHER DIAGNOSTIC ASSESSMENT

An electrocardiogram (ECG) is also performed. The ECG may demonstrate ventricular hypertrophy, dysrhythmias, and any degree of myocardial ischemia, injury, or infarction. It is not helpful in determining the presence or extent of heart failure.

Echocardiography is useful in diagnosing cardiac valvular changes, pericardial effusion, chamber enlargement, and ventricular hypertrophy. Radionuclide studies (thallium imaging or technetium pyrophosphate scanning) can also indicate the presence and cause of heart failure. Multigated angiographic (MUGA) scans provide information about left ventricular ejection fraction and velocity, which is typically low in clients with heart failure.

Pulmonary artery catheters allow the assessment of cardiac function and volume status in acutely ill clients. These measurements can confirm the diagnosis and guide the management of heart failure. Right atrial pressure may be normal or elevated in left ventricular failure and is elevated in right ventricular failure. Pulmonary artery pressure and pulmonary artery wedge pressure (PAWP) are elevated in left-sided heart failure because volumes and pressures are increased in the left ventricle. (See Chapter 33 for a more detailed description of these diagnostic assessments.)

Analysis

COMMON NURSING DIAGNOSES AND COLLABORATIVE PROBLEMS

The following are common nursing diagnoses for clients with heart failure:

1. Impaired Gas Exchange related to inadequate cardiac pump function
2. Decreased Cardiac Output related to a reduction in stroke volume as a result of mechanical malfunctions
3. Activity Intolerance related to an imbalance between oxygen supply and demand, fatigue, or an electrolyte imbalance

The primary collaborative problem is Potential for Pulmonary Edema.

ADDITIONAL NURSING DIAGNOSES AND COLLABORATIVE PROBLEMS

In addition to the common nursing diagnoses and collaborative problems, clients with heart failure may have one or more of the following:

- Ineffective Therapeutic Regimen Management related to failed social support systems, inadequate follow-up, inadequate discharge planning, or knowledge deficit
- Ineffective Coping related to physical inactivity, major changes in lifestyle, loss of control over body function, or fear of death
- Acute Confusion related to impaired gas exchange
- Impaired Physical Mobility related to fatigue and activity intolerance

Some clients are also at risk for the following collaborative problems:

- Potential for Pneumonia
- Potential for Dysrhythmias
- Potential for Renal Dysfunction secondary to decreased renal perfusion

Planning and Implementation

IMPAIRED GAS EXCHANGE

NOC **PLANNING: EXPECTED OUTCOMES.** The client with heart failure is expected to have (1) a normal rate, rhythm, and depth of respiration, (2) an oxygen saturation within normal limits (WNL), and (3) no dyspnea at rest.

INTERVENTIONS. The purpose of care is to promote an optimal spontaneous breathing pattern that maximizes oxygen and maintains a normal carbon dioxide level in the lungs (Chart 35-3).

NIC **VENTILATION ASSISTANCE.** The nurse or assistive nursing personnel monitors the client's respiratory rate, rhythm, and character every 1 to 4 hours and auscultates breath sounds. The oxygen content of the blood is often markedly reduced in clients who are experiencing pulmonary congestion. The nurse may titrate the amount of supplemental oxygen delivered to the client within a range prescribed by the health care provider to maintain oxygen saturation at 92% or greater.

If the client is experiencing respiratory difficulty, the nurse or assistive nursing personnel places him or her in a high Fowler's position with pillows under each arm to maximize chest expansion and improve oxygenation. Repositioning and performing coughing and deep breathing exercises every 2 hours helps to improve oxygenation and prevent atelectasis.

CHART 35-3

NIC INTERVENTION ACTIVITIES *for* The Client with Heart Failure

Ventilation Assistance: *Promotion of the optimal spontaneous breathing pattern that maximizes oxygen and carbon dioxide exchange in the lungs*
- Monitor respiratory and oxygenation status.
- Initiate and maintain supplemental oxygen, as prescribed.
- Position to alleviate dyspnea.
- Auscultate breath sounds, noting areas of decreased or absent ventilation, and presence of adventitious sounds.
- Position to minimize respiratory efforts (e.g., elevate the head of the bed and provide overbed table for client to lean on).
- Monitor the effects of position change on oxygenation: ABG, Sao_2, Svo_2, end tidal CO_2, Q_{sp}/Q_t, A-aDO_2 levels.

Hemodynamic Regulation: *Optimization of heart rate, preload, afterload, and contractility*
- Monitor and document heart rate, rhythm, and pulses.
- Monitor peripheral pulses, capillary refill, and temperature and color of extremities.
- Monitor pulmonary capillary pressure/pulmonary artery wedge pressure and central venous/right atrial pressure, if appropriate.
- Administer vasodilator and/or vasoconstrictor medication, as appropriate.
- Administer positive inotropic/contractility medications.
- Maintain fluid balance by administering IV fluids or diuretics, as appropriate.
- Monitor intake/output, urine output, and client weight, as appropriate.
- Monitor electrolyte levels.
- Evaluate side effects of negative inotropic medications.

Energy Management: *Regulating energy use to prevent fatigue and optimize function*
- Monitor cardiorespiratory response to activity (e.g., tachycardia, other dysrhythmias, dyspnea, diaphoresis, pallor, hemodynamic pressures, and respiratory rate).
- Determine client's physical limitations.
- Encourage alternate rest and activity periods.
- Arrange physical activities to reduce competition for oxygen supply to vital body functions (e.g., avoid activity immediately after meals).
- Encourage physical activity (e.g., ambulation or performance of activities of daily living, consistent with client's energy resources).
- Monitor client's oxygen response (e.g., pulse rate, cardiac rhythm, and respiratory rate) to self-care or nursing activities.
- Teach client and significant other techniques of self-care that will minimize oxygen consumption (e.g., self-monitoring and pacing techniques for performance of activities of daily living).

NIC intervention activities selected from McCloskey, J.C., & Bulechek, G.M. (Eds.). (2000). *Nursing interventions classification (NIC)* (3rd ed.). St. Louis: Mosby. No part of this work is to be altered without prior written permission from the Publisher.

ABG, Arterial blood gas, *CO_2,* carbon dioxide, *Sao_2,* saturation of arterial oxygen, *Svo_2,* saturation of venous oxygen, Q_{sp}/Q_t, physiologic blood flow per minute/cardiac output per minute; *A-aDO_2,* alveolar-arterial oxygen pressure difference.

DECREASED CARDIAC OUTPUT

NOC **PLANNING: EXPECTED OUTCOMES.** The client with heart failure is expected to resume and maintain an adequate cardiac output, as indicated by (1) a heart rate in expected range (IER), (2) a cardiac index IER, (3) dysrhythmia not present, (4) abnormal heart sounds not present, and (5) peripheral pulses strong.

INTERVENTIONS. The purpose of care is to optimize afterload, preload, and contractility, thus improving cardiac output. Therapy may be directed toward optimizing the two major components of cardiac output: stroke volume (determined by preload, afterload, and contractility) and heart rate (see Chart 35-3). (See Chapter 33 for a further explanation of these concepts.)

NIC **HEMODYNAMIC REGULATION.** Interventions to optimize stroke volume include reducing afterload, reducing preload, and improving cardiac muscle contractility.

REDUCING AFTERLOAD. By relaxing the arterioles, arterial vasodilators can reduce the resistance to left ventricular ejection (afterload) and improve cardiac output. These drugs do not cause excessive vasodilation but reverse some of the inappropriate or excessive vasoconstriction common in heart failure.

Clients with even mild heart failure resulting from left ventricular dysfunction should be given a trial of angiotensin-converting enzyme (ACE) inhibitors. ACE inhibitors are a group of arterial vasodilators such as enalapril (Vasotec), moexipril (Univasc), and captopril (Capoten). In general, these drugs prolong and improve the quality of life for clients with heart failure (Chart 35-4). They enhance functional status, with 40% to 80% of clients showing an improvement in the New York Heart Association (NYHA) class.

ACE inhibitors suppress the renin-angiotensin-aldosterone system, which is activated in response to decreased renal blood flow. ACE inhibitors benefit clients by reducing arterial resistance, decreasing pulmonary artery wedge pressure, and increasing stroke volume and cardiac output.

The health care provider usually starts doses of ACE inhibitors slowly and cautiously. The first dose of an ACE inhibitor is sometimes associated with a rapid drop in blood pressure. Clients at risk for hypotension following ACE inhibitor administration have initial systolic blood pressures less than 100 mm Hg, are older than 75 years of age, have a serum sodium level less than 135 mEq/L, or are volume depleted. Blood pressure is monitored for several hours after the initial dose and each time the dose is increased.

The nurse clarifies with the health care provider the guidelines for administering the vasodilator. For example, many clinicians maintain clients with heart failure at systolic blood pressures ranging from 90 to 110 mm Hg. When such a blood pressure is the maintenance level, the client is assessed for orthostatic hypotension, confusion, poor peripheral perfusion, and reduced urine output. While the client is receiving ACE inhibitors, the nurse monitors serum potassium levels for hyperkalemia, serum creatinine for renal dysfunction, and the client for development of a cough. Table 35-2 compares the effects of selected agents that reduce preload and afterload. Intravenous (IV) medications

CHART 35-4

DRUG THERAPY *for* Cardiac Failure

Drug	Usual Dosage	Nursing Interventions	Rationale
DRUGS COMMONLY USED PRIMARILY TO REDUCE AFTERLOAD			
Angiotensin-Converting Enzyme Inhibitors			
Captopril (Capoten)	To start: 6.25-12.5 mg tid PO May increase to 50-100 mg tid PO	Monitor the client's blood pressure closely for several hours after the first dose. Consult with the health care provider to determine the desired range for blood pressure.	Hypotension may occur as a first-dose effect. It is most common in sodium- or volume-depleted clients.
		Monitor the serum creatinine and potassium levels carefully	Clients with impaired renal function may develop hyperkalemia.
		Report fever and sore throat to the health care provider. Monitor the results of the complete blood count.	Neutropenia, although rare, can be a hazardous complication.
		Report cough to the health care provider	Cough is a side effect of the drug.
Enalapril maleate (Vasotec)	To start: 2.5-5 mg/day May increase to 10-40 mg/day as a single dose or divided doses	Administer 1 hr before or 2 hr after meals.	Administration on an empty stomach enhances absorption.
		Enalapril is similar to captopril but may be administered less frequently.	Enalapril has a longer half-life than captopril.
DRUGS COMMONLY USED PRIMARILY TO REDUCE PRELOAD			
Loop Diuretics			
Furosemide (Lasix, Furoside✤)	40 mg qd or bid PO 40 mg qd IV push (may increase to 80 mg and repeat × 1 in 30 min in acute situations) Older adults may be more sensitive to the effects of the usual adult dose	Administer once daily when the client arises.	The volume and frequency of urination increase for 6-8 hr after an oral dose.
		Assess the client for adequate diuresis. Obtain daily weights. Note changes in breath sounds and edema.	Weight is the most accurate noninvasive measurement of volume status.
		Monitor the client's serum electrolytes (especially K^+, Na^+, and Cl^-). Provide K^+ supplementation is prescribed.	Loop diuretics may produce an excessive loss of these electrolytes.
		Monitor the client for signs of dehydration (hypotension, dry mucous membranes, poor skin turgor, thirst, and oliguria).	Loop diuretics continue to cause diuresis even after the excessive fluid has been removed.
		Note any report of ringing in the ears.	Tinnitus may indicate toxicity.
Nitrates			
Isosorbide dinitrate (Isordil, Sorbitrate, Coronex✤, Novosorbide✤	PO (tablet): 15-30 mg q6h PO (sustained release): 40 mg q6-12h	Observe the client for postural hypotension. Supervise ambulation until the dose response is determined.	Relaxation of venous smooth muscle causes blood to pool in the veins when the client stands.
Nitroglycerin (Nitro-Dur)	Transdermal ointment: starting dose of ½ inch q4-8h increasing to 2 inches q4-8h	Assess the client for headache. Inform the physician and provide relief.	Headache diminishes with tolerance. Mild analgesics and administration with food should provide relief until then.

Continued

CHART 35-4

DRUG THERAPY *for* Cardiac Failure—cont'd

Drug	Usual Dosage	Nursing Interventions	Rationale
DRUGS COMMONLY USED PRIMARILY TO REDUCE PRELOAD—cont'd			
Nitroglycerin (Nitrodisc)	Transdermal patch: 2.5-15 mg/12-18 hr	Administer PO dose 30 min before or 2 hr after meals. Make sure the client does not chew.	Oral nitrates are most rapidly absorbed from an empty stomach.
		Administer the ointment on a hairless part of the body in a uniform layer using an applicator.	Proper administration ensures consistent dose administration.
		If so prescribed, allow an 8-12-hr nitrate-free period at night.	A nitrate-free period prevents the development of tolerance to the vasodilating effect of nitrates.
		Rotate the skin sites of transdermal nitrate administration.	Nitrates cause skin irritation.
		Remove transdermal nitrates before defibrillation.	Skin burns have occurred, and explosion is possible.
Cardiac Glycosides			
Digoxin (Lanoxin, Novodigoxin✱)	Loading dose of 1 mg divided over 24 hr Then maintenance 0.125-0.5 mg qd PO Usually 0.25-0.375 mg qd IV	Ask the client about previous use of digitalis; provide the preparation previously taken. (Do not substitute one preparation for another.)	Dosages, absorption rates, and duration of effects differ among drugs.
Digitoxin (Crystodigin) (infrequently used)	Loading dose of 1.2-1.6 mg divided during 24 hr Then 0.1 mg daily IV or PO	Be alert for the following: • Myocardial infarction • Hypokalemia • Renal or hepatic disorders • Diuretic therapy • Diarrhea • Advanced age • Metabolic alkalosis	Any of these factors may result in an increased sensitivity to digitalis and increase the risk of toxicity.
		Monitor serum potassium levels and electrocardiograms.	Hypokalemia is often associated with digitalis toxicity and dysrhythmias.
		Take the apical pulse or check the cardiac monitor pattern before administering each dose of digitalis.	Changes in pulse rate and rhythm may signify digitalis toxicity.
		Monitor serum levels of digitalis. The therapeutic digoxin level is 0.9-1.2 ng/mL.	There is a narrow margin between therapeutic and toxic doses of digitalis. Toxicity occurs in approximately 10%-20% of clients receiving digitalis.
		Observe for signs of digitalis toxicity, and notify the physician if any occur: • Confusion • Dysrhythmias • Anorexia • Fatigue • Muscle weakness	
Beta Blockers			
Carvedilol (Coreg)	Starting dose: 3.125 mg twice daily 12.5 mg at bedtime (¼ tablet) Both doses should be doubled every 2-4 wk	BP and pulse are monitored during the initiation of therapy and with each increase in dose.	Hypotension and bradycardia may occur during initiation or increase in beta-blocker therapy.
		Perform weekly checks for BP, pulse, activity tolerance, and orthopnea.	Beta-blocker therapy may increase the symptoms of heart failure.
		Teach client to weigh self daily and never to stop medication suddenly or without health care provider's advice.	Stopping beta-blocker therapy quickly may cause angina or myocardial infarction.

TABLE 35-2 • EFFECTS OF VASODILATORS*

Drug	Preload Reduction (Vasodilates Peripheral Veins)	Afterload Reduction (Vasodilates Arterioles)
Nitrates (nitroglycerin, isosorbide dinitrate)	+++	+
Hydralazine hydrochloride (Apresoline)	0	+++
Nifedipine (Procardia)	0	++
Sodium nitroprusside (Nitropress)	+++	+++
Captopril (Capoten)	+	++
Prazosin (Minipress)	++	+

*0, no effect; +, mild effect; ++, moderate effect; +++, maximal effect.

used to decrease preload and afterload are described in Chapter 38.

REDUCING PRELOAD. Ventricular fibers contract less forcefully when they are overstretched, such as in a failing heart. Interventions aimed at reducing preload attempt to decrease volume and pressure in the left ventricle, optimizing ventricular muscle stretch and contraction. Preload reduction is appropriate for heart failure accompanied by congestion with total body sodium and water overload.

Diet Therapy. In heart failure, diet therapy is aimed at reducing sodium and water retention.

Sodium Restriction. In collaboration with the dietitian, the health care provider may restrict sodium intake in an attempt to decrease fluid retention. Many clients with heart failure need to omit only table salt (ingest no added salt) from their diet, thus reducing sodium intake to approximately 3 g/day.

If salt intake must be reduced further, the client may need to eliminate all salt in cooking as well as high-sodium foods, thus reducing sodium intake to 2.0 g/day. A dietitian is essential in helping to select foods that meet such a restricted therapeutic diet. Approximately 25% of hospital admissions for clients with heart failure are due to excessive sodium intake. Therefore all clients must be advised to maintain an appropriate sodium restriction and avoid bingeing on high sodium foods (e.g., pickles). Table 11-6 lists the sodium contents of some common foods.

Fluid Volume Restriction. Few clients are placed on severe fluid restrictions. However, clients with excessive aldosterone secretion may experience thirst and drink 3 to 5 L of fluid each day. As a result, their fluid intake may be limited to a more normal 2 L/day. Compliance with these simple strategies may be high, especially if the client experiences relief of any of the symptoms of volume excess. When a fluid restriction is imposed on the hospitalized client, the nurse adjusts oral and IV therapy accordingly.

The nurse or assistive nursing personnel weighs the client daily (1 kg of weight gain or loss equals 1 L of retained or lost fluid, respectively) and keeps accurate records of fluid intake and output. The same scale should be used every morning before breakfast for the most accurate assessment of weight.

Drug Therapy. Common drugs prescribed to reduce preload are diuretics and venous vasodilators.

Diuretics. The health care provider adds diuretics to the regimen when diet and fluid restriction have not been effective in managing the symptoms of systemic or pulmonary congestion associated with heart failure. Diuretics enhance the renal excretion of sodium and water by reducing circulating blood volume, decreasing preload, and reducing systemic and pulmonary congestion.

The type and dosage of diuretic prescribed depend on the degree of heart failure and renal function. High-ceiling (loop) diuretics, such as furosemide (Lasix, Furoside🍁), torsemide (Demadex), and ethacrynic acid (Edecrin), are most effective for treating fluid volume overload. The practitioner may initially use a thiazide diuretic, such as hydrochlorothiazide (HydroDIURIL, Urozide🍁) and metolazone (Zaroxolyn), for older clients with mild volume overload. The action of thiazide diuretics is self-limiting (i.e., diuresis decreases after edema fluid is lost), thus the excessive diuresis and dehydration that may occur with loop diuretics are uncommon occurrences with thiazide diuretics. Clients often prefer thiazide diuretics because of the gradual onset of diuresis. However, loop diuretics are needed to ensure effective diuresis for many clients in heart failure.

As heart failure progresses, many clients develop diuretic resistance with refractory edema. The health care provider may choose to treat this problem by administering two types of diuretics, most commonly a loop diuretic and a thiazide diuretic such as metolazone.

The nurse also needs to monitor for and prevent potassium deficiency (hypokalemia) from diuretic therapy. The signs of hypokalemia are nonspecific neurologic and muscular complaints such as generalized weakness, depressed reflexes, and irregular heart rate. Therefore the physician, nurse, and dietitian monitor serum potassium levels to accurately identify hypokalemia.

If the client's serum potassium level is less than 4.0 mEq/L, the health care provider has several alternatives:

- Add a potassium-sparing diuretic to the regimen
- Request that clients increase their dietary intake of potassium-rich foods
- Prescribe a potassium supplement

Clients being treated simultaneously with ACE inhibitors and diuretics may not experience hypokalemia. If their kidneys are not functioning well, they may develop hyperkalemia (elevated serum potassium level). The nurse should review the client's serum creatinine level. If the creatinine is greater than 1.8, the nurse should notify the health care provider before administering supplemental potassium.

CONSIDERATIONS FOR OLDER ADULTS

Older clients receiving loop diuretics are very prone to dehydration, especially if they have type 2 diabetes mellitus. The nurse checks orthostatic blood pressures in the client receiving loop diuretics to detect volume depletion. The client is weighed daily to detect the development of a slow, progressive weight loss despite an adequate diet. The nurse also examines for flat neck veins when the client is supine and for a loss of skin turgor. All of these signs, plus disorientation in a very old client, may indicate excessive diuresis and volume depletion (Chart 35-5).

CHART 35-5

NURSING FOCUS *on the* OLDER ADULT
Heart Failure

- Assess older clients with confusion for indications of heart failure. People older than 80 years often experience restlessness or confusion as the initial manifestation of heart failure.
- Auscultate the lungs carefully, recognizing that dependent crackles may not be an indication of heart failure in the older adult.
- Do not expect crackles to clear rapidly after treatment. Crackles may persist in the lung bases of older adults for an extended period after pulmonary congestion has decreased.
- Be especially alert for the signs of digitalis toxicity in the older client, because it is common.
- If loop diuretics are used for diuresis, monitor the client closely for signs of excessive diuresis, dehydration, and hypokalemia.
- In older clients receiving drug therapy for heart failure, monitor for orthostatic hypotension. Cardiovascular changes associated with aging make this likely to develop.

Venous Vasodilators. The health care provider may prescribe venous vasodilators. (e.g., nitrates) for the client with heart failure and persistent dyspnea. Significant constriction of venous and arterial blood vessels occurs to compensate for reduced cardiac output. This reduces the volume of fluid that the vascular bed can hold and increases preload. Venous vasodilators may benefit by:

- Returning venous vasculature to a more normal capacity
- Decreasing the volume of blood returning to the heart
- Improving left ventricular function

Some of the most common vasodilators are summarized in Table 35-2.

Nitrates may be administered intravenously, orally, or topically. These drugs cause primarily venous vasodilation but also a significant amount of arteriolar vasodilation. It is essential for the nurse to monitor the client's blood pressure when initiating nitrate therapy or increasing the dosage. Clients may initially report headache, but they are assured that they will develop a tolerance to this effect and that the headache will cease or diminish.

Unfortunately, clients may develop tolerance to the vasodilating effects when nitrates are uniformly administered during 24 hours. To prevent such tolerance, the health care provider may order at least one 12-hour nitrate-free period out of every 24 hours (usually overnight). Clients whose major complaint is nocturnal dyspnea may experience relief when nitroglycerin ointment is applied at bedtime and removed during the day.

ENHANCING CONTRACTILITY. Contractility of the heart can also be enhanced with drug therapy. The preferred drug is digitalis.

Digitalis. Digoxin (Lanoxin), a cardiac glycoside, has been demonstrated to provide benefits for clients in heart failure with sinus rhythm and atrial fibrillation. "Dig" therapy reduces exacerbations of heart failure and hospitalizations, resulting in an estimated annual savings of $406 million. When added to a regimen of angiotensin-converting enzyme (ACE) inhibitors and diuretics, digoxin increases functional capacity and improves hemodynamic parameters in clients with New York Heart Association (NYHA) class III and IV heart failure resulting from left systolic dysfunction.

The potential benefits of digitalis derivatives include an increase in contractility, a reduction in heart rate, a slowing of conduction through the atrioventricular node, and an inhibition of sympathetic activity while enhancing parasympathetic activity. Digitalis also may have a mild diuretic effect. Increased automaticity occurs with toxic digitalis levels or in the presence of hypokalemia (which increases sensitivity to digitalis), and ectopic beats (premature ventricular contractions [PVCs]) may result.

The most commonly prescribed cardiac glycoside is digoxin (Lanoxin, Novodigoxin♣). Digoxin is erratically absorbed from the gastrointestinal tract. Many medications, especially antacids, interfere with its absorption. It is eliminated primarily by renal excretion.

CONSIDERATIONS FOR OLDER ADULTS

The half-life of digoxin in middle-aged adults is 36 hours; in older adults, who typically have diminished renal function, the half-life may be 48 hours or longer. Thus older clients are particularly susceptible to digoxin toxicity. Toxicity occurs in 10% to 20% of all clients taking digoxin, more commonly in elders and clients with hypokalemia. Toxicity in older, hypokalemic clients may be fatal.

Digitalis Toxicity. The presentation of **digitalis toxicity** is often vague and nonspecific and includes anorexia, fatigue, and mental status changes. Toxicity may cause nearly any dysrhythmia, but premature ventricular contractions (PVCs) are most commonly noted. The nurse or nursing staff member carefully monitors the apical pulse rate and heart rhythm of clients receiving digoxin. A resting heart rate of less than 60 beats/min or greater than 100 beats/min is reported to the health care provider. It is equally important to report the development of either an irregular rhythm in a client with a previously regular rhythm or a regular rhythm in a client with a previously irregular one. The nurse also monitors serum digoxin and potassium levels (hypokalemia potentiates digitalis toxicity) to identify toxicity. Chart 35-4 presents information about selected cardiac glycosides.

Any medication that increases the workload of the failing heart also increases its oxygen requirement. The nurse should be alert for the possibility that the client may experience angina (chest pain) in response to digoxin. IV medications that increase contractility are described in Chapter 38.

Beta-Adrenergic Blockade. Although it is not completely clear how they accomplish their effect, beta blockers improve the condition of some clients in heart failure. It appears that prolonged exposure to increased levels of sympathetic stimulation and catecholamines worsens cardiac function. Beta-adrenergic blockade reverses this effect, improving morbidity, mortality, and quality of life for clients in heart failure.

Beta blockers must be started and used with great caution for heart failure. In most cases, clients in heart failure should not be started on a beta blocker until their ACE inhibitor and diuretic doses have been stabilized for 2 weeks. Carvedilol (Coreg) is the only beta blocker approved for treatment of heart failure, but metoprolol (Lopressor, Betaloc♣, Novometoprol♣) is also often used. The first dose is extremely low, and the client is monitored either in the hospital or the health care provider's office to detect bradycardia or hypotension.

The nurse instructs the client to weigh daily while taking the beta blocker and to report any signs of worsening heart failure immediately. The health care provider gradually titrates the drug dose upward, and the client is evaluated at least weekly for changes in blood pressure, pulse, activity tolerance, and orthopnea. A modest drop in blood pressure is acceptable if the client remains asymptomatic and can stand without experiencing dizziness or a further drop in blood pressure. The resting heart rate should remain between 55 and 60 and increase slightly with exercise. The client's activity tolerance should improve, and he or she should not experience orthopnea. Most clients with mild and moderate heart failure demonstrate improved ejection fraction, decreased hospital admissions, and improvement in symptoms when beta blockers are added to their treatment regimens. Clients should be advised that the benefits of beta-blocker therapy accrue over a long period, not immediately.

CRITICAL THINKING CHALLENGE

You are a home care nurse visiting a 76-year-old former nurse who is recovering at home following hospitalization for heart failure. She is taking the following medications: Lasix, Prinivil, digoxin, and Coumadin. She occasionally uses oxygen at night and sleeps sitting up in a lounge chair.

You note that she occasionally takes a Theo-Dur tablet when she feels she is having difficulty breathing. Her vital signs are as follows: blood pressure, 110/72; pulse, 60 and irregular; and respirations, 28. She is short of breath after walking 20 to 30 feet and is unable to climb stairs; her legs are edematous to her knees, even though she is wearing elastic stockings.

- What additional information do you need to obtain?
- What actions should you take at this time?

For suggested answer guidelines, go to SIMON http://www.wbsaunders.com/SIMON/Iggy/.

ACTIVITY INTOLERANCE

NOC **PLANNING: EXPECTED OUTCOMES.** The client with heart failure is expected to (1) perform activities of daily living, (2) walk at least two blocks without experiencing dyspnea or excessive fatigue, (3) have energy restored after rest, and (4) perform usual routine.

INTERVENTIONS. The purpose of interdisciplinary interventions is to regulate energy to prevent fatigue and optimize function (see Chart 35-3).

NIC **ENERGY MANAGEMENT.** The client in severe heart failure initially requires physical and emotional rest. On the first day of hospitalization, he or she may sit up in a chair for meals and perform basic leg exercises while out of bed. Nursing care should be organized to allow periods of rest. The interdisciplinary team observes and documents the client's physiologic response to activity.

As the condition improves, the physical therapist (PT) initiates ambulation, usually on hospital day 2. The nurse checks the blood pressure, pulse, and oxygen saturation before and after the activity. A blood pressure change of more than 20 mm Hg or a pulse increase of more than 20 beats/min may indicate that the activity is too stressful. Other indications of activity intolerance include dyspnea, fatigue, and chest pain. A client displaying any of these symptoms is asked to rate how hard he or she has been working on a scale of 1 to 20, with 20 being the maximum perceived exertion. If the client rates the exertion higher than 12, the nurse counsels him or her to slow down. If the client tolerates the activity, the PT steadily increases the activity level until the client is ambulating 200 to 400 feet several times a day.

If the client is able, the PT (or assistive nursing or PT personnel) might time him or her for 6 minutes while walking at a comfortable pace. The distance the client can walk can be used to determine his or her functional level and activity plan.

POTENTIAL FOR PULMONARY EDEMA

PLANNING: EXPECTED OUTCOMES. The client with heart failure is expected to be free of pulmonary edema.

INTERVENTIONS. The nurse monitors for acute pulmonary edema, a life-threatening event that can result from severe heart failure. In pulmonary edema, the left ventricle fails to eject sufficient blood, and pressure increases in the lungs because of the accumulated blood. The increased pressure causes fluid to leak across the pulmonary capillaries and into the pulmonary interstitium.

The nurse assesses for early signs and symptoms of pulmonary edema (e.g., crackles in the lung bases, dyspnea at rest, disorientation, and confusion), especially in older clients. Documentation of the precise location of the crackles is crucial, because the level of the fluid ascends as the pulmonary edema worsens. The client in acute pulmonary edema is also extremely anxious, tachycardiac, and struggling for air. As pulmonary edema becomes more severe, he or she may have a moist cough productive of frothy, blood-tinged sputum, and his or her skin may be cold, clammy, or cyanotic.

The client diagnosed with pulmonary edema is admitted to the acute care hospital. The physician prescribes rapid-acting diuretics, such as furosemide (Lasix, Furoside♣). Furosemide is given intravenously over 1 to 2 minutes, usually at a starting dose of 40 mg, with another 40 mg repeated if needed in 30 minutes.

Oxygen is always ordered, and the client is placed in a high Fowler's position. IV morphine sulfate may be prescribed, 1 to 2 mg at a time, to reduce venous return (preload), decrease anxiety, and reduce the work of breathing. The nurse should monitor respiratory rate and blood pressure closely. Nitroglycerin may be administered sublingually, and the blood pressure should be monitored closely.

The nurse or assistive nursing personnel inserts a Foley catheter, if ordered, to assess urine output after diuretic administration and to minimize exertion related to voiding. Diuresis normally begins within 5 minutes of the administration of IV furosemide and peaks at 30 minutes. Chart 35-6 summarizes the care of the client with acute pulmonary edema.

Clients often respond dramatically and quickly to these interventions, but their condition can also deteriorate rapidly because of pulmonary congestion and severe hypoxemia. Clients occasionally require biPAP or intubation and ventilation to survive the acute episode. A skilled nurse is needed to assist with intubation. If a client does not respond to other methods, vasodilators such as nitroglycerin or sodium nitroprusside may be administered intravenously, or inotropic sup-

CHART 35-6

BEST PRACTICE *for* Care of the Client with Pulmonary Edema

- Identify the client's chief complaint.
- If the client's blood pressure is adequate, place the client in a high Fowler's position.
- Auscultate the client's lungs briefly (posterior assessment).
- Ensure that vascular access is present, and check for patency.
- Provide oxygen as ordered.
- Provide an IV diuretic (usually furosemide) as prescribed.
- Anticipate urine output 5 to 15 minutes after diuretic administration; catheterize if ordered.
- Monitor blood pressure, respiratory rate, pulse oximetry, pulse, cardiac rhythm, and the client's subjective feelings of ability to breathe.
- Provide additional medications as prescribed (usually morphine sulfate or nitroglycerin).
- Provide comfort measures and reassurance.
- Notify the health care provider if the client does not experience a rapid improvement and diuresis.

port may be required. Such a client should be in an emergency department or intensive care unit (ICU), where the medications are carefully titrated via continuous infusion pumps and the client is closely assessed. Management of the client who is critically ill with heart failure is detailed in Chapter 38.

Community-Based Care

CASE MANAGEMENT

Clients who have not been adequately prepared for discharge or who do not have good community support and follow-up are at high risk for recurrent hospital admissions for heart failure. In a case management system, the case manager or care coordinator assesses the client's needs for health care resources and facilitates appropriate placement. It is imperative that the case manager assess the available social supports. An inability to obtain help in activities such as food shopping and obtaining medications is a major contributor to hospital readmission. If home support is available, the client may be discharged home in the care of a family member or other caregiver. Home care nurses may direct the care, and aides may provide assistance with activities of daily living (ADLs).

If the client has multiple health problems or has been severely compromised by heart disease, he or she may require admission to a subacute unit or traditional nursing home for either transitional or long-term care. Home care services cost about $125 per nursing visit compared with $150 to $300 per day in a traditional nursing home and up to $1000 per day for hospital care. A variety of nontraditional approaches to the ambulatory care of clients with heart failure have been demonstrated to decrease rehospitalization rates. Successful programs use weekly evaluations in the home by a primary care provider; weekly telephone monitoring by nurses; intensive education after discharge by nurses, dietitians, and pharmacists; and weekly educational mailings. Such programs decrease rehospitalization rates at 60 and 90 days by 50% to 87% (Albert, 1999).

HEALTH TEACHING

Clients in heart failure and their nurses may have different priorities for health teaching. The Evidence-Based Practice for Nursing box on p. 701 describes a study that examined the perceived learning needs of clients with heart failure.

ACTIVITY SCHEDULE. Medicare usually provides reimbursement for assessment and teaching so that a home care nurse can continue teaching and assessment when the client returns home. The nurse encourages clients with heart failure to stay as active as possible and to develop a regular exercise regimen. Clients who are more active appear to have better outcomes. The primary outcome is development of a regular exercise routine (probably a home walking program) several times a week. Medicare and third-party payers typically do not reimburse for cardiac rehabilitation for heart failure clients, and paying for a cardiac rehabilitation program out of pocket is expensive.

Although most clients with heart failure appear to benefit from exercise programs, those with persistent crackles and uncontrolled edema despite medical therapy are not encouraged to exercise until their heart failure is stabilized. When exercise is indicated, the nurse teaches the client to begin walking 200 to 400 feet/day. At home, the client should try to walk at least three times a week and should slowly increase the amount of time walked (perhaps 2 minutes a week) over several months. If he or she experiences chest pain or pronounced dyspnea while exercising or experiences fatigue the next day, he or she is probably advancing the activity too quickly and should slow down. The home care nurse encourages the client to keep an exercise diary that documents the time and duration of each exercise session as well as heart rate and any symptoms that occur with exercise.

INDICATIONS OF WORSENING HEART FAILURE. Many clients who are readmitted to hospitals for treatment of heart failure fail to seek medical attention promptly when symptoms recur. The nurse instructs the client and caregiver to immediately report to the health care provider the occurrence of any of the following symptoms of worsening heart failure:

- Rapid weight gain (3 pounds in a week)
- Decrease in exercise tolerance lasting 2 to 3 days
- Cold symptoms (cough) lasting more than 3 to 5 days
- Excessive awakening at night to urinate
- Development of dyspnea or angina at rest or worsening angina

DRUG THERAPY. The health care provider or nurse provides oral and written instructions about the medication regimen. If the client is taking digoxin, the caregiver and client are taught how to count a pulse rate. The nurse assesses their ability to accurately take and record the pulse rate. Chart 35-7 lists instructions for the client taking digoxin at home.

The nurse advises clients taking diuretics to take them in the morning to avoid waking during the night for voiding. After determining if the client has a weight scale and can use it, he or she is instructed to weigh each morning. Although this simple intervention can greatly assist in managing heart failure, most clients do not weigh themselves regularly. The nurse should emphasize the relationship between weight gain, fluid retention, and heart failure. Daily weights indicate whether the client is losing or retaining fluid. Some motivated clients are taught to use a sliding scale to adjust their daily diuretic dose depending on their daily weight—similar to the way a diabetic client adjusts an insulin dose based on the cap-

CHART 35-7

CLIENT EDUCATION GUIDE
Digoxin Therapy

- Noon is the best time of day to take this medication if you can remember to take it then.
- Continue taking this medication unless your health care provider tells you to stop.
- Do not take digoxin at the same time as antacids or cathartics (laxatives).
- Take your pulse rate before taking each dose of digoxin. Notify your health care provider of a change in pulse rate (60-100 beats/min is normal) or rhythm, as well as increasing fatigue, muscle weakness, confusion, or loss of appetite (signs of digitalis toxicity).
- If you forget to take a dose, it may be delayed a few hours. However, if you do not remember it until the next day, you should take only your usual daily dose.
- Report for scheduled laboratory tests (such as potassium and digoxin levels).
- If potassium supplements are prescribed, continue the dose until told to stop by your health care provider.

illary glucose level. The home care nurse may reliably assess volume status by checking the pattern of daily weights.

Clients receiving angiotensin-converting enzyme (ACE) inhibitors should be taught to move slowly when changing positions, especially from a lying to a sitting position. Dizziness, lightheadedness, and cough need to be reported to the health care provider.

Clients taking diuretics and ACE inhibitors require that their serum potassium level and renal function be monitored at least every few months. Diuretics, especially loop diuretics such as furosemide, deplete potassium and often cause hypokalemia. Conversely, ACE inhibitors may result in potassium retention. If potassium levels drop below 4.0 mEq/L, the primary care physician may prescribe potassium supplementation or a potassium-sparing diuretic such as spironolactone (Aldactone). Depending on the client's third-party payer, a dietitian may be consulted to provide information about potassium-rich foods to include in the diet.

DIET THERAPY. Clients with chronic heart failure are advised to restrict their dietary sodium. The home care nurse or dietitian provides written instructions on low- or restricted-sodium diets. A 3-g sodium diet is recommended for mild or moderate failure. Clients are asked to avoid salty foods and table salt but usually find this diet palatable and fairly easy to follow.

A 2-g sodium diet may be attempted for clients with severe heart failure. These clients are told not to add salt during or after meal preparation, to avoid milk and milk products, to use few canned or prepared foods, and to read food labels to determine sodium content. This diet is unpalatable, and for many clients the cost of low-sodium foods is a financial burden. Therefore the home care nurse or dietitian should assess the client for compliance.

Clients are instructed to confer with their health care provider if they want to use commercial salt substitutes. Most salt substitutes contain potassium, and the client's renal status and serum potassium level need to be considered before these products can be recommended. Clients may use lemon, garlic, and herbs to enhance the flavor of low-salt foods.

ADVANCE DIRECTIVES. Approximately 50% of deaths from heart failure are sudden—many without any warning or worsening of symptoms. Because the majority of these deaths occur at home, it is important for the health care provider or home care nurse to discuss advance directives with the client and family. The family should be prepared to act in accordance with the client's wishes in the event of cardiac arrest. If the client desires resuscitation, the family should know how to activate the Emergency Medical System (EMS) and how to provide cardiopulmonary resuscitation (CPR) until an ambulance arrives. If the client does not wish to receive CPR, the client, family, and nurse should plan how the family will respond.

CHART 35-8

FOCUSED ASSESSMENT *of*
Home Care Clients with Heart Failure

Assess for signs of heart failure, including the following:
- Changes in vital signs (heart rate >100 beats/min at rest, new atrial fibrillation, BP <90 or >150 systolic)
- Indications of poor tissue perfusion
  - Fatigue
  - Angina
  - Activity intolerance
  - Changes in mental status
  - Pallor or cyanosis
- Indications of congestion
  - Presence of cough or dyspnea
  - Weight gain
  - Jugular venous distention and peripheral edema

Assess functional ability, including the following:
- Performance of activities of daily living
- Mobility and ambulation (review frequency and duration of walking, development of symptoms, and pulse rate)
- Cognitive ability

Assess nutritional status, including the following:
- Food and fluid intake
- Intake of sodium-rich foods
- Alcohol consumption
- Skin turgor

Assess home environment, including the following:
- Safety hazards, especially related to oxygen therapy
- Structural barriers affecting functional ability
- Social support (family, home health services)

Assess client's compliance and understanding of illness and its treatment, including the following:
- Signs and symptoms to report to health care provider
- Dosages, effects, and side or toxic effects of medications
- When to report for laboratory and health care provider visits
- Ability to accurately weigh self on scale
- Presence of advanced directive
- Use of home oxygen, if appropriate

Assess client and caregiver coping skills

HOME CARE MANAGEMENT

The focus of the home care nurse's interventions is assessment and health teaching, which is reimbursable by Medicare and other third-party payers. Chart 35-8 lists the major areas of assessment.

Clients with chronic heart failure must make many adjustments in their lifestyles. They must adhere to a medical regimen that includes dietary restrictions, activity prescriptions, and drug therapy. They need careful, concise explanations of the treatment plan. The community-based nurse in any setting encourages the client to verbalize fears and concerns about his or her illness and assists in exploring the appropriate coping skills. Client participation in treatment can help alleviate and control symptoms.

CRITICAL THINKING CHALLENGE

The 76-year-old former nurse with congestive heart failure is rehospitalized for pulmonary edema. Her medications (Lasix, Prinivil, digoxin, and Coumadin) are readjusted when carvedilol (Coreg) is added to her regimen. When preparing for discharge, her blood pressure is 95/60, and her heart rate is 56 and irregular.

- What information should you obtain before discharging the client to her home?
- What essential teaching should you provide for her before she is discharged?

For suggested answer guidelines, go to SIMON http://www.wbsaunders.com/SIMON/Iggy/.

HEALTH CARE RESOURCES

A home care nurse may be needed to assess the client's adherence to medication and diet therapy and to monitor for worsening heart failure. Clients with activity limitations benefit from the services of a home care aide. A dietitian might be consulted to assist with menu planning and teaching. Although participation in structured cardiac rehabilitation programs has been shown to be beneficial, referrals to such programs are not widespread because coverage is usually not provided by third-party payers.

In addition to home care support, other resources are available for client education and family support. The American Heart Association is an excellent community resource for pamphlets, books, cookbooks, and videotapes related to heart failure and heart disease. The organization also provides referrals to various local support groups for clients and their caregivers.

For equipment needs (e.g., home oxygen therapy, hospital bed), medical supply companies provide setup and maintenance services. Chapter 28 provides a detailed description of home oxygen therapy.

Evaluation: Outcomes

NOC The nurse evaluates the care of the client with heart failure on the basis of the identified nursing diagnoses and collaborative problems. The expected outcomes include that the client will:

- Have a normal rate, rhythm, and depth of respiration
- Have an oxygen saturation within normal limits (WNL)
- Have no dyspnea at rest
- Resume and maintain an adequate cardiac output as demonstrated by a proportional pulse pressure greater than 25%, a blood pressure greater than 90 or 100 without orthostatic changes, and a heart rate within acceptable parameters
- Have a cardiac index in expected range (IER)
- Not have dysrhythmias or abnormal heart sounds
- Have strong peripheral pulses
- Perform activities of daily living and usual routine without dyspnea or excessive fatigue
- Have energy restored after rest
- Be free of pulmonary edema

VALVULAR HEART DISEASE

OVERVIEW

Approximately 5 million Americans have some form of valvular heart disease. Valvular heart disease occurs when the heart valves cannot open fully (valvular stenosis) or close completely (valvular insufficiency or regurgitation). Acquired valvular dysfunctions most often involve the left side of the heart, especially the mitral valve. Acquired valvular dysfunctions, in decreasing order of occurrence, are mitral stenosis, mitral regurgitation, mitral valve prolapse, aortic stenosis, and aortic regurgitation (Chart 35-9).

The tricuspid valve is affected infrequently—primarily following endocarditis in IV drug abusers. The pulmonic valve is rarely involved. Stenosis and regurgitation often occur simultaneously in a defect called a mixed lesion.

Mitral Stenosis

Mitral stenosis usually results from rheumatic carditis, which can cause valve thickening by fibrosis and calcifica-

CHART 35-9

KEY FEATURES *of* Valvular Heart Disease

Mitral Stenosis	Mitral Insufficiency	Mitral Valve Prolapse	Aortic Stenosis	Aortic Insufficiency
Fatigue Dyspnea on exertion Orthopnea Paroxysmal nocturnal dyspnea Hemoptysis Hepatomegaly Neck vein distention Pitting edema Atrial fibrillation Rumbling, apical diastolic murmur	Fatigue Dyspnea on exertion Orthopnea Palpitations Atrial fibrillation Neck vein distention Pitting edema High-pitched holosystolic murmur	Atypical chest pain Dizziness, syncope Palpitations Atrial tachycardia Ventricular tachycardia Systolic click	Dyspnea on exertion Angina Syncope on exertion Fatigue Orthopnea Paroxysmal nocturnal dyspnea Harsh, systolic crescendo-decrescendo murmur	Palpitations Dyspnea Orthopnea Paroxysmal nocturnal dyspnea Fatigue Angina Sinus tachycardia Blowing, decrescendo diastolic murmur
S_1 S_2 S_1 S_2 S_1	S_1 S_2S_3 S_1 S_2S_3	click click S_1 S_2 S_1 S_2	S_1 S_2 S_1 S_2	S_1 S_2 S_1 S_2 S_1

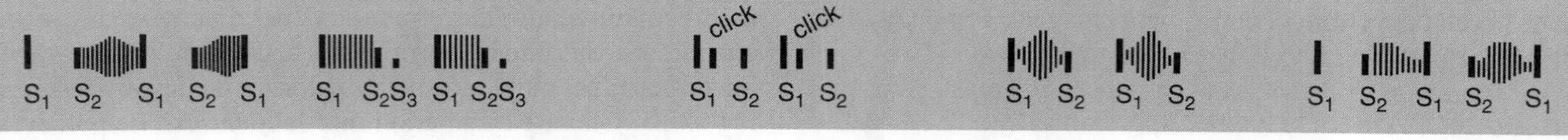

tion. Rheumatic fever is the most common cause of mitral stenosis. Nonrheumatic causes include atrial myxoma (tumor), calcium accumulation, and thrombus formation.

In this condition, the valve leaflets fuse and become stiff, and the chordae tendineae contract and shorten. The valvular orifice narrows, preventing normal blood flow from the left atrium to the left ventricle. As a result of these changes, left atrial pressure rises, the left atrium dilates, pulmonary artery pressures increase, and the right ventricle hypertrophies.

Pulmonary congestion and right-sided heart failure initially occur. Later, when the left ventricle receives insufficient blood volume, preload is decreased and cardiac output falls.

Clients with mild mitral stenosis are usually asymptomatic. As the valvular orifice narrows and pressure in the lungs increases, the client experiences dyspnea on exertion, orthopnea, paroxysmal nocturnal dyspnea (sudden dyspnea at night), and dry cough. Hemoptysis and pulmonary edema appear as pulmonary hypertension and congestion progress. Right-sided heart failure can cause hepatomegaly, neck vein distention, and pitting edema late in the disorder.

On palpation, the pulse may be normal, tachycardiac, or irregularly irregular (as in atrial fibrillation). Because the development of atrial fibrillation indicates that the client may decompensate, the physician should be notified immediately of the development of an irregularly irregular rhythm. On auscultation, the nurse notes a rumbling, apical diastolic murmur.

WOMEN'S HEALTH CONSIDERATIONS

Two thirds to three fourths of all clients with mitral stenosis are women. Approximately two thirds of the women with rheumatic mitral stenosis are younger than 45 years of age.

Mitral Regurgitation (Insufficiency)

The fibrotic and calcific changes occurring in **mitral regurgitation** prevent the mitral valve from closing completely during *systole.* Incomplete closure of the valve allows the backflow of blood into the left atrium when the left ventricle contracts. During *diastole,* regurgitant output again flows from the left atrium to the left ventricle along with the normal blood flow. This increases the volume that must be ejected during the next systole. To compensate for the increased volume and pressure, the left atrium and ventricle dilate and hypertrophy.

Mitral insufficiency usually progresses slowly; clients may remain symptom free for decades. Symptoms begin to occur when the left ventricle fails in response to increased blood volumes. The client most often reports fatigue and chronic weakness as a result of reduced cardiac output. Dyspnea on exertion and orthopnea develop later. A significant number of clients complain of anxiety, atypical chest pains, and palpitations. Nursing assessment may reveal normal blood pressure, atrial fibrillation (an irregularly irregular rhythm occurring in 75% of clients), or changes in respirations characteristic of left ventricular failure.

When right-sided heart failure develops, the neck veins become distended, the liver enlarges (hepatomegaly), and pitting edema is noted. On auscultation, the nurse hears a high-pitched systolic murmur at the apex, with radiation to the left axilla. Severe regurgitation often exhibits a third heart sound.

Rheumatic heart disease is the predominant cause of mitral insufficiency. When mitral insufficiency results from rheumatic heart disease, it usually coexists with some degree of mitral stenosis. Nonrheumatic causes include papillary muscle dysfunction or rupture resulting from ischemic heart disease, infective endocarditis, and a congenital anomaly. Mitral regurgitation resulting from rheumatic heart disease is more common in women than in men. Mitral regurgitation of a nonrheumatic etiology occurs more often in men.

Mitral Valve Prolapse

Mitral valve prolapse occurs because the valvular leaflets enlarge and prolapse into the left atrium during systole. This abnormality is usually benign but may progress to pronounced mitral regurgitation.

Most clients with mitral valve prolapse are asymptomatic. However, they may report chest pain, palpitations, or exercise intolerance. Chest pain is usually atypical, with clients describing a sharp pain localized to the left side of the chest. Dizziness, syncope, and palpitations may be associated with atrial or ventricular dysrhythmias.

The nurse usually finds a normal heart rate and blood pressure on physical examination. A midsystolic click and a late systolic murmur may be audible at the apex.

The etiology of mitral valve prolapse is variable and has been associated with conditions such as Marfan's syndrome and other congenital cardiac defects (see Chapter 21 for a discussion on Marfan's syndrome). However, most of the time no other cardiac abnormality is found. A familial occurrence is well established.

Mitral valve prolapse affects 5% to 10% of people. Although it is present in all age-groups, it is most common in women between 20 and 54 years of age.

Aortic Stenosis

In **aortic stenosis,** the aortic valve orifice narrows and obstructs left ventricular outflow during systole. This increased resistance to ejection or afterload results in ventricular hypertrophy. As stenosis progresses, cardiac output becomes fixed and unable to increase to meet the demands of the body during exertion, and symptoms develop. Eventually the left ventricle fails, volume backs up in the left atrium, and the pulmonary system becomes congested. Right-sided heart failure can occur late in the disease.

The classic symptoms of aortic stenosis result from the fixed cardiac output: dyspnea, angina, and syncope occurring on exertion. When cardiac output falls in the late stages of the disease, the client experiences marked fatigue, debilitation, and peripheral cyanosis. A narrow pulse pressure is noted when the blood pressure is examined. A diamond-shaped, systolic crescendo-decrescendo murmur is usually noted on auscultation.

Congenital valvular disease or malformation is the predominant etiologic factor in aortic stenosis. Bicuspid or unicuspid aortic valves are the primary reason for aortic stenosis in clients younger than 30 years and account for about 50% of the disease in clients 30 to 70 years of age. Rheumatic aortic stenosis is always concomitant with rheumatic disease of the mitral valve and develops in clients between 30 and 70 years of age. Atherosclerosis and degenerative calcification of the aortic valve are the predominant factors in people older than age 70. Aortic stenosis has become the most common valvular disorder in countries with aging populations. Of clients with aortic stenosis, 80% are men.

Aortic Regurgitation (Insufficiency)

In clients with **aortic regurgitation,** the aortic valve leaflets do not close properly during diastole, and the annulus (the valve ring that attaches to the leaflets) may be dilated, loose, or deformed. This allows regurgitation of blood from the aorta back into the left ventricle during diastole. The left ventricle, in compensation, dilates to accommodate the greater blood volume and eventually hypertrophies.

Clients with aortic regurgitation remain asymptomatic for many years because of the compensatory mechanisms of the left ventricle. As the disease progresses and left ventricular failure occurs, the principal concerns are exertional dyspnea, orthopnea, and paroxysmal nocturnal dyspnea. Palpitations may be noted with severe disease, especially while lying on the left side. Many clients with aortic regurgitation experience nocturnal angina with diaphoresis.

On palpation, the nurse notes a "bounding" arterial pulse. The pulse pressure is usually widened, with an elevated systolic pressure and diminished diastolic pressure. The classic auscultatory finding is a high-pitched, blowing, decrescendo diastolic murmur.

Aortic insufficiency usually results from nonrheumatic conditions such as infective endocarditis, congenital anatomic aortic valvular abnormalities, hypertension, and Marfan's syndrome (a rare, generalized, systemic disease of connective tissue). Approximately 75% of clients with aortic regurgitation are men.

COLLABORATIVE MANAGEMENT

Assessment

A client with valvular disease may suddenly become ill or may slowly develop symptoms over many years. Information is collected about the client's family health history, including valvular or other forms of heart disease to which he or she may be genetically predisposed. The nurse questions about attacks of rheumatic fever, the specific dates when these occurred, and the use of antibiotic prophylaxis against the recurrence of rheumatic fever. The client should also be questioned about a history of IV drug abuse. The client's fatigue level and tolerated activity level, the presence of angina or dyspnea, and the occurrence of palpitations, if present, are also discussed.

As part of the physical assessment, the nurse obtains the client's vital signs, inspects for signs of edema, palpates and auscultates the heart and lungs, and palpates the peripheral pulses. Findings consistent with valvular malformation are summarized in Chart 35-9.

In clients with mitral stenosis, the chest x-ray study shows left atrial enlargement, prominent pulmonary arteries, and an enlarged right ventricle. In those with mitral regurgitation, the chest x-ray study reveals an increased cardiac shadow, indicating left ventricular and left atrial enlargement.

In the later stages of aortic stenosis, the chest x-ray study may show left ventricular enlargement and pulmonary congestion. Left atrial and left ventricular dilation appear on the chest x-ray film of clients with aortic *insufficiency.* If heart failure is present, pulmonary venous congestion is also evident.

For clients with valvular heart disease, echocardiography is the diagnostic procedure of choice because it is an excellent noninvasive tool for defining cardiac structure, movement of the valve leaflets, and size and function of the cardiac chambers. Exercise tolerance testing (ETT) is sometimes performed to evaluate symptomatic response, assess functional capacity, and enhance auscultatory findings. In clients with either mitral or aortic stenosis, cardiac catheterization is often indicated to assess the severity of the stenosis and its other effects on the heart.

The health care provider also orders an electrocardiogram (ECG) to assess abnormalities such as left ventricular hypertrophy, as seen with mitral regurgitation and aortic regurgitation, or right ventricular hypertrophy, as seen in severe mitral stenosis. Atrial fibrillation is a common finding in both mitral stenosis and mitral regurgitation and may develop in aortic stenosis because of left atrial dilation.

Interventions

Management of valvular heart disease depends on which valve is affected and the degree of valve impairment. Some clients can be managed with yearly monitoring and medications, whereas other clients require invasive procedures or heart surgery.

NONSURGICAL MANAGEMENT. Nonsurgical management focuses on drug therapy and rest. During the course of valvular disease, clients may develop left ventricular failure with pulmonary or systemic congestion. Diuretics, digoxin, and oxygen are often administered to improve the symptoms of heart failure (see Chart 35-4). Nitrates are administered cautiously to clients with aortic stenosis because of the potential for syncope associated with a reduction in left ventricular volume (preload). Vasodilators such as nifedipine (Adalat, Procardia) may be used to reduce the regurgitant flow for clients with aortic or mitral stenosis.

Prophylactic antibiotic therapy is required for all clients with valve disease before any invasive procedure. Procedures for which clients require antibiotic coverage include bronchoscopy, endoscopy, sigmoidoscopy, colonoscopy, genitourinary instrumentation, surgery, and dental procedures of any type.

A major concern in valvular heart disease is maintaining cardiac output should atrial fibrillation develop. With mitral valvular disease, left ventricular filling is especially dependent on atrial contraction. When atrial fibrillation develops, there is no longer a single, coordinated atrial contraction. Cardiac output can decrease by 25% to 30%, and heart failure may occur. Ineffective atrial contraction may also lead to the stasis of blood and thrombi in the left atrium. The nurse monitors the client for the development of an irregularly irregular rhythm and notifies the primary care provider should it develop. (See Chapter 34 for a detailed explanation of atrial fibrillation.)

The primary care provider usually institutes therapy to restore normal sinus rhythm or, if that is unsuccessful, to slow ventricular rate. The physician might elect to convert a client from atrial fibrillation to sinus rhythm using IV diltiazem (Cardizem). The client should be on a unit where nurses are able to monitor cardiac rhythm and blood pressure closely. Synchronized countershock (cardioversion) may be attempted if atrial fibrillation is rapid and the client is unresponsive to medical treatment (see Chapter 34).

Whether the client is converted to sinus rhythm or remains in an atrial fibrillation, digoxin is often prescribed to slow ventricular rate and increase the force of contraction. If atrial fibrillation does not resolve, quinidine gluconate (Quinaglute, Quinate✱) or procainamide hydrochloride (Pronestyl hydrochloride, Procanbid) may be added to the regimen. A beta-blocking agent, such as propranolol hydrochloride (Inderal, Apo-Propranolol✱), or a calcium channel blocker, such as verapamil hydrochloride (Calan), may also be considered to slow the ventricular response.

For valvular heart disease and chronic atrial fibrillation, anticoagulation with sodium warfarin (Coumadin, Warfilone✱) is usually a part of the medical treatment plan to prevent thrombus formation. Thrombi may form in the atria or on defective valve segments, resulting in systemic emboli. As a result, one or more strokes may occur. Therefore the nurse assesses the client's baseline neurologic status and regularly reassesses for neurologic changes.

Rest is often an important part of treatment. Activity may be limited because cardiac output cannot meet increased metabolic demands, and angina or heart failure can result.

SURGICAL MANAGEMENT. Surgical repair or replacement of heart valves has a major effect on the prognosis of valvular heart disease. Correct timing is crucial. Repair or replacement of the valve is usually performed after symptoms of left ventricular failure have developed but before irreversible dysfunction occurs. Surgical therapy is the only definitive treatment of aortic stenosis and is recommended when angina, syncope, or dyspnea on exertion develop.

REPARATIVE PROCEDURES. Reparative procedures are gaining in popularity because of continuing problems with thrombi, endocarditis, and left ventricular dysfunction after valvular replacement. Reparative procedures do not result in a normal valve, but they usually "turn back the clock." This results in a more functional valve and an improvement in cardiac output. Turbulent blood flow through the valve may persist, and degeneration of the repaired valve is possible.

Balloon Valvuloplasty. **Balloon valvuloplasty,** an invasive nonsurgical procedure, is possible for stenotic mitral and aortic valves. Careful selection of clients is necessary. Valvuloplasty may be the initial treatment of choice for people with noncalcified, mobile, mitral valves. Clients selected for aortic valvuloplasty are usually older and are at high risk for surgical complications or have refused operative treatment. The benefits of aortic valvuloplasty for aortic stenosis tend to be short lived, rarely lasting longer than 6 months.

When performing mitral valvuloplasty, the physician passes a balloon catheter from the femoral vein, through the atrial septum, and to the mitral valve. The balloon is inflated to enlarge the mitral orifice. For aortic valvuloplasty, the physician inserts the catheter through the femoral artery and advances it to the aortic valve, where it is inflated to enlarge the orifice. Valvuloplasty usually offers immediate relief of symptoms because the balloon has dilated the orifice and improved leaflet mobility. The results are comparable with those of surgical commissurotomy for appropriately selected clients.

After the procedure, the nurse observes the client closely for bleeding from the catheter insertion site and institutes precautions for arterial puncture if appropriate. Bleeding is likely after valvuloplasty because of the large size of the catheter. The nurse also observes for signs of a regurgitant valve by closely monitoring heart sounds, cardiac output, and heart rhythm. Because vegetations (thrombi) may have been dislodged from the valve, the nurse observes for any indication of systemic emboli (see Infective Endocarditis, p. 718).

Direct, or Open, Commissurotomy. **Direct commissurotomy** is accomplished with cardiopulmonary bypass during open heart surgery. The surgeon visualizes the valve, removes thrombi from the atria, incises the fused commissures (leaflets), and debrides calcium from the leaflets, widening the orifice.

Mitral Valve Reconstruction. **Mitral valve reconstruction** is the reparative procedure of choice for most clients with acquired mitral insufficiency. To make the annulus (the valve ring that attaches to and supports the leaflets) smaller, the physician may suture the leaflets to an annuloplasty ring or take tucks in the client's annulus. Leaflet repair is often performed at the same time. Elongated leaflets may be shortened, and shortened leaflets may be repaired by lengthening the chordae that bind them in place. Perforated leaflets may be patched with synthetic grafts.

Annuloplasty and leaflet repair result in an annulus of the appropriate size and in leaflets that can close completely. Thus regurgitation is eliminated or markedly reduced.

REPLACEMENT PROCEDURES. The development of prosthetic (synthetic) and biologic (tissue) valves has improved the surgical therapy and prognosis of valvular heart disease. Prosthetic valves come in a wide variety (Figure 35-2). Although prosthetic valves are very durable, all clients must receive oral anticoagulation for the rest of their lives because of the possibility of clot formation.

Biologic valves may be **xenograft** (from other species), such as a porcine valve (from a pig) (Figure 35-3) or a bovine valve (from a cow). Because tissue valves are associated with little risk of clot formation, long-term anticoagulation is not indicated. However, xenografts are not as durable as prosthetic valves and usually must be replaced every 7 to 10 years. The durability of a xenograft is related to the age of the recipient. Calcium in the blood, which is present in larger quantities in younger clients, breaks down the valves. The older the client, the longer the xenograft will last. Valves donated from human cadavers and **pulmonary autographs** (relocation of the client's own pulmonary valve to the aortic position) are also being used for valve replacement, especially in younger clients.

The mitral valve should be replaced if the leaflets are calcified and immobile. The surgeon excises the valve during cardiopulmonary bypass surgery, and the new biologic or prosthetic valve is sutured into place.

An aortic valve is replaced for most symptomatic adults with aortic stenosis and aortic insufficiency. As with mitral valve replacement, the surgeon excises the aortic valve during cardiopulmonary bypass surgery and sutures the new valve into place.

PREOPERATIVE CARE. Clients undergoing valve surgery have open heart surgery similar to the procedure for a coronary artery bypass graft (CABG) (see Chapter 38). Ideally, surgery is an elective and planned procedure. Therefore the nurse can assist in preparing the client by instructing the client and family members or a significant other about the management of postoperative pain, incision care, and strategies to prevent respiratory complications (see Chapters 17 and 19).

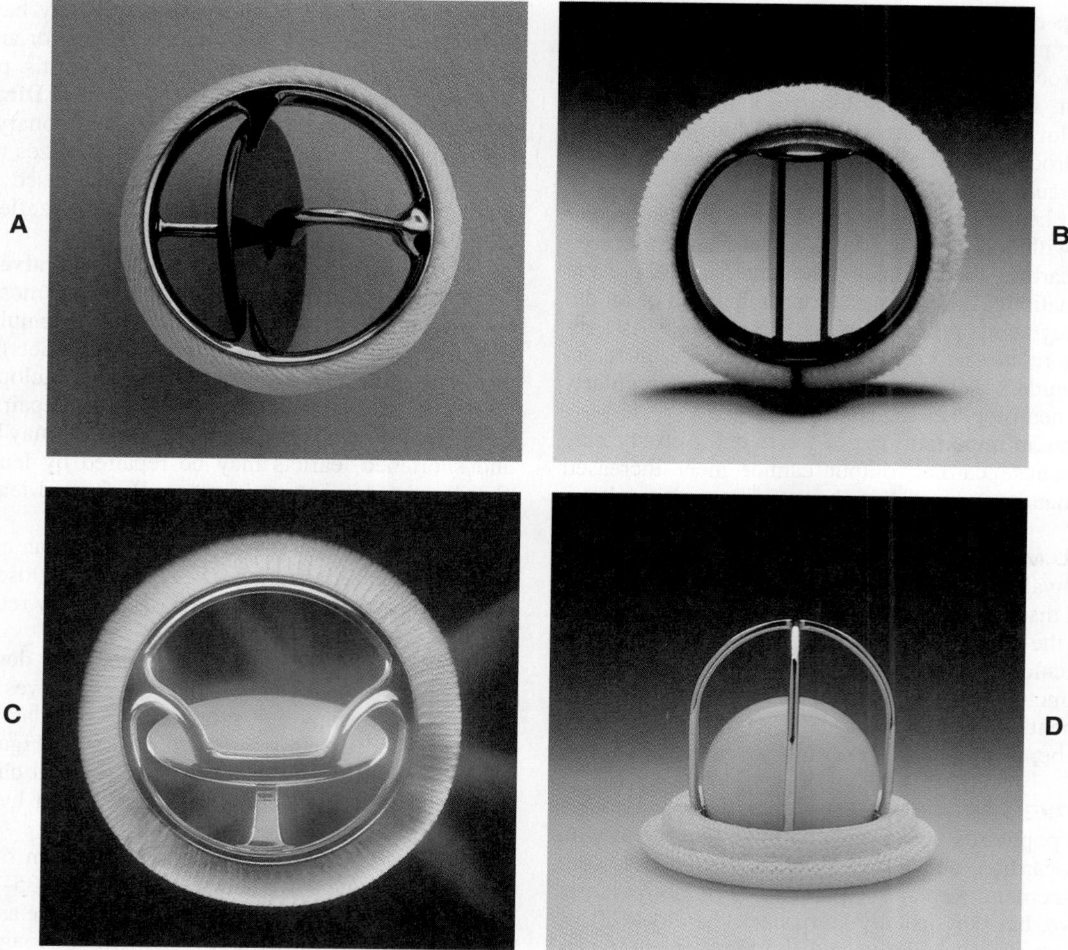

Figure 35-2 ● Examples of prosthetic (synthetic) heart valves. **A,** Medtronic Hall, a tilting-disk valve. **B,** St. Jude Medical mechanical heart valve. **C,** Monostrat mechanical heart valve. **D,** Starr-Edwards Silastic ball valve. (**A** courtesy Medtronic, Inc., Minneapolis, MN; **B** courtesy St. Jude Medical, Inc. All rights reserved. St. Jude Medical is a registered trademark of St. Jude Medical, Inc.; **C** courtesy Alliance Medical Products, Irvine, CA; **D** courtesy Baxter Healthcare Corporation, Edwards CVS Division, Santa Ana, CA.)

The nurse may also introduce the client and the family or significant other to the staff and the environment of the surgical critical care unit (where the client will be transferred after surgery). Clients receiving oral anticoagulants stop taking them at least 72 hours before the procedure.

POSTOPERATIVE CARE. Nursing interventions for clients undergoing open heart surgery for valve disorders are similar to those for a CABG (see Chapter 38). However, a few significant differences depend in part on the type of valvular surgery. Clients with mitral stenosis often have pulmonary hypertension and stiff lungs. The nurse monitors respiratory status and watches the client closely during weaning from the ventilator. Aortic valve replacements pose a higher risk for postoperative hemorrhage, and the nurse is especially vigilant for indications of bleeding.

Clients with valve replacements are also more likely to experience significant reductions in cardiac output after surgery, especially those with aortic stenosis or left ventricular failure from mitral valve disease. The nurse is particularly attentive in monitoring the client's cardiac output and identifying any indications of pump failure. High filling pressures (pulmonary artery wedge pressure greater than 18 mm Hg) may be required to maintain an acceptable cardiac output in the immediate postoperative period. The physician may prescribe digoxin (Lanoxin, Novodigoxin♣) for 3 to 6 months postoperatively to maintain cardiac output and prevent atrial fibrillation. Clients who have had valve replacements with prosthetic valves require lifetime prophylactic anticoagulation therapy to prevent thrombus formation.

Community-Based Care

The client with valvular heart disease may be discharged home on medical therapy or postoperatively after valve repair or replacement. Because fatigue is a common problem for clients with valve disorders, the nurse helps the client and family ensure that the home environment is conducive to providing rest. Older clients with aortic stenosis may reside in long-term care.

A

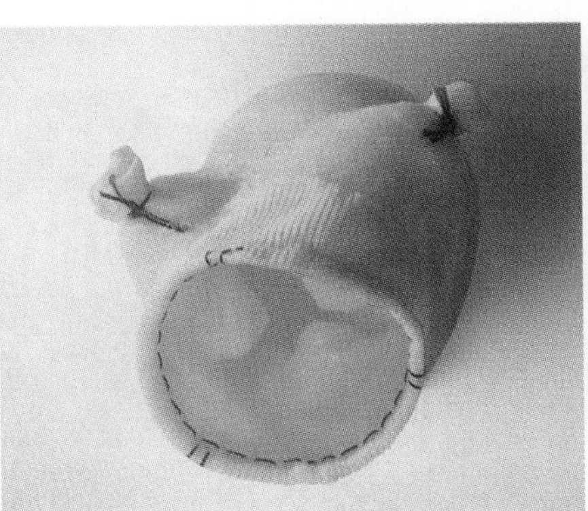

B

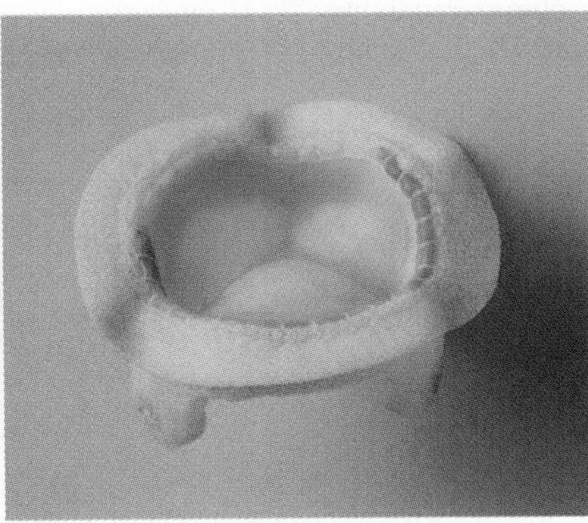

C

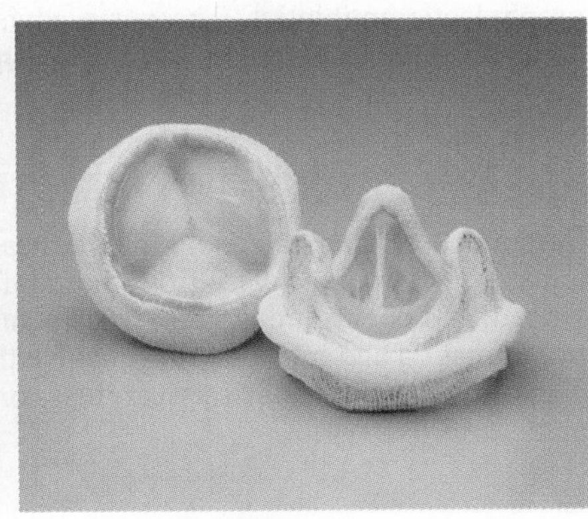

Figure 35-3 ● Examples of biologic (tissue) heart valves. **A,** Freestyle, a stentless pig valve with no frame. **B,** Hancock II, a stented pig valve. **C,** Carpentier-Edwards pericardial bioprosthesis. (**A** and **B** courtesy Medtronic, Inc., Minneapolis, MN; **C** courtesy Baxter Healthcare Corporation, Edwards CVS Division, Santa Ana, CA.)

HEALTH TEACHING

The teaching plan for the client with valvular heart disease includes the following:

- The disease process
- Medications, including diuretics, vasodilators, cardiac glycosides, antibiotics, and anticoagulants
- The prophylactic use of antibiotics
- A plan of work, activity, and rest to conserve energy
- The purpose and nature of surgical intervention, if appropriate

Because clients with defective or repaired valves are at risk for infective endocarditis, the nurse teaches them to adhere to the precautions described for endocarditis. The nurse instructs clients to inform all health care providers of the valvular heart disease history; they are also told that they require antibiotic administration before all invasive procedures and tests. Instructions for the client are described in Chart 35-10.

The nurse teaches clients taking anticoagulants how to manage their drug therapy successfully, including dietary considerations (if taking warfarin) and prevention of bleeding. For example, the client should be taught to avoid foods high in vitamin K and to use an electric razor to avoid skin cuts. The client should report any bleeding or excessive bruising to the health care provider. (See Chapter 38 for more information on anticoagulants.)

The nurse teaches clients who have undergone valve surgery how to care for the sternal incision and instructs them to watch for and report any fever or drainage or redness at the site. Clients can usually return to normal activity after 6 weeks but should avoid heavy physical labor with their upper extremities for 3 to 6 months to allow the sternotomy incision to heal. Clients who have had valvular surgery should also avoid any dental procedures for 6 months because of the potential for endocarditis. Those with prosthetic valves need to avoid any procedure using magnetic resonance technology.

Clients with valvular heart disease may have complicated medication schedules as well as long-term antibiotic or anticoagulant therapy. These circumstances may potentially lead to noncompliance. The nurse provides clear, concise instructions about medication schedules.

CHART 35-10

CLIENT EDUCATION GUIDE
Valvular Heart Disease

- Notify all of your health care providers that you have a defective heart valve.
- Remind the health care provider of your valvular problem when you have any dental work (cleaning, filling, or extraction), any examination by instrument (cystoscopy, endoscopy, or sigmoidoscopy), or any other invasive procedure (arteriogram, surgery).
- Request antibiotic prophylaxis before and after these procedures if the health care provider does not offer it.
- Clean all wounds and apply antibiotic ointment to prevent infection.
- Notify your health care provider immediately if you experience fever, petechiae (pinpoint red dots on your skin), or shortness of breath.

The psychologic response to valve surgery is similar to that following coronary artery bypass surgery. Clients may experience an altered self-image as a result of the required lifestyle changes or the visible medial sternotomy incision. In addition, clients with prosthetic valves may need to adjust to a soft but audible clicking sound of the prosthetic valve. The nurse encourages them to verbalize their feelings about the sternotomy incision and the prosthetic heart valve.

HOME CARE MANAGEMENT

A home care nurse may be needed to help the client adhere to medication and activity schedules and to detect any problems, particularly with anticoagulant therapy. Clients who have undergone surgery may require a nurse for assistance with incision care. A home care aide may assist with activities of daily living.

HEALTH CARE RESOURCES

The American Heart Association is a community resource that provides information about valvular heart disease. A wallet-sized card can be obtained to identify the client as needing prophylactic antibiotics. The nurse advises clients receiving anticoagulants to obtain an identification bracelet that states the name of the drug they are taking.

INFLAMMATIONS AND INFECTIONS

Inflammations and infections of the heart often follow systemic infections. Recovery from these infections is often prolonged, and clients are at great risk for future heart problems. Inflammation and infection may involve the endocardium (endocarditis), pericardium (pericarditis), or entire heart (rheumatic carditis).

Infective Endocarditis

OVERVIEW

Pathophysiology

Infective endocarditis (previously called *bacterial endocarditis*) refers to a microbial infection involving the endocardium. A defective or prosthetic valve is most commonly affected, but infection may also occur in apparently healthy endocardium or in septal defects. Current classification of infective endocarditis is by site of involvement, type of pathogen, and definitiveness of the diagnosis.

Etiology

Infective endocarditis occurs primarily in clients who abuse IV drugs, have had valve replacements, or have structural cardiac defects.

With a cardiac defect, blood may flow rapidly from a high-pressure area to a low-pressure zone, eroding a section of endocardium. Platelets and fibrin adhere to the denuded endocardium, forming a vegetative lesion. During bacteremia, bacteria become trapped in the low-pressure "sinkhole" and are deposited in the vegetation. Additional platelets and fibrin are deposited, which causes the vegetative lesion to grow; the endocardium and valve are destroyed. Valvular insufficiency may result when the lesion interferes with normal alignment of the valve. If vegetations become so large that blood flow through the valve is obstructed, the valve appears stenotic.

Possible ports of entry for infecting organisms include the following:

- The oral cavity (especially if dental procedures have been performed)
- Skin rashes, lesions, or abscesses
- Infections (cutaneous, genitourinary, or gastrointestinal)
- Surgery or invasive procedures, including IV line placement

Incidence/Prevalence

The incidence of infective endocarditis is estimated to be 5 out of every 100,000 people, with men having a higher incidence than women. Mortality rates for infective endocarditis have remained high—12% to 15% despite antibiotic therapy. In 1995 approximately 2000 people died from endocarditis, and 16,000 people were discharged from hospitals with the primary diagnosis of endocarditis (AHA, 1998).

CHART 35-11

KEY FEATURES *of* Infective Endocarditis

- Fever associated with chills, night sweats, malaise, and fatigue
- Anorexia and weight loss
- Cardiac murmur (newly developed or change in existing)
- Development of heart failure
- Evidence of systemic embolization
- Petechiae
- Splinter hemorrhages
- Osler's nodes
- Janeway's lesions

COLLABORATIVE MANAGEMENT

Assessment

Because mortality remains high, early detection of infective endocarditis is essential. Unfortunately, many clients (especially older adults) are misdiagnosed. Clinical manifestations usually occur within 2 weeks of a bacteremia (Chart 35-11).

Assessment usually reveals a recurrent fever. Most clients have temperatures from 99° to 103° F (37.2° to 39.4° C). Many older adults remain afebrile. The severity of symptoms may depend on the virulence of the infecting organism.

CARDIOVASCULAR MANIFESTATIONS

The nurse assesses the client's cardiovascular status. More than 90% of clients with infective endocarditis develop murmurs. The nurse carefully auscultates the precordium, noting and documenting any new murmurs (usually regurgitant in nature) or any changes in the intensity or quality of an old murmur. An S_3 or S_4 heart sound may also be heard.

Heart failure is the most common complication of infective endocarditis. The nurse assesses for right-sided heart failure (as evidenced by peripheral edema, weight gain, and anorexia) and left-sided heart failure (as evidenced by fatigue, shortness of breath, and crackles on auscultation of breath sounds).

EMBOLIC COMPLICATIONS

Arterial embolization is a major complication in up to 50% of clients with infective endocarditis. Fragments of vegetation break loose and travel randomly through the circulation. When the left side of the heart is involved, vegetation fragments are carried to the spleen, kidneys, gastrointestinal (GI) tract, brain, and extremities. When the right side of the heart is involved, emboli enter the pulmonary circulation.

Clients with splenic infarction describe sudden abdominal pain with radiation to the left shoulder. When performing an abdominal assessment, the nurse notes rebound tenderness on palpation. The classic pain described with renal infarction is flank pain that radiates to the groin and is accompanied by hematuria or pyuria. Mesenteric emboli may result in the client complaining of diffuse abdominal pain, often after eating, and abdominal distention.

Emboli to the central nervous system cause either transient ischemic attacks (TIAs) or a stroke. The client may appear confused, experience reduced concentration and aphasia, or have dysphagia. Pleuritic chest pain, dyspnea, and cough are

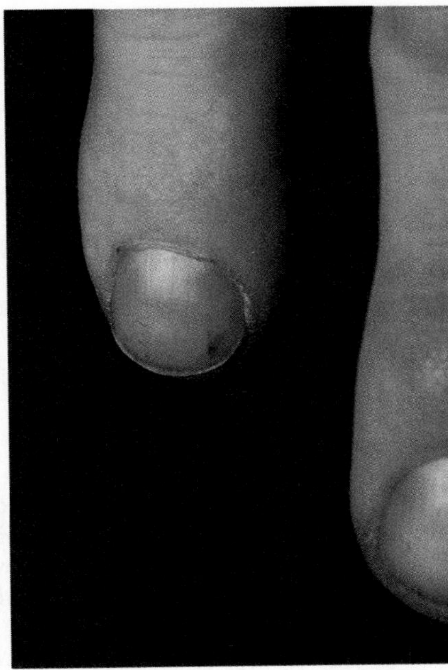

Figure 35-4 ● Splinter hemorrhage lesions in endocarditis. (From Callen, J.P., et al. [1993]. *Color atlas of dermatology.* Philadelphia: W.B. Saunders.)

often described by the client who is experiencing pulmonary infarction related to embolization.

PERIPHERAL MANIFESTATIONS

Petechiae (pinpoint red spots) occur in up to 40% of clients with endocarditis. The nurse examines the mucous membranes, the palate, the conjunctivae, and the skin above the clavicles for small, red, flat lesions. The nurse also examines the distal third of the nail bed for **splinter hemorrhages,** which appear as black longitudinal lines or small red streaks (Figure 35-4).

Osler's nodes and **Janeway's lesions** are considered classic manifestations of endocarditis but may occur with other conditions. The nurse inspects the pads of the fingers, hands, and toes for Osler's nodes, a late sign, which are reddish tender lesions with a white center. Janeway's lesions, an early sign (Figure 35-5), are nontender, hemorrhagic lesions on the fingers, toes, nose, or earlobes. Splenomegaly and clubbing of the fingers may occur in clients who have had infective endocarditis for longer than 6 weeks.

DIAGNOSTIC ASSESSMENT

A positive blood culture is of prime diagnostic and therapeutic importance. Both aerobic and anaerobic specimens are obtained for culture. Some slow-growing organisms may take 3 weeks and require a specialized medium to isolate. Therefore cultures should be monitored by the laboratory for 3 to 4 weeks. Low hemoglobin and hematocrit levels may also be found.

Echocardiography has improved the ability to accurately diagnose infective endocarditis. Transesophageal echocardiography (TEE) allows visualization of cardiac structures that are difficult to see with transthoracic echocardiography (TTE). TEE provides good resolution and is very sensitive for

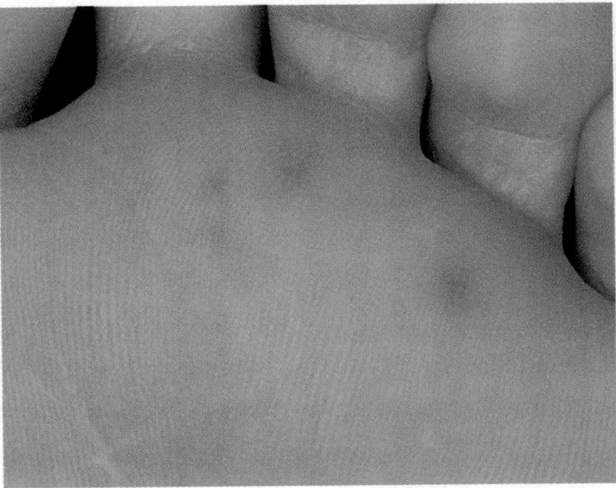

Figure 35-5 ● Janeway's lesions on the sole of the foot. (From Zitelli, B.J., & Davis, H.W. [1997]. *Atlas of pediatric physical diagnosis* [3rd ed.]. St. Louis, Mosby.)

discovering valvular abnormalities, thereby enabling the clinician to diagnose infective endocarditis more accurately (see Chapter 33).

The most reliable criteria for diagnosing endocarditis include positive blood cultures, a new regurgitant murmur, and evidence of endocardial involvement by echocardiography.

Interventions

Care of the client with endocarditis usually includes antibiotics, rest, and supportive therapy for heart failure. If these interventions are successful, surgery is usually not required.

NONSURGICAL MANAGEMENT. The major component of treatment for endocarditis is drug therapy. Other interventions help to prevent the life-threatening complications.

DRUG THERAPY. Antibiotics are the mainstay of treatment, with the choice of antibiotics depending on the specific organism involved. Because vegetations surround and protect the bacteria, an appropriate antibiotic must be given in a sufficiently high dose to ensure a bactericidal effect. Antibiotics are most often given intravenously, with the course of treatment lasting 4 to 6 weeks. In most cases, the ideal antibiotic is one of the penicillins.

Until recently, clients with endocarditis were hospitalized for up to 6 weeks for IV antibiotic therapy. Now they are hospitalized for 5 to 7 days to institute IV therapy and then are discharged for continued IV therapy at home. During hospitalization, the nurse assesses the client's response to therapy. Clients are responding to antimicrobial therapy and may be considered for home therapy when they have been afebrile for 3 to 4 days, have negative blood cultures, and have no signs of heart failure or embolization.

Anticoagulants are of no value in preventing embolization from vegetations. Because they may result in bleeding, they are avoided unless they are required to prevent thrombus formation on a prosthetic valve.

OTHER INTERVENTIONS. Complete bedrest need not be enforced unless clients have fever or signs of heart failure.

TABLE 35-3 • ANTIBIOTIC PROPHYLAXIS* FOR CLIENTS SUSCEPTIBLE TO INFECTIVE ENDOCARDITIS

Procedure	Standard Regimen	For Clients Allergic to Penicillin
Dental, oral, upper respiratory tract, or esophageal procedures and surgery	One of the following: Amoxicillin 2 g PO Ampicillin 2 g IM or IV	One of the following: Clindamycin (Cleocin) 600 mg PO or IV Cephalexin (Keflex) 2 g PO Azithromycin (Zithromax) 500 mg PO Clarithromycin (Biaxin) 500 mg PO Cefazolin (Ancef) 1 g IM or IV within 30 min of the procedure
Genitourinary tract and gastrointestinal tract surgery or instrumentation	One of the following: Ampicillin 2 g PO, IM, or IV	Vancomycin 1 g IV given over 1-2 hr to be completed 30 min before starting procedure

*PO doses are given 1 hr before the procedure; IM or IV doses are given or completed 30 min before the procedure.

However, activities are monitored to allow adequate rest. The nurse explains proper oral and general body hygiene and consistently uses appropriate aseptic technique to protect the client from contact with potentially infective organisms. Nursing assessment for signs of heart failure (including rapid pulse, fatigue, cough, and dyspnea; new heart murmurs; and early signs of embolization) continues throughout the antibiotic regimen.

SURGICAL MANAGEMENT. The cardiac surgeon may be consulted if antibiotic therapy is ineffective in sterilizing a valve, if refractory heart failure develops secondary to a defective valve, if large valvular vegetations are present, or if multiple embolic events occur. Current surgical interventions for infective endocarditis include the following:

- Removing the infected valve (either biologic or prosthetic)
- Repairing or removing congenital shunts
- Repairing injured valves and chordae tendineae
- Draining abscesses in the heart or elsewhere

Preoperative and postoperative care of clients having surgery involving the valves is similar to that described earlier for valve replacement (pp. 715 and 716).

Community-Based Care

Community-based care for clients with infective endocarditis is essential to resolve the problem and avoid complications. Clients and families need to be motivated and have the knowledge, physical ability, and resources to administer IV antibiotics at home. The home care nurse may be contacted to complete teaching started in the acute care institution and to monitor client compliance and health status.

The home care nurse and pharmacist arrange for appropriate supplies to be available to the client at home. Supplies include the prepared antibiotic, IV pump with tubing, alcohol wipes, IV access device, normal saline solution, and a heparin or saline lock flush solution drawn up in syringes. A heparin or saline lock, peripherally inserted central catheter (PICC line), or central catheter is positioned at a new venous site that is easily accessible to the client or a family member.

The nurse teaches the client, family members, or a significant other how to administer the antibiotic and care for the infusion site while maintaining aseptic technique. The client or family member demonstrates this technique before the client is discharged from the hospital. The nurse emphasizes the importance of maintaining a blood level of the antibiotic by administering the antibiotics as scheduled. After stabilization at home, the health care provider contacts the client every 3 to 7 days to determine if he or she is able to comply with and benefit from the IV antibiotic therapy.

The nurse encourages proper hygiene, particularly oral hygiene. Clients are advised to use a soft toothbrush, to brush their teeth at least twice a day, and to rinse the mouth with water after brushing. They should not use irrigation devices or floss the teeth because bacteremia may result. The nurse instructs clients to wash lacerations well and apply an antibiotic ointment.

Clients must remind health care providers (including their dentists) of their endocarditis and request prophylactic antibiotic coverage for every invasive procedure, including dental care (Table 35-3). This protection is essential because studies have documented low compliance with prophylaxis regimens by health care providers.

The nurse teaches clients self-monitoring for the manifestations of endocarditis, including the complications of heart failure and embolic phenomena. They are instructed to monitor their temperature daily and record it for up to 6 weeks. They are also taught to report fever, chills, malaise, weight loss, increased fatigue, or dyspnea to their primary care provider.

Pericarditis

OVERVIEW

Pericarditis is an inflammation or alteration of the pericardium, the membranous sac that encloses the heart. There are two general types of pericarditis: acute pericarditis and chronic constrictive pericarditis.

Acute pericarditis may be fibrous, serous, hemorrhagic, purulent, or neoplastic. Acute pericarditis is most commonly associated with the following:

- Malignant neoplasms
- Idiopathic causes
- Infective organisms (bacteria, viruses, or fungi)
- Postmyocardial infarction (MI) syndrome (Dressler's syndrome)
- Postpericardiotomy syndrome
- Systemic connective tissue disease
- Renal failure

The cause of the pericarditis determines its presentation. Acute viral pericarditis commonly follows a respiratory infection and is more common in men between 20 and 50 years of age. In 5% to 15% of clients who experience an MI, Dressler's syndrome occurs from 1 to 12 weeks after the infarction. This syndrome is characterized by pericarditis, fever, and pericardial and pleural effusions. **Postpericardiotomy syndrome** occurs in 10% to 40% of clients after cardiac surgery.

Chronic constrictive pericarditis occurs when chronic pericardial inflammation causes a fibrous thickening of the pericardium. It is caused by tuberculosis, radiation therapy, trauma, renal failure, or metastatic cancer. In chronic constrictive pericarditis, the pericardium becomes rigid, preventing adequate filling of the ventricles and eventually resulting in cardiac failure.

COLLABORATIVE MANAGEMENT

Assessment

Assessment findings include substernal precordial pain that radiates to the left side of the neck, the shoulder, or the back. Pain is classically grating and oppressive and is aggravated by breathing (mainly on inspiration), coughing, and swallowing. The pain is worse when the client is in the supine position and may be relieved by sitting up and leaning forward. The nurse asks all of the questions to evaluate chest discomfort because it is important that the pain of pericarditis be differentiated from that of an acute MI (see Chapter 33).

The nurse may hear a pericardial friction rub with the diaphragm of the stethoscope positioned at the left lower sternal border. This scratchy, high-pitched sound is produced when the inflamed, roughened pericardial layers create friction as their surfaces rub together.

Clients with acute pericarditis may have an elevated white blood cell count. Electrocardiogram (ECG) changes consisting of an ST-T wave elevation in all leads develop concurrently with the onset of the chest pain. Later with treatment and as the pain diminishes and after ST segments return to baseline, the T waves become inverted in most leads. Clients with infectious pericarditis usually have fever. Blood specimens for culture may be obtained to assess for possible bacterial infection. Echocardiograms may demonstrate a pericardial effusion.

Clients with chronic constrictive pericarditis show signs of right-sided heart failure, elevated systemic venous pressure with jugular distention, hepatic engorgement, and dependent edema. Exertional fatigue and dyspnea are common complications. These clients may have thickening of the pericardium on echocardiography or a computed tomography (CT) scan. ECG changes include inverted or flat T waves. Atrial fibrillation is common.

Interventions

MEDICAL THERAPY. The client with acute pericarditis may be hospitalized for diagnostic evaluation, observation for complications, and symptom relief. The health care provider usually prescribes nonsteroidal anti-inflammatory drugs for the relief of pain. Clients who do not obtain pain relief within 48 to 96 hours and who do not have bacterial pericarditis may receive corticosteroid therapy. The nurse assesses for pain relief and assists the client to assume positions of comfort—usually sitting upright and leaning slightly forward. If the pain is not relieved within 24 to 48 hours, the nurse notifies the primary care provider.

CHART 35-12

BEST PRACTICE *for* Care of the Client with Pericarditis

- Assess the nature of the client's chest discomfort. (Pericardial pain is typically substernal; it is worse on inspiration and decreases when the client leans forward.)
- Auscultate for a pericardial friction rub.
- Assist the client to a position of comfort.
- Provide anti-inflammatory agents as prescribed.
- Explain that anti-inflammatory agents usually decrease the pain within 48 hours.
- Avoid the administration of aspirin and anticoagulants because these may increase the possibility of tamponade.
- Ausculate the blood pressure carefully to detect paradoxical blood pressure (pulsus paradoxus), a sign of tamponade.
  - Palpate the blood pressure and inflate the cuff above the systolic pressure.
  - Deflate the cuff gradually, and note when sounds are first audible on expiration.
  - Identify when sounds are also audible on inspiration.
  - Subtract the inspiratory pressure from the expiratory pressure to determine the amount of pulsus paradoxus (>10 mm Hg is an indication of tamponade).
- Inspect for other indications of tamponade, including jugular venous distention with clear lungs, muffled heart sounds, and decreased cardiac output.
- Notify the physician if tamponade is suspected.

The various causes of pericarditis require specific therapies. For example, bacterial pericarditis (acute) usually requires antibiotics and pericardial drainage. The usual clinical course of acute pericarditis is short term (2 to 6 weeks), but episodes may recur. Chronic pericarditis caused by malignant disease may be treated with radiation or chemotherapy, whereas uremic pericarditis is treated by hemodialysis.

The definitive treatment for chronic constrictive pericarditis is surgical excision of the pericardium **(pericardiectomy).**

MONITORING FOR COMPLICATIONS OF PERICARDITIS. A significant complication of pericarditis is pericardial effusion, which occurs when the space between the parietal and visceral layers of the pericardium fills with fluid. Pericardial effusion puts the client at risk for cardiac tamponade, or excessive fluid within the pericardial cavity. Tamponade, which occurs in 15% of clients with acute pericarditis, restricts diastolic ventricular filling, and cardiac output drops. Findings of cardiac tamponade include the following:

- Jugular venous distention
- Paradoxical pulse (systolic blood pressure 10 mm Hg higher or more on expiration than on inspiration) (Chart 35-12)
- Decreased cardiac output
- Muffled heart sounds

MANAGEMENT OF ACUTE CARDIAC TAMPONADE. **Acute cardiac tamponade** may occur when small volumes (20 to 50 mL) of fluid accumulate rapidly in the pericardium. If the fluid accumulates slowly, the pericardium may stretch to accommodate several hundred milliliters of fluid. The nurse reports any suspicion of this complication to the physician immediately. The physician may initially manage the decreased cardiac output with increased fluid volume administration while awaiting a chest x-ray study or echocardiogram to confirm the diagnosis. Unfortunately, these tests are not always helpful because the fluid volume around the heart may be too small to visualize. Hemodynamic monitoring in a specialized critical care unit usually demonstrates compression of the heart, with all pressures (right atrial, pulmonary artery, and wedge) being similar and elevated (plateau pressures).

The physician may elect to perform a **pericardiocentesis** to relieve the pressure on the heart. Under echocardiographic or fluoroscopic and hemodynamic monitoring, the cardiologist inserts an 8-inch (20.3-cm), 16- or 18-gauge pericardial needle into the pericardial space. The physician and the nurse monitor the needle's position, recognizing that ST-wave and T-wave changes indicate myocardial injury and that the needle must be withdrawn slightly. When the needle is properly positioned, a catheter is inserted and all available pericardial fluid is withdrawn. The nurse monitors the pulmonary artery, wedge, and right atrial pressures during the procedure. The pressures should return to normal as the fluid compressing the heart is removed, and the clinical manifestations of tamponade should resolve. In situations in which the cause of the effusion is unknown, pericardial fluid specimens may be sent to the laboratory for cell count, culture and sensitivity tests, and cytology.

After the pericardiocentesis, the nurse closely monitors for the recurrence of tamponade. Pericardiocentesis alone often does not resolve acute tamponade. The nurse should be prepared to provide adequate fluid volumes to increase cardiac output and to prepare the client for emergency sternotomy if tamponade recurs.

If the client experiences a recurrence of tamponade or recurrent effusions or adhesions from chronic pericarditis, a portion or all of the pericardium may need to be removed to allow adequate ventricular filling and contraction. The surgeon may perform a pericardial window, which involves removing a portion of the pericardium to permit excessive pericardial fluid to drain into the pleural space. In more severe cases, removal of the toughened encasing pericardium (pericardiectomy) may be necessary.

Rheumatic Carditis

OVERVIEW

Rheumatic carditis occurs in about 40% of clients with rheumatic fever and affects more than 1 million Americans. It is a sensitivity response that develops after an upper respiratory tract infection with group A beta-hemolytic streptococci. The precise mechanism by which the infection causes inflammatory lesions in the heart is not established. However, inflammation is evident in all layers of the heart. The inflammation results in impaired contractile function of the myocardium, thickening of the pericardium, and valvular damage.

Rheumatic carditis is characterized by the formation of Aschoff's bodies, small nodules in the myocardium that are replaced by scar tissue. A diffuse cellular infiltrate also develops and appears to be responsible for the heart failure. The pericardium becomes thickened and covered with exudate, and a serosanguineous pleural effusion may develop. The most serious damage occurs to the endocardium, with inflammation of the valve leaflets developing. Hemorrhagic and fibrous lesions form along the inflamed surfaces of the valves, resulting in stenosis or regurgitation primarily of the mitral and aortic valves.

Rheumatic fever may be a complication of 3% of group A beta-hemolytic throat infections. Although the primary attacks occur most often in childhood, rheumatic fever may occur in adulthood. The incidence of rheumatic carditis had been decreasing consistently until the mid-1980s. At that time, a resurgence of rheumatic fever began in both the United States and Europe.

➤ COLLABORATIVE MANAGEMENT

Rheumatic carditis is one of the major indicators of rheumatic fever. The following are common clinical manifestations:

- Tachycardia
- Cardiomegaly
- Development of a new murmur or a change in an existing murmur
- Pericardial friction rub
- Precordial pain
- Electrocardiogram (ECG) changes (prolonged PR interval)
- Indications of heart failure
- Evidence of an existing streptococcal infection

Primary prevention is extremely important. The nurse teaches all clients to consult their health care providers and receive appropriate antibiotic therapy if they develop the following indications of streptococcal pharyngitis: moderate to high fever, abrupt onset of a sore throat, a reddened throat with exudate, and enlarged and tender lymph nodes. Penicillin is the antibiotic of choice for treatment. Erythromycin (Eryc, Erythromid✦) is the alternative for penicillin-sensitive clients.

The signs of rheumatic carditis must be recognized promptly, and antibiotic therapy must be instituted immediately for secondary prevention. The client is urged to continue the antibiotic administration for the full 10 days to prevent reinfection. The nurse suggests ways to manage the fever, such as maintaining hydration and administering antipyretics. The nurse encourages the client to obtain adequate rest.

The nurse emphasizes tertiary prevention in client education, explaining that a recurrence of rheumatic carditis is probable with reinfection by a streptococcal organism. Thus antibiotic therapy is essential for streptococcal infection. The nurse also informs the client that antibiotic prophylaxis is necessary for the rest of his or her life to prevent infective endocarditis (see Infective Endocarditis, p. 718).

CARDIOMYOPATHY

OVERVIEW

Cardiomyopathy is a subacute or chronic enlargement of cardiac muscle. It is not common, occurring in only 10 to 20 per 100,000 population and resulting in about 27,000 deaths each year in the United States. The cause is usually unknown.

Treatment is usually palliative, not curative, and approximately 50% of clients die within 5 years of diagnosis. Clients need to deal with a shortened life span along with numerous lifestyle changes.

Cardiomyopathies are classified into three categories on the basis of abnormalities in structure and function: dilated cardiomyopathy, hypertrophic cardiomyopathy, and restrictive cardiomyopathy (Table 35-4).

Dilated Cardiomyopathy

Dilated cardiomyopathy (DCM) is the structural abnormality in 87% of cardiomyopathy cases. DCM involves exten-

TABLE 35-4 • PATHOPHYSIOLOGY, SIGNS AND SYMPTOMS, AND TREATMENT OF CARDIOMYOPATHIES

Dilated Cardiomyopathy	Hypertrophic Cardiomyopathy: Nonobstructed	Hypertrophic Cardiomyopathy: Obstructed	Restrictive Cardiomyopathy
PATHOPHYSIOLOGY			
Fibrosis of myocardium and endocardium Dilated chambers Mural wall thrombi prevalent	Hypertrophy of all walls Hypertrophied septum Relatively small chamber size	Same as for nonobstructed except for obstruction of left ventricular outflow tract associated with the hypertrophied septum and mitral valve incompetence	Mimics constrictive pericarditis Fibrosed walls cannot expand or contract Chambers narrowed; emboli common
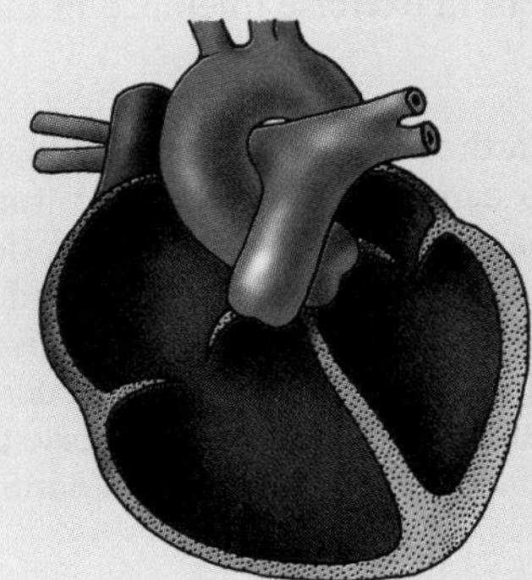	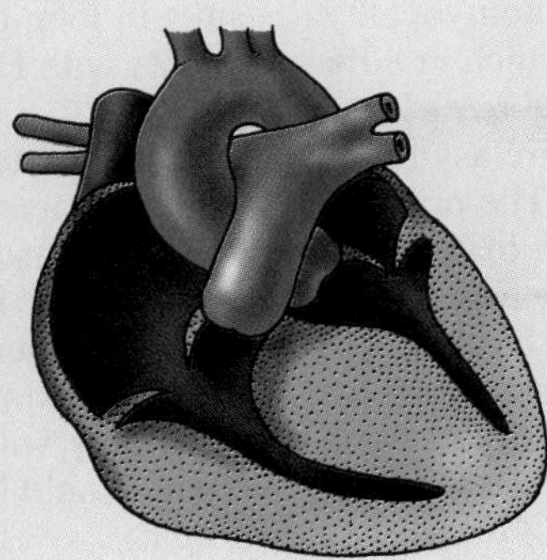		
SIGNS AND SYMPTOMS			
Fatigue and weakness Heart failure (left side) Dysrhythmias or heart block Systemic or pulmonary emboli S_3 and S_4 gallops Moderate to severe cardiomegaly	Dyspnea Angina Fatigue, syncope, palpitations Mild cardiomegaly S_4 gallop Ventricular dysrhythmias Sudden death common Heart failure	Same as for nonobstructed except with mitral regurgitation murmur Atrial fibrillation	Dyspnea and fatigue Heart failure (right-sided) Mild to moderate cardiomegaly S_3 and S_4 gallops Heart block Emboli
TREATMENT			
Symptomatic treatment of heart failure Vasodilators Control of dysrhythmias Surgery: heart transplant	For both: Symptomatic treatment Beta blockers Conversion of atrial fibrillation Surgery: ventriculomyotomy or muscle resection with mitral valve replacement Digitalis, nitrates, and other vasodilators **contraindicated** with the obstructed form		Supportive treatment of symptoms Treatment of hypertension Conversion from dysrhythmias Exercise restrictions Emergency treatment of acute pulmonary edema

Data from Wynne, J., & Braunwald, E. (1992). The cardiomyopathies and myocarditis. In E. Braunwald (Ed.), *Heart disease: A textbook of cardiovascular medicine* (3rd ed.). Philadelphia: W.B. Saunders.

sive damage to the myofibrils and interference with myocardial metabolism. There is normal ventricular wall thickness but a dilation of both ventricles and impairment of systolic function. Decreased cardiac output from inadequate pumping of the heart causes the client to experience dyspnea on exertion, decreased exercise capacity, fatigue, and palpitations. With the exception of peripartum cardiomyopathy, DCM is twice as common in men as in women and occurs most often in middle age. Causes may include alcohol abuse and chemotherapy.

Hypertrophic Cardiomyopathy

The cardinal features of hypertrophic cardiomyopathy (HCM) are asymmetric ventricular hypertrophy of the left ventricle and disarray of the myocardial fibers. Left ventricular hypertrophy leads to a hypercontractile left ventricle with rigid ventricular walls. Obstruction in the left ventricular outflow tract is seen in 75% to 80% of clients with HCM. The abnormal stiffness of the ventricle in HCM results in diastolic filling abnormalities. In approximately 50% of clients, HCM is transmitted as a single-gene autosomal dominant trait. The American Heart Association (1998) reports that approximately 36% of young athletes who die suddenly probably had hypertrophic cardiomyopathy.

Restrictive Cardiomyopathy

Restrictive cardiomyopathy, the rarest of the three cardiomyopathies, results in restriction of filling of the ventricles. It is caused by endocardial and/or myocardial disease and produces a clinical picture similar to that of constrictive pericarditis.

COLLABORATIVE MANAGEMENT

Assessment

Findings in cardiomyopathy depend on the structural and functional abnormalities. Left ventricular or biventricular failure is characteristic of *dilated* cardiomyopathy (DCM). Some clients with DCM are asymptomatic for months to years and have left ventricular dilation identified on x-ray examination. Other clients experience sudden, pronounced symptoms of left ventricular failure, such as progressive dyspnea on exertion, orthopnea, palpitations, and activity intolerance. Right-sided heart failure develops late in the disease and is associated with a poor prognosis. Atrial fibrillation occurs in 25% of clients and is associated with embolism.

The clinical picture of *hypertrophic* cardiomyopathy (HCM) results from the hypertrophied septum, which in 80% of cases causes a mechanical obstruction and thereby reduces stroke volume and cardiac output. Most clients are asymptomatic until late adolescence or early adulthood. The primary symptoms of HCM are exertional dyspnea (90% of clients), angina (75% of clients), and syncope. The chest pain is atypical in that it usually occurs at rest, is prolonged, has no relation to exertion, and is not relieved by the administration of nitrates. A high incidence of ventricular dysrhythmias is associated with HCM. Sudden death occurs and may be the first manifestation of the disease.

The earliest clinical finding in *restrictive* cardiomyopathy is exertional dyspnea. Cardiac output cannot increase during periods of exertion because of the fixed ventricular volume. The client also reports weakness, exercise intolerance, palpitations, and syncope.

Echocardiography, radionuclide imaging, and angiocardiography during cardiac catheterization are performed to diagnose and differentiate cardiomyopathies.

Interventions

The treatment of choice for the client with cardiomyopathy varies with the type of cardiomyopathy and may include both medical and surgical interventions.

NONSURGICAL MANAGEMENT. The care of clients with dilated or restrictive cardiomyopathy is initially the same as for heart failure. Drug therapy includes the use of diuretics, vasodilating agents, and cardiac glycosides to increase cardiac output. Because clients are at risk for sudden death, the nurse urges them to report any palpitations, dizziness, or fainting, which might indicate a dysrhythmia. Antidysrhythmic drugs or implantable cardiac defibrillators may be used to control life-threatening dysrhythmias. Beta blockers (e.g., metoprolol) are used experimentally for clients with excessive sympathetic stimulation and resting tachycardia. If cardiomyopathy has developed in response to a toxin, clients are instructed to avoid further exposure to that toxin. The nurse teaches all clients with cardiomyopathy to abstain from alcohol ingestion because of its cardiac depressant effects.

Management of obstructive HCM includes administering negative inotropic agents such as beta-adrenergic blocking agents (carvedilol) and calcium antagonists (diltiazem). They decrease the outflow obstruction that accompanies exercise and also decrease heart rate, resulting in less angina, dyspnea, and syncope. Vasodilators and cardiac glycosides are contraindicated in clients with obstructive HCM because vasodilating and positive inotropic effects may augment the obstruction. Strenuous exercise is also prohibited because it can increase the risk of sudden death.

SURGICAL MANAGEMENT. The type of surgery performed depends on the type of cardiomyopathy.

EXCISION OF HYPERTROPHIED SEPTUM. Surgery may be considered for the small percentage of clients with obstructive HCM who do not respond to medical therapy. The most commonly used surgical treatment (ventriculomyomectomy) includes excising a portion of the hypertrophied ventricular septum to create a widened outflow tract. Surgery results in long-term improvement in exercise tolerance in most clients with HCM.

CARDIOMYOPLASTY. Cardiomyoplasty is used for some clients with DCM who cannot undergo cardiac transplantation and are asymptomatic at rest. The latissimus dorsum muscle is dissected free of its distal insertion and is wrapped around the heart. For the next 2 months, the muscle is stimulated with increasing frequency until it can contract in synchrony with each heartbeat. Six months after surgery, the client should begin to feel the effects of an enhanced cardiac output.

HEART TRANSPLANTATION. **Heart transplantation** is the treatment of choice for clients with severe DCM and may be considered for clients with restrictive cardiomyopathy. Each year about 2300 clients in the United States receive cardiac transplants—most for DCM (see the Legal/Ethical Issues in Health Care box on p. 725). Criteria for candidate selection include the following:

- Life expectancy less than 1 year
- Age generally less than 65 years
- New York Heart Association (NYHA) class III or IV
- Normal or only slightly increased pulmonary vascular resistance
- Absence of active infection
- Stable psychosocial status
- No evidence of drug or alcohol abuse

The surgeon transplants a heart from a donor with a comparable body weight and ABO compatibility into a recipient less than 6 hours after procurement. In the most common procedure **(orthotopic transplantation),** the surgeon removes the diseased heart and leaves the posterior walls of the client's atria. The remnant atria serve as the anchor for the donor heart. Anastomoses are made between the recipient and donor atria, aorta, and pulmonary arteries (Figure 35-6). Because the remaining remnant of the recipient's atria contains the sinoatrial node, two unrelated P waves are visible on the ECG.

The postoperative care of the heart transplant recipient is similar to that for conventional cardiac surgery. However, the nurse must be especially vigilant to identify occult bleeding into the pericardial sac with the potential for tamponade. The recipient's pericardium has usually stretched considerably to accommodate the diseased, hypertrophied heart. This predisposes the client to concealed postoperative bleeding.

The transplanted heart is denervated and is unresponsive to vagal stimulation. The client's heart rate approximates 100 beats/min, responding slowly to exercise, stress, or position change with increases in heart rate, contractility, and cardiac output. In the early postoperative phase, the nurse may titrate isoproterenol (Isuprel) to support the heart rate and maintain cardiac output. Atropine, digitalis, and carotid sinus pressure are not used because they do not have their usual effects on the denervated heart. Denervation of the heart may cause pronounced orthostatic hypotension in the immediate postoperative phase, and the nurse cautions the client to change position slowly.

To suppress natural defense mechanisms and prevent transplant rejection, clients require immunosuppressant therapy for the rest of their lives. Most commonly, the physician prescribes therapy with cyclosporine (Sandimmune) and azathioprine (Imuran). Nurses must be vigilant about handwashing and aseptic technique because clients are immunosuppressed and infection is the major cause of death. Infection usually develops in the immediate post-transplant period or during treatment for acute rejection.

Most clients experience their initial episode of acute rejection in the first 3 months after heart transplantation. Symptoms of rejection are nonspecific and occur late in the rejection process. They include cardiac dysrhythmias (especially

Legal/Ethical Issues in Health Care

TO WHOM SHOULD DONATED HEARTS BE ALLOCATED FOR TRANSPLANTATION?

Each year approximately 16,000 Americans younger than 55 years of age are waiting for a heart transplant. This number increases to 40,000 if Americans younger than 65 years old are considered. However, only about 2300 heart transplants are performed each year because of a limited number of donor hearts. In the past, human organ allocation was both by recipient need and by region of the country. The Department of Health and Human Services (DHHS) has now ruled that the person who is the best match and has the greatest need anywhere in the nation should receive a donated heart.

Critics temporarily blocked enactment of the ruling, stating there were serious ethical concerns. First, they noted that donating the heart to the most critically ill person does not always represent good stewardship of resources. The survival rate for heart transplant recipients is better (approximately 70% at 4 years) when the recipient requires a heart transplant but is not critically ill. Critics of the DHHS policy contend that transplanting organs into clients who are too ill to benefit would waste a very precious resource from which someone else could have benefited. The transplant procedure is also expensive, costing approximately $253,000 in the first year. That money would also be wasted if the recipient was too ill to benefit and died after receiving the transplant.

Critics also argue that a national allocation of transplants would result in less local publicity about transplant recipients. They ask what will happen to the already low rate of donations when people are unable to perceive an immediate and local benefit. They fear that only the largest urban transplant centers will survive and that donation rates will drop still further, worsening the scarcity.

The question of how best to allocate donated hearts remains controversial. Should donated hearts be allocated to the sickest person in the nation who is a match? Or should the heart be provided to a person who lives in the region, matches the donor, and is most likely to benefit? The ethical issue is: How do we decide what is a just or fair way to distribute scarce health care resources? Do we distribute to the person with the greatest need or to the person who is most likely to benefit? Should concerns about how to secure a continuing supply of the scarce resource deserve consideration when deciding how to allocate the resource?

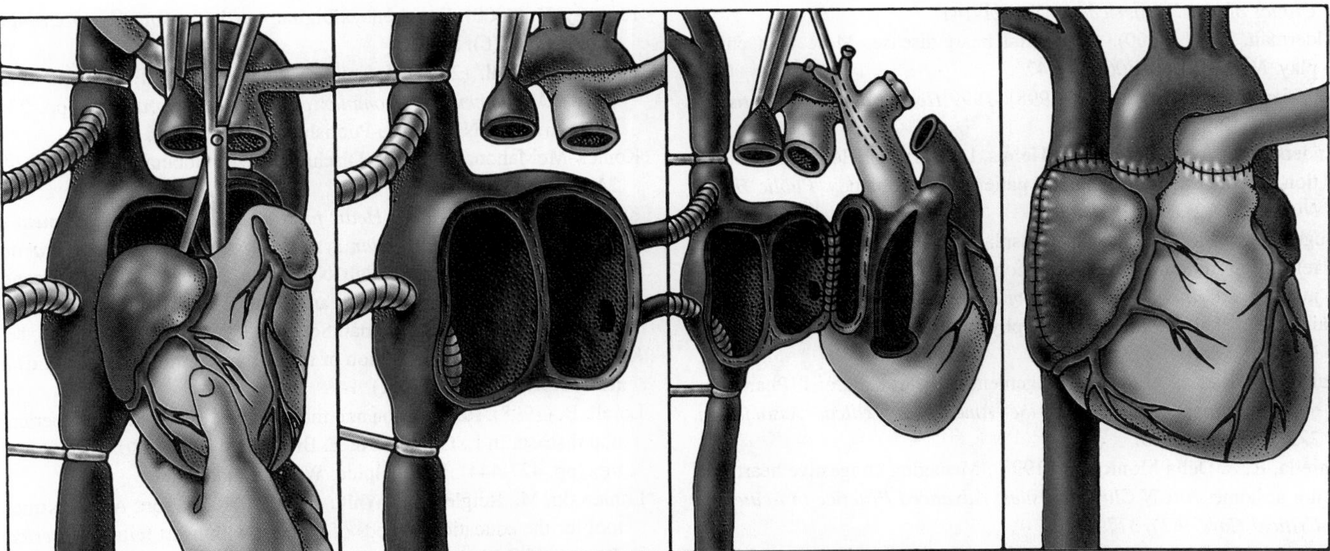

Figure 35-6 ● Heart transplantation.

atrial dysrhythmias), hypotension, weakness, fatigue, and dizziness. To detect rejection, the surgeon performs right endomyocardial biopsies at regularly scheduled intervals and whenever symptoms occur.

Approximately 75% of clients survive 3 years after transplantation; most return to NYHA class I or II status (AHA, 1998). Five years after transplantation, many of the surviving clients (20% to 40%) have evidence of coronary artery disease (CAD) presenting as diffuse plaque in the arteries of the donor heart. Because the heart is denervated, clients do not usually experience angina, and regularly scheduled exercise tolerance tests and angiography are required to identify CAD.

To delay the development of CAD, clients are encouraged to follow a prudent lifestyle similar to clients with CAD (see Chapter 38). The physician may prescribe a calcium channel blocker such as diltiazem (Cardizem) to decrease the rate of coronary artery narrowing. The nurse stresses the importance of compliance with dietary modifications and medication regimens. The client is encouraged to participate in a regular exercise program but is cautioned to allow at least 10 minutes of warm up and cool down for the denervated heart to adjust to changes in activity level.

ONLINE RESOURCES

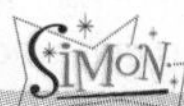

For suggested readings and Internet resources, go to http://www.wbsaunders.com/SIMON/Iggy/.

SELECTED BIBLIOGRAPHY

Asterisk indicates a classic or definitive work on this subject.

Acute care decisions: Patient education. CHF education saved this hospital $173,000. (1998). *RN, 61*(11), 24C-D.

Albert, N.M. (1999). Manipulating survival and life quality outcomes in heart failure through disease state management. *Critical Care Nursing Clinics of North America, 11*(2), 121-141.

Alderman, L.M. (2000). Congenital heart disease: More than child's play. *Nursing2000, 30*(5), 41-47.

American Heart Association. (1998). *1999 Heart and Stroke Statistical Update.* Dallas: Author.

Anderson, M.A., Pena, R.A., & Helms, L.B. (1998). Home care utilization by congestive heart failure patients: A pilot study. *Public Health Nursing, 15*(2), 146-162.

Augustine, S.M. (2000). Heart transplantation: Long-term management related to immunosuppression, complications, and psychosocial adjustments. *Critical Care Clinics of North America, 12*(1),79-85.

Baig, M.K., et al. (1999). The pathophysiology of advanced heart failure. *Heart and Lung, 28*(2), 87-101.

*Baker, D.W., et al. (1994). Management of heart failure: I. Pharmacologic treatment. *Journal of the American Medical Association, 272*(17), 1361-1365.

Barella, P., & Della Monica, E. (1998). Managing congestive heart failure at home. *AACN Clinical Issues: Advanced Practice in Acute and Critical Care, 9*(3), 377-388.

Bennett, S.J., et al. (1999). Cost of hospitalizations for heart failure: Sodium retention versus other decompensating factors. *Heart and Lung, 28*(2), 102-108.

Branum, K. (1999). Using beta blockers in the treatment of heart failure. *The Nurse Practitioner, 24*(7), 75-83.

Braunwald, E. (1997). *Heart disease: A textbook of cardiovascular medicine* (5th ed.). Philadelphia: W.B. Saunders.

Cambell, R.L., Konick-McMahan, J., & Naylor, M.D. (1998). Discharge planning and home follow-up for the elderly patient with heart failure. *Nursing Clinics of North America, 33*(3), 497-513.

Carabello, B.A. (1998). Recognition and management of patients with valvular heart disease. In L. Goldman & E. Braunwald (Eds.), *Primary cardiology* (pp. 257-283). Philadelphia: W.B. Saunders.

A CHF program that focuses on best practices and benchmarks. (1998). *RN, 61*(3), 24AA-24BB.

Chin, M.H., & Goldman, L. (1997). Factors contributing to the hospitalization of patients with congestive heart failure. *American Journal of Public Health, 87*(4), 643-647.

Clinical update. Cardiac care: Heart failure: Widely undertreated. (1999). *Nursing99, 29*(4), 68.

Colletti, C. (1999). Emergency pericarditis. *American Journal of Nursing, 99*(10), 35.

Cupples, S.A., & Spruill, L.C. (2000). Evaluation criteria for the pretransplant patient. *Critical Care Clinics of North America, 12*(1), 35-47.

Dahl, J., & Penque, S. (2000). The effects of an advanced practice nurse-directed heart failure program. *Nurse Practitioner, 25*(3), 61-62, 65-66, 68.

Dec, G.W. (1998). Recognition and management of patients with cardiomyopathies. In L. Goldman & E. Braunwald (Eds.), *Primary cardiology* (pp. 487-508). Philadelphia: W.B. Saunders.

Dugan, K.J. (1998). Caring for patients with pericarditis. *Nursing98, 28*(3), 50-51.

Guido, G.W. (2000). Heart transplant from an ethical perspective. *Critical Care Clinics of North America, 12*(1),111-119.

Hines, S.E. (2000). Update on mitral prolapse. *Patient Care Nurse Practitioner, 3*(3), 35-37, 41-42, 45-46.

Hoffmann, R.L., & Reeder, S.J. (1998). Applied pharmacology: Angiotensin-converting enzyme inhibitors and left ventricular remodeling: Implications for nurses. *Dimensions of Critical Care Nursing, 17*(5), 256-263.

Karchener, A.W. (1998). Approach to the patient with infective endocarditis. In L. Goldman & E. Braunwald (Eds.), *Primary cardiology* (pp. 201-218). Philadelphia: W.B. Saunders.

Kearney, K. (2000). Emergency: Digitalis toxicity. *American Journal of Nursing, 100*(6), 51-52.

Khai, P.G., et al. (2000). Infective endocarditis. In T. Nguyen, et al. (Eds.). *Management of complex cardiovascular problems* (pp. 235-250). Armonk, NY: Futura Publishing.

Konick-McMahon, J. (1997). Discharged with dobutamine. *RN, 60*(4), 24-28.

*Konstam, M., et al. (1994). *Heart failure: Evaluation and treatment of patients with left ventricular systolic dysfunction. Clinical practice guideline No. 11.* AHCPR Pub. No. 94-0612. Rockville, MD: Agency for Health Care Policy and Research, Public Health Service, U.S. Department of Health and Human Services.

Krau, S.D. (2000). The evolution of heart transplant. *Critical Care Clinics of North America, 12*(1), 1-9.

Lorell, B. (1998). Recognition and management of patients with pericardial disease. In L. Goldman & E. Braunwald (Eds.), *Primary cardiology* (pp. 427-444). Philadelphia: W.B. Saunders.

*Luniewski, M., Reigle, J., & White, B. (1990). Card sort: An assessment tool for the educational needs of patients with heart failure. *American Journal of Critical Care, 8*(5), 297-302.

Martensson, J., Karlsson, J., & Fridlund, B. (1998). Female patients with congestive heart failure: How they conceive their life situation. *Journal of Advanced Nursing, 28*(6), 1216-1224.

Martens, K.H., & Mellor, S.D. (1997). A study of the relationship between home care services and hospital readmission of patients with congestive heart failure. *Home Healthcare Nurse, 15*(2), 123-129.

McCloskey, J.C., & Bulechek, G.M. (Eds.). (2000). *Nursing intervention classification (NIC),* (3rd ed.). St. Louis: Mosby.

McGrath, D. (1997). Clinical snapshot: Mitral valve prolapse. *American Journal of Nursing, 97*(5), 40-41.

Moccia, J.M. (1997). Unmasking pericarditis. *Nursing97, 27*(12), 32cc1-4.

Moons, P., et al. (1998). Symptom experience associated with maintenance immunosuppression after heart transplant: Patient appraisal of side effects. *Heart and Lung, 27*(5), 315-325.

Moser, D.K. & Worster, P.L. (1999). The role of the critical care nurse in preventing heart failure after myocardial infarction. *Critical Care Nurse, 19*(5 Suppl.), 11-15.

Nagle, B.M., & O'Keffe, L.M. (1999). Closing in on mitral valve disease. *Nursing99, 29*(4), 32cc1-32cc7.

Nagle, B.M., & Taylor, J. (1998). Getting to the heart of aortic valve disease. *Nursing99, 28*(5), 32cc8-32cc12.

O'Connor, C.M., Gattis, W.A., & Swenberg, D. (1998). Current and novel pharmacologic approaches in advanced heart failure. *Heart and Lung, 28*(4), 227-239.

O'Gara, P.T. (1998). Approach to the patient with cardiac enlargement. In L. Goldman & E. Braunwald (Eds.), *Primary cardiology* (pp. 174-187). Philadelphia: W.B. Saunders.

O'Rourke, R.A. (1998). Approach to the patient with a heart murmur. In L. Goldman & E. Braunwald (Eds.), *Primary cardiology* (pp. 155-173). Philadelphia: W.B. Saunders.

Paul, S. (2000). Impact of a nurse-managed heart failure clinic: A pilot study. *American Journal of Critical Care, 9*(2), 140-146.

Pawsat, D.E., & Lee, J.Y. (1998). Inflammatory disorders of the heart: Pericarditis, myocarditis, and endocarditis. *Emergency Medical Clinics of North America, 16*(3), 665-681.

Piano, M.J. (1999). Familial hypertropic cardiomyopathy. *Journal of Cardiovascular Nursing, 13*(4), 46-58.

Reeder, D.E., et al. (2000). The impact of angiotensin-converting enzyme inhibitors on managed care: Economic, clinical, and humanistic outcomes. *American Journal of Managed Care, 6*(3 Suppl.): S112-131.

Rockett, J. (1999) Endothelial dysfunction and the promise of ACE inhibitors. *American Journal of Nursing, 99*(10), 44-49.

Ross, G.K., & DeJong, M.J. (1999). Emergency! Pericardial tamponade. *American Journal of Nursing, 99*(2), 35.

Sanderson, J.E. (2000). Heart failure. In T. Nguyen, et al. (Eds.). *Management of complex cardiovascular problems* (pp. 235-250). Armonk, NY: Futura Publishing.

Scorde, K.A.B. (1998). Mitral valve prolapse syndrome: Interventions for symptom control. *Dimensions of Critical Care Nursing, 17*(4), 177-186.

Sparacino, P. (1999). Cardiac infections: Medical and surgical therapies. *Journal of Cardiovascular Nursing, 13*(2), 49-65.

Strimike, C.L., & Wojcik, J. (2000). Getting the facts on heart failure treatment. *Nursing2000, 30*(5), 32hn18-32hn20.

Tasota, F.J., & Tate, J. (2000). Assessing digoxin levels. *Nursing2000, 30*(3), 24.

Thomas, D.J.G., & Harrah, B.F. (2000). *Home Healthcare Nurse, 18*(3), 164-171.

*United Network for Organ Sharing. (1996). *Donation and transplantation: Nursing curriculum.* Richmond, VA: Author.

*U.S. Department of Health and Human Services, Agency for Health Care Policy and Research. (1994). *Heart failure: Evaluation and care of patients with left-ventricular systolic dysfunction.* Rockville, MD: Agency for Health Care Policy and Research, Public Health Service, U.S. Department of Health and Human Services.

Wallace, C.J. (1998). Emergency! Acute pulmonary edema. *RN, 61*(1), 36-41.

Wehby, D., Brenner, P.S. (1999). Perceived learning needs of patients with heart failure. *Heart and Lung, 28*(1), 31-40.

Wilkinson, J.M. (2000). *Nursing diagnosis handbook: NIC interventions and NOC outcomes.* Upper Saddle River, NJ: Prentice Hall Health.

CHAPTER 36

Interventions for Clients with Vascular Problems

DOROTHY J. HAMILTON • DONNA D. IGNATAVICIUS

Learning Objectives

After studying this chapter, you should be able to:

1. Explain the pathophysiology of arteriosclerosis and atherosclerosis, including the factors that cause arterial injury.
2. Discuss the role of diet therapy in the management of clients with arteriosclerosis.
3. Describe the differences between essential and secondary hypertension.
4. Develop a plan of care for a client with essential hypertension.
5. Compare drug classifications used to treat hypertension.
6. Identify cultural considerations when caring for clients with hypertension.
7. Evaluate the effectiveness of interdisciplinary interventions to improve hypertension.
8. Compare and contrast assessment findings typically present in clients with peripheral arterial and peripheral venous disease.
9. Prioritize postoperative care for clients who have undergone peripheral bypass surgery.
10. Develop a continuing care plan for a client who has undergone an abdominal aortic aneurysm repair.
11. Compare and contrast Raynaud's disease and Buerger's disease.
12. Describe the nurse's role in monitoring clients who are receiving anticoagulants, including unfractionated heparin, low–molecular weight heparin, and warfarin.

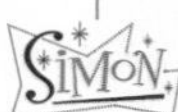

Go to http://www.wbsaunders.com/SIMON/Iggy/ for self-assessment questions related to these Learning Objectives.

The leading cause of death in the United States is disease associated with atherosclerosis. Nearly 1 million people die of heart and blood vessel diseases each year in the United States (American Heart Association, 1999). Atherosclerosis is a common link between cardiovascular disease, cerebrovascular disease, and peripheral vascular disease (PVD). People with atherosclerosis have an increased risk of developing one or more of these diseases.

Disorders of the vascular system cause many problems and may lead to complete shutdown of all body organs and eventually death. Although vascular disease can affect any portion of the human body, such as the heart, brain, and kidneys, the peripheral vascular system and its associated diseases are described here.

ARTERIOSCLEROSIS AND ATHEROSCLEROSIS

OVERVIEW

Arteriosclerosis is a thickening, or hardening, of the arterial wall. **Atherosclerosis,** a type of arteriosclerosis, involves the formation of plaque within the arterial wall. Atherosclerosis is the most common cause of arterial obstruction.

Pathophysiology

The exact pathophysiology of atherosclerosis is not known, but the condition is thought to occur in the following way (Figure 36-1). A fatty streak appears on the intimal surface (inner lining) of the artery. At this stage, the fatty streak may appear flattened or elevated, but it generally does not affect the integrity of the arterial wall.

Next, a fibrous plaque develops. This plaque is described as a white, glistening, fibrous elevation that covers a lipid core. At this stage, the plaque is elevated enough to partially or completely occlude the blood flow of an artery.

In the final stage, the fibrous lesions become calcified, hemorrhagic, ulcerated, or thrombosed. The rate of progression of this process may be influenced by genetic factors; certain chronic diseases, such as diabetes mellitus; and lifestyle habits, including smoking, eating habits, and level of exercise.

Etiology

THEORIES

The exact etiology of atherosclerosis is unknown, but several theories attempt to explain its cause. It is believed that an injury to the intimal layer of the artery may initiate the devel-

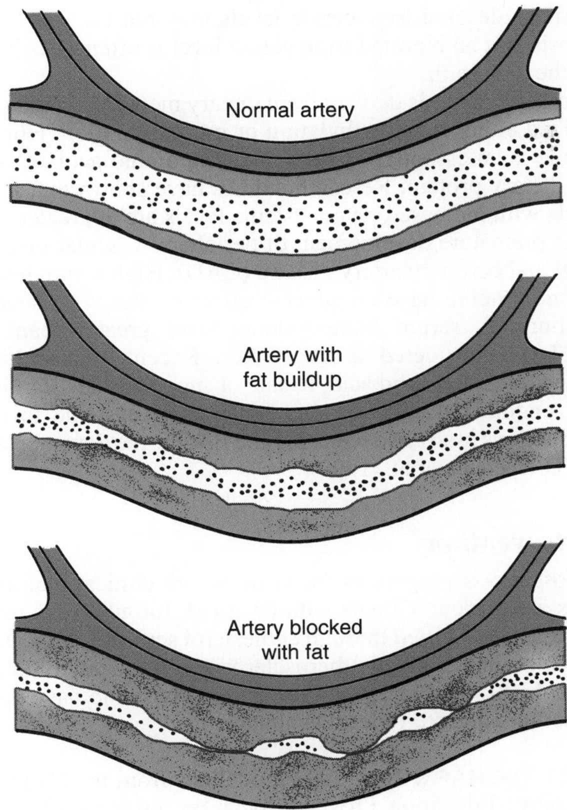

Figure 36-1 ● Pathophysiology of atherosclerosis.

opment of atherosclerosis. One popular theory, known as platelet aggregation, is that after the intimal injury has occurred, platelets form a cluster at the arterial wall and produce a peptide that stimulates the proliferation of the smooth muscle cells of the intima. Eventually, this proliferation can narrow the artery enough to compromise the flow of blood or completely occlude arterial blood flow.

Another theory, the *lipid hypothesis,* assumes that after an intimal injury, a group of blood lipids (fats) accumulate. Again, this accumulation can partially or completely occlude arterial blood flow. The principal lipids involved are cholesterol and triglyceride.

Many theorists believe that a combination of these two events provides the most appropriate explanation of the atherosclerotic process and that this process can occur in any arterial wall of the body. Usually the disease affects the larger arteries, such as the coronary artery beds, the major branches of the aorta, the visceral branches of the aorta, the terminal abdominal aorta, the carotid and vertebral arteries, or any combination of these.

FACTORS CAUSING ARTERIAL INJURY

Intimal injury of the major arteries of the body can be attributed to many factors. Hypertension can cause a mechanical injury, whereas elevated levels of low-density lipoproteins (LDLs) and decreased levels of high-density lipoproteins (HDLs) can cause chemical injuries to the intimal wall. Chemical injury can also be caused by elevated levels of toxins in the bloodstream, which may occur with renal failure or by carbon monoxide circulating in the bloodstream from cigarette smoking. The intimal wall can be weakened by the natural process of aging or by physiologic disorders, such as diabetes.

Genetic predisposition and diabetes have a fairly direct effect on the development of atherosclerosis. Some families demonstrate inherited hyperlipidemia, an elevation in levels of blood lipids. In these people the liver makes excessive cholesterol, which accounts for the development of atherosclerosis. In some people with hereditary atherosclerosis, however, the blood cholesterol level is normal. The reason for the development and progression of plaque in these people is not understood.

People with severe diabetes mellitus frequently have premature and severe atherosclerosis, often involving the microvasculature. This occurs because diabetes promotes an increase in LDL in plasma. In addition, intimal arterial damage may result from the effect of hyperglycemia.

Factors indirectly related to atherosclerosis include obesity, a sedentary lifestyle, and stress. Clients who are obese are at greater risk, most often because of concomitant elevations in cholesterol levels. Long-term physical activity is important in maintaining ideal body weight; it is also thought to help in maintaining optimal blood pressure and cholesterol levels and improved glucose tolerance. The effect of stress may be due to its effect on the sympathetic and parasympathetic release of catecholamines and an acute rise in blood pressure. (See Chapter 38 for further discussion of these and other risk factors for heart disease.)

Incidence/Prevalence

It is not known exactly how many people have atherosclerosis, but small plaques are almost always present in the arteries of young adults. The incidence can be better quantified by assessing diseases that result from this process. However, it is estimated that peripheral atherosclerosis affects 5% of Americans over 60 years of age and up to 25% of those over 75 years of age (Meyerson & Schwartz, 1999). It is predicted that these numbers will increase as a result of the increasing population of older adults.

WOMEN'S HEALTH CONSIDERATIONS

Although the process of atherosclerosis does not appear to differ between men and women, coronary artery disease (CAD) is much less common in premenopausal women than in age-matched men because of the lipid-lowering effect of estrogen. The rates of CAD in postmenopausal women are similar to those of men in the same age-group. People in the United States have a higher incidence of CAD related to atherosclerosis than people in other industrialized nations (American Heart Association, 1999).

➤ COLLABORATIVE MANAGEMENT

● Assessment

VITAL SIGNS

Because of the high incidence of hypertension in clients with atherosclerosis, the nurse assesses the blood pressure in both arms. The heart is also thoroughly assessed because concomitant cardiac disease is often present.

The nurse may palpate pulses at all of the major sites on the body and note any differences. Carotid arteries are palpated separately because of the risk of inadequate cerebral perfusion. The nurse also palpates for temperature differences in the lower extremities and checks capillary filling. Prolonged capillary filling (>3 seconds in young to middle-aged adults; >5 seconds in older adults) generally indicates poor circulation. An extremity in a person with significant atherosclerotic disease may be cool or cold, with a diminished or absent pulse.

ASSESSMENT FOR BRUITS

After palpating the pulses, the nurse may auscultate each large artery from the carotid to the dorsalis pedis with a stethoscope or a Doppler probe. Many clients with vascular disease have a **bruit** in the larger arteries. A bruit is described as a turbulent, swishing sound, which can be soft or loud in pitch. The mere existence of a bruit is considered abnormal, but the role it plays in indicating the severity of vascular disease is not understood. The nurse should document the location of bruits. They often occur in the carotid, aortic, femoral, and popliteal arteries and usually indicate some degree of narrowing of the arterial wall. The rate and intensity of the pulse in each artery during auscultation is also noted. A decrease in intensity and audibility or a complete loss of a pulse may indicate an arterial occlusion.

LABORATORY ASSESSMENT

Total serum cholesterol levels are often elevated in clients with atherosclerosis. Clients should keep their total serum cholesterol levels below 200 mg/dL. The National Cholesterol Education Program has recommended screening guidelines based on the following:

- Total serum cholesterol and high-density lipoprotein (HDL) cholesterol levels in individuals without evidence of cardiac or vascular disease
- Total serum cholesterol and HDL cholesterol levels in individuals with risk factors (Table 36-1)

Elevated cholesterol levels must be validated by HDL and LDL determinations. Elevated LDL cholesterol levels indicate that a person is at an increased risk for atherosclerosis. Low or normal HDL cholesterol levels also indicate an increased risk. A desirable LDL level is one below 100 mg/dL for all individuals. A desirable HDL level is 35 mg/dL or above. In some people, particularly women, an elevated cholesterol level may be due to an elevated HDL level, which is not considered a risk.

Triglyceride levels may also be elevated with atherosclerosis. A level of 200 mg/dL or above indicates hypertriglyceridemia. Elevated triglyceride levels may not cause atherosclerosis, but an elevated triglyceride level is often associated with the condition.

Homocysteine is derived from dietary methionine and metabolized either by remethylation or transsulfuration. Homocysteine is an essential sulfur-containing amino acid derived from dietary protein. Research studies have shown that individuals with increased homocysteine levels are at greater risk for the premature development of peripheral vascular disease (PVD) and coronary artery disease (CAD). High serum levels of homocysteine have an adverse effect on the vascular endothelium. A serum homocysteine level greater than 15 μmol/L is considered a risk factor. Recent studies have demonstrated that folic acid, usually 1 mg every day, can improve endothelial function and lower homocysteine levels. These actions assist in decreasing the risk for the development of PVD (Jacques et al., 1999).

Interventions

Atherosclerosis progresses for years before clinical manifestations are evident. Clients with or at risk for atherosclerosis can often be identified through cholesterol screening. Because of the high incidence of atherosclerosis in the United States, all people 20 years of age and older are advised to have their total serum cholesterol level evaluated.

DIET THERAPY. New 2001 guidelines from the National Cholesterol Education Program focus on an aggressive approach to lowering low-density lipoprotein (LDL) values. Having an LDL value of less than 100 mg/dL is optimal; values of 100 to 129 mg/dL are near or above optimal. Clients with LDL values of 130 to 159 mg/dL (borderline high) are advised to follow a fat-modified diet. In collaboration with the dietitian, the nurse instructs clients with LDL values of 160 mg/dL or greater (high or very high) to follow a more structured diet aimed at decreasing saturated fat and cholesterol and, if appropriate, promoting weight loss. A decrease in fat, particularly saturated fat, is considered more important than simply decreasing the cholesterol number because saturated fat is one of the main determinants of cholesterol synthesis in the body.

In the United States, 37% of the total caloric intake in the diets of many people is made up of fat, and this overconsumption of fat and cholesterol leads to **hypercholesterolemia,** an elevated total blood cholesterol level. On the other hand, elevated cholesterol levels can often be decreased if fat in the diet is limited to no more than 30% of the caloric intake.

To assess what 30% of the caloric intake is, clients first need to determine their ideal daily caloric intake. They can then cal-

TABLE 36-1 • SERUM CHOLESTEROL AND HIGH-DENSITY LIPOPROTEIN LEVELS IN INDIVIDUALS WITHOUT EVIDENCE OF CARDIAC OR VASCULAR DISEASE (PRIMARY PREVENTION)

Total Serum Cholesterol <200		Total Cholesterol = 200-239	
HDL <35: Perform full fasting lipoprotein analysis.	HDL >35: Repeat total and HDL cholesterol testing in 5 years or with physical examination.	HDL <35 or more than two other risk factors: Perform full fasting lipoprotein analysis.	HDL >35 and fewer than two other risk factors: monitor at least every year.

HDL, High-density lipoprotein.

culate their fat limit in grams. In addition to tracking fat in grams, people need to assess the fatty acid content of foods.

STEP ONE DIET. The Step One diet of the American Heart Association, which is often recommended to decrease the serum cholesterol level, calls for a total fat intake of less than 30% of total calories, with less than 10% of total caloric intake coming from saturated fat, up to 10% of total calories coming from polyunsaturated fat, and 10% to 15% coming from monounsaturated fat. Cholesterol intake with this diet is limited to less than 300 mg daily.

In collaboration with the dietitian, the nurse educates the client about the fat content of foods in terms of the total degree of fat and saturation. Meats and eggs contain mostly saturated fats. Because canola (rapeseed) oil is rich in monounsaturated fat and safflower and sunflower oil are rich in polyunsaturated oils, they are recommended over highly saturated oils, such as palm or coconut oil. Cholesterol is found only in animal sources, such as meat and eggs, which are also high in saturated fats.

STEP TWO DIET. The client's serum cholesterol levels are retested 6 and 12 weeks after the initial dietary intervention. If the cholesterol level has not significantly decreased, the client may be referred to a registered dietitian for instruction on a more restricted diet, such as the Step Two diet. The Step Two diet limits saturated fat to less than 7% of total calories and cholesterol to less than 200 mg/day.

In addition to elevated LDL values, other variations of hyperlipidemias put clients at risk for atherosclerosis. A low-fat, low-cholesterol diet, however, can play a significant role in improving a lipid profile, regardless of the lipid alteration.

SMOKING CESSATION. Cigarette smoking lowers levels of high-density lipoprotein (HDL) cholesterol and dramatically increases the rate of progression of atherosclerosis. The nurse can play an important role in helping clients stop smoking (see the Evidence-Based Practice for Nursing box at right).

The nurse advises all clients who smoke to stop smoking and all clients to avoid secondhand smoke. The nurse describes the relationship of smoking to atherosclerosis and assesses the client's willingness to change this behavior. Nurses and other health care providers can refer to the Agency for Healthcare Research and Quality's Practice Guidelines on Smoking Cessation (formerly the Agency for Health Care Policy and Research). This reference provides strategies to assist clients in quitting smoking. A smoking cessation group, such as the American Cancer Society's Fresh Start, may help with this difficult process. Most formal programs encourage people to stop smoking "cold turkey."

Johns Hopkins Hospital in Baltimore has developed a stage-of-readiness model that classifies clients into one of six stages (Stillman, 1995). The nurse can assess the client's readiness to stop smoking using this model (Table 36-2).

Clients may consider using a nicotine patch (Nicoderm, Habitrol, Prostep), which helps relieve nicotine withdrawal symptoms. The patch is about 50% effective in helping clients to stop smoking and is available over the counter. The dose is determined by the client's weight and the extent to which he or she smokes. Clients are urged to stop smoking completely when the nicotine patch is initiated. The nurse informs clients that if they continue to smoke while using the patch, their risks for adverse effects are increased because the peak levels of nicotine are higher than those experienced from smoking alone. Serious cardiovascular effects, such as angina and dysrhythmias, may result from the patch, although the most common side effect is skin irritation. Many health insurance programs will not cover the costs associated with nicotine patches unless the client is enrolled in a smoking cessation program.

Nicotine gum (Nicorette) also may be used if a client feels the need to smoke. Clients should not chew more than 30 pieces of gum per day.

Some clients need an oral medication, such as bupropion (Wellbutrin, Zyban), to help decrease the urge to

EVIDENCE-BASED PRACTICE FOR NURSING

How effective are smoking cessation interventions directed by nurses?

Johnson, J.L., et al. (1999). Evaluation of a nurse-delivered smoking cessation intervention for hospitalized patients with cardiac disease. *Heart and Lung, 28*(1), 55-64.

The purpose of this quasi-experimental study was to evaluate the effectiveness of a nurse-delivered smoking cessation intervention for clients with cardiac disease in a hospital setting. The study group consisted of cardiac clients admitted to inpatient cardiac units for medical or surgical treatment. The subjects recruited for the study were clients who reported smoking for more than 1 year, were medically stable, and had a hospital stay longer than 3 days. There were 102 subjects in the study—52 in the control group and 50 in the treatment group.

The treatment group received a series of interventions provided by nurses. The first nursing intervention consisted of the subjects viewing a 19-minute video entitled *The Smoke-Free Habit,* in which the effects of smoking, the importance of smoking cessation, the smoking cessation process, and smoking triggers were presented. While viewing the video, subjects were prompted to answer key questions about their smoking habits, and they documented their responses on an answer sheet. After viewing the video, the nurses answered questions about smoking and encouraged subjects to set a firm date to quit smoking. At the time of discharge from the hospital, subjects viewed the second part of the video, in which approaches to smoking cessation were viewed and reinforced. Subjects were followed with weekly telephone calls for 1 month and then monthly telephone calls for 2 months. The subjects received a total of six telephone calls. The nurses provided positive reinforcement for all efforts made to quit smoking during the telephone calls. Clients completed a questionnaire at the start of the study and at 6 months.

At the completion of the study, there were 42 subjects in the intervention group and 44 subjects in the control group. Of the initial 102 subjects, 5 subjects were deceased at 6 months and 11 subjects were lost to follow-up. The results of the study showed that the intervention group had a higher rate of nonsmoking compared with the control group. This research suggests that a nurse-delivered smoking cessation intervention may improve the smoking cessation rate in clients with cardiac disease.

Critique. This is an excellent study in which nurses provide strategies and support for cardiac clients to quit smoking. This study should be repeated with a larger sample size, including clients with vascular, as well as cardiac, problems and following clients for 1 year.

Implications for Nursing. Smoking has been identified as a strong risk factor for the development and acceleration of peripheral vascular disease (PVD). Even though this study was done in clients with cardiac problems, nurses caring for people with vascular disease need to identify smokers. Nurses should provide information related to smoking cessation interventions and smoking cessation programs. This is an area in which nurses truly can make a positive impact on client outcomes.

TABLE 36-2 • STAGE-OF-READINESS MODEL FOR SMOKING CESSATION

Description of Stage	Nursing Strategies
PRECONTEMPLATION	
Clients have no desire to quit smoking.	Teach negative effects of smoking; reassure client that feelings are part of addiction process; deliver a "fear" message related to poor health consequences.
CONTEMPLATION	
Clients have thought about smoking cessation but have taken no action.	Provide specific examples of how smoking is affecting the client; stress health benefits if client quits smoking.
PREPARATION	
Client has taken some steps to quit smoking.	Provide behavioral reinforcement; help the client identify cues that lead to smoking, such as after eating; help the client identify coping strategies.
ACTION	
Client quits smoking.	Provide positive reinforcement to prevent relapse.
MAINTENANCE	
Client has not smoked for 6 months.	Continue with positive reinforcement.

Data from Stillman, F.A. (1995). Smoking cessation for the hospitalized cardiac patient: Rationale for and report of a model program. *Journal of Cardiovascular Nursing*, 9, 25-36.

smoke. Because these drugs depress the central nervous system, clients taking them are carefully monitored by a health care provider.

COMPLEMENTARY AND ALTERNATIVE THERAPIES. Some clients try other methods to help them stop smoking, including acupuncture, acupressure, hypnosis, and biofeedback. Chapter 4 describes these modalities in more detail.

CULTURAL CONSIDERATIONS

African Americans have a higher prevalence of smoking than other ethnic groups. African-American women are less likely to stop smoking than Caucasian women. The reason for this difference is not known (Allen & Phillips, 1997).

EXERCISE. Regular exercise is recommended to promote optimal lipid levels and can actually prevent atherosclerosis. Exercise can also lead to regression of atherosclerotic plaque and the building of collateral circulation in people with atherosclerosis. The level of exercise required to provide protection from atherosclerotic disease has not been well established, but it is recommended that individuals get 30 minutes of moderate to vigorous exercise at least three to four times a week. The nurse should instruct clients with heart disease and other comorbid conditions, such as hypertension, vascular disease, or diabetes, to undergo an exercise tolerance (treadmill or stress) test before undertaking an exercise program (e.g., aerobics, walking, or running).

DRUG THERAPY. Clients with elevated total and LDL cholesterol levels that do not respond adequately to dietary intervention are started on a regimen of lipid-lowering agents (Chart 36-1). Drug choice is dependent on the triglyceride levels. Because most of these drugs can produce major side effects, they are generally given only when nonpharmacologic management has been unsuccessful. Bile acid–binding resins, such as cholestyramine (Questran) or colestipol (Colestid), may be recommended initially because of their low toxicity. Medications such as lovastatin (Mevacor), simvastatin (Zocor), atorvastatin (Lipitor), and fluvastatin (Lescol) lower both LDL and triglyceride levels. These statins are contraindicated in clients with active liver disease or during pregnancy, since they can cause muscle myopathies and marked increases in liver function. Nicotinic acid lowers LDL and very low-density lipoprotein (VLDL) cholesterol levels and increases HDL cholesterol levels. It is used as a single agent or in combination with an acid-binding resin drug or a statin. Low doses (1.0 to 1.5 g/day) are generally well tolerated, but higher doses can result in an elevation of hepatic enzymes and various other side effects. Gemfibrozil (Lopid) raises HDL and lowers triglyceride and VLDL levels, but it is not as effective in lowering LDL levels.

GENE THERAPY. As the U.S. population continues to age, it is predicted that more people will need some type of vascular intervention. Ongoing clinical trials are examining the effectiveness of gene therapy in treating vascular disease. In addition, vascular endothelial growth factor (VEGF) is being used to stimulate new blood vessel growth through angiogenesis in clients with end-stage peripheral ischemia (Meyerson & Schwartz, 1999). As clinical research continues in this area, more options will be available for people with vascular disease.

HYPERTENSION

OVERVIEW

Hypertension is generally defined as a systolic blood pressure greater than or equal to 140 mm Hg and/or a diastolic blood pressure greater than or equal to 90 mm Hg in individuals who do not have diabetes. In individuals with diabetes and/or renal impairment, hypertension is considered to be a systolic blood pressure of 130 mm Hg and/or a diastolic blood pressure of 85 mm Hg or higher (Joint National Committee, 1997). Generally, hypertension is determined by two separate readings (Figure 36-2). However, if the client has risk factors for hypertension, lifestyle changes can be recommended before the second evaluation.

Hypertension is classified into three stages (Table 36-3). The significance of this disease is that it is a major risk factor for coronary, cerebral, renal, and peripheral vascular disease. However, control of hypertension has resulted in significant decreases in cardiovascular morbidity and mortality.

Although mortality rates have declined over the last 20 years, hypertension costs more than $500 million per year and

CHART 36-1

DRUG THERAPY *for* Hyperlipidemia

Drug	Usual Dosage	Nursing Interventions	Rationale
Bile acid sequestrants			
Cholestyramine (Questran)	4 g ac and hs; not to exceed 32 g/day	Encourage clients to increase fluid intake and consider stool softeners/psyllium if needed.	Cholestyramine is constipating.
Colestipol (Colestid)	2-16 g/day in divided doses		
Nicotinic acid (Nicobid, Nicolar, Nia-Bid [niacin])	1.5-3 g/day, with maximum dose of 6 g/day	Encourage clients to take with meals. Increase dose gradually.	Flushing of skin and pruritus are common side effects, which can be minimized when drug is taken with meals.
Fibric acid derivatives			
Gemfibrozil (Lopid)	600 mg bid	Instruct clients to take with meals if nausea or gastrointestinal (GI) discomfort occurs.	Although well tolerated, nausea and GI discomfort may occur and can be prevented if drug is taken with meals.
Fenofibrate (Tricor)	67 mg qd		
HMG-CoA reductase inhibitors			
Lovastatin (Mevacor)	20 mg qd; may increase to 40-80 mg/day	Instruct clients to report muscle tenderness. Tell clients to take with evening meal. Monitor liver enzymes.	Although rare, myopathy has occurred as a side effect, especially when taken with fibric acid. GI disturbances, such as diarrhea, nausea, and vomiting, are common. Minor liver enzyme elevations can occur but are rare.
Simvastatin (Zocor)	5-10 mg qd; may increase to 40 mg/day		
Fluvastatin (Lescol)	20-40 mg qd; not to exceed 80 mg/day		
Atorvastatin (Lipitor)	10 mg qd; increased to 80 mg qd		
Pravastatin (Pravachol)	10-40 mg qd at hs		

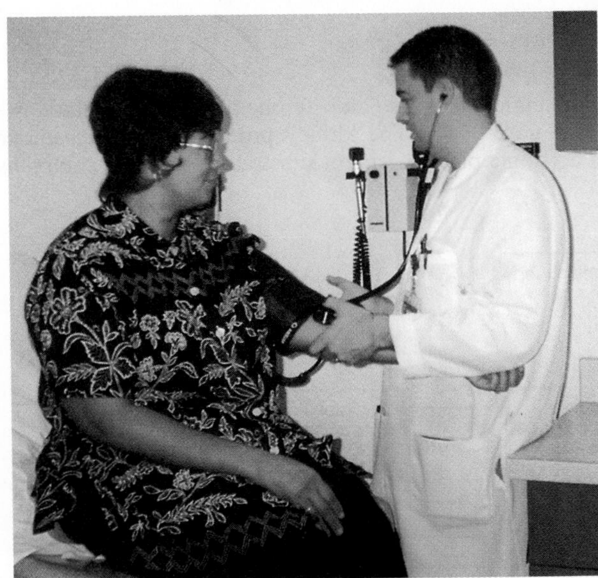

Figure 36-2 ● Blood pressure screening during routine history and physical examination.

accounts for the largest number of health care provider visits per year, as well as the largest consumption of prescription drugs (Eaton, Buck, & Catanzaro, 1996). To achieve the Healthy People 2010 objective of increased blood pressure control among clients with hypertension, nurses must be able

TABLE 36-3 • STAGES OF HYPERTENSION

Stage 1	Systolic, 140–159 mm Hg Diastolic, 90–99 mm Hg
Stage 2	Systolic, 160–179 mm Hg Diastolic, 100–109 mm Hg
Stage 3	Systolic, >180 mm Hg Diastolic, >110 mm Hg

From U.S. Department of Health and Human Services. (1997). *The fifth report of the Joint National Committee on Detection, Evaluation, and Treatment of High Blood Pressure.* NIH Publication. Washington, DC: U.S. Government Printing Office.

to assess and intervene appropriately in their care (see the Meeting Healthy People 2010 Objectives box on p. 734).

Pathophysiology

The systemic arterial pressure is a product of the cardiac output and the total peripheral resistance (Figure 36-3). Cardiac output is determined by the stroke volume and heart rate. Control of peripheral resistance is maintained by the autonomic nervous system and circulating hormones, such as norepinephrine and epinephrine. Consequently, any factor producing an alteration in peripheral resistance, heart rate, or stroke volume affects the systemic arterial pressure.

REGULATION OF BLOOD PRESSURE

Stabilizing mechanisms exist in the body to exert an overall regulation of systemic arterial pressure and to prevent circu-

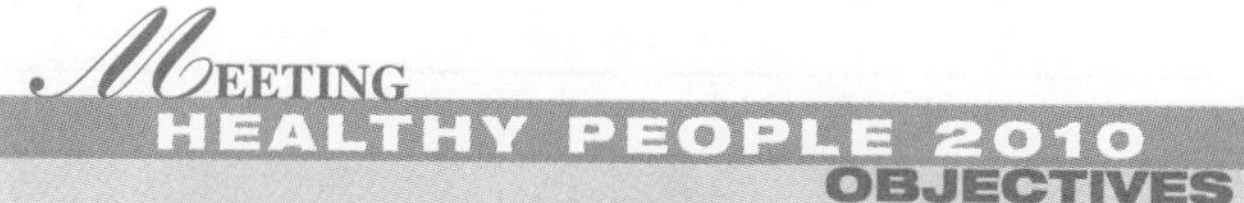

BLOOD PRESSURE

Objective 12.11: Increase the proportion of adults with high blood pressure who are taking action to help control their blood pressure.

- Teach adults with high blood pressure the importance of controlling sodium intake, including reading food labels for sodium content and avoiding high-sodium foods, such as bacon, ham, and processed snacks.
- Refer overweight adults to a support group or weight reduction program.
- Teach about the importance of exercise and increased physical activity to reduce blood pressure.
- For the adult who smokes, teach about the relationship between cardiovascular disease and smoking; refer the individual to a smoking cessation program.
- Participate in community or health care agency health fairs to screen for hypertension and provide community education.
- Teach all adults to have their blood pressure taken at least once every 2 years; for those with hypertension, monitor blood pressure as recommended by the health care provider.

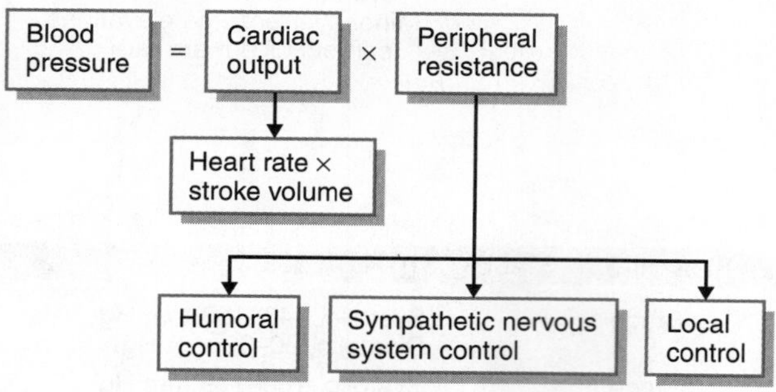

Figure 36-3 ● The components of blood pressure.

latory collapse. Four control systems play a major role in maintaining blood pressure: the arterial baroreceptor system, regulation of body fluid volume, the renin-angiotensin-aldosterone system, and vascular autoregulation.

ARTERIAL BARORECEPTORS

The arterial baroreceptors are found primarily in the carotid sinus but also in the aorta and the wall of the left ventricle. These baroreceptors monitor the level of arterial pressure. The baroreceptor system counteracts a rise in arterial pressure through vagally mediated cardiac slowing and vasodilation with decreased sympathetic tone. Therefore reflex control of circulation elevates the systemic arterial pressure when it falls and lowers it when it rises. Why this control fails in hypertension is unknown. There is evidence for upward resetting of baroreceptor sensitivity so that pressure rises are inadequately sensed even though pressure decreases are not.

REGULATION OF BODY FLUID VOLUME

Changes in fluid volume also affect the systemic arterial pressure. If there is an excess of salt and water in a person's body, the blood pressure rises through complex physiologic mechanisms that change the venous return to the heart, producing a rise in cardiac output. If the kidneys are functioning adequately, a rise in systemic arterial pressure produces diuresis and a fall in pressure. Pathologic conditions that change the pressure threshold at which the kidneys excrete salt and water alter the systemic arterial pressure.

RENIN-ANGIOTENSIN-ALDOSTERONE SYSTEM

Renin, angiotensin, and aldosterone also regulate blood pressure (Figure 36-4). The kidney produces renin, an enzyme that acts on a plasma protein substrate to split off angiotensin

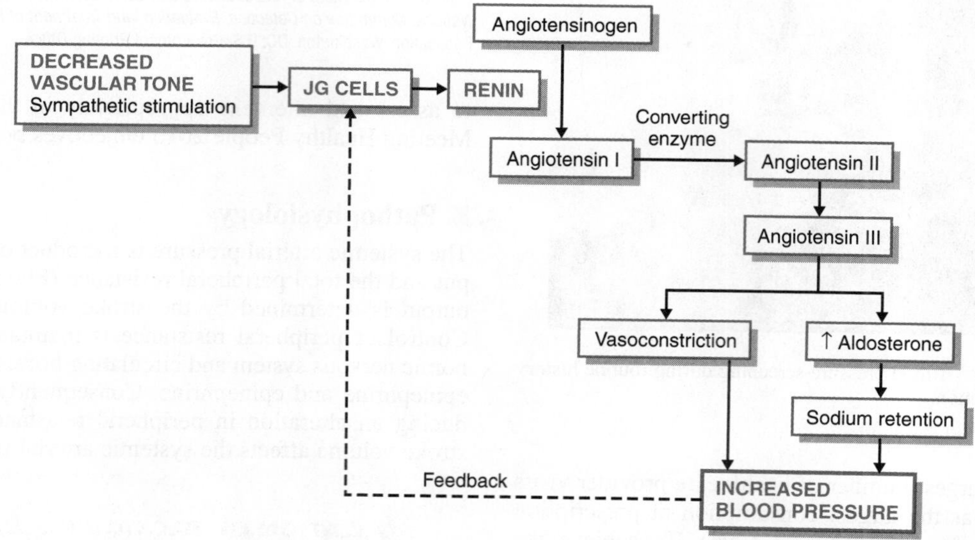

Figure 36-4 ● The effect of the renin-angiotensin system on blood pressure control. (From Copstead, L.E.C. [1995]. *Perspectives on pathophysiology.* Philadelphia, W.B. Saunders.)

I, which is converted by an enzyme in the lung to form angiotensin II. Angiotensin II has strong vasoconstrictor action on blood vessels and is the controlling mechanism for aldosterone release. The significance of aldosterone in hypertension is most evident in primary aldosteronism. By increasing the activity of the sympathetic nervous system, angiotensin II also appears to inhibit sodium excretion, resulting in an elevation in blood pressure.

Inappropriate secretion of renin may cause increased peripheral vascular resistance in essential (primary) hypertension. In high blood pressure, renin levels should be expected to fall because the increased renal arteriolar pressure should inhibit renin secretion. In most people with essential hypertension, however, renin levels are normal.

VASCULAR AUTOREGULATION

The process of vascular autoregulation, which keeps perfusion of tissues in the body relatively constant, appears to be important in causing hypertension accompanying salt and water overload. This mechanism is poorly understood.

COMPLICATIONS OF HYPERTENSION

Sustained blood pressure elevation in clients with essential (primary) hypertension results in damage to blood vessels in vital organs. Essential hypertension produces medial hyperplasia (thickening) of the arterioles. As the blood vessels thicken and perfusion decreases, body organs are damaged; these changes can result in myocardial infarctions, strokes, PVD, or renal failure.

Malignant hypertension is a severe type of elevated blood pressure that is rapidly progressive. A person with malignant hypertension usually has symptoms such as morning headaches, blurred vision, and dyspnea and/or symptoms of uremia (accumulation in the blood of substances ordinarily eliminated in the urine). Clients are often in their 30s, 40s, or 50s. The systolic blood pressure is greater than 200 mm Hg. The diastolic blood pressure is greater than 150 mm Hg, or greater than 130 mm Hg when there are pre-existing complications. Unless intervention occurs promptly, a client with malignant hypertension may experience renal failure, left ventricular failure, or stroke.

Etiology

Hypertension can be essential (primary) or secondary (Table 36-4). Essential hypertension accounts for 90% of all cases (Dumas, 1999).

ESSENTIAL HYPERTENSION

Although there is no known cause for essential hypertension, several associated risk factors have been discovered on the basis of common characteristics of people with this disease:

- Age greater than 60 years
- A family history of hypertension
- Excessive calorie consumption
- Physical inactivity
- Excessive alcohol intake
- Hyperlipidemia
- African-American ethnicity
- High intake of salt or caffeine; reduced intake of potassium, calcium, or magnesium
- Obesity
- Smoking
- Stress

A family history of hypertension is a major risk factor. In families with hypertension, there may be a defect in renal secretion of sodium or a heightened sympathetic nervous system response to stress.

The stress of caregiving by family members can also accelerate the risk of hypertension. Shaw et al. (1999) found that hypertension was more common in spouses of clients with Alzheimer's disease when compared with similar subjects who did not have caregiving responsibilities. The researchers concluded that the chronic stress of caregiving contributed to the incidence of high blood pressure.

TABLE 36-4 • ETIOLOGY OF HYPERTENSION

ESSENTIAL (PRIMARY)
- No known cause
- Associated risk factors
  - Family history of hypertension
  - High sodium intake
  - Excessive calorie consumption
  - Physical inactivity
  - Excessive alcohol intake
  - Low potassium intake

SECONDARY
- Renal vascular and renal parenchymal disease
- Primary aldosteronism
- Pheochromocytoma
- Cushing's disease
- Coarctation of the aorta
- Brain tumors
- Encephalitis
- Psychiatric disturbances
- Pregnancy
- Medications
  - Estrogen (e.g., oral contraceptives)
  - Glucocorticoids
  - Mineralocorticoids
  - Sympathomimetics

SECONDARY HYPERTENSION

Specific disease states and medications can increase a person's susceptibility to hypertension; a person with this type of elevation in blood pressure has secondary hypertension.

DISEASES. Renal vascular and renal parenchymal diseases are two of the most common causes of secondary hypertension. Hypertension can develop when there is any sudden damage to the kidneys. Renovascular hypertension is associated with narrowing of one or more of the main arteries carrying blood directly to the kidneys. Renal parenchymal diseases are related to infection, inflammation, and changes in kidney structure and function.

Dysfunction of the adrenal medulla or the adrenal cortex can cause secondary hypertension. Adrenal-mediated hypertension is due to primary excesses of aldosterone, cortisol, and catecholamines. In *primary aldosteronism,* excessive aldosterone causes hypertension and hypokalemia (low potassium levels). Primary aldosteronism usually arises from benign adenomas of the adrenal cortex. *Pheochromocytomas* originate most commonly in the adrenal medulla and result in excessive secretion of catecholamines. In *Cushing's syndrome,* excessive glucocorticoids are excreted from the adrenal cortex. The cause of Cushing's syndrome may be either adrenocortical hyperplasia or adrenocortical adenoma (see Chapter 63).

Coarctation of the aorta is a congenital narrowing of the aorta that may cause hypertension. Occurring at any level of the thoracic or abdominal aorta, the narrowing restricts blood flow through the aortic arch, resulting in an elevated blood pressure above the constriction. After surgical repair, the elevation in blood pressure eventually subsides.

Secondary hypertension is also associated with other neurogenic disturbances, such as brain tumors, encephalitis, and psychiatric disturbances.

MEDICATIONS. Medications that can cause secondary hypertension include estrogen, glucocorticoids, mineralocorticoids, sympathomimetics, cyclosporine, and erythropoietin. The use of estrogen-containing oral contraceptives is probably the most common cause of secondary hypertension in women. Discontinuation of medications capable of causing hypertension often reverses this problem.

Incidence/Prevalence

It is estimated that 50 million Americans, or 1 in every 4 adults, have high blood pressure or are currently being treated for hypertension.

CONSIDERATIONS FOR OLDER ADULTS

As adults age, they are more likely to develop hypertension. In fact, the most prevalent cardiovascular disease in older adults is hypertension, a significant risk factor for death in that population (Matteson, McConnell, & Linton, 1997).

CULTURAL CONSIDERATIONS

In the United States the incidence of hypertension among African Americans is two times greater than that for Caucasians. Hypertension is more prevalent in African Americans and Caucasians living in the southeastern United States than in African Americans and Caucasians living in other parts of the country.

WOMEN'S HEALTH CONSIDERATIONS

African-American women have a higher incidence of hypertension than Caucasian women, Hispanic women, Caucasian men, and African-American men. Studies are beginning to show that hypertension is being found in African-American teenage girls, especially those who are obese (Allen & Phillips, 1997).

COLLABORATIVE MANAGEMENT

SIMON Activity Link

Assessment

HISTORY

During history taking, the client's risk factors for hypertension are reviewed. The nurse ascertains the client's age; ethnic origin or race; family history of hypertension; average dietary intake of calories, sodium- and potassium-containing foods, and alcohol; and exercise habits. Any past and/or present history of renal or cardiovascular disease and current use of medications are also assessed.

PHYSICAL ASSESSMENT/CLINICAL MANIFESTATIONS

When a diagnosis of hypertension is made, most clients have no symptoms; however, they may experience headaches, dizziness, or fainting as a result of the elevated blood pressure. The nurse obtains blood pressure readings in both arms. Two or more readings are taken at each visit, with the average of the readings used as the value for the visit. To detect postural (orthostatic) changes, the nurse should also take readings with the client in the supine (lying) or sitting position and at least 2 minutes later with the client standing.

Funduscopic examination of the eyes is done by a skilled practitioner to observe vascular changes in the retina. The appearance of the retina can be a reliable index of the severity and prognosis of hypertension. The Keith-Wagener (KW) classification of retinal changes in hypertension is commonly used to stage changes:

- Stage I is characterized by minimal arteriolar narrowing.
- Stage II involves more marked narrowing of arterioles and arteriovenous nicking (changes at the arteriovenous crossings).
- Stage III shows circular or flame-shaped hemorrhages and fluffy, "cotton wool" exudates.
- Stage IV, the most severe, is the same as stage III but with the addition of papilledema (malignant hypertension is always associated with papilledema).

Physical assessment is helpful in diagnosing several conditions that produce secondary hypertension. The presence of abdominal bruits is typical of clients with renovascular disease. Tachycardia, sweating, and pallor suggest a pheochromocytoma or adrenal medulla tumor. Coarctation of the aorta is often characterized by elevation of blood pressure in the arms, with normal or low blood pressure in the lower extremities. Femoral pulses are also delayed or absent.

PSYCHOSOCIAL ASSESSMENT

The nurse assesses for psychosocial stressors that can worsen hypertension and that may affect the client's ability to collaborate in treatment. Job-related, economic, and other life stressors are evaluated, as well as the client's response to these stressors.

Some clients may have difficulty coping with the lifestyle changes needed to control hypertension. The nurse assesses the client's past coping strategies.

LABORATORY ASSESSMENT

Although no laboratory tests are diagnostic of essential hypertension, several laboratory tests can assess possible causes of secondary hypertension. The presence of protein, red blood cells, pus cells, and casts in the urine; elevated levels of blood urea nitrogen (BUN); and elevated serum creatinine levels indicate renal disease. In clients with a pheochromocytoma (tumor of the adrenal medulla), urinary test results are positive for the presence of catecholamines. An elevation in levels of serum corticoids and 17-ketosteroids in the urine is diagnostic of Cushing's disease.

RADIOGRAPHIC ASSESSMENT

No specific x-ray studies can diagnose hypertension. Routine chest radiography may be of assistance in recognizing left ventricular hypertrophy that results from hypertension.

Intravenous pyelography (IVP) is performed when clinical findings suggest renovascular hypertension. Renal arteriography is undertaken to establish the exact location and the extent of any lesions, the degree of obstruction, and the basic pathologic change in the renal arteries.

OTHER DIAGNOSTIC ASSESSMENT

An electrocardiogram (ECG) is of value in determining the degree of cardiac involvement. Left atrial abnormality is the first ECG sign of cardiac involvement resulting from hypertension.

Analysis

COMMON NURSING DIAGNOSES AND COLLABORATIVE PROBLEMS

The following are common nursing diagnoses for clients with hypertension:

1. Deficient Knowledge related to information misinterpretation or unfamiliarity with information resources
2. Risk for Ineffective Therapeutic Regimen Management related to noncompliance with treatment

ADDITIONAL NURSING DIAGNOSES AND COLLABORATIVE PROBLEMS

In addition to the common nursing diagnoses, clients with hypertension may have one or more of the following:

- Ineffective Tissue Perfusion (Renal, Cerebral, Cardiopulmonary, and Peripheral) related to decreased blood flow
- Imbalanced Nutrition: Risk for More Than Body Requirements related to learned eating behaviors, ethnic and cultural values, lack of social support for weight loss, and/or imbalance between the activity level and caloric intake
- Fatigue related to altered body chemistry (medications)
- Ineffective Sexuality Patterns related to effects of medical treatment (drugs)
- Ineffective Coping related to effects of chronic illness and major changes in lifestyle
- Risk for Noncompliance with treatment regimen

The following collaborative problems may also occur in some clients with hypertension:

- Potential for Cerebrovascular Hemorrhage
- Potential for Retinal Hemorrhage

Planning and Implementation

DEFICIENT KNOWLEDGE

PLANNING: EXPECTED OUTCOMES. The client with hypertension is expected to verbalize an understanding of the management of hypertension.

INTERVENTIONS. For the client with essential hypertension, the nurse initially recommends the following lifestyle modifications:

- Sodium restriction
- Weight reduction
- Moderation of alcohol intake
- Exercise
- Relaxation techniques
- Tobacco avoidance

If these modifications, which are considered the foundation of hypertension control, are unsuccessful, the health care provider considers the use of antihypertensive drugs (see the Concept Map on p. 738).

There is no surgical treatment for essential hypertension. However, surgery may be indicated for certain causes of secondary hypertension, such as renal vascular disease, coarctation of the aorta, and pheochromocytoma.

SODIUM RESTRICTION. In collaboration and consultation with the dietitian, the nurse advises all clients with hypertension to decrease their sodium chloride intake from the average of 150 mmol/L (150 mEq/L) to less than 100 mmol/L (100 mEq/L; less than 2.3 g of sodium) per day. To accomplish this goal, clients should avoid adding salt at the table, avoid cooking with salt, avoid adding seasonings that contain sodium, and limit consumption of canned, frozen, or other processed foods.

The dietitian reviews a 3-day dietary recall with the client to identify whether sodium intake has been excessive. In collaboration with the dietitian, the nurse suggests spices, herbs, fruits, and other non–salt-containing substances, such as powdered garlic and onion, to enhance the flavor of meat, chicken, seafood, and snacks. The nurse and dietitian instruct clients to read the labels on processed foods and to avoid those that are high in sodium. Salt substitutes are an alternative to salt, but a physician's order is needed before using them. This order is necessary because salt substitutes are high in potassium, and the client may have hyperkalemia (high potassium levels) associated with a concomitant problem, such as renal impairment. Although hyperkalemia is unusual, it can also occur in clients who are taking potassium-sparing diuretics.

Whereas salt is restricted, the client should include recommended daily allowances of potassium, calcium, and magnesium in the diet. Studies are not conclusive, but data suggest that low levels of these electrolytes are associated with high blood pressure.

WEIGHT REDUCTION. If a client's body mass index (BMI) is 27 or higher, the nurse and dietitian encourages weight loss. The dietitian discusses the rationale for reducing or maintaining weight and plans a weight reduction diet with the client. He or she may be referred to a group or organization for weight reduction.

Because of the relationship of saturated fat and cholesterol to weight, a weight reduction plan is formulated with the following limits:

- Total fat: less than 30% of daily caloric intake
- Saturated fat: less than 10%
- Cholesterol: less than 300 mg/day

Table 36-5 describes how to calculate grams of fat.

MODERATION OF ALCOHOL INTAKE. The nurse instructs clients to limit alcohol intake to no more than 1 ounce of ethanol (2 ounces of liquor, 8 ounces of wine, or 24 ounces of beer) daily. The client is taught that alcohol consumption may elevate arterial blood pressure and can add "empty" calories.

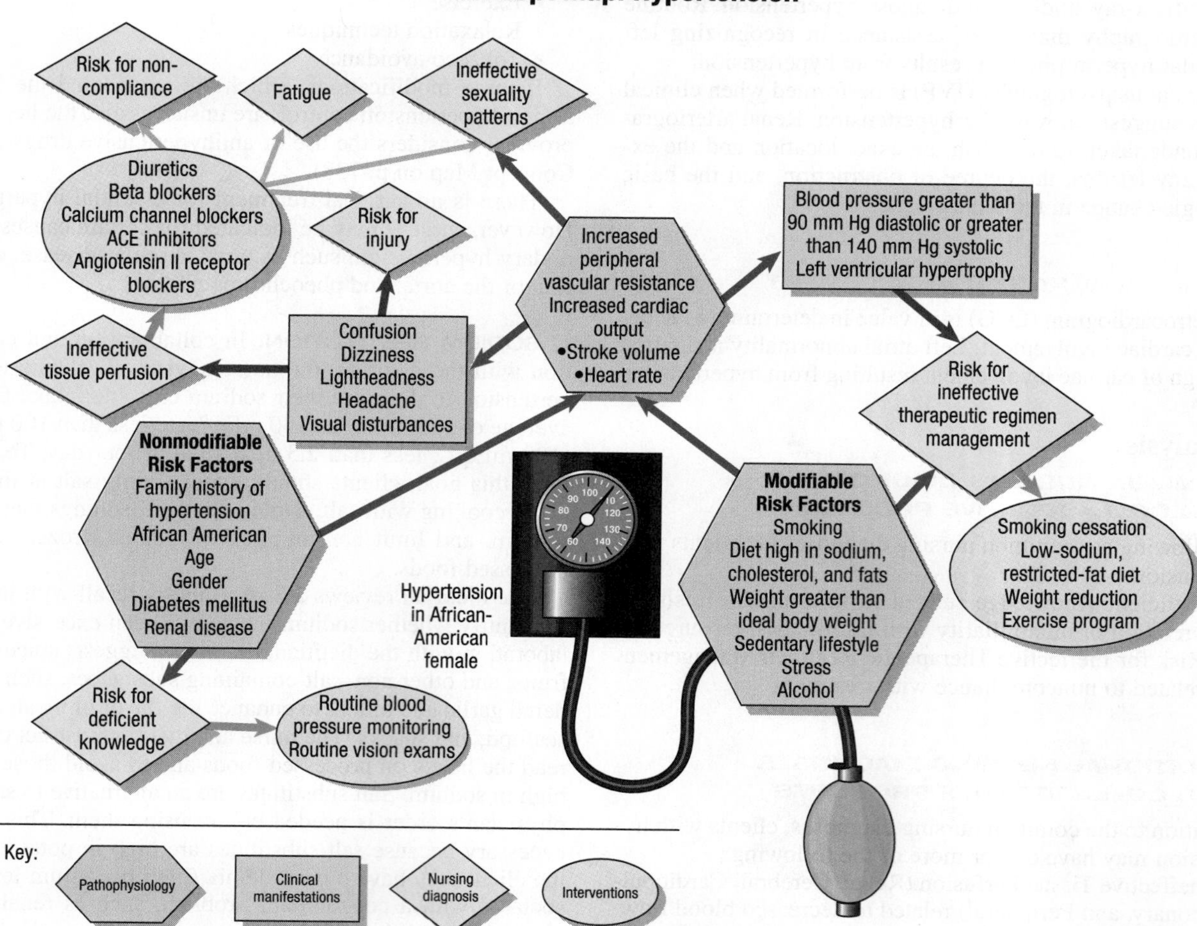

TABLE 36-5 • HOW TO DETERMINE DIETARY FAT LIMITS

Procedure	Example
1. Begin with the number of calories consumed in a day.	1800 kcal
2. Multiply the number of calories by 0.3 (30% of total calories) to determine the maximum number of calories that should be obtained from fat.	$1800 \times 0.30 = 540$ kcal/day from fat
3. Divide by 9 (1 g of fat contains 9 kcal) to determine the maximum number of grams of fat in the diet per day.	$540 \div 9 = 60$ g/day of fat (To limit fat intake to no more than 30% of calories, the client must take in no more than 60 g of fat daily.)

EXERCISE. With the physician's approval and in collaboration with the physical therapist, the nurse can help the client develop a regular exercise program. The therapist usually recommends regular aerobic exercise, such as brisk walking, running, cycling, swimming, or stair climbing, 30 to 45 minutes three to five times a week. The client should initiate exercise gradually and should stop and notify the physician if severe shortness of breath, fainting, or chest pain occurs. Clients should avoid muscle-building isometric exercise (weight lifting, wrestling, rowing) because it may raise the blood pressure to dangerous levels.

NIC **SMOKING CESSATION ASSISTANCE.** Although cigarette smoking is not directly related to hypertension, it is a major risk factor for cardiovascular disease. Therefore the client who smokes is strongly urged to stop (Chart 36-2). With input from the nurse and physician, the client plans a smoking cessation program that best fits into his or her lifestyle. The nurse explains use of the nicotine patch and smoking cessation programs and implements follow-up to assess the client's plans for quitting (see the earlier discussion of smoking cessation on p. 731).

COMPLEMENTARY AND ALTERNATIVE THERAPIES. In addition to exercise, complementary modalities are often used by clients to reduce stress and thus decrease blood pressure. Examples include yoga, massage, biofeedback, music therapy, and hypnosis. Information on these therapies is found in Chapter 4.

DRUG THERAPY. Drug therapy is individualized for each client, with consideration given to the client's culture, age, concomitant illness, severity of blood pressure elevation, and cost of drugs and follow-up.

Treatment of hypertension generally begins with a single drug. Once-a-day drug therapy is best, because the more doses required each day, the higher the risk that a client will not follow the treatment regimen. Several classifications of medications are available to control hypertension. Examples of commonly used drugs for hypertension are listed in Chart 36-3.

DIURETICS. Three basic types of diuretics are used to decrease blood volume and lower blood pressure:

- Thiazide diuretics, such as hydrochlorothiazide (HydroDiuril, Urozide✱), prevent sodium and water reabsorption in the distal tubules while promoting potassium excretion.
- Loop (high-ceiling) diuretics, such as furosemide (Lasix, Furoside✱), depress sodium reabsorption in the ascending loop of Henle and promote potassium excretion.
- Potassium-sparing diuretics, such as spironolactone (Aldactone, Novospiroton✱), act on the distal tubule to inhibit reabsorption of sodium ions in exchange for potassium, thereby retaining potassium.

Diuretics are the drugs of choice for clients who have asthma, chronic airway limitation, and chronic renal disease and for selected clients with congestive heart failure. They are particularly effective for African Americans.

Diuretics are relatively inexpensive, and adherence to the medication regimen is enhanced because the drug can usually be prescribed on a once-a-day or, at most, twice-a-day schedule.

CHART 36-2

NIC INTERVENTION ACTIVITIES *for* The Client with Vascular Disease and Risk Factor of Smoking

Smoking Cessation Assistance: *Helping another to stop smoking*

- Record current smoking status and smoking history.
- Give smoker clear, consistent advice to quit smoking.
- Help motivated smokers to set a quit date.
- Refer to group programs or individual therapists, as appropriate.
- Assist client with any self-help methods.
- Help client plan specific coping strategies and resolve problems that result from quitting.
- Advise to avoid dieting while trying to give up smoking because it can undermine chances of quitting.
- Advise to work out a plan to cope with others who smoke and to avoid being around them.
- Inform client that dry mouth, cough, scratchy throat, and feeling on edge are symptoms that may occur after quitting; the patch or gum may help with cravings.
- Advise to keep a list of "slips" or near slips, what causes them, and what client learned from them.
- Contact national and local resource organizations for resource materials.
- Encourage the relapsed client to try again.

NIC intervention activities selected from McCloskey J.C., & Bulechek, G.M. (2000). *Nursing interventions classification (NIC)* (3rd ed.). St. Louis: Mosby. No part of this work is to be altered without prior written permission from the Publisher.

CHART 36-3

DRUG THERAPY *for* Hypertension

Drug	Usual Dosage	Nursing Interventions	Rationale
DIURETICS			
Thiazides			
Chlorothiazide (Diuril)	125-500 mg/day	Monitor potassium levels and watch for muscle weakness or irregular pulse	Hypokalemia is a common occurrence.
Hydrochlorothiazide (Esidrix, HydroDiuril)	12.5-50 mg/day	Encourage intake of foods high in potassium (e.g., bananas and orange juice).	Depleted potassium needs to be replaced.
Loop Diuretics			
Furosemide (Lasix, Furoside✱)	20-40 mg/day	Same as for thiazide diuretics.	Same as for chlorothiazide.
Ethacrynic acid (Edecrin)	25-100 mg/day		
Potassium-Sparing Diuretics			
Spironolactone (Aldactone)	25-100 mg/day	Monitor potassium levels and watch for muscle weakness or irregular pulse.	Hypokalemia or hyperkalemia may occur.
Triamterone (Dyrenium)	50-100 mg/day		
BETA-BLOCKING AGENTS			
Propranolol (Inderal, Apo-Propranolol✱)	40-240 mg/day	Monitor pulse rate.	A drop in pulse is expected, and bradycardia may occur.
		Watch for shortness of breath or cough.	Bronchospasm caused by blockage of beta receptors in the lungs may occur.
Atenolol (Tenormin)	25-100 mg qd	Instruct client to report any difficulty in sexual function, fatigue, weakness, or depression.	Although these are common side effects, newer beta-blocking agents may be more "selective" in terms of side effects.
Nadolol (Corgard)	20-240 mg/day		
Metoprolol (Lopressor)	50-200 mg/day	Instruct clients with diabetes to monitor blood glucose levels.	Hypoglycemic symptoms may be blocked in clients taking beta-blocking agents.

Continued

CHART 36-3

DRUG THERAPY *for* Hypertension—cont'd

Drug	Usual Dosage	Nursing Interventions	Rationale
CALCIUM CHANNEL BLOCKERS			
Nifedipine (Procardia, Adalat)	10-30 mg tid	Monitor blood pressure. Assess for dizziness.	A drop in blood pressure occurs within 30 min after oral administration.
		Assess lower extremities.	Pedal edema can occur as a result of peripheral vasodilation.
Verapamil (Calan, Isoptin)	40-80 mg q8h, 240 mg qd SR	Monitor blood pressure and pulse.	Hypotension and decreased heart rate may occur.
		Encourage intake of foods high in fiber.	Constipation is a common side effect.
Diltiazem hydrochloride (Cardizem)	30-60 mg q8h	Monitor blood pressure and pulse.	Hypotension and decreased heart rate may occur.
ANGIOTENSION-CONVERTING-ENZYME INHIBITORS			
Captopril (Capoten)	6.25 mg tid initially, increased to 50 mg tid	Instruct client to stay in bed for 3 hr after the first dose.	Severe hypotension may follow the first dose.
Enalapril (Vasotec)	2.5 mg/day initially, increased to 10-40 mg/day	Monitor blood pressure.	Hypotension needs to be detected promptly.
Lisinopril (Zestil, Prinvil)	5 mg/day initially, increased to 10-40 mg/day	Monitor renal function tests.	
CENTRAL ALPHA AGONISTS			
Clonidine hydrochloride (Catapres)	0.1-1.2 mg hs or 0.1-0.3 mg once a week transdermally	Administer at bedtime.	Sedation is a common side effect.
		Instruct client to report rash associated with transdermal route.	Bothersome skin rashes occur in about 25% of clients using a transdermal patch.
Methyldopa (Aldomet)	250-500 mg qid	Instruct client to sit on the side of the bed for several minutes before arising and to avoid changing position suddenly.	Postural hypotension is a common complication.
		Warn clients that sedation can occur when drug is initiated and dose is increased.	This information can assist clients in planning activity and rest periods.
		Instruct male clients to report any difficulty in sexual functions.	Impotence is a common side effect.
VASODILATORS			
Hydralazine (Apresoline)	10-50 mg qid	Monitor pulse rate.	Tachycardia may occur as a result of reflex increase in sympathetic activity.
Alpha$_1$-receptor blockers Doxazosin (Cardura)	1.0-16 mg/day	Monitor blood pressure.	A drop in blood pressure can occur between 2 and 6 hr after initial dose or dose increases.
Terazosin (Hytrin)	1.0-20 mg/day	Assess for dizziness.	Give first dose at bedtime to avoid postural hypotension.

However, the frequent voiding that occurs after a person takes a diuretic may interfere with daily activities. The most frequent side effect associated with diuretics is hypokalemia (low potassium levels). The nurse monitors the serum potassium level and assesses for signs and symptoms of irregular pulse and muscle weakness, which may indicate hypokalemia. Clients receiving potassium-depleting diuretics should eat foods high in potassium, such as bananas and orange juice. However, the client may need a potassium supplement to maintain adequate serum potassium levels (see Chapter 13). The nurse assesses for hypokalemia and hyperkalemia in clients taking potassium-sparing diuretics. Both of these electrolyte disturbances are characterized by weakness and an irregular pulse.

BETA-ADRENERGIC BLOCKING AGENTS. Beta blockers lower blood pressure by blocking beta receptors in the heart and peripheral vessels, reducing the cardiac rate and output. By blocking beta-adrenergic receptors in the heart, these drugs cause a decrease in the heart rate and decreased contractility. Bradycardia (slow heart rate) and heart failure may result. Beta blockers can also prohibit bronchodilation by blocking beta receptors in the lungs. Therefore clients with a history of asthma or bronchospasm are generally not given these drugs, and all clients taking these drugs must be monitored for shortness of breath and wheezing.

Common side effects of beta blockers include fatigue, weakness, depression, and sexual dysfunction, although the potential for side effects depends on the "selective" blocking effects of the drug. A variety of drugs are available, and they differ from each other in terms of their cardioselectivity (primarily $beta_1$ effects, with lesser $beta_2$ effects), lipid solubility, and sympathomimetic activity throughout the body.

Clients with diabetes who take beta blockers may not have the usual signs and symptoms of hypoglycemia because the sympathetic nervous system is blocked. Counterregulatory responses to hypoglycemia, such as gluconeogenesis, may also be inhibited by certain beta blockers.

CALCIUM CHANNEL-BLOCKING AGENTS. Calcium channel blockers, such as verapamil hydrochloride (Calan), nifedipine (Procardia, Adalat), and diltiazem (Cardizem), lower blood pressure by interfering with the transmembrane flux of calcium ions, resulting in reduced vasoconstriction.

CULTURAL CONSIDERATIONS

Calcium channel blockers are thought to be particularly effective for older clients and African Americans. Verapamil and diltiazem can affect atrial-ventricular conduction and often lower the heart rate. Oral nifedipine can reduce blood pressure quickly, often decreasing it by 25% within 30 minutes. Nifedipine, given by puncturing the capsule and placing the liquid contents under the tongue, acts within 10 to 15 minutes.

ANGIOTENSIN-CONVERTING ENZYME INHIBITORS. Angiotensin-converting enzyme (ACE) inhibitors are also used as single or combination agents in the treatment of hypertension. The angiotensin-converting enzyme converts angiotensin I to angiotensin II, one of the most powerful vasoconstrictors in the body. ACE inhibitors include captopril (Capoten), enalapril (Vasotec), and lisinopril (Prinivil).

The client receiving an ACE inhibitor for the first time is instructed to stay in bed for 3 to 4 hours to avoid the severe hypotensive effect that can occur with initial use. The nurse monitors the blood pressure every 15 minutes after this first dose. **Postural (orthostatic) hypotension** may occur with subsequent doses, but it is less severe. Postural hypotension is assessed by taking the blood pressure when the client is lying, sitting, and standing. If there is a significant decrease in the systolic blood pressure (<20 mm Hg), the nurse notifies the physician.

CONSIDERATIONS FOR OLDER ADULTS

The older client is at the greatest risk for postural hypotension because of the cardiovascular changes associated with aging (Chart 36-4).

CULTURAL CONSIDERATIONS

ACE inhibitors are most effective in young Caucasian adults. They are less effective in African Americans or older adults.

ANGIOTENSIN II RECEPTOR ANTAGONISTS. Angiotensin II receptor antagonists make up a new group of drugs that selectively block the binding of angiotensin II in the vascular and adrenal tissues by competing directly with angiotensin II but not inhibiting ACE. Examples of drugs in this group are candesartan (Atacand), losartan (Cozaar), and telmisartan (Micardis). Angiotensin II receptor antagonists can be used alone or in combination with other antihypertensive drugs. They are excellent options for clients who complain of cough associated with ACE inhibitors and for those with hyperkalemia. In addition, these drugs do not require initial adjustment of the dose for older adults or for clients with renal impairment. However, these drugs may be less effective in African Americans (Dumas, 1999).

CHART 36-4

NURSING FOCUS *on the* OLDER ADULT
Hypertension

- Before initiating drug therapy, obtain blood pressure measurements with the client lying, sitting, and standing to assess for postural changes.
- Monitor the client's standing blood pressure during treatment.
- Instruct the client to avoid caffeine and nicotine for 1 hour before blood pressure measurements to obtain accurate readings.
- Teach the client that dizziness is a symptom of hypotension that should be reported.
- Instruct clients how to avoid orthostatic (postural) hypotension by avoiding sudden changes in position. Clients should arise from bed in three stages: sit in bed for 1 minute; sit on the side of the bed with legs dangling for 1 minute; and stand, holding onto a nonmovable object for 1 minute before walking. Clients should also be cautious about heat exposure (hot tub), alcohol intake, and exercise, which can lead to orthostatic hypotension.

CENTRAL ALPHA AGONISTS. Central alpha agonists act on the central nervous system, preventing reuptake of norepinephrine, resulting in a lowering of peripheral vascular resistance and blood pressure. Common central alpha agonists include clonidine (Catapres) and methyldopa (Aldomet, Apo-Methyldopa♣). Methyldopa can cause unique side effects, such as hemolytic anemia and inflammatory disorders of the liver, although they happen rarely. Because of this potential, clonidine is the more commonly used central alpha agonist. Clonidine can also be given as a transdermal patch, providing control of blood pressure for as long as 7 days. Side effects common to clonidine and methyldopa include sedation, postural hypotension, and impotence.

VASODILATORS. Vasodilators lower blood pressure by relaxing vascular smooth muscle tone, thus reducing total peripheral resistance. Vasodilators include minoxidil (Loniten), nitroglycerin (Nitro-Bid), and nitroprusside (Nitropress).

ALPHA-ADRENERGIC RECEPTOR AGONISTS. Alpha-adrenergic agonists, such as prazosin (Minipress), dilate the arterioles and veins. These drugs can lower blood pressure quickly, but their use is limited because of frequent and bothersome side effects.

• • •

The Joint National Committee on Prevention, Detection, Evaluation, and Treatment of High Blood Pressure (1997) has recommended that initial therapy for hypertension include either a diuretic or a beta blocker unless these drugs are contraindicated or ineffective, or there are special indications for agents such as calcium antagonists or ACE inhibitors. If after 1 to 3 months blood pressure does not decrease adequately in response to initial therapy, the health care provider may increase the dose of the drug, substitute a drug from another class of antihypertensives, or add a second drug from another class. Because of changes in recommendations and the availability of more drug options and more information on drug tolerance, the nurse sees a variety of drug protocols used by the health care provider to meet the individual needs of clients with hypertension.

RISK FOR INEFFECTIVE THERAPEUTIC REGIMEN MANAGEMENT

PLANNING: EXPECTED OUTCOMES. The client with hypertension is expected to adhere to the therapeutic regimen, thus minimizing the risk of target organ damage.

INTERVENTIONS. Clients who require pharmacologic treatment to control essential hypertension usually need to take medication for the rest of their lives. Frequently, however, clients stop taking antihypertensive medications because they have no symptoms. They may also discontinue medication because of cost or side effects.

In collaboration with the pharmacist, the nurse and client discuss the goals of therapy, including potential side effects, to help identify potential problems. The nurse then assists the client in tailoring the therapeutic regimen to his or her activities of daily living (ADLs).

Clients who do not comply with antihypertensive treatment are at great risk for target organ damage and hypertensive crisis (malignant hypertension). Clients in hypertensive crisis are admitted to critical care units, where they receive intravenous (IV) antihypertensive therapy, such as nitroprusside (Nitropress), nitroglycerin (Nitro-Bid IV, Tridil), labetalol (Normodyne), or diazoxide (Hyperstat IV), or sublingual nifedipine (Procardia, Adalat) (Chart 36-5). Hospitalization for complications of hypertension can be financially costly both in medical expenses and in lost income.

CHART 36-5

BEST PRACTICE *for*
Assessment and Management of Hypertensive Crisis

Assess
- Severe headache
- Extremely high blood pressure
- Dizziness
- Blurred vision
- Disorientation

Intervene
- Place client in a semi-Fowler's position.
- Administer oxygen.
- Administer IV nitroprusside (Nitropress) or other infusion drug as ordered (for nitroprusside, cover infusion bag to prevent drug breakdown by light).
- Monitor blood pressure every 5 to 15 minutes until the diastolic pressure is also below 90 and not less than 75; then monitor blood pressure every 30 minutes.
- Observe for neurologic or cardiovascular complications, such as seizures; numbness, weakness, or tingling of extremities; dysrhythmias; or chest pain.

CRITICAL THINKING CHALLENGE

A middle-aged man visits the community health fair where you are volunteering and asks to have his blood pressure taken. He tells you that he gets "white coat syndrome," which makes his blood pressure increase when he is in a physician's office. He also states that he is concerned about his blood pressure because his father had hypertension and died from a stroke last year. When you take his blood pressure, it is 188/124 on the first reading and 182/120 on the second reading.
- What should you do at this time?
- What other information about the man's lifestyle would be helpful to know?
- What options for management of his blood pressure might be available for him?

For suggested answer guidelines, go to SIMON http://www.wbsaunders.com/SIMON/Iggy/.

Community-Based Care

Clients who require pharmacologic treatment to control essential hypertension usually need to take medication for the rest of their lives. Studies have shown that within the first year of therapy, more than 50% of clients discontinue their treatment (Eaton, Buck, & Catanzaro, 1996). They often stop taking antihypertensive medications with the assumption that the hypertension is under control because they have no symptoms. Clients may assume that if their blood pressure returns to normal levels with antihypertensives, they no longer need them. They may also stop taking antihypertensives because of adverse side effects or cost.

HOME CARE MANAGEMENT

If possible, the client should obtain a blood pressure monitor for use at home so that the pressure can be checked periodically. The nurse evaluates the client's ability to learn how to check his or her blood pressure. If the client cannot monitor the blood pressure, a family member or significant other may be taught how to perform this procedure. If weight reduction is a goal, the nurse suggests having a scale in the home for weight monitoring.

HEALTH TEACHING

The client is instructed about sodium restriction, weight maintenance or reduction, alcohol restriction, stress management, and exercise (see Interventions [Arteriosclerosis and Atherosclerosis], p. 730). If necessary, the nurse also explains about the need to stop smoking. Older adults can also benefit from lifestyle modifications (Matteson, McConnell, & Linton, 1997).

For clients taking medication for hypertension, the nurse provides oral and written information about the indications, dosage, times of administration, side effects, and drug interactions (see Chart 36-3). The nurse stresses that the medication must be taken as prescribed and that when all of it has been consumed, the prescription must be renewed on a continual basis. Abrupt discontinuation of medications such as beta blockers can result in angina (chest pain) or myocardial infarction.

The nurse also urges clients to report unpleasant side effects, such as sexual dysfunction. In many instances, an alternative medication can be prescribed to minimize certain side effects.

Hypertension is a chronic illness, and clients may not be prepared to accept this fact. The nurse allows clients to verbalize feelings about this disease and its treatment. They are advised that their involvement in the treatment can lead to control of this disease and can prevent complications.

HEALTH CARE RESOURCES

A home care nurse may be needed for follow-up to monitor the blood pressure. The nurse evaluates the ability of the client or the family to obtain accurate blood pressure measurements and assesses their compliance with treatment. If clients cannot purchase equipment to monitor their blood pressure, the American Heart Association, the Red Cross, or a local pharmacy may be used for free blood pressure checks.

Evaluation: Outcomes

The nurse evaluates the care of the client with hypertension on the basis of the identified nursing diagnoses and collaborative problems. The expected outcomes are that the client will:

- Explain the rationale for treatment of hypertension
- Maintain a blood pressure of less than 130/85 mm Hg for clients with diabetes and less than 140/90 mm Hg for clients without diabetes
- Demonstrate no signs or symptoms of target organ damage, such as renal or heart disease

PERIPHERAL ARTERIAL DISEASE

OVERVIEW

Peripheral vascular disease (PVD) includes disorders that alter the natural flow of blood through the arteries and veins of the peripheral circulation. PVD affects the lower extremities much more frequently than the upper extremities. Generally, a client with a diagnosis of PVD has arterial disease (peripheral arterial disease [PAD]) rather than venous involvement. Some clients have both arterial and venous disease.

Pathophysiology

PAD is a chronic condition in which partial or total arterial occlusion deprives the lower extremities of oxygen and nutrients. PAD of the lower extremities is sometimes referred to as lower extremity arterial disease (LEAD). Body tissues cannot live without an adequate oxygen and nutrient supply, and tissue eventually dies. Atherosclerosis is the most common cause of chronic altered blood flow. Fatty substances accumulate at the site of vessel wall injury and alter or totally occlude blood flow within the arteries. Tissue damage generally occurs below the arterial obstruction.

Obstructions are classified as inflow or outflow, according to the arteries involved and their relationship to the inguinal ligament (Figure 36-5). *Inflow* obstructions involve the distal end of the aorta and the common, internal, and external iliac arteries. They are located above the inguinal ligament. *Outflow* obstructions involve infrainguinal arterial segments (the femoral, popliteal, and tibial arteries) and are below the superficial femoral artery (SFA). Gradual inflow occlusions may not cause significant tissue damage; gradual outflow occlusions typically do.

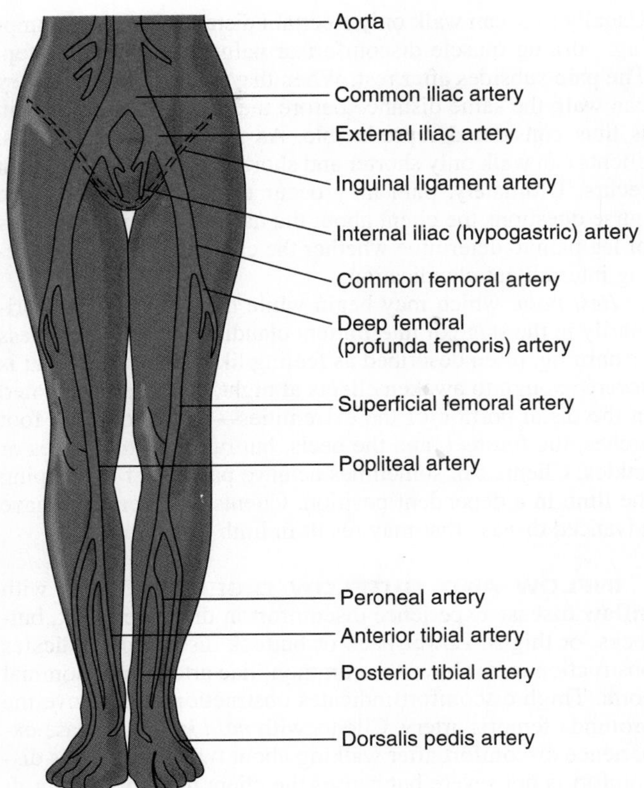

Figure 36-5 ● Common locations of inflow and outflow lesions.

Etiology

Because atherosclerosis is the most common cause of chronic arterial obstruction, the risk factors for atherosclerosis apply to PAD as well. These include hypertension, hyperlipidemia, diabetes mellitus, cigarette smoking, obesity, and familial predisposition. Advancing age also increases the risk of disease related to atherosclerosis.

Incidence/Prevalence

Approximately 8 million people in the United States have PAD. At least 10% of people over 70 years of age and 2% of people 37 to 69 years of age have symptomatic, chronic PAD (American Heart Association, 1999). PAD generally occurs in men older than 45 years of age and in postmenopausal women. The costs of vascular disease to society are astounding (see the Cost of Care box on p. 744).

COLLABORATIVE MANAGEMENT

Assessment

HISTORY

The clinical course of chronic peripheral arterial disease (PAD) can be divided into four stages (Chart 36-6). Clients do not experience symptoms in the early stages of disease.

PAIN ASSESSMENT. Most clients initially seek treatment for a characteristic leg pain known as **intermittent claudication** (a term derived from a word meaning "to limp").

Usually they can walk only a certain distance before a cramping, burning muscle discomfort or pain forces them to stop. The pain subsides after rest. When they resume walking, they can walk the same distance before the pain returns. The pain is thus considered reproducible. As the disease progresses, clients can walk only shorter and shorter distances before pain recurs. Ultimately, pain may occur even while at rest. The nurse questions the client about the nature and characteristics of leg pain to determine whether the client may be experiencing intermittent claudication.

Rest pain, which may begin while the disease is still primarily in the stage of intermittent claudication, is a numbness or burning, often described as feeling like a toothache, that is severe enough to awaken clients at night. It is usually located in the distal portion of the extremities—in the toes, the foot arches, the forefeet, and the heels, but rarely in the calves or ankles. Clients can sometimes achieve pain relief by keeping the limb in a dependent position. Clients with rest pain have advanced disease that may result in limb loss.

INFLOW AND OUTFLOW DISEASE. Clients with **inflow disease** experience discomfort in the lower back, buttocks, or thighs. Lower back or buttock discomfort indicates obstruction at or above the common iliac artery or abdominal aorta. Thigh discomfort indicates obstruction at or above the profunda femoris artery. Clients with *mild* inflow disease experience discomfort after walking about two blocks. This discomfort is not severe but causes the client to stop walking. It is relieved with rest. Clients with *moderate* inflow disease experience pain in these areas after walking about one or two blocks. The discomfort is described as being more like pain, but it subsides with rest most of the time. *Severe* inflow disease causes the client severe pain after walking less than one block. These clients usually have rest pain.

Clients with **outflow disease** describe burning or cramping in the calves, ankles, feet, and toes. Calf discomfort usually indicates arterial obstruction at or below the superficial femoral or popliteal artery. Instep or foot discomfort indicates an obstruction below the popliteal artery. Clients with *mild* outflow disease experience discomfort after walking about five blocks. This discomfort is relieved by rest. Clients with *moderate* outflow disease have pain after walking about two blocks. Intermittent rest pain may be present. Clients with *severe* outflow disease are usually unable to walk more than one-half block and usually experience rest pain. They may hang their feet off the bed at night for comfort. Clients with outflow disease complain more frequently of rest pain than do those with inflow disease.

WOMEN'S HEALTH CONSIDERATIONS

Women suffer serious problems related to PVD of the lower extremities after menopause. In fact, 25% of women 55 to 74 years of age develop PVD (Gerhard, Baum, & Raby, 1995). The major risk factors for women with PVD are cigarette smoking, diabetes mellitus, hypertension, hyperlipidemia, and menopause.

Conservative treatment for women includes exercise training and quitting smoking. Estrogen replacement therapy and cholesterol-lowering drugs may slow the development of arteriosclerosis in the lower extremities in women. Women appear to be at higher risk for amputation than men and should be encouraged to adhere to conservative therapy recommendations to prevent progression of the disease.

COST OF CARE IMPLICATIONS FOR NURSING

PERIPHERAL VASCULAR DISEASE

Cost of Care

- Each year, vascular disorders result in disability or death, and the financial impact on society is overwhelming.
- The cost of cardiovascular disease in 1999 is estimated at $287 billion according to the National Heart, Lung, and Blood Institute and the American Heart Association. This includes direct and indirect health care costs for expenditures such as health care provider fees, hospital care, nursing home services, medications, home care services, durable medical equipment, and loss of productivity to the client, family, and society.
- Case management and the use of critical care pathways by all health care providers decreases the cost of hospital care and helps to decrease the length of stay for hospitalized clients.

Implications for Nursing

The medical and nursing management of clients with cardiovascular disease is costly. Research has identified certain risk factors that contribute to the development of cardiac and vascular disease. Nurses should be committed to identifying clients at risk and providing teaching and support toward reducing risk factors. Nurses need to be involved in programs related to smoking cessation, weight reduction, lipid screening, stress reduction, and promoting healthy living behaviors.

Data from American Heart Association. (1999). *Heart and stroke facts: 1999 statistical supplement* (pp. 1-28), Dallas: Author; and National Heart, Lung, and Blood Institute. (1996). *Morbidity and mortality 1996 chartbook on cardiovascular lung and blood diseases* (pp. 5-116). Washington, DC: National Institutes of Health, Public Health Service, U.S. Department of Health and Human Services.

PHYSICAL ASSESSMENT/CLINICAL MANIFESTATIONS

Specific findings for PAD depend on the severity of the disease. The nurse may observe loss of hair on the lower calf, ankle, and foot; dry, scaly, dusky, pale, or mottled skin; and

CHART 36-6

KEY FEATURES *of* Chronic Peripheral Arterial Disease

Stage I: Asymptomatic
- No claudication is present.
- Bruit or aneurysm may be present.
- Pedal pulses are decreased or absent.

Stage II: Claudication
- Muscle pain, cramping, or burning occurs with exercise and is relieved with rest.
- Symptoms are reproducible with exercise.

Stage III: Rest Pain
- Pain while resting commonly awakens the client at night.
- Pain is described as numbness, burning, toothache-type pain.
- Pain usually occurs in the distal portion of the extremity—toes, arch, forefoot, or heel—rarely in the calf or the ankle.
- Pain is relieved by placing the extremity in a dependent position.

Stage IV: Necrosis/Gangrene
- Ulcers and blackened tissue occur on the toes, the forefoot, and the heel.
- Distinctive gangrenous odor is present.

thickened toenails. With severe arterial disease, the extremity is cold and gray-blue (cyanotic) or darkened. Pallor may occur when the extremity is elevated; dependent **rubor** may occur when the extremity is lowered. Muscle atrophy can accompany prolonged chronic arterial disease.

The nurse palpates all pulses in both legs. The most sensitive and specific indicator of arterial function is the quality of the posterior tibial pulse. The pedal pulse is not palpable in a small percentage of people. The strength of the pulse should be compared bilaterally. Several scales are available for grading pulse strength. A popular system is presented in Table 36-6.

TABLE 36-6 • PULSE GRADING SCALE

Value	Characteristic
0	No detectable pulse (0/4)
1	Pulse thready, weak, difficult to detect; may fade in and out; easily obliterated by pressure (1/4)
2	Pulse difficult to palpate, hypokinetic, and may be obliterated by pressure; light palpation recommended (2/4)
3	Pulse easily palpable and not easily obliterated by pressure; considered normal in volume (3/4)
4	Pulse strong, bounding, hyperkinetic, easily palpated and not obliterated by pressure; may be pathologic if aortic regurgitation is present (4/4)

The nurse may also note early signs of ulcer formation or complete ulcer formation, a complication of PAD. Arterial and venous stasis ulcers differ from diabetic ulcers (Chart 36-7).

Initially, **arterial ulcers** are painful and develop on the toes (often the great toe), between the toes, or on the upper aspect of the foot. With prolonged occlusion, the toe(s) can become gangrenous. **Diabetic ulcers** develop on the plantar surface of the foot, over the metatarsal heads, and on the heel anywhere that pressure is exerted. Diabetic ulcers may not be painful because of diabetic neuropathy. **Venous stasis ulcers** cause minimal pain and occur in the ankle area. The foot is warm, and distal pulses are palpable. The nurse notes discoloration of the lower extremity at the ulcer site. Skin lesions are discussed in further detail in Chapter 67.

CULTURAL CONSIDERATIONS

In clients with dark skin, the soles of the feet and the toenails enable the nurse to detect cyanosis or duskiness in the lower extremities because these areas are less pigmented.

CHART 36-7

KEY FEATURES *of* Lower Extremity Ulcers

Feature	Arterial Ulcers	Venous Ulcers	Diabetic Ulcers
History	Client complains of claudication after walking approximately 1-2 blocks Rest pain usually present Pain at ulcer site Two or three risk factors present	Chronic nonhealing ulcer No claudication or rest pain Moderate ulcer discomfort Client complains about ankle or leg swelling	Diabetes Peripheral neuropathy No complaints of claudication
Ulcer location and appearance	End of the toes Between the toes Deep Ulcer bed pale, with even edges Little granulation tissue	Ankle area Brown pigmentation Ulcer bed pink Usually superficial, with uneven edges Granulation tissue present	Plantar area of foot Metatarsal heads Pressure points on feet Deep Pale, with even edges Little granulation tissue
		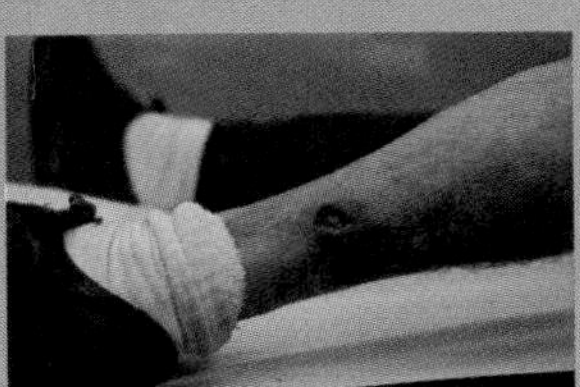	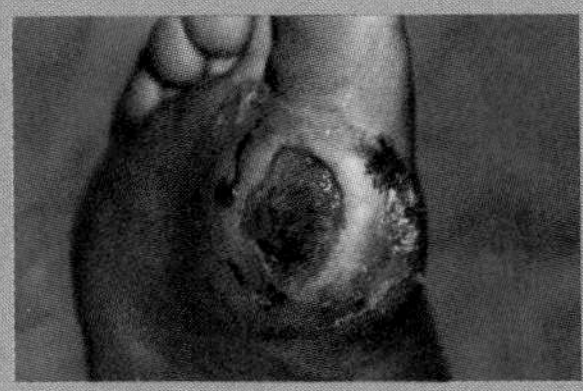
Other assessment findings	Cool or cold foot Decreased or absent pulses Atrophy of skin Hair loss Pallor with elevation Dependent rubor Possible gangrene When acute, neurologic deficits noted	Ankle discoloration and edema Full veins when leg slightly dependent No neurologic deficit Pulses present May have scarring from previous ulcers	Pulses usually present Cool or warm foot Painless
Treatment	Treat underlying cause (surgical, revascularization) Prevent trauma and infection Client education, stressing foot care	Long-term wound care (Unna boot, damp-to-dry dressings) Elevate extremity Client education Prevent infection	Rule out major arterial disease Control diabetes Client education regarding foot care Prevent infection

Photographs of arterial ulcer and diabetic ulcer from Callen, J.P., et al. (1993). *Color atlas of dermatology: Slide set.* Philadelphia: W.B. Saunders.

RADIOGRAPHIC ASSESSMENT

The most common x-ray study for PAD is arteriography of the lower extremities. Because arteriography involves injecting contrast medium into the arterial system, the risks, which include hemorrhage, thrombosis, embolus, and death, are serious. Arteriography is often performed before surgery to pinpoint the exact location of the occlusion. The nurse prepares the client for the procedure and carefully implements follow-up care.

OTHER DIAGNOSTIC ASSESSMENT

The advent of noninvasive evaluation of arterial disease has become a popular method of diagnosis. Noninvasive testing provides information about the arterial system with minimal risk to the client.

SEGMENTAL SYSTOLIC BLOOD PRESSURE MEASUREMENTS. Segmental systolic blood pressure measurements of the lower extremities at the thigh, calf, and ankle are a noninvasive method of assessing PAD. Normally, blood pressure readings in the thigh and calf are higher than those in the upper extremities. With the presence of arterial disease, these pressures are lower than the brachial pressure.

With *inflow* disease, pressures taken at the thigh level indicate the severity of disease. Mild inflow disease may cause a difference of only 10 to 30 mm Hg in pressure on the affected side compared with the brachial pressure. Severe inflow disease can cause a pressure difference of greater than 40 to 50 mm Hg. The ankle pressure is normally equal to or greater than the brachial pressure.

To evaluate *outflow* disease, the nurse compares ankle pressure with the brachial pressure, which provides a ratio known as the **ankle-brachial index (ABI).** This value can be derived by dividing the ankle blood pressure by the brachial blood pressure.

With mild outflow disease, the client has an ankle/brachial index of 0.8 to 1.0; pressures are decreased by about 10 to 30 mm Hg. The client with moderate outflow disease has an ankle/brachial index of 0.5 to 0.8, with pressure differences of 20 to 40 mm Hg. An ankle/brachial index of less than 0.5 indicates severe outflow disease.

EXERCISE TOLERANCE TESTING. Exercise tolerance testing (by stress test or treadmill) may give valuable information about clients who are experiencing claudication (muscle pain) without rest pain. The nurse or technician obtains resting pulse volume recordings and has the client walk on a treadmill until the symptoms are reproduced. At the time of symptom onset or after approximately 5 minutes, the nurse or technician obtains another pulse volume recording. Normally, there may be an increased waveform with minimal, if any, drop in the ankle pressure. In clients with arterial disease, the waveforms are decreased (dampened) and there is a decrease in the ankle pressure of 40 to 60 mm Hg for 20 to 30 seconds in the affected limb. If the return to normal pressure is delayed (longer than 10 minutes), the results suggest abnormal arterial flow in the affected limb.

PLETHYSMOGRAPHY. Plethysmography can also be performed to evaluate arterial flow in the lower extremities. This measurement provides graphs or tracings of arterial flow in the limb. If an occlusion is present, the waveforms are dampened to flattened, depending on the degree of occlusion.

Interventions

The nurse first determines whether the altered tissue perfusion is of arterial or venous origin. An accurate assessment often provides this information, but in some people both conditions may exist. In this case, each disease must be considered separately when appropriate interventions are planned.

NONSURGICAL MANAGEMENT. The interventions of exercise, position changes, promotion of vasodilation, drug therapy, and invasive nonsurgical procedures are used to increase arterial flow to the affected limb.

EXERCISE. Exercise may improve arterial blood flow to the affected limb through buildup of the *collateral* circulation. (Collateral circulation provides blood to the affected area through smaller vessels that develop and compensate for the occluded vessels.) Exercise is individualized for each client, but people with severe rest pain, venous ulcers, or gangrene should not participate. Other clients with peripheral arterial disease (PAD) can benefit from exercise that is initiated gradually and is slowly increased; walking is an excellent exercise (Braun, Colucci, & Patterson, 1999). The nurse instructs the client to walk until the point of claudication, stop and rest, and then walk a little farther. Eventually, clients are able to walk longer distances as collateral circulation develops. The nurse collaborates with the health care provider and physical therapist in determining an appropriate exercise program.

POSITIONING. Positioning of the client to promote circulation has been somewhat controversial. Some clients have swelling in their extremities. Because swelling prevents arterial flow, they should elevate their feet at rest, but the nurse teaches them to refrain from raising their legs above the heart level. Extreme elevation *slows* arterial blood flow to the feet.

In severe cases, clients with PAD and swelling may sleep with the affected limb hanging from the bed, or they may sit upright in a chair for comfort. The nurse instructs all clients with PAD to avoid crossing their legs, which may interfere with blood flow.

PROMOTING VASODILATION. Vasodilation can be achieved by providing warmth to the affected extremity and preventing long periods of exposure to cold. The nurse encourages the client to maintain a warm environment at home and to wear socks or insulated shoes at all times. The client is cautioned *never* to apply direct heat to the limb, such as with the use of heating pads or extremely hot water. Sensitivity is decreased in the affected limb, and the client may get burned without feeling it.

The nurse encourages clients to prevent exposure of the affected limb to the cold because cold temperatures cause vasoconstriction (decreasing of the diameter of the blood vessels) and therefore decrease arterial blood flow. Emotional stress, caffeine, and nicotine also can cause vasoconstriction. The nurse emphasizes that complete abstinence from smoking or chewing tobacco is the most effective method of preventing vasoconstriction. The vasoconstrictive effects of each cigarette may last up to 1 hour after the cigarette is smoked.

DRUG THERAPY. For clients with chronic PAD, prescribed drugs include hemorheologic and antiplatelet agents. Pentoxifylline (Trental) is a hemorheologic agent that increases the flexibility of red blood cells; it decreases blood viscosity by inhibiting platelet aggregation and decreasing fibrinogen and thus increases blood flow in the extremities. Many clients report limited improvement in their daily lives after taking pentoxifylline. Moreover, clients with extremely limited endurance for walking have reported improvement to the point that they can perform some activities (e.g., walk to the mailbox or dining room) that were previously impossible.

Antiplatelet agents, such as aspirin (acetylsalicylic acid, Ancasal🍁) and clopidogrel (Plavix), are commonly used for clients with PAD. Aspirin 325 or 81 mg/day is typically recommended for all clients with chronic PAD. In a trial of *c*lopidogrel versus *a*spirin in *p*atients at *r*isk of *i*schemic *e*vents (CAPRIE), clopidogrel demonstrated improvement over aspirin for risk reduction for myocardial infarction, ischemic stroke, and vascular death, but the difference was slight. Therefore clients with peripheral vascular disease (PVD) with no contraindications to platelet therapy should receive either aspirin or clopidogrel.

Controlling hypertension can improve tissue perfusion by maintaining pressures that are adequate to perfuse the periphery but not vasoconstrict the vessels. Nurses should make clients aware of the effect of blood pressure on the circulation and should instruct them in methods of control. For example, clients taking beta blockers may experience drug-related claudication or an exacerbation of their symptoms. The health care provider closely monitors clients with PAD who are receiving beta blockers.

PERCUTANEOUS TRANSLUMINAL ANGIOPLASTY. Another nonsurgical but invasive method of improving arterial flow is **percutaneous transluminal angioplasty (PTA)** (Figure 36-6). One or more arteries are dilated with a balloon catheter advanced through a cannula, which is inserted into or above an occluded or stenosed artery. When the procedure is successful, it opens the vessel lumen and improves arterial blood flow, creating a smooth inner-vessel surface. In addition, a stent (wirelike device) may be used along with the PTA to help keep the vessel open. Clients who are candidates for PTA must have occlusions or stenoses that are accessible to the catheter. The physician often uses (PTA) for clients who are poor surgical candidates who cannot withstand general anesthesia or for whom amputation may be inevitable. Reocclusion may occur after this procedure, and the procedure may be repeated. Some clients are occlusion free for up to 3 to 5 years, whereas others may experience reocclusion within a year.

During PTA, intravascular stents may be placed to ensure adequate blood flow in a stenosed vessel. Candidates for this type of procedure are individuals with stenosis of the common or external iliac arteries. This type of procedure is cost-effective and results in shorter hospital stays and earlier recoveries.

LASER-ASSISTED ANGIOPLASTY. Another invasive procedure is **laser-assisted angioplasty.** A laser probe is advanced through a cannula similar to that used for PTA. Laser-assisted angioplasty is usually reserved for clients with smaller occlusions in the distal superficial femoral, proximal popliteal, and common iliac arteries. Heat from the laser vaporizes the arteriosclerotic plaque to open the occluded or stenosed artery. If significant stenosis remains after the artery is opened, a balloon catheter may be inserted to further dilate the artery.

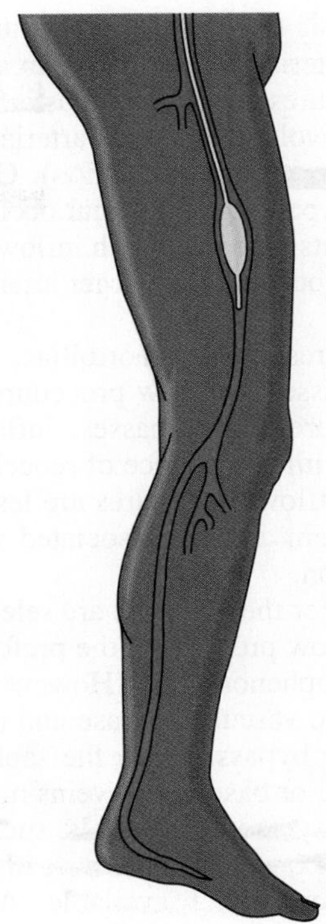

Figure 36-6 ● Percutaneous transluminal angioplasty.

Preparation of the client for PTA or laser-assisted angioplasty is similar to that for diagnostic angiography. The client must have nothing by mouth (NPO) after midnight. The surgeon may require that the client scrub the groin area with an antiseptic solution.

Postprocedure nursing care involves observing for bleeding at the puncture site. The nurse or assistive nursing personnel closely observes vital signs and frequently checks the distal pulses in both limbs. These clients are typically restricted to bedrest, with the limb straight for approximately 6 to 8 hours before ambulation. Many receive anticoagulant therapy, such as heparin, during the procedure and for a short time after the procedure. Some type of antiplatelet drug is provided for 1 to 3 months after the procedure. Clients usually take aspirin on a permanent basis.

ATHERECTOMY. The technique of mechanical rotational abrasive **atherectomy** is used to improve blood flow to ischemic limbs in people with PAD. The rotational atherectomy device (Rotablator) is a high-speed rotary, metal bur ranging in size from 1.25 to 4.5 mm in diameter. The distal half of the bur is embedded with fine abrasive bits, which at rotational speeds of 100,000 to 120,000 rotations per minute result in fine-particle destruction of tissue. The Rotablator is designed to preferentially scrape "hard" surfaces (such as plaque) while minimizing damage to the vessel surface.

SURGICAL MANAGEMENT. Clients with severe rest pain or claudication that interferes with the ability to work or threatens loss of a limb become surgical candidates. **Arterial**

revascularization is the surgical procedure most commonly used to increase arterial blood flow in an affected limb.

Surgical procedures are classified as inflow or outflow. Inflow procedures involve bypassing arterial occlusions above the superficial femoral arteries (SFAs). Outflow procedures involve surgical bypassing of arterial occlusions at or below the SFAs. For clients who have both inflow and outflow problems, the inflow procedure (for larger arteries) is done before the outflow repair.

Inflow procedures include aortoiliac, aortofemoral, and axillofemoral bypasses. Outflow procedures include femoropopliteal and femorotibial bypasses. Inflow procedures are more successful, with less chance of reocclusion or postoperative ischemia. Outflow procedures are less successful in relieving ischemic pain and are associated with a higher incidence of reocclusion.

Graft materials for the bypasses are selected on an individual basis. For outflow procedures the preferred graft material is an autogenous saphenous vein. However, these clients can experience systemic vascular disease and may need this vein for coronary artery bypass. When the saphenous vein is not usable, the cephalic or basilic arm veins may be used.

Grafts made of synthetic materials, such as polytetrafluoroethylene, Gore-Tex, and Dacron, have also been used when autogenous veins were not available. Although synthetic grafts have achieved adequate patency in arteries above the knee, they have failed to achieve satisfactory results in infrapopliteal outflow vessels. In addition, autogenous veins are often not long enough for use in these vessels. Composite grafts constructed from multiple vein segments offer even better patency to arteries below the knee.

PREOPERATIVE CARE. Preparing the client for surgery is similar to that described for general or epidural anesthesia (see Chapter 17). Documentation of vital signs and peripheral pulses provides a baseline of information for comparison during the postoperative phase. Depending on the surgical procedure, the client may have an intravenous (IV) line, urinary catheter, central venous catheter, and/or arterial line. To prevent postoperative infection, clients typically receive antibiotic therapy before the procedure.

OPERATIVE PROCEDURES. The anesthesiologist or nurse anesthetist places the client under general, epidural, or spinal anesthesia. Epidural or spinal induction is preferred for older adults to decrease the risk of cardiopulmonary complications in this age-group. If arterial bypass is to be accomplished by autogenous grafts, the surgeon excises the appropriate veins through an incision. The occluded artery is then exposed through an incision, and the conduit veins or synthetic graft material is sutured above and below the occlusion to facilitate blood flow around the occlusion.

For *aortoiliac* and *aortofemoral* bypass surgery, the surgeon makes a midline incision into the abdominal cavity to expose the abdominal aorta, with additional incisions into each groin (Figure 36-7). Graft material is tunneled from the aorta to the groin incisions, where it is sutured in place.

In an *axillofemoral* bypass (Figure 36-8), the surgeon makes an incision beneath the clavicle and tunnels graft material subcutaneously with a catheter from the chest to the iliac crest, into a groin incision, where it is sutured in place. Neither the thoracic nor the abdominal cavity is entered. For this reason, the axillofemoral bypass is used for high-risk clients who cannot tolerate a procedure requiring abdominal surgery.

POSTOPERATIVE CARE. Graft occlusion often occurs within the first 24 hours. Therefore astute nursing care is cru-

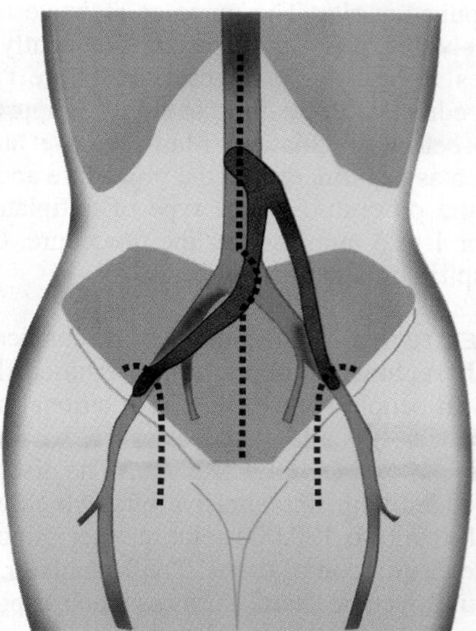

Figure 36-7 ● In aortoiliac and aortofemoral bypass surgery, a midline incision into the abdominal cavity is required, with an additional incision in each groin.

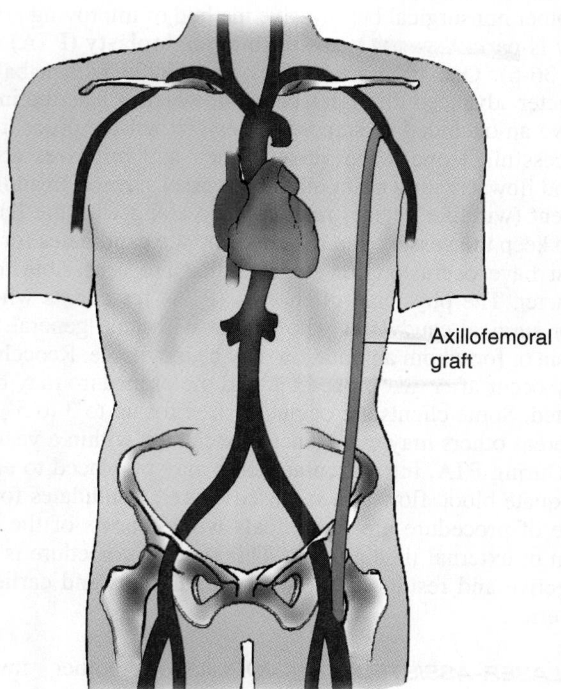

Figure 36-8 ● An axillofemoral bypass graft.

cial. The Client Care Plan below highlights the most important aspects of postoperative care.

Assessment for Graft Occlusion. The nurse monitors the patency of the graft by checking the extremity every 15 minutes for the first hour, then hourly, for changes in color, temperature, and pulse intensity. Warmth, redness, and edema of the affected extremity are often expected outcomes of surgery as a result of increased blood flow. Immediately postoperatively, the operating room or postanesthesia care unit (PACU) nurse marks the site where the distal (dorsalis pedis or posterior tibial) pulse is best palpated or heard by Doppler ultrasonography. The nurse communicates this information to the nursing staff on the unit where the client will be sent.

Pain is frequently the first indicator of postoperative graft occlusion. Many people experience a throbbing pain caused by the increased blood flow to the extremity. This sensation is different from ischemic pain, and the nurse must assess the type of pain that the client is experiencing. If graft occlusion occurs, the client will experience a sharp increase in ischemic pain, described as similar to the pain felt before surgery. The nurse reports severe pain to the surgeon immediately.

Promotion of Graft Patency. To promote graft patency, the nurse monitors the client's blood pressure and notifies the surgeon if the pressure increases or decreases beyond normal limits. Hypotension may indicate hypovolemia, which can increase the risk of clotting. Range of motion of the affected limb is usually limited, with bending of the hip and knee contraindicated. The nurse consults with the surgeon on a case-by-case basis regarding limitations of movement, including turning. Clients are restricted to bedrest for at least 24 hours postoperatively.

The nurse instructs all clients to cough and deep breathe every 1 to 2 hours and to use an incentive spirometer. Clients who have undergone aortoiliac or aortofemoral bypass are allowed nothing by mouth for at least 1 day postoperatively. Those who have undergone bypass surgery of the lower extremities not involving the aorta or abdominal wall (femoropopliteal or femorotibial bypass) may be on NPO status the night of surgery but are often allowed clear liquids the morning after surgery.

Treatment of Graft Occlusion. If manifestations of graft occlusion occur, the nurse notifies the surgeon immediately. Perfusion through the graft must be resolved promptly to avoid ischemic injury to the limb. Emergency *thrombectomy* (removal of the clot), which the surgeon may perform at the bedside, is the most common treatment for acute graft occlusion. Thrombectomy is associated with excellent results in prosthetic grafts but variable results in autogenous vein grafts, which often necessitate graft revision and even replacement.

Local intra-arterial thrombolytic therapy with an agent such as tissue plasminogen activator (t-PA), or an infusion of a platelet inhibitor such as abciximab (ReoPro), may be used for acute graft occlusions in selected clients in settings where health care providers are experts on its use. The physician considers these therapies when the surgical alternative (e.g., thrombectomy with or without graft revision or replacement) carries high morbidity or mortality or when surgery for this type of occlusion has traditionally yielded poor results. When the physician uses thrombolytic therapy, the

CLIENT CARE PLAN • THE CLIENT WHO HAS UNDERGONE PERIPHERAL ARTERIAL REVASCULARIZATION (BYPASS) SURGERY

NURSING DIAGNOSIS NO. 1 • Altered Tissue Perfusion (Peripheral)

Expected Outcomes	Nursing Interventions	Rationale
The client will maintain an increase in arterial blood flow to an extremity previously deprived of arterial blood flow.	Assess color, temperature, and pulse intensity of the affected extremity hourly. Notify the surgeon of a significant change.	Color, temperature, and pulse intensity immediately postoperatively indicate optimal arterial flow achieved with revascularization. Any increase in pallor or cyanosis or decrease in temperature or pulse intensity indicates postoperative graft occlusion.
	Assess the client for pain in the affected extremity, and report if described as "severe, similar to the pain before surgery."	Severe pain, similar to the pain felt before surgery, is frequently the first indicator of postoperative graft occlusion.
	Monitor the client's blood pressure, and report if it is increased or decreased beyond the client's normal limits. D	Hypotension may indicate hypovolemia, which can increase the risk of clotting. Hypertension may put stress on the graft.
	Instruct the client to keep the affected extremity straight, limit movement, and avoid flexion of the knee and hip. Consult with the surgeon about turning the client.	Pressure on the graft can facilitate clot formation.
	Assess the incision for drainage, edema, and temperature.	Edema of the affected extremity is an expected outcome, but excessive edema should be reported. A small amount of bloody drainage is expected, but excessive bleeding is abnormal. Warmth, erythema, or a hard, tender area around the incision may indicate infection.

D indicates tasks that can be delegated to assistive nursing personnel.

nurse closely assesses the client for signs and symptoms of bleeding.

Monitoring for Compartment Syndrome. Compartment syndrome occurs when tissue pressure within a confined body space becomes elevated and restricts blood flow. The resultant ischemia can lead to tissue damage and eventually tissue death. The nurse assesses the motor and sensory function of the affected extremity. The extremity should also be assessed for worsening pain, fullness, swelling, and tenseness. These symptoms should be reported to the health care provider immediately. When compartment syndrome is suspected, the nurse continues to assess the extremity, removes or loosens the dressings, and places the extremity at the level of the heart. A complete discussion of compartment syndrome is found in Chapter 52.

Assessment for Infection. Graft or wound infections can be life threatening and can endanger the client's limb. The nurse uses sterile technique when in contact with the incision and observes for symptoms of infection at or around the graft and incision sites. If the area over the graft becomes hard, tender, red, or warm, the client may have an infection. The nurse notifies the surgeon if any of these symptoms occur.

Community-Based Care

CASE MANAGEMENT

Peripheral arterial disease (PAD) is a chronic, long-term problem with frequent complications. Clients with PAD may benefit from a case manager who can follow them across the continuum of care. The goal is to maintain the client in the home environment.

HOME CARE MANAGEMENT

Managing the client at home often requires an interdisciplinary team approach. Chart 36-8 outlines the assessment highlights for home care clients with peripheral vascular disease (PVD). The clinical guide in Figure 36-9 shows how one home care agency documents care for homebound clients with PAD.

HEALTH TEACHING

The nurse instructs all clients on methods to promote vasodilation. They are taught to avoid raising their legs above the level of the heart unless they also have venous stasis. The nurse provides written and oral instructions on foot care and methods to prevent injury and ulcer development for all clients (Chart 36-9).

Clients who have had surgery require additional instruction on incision care (see Chapter 19). The nurse encourages all clients to avoid smoking and to limit dietary fat intake to less than 30% of the total daily calories.

Clients with chronic arterial obstruction may fear recurrent occlusion or further narrowing of the artery. They often fear that they might lose a limb or become debilitated in other ways. Indeed, chronic PAD may worsen, especially in clients with diabetes mellitus. The nurse, however, reassures clients that their participation in prescribed exercise, diet, and pharmacologic therapy, along with cessation of smoking, can limit further formation of atherosclerotic plaques.

CONSIDERATIONS FOR OLDER ADULTS

Older clients with PVD may have visual or mobility problems that impede their ability to effectively provide foot care. The nurse can suggest using magnifying mirrors to check the feet and toes for cracks or blisters. Before washing the feet with mild soap and warm water, the temperature of the water should be tested with a thermometer or elbow, not the hand. Older adults may be at increased risk for trauma or self-inflicted injury. They should be advised never to go barefoot, to wear cotton socks, and to wear protective shoes. They should also be advised to see a podiatrist to trim their toenails and manage corns or calluses.

CHART 36-8

FOCUSED ASSESSMENT *of* Home Care Clients with Peripheral Vascular Disease

Assess tissue perfusion to affected extremity(ies), including:
- Distal circulation, sensation, and motion
- Presence of pain, pallor, paresthesias, pulselessness, paralysis, poikilothermia (coolness)
- Ankle/brachial index

Assess adherence to therapeutic regimen, including:
- Following foot care instructions
- Quitting smoking
- Maintaining dietary restrictions
- Participating in exercise regimen
- Avoiding exposure to cold and constrictive clothing

Assess ability to manage wound care and prevent further injury, including:
- Use of compression stockings or compression pumps as directed
- Use of various dressing materials
- Signs and symptoms to report to nurse

Assess coping ability of client and family members.

Assess home environment, including:
- Safety hazards, especially related to falls

CHART 36-9

CLIENT EDUCATION GUIDE
Foot Care for the Client with Peripheral Vascular Disease

- Keep your feet clean by washing them with a mild soap in room-temperature water.
- Keep your feet dry, especially between the toes and ankles.
- Avoid injury to your feet and ankles. Wear comfortable, well-fitting shoes. Never go without shoes.
- Keep your toenails clean and filed. Have someone cut them if you cannot see them clearly. Cut your toenails straight across.
- To prevent dry, cracked skin, apply a lubricating lotion to your feet.
- Prevent exposure to extreme heat or cold. Never use a heating pad on your feet.
- Avoid constricting garments.
- If a problem develops, see a podiatrist or physician.
- Avoid extended pressure on your feet or ankles, such as occurs when you lean against something.

Text continued on page 755

Multidisciplinary Clinical Guide
Visit Summary

Instructions: Associate Nurse or Practitioner of an Associated Discipline, please complete this visit summary and transmit to the Nursing Case Manager within 24 hours of the completion of each visit.

Date: ___________ Name of Patient: ___________________________ and/or Caregiver: ______________

Medical Diagnoses: ____

Discipline of Professional Making Visit: ____

Discharge Planning Started: ____

Discipline-Specific Diagnoses Treated at this visit:

____

____

Discipline-Specific Goals: (Note any change in goal[s] with reason for change)

____

____

Assessment Changes to Be Noted by Case Manager:

____

____

Variances from POC Detected: (use key numbers and explain if needed)

____

____

____

Note follow-up care needed or plan for discharge:

____

____

Physician Contacted: ____

New Orders: ____

Signature: ___________________________ Date: ________________

Variances:

Key

1. Psychosocial
2. Environment
3. Physiologic
4. Health-related behaviors
5. Other

Figure 36-9 ● Multidisciplinary clinical guide visit summary. (From Wills, E.M., & Sloan, H.L. [1996]. Assessing peripheral arterial disorders in the home: A multidisciplinary clinical guide. *Home Healthcare Nurse, 14*[9], 670-674.)

Continued

Criterion		Admission Date:	V	V	V	V	V
KNOWLEDGE	**Assessment Data Key:** 1 = none; 2 = minimal; 3 = basic; 4 = adequate; 5 = superior						
Patient/family	General knowledge about PAD (include smoking)						
Caregiver able to:	1. Inspect daily: blisters, itching, cuts, lesions, redness, pain, swelling, heat, dryness, calluses, corns 2. Administer hygiene: a. Wash daily with warm water b. Dry carefully between toes c. Change socks, shoes daily						
Selecting footwear	1. Shoes (leather, avoids synthetic) a. Style (wide toe, avoids sandals) b. Inside condition (no foreign objects, nail points, lining intact, no rough areas) c. Wears shoes indoors and outdoors d. Correctly breaks in new shoes (wear for 20-30 minutes daily)						
Skin care	1. Corn/callus care a. No chemical products used b. Pumice stone if sensitive 2. Dry skin care a. Uses superfatted soap b. Water temp 90°-105° F c. Emollient to dry areas before drying skin (none between toes)						
Professional care	1. Identifies need for care 2. Reports problems (skin breakdown, edema, ingrown toenails, inability to trim nails safely, shoe problems, rest or night pain) 3. Has routine foot assessment quarterly						
Medications	1. Identifies name and dose 2. Verbalizes reason for use 3. Avoids over-the-counter drugs (interactions with prescriptions)						
Monitors pain and complications	1. Degree and type of pain 2. Identifies one complication (ulcer, gangrene, amputation, functional limitations)						
Exercise/rest	1. Exercise patterns 2. Control of symptoms						
Diet	Knows diet. Type: Activate teaching plan if necessary						

Figure 36-9, cont'd ● Multidisciplinary clinical guide visit summary. (From Wills, E.M., & Sloan, H.L. [1996]. Assessing peripheral arterial disorders in the home: A multidisciplinary clinical guide. *Home Healthcare Nurse, 14*[9], 670-674.)

Criterion		Admission Date:	V	V	V	V	V
KNOWLEDGE *(continued)*	**Assessment Data Key:** 1 = none; 2 = minimal; 3 = basic; 4 = adequate; 5 = superior						
Discipline-specific diagnoses and goal dates:	1. Goal date:	Met? (y/n)					
Discipline: Specify							
Goal achieved (y/n) Variances: Key 1. Psychosocial 2. Environment 3. Physiologic 4. Health-related behaviors 5. Other							
Comments							
BEHAVIOR	**Behavior displayed is appropriate:** **Key:** 1 = not; 2 = rarely; 3 = inconsistently; 4 = usually; 5 = consistently						
Diet	Type of diet:	Follows diet:					
Smoking	Changes in smoking behavior:						
Medications List:	Medications taken correctly						
Problem solving	Identifies preferences, assists nurse to individualize plan of care (POC)						
Community resources	Needs referrals for: a. Meal preparation b. Transportation c. Personal care	d. Health care funding e. Support groups f. Shoe fitting, care					
Coping skills	Identifies ways to deal with pain, loss of function						
Beliefs/self-efficacy	a. Identifies beliefs about ability to follow POC b. Beliefs about insensitive feet 1. no pain = no problem 2. no pain means no care is required c. Nurse may need to reinterpret signs and symptoms for client						
Motivation	Client/family motivation to follow POC?						
Diagnoses and goal dates:	1. Goal date:	Met? (y/n)					

Figure 36-9, cont'd ● Multidisciplinary clinical guide visit summary. (From Wills, E.M., & Sloan, H.L. [1996]. Assessing peripheral arterial disorders in the home: A multidisciplinary clinical guide. *Home Healthcare Nurse, 14*[9], 670-674.)

Continued

Criterion		Admission Date:	V	V	V	V	V
BEHAVIOR *(continued)*	**Behavior displayed is appropriate:** **Key:** 1 = not; 2 = rarely; 3 = inconsistently; 4 = usually; 5 = consistently						
Discipline(s): Specify with diagnosis							
Goal achieved (y/n) Variances: Key 1. Psychosocial 2. Environment 3. Physiologic 4. Health-related behaviors 5. Other							
Comments							
STATUS	**Assessment Data Key: Signs & Symptoms:** 1 = extreme; 2 = severe; 3 = moderate; 4 = minimal; 5 = none						
Foot assessment Nails Hygiene Footwear	Inspection: 1. Nails cut straight across or slightly rounded 2. Rate hygiene good, fair, poor 3. Footwear adequate or inadequate a. Socks (materials: cotton, wool, polyester blend) Cautions: nonrestricting fit, no circular garters or constricting clothes, no knee-highs b. Shoes (check type, fit, condition)						
Skin	1. Color (rubor, pallor, cyanosis, blackened areas) 2. Temperature (check both extremities, note differences) 3. Edema (pitting/nonpitting Grade [1-4]/4)						
Atrophy	Skin (shiny, pale, translucent)						
Changes to foot	1. Toenails (label as thickened, discolored, deformed) 2. Corns/calluses (describe location, size) 3. Deformities (describe in nurse's note; presence of hammer toes, claw toes, bunions)						
Vital signs Post, tibial pulse Blood pressure	Grade pulse (use 0-4/4 [0 = not palpable, 1 = easily obliterated, 2 = easily palpable, 3 = not easily obliterated, 4 = strong, bounding]) Both arms and do orthostatic if possible						
Ulcerations (location)	Describe completely in nurse's notes and on wound flow sheet						

Figure 36-9, cont'd ● Multidisciplinary clinical guide visit summary. (From Wills, E.M., & Sloan, H.L. [1996]. Assessing peripheral arterial disorders in the home: A multidisciplinary clinical guide. *Home Healthcare Nurse, 14*[9], 670-674.)

Criterion		Admission Date:	V	V	V	V	V
STATUS (continued)	**Assessment Data Key: Signs & Symptoms:** 1 = extreme; 2 = severe; 3 = moderate; 4 = minimal; 5 = none						
Complication potential (Evaluate on admission and every 60 days)	Ulcer, ischemia, gangrene, functional limitations						
ABI on admission (Reassess if post-tibial pulse changes)	1. Blood pressure at brachial and ankle locations bilaterally 2. Use Doppler if possible 3. Calculate index from highest readings (A/B = ABI)						
Protective sensation	Measure with Semmes/Weinstein Monofilament (10 g/0.5). Apply to feet and ankles and random areas (present or not).						
Discipline-specific diagnoses and goal dates:	1. Goal date: Met? (y/n)						
Discipline: Specify							
Goal achieved (y/n) Variances: Key 1. Psychosocial 2. Environment 3. Physiologic 4. Health-related behaviors 5. Other							
Comments							

Figure 36-9, cont'd ● Multidisciplinary clinical guide visit summary. (From Wills, E.M., & Sloan, H.L. [1996]. Assessing peripheral arterial disorders in the home: A multidisciplinary clinical guide. *Home Healthcare Nurse, 14*[9], 670-674.)

HEALTH CARE RESOURCES

Clients with arterial compromise may need assistance with activities of daily living (ADLs) if activity is limited by pain. They may need to limit or avoid stair climbing, depending on the severity of disease. Clients who have undergone surgery usually need temporary help with ADLs.

Clients who must limit activity because of PAD may benefit from the assistance of a home care aide. Those who has undergone surgery may require a home care nurse to assist with incision care. The nurse or case manager arranges for home care resources before the client is discharged.

Acute Peripheral Arterial Occlusion

OVERVIEW

Although chronic peripheral arterial disease (PAD) progresses slowly, the onset of **acute arterial occlusions** may be sudden and dramatic. An embolus is the most common cause of peripheral occlusions, although a local thrombus may be the cause. Occlusion may affect the upper extremities, but it is more common in the lower extremities. Emboli originating from the heart are the most common cause of acute arterial occlusions. Most clients with an embolic occlusion have had an acute myocardial infarction and/or atrial fibrillation within the preceding weeks.

COLLABORATIVE MANAGEMENT

Assessment

Clients with an acute arterial occlusion describe severe pain below the level of the occlusion that occurs even at rest. The affected extremity is cool or cold, pulseless, and mottled. Minute areas on the toes may be blackened or gangrenous. Clients with acute arterial insufficiency often present with the "six *P*'s" of ischemia: *p*ain, *p*allor, *p*ulselessness, *p*aresthesia, *p*aralysis, and *p*oikilothermia (coolness) of the involved extremity.

Interventions

The health care provider must initiate treatment promptly to avoid permanent damage or loss of an extremity. Anticoagulant therapy with unfractionated heparin (UFH; Hepalean🍁) is usually the first intervention to prevent further clot formation. A bolus of up to 10,000 units may be ordered. The client may also undergo angiography.

A surgical thrombectomy or embolectomy with local anesthesia may be performed to remove the occlusion. The physician makes an incision, which is followed by an arteriotomy (a surgical opening into an artery). The physician then inserts a Fogarty catheter into the artery and retrieves the embolus. It may be necessary to close the artery with a patch graft.

Postoperatively, the nurse monitors the affected extremity for improvement in color, temperature, and pulse, as well as other extremities for signs and symptoms of new thrombi or emboli. Pain should significantly diminish after the surgical procedure, although mild incisional pain remains. The nurse watches closely for complications caused by reperfusing the artery after thrombectomy or embolectomy, which include spasms and swelling of the skeletal muscle. Swelling of the skeletal muscles is characterized by edema, pain on passive movement, poor capillary refill, numbness, and muscle tenseness. Fasciotomy (surgical opening into the tissues) may be necessary to prevent further injury and save the limb.

The use of systemic thrombolytic therapy for acute arterial occlusions has been disappointing because bleeding complications have outweighed the benefits obtained. Local intra-arterial thrombolytic therapy with alteplase (Activase) or t-PA and the use of platelet inhibitors, such as abciximab (ReoPro), have emerged as alternatives to surgical treatment in selected clients in settings where health care providers are familiar with their use and complications. When thrombolytics are given, the nurse monitors for signs and symptoms of bleeding, bruising, or hematoma. When a client receives abciximab (ReoPro), platelet counts need to be monitored for the first 3, 6, and 12 hours after the start of the infusion. If the platelet count decreases to below 100,000, the abciximab infusion needs to be readjusted or discontinued. If any of these complications occur, the nurse notifies the physician immediately.

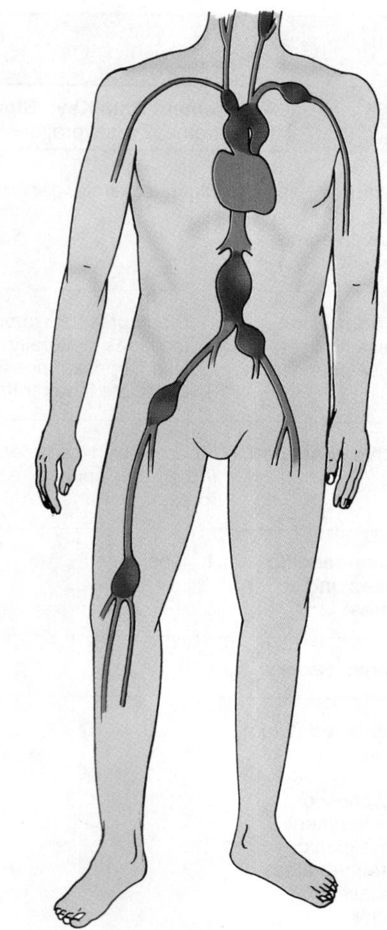

Figure 36-10 ● Common anatomic sites of arterial aneurysms.

ANEURYSMS

OVERVIEW

An **aneurysm** is a permanent localized dilation of an artery, which enlarges the artery to at least two times its normal diameter.

Types of Aneurysms

An aneurysm may be described as *fusiform* (a diffuse dilation affecting the entire circumference of the artery) or *saccular* (an outpouching affecting only a distinct portion of the artery). Aneurysms may also be described as true or false. In true aneurysms the arterial wall is weakened by congenital or acquired problems. False aneurysms occur as a result of vessel injury or trauma to all three layers of the arterial wall.

Dissecting hematomas, traditionally called *dissecting aneurysms,* are more accurately described as *aortic dissections* (see the later discussion on p. 760). Aortic dissections differ from aneurysms in that they are formed when blood accumulates in the wall of an artery.

Aneurysms tend to occur at specific anatomic sites (Figure 36-10), most commonly in the abdominal aorta. Aneurysms often occur at a point where the artery is not supported by skeletal muscles or on the lines of curves or flexion in the arterial tree.

Pathophysiologic Process

An aneurysm forms when the middle layer (media) of the artery is weakened, producing a stretching effect in the inner layer (intima) and outer layers (adventitia) of the artery. As the artery widens, tension in the wall increases and further widening occurs, thus enlarging the aneurysm. Hypertension (high blood pressure) produces more tension and enlargement within the artery. As the aneurysm grows, the risk of arterial rupture increases.

Abdominal aortic aneurysms (AAAs) account for approximately 75% of all aneurysms. Most of these aneurysms are located between the renal arteries and the aortic bifurcation. Of all AAAs greater than 6 cm in diameter, 50% rupture within 1 year; of those aneurysms smaller than 6 cm in diameter, 15% to 20% rupture.

Thoracic aortic aneurysms account for approximately 25% of all aneurysms and are frequently misdiagnosed (McClarren-Curry & Shaughnessy, 1999). They commonly develop between the origin of the left subclavian artery and the diaphragm. They are located in the descending, ascending, and transverse sections of the aorta.

Aneurysms can cause symptoms by exerting pressure on surrounding structures or by rupturing. Rupture of an aneurysm is the most frequent complication and is life threatening because abrupt and massive hemorrhagic shock occurs with the rupture. Thrombi within the wall of an aneurysm can also be the source of emboli in distal arteries below the aneurysm.

Atherosclerosis is the most common cause of all aneurysms, with hypertension and cigarette smoking being contributing factors. Syphilis (a sexually transmitted disease) and Ehlers-Danlos syndrome (a rare genetic disorder) are other causes of AAAs.

The incidence of AAAs, estimated to be between 30 and 66 per 1000 persons, is increasing in the Western world. Approximately 15,000 people in the United States die annually from abdominal aneurysms, making it the thirteenth leading cause of death in the United States. Thoracic aortic aneurysms occur most often in older adults and have a 50% mortality rate even with surgical intervention (McClarren-Curry & Shaughnessy, 1999). AAAs are more common in men than in women (with a ratio of 4:1).

COLLABORATIVE MANAGEMENT

Assessment

Most clients with abdominal or thoracic aneurysms are asymptomatic when their aneurysms are first discovered by routine examination or during radiographic study performed for another reason.

ABDOMINAL AORTIC ANEURYSMS

Because there may be symptoms, the nurse assesses clients with a known or suspected abdominal aortic aneurysm (AAA) for abdominal, flank, or back pain. Pain related to an AAA is usually steady with a gnawing quality, is unaffected by movement, and may last for hours or days.

A pulsation in the upper abdomen slightly to the left of the midline between the xiphoid process and the umbilicus may be present. A detectable aneurysm is at least 5 cm in diameter. The nurse auscultates for a bruit over the mass but avoids palpating the mass because it may be tender and there is a risk of rupture.

Although some clients have symptoms when the aneurysm is intact, many are asymptomatic until the time of rupture. If expansion and impending rupture of an AAA are suspected, the nurse assesses for severe pain of sudden onset in the back or lower abdomen, which may radiate to the groin, buttocks, or legs.

Clients with a rupturing AAA are critically ill and in hemorrhagic (hypovolemic) shock. Signs include hypotension, diaphoresis, mental obtundation, oliguria, and dysrhythmias. Retroperitoneal hemorrhage is manifested by hematomas in the flanks. Rupture into the abdominal cavity causes abdominal distention.

> **CRITICAL THINKING CHALLENGE**
>
> While you are obtaining a nursing health history from your client, she tells you that she has a sharp pain across her back. She has a history of hypertension and a pulsating mass in her abdominal area.
>
> - What might you expect to find on your physical assessment?
> - How are you going to treat her pain?
> - Why is the history of hypertension important?

For suggested answer guidelines, go to SIMON http://www.wbsaunders.com/SIMON/Iggy/.

THORACIC AORTIC ANEURYSMS

When a thoracic aortic aneurysm is suspected, the nurse assesses the client for back pain and manifestations of compression of the aneurysm on adjacent structures. Signs include shortness of breath, hoarseness, and difficulty swallowing. Thoracic aneurysms are not often detected by physical assessment, but occasionally a mass may be visible above the suprasternal notch.

The client with suspected rupture of a thoracic aneurysm is assessed for sudden and excruciating back or chest pain. Rupture of a thoracic aneurysm is also indicated by hemorrhagic shock (see Chapter 37).

RADIOGRAPHIC ASSESSMENT

An abdominal x-ray film or a lateral x-ray film of the spine often shows an AAA. The "eggshell" appearance of the aneurysm is essentially diagnostic.

Computed tomographic (CT) scanning is the standard tool for assessing the size and location of an abdominal or thoracic aneurysm. A thoracic aneurysm can be diagnosed by chest x-ray examination. Aortic arteriography is usually performed for clients who are to undergo surgical repair of a thoracic aneurysm.

OTHER DIAGNOSTIC ASSESSMENT

Ultrasonography is a noninvasive technique that provides an accurate diagnosis, as well as information about the size and location of an AAA.

Interventions

The size of the aneurysm and the presence of symptoms are the most important parameters in the determination of treatment.

NONSURGICAL MANAGEMENT. The goal of nonsurgical management is to monitor the growth of the aneurysm and maintain the blood pressure at a normal level to decrease the risk of rupture.

Because elevated blood pressure can increase the rate of aneurysmal enlargement, hypertension is an important risk factor for rupture. Clients with hypertension are treated with antihypertensives to decrease the rate of enlargement and the risk for early rupture.

For clients with small or asymptomatic aneurysms, frequent CT scans are necessary to monitor the growth of the aneurysm. The nurse emphasizes the importance of following through with scheduled tests to monitor the growth. The nurse also explains the clinical manifestations of aneurysms that need to be promptly reported.

SURGICAL MANAGEMENT. Surgical management of an aneurysm may be an elective or an emergency procedure. For clients with either a rupturing abdominal aortic or a thoracic aneurysm, emergency surgery is performed.

Clients with an abdominal aortic aneurysm (AAA) 6 cm in diameter or wider undergo elective surgery. Some surgeons favor surgical treatment for clients with aneurysms 4 to 6 cm in diameter if the client is in good health. Clients in good health with aneurysms smaller than 4 cm and clients in poor health with aneurysms 4 to 6 cm in diameter undergo nonsurgical treatment until the aneurysm reaches 6 cm.

Clients with thoracic aortic aneurysms measuring 7 cm or more in diameter and clients with smaller aneurysms that are producing symptoms are advised to have elective surgery. Clients with aneurysms smaller than 7 cm in diameter that are not causing symptoms are treated nonsurgically until symptoms occur or the aneurysm enlarges to 7 cm.

The most common procedure performed for clients with an AAA has traditionally been an AAA resection or repair (aneurysmectomy). The mortality rate for elective AAA resection is 2% to 5%. The mortality rate for emergency surgery for expanding AAAs is 5% to 15% and 50% for those that have ruptured.

Newer technology, such as endothelial stent grafts, has improved mortality rates and shortened the hospital stay for selected clients who need aneurysm repair.

ABDOMINAL AORTIC ANEURYSM RESECTION. In an AAA resection, the physician excises the aneurysm from the abdominal aorta to prevent or repair the rupture. The goal is to secure stable aortic integrity and tissue perfusion throughout the body.

Preoperative Care. Interventions are similar to those for clients undergoing surgery with general anesthesia (see Chapter 17). A bowel preparation and emphasis on coughing and deep breathing are very important. Because significant blood loss often occurs during AAA resection, clients planning elective surgery may be advised to bank their blood for autologous (self) transfusions postoperatively.

The nurse assesses all peripheral pulses to serve as a baseline for comparison postoperatively. The nurse may mark where the pulse is palpated or heard by Doppler ultrasonography to facilitate locating the pulse postoperatively.

Clients with ruptured aneurysms are brought to the operating suite directly from the emergency department. Preoperative care of clients with ruptured aneurysms involves administration of large volumes of intravenous IV fluids to maintain tissue perfusion.

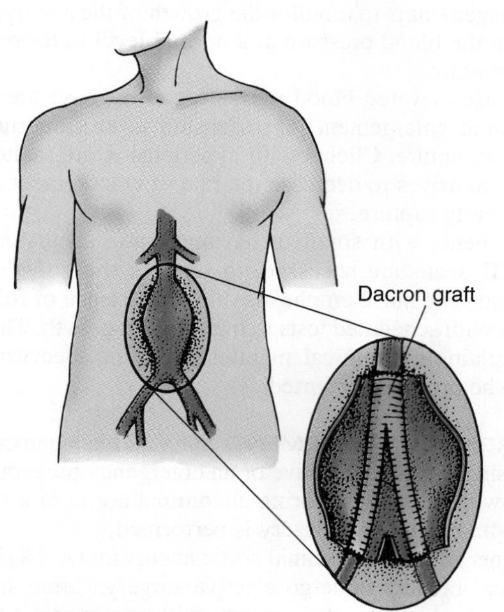

Figure 36-11 ● Surgical repair of abdominal aortic aneurysm with a woven Dacron graft.

Operative Procedure. The surgeon makes a midline abdominal incision from the xiphoid process to the symphysis pubis, or a wide transverse incision from flank to flank, to expose the aneurysm. Clamps are applied just above and just below the aneurysm, the aneurysm is excised, and a preclotted Dacron graft is sutured in an end-to-end fashion (Figure 36-11).

Postoperative Care. Immediately postoperatively, the client is typically admitted to a critical care unit for 24 to 48 hours, depending on his or her the age and condition. In addition to providing the routine postoperative care discussed in Chapter 19, the nurse assesses for and assists in prevention of the postoperative complications that can occur after an AAA repair. These complications include myocardial infarction, graft occlusion or rupture causing hemorrhage, hypovolemia and/or renal failure, respiratory distress, and paralytic ileus.

Myocardial Infarction. During the immediate postoperative period, the client's blood pressure is monitored with an arterial catheter. Continuous cardiac monitoring is used to detect any dysrhythmias. Using hemodynamic monitoring, the nurse monitors for low cardiac output and other findings consistent with an acute myocardial infarction. Other signs of myocardial infarction, include chest pain, shortness of breath, complaints of dyspnea, diaphoresis, anxiety, and restlessness.

Graft Occlusion or Rupture. The nurse or assistive nursing personnel assesses vital signs and circulation every 15 minutes for the first hour, then hourly, with assessment of pulses distal to the graft site (including the posterior tibial and dorsalis pedis pulses). Signs of graft occlusion or rupture are reported, including the following:

- Changes in pulses
- Cool to cold extremities below the graft
- White or blue extremities or flanks
- Severe pain
- Abdominal distention

The nurse limits elevation of the head of the bed to 45 degrees to avoid flexion of the graft.

Hypovolemia or Renal Failure. Hypovolemia and renal failure may occur because of blood loss during surgery or before if rupture occurred. The nurse assesses urine output via a Foley catheter hourly. If urine output is less than 50 mL/hr, the nurse notifies the surgeon. Although advances in surgical technique have decreased the risk of renal failure after clamping during surgery, renal failure may occur. Renal failure caused by acute tubular necrosis is more common after emergency surgery. In addition to monitoring urine output, the nurse and physician monitor serum creatinine and blood urea nitrogen (BUN) levels daily.

Respiratory Distress. The nurse assesses the respiratory rate and depth every hour and auscultates breath sounds every 4 hours to monitor for respiratory complications. Often, the client is maintained on a ventilator at least overnight to facilitate respiratory exchange. Opioids are administered for pain, as ordered, and the client is turned and suctioned as needed. The nurse provides firm abdominal support of the incision with a pillow or bath blanket while the client is coughing to prevent the incision from separating. After the client is extubated, he or she should continue to turn, cough, and deep breathe every 1 to 2 hours, and increase his or her mobility as ordered.

Paralytic Ileus. Paralytic ileus after AAA repair is expected for 2 to 3 days. Clients have a nasogastric tube set to low suction until bowel sounds return. The nurse listens for bowel sounds every 8 hours and reports their return to the physician. Prolonged absence of bowel sounds and distention may indicate a prolonged ileus or a bowel infarction.

THORACIC AORTIC ANEURYSM REPAIR. Repair of thoracic aneurysms is tailored to each client; the procedure depends on the type and location of the aneurysm. Total cardiopulmonary bypass (CPB) is necessary for excision of aneurysms in the ascending aorta, and partial bypass is often used during excision of aneurysms in the descending aorta.

Preoperative Care. The care of the client undergoing thoracic aneurysm resection is similar to that provided for the client having thoracic surgery.

Operative Procedure. The surgeon uses either a thoracotomy or a median sternotomy approach to enter the thoracic cavity. The surgeon exposes the aneurysm and excises it. After excising the aneurysm, the surgeon usually sews a Dacron graft or prosthesis onto the aorta. Saccular aneurysms, which have an outpouching from a distinct portion of the arterial wall, can sometimes be removed without resection of the aorta.

Postoperative Care. The care of a client who has undergone thoracic aneurysm repair is similar to that after other chest surgery. Clients who have undergone CPB receive care similar to that described in Chapter 35. The nurse assesses for and assists in the prevention of postoperative complications that can occur after a thoracic aneurysm repair. These complications include hemorrhage, ischemic colitis, spinal cord ischemia resulting in paraplegia, respiratory distress, and cardiac dysrhythmias.

Hemorrhage. The nurse assesses vital signs at least hourly, reporting any signs of hemorrhage (e.g., a decrease in blood pressure, an increase in pulse rate, rapid respirations, diaphoresis) to the physician immediately. The nurse assesses for bleeding or separation at the graft site by noting significant increases in chest drainage from the chest tubes.

Paraplegia. Inadvertent interruption of the blood supply to the spinal cord during thoracic aneurysm repair can result in paraplegia. The nurse assesses the client hourly for sensation and motion in all extremities and reports deficits immediately.

Respiratory Distress. After thoracic aneurysm repair, clients are especially susceptible to respiratory distress from atelectasis or pneumonia. This problem occurs as a result of both CPB and incisional discomfort. Both atelectasis and pneumonia may cause shallow breathing and poor cough effort. These clients are often maintained on a ventilator, at least overnight, after surgery. For clients with a median sternotomy, the surgeon firmly splints the incision to prevent separation of the sternum.

Cardiac Dysrhythmias. The nurse assesses all clients recovering from thoracic aneurysm repair for cardiac dysrhythmias. The stress of the thoracic surgery, added to the increased incidence of arteriosclerosis in this group, may predispose these clients to a myocardial infarction, cardiac dysrhythmias, or heart failure.

ENDOVASCULAR REPAIR OF ABDOMINAL AORTIC ANEURYSMS. The repair of AAAs with **endovascular stent grafts** provides an alternative choice for some clients. Clients selected for endovascular repair of AAAs are generally at high risk for major abdominal surgery. However, some clients with AAAs may be referred for endovascular repair before the aneurysm reaches the recommended diameter for elective surgery.

There are different designs of endovascular stent grafts for use, depending on the anatomic involvement of the aneurysm. The stent graft is flexible with either Dacron or polytetrafluoroethylene (PTFE) material. It is inserted through a skin incision into the femoral artery by way of a catheter-based system. The catheter is advanced to a level above the aneurysm, away from the renal arteries. The graft is released from the catheter, and the stent graft is deployed into place with a series of hooks. A defined proximal and distal neck is needed for tight seating of the stent to prevent leakage. This procedure is done in collaboration with the vascular surgeon, interventional radiologist, operating room team, and at some centers, vascular medicine physician.

The endovascular repair of AAAs has decreased the length of hospital stay for clients requiring repair of abdominal aneurysms from 7 to 9 days to 5 to 6 days or less; however, the client needs to be closely monitored, in the hospital and at home, for the development of complications following the procedure. Expert nursing care is required to allow for early identification of problems and complications that can be resolved in a timely fashion. In addition, expert nursing skills are needed for the coordination and collaboration required for discharge planning and follow-up care for clients at home (see the Clinical Pathway on p. 1838).

Endovascular stent repair is not without its complications. Complications include the need for conversion from an endovascular repair to open surgical repair of the aneurysm, bleeding, aneurysm rupture, peripheral embolization, and misdeployment of the stent graft. All of these complications require surgical interventions.

Community-Based Care

Most clients are discharged to home after aneurysm repair. In rare instances, in the absence of family or other support systems, the postoperative client may be discharged to an extended (long-term) care facility for rehabilitation.

HOME CARE MANAGEMENT

If discharged to home, the client must follow the instructions provided by the nurse regarding activity level and incisional care. Because stair climbing may be restricted initially, the client may need a bedside commode if the bathroom is inaccessible.

HEALTH TEACHING

For clients who have not undergone surgical aneurysm repair, the teaching plan emphasizes the importance of compliance with the schedule of computed tomography (CT) scanning to monitor the size of the aneurysm. The nurse educates the client receiving treatment for hypertension about the importance of continuing to take prescribed medication. The client and family or significant others are instructed about signs and symptoms that they must promptly report to the health care provider:

- Clients with abdominal aortic aneurysms (AAAs) must report abdominal fullness or pain, or back pain.
- Clients with thoracic aneurysms must report chest or back pain, shortness of breath, difficulty swallowing, or hoarseness.

The nurse teaches the client who has undergone repair of the aneurysm about activity restrictions, wound care, and pain management. Clients may not engage in activities that involve lifting heavy objects (usually more than 15 to 20 pounds [6.8 to 9.1 kg]) for 6 to 12 weeks postoperatively. The nurse advises them to use discretion in activities that involve pulling, pushing, or straining, such as vacuuming, changing bed linens, moving furniture, mopping or sweeping, raking leaves, mowing grass, and chopping wood. Clients should temporarily avoid such hobbies as tennis, swimming, horseback riding, and golf, although putting practice is allowed. Because of postoperative weakness, they are usually restricted from driving a car for several weeks after discharge.

Clients who have not undergone aneurysm repair may fear rupture and subsequent death. The nurse reinforces the rationales for CT monitoring of the size of the aneurysm and for controlling hypertension and encourages clients to verbalize their fears.

HEALTH CARE RESOURCES

In collaboration with the case manager or social worker, the nurse assesses the availability of transportation to and from appointments for clients needing CT monitoring. Clients who have undergone surgery may require the services of a home care nurse for assistance with dressing changes. A home care aide may be needed to assist with activities of daily living (ADLs).

Aneurysms of the Peripheral Arteries

OVERVIEW

Although femoral and popliteal aneurysms are relatively uncommon, they are often associated with an aneurysm in another location of the arterial tree. To detect a popliteal aneurysm, the nurse observes a pulsating mass in the popliteal space. To detect a femoral aneurysm, the nurse observes a pulsatile mass over the femoral artery. Both extremities are evaluated because more than one femoral or popliteal aneurysm may be present.

COLLABORATIVE MANAGEMENT

The client may exhibit symptoms of limb ischemia, including diminished or absent pulses, cool to cold skin, and pain. Pain may also be present if an adjacent nerve is compressed. The recommended treatment for either type of aneurysm, regardless of the size, is surgery because of the risk of thromboembolic complications associated with their presence.

To treat a femoral aneurysm, the physician excises the aneurysm and restores circulation using a Dacron graft or an autogenous saphenous vein graft. Most surgeons prefer to bypass rather than resect a popliteal aneurysm.

Postoperatively, the nurse monitors for lower limb ischemia. The nurse palpates pulses below the graft to assess graft patency. Often, Doppler ultrasonography is necessary to assess blood flow when pulses are not palpable. Sudden development of pain or discoloration of the extremity is reported immediately to the physician because it may indicate graft occlusion.

AORTIC DISSECTION

OVERVIEW

Aortic dissection has traditionally been referred to as a dissecting aneurysm. However, because this condition is more accurately described as a dissecting hematoma, the term *aortic dissection* has gained favor.

Aortic dissection is thought to be caused by a sudden tear in the aortic intima, opening the way for blood to enter the aortic wall. Degeneration of the aortic media might be a prerequisite for this condition, with hypertension an important contributing factor.

Aortic dissection is a relatively common event, occurring in at least 2000 people in the United States annually. It is frequently associated with connective tissue disorders such as Marfan's syndrome (see Chapter 21). It also occurs in older people, peaking in adults in their 50s and 60s, and in women in their third trimester of pregnancy.

Because the circulation of any major artery arising from the aorta can be impaired in clients with aortic dissection, this condition is highly lethal and represents an emergency situation.

Dissections are classified in various ways (Goldman & Braunwald, 1998). Debakey's classification contains three groups:

- *Type 1:* Characterized by an intimal tear in the ascending (proximal) aorta, with extension of the dissection into the descending (distal) aorta
- *Type 2:* Originates in and is limited to the ascending (proximal) aorta
- *Type 3:* Arises within the descending (distal) thoracic aorta and often progresses distally

Proximal dissections occur almost twice as often as distal dissections. Although the ascending aorta and descending thoracic aorta are the most common sites, dissections can also occur in the abdominal aorta and other arteries.

COLLABORATIVE MANAGEMENT

The most common presenting symptom of aortic dissection is pain, with painless dissection occurring rarely. The pain is described as "tearing," "ripping," and "stabbing" and tends to move from its point of origin. Depending on the site of dissection, the client may feel pain in the anterior chest, back, neck, throat, jaw, or teeth.

Diaphoresis, nausea, vomiting, faintness, and apprehension are also common. Blood pressure is usually elevated unless complications, such as cardiac tamponade or rupture, have occurred. A decrease or absence of peripheral pulses is common, as is aortic regurgitation, which is characterized by a musical murmur better heard along the right sternal border. Neurologic deficits, such as an altered level of consciousness, paraparesis, and strokes, can also occur.

Chest x-ray examination, Doppler echocardiogram, computed tomography (CT), and aortic angiography are commonly used to confirm the diagnosis.

The following are goals of emergency treatment:

- The elimination of pain
- A reduction of blood pressure to 100 to 120 mm Hg
- A decrease in the velocity of left ventricular ejection

The physician prescribes IV sodium nitroprusside (Nitropress) by continuous drip initially to lower the blood pressure.

If this regimen is ineffective, nicardipine hydrochloride (Cardene) may be used. Propranolol (Inderal, Apo-Propranolol♣) is given in increments of 1 mg intravenously to decrease left ventricular ejection.

Subsequent treatment depends on the location of the dissection. Generally, clients receive continued medical treatment for uncomplicated distal dissections and surgical treatment for proximal dissections.

For clients receiving long-term medical treatment, the systolic blood pressure must be maintained at or below 130 to 140 mm Hg. Beta blockers (propranolol) and calcium channel antagonists are indicated.

Clients receiving surgical intervention for a proximal dissection always require cardiopulmonary bypass (CPB) (see Chapter 38). The surgeon excises the intimal tear and obliterates entry in the false opening by suturing edges of the dissected aorta. Usually, a prosthetic graft is used.

BUERGER'S DISEASE

OVERVIEW

Buerger's disease (thromboangiitis obliterans) is a relatively uncommon occlusive disease limited to the medium and small arteries and veins. The distal upper and lower limbs are the most frequently affected. Typically, Buerger's disease is identified in young adult men who smoke. Larger arteries, such as the femoral and brachial, become involved in the late stages of the disease. The veins are less commonly involved.

The disease often extends into the perivascular tissues, resulting in fibrosis and scarring that binds the artery, vein, and nerve firmly together. For people who have this disease, cessation of cigarette smoking usually arrests the disease process, but persistence in smoking causes occlusion in the more proximal vessels.

The cause of Buerger's disease is unknown, although there is a strong association with tobacco smoking. A familial or genetic predisposition and autoimmune etiologic factors are also possible.

COLLABORATIVE MANAGEMENT

Assessment

The first clinical manifestation of Buerger's disease is usually claudication (pain in the muscles resulting from an inadequate blood supply) of the arch of the foot. Intermittent claudication may occur in the lower extremities. The pain may be ischemic, occurring in the digits while the client is at rest. Often, there is an aching pain that is more severe at night. Paroxysmal shocklike pain can be the result of ischemic neuropathy. Clients often experience increased sensitivity to cold and complain of coldness and numbness. On physical examination, the nurse notes that the pulses are often diminished in the distal extremities, and the extremities are cool and red or cyanotic in the dependent position.

A diagnosis of Buerger's disease is commonly based on a physical finding of peripheral ischemia, often in association with migratory superficial phlebitis. Ulcerations and gangrene may be seen in the digits. The ulcerations are usually sharply demarcated. The gangrenous lesion can be small or can affect the entire digit.

Arteriograms can be useful in delineating the degree of disease in the arteries. Commonly, arteriography reveals multiple segmental occlusions in the smaller arteries of the forearm, hand, leg, and foot. Plethysmographic studies of the fingers or toes may be diagnostic of the disease in the early stages. These studies can also be useful in following the progression of the disease in more proximal arteries.

Interventions

Nursing interventions are directed at:

- Preventing the progression of the disease
- Avoiding vasoconstriction
- Promoting vasodilation
- Relieving pain
- Treating ulceration and gangrene

To prevent the progression of Buerger's disease, complete abstinence from tobacco in all forms is essential. The client is instructed to avoid extreme or prolonged exposure to cold to prevent vasoconstriction. The nurse instructs the client about medications that are prescribed for vasodilation, such as nifedipine (Procardia, Adalat). (See Chapter 7 for interventions and nursing management for pain relief.)

The treatment of clients with Buerger's disease is similar to that for peripheral arterial disease (PAD) (see Interventions [Peripheral Arterial Disease], p. 746).

CRITICAL THINKING CHALLENGE

You are assigned to care for a 34-year-old man with Buerger's disease. The client was admitted to the hospital for a below-the-knee amputation on the right side. While completing the nursing health history form, the client tells you that he smokes 2 packs of cigarettes a day. He informs you that he has tried to quit smoking in the past.

- What might you expect to find from your psychosocial assessment?
- What information would you provide for the client in regard to smoking?
- When is the appropriate time to discuss smoking cessation with him to improve outcomes?

For suggested answer guidelines, go to SIMON http://www.wbsaunders.com/SIMON/Iggy/.

SUBCLAVIAN STEAL

OVERVIEW

Subclavian steal occurs in the upper extremities from a subclavian artery occlusion or stenosis. The result is altered blood flow and ischemia in the arm. Subclavian steal can occur in people at any age but is more common in those with risk factors for atherosclerosis. Symptoms include tiredness in the arm with exertion, paresthesias, dizziness, and exercise-induced pain in the forearm when the arms are elevated.

COLLABORATIVE MANAGEMENT

Physical examination usually reveals a significant difference in the blood pressures between the arms. A difference greater than 20 mm Hg is considered significant. Another important finding is a subclavian bruit, which can occur on the affected side. The subclavian pulse may be decreased on the occluded side compared with the opposite side. The client's arm may also be discolored or cyanotic; however, this finding generally occurs only in severe cases.

Surgery is the recommended intervention when a client has cyanosis or pain. One of three procedures may be used: endarterectomy of the subclavian artery, carotid-subclavian bypass, or dilation of the subclavian artery with placement of a vascular stent.

Nursing care encompasses postoperative care of the client and monitoring of the arterial flow in the affected arm. The nurse should check brachial and radial pulses frequently and observe for ischemic changes. The nurse also observes the arm for edema, redness, or any other signs.

THORACIC OUTLET SYNDROME

OVERVIEW

Thoracic outlet syndrome is a compression of the subclavian artery at the thoracic outlet by anatomic structures, such as a rib or muscle. The arterial wall may be damaged, producing thrombosis or embolization to distal arteries of the arms. The three common sites of compression in the thoracic outlet are as follows:

- The interscalene triangle
- Between the coracoid process of the scapula and the pectoralis minor tendon
- Most commonly, the costoclavicular space

COLLABORATIVE MANAGEMENT

Thoracic outlet syndrome is more common in females and in people whose occupations require holding their arms up or leaning over, such as baseball players, golfers, or swimmers. It is also seen in clients who have had trauma such as whiplash or after clavicular fracture. Clients generally complain of neck, shoulder, and arm pain that may be intermittent. They may also have numbness and moderate edema of the extremity. The pain and numbness are worse when the arm is placed in certain positions, such as over the head or out to the side. Clients may have overdeveloped neck and shoulder muscles, and the affected arm may appear cyanotic.

Treatment includes physical therapy, exercises, and avoiding aggravating positions, such as elevating the arms. Surgical treatment involves resection of the anatomic structure that is compressing the artery. Surgery is performed only if a client has severe pain, has lost hand function, or is responding poorly to conservative treatment.

RAYNAUD'S PHENOMENON

OVERVIEW

Raynaud's phenomenon is caused by vasospasm of the arterioles and arteries of the upper and lower extremities, usually unilaterally. *Raynaud's disease* occurs bilaterally. The two terms are sometimes used interchangeably, but although they are related, there are some differences. Raynaud's phenomenon usually occurs in people older than 30 years of age; Raynaud's disease can occur between the ages of 17 and 50 years. Raynaud's phenomenon can occur in either sex, but Raynaud's disease is more common in women.

The pathophysiology is the same for both entities. The etiology is unknown. Clients often have an associated systemic connective tissue disease, such as systemic lupus erythematosus or progressive systemic sclerosis (see Chapter 21).

As a result of vasospasm, the cutaneous vessels are constricted and blanching of the extremity occurs, followed by cyanosis. When the vasospasm is relieved, the tissue becomes reddened or hyperemic. The client's extremities are numb and cold, and he or she may complain of pain and swelling. Ulcers may also be present. These attacks are intermittent and can be aggravated by cold or stress. In severe cases, the attack lasts longer and gangrene of the digits can occur.

COLLABORATIVE MANAGEMENT

Treatment involves relieving or preventing the vasoconstriction by drug therapy. Commonly prescribed drugs are nifedipine (Procardia), cyclandelate (Cyclospasmol), and phenoxybenzamine (Dibenzyline). These vasodilating agents may help to relieve the symptoms, but they can cause uncomfortable side effects, such as facial flushing, headaches, hypotension, and dizziness.

For severe symptoms that cannot be alleviated by drugs, a lumbar sympathectomy can be performed. The physician cuts the sympathetic nerve fibers that cause vasoconstriction of blood vessels in the lower extremities. This method is effective when clients are experiencing foot symptoms. For the upper extremities, a similar procedure—sympathetic ganglionectomy—may provide symptom relief. The long-term effectiveness of these treatments is questionable.

Education of the client is important in prevention of complications. The nurse explains methods to prevent vasoconstriction, such as minimizing exposure to cold and decreasing stress. The client is instructed to wear warm clothes, socks, or gloves when exposed to cool or cold temperatures. He or she should keep the homes at a comfortably warm temperature. The nurse helps the client to identify stressors and provides suggestions for reducing them. (See Chapter 21 for further discussion of Raynaud's disease as it relates to connective tissue disease.)

POPLITEAL ENTRAPMENT

Popliteal entrapment causes ischemic symptoms in the affected leg or foot because of anatomic compression of the popliteal artery. Popliteal entrapment occurs in young people, most often in men complaining of intermittent claudication of one or both extremities.

Physical examination may reveal ischemic changes of the affected extremity, with normal function of the unaffected limb. When the client is at rest, the nurse may note diminished distal pulses, although this is a rare finding.

Diagnosis of popliteal entrapment is possible only after an accurate client history, physical examination, and arteriography.

The recommended treatment is surgical repair of the anatomic compression. Reconstruction of the popliteal artery may be necessary to restore arterial blood flow to the limb.

Nursing care involves preventing general postoperative complications and evaluating the patency of the graft or artery postoperatively. The nurse observes for ischemic changes and evaluates distal pulses frequently postoperatively.

PERIPHERAL VENOUS DISEASE

To function properly, veins must be patent (unobstructed) with competent valves. Vein function also necessitates the assistance of the surrounding muscle beds to help pump blood toward the heart. If one or more veins are not operating efficiently, they become distended and clinical manifestations occur.

Two distinct phenomena alter the blood flow in veins:

- Thrombus formation *(venous thrombosis)* can lead to pulmonary embolism, a life-threatening complication (see Chapter 30).
- Defective valves lead to *venous insufficiency* and *varicose veins,* which are not life threatening but are problematic.

Venous Thrombosis

OVERVIEW

Thrombus formation constitutes one of health care's greatest challenges. A thrombus (also called a thrombosis) is a blood clot believed to result from an endothelial injury, venous stasis, or hypercoagulability. The thrombosis may not be specifically attributable to one element, or it may involve all three elements. Thrombosis is often associated with an inflammatory process. When a thrombus develops, inflammation can occur around the thrombus, thickening the vein wall and consequently leading to embolization (the formation of an embolus).

Thrombophlebitis refers to a thrombus that is associated with inflammation; *phlebothrombosis* is a thrombus without inflammation. Thrombophlebitis can occur in superficial veins; however, it most frequently occurs in the deep veins of the lower extremities.

Deep vein thrombophlebitis, commonly referred to as **deep vein thrombosis (DVT),** not only is more common but also is more serious than superficial thrombophlebitis because it presents a greater risk for *pulmonary embolism (PE),* in which a dislodged blood clot travels to the pulmonary artery. Clients with DVT account for up to 600,000 hospitalizations each year in the United States. Of these, between 50,000 and 200,000 clients experience PE, causing up to 25% of all hospital deaths (Church, 2000).

Thrombus formation has been associated with stasis of blood flow, endothelial injury, and/or hypercoagulability, known as **Virchow's triad.** The precise cause of these events remains unknown; however, a few predisposing factors have been identified. Thrombosis has commonly occurred in people undergoing certain surgical procedures. The highest incidence of clot formation occurs in clients who have undergone hip surgery or open prostate surgery. Other conditions that seem to promote thrombus formation are pregnancy, ulcerative colitis, and heart failure.

Immobility can predispose a person to thrombosis. This can occur during prolonged bedrest, such as when a client is confined to bed during the perioperative period. **Phlebitis** (vein inflammation) associated with invasive procedures, such as IV therapy, can predispose clients to thrombosis. Severe infections, systemic lupus erythematosus, polycythemia vera, oral contraceptives, and trauma have also been linked to thrombosis.

COLLABORATIVE MANAGEMENT

Assessment

Clients with DVT may have symptoms or may be asymptomatic. The classic signs and symptoms of DVT are calf or groin tenderness and pain, and sudden onset of unilateral swelling of the leg. Pain in the calf on dorsiflexion of the foot (positive Homan's sign) appears in only 10% of clients with DVT, and false-positive findings are common (Church, 2000). *Therefore checking a Homan's sign is not advised!* The nurse examines the area described as painful, comparing this site with the contralateral limb. The nurse gently palpates the site, observing for warmth and edema. Signs and symptoms, however, may be absent with thrombophlebitis. Because there are often silent clinical findings, the nurse must have a high index of suspicion for this disorder when caring for clients at high risk.

Localized edema in one extremity may suggest thrombophlebitis. The nurse can measure and compare right and left calf and thigh circumferences for changes over time as an indicator of DVT or venous insufficiency. However, serial leg measurements may not be the most reliable indicator of DVT.

Although diagnostic tests for DVT are available, physical examination findings are often adequate for diagnosis. If a definitive diagnosis is lacking from physical examination alone, other diagnostic tests may be performed, such as contrast venography, duplex ultrasonography, Doppler flow studies, and impedance plethysmography.

Venography with contrast medium visualizes clot formation in approximately 95% of people with DVT. However, this study is generally not performed, because it may precipitate thrombosis and is very painful.

Duplex ultrasonographic scanning, a noninvasive test, is the preferred diagnostic test for DVT if a definitive diagnosis cannot be made by physical examination. Doppler flow studies may also be useful in the diagnosis of DVT, but they are more sensitive in detecting proximal rather than distal DVT. Normal venous circulation is characterized by audible signals, whereas thrombosed veins produce little or no flow.

Impedance plethysmography assesses venous outflow and can detect more than 90% of DVTs that are located above the popliteal vein. However, it is not helpful in locating clots in the calf and is less sensitive than Doppler studies (Church, 2000).

Interventions

The focus of treatment for thrombophlebitis is to prevent complications, such as pulmonary emboli, and to prevent an increase in size of the thrombus. Deep venous thrombophlebitis (thrombosis) is the most common type of thrombophlebitis. Clients with deep vein thrombosis (DVT) are often hospitalized for treatment, although this practice is changing as a result of the use of newer drugs.

NONSURGICAL MANAGEMENT. DVT is most often treated medically, using a combination of rest, drug therapy, and preventive measures.

REST. Supportive therapy for DVT includes bedrest and elevation of the extremity. Some health care providers order intermittent or continuous warm, moist soaks to the affected area. All clients are evaluated for signs and symptoms of pulmonary embolism (PE), which include shortness of breath and chest pain. Emboli may also travel to the brain or heart, but these complications are not as common as PE.

DRUG THERAPY. Anticoagulants are the drugs of choice for a client with DVT and for clients at risk for DVT. The conventional treatment has been IV unfractionated heparin followed by oral anticoagulation with warfarin (Coumadin). However, unfractionated heparin can be problematic because each client's response to the drug is unpredictable, and hospital admission is usually required for laboratory monitoring and dose adjustments. Today the use of low–molecular weight heparin is changing the management of both DVT and PE.

Unfractionated Heparin Therapy. Many clients with a confirmed diagnosis of an existing blood clot are started on a regimen of IV unfractionated heparin (UFH; Hepalean✱) therapy. UFH is an anticoagulant agent that at low doses interacts with antithrombin III to produce selective inhibition of clotting factors IIa (thrombin) and Xa. At higher doses it inhibits practically all clotting factors. The ultimate result is inhibition of fibrin formation; the drug does nothing to the existing clot. The physician prescribes UFH to prevent the formation of other clots, which often develop in the presence of an existing clot, and to prevent enlargement of the existing clot. Over a long period of time, the existing clot is slowly absorbed by the body.

Before UFH administration the client requires a baseline prothrombin time (PT), activated partial thromboplastin time (aPTT), International Normalized Ratio (INR), complete blood count (CBC) with platelet count, urinalysis, stool for occult blood, and creatinine level.

UFH is initially given in a bolus IV dose of approximately 100 units/kg of body weight, followed by constant infusion. The infusion is regulated by a reliable electronic infusion device that protects against accidental free flow of solution. The physician or clinical pharmacist orders concentrations of UFH (in 5% dextrose in water) and the number of units or milliliters per hour needed to maintain a therapeutic aPTT. aPTTs are obtained daily, or more frequently, and are reported to the health care provider as soon as the results are available to allow adjustment of heparin dosage. Therapeutic levels of aPTTs are usually one to two times normal control levels. The nurse assesses clients for signs and symptoms of bleeding, which include hematuria, frank or occult blood in the stool, ecchymosis (bruising), petechiae, an altered level of consciousness, or pain.

UFH can also decrease platelet counts. Mild reductions are common and are resolved with continued heparin therapy. Severe platelet reductions, although rare, result from the development of antiplatelet bodies within 6 to 14 days after the beginning of treatment. Platelets aggregate into "white clots" that can cause thrombosis, usually in the form of an acute arterial occlusion (Simko & Lockhart, 1996). The provider discontinues heparin administration if severe **heparin-induced thrombocytopenia and thrombosis (HITT)** (>100,000 mm^3), or "white clot syndrome," occurs. An oral anticoagulant may then be substituted for heparin if necessary.

The nurse also ensures that protamine sulfate, the antidote for heparin, is available, if needed, for excessive bleeding. Chart 36-10 highlights information important to nursing care and client education associated with anticoagulant therapy.

CHART 36-10

BEST PRACTICE *for*
The Client Receiving Anticoagulant Therapy

- Carefully check the dosage of anticoagulant to be administered, even if the pharmacy prepared the medication.
- Monitor the client for signs and symptoms of bleeding, including hematuria, frank or occult blood in the stool, ecchymosis, petechiae, altered mental status (indicating possible cranial bleeding), or pain (especially abdominal pain, which could indicate abdominal bleeding).
- Monitor vital signs frequently for decreased blood pressure and increased pulse (indicating possible internal bleeding).
- Have antidotes available as needed (e.g., protamine sulfate for heparin and vitamin K for warfarin [Coumadin, Warfilone✱]).
- Monitor activated partial thromboplastin time (aPTT) for clients receiving unfractionated heparin; monitor prothrombin time (PT) or International Normalized Ratio (INR) for clients receiving warfarin or low–molecular weight heparin (LMWH).
- Apply prolonged pressure over venipuncture sites and injection sites.
- When administering *subcutaneous* heparin, apply pressure over the site and do not massage.
- Teach the client going home while taking an anticoagulant to:
  - Use only an electric razor
  - Take precautions to avoid injury; for example, do not use tools such as hammers or saws, where accidents commonly occur
  - Report signs and symptoms of bleeding, such as blood in the urine or stool, nosebleeds, ecchymosis, or altered mental status
  - Take the prescribed dosage of medication at the precise time that it was ordered to be given
  - Not stop taking the medication abruptly; the physician usually tapers the anticoagulant gradually

To *prevent* DVT, heparin may be given in low doses subcutaneously for high-risk clients, especially after orthopedic surgery. Other pharmacologic agents that may be used for prophylaxis are as follows:

- Low–molecular weight heparin (e.g., enoxaparin [Lovenox])
- Dextran, an IV plasma expander
- Dihydroergotamine (DHE)
- Warfarin (Coumadin, Warfilone✱)
- Aspirin (ASA)

Prevention of DVT also includes early ambulation and mobilization, thigh-high graduated compression elastic stockings (such as TED stockings), and external intermittent or sequential compression devices (SCDs) (Church, 2000). The nurse ensures that the compression devices fit properly and do not restrict blood flow.

Low-Molecular Weight Heparin. Subcutaneous low–molecular weight heparins (LMWHs), such as enoxaparin (Lovenox), dalteparin (Fragmin), and ardeparin (Normiflo), have a consistent action and are approved for prevention and treatment of DVT. Danaparoid (Orgaran) is also classified as an LMWH but is actually a heparinoid. LMWHs bind less to plasma proteins, blood cells, and vessel walls, resulting in a longer half-life and more predictable response. Clients may be safely managed at home with daily visits from a home care nurse. They must be willing to learn self-injection or have a family member, friend, or home care nurse administer the subcutaneous injections.

Some health care providers place the client on a regimen of IV unfractionated heparin (UFH) for several days, then follow up with an LMWH. In this case, the UFH is discontinued at least 30 minutes before the first LMWH injection. The usual dose of enoxaparin is 1 mg/kg of body weight, not to exceed 90 mg, and is repeated every 12 hours. If the client's creatinine level is greater than 2 mg/dL (indicating renal insufficiency), the health care provider lowers the dose. Dalteparin can be given once a day at 200 units/kg of body weight and does not require dose adjustment for renal insufficiency. The usual dose of ardeparin is 50 units/kg of body weight and is given every 12 hours.

The nurse monitors the INR and stools daily for occult blood. aPTTs are not checked on an ongoing basis, because the doses of LMWH are not adjusted.

Warfarin Therapy. If the client is receiving continuous UFH, warfarin (Coumadin) is added at least 5 days later. Clients receiving LMWH are placed on a regimen of warfarin after the first dose. Warfarin works in the liver to inhibit synthesis of the four vitamin K–dependent clotting factors and takes 3 to 4 days before it can exert therapeutic anticoagulation. The heparin continues to provide therapeutic anticoagulation until this effect is achieved with warfarin. IV heparin is then discontinued at that time.

Therapeutic levels of warfarin are monitored by measuring prothrombin time (PT) and/or the International Normalized Ratio (INR). Because PTs are often inconsistent and misleading, the INR was developed. Most laboratories report both results. Most clients receiving warfarin for DVT should have an INR between 2.0 and 3.0 (Coyne, 1997).

Warfarin therapy should be started with low doses, at least 5 mg, and gradually titrated up according to the INR. Clients usually receive warfarin for 3 to 6 months after an episode of DVT.

Nursing assessment for bleeding is similar to that described for clients receiving heparin. The nurse ensures that vitamin K, the antidote for warfarin, is available in case of excessive bleeding (see Chart 36-10).

Thrombolytic Therapy. The use of systemic thrombolytic therapy for DVT is effective in dissolving thrombi quickly and completely. The greatest advantage is thought to be the prevention of valvular damage and consequential venous insufficiency, or "postphlebitis syndrome." However, thrombolytic therapy is contraindicated postoperatively, during pregnancy, and after childbirth, trauma, brain attacks, or spinal injuries. To be most effective, thrombolytic therapy must be initiated within 5 days after the onset of symptoms.

Thrombolytic agents such as streptokinase and recombinant tissue plasminogen activator (t-PA), as well as platelet inhibitors such as abciximab (ReoPro), may be effective in dissolving a clot or preventing new clots during the first 24 hours. Nurses caring for clients receiving these agents must monitor closely for signs and symptoms of bleeding.

CRITICAL THINKING CHALLENGE

An older adult who had a total hip replacement 3 days ago was diagnosed as having DVT of the operative leg calf. She plans to return home while receiving low-molecular weight heparin (LMWH) injections, but she lives alone.

- What teaching will the client require?
- What resources will she need at home during her recovery?
- What laboratory tests will need to be monitored while she is receiving LMWH?

For suggested answer guidelines, go to SIMON http://www.wbsaunders.com/SIMON/Iggy/.

PREVENTION AND TREATMENT OF PERIPHERAL EDEMA. The client's legs should be elevated when in bed and when in a chair. To help prevent chronic venous insufficiency, clients with active and resolving DVT are often instructed to wear knee- or thigh-high compression or elastic stockings.

SURGICAL MANAGEMENT. A deep vein thrombus is rarely removed surgically unless there is a massive occlusion that does not respond to medical treatment and the thrombus is of recent (1 to 2 days) onset. **Thrombectomy** is the most common surgical procedure for removing the thrombus. Preoperative and postoperative care of clients undergoing thrombectomy are similar to that for clients undergoing arterial surgery (see earlier discussion under Acute Peripheral Arterial Occlusion, p. 755).

INFERIOR VENA CAVAL INTERRUPTION. For clients with recurrent deep vein thrombosis (DVT) or pulmonary emboli that do not respond to medical treatment and for clients who cannot tolerate anticoagulation, **inferior vena caval interruption** may be indicated to prevent pulmonary emboli.

Preoperative care is similar to that provided for clients receiving local anesthesia (see Chapter 17). If clients have recently been taking anticoagulants, such as warfarin (Coumadin, Warfilone✤) or heparin (Hepalean✤), the nurse consults with the physician about interrupting this therapy in the preoperative period to avoid hemorrhage.

The surgeon inserts a filter device, or "umbrella," percutaneously into the inferior vena cava (Figure 36-12). The device is meant to trap emboli in the inferior vena cava before they progress to the lungs. Holes in the device allow blood to pass through, thus not significantly interfering with the return of blood to the heart. Popular inferior vena caval filters include the bird's-nest filter and the Greenfield filter.

Postoperatively, the nurse inspects the incision on the right side of the chest for bleeding and signs or symptoms of infection. Other postoperative nursing care is similar to that for any client undergoing surgery (see Chapter 19).

LIGATION OR EXTERNAL CLIPS. If an inferior vena caval filter is not successful in preventing pulmonary emboli, or if the filter becomes blocked with thrombi, the surgeon may perform ligation or insert external clips on the inferior vena cava to prevent pulmonary emboli.

Preoperative care for clients undergoing ligation of the vena cava or placement of an external clip is similar to that for an abdominal laparotomy. If the client is receiving anticoagulation therapy, the nurse consults with the surgeon about temporary interruption of therapy.

Ligation and insertion of external clips in the inferior vena cava are often performed by means of an abdominal laparotomy. In a ligation, the surgeon ties off the inferior vena cava to block emboli. Application of an external clip, such as the Adams-DeWeese clip, narrows the inferior vena cava to four serrated transverse slits, 3 to 5 mm in diameter. If laparotomy is performed, the external clip procedure is preferred because there are fewer hemodynamic or venous complications and a low frequency of recurrent pulmonary emboli associated with its use.

Postoperative care for the client with inferior vena caval ligation or external clip placement is similar to that for an abdominal laparotomy.

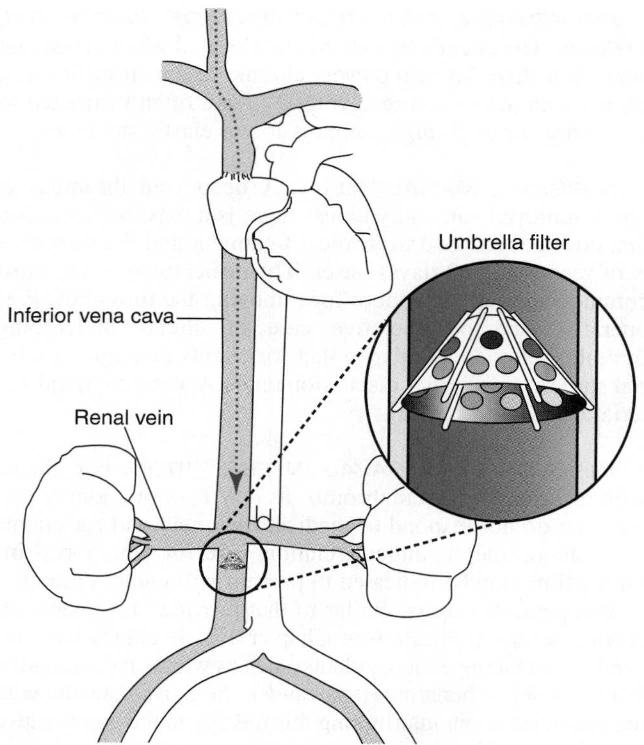

Figure 36-12 ● An inferior vena caval filter.

Community-Based Care

Clients recovering from thrombophlebitis or deep vein thrombosis (DVT) are usually ambulatory when they are discharged from the hospital. The primary focus of planning for discharge is to educate the client about the hazards of anticoagulation therapy (see Chart 36-10).

HOME CARE MANAGEMENT

The nurse helps the client identify situations and equipment that might cause trauma, such as the use of a straight-edged razor. The nurse helps the client and family or significant others to make arrangements to avoid hazardous situations and to procure alternative types of equipment if needed, such as an electric razor.

HEALTH TEACHING

The nurse teaches clients recovering from DVT to stop or avoid smoking and to avoid the use of oral contraceptives to decrease the risk of recurrence. Most clients are discharged on a regimen of warfarin (Coumadin, Warfilone✦) or low–molecular weight heparin (LMWH). The nurse instructs clients and their families to avoid potentially traumatic situations, such as participation in contact sports. The nurse provides written and oral information about the signs and symptoms of bleeding (see Chart 36-10). The client must report any of these manifestations to the health care provider immediately.

The anticoagulant effect of warfarin may be reversed by the omission of one or two doses of the drug or by the administration of vitamin K. In case of injury, clients are directed to apply pressure to bleeding wounds and to seek medical assistance immediately. The nurse encourages them to carry an identification card or wear a medical alert bracelet that states that they are taking warfarin.

The nurse also instructs clients to inform their dentist and other health care providers that they are taking warfarin before receiving treatment or prescriptions. Prothrombin times are affected by many prescription and over-the-counter medications, such as antacids, antihistamines, aspirin, mineral oil, oral contraceptives, and large doses of vitamin C. The action of warfarin is also affected by high-fat and vitamin K–rich foods, such as cabbage, cauliflower, broccoli, asparagus, turnips, spinach, kale, fish, and liver. Clients are therefore instructed to eat a well-balanced diet and to avoid taking additional medications without consulting a health care provider. The nurse arranges for clients to have prothrombin time (PT) and International Normalized Ratio (INR) determinations made 1 to 2 weeks after discharge.

Clients receiving subcutaneous LMWH injections at home need instruction on self-injection. If family members or friends are administering the injections, the nurse teaches the appropriate caregiver.

CONSIDERATIONS FOR OLDER ADULTS

Warfarin is used with caution with older adults or debilitated clients. A reduced dose is often recommended in an effort to prevent spontaneous intracranial bleeding or excessive bleeding related to trauma. Many older adults may have reduced kidney or liver function and a decreased ability to metabolize and excrete the drug. For this reason, it is usually used only when the benefits outweigh the risks. The older adult may have problems adhering to the routine laboratory tests required to monitor the medication's effectiveness.

Clients who have experienced DVT may fear recurrence of a thrombus and may also be concerned about treatment with warfarin and the risk for bleeding. The nurse assures them that participation in the prescribed treatment frequently helps in resolving this problem and that ongoing assessment of PTs and INRs should minimize the risks of bleeding.

HEALTH CARE RESOURCES

Clients discharged on a regimen of warfarin need access to a pharmacy to renew prescriptions and, if feasible, obtain a medical alert bracelet. They also need access to a laboratory for frequent monitoring of PTs and INRs.

Venous Insufficiency

OVERVIEW

Venous insufficiency occurs as a result of prolonged venous hypertension, which stretches the veins and damages the valves. This can lead to a backup of blood and further venous hypertension, resulting in edema. Edema occurs as the by-products of red blood cells break down and infiltrate the surrounding tissues. Because the client cannot eliminate waste products, they accumulate within the tissues. With time, this stasis (stoppage) results in venous stasis ulcers, swelling, and cellulitis.

Venous efficiency is altered when thrombosis occurs or when valves are not functioning correctly. Defective valves can result from prolonged venous hypertension, which stretches the veins and damages valves. This can occur in people who stand or sit in one position for long periods, such as teachers and office personnel. Pregnancy and obesity can also cause chronically distended veins, which lead to damaged valves. Thrombus formation can contribute to valve destruction. Chronic venous insufficiency often occurs in clients who have had thrombophlebitis.

COLLABORATIVE MANAGEMENT

Assessment

Clients with venous insufficiency may have edema in both extremities. There may be **stasis dermatitis** or discoloration along the ankles, extending up to the calf. In people with long-term venous insufficiency or stasis, *ulcers* often form. Ulcer formation can result from the edema or from minor injury to the limb. Venous ulcers typically occur over the malleolus, more often medially than laterally. The ulcer usually has irregular borders. Generally, these ulcers are chronic and difficult to heal (see Chart 36-7). Many clients live with ulcers for years, and recurrence is common. Some may lose one or both limbs if ulcers are not controlled.

Interventions

The focus of treating venous insufficiency is to decrease edema and promote venous return from the affected extremity. Clients are not usually hospitalized for venous insufficiency alone unless it is complicated by an ulcer or another disorder is occurring simultaneously.

NONSURGICAL MANAGEMENT. Treatment of chronic venous insufficiency is primarily nonsurgical, unless it is complicated by a venous stasis ulcer that requires surgical debridement. The goal of managing venous stasis ulcers is twofold: to heal the ulcer and to prevent stasis with recurrence of ulcer formation.

TREATMENT OF EDEMA. Clients with chronic venous insufficiency wear elastic or compression stockings, which fit from the middle of the foot to just below the knee or to the thigh. Clients should wear the stockings during the day and evening. The nurse instructs them to elevate their legs for at least 20 minutes four or five times per day and to avoid long periods of sitting or standing in place. When the client is in bed, the legs should be elevated above the level of the heart (Chart 36-11).

The nurse and physician should also confer about the use of intermittent sequential pneumatic compression of the lower extremities for clients with past or present venous stasis ulcers. If the client is being treated for an open venous ulcer, the device is applied over a dressing such as an Unna boot. The nurse instructs the client to apply the pump as directed during the period of healing. Because of the high incidence of venous ulcer recurrence, clients with chronic venous insufficiency whose ulcers have healed are encouraged to continue compression therapy for life.

CHART 36-11

CLIENT EDUCATION GUIDE
Venous Insufficiency

Elastic Stockings
- Wear elastic stockings as prescribed, usually during the day and evening.
- Put the stockings on upon awakening and before getting out of bed.
- When applying the stockings, do not "bunch up" and apply like socks. Instead, place your hand inside the stocking and pull out the heel. Then place the foot of the stocking over your foot and slide the rest of the stocking up. Be sure that rough seams on the stocking are on the outside, not next to your skin.
- Do not push stockings down for comfort, because they may function like a tourniquet and further impair venous return.
- Put on a clean pair of stockings each day. Wash them by hand (not in a washing machine) in a gentle detergent and warm water.
- If the stockings seem to be "stretched out," replace them with a new pair.

Do's and Dont's
- Elevate your legs for at least 20 minutes four or five times a day. When in bed, elevate your legs above the level of your heart.
- Avoid prolonged sitting or standing.
- Do not cross your legs; crossing at the ankles is acceptable for short periods of time.
- Do not wear tight, restrictive pants; avoid girdles and garters.

TREATMENT OF VENOUS STASIS ULCERS. Venous stasis ulcers are slightly more manageable than ulcers resulting from arterial disease. They are chronic in nature, with some clients manifesting the same ulcer for years. Ulcers often heal, only to recur in the same area. The client may have simultaneous ulcers for several years.

Dressings. Two types of occlusive dressings are used for venous stasis ulcers: oxygen permeable dressings and oxygen impermeable dressings. Because the role of atmospheric oxygen in wound healing is controversial, opinions vary with regard to which type of dressing is preferred. An oxygen-permeable polyethylene film and an oxygen-impermeable hydrocolloid dressing (e.g., DuoDerm) are common. Hydrocolloid dressings are left in place for a minimum of 3 to 5 days for best effect.

A cultured, bi-layered human skin equivalent has recently become available for difficult-to-heal venous leg ulcers. This graft was approved first in Canada, and research on its success has been very promising (Dolynchuk et al., 1999).

CONSIDERATIONS FOR OLDER ADULTS
A potential problem is that some occlusive dressings stick to the skin and can cause more damage to friable skin, especially in older clients. Newer dressings have calcium alginate (e.g., Sorbsan), which prevents maceration of healthy tissue.

If the client is ambulatory, an **Unna boot** may be used. This dressing is constructed of gauze that has been moistened with zinc oxide. The health care provider applies the boot to the affected limb, from the toes to the knee, after the ulcer has been cleaned with normal saline solution. Povidone-iodine (Betadine) and hydrogen peroxide are not used, because they destroy granulation tissue. The Unna boot is then covered with an elastic wrap and hardens like a cast; this promotes venous return and prevents stasis. The Unna boot also forms a sterile environment for the ulcer. The physician or advanced-practice nurse should change the boot approximately once a week. The nurse instructs the client about what to look for if arterial occlusion should occur from an Unna boot that is too tight.

Drug Therapy. The provider may prescribe topical agents, such as Accuzyme, to chemically debride the ulcer, eliminating necrotic tissue and promoting healing. If an infection or cellulitis develops, systemic antibiotics are necessary.

SURGICAL MANAGEMENT. Surgery for chronic venous insufficiency is not usually performed, because historically it has not been successful. Attempts at transplanting vein valves have had limited success. Surgical debridement of venous ulcers is similar to that performed for arterial ulcers (see Chapter 67).

Community-Based Care

The goal for the client with chronic venous insufficiency is to be managed in the home. For clients with frequent acute complications and repeated hospital admissions, case management can help to meet appropriate clinical and cost outcomes.

HOME CARE MANAGEMENT

The nurse helps clients with chronic venous insufficiency to plan for opportunities and facilities that allow for elevation of the lower extremities in and outside the home. In addition, clients with venous stasis ulcers need to plan for care of the ulcers.

HEALTH TEACHING

The nurse instructs clients with chronic venous stasis to:

- Avoid standing still if possible
- Elevate their legs when sitting
- Avoid crossing their legs
- Avoid wearing tight girdles, tight pants, and narrow-banded knee-high socks

The physician prescribes support hose or antiembolism stockings. The nurse teaches clients to apply these stockings before they get out of bed in the morning and to remove them just before going to bed at night (see Chart 36-11). The nurse also advises them that they will probably need to wear these stockings for the rest of their lives.

To improve circulation and aid in weight reduction, the nurse prescribes an exercise program on an individual basis with health care provider input. The nurse encourages all clients to maintain an optimal weight and may consult with the dietitian to plan a weight reduction diet. The nurse instructs clients with venous stasis ulcers how to care for the ulcers at home.

Clients with venous stasis disease, especially those with venous stasis ulcers, may require long-term emotional support to assist them in meeting chronic needs. They may also need assistance in coping with necessary lifestyle adjustments, such as changes in occupation.

HEALTH CARE RESOURCES

Clients with venous stasis ulcers may need the assistance of a home care nurse to perform dressing changes. Clients with Unna boots need weekly transportation to their health care provider for dressing changes. The nurse arranges for a sequential compression device in the home if the health care provider prescribes one.

Varicose Veins

OVERVIEW

Varicose veins are distended, protruding veins that appear darkened and tortuous. They can occur in anyone, but they are common in clients older than 30 years of age whose occupations require prolonged standing. Varicose veins are also frequently seen in pregnant women, clients with systemic problems (such as heart disease), obese clients, and clients with a family history of varicose veins.

As the vein wall weakens and dilates, venous pressure increases and the valves become incompetent (defective). The incompetent valves enhance the vessel dilation, and the veins become tortuous and distended. The client may complain of pain, especially after standing, and may experience a fullness in the legs. Nursing assessment reveals distended, protruding veins.

The Trendelenburg test assists with the diagnosis. The client is placed in a supine position with elevated legs. As the client sits up, the veins would normally fill from the distal end; however, if there are varicosities, the veins fill from the proximal end.

COLLABORATIVE MANAGEMENT

Conservative measures are the treatment of choice. These involve wearing elastic stockings and elevating the extremities as much as possible. Clients who continue to have pain or unsightly veins, despite this treatment, may opt for either sclerotherapy or surgical removal of the vein.

Sclerotherapy is performed on small or a limited number of varicosities. The physician injects a solution, such as sodium tetradecyl, directly into the vein, or he or she may use a laser device. A pressure dressing may be applied over the sclerosed vein to keep vessels free of blood for 24 to 72 hours. The surgeon performs an incision and drainage of trapped blood in the sclerosed vein 14 to 21 days after injection, followed by application of a second pressure dressing for 12 to 18 hours.

Varicose veins are surgically removed when they are larger than 4 mm in diameter or are in clusters. The stab avulsion technique may be used if the saphenous veins are competent. The surgeon exposes varices through 2- to 3-mm stab incisions, grasping the veins with hooks, and dividing and avulsing each vein.

The surgeon may need to strip (remove) affected veins if the saphenous vein is incompetent. The surgeon threads a long wire through an incision above an affected vein, pulling it down through the vein and out through an incision below the vein. After this procedure, the client's legs are bandaged with firm elastic (Ace) bandages.

Postoperatively, the nurse assesses the groin and entire leg for bleeding through the elastic bandage. The nurse instructs the client to keep the legs elevated and to perform range-of-motion exercises of the legs at least hourly. Clients are ambulatory and are often discharged from the hospital by the first postoperative day. At this time, the nurse instructs clients to continue to wear elastic stockings, walk, limit sitting, avoid standing in one place, and elevate their legs when sitting.

PHLEBITIS

Phlebitis is an inflammation of the superficial veins caused by an irritant, such as IV therapy (see Chapter 14). The client has a reddened, warm area radiating up an extremity, commonly an arm. The client may also experience pain, soreness, and swelling of the extremity.

Treatment involves application of warm, moist soaks, which dilate the vein and promote circulation. Sometimes a heating unit is used to keep the soaks warm. Rarely, ice packs are used. The nurse applies the soaks, making sure that the temperature is not hot enough to burn the client, and assesses for complications, such as tissue necrosis, infection, or pulmonary embolus. After a few days of conservative therapy, the inflammation usually subsides.

VASCULAR TRAUMA

OVERVIEW

Many types of trauma can result in vascular injury. Injuries to the blood vessels in the upper and lower extremities account for approximately 70% of all vascular injuries to the human body. Vascular injuries to the blood vessels include punctures, lacerations, and transections. Acute blunt or penetrating trauma may result in a false aneurysm or hematoma. Arteriovenous fistulas may be seen after penetrating injuries. The more common causes of penetrating injuries to the blood vessels are gunshot and knife wounds.

Blunt trauma, which is less common, can result from high-speed automobile accidents as a result of the shearing force of rapid deceleration. Vascular trauma can also occur during arterial puncture for arteriographic or hemodynamic studies in which a dissection, hematoma, or occlusive lesion occurs.

COLLABORATIVE MANAGEMENT

The history and physical examination aid in establishing the diagnosis in the client with vascular injury. The nurse questions the client or family about the mechanism of injury, the site of injury, the amount of blood loss, and symptoms present after the injury.

The nurse assesses for circulatory, sensory, or motor impairment but is aware that, despite significant trauma, impairment may not be apparent, especially if deep vessels have been injured. Arteriography provides essential information about the vascular injury. Emergency or urgent surgical intervention is warranted for clients with ischemia to maximize successful revascularization.

Management of vascular injuries is often initiated in a hospital emergency department. Careful triage by the nurse is crucial. The most important principles in the management of vascular trauma are establishment of a patent airway, control of bleeding, and restoration of blood flow.

The method of repair varies with the type of vascular injury. Techniques include vein bypass grafting, lateral suture repair, thrombectomy (excision of blood clot), resection with end-to-end anastomosis, and vein patch grafting.

ONLINE RESOURCES

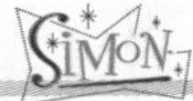

For suggested readings and Internet resources, go to http://www.wbsaunders.com/SIMON/Iggy/.

SELECTED BIBLIOGRAPHY

Asterisk indicates a classic or definitive work on this subject.

Allen, K.M., & Phillips, J.M. (1997). *Women's health across the lifespan.* Philadelphia: J.B. Lippincott.

*Allen, S.L. (1995). Perioperative nursing interventions for intravascular stent placement. *AORN Journal, 61*(4), 689-709.

American Heart Association. (1999). *Heart and stroke facts;* www.americanheart.org.

Ayello, E.A. (2000). On the lookout for peripheral vascular disease. *Nursing2000, 30*(6), 64hh1-64hh4.

Babaritio, C. (1998). Emergency! Hypertension-induced epistaxis. *American Journal of Nursing, 98*(2), 48.

Braun, C.M., Colcucci, A.M., & Patterson, R.B. (1999). Components of an optimal exercise program for the treatment of patients with claudication. *Journal of Vascular Nursing, 17*(2), 32-36.

Christman, S.K., et al. (1998). Stepping as an exercise modality for improving fitness and function. *Applied Nursing Research, 11*(2), 49-54.

Church, V. (2000). Staying on guard for DVT and PE. *Nursing2000, 30*(2), 34-44.

Conley, K., & Letizia, M. (1999). Heparin-induced thrombocytopenia. *MEDSURG Nursing, 8*(6), 355-357.

Coyne, N. (1997). Current concepts in anticoagulant therapy. *Journal of Care Management, 3*(4), 28-46, 73.

Dolynchuk, K., et al. (1999). The role of Apligraf in the treatment of venous leg ulcers. *Ostomy/Wound Management, 45*(1), 34-43.

*Dumas, M.A. (1995). Intermittent claudication. *American Journal of Nursing, 95*(12), 34.

Dumas, M.A. (1999). Hypertension in primary care. *American Journal for Nurse Practitioners, 3*(2), 7-32.

*Eaton, L.E., Buck, E.A., & Catanzaro, J.E. (1996). The nurse's role in facilitating compliance in clients with hypertension. *MEDSURG Nursing, 5,* 339-345, 359.

Engen, C. (1998). A case management primer for clinical and economic issues surrounding extended prophylaxis against deep vein thrombosis and pulmonary embolism. *Journal of Care Management, 4*(5), 33-41.

Fahey, V.A. (1999). *Vascular nursing* (3rd ed.). Philadelphia: W.B. Saunders.

Finlayson, S.R., et al. (1999). Should endovascular surgery lower the threshold for repair of abdominal aortic aneurysms? *Journal of Vascular Surgery, 29,* 973-985.

*Gerhard, M., Baum, P., & Raby, K.E. (1995). Peripheral arterial vascular disease in women: Prevalence, prognosis, and treatment. *Cardiology, 86,* 349-355.

Giobson, J.M., & Kenrick, M. (1998). Pain and powerlessness: The experience of living with peripheral vascular disease. *Journal of Advanced Nursing, 27*(4), 737-745.

Goldman, L., & Braunwald, E. (1998). *Primary cardiology.* Philadelphia: W.B. Saunders.

*Harris, A.H., Brown-Etris, M., & Troyer-Caudle, J. (1996a). Managing vascular leg ulcers: Part 1. Assessment. *American Journal of Nursing, 96*(1), 38-43.

*Harris, A.H., Brown-Etris, M., & Troyer-Caudle, J. (1996b). Managing vascular leg ulcers: Part 2. Treatment. *American Journal of Nursing, 96*(2), 40-46.

Huber, T.S., et al. (1999). Impact of race on the treatment for peripheral arterial occlusive disease. *Journal of Vascular Surgery, 30*(3), 417-425.

Jacques, P.F., et al. (1999). The effect of folic acid fortification on plasma folate and total homocysteine concentrations. *New England Journal of Medicine, 340*(19), 1449-1454.

Johnson, J.L., et al. (1999). Evaluation of a nurse-delivered smoking cessation intervention for hospitalized patients with cardiac disease. *Heart and Lung, 28*(1), 55-64.

Joint National Committee. (1997). The sixth report of the Joint National Committee on Prevention, Detection, Evaluation, and Treatment of High Blood Pressure. *Archives of Internal Medicine, 157*, 2413-2446.

Judelson, D.R. (1999). Gender gap: Women and coronary heart disease. *ADVANCE for Nurse Practitioners, 7*(11), 43-48.

Kirk, J.K. (1999). Angiotensin-II receptor antagonists: Their place in therapy. *American Family Physician, 59*(11), 3140-3148.

Kuncl, N., & Nelson, K.M. (1997). Antihypertensive drugs: Balancing risks and benefits. *Nursing97, 27*(8), 46-49.

Kuncl, N., & Nelson, K.M. (2000). Getting the skinny on lipid-lowering drugs. *Nursing2000, 30*(7), 52-53.

Lechner, D.L. (1998). Sizing up your patient for heparin therapy. *Nursing98, 27*(8), 36-42.

Matteson, M.A., McConnell, E.S., & Linton, A.D. (1997). *Gerontological nursing: Concepts and practice* (2nd ed.). Philadelphia: W.B. Saunders.

McClarren-Curry, C., & Shaughnessy, K. (1999). Acute thoracic aortic dissection: How to diffuse a time bomb. *Dimensions of Critical Care Nursing, 18*(4), 26-29.

Meyerson, S.L., & Schwartz, L.B. (1999). Gene therapy as a therapeutic intervention for vascular disease. *Journal of Cardiovascular Nursing, 13*(4), 91-109.

Miller, C.A. (1999). Update on hypertension management. *Geriatric Nursing, 20*(4), 218-219.

*Nunnelee, J.D. (1995). Minimize the risk of DVT. *RN*, December, pp 28-31.

Oertel, L.B. (1999). Monitoring warfarin therapy—How the INR keeps your patient safe. *Nursing99, 29*(11), 41-44.

Patel, S.T., et al. (1999). The cost-effectiveness of endovascular repair versus open surgical repair of abdominal aortic aneurysms: A decision analysis model. *Journal of Vascular Surgery, 29*(6), 958-972.

Phillips, J.K. (1998). Abdominal aortic aneurysm. *Nursing98, 28*(5), 34-40.

Schwartz, L.B. (1998). Conventional and alternative therapies for acute deep vein thrombosis. *Journal of Care Management, 4*(Suppl.), 9-13.

Shaw, W.S., et al. (1999). Accelerated risk of hypertensive blood pressure recordings among Alzheimer's caregivers. *Journal of Psychosomatic Research, 46*(3), 215-227.

*Simko, L.C., & Lockhart, J.S. (1996). Action stat: Heparin-induced thrombocytopenia and thrombosis. *Nursing96, 26*(3), 33.

*Sparks, K.S. (1996). Are you up to date on weight-based heparin dosing? *American Journal of Nursing, 96*(4), 33-36.

*Stillman, F.A. (1995). Smoking cessation for the hospitalized cardiac patient: Rationale for and report of a model program. *Journal of Cardiovascular Nursing, 9*, 25-36.

Sullivan, J.A. (1998). Hypertension in the elderly: Don't treat too quickly! *Journal of Emergency Nursing, 24*(1), 20-23, 24-25.

Tobin, L.J. (1999). Evaluating mild to moderate hypertension. *Nurse Practitioner, 24*(5), 22-40.

*Wills, E., & Sloan, H.L. (1996). Assessing peripheral arterial disorders in the home: A multidisciplinary clinical guide. *Home Healthcare Nurse, 14*(9), 670-674.

Wipke-Tevis, D.D. (1999). Vascular infections: Medical and surgical therapies. *Journal of Cardiovascular Nursing, 13*(2), 70-81.

CHAPTER 37

Interventions for Clients with Shock

M. LINDA WORKMAN

Learning Objectives

After studying this chapter, you should be able to:

1. Describe the clinical manifestations associated with the compensatory mechanisms for shock.
2. Identify clients at risk for hypovolemic shock.
3. Use laboratory data and clinical manifestations to determine the effectiveness of therapy for shock.
4. Explain the basis for crystalloid versus colloid intravenous therapy for shock.
5. Explain the expected client responses to the drugs used in the treatment of shock.
6. Prioritize nursing care for the client experiencing the nonprogressive stage of hypovolemic shock.
7. Compare and contrast the pathophysiology and clinical manifestations of the hyperdynamic and hypodynamic phases of septic shock.
8. Identify clients at risk for septic shock.
9. Develop an educational plan for prevention for the client at risk for septic shock who lives at home.

SIMON

Go to http://www.wbsaunders.com/SIMON/Iggy/ for self-assessment questions related to these Learning Objectives.

Shock, the whole-body response to poor tissue oxygenation, is a condition rather than a disease state. Any situation that impairs oxygen delivery to tissues and organs can start a syndrome of shock and lead to a life-threatening emergency. Clients in acute care settings are at high risk for conditions that lead to shock, but shock can occur in any setting. When compensation or interventions are ineffective and shock progresses, extensive hypoxia can lead to the complication of **multiple organ dysfunction syndrome (MODS)** and death. Table 37-1 lists important concepts related to shock.

OVERVIEW

Body organs, tissues, and cells need a continuous supply of oxygen for proper metabolism and function. The pulmonary system initially supplies oxygen to the body. The cardiovascular system delivers oxygen to all tissues and removes cellular wastes. The units of the cardiovascular system are the blood, blood vessels, and heart. When any component of the cardiovascular system does not function properly for any reason, shock can result.

Shock, a pathologic condition, is started by abnormal cellular metabolism that occurs when too little oxygen is delivered to the tissues (Guyton & Hall, 2000). Shock used to be classified as hypovolemic, cardiogenic, vasogenic, or septic, which indicated the origin of the problem causing the shock. Shock is now classified by the specific functional impairment caused: **hypovolemic shock, cardiogenic shock, distributive shock,** and **obstructive shock** (Effron & Chernow, 1992). Table 37-2 compares the old and new classification systems and common conditions causing each category of shock. The functional classification is used by researchers and guides clinicians and therefore is used in this chapter.

Many clinical manifestations of shock are similar regardless of what starts the process or which tissues are affected first. These common clinical manifestations are due to physiologic compensatory mechanisms. Manifestations unique to any one type of shock result from specific tissue dysfunction. The common clinical features of shock are listed in Chart 37-1.

Physiology Review

Oxygenation of any organ or tissue depends on how much oxygenated arterial blood perfuses the organ or tissue. Organ perfusion is related to **mean arterial pressure (MAP).** Because the cardiovascular system is a closed but continuous circuit, the factors that influence MAP include the following:

- Total blood volume
- Cardiac output
- Size of the vascular bed

Total blood volume and cardiac output are directly related to MAP—increases in either total blood volume or cardiac output usually raise MAP. Decreases in either total blood volume or cardiac output eventually lower MAP.

The size of the vascular bed is inversely (negatively) related to MAP—increases in the size of the vascular bed lower MAP, and decreases raise MAP (Figure 37-1). Blood vessels, especially small arteries and veins connected directly to capillaries, can increase in diameter by relaxing the smooth muscle in vessel walls (dilating) or decrease in diameter by contracting the muscle (vasoconstriction). When blood vessels dilate and total blood volume remains the same, blood pressure decreases and blood flow is slower. When blood vessels constrict and total blood volume remains the same, blood pressure increases and blood flow is faster.

Blood vessels contain nerves from the sympathetic division of the autonomic nervous system. Some nerves continuously stimulate vascular smooth muscle so that the blood vessels are normally partially constricted. This state of partial blood vessel constriction is called **sympathetic tone.** An increase in sympathetic stimulation causes the smooth muscle of the blood vessels to constrict further, raising MAP; a decrease in sympathetic stimulation causes the smooth muscle of the blood vessels to relax, dilating them and lowering MAP.

Blood flow to body organs varies and adjusts to changes in tissue oxygen needs. The body can selectively increase blood flow to some areas while reducing blood flow to others. Some organs, such as the skin and skeletal muscles, can tolerate low levels of oxygen for hours without dying or being damaged. Other organs (e.g., heart, brain, and liver) tolerate **hypoxic** conditions (low levels of tissue oxygenation) poorly, and even just a few minutes without adequate oxygen results in serious or permanent damage.

TABLE 37-1 • KEY CONCEPTS RELATED TO SHOCK

- Shock results when too little oxygen reaches the cells and tissues.
- Anyone is susceptible to shock.
- Shock progresses in a predictable, orderly fashion.
- Shock is reversible when the compensatory mechanisms are supported and the underlying causes are eliminated.
- Most clinical manifestations of shock are related to the body's compensatory responses to shock—not to the cause of shock.
- The nurse always considers the possibility and probability of shock development.
- Subtle changes in heart rate, diastolic blood pressure, level of consciousness, and behavior may herald the onset of shock.
- Clients experiencing the early phase of sepsis-induced distributive shock may be warm and pink and have a high cardiac output.
- Oxygen administration is an appropriate therapy for any type of shock.
- Changes in systolic blood pressure are not reliable indicators of initial and nonprogressive stages of shock.
- One consequence of shock is multiple organ dysfunction syndrome (MODS); leading to death.

Pathophysiology

The underlying problems common to all types of shock, regardless of cause, are the effects of **anaerobic cellular metabolism** (metabolism without oxygen). These effects result from inadequate tissue oxygenation and cause adverse changes in tissue function. The body begins to compensate in an attempt to maintain or restore tissue perfusion and oxygenation—even while the causes of shock are still present.

When the conditions that cause shock remain uncorrected, shock progresses through the following predictable stages:

1. Initial stage
2. Nonprogressive stage
3. Progressive stage
4. Refractory stage

TABLE 37-2 • COMPARISON OF NEW AND OLD SHOCK CLASSIFICATION SYSTEMS

CLASSIFICATION BY FUNCTIONAL IMPAIRMENT

Hypovolemic	*Cardiogenic*	*Distributive*	*Obstructive*
Total body fluid decreased (in all fluid compartments) • Hemorrhage • Dehydration	Direct pump failure Fluid volume not affected • Myocardial infarction • Valvular problems Stenosis Incompetence • Myopathies • Dysrhythmias • Cardiac arrest	Fluid shifted from central vascular space Total body fluid volume normal or increased • Neural-induced loss of vascular tone • Chemical-induced loss of vascular tone Sepsis Anaphylaxis Capillary leak	Cardiac function decreased by noncardiac factors Total body fluid volume not affected Central volume decreased • Pulmonary hypertension • Tension pneumothorax • Pericarditis • Thoracic tumor • Tamponade

CLASSIFICATION BY SITE OF ORIGIN

Hypovolemic	*Cardiogenic*	*Vasogenic*	*Septic*
Central vascular volume decreased Total body fluid may or may not be decreased • Hemorrhage • Dehydration • Fluid shifts Trauma Burns Anaphylaxis	Direct pump failure Indirect pump failure Decreased cardiac output Total body fluid not decreased • Valvular problems Stenosis Incompetence • Myocardial infarction • Myopathies • Dysrhythmias • Cardiac arrest • Tamponade • Pericarditis • Pulmonary hypertension • Pulmonary emboli	Loss of vascular tone Total body fluid not decreased • Neurogenic Head trauma Vasovagal response • Vessel dilation Anaphylaxis Inflammation	Loss of vascular tone Eventual reduced cardiac output Seen as a more intense type of vasogenic shock • Infection

CHART 37-1

KEY FEATURES *of* Shock

Cardiovascular Manifestations
- Decreased cardiac output
- Increased pulse rate
- Thready pulse quality
- Decreased blood pressure
- Narrowed pulse pressure
- Postural hypotension
- Low central venous pressure
- Flat neck and hand veins in dependent positions
- Slow capillary refill in nail beds
- Diminished peripheral pulses

Respiratory Manifestations
- Increased respiratory rate
- Shallow depth of respirations
- Decreased $Paco_2$
- Decreased arterial Pao_2
- Cyanosis, especially around lips and nail beds

Neuromuscular Manifestations
- Early
  - Anxiety
  - Restlessness
- Late
  - Decreased central nervous system activity (lethargy to coma)
  - Generalized muscle weakness
  - Diminished or absent deep tendon reflexes
  - Sluggish pupillary response to light

Renal Manifestations
- Decreased urine output
- Increased specific gravity
- Sugar and acetone present in urine

Integumentary Manifestations
- Cool to cold
- Pale to mottled to cyanotic
- Moist, clammy
- Mouth dry; paste-like coating present

Gastrointestinal Manifestations
- Decreased motility
- Diminished or absent bowel sounds
- Nausea and vomiting
- Constipation
- Increased thirst

$Paco_2$, Partial pressure of arterial carbon dioxide; *Pao_2*, partial pressure of arterial oxygen.

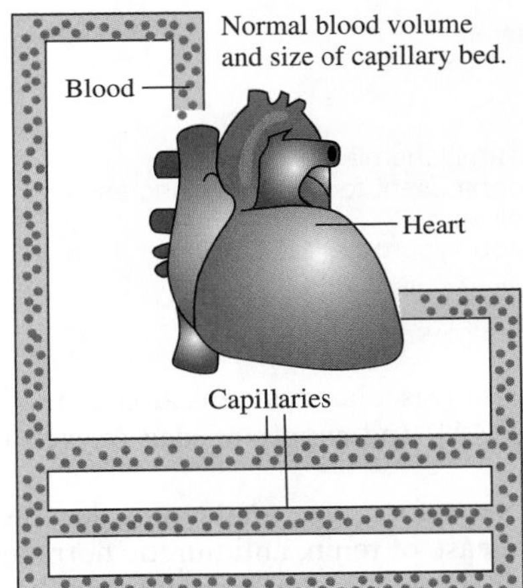

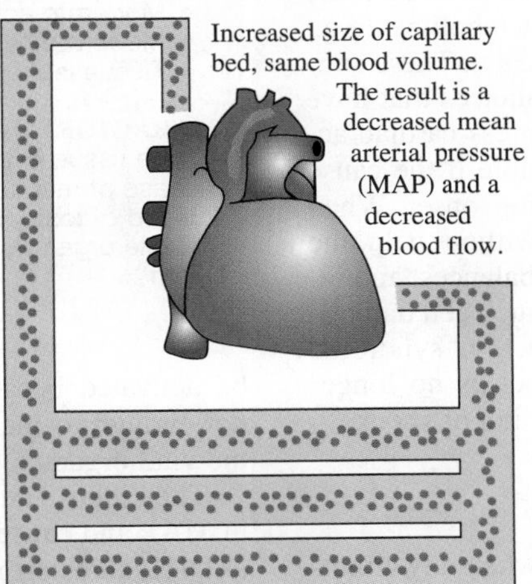

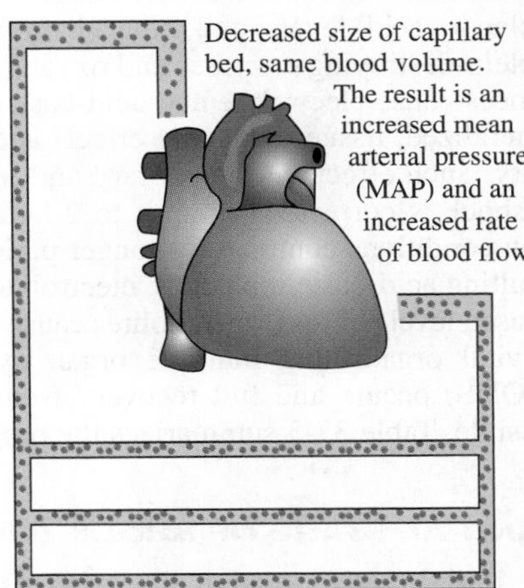

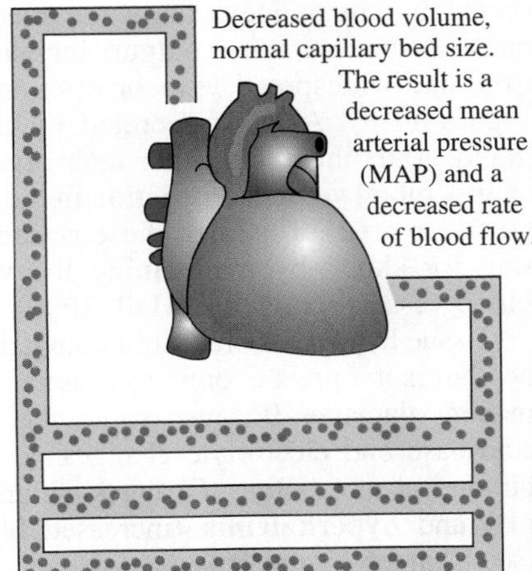

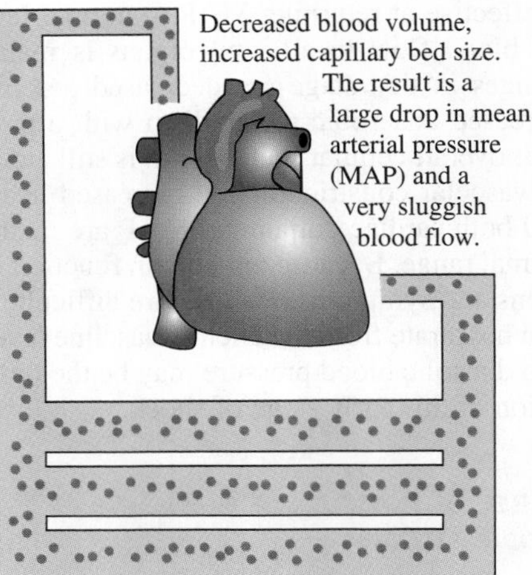

Figure 37-1 ● Interaction of blood volume and size of the capillary bed affecting mean arterial pressure.

The stages of shock are identified on the basis of the following:

- How well the client's compensatory mechanisms are working
- The severity of the clinical manifestations
- Whether tissue damage is reversible

The main trigger leading to the recognizable picture of shock is a sustained decrease in mean arterial pressure (MAP) that results from decreased cardiac output, decreased circulating blood volume, or expansion of the vascular bed. A decrease in MAP of 5 to 10 mm Hg below the client's baseline value is immediately detected by pressure-sensitive nerve receptors **(baroreceptors)** in the aortic arch and carotid sinus (Guyton & Hall, 2000). This information is transmitted to brain centers, which stimulates **compensatory mechanisms.** These mechanisms ensure continued blood flow and oxygen delivery to vital organs while limiting blood flow to less vital areas. Moving blood into selected areas while bypassing others **(shunting)** causes the physiologic changes and clinical manifestations of shock.

If the events that caused the initial decrease in MAP are halted at this point, the compensatory mechanisms can return the body to a normal perfused and oxygenated state, even without outside intervention. However, if the initiating events continue and MAP decreases further, some tissues function under anaerobic conditions. This condition creates an increase in lactic acid levels and other harmful metabolites (e.g., protein-destroying enzymes and oxygen radicals). These substances cause electrolyte and acid-base imbalances that have generalized, tissue-damaging effects and depress cardiac activity. Such effects are temporary and reversible if the cause of shock is corrected within 1 to 2 hours after onset. When such conditions continue for longer periods without help, the resulting acid-base imbalance, electrolyte imbalances, and increased levels of toxic metabolites cause so much cell damage in vital organs that multiple organ dysfunction syndrome (MODS) occurs and full recovery from shock is no longer possible. Table 37-3 summarizes the progression of shock.

TABLE 37-3 • PHYSIOLOGIC EVENTS DURING SHOCK

INITIAL STAGE

Decrease in baseline mean arterial pressure (MAP) of 5-10 mm Hg

Increased sympathetic stimulation

- Mild vasoconstriction
- Increase in heart rate

NONPROGRESSIVE STAGE

Decrease in MAP of 10-15 mm Hg from the client's baseline value

Continued sympathetic stimulation

- Moderate vasoconstriction
- Increased heart rate
- Decreased pulse pressure

Chemical compensation

- Renin, aldosterone, and antidiuretic hormone secretion
  - Increased vasoconstriction
  - Decreased urine output
  - Stimulation of the thirst reflex

Some anaerobic metabolism in nonvital organs

- Mild acidosis
- Mild hyperkalemia

PROGRESSIVE STAGE

Decrease in MAP of >20 mm Hg from the client's baseline value

Anoxia of nonvital organs

Hypoxia of vital organs

Overall metabolism is anaerobic

- Moderate acidosis
- Moderate hyperkalemia
- Tissue ischemia

REFRACTORY STAGE

Severe tissue hypoxia with ischemia and necrosis

Release of myocardial depressant factor from pancreas

Buildup of toxic metabolites

Multiple organ dysfunction syndrome (MODS)

Death

INITIAL STAGE OF SHOCK (EARLY STAGE)

The **initial** (early) stage of shock is present when any condition causes MAP to decrease from the client's baseline level by less than 10 mm Hg. During this stage, active compensatory mechanisms are so effective at returning MAP to normal levels that oxygenated blood flow to all vital organs is maintained. Cellular changes in this stage are decreased aerobic metabolism and increased anaerobic metabolism with a production of lactic acid; overall cellular metabolism is still aerobic. Compensation (vascular constriction and increased heart rate) is effective, and both cardiac output and MAP are maintained within the normal range. Because vital organ function is not disrupted, the signs and symptoms of shock are difficult to detect. An increase in heart rate from the client's baseline level or a slight increase in diastolic blood pressure may be the only objective manifestation of this early stage of shock.

NONPROGRESSIVE STAGE OF SHOCK (COMPENSATORY STAGE)

The **nonprogressive** (compensatory) stage of shock occurs when conditions decrease MAP 10 to 15 mm Hg from baseline. Kidney and chemical compensatory mechanisms need to be activated because cardiovascular compensation alone is not enough to maintain MAP and supply needed oxygen to the vital organs.

The kidneys and baroreceptors sense an ongoing decrease in MAP and cause the release of renin, antidiuretic hormone (ADH), aldosterone, epinephrine, and norepinephrine. Kidney compensation occurs through the actions of renin, aldosterone, and ADH (see Chapter 11). Renin, which is secreted by the kidney, starts the reactions that eventually cause decreased urine output, increased sodium reabsorption, and widespread vasoconstriction (see Chapter 11 and Figure 11-8). ADH is secreted by the posterior pituitary gland. ADH increases water reabsorption in the kidney and causes blood vessel constriction in the skin and other less vital tissue areas. Together, these actions attempt to compensate for shock by maintaining the volume in the central blood vessels (Guyton & Hall, 2000).

Tissue hypoxia is present in nonvital organs and in the kidney but is not great enough to cause severe symptoms or permanent damage. Because some metabolism is anaerobic, acid-base and electrolyte changes occur in response to the buildup of metabolites. Changes include **acidosis** (low blood pH) and **hyperkalemia** (increased blood potassium level) (see Chapter 13 and 16).

If the client's condition is stable and compensatory mechanisms are supported by medical and nursing interventions, he or she can remain in this stage for hours without experiencing permanent damage. Stopping the conditions that started the shock and providing supportive interventions can prevent the shock from progressing and reverse the effects of this stage.

PROGRESSIVE STAGE OF SHOCK (INTERMEDIATE STAGE)

The **progressive** stage of shock results when there is a sustained decrease in MAP of more than 20 mm Hg from baseline. In this stage, compensatory mechanisms are functioning but are no longer able to deliver sufficient oxygen, even to vital organs. Compensatory mechanisms use large amounts of oxygen in certain tissues, which worsens the problem of general inadequate oxygenation. Vital organs develop hypoxia, and less vital organs experience **anoxia** (no oxygen) and **ischemia** (cell dysfunction or death from lack of oxygen). As a result of inadequate oxygenation and a buildup of toxic metabolites, some tissues experience extensive cell damage and ultimately die.

The progressive stage of shock is a life-threatening emergency. Vital organs can tolerate this situation for only a short time before being permanently damaged. Immediate interventions are needed to reverse the effects of this stage of shock. Tolerance varies from person to person and depends greatly on pre-existing health. Usually the client's life can be saved if the conditions causing shock are corrected within 1 hour of the onset of the progressive stage.

REFRACTORY STAGE OF SHOCK (IRREVERSIBLE STAGE)

Formerly called the irreversible stage, the **refractory** stage of shock occurs when too much cell death and tissue damage results from too little oxygen reaching the tissues. As a result, the vital organs experience overwhelming changes. This stage is termed *refractory* because the body is unable to respond effectively to interventions, and the syndrome of shock continues. The remaining cells perform their metabolic functions anaerobically. *Therapy is ineffective in saving the client's life, even if the underlying cause of shock is corrected and MAP temporarily returns to normal.* So much tissue damage has occurred, causing widespread release of toxic metabolites and destructive enzymes, that cell deterioration in vital organs continues.

MULTIPLE ORGAN DYSFUNCTION SYNDROME

The sequence of cell damage caused by the massive release of toxic metabolites and enzymes is termed **multiple organ dysfunction syndrome (MODS).** Once the damage has started, the sequence of events becomes a vicious cycle as more dead or dying cells break open and release more harmful metabolites. The metabolites cause the formation of small clots **(microthrombi);** this blocks tissue oxygenation and damages more cells, thus continuing the devastating cycle. MODS occurs first in the liver, heart, brain, and kidney. In sepsis-induced distributive shock, the lungs also are affected. The most profound change is deterioration of the heart muscle. One contributing factor is the release of **myocardial depressant factor (MDF)** from the ischemic pancreas.

TABLE 37-4 • CAUSES OF SHOCK

HYPOVOLEMIC SHOCK ***Overall Cause*** Body fluid depletion Hemorrhage • Trauma • Gastrointestinal ulcer • Surgery • Inadequate clotting Hemophilia Liver disease Malnutrition Bone marrow suppression Cancer Anticoagulation therapy Dehydration • Vomiting • Diarrhea • Heavy diaphoresis • Diuretic therapy • Nasogastric suction • Diabetes insipidus • Hyperglycemia	**DISTRIBUTIVE SHOCK** ***Overall Cause*** Decreased vascular volume or tone ***Specific Cause or Risk Factors*** Neural-induced • Pain • Anesthesia • Stress • Spinal cord injury • Head trauma Chemical-induced • Anaphylaxis • Sepsis • Capillary leak Burns Extensive trauma Hepatic dysfunction Hypoproteinemia
CARDIOGENIC SHOCK ***Overall Cause*** Direct pump failure ***Specific Cause or Risk Factors*** Myocardial infarction Cardiac arrest Ventricular dysrhythmias • Fibrillation • Tachycardia Cardiac amyloidosis Cardiomyopathies • Viral • Toxic Myocardial degeneration	**OBSTRUCTIVE SHOCK** ***Overall Cause*** Indirect pump failure ***Specific Cause or Risk Factors*** Cardiac tamponade Arterial stenosis Pulmonary embolus Pulmonary hypertension Constrictive pericarditis Thoracic tumors Tension pneumothorax

Etiology

Because shock is a manifestation of a pathologic condition rather than a disease state, its causes vary. Specific conditions leading to hypovolemic, cardiogenic, distributive, and obstructive shock are listed in Table 37-4. *More than one type of shock can be present at the same time.* For example, trauma caused by an automobile accident may trigger hemorrhage (leading to hypovolemic shock) and a myocardial infarction (leading to cardiogenic shock).

HYPOVOLEMIC SHOCK

Hypovolemic shock occurs when too little circulating blood volume causes a MAP decrease so that the body's total need for tissue oxygenation is not met. The most common conditions leading to hypovolemic shock are hemorrhage (external or internal) and dehydration.

Hypovolemic shock caused by external hemorrhage is common after trauma, wounds, and surgery. Hypovolemic shock caused by internal hemorrhage occurs with blunt trauma, gastrointestinal (GI) ulcers, and poor control of surgical bleeding. External and internal hemorrhage can be caused by any health problem that reduces the levels of clotting factors (see Table 37-4).

Hypovolemia as a result of dehydration can be caused by any condition that decreases fluid intake or increases fluid loss (see Table 37-4).

CARDIOGENIC SHOCK

Cardiogenic shock occurs when the actual heart muscle is unhealthy and contraction is directly impaired. Table 37-4 lists the common causes of direct pump failure. These conditions decrease cardiac output and afterload, thus reducing MAP. Chapter 38 provides an in-depth discussion of cardiogenic shock resulting from myocardial infarction.

DISTRIBUTIVE SHOCK

Distributive shock is caused by a loss of sympathetic tone, blood vessel dilation, pooling of blood in venous and capillary beds, and increased blood vessel permeability (leak). All of these factors can decrease mean arterial pressure (MAP) and may be induced either neurogenically or chemically.

NEURAL-INDUCED DISTRIBUTIVE SHOCK. Neural-induced loss of MAP occurs when sympathetic stimulation of the nerves controlling blood vessel smooth muscle is decreased and the smooth muscles of blood vessels relax, causing vasodilation. This blood vessel dilation can be a normal local response to injury, but shock results when the vasodilation is widespread or systemic. Common conditions that can cause a systemic loss of sympathetic tone are listed in Table 37-4.

CHEMICAL-INDUCED DISTRIBUTIVE SHOCK. Chemical-induced distributive shock has three common origins: anaphylaxis, sepsis, and capillary leak syndrome. Chemical-induced distributive shock occurs when certain chemicals or foreign substances within the blood and blood vessels start widespread changes in blood vessel walls. The chemicals are usually **exogenous** (originate outside the body), but this type of shock can be induced by substances normally found in the body **(endogenous).**

ANAPHYLAXIS. Anaphylaxis is one result of type I allergic reactions (see Chapter 23). It usually begins within seconds to minutes after exposure to a specific allergen. However, it is termed *delayed* because this type of reaction rarely occurs the first time a person encounters the allergen. It occurs on repeated exposure to the same allergen (Guyton & Hall, 2000). Table 23-2 lists common allergens that can cause anaphylaxis.

Anaphylaxis is due to an antigen-antibody reaction that occurs in blood vessels throughout the body in response to contact with a substance to which the person has a severe allergy **(hypersensitivity).** This widespread reaction involves the interaction of the allergen, immunoglobulin E (IgE), basophils, and mast cells. It occurs within the walls of blood vessels, heart muscle cells, and bronchial tubes (see Chapters 20 and 23).

Anaphylaxis damages cells and causes the release of large amounts of histamine and other inflammatory chemicals. These substances move rapidly throughout the circulatory system, causing massive blood vessel dilation and increased capillary permeability. These responses result in severe hypovolemia and vascular collapse. Decreased cardiac contractility and dysrhythmias occur during anaphylaxis. These symptoms may be the direct result of heart muscle changes induced by the antigen-antibody reaction, or they may result from the profound hypovolemia. Antigen-antibody reactions in the bronchial tissues cause severe edema and pulmonary obstruction, which greatly reduce gas exchange. The pulmonary problems, together with inadequate circulation, cause extreme whole-body hypoxia. *Without intervention, this condition results in death.*

TABLE 37-5 • CONDITIONS PREDISPOSING TO SEPSIS-INDUCED DISTRIBUTIVE SHOCK (SEPTIC SHOCK)

- Malnutrition
- Immunosuppression
- Large, open wounds
- Mucous membrane fissures in prolonged contact with bloody or drainage-soaked packing
- Gastrointestinal ischemia
- Loss of gastrointestinal integrity
- Exposure to invasive procedures
- Malignancy
- Over 85 years of age
- Infection with resistant microorganisms

SEPSIS. Sepsis leading to distributive shock occurs when microorganisms are present in the blood. This form of shock is most commonly called **septic shock** in clinical situations. Sepsis is often associated with **disseminated intravascular coagulation (DIC).** Distributive shock (septic shock) is more often associated with bacterial infection and has also been reported among clients with viral and yeast sepsis. Organisms often causing sepsis include gram-negative bacteria (*Pseudomonas aeruginosa, Escherichia coli,* and *Klebsiella pneumoniae*) and gram-positive bacteria (*Staphylococcus* and *Streptococcus*). Table 37-5 lists some of the conditions that put the client at risk for septic shock (sepsis-induced distributive shock).

Septic shock results when large amounts of toxins and endotoxins produced by bacteria are secreted into the blood, causing a whole-body inflammatory reaction. These toxins and endotoxins react with blood vessels and cell membranes. Through the activity of white blood cells, the resulting reactions start inflammatory and immune events known as the **systemic inflammatory response syndrome (SIRS).** These toxin-host interactions activate complement, alter microcirculation within the vital organs (including selective coagulation and thrombus formation), increase capillary **permeability** (leakiness), cause cell injury, and increase cell metabolism (in combination with a decreased ability of some cells to take up needed oxygen). Metabolism becomes anaerobic because of decreased MAP, clot formation in capillaries, and poor cell uptake of oxygen.

CAPILLARY LEAK SYNDROME. Capillary leak syndrome leading to distributive shock occurs when there is a fluid shift from the blood to the interstitial space. Such shifts are caused by increased capillary permeability, loss of plasma osmolarity, and increased hydrostatic pressure in the blood. Specific conditions causing fluid shifts include severe burns, bullous skin disease, liver disorders, abdominal ascites, acute peritonitis, paralytic ileus, severe malnutrition, surgical wounds, hyperglycemia, kidney disease, hypoproteinemia, and trauma.

OBSTRUCTIVE SHOCK

Obstructive shock is caused by conditions that affect the ability of the normal heart muscle to pump effectively. The heart itself is normal, but conditions outside the heart prevent either adequate filling of the heart or adequate contraction of the healthy heart muscle. Common causes of obstructive shock are listed in Table 37-4.

Incidence/Prevalence

The exact incidence of shock is not known because it is a response rather than a separate disease entity. Some degree of shock is a common complication among hospitalized clients. Hypovolemic shock is the most common type experienced by clients in emergency departments and after surgery or invasive procedures. Cardiogenic shock is the most common complication of myocardial infarction in clients who experience damage to 40% or more of the heart muscle. The frequency of distributive shock as a result of sepsis, which has a 40% to 85% mortality rate, is increasing among clients who are immunocompromised or have infections (Ackerman, 1994; Clochesy, 1996).

This chapter presents the collaborative management of clients experiencing hypovolemic shock caused by hemorrhage and distributive shock caused by sepsis. Chapter 23 discusses interventions for anaphylaxis, and Chapter 38 discusses care of the client experiencing cardiogenic shock as a result of myocardial infarction.

COLLABORATIVE MANAGEMENT: HYPOVOLEMIC SHOCK

The Concept Map on p. 778 addresses assessment and nursing care issues related to clients with hypovolemic shock.

Assessment

HISTORY

The nurse collects data on risk factors and causative factors related to hypovolemic shock. *Age* is important because hypovolemic shock associated with trauma is more common in young adults, whereas sepsis is more common among older adults. Clients are asked specific questions about recent illness, trauma, procedures, or chronic conditions that may lead to shock. Such conditions include gastrointestinal ulcers, general surgery, hemophilia, liver disorders, prolonged vomiting, and prolonged diarrhea. Medications such as aspirin, diuretics, and antacids may cause changes leading to hypovolemic shock or may indicate the presence of a problem that can contribute to hypovolemic shock.

The nurse asks about fluid intake and output during the previous 24 hours. *Information about urine output is especially important because the first stages of shock are characterized by a reduced urine output, even when fluid intake is normal.*

The nurse assesses the client and the immediate environment for obvious signs of factors leading to shock. Areas to examine for signs of hemorrhage include the gums, wounds, and sites of dressings, drains, and vascular access. The nurse observes for any swelling, skin discoloration, or manifestations of pain that may indicate an internal hemorrhage.

PHYSICAL ASSESSMENT/CLINICAL MANIFESTATIONS

Most of the visible signs of hypovolemic shock are caused by the changes resulting from compensatory efforts. **Compensation** or **compensatory mechanisms** are physiologic responses that try to keep an adequate blood flow to vital organs. Signs of shock are first evident as changes in cardiovascular function. As shock progresses, changes in the kidney, respiratory, integumentary, musculoskeletal, and central nervous systems become evident.

CARDIOVASCULAR MANIFESTATIONS. Shock involves a decrease of mean arterial pressure (MAP), and the resulting early compensation is cardiovascular. Therefore the earliest clinical signs of hypovolemic shock are also cardiovascular.

PULSE. The nurse or assistive nursing personnel assesses the central and peripheral pulses for rate and quality. In the initial stage of hypovolemic shock, the pulse rate increases to keep cardiac output and MAP at normal levels, even though the actual **stroke volume** (amount of blood pumped out from the heart) per beat is usually decreased. Because stroke volume is decreased, the peripheral pulses are more difficult to palpate and are easily blocked with light pressure. As hypovolemic shock progresses, superficial peripheral pulses may be absent.

BLOOD PRESSURE. Changes in systolic blood pressure are not always present in the initial stage of hypovolemic shock. When assessing the blood pressure of a client at risk for shock, the nurse considers the client's normal baseline blood pressure level. Although a blood pressure of 90/50 may indicate severe shock in one person, it may be the normal blood pressure value for another healthy adult.

When vasoconstriction is present, diastolic pressure increases but systolic pressure remains the same. As a result, the **pulse pressure,** or the difference between the systolic and diastolic pressures, is smaller. The blood pressure is monitored for changes from baseline levels and for changes from the previous measurement. For accuracy, the same equipment is used on the same extremity. When possible, the nurse measures blood pressure with the client in the lying, sitting, and standing positions.

Systolic pressure decreases as shock progresses and cardiac output decreases; this reduces the pulse pressure even further. When shock continues and interventions are not adequate, compensation fails and systolic and diastolic pressures decrease. At this stage, blood pressure is difficult to hear. Palpation or a Doppler device may be needed to detect the systolic blood pressure.

OXYGEN SATURATION. Peripheral oxygen saturation is assessed through pulse oximetry. Hemoglobin oxygen saturation values between 90% and 95% are associated with the nonprogressive stage of shock, and values between 75% and 80% are associated with the progressive stage of shock. *Any value below 70% is considered a life-threatening emergency and may signal the refractory stage of shock.*

INTEGUMENTARY MANIFESTATIONS. Skin changes occur in shock because of decreased perfusion. An early compensatory mechanism for hypovolemic shock is vasoconstriction in the skin, which results in minimal perfusion. This allows more blood to circulate to the vital organs, which cannot tolerate low oxygen levels.

The skin is assessed for temperature, color, and degree of moisture. It feels cool or cold to the touch, and the color is

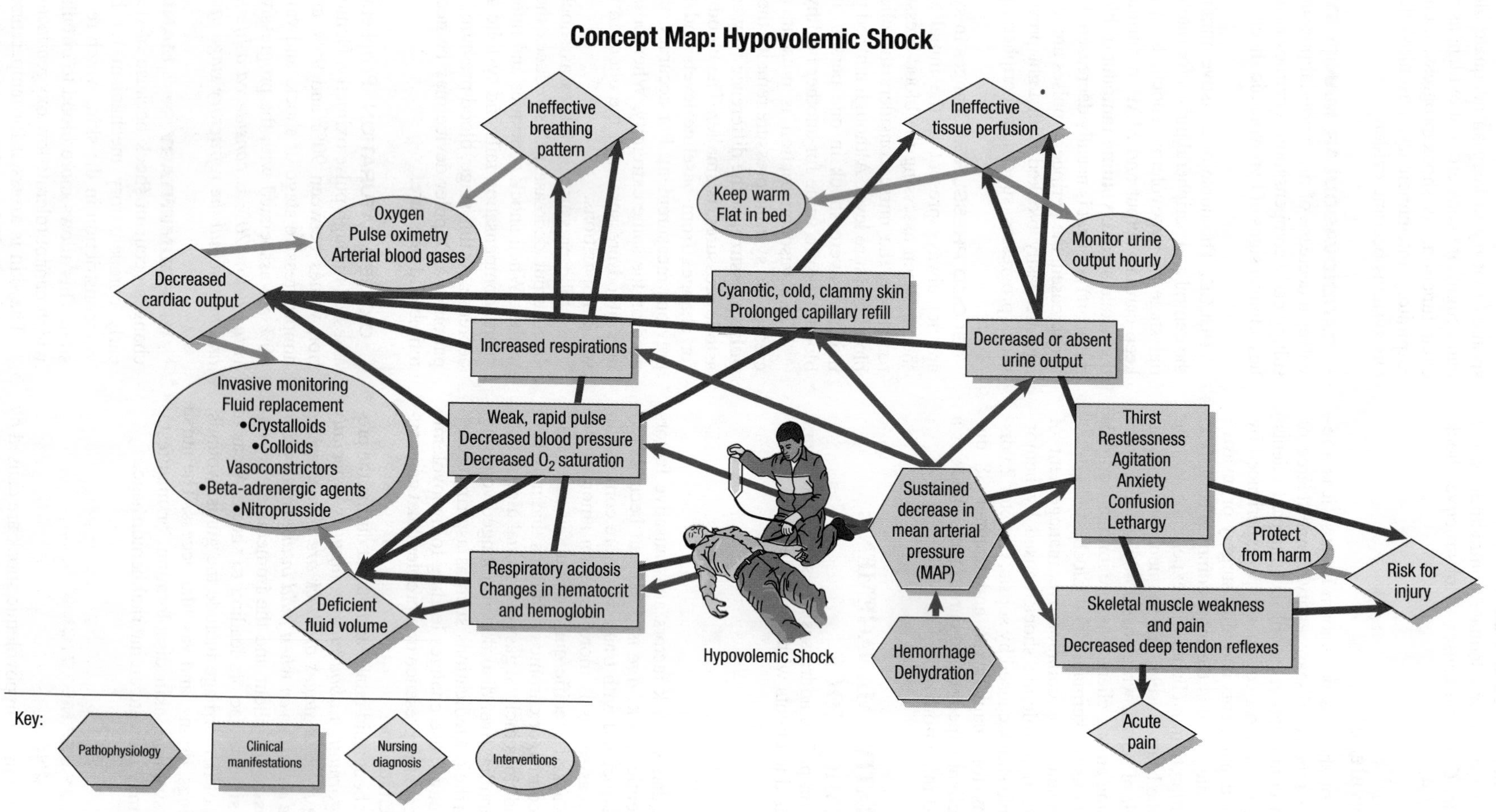
Concept Map: Hypovolemic Shock
Hemorrhage
Dehydration
Sustained decrease in mean arterial pressure (MAP)
Hypovolemic Shock
Weak, rapid pulse
Decreased blood pressure
Decreased O_2 saturation
Respiratory acidosis
Changes in hematocrit and hemoglobin
Increased respirations
Cyanotic, cold, clammy skin
Prolonged capillary refill
Decreased or absent urine output
Thirst
Restlessness
Agitation
Anxiety
Confusion
Lethargy
Skeletal muscle weakness and pain
Decreased deep tendon reflexes
Ineffective breathing pattern
Ineffective tissue perfusion
Decreased cardiac output
Deficient fluid volume
Risk for injury
Acute pain
Oxygen
Pulse oximetry
Arterial blood gases
Keep warm
Flat in bed
Monitor urine output hourly
Protect from harm
Invasive monitoring
Fluid replacement
•Crystalloids
•Colloids
Vasoconstrictors
•Beta-adrenergic agents
•Nitroprusside
Key:
Pathophysiology
Clinical manifestations
Nursing diagnosis
Interventions

pale to cyanotic. Color changes are first evident in the mucous membranes and in the skin around the mouth. Pallor or cyanosis may be difficult to observe in many areas in dark-skinned clients, and the nurse particularly assesses color changes in oral mucous membranes. As shock progresses, color changes in clients with lighter skin are noted first in the extremities and then in the central trunk area. The skin also feels clammy or moist to the touch, not because sweating increases but because the normal fluid lost through the skin does not evaporate quickly on cold skin.

Capillary refill time is evaluated by pressing on the client's fingernail until it blanches and then observing how fast the nail bed resumes color when pressure is released. Normally the nail bed capillaries resume color as soon as pressure is released. With shock, capillary refill is usually slow and is sometimes absent.

RESPIRATORY MANIFESTATIONS. The nurse assesses the rate, depth, and ease of respiration and also auscultates the lungs for abnormal breath sounds. Respiratory rate increases during hypovolemic shock. This increase is a compensatory mechanism to provide adequate oxygen to the critical tissues. When shock progresses to the stage at which lactic acidosis is present, the depth of respiration also increases.

KIDNEY/URINARY MANIFESTATIONS. The renal system compensates for decreased MAP by conserving body water through decreased filtration and increased water reabsorption. Urine is assessed for color, specific gravity, and the presence of blood or protein. The nurse or assistive nursing personnel measures urine output every hour. In severe shock, urine output is decreased (compared with fluid intake) or even absent. Of the four vital organs (heart, brain, liver, and kidney), only the kidney can tolerate hypoxia and anoxia for up to 1 hour without permanent damage. When hypoxic or anoxic conditions persist beyond this time, clients are at grave risk for **acute tubular necrosis (ATN)** and renal failure.

CENTRAL NERVOUS SYSTEM MANIFESTATIONS. Clients in hypovolemic shock are thirsty. This sensation is caused by stimulation of the osmoreceptors in the brain in response to decreased blood volume (see Chapter 11).

The nurse assesses the client's level of consciousness (LOC) and orientation to person, time, and place. Most causes of hypovolemic shock do not interfere with the transmission of nerve impulses. The central nervous system manifestations of hypovolemic shock are instead associated with cerebral hypoxia. In the initial and nonprogressive stages, clients may be restless or agitated and may be anxious or have a feeling of impending doom that has no obvious cause. As hypoxia progresses, clients become confused and lethargic. Lethargy progresses to somnolence and loss of consciousness as cerebral hypoxia worsens.

MUSCULOSKELETAL MANIFESTATIONS. Tissue hypoxia, anaerobic metabolism, and lactic acidosis cause weakness and pain in skeletal muscle. This weakness is generalized and has no specific pattern. The electrolyte disturbances in the progressive and refractory stages of shock worsen muscle weakness by interfering with action potentials. In this situation, deep tendon reflexes are decreased or absent.

The nurse assesses muscle strength by having the client squeeze the nurse's hand and try to keep the arms flexed while the nurse pulls downward on the lower arms. Deep tendon reflexes are assessed by lightly tapping the patellar tendons and Achilles tendons with a reflex hammer and observing the degree of reflexive movement.

PSYCHOSOCIAL ASSESSMENT

Changes in mental status and behavior may be early signs of hypovolemic shock. The nurse observes the client closely and documents behavior. The nurse assesses current mental status by evaluating LOC and noting whether the client is asleep or awake. If the client is asleep, the nurse attempts to awaken him or her and documents how easily he or she is aroused. If the client is awake, the nurse establishes whether he or she is oriented to person, time, and place. Questions that can be answered with a "yes" or a "no" response are avoided. The following points are considered during evaluation:

- Is it necessary to repeat questions to obtain a response?
- Does the response answer the question asked?
- Does the client have difficulty making word choices?
- Is the client irritated or upset by the questions?
- Can the client concentrate on a question long enough to answer appropriately, or is attention span limited?

If possible, the nurse questions family members or a significant other to determine whether the client's behavior and mental status are typical.

LABORATORY ASSESSMENT

Although no single laboratory finding confirms or rules out the presence of shock, changes in laboratory data may support the diagnosis of hypovolemic shock. (Chart 37-2 lists the common laboratory findings associated with hypovolemic shock.) As shock progresses, arterial blood gas values become abnormal. The pH usually decreases, the partial pressure of arterial oxygen (Pa_{O_2}) decreases, and the partial pressure of arterial carbon dioxide (Pa_{CO_2}) increases. Changes in other laboratory values may be associated with specific causes of hypovolemic shock.

Hematocrit and hemoglobin concentrations decrease if hypovolemic shock is caused by hemorrhage. When hypovolemic shock is the result of dehydration or a fluid shift, hematocrit and hemoglobin values are elevated.

Interventions

Interventions for clients in hypovolemic shock are focused on reversing the shock, restoring fluid volume, and preventing ischemic complications through supportive and drug therapies. Surgery may be necessary to correct the underlying problem leading to hypovolemic shock. Chart 37-3 summarizes best practices for clients in hypovolemic shock. Chart 37-4 lists selected interventions based on the Nursing Interventions Classification (NIC) for clients with hypovolemic shock.

NONSURGICAL MANAGEMENT. The goals of intervention are to maintain tissue oxygenation, increase body fluid compartment volumes to normal ranges, and support operating compensatory mechanisms. Oxygen therapy, intravenous

CHART 37-2

LABORATORY PROFILE
Hypovolemic Shock

Test	Normal Range for Adults	Significance of Abnormal Findings
pH (arterial)	7.35-7.45	Decreased: insufficient tissue oxygenation causing anaerobic metabolism and acidosis
Pao_2	80-100 mm Hg	Decreased: anaerobic metabolism
$Paco_2$	35-45 mm Hg	Increased: anaerobic metabolism
Lactic acid (arterial)	0.9-1.7 mmol/L	Increased: anaerobic metabolism with buildup of metabolites
Hematocrit	Females: 37%-47% Males: 42%-52%	Increased: fluid shift, dehydration Decreased: hemorrhage
Hemoglobin	Females: 12-16 g/dL Males: 14-18 g/dL	Increased: fluid shift, dehydration Decreased: hemorrhage
Potassium	3.5-5.0 mEq/L or mmol/L	Increased: dehydration, acidosis

Data from Pagana, K., & Pagana, T. (1999). *Diagnostic testing and nursing implications: A case study approach* (5th ed.). St. Louis: Mosby.
Pao_2, Partial pressure of arterial oxygen; *$Paco_2$*, partial pressure of arterial carbon dioxide.

CHART 37-3

BEST PRACTICE *for*
The Client in Hypovolemic Shock

- Ensure a patent airway.
- Start an IV catheter or maintain an established catheter.
- Administer oxygen.
- Elevate the client's feet, keeping his or her head flat or elevated to a 30-degree angle.
- Examine the client for overt bleeding.
- If overt bleeding is present, apply direct pressure to the site.
- Take the client's vital signs every 5 minutes until stable.
- Administer medications as ordered.
- Increase the rate of IV fluid delivery.
- Do not leave the client.

CHART 37-4

NIC INTERVENTION ACTIVITIES *for*
The Client with Hypovolemic Shock

Shock Management Volume: *Promotion of adequate tissue perfusion for a client with severely compromised intravascular volume*

- Monitor for signs and symptoms of persistent bleeding (e.g., check all secretions for frank or occult blood).
- Monitor the client closely for hemorrhage.
- Prevent blood volume loss (e.g., apply pressure to site of bleeding).
- Administer IV fluids, as appropriate.
- Note hemoglobin/hematocrit level before and after blood loss, as indicated.
- Administer blood products (e.g., platelets or fresh frozen plasma), as appropriate.
- Monitor coagulation studies, including prothrombin time (PT), partial thromboplastin time (PTT), fibrinogen, fibrin degradation/split products, and platelet counts, as appropriate.

NIC intervention activities selected from McCloskey, J.C., & Bulechek, G.M. (Eds.). (2000). *Nursing interventions classification (NIC)* (3rd ed.). St. Louis: Mosby.

(IV) therapy, fluid replacement therapy, and drug therapies are the management choices for this problem.

OXYGEN THERAPY. Oxygen therapy is useful whenever shock is present. Oxygen can be administered by mask, hood, nasal cannula, nasopharyngeal tube, endotracheal tube, and tracheostomy tube. Oxygen is administered in liters per minute (for administration via cannula) or concentration by percentage (for administration by mask), as specified by the health care provider's order.

INTRAVENOUS THERAPY. Colloids and crystalloids are the two types of fluids commonly used for volume replacement during hemorrhagic hypovolemia. IV colloid solutions are used to restore plasma volume and colloidal osmotic pressure and contain large molecules (usually proteins or starches) (see Chapter 11). IV crystalloid solutions are given for fluid and electrolyte replacement and contain nonprotein substances (e.g., minerals, salts, and sugars). A current controversy involves the infusion rate of fluids when hypovolemia is a result of hemorrhage that has not yet been controlled. A consideration is that the rapid infusion of large-volume IV fluids can increase blood pressure and may actually increase the rate of blood loss (see the Evidence-Based Practice for Nursing box on p. 781).

Colloid Fluid Replacement. Protein-containing colloid fluids are good for restoring vascular osmotic pressure and fluid volume. Blood and blood products are often used for this purpose and are the treatment of choice for hypovolemia caused by blood loss. These products include whole blood, packed red blood cells, plasma, plasma fractions, and synthetic plasma expanders.

Whole blood and packed red blood cells increase hematocrit and hemoglobin concentrations as well as vascular fluid volume. Whole blood is used to replace large volumes of blood loss because it provides increased intravascular volume while improving the oxygen-carrying capacity of the blood. Packed red cells are given for moderate blood loss because they replenish the red blood cell deficit and improve oxygen-carrying capacity without adding excessive fluid volume. Chapter 40 discusses nursing care issues in blood and blood product administration.

Human plasma, an acellular blood product containing some clotting factors, is given to correct plasma deficits and restore osmotic pressure when hematocrit and hemoglobin levels are within normal ranges. Plasma protein fractions

EVIDENCE-BASED PRACTICE FOR NURSING

Infusion of increased intravenous fluid volume during hemorrhagic shock may have more risk than benefit

Smail, N., et al. (1998). Resuscitation after uncontrolled venous hemorrhage: Does increased resuscitation volume improve regional perfusion? *Journal of Trauma: Injury, Infection, and Critical Care, 44*(4), 701-708.

A routine intervention for hypovolemic shock is the rapid infusion of large volumes of crystalloidal and/or colloidal IV fluids in an attempt to increase mean arterial pressure (MAP) and improve regional perfusion. The investigators hypothesized that increasing MAP by increasing IV fluid volume before the cause of hemorrhage is identified and corrected may not improve regional blood flow and could result in an increased rate of bleeding.

The investigators used an animal model to test this theory. After inflicting a standardized injury consisting of bilateral severing of the lumbar veins, rats were assigned to one of three interventions groups: no resuscitation, moderate-volume infusion of Ringer's lactate (10 mL/hr), and large-volume infusion of Ringer's lactate (30 mL/hr). Pair-matched control animals underwent anesthesia and surgery without hemorrhage or resuscitation. The variables of cardiac output and regional blood flow in various organs were measured immediately and 1.5 hours later in all animals.

Rats receiving moderate volume infusions temporarily improved cardiac output and MAP while also improving blood flow to the liver. Large-volume infusions did not improve either hemodynamic values or regional blood flow.

Critique. The study was well controlled and conducted under ideal laboratory conditions in that all rat subjects were as similar as possible for most variables. Although animal models have been used successfully to mimic human responses to trauma and interventions for trauma, a major limitation of the study is the size of the animal model. Replication of the study using a larger animal model more comparable to humans is warranted.

Implications for Nursing. The results of this study indicate that, although IV access and infusion should be a mainstay of intervention for clients with hypovolemic shock, the infusion volume and rate should not be excessive when hemorrhage is suspected. It is imperative that the health care provider assess all indicators of hemorrhage for response to the infusion therapy.

(e.g., Plasmanate) and synthetic plasma expanders (e.g., hetastarch [hydroxyethyl starch, Hespan]) increase plasma volume and are often used as early treatment for hypovolemic shock before a cause has been established.

Crystalloid Fluid Replacement. Crystalloid solutions are given to help establish and maintain an adequate fluid and electrolyte balance. Two common crystalloid solutions are Ringer's lactate and normal saline. Ringer's lactate contains physiologic concentrations of sodium, chloride, calcium, potassium, and lactate dissolved in water. This isotonic solution is a good volume expander, and the lactate is a buffer in the presence of acidosis. Normal saline (0.9% sodium chloride in water) is a fluid replacement used to increase plasma volume when there has been no loss of red blood cells.

DRUG THERAPY. Medications may be necessary if the volume deficit is severe and the client does not respond sufficiently to the replacement of fluid volume and blood products. The actions of drugs for shock increase venous return, improve cardiac contractility, or ensure adequate cardiac perfusion through dilation of the coronary vessels. Chart 37-5 lists the drugs commonly used to treat hypovolemic shock.

Vasoconstricting Agents. Many drugs stimulate venous return by causing vasoconstriction and decreasing venous pooling of blood. These actions increase cardiac output and mean arterial pressure (MAP), which helps to improve tissue perfusion and oxygenation. Examples of such agents include dopamine (Intropin, Revimine✱) and norepinephrine (Levophed). Most of these drugs produce serious side effects, and their dosages must be carefully calculated on the basis of the client's size and degree of response (see Chart 37-5).

Agents Enhancing Myocardial Contractility. Some drugs directly stimulate adrenergic receptor sites on the heart muscle (especially $beta_1$ receptors) and increase the contraction of the cardiac muscle cells. Other agents enhance cardiac contractility—they slow heart rate by altering electrical conduction and allowing the left ventricle a longer filling time. When filling time is increased, more blood enters the left ventricle and stretches the muscle fibers. Thus greater recoil is achieved, and more blood leaves the left ventricle during contraction. Some of these drugs also stimulate the ventricles. Agents with these types of actions include digoxin (Lanoxin) and dobutamine (Dobutrex).

Agents Enhancing Myocardial Perfusion. The treatment of shock includes giving agents that cause systemic vasoconstriction to help enhance venous return and increase MAP. It is important to ensure that the heart is well perfused so that aerobic metabolism is maintained in the cardiac cells and maximum contractility can be achieved. Agents that dilate coronary blood vessels while causing minimal systemic vasodilation are used for this purpose. A common agent with this action is sodium nitroprusside (Nitropress, Nipride✱). Care is taken because higher dosages can cause some systemic vasodilation and increase shock.

MONITORING. A major nursing responsibility in caring for the client in hypovolemic shock is monitoring his or her vital signs and level of consciousness (LOC). On the acute nursing unit, the nurse monitors the client's:

- Pulse
- Blood pressure
- Pulse pressure
- Central venous pressure
- Respiratory rate
- Skin and mucosal color
- Oxygen saturation

These parameters are assessed at least every 15 minutes until the shock is under control and the client's condition improves. More extensive monitoring of cardiac output (hemodynamic monitoring) occurs in critical care settings and includes intra-arterial monitoring, mixed venous oxygen saturation (Svo_2), and pulmonary artery wedge pressures.

Clients in shock are transported to a critical care unit if they require more invasive monitoring such as central venous pressure (CVP), pulmonary artery pressure (PAP), and pulmonary artery wedge pressure (PAWP). Table 37-6 compares the changes in hemodynamic patterns seen with different types of shock.

Insertion of a CVP catheter allows pressure to be monitored in the client's right atrium or superior vena cava while providing venous access. Changes in CVP reflect hypovolemic shock. As circulating volume decreases, the amount of blood returning to the right atrium also decreases, causing the CVP to decrease from baseline levels.

CHART 37-5

DRUG THERAPY *for* Hypovolemic Shock

Drug	Usual Dosage	Nursing Interventions	Rationale
VASOCONSTRICTORS			
Dopamine hydrochloride (Intropin, Revimine✱)	5-30 µg/kg/min IV (for hypotension) 2-5 µg/kg/min IV (for renal perfusion)	Assess the client for chest pain.	Dopamine increases myocardial oxygen consumption.
		Monitor urine output hourly.	Higher doses decrease renal perfusion and urine output.
		Assess blood pressure every 15 minutes.	Hypertension is a symptom of overdose.
		Assess the client for headache.	Headache is an early symptom of drug excess.
Epinephrine (Adrenalin)	0.5-1 mg IV initially, followed by 0.5 mg q5min May also be given by intracardiac injection	Monitor the client for dysrhythmias.	Epinephrine may cause ventricular tachyarrhythmias.
		Assess the client for chest pain.	Vasoconstriction may impair cardiac oxygenation.
Norepinephrine (Levophed)	0.5-1.0 µg/kg/min continuous IV infusion to maintain blood pressure at 90-100 mm Hg	Assess for extravasation.	Norepinephrine can cause severe tissue damage and necrosis.
		Observe the client's extremities for color and perfusion.	Norepinephrine can cause such vasoconstriction that peripheral ischemia may result.
Phenylephrine (Neo-Synephrine)	80-200 µg/min IV	Assess for chest pain.	Vasoconstriction may impair cardiac oxygenation.
AGENTS ENHANCING CONTRACTILITY			
Amrinone (Inocor)	0.75-1.5 mg/kg bolus 5-20 µg/kg/min continuous IV infusion	Assess blood pressure every 15 minutes.	Hypertension is a symptom of overdose.
		Do not administer through the same tubing as furosemide	Amrinone and furosemide form a precipitate.
Atropine sulfate	0.5-1 mg IV q5min, up to a total of 2 mg	Take pulse every 5 minutes.	Atropine sulfate may cause a rebound tachycardia.
		Monitor urine output every 30 minutes.	Atropine sulfate may cause urinary retention.
		Administer cautiously to clients with glaucoma.	Atropine sulfate may precipitate an episode of acute angle-closure glaucoma.
Dobutamine hydrochloride (Dobutrex)	2.5-20 µg/kg/min continuous IV infusion	Assess the client for chest pain.	Dobutamine increases myocardial oxygen consumption.
		Assess blood pressure every 15 minutes.	Hypertension is a symptom of overdose.
AGENTS ENHANCING MYOCARDIAL PERFUSION			
Sodium nitroprusside (Nitropress, Nipride✱)	0.5-10 µg/kg/min continuous IV infusion	Assess blood pressure every 15 minutes.	Hypotension may result from the systemic dilation of veins and arteries.

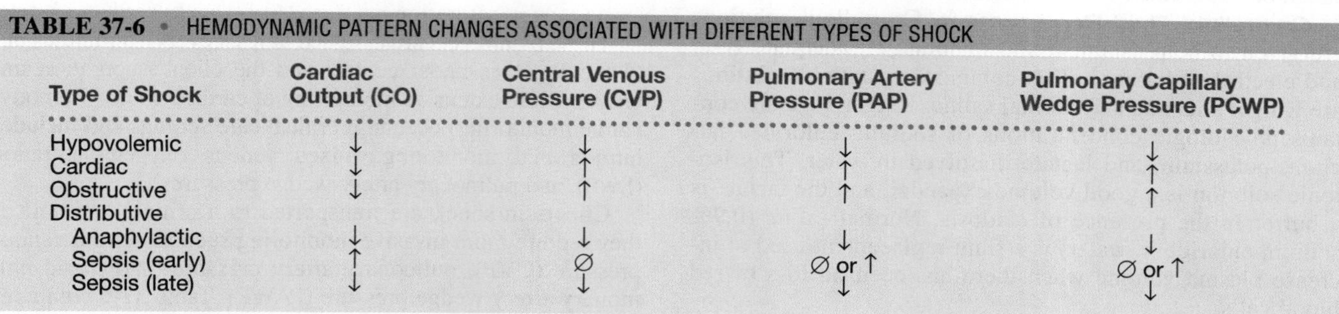

TABLE 37-6 • HEMODYNAMIC PATTERN CHANGES ASSOCIATED WITH DIFFERENT TYPES OF SHOCK

Type of Shock	Cardiac Output (CO)	Central Venous Pressure (CVP)	Pulmonary Artery Pressure (PAP)	Pulmonary Capillary Wedge Pressure (PCWP)
Hypovolemic	↓	↓	↓	↓
Cardiac	↓	↑	↑	↑
Obstructive	↓	↑	↑	↑
Distributive				
Anaphylactic	↓	↓	↓	↓
Sepsis (early)	↑	∅	∅ or ↑	∅ or ↑
Sepsis (late)	↓	↓	↓	↓

Data from Jones, K. (1996). Shock. In J. Clochesy, et al. (Eds.), *Critical care nursing* (2nd ed., pp. 1371–1381). Philadelphia: W.B. Saunders.

↑, Increased; ↓, decreased; ∅, normal or unchanged.

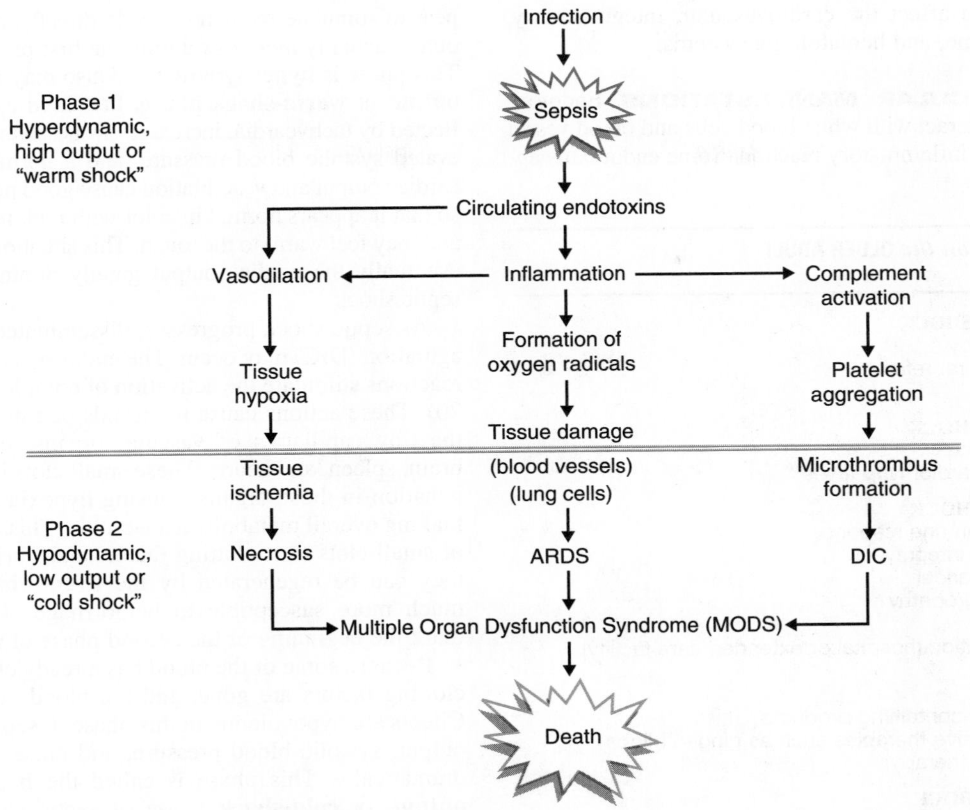

Figure 37-2 ● The sequence of sepsis-induced distributive shock—septic shock. (*ARDS,* Acute respiratory distress syndrome; *DIC,* disseminated intravascular coagulation.)

Intra-arterial catheter placement provides a means of monitoring blood pressure continuously and serves as an access for arterial blood sampling. Intra-arterial catheters are inserted into an artery (radial, brachial, femoral, or dorsalis pedis). The arterial catheter is attached to pressure tubing and a transducer. The transducer converts pressure in the artery (mechanical energy) into an electrical signal that is expressed as a visible waveform on an oscilloscope, and a digital numeric value is displayed.

SURGICAL MANAGEMENT. The nurse monitors fluid loss and uses the nonsurgical interventions described on pp. 779-781 to stabilize the client's hemodynamic status. After a cause has been established, surgical intervention may be necessary to correct the underlying problem. Such interventions include vascular repair or revision, surgical hemostasis of major wounds, closure of bleeding ulcers, and chemical scarring (chemosclerosis) of varicosities.

SIMON Activity Link

COLLABORATIVE MANAGEMENT: SEPSIS-INDUCED DISTRIBUTIVE SHOCK (SEPTIC SHOCK)

Assessment

Distributive shock caused by sepsis does not resemble other types of shock in that it has two distinctive phases (Figure 37-2). The first phase is relatively long, often lasting from hours to a day or longer. The clinical manifestations during this phase are subtle. The chance for recovery is good when the client is recognized as being in the first phase of septic shock and the appropriate interventions are made. The second phase of septic shock has a sudden onset and a rapid downhill course. If septic shock progresses without intervention to the second phase, chances for recovery are slim. Identification of the first phase of sepsis-induced distributive shock can make the greatest difference in survival.

HISTORY

The nurse collects data about risk factors and causative factors related to septic shock. Age is important because sepsis can develop more easily among older, debilitated people with any degree of immunosuppression. Chart 37-6 lists some of the factors that increase the older adult's risk for shock. Clients are asked specific questions about recent illness, trauma, or procedures or chronic conditions that may lead to sepsis and distributive shock. The use of some medications may directly cause changes leading to shock. A medication regimen may also indicate a disease or problem that can contribute to septic shock. Such medications include aspirin and aspirin-containing drugs, antibiotics, and chemotherapeutic agents.

PHYSICAL ASSESSMENT/CLINICAL MANIFESTATIONS

Many of the clinical manifestations of the first phase are unique to septic shock and are often opposite from those associated with all other types of shock. Chart 37-7 summarizes the clinical manifestations of the first (hyperdynamic) phase of septic shock. These findings result from the body's reaction to endotoxins and affect the cardiovascular, integumentary, pulmonary, immune, and hematologic systems.

CARDIOVASCULAR MANIFESTATIONS. Endotoxins in the blood interact with white blood cells and blood vessel walls to trigger an inflammatory reaction. Some endotoxins appear to stimulate the heart muscle directly. As a result, cardiac output actually *increases* during the first phase of septic shock. This phase is **hyperdynamic** and also may be called the **high-output** or **warm-shock phase.** Increased cardiac output is reflected by tachycardia, increased stroke volume, a normal-to-elevated systolic blood pressure, and a normal CVP. Increased cardiac output and vasodilation cause good perfusion of the skin so that it appears normal in color with pink mucous membranes and may feel warm to the touch. This situation is temporary, and eventually the cardiac output greatly diminishes in clients in septic shock.

As septic shock progresses, disseminated intravascular coagulation (DIC) may occur. The endotoxins and inflammatory reactions stimulate the activation of complement (see Chapter 20). These actions cause thousands of small clots to form in the tiny capillaries of vascular organs (e.g., liver, kidney, brain, spleen, and heart). These small clots interfere with oxygenation in those organs, causing hypoxia and ischemia and making overall metabolism anaerobic. This enormous number of small clots uses clotting factors and fibrinogen faster than they can be regenerated by the liver, which makes clients much more susceptible to hemorrhage. These occurrences mark the beginning of the second phase of septic shock.

Because some of the blood has already clotted, most of the clotting factors are gone, and the blood vessels are dilated. Clients are hypovolemic in this phase of septic shock. Cardiac output, systolic blood pressure, and pulse pressure decrease dramatically. This phase is called the **hypodynamic, low-output,** or **cold-shock** phase of septic shock. The clinical manifestations of this phase resemble those of the later stages of all forms of shock.

CHART 37-6

NURSING FOCUS *on the* OLDER ADULT
Risk Factors for Shock

HYPOVOLEMIC SHOCK
- Diuretic therapy
- Diminished thirst reflex
- Immobility

CARDIOGENIC SHOCK
- Diabetes mellitus
- Presence of cardiomyopathies

DISTRIBUTIVE SHOCK
- Diminished immune response
- Reduced skin integrity
- Presence of cancer
- Peripheral neuropathy
- Strokes
- Institutionalization (hospital or extended care facility)
- Malnutrition
- Anemia
- Use of aspirin-containing products
- Use of integrative therapies such as gingko biloba
- Anticoagulant therapy

OBSTRUCTIVE SHOCK
- Pulmonary hypertension
- Presence of cancer

CHART 37-7

KEY FEATURES *of*
Hyperdynamic Phase of Sepsis-Induced Distributive Shock (Septic Shock)

Assessment	Findings
General	
Assess the mental status and level of consciousness.	Irritability, restlessness, lethargy, disorientation, and inappropriate euphoria
Check the oral temperature.	Normal, subnormal, or elevated temperature
Cardiovascular System	
Check the pulse and blood pressure. Document the pulse pressure with each blood pressure reading.	Tachycardia: normal mean arterial blood pressure; widening pulse pressure
Check peripheral pulses.	"Bounding" peripheral pulses
Auscultate heart sounds at four valvular sites, and record the onset of murmur or gallop.	No murmur or gallop
Respiratory System	
Observe the rate, rhythm, and effort of breathing. Observe the symmetry of chest expansion.	Tachypnea, hyperventilation
Percuss and auscultate the lungs. Note the onset of adventitious sounds.	Crackles and decreased breath sounds
Check blood gas levels.	Respiratory alkalosis
Integumentary System	
Inspect and palpate the skin. Note color, vascularity, moisture, temperature, texture, thickness, mobility, and turgor. Assess the oral mucosa.	Warm, flushed skin and peripheral edema
Immune System	
Check complete white blood count with differential.	Abnormal total white blood cell count "Left shift" (decreasing segmented neutrophils; rising band neutrophils)
Hematologic System	
Check platelets and clotting factors.	Decreasing fibrinogen levels Decreasing platelet levels

RESPIRATORY MANIFESTATIONS. In the hyperdynamic phase of septic shock, respiratory rate and depth are increased. Clients often experience a respiratory alkalosis.

When septic shock progresses to the hypodynamic phase, the possible life-threatening pulmonary complication of acute respiratory distress syndrome (ARDS) may occur. Although this complication has many causes, ARDS in cases of sepsis is thought to be related to the formation of oxygen free radicals, which damage the pulmonary cells. Oxygen free radicals can form as a result of oxygen therapy and in response to cellular destruction and the subsequent release of oxidizing enzymes. *The presence of ARDS in a client with septic shock is an ominous clinical sign and is associated with a high mortality rate.*

INTEGUMENTARY MANIFESTATIONS. Clients in the hyperdynamic phase of septic distributive shock often are not recognized as having a problem. The appearance of the skin and mucous membranes leads health care professionals to believe that circulation is unimpaired. Clients feel warm to the touch, and their lips and mucous membranes appear well oxygenated.

When septic shock progresses so that circulation is compromised in the hypodynamic phase, the skin is cool and clammy, and pallor or cyanosis is present. In clients with DIC, petechiae and ecchymoses can occur anywhere. Blood may ooze from the gums, other mucous membranes, and venipuncture sites, as well as around IV catheters.

PSYCHOSOCIAL ASSESSMENT

The indicator that all is not well with clients at the beginning of septic shock is often a change in affect or behavior. The nurse compares the client's presenting behavior, verbal responses, and general affect with those assessed earlier in the day or the day before and notes changes. Clients may seem just slightly different in their reactions to greetings, comments, or jokes. They may be less patient than usual or act restless or fidgety. They may verbalize feelings such as, "I feel as if something is wrong, but I don't know what." If this behavior represents a change from prior assessments, the nurse always considers the possibility of sepsis and shock.

LABORATORY ASSESSMENT

The presence of bacteria in the blood and other extracellular fluids supports the diagnosis of sepsis. The nurse obtains specimens of urine, blood, sputum, and any drainage for culture to identify the causative organisms for both diagnostic and therapeutic purposes. Other abnormal laboratory findings associated with septic shock include changes in the white blood cell count; the differential leukocyte count may demonstrate a left shift (see Chapter 20). Changes in hematocrit and hemoglobin levels usually are not evident until late in septic shock, when the client is hemorrhaging. At that point, the hematocrit and hemoglobin levels, fibrinogen levels, and platelet count are low.

CRITICAL THINKING CHALLENGE

Your client is a 78-year-old man who underwent a bowel resection 2 days ago. He has slept poorly and states that he is nauseated and "feels nervous." His vital signs were taken 1 hour ago and are as follows: temperature, 97.7° F (36.4° C); pulse, 88; respirations, 22; blood pressure, 142/66. You are concerned that he may be developing septic shock.

- Which vital sign(s) support(s) this suspicion?
- What should be your first nursing action?
- What laboratory data would be the most important in monitoring for indications of progression or resolution of the condition?

For suggested answer guidelines, go to SIMON http://www.wbsaunders.com/SIMON/Iggy/.

Analysis

A common collaborative problem for clients with septic shock is Potential for Multiple Organ Dysfunction Syndrome (MODS).

Planning and Implementation

PLANNING: EXPECTED OUTCOMES. The client in septic shock is expected to have normal arterial blood gases, maintain a urine output of at least 20 mL/hr, and have a mean arterial blood pressure within 10 mm Hg of baseline.

INTERVENTIONS. Interventions for the client experiencing septic shock focus on correcting the conditions causing shock and on preventing complications. Chart 37-8 summarizes the best practices for clients experiencing septic shock.

Control of fluid volume deficit associated with septic shock is accomplished through supportive and drug therapies. IV therapy is the same as for hypovolemic shock.

OXYGEN THERAPY. Oxygen therapy is useful whenever inadequate tissue perfusion and inadequate oxygenation are present, such as during distributive shock. Oxygen therapy for septic shock is administered in the same ways as for hypovolemic shock.

DRUG THERAPY. The same agents used to enhance cardiac output and restore vascular volume in hypovolemic shock are used for septic shock. A major focus is the administration of antibiotics to combat sepsis. In addition, agents to

CHART 37-8

BEST PRACTICE *for*
The Client in Sepsis-Induced Distributive Shock (Septic Shock)

- Ensure a patent airway.
- Start or maintain an established IV catheter.
- Administer oxygen.
- Administer antibiotics.
- Obtain specimens of blood, urine, wound drainage, and sputum for culture.
- Increase the rate of IV fluid delivery.
- Use aseptic technique for any invasive procedure.
- Handle the client gently.
- Examine the client for overt bleeding, especially of gums, injection sites, and IV sites.
- Elevate the client's feet, keeping his or her head flat or elevated to a 30-degree angle.
- Take the client's vital signs every 5 minutes until they are stable.
- Administer medications as ordered:
  - Heparin during phase I
  - Clotting factors, platelets, and plasma during phase 2
- Do not leave the client.

counteract disseminated intravascular coagulation (DIC) may be required. Septic shock and DIC have two distinctly different phases, and the drug therapies for each phase of septic shock are different. Drug therapy in the first phase is aimed at preventing coagulation and usually consists of heparin administration. Drug therapy in the second, late phase of septic shock is aimed at increasing the blood's ability to clot and usually consists of the administration of clotting factors, plasma, platelets, or other blood products.

ANTIBIOTICS. Although sepsis and distributive shock can be caused by any microorganism, the most common agents are gram-negative bacteria. When blood cultures have identified specific bacteria, IV antibiotics with known activity against the bacteria are administered. Multiple agents with wide activity are prescribed when the causative agent is not known. A common "triple-antibiotic" regimen includes vancomycin, one of the aminoglycosides (e.g., amikacin, streptomycin, kanamycin, gentamicin), and a systemic penicillin or cephalosporin.

ANTIBODIES. Antibodies against the body's mediators for inflammation are being tested for their effectiveness in septic shock. Antibodies have been developed against the different substances produced by white blood cells to stimulate the inflammatory response. The mediators thought to start the inflammatory responses in blood vessels and lead to the cascade of septic shock are interleukin-1 (IL-1), interleukin-6 (IL-6), and tumor necrosis factor (TNF). This experimental therapy shows promise in reducing the extensive mortality associated with septic shock (Clochesy, 1996; Workman, 1995).

ANTICOAGULANTS. When clients are identified as being in the early phase of septic shock and are beginning to form numerous small clots, heparin is given to limit unnecessary clotting and to prevent the consumption of clotting factors.

CLOTTING FACTORS AND BLOOD PRODUCTS. When septic shock progresses to the point that small clots have formed to such an extent that the client no longer has sufficient clotting factors to prevent hemorrhage, clotting factors are given intravenously. These factors are obtained from pooled human serum. Infusing fresh frozen plasma also helps to replace clotting factors. In addition, platelets or other blood products may be needed.

PROVIDING A SAFE ENVIRONMENT. Primary prevention is possible for some types of shock by identifying clients at risk for conditions and complications leading to sepsis and preventing those complications. Strict adherence to aseptic technique during invasive procedures and during the manipulation of nonintact skin and mucous membranes in immunocompromised clients can help to prevent or limit sepsis and septic shock.

Early detection of the clinical manifestations of shock is a major nursing responsibility. Because shock is a common complication of many conditions found in acute care settings, the nurse always considers the possibility of septic shock. For early detection, the nurse frequently assesses vital signs for specific changes from normal values or from baseline levels. After distributive shock is recognized, health care providers rapidly take action to halt or change the conditions contributing to shock, to support the physiologic compensatory mechanisms, and to prevent life-threatening complications.

CRITICAL THINKING CHALLENGE

The health care provider prescribes the following for your previously described client: nothing by mouth, chest x-ray examination, initiation of venous access, IV antibiotics, blood culture, urine culture, wound culture, rapid blood test for endotoxin antibodies, and dressing change with wound care.

- In what order should you carry out the prescription?
- What size venous access device should you select, and where should it be placed?

For suggested answer guidelines, go to SIMON http://www.wbsaunders.com/SIMON/Iggy/.

Community-Based Care

For most clients, shock is a complication of another condition and is resolved before they are discharged from the emergency department or acute care setting. Because more clients are receiving treatment on an outpatient basis and are being discharged earlier from acute care settings, more

CHART 37-9

CLIENT EDUCATION GUIDE
Infection Precautions

- Avoid crowds and other large gatherings of people, who might be ill.
- Do not share eating utensils or personal toilet articles (e.g., toothbrushes, toothpaste, washcloths, or deodorant sticks) with others.
- If possible, bathe daily.
- Wash the armpits, groin, genitals, and rectal area at least twice a day with an antimicrobial soap.
- Clean your toothbrush daily by either running it through the dishwasher or rinsing it in liquid laundry bleach.
- Wash your hands thoroughly with an antimicrobial soap before you eat or drink, after touching a pet, after shaking hands with anyone, as soon as you come home from any outing, and after using the toilet.
- Wash dishes between use with hot, sudsy water, or use a dishwasher.
- Do not drink water that has been standing for longer than 15 minutes.
- Do not reuse cups and glasses without washing them.
- Do not change pet litter boxes.
- Take your temperature at least once a day.
- Refrigerate and prepare food appropriately. Do not eat raw or undercooked meat, fish, poultry, or eggs.
- Report any of the following signs or symptoms of infection to your physician immediately:
  - Temperature greater than 100° F (38° C)
  - Persistent cough (with or without sputum)
  - Pus or foul-smelling drainage from any open skin area or normal body opening
  - Presence of a boil or abscess
  - Urine that is cloudy or foul-smelling or causes burning on urination
- Do not dig in the garden or work with houseplants.
- Use antibacterial cleansers to clean kitchen and bathroom surfaces at least twice each week. If you clean these areas yourself, wear rubber or vinyl work gloves while cleaning.
- Use a condom when having sex.
- Take all prescribed medications as the physician has ordered.

clients at home are at increased risk for infection and septic shock.

HEALTH TEACHING

Protecting vulnerable clients from infection and sepsis at home is an important nursing function. The nurse instructs clients about the importance of self-care strategies, such as good hygiene, handwashing, balanced diet, rest, and exercise, skin care, and mouth care. If clients or family members do not know how to take a temperature or read a thermometer, the nurse provides instruction and obtains a return demonstration. Clients are instructed to avoid crowds or other people with known illnesses and to notify the health care provider immediately if experiencing any fever or other sign of infection. Specific recommendations for infection precautions are listed in Chart 37-9.

> **CRITICAL THINKING CHALLENGE**
>
> You understand that the source of your client's sepsis-induced distributive shock was a gastrointestinal wound. With this source in mind, what three areas should you stress specifically in health teaching for this client at home?

For suggested answer guidelines, go to SIMON http://www.wbsaunders.com/SIMON/Iggy/.

HOME CARE MANAGEMENT

The nurse or home care aide evaluates the home environment for safety regarding infection hazards. General cleanliness is noted, and particular attention is given to the kitchen and bathrooms. Chart 37-10 lists focused client and environmental assessment data to obtain during a home visit.

Evaluation: Outcomes

NOC The nurse evaluates the care of the client with sepsis-induced distributive shock. The expected outcomes are that the client:

- Maintains oxygen saturation (as measured by pulse oximetry) of at least 85%
- Maintains a urine output of at least 20 mL/hr

CHART 37-10

FOCUSED ASSESSMENT *of* Home Care Clients at Risk for Sepsis

Assess the client for any clinical manifestations of infection, including:
- Temperature, pulse, respiration, and blood pressure
- Color of skin and mucous membranes
- The mouth and perianal area for fissures or lesions
- Any nonintact skin area for the presence of exudates, redness, increased warmth, swelling
- Any pain, tenderness, or other discomfort anywhere
- Cough or any other symptoms of a cold or the flu
- Urine; or ask client whether urine is dark or cloudy, has an odor, or causes pain or burning during urination

Assess client's and caregiver's compliance with and understanding of infection prevention techniques

Assess home environment, including:
- General cleanliness
- Kitchen and bathroom facilities, including refrigeration
- Availability and type of soap for handwashing
- Presence of pets, especially cats, rodents, or reptiles

- Has arterial blood gas values within the normal range
- Has a mean arterial pressure within 10 mm Hg of baseline
- Does not experience multiple organ dysfunction syndrome (MODS)
- Correctly states measures to reduce the risk for sepsis

ONLINE RESOURCES

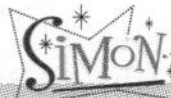

For suggested readings and Internet resources, go to http://www.wbsaunders.com/SIMON/Iggy/.

SELECTED BIBLIOGRAPHY

Asterisk indicates a classic or definitive work on this subject.

*Ackerman, M. (1994). The systemic inflammatory response, sepsis and multiple organ dysfunction: New definitions for an old problem. *Critical Care Clinics of North America, 6*(2), 243-250.

Atassi, K., & Harris, M. (2001). Action stat: Disseminate intravascular coagulation. *Nursing 2001, 31*(3), 64.

Bannon, J., Visvanathan, K., & Zabriskie, J. (1999). Structure and function of streptococcal and staphylococcal superantigens in septic shock. *Infectious Disease Clinics of North America, 13*(2), 387-396.

Carroll, P. (1999). Monitoring the gut to prevent MODS. *RN, 62*(10), 34-37.

*Chernow, B. (1996). New advances in the pharmacologic approach to circulatory shock. *Journal of Clinical Anesthesiology, 8*(Suppl. 3), 67s-69s.

*Clochesy, J. (1996). Patients with systemic inflammatory response syndrome. In J. Clochesy et al. (Eds.), *Critical care nursing* (2nd ed., pp. 1359-1370). Philadelphia: W.B. Saunders.

Copelin, C. (1998). Practical points in the use of albumin for hypovolemia. *Journal of PeriAnesthesia Nursing, 13*(2), 118-120.

Cotran, R., Kumar, V., & Collins, T. (1999). *Robbins pathologic basis of disease* (6th ed.). Philadelphia: W.B. Saunders.

deGuzman, E., Shankar, M., & Mattox, K. (1999). Limited volume resuscitation in penetrating thoracoabdominal trauma. *AACN Clinical Issues: Advanced Practice in Acute and Critical Care, 10*(1), 61-66.

DeJong, M. (1997). Clinical snapshot: Cardiogenic shock. *American Journal of Nursing, 97*(6), 40-41.

*Effron, M., & Chernow, B. (1992). Shock. In E. Rubenstein & D. Federman (Eds.), *Scientific American: Medicine* (pp. I card III Shock 1-12). New York: Scientific American.

Fink, K. (1999). Is Trendelenburg a wise choice? *Journal of Emergency Nursing, 25*(1), 60-62.

Gordon, L. (1999). The sepsis continuum from systemic inflammatory response syndrome to multiple organ dysfunction syndrome. *Nursing in Critical Care, 4*(5), 238-244.

Grap, M. (1998). Pulse oximetry. *Critical Care Nurse, 18*(1), 94-99.

Guyton, A., & Hall, J. (2000). *Textbook of medical physiology* (10th ed.). Philadelphia: W.B. Saunders.

Heckbert, S., et al. (1998). Outcome after hemorrhagic shock in trauma patients. *Journal of Trauma: Injury, Infection, and Critical Care, 45*(3), 545-549.

*Jones, K. (1996). Shock. In J. Clochesy et al. (Eds.), *Critical care nursing* (2nd ed., p. 1371). Philadelphia: W.B. Saunders.

McCloskey, J., & Bulechek, G. (2000). *Nursing interventions classification (NIC)* (3rd ed.). St. Louis: Mosby.

McGrath, A., & Cox, C. (1998). Cardiac and circulatory assessment in intensive care units. *Intensive and Critical Care Nursing, 14*, 283-287.

*Miller, L. (1996). Hemodynamic monitoring. In J. Clochesy et al. (Eds.), *Critical care nursing* (2nd ed., pp. 203-234). Philadelphia: W.B. Saunders.

Mower-Wade, D., Bartley, M., & Chiari-Allwein, J. (2001). How to respond to shock. *Dimensions in Critical Care Nursing, 20*(2), 22-27.

Pagana, K., & Pagana, T. (1999). *Diagnostic testing and nursing implications: A case study approach* (5th ed.). St. Louis: Mosby.

Robb, W. (1999). Massive transfusion in trauma. *AACN Clinical Issues: Advanced Practice in Acute and Critical Care, 10*(1), 69-84.

Sandrock, J. (1998). Treating traumatic hypovolemia: Which fluid to choose? *Nursing98, 28*(1), 32cc1-32cc4.

Septic shock therapy remains elusive. (1998). *Nursing98, 98*(7), 66.

Shock. (1999). *Nursing Times, 95*(28), 46.

*Shoemaker, W. (1994). Pathophysiology, monitoring and therapy of acute circulatory problems. *Critical Care Clinics of North America, 6*(2), 295-307.

Smail, N., et al. (1998). Resuscitation after uncontrolled venous hemorrhage: Does increased resuscitation volume improve regional perfusion? *Journal of Trauma: Injury, Infection, and Critical Care, 44*(4), 701-708.

*Stengle, J., & Dries, D. (1994). Sepsis in the elderly. *Critical Care Nursing Clinics of North America, 6*(2), 421-427.

Tangredi, M. (1998). Clinical snapshot: Septic shock. *American Journal of Nursing, 98*(3), 46-47.

Watson, H. (1999). How safe is our blood supply? *Registered Nurse, 11*(3), 10-11.

*Workman, M.L. (1995). Essential concepts of inflammation and immunity. *Critical Care Clinics of North America, 7*(4), 601-615.

CHAPTER 38

Interventions for Critically Ill Clients with Coronary Artery Disease

KATHLEEN OUIMET PERRIN

Learning Objectives

After studying this chapter, you should be able to:

1. Explain the pathophysiology of coronary artery disease (CAD).
2. Compare and contrast stable angina, unstable angina, and myocardial infarction (MI).
3. Identify modifiable and nonmodifiable risk factors for CAD.
4. Interpret physical and diagnostic assessment findings in clients who have CAD.
5. Describe the psychosocial aspects of CAD.
6. Prioritize nursing care for clients who have CAD.
7. Explain the advantages of thrombolysis for a client experiencing an MI.
8. Identify the life-threatening complications of CAD.
9. Describe the postprocedure care for the client who has undergone a percutaneous transluminal coronary angioplasty.
10. Describe the postoperative care for the client who has undergone coronary artery bypass graft (CABG) surgery.
11. Discuss the differences between CABG surgery, minimally invasive direct coronary artery bypass, and transmyocardial laser revascularization.
12. Develop a discharge plan for the client with CAD.

SIMON Go to http://www.wbsaunders.com/SIMON/Iggy/ for self-assessment questions related to these Learning Objectives.

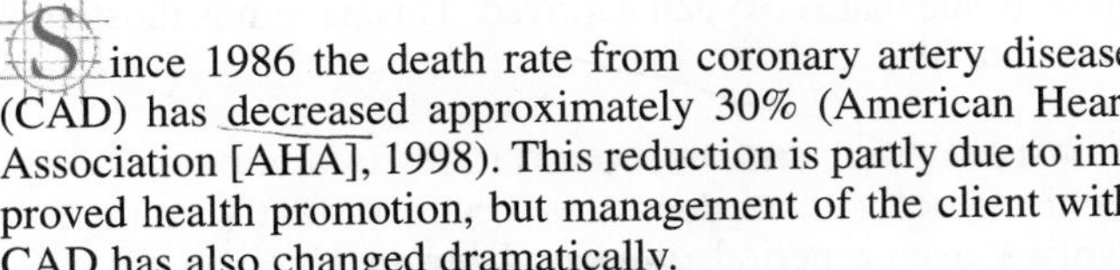

Since 1986 the death rate from coronary artery disease (CAD) has decreased approximately 30% (American Heart Association [AHA], 1998). This reduction is partly due to improved health promotion, but management of the client with CAD has also changed dramatically.

Most deaths today from myocardial infarction (MI) ("heart attack") are due to dysrhythmias that occur before the client reaches the hospital. During the past 10 years, in-hospital mortality from MI has decreased from 15% to 5%. Advances in cardiac care, especially new strategies for opening and maintaining the patency of obstructed coronary vessels, have contributed to this decline.

OVERVIEW

Coronary artery disease (CAD) is still the leading cause of death in the United States. This disease affects the arteries that provide blood, oxygen, and nutrients to the myocardium. When blood flow through the coronary arteries is partially or completely blocked, ischemia and infarction (necrosis) of the myocardium may result. **Ischemia** occurs when insufficient oxygen is supplied to meet the requirements of the myocardium. Infarction occurs when severe ischemia is prolonged and irreversible damage to tissue results.

Pathophysiology

Atherosclerosis is the leading contributor to CAD and death in Western civilizations. Three basic processes occur in atherosclerosis:

- Overgrowth of intimal smooth muscle cells with accumulation of macrophages and T cells
- Formation of a connective tissue matrix in the vessel intima
- Accumulation of lipids, especially cholesterol, in the connective tissue

These processes narrow the vessel lumen (Figure 38-1). Blood flow through the restricted lumen may be adequate to perfuse myocardial tissue when the client is at rest but inadequate to meet oxygen requirements during activity. The heart extracts a larger amount of oxygen (75%) from its blood flow than does any other major organ in the body, even at rest.

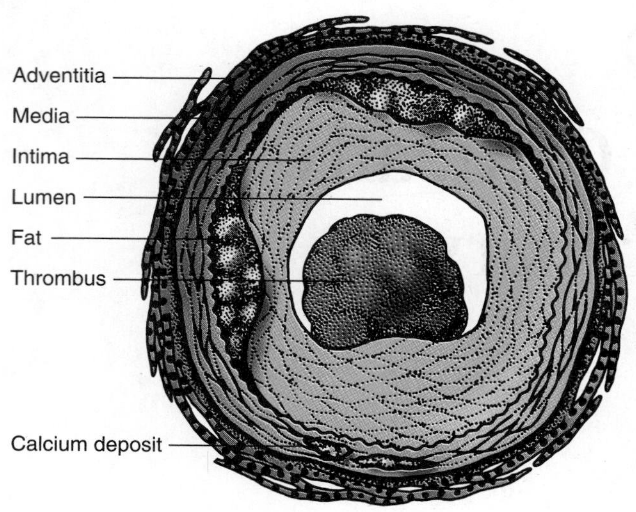

Figure 38-1 ● A cross section of an atherosclerotic coronary artery.

When additional oxygen is needed to meet increased tissue demands, an increase in coronary artery blood flow is also required. Once the lumen of a coronary artery is obstructed by more than 70%, blood flow may not be able to increase in response to tissue demands. Increases in myocardial oxygen requirements (e.g., exercise or aortic stenosis) or transient reductions in blood flow (e.g., hypotension or coronary spasm) may result in inadequate oxygen supply to and ischemia of the myocardium. Ischemic myocardium is oxygen-deprived myocardium, and the client typically experiences angina.

STABLE ANGINA PECTORIS

Angina pectoris, a term derived from a Latin phrase, means "strangling of the chest." Angina is a temporary imbalance between the coronary arteries' ability to supply oxygen and the cardiac muscle's demand for oxygen. Ischemia that occurs with angina is limited in duration, and it does not cause permanent damage of myocardial tissue.

Angina may be of two predominant types: stable angina and unstable angina. **Stable angina** is chest discomfort that occurs with moderate to prolonged exertion in a pattern that is familiar to the client; the frequency, duration, and intensity of symptoms have not increased over the past several months. Stable angina results in only slight limitation of activity. This condition is usually associated with a stable atherosclerotic plaque. Stable angina is usually relieved by nitroglycerin or rest. It is often managed by medical means such as calcium channel blockers and beta-blocking medications; rarely, however, it requires aggressive treatment.

WOMEN'S HEALTH CONSIDERATIONS

Many women experience atypical angina; they may describe angina as a choking sensation that occurs with exertion. Angina is more likely to be the primary presenting symptom of CAD in women (56%) than in men (46%) and is twice as common as MI in women. For 86% of women, compared with 56% of men, angina does not progress to MI (Halm & Penque, 1999).

ACUTE CORONARY SYNDROMES

Unstable angina is chest pain or discomfort that occurs at rest or with minimal exertion and causes marked limitation of activity. An increase in the number of attacks and an increase in the intensity of the pain characterize unstable angina. The pain may last longer than 15 minutes or be poorly relieved by rest or nitroglycerin. Unstable angina describes a broad spectrum of disorders, including *new-onset angina, variant (Prinzmetal's) angina, preinfarction angina,* and *crescendo angina.* A newer way to describe the disorders that make up unstable angina, subendocardial MI, and MI is to call them acute coronary syndromes.

In **acute coronary syndromes,** it is believed that the atherosclerotic plaque in the coronary artery ruptures, resulting in platelet aggregation, thrombus formation, and vasoconstriction. The amount of disruption of the atherosclerotic plaque determines the degree of obstruction of the coronary artery and the specific disease process (unstable angina, subendocardial MI, or MI). Between 10% and 30% of clients with unstable angina progress to having an MI in 1 year, and 29% die from MI in 5 years.

MYOCARDIAL INFARCTION

Myocardial infarction (MI) occurs when myocardial tissue is abruptly and severely deprived of oxygen. When blood flow is acutely reduced by 80% to 90%, ischemia develops. Ischemia can lead to necrosis of myocardial tissue if blood flow is not restored. Most MIs are the result of atherosclerosis of a coronary artery, rupture of the plaque, subsequent thrombosis, and occlusion of blood flow. However, other factors may be implicated, such as coronary artery spasm, platelet aggregation, and emboli from mural thrombi (thrombi lining the walls of the cardiac chambers).

MIs often begin with infarction (necrosis) of the subendocardial layer of cardiac muscle. This layer has the longest myofibrils in the heart, the greatest oxygen demand, and the poorest oxygen supply. Around the initial area of infarction in the subendocardium are two zones: (1) the zone of injury, tissue that is injured but not necrotic, and (2) the zone of ischemia, tissue that is oxygen deprived. This pattern is illustrated in Figure 38-2.

PROCESS OF INFARCTION. Infarction is a dynamic process that does not occur instantly; rather, it evolves over a period of several hours. Hypoxia from ischemia may lead to local vasodilation of blood vessels and acidosis. Imbalances of potassium, calcium, and magnesium, as well as acidosis at the cellular level, may lead to suppression of normal conduction and contractile functions. Automaticity and ectopy are enhanced. Catecholamines released in response to hypoxia and pain may increase the heart's rate and force of contraction. These factors increase oxygen requirements in tissue that is already oxygen deprived. The area of infarction may extend into the zones of injury and ischemia.

The actual extent of the zone of infarction depends on three factors: collateral circulation, anaerobic metabolism, and workload demands on the myocardium.

The infarction may involve only the subendocardium (called a **subendocardial MI**), or it may spread to the epi-

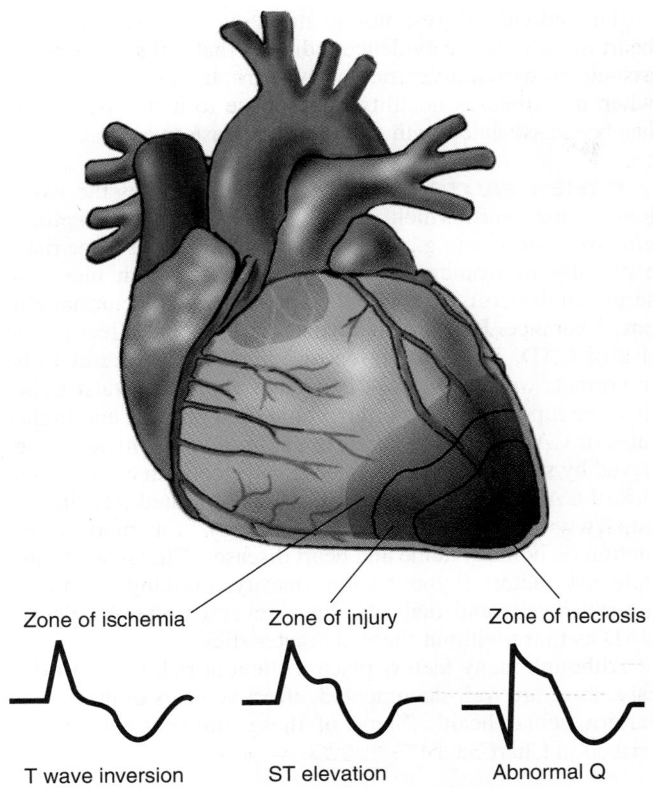

Figure 38-2 ● ECG changes seen in myocardial infarction.

cardium or to all three layers of cardiac muscle. When all three layers are involved, the MI is termed *transmural.* Subendocardial MIs have less effect on wall motion and cardiac output than transmural infarctions do.

PHYSIOLOGIC RESPONSE TO THE INFARCTION. Obvious physical changes do not occur in the heart until 6 hours after the infarction, when the infarcted region appears blue and swollen. After 48 hours, the infarct turns gray with yellow streaks as neutrophils invade the tissue and begin to remove the necrotic cells. By 8 to 10 days after infarction, granulation tissue forms at the edges of the necrotic tissue. Over a 2- to 3-month period, the necrotic area eventually develops into a shrunken, thin, firm scar. Scar tissue permanently changes the size and shape of the entire left ventricle (ventricular remodeling). Remodeling may decrease left ventricular function, cause heart failure, and increase morbidity and mortality.

CLASSIFICATION OF MYOCARDIAL INFARCTION BY LOCATION. The client's response to an MI also depends on which coronary artery or arteries were obstructed and which part of the left ventricle wall was damaged: anterior, lateral, septal, inferior, or posterior. Figure 38-3 details the major coronary arteries, and Table 38-1 describes the structures they perfuse.

Clients with obstruction of the left anterior descending (LAD) artery usually have anterior or septal MIs because the LAD artery perfuses the anterior wall and most of the septal wall of the left ventricle. Anterior wall MIs account for 25% of all MIs and, at 25%, have the highest mortality rate. Clients with anterior MIs are most likely to experience left ventricular heart failure and ventricular dysrhythmias, because a large segment of the left ventricle wall may have been damaged.

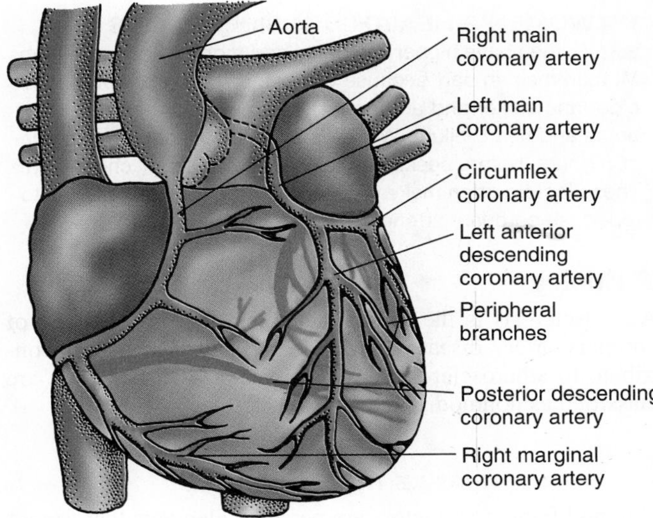

Figure 38-3 ● Coronary arterial system.

TABLE 38-1 • MAJOR CORONARY VESSELS AND THE STRUCTURES THEY PERFUSE

LEFT ANTERIOR DESCENDING CORONARY ARTERY
- Most of the left ventricular muscle mass and septum

LEFT CIRCUMFLEX CORONARY ARTERY
- Posterior wall of the left ventricle
- SA node in 39% of clients
- AV node in 12% of clients
- Left ventricular muscle in 10% of clients

RIGHT CORONARY ARTERY
- Right ventricle
- Inferior portion of the left ventricle
- SA node in 59% of clients
- AV node in 88% of clients

SA, Sinoatrial; *AV*, atrioventricular.

The circumflex artery supplies the lateral wall of the left ventricle and possibly portions of the posterior wall or the sinoatrial (SA) and atrioventricular (AV) nodes. Clients with obstruction of the circumflex artery may experience a posterior wall MI (2% of MIs) or a lateral wall MI (3% of MIs) and sinus dysrhythmias.

In most people, the right coronary artery perfuses the SA and AV nodes, as well as the inferior or diaphragmatic portion of the left ventricle. Clients with obstruction of the right coronary artery often have inferior MIs. Inferior wall MIs account for approximately 17% of all MIs and have a mortality rate of about 10%. Clients are most likely to experience bradydysrhythmias or AV conduction defects, especially transient second-degree heart blocks. About one third of clients with inferior MIs have a right ventricular MI and right ventricular failure (Braunwald, 1998a).

WOMEN'S HEALTH CONSIDERATIONS

Women have higher morbidity and mortality rates after an MI than men, in part because when an MI occurs, women are older and sicker and are more likely to have pre-existing diabetes and heart failure. Women also delay longer, an average of 5 hours, before seeking medical assistance for chest pain. These factors often make women ineligible for interventions to reperfuse coronary arteries.

Etiology

Atherosclerosis is the primary factor in the development of coronary artery disease (CAD). Numerous risk factors contribute to atherosclerosis (see Chapter 36). Risk factors are classified as nonmodifiable and modifiable.

NONMODIFIABLE RISK FACTORS

Nonmodifiable risk factors are personal elements that cannot be altered or controlled. These risk factors, which interact with each other, include age, gender, family history, and ethnic background. The risk of CAD increases with age; 55% of clients who experience a myocardial infarction (MI) are 65 years of age or older.

Premenopausal women have a lower incidence of MI than men do. However, for postmenopausal women in their 70s, the incidence of MI equals that of men. Family history is also a risk factor; people whose parents had CAD are more susceptible.

MODIFIABLE RISK FACTORS

Modifiable risk factors include elevated serum cholesterol levels, cigarette smoking, hypertension, impaired glucose tolerance, obesity, physical inactivity, and stress.

ELEVATED SERUM CHOLESTEROL LEVELS. The risk of CAD rises as serum cholesterol levels increase. The American Heart Association (AHA) estimates that 52% of Americans have serum cholesterol levels greater than 200 mg/dL and that 20% have levels above 240 mg/dL, putting them at risk for CAD. A 1% reduction in serum cholesterol has been associated with a 2% reduction in CAD. Elevated levels of low-density lipoprotein (LDL) combined with low levels of high-density lipoprotein (HDL) increase the risk further. HDL levels less than 37 mg/dL for men and 47 mg/dL for women are considered to be risk factors for CAD. HDL levels greater than 53 mg/dL for men and 67 mg/dL for women *decrease* the risk of CAD.

CIGARETTE SMOKING. Cigarette smokers have twice the risk of MI that nonsmokers have and two to four times the risk of sudden cardiac death (Andrews, 1998). An estimated 26.7% of men and 22.8% of women in the United States are smokers (AHA, 1998). Reducing the tar and nicotine content of the cigarettes smoked does not reduce the risk of CAD.

PHYSICAL INACTIVITY. Physical inactivity may be the most important risk factor for the general population because between 40% and 60% of Americans are sedentary. Regular physical activity helps maintain body weight and muscle mass while optimizing blood pressure and lipid values.

The individual's response to stress may be associated with heart disease. Some evidence indicates that job stress may be associated with left ventricular hypertrophy. *Type A behavior,* when described as hostility in response to a stressful event, has been associated with a twofold increase in angina.

OTHER FACTORS. *Hypertension* increases the workload of the heart, which increases the risk of MI. *Impaired glucose tolerance* (e.g., diabetes) seriously increases the risks, especially in women. *Obesity* is associated with increased serum cholesterol, elevated blood pressure, and abnormal glucose tolerance. It may also have an independent effect on the risk of CAD. The distribution of adipose tissue seems to be important; women with fat deposited about the waist rather than the hips often have unfavorable lipid profiles and higher rates of CAD. Elevated levels of serum *homocysteine* are believed by some researchers to be associated with an increased risk of CAD. (See Chapter 33 and the Suggested Readings at http://www.wbsaunders.com/SIMON/Iggy/ for more information on homocysteine and heart disease.) Clients with multiple risk factors (hypertension, obesity, smoking, high cholesterol levels, and diabetes) have several times the risk of CAD as those without these characteristics.

Although many factors place a client at risk for heart disease, there are well-documented, effective ways of promoting cardiovascular health. Some of these interventions are described in Chart 38-1.

CULTURAL CONSIDERATIONS

Modifiable risk factors vary for people of different racial and ethnic backgrounds. African Americans do not have significantly higher overall heart disease rates than other groups. However, among African Americans the incidence of diabetes is 33% higher, and hypertension develops at an earlier age and is more severe at every decade of life. Obesity is significantly more common in African-American women than in Caucasian women (U.S. Department of Health and Human Services [USDHHS], 1999).

Hispanics have lower death rates from heart disease than non-Hispanics. Above-normal weight is more of a problem for Hispanic women, especially Mexican-American women (AHA, 1998), and may be associated with less-than-average physical activity. As many as 67% of Mexican-American men and women are overweight, with 23% of men and 34% of women classified as obese (AHA, 1998; USDHHS, 1999)

Tremendous diversity among the Asian and Pacific Island American populations makes generalizations difficult. However, Filipino-Americans seem to have an increased incidence of hypertension, and more than 60% of native Hawaiians are overweight.

The major modifiable cardiovascular risk factors for Native Americans seem to be obesity and diabetes. The increase in obesity in Native Americans has paralleled the increase in diabetes (USDHHS, 1999). In many tribes, more than 40% of the members have diabetes (AHA, 1998).

Incidence/Prevalence

Approximately 1,100,000 people experience MIs each year in the United States, and about one third of these people die (AHA, 1998). MI is the single largest cause of death for both

CHART 38-1

CLIENT EDUCATION GUIDE
Prevention of Coronary Artery Disease

Smoking
- If you smoke, quit.
- If you don't smoke, don't start.

Diet
- Follow a prudent daily diet.
- Consume sufficient calories for your body: you must obtain:
  - 50% to 55% of your calories from carbohydrates
  - 30% to 35% of your calories from complex carbohydrates
  - 10% of your calories from simple sugars
  - Less than 30% of your calories from fat
  - 15% of your calories from monounsaturated fat
  - 10% of your calories from polyunsaturated fat
  - The remainder of your calories (5% to 10%) from saturated fat
  - 12% to 20% of your calories from protein
- Limit your cholesterol intake to less than 300 mg daily.
- Limit your sodium intake to less than 130 mEq daily.

Cholesterol
- Have your cholesterol and low-density lipoprotein (LDL) levels checked regularly.
- If your cholesterol and LDL levels are elevated, follow your health care provider's advice.

Physical Activity
- If you are middle-aged or older or have a history of medical problems, check with your health care provider before starting an exercise program.
- Appropriate exercise should be enjoyable; burn 400 calories per session, and sustain a heart rate of 120 to 150 beats/min, depending on your age.
- Exercise moderately at least three times each week, preferably five.
- Exercise periods should be at least 20 to 30 minutes long with 10-minute warm-up and 5-minute cool-down periods.
- If your are unable to exercise moderately three to five times each week, walk daily for 30 minutes at a comfortable pace.
- If you are unable to walk 30 minutes daily, walk any distance you can (e.g., park further away from a site than necessary; use the stairs, not the elevator, to go one floor up or two floors down).

Diabetes
- Manage your diabetes with your health care provider.

Blood Pressure
- Have your blood pressure checked regularly.
- If your blood pressure is elevated, follow your health care provider's advice.
- Continue to monitor your blood pressure at regular intervals.

Obesity
- Avoid severely restricted or fad diets.
- Consider a restriction in intake of saturated fats, simple sugars, and cholesterol-rich foods.
- Increase your physical activity.

men and women. Approximately half of the deaths from MI occur in the first hour before reaching the hospital.

Approximately 350,000 people experience angina for the first time each year. The AHA estimates that more than 6 million people who have experienced angina or an MI are still living (AHA, 1998). The estimated cost of caring for people with CAD is slightly less than $150 billion yearly (see the Cost of Care box above, right).

COST OF CARE
IMPLICATIONS FOR NURSING

CORONARY ARTERY DISEASE

Cost of Care
- In 1996 for people younger than 65 years of age, the average cost of a coronary event from hospital admission to discharge was $22,720, with an average length of stay of 4.3 days. In 1995, $9.8 billion (a range of $3769 to $11,110 per discharge) was paid to Medicare beneficiaries for coronary heart disease.
- The average cost of coronary artery bypass surgery in 1995 was $44,820 (AHA, 1998).
- Goldman (1998) evaluated the cost-effectiveness of cardiac interventions. The following were described as highly cost-effective:
  - Lovastatin for cholesterol levels greater than 250 for men 25 to 54 years of age (saves both money and lives)
  - Nurse counseling and manual for smoking cessation (cost $250 per year of life saved)
  - Physician counseling for smoking cessation (cost $1300 per year of life saved)
  - Administration of beta blockers following myocardial infarction (MI) (cost $1300 per year of life saved)
  - Percutaneous transluminal coronary angioplasty (PTCA) for severe angina (cost $8700 to $10,200 per year of life saved)
  - Coronary artery bypass grafting (CABG) for severe angina and left anterior descending (LAD) artery disease (cost $9200 per year of life saved)
- Interventions determined by Goldman (1998) to be very expensive per year of life saved included the following:
  - PTCA for mild angina and two-vessel disease (cost $109,000 per year of life saved)
  - Electrocardiogram (ECG) testing for asymptomatic 40-year-old men (cost $148,000 per year of life saved)
  - CABG for mild angina (cost $2,204,800 per year of life saved)

Implications for Nursing
Nurses have demonstrated they can save lives at a minimal cost by counseling clients about prevention of coronary artery disease (CAD). Since the same intervention may be cost-effective for one group of clients and not for another, nurses need to become aware of which cardiac interventions are cost-effective for which group of clients and which represent major investments with minimal expectation of improvement in client outcomes.

COLLABORATIVE MANAGEMENT

Assessment

HISTORY

If chest discomfort is present at the time of the interview, the nurse delays collection of historical data until interventions for pain, vital sign instability, and dysrhythmias are initiated and the discomfort resolves. The nurse obtains information about how the client has managed the current episode of chest discomfort and which medications he or she is taking. When the client is *pain free,* information about family history and modifiable risk factors, including eating habits, lifestyle, and physical activity levels, is obtained.

PHYSICAL ASSESSMENT/CLINICAL MANIFESTATIONS

The nurse asks clients to describe the immediate concern. The presence of chest, epigastric, jaw, back, or arm discomfort is noted. The client is asked to rate the discomfort on a scale of 0 to 10, with 10 being the highest level of discomfort. Clients often describe the discomfort as tightness, a burning sensa-

CHART 38-2

KEY FEATURES *of* Angina and Myocardial Infarction

Angina	Myocardial Infarction
Substernal chest discomfort	Substernal chest pressure
• Radiating to the left arm	• Radiating to the left arm, back, or jaw
• Precipitated by exertion or stress	• Occurring without cause, primarily early in the morning
• Relieved by nitroglycerin or rest	• Relieved only by opioids
• Lasting <15 min	• Lasting 30 min or more
• Few associated symptoms	• Frequent associated symptoms: Nausea, Diaphoresis, Dyspnea, Feelings of fear and anxiety, Dysrhythmias

tion, pressure, or indigestion. The nurse asks them what they have already done to try to relieve the pain. Pain management is described in detail in Chapter 7.

PAIN ASSESSMENT. The nurse rapidly yet completely assesses the client with ongoing chest pain. Because chest discomfort may occur from a variety of causes and only 30% of people experiencing chest pain are having a myocardial infarction (MI), it is important to differentiate among the types of chest pain and to identify the source (see Table 33-1). Both the physician and the nurse may question the client to determine the characteristics of the discomfort. Appropriate questions for the nurse to ask concerning the discomfort include onset, location, radiation, intensity, duration, and precipitating and relieving factors.

Chart 38-2 compares and contrasts anginal and infarction pain. Because anginal pain is ischemic pain, it usually improves when the disparity between oxygen supply and demand is resolved. For example, rest reduces tissue demands, and nitroglycerin improves oxygen supply. Discomfort from an MI does not usually resolve with such simple measures. The nurse also notes the presence of any associated symptoms, including nausea, vomiting, diaphoresis, dizziness, weakness, palpitations, and shortness of breath.

WOMEN'S HEALTH CONSIDERATIONS

Chest discomfort is often not the initial symptom reported by women experiencing an MI. Women may initially complain of atypical symptoms such as heart "flutters" without pain, shortness of breath, fatigue, or depression (Halm & Penque, 1999). As the MI progresses, women usually report typical chest discomfort, arm and shoulder pain, back pain, or an aching jaw, neck, or tooth.

CULTURAL CONSIDERATIONS

African Americans experience longer delays in seeking treatment for MI and higher mortality rates than Caucasians. One factor thought to contribute to this delay is a greater incidence of dyspnea as an acute symptom of MI among both male and female African Americans rather than the more classic chest discomfort.

CONSIDERATIONS FOR OLDER ADULTS

The presence of the associated symptoms without chest discomfort is also significant. In 15% to 25% of all clients with MI, primarily older adults and clients with diabetes, chest pain or discomfort may be mild or absent, and clients may complain primarily of the associated symptoms. Some elders may think they are experiencing indigestion and therefore not recognize that they are having an MI. Twenty-five percent of older adults experiencing an MI complain only of shortness of breath. The major manifestation of MI in clients older then 80 years of age may be disorientation or confusion due to poor cardiac output.

CARDIOVASCULAR ASSESSMENT. The nurse immediately obtains a blood pressure measurement, determines the heart rate, interprets the cardiac rhythm, and assesses for dysrhythmias. Sinus tachycardia with premature ventricular contractions (PVCs) frequently occurs in the first few hours after an MI. If an intravenous (IV) access is available, the nurse ensures that it is patent, because the client will most likely receive IV fluids and medications. If an access is not available, one or preferably two IV accesses are initiated. The nurse may administer oxygen, titrating the fraction of inspired oxygen (FIO_2) to the arterial oxygen saturation (SaO_2) according to protocols or the physician's order.

Next, the nurse assesses distal peripheral pulses and skin temperature. The skin should be warm, with all pulses palpable. In the client with unstable angina or MI, poor cardiac output may be manifested by cool, diaphoretic skin and diminished or absent pulses.

The nurse auscultates for an S_3 gallop, which often indicates heart failure, a serious and common complication of MI. The nurse also assesses the respiratory rate and breath sounds for signs of heart failure. An increased respiratory rate is common because of anxiety and pain, but crackles or wheezes may indicate heart failure. Auscultation of an S_4 heart sound is a common finding in the client who has had a previous MI or hypertension.

The client with MI may experience a temperature elevation for several days after infarction. Temperatures as high as 102°F (38.9° C) may occur in response to myocardial necrosis.

PSYCHOSOCIAL ASSESSMENT

Denial is a common early reaction to chest discomfort associated with angina or MI. On average, the client with an acute MI waits more than 2 hours before seeking medical attention. Often the client rationalizes that symptoms are due to indigestion or overexertion. In some situations, denial is a normal part of adapting to a stressful event. However, denial that interferes with identification of a symptom, such as chest discomfort, can be harmful. The nurse explains the significance of reporting any discomfort, emphasizing that health care provisions attempt to relieve the discomfort immediately.

Fear, anxiety, and anger are other common reactions of clients and families. Nursing assessment focuses on assisting the client and family members in identifying these feelings. The nurse allows the client and family time to explain their understanding of the event and clarifies any misconceptions.

LABORATORY ASSESSMENT

SERUM MARKERS OF MYOCARDIAL DAMAGE: CARDIAC ENZYMES. An MI can be confirmed by abnormally high blood levels of cardiac enzymes and isoenzymes. Of all the cardiac enzymes, **creatine kinase (CK)** is considered the most sensitive and reliable indicator for diagnosis of MI. Total CK levels rise within 3 hours after the onset of chest pain and peak within 24 hours after damage and death of cardiac tissue. Because total CK also rises with brain or muscle injury, an elevation is not specific for myocardial damage.

When cardiac muscle tissue dies, the CK specific to myocardial cells (CK-MB isoenzyme) enters the bloodstream (serum does not normally contain CK-MB isoenzyme). Peak elevation of CK-MB isoenzyme levels occurs approximately 12 to 24 hours after the onset of chest pain; levels return to normal 48 to 72 hours later. Confirmation of myocardial damage within 2 hours of emergency department admission is possible with the use of stat determinations of CK and CK subforms. These are gaining popularity as a result of the need to confirm or rule out MI rapidly.

The physician may also use serum measurement of lactate dehydrogenase (LDH) to confirm MI. However, identification of LDH is not as reliable as that of CK-MB. LDH levels start to rise within 12 to 24 hours after an MI, peak between 48 and 72 hours, and fall to normal in 7 days. Thus they may be useful in diagnosing an MI in a client who has delayed seeking medical help for several days after the onset of chest discomfort. Serum levels of LDH_1 isoenzyme rise higher than serum levels of LDH_2 in the presence of MI. Newer measurements for detection of cardiac damage, such as troponins T and I, are gaining in popularity for this purpose, since they are more sensitive and specific than LDH. (See Chapter 33 for a more detailed discussion of cardiac enzymes.)

OTHER SERUM MARKERS OF MYOCARDIAL DAMAGE. **Myoglobin** is a heme protein found in both skeletal and cardiac muscle. It is released rapidly following myocardial damage and can be detected in the serum in 2 to 3 hours following an MI. Since myoglobin always elevates within 3 to 6 hours following an MI, if it has not increased by 6 hours, it can be determined that an MI has not occurred.

Troponins T and I are basic components of the myocardium that are not found in significant levels in the blood of healthy adults. They begin to elevate 3 to 6 hours after an MI and remain elevated for 5 to 7 days. Elevation of troponin T is specific for acute coronary syndromes, identifying the development of unstable angina, subendocardial MI, or MI. Rapid bedside assays are becoming available for the measurement of troponins T and I.

No laboratory test can confirm the diagnosis of stable angina. Serum enzyme determinations are not useful in assessing the presence of angina. However, serum markers of myocardial damage remaining within normal limits are an indication that the client has not had an acute MI.

The **C-reactive protein (CRP)** test is also helpful in determining whether the client has had an acute MI. The level of CRP (normal is 0) correlates with CK-MB levels, but CRP peaks several days later. Levels of CRP are not elevated in clients who have angina.

OTHER LABORATORY TESTS. The finding of an elevated white blood cell count (10,000 to 20,000 cells/mm^3) helps in the diagnosis of MI. It typically appears on the second day and lasts up to a week.

RADIOGRAPHIC ASSESSMENT

Unless there is associated cardiac dysfunction (e.g., valvular disease) or heart failure, a chest x-ray film is not diagnostic for angina or MI.

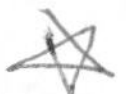

OTHER DIAGNOSTIC ASSESSMENT

ELECTROCARDIOGRAPHY. Twelve-lead electrocardiograms (ECGs) allow the health care provider to examine the heart from varying perspectives and note both the occurrence and the location of ischemia (angina) or necrosis (infarction).

Ischemic myocardium does not repolarize normally. Thus 12-lead ECGs obtained during an anginal episode reveal ST depression, T-wave inversion, or both. **Variant angina,** caused by coronary spasm, usually causes elevation of the ST segment during anginal attacks. These ST- and T-wave changes usually subside when the ischemia is resolved and the pain is relieved. However, the T wave may remain flat or inverted for a period of time. If the client is not experiencing angina at the moment of the test, the ECG for the client with angina is usually normal.

When infarction occurs, three ECG changes are usually observed: ST-segment elevation, T-wave inversion, and an abnormal Q wave (wider than 0.04 seconds or more than one third the height of the QRS complex). Figure 38-2 displays the typical ECG changes seen in MI.

The Q wave develops because necrotic cells do not conduct electrical stimuli. Hours to days after the MI, the ST-segment and T-wave changes will return to normal, but the Q wave usually remains permanently. By identifying the lead in which the ECG changes are occurring, the health care provider can identify the extent and location of the infarction.

STRESS TEST. After the acute stages of an anginal episode or MI, the health care provider often orders an **exercise tolerance test (stress test)** to assess for ECG changes consistent with ischemia, evaluate medical therapy, and identify clients who might benefit from referral for invasive therapy.

SCANS. *Thallium* scans use radioisotope imaging to assess for ischemia or necrotic muscle tissue related to angina or MI. Areas of decreased or absent perfusion, referred to as cold spots, identify ischemia or infarction. *Multigated acquisition* (MUGA) scans may be used to evaluate left ventricular function.

CARDIAC CATHETERIZATION. This procedure may be performed to determine the extent and location of obstructions of the coronary arteries. Cardiac catheterization, the "gatekeeper" to invasive management, allows the cardiologist and cardiac surgeon to identify clients who might benefit from percutaneous transluminal angioplasty (PCTA) or coronary artery bypass grafting (CABG). Each of these tests is described in detail in Chapter 33.

Analysis

The client with coronary artery disease (CAD) may have either angina or myocardial infarction (MI). If MI is suspected or cannot be completely ruled out, the client is admitted to a coronary or critical care unit for continuous monitoring.

COMMON NURSING DIAGNOSES AND COLLABORATIVE PROBLEMS

The following are common nursing diagnoses for clients with CAD:

1. Acute Pain related to imbalance between myocardial oxygen supply and demand
2. Ineffective Tissue Perfusion (Cardiopulmonary) related to interruption of blood flow
3. Activity Intolerance related to imbalance between oxygen supply and demand
4. Ineffective Coping related to effects of acute illness, major changes in lifestyle, or loss of control over a body part

For the client experiencing an MI, the following are the most important collaborative problems:

1. Potential for Dysrhythmias
2. Potential for Heart Failure
3. Potential for Recurrent Chest Discomfort and Extension of Injury

ADDITIONAL NURSING DIAGNOSES AND COLLABORATIVE PROBLEMS

In addition to the common nursing diagnoses and collaborative problems, clients with CAD may have one or more of the following:

- Fear related to threat of death
- Ineffective Sexuality Patterns related to pain and effects of illness
- Impaired Physical Mobility related to pain or fear of movement

Planning and Implementation

ACUTE PAIN

NOC **PLANNING: EXPECTED OUTCOMES.** The client with CAD is expected to state that chest discomfort is alleviated.

INTERVENTIONS. The objective of management is to eliminate chest discomfort by providing pain relief, decreasing myocardial oxygen demand, and increasing myocardial oxygen supply.

NIC **PAIN MANAGEMENT.** The nurse evaluates the chest pain, obtains vital signs, ensures the patency of IV accesses, and notifies the physician of the client's condition. Chart 38-3 summarizes appropriate interventions for the client with chest discomfort.

CHART 38-3

BEST PRACTICE *for* Managing the Client with Chest Discomfort

- Obtain the client's description of the chest discomfort.
- Obtain the client's vital signs (blood pressure, pulse, respiration).
- Assess the client's vascular access.
- Consult standing orders or notify the physician for specific intervention.
- Obtain a 12-lead electrocardiogram if indicated.
- Provide pain relief medication and aspirin (ASA) as ordered.
- Administer oxygen therapy as prescribed.
- Remain calm; stay with the client if possible.
- Assess the client's vital signs and intensity of pain 5 minutes after administration of medication.
- Remedicate (if vital signs remain stable), and check the client every 5 minutes.
- Notify the physician if vital signs deteriorate or pain is not relieved after three doses of nitroglycerin.

DRUG THERAPY. If appropriate, the nurse may administer the prescribed pain medication. One of the initial medications prescribed for chest pain is usually sublingual nitroglycerin (Chart 38-4). Aspirin 325 mg also may be administered orally (chewed) immediately if the client is believed to be experiencing an acute coronary syndrome.

Nitroglycerin. **Nitroglycerin,** a nitrate often referred to as "nitro," increases collateral blood flow, redistributes blood flow toward the subendocardium, and causes dilation of the coronary arteries. The nurse instructs the client to hold the tablet under the tongue and provides 5 mL of water, if necessary, to allow the tablet to dissolve. Pain relief should begin within 1 or 2 minutes and be clearly evident in 3 to 5 minutes. After 5 minutes, the nurse rechecks the client's pain intensity and vital signs. If the blood pressure is less than 100 mm Hg systolic or 25 mm Hg lower than the previous reading, the nurse lowers the head of the bed and notifies the physician. If the client is experiencing some but not complete relief and vital signs remain stable, another nitroglycerin tablet may be used. A total of 3 tablets may be administered in an attempt to relieve anginal pain.

Angina usually responds to nitroglycerin. The client typically states that the pain is relieved or markedly diminished. When simple measures, such as taking three sublingual nitroglycerin tablets one after the other, do not relieve chest discomfort, the client may be experiencing an MI. The nurse should inform the physician immediately and prepare the client for transfer to a specialized unit where he or she can be closely monitored and appropriately managed.

In a specialized unit the physician may prescribe IV nitroglycerin for management of the chest pain. The nurse begins the nitroglycerin infusion slowly, checking the blood pressure and pain level every 3 to 5 minutes. The nitroglycerin dose is increased until the pain is relieved, the blood pressure falls excessively, or the maximum prescribed dose is reached. The blood pressure is continuously monitored (Chart 38-5).

Morphine Sulfate. The physician may prescribe morphine sulfate (MS) to relieve chest discomfort that is unresponsive to nitroglycerin. Morphine relieves MI pain, decreases myocardial oxygen demand, and reduces circulating catecholamines. It is usually administered in 2- to 5-mg increments intravenously every 5 to 15 minutes until the maximum prescribed dose is reached or until the client experiences relief or signs of toxicity. Signs of morphine toxicity include respiratory depression, hypotension, and severe vomiting.

The nurse monitors the client's vital signs and cardiac rhythm every few minutes. These strategies are often enough to relieve the pain. If these methods are not adequate, additional interventions, identified later under Ineffective Tissue Perfusion (Cardiopulmonary), p. 798, may be attempted.

OTHER INTERVENTIONS. Several interventions may assist in relieving chest pain. Supplemental oxygen may increase

CHART 38-4

DRUG THERAPY *for* Coronary Artery Disease

Drug	Usual Dosage	Nursing Interventions	Rationale
NITRATES			
Nitroglycerin (Nitrostat, Tridil)	0.3-0.4 mg q5min sublingually, up to 3 tablets	Instruct the client to lie down with the head of the bed at a level of comfort when taking the sublingual form.	Hypotension can be dramatic, immediate, and intensified by the upright position.
		Monitor blood pressure. Pay attention to orthostatic changes.	A decrease in blood pressure occurs with vasodilation.
		Instruct the client to allow the sublingal tablet to dissolve and to avoid swallowing the tablet.	The sublingual dose is absorbed through the sublingual mucous membranes.
		Check the expiration date on sublingual tablets. Tablets should be replaced every 3-5 mo.	The efficacy of the tablets decreases with time.
		Determine whether pain is relieved.	Additional medication may be required to relieve pain.
		Monitor for headache.	Vasodilation is generalized.
Isosorbide dinitrate (Isordil, Iso-Bid)	2.5 mg q4-6h sublingually 5-30 mg qid PO	Instruct the client taking sublingual forms to lie down before administration.	The hypotensive effect can be dramatic and immediate with sublingual administration.
	40-mg sustained-release tablet 2-3 times daily	Monitor blood pressure and assess for dizziness.	A decrease in blood pressure occurs with vasodilation.
Isosorbide mononitrate	60-mg extended-release tablet qd	Schedule sustained-release form with an 8 to 12 hr dose-free interval.	Tolerance may develop.
Nitroglycerin patch (Nitro-Bid Patch)	Transdermally started at 5 mg/24 hr (10-cm^2 system)	Remove the patch from the client before defibrillation.	The client may develop a burn.
		Rotate application sites.	Rotation prevents skin irritation.
		Apply the patch to a clean, dry, hairless area.	The drug is better absorbed when the skin is clean, dry, and hairless.
		Remove patch for 8-12 hr each day.	Tolerance will develop.
BETA BLOCKERS			
Propranolol (Inderal)	10-80 mg bid-qid to 240 mg/day PO 1-3 mg at rate not to exceed 1 mg/min IV	Assess heart rate before administration.	Beta-blocking effects cause a decrease in heart rate.
		Monitor blood pressure.	The hypotensive effect is due to a decrease in cardiac output, suppressed renin activity, and beta-blocking effects.
		Observe for signs of heart failure.	Heart failure may occur as a result of a decrease in cardiac output.
		Assess for shortness of breath and wheezing.	Beta$_2$-blocking effects in the lungs can cause bronchoconstriction.
Metoprolol (Lopressor, Betaloc🍁), a cardioselective beta-adrenergic blocker	100-450 mg/day PO 5 mg IV over 2 min may be repeated twice for a total of 15 mg	Assess heart rate before administration; do not administer if heart rate <50.	Beta blockers may cause further decreases in heart rate.
		Monitor BP and hold for systolic <90.	Decreased blood pressure is an anticipated effect.
		Assess client for cough, shortness of breath, edema, and weight gain.	These are indications of heart failure.
CALCIUM CHANNEL BLOCKERS			
Nifedipine (Procardia, Adalat)	10-30 mg tid PO or sublingually	Monitor blood pressure and assess for dizziness.	Vasodilation can cause dramatic hypotension, which occurs within minutes, especially after sublingual administration.
		Assess for headache and edema of the lower extremities.	These are common side effects.

SA, Sinoatrial; *AV*, atrioventricular.

Continued

CHART 38-4

DRUG THERAPY *for* Coronary Artery Disease—cont'd

Drug	Usual Dosage	Nursing Interventions	Rationale
Verapamil hydrochloride (Calan, Isoptin)	40-80 mg qid PO or 120- to 240-mg sustained-release tablet once a day	Monitor heart rate.	This agent slows SA and AV node conduction.
	5-10 mg over 2 min IV	Monitor blood pressure and assess for dizziness.	Vasodilation decreases blood pressure.
		Assess for constipation.	This is a common side effect.
Diltiazem hydrochloride (Cardizem)	30-60 mg qid PO or 120- to 480-mg sustained-release tablet once a day; increase dose slowly	Monitor blood pressure and assess for dizziness.	Vasodilation decreases blood pressure.
		Monitor heart rate.	This drug slows SA and AV node conduction, but the decrease is not as great as that which occurs with verapamil.
ANTIPLATELET AGENTS			
Aspirin (Empirin, Apo-ASA✤)	80-325 mg PO	Suggest that the client take the daily dose with food.	Gastric irritation may occur.
		Question the client about ringing in the ears.	Tinnitus may occur with aspirin toxicity.
		Emphasize to the client that aspirin is an important cardiac medication and should be continued unless the client is told to stop.	Studies document significantly better survival rates for clients with coronary artery disease receiving aspirin.

SA, Sinoatrial; *AV,* atrioventricular.

the amount of oxygen available to myocardial tissue. Therefore oxygen is often prescribed and administered at a flow of 2 to 4 L/min by nasal cannula titrated to maintain an arterial oxygen saturation (Sa_{O_2}) greater than 92%. If the blood pressure is stable, the nurse may assist the client in assuming any position of comfort. Placing the client in semi-Fowler's position often enhances comfort and tissue oxygenation. A quiet, calm environment and explanations of interventions often reduce anxiety and assist in relief of chest pain.

When the pain has subsided and the client is stabilized, the physician may change the medication to an oral or topical nitrate. During administration of long-term oral and topical nitrates, a 12-hour nitrate-free period should be maintained to prevent tolerance. The client may complain initially of headache. The physician may prescribe acetaminophen (Tylenol, Exdol✤) to be taken before the nitrate to prevent some of this discomfort.

CRITICAL THINKING CHALLENGE

A 45-year-old businessman arrives in the emergency department complaining of severe chest pain (9 on a scale of 0 to 10) radiating down his left arm. The pain began in the left antecubital space and spread to the left side of his chest. He received 2 nitroglycerin tablets and 1 aspirin in the ambulance during transport.

- What are the essential elements of the initial assessment?
- What are the priorities for care at this time?

For suggested answer guidelines, go to SIMON http://www.wbsaunders.com/SIMON/Iggy/.

INEFFECTIVE TISSUE PERFUSION (CARDIOPULMONARY)

NOC **PLANNING: EXPECTED OUTCOMES.** The client with coronary artery disease (CAD) is expected to exhibit (1) relief of chest discomfort, (2) resolution of ST-segment and T-wave changes, (3) sinus rhythm (or normal rhythm for the client) of approximately 60, and (4) blood pressure within an acceptable range.

INTERVENTIONS. Because myocardial infarction (MI) is a dynamic process, restoration of perfusion to the injured area often reduces the size of the infarct and improves left ventricular function. Complete, sustained reperfusion of coronary arteries in the first few hours after an MI has decreased mortality in clients with MI.

THROMBOLYTIC THERAPY. Fibrinolytics are used to dissolve thrombi in the coronary arteries and restore myocardial blood flow. Examples of these agents, which target the fibrin component of the coronary thrombosis, include tissue plasminogen activator (t-PA, alteplase [Activase]), anisoylated plasminogen-streptokinase activator complex (APSAC), and reteplase (Retavase). The physician may order the administration of fibrinolytics intravenously or by the intracoronary route during cardiac catheterization. Thrombolytic agents are most effective when administered within the first 6 hours of the coronary event. Thrombolytics are underused nationwide in men and women, young and old.

Thrombolytic therapy should be given in a unit where the client can be continuously monitored. It is indicated for clients who have chest pain of greater than 30 minutes' duration that is unrelieved by nitroglycerin, with indications of transmural ischemia and injury as shown by the ECG. Contraindications include recent abdominal surgery or stroke, because bleeding may occur when fresh clots are lysed (broken down). Table 38-2 lists the current contraindications to thrombolytic therapy.

Before thrombolytic administration, the nurse may need to apply pressure dressings to IV puncture sites or wounds to limit bleeding. Clients who weigh less than 65 kg may need to have their dose of thrombolytic weight adjusted to lessen the likeli-

CHART 38-5

DRUG THERAPY *with* Commonly Used Intravenous Vasodilators and Inotropes

Drug	Usual Dosage	Nursing Interventions	Rationale
Nitroprusside sodium (Nipride, Nitropress)	IV only by infusion device Begin with 0.2 μg/kg/min May increase gradually to 10 μg/kg/min	Monitor BP q2-5 min when initiating therapy. If BP drops excessively, elevate the legs, decrease the dose, and increase fluids per unit policy.	This agent is a potent, rapidly reversible vasodilator acting on both peripheral venous and arterial musculature. BP may drop in 2 min.
		Monitor PAWP, SVR, BP, heart rate, and urine output frequently.	
		Titrate medication to obtain the desired effect.	
		Protect from light.	This agent is light sensitive.
		Maintain dose at less than 3 μg/min if possible.	Doses >3 μg/min are associated with thiocyanate or cyanide toxicity.
		In clients requiring doses >3 μg/min for >24-36 hr, monitor for metabolic acidosis, confusion, or hyperreflexia. Examine blood thiocyanate level.	These are indications of the toxic effects of cyanide.
Nitroglycerin (Tridil)	IV only by infusion device started at 0.3 μg/min and gradually increased in increments of 3 μg/min until maximum of 20 μg/min	Monitor BP q1-3min when initiating therapy. If BP drops excessively, elevate the legs and decrease the dose according to unit policies.	This agent dilates coronary arteries. It is a more potent systemic venodilator than an arterial vasodilator. BP may drop in 1 min.
		Monitor RAP, PAWP, SVR, BP, heart rate, and urine output frequently.	
		Titrate medication to obtain the desired effect.	
		Intermittent administration of IV nitroglycerin should be considered.	Tolerance may develop rapidly to nitroglycerin administered by continuous IV.
		Monitor the client for headache.	Headache is a frequent side effect of initial nitroglycerin therapy.
SYMPATHOMIMETICS			
Dopamine (Intropin)	IV only by infusion device Starting dose 2-5 μg/kg/min Titrate up to 20 μg/kg/min	Determine the reason for use and the expected result.	This agent is a dose-dependent activator of alpha, beta, and dopaminergic receptors.
		Observe the client's heart rate, ECG, BP, PAWP, SVR, CO, and urine output q5min to q1h.	2-5 μg/kg/min stimulates dopaminergic receptors, which promotes renal and mesenteric blood flow.
		Titrate the dose carefully to maintain the dose range and obtain the desired effect.	5 μg/kg/min stimulates beta receptors. This increases heart rate and contractility. >10-15 μg/kg/min, alpha effects predominate. This causes peripheral constriction.
		Infuse through a central catheter.	Extravasation can cause tissue necrosis and sloughing.
		Monitor the client for ectopy and angina.	These are adverse effects.
Dobutamine (Dobutrex)	IV only by infusion device, 2-10 μg/kg/min	Observe the client continuously during administration.	This agent is a very strong $beta_1$-receptor activator and a moderately strong $beta_2$ activator.
		Titrate the drug on the basis of heart rate, ECG findings, BP, PAWP, CO, SVR, and urine output.	
		Monitor for atrial and ventricular ectopy.	Dysrhythmias are an adverse effect.

PAWP, Pulmonary artery wedge pressure; *SVR,* systemic vascular resistance; *RAP,* right atrial pressure; *ECG,* electrocardiogram; *CO,* cardiac output.

TABLE 38-2 • CONTRAINDICATIONS TO THROMBOLYTIC THERAPY

ABSOLUTE
- Active internal bleeding
- Cerebrovascular processes
  - Recent stroke (within 2 months)
  - Recent spinal or cerebral surgery
  - Cranial neoplasm
- Prolonged cardiopulmonary resuscitation (CPR)

RELATIVE
- Endocarditis or pericarditis
- Hemostatic defects
- Severe uncontrolled hypertension
- Pregnancy or recent delivery
- Trauma within last 10 days
- Surgery within last 10 days

hood of bleeding. During administration, the nurse immediately reports any indications of bleeding to the physician. After administration, the nurse observes for signs of bleeding by:

- Documenting the client's neurologic status
- Observing all IV sites
- Monitoring clotting studies
- Observing for signs of internal bleeding (watching hemoglobin and hematocrit)
- Testing stools, urine, and emesis for occult blood

Some concerns in thrombolytic administration are associated with the specific agent. For example, *streptokinase,* a first-generation thrombolytic agent, is not fibrin specific; thus it may create systemic bleeding problems. Because it is a bacterial protein, streptokinase can cause a hypersensitivity reaction in the client who has had previous exposure. Therefore the nurse questions the client about streptococcal infections or doses of streptokinase within the past year. To prevent an allergic reaction, the physician may prescribe steroids or antihistamines before the administration of streptokinase. During administration, the nurse observes the client closely for hives and shivering, the most common responses. The half-life of the drug is 16 minutes.

Second- and third-generation fibrinolytics include tissue plasminogen activator (t-PA, alteplase [Activase]), anisoylated plasminogen-streptokinase activator complex (APSAC; Eminase), reteplase (Retavase), and lanoteplase (n-PA). t-PA is fibrin specific, has a short half-life (3 to 5 minutes), and lacks antigenicity. Because some studies have associated t-PA with a more frequent occurrence of cerebrovascular bleeding, the nurse carefully documents neurologic findings. t-PA is also much more expensive than streptokinase. Reteplase can be given in two boluses ½ hour apart, need not be weight adjusted, and results in greater rates of reperfusion than t-PA. APSAC is a streptokinase derivative; it has a longer half-life (90 to 105 minutes) than streptokinase but has the same antigenic properties.

Tenecteplase (TNKase) is the most recent fibrinolytic to be approved for use in clients with MIs. This drug appears to have some advantages over other fibrinolytics. First, it can be easily administered as a single bolus over 5 seconds. Tenecteplase also targets clots more specifically than other fibrinolytics, resulting in slightly less overall bleeding. However, bleeding is still possible, and nursing considerations are similar to the other fibrinolytics. Dosage is based on the client's weight.

GLYCOPROTEIN IIB/IIIA INHIBITORS. Glycoprotein (GP) IIb/IIIa inhibitors target the platelet component of the thrombus. Abciximab (ReoPro), eptifibatide (Integrilin), and tirofiban (Aggrastat) may be administered intravenously to prevent fibrinogen from attaching to activated platelets at the site of a thrombus. These medications have been used in acute coronary syndromes (especially unstable angina and non–Q-wave MI) during and before percutaneous transluminal coronary angioplasty (PTCA) to ensure patency of the newly opened artery and in conjunction with fibrinolytic agents following MI. If the GP IIb/IIIa inhibitors are used with a fibrinolytic agent, then the dose of the thrombolytic should be reduced by 25% to 50% to decrease the likelihood of bleeding. Combining a GP IIa/IIIb inhibitor with a fibrinolytic agent following MI appears to improve coronary flow without increasing the risk of hemorrhagic events (Roberts, 1999). During the administration of GP IIa/IIIb inhibitors, the nurse assesses the client closely for indications of bleeding or hypersensitivity reactions. If either occurs, the health care provider is notified immediately regarding administration of the appropriate medications (e.g., antihistamines or corticosteroids) for a hypersensitivity response.

For some clients experiencing an MI, primary PTCA may be used to reopen the thrombosed coronary artery. PTCA has been associated with excellent return of blood flow through the coronary artery when it can be performed within 70 minutes of the onset of chest discomfort by a highly experienced practitioner. However, most community hospitals are not capable of performing emergent PTCA. When primary PTCA is not available, the client with MI should receive immediate thrombolytic agents if he or she is an appropriate candidate. PTCA is described in detail later in this chapter.

IDENTIFICATION OF CORONARY ARTERY REPERFUSION. The nurse monitors the client for indications that the clot has been lysed and the artery reperfused. These indications include the following:

- Abrupt cessation of chest pain
- Sudden onset of ventricular dysrhythmias
- Resolution of ST-segment depression
- A peak at 12 hours of markers of myocardial damage

After clot lysis with thrombolytics, large amounts of thrombin are released into the system, increasing the risk of vessel reocclusion. To maintain the patency of the coronary artery after thrombolytic therapy, the physician usually prescribes aspirin and IV heparin. The nurse monitors the activated partial thromboplastin time (aPTT)—the usual appropriate range is 1½ to 2½ times the control sample)—and maintains the heparin infusion for 3 to 5 days, as prescribed. Low–molecular weight heparin (enoxaparin) may be substituted for IV heparin.

CRITICAL THINKING CHALLENGE

A client diagnosed with an MI has ST-segment elevations in anterior and lateral wall leads. The physician offers him a choice of emergent PTCA or thrombolytic therapy. The client is in severe pain, afraid, and unable to decide what to do.

- What are the advantages and contraindications to immediate thrombolysis?
- What are the advantages and disadvantages of primary PTCA for the client?

See the Legal/Ethical Issues in Health Care box on p. 801 for a discussion of the dilemma of requiring a client to provide informed consent under such stressful conditions.

For suggested answer guidelines, go to SIMON http://www.wbsaunders.com/SIMON/Iggy/.

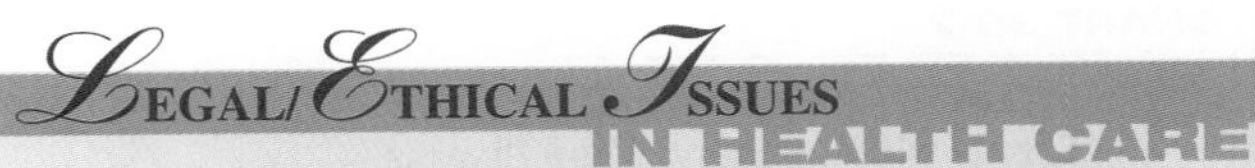

IS INFORMED CONSENT POSSIBLE IN EMERGENT SITUATIONS?

Twenty-five years ago, physicians consistently provided care with a paternalistic, "father knows best," approach. They decided what care was best for their clients and provided it with little input from them. For the past 15 years, there has been a movement toward client autonomy—the belief that clients should have the final say in their medical care. To ensure that they understand their options, many ethicists, lawyers, and health care providers have supported the concept of informed consent.

Informed consent has three important components: the client must be competent, must understand his or her treatment options, and must make his or her choice freely without coercion by family or health care providers. The information provided to the client should include the following:

- Nature and purpose of the proposed treatment
- Expected outcome and likelihood of success
- Risks involved
- Alternatives to treatment
- Effect of no treatment

Unfortunately, health care is frequently provided in an emotionally charged atmosphere with clients in pain, hypoxic, or incapacitated. In addition, care to clients experiencing an MI must be provided almost immediately, and there is little opportunity for them to weigh and evaluate options.

Some ethicists would argue that asking a client experiencing pain and anxiety to make a decision about care represents a distortion of informed consent. They might argue that the client had presented himself for emergent care and was therefore implying consent to standard treatment for that emergency. Benjamin and Curtis (1992) contend that it is appropriate for health care providers to act paternalistically and make health care decisions for clients in the following limited situations:

- If the client is incompetent or incapacitated and unable to make a rational decision
- If there is likely to be significant harm to the client if a decision is not made
- If the client is likely to approve of the decision when and if his or her capacity to make rational decisions is restored

The client would meet Benjamin and Curtis's criteria for a paternalistic decision.

Implications for Nursing

In collaboration with the health care provider, it is the nurse's responsibility to be sure that the client desires and comprehends the medical and nursing care that is being provided. That usually entails ensuring that the client is fully informed and voluntarily consenting to the treatment. However, in some emergent situations or incapacitated clients, fully informed consent may not be reasonable or possible. In such situations, Benjamin and Curtis's criteria for making a paternalistic decision might be applied.

DRUG THERAPY. Clients who have had an MI, whether receiving thrombolytics or not, should begin aspirin therapy unless contraindicated. They may receive a chewable aspirin immediately and then an enteric-coated aspirin (Ancasal🍁, Ecotrin) 80 to 325 mg daily or every other day to prevent platelet aggregation at the site of the obstruction.

Beta-adrenergic blocking agents (e.g., metoprolol [Lopressor, Betaloc🍁]) decrease the size of the infarct, ventricular dysrhythmias, and mortality rates in clients with MI. The physician usually prescribes a cardioselective beta-blocking agent within the first 24 hours after an MI. Beta blockers slow the heart rate and decrease the force of cardiac contraction. Thus these agents prolong the period of diastole and increase myocardial perfusion while reducing the force of myocardial contraction. With beta blockade, the heart is capable of performing 25% to 30% more work without ischemia. During beta-blocking therapy, the nurse:

- Monitors the heart rate (bradycardia is common)
- Checks the blood pressure
- Measures the PR interval
- Checks the level of consciousness
- Monitors for any chest discomfort

The nurse assesses the lungs for crackles (indicative of heart failure) and wheezes (indicative of bronchospasm). Hypoglycemia, depression, nightmares, and forgetfulness are also problems with beta blockade, especially in older clients (see Chart 38-6).

Physicians frequently prescribe angiotensin-converting enzyme (ACE) inhibitors within 48 hours of an MI to prevent ventricular remodeling and the development of heart failure. ACE inhibitors have been demonstrated to increase survival after an MI. The nurse monitors the client for hypotension, cough, and changes in serum potassium, creatinine, and blood urea nitrogen. (See Chapter 35 for a more detailed discussion of ACE inhibitors.)

For clients with angina, the health care provider may prescribe calcium channel blockers to enhance vasodilation and myocardial perfusion. Calcium channel blockers are indicated for clients with variant angina or for those who are hypertensive and continue to have angina despite therapy with beta blockers. They are not indicated after an MI. The nurse monitors the client receiving calcium channel blockers for hypotension and headaches and reviews the frequency of anginal episodes.

The recent Clopidogrel in Unstable Angina to Prevent Recurrent Ischemic Events (CURE) study showed that the combination of clopidogrel (Plavix) and aspirin was more effective in reducing death, MI, and stroke when compared to aspirin alone. The risk of bleeding from using two antiplatelet agents together was not significantly increased (Palatnik, 2001).

ACTIVITY INTOLERANCE

NOC **PLANNING: EXPECTED OUTCOMES.** The client with coronary artery disease (CAD) is expected to walk at least 200 feet four times a day without chest discomfort or shortness of breath.

INTERVENTIONS. Activity intolerance is reduced by a planned program of cardiac rehabilitation implemented primarily by the nurse and physical therapist.

NIC **CARDIAC CARE REHABILITATION. Cardiac rehabilitation** is the process of actively assisting the client with cardiac disease in achieving and maintaining a vital and productive life while remaining within the limits of the heart's ability to respond to increases in activity and stress. It can be divided into three phases. *Phase 1* begins with the acute illness and ends with discharge from the hospital. *Phase 2* begins after discharge and continues through convalescence at home. *Phase 3* refers to long-term conditioning.

In the acute phase (phase 1), the nurse promotes rest and yet ensures some limited mobility. Assistance is provided for some activities of daily living (ADLs), such as bathing and toileting. Clients progress at their own rate to increasing levels of activity, depending on their clinical status, age, and physical capabilities. For example, for the first 24 hours, the client may be restricted to bedrest but allowed to stand to void or to use the bedside commode. The second day, the client

CHART 38-6

NURSING FOCUS *on the* OLDER ADULT
Coronary Artery Disease

- Recognize that chest pain may not be evident in the older client; associated symptoms, such as dyspnea and confusion, may prevail.
- Although older adults have a greater reduction in mortality from myocardial infarction (MI) with the use of thrombolytics, they also have the most severe side effects. Monitor older clients receiving thrombolytics extremely carefully.
- Dysrhythmia may be a normal age-related change rather than a complication of MI. Determine whether the dysrhythmia is causing significant symptoms, then notify the physician.
- If beta blockers are used, assess the client carefully for the development of side effects. Exacerbation of the depression already present in older adults is a significant problem with beta blockade.
- Plan slow, steady increases in activity. Older adults with minimal previous exercise show particular benefit from a gradual increase in activity.
- Older adults should plan longer warm-up and cool-down periods when participating in an exercise program. Their pulse rates may not return to baseline until 30 minutes or longer after exercise.

may be out of bed sitting in a chair as tolerated, usually for 30 minutes three times a day.

The next step in phase 1 is ambulation of the client in the room and to the bathroom. The nurse encourages progressive ambulation in the hallway, usually 50, 100, and then 200 feet three times a day. In addition, the client may begin showering for 5 or 10 minutes with warm water; a stool should be available for him or her to sit on if necessary.

The nurse assesses the client's heart rate, blood pressure, respiratory rate, and level of fatigue with each higher level of activity. Decreases greater than 20 mm Hg in the systolic blood pressure, changes of 20 beats/min in the pulse rate, and complaints of dyspnea or chest pain indicate intolerance of activity. When such signs and symptoms develop, the nurse notifies the physician and does not advance the client to the next level. Older adults with CAD often have needs and concerns different from those of younger adults (Chart 38-6).

CHART 38-7

NIC INTERVENTION ACTIVITIES *for* Clients with Coronary Artery Disease

Pain Management: *Alleviation of pain or reduction of pain to a level of comfort that is acceptable to the patient*
- Perform a comprehensive assessment of pain to include location, characteristics, onset/duration, frequency, quality, intensity or severity of pain, and precipitating factors.
- Verify level of discomfort with client, note changes in the medical record, inform other health professionals working with the client.
- Ensure that the client receives attentive analgesic care.
- Determine the needed frequency of making an assessment of client comfort and implement monitoring plan.
- Evaluate the effectiveness of the pain control measures used through thorough ongoing assessment of the pain experience.

Cardiac Care: Rehabilitative: *Promotion of maximum functional activity level for a client who has suffered an episode of impaired cardiac function that resulted from an imbalance between myocardial oxygen supply and demand*
- Monitor the client's activity tolerance.
- Maintain ambulation schedule, as tolerated.
- Instruct the client and family on the exercise regimen, including warm-up, endurance, and cool-down as appropriate.
- Instruct the client and family on any lifting/pushing weight limitations, if appropriate.
- Encourage realistic expectations for the client and family.

Coping Enhancement: *Assisting a client to adapt to perceived stressors, changes, or threats that interfere with meeting life demands and roles*
- Appraise the client's understanding of the disease process.
- Use a calm, reassuring approach.
- Provide an atmosphere of acceptance.
- Assist the client in developing an objective appraisal of the event.
- Help client to identify the information he or she is most interested in obtaining.
- Provide factual information concerning diagnosis, treatment, and prognosis.
- Foster constructive outlets for anger and hostility.
- Explore with the client previous methods of dealing with life problems.
- Support the use of appropriate defense mechanisms.

NIC intervention activities selected from McCloskey, J.C., & Bulechek, G.M. (2000). *Nursing interventions classification (NIC)* (3rd ed.). St. Louis: Mosby.

INEFFECTIVE COPING

PLANNING: EXPECTED OUTCOMES. The client with CAD is expected to indicate a reduction in anxiety and recognize the beginning of control over life.

INTERVENTIONS. The nurse assesses the client's level of anxiety while allowing him or her to express any anxiety and attempt to define its origin. Simple, repeated explanations of therapies, expectations, and surroundings may help relieve anxiety.

NIC **COPING ENHANCEMENT.** During the acute phase of illness, the physician may prescribe anxiolytic (antianxiety) medications, such as alprazolam (Xanax). The nurse identifies the client's current coping mechanisms; the most common are denial, anger, and depression.

Denial allows the client to minimize a threat and use problem-focused coping mechanisms. He or she may avoid discussing what has happened yet comply with treatment regimens. This type of denial decreases anxiety, and the nurse should not discourage it. However, denial that results in a client's "acting out" and refusing to follow treatment regimens can be harmful. Because this behavior is usually due to extreme anxiety or fear, threats only worsen the behavior. The nurse remains calm and avoids confronting the client but clearly indicates when a behavior is not acceptable and is potentially harmful.

Anger may represent an attempt to regain control of life. The nurse encourages the client to verbalize the source of frustration and provides opportunities for decision making and control.

Depression may be a client's response to grief and loss of function. The nurse listens as the client verbalizes feelings of loss, being careful not to offer false or general reassurances. Depression is acknowledged, but the client is expected to perform ADLs and other activities within restrictions. The nurse identifies all improvements in the client's condition and shares them with him or her. Chart 38-7 summarizes the major NIC intervention activities for clients with CAD.

POTENTIAL FOR DYSRHYTHMIAS

PLANNING: EXPECTED OUTCOMES. The client with CAD is expected to resume a normal sinus rhythm or normal rhythm for the client and be hemodynamically stable.

INTERVENTIONS. Dysrhythmias are the cause of death in most clients with myocardial infarction (MI) who die before they can be hospitalized. Even in the early period of hospitalization, 70% to 90% of clients with MI experience some abnormality of cardiac rhythm. Whenever a dysrhythmia develops in a client with CAD, the cardiac nurse:

- Identifies the dysrhythmia
- Assesses the client's hemodynamic status
- Evaluates the client for chest discomfort

Dysrhythmias are treated when they are causing hemodynamic compromise, are increasing myocardial oxygen requirements, or predispose to lethal ventricular dysrhythmias.

INFERIOR MYOCARDIAL INFARCTION. Typical dysrhythmias for the client with an *inferior* MI are bradycardias and second-degree AV blocks resulting from ischemia of the AV node. These rhythms tend to be transient. The nurse monitors the cardiac rhythm and rate, and the hemodynamic status. If the client becomes hemodynamically unstable, a temporary pacemaker may be necessary.

ANTERIOR MYOCARDIAL INFARCTION. The client with an *anterior* MI is likely to exhibit ventricular irritability (premature ventricular contractions [PVCs]). Third-degree or bundle branch block is a serious complication in the client with an anterior MI, because it indicates that a large portion of the left ventricle is involved. The physician may insert a pacemaker. The nurse should observe the client closely to detect the development of heart failure. Appropriate interventions for dysrhythmias are described in Chapter 34.

POTENTIAL FOR HEART FAILURE

PLANNING: EXPECTED OUTCOMES. The client with coronary artery disease (CAD) is expected to regain hemodynamic stability as evidenced by the following:

- Blood pressure and pulse rate within the client's acceptable range
- Adequate urine output
- Mental alertness
- Clear lungs on auscultation
- Palpable peripheral pulses

INTERVENTIONS. Decreased cardiac output related to heart failure is a relatively common complication after an MI. After an MI the client may experience heart failure as a result of left ventricular dysfunction, rupture of the intraventricular septum, papillary muscle rupture with valvular dysfunction, or right ventricular infarction. The most severe form of heart failure, *cardiogenic shock* (described on p. 804), accounts for most in-hospital deaths after an MI. The type of management used to increase cardiac output depends on the location of the MI and the type of heart failure that resulted from the infarction.

MANAGING LEFT VENTRICULAR FAILURE. When a client with MI experiences damage to the left ventricle, rupture of the intraventricular septum, or tear of a papillary muscle, a reduction occurs in the amount of blood that the heart can eject. This reduction in ejection fraction results in a decreased cardiac output and greater left ventricular residual volumes. Volume and pressure increase first in the left ventricle and eventually in the pulmonary vasculature. When volume and pressure are markedly increased in the pulmonary vasculature, pulmonary complications develop.

TABLE 38-3 • KILLIP CLASSIFICATION OF HEART FAILURE

Class	Description
I	Absent crackles and S_3
II	Crackles in the lower half of the lung fields and possible S_3
III	Crackles more than halfway up the lung fields and frequent pulmonary edema
IV	Cardiogenic shock

NURSING ASSESSMENT AND MONITORING. The development of left ventricular failure and pulmonary edema is assessed by auscultating for crackles and identifying their location in the lung fields. Wheezing, tachypnea, and frothy sputum may also occur with pulmonary edema. The nurse auscultates the heart, paying particular attention to the presence of an S_3 heart sound. The nurse monitors for the following signs of poor organ perfusion that may result from decreased cardiac output:

- A change in orientation or mental status
- Urine output less than 1 mL/kg/hr or less than 30 mL/hr
- Cool, clammy extremities with decreased or absent pulses
- Unusual fatigue
- Recurrent chest pain

In specialized units, hemodynamic monitoring may be instituted to assess the client's preload, afterload, and cardiac output. Hemodynamic monitoring in the hospital requires the insertion of a pulmonary artery catheter (see Chapter 33). The cardiac nurse obtains and records hemodynamic measurements, which include right atrial pressure, pulmonary artery systolic and diastolic pressures, pulmonary artery wedge pressure (PAWP) (a measure of preload), systemic vascular resistance (a measure of afterload), cardiac output, and cardiac index. Single values of these measurements are less significant than the trend of values combined with the client's clinical manifestations. These measurements help both the nurse and the physician to identify heart failure and guide the administration of fluids and vasoactive drugs.

CLASSIFICATION OF POSTMYOCARDIAL INFARCTION HEART FAILURE. Killip categorized heart failure after an MI into four classes based on prognosis (Table 38-3).

Class I. Clients with class I heart failure often respond well to reduction in preload with IV diuretics. The nurse monitors the urine output hourly, checks vital signs hourly, continues to assess for signs of heart failure, and reviews the serum potassium level.

Class II and Class III. Clients with class II and class III heart failure may require diuresis and more aggressive medical intervention, such as reduction of afterload or enhancement of contractility. IV nitroprusside or nitroglycerin may be used to decrease both preload and afterload. These drugs are administered as continuous infusions in specialized units where the PAWP and blood pressure can be closely monitored. The blood pressure can drop in response to excessive vasodilation (see Chart 38-5).

Positive inotropes, such as dopamine (Intropin), dobutamine (Dobutrex), and amrinone (Inocor), increase the force of cardiac contraction. They are administered by continuous IV infusion. The effects of these drugs on the vasculature and heart rate vary and may be dose dependent. The nurse must understand the anticipated effect of the drug and the desired dosage range. The infusions are titrated to optimize cardiac output. The nurse uses caution when administering these drugs because of the potential risk of increasing myocardial oxygen consumption and further decreasing cardiac output. The client is frequently monitored, paying particular attention to the development of chest pain.

Class IV: Cardiogenic Shock. Class IV heart failure is cardiogenic shock. In **cardiogenic shock,** necrosis of more than 40% of the left ventricle has occurred. Most clients have a stuttering pattern of chest pain, resulting in piecemeal extension of the MI. Manifestations of cardiogenic shock include the following:

- Tachycardia
- Hypotension
- Blood pressure less than 90 mm Hg, or 30 mm Hg less than the client's baseline
- Urine output less than 30 mL/hr
- Cold, clammy skin with poor peripheral pulses
- Agitation, restlessness, or confusion
- Pulmonary congestion
- Tachypnea
- Continuing chest discomfort

Early detection is essential because established cardiogenic shock has a mortality rate of 65% to 100%.

MEDICAL MANAGEMENT. Medical interventions aim to relieve pain and decrease myocardial oxygen requirements through preload and possibly afterload reduction (see Chart 38-5). The physician orders IV morphine, which is used to decrease pulmonary congestion and relieve pain. Oxygen is administered; intubation and ventilation may be necessary. The nurse uses the information gained from hemodynamic monitoring to titrate drug therapy. Preload reduction may be cautiously attempted with diuretics, nitroglycerin, or nitroprusside, as described for clients with Killip class III heart failure. (See Chapter 35 for a complete discussion of preload and afterload.) Because vasodilation may result in a further decline in blood pressure, the nurse monitors systolic pressure constantly. Vasopressors and positive inotropes may be used to maintain organ perfusion, but such drugs increase myocardial oxygen consumption and can worsen ischemia.

Use of an Intra-Aortic Balloon Pump. When clients do not respond to drug therapy with improved tissue perfusion, decreased workload of the heart, and increased cardiac contractility, an **intra-aortic balloon pump (IABP)** may be inserted. Insertion of an intra-aortic counterpulsation device, such as the IABP, is an invasive intervention that is used to improve myocardial perfusion during an acute MI, reduce afterload, and facilitate left ventricular emptying.

The physician can insert an IABP percutaneously or through surgical cutdown. Inflation of the IABP during diastole increases the diastolic pressure and improves coronary perfusion. Deflation of the balloon just before systole reduces afterload at the time of systolic contraction. This facilitates emptying of the left ventricle and improves cardiac output. The balloon catheter is attached to a pump console, which is triggered by an electrocardiogram (ECG) tracing and arterial waveform (Figure 38-4).

Immediate Reperfusion. Immediate reperfusion is an invasive intervention that shows some promise for clients with cardiogenic shock. The client is taken to the cardiac catheterization laboratory, and an emergency left-sided heart catheterization is performed. If the client has a treatable lesion or lesions, the surgeon performs an immediate percutaneous transluminal coronary angioplasty (PTCA) in the catheterization laboratory, or the client is transferred to the operating suite for a coronary artery bypass graft (CABG).

MANAGING RIGHT VENTRICULAR FAILURE. Conditions other than left ventricular failure may result in decreased cardiac output after an MI. In approximately 30% of clients with inferior MIs, right ventricular infarction and failure develop. In this instance, the right ventricle fails independently of the left. Decreased cardiac output with a paradoxical pulse, clear lungs, and jugular venous distention results when the client is in semi-Fowler's position.

A right ventricular MI may be documented by echocardiography and by an ECG using right-sided precordial leads. The goal of medical management is to improve right ventricular stroke volume by increasing right ventricular fiber stretch or preload. To enhance right ventricular preload, the nurse administers sufficient fluids (as much as 200 mL/hr) to increase right atrial pressure to 20 mm Hg, as ordered. The cardiac nurse monitors the pulmonary artery wedge pressure (PAWP) (attempting to maintain it below 15 to 20 mm Hg) and auscultates the lungs to ensure that left-sided failure is not developing. The client's cardiac output is monitored to ensure that fluid administration is having the desired effect.

POTENTIAL FOR RECURRENT CHEST DISCOMFORT AND EXTENSION OF INJURY

PLANNING: EXPECTED OUTCOMES. The client with coronary artery disease (CAD) is expected to experience minimal angina while engaging in activities of daily living (ADLs) and an exercise program.

INTERVENTIONS. Recurrent chest discomfort despite medical therapy is one of the major indications for surgical management of CAD. Clients who continue to have chest discomfort despite medical therapy or ischemia during a stress test may require invasive correction by PTCA or CABG to resolve angina or prevent myocardial infarction (MI). Before invasive treatment, a left-sided cardiac catheterization with coronary angiogram (see Chapter 33) is performed to document that the lesions are correctable and that left ventricular pump function is adequate.

PERCUTANEOUS TRANSLUMINAL CORONARY ANGIOPLASTY. **Percutaneous transluminal coronary angioplasty (PTCA)** is an invasive but technically nonsurgical technique. It is performed to reduce the frequency and sever-

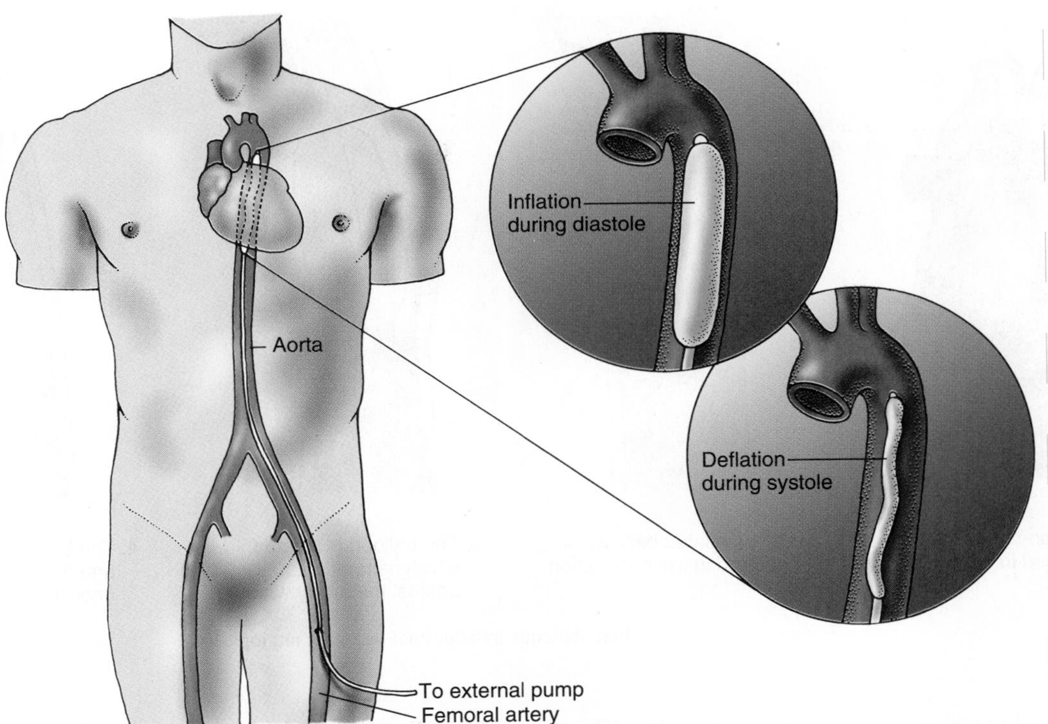

Figure 38-4 ● Intra-aortic balloon pumping. An intra-aortic balloon catheter is inserted into the femoral artery and advanced into the descending aorta. The polyethylene balloon lies just distal to the left subclavian artery. Immediately after it is inserted, the catheter is connected to the external pump.

ity of chest discomfort for clients with angina. The risk of complications is not significant.

INDICATIONS. Clients who are most likely to benefit from PTCA have single- or double-vessel disease with discrete, proximal, noncalcified lesions. When identifying which lesions are treatable with PTCA, the cardiologist considers the lesion's complexity and location, as well as the amount of myocardium at risk. PTCA often will not open complex lesions. Treating lesions located in the left main artery would place a large amount of myocardial tissue at risk should the vessel close acutely; therefore these lesions are rarely treated with PTCA.

PTCA may also be used for the client with an evolving acute MI, either alone or in conjunction with thrombolytic therapy or GP IIa/IIIb inhibitor, to reperfuse the damaged myocardium. Approximately 50% of clients needing revascularization are initially treated with PTCA.

PROCEDURE. The physician performs PTCA under fluoroscopic guidance in the cardiac catheterization laboratory. A balloon-tipped catheter is introduced through a guidewire to the occlusion in the coronary vessel. The physician activates a compressor that inflates the balloon at 4 to 14 atmospheres of pressure. This process compresses the plaque against the vessel wall and reduces or eliminates the occluding lesion (Figure 38-5). Balloon inflation may be repeated until angiography indicates a decrease in the stenosis (narrowing) to less than 50% of the vessel's diameter.

IV heparin is administered in a continuous infusion to prevent thrombus formation; IV or intracoronary nitroglycerin or sublingual nifedipine is given to prevent coronary spasm. PTCA initially reopens the vessel in more than 90% of appropriately selected clients. However, restenosis occurs in a large number of these clients. Glycoprotein (GP) IIa/IIIb inhibitors have demonstrated benefit in preventing restenosis and maintaining the patency of the artery, reducing nonfatal MIs, and preventing deaths following PTCA and are usually administered.

Other techniques being used to ensure continued patency of the vessel are laser angioplasty, arthrectomy, and stents. Lasers may be used alone to remove atherosclerotic material from coronary arteries, or they may be used in conjunction with balloon angioplasty to create a smooth lumen about the size of the balloon. Arthrectomy devices can either excise and retrieve plaque or emulsify it. One of the advantages of arthrectomy is that it creates a less bulky vessel with better elastic recoil. **Stents** are used to maintain the patent lumen obtained by angioplasty or arthrectomy. By providing a supportive scaffold, stents prevent acute closure of the vessel from arterial dissection or vasospasm. Figure 38-6 depicts a stent positioned in a coronary artery.

POSTPROCEDURE CARE. The nurse monitors for potential problems, which include acute closure of the vessel, bleeding from the insertion site, reaction to the dye used in angiography, hypotension, hypokalemia, and dysrhythmias.

The physician usually prescribes a long-term nitrate, calcium channel blocker, and aspirin therapy for clients after PTCA. A beta blocker and an angiotensin-converting enzyme (ACE) inhibitor may be added for clients who have had primary angioplasty following an MI. Many clients continue to have infusions

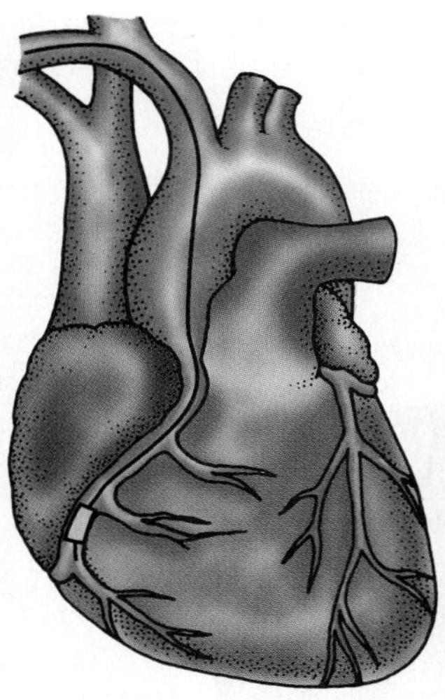

1. The balloon-tipped catheter is positioned in the artery.

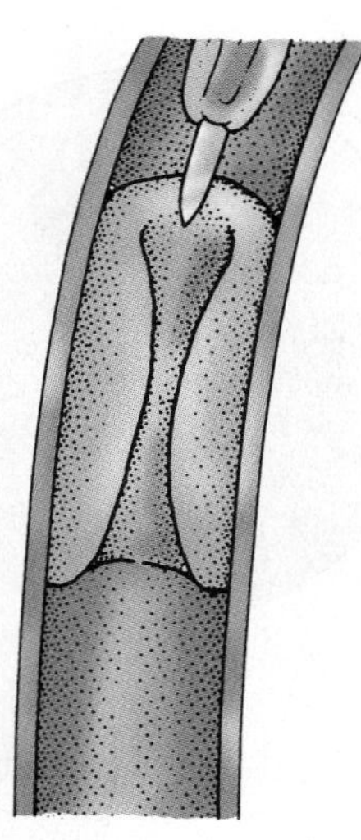

2. The uninflated balloon is centered in the obstruction.

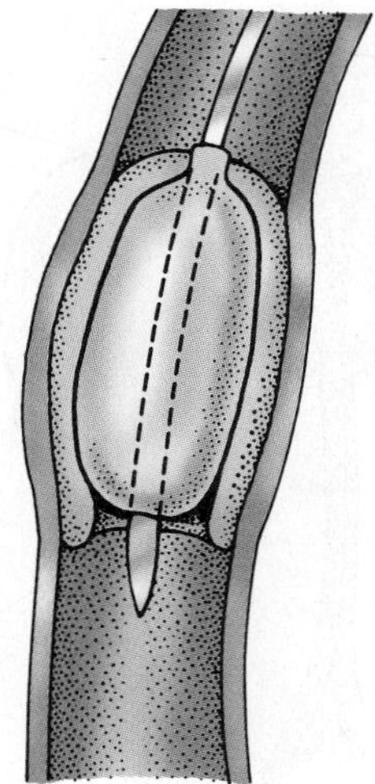

3. The balloon is inflated, which flattens plaque against the artery wall.

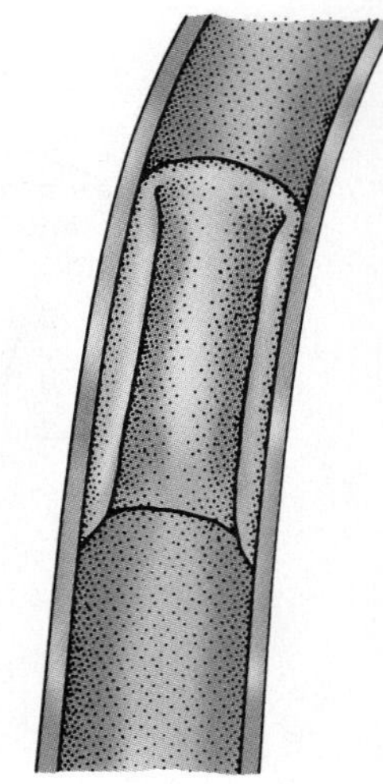

4. The balloon is removed, and the artery is left unoccluded.

Figure 38-5 ● Percutaneous transluminal coronary angioplasty.

of GP IIa/IIIb inhibitors during the initial hours after PTCA. Clients may experience hypokalemia after the procedure and require careful monitoring and supplementation of potassium. Clients who have intracoronary stents inserted may require anticoagulation with warfarin (Coumadin) for 1 to 3 months until an endothelial covering is laid over the stent. The nursing interventions for clients receiving these medications are described in Chart 38-4. The nurse provides careful explanations of drug therapy and any recommended lifestyle changes.

CRITICAL THINKING CHALLENGE

A client has undergone primary PTCA with stenting of a large stenotic lesion in his left anterior descending (LAD) coronary artery. Following treatment, he is returned to his hospital room. Continuous IV infusions include lidocaine (following a run of ventricular tachycardia during reperfusion), abciximab (ReoPro), and heparin. He has also received metoprolol (Lopressor) and aspirin.

- What are the most important nursing assessments following PTCA?
- What are the priorities for your nursing care?
- The client complains of pain near the IV site in his left antecubital space. What should you do at this time?

For suggested answer guidelines, go to SIMON http://www.wbsaunders.com/SIMON/Iggy/.

CORONARY ARTERY BYPASS GRAFT SURGERY. Approximately 598,000 **coronary artery bypass graft (CABG)** surgeries were performed in the United States in 1996. This represents a 424% increase since 1979. CABG is the most common type of cardiac surgery and the most common procedure for older adults; more than 44% of all CABGs are performed on clients older than 65 years of age. The occluded coronary arteries are bypassed with the client's own venous or arterial blood vessels or synthetic grafts. The internal mammary artery (IMA) is the current graft of choice because it has a 90% patency rate at 12 years after the procedure.

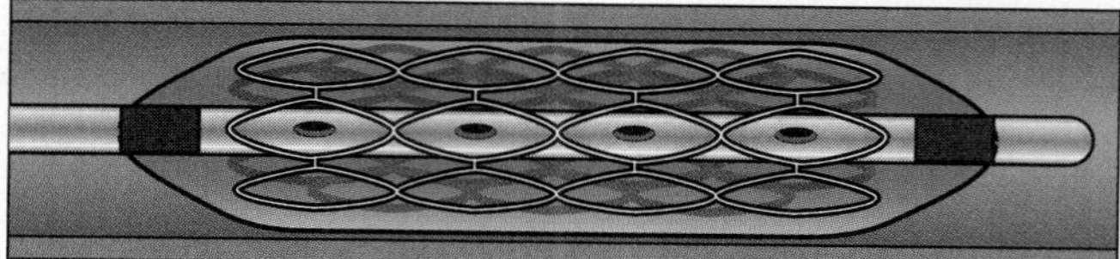

Figure 38-6 ● A coronary stent open after balloon inflation.

CABG is indicated when clients do not respond to medical management of CAD or when disease progression is evident. The decision for surgery is based on the client's symptoms and the results of cardiac catheterization.

- Candidates for surgery are clients who have the following:
- Angina with greater than 50% occlusion of the left main coronary artery
- Unstable angina with severe two-vessel or moderate three-vessel disease
- Ischemia with heart failure
- Acute MI
- Signs of ischemia or impending MI after angiography or PTCA

The vessels to be bypassed should have proximal lesions occluding more than 70% of the vessel's diameter but good distal runoff. Bypass of less occluded vessels may result in poor perfusion through the graft and early obstruction. CABG is most effective when good ventricular function remains and the ejection fraction is more than 40% to 50%. Clients with lower ejection fractions are poorer risks.

For most clients, the risk is low and the benefits of bypass surgery are clear. Surgical treatment of CAD does not appear to affect the life span. Early mortality rates are 1% to 2%. Left ventricular function is the most important long-term indicator of survival. CABG does improve the quality of life for most clients; 80% to 90% of clients are pain free at 1 year after CABG, and 70% remain pain free at 5 years after the proce-

TABLE 38-4 • MEDICATION ADMINISTRATION BEFORE CORONARY ARTERY BYPASS GRAFT SURGERY

MEDICATIONS OFTEN DISCONTINUED
- Digitalis 12 hours before surgery
- Diuretics 2 to 3 days before surgery
- Aspirin and anticoagulants 1 week before surgery

MEDICATIONS OFTEN ADMINISTERED
- Potassium chloride to maintain potassium between 3.5 and 4.0
- Scheduled beta blockers
- Scheduled calcium channel blockers
- Scheduled antidysrhythmics
- Scheduled antihypertensives
- Prophylactic antibiotic 20 to 30 minutes before surgery

dure. The percentage of clients experiencing some pain increases sharply after 5 years.

PREOPERATIVE CARE. CABG surgery may be planned as an elective procedure or performed on an emergency basis. Clients undergoing elective surgery are often admitted on the morning of the surgery. Preoperative preparations and teaching are completed during prehospitalization interviews (see the Clinical Pathway on pp. 1834-1837). Clients must understand that some medication will need to be adjusted because of the surgery. The nurse ensures that appropriate medications have been discontinued preoperatively and that the necessary ones have been administered (Table 38-4).

Prehospital Preparation. The nurse familiarizes the client and family with the cardiac surgical critical care environment and prepares the client for postoperative care. The nurse demonstrates and has the client return a demonstration of how to splint the chest incision, cough, deep breathe, and perform arm and leg exercises (see Chapter 17). The nurse stresses the following:

- The client should identify any pain to the nursing staff.
- Most of the pain will be in the sternal incision.
- Pain medication will be available.

The nurse explains that the client should expect to have a sternal incision, possibly a leg incision, one or two chest tubes, a Foley catheter, and several IV fluid catheters postoperatively. An endotracheal tube will be connected to a ventilator for several hours postoperatively. The client and family must understand that the client will not be able to talk while the endotracheal tube is in place. The client should breathe with the ventilator and not fight it. When describing the postoperative course, the nurse emphasizes that close monitoring and the use of sophisticated equipment are standard treatment.

Psychosocial Preparation. Preoperative anxiety is common. Clients often wait 1 to 6 weeks for CABG surgery to be scheduled and performed. As the length of the wait increases, anxiety may increase. An appropriate nursing assessment should identify the level of anxiety and the coping methods clients have used successfully in the past. Some clients may find it helpful to define their fears. Common sources of fear include fear of the unknown, fear of bodily harm, and fear of death.

Clients may benefit from detailed information about the surgery, or they may feel overwhelmed by so much material. Some need to discuss their feelings in detail or describe the experiences of people they know who have undergone CABG. The nurse assesses clients' anxiety level and helps them to cope. Preoperative anxiety has been positively associated with postpericardiotomy delirium.

OPERATIVE PROCEDURE. Coronary artery bypass surgery is performed with the client under general anesthesia and undergoing cardiopulmonary bypass. The anesthesiologist or nurse anesthetist administers anesthesia and intubates the client. Once the client is anesthetized, one surgical team may begin harvesting the saphenous vein if it is to be used for the graft. The cardiac surgical team begins the procedure with a median sternotomy incision and visualization of the heart and great vessels.

Cardiopulmonary bypass (CPB) is accomplished by cannulation of the inferior and superior venae cavae. The purpose of CPB is to provide oxygenation, circulation, and hypothermia during induced cardiac arrest. Blood is diverted from the heart to the bypass machine, where it is heparinized, oxygenated, and returned to the circulation through a cannula placed in the ascending aortic arch or femoral artery (Figure 38-7). During bypass, the client's core temperature is cooled to 82.6° to 89.6° F (28° to 32° C). Cooling decreases the rate of metabolism and demand for oxygen. The heart is perfused with a cardioplegic solution containing potassium, which decreases myocardial oxygen consumption and causes the heart to stop during diastole. This process ensures a still operative field and prevents myocardial ischemia.

Once the heart is arrested, the grafting procedure can begin. The surgeon uses the internal mammary artery (IMA), a saphenous vein, or both, or a radial artery to bypass lesions in the coronary arteries (Figure 38-8). The distal end of the IMA is dissected and attached below the lesion on the coronary artery. If the surgeon uses a venous graft or the radial artery, it is anastomosed (sutured) proximally to the aorta and distally to the coronary artery just beyond the occlusion. Thus myocardial perfusion is improved. After flow rates through the grafts are measured, the heart is rewarmed slowly. The cardioplegic solution is flushed from the heart. The heart regains its rate and rhythm, or it may be defibrillated to return it to a normal rhythm. When the procedure is completed, the client is rewarmed by CPB and weaned from the bypass machine while the grafts are observed for patency and leakage. The surgeon then places atrial and ventricular pacemaker wires and mediastinal chest tubes. Finally, the surgeon closes the sternum with wire sutures.

POSTOPERATIVE CARE. After surgery, the client is transported to a post–open heart surgery unit. There the client undergoes mechanical ventilation for 3 to 6 hours. The client requires highly skilled nursing care from a nurse qualified to provide post–cardiac surgery care. The nurse connects mediastinal tubes to water seal drainage systems and grounds the epicardial pacer wires and connects them to the pacemaker box. The nurse monitors pulmonary artery and arterial pressures, as well as the heart rate and rhythm, which are displayed on a monitor (see the Clinical Pathway on pp. 1834-1837).

The nurse closely assesses the client for dysrhythmias, such as ventricular ectopic rhythms, bradydysrhythmias, or heart block. The nurse treats symptomatic dysrhythmias according to unit protocol or the physician's order. If the client has symptomatic bradydysrhythmias or heart block, the nurse turns on the pacemaker and adjusts the pacemaker settings as ordered

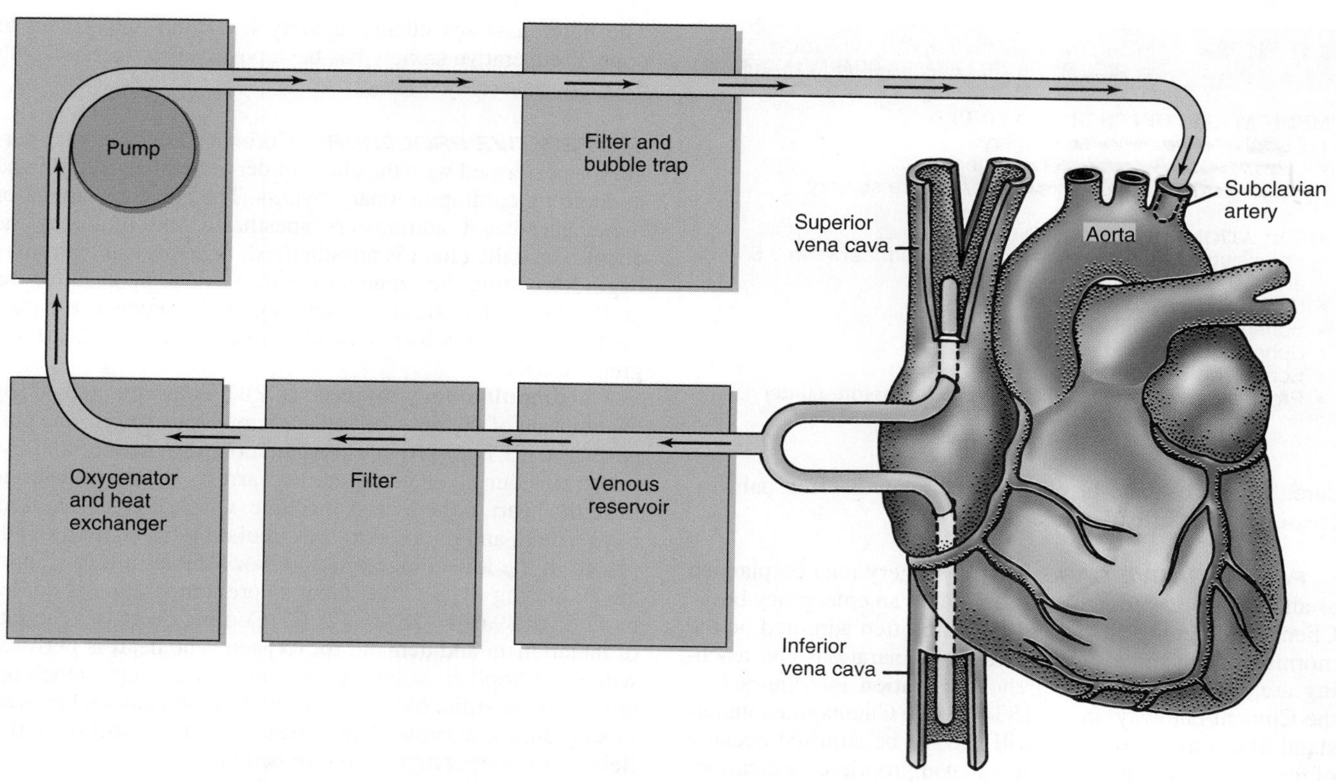

Figure 38-7 ● Heart-lung bypass circuitry used during cardiopulmonary bypass.

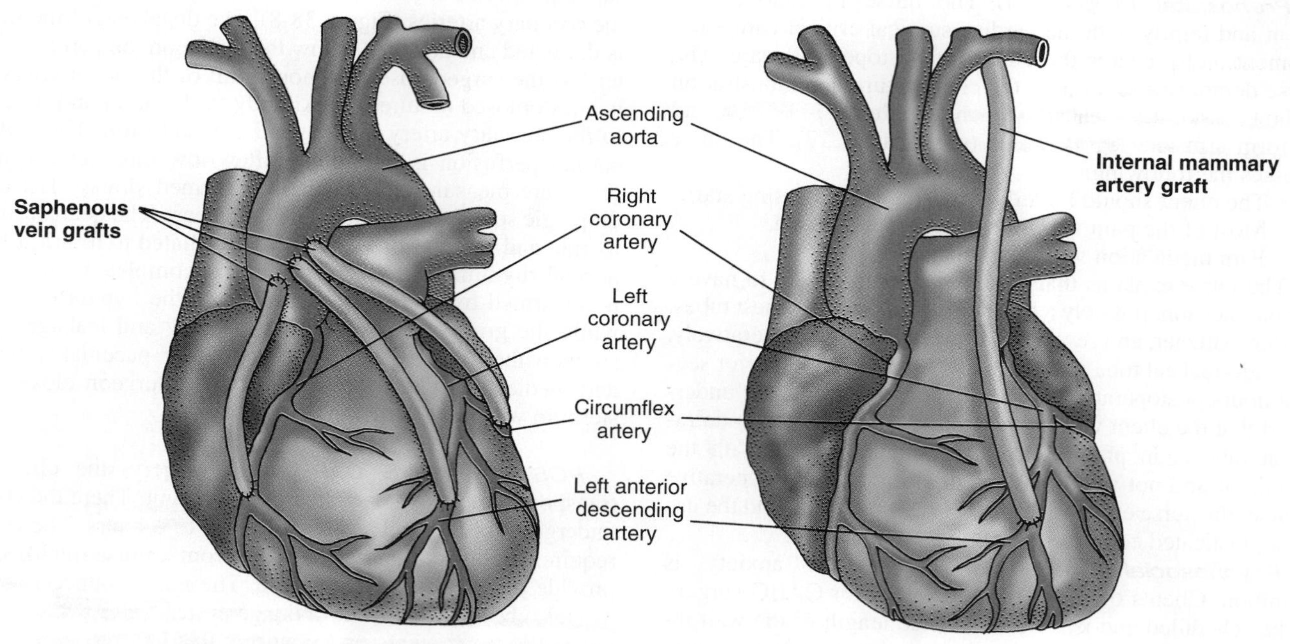

Figure 38-8 ● Two methods of coronary artery bypass grafting. The procedure used depends on the nature of the coronary artery disease, the condition of the vessels available for grafting, and the client's health status.

(see Chapter 34). The nurse also monitors for other complications of CABG, including fluid and electrolyte imbalance, hypotension, hypothermia, hypertension, bleeding, cardiac tamponade, and altered cerebral perfusion. Table 38-5 lists some of the possible postoperative complications of CABG.

Management of Fluid and Electrolyte Imbalance. Assessing fluid and electrolyte balance is a high priority in the early postoperative period. Clients usually have edema, and fluids may be limited to 1500 to 2000 mL. However, decisions concerning fluid administration are made on the basis

TABLE 38-5 • POSSIBLE POSTOPERATIVE COMPLICATIONS OF CORONARY ARTERY BYPASS GRAFT SURGERY

DECREASED CARDIAC OUTPUT
- Reduced preload
  - Hypovolemia
  - Hemorrhage
- Increased preload
  - Heart failure
  - Cardiogenic shock
- Increased afterload
  - Hypothermia
  - Increased sympathetic activity
- Dysrhythmias
  - Bradydysrhythmias
  - Conduction defects
  - Tachydysrhythmias
- Myocardial infarction

PULMONARY DYSFUNCTION
- Atelectasis
- Pneumonia
- Pulmonary edema
- Hemothorax/pneumothorax

NEUROLOGIC DYSFUNCTION
- Transient neurologic deficits
- Postpericardiotomy delirium
- Cerebrovascular accident

ACUTE RENAL FAILURE

GASTROINTESTINAL DYSFUNCTION
- Stress ulcer
- Paralytic ileus

INFECTION

of the blood pressure, pulmonary artery wedge pressure (PAWP), right atrial pressure, cardiac output, cardiac index, systemic vascular resistance, and urine output. An experienced nurse interprets assessment findings and adjusts fluid administration on the basis of standing unit policies or specific orders from the physician.

Serum electrolytes (especially calcium, magnesium, and phosphorus) may be reduced postoperatively and are monitored carefully by both the physician and the nurse. Because the serum potassium level can fluctuate dramatically, electrolyte levels are checked frequently. Potassium depletion is common and may result from hemodilution, diuretic therapy, and nasogastric suction. To prevent dysrhythmias, potassium concentrations are maintained between 4 and 5 mEq/L.

If the serum potassium level is depleted, the physician may order IV potassium replacement. The dose of potassium administered exceeds the usual recommended level of no more than 20 mEq of potassium per hour. For a potassium bolus, as much as 40 to 80 mEq may be mixed in 100 mL of IV solution and given at a rate as high as 40 mEq/hr. The drug must be given through a central catheter, and the rate of administration controlled by an infusion pump. The client must be on a cardiac monitor for extremely careful observation.

Management of Hypotension. Hypotension (systolic blood pressure less than 90 mm Hg) is a significant problem because it may result in the collapse of a vein graft. The nurse reviews the assessment parameters to identify what might be causing the hypotension. Decreased preload (decreased PAWP) can result from hypovolemia or vasodilation. If the client is hypovolemic, it might be appropriate to increase fluid administration or administer blood. The physician may treat the client with a low PAWP, decreased systemic vascular resistance, and vasodilation with vasopressor therapy to increase the blood pressure. However, if hypotension is the result of left ventricular failure (increased PAWP), IV inotropes might be necessary.

Management of Hypothermia. Although the client is rewarmed to 98.6° F (37° C) before being removed from bypass, it is not uncommon for the body temperature to drift downward after the client leaves the surgical suite. The nurse monitors the body temperature and institutes rewarming procedures should the temperature drop below 96.8° F (36° C). Rewarming may be accomplished with warm blankets, rewarming lights, or thermal blankets. The danger of rewarming a client too quickly is that he or she may begin shivering, resulting in metabolic acidosis and hypoxia. To prevent shivering, rewarming should proceed at a rate no faster than 1.8° F (1° C)/hr. The nurse discontinues rewarming when the body temperature approaches 98.6° F (37° C) and the client's extremities feel warm.

Management of Hypertension. Hypothermia is a significant risk for the client following CABG surgery because it promotes vasoconstriction and hypertension. Other factors contributing to hypertension in the CABG client include CPB, medications, and the client's own sympathetic activity.

Most CABG clients experience hypertension (if hypertension is defined as a systolic blood pressure greater than 140 to 150 mm Hg). Hypertension is dangerous because increased pressure promotes leakage from suture lines and may cause bleeding. To return the blood pressure to acceptable limits, the nurse titrates IV nitroprusside or nitroglycerin (see Chart 38-4).

Management of Bleeding. Bleeding occurs to a limited extent postoperatively in all clients. Mediastinal and chest tube drainage is measured at least hourly, and drainage exceeding 150 mL/hr is reported to the surgeon. Clients with IMA grafts may have more chest drainage. The nurse may autotransfuse the chest drainage to assist with volume management when 500 mL has accumulated or 4 hours has elapsed, depending on the clinical pathway or the physician's order. The nurse must maintain the patency of the mediastinal and chest tubes. One effective way of promoting chest tube drainage is to prevent a dependent loop from forming in the tubing.

Management of Cardiac Tamponade. If the client is bleeding and the mediastinal tubes are not kept patent, blood may accumulate around the heart. The myo-cardium is compressed, and **cardiac tamponade** results. The fluid accumulating around the heart compresses the atria and ventricles, prevents them from filling adequately, and reduces cardiac output. The following are hallmarks of cardiac tamponade:

- Sudden cessation of previously heavy mediastinal drainage
- Jugular venous distention but clear lung sounds
- Pulsus paradoxus (blood pressure greater than 10 mm Hg higher on expiration than on inspiration)
- An equalizing of PAWP and right atrial pressure

Tamponade can be confirmed by echocardiogram or chest x-ray study. Pericardiocentesis (see Chapter 35) may not be appropriate for tamponade after CABG, because the blood in the pericardium may have clotted. Volume expansion and emergency sternotomy with drainage are then the treatments of choice.

Management of Altered Levels of Consciousness. The client may demonstrate changes in the level of consciousness, which may be permanent or transient. Transient changes related to anesthesia, CPB, air emboli, or hypothermia occur in as many as 75% of clients. Transient neurologic deficits may include slowness to arouse, memory loss, and confusion.

Clients with transient neurologic deficits usually return to baseline neurologic status within 4 to 8 hours. Permanent deficits may be associated with a stroke during surgery. The client may demonstrate the following:

- Abnormal pupillary response
- Failure to awaken from anesthesia
- Seizures
- Absence of sensory or motor function

The nurse checks the client's neurologic status every 30 to 60 minutes until the client has awakened from anesthesia; the nurse then checks every 2 to 4 hours.

Pain Management. The nurse must differentiate between sternotomy pain, which is expected after CABG, and anginal pain, which might indicate graft failure. Typical sternotomy pain is localized, does not radiate, and often becomes worse when the client coughs or breathes deeply. The client may describe the pain as sharp, aching, or burning. Pain may stimulate the sympathetic nervous system, which increases the heart rate and vascular resistance while decreasing cardiac output. The nurse administers the prescribed medication, in adequate doses, frequently enough to limit pain. However, during the process of weaning the client from mechanical ventilation, it may be necessary to use short-acting analgesics and to limit pain medication because of the respiratory depressant effects of analgesia.

Transfer from the Special Care Unit. Ventilation is usually provided for 3 to 6 hours postoperatively, until the client is breathing adequately and is hemodynamically stable. During the first day, the client usually has pacer wires, hemodynamic monitoring lines, and mediastinal tubes removed and is transferred to an intermediate care unit. All CABG clients, but especially those with IMA grafts, are at high risk for atelectasis, so the nurse encourages the client to splint, cough, turn, and deep breathe to raise secretions. The nurse guides him or her in a gradual resumption of activity. Two hours after extubation, the client should be dangled as tolerated and turned side to side. Within 4 to 8 hours after extubation, the client should be out of bed in a chair. By the first day after surgery, the client should be out of bed in a chair and ambulating 25 to 100 feet three times a day as tolerated. The nurse continues to monitor for decreased cardiac output, pain, dysrhythmias, and infection.

The nurse assesses the neurovascular status of the donor arm of clients who have had the radial artery used as a conduit in CABG. Every hour initially, and eventually every 4 hours, the nurse assesses the hand color, temperature (pulse both ulnar and radial stump), and capillary refill. In addition, the fingertips, hand, and arm are assessed for sensation and mobility at least every 4 hours.

Approximately one third of clients with CABG and two thirds of those with valve replacements experience supraventricular dysrhythmias (especially atrial fibrillation) during the postoperative period, most commonly on the second or third postoperative day. The nurse examines the monitor pattern for atrial fibrillation. When auscultating the heart, the nurse listens for an irregular rhythm. (See Chapter 34 for interventions for atrial fibrillation.)

Sternal wound infections develop between 5 days and several weeks postoperatively in about 2% of clients and represent a significant complication (Hussey & Leeper, 1998). The nurse is alerted to the presence of *mediastinitis* by the following:

- Fever continuing beyond the first 4 days after CABG
- Instability (bogginess or stepping) of the sternum
- Redness or purulent drainage from suture sites
- An increased white blood cell count

CHART 38-8

NURSING FOCUS *on the* OLDER ADULT
Coronary Artery Bypass Graft Surgery

- Be aware that perioperative mortality rates are higher for the older client (4% to 9%) than for the client younger than 60 years of age (1% to 2%).
- Monitor neurologic and mental status carefully because older adults are more likely to have transient neurologic deficits after coronary artery bypass graft (CABG) surgery than younger adults are.
- Observe for side effects of cardiac drugs because elders are more likely to develop toxic effects from positive inotropes (dobutamine) and potent antihypertensives (nitroglycerin or nitroprusside).
- Monitor the client closely for dysrhythmias because older adults are more likely to have dysrhythmias, such as atrial fibrillation or supraventricular tachycardia, after CABG surgery.
- Be aware that recuperation after CABG surgery is slower for older clients and that their average length of hospital stay is longer.
- Teach the client and family that during the first 2 to 5 weeks after discharge, fatigue, chest discomfort, and lack of appetite may be particularly bothersome for older clients.

The physician may perform a needle biopsy to confirm a sternal infection. Surgical debridement, antibiotic wound irrigation, and IV antibiotics are usually indicated. Four to 6 weeks of IV antibiotics are required if sternal osteomyelitis has developed.

Postpericardiotomy syndrome is a source of chest discomfort in 10% to 40% of post–cardiac surgery clients. The syndrome is characterized by pericardial and pleural pain, pericarditis, a friction rub, an elevated temperature and white blood cell count, and dysrhythmias. Postpericardiotomy syndrome may occur days to weeks after surgery and seems to be associated with blood remaining in the pericardial sac. The nurse observes for the development of pericardial or pleural pain. For most clients, the syndrome is mild and self-limiting. However, the client may require treatment similar to that for pericarditis. The nurse should be prepared to detect pericardial tamponade (see Chapter 35).

Older adults may have different needs and experience slightly different problems after CABG. Nursing concerns related to the older CABG client are detailed in Chart 38-8.

MINIMALLY INVASIVE DIRECT CORONARY ARTERY BYPASS. The **minimally invasive direct coronary artery bypass (MIDCAB)** may be indicated for clients with a lesion of the left anterior descending (LAD) artery. In one of the most common MIDCAB procedures, after a 2-inch left thoracotomy incision is made and the fourth rib removed, the left internal mammary artery (IMA) is dissected and attached to the still-beating heart below the level of the lesion in the LAD. Cardiopulmonary bypass (CPB) is not required. Nurses must assess postoperatively for chest pain and electrocardiogram (ECG) changes (Q waves and ST-segment and T-wave changes in leads V_2 to V_6) because occlusion of the IMA graft occurs acutely in 10% of clients. If there is any question of acute graph closure, the nurse notifies the surgeon immediately. Clients tend to have more incisional pain after MIDCAB than after traditional CABG surgery, but the pain can usually be managed with oxycodone or codeine. Because they

CHART 38-9

FOCUSED ASSESSMENT *of* Home Health Clients Who Have Had a Myocardial Infarction

Assess cardiovascular function, including:
- Current vital signs (compare with previous to identify changes)
- Recurrence of chest discomfort (characteristics, frequency, onset)
- Indications of heart failure (weight gain, crackles, cough, or dyspnea)
- Adequacy of tissue perfusion (mentation, skin temperature, peripheral pulses, urine output)
- Indications of serious dysrhythmia (very irregular pulse, palpitations with fainting or near fainting)

Assess coping skills, including:
- Is client displaying denial, anger, or fear?
- Is caregiver providing adequate support?
- Are client and caregiver having disagreements about treatment?

Assess functional ability, including:
- Activity tolerance (examine client's activity diary: review distance, duration, frequency, symptoms occurring during exercise)
- Activities of daily living (is any assistance needed?)
- Household chores (who performs them?)
- Does client plan to return to work? When?

Assess nutritional status, including:
- Food intake (review client's intake of fats and cholesterol)

Assess client's understanding of illness and its treatment, including:
- How to treat chest discomfort
- Signs and symptoms to report to health care provider
- Dosage, effects, and side effects of medications
- How to advance and when to limit activity
- Modification of risk factors for coronary artery disease

have a thoracotomy incision and a chest tube or smaller lumen vacuum chest device, clients are encouraged to cough, deep breathe, and use an incentive spirometer for a week postoperatively. Most clients spend less than 6 hours in a critical care unit and are discharged in 2 or 3 days.

TRANSMYOCARDIAL LASER REVASCULARIZATION. **Transmyocardial laser revascularization** is a new procedure for clients with unstable angina and inoperable CAD with areas of reversible myocardial ischemia. After a single-lung intubation, a left anterior thoracotomy is performed and the heart is visualized. A laser is used to create 20 to 24 long, narrow channels through the left ventricular muscle to the left ventricle. These channels will eventually allow oxygenated blood to flow during diastole from the left ventricle to nourish the muscle. After the surgery, the client is transported to a critical care unit, where the nurse institutes hemodynamic monitoring and monitors for anginal episodes and bleeding disturbances. Although many clients report decreases in anginal episodes following the procedure, researchers have been unable to document why clients experience such an improvement.

Community-Based Care

CASE MANAGEMENT

Case management is most appropriate for clients who meet high-cost, high-volume, and high-risk criteria. Clients with coronary artery disease (CAD) clearly meet all of these criteria. Clinical pathways and case management programs for clients who have CAD are in effect in most U.S. hospitals. By focusing on cardiovascular risk reduction and improving the continuity of care, health care professionals have reduced the length and cost of hospital stays. Posthospital case management should reduce hospital readmission rates and improve client health.

EVIDENCE-BASED PRACTICE FOR NURSING

What factors predict readmission to the hospital following cardiac surgery?

Sabourin, C.B., & Funk, M. (1999). Readmission of patients after coronary artery bypass graft surgery. *Heart and Lung, 28*(4), 243-250.

The purpose of this study was to assess the rates, reasons, and predictors of hospital readmission following coronary artery bypass surgery. This is important, since the length of stay following cardiac surgery has decreased dramatically with the advent of fast tracking. Hospital readmissions following fast-tracked discharge can result in substantial financial losses for both the hospital and the insurer.

This study was a portion of a larger one conducted by the Center for Outcome and Evaluation Research at Yale University Medical Center. Within 6 weeks of hospital discharge, 9.7% of the sample sought care in an emergency department and 18.5% of the sample was readmitted unexpectedly to a hospital. Women who were older, unmarried, lived alone, and had a history of heart failure were more likely to be readmitted, as were obese clients. These findings corroborated findings from other studies.

Critique. It was unclear how participants were chosen for this research. In addition, only 51% of the people who consented to participate in the study returned their questionnaires. No attempt was made to determine if those who did not return their questionnaires were significantly different from those who did. If those who did not answer differed in some important way (perhaps many of them were hospitalized), it could change the results of the study.

Implications for Nursing. Since this study corroborates the findings of other studies, nurses might want to pay particular attention to obtaining the assistance of a social worker and developing social supports when planning for the hospital discharge of older, unmarried women who live alone. When doing discharge teaching, the nurse should provide information about management of heart failure to clients, especially women who have had heart failure in the past, and skin and suture line care should be emphasized for obese clients.

HOME CARE MANAGEMENT

Clients who have experienced a myocardial infarction (MI), angina, or coronary artery bypass graft (CABG) surgery are usually discharged to home or to a subacute care setting with pharmacologic therapy and specific activity prescriptions. Hospital stays are approximately 5 to 7 days for clients with MI or those undergoing CABG, and only 2 days for those undergoing percutaneous transluminal coronary angioplasty (PTCA); therefore clients are still recovering when they are discharged. They may require a home care nurse for assessment and teaching following discharge and an aide for assistance with activities of daily living (ADLs) if they are older or weaker (Chart 38-9). In addition, women, who tend to be older and living alone when coronary events occur, may have a greater need for home assistance after CABG surgery (see the Evidence-Based Practice for Nursing box above). Clients who were residents in long-term care may be returned there after hospitalization for unstable angina, MI, or CABG surgery.

Cardiac rehabilitation is available in many communities for clients after an MI or CABG surgery, but only 10% to 30% of clients participate in structured rehabilitation programs. The most frequently cited reasons for nonparticipation are lack of insurance coverage, a physician's directive that it is unnecessary, and the client's decision that it is not necessary. Clients who participate in structured rehabilitation programs report greater improvement in exercise tolerance and improved ability to control stress. However, there is no difference in their return to work.

HEALTH TEACHING

Because hospital stays are short and clients are quite ill during hospitalization, most in-hospital education programs concentrate on the skills essential to self-care after discharge. As part of home visits or a cardiac rehabilitation program, the nurse identifies the additional educational needs of the client and family, as well as their readiness to learn. The nurse then develops a teaching plan, which usually includes education about the normal anatomy and physiology of the heart, the pathophysiology of angina and MI, risk factor modification, activity and exercise protocols, cardiac medications, and when to seek medical assistance.

The nurse informs the client about the normal function of the heart and coronary arteries and explains angina and MI. Clients are taught that myocardial healing after an MI begins early and is usually complete in 6 to 8 weeks. Clients who have undergone CABG are told that the sternotomy heals in about 6 to 8 weeks.

Clients who have undergone CABG require instruction on incisional care for the sternum and the graft site. They should inspect the incisions daily for any redness, swelling, or drainage. The leg of a saphenous vein donor site is often edematous. The nurse instructs clients to avoid crossing legs, to wear elastic stockings until the edema subsides, and to elevate the surgical limb when sitting in a chair. Clients who have had a radial artery graft are instructed to open and close the hand vigorously 10 times every 2 hours.

RISK FACTOR MODIFICATION. Modification of risk factors is a necessary part of a client's management and involves changing his or her health maintenance patterns. Such modifications may include smoking cessation, altered dietary habits, regular exercise, blood pressure control, and blood glucose control.

SMOKING CESSATION. For clients who smoke, the nurse explains the detrimental effects on the cardiovascular system of smoking tobacco, especially cigarettes. Many clients spontaneously quit smoking soon after an MI. Nurse counseling has been demonstrated to be a cost-effective way to assist clients in stopping smoking. Clients who use nicotine replacement are two to three times more likely to be successful in abstaining from cigarettes permanently. However, the nurse advises the client that nicotine replacement is not recommended for those who have acute coronary syndromes or recently experienced an MI. If the client relapses and begins smoking again, the nurse reassures him or her that most former smokers relapsed several times before quitting permanently.

Other methods of smoking cessation include acupuncture, acupressure, and hypnosis (see Chapter 4).

CHOLESTEROL CONTROL. The mainstays of cholesterol control are diet therapy and administration of antihyperlipidemic agents.

DIET THERAPY. The nurse collaborates with the dietitian to encourage the client to follow a prudent diet. Less than 30% of the calories in the diet should be from fat, and the fat consumed should be primarily monounsaturated or polyunsaturated. Clients should avoid saturated fats and foods rich in cholesterol. The nurse or dietitian also instructs the client not to add salt at the table. Booklets and cookbooks that can assist the client in learning to cook with reduction of fats, oils, and salt are available from the American Heart Association (AHA). Merely making such printed information available for clients to peruse has been demonstrated to result in decreased consumption of fat and increased fiber intake (Bereford et al., 1997).

Weight reduction can normalize plasma lipid and lipoprotein levels in overweight clients. The cardiac rehabilitation nurse collaborates with the dietitian and physical therapist to provide multifactorial rehabilitation, including nutrition education, counseling, behavior modification, and exercise training, to help the overweight client lose weight permanently.

ANTIHYPERLIPIDEMIC AGENTS. Reduction of cholesterol levels with antihyperlipidemic agents, such as pravastatin (Pravachol), has been demonstrated to reduce significantly the risk of further CAD (including recurrent MI), death from CAD, and the need for revascularization procedures. Thus many clients with both normal and high cholesterol levels are encouraged to take these agents after CAD develops.

An area of controversy is the use of antioxidants (such as vitamin E). Some researchers report that the use of such agents counteracts the adverse effects of oxygen free radicals (derived from high cholesterol levels) on blood vessels and protects arteries. Other reports point out that excessive vitamin E increases the risk for liver damage and that the long-term effects of antioxidants are not known.

PHYSICAL ACTIVITY. The nurse collaborates with the physical therapist to establish an activity and exercise schedule as part of client rehabilitation. The nurse instructs the client to remain near home during the first week after discharge and to continue a walking program. The client may engage in light housework or any activity done while sitting and that does not precipitate angina. During the second week, he or she is encouraged to increase social activities and possibly to return to work part time. By the third week, he or she may begin to lift objects as heavy as 15 pounds (such as 2 gallons of milk) but should avoid lifting or pulling heavier objects for the first 6 to 8 weeks. Chart 38-10 lists suggested instructions for exercise.

The client may begin a simple walking program by walking 400 feet twice a day at the rate of 1 mile/hr the first week after discharge and increasing the distance and rate as tolerated, usually weekly, until he or she can walk 2 miles at 3 to 4 miles/hr. The nurse instructs the client to take a pulse reading before, halfway through, and after exercise. The client should stop exercising if the target pulse rate is exceeded or if dyspnea or angina develops.

After a limited exercise tolerance test, the physical therapist or nurse encourages the client to join a formal exercise program, ideally one that assists the client in monitoring cardiovascular progress. The program should include 5- to 7-minute warm-up and cool-down periods, as well as 30 minutes of aerobic exercise. The client should engage in aerobic exercise a minimum of three (and preferably five) times a week.

CHART 38-10

CLIENT EDUCATION GUIDE
Activity for the Client with Coronary Artery Disease

- Begin by walking the same distance at home as in the hospital (usually 400 feet) three times each day.
- Carry nitroglycerin with you.
- Check your pulse before, during, and after the exercise.
- Stop the activity for a pulse increase of more than 20 beats/min, shortness of breath, angina, or dizziness.
- Exercise outdoors when the weather is good.
- Gradually increase the walking until the distance is 1/4 mile twice daily (usually the end of the second week).
- After an exercise tolerance test and with your physician's approval, walk at least three times each week, increasing the distance by 1/2 mile every other week, until the total distance is 2 miles.
- Avoid straining (lifting, pushups, pull-ups, and straining at bowel movements).

COMPLEMENTARY AND ALTERNATIVE THERAPIES. Additional therapies can aid in reducing the client's anxiety about progressive activity both in the immediate postoperative period and during the rehabilitation phase. Such techniques as progressive muscle relaxation, guided imagery, and music therapy have been shown to decrease anxiety, reduce depression, and increase compliance with activity/exercise regimens after CABG (see Chapter 4).

SEXUAL ACTIVITY. Sexual activity is often a subject of great concern to clients and their partners. The nurse informs the client and partner that engaging in their usual sexual activity is unlikely to cause any damage to the heart. Clients can resume sexual intercourse on the advice of the physician, usually after exercise tolerance is assessed. The client who can walk one block or climb two flights of stairs without symptoms can usually safely resume sexual activity.

The nurse suggests that initially clients schedule intercourse after a period of rest. They might try having intercourse in the morning when they are well rested or wait 1½ hours after exercise or a heavy meal. The position selected should be comfortable for both the client and his or her partner (e.g., side-lying position) so that no undue stress is placed on the heart or suture line.

BLOOD PRESSURE CONTROL. The nurse may make arrangements for the client to have blood pressure measurements taken at regular intervals and collaborates with the primary care provider to establish parameters for reporting the blood pressure to the provider. Lifestyle modifications such as weight reduction, physical activity, and reduced-sodium diets may assist in the management of hypertension. If the client is taking medication, the nurse assesses his or her compliance with the medication regimen.

BLOOD GLUCOSE CONTROL. Clients with diabetes mellitus are assessed for their participation in efforts to control hyperglycemia. The nurse reviews the prescribed dosage of insulin or oral hypoglycemic agents with the client and family. The client should demonstrate accurate testing of blood for glucose levels.

CARDIAC MEDICATIONS. The nurse assists the client in understanding the type of cardiac medications prescribed, the benefit of each drug, potential side effects to watch for, and the correct dosage and time of day to take each drug. Medication regimens vary considerably among clients. However, many clients with angina are discharged while taking aspirin, a beta blocker, a calcium channel blocker, an antihyperlipidemic agent, and a nitrate. Clients who have experienced an MI may require aspirin, a beta blocker, an antihyperlipidemic agent, and an angiotensin-converting enzyme (ACE) inhibitor. The regimen can be complex. The nurse must determine that the client can comply with the instructions.

Use of sublingual nitroglycerin deserves special attention. The nurse instructs the client to carry nitroglycerin tablets at all times and to keep the tablets in a light-resistant container. Nitroglycerin tablets should be replaced every 3 to 5 months, before they lose their potency and stop producing a tingling sensation when placed under the tongue. Chart 38-11 gives instructions for clients concerning management of chest discomfort at home.

CHART 38-11

CLIENT EDUCATION GUIDE
Management of Chest Pain at Home

- Keep fresh nitroglycerin available for immediate use.
- At the first indication of chest discomfort, cease activity and sit or lie down.
- Place 1 nitroglycerin tablet under your tongue and allow it to dissolve.
- Wait 5 minutes for relief.
- If no relief results, repeat the nitroglycerin and wait 5 more minutes.
- If there is no relief, repeat and wait 5 more minutes.
- If there is still no relief, call for transportation to a health care facility.

SEEKING MEDICAL ASSISTANCE. Clients are encouraged to notify their health care provider if they experience the following:

- Heart rate remaining less than 50 after arising
- Wheezing or difficulty breathing
- Weight gain of 3 pounds in 1 week
- Slow persistent increase in nitroglycerin use
- Dizziness, faintness, or shortness of breath with activity

Clients are encouraged to call for transportation to the hospital if they experience the following:

- Chest discomfort that does not improve after 20 minutes or 3 nitroglycerin tablets
- Extremely severe chest discomfort with weakness, nausea, or fainting.

WOMEN'S HEALTH CONSIDERATIONS

Women with coronary artery disease (CAD) report requiring more assistance from friends and extended family than men require. Male spouses of clients with CAD may be unaccustomed to assuming a caregiving role, and the older woman, who may be widowed or divorced, may live alone. If a woman is able to develop two or more sources of emotional support, her chance of surviving 5 years is three times higher than if she remains isolated and alone. The cardiac rehabilitation nurse should assess the emotional support available to women with CAD. If adequate support is not available, the nurse should provide it or arrange for the client to participate in a support group.

Women are less likely to enroll and stay in structured cardiac rehabilitation programs or participate in home walking programs than men. Most cite family and domestic responsibilities as reasons for not participating. Although housework is important to the role satisfaction of many older women, it is a poor choice for cardiovascular activity. The home health or cardiac rehabilitation nurse should assess the activity level of the woman with CAD and encourage her to participate in an appropriate exercise program.

HEALTH CARE RESOURCES

The AHA is an excellent source for booklets, films, video cassettes, cookbooks, and professional service referrals for the client with CAD. Many local affiliates have their own cardiac rehabilitation programs.

Within the community, cardiac rehabilitation programs may be affiliated with local hospitals, community centers, or other facilities, such as clinics. Many shopping malls open before shopping hours to allow a measured walking program indoors; this is particularly popular with older clients and also provides a good support group.

Mended Hearts is a nationwide program with local chapters that provides education and support to CABG clients and their families. Smoking cessation programs and clinics, as well as weight reduction programs, are found within the community. Many hospitals sponsor health fairs, blood pressure screening, and risk factor modification programs as well.

Evaluation: Outcomes

NOC The nurse evaluates the client with CAD on the basis of the identified nursing diagnoses and collaborative problems. The expected outcomes are that the client will:

- State that the chest discomfort is alleviated, appear comfortable, and have resolution of ST-segment and T-wave changes
- Remain hemodynamically stable: maintain a normal sinus rhythm or normal rhythm for the client at a rate of approximately 60, as well as maintain blood pressure within an acceptable range, adequate urine output, mental alertness, palpable pedal pulses, and clear lungs on auscultation
- Walk 200 feet four times a day without chest discomfort or shortness of breath
- Indicate decreased anxiety
- Indicate a sense of having some control over life
- Experience minimal angina while engaging in activities of daily living (ADLs) or an exercise program

ONLINE RESOURCES

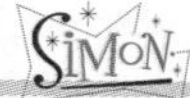

For suggested readings and Internet resources, go to http://www.wbsaunders.com/SIMON/Iggy/.

SELECTED BIBLIOGRAPHY

Asterisk indicates a classic or definitive work on this subject.

Acute care decisions: EKG and MI: How to rely on an EKG in detecting an MI. (1998). *RN, 61*(7), 24A, 24C.

Allen, J.K. (2000). Cholesterol management: An opportunity for nurse case managers. *Journal of Cardiovascular Nursing, 14*(2), 50-58.

American Heart Association. (1998). *1999 heart and stroke statistical update.* Dallas: Author.

Anderson, B., Higgins, L., & Rzmus, C. (1999). Critical pathways: Application to selected patient outcomes following coronary artery bypass graft. *Applied Nursing Research, 12*(4), 168-174.

Andrews, J. (1998). Optimizing smoking cessation strategies. *Nurse Practitioner, 23*(8), 47-65.

Beattie, S. (1999). Management of chronic stable angina. *Nurse Practitioner, 24*(5), 44-61.

*Benjamin, M., & Curtis, J. (1992). *Ethics in nursing.* New York: Oxford University Press.

Bereford, S.A., et al. (1997). A dietary intervention in primary care practice: The Eating Patterns Study. *American Journal of Public Health, 84*(4), 610-616.

Bernat, J. (1997). Smoothing the CABG patient's road to recovery. *American Journal of Nursing, 97*(2), 23-27.

Braunwald, E. (1998a). Recognition and management of patients with acute myocardial infarction. In L. Goldman & E. Braunwald (Eds.), *Primary cardiology* (pp. 257-283). Philadelphia: W.B. Saunders.

Braunwald, E. (1998b). Recognition and management of patients with unstable angina. In L. Goldman & E. Braunwald (Eds.), *Primary cardiology* (pp. 284-295). Philadelphia: W.B. Saunders.

*Braunwald, E., et al. (1994). *Diagnosing and managing unstable angina. Quick reference guide for clinicians, No. 10.* AHCPR Pub. No. 94-0603. Rockville, MD: Agency for Health Care Policy and Research, Public Health Service, U.S. Department of Health and Human Services.

Bridges, E.J., & Woods, S.L. (1998). Cardiovascular chronobiology: Implications for critical care nursing. *Critical Care Nurse, 18*(4), 49-66.

Chattterjee, K. (1998). Recognition and management of patients with stable angina pectoris. In L. Goldman & E. Braunwald (Eds.), *Primary cardiology* (pp. 234-256). Philadelphia: W.B. Saunders.

Clark, J.A., Kotyra, L.G., & Brocious, T. (1999). Rapid progression following cardiac surgery. *Critical Care Nursing Clinics of North America, 11*(2), 159-175.

Collins, J., & Rice, V. (1997). Effects of relaxation intervention in phase II cardiac rehabilitation: Replication and extension. *Heart and Lung, 26*(1), 31-44.

Cronin, S.N., et al. (2000). Recovery after percutaneous transluminal coronary angioplasty: Assessment after discharge. *Critical Care Nurse, 20*(2), 70-84.

Crumlish, C.M., et al. (2000). When time is muscle. *American Journal of Nursing, 100*(1), 26-34.

Daly, J., et al. (2000). Health status, perceptions of coping, and social support immediately after discharge of survivors of acute myocardial infarction. *American Journal of Critical Care, 9*(1), 62-69.

Dracup, K.A., & Cannon, C.P. (1999). Combination treatment strategies for management of acute myocardial infarction: New directions with current therapies. *Critical Care Nurse* (Suppl.), April, pp. 3-17.

Drew, B.J., & Kruchoff, M.W. (1999). Multilead ST segment monitoring in patients with acute coronary syndrome: Consensus statement for health care professionals. *American Journal of Critical Care, 8*(6), 372-386.

Drew, B.J., et al. (1998). Twelve-lead ST-segment monitoring vs single lead maximum ST-segment monitoring for detecting ongoing ischemia in patients with unstable coronary syndromes. *American Journal of Critical Care, 7*(5), 355-363.

Edgar, W.F., Ebersole, N., & Mayfield, M.G. (1999). MIDCAB. *American Journal of Nursing, 99*(7), 40-50.

Furry, B., & House-Fancher, M.A. (2000). Reviewing the drug lineup against AMI. *Nursing2000, 30*(7), 32hn1-32hn3.

Futterman, L.G., & Lemberg, L. (2000). Update on management of acute myocardial infarction: Facilitated percutaneous coronary intervention. *American Journal of Critical Care, 9*(1), 70-76.

Gentz, C.A. (2000). Perceived learning needs of the patient undergoing coronary angioplasty: An integrative review of the literature. *Heart and Lung, 29*(3), 161-172.

Goldman, L. (1998). Approach to the patient with chest pain. In L. Goldman & E. Braunwald (Eds.), *Primary cardiology* (pp. 70-82). Philadelphia: W.B. Saunders.

*Gortner, S.R., Dirks, J., & Wolfe, M.M. (1992). The road to recovery for elders after CABG. *American Journal of Nursing, 92*(8), 44-49.

Gulanich, M., et al. (1997). Patients' responses to the angioplasty experience: A qualitative study. *American Journal of Critical Care, 6*(1), 25-32.

Halm, M.A., & Penque, S. (1999). Heart disease in women. *American Journal of Nursing, 99*(4), 26-32.

Harrell, J.S., & Gore, S.V. (1998). Cardiovascular risk factors and socioeconomic status in African-American and Caucasian women. *Research in Nursing and Health, 21*(4), 285-295.

Hill, B., & Geraci, S.A. (1998). A diagnostic approach to chest pain based on history and ancillary evaluation. *Nurse Practitioner, 23*(4), 22-24, 29-30.

Huerta-Torres, V. (1998). Preparing patients for early discharge after CABG. *American Journal of Nursing, 98*(5), 49-51.

Hussey, L., & Leeper, B. (1998). Sternal wound infection: A case study of a devastating postoperative complication. *Critical Care Nurse, 18*(1), 31-39.

Jairath, N. (1999). Myocardial infarction patients' use of metaphors to share meaning and communicate their underlying frames of experience. *Journal of Advanced Nursing, 29*(2), 283-289.

Jensen, L., & King, K. (1997). Women and heart disease. *Critical Care Nurse, 17*(2), 45-52.

Juran, N.B, et al. (1999). Nursing interventions to decrease bleeding at the site after percutaneous coronary intervention. *American Journal of Critical Care, 8*(5), 303-313.

Kettunen, S., et al. (1999). Myocardial infarction, spouses' reactions and their need of support. *Journal of Advanced Nursing, 30*(2), 479-488.

Kline-Rogers, E., Martin, J.S., & Smith, D.D. (1999). New era of reperfusion in acute myocardial infarction. *Critical Care Nurse, 19*(1), 21-31.

Kneeshaw, M.F., Considine, R.M., & Jennings, J. (1999). Mutuality and preparedness of family caregivers for elderly women after bypass surgery. *Applied Nursing Research, 12*(3), 128-135.

Kosnik, L. (1999). Treatment protocols and pathways: Improving the process of care. *Critical Care Nurse, 19*(5 Suppl.), 3-7.

Lai, S.C., & Cohan, M.N. (1999). Promoting lifestyle changes. *American Journal of Nursing, 99*(4), 63-67.

Laosa, J.C. (1998). Cholesterol and atherosclerosis: A controversy resolved. *ADVANCE for Nurse Practitioners*, May, pp. 37-48.

Maglish, B., Schwartz, J.L., & Methany, R.G. (1999). Outcomes improvement following minimally invasive direct coronary artery bypass surgery: The nursing role in critical care and cardiovascular risk factor reduction. *Critical Care Nursing Clinics of North America, 11*(2), 177-188.

McAvoy, J.A. (2000). Cardiac pain: Discover the unexpected. *Nursing2000, 30*(3), 34-40.

McCloskey, J.C., & Bulechek, G.M. (Eds.). (2000). *Nursing interventions classification (NIC)* (3rd ed.). St. Louis: Mosby.

Moser, D. (1997). Correcting misconceptions about women and heart disease. *American Journal of Nursing, 97*(4), 26-33.

Murphy, M.J., & Berding, C.B. (1999). Use of measurements of myoglobin and cardiac troponins in diagnosis of acute myocardial infarctions. *Critical Care Nurse, 19*(1), 58-65.

Nguyen, T., et al. (2000). Catheter based interventions in acute myocardial infarction. In T. Nguyen et al. (Eds.), *Management of complex cardiovascular problems* (pp. 37-56). Armonk, NY: Futura Publishing.

Palatnik, A.M. (2001). Acute coronary syndrome: New advances and nursing strategies. *Nursing 2001, 31*(5), 32cc1-32cc6.

Parson, C. (1999). Evidence-based clinical outcome in interventional cardiology. *Critical Care Nursing Clinics of North America, 11*(2), 143-157.

Patterson, S., Citro, K., & Gillium, N. (1999). Percutaneous myocardial revascularization: New treatment option for patients with angina. *Critical Care Nurse, 19*(5), 27-36.

Peterson, D.A. (2000). Managing hypotension after cardiac surgery: An algorithm for treatment. *Critical Care Nurse, 20*(2), 36-49.

Redeker, N.S., & Wykpisz, E. (1999). Effects of age on activity patterns after coronary artery bypass surgery. *Heart and Lung, 28*(1), 5-14.

Reger, T.B., & Vargas, G. (1999). The return of radial artery in CABG. *American Journal of Nursing, 99*(9), 26-31.

Richards, S.B., Funk, M., & Milner, K.A. (2000). Differences between blacks and whites with coronary artery disease in initial symptoms and delay in seeking care. *American Journal of Critical Care, 9*(4), 237-244.

Roberts, C. (1999). Have we reached the therapeutic ceiling in acute myocardial infarction? *Critical Care Nurse, 19*(5 Suppl.), 7-11.

Robinson, A.W. (1999). Getting to the heart of denial, *American Journal of Nursing, 99*(5), 38-43.

Ryan, D. (2000). Is it an MI? A lab primer for myocardial infarction. *RN,* 63(1), 26-31.

Sabourin, C.B., & Funk, M. (1999). Readmission of patients after coronary artery bypass graft surgery. *Heart and Lung, 28*(4), 243-250.

Sakallaris, B.R., et al. (2000). Same-day transfer of patients to the cardiac telemetry unit after surgery: The Rapid After Bypass Back into Telemetry (RABBIT) program. *Critical Care Nurse, 20*(2), 50-68.

Savage, L.S., & Grap, M.J. (1999). Telephone monitoring after early discharge of cardiac surgery patients. *American Journal of Critical Care, 8*(3), 154-159.

Solomon, A.J., & Gersh, B.J. (2000). Unstable coronary artery disease. In T. Nguyen et al. (Eds.), *Management of complex cardiovascular problems* (pp. 1-14). Armonk, NY: Futura Publishing.

Sox, H.C. (1998). Screening for coronary artery disease and its risk factors. In L. Goldman & E. Braunwald (Eds.), *Primary cardiology* (pp. 57-69). Philadelphia: W.B. Saunders.

Tahan, H.A. (1998). Patients waiting for heart transplant: An analysis of vulnerability. *Critical Care Nurse, 18*(4), 40-48.

Tobin, L.J. (1999). Evaluating mild to moderate hypertension. *Nurse Practitioner, 24*(5), 22-41.

*U.S. Department of Health and Human Services. (1999). *Healthy people 2000: National health promotion and disease prevention objectives: Healthy people 2000 review 1998-1999.* Washington, DC: U.S. Government Printing Office.

Walton, J. (1998). Nursing interventions to reduce perioperative cardiac morbidity and mortality. *Dimensions of Critical Care Nursing, 17*(6), 282-292.

Warren, C. (1999). What is homocysteine? *American Journal of Nursing, 99*(10), 39-41.

Wenger, N.K. (1998). Cardiovascular disease in the elderly and in women. In L. Goldman & E. Braunwald (Eds.), *Primary cardiology* (pp. 70-82). Philadelphia: W.B. Saunders.

*Wenger, N.K., et al. (1995). *Cardiac rehabilitation as secondary prevention. Clinical practice guideline. Quick reference guide for clinicians, No. 17.* AHCPR Pub. No. 96-0673. Rockville, MD: Agency for Health Care Policy and Research and National Heart, Lung, and Blood Institute, Public Health Service, U.S. Department of Health and Human Services.

Wilkinson, J.M. (2000). *Nursing diagnosis handbook: NIC interventions and NOC outcomes.* Upper Saddle River, NJ: Prentice Hall.

UNIT

8

PROBLEMS OF TISSUE PERFUSION

Management of Clients with Problems of the Hematologic System

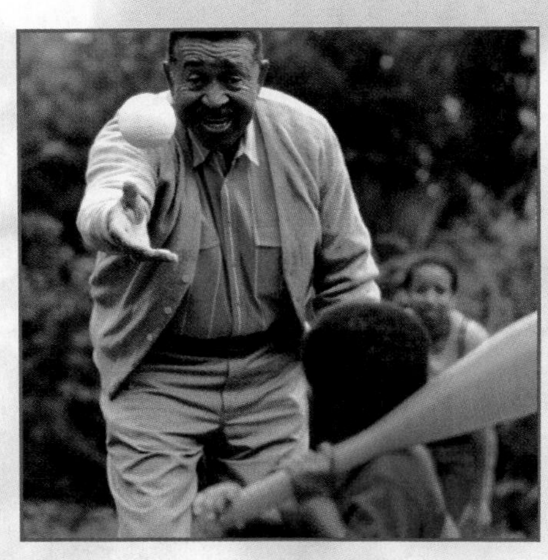

UNIT 8

PROBLEMS OF TISSUE PERFUSION: HEMATOLOGIC SYSTEM ■ Core Concepts Grid

Anatomy	Physiology	Pathophysiology	History	Physical Exam	Diagnostic Tests	Interventions	Pharmacology
• Blood cells • Plasma • Lymph system • Bone marrow	• Oxygen transport • Hematopoesis • Phagocytosis • Blood-clotting mechanism	• Hemolysis • Insufficient production • Hyperproduction • Active loss • Defective cells • Hypoxia • Hypoxemia	• History of bleeding • Fatigue • Bruising • Weakness • Weight loss • Behavioral changes • Anorexia	• Bruising • Pallor • Tachycardia • Tachypnea • Hypotension • Pain • Swelling • Purpura • Infection • Decreased level of consciousness • Skin ulcers • Jaundice • Glossitis • Paresthesias	• Hemoglobin • Hematocrit • Red blood cell count (RBC) • White blood cell count (WBC) • Platelet count • Erythrocyte sedimentation rate (ESR) • WBC differential • Prothrombin time (PT) • Partial thromboplastin time (PTT) • Activated partial thromboplastin time (aPPT) • International Normalized Ratio (INR) • Bone marrow biopsy • Iron	• Blood transfusions • Phlebotomy • Radiation • Chemotherapy • Diet modification • Pain control • Fluids (oral and parenteral) • Bone marrow transplantation • Bleeding precautions • Energy conservation • Health teaching	• Iron supplements • Chemotherapy • Anticoagulants • Opioids • Antivirals • Antifungals • Antibiotics

CHAPTER 39

Assessment of the Hematologic System

M. LINDA WORKMAN

Learning Objectives

After studying this chapter, you should be able to:

1. Describe hematologic changes associated with aging.
2. Explain the process of erythrocyte maturation.
3. Describe the role of platelets in hemostasis.
4. Compare and contrast the structure and function of platelet plugs and fibrin clots.
5. Interpret blood cell counts and clotting tests to assess the client's hematologic status.
6. Compare and contrast the actions and uses of anticoagulants and thrombolytics.
7. Prioritize nursing care for the client after bone marrow aspiration.

SIMON Go to http://www.wbsaunders.com/SIMON/Iggy/ for self-assessment questions related to these Learning Objectives.

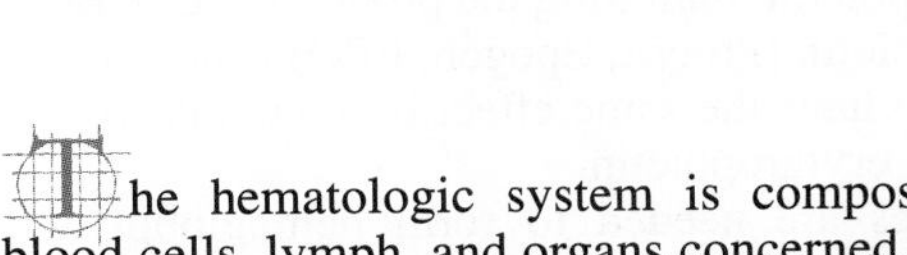

The hematologic system is composed of the blood, blood cells, lymph, and organs concerned with blood formation or blood storage. Because all systems depend on circulation and lymph flow, any problem of the hematologic system has widespread consequences for health and well-being. This chapter and Chapter 20 review the normal physiology of the hematologic system and the assessment of hematologic status.

ANATOMY AND PHYSIOLOGY REVIEW

Bone Marrow

Bone marrow is the blood-forming **(hematopoietic)** organ. It produces most of the cellular elements of the blood, including **red blood cells (RBCs, erythrocytes),** white blood cells (WBCs), and platelets. Bone marrow also is involved in some aspects of the immune response (see Chapter 20).

Each day, the bone marrow in a healthy adult produces and releases approximately 2.5 billion RBCs, 2.5 billion platelets, and 1 billion white blood cells **(leukocytes)** per kilogram of body weight.

In the fetus, blood components are formed in the liver and spleen and, by the last trimester, in the bone marrow. At birth, blood-producing marrow is present in every bone. The flat bones (sternum, skull, pelvic and shoulder girdles) contain active blood-producing marrow throughout life. As a person ages, the amount of functional bone marrow decreases in the long bones and in small, irregularly shaped bones. By age 18 blood production is limited to the ends of the long bones. During adulthood, fatty tissue replaces inactive bone marrow. In older adults, the proportion of fatty marrow increases to approximately one half of the marrow found in the sternum and ribs, and only a relatively small portion of the remaining marrow continues active blood production.

The bone marrow produces all blood cells, which initially start out as **stem cells.** Bone marrow contains ***pluripotent stem cells.*** Pluripotent stem cells are immature and undifferentiated cells that are capable of maturing into any one of several types of blood cells: RBCs, WBCs, or platelets, depending on the body's needs (Figure 39-1).

The next stage in cell development is the committed stem cell (also called the precursor cell or unipotent stem cell). A committed stem cell has one specific maturational pathway and matures or differentiates into only one cell type. Committed stem cells actively divide but require the presence of a specific growth factor for further development and maturation. For example, **erythropoietin** is a growth factor made in the kidneys that is specific for the red blood cell line. Many different growth factors influence the maturation of white blood cells and platelets (see Chapters 20, 25, and 40).

Blood Components

Blood is composed of plasma and cells. Plasma, part of the extracellular fluid of the body, is similar to the interstitial fluid found between tissue cells. Plasma, however, contains about three to four times more protein than does interstitial fluid. There are three major types of plasma proteins: albumin, globulins, and fibrinogen.

The primary function of **albumin** is to increase the osmotic pressure of the blood, which prevents plasma from leaking into the tissues (see Chapter 11). **Globulins** perform many functions, such as transporting other substances and protecting the body against infection. Globulins are also the main component of antibodies. **Fibrinogen** is a protein molecule that can be activated to form fibrin. Individual molecules of **fibrin** assemble to form large structures important in the blood-clotting process.

The cells of the blood include RBCs, WBCs, and platelets. These blood cells differ in structure, site of maturation, and function.

RED BLOOD CELLS (ERYTHROCYTES)

Red blood cells (RBCs), or erythrocytes, make up the largest proportion of blood cells. Mature RBCs have no nucleus and have a biconcave disk shape. Together with a flexible membrane, this feature allows RBCs to change their shape without breaking as they pass through narrow, winding capillaries. The number of RBCs a person has varies according to gender, age, and general health, but the normal range is from 4.4 to 5.5 million/mm^3.

As shown in Figures 39-1 and 39-2, RBCs start out as pluripotent stem cells, enter the myeloid pathway, and progress in stages to the mature RBC (the erythrocyte). Healthy, mature RBCs have a life span of approximately 120 days after being released into the blood from the bone marrow. As RBCs age, their membranes become more fragile. These old cells are trapped and destroyed by fixed macrophages in the tissues, spleen, and liver. Some parts of destroyed RBCs (e.g., iron) are recycled and used in the formation of new RBCs.

RBCs are responsible for producing hemoglobin (Hgb). Each normal, mature RBC contains many thousands of hemoglobin molecules (Guyton & Hall, 2000). The heme part of each hemoglobin molecule requires a molecule of iron. Only when the heme molecule is complete with iron can it transport up to four molecules of oxygen. *Therefore iron is a critical component of hemoglobin.* The globin portion of the hemoglobin molecule carries carbon dioxide. RBCs also serve as a buffer and help maintain acid-base balance.

The most important feature of the hemoglobin molecule is its ability to combine loosely with oxygen. With only a small drop in oxygen concentration at the tissue level, a greater increase in the transfer of oxygen from hemoglobin to the tissues occurs. This transfer is also known as **oxygen dissociation.** Some pathologic conditions change the speed and amount of oxygen released to the tissues.

The total number of RBCs is carefully controlled through **erythropoiesis** (selective maturation of stem cells into mature erythrocytes). This process ensures that enough RBCs are present for good oxygenation without having an excess concentration, which could "thicken" the blood and slow its flow. The trigger for control of erythropoiesis is tissue oxygenation. The kidney produces the RBC growth factor erythropoietin at the same rate as RBC destruction to maintain a constant normal level of circulating RBCs. When tissue oxygenation is less than normal **(hypoxia),** the kidney increases the production and release of erythropoietin. This growth factor stimulates the bone marrow to increase RBC production. When tissue oxygenation is excessive, the kidney decreases the production erythropoietin, inhibiting the production of RBCs. Synthetic erythropoietin (Procrit, Epogen, EPO) is now available and appears to have the same effect on bone marrow as naturally occurring erythropoietin.

Many substances are needed to form hemoglobin and RBCs, including iron, vitamin B_{12}, folic acid, copper, pyridoxine, cobalt, and nickel. A lack of any of these substances can lead to **anemia.** Anemia is the result of any condition in which either the function or the number of erythrocytes is inadequate to meet tissue oxygen demands (see Chapter 40).

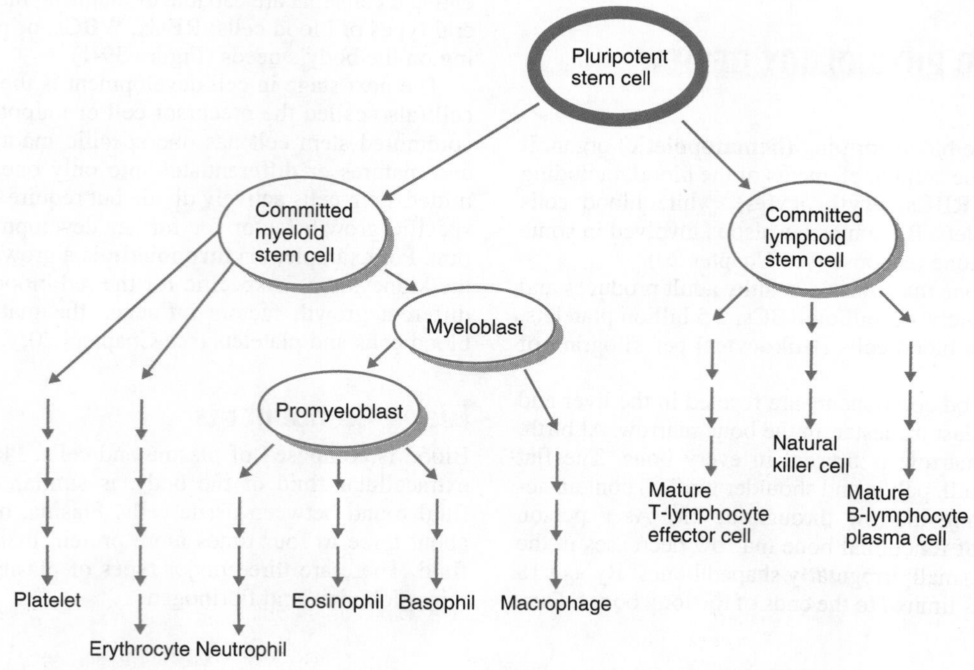

Figure 39-1 ● Bone marrow cell differentiation and maturational pathways.

WHITE BLOOD CELLS (LEUKOCYTES)

White blood cells (WBCs), or leukocytes, are the second category of blood cells. There are many types of leukocytes, and each type performs at least one specific action critical to inflammation or immunity (Table 39-1). Most WBCs are formed in the bone marrow and are considered part of the hematopoietic system. A detailed discussion of leukocyte anatomy and function is presented in Chapter 20, because these cells provide immunity and protect against the effects of invasion, infection, and injury.

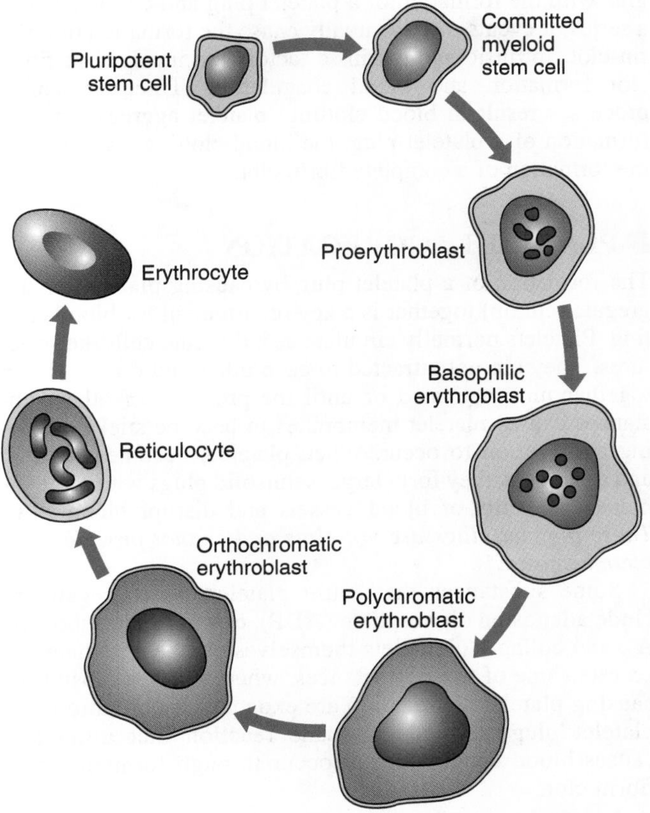

Figure 39-2 ● Erythrocyte maturational pathway.

PLATELETS

Platelets are the third type of blood cells. They are the smallest of the blood cells and are formed as fragments of a giant precursor cell in the bone marrow, the **megakaryocyte.** Figure 39-1 shows the overall developmental pathway of blood cells, and Figure 39-3 shows specific platelet development.

Platelets stick to injured blood vessel walls and form platelet plugs that can stop the flow of blood from the injured site. They also produce substances important to coagulation. Platelets maintain blood vessel integrity by beginning the repair of damage to small blood vessels. They perform most of their functions by **aggregation** (clumping).

Platelet production in the bone marrow also is precisely controlled by growth factors (thrombopoietin). After platelets leave the bone marrow, they are taken up by the spleen for storage and are released slowly according to the body's needs. Normally, 80% of platelets circulate and 20% are stored in the spleen. Each platelet has a life span of 1 to 2 weeks, after which it is gradually used up or destroyed during normal clotting activities.

Accessory Organs of Hematopoiesis

The spleen and liver are important accessory organs of the hematopoietic system. They help regulate the maturation of blood cells to help maintain hematologic homeostasis.

SPLEEN

The spleen is located under the diaphragm to the left of the stomach. It contains three types of tissue—white pulp, red pulp, and marginal pulp—all of which help to balance blood cell production with blood cell destruction and assist with immunologic defensive mechanisms. White pulp is filled with

TABLE 39-1 • FUNCTIONS OF SPECIFIC LEUKOCYTES

Leukocyte	Function
INFLAMMATION	
Neutrophil	Nonspecific ingestion and phagocytosis of microorganisms and foreign protein
Macrophage	Nonspecific recognition of foreign proteins and microorganisms; ingestion and phagocytosis
Monocyte	Destruction of bacteria and cellular debris; matures into macrophage
Eosinophil	Weak phagocytic action; releases vasoactive amines during allergic reactions
Basophil	Releases histamine and heparin in areas of tissue damage
ANTIBODY-MEDIATED IMMUNITY	
B-lymphocyte	Becomes sensitized to foreign cells and proteins
Plasma cell	Secretes immunoglobulins in response to the presence of a specific antigen
Memory cell	Remains sensitized to a specific antigen and can secrete increased amounts of immunoglobulins specific to the antigen
CELL-MEDIATED IMMUNITY	
T-lymphocyte helper/inducer T-cell	Enhances immune activity through the secretion of various factors, cytokines, and lymphokines
Cytotoxic-cytolytic T-cell	Selectively attacks and destroys non-self cells, including virally infected cells, grafts, and transplanted organs
Natural killer cell	Nonselectively attacks non-self cells, especially body cells that have undergone mutation and become malignant; also attacks grafts and transplanted organs

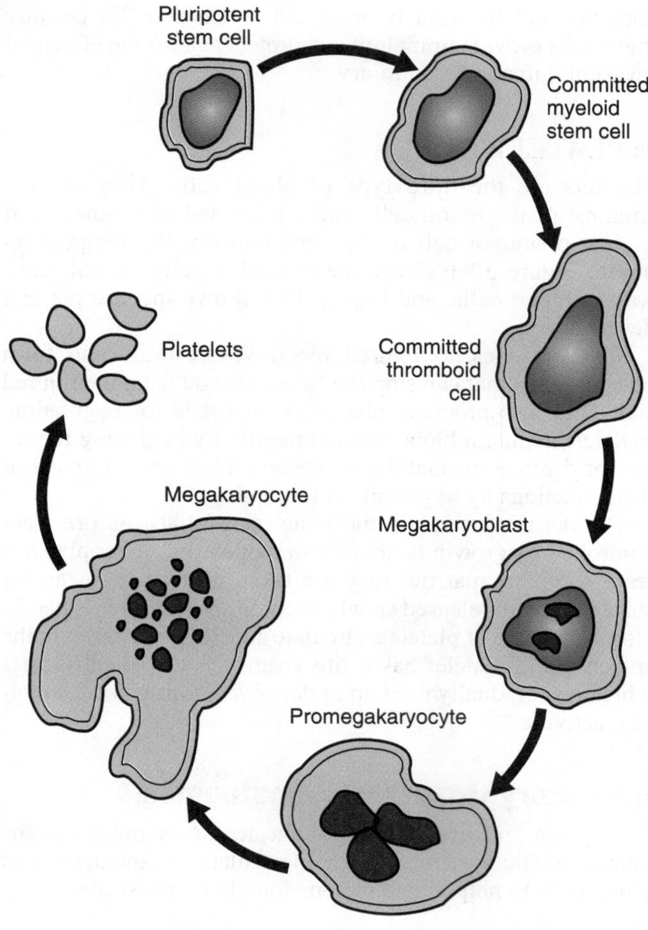

Figure 39-3 ● Platelet maturational pathway.

lymphocytes and macrophages. As whole blood circulates and filters through the white pulp, unwanted cells (e.g., bacteria and old RBCs) are removed. Red pulp is composed of vascular enlargements **(sinuses)** that are storage sites for RBCs and platelets. Marginal pulp contains the ends of many arteries and other blood vessels.

During blood formation, the spleen destroys old or imperfect RBCs, assists in iron metabolism by breaking down the hemoglobin released from these destroyed cells, stores platelets, and filters antigens. A client who has undergone a splenectomy experiences an impairment of some immune functions. Thus after a splenectomy, the body is not efficient at disposing of many bloodborne pathogenic microorganisms and is at a greatly increased risk for infection and sepsis (Workman, 1998).

LIVER

The liver is important for normal erythropoiesis and is the primary production site for prothrombin and most of the blood-clotting factors. In addition, proper liver function and bile production are critical to the formation of vitamin K in the intestinal tract. (Vitamin K is essential in the formation of blood-clotting factors VII, IX, and X and prothrombin.) Large quantities of whole blood and blood cells can be stored in the liver. The liver also converts bilirubin (one end-product of hemoglobin breakdown) to bile and stores extra iron within a storage protein called ferritin. Small amounts of erythropoietin are produced in the liver.

Hemostasis/Blood Clotting

In hemostasis, selective localized blood clotting occurs in damaged blood vessels while blood circulation to all other areas is maintained. Hemostasis is a complex process that balances the production of clotting and dissolving factors. It begins with the formation of a platelet plug and continues with a series of events that eventually cause the formation of a fibrin clot. Intrinsic and extrinsic factors are involved in fibrin clot formation and blood coagulation. Three sequential processes result in blood clotting: platelet aggregation with formation of a platelet plug, the blood-clotting cascade, and the formation of a complete fibrin clot.

PLATELET AGGREGATION

The formation of a platelet plug by causing platelets to aggregate (clump) together is a key requirement for blood clotting. Platelets normally circulate as individual cell-like structures. They are not attracted to each other and do not clump together until activated or until the presence of other substances causes platelet membranes to become sticky, allowing aggregation to occur. When platelets become activated and aggregate, they form large, semisolid plugs within the lumens and walls of blood vessels and disrupt blood flow. *These platelet plugs are not clots and cannot provide complete hemostasis.*

Some substances that cause platelets to aggregate include adenosine diphosphate (ADP), calcium, thromboxane A_2, and collagen. Platelets themselves can be stimulated to secrete some of these substances, whereas other substances causing platelet aggregation are exogenous. Formation of a platelet plug starts the cascade reaction that ultimately causes blood coagulation to occur through formation of a fibrin clot.

THE BLOOD-CLOTTING CASCADE

The blood-clotting cascade is triggered by the formation of a platelet plug. Platelet plug formation results from intrinsic or extrinsic factors. The beginning of this cascade is rapidly amplified or enhanced, with the final result much larger than the triggering event. Cascades work like a landslide. A few small pebbles rolling down a steep hillside can dislodge large rocks and pieces of soil, causing a final enormous movement of earth. As with landslides, cascade reactions are hard to stop once set into motion.

Intrinsic Factors

Intrinsic factors are problems or substances directly in the blood itself that first make platelets aggregate and then proceed to activate the blood-clotting cascade (Figure 39-4). Intrinsic events that stimulate platelet aggregation include antigen-antibody reactions, circulating debris, prolonged venous stasis, and bacterial endotoxins. Continuation of the cascade to the point of fibrin clot formation depends on the presence of sufficient amounts of all the various clotting factors and cofactors (Table 39-2).

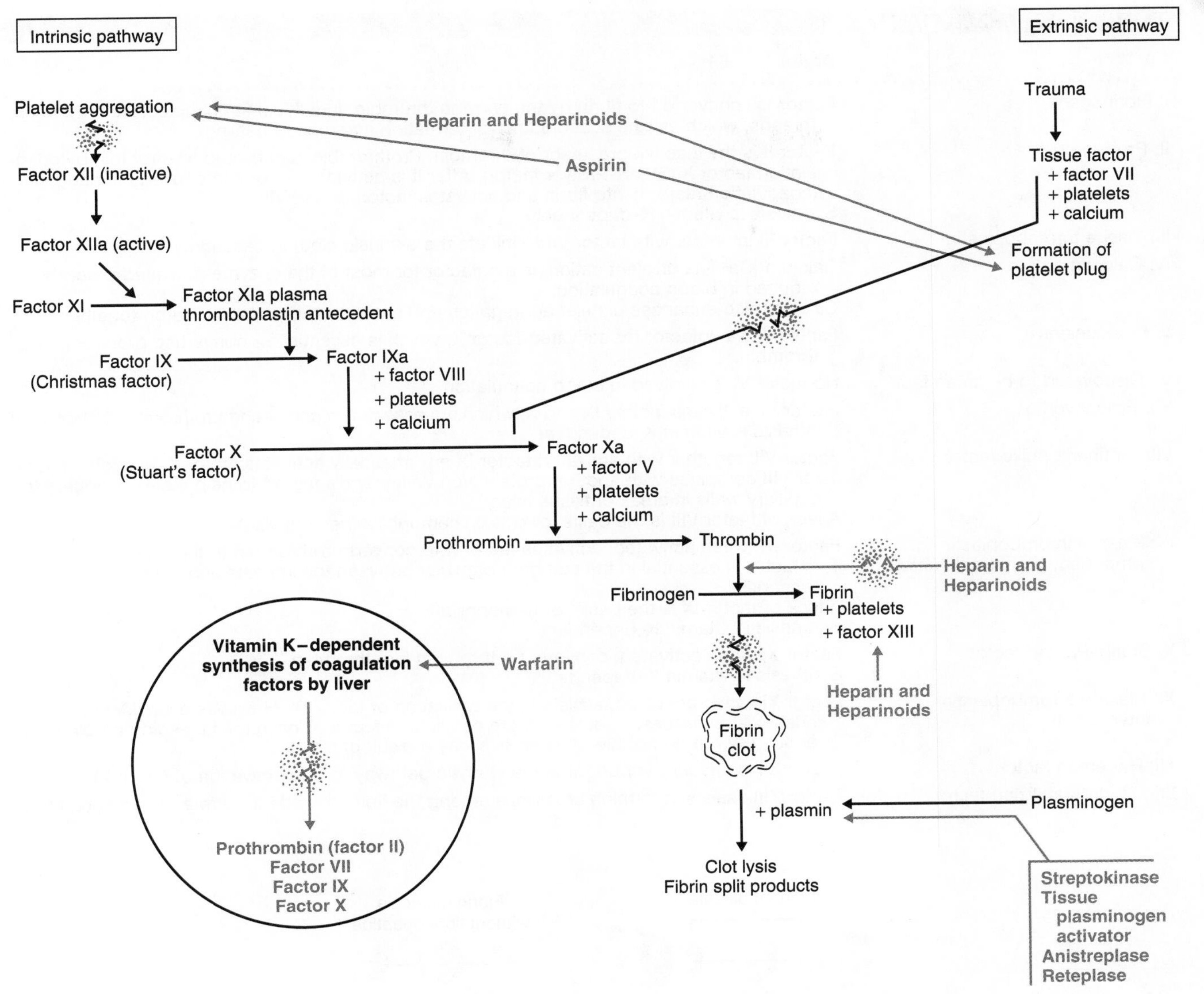

Figure 39-4 ● Summary of blood-clotting cascade.

Extrinsic Factors

Platelet plugs can begin to form as a result of changes in the blood vessels rather than changes in the blood. When platelet plugs form in response to blood vessel changes, the response is said to be caused by **extrinsic factors** (extrinsic to the blood). The most common extrinsic events are trauma to tissues and damage to blood vessels, which exposes the platelets to collagen and stimulates aggregation. The platelet plug is formed within seconds of the trauma. The blood-clotting cascade is started sooner by the extrinsic pathway than by the intrinsic pathway because some of the steps of the intrinsic pathway are bypassed.

Whether the platelet plugs were formed because of abnormal blood (intrinsic factors) or by exposure of substances from damaged blood vessels (extrinsic factors), the end result of the cascade is the same: *formation of a fibrin clot and coagulation.* The many steps of the cascade between the formation of a platelet plug and the formation of a fibrin clot are dependent on the presence of specific **clotting factors,** calcium, and more platelets.

Clotting factors (see Table 39-2) are actually inactive proteins that become activated in a sequence to activate fibrinogen into fibrin. At each step, the activated protein from the previous step allows activation of the next protein. The last two steps in the cascade are the activation of thrombin from prothrombin and the conversion (by thrombin) of fibrinogen into fibrin. Only fibrin molecules can begin the formation of a true clot.

FIBRIN CLOT FORMATION

Fibrinogen is a large, inactive protein molecule made in the liver and secreted into the blood. Thrombin, an enzyme, removes the end portions of fibrinogen and converts it to the active fibrin molecule. Individual fibrin molecules link together to form fibrin threads. The fibrin threads make a lattice-like meshwork that forms the base of a blood clot (Figure 39-5).

TABLE 39-2 • THE CLOTTING FACTORS

Factor	Action
I: Fibrinogen	Factor I is converted to fibrin by the enzyme thrombin. Individual fibrin molecules form fibrin threads, which are the scaffold for clot formation and wound healing.
II: Prothrombin	Factor II is the inactive precursor of thrombin. Prothrombin is activated to thrombin by coagulation factor X (Stuart-Prower factor). After it is activated, thrombin converts fibrinogen (coagulation factor I) into fibrin and activates factors V and VIII. Synthesis is vitamin K–dependent.
III: Tissue thromboplastin	Factor III interacts with factor VII to initiate the extrinsic clotting cascade.
IV: Calcium	Calcium (Ca^{2+}), a divalent cation, is a cofactor for most of the enzyme-activated processes required in blood coagulation. Calcium also enhances platelet aggregation and makes red blood cells clump together.
V: Proaccelerin	Factor V is a cofactor for activated factor X, which is essential for converting prothrombin to thrombin.
VI: Discovered to be an artifact	No factor VI is involved in blood coagulation.
VII: Proconvertin	Factor VII activates factors IX and X, which are essential in converting prothrombin to thrombin. Synthesis is vitamin K–dependent.
VIII: Antihemophilic factor	Factor VIII together with activated factor IX enzymatically activates factor X. In addition, factor VIII combines with another protein (von Willebrand's factor) to help platelets adhere to capillary walls in areas of tissue injury. A lack of factor VIII is the basis for classic hemophilia (hemophilia A).
IX: Plasma thromboplastin component (Christmas factor)	Factor IX, when activated, activates factor X to convert prothrombin to thrombin. This factor is essential in the common pathway between the intrinsic and extrinsic clotting cascades. A lack of factor IX is the basis for hemophilia B. Synthesis is vitamin K–dependent.
X: Stuart-Prower factor	Factor X, when activated, converts prothrombin into thrombin. Synthesis is vitamin K–dependent.
XI: Plasma thromboplastin antecedent	Factor XI, when activated, assists in the activation of factor IX. However, a similar factor must exist in tissues. People who are deficient in factor XI have mild bleeding problems after surgery but do not bleed excessively as a result of trauma.
XII: Hageman factor	Factor XII is critically important in the intrinsic pathway for the activation of factor XI.
XIII: Fibrin-stabilizing factor	Factor XIII assists in forming crosslinks among the fibrin threads to form a strong fibrin clot.

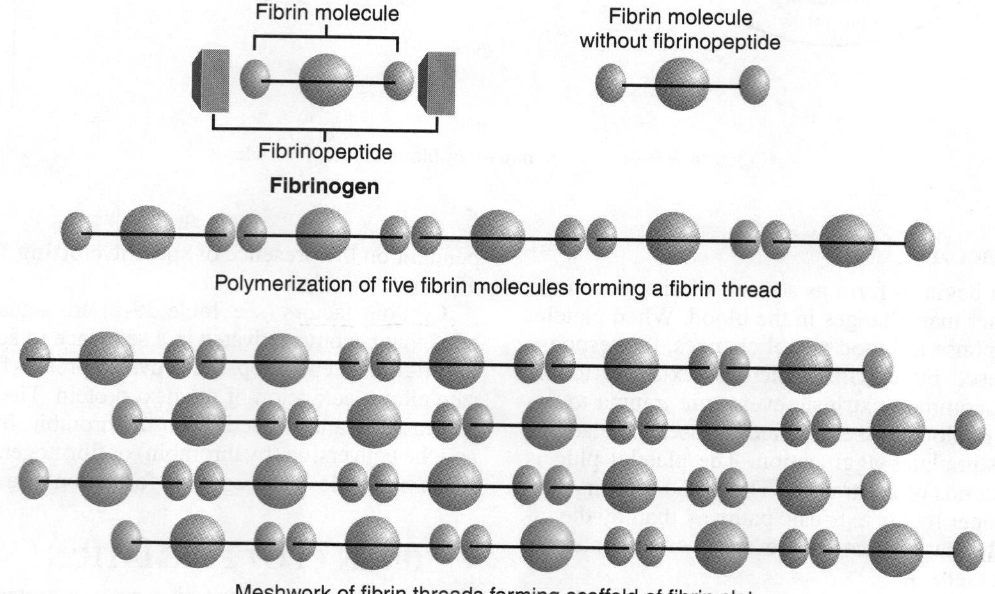

Figure 39-5 • Activation and polymerization of fibrin to form fibrin clot.

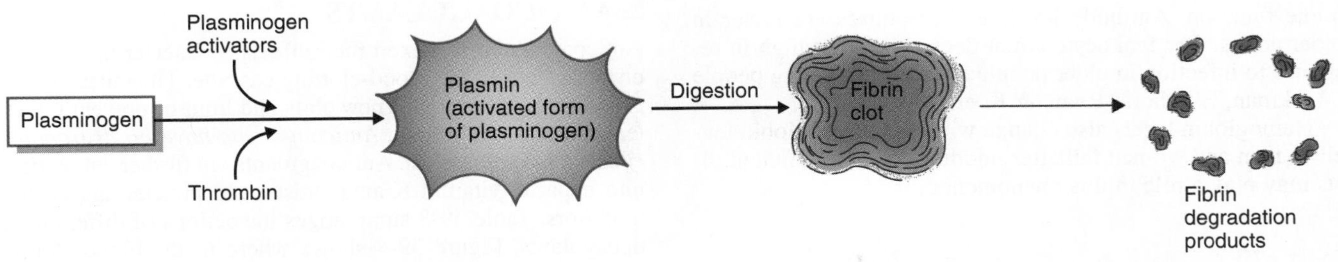

Figure 39-6 ● The process of fibrinolysis.

CHART 39-1

NURSING FOCUS *on the* OLDER ADULT
Hematologic Assessment

Findings in Hematologic Disorders	Normal Changes in the Older Adult	Significance/Alternatives
NAIL BEDS (FOR CAPILLARY REFILL) Pallor or cyanosis may indicate a hematologic disorder.	Thickened or discolored nails make visualization of skin color beneath the nails impossible.	Use another body area, such as the lip, to assess central capillary refill.
HAIR DISTRIBUTION Thin or absent hair on the trunk or extremities may indicate poor circulation to a particular area.	Progressive loss of body hair is a normal facet of aging.	A relatively even pattern of hair loss that has occurred over an extended period is not significant.
SKIN MOISTURE Skin dryness may indicate any of a number of hematologic disorders.	Skin dryness is a normal result of aging.	Skin moisture is not usually a reliable indicator of an underlying pathologic condition in the older adult.
SKIN COLOR Skin color changes, especially pallor and jaundice, are associated with some hematologic disorders.	Pigment loss and skin yellowing are common changes associated with aging.	Pallor in an older adult may not be a reliable indicator of anemia; laboratory testing is required. Yellow-tinged skin in an older adult may not be a reliable indicator of increased serum bilirubin levels; laboratory testing is required.

After the fibrin mesh is formed, a stabilizing factor (clotting factor XIII) tightens up the mesh, making it more dense. Additional platelets stick to the threads of the mesh and attract other blood cells and proteins to form an actual blood clot. As this clot retracts, the **serum** (plasma without the clotting factors) is excreted, and clot formation is complete.

FIBRINOLYSIS

Because blood coagulation occurs through a rapid cascade process, in theory it keeps forming fibrin clots whenever the cascade is set into motion until all blood throughout the entire body has coagulated. Such widespread coagulation is not compatible with life. Therefore, when the blood-clotting cascade is started, counterclotting or **anticoagulant** forces are also started to limit clot formation to only damaged areas; normal blood flow is maintained everywhere else. When blood clotting and anticlotting actions are appropriately balanced, coagulation occurs only where needed, and normal circulation is maintained.

The fibrinolytic system dissolves the fibrin clot with special enzymes (Figure 39-6). The key event of fibrinolysis is the conversion of plasminogen to plasmin. Plasmin, an active enzyme, digests fibrin, fibrinogen, prothrombin, and factors V, VIII, and XII, thus breaking down the fibrin clot.

Hematologic Changes Associated with Aging

Aging changes the cellular and plasma components of blood, making accurate assessment of the hematologic system in older adults more difficult. Chart 39-1 lists assessment tips for this population. Several factors cause a decreased blood volume in older people. Total body water is decreased among older adults. In addition, they tend to have a lower concentration of plasma proteins and a decreased plasma osmotic pressure (possibly related to a decreased dietary intake of proteins), which also causes some loss of blood volume into the interstitial space.

Bone marrow produces fewer blood cells as it ages. Total red blood cell (RBC) and white blood cell (WBC) counts (especially lymphocyte counts) are lower among older adults. Platelet counts do not appear to change with age. Lymphocytes become less reactive to antigens and have a loss of immune function. Antibody levels and responses are lower in older adults. The leukocyte count does not rise as high in response to infection in older people as it does in young people (Workman, Ellerhorst-Ryan, & Koertge, 1993).

Hemoglobin levels also change with age. Hemoglobin levels in men and women fall after middle age. Iron-deficient diets may play a role in this phenomenon.

Anticoagulants and Thrombolytics

Drug therapy is commonly used to alter clotting ability or to destroy existing clots when circulation is at risk. The two broad categories of drugs are anticoagulants and thrombolytics. Both categories of agents are used widely to treat excessive or inappropriate clot formation, but their actions, side effects, and precautions are very different.

ANTICOAGULANTS

Anticoagulant drugs exert their effects by interfering with one or more steps in the blood-clotting cascade. Thus these agents *prevent* the formation of new clots and limit or prevent the extension of formed clots. *Anticoagulants have no degradative effects on existing clots.* Anticoagulants are further categorized into heparin, vitamin K antagonists, and platelet aggregation inhibitors. Table 39-3 summarizes the actions of different anticoagulants. Figure 39-4 shows where in the blood-clotting cascade these agents exert their anticlotting effects.

THROMBOLYTICS

Thrombolytic agents preferentially degrade fibrin threads already present in the formed blood clot. The four most extensively used agents are tissue plasminogen activator (t-PA),

TABLE 39-3 • ANTICOAGULANTS AND THROMBOLYTICS

Agent	Mechanism of Action	Nursing Implications
ANTICOAGULANTS		
Heparin (Calciparine, Hepalean♣, Liquaemin)	Potentiates the inhibiting actions of antithrombin III Interferes with thrombin formation Prevents conversion of fibrinogen to fibrin Prevents stabilization of fibrin clots	Prevents clot formation Has no effect on existing clots Must be given parenterally Antidote is protamine sulfate Half-life is 1 to 6 hours Can be allergenic
Low–Molecular Weight Heparins		
Enoxaparin (Lovenox)	Same as heparin	Same as for heparin, but less allergenic Must be administered as a deep subcutaneous injection **Do not administer intravenously or intramuscularly** Does not require monitoring of drug levels or PTT
Dalteparin (Fragmin)	Similar to heparin Most activity involves the inhibition of clotting factor Xa	Same as for enoxaparin
Warfarin (Coumadin, Warfilone♣)	Disrupts liver synthesis of vitamin K–dependent clotting factors (factors II, VII, IX, X)	Requires 48-96 hours to peak effect May be started while the client is still receiving heparin Requires 1 week to clear after drug is discontinued Instruct client **not** to take aspirin, any nonsteroidal anti-inflammatory drug, or Ginkgo biloba Antidote is vitamin K
THROMBOLYTICS		
Reteplase (Retavase)	Breaks plasminogen, activating it into plasmin; plasmin then breaks the fibrin meshwork of a clot, causing it to disintegrate	Avoid venipunctures during and for 1 hour following administration May induce intracranial hemorrhage in older clients Affects all existing clots <24 hours old Half-life is approximately 15-20 minutes
Anistreplase (Eminase)	Binds with plasminogen to form an anistreplase-plasminogen complex that converts to an anistreplase-plasmin complex, which then digests fibrin	Avoid venipunctures during and for 4 hours following administration May induce intracranial hemorrhage in older clients Affects all existing clots <24 hours old Half-life is approximately 70-120 minutes
Alteplase (Activase)	Same as for reteplase	Avoid venipunctures during and for 2 hours following administration May induce intracranial hemorrhage in older clients Affects all existing clots <12 hours old Half-life is approximately 35 minutes
Streptokinase (Streptase)	Same as for anistreplase	Made from exogenous substances and is allergenic; anaphylaxis possible Not clot specific; also disrupts clotting cascade; greater risk for hemorrhage May not be effective in clients who have antibodies to streptococcal microorganisms Half-life is approximately 23 minutes

Data from *United States Pharmacopeia Dispensing Information (USP DI): Volume I. Drug information for the health care professional* (20th ed.). (2000). Englewood, CO: Micromedix.
PTT, Partial thromboplastin time.

streptokinase (SK), reteplase, and anistreplase. The mechanism to start fibrin degradation is the activation of the inactive tissue protein **plasminogen** to its active form, **plasmin.** Plasmin directly attacks and degrades the fibrin molecule and has fewer effects on the fibrinogen molecule. The general action of all these thrombolytic agents is the selective degradation of formed fibrin clots with minimal effect on clot formation.

In general, the administration of thrombolytic agents results in clot breakdown with less disruption of blood clotting. Thrombolytic agents are the first-line therapy for conditions caused by existing small or localized formed clots, such as myocardial infarction, limited arterial thrombosis, thrombotic strokes, and occluded shunts. For some conditions (e.g., myocardial infarction), these drugs are given only within the first 6 hours after the onset of symptoms. This time limitation is not related to drug activity, because thrombolytic agents can break down clots older than 6 hours. Rather, tissue that has been anoxic for more than 6 hours is not likely to benefit from this therapy, making the risks to the client greater than the advantages.

Thrombolytic therapy has a very limited role when clotting is extensive, such as in deep vein thrombophlebitis within the pelvis or massive pulmonary emboli. In these situations clots are very large compared to their usual size in the coronary arteries. The amount of drug and duration of therapy needed for the effective breakdown of such clots is both cost prohibitive and physiologically risky. Many of these clots are not easily accessed for direct infusion of the thrombolytic agent. In addition, these clots are large, and the danger of releasing large-sized particles from the clots during breakdown and having them occlude other blood vessels is much greater than the thrombolytic therapy of smaller arterial clots.

ASSESSMENT TECHNIQUES

History

DEMOGRAPHIC DATA

Chart 39-2 lists questions based on Gordon's Functional Health Patterns to ask during the assessment of hematologic function. Age and gender are important variables to obtain when assessing the client's hematologic status. Bone marrow and immune activity diminish with age.

WOMEN'S HEALTH CONSIDERATIONS

At all ages, women have lower blood cell counts than men. This difference is greater during the menstrual years. This gender difference may be related to a dilutional effect of female hormones, which causes fluid retention, or to differences in bone marrow activity.

It is also important for the nurse to collect information on the client's occupation, hobbies, and location of housing. This information may indicate an exposure to agents or chemicals that affect bone marrow growth and hematologic function.

PERSONAL AND FAMILY HISTORY

Obtaining an accurate family history is important because many bleeding disorders are inherited. The nurse asks whether anyone in the family has had hemophilia, frequent nosebleeds, postpartum hemorrhages, excessive bleeding after tooth extractions, or continuous heavy bruising in response to relatively mild trauma. Family information about sickle cell disease or sickle cell traits also is obtained. Although sickle cell disease is seen primarily among African Americans, anyone may have the trait.

Personal factors to be included in the hematologic assessment are liver function, the presence of known immunologic or hematologic disorders, and current medication use. Because liver function is important in the synthesis of clotting factors, the nurse also asks about jaundice, anemia, and gallstones.

The client is asked about use of blood "thinners" such as sodium warfarin (Coumadin, Warfilone♣), aspirin, and other nonsteroidal anti-inflammatory drugs (NSAIDs). A person who takes aspirin on a daily basis may have bleeding problems, and many over-the-counter medications contain aspirin or other salicylates that disrupt platelet aggregation. The nurse determines all medications that the client is using or has used in the past 3 weeks. Clients are also asked about the use of antibiotics, because prolonged antibiotic therapy can lead to coagulopathies or bone marrow depression. Table 39-4 lists drugs known to alter hematologic function. Previous radiation therapy may result in some permanent impairment of hematologic function, especially if marrow-forming bones were in the path of the radiation.

DIET HISTORY

Dietary pattern can alter cell quality and affect blood clotting. The nurse asks clients to record everything eaten during the previous week. This information is helpful in determining the causes of anemias and of protein, mineral, or vitamin deficiencies. Diets high in fat and carbohydrates and low in protein, iron, and vitamins can cause many types of anemia and decrease the functions of all blood cells.

CHART 39-2

HEMATOLOGIC ASSESSMENT
Using Gordon's Functional Health Patterns

Activity-Exercise Pattern
How does your energy level seem to you compared to last year at this time?
Do you feel rested after a typical night's sleep?
Have you experienced any dizziness or lightheadedness?
Does your heart ever seem to pound?
How much exercise do you get? How often? What type?
Do you feel you have enough energy to do what you want or need to do?

Nutrition-Metabolic Pattern
Have you noticed any change in your skin lately?
How easily do you bruise?
Do your gums ever bleed? Under what conditions?
How much meat do you eat in a week?
How often do you eat salads or other green leafy vegetables?
Are you taking any vitamin or mineral supplements?
Do your feet and hands usually feel warm or cold?
Has your weight changed by 5 pounds or more this year?
How often do you take aspirin or any other nonsteroidal anti-inflammatory drug?
What medications do you take daily?

Based on Gordon, M. (2000). *Manual of nursing diagnosis* (9th ed.). St. Louis: Mosby.

TABLE 39-4 • DRUGS IMPAIRING THE HEMATOLOGIC SYSTEM

Generic Name	Common Trade Names
DRUGS CAUSING BONE MARROW SUPPRESSION	
Altretamine	Hexalen, Hexastat♣
Amphotericin B	Fungizone
Azathioprine	Imuran
Chemotherapeutic agents*	
Chloramphenicol	Chloromycetin, Novochlorocap♣
Chromic phosphate	Phosphocol
Colchicine	(Generic only)
Didanosine	Videx
Eflornithine	Ornidyl
Foscarnet sodium	Foscavir
Ganciclovir	Cytovene
Interferon alfa	Actimmune, Alferon, Intron-A, Roferon-A, Wellferon
Pentamidine	Pentam 300, NebuPent, Pentacarinat♣
Sodium iodide	Iodopen
Zalcitabine	HIVID
Zidovudine	AZT, Retrovir, Novo-AZT♣
DRUGS CAUSING HEMOLYSIS	
Acetohydroxamic acid	Lithostat
Chlorpropamide	Diabinese, Glucamide, Novo-Propamide♣
Doxapram	Dopram
Glyburide	DiaBeta, Micronase, Euglucon♣
Mefenamic acid	Ponstel, Ponstan♣
Menadiol diphosphate	Synkayvite
Methyldopa	Aldomet, Dopamet♣
Nitrofurantoin	Macrodantin, NovoFurantoin♣
Amoxicillin	Amoxil, Augmentin, Apo-Amoxi♣
Penicillin G benzathine	Bicillin, Crystapen
Penicillin V	Pen-Vee K, Pen Vee, Nu-Pen-VK♣
Primaquine	(Generic only)
Procainamide hydrochloride	Procan-SR, Promine, Pronestyl
Quinidine polygalacturonate	Cardioquin, Quinalan, Novoquinidin♣
Quinine	Legatrin, Quindan
Sulfonamides	Sulfamethoxazole (Gantanol), sulfisoxazole (Gantrisin, Novo-Soxazole♣)
Tolbutamide	Oramide, Orinase, Apo-Tolbutamide♣, Mobenol♣
Vitamin K	AquaMEPHYTON, Konakion
DRUGS DISRUPTING PLATELET ACTION	
Aspirin	Anacin, Ascriptin, Bufferin, Ecotrin, Entrophen♣, Riphen♣, Triaphen♣
Carbenicillin	Geopen, Pyopen♣
Carindacillin	Geocillin
Dipyridamole	Persantine, Apo-Dipyridamole♣, Novodipiradol♣
Moxalactam	Moxam
Pentoxifylline	Trental
Sulfinpyrazone	Anturane, Antazone♣, Novopyrazone♣
Ticarcillin	Ticar
Ticlopidine	Ticlid
Valproic acid	Dalpro, Depakene, Epival♣

Data from United States Pharmacopeia *Dispensing Information (USP DI): Vol. I. Drug information for the health care professional* (20th ed.). Englewood, CO: Micromedix.
*General categories of chemotherapeutic agents include alkylating agents, antimitotics, antitumor antibiotics, and antimetabolites.

Clients are asked about alcohol consumption. Chronic alcoholism is associated with nutritional deficiencies and liver impairment, both of which can decrease the ability of the blood to clot.

Certain dietary habits can enhance blood clotting. Diets high in vitamin K may increase the rate of blood coagulation. The nurse assesses the amount of raw, leafy green vegetables that the client consumes and whether he or she routinely takes supplemental vitamins. The amount of calcium consumed within the diet or in supplements is also assessed.

SOCIOECONOMIC STATUS

The nurse assesses the client's ability to understand and follow instructions related to proper diet, specific procedures and tests, and therapeutic regimens. Personal resources, such as finances and social support, are determined. A person with a marginal income may have a diet low in iron and protein. The nurse also notes the client's occupation and asks about potential exposure to chemicals.

CURRENT HEALTH PROBLEMS

The nurse determines whether the client has experienced swelling of the lymph nodes or excessive bruising or bleeding and whether the bleeding was spontaneous or induced by trauma. The client is asked about the amount and duration of bleeding after routine dental work. Women are asked about the presence of **menorrhagia** (excessive menstrual flow). They are asked to estimate the number of pads or tampons used during the most recent menstrual cycle and whether this amount represents a change from their usual pattern of menstrual flow. The nurse asks whether clots are present in menstrual blood. Clot size is estimated using coins or fruit for comparison ("clots are dime sized" or "clots are the size of lemons").

The nurse determines whether the client experiences dyspnea on exertion, palpitations, frequent infections, fevers, recent weight loss, headaches, or paresthesias. Any or all of these symptoms may accompany hematologic disease.

The single most common symptom of anemia is fatigue. Clients are asked about feeling tired, needing more rest, or losing endurance during normal activities. They are asked to compare the extent and intensity of their activities during the past month with those of the same month a year ago. The nurse asks about other symptoms associated with anemia, such as vertigo, tinnitus, anorexia, dysphagia, and a sore tongue.

Physical Assessment

The nurse performs a comprehensive physical assessment, because hematologic dysfunction affects the whole body. Certain problems are specific for hematologic assessment in older clients (see Chart 39-1).

SKIN ASSESSMENT

The nurse inspects the color of the skin for pallor or jaundice and of the mucous membranes and nail beds for pallor or cyanosis. Pallor of the gums, conjunctivae, and palmar creases indicates decreased hemoglobin levels. The gums are also assessed for active bleeding in response to light pressure or brushing the teeth with a soft-bristled brush, and any lesions or draining areas are noted. The nurse assesses for signs of bleeding in the form of petechiae and large bruises **(ecchymoses). Petechiae** are pinpoint hemorrhagic lesions in the skin. Bruises may be confluent or clustered. For hospitalized clients, the nurse determines if there is bleeding from sites such as nasogastric tubes, endotracheal tubes, central lines, peripheral intravenous sites, or Foley catheters. Skin turgor and itching are noted, because dry skin or intense itching can indicate hematologic disease.

CULTURAL CONSIDERATIONS

The nurse may have difficulty assessing people with darker skin for pallor, jaundice, petechiae, and bruising. Pallor and cyanosis are more easily detected in the oral mucous membranes and the conjunctiva of the eye. Jaundice can be seen more easily on the roof of the mouth. Petechiae may be visible only on the palms of the hands or the soles of the feet. Bruises can be seen as darker areas of skin and palpated as slight swellings or irregular skin surfaces. The nurse asks the client about pain when skin surfaces are touched lightly or palpated. Chapter 66 provides additional information on accurate assessment techniques for darker skin.

HEAD AND NECK ASSESSMENT

The nurse notes pallor or ulceration of the oral mucosa. The tongue may be completely smooth in pernicious anemia and iron deficiency anemia or smooth and red in nutritional deficiencies. These manifestations may be accompanied by fissures at the corners of the mouth. The nurse also observes for jaundice of the sclera.

All lymph node areas are inspected and palpated. Any lymph node enlargement is documented, including whether palpation of the enlarged node causes pain. It is important to determine whether the enlarged node moves or remains fixed with palpation.

RESPIRATORY ASSESSMENT

The rate and depth of respiration are assessed while the client is at rest, as well as during and after mild physical activity (e.g., walking 20 steps in 10 seconds). The nurse notes whether the client can complete a 10-word sentence without stopping for a breath. The nurse assesses whether the client is fatigued easily, experiences shortness of breath at rest or on exertion, or requires additional pillows to sleep comfortably at night. Many anemias cause these symptoms.

CARDIOVASCULAR ASSESSMENT

The nurse observes for heaves, distended neck veins, edema, or signs of phlebitis. He or she also auscultates for murmurs, gallops, irregular rhythms, and abnormal blood pressure. Systolic blood pressure tends to be lower than normal in clients with anemia. In conditions of hypercellularity, blood pressure is greater than normal. Severe anemias can cause right-sided ventricular hypertrophy and heart disease.

RENAL AND URINARY ASSESSMENT

The kidneys are extremely vascular, and bleeding problems may manifest as overt or occult **hematuria** (blood in the urine). The nurse inspects a voided sample of urine for color. Hematuria may be detected by grossly, bloody red or dark, brownish gold urine. The urine is tested for proteins with a urine test dipstick because hematologic problems may increase the protein content of urine. The urine sample also is tested for occult blood (Hemoccult test).

MUSCULOSKELETAL ASSESSMENT

Rib or sternal tenderness is an important sign of hematologic malignancy. The nurse examines the superficial surfaces of all bones, including the ribs and sternum, by applying intermittent firm pressure with the fingertips. The client's range of joint motion is assessed, and any swelling or joint pain is documented.

ABDOMINAL ASSESSMENT

The normal adult spleen is usually not palpable. An enlarged spleen is associated with many hematologic problems. An enlarged spleen may be detected by percussion, but palpation is more reliable. The spleen lies just beneath the abdominal wall and is identified by its movement during respiration. During palpation, the client lies in a relaxed, supine position while the nurse stands on the client's right side and palpates the left upper quadrant. *The nurse palpates gently and cautiously, because an enlarged spleen may be tender and easily ruptured.*

Palpating the edge of the liver in the right upper quadrant of the abdomen can detect hepatic enlargement, which is often associated with hematologic problems. A normal liver may be palpable as much as 4 to 5 cm below the right costal margin but is usually not palpable in the epigastrium.

A common cause of anemia among older adults is a chronically bleeding gastrointestinal lesion. If the lesion or open area is located in the stomach or small intestine, obvious blood may not be visible in the stool, or such a small amount is passed each day that the client is not aware of it. Therefore a stool specimen is obtained for occult blood testing.

CENTRAL NERVOUS SYSTEM ASSESSMENT

A thorough examination of the cranial nerves and neurologic function is necessary in many clients with hematologic disease. Vitamin B_{12} deficiency impairs cerebral, olfactory, spinal cord, and peripheral nerve function, and severe chronic deficiency may lead to irreversible neurologic degeneration. Many neurologic problems may develop in clients who have hematologic malignancies as a consequence of bleeding, infection, or tumor spread. When the client has a known or suspected bleeding disorder and has experienced any head trauma, the nurse expands the physical assessment to include frequent neurologic checks and mental status examinations (see Chapter 41).

Other important clinical manifestations associated with impaired hematologic function include fever, chills, and night sweats.

Psychosocial Assessment

The person with hematologic abnormalities may have a chronic illness (e.g., hemophilia or cancer) or an acute exacerbation of a chronic disease (e.g., pernicious anemia). In either instance each person brings his or her own coping style to the illness. After developing a rapport with the client, the nurse can learn what coping mechanisms he or she has used successfully during past illness or crises.

The nurse also asks the client and family members about social support networks, community resources, and financial health. A problem in any of these areas can interfere with compliance with therapy and, ultimately, recovery.

CRITICAL THINKING CHALLENGE

The client is a very active 62-year-old woman who is seen for an annual physical examination. Her complete blood count indicates a total white blood count of 22,000, a erythrocyte count of 100,000 and a platelet count of 55,000.

- Are these counts considered normal or abnormal? If any are abnormal, are they high or low?
- What specific questions regarding family history, recent health history, diet history, and personal history should you ask?

For suggested answer guidelines, go to SIMON http://www.wbsaunders.com/SIMON/Iggy/.

Diagnostic Assessment

LABORATORY TESTS

In hematologic disease, the most definitive signs are often the laboratory test results. Chart 39-3 lists laboratory data associated with hematologic function.

Tests of Cell Number and Function

COMPLETE BLOOD COUNT

A complete blood count (CBC) includes a number of studies: red blood cell (RBC) count, white blood cell (WBC) count, hematocrit, and hemoglobin level. The RBC count measures circulating RBCs in 1 mm^3 of venous blood, and the WBC count measures all leukocytes present in 1 mm^3 of venous blood. To determine the percentages of different types of leukocytes circulating in the blood, a WBC count with differential leukocyte count is performed (see Chapter 20). The hematocrit (Hct) is calculated as the percentage of RBCs in the total blood volume, and the hemoglobin level represents the total amount of hemoglobin in the peripheral blood.

The CBC can measure other variables of the circulating cells, including mean corpuscular volume (MCV), mean corpuscular hemoglobin (MCH), and mean corpuscular hemoglobin concentration (MCHC). MCV measures the average volume or size of a single RBC and is useful for classifying anemias. When MCV is elevated, the cell is said to be abnormally large **(macrocytic),** as seen in megaloblastic anemias. When MCV is decreased, the cell is abnormally small **(microcytic),** as seen in iron deficiency anemia. MCH is the average amount of hemoglobin in a single RBC. MCHC measures the average concentration of hemoglobin in a single RBC. When the MCHC is decreased, the cell has a hemoglobin deficiency and is hypochromic, as in iron deficiency anemia.

RETICULOCYTE COUNT

Another hematologic test helpful in determining bone marrow function is the reticulocyte count. A reticulocyte is an immature RBC. An elevated reticulocyte count indicates increased RBC production by the bone marrow. Normally about 2% of circulating RBCs are reticulocytes. An elevated reticulocyte count is desirable in an anemic client or after hemorrhage, because this indicates that the bone marrow is responding appropriately to a decrease in the total RBC mass. An elevated reticulocyte count without a precipitating cause may indicate a pathologic condition, such as polycythemia vera.

HEMOGLOBIN ELECTROPHORESIS

Hemoglobin electrophoresis detects abnormal forms of hemoglobin, such as hemoglobin S in sickle cell disease. Hemoglobin A is the major component of hemoglobin in the normal RBC. Decreased levels of hemoglobin A with increasing levels of other types of hemoglobin are typical of some hematologic problems, such as sickle cell disease.

LEUKOCYTE ALKALINE PHOSPHATASE

Leukocyte alkaline phosphatase (LAP) is an enzyme produced by normal mature neutrophils. Elevated LAP levels occur during episodes of infection or stress. An elevated neutrophil count without an accompanying elevation in LAP level is associated with chronic myelogenous leukemia.

COOMBS' TEST

The two Coombs' tests (direct and indirect) are used for blood typing. The direct test detects the presence of antibodies (also called antiglobulins) against RBCs that may be attached to the RBCs. Although healthy people can make these antibodies, certain diseases (e.g., systemic lupus erythematosus, mononucleosis, and lymphomas) are associated with the production of antibodies directed against the body's own RBCs. The presence of these antibodies usually causes a hemolytic anemia.

The indirect Coombs' test detects the presence of circulating antiglobulins. The test is used to determine whether the client has serum antibodies to the type of RBCs he or she is about to receive by blood transfusion.

SERUM FERRITIN, TRANSFERRIN, AND TOTAL IRON-BINDING CAPACITY

Serum ferritin, transferrin, and total iron-binding capacity (TIBC) tests measure iron levels. Abnormal levels of iron and TIBC are associated with many hematologic problems, including iron deficiency anemia.

The serum ferritin test measures the quantity of iron present as free iron in the plasma. The amount of serum ferritin is proportionally related to the amount of intracellular iron and represents 1% of the total body iron stores. Therefore the serum ferritin level provides a means to assess total iron stores. People with serum ferritin levels within 10 g of the normal range for their gender have adequate iron stores; people with levels 10 g or more lower than the normal range have inadequate iron stores and have difficulty recovering from any hemorrhagic event.

CHART 39-3

LABORATORY PROFILE
Hematologic Assessment

Test	Reference Range		International Reference Units	Significance of Abnormal Findings
Red blood cell (RBC) count	18-44 yr	F: 3.8-5.1 million/μL M: 4.3-5.7 million/μL	$3.8\text{-}5.1 \times 10^{12}$ cells/L $4.3\text{-}5.7 \times 10^{12}$ cells/L	*Decreased levels* indicate possible anemia or hemorrhage *Increased levels* indicate possible chronic anoxia or polycythemia vera
	45-64 yr	F: 3.8-5.3 million/μL M: 4.2-5.6 million/μL	$3.8\text{-}5.3 \times 10^{12}$ cells/L $4.2\text{-}5.6 \times 10^{12}$ cells/L	
	>64 yr	F: 3.8-5.2 million/μL M: 3.8-5.8 million/μL	$3.8\text{-}5.2 \times 10^{12}$ cells/L $3.8\text{-}5.8 \times 10^{12}$ cells/L	
Hemoglobin (Hgb)	18-44 yr	F: 11.7-15.5 g/dL M: 13.2-17.3 g/dL	117-155 g/L 132-173 g/L	Same as for RBC
	45-64 yr	F: 11.7-16.0 g/dL M: 13.1-17.2 g/dL	117-160 g/L 131-172 g/L	
	>65 yr	F: 11.7-16.1 g/dL M: 12.6-17.4 g/dL	117-161 g/L 126-174 g/L	
Hematocrit	18-44 yr	F: 34%-45% M: 39%-49%	0.34-0.45 fraction 0.39-0.49 fraction	Same as for RBC
	45-64 yr	F: 35%-47% M: 39%-50%	0.35-0.47 fraction 0.39-0.50 fraction	
	>65 yr	F: 35%-47% M: 37%-51%	0.35-0.47 fraction 0.37-0.51 fraction	
Mean cell volume (MCV)		80-100 fL	Same as reference range	*Increased levels* indicate macrocytic cells, possible anemia *Decreased levels* indicate microcytic cells, possible iron deficiency anemia
Mean cell hemoglobin (MCH)		26-35 pg/cell	Same as reference range	Same as for MCV
Mean cell hemoglobin concentration (MCHC)		31-37 g/dL cells	310-370 g/L	*Increased levels* may indicate spherocytosis or anemia *Decreased levels* may indicate iron deficiency anemia or a hemoglobinopathy
White blood cell (WBC) count		4500-11,000/μL	$4.5\text{-}11.0 \times 10^9$ cells/L	*Increased levels* are associated with infection, inflammation, autoimmune disorders, and leukemia *Decreased levels* may indicate prolonged infection or bone marrow suppression
Reticulocyte count		0.5%-1.5% of RBCs	0.005-0.015 fraction	*Increased levels* may indicate chronic blood loss *Decreased levels* indicate possible inadequate RBC production
Total iron binding capacity (TIBC)		250-425 μg/dL	44.8-76.1 μmol/L	*Increased levels* indicate iron deficiency *Decreased levels* may indicate anemia, hemorrhage, hemolysis
Serum haptoglobin		40-240 mg/dL	0.4-2.5 g/L	*Increased levels* indicate possible inflammatory disease *Decreased levels* may indicate liver disease or hemolytic disease
Iron (Fe)		F: 50-170 μg/dL M: 65-175 μg/dL	9.0-30.4 μmol/L 11.6-31.3 μmol/L	*Increased levels* indicate iron excess, hemochromocytosis, liver disorders, megaloblastic anemia *Decreased levels* indicate possible iron deficiency anemia, hemorrhage
Serum ferritin		F: 10-120 ng/mL M: 20-250 ng/mL	Same as reference range	Same as for iron
Platelet count		150,000-400,000/μL	$150\text{-}400 \times 10^9$/L	*Increased levels* may indicate polycythemia vera or malignancy *Decreased levels* may indicate bone marrow suppression, autoimmune disease, hypersplenism

Continued

Data from Tietz, N. (1995). *Clinical guide to laboratory tests* (3rd ed.) Philadelphia: W.B. Saunders.
F, Female; *M,* male, *fL,* femtoliter; *pg,* picogram; *INR,* International Normalized Ratio.

CHART 39-3

LABORATORY PROFILE
Hematologic Assessment—cont'd

Test	Reference Range	International Reference Units	Significance of Abnormal Findings
Hemoglobin electrophoresis	Hgb A_1: >95% Hgb A_2: 1.5%-3.7% Hgb F: <2% Hgb S: 0% Hgb C: 0%	>0.95 fraction 0.015-0.037 fraction <0.02 fraction 0.0 fraction 0.0 fraction	*Variations* indicate hemoglobinopathies
Direct Coombs' and indirect Coombs' test	Negative	Negative	*Positive findings* indicate antibodies to RBCs
Prothrombin time (PT)	11-15 sec	Patient PT/normal/PT (INR)	*Increased time* indicates possible deficiency of clotting factors V and VII *Decreased time* may indicate vitamin K excess
Bleeding time	2-7 min	Same as reference range	*Increased time* may indicate inadequate platelet function or number, clotting factor deficiencies
Euglobin lysis time	2-4 hr	Same as reference range	*Decreased time* may indicate possible fibrinolysis
Fibrin degradation products	<10 μg/mL	<10 mg/L	*Increased levels* may indicate disseminated intravascular coagulation of fibrinolysis

Data from Tietz, N. (1995). *Clinical guide to laboratory tests* (3rd ed.), Philadelphia: W.B. Saunders.
F, Female; *M,* male, *fL,* femtoliter; *pg,* picogram; *INR,* International Normalized Ratio.

Transferrin is a protein that transports iron from the gastrointestinal tract to cell storage sites. It is not easy to measure the amount of transferrin. However, measuring the amount of iron that can be bound to serum transferrin indirectly determines whether an adequate amount of transferrin is present. This test is the TIBC test. In healthy people, only about 30% of the transferrin is bound to iron in the blood. TIBC is measured by taking a sample of blood and adding measured amounts of iron to it. TIBC is calculated when the blood no longer binds the iron but allows it to precipitate. TIBC increases when a person is deficient in serum iron and stored iron levels. Such a value indicates that an adequate amount of transferrin is present but that less than 30% of it is bound to serum iron.

Tests Measuring Bleeding and Coagulation

CAPILLARY FRAGILITY TEST

The capillary fragility test, or Rumpel-Leede test, measures vascular hemostatic function by increasing intracapillary pressure in the arm. This is done by occluding venous outflow or by applying controlled negative pressure to a skin area. A blood pressure cuff is usually inflated to a pressure halfway between the systolic and diastolic pressures. This pressure is maintained for 5 minutes, and the petechiae that appear distal to the cuff are counted. Normally, five to ten petechiae appear. The capillary fragility test can help determine whether excessive bleeding or bruising results from increased capillary fragility or impaired platelet action.

BLEEDING TIME TEST

The bleeding time test evaluates vascular and platelet activity during hemostasis. A special spring-loaded lancet that ensures uniform wound depth is used to make a small incision in the forearm while a blood pressure cuff remains inflated at 40 mm Hg. Blood is blotted from the site at 30-second intervals, and the time required for the bleeding to stop is recorded. Normal bleeding time ranges from 1 to 9 minutes.

PROTHROMBIN TIME

Prothrombin time (PT) is a measurement of how long blood takes to clot. This test reflects how much of the clotting factors II, V, VII, and X is present and how well they are functioning. When sufficient amounts of these clotting factors are present and functioning, the PT shows blood clotting between 11 and 13 seconds, or within 85% to 100% of the time needed for a control sample of blood to clot. PT is prolonged when one or more clotting factors is deficient, or when liver disease is present. Sodium warfarin (Coumadin, Warfilone🍁) therapy is also monitored using PT levels. Appropriate warfarin therapy prolongs PT by 1.5 to 2 times the client's normal PT value.

Facilities are using the PT test less often to assess blood clotting because control blood is taken from different people and may not be the same from one day to the next, even in a single laboratory. To eliminate PT errors resulting from variations in control blood or in some of the chemicals used in the test, the **International Normalized Ratio (INR)** is used more often to assess clotting time.

INTERNATIONAL NORMALIZED RATIO

The INR measures the same process as the PT but in a slightly different way—by establishing a normal mean or standard for PT. The INR is calculated by dividing the client's PT by the established standard PT. A normal INR ranges between 0.7

and 1.8. When using the INR to monitor warfarin therapy, it should be maintained between 2.0 and 3.0 regardless of the actual PT in seconds.

PARTIAL THROMBOPLASTIN TIME

Partial thromboplastin time (PTT) assesses the intrinsic coagulation cascade and evaluates the presence of factors II, V, VIII, IX, XI, and XII. PTT is prolonged whenever any of these factors is deficient, such as in hemophilia or disseminated intravascular coagulation (DIC). Because factors II, IX, and X are vitamin K dependent and are produced in the liver, liver disease can decrease their concentration and prolong PTT. Heparin (Calciparine, Liquaemin, Hepalean✤) therapy is monitored by PTT. The desired ranges for therapeutic anticoagulation are 1.5 to 2.5 times the normal values.

Controversy exists regarding whether this test is accurate when the blood sample is obtained through an existing vascular access device (e.g., arterial line or normal saline lock) instead of through a separate new venipuncture. Clinical studies have shown that with an appropriate discard, samples obtained through existing vascular access devices do accurately reflect the client's activated partial thromboplastin time (see the Evidence-Based Practice for Nursing box at right).

PLATELET AGGLUTINATION/AGGREGATION

Platelet aggregation, or the ability to clump, can be tested by mixing the client's plasma with a substance called ristocetin. The degree of aggregation is noted. Aggregation can be impaired in von Willebrand's disease and during the use of drugs such as aspirin, anti-inflammatory agents, and psychotropic agents.

RADIOGRAPHIC EXAMINATIONS

Assessment of the client with a suspected hematologic abnormality can include radioisotopic imaging. Isotopes are used to evaluate the bone marrow for sites of active blood cell formation and sites of iron storage. Radioactive colloids are routinely used to determine organ size and liver and spleen function.

The client is given a radioactive isotope intravenously approximately 3 hours before the procedure. The client is taken to the nuclear medicine department for the scan, where he or she must lie still for approximately 1 hour. No special client preparation or follow-up care is needed for these tests.

Standard x-ray studies may be used to diagnose certain hematologic disorders. For example, multiple myeloma causes characteristic bone destruction, with a "Swiss cheese" appearance on the x-ray film.

BONE MARROW ASPIRATION AND BIOPSY

A bone marrow aspiration or biopsy is often performed to evaluate the client's hematologic status when other tests show persistent abnormal findings. Results can provide important information about bone marrow function, including the production of red blood cells (RBCs), white blood cells (WBCs), and platelets. Bone marrow aspiration and bone marrow biopsy are similar invasive procedures. In a bone marrow aspiration, cells and fluids are suctioned from the bone marrow. In a bone marrow biopsy, solid tissue and cells are obtained by coring out an area of bone marrow with a large-bore needle.

A physician's order and a signed, informed consent are obtained from the client before a bone marrow aspiration or biopsy is performed. Bone marrow aspiration may be performed by a physician, sanctioned clinical nurse specialist, nurse practitioner, or physician assistant, depending on the agency's policy and regional law. The procedure may be performed at the client's bedside, in an examination room, in a laboratory, or in a clinic setting.

On learning what specific tests will be performed on the marrow, the nurse checks the facility's procedure manual and checks with the hematology laboratory to determine how to handle the specimen. Some tests require the addition of heparin or other special solutions to the specimen.

CLIENT PREPARATION. Most clients experience anxiety or fear before a bone marrow aspiration. Clients who have experienced a bone marrow aspiration may have less anxiety or more anxiety depending on their previous experience. The nurse can help reduce anxiety and allay fears by providing accurate information and continuous emotional support. Some clients like to have their hand held during the procedure; other clients may want the nurse to hug or hold their entire upper body.

The nurse explains the procedure to the client and says that he or she will stay during the entire procedure. Occasionally, a friend or family member is permitted to be pres-

EVIDENCE-BASED PRACTICE FOR NURSING

Discard blood to increase accuracy

Powers, J. (1999). Obtaining blood samples for coagulation studies from a normal saline lock. *American Journal of Critical Care, 8*(4), 250-253.

This prospective, descriptive clinical study sought to determine whether blood samples drawn through existing vascular access devices paralleled the activated partial thromboplastin time (aPPT) results obtained from fresh venipunctures of the same clients. Blood samples were obtained from 32 clients both by direct venipuncture and through a normal saline lock. A total of 4 samples through the normal saline lock were obtained from all subjects: using no discard, a discard of 2 times the device dead space (3 mL), a discard of 4 times the device dead space (6 mL), and a discard of 6 times the dead space (9 mL).

When no blood was discarded from the samples drawn from the normal saline lock, the aPTTs were significantly different from those obtained by direct venipuncture. When blood was discarded representing twice or more of the device dead space, the aPTT results were not different from those obtained by direct venipuncture.

Critique. This study was well controlled and used clearly defined measurement parameters. Sample size was adequate for the design, and the results were consistent with those from other clinical studies with similar designs.

Implications for Nursing. If the volume of dead space is known and accurate, nurses could use only a minimal discard (twice the device dead space) when obtaining blood samples from existing vascular access devices to monitor aPTT levels. The primary outcome of this change in practice would be the avoidance of an unnecessary needle stick to the client. Possible secondary outcomes include a decreased blood loss for the client and a decrease in cost for the procedure by reducing the amount of venipuncture equipment used.

ent to hold the client's hand and provide additional emotional support. If a local anesthetic is used, the nurse explains that the injection will feel like a stinging or burning sensation. The nurse tells the client to expect a heavy sensation of pressure and pushing while the needle is being inserted. Some clients also can hear a crunching sound or feel a scraping sensation as the needle punctures the bone. The nurse explains that a brief sensation of painful pulling will be experienced as the marrow is aspirated by mild suction in the syringe. If a biopsy is performed, the client may feel more pressure and discomfort as the needle is rotated into the bone.

The client is assisted onto an examining table, and the site (most commonly the iliac crest) is exposed. If this site is not available or if more marrow is needed, the sternum can be used. If the iliac crest is being used, the client is usually placed in the prone position or occasionally in the side-lying position. Depending on the tests to be performed on the specimen, a laboratory technician may also be present to ensure appropriate handling of the specimen.

PROCEDURE. The procedure usually lasts from 5 to 15 minutes. Clients may be uncomfortable and may experience pain. The type and amount of anesthesia or sedation used depends on the physician's preference, the client's preference and previous experience with bone marrow aspiration and biopsy, and the setting.

A local anesthetic solution may be injected into the skin around the site. The client may also receive a mild tranquilizer or a rapid-acting sedative, such as midazolam hydrochloride (Versed) or lorazepam (Ativan, Apo-Lorazepam✤, Novo-Lorazem✤). Some clients do well with guided imagery or autohypnosis.

Aspiration or biopsy procedures are invasive, and sterile precautions are observed. The skin over the site is cleaned with a disinfectant solution. For an aspiration, the needle is inserted with a twisting motion, and the marrow is aspirated by pulling back on the plunger of the syringe. When sufficient marrow has been aspirated to ensure accurate analysis, the needle is carefully and rapidly withdrawn while the tissues are supported at the site. For a biopsy, a small skin incision is made, and the biopsy needle is inserted through the skin opening. Pressure and several twisting motions are performed to ensure coring and loosening of an adequate amount of marrow tissue. External pressure is applied to the site until hemostasis is ensured. A pressure dressing or sandbags may be applied to minimize bleeding at the site.

FOLLOW-UP CARE. The site is covered with a dressing after hemostasis is achieved and is observed closely for 24 hours for signs of bleeding and infection. A mild analgesic (aspirin-free) is prescribed for discomfort, and ice packs are applied over the site to limit bruising. The nurse instructs the client to inspect the site every 2 hours for the first 24 hours and to note the presence of active bleeding or bruising. The client is advised to avoid contact sports or any activity that might result in trauma to the site for 48 hours.

Information obtained from bone marrow aspiration or biopsy reflects the degree and quality of bone marrow activity. The counts made on a marrow specimen can indicate whether stem cells, blast cells, committed cells, and more mature cell forms are present in the expected quantities and proportions. In addition, bone marrow aspiration or biopsy can confirm the spread of cancer cells from other tumor sites.

CRITICAL THINKING CHALLENGE

The client is a 62-year-old woman who is scheduled to have a bone marrow aspiration in 1 week to help determine the cause of abnormal WBC and RBC counts. This client cleans her own house, does her own shopping, eats lunch out with her friends once each week, volunteers in a soup kitchen one day per week, plays cards once each week, plays golf once each week, and plays bingo three times each week. She also drinks one glass of wine with dinner each day and bakes her own bread. Her medications include a daily multiple vitamin, 400 mg of Advil (ibuprofen) twice a day for joint pain, and conjugated estrogen (Premarin) daily. She is very concerned about the pain associated with this procedure.

- What is your teaching priority for this client?
- What will you tell her regarding pain or pain management?
- Which activities should she continue and which activities should she avoid for the first 24 hours and for the first week following the procedure?

For suggested answer guidelines, go to SIMON http://www.wbsaunders.com/SIMON/Iggy/.

ONLINE RESOURCES

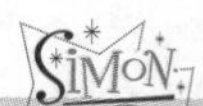

For suggested readings and Internet resources, go to http://www.wbsaunders.com/SIMON/Iggy/.

SELECTED BIBLIOGRAPHY

Asterisk indicates a classic or definitive work on this subject.

Bennett, J., DiMichele, D., & Haire, W. (1998). Clotting and bleeding: A new understanding. *Patient Care, 32*(11), 87-88.

*Beutler, E., et al. (1995). *William's hematology* (5th ed.). New York: McGraw-Hill.

Field, D. (1998). Assessment of haemostasis. *Nursing Times, 94*(29), 54-56.

Frizzell, J. (1998). Avoiding lab test pitfalls. *American Journal of Nursing, 98*(2), 34-38.

Gordon, M. (2000). *Manual of nursing diagnosis* (9th ed.). St. Louis: Mosby.

Guyton, A., & Hall, J. (2000). *Textbook of medical physiology* (10th ed.). Philadelphia: W.B. Saunders.

*Hays, K. (1990). Physiology of normal bone marrow. *Seminars in Oncology Nursing, 6*(1), 3-8.

Hirsh, J., Dalen, J., & Guyatt, G. (2001 supplement). Oral anticoagulants: Mechanisms of action, clinical effectiveness, and optimal therapeutic range. *Chest, 119*(1), 8S-21S.

Keen, M. (1998). Hemoglobin and hematocrit: An analysis of clinical accuracy. *American Nephrology Nurses Association Journal, 25*(1), 83-86.

Lechner, D. (1998). Sizing up your patient for heparin therapy. *Nursing98, 28*(8), 36-41.

Levine, M. et al. (2001 supplement). Hemorrhagic complications of anticoagulant treatment. *Chest, 119*(1), 108S-121S.

Oertel, L. (1999). Monitoring warfarin therapy: How the INR keeps your patient safe. *Nursing99*, 29(11), 41-45.

Pinkowish, M. (1998). Anticoagulation: Promises and pitfalls. *Patient Care Nurse Practitioners, 1*(2), 44-55.

Powers, J. (1999). Obtaining blood samples for coagulation studies from a normal saline lock. *American Journal of Critical Care, 8*(4), 250-253.

Seay, R. (1998). Frequently asked questions about warfarin sodium. *Home Healthcare Nurse, 16*(5), 328-329.

Then, K., & Rankin, J. (1999). The Internationalized Normalized Ratio: A review. *Canadian Journal of Cardiovascular Nursing, 10*(1-2), 40-42.

*Tietz, N. (1995). *Clinical guide to laboratory tests* (3rd ed.). Philadelphia: W.B. Saunders.

United States Pharmacopeia Dispensing Information (USP DI): Vol. I. *Drug information for the health care professional* (20th ed.). (2000). Englewood , CO: Micromedix.

*Weitz, J., & Hirsh, J. (2001 supplement). New anticoagulant drugs. *Chest, 119*(1), 95S-107S.

Williams, W. (1995). Hematology in the aged. In E. Beutler et al. (Eds.), *Williams hematology* (5th ed., pp. 72-77). New York: McGraw-Hill.

Workman, M. (1998). The lymphoid system and its role in maintaining immunocompetence. *Seminars in Oncology Nursing, 14*(4), 248-255.

*Workman, M., Ellerhorst-Ryan, J., & Koertge, V. (1993). *Nursing care of the immunocompromised patient.* Philadelphia: W.B. Saunders.

CHAPTER 40

Interventions for Clients with Hematologic Problems

SUSAN M. SCHNEIDER

Learning Objectives

After studying this chapter, you should be able to:

1. Identify three clinical manifestations common to clients who have any type of anemia.
2. Explain the pattern of inheritance for sickle cell disease.
3. Prioritize nursing care for the client who has sickle cell disease.
4. Plan a diet for a client who has iron deficiency anemia or vitamin B_{12} deficiency anemia.
5. Explain the mechanism of action and potential side effects of epoetin alpha therapy.
6. Compare and contrast the pathologic mechanisms of hemolytic anemia versus aplastic anemia.
7. Compare and contrast leukemia and lymphoma for etiology, pathophysiology, and clinical manifestations.
8. List four risk factors for the development of leukemia.
9. Analyze laboratory data and clinical manifestations to determine the presence of infection in a client who has neutropenia.
10. Compare the purposes and scheduling of induction therapy, consolidation therapy, and maintenance therapy for leukemia.
11. Prioritize nursing interventions for the client with neutropenia.
12. Prioritize nursing interventions for the client with thrombocytopenia.
13. Develop a teaching plan for a client with thrombocytopenia who is at home.
14. Prioritize nursing responsibilities during transfusion therapy.
15. Identify clients at risk for complications of transfusion therapy.

SIMON

Go to http://www.wbsaunders.com/SIMON/Iggy/ for self-assessment questions related to these Learning Objectives.

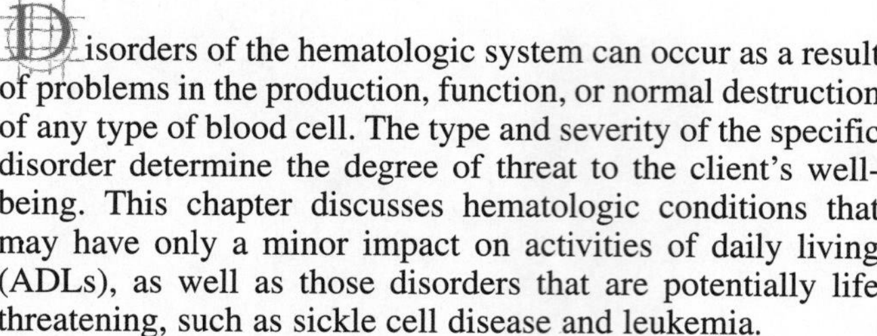

Disorders of the hematologic system can occur as a result of problems in the production, function, or normal destruction of any type of blood cell. The type and severity of the specific disorder determine the degree of threat to the client's well-being. This chapter discusses hematologic conditions that may have only a minor impact on activities of daily living (ADLs), as well as those disorders that are potentially life threatening, such as sickle cell disease and leukemia.

RED BLOOD CELL DISORDERS

The major cellular population of the blood consists of red blood cells (RBCs), or erythrocytes. Adequate tissue oxygenation depends on maintaining the circulating number of RBCs within the normal range for the person's age and gender and ensuring that the cells can perform their normal functions. RBC disorders include problems in production, function, and destruction. These problems may result in an insufficient number or insufficient function of RBCs **(anemia)** or an excess of RBCs **(polycythemia).**

Anemia is a reduction in either the number of RBCs, the quantity of hemoglobin, or the hematocrit (percentage of packed RBCs per deciliter of blood). Anemia is a clinical sign, not a diagnosis, because it is a manifestation of a number of abnormal conditions. Anemia can result from dietary deficiencies, hereditary disorders, bone marrow disease, or bleeding.

There are many types and causes of anemia. Some anemias are caused by a deficiency in one or more of the components needed to make fully functional RBCs. Such anemias can be caused by deficiencies of iron, vitamin B_{12}, folic acid, or intrinsic factor. Additional causes include a decreased rate of erythrocyte production and increased destruction of RBCs. Table 40-1 lists common causes of various types of anemia. Despite the many causes of anemia, the effects of anemia on the client (Chart 40-1) and the corresponding nursing care are similar for all types of anemia.

TABLE 40-1 • COMMON CAUSES OF ANEMIA

Type of Anemia	Common Causes
Sickle cell disease	Autosomal recessive inheritance of two defective genes for hemoglobin synthesis
Glucose-6-phosphate dehydrogenase (G6PD) deficiency anemia	X-linked recessive deficiency of the enzyme G6PD
Autoimmune hemolytic anemia	Abnormal immune function in which a person's immune reactive cells fail to recognize his or her own red blood cells as self cells
Iron deficiency anemia	Inadequate iron intake caused by: • Iron-deficient diet • Chronic alcoholism • Malabsorption syndromes • Partial gastrectomy Rapid metabolic (anabolic) activity caused by: • Pregnancy • Adolescence • Infection
Vitamin B_{12} deficiency anemia	Dietary deficiency Failure to absorb vitamin B_{12} from intestinal tract as a result of: • Partial gastrectomy • Pernicious anemia
Folic acid deficiency anemia	Dietary deficiency Malabsorption syndromes Drugs • Oral contraceptives • Anticonvulsants • Methotrexate
Aplastic anemia	Exposure to myelotoxic agents • Radiation • Benzene • Chloramphenicol • Alkylating agents • Antimetabolites • Sulfonamides • Insecticides Viral infection (unproven) • Epstein-Barr virus • Hepatitis B • Cytomegalovirus

CHART 40-1

KEY FEATURES *of* Anemia

Integumentary Manifestations
- Pallor, especially of the ears, the nail beds, the palmar creases, the conjunctiva, and around the mouth
- Cool to the touch
- Intolerance of cold temperatures
- Nails become brittle and may lose the normal convex shape; over time, nails become concave and fingers assume clublike appearance

Cardiovascular Manifestations
- Tachycardia at basal activity levels, increasing with activity and during and immediately after meals
- Murmurs and gallops heard on auscultation when anemia is severe
- Orthostatic hypotension

Respiratory Manifestations
- Dyspnea on exertion
- Decreased oxygen saturation levels

Neurologic Manifestations
- Increased somnolence and fatigue
- Headache

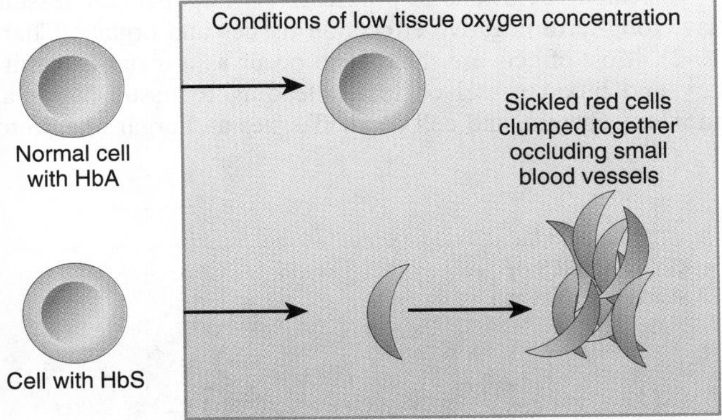

Figure 40-1 ● Red blood cell actions under conditions of low tissue oxygenation. (*HbS,* Hemoglobin S; *HbA,* hemoglobin A.)

ANEMIAS RESULTING FROM INCREASED DESTRUCTION OF RED BLOOD CELLS

Sickle Cell Disease

OVERVIEW

Sickle cell disease is a condition in which chronic anemia is one of many problems causing pain, disability, increased risk for disease, and early death. Once considered a childhood disorder, clients with sickle cell disease who receive appropriate supportive care may live into their 30s and 40s. In addition, there is great variation among clients in the severity of the disease and the onset of complications.

Pathophysiology

The primary problem in this hereditary disorder is the formation of abnormal beta chains in the hemoglobin molecule. The hemoglobin molecule of adults is composed partially of the globin protein, consisting of two alpha chains and two beta chains of amino acids. This normal adult hemoglobin is called **hemoglobin A (HbA).** The total hemoglobin of normal healthy adults is usually 98% to 99% HbA, with a small percentage of a fetal form of hemoglobin (HbF).

In sickle cell disease, at least 40% of the total hemoglobin contains an abnormality of the beta chains, known as hemoglobin S (HbS). HbS is sensitive to changes in the oxygen content of the RBC. When RBCs containing large amounts of HbS are exposed to conditions of decreased oxygen, the abnormal beta chains contract and pile together within the cell, distorting the overall shape of the RBC. These cells assume a sickle shape, become rigid, clump together, and form clusters that block capillary blood flow (Figure 40-1). Capillary obstruction leads to further tissue **hypoxia** (reduced oxygen supply) and more sickling, causing blood vessel obstructions and infarctions in the locally affected tissues. Situations that lead to sickling include hypoxia, dehydration, infections, vascular stasis, low environmental or body temperatures, acidosis, strenuous exercise, and anesthesia.

Usually, sickled cells resume a normal shape when the precipitating condition is removed and proper oxygenation occurs. However, although the outward appearance of the RBCs is normal, at least some of the hemoglobin remains twisted, decreasing cell flexibility. The membranes of the cells become damaged over time, and cells become irreversibly sickled. In addition, the membranes of cells with HbS are more fragile and more easily destroyed in the spleen and in other organs that have long, twisted capillary pathways. The average life span of an RBC containing 40% or more of HbS is approximately 20 days, considerably less than the 120-day life span of RBCs containing only HbA. This reduced life span is responsible for **hemolytic** (blood cell–destroying) anemia in clients with sickle cell disease.

The client with sickle cell disease experiences periodic episodes of extensive cellular sickling, or **crises.** The crises have a sudden onset and can occur as frequently as weekly or as seldom as once a year. Many clients are in good health much of the time, with crises occurring sporadically in response to precipitating conditions that stimulate local or systemic **hypoxemia** (deficient oxygen in the blood).

Repeated occlusions of progressively larger blood vessels have long-term negative effects on tissues and organs (Chart 40-2). Most effects are thought to occur as a result of capillary and blood vessel occlusion leading to tissue hypoxia, anoxia, ischemia, and cell death. Tissues and organs begin to have small infarcted areas that eventually destroy all healthy cells and lead to organ failure. Tissues and organs most commonly affected in this way are the spleen, liver, heart, kidney, brain, bones, and retina.

CHART 40-2

KEY FEATURES *of* Sickle Cell Disease

Hematologic Manifestations
- Fragile red blood cells that sickle and clump under conditions of low tissue oxygenation, venous stasis, lower environmental or body temperature
  - Anemia
- Tissue hypoxia and ischemia
  - Pain
  - Hardened, enlarged spleen

Respiratory Manifestations
- Pulmonary infarcts
  - Chest pain
  - Pneumonia

Genitourinary Manifestations
- Renal ischemia
  - Decreased urine concentration
- Priapism

Cardiovascular Manifestations
- Cardiac ischemia
  - Myocardial infarctions
  - Chest pain
  - Congestive heart failure
- Strokes

Musculoskeletal Manifestations
- Necrosis of femur head
- Pain in extremities with moderate physical exercise
- Delayed growth—small stature

Integumentary Manifestations
- Leg ulcers
- Pale, cyanotic skin

Etiology

Sickle cell disease is a genetic disorder with an autosomal recessive pattern of inheritance. The formation of the beta chains of the hemoglobin molecule is dependent on a pair of genes. A mutation in these genes leads to the formation of HbS instead of HbA. When the client inherits one abnormal gene of this pair, the condition is called **sickle cell trait.** The client can pass the condition on to his or her children, but the client has only mild manifestations of the disease under severe precipitating conditions because less than about 30% of the hemoglobin is abnormal. When the client inherits two abnormal genes, the condition is called **sickle cell disease** (formerly sickle cell anemia), and the client has severe manifestations of the disease even under relatively mild precipitating conditions. In addition, if the client has children, each child will inherit one of the two abnormal genes and at least have sickle cell trait.

Incidence/Prevalence

Sickle cell trait and different forms of sickle cell disease occur in people of all races and ethnicities but less often among Caucasians.

CULTURAL CONSIDERATIONS

Sickle cell disease occurs most often in African Americans, as well as in African, Mediterranean, Caribbean, Middle Eastern, and Central American populations. Approximately 1 of every 12 African Americans has the sickle cell trait. One of every 345 African-American infants inherits two abnormal genes (one from each parent) and has overt sickle cell disease (Larsen, Neverett, & Larsen, 2001; Mitchell, 1999).

COLLABORATIVE MANAGEMENT

Assessment

HISTORY

An adult with sickle cell disease has a long-standing diagnosis of the disorder. An adult who has sickle cell trait, however, may have had such mild clinical manifestations that he or she is unaware of the problem until it is diagnosed with an accompanying disorder or when anesthesia is administered.

The nurse asks the client about previous crises, including precipitating events, severity, and usual treatments. Recent activities and situations are explored to determine the probable precipitating condition or event. The nurse also reviews all activities and events during the previous 24 hours, including food and fluid intake, exposure to temperature extremes, types of clothing worn, medications taken, exercise, trauma, stress, and ingestion of alcohol or other recreational drugs. This activity review provides important information about fatigue, activity tolerance, and participation in activities of daily living (ADLs).

The client is asked about changes in sleep and rest patterns, ability to climb stairs, and any activity that induces shortness of breath. Obtaining a subjective baseline assessment of the client's perceived energy level using a scale ranging from 0 to 10 (0 = not tired with plenty of energy; 10 = total exhaustion) can be useful in evaluating the degree of fatigue and the effectiveness of later treatments.

PHYSICAL ASSESSMENT/CLINICAL MANIFESTATIONS

Pain is the most common symptom experienced during sickle cell crisis. Jaundice may also be present as a result of increased red blood cell (RBC) destruction and release of bilirubin. Other clinical manifestations vary with the site of tissue damage.

CARDIOVASCULAR ASSESSMENT. The nurse assesses the client's cardiovascular and peripheral vascular status by comparing peripheral pulses, temperature, and capillary refill in all extremities. Extremities distal to blood vessel occlusion are cool to the touch with slow capillary refill and may have diminished or absent pulses. The heart rate may be rapid and the blood pressure low to average, with a decreased pulse pressure because breakage of RBCs leads to anemia.

INTEGUMENTARY ASSESSMENT. The skin may be pale or cyanotic as a result of decreased perfusion and anemia. The nurse examines the lips, tongue, nail beds, conjunctivae, palms, and soles at regular intervals for subtle color changes. With cyanosis, the lips and tongue are gray, and the palms, soles, conjunctivae, and nail beds have a bluish tinge.

Another skin manifestation associated with sickle cell disease is jaundice. Bilirubin, a major component of RBCs, is released when fragile cells are damaged, leading to jaundice. The nurse assesses for jaundice in clients with darker skin by inspecting the oral mucosa, especially the hard palate, for yellow discoloration. Inspection of the conjunctivae and adjacent sclera may be misleading because of normal deposits of subconjunctival fat that produce a yellowish hue when seen in contrast to the dark periorbital skin. Therefore the nurse examines the sclera closest to the cornea to diagnose jaundice more accurately. Similarly, the palms and soles of dark-skinned clients may appear yellow if callused and should not be mistaken for jaundice. Jaundice from excessive bilirubin may also cause intense itching.

In spite of the anemia, clients with sickle cell disease usually are not deficient in iron. In fact, with increased RBC production and destruction, iron released from the cells may increase the pigmentation of the skin.

As many as 75% of adult clients with sickle cell disease have stasis ulcers or pressure ulcers on the lower extremities. The ulcers usually occur on the lower portion of the legs (Rausch & Pollard, 1998). The outer sides and inner aspect of the ankle or the shin are common sites. The nurse inspects the legs and feet for open lesions or darkened areas that may indicate necrotic tissue. Infections of these lesions occur frequently.

ABDOMINAL ASSESSMENT. Abdominal organs are usually the first to be damaged as a result of multiple episodes of hypoxia and ischemia. The nurse inspects the abdomen for asymmetry or bulging areas, gently palpating it. Affected organs, such as the liver or spleen, may be firm and enlarged with a nodular texture in later stages of the disease.

MUSCULOSKELETAL ASSESSMENT. Extremities are a common site of vascular occlusion among clients who have sickle cell disease. In addition, joints may be damaged from frequent hypoxic episodes and undergo necrotic degeneration. The nurse inspects the extremities for symmetry and records any areas of swelling or color difference. Clients are asked to move all joints, and the nurse notes the range of motion and any accompanying pain.

CENTRAL NERVOUS SYSTEM ASSESSMENT. Changes in central nervous system (CNS) function may occur directly or indirectly in sickle cell disease. During crises, clients may have a low-grade fever. If the CNS sustains infarcts or repeated episodes of hypoxia, they may have seizure activity or clinical manifestations of a stroke. Hand grasps are assessed bilaterally. The nurse assesses gait and coordination in those clients who are permitted to walk.

PSYCHOSOCIAL ASSESSMENT

Psychosocial assessment is important because behavioral changes may be the first observable clinical manifestations of cerebral hypoxia. The nurse observes the client and documents presenting behavior. Family members or significant others are questioned to determine whether the presenting behavior and mental status are typical.

Sickle cell disease represents a chronic, painful, life-limiting disorder that can be passed on to one's children. The nurse assesses the client's psychosocial needs in terms of new factors, established support systems, previous and current coping patterns, and disease progression. The client is asked how he or she views the disease and what adjustments in lifestyle have been made to accommodate limitations.

LABORATORY ASSESSMENT

The primary laboratory finding associated with sickle cell disease is the large percentage of hemoglobin S (HbS) present on electrophoresis. A person who has sickle cell trait usually expresses less than 40% HbS, and the client with sickle cell disease may express 85% to 95% HbS. *This percentage does not change during crises.* Another indicator of sickle cell disease is the percentage of RBCs showing irreversible sickling. This value is less than 1% among people who do not have sickle cell disease, is 5% to 50% among people with sickle cell trait, and may exceed 90% among clients with sickle cell disease.

A variety of other laboratory tests reflect the problems associated with sickle cell disease, especially during crises. The hematocrit of clients with sickle cell disease is usually low (between 20% and 30%). This value decreases even more dramatically during vascular occlusive crises, or **aplastic crises,** when the bone marrow temporarily fails to produce cells during stressful periods (such as infection). The reticulocyte count is elevated, indicating anemia of long duration. Often the mean corpuscular hemoglobin concentration (MCHC) and total bilirubin level are elevated in the client who has sickle cell disease.

The total white blood cell (WBC) count is usually above normal among clients who have sickle cell disease. It is thought that this elevation is related to chronic inflammation resulting from tissue hypoxia and ischemia.

RADIOGRAPHIC ASSESSMENT

Bone changes occur as a result of chronically stimulated marrow and hypoxic bone tissue. The skull may show radiographic changes resulting from chronic bone surface resorption and regeneration, giving the skull a "crew cut" appearance. Joint necrosis and degeneration also are obvious on x-ray examination.

OTHER DIAGNOSTIC ASSESSMENT

Electrocardiographic (ECG) changes document cardiac infarcts and tissue damage. Specific ECG changes are related to the area of the myocardium sustaining the damage. Ultrasonography, computed tomography (CT), positron emission tomography (PET), and magnetic resonance imaging (MRI) may reveal soft-tissue and organ degenerative changes resulting from inadequate oxygenation and chronic inflammation.

CHART 40-3

BEST PRACTICE *for* Care of the Client in Sickle Cell Crisis

- Administer oxygen.
- Administer pain medication as ordered.
- Hydrate the client with normal saline intravenously and with beverages of choice (without caffeine) orally.
- Remove any constrictive clothing.
- Encourage the client to keep extremities extended to promote venous return.
- Do not raise the knee gatch of the bed.
- Elevate the head of the bed no more than 30 degrees.
- Keep room temperature at or above 72°F (22.2°C).
- Avoid taking blood pressure with external cuff.
- Check circulation in extremities every hour:
  - Pulse oximetry of fingers and toes
  - Capillary refill
  - Peripheral pulses
  - Toe temperature

Interventions

The most common health problems for the client with sickle cell disease are pain, the potential complications of sepsis, and multiple organ dysfunction. Interventions are aimed at reducing or preventing these problems.

PAIN. The most prominent clinical manifestation of sickle cell disease is pain. More than one fifth of clients experience frequent painful episodes and may have as many as 40 episodes per year (Rausch & Pollard, 1998). The pain associated with sickle cell crisis is the result of ischemic tissue injury caused by obstructed blood flow. The pain is often severe enough to require hospitalization and large doses of opioid analgesics. Pain is chronic with acute episodes and can occur anywhere in the body, often where circulation is impaired. It is sudden and is often described as gnawing or throbbing. Subjective reports of pain may be the only evidence, because the chronic nature of the pain may make physiologic changes less obvious.

The subjective nature of the pain, racial prejudice, and concern for addiction often cause the client with sickle cell disease to be labeled as difficult (Gorman, 1999). Health care providers must be aware of their own attitudes when caring for this population and must realize that lack of knowledge, in addition to concern for addiction, often prevents proper pain management of clients with sickle cell disease. Use of a pain rating scale by all nursing personnel can promote proper pain management. The nurse asks the client to rate pain on a scale ranging from 0 to 10 and evaluates the effectiveness of interventions based on the ratings. Use of contracts for pain control can also be helpful.

DRUG THERAPY. Clients in acute sickle cell crisis often require at least 48 hours of parenteral analgesics. (Chart 40-3 highlights best practices for nursing care of the client in sickle cell crisis.) Morphine and hydromorphone (Dilaudid) are the medications of choice (Gorman, 1999). For sickle cell crisis, these agents should be administered intravenously on a routine schedule. Once relief is obtained, the intravenous (IV) dose can be tapered and then administered orally (Rausch & Pollard, 1998). Meperidine (Demerol) is also used for sickle cell crisis, but long-term use of this agent can cause neurologic symptoms, including anxiety and seizures (Gorman, 1999). "As needed" (prn) schedules are discouraged because they do not provide adequate relief, and intramuscular (IM) injections are avoided because frequent injections lead to sclerosing of tissue (and absorption may be impaired by poor circulation). Moderate pain may be treated with oral doses of codeine, morphine sulfate, or nonsteroidal anti-inflammatory drugs (NSAIDs). (See Chapter 7 for more information on pain management.)

COMPLEMENTARY AND ALTERNATIVE THERAPIES. Complementary therapies and other nonpharmacologic measures, such as keeping the room warm, using distraction and relaxation techniques, proper positioning with support for painful areas, aroma therapy, therapeutic touch, and warm soaks or compresses, have all been useful in decreasing pain. *The nurse must not assume, however, that these methods alone will provide adequate pain relief. Analgesics are required to treat sickle cell pain.*

POTENTIAL FOR SEPSIS. The client with sickle cell disease is more susceptible to bloodborne infections and infection by encapsulated microorganisms, such as *Streptococcus pneumoniae* and *Haemophilus influenzae,* as a result of decreased spleen function. Interventions aim at preventing or halting the process of infection, controlling infection, and initiating early, effective treatment regimens for specific infections.

PREVENTION/EARLY DETECTION. A major objective is to protect the client in sickle cell crisis from infection. Frequent, thorough handwashing is of the utmost importance. Any person with an upper respiratory tract infection who must enter the client's room wears a mask. Strict aseptic technique is used for all invasive procedures.

The nurse continually assesses the client for the presence of infection and monitors a daily complete blood count (CBC) with differential WBC count. The oral mucosa is inspected during every nursing shift for lesions indicating fungal or viral infection. The lungs are auscultated every 8 hours for crackles, wheezes, or diminished breath sounds. Each time the client voids, assistive nursing personnel inspect the urine for odor and cloudiness, and the client is asked about any sensation of urgency, burning, or pain during urination. Vital signs are taken at least every 4 hours to assess for fever.

DRUG THERAPY. Drug therapy is a primary defense against the infections that develop in the client with sickle cell disease. Prophylactic therapy with twice-daily administration of oral penicillin in the penicillin-tolerant client has resulted in dramatic reductions in the number of pneumonia and other streptococcal infections. Yearly vaccination for influenza is advocated (Rausch & Pollard, 1998). Drug therapy for an actual infection can control infection and prevent complications associated with sepsis. Agents used depend on the sensitivity of the specific organism causing the infection, as well as the extent of the infection.

POTENTIAL FOR MULTIPLE ORGAN DYSFUNCTION. The threat of multiple organ dysfunction arises from continued vascular occlusions after clumping of sickled cells. Management of sickle cell disease focuses on prevention of vascular occlusion and promotion of adequate oxygenation.

The client in sickle cell crisis is admitted to the acute care hospital. The nurse assesses for adequacy of circulation to all body areas. Restrictive clothing is removed, and the client is instructed to avoid keeping the hips or knees in a flexed position.

Dehydration perpetuates cell sickling and must be avoided. Nursing personnel assist the client in maintaining an adequate hydration status. The client in crisis requires an oral or parenteral intake of at least 200 mL/hr.

Oxygen is ordered, and the nurse ensures that oxygen therapy is delivered appropriately, including nebulization to prevent dehydration. Transfusion therapy has been used to decrease the incidence of organ dysfunction and stroke. RBC transfusions are therapeutic because levels of hemoglobin A (HbA) are sustained, whereas levels of hemoglobin S (HbS) are diluted. Transfusions also suppress erythropoiesis, thereby decreasing the production of sickle cells. Transfusions may be administered in either the acute care or clinic setting by a registered nurse. The nurse monitors the client closely for complications of transfusion therapy (discussed under Transfusion Reactions, p. 866).

In some treatment centers, bone marrow transplantation is being performed to correct abnormal hemoglobin permanently. Because bone marrow transplantation is expensive and may result in chronic and life-threatening complications, its risks and benefits need to be seriously considered for each client.

CRITICAL THINKING CHALLENGE

It is winter in Minnesota. You are working in the emergency department of a local hospital and are informed that there has been a motor vehicle accident. The emergency technicians (EMTs) are bringing in a woman who has been out in the cold for several hours. The woman has no obvious injuries but is complaining of severe pain. An EMT notifies you that the client is wearing a medical alert bracelet indicating that she has sickle cell disease.

- What should you include in your initial assessment?
- What measures would be appropriate for management of this individual's pain?

For suggested answer guidelines, go to SIMON http://www.wbsaunders.com/SIMON/Iggy/.

Community-Based Care

Sickle cell disease is a progressive disorder with periods of varying degrees of exacerbation. Rarely is there a true remission, although crisis episodes may be infrequent. Care focuses on prevention of complications, an ongoing daily necessity for the client with sickle cell disease. The client with sickle cell disease may be cared for in a variety of settings, including acute care, subacute care, extended or assistive care, and home care.

The client is taught to avoid specific activities that lead to hypoxia and hypoxemia. Recognition of the early signs and symptoms of crisis is emphasized, so that appropriate treatment can be initiated early to prevent undue pain, complications, and permanent tissue damage. The client is often given opioid analgesics for self-management of sickle cell crises at home; the nurse teaches clients and families about the correct administration. In addition, clients are counseled about the hereditary aspects of sickle cell disease, and information concerning prenatal diagnosis, birth control methods, and pregnancy options is offered.

WOMEN'S HEALTH CONSIDERATIONS

Pregnancy in women with sickle cell disease presents special physiologic challenges and may be life threatening. Clients who show evidence of damage to vital organs are advised against becoming pregnant. Usually, barrier methods of contraception (cervical cap, diaphragm, or condoms with or without spermicide) are recommended for women with sickle cell disease. The use of oral contraceptives among these women is controversial. Oral contraceptives may increase susceptibility to occlusion by increasing clot formation, especially among smokers. However, the use of oral contraceptives also can reduce menstrual blood loss, thus decreasing the degree of anemia. Therefore the determination of risks versus benefits of oral contraceptives must be individualized.

Glucose-6-Phosphate Dehydrogenase Deficiency Anemia

OVERVIEW

Many forms of congenital **hemolytic** (blood cell–destroying) anemia result from defects or deficiencies of one or more enzymes within the red blood cell (RBC). More than 200 such disorders have been identified. Most of these enzymes are needed to complete some critical step in cellular energy production. The most common type of congenital hemolytic anemia is associated with a deficiency of the enzyme glucose-6-phosphate dehydrogenase (G6PD). This disease is inherited as an X-linked recessive disorder and affects about 10% of all African Americans (Cotran, Kumar, & Robbins, 1999).

G6PD stimulates critical reactions in the glycolytic pathway. RBCs contain no **mitochondria** (sites of high-efficiency production of the energy compound **adenosine triphosphate [ATP]**), so active glycolysis is essential for energy metabolism. Newly produced RBCs from clients with G6PD deficiency have relatively sufficient quantities of G6PD; however, as the cells age, the concentration diminishes drastically. Cells that have reduced amounts of G6PD are more susceptible to breaking during exposure to specific drugs (e.g., phenacetin, sulfonamides, aspirin [acetylsalicylic acid], quinine derivatives, thiazide diuretics, and vitamin K derivatives) and toxins.

After exposure to any of these agents, clients experience acute intravascular hemolysis lasting from 7 to 12 days. During this acute phase, anemia and jaundice develop. The hemolytic reaction is self-limited because only older erythrocytes, containing less G6PD, are destroyed.

➤ COLLABORATIVE MANAGEMENT

It is critical that the precipitating drug or the agent responsible for the hemolytic reaction be identified and totally removed. People should be screened for this deficiency before donating blood, because administration of cells deficient in G6PD can be hazardous for the recipient.

During and immediately after an episode of hemolysis, adequate hydration is essential to prevent precipitation of cellular debris and hemoglobin in the kidney tubules, which can lead to acute tubular necrosis. Osmotic diuretics, such as mannitol (Osmitrol), may assist in preventing this complication. Transfusion therapy is indicated when anemia is present and kidney function is normal. Table 40-2 lists indications for transfusion with various types of blood components.

Immunohemolytic Anemia

OVERVIEW

Increased RBC destruction through hemolysis can occur in response to many situations, including trauma, infection (especially malarial infections), and autoimmune reactions. All increase the rate at which RBCs are destroyed by causing lysis (breakage) of the RBC membrane. The most common types of hemolytic anemias in industrialized countries are the immunohemolytic anemias, also referred to as autoimmune hemolytic anemias (Cotran, Kumar, & Robbins, 1999).

In immunohemolytic anemia, immune system components attack a person's own RBCs. The exact mechanism that causes immune components to no longer recognize blood cells as self and to initiate destructive processes against RBCs is not known. Some hemolytic anemias are present with other autoimmune disorders (such as systemic lupus erythematosus) or lymphoproliferative disorders. Regardless of the cause, RBCs are viewed as non-self by the immune system and are destroyed.

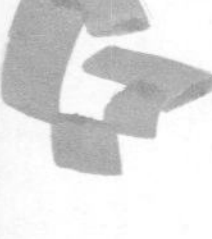

There are two types of immunohemolytic anemia: warm antibody anemia and cold antibody anemia. **Warm antibody anemia** is usually associated with immunoglobulin G (IgG) antibody excess. These antibodies are most active at 98° F (37° C) and may be stimulated by drugs, chemicals, or other autoimmune problems. **Cold antibody anemia** is associated with fixation of complement proteins on immunoglobulin M (IgM) and occurs best at 86° F (30° C). This problem is commonly associated with a Raynaud-like response in which the arteries in the distal extremities constrict profoundly in response to cold temperatures or stress.

➤ COLLABORATIVE MANAGEMENT

Treatment depends on clinical severity. Steroid therapy for mild to moderate immunosuppression is the first line of treatment and is temporarily effective in most clients. Splenectomy and more intensive immunosuppressive therapy with cyclophosphamide (Cytoxan, Procytox✤) and azathioprine (Imuran) may be instituted if steroid therapy fails. Plasma exchange therapy to remove attacking antibodies is effective for clients who do not respond to immunosuppressive therapy.

ANEMIAS RESULTING FROM DECREASED PRODUCTION OF RED BLOOD CELLS

Anemias associated with decreased red blood cell (RBC) production can result from alterations in any of a variety of physiologic mechanisms. Some anemias are caused by failure or inability of the bone marrow to properly produce RBCs; others are caused by failure of the body to make or absorb a specific component necessary for RBC production.

CONSIDERATIONS FOR OLDER ADULTS

Older clients often have restricted diets and may be unable to consume enough meat because of poor dentition or economic reasons and thus are at risk for iron deficiency anemia (Cotran, Kumar, & Robbins, 1999). The nurse asks about a family history of anemia. Vitamin B_{12} deficiency anemia often occurs in individuals 50 to 80 years of age and may be genetically transmitted.

Iron Deficiency Anemia

OVERVIEW

The adult body contains between 2 and 6 g of iron, depending on the size of the person and the amount of hemoglobin in the cells. Approximately two thirds of this iron is contained in hemoglobin; the other third is stored in the bone marrow, spleen,

TABLE 40-2 • INDICATIONS FOR TREATMENT WITH BLOOD COMPONENTS

Component	Volume	Infusion Time	Indications
Packed red blood cells (PRBCs)	200-250 mL	2-4 hr	Anemia; hemoglobin <6 g/dL, 6-10 g/dL, depending on symptoms
Washed red blood cells (WBC-poor PRBCs)	200 mL	2-4 hr	History of allergic transfusion reactions Bone marrow transplant clients
Platelets			
Pooled	Approximately 300 mL	15-30 min	Thrombocytopenia platelet count <20,000 Clients who are actively bleeding with a platelet count <80,000
Single donor	200 mL	30 min	History of febrile or allergic reactions
Fresh frozen plasma	200 mL	15-30 min	Deficiency in plasma coagulation factors Prothrombin or partial thromboplastin time 1.5 times normal
Cryoprecipitate	10-20 mL/unit	15-30 min	Hemophilia VIII or von Willebrand's disease Fibrinogen levels <100 mg/dL
White blood cells (WBCs)	400 mL	1 hr	Sepsis, neutropenic infection not responding to antibiotic therapy

liver, and muscle (see Chapter 39). If a person has an iron deficiency, the iron stores are depleted first, followed by the hemoglobin stores. As a result, RBCs are small **(microcytic),** and the client has relatively mild manifestations of anemia, including weakness and pallor. In iron deficiency anemia, serum ferritin values are less than 12 g/L.

Iron deficiency anemia is the most common type of anemia and can result from blood loss, increased energy demands, gastrointestinal malabsorption, and dietary inadequacy. The basic problem of iron deficiency anemia is a decreased supply of iron for the developing RBC. Iron deficiency anemia can occur at any age but is more frequent in women, older adults, and people with poor diets.

➤ COLLABORATIVE MANAGEMENT

The primary treatment of clients with iron deficiency anemia is to increase the oral intake of iron from common food sources (Table 40-3). An adequate diet supplies a person with about 10 to 15 mg of iron per day, of which only 5% to 10% is absorbed in the stomach, duodenum, and upper jejunum (Worrall, Tompkins, & Rust, 1999). This amount is sufficient to meet the needs of healthy men and healthy women after childbearing age but is not sufficient to supply the greater needs of menstruating women and adolescents during growth spurts. Fortunately, if iron intake is inadequate, or if bleeding or pregnancy occurs, the gastrointestinal tract is capable of increasing the absorption of iron to about 20% to 30% of the total daily intake (Cotran, Kumar, & Robbins, 1999).

When iron deficiency anemia is severe, iron preparations can be administered intramuscularly. Such preparations are administered using the Z-track best practice method outlined in Chart 40-4.

Vitamin B_{12} Deficiency Anemia

OVERVIEW

Proper production of RBCs depends on adequate **deoxyribonucleic acid (DNA)** synthesis in the precursor cells so that cell division and maturation into functional RBCs can occur. All DNA synthesis requires adequate amounts of **folic acid (folate)** to ensure the availability of the nucleotide thymidine, which stimulates DNA synthesis. One function of vitamin B_{12} is to serve as a cofactor to activate the enzyme system responsible for transporting folic acid into the cell, where DNA synthesis occurs. Thus a deficiency of vitamin B_{12} indirectly causes anemia by inhibiting folic acid transportation and limiting DNA synthesis in RBC precursor cells. These precursor cells then undergo improper DNA synthesis and increase in size. Only a few are released from the bone marrow. This type of anemia is called **megaloblastic (macrocytic)** because of the large size of these abnormal cells.

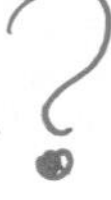

Vitamin B_{12} deficiency can result from inadequate intake (dietary deficiency). This can occur with strict vegetarian diets or diets lacking sufficient dairy products. Conditions such as small bowel resection, diverticula, tapeworm, or overgrowth of intestinal bacteria can lead to poor absorption of vitamin B_{12} from the intestinal tract (Worrall, Tompkins, & Rust, 1999). Anemia caused by failure to absorb vitamin B_{12} **(pernicious anemia)** can also result from a deficiency of **intrinsic factor** (a substance normally secreted by the gastric mucosa), which is necessary for intestinal absorption of vitamin B_{12}.

Vitamin B_{12} deficiency anemia may be mild or severe, usually develops slowly, and produces few symptoms. Clients usually have pallor and jaundice, as well as **glossitis** (a smooth, beefy-red tongue), fatigue, and weight loss. Because vitamin B_{12} also is necessary for normal nervous system functioning, especially of the peripheral nerves, clients with pernicious anemia may also have neurologic abnormalities, such as **paresthesias** (abnormal sensations) in the feet and hands and disturbances of balance and gait (Chart 40-5).

➤ COLLABORATIVE MANAGEMENT

When anemia is caused by a dietary deficiency, the client must increase the intake of foods rich in vitamin B_{12} (animal proteins, eggs, dairy products). Vitamin supplements may be prescribed when anemia is severe. For clients who have anemia as

TABLE 40-3 • COMMON FOOD SOURCES OF IRON, VITAMIN B_{12}, AND FOLIC ACID

IRON	VITAMIN B_{12} / FOLIC ACID
• Liver (especially pork and lamb)	• Liver
• Red meat	• Organ meats
• Organ meats	• Dried beans
• Kidney beans	• Nuts
• Whole-wheat breads and cereals	• Green leafy vegetables
• Leafy green vegetables	• Citrus fruit
• Carrots	• Brewer's yeast
• Egg yolks	**FOLIC ACID**
• Raisins	• Liver
	• Organ meats
	• Eggs
	• Cabbage
	• Broccoli
	• Brussels sprouts

Data from Pennington, J. (1998). *Bowe's and Church's food values of portions commonly used* (17th ed.). Philadelphia: J.B. Lippincott.

CHART 40-4

BEST PRACTICE *for* Administering Intramuscular Medications by the Z-Track Method

- Draw the medication up into the syringe using aseptic technique.
- Add 0.25 mL of air to the syringe.
- Discard the needle used to draw up the medication.
- Place a new needle (22-gauge, 2 to 3 inches long) on the syringe.
- Make certain that the injection site is in bright light.
- *Select the dorsal gluteal site only.*
- Identify appropriate landmarks for administration into the upper, outer quadrant.
- Once the site is selected, pull the skin and subcutaneous tissues sideways away from the muscle.
- Clean the site while holding the skin and subcutaneous tissues off to the side.
- Insert the needle deeply into the muscle tissue.
- Aspirate to determine needle placement.
- Iron dextran is black; look very closely to determine whether or not blood is being aspirated into the syringe.
- If blood is aspirated, withdraw the needle and begin the procedure again from the first step.
- If no blood is aspirated, inject the medication slowly, followed by injection of the air bubble.
- Quickly withdraw the needle.
- Release the skin and subcutaneous tissue.
- *Do not massage the injection site.*

CHART 40-5

KEY FEATURES *of* Vitamin B_{12} Deficiency Anemia

- Severe pallor
- Slight jaundice
- Smooth, beefy red tongue
- Fatigue
- Weight loss
- Paresthesias of the hands and feet
- Difficulty with gait

a result of a deficiency of intrinsic factor, vitamin B_{12} must be administered parenterally on a regular schedule (usually weekly for initial treatment, then monthly for maintenance).

Folic Acid Deficiency Anemia

OVERVIEW

Primary folic acid deficiency can also cause megaloblastic anemia. Clinical manifestations are similar to those of vitamin B_{12} deficiency without the accompanying nervous system manifestations, because folic acid does not appear to affect nerve function. The absence of neurologic problems is an important diagnostic finding to differentiate folic acid deficiency from vitamin B_{12} deficiency. The disease develops slowly, and symptoms may be attributed to other problems or diseases.

The three common causes of folic acid deficiency are poor nutrition, malabsorption, and drugs. Poor nutrition, especially a diet lacking green leafy vegetables, liver, yeast, citrus fruits, dried beans, and nuts, is the most common cause. Chronic alcohol abuse and parenteral alimentation without folic acid supplementation are other dietary causes. Malabsorption syndromes, such as Crohn's disease, are the second most common cause.

Specific drugs impede the absorption and conversion of folic acid to its active form and can also lead to folic acid deficiency and anemia. Such drugs include methotrexate, some anticonvulsants, and oral contraceptives.

➤ COLLABORATIVE MANAGEMENT

Prevention of folic acid deficiency anemia is aimed at identifying high-risk clients, such as older, debilitated clients with alcoholism; clients prone to malnutrition; and those with increased folic acid requirements. A diet high in folic acid and vitamin B_{12} prevents a deficiency (see Table 40-3). By routinely including assessment of dietary habits in a health history, the nurse can determine which clients are at risk for diet-induced anemias and provide appropriate follow-up. For the client diagnosed with this type of anemia, management includes oral folic acid 1 mg daily or intramuscular administration of folic acid for clients with absorption problems (Worrall, Tompkins, & Rust, 1999).

Aplastic Anemia

OVERVIEW

Aplastic anemia is a deficiency of circulating erythrocytes resulting from arrested development of RBCs within the bone marrow. It is caused by an injury to the hematopoietic precursor cell, the **pluripotent stem cell.** Although aplastic anemia sometimes occurs alone, it is usually accompanied by **agranulocytopenia** (a reduction in leukocytes) and **thrombocytopenia** (a reduction in platelets). These three problems occur at the same time because the bone marrow produces not only RBCs but also white blood cells (WBCs) and platelets. Consequently, if the bone marrow is abnormal for any reason or if it has been exposed to a toxic substance that can damage bone marrow cells, production of erythrocytes, leukocytes, and thrombocytes slows greatly. **Pancytopenia** (a deficiency of all three cell types) is common in aplastic anemia. The onset of aplastic anemia may be insidious or rapid.

The development of aplastic anemia, although relatively rare, is associated with chronic exposure to several toxic agents (see Table 39-4). In about 50% of cases, the cause of aplastic anemia is unknown. Aplastic anemia may occur as an aftermath of viral infection (Cotran, Kumar, & Robbins, 1999), but the mechanism of bone marrow damage is unknown.

➤ COLLABORATIVE MANAGEMENT

Blood transfusions are the mainstay of treatment for clients with aplastic anemia. Transfusion is indicated only when the anemia causes real disability or when bleeding is life threatening because of thrombocytopenia. Unnecessary transfusion, however, increases the opportunity for the development of immune reactions to platelets, shortens the life span of the transfused cell, and may increase the rate of rejection of transplanted marrow cells. Thus transfusions are discontinued as soon as the bone marrow begins to produce RBCs.

Because clients with some types of aplastic anemia have a disease course similar to that of autoimmune problems, immunosuppressive therapy may be helpful. Agents that selectively suppress lymphocyte activity, such as antilymphocyte globulin (ALG), antithymocyte globulin (ATG), and cyclosporine (Sandimmune), have brought about partial or complete remissions. In more severe cases, general immunosuppressive agents, such as prednisone and cyclophosphamide (Cytoxan, Procytox✤), have been effective.

Splenectomy (removal of the spleen) is considered in clients with an enlarged spleen that is either destroying normal RBCs or suppressing their development. Bone marrow transplantation, which replaces defective stem cells, has also resulted in a cure for some clients (Cotran, Kumar, & Robbins, 1999). Cost, availability, and complications limit this technique for treatment of aplastic anemia, however.

POLYCYTHEMIA

In polycythemia, the number of red blood cells (RBCs) in whole blood is greater than normal. The blood of a client with polycythemia is **hyperviscous** (thicker than normal blood). The problem may be temporary (occurring as a result of other conditions) or chronic. One type of polycythemia, polycythemia vera, is fatal if left untreated.

Polycythemia Vera

OVERVIEW

Polycythemia vera (PV) is characterized by a sustained increase in blood hemoglobin concentration to 18 g/dL, an RBC count of 6 million/mm^3, or a hematocrit increase to 55% or greater. PV is a cancer of the RBCs with three major hall-

CHART 40-6

KEY FEATURES *of* Polycythemia Vera

- Persistently elevated hematocrit value (>55%)
- Hypertension
- Dark, flushed appearance of the hands and face
- Distention of superficial veins
- Weight loss
- Fatigue
- Intense itching
- Enlarged hemorrhoids
- Swollen, painful joints
- Enlarged, firm spleen
- Infarctions of the heart
    - Chest pain
    - Congestive heart failure
- Strokes
- Bleeding tendency

CHART 40-7

CLIENT EDUCATION GUIDE Polycythemia Vera

- Drink at least 3 L of liquids each day.
- Avoid tight or constrictive clothing, especially garters or girdles.
- Wear gloves when outdoors in temperatures lower than 50°F (10°C).
- Keep all health care–related appointments.
- Contact your physician at the first sign of infection.
- Take anticoagulants as ordered.
- Wear support hose or stockings while you are awake and up.
- Elevate your feet whenever you are seated.
- Exercise slowly and only on the advice of your physician.
- Stop activity at the first sign of chest pain.
- Use an electric razor, not a manual one.
- Use a soft-bristled toothbrush to brush your teeth.
- Do not floss between your teeth.

marks: continuous production of massive numbers of RBCs, excessive leukocyte production, and overproduction of thrombocytes. As described in Chart 40-6, extreme **hypercellularity** (cell excess) of the peripheral blood occurs in people with PV.

The skin, especially facial, and mucous membranes have a dark, flushed **(plethoric)** appearance. These areas may appear purplish or cyanotic because the blood in these tissues is incompletely oxygenated. Most clients experience intense itching related to vasodilation and variation in tissue oxygenation. Blood viscosity is also greatly increased, causing a corresponding increase in peripheral resistance. Superficial veins are visibly distended. Blood moves more slowly through all tissues and thus places increased demands on the pumping action of the heart, resulting in hypertension. In some highly vascular areas, blood flow may become so slow that vascular stasis occurs. Vascular stasis causes **thrombosis** (clot formation) within the smaller vessels to the extent that the vessels are occluded and the surrounding tissues experience hypoxia, progressing to anoxia and further to infarction and necrosis. Tissues most prone to this complication are the heart, spleen, and kidneys, although infarction with loss of tissue and organ function can occur in any organ or tissue.

Because the actual number of cells in the blood is greatly increased and the cells are not completely normal, individual cell life spans are shorter. The shorter life spans, coupled with increased cell production, result in a rapid turnover of peripheral blood cells. This rapid turnover increases the amount of intracellular products (released when cells die) in the blood, adding to the general "sludging" of the blood. These products include uric acid and potassium, which cause the symptoms of gout and **hyperkalemia** (elevated serum potassium level).

Later clinical manifestations of PV are related to abnormal blood cells. Even though the number of circulating erythrocytes is greatly increased, their oxygen-carrying capacity is impaired, and clients experience severe generalized hypoxia. In spite of the RBC excess, most clients with PV are susceptible to bleeding problems because of an associated platelet dysfunction (Cotran, Kumar, & Robbins, 1999).

➤ COLLABORATIVE MANAGEMENT

Polycythemia vera is a malignant disease that progresses in severity over time. If left untreated, few people with PV live longer than 2 years. Conservative management with repeated phlebotomies (two to five times per week) can prolong life for 5 to 10 years. (**Phlebotomy** is the collection of the client's RBCs to decrease the number of RBCs and diminish blood viscosity.) Maintaining adequate hydration and promoting venous return are essential to prevent thrombus formation. Therapy aims to prevent clot formation and includes the use of anticoagulants. Chart 40-7 lists preventive tips for clients with PV.

As the disease progresses, clients need more intensive therapies that suppress bone marrow activity, including oral alkylating agents and/or irradiation with injections of radioactive phosphorus. Bone marrow transplantation, an experimental treatment, is promising, but the results are too limited to determine its application to PV.

WHITE BLOOD CELL DISORDERS

As discussed in Chapter 20, white blood cells (WBCs), or **leukocytes,** provide protection from invading non-self cells and cancer cells in several ways. These protective functions depend on maintaining normal numbers and ratios of many specific mature, circulating leukocytes. When any one type of WBC is present in either abnormally high or abnormally low amounts, hematopoietic function and immune function may be altered to some degree, placing clients at risk for specific complications. This section covers the pathologic changes and nursing care requirements for clients with disorders involving overgrowth of specific types of WBCs. (See Chapter 22 for the pathologic alterations and care requirements for clients with leukocyte-related problems of immunodeficiency.)

LEUKEMIA

OVERVIEW

The leukemias are a group of malignant disorders involving abnormal overproduction of a specific WBC type, usually at an immature stage, in the bone marrow. **Leukemia** may be **acute,** with a sudden onset and short duration, or **chronic,** with a slow onset and persistent symptoms over a period of years.

Leukemias are categorized by the specific maturational pathway from which the abnormal cells arise (Dietz, 1999). Leukemias in which the abnormal cells arise from within the committed lymphoid maturational pathways (see Figure 20-3) are **lymphocytic** or **lymphoblastic.** Leukemias in which the abnormal cells arise within the committed myeloid maturational pathways are **myelocytic** or **myelogenous.** Several subtypes exist for each of these diseases, which are classified according to the degree of maturity of the abnormal cell and the specific cell type involved (Table 40-4).

Pathophysiology

The basic problem in leukemia is a malignant transformation of the stem cells or early committed precursor leukocyte cells, causing an abnormal proliferation of a specific type of leukocyte. The functionally and structurally abnormal immature leukocytes, produced in excessive quantities in the bone marrow, essentially shut down normal bone marrow production of erythrocytes, platelets, and other mature leukocytes. This situation leads to anemia, thrombocytopenia, and leukopenia of the unaffected WBC types, even though the number of immature, abnormal WBCs in the circulation is greatly elevated (Dietz, 1999). Without treatment, the client usually dies of infection or hemorrhage. For clients with acute leukemias, these pathologic changes occur rapidly and, without intervention, progress quickly to death. Chronic leukemia may be present for many years before overt pathologic changes occur (Pittinger, 1999).

Etiology

Epidemiologic studies suggest that many different genetic and environmental factors may be involved in the development of leukemia. Although only a few of these factors have been positively identified, the basic mechanism appears to involve gene damage of cells, changing those cells from a normal to a **malignant** (cancer) state. The following conditions or substances are possible risk factors: ionizing radiation, chemicals and drugs, marrow **hypoplasia** (slow functioning with less than the normal production rate of blood cells), environmental interactions, genetic factors, viral factors, immunologic factors, and the interaction of these factors (Dietz, 1999).

Ionizing radiation exposure in large quantities appears to be a major risk factor. Exposures ranging from therapeutic irradiation (for such diseases as ankylosing spondylitis and Hodgkin's lymphoma) to environmental irradiation (such as the atomic bomb at Hiroshima or the nuclear accident at Chernobyl) have been associated with leukemia.

Chemicals and drugs have been linked to the development of leukemia. Table 39-3 lists many common offenders.

Marrow hypoplasia can increase the risk of leukemia. A reduction or alteration in the production of hematopoietic cells may be responsible. Examples of conditions associated with the later development of leukemia include Fanconi's syndrome, paroxysmal nocturnal hemoglobinuria during its aplastic phase, and myelodysplastic syndromes.

Genetic factors are suspected as a cause of leukemia because of the increased frequency of leukemia in the following populations: identical twins of clients with leukemia, as well as people with Down syndrome, Bloom syndrome, Fanconi's syndrome, and Klinefelter's syndrome. Chromosomal aberration may be an important factor in these syndromes (Dietz, 1999).

Immunologic factors, especially immune deficiencies, may also favor the development of leukemia. Leukemia among im-

TABLE 40-4 • DIFFERENTIATING CHARACTERISTICS OF THE FOUR TYPES OF LEUKEMIA

Age at Onset (yr)	Gender Predilection	Racial Predilection	Cell of Origin	Specific Markers	Comments
ACUTE LYMPHOCYTIC (ALL)					
<15	Males	Caucasian	B-cell	CALLA+ Hyperdiploidy TDT+	Prognosis poorer for adults than for children Prognosis better than in AML Curable in children
ACUTE MYELOGENOUS (AML)					
15-39	Equal incidence	None	Myeloblast Myelocyte Promyelocyte Myelomonocyte	TDT− t(9;22) t(15;17)	Prognosis generally poor Heterogeneous tumor cell populations Best prognosis with bone marrow transplant
CHRONIC MYELOGENOUS (CML)					
>50	Males	None	Myeloid cell	Ph^1 chromosome	Prognosis generally poor; worse if no Ph^1 chromosome No blockage of maturation of nonmalignant leukocytes Blastic crisis indicative of more acute disease
CHRONIC LYMPHOCYTIC (CLL)					
>50	Males	Caucasian	B-cell	Trisomy 12	Prognosis poor Long (4-10 yr) course with rare conversion to acute form Only leukemia with a possible genetic predisposition

munodeficient people may be a result of immunosurveillance failure, or the pathologic mechanisms that cause the immune deficiency may also trigger cancer in the WBC population.

Interaction of multiple host and environmental factors may result in leukemia. Because each person tolerates the interaction of these factors differently, it is difficult to determine the origin of any specific leukemia.

Incidence/Prevalence

The leukemias account for 2% of all newly diagnosed cases of cancer and for 4% of all deaths from cancer (American Cancer Society, 2001). The incidence and the frequency of leukemia depend on many factors, including the type of WBC affected, age, gender, race, and geographic locale.

In the United States an estimated 28,800 new cases of leukemia were projected for 2001 (American Cancer Society, 2000). In this country, leukemia is categorized into any one of four basic types based on the cell type affected and the rate of progression of the leukemia:

- *Acute myelogenous leukemia (AML)* occurs with similar frequency in all ages and is the most common form of leukemia in adults.
- *Acute lymphocytic leukemia (ALL)* constitutes about 10% of adult leukemias but is most common in children.
- *Chronic myelogenous leukemia (CML)* constitutes about 20% of adult leukemias, occurring more often in people older than 50 years of age.
- *Chronic lymphocytic leukemia (CLL)* is the rarest type of leukemia, occurring primarily in people older than 50 years of age.

Characteristics and risk factors associated with these four types of leukemia are presented in Table 40-4.

COLLABORATIVE MANAGEMENT

SIMON Activity Link

Assessment

HISTORY

The nurse asks the client about risk factors and causative factors. Age is important because the incidence of adult leukemia increases with age. Occupation and hobbies may also reveal specific environmental exposures that increase the risk of leukemia. Previous illnesses and the medical history may indicate exposure to ionizing radiation or medications that increase risk.

Because of leukemia-related alterations of immune function, the risk for infection is increased in the client with leukemia. The nurse asks about the frequency and severity of infectious processes (such as colds, influenza, pneumonia, bronchitis, or unexplained episodes of fever) during the preceding 6 months (Pittinger, 1999).

Because platelet function may be diminished in people with leukemia, the client is asked about any overt or hidden excessive bleeding episodes, such as the following:

- A tendency to bruise easily
- Nosebleeds
- Increased menstrual flow
- Bleeding from the gums
- Rectal bleeding
- Hematuria (blood in the urine)
- Prolonged bleeding after minor abrasions or lacerations

If the client has experienced such an episode, the nurse asks whether this type and extent of bleeding constitute the usual response to injury or represent a change.

The client with leukemia often experiences weakness and fatigue resulting from anemia and increased metabolic and energy demands of the leukemic cells. The client is asked whether he or she has experienced any of the following:

- Headaches
- Behavior changes
- Increased somnolence
- Decreased alertness
- Decreased attention span
- Lethargy, muscle weakness
- Diminished appetite
- Weight loss
- Increased fatigue

Listing activities in the previous 24 hours may disclose additional information about activity intolerance, changes in behavior, and unexplained fatigue. The nurse determines how long the client has had any of these debilitating symptoms.

PHYSICAL ASSESSMENT/CLINICAL MANIFESTATIONS

Because leukemia affects all blood cells, and blood influences the health and functional capacity of all organs and systems, many areas remote from the actual site of origin of malignant cells may be affected (Chart 40-8). The following clinical manifestations are associated with the acute leukemias (Cotran, Kumar, & Robbins, 1999). Some of these findings may also be present in the client with chronic leukemia in the blast phase.

CHART 40-8

KEY FEATURES *of* Acute Leukemia

Integumentary Manifestations
- Ecchymoses
- Petechiae
- Open infected lesions
- Pallor of the conjunctiva, nail beds, palmar creases, and around the mouth

Gastrointestinal Manifestations
- Bleeding gums
- Anorexia
- Weight loss
- Enlarged liver and spleen

Renal Manifestations
- Hematuria

Cardiovascular Manifestations
- Tachycardia at basal activity levels
- Orthostatic hypotension
- Palpitations

Respiratory Manifestations
- Dyspnea on exertion

Neurologic Manifestations
- Fatigue
- Headache
- Fever

Musculoskeletal Manifestations
- Bone pain
- Joint swelling and pain

CARDIOVASCULAR MANIFESTATIONS. Cardiovascular manifestations are usually related to anemia. The heart rate may be increased and blood pressure decreased. **Murmurs** (abnormal blood flow sounds through the heart) and **bruits** (abnormal blood flow sounds heard over arteries) may be present. Capillary filling time is increased.

RESPIRATORY MANIFESTATIONS. Respiratory manifestations are primarily associated with anemia and infectious complications. The respiratory rate increases as the degree of anemia becomes greater. If respiratory tract infections are present, the client may experience signs and symptoms of pneumonia, including cough and shortness of breath. Abnormal breath sounds are present on auscultation.

INTEGUMENTARY MANIFESTATIONS. The skin and mucous membranes may manifest abnormalities. The skin may be pale and cool to the touch as a result of accompanying anemia. Pallor is especially evident on the face, around the mouth, and in the nail beds. The conjunctiva of the eye also is pale, as are the creases on the palm of the hand (most evident when the skin over the palm of the hand is stretched). **Petechiae** (raised red spots) may be present on any area of skin surface, especially the lower extremities (Dietz, 1999). The petechiae may be unrelated to any obvious trauma. The nurse carefully inspects for any skin infections or traumatized areas that have failed to heal. The mouth is inspected for evidence of bleeding from the gums and any sore or lesion of the oral cavity indicating infection.

GASTROINTESTINAL MANIFESTATIONS. Gastrointestinal manifestations may be related to an increased tendency toward bleeding and to fatigue. Weight loss, nausea, and anorexia are common. The nurse examines the rectal area for fissures and tests the stool for occult blood. Many clients with leukemia have diminished bowel sounds and constipation. Enlargement of the liver and spleen and abdominal tenderness also may be present from leukemic infiltration of abdominal viscera (Chielens, 1999).

CENTRAL NERVOUS SYSTEM MANIFESTATIONS. Cranial nerve disturbances, headache, papilledema as a result of leukemic infiltration of the meninges or central nervous system (CNS), and in advanced cases, seizure activity and coma may occur. Although clients often have fever, this manifestation may be more a response to infection than to malignant changes in the CNS.

MISCELLANEOUS MANIFESTATIONS. Other manifestations include bone and joint tenderness as a result of marrow involvement and bone resorption. Leukemic cell growth or infiltration may produce enlarged lymph nodes or masses.

PSYCHOSOCIAL ASSESSMENT

The client with newly diagnosed leukemia is extremely anxious, because the average layperson equates a diagnosis of any cancer with a death sentence (Dietz, 1999). Current therapies have greatly improved the prognoses of most cancers, yet the public is largely unaware of these advances. The nurse spends time with the client and family to ascertain what the diagnosis means to them and what they expect from the future. Without knowing the client's expectations and feelings, the nurse cannot educate and provide support in an individualized manner or develop a meaningful plan of care.

A diagnosis of leukemia has dramatic implications for a person's lifestyle. Hospitalization for initial treatment often lasts several weeks and may result in boredom, loneliness, and isolation. The nurse assesses coping patterns, including activities that the client finds enjoyable and methods that help the client to relax. A plan of care to prevent diversional activity deficit is particularly beneficial. After initial therapy, the client may be able to resume work, depending on his or her occupation. However, he or she often must make adjustments to accommodate changes in functional status. Repeated hospitalizations may also be necessary.

LABORATORY ASSESSMENT

The client with acute leukemia usually has decreased hemoglobin and hematocrit levels, a decreased platelet count, and an altered white blood cell (WBC) count. The WBC count may be low, normal, or elevated but usually is quite elevated; counts of 20,000 to 100,000 are common. The client with a higher WBC count on diagnosis has a poorer prognosis (Dietz, 1999).

The definitive test for leukemia includes various examinations of cells obtained from bone marrow aspiration and biopsy. The bone marrow is full of leukemic **blast phase cells** (immature cells that are dividing). The composition of various proteins **(antigens)** on the surfaces of the leukemic cells helps diagnose the type of leukemia (Scheinberg, Mazslak, & Weiss, 1997). Such markers include the T11 protein, the enzyme **terminal deoxynucleotidyl transferase (TDT),** and the **common acute lymphoblastic leukemia antigen (CALLA).** These markers also indicate the prognosis.

Blood-clotting times and factors are usually abnormal for the client with acute leukemia. Reduced levels of fibrinogen and other coagulation factors are typical. Whole blood–clotting time (Lee-White clotting test) is increased, as is the activated partial thromboplastin time (aPTT).

Chromosome analysis of the malignant bone marrow cells may identify specific marker chromosomes to assist in the diagnosis of the type of leukemia, predict the prognosis, and determine the effectiveness of therapy. An example is the Philadelphia chromosome, which is important in the diagnosis of chronic myelogenous leukemia (CML) (Chielens, 1999).

RADIOGRAPHIC ASSESSMENT

Specific symptoms determine the need for specific tests. For example, in a client with dyspnea, a chest x-ray study is needed to determine whether leukemic infiltrates are present in the lung. Skeletal x-ray films may help to determine whether bone **resorption** (loss of bone minerals and density) is present.

Analysis

COMMON NURSING DIAGNOSES AND COLLABORATIVE PROBLEMS

The following are common nursing diagnoses for adult clients with acute myelogenous leukemia (AML), the most common type of adult leukemia:

1. Risk for Infection related to decreased immune response
2. Risk for Injury related to thrombocytopenia
3. Fatigue related to decreased tissue oxygenation and increased energy demands

The primary collaborative problem is Potential for Antineoplastic Therapy Adverse Effects.

ADDITIONAL NURSING DIAGNOSES AND COLLABORATIVE PROBLEMS

In addition to the common nursing diagnoses and collaborative problems, clients with AML may have one or more of the following:

- Impaired Skin Integrity related to prolonged immobility
- Impaired Oral Mucous Membrane related to effects of chemotherapy and pancytopenia
- Self-Care Deficit (Total) related to progressive debilitation and weakness
- Imbalanced Nutrition: Less Than Body Requirements related to anorexia, nausea, and vomiting
- Anxiety related to fear of death
- Powerlessness related to an inability to control disease progression
- Interrupted Family Processes related to acute, life-threatening illness of a family member
- Ineffective Role Performance related to perceived inability to fulfill parental and other family roles and prolonged hospitalization
- Deficient Diversional Activity related to prolonged hospitalization.

Planning and Implementation

RISK FOR INFECTION

PLANNING: EXPECTED OUTCOMES. The client with leukemia is expected to:

- Remain free of cross-contamination–induced infection
- Remain free of autocontamination-induced infection
- Not experience sepsis

INTERVENTIONS. Infection is a major cause of death in the immunosuppressed client, and septicemia is a common complication (Pittinger, 1999). Infection of the client with leukemia occurs through both **autocontamination** (normal flora overgrows and penetrates the internal environment) and **cross-contamination** (microorganisms from another person or the environment are transmitted to the client). The three most common sites of infection are the skin, respiratory tract, and gastrointestinal tract.

Gram-negative bacteria are most often the cause of infection, although gram-positive and fungal infections do occur. Interventions aim to interrupt or halt the process of infection and control specific infections early. Chart 40-9 emphasizes the importance of thorough assessment for the client at risk for infection.

DRUG THERAPY FOR LEUKEMIA. Drug therapy for clients with AML is divided into three distinctive phases: induction, consolidation, and maintenance.

INDUCTION THERAPY. Induction therapy is intensive and consists of combination chemotherapy initiated at the time of diagnosis. This therapy is aimed at achieving a rapid, complete remission of all manifestations of disease. Institutions and physicians differ in agents used and the treatment schedule, but a typical course of aggressive chemotherapy includes IV administration of cytosine arabinoside for 7 days with concomitant administration of daunorubicin for the first 3 days (Dietz, 1999).

A major side effect of these agents is severe bone marrow suppression. As a result, the client becomes even more vulnerable to infection than before the treatment started. Prolonged hospitalizations are common while the client is immunosuppressed. Recovery of bone marrow function requires at least 2 to 3 weeks, during which time the client must be protected from life-threatening infections. Other adverse reactions include nausea, vomiting, diarrhea, **alopecia** (hair loss), **stomatitis** (mouth sores), kidney toxicity, liver toxicity, and cardiac toxicity. (See Chapter 25 for information on nursing management of adverse reactions to anticancer agents.)

CONSOLIDATION THERAPY. Consolidation therapy usually consists of another course of either the same agents used for induction at a different dosage or a different combination of chemotherapeutic agents (Dietz, 1999). This treatment occurs early in remission, and its intent is to cure. At some institutions, consolidation therapy is a single course of chemotherapy; at others, it involves regularly scheduled, repeated courses of chemotherapy for 1 to 2 years.

MAINTENANCE THERAPY. Maintenance therapy may be prescribed for months to years after successful induction and consolidation therapies. It is commonly indicated for clients with acute lymphocytic leukemia (ALL). The purpose is to maintain the remission achieved through induction and consolidation. Maintenance agents are milder and are often given orally for 2 to 5 years. There are conflicting data regarding the effectiveness of maintenance therapy. Maintenance therapy is not beneficial for clients with AML (Dietz, 1999).

WOMEN'S HEALTH CONSIDERATIONS

Pregnancy may increase a woman's risk for developing leukemia, although the current data are inconclusive. The diagnosis of acute leukemia during pregnancy forces a woman to face a difficult ethical dilemma regarding treatment (Wallace, Wiegand, & Warren, 1997). AML is fatal for the mother if she is not treated aggressively with chemotherapeutic agents, many of which are harmful and potentially lethal to the fetus (see the Legal/Ethical Issues in Health Care box on p. 850). A review of the current literature suggests the following findings regarding chemotherapy treatment for AML during pregnancy (Ramirez-Smiley & Ingle, 1995):

- Certain chemotherapeutic and supportive agents may be used judiciously in pregnant women.
- First-trimester treatment can cause severe fetal malformation or miscarriage.
- Normal live births to mothers treated after the first trimester are well documented.
- Infants born to mothers treated during the second and third trimesters did not differ from those born to healthy mothers.
- Side effects experienced by the mother, such as malnutrition, infection, and death, may harm the fetus.

Nursing care for the pregnant client with leukemia focuses on prevention of infection, bleeding, injury, and premature delivery. The nurse assists in maintaining adequate nutrition and provides resources to help cope with a diagnosis that can be fatal to both the mother and the fetus.

CHART 40-9

FOCUSED ASSESSMENT *of*
Hospitalized or Home Care Clients with Potential or Actual Risk for Infection

General Condition
Age, fatigue, malaise
History of allergies
History of chemotherapy, radiation therapy, or other immunosuppressive therapies, such as steroid use
Chronic diseases
History of febrile neutropenia and associated symptoms
Nutritional status
Functional status—problems with immobility
Tobacco use—cigarettes, pipe, cigars, oral
Recreational drug use
Alcohol use
Prescribed and over-the-counter medication use
Baseline and ongoing viral signs—blood pressure, heart rate, respiratory rate, and temperature

Skin and Mucous Membranes
Thorough inspection of all skin surfaces with special attention to axilla, perineum (particularly the anorectal area), and under breasts; inspection of skin for color, vascularity, bleeding, lesions, edema, moist areas, excoriation, irritation, erythema; general condition of hair and nails, pressure areas, swelling, pain, tenderness, biopsy or surgical sites, wounds, enlarged lymph nodes, catheters, or other devices
Inspection of oral cavity, including lips, tongue, mucous membranes, gingiva, teeth, and throat—color, moisture, bleeding, ulcerations, lesions, exudate, mucositis, stomatitis, plaque, swelling, pain, tenderness, taste changes, amount and character of saliva, ability to swallow, changes in voice, dental caries, client's oral hygiene routine
History of current skin disorders or problems with mucous membranes

Head, Eyes, Ears, Nose
Pain, tenderness, exudate, crusting, enlarged lymph nodes

Cardiopulmonary
Respiratory rate and pattern, breath sounds (presence/absence, adventitious sounds), quantity and characteristics of sputum, shortness of breath, use of accessory muscles, dysphagia, diminished gag reflex, tachycardia, blood pressure

Gastrointestinal
Pain, diarrhea, bowel sounds, character and frequency of bowel movements, constipation, rectal bleeding, hemorrhoids, change in bowel habits, sexual practices, erythema, ulceration

Genitourinary
Dysuria, frequency, urgency, hematuria, pruritus, pain, vaginal or penile discharge, vaginal bleeding, burning, lesions, ulcerations, characteristics of urine

Central Nervous System
Cognition, level of consciousness, personality, behavior

Musculoskeletal
Tenderness, pain, loss of function

Modified from Dean, G.E., Haeuber D., & Rivera, L.M. (1996). Infection. In R. McCorkle et al. (Eds.), *Cancer nursing: A comprehensive textbook* (2nd ed., p. 975). Philadelphia: W.B. Saunders.

LEGAL/ETHICAL ISSUES IN HEALTH CARE

TREATMENT DECISIONS FOR A PREGNANT WOMAN WITH LEUKEMIA

When a woman diagnosed with leukemia is pregnant, careful consideration is required regarding treatment decisions. An ethical dilemma arises when there is a conflict between ethical principles. In this situation, treatment decisions that may be beneficent and nonmaleficent to the mother may not be beneficent to the fetus (Wallace, Wiegand, & Warren, 1997).

Decisions are best made on a case-by-case basis. Possible options include the following: continue the pregnancy without treating the mother, continue the pregnancy and begin treating the mother, deliver the fetus early and begin treating the mother, or delay delivery of the fetus until lung maturity and then begin treating the mother. Informed consent involves careful consideration of all available options. The mother must decide what is best for herself and the fetus. Factors to consider include cultural values, religious beliefs, quality of life, and effects of treatment on both maternal and fetal health.

Data from Wallace, R., Wiegand, F., & Warren, C. (1997). Beneficence toward whom? Ethical decision making in a maternal-fetal conflict. *AACN Clinical Issues: Advanced Practice in Acute and Critical Care, 8*(4), 586-594.

DRUG THERAPY FOR INFECTION. Drug therapy is the primary defense against infections that develop in clients undergoing therapy for AML. Agents used depend on the sensitivity of the specific organism causing the infection, as well as the extent of the infection, and are categorized by specificity as antibacterial, antiviral, or antifungal. Figure 40-2 outlines pharmacologic management of the febrile neutropenic client.

ANTIBIOTIC AND ANTIBACTERIAL AGENTS. Antibiotic and antibacterial agents used for prophylaxis or treatment of infection in clients with AML usually include at least one of the aminoglycoside antibiotics (amikacin, gentamicin, and tobramycin) and a systemic penicillin. Additional, powerful antibiotics used may include vancomycin and drugs from the tetracycline and third-generation cephalosporin classes.

ANTIFUNGAL AGENTS. Systemic antifungal agents, used when a fungal infection has been diagnosed or is strongly suggested, include amphotericin B, ketoconazole (Nizoral), and

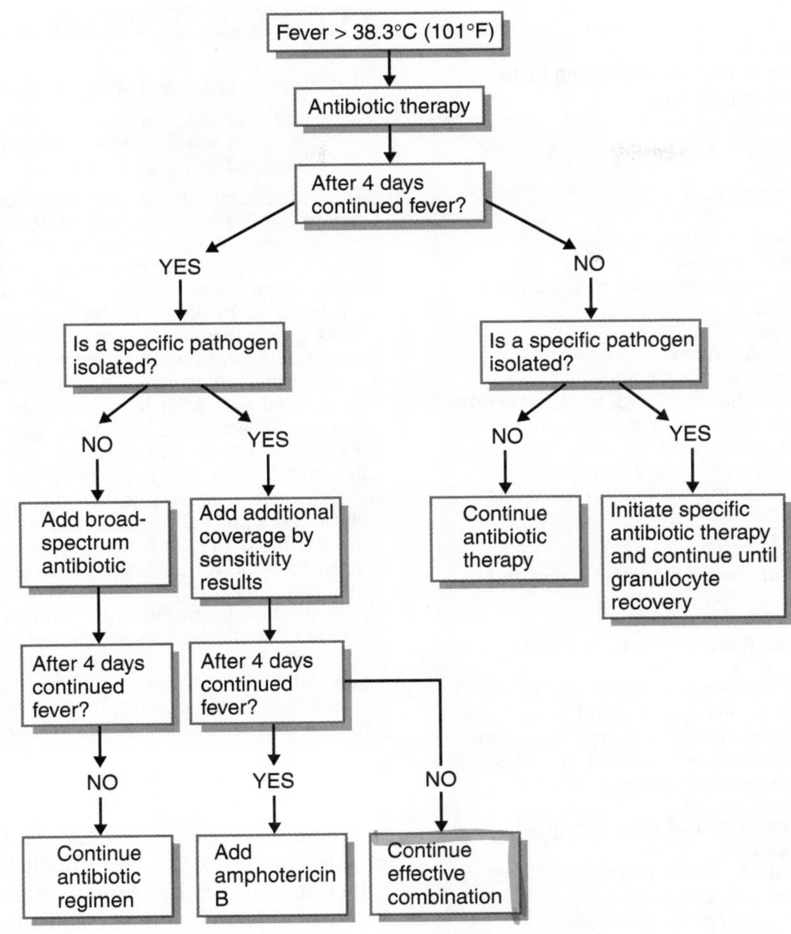

Figure 40-2 ● Example of antibiotic management for fever in the neutropenic client.

nystatin (Mycostatin, Nadostine✤, Nilstat). In neutropenic clients, antifungal creams (e.g., miconazole nitrate) are administered intravaginally to prevent yeast infections.

ANTIVIRAL AGENTS. Antiviral agents are commonly used in clients with leukemia to prevent and treat viral infections. Acyclovir is administered either orally or parenterally before the initiation of antineoplastic agents, especially in clients who are cytomegalovirus (CMV) positive. If a viral infection is suspected or diagnosed with positive cultures, pharmacologic treatments may include ganciclovir, foscarnet, or steroids. The antivirals, although helpful in combating severe infections, are associated with a wide range of serious adverse effects, especially **ototoxicity** (disruption of hearing and/or balance) and **nephrotoxicity** (disruption of kidney function). The nurse carefully monitors the client treated with such drugs for signs of hearing impairment and renal insufficiency.

NIC **INFECTION PROTECTION.** A major objective in caring for the client with leukemia is protection from infection (Chart 40-10). Nurses and all assistive nursing personnel must use extreme care during all nursing procedures. Frequent, thorough handwashing is of the utmost importance. Anyone with an upper respiratory tract infection who must enter the client's room must wear a mask. Nurses must also observe strict procedures when performing dressing changes or when helping a physician to insert a central venous catheter. The nurse maintains strict aseptic technique in the care of these catheters at all times.

If possible, the nurse ensures that the client is in a private room to minimize cross-contamination. Because infection in the immunosuppressed person is most commonly caused by normal body microorganisms, **protective (reverse) isolation** has been eliminated from the Centers for Disease Control and Prevention (CDC) guidelines for infection control (see the Evidence-Based Practice for Nursing box on p. 852). However, other environmental precautions are heeded, such as allowing no standing collections of water in vases, denture cups, or humidifiers in the client's room, because they are excellent breeding grounds for microorganisms.

Some institutions prescribe a "minimal bacteria diet" during the neutropenic period. Any uncooked foods, such as raw fruits and vegetables, and pepper are eliminated from the diet because they contain large numbers of microorganisms. Whether clients benefit from this diet is controversial.

In some institutions, the immunosuppressed client is placed in a room with a high-efficiency particulate air (HEPA) filtration or laminar airflow system. These systems decrease the number of airborne pathogens. Again, whether these restrictions benefit clients is debatable.

CHART 40-10

NIC INTERVENTION ACTIVITIES *for* Clients with Leukemia or Clients Undergoing Bone Marrow/Stem Cell Transplantation

Infection Protection: *Prevention and early detection of infection in client at risk*
- Monitor absolute granulocyte count, WBC, and differential results.
- Screen all visitors for communicable disease.
- Maintain asepsis for client at risk.
- Inspect skin and mucous membranes for redness, extreme warmth, or drainage.
- Obtain cultures, as needed.
- Promote sufficient nutritional intake.
- Encourage fluid intake, as appropriate.
- Encourage deep breathing and coughing, as appropriate.
- Instruct client to take antibiotics as prescribed.
- Teach client/family about signs, symptoms of infection and when to report them to health care provider.
- Remove fresh flowers and plants from client areas, as appropriate.
- Provide private room, as needed.

Bleeding Precautions: *Reduction of stimuli that may induce bleeding or hemorrhage in at-risk clients*
- Monitor the client closely for hemorrhage.
- Note hemoglobin/hematocrit levels before and after blood loss, as indicated.
- Monitor for signs and symptoms of persistent bleeding (e.g., check all secretions for frank or occult blood).
- Monitor coagulation studies, including prothrombin time (PT), partial thromboplastin time (PTT), fibrinogen, fibrin degradation/split products, and platelet counts, as appropriate.
- Administer blood products (e.g., platelets and fresh frozen plasma), as appropriate.
- Protect the client from trauma, which may cause bleeding.
- Avoid injections (IV, IM, or SQ), as appropriate.
- Use soft toothbrush or toothettes for oral care.
- Use electric razor, instead of straight-edge, for shaving.
- Instruct client to avoid aspirin or other anticoagulants.
- Instruct client to increase intake of foods rich in vitamin K.
- Avoid constipation (e.g., encourage fluid intake and stool softeners), as appropriate.
- Instruct the client/and or family on signs of bleeding and appropriate actions (e.g., notify the nurse), should bleeding occur.

Energy Management: *Regulating energy use to treat or prevent fatigue and optimize function*
- Determine client's/significant other's perception of causes of fatigue.
- Encourage verbalization of feelings about limitations.
- Monitor nutritional intake to ensure adequate energy resources.
- Monitor/record client's sleep pattern and number of sleep hours.
- Limit number of and interruptions by visitors, as appropriate.
- Provide calming diversional activities to promote relaxation.
- Encourage an afternoon nap, if appropriate.
- Avoid care activities during scheduled rest periods.
- Plan activities for periods when the client has the most energy.
- Monitor client's oxygen response (e.g., pulse rate, cardiac rhythm, and respiratory rate) to self-care or nursing activities.
- Instruct client/significant other to recognize signs and symptoms of fatigue that require reduction in activity.
- Monitor location and nature of discomfort or pain during movement/activity.

NIC intervention activities selected from McCloskey, J.C., & Bulechek, G.M. (2000). *Nursing interventions classification (NIC)* (3rd ed.). St. Louis: Mosby. No part of this work is to be altered without prior written permission from the Publisher.
WBC, White blood cell.

EVIDENCE-BASED PRACTICE FOR NURSING

Does wearing gowns and shoe covers prevent infection?

Duquette-Petersen, L., et al. (1999). The role of protective clothing in infection prevention in patients undergoing autologous bone marrow transplant. *Oncology Nursing Forum*, 26(8), 1319-1333.

The purpose of this randomized two-group clinical trial was to determine the effectiveness of cover gowns and shoe covers in preventing infection in autologous bone marrow transplant clients. Forty men and women undergoing autologous bone marrow transplantation at a university teaching hospital were randomized to either the control group, in which caregivers wore gowns and shoe covers, or the experimental group, in which caregivers wore no protective clothing. Data were collected from the client's medical records to determine the time to the first antibiotic treatment and the duration of antibiotic therapy. There were no statistical differences in the above measures between the two groups of clients. Use of protective clothing by caregivers provided no benefit.

Critique. This was a well-designed study. Limitations include the small sample size and the fact that caregivers could not be blind to group assignment. Findings do support the need to conduct a similar study with a larger sample using multiple sites.

Implications for Nursing. The use of protective clothing to prevent infection is a practice that has not been supported by research. This practice is costly in both supplies and nursing care time. The estimated savings for the group in this study was $70,000. In addition, the use of protective clothing often makes clients feel more isolated and fearful.

The nurse continually assesses the client for the presence of infection. This task is difficult because manifestations of infection may not be obvious in the client with leukopenia. The development of fever and the formation of pus (both common indicators of infection) depend on the presence of leukocytes. Therefore the client with leukopenia may have a severe infection without pus and with a relatively low fever.

The nurse monitors the client's daily complete blood count (CBC) with differential white blood cell (WBC) count. The oral mucosa is inspected during every nursing shift for lesions indicating fungal or viral infection. The nurse also auscultates the lungs every 8 hours for crackles, wheezes, or diminished breath sounds. Each time the client voids, the urine is assessed for odor and cloudiness. The client is asked about any urgency, burning, or pain present on urination.

Vital signs are taken at least every 4 hours to assess for fever. A temperature elevation of even 0.5° F (or 0.5° C) above baseline is significant for a client with leukopenia and indicates infection until it has been proved otherwise.

Many hospital units that specialize in the care of clients with neutropenia have specific protocols for antibiotic therapy if infection is suspected. Usually, physicians are notified immediately, and specific specimens are obtained for culture. Blood for bacterial and fungal cultures is obtained from peripheral sites and from the central venous catheter. Urine specimens, sputum specimens, and specimens from open lesions are taken for culture, and chest x-ray films are taken. After the specimens are obtained, the client begins a regimen of IV antibiotics.

SKIN CARE. Skin care is important for preventing infection in the client with leukemia. The skin may be the only intact defense. The nurse teaches the ambulatory client thorough hygiene care and encourages daily bathing. If the client is immobile, turning is necessary every hour and skin lubricants are applied.

RESPIRATORY CARE. Respiratory care, including pulmonary hygiene, is performed every 2 to 4 hours. The nurse auscultates the lungs for crackles, wheezes, or diminished breath sounds. The client is encouraged to cough and deep breathe or to perform sustained maximal inhalations every hour while awake.

BONE MARROW TRANSPLANTATION. Once viewed as a treatment of last resort, bone marrow transplantation (BMT) is now considered a standard treatment for the client with leukemia. This treatment modality began more than 25 years ago (Johns, 1998). BMT is the treatment of choice for the client with leukemia who has a closely matched donor and who is experiencing temporary remission with induction therapy. Because of the success of BMT in the client with leukemia, this therapy is now being used for lymphoma, aplastic anemia, inborn errors of metabolism, and many solid tumors (Wolf, 1999).

The bone marrow is the actual site of production of leukemic cells. Because it can be difficult to ensure that all leukemic cells have been eradicated during induction therapy, the goal is for extremely high doses of chemotherapy to destroy all of the affected marrow. The new, healthy marrow then begins the process of hematopoiesis, which results in normal, properly functioning cells and, it is hoped, a permanent cure.

For many malignant disorders, the dose-limiting toxicity of treatments is bone marrow suppression. The aim of bone marrow or stem cell transplantation is to rid the client of all leukemic or other malignant cells through high doses of chemotherapy, often in conjunction with whole-body irradiation. These treatments are lethal to the bone marrow, and without replacement of bone marrow function through transplantation of progenitor cells of the hematopoietic system, the client would die of infection or hemorrhage.

Advances in the field of transplantation have been remarkable. Even as recently as the late 1980s, the client undergoing transplantation would have been seen only in major medical centers. Today, transplant units are becoming commonplace, even in community hospital settings. With long-term survival after transplantation increasing, nurses can expect to be caring for these people, if not during the actual transplantation or recovery period, then during the post-transplantation period, in a variety of health care settings.

SOURCES OF STEM CELLS. BMT originated with the use of **allogeneic bone marrow transplantation** (transplantation of identical bone marrow from a sibling) and has advanced to the use of human leukocyte antigen (HLA)–matched stem cells from the umbilical cords of unrelated donors (Wolf, 1999).

Transplants can be classified based on the source of stem cells. In **autologous transplants,** the clients receive their own stem cells, which were collected before therapy. **Syngeneic transplants** are rare and involve the client's own identical twin as the donor of stem cells. In **allogeneic transplants,** a closely HLA-matched sibling or an unrelated donor provides the stem cells. Stem cells for transplantation may be obtained by one of the following methods: bone marrow harvest, peripheral stem cell pheresis, or umbilical cord blood stem cell banking. Table 40-5 provides an overview of the types of transplants.

TABLE 40-5 • CLASSIFICATION OF TRANSPLANTS

Type of Transplant	Sources of Stem Cells
AUTOLOGOUS	
Self-donation	Bone marrow harvest Peripheral stem cell pheresis Umbilical cord blood
SYNGENEIC	
Client's HLA identical twin	Bone marrow harvest Peripheral stem cell pheresis
ALLOGENEIC	
HLA-matched relative, usually a sibling Unrelated HLA-matched donor Mismatched or partially HLA-matched family member or unrelated donor (donor registries)	Bone marrow harvest Peripheral stem cell pheresis Umbilical cord blood

HLA, Human leukocyte antigen.

• • •

Transplantation procedures have five phases: stem cell procurement, conditioning regimen, transplantation, engraftment, and post-transplantation recovery.

OBTAINING STEM CELLS. Stem cells for transplantation are obtained either by harvest of bone marrow, by pheresis for peripheral blood stem cells, or by collection of umbilical cord stem cells.

Bone marrow is harvested either from the client directly (autologous marrow) or from an HLA-matched person (allogeneic marrow). For allogeneic marrow, a suitable donor is selected after family members are tested for HLA type. Preferred transplantations are those between HLA-identical siblings, but transplantation can also be successful between those with closely matched HLA types. The chance of matching with any given sibling is 25%. Several donor registries have been formed that keep records of people willing to donate marrow to provide marrow for clients who do not have a family member HLA match. The chance of matching with an unrelated donor is one in 5000 (Alcoser & Burchett, 1999).

CULTURAL CONSIDERATIONS

Approximately 70% of individuals on the bone marrow donor lists are Caucasian. It is estimated that the chance of finding an HLA-matched unrelated donor is 30% to 40% for Caucasians but less than 20% for African Americans (Wolf, 1999). Nationally, efforts have been made to publicize the need for donors from all cultural backgrounds. It is estimated that of the 10,000 to 15,000 people each year who search for an unrelated marrow donor, only 25% find a suitable match (Wolf, 1999).

After a suitable donor is identified by tissue typing, the donor is taken to the operating room, where sufficient marrow for transplant is harvested through multiple aspirations from the iliac crests. About 500 to 1000 mL of marrow is aspirated; this amount is approximately 5% to 10% of the donor's marrow supply and will be replenished in a few weeks (Poliquin, 1997). The marrow is then filtered and may be further processed to purge the autologous marrow of any residual cancer cells or to deplete the allogeneic marrow of T-cells, which may later cause **graft-versus-host disease (GVHD)** (see p. 855). Allogeneic marrow is transfused into the recipient immediately; autologous marrow is frozen for later use.

The nurse monitors the donor for signs and symptoms of fluid loss, assesses for complications of anesthesia, and manages postoperative pain. During surgery, donors may lose a significant amount of fluid in addition to the volume of marrow donated. Donors are often hydrated with saline infusions before and immediately after surgery. Occasionally the donor may require an infusion of autologous salvaged red blood cells (RBCs) (Poliquin, 1997). The nurse assesses the harvest sites to ensure that the dressings are dry and intact and that the donor is not bleeding excessively.

Marrow donation is usually a same-day surgical procedure. At home the donors are taught to inspect the harvest sites for bleeding and to take analgesics for pain. Pain is often experienced at the harvest sites (hip) and is usually managed effectively with oral non–aspirin-containing analgesics. Individual differences do occur, however. Some donors refuse pain medication, but others require opioid analgesics.

There are three phases to obtaining **peripheral blood stem cells (PBSCs):** mobilization, collection, and reinfusion. During the mobilization phase, chemotherapy or hematopoietic growth factors are administered to the client (Wagner & Quinones, 1998). These agents cause stem cells to circulate in the peripheral blood and the number of WBCs to increase. The stem cells are then collected by **pheresis** (withdrawing whole blood, filtering out the cells, and returning the plasma to the client). One to five pheresis procedures, each lasting 2 to 4 hours, are usually required to obtain enough stem cells for PBSC transplantation. The stem cells are then frozen and stored for reinfusion after the conditioning regimen (Wolf, 1999).

The nurse must monitor the client closely during pheresis. Common complications include catheter clotting, which may delay pheresis, and hypocalcemia caused by anticoagulants (Poliquin, 1997). The client with hypocalcemia may experience chills, paresthesia, abdominal or muscle cramping, or chest pain, and the nurse may need to administer oral calcium supplements to manage these symptoms. The nurse must also monitor vital signs frequently. The client may experience hypotension as a result of fluid volume changes during the procedure.

Stem cells may also be obtained from umbilical cords. The first cord blood transplant was done in France in 1988 (Wolf, 1999). Umbilical stem cells are obtained via a simple phlebotomy procedure. After birth, before the placenta detaches, a syringe is used to withdraw 40 to 150 mL of blood from the umbilical vein. The syringes are placed in a kit, which is returned to the Cord Blood Registry for processing and storage (Wolf, 1999). The stem cells may be used later for an unrelated recipient or stored in case the infant develops a serious illness later in life and needs them. The cost of banking and processing umbilical cord stem cells is approximately $1500, with an additional charge of $100 per year for storage. Umbilical stem cells can last for years when stored properly in liquid nitrogen. The oldest viable sample is nearly 20 years old (Wolf, 1999).

CONDITIONING REGIMEN. Figure 40-3 outlines the timing and steps typically involved in BMT. The day the client receives the bone marrow is considered day T-0. Pretransplantation conditioning days are counted in reverse chronologic order from T-0, just like a rocket countdown. Post-transplantation days are counted in chronologic order from the day of transplantation.

The client must first undergo a conditioning regimen, which varies with the diagnosis and type of transplant to be received. The conditioning regimen serves two purposes: (1) to obliterate, or "wipe out," the client's own bone marrow, thus preparing the client for optimal graft take, and (2) to give higher than normal doses of chemotherapy and/or radiotherapy to obliterate, or wipe out, a malignancy, such as breast cancer. Usually a period of 5 to 10 days is required. The conditioning regimen always includes intensive chemotherapy and sometimes includes radiotherapy, usually total-body irradiation (TBI). Each conditioning regimen is individually tailored, with the client's specific disease, overall health, and previous treatment taken into account (Poliquin, 1997).

A typical conditioning regimen for an adult client receiving an allogenic BMT for treatment of acute myelogenous leukemia (AML) is as follows:

- *Days T-7 through T-5:* High-dose chemotherapy to obliterate the client's own bone marrow cells and to eradicate any remaining leukemic cells. Specific agents include busulfan, carmustine, cyclophosphamide, cytosine arabinoside, etoposide, and melphalan. The dosages are many times higher than those used for normal chemotherapy.

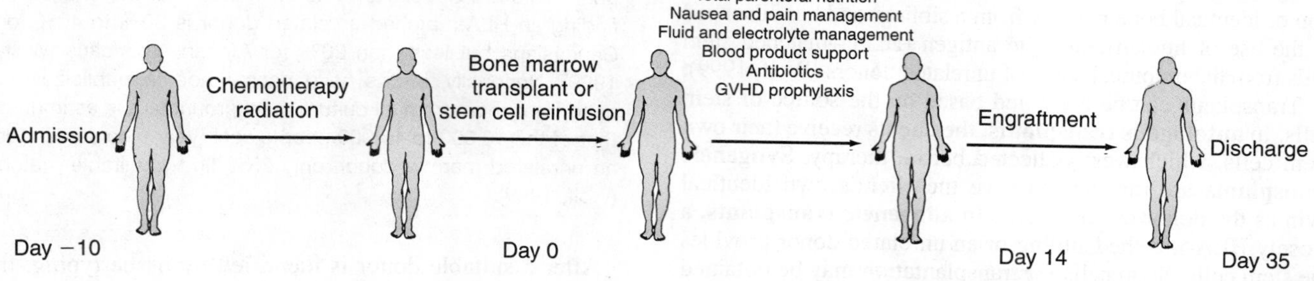

Figure 40-3 ● Timing and steps of allogeneic bone marrow transplantation. (*GVHD,* Graft-versus-host disease.)

- *Days T-4 through T-2:* Delivery of fractionated TBI (smaller doses of radiation given over a period of time instead of one larger dose). The typical radiation dose for TBI is 1200 rad. The client usually receives no cell-killing treatment on day T-1.

During conditioning, bone marrow and normal tissues begin to respond immediately to the chemotherapy and radiotherapy. The client experiences all of the expected side effects associated with both therapies. Because the chemotherapy is administered in such high doses, these side effects are much more intense than those seen with either standard chemotherapy or radiation. These side effects include severe nausea and vomiting, mucositis, capillary leak syndrome, diarrhea, and bone marrow suppression (Poliquin, 1997).

Late effects from the conditioning regimen are also common, occurring as late as 3 to 10 years after transplantation, and include **veno-occlusive disease (VOD),** skin toxicities, cataracts, fibrotic pulmonary disease, secondary malignancies, cardiomyopathy, endocrine complications, and neurologic complications (Poliquin, 1997).

TRANSPLANTATION. Day T-0, the day of transplantation, is separated from the chemotherapy conditioning by at least 2 days to ensure that the chemotherapeutic agent has cleared and will not exert any cytotoxic effects on the transplanted stem cells. The client should have few, if any, circulating white blood cells (WBCs) at this point, indicating successful conditioning.

The transplantation itself is very simple. Frozen marrow, PBSCs, or umbilical cord blood cells are thawed in a temperature-controlled warm water bath (D'Andrea et al., 1997). The bone marrow is administered through the client's central catheter like an ordinary blood transfusion, but not using blood administration tubing. Usually the marrow is infused over a 30-minute period, although it may also be administered by IV push directly into the central catheter with syringes.

Side effects of all types of stem cell transfusions are similar. The client may experience fever and hypertension as a result of a reaction to the preservative used for storage of stem cells (D'Andrea et al., 1997). To prevent these reactions, the nurse administers acetaminophen (Tylenol), hydrocortisone, and diphenhydramine (Benadryl) before the transfusion (Johns, 1998). Antihypertensives or diuretics may also be required to treat fluid volume changes. The client may experience red urine secondary to hemolysis of erythrocytes in the infused product.

ENGRAFTMENT. The transfused PBSCs and marrow cells circulate only briefly in the peripheral blood. Most of the cells, especially the stems cells, find their way to the marrow-forming sites of the recipient's bones and establish residency there. The mechanism by which the donated marrow cells "home in" on the appropriate sites is not yet understood.

Engraftment, successful "take" of the transplanted cells in the recipient's bone marrow, is key to the whole transplantation process. For the donated marrow or stem cells to "rescue" the client after large doses of chemotherapy and/or radiotherapy wipe out his or her own bone marrow, the transfused stem cells must survive and grow in the clients' bone marrow sites. The engraftment process takes 8 to 12 days for peripheral blood stem cells and 12 to 28 days for bone marrow stem cells (Poliquin, 1997). To facilitate engraftment, hematopoietic growth factors, such as granulocyte colony-stimulating factor or granulocyte-macrophage colony-stimulating factor, may be administered (Alcoser & Burchett, 1999). When engraftment is successful, the client's WBC, erythrocyte, and platelet counts begin to rise.

PREVENTION OF COMPLICATIONS. The post-transplantation period is difficult. Because the client remains without any natural immunity until the transfused stem cells begin to proliferate and engraftment occurs, infection and severe thrombocytopenia are major problems. The nursing care requirements for this client are virtually identical to those for the client undergoing aggressive induction therapy for AML. Helping the client to maintain hope through this long recovery period is difficult (Campbell, 1999). Complications are often severe and life threatening. The nurse should try to encourage the client to maintain a positive attitude and be involved in his or her own recovery.

In addition to the problems related to the period of **pancytopenia** (too few circulating blood cells), other immediate hazards associated with BMT include failure to engraft, development of GVHD, and VOD.

Failure to Engraft. Sometimes the donated marrow or stem cells fail to engraft. This possibility is discussed in advance with the client and the donor. Failure to engraft occurs more often among allogeneic stem cell recipients than among autologous stem cell recipients. The causes may be related to insufficient numbers of cells transplanted, attack or rejection of donor cells by the remaining immunologically competent recipient cells, infection of transplanted cells, and unknown biologic factors. If the transplanted stem cells fail to engraft, the client will die unless another transplantation is successful.

Graft-Versus-Host Disease. Graft-versus-host disease (GVHD) is an immunologic event that occurs in allogeneic transplants. The immunocompetent cells of the donated marrow recognize the client's (recipient) cells, tissues, and organs as foreign and mount an immune offense against them. The graft is actually trying to attack the host (Alcoser & Burchett, 1999).

Although all host tissues can be attacked and harmed, the tissues most commonly damaged are the skin, gastrointestinal tract, and liver. Approximately 25% to 50% of all allogeneic BMT recipients experience some degree of GVHD, and more than 15% of the clients who experience GVHD die of its complications (Johns, 1998). The presence of GVHD indicates that the transplanted cells are competent and have successfully engrafted.

Management of GVHD is achieved by limiting the activation of donor T-lymphocytes through the administration of immunosuppressive agents such as cyclosporine, methotrexate, corticosteroids, and antithymocyte globulin (Alcoser & Burchett, 1999). Care is taken to avoid suppressing the new immune system to the extent that either the client becomes more susceptible to infection or the transplanted cells stop engrafting.

Veno-occlusive Disease. Veno-occlusive disease (VOD) involves occlusion of the hepatic blood vessels by clotting and inflammation **(phlebitis).** This condition occurs in up to 20% of clients who receive either an autologous or an allogeneic transplant, and symptoms usually occur within the first 30 days after transplantation (Johns, 1998). Clients who have received high doses of chemotherapy, especially alkylating agents, are at risk for life-threatening hepatic complications. Clinical signs include jaundice, pain in the right upper quadrant, ascites, weight gain, and liver enlargement.

Because there is no known way of opening the hepatic vessels, treatment is supportive. Early detection enhances the chances of survival. Fluid management is also crucial. The nurse assesses the client daily for weight gain, fluid accumulation, increases in abdominal girth, and hepatomegaly.

RISK FOR INJURY

Because normal bone marrow production is severely limited with acute myelogenic leukemia (AML), the number of circulating platelets is severely diminished, causing **thrombocytopenia.** This condition puts the client with AML at a greatly increased risk for excessive bleeding in response to minimal trauma. Thrombocytopenia can also be induced by induction therapy for AML or high-dose chemotherapy for transplantation (Rust, Wood, & Battiato, 1999).

PLANNING: EXPECTED OUTCOMES. The client with leukemia is expected to remain free from bleeding.

INTERVENTIONS. As a result of chemotherapy-induced pancytopenia, the client's platelet count is decreased. During the period of greatest bone marrow suppression (the nadir), the platelet count may be extremely low (<10,000/mm^3). The client is at great risk for bleeding once the platelet count falls below 50,000/mm^3, and spontaneous bleeding often occurs when the platelet count is lower than 20,000 (Harrahill & DeLoughery, 1998).

NIC **BLEEDING PRECAUTIONS.** The nurse's major objectives are to protect the client from situations that could lead to bleeding and to closely monitor any bleeding that does occur (see Chart 40-10). The nurse assesses the client frequently for evidence of bleeding: oozing, confluent ecchymoses, petechiae, or purpura. All stools, urine, nasogastric drainage, and vomitus are examined visually for blood and tested for occult blood. The nurse measures any blood loss as accurately as possible and measures the client's abdominal girth daily. Increases in abdominal girth can indicate internal hemorrhage. Bleeding precautions are instituted (Chart 40-11).

The nurse also monitors laboratory values daily. Complete blood count (CBC) results are reviewed daily to determine the risk for bleeding, as well as actual blood loss. The client with a platelet count below 20,000/mm^3 may need a platelet transfusion. An alternative treatment is the administration of oprelvekin (Neumega), a platelet **(thrombopoietic)** growth factor. The recommended dose is 50 μg/kg/day subcutaneously starting 6 to 12 hours after the completion of chemotherapy (Rust, Wood, & Battiato, 1999). For the client with severe blood loss, packed RBCs may be ordered (see later discussion under Red Blood Cell Transfusions, p. 864).

FATIGUE

Because normal bone marrow production is severely limited in leukemia, the number of circulating erythrocytes is severely diminished, creating a condition of anemia, leading in turn to fatigue. Because leukemic cells tend to have higher rates of metabolism and greater utilization of oxygen, the anemic client with leukemia is at risk for severe fatigue. Anemia also occurs secondary to chemotherapy treatment (Richardson, Ream, & Wilson-Barnett, 1998).

CHART 40-11

BEST PRACTICE *for* The Client with Thrombocytopenia

- Handle the client gently.
- Use a lift sheet when moving and positioning in bed.
- Avoid intramuscular injections and venipunctures.
- When injections or venipunctures are necessary, use the smallest-gauge needle for the task.
- Apply firm pressure to the needle stick site for 10 minutes or until the site no longer oozes blood.
- Apply ice to areas of trauma.
- Test all urine and stool for the presence of occult blood.
- Observe IV sites every 2 hours for bleeding.
- Avoid trauma to rectal tissues:
  - Do not take temperatures rectally.
  - Do not give enemas.
  - Administer well-lubricated suppositories with caution.
  - Advise client not to have anal intercourse.
- Measure abdominal girth daily.
- Teach the client to use an electric razor.
- Teach the client to avoid mouth trauma:
  - Use soft-bristled toothbrush or tooth sponges.
  - Do not floss between teeth.
  - Avoid dental work, especially extractions.
  - Avoid hard foods.
  - Make sure that dentures fit and do not rub.
- Encourage the client not to blow the nose or insert objects into the nose.
- Teach the client to avoid contact sports.
- Teach client to wear shoes with firm soles whenever ambulating.

NOC **PLANNING: EXPECTED OUTCOMES.** The client with leukemia is expected to:

- Experience no increase in fatigue
- Recognize symptoms of fatigue and alter activity before fatigue becomes excessive

INTERVENTIONS

NIC **ENERGY MANAGEMENT.** Energy management aims at decreasing the effects of anemia and conserving energy expenditure (see Chart 40-10).

DIET THERAPY. Diet therapy is indirectly related to fatigue and subsequent activity intolerance. The client must ingest enough calories to meet at least basal energy requirements, but increasing dietary intake can be difficult when the client is extremely fatigued. The nurse thus provides small, frequent meals high in protein and carbohydrates. Food items that are liquid or easy to chew also require less effort to eat.

BLOOD REPLACEMENT THERAPY. Blood transfusions are sometimes indicated for the client with fatigue. Transfusions increase the blood's oxygen-carrying capacity and replace missing red blood cells (RBCs) and some coagulation factors (see Table 40-2). For the client with leukemia who is experiencing fatigue related to anemia, packed RBCs are usually the blood component of choice. (See Transfusion Therapy, p. 862, for a discussion of nursing care during transfusions.)

DRUG THERAPY. Clients may receive subcutaneous injections of epoetin alfa (Epogen or Procrit) 50 to 100 units/kg three times per week (Cella & Bron, 1999). This growth factor is naturally secreted by the kidney and boosts the production of RBCs. Epoetin alfa has previously been used in anemia associated with chronic renal failure and in clients with human immunodeficiency virus (HIV) who are receiving zidovudine and is now approved for use in anemia associated with chemotherapy. The nurse administers injections three times a week and assesses for side effects such as hypertension, headaches, fever, **myalgia** (muscle aches), and rashes. (See Chapter 25 for more information on hematopoietic growth factors.)

CONSERVATION OF ENERGY. The nurse examines the hospitalized client's schedule of prescribed and routine activities. Those activities that do not have a direct positive effect on the client's condition are assessed in terms of their usefulness. If the actual or potential benefit of an activity is less than its actual or potential worsening of fatigue, the nurse consults with other members of the health care team about eliminating or postponing it. Candidates for cancellation or postponement include physical therapy and certain invasive diagnostic tests not required for assessment or treatment of current problems.

Community-Based Care

The client with leukemia is discharged after induction chemotherapy and recovery of blood cell–producing function. Follow-up care is provided on an outpatient basis. Although the majority of transplant centers discharge clients following engraftment, some centers administer high-dose chemotherapy and stem cell infusion on an outpatient basis. This plan involves daily clinic visits and frequent follow-up by nurses in the home care setting (D'Andrea et al., 1997).

HOME CARE MANAGEMENT

Planning for home care for the client with leukemia begins as soon as a client achieves remission. He or she will need assistance at home until the condition improves. The nurse assesses the available support mechanisms. Many clients require the services of a visiting nurse to assist with dressing changes for central venous catheters, to assist with hyperalimentation infusions, to transfuse platelets, and to answer questions. Occasionally they may also require home transfusion therapy for one or more blood components (Bean, 1998).

The home care team is critical for the client receiving stem cell transplantation in the home setting. Potential candidates are evaluated in advance. Criteria include a knowledgeable caregiver, a clean home environment, close proximity to the hospital, telephone access, and emotional stability on the part of the client and caregiver (Herrmann et al., 1998).

In one sample program, clients receive their daily dose of chemotherapy in the outpatient clinic in the morning and then receive a home visit in the evening. Home care nurses administer chemotherapy and monitor the client for complications. Nurses visit the client once or twice a day and spend between 4 and 8.5 hours per day in the home (D'Andrea et al., 1997). The client receives the stem cell transplant infusion in the outpatient clinic. Nursing care is similar to that provided in the hospital. If serious complications such as sepsis or veno-occlusive disease occur, the client is admitted to the inpatient facility.

CHART 40-12

CLIENT EDUCATION GUIDE
Home Care of the Central Venous Catheter

- To maintain patency, flush the catheter briskly with heparinized saline (10 units/mL) once a day and after completing infusions.
- Change the Luer-Lok cap on each catheter lumen weekly.
- Change the dressing every other day:
  - Use clean technique with thorough handwashing.
  - Clean the exit site with alcohol and povidone-iodine (Betadine).
  - Apply antibacterial ointment to the site.
  - Cover the site with dry sterile gauze dressing, taped securely, or with transparent adherent dressing.
- To prevent tension, always tape the catheter to yourself.
- Look for and report any signs of infection (redness, swelling, or drainage at the exit site).
- In case of a break or puncture in the catheter lumen, immediately clamp the catheter between yourself and the opening. *Notify your physician immediately.*

HEALTH TEACHING

The client and the family need to be educated about the importance of continuing therapy and appropriate medical follow-up, despite the unpleasant side effects of therapy. Many clients go home with a central venous catheter in place and require instructions about its care and maintenance (Bean, 1998). Chart 40-12 lists general guidelines for central venous catheter care at home. These guidelines may be altered depending on the home setting, assistance available, and agency policy.

Protecting the client from infection after discharge from the hospital is just as important as it was during hospitalization. (See Chart 40-9 for focused assessment for the client at risk for infection.) The nurse urges the client to use proper hygiene and to avoid crowds or others with infections. Neither the client nor any household member should receive live virus immunization (poliomyelitis, measles, or rubella) for 2 years after transplantation (Alcoser & Burchett, 1999). The client should continue mouth care regimens at home. The nurse emphasizes that the client should immediately notify the physician if he or she experiences fever or any other sign of infection. Chart 40-13 lists guidelines for clients for the prevention of infection.

Because platelet recovery is usually slower than recovery of white blood cells (WBCs), many clients return home still at risk for bleeding. Thrombocytopenia may be present for 6 months following transplantation (Hurley, 1997). The nurse reinforces the safety and bleeding precautions initiated in the hospital, emphasizing that the client must follow these precautions until the platelet count is above 50,000. The client and family are instructed to assess for petechiae, avoid trauma and sharp objects, apply pressure to wounds for 10 minutes, and report any unusual symptoms, including blood in the stool or urine, or headache that does not respond to acetaminophen. Chart 40-14 lists guidelines for clients at risk for bleeding.

PSYCHOSOCIAL PREPARATION

The nurse's responsibility in psychosocial preparation of the client before discharge is very important. A diagnosis of leukemia threatens self-esteem and the family role. The client is confronted with the reality of death, and treatment causes major adjustments in self-image. The client and family also

CHART 40-13

CLIENT EDUCATION GUIDE
Prevention of Infection

- Avoid crowds and other large gatherings of people who might be ill.
- Do not share personal toilet articles, such as toothbrushes, toothpaste, washcloths, or deodorant sticks, with others.
- If possible, bathe daily.
- Wash the armpits, groin, genitals, and anal area at least twice a day with an antimicrobial soap.
- Clean your toothbrush daily by either running it through the dishwasher or rinsing it in liquid laundry bleach and water.
- Wash your hands thoroughly with an antimicrobial soap before you eat or drink, after touching a pet, after shaking hands with anyone, as soon as you come home from any outing, and after using the toilet.
- Eat a low-bacteria diet, and avoid salads, raw fruits and vegetables, undercooked meat, pepper, and paprika.
- Wash dishes between use with hot, sudsy water, or use a dishwasher.
- Do not drink water that has been standing for longer than 15 minutes.
- Do not reuse cups and glasses without washing.
- Avoid changing pet litter boxes. If unavoidable, use gloves or wash hands immediately.
- Avoid keeping turtles and reptiles as pets.
- Do not feed pets raw or undercooked meat.
- Take your temperature at least twice a day.
- Report any of the following signs or symptoms of infection to your physician immediately:
  - Temperature greater than 100°F (38°C)
  - Persistent cough (with or without sputum)
  - Pus or foul-smelling drainage from any open skin area or normal body opening
  - Presence of a boil or abscess
  - Urine that is cloudy or foul smelling, or burning on urination
- Take all prescribed medications as ordered.
- Do not dig in the garden or work with houseplants.
- Avoid travel to areas of the world with poor sanitation or less-than-adequate health care facilities.

experience changes in the client's body image, level of independence, and lifestyle. Some feel threatened by their environment, seeing everything as potentially infectious. Clients who are cared for in protective isolation may experience loneliness and loss of contact with the outside world (Campbell, 1999). The nurse helps the client and family redefine priorities, understand the illness and its treatment, and find hope. The nurse makes referrals to support groups sponsored by organizations such as the American Cancer Society ("I Can Cope" and "Make Today Count"), which can be enormously beneficial to both the client and the family.

HEALTH CARE RESOURCES

The client with limited social support may need assistance at home until strength and energy return. A home care aide may suffice for some clients, whereas for others a visiting nurse may be needed to reinforce teaching. The client may also need equipment to facilitate activities of daily living (ADLs) and ambulation. Financial resources are assessed. Treatment of cancer is expensive, and the nurse works closely with the local social services department to ensure that insurance is adequate. If the client is uninsured, other sources, such as drug company–sponsored compassionate aid programs, are explored. The Leukemia Society of America offers limited financial assistance for clients with leukemia, sponsors support groups, and provides publications for clients and health care providers.

Prolonged outpatient contact and follow-up will be necessary, and clients will need transportation to the outpatient facility. Many local divisions of the American Cancer Society offer free transportation to clients with cancer, including leukemia.

CHART 40-14

CLIENT EDUCATION GUIDE
The Client at Risk for Bleeding

- Use an electric razor.
- Use a soft-bristled toothbrush, and do not floss.
- Do not have dental work done without consulting your doctor.
- Do not take aspirin or any aspirin-containing products. Read the label to be sure that the product does not contain aspirin or salicylates.
- Do not participate in contact sports or any activity likely to result in your being bumped, scratched, or scraped.
- If you are bumped, apply ice to the site for at least 1 hour.
- Notify your doctor if you:
  - Experience an injury and persistent bleeding results
  - Have excessive menstrual bleeding
  - See blood in your urine or bowel movement
  - Have a headache that does not respond to acetaminophen.
- Avoid anal intercourse.
- Take a stool softener to prevent straining during a bowel movement.
- Do not use enemas or rectal suppositories.
- Avoid bending over at the waist.
- Do not wear clothing or shoes that are tight or that rub.
- Avoid blowing your nose or placing objects in your nose. If you must blow your nose, do so gently without blocking either nasal passage.

Evaluation: Outcomes

NOC The nurse evaluates the care of the client with leukemia on the basis of the identified nursing diagnoses and collaborative problems. The expected outcomes include that the client will:

- Remain free of cross-contamination–induced infection
- Remain free of autocontamination-induced infection
- Not experience sepsis
- Remain free of episodes of bleeding
- Balance activity and rest
- Use energy conservation techniques
- Adapt lifestyle to energy level

MALIGNANT LYMPHOMA

Malignant lymphomas occur as a result of abnormal overgrowth of one type of leukocyte (lymphocytes); they differ from the leukemias in the degree of maturation of the affected cells and the location of cell production. Lymphomas are malignancies characterized by a proliferation of committed lymphocytes rather than stem cell precursors (as in leukemia). This proliferation occurs not in bone marrow but in other lymphoid tissues scattered throughout the body, especially the lymph nodes and spleen. Lymphomas are actually solid tumors rather than cellular suspensions within the blood and bone marrow, and they fall into two major categories among adults: Hodgkin's lymphoma and non-Hodgkin's lymphoma.

Hodgkin's Lymphoma

OVERVIEW

Hodgkin's lymphoma is a cancer that can affect any age-group, although incidence peaks first in people in their mid-to-late 20s and then in people older than 50 years of age (Callaghan, 1998). Men and women are affected equally in the first group, but the disease is more prevalent in men in the older group.

Factors implicated as possible causes of Hodgkin's lymphoma include viral infections and previous exposure to alkylating chemical agents. This cancer usually originates in a single lymph node or a single chain of nodes. The lymphoid tissues within the node undergo malignant transformation, usually initiating some inflammatory processes. These nodes contain a specific transformed cell type, the **Reed-Sternberg cell,** a marker for Hodgkin's lymphoma. The disease first **metastasizes** (spreads) to other nearby lymphoid structures and eventually invades nonlymphoid tissues.

COLLABORATIVE MANAGEMENT

Assessment

Assessment most often reveals a greatly enlarged but painless lymph node or nodes, usually the earliest manifestation of Hodgkin's lymphoma. The client also often experiences fever, malaise, and night sweats (Table 40-6). More specific clinical manifestations depend on the site (or sites) of malignancy and the extent of disease.

Diagnosis and grade are established when biopsy of a node or mass reveals Reed-Sternberg cells (Callaghan, 1998). The client then undergoes extensive staging procedures to determine the exact extent of disease. Staging must be detailed and accurate because the treatment regimen is determined by the extent of disease (DeVita, Mauch, & Harris, 1997). Staging procedures for Hodgkin's lymphoma include biopsies of distant lymph nodes, computed tomography (CT) of the thorax and abdomen, staging laparotomy, a complete blood count (CBC), liver function studies, and bilateral bone marrow biopsies.

TABLE 40-6 • MANIFESTATIONS AND STAGING CRITERIA FOR HODGKIN'S LYMPHOMA

STAGE Ia
Disease is confined to a single lymph node region or only one extranodal site.

STAGE Ib
Disease is confined to a single lymph node region or only one extranodal site. The client also experiences some or all of the following systemic symptoms: persistent fever, night sweats, and significant weight loss (>10%).

STAGE IIa
Disease is confined to either two or more lymph node regions on the same side of the diaphragm or contiguous extranodal sites on the same side of the diaphragm.

STAGE IIb
Disease is confined to either two or more lymph node regions on the same side of the diaphragm or contiguous extranodal sites on the same side of the diaphragm. Client also experiences some or all of the following systemic symptoms: persistent fever, night sweats, and significant weight loss (>10%).

STAGE IIIa
Disease extends to lymph node regions on both sides of the diaphragm.

STAGE IIIb
Disease extends to lymph node regions on both sides of the diaphragm. The client also experiences some or all of the following systemic symptoms: persistent fever, night sweats, and significant weight loss (>10%).

STAGE IIIc
Disease extends to lymph node regions on both sides of the diaphragm. The client also experiences some or all of the following systemic symptoms: persistent fever, night sweats, and significant weight loss (>10%). The spleen is also involved in disease.

STAGE IV
Disease has widely disseminated foci of involvement, including one or more extranodal tissues and organs.

Interventions

Such great progress has been made in treatment regimens that Hodgkin's lymphoma is now one of the most curable types of cancer (Callaghan, 1998). Generally, for stage I and stage II disease without mediastinal node involvement, the treatment of choice is extensive external radiation of involved lymph node regions. With more extensive disease, radiation coupled with an aggressive multiagent chemotherapy regimen is most effective in achieving a cure (DeVita, Mauch, & Harris, 1997). (See Chapter 25 on general care of clients receiving radiation and/or chemotherapy.)

Specific nursing management of the client undergoing treatment for Hodgkin's lymphoma focuses on the side effects of therapy, especially the following:

- Drug-induced pancytopenia, which results in increased risk for infection, bleeding, and anemia
- Severe nausea and vomiting
- Skin irritation and breakdown at the site of radiation
- Impaired hepatic function either by metastasis to the liver or by multiagent chemotherapy
- Permanent sterility for male clients receiving radiation to the abdominopelvic region in the pattern of an inverted Y in combination with specific chemotherapeutic agents (the client should be informed of this side effect and given the option to store sperm in a sperm bank before treatment)
- Secondary malignancies for clients receiving radiation alone or chemotherapy (Long-term follow-up should include screening for recurrence, as well as the possible development of a secondary cancer.)

Non-Hodgkin's Lymphoma

OVERVIEW

Non-Hodgkin's lymphoma is the classification for all cancers originating from lymphoid tissues that are not diagnosed as Hodgkin's lymphoma. There are more than 12 subtypes of non-Hodgkin's lymphoma, including low-grade, intermediate, and high-grade lymphomas.

The low-grade lymphomas usually arise from B-cell lymphocytes and progress slowly. Although clients with low-grade lymphomas have longer survival rates, the diseases are less responsive to treatment and, consequently, cures are rare (Bilodeau & Fessele, 1998).

At the other end of the spectrum are the high-grade lymphomas, which are aggressive tumors of usually mixed cellularity with rapid doubling times. High-grade lymphomas are more responsive to chemotherapy, and the chances for a long-term cure are greater.

Non-Hodgkin's lymphoma is ranked as the sixth most common cause of cancer-related death in the United States. The disease is more prevalent in men, Caucasians, and individuals older than 50 years of age. The long-term prognosis is better for women and clients younger than 65 years of age (Bilodeau & Fessele, 1998). Most non-Hodgkin's lymphomas arise from lymph nodes, but they can originate in virtually any tissue or organ. A low-grade lymphoma also can convert to a higher-grade lymphoma. Definitive causes are unknown, but viral infection, exposure to ionizing radiation, autoimmune disorders, and exposure to toxic chemicals have all been implicated.

➤ COLLABORATIVE MANAGEMENT

Because lymphomas may arise from lymphoid cells in any tissue and because the malignancy can spread to any organ, assessment reveals no specific clinical manifestations other than lymphadenopathy common to all types of lymphoma. Diagnosis is made from the histologic features apparent on biopsy of any suspicious node or mass. Classification of the specific lymphoma subtype is based on a complex grading of surface markers, cytogenetic features, cell size, and expression of viral antigens (Bilodeau & Fessele, 1998). Staging is similar to that for Hodgkin's lymphoma (see Table 40-6).

Treatment consists of radiation therapy and multiagent chemotherapy. Nursing care needs are similar to those for clients with Hodgkin's lymphoma, with additional organ-specific problems taken into account if the disease is widely disseminated.

COAGULATION DISORDERS

Coagulation disorders are synonymous with bleeding disorders and are characterized by abnormal or increased bleeding resulting from defects in one or more components regulating hemostasis. Bleeding disorders may be spontaneous or traumatic, localized or generalized, lifelong or acquired. They can originate from a defect in the hemostatic processes at the vascular, platelet, or clotting factor level. Figure 40-4 outlines blood-clotting cascades and sites where specific defects and drugs disrupt the hemostatic processes.

PLATELET DISORDERS

Platelets play a vital role in hemostasis. For both the intrinsic and the extrinsic pathways, blood clotting starts with platelet adhesion and the formation of a platelet plug. Any condition that either reduces the number of platelets or interferes with their ability to adhere (to one another, blood vessel walls, collagen, or fibrin threads) can be manifested as increased bleeding. Platelet disorders can be inherited, acquired, or temporarily induced by the ingestion of substances that limit platelet production or inhibit aggregation.

A drop in the number of platelets below the level needed for normal coagulation is called **thrombocytopenia.** Thrombocytopenia may occur as a result of other conditions or treatments that suppress general bone marrow activity. It also can occur through processes that specifically limit platelet formation or increase the rate of platelet destruction. The two thrombocytopenic conditions affecting adults are autoimmune thrombocytopenic purpura and thrombotic thrombocytopenic purpura.

Autoimmune Thrombocytopenic Purpura

OVERVIEW

Before the underlying cause of autoimmune thrombocytopenic purpura was identified, this condition was known as idiopathic thrombocytopenic purpura (ITP). Although the cause is now thought to be an autoimmune reaction, the condition is still commonly known as ITP. The total number of circulating platelets is greatly reduced in ITP, even though platelet production in the bone marrow is normal.

Clients with idiopathic thrombocytopenic purpura make an antibody directed against the surface of their own platelets (an antiplatelet antibody). This antibody coats the surface of the platelets, making them more susceptible to attraction and destruction by phagocytic leukocytes, especially macrophages (see Chapter 20). Because the spleen contains a large concentration of macrophages and because the blood vessels of the spleen are long and twisted, antibody-coated platelets are destroyed primarily in the spleen. When the rate of platelet destruction exceeds that of production, the number of circulating platelets decreases and blood clotting slows.

Although the cause of this disorder appears to be autoimmune, the exact mechanism initiating the production of autoantibodies is unknown. ITP is most common among women between the ages of 20 and 40 and among people with a preexisting autoimmune condition, such as systemic lupus erythematosus (Cotran, Kumar, & Robbins, 1999).

➤ COLLABORATIVE MANAGEMENT

• Assessment

Clinical manifestations associated with ITP are generally limited to the skin and mucous membranes: large **ecchymoses** (bruises) on the arms, legs, upper chest, and neck or a petechial rash. Mucosal bleeding occurs easily. If the client has experienced significant blood loss, signs of anemia may also be present.

A rare complication is an intracranial bleeding–induced stroke. The nurse assesses for neurologic function and mental status (see Chapter 41). Family members or significant others are asked if the client's behavior and responses to the mental status examination are typical or represent a change from usual reactions.

Idiopathic thrombocytopenic purpura is diagnosed by a decreased platelet count and large numbers of megakaryocytes in the bone marrow. Antiplatelet antibodies may be present in detectable levels in peripheral blood. If the client experiences any episodes of bleeding, hematocrit and hemoglobin levels also are low.

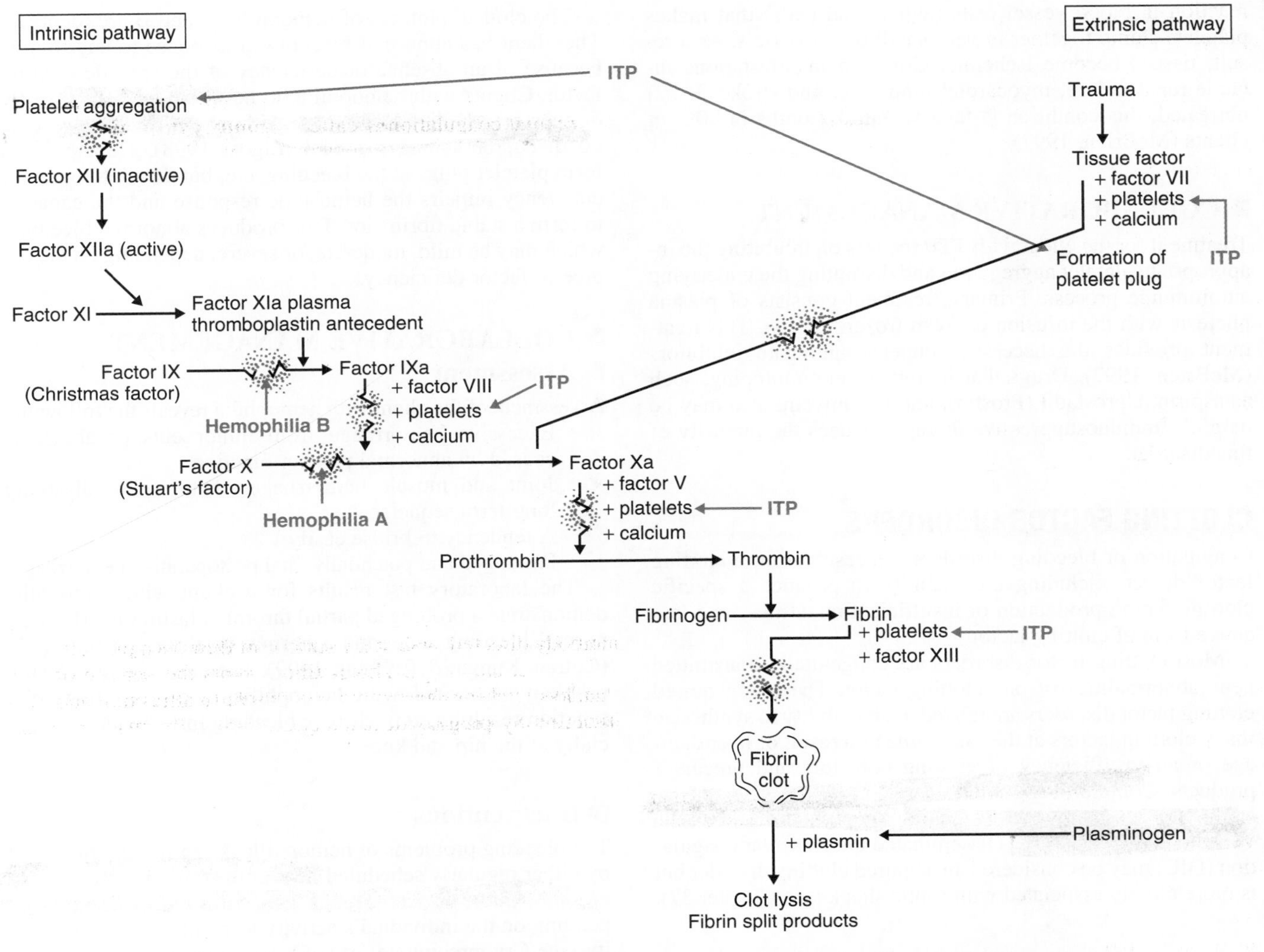

Figure 40-4 ● Sites of disruption of the coagulation mechanisms by disease. (*ITP,* Idiopathic thrombocytopenic purpura.)

Interventions

NONSURGICAL MANAGEMENT. As a result of the decreased platelet count, the client is at great risk for bleeding. Interventions include therapy for the underlying condition, as well as protection from trauma-induced bleeding episodes.

DRUG THERAPY. Agents used to control ITP include drugs that suppress immune function to some degree. The premise for the use of agents such as corticosteroids and azathioprine (Imuran) is to inhibit immune system synthesis of antiplatelet autoantibodies. More aggressive therapy can include low doses of chemotherapeutic agents, such as the antimitotic agents and cyclophosphamide.

BLOOD REPLACEMENT THERAPY. For the client with a platelet count of less than 20,000/mm^3 who is experiencing an acute life-threatening bleeding episode, a platelet transfusion may be required. Platelet transfusions are not performed routinely, because the donated platelets are just as rapidly destroyed by the spleen as the client's own platelets (see later discussion under Platelet Transfusions, p. 865).

MAINTAINING A SAFE ENVIRONMENT. The nurse's major objectives are to protect the client from situations that can lead to bleeding and to closely monitor the amount of bleeding that is occurring. (For nursing care actions, see Risk for Injury [Leukemia], p. 856.)

SURGICAL MANAGEMENT. For the client who does not respond to drug therapy, splenectomy may be the treatment of choice. Because the leukocytes in the spleen perform many different immunodefensive functions, the client who has undergone a splenectomy is at increased risk for infection.

Thrombotic Thrombocytopenic Purpura

OVERVIEW

Thrombotic thrombocytopenic purpura (TTP) is a rare disorder in which platelets clump together inappropriately in the microcirculation and insufficient platelets remain in the systemic circulation. The client experiences inappropriate clotting, yet the blood fails to clot properly when trauma occurs. The underlying cause of TTP appears to be an autoimmune reaction in blood vessel cells (endothelial cells) that makes platelets clump together in very small blood vessels. As a result, tissues become ischemic. Common manifestations include renal failure, myocardial infarction, and stroke. If left untreated, this condition is fatal within 3 months in 90% of clients (McBrien, 1997).

➤ COLLABORATIVE MANAGEMENT

Treatment for the client with TTP focuses on inhibiting the inappropriate platelet aggregation and disrupting the underlying autoimmune process. Primary treatment consists of plasma pheresis with the infusion of fresh frozen plasma. This treatment provides the necessary platelet aggregate inhibitors (McBrien, 1997). Drugs that inhibit platelet clumping, such as aspirin, alprostadil (Prostin), and plicamycin, also may be helpful. Immunosuppressive therapy reduces the intensity of this disorder.

CLOTTING FACTOR DISORDERS

Coagulation or bleeding disorders can result from a clotting factor defect, including the inability to produce a specific clotting factor, production of insufficient quantities, or a less active form of clotting factor.

Most clotting factor disorders are congenitally transmitted gene abnormalities of one clotting factor. The few acquired clotting factor disorders are related to an inability to synthesize many clotting factors at the same time as a result of liver damage or an insufficiency of clotting cofactors and precursor products. Common congenital disorders that result in defects at the clotting factor level include hemophilias A and B and von Willebrand's disease. Disseminated intravascular coagulation (DIC) may be considered an acquired clotting disorder but is more closely associated with septic shock (see Chapter 37).

Hemophilia

OVERVIEW

Hemophilia comprises two hereditary bleeding disorders resulting from deficiencies of specific clotting factors. Hemophilia A (classic hemophilia) results from a deficiency of factor VIII and accounts for 80% of cases of hemophilia. Hemophilia B (Christmas disease) is a deficiency of factor IX and accounts for 20% of cases.

The incidence of both is 1 in 10,000. Hemophilia is an X-linked recessive trait. Female carriers have a 50% chance of transmitting the gene for hemophilia to their daughters (who then are carriers) and to their sons (who will have overt hemophilia). Hemophilia A is, with rare exceptions, a disease affecting males, none of whose sons will have the gene for hemophilia and all of whose daughters will be **carriers** (able to pass on the gene without actually having the disorder). In about 30% of clients with hemophilia, there is no family history, and it is presumed that their disease is the result of a new mutation (Cotran, Kumar, & Robbins, 1999).

The bleeding disorder associated with hemophilia A is so severe that before blood transfusions were available, children with hemophilia rarely survived past age 3 years. With the availability of blood transfusion and factor VIII therapy, mean survival time has increased so greatly that hemophilia now is commonly seen among adult clients.

The clinical pictures of hemophilia A and B are identical. The client has abnormal bleeding in response to any trauma because of an absence or deficiency of the specific clotting factor. Clients with hemophilia do not bleed more frequently or even more rapidly that those without the disease, but they do bleed for a longer period (Ligda, 1998). Hemophiliacs form platelet plugs at the bleeding site, but the clotting factor deficiency impairs the hemostatic response and the capacity to form a stable fibrin clot. This produces abnormal bleeding, which may be mild, moderate, or severe, depending on the degree of factor deficiency.

➤ COLLABORATIVE MANAGEMENT

Assessment

Assessment of the client with hemophilia reveals the following:

- Excessive hemorrhage from minor cuts or abrasions caused by abnormal platelet function
- Joint and muscle hemorrhages that lead to disabling long-term sequelae
- A tendency to bruise easily
- Prolonged and potentially fatal postoperative hemorrhage

The laboratory test results for a client with hemophilia demonstrate a prolonged partial thromboplastin time (PTT), a normal bleeding time, and a normal prothrombin time (PT) (Cotran, Kumar, & Robbins, 1999). The most common health problem associated with hemophilia is degenerating joint function resulting from chronic bleeding into the joints, especially at the hip and knee.

Interventions

The bleeding problems of hemophilia A can be well managed by either regularly scheduled IV administration of factor VIII cryoprecipitate or intermittent administration as needed, depending on the individual's activity level and injury probability (see Cryoprecipitate, p. 865). However, the cost of cryoprecipitate is prohibitive for many people with hemophilia. In addition, because the precipitated clotting factors are derived from pooled human serum, a risk of viral contamination remains, even with the use of heat-inactivated serum (Ligda, 1998). Major complications of hemophilia therapy during the 1980s were infection with hepatitis B virus, cytomegalovirus, and human immunodeficiency virus (HIV). Although heat-inactivated serum and the elimination of HIV-positive donors have reduced these risks, they have not yet been eliminated (see the Cost of Care box on p. 863).

TRANSFUSION THERAPY

Any blood component may be removed from a donor and transfused to benefit a recipient. Components may be transfused individually or collectively, with varying degrees of benefit to the recipient.

PRETRANSFUSION RESPONSIBILITIES

Nursing actions during transfusions aim largely at prevention or early recognition of adverse transfusion reactions. Preparation of the client for transfusion therapy is imperative, and in-

COST OF CARE IMPLICATIONS FOR NURSING

HEMOPHILIA

Cost of Care

- Hemophilia is among the eight most costly diseases to treat. The yearly cost to manage this disease is nearly $100,000.
- The average wholesale cost of 2000 units of recombinant factor is $2360.
- The cost of an emergency department visit for a bleeding episode for an average man is approximately $5620. The majority of the expense is related to the cost of an initial and 12-hour follow-up infusion of 2000 units of recombinant factor. Other expenses include the emergency department charge ($350), laboratory tests ($150), and the physician's fee ($200).
- The cost of self-care management of a bleeding episode for an average man is approximately $1186. This involves immediate self-infusion of 1000 units of recombinant factor. No follow-up infusion is required.
- Self-care programs reduce the number of emergency department visits (0 to 5 per year) as compared with traditionally treated clients (10 to 15 per year).

Implications for Nursing

Research demonstrated that clients who participated in a self-care model for the management of hemophilia bleeding episodes spent significantly less to manage their disease than the national average. Programs developed and run by a nurse case manager can help promote client independence, prevent serious complications, and improve cost outcomes.

Data from Ligda, D.S. (1998). Hemophilia case management. *Journal of Care Management* 4(3), 12-24.

stitutional blood product administration procedures should be carefully followed. Before administering any blood product, the nurse reviews the agency's policies and procedures. Chart 40-15 presents best practices for transfusion therapy.

Legally, a physician's order is needed to administer blood or its components. The order specifies the type of component to be delivered, the volume to be transfused, and any special conditions the physician judges to be important. The nurse verifies the order for accuracy and completeness. The nurse also evaluates the need for transfusion, considering both the client's clinical condition and the laboratory values. In many hospitals a separate consent form must be obtained for the administration of blood products before a transfusion is performed.

A blood specimen is obtained for crossmatching (testing of the donor's blood and the recipient's blood for compatibility). The procedure and responsibility for obtaining this specimen are specified by hospital policy. The laboratory requires at least 45 minutes to complete the crossmatch testing. In most hospitals a new crossmatching specimen is required at least every 48 hours (Dreger & Tremback, 1998).

Because of the viscosity of blood components, a 19-gauge needle or larger is used, whenever possible, for venous access. Both Y-tubing and straight tubing sets are available for blood component administration. A blood filter (approximately 170 μm) to remove aggregates from the stored blood products is included with component administration equipment and must be used to transfuse all blood products. In massive transfusion, a microaggregate filter (20 to 40 μm) may be used.

CHART 40-15

BEST PRACTICE *for* Transfusion Therapy

NURSING ACTIONS	RATIONALE
Before Infusion	
1. Assess laboratory values.	Many institutions have specific guidelines for blood product transfusions (i.e., platelet count <20,000 or hemoglobin <6 g/dL).
2. Verify the medical order.	Legally, a physician's order is required for transfusions. The order should state the type of product, dose, and transfusion time.
3. Assess the client's vital signs, urine output, skin color, and history of transfusion reactions.	Determine whether the client can tolerate infusion. Baseline information may be needed to help identify transfusion reactions.
4. Obtain venous access. Use a central catheter or 19-gauge needle if possible.	The larger-bore needle allows cells to flow more easily without occluding the lumen of the catheter.
5. Obtain blood products from a blood bank. Transfuse immediately.	Once a blood product has been released from the blood bank, the product should be transfused as soon as possible (e.g., red blood cell transfusions should be completed within 4 hours of removal from refrigeration).
6. With another registered nurse, verify the client by name and number, check blood compatibility, and note expiration time.	Human error is the most common cause of ABO incompatibility reactions.
7. Administer the blood product using the appropriate filtered tubing.	Filters are needed to remove aggregates and possible contaminants.
8. If the blood product needs to be diluted, use only normal saline solution.	Hemolysis occurs if any other IV solution is used.
9. Remain with the client during the first 15 to 30 minutes of the infusion.	Hemolytic reactions occur most often within the first 50 mL of the infusion.
10. Infuse the blood product at the ordered rate.	Fluid overload is a potential complication of rapid infusion.
11. Monitor vital signs.	Vital sign changes often indicate transfusion reactions.
12. When the transfusion is completed, discontinue infusion and dispose of the bag and tubing properly.	Bloodborne pathogens may be spread inadvertently through improper disposal.
13. Document.	The client record should indicate the type of product infused, product number, volume infused, time of infusion, and any adverse reactions.

Normal saline is the solution of choice for administration. Ringer's lactate and dextrose in water are contraindicated for administration with blood or blood products because they cause clotting or hemolysis of blood cells. *Medications are never added to blood products.*

Before the transfusion is initiated, it is essential to determine that the blood component delivered is correct. Two registered nurses simultaneously check the physician's order, the client's identity, and whether the hospital identification band name and number are identical to those on the blood component tag. The blood bag label, the attached tag, and the requisition slip are examined to ensure that the ABO and Rh types are compatible. The expiration date is also checked, and the product is inspected for discoloration, gas bubbles, or cloudiness—indicators of bacterial growth or hemolysis.

TRANSFUSION RESPONSIBILITIES

The nurse takes the vital signs, including temperature, immediately before initiating the transfusion. Infusion begins slowly. A nurse remains with the client for the first 15 to 30 minutes. Any severe reaction usually occurs with administration of the first 50 mL of blood. The nurse assesses vital signs 15 minutes after initiation of the transfusion to detect signs of a reaction. If there are none, the infusion rate can be increased to transfuse 1 unit in about 2 hours (depending on the client's cardiovascular status). The nurse takes the vital signs every hour throughout the transfusion or as specified by agency policy.

Blood components without large amounts of red blood cells (RBCs) can be infused more quickly. The identification checks are the same as for RBC transfusions. Physiologic changes in older clients may necessitate that blood products be transfused at a slower rate. Best practices related to the nursing care needs of older clients undergoing transfusion therapy are provided in Chart 40-16.

TYPES OF TRANSFUSIONS

Red Blood Cell Transfusions

RBCs are administered to replace erythrocytes lost as a result of trauma or surgical interventions. Clients with clinical conditions that result in the destruction or abnormal maturation of RBCs may also benefit from RBC transfusions. Packed RBCs, supplied in 250-mL bags, are a concentrated source of RBCs and are the most common component administered to RBC-deficient clients (Dreger & Tremback, 1998). Packed RBCs are administered to individuals with a hemoglobin concentration less than 6 g/dL (or a hemoglobin value of 6 to 10 g/dL if clinical symptoms are present) (Kennedy, 1999).

Blood transfusions are actually transplantations of tissue from one person to another. The donor and recipient blood must thus be carefully checked for compatibility to prevent potentially lethal reactions (Table 40-7). Compatibility is determined by two different types of antigen systems (cell surface proteins): the ABO system antigens and the Rh antigen, present on the membrane surface of RBCs (Dreger & Tremback, 1998).

RBC antigens are inherited. For the ABO antigen system, a person inherits one of the following:

- A antigen (type A blood)
- B antigen (type B blood)
- Both A and B antigens (type AB blood)
- No antigens (type O blood)

CHART 40-16

BEST PRACTICE *for*
The Older Adult Receiving a Transfusion

- Assess the client's circulatory, renal, and fluid status before initiating the transfusion.
- Use no larger than a 19-gauge needle.
- Try to use blood that is less than 1 week old. (Older blood cell membranes are more fragile, break easily, and release potassium into the circulation.)
- Take vital signs (especially pulse, blood pressure, and respiratory rate) every 15 minutes throughout the transfusion. Changes in these parameters can indicate fluid overload and may also be the only indicators of adverse transfusion reactions.

Overload
- Rapid bounding pulse
- Hypertension
- Swollen superficial veins

Transfusion Reaction
- Rapid thready pulse
- Hypotension
- Increased pallor, cyanosis
- Administer blood slowly, taking 2 to 4 hours for each unit of whole blood, packed red blood cells, or plasma.
- Avoid concurrent fluid administration into any other IV site.
- If possible, allow 2 full hours after the administration of 1 unit of blood before administering the next unit.

TABLE 40-7 • COMPATIBILITY CHART FOR RED BLOOD CELL TRANSFUSIONS

	Recipient			
Donor	A	B	AB	O
A	X		X	
B		X	X	
AB			X	
O	X	X	X	X

Within the first few years of a child's life, circulating antibodies develop against the blood type antigens that were not inherited. For example, a child with type A blood will form antigens against type B blood. A child with type O blood has not inherited either A or B antigens and will form antibodies against RBCs that contain either A or B antigens. If erythrocytes that contain a foreign antigen are infused into a recipient, the donated tissue can be recognized by the immune system of the recipient as non-self, and the client may have a reaction to the transfused products.

The mechanism of the Rh antigen system is slightly different. An Rh-negative person is born without the antigen and does not form antibodies unless he or she is specifically sensitized to it. Sensitization can occur with RBC transfusions from an Rh-positive person or from exposure during pregnancy and birth. Once an Rh-negative person has been sensitized and antibody development has occurred, any exposure to Rh-positive blood can cause a transfusion reaction. Antibody development can be prevented by administration of Rh-immune globulin as soon as exposure to the Rh antigen is suspected. People who have Rh-positive blood can receive an RBC transfusion from an Rh-negative donor, but Rh-negative people must never receive Rh-positive blood.

Platelet Transfusions

Platelets are administered to clients with platelet counts below 20,000 mm^3 and to clients with thrombocytopenia who are actively bleeding or are scheduled for an invasive procedure (Dreger, & Tremback, 1998). Platelet transfusions are usually pooled from as many as 10 donors and do not have to be of the same blood type as the client. For clients who are candidates for bone marrow transplantation (BMT) or who require multiple platelet transfusions, single-donor platelets may be ordered. Single-donor platelets are obtained from one person and decrease the amount of antigen exposure to the recipient, helping prevent the formation of platelet antibodies. The chances of allergic transfusion reactions to future platelet transfusions are thus reduced.

Platelet infusion bags usually contain 300 mL for pooled platelets and 200 mL for single-donor platelets. Because the platelet is a fragile cell, platelet transfusions are administered rapidly after being brought to the client's room, usually over a 15- to 30-minute period. A special transfusion set with a smaller filter and shorter tubing is used.

Standard transfusion sets are not used with platelets because the filter traps the platelets, and the longer tubing increases platelet adherence to the lumen. Additional platelet filters help remove white blood cells (WBCs) in the platelet concentrate. These filters are connected directly to the platelet transfusion set and are used for clients who have a history of febrile reactions or who will require multiple platelet transfusions.

The nurse takes the vital signs before the infusion, 15 minutes after the infusion is initiated, and at its completion. The client may be premedicated with meperidine (Demerol) or hydrocortisone to minimize the chances of a reaction. He or she can become febrile and experience **rigors** (severe chills) during transfusion, but these symptoms are not considered a true transfusion reaction. IV administration of amphotericin B (Amphotec, Fungizone), an antifungal agent given to many clients with leukemia, is discontinued during platelet transfusion and not resumed for at least 1 hour after transfusion. Amphotericin B can cause severe allergic reactions that are difficult to distinguish from transfusion reactions.

Plasma Transfusions

Historically, plasma infusions have been administered to replace blood volume, and they are occasionally still used for this purpose. It is more common for plasma to be frozen immediately after donation. Freezing preserves the clotting factors, and the plasma can then be used for clients with clotting disorders (Kennedy, 1999). **Fresh frozen plasma (FFP)** is infused immediately after thawing while the clotting factors are still viable. Clients who are actively bleeding with a prothrombin time (PT) or partial thromboplastin time (PTT) greater than 1.5 times normal are candidates for an FFP infusion (Harrahill & DeLoughery, 1998).

ABO compatibility is required for transfusion of plasma products. The volume of the infusion bag is approximately 200 mL. The infusion takes place as rapidly as the client can tolerate, generally over a 30- to 60-minute period, through a regular Y-set or straight-filtered tubing.

Cryoprecipitate

Cryoprecipitate is a product derived from plasma. Clotting factors VIII and XIII, von Willebrand's factor, fibronectin, and fibrinogen are precipitated from pooled plasma to produce cryoprecipitate. Clients with a fibrinogen level less than 100 mg/dL are candidates for a cryoprecipitate infusion (Harrahill & DeLoughery, 1998). This highly concentrated blood product is administered to clients with clotting factor disorders at a volume of 10 to 15 mL/unit. Although cryoprecipitate can be infused, it is usually given by IV push within 3 minutes. Dosages are individualized, and it is best if the cryoprecipitate is ABO compatible.

Granulocyte Transfusions

At some centers, neutropenic clients with infections receive granulocyte transfusions for WBC replacement. However, this practice is highly controversial because the potential benefit to the client must be weighed against the potential severe reactions that often accompany granulocyte transfusions. The surfaces of granulocytes contain numerous antigens that can cause severe antibody-antigen reactions when infused into a recipient whose immune system recognizes these antigens as non-self. In addition, transfused granulocytes have a very short life span and are probably of minimal benefit to the client (see Chapter 20). There is some evidence that treatment with antibiotics alone results in better survival rates.

Granulocytes are suspended in 400 mL of plasma and should be transfused over a 45- to 60- minute period. Institutional policies often require more stringent monitoring of clients receiving granulocytes. A physician may need to be present in the hospital unit, and vital signs may need to be taken every 15 minutes throughout the transfusion. Administration of amphotericin B and granulocyte transfusions should be separated by 4 to 6 hours.

CULTURAL CONSIDERATIONS

Although transfusion with blood products is relatively common in acute care settings, the nurse remains sensitive to those clients who view receiving blood or blood products of others as repugnant or even sinful. Approximately 800,000 Jehovah's Witnesses live in the United States. The tenets of this religion include that blood removed from the body should be discarded (Dreger & Tremback, 1998). A belief of Jehovah's Witnesses is that receiving autotransfusion or donated blood is the same as "consuming" blood, an act specifically prohibited in the Old Testament. Often, Jehovah's Witnesses will accept the use of dialysis and heart-lung equipment, as well as intraoperative blood salvage, if the blood outside the body remains intact with the circulatory system (Dreger & Tremback, 1998). Whenever possible, transfusion therapy with human blood products is avoided for this group. If in an emergency situation, clients are transfused with blood products against their will, the nurse shows respect for the client's distress and religious beliefs.

Some of the newer therapies for clients with anemia or hypovolemia may reduce the need for transfusion of human or animal blood products. One such therapy is the increasing use of hemoglobin substitutes, also known as "artificial blood." These agents increase the oxygen-carrying and oxygen-releasing power of the client's own blood. In addition, pretreating or treating these clients with synthetic erythropoietin can reduce the time it takes for them to recover from blood loss without transfusion.

TRANSFUSION REACTIONS

Clients can experience any of the following transfusion reactions: hemolytic, allergic, febrile, or bacterial reactions; circulatory overload; or transfusion-associated graft-versus-host disease (GVHD). The nurse is vigilant to prevent serious complications through early detection and initiation of appropriate treatment.

Hemolytic Transfusion Reactions

Hemolytic transfusion reactions are caused by blood type or Rh incompatibility. When blood containing antibodies against the recipient's blood is infused, antigen-antibody complexes are formed and released into the circulation. These complexes can destroy the transfused cells and initiate inflammatory responses in the recipient's blood vessel walls and organs. The ensuing reaction may be mild, with fever and chills, or life threatening, with disseminated intravascular coagulation (DIC) and circulatory collapse (Robb, 1999). Other clinical signs include the following:

- Apprehension
- Headache
- Chest pain
- Low back pain
- Tachycardia
- Tachypnea
- Hypotension
- Hemoglobinuria
- A sense of impending doom

The onset of a hemolytic transfusion reaction may be immediate or may not occur until subsequent units have been transfused.

Allergic Transfusion Reactions

Allergic transfusion reactions are most often seen in clients with a history of allergy. They may have urticaria, itching, bronchospasm, or occasionally anaphylaxis. Onset of this type of reaction usually occurs during or up to 24 hours after the transfusion. Clients with a history of allergy can be given buffy coat–poor or washed red blood cells (RBCs) in which the white blood cells (WBCs) and plasma have been removed. This procedure minimizes the possibility of an allergic reaction.

Febrile Transfusion Reactions

Febrile transfusion reactions occur most commonly in the client with anti-WBC antibodies, a situation seen after multiple transfusions. The recipient experiences the following:

- Sensations of cold
- Tachycardia
- Fever
- Hypotension
- Tachypnea

Again, the physician can order buffy coat–poor RBCs or single-donor HLA-matched platelets. Leukocyte filters may also be used to trap WBCs and prevent their transfusion into the client.

Bacterial Transfusion Reactions

Bacterial transfusion reactions are seen after transfusion of contaminated blood products. Usually a gram-negative organism is the source because these bacteria grow rapidly in blood stored under refrigeration. Symptoms include the following:

- Tachycardia
- Hypotension
- Fever
- Chills
- Shock

The onset of a bacterial transfusion reaction is rapid. (See Chapter 37 for care of the client experiencing septic shock.)

Circulatory Overload

Circulatory overload can occur when a blood product is administered too quickly (Goldy, 1998). This complication is most common with whole-blood transfusions or when the client requires multiple transfusions. Older adults are most at risk for this condition (see Chart 40-16). Symptoms include the following:

- Hypertension
- Bounding pulse
- Distended jugular veins
- Dyspnea
- Restlessness
- Confusion

The nurse can both manage and prevent this complication by monitoring intake and output, transfusing blood products more slowly, and administering diuretics. (See Chapter 12 for management of clients with fluid overload.)

Transfusion-Associated Graft-Versus-Host Disease

Transfusion-associated graft-versus-host disease (TA-GVHD) is an infrequent but life-threatening complication that can occur in both immunosuppressed and immunocompetent clients. Its cause in immunosuppressed clients is similar to that of GVHD associated with allogeneic bone marrow transplantation (BMT), discussed on p. 855, in which donor T-cell lymphocytes attack host tissues.

The cause of TA-GVHD in immunocompetent hosts is uncertain. Reactions are more common when the host and donor share similar human leukocyte antigens (HLAs), such as in first-degree relatives or individuals with a similar ethnic background. Symptoms typically occur within 1 to 2 weeks and include thrombocytopenia, anorexia, nausea, vomiting, chronic hepatitis, weight loss, and recurrent infection.

TA-GVHD has a 90% mortality rate but can be prevented by using irradiated blood products, which destroy T-cells and their cytokine products (Dreger & Tremback, 1998).

CRITICAL THINKING CHALLENGE

A client of yours is receiving a unit of packed RBCs in the postanesthesia unit. Her vital signs were normal before the transfusion, although her pulse was slightly rapid at 100 beats/min. Within the first 20 minutes of the infusion, the client begins to shake and complains that she is cold; her temperature is now 100.2° F (37.9° C).

- What should you do first?
- What type of reaction is this client most likely to be experiencing?
- What other symptoms might you expect?

For suggested answer guidelines, go to SIMON http://www.wbsaunders.com/SIMON/Iggy/.

AUTOLOGOUS BLOOD TRANSFUSIONS

Autologous blood transfusions involve collection and transfusion of the client's own blood. Advantages of this type of transfusion are guaranteed compatibility and elimination of the risk of transmitting diseases such as hepatitis or HIV. The four types of autologous blood transfusions are preoperative autologous blood donation, acute normovolemic hemodilution, intraoperative autologous transfusion, and postoperative blood salvage.

Preoperative autologous blood donation, the most common type of autologous blood transfusion, involves collection of whole blood from the client, division into components, and then storage for later use (such as after a scheduled surgical procedure). As long as hematocrit and hemoglobin levels are within a safe range, the client can donate blood on a weekly basis until the prescribed amount of blood is obtained. Fresh packed RBCs may be stored for 42 days. For individuals with rare blood types, blood may be frozen for up to 10 years. Platelets and plasma may be collected via pheresis. Some cardiovascular problems and bacteremia are contraindications for autologous blood donation.

Acute normovolemic hemodilution involves withdrawal of a client's RBCs and volume replacement just before a surgical procedure. The goal is to decrease RBC loss during surgery. The blood is stored at room temperature for up to 6 hours and reinfused after surgery. This type of autologous transfusion is appropriate for healthy clients but is contraindicated for individuals who are anemic or who have poor renal function.

Intraoperative autologous transfusion and postoperative blood salvage involve the recovery and reinfusion of a client's own blood, collected either from an operative field or postoperatively from a wound. Several commercial products are available that collect, filter, and drain the blood into a transfusion bag. This autologous blood is often used for trauma or surgical clients with severe blood loss and must be reinfused within 6 hours.

The nurse transfuses autologous blood products using the guidelines previously described. Although the client receiving autologous blood is not at risk for most types of transfusion reactions, the nurse must still assess for circulatory overload or bacterial transfusion reactions that can occur as a result of contamination.

ONLINE RESOURCES

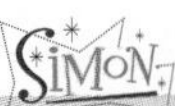

For suggested readings and Internet resources, go to http://www.wbsaunders.com/SIMON/Iggy/.

SELECTED BIBLIOGRAPHY

Asterisk indicates a classic or definitive work on this subject.

Alcoser, P.W., & Burchett, S. (1999). Bone marrow transplantation: Immune system suppression and reconstitution. *American Journal of Nursing, 99*(6), 26-32.

American Cancer Society. (2001). *Cancer facts and figures—2001.* Report No. 01-300M-No. 5008.01. Atlanta: Author.

Anastasia, P. (2001). Nursing considerations for managing topotecan-related hematologic side effects. *Clinical Journal of Oncology Nursing, 5*(1), 9-13.

Baker, F., et al. (1999). Reintegration after bone marrow transplantation. *Cancer Practice, 7*(4), 190-197.

Bean, C.A. (1998). High-tech homecare infusion therapies. *Critical Care Nursing Clinics of North America, 10*(3), 287-303.

Bilodeau, B.B., & Fessele, K.L. (1998). Non-Hodgkin's lymphoma. *Seminars in Oncology Nursing, 14*(4), 273-283.

Callaghan, M. (1998). Hodgkin's disease. *Seminars in Oncology Nursing 14*(4), 262-272.

Campbell, T. (1999). Feelings of oncology patients about being nursed in protective isolation as a consequence of cancer chemotherapy treatment. *Journal of Advanced Nursing 30*(2) 439-447.

Cella, D., & Bron, D. (1999). The effect of epoetin alfa on quality of life in anemic cancer patients. *Cancer Practice, 7*(4), 177-182.

Chielens, D. (1999). Chronic myelogenous leukemia. In C. Miaskowski & P. Buchsel (Eds.), *Oncology nursing: Assessment and clinical care* (pp. 1239-1250). St. Louis: Mosby.

Clark, P. & Gomez, E. (2001). Details on demand: Consumers, cancer information, and the Internet. *Clinical Journal of Oncology Nursing, 5*(1), 19-26.

Cook, L. (2000). A simple case of anemia: Pathophysiology of a common symptom. *Journal of Intravenous Nursing, 23*(5), 271-281.

Cotran, R., Kumar, V., & Robbins, S. (1999). *Robbins pathologic basis of disease* (6th ed.). Philadelphia: W.B. Saunders.

D'Andrea, B., et al. (1997). High-dose chemotherapy followed by stem cell transplant: The clinical/home care experience. *Journal of Care Management, 3*(2), 46-58, 80-85.

DeVita, V.T., Mauch, P., & Harris, N.L. (1997). Hodgkin's disease. In V.T. DeVita et al. (Eds.), *Cancer: Principles and practice of oncology* (5th ed., pp. 2242-2283). Philadelphia: Lippincott-Raven.

Dietz, K. (1999). Acute leukemia. In C. Miaskowski & P. Buchsel (Eds.), *Oncology nursing: Assessment and clinical care* (pp. 1223-1237). St. Louis: Mosby.

Dreger, V., & Tremback, T. (1998). Blood and blood product use in perioperative patient care. *AORN Journal 67*(1), 154-190.

Duquette-Petersen, L., et al. (1999). The role of protective clothing in infection prevention in patients undergoing autologous bone marrow transplant. *Oncology Nursing Forum, 26*(8), 1319-1333.

Goldy, D. (1998). Emergency! Circulatory overload secondary to blood transfusion. *American Journal of Nursing 98*(7), 33.

Gorman, K. (1999). Sickle cell disease: Do you doubt your patient's pain? *American Journal of Nursing 99*(3), 38-44.

Harrahill, M., & DeLoughery, T. (1998). Transfusion and blood component therapy: Key facts. *Journal of Emergency Nursing 24*(4), 368-370.

Herrmann, R.P., et al. (1998). Clinical care for patients receiving autologous hematopoietic stem cell transplantation in the home setting. *Oncology Nursing Forum, 25*(8), 1427-1432.

Horrell, C., & Rothman, J. (2000). Establishing the etiology of thrombocytopenia. *The Nurse Practitioner, 25*(6), 68-77.

Hurley, C. (1997). Ambulatory care after bone marrow or peripheral blood stem cell transplantation. *Clinical Journal of Oncology Nursing, 1*(1), 19-21.

Johns, A. (1998). Overview of bone marrow and stem cell transplantation. *Journal of Intravenous Nursing, 21*(6), 356-360.

Kennedy, M.S. (1999). Undertransfusion or the prudent, cautious, and wise use of blood? *Journal of Intravenous Nursing, 22*(3), 131-135.

Larsen, L., Neverett, S., & Larsen, R. (2001). Clinical nurse specialist as facilitator of interdisciplinary collaborative program for adult sickle cell population. *Clinical Nurse Specialist, 15*(1), 15-22.

Ligda, D.S. (1998). Hemophilia case management. *The Journal of Care Management 4*(3), 12-24.

Maloy, B. (2000). Hematopoiesis, stem cells, and transplantation. *Journal of Intravenous Nursing, 23*(5), 298-303.

McBrien, N.J. (1997). Thrombotic thrombocytopenic purpura. *American Journal of Nursing, 97*(2), 28-29.

Mitchell, R. (1999). Sickle cell anemia. *American Journal of Nursing, 99*(5), 36-37.

Mower-Wade, D., Bartley, M., & Chiari-Allwein, J. (2001). How to respond to shock. *Dimensions of Critical Care Nursing, 20*(2), 22-27.

Pittinger, C.K. (1999). Chronic lymphocytic leukemia. In C. Miaskowski & P. Buchsel (Eds.), *Oncology nursing: Assessment and clinical care* (pp. 1251-1261). St. Louis: Mosby.

Poliquin, C. (1997). Overview of bone marrow and peripheral blood stem cell transplantation. *Clinical Journal of Oncology Nursing, 1*(1), 11-17.

*Ramirez-Smiley, M., & Ingle, B. (1995). Leukemia during pregnancy. *Oncology Nursing Forum, 22*(9), 1363-1367.

Rausch, M., & Pollard, D. (1998). Management of the patient with sickle cell disease. *Journal of Intravenous Nursing, 21*(1), 27-40.

Richardson, A., Ream, E., & Wilson-Barnett, J. (1998). Fatigue in patients receiving chemotherapy: Patterns of change. *Cancer Nursing, 21*(1), 17-30.

Robb, W.J. (1999). Massive transfusion in trauma. *AACN Clinical Issues: Advanced Practice in Acute and Critical Care, 10*(1), 69-84.

Rust, D.M., Wood, L.S., & Battiato, L.A. (1999). Oprelvekin: An alternative treatment for thrombocytopenia. *Clinical Journal of Oncology Nursing, 3*(2), 57-62.

Scheinberg, D., Mazslak, P., & Weiss, M. (1997). Acute leukemias. In V.T. DeVita, S. Hellman, & S.A. Rosenberg (Eds.), *Cancer: Principles and practice of oncology* (5th ed.). Philadelphia: Lippincott-Raven.

Stevens, S. (2000). Heparin-induced thrombocytopenia. *Journal of Vascular Nursing, 18*(2), 54-68.

Vernon, S., & Pfeifer, G. (1997). Are you ready for bloodless surgery? *American Journal of Nursing, 97*(9), 40-46.

Wagner, N.D., & Quinones, V.W. (1998). Allogeneic peripheral blood cell transplantation: Clinical overview and nursing implications. *Oncology Nursing Forum, 25*(6), 1049-1055.

Wallace, R., Wiegand, F., & Warren, C. (1997). Beneficence toward whom? Ethical decision-making in a maternal-fetal conflict. *AACN Clinical Issues: Advanced Practice in Acute and Critical Care, 8*(4), 586-594.

Wolf, S.A. (1999). Cord blood stem cell banking. *American Journal of Nursing, 99*(8), 60, 62, 65, 66, 68, 69.

Worrall, L.M., Tompkins, C.A., & Rust, D.M. (1999). Recognizing and managing anemia. *Clinical Journal of Oncology Nursing, 3*(4), 153-160.

Young, J. (2000). Transfusion reaction. *Nursing2000, 30*(12), 33.

UNIT

9

Problems of Mobility, Sensation, and Cognition

Management of Clients with Problems of the Nervous System

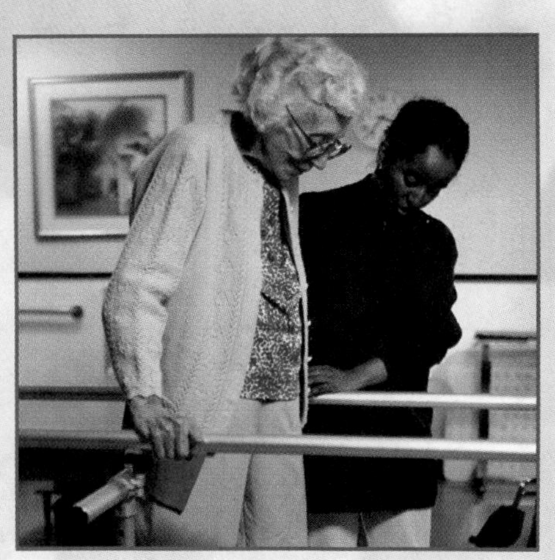

PROBLEMS OF MOBILITY, SENSATION, AND COGNITION: NERVOUS SYSTEM ■ Core Concepts Grid

Anatomy	Physiology	Pathophysiology	History	Physical Exam	Diagnostic Tests	Interventions	Pharmacology
• **Central system** Brain Cerebrum Cerebellum Limbic system Brainstem Reticular activating system (RAS) Spinal cord Meninges Ventricles Sensory pathways Motor pathways Reflex arcs • **Peripheral system** Cranial nerves Autonomic nervous system	• **Coordination** Movement Equilibrium • **Regulation** • **Mental activity** Consciousness Memory Thinking • **Nerve impulse** Transmission • **Sensation**	• **Infection** • **Inflammation** • **Obstruction** • **Seizure activity** • **Paralysis** • **Paresis** • **Fasciculations** • **Increased intracranial pressure (ICP)** • **Bradykinesia** • **Tremors** • **Hemorrhage** • **Ischemia** • **Plaques and tangles** • **Tumors**	• **Past history of neurologic symptoms** • **Past history of neurologic trauma, infections** • **Family history** Familial neurologic diseases • **Social history** Drugs Occupation Age	• **Mental status** General appearance Orientation Mood/affect Thought content Intelligence Recent/remote memory • **Cranial nerves** • **Motor system** Muscles Balance Coordinated movement • **Sensory system** Light touch Pain Temperature Vibration Position Recognition • **Reflexes** • **Other** Romberg's test Brudzinski's sign Kernig's sign • **Functional assessment** • **Speech and language ability**	• **Radiologic** Skull, spine Computed tomography (CT) • **Magnetic resonance imaging (MRI)** • **Electroencephalogram (EEG)** • **Lumbar puncture (LP)** • **Cerebrospinal fluid** • **Toxic drug levels**	• **Environmental modification** Quiet Dim light Padded rails • **Bladder training** • **Bowel training** • **Positioning** • **Nutrition** • **Airway management** • **Lifestyle modification** • **Imunosuppressive therapy** • **Intracranial pressure (ICP) monitoring** • **Rehabilitation (physical and vocational)**	• **Anticonvulsants** • **Antispasmotics** • **Dopaminergics** • **Anticholinergics** • **Dopamine agonists** • **Anticholinesterases** • **Antibiotics** • **Cholinergics**

CHAPTER 41

Assessment of the Nervous System

DEBORAH WRIGHT SHPRITZ

Learning Objectives

After studying this chapter, you should be able to:

1. Explain the function of the major divisions of the nervous system.
2. Identify common physiologic changes associated with aging that affect the nervous system.
3. Perform a neurologic history based on Gordon's Functional Health Patterns.
4. Perform a basic neurologic physical assessment.
5. Perform a rapid neurologic assessment.
6. Plan pretest and follow-up care for clients undergoing common neurologic diagnostic tests.

SIMON **Go to http://www.wbsaunders.com/SIMON/Iggy/ for self-assessment questions related to these Learning Objectives.**

The nervous system is the center of thinking, memory, judgment, sensation, movement, cognition, communication, behavior, and personality. In addition to its direct control over many processes, the nervous system innervates many other body systems and thus indirectly influences their functions. For example, damage to the spinal nerves that innervate the diaphragm may result in respiratory arrest.

ANATOMY AND PHYSIOLOGY REVIEW

The major divisions of the nervous system are the central nervous system (CNS) and the peripheral nervous system (PNS).

The brain and spinal cord are the major components of the CNS. The PNS is composed of 12 pairs of cranial nerves, 31 pairs of spinal nerves, and the autonomic nervous system. The autonomic nervous system is further subdivided into sympathetic and parasympathetic fibers.

The nervous system contains two types of cells: neurons, which transmit or conduct nerve impulses, and neuroglial cells, which have an interdependent role with the neuron.

Nervous System Cells

NEURONS

Structure

The basic unit of the nervous system, the neuron, functions to transmit impulses. Some neurons are motor (facilitating movement), and some are sensory (facilitating sensation). Some process information, and some retain information. When a neuron receives an impulse from another neuron, the effect may be excitation or inhibition as well as conduction of the impulse. Each neuron has a cell body, or soma; short, branching processes called a dendrite; and a single axon (Figure 41-1).

Dendrites may have many branches or few. Each dendrite synapses with another cell body, axon, or dendrite and brings information to the cell body from other neurons. The dendritic process is described as an afferent pathway. The axonal process, called the efferent pathway, transmits impulses from its cell body to other neurons. Although only one axon extends from each neuron, it may extend long distances.

Many (but not all) axons are covered by a myelin sheath, a white, lipid covering. Myelinated axons appear whitish and therefore are also called white matter. Nonmyelinated axons have a grayish cast and are called gray matter. Myelinated axons have gaps in the myelin called nodes of Ranvier. The nodes of Ranvier play a major role in impulse conduction (see Figure 41-1). The enlarged, distal end of each axon is called the synaptic, or terminal, knob. Within the synaptic knobs are the mechanisms for manufacturing, storing, and releasing a transmitter substance. Each neuron produces a specific transmitter substance (e.g., acetylcholine or serotonin) that is capable of either enhancing or inhibiting the impulse, but not both.

Mechanism for Nerve Impulse Conduction

Sodium (Na^+) and chloride (Cl^-) ions are heavily concentrated in the area outside of the cell (interstitial space). Potassium ions (K^+) and other organic material are present within the cell (intracellular space). The inside of the cell is negatively charged compared with the interstitial space. Because of the different concentration of Na^+ and K^+, a neuron is constantly charged, even at rest.

When a stimulus is strong enough, the permeability of the cell membrane to Na^+ and K^+ is changed, and depolarization

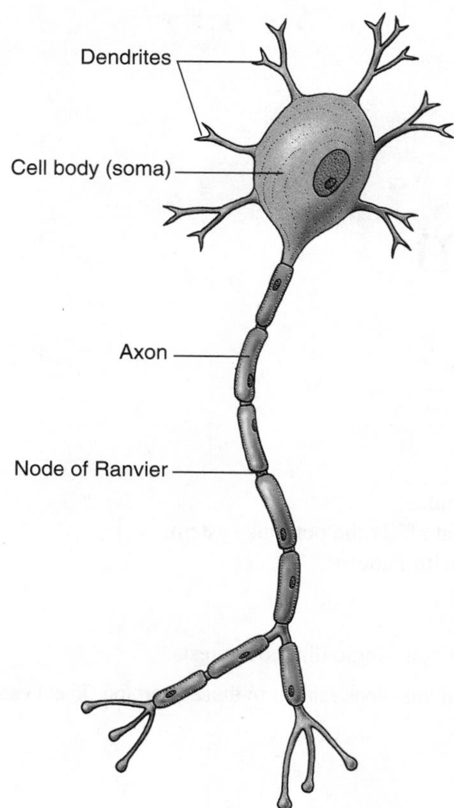

Figure 41-1 ● The structure of a typical neuron.

(impulse conduction) begins. Certain proteins within the membrane function as gates, or channels, that open for either sodium or potassium. With depolarization, sodium diffuses through the membrane first. It is believed that calcium plays a part in controlling the amount of sodium that diffuses through the membrane by controlling the gates. After sodium has entered the cell, potassium begins to leave the cell. Sodium is actively pumped out of the cell, and repolarization (return to baseline) occurs in preparation for another impulse. As an action potential or impulse occurs at one point on the cell membrane, the impulse excites adjacent cells so the impulse is conducted all along the nerve fiber membrane. If the impulse is not of sufficient strength, there will be no action potential.

Synapses

Impulses are transmitted to their eventual destination through synapses. There are two distinct types of synapses: *neuron to neuron* and *neuron to muscle* (or gland). Between the terminal knob and the next cell is a small space called the synaptic cleft. The knob, the cleft, and the portion of the cell to which the impulse is being transmitted constitute the synapse.

Factors Affecting Transmission

Several factors affect the transmission of an impulse. Distance is one of the established factors. Synapses on or near the body of the cell have greater influence than those farther along the dendrite. The strength of the stimulus can also be influenced by other mechanisms, such as inhibition by another neuron, inadequate supply of transmitter substance, and extracellular fluid (ECF) changes. Lack of oxygen or the effects of hypnotics and anesthetics can quickly depress nerve cell activity.

Changes in the pH of ECF also affect neuron transmission. For example, acidosis depresses nerve cell activity. Alkalosis, on the other hand, excites nerve cells. Increased nerve cell activity occurs with the use of some drugs, such as caffeine (in coffee), theophylline (in tea and asthma drugs), and theobromine (in cocoa).

Neurotransmitters

Neurotransmitters are chemical substances that enhance or inhibit nerve impulses. These include the following:

- Acetylcholine
- Serotonin
- Dopamine
- Norepinephrine
- Gamma-amino butyric acid (GABA)
- Substance P
- Endorphins and enkephalins

Other substances, although not specifically identified as transmitters, are considered probable transmitters. Table 41-1 summarizes what is currently known about them.

NEUROGLIAL CELLS

Neuroglial cells, which vary in size and shape, provide protection, structure, and nutrition for the neurons. There are 5 to 10 times more neuroglial cells than neurons in the central nervous system (CNS), and they account for 40% of the CNS cell mass. Neuroglial cells are classified into four types: astroglial cells, ependymal cells, oligodendrocytes, and microglial cells. Microglial cells play a scavenger role by responding to infection in the CNS or trauma to the CNS. Astroglial (star-shaped) cells provide the physical support for the neurons, regulate the chemical environment, and nourish the neurons. Oligodendrocytes form myelin sheaths around the axons. Ependymal cells form the lining of ventricles and the central canal of the spinal cord. They are also part of the blood-brain barrier and help regulate the composition of cerebrospinal fluid (CSF).

Central Nervous System

The central nervous system (CNS) is composed of the brain, which directs the regulation and function of the nervous system and all other systems of the body, and the spinal cord, which initiates reflex activity and transmits impulses to and from the brain.

BONE

The brain and spinal cord are encased in the cranium and vertebral column, respectively. For the most part, they are well protected. However, there are some areas of vulnerability, such as the nasal sinuses, the palate of the throat, the ears, and the cervical spine. The upright position of humans creates additional strain on the vertebrae and musculature. There are 7 cervical, 12 thoracic, 5 lumbar, 5 fused sacral, and 4 fused coccygeal vertebrae. Although there are some differences in structure, all of the vertebrae protect the spinal cord and give structure to the body.

TABLE 41-1 • SITES, FUNCTIONS, AND ACTIONS OF TRANSMITTERS, PROBABLE TRANSMITTERS, AND NEUROMODULATORS

Transmitter Substance	Site	Function/Comments	Action
Acetylcholine	Brain, brainstem, basal ganglia, autonomic nervous system	Nerve and muscle transmission Parasympathetic and preganglionic sympathetic system	Excitatory, but some inhibitory
Serotonin	Medial brainstem, hypothalamus, dorsal horn of spinal cord	Possible onset of sleep, mood control; pain pathway inhibitor in spinal cord	Inhibitory
CATECHOLAMINES			
Dopamine	Substantia nigra to basal ganglia	Complex movements, emotional response regulation, attention	Usually inhibitory
Norepinephrine (epinephrine parallels)	Hypothalamus, brainstem, reticular formation, cerebellum, sympathetic nervous system	Maintenance of arousal, reward system, dreaming sleep, mood regulation	Mainly excitatory
AMINO ACIDS			
Aspartate	Brain, spinal cord interneurons	Sensation	Excitatory
Gamma-aminobutyric acid (GABA)	Brain, brainstem, basal ganglia, spinal cord, cerebellum	Nerve and muscle transmission Possibly one third of brain neurons	Inhibitory
Glutamate	Sensory pathways	Sensation	Excitatory
Glycine	Spinal cord interneurons	Muscle control	Inhibitory
PEPTIDES*			
Substance P	Brain, neurons in spinal cord	Pain transmission	Excitatory
Endorphins, enkephalins	Thalamus, hypothalamus, spinal cord, pituitary	Pleasure sensation, reward system, analgesia, (inhibits release of substance P), released with ACTH (corticotropin) during stress	Probably excitatory
GASES			
Nitric acid	Neurons	Not stored in specific site; made by enzymes as needed; released by diffusion	Excitatory
Carbon monoxide	Neurons		Questionable

*Other peptides under investigation as probable transmitters are vasopressin (ADH), gastrin, cholecystokinin, glucagon, insulin, somatostatin, angiotensin, melanocyte-stimulating hormone (MSH), luteinizing hormone–releasing hormone (LH-RH), and thyrotropin-releasing hormone (TRH). Prostaglandins, also under investigation, are thought to be modulators.

BRAIN

Meninges

The meninges form the immediate protective covering of the brain and the spinal cord:

- The pia mater is a thin, delicate, and vascular membrane that adheres to the brain and the spinal cord.
- The arachnoid, the next layer, is thin and delicate but is also fibrous. Cerebrospinal fluid (CSF) fills the weblike tissue.
- The dura mater, the outer layer, is heavy, fibrous, and nonelastic. There are actually two layers of dura. The outer layer adheres to the cranium and becomes the periosteum. The inner layer covers the brain.

Situated between the arachnoid and pia mater is the subarachnoid space, where CSF circulates. The subdural space is located between the inner dura and the arachnoid. A *potential* space, referred to as the epidural space, is located between the skull and the outer layer of the dura. This area also extends down the spinal cord and is important in the delivery of epidural analgesia.

Between the two layers of dura are the venous sinuses. The inner layer of dura dips down between the two hemispheres and is called the falx. The dura also lies between the cerebral hemispheres and the cerebellum and is called the tentorium. The falx and the tentorium decrease or prevent the transmission of force from one hemisphere to another and protect the lower brainstem. Clinical references may be made to a lesion (e.g., a tumor) as being *supratentorial* (above the tentorium) or *infratentorial* (below the tentorium).

Cerebrum

The right and left hemispheres of the cerebrum are joined by the corpus callosum. The *left* hemisphere is the dominant hemisphere in most people (even in many left-handed people). Within the deeper structures of the cerebrum are the right and left lateral ventricles. At the base of the cerebrum near the ventricles is a group of neurons called the basal ganglia. Composed of the caudate nucleus, putamen, and globus pallidus, the basal ganglia regulate movement and body tone.

The motor cortex, which is located anterior to the central fissure of Rolando of the cerebrum, controls voluntary movement. Corticospinal tracts, also called pyramidal tracts, begin in the motor cortex and travel through the internal capsule and diencephalons and cross at the decussation of the pyramids in the medulla. Nerve fibers continue to the target muscle to ini-

TABLE 41-2 • BRAIN LOBE FUNCTIONS

FRONTAL LOBE
- The primary motor area (also known as the motor "strip" or cortex)
- Broca's speech center on the dominant side
- Voluntary eye movement
- Access to current sensory data
- Access to past information or experience
- Affective response to a situation
- Regulates behavior based on judgment and foresight
- Judgment
- Ability to develop long-term goals
- Reasoning, concentration, abstraction

PARIETAL LOBE
- Understand sensation, texture, size, shape, and spatial relationships
- Three-dimensional (spatial) perception
- Important for singing, playing musical instruments, and processing nonverbal visual experiences
- Perception of body parts and body position awareness
- Taste impulses for interpretation

TEMPORAL LOBE
- Auditory center for sound interpretation
- Complicated memory patterns
- Wernicke's area for speech

OCCIPITAL LOBE
- Primary visual center

LIMBIC LOBE
- Emotional and visceral patterns connected with survival
- Learning and memory

tiate movement on each side of the body. The crossing of the fibers in the medulla (decussation of the pyramids) is responsible for the contralateral control of motor movement. In the motor cortex the motor homunculus is the spatial arrangement of motor nuclei controlling voluntary muscles of the body. The nuclei controlling the feet are located in the area of the longitudinal fissure, whereas the nuclei for face muscles are located on the opposite end of the homunculus. The large areas dedicated to the mouth and hands are indicative of the multiple functions and importance of these structures.

The cerebrum is divided into lobes by sulci (fissures) and are given the same name as the overlying bone, with the exception of the limbic lobes. The name and function of each lobe can be found in Table 41-2.

Since the early 1900s, attempts have been made to classify neurons by their cellular structure and then relate that to function. Brodmann mapped the cortical areas of the brain based on histologic cell differences. Almost 100 areas have been identified (Figure 41-2).

Two important speech areas of the cerebrum are *Broca's area* and *Wernicke's area.* Broca's area, located in the frontal lobe, is composed of neurons responsible for the formation of words, or speech. This requires respiratory activation of the vocal cords, which must occur at the same time as tongue and mouth movements. This association area, Wernicke's area, is located in the temporal lobe and plays a significant role in higher-level brain function. It enables processing of words into coherent thought and recognition of the idea behind written or printed words (language).

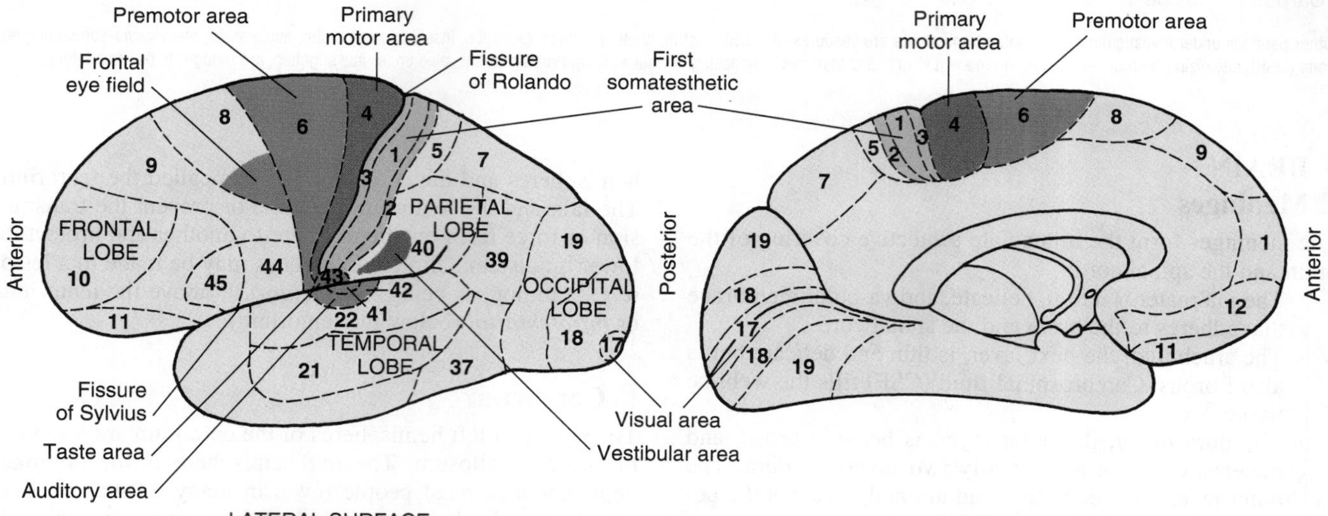

Figure 41-2 ● The functions of the brain according to Brodmann's map. *1-3,* Primary somatic sensory area (overlap with *4*). *4,* Primary motor area. *5,* Somatesthetic association cortex. *6,* Premotor area. *7,* Somatesthetic association cortex. *8,* Frontal eye field. *9-14,* Prefrontal or orbitofrontal association cortex (judgment, foresight, behavior), autonomic centers (respiratory, circulatory, renal, gastrointestinal); *11* and *12* have no clearly assigned function. *17,* Visual area. *18* and *19,* Visual association cortex. *21* and *22,* Ideation, sensory, language (also *37,* posterior part: auditory association cortex [Wernicke's area]). 39 and *40,* Ideation, sensory, language, angular gyrus. *41,* Auditory area. *42,* May also function as auditory area. *43,* Taste area. *44* and *45,* Dominant hemisphere (motor speech centers and related functions), lips, and tongue (Broca's center). *47,* No clearly assigned function. (Modified from Barr, M.L., & Kiernan, J.A. [1988]. *The human nervous system: An anatomical viewpoint* [5th ed.]. Philadelphia: J.B. Lippincott.)

The general interpretive area, which is located where the temporal, parietal and occipital lobes meet at the junction of the lateral fissure, enables a person to process complex thoughts, remember the notes of music, recite a speech heard or read long ago, recall childhood experiences, and so forth. Damage to this area on the dominant side after 5 years of age is catastrophic.

Diencephalon

The diencephalon, which lies below the cerebrum, includes the thalamus, hypothalamus, and epithalamus (Figure 41-3).

The thalamus is the major "relay station," or "central switchboard," for the CNS. The hypothalamus is an integral part of the autonomic nervous system control and plays an essential role in intellectual function. The epithalamus contains the roof of the third ventricle and the pineal gland. See Table 41-3 for additional information concerning the diencephalon.

Hypophysis (Pituitary Gland)

The hypophysis is situated in the sella turcica of the ethmoid bone and is connected to the hypothalamus by tissue called the hypophyseal stalk. The hypophysis has two lobes, each releasing specific hormones into the circulation under the regulation of the hypothalamus. The pituitary is often referred to as the "master gland" because of its control of numerous hormonal functions.

Brainstem

The brainstem (see Figure 41-3) includes the midbrain, pons, and medulla. The functions of these structures are presented in Table 41-4.

Throughout the brainstem are special cells that constitute the *reticular activating system (RAS),* which controls awareness and alertness. For example, this tissue awakens a person from sleep when presented with a noxious stimuli, when there is pain, or when it is time to rise. Many sensory fibers branch and terminate here. The reticular formation area has abundant connections with the cerebrum, the rest of the brainstem, and the cerebellum. Within the reticular formation tissue, groups of specific neurons have functions other than controlling alertness. These neurons are referred to as brainstem nuclei.

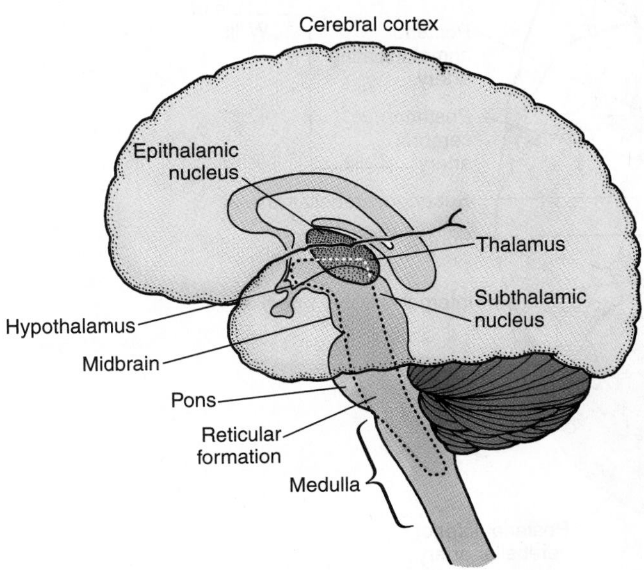

Figure 41-3 • The structures of the brainstem and diencephalon.

Cerebellum

The cerebellum receives instantaneous and continuous information about the condition of the muscles, joints, and tendons. Cerebellar function enables a person to do the following:

- Keep a moving part from overshooting the intended destination
- Move from one skilled movement to another in an orderly sequence

TABLE 41-3 • DIENCEPHALON FUNCTIONS

THALAMUS
- All sensation except smell
- Sensation perceived at the thalamic level is crude and cannot be localized or quantified

HYPOTHALAMUS
- Regulates water metabolism, appetite, sleep-wake cycle, temperature control, and thirst
- Hormonal activity
- Posterior pituitary hormones, such as vasopressin and oxytocin
- Anterior pituitary hormone excretion
- Growth, thyrotropin, and follicle-stimulating hormones, prolactin and corticotropin
- Emotions and drives basic to self-preservation

EPITHALAMUS
- Often calcified by young adulthood and is radiopaque
- Used as a point of reference on an x-ray film or a computed tomography scan

SUBTHALAMUS
- Contains sensory tracts
- Connections to basal ganglia

TABLE 41-4 • BRAINSTEM STRUCTURE FUNCTIONS

MEDULLA
- Cardiac-slowing center
- Respiratory center
- Cranial nerves IX (glossopharyngeal), X (vagus), XI (accessory), and XII (hypoglossal) emerge from the medulla, as do portions of cranial nerves VII (facial) and VIII (acoustic)

PONS
- Cardiac acceleration and vasoconstriction centers
- Pneumotaxic center helps control respiratory pattern and rate
- Four cranial nerves originate from the pons: V (trigeminal), VI (abducens), VII (facial), and VIII (acoustic)

MIDBRAIN
- Contains the cerebral aqueduct or aqueduct of Sylvius
- Location of periaqueductal gray, which may abolish pain when stimulated
- Cranial nerve nuclei III (oculomotor) and IV (trochlear) located here

- Predict distance or gauge the speed with which one is approaching an object
- Control voluntary movement
- Maintain equilibrium

Cerebellar control of the body is *ipsilateral* (situated on the same side). The right side of the cerebellum controls the right side of the body, and the left cerebellum controls the left side of the body.

Cerebral Circulation

Circulation in the brain originates from the carotid and vertebral arteries (Figure 41-4). The internal carotid arteries branch into the anterior cerebral artery (ACA) and middle cerebral arteries (MCA). The two posterior vertebral arteries become the basilar artery, which then divides into two posterior cerebral arteries. The anterior, middle, and posterior cerebral arteries are joined together by small communicating arteries to form a ring at the base of the brain known as the circle of Willis.

The circle of Willis is located at about the level of the pons, or the general level of the upper nose and lower border of the eye. The middle cerebral artery supplies the lateral surface of the cerebrum from about the mid-temporal lobe upward (i.e., the area for hearing and upper body motor and sensory neurons). The anterior cerebral artery supplies the midline, or medial, aspect of the same area (i.e., the lower body motor and sensory neurons). The posterior cerebral arteries supply the area from the mid-temporal region down and posteriorly (occipital lobe), as well as much of the brainstem. Table 41-5 identifies the distribution of blood supply to the brain.

Venous drainage occurs through the cerebral veins into the dural sinuses, which are large venous reservoirs between the inner and outer dura mater. From the dural sinuses, the blood drains into the jugular vein and then into the superior vena cava. Because cerebral veins have no valves, intracranial pressure (ICP) can be affected by central venous pressure (CVP).

Two sinuses are of particular importance: the superior sagittal sinus (SSS) and the cavernous sinus. The superior sagittal sinus receives cerebrospinal fluid after it circulates through the ventricular system. The cavernous sinus is located near the eye and receives venous blood from the eye. In addition, the carotid artery passes through the cavernous sinus (the only place in the body where an artery passes through a vein); thus the potential exists for development of a fistula between an artery and a vein (usually from trauma).

Blood-Brain Barrier

The blood-brain barrier (BBB) seems to exist because the endothelial cells of the cerebral capillaries (along with ependymal cells) are joined tightly together. This keeps some substances in the plasma out of the cerebrospinal circulation and out of brain tissue. Substances that can pass through the blood-brain barrier include oxygen, glucose, carbon dioxide, alcohol, anesthetics, and water. Large molecules such as albumin, any substance bound to albumin, and many antibiotics are prevented from crossing the blood-brain barrier.

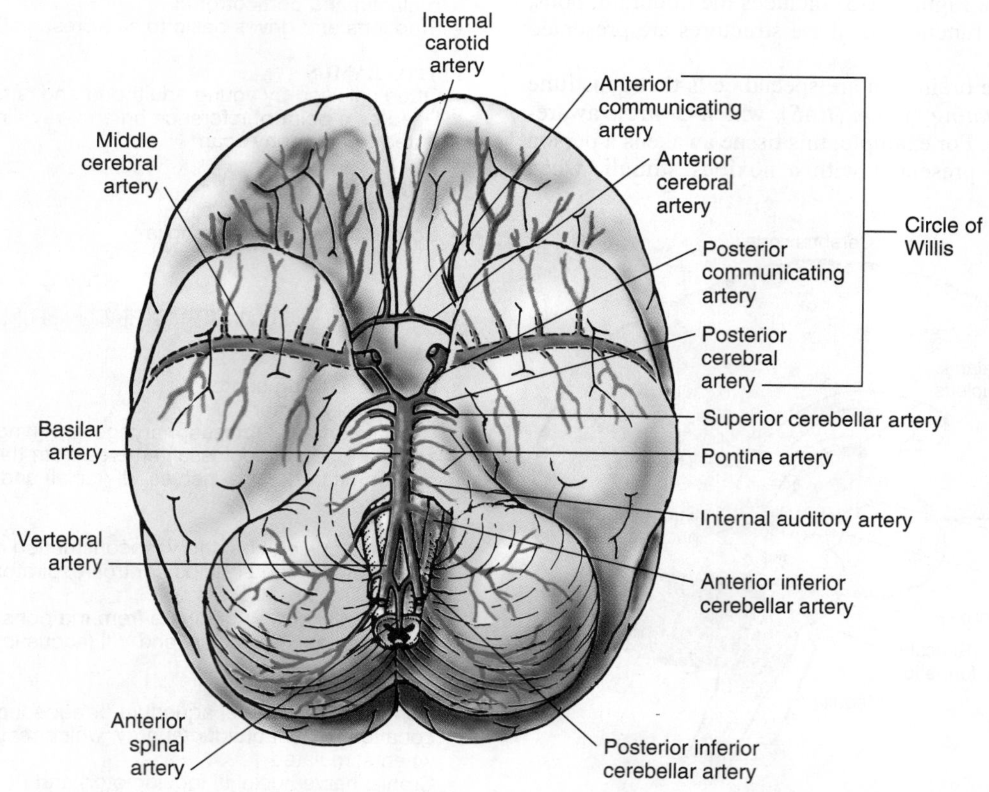

Figure 41-4 ● Cerebral circulation and the circle of Willis at the base of the brain.

Cerebrospinal Fluid Circulation

Cerebrospinal fluid (CSF) surrounds and cushions the brain and spinal cord. While circulating through the subarachnoid space, the fluid is continuously produced by the choroid plexus, reabsorbed by the arachnoid villi, and then channeled into the superior sagittal sinus (Figure 41-5). Expanded areas of subarachnoid space, where there are large amounts of CSF, are called *cisterns.* The largest cistern is the lumbar cistern, the site of lumbar puncture, from the level of the second lumbar vertebrae to the second sacral vertebrae (L2-S2).

TABLE 41-5 • BLOOD DISTRIBUTION TO THE BRAIN

Artery	Distribution
INTERNAL CAROTID ARTERY BRANCHES	
Hypophyseal	Posterior pituitary
Ophthalmic	Eye, frontal scalp, frontal and ethmoid sinuses
Anterior choroidal	Choroid plexus (lateral), optic tract, uncus, amygdaloid body, hippocampus, globus pallidus, lateral geniculate nucleus, internal capsule
Middle cerebral	Insula; lateral frontal, parietal, occipital, and temporal lobes (major motor and sensory areas)
Lenticulostriate	Putamen, caudate nucleus, globus pallidus, internal capsule, corona radiata
Other	Choroid plexus (lateral ventricles), hippocampus, globus pallidus
Anterior cerebral	Medial surface of frontal and parietal lobes, corpus callosum, superior or lateral strip of frontal and parietal lobes
VERTEBRAL ARTERY BRANCHES	
Posterior cerebellar	Medulla Posterior cerebellum, inferior vermis, cerebellar nuclei, choroid plexus (fourth ventricle), posterolateral medulla
BASILAR ARTERY BRANCHES	
Anterior inferior cerebellar	Cortex and inferior surface cerebellum, cerebellar nuclei, upper medulla, lower pons
Internal auditory	Inner ear
Pontine	Pons
Superior cerebellar	Cortex, white matter and nuclei of cerebellum, pons, superior cerebellar peduncle, inferior peduncle, inferior colliculus
POSTERIOR CEREBRAL ARTERY BRANCHES	
Posterior cerebral	Medial, inferior temporal, and occipital lobes
Calcarine	Visual cortex
Other	Posterior and lateral thalamus, subthalamus, pituitary, mammillary bodies, and midbrain; choroid plexus of lateral and third ventricle, dorsal thalamus
Circle of Willis	Hypothalamus, caudate nucleus, putamen, globus pallidus, internal capsule, external capsule thalamus, subthalamus, cerebral peduncles

SPINAL CORD

The spinal cord controls body movement; regulates visceral function; processes sensory information from the extremities, trunk, and many internal organs; and transmits information to and from the brain. It contains H-shaped gray matter (neuron cell bodies) that is surrounded by white matter (myelinated axons). The white matter is divided into posterior, lateral, and anterior columns. Groups of cells in the white matter (ascending and descending tracts) have been fairly well identified (Figure 41-6). The gray matter divisions are posterior, intermediolateral, and anterior.

Ascending Tracts

As a general rule, ascending tracts originate in the spinal cord and end in the brain. Three ascending tracts are important for understanding the client with neurologic problems: spinothalamic tracts, spinocerebellar tracts, and fasciculi gracilis and cuneatus (posterior white columns).

SPINOTHALAMIC TRACTS

As the name indicates, spinothalamic tracts begin in the spinal cord and end primarily in the thalamus. These tracts carry sensations of pain, temperature, light touch, and pressure. The axon fibers from the cells decussate (cross) the anterior white and gray commissures to the opposite side and become the contralateral (situated on the opposite side) spinothalamic tract. These fibers continue up to the thalamus. Some branches terminate in the reticular formation of the medulla and pons.

A pain or temperature impulse enters the posterior horn on the same side on which the sensation occurs. It is transmitted to other cells in several laminae, is further propelled to the opposite spinothalamic tract, and continues up to its ultimate destinations—the thalamus and the parietal lobe (Figure 41-7).

POSTERIOR AND ANTERIOR SPINOCEREBELLAR TRACTS

Spinocerebellar tracts begin in the spinal cord and end in the cerebellum. The *posterior* spinocerebellar tract transmits impulses of proprioception (awareness of position and movements of body parts) or kinesthesia, mostly from the lower extremities. The impulses enter the posterior gray horn and synapse with tract cells in lamina VII. Spinocerebellar axons then form the tract on the *same,* or ipsilateral, side. This tract begins at the second lumbar level and ascends to the medulla and then to the cerebellum.

The *anterior* spinocerebellar tract begins lower in the lumbar spine than does the posterior tract. These fibers cross immediately and ascend as a contralateral tract, transmitting proprioceptive impulses from the lower extremities. The fibers cross again in the midbrain on their way to the cerebellum. Because these fibers have crossed the midline twice,

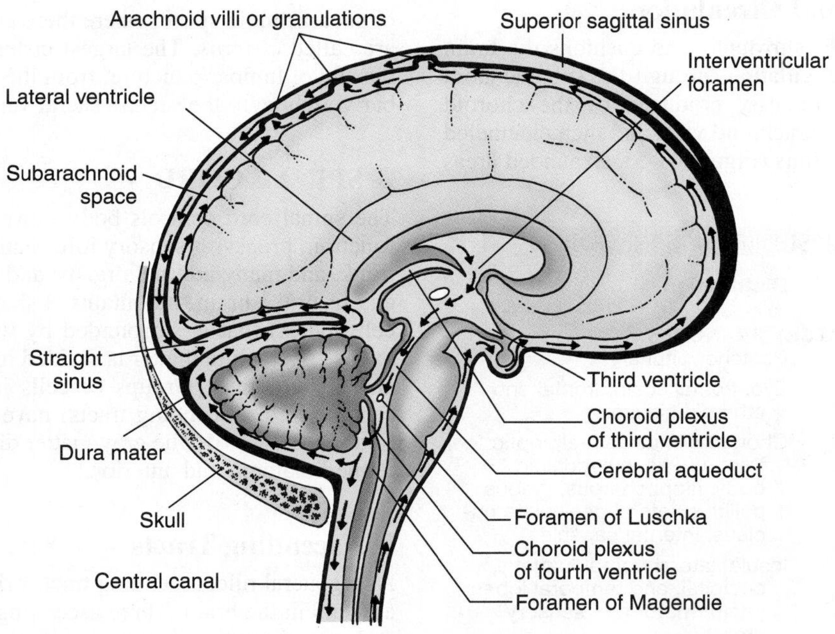

Figure 41-5 ● Circulation of cerebrospinal fluid. Note that the fluid also extends down into the spinal column.

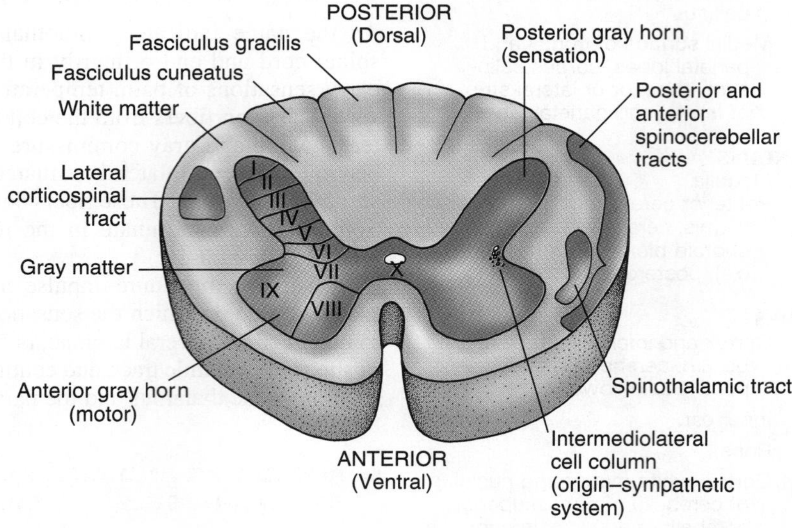

Figure 41-6 ● A cross section of the spinal cord showing the common tracts.

the sensations terminate on the side on which they originated. The *right* cerebellum receives information about the *right* side of the body, and the *left* cerebellum receives data about the *left* side.

FASCICULUS GRACILIS AND FASCICULUS CUNEATUS (POSTERIOR WHITE COLUMNS)

The posterior white columns transmit the following information to the thalamus:

- The sensation of proprioception from muscles, joints, and tendons
- Vibratory sense
- Light touch from the skin
- Discrete localization
- Two-point discrimination

Most of the fibers ascend on the *same* side as their origin to the medulla, where they cross and then synapse in the thalamus, with termination in the parietal lobe. This tract enables identification of the exact point of pressure on the skin. Recognition of pressure includes the shape of an object (with eyes closed), movement across the skin (a number being written), and acknowledgment of two points of touch close together.

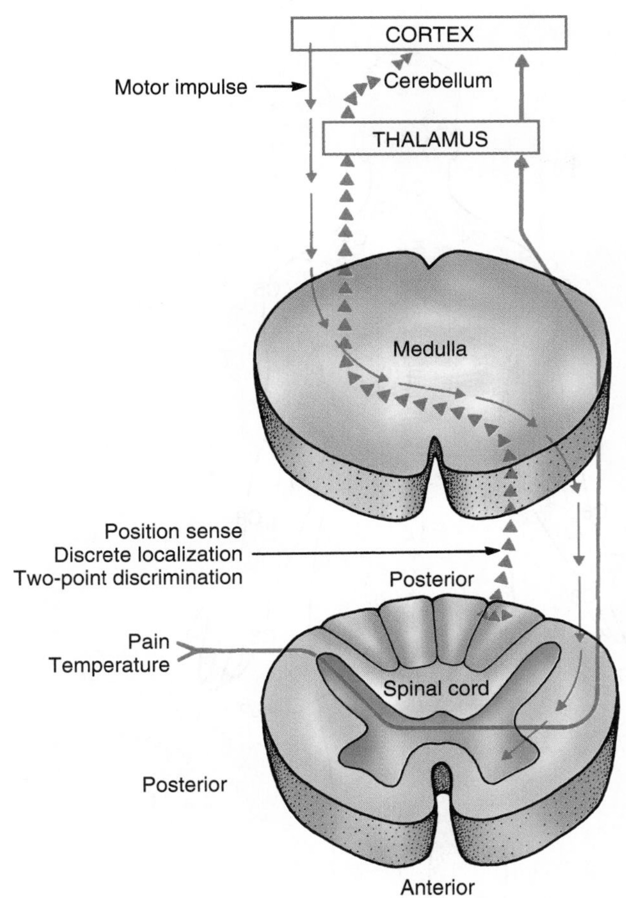

Figure 41-7 ● Examples of common spinal tract pathways.

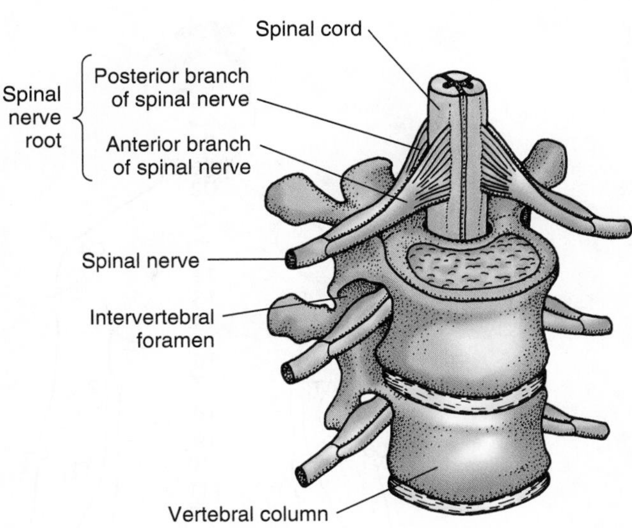

Figure 41-8 ● Spinal nerve branches exiting from the spinal cord through the intervertebral foramen of a vertebra.

Descending Tracts

Descending tracts *begin* in the brain and *end* in the spinal cord. The major descending tract of importance for understanding neurologic problems is the lateral corticospinal, or pyramidal, tract. The corticospinal tract originates in the motor cortex of the frontal lobe and portions of the parietal lobe. The lateral tract fibers cross to the opposite side at the level of the medulla. After crossing, the fibers descend to a predetermined level and synapse with interneurons of the gray matter. A few fibers connect directly with lower motor neurons (LMNs). The cervical area has a high concentration of fibers synapsing with interneurons, which possibly reflects the complexity of hand and finger movements.

The motor neurons of the other descending tracts and the basal ganglia used to be referred to as an extrapyramidal system. It was thought that pyramidal neurons initiated voluntary muscle activity and that extrapyramidal neurons initiated automatic or nonvoluntary muscle action. The descending tracts and the basal ganglia are necessary for the smooth function of all motor activity. The term *extrapyramidal* is still often used clinically to connote the origin of abnormal spontaneous movement.

Spinal Cord Circulation

The blood supply for the spinal cord comes from three main arteries. The anterior spinal artery originates from a branch of the vertebral arteries. The two posterior spinal arteries originate from either the vertebral or posterior inferior cerebellar artery. Additional circulation is supplied by branches of the descending aorta.

Peripheral Nervous System

The peripheral nervous system (PNS) is composed of the spinal nerves, cranial nerves, and autonomic nervous system.

SPINAL NERVES

There are 31 pairs of spinal nerves (8 cervical, 12 thoracic, 5 lumbar, 5 sacral, and 1 coccygeal) exiting from the spinal cord. Each of the nerves has a posterior and an anterior branch (Figure 41-8). The posterior branch carries sensory information to the cord (afferent pathway). The anterior branch transmits motor impulses to the muscles of the body (efferent pathway).

Each spinal nerve is responsible for the muscle innervation and sensory reception of a given area of the body. The cervical and thoracic spinal nerves are relatively close to their areas of responsibility, whereas the lumbar and sacral spinal nerves are some distance from theirs. Because the spinal cord ends between L1 and L2, the axons of the lumbar and sacral cord extend downward before exiting the appropriate intervertebral foramen. The area controlled by each spinal nerve is roughly reflected in the dermatomes. Dermatomes represent sensory input from spinal nerves to specific areas of the skin (Figure 41-9). For example, the client with an injury to cervical spinal nerve root C6 and C7 exhibits sensory changes in the thumb, index finger, middle finger, middle of the palm, and back of the hand.

SENSORY RECEPTORS

Sensory receptors throughout the body monitor and transmit impulses of pain, temperature, touch, vibration, pressure, visceral sensation, and proprioception. Sensory receptors also

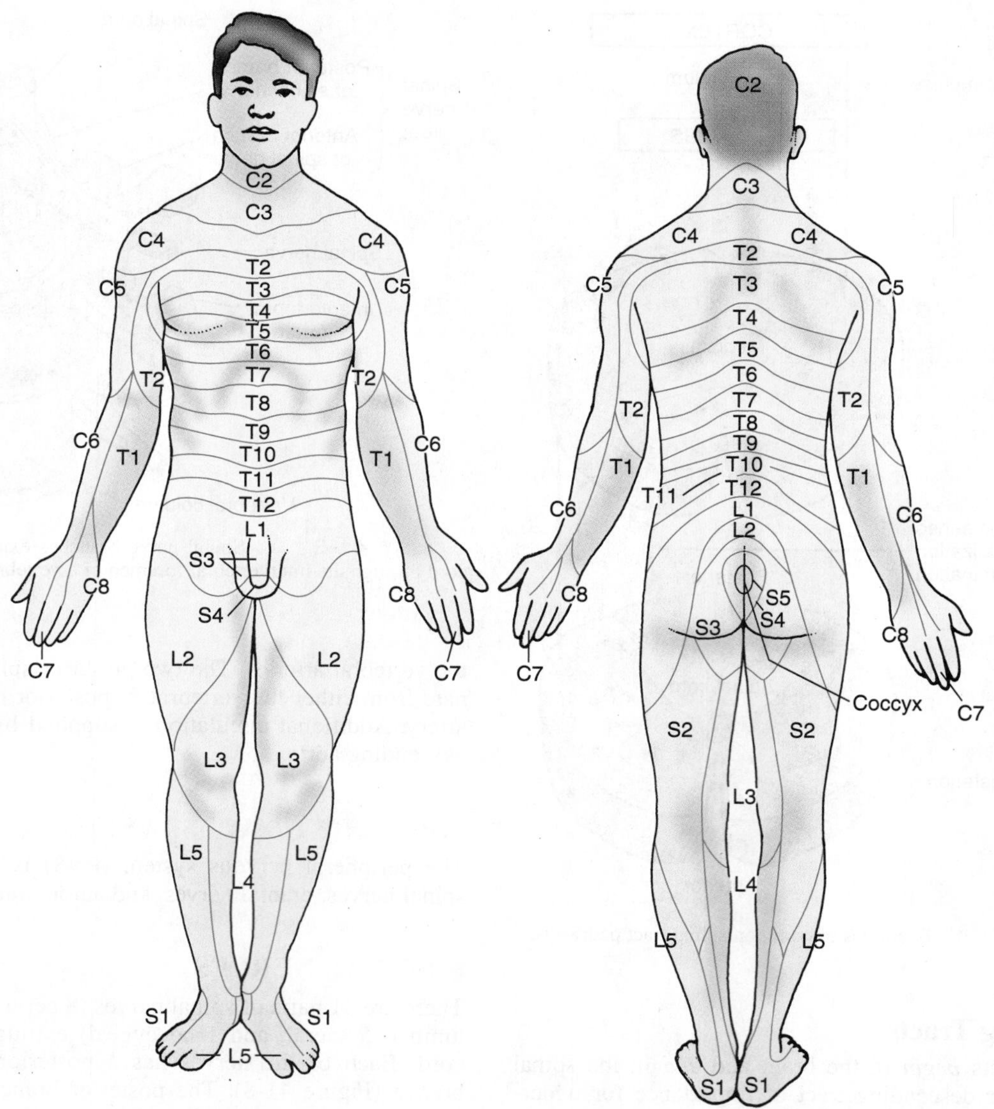

Figure 41-9 ● Dermatomes (cutaneous innervation of spinal nerves).

monitor and transmit the sensations of the special senses—vision, taste, smell, and hearing.

LOWER MOTOR NEURONS AND PLEXUSES

The cell bodies of the anterior spinal nerves are located in the anterior gray matter (anterior horn) of each level in the spinal cord. The anterior motor neurons are also referred to as lower motor neurons. As each nerve axon leaves the spinal cord, it joins other spinal nerves to form plexuses (clusters of nerves). Plexuses continue as trunks, divisions, and cords and finally branch into individual peripheral nerves.

The major plexuses are cervical, brachial, lumbar, and sacral. The latter two plexuses are also referred to as lumbosacral. An awareness of the location of the plexuses is helpful because a major concentration of nerves is present. In addition, the nerves of each plexus pass through or are surrounded by bone. Injury to the area or entrapment of a nerve by bone can cause multiple problems.

REFLEXES

Reflexes consist of sensory input from the following (Figure 41-10):

- The muscles, tendons, skin, organs, and special senses
- Small cells in the spinal cord lying between the posterior and anterior gray matter (interneurons)
- The anterior motor neurons, along with the muscles they innervate

Sensory data from a specific peripheral location account for a change in the motor impulses going to that location. This closed circuit, which requires no mediation in the cerebral cortex, is called the reflex arc.

Muscle tone is achieved by special fibers in the middle of the muscle. These special fibers, called muscle spindles or in-

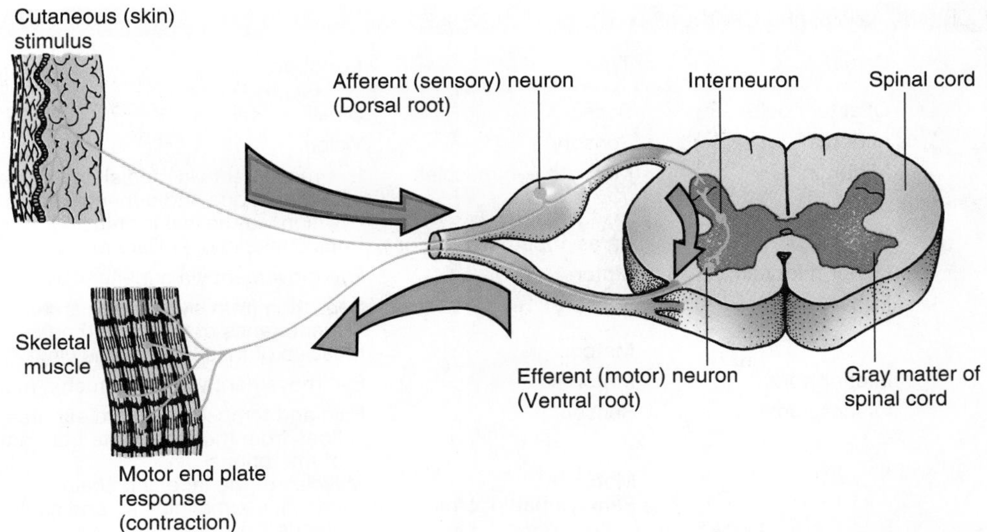

Figure 41-10 ● An example of reflex activity. Stimulation of skin results in involuntary muscle contraction (reflex arc).

trafusal fibers, are attached to the surrounding muscle and are able to contract only at their ends. The contractible ends are innervated by special motor fibers from the anterior horn. The middle portion of the intrafusal fibers contains special receptors that measure the degree of stretch of the muscle.

CRANIAL NERVES

There are 12 cranial nerves. The name, number, origin, type, and function of the cranial nerves are summarized in Table 41-6.

Autonomic Nervous System

The autonomic nervous system (ANS) is composed of two parts: the sympathetic nervous system (SNS) and the parasympathetic nervous system (PNS). Through the use of biofeedback and other mechanisms, some ANS functions can be brought under conscious control.

SYMPATHETIC NERVOUS SYSTEM

The cells of origin for the sympathetic nervous system are located in the gray matter of the spinal cord from T1 and through L2 or L3. This part of the ANS is considered *thoracolumbar* because of its anatomic location.

Structure

Lying on either side of the spinal cord is a chain of ganglia extending the length of the cord. This chain of ganglia is called the sympathetic chain. Sympathetic axons leave the spinal nerve immediately and enter the sympathetic chain. Some fibers synapse within the sympathetic chain, and others do not.

Function

If almost any portion of the sympathetic nervous system is stimulated, the whole system responds (the fight-or-flight response). The following occurs during periods of excessive sympathetic stimulation:

- Skeletal muscle vessels dilate.
- The heart pumps faster.
- The liver releases extra glucose.
- The thyroid is stimulated.
- Sweating increases.
- Kidney vessels constrict.

During true emergencies, this is a helpful mechanism; with false emergencies (e.g., being unduly anxious), this mechanism wastes resources.

PARASYMPATHETIC NERVOUS SYSTEM

The cells of origin for the PNS are located in the gray matter of the sacral area of the spinal cord (from S2 to S4) plus portions of cranial nerves III, VII, IX, and X. The PNS conserves the body's resources.

Parasympathetic fibers to the viscera have some sensory ability in addition to motor function. Sensations of irritation, stretching of an organ, or a decrease in tissue oxygen are transmitted to the thalamus through pathways not yet fully understood. Because pain from internal organs is often felt below the body wall innervated by the spinal nerve, it is presumed that there are connections between the viscera and body structure that relay pain sensations. Table 41-7 compares the action of sympathetic and parasympathetic systems in the body.

Neurologic Changes Associated with Aging

MOTOR/SENSORY ABILITY

Motor changes in late adulthood are interrelated with sensory function and musculoskeletal status (Chart 41-1). Any problems that affect the nerves, bones, muscles, or joints also affect motor ability. The older adult may have tremors without rigidity, and deep tendon reflexes may be hypoactive. Balance and coordination may be impaired as a result.

Sensory changes in older adults can affect their daily activities. Pupils decrease in size, which restricts the amount of

TABLE 41-6 • ORIGINS, TYPES, AND FUNCTIONS OF THE CRANIAL NERVES

Cranial Nerve	Origin	Type	Function
I: Olfactory	Olfactory bulb	Sensory	Smell
II: Optic	Midbrain	Sensory	Vision
III: Oculomotor	Midbrain	Motor to eye muscles	Eye movement via medial and lateral rectus and inferior oblique and superior rectus muscles; lid elevation via the levator muscle
		Parasympathetic-motor	Pupil constriction; ciliary muscles
IV: Trochlear	Lower midbrain	Motor	Eye movement via superior oblique muscles
V: Trigeminal	Pons	Sensory	Sensation from skin of face and scalp and mucous membranes of mouth and nose
		Motor	Muscles of mastication (chewing)
VI: Abducens	Inferior pons	Motor	Eye movement via lateral rectus muscles
VII: Facial	Inferior pons	Sensory	Pain and temperature from ear area; deep sensations from the face; taste from anterior two thirds of the tongue
		Motor	Muscles of the face and scalp
		Parasympathetic-motor	Lacrimal, submandibular, and sublingual salivary glands
VIII: Vestibulocochlear	Pons-medulla junction	Sensory	Hearing Equilibrium
IX: Glossopharyngeal	Medulla	Sensory	Pain and temperature from ear; taste and sensations from posterior one third of tongue and pharynx
		Motor	Skeletal muscles of the throat
		Parasympathetic-motor	Parotid glands
X: Vagus	Medulla	Sensory	Pain and temperature from ear; sensations from pharynx, larynx, thoracic and abdominal viscera
		Motor	Muscles of the soft palate, larynx, and pharynx
		Parasympathetic-motor	Thoracic and abdominal viscera; cells of secretory glands; cardiac and smooth muscle innervation to the level of the splenic flexure
XI: Accessory	Medulla (anterior gray horn of the cervical spine)	Motor	Skeletal muscles of the pharynx and larynx and sternocleidomastoid and trapezius muscles
XII: Hypoglossal	Medulla	Motor	Skeletal muscles of the tongue

light entering the eye. The pupils also adapt more slowly. Touch sensation decreases, which may precipitate falls because the older person may not feel pebbles or small objects underfoot. Vibration sense may be lost in the ankles and feet. (See also the discussion on fall prevention in Chapter 5.) Hearing also decreases, especially for high-pitched sounds (presbycusis).

MENTAL STATUS

Intellect does not decline as a result of aging; however, a person with certain pathologic conditions may experience a decrease in intellectual level caused by drug interactions or an insufficient oxygen supply to the brain. Some older adults may need more time than a younger person to process questions, learn new information, solve problems, or complete analogies.

Subtle memory changes are typical for many older people. Long-term memory seems better than recall (recent) or immediate (registration) memory. Older adults may need more time to retrieve information. These changes may be partly due to the loss of cerebral neurons, which is associated with the aging process.

Insomnia, anxiety, and depression in late adulthood may cause some changes in mental status. Circadian rhythm disorders may lead to wakefulness until later at night, with extended sleeping in the morning (a pattern opposite that of most health care facility routines). Many older adults require less sleep than do their younger counterparts.

Mental status may also be compromised as the result of infection. Many times this change in mental status is a key early sign of an infectious process in the older client.

ASSESSMENT TECHNIQUES

History

The neurologic history and assessment begin the moment the nurse firsts meets the client. During the introduction, the nurse notes the client's appearance and assesses his or her speech, affect, and motor function. The nurse provides privacy and as much comfort as possible. If the client appears to have cognitive deficits or has trouble speaking or hearing, the nurse asks a family member or significant other to stay during the history taking to help secure accurate information. Charts 41-2 and 41-3 elaborate on the information the nurse obtains from the client or family.

PERSONAL AND FAMILY HISTORY

Questions about the client's medical history and the family and dietary history are necessary for any bearing they might have on the present problem. Ethnic and cultural background

TABLE 41-7 • EFFECTS OF THE AUTONOMIC NERVOUS SYSTEM ON VARIOUS ORGANS OF THE BODY

Organ	Effect of Sympathetic Stimulation	Effect of Parasympathetic Stimulation
Eye		
Pupil	Dilated	Constricted
Ciliary muscle	Slight relaxation	Constricted
Glands		
Nasal Lacrimal Parotid Submandibular Gastric Pancreatic	Vasoconstriction and slight secretion	Stimulation of copious (except pancreas) secretion (containing many enzymes for enzyme-secreting glands)
Sweat glands	Copious sweating (cholinergic)	Sweating of the palms of the hands
Apocrine glands	Thick, odoriferous secretion	None
Heart		
Muscle	Increased rate Increased force of contraction	Slowed rate Decreased force of contraction
Coronary arteries	Dilated ($beta_2$); constricted (alpha)	Dilated
Lungs		
Bronchi	Dilated	Constricted
Blood vessels	Mildly constricted	? Dilated
Gut		
Lumen	Decreased peristalsis and tone	Increased peristalsis and tone
Sphincter	Increased tone (most times)	Relaxed (most times)
Liver	Glucose released	Slight glycogen synthesis
Gallbladder and bile ducts	Relaxed	Contracted
Kidney	Decreased output and renin secretion	None
Bladder		
Detrusor	Relaxed (slight)	Excited
Trigone	Contracted	Relaxed
Penis	Ejaculation	Erection
Systemic arterioles		
Abdominal	Constricted	None
Muscle	Constricted (alpha-adrenergic) Dilated ($beta_2$-adrenergic) Dilated (cholinergic)	None
Skin	Constricted	None
Blood		
Coagulation	Increased	None
Glucose	Increased	None
Lipids	Increased	None
Basal metabolism	Increased up to 100%	None
Adrenal medullary secretion	Increased	None
Mental activity	Increased	None
Piloerector muscles	Contracted	None
Skeletal muscle	Increased glycogenolysis Increased strength	None
Fat cells	Lipolysis	None

From Guyton, A.C. (1991). *Textbook of medical physiology* (8th ed.). Philadelphia: W.B. Saunders.

may be an influence depending on the degree of socialization to the health care system.

Questions about the client's level of activities of daily living (ADLs) may highlight subtle changes in neurologic function. Knowing the level of daily activity also helps the nurse establish a baseline for later comparison with changes resulting from improving or worsening neurologic function. The nurse asks whether the client is right-handed or left-handed. This information is important for several reasons:

- The client may be somewhat stronger on the dominant side, and this is expected.
- The client has a greater degree of independence if the dominant hand and arm can be free of tubing and tape.
- The effects of cerebral injury or disease are more pronounced if the dominant hemisphere is involved.

CURRENT HEALTH PROBLEMS AND SOCIAL HISTORY

The nurse obtains information from the client as outlined in Charts 41-2 and 41-3.

CHART 41-1

NURSING FOCUS *on the* OLDER ADULT
Changes in the Nervous System Related to Aging

Physiologic Changes	Nursing Implications	Rationale
Recent memory loss	Reinforce teaching by repetition and written teaching aids.	Intellect is not impaired, but the learning process is slowed. Repetition helps the client learn new information and recall it when needed.
Decreased touch sensation	Remind the client to look where his or her feet are placed when walking. Instruct the client to wear shoes that provide good support when walking. If the client is unable, change his or her position frequently (every hour) while he or she is in bed or the chair.	Decreased sensation may cause the client to fall.
Change in perception of pain	Ask the client to describe the nature and specific characteristics of pain. Monitor additional assessment variables to detect possible health problems.	Accurate and complete nursing assessment ensures that the interventions will be appropriate for the older adult (see Chapter 7).
Change in sleep patterns	Ascertain sleep patterns and preferences. Adjust the client's daily schedule to his or her sleep pattern and preference as much as possible (e.g., evening versus morning bath).	Most older adults require less sleep than do younger adults. However, frequent rest periods are needed.
Altered balance or coordination	Instruct the client to move slowly when changing positions. If needed, advise the client to hold on to handrails when ambulating. Assess the need for an ambulatory aid, such as a cane.	The client may fall if moving too quickly. Assistive and adaptive aids provide support and prevent falls.

CHART 41-2

BEST PRACTICE *for*
Establishing a Nursing Database: History

Demographic Data
Age
Sex

Past Medical History
Client's medical history
Family's medical history
Previous injuries or congenital problems
Chronic diseases
- Hypertension
- Diabetes mellitus
- Lung disease

Previous neurologic problems
- Headaches
- Seizures
- Head or spine trauma
- Eye problems

Current History
Current symptoms
- Blurred vision
- Headache
- Speech or swallowing difficulty
- Numbness, tingling
- Weakness, clumsiness
- Bowel or bladder difficulties
- Nausea or vomiting
- Personality seizures

Allergies
- Food
- Medications
- Environment

Pain tolerance
- Medications taken for pain
- Behaviors to reduce pain

Medications
- Prescribed
- Illicit
- Over-the-counter

Activities of daily living

Social History
Usual recreational activities
Level of physical activity each day
Hobbies
Alcohol consumption and use of recreational drugs
Smoking, use of any tobacco products
Sleep habits
- Changes in pattern, duration, or intensity

Work history
- Exposure to toxic agents

Ethnic and cultural background
Handedness (right or left)
Educational background

CHART 41-3

NEUROLOGIC ASSESSMENT
Using Gordon's Functional Health Patterns

Health Perception-Health Management Pattern
How would you describe your general health?
Has your health changed significantly over the past few weeks or months?
Have you had to miss any work because of changes in your health?

Cognitive-Perceptual Pattern
Have you noticed any changes in your vision? Hearing? Memory?
Do you feel you are having any difficulty in making decisions? In learning?
Are you experiencing any discomfort? Pain? Weakness?

Activity-Exercise Pattern
Do you have enough energy for your activities?
What is your perceived ability for the following (code for level according to key below):

Feeding?
Bathing?
Toileting?
Bed mobility?
Dressing?
Grooming?
General mobility?
Cooking?
Home maintenance?
Shopping?

Level 0: Full self-care
Level I: Requires use of equipment or device
Level II: Requires assistance or supervision of another person
Level III: Requires assistance or supervision of another person and equipment or device
Level IV: Is dependent and does not participate

Based on Gordon, M. (2000). *Manual of nursing diagnosis* (9th ed.). St. Louis: Mosby.

Physical Assessment

The complete neurologic examination may be performed by the health care provider—the physician or advance practice nurse. Most nurses, however, perform focused assessments based on the client's presenting symptoms or diagnosis. The establishment of baseline data is most important. Nurses must constantly make comparisons with each assessment (e.g., to findings 5 minutes or an hour earlier, to the client's baseline, between the right and left sides, between upper and lower extremities, and to the expected progression for the client). Much of the neurologic assessment can be performed with the client sitting or lying down.

ASSESSMENT OF MENTAL STATUS

While collecting the history data, the nurse makes observations about the client's mental status, speech, and behavior:

- Are the client's answers appropriate?
- Is the client's behavior appropriate?
- Is the speech pattern of normal tone, rate, rhythm, and volume?
- Are the answers complete?
- Is the client's appearance neat or untidy; appropriate for age and weather conditions?
- Is the client cooperative, hostile, anxious, withdrawn, or guarded?

Although the mental status examination is often left until last, it may be better to complete it as part of the initial physical assessment, especially if neurologic problems have been noted.

CONSIDERATIONS FOR OLDER ADULTS

Normal mental status in older adults varies, but the nurse should be aware of some general considerations during the mental status assessment. These clients may take longer to process and answer questions, particularly if they do not understand the relevancy. Their attention span may be short, and they may be guided by internal rather than external motivation. Depending on age, previous occupation, and retirement activities, a client may find some of the cognitive tests difficult or impossible to perform. The nurse should then change the questions to focus on the client's immediate life. If his or her behavior seems appropriate, the mental status assessment can be shortened. If his or her behavior is not appropriate, the nurse performs an in-depth mental status assessment; a tool such as the Mini-Mental State Exam (MMSE), described in Chapter 42, is used for this assessment. The MMSE is an organized way to assess memory, attention, speech, language, and cognition, described in more detail in the next section.

Level of Consciousness and Orientation

The nurse determines **level of consciousness (LOC)** by observing the client's level of responsiveness to the environment. A change in LOC is the first indication that central neurologic function has declined. The client who is alert is awake and responsive. Clients who are less than alert are labeled lethargic (sleepy but arousable), stuporous (arousable with difficulty), or comatose (not arousable). Assessment of the client who is less than alert because of trauma or surgery, for example, is discussed in Chapters 42 and 45.

To better identify the client's level of cognitive function or exact state of consciousness, the nurse describes behavior in response to stimulation. The client is asked questions that indicate orientation to *person, place,* and *time.* Varying the sequence of questioning on repeated assessments prevents the client from memorizing the answers. During the history taking, responses that indicate orientation to person, place, and time include the following:

- The client's ability to relate the onset of symptoms
- The name of his or her physician/nurse practitioner/nurse
- The year and month
- His or her address
- The name of the referring physician or health care agency

Advanced age, time of day, medications, and the need for sleep affect responses.

CRITICAL THINKING CHALLENGE

You are caring for an older adult who has been admitted to the hospital for a possible brain attack (stroke). The client's daughter states that her father has been living independently at home and previously had no problems with mental status. She is now concerned that he seems very confused.

- What is your priority in performing a neurologic assessment of this client?
- What are some possible explanations for the client's apparent change in mental status?
- What should you tell the daughter to address her concerns about her father?

For suggested answer guidelines, go to SIMON http://www.wbsaunders.com/SIMON/Iggy/.

Memory

Memory is one of the most important criteria for neurologic assessment. If the client cannot remember, most of the verbal assessment tests are either not feasible or are at best unreliable. Loss of memory, especially recent memory, tends to be an *early* sign of neurologic problems. Three facets of memory are tested: long-term (remote) memory, recall (recent) memory, and immediate memory. Some older clients may not be as capable with recall or immediate memory, and this may be acceptable for that person.

The nurse can test **remote,** or long-term, **memory** by asking clients about their birth date, schools attended, the city of birth, or anything from the past that can be verified. Nurses often ask the maiden name of the client's mother; this is sometimes listed on the admission form and can be checked.

Recall (recent) **memory** can be tested fairly well during the history taking by assessing the following:

- The accuracy of the medical history
- Dates of clinic or physician appointments
- The time of admission
- Health care providers seen within the past few days
- Mode of transportation to the hospital or clinic

The nurse may test **immediate** (new) **memory** by giving the client two or three unrelated words, such as "apple," "street," and "chair," and asking him or her to repeat the words to make sure they were heard. After about 5 minutes, while continuing with the examination, the nurse asks the client to repeat the words. A person normally should be able to do this correctly. An alternative to this method is to give a three-step command that is carried out correctly.

Attention

To assess attention, the nurse may ask the client to repeat three numbers, such as 4, 7, and 3. The series is increased by one number with each successful repetition until seven or eight digits are achieved. If the client has difficulty at any level (cannot repeat the series), the nurse repeats the numbers. If the client cannot repeat, then the nurse stops the procedure. Next, the nurse asks the client to repeat the numbers backward, starting again with three digits and increasing by one each time. Normally, a person should be able to repeat five to eight digits forward and four to six backward. Education, occupation, interest, culture, anxiety, and depression affect mental status, and what is considered normal may not be so for a particular client.

The nurse can also use the serial seven test to test attention. The client is asked to count backward from 100 by 7 (the examiner stops when the client reaches 65 successfully). Depending on education and other factors, it may be better to ask the person to subtract by three or to add forward by five. The nurse must use judgment in deciding which of these tests to use.

Language and Copying

If desired, the nurse can assess most language and copying skills during the initial interview. The client demonstrates language comprehension by following the nurse's directions on admission (e.g., getting undressed and providing a urine specimen). Was there any hesitancy in speech, indicating that the client groped for words? If so, the nurse points to items and asks the client to name them, such as a drinking glass, the door, or the bed.

The advance practice nurse or speech and language pathologist tests reading comprehension by writing a simple command and giving it to the client (e.g., "close your eyes"). Writing can be tested by asking the client to write a sentence. The practitioner must remember that some clients are not able to read or write and modify the examination accordingly. The practitioner usually tests copying ability by having the client copy something the nurse has drawn, such as a cross, circle, diamond, or square.

Cognition

The nurse assesses higher intellectual function by asking about favorite hobbies, current events, the names of the last few presidents, or the meaning of a statement. The nurse can evaluate abstract reasoning by asking the meaning of proverbs (e.g., "A stitch in time saves nine" or "A rolling stone gathers no moss"). Nurses can also assess the client's judgment, at least partially, during the interview. Did he or she make rational decisions in dealing with his or her symptoms? The nurse can evaluate judgment by asking questions such as, "What would you do if stopped for speeding?" and "What would you do if there was a fire in the wastepaper basket?" The nurse should remember that testing of cognition (general knowledge, abstraction, and judgment) is influenced by culture.

ASSESSMENT OF CRANIAL NERVES

Cranial nerves are typically tested to establish a baseline from which to compare progress or deterioration. However, they are not routinely tested unless the client has a suspected problem affecting one or more of the cranial nerves (see Table 41-6). The testing of cranial nerve III is usually a part of the rapid neurologic assessment described on p. 889. Adding the specific cranial nerves to be tested on the flowsheet of a client with a problem affecting the cranial nerves helps ensure continued comparison and evaluation.

ASSESSMENT OF SENSORY FUNCTION

For the most part, the assessment of sensory function is reserved for clients with problems affecting the spinal cord or spinal nerves, such as trauma, intervertebral disk disease, Guillain Barré syndrome (GBS), neoplasm, infection, stenosis, or transverse myelitis. Components of the sensory assessment include pain, superficial and deep sensation, light touch, and proprioception. Pain and light touch are the most commonly assessed component of sensory function. Sensory assessment of the face may be completed with testing of the trigeminal nerve.

The acuity level of the client will determine the frequency of the sensory assessment and the targeted sensory parameter. Clients with acute spinal cord trauma or GBS should be assessed every hour until stable, then every 4 hours. As the condition improves, sensory assessment may be needed only once each shift. Findings of the sensory assessment are documented according to agency protocol. A special spinal cord assessment flowsheet may be used to document sensory and/or motor findings for the client with a spinal cord injury.

Pain and Temperature

Pain and temperature sensations are transmitted by the same nerve endings. Therefore if one sensation is tested and found to be intact, it can safely be assumed that the other is intact. Testing temperature sensation can usually be accomplished using a cold reflex hammer and the warm touch of the hand for clients with known or suspected spinal problems. Testing pain sensation is relatively easy and more reliable.

The nurse may assess for pain sensation with any object perceived as being sharp or dull. A cotton-tipped applicator or paper clip has a sharp end and a dull end. The nurse instructs the client to keep the eyes closed and to indicate whether the touch is sharp or dull. It is necessary to demonstrate what will be done while the client's eyes are open. The sharp and dull stimuli should be interchanged at random so the client does not anticipate the type of the next stimulus. Not all areas need to be tested unless the client has suffered a spinal cord injury. If testing begins on the hands and feet, there is no need to test the more proximal parts of the extremities because the tracts transmitting pain and temperature sensations are intact. The nurse compares reactions on each side. A sensation reported as dull when the stimulus was actually sharp necessitates more finite testing. A client with sensory loss as a result of diabetes mellitus or peripheral vascular disease may or may not be aware of the loss until tested. Some clients may in fact point out their sensory loses to the nurse.

Touch

Light touch discrimination is likely to be normal if pain and temperature sensations are intact. Touch discrimination and two-point discrimination are performed as part of a complete neurologic examination by the health care provider.

For testing **touch discrimination,** the client closes his or her eyes. The practitioner touches him or her with a finger and asks that he or she point to the area touched. This procedure is repeated on each extremity at random rather than at sequential points. Next, the practitioner touches the client on each side of the body on corresponding sites at the same time. The client should be able to point to both sites. An inability to sense touch on one side is called the extinction phenomenon and is a subtle test for sensory loss.

The practitioner then touches the client in two places on the same extremity with two objects, such as cotton-tipped applicators. A person can normally identify two points fairly close together depending on the location of the stimuli. The more nerve innervation in an area, the closer the two-point discrimination.

Abnormal Sensory Findings

Abnormal sensory findings may have a peripheral nervous system (PNS) or a central nervous system (CNS) cause. The neuropathies of diabetes, malnutrition, and vascular problems are attributable to a PNS cause and generally involve the entire extremity or both extremities. Damage to a specific spinal nerve may not result in significant sensory loss because the spinal nerves overlap. Injury to several adjacent spinal nerves is manifested as decreased or absent sensation in the dermatomes of those nerves.

CNS problems can occur within the spinal cord, the brainstem, the cerebellum, and the cerebral cortex. Sensory deficits attributable to spinal cord damage vary with the location of the damage. Involvement of only the posterior column leads to lost proprioception below the level of the damage on the same side or on both sides (if both the right and left posterior columns are involved). A lesion involving only the right spinothalamic tract results in a loss of pain and temperature sensation below the lesion on the *left* side. Problems in the brainstem, thalamus, and cortex generally result in loss of sensation on the *contralateral* (opposite) side of the body. Cerebellar lesions affect sensation on the *same* side of the body.

ASSESSMENT OF MOTOR FUNCTION

Throughout the physical assessment, the nurse observes the client for involuntary tremors or movements. Such movements need to be characterized as accurately as possible, such as "pill rolling with the thumbs and fingers at rest" or "intention tremors of both hands" (tremors that occur when the client tries to do something).

Muscle Strength

The nurse measures hand strength by asking the client to grasp and squeeze two fingers of each of the nurse's hands. The nurse then compares the grasps for equality of strength. As another means of evaluating strength, the nurse tries to withdraw the fingers from the client's grasp and compares the ease or difficulty. The client should release the grasps on command—another assessment of consciousness and the ability to follow commands.

The nurse usually tests the client's strength against resistance by asking him or her to resist the nurse's bending or straightening of the arm, hand, leg, or foot being tested (Figure 41-11). A five-point rating scale is commonly used (see Chapter 50, Table 50-1). Test results are sometimes recorded as 5/5, 3/5, and so forth, indicating the criteria that were used and the status of the client at that testing. The nurse must evaluate and compare strength on each side. Later testing results are compared with previous results to indicate progress or regression.

Cerebral/Brainstem Integrity

Cerebral motor or brainstem integrity may also be assessed. The nurse asks the client to close the eyes and hold the arms perpendicular to the body with the palms up for 15 to 30 seconds. If there is a cerebral or brainstem reason for muscle weakness, the arm on the weak side will start to fall, or "drift," with the palm pronating (turning inward). This is called a "pronator drift." The same can be done for the lower extremities, with the client lying on his or her stomach with the legs bent upward at the knees. However, it is easier for most clients to sit on the side of the bed and extend the legs outward.

Abnormal Motor Findings

Peripheral motor problems are caused by injury, neuropathies, vascular problems, or a localized lesion in the opposite motor cortex. Tremors, unintentional movements, and changes in gait or posture represent problems in the basal ganglia or specialized nuclei of the brainstem or cerebellum. Motor cortex lesions, such as strokes, cause weakness or paralysis on the contralateral side of the body.

ASSESSMENT OF CEREBELLAR FUNCTION

Coordination

Most of the assessment of cerebellar function can be performed with the client sitting on the side of the bed or examining table. Fine coordination of muscle activity is tested. The

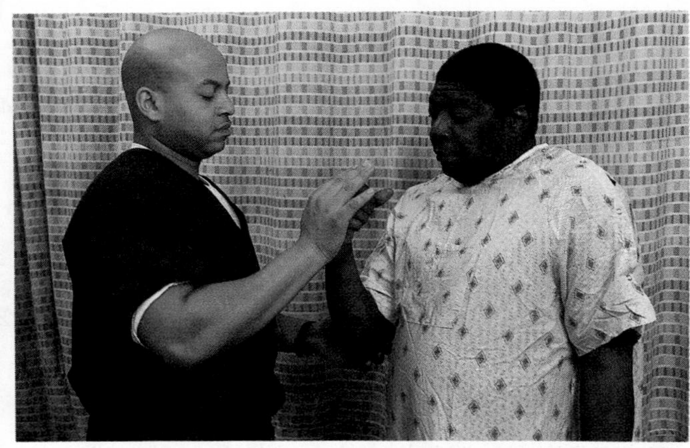

Figure 41-11 ● Testing for strength against resistance.

health care provider asks the client to perform the following with his or her eyes closed:

- Run the heel of one foot down the shin of the other leg, and repeat with the other leg (the client should be able to do this smoothly and keep the heel on the shin).
- Place the hands palm-up and then palm-down on each thigh, repeating as fast as possible (this can normally be done rapidly).
- With arms out at the side, touch the finger to the nose two or three times, with eyes open and then with eyes closed (this can be done with alternating arms or with each arm individually).

Gait and Equilibrium

For the last part of the cerebellar assessment, the ambulatory client stands for testing of gait and equilibrium. Gait and equilibrium are usually tested at the end of the entire neurologic assessment. First, the practitioner asks the client to walk across the room, turn, and return. The client is observed for inequality in steps, difficulty maneuvering, and so forth. To evaluate balance, the client is asked to stand on one foot and then on the other. Tiptoe walking and heel-to-toe walking can also demonstrate gait problems.

To test equilibrium, the client is asked to stand with arms at the sides, feet and knees close together, and eyes open. The practitioner checks for swaying and then asks the client to close his or her eyes and maintain position. The examiner should be close enough to prevent falling if the client cannot stay erect. If the client sways with the eyes closed but not when the eyes are open (the **Romberg sign**), the problem is probably **proprioceptive** (awareness of body position). If the client sways with the eyes both open and closed, the neurologic disturbance is probably *cerebellar* in origin.

If the client is not able to perform any of these activities smoothly, the problem is manifested on the same side as the cerebellar lesion. If both lobes of the cerebellum are involved, the incoordination is bilateral.

ASSESSMENT OF REFLEX ACTIVITY

Procedure

The health care provider assesses deep tendon reflexes (DTRs) and superficial (cutaneous) reflexes (Table 41-8). The *deep tendon reflexes* of the biceps, triceps, brachioradialis, and quadriceps muscles and of the Achilles tendon can be tested as part of the routine neurologic assessment. Striking the tendon with the hammer should cause contraction of the muscle (Figure 41-12). The appropriate muscle contraction indicates an intact reflex arc. The tendon is tapped quickly but not with too much force. If the client is tensing the muscle, the reflexes cannot be elicited. Having the client interlock his or her hands and pull outward will help to decrease muscle tensing so the reflex can be tested.

The *cutaneous* (superficial) reflexes usually tested are the plantar reflexes and sometimes the abdominal reflexes. The plantar reflex is tested with a pointed (but not sharp) object, such as the handle end of the reflex hammer or the rounded end of bandage scissors. The sole of the client's foot is stroked from the heel, up the lateral side, and then across the ball of the foot to the medial side. The normal response is plantar flexion of all

TABLE 41-8 • DEEP TENDON AND SUPERFICIAL REFLEXES

DEEP TENDON REFLEXES	SUPERFICIAL REFLEXES
• Jaw closure	• Corneal
• Biceps	• Palatal
• Triceps	• Pharyngeal
• Brachioradialis	• Abdominal (upper and lower)
• Patellar	• Cremasteric
• Achilles	• Gluteal
	• Plantar
	• Gag

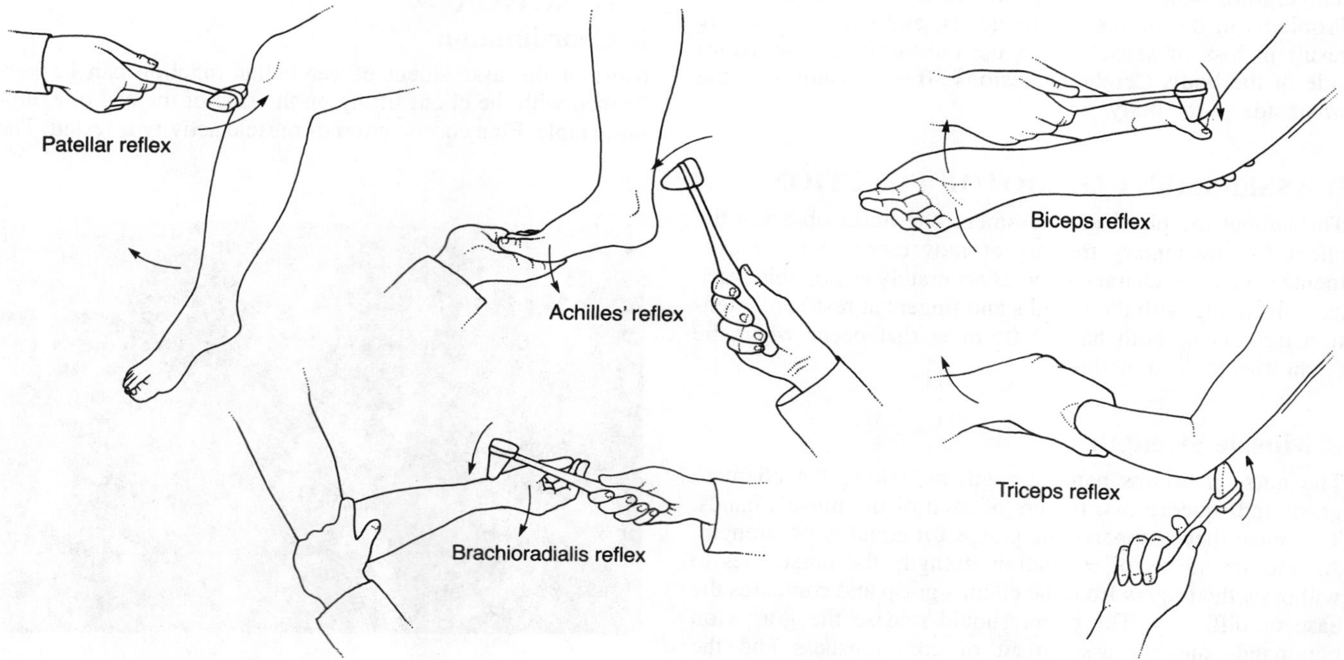

Figure 41-12 • Procedures for testing deep tendon reflexes.

toes. Dorsiflexion of the great toe and fanning of the other toes (Babinski's sign) is abnormal in anyone older than 2 years and represents the presence of central nervous system (CNS) disease. The term "positive Babinski's sign" (abnormal response) and "negative Babinski's sign" (normal response) are clinically used terms but are not correct. Babinski's sign is a pathologic reflex. Health care providers may also use the terms "upgoing" or "downgoing" to refer to the toes of the stimulated foot. "Upgoing" toes is an abnormal response that indicates the presence of pathology in the CNS. Babinski's sign can occur with drug and alcohol intoxication or after a seizure.

To test the abdominal reflex, the practitioner strokes the client's abdomen in all four quadrants diagonally toward the umbilicus. The umbilicus should deviate toward the stimulus, but obesity may mask the reflex. The abdominal reflex can be absent in both upper and lower motor neuron disease.

Abnormal Reflex Findings

Hyperactive reflexes indicate possible upper motor neuron disease, tetanus, or hypocalcemia. Hypoactive reflexes may result from lower motor neuron disease (damage to the spinal cord), disease of the neuromuscular junction, muscle disease, or metabolic diseases such as diabetes mellitus, hypothyroidism, or hypokalemia.

Although people can display hyperactive, hypoactive, or even absent reflexes, *asymmetry* is an important finding because it probably indicates a disease process. The results of reflex testing are recorded by the use of a stick figure and a scale of 0 to 4 (Figure 41-13). A score of 2 (++) is considered normal, although scores of 1 (hypoactive) or 3 (stronger than normal) may be normal for a particular client. **Clonus** is the sudden, brief, jerking contraction of a muscle or muscle group often seen in seizures.

RAPID NEUROLOGIC ASSESSMENT

The nurse performs a neurologic assessment when the client is admitted to a health care facility on an emergent basis. The nurse may perform a rapid neurologic "neuro" assessment as part of the client's routine or ongoing assessment or in the event of a sudden change in neurologic status.

A form of the Glasgow Coma Scale (GCS) (Figure 41-14) is used in many health care agencies. This tool has been shown to be reliable as one measure of neurologic assessment. Some agencies may use the GCS along with other assessment findings for a more comprehensive picture of the client's condition.

The GCS establishes baseline data in each of the following areas: eye opening, motor response, and verbal response. The client is assessed and assigned a numerical score for each of these areas. A score of 15 represents normal neurologic functioning; a score of 3 represents a deep coma state.

The nurse must use the most appropriate stimulus for eliciting a response. If the client is not awake and responding to commands, it may be necessary to use painful stimuli to obtain the best response. The client's response to central pain (brain response) is assessed first. On the basis of this response, peripheral pain may be assessed. Failure to apply painful stimuli appropriately may lead to an erroneous conclusion about the client's neurologic status.

Response to Painful Stimuli

To apply painful stimuli, the nurse starts with the least noxious irritation or pressure and proceeds to more painful stimulation if the client does not respond. The nurse begins each phase of the assessment by speaking to the client in a normal voice; if no response is obtained, the nurse uses a loud voice.

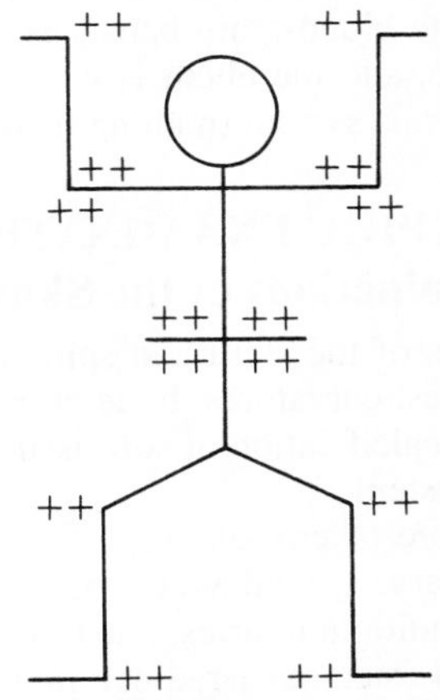

0	Absent, no response
1 (+)	Weaker than normal, hypoactive
2 (++)	Normal
3 (+++)	Stronger or more brisk than normal
4 (++++)	Hyperactive
	(Note: 1 and 3 may be normal for some individuals)

Figure 41-13 ● A stick figure and scale for recording reflex activity.

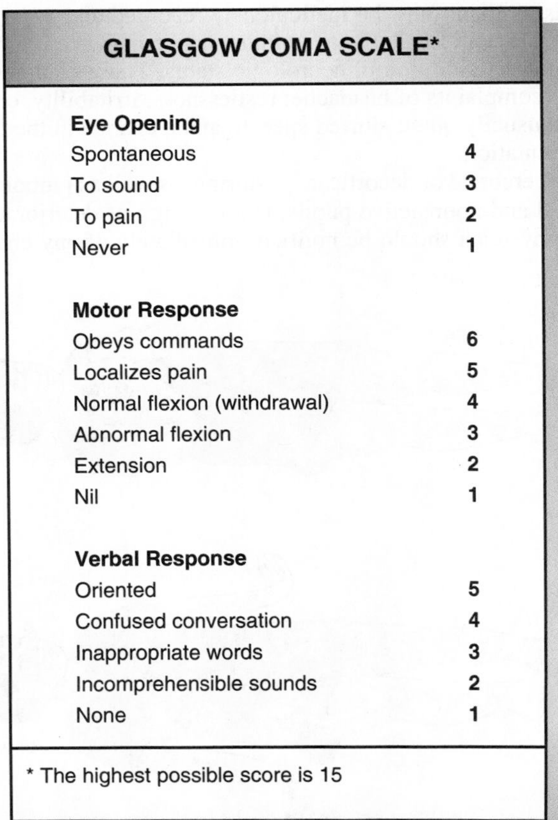

GLASGOW COMA SCALE*	
Eye Opening	
Spontaneous	4
To sound	3
To pain	2
Never	1
Motor Response	
Obeys commands	6
Localizes pain	5
Normal flexion (withdrawal)	4
Abnormal flexion	3
Extension	2
Nil	1
Verbal Response	
Oriented	5
Confused conversation	4
Inappropriate words	3
Incomprehensible sounds	2
None	1

* The highest possible score is 15

Figure 41-14 ● The Glasgow Coma Scale. The highest possible score is 15.

If the client does not respond, the nurse gently shakes him or her. The shaking should be similar to that used in attempting to wake up a child. If that is unsuccessful, painful stimuli are applied. First, the nurse applies supraorbital pressure by placing a thumb under the orbital rim in the middle of the eyebrow and pushing upward. This technique is not used if the client has orbital or facial fractures.

A second technique to elicit pain is to pinch the trapezius muscle located at the angle of the shoulder and neck muscle. If the client remains unresponsive, the nurse rubs the sternum. The nurse makes a fist and rubs the knuckles of the hand against the sternum in a twisting motion. The tissue in this area is tender, and bruising is not unusual. Therefore the nurse must exercise judgment regarding the value of the information gained from frequent or prolonged sternal rubs.

The client may respond to painful stimuli in several ways. Although the initial response to pain may be abnormal flexion or extension, continued application of pain for no more than 20 to 30 seconds may demonstrate that he or she can localize or withdraw. If the client does not respond after 20 to 30 seconds, it is not necessary to continue applying the painful stimulus.

If the client responds by moving, but not all extremities move, the nurse assesses the peripheral response to pain. The nurse places a pen or pencil on top of the client's nail bed at the base of the cuticle and applies pressure. This maneuver is performed only on the extremity that did not move.

Level of Consciousness

In addition to using the Glasgow Coma Scale, the nurse assesses the client's level of consciousness (LOC). This area of the assessment must be meticulously recorded and described as a change in LOC. Even a subtle change is the first indicator of a deterioration in neurologic status. These changes include complaints of headache; restlessness, irritability, or being unusually quiet; slurred speech; and a change in the level of orientation.

Decerebrate or decorticate posturing, as well as pinpoint or dilated and nonreactive pupils, is a late sign of deterioration. The physician should be notified immediately of any change in the client's status. Decortication is abnormal posturing seen in the client with lesions that interrupt the corticospinal pathways (Figure 41-15, *A*). The client's arms, wrists, and fingers are flexed with internal rotation and plantar flexion of the legs. Decerebration is abnormal posturing and rigidity characterized by extension of the arms and legs, pronation of the arms, plantar flexion, and opisthotonos (Figure 41-15, *B*). Decerebration is usually associated with dysfunction in the brainstem area.

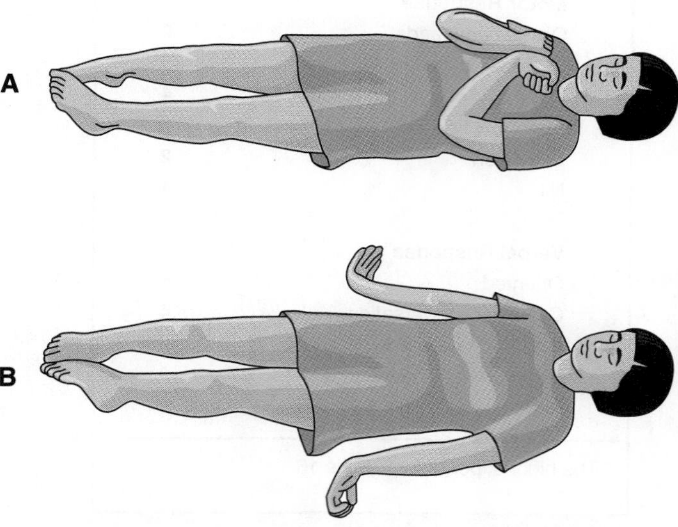

Figure 41-15 ● Posturing. **A,** Decorticate posturing. **B,** Decerebrate posturing.

Pupil Assessment

The client's pupils are assessed as part of ongoing "neuro" checks. Pupil constriction is a function of cranial nerve III. *P*upils should be *e*qual in size, *r*ound and *r*egular in shape, and react to *l*ight and *a*ccommodation (PERRLA). The nurse estimates the size of both pupils using a millimeter ruler. Clients who have had eye surgery for cataracts or glaucoma often have irregularly shaped pupils. Clients using eyedrops for either cataracts or glaucoma may have unequal pupils if only one eye is being treated, and the pupillary response may be altered.

To test for pupil constriction, the client should be asked to close his or her eyes. The nurse brings a penlight in from the side of the client's head and shines the light in the eye being tested as soon as the client opens his or her eyes. The pupil should constrict **(direct response);** the other eye should also constrict slightly **(consensual response).** To test accommodation, the client focuses on a distant object and then immediately focuses on an object 4 to 5 inches from the nose. The eyes should converge, and the pupils should constrict.

Diagnostic Assessment

LABORATORY TESTS

For clients with a neurologic problem resulting from or concomitant with systemic infection, blood cultures are necessary to identify the causative agent of the infection. Although the cause of infection must be determined for any client, this is especially true for clients with central nervous system (CNS) disease. The blood-brain barrier is often not intact in neurologic disease, and the client is more susceptible to infection of the nervous system (meningitis or encephalitis).

RADIOGRAPHIC EXAMINATIONS

X-Ray Examinations of the Skull and Spine

Plain x-ray studies of the skull and spine are used to determine bony fractures, curvatures, bone erosion, bone dislocation, and possible calcification of soft tissue, which can damage the nervous system.

Several views are taken—anteroposterior, lateral, oblique and, when necessary, special views of the facial bones. In head trauma and multiple injuries, one of the first priorities is to rule out cervical fracture by radiography.

The nurse explains that the x-ray procedure for the skull and spine is similar to that for a chest x-ray procedure, that the client will need to remain still during the procedure, and that the exposure to radiation is minimal. If the client is in traction and a portable x-ray unit is not available, the nurse may need to accompany him or her to assist with positioning. Any client who cannot walk from a wheelchair to the x-ray table should go to the radiology department on a stretcher. The client is positioned for each of the desired views and is asked not to move just before each x-ray. Follow-up care is not required.

Cerebral Angiography

Cerebral angiography (arteriography) illuminates the cerebral, carotid, and vertebral circulation. Contrast medium is injected into an artery (usually the femoral), and x-rays are taken sequentially as the contrast medium flows with the blood. The test is used to diagnose vascular aneurysms, arteriovenous malformations, displacements, and occluded or leaking blood vessels. It is not used as often today as other, less invasive tests.

CONTRAST MEDIA METHOD

CLIENT PREPARATION. The nurse ascertains that the client has no allergies to contrast agents, shellfish, or iodine. The procedure is initially explained to the client by the person obtaining the written consent, usually the radiologist. The nurse can clarify the explanation by answering questions and reinforcing the following important points:

- The necessity for not moving during the procedure
- The necessity for immobilization of the head
- The expectation of burning or heat sensation from the contrast medium as it is injected

The sensation lasts just a few seconds and is often noted behind the eyes or in the face. The client is allowed nothing by mouth for 8 to 12 hours before the test. Most hospitals require that the nurse complete a preoperative checklist. The nurse:

- Removes the client's hairpins, jewelry, hearing aids, and/or dentures
- Records neurologic and vital signs
- Asks the client to empty his or her bladder before the procedure
- Administers the preangiography hypnotic, sedative, or analgesic as ordered by the physician

PROCEDURE. The client is placed on an examining table and secured with straps. His or her head is placed in a headrest device or immobilized with tape. The radiologist locates the artery to be used either by cutdown or palpation and threads a catheter into the artery. Although the carotid or vertebral artery can be used, the femoral or brachial artery is preferred because there are fewer complications. Patency of the catheter is maintained with intravenous (IV) fluid.

The radiologist injects the contrast medium (usually 40 to 50 mL), and images are automatically taken as the contrast material moves through the circulation. The major risks are allergic response to the contrast medium and vasospasm, either of which may end the test. Vasospasm may be severe enough to cause occlusion and subsequent ischemia or infarction. The resultant tissue ischemia can cause hemiparesis, paralysis, or speech difficulties depending on the artery in spasm. This risk is about 0.5% to 1%. If the client has a history of allergic reactions, antihistamines or steroids may be given prophylactically before and after the test. After the catheter is removed, pressure is maintained over the puncture site for at least 5 to 10 minutes to prevent arterial bleeding.

FOLLOW-UP CARE. The nurse obtains the client's vital signs, "neuro" signs, and neurovascular checks according to hospital policy. The client is usually restricted to bedrest for several hours. The extremity into which the contrast medium was injected is kept straight and immobilized for approximately the length of the bedrest. The nurse checks the extremity for adequate circulation, which is demonstrated by the following:

- Skin color and temperature
- Pulses distal to the injection site
- Capillary refill

The nurse inspects the injection site frequently for evidence of bleeding. A pressure dressing, sandbag, ice bag, or combination of the three may be maintained over the site for at least 6 hours to prevent bleeding, swelling, or hematoma formation. The nurse checks the neurologic and vital signs frequently (every 15 to 20 minutes) for the first hour or two and compares them with the preangiography signs. If fluids are not contraindicated, oral or IV fluid intake is increased to help the client excrete the contrast material, which takes approximately 24 hours.

DIGITAL SUBTRACTION ANGIOGRAPHY

Digital subtraction angiography (DSA) is a refinement of the angiographic technique using digital computer enhancement to produce images of cerebral circulation. This technique eliminates surrounding and interfering anatomic structures.

CLIENT PREPARATION. The nurse determines whether the client has allergies to contrast agents, shellfish, or iodine. Food intake is restricted for 2 hours before the test, but fluids are not. The nurse instructs the client to remain still during the test (as for the contrast media method). A signed consent form and preoperative or preprocedural checklist is necessary. The client must empty his or her bladder. Preprocedure medication may be given to help the client relax. The nurse takes and records neurologic and vital signs before the procedure.

PROCEDURE. Because DSA is performed through the IV route, it has the advantage of causing a lower risk for bleeding or spasm. DSA can be an outpatient procedure. The radiologist threads a large angiocatheter into the brachial vein (usually) and positions it in the superior vena cava near the right atrium. IV fluid is given via a catheter. An initial x-ray image is taken and is placed in a computer as a reference for subsequent images. The radiologist then injects the contrast medium. As subsequent images appear on a screen and are transferred to the computer, the original reference image is subtracted from the later images. DSA is less invasive, is safer, poses less client risk, is more economical, and can be used in place of conventional angiography.

FOLLOW-UP CARE. The client's vital signs and neurologic signs are checked frequently. As outlined for the contrast media method, the nurse checks the extremity into which the contrast medium was injected for adequate circulation. The nurse checks the IV injection site for any bloody drainage because of the large size of the catheter. Unless it is contraindicated, the nurse encourages the client to increase fluid intake for 24 hours after the procedure to help excrete the contrast medium. There are no activity restrictions.

MYELOGRAPHY

To perform a **myelogram,** a water-based or oil-based contrast medium or dye is inserted into the subarachnoid space of the spine. A lumbar puncture is the usual insertion site. Myelography enables the vertebral column, intervertebral disks, spinal nerve roots, and blood vessels to be visualized.

After the procedure, the client is usually managed in the same manner as the client who had a lumbar puncture, which is described on p. 893. Although this test is still performed, it is becoming less popular as computed tomography (CT) and magnetic resonance imaging (MRI) replace such invasive diagnostic techniques. This procedure is usually performed as an ambulatory procedure.

Computed Tomography

Computed tomography (CT) scanning is relatively accurate and is the quickest, easiest, and least expensive method of diagnosing neurologic problems. With the aid of a computer, pictures are taken at many horizontal levels, or slices, of the brain or spinal cord. The cross-sectional slices build up three-dimensional pictures of the brain or spinal cord. A contrast medium may be used to enhance the image. CT scans distinguish bone, soft tissue (e.g., the brain, vascular system, and ventricular system), and fluids such as cerebrospinal fluid or blood. Tumors, infarctions, hemorrhage, hydrocephalus, and bone malformations can be identified.

CLIENT PREPARATION. The nurse explains the procedure and ascertains whether the client has allergies to contrast media, shellfish, or iodine. The nurse instructs the client to remove hairpins, hairpieces, or wigs. If a contrast medium is used, food is withheld for 4 to 6 hours before the test. Fluids are generally not withheld. The nurse alerts the physician if the client seems unduly anxious, fearful, or unable to cooperate. A preprocedure sedative may be ordered, although it is not usually necessary. A consent form is obtained by the health care provider.

PROCEDURE. The client is placed on a movable table. His or her head is positioned in a holding device, which is then secured. The client must remain completely still during the test, which may be difficult. The angles for the desired pictures are determined by the x-ray technician. The table is then positioned within the machine, a large cylinder-type structure. Some clients are fearful of the machine or of being confined in a small space. A noncontrast series of pictures is taken first. Contrast media enhance the visualization of the vascular system and are commonly used. Except for the IV injection of contrast media, the procedure is noninvasive. The entire procedure takes 10 minutes or less with the newer machines and 40 minutes with older machines or the use of contrast media.

FOLLOW-UP CARE. The nurse checks for a delayed allergic response to the contrast medium if it was used. If a contrast medium was used, the resultant diuresis may require the administration of replacement fluids.

Positron Emission Tomography/Single-Photon Emission Computed Tomography

Positron emission tomography (PET) scanning is a diagnostic tool currently available only in large medical centers. Its benefit over a computed tomography (CT) scan or magnetic resonance imaging (MRI) is that it provides information about the *function* of the brain, specifically glucose and oxygen metabolism and cerebral blood flow. Current CT scans and MRIs provide information about the *structure* of the central nervous system.

The physician or technician injects the client with the molecule deoxyglucose, which is tagged to an isotope. The isotope emits activity in the form of positrons, which are scanned and converted into a color image by computer. The more active a given part of the brain, the greater the glucose uptake. This test is used to evaluate drug metabolism and detect areas of metabolic alteration that occur in dementia, epilepsy, psychiatric and degenerative disorders, neoplasms, and Alzheimer's disease. The level of radiation is equivalent to that of five or six x-rays but much less than exposure during CT. Because the radioisotopes have such a short half-life, an on-site cyclotron is needed to prepare them. This need limits the number of medical centers able to offer the test.

This limitation of PET may be overcome through the use of **single-photon emission computed tomography (SPECT).** With SPECT, radionuclides that emit gamma rays are administered by IV injection or inhalation. Gamma-emitting radionuclides have longer half-lives, therefore eliminating the need for a cyclotron near the scanner. Although SPECT is less expensive than PET, the resolution of the images is limited. SPECT is particularly useful in studying cerebral blood flow, stroke, dementia, acquired immunodeficiency syndrome (AIDS), amnesia, neoplasms, trauma, seizures, a persistent vegetative state, brain death, and psychiatric disorders.

CLIENT PREPARATION. The nurse explains the test and instructs the client to withhold caffeine, alcohol, and tobacco for 24 hours before the test, according to agency policy. The client is on NPO status (nothing by mouth) for 6 to 12 hours before the procedure (if the client is diabetic, no insulin is given before the test). The nurse withholds glucose solutions and any other drugs that alter glucose metabolism.

PROCEDURE. The client is placed on a stretcher. An IV line is started to inject the isotope. An arterial line may be used to obtain blood samples. The client may be blindfolded and have earplugs inserted for all or part of the test. The total procedure takes 2 to 3 hours. The client is asked to perform certain mental functions to activate different areas of the brain.

FOLLOW-UP CARE. The radioisotope is eliminated in the urine and requires no special precautions. However, the client is encouraged to increase fluid intake. Follow-up care is not required.

OTHER DIAGNOSTIC TESTS

Magnetic Resonance Imaging

Magnetic resonance imaging (MRI) produces images considered superior to the CT scan. It does not use ionizing radiation but instead relies on magnetic fields. Considered to be the most sensitive technology for detecting abnormalities of the brain and spinal cord, MRI is often more accurate in making diagnoses. Images may be enhanced with the use of gadolinium, a non–iodine based contrast. MRIs of the spine have replaced CT scans and myelography in most instances (see Chapter 50).

CLIENT PREPARATION. A signed consent form is obtained; no food or fluid restrictions are necessary. The nurse tells the client that the procedure is noisy and that earplugs are available. In addition, the client should know that he or she will be asked to lie on a hard, cold surface inside a hollow tube. If the client is claustrophobic, a mild sedative may be administered before the procedure.

Newer, open-sided units now produce images equivalent to those of the closed units. MRI is contraindicated in clients who are confused, pregnant, or agitated; have unstable vital signs; are on continuous life support; or have implanted ferromagnetic devices (e.g., prostheses, clips, or pacemakers) or tattoos. The client is asked to remove any metals, such as watches, rings, earrings, or necklaces.

PROCEDURE. MRI uses magnets, hydrogen nuclei (protons), and the body's response to the magnetic fields to align the cells. Radiofrequency waves applied to aligned cells cause them to spin; this is known as resonance. When nuclei relax and return to their original position, small radiofrequency signals are produced. These signals are detected and interpreted by the computer and translated into cross-sectional images.

FOLLOW-UP CARE. No special postprocedure or follow-up care is required.

Lumbar Puncture

Lumbar puncture (spinal tap) is the insertion of a spinal needle into the subarachnoid space between the third and fourth (sometimes the fourth and fifth) lumbar vertebrae. A lumbar puncture is used to do the following:

- Obtain pressure readings with a manometer
- Obtain cerebrospinal fluid (CSF) for analysis
- Check for spinal blockage attributable to a spinal cord lesion
- Inject contrast medium or air for diagnostic study
- Inject spinal anesthetics
- Inject certain medications
- Reduce mild to moderate increased intracranial pressure in certain conditions

Because of the danger of sudden release of CSF pressure, a lumbar puncture is contraindicated in clients with symptoms suggestive of increased intracranial pressure (ICP). The sudden release of CSF pressure causes a sudden shift of cranial tissue known as *uncal herniation,* which results in more brain damage. The procedure is also contraindicated in clients with skin infections at or near the puncture site because of the danger of introducing infective organisms into the CSF.

CLIENT PREPARATION. An informed consent form is signed by the client. The nurse explains the procedure, noting that some discomfort may be felt when the local anesthetic is injected. Some clients experience pain in the leg when the spinal needle is inserted. The nurse asks the client to empty his or her bladder as a comfort measure. The nurse then positions the client on whichever side he or she is most comfortable, with his or her back close to the edge of the bed or examining table. When the physician or nurse practitioner is ready, the nurse asks the client to bring the knees up as close as possible to the trunk and to assume a "fetal" position (using the arms to hold the knees in place) with the head bent forward. Some clients need help in achieving and maintaining this position. To help maintain the position, the nurse grasps the client behind the knees and the back of the lower neck. A pillow under the head and between the knees aids body alignment.

PROCEDURE. The health care provider cleans the skin site thoroughly. The injection site is determined, and the local anesthetic is injected. In a few minutes, the health care provider inserts a spinal needle between the third and fourth lumbar vertebrae. The nurse instructs the client to inform the provider if there is shooting pain or a tingling sensation. After determining proper placement in the subarachnoid space by removing the stylet and seeing CSF, the client is asked to relax a little so the pressure reading will be more accurate. Opening and closing pressure readings are taken and recorded. Three to five test tubes of CSF are usually collected and numbered sequentially. After specimen collection, the needle is withdrawn, slight pressure is applied, and an adhesive bandage strip is placed over the insertion site. The nurse may or may not be able to help with the collection and numbering of the specimens, depending on the client's ability to remain quiet. If the client is restless or unable to cooperate, two people may need to assist instead of one. The nurse considers this possibility before beginning the procedure.

Examination of CSF has been a useful diagnostic tool for some time, and recent technical advances are increasing the number of analyses that can be done on CSF. The normal characteristics of CSF and some of the more common abnormalities are given in Table 41-9. Gram stain smears can test for particular types of meningitis, such as tubercular meningitis. CSF can be cultured, and sensitivity studies determine the best choice of antibiotic if an infection is diagnosed. A specific test for neurosyphilis is the fluorescent treponemal antibody absorption (FTA-ABS) test. Cytologic studies of CSF can identify tumor cells.

FOLLOW-UP CARE. After lumbar puncture, the client is restricted to bedrest in a flat position for 4 to 8 hours as prescribed by the physician or as determined by hospital policy. This prevents CSF leakage from the puncture site. In some centers today, bedrest is no longer required. The nurse instructs the client to increase fluid intake (to 3000 mL if possible) for 24 to 48 hours to facilitate CSF production. A decrease in CSF may cause a severe, throbbing headache (also called a spinal headache). The nurse administers analgesics as ordered for headache if it occurs. If the lumbar puncture was done to reduce intracranial pressure, neurologic signs (especially level of consciousness) are assessed more frequently until stability is ensured. Complications of lumbar puncture, although uncommon, include infection, CSF leakage, and hematoma formation.

Electroencephalography

Electroencephalography (EEG) records the electrical activity of the cerebral hemispheres. Each graphic recording represents the voltage changes in various areas of the brain (determined by recording the difference between two electrodes). The EEG may be normal even when a pathologic condition is present. The test is performed to:

- Determine the general activity of the cerebral hemispheres
- Determine the origin of seizure activity (epilepsy)

TABLE 41-9 • SIGNIFICANCE OF CEREBROSPINAL FLUID FINDINGS

Findings	Significance
PRESSURE	
70-180 mm H_2O (5-13 mm Hg)	Normal range
68-195 mm H_2O (4-15 mm Hg)	Upper limits of normal
COLOR/APPEARANCE	
Clear, colorless	Normal
Pink-red to orange	Red blood cells present
Yellow	Bilirubin present owing to hemolysis of red blood cells; possible causes include subarachnoid hemorrhage, jaundice, increased cerebrospinal fluid (CSF) protein, hypercarotenemia, or hemoglobinemia
Brown	Methemoglobin present, indicating previous meningeal hemorrhage
Unclear or hazy	Cell count greater than 200/mL
CELLS	
0-5 small lymphocytes/mm^3	Normal
More than 5 lymphocytes/mm^3	Reaction to infection, tumor, chemical substance, or blood
PROTEINS	
Total	
15-45 mg/100 mL (or less than 1% of serum levels)	Normal
45-100 mg/100 mL	Paraventricular tumor
50-200 mg/100 mL	Viral infection
More than 500 mg/100 mL	Bacterial infection, Guillain-Barré syndrome
Less than 15 mg/100 mL	Meningismus, pseudotumor cerebri, hyperthyroidism, normal finding after lumbar puncture
Immune Gamma Globulin (IgG, the most important protein)	
3%-12% of *total* protein	Normal
More than 3%-12% of total protein	Multiple sclerosis, neurosyphilis, or viral infection
Albumin/Globulin Ratio	
8:1	Normal
GLUCOSE	
45-80 mg/100 mL (dL)	Normal
Less than 45 mg/100 mL (usually accompanied by the presence of pathologic organisms)	Bacterial, fungal, or viral meningitis; central nervous system (CNS) leukemia; or cancer
ELECTROLYTES AND MINERALS	
Sodium	
144-154 mEq/L	Normal (abnormal values are not disease specific)
Potassium	
2.4-3.1 mEq/L	Normal (abnormal values are not disease specific)
Chloride	
118-132 mEq/L	Normal (abnormal values are not disease specific)
Calcium	
2.1-2.7 mEq/L	Normal (abnormal values are not disease specific)
OTHER CHARACTERISTICS	
Lactic Acid	
10-20 mg/100 mL	Normal
More than 10-25 ml/100 mL	Systemic acidosis or increased CSF glucose metabolism
Urea	
10-15 mg/100 mL	Normal
More than 10-15 mg/100 mL	Uremia, meningitis, or urea administration
Glutamine	
Less than 20 mg/100 mL	Normal
More than 20 mg/100 mL	Hepatic coma or cirrhosis of liver
Lactate Dehydrogenase	
10% of serum level	Normal
More than 10% of serum level	Bacterial meningitis, inflammatory diseases of CNS

- Determine cerebral function in pathologic conditions other than epilepsy, such as tumors, abscesses, cerebrovascular disease, hematomas, injury, metabolic diseases, degenerative brain disease, and drug intoxication
- Differentiate between organic and hysterical or feigned blindness or deafness
- Monitor cerebral activity during surgical anesthesia
- Diagnose sleep disorders (all-night EEG)
- Determine brain death

CLIENT PREPARATION. This test is done on an ambulatory (outpatient) basis. Chart 41-4 lists instructions for the client preparing to have an EEG.

The nurse explains the purpose of and procedure for the test. If the EEG is ordered with the client "sleep deprived," he or she should be kept awake from about 2 to 3 AM through the rest of the night. CNS depressants and stimulants are usually not administered for 24 hours before the test. The physician indicates whether anticonvulsants are to be withheld. If anticonvulsants are withheld, the nurse monitors the client for signs of seizure activity. Coffee, tea, and other stimulants are avoided, but food and other fluids may be consumed because hypoglycemia affects brain activity. The client's hair should be shampooed, clean, and free from hairpins, sprays, or oils.

PROCEDURE. The client is placed on a reclining chair or bed. According to an internationally accepted procedure, 16 to 24 electrodes are usually attached to the scalp with a jelly-like substance and connected to the machine. The physician or EEG technician places glue over the electrodes to prevent slippage. The client must lie still with his or her eyes closed during the initial recording. The rest of the test engages the client in certain activities: hyperventilation, photic stimulation, and sleep. A portable EEG may be performed at the bedside if necessary, but the preference is for the EEG to be done in a room devoid of stimuli.

Hyperventilation produces cerebral vasoconstriction and alkalosis, which increases the likelihood of seizure activity. The client is asked to breathe deeply 20 to 30 times for 3 minutes.

In *photic stimulation,* a strobe light (bright light) is placed in front of the client. Frequencies of 1 to 20 flashes per second are used with the client's eyes open and then closed. The client's seizures are photosensitive in origin. The EEG will show waves corresponding to each flash of light or waves indicating seizure activity.

Sleep is either natural or induced by an oral or IV sedative. EEG waves indicative of temporal lobe epilepsy can be demonstrated best during sleep.

Throughout the test, which takes 40 to 60 minutes, the technician watches the client closely and records any movement. These movements alter the record and must be labeled as artifacts. Examples of artifacts are tongue movement, eye blinking, muscle tenseness, and nervousness.

FOLLOW-UP CARE. If not removed in the EEG laboratory, the client removes the jelly-like substance and glue from the scalp and hair with acetone and then with shampoo. Any medications that were withheld are reinstituted. The client may need a nap if he or she was deprived of sleep before the test.

CHART 41-4

BEST PRACTICE *for* The Client Having an Electroencephalogram

- Thoroughly explain the procedure to the client.
- If the order is for the client to be "sleep deprived," tell the client to awaken about 2 to 3 AM and stay awake for the rest of the night.
- Instruct the client to avoid central nervous system depressants or stimulants; withhold anticonvulsants only if instructed by the physician.
- Tell the client not to drink caffeine-containing fluids, such as coffee or tea, on the day of the test.
- Reassure the client that the test is not dangerous or uncomfortable.
- Ask the client to wash his or her hair on the morning of the test and to remove all hairpins, sprays, or oils.
- Inform the client that the hair will need to be washed again after the test to remove the electrode glue.

Electromyography

Electromyography (EMG) records the electrical activity of peripheral nerves by testing muscle activity (see Chapter 50 for a description of client preparation, procedure, and follow-up care). Electromyography and electroneurography or nerve conduction velocity studies (NCVS) are usually used together and are referred to as electromyoneurography.

Cerebral Blood Flow Evaluation

Cerebral blood flow (CBF) can be measured in many areas of the brain with the use of radioactive substances. It is particularly useful in evaluating cerebral vasospasm. The nurse explains the test and, if drugs have previously been ordered, withholds central nervous system (CNS) depressants and stimulants for 24 hours before the test.

Because xenon readily diffuses into brain tissue, it is the most common choice as an inhaled or injected tracer. The xenon travels through the vasculature to the brain, where it is detected by external scintillation counters placed on the skull. Normal CBF is 50 to 55 mm/min/100 g of cerebral tissue. The client receives various stimuli during the test. Increases in local blood flow can be seen with any neuronal activity, such as reading, hand movement, seizures, and temperature elevation (up to 107.6° F [42° C]). Local blood flow decreases with degenerative disease, comas of metabolic origin, increased intracranial pressure, or subarachnoid hemorrhage. Follow-up care for this test is not required.

Brain Scan

The **brain scan** is a radionuclide imaging study. A radioactive substance is injected to detect certain pathologic conditions. The test is especially useful in evaluating vascular abnormalities such as aneurysms and in locating tumors, hematomas, and abscesses. As technologic advances in diagnostic testing continue, this test is being performed less frequently.

The nurse explains the test and asks the client to empty the bladder as a comfort measure. A signed consent form may be necessary, depending on agency policy.

During the procedure, the physician injects the client with a radioactive isotope, usually technetium (Tc 99m). There is a delay in the test of up to 2 hours while the brain absorbs the isotope. The client is placed on a table and must remain still with the hands at his or her side for the duration of the test. The test takes 1 to 2 hours, depending on the number of scannings used.

For follow-up care, the nurse provides fluid to promote elimination of the isotope (urine does not need special handling).

Transcranial Doppler

Intracranial hemodynamics can be evaluated through the use of the **Transcranial Doppler (TCD).** TCD does not measure cerebral blood flow or visualize the vessels, but it does measure the time needed for pulse waves to travel a specific depth and return to the skull's surface. It is particularly valuable in evaluating cerebral vasospasm. TCD is safe and repeatable and is an inexpensive alternative to angiography.

ONLINE RESOURCES

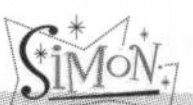

For suggested readings and Internet resources, go to http://www.wbsaunders.com/SIMON/Iggy/.

SELECTED BIBLIOGRAPHY

Asterisk indicates a classic or definitive work on this subject.

Adams, R.D., Victor, M., & Ropper, A.H. (1997). *Principles of neurology* (6th ed.). New York: McGraw-Hill.

*Bentson, J.R. (1996). Magnetic resonance imaging. In J.R. Youmans (Ed.), *Neurological surgery* (4th ed., Vol. 1). Philadelphia: W.B. Saunders.

Darovic, G. (1997). Assessing pupillary responses. *Nursing97, 27*(2), 49.

Gordon, M. (2000). *Manual of nursing diagnosis* (9th ed.). St. Louis: Mosby.

Hickey, J. (2000). *The clinical practice of neurological and neurosurgical nursing.* Philadelphia: J.B. Lippincott.

Jarvis, C. (2000). *Physical examination and health assessment* (3rd ed.). Philadelphia: W.B. Saunders.

*Martin, H.H. (1996). *Neuroanatomy text and atlas.* Philadelphia: W.B. Saunders.

Minton, M., & Hickey, J. (1999). A primer of neuroanatomy and neurophysiology. *Nursing Clinics of North America, 34*(3), 555-572.

Neatherlin, J.S. (1999). Foundation for practice: Neuroassessment for neuroscience nurses. *Nursing Clinics of North America, 34*(3), 573-592.

O'Hanlon-Nichols, T. (1999). Neurologic assessment. *American Journal of Nursing, 99*(6), 44-50.

*Raila, F.A. (1996). Radiology of the skull. In J.R. Youmans (Ed.), *Neurological surgery* (4th ed., Vol. 1). Philadelphia: W.B. Saunders.

Shpritz, D. (1999). Neurodiagnostic studies. *Nursing Clinics of North America, 34*(3), 593-606.

*Stewart, N. (1996). Neurological observation. *Professional Nurse, 11*(6), 377-378.

*Weisberg, L.A., Garcia, C., & Strub, R. (1996). *Essentials of clinical neurology.* St. Louis: Mosby.

*Wooten, C. (1996). The top ten ways to detect deteriorating central neurological status. *Journal of Trauma Nursing, 3*(1), 25-27.

*Youmans, J.R. (1996). *Neurological surgery* (4th ed., Vol. 1). Philadelphia: W.B. Saunders.

CHAPTER 42

Interventions for Clients with Problems of the Central Nervous System

The Brain

DEBORAH WRIGHT SHPRITZ

Learning Objectives

After studying this chapter, you should be able to:

1. Compare migraine and cluster headaches in terms of assessment findings.
2. Develop a teaching plan for a client diagnosed with migraine headaches.
3. Differentiate the common types of seizures, including presenting clinical manifestations and management.
4. Explain the nurse's role in implementing seizure precautions.
5. Plan and document care for a client experiencing a seizure.
6. Identify collaborative management options for treating clients diagnosed with epilepsy.
7. Outline the priorities for care of clients with meningitis and encephalitis.
8. Describe the pathophysiology of Parkinson's disease.
9. Develop a community-based plan of care for a client with Parkinson's disease.
10. Outline realistic expected outcomes for clients with Alzheimer's disease.
11. Explain the use of drug therapy for clients with Alzheimer's disease.
12. Develop a teaching plan for caregivers of clients with Alzheimer's disease in community-based settings.
13. Analyze legal/ethical concerns related to genetic counseling of children with Huntington's disease.

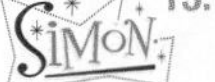

Go to http://www.wbsaunders.com/SIMON/Iggy/ for self-assessment questions related to these Learning Objectives.

Dysfunction of the brain may be a mild disorder that a person can learn to live with or a devastating disorder that drastically affects the client and the family. With newer diagnostic tools and treatment methods, the rate and the quality of recovery and rehabilitation are improving steadily. Neurologic impairment tends to involve many aspects of the person's life: the neurologic problem itself, family life alteration or disruption, occupational changes, body image and self-worth conflicts, and often, the realization of a continuous need for numerous resources.

HEADACHES

Probably few people have not experienced a headache. Headaches occur when pain-sensitive areas of the head have been stimulated, although much of the brain is not pain sensitive. In addition to a neurologic assessment of the client having a headache, psychosocial issues should be addressed because depression can be manifested as chronic headache. Two of the most common types of headaches are migraine headaches and cluster headaches. Clients are managed in the ambulatory care setting by the primary health care provider.

Migraine Headache

OVERVIEW

A **migraine headache** is an episodic familial disorder manifested by unilateral, frontotemporal, throbbing pain in the head, which is often worse behind one eye or ear. It is often accompanied by a sensitive scalp, anorexia, photophobia, and nausea with or without vomiting. Clients tend to have the same clinical manifestations each time they have a migraine headache. Some may have to refrain from regular activities for several days if they cannot control or relieve the pain in its early stage.

WOMEN'S HEALTH CONSIDERATIONS

Migraine headaches ("migraines") affect between 23 and 25 million people each year in the United States. Attacks begin in early childhood or near puberty, affect primarily females (3-to-1 predominance over males), and continue periodically, with diminishing severity, until middle age (Deraps, 2000). Menopause may cause an exacerbation. People may continue to have migraine headaches as they age, although this is not typical. Classic migraine episodes tend to increase in frequency during pregnancy, although the usual migraine incidence decreases in most pregnant women.

Several theories have emerged regarding the causes of migraines. The first, well-accepted theory is that these headaches have a vascular cause. Blood vessels in the brain dilate, causing vascular, pulsating pain. Recently, reanalysis of this theory has led to other theories suggesting a neuronal component. The pain and aura of migraines may be the result of neuronal hyperexcitability. Those neurons in the brain containing **serotonin** (5-hydroxytryptamine [5-HT]), as well as norepinephrine, are activated and start the events leading to the headache. This theory is supported by the success of medication that affects 5-HT in the brain (Deraps, 2000).

COLLABORATIVE MANAGEMENT

Assessment

The International Headache Society developed diagnostic criteria for headaches (Deraps, 2000). Migraines fall into three categories: migraines with aura, migraines without aura, and complicated migraines. *Migraines with aura,* or "classic" migraines, usually occur in three phases. *Migraines without aura,* also referred to as "neurologic" migraines, begin without an **aura** before the onset of the headache, or if present, the aura may be unrecognized as such. The signs and symptoms of both types of migraines are found in Chart 42-1. *Complicated migraines* are less common and include menstrual and cluster migraines. Menstrual migraines typically develop in a woman's early 20s and continue throughout the reproductive years. Cluster migraines occur in a series lasting 4 to 8 weeks and are separated by months or years of remission.

CHART 42-1

KEY FEATURES *of* Migraine Headaches

Phases of Migraine with Aura

First, or Prodromal, Phase

- Aura develops over a period of several minutes and lasts no more than 1 hour.
- Well-defined transient focal neurologic dysfunction exists.
- Pain may be preceded by:
  - Visual disturbances
  - Flashing lights
  - Lines or spots
  - Shimmering or zigzag lights
- Pain may be preceded by a variety of neurologic changes, including:
  - Numbness, tingling of the lips or tongue
  - Acute confusional state
  - Aphasia
  - Vertigo
  - Unilateral weakness
  - Drowsiness

Second Phase

- Headache is accompanied by nausea and vomiting.
- Pain usually begins in the temple; it increases in intensity and becomes throbbing within 1 hour.

Third Phase

- Pain changes from throbbing to dull.
- Headache, nausea, and vomiting usually last from 4 to 72 hours. (Older clients may have aura without pain, known as a visual migraine.)

Migraine Without Aura

- Migraine begins without an aura before the onset of the headache.
- Early warning is usually a mood change, such as:
  - Depression
  - Lethargy
  - Hyperactivity
  - Craving for foods
- The pain has two of four characteristics:
  - Unilateral site
  - Pulsating quality
  - Associated nausea, **photophobia** (light sensitivity), and **phonosensitivity** (sound sensitivity)
  - Headache that lasts for 4 to 72 hours
- Migraine often occurs in the early morning hours, during periods of stress, or in those with premenstrual tension or fluid retention.

Complicated Migraine

- Headache occurs with the menstrual cycle.
- Menstrual headaches occur at the time of menstruation, during the late luteal phase as the estrogen levels decrease, or at ovulation.

Interventions

The priority for interdisciplinary care of the client experiencing a migraine is pain management, which may be achieved by drug therapy and nondrug measures initiated by the health care provider or nurse.

MODIFICATION OF POTENTIAL TRIGGERING FACTORS. The nurse collaborates with the client and other health care providers to determine which factors, if any, may trigger the development of a headache. For example, monosodium glutamate, aged cheese, caffeine, chocolate, nitrites or nitrates, and red wine often trigger headaches. Many clients are sensitive to odors from cigarette or cigar smoke, paint or gasoline fumes, perfumes, or aftershave lotion.

The nurse teaches that lifestyle changes may be necessary, including regular mealtimes, sleep patterns, and exercise. Clients may also need to modify their lifestyle to decrease stress if stress is a contributing factor to migraine attacks.

DRUG THERAPY. The health care provider may prescribe drug therapy to prevent and treat (abort) migraine headaches. Headaches that occur more frequently than two to three times a month require preventive therapy.

PREVENTIVE THERAPY. Unless otherwise contraindicated, the health care provider may initially prescribe a nonsteroidal anti-inflammatory drug (NSAID), a beta-adrenergic blocker, or a calcium channel blocker. Propranolol (Inderal, Apo-Propranolol✤, Novopranol✤) and timolol (Blocadren, Apo-Timol✤) are the only beta blockers approved for migraine prophylaxis, but others are also effective (Table 42-1).

TABLE 42-1 • COMMONLY USED DRUGS FOR MIGRAINE HEADACHE

PREVENTIVE (PROPHYLACTIC) DRUGS	ABORTIVE DRUGS
Nonsteroidal Anti-inflammatory Drugs (NSAIDs) • Aspirin • Ibuprofen • Naproxen • Flurbiprofen	*Analgesics* • Aspirin • Acetaminophen
Beta Blockers • Propranolol • Timolol • Metoprolol • Nadolol	*NSAIDs* • Naproxen • Ibuprofen • Flurbiprofen
Calcium Channel Blockers • Verapamil • Nifedipine	*Ergotamine Preparations* • Ergotamine with caffeine (oral or suppository) • Ergotamine metered dose inhaler (MDI) or sublingual (SL) • Dihydroergotamine (DHE)
Antidepressants • Amitriptyline • Fluoxetine • Nortriptyline	*Triptan Preparations* • Sumatriptan tablets, injection, or nasal spray • Naratriptan • Rizatriptan • Zolmitriptan

TREATMENT OF HEADACHES. Abortive drugs aimed at alleviating pain after the headache has started include ergotamine tartrate (Cafergot), acetaminophen (Tylenol, Abenol♣), and NSAIDs, such as naproxen (Naprosyn, Novo-Naprox♣). The health care provider may order antiemetics, such as prochlorperazine (Compazine), to help control nausea and vomiting.

The triptan preparations are the newest group of drugs used for migraines. These drugs activate the 5-HT (serotonin) receptors on the cranial arteries, the basilar artery, and the vasculature of the dura mater to produce a vasoconstrictive effect. Sumatriptan succinate (Imitrex) is given or self-administered for acute migraine relief. It is available in tablets, as a subcutaneous injection, or as a nasal spray. Newer drugs in this category include rizatriptan (Maxalt), naratriptan (Naramig♣), and zolmitriptan (Zomig)—all available as tablets. For many clients, these drugs are highly effective for pain, nausea, vomiting, and light and sound sensitivity with few side effects. Most are contraindicated in clients with actual or suspected ischemic heart disease or in those with Prinzmetal's angina because of the potential of coronary vasospasm.

Dihydroergotamine (DHE) may be given intravenously or intramuscularly, along with an antiemetic, if satisfactory pain control and relief of nausea is not achieved with other medications. Table 42-1 lists commonly used medications for migraine headaches. This table is not inclusive; new medications are introduced on the market regularly.

COMPLEMENTARY AND ALTERNATIVE THERAPIES. At the beginning of a migraine attack, clients may be able to alleviate pain if they lie down and darken the room. They may want their eyes covered as well and should be allowed to sleep undisturbed until awakening.

The nurse explores the possibility of using behavior therapy in conjunction with drug therapy. Behavior therapy includes biofeedback, exercise classes, and relaxation techniques, which are generally offered in a center such as a specialized headache clinic (see Chapter 4). Often a combination of these alternative methods is recommended for best results. These resources are becoming more available and may be paid for by managed care companies. The programs enable clients to actively participate in their pain control and usually give them a chance to interact with others with the same or similar problems. Knowing that they are not alone may help relieve fear and allow them an opportunity to exchange ideas with others.

A number of herbs are also used for headaches, both for prevention and pain management. Table 42-2 describes commonly used herbs for migraines.

TABLE 42-2 • COMMONLY USED HERBS FOR MIGRAINE HEADACHES

- Feverfew *(Tanacetum pathenium)*
- Bay *(Laurus nobilis)*
- Willow *(Salix)*
- Ginger *(Zingiber officinale)*
- Red pepper *(Capsicum)*
- Lemon balm *(Melissa officinalis)*
- Purslane *(Portulaca oleracea)*

MIGRAINE MENTORS PROGRAM. In an effort to help women receive an earlier diagnosis and relief from migraines, the National Headache Foundation and AstraZeneca created the Migraine Mentors program. Although not available throughout the United States, this unique program brings together women with migraines through education, public outreach, and support.

Cluster Headache

OVERVIEW

The **cluster headache,** also referred to as histamine cephalalgia, is less common than the migraine headache. It occurs six times more frequently in young adult men between 20 and 50 years of age than in women, and it generally begins in the third or fourth decade of life.

The pain of these unilateral (one-sided), oculotemporal, or oculofrontal headaches is often described as excruciating, boring, and nonthrobbing. The intense pain is felt deep in and around the eye. The headaches occur every 8 to 12 hours and up to 24 hours daily at the same time for about 6 to 8 weeks (hence the term *cluster*), followed by a period of remission for 9 months to a year. This episodic form is the most common, although there is a chronic form in which there may not be a remission for more than a year. The average duration of each headache is 10 to 45 minutes.

The headache is accompanied by **ipsilateral** (same side) tearing of the eye, **rhinorrhea** ("runny nose") or congestion, ptosis (drooping eyelid), eyelid edema, facial sweating, and miosis (abnormal constriction of pupils). The ptosis may become permanent. There may be bradycardia, flushing or pallor of the face, increased intraocular pressure, and increased skin temperature.

The pain may radiate to the forehead, temple, or cheek; it may also radiate, but to a lesser extent, to the ear, occiput, and neck. The temporal artery may be prominent and tender. Physical activity during the attack consists of pacing, walking, or sitting and rocking. A cluster is the only headache type in which this behavior occurs. During periods of remission, alcohol does not induce a headache (as it does during the headache period). The onset of the headache is associated with relaxation, napping, or rapid eye movement (REM) sleep.

The cause and mechanism of cluster headaches is unknown. There is no genetic or family link, diet has no effect, and the disorder is unrelated to personality type.

➤ COLLABORATIVE MANAGEMENT

The nurse asks the client about prescribed and nonprescribed drugs for both the prevention and the alleviation of the headache, as well as over-the-counter drugs he or she may be taking. Interventions used by the client may include relaxation techniques, meditation, acupuncture, or massage therapies. The client is asked to recall a typical week's activities and any recent changes in lifestyle, and specifically to identify bedtimes and waking times, which helps the nurse assess changes in activity or lack of continuity in the sleep-wake cycle.

Pain control may be accomplished by drug and nondrug measures initiated by the nurse. The client's understanding of the preventive measures is important in the management of cluster headaches.

Drug Therapy

The health care provider typically prescribes the same types of drugs used for migraines. Because an informed person is better able to comply with the therapeutic plan, the nurse instructs the client in all aspects of the drugs being taken.

Other Pain Relief Measures

During the periods of attack, the nurse instructs the client to wear sunglasses and to sit facing away from the window, which helps to decrease exposure to light and glare. If the health care provider orders oxygen, the nurse or assistive nursing personnel gives 100% oxygen via mask at 5 L/min with the client in a sitting position. The oxygen is administered for no longer than 15 minutes and is discontinued when the headache is relieved. Oxygen reduces cerebral blood flow and inhibits activity of the carotid bodies, which are sensitive to oxygen levels in the body. To prevent future attacks brought on by precipitating factors, the nurse discusses the relationship among such factors (bursts of anger, prolonged anticipation, excessive physical activity, and excitement), the postactivity period, and the onset of cluster headaches. The nurse also explains the necessity and importance of a consistent sleep-wake cycle.

EPILEPSY

OVERVIEW

Epilepsy is a chronic disorder characterized by recurrent, unprovoked seizure activity and may be inherited. It is the result of brain or central nervous system (CNS) irritation. A **seizure** is an abnormal, sudden, excessive discharge of electrical activity within the brain. Epilepsy affects 2.3 million Americans, with the highest incidence in older adults and children (Hickey, 1997). In spite of intense public education programs, social barriers and discriminatory practices against people who have seizures continue to exist.

Primary or idiopathic epilepsy is not associated with any identifiable brain lesion. Secondary epilepsy results from an underlying brain lesion, most commonly a tumor or trauma. Seizures may also be caused by metabolic disorders, acute alcohol withdrawal, electrolyte disturbances (e.g., hyperkalemia, water intoxication, hypoglycemia), and heart disease. Seizures resulting from these problems are not considered epilepsy (McNew, Hunt, & Warner, 1997). Certain risk factors can trigger a seizure, such as increased physical activity, emotional stress, excessive fatigue, alcohol or caffeine consumption, or certain foods or chemicals.

Types of Seizures

The International Classification of Epileptic Seizures recognizes three broad categories of seizure disorders: generalized seizures, partial seizures, and unclassified seizures (Table 42-3).

GENERALIZED SEIZURES

Six types of **generalized seizures** may occur and involve both cerebral hemispheres. The **tonic-clonic seizure** (formerly called a *grand mal* seizure), lasting 2 to 5 minutes, begins with a tonic phase that is characterized by stiffening or rigidity of the muscles, particularly of the arms and legs, and immediate loss of consciousness. It is followed by clonic or rhythmic jerking of all extremities. The client may bite his or her tongue and may become incontinent of urine or feces. Fatigue, confusion, and lethargy may last up to an hour after the seizure.

Occasionally, only tonic or clonic movement may occur. Tonic seizures are characterized by an abrupt increase in muscle tone, loss of consciousness, and loss of autonomic signs lasting from 30 seconds to several minutes. The clonic seizure lasts several minutes and is characterized by muscle contraction and relaxation.

The **absence seizure,** previously referred to as a *petit mal* seizure, is more common in children. It consists of brief (often just seconds) periods of loss of consciousness and blank staring, as though the person is daydreaming. The client returns to baseline immediately after the seizure.

The **myoclonic seizure** is characterized by a brief jerking or stiffening of the extremities, which may occur singly or in

TABLE 42-3 • CLASSIFICATION OF SEIZURE DISORDERS

GENERALIZED SEIZURES
- Absence (petit mal)
- Generalized tonic-clonic (grand mal)
- Myoclonic
- Atonic
- Clonic
- Tonic

PARTIAL SEIZURES (FOCAL SEIZURES)
- Simple partial
- Complex partial

UNCLASSIFIED SEIZURES*

*Incomplete data.

groups. Lasting for just a few seconds, the contractions may be symmetric or asymmetric.

The ***atonic (akinetic) seizure*** (formerly known as a drop attack), is characterized by a sudden loss of muscle tone, lasting for seconds, followed by postictal confusion. In most cases, these seizures cause the client to fall.

PARTIAL SEIZURES

Partial seizures, also called *focal* seizures, begin in a part of one cerebral hemisphere. They are further subdivided into two main classes: complex partial seizures and simple partial seizures. They are most often seen in adults and generally are less responsive to medical treatment.

Complex partial seizures cause the client to lose consciousness, or black out, for 1 to 3 minutes. Characteristic behavior known as automatisms (the client is not aware of the behavior) may occur, such as lip smacking, patting, picking at clothes, and so forth. In the period after the seizure, the client may experience amnesia. Because the area of the brain most often involved in this type of epilepsy is the temporal lobe, complex partial seizures are often called *psychomotor* seizures or *temporal lobe* seizures.

The client with a simple partial seizure remains conscious throughout the episode. He or she often reports an aura (unusual sensation) before the seizure takes place. This may consist of a deja vu phenomenon, perception of an offensive smell, or sudden onset of pain. During the seizure, the client may have unilateral movement of an extremity, experience unusual sensations, or have autonomic or psychic symptoms. Autonomic changes include a change in heart rate, skin flushing, and epigastric discomfort.

UNCLASSIFIED SEIZURES

Unclassified, or idiopathic, seizures account for about half of all seizure activity. They occur for no known reason and do not fit into the generalized or partial classifications.

COLLABORATIVE MANAGEMENT

Assessment

A complete description of the type of seizure activity that occurs and events surrounding the seizure assists in determining the best treatment plan. The nurse or other health care provider obtains information from the client and family or significant others regarding the presence of an aura before the seizure **(preictal phase).**

Interventions

Secondary epilepsy and seizures that are not considered epileptic are managed by removing or treating the underlying condition or cause of the seizure. In most cases, primary epilepsy is managed through drug therapy.

NONSURGICAL MANAGEMENT. Most seizures can be completely or almost completely controlled through the administration of antiepileptic drugs (AEDs), sometimes referred to as anticonvulsants, for specific types of seizures. The nurse plays an important role in drug therapy and seizure management.

DRUG THERAPY. Drug therapy is the major component of management (Chart 42-2). Generally, the health care provider introduces one drug at a time to achieve seizure control. If the chosen drug is not effective, the dosage may be increased or another drug introduced. At times, seizure control is achieved only through a combination of medications. The dosage of medications is adjusted to achieve therapeutic blood levels without causing major side effects.

The nurse administers the medications on time to maintain therapeutic blood levels and maximal effectiveness. The client is instructed to avoid drugs and foods that might interfere with the absorption or metabolism of the AED. For instance, warfarin (Coumadin, Warfilone✤) should not be given with phenytoin (Dilantin). In addition, the nurse observes for side and adverse effects of the prescribed medications.

CONSIDERATIONS FOR OLDER ADULTS

Epilepsy is especially likely to affect older adults secondary to cerebrovascular disease, metabolic changes, and head trauma. It is especially important to monitor older clients' medication closely because of changes in metabolism and elimination of epileptic drugs associated with aging. Older adults are at risk for adverse drug reactions from the epilepsy medication itself or other medications prescribed to treat concurrent medical problems.

SEIZURE PRECAUTIONS. When a client has a history of seizures, the nurse takes precautions to prevent him or her from injury if a seizure occurs. Seizure precautions vary, depending on health care agency policy. In most agencies it is recommended that oxygen and suctioning equipment with an airway be readily available. It is also appropriate to insert a saline lock in hospitalized clients who do not have an intravenous (IV) access and are at significant risk for generalized tonic-clonic seizures. The saline lock provides ready access if IV medication must be given to stop the seizure.

The use of padded siderails is controversial. Although the siderails are rarely the source of significant injury, they should be in the "up" position at all times. More important, padded siderails may embarrass the client and the family. The bed is kept in the lowest position in case the client falls out of bed.

Padded tongue blades do not belong at the bedside and should never be inserted into the client's mouth after a seizure begins, because the jaw may clench down as soon as the seizure begins. Forcing a tongue blade or airway into the mouth is more likely to chip the teeth and increase the risk of aspiration of tooth fragments than to prevent the client from biting the tongue. Furthermore, improper placement of a padded tongue blade can obstruct the airway.

SEIZURE MANAGEMENT. The actions taken by the nurse should be appropriate for the type of seizure. For example, for a simple partial seizure, the nurse may only have to observe, document, and time the length of the seizure. The client engaged in activities that may cause harm is directed away from the activity. The client who loses consciousness during a seizure, usually during a generalized tonic-clonic or complex partial seizure, should be turned on the side (Chart 42-3). If possible, the nurse turns the client's head to the side to prevent aspiration and allow secretions to drain. The nurse removes any objects that might injure the client.

CHART 42-2

DRUG THERAPY *for* Commonly Used Antiepileptic Drugs

Drug	Indication for Use	Nursing Implications
Carbamazepine (Tegretol, Tegretol-XR, Carbatrol)	Partial, generalized tonic-clonic seizures	Give with meals. Monitor for headache, dizziness, diplopia or blurred vision, N/V, and leukopenia. Monitor CBC. Do not crush or chew sustained-release capsules.
Valproate (Depakote); valproate sodium injection (Depacon)	Simple and complex absence seizures Adjunct therapy for partial complex and generalized tonic-clonic seizures	Monitor for hair loss, tremor, increased liver enzymes, bruising, and N/V Monitor CBC, PT, PTT, AST.
Diazepam (Valium, Apo-Diazepam✤); lorazepam (Ativan); diastat (Valium rectal gel delivery system)	Status epilepticus	Monitor for respiratory distress if given IV. Monitor VS carefully.
Divalproex (Depakote); valproic acid (Depakene)	All types of seizures	Monitor for hair loss, tremor, increased liver enzymes, bruising, and N/V. Monitor CBC, PT, PTT, and AST.
Ethosuximide (Zarontin)	Absence seizures	Watch for N/V, skin rash, lethargy, and anorexia. Monitor CBC and liver function tests. (Used infrequently.)
Felbamate (Felbatol)	Adjunct therapy for intractable complex partial seizures	Aplastic anemia and liver failure are major sequelae of treatment. Client must sign consent for use, acknowledging risk for aplastic anemia and liver failure. Monitor CBC. Monitor liver function tests. Watch for anorexia and weight loss.
Gabapentin (Neurontin)	Partial seizures	Watch for increased appetite and weight gain. Monitor for ataxia, irritability, dizziness, and fatigue.
Lamotrigine (Lamictal)	Partial seizures	Watch for diplopia, headaches, dizziness, drowsiness, ataxia, N/V, and life-threatening rash when given with valproic acid.
Phenobarbital (Barbita, Luminal)	Generalized tonic-clonic seizures, partial seizures	Less desirable than other antiepileptic drugs (AEDs) because of sedation. Overdose can be fatal. Monitor for drowsiness, sleep disturbances, cognitive impairment, and depression.
Phenytoin (Dilantin); fosphenytoin (Cerebyx)	All types, except absence, myoclonic, and atonic seizures; for status epilepticus	Monitor for gastric distress, gingival hyperplasia, anemia, ataxia, and nystagmus. Check CBC and calcium levels. For IV phenytoin, flush catheter with saline before and after administration. For fosphenytoin, use phenytoin equivalent for dosing.
Primidone (Mysoline, Sertan✤)	Partial seizures, generalized tonic-clonic seizures	Monitor for vertigo and lethargy. Watch for drug interactions with phenobarbital and isoniazid.
Topiramate	Adjunct therapy for intractable partial seizures	Monitor for ataxia, confusion, dizziness, and fatigue. Increased risk for renal calculi.
Tiagabine (Gabatril)	Partial seizures	Monitor for dizziness, weakness, nervousness, psychomotor slowing, nystagmus, and paresthesias. Administer with food.

N/V, Nausea and vomiting; *CBC,* complete blood count; *PT,* prothrombin time; *PTT,* partial thromboplastin time; *AST,* aspartate aminotransferase.

It is not unusual for the client to become cyanotic during a generalized tonic-clonic seizure. The cyanosis is generally self-limiting, and no treatment is needed. Some health care providers prefer to give the high-risk client (e.g., older adult; critically ill or debilitated client) oxygen by nasal cannula or face mask during the **postictal phase.** He or she is not restrained, because this may cause injury and may exacerbate (worsen) the situation, causing more seizure activity. However, the client with atonic seizures may benefit from wearing a protective vest to keep from falling when sitting in a chair. For any type of seizure, the nurse carefully observes the seizure and documents assessment findings (Chart 42-4).

ACUTE SEIZURE AND STATUS EPILEPTICUS MANAGEMENT. Seizures occurring in greater intensity, number, or length than the client's usual seizures are considered acute. They may also appear in clusters that are different from the client's typical seizure pattern (Shafer, 1999). Treatment with

CHART 42-3

BEST PRACTICE *for*
Care of the Client During a Tonic-Clonic or Complete Partial Seizure

- Protect the client from injury.
- Do not force anything into the client's mouth.
- Turn the client to the side.
- Loosen any restrictive clothing the client is wearing.
- Maintain the client's airway and suction as needed.
- Do not restrain the client; guide the client's movements if necessary.
- At the completion of the seizure:
  - Take the client's vital signs.
  - Perform neurologic checks.
  - Keep the client on his or her side.
  - Allow the client to rest.
  - Document the seizure (see Chart 42-4).

CHART 42-4

FOCUSED ASSESSMENT *of*
Seizures: Nursing Observations and Documentation

How often the seizures occur
- Date, time, and duration of the seizure

Description of each seizure
- Tonic, clonic
- Staring spells, blinking
- Automatism

Whether more than one type of seizure occurs

Sequence of seizure progression
- Where the seizure began
- Body part first involved

Observations during the seizure
- Changes in pupil size and any eye deviation
- Level of consciousness
- Presence of apnea, cyanosis, and salivation
- Incontinence of bowel or bladder during the seizure
- Eye fluttering
- Movement and progression of motor activity
- Lip smacking or other automatism
- Tongue or lip biting

How long the seizures last

When the last seizure took place

Whether the seizures are preceded by an aura
- Dizziness, numbness, or visual disturbances
- Gustatory or auditory disturbances

What the client does after the seizure
- Feels drowsy or weak
- May resume normal behavior
- May be unaware that the seizure took place

How long it takes for the client to return to preseizure status

lorazepam (Ativan, Apo-Lorazepam✤) or diazepam (Valium, Meval✤, Vivol✤, Diastat [rectal diazepam gel]) may be given to stop the clusters to prevent the development of status epilepticus.

Status epilepticus is seizure activity that lasts longer than 30 minutes or a series of seizures that occur in rapid succession. It is a potential complication of all types of seizures. The usual causes of status epilepticus include the following:

- Sudden withdrawal from anticonvulsant medication
- Infections
- Acute alcohol withdrawal
- Head trauma
- Cerebral edema
- Metabolic disturbances

CHART 42-5

BEST PRACTICE *for*
Care for the Client in Status Epilepticus

- Support the ABCs (airway, breathing, and circulation).
  - Prepare for possible intubation.
  - Protect the client from injury.
- Do not force an airway into the client's mouth; provide oxygen via nasal cannula or face mask.
- Establish IV access if not already available, and begin infusion of 0.9% saline.
  - Administer drugs as ordered, and observe the client for side effects or signs of toxicity from the medications.
  - Monitor vital signs and cardiac rhythm.

Status epilepticus is characterized by prolonged seizures lasting more than 10 minutes or repeated seizures over the course of 30 minutes. Convulsive status epilepticus is a neurologic emergency and must be treated promptly to prevent irreversible brain damage and possibly death from hypoxia, cardiac dysrhythmias, or lactic acidosis. The nurse notifies the physician immediately if this condition occurs and establishes an adequate airway promptly. (Intubation by an anesthesiologist or nurse anesthetist may be necessary.) Oxygen is given as indicated by the client's condition. If not already in place, IV access is established, and the client should receive 0.9% sodium chloride (Chart 42-5).

Medications that the physician uses to treat status epilepticus include IV diazepam (Valium, Meval✤, Vivol✤), IV lorazepam (Ativan, Apo-Lorazepam✤), diazepam rectal gel (Diastat), or IV valproate (Depacon) to stop motor movement, followed by phenytoin (Dilantin) or fosphenytoin (Cerebyx) to prevent recurrence (McNew, Hunt, & Warner, 1997). Fosphenytoin can be administered intramuscularly, as well as intravenously, and is compatible with most IV solutions. After administration, fosphenytoin converts to phenytoin in the body. Therefore the Food and Drug Administration (FDA) requires the dosage to be written as a phenytoin equivalent (PE); 150 mg of fosphenytoin equals 100 mg of phenytoin. Fosphenytoin should never be given at a faster rate than 50 mg/min, because rapid administration may lead to cardiac dysrhythmias. General anesthesia may be used as a treatment of last resort to stop the seizure activity. The nurse, physician, or clinical pharmacist monitors serum drug levels closely for the first 3 days after the start of the anticonvulsant medication and thereafter as indicated.

VAGAL NERVE STIMULATION. Vagal nerve stimulation (VNS) was recently approved for control of medically intractable simple or complex partial seizures with or without secondary generalization. Clients with multifocal or bihemisphere seizure foci, who are not candidates for surgical excision (because this may result in severe neurologic deficits), and those in whom other, less invasive treatment options are not effective may also qualify for the use of VNS. The NeuroCybernetic Prosthesis system has received FDA approval as a means of providing VNS. The stimulating device is surgically implanted in the left chest wall. An electrode lead is attached to the left vagus nerve, tunneled under the skin, and connected to a generator (Shafer, 1999). The procedure usually takes 2 hours with the client under general anesthesia. The stimulator is activated to deliver intermittent VNS. Programming is titrated gradually over a period of time. The pattern of stimulation is individualized to the client's tolerance. The client can activate the VNS with a handheld magnet when experiencing an aura, thus aborting the seizure. The battery life is 3 to 5 years.

Clients experience a change in voice quality, which signifies that the vagus nerve has been stimulated. They report a relief in intensity and duration of seizures and an improved quality of life.

SURGICAL MANAGEMENT. A small percentage of clients with epilepsy cannot be fully controlled with medications or VNS. When all other treatment options are exhausted, surgery may be indicated to improve the quality of life.

Care is similar to that described for clients undergoing a craniotomy (see Chapter 45). Preoperative diagnostic tests include magnetic resonance imaging (MRI) and single-photon emission computed tomography (SPECT)/positron emission tomography (PET) scans as described in Chapter 41. An intracarotid amobarbital test (Wada test) and neuropsychologic testing are also done. The Wada test assesses hemispheric lateralization of language and memory after intracarotid injection of amobarbital, a short-acting anesthetic. This procedure establishes the safety of surgery in terms of language preservation and memory. Neuropsychologic testing evaluates memory, visuospatial function, language function, and intelligence quotient to identify deficiencies in a restricted brain region that might correspond to areas believed to be the epileptogenic region. It is also used to compare preoperative and postoperative cognitive functioning.

CONVENTIONAL SURGICAL PROCEDURES. Clients with seizures that do not respond to medication may benefit from surgical excision of the seizure area of the brain. The procedure involves continuous electroencephalogram (EEG) recording, close observation, and in many hospitals, video monitoring of the client at all times except during personal care activities. After the seizure area is identified, electrodes are surgically implanted into the brain tissue to identify the extent of the focal area. This step is followed by additional continuous EEG and video monitoring at all times (except during personal care), as well as close observation by the nursing staff. The area is excised if it can be safely removed without affecting vital areas of brain function.

Anterior temporal lobe resection is the safest and most effective procedure for complex partial seizures of temporal origin. Multiple suboccipital transection done over all areas of seizure foci, as well as over other stereotactic volumetric radiofrequency lesions of the intracranial structures, may be performed.

The more traditional surgical approach, the **corpuscallosotomy,** is used to treat tonic-clonic or atonic seizures in clients who are not candidates for other surgical procedures. The surgeon sections the anterior two thirds of the corpus callosum, preventing neuronal discharges from passing between the two hemispheres of the brain. This surgery usually reduces the number and severity of the seizures, making them more amenable to more conventional drug therapy.

CLIENT AND FAMILY EDUCATION. An educational program is provided for the client and family or significant others in a manner that can be easily understood (Chart 42-6).

CHART 42-6

CLIENT EDUCATION GUIDE
Instructions for the Client with Epilepsy

- Avoid alcohol consumption and excessive fatigue.
- Do not take any medication, including over-the-counter drugs, without asking your physician.
- Wear a medical alert bracelet or necklace.
- Contact the Epilepsy Foundation of America or other organized epilepsy group.
- Investigate your local state laws covering driving and operating machinery as an epileptic.
- Medication information:
  - Name, dosage, time of administration
  - Actions to take if side effects occur
  - Importance of taking as prescribed and not missing a dose
  - What to do if a medication is missed or cannot be taken

The nurse ascertains what they understand about the disorder, corrects any misinformation, and presents new information as the client and family are able to understand it.

The nurse emphasizes that antiepileptic drugs (AEDs) must not be stopped, even if the seizures have stopped. Discontinuing AEDs can lead to the recurrence of seizures or the life-threatening complication of status epilepticus. Some clients may stop taking their medications simply because they do not have the money to purchase them. The nurse refers limited-income clients to the social services department for financial assistance or to a case manager to locate other resources.

All states prohibit discrimination against people who have epilepsy. Clients who work in occupations in which a seizure might cause serious harm to themselves or others (e.g., construction workers, operators of dangerous equipment, pilots, railroad engineers) may need to find alternative employment. They may need to curtail or modify strenuous or potentially dangerous physical activity to avoid harm, although this varies with the individual.

CRITICAL THINKING CHALLENGE

You are shopping in your local mall when you notice a small crowd of people hovering over a young woman on the floor having a seizure. She is making jerking movements and seems to be unconscious.

- What other assessment data should you note during the woman's seizure?
- What type of seizure do you think she may be having?
- What should you do first to help manage this woman?

For suggested answer guidelines, go to SIMON http://www.wbsaunders.com/SIMON/Iggy/.

INFECTIONS

Meningitis

OVERVIEW

Meningitis is an inflammation of the arachnoid and pia mater of the brain and spinal cord and the cerebrospinal fluid (CSF). Bacterial and viral organisms are most often responsible for meningitis, although fungal meningitis and protozoal meningitis also occur. Bacterial meningitis occurs most frequently; early detection and treatment are associated with a more favorable outcome. Viral meningitis is usually self-limiting, and

TABLE 42-4 • COMMON BACTERIA THAT CAUSE MENINGITIS

- *Haemophilus influenzae*
- *Neisseria meningitidis* (meningococcal)
- *Diplococcus pneumoniae* (pneumococcal)
- Streptococci, group A
- *Staphylococcus aureus*
- *Escherichia coli*
- *Klebsiella*
- *Proteus*
- *Pseudomonas*

the client has a complete recovery. It is not considered as serious or potentially life threatening. Regardless of the causative organism, symptoms are the same.

The organisms responsible for meningitis enter the central nervous system (CNS) via the bloodstream at the blood-brain barrier. Direct routes of entry occur as a result of penetrating trauma, surgical procedures, or a ruptured cerebral abscess. **Otorrhea** (ear discharge) or **rhinorrhea** (nasal discharge, or "runny nose"), which may be caused by a basilar skull fracture, may lead to meningitis as a result of the direct communication of CSF with the environment. The invading organisms migrate throughout the CNS via the subarachnoid space. The presence of the organism in the subarachnoid space produces an inflammatory response in the pia mater, the arachnoid, the CSF, and the ventricles. The exudate formed may spread to both cranial and spinal nerves, causing further neurologic deterioration.

Bacterial Meningitis

Bacterial meningitis is seen most often in fall and winter, when upper respiratory tract infections commonly occur. The most frequently involved organisms responsible for bacterial meningitis include *Streptococcus pneumoniae* (pneumococcal disease), *Neisseria meningitides,* and *Haemophilus influenzae* (Table 42-4).

Meningococcal meningitis is the only type of bacterial meningitis that occurs in outbreaks, and it is most likely to occur in areas of high population density, such as college dormitories, military barracks, crowded living areas, and prisons. The number of outbreaks on college campuses has been increasing over the past few years (Harrison et al., 1999), prompting some states to require students to be vaccinated against meningitis. A meningitis polysaccharide vaccine (Menomune) is available to prevent infection by certain groups of meningococcal bacteria.

Most often, the client has a predisposing condition, such as otitis media, pneumonia, acute sinusitis, or sickle cell anemia, that increases the likelihood of meningitis. A fractured skull or brain or spinal surgery may also contribute to the development of meningitis. Vulnerable populations include clients who are immunosuppressed, have immunocompromised disorders, or have infections elsewhere in the body, and older adults, especially those with chronic debilitating diseases.

Viral Meningitis

Viral meningitis is sometimes referred to as aseptic meningitis. It often occurs as a sequela to a variety of viral illnesses, including measles, mumps, herpes simplex, and herpes zoster. The formation of exudate that is common in bacterial meningitis does not occur, and no organisms are obtained for culture from the CSF. Inflammation occurs over the cerebral cortex, the white matter, and the meninges. The susceptibility of the brain tissue to the virus varies, depending on which type of cell is involved. The herpes simplex virus alters cellular metabolism, which quickly results in necrosis of the cells. The coxsackie and echovirus families also may cause viral meningitis. Other viruses cause an alteration in the production of enzymes or neurotransmitters, which results in dysfunction of the cells and possible neurologic defects.

CHART 42-7

FOCUSED ASSESSMENT *of* The Client with Meningitis

Level of consciousness
Orientation to person, place, and year
Pupil reaction and eye movements
- Photophobia
- Nystagmus
- Abnormal eye movements

Motor response
- Normal early in disease process
- Hemiparesis, hemiplegia, and decreased muscle tone may occur later.
- Cranial nerve dysfunction
  - Cranial nerves III, IV, VI, VII, VIII
- Memory changes
- Attention span (usually short)
- Personality and behavior changes
  - Bewilderment
- Severe, unrelenting headaches
- Generalized muscle aches and pain
- Nausea and vomiting
- Fever and chills
- Tachycardia
- Red macular rash (meningococcal meningitis)

Fungal Meningitis

Cryptococcus neoformans meningitis is the most commonly seen fungal infection that affects the CNS of clients with acquired immunodeficiency syndrome (AIDS). Fulminant invasive fungal sinusitis is also a recognized cause of fungal meningitis. The clinical manifestations vary among people because of their compromised immune system, which affects the inflammatory response. For example, some clients have fever and others do not. Almost all clients have headache, nausea, and vomiting and show a decline in mental status.

COLLABORATIVE MANAGEMENT

Assessment

The nurse performs a complete neurologic assessment to detect changes associated with a diagnosis of meningitis or suspected meningitis as outlined in Chart 42-7.

MENINGEAL IRRITATION

Meningeal irritation is indicated by nuchal rigidity and positive Kernig's and Brudzinski's signs. **Nuchal rigidity** is manifested by a stiff neck and soreness, particularly when the neck is flexed. The nurse may elect to test for both Kernig's and Brudzinski's signs. A positive response occurs in the presence of bacterial meningitis but is absent in viral meningitis. The client lies supine in bed for both tests.

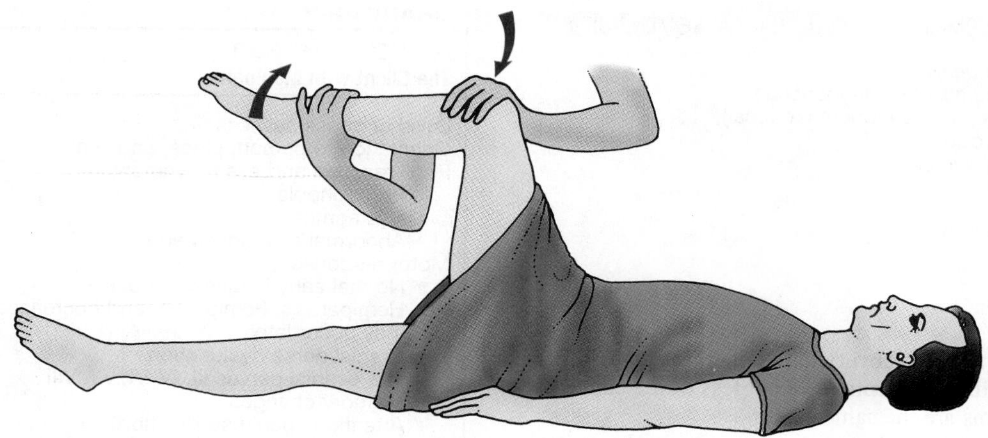

Figure 42-1 ● Kernig's sign, which indicates meningitis. Flexion of the hip and knee causes pain.

To elicit **Kernig's sign,** the nurse flexes the client's leg at the hip, brings the knee to a 90-degree angle (Figure 42-1), and then attempts to extend the knee. If meningitis is present, the client will experience pain and spasm of the hamstring muscle when the leg is straightened. Pain occurs secondary to meningeal irritation and spinal nerve root inflammation (from exudate around the roots).

To test the **Brudzinski reflex,** the nurse gently flexes the client's head and neck onto the chest. A positive response is indicated by flexion of the hips and knees.

INCREASED INTRACRANIAL PRESSURE

The nurse also assesses the client for complications that may occur, including increased intracranial pressure (ICP) resulting from the presence of exudate, which can lead to hydrocephalus and cerebral edema. Left untreated, increased ICP can lead to herniation of the brain and death (see Chapter 45).

Seizure activity may be caused by irritation of the cerebral cortex. Because of abnormal stimulation of the hypothalamic area, excessive amounts of antidiuretic hormone (ADH) (vasopressin) are produced. This results in water retention and dilution of serum sodium attributable to increased excretion of sodium by the kidneys. This syndrome of inappropriate antidiuretic hormone (SIADH) production may lead to further increases in ICP (see Chapter 45).

VASCULAR DYSFUNCTION

To assess the client's vascular status, the nurse:

- Observes the color and temperature of the extremities
- Determines the presence of peripheral pulses
- Identifies any indicators of abnormal bleeding

Septic emboli in the blood may block circulation in the small vessels of the hands and feet, leading to gangrene. Excessive fibrinolysis that occurs in bacteremia and infections from viruses, fungi, or protozoa may lead to disseminated intravascular coagulation (DIC). Vascular involvement of the cerebral arteries, veins, and venous sinuses may lead to seizures and hemiparesis.

TABLE 42-5 • CEREBROSPINAL FLUID FINDINGS IN MENINGITIS

Finding	Bacterial Meningitis	Viral Meningitis
Appearance	Cloudy, turbid	Clear
White blood cells	Increased	Increased
Protein	Increased	Increased, slightly elevated
Glucose	Decreased	Normal
CSF pressure	Elevated	Varies

LABORATORY ASSESSMENT

The most significant laboratory test used in the diagnosis of meningitis is the analysis of the cerebrospinal fluid (CSF). A lumbar puncture is usually not done in the presence of increased ICP. The CSF is analyzed for cell count and protein. Glucose concentrations are determined, and culture, sensitivity, and Gram stain studies are performed.

Counterimmunoelectrophoresis (CIE) may be performed to determine the presence of viruses or protozoa in the CSF. CIE is also indicated if the client has received antibiotics before the CSF was obtained. To identify a possible bacterial source of infection, specimens for culture are obtained and Gram stains of the blood, urine, throat, and nose are performed. Table 42-5 compares CSF findings in bacterial meningitis and in viral meningitis.

Polymerase chain reaction may be used to detect viral deoxyribonucleic acid (DNA) or ribonucleic acid (RNA) in the CSF. Specificity and sensitivity in diagnosing encephalitis are excellent, especially with herpes simplex virus (HSV). The test is rapid and noninvasive, replacing the brain biopsy for diagnosis.

A complete blood count (CBC) is performed, with attention to the white blood cell (WBC) count, which is generally elevated well above the normal value. Serum electrolyte values are also assessed with attention to the sodium value. Dilutional hyponatremia may occur secondary to SIADH, a complication of bacterial meningitis.

CHART 42-8

BEST PRACTICE *for* Care of the Client with Meningitis

- Take vital signs and perform neurologic checks every 2 to 4 hours, as ordered.
- Perform nerve assessments, with particular attention to cranial nerves III, IV, VI, VII, and VIII, and monitor for changes.
- Manage pain through drug and nondrug methods.
- Provide interventions to treat or prevent increased intracranial pressure.
- Perform vascular assessment and monitor for changes.
- Give medications as ordered, and document the client's response.
- Protect the client from injury; use seizure precautions.
- Maintain isolation precautions per hospital policy.

TABLE 42-6 • EMPIRIC THERAPY OF MENINGITIS

Organism	Antibiotic
Staphylococcus	Vancomycin Ceftazidime
Haemophilus influenzae	Cefotaxime Ceftriaxone
Streptococcus	Third-generation cephalosporins Rifampin Vancomycin
Neisseria meningitidis	Cephalosporins
Fungus	Amphotericin B Flucytosine Fluconazole
Virus	Acyclovir

OTHER DIAGNOSTIC ASSESSMENT

X-ray films of the chest, air sinuses, and mastoids are taken to determine the presence of infection. A computed tomography (CT) or magnetic resonance imaging (MRI) scan may be performed to identify increased ICP, the presence of a brain abscess, or developing hydrocephalus.

Interventions

The most important nursing intervention for clients with meningitis is the accurate monitoring and recording of their neurologic status, vital signs, and vascular assessment. Other areas of nursing care are found in Chart 42-8.

NEUROLOGIC STATUS AND VITAL SIGNS MONITORING. The client's neurologic status and vital signs are assessed at least every 4 hours or more often if clinically indicated. The nurse assesses for neurologic changes indicative of cerebral complications, especially increased ICP. The health care team provides interventions for the client with increased ICP as discussed in Chapter 45. The client is at risk for seizure activity, and care should be provided as discussed under Interventions (Epilepsy), p. 901.

The specialty or advanced-practice nurse includes complete cranial nerve testing as part of the routine neurologic assessment because of possible cranial nerve involvement. Particular attention is given to cranial nerves III, IV, VI, VII, and VIII (see Chapter 41). A sixth cranial nerve defect (inability to move the eyes laterally) may indicate the development of hydrocephalus. Other indicators of hydrocephalus include the usual signs of increased ICP and the presence of urinary incontinence in the previously continent client. Urinary incontinence occurs secondary to the decreasing level of consciousness (LOC).

MONITORING FOR COMPLICATIONS. The nurse performs a complete vascular assessment during each nursing shift or more often, if indicated, to prevent and detect early vascular compromise from septic emboli. This severe complication is most often seen in circulation to the hand. The nurse assesses the client's temperature, color, pulses, and capillary refill (by applying pressure to the nail bed and looking for blood return). Normal capillary refill occurs within 3 seconds. If vascular compromise is left unrecognized and untreated, gangrene can develop quickly, possibly leading to loss of the involved extremity. The health care team monitors the client for other complications, including shock, coagulation disorders, septic complications (bacterial endocarditis), and prolonged fever.

DRUG THERAPY. To avoid life-threatening complications, the health care provider usually prescribes a broad-spectrum antibiotic until the results of the culture and Gram stain are available. After this information is available, the specific antibiotic to treat the specific type of meningitis is given. Table 42-6 lists some of antibiotics commonly used. The nurse begins the medication within 1 to 2 hours after it is ordered and monitors and documents the client's response.

The client with bacterial meningitis may experience increased ICP, and seizure activity may occur. Medications used by the physician to treat these complications include hyperosmolar agents, steroids, and anticonvulsants. People who have been in close contact with a client who has meningococcal meningitis must have prophylaxis treatment with rifampin.

CRITICAL THINKING CHALLENGE

You are working part-time in the college infirmary when a student reports to you that he has had a severe headache for 2 days and is unable to "keep anything down." He also complains that he is having difficulty concentrating on his homework and has been more forgetful than usual. Two other students on campus have recently been diagnosed with bacterial meningitis.

- What history questions should you ask the student?
- What other assessments should you perform?
- If you suspect meningitis based on your assessment, what should you do at this time?

For suggested answer guidelines, go to SIMON http://www.wbsaunders.com/SIMON/Iggy/.

Encephalitis

OVERVIEW

Encephalitis is an inflammation of the brain parenchyma (brain tissue) and often the meninges. It affects the cerebrum, the brainstem, and the cerebellum. The incidence of encephalitis is 1 in 200,000 people (Hickey, 1997). It is most often caused by a viral agent, although bacteria, fungi, or parasites may also be involved (e.g., malaria). Viral encephalitis is almost always preceded by a viral infection. The virus gains access to the central nervous system (CNS) via the bloodstream, along peripheral or cranial nerves, or in the meninges (e.g., varicella zoster).

After the virus invades the brain tissue, it begins to reproduce, causing an inflammatory response. Unlike with meningitis, this response does not cause exudate formation. Inflammation extends over the cerebral cortex, the white matter, and the meninges, causing degeneration of the neurons of the cortex. Demyelination of axons occurs in the involved area because the white matter is destroyed. This leads to hemorrhage, edema, necrosis, and the development of small lacunae (hollow cavities) within the cerebral hemispheres. Widespread edema can cause compression of blood vessels, leading to a further increase in intracranial pressure (ICP). Death may occur from herniation and increased ICP.

Arboviruses

Arboviruses can be transmitted to humans through the bite of an infected mosquito or tick. The most common types of encephalitis caused by arboviruses are eastern or western equine encephalitis, St. Louis encephalitis, and California encephalitis.

A New York encephalitis outbreak in 1999 involved 61 confirmed cases and 7 deaths due to the West Nile virus, an arbovirus typically affecting animals, especially birds (Centers for Disease Control and Prevention [CDC], 2000). Since that time, the virus has been found in a variety of birds along the East Coast of the United States. It is expected to spread throughout the country in 3 to 5 years. West Nile virus primarily affects older adults and can result in long-term residual fatigue and weakness, as well as death. Clients who have a mosquito or other insect bite that is large and reddened or that becomes infected should be monitored for symptoms of encephalitis.

Encephalitis associated with tick bites tends to occur more frequently in the spring; encephalitis associated with mosquitoes occurs in middle to late summer. The incubation period for both types is 5 to 15 days. Summer is also the peak time for encephalitis caused by the enteroviruses, except the mumps virus, which is more prevalent in early winter. The incubation period varies, depending on the virus involved. Because clients are often unaware of tick bites, the nurse asks about outdoor activities.

Enteroviruses

Echovirus, coxsackievirus, poliovirus, herpes zoster, and viruses that cause mumps and chickenpox are the common enteroviruses associated with encephalitis.

Herpes Simplex Virus Type 1

Herpes simplex virus type 1 (HSV1) encephalitis is the most common nonepidemic type of encephalitis in North America. Clients with herpes encephalitis often have a history of cold sores. Mortality rates for HSV1 encephalitis can be as high as 80%, whereas mortality for the other types is much lower (Hickey, 1997).

Amebae

Amebic meningoencephalitis is caused by the amebae *Naegleria* and *Acanthamoeba.* Both are found in warm freshwater areas and can enter the nasal mucosa of people swimming in ponds or lakes. The amebae may also be found in soil and decaying vegetation. Although this infection has not often been seen in the past, the incidence in North America is increasing, perhaps because the ponds and lakes are becoming more polluted.

➤ COLLABORATIVE MANAGEMENT

Assessment

The typical client with encephalitis has a fever and complains of nausea, vomiting, and a stiff neck. Other signs and symptoms include the following:

- Changes in the level of consciousness (LOC) and mental status
- Motor dysfunction
- Focal neurologic deficits
- Fatigue
- Symptoms of increased intracranial pressure (ICP)

The nurse assesses the LOC using the Glasgow Coma Scale (see Chapter 41). The client may be lethargic, stuporous, or comatose. Mental status changes include acute confusion, irritability, and personality and behavior changes (especially noted in the presence of herpes simplex). The nurse examines for signs of meningeal irritation by assessing for the presence of nuchal rigidity and Kernig's or Brudzinski's sign (described earlier under Meningeal Irritation, pp. 905 and 906). Motor changes may vary from a mild weakness to hemiplegia. The client may have muscle tremors, spasticity, an ataxic gait (postencephalitic parkinsonism), myoclonic jerks, and increased deep tendon reflexes. Seizure activity is not uncommon. He or she often experiences fever, nausea, vomiting, headache, and vertigo.

Cranial nerve involvement is exhibited by ocular palsies, facial weakness, and nystagmus. The herpes zoster lesion affects cranial and spinal nerve root ganglia, which is clinically manifested by a rash, severe pain, itching, burning, or tingling in the areas innervated by these nerves.

In severe cases of encephalitis, the client may exhibit increased ICP resulting from cerebral edema, hemorrhage, and necrosis of brain tissue. The nurse observes the vital signs for indications of a widened pulse pressure, bradycardia, and irregular respirations. The pupils become increasingly dilated and less responsive to light. Left untreated, increased ICP leads to herniation of the brain tissue and possibly death.

Interventions

Nursing interventions for encephalitis are similar to those for meningitis, with the exception of drug therapy. Supportive nursing care and prompt recognition and treatment of increased ICP are essential components of management. The nurse also maintains a patent airway to prevent the development of atelectasis or pneumonia, which can lead to further brain hypoxia from inadequate amounts of oxygen in the circulating blood.

The nurse or assistive nursing personnel encourages and helps the client to turn, cough, and deep breathe at least every 2 hours. Deep tracheal suctioning may be performed, even in the presence of increased ICP, if the findings of the respiratory assessment indicate that respiratory status is compromised, possibly causing cerebral hypoxia.

The nurse also checks vital signs and neurologic signs every 2 hours or more frequently if clinically indicated. The head of the bed is elevated 30 to 45 degrees unless this is contraindicated (e.g., after lumbar puncture or in the client with severe hypotension).

Acyclovir (Zovirax) is the drug of choice for the treatment of herpes encephalitis and is associated with a significantly lower mortality rate than vidarabine (Vira-A). Drug therapy is most effective if begun early, before the client becomes stuporous or comatose. This usually occurs within 4 to 6 days after the appearance of the initial neurologic symptoms. No specific drug therapy is available for infection by arboviruses or enteroviruses.

If there are permanent neurologic disabilities, the client with encephalitis is usually discharged to a rehabilitation setting or a long-term care facility. The client with minimal neurologic problems is discharged to the home setting.

PARKINSON'S DISEASE

OVERVIEW

Parkinson's disease (PD), also referred to as paralysis agitans, is the second most common neurologic degenerative disease. PD has a large economic impact in the form of direct medical costs, as well as indirect costs, such as lost wages and decreased productivity. It is a debilitating disease affecting motor ability and is characterized by three cardinal symptoms: muscle rigidity, **bradykinesia** (slow movement), and tremor. Although the exact cause of PD is not known, evidence suggests it might be related to a genetic defect of chromosome 4.

PD is generally a disease of older adults, but with the admission by actor Michael J. Fox that he has had PD since age 30, the focus on the disease has increased. It occurs most often in people older than 50 years of age. Parkinson's syndrome may be seen in those younger than 40 years, secondary to certain medications or as result of trauma or ischemia to the substantia nigra.

For motor activity to occur, the actions of the cerebral cortex, basal ganglia, and cerebellum must be integrated. The basal ganglia are a group of neurons located deep within the cerebrum at the base of the brain near the lateral ventricles. When the basal ganglia is stimulated, muscle tone in the body is inhibited and voluntary movements are refined. This process is accomplished by the secretion of two neurotransmitters: dopamine and acetylcholine (ACh).

Dopamine is produced in the substantia nigra, as well as in the adrenal glands, and is transmitted to the basal ganglia along a connecting neural pathway for secretion when needed. ACh is produced and secreted by the basal ganglia, as well as in the nerve endings in the periphery of the body. ACh-producing neurons transmit excitatory messages throughout the basal ganglia. Dopamine inhibits the function of these neurons, allowing control over voluntary movement. This system of checks and balances allows for refined, coordinated movement, such as picking up a pencil and writing.

PD is caused by widespread degeneration of the substantia nigra, a part of the basal ganglia, leading to a decrease in the amount of dopamine. Dopamine produced in the adrenal glands is not available, because it is quickly metabolized in

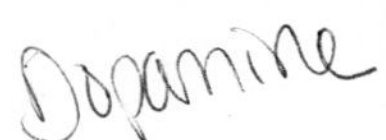

TABLE 42-7 • STAGES OF PARKINSON'S DISEASE

STAGE 1: INITIAL STAGE • Unilateral limb involvement • Minimal weakness • Hand and arm trembling	**STAGE 3: MODERATE DISEASE** • Gait disturbances increase
STAGE 2: MILD STAGE • Bilateral limb involvement • Masklike facies • Slow, shuffling gait	**STAGE 4: SEVERE DISABILITY** • Akinesia • Rigidity **STAGE 5: COMPLETE DEPENDENCE**

the body. When dopamine levels are decreased, a person loses the ability to refine voluntary movement. The large number of excitatory ACh-secreting neurons remains active, creating an imbalance between excitatory and inhibitory neuronal activity. The resulting excessive excitation of neurons prevents a person from controlling or initiating voluntary movement.

In addition to changes in voluntary movement, some clients experience autonomic nervous system symptoms, such as excessive perspiration and orthostatic hypotension; however, the cause of these symptoms is unclear. Some also experience dementia later as the disease progresses.

PD is separated into stages according to the symptoms and degree of disability (Table 42-7). Stage 1 is mild disease with unilateral limb involvement. Bilateral limb involvement occurs in stage 2. In stage 3, the client exhibits significant gait disturbances and moderate generalized disability. Stage 4 is characterized by severe disability, akinesia (no initiation of movement), and muscle rigidity. The client with stage 5 disease is completely dependent in all activities of daily living (ADLs). Other classifications refer simply to mild, moderate, and severe disease.

COLLABORATIVE MANAGEMENT

Assessment

The nurse collects data related to the time and progression of symptoms noticed by the client or the family. Early signs and symptoms, such as fatigue, slight tremor, and problems with manual dexterity, may be ignored, especially by the older adult, who may assume that these behaviors are normal changes associated with aging. Other signs and symptoms are found in Chart 42-9, which summarizes the clinical manifestations of Parkinson's disease (PD).

The nurse begins the assessment by checking for evidence of **rigidity,** or resistance to passive movement of the extremities. Rigidity is evaluated as the nurse performs passive range of motion (ROM) of the extremities. Rigidity is classified as follows:

- Cogwheel, manifested by a rhythmic interruption of the muscle movement
- Plastic, defined as mildly restrictive movement
- Lead pipe, or total resistance to movement

Rigidity is present early in the disease process and progresses over time. The nurse further observes the client's ability to relax a muscle or move a selected muscle group.

CHART 42-9

KEY FEATURES *of* Parkinson's Disease

Posture
- Stooped posture
- Flexed trunk
- Fingers abducted and flexed at the metacarpophalangeal joint
- Wrist slightly dorsiflexed

Gait
- Slow and shuffling
- Short, hesitant steps
- Propulsive gait
- Difficulty stopping quickly

Motor
- Bradykinesia
- Akinesia
- Tremors
- "Pill-rolling" movement
- Masklike facies
- Difficulty chewing and swallowing
- Uncontrolled drooling, especially at night
- Fatigue
- Difficulty getting in and out of bed
- Little arm swinging when walking
- Change in handwriting (micrographia, or gets smaller)

Speech
- Soft, low-pitched voice
- Dysarthric
- Echolalia (automatic repetition of what another person says) and repetition of sentences
- Change in voice volume, phonation, or articulation

Autonomic Dysfunction
- Orthostatic hypotension
- Excessive perspiration
- Oily skin
- Seborrhea
- Flushing
- Changes in skin texture
- Blepharospasm (eyelid spasm)

Psychosocial Assessment
- Emotionally labile
- Depression
- Paranoia
- Easily upset
- Rapid mood swings
- Cognitive impairments (i.e., dementia)
- Delayed reaction time
- Sleep disturbances

Changes in facial expression or a masklike facies with wide-open, fixed, staring eyes is caused by rigidity of the facial muscles (Figure 42-2). This rigidity can lead to difficulties in chewing and swallowing, particularly if the pharyngeal muscles are involved. Uncontrolled drooling may occur.

A diagnosis of PD is made on the basis of the clinical findings and after other neurologic diseases are eliminated. There are no specific diagnostic tests. Analysis of cerebrospinal fluid (CSF) may show a decrease in dopamine levels, although the results of other studies are usually normal.

Interventions

Drug therapy, physical or occupational therapy, and as a last resort, palliative surgery may be performed to assist the client in remaining mobile for as long as possible. Chart 42-10 provides best practices for nursing management of the client with PD.

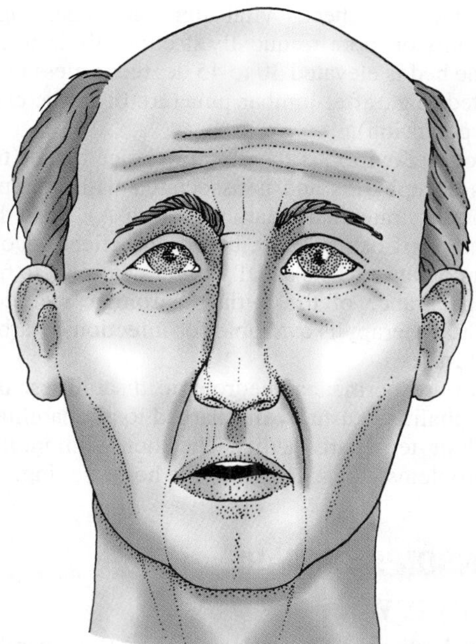

Figure 42-2 ● The masklike facial expression typical of clients with Parkinson's disease.

CHART 42-10

BEST PRACTICE *for* Care of the Client with Parkinson's Disease

- Administer medications promptly on schedule to maintain continuous therapeutic drug levels.
- Monitor for side effects of medications, especially orthostatic hypotension, hallucinations, and acute confusional state.
- Collaborate with physical and occupational therapists to keep the client as mobile and as independent as possible in activities of daily living.
- Allow the client time to perform activities of daily living and mobility skills.
- Implement interventions to prevent complications of immobility, such as constipation, pressure ulcers, and contractures.
- Schedule appointments and activities late in the morning to prevent rushing the client, or schedule them at the time of the client's optimal level of functioning.
- Teach the client to speak slowly and clearly; use alternative communication methods, such as a communication board.
- Monitor the client's ability to eat and swallow; monitor actual food and fluid intake.
- Provide high-protein, high-calorie foods or supplements to maintain weight.
- Recognize that Parkinson's disease affects the client's body image; focus on the client's strengths.
- Assess for depression and anxiety.

NONSURGICAL MANAGEMENT

DRUG THERAPY. A variety of medications are used to control tremor and rigidity, usually within 2 years after diagnosis. Many questions and controversies remain about which drugs to use, when to start therapy, and how to prevent complications. Medication administration is closely monitored, and the physician adjusts the dosage or changes the medication as the client's condition warrants. The nurse ensures that the drug is given at the prescribed times to keep the serum level of the drug constant.

Types of Drugs. The drugs of choice used by many health care providers to treat rigidity are the **dopaminergics,** precursors to dopamine, such as carbidopa/levodopa (Sinemet). These drugs are typically the most effective during the first 3 to 5 years of use. At this point, there is a loss of response to the medication, resulting in the "on-off" phenomena, which is characterized by periods of good mobility ("on") alternating with periods of poor mobility ("off"). Long-term use of these medications is associated with side effects (e.g., **dyskinesias** [abnormal movements], hallucinations, and severe orthostatic hypotension). Sinemet CR has been demonstrated to prevent motor fluctuations and is safe and well tolerated.

Anticholinergic drugs, such as trihexyphenidyl (Artane) and benztropine (Cogentin), extend the effects of levodopa therapy and particularly benefit the client whose primary symptom is tremor. The health care provider prescribes anticholinergic drugs less frequently today than previously because newer drugs are available. However, small doses may be prescribed to younger clients when tremor is the main problem.

When the classic dopaminergics and anticholinergics fail or are no longer effective, bromocriptine mesylate (Parlodel) or pergolide may be prescribed to activate the release of dopamine. They may be used alone or in combination with carbidopa/levodopa (Sinemet). Some providers may prescribe bromocriptine mesylate early in the course of treatment. It is especially useful in the client who has experienced side effects such as dyskinesias or orthostatic hypotension while receiving levodopa.

Additional therapeutic strategies used for PD include the administration of monoamine oxidase (MAO) inhibitors, such as selegiline (Eldepryl), to reduce the metabolic breakdown of dopamine and catechol *O*-methyltransferase inhibitors to retard the breakdown of levodopa. The use of dextromethorphan glial-derived neurotrophic factor administered directly into the brain is undergoing clinical trials (Hickey, 1997).

Catechol *O*-methyltransferase (COMT) inhibitors received Food and Drug Administration (FDA) approval in 1998. COMT is an enzyme that inactivates dopamine. Therefore COMT inhibitors block this activity, thus increasing the effectiveness of levodopa. For example, entacapone (Comtan) has received FDA approval for use in combination with levodopa and carbidopa.

Studies are ongoing to search for more effective ways of delivering the best medications. For example, topical patches may be available rather than pills to treat PD. Neuroprotective drugs, such as coenzyme Q10, may replace traditional drug therapy for some clients (Simon & Strandaert, 1999).

Drug Toxicity. For the client on long-term drug therapy regimens, drug tolerance or drug toxicity often develops. Drug toxicity is evidenced by delirium, cognitive impairment, decreased effectiveness of the drug, or hallucinations. Delirium may be difficult to assess in the client who is already suffering from chronic dementia as a result of PD or another disease. If possible, the nurse compares the client's current cognitive and behavioral status with his or her baseline before drug therapy began.

When drug tolerance is reached, the drug's effects do not last as long as previously. The treatment of drug toxicity or tolerance includes the following:

- A reduction in medication dosage
- A change of medications or in the frequency of administration
- A drug holiday (particularly with levodopa therapy)

During a drug holiday, which typically lasts up to 10 days, the client receives no medications. He or she must be carefully monitored during this time.

EXERCISE/AMBULATION. Nontraditional exercise programs, such as yoga and tai chi, may help to elevate mood, as well as improve mobility, in the early stage of the disease. As the disease progresses, physical and occupational therapists may need to plan and implement a program incorporating active and passive range-of-motion (ROM) exercises, muscle stretching, and activity. The prescribed program may include exercises for the muscles of the face and tongue to facilitate swallowing and speech. A speech and language pathologist (SLP) may also be needed.

Because of the potential for respiratory problems, the nurse or respiratory therapist teaches the client how to perform breathing exercises, including diaphragmatic and abdominal exercises. The nurse instructs the client with orthostatic hypotension to wear elastic stockings and change positions slowly, especially when moving from a sitting to a standing position, to allow for adequate cerebral blood flow.

SELF-CARE. In collaboration with the rehabilitation team, the nurse encourages the client to participate as much as possible in the performance of self-care or activities of daily living (ADLs). The team makes the environment conducive to independence in activity and as stress free and safe as possible. Consultations with occupational and physical therapists are obtained for training in ADLs and the use of adaptive devices, if needed, to facilitate independence.

NUTRITION. If intake is not sufficient, the client is weighed weekly. Food intake is recorded daily or as needed. The nurse consults the dietitian for calorie calculation and diet planning. Supplemental feedings with high-protein, high-calorie liquids or puddings may be given several times a day to maintain weight. (See Chapter 61 for additional interventions for clients with undernutrition.) The nurse and dietitian carefully monitor swallowing and chewing abilities, as well as the ability to feed independently. The client who attempts self-feeding may drop a large portion of the food on the lap instead of getting the food into the mouth. The nurse carefully monitors actual food intake. Usually a soft diet or thick, cold fluids, such as milk shakes, are more easily tolerated. Smaller, more frequent meals or a commercial powder, such as Thick-It, added to liquids may assist the client who has difficulty swallowing. The client is positioned properly with the head elevated to facilitate swallowing and prevent aspiration. The SLP can be very helpful in evaluating swallowing ability and recommending specific strategies to use.

When possible, the nurse schedules medications so that peak action occurs during mealtime, facilitating independence in feeding. Taking levodopa with meals can prevent nausea.

COMMUNICATION. The nurse instructs the client to speak slowly and clearly and to pause and take deep breaths at appropriate intervals during each sentence. Unnecessary environmental noise should be eliminated, if possible, to maximize the listener's ability to hear and understand the client. The nurse and the family ask the client to repeat words they do not understand, and they watch his or her lips and nonverbal expressions for cues as to the meaning of conversation. The nurse instructs him or her to organize thoughts before speaking and encourages the use of facial expression and gestures, if possible, to assist with communication. In addition, the client should exaggerate words to increase the listener's ability to understand.

If the client cannot communicate verbally, he or she must use alternative methods of communication, such as a communication board, mechanical voice synthesizer, or computer. The SLP assesses the client's ability to use these devices before a decision is made about the method to use.

PSYCHOSOCIAL SUPPORT. Although not all clients with PD have dementia, impaired cognitive function and memory deficits are common. Clients may also experience changes in gait and tremors that are uncontrollable. In the late stages of the disease, they cannot move without assistance, have difficulty with articulation, have minimal facial expression, and may drool. Clients often state that they are embarrassed, and they tend to avoid social events or groups of people. They should not be forced into situations in which they feel ashamed of their appearance. They should be encouraged to undertake activities that do not require small-muscle dexterity, such as light, modified aerobic exercises.

The nurse emphasizes the client's abilities or strengths and provides positive reinforcement when he or she meets the daily goals. The client, the family or significant others, and the rehabilitation team mutually set realistic goals that can be achieved. Assisting the client with grooming and hygiene is also important in maintaining a positive body image.

The long-term management of PD presents a special challenge in the home care setting. A case manager may be required to coordinate interdisciplinary care and provide support for the client and family (Vickers & O'Neill, 1998). Impaired mobility affects the daily lifestyle, including sexuality. The case manager or home care nurse uses a holistic approach to ensure that psychosocial, as well as physical, needs are addressed.

SURGICAL MANAGEMENT. Several options are available if surgery for the client with Parkinson's disease (PD) is needed. Surgery is a last resort when drugs are ineffective in symptom management. The most common surgeries are stereotactic pallidotomy and thalamotomy, although newer surgical procedures are being tried.

STEREOTACTIC PALLIDOTOMY/THALAMOTOMY. **Stereotactic pallidotomy** can be a very effective treatment for controlling the symptoms associated with PD (Eller & Dan, 1997). First, the target area within the pallidum is identified via a computed tomography (CT) or magnetic resonance imaging (MRI) scan. Next, the stereotactic head frame is placed on the client. IV sedation is given, and a burr hole is made into the cranium; an electrode or cylindric rod is inserted into the target area. The target area receives a mild electrical stimulation, and the client's reaction is assessed for reduction of tremor and rigidity. If this result does not occur, or if unexpected visual, motor, or sensory symptoms appear, the probe is repositioned. When the probe is in the ideal location, a temporary lesion is made. If this is successful, the permanent lesion is made. The client is monitored in the postanesthesia care unit (PACU) for about 1 hour and is then returned to the inpatient unit for continuing postoperative care.

As an alternative to stereotactic pallidotomy, the surgeon may perform a **thalamotomy** for treatment of tremor through thermocoagulation of brain cells. Because bilateral procedures have increased surgical complication rates, only unilateral surgery is done to benefit the side of the body that is most affected by the disease.

DEEP BRAIN STIMULATION. Deep brain stimulation (DBS) has recently been approved for unilateral procedures. An electrode is implanted in the thalamus and connected to a "pacemaker" that delivers electrical current to interfere with "tremor" cells. DBS has the advantage of adjustable pacemaker settings as the disease progresses (Arle & Alterman, 1999).

FETAL TISSUE TRANSPLANTATION. Fetal tissue transplantation is an experimental and highly controversial procedure. Fetal substantia nigra tissue, either human or pig, is transplanted into the caudate nucleus of the brain. Preliminary reports suggest that clients show substantial clinical improvement in motor symptoms without dyskinesias after receiving the transplanted tissue. Long-term results are yet to be seen (Ross, 1999).

CRITICAL THINKING CHALLENGE

One of the residents on your unit in the nursing home has a long history of PD. She requires assistance with most of her ADLs, but she is alert and oriented most of the time. Today she complains of feeling dizzy when sitting in her wheelchair. She also tells you that she has been seeing spiders in her room at night, which disturbs her sleep. When you check her chart, you note that she has been taking carbidopa/levodopa (Sinemet) for more than 5 years and has had a low blood pressure for the last 3 days.

- What additional assessment should you perform at this time?
- What are the possible explanations for the resident's new symptoms?
- What interventions should you implement at this time?

For suggested answer guidelines, go to SIMON http://www.wbsaunders.com/SIMON/Iggy/.

ALZHEIMER'S DISEASE

OVERVIEW

Alzheimer's disease (AD), also known as dementia, Alzheimer's type (DAT), is a chronic, progressive, degenerative disease that accounts for 60% of the dementias occurring in people older than 65 years of age. It may also be seen less commonly in people in their 40s and 50s, which is referred to as early dementia, Alzheimer's type, or presenile dementia, Alzheimer's type. It is characterized by loss of memory, judgment, and visuospatial perception, and by a change in personality. Over time, the client becomes increasingly cognitively impaired; severe physical deterioration takes place and death occurs as a result of complications of immobility.

Studies have shown that lay caregivers and health care providers lack a thorough understanding of the difference between changing memory associated with aging and AD. Ongoing public and professional education is needed for recognition and early diagnosis of this disease.

The cost of care for clients with AD is tremendous, making it the third most expensive disease in the United States (see the Cost of Care box below). Loss of wages and productivity in society adds to the increasing costs of health care.

Pathophysiology

STRUCTURAL CHANGES IN THE BRAIN

The brain of the older adult weighs less and occupies less space in the cranial vault than does the brain of a younger person. Other changes in the brain that occur with aging include widening of the cerebral sulci, narrowing of the gyri, and enlargement of the ventricles. In the presence of AD, these normal changes are greatly accelerated. Brain weight is reduced further, and there is marked cerebral atrophy. The cerebral sulci and fissures, as well as the ventricles, are enlarged more than those of persons of the same age without AD. The following areas of the brain are particularly affected:

- Precentral gyrus of the frontal lobe
- Superior temporal gyrus
- Hippocampus
- Substantia nigra

Microscopic changes of the brain found in people with AD include **neurofibrillary tangles,** senile or **neuritic plaques,** and granulovascular degeneration.

COST OF CARE IMPLICATIONS FOR NURSING

CLIENTS WITH ALZHEIMER'S DISEASE

Cost of Care

- Average annual cost per client is $47,000, not including indirect costs such as productivity or wages.
- Overall cost of a lifetime of care for a client with Alzheimer's disease (AD) is staggering; average lifetime cost per client is $174,000.
- AD is the third most expensive disease in the United States, after heart disease and cancer.
- U.S. society spends at least $100 billion per year on AD.
- Lost productivity of caregivers averages $26 billion.
- $7 billion is spent annually on health and long-term care.
- Half of all nursing home clients suffer from AD; average cost per client for nursing home care is $42,000 per year, but cost can exceed $70,000 in some geographic areas.
- In 1999 the federal government spent approximately $400 million for AD research.

Implications for Nursing

It is important for all health care providers to understand the staggering costs of caring for clients with AD, not only the monetary cost but also the psychologic and emotional costs to the family and caregivers. Despite increasing research dollars, no cure for AD has been found. Care continues to be symptomatic; thus costs of providing care for clients increase as they progress through the stages of the disease. Clients often require nursing home care and specialized equipment as the disease progresses.

Data from National Institute on Aging (1998). Progress Report on Alzheimer's Disease, 1998; and Alzheimer's Association (1999). Statistics/Prevalence of Alzheimer's Disease.

Neurofibrillary tangles are a classic finding at autopsy in the brains of clients with AD. They consist of tangled masses of fibrous elements throughout the neurons. The same tangles and chemical changes are found in people with Down syndrome.

Senile plaques are composed of degenerating nerve terminals and are found particularly in the hippocampus, an important part of the limbic system. Deposited within the plaques are increased amounts of an abnormal protein called **amyloid.** When amyloid infiltrates body tissue, it causes the tissue to decrease or lose function.

Although vascular degeneration occurs in the normally aging brain, its presence is significantly increased in clients with AD. Vascular degeneration accounts for at least partial loss of the ability of nerve cells to function properly. This pathologic change contributes to the mortality associated with this disorder.

CHEMICAL CHANGES IN THE BRAIN

In addition to the structural changes in the brain associated with AD, abnormalities in the neurotransmitters (acetylcholine [ACh], norepinephrine, dopamine, serotonin) may occur. ACh in the brain is reduced by as much as 75%, which leads to a decrease in the amount of acetyltransferase in the hippocampus. This loss is significant because the decrease in acetyltransferase interferes with cholinergic innervation to the cerebral cortex. This results in dysfunction of cognition, recent memory, and the ability to acquire new memories. The exact role of the reduction of neurotransmitters in the development of AD is not well understood.

Etiology

The exact cause of AD is unknown. Several theories and risk factors have been proposed: genetics, chemical imbalances, environmental agents, and immunologic changes.

There is little doubt that for many clients with AD there is a genetic predisposition to the development of the disease. Studies of families are ongoing to determine the exact genetic pathway that is responsible. Currently, the following four genes are associated with an increased risk of AD (Schutte, 1998):

- Presenilin I gene on chromosome 14
- Presenilin gene on chromosome 1
- Apolipoprotein E (Apo E) gene on chromosome 19
- Amyloid precursor protein gene on chromosome 21

People with Down syndrome often develop dementia with characteristic features of AD.

Chemical changes in the brain, particularly in relation to ACh and amyloid, are also being studied. Clients with AD may have a shortage of the neurotransmitter ACh and an abnormal buildup of amyloid. The abnormal buildup of amyloid appears to be directly related to the lack of ACh. An Alzheimer vaccine that could ultimately prevent AD is being tested with animals. This new experimental compound, currently called AN-1792, prevented amyloid plaques in mice (Alzheimer's Association, 1999).

Environmental agents, especially certain viruses such as herpes zoster and herpes simplex, as well as aluminum toxicity, have also been suggested as causes. Clients who have experienced a head injury may be more at risk for AD, and at an earlier age, than others.

Incidence/Prevalence

AD may affect anyone older than 40 years of age, although it occurs more often in those older than 65 years of age.

WOMEN'S HEALTH CONSIDERATIONS

When AD occurs in old age, it tends to affect women three times as often as men, perhaps in part because many women outlive men. Worldwide, AD occurs in more than 20 million people; some 5 million people in the United States older than 65 years of age have the disease. It is the fourth leading cause of death, after heart attacks, cancer, and strokes. The cost of care for those with the disease is estimated at more than $60 billion annually (Ross, 1999).

COLLABORATIVE MANAGEMENT

Assessment

The client with Alzheimer's disease (AD) often presents with cognitive impairment, although many other disorders, drugs, and environmental factors can cause changes in cognition as well. A thorough history and physical examination are necessary to differentiate AD from other, possibly reversible causes (Table 42-8). The nurse obtains information from family members or significant others, as well as from the client, because the client may be unaware of the problems, denying their existence or covering them up.

The most important information to be obtained concerns the onset, duration, progression, and course of the symptoms obtained. The nurse questions the client and the family about changes in memory or increasing forgetfulness and about the ability to perform activities of daily living (ADLs). Further information obtained includes current employment status, work history, and ability to fulfill household responsibilities, including cleaning, grocery shopping, and preparing meals. The nurse elicits a history concerning changes in driving ability, ability to handle routine financial transactions, and language and communication skills. In addition, any changes in personality and behavior are recorded.

The history taking concludes with a review of the client's medical history. The nurse asks about any history of head trauma, viral illness, or exposure to metal or toxic waste, as well as any family history of AD or Down syndrome.

PHYSICAL ASSESSMENT/CLINICAL MANIFESTATIONS

STAGES OF ALZHEIMER'S DISEASE. The clinical manifestations associated with AD can be grouped into three broad stages on the basis of the progress of the disease (Chart 42-11). The client does not necessarily progress from one stage to the next in an orderly fashion. A stage may be bypassed, or he or she may exhibit symptoms of one or several stages. Each client exhibits different disease stages and clinical manifestations. Consequently, some authorities now use broader terms, such as early (mild), middle (moderate), and late (severe) stages.

The primary focus of the nurse's neurologic assessment of clients with AD is to identify abnormalities in cognition, including language, personality, and behavior. Physical manifestations of neurologic impairment (seizures, tremors, or ataxia) tend to occur late in the disease process.

CHANGES IN COGNITION. **Cognition** refers to the ability of the brain to process, store, retrieve, and manipulate in-

TABLE 42-8 • CAUSES OF COGNITIVE IMPAIRMENT IN THE OLDER ADULT

NEUROLOGIC CAUSES
- Vascular insufficiency
- Infections
- Trauma
- Tumors
- Normal-pressure hydrocephalus

CARDIOVASCULAR CAUSES
- Myocardial infarction
- Dysrhythmias
- Congestive heart failure
- Cardiogenic shock
- Endocarditis

PULMONARY CAUSES
- Infection
- Pneumonia
- Hypoventilation

METABOLIC CAUSES
- Electrolyte imbalance
- Acidosis/alkalosis
- Hypoglycemia/hyperglycemia
- Acute and chronic renal failure
- Fluid volume deficit
- Hepatic failure

DRUG INTOXICATION
- Misuse of prescribed medications
- Side effects of medications
- Incorrect use of over-the-counter medications
- Ingestion of heavy metals

NUTRITIONAL DEFICIENCIES
- B vitamins
- Vitamin C
- Hypoproteinemia

ENVIRONMENTAL CAUSES
- Hypothermia/hyperthermia
- Unfamiliar environment
- Sensory deprivation/overload

PSYCHOLOGIC CAUSES
- Depression
- Anxiety
- Pain
- Fatigue
- Grief
- Paranoia

CHART 42-11

KEY FEATURES *of* Alzheimer's Disease

Early, or Stage I
- Forgets names; misplaces household items
- Mild memory loss
- Short attention span
- Subtle changes in personality and behavior
- No social or employment problems
- Cognitive impairment, problems with judgment
- Decreased performance, especially when stressed
- Unable to travel alone to new destinations
- Decreased knowledge of current events
- Loss of judgment
- Wandering

Middle, or Stage II
- Severe impairment of all cognitive functions
- Gross intellectual impairments
- Complete disorientation to time, place, and event
- Possible depression, agitated
- Physical impairment
- Loss of ability to care for self
- Visuospacial deficits
- Speech and language deficits
- Incontinent
- Wandering

Late, or Stage III
- Completely incapacitated
- Totally dependent in activities of daily living
- Motor and verbal skills lost
- General and focal neurologic deficits

formation. Therefore the nurse assesses the client for deficits in the following abilities:

- Attention and concentration
- Judgment and perception
- Learning and memory
- Communication and language
- Speed of information processing

Typical symptoms experienced by the client include memory impairment, as well as new memory, and defects in information retrieval resulting from dysfunction in the hippocampal, frontal, or parietal region. Alterations in communication abilities, such as **apraxia** (inability to use objects appropriately), **aphasia** (inability to speak or understand), **anomia** (inability to find words), and **agnosia** (loss of sensory comprehension), are due to dysfunction of the temporal and parietal lobes. Frontal lobe impairment produces difficulties with judgment, inability to make decisions, decreased attention span, and diminished ability to concentrate. As the disease progresses, the client loses all cognitive abilities, is totally unable to communicate, and becomes less aware of the environment.

To assess the presence of cognitive impairment, the nurse or other health care provider can use one of several assessment tools. One of the most popular tools is Folstein's Mini-Mental State Examination (MMSE), also known as the "mini-mental" (Folstein, Folstein, & McHugh, 1975). The MMSE assesses five major areas—orientation, registration, attention and calculation, recall, and speech/language (including reading). Figure 42-3, *A* lists examples of the questions asked on this test. The client performs certain cognitive tasks that are scored and added together for a total score of 0 to 30. The lower the score, the greater the severity of the dementia. It is not unusual for a client with advanced AD to score below 5.

Although the MMSE is used very frequently, the client must be able to read. For the client who cannot read, or for a quicker screening test, the nurse can use a SET test, which is especially useful for the older adult. The nurse asks the client to name 10 items in each of four categories: fruits, animals, colors, and towns (FACT). Other categories can be used, if necessary. The client receives 1 point for each item, for a possible maximum score of 40. Clients who score above 25 do not have dementia. Although this assessment is more comprehensive and easy to administer, it should not be used for clients with hearing impairments or aphasia. References describing other available tests to measure cognitive impairment may be found in the Selective Bibliography.

CHANGES IN BEHAVIOR AND PERSONALITY. One of the most difficult aspects of AD that families, significant others, and health care professionals cope with are the behavioral

Orientation to Time
"What is the date?"

Registration
"Listen carefully, I am going to say three words. You say them back after I stop. Ready? Here they are...
HOUSE (pause), CAR (pause), LAKE (pause). Now repeat those words back to me." [Repeat up to 5 times, but score only the first trial.]

Naming
"What is this?" [Point to a pencil or pen.]

Reading
"Please read this and do what it says." [Show examinee the words on the stimulus form.]
CLOSE YOUR EYES

A

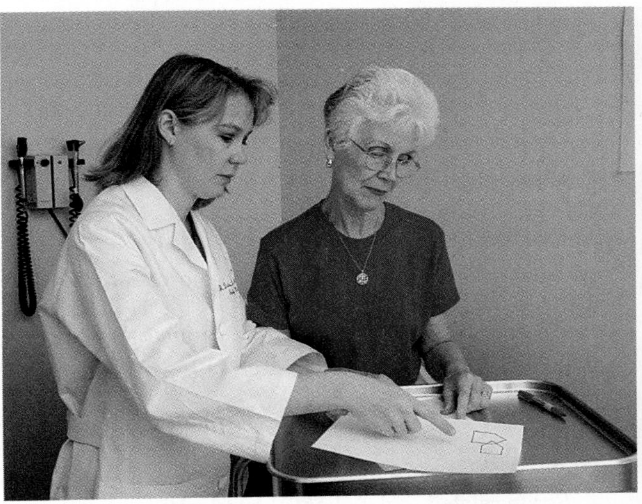

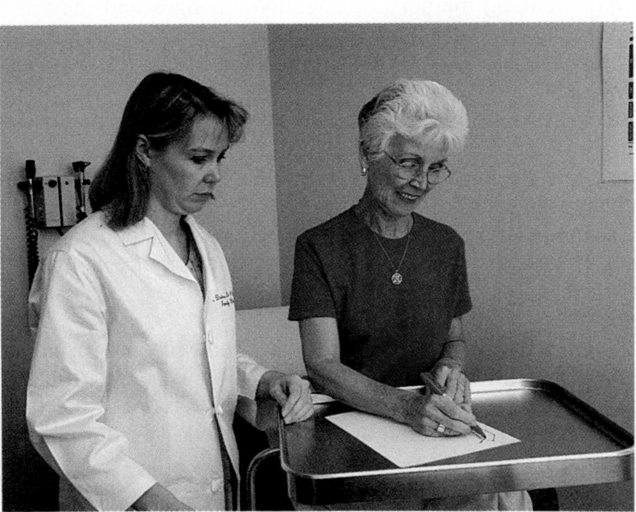

B

Figure 42-3 ● **A,** Examples of questions that are asked on the Mini-Mental State Examination. **B,** Copying is one of the tasks on the MMSE. (**A** from Mini-Mental State Examination © 1975, 1998, 2001 by MiniMental, LLC. All rights reserved. Published 2001 by Psychological Assessment Resources, Inc. May not be reproduced in whole or in part in any form or by any means without written permission of Psychological Assessment Resources, Inc., P.O. Box 998, Odessa, FL 33556; (800) 331-8378 or (813) 968-3003. **B** from Seidel, H.M., et al. (1999). *Mosby's guide to physical examination* (4th ed.). St. Louis: Mosby.)

changes that can occur in advanced disease. The nurse assesses for the following:

- Aggressiveness, especially verbal and physical abusive tendencies
- Rapid mood swings
- Increased confusion at night **(sundowning)** or in excessively fatigued clients

If the client is not too ill to ambulate, he or she may also wander and become lost or may go into other rooms to rummage through another's belongings. Hoarding objects such as washcloths is also common.

For some clients with dementia, emotional and behavioral problems accompany the primary disease. Some clients experience paranoia, delusions, hallucinations, and depression. The nurse assesses for these behaviors and documents their occurrence. (Refer to a mental health/behavioral health nursing textbook for a complete discussion of these disorders.)

Although drug therapy is not effective in treating dementia, certain drugs may help to control the emotional and psychiatric manifestations, such as depression, anxiety, paranoia, and aggression, associated with the primary disease.

CHANGES IN SELF-CARE SKILLS. Changes in the client's self-care skills that may be observed by the family, significant others, or nurse include the following:

- Decreased interest in personal appearance
- Selection of clothing that is inappropriate for the weather or event
- Loss of bowel and bladder control
- Decreased appetite or ability to eat

Over time, the client becomes less mobile and muscle contractures develop; the he or she eventually becomes totally immobile and requires total physical care.

PSYCHOSOCIAL ASSESSMENT

In people with AD, the cognitive changes, as well as biochemical and structural dysfunctions, affect personality and behavior. In the early stage, clients often recognize that they are experiencing memory or cognitive changes and may attempt to hide the problems, deny them, or become depressed over the changes. Older clients typically attribute the changes to "old age."

As the disease progresses, clients begin to display major changes in emotional and behavioral affect. Of particular importance is the need for the nurse to assess clients' reactions to changes in routine or environment. For example, a hospital admission is very traumatic for most clients with dementia. It is not unusual for them to exhibit a catastrophic response or overreact to any change by becoming excessively aggressive or abusive.

As clients become unaware of their behavior, the focus of the psychosocial assessment shifts to the family or significant others. The nurse assesses their ability to cope with the chronicity and progression of the disease and identifies possible support systems.

LABORATORY ASSESSMENT

No laboratory tests exist to confirm the diagnosis of AD. Diagnosis is made on the basis of brain tissue examination at autopsy, which confirms the presence of neurofibrillary tangles and neuritic plaques.

Genetic testing, specifically for apolipoprotein E (Apo E), may be helpful as an ancillary test (not a predictive test) for the differential diagnosis of AD. Four genes have been found to be associated with AD (see earlier discussion under Etiology, p. 913). Three are associated with early onset (before age 65), and one gene (Apo E) is associated primarily with late onset.

A variety of laboratory tests may be performed to rule out other treatable causes of dementia or delirium, including the following:

- A complete blood count (CBC)
- Determination of serum electrolyte levels, blood urea nitrogen, and glucose
- Determination of vitamin B_{12} levels
- Determination of folate levels
- Thyroid and liver function tests
- A serologic test for syphilis
- Drug toxicity screening tests (over-the-counter and illegal drugs)
- Alcohol screening tests

RADIOGRAPHIC ASSESSMENT

Computed tomography (CT) and positron emission tomography (PET) may be performed to rule out other causes of neurologic disease. The CT scan typically shows cerebral atrophy and ventricular enlargement, wide sulci, and shrunken gyri in the later stages of the disease. The PET scan, which measures glucose in living cells, shows a significant decrease in metabolic activity in the brains of people with AD.

OTHER DIAGNOSTIC ASSESSMENT

Magnetic resonance imaging (MRI) can also rule out other causes of neurologic disease. The electroencephalogram (EEG) shows slow-wave delta activity indicative of dementia in the second and third stages of AD.

In an effort to identify clearly the nature and extent of the client's cognitive dysfunction, several neuropsychologic tests are administered by the physician, usually a neurologist. The tests used depend on physician preference and the ability of the client to participate in testing. All of the tests focus on cognitive ability and may be repeated over time to measure changes.

• Analysis

COMMON NURSING DIAGNOSES AND COLLABORATIVE PROBLEMS

The following are common nursing diagnoses for clients with Alzheimer's disease (AD):

1. Chronic Confusion related to a limited attention span, loss of memory, and/or exposure to an unfamiliar environment
2. Risk for Injury related to memory loss, wandering, behavior changes, and/or seizure activity
3. Compromised Family Coping and Caregiver Role Strain related to the client's deteriorating condition and care demands
4. Disturbed Sleep Pattern related to an unfamiliar environment, overstimulation, and/or confusion

ADDITIONAL NURSING DIAGNOSES AND COLLABORATIVE PROBLEMS

In addition to the common nursing diagnoses, clients with AD may have one or more of the following:

- Impaired Verbal Communication related to aphasia, anomia, agnosia, and/or apraxia
- Imbalanced Nutrition: Less Than Body Requirements related to self-care deficit and/or anorexia
- Total Urinary Incontinence and Bowel Incontinence related to cognitive and self-care deficits
- Social Isolation related to personality and behavior changes
- Impaired Physical Mobility related to contractures and other effects of debilitating disease
- Risk for Impaired Skin Integrity related to immobility and/or impaired nutritional status
- Self-Care Deficit (Total) related to cognitive deficit
- Risk for Other-Directed Violence and Risk for Self-Directed Violence related to behavior changes
- Hopelessness related to inability to control the progression of disease

Planning and Implementation

CHRONIC CONFUSION

NOC **PLANNING: EXPECTED OUTCOMES.** The client with AD is expected to (1) be reoriented to person, place, or time in early AD or (2) have no or decreased episodes of agitation in middle to late AD.

INTERVENTIONS. The client with memory problems benefits from a structured and consistent environment. Many variables, including physical illness and environmental factors, can worsen or exacerbate the clinical manifestations of AD (Table 42-9). The nurse assesses for the presence of these factors so that they can be addressed if present.

NIC **COGNITIVE THERAPY.** The purpose of cognitive therapy is to reinforce or promote desirable cognitive function or alterations in undesirable cognitive function (Chart 42-12).

STRUCTURING THE ENVIRONMENT. The health care team collaborates to identify conditions in the environment that can be modified to increase the client's ability to function. The two most important actions that are necessary for the client with AD are preventing overstimulation and providing a structured and orderly environment.

PREVENTING OVERSTIMULATION. When a client is admitted to a new setting or environment (hospital, assisted-living, or long-term care facility), the staff works with the admitting department to select a room that is in the quietest area of the unit and away from obvious exits, if possible. A private room may be needed if the client has a history of agitation or wandering. The television should remain off unless the client turns it on or requests that it be turned on.

In addition to disturbed sleep, other negative effects of high noise levels include decreased nutritional intake, changes in blood pressure and pulse rates, and feelings of increased stress and anxiety. The client with AD is especially susceptible to these changes and needs to have as much undisturbed sleep at night as possible. Fatigue increases confusion and behavioral manifestations such as agitation and aggressiveness.

The nurse also assesses the client's assigned room for pictures on the wall that could be misinterpreted as people or animals that could harm the client. An abstract painting or wallpaper might look like a fire or an explosion and might scare the client. The nurse checks all areas of the room for adequate, nonglare lighting and potentially frightening shadows.

TABLE 42-9 • FACTORS THAT CAN WORSEN ALZHEIMER'S DISEASE

- Stroke
- Subdural hematoma
- Space-occupying lesion
- Decrease in blood supply to the brain
- Myocardial infarction
- Dysrhythmias
- Hypoglycemia
- Impaired renal function
- Impaired hepatic function
- Infection
- Impaired vision and hearing
- Sudden changes in surroundings
- Pain and discomfort
- Drugs
- Physical restraint

CHART 42-12

NIC INTERVENTION ACTIVITIES *for* The Client with Alzheimer's Disease

Cognitive Restructuring: *Challenging a client to alter distorted thought patterns and view self and the world more realistically*

- Help the client accept the fact that self-statements mediate emotional arousal.
- Help client understand the inability to attain desirable results from irrational self-statements.
- Point out styles of dysfunctional thinking (e.g., polarized thinking, overgeneralization, magnification, personalization).
- Assist client in labeling the painful emotion (e.g., anger, anxiety, hopelessness) that he or she is feeling.
- Assist client in identifying the perceived stressors (e.g., situations, events, interactions with other people) that contributed to his or her stress.

Memory Training: *Facilitation of memory*

- Discuss with client/family any practical memory problems experienced.
- Stimulate memory by repeating client's last expressed thought, as appropriate.
- Reminisce about past experiences with client, as appropriate.
- Implement appropriate memory techniques such as visual imagery, mnemonic devices, memory games, memory cues, association techniques, making lists, using computers, using name tags, or rehearsing information.
- Provide for orientation training, such as client rehearsing personal information and dates, as appropriate.
- Provide for picture recognition memory, as appropriate.
- Encourage client to participate in group memory training programs, as appropriate.
- Monitor client's behavior during therapy.

NIC intervention activities selected from McCloskey, J.C., & Bulechek, G.M. (2000). *Nursing interventions classification (NIC)* (3rd ed.). St. Louis: Mosby.

PROVIDING CONSISTENCY. The nurse plans ways to provide consistency for the client. For example, objects such as furniture, a hairbrush, and eyeglasses should be kept in the same place. A daily routine is established and followed as much as possible. In some settings, each room has a communication board on which scheduled activities and other data to promote orientation are listed, such as the day of the week, the month, and the year. Pictures of people familiar to the client can be placed on this board.

ORIENTATION AND VALIDATION THERAPY. The nurse explains changes in routine before the occurrence, repeating the explanation immediately before the changes take place. Clocks and single-date calendars also help the client maintain day-to-day orientation to the environment in the early stages of the disease process. For the client with early disease, **reality orientation** is usually appropriate. Family members and health care professionals should frequently reorient the client to the environment.

For the client in the later stages of AD, reality orientation is ineffective and often increases agitation. The health care team uses validation therapy for the client with moderate or severe AD. In **validation therapy,** the staff member recognizes and acknowledges the client's feelings and concerns. For example, rather than argue with the client who insists that he or she has not had breakfast (even though the nurse saw the client eat it), the nurse obtains juice, toast, or another food item.

PROMOTING INDEPENDENCE IN ACTIVITIES OF DAILY LIVING. As the disease progresses, altered thought processes affect the ability to perform activities of daily living (ADLs). The nurse allows the client to perform as much self-care as possible. The nurse also teaches the family or significant others that every effort should be made to allow the client to maintain independence in daily living skills as long as possible. For example, in the home setting, complete clothing outfits that can be easily removed and put on (e.g., shirt, slacks, underwear, and socks) can be placed on a single hanger; the client selects from these groupings. When possible, the client should participate in meal preparation, grocery shopping, and other household routines.

The nurse may need to consult with the occupational therapist for a complete evaluation and assistance in helping the client become more independent. Adaptive devices, such as grab bars in the bathtub or shower area, an elevated commode, and adapted eating utensils, may enable the client to maintain independence in grooming, toileting, and feeding.

PROMOTING BOWEL AND BLADDER CONTINENCE. The client may remain continent of bowel and bladder for long periods if taken to the bathroom or given a bedpan or urinal every 2 hours or more often during the day and possibly less frequently at night. The staff encourages him or her to drink adequate fluids to promote optimal voiding. A client may refuse to drink enough fluids because of a fear of incontinence. The staff assures the client that he or she will be toileted on a regular schedule to prevent incontinent episodes.

When clients with AD are in the hospital or other unfamiliar place, they may get out of bed unassisted during the night and fall while trying to locate the bathroom. In some hospitals, the siderails on beds are required to be up for all clients older than 60 or 65 years of age. However, if the client climbs over the siderail and falls, the injury is likely to be worse than if the bed had been left in the lowest position and the siderail left down (preferably the lower rail in a split rail system). The nurse maintains an unobstructed path between the bed and bathroom at all times. For clients who are too weak to walk to the bathroom, a bedside commode may be used. (See Chapter 5 for further discussion on fall prevention.)

Some clients may void in inappropriate places, such as the sink or a wastebasket. As a reminder of where they should toilet, the nurse may place a picture of the commode on the bathroom door. Depending on written signs for identification is useless because most clients lose their ability to read as the disease progresses.

ASSISTING WITH FACIAL RECOGNITION. As the disease progresses, the client may experience **prosopagnosia,** an inability to recognize oneself and other familiar faces (see the Evidence-Based Practice for Nursing box below). The nurse encourages the family to provide pictures of family members and close friends that are labeled with the person's name on the picture. In addition, the nurse advises the family to reminisce with the client about pleasant experiences from the past. The nurse may also conduct reminiscence therapy while assisting the client with ADLs or performing a treatment or assessment. Referring to a personal item in the room may help the client begin to talk about its meaning in the present and in the past.

It is not unusual for the client to talk to his or her image in the mirror. This behavior should be allowed as long as it is not harmful. If the client becomes frightened by the mirror image, the nurse covers the mirror. In some health care settings, a

EVIDENCE-BASED PRACTICE FOR NURSING

Do clients with mild to moderate Alzheimer's disease retain personal identity?

Tappen, R.M., et al. (1999). Persistence of self in advanced Alzheimer's disease. *Image: The Journal of Nursing Scholarship 31*(2), 121-131.

The purpose of this qualitative study was to determine if there is evidence of the persistence of a sense of self or personal identity in people with mild to moderate Alzheimer's disease (AD). Literature on AD indicates the theme of a diminishing sense of self occurring in the late stages of the disease. Analysis of 45 conversations with 23 subjects was conducted to search for the use of the first-person pronoun, self-reference, or indications of personal identity. Evidence to counter the idea of a sense of self was also explored.

The researchers found that the clients used the first-person pronoun freely, frequently, and coherently, thus supporting the notion that clients with mild to moderate AD are very much aware of their personal identity. Clients were also aware of the changes in their cognitive function and struggled to find an explanation for it.

Critique. This study provides valuable information for anyone associated with clients with AD. It is important to remember that a qualitative study cannot be judged by the sample number but should be viewed in the context of interpretation of meaning. The researchers note that one subject spoke in a combination of Yiddish and English that neither the project staff nor a native Yiddish speaker could accurately transcribe.

Implications for Nursing. Health care providers and caregivers need to have an understanding of the experience of clients with AD. This knowledge can lead to the development of more holistic and humanistic approaches to care, to preserve the personhood and individuality of the client with AD.

picture of the client is placed on the room door to help with facial recognition and to help the client locate his or her room. This picture also helps the staff to locate the client in case of elopement (running away). A nursing study by Tappen et al. (1999) found that clients in the mild and moderate stages of AD continue to be aware of self (see the Evidence-Based Practice for Nursing box on p. 918).

PROMOTING COMMUNICATION. With the intervention known as **redirection,** the nurse assists the client with communication problems and nonlistening behaviors by attracting his or her attention before conversing, The environment should be as free of distractions as possible. The nurse speaks directly to the client in a slow and distinct manner. Sentences should be clear and short. The client is asked to perform one task at a time, and sufficient time must be allowed for completion. It may be necessary to break each task down into many small steps.

As the disease progresses, the client is unable to perform tasks when asked. The nurse shows what needs to be done or provides cues to remind the client how to perform the task. For example, if the nurse wishes to clean the client's dentures but the client refuses to remove them from the mouth, the nurse leaves a denture cup, which may trigger the client's memory about the need to remove and clean the dentures. When possible, the nurse explains and demonstrates the task that the client is asked to perform.

DRUG THERAPY. Acetylcholinesterase inhibitors, such as galantamine (Reminyl), donepezil (Aricept), and rivastigmine (Exelon), are drugs approved for symptomatic treatment of AD. These drugs improve cholinergic neurotransmission in the central nervous system (CNS) by delaying the destruction of acetylcholine (ACh) by acetylcholinesterase, thus delaying the onset of cognitive decline. None of these drugs affects the course of the disease. They have side effects that include gastrointestinal upset and liver toxicity. Liver function tests should be monitored frequently. Additional side effects include dizziness, unsteadiness, and clumsiness. Tacrine seems to cause more problems than other drugs in its class and therefore is no longer commonly used. Side effects have been noted to occur more often with women and with advancing age.

Investigational drugs for AD include metrifonate (ProMem), lazabemide (Tempium), physostigmine (Synapton), idebenon, propentofylline (HWA-285), and galantamine (Reminyl). Most of these drugs work like donepezil.

Some clients with AD experience depression and may be treated with fluvoxamine (Luvox), sertraline (Zoloft), desipramine (Norpramin), maprotiline (Ludiomil), or trazodone (Desyrel). Antidepressants such as amitriptyline (Elavil, Levate🍁) should not be used because of their anticholinergic effect. The nurse observes for therapeutic effects of these medications and reports side effects, such as increased delirium, drowsiness, orthostatic hypotension, and urinary retention, to the health care provider as soon as possible.

Psychotropic drugs, also called antipsychotic and neuroleptic drugs, should be reserved for clients with emotional and behavioral health problems that sometimes accompany dementia, such as hallucinations and delusions. In clinical practice, however, the nurse may find that these drugs are sometimes inappropriately used for agitation, combativeness, or restlessness.

Psychotropic drugs are considered chemical restraints because they decrease mobility and clients' ability to care for themselves. Therefore most geriatricians recommend that these medications be used as a last resort and with caution in low doses for a specific emotional or behavioral health problem, because most clients with dementia are in late adulthood (see Chapter 5). The specific drug prescribed depends on side effects, the condition of the client, and anticipated outcomes. For example, some geriatricians favor thioridazine (Mellaril, Novo-Ridazine🍁) over haloperidol (Haldol, Peridol🍁), a commonly prescribed medication for older adults, because of haloperidol's potency and tendency to be overprescribed. The nurse observes for drug side effects, including increased confusion and extrapyramidal symptoms (e.g., rigidity, tremors), drooling, constipation, and urinary retention, and promptly reports these effects to the health care provider.

COMPLEMENTARY AND ALTERNATIVE THERAPIES. A number of complementary and alternative therapies are being researched that may prevent AD, slow its occurrence, or slow its progression in older adults. Examples of these therapies include vitamin E and selegiline (antioxidants), ibuprofen, estrogen, melatonin, and nicotine patches (Schweiger & Huey, 1999).

Art, massage, dance, and music therapy are often used in long-term care settings to minimize agitation. Rowe and Alfred (1999) found that expressions of agitation among clients with AD increased in a linear pattern from dawn until dusk. Although verbal displays of agitation were not affected, slow-stroke massage decreased the more physical expressions, such as pacing, wandering, and resisting care. Another nursing study found that expressive physical touch with verbalization was effective in decreasing anxiety and dysfunctional behavior of clients with AD (Kim & Buschmann, 1999).

RISK FOR INJURY

PLANNING: EXPECTED OUTCOMES. The client with Alzheimer's disease (AD) is expected to remain free from physical harm and not injure anyone else.

INTERVENTIONS. Many clients with AD tend to wander and may easily become lost. In later stages of the disease, some clients may become severely agitated and physically or verbally abusive to others.

COPING WITH RESTLESSNESS AND WANDERING. The nurse teaches the home caregiver that the client should always wear an identification badge or bracelet. In an inpatient setting the client is checked frequently and placed in a room that can be monitored easily. The room may need to be close to the nurses' station (if the noise level in the nurses' station can be managed) and away from exits and stairs. Some health care agencies place large stop signs or red tape on the floor in front of exits. Others have installed alarm systems to indicate when a client is opening the door.

Restlessness may be decreased if the client is taken for frequent walks. If the client begins to wander, the nurse redirects him or her and tries to determine where he or she is trying to go. For example, if the client insists on going shopping for clothes, the nurse or other caregiver might redirect the client to his or her closet to select clothing that will not be recognized as his or her own. This type of activity can be repeated a number of times because the client has lost short-term memory.

In any setting, clients should be kept busy with structured activities. In a health care agency an activity or recreational therapist may work with clients as a group or individually to determine the type of activity that is appropriate for the stage of the disease. Puzzles, board games, and art activities are often appropriate. Music and art therapy are becoming very popular in acute and long-term care for clients with dementia (Clark, Lipe, & Bilbrey, 1998).

Physical restraints, such as protective vests and geri-chairs with lap boards, should be used only as a last resort because they often increase the restlessness and cause agitation. Federal regulations in long-term care facilities in the United States mandate that all residents have the right to be free of both physical and chemical restraints. In addition, agencies accredited by the Joint Commission on Accreditation of Healthcare Agencies (JCAHO) are required to minimize the use of restraints and use alternatives (see Chapter 5).

ENSURING SAFETY. Clients with AD may become injured because they cannot recognize objects or situations as harmful. All potentially dangerous objects (e.g., knives, needles, and cleaning solutions) are removed or secured. Clients are often unaware that their driving ability is impaired and usually want to continue this activity even if their driver's license has been suspended secondary to the disease. Automobile keys must be secured, and the client appropriately informed.

Late in the disease process, the client may experience seizure activity. The nurse institutes seizure precautions and takes appropriate action during a seizure episode (see earlier discussion under Interventions [Epilepsy], p. 901).

MINIMIZING AGITATION. In the event of agitated behavior, the nurse talks calmly and softly and attempts to redirect the client to a more positive behavior or activity. If the client remains agitated, the nurse ensures the client's safety and leaves the room after explaining that he or she will return later. Frequent visual checks must be done during this time.

If the client is connected to any type of tubing or other device, he or she may try to disconnect it or pull it out. These devices should be used sparingly in the client with dementia. If IV access, for example, is needed, the nurse places the catheter or cannula in an area that the client cannot easily see. Some health care agencies recommend covering the site with a transparent protective device such as the I.V. House (see Chapter 14).

Another way to manage this problem is to provide a diversion. For example, if the client is doing an activity or holding an item such as a stuffed animal or doll, he or she might be less likely to pay attention to medical devices. The nurse asks the family or significant others to provide the client's favorite keepsake, which may help to divert the client's attention. Some nursing units keep items on hand for this purpose.

COMPROMISED FAMILY COPING/CAREGIVER ROLE STRAIN

PLANNING: EXPECTED OUTCOMES. The family or other caregivers of the client with Alzheimer's disease (AD) are expected to obtain appropriate support services to enable them to adjust and cope with the client's physical and mental problems.

INTERVENTIONS. The client with AD requires continual, 24-hour supervision and caregiving. Severe cognitive changes leave the client unable to manage finances, property, or personal care. The nurse advises the family to seek legal counsel regarding the client's competency and the need to obtain guardianship or a durable medical power of attorney. The family can be referred to the local AD support group for literature and information concerning the disease and related problems.

The nurse establishes a supportive environment for family members and encourages them to express their feelings to other family members. They are also encouraged to maintain their own social network and obtain respite from care of the client. In a study of African-American caregivers by Sterritt and Pokorny (1998), four major themes emerged:

- Caregiving is a traditional family value.
- Caregiving is an act of love.
- Social support is a mediator of the caregiver burden.
- Caregiving is a female role.

Buffam and Brod (1998) found that humor improved the well-being of 96 older spouse caregivers of community-dwelling clients with AD. Caregivers of clients with advanced disease used less humor and had more psychologic distress than caregivers of clients who had early-stage disease.

DISTURBED SLEEP PATTERN

NOC **PLANNING: EXPECTED OUTCOMES.** The client with AD is expected to sleep through the night and be awake at appropriate times.

INTERVENTIONS. The client with AD often has difficulty sleeping at night but tends to nap frequently during the day. One way to establish the usual day-night pattern is to keep the client very active during the day. A daily routine that consists of a balance between passive activities and those requiring more strenuous exercise, such as walking or stretching activities, usually facilitates sleep at night. The client may want to take a nap in the late afternoon, but this should be discouraged if possible. In the last stage of the disease, the client may sleep during much of the day and night.

To facilitate sleep, a before-bedtime ritual is established. The routine usually consists of personal hygiene activities (e.g., bathing, toileting, brushing teeth) and environmental control measures to reduce noise and eliminate distractions. A back rub or small snack may help the client prepare for sleep.

The nurse adjusts the client's treatment and medication schedule to provide for uninterrupted sleep. If more conventional measures fail to induce sleep, the health care provider may prescribe a mild antianxiety agent or hypnotic.

Community-Based Care

HOME CARE MANAGEMENT

Alzheimer's disease (AD) is a chronic, progressive condition that eventually leaves the client completely disoriented and totally dependent on others for all aspects of care. In the early stages, clients may be cared for at home with little need for outside intervention. Whenever possible, the client and family should be assigned to a case manager, who can assess their needs for health care resources and facilitate appropriate placement throughout the continuum of care.

The client usually begins to withdraw from friends and social events as memory impairment and personality and behavior changes become more apparent. This increases the family's responsibilities to minimize the impact of social isolation and decreased activity. The family may begin to decrease their own social activities as the demands of the client's care take more of their time. The nurse should emphasize to the family the importance of maintaining their own social contacts and leisure activities. Many family members experience caregiver stress, which affects their physical, mental, and emotional health. Chart 42-13 lists strategies for reducing caregiver stress. (See Chapter 5 for further discussion on caregiver role strain and interventions.)

It is now possible in most areas of the United States for the family to arrange respite care. The client may be placed in a respite facility or nursing home for the weekend or for several weeks to give the family a rest from the constant care demands. The family may also be able to obtain respite care in the home through a home care agency or the Alzheimer's Disease and Related Disorders Association (often called the Alzheimer's Association). The nurse stresses that respite care is for a short period of time; it is not a permanent placement. Some health care agencies have opened adult day care centers or specialty units for clients with AD. In the day care center, clients spend all or part of the day at the facility and participate in activities as their condition permits. Although these centers are usually open only on weekdays, this arrangement allows the caregiver to work or participate in other activities.

The nurse teaches the family to be prepared in the event that the client becomes restless, agitated, abusive, or combative. In addition, the family can learn how to use reality orientation or validation therapy, depending on the stage of the disease.

HEALTH TEACHING

Usually the client with AD is cared for in the home until late in the disease process. Because health insurance coverage in the United States and family finances are usually insufficient to cover the services of a private duty nurse or home care aide, the care is typically provided by family members. The client care plan developed by the nurse or case manager, in conjunction with the family, must be reasonable and realistic for the family to implement.

CHART 42-13

CLIENT EDUCATION GUIDE
Reducing Caregiver Stress

- Maintain realistic expectations for the person with Alzheimer's disease (AD)
- Take each day one at a time.
- Try to find the positive aspects of each incident or situation.
- Use humor with the person who has AD.
- Set aside time each day for rest or recreation away from the client, if possible.
- Seek respite care periodically for longer periods of time.
- Use the resources of the Alzheimer's Association, including attending local support group meetings.
- Explore alternative care settings early in the disease process for possible use later.
- Establish advance directives with the AD client early in the disease process.

The nurse teaches the family how to assist with bathing, dressing, toileting, and other self-care activities. The occupational therapist teaches the family and the client how to use adaptive equipment, such as a brace, a sling, a cane, or modified eating utensils. The client may have difficulty chewing, swallowing, or tasting foods and may not be able to eat without assistance. The nurse, the family, and the dietitian should develop a diet plan to maximize the client's nutritional intake. In the late stage of AD, the client's intake often decreases, and he or she loses weight.

The nurse also teaches the family what to do in the event of a seizure and how to protect the client from injury. The family is instructed to notify the health care provider if the seizure is prolonged or if the client's seizure pattern changes.

DRUG THERAPY. The nurse explains the name, time, and route of administration; the dosage; and the side effects of all medications to the family or other caregiver. The family is instructed to check with the health care provider before using any over-the-counter medications because they may interact with prescribed medication.

EXERCISE. The nurse emphasizes the need for the client to have an established exercise program to maintain mobility as long as possible, as well as to prevent complications of immobility. In collaboration with the family, the physical therapist develops an individualized exercise program. The physical therapist may continue to work with the client at home until goals are achieved, depending on the payer source.

SAFETY. The nurse instructs the family or other caregiver to take special precautions to maintain the client safely at home. The environment must be uncluttered, consistent, and structured. All hazardous items (e.g., cleaning fluids, power tools, insect spray) are removed or secured. All electrical sockets not in use should be covered with safety plugs. Handrails and grab bars should be installed in the bathroom; handrails should be along all stairways, and a guardrail should be placed around porches or open stairwells. Because the client may have a tendency to wander, especially at night, the family may want to install alarms to all outside doors, the basement, and the client's bedroom. All outside and basement doors should have deadbolt locks to prevent the client from going outside unsupervised. The temperature of the water heater should be adjusted to prevent accidental burns. Night-lights should be used in the client's bedroom, hallway, and bathroom.

HEALTH CARE RESOURCES

When the client can no longer be cared for at home, referral to an assisted-living or long-term care facility may be needed. Early in the course of the disease, the nurse should advise the family that placement may be needed in the late stages of the disease. This allows the family to begin the search process for an appropriate facility before a crisis develops and immediate placement is needed. A number of facilities specialize in the care of clients with AD and other dementias. These units generally have a high staff-client ratio and are architecturally designed to meet the special needs of this type of client. The national office of the Alzheimer's

Association has a publication that outlines criteria for a dementia unit.

All families should be referred to their local chapter of the Alzheimer's Association. This organization provides information and support services to clients and their families, including seminars, audiovisual aids, and publications.

> **CRITICAL THINKING CHALLENGE**
>
> When making a home visit, a caregiver wife tells you that she is having problems managing her husband, who has AD, at home. He frequently gets up at night and wanders outside and has begun urinating in various parts of the house, most often in a wastebasket. She confides in you that she feels guilty for complaining, but she is afraid that she may not be able to keep him safe.
>
> - What stage of AD does the client have?
> - What are realistic outcomes for the husband in this stage of the disease?
> - What options does the wife have if she wishes to keep him at home?
> - What community resources might she explore for him now and perhaps later, when his disease progresses?

For suggested answer guidelines, go to SIMON http://www.wbsaunders.com/SIMON/Iggy/.

Evaluation: Outcomes

NOC The nurse evaluates the care of the client with Alzheimer's disease (AD) on the basis of the identified nursing diagnoses and collaborative problems. The expected outcomes include that the client will:

- Remain at home for as long as possible
- Maintain independence in activities of daily living (ADLs) and self-care skills as long as possible to preserve quality of life
- Remain free of injury from falls, seizure activity, and environmental hazards
- Be reoriented to person, place, or time in early AD
- Sleep through the night and be awake at appropriate times

HUNTINGTON'S DISEASE

OVERVIEW

Huntington's disease (HD), formerly called Huntington's chorea, is a hereditary disorder transmitted as an autosomal dominant trait at the time of conception. The causative gene is located on chromosome number 4. The offspring of a parent with the disease has a 50% chance of eventually manifesting the disease. It is estimated that 25,000 people in the United States have the disease, and another 20,000 to 50,000 are thought to carry the gene (Hickey, 1997). Men and women are equally affected, and symptoms begin between 30 and 50 years of age, striking at a highly productive time in life. The clinical onset of HD is gradual. The two main symptoms of the disease are progressive mental status changes, leading to dementia, and choreiform movements (rapid, jerky movements) in the limbs, trunk, and facial muscles. Dementia is related to the destruction of neurons within the cerebral cortex; it may also be associated with excessive amounts of dopamine found within the cerebral cortex and limbic systems of those affected.

Two structures within the basal ganglia are involved in the development of HD: the caudate nucleus and the putamen. Both structures have close connections to the cerebral cortex and are closely associated with neurotransmitters. Neurotransmitters are secreted at the synapse, or junction, of one neuron with another, and it is through their specific excitation or inhibition of neurons that fine, controlled, integrated motor activity occurs.

In the presence of HD, there is a decrease in the amount of gamma-aminobutyric acid (GABA) and acetylcholine (ACh), both excitatory neurotransmitters. Dopamine is not affected. This shift in balance between dopamine (an inhibitory neurotransmitter) and GABA at the synapse leads to uninhibited motor activity. The result is brisk, jerky, purposeless movements, particularly of the hands, face, tongue, and legs, which the client is unable to stop.

There are three stages of HD, each lasting roughly 5 years, corresponding to the average 15-year course of the disease. Stage 1 is the onset of neurologic or psychologic symptoms; stage 2 is characterized by an increasing dependence on others for care; stage 3 results in loss of independent function.

The diagnosis of HD is made on the basis of a family history of the disease and clinical assessment. The triad of dominant inheritance, choreoathetosis, and dementia are hallmarks of the disease. Clinical manifestations include chorea, poor balance, hesitant or explosive speech, dysphagia, impaired respiration, and bowel and bladder incontinence. Mental status changes include decreased attention span, poor judgment, memory loss, personality changes, and dementia (later in the disease process).

> **CULTURAL CONSIDERATIONS**
>
> HD is most prevalent in people of western European ancestry (Adams et al., 1997).

COLLABORATIVE MANAGEMENT

There is no known cure or treatment for HD. The only way to prevent transmission of the gene is for those affected to refrain from having children. Genetic counseling is important for children of clients with the disease. It is now possible to test people at risk for the disease to determine whether or not the gene is present on chromosome 4 (see the Legal/Ethical Issues in Health Care box on p. 923). Before the testing procedure is undertaken, counseling is necessary to ensure that the client has voluntarily decided in favor of testing and is not being pressured by family or friends. In addition, counseling helps to determine whether the benefits of knowing the results outweigh the risks of a positive result (e.g., depression or suicide).

Management is symptomatic. Some symptoms can be managed with medications, but there is no cure. The client's status deteriorates, and death occurs from complications of immobility, such as pneumonia, sepsis, or heart disease, within 15 years of the onset of symptoms. Haloperidol (Haldol) is most effective in suppressing the movement disorder, but it is used only when the movements are functionally disabling.

LEGAL/ETHICAL ISSUES IN HEALTH CARE

PRESYMPTOMATIC GENE TESTING FOR HUNTINGTON'S DISEASE

Predicting whether a person will develop an inherited disease in the future is termed presymptomatic testing. Although it may seem that knowing whether or not one may develop a disease could be advantageous in terms of prior planning and decision making in health and end-of-life care and relief of uncertainty, this is not always the case. Advances in technology allow scientists to conduct presymptomatic testing of healthy people with a family history of Huntington's disease (HD) to determine if they have the gene mutation for the disease. The psychosocial outcomes of presymptomatic testing for HD, an incurable, progressive, and neurodegenerative disorder, are enormous. Carriers and noncarriers of the gene may experience a wide variety of emotional reactions following disclosure of the results. Participants seeking such information should consider the effect of the knowledge on themselves and their families. The possibility that discrimination in employment or insurance limitations may occur often contributes to participants' not obtaining the results of the testing. Risk identification and genetic counseling are essential to facilitate decision making regarding this issue.

From Williams, J.K., et al. (1999). Adults seeking presymptomatic gene testing for Huntington disease. *Image: The Journal of Nursing Scholarship 31*(2), 109-113.

ONLINE RESOURCES

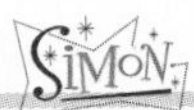

For suggested readings and Internet resources, go to http://www.wbsaunders.com/SIMON/Iggy/.

SELECTED BIBLIOGRAPHY

Asterisk indicates a classic or definitive work on this subject.

Abudi, S., et al. (1997). Parkinson's disease symptoms—Patient's perspective. *Journal of Advanced Nursing, 25*(1), 54-59.

Adams, R.D., et al. (1997). *Principles of neurology* (6th ed.). New York: McGraw-Hill.

Allen, L.A. (1999). Treating agitation without drugs. *American Journal of Nursing, 99*(4), 36-42.

Alzheimer's Association. (1999). A vaccine for Alzheimer's? *Advances, 19*(3), 1, 4.

American Association of Neuroscience Nurses. (1997). *Clinical guidelines series: Seizure assessment.* Chicago: Author.

Arle, J., & Alterman, R. (1999). Surgical options in Parkinson's disease. *Medical Clinics of North America, 83*(2), 483-498.

Blacker, D., et al. (1997). Apo E-4 and the age of onset of Alzheimer's disease. *Neurology, 48*(1), 139-141.

Brown University. (1999). Psychotropic drugs in phase III development: Alzheimer's disease and other dementias. *GeroPsych Report, 3*(11), 6.

Buckwalter, K.C. (1997). What's hot, what's not, in dementia drugs? Part 1. Cholinergic therapies. *Journal of Gerontological Nursing, 23*(9), 52-54.

Buffam, M.D., & Brod, M. (1998). Humor and well-being in spouse caregivers of patients with Alzheimer's disease. *Applied Nursing Research, 11*(1), 12-18.

Burgener, S.C., et al. (1998). Effective caregiving approaches for patients with Alzheimer's disease. *Geriatric Nursing, 19*(3), 121-126.

Campbell, J.M., Linc, L., & Mutersbaugh, K. (1998). Viral encephalitis: A challenging diagnosis in an ICU. *Critical Care Nurse, 18*(3), 58-65.

Centers for Disease Control and Prevention. (2000). Guidelines for surveillance, prevention, and control of West Nile virus infection—United States. *Morbidity and Mortality Weekly Report, 49*(1), 25-28.

Chiocca, E. (1997). Action stat—bacterial meningitis. *Nursing97, 27*(9), 33.

*Chisholm, A.H. (1996). Fetal tissue transplantation for the treatment of Parkinson's disease: A review of the literature. *Journal of Neuroscience Nursing, 28*(5), 329-338.

Clark, M.E., Lipe, A.W., & Bilbrey, M. (1998). Use of music to decrease aggressive behaviors in people with dementia. *Journal of Gerontological Nursing, 24*(7), 10-17.

Cleeland, E.A., & Davis, L.L. (1997). Depression in elders with dementia: Implications for home healthcare practice. *Home Healthcare Nurse, 15*(11), 780-787.

Deraps, P.K. (2000). Managing migraines. *Advance for Nurses, 2*(4), 11-13.

Eller, T.W., & Dan, D.A. (1997). Stereotactic pallidotomy for treatment of Parkinson's disease. *AORN Journal, 65*(5), 903-904, 907-916.

*Folstein, M.F., Folstein, S.E., & McHugh, P.R. (1975). "Mini-mental state": A practical method for grading the cognitive state of patients for the clinician. *Journal of Psychiatric Research, 12*(3), 189-198.

Forbes, D.A. (1998). Strategies for managing behavioural symptomatology associated with dementia for the Alzheimer type: A systematic overview. *Canadian Journal of Nursing Research, 30*(2), 67-86.

Fowler, S. (1997). Hope and a health promoting lifestyle in persons with Parkinson's disease. *Journal of Neuroscience Nursing, 29*(2), 111-116.

Gilbert, K. (1999). An algorithm for diagnosis and treatment of status epilepticus in adults. *Journal of Neuroscience Nursing, 31*(1), 27-36.

*Gilbert, M., Counsell, C.M., & Snively, C. (1996). Pallidotomy: A surgical intervention for control of Parkinson's disease. *Journal of Neuroscience Nursing, 28*(4), 215-221.

Habermann, B. (1999). Continuity challenges of Parkinson's disease in middle life. *Journal of Neuroscience Nursing, 31*(4), 200-207.

Harrison, L.H., et al. (1999). Risk of meningococcal infection in college students. *Journal of the American Medical Association, 281*(20), 1906-1910.

Hickey, J.V. (1997). *The clinical practice of neurological and neuroscience nursing* (4th ed.). Philadelphia: Lippincott-Raven.

Hoffman, N. (1999). Understanding the neuropsychiatric symptoms of Huntington's disease. *Journal of Neuroscience Nursing, 31*(5), 309-313.

Jacobs, L.A., & Deatrick, J.A. (1999). The individual, the family, and genetic testing. *Journal of Professional Nursing, 15*(5), 313-324.

Kim, E.J., & Buschmann, M.T. (1999). The effect of expressive physical touch on patients with dementia. *International Journal of Nursing Studies, 36*(3), 235-243.

Kovach, C.R., & Magliocco, J.S. (1998). Late-stage dementia and participation in therapeutic activities. *Applied Nursing Research, 11*(4), 167-173.

Lewis, A.M. (1999). Neurologic emergency! *Nursing99, 29*(10), 54-56.

Lloyd, M., Matthews, M., & Mulholland, H. (1999). Parkinson's disease: What a nurse should know. *Nursing Spectrum,* November 29, pp. 14-15.

Marin, P. (1998). Pharmacologic management of migraine. *Journal of the American Academy of Nurse Practitioners, 10*(9), 407-410.

McNew, C.D., Hunt, S., & Warner, L.S. (1997). How to help your patient with epilepsy. *Nursing97, 27*(9), 57-63.

Montagna, P., et al. (1997). Male preponderance: Similar pathway to migraine. *Neurology, 48*(1), 113-118.

*Neal, L.J. (1996a). The home care client with Alzheimer's disease: Part 1. Assessment tool for activities of daily living. *Home Healthcare Nurse, 14*(3), 175-178.

*Neal, L.J. (1996b). The home care client with Alzheimer's disease: Part 2. Interventions. *Home Healthcare Nurse, 14*(4), 265-267.

Nuorti, J., et al. (2000). Cigarette smoking and invasive pneumococcal disease. *New England Journal of Medicine, 342*(10), 681-689.

Ozuna, J. (1997a). Action stat–Status epilepticus. *Nursing97, 27*(12), 47.

Ozuna, J. (1997b). Pharmacologic management of epilepsy: An update, *Journal of Neuroscience Nursing 29*(5), 330-337.

Patil, A.A., Andrews, R., & Torkelson, R. (1997). Surgical treatment of intractable seizures with multilobar or bi-hemispheric seizure focus. *Surgical Neurology, 41*(1), 72-78.

Ross, A.P. (1999). Neurologic degenerative diseases. *Nursing Clinics of North America, 34*(3), 725-742.

Rowe, M., & Alfred, D. (1999). The effectiveness of slow-stroke massage in diffusing agitated behaviors in individuals with Alzheimer's disease. *Journal of Gerontological Nursing, 25*(6), 22-34.

Schlicher, M.L. (1998). Dilantin jeopardy: Avoiding the dangers of phenytoin. *MEDSURG Nursing, 7*(6), 343-347, 356.

Schutte, D.L. (1998). The impact of Alzheimer disease genetics on expert and advanced gerontological nursing practice. *AACN Clinical Issues: Advanced Practice in Acute and Critical Care, 9*(4), 513-523.

Schweiger, J.L., & Huey, R.A. (1999). Alzheimer's disease—Your role in the caregiving equation. *Nursing99, 29*(6), 34-41.

Shafer, P.O. (1999). New therapies in the management of acute or cluster seizures and seizure emergencies. *Journal of Neuroscience Nursing, 31*(4), 224-230.

Shikiar, R., et al. (2000). The impact of metrifonate therapy on caregivers of patients with Alzheimer's disease: Results from the MALT clinical trial. *Journal of the American Geriatrics Society, 48,* 268-274.

Simon, D., & Strandaert, D. (1999). Neuroprotective therapies. *Medical Clinics of North America, 83*(2), 509-523.

Snively, C., Counsell, C., & Lilly, D. (1998). Vagus nerve stimulator as a treatment for intractable epilepsy. *Journal of Neuroscience Nursing, 30*(5), 286-289.

Sterritt, P.F., & Pokorny, M.E. (1998). African-American caregiving for a relative with Alzheimer's disease. *Geriatric Nursing, 19*(3), 133-134.

Tappen, R.M., et al. (1999). Persistence of self in advanced Alzheimer's disease. *Image: The Journal of Nursing Scholarship, 31*(2), 121-131.

Vickers, L.F., & O'Neill, C.M. (1998). An interdisciplinary home healthcare program for patients with Parkinson's disease. *Rehabilitation Nursing, 23*(6), 286-289, 299.

Wallhagen, M.I., & Brod, M. (1997). Perceived control and well-being in Parkinson's disease. *Western Journal of Nursing Research, 19*(11), 11-31.

Williams, J.K., et al. (1999). Adults seeking presymptomatic gene testing for Huntington disease. *Image: The Journal of Nursing Scholarship, 31*(2), 109-113.

Winkelman, C. (1999). A review of pharmacodynamics and pharmacokinetics in seizure management. *Journal of Neuroscience Nursing, 31*(1), 50-53.

Wright, L.K., et al. (1999). Emotional and physical health of spouse caregivers of persons with Alzheimer's disease and stroke. *Journal of Advanced Nursing, 30*(3), 552-563.

Yen, P.K. (1997). Weight loss resulting from Alzheimer's disease. *Geriatric Nurse, 18*(3), 132-133.

CHAPTER 43

Interventions for Clients with Problems of the Central Nervous System

The Spinal Cord

DEBORAH WRIGHT SHPRITZ

Learning Objectives

After studying this chapter, you should be able to:

1. Identify risk factors that contribute to back pain.
2. Explain ways to prevent back pain.
3. Plan care for the client having a diskectomy, laminectomy, and/or spinal fusion.
4. Analyze the common nursing diagnoses and collaborative problems for the client with an acute spinal cord injury (SCI).
5. Describe typical medical complications that are experienced by clients with an SCI.
6. Prioritize the nursing care of the client with an SCI.
7. State the expected outcomes for the client with an SCI.
8. Develop a community-based teaching plan for clients who have an SCI.
9. Identify the clinical manifestations associated with spinal cord tumors.
10. Explain the pathophysiology of multiple sclerosis (MS), including the six basic types.
11. Discuss the role of medications in treating clients with MS.
12. Develop a community-based teaching plan for the client with MS.
13. Compare and contrast the clinical manifestations of MS and amyotrophic lateral sclerosis.

SIMON

Go to http://www.wbsaunders.com/SIMON/Iggy/ for self-assessment questions related to these Learning Objectives.

Problems of the spinal cord may be either acute or chronic and either short term or long term. Some problems require surgery, whereas others require extensive rehabilitation. Spinal cord neurons do not regenerate, and damage to neuronal fibers is permanent.

BACK PAIN

OVERVIEW

Back pain is one of the most common reasons for visiting a health care provider. Back problems are very costly in terms of time lost from work and medical treatment, and they are the most common cause of disability for persons younger than 43 years of age. Disabling low back pain is the single greatest cause of compensable injury in the working population. Eighty percent of the U.S. population has low back pain at some time. It is estimated that 85% to 90% of adults over 50 years of age have degenerative disk disease. The cervical (upper back) vertebrae and lumbosacral (lower back) vertebrae are most commonly affected.

Pathophysiology

CERVICAL BACK PAIN

Cervical involvement usually results from a herniation of the nucleus pulposus in an intervertebral disk (also spelled *disc*). As seen in Figure 43-1, the herniation usually occurs laterally where the annulus fibrosus is weakest and the posterior longitudinal ligament is thinned. The result is spinal nerve root compression, with subsequent motor and sensory manifestations, typically in the neck and down the affected arm. The disk between the fifth and sixth cervical vertebrae (C5-6) is affected most often.

If the disk does not rupture, nerve compression may be caused by osteophyte (bony outgrowth) formation from degen-

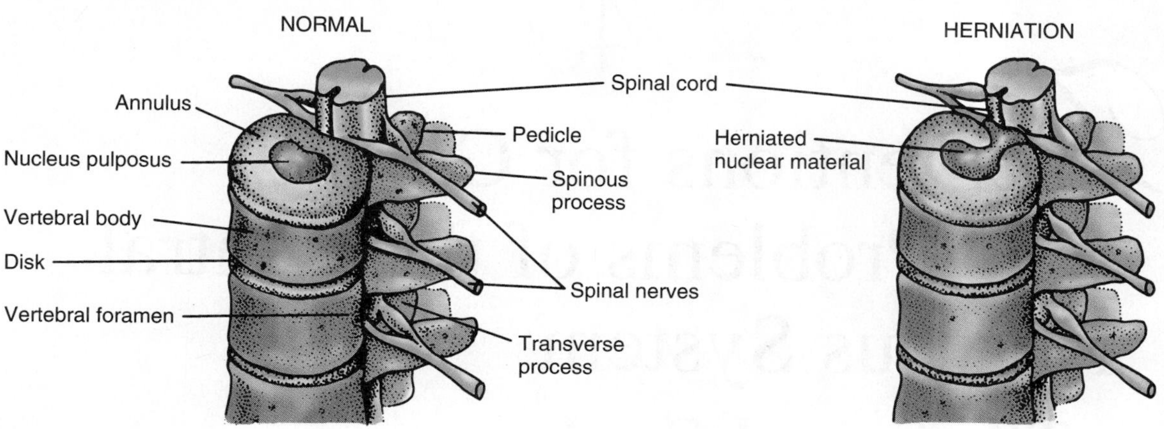

Figure 43-1 ● Herniation of the nucleus pulposus.

CHART 43-1

NURSING FOCUS *on the* OLDER ADULT
Factors Contributing to Low Back Pain

- Changes in support structures
  - Spinal stenosis
  - Hypertrophy of the intraspinal ligaments
  - Arthritis
- Changes in vertebral support and malalignment
  - Scoliosis
  - Lordosis
- Vascular changes
  - Diminished blood supply to the spinal cord or cauda equina caused by arteriosclerosis
  - Blood dyscrasias
- Intervertebral disk degeneration

erative joint disease. The osteophyte presses on the intervertebral foramen, which results in a narrowing of the disk and pressure on the nerve root. A client with nerve compression may experience either continuous or intermittent chronic pain. When the disk herniates centrally, pressure on the spinal cord occurs.

Cervical pain—acute or chronic—may also occur from muscle strain or ligament sprain. If these injuries occur in the workplace, the client may be eligible for workers' compensation benefits.

LUMBOSACRAL BACK PAIN

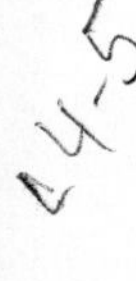

Lumbosacral back pain, referred to as **low back pain (LBP),** is more common than cervical pain. Acute pain is caused by muscle strain or spasm, ligament sprain, disk degeneration, or herniation of the nucleus pulposus from the center of the disk. Herniated disks occur most often between the fourth and fifth lumbar vertebrae (L4-5) but may occur at other levels. A **herniated nucleus pulposus (HNP)** in the lumbosacral area can press on the adjacent spinal nerve (usually the sciatic nerve), causing severe, burning, or stabbing pain down into the leg or foot. The HNP may press on the spinal cord itself, causing leg weakness and bowel and bladder dysfunction. The specific area of pain depends on the level of herniation.

Muscle spasms of the affected leg may also occur. The pain is usually aggravated by sneezing, coughing, or straining. If LBP continues for 3 months or if repeated episodes of pain occur, the client has chronic back pain.

Etiology

Acute back pain usually results from trauma. The client typically hyperflexes or twists the back during a vehicular accident, or the injury occurs when the client lifts a heavy object. Obesity places increased stress on the back muscles and typically contributes to the occurrence or severity of back pain. Smoking has been linked to disk degeneration. Congenital spinal conditions and scoliosis can also lead to back discomfort.

CONSIDERATIONS FOR OLDER ADULTS

For older adults, the cause of back pain is usually degenerative joint disease, a type of arthritis seen with aging. Cervical pain is common in clients with advanced rheumatoid arthritis who experience cervical disk subluxation (dislocation), most often at the C1-2 level. Other factors contributing to back pain in older adults are presented in Chart 43-1.

WOMEN'S HEALTH CONSIDERATIONS

Chronic back pain in women often results from having poor posture or from wearing high-heeled shoes. Excessively high heels cause the body to compensate to maintain balance. The lower back becomes more lordotic (anteriorly curved), which strains the back muscles.

Many of the problems related to acute back pain can be prevented by recognizing the causes of back pain and taking appropriate action. For example, good posture, proper lifting techniques, and exercise can significantly decrease the incidence of low back pain. Chart 43-2 summarizes ways to prevent low back pain.

COLLABORATIVE MANAGEMENT

Assessment

PHYSICAL ASSESSMENT/CLINICAL MANIFESTATIONS

The nurse assesses the client's posture and gait. Some clients have so much pain that they walk in a stiff, flexed state, or they may be unable to bend at all. If a client has low back pain, the nurse may note a limp, which may indicate sciatic

CHART 43-2

CLIENT EDUCATION GUIDE
Prevention of Low Back Pain

- Use proper body mechanics, with specific attention to bending, lifting, and sitting.
- Assess the need for assistance with your household chores or other activities.
- Participate in a regular exercise program, especially one that promotes back strengthening, such as swimming and walking.
- Do not wear high-heeled shoes.
- Use good posture when sitting, standing, or walking.
- Avoid prolonged sitting or standing. Use a foot stool and ergonomic chairs and tables to lessen back strain.
- Keep weight within 10% of ideal body weight. Ensure adequate calcium intake.
- Stop smoking. If you are not able to stop, cut down on the number of cigarettes or decrease the use of other forms of tobacco.

nerve impairment. Walking on the heels or toes often causes severe pain in the affected leg, the back, or both.

The nurse inspects the back for vertebral alignment and swelling caused by muscle spasm. Local muscle spasm is common in clients with back pain, and muscle spasm in the affected extremity is not uncommon. It is thought that a compressed nerve becomes inflamed and irritates adjacent muscle tissue. Clients complain of stabbing, continuous pain in the muscle close to the affected disk. In clients with cervical injury, pain radiates down one arm; in clients with lumbosacral involvement, pain radiates down the posterior leg. The pain usually does not extend the entire length of the limb. Clients with low back pain report sharp, burning posterior thigh or calf pain that may radiate to the ankle or toes. They may also report the same type of pain in the middle of one buttock.

The nurse palpates the back and the involved extremity for tenderness, which is often present. The client is asked whether there is **paresthesia** (tingling sensation) or numbness in the involved limb. Both extremities may be checked for sensation by using a pin or paper clip and a cotton ball for comparison of light and deep touch. The client may feel sensation in both limbs but may experience a stronger sensation on the unaffected side. The client with a severe case may lose both bowel and bladder control from spinal nerve involvement.

If the sciatic nerve is compressed, the client reports severe pain when raising a straight leg. Foot, ankle, and leg weakness may accompany the pain. To complete the neurologic assessment, the nurse evaluates muscle tone and strength. Muscles in the extremity or in the back atrophy in severe, chronic conditions. The client has difficulty with movement, and certain movements elicit more pain than others. The client with cervical pain may lose handgrip strength and may be unable to carry as much weight as before the injury.

DIAGNOSTIC ASSESSMENT

The health care provider often orders magnetic resonance imaging (MRI), performed with or without contrast media enhancement, to visualize the herniated disk and pressure on the nerve root or spinal cord. Less often, the caregiver may order a myelogram, an invasive procedure that may or may not detect the problem.

Electrodiagnostic studies, such as electromyography (EMG) and nerve conduction studies, may help differentiate motor neuron diseases, peripheral neuropathies, peripheral nerve entrapment, and radiculopathies. These are especially useful in chronic diseases because it takes at least 3 weeks for pathologic changes to produce symptoms. Chapter 41 describes these tests in more detail.

Interventions

Management of clients with back pain varies with the severity and chronicity of the problem. Most clients with acute low back pain (LBP) need only a short-term treatment regimen. The client, family members, and nurse can become frustrated if treatment measures are ineffective. The health care provider initially implements conservative measures; if these are unsuccessful, surgery may be indicated.

NONSURGICAL MANAGEMENT. Nonsurgical management of back pain may include proper positioning, exercise, anti-inflammatory analgesics, heat or ice therapy, and other pain relief measures and preventive measures in the work setting.

POSITIONING. The **Williams position** is typically more comfortable and therapeutic for the client with low back pain. In this position, the client lies in the semi-Fowler's position and flexes the knees to relax the muscles of the lower back and relieve pressure on the spinal nerve root.

A firm mattress or a back board placed under a soft mattress provides back support. A flat position is particularly helpful for the client with a muscle injury. For a herniated disk causing spinal nerve root compression in the lumbar spine, a flat position may aggravate the pain. The client usually gains pain relief from reclining or sleeping in the Williams position.

EXERCISE. Exercises are used to strengthen the back, relieve pressure on compressed nerves, and protect the back from reinjury. A variety of exercise programs are available to treat low back pain. Isometric exercises are generally the most effective.

The physical therapist (PT) works with the client to develop an individualized exercise program. The type of exercises prescribed depends on the location and nature of the injury and the type of pain. The client does not begin exercises until acute pain is reduced by other means. Several specific exercises for low back pain are provided in Chart 43-3.

DRUG THERAPY. The health care provider often prescribes muscle relaxants, such as cyclobenzaprine hydrochloride (Flexeril), and nonsteroidal anti-inflammatory drugs, such as aspirin and ibuprofen (Motrin). Opioid analgesics are no more effective than nonsteroidal analgesics and should be avoided if at all possible. If they must be used, the course of therapy should be short to prevent adverse side effects or possible addiction. An epidural or local steroid injection may also be helpful. Short-term oral steroids may be prescribed for some clients. Chapter 7 describes in detail the drug therapy and nursing implications for the care of clients in acute or chronic pain.

HEAT AND ICE THERAPY. Some clients with back pain experience temporary relief from the application of heat. Heat

CHART 43-3

CLIENT EDUCATION GUIDE
Typical Exercises for Chronic or Postoperative Low Back Pain

Extension Exercises
Stomach lying: Lie face down with a pillow under your chest; lift legs straight up (alternate legs).
Upper trunk extension: Lie face down with your arms at your sides, and lift your head and neck.
Prone pushups: Lie face down on a mat and, keeping your body stiff, push up to extend your arms.

Flexion Exercises
Pelvic tilt: Lying on your back with your knees bent, tighten your abdominal muscles to push your lower back against the mat.
Semi–sit-ups: Lying on your back with your knees bent, raise your upper body at a 45-degree angle, and hold this position for 5-10 seconds.
Knee to chest: Lying on your back with your knees bent, tighten your abdominal muscles to push your lower back against the mat. Now bring one or both knees to your chest and hold this position for 5 to 10 seconds.

increases blood flow to the affected area and promotes the healing of injured nerves. The nurse or therapist recommends moist heat in the form of heat packs or hot towels for 20 to 30 minutes at least four times a day. Hot showers or baths are also often beneficial. The physical therapist may administer deep heat therapy, such as ultrasound treatments and diathermy. The therapist and nurse monitor the effects of heat treatment by assessing the client's skin condition and the relief of pain.

Some clients prefer ice instead of heat to relieve pain and inflammation. Ice therapy using ice packs or ice massage may be applied over the affected area for 10 to 15 minutes every 1 to 2 hours. For some clients, a course of alternating ice and heat applications may be effective.

DIET THERAPY. Weight control often helps to reduce chronic back pain by decreasing the work on the vertebrae caused by excess weight. If the client's weight exceeds the ideal by more than 10%, caloric restriction is necessary.

Health care providers must be sensitive when reinforcing the need for clients to lose weight to prevent or to lessen chronic back pain. The nurse collaborates with the dietitian to plan and implement an appropriate calorie-restricted diet plan. Positive reinforcement and self-esteem building are integral to the diet plan.

OTHER PAIN RELIEF MEASURES. Physical therapy with manipulation of the lower back during the first month of symptoms may be beneficial. Shoe insoles may also help decrease pain when standing for prolonged periods of time. Preventive measures for the occupational setting may include a corset, supportive back belt, and ergonomic office furniture. A structured educational program about low back problems in the work setting has also been helpful in decreasing both injuries and time lost from work.

COMPLEMENTARY AND ALTERNATIVE THERAPIES. The client may find that other nontraditional and complementary therapies provide short-term pain relief. Distraction, imagery, magnetic field therapy, and music therapy are examples of pain-relief therapies. Chapters 4 and 7 describe these techniques in detail.

PERCUTANEOUS LASER DISK DECOMPRESSION. A new nonsurgical procedure, known as percutaneous laser disk decompression (PLDD), relieves the pain of a herniated disk by drawing the herniated portion away from the nerve root. This treatment is performed in special spinal centers around the United States and throughout the world.

Using advanced laser technology and a local anesthetic, a thin needle is inserted under fluoroscopy. An optical fiber is placed through the needle to enable laser energy to travel and vaporize the disk nucleus. Most clients walk away from this half-hour procedure pain free and with just a small bandage. Most physicians prescribe 24 hours of bedrest after the procedure before beginning progressive ambulation. Depending the type of work, most clients can resume work within a week.

SURGICAL MANAGEMENT. Surgery is usually performed when conservative measures fail to relieve back pain after 1 month or if neurologic deficits progress.

CONVENTIONAL OPERATIVE PROCEDURES. The most common conventional operative procedures are diskectomy, laminectomy, and spinal fusion. These open surgical procedures can cause major complications, including nerve injuries, diskitis, and dural tears.

In a conventional **diskectomy,** the spinal nerve is usually lifted to remove the offending portion of the disk. A **laminectomy** is the removal of one or more vertebral laminae plus osteophytes, if present, and the herniated nucleus pulposus. Both procedures are performed through a 3- to 4-inch (7.5- to 10-cm) longitudinal incision. The standard hospital stay is 2 to 3 days but may be shorter or longer depending on the client's condition and the reimbursement source.

When repeated laminectomies are performed or the spine is unstable, the surgeon may perform a spinal fusion (arthrodesis) to stabilize the affected area. Chips of bone are removed, typically from the iliac crest or from donor bone, and are grafted between the vertebrae for support and to strengthen the back.

For clients who may be difficult to fuse, implantable direct current stimulation (DCS) may be used to promote bone fusion. Studies show that DCS has a success rate of 90% or more (Kahanovitz & Pashos, 1996). External bone stimulators may also be effective for healing bone fusions.

ALTERNATIVE OPERATIVE PROCEDURES. Three alternatives to a laminectomy that have varying degrees of popularity are **percutaneous lumbar diskectomy, microdiskectomy,** and laser-assisted **laparoscopic lumbar diskectomy.** The primary advantage of these surgical procedures is a shortened hospital stay and the possibility of an ambulatory procedure. Spinal cord complications are also less likely. Newer procedures (e.g., laproscopic lumbar fusion) and intervertebral body fusion devices (e.g., titanium-threaded and mesh interbody cages) are more commonly used today (Rauzzino et al., 1999).

Percutaneous Lumbar Diskectomy. Using a local anesthetic for this procedure, the surgeon uses fluoroscopy to

CHART 43-4

BEST PRACTICE *for*
Assessing and Managing the Client with Major Complications of Lumbar Spinal Surgery

COMPLICATION	ASSESSMENT/INTERVENTIONS
Cerebrospinal fluid (CSF) leakage	Observe for clear fluid on or around the dressing. If CSF is present, test for glucose. (The test result is positive if glucose is present.) Report CSF leakage immediately to the surgeon. (The client is usually kept on flat bedrest for 7 to 10 days while the dural tear heals.)
Fluid volume deficit	Monitor vital signs carefully for hypotension and tachycardia. Monitor intake and output; monitor drain output, which should not be more than 250 mL in 8 hours during the first 24 hours. Drainage should taper within 12 hours after surgery. (The surgeon removes the drain in 24 to 36 hours.)
Acute urinary retention	Assist the client to the bathroom or a bedside commode as soon as possible postoperatively. Assist male clients to stand at the bedside as soon as possible postoperatively. Give bethanechol (Urecholine) chloride as ordered to stimulate the detrusor muscle of the bladder.
Paralytic ileus	Monitor for the return of bowel sounds. Assess for abdominal distention, nausea, and vomiting.
Fat embolism syndrome (FES) (more common in people with spinal fusion)	Observe for and report chest pain, dyspnea, anxiety, and mental status changes (particularly common in older adults). Note petechiae around the neck, upper chest, buccal membrane, and conjunctiva. Monitor arterial blood gas values for decreased Pa_{O_2}.
Persistent or progressive lumbar radiculopathy (nerve root pain)	Report pain not responsive to opioids. Document the location and nature of pain. Administer analgesics as ordered.
Infection (e.g., wound diskitis, hematoma)	Monitor the client's temperature carefully (a slight elevation is normal). Increased temperature elevation or a spike after the second postoperative day is possibly indicative of infection. Report increased pain at the wound site or in the legs. Give antibiotics as ordered. Use sterile technique for dressing changes.

Pa_{O_2}, Partial pressure of arterial oxygen.

insert a metal cannula, or endoscope, adjacent to the affected disk. A special cutting tool is threaded through the cannula for removal of disk pieces that are compressing the nerve root.

Microdiskectomy. A microdiskectomy involves microscopic surgery through a 1-inch incision. This procedure allows for easier identification of anatomic structures, improved precision in removing small fragments, and decreased tissue trauma and pain.

Laser-Assisted Laparoscopic Lumbar Diskectomy. This procedure combines a laser with modified standard disk instruments inserted periumbilically through the laparoscopic cannula. It may be used to treat herniated disks that, although bulging, have not encroached the vertebral canal. The primary risks of this surgery are infection and nerve root injury. The client is typically discharged in 24 to 48 hours but may be discharged the same day.

Disk Prosthesis. A new experimental treatment involves a hard plastic prosthesis that replaces the client's natural disk. The disk is shaped to allow full spinal movement. If approved for widespread use, this device could revolutionize care for clients with herniated disks.

PREOPERATIVE CARE. Because lumbar back surgery is performed more often than cervical back surgery, preoperative and postoperative care for lumbar procedures is described here. Preoperative care of the client preparing for a laminectomy is similar to that for any client undergoing surgery (see Chapter 17). The nurse and physical therapist teach the client what to expect postoperatively and how to move in bed. The client should be warned that various sensations, such as numbness and tingling, may be experienced in the affected leg or in both legs because of the manipulation of nerves and muscles during surgery.

The client who has undergone a spinal fusion is usually braced postoperatively. This brace is fitted by the physical therapist before surgery. The nurse in the surgeon's office or clinic teaches about the importance of wearing the brace as instructed during the healing process.

The surgeon explains where the bone for grafting will be obtained. The client's own bone is used whenever possible, but supplemental bone from a bone bank may be needed. The surgeon provides verbal and written information about the type and the source of bone for surgery. The client signs an informed consent form before surgery.

POSTOPERATIVE CARE. Early postoperative nursing care focuses on preventing and assessing complications that might occur in the first 24 to 48 hours (Chart 43-4). As for any client undergoing surgery, the nurse or assistive nursing personnel measures the vital signs at least every 4 hours during the first 24 hours to assess for fever and for hypotension, which could indicate bleeding or severe pain. The nurse also performs a complete neurologic assessment every 4 hours. Of particular importance is the client's ability to move and feel sensation in the extremities.

The nurse carefully checks the client's ability to void. Pain and a flat position in bed make voiding difficult, especially for men. An inability to void may indicate damage to the sacral spinal nerves, which control the detrusor muscle in the bladder. The client with a diskectomy or laminectomy typically gets out of bed with assistance on the evening of surgery, which may facilitate voiding.

Pain control may be achieved with intramuscular opioid analgesia or patient-controlled analgesia (PCA). Morphine may be used during the first 24 hours, depending on the client's age and mental status. The health care provider prescribes oral opioids after the parenteral drug administration is discontinued. The client is assured that pain should decrease as the incision area heals.

The nurse inspects the surgical dressing for blood or any other type of drainage. Clear drainage may mean cerebrospinal fluid (CSF) leakage, and the nurse must report such a finding to the surgeon immediately. Bulging at the incision site may be due to a CSF leak or a hematoma, both of which are reported to the surgeon.

The nurse or assistive nursing personnel also empties and measures the drainage from the surgical drain, usually a Jackson-Pratt or Hemovac drain. Because the drainage is usually minimal, the surgeon usually removes the drain in 24 to 36 hours.

Correct turning of the client in bed is especially important. The nurse or assistive nursing personnel logrolls the client every 2 hours from side to back and vice versa. In **logrolling,** the client turns all at once while his or her back is kept as straight as possible. A turning sheet may be used for large clients. Either turning method may require additional assistance, depending on how much the client can assist. When the nurse or assistive nursing personnel helps the client get out of bed, the client's back is kept straight, and he or she is placed in a straight-backed chair with the feet resting comfortably on the floor.

As after any surgery, the nurse instructs the client to deep breathe every 2 hours to prevent atelectasis and pneumonia. Until the client can ambulate independently, he or she wears graduated compression stockings, sequential compression devices (SCDs), or pneumatic compression boots (PCBs) to prevent deep venous thrombosis (DVT) and possible pulmonary emboli. Older adults are especially susceptible to these complications of immobility.

When a spinal fusion is performed in addition to a laminectomy, more care is taken with mobility and positioning. The client usually stays in bed for 24 hours, with the nurse or assistive nursing personnel logrolling him or her every 2 hours. The nurse inspects both the iliac and spinal incision areas for problems, as described earlier in this section.

A brace or other type of thoracolumbar support is worn when the client is out of bed. The nurse discourages prolonged sitting or standing.

Community-Based Care

The client with back pain who does not undergo surgery is typically managed at home. If back surgery is performed, the client is usually discharged to home with support from family or significant others. For older adults without a community support system, a short-term stay in a nursing home or subacute unit may be needed. The case manager or discharge planner collaborates with the health care team, client, and family to determine the most appropriate placement.

HOME CARE MANAGEMENT

The nurse informs the client and family members or significant other that the client should have a firm mattress to provide support for the entire vertebral column. A bed board or large piece of plywood placed under a soft mattress may suffice. After back surgery, the client may not be allowed to climb stairs for several weeks. It is essential that facilities to meet personal needs be on one level in the home. The client can usually return to work in 2 to 6 weeks, depending on the nature of the job and the extent and type of surgery. Weight that may be lifted is initially limited to 5 pounds. The amount is gradually increased as healing occurs.

HEALTH TEACHING

In collaboration with the dietitian and physical therapist, the nurse instructs the client to do the following:

- Continue with a weight-reduction diet, if needed
- Stop smoking
- Use moist heat as needed
- Perform strengthening exercises as initiated in the hospital setting

The physical therapist reviews and demonstrates the principles of body mechanics and muscle-strengthening exercises. The client is then asked to demonstrate these principles (Chart 43-5).

The health care provider may want the client to continue taking medications such as anti-inflammatory drugs and muscle relaxants. The nurse reminds the client and family about the possible side effects of drugs and what to do if they occur. If the client has a spinal fusion, he or she may need to wear a brace or thoracolumbar support for 3 to 6 months while the fusion heals completely. The client may not be able to return to full functioning for 6 to 12 months after a spinal fusion.

The client with an acute episode of back pain typically returns to his or her usual activities but may fear a recurrence. The nurse reminds the client that he or she may never have another episode if caution is used. However, continuous or repeated pain can be frustrating and tiring. If pain is unremitting, surgery is indicated. The nurse encourages the client and family members to set short-term goals and to take steps toward recovering slowly.

In a few clients, back surgery may not be successful. This situation, referred to as failed back surgery syndrome (FBSS), is a complex combination of organic, psychologic, and socioeconomic factors. Repeated surgical procedures often discourage these clients, who must continue nonsurgical management of pain after multiple operations. Nerve blocks and other pain management modalities may be needed on a long-term basis (see Chapter 7).

CHART 43-5

CLIENT EDUCATION GUIDE

Use of Proper Body Mechanics to Prevent Back Injury

- Size up the load to determine the number of persons needed to perform the task.
- When lifting an object, keep your back straight and do not bend at the waist; lift with your large thigh muscles.
- Push objects rather than pull them.
- Do not twist your back.
- Avoid prolonged sitting or standing. Use a footstool to lessen back strain.
- Sit in chairs with good support; sleep on a firm mattress.
- Avoid shoulder stooping; use proper posture.
- Do not walk or stand in high-heeled shoes for prolonged periods (for women).

HEALTH CARE RESOURCES

The nurse identifies support systems (e.g., family, church groups, and clubs) for the client after back surgery or FBSS. For example, a spouse may help the client with exercises or may perform the exercises with the client. Members of a church group may help run errands and do household chores.

The client with back pain may continue physical therapy on an ambulatory basis after discharge. For unresolved pain, the client may be referred to pain specialists or clinics, which are usually found in large metropolitan hospitals. A case manager may be assigned to the client to help with resource management and utilization.

SPINAL CORD INJURY

OVERVIEW

Spinal cord injury (SCI) has received increased public attention and research as a result of actor Christopher Reeve's spinal cord trauma. Despite this increased awareness and the sophistication of treatment for spinal cord injury, the effects of the initial injury still cannot be reversed. The cost of care for clients with an SCI varies with the neurologic deficit. Clients experiencing **quadriplegia** (paralysis from the neck down) are the most expensive for society in terms of both health care and living expenses (see the Cost of Care box below).

COST OF CARE IMPLICATIONS FOR NURSING

SPINAL CORD INJURIES

Cost of Care

- The average annual cost (health care and living expenses) and the estimated lifetime costs for a client with a spinal cord injury (SCI) varies greatly with the severity of injury.
- The cost of care for a C1-C4 quadriplegic is $549,800 for the first year; each subsequent year the cost is $98,483.
- The cost of care for a paraplegic is $200,897 for the first year and $19,694 for each subsequent year.
- Estimated lifetime costs for a C1-C4 quadriplegic, 25 years old, is $2,100,185; 50 years old, $1,236,390.
- Cost-of-care estimates do not include loss of income, fringe benefits, and productivity, which could average $46,000 depending on education and occupation and pre-employment work history.
- The average length of stay in the acute setting in 1974 was 26 days; in 1998 it was 15 days. The average length of stay in the rehabilitation setting has decreased from 115 to 44 days. Clients with more neurologically complete injuries require longer acute and rehabilitation stays.
- Only 4% of clients with an SCI are discharged to nursing homes; 91.3% are sent to noninstitutional residences, usually their home. The remaining SCI clients are discharged to hospitals, group living situations, or other places.

Implications for Nursing

The high cost of care for quadriplegic clients requires nurses to be more vigilant in the prevention of complications of immobility that would extend the average length of stay, increase morbidity, and increase the cost of care. Inherent in this preventive strategy is the need to thoroughly educate the client and family on potential complications that would lengthen recovery and delay discharge to rehabilitation. The use of rehabilitation principles from the time of admission would facilitate earlier discharge and a smoother transition back into society.

Data from Spinal Cord Injury Information Network. Spinal cord injury facts and figures at a glance; www.spinalcord.uab.edu.

Loss of motor function, sensation, reflex activity, and bowel and bladder control often result from an SCI. In addition, the client may experience significant behavior and emotional problems as a result of changes in body image, role performance, and self-concept.

SCIs are classified as complete or incomplete. A complete injury is one in which the spinal cord has been severed or damaged in a way that eliminates all innervation below the level of the injury. Injuries that allow some function or movement below the level of the injury are described as incomplete.

Pathophysiology

AUTONOMIC NERVOUS SYSTEM SYNDROMES

Specific syndromes seen after spinal cord injury (SCI) and damage to the autonomic nervous system (ANS) are spinal shock and autonomic dysreflexia.

Spinal shock occurs immediately after injury as a result of disruption in the communication pathways between upper motor neurons and lower motor neurons. This condition, also known as **neurogenic shock,** is characterized by the following:

- Flaccid paralysis
- Loss of reflex activity below the level of the lesion
- Bradycardia
- Paralytic ileus (occasionally)
- Hypotension

Spinal shock may last from a few days to several months; its reversal is indicated by the return of reflex activity.

Autonomic dysreflexia, or **hyperreflexia,** is usually seen in injuries above the level of the sixth thoracic vertebra. It generally occurs after the period of spinal shock has completed. This syndrome results from uninhibited sympathetic discharge; that is, the sympathetic nervous system (SNS) is no longer controlled by higher centers in the cerebral cortex because of the disruption in impulse transmission. Chart 43-6 summarizes the key features of this life-threatening complication.

MECHANISMS OF INJURY

When sufficient force is applied to the spinal cord, damage results in neurologic deficits. Sources of force include injury to the vertebral column (fracture, dislocation, and subluxation) or penetrating trauma (gunshot or knife wounds). Although in some cases the cord itself may remain intact, at other times the cord undergoes a destructive process caused by a contusion, compression, or concussion.

Four mechanisms may result in an SCI: hyperflexion; hyperextension; axial loading, or vertical compression; and ex-

CHART 43-6

KEY FEATURES *of* Autonomic Dysreflexia

- Severe, rapidly occurring hypertension
- Bradycardia
- Flushing above level of lesion
- Severe, throbbing headache
- Nasal stuffiness
- Sweating
- Nausea
- Blurred vision

cessive rotation. Penetrating injuries to the cord may also occur.

A hyperflexion injury occurs when the head is suddenly and forcefully accelerated forward, causing extreme flexion of the neck (Figure 43-2). This type of injury often occurs in head-on collisions and diving accidents. Flexion injury to the lower thoracic and lumbar spine may occur when the trunk is suddenly flexed on itself, such as occurs in a fall on the buttocks. The posterior ligaments can be stretched or torn, or the vertebrae may fracture or dislocate. Either process may disrupt the integrity of the spinal cord, causing hemorrhage, edema, and necrosis.

Hyperextension injuries occur most often in automobile accidents in which the client's vehicle is struck from behind or during falls when the client's chin is struck (Figure 43-3). The head is suddenly accelerated and then decelerated. This stretches or tears the anterior longitudinal ligament, fractures or subluxates the vertebrae, and perhaps ruptures an intervertebral disk. As with flexion injuries, the spinal cord may easily be damaged.

Diving accidents, falls on the buttocks, or a jump in which a person lands on the feet can cause many of the injuries attributable to axial loading (vertical compression) (Figure 43-4). The blow to the top of the head causes the vertebrae to shatter. Pieces of bone enter the spinal canal and damage the cord. Rotation injuries are caused by turning the head beyond the normal range.

Penetrating injuries to the spinal cord are classified by the velocity of the vehicle (e.g., knife or bullet) causing the injury. Low-velocity, or low-impact, injuries cause damage directly at the site or localized damage to the spinal cord or spinal nerves. In contrast, high-velocity injuries that occur from gunshot wounds cause both direct and indirect damage.

As mentioned earlier, the spinal cord may be contused, lacerated, or compressed as a result of injury. Petechial hemorrhage into the central gray matter, and later into the white matter, can be caused by a contusion and laceration of the spinal cord. Spinal cord edema occurs as a result of cord compression by hemorrhage, bony fragments, or laceration. Necrosis of the spinal cord occurs from compromised capillary circulation and venous return.

EXTENT OF INJURY

Incomplete SCIs are more common than complete lesions. A client experiencing an incomplete lesion typically has preservation of a mixed pattern of motor, sensory, and reflex function. Specific syndromes result from incomplete lesions (Figure 43-5). A "pure" syndrome may not be seen. Cervical injuries may produce anterior cord syndrome, posterior cord syndrome, Brown-Séquard syndrome, or central cord syndrome. Conus medullaris and cauda equina syndromes are associated with injuries to the lumbar and sacral cord.

CERVICAL INJURIES. Anterior cord syndrome results from damage to the anterior portion of both gray and white matter of the spinal cord, usually as a result of decreased blood supply. Although motor function and pain and temperature sensation are lost below the level of injury, the sensations of touch, position, and vibration remain intact. More than 50% of the clients with this syndrome are older than 40 years of age, with the majority between 50 and 70 years of

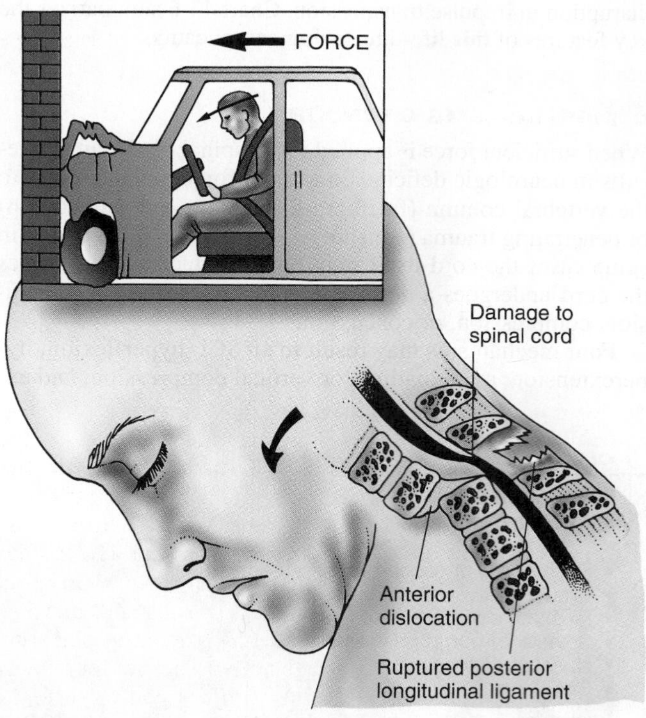

Figure 43-2 ● Hyperflexion injury of the cervical spine.

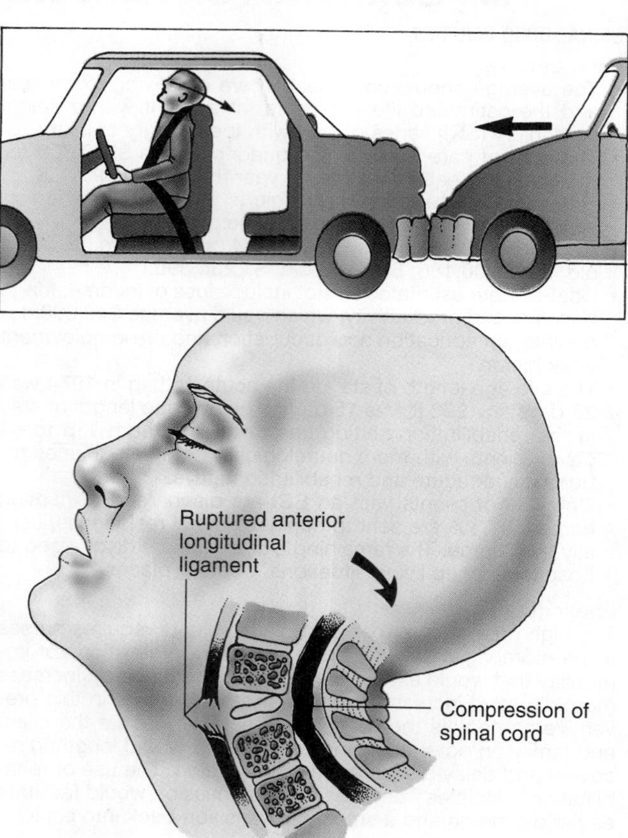

Figure 43-3 ● Hyperextension injury of the cervical spine.

age. Functional motor control is recovered in 10% to 20% of clients with cervical spine injuries.

Just the opposite transpires in a rarely encountered posterior cord lesion, which also occurs from damage to the posterior gray and white matter of the spinal cord. Motor function remains intact, but the client experiences a loss of vibratory sense, crude touch, and position sensation.

Brown-Séquard syndrome generally results from penetrating injuries that cause hemisection of the spinal cord or injuries that affect half of the spinal cord. Motor function, proprioception, vibration, and deep touch sensations are lost on the same side of the body as the lesion (ipsilateral). On the opposite side of the body (contralateral) from the injury, the sensations of pain, temperature, and light touch are affected.

Lesions of the central portion of the spinal cord produce a central cord syndrome. Loss of motor function is more pronounced in the upper extremities than in the lower extremities. Varying degrees and patterns of sensation remain intact.

LUMBOSACRAL INJURIES. Damage to the cauda equina or conus medullaris produces a variable pattern of motor or sensory loss, because the peripheral nerves have the potential for recovery and regrowth. In addition, this injury usually results in a neurogenic bowel and bladder.

Etiology

Trauma is the leading cause of SCIs; almost 50% result from motor vehicle accidents. The second leading cause is falls, acts of violence, and sports accidents. Spinal cord damage can also result from diseases such as polio, spina bifida, and tumors.

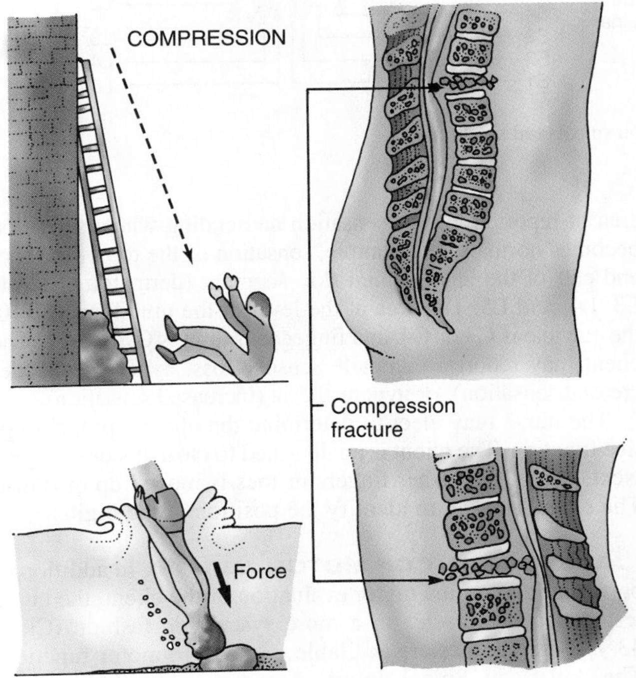

Figure 43-4 ● Axial loading (vertical compression) injury of the cervical spine and the lumbar spine.

Incidence/Prevalence

More than 200,000 persons in the United States have SCIs, and 8000 to 10,000 new injuries occur each year (Buckley & Guanci, 1999). The client may be hospitalized for 3 months or longer, including acute care and rehabilitation. Life expectancy has increased but is still below that of individuals without an SCI.

A typical client with an SCI is an unmarried man between 15 and 30 years of age (median age, 19 years). Peak incidence of injury occurs in the summer or warmer months. Men comprise 81% of SCI clients, and the majority are Caucasian. Most injuries are cervical.

COLLABORATIVE MANAGEMENT

Assessment

HISTORY

When obtaining a history from a client with a spinal cord injury (SCI), the nurse gathers as much data as possible about how the accident occurred and the probable mechanism of injury. The nurse specifically asks about the position of the client immediately after the injury, the symptoms that occurred after the injury, and the changes that have occurred since the initial appearance of signs and symptoms. If possible, prehospital rescue personnel are questioned about the type of immobilization devices used and whether any problems occurred during stabilization and transport to the hospital. The nurse asks about the medical treatment given at the scene of injury or in the emergency department (e.g., medications and intravenous [IV] fluids).

The nurse also determines the client's medical history, including a history of arthritis of the spine, congenital deformities, osteoporosis or osteomyelitis, cancer, and previous injury or surgery of the neck or back. These health problems may cause or contribute to an SCI. If the client has experienced a cervical SCI, the nurse documents a detailed history of any respiratory problems.

PHYSICAL ASSESSMENT/CLINICAL MANIFESTATIONS

INITIAL ASSESSMENT. The first priority for the client with an SCI is assessing the respiratory pattern and ensuring an adequate airway. The client with a cervical SCI is at high risk for respiratory compromise because the cervical spinal nerves (C3 through C5) innervate the phrenic nerve, which controls the diaphragm. Endotracheal intubation may be necessary to prevent respiratory arrest.

The nurse also assesses the client for indications of intra-abdominal hemorrhage or hemorrhage or bleeding around fracture sites. Other indicators of hemorrhage include hypotension and tachycardia with a weak and thready pulse.

The client's level of consciousness (LOC) is usually assessed by the Glasgow Coma Scale (see Chapter 41 for a description of this tool). Cognitive impairment as a result of an associated traumatic brain injury (TBI) or substance abuse is seen in about half of all traumatic SCIs. The nurse performs a detailed assessment of the client's motor and sensory status to assist in determining the level of injury and to serve as baseline data for future comparison. The level of injury is the lowest neurologic segment with intact or normal motor and

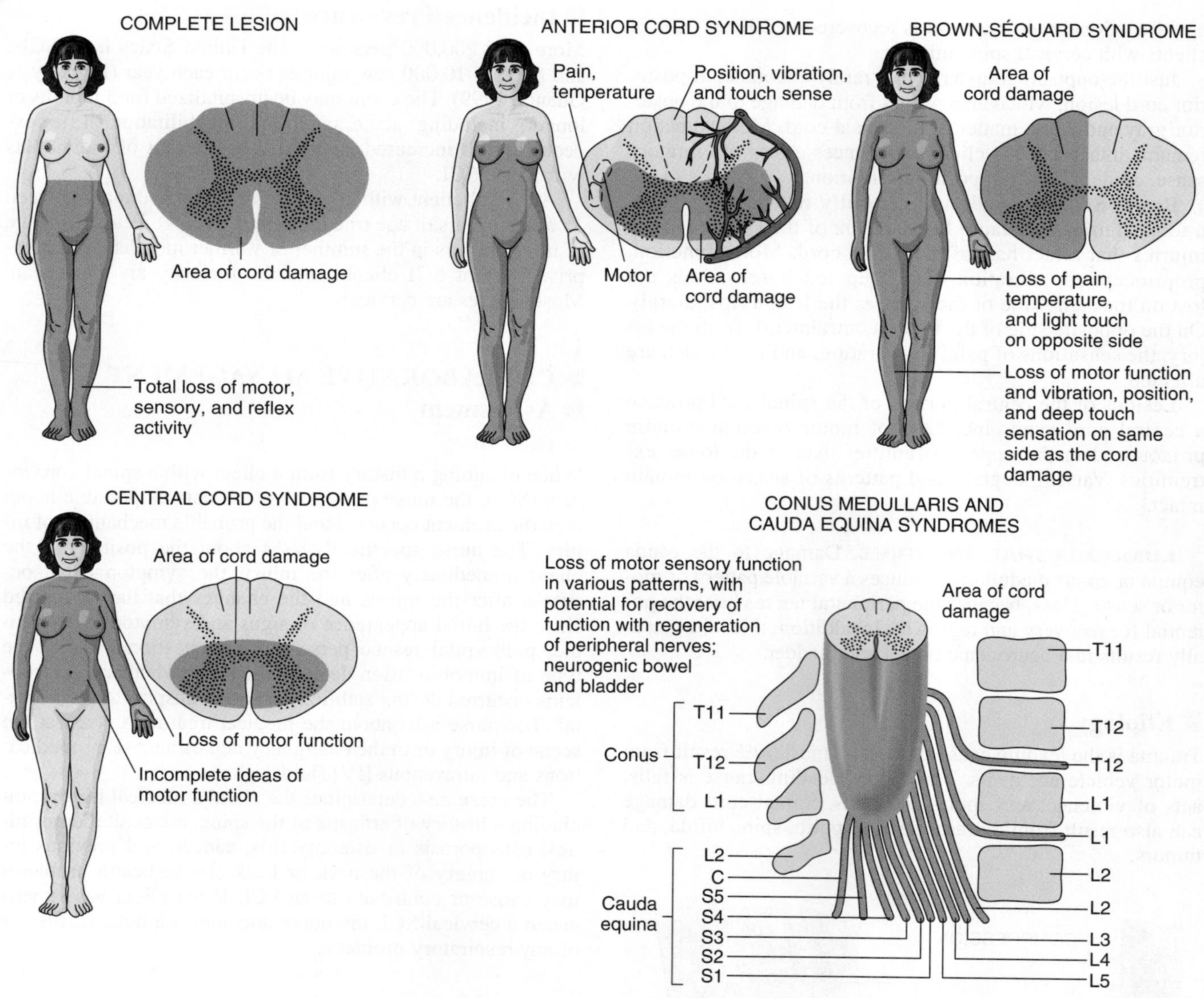

Figure 43-5 ● Common spinal cord syndromes.

sensory function. **Quadriplegia,** also called **tetraplegia** (paralysis), and **quadriparesis** (weakness) involve all four extremities, as seen with cervical cord injury. **Paraplegia** (paralysis) and **paraparesis** (weakness) involve only the lower extremities, as seen in lower thoracic and lumbosacral injuries or lesions.

ASSESSMENT OF SENSATION. Sensation is carried from the peripheral nerves to the spinal cord and up to the cerebral cortex via a variety of sensation-specific tracts. Injury to the spinal cord may prohibit sensory impulses from reaching the brain. To test sensory abilities, the specialty or advanced practice nurse first asks the client to close his or her eyes. Next, the nurse touches the skin with a clean safety pin or cotton-tipped applicator and asks the client whether he or she can feel the pinprick or light touch. Bilateral responses are compared. The nurse follows the sensory distribution of the skin dermatomes (see Figure 41-9), beginning the examination in the area of reported loss of sensation and ending where sensation becomes normal. For example, sensation of the top of the foot and calf of the leg is spinal skin segment (dermatome) levels L3, L4, and L5. The area at the level of the umbilicus is T10, the clavicle is C3 or C4, and finger sensation is C7 and C8. The client may report a complete sensory loss, hypoesthesia (decreased sensation), or hyperesthesia (increased sensation).

The nurse may elect to determine the client's proprioceptive function. The client is again asked to close his or her eyes. Next, one of his or her fingers or toes is moved up or down. The client is asked to identify the position of the digits.

ASSESSMENT OF MOTOR ABILITY. In addition to performing a routine motor evaluation of the client, the nurse tests selected muscles in a more systematic fashion (Chart 43-7). Many scales are available to measure motor function. The American Spinal Injury Association (ASIA) recommends a five-point grading scale, with 0 being no movement

CHART 43-7

FOCUSED ASSESSMENT *of*
Motor Function in the Client with a Spinal Cord Injury

- To assess C4-C5, apply downward pressure while the client shrugs his or her shoulders upward.
- To assess C5-C6, apply resistance while the client pulls up his or her arms.
- To assess C7, apply resistance while the client straightens his or her flexed arms.
- To assess C8, make sure the client is able to grasp an object and form a fist.
- To assess L2-L4, apply resistance while the client lifts his or her legs from the bed.
- To assess L5, apply resistance while the client dorsiflexes his or her feet.
- To assess S1, apply resistance while the client plantar flexes his or her feet.

CHART 43-8

BEST PRACTICE *for*
Emergency Care of the Client Experiencing Autonomic Dysreflexia

- Raise the head of the bed to a high Fowler's position.
- Call the physician and notify him or her of the emergency.
- Loosen tight clothing on the client.
- Check the Foley catheter tubing (if present) for kinks or obstruction.
- If a Foley catheter is not present, check for bladder distention and catheterize immediately.
- Check the client for fecal impaction; if present, disimpact immediately using anesthetic ointment.
- Check the room temperature to ensure that it is not too cool or drafty.
- Monitor blood pressures every 10 to 15 minutes.
- Give nitrates or hydralazine (Apresoline, Novo-Hylazin♣) as ordered.

and 5 being normal strength (Buckley & Guanci, 1999). The nurse asks the client to flex and extend the elbows, elevate both arms off the bed, flex and extend the wrists and fingers, and touch each finger to the thumb. The client with spinal injuries at the fifth or sixth cervical vertebra are often able to flex but not extend their arms. Next, the nurse observes the client's ability to move the lower extremities. He or she is asked to wiggle the toes, flex and extend the feet and knees, and move one or both hips.

The advanced practice nurse or health care provider may also test deep tendon reflexes (DTRs), including the biceps (C5), triceps (C7), patella (L3), and ankle (S1). It is not unusual for these reflexes, as well as all motor function or sensation, to be absent immediately after the injury because of spinal shock. After spinal shock has resolved, the reflexes may return if the lesion is incomplete or involves upper motor neurons.

CARDIOVASCULAR ASSESSMENT. Cardiovascular dysfunction is usually the result of disruption of the autonomic nervous system, especially if the injury is above the sixth thoracic vertebra. Bradycardia, hypotension, and hypothermia result from a loss of sympathetic input and may lead to cardiac dysrhythmias. In addition, the lack of sympathetic or hypothalamic control causes the client to lose thermoregulatory functions; as a result, the body tends to assume the temperature of the environment.

The nurse must continually observe for signs of autonomic dysreflexia. Dysreflexia is characterized by severe hypertension, bradycardia, severe headache, nasal stuffiness, and flushing (see Chart 43-6). The cause of this syndrome is a noxious stimulus, most often a distended bladder or constipation. This is a neurologic emergency and must be promptly treated to prevent a hypertensive stroke. Chart 43-8 lists emergency care for autonomic dysreflexia.

RESPIRATORY ASSESSMENT. A client with a cervical SCI is at risk for respiratory problems resulting from immobility or from an interruption of spinal innervation to the respiratory muscles. Some clients require intubation and mechanical ventilation. The nurse performs a complete respiratory assessment in collaboration with the respiratory therapist, if available. The respiratory therapist should evaluate vital capacity and minute volume as part of the assessment. Periodic repetition of these tests should be performed as the client's clinical status indicates.

During the hospital stay, the nurse observes for life-threatening respiratory complications such as impaired gas exchange resulting from pneumonia, pulmonary emboli, and atelectasis. Pneumonia and pulmonary emboli decrease the life expectancy of SCI clients and have replaced renal failure as the leading cause of death.

GASTROINTESTINAL AND GENITOURINARY ASSESSMENT. The nurse assesses the client's abdomen for indications of hemorrhage, distention, or paralytic ileus. Hemorrhage may result from the trauma, or it may occur later from a stress ulcer or the administration of steroids. Paralytic ileus may develop within 72 hours of hospital admission. During the period of spinal shock, peristalsis decreases, leading to a loss of bowel sounds and gastric distention. This lack of or interference with autonomic innervation may lead to a reflex or hypotonic bowel. The nurse should also assess the client's nutritional status.

Autonomic dysfunction initially causes an areflexic bladder, which later leads to urinary retention and a neurogenic bladder. The client is at risk for urinary tract infection from an indwelling urinary catheter, from intermittent catheterizations, or from bladder distention, stasis, and overflow.

MUSCULOSKELETAL ASSESSMENT. The nurse assesses the client's muscle tone and size. Muscle wasting results from the long-term flaccid paralysis seen in clients with lower motor neuron (LMN) lesions. Incomplete lesions or upper motor neuron (UMN) lesions may cause muscle spasticity, which can lead to contractures after spinal shock has resolved.

The nurse assesses the condition of the client's skin, especially over pressure points, at least twice daily. Any reddened area is carefully assessed and monitored for change. A pressure-reducing mattress or special bed are used to prevent skin breakdown.

Another complication of prolonged immobility is heterotopic ossification (bony overgrowth, often into muscle). It is evidenced by swelling, redness, warmth, and decreased range of motion (ROM) of the involved extremity. Changes in the bony structure are not evident until several weeks after initial symptoms appear.

PSYCHOSOCIAL ASSESSMENT

If possible, the nurse assesses the client's preinjury psychosocial status by obtaining information about his or her usual methods of coping with illness, difficult situations, and disappointments. The nurse determines his or her level of independence or dependence and his or her comfort level in discussing feelings and emotions with family members or close friends. Clients who are emotionally secure and have a positive self-image, supportive family, and financial and job security often adapt to their injury. Information about the client's religious beliefs or cultural background also assists the nurse in developing the plan of care. The client with an SCI must cope with changes in body image, self-esteem, independence, role relationships, and sexuality.

In addition, the nurse assesses family members or significant others to determine how well they are coping with the client's injury and their role changes. The client and significant others must be prepared for extensive rehabilitation and changes in lifestyle. Financial constraints may pose additional stress.

LABORATORY ASSESSMENT

The health care provider orders routine laboratory studies for the client with an SCI to establish baseline data or to prepare for surgery. A urinalysis is used to check for the presence of blood in the urine after trauma. Arterial blood gas analysis is used to monitor the respiratory status of a client at risk for respiratory insufficiency. The findings should be within normal limits unless the client has a history of heavy smoking or preinjury pulmonary disease or is experiencing respiratory failure as indicated by decreased oxygen levels, increased carbon dioxide levels, and respiratory acidosis.

DIAGNOSTIC ASSESSMENT

The physician orders a complete radiographic series of the spine to identify vertebral fractures, subluxation, or dislocation. Computed tomography (CT) or magnetic resonance imaging (MRI) may be performed to determine the degree and extent of damage to the spinal cord and to detect the presence of blood and bone within the spinal column.

Analysis

COMMON NURSING DIAGNOSES AND COLLABORATIVE PROBLEMS

The following are the most common nursing diagnoses for clients with a spinal cord injury (SCI):

1. Ineffective Tissue Perfusion (Spinal Cord) related to compression, contusion, and/or edema
2. Ineffective Airway Clearance, Ineffective Breathing Pattern, and Impaired Gas Exchange related to decreased innervation to muscles of respiration or immobility
3. Impaired Physical Mobility and/or Self-Care Deficit (the level depends on the extent and level of the injury) related to quadriplegia, quadriparesis, paraplegia, or paraparesis
4. Impaired Urinary Elimination and Constipation related to neurogenic bowel and bladder
5. Impaired Adjustment related to depression, fear, a change in body image, or altered role performance

ADDITIONAL NURSING DIAGNOSES AND COLLABORATIVE PROBLEMS

In addition to the common nursing diagnoses, clients with an SCI may have one or more of the following:

- Risk for Impaired Skin Integrity related to immobility
- Ineffective Sexuality Patterns and Sexual Dysfunction related to decreased or absent innervation of the reproductive system
- Acute Pain related to trauma, spasticity, and/or immobility
- Risk for Injury related to immobility and decreased sensation
- Imbalanced Nutrition: Less Than Body Requirements related to paralytic ileus

Collaborative problems include the following:

- Potential for Deep Vein Thrombosis (DVT)
- Potential for Sepsis
- Potential for Hypoxemia
- Potential for Atelectasis, Pneumonia

Planning and Implementation

INEFFECTIVE TISSUE PERFUSION (SPINAL CORD)

PLANNING: EXPECTED OUTCOMES. The client with an SCI is expected to demonstrate adequate spinal cord tissue perfusion as evidenced by no further deterioration in neurologic status.

INTERVENTIONS. If the client has a fractured vertebrae, the primary concern of the health care team is to reduce and immobilize the fracture to prevent further damage to the spinal cord from bone fragments. The health care provider typically uses nonsurgical techniques with traction or external fixation, but surgery may be necessary to stabilize the spine and prevent further spinal cord damage.

NONSURGICAL MANAGEMENT. The nurse assesses the client's vital signs and neurologic status, especially respiratory function and motor and sensory changes in the extremities, every 4 hours or more often if clinically indicated. In the first 24 hours after injury, the client is at risk for neurogenic shock as manifested by hypotension and bradycardia. Neurogenic shock is most often associated with cervical spinal injuries and is caused by a loss of autonomic function.

NIC ***POSITIONING: NEUROLOGIC.*** Regardless of the level of SCI, the nurse keeps the client in optimal body alignment to prevent further cord injury or irritability (Chart 43-9). Devices such as traction, orthoses, or collars may be used to keep the spine immobilized during healing and rehabilitation.

Immobilization: Cervical Injuries. The client with a cervical spine injury is usually placed in fixed skeletal traction to realign the vertebrae, facilitate bone healing, and prevent further injury. The most commonly used devices for immobilization are the halo fixation device and cervical tongs (Gardner-Wells, Barton, or Crutchfield tongs), which may be used in conjunction with a Stryker frame or kinetic treatment table. Either device is inserted by the physician into the outer aspect of the skull and may be used with a Stryker frame or kinetic treatment table to maintain spinal alignment and allow frequent turning. The addition of traction to the cervical tongs

CHART 43-9

NIC INTERVENTION ACTIVITIES *for* Clients with a Spinal Cord Injury

Positioning: Neurologic: *Achievement of optimal, appropriate body alignment for the client experiencing or at risk for spinal cord injury or vertebral irritability.*
- Immobilize or support the affected body part, as appropriate.
- Place in the designated therapeutic position.
- Maintain proper body alignment.
- Position with head and neck in alignment.
- Turn using the logroll technique.
- Apply an orthosis collar.
- Instruct on orthosis collar care, as needed.
- Apply and maintain a splinting or bracing device.
- Monitor skin integrity under bracing device/orthosis collar.
- Instruct on pin site care, as needed.
- Monitor traction pin insertion site.
- Perform traction/orthosis device pin insertion site care.
- Monitor traction device setup.

Airway Management: *Facilitation of patency of air passages*
- Position client to maximize ventilation potential.
- Identify client requiring actual/potential airway insertion.
- Insert oral or nasopharyngeal airway, as appropriate.
- Perform chest physical therapy, as appropriate.
- Remove secretions by encouraging coughing or suctioning.
- Encourage slow, deep breathing; turning; and coughing.
- Instruct how to cough effectively.
- Assist with incentive spirometer, as appropriate.
- Auscultate breath sounds, noting areas of decreased or absent ventilation and presence of adventitious sounds.
- Perform endotracheal or nasotracheal suctioning, as appropriate.
- Administer humidified air or oxygen, as appropriate.
- Regulate fluid intake to optimize fluid balance.
- Position to alleviate dyspnea.
- Monitor respiratory and oxygenation status, as appropriate.

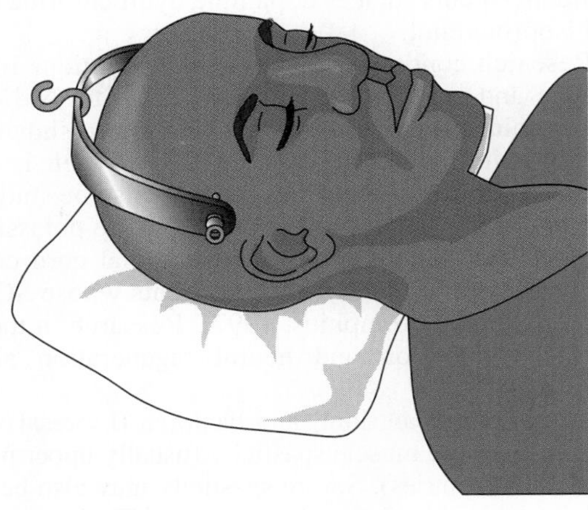

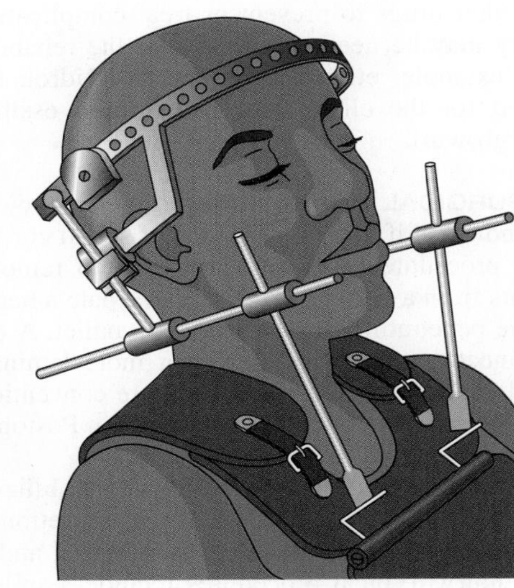

Figure 43-6 ● Types of cervical spine traction.

assists in reducing the fracture. Traction may or may not be used with the halo fixator. Traction weights may be ordered by the physician.

The halo fixator is a static traction device. Four pins (or screws) are inserted into the skull. The metal halo ring may be attached to a plastic vest or cast when the spine is stable, allowing increased client mobility. The client should never be moved or turned by holding or pulling on the halo device. The client's skin is checked frequently to ensure that the jacket or cast is not causing pressure. The nurse should be able to insert one finger easily under the jacket or cast.

The nurse monitors the client's neurologic status for changes in movement or decreased strength. The weights of the traction should hang freely at all times. Releasing the traction could cause further neurologic damage. The nurse maintains the client in alignment and ensures that the ropes for the traction remain within the pulley and hang freely. The insertion sites of the tongs or halo device are monitored for signs of infection. The nurse follows hospital policy for pin site care, which may specify the use of solutions such as hydrogen peroxide and saline (Figure 43-6).

Immobilization: Thoracic and Lumbar/Sacral Injuries. The client with a thoracic injury is placed on bedrest; immobilization with a fiberglass or plastic body cast may be done (see also Chapter 52). For lumbar and sacral injuries, immobilization of the spine is typically accomplished with a brace or a corset worn when the client is out of bed. Newer lightweight, custom-fit thoracic lumbar sacral orthoses (TLSOs) are preferred over heavier braces or splints, such as the Taylor splint.

DRUG THERAPY. Methylprednisolone (Solu-Medrol) given within 8 hours of injury is now the widely recognized first course of treatment for spinal cord injury (SCI). Initially, 30 mg/kg is given intravenously, followed by a 45-minute rest period; 5.4 mg/kg is then given as a continuous infusion for 23 hours. Clients receiving this medication usually show improvement in motor and sensory function. Dextran, a plasma expander, may be used to increase capillary blood flow within the spinal cord and to prevent or treat hypotension. Atropine sulfate is used to treat bradycardia if the pulse rate falls below 50 to 60 beats/min. Hypotension, if severe, is treated with inotropic and sympathomimetic agents such as dopamine hydrochloride (Intropin) and isoproterenol.

Research continues to explore interventions in pharmacologic and surgical management of SCIs. Naloxone and thyrotropin-releasing hormone (TRH) have shown promise in improving spinal cord blood flow. Sygen is being researched for use in acute SCI but may also be studied for its use for chronic SCI. Another drug, 4-AP, a potassium channel blocker, is thought to improve spinal cord conduction and remains in clinical trials for clients whose SCI is older than 18 months (Tompkins, 1997). Research in the areas of muscle stimulation and neural regeneration also show promise.

Dantrolene (Dantrium) and baclofen (Lioresal) may help to control severe muscle spasticity (usually upper motor neuron [UMN] injuries). Severe spasticity may also be managed with intrathecal baclofen (ITB) therapy. The drug is administered through a programmable infusion pump and intrathecal catheter directly into the cerebrospinal fluid (Leslie & Ahrendt, 1999).

Other drugs to prevent or treat complications of immobility may be needed later during the rehabilitative phase. For example, etidronate disodium (Didronel) may be ordered for the client with **heterotopic ossification** (bony overgrowth).

SURGICAL MANAGEMENT. Emergency surgery may be indicated if there is evidence of spinal cord compression. The procedure is usually necessary to remove bone fragments from a vertebral fracture, evacuate a hematoma, or remove penetrating objects such as a bullet. A decompressive laminectomy (removal of one or more laminae) allows for cord expansion from edema if more conventional measures fail to prevent neurologic deterioration. Postoperative care is discussed on pp. 929 and 930.

Additional surgical procedures to stabilize and support the spine may be performed at the discretion of the physician, depending on the client's condition and the extent of the injury. Typical procedures include a spinal fusion and the insertion of metal or steel rods, such as Harrington rods, to stabilize thoracic spinal injuries. After surgery, the client usually wears a brace, a corset, or lumbosacral support (TLSO) to keep the operative area immobilized during recovery. (See also Chapter 51, Collaborative Management of Scoliosis.)

Postoperatively, the nurse assesses the client's neurologic status and vital signs at least every hour for the first 4 to 6 hours after surgery and then, if the client is stable, every 4 hours. Complications of surgery, such as hematoma and edema, are manifested by a deterioration in neurologic status.

The client is also at risk for cardiovascular instability because of a loss of sympathetic innervation. In some cases the client may require a pacemaker. The client is logrolled when being moved to maintain skeletal alignment or placed on a special bed such as a kinetic treatment table. The nurse monitors the client's cardiovascular status carefully, especially with position changes. A complete discussion of postoperative nursing care is found in Chapter 19.

INEFFECTIVE AIRWAY CLEARANCE; INEFFECTIVE BREATHING PATTERN; IMPAIRED GAS EXCHANGE

NOC **PLANNING: EXPECTED OUTCOMES.** The client with an SCI is expected to (1) maintain a patent airway, (2) have respiratory rate and rhythm in expected range (IER), (3) have no adventitious breath sounds, and (4) not experience respiratory complications, such as pneumonia, atelectasis, and aspiration.

INTERVENTIONS. Clients with injuries at or above the sixth thoracic vertebra are especially at risk for respiratory complications (e.g., pneumonia) and pulmonary embolus as a result of impaired functioning of the intercostal muscles. Depending on the level of injury, intubation or tracheotomy with mechanical ventilation may be needed.

NIC **AIRWAY MANAGEMENT.** The nurse or assistive nursing personnel turns the client at least every 2 hours and instructs the client to breathe as deeply as possible. The nurse can assist quadriplegic clients to cough by placing his or her hands on either side of the rib cage or upper abdomen below the diaphragm. This technique is sometimes called "assisted coughing," "quad cough," or "cough assist." As the client inhales, the nurse pushes upward to help the client expand the lungs and cough.

The nurse also encourages the client to use an incentive spirometer. The nurse or respiratory therapist performs a respiratory assessment every 8 hours to determine the effectiveness of these strategies. In some cases it may be necessary to perform oral or nasal suctioning if the client cannot clear the airway of secretions effectively (see Chart 43-9).

IMPAIRED PHYSICAL MOBILITY; SELF-CARE DEFICIT

NOC **PLANNING: EXPECTED OUTCOMES.** The client with an SCI is expected to be free from complications of immobility and perform the most basic physical tasks and personal care activities as independently as possible.

INTERVENTIONS. The client with an SCI is especially at risk for pressure ulcers, contractures, and deep vein thrombosis (DVT) or pulmonary emboli. Proper positioning not only helps prevent complications but also provides alignment to prevent further spinal cord injury or irritability, as described under Positioning: Neurologic, p. 936.

PREVENTING COMPLICATIONS OF IMMOBILITY. To decrease the high risk of pressure ulcers, the nurse or assistive nursing personnel turns and repositions the client in bed at least every 2 hours. When sitting in a chair, the client is repositioned or taught to reposition himself or herself more often than every 2 hours, because in the sitting position most of the weight is placed on one area, the ischial tuberosities. Special pressure-relief devices, such as gel pads, may be used in the wheelchair or the bed, but these do not eliminate the need for regular turning and repositioning.

The nurse inspects (and teaches the client to inspect) the skin frequently to determine the client's tolerance for sitting and to detect reddened areas. The nurse presses on the reddened areas over the ischial tuberosities and looks for blanching. If blanching does not occur, the area is vulnerable to skin breakdown.

To decrease the risk of contractures as a result of immobility, the nurse or assistive nursing personnel performs range-of-motion (ROM) exercises at least once every 8 hours. The physical therapist and the occupational therapist:

- Determine the most appropriate positioning and exercise techniques
- Assess the need for hand and wrist splints
- Develop a plan to prevent footdrop (usually clients wear high-topped tennis shoes for prevention)

The nurse assesses the client's lower extremities for indications of DVT. Signs and symptoms include leg or calf pain, localized tenderness, swelling, and redness. Some clients may be totally asymptomatic. Graduated compression stockings (GCSs), also called sequential compression devices (SCDs), or pneumatic compression boots (PCBs) are typically ordered. Sodium heparin, 5000 units every 12 hours subcutaneously, or sodium warfarin (Coumadin, Warfilone✤) in therapeutic dosages may be ordered to prevent DVT or embolus formation. Low–molecular weight (LMW) heparin (e.g., enoxaparin [Lovenox]) has begun to replace sodium heparin as a more common treatment. Lovenox provides the same level of antithrombotic activity as heparin but may decrease the risk for hemorrhage. (See Chapter 10 for further discussion of measures to prevent complications of immobility.)

PREVENTING ORTHOSTATIC HYPOTENSION. Clients with cervical cord injuries are especially at high risk for orthostatic (postural) hypotension, but any client who is immobilized may have this problem. If the client moves from a lying position to a sitting or standing position too quickly, he or she may experience hypotension, which could result in dizziness and falls. Because of interrupted autonomic innervation, the blood vessels do not constrict quickly enough to push blood up into the brain; this causes the dizziness or lightheadedness often experienced by these clients.

The nurse observes the client carefully for indications of orthostatic hypotension when the head of the bed is raised and when the client is permitted to dangle the legs over the side of the bed or get up in a chair. Blood pressure is measured in each position.

To help prevent orthostatic hypotension, the nurse teaches the client to change positions slowly. Some clients wear elastic corsets around the trunk to help facilitate blood flow. Thigh-high antiembolism stockings or elastic (Ace) wraps around both legs may also be used. A tilt table may be used to help the client get used to postural changes. Chart 43-10 summarizes the most important aspects of care for clients with an SCI.

PROMOTING SELF-CARE. The most important part of promoting self-care is setting realistic goals on the basis of the client's potential functional level. Even clients with a cervical SCI may be able to learn how to perform most ADLs independently. The nurse collaborates with the physical therapist and occupational therapist to evaluate how the client can best transfer from a bed to the wheelchair and feed, dress, and bathe. Various assistive/adaptive devices are available to help clients regain their independence.

Many clients with an SCI can no longer ambulate. They become wheelchair dependent and must learn new skills. The physical therapist carefully measures the client and orders a custom-made wheelchair. If the client is unable to self-propel the chair manually, electronic devices are available so he or she can use the mouth, neck, or upper arm to ambulate in the chair.

CHART 43-10

BEST PRACTICE *for*
Care of the Client with a Spinal Cord Injury

- Assess the client's respiratory status; monitor for atelectasis, pneumonia, and pulmonary embolus.
- Take vital signs every 4 hours, or more often if clinically indicated; monitor for orthostatic hypotension.
- Perform neurologic status checks every 4 hours, or more often if clinically indicated.
  - Notify the physician immediately of a deterioration in motor status.
  - Watch for and immediately treat autonomic dysreflexia.
- Give pain medication as ordered; document the client's response.
- Prevent immobility complications.
  - Have the client TCDB every 2 hours.
  - Use pneumatic compression boots or gradiated compression stockings.
  - Check the skin and bony prominences for redness and breakdown.
- Assess bladder function.
  - Palpate the abdomen for distention.
  - Begin a bladder retraining program as appropriate.
  - Assess intake and output.
- Assess bowel function.
  - Auscultate bowel sounds.
  - Palpate for distention.
  - Chart stool frequency.
  - Begin a bowel program as appropriate.
- Monitor nutritional status, including a calorie count, and collaborate with the dietitian to identify an appropriate diet.
- Assess psychologic status.
  - Communicate with the client.
  - Answer questions honestly; refer questions that you cannot answer to someone who can.
  - Assess for signs of depression or anger.

TCDB, Turn, cough, and deep breathe.

CRITICAL THINKING CHALLENGE

A young male client is admitted to your unit with a diagnosis of a complete C5-C6 SCI as a result of a diving accident. When you talk with him, he seems very anxious about his future. His respirations are shallow and rapid, but otherwise his vital signs are within normal limits.

- What is the most important assessment needed for this client?
- What response will you provide if he asks if his condition is permanent?
- What members of the health care team will need to collaborate for his care?
- What is a realistic long-term outcome for him?

For suggested answer guidelines, go to SIMON http://www.wbsaunders.com/SIMON/Iggy/.

IMPAIRED URINARY ELIMINATION; CONSTIPATION

NOC **PLANNING: EXPECTED OUTCOMES.** The client with an SCI is expected to achieve control of urine and stool, as indicated by urinary continence (depending on SCI level), complete emptying of bladder, absence of urinary tract infection, and no constipation.

INTERVENTIONS. Clients with SCIs have reflex or neurogenic loss of bowel and bladder control. Many can become continent if they rigorously adhere to an established program. The type of program depends on the usual elimination pattern and whether the injury involved upper motor neurons (UMNs) or lower motor neurons (LMNs). A urologic evaluation may be needed to identify bladder type.

ESTABLISHING A BLADDER RETRAINING PROGRAM. As soon as the client is medically stable, the indwelling Foley catheter is removed. Initially, the physician may prescribe an intermittent catheterization program. The nurse typically catheterizes the client every 4 hours as ordered and more frequently if the urinary output is greater than 500 mL. Over time, the intervals between catheterizations are increased and adjusted to the client's fluid intake and sleep times. A bedside bladder ultrasound device may be used to measure bladder residual.

After the acute care phase has passed, the client may be able to initiate voiding by using specific techniques. Clients with UMN (spastic) bladder problems (injury above the sacrum) may be able to stimulate voiding by doing the following:

- Stroking the inner thigh
- Pulling on pubic hair and hair of the upper thigh
- Pouring warm water over the perineum
- Tapping the bladder area to stimulate the detrusor muscle

Some health care providers prescribe a drug to stimulate voiding, such as bethanechol chloride (Urecholine). Bethanechol is a cholinergic agent that facilitates contraction of the detrusor muscle and is usually given two to four times daily about 1 hour before attempts to void.

Clients with injuries to the lumbosacral area usually have an LMN (flaccid) bladder. Clients with flaccid bladders may achieve emptying of the bladder by performing a Valsalva maneuver or tightening the abdominal muscles. These techniques are not successful for all LMN injuries. To ascertain the effectiveness of these maneuvers, the nurse catheterizes the client for residual urine after voiding. Some clients rely solely on catheterization two or three times daily to empty the bladder. All clients are encouraged to drink 2000 to 2500 mL of fluid each day to prevent urinary tract infection and calculus formation. Clients with an LMN injury may decrease fluid intake after 6 or 7 PM each evening to prevent the need for catheterization in the middle of the night.

The client with any SCI is at risk for pyelonephritis, hydronephrosis, renal failure, and kidney stones (see Chapters 71 and 72).

ESTABLISHING A BOWEL RETRAINING PROGRAM. The following are essential elements of a bowel program:

- A consistent time for bowel elimination
- A high fluid intake (at least 2000 mL/day) unless fluid intake is restricted
- A high-fiber diet
- Rectal stimulation with or without suppositories
- If needed, stool softener medications such as docusate sodium (Colace) and docusate sodium and casanthranol (Peri-Colace)

If the client has sustained an LMN injury, the resulting flaccid large bowel may require the client to perform or undergo manual disimpaction. Additional stimuli to facilitate a bowel movement include scheduling toileting 30 minutes to 1 hour after meals to optimize the gastrocolic reflex and teaching the client to perform a Valsalva maneuver. Massaging the abdomen from right to left along the outline of the large intestine may also be helpful. Additional information about bladder and bowel retraining is provided in Chapter 10.

IMPAIRED ADJUSTMENT

NOC **PLANNING: EXPECTED OUTCOMES.** The client with an SCI is expected to demonstrate an ability to cope with the changes caused by the injury and verbalize acceptance of the injury and changes in lifestyle.

INTERVENTIONS. The nurse uses the information obtained from the psychosocial assessment to identify strategies to help the client adjust to the disability. The client is invited to ask questions, which the nurse should answer openly and honestly. The nurse should refer questions about prognosis and potential for complete recovery to the health care provider, because the timing and extent of recovery vary for each client.

The client is encouraged to discuss his or her perceptions of the situation and the coping strategies that can be used. He or she should feel free to express personal feelings and emotions in an acceptable manner. He or she may behave in a socially unacceptable manner (excessive anger, verbal abuse, use of illegal drugs), and the nurse attempts to redirect this behavior. In addition, the nurse begins a client education program to clarify misconceptions and provide health teaching. Referrals to clergy, rabbis, other spiritual leaders, or a psychologist or psychiatric liaison nurse may be needed to help clients adjust to their unexpected life change. Support groups are available for clients and families.

Clients with SCIs should be referred to a social worker or financial counselor for a review of their insurance and financial status and also referred to the appropriate social service agencies as necessary. Many insurance policies do not provide coverage for rehabilitation.

Community-Based Care

Case managers are ideal care coordinators to act as SCI client advocates. In some settings, case managers begin working with clients in the emergency department to establish a positive image of SCI rehabilitation (Hesslegrave, 1997). Rehabilitation begins in the critical care unit when clients are hemodynamically stable and spinal shock has subsided. They are usually transferred from the acute care setting to a rehabilitation setting, where they learn more about self-care, mobility skills, and bladder and bowel retraining. The length of stay in the rehabilitation hospital or unit is typically 1 to 3 months, depending on the medical complications that may occur, such as infections.

CRITICAL THINKING CHALLENGE

A quadriplegic client on your rehabilitation unit complains that he gets dizzy when transferring from the bed to his wheelchair. He has been told that his blood pressure drops when he changes position. However, last week he had an episode of very high blood pressure, skin flushing, and severe headache. The client does not understand why he is experiencing such fluctuations in his blood pressure.

- What explanation should you give him to explain his increase and decrease in blood pressure?
- What precautions should he take to help prevent these events from recurring?

For suggested answer guidelines, go to SIMON http://www.wbsaunders.com/SIMON/Iggy/.

HOME CARE MANAGEMENT

If the client is discharged home or returns home for a weekend visit from the rehabilitation setting, the environment must be assessed to ensure that it is free from hazards and can accommodate the client's special needs (e.g., a wheelchair). The occupational or physical therapist, in collaboration with rehabilitation and the home care nurse, usually assesses the client's temporary or permanent home environment. Ease of accessibility is particularly important at the entrance of the home as well as the bathroom, kitchen, and bedroom. The height of the client's bed may need to be adjusted to facilitate a smooth transfer into or out of the bed.

All adaptive devices that the client will use at home should be ordered and delivered to the rehabilitation facility. This enables the nurse and other therapists to ensure that the items fit correctly and that the client and family know how to use them correctly.

HEALTH TEACHING

The teaching plan for the client with an SCI includes the following:

- Physical mobility and activity skills
- Activities of daily living (ADLs) skills
- Bowel and bladder retraining program
- Skin care
- Medication regimen
- Sexuality education

This information should be reinforced with written handouts or other client education material that the client, family members, or significant others can use after discharge to the home.

It is important that the client learn mobility skills so he or she can negotiate movement on sidewalks, carpeting, and other flooring surfaces. The client must also be able to negotiate sidewalk curbs while walking independently with crutches or a cane or while in a wheelchair.

Some clients are discharged home or to a rehabilitation setting with a halo vest. A halo vest has a significant physical and psychologic impact on clients. Physically, clients find it difficult to perform mobility skills and ADLs independently, especially dressing, bathing, and feeding. From a psychologic perspective, clients perceive an altered body image. The nurse teaches the client going home or to a rehabilitation setting how to care for and adjust to the halo device (Chart 43-11).

ADL training for the client with an SCI includes a structured exercise program to promote strength and endurance. The occupational therapist instructs the client in the correct use of all adaptive equipment. In collaboration with the therapists, the nurse instructs family members or the caregiver in transfer skills, feeding, bathing, dressing, positioning, and skin care as appropriate. The nurse collaborates with the dietitian to help the client maintain an ideal body weight and to promote bowel and bladder elimination. The nurse also reinforces the need to follow the client's individualized bowel and bladder program. The client is instructed in the procedures to follow if problems develop.

CHART 43-11

CLIENT EDUCATION GUIDE
Use of a Halo Device*

- Be aware that the weight of the halo device alters balance. Be careful when leaning forward or backward.
- Wear loose clothing, preferably with hook and loop (Velcro) fasteners or large openings for head and arms.
- Bathe in the bathtub or sponge bathe. (Some physicians allow showers.*)
- Wash under the lamb's wool liner of the vest to prevent rashes or sores; use powders or lotions sparingly under the vest.
- Have someone change the liner if it becomes odorous.
- Support the head with a small pillow when sleeping to prevent unnecessary pressure and discomfort.
- Try to resume usual activities to the extent possible; keep as active as possible. (The weight of the device may cause fatigue or weakness.) Avoid contact sports or swimming, however.
- Do not drive, because vision is impaired with the device.
- Keep straws available for drinking fluids.
- Cut meats and other food into small pieces to facilitate chewing and swallowing.
- If going outside in cold temperatures, wrap the pins with cloth to prevent the metal from getting cold.
- Have someone clean the pin sites as recommended by physician or hospital protocol.
- Observe the pin sites daily for redness, drainage, or loosening; report changes to the physician.
- Increase fluids and fiber in the diet to prevent constipation.
- Use a position of comfort during sexual activity.

*Home care instructions may vary depending on hospital or physician preference.

The nurse teaches about the name, purpose, dosage, timing of administration, and side effects of all medications. The client should understand the possible interaction of prescribed medications with over-the-counter medications or alcohol and illegal drugs.

The goal of sexuality education is to answer questions and correct any misinformation. Unless the nurse has specific training or experience in sexuality counseling of people with SCIs, detailed questions should be directed to a sexuality counselor.

CONSIDERATIONS FOR OLDER ADULTS

Many clients with an SCI are living into middle and older adulthood. Thinking and planning about preventive health care for the future is an important part of health teaching. Chart 43-12 outlines important interventions for maintaining health in older adults with an SCI.

PSYCHOSOCIAL PREPARATION

Psychosocial adaptation is one of the critical factors in determining the success of rehabilitation. The case manager or acute care nurse can help the client prepare for discharge or transfer to a rehabilitation hospital. The nurse assists the client to verbalize feelings and fears about body image, self-concept, role performance, and self-esteem. The client should be told about the expected reactions of those outside the security of the hospital environment. In the acute care setting, the nurse, family members, or friends can take the client to the hospital lobby or, if permitted, to the cafeteria or outside on

CHART 43-12

NURSING FOCUS *on the* OLDER ADULT
What Clients Need to Know About Aging with Spinal Cord Injury

Nursing Intervention	Rationale
Get flu shots annually, tetanus shots every 10 years, and the pneumonia vaccine as required.	Respiratory complications are the most common cause of death following spinal cord injury (SCI).
For women, have annual Papanicolaou (Pap) smears and mammograms.	Limitations in movement may make breast self-examination difficult. All older women should have an annual Pap smear.
Take measures to prevent osteoporosis, such as increasing calcium intake, exercising, and avoiding caffeine and smoking.	Women over 50 years of age often lose bone density, which can result in fractures.
Practice meticulous skin care, including moisturizing and drinking plenty of water.	As a person ages, skin becomes dry and less elastic, predisposing the client to pressure ulcers.
Take measures to prevent constipation, such as drinking adequate fluids, eating a healthy diet with fiber, and exercising.	Constipation is a problem for most clients with SCI, and they are more likely to develop the problem later in life.
Modify activities if joint pain occurs; use a powered rather than a manual wheelchair. Ask the health care provider about treatment options.	Arthritis occurs in more than half of people over 65 years of age. Clients with SCI are more likely to develop arthritis due to added stress on the upper extremities when using a wheelchair.

the hospital grounds. The nurse should tactfully and nonjudgmentally let the client know when behavior is unacceptable for the time and place in which it occurs and should encourage more positive behaviors. Role-playing or anticipating responses to potential problems is helpful. For example, the client can practice answering questions from children about why he or she is in a wheelchair or cannot move certain parts of the body.

HEALTH CARE RESOURCES

The nurse or case manager refers the client and family or significant others to the local, state or province, and national organizations for those with SCIs. These organizations include the National Spinal Cord Injury Association and the Spinal Cord Injury Hotline. Many consumer-oriented books, journals, and films are also available. Support groups may help the client and family adjust to a changed lifestyle and provide solutions to commonly encountered problems.

A full-time caretaker or personal assistant is usually required if the quadriplegic client returns home. The caretaker may be a family member or a nursing assistant employed to help provide care and companionship. A paraplegic client is often able to function without assistance after an appropriate rehabilitation program.

Evaluation: Outcomes

NOC The nurse evaluates the care of the client with an SCI on the basis of the identified nursing diagnoses and collaborative problems. The expected outcomes are that the client:

- Exhibits no deterioration in neurologic status
- Maintains a patent airway and experiences no respiratory complications
- Is free from complications of immobility
- Performs ADLs as independently as possible with or without the use of assistive/adaptive devices
- Achieves continence of stool and urine
- Demonstrates the ability to cope with the change caused by the injury

SPINAL CORD TUMORS

OVERVIEW

Spinal cord tumors occur most often in the thoracic area, followed by an almost equal distribution in the lumbar and cervical region. Signs and symptoms depend on the location of the tumor and its speed of growth.

The pathologic effects of a spinal cord tumor are more often related to compression of the cord than to invasion of the spinal cord itself. As the tumor expands within the vertebral column, it compresses the cord or the spinal nerve roots. Further growth leads to displacement of the cord. In addition, a large tumor may disrupt the vascular supply to the cord by compression or obstruct the normal flow of cerebrospinal fluid (CSF). Venous occlusion by the tumor may lead to spinal cord congestion and infarction.

The appearance of neurologic signs and symptoms is related to the rate of tumor growth. The spinal cord can often accommodate a slowly growing lesion. With time, the cord may become significantly misshapen and displaced, but the client has surprisingly few symptoms. On the other hand, a rapidly growing tumor quickly leads to spinal cord compression and edema and the development of neurologic symptoms, such as numbness and paralysis.

Primary spinal cord tumors arise from the epidural vessels, spinal meninges, or glial cells of the cord. Their cause is unknown. Approximately 20% to 30% of spinal cord tumors develop as a consequence of metastatic tumors from the lungs, breasts, prostate, colon, and uterus.

Anatomically, spinal cord tumors may be extramedullary or intramedullary. **Intramedullary tumors** account for 10% of spinal cord tumors and are usually malignant. They originate within the spinal cord itself, in the central gray matter and the anterior commissure. **Extramedullary tumors,** 90% of spinal cord tumors, are found within the spinal dura but outside the cord. They are further defined anatomically as extradural and intradural tumors. Extradural or epidural tumors occur between the vertebrae and the spinal dura. They develop in the surrounding bone and cause destruction of the vertebral bodies. Intradural tumors are located within the dura and originate from the pia-arachnoid, spinal roots, or denticulate ligaments.

Spinal cord tumors account for only about 0.5% of all tumors in adults and 10% to 15% of primary central nervous system (CNS) tumors. Thoracic tumors account for 50% of all spinal cord tumors. Cervical tumors occur 30% of the time, followed by lumbosacral tumors (20%). The majority of tumors are benign. They occur equally in both men and women between 20 and 60 years of age.

COLLABORATIVE MANAGEMENT

Assessment

PHYSICAL ASSESSMENT/CLINICAL MANIFESTATIONS

The clinical manifestations of a spinal cord tumor depend on its location (Chart 43-13) and rate of growth. The most common complaint of the client with a spinal cord tumor is pain. Pain results from spinal cord compression, infiltration of the spinal tracts, or irritation of the spinal roots. The nurse assesses the quality, severity, and intensity of the pain. In addition, the nurse asks the client to describe factors that exacerbate and relieve the pain. Radicular (nerve root) pain is described as stabbing or dull, with intermittent episodes of sharp, piercing pain. The pain may be increased when coughing, straining, or sneezing. Lying flat may increase the pain as a consequence of stretching the involved spinal nerve roots.

Involvement of the corticospinal tract may lead to motor deficits. The nurse assesses for weakness, clumsiness, spasticity, and hyperactive reflexes and compares the responses on both sides of the body. Other presenting signs include ataxia, hypotonia, and a positive Babinski's reflex. Spastic paralysis is seen most often, although a flaccid paralysis may be seen in a tumor that affects the spinal roots, in an intramedullary tumor in the enlargements of the cervical or lumbar area, or in an extramedullary tumor complicated by spinal shock. A flaccid paralysis may also be noted in the presence of a cauda equina lesion.

The nurse also assesses for sensory loss on each side of the body and compares the responses. Early symptoms of sensory loss include a slowly progressive numbness or tingling, pain, and temperature loss. The sensory deficit is further marked by a decreased appreciation of touch, an inability to sense vibration, and a loss of position sense. The client often reports a tight, bandlike feeling around the trunk. Brown-Séquard syndrome or central cord syndrome may be manifested (see Extent of Injury [Spinal Cord Injury], p. 932).

Loss of bladder control often precedes a loss of bowel control in the client with a spinal cord tumor. Typically, bladder dysfunction is manifested by hesitancy, dribbling, incontinence, urgency, or acute retention. Bowel dysfunction is manifested by constipation. The nurse must remember that the client is often embarrassed to admit to bladder or bowel dysfunction.

A lesion in the sacral area may cause a decrease in genital sensation and thus impair the client's sexual function and enjoyment. Men may be unable to have an erection or to ejaculate.

CHART 43-13

KEY FEATURES *of* Spinal Cord Tumors

General Manifestations
- Pain
- Sensory loss or impairment
- Motor loss or impairment
- Sphincter disturbance (bladder before bowel)

Cervical Manifestations
- High cervical
  - Respiratory distress
  - Diaphragm paralysis
  - Occipital headache
  - Quadriparesis
  - Stiff neck
  - Nystagmus
  - Cranial nerve dysfunction
- Low cervical
  - Pain in the arms and the shoulders
  - Weakness
  - Paresthesia
  - Motor loss
  - Horner's syndrome
  - Increased reflexes

Thoracic Manifestations
- Sensory loss
- Spastic paralysis
- Positive Babinski's sign
- Bladder and bowel dysfunction
- Pain in the chest and the back
- Muscle atrophy
- Muscle weakness in the legs
- Foot drop

Lumbosacral Manifestations
- Low back pain
- Paresis
- Spastic paralysis
- Sensory loss
- Bladder and bowel dysfunction
- Sexual dysfunction
- Decreased-to-absent ankle and knee reflexes

DIAGNOSTIC ASSESSMENT

Routine x-ray examinations or tomographic scans of the spine are obtained to detect a narrowing of the spinal canal, destruction of the vertebrae, or the presence of calcification. A myelogram is useful when a block is incomplete; it indicates the level, extent, and boundaries of a tumor.

A magnetic resonance imaging (MRI) scan with and without enhancement provides more detail of the pathologic condition of the spinal cord than either a computed tomography (CT) scan or myelography. Electromyography may help make a differential diagnosis to rule out multiple sclerosis or amyotrophic lateral sclerosis (ALS).

Interventions

Nursing care of the client with a spinal cord tumor includes obtaining the vital signs and checking neurologic status at least every 4 hours and more often as clinically indicated. As for any client with a spinal cord problem, the nurse must pay meticulous attention to motor and sensory status. The nurse reports any changes immediately to the physician.

SURGICAL MANAGEMENT. The primary management of a spinal cord tumor is surgery. The goal of surgical intervention is to remove as much of the tumor as possible. Often this is not feasible and other treatment is indicated (e.g., radiation therapy). Emergency surgery is indicated if the client experiences a rapid loss of motor and sensory function and/or a loss of bladder and bowel control. Surgical decompression may be performed to maintain bladder, bowel, or motor function and to preserve quality of life—even with a poor prognosis. Table 43-1 summarizes the treatment of spinal cord tumors of various types and locations.

General preoperative care is performed (see Chapter 17). The nurse devotes particular attention to detailed documentation of the client's motor and sensory status.

The neurosurgeon performs a laminectomy and surgical decompression and total or partial resection of the tumor. Depending on the extent of the tumor, a spinal fusion may be necessary. Rarely, a cordotomy or a palliative sectioning of sensory roots is done to control intractable pain. Laminectomies are discussed under Surgical Management (Back Pain), p. 928.

General postoperative care is provided (see Chapter 19). After surgery, the nurse assesses the client's vital signs and neurologic status every 1 to 2 hours until they are stable and then every 4 hours. The client is logrolled (turned as a unit) and repositioned every 2 hours. The nurse inspects the incision site for drainage, especially of cerebrospinal fluid (CSF), and signs of infection. The client with a cervical cord tumor must also be carefully monitored for respiratory compromise. Postoperative nursing care for a client undergoing a

TABLE 43-1 • LOCATION AND TREATMENT OF SPINAL CORD TUMORS

Type	Location	Symptoms	Treatment
EXTRAMEDULLARY TUMORS			
Vertebral hemangioma	Thoracic or lumbar spine (more common in women; this type of tumor is essentially an atrioventricular shunt fed by the intercostal and lumbar arteries)	Back pain Paraparesis Radicular pain	Embolization of the mass followed by surgical excision
Meningioma	Cervical or thoracic area (more common in women)	Vague sensory loss Midline back pain	Resection of tumor Radiation therapy
Chordoma	Cervical or sacrococcygeal area	Slow growing; locally invasive Low back pain Bowel or bladder dysfunction	Resection of tumor Unresponsive to radiation therapy
Schwannoma and neurofibroma	Thoracic or cervical area	Radicular pain Motor weakness	Surgical resection Unresponsive to radiation therapy
Hemangioblastoma	Thoracic area	Progressive neurologic dysfunction Motor weakness Sensory dysfunction	Surgical excision (prognosis is good)
INTRAMEDULLARY TUMORS			
Astrocytoma type I or II	Cervical or thoracic area (slightly more common in men)	Slowly progressive May mimic multiple sclerosis Back or neck pain Paresthesia Paresis	Surgical excision and drainage of the cyst Radiation therapy
Malignant astrocytoma		Rapid neurologic deterioration Pain Paralysis Sensory impairment	Surgical excision Radiation therapy Chemotherapy (prognosis is poor)
Ependymoma	Cauda equina or cervical area (more common in men)	Slowly progressive, gradual onset Back pain, worse at night Radicular pain Motor weakness Sensory dysfunction	Surgical excision Radiation therapy (prognosis is good with total excision of the tumor)
SPINAL CYSTS			
Dermoid and epidermoid	Conus medullaris or thoracic area (slightly more common in men)	Back pain Saddle anesthesia Leg weakness Sphincter dysfunction	Surgical excision May recur
Teratoma	Lumbar area	Progressive spastic paralysis	Surgical excision
Lipoma	Cervical and thoracic areas	Sensory dysfunction	Surgical excision

laminectomy was discussed under Postoperative Care (Back Pain), pp. 929 and 930.

NONSURGICAL MANAGEMENT

RADIATION THERAPY. Radiation therapy may be necessary depending on the tumor type. It is usually used with low-grade malignant tumors that are not completely resected, metastatic tumors, or with recurrent tumors when there is no other treatment option. The spinal cord cannot tolerate high doses of radiation. Overexposure to radiation may lead to radiation myelopathy, which develops over 6 to 12 months. It is manifested by progressive spinal cord degeneration and neurologic deficits such as Brown-Séquard syndrome. With time, the client experiences spastic paralysis, loss of sensation, and bowel and bladder dysfunction; death may occur. Care of the client undergoing radiation therapy is described in detail in Chapter 25.

CHEMOTHERAPY. The use of chemotherapy in the treatment of spinal cord tumors is very limited. There are no reports of clinical trials with chemotherapy for primary spinal cord tumors. However, chemotherapy may be used as an adjunctive therapy for tumors metastasized to the spinal cord from other primary sites, such as the breast. Leptomeningeal involvement may benefit from intrathecal chemotherapy.

PAIN CONTROL. Pain control may be accomplished by pharmacologic and nonpharmacologic measures. Patient-controlled analgesia (PCA) with morphine is often used to provide immediate postoperative pain relief. The client is gradually switched to oral analgesics before discharge. The nurse assesses the client's level of pain, provides appropriate pain relief medication, and documents the response to the medication. If drug therapy does not provide pain relief, the nurse collaborates with the health care provider to identify a more effective medication.

Turning and proper positioning of the client often enhances pain relief. The nurse or assistive nursing personnel provides range-of-motion (ROM) exercises to prevent atrophy and contractures, which can increase pain. Hypnosis, music therapy, and imagery techniques are other methods of pain relief (see Chapters 4 and 7).

PREVENTING COMPLICATIONS OF IMMOBILITY. The client who is immobilized from a spinal cord tumor or spinal surgery is especially at risk for pressure sores and deep vein thrombosis (DVT) or pulmonary emboli. The nurse or assistive nursing personnel turns the client in bed at least every 2 hours. When the client is sitting in a chair, he or she is repositioned every 30 to 60 minutes.

The nurse inspects the client's skin frequently to determine tolerance for sitting and to detect the presence of reddened areas. The nurse presses on the reddened areas over the ischial tuberosities and looks for blanching. If blanching does not occur, the area is vulnerable to skin breakdown. The physical and occupational therapists determine the most appropriate positioning and exercise techniques and assess the need for assistive devices. It may be necessary for the client to be placed on a water bed or an air bed to prevent or treat pressure ulcers.

The nurse assesses the client's lower extremities for indications of DVT. Sequential compression devices may be used in place of or as an adjunct to graduated compression stockings. The health care provider may order sodium heparin 5000 units every 12 hours subcutaneously, low-molecular-weight heparin (enoxaparin [Lovenox]), or sodium warfarin (Coumadin, Warfilone🍁) in therapeutic dosages to help prevent DVT or embolus formation.

BOWEL AND BLADDER PROGRAM. The nurse asks the client about his or her normal defecation pattern. On the basis of this information, the nurse establishes a bowel program. The following are the essential elements of this program:

- A consistent time for bowel elimination
- A high fluid intake (2000 mL/day) unless fluid intake is restricted
- A high-fiber diet
- Rectal stimulation with or without suppositories
- If needed, stool softener medications, such as docusate sodium (Colace) and docusate sodium and casanthranol (Peri-Colace)

Manual disimpaction may be necessary if the client has lower motor neuron (LMN) symptoms.

The client's bladder program is determined by the specific dysfunction, usually urinary retention. The nurse or assistive nursing personnel monitors the voiding pattern and strictly measures and records intake and output. The nurse assesses for suprapubic distention and other indications of retention, such as overflow and dribbling. The client is encouraged to empty the bladder every 2 hours.

Community-Based Care

HOME CARE MANAGEMENT

The nurse collaborates with the client and family members or significant others to identify and suggest corrections for potential hazards in the home. If necessary, referral is made to a home care nurse, social worker, or case manager to assess the need for structural alterations to the home. Structural alterations may be needed to accommodate ambulatory aids (e.g., a walker) and to enable the client to perform activities of daily living (ADLs).

Some clients may be discharged from the acute care hospital to a rehabilitation setting, where they can learn to function as independently as possible. Chapter 10 describes rehabilitation in detail.

HEALTH TEACHING

The teaching plan for the client with a spinal cord tumor depends on the level of dysfunction present. With decompression of the tumor, the severity of the client's symptoms often lessens. Deficits that may remain include mobility and sensory loss. Learning mobility skills can enable the client to negotiate movement on sidewalks, carpeting, and other flooring surfaces. The client must also be able to negotiate sidewalk curbs independently. The physical or occupational therapist instructs the client in the correct use of all adaptive equipment. The nurse reinforces the individualized bowel and bladder program.

The goal of sexuality education in the acute care setting is to answer questions and correct any misinformation. Unless the nurse has had specific training or experience in sexuality counseling of people with spinal cord tumors or injuries, more detailed questions should be directed to a sexuality counselor.

PSYCHOSOCIAL PREPARATION

The prognosis for the client with malignant tumors or secondary tumors is poor. The nurse determines what the physician and family members have told the client about diagnosis and prognosis. The client is encouraged to verbalize feelings and fears about prognosis, body image, self-concept, role performance, and self-esteem.

HEALTH CARE RESOURCES

Clients and family members or significant others should be referred to local, state or province, and national organizations for people with spinal cord injuries, which are applicable to spinal cord tumors. These groups often have information for clients with spinal cord tumors. Clients with a malignancy are referred to the American Cancer Society. Referral to support groups may also assist clients and family with adapting to lifestyle changes.

MULTIPLE SCLEROSIS

OVERVIEW

Multiple sclerosis (MS) is a progressive, degenerative disease that affects the myelin sheath and conduction pathway of the central nervous system (CNS). It is one of the leading causes of neurologic disability in persons 20 to 40 years of age. This chronic disease is characterized by periods of remission and **exacerbation** (flare). As the severity and the duration of the disease progress, the periods of exacerbation become more frequent. MS has received more public attention since actress Annette Funicello and talk show host Montel Williams have been diagnosed with the disease.

Pathophysiology

Nerve impulses are transmitted from one nerve cell to another along unmyelinated fibers or via the nodes of Ranvier in myelinated axon fibers. In the presence of MS, the myelin sheath is damaged, causing an inflammatory response. This inflammation reduces the thickness of the myelin sheath. Impulses are still transmitted but are not as effective as before. The damaged myelin is then removed by astrocytes (scavenger cells). These cells form scar tissue, known as plaque, which interferes with normal pulse transmission.

The white fiber tracts that connect the neurons in the brain and spinal cord are generally involved in MS. The areas particularly affected include optic nerves, pyramidal tracts, posterior columns, brainstem nuclei, and the periventricular region of the brain. Although the myelin surrounding the axon is involved, the axon itself is relatively spared until late in the disease process, when scarring occurs. Initially, recovery of the myelin occurs with the remission of symptoms. Eventually, with repeated exacerbations of the disease, damage becomes permanent.

Six types of MS are seen (Smeltzer & Kelley, 2000):

- Benign
- Relapsing-remitting
- Progressive-relapsing
- Primary progressive
- Secondary progressive
- Malignant

Of clients with MS, 10% have the benign type and demonstrate no active disease or clinical deterioration in the preceding year. Those with benign MS present with a few episodes of mild attacks; there is minimal or no disability.

The classic picture of the relapsing-remitting type of MS occurs in 65% of cases and is characterized by increasingly frequent attacks. The course of the disease may be mild or moderate, depending on the degree of disability. Relapses develop over 1 to 2 weeks, and resolve over 4 to 8 months, after which the client returns to baseline.

Progressive-relapsing MS occurs less often and is similar to the relapsing-remitting MS. It is characterized by the absence of periods of remission, and the client's condition does not return to baseline. Progressive, cumulative symptoms and deterioration occur over several years.

Primary progressive MS involves a gradual neurologic deterioration without remission of symptoms. Clients with this type of MS tend to be between 40 and 60 years of age at onset of the disease.

Secondary progressive MS is also gradual, but the client may or may not have acute relapses.

Etiology

The exact cause of MS remains unknown. Research continues on viral, immunologic, and genetic etiologic factors. The viral theory suggests that MS is caused by a slow virus that has been dormant for many years.

The immune theory suggests that an unidentified factor (probably a virus) triggers an autoimmune response in the CNS. Both humoral and cell-mediated immune system dysfunction have been implicated. This theory is supported by research data that shows elevated immunoglobulin G (IgG) and oligoclonal bands in the CSF of clients with MS.

Genetics may play a role in determining susceptibility to MS. HLA or a major histocompatibility complex on chromosome 6, which influences the immune system, is found more often in clients with MS. Chromosomes 2, 3, 7, 11, 17, 19, and X also contain possible genes involved in the development of MS. The risk is greater if an identical twin has MS.

Incidence/Prevalence

Multiple sclerosis (MS) usually occurs in people between the ages of 20 and 40 years, but cases may occur in those younger than 15 years and older than 50 years. It is known as the disease of young adults. Only 20% of clients with MS report that their first symptom occurred in their 40s or 50s. Approximately 500,000 people in the United States are currently affected. Women are affected slightly more often than men (1.5:1). The incidence in first-degree relatives of persons with MS is 15 times greater than in the general population (Hickey, 1997).

MS is seen more often in the colder climates of the northeastern, Great Lakes, and Pacific northwestern states. In Canada, the prevalence rate is about 100 per 100,000 people (Koopman & Schweitzer, 1999). Studies have indicated that if one relocates after the age of 15 years from an area of high incidence to one of a lower incidence, the risk factor of the higher area is carried. For people younger than 15 years, the risk factor is not carried. These studies suggest that the risk factor for MS occurs at about 15 years of age. The life expectancy for those with MS is about 85% of that of the general population, or about 35 years after the onset of symptoms (Hickey, 1997).

COLLABORATIVE MANAGEMENT

Assessment

HISTORY

Multiple sclerosis (MS) often mimics other neurologic diseases, which often makes the diagnosis difficult and prolonged (see the Evidence-Based Practice for Nursing box below). Therefore obtaining a thorough history is essential for accurate diagnosis. The nurse begins by asking the client for a history of vision changes, motor skills, and sensations, all of which are early indicators of MS. The symptoms are often vague and nonspecific in the early stages of the disease. Of significance is the client's report that symptoms were first noticed several years earlier but that medical attention was not sought because the symptoms disappeared. The nurse questions about the progression of symptoms, with particular attention given to determining whether the symptoms are intermittent or are becoming progressively worse. The nurse should find out the date (month and year) when the client first noticed the clinical manifestations.

Next, the nurse questions about factors that aggravate the symptoms, such as fatigue, stress, overexertion, temperature extremes, or a hot shower or bath. The client and the family are questioned about any personality or behavioral changes that have occurred (e.g., euphoria, poor judgment, inattentiveness). In addition, they are questioned about a family history of MS.

EVIDENCE-BASED PRACTICE FOR NURSING

What is it like to have symptoms of an illness and then be told the illness is multiple sclerosis?

Koopman, W., & Schweitzer, A. (1999). The journey to multiple sclerosis: A qualitative study. *Journal of Neuroscience Nursing, 31*(1), 17-26.

The path to the final diagnosis of multiple sclerosis (MS) is often long, frightening, and stressful for the client and family. It may take years to reach a definitive diagnosis of MS, often resulting in relief for the client and family because there *is* a diagnosis. The purpose of this qualitative study was to explore the individual experiences of having symptoms of a neurologic illness for a period of time and finally being told that the illness is MS. Four major themes, using the metaphor of a labyrinth of voices, emerged from the study: Whispered Beginnings (listening for meanings and creating possible answers), Echoes of Silence (worrying, wondering, and waiting), The Spoken Word (hearing the sentence and telling others their story), Recreating Voice (claiming and refocusing).

Critique. In keeping with the methodology of the study, the meaning and the importance of the results of this study rely on individual interpretation to uncover the meanings of the participants' words. Many nurses may be reluctant to read beyond the abstract because the terms used by the researchers in describing the themes obscure the value of the information presented and may minimize its value as perceived by nurses. This would be unfortunate, because clients with MS have much to offer health care providers in understanding how they cope with a chronic illness.

Implications for Nursing. This study provides valuable insight and information for health care providers about the experience of being diagnosed with MS after months, or even years, of unexplained neurologic symptoms. The willingness of participants to share their journey with the researchers and the health care community contributes to the understanding of the experience of chronic illness.

PHYSICAL ASSESSMENT/CLINICAL MANIFESTATIONS

MS produces a wide variety of signs and symptoms. Any myelinated fibers of the brain and spinal cord may be affected. To determine a client's specific manifestations, the nurse performs a complete neurologic assessment.

MOTOR ASSESSMENT. The nurse first assesses the client's motor status. The client often reports increased fatigue and stiffness of the extremities, particularly the legs. Flexor spasms at night may awaken the client from sleep. Further examination reveals increased, or hyperactive, deep tendon reflexes; clonus; positive Babinski's reflex; and absent abdominal reflexes. Gait may be unsteady because of leg weakness and spasticity.

Significant cerebellar findings include **intention tremor** (tremor when performing an activity), **dysmetria** (inability to direct or limit movement), and dysdiadochokinesia (inability to stop one motor impulse and substitute another). Motor movements are often clumsy; the client may lose balance easily and may exhibit signs of poor coordination.

During examination of the cranial nerves and brainstem function, the client may report tinnitus, vertigo, and hearing loss. The client may show indications of facial weakness and have dysphagia. Speech problems include dysarthria, ataxia, and slow, scanning speech.

Typical clinical findings from assessment of the client's visual acuity, visual fields, and pupils include the following:

- Blurred vision
- **Diplopia** (double vision)
- Decreased visual acuity
- **Scotomas** (changes in peripheral vision)
- **Nystagmus** (involuntary, rapid eye movements)

SENSORY ASSESSMENT. Sensory findings include hypalgesia (diminished sensitivity to pain), paresthesia, facial pain, and decreased temperature perception. The client may report numbness, tingling, burning, or crawling sensations.

If demyelination of the spinal cord has occurred, the client may experience bowel and bladder dysfunctions as well as alterations in sexuality. The client may have an areflexic bladder or experience frequency, urgency, or nocturia. Bowel problems include altered rectal tone, constipation, and incontinence. Problems with sexuality include impotence, difficulty sustaining an erection, and decreased vaginal secretion.

COGNITIVE ASSESSMENT. Finally, the nurse examines the client for mental status changes. Cognitive changes are usually seen late in the course of the disease and include decreased short-term memory, decreased concentration, decreased ability to perform calculations, inattentiveness, and impaired judgment. Chart 43-14 summarizes the common clinical manifestations of MS.

PSYCHOSOCIAL ASSESSMENT

After the initial diagnosis of MS, the client is often anxious. Apathy, emotional lability, and depression are fairly common.

CHART 43-14

KEY FEATURES *of* Multiple Sclerosis

- Muscle weakness and spasticity
- Fatigue
- Intention tremors
- Dysmetria (inability to direct or limit movement)
- Numbness or tingling sensations (paresthesia)
- Hypalgesia
- Ataxia (decreased motor coordination)
- Dysarthria (slurred speech)
- Dysphagia (difficulty swallowing)
- Diplopia (double vision)
- Nystagmus (involuntary eye movements)
- Scotomas (changes in peripheral vision)
- Decreased visual and hearing acuity
- Tinnitus, vertigo (ringing in the ears, dizziness)
- Bowel and bladder dysfunction
- Alterations in sexual function, such as impotence
- Cognitive changes, such as memory loss, impaired judgment, and decreased ability to solve problems or perform calculations

The client may be euphoric or giddy, either as a result of the disease itself or because of the medications used to treat the disease. The nurse assesses the client's previously used coping and stress management skills in preparing him or her for a chronic, usually debilitating disease.

LABORATORY ASSESSMENT

No one specific procedure is definitively diagnostic for MS. However, the collective results of a variety of tests are usually conclusive. Changes may be evident during an acute attack. Abnormal cerebrospinal fluid (CSF) findings include an elevated protein level and a slight increase in the white blood cell count. CSF electrophoresis reveals an increase in the myelin basic protein and the presence of oligoclonal (IgG) bands. IgG bands are seen in most clients with MS.

OTHER DIAGNOSTIC ASSESSMENT

The health care provider usually orders a computed tomography (CT) scan, which may show an increased density in the white matter and MS plaques. Magnetic resonance imaging (MRI) demonstrates the presence of plaques and is considered diagnostic for MS. A complete diagnostic evaluation is necessary to exclude other disease.

Results of visual, auditory, and brainstem-evoked potential studies are often abnormal. Electromyogram findings may be grossly abnormal in people with advanced disease.

The diagnosis of MS is made by the exclusion of other neurologic diseases, laboratory and neuroimaging assessment, and on specific diagnostic criteria, including the presence of neurologic dysfunction that occurs over time and in more than one area of the central nervous system (CNS).

CRITICAL THINKING CHALLENGE

A young, married woman comes to the neurologic clinic with vague symptoms of weakness and spasticity. The neurologist suspects MS and schedules her for an MRI of the spine. She has three children under 3 years of age.

- What are the most important assessments that you need to make at this time?
- What client education is needed at this time?
- What nursing diagnoses are likely for this client?

For suggested answer guidelines, go to SIMON http://www.wbsaunders.com/SIMON/Iggy/.

Interventions

The client with MS is often weak and easily fatigued. The Concept Map on p. 949 illustrates the common problems and interventions for the client with MS. The nurse teaches the client the importance of planning activities and allowing sufficient time to complete activities. For example, the client should check that all items needed for work are gathered before leaving the house. Items used on a daily basis should be easily accessible.

EXERCISE PROGRAM. In collaboration with physical and occupational therapists, an exercise program is developed and includes range-of-motion (ROM) exercises and stretching and strengthening exercises. The nurse encourages the client to ambulate as tolerated and to use assistive ambulation devices as needed, including a cane, walker, wheelchair, or electric cart (Amigo). Additional assistive/adaptive devices may be needed to enable the client with tremor, spasticity, and weakness to remain independent in activities of daily living (ADLs). Chapter 10 describes additional interventions to increase physical mobility and promote ADL independence.

The nurse emphasizes the importance of avoiding rigorous activities that increase body temperature. Increased body temperature may lead to increased fatigue, diminished motor ability, and decreased visual acuity resulting from changes in the conduction abilities of the injured axons.

DRUG THERAPY. A variety of medications are used to treat and control the disease, decrease specific symptoms, and attempt to slow its progression.

STEROID THERAPY. The health care provider may use methylprednisolone (Solu-Medrol) to reduce edema and the inflammatory response in acute exacerbations. One gram is administered intravenously daily for 3 to 14 days depending on the provider and the extent of the client's symptoms. A course of oral prednisone 60 mg every day for 5 to 7 days, may be used following the methylprednisolone. Adrenocorticotropic hormone (ACTH), 25 to 60 IU IV or IM, may be given instead of methylprednisolone and tapered gradually over 2 to 4 weeks.

Common nursing interventions while the client is receiving these medications include the following:

- Carefully monitoring fluid and electrolyte levels
- Testing the client's serum glucose concentration
- Providing dietary or supplemental potassium
- Observing for indications of gastrointestinal (GI) bleeding, such as gastric pain or blood in the stool
- Documenting any changes in personality (e.g., euphoria and insomnia)
- Minimizing the client's exposure to people with communicable or infectious diseases

IMMUNOSUPPRESSIVE THERAPY. Because multiple sclerosis (MS) is now considered an autoimmune disease, im-

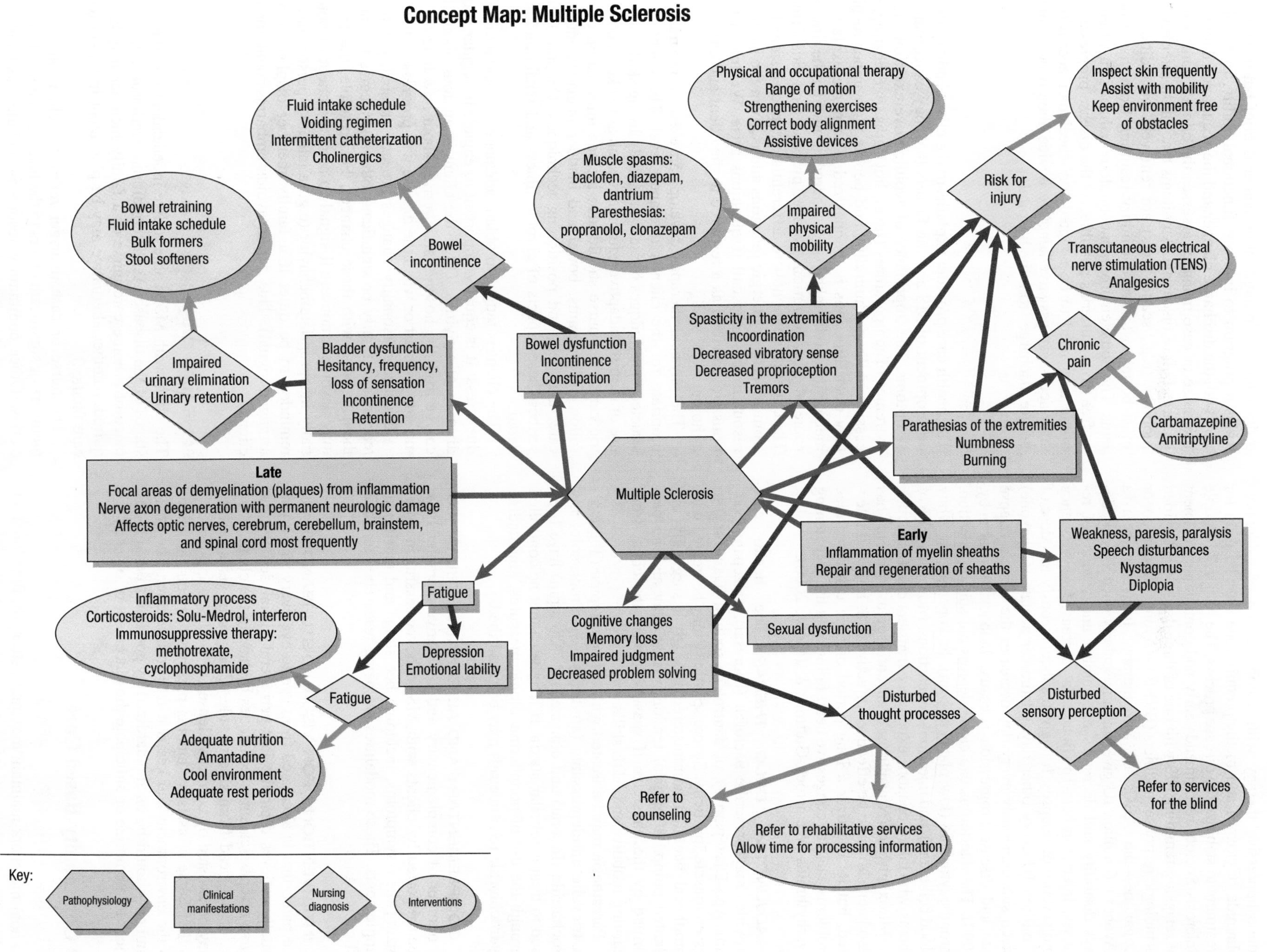
Concept Map: Multiple Sclerosis
Bowel retraining
Fluid intake schedule
Bulk formers
Stool softeners
Fluid intake schedule
Voiding regimen
Intermittent catheterization
Cholinergics
Bowel incontinence
Impaired urinary elimination
Urinary retention
Bladder dysfunction
Hesitancy, frequency, loss of sensation
Incontinence
Retention
Bowel dysfunction
Incontinence
Constipation
Muscle spasms: baclofen, diazepam, dantrium
Paresthesias: propranolol, clonazepam
Physical and occupational therapy
Range of motion
Strengthening exercises
Correct body alignment
Assistive devices
Impaired physical mobility
Spasticity in the extremities
Incoordination
Decreased vibratory sense
Decreased proprioception
Tremors
Inspect skin frequently
Assist with mobility
Keep environment free of obstacles
Risk for injury
Transcutaneous electrical nerve stimulation (TENS)
Analgesics
Chronic pain
Carbamazepine
Amitriptyline
Parathesias of the extremities
Numbness
Burning
Late
Focal areas of demyelination (plaques) from inflammation
Nerve axon degeneration with permanent neurologic damage
Affects optic nerves, cerebrum, cerebellum, brainstem, and spinal cord most frequently
Multiple Sclerosis
Early
Inflammation of myelin sheaths
Repair and regeneration of sheaths
Weakness, paresis, paralysis
Speech disturbances
Nystagmus
Diplopia
Fatigue
Depression
Emotional lability
Inflammatory process
Corticosteroids: Solu-Medrol, interferon
Immunosuppressive therapy: methotrexate, cyclophosphamide
Fatigue
Adequate nutrition
Amantadine
Cool environment
Adequate rest periods
Cognitive changes
Memory loss
Impaired judgment
Decreased problem solving
Sexual dysfunction
Disturbed thought processes
Disturbed sensory perception
Refer to counseling
Refer to rehabilitative services
Allow time for processing information
Refer to services for the blind
Key:
Pathophysiology
Clinical manifestations
Nursing diagnosis
Interventions

munosuppressive therapy with a combination of cyclophosphamide (Cytoxan) and methylprednisolone may be used for treatment to stabilize the disease process. The National Multiple Sclerosis Society recommends early and continuous treatment of relapsing-remitting MS with one of three drugs, all classified as biologic response modifiers (BRMs)—Avonex, Betaseron, or Copaxone—the ABCs of MS therapy. Interferon beta-1a (Avonex), 6 million IU given intramuscularly once a week, delays disability and decreases the number and severity of relapses. Interferon beta-1b (Betaseron) decreases the frequency and severity of relapses. It is given subcutaneously in a dose of 8 million IU every other day. Glatiramer acetate (Copaxone) given subcutaneously every day decreases the clinical relapse rate and disease progression (Lesaux, Jadbäck, & Harfagby, 1999). The interferons can cause depression, suicidal ideation, thrombocytopenia (low platelet count), leukopenia (low white blood cell count), and injection site reactions. More than 20% of clients who take Copaxone experience transient chest pain.

Mitoxantrone (Novantrone), an antineoplastic agent, has also been shown to be effective for active MS. It is well tolerated, but its use over a long period of time causes cardiac problems, such as congestive heart failure and life-threatening dysrhythmias (Weinstock-Guttman & Jacobs, 2000).

ADJUNCTIVE DRUG THERAPY. The health care provider may prescribe baclofen (Lioresal), diazepam (Valium, Apo-Diazepam✤), or dantrolene sodium (Dantrium) to lessen muscle spasticity. Severe spasticity may be treated with intrathecal baclofen administered through a surgically implanted pump. A surgical tendon release may also be performed by the physician if spasms prevent the client from learning mobility and ADL skills.

Paresthesia may be treated with carbamazepine (Tegretol) or tricyclic antidepressants (amitriptyline). Propranolol hydrochloride (Inderal) and clonazepam (Klonopin) have been used to treat cerebellar ataxia. If fatigue cannot be controlled through the use of nonpharmacologic measures, amantadine hydrochloride (Symmetrel) may be prescribed.

COMPLEMENTARY AND ALTERNATIVE THERAPIES. A number of complementary and alternative therapies have been reported by clients with MS to be successful in minimizing their symptoms, including bee stings and nutritional supplements. These modalities are being researched for their efficacy.

INTERVENTIONS FOR VISUAL DISTURBANCES. An eye patch that is alternated from eye to eye every few hours usually relieves diplopia. For peripheral visual deficits, the nurse teaches scanning techniques by having the client move his or her head from side to side. Changes in visual acuity may be assisted by corrective lenses.

The nurse or assistive nursing personnel orients the client to the environment and keeps it free from clutter. The environment should be as standardized as possible to enable the client to memorize or anticipate the placement of objects.

Community-Based Care

HOME CARE MANAGEMENT

To help the client maintain maximum strength, function, and independence, continuity of care through an interdisciplinary team in both the rehabilitation and home setting is necessary. Admission to a rehabilitation center is brief but usually provides a program to improve functional ability. In collaboration with the discharge planner and the occupational therapist, the nurse or case manager assesses the client's home for any hazards before discharge. Any items that might interfere with mobility (e.g., scatter rugs) are removed. In addition, care must be taken to prevent injury resulting from visual problems. The home environment should remain as structured and as free from clutter as possible. As the disease progresses, the home may need to be adapted for wheelchair accessibility. Any necessary assistive/adaptive device should be available before discharge from the hospital.

HEALTH TEACHING

The health care provider explains to the client and family the development of MS and the factors that may exacerbate the symptoms. The importance of avoiding overexertion, stress, extremes of temperatures (fever, hot baths, overheating, excessive chilling), humidity, and people with upper respiratory tract infections is emphasized. The nurse explains all medications to be taken on discharge, including the time and route of administration, dosage, purpose, and side effects. The client is taught how to differentiate expected side effects from adverse or allergic reactions and is given the name of a resource person to call if questions arise. Written instructions are provided as a resource to the client and caregivers at home.

The physical therapist develops an exercise program appropriate for the client's tolerance level. The client is instructed in techniques for self-care, daily living skills, and the use of required adaptive equipment, such as walkers and electric carts. The nurse should also include information on the following programs: bowel and bladder management, skin care, nutrition, and positioning techniques. Chapter 10 describes these aspects of chronic illness and rehabilitation in detail.

The client is taught to obtain adequate rest and avoid undue stress. It is equally important to engage in regular social diversional activities. Often the client is anxious about discharge from the hospital and worries about how long the remission will last or when the disease will progress further.

Because personality changes are not unusual, the nurse teaches the family or significant others strategies to enable them to cope with these changes. For example, the family may develop a nonverbal signal to alert the client to potentially inappropriate behavior (e.g., a talkative person may be reminded to be quiet if a family member displays a prearranged signal). This action avoids embarrassment for the client.

HEALTH CARE RESOURCES

The client with MS is able to live independently in the early stages of the disease. As the condition deteriorates, the assistance of a home care nurse or a family member may be required. Another alternative may be placement in a long-term care facility.

The nurse or case manager refers the client and family members or significant others to the local and national MS societies. Other community resources include meal delivery services (e.g., Meals on Wheels), transportation services for the disabled, and homemaker services.

AMYOTROPHIC LATERAL SCLEROSIS

OVERVIEW

Amyotrophic lateral sclerosis (ALS), also known as Lou Gehrig's disease, is a progressive and degenerative disease that involves the motor system. It is characterized by atrophy of the hands, forearms, and legs. ALS results in paralysis and death. There is no known cause, no cure, no specific treatment, no standard pattern of progression, and no method of prevention. Unlike with many other neural degenerative diseases, the sensory and autonomic nervous systems are not involved. Mental status changes do not result from the disease.

ALS may occur at any age. The incidence in the United States is 4.6 per 100,000. The usual age of onset is between 40 and 70 years; the incidence increases with each decade of life. ALS is more prevalent in men than in women. Death typically occurs within 2 to 5 years after the onset of symptoms and is attributable to respiratory failure (Hickey, 1997).

The cause of the disease is unknown. Researchers are exploring genetic, viral, and environmental factors as potential causes (Ross, 1999).

COLLABORATIVE MANAGEMENT

Assessment

The clinical manifestations of ALS include fatigue, muscle atrophy, and weakness. Early symptoms include the following:

- Fatigue while talking
- Tongue atrophy
- Dysphagia
- Weakness of the hands and arms
- Fasciculations of the face
- Nasal quality of speech
- Dysarthria

As the disease progresses, muscle atrophy, particularly of the trapezius and sternocleidomastoid muscles, develops. Muscle weakness and atrophy extend until a flaccid quadriplegia develops. Eventually the respiratory muscles become involved, leading to respiratory compromise, pneumonia, and death.

Diagnosis is based on clinical and diagnostic test findings and by ruling out other causes of the motor changes. There is no specific test to diagnose ALS, but creatine kinase (CK) is increased. The electromyogram demonstrates fibrillations and fasciculations of the muscles. A muscle biopsy specimen typically demonstrates small, angulated, atrophic fibers. Other diagnostic studies reveal motor strength deficits in serial muscle testing; abnormal pulmonary function test results, such as a decreased vital capacity (less than 2 L); and dysphagia.

Interventions

There is no known cure for ALS, but an interdisciplinary approach is needed for maintaining optimum functioning. Riluzole (Rilutek) was approved by the Food and Drug Administration as the only drug for use with ALS clients. It is not a cure, but it does extend survival time. The usual dose is 50 mg twice daily on an empty stomach. The client is monitored for liver toxicity from the drug by frequent measures of liver enzymes, such as alanine aminotransferase (ALT) and aspartate aminotransferase (AST).

Other nursing interventions are directed toward preventing complications of immobility and promoting comfort. In addition, the nurse provides ongoing support and counseling to the client and the family as they begin to cope with the impact of this terminal disease. The client should be informed about the need for advance directives, such as a living will. Community resources include clinics and other support services run by the ALS Association or the Muscular Dystrophy Association.

ONLINE RESOURCES

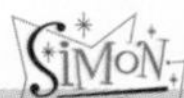

For suggested readings and Internet resources, go to http://www.wbsaunders.com/SIMON/Iggy/.

SELECTED BIBLIOGRAPHY

Asterisk indicates a classic or definitive work on this subject.

Adams, R.D., Victor, M. & Ropper, A.H. (1997). *Principles of neurology* (6th ed.). New York: McGraw-Hill.

*American Association of Neuroscience Nurses. (1996). *Core curriculum for neuroscience nursing.* Chicago: Author.

Buckley, D.A., & Guanci, M.M. (1999). Spinal cord trauma. *Nursing Clinics of North America, 34*(3), 661-687.

Cerrata, E. (1998). The role of magnetic resonance imaging studies in multiple sclerosis. *Journal of Neuroscience Nursing, 30*(5), 290-301.

Coric, D., & Branch, C.L. (1997). Posterior lumbar interbody fusion in the treatment of symptomatic spinal stenosis. *Neurosurgery Focus, 3*(2); http://www.neurosurgery.org/focus/august97/3-2-5.html.

Halper, J. (1998). The nurse case manager in multiple sclerosis. *The Journal of Care Management, 4*(1), 12-24.

*Halper, J., & Holland, N.J. (1996). *Comprehensive nursing care in multiple sclerosis.* New York: Demos Vermande.

Hesslegrave, B. (1997). Case management and spinal cord management. *The Case Manager, 8*(3), 89-94.

Hickey, J. (1997). *Clinical practice of neurological and neurosurgical nursing* (4th ed.). Philadelphia: J.B. Lippincott.

*Kahanovitz, N., & Pashos, C.L. (1996). The role of implantable direct current stimulation in the critical pathway for lumbar spinal fusion. *The Journal of Care Management, 2*(6), 46-48, 53-54, 56, 58.

*Kelley, C.L. (1996). The role of interferon in the treatment of MS. *Journal of Neuroscience Nursing, 28*(2), 114-120.

Kinney, M.R., et al. (1998). *AACN: Clinical reference for critical care nursing* (4th ed.). St. Louis: Mosby.

Koopman, W., & Schweitzer, A. (1999). The journey to multiple sclerosis: A qualitative study. *Journal of Neuroscience Nursing, 31*(1), 17-26.

Lesaux, J., Jadbäck, G., & Harfagby, C.E. (1999). Improving the convenience of home-based interferon beta-1a therapy for multiple sclerosis. *Journal of Neuroscience Nursing, 31*(2), 174-179.

Leslie, D.P. & Ahrendt, L. (1999). Managing severe spasticity with Intrathecal Baclofen (ITB) Therapy. *The Journal of Care Management,* Special edition, pp. 21-26.

Lucke, K. (1998). Pulmonary management following acute SCI. *Journal of Neuroscience Nursing, 30*(2), 91-104.

Miller, C.M. (1997). The lived experience of relapsing multiple sclerosis: A phenomenological study. *Journal of Neuroscience Nursing, 29*(5), 294-304.

Rauzzino, M.J., et al. (1999). Anterior lumbar fusion with titanium threaded and mesh interbody cages. *Neurosurgery Focus, 7*(6); http://www.neurosurgery.org/focus/dec99/7-6-7.html.

Ross, A.P. (1999). Neurologic degenerative disorders. *Nursing Clinics of North America, 34*(3), 725-742.

*Shpritz, D.W. (1996). *Rapid nursing intervention: Neurological nursing.* Albany, NY: Delmar.

Smeltzer, S.C. & Kelley, L. (2000). Multiple sclerosis. *Advance for Nurses, DC/Baltimore, 2*(15), 10-12.

Stuifbergen, A., et al. (1999). Promoting wellness for women with multiple sclerosis. *Journal of Neuroscience Nursing, 31*(2), 73-79.

Tompkins, J.A. (1997). High- and low-tech case management for the spinal cord injured patient. *The Case Manager, 8*(3), 83-88.

Weinstock-Guttman, B., & Jacobs, L.D. (2000). What is new in the treatment of multiple sclerosis? *Drugs 2000, 59*(3), 401-410.

Werner, P. (1997). New medications for brain and spinal cord injury: Minimizing the second injury. *The Journal of Care Management, 3*(1), 46-56.

White, C.L., Pokrupa, R.P. & Chan, M.H. (1998). An evaluation of the effectiveness of patient-controlled analgesia after spinal surgery. *Journal of Neuroscience Nursing, 30*(4), 225-232.

CHAPTER 44

Interventions for Clients with Problems of the Peripheral Nervous System

DEBORAH WRIGHT SHPRITZ

Learning Objectives

After studying this chapter, you should be able to:

1. Compare and contrast the pathophysiology and etiology of Guillain-Barré syndrome (GBS) and myasthenia gravis.
2. Analyze assessment data for a client with GBS to determine common nursing diagnoses.
3. Prioritize nursing care for the client with GBS.
4. Evaluate nursing care for the client with GBS based on expected outcomes.
5. Identify common clinical manifestations associated with myasthenia gravis (MG).
6. Differentiate between a myasthenic crisis and a cholinergic crisis.
7. Develop a community-based plan of care for the client with MG.
8. Develop a teaching plan for the client with peripheral neuropathy.
9. Prioritize postoperative care for the client undergoing peripheral nerve repair.
10. Compare and contrast trigeminal neuralgia and facial paralysis.
11. Discuss the role of drug therapy in managing the client with trigeminal neuralgia and facial paralysis.
12. Explain the purpose of surgery for clients with trigeminal neuralgia.

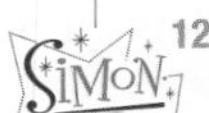

Go to http://www.wbsaunders.com/SIMON/Iggy/ for self-assessment questions related to these Learning Objectives.

Peripheral nervous system (PNS) disorders range in severity from potentially life-threatening conditions, such as Guillain-Barré syndrome, to relatively benign (but often painful) conditions, such as polyneuritis. Although hospitalization is rarely required for these less serious dysfunctions, the nurse may encounter them as secondary disorders in hospitalized clients as well as in clients in ambulatory care, long-term care, or community settings.

GUILLAIN-BARRÉ SYNDROME

OVERVIEW

Guillain-Barré syndrome (GBS) is an acute inflammatory process characterized by varying degrees of motor weakness and paralysis. It may be referred to by a variety of other names, such as *acute idiopathic polyneuritis* and *polyradiculoneuropathy.*

In GBS, the client's life and ultimate potential for rehabilitation depend on appropriate interventions and the effectiveness of nursing care. The nurse's expertise in providing care, monitoring for and preventing complications, and offering emotional support to the client and significant others is essential. With skilled care, the mortality rate can be very low. Mortality generally results from complications of respiratory compromise, such as pulmonary emboli or respiratory arrest.

Pathophysiology

In GBS, the immune system starts to destroy the myelin sheath that surrounds the axons. Segmental demyelination (the destruction of myelin between the nodes of Ranvier) is the major pathologic finding in GBS. This destruction affects saltatory conduction, or the leaping of impulses from node to node. The result is dispersion of impulses and slow conduction velocities or conduction block in the late stages of the disease. Although the heavily myelinated cranial and motor nerves are affected more often than are the thinly myelinated pain, touch, and temperature nerve fibers, sensory function is often affected. In addition, the brain may receive inappropriate sensory signals, resulting in tingling, "crawling skin," or pain.

On microscopic examination, aggregates of lymphocytes are seen at the points of myelin breakdown, yet the axons usually remain intact. In some instances there may be secondary damage to the cell body, the neurilemma, or the axon; this can delay recovery or result in permanent deficits.

Three stages make up the *acute* course of GBS:

- The *initial period* (1 to 3 weeks), which begins with the onset of the first definitive symptoms and ends when no further deterioration is noted
- The *plateau period* (several days to 2 weeks)
- The *recovery phase* (4 to 6 months), which is thought to coincide with remyelination and axonal regeneration

Chronic inflammatory demyelinating polyneuropathy (CIDP) is an unusual type of GBS that progresses over a longer period; complete recovery rarely occurs. The uncommon condition in which relapsing attacks of GBS occur is called chronic relapsing polyneuropathy.

Etiology

The cause of GBS remains obscure. Most of the evidence implicates a cell-mediated immunologic reaction. Research suggests that the humoral immune system is also involved. Defects of T-lymphocytes (T-cells) and B-lymphocytes (B-cells) of the lymphatic system may be the basis of the syndrome. T-cells are responsible for cell-mediated immunity and the phagocytosis of bacteria. B-lymphocytes produce and secrete immunoglobulin, which form the humoral part of the immune system. Normally these antibodies combine with antigens, such as viruses, and prevent the organisms from having a harmful effect. This antigen-antibody combination also induces an inflammatory reaction by attracting T-cells.

The client with GBS often relates a history of acute illness, trauma, surgery, or immunization 1 to 8 weeks before the onset of neurologic signs and symptoms. Other risk factors identified in epidemiologic studies include an upper respiratory tract infection or gastrointestinal (GI) illness (50% of cases) and positive antibodies to cytomegalovirus or Epstein-Barr virus (EBV). It is believed that the prodromal (earlier) event causes a limited malfunction of the immune system, which sensitizes the T-cells to the client's myelin. In response to several antigens, some clients apparently form a demyelinating antibody that has a direct toxic effect on nerves or attracts a cellular immune response; this ultimately destroys the myelin (Hickey, 1997).

Incidence/Prevalence

The annual incidence of GBS in the United States is approximately 0.4 to 1.7 cases per 100,000 population. It generally affects people between 30 and 50 years of age; women are more susceptible. The mortality rate in older adults is 5% higher than in the general population. GBS is seen more often in clients with Hodgkin's disease, systemic lupus erythematosus, and human immunodeficiency virus (HIV) infection. In 3% to 10% of cases, a chronic or recurrent GBS develops (Hickey, 1997).

CULTURAL CONSIDERATIONS

GBS has worldwide distribution, is not seasonal, and affects people of all races and ages. Higher rates have been noted in people 45 years of age or older. The incidence of the disease is 50% to 60% higher in Caucasians than in African Americans (Adams, Victor, & Ropper, 1997).

COLLABORATIVE MANAGEMENT

Assessment

HISTORY

In addition to biographic data (e.g., age, sex, cultural background), the nurse collects a complete medical and surgical history. Any antecedent illness (infection or other illness) 1 to 8 weeks before the onset of Guillain-Barré syndrome (GBS) is explored. The nurse asks the client to describe the symptoms in chronologic order, if possible.

PHYSICAL ASSESSMENT/CLINICAL MANIFESTATIONS

Manifestations of GBS depend on the degree of weakness and the progression of symptoms.

COMMON CLINICAL MANIFESTATIONS. Although features may vary (Chart 44-1), most people with GBS relate an abrupt onset. Typically, GBS does not affect level of consciousness, cerebral function, or pupillary signs.

CLINICAL VARIATIONS. The clinical variations of GBS reflect the areas of earliest or most severe involvement. *Ascending* GBS is the most common clinical pattern. Weakness and paresthesia begin in the lower extremities and progress upward to include the trunk and arms or affect the cranial nerves. The client may exhibit symptoms of an ascending flaccidity or weakness that evolves over hours to several days (1 to 10 days). The extent of the motor deficit ranges from mild paresis to total quadriplegia. About half of the clients with GBS experience some degree of respiratory compromise. Although they may be diminished during the initial assessment, deep tendon reflexes are absent in limbs that become paralyzed. *Pure motor* GBS is identical to the ascending variant, except sensory signs and symptoms are absent.

In clients with *descending* GBS, the nurse initially observes weakness of the face or bulbar muscles of the jaw, the

CHART 44-1

KEY FEATURES *of* Guillain-Barré Syndrome

Motor Manifestations
- Ascending symmetric muscle weakness → flaccid paralysis without muscle atrophy
- Decreased or absent deep tendon reflexes (DTRs)
- Respiratory compromise (dyspnea, diminished breath sounds, decreased tidal volume and vital capacity) and respiratory failure
- Loss of bowel and bladder control (less common)

Sensory Manifestations
- Paresthesias
- Pain (cramping)

Cranial Nerve Manifestations
- Facial weakness
- Dysphagia
- Diplopia
- Difficulty speaking

Autonomic Manifestations
- Labile blood pressure
- Cardiac dysrhythmias
- Tachycardia

sternocleidomastoid muscles (head rotators), and the muscles of the tongue, pharynx, and larynx. Weakness progresses downward to involve the limbs. This type of GBS may quickly affect the respiratory function. The nurse carefully monitors the client for breathlessness during speech, shallow respirations, dyspnea, and decreased tidal volume.

Descending GBS often includes ophthalmoplegia (paralysis or weakness of the eye muscles), causing diplopia. If the pupillary response to light is affected, functional blindness may result. Thus the nurse assesses visual function while providing information, explanation, and support to the client experiencing visual disturbances. In this variation, numbness is more common in the hands than in the feet. Deep tendon reflexes are decreased or absent.

The *Miller Fisher variant* consists of a triad of ophthalmoplegia (paralysis of ocular [eye] muscles), areflexia (absence of reflexes), and severe ataxia (defective muscle coordination). Motor strength and sensory function are normal. The pupillary response to light is occasionally affected by the ophthalmoplegia, which results in functional blindness. Although respiratory complications are rare in clients with this variant, respiratory function is monitored frequently.

With any of the variants, *cranial nerve* involvement most often affects the facial nerve (cranial nerve VII). Involvement of the facial nerve results in the inability to smile, frown, whistle, or drink from a straw. In addition to monitoring the functions of cranial nerve VII, the nurse assesses the client for dysphagia and paralysis of the larynx. Less frequently affected cranial nerves include the glossopharyngeal (IX), vagus (X), accessory (XI), and hypoglossal (XII) nerves. The client's inability to cough, gag, or swallow results from the involvement of cranial nerves IX and X. The nurse monitors closely for varying blood pressure (hypertensive and hypotensive episodes or postural hypotension) and tachycardia. These symptoms are characteristic of *autonomic dysfunction,* which is linked to vagus nerve (X) deficit. The nurse may assess cranial nerve XI (accessory) by asking the client to perform shoulder shrugs. Hypoglossal nerve (XII) deficit is evidenced by deviation or paralysis of the tongue.

PSYCHOSOCIAL ASSESSMENT

In addition to determining the usual roles and responsibilities, occupation, motivation, and available support systems, the nurse assesses the client's ability to cope with this devastating illness and the accompanying fear and anxiety. In general, GBS is self-limiting and the paralysis temporary.

LABORATORY ASSESSMENT

Although no single clinical or laboratory finding confirms the diagnosis of Guillain-Barré syndrome (GBS), the health care provider may perform a lumbar puncture (LP) to evaluate cerebrospinal fluid (CSF). An increase in CSF protein level without an increase (or only a slight to moderate increase) in cell count is a distinguishing feature of GBS. However, high protein levels may not be noted until after 1 to 2 weeks of illness, reaching a peak in 4 to 6 weeks. The CSF lymphocyte count is normal.

Peripheral blood tests may show a moderate leukocytosis early in the illness. The number of leukocytes rapidly returns to normal in the absence of complications or concurrent illness.

OTHER DIAGNOSTIC ASSESSMENT

Electrophysiologic studies demonstrate demyelinating neuropathy. The degree of abnormality found on testing does not always correlate with clinical severity. Within 3 weeks of symptoms, nerve conduction velocities are depressed. In some cases, denervated potentials (fibrillations) develop later in the illness. Electromyographic (EMG) findings, which reflect peripheral nerve function, are normal early in the illness. Electrophysiologic changes appear only after denervation of muscle has been present for 4 weeks or longer.

Respiratory function is often compromised in clients with GBS. Vital capacity may be decreased, and arterial blood gas (ABG) values may be abnormal (decreased partial pressure of arterial oxygen [$Pa{O_2}$], increased partial pressure of arterial carbon dioxide [$Pa{CO_2}$], or increased pH).

Analysis

COMMON NURSING DIAGNOSES AND COLLABORATIVE PROBLEMS

The following are common nursing diagnoses for clients with GBS:

1. Ineffective Breathing Pattern, Ineffective Airway Clearance, and Impaired Gas Exchange related to respiratory muscle weakness or paralysis, inability to cough and deep breathe effectively, and immobility
2. Impaired Physical Mobility related to weakness, paralysis, and ataxia
3. Acute Pain related to paresthesia
4. Impaired Verbal Communication related to intubation or paralysis of the muscles required for speech
5. Powerlessness related to the inability to perform activities of daily living (ADLs) and usual role responsibilities
6. Anxiety related to powerlessness, uncertain prognosis, and fear of the unknown
7. Anticipatory Grieving related to loss of function and an inability to perform usual roles and responsibilities
8. Self-Care Deficit (level depends on extent and stage of disease) related to weakness or paralysis

ADDITIONAL NURSING DIAGNOSES AND COLLABORATIVE PROBLEMS

In addition to the common nursing diagnoses, clients with GBS may have one or more of the following:

- Impaired Home Maintenance related to lack of knowledge or inadequate support systems
- Disturbed Sensory Perception (Tactile, Kinesthetic, and Visual) related to paresthesia and diplopia
- Risk for Impaired Skin Integrity related to altered sensation, altered nutrition, or immobility
- Disturbed Body Image and Situational Low Self-Esteem related to loss of body function, physical changes, and dependency
- Imbalanced Nutrition: Less than Body Requirements related to difficulty chewing, dysphagia, paralysis of the extremities, anxiety, or depression
- Risk for Deficient Fluid Volume related to cranial nerve paralysis, dysphagia, and paralysis of the extremities
- Constipation, Diarrhea, or Bowel Incontinence related to inadequate oral intake, immobility, and impaired communication

- Decreased Cardiac Output related to autonomic dysfunction
- Deficient Knowledge related to understanding the disease process and expectations

A possible collaborative problem is Potential for Respiratory Paralysis, which results in death if the disorder is not managed.

Planning and Implementation

INEFFECTIVE BREATHING PATTERN; INEFFECTIVE AIRWAY CLEARANCE; IMPAIRED GAS EXCHANGE

NOC **PLANNING: EXPECTED OUTCOMES.** The client is with Guillain-Barré syndrome (GBS) expected to have an effective air exchange as indicated by a vital capacity in expected range (IER) and arterial blood gas levels within normal limits (WNL).

INTERVENTIONS. In the acute (initial) phase, the nurse monitors the client closely (usually in a critical care unit) for signs of respiratory distress, such as dyspnea, air hunger, confusion (resulting from hypoxia), and cyanosis. In addition, the nurse monitors respiratory rate, rhythm, and depth every 1 to 4 hours; checks the client's vital capacity every 2 to 4 hours; and auscultates the lungs at 4-hour intervals.

NIC **AIRWAY MANAGEMENT.** The purpose of airway management is to promote airway patency and gas exchange (Chart 44-2). Arterial blood gas values are monitored for acid-base abnormalities and decreasing oxygen saturation. Deterioration of vital capacity to less than 15 to 20 mL/kg and the inability to clear secretions may be indications for elective intubation. Equipment for performing an endotracheal intubation is kept at the bedside, and a ventilator is readily available in case of respiratory emergency.

The nurse maintains (or assists the client to maintain) a patent airway by correctly positioning the client, suctioning, and adjusting the endotracheal or nasotracheal airways. To prevent infection, sterile technique is maintained in suctioning the client. The color, consistency, and amount of secretions are monitored. Chest physiotherapy (performed by the respiratory therapist or nurse) and frequent position changes are combined with breathing exercises (coughing and deep breathing) to prevent pneumonia and atelectasis. Oxygen may be administered by nasal cannula at a flow rate prescribed by the health care provider.

DRUG THERAPY. The treatment of GBS depends on ventilatory assistance and supportive nursing care. In most cases, the disease is self-limiting and recovery is complete. Treatment with immunoglobulins has been shown to be as effective as plasmapheresis, and it is safer and immediately available. Side effects of immunoglobulin therapy include minor annoyances (e.g., mild fever, myalgia, and headache) to major complications (e.g., aseptic meningitis, retinal necrosis, and acute renal failure).

PLASMAPHERESIS. **Plasmapheresis** removes the circulating antibodies thought to be responsible for the disease. In this procedure, plasma is selectively separated from whole blood. The blood cells are returned to the client without the plasma. Plasma usually replaces itself, or the client is transfused with normal plasma or a colloidal substitute. This procedure must be started 7 to 14 days after the onset of the illness. The client usually receives 3 to 4 treatments, 1 to 2 days apart. Some clients may require a second round of treatment if they deteriorate after the first plasmapheresis.

Nursing responsibilities for the client undergoing plasmapheresis include providing information and reassurance to the client, weighing the client before and after the procedure, and administering proper care to the shunt. Proper shunt care includes maintaining shunt patency, checking for bruits every 2 to 4 hours, keeping double bulldog clamps at the bedside, and observing the puncture site for bleeding or ecchymosis (bruising). The nurse also monitors the client's vital signs and observes for signs of complications throughout the procedure (Chart 44-3).

CHART 44-2

NIC INTERVENTION ACTIVITIES *for* The Client with Guillain-Barré Syndrome

Respiratory Monitoring: *Collection and analysis of client data to ensure airway patency and adequate gas exchange.*
- Monitor rate, rhythm, depth, and effort of respirations.
- Monitor breathing patterns: bradypnea, tachypnea, hyperventilation, Kussmaul respirations, Cheyne-Stokes respirations, apneustic, Biot, and ataxic patterns.
- Auscultate breath sounds, noting areas of decreased/absent ventilation and presence of adventitious sounds.
- Monitor PFT values, particularly vital capacity, maximal inspiratory force, forced expiratory volume in 1 second (FEV_1), and FEV_1/FVC, as available.
- Monitor mechanical ventilator readings, noting increases in inspiratory pressures and decreases in tidal volume, as appropriate.
- Monitor for increased restlessness, anxiety, and air hunger.
- Note changes in Sao_2, Svo_2, end tidal CO_2, and changes in ABG values, as appropriate.
- Monitor client's ability to cough effectively.
- Monitor for dyspnea and events that improve and worsen it.
- Monitor chest x-ray reports.
- Place the client on side, as indicated, to prevent aspiration; logroll if cervical aspiration suspected.
- Institute respiratory therapy treatments (e.g., nebulizer), as needed.

Airway Management: *Facilitation of patency of air passages*
- Position the client to maximize ventilation potential.
- Identify client requiring actual/potential airway insertion.
- Perform chest physical therapy, as appropriate.
- Remove secretions by encouraging coughing or suctioning.
- Instruct how to cough effectively.
- Auscultate breath sounds, noting areas of decreased or absent ventilation and presence of adventitious sounds.
- Perform endotracheal or nasotracheal suctioning, as appropriate.
- Administer humidified air or oxygen, as appropriate.
- Administer aerosol treatments, as appropriate.
- Administer ultrasonic nebulizer treatments, as appropriate.
- Position to alleviate dyspnea.
- Monitor respiratory and oxygenation status, as appropriate.

NIC intervention activities selected from McCloskey, J.C., & Bulechek, G.M. (Eds.). (2000). *Nursing interventions classification (NIC)* (3rd ed.). St. Louis: Mosby. No part of this work is to be altered without prior written permission from the Publisher.

PFT, Pulmonary function test; *FEV_1,* forced expiratory volume in 1 second; *FVC,* forced vital capacity; *Svo_2,* venous oxygen saturation; *Sao_2,* arterial oxygen saturation; *CO_2,* carbon dioxide; *ABG,* arterial blood gas.

CHART 44-3

BEST PRACTICE *for* Managing Complications of Plasmapheresis

COMPLICATION	NURSING INTERVENTIONS
Trauma or infection at vascular access site	Keep the site clean and dry. Monitor the site for redness, swelling, drainage, or other signs of infection.
Hypovolemia with resultant hypotension, tachycardia, dizziness, and diaphoresis	Monitor fluid and electrolyte status and vital signs. Administer fluids as prescribed. Provide an explanation of side effects, and reassure the client.
Hypokalemia and hypocalcemia	Monitor fluid and electrolyte balance. Administer replacement electrolytes, as ordered. Observe for cardiac dysrhythmias.
Temporary circumoral and distal extremity paresthesias, muscle twitching, nausea, and vomiting related to administration of citrated plasma	Add calcium gluconate or calcium chloride to exchange fluids, as prescribed. Provide explanations, comfort measures, and reassurance.

IMPAIRED PHYSICAL MOBILITY

NOC **PLANNING: EXPECTED OUTCOMES.** The client with GBS is expected to (1) perform ambulation, transfers, and bed mobility skills; and (2) not experience physiologic immobility consequences, such as pressure ulcers, constipation, and pulmonary emboli.

INTERVENTIONS. Symptoms may develop rapidly during the initial period. Therefore the nurse assesses motor (muscle) function every 2 to 4 hours. A reproducible method that is readily understood by all members of the health care team is used for this assessment, such as Lovett's scale for determining muscle strength (see Table 50-1). Nursing interventions to provide for mobility and prevent complications depend on the degree of motor deficit. To ensure the client's safety, the nurse assists with ambulation, transfers from bed to chair, position changes, and maintenance of proper body alignment. Maximal independence is always encouraged. Range-of-motion (ROM) exercises are performed actively or passively every 2 to 4 hours. The nurse instructs family members in these techniques. (See Chapter 10 for measures to improve physical mobility and prevent immobility consequences).

Because pulmonary emboli are common complications of immobility, the health care provider may prescribe subcutaneous heparin injections every 12 hours. Antiembolism stockings and sequential compression stockings may be used to promote venous return. The nurse or assistant nursing personnel removes the stockings at least once every 24 hours for 15 to 30 minutes and observes the client's skin condition and circulation. Other prevention measures are determined by agency policy or health care provider preference.

CRITICAL THINKING CHALLENGE

A client is admitted to the critical care unit with a possible diagnosis of ascending GBS. On assessment you note that the client has weakness in both legs, causing her to be very apprehensive.

- What is the priority potential problem for the client during the hospital stay?
- What assessments will you perform to determine if the problem occurs?
- What is this client's prognosis?
- What psychosocial support will you provide?

For suggested answer guidelines, go to SIMON http://www.wbsaunders.com/SIMON/Iggy/.

ACUTE PAIN

NOC **PLANNING: EXPECTED OUTCOMES.** The client with Guillain-Barré syndrome (GBS) is expected to experience adequate pain relief as indicated by client report.

INTERVENTIONS. The nurse assesses the severity and nature of the client's pain, which is often worse at night. The typical pain experienced is often not relieved by medication other than opiates, which can be administered via a patient-controlled analgesia (PCA) pump or continuous intravenous (IV) drip. The nurse documents the client's response to the pain medication and notifies the health care provider if pain relief is not sufficient. Other pain relief measures include frequent repositioning, relaxation techniques, guided imagery, and distractions (e.g., music or visitors). Chapter 7 discusses these pain relief measures in detail.

IMPAIRED VERBAL COMMUNICATION

NOC **PLANNING: EXPECTED OUTCOMES.** The client with Guillain-Barré syndrome (GBS) is expected to receive, interpret, and express written and nonverbal messages to and from the staff, family, and/or significant others.

INTERVENTIONS. The client may have difficulty communicating because the muscles required for the production of speech are weak, or the client may be on a mechanical ventilator because the respiratory muscles are paralyzed. In either case, the nurse collaborates with the speech and language pathologist in developing a communication system. A simple technique involves eye blinking or moving a finger to indicate "yes" and "no." A communication board can be developed with the letters of the alphabet or a list of common requests, such as the need to be repositioned or the need for pain medication. Both the staff and the visitors must know how the client's communication system operates.

POWERLESSNESS

NOC **PLANNING: EXPECTED OUTCOMES.** The client with GBS is expected to (1) increase the ability to identify factors that are under independent control; (2) make decisions regarding care, treatment options, and the future when possible; and (3) participate in care within the limitations of the illness.

INTERVENTIONS. The nurse assesses feelings of powerlessness by encouraging the client to verbalize feelings about the illness and its effects. Previous decision-making patterns, roles, and responsibilities are examined. By asking the client and the family to describe their usual lifestyles and the situations in which they coped both effectively and ineffectively, the nurse may identify factors that influence coping ability.

The nurse provides information about the pathophysiology and natural progression of the syndrome and describes tests, procedures, and routines to increase the client's knowledge and sense of control. The client is encouraged to make choices and to participate in care as much as possible, and he or she is given positive feedback for doing so.

The client's own cosmetics, personal hygiene items, and clothing are used whenever feasible to provide a sense of control and of the familiar. The nurse ensures environmental control by keeping the call light, television control, telephone, and other necessary items within the client's reach. Alternative communication methods (e.g., pad and pencil or computer) may be needed if the client cannot verbally express his or her needs.

ANXIETY; ANTICIPATORY GRIEVING

NOC **PLANNING: EXPECTED OUTCOMES.** The client with GBS is expected to (1) use actions to manage stressors and adapt to the changes in roles and responsibilities associated with the disease process, and (2) communicate feelings related to anxiety, fear, and grief.

INTERVENTIONS. The nurse assesses the client and family or significant others for verbal and nonverbal behaviors that indicate anxiety, fear, and grieving. Sadness, depression, anger, guilt, crying (or the inability to cry), denial, and withdrawal may be noted. The nurse helps establish a trusting, therapeutic nurse/client relationship. The client and the family or significant other are encouraged to discuss their fears and concerns. The client's usual coping strategies and remaining strengths are identified and capitalized on. The family is encouraged to spend time with the client and to assist with care by providing range-of-motion (ROM) exercises, massages, and other comfort measures. The nurse provides as much information as needed and, if indicated, initiates referrals to the social services department, hospital chaplain or appropriate spiritual resource, and local support groups.

SELF-CARE DEFICIT

PLANNING: EXPECTED OUTCOMES. The client with GBS is expected to adapt to his or her deficits and plan for an optimal ability to perform daily living skills, such as ambulation, eating, dressing, and hygiene.

INTERVENTIONS. The nurse assesses the client's ability to perform activities of daily living (ADLs). While monitoring the client's emotional and mental status, the nurse determines his or her level of acceptance of the disability. Assistance is offered as necessary, but the client is encouraged to perform ADLs independently, if possible. The nurse or assistive nursing personnel monitors responses to or tolerance of activity and provide adequate rest periods between activities and therapy sessions. Activities are coordinated with the interventions of other health care team members (occupational, speech, and physical therapists). Assistive devices and instructions for their use are provided for the client. The nurse freely gives positive feedback for any gains noted in self-care activities. The family or significant other is encouraged to become involved in all aspects of the rehabilitation process.

Community-Based Care

The severity and course of Guillain-Barré syndrome (GBS) are extremely variable, which makes it difficult to predict the prognosis. By the time the client is discharged from the hospital, major problems (e.g., respiratory paralysis) are resolved. The most likely residual effects at discharge are related to motor status and mobility, self-care, and perhaps sensory alteration and disturbed self-concept. For clients who experience total quadriparesis or respiratory paralysis, the course of the rehabilitation phase is even more variable and may require weeks to years.

Planning for discharge begins on admission. The client may be discharged to home or to a rehabilitation unit. The nurse, discharge planner, or case manager makes appropriate referrals to a home care agency and community agencies for assistance in the home setting after discharge. Clients who require more intensive physical and occupational therapy may be discharged to a skilled nursing facility or rehabilitation setting before returning home.

HEALTH TEACHING

The nurse or case manager provides oral and written information and reinforces the teaching provided by the interdisciplinary health care team. A family member or significant other is included in the education process throughout the client's hospitalization.

The client and family are given both oral and written instructions in techniques to facilitate mobility and prevent skin breakdown. If mobility remains markedly impaired, the nurse and physical therapist emphasize the need for ROM exercises, positioning and frequent turning techniques, and prevention of skin breakdown.

The nurse and rehabilitation team ensure that the client and family understand how to use assistive devices safely and properly; written instructions and diagrams are provided as necessary. If paresthesia persists, the nurse instructs the client and family to visually examine the affected limbs several times daily. After discharge, the client must be monitored by the physician for recurring disease.

The psychosocial adjustment needed may be minimal or dramatic depending on the client's residual deficit, age, sex, usual roles and responsibilities, usual coping strategies, available support systems, and occupation. It is likely that self-concept will improve as the client begins to function in familiar surroundings. Residual deficits rarely require permanent changes in lifestyles or roles. To provide the necessary support, the nurse encourages the client and family to discuss their feelings with one another. The nurse helps the client identify other support systems, such as church members, social club members, or spiritual resources.

HOME CARE MANAGEMENT

If the client is discharged to home while still dependent on assistive devices, the interdisciplinary health care team makes certain that the necessary equipment has been delivered after evaluation of the home setting. These activities may be coordinated by the case manager. The occupational therapist checks to see that grab bars for bathtub and toilet transfers, if needed, are properly installed. Any modifications to the home need to be completed before the client's arrival. Throw rugs are removed if they pose a hazard. Ramps are installed, doorways are widened, and commodes are provided if the client remains wheelchair dependent.

HEALTH CARE RESOURCES

Self-help groups for clients with chronic illness are common. The nurse consults with the client and the health care provider and seeks referrals to these groups if indicated. The Guillain-Barré Foundation provides information about local resources and information for clients and their families.

Evaluation: Outcomes

NOC The nurse evaluates the care of the client with GBS on the basis of the identified nursing diagnoses and collaborative problems. The expected outcomes include that the client will:

- Have an effective respiratory rate, cough effectively, and have adequate gas exchange in the lungs
- Participate in mobilization to the greatest extent possible to prevent complications of immobility
- Verbalize relief from pain and be able to use relaxation and imaging techniques to reduce pain
- Perform ADLs as independently as possible
- Verbalize feelings relative to emotional status and coping abilities, using family members, the nurse, and other sources for support (with the family or significant others)
- Develop appropriate coping strategies on the basis of personal strengths and previous experiences (with the family or significant others)

MYASTHENIA GRAVIS

OVERVIEW

Myasthenia gravis (MG) means "grave muscle weakness" or weakness of the voluntary or striated muscles. It is an autoimmune disease of the neuromuscular junctions and may take many forms—from mild disturbances of the ocular muscles to a rapidly developing, generalized weakness that may lead to death from respiratory failure. It is characterized by remissions and exacerbations (worsening). MG is a chronic, neuromuscular, autoimmune disease that involves a decrease in the number and effectiveness of acetylcholine (ACh) receptors at the neuromuscular junction.

Pathophysiology

The major pathologic defect in MG is that nerve impulses are not transmitted to the skeletal muscle at the neuromuscular junction. Clients with MG develop specific antibodies to one or more ACh receptor sites, possibly because of autoimmune injury. These antibodies accelerate the degeneration of ACh receptors.

There is no evidence of central or peripheral nervous system disease in MG. The muscle appears normal macroscopically, and there is usually no evidence of atrophy. On microscopic examination, lymphocytic infiltrates may be seen within muscles and other organs, but such findings have been inconsistent.

The thymus gland is often abnormal. Thymoma (encapsulated thymus gland tumor) occurs in approximately 15% of cases, and 70% of the remaining cases show hyperplasia of the thymus. There is also a very strong association between MG and hyperthyroidism. Genetic factors may play a role in the development of MG (Ross, 1999).

Etiology

Although the precipitating event remains unclear, research strongly suggests that MG is caused by antibodies to the ACh receptors. Evidence also suggests a relationship between MG and hyperplasia of the thymus gland.

Incidence/Prevalence

The incidence of MG in the United States is estimated to be 0.5 per 100,000 population. It is not hereditary, but there is a 5% familial incidence. Although it may begin at any age, the onset of MG before 10 years of age or after 60 years of age is rare. The peak age at onset is between 20 and 30 years of age. Before 40 years of age, women are affected three times more often than are men (Ross, 1999).

> **CONSIDERATIONS FOR OLDER ADULTS**
> In later life, the incidence of MG is about equal in men and women. Men predominate among myasthenic clients with thymoma, and these men tend to be 50 to 60 years of age.

COLLABORATIVE MANAGEMENT

Assessment

In addition to the biographic data and nursing history, the nurse assesses the client with MG for the rapid onset of fatigue. Subjective complaints of muscle weakness that increases on exertion or as the day wears on and improves with rest are noted. The nurse asks the client to describe his or her symptoms, specifically noting the affected muscle groups and any limitation or inability in performing activities of daily living (ADLs).

Additional areas of inquiry include any history of **ptosis** (drooping eyelids) or **diplopia** (double vision), difficulty chewing or swallowing, and the type of diet best tolerated. Signs and symptoms of respiratory difficulty, choking, or weakness of the voice are also elicited. The client is asked about any difficulty holding up the head, brushing the teeth, combing the hair, or shaving. The nurse inquires about the presence of paresthesia or aching in weakened muscles. Finally, any history of thymus gland tumor is elicited.

Although the onset of MG is usually insidious, some instances of fairly rapid development have been preceded by infection, emotional upset, pregnancy, or anesthesia. Thus the nurse inquires about any history of these events. A temporary increase in weakness may be noted after vaccination, menstruation, and exposure to extremes in environmental temperature.

PHYSICAL ASSESSMENT/CLINICAL MANIFESTATIONS

If the client can cooperate fully, MG may be diagnosed after the demonstration of *progressive* paresis of affected muscle groups that is resolved, at least in part, by rest (Chart 44-4). The most common symptoms (exhibited by more than 90% of clients) are related to involvement of the levator palpebrae or extraocular muscles. The nurse assesses the client for ocular palsies, ptosis, diplopia, and weak or incomplete eye closure. These symptoms may last only a few days at the onset and then resolve—only to return weeks or months later. Normal pupillary responses to light and accommodation are present.

For most clients, the muscles of facial expression, chewing, and speech are affected. The nurse notes the client's smile, which may be transformed into a snarl; the jaw may hang so that the client must prop it up with the hand. Chewing and swallowing difficulties, choking, and regurgitation of fluids through the nose may lead to considerable weight loss. The nurse inquires about the client's nutritional status and any recent weight loss. It may be more difficult for the client to eat after talking. After extended conversations, the voice may become weaker or exhibit a nasal twang. In some clients, the tongue has one central and two lateral longitudinal fissures.

Less often involved are the muscles of the shoulders, the flexors of the neck, and the hip flexors. Because limb weakness is more often *proximal,* the client may have difficulty climbing stairs, lifting heavy objects, or raising the arms overhead. Neck weakness may be mild or severe enough to cause difficulty in holding the head erect. Among the trunk muscles, the erector spinae are most commonly affected. This results in difficulty sustaining a sitting or walking posture.

In the most advanced cases of MG, all muscles are weakened, including those associated with respiratory function and the control of bladder and bowel function. In severe cases, the nurse inquires about bowel and bladder function. Respiratory function is assessed regularly.

CHART 44-4

KEY FEATURES *of* Myasthenia Gravis

Motor Manifestations
- Progressive muscle weakness (proximal) that usually improves with rest
- Poor posture
- Ocular palsies
- Ptosis
- Weak or incomplete eye closure
- Diplopia
- Respiratory compromise
- Loss of bowel and bladder control
- Fatigue

Sensory Manifestations
- Muscle achiness
- Paresthesias
- Decreased smell and taste

Muscle atrophy, although rarely marked in degree, occurs in a small percentage of clients with myasthenia gravis (MG). The client's tendon reflexes should be assessed, but they are not often affected. The nurse assesses for pain, which is seldom a major complaint. However, many clients report some aching of the weakened muscles. Paresthesia affecting the muscles of the face, hands, and thighs is not associated with any loss of sensation. Lost or decreased sensations of smell and taste have been reported. There is no alteration of consciousness.

In *Eaton-Lambert syndrome,* a special form of myasthenia often observed in combination with small cell carcinoma of the lung, the muscles of the trunk and the pelvic and shoulder girdles are most commonly affected. Although weakness increases after exertion, there may be a temporary increase in muscle strength during the first few contractions, followed by rapid decrements. Diagnosis is confirmed by electromyography. Treatment includes removing the tumor, managing the cancer, and administering medications to release acetylcholine (ACh). Additional therapies may include plasmapheresis and immunosuppressive therapy.

LABORATORY ASSESSMENT

In virtually all cases of MG, the diagnosis is obvious from the history and physical examination findings. MG may be immediately confirmed by the client's response to cholinergic drugs. A standard series of laboratory studies is usually performed for clients with known or suspected MG. Thyroid function should be tested. Serum protein electrophoresis evaluates the client for immunologic disorders. Thyrotoxicosis (excessive thyroid hormone) is present in approximately 5% of myasthenic clients. Rheumatoid arthritis, systemic lupus erythematosus, and polymyositis are also associated with the disease.

Testing for acetylcholine receptor antibodies (AchR) has become an important diagnostic criterion, because 80% to 90% of clients with MG have elevated AchR. A positive antibody test result confirms the diagnosis, but a negative finding does not exclude the disease (Ross, 1999).

RADIOGRAPHIC ASSESSMENT

Some clients with MG have a thymoma, and therefore clients are assessed for this condition. The thymus, an H-shaped gland located in the upper mediastinum beneath the sternum, is one organ in which ACh receptor antibodies are formed. Although a thymoma can often be seen on routine frontal and lateral chest x-ray films, special studies should be performed for any area suggestive of thymoma in the anterior mediastinum. The nurse prepares the client for these tests or for a computed tomography (CT) scan by explaining the equipment and what to expect during the tests.

OTHER DIAGNOSTIC ASSESSMENT

TENSILON TESTING. Pharmacologic tests with the cholinesterase inhibitors edrophonium chloride (Tensilon) and neostigmine bromide (Prostigmin) have been in use since the 1950s. Tensilon is used more often because of its rapid onset and brief duration of action. This drug inhibits the breakdown of ACh at the postsynaptic membrane, which increases the availability of ACh for excitation of postsynaptic receptors. To perform the test, the physician first estimates the strength of certain cranial muscles. Initially, 2 mg (0.2 mL) is injected intravenously; if this is tolerated, an additional 8 mg (0.8 mL) is injected after 30 seconds. Within 30 to 60 seconds of the first dose, most myasthenic clients show a marked improvement in muscle tone that lasts 4 to 5 minutes. False-positive test results may be caused by increased muscle effort by the client. False-negative findings may be seen if the tested muscle is extremely weak or refractory to the drug.

This test may also be used to help determine whether increasing weakness in the previously diagnosed myasthenic client is due to a *cholinergic crisis* (overmedication with anticholinesterase drugs) or a *myasthenic crisis* (undermedication with cholinesterase inhibitors). In a cholinergic crisis, muscle tone does not improve after the administration of Tensilon. Instead, weakness may actually increase, and fasciculations (muscle twitching) may be noted around the eyes and face. The Tensilon test poses a danger of ventricular fibrillation and cardiac arrest, but these reactions rarely occur. Atropine sulfate is the antidote for Tensilon and must be available in case these complications occur.

ELECTROMYOGRAPHY. A common diagnostic test performed by the physician or technician is electromyography (EMG). Although electrical testing of the normal neuromuscular junction produces no change in the amplitude of muscle contraction, the amplitude of the muscle's response diminishes with progressive stimulation. A decrease in amplitude of more than 10% between the first and fifth responses generally indicates the defective neuromuscular transmission characteristic of, but not unique to, MG. Several muscles may be tested to increase the likelihood of detecting an abnormality. Testing may be performed after exercise or exposure of the muscle to curare or to ischemia.

Single-fiber EMG is even more sensitive in detecting defects of neuromuscular transmission. This test compares the stability of the firing of one muscle fiber with that of another fiber innervated by the same motor neuron. The time interval between the two firings normally shows a minor degree of variability, called jitter. Defective transmission increases jitter or actually blocks successive discharges.

Interventions

The hallmark of MG is muscle weakness that increases when the client is fatigued and limits the client's mobility and ability to participate in activities. Treatment efforts for this disease fall into two categories:

- Treatment that affects the symptoms of MG without influencing the actual course of the disease (anticholinesterases or cholinergic drugs)
- Therapeutic efforts for inducing remission, such as the administration of immunosuppressive drugs or corticosteroids, plasmapheresis, and thymectomy (removal of the thymus gland)

NONSURGICAL MANAGEMENT. The nurse assesses the client's motor strength before and after periods of activity. Assistance is provided as necessary to prevent the client from becoming fatigued. The nurse teaches the client to participate in activities early in the day or during the energy peaks that follow the administration of medications. The client is assisted in planning the periods of rest necessary for avoiding excess fatigue.

PROVIDING ASSISTANCE WITH ACTIVITIES. During periods of maximal weakness, the nurse or assistive nursing personnel may need to provide assistance with ambulation, transfers from bed to chair or toilet/commode, position changes, and maintenance of body alignment. Active or passive range-of-motion (ROM) exercises are performed every 2 to 4 hours. The nurse assesses skin integrity and instructs family members or significant others in this skill. The client is repositioned, and bony prominences are assessed at least every 2 hours for skin breakdown and contractures. Pressure-reducing devices or mattresses are used to prevent pressure ulcers. The nurse collaborates with the physical and occupational therapy departments for assistance with mobility, self-care, and energy conservation techniques.

DRUG THERAPY. Three groups of drugs are typically prescribed for the treatment of myasthenia gravis (MG): anticholinesterases, corticosteroids, and immunosuppressants. The nurse is responsible for administering these medications *on time* to maintain blood levels and thus facilitate increased muscle strength. The nurse also monitors and documents the client's responses. The nurse instructs the client and the family about the indications for, effectiveness of, and side effects of the drugs used in the treatment of MG.

Cholinesterase Inhibitor Drugs. Cholinesterase (ChE) inhibitor drugs are the first-line management of MG. These drugs are also referred to as anticholinesterase drugs or antimyasthenics. They enhance neuromuscular impulse transmission by preventing the degradation of AcH by the enzyme ChE, thus increasing the response of the muscles to nerve impulses and improving muscle strength. The ChE drug of choice is pyridostigmine (Mestinon, Regonol). The nurse may expect day-to-day variations in dosage depending on the client's fluctuating symptoms.

A potential side effect of these medications is cholinergic crisis. This effect is generally treated with atropine sulfate. The nurse must administer these medications on time to maintain consistent blood levels. The nurse administers the medications with a small amount of food to help alleviate gastrointestinal side effects and instructs the client to eat meals 45 minutes to 1 hour after taking these medications. This is very important if the client has bulbar involvement to avoid aspiration. Drugs containing magnesium, morphine or its derivatives, curare, quinine, quinidine, procainamide, and hypnotics or sedatives should be avoided because they may increase the client's weakness. Antibiotics such as neomycin, kanamycin, polymyxin B, and certain tetracyclines impair transmitter release and also increase myasthenic symptoms.

Sudden increases in weakness and the inability to clear secretions, swallow, or breathe adequately indicate that the client is experiencing crisis. There are two types of crises:

- **Myasthenic crisis**—an exacerbation of the myasthenic symptoms caused by undermedication with anticholinesterase drugs
- **Cholinergic crisis**—an acute exacerbation of muscle weakness caused by overmedication with cholinergic (anticholinesterase) drugs

Myasthenic crisis is often preceded by some type of infection. In either crisis, an adequate airway and artificial respiration must be maintained. Because myasthenic and cholinergic crises have many common characteristics, the type of crisis the client is experiencing must be identified for effective treatment to be provided (Table 44-1). In many clients, increasing myasthenic symptoms leads to an overdose of anticholinesterase drugs. As a result, the client may experience a *mixed* crisis. The Tensilon test (described on p. 960), although not always conclusive, is an important procedure for differentiation. Tensilon produces a temporary improvement in myasthenic crisis but no improvement or worsening of symptoms in cholinergic crisis.

Nursing management of the client in myasthenic crisis is directed at early detection and the maintenance of adequate respiratory function. The acutely ill client may need intensive nursing care for monitoring and maintenance of body functions. The client may require mechanical ventilation. Cholinesterase-inhibiting drugs are withheld because they increase respiratory secretions and are usually ineffective for the first few days after the crisis begins. Medications are reinstituted gradually and at lower dosages.

In *cholinergic* crisis, anticholinergic drugs are withheld while the client is maintained on a ventilator. Atropine (1 mg intravenously) may be given and repeated, if necessary. When atropine is ordered, the nurse must observe the client carefully; secretions are thickened by the drug, which causes more difficulty with airway clearance and possibly the development of mucous plugs. Unless complications such as pneumonia or aspiration develop, the client in crisis improves rapidly after the appropriate drugs have been given. The nurse continues to provide assistance as necessary, because the client tires easily after minimal exertion.

Immunosuppression. Immunosuppression may be accomplished with the use of prednisone (Deltasone, Winpred✱), azathioprine (Imuran), or cyclophosphamide (Cytoxan, Procytox✱). Prednisone is used initially to reduce remission and to control and improve symptoms. The drug is tapered over a period of weeks to months. Some clients may need continuous lowest-dose therapy because of exacerbations of symptoms. Azathioprine and cyclophosphamide are used for long-term management. Cyclophosphamide is reserved for clients who are refractory to other treatments. IV immunoglobulins may also be used for acute disease management or as a long-term option for clients refractory to other treatment.

TABLE 44-1 • CHARACTERISTICS OF MYASTHENIC AND CHOLINERGIC CRISES

Myasthenic Crisis	Cholinergic Crisis	Mixed Crisis
Increased pulse and respiration	Nausea	Apprehension
Rise in blood pressure	Vomiting	Restlessness
Anoxia	Diarrhea	Dyspnea
Cyanosis	Abdominal cramps	Dysphagia
Bowel and bladder incontinence	Blurred vision	Dysarthria
Decreased urine output	Pallor	Increased lacrimation
Absence of cough and swallow reflex	Facial muscle twitching	Increased salivation
	Pupillary miosis	Diaphoresis
	Hypotension	Generalized weakness

PLASMAPHERESIS. Plasmapheresis is a method by which antibodies are removed from the plasma. It may be used to decrease symptoms. Six exchanges occur over a 2-week period, with follow-up exchanges weekly or monthly as needed. This is usually done on an ambulatory care basis. Nursing management of the client undergoing plasmapheresis are presented in the earlier discussion of Guillain-Barré syndrome, p. 956.

RESPIRATORY SUPPORT. Although not all clients with MG experience respiratory compromise, the nurse must provide ongoing assessment and maintenance of respiratory function. Both myasthenic crisis (undermedication) and cholinergic crisis (overmedication) increase muscle weakness and the client's risk for respiratory compromise. The diaphragm and the respiratory and intercostal muscles may be affected, which inhibits the client's ability to maintain adequate ventilation, breathe deeply, and cough effectively. In addition, dysphagia may result in the aspiration of foods, fluids, or saliva, which compounds the respiratory problems. Because of their respiratory muscle involvement, many of these clients have an increased risk of pulmonary infections.

The client who cannot cough effectively may require oropharyngeal or nasopharyngeal suctioning. The nurse may need to teach the assisted cough technique, similar to that used by clients who are quadriplegic (see Chapter 43). Chest physiotherapy consisting of postural drainage, percussion, and vibration mobilizes secretions and helps prevent pneumonia and atelectasis. The nurse keeps an Ambu bag, equipment for oxygen administration, and endotracheal intubation equipment at the bedside in case of respiratory distress.

Because breathing difficulty or the inability to breathe easily is frightening, the nurse should be aware of the client's mental and emotional status during periods of respiratory compromise. While monitoring and documenting the client's response, the nurse administers the medications prescribed for muscle weakness, bronchodilation, and pulmonary congestion.

SELF-CARE. Generalized weakness and fatigue affect the client's ability to participate in activities of daily living (ADL). Impaired fine motor control and shoulder weakness, which result in difficulty raising the arms, often compound the problem. Self-care deficits may be complete or partial depending on the severity of the illness, the client's response to drugs, and the client's ability to tolerate activity without excessive fatigue.

To establish abilities and limitations, the nurse assesses the client's ability to perform ADLs. Although the client is encouraged to perform activities as independently as possible, assistance is provided as necessary to avoid undue frustration and fatigue. For maximizing independence and making attempts at self-care successful, activities are planned to follow the administration of medication. The nurse monitors and documents the client's response to or tolerance of activity, providing alternating periods of activity and rest. Rest is critical because increased fatigue can precipitate a crisis. In addition, occupational and physical therapists evaluate the client for assistive/adaptive devices. In collaboration with the nurse, they teach the client and family energy conservation techniques and ideas for making work and self-care easier after discharge from the hospital.

ASSISTANCE WITH COMMUNICATION. Weakness of the speech and facial muscles often results in dysarthric and nasal speech. Thus it may be difficult for myasthenic clients to make their speech understood by others.

In collaboration with the speech and language pathologist, the nurse determines the client's ability to communicate. The client is instructed to speak slowly while the nurse attempts to lip-read. The nurse repeats the information to verify that it is correct. Questions that can be answered with "yes" or "no" or by gestures may be used along with alternative communication systems such as eye blinking, flash cards, magic slates, notebook and pencil, and picture, letter, or word boards.

NUTRITIONAL SUPPORT. The client with myasthenia gravis (MG) may have difficulty maintaining an adequate intake of food and fluid because the muscles needed for chewing and swallowing become weakened and tire easily. In collaboration with the dietitian, occupational therapist, and speech and language pathologist, the client's nutritional status and his or her ability to receive adequate oral nutrition are evaluated. Small, frequent meals and high-calorie snacks are often well tolerated. The nurse and assistive nursing personnel monitors the effectiveness of the nutrition program by recording calorie counts, intake and output, serum albumin levels, and daily weights (Chart 44-5). If the client is not able to swallow, a feeding tube may be used.

EYE PROTECTION. The client's inability to completely close the eyes may lead to corneal abrasions and further compromise vision and comfort. During the day, the nurse or family member applies artificial tears to keep the corneas moist and free from abrasion. A lubricant gel and shield may be applied to the eye at bedtime to provide more extensive coverage. To help relieve diplopia, the eyes should be alternately covered with a patch for 2 to 3 hours at a time.

SURGICAL MANAGEMENT. For clients with MG, thymectomy is an alternative method of treatment and is usually performed early in the disease. The procedure is not always immediately effective, and it may take several years for remission to occur—if it occurs at all. Clients who have the surgery within 2 years of the onset of myasthenic symptoms show the most improvement.

PREOPERATIVE CARE. The nurse teaches the client coughing and deep-breathing exercises and the use of incentive spirometry. The nurse demonstrates airway suctioning and discusses wound care, IV infusions, and the critical care unit environment (if indicated). Because there is no way to predict whether remission or improvement will occur, it is important to avoid making promises, although optimism is warranted.

Immediately before surgery, the nurse may administer pyridostigmine (Mestinon), as ordered, with a small amount of water to keep the client stable during and after surgery. If steroids have been used, they are also given before surgery and are tapered during the postoperative period. The nurse also administers antibiotics immediately before and for several days after surgery. Plasmapheresis may be used preoperatively and postoperatively to decrease circulative antibodies more quickly.

OPERATIVE PROCEDURE. One of two surgical approaches may be used: the transcervical incision or the sternal split. Advocates of the transcervical approach claim a lower morbidity rate and more rapid recovery with less postoperative discomfort. The client often requires only a small dressing and an IV line. However, the sternal split allows the surgeon to directly visualize the mediastinum. Because more precise and complete removal of all thymic tissue is ensured, this may be the approach of choice.

When thymoma is present, all contiguous involved structures (e.g., the pericardium, the innominate vein, a portion of the superior vena cava, and a portion of the lung) are removed. A single chest tube is placed in the anterior mediastinum. The client may be admitted to the critical care unit postoperatively.

POSTOPERATIVE CARE. Although clients with adequate respiratory function may be extubated immediately after the procedure, most clients require a gradual weaning from the ventilator. Prolonged ventilatory assistance is rare. After the client is extubated, the nurse pays conscientious attention to pulmonary hygiene. Suctioning is performed as necessary, and the client is encouraged to turn, cough, and breathe deeply and to use incentive spirometry every 2 hours. In addition to observing respiratory function and providing bronchial hygiene, the nurse observes the client for signs of pneumothorax or hemothorax, such as the following:

- Chest pain
- Sudden shortness of breath
- Diminished or delayed chest wall expansion
- Diminished or absent breath sounds
- Restlessness or a change in vital signs (decreasing blood pressure or a weak, rapid pulse)

For the sternal surgical technique, the nurse provides chest tube care (see Chapter 30). Both surgical approaches require meticulous wound care. The nurse also observes for signs of infection, such as increasing or purulent drainage; redness, warmth, or swelling around the wound; and elevated temper-

CHART 44-5

BEST PRACTICE *for*
Improving Nutrition in Clients with Myasthenia Gravis

- Assess the client's gag reflex and ability to chew and swallow.
- Provide frequent oral hygiene as needed.
- Collaborate with the dietitian, speech and language pathologist, and occupational therapist to plan and implement meals that the client can eat and enjoy.
- Offer small, frequent meals.
- Cut food into small bites, and encourage the client to eat slowly.
- Observe client for choking, nasal regurgitation, and aspiration.
- Provide high-calorie snacks or supplements (e.g., puddings).
- Keep the head of the bed elevated during meals and for 30 to 60 minutes after the client eats.
- Avoid liquids because they can easily cause choking and aspiration; provide a soft diet.
- Monitor food intake carefully.
- Weigh the client daily.
- Monitor serum transferrin and albumin levels.
- Administer anticholinesterase drugs, as ordered: 30 to 60 minutes before meals.

ature. Appropriate client and family teaching is needed before discharge from the hospital.

Community-Based Care

The client with myasthenia gravis (MG) may be cared for in a variety of settings, including the home, subacute unit, rehabilitation setting, or long-term care facility. The client discharged from the hospital may be weak and may require the assistance of a family member, home care nurse, physical therapist, occupational therapist, and/or home care aide.

HEALTH TEACHING

The more the client and family know about the disease and the drugs used for treatment, the less likely it is that complications will develop.

DISEASE PROCESS. The client and the family are encouraged to ask questions. The nurse discusses the episodic nature (exacerbations and remissions) of the disease, including factors that predispose the client to exacerbation, such as infection, stress, surgery, hard physical exercise, sedatives, and enemas or strong cathartics (Table 44-2). The client is instructed to collaborate with the health care provider to monitor muscle strength, ability to perform activities of daily living (ADL), and the need to adjust medications.

LIFESTYLE CHANGES. The nurse stresses the importance of lifestyle adaptations such as avoiding heat (e.g., sauna, hot tubs, and sunbathing), crowds, overeating, erratic changes in sleep habits, or emotional extremes. The nurse describes the signs of exacerbation, such as increased weakness, increased diplopia, ptosis, and problems with chewing or swallowing. The client is instructed to plan activities to allow for rest periods and to conserve energy (see the Evidence-Based Practice for Nursing box at right).

DRUG THERAPY. The medication regimen is provided in a written format that includes the names, purposes, dosages, scheduled administration times, administrative routes, and side effects of the drugs. The nurse explains that the drugs are normally taken before activities such as eating, participating in sports, or engaging in work. The importance of maintaining therapeutic blood levels by taking the medications on time and as prescribed and not missing or postponing doses is stressed. In addition, the nurse informs the client of the side effects of anticholinesterase drugs.

The nurse advises the client to avoid medications such as morphine, curare, quinine, quinidine, procainamide, mycin-type antibiotics, and drugs containing magnesium. These agents markedly increase muscle weakness.

Additional health teaching regarding medications is found in Chart 44-6.

In preparing the client for discharge, the nurse explains the signs and symptoms of myasthenic and cholinergic crises and the need to contact the physician or other health care professional whenever either type of crisis is suspected. Because respiratory compromise often occurs in myasthenic clients, family members are encouraged to gain skills in resuscitation procedures. An Ambu bag, suctioning equipment, and oxygen should be available in the home for clients susceptible to crisis. Family members should be instructed in the proper use of equipment.

PSYCHOSOCIAL PREPARATION. The episodic nature of MG, the potential or actual loss of independence, and body image changes (e.g., the inability to smile) affect the

TABLE 44-2 • FACTORS PRECIPITATING OR WORSENING MYASTHENIA GRAVIS

Various medications, including the following:
- Antidysrhythmics
- Beta-blocking agents
- Antibiotics
- Antirheumatic drugs
- Antispasmodics
- Antihistamines
- Opioids
- Phenytoin (Dilantin)
- Antidepressants (tricyclics)

Rheumatoid arthritis
Alcohol
Hormonal changes
Stress
Infection
Seasonal temperature changes
Heat
Surgery

EVIDENCE-BASED PRACTICE FOR NURSING

How do clients with myasthenia gravis manage fatigue?

Grohar-Murray, M.E., et al. (1998). Self-care actions to manage fatigue among myasthenia gravis patients. *Journal of Neuroscience Nursing 30*(3), 191-199.

The purpose of this study was to describe self-care activities used by clients with myasthenia gravis (MG) to manage their fatigue. A nonexperimental design was used via mail to survey 250 MG clients from the National Myasthenia Gravis Foundation. Two structured instruments were used in the survey: The Fatigue Survey (adapted by the authors with permission) and the Myasthenia Gravis Fatigue Scale. Three data sets were collected: an estimation of the psychometric properties of the instruments, a fatigue score and characteristics of MG fatigue, and reports of self-care actions taken by clients to manage the fatigue of MG. The researchers found that effective self-care actions include stress-reduction techniques, the pacing of all activities, and increased rest and sleep. A small number ($n = 36$) reported using aerobic exercise—usually contraindicated with MG—to relieve fatigue. These respondents also reported the highest functional status.

Critique. Drawing a study sample from the National Myasthenia Gravis Foundation contributes to responder bias, because the results of the study may be influenced by those with a vested interest in the topic. There is no way to know whether those who did not have the opportunity to respond to the instruments would have answered in a manner similar to those who did. The study is further limited by a 46% response rate and the use of mailed surveys. Despite the limitations of this study, the researchers have contributed to the body of knowledge that can be used to develop protocols to manage fatigue in clients with MG.

Implications for Nursing. Because fatigue is the most troublesome and prominent symptom reported by clients with MG, this study makes an important contribution to the nursing management of these clients. Fatigue in MG is a very complex symptom with no specific protocols to guide its clinical management. It is essential that clients with MG recognize their fatigue early on and identify actions that can conserve their energy and potentially contribute to an increased quality of life. Information from MG clients themselves about how they manage fatigue is an important contribution to the care of all clients with MG.

client's adjustment. During discharge planning, the case manager (CM) considers factors such as age, sex, usual roles and responsibilities, available support systems, occupation, and financial status. Because the client's and family's need for psychosocial adjustment may range from minimal to dramatic, the CM remains sensitive to their needs and provides information and support. The CM encourages family members or significant others to discuss their feelings with one another.

HOME CARE MANAGEMENT

Clients with MG are usually managed at home. Hospitalization is restricted to the diagnostic and evaluation processes, myasthenic or cholinergic crisis resulting in respiratory failure, or periods of exacerbation when respiratory function is threatened.

Unless the client requires assistive devices, little preparation of the home setting is required. In consultation with physical and occupational therapists, the CM makes certain that the necessary equipment has been delivered and properly installed. In addition, the CM makes sure that the client and family members can use the equipment safely. If the client becomes wheelchair dependent, the discharge planner or CM ensures that any necessary modifications to the home (e.g., the installation of ramps or widening of doorways) have been completed before the client's discharge from the hospital.

HEALTH CARE RESOURCES

In consultation with the health care provider, client, and family, the staff nurse or CM may initiate referrals to home care agencies and to local self-help groups for people who have chronic illnesses and for their families. The Myasthenia Gravis Foundation, headquartered in New York City, has education and research programs and provides assistance with financial aid and community resources. The CM encourages the client to obtain and wear a medical alert (MedicAlert) bracelet or necklace and to carry identification at all times.

POLYNEURITIS AND POLYNEUROPATHY

OVERVIEW

Systemic diseases, vitamin B_{12} deficiency, drug toxicity, infections, trauma, vascular or metabolic disturbances, and exogenous substances such as alcohol, medications, industrial agents, and heavy metals may damage cranial and peripheral nerves. Although the term **polyneuritis** implies an inflammatory process, it may also denote noninflammatory lesions. Thus the terms *polyneuritis,* **polyneuropathy,** and **peripheral neuropathy** may describe syndromes whose clinical hallmarks are muscle weakness with or without atrophy, pains and paresthesia or loss of sensation, impaired reflexes, autonomic manifestations, or combinations of these symptoms.

The most common type of neuropathy is a symmetric polyneuropathy in which the client experiences decreased sensation along with the feeling that an extremity is asleep. Tingling, burning, tightness, or aching sensations generally start in the feet and progress to the level of the knee before being noted in the hands (glove and stocking neuropathy). Other clients may complain of unsteadiness, clumsiness, an inability to recognize objects by feel, and injury without pain. Diabetic neuropathy is a common example, as are the neuropathies resulting from renal or hepatic failure, alcoholism, acquired immunodeficiency syndrome (AIDS), and drug or toxic exposures. Common factors associated with polyneuropathy are presented in Table 44-3.

COLLABORATIVE MANAGEMENT

Assessment

Although peripheral neuropathy rarely necessitates hospitalization, the nurse is likely to encounter clients with this condition in a variety of settings, particularly among older adults or in clients with a related illness. Nursing assessment includes an examination of the client's sensory and motor abilities. The client can often outline a specific area of sensory deficit. Because the client may be unaware of decreased sensation, the nurse or nurse practitioner may assess the distal extremities for light touch using cotton balls or cotton-tipped applicators and for pain using a safety pin. The nurse assesses position sense, or kinesthetic sensation, by gently grasping the involved digit or extremity on its sides. With the client's eyes closed, the nurse changes the position of the digit or extremity, and the client is asked to describe how the position was changed. The client should be able to acknowledge even slight movements. A tuning fork may be placed on bone

CHART 44-6

CLIENT EDUCATION GUIDE
Helpful Hints for Medication Teaching of Clients with Myasthenia Gravis

- Keep medications and a glass of water at your bedside if you are weak in the morning.
- Wear a watch with an alarm function (or beeper) to remind you to take your medications.
- Post your medication schedule so others know it.
- Plan strenuous activities, when possible, when the medication peaks.
- Keep an extra supply of medications in your car or at work. Be sure they are secured.
- Do not take any over-the-counter medications without checking with your health care provider.

TABLE 44-3 • FACTORS ASSOCIATED WITH POLYNEUROPATHY

DISEASES
- Amyloidosis
- Alcoholism
- Carcinomas
- Diabetes mellitus
- Diphtheria
- Hepatic failure
- Malabsorption or malnutrition
- Porphyria
- Renal failure (uremia)
- Trauma
- Vascular disease

VITAMIN DEFICIENCIES
- Vitamin B_1 (thiamine)
- Vitamin B_6 (pyridoxine)
- Vitamin B_2 (riboflavin)
- Vitamin B_c (folic acid)
- Vitamin B_{12}
- Niacin

DRUG USE
- Nitrofurantoin
- Vincristine
- Isoniazid
- Phenytoin
- Amitriptyline
- Hydralazine

ENVIRONMENTAL EXPOSURES
- Heavy metals
- Industrial solvents

prominences to test for sensitivity to vibration. The examination is started at the distal sites. More proximal areas are tested only if the client fails to perceive the duration of vibration at the distal site.

The nurse examines the extremities for any signs of injury of which the client may be unaware. The client is also assessed for the following:

- Orthostatic hypotension
- Abnormal sweating
- Miosis (abnormal constriction of the pupil)
- Sphincter disturbances, such as loss of bowel and bladder control
- Other autonomic dysfunctions that may accompany the neuropathy

All abnormal findings are documented and brought to the health care provider's attention.

Interventions

Medical management of clients with peripheral neuropathy consists of the removal or treatment of the underlying cause and symptomatic therapy, including supportive care and physiotherapy. The diet is generally supplemented with vitamins, especially if vitamin deficiency is an underlying cause. However, there is no evidence that vitamins in excess of those contained in a well-balanced diet have any effect on the forms of polyneuropathy unrelated to vitamin deficiency.

With removal of the toxic agent or correction of the metabolic defects, recovery may be rapid if the continuity of the nerves has not been interrupted. If there has been axonal destruction, recovery may require several months. After severe degeneration, there may be permanent weakness, atrophy, decreased reflexes, and sensory deficits.

Extensive client teaching is essential. For clients with decreased sensation in their feet and legs, the nurse explains the importance of proper foot care (Chart 44-7). In addition, the nurse assists the client who has decreased sensation to recognize potential hazards, such as the following:

- Exposure to extremes of environmental temperature (e.g., frostbite)
- Bathwater or dishwater that may be too hot
- Contact of the feet with heat sources (e.g., heating pads, radiators) while sleeping
- Burns associated with cooking

Smoking is discouraged because the resulting vasoconstriction may worsen the neuropathy. The nurse may need to refer the client to a smoking cessation program. The importance of maintaining adequate nutrition is emphasized. Clients with postural hypotension are taught to arise slowly and wear support or elastic stockings to minimize the pooling of blood in the legs.

Many clients, especially those with the acute forms of polyneuropathy associated with drugs or exposure to toxic substances, experience anxiety, impaired coping, and changes in family processes such as role responsibilities and sexual functioning. Thus it is vital for the nurse to establish a trusting nurse/client relationship and to provide psychosocial support. In consultation with the physician, social worker, chaplain or religious leader, and physical and occupational therapists, the nurse focuses on the client's abilities and strengths and helps identify new ways of coping, meeting needs, and restructuring activities.

CHART 44-7

CLIENT EDUCATION GUIDE
Peripheral Neuropathy of the Lower Extremities

- Wash your feet and legs with mild soap each day; rinse and dry them well.
- Apply lanolin or lubricating lotion to your feet and legs once or twice daily.
- Inspect your feet and legs daily; report skin changes or open areas to your physician or other health care provider.
- Wear white or colorfast stockings or socks, and change them daily.
- Check the temperature of your bathwater with a thermometer before putting your feet into the water.
- Do not use heating pads or other heat sources on your feet.
- Do not use sharp devices to remove corns or calluses (use a pumice stone) or to cut nails. Seek professional podiatry care on a regular basis.
- Wear support or elastic stockings if you have orthostatic hypotension or dependent edema.
- Wear well-fitted shoes; avoid going barefoot.

PERIPHERAL NERVE TRAUMA

OVERVIEW

The peripheral nerves are subject to injuries associated with mechanical or vehicular accidents, certain sports, the injection of particular drugs, military conflicts or wars, and acts of violence (e.g., knife or gunshot wounds). Specific mechanisms of injury include the following:

- Partial or complete severance of a nerve or nerves
- Contusion, stretching, constriction, or compression of a nerve or nerves
- Ischemia
- Electrical, thermal, or radiation injury

Most commonly affected are the median, ulnar, and radial nerves of the arms and the peroneal, femoral, and sciatic nerves of the legs (Figure 44-1).

After a nerve is transected, the nerve distal to the injury degenerates and retracts within 24 hours. Motor and sensory dysfunction distal to the lesion coincide with the loss of electrical excitability as the nerve fibers degenerate. Recovery occurs as Schwann cells of the neurilemma proliferate from both the proximal and distal stumps. Dividing mitotically, these cells form neurilemmal cords, which act as guidelines for the regenerating axon. Tiny unmyelinated sprouts are generated at the proximal axon and grow 1 to 4 mm each day. Some can cross the transected gap through guidance by the neurilemma to find their way to the distal stump. The better aligned the union, the more normal the functional return (Figure 44-2).

Successfully realigned nerves remyelinate, grow to their former size, and eventually claim conduction velocities of 80% of their former capacity (Hickey, 1997). Successful reinnervation is adversely affected by the loss of anatomic continuity of the nerve, infection, and increasing age. Disorganization of the nerve or mismatched realignments may result in functional weakness, unintentional muscle movements, and poor sensory discrimination and localization of stimuli.

Some sensory function may return before the regeneration process can occur. This is because nerves proximal to the injured neurons are stimulated to produce collateral innervation to the affected areas. These collaterals provide some innervation before the axon itself has regenerated sufficiently.

COLLABORATIVE MANAGEMENT

Assessment

The primary nursing considerations for the client with peripheral nerve trauma are assessment of function, maintenance of function, and rehabilitation.

The client may relate a history of extremity or pelvic trauma, penetrating injury, recent surgery, the use of crutches, or pain after medication injections. In addition to weakness or flaccid paralysis, the client may complain of burning sensations distal to the trauma or pain that increases with tactile or environmental stimulation. Skin and nail changes of the affected extremities may also be noted by the client.

The nurse performs a physical assessment to determine which neurologic functions are intact. In acute trauma, the injury should first be evaluated by the physician to determine whether movement is contraindicated. If movement is not contraindicated, the nurse assesses motor function by asking the client to put the limb through the normal range of motion. Any abnormal movements, tremor, atrophy, contractions, paresis or paralysis, and weak or absent deep tendon reflexes are documented. The nurse questions the client about abnormal sensations.

After complete denervation, the extent of vasomotor function is reflected in skin temperature, skin color, and edema. A warm phase and a cold phase have been identified. During the *warm phase,* the extremity is warm, and the skin appears flushed or rosy. Over 2 to 3 weeks, this phase is gradually superseded by a *cold phase,* during which the skin appears cyanotic, mottled, or reddish blue and feels cool compared with the contralateral, unaffected extremity. The nurse uses the dorsal surface of the hand to compare skin temperatures because the abundance of temperature receptors in this area facilitates more accurate assessments. The nurse may note edema immediately after injury or later as a result of surgical procedures. Any evidence of trophic changes (e.g., scaling of skin, brittleness of nails, or loss of body hair) is recorded. This initial assessment serves as the baseline for comparison during subsequent examinations, which are performed every 2 to 4 hours or less frequently as the client's condition indicates.

Interventions

Interventions for the client with peripheral nerve trauma depend on the location as well as the type and degree of injury.

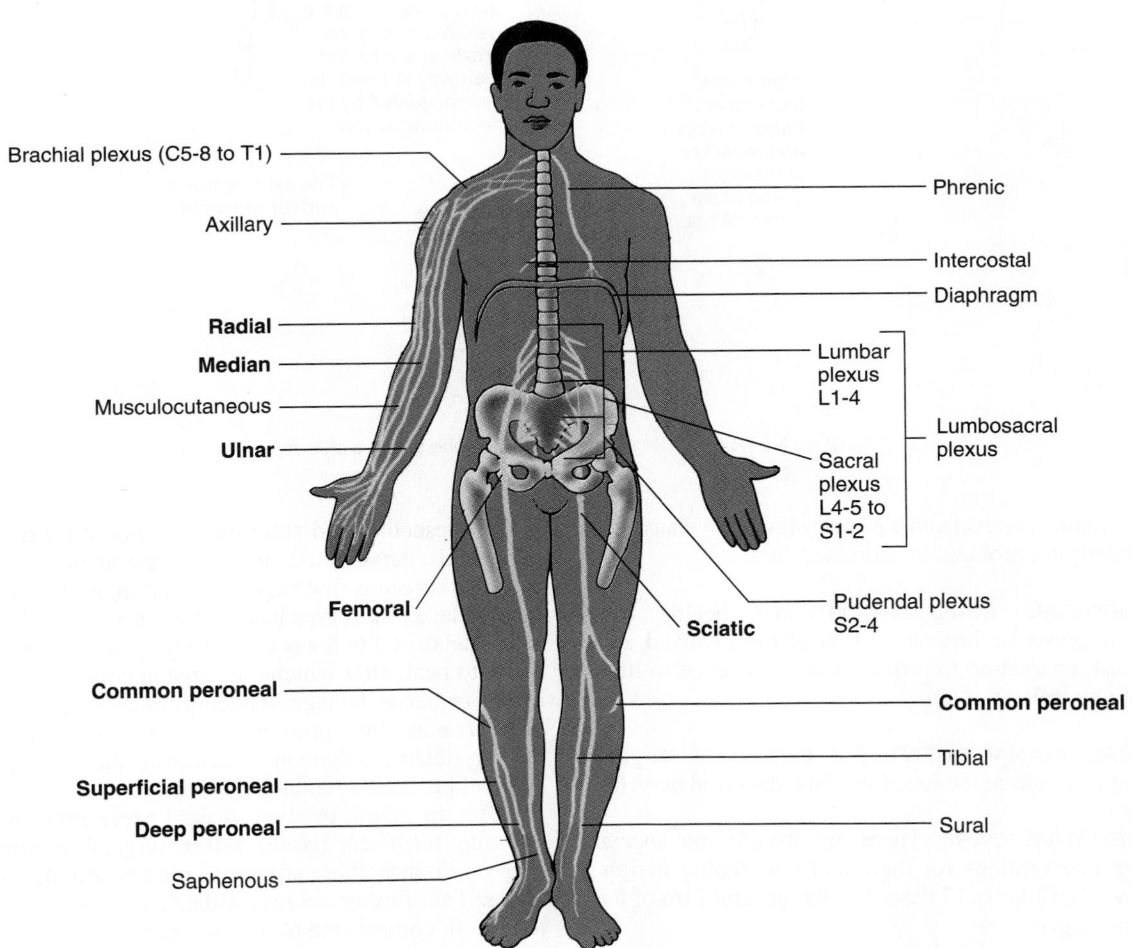

Figure 44-1 ● Distribution of selected peripheral nerves in the body. The nerves most commonly affected by trauma are highlighted in **bold** type.

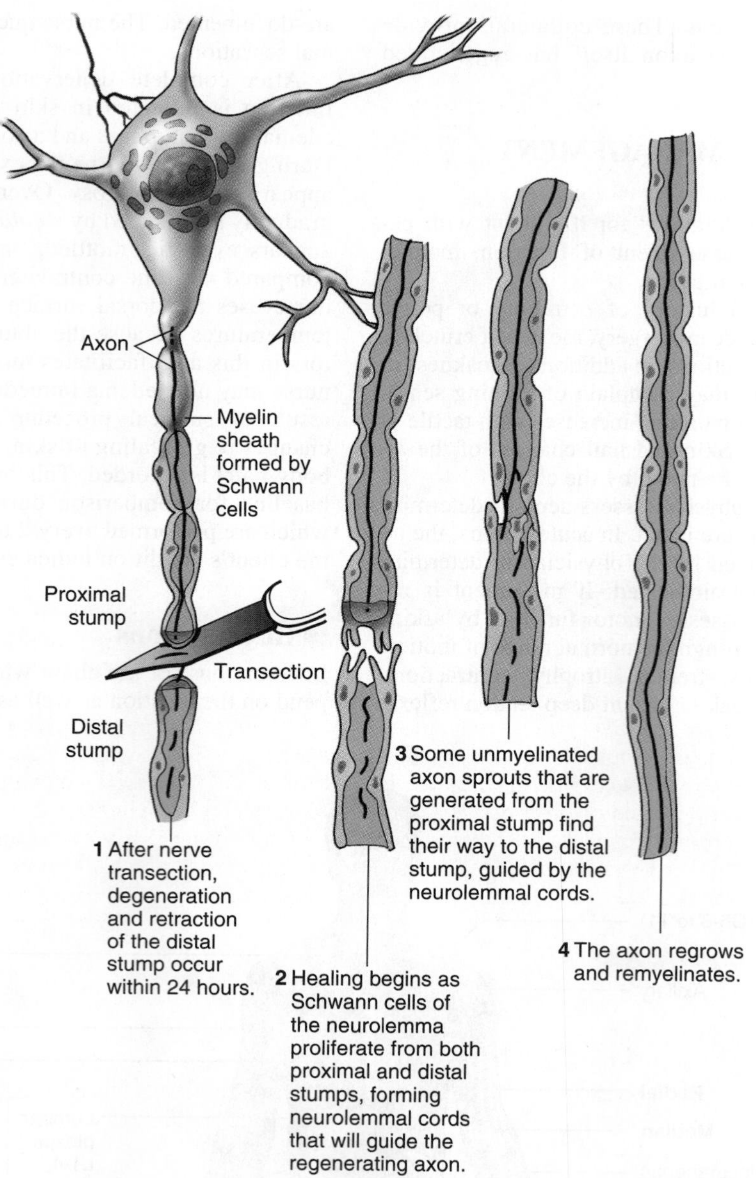

Figure 44-2 ● Regeneration of a peripheral nerve after injury.

If the nerve trauma results from a primary lesion, such as a tumor, the underlying problem is addressed first.

NONSURGICAL MANAGEMENT. The health care provider may prescribe immobilization of the involved area by splint, cast, or traction to provide the rest needed to limit and resolve any inflammation.

SURGICAL MANAGEMENT. The purpose of surgical management is to restore the function of the damaged nerve(s).

PREOPERATIVE CARE. There are usually no special preoperative interventions for the client undergoing peripheral nerve repair. Chapter 17 describes the general care of the client before surgery.

OPERATIVE PROCEDURE. If the nerve is lacerated or transected, surgery may be indicated. Restorative procedures include resecting and suturing to reapproximate the severed nerve ends, nerve grafts, and nerve and tendon transplants.

Since surgeons first began to repair injured nerves, the timing of these procedures has been controversial. In the past, a repair delay of 3 to 8 weeks after injury allowed associated injuries to heal, after which the surgeon could better assess the extent of nerve damage. Although microsurgery and the use of lasers now allow primary nerve repair at the time of injury, the physician's judgment in selecting the optimal time and surgical procedure remains crucial.

After an injury, the two severed nerve segments contract and may form scar tissue. Before surgical anastomosis, the surgeon dissects these stumps to remove any damaged nerve tissue. This further decreases the lengths of the ends to be joined. To compensate for this shortening and to avoid excessive tension on the sutured nerve, the involved extremity is positioned in exaggerated flexion. The surgeon aligns the segments under magnification, bringing proximal motor and sensory fibers to distal motor and sensory fibers, and then sutures the nerve tissue.

POSTOPERATIVE CARE. After suturing, the extremity is placed in a cast to maintain the flexed position and to avoid tension on the suture line. Ten to 14 days after nerve repair, the entire dressing is removed, the joint flexion is eased, and a new splint may be applied for an additional 2 weeks. At that time, a removable splint may be applied and physiotherapy begun. Protection of the nerve sutures is continued for a minimum of 6 weeks.

If a large segment of nerve has been damaged and direct anastomosis would be impossible without stretching the nerve more than 10% to 15% of its total length, the surgeon may interpose a nerve graft. Motor and sensory axons may regenerate through the graft, joining proximal and distal segments through the two sites of anastomosis. The amount of sensory and motor regeneration depends on the length of the graft, the type of nerve involved, the condition of the end plates, and the number of axons able to traverse the graft and suture sites. Thus the results are not usually as favorable as with direct reanastomosis. In the case of grafted nerve repairs, maintenance of the flexed position is less essential, although immobilization by splints or casts to facilitate healing of the surgical sites remains imperative.

Splints are usually held in place with elastic (Ace) wrapping or hook-and-loop (Velcro) closures, which can become too tight if edema develops. The nurse checks the skin around the splints and casts frequently (hourly, initially) for tightness, warmth, and color. If the client complains of discomfort, tingling, or coolness or if the color is blanched, the cast or splint may be too tight; the nurse promptly informs the physician. The nurse immediately reports any indication of drainage under a splint or cast.

Skin care is essential. Atrophy of the epidermis and underlying tissue causes the skin to become more fragile and more susceptible to injury and breakdown. The decreased skin nutrition and decreased vascularity associated with denervation cause delayed healing, which further compounds the problem. The nurse thoroughly examines the skin for evidence of irritation or injury and assists or instructs the client to wash and dry the involved areas carefully. If the skin is dry, lanolin or cocoa butter may be used as a lubricant. Because sensation may be absent or inhibited, the nurse instructs the client to protect the involved areas from temperature extremes or other sources of potential trauma.

REHABILITATION. Physiotherapy is the major approach for rehabilitation after surgical repair. The nurse reinforces and helps the client perform the exercises learned in these sessions. Because the regeneration of nerves and subsequent return of sensory and motor function may be extremely slow and produce pain, the client may become discouraged and depressed. If the disability is permanent, the client needs encouragement and assistance to cope with the changes in body image, self-esteem, and lifestyle.

RESTLESS LEGS SYNDROME

OVERVIEW

Restless legs syndrome (RLS) is characterized by leg paresthesia associated with an irresistible urge to move. It affects between 5% and 15% of the U.S. population, but most health care providers do not identify it. The incidence may be higher in nursing home and home care clients, who often have diabetes and renal failure—two conditions correlated with RLS (Boucher, 1997). The incidence is equal in men and women.

The client with RLS complains of intense burning or "crawling-type" sensations in the limbs and subsequently feels the need to move the limbs repeatedly. These symptoms are worse at night and when the client is still for a period of time. Clients feel they need to move to relieve the symptoms. For that reason, clients with RLS often refer to themselves as "night walkers."

➤ COLLABORATIVE MANAGEMENT

Diagnosis is made on the history; there is no known etiology. Potential contributing factors include vitamin and mineral deficiencies, anemias, polyneuropathies, diabetes mellitus, pregnancy, peripheral nerve disease, pinched nerves, lumbar surgical procedures, renal failure, and substances such as caffeine, alcohol, tricyclics, and beta blockers.

The management of RLS is symptomatic and involves treating the underlying cause or contributing factor, if known. The nurse recommends measures for promoting sleep. For some clients, the health care provider orders medications that have proven to be effective for some clients, such as clonidine hydrochloride (Catapres, Dixarit🍁), carbamazepine (Tegretol, Mazepine🍁), clonazepam (Klonopin, Rivotril🍁), and pain relievers such as acetaminophen (Tylenol) (Boucher, 1997). More recently, dopaminergic agents such as levodopa, pergolide (Permax), and pramipexole (Mirapex) have been used to relieve symptoms (Montplaisir et al., 1999; Wetter et al., 1999). The Restless Legs Foundation is an excellent resource for information and client and family support.

DISEASES OF THE CRANIAL NERVES

The nurse may encounter clients with cranial nerve disease in various practice settings. The cranial nerves may be affected in association with other disorders of the nervous system or as a result of trauma. The most common disorders, those affecting cranial nerves V (trigeminal) and VII (facial), are discussed here.

Trigeminal Neuralgia

OVERVIEW

Trigeminal neuralgia *(tic douloureux):*

- Entails a specific type of facial pain, which occurs in abrupt, intense paroxysms
- Is usually provoked by minimal stimulation of a trigger zone
- Is unilateral and confined to the area innervated by the trigeminal nerve, most often the second and third branches (Figure 44-3)

> **CONSIDERATIONS FOR OLDER ADULTS**
> Trigeminal neuralgia usually appears in people older than 50 years of age. Older adults are affected at a frequency of 15 cases per 100,000, with a female-to-male ratio of 2:1 (Weisberg, Garcia, & Strub, 1996).

Clients younger than 30 years of age with pain in more than one branch of the trigeminal nerve may be further evaluated to rule out the possibility of a tumor or multiple sclerosis.

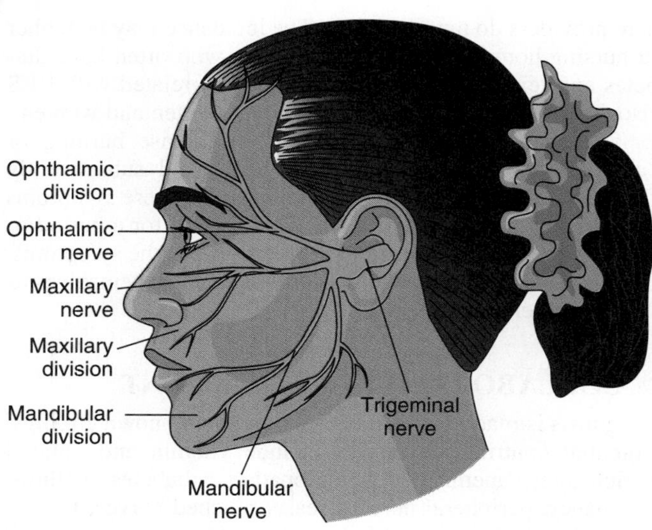

Figure 44-3 ● Distribution of the trigeminal nerve and its three divisions: ophthalmic, maxillary, and mandibular.

When describing the pain, clients use terms such as "excruciating," "sharp," "shooting," "piercing," "burning," and "jabbing." Between bursts of pain, which last from seconds to minutes, there is usually no pain. The nurse usually finds no sensory or motor deficits on examination, but the condition can be agonizing for the client. The fear of precipitating attacks often causes clients to avoid talking, smiling, eating, or attending to hygienic needs such as shaving, washing the face, and brushing the teeth.

The cause of trigeminal neuralgia is thought to be related to impaired inhibitory mechanisms in the brainstem caused by excessive firing of irritated fibers in the trigeminal nerve. In addition, trauma and infection of the teeth, jaw, or ear may be contributing factors.

The course of trigeminal neuralgia is characterized by bouts of pain for several weeks or months followed by spontaneous remissions. The length of these remissions may vary from days to years, but attack-free periods tend to become shorter as the client grows older. Symptoms rarely disappear permanently.

➤ COLLABORATIVE MANAGEMENT

Management of the client with trigeminal neuralgia is determined by the amount of pain the client is experiencing. Conservative measures are usually tried first.

NONSURGICAL MANAGEMENT. Medical management is accomplished with the use of drugs such as carbamazepine (Tegretol, Apo-Carbamazepine✤, Mazepine✤), phenytoin (Dilantin), baclofen (Lioresal) and, occasionally, amitriptyline (Elavil, Meravil✤) or diazepam (Valium, E-Pam✤). Initial therapy should always be nonsurgical, and drugs may be used singly or in combination. Surgical management may be considered if the client and the physician agree that the pain or the toxic effects of drug therapy are worse than the risk of surgery.

Approximately 70% of clients respond to carbamazepine, 20 to 1200 mg daily, alone or in combination with phenytoin in average daily doses of 200 to 400 mg. Fosphenytoin (Cerebyx) may also be given intravenously to abort an acute attack. Phenytoin and fosphenytoin are anticonvulsants believed to decrease the paroxysmal afferent impulses in much the same way as when they are used to treat seizure disorders.

Injection of alcohol or phenol into the affected branch of the trigeminal nerve may relieve pain for up to 16 months. Injection into the gasserian ganglion, where sensory root fibers arise, may provide permanent pain control but carries with it a greater risk of extraocular palsies, keratitis, blindness, or masticatory paralysis. In both blocking procedures, there is complete anesthesia to the portion of the face innervated by the injected branch.

SURGICAL MANAGEMENT. The primary purpose of surgery is to relieve the client's pain.

PREOPERATIVE CARE. In addition to the general preoperative care provided to all clients (see Chapter 17), the surgeon thoroughly explains the surgical benefits and any expected neurologic deficits. The nurse reinforces the information provided by the surgeon.

OPERATIVE PROCEDURE. In some clients, a small artery compresses the trigeminal nerve as it enters the pons. Surgical relocation of this artery may relieve the pain of trigeminal neuralgia without compromising facial sensation. The *Jannetta procedure* accomplishes this through a posterior fossa craniotomy. Under microscopic vision, the surgeon carefully lifts the loop of artery off the nerve and places a small silicone (Silastic) sponge between the vessel and the nerve. In a similar microvascular procedure, one or all branches of the trigeminal nerve are visualized and dissected.

Radiofrequency percutaneous electrocoagulation may provide lasting relief of pain without compromising touch or motor function. During this procedure, the client is sedated with small doses of diazepam, midazolam hydrochloride (Versed), or fentanyl (Sublimaze) but is alert and able to respond verbally to questions. The physician inserts a needle electrode and, under radiographic control, advances it to the appropriate area, where a heat lesion is made. After each needle insertion, the corneal and ciliary reflexes, as well as sensation in the face, are checked. The advantages of this procedure include the following:

- Long-term pain relief
- Relatively short hospital stays
- Tolerance by older adults
- Absence of facial paralysis
- Preservation of the sensation of touch

The possibility of puncturing the internal carotid artery and the occurrence of anesthesia dolorosa are disadvantages (Hickey, 1997). The affected side is permanently insensitive to pain.

POSTOPERATIVE CARE. In addition to general post-craniotomy care, the nurse monitors for complications associated with these procedures, including headache, permanent cranial nerve dysfunction, and hemorrhage. The nurse assesses the client's corneal reflex, extraocular muscles, and facial nerve. The nurse tests the corneal reflex by making a threatening motion with the hand close to the eye. The client will blink if the reflex is intact. Extraocular muscles are assessed by asking the client to follow a finger through the six cardinal positions while observing for conjugate eye movements. To assess the facial nerve, the nurse asks the client to wrinkle the forehead, frown, wink, squeeze the eyes closed, whistle, and blow air out of the cheeks. Last, the client is evaluated for abnormal sensations and pain and for the ability to chew. The nurse documents any abnormal findings and reports them to the physician.

The nurse or assistive nursing personnel applies an ice pack to the operative site on the jaw for 4 hours. A soft diet is prescribed, and the client is discouraged from chewing on the affected side until the paresthesia is abated. The nurse instructs the client to avoid rubbing the eye on the affected side because the protective mechanism of pain will no longer warn of injury. The client should inspect the eye daily for redness or irritation and report any change or blurred vision to the physician. The nurse encourages the client to schedule regular dental examinations because the absence of pain may not warn of potential problems.

Psychosocial considerations for the client with trigeminal neuralgia include disappointment with ineffective drug protocols or surgical procedures, as well as the fear that the pain may recur with any activity. The client may fail to move the face in an attempt to prevent pain. This behavior may be misinterpreted by others as withdrawal, antisociability, or depression. The nurse's goal is to help the client cope with the condition and to develop strategies for dealing with identified problems.

Facial Paralysis

OVERVIEW

Facial paralysis, or *Bell's palsy* (acute paralysis of cranial nerve VII), was first described by Sir Charles Bell of England in 1821. The incidence is 23 persons per 100,000 population; men and women are equally affected (Hickey, 1997). Although the incidence may be slightly higher among people with diabetes, the condition occurs in all ages and at all times of the year.

The onset of Bell's palsy is acute. Maximal paralysis is attained within 48 hours in about half the clients and within 5 days in almost all clients. Pain behind the ear or on the face may precede paralysis by a few hours or days. The disorder is characterized by a drawing sensation and paralysis of all facial muscles on the affected side. The client cannot close the eye, wrinkle the forehead, smile, whistle, or grimace. The face appears masklike and sags. Taste is usually impaired to some degree, but this symptom seldom persists beyond the second week of paralysis.

Although the cause of Bell's palsy remains obscure, it may be the result of an inflammatory process. Clients with Bell's palsy are rarely hospitalized, but the nurse may encounter them in community-based settings such as clinics, physicians' offices, or emergency departments.

COLLABORATIVE MANAGEMENT

Medical management consists of the administration of prednisone (Deltasone, Winpred✱), 30 to 60 mg daily, during the first week after the onset of symptoms. Analgesics may help relieve the pain. Nursing care is directed toward managing the major neurologic deficits and providing psychosocial support. Because the eye does not close, the cornea must be protected from drying and subsequent ulceration or abrasion. The nurse instructs the client to manually close the eyelid at intervals and to instill artificial tears four times daily. The eye may be patched or taped closed at bedtime.

The client may be unable to chew, sip fluids through a straw, or control drooling on the affected side. Thus mealtime may become a problem. The nurse encourages the client to eat and drink using the unaffected side of the mouth. The nurse may be needed to provide emotional support and suggestions for coping and adapting. Frequent, small meals may be better tolerated, and clients may require a soft diet. The nurse explains simple techniques of massage; the application of warm, moist heat; and facial exercises.

A facial sling may prevent drooping of the affected side. As muscle tone improves, the nurse instructs the client to grimace, wrinkle the brow, force the eyes closed, whistle, and blow air out of the cheeks three or four times daily for 5 minutes in front of a mirror.

Although 80% of clients recover fully within a few weeks or months, approximately 15% to 20% experience some residual weakness; a few have permanent neurologic deficits (Hickey, 1997). These clients require a great deal of support because body image and self-esteem are drastically affected. The nurse is a valuable source of both information and psychosocial support.

ONLINE RESOURCES

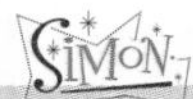

For suggested readings and Internet resources, go to http://www.wbsaunders.com/SIMON/Iggy/.

SELECTED BIBLIOGRAPHY

Asterisk indicates a classic or definitive work on this subject.

Adams, R.D., Victor, M., & Ropper, A.H. (1997). *Principles of neurology* (6th ed.). New York: McGraw-Hill.

Anderson, L. (1998). Miracles do happen. *Rehabilitation Nursing, 23*(5), 269.

*Barker, F.G., et al. (1996). Long-term outcomes after microvascular decompression for trigeminal neuralgia. *New England Journal of Medicine, 334*(5), 1077-1083.

Boucher, M.A. (1997). Restless legs syndrome in home healthcare. *Home Healthcare Nurse, 15*(8), 550-556.

Costa, M.E. (1998). Clinical snapshot: Trigeminal neuralgia. *American Journal of Nursing, 98*(6), 42-43.

Giger, J.N., & Davidhizar, R.E. (1999). *Transcultural nursing: Assessment and intervention* (3rd ed.). St. Louis: Mosby.

Grohar-Murray, M.E., et al. (1998). Self-care actions to manage fatigue among myasthenia gravis patients. *Journal of Neuroscience Nursing, 30*(3), 191-199.

Hickey, J.V. (1997). *The clinical practice of neurological and neurosurgical nursing.* Philadelphia: J.B. Lippincott.

*Kernich, C.A. (1996). Myths and facts about myasthenia gravis. *Nursing96, 26*(7), 21.

McMahon-Parkes, K. (1997). Guillain-Barré syndrome: Biological basis, treatment, and care. *Critical Care Nurse, 13*(1), 42-48.

*Midroni, G. (1996). Chronic inflammatory polyradicular demyelinating neuropathy: Unusual clinical features and therapeutic response. *Neurology, 46*(5), 1206-1212.

Montplaisir, J., et al. (1999). Restless legs syndrome improved by pramipexole: A double-blind randomized trial. *Neurology, 52*(5), 938-943.

*Pascuzzi, R.M., & Fleck, J.D. (1999). Acute peripheral neuropathy in adults: Guillain-Barré syndrome and related disorders. *Neurology Clinics, 15*(3), 529-547.

Petit, J., & Barkhaus, P.E. (1997). Evaluation and management of polyneuropathy: A practical approach. *Nurse Practitioner, 22*(5), 131-133, 136-138, 141-143.

Ross, A.P. (1999). Neurologic degenerative diseases. *Nursing Clinics of North America, 34*(3), 725-742.

*Shpritz, D. (1996). *Rapid nursing intervention: Neurologic.* Albany, NY: Delmar.

Sorrell, J. (1999). Taking steps to calm restless legs syndrome. *Nursing99, 29*(9), 60-61.

*Taha, J.M., & Tew, J.M. (1996). Comparison of surgical treatments for trigeminal neuralgia: Reevaluation of radiofrequency rhizotomy. *Neurosurgery, 38*(5), 865-871.

*Weisberg, L.A., Garcia, C., & Strub, R. (1996). *Essentials of clinical neurology.* St. Louis: Mosby.

Wetter, T.C., et al. (1999). A randomized controlled study of pergolide in patients with restless legs syndrome. *Neurology, 52*(5), 944-950.

CHAPTER 45

Interventions for Critically Ill Clients with Neurologic Problems

DEBORAH WRIGHT SHPRITZ

Learning Objectives

After studying this chapter, you should be able to:

1. Identify the common types of strokes.
2. Discuss risk factors that increase the likelihood of strokes.
3. Describe typical clinical manifestations associated with stroke.
4. Analyze assessment data to determine common nursing diagnoses that are pertinent to clients with strokes.
5. Identify the purpose of intracranial pressure (ICP) monitoring and signs of increasing ICP.
6. Explain the role of drug therapy in managing clients with strokes.
7. Prioritize nursing care for a client who has experienced a stroke.
8. Discuss the purpose of rehabilitation for the client with a stroke.
9. Develop a teaching plan for the client who has experienced a stroke.
10. Differentiate the common types of traumatic brain injury (TBI).
11. Explain the pathophysiologic changes that can result from moderate or severe TBI.
12. Describe the psychosocial and behavioral manifestations associated with TBI.
13. Prioritize nursing care for the client with TBI.
14. Describe common complications of brain tumors.
15. Develop a postoperative plan of care for a client having a craniotomy.

SIMON

Go to http://www.wbsaunders.com/SIMON/Iggy/ for self-assessment questions related to these Learning Objectives.

Certain neurologic problems can cause clients to become critically ill or die. Stroke, head injury, brain tumor, and brain abscess can cause increased intracranial pressure (ICP), a life-threatening complication. Permanent neurologic dysfunction or death may be prevented by prompt recognition and aggressive management of this complication by the interdisciplinary health care team.

STROKE

OVERVIEW

A **stroke** is a disruption in the normal blood supply to the brain. Formerly called cerebrovascular accident (CVA), the National Stroke Association now uses the term "brain attack" to describe a stroke. A stroke is a medical emergency that strikes suddenly, and it should be treated immediately to prevent neurologic deficit and permanent disability.

Although the number of stroke deaths has decreased during the past several years, stroke remains the third most common cause of death in the United States and the primary cause of adult disability. The direct and indirect costs of stroke are more than $41 billion annually (see the Cost of Care box on p. 974).

Pathophysiology

PATHOPHYSIOLOGIC CHANGES IN THE BRAIN

The brain is unable to store oxygen or glucose and therefore must receive a constant flow of blood to function normally. In addition, blood flow is important for the removal of metabolic waste, carbon dioxide, and lactic acid. If deprived of its blood flow, the brain can be permanently damaged within a few minutes.

Through the processes of cerebral autoregulation, blood flow is maintained at a fairly constant rate of 1000 mL/min. The cerebral arteries dilate or constrict in response to blood pressure changes or changes in carbon dioxide tension.

In a stroke, ischemia occurs in the brain tissue supplied by the affected artery, and brain dysfunction results. Ischemia leads to hypoxia or anoxia and hypoglycemia. These processes then cause infarction or death of neurons, glia, and the involved area of the brain. In addition, brain metabolism after a stroke is affected in the involved area as well as in the contralateral (opposite side) hemisphere.

Small lacunar infarcts may also occur. Lacunae are small, deep cavities within the brain that result from occlusion of a small vessel. This occlusion leads to infarct and necrosis of the area of the brain supplied by the affected vessel. Lacunar infarcts occur almost exclusively in the internal capsule, basal ganglia, and thalamus. They produce either a pure motor deficit (internal capsule) or a pure sensory deficit (thalamus). A lacunar infarct is generally regarded as a type of ischemic stroke, which is described in the next section.

COST OF CARE IMPLICATIONS FOR NURSING

STROKE

Cost of Care

- The direct and indirect costs of stroke is $41 billion annually, including medical care, lost wages, and lost productivity.
- The cost of rehabilitation is $30,000 to $50,000 per client.
- Clinical pathways for clients with strokes decrease the length of stay and costs.
- The use of specialized stroke teams to enhance the rapid diagnosis and treatment of stroke improves outcomes and decreases morbidity and mortality.

Implications for Nursing

The institution of specialized stroke teams has had a significant impact on clients with ischemic stroke. A decreased length of stay and improved outcomes has significantly affected the cost of care. Nurses must be aware of the revised focus of stroke as an emergency (much like a myocardial infarction) and the valuable contributions of the stroke team to improve client outcomes.

Data from Gonzaga-Camfield., R. (1999). Developing an emergency department team for treatment of stroke with recombinant tissue plasminogen activator. *Critical Care Nursing Clinics of North America, 11*(2), 261-268; and Hickman, J.L. (1998). Outcomes management for stroke patients using thrombolytics. *Critical Care Nursing Clinics of North America, 10*(1), 101-115.

TYPES OF STROKES

Strokes are generally classified as ischemic (occlusive) or hemorrhagic. Ischemic strokes are further divided into thrombotic strokes and embolic strokes (Table 45-1).

ISCHEMIC STROKE. An **ischemic stroke** is caused by the occlusion of a cerebral artery by either a thrombus or an embolus (Figure 45-1). A stroke that is caused by a thrombus is referred to as a thrombotic stroke, whereas a stroke caused by an embolus is referred to as an embolic stroke.

THROMBOTIC STROKE. **Thrombotic strokes** account for more than half of all strokes and are commonly associated with the development of atherosclerosis of the blood vessel wall (see Figure 45-1). Atherosclerosis is a noninflammatory degenerative disease that can affect almost any cerebral blood vessel. As a result of plaques or atheromatous deposits that gradually build up on the interior of the vessel wall, the artery loses its elasticity and hardens. The thrombus extends along the interior of the artery, gradually occluding the lumen of the artery. This process may occur over many years, and often collateral circulation to the involved area develops. As the artery becomes completely occluded, blood flow to the area is markedly diminished. Decreased blood flow causes transient ischemia, which progresses to complete ischemia and infarc-

TABLE 45-1 • DIFFERENTIAL FEATURES OF THE TYPES OF STROKE

	Ischemic		
Feature	Thrombotic	Embolic	Hemorrhagic
Evolution	Intermittent or stepwise improvement between episodes of worsening Completed stroke	Abrupt development of completed stroke Steady progression	Usually abrupt onset
Onset	Daytime (10 AM to 12 PM) Gradual (minutes to hours)	Daytime Sudden	Daytime Sudden, may be gradual if caused by hypertension
Level of consciousness	Preserved (client is awake)	Preserved (client is awake)	Deepening stupor or coma
Contributing associated factors	Hypertension Atherosclerosis	Cardiac disease	Hypertension Vessel disorders
Prodromal symptoms	Transient ischemic attack		
Neurologic deficits	Deficits during the first few weeks Slight headache Speech deficits Visual problems Confusion	Maximal deficit at onset Paralysis Expressive aphasia	Focal deficits Severe, frequent
Cerebrospinal fluid	Normal; possible presence of protein	Normal	Bloody
Seizures	No	No	Usually
Duration	Improvements over weeks to months Permanent deficits possible	Rapid improvements	Variable Permanent neurologic deficits possible

tion of the brain tissue. Within 72 hours, the area is edematous and necrotic, and cavities develop. The bifurcation (point of division) of the common carotid artery and the vertebral arteries at their junction with the basilar artery are the most common sites involved. Because of the gradual occlusion of the arteries, thrombotic strokes tend to have a slow onset.

A **lacunar stroke** is another type of thrombotic stroke. A lacunar stroke causes a soft area or cavity to develop in the white matter or deep gray matter of the brain. This type of stroke may result in significant neurologic dysfunction if it damages a critical area in the brain.

EMBOLIC STROKE. An **embolic stroke** is caused by an embolus or a group of emboli that break off from one area of the body and travel to the cerebral arteries via the carotid artery (see Figure 45-1). The usual sources of emboli are cardiac. Emboli can occur in clients with nonvalvular atrial fibrillation, ischemic heart disease, rheumatic heart disease, and mural thrombi following a myocardial infarction (MI) or insertion of a prosthetic heart valve. Another source of emboli may be plaque that breaks off from the carotid sinus or internal carotid artery. Emboli tend to become lodged in the smaller cerebral blood vessels at their point of bifurcation or where the lumen narrows. Embolic strokes account for about one third of all strokes.

The middle cerebral artery (MCA) is most commonly involved in an embolic stroke. As the emboli occlude the vessel, ischemia develops, and the client experiences the clinical manifestations of the stroke. However, the occlusion is often temporary, and the embolus breaks into smaller fragments, enters smaller blood vessels, and is absorbed. For these reasons, embolic strokes are characterized by the sudden development and rapid occurrence of focal neurologic deficits, followed by clearing of the symptoms over several hours or a few days. A cerebral hemorrhage may result if significant damage to the wall of the involved vessel has occurred.

TRANSIENT ISCHEMIC ATTACK AND REVERSIBLE ISCHEMIC NEUROLOGIC DEFICIT. Ischemic strokes are often preceded by warning signs, such as a **transient ischemic attack (TIA),** also called a "silent" stroke (Chart 45-1), or a **reversible ischemic neurologic deficit (RIND).** Both warning signs cause transient focal neurologic dysfunction due to a brief interruption in cerebral blood flow, possibly resulting from cerebral vasospasm or transient systemic arterial hypertension. The difference between a TIA and an RIND is the length of time the client is symptomatic. A TIA lasts a few minutes to fewer than 24 hours, whereas RIND symptoms last longer than 24 hours but less than a week. Both TIAs and RINDs damage the brain tissue, as evidenced by magnetic resonance imaging (MRI) or computed tomography (CT). Multiple TIAs increase the risk of major stroke.

HEMORRHAGIC STROKE. The second major classification of stroke is **hemorrhagic stroke** (see Figure 45-1). In this type of stroke, vessel integrity is interrupted, and bleeding occurs into the brain tissue or into the spaces surrounding the brain (ventricular, subdural, subarachnoid). Hemorrhage into the brain tissue generally results from a ruptured saccular (berry) aneurysm, rupture of an arteriovenous malformation or, more commonly, hypertension. Although the exact mechanisms involved are unknown, it is hypothesized that elevated systolic and diastolic pressures cause changes within the arterial wall that leave it susceptible to rupture. An intracerebral hemorrhage occurs when the vessel ruptures.

A ruptured cerebral aneurysm is another cause of hemorrhagic stroke. An aneurysm is an abnormal ballooning or blister on the involved artery (Figure 45-2). Aneurysms may be congenital or traumatic. A congenital aneurysm is a developmental defect in the media and elastica of the vessel wall. Both etiologies weaken the vessel wall. Continued force on the weakened vessel wall from elevated blood pressure stretches and thins the vessel wall. Although the rupture may occur at any time, it usually happens during activity. Aneurysms are often found at the branchings of major cerebral arteries (Figure 45-3).

Rupture of the aneurysm causes the development of an intracerebral hematoma, bleeding into the subarachnoid space, or bleeding directly into the ventricles. Vasospasm, a sudden and transient constriction of a cerebral artery, often occurs after a cerebral hemorrhage. Blood flow to distal areas of the brain supplied by the artery is markedly diminished, which

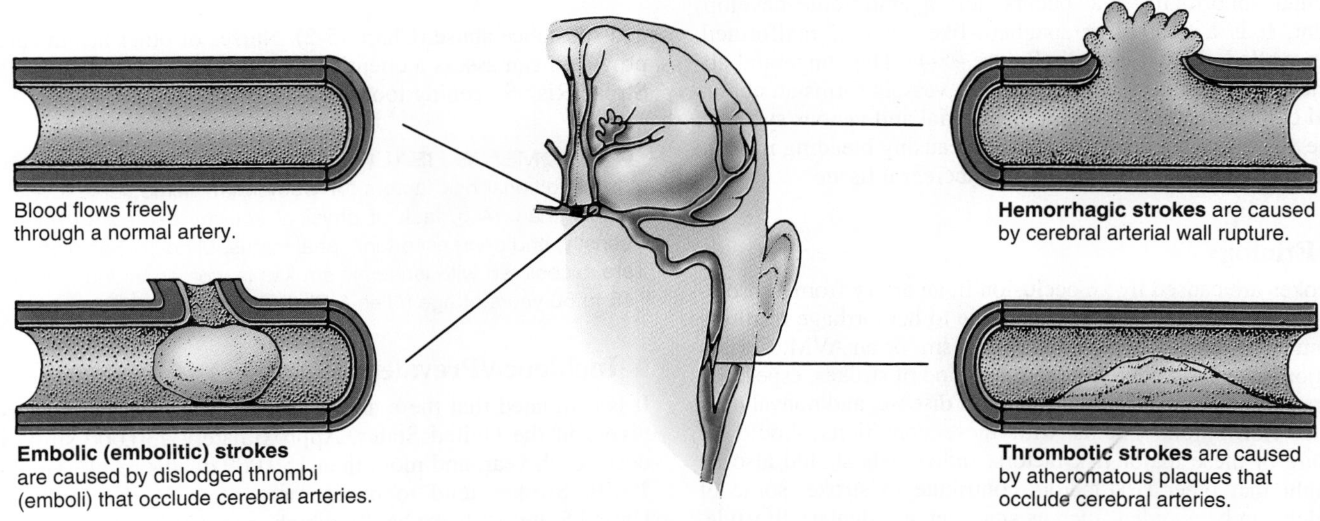

Figure 45-1 ● The types of stroke.

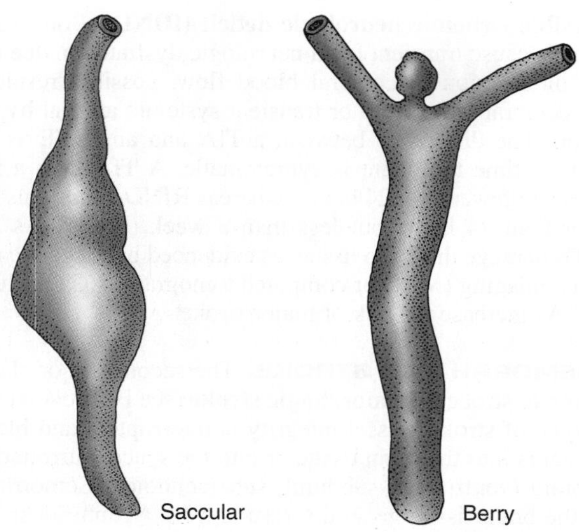

Figure 45-2 ● Two common types of cerebral aneurysms.

CHART 45-1

KEY FEATURES *of* Transient Ischemic Attack

Visual Deficits
- Blurred vision
- Diplopia (double vision)
- Blindness in one eye
- Tunnel vision

Motor Deficits
- Transient weakness (arm, hand, or leg)
- Gait disturbance (ataxic)

Sensory Deficits
- Transient numbness (face, arm, or hand)
- Vertigo

Speech Deficits
- Aphasia
- Dysarthria (slurred speech)

leads to cerebral ischemia and infarction and further neurologic dysfunction.

An **arteriovenous malformation (AVM)** is a developmental abnormality that occurs during embryonic development. It is a tangled or spaghetti-like mass of malformed, thin-walled, dilated vessels (Figure 45-4). The congenital absence of a capillary network in these vessels forms an abnormal communication between the arterial and venous systems. The vessels may eventually rupture, causing bleeding into the subarachnoid space or into the intracerebral tissue.

Etiology

Strokes are caused by an occlusion in an artery from a thrombus or an embolus; they are also due to hemorrhage resulting from hypertension, a ruptured aneurysm, or an AVM. Certain major risk factors increase the likelihood of strokes, especially hypertension, diabetes mellitus, heart disease, and nonvalvular atrial fibrillation. Clients with these conditions should be aware of these major risk factors. Individuals should also be taught that other risk factors contribute to stroke, some of which can be avoided, such as smoking, a sedentary lifestyle, and substance abuse (Chart 45-2). Nurses or other health care providers can assess a client's risk for stroke by completing a Stroke Risk Screening tool (Figure 45-5).

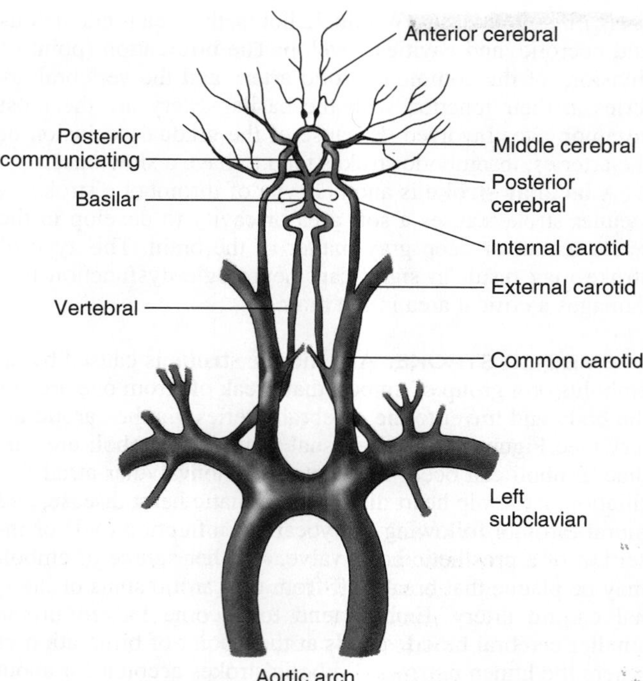

Figure 45-3 ● Common locations for cerebral aneurysms.

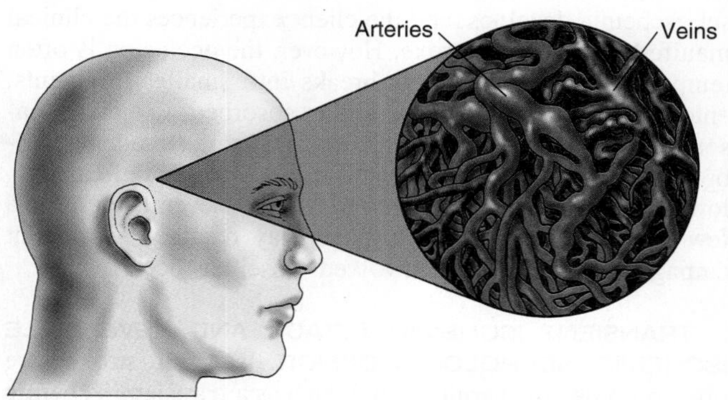

Figure 45-4 ● Appearance of an arteriovenous malformation. Note the dilated, entangled blood vessels.

WOMEN'S HEALTH CONSIDERATIONS

Additional risk factors for women are hemoglobin levels higher than 14 g, lack of physical activity, decreased bone density, and decreased functional status. Migraine headaches are associated with ischemic strokes in women younger than 45 to 50 years of age (Allen & Phillips, 1997).

Incidence/Prevalence

It is estimated that there are more than 3 million stroke survivors in the United States. Approximately 730,000 strokes occur each year, and more than 150,000 deaths result (Hock, 1999). Strokes tend to occur more often in the southern United States ("stroke belt"), which is probably related to the

CHART 45-2

CLIENT EDUCATION GUIDE
Common Risk Factors for Developing a Stroke

- Atrial fibrillation or heart murmur
- Myocardial infarction
- Previous stroke or transient ischemic attack (TIA)
- Heart surgery
- Diabetes mellitus
- Smoking
- Substance abuse (particularly cocaine)
- Obesity
- Sedentary lifestyle
- Oral contraceptive use
- Elevated serum cholesterol, lipoprotein, triglyceride, low-density lipoprotein (LDL) and high-density lipoprotein (HDL) levels
- Previous stroke or TIA
- Heavy alcohol use
- Sudden discontinuation of antihypertensive medications (causes hemorrhagic stroke)
- Heredity/familial tendency
- Migraines
- Older age
- Male
- African American heritage
- Sickle cell anemia
- Use of phenylpropanolamine (PPA), which is found in antihistamine drugs (causes catastrophic strokes, primarily in young and middle-aged women)
- Hypercoagulable states

geographic distribution of the older population, an increased use of tobacco, increased obesity, and a diet higher in fats. The number of strokes occurring in the younger population is increasing as a result of chronic intravenous (IV) drug abuse. Those using crack cocaine experience an increased incidence of stroke due to changes in the clotting mechanism caused by the drugs or the sudden increase in systolic blood pressure.

CONSIDERATIONS FOR OLDER ADULTS

Strokes may occur at any age. However, they usually occur in people older than 60 years, with an increased frequency in people older than 65 years. After 65 years, the incidence doubles in each successive decade (Hock, 1999). Males have a higher rate of stroke than females by a 3:1 ratio.

CULTURAL CONSIDERATIONS

African Americans are affected by stroke more often than other groups, possibly as a result of the high frequency of hypertension and diabetes in this group. A study of 660,000 medical records of clients 15 to 44 years of age found that ischemic strokes were twice as common in African Americans as in Caucasians; hemorrhagic strokes were three times more common among African Americans (Allen & Phillips, 1997).

SIMON Activity Link

COLLABORATIVE MANAGEMENT

Assessment

HISTORY

An accurate history is important in the diagnosis of a stroke. The information obtained assists in identifying the area of the brain involved as well as the cause. The nurse obtains a history of the client's activity when the stroke began. Ischemic strokes often occur during sleep, whereas hemorrhagic strokes tend to occur during activity. Next, the nurse asks the client or a family member how the symptoms progressed. The nurse also elicits a history of the onset of the stroke. Symptoms of an embolic or hemorrhagic stroke tend to occur abruptly, whereas thrombotic strokes generally have a more gradual progression. The nurse must also determine the severity of the symptoms, such as whether they worsened after the initial onset (hemorrhagic stroke) or began to improve (embolic stroke). It is important to determine whether the symptoms come and go, possibly indicating a transient ischemic attack (TIA) or a reversible ischemic neurologic deficit (RIND).

During the interview, the nurse observes the client's level of consciousness (LOC) and assesses for indications of intellectual or memory impairments or difficulties with speech or hearing. The client or family member is questioned about the presence of any sensory or motor changes, visual problems, problems with balance or gait, and changes in reading or writing abilities.

In addition, the nurse asks about the client's medical history, with specific attention directed toward a history of head trauma, diabetes, hypertension, heart disease, anemia, obesity, and headache. The nurse also obtains a list of current medications, including prescribed, over-the-counter, and recreational (illicit) drugs. Medications that could contribute to stroke include anticoagulants, aspirin, vasodilators, and illegal drugs. To complete the history, the nurse obtains data about the client's social history, including education, employment, travel, leisure activities, and personal habits (e.g., smoking, diet, exercise pattern, and drug and alcohol use).

PHYSICAL ASSESSMENT/CLINICAL MANIFESTATIONS

NEUROLOGIC ASSESSMENT. The nurse performs a neurologic assessment of the client. Specific neurologic signs and other signs and symptoms depend on the extent and location of the ischemia and the arteries involved (Chart 45-3).

COGNITIVE CHANGES. The client may exhibit a variety of cognitive problems in addition to changes in LOC. LOC may vary depending on the extent of increased intracranial pressure (ICP) caused by the stroke. The nurse assesses for indications of denial of the illness; neglect syndrome or hemiparesis; spatial and proprioceptive (awareness of body position in space) dysfunction; impairment of memory, judgment, or problem-solving and decision-making abilities; and decreased ability to concentrate and attend to tasks. Dysfunction in one or more of these areas may be more pronounced, depending on the hemisphere involved (Chart 45-4).

The right cerebral hemisphere is more involved with visual and spatial awareness and proprioception. A person who has a stroke involving the right cerebral hemisphere is often unaware of any deficits and may be disoriented to time and place. Personality changes include impulsivity and poor judgment. The left cerebral hemisphere, the dominant hemisphere in all but about 15% to 20% of the population, is the center for language, mathematic skills, and analytic thinking. Therefore a left hemisphere stroke results in **aphasia** (inability to use or comprehend language), **alexia** (reading problems), and **agraphia** (difficulty

STROKE RISK SCREENING

Site and address of Screening ________________________________ Date:____/____/____

PART I - DEMOGRAPHICS, AGE AND ETHNICITY

Name: (last)________________________ (first) ________________________ (middle initial)____

Gender: __ Male __Female Highest Level of Education: ___ High School or less ___ College ___ Graduate School

Address:________________________(city)__________(state)______(zip)_____(county)______

Phone: Home (___)__________ Work (___)__________ Date of Birth:___/___/___ Age today_____

Do you have a primary health care provider? .... _____Yes_____No

Have you seen a health care provider in the past year? .... _____Yes_____No

Do you have medical insurance? .... _____Yes_____No

Ethnicity/Race: ____ African American ____Caucasian ____Hispanic White ____ Hispanic Non-White

____ Asian/Pacific Islander ____ American Indian or Alaskan Native ____ Other or Unknown

PART II - HISTORY FOR KNOWN AND ESTABLISHED HIGH RISK FACTORS FOR STROKE

1. Have you ever been told that you have high blood pressure? .... _____Yes_____No
2. Do you take medication for high blood pressure? .... _____Yes_____No
3. Do you have a history of abnormal heart rate or rhythm called atrial fibrillation? .... _____Yes_____No
4. Have you ever been checked for or been told that you have narrowing of the arteries to the brain? .... _____Yes_____No
5. Have you had a heart attack, heart bypass surgery, angioplasty or another disease of the heart? .... _____Yes_____No
6. Have you had a previous stroke, mini-stroke or TIA? .... _____Yes_____No
7. Do you have diabetes mellitus (DM) or are you on insulin or medication for high blood sugar? .... _____Yes_____No
8. Have you ever smoked cigarettes? .... _____Yes_____No
9. Do you currently smoke cigarettes? .... _____Yes_____No

PART III - HISTORY FOR SIGNIFICANT BUT SLIGHTLY LOWER RISK FACTORS FOR STROKE

10. Has a family member had a stroke or heart attack when they were less than 45 years of age? .... _____Yes_____No
11. Do you consume more than two ounces of alcohol per day on a daily basis? .... _____Yes_____No
12. Do you have a cholesterol level greater than 200? .... _____Yes_____No

PART IV - HISTORY OF OTHER/UNCOMMON IMPORTANT RISK FACTORS FOR STROKE

13. Do you smoke cigarettes and take birth control pills? .... _____Yes_____No
14. Do you have Sickle Cell Anemia? .... _____Yes_____No
15. Do you use one or more of the following drugs: Cocaine, Crack, Heroin, Amphetamines? .... _____Yes_____No
16. Are you overweight or obese? .... _____Yes_____No
17. Do you consider your activity level as generally inactive? .... _____Yes_____No

Figure 45-5 ● Stroke Risk Screening Tool.

PART V - BLOOD PRESSURE AND PULSE

Blood Pressure (BP) recorded sitting ____________(Systolic)__________(Diastolic) ______ Right Arm ______Left Arm

Radial Pulse rate for 60 seconds (beats/minute) ______________________ Irregular pulse rate?________Yes______No

PART VI - IDENTIFICATION OF RISK FOR STROKE AND RECOMMENDATION

1. ______ **Low Risk for Stroke:**

Under the age of 55, responded "**NO**" to questions 1-17 (self-reported risk factors) and was not identified to have an irregular pulse rate or a measured Systolic BP equal to or greater than or equal to 140 or Diastolic equal to or greater than 90.

RECOMMENDATION: Take this completed screening form to your health care provider at your next appointment.

2. ______ **Moderate Risk for Stroke:**

Age equal to or greater than 55 with no self-reported risk factors and no risk factors identified on screening

OR - Age up to 64 with one self-reported risk factor, or an irregular pulse rate or a measured Systolic BP equal to or greater than 140 or a Diastolic equal to or greater than 90.

RECOMMENDATION: Notify your health care provider within a week with the results of your screening and request an appointment for an evaluation and care to prevent a stroke.

3. ______ **High Risk for Stroke:**

Age equal to or greater than 65 with one self-reported risk factor, or irregular pulse, or a measured Systolic BP equal to or greater than 140 or a Diastolic BP equal to or greater than 90.

OR - Any age with **two or more risk factors**, either self-reported and/or identified on measurement of an irregular pulse or Systolic BP equal to or greater than 140 or a Diastolic equal to or greater than 90.

RECOMMENDATION: Notify your health care provider TODAY with the results of your screening and request an appointment for an evaluation of your risks for stroke and care to prevent a stroke.

4. ______ **PRESENTS WITH WARNING SIGNS OF STROKE, OR TIA (MINI-STROKE)**
RECOMMENDATION: CALL OR HAVE SOMEONE CALL 9-1-1 IMMEDIATELY!

PART VII - THE EARLY WARNING SIGNS OF STROKE

*** SUDDEN WEAKNESS, NUMBNESS, OR PARALYSIS OF THE FACE, ARM OR LEG, ON ONE OR BOTH SIDES OF THE BODY**

*** SUDDEN BLURRED VISION OR BLINDNESS IN ONE OR BOTH EYES**

*** SUDDEN DIFFICULTY SPEAKING, SLURRING OF SPEECH OR DIFFICULTY UNDERSTANDING**

*** SUDDEN SEVERE HEADACHE WITH SUDDEN ONSET THAT OCCURS WITHOUT APPARENT REASON**

*** SUDDEN LOSS OF BALANCE, DIZZINESS, OR FALLING WITHOUT ANY APPARENT REASON**

CALL 9-1-1 IMMEDIATELY IF YOU EXPERIENCE ANY OF THESE SYMPTOMS

I have received a screening for the risk of stroke and agree to follow up with the recommendations. I understand this is only a screening. I agree that this data can be entered into a database for research without identifying me by name.

(Signature of Participant)____________________**Signature of Health care provider**____________________

The **Stroke Risk Screening** was developed in 1999 jointly by the Division on Research, Delaware Nurses Association and Ellen Barker, MSN, RN, CNRN, Neuroscience Nursing Consultants, Wilmington, Delaware. Marian P. LaMonte, M.D., M.S.N., Assistant Professor of Neurology and Co-Director of the Maryland Brain Attack Center, University of Maryland Medical Center, Baltimore, Maryland, served as Nurse/Neurologist advisor. There is no Copyright and permission is not needed to duplicate this form.

Figure 45-5, cont'd ● Stroke Risk Screening Tool.

CHART 45-3

KEY FEATURES *of* Stroke Syndromes

Middle Cerebral Artery Strokes
- Contralateral hemiparesis: arm > leg
- Contralateral sensory deficit
- Homonymous hemianopsia
- Unilateral neglect or inattention
- Aphasia, anomia, alexia, agraphia, and acalculia
- Impaired vertical sensation
- Spatial deficit
- Perceptual deficit
- Visual field deficit
- Altered level of consciousness: drowsy to comatose

Posterior Cerebral Artery Strokes
- Perseveration
- Aphasia, amnesia, alexia, agraphia, visual agnosia, and ataxia
- Loss of deep sensation
- Decreased touch sensation
- Possible choreoathetoid movements
- Stupor; coma

Internal Carotid Artery Strokes
- Contralateral hemiparesis
- Sensory deficit
- Hemianopsia, blurred vision, blindness
- Aphasia (dominant side)
- Headache
- Bruit

Anterior Cerebral Artery Strokes
- Contralateral hemiparesis: leg > arm
- Bladder incontinence
- Personality and behavior changes
- Aphasia, gait apraxia, and amnesia
- Positive grasp and sucking reflex
- Perseveration
- Sensory deficit (lower extremity)
- Memory impairment
- Apraxic gait

Vertebrobasilar Artery Strokes
- Headache and vertigo
- Coma
- Memory loss and confusion
- Flaccid paralysis
- Areflexia, ataxia, and vertigo
- Cranial nerve dysfunction
- Dysconjugate gaze
- Visual deficits (uniorbital) and homonymous hemianopsia
- Sensory loss: numbness

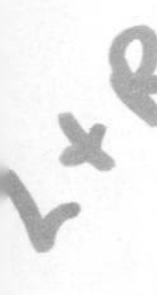

CHART 45-4

KEY FEATURES *of* Left and Right Hemisphere Strokes

Feature	Left Hemisphere*	Right Hemisphere
Language	Aphasia Agraphia Alexia (word blindness)	Impaired sense of humor
Memory	Possible deficit	Disorientation to time, place, and person Inability to recognize faces
Vision	Inability to discriminate words and letters Reading problems Deficits in the right visual field	Visual spatial deficits Neglect of the left visual field Loss of depth perception
Behavior	Slowness Cautiousness Anxiety when attempting a new task Depression or a catastrophic response to illness Sense of guilt Feeling of worthlessness Worries over future Quick anger and frustration Intellectual impairment	Impulsiveness Lack of awareness of neurologic deficits Confabulation Euphoria Constant smiling Denial of illness Poor judgment Overestimation of abilities (risk for injury)
Hearing	No deficit	Loss of ability to hear tonal variations

*Location for speech in all but 15% to 20% of people.

with writing). Persons with left-hemisphere strokes tend to be slow and cautious.

MOTOR CHANGES. The motor examination provides information about which cerebral hemisphere is involved. A right **hemiplegia** (paralysis on one side of the body) or **hemiparesis** (weakness on one side of the body) indicates a stroke involving the left cerebral hemisphere, because the motor nerve fibers cross in the medulla before entering the spinal cord and periphery. Conversely, a left hemiplegia or hemiparesis indicates a stroke in the right cerebral hemisphere.

In collaboration with the physical and occupational therapist, the nurse gauges the client's muscle tone. The client with hypotonia, or flaccidity, is unable to overcome the forces of gravity, and the extremities tend to fall to the side. The extremities feel heavy, and muscle tone is inadequate for balance, equilibrium, or protective mechanisms. Hypertonia (spastic paralysis) tends to cause fixed positions or contractures of the involved extremities. Range of motion (ROM) of the joints is restricted, and shoulder subluxation may easily occur from either spasticity or flaccidity. The nurse also assesses proprioception (position sense), head and trunk control, balance, coordination, and gait.

Loss of inhibitory nervous control from the cerebral cortex results in a spastic (upper motor neuron), uninhibited bladder. Bowel function may also be affected.

SENSORY CHANGES. The sensory examination evaluates the client's response to touch and painful stimuli. The client who has had a stroke may be unable to write, comprehend reading material, use an object correctly **(agnosia),** or carry out a purposeful motor activity **(apraxia).**

The nurse also evaluates for indications of **neglect syndrome,** which is particularly evident with strokes in the right

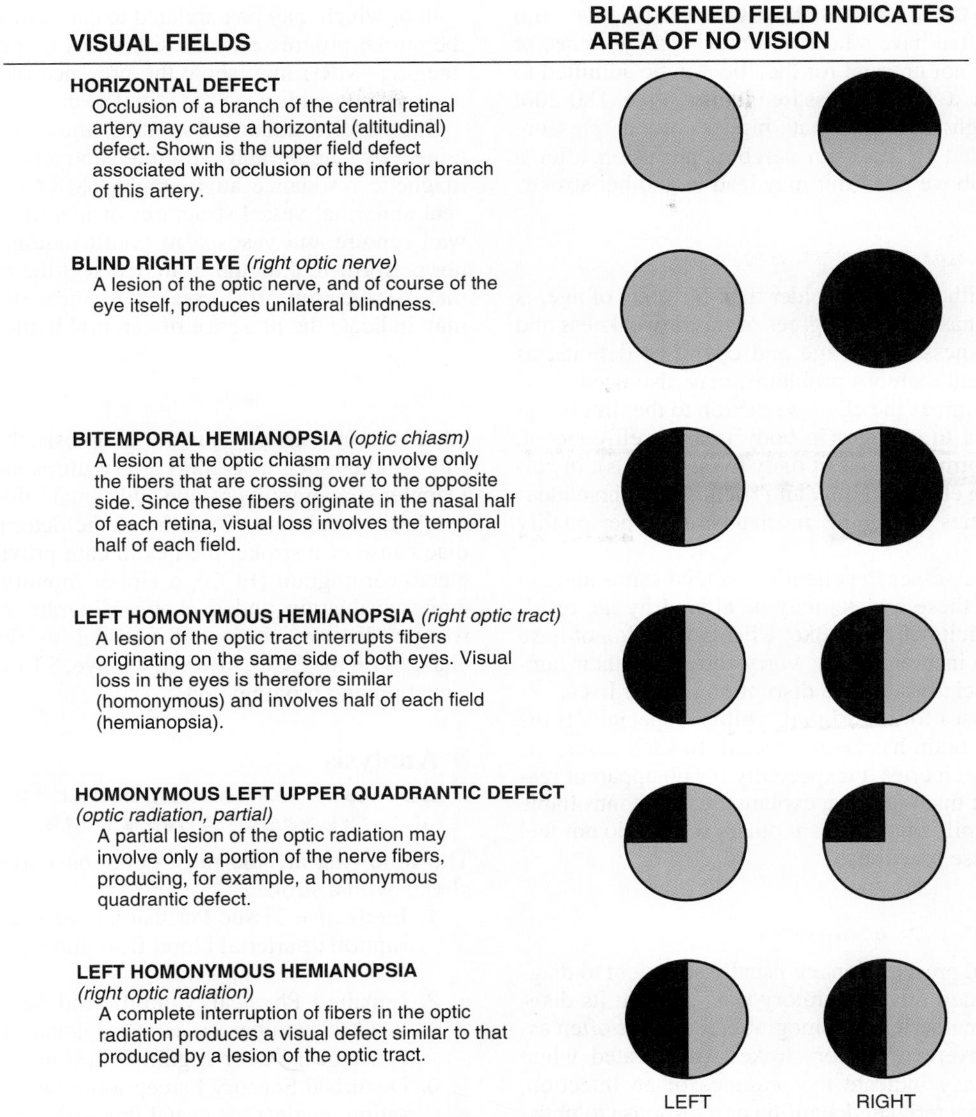

VISUAL FIELDS	BLACKENED FIELD INDICATES AREA OF NO VISION
HORIZONTAL DEFECT Occlusion of a branch of the central retinal artery may cause a horizontal (altitudinal) defect. Shown is the upper field defect associated with occlusion of the inferior branch of this artery.	
BLIND RIGHT EYE *(right optic nerve)* A lesion of the optic nerve, and of course of the eye itself, produces unilateral blindness.	
BITEMPORAL HEMIANOPSIA *(optic chiasm)* A lesion at the optic chiasm may involve only the fibers that are crossing over to the opposite side. Since these fibers originate in the nasal half of each retina, visual loss involves the temporal half of each field.	
LEFT HOMONYMOUS HEMIANOPSIA *(right optic tract)* A lesion of the optic tract interrupts fibers originating on the same side of both eyes. Visual loss in the eyes is therefore similar (homonymous) and involves half of each field (hemianopsia).	
HOMONYMOUS LEFT UPPER QUADRANTIC DEFECT *(optic radiation, partial)* A partial lesion of the optic radiation may involve only a portion of the nerve fibers, producing, for example, a homonymous quadrantic defect.	
LEFT HOMONYMOUS HEMIANOPSIA *(right optic radiation)* A complete interruption of fibers in the optic radiation produces a visual defect similar to that produced by a lesion of the optic tract.	LEFT RIGHT

Figure 45-6 ● Visual field defects produced by selected lesions in the visual pathways. (Modified from Bates, B. [2000]. *Bates' guide to physical examination and history taking* [7th ed.]. Philadelphia: J.B. Lippincott.)

cerebral hemisphere. In this syndrome, the client is unaware of the existence of his or her left or paralyzed side. The typical picture is that of the client sitting in a wheelchair, leaning to the left with the arm caught in the wheelchair wheel. When questioned, the client often states that everything is fine and believes that he or she is sitting up straight in the chair. Another typical example of neglect syndrome is the client who washes or dresses only one side of the body.

Another important part of the nursing assessment focuses on visual ability. Infarction or ischemia involving the carotid artery may cause pupillary abnormalities, **ptosis** (eyelid drooping), visual field deficits, or pallor and petechiae of the conjunctiva. **Amaurosis fugax,** a brief episode of blindness in one eye, results from retinal ischemia caused by ophthalmic or carotid artery insufficiency. **Hemianopsia,** or blindness in half of the visual field, results from damage to the optic tract or occipital lobe. Most often this deficit occurs as homonymous hemianopsia, in which there is blindness in the same side of both eyes (Figure 45-6). The client with this condition must turn his or her head to scan the complete range of vision. Otherwise, he or she does not see half of the visual field. For example, the client eats only half of a meal because that is the only portion seen.

CRANIAL NERVE INTACTNESS. The nurse conducts an assessment of the client's ability to chew (cranial nerve [CN] V) and swallow (CNs IX and X). In addition, the nurse notes any facial paralysis or paresis (CN VII), absent gag reflex (CN IX), or impaired tongue movement (CN XII). The client who has difficulty chewing or swallowing foods and liquids is at risk for aspiration pneumonia and may become constipated from inadequate fluid intake.

CARDIOVASCULAR ASSESSMENT. Clients with embolic strokes often have a heart murmur, dysrhythmias, or hypertension. It is not unusual for the client to be admitted to the hospital with a blood pressure greater than 180-200/110-120. Although a somewhat higher blood pressure (150/100) is needed to maintain cerebral perfusion after a stroke, pressures above this limit may lead to another stroke.

PSYCHOSOCIAL ASSESSMENT

A typical client with a stroke is older than 60 years of age, is hypertensive, and has varying degrees of motor weakness and level of consciousness. Language and cognitive deficits, as well as behavior and memory problems, may also occur.

The nurse determines the client's reaction to the illness, especially in relation to changes in body image, self-concept, and ability to perform activities of daily living (ADLs). In collaboration with the client's family and friends, the nurse identifies any difficulties in coping mechanisms or personality changes.

The nurse also assesses the client's financial status and occupation, because these aspects may be altered by the residual neurologic deficits of the stroke. Clients who do not have disability or health insurance may worry about how their family will cope financially with the disruption in their lives.

The nurse assesses for **emotional lability,** especially if the frontal lobe of the brain has been affected. In such cases, the client laughs and then cries unexpectedly for no apparent reason. It is important that the nurse explain these uncontrollable emotions to the family or significant others so they do not feel responsible for these reactions.

LABORATORY ASSESSMENT

Clinical history and presentation are usually sufficient to diagnose a stroke. No definitive laboratory tests confirm its diagnosis. Elevated hematocrit and hemoglobin levels are often associated with a severe or major stroke. An elevated white blood cell count may indicate the presence of an infection, possibly subacute bacterial endocarditis or a response to physiologic stress. The health care provider typically orders a prothrombin time (PT) or International Normalized Ratio (INR), as well as a partial thromboplastin time (PTT), to establish baseline coagulation information in case anticoagulation therapy is initiated. These diagnostic tests may also provide supportive evidence that a hemorrhagic stroke has occurred. If there is no indication of increased intracranial pressure (ICP), a lumbar puncture may be performed to obtain cerebrospinal fluid (CSF) for analysis. Blood in the spinal fluid or a high red blood cell count in the CSF is indicative of a subarachnoid hemorrhage.

RADIOGRAPHIC ASSESSMENT

Computed tomography (CT) assists in the differential diagnosis of a stroke. The primary purpose of the initial scan is to identify the presence of a hemorrhage or cerebral aneurysm. This diagnostic test shows the presence of ischemia and is invaluable in establishing baseline information for future comparison in case the client's condition deteriorates. In addition, the scans enable the physician to identify pathologic changes that may mimic a stroke, such as a brain tumor or a hematoma, both of which may be unrelated to cerebrovascular disease. As the stroke progresses, later CT scans or magnetic resonance imaging (MRI) may show the presence of edema and tissue necrosis not evident on the initial scan.

Information about the status of the cerebral vessels is obtained by angiography, digital subtraction angiography, or magnetic resonance angiography (MRA). These studies reveal abnormal vessel structures or identify the area of vessel wall rupture and vasospasm. Skull radiography is generally not performed, although it may detect the presence of abnormal calcification of a vessel or a pineal shift, both of which may indicate the presence of cerebral hemorrhage.

OTHER DIAGNOSTIC ASSESSMENT

An MRI may assist with the diagnosis. Noninvasive blood flow studies such as carotid artery ultrasound or transcranial Doppler sonography provide additional information about the cerebral vasculature. To assist in the determination of a cardiac cause of a stroke, the health care provider may order an electrocardiogram (ECG), a Holter monitor test, cardiac enzymes evaluation, and an echocardiogram. As with other neurologic diseases, it is not unusual to find the following changes on the ECG: inverted T wave, ST depression, and QT elevation and prolongation.

Analysis

COMMON NURSING DIAGNOSES AND COLLABORATIVE PROBLEMS

The following are the most common nursing diagnoses for clients with a stroke:

1. Ineffective Tissue Perfusion (Cerebral) related to interruption of arterial blood flow and a possible increase in ICP
2. Impaired Physical Mobility and Self-Care Deficit related to hemiparesis or hemiplegia, decreased level of consciousness, or cognitive dysfunction
3. Disturbed Sensory Perception related to decreased sensation, neglect, or visual impairment
4. Unilateral Neglect related to right cerebral hemisphere dysfunction or hemianopsia
5. Impaired Verbal Communication related to decreased circulation in the brain
6. Impaired Swallowing related to weakness of the muscles necessary for swallowing and a decreased gag reflex
7. Total Urinary Incontinence and Bowel Incontinence related to neurologic dysfunction, decreased sensation, cognitive dysfunction, immobility, or expressive aphasia

ADDITIONAL NURSING DIAGNOSES AND COLLABORATIVE PROBLEMS

In addition to the common nursing diagnoses, clients with stroke may have one or more of the following:

- Risk for Aspiration related to impaired swallowing
- Disturbed Body Image related to physical or cognitive disability
- Ineffective Role Performance related to a change in physical capacity to perform role
- Risk for Injury related to neglect syndrome, visual disturbances, and paralysis or weakness

- Sexual Dysfunction related to altered body function
- Constipation related to lack of adequate fluid intake, immobility, or lack of physical activity

Additional collaborative problems include the following:

- Potential for Deep Vein Thrombosis
- Potential for Increased Intracranial Pressure
- Potential for Seizures
- Potential for Hypoxemia
- Potential for Atelectasis and Pneumonia

CRITICAL THINKING CHALLENGE

An older adult is admitted to the emergency department with complaints of a severe headache and dizziness. He states that he was doing yard work when he started feeling "strange" and lightheaded. He has a history of hypertension and has been taking medication for it.

- What other information will you need to collect to complete his history?
- What physical assessment findings should you monitor for?
- During his interview, the client begins to get drowsy and vomits in a projectile manner. What pathologic change do you suspect, and what should you do now?

For suggested answer guidelines, go to SIMON http://www.wbsaunders.com/SIMON/Iggy/.

Planning and Implementation

INEFFECTIVE TISSUE PERFUSION (CEREBRAL)

NOC **PLANNING: EXPECTED OUTCOMES.** The client with a stroke is expected to maintain intracranial pressure within normal limits (WNL), maintain or improve level of consciousness, and not experience additional neurologic problems (e.g., seizures).

INTERVENTIONS. Interventions are primarily determined by the type and extent of the stroke (see the Clinical Pathway for ischemic cerebral infarction [mild to moderate] on pp. 1839-1847). For selected clients with ischemic strokes, early intervention with thrombolytic therapy to dissolve the clot can prevent neurologic deficits if implemented within 3 hours of the onset of stroke.

Unless major medical complications occur, the health care provider manages the client conservatively with drug therapy and aggressive rehabilitation to promote an optimal level of well-being and function. In some cases, the physician may need to intervene surgically to prevent further neurologic dysfunction.

NONSURGICAL MANAGEMENT. Nursing interventions are initially aimed at monitoring for neurologic changes or complications associated with stroke. The client is at risk for continued progression of the stroke or increased intracranial pressure (ICP) (Chart 45-5). The nurse performs a neurologic assessment when the client is admitted to the hospital and at the beginning of each nursing shift. Periodic neurologic checks using the Glasgow Coma Scale (GCS) (see Chapter 41) or other neurologic assessment tools are indicated at least every 4 hours or more, depending on the client's condition.

NIC ***INTRACRANIAL PRESSURE MONITORING.*** The client is most at risk for increased ICP resulting from edema during the first 72 hours after onset of the stroke (Chart 45-6). The nurse must be alert for symptoms of increased ICP and report any deterioration in the client's neurologic status to the health care provider.

CHART 45-5

KEY FEATURES *of* Increased Intracranial Pressure

- Decreased level of consciousness (lethargy to coma)
- Behavior changes: restlessness, irritability, and confusion
- Headache
- Nausea and vomiting
- Change in speech pattern
- Aphasia
- Slurred speech
- Change in sensorimotor status
- Pupillary changes: dilated and nonreactive or constricted and nonreactive pupils
- Cranial nerve dysfunction
- Ataxia
- Seizures
- Cushing's triad
- Abnormal posturing
  - Decerebrate
  - Decorticate

CHART 45-6

NIC INTERVENTION ACTIVITIES *for* The Client with a Stroke

Intracranial Pressure Monitoring: *Measurement and interpretation of client data to regulate intracranial pressure*

- Assist with ICP monitoring device insertion.
- Provide information to family/significant others.
- Calibrate and level the transducer.
- Set alarms.
- Record ICP pressure readings and analyze waveforms.
- Note client's change in response to stimuli.
- Monitor cerebral perfusion pressure.
- Monitor client's ICP and neurological response to care activities.
- Monitor intake and output.
- Monitor insertion site for infection.
- Monitor temperature and WBC count.
- Administer pharmacologic agents to maintain ICP within specified range.
- Space nursing care to minimize ICP elevation.
- Notify health care provider for elevated ICP that does not respond to treatment protocols.

NIC intervention activities selected from McCloskey, J.C., & Bulechek, G.M. (Eds.). (2000). *Nursing interventions classification (NIC)* (3rd ed.). St. Louis: Mosby. No part of this work is to be altered without prior written permission from the Publisher.
ICP, Intracranial pressure; *WBC,* white blood cell.

The nurse elevates the head of the client's bed to 30 degrees (or as ordered) and maintains the head in a midline, neutral position to facilitate venous drainage from the brain. In collaboration with the health care team, the nurse plans care to avoid activities and procedures that may increase ICP, particularly if the client has focal neurologic deficits and indications of cerebral edema. Extreme hip and neck flexion should be avoided. Extreme hip flexion may increase intrathoracic pressure, whereas extreme neck flexion prohibits venous drainage from the brain.

Additional management measures include avoiding the clustering of nursing procedures (e.g., giving a bath followed immediately by changing the bed linen) and hyperoxygenating the client before suctioning (if needed). The nurse should fully assess the need for suctioning because it may increase ICP. A quiet environment is particularly important for the client experiencing a headache, which is common with an aneurysm or increased ICP. The client may have **photophobia** (sensitivity to light); therefore the nurse or assistive nursing personnel should keep the room lights lowered.

Vital signs are monitored closely, at least every 4 hours. The nurse notifies the health care provider if the blood pressure exceeds acceptable levels. Generally, the health care provider allows the client to be slightly hypertensive (150/100) to facilitate adequate cerebral tissue perfusion. A higher blood pressure could lead to a hemorrhagic stroke or rebleeding of an aneurysm (if present).

Clients admitted to a critical care unit are connected to a cardiac monitor and observed for dysrhythmias. The nurse performs a cardiac assessment, with particular attention directed toward auscultation of heart sounds to identify the presence of cardiac murmurs or atrial fibrillation (AF). Murmurs or AF may place the client at increased risk for emboli. Hemodynamic monitoring may be needed to monitor and evaluate physiologic stability and response to therapy. (See also Chapter 33 for a discussion of AF.)

DRUG THERAPY. The types of medications prescribed by the health care provider for a stroke depends on the type of stroke and the resulting neurologic dysfunction (see Chart 45-6). In general, the goals of drug therapy are to prevent further thrombotic episodes (anticoagulation), increase blood flow, and protect the neurons (cytoprotection).

Thrombolytic Therapy. Thrombolytic therapy for an acute ischemic stroke (AIS) dissolves the cerebral artery occlusion to reestablish blood flow and prevent cerebral infarction. Recombinant tissue plasminogen activator (rt-PA) is the first definitive drug with Food and Drug Administration (FDA) approval for the treatment of acute ischemic stroke (Hock, 1999). Clients must meet strict eligibility criteria for rt-PA administration. Stroke or serious head injury in the past 3 months, hemorrhagic stroke, recent myocardial infarction (MI), increased partial thromboplastin time (PTT), anticoagulant therapy, or pregnancy excludes clients from rt-PA administration. The stroke should be verified by CT imaging, and the rt-PA should be given within 3 hours of the onset of symptoms (Adams et al., 1996; Hock, 1999).

Anticoagulants. The use of anticoagulants and antiplatelet agents to treat stroke is also controversial and depends on the health care provider's preference. The principal drugs used are aspirin, heparin, low–molecular weight heparin (enoxaparin [Lovenox]), and warfarin (Coumadin). If the client received a thrombolytic, an IV anticoagulant is usually ordered as a follow-up treatment.

The provider typically orders sodium heparin (Hepalean🍁) subcutaneously or via a continuous IV infusion to prevent the progression of transient ischemic attacks (TIAs) or evolving strokes. Baseline prothrombin time (PT) and partial thromboplastin time (PTT) values are usually obtained before the initiation of heparin therapy, 6 to 8 hours after the start of the infusion, and every morning while the client is receiving heparin therapy. The therapeutic goal is to achieve 1.5 to 2 times the client's normal baseline PT and PTT values. PT is used to monitor oral anticoagulant therapy, whereas PTT is used to monitor heparin therapy. The World Health Organization advocates the use of the International Normalized Ratio (INR) to monitor warfarin therapy. The target INR value for most clients with strokes is 2.0 to 3.0; for strokes of cardiac origin, the goal is usually 3.0 to 4.5.

Sodium heparin and other anticoagulants, such as warfarin (Coumadin, Warfilone🍁), may cause bleeding. The nurse observes for signs of blood in the urine or stool, epistaxis, bleeding gums, and easy bruising. Anticoagulant therapy is contraindicated in clients who have ulcers, uremia, or hepatic failure.

Enteric-coated or other forms of aspirin (Ancasal🍁) have proved useful primarily in the prevention of recurrent stroke or embolic stroke. These drugs prevent blood clotting by reducing platelet adhesiveness. Other commonly used **antiplatelet medications** include ticlopidine hydrochloride (Ticlid), clopidogrel (Plavix), and dipyridamole (Persantine, Apo-Dipyridamole🍁). These agents can cause bruising, hemorrhage, and liver disease. The nurse teaches the client to report any unusual bruising or bleeding to the health care provider. Liver function and coagulation studies are carefully monitored during the course of drug therapy. Plavix should be taken with food to prevent gastric distress.

Other Drugs. The health care provider may prescribe antiepileptic drugs (AEDs), such as phenytoin (Dilantin), gabapentin (Neurontin), or topiramate (Topamax), to treat seizures if they occur. Calcium channel blockers (e.g., nimodipine [Nimotop]) are used to treat cerebral vasospasm, which usually occurs between 4 and 14 days after the stroke, inhibits blood flow to the area, and worsens ischemia. These drugs work by relaxing the smooth muscles of the vessel wall and reducing the incidence and severity of the spasm, thus improving neurologic functioning. In addition, calcium channel blockers possibly dilate collateral vessels to ischemic areas of the brain. Stool softeners, analgesics for pain, and antianxiety drugs may also be ordered.

MONITORING FOR OTHER COMPLICATIONS. The client with an aneurysm or AVM must be monitored for the presence of hydrocephalus and vasospasm. Hydrocephalus (increased cerebrospinal fluid within the brain) may occur as a consequence of blood in the cerebrospinal fluid, which prevents it from being reabsorbed properly by the arachnoid villi. Eventually the ventricles become enlarged and, if hydrocephalus is left untreated, increased intracranial pressure occurs. The nurse observes for the clinical manifestations of hydrocephalus, which include a change in the level of consciousness (LOC) (drowsy to coma), gait disturbances, and behavior changes.

Vasospasm, or a narrowing of the cerebral vessels, leads to cerebral ischemia and infarction. It is characterized by a decreased level of consciousness, motor and reflex changes, and increased neurologic deficits (e.g., cranial nerve dysfunction and aphasia). The symptoms may fluctuate with the occurrence of vasospasm.

Rebleeding or rupture is a common complication for the client with an aneurysm or AVM. It tends to occur within 24 hours of the initial bleed or rupture and 7 to 10 days later. It is manifested by severe headache, nausea and vomiting, a decreased level of consciousness, and additional neurologic deficits.

OTHER NONSURGICAL TECHNIQUES. New early techniques are being tried for clients who are not candidates for thrombolytic therapy. For example, hypothermia treatment started during the first few hours after the onset of a stroke has shown some success in reversing neurologic deficits. Cytoprotective drugs such as sodium channel blockers, opioid antagonists, free radical scavengers, glutamate receptor antagonists, calcium channel blockers, and membrane stabilizers are being tested as a therapy for stroke. No conclusive results have been demonstrated.

SURGICAL MANAGEMENT. The surgical procedure depends on the cause of the stroke.

ENDARTERECTOMY. **Carotid endarterectomy** is the most widely used surgical procedure to prevent progressing stroke in symptomatic clients with recurrent TIAs or carotid stenosis (Hock, 1999). The purpose of an endarterectomy is to remove atherosclerotic plaque from the inner lining of the carotid artery. It is hoped that this will open the artery enough to re-establish blood flow.

EXTRACRANIAL-INTRACRANIAL BYPASS. In an extracranial-intracranial bypass, the surgeon performs a craniotomy and bypasses the blocked artery by making a graft or a bypass from the first artery to the second artery. This procedure establishes blood flow around the blocked artery and re-establishes blood flow to the involved areas. Clinical trials have shown little or no differences in the effectiveness and benefit of this procedure in preventing stroke. Despite this finding, this procedure continues to be performed. The two most common techniques are the superficial middle temporal artery–to–middle cerebral artery (STA-MCA) graft and the occipital–to–posterior inferior cerebellar artery (PICA) bypass. These procedures are used only for selected clients in whom it is believed that more conservative therapy would not be beneficial.

MANAGEMENT OF ARTERIOVENOUS MALFORMATIONS. The usual treatment of an arteriovenous malformation (AVM) is interventional therapy to occlude abnormal arteries or veins. The same procedure may be performed to occlude the vessels surrounding an aneurysm. The physician inserts a microcatheter into the carotid artery, or more often into the femoral artery, and threads it to the vessel to be embolized. The physician then injects an embolic agent, such as platinum coils, detachable silicone balloons, liquid acrylic, or polyvinyl alcohol, to embolize the involved arteries (Figure 45-7). If the AVM is large, the physician may elect to occlude the artery gradually to allow a gradual change in the blood supply to the surrounding brain. In this case, the embolization procedure is carried out over 1 to 2 weeks. Whenever possible, the involved vessels are totally removed surgically. The surgeon ligates the vessels and removes the defect. Gamma radiation delivered through the gamma knife produces sloughing of the endothelial lining of the vessels to prevent further vessel enlargement. Improved microsurgical techniques have significantly reduced morbidity and mortality rates, and these procedures are becoming the treatment of choice in many medical centers.

MANAGEMENT OF CEREBRAL ANEURYSMS. Cerebral aneurysms are repaired via a craniotomy as soon as the client's condition is stabilized. Surgery may be postponed for clients with a Hunt and Hess grade IV or V ruptured aneurysm (Table 45-2) because their condition makes them high-risk surgical candidates. During surgery, the aneurysm is clipped or a clamp is placed at the base, or neck, of the aneurysm to prevent blood from entering the area. If the aneurysm does not have a neck, it may be wrapped with muscle, muslin, or a plas-

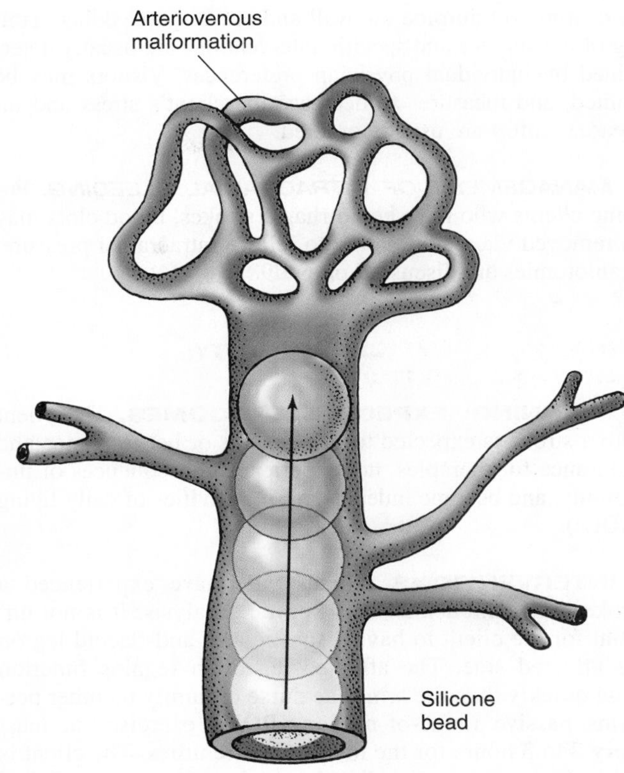

Figure 45-7 ● Embolization procedure to treat an arteriovenous malformation. The embolic agent travels to the area to cause vessel thrombosis.

TABLE 45-2 ● MODIFIED HUNT AND HESS CLASSIFICATION OF SUBARACHNOID HEMORRHAGE

Grade	Amount of Bleeding	Neurologic Findings
I	Minimal	Neurologically intact Slight headache and stiff neck
II	Mild	Minimal neurologic deficit Alert state Severe headache Stiff neck
III	Moderate	Facial deficits Drowsy, sleepy Headache, stiff neck
IV	Moderate to severe	Hemiparesis Increasing neurologic deficits Stuporous, obtunded
V	Severe	Comatose Decorticate or decerebrate posturing

Data from Adams, R.D., Victor, M., & Ropper, A.H. (1997). *Principles of neurology* (6th ed.). New York: McGraw-Hill.

tic coating to reinforce the wall and prevent rebleeding. Timing of the surgery and specific interventions are usually determined by individual physician preferences. Visitors may be limited, and measures to decrease the client's stress and increase comfort are usually ordered.

MANAGEMENT OF INTRACRANIAL BLEEDING. For some clients who have hemorrhagic strokes, blood clots may be removed via a craniotomy to relieve intracranial pressure. Craniotomies are discussed on p. 998.

IMPAIRED PHYSICAL MOBILITY; SELF-CARE DEFICIT

NOC **PLANNING: EXPECTED OUTCOMES.** The client with a stroke is expected to increase his or her tolerance and endurance for therapies, not experience consequences of immobility, and become independent in activities of daily living (ADLs).

INTERVENTIONS. Clients who have experienced a stroke may exhibit flaccid or spastic paralysis. It is not unusual for the client to have a spastic arm and flaccid leg on the affected side. The affected leg often regains function more quickly than the arm. The nurse or family member performs passive range-of-motion (ROM) exercises at least every 2 to 3 hours for the involved extremities. The client is taught how to do active ROM exercises for the unaffected side. When able, he or she may perform passive exercises on the affected side.

Careful positioning is necessary to maintain proper body alignment and decrease spasticity or increase muscle tone in flaccid extremities. The affected hand or lower leg may need splinting to prevent contractures. The nurse collaborates with the physical and occupational therapists to determine the most appropriate splinting technique and client positions when lying, sitting, and transferring from the bed to a chair.

A major complication of immobility is the development of deep vein thrombosis (DVT). The nurse provides care to prevent this complication by the application of sequential compression stockings or pneumatic compression boots, frequent positioning changes, and mobilization of the client. The nurse reports any indications of DVT to the health care provider and documents the finding in the client's chart.

DISTURBED SENSORY PERCEPTION

PLANNING: EXPECTED OUTCOMES. The major concern of clients with sensory or perceptual changes is learning to adapt to the deficits. Therefore the client with stroke is expected to adapt to sensory or perceptual changes in vision, proprioception, and sensation and to be free from injury.

INTERVENTIONS. Clients with right hemisphere brain damage typically have difficulty with visual-perceptual or spatial-perceptual tasks. They have problems with depth and distance perception and with discrimination of right from left or up from down. Because of these problems, they have difficulty performing routine activities of daily living (ADLs). The nurse and significant others help the client adapt to these disabilities by using frequent verbal and tactile cues and by breaking down tasks into discrete steps. The nurse or assistive nursing personnel approaches the client from the unaffected side, which should face the door of the room.

The client who has experienced a stroke may have difficulties with ambulating, lack depth perception, and have altered **proprioception** (position sense). The nurse teaches the client with visual field deficits to turn his or her head from side to side and to scan with the eyes to compensate for the disability. Objects should be placed within the client's field of vision; a mirror may help in visualizing more of the environment. If the client has diplopia (double vision), a patch may be placed over the affected eye. The nurse or assistive nursing personnel ensures a safe environment by removing clutter from the room.

The client with a left hemisphere lesion generally experiences memory deficits and may show significant changes in the ability to carry out simple tasks. To assist with memory problems, the nurse reorients the client to the month, year, day of the week, and circumstances surrounding hospital admission. The nurse establishes a routine or schedule that is as structured, repetitious, and consistent as possible. Information is presented in a simple, concise manner. A step-by-step approach is often most effective because the client can master one step before moving to the next. When possible, the family or significant other should bring in pictures and other familiar objects.

The client may be unable to plan and execute tasks in an organized manner. Apraxia, or the inability to perform previously learned motor skills or commands, may be present. Typically, the client with apraxia exhibits a slow, cautious, and hesitant behavior style.

UNILATERAL NEGLECT

PLANNING: EXPECTED OUTCOMES. The client with stroke is expected to adjust and use techniques to compensate for one-sided neglect.

INTERVENTIONS. Unilateral neglect, or neglect syndrome, occurs most commonly in clients who have had a right cerebral stroke. However, it can occur in any client who experiences hemianopsia, in which the vision of one or both eyes is affected. This problem places the client at additional risk for injury because of an inability to recognize his or her physical impairment or because of a lack of proprioception.

The primary role of the nurse is to teach the client to touch and use both sides of the body. For example, the nurse or assistive nursing personnel encourages the client to wash both the affected and unaffected sides of the body. When dressing, the nurse reminds the client to dress the affected side first. If hemianopsia is present, the nurse also teaches the client to turn his or her head from side to side to expand the visual field. This scanning technique is also useful when the client is eating or ambulating.

IMPAIRED VERBAL COMMUNICATION

PLANNING: EXPECTED OUTCOMES. The client with a stroke is expected to develop strategies for alternative methods of communication, such as pictures or nonverbal language.

INTERVENTIONS. Language or speech problems are usually the result of a stroke involving the dominant hemisphere. The left cerebral hemisphere is the speech center in all but 15% to 20% of the population. Speech and language problems may be the result of aphasia or dysarthria. Although aphasia is caused by cerebral hemisphere damage, **dysarthria** is due to a loss of motor function to the tongue or to the muscles of speech, causing slurred speech.

Aphasia can be classified in a number of ways. Most commonly, aphasia is classified as expressive, receptive, or global (mixed) (Table 45-3). **Expressive (Broca's, or motor) aphasia** is the result of damage in Broca's area of the frontal lobe. It is a motor speech problem in which the client generally understands what is said but is unable to communicate verbally. He or she also has difficulty writing. Rote speech and automatic speech, such as responses to a greeting, are often intact. The client is aware of the deficit and may become frustrated and angry.

Receptive (Wernicke's, or sensory) aphasia is due to injury involving Wernicke's area in the temporoparietal area. The client is unable to understand the spoken and often the written word. Although he or she may be able to talk, the language is often meaningless. Neologisms (made-up words) are common parts of speech.

More often, the client exhibits dysfunction in both the areas of expression and reception; this is known as a global, or mixed, aphasia. Reading and writing ability are equally affected. Few clients exhibit either expressive *or* receptive aphasia. In most cases, one type is dominant but two or more types are present.

The nurse collaborates with the speech-language pathologist (SLP) in working with the client who has aphasia or dysarthria. The aphasic client requires repetitive directions to understand or complete a task. Each task should be broken down into component parts and given one step at a time. The nurse faces the client and speaks slowly and clearly. The client should be given sufficient time to understand and process the information and to respond. The nurse encourages the client to communicate and reinforces this behavior positively.

Family members or significant others and staff repeat the names of objects used on a routine basis. For example, the nurse states, "This is the toothbrush" when assisting the client to brush his or her teeth. If necessary, a picture board or communication board should be developed by the SLP for the client with Broca's aphasia. This board consists of a picture of an activity (e.g., someone eating) and the printed description below. The client can point to the activity or object desired.

TABLE 45-3 • TYPES OF APHASIA

EXPRESSIVE
- Referred to as Broca's, or motor, aphasia
- Difficulty speaking
- Difficulty writing

RECEPTIVE
- Referred to as Wernicke's, or sensory, aphasia
- Difficulty understanding spoken words
- Difficulty understanding written words
- Speech often meaningless
- Neologisms

GLOBAL (MIXED)
- Combination of difficulty understanding words and speech
- Difficulty with reading and writing

It is difficult to understand a client with dysarthria. The same techniques used by the nurse for the client with aphasia can be used for dysarthria. Facial muscle exercises may be performed to strengthen the muscles used for speech. Many clients who are dysarthric are also aphasic.

IMPAIRED SWALLOWING

NOC **PLANNING: EXPECTED OUTCOMES.** The client with a stroke is expected to eat meals and drink fluids without aspiration and maintain or attain his or her ideal or usual body weight.

INTERVENTIONS. Before feeding, the nurse assesses the client's ability to swallow. The nurse observes for facial drooping, drooling, and a weak, hoarse voice. To assess the swallowing reflex, the nurse places the thumb and the index finger on either side of the client's Adam's apple, or laryngeal protuberance, and asks him or her to swallow. The nurse should be able to feel the larynx elevate. Next, the nurse checks the gag and cough reflex. The nurse collaborates with the speech-language pathologist, who specializes in swallowing evaluation, to determine the extent of the swallowing problem. In some cases, the health care provider may order a barium swallow to detect the specific cause of the swallowing problem.

Positioning the client to facilitate the swallowing process is extremely important. He or she should eat all meals sitting in a chair or sitting straight up in bed. The head and neck are positioned slightly forward and flexed. In general, clients with swallowing problems are able to tolerate or swallow soft or semisoft foods and fluids (mechanically soft or dental diet, junior baby foods, custards, scrambled eggs) better than thin liquids (water, juice, or milk) or a regular meal. Powdered thickener (Thick-It) may be added to thicken foods to a more manageable consistency.

The nurse collaborates with the dietitian to find an appropriate diet for the client with dysphagia. The nurse monitors the client's weight at least twice a week to ensure that he or she is receiving adequate nutrition. Supplements such as milkshakes and Ensure may be needed to meet caloric and protein requirements. Calorie counts may be necessary to evaluate nutritional intake fully.

Foods that stimulate saliva production and thus facilitate swallowing include beef broth and sweet, sour, or salty foods. The nurse instructs the client to place food in the back of the mouth on the unaffected side to prevent trapping food in the affected cheek.

Some clients are able to swallow without difficulty but are at risk for aspiration because they are easily distracted and impulsive. These clients require a distraction-free environment with minimal disruption from television, visitors, or environmental noise. The nurse observes for indications of fatigue because this can significantly interfere with the desire and ability to eat.

TOTAL URINARY INCONTINENCE; BOWEL INCONTINENCE

NOC **PLANNING: EXPECTED OUTCOMES.** The client with a stroke is expected to become continent of urine and stool.

INTERVENTIONS. The client may be incontinent of urine and stool because of an altered level of consciousness, impaired innervation, or an inability to communicate the need to urinate or defecate. Before beginning an education program to correct these problems, the cause must first be established. Typically, the client who has had a stroke can relearn both bowel and bladder control. To begin a bladder training program, the nurse places the client on the bedpan or the commode or offers the urinal every 2 hours. The nurse encourages a total fluid intake of at least 2000 mL/day unless contraindicated. Catheterizations to check for residual urine after voiding (postvoiding residuals) may be done in the early part of the bladder retraining program to ensure that the client is emptying the bladder. Retained urine can lead to a urinary tract infection.

Before establishing a bowel training program, the nurse determines the client's normal time for bowel elimination and any routine that helps to ensure an acceptable evacuation. This routine is followed if possible, and the client is placed on the bedpan or commode at the same time as the previous schedule at home. The nurse collaborates with the dietitian to provide a diet high in bulk and fiber. The nurse encourages the client to drink apple or prune juice to help promote bowel elimination. A stool softener (Colace) may be ordered. Suppositories or digital stimulation may also assist in re-establishing a bowel routine. Chapter 10 provides a complete discussion of bowel and bladder training programs.

CRITICAL THINKING CHALLENGE

You are visiting your parents when your father begins to slur his speech and complain of numbness in his right arm. He is a diabetic (Type II) but otherwise has no significant medical history. His symptoms progress for the next hour, at which point you call 911 for a suspected "brain attack."

- What options for management might he have?
- What are his priority nursing diagnoses at this time?
- The emergency department physician determines that your father is having an evolving thrombotic stroke and wants to give him thrombolytic therapy. What are the benefits and hazards of this treatment?

For suggested answer guidelines, go to SIMON http://www.wbsaunders.com/SIMON/Iggy/.

Community-Based Care

The client with a stroke without complications may be discharged within 4 days to home, a rehabilitation center, or a long-term care facility, depending on the extent of the disability and the availability of family or caregiver support. Some clients experience no significant neurologic dysfunction and are able to return home and live independently or with minimal support. Other clients are able to return home but require ongoing assistance with activities of daily living, as well as supervision to prevent accidents or injury. Speech, physical, or occupational therapy may continue in the home or on an ambulatory care basis. Clients admitted to a rehabilitation or long-term care facility require continued or more complex nursing care as well as extensive physical, occupational, recreational, speech-language, or cognitive therapy, which is coordinated by a case manager. The goal of rehabilitation is to maximize the client's abilities in all aspects of life.

HEALTH TEACHING

The teaching plan for the client with a stroke includes the medication schedule, mobility transfer skills, communication skills, safety precautions, dietary management, activity levels, and self-care skills. Health teaching should focus on tasks that must be performed by the client and the family after hospital discharge. The nurse should provide both written and verbal instruction. Return demonstrations assist the nurse in evaluating the family members' competency in tasks required for the client's care.

The client must take the prescribed medication to prevent another stroke and to keep hypertension under control. The nurse teaches the client and the family the name of the drug, the dosage, the timing of administration and how to take it, and possible side effects. In collaboration with the physical and occupational therapists, the nurse teaches the client how to climb stairs safely, if able; transfer from the bed to a chair; get into and out of a car; and use any aids to mobility. Finally, the client and family members are taught how to use any equipment needed to increase independence in self-care skills. The most important information the nurse provides is what to do in an emergency and whom to call for nonemergency questions.

It is not unusual for clients, particularly older Caucasian men, to become depressed within 6 months after discharge. In general, this depression is self-limiting, but the client may require antidepressants for a short time. Emotional lability is also common. The family is advised to avoid being overprotective and is assisted to establish realistic and achievable goals.

Families may feel overwhelmed by the continuing demands placed on them. Depending on the location of the lesion, the client may be anxious, slow, cautious, hesitant, and lack initiative (left hemisphere lesions), or he or she may be impulsive and seemingly unaware of any deficit. Family members and other caregivers need to spend time away from the client on a routine basis to continue to provide full-time care without sacrificing their own physical and emotional health. The nurse may refer the family to a social worker for further support and counseling.

HOME CARE MANAGEMENT

Collaboration with the case manager is needed if the client is discharged to the home setting. Needs for assistive or adaptive and safety equipment must be identified. The extent of this assessment depends on the disabilities experienced by the client. The home of the client with hemiparesis should be free from scatter rugs or other obstacles in the walking pathways. The bathtub and toilet should be equipped with grab bars. Antiskid patches or strips should be placed in the bathtub to prevent slipping. The physical or occupational therapist works with the client and the family or significant others to obtain all needed assistive devices *before* discharge from the hospital, rehabilitation setting, or long-term care facility. Appointments for outpatient speech, physical, and occupational therapy must also be arranged before discharge.

HEALTH CARE RESOURCES

Available resources include a variety of publications from the American Heart Association, including *Stroke: A Guide for*

Families and *Stroke: Why Do They Behave That Way?* The National Stroke Association also provides publications and videotapes for caregivers and clients. *Recovering After a Stroke: A Patient and Family Guide* is available from the Agency for Healthcare Research and Quality (http://www.ahrq.gov), formerly the Agency for Health Care Policy and Research. The nurse refers the client and family members or significant others to local stroke support groups.

Evaluation: Outcomes

NOC The nurse evaluates the care of the client with stroke on the basis of the identified nursing diagnoses and collaborative problems. The expected outcomes are that the client:

- Maintains intracranial pressure within normal limits (WNL)
- Maintains or improves his or her level of consciousness
- Experiences no additional neurologic problems, such as seizures
- Adapts to sensory or perceptual changes in vision, proprioception, and sensation
- Increases tolerance and endurance for therapies
- Uses assistive or adaptive devices as needed
- Exhibits no consequences of immobility
- Is free from injury
- Becomes independent in activities of daily living (ADLs)
- Develops strategies for alternative methods of communication
- Eats and drinks fluids without aspiration
- Maintains or attains ideal or usual body weight
- Is continent of urine and stool

TRAUMATIC BRAIN INJURY

OVERVIEW

Traumatic brain injury (TBI) occurs as a result of an external physical force that may produce a diminished or altered state of consciousness. TBI may result in the impairment of cognitive abilities or physical functioning as well as a disturbance of behavior or emotional functioning. These impairments may be either temporary or permanent and cause partial or total functional disability or psychosocial maladjustment. In the United States, TBI has taken more lives of people 18 to 34 years of age than all other causes combined for that age-group. The annual cost of care for TBI survivors in the United States is estimated to be $48 billion to $83.5 billion, including direct costs (hospitalization and rehabilitation) and indirect costs (lost wages and productivity) (McNair, 1999).

Pathophysiology

Various terms are used to describe the brain injuries that occur when a mechanical force is applied either directly or indirectly to the brain. A force produced by a blow to the head is a direct injury, whereas a force applied to another body part with a rebound effect to the brain is an indirect injury. The brain responds to these forces by forward movement within the rigid cranial vault. The brain may also rebound or rotate on the brainstem, causing diffuse axonal injury (shearing injuries). The moving brain may be contused or lacerated as it moves over the inner surfaces of the cranium, which is irregularly shaped and sharp. Damage most commonly occurs to the frontal and temporal lobes of the brain, especially the raised surfaces of the gyri.

PRIMARY BRAIN INJURY

Primary brain damage results from the physical stress (force) within the brain tissue caused by open or closed trauma. An open head injury occurs when there is a skull fracture or when the skull is pierced by a penetrating object. The integrity of the brain and the dura is violated, and there is exposure to outside, or environmental, contaminants. Damage may occur to the underlying vessels, dural sinus, brain, and cranial nerves. A closed head injury is the result of blunt trauma; the integrity of the skull is not violated. It is the more serious of the two types of injury, and the damage to brain tissue depends on the degree and mechanisms of injury.

Injury may also be described as mild, moderate, or severe. A Glascow Coma Scale (GCS) score of 13 to 15 and the appearance of signs and symptoms such as mild confusion and unsteady gait characterize a mild TBI. A moderate TBI often includes a period of loss of consciousness and may be accompanied by other systemic injury and a GCS score of 9 to 12. A short critical care stay maybe needed for close monitoring. After injury, these clients may have difficulty with work, learning, and role function. Severe head injury (GCS score of 3 to 8) is more serious and requires management in critical care with ongoing monitoring of multiple physiologic parameters.

OPEN HEAD INJURY. The types of fractures associated with an open head injury are linear, depressed, open, and comminuted. A **linear fracture** is a simple, clean break in which the impacted area of bone bends inward and the area around it bends outward; linear fractures account for about 80% of all skull fractures. In a **depressed fracture,** the bone is pressed inward into the brain tissue to at least the thickness of the skull. In an **open fracture,** the scalp is lacerated, creating a direct opening to the brain tissue. A **comminuted fracture** involves fragmentation of the bone, with depression of bone into the brain tissue.

A unique fracture is a basilar skull fracture. It occurs at the base of the skull, usually extending into the anterior, middle, or posterior fossa, and results in cerebrospinal fluid (CSF) leakage from the nose or ears. Of significance with this fracture is the potential development of hemorrhage caused by damage to the internal carotid artery; damage to cranial nerves I, II, VII, and VIII; and infection.

The majority of penetrating injuries to the skull are caused by gunshot wounds and knife injuries. The degree of injury to brain tissue depends on the velocity, mass, shape, and direction of impact. High-velocity injuries produce the greatest damage to brain tissue. As with any open head injury, the client with a penetrating injury is at high risk for infection from the object that pierced the skull and from other environmental contaminants.

CLOSED HEAD INJURY. Closed head injuries are caused by blunt trauma and lead to concussions, contusions, and lacerations of the brain. The damage to the brain may be mild, as occurs in a concussive injury, or it may be more severe, causing diffuse axonal injury or widespread injury to the white matter of the brain. A **concussion** is characterized by a brief loss of consciousness. Damage occurs to the gray matter of the cerebral cortex or possibly to the diencephalon or brainstem. The damage to the axons is functional, not structural, which is why permanent neurologic dysfunction is generally not seen. (However, some authorities believe that both functional and structural damage are involved.) A **contusion** is a bruising of the brain tissue and is most commonly found at the site of impact (coup injury) or in a line opposite the site of impact (contrecoup injury) (Figure 45-8). The base of the frontal and temporal lobes is most often involved. A **laceration** causes actual tearing of the cortical surface vessels, which may lead to secondary hemorrhage; therefore this condition is more serious than a contusion.

TYPES OF FORCE

Other factors that must be considered in the dynamics of head injury are the type of force and the mechanisms of injury involved (Figure 45-9). An acceleration injury is caused by the head in motion. A deceleration injury occurs when the head is suddenly stopped or hits a stationary object. These forces may be sufficient to cause the cerebrum to rotate about the brainstem, resulting in shearing, straining, and distortion of the brain tissue, particularly of the axons in the brainstem and cerebellum. Small areas of hemorrhage may develop around the blood vessels that sustain the impact of these forces (stress), with destruction of adjacent brain tissue. Particularly affected are the basal nuclei and the hypothalamus.

SECONDARY RESPONSES AND INSULTS

Secondary responses to brain injury include any neurologic damage that occurs after the initial injury. Secondary injuries or responses increase the morbidity and mortality after head trauma. The most common response is the development of increased intracranial pressure (ICP) attributable to edema, hemorrhage, hematoma development, impaired cerebral autoregulation, or hydrocephalus. Hypoxemia, hypercapnia, or systemic hypotension may precipitate increased ICP. Damage to the brain tissue occurs primarily because the delivery of oxygen and glucose to the brain is interrupted.

INCREASED INTRACRANIAL PRESSURE. The cranial contents include brain tissue, blood, and cerebrospinal fluid (CSF). These components are encased in the relatively rigid skull. Within this space, there is little room for any of the components to expand or increase in volume. Through the processes of accommodation and compliance, ICP is maintained at its normal level of 10 to 15 mm Hg despite transient increases in pressure that occur with straining during defecation, coughing, or sneezing. According to the Monro-Kellie hypothesis, any increase in the volume of one component must be compensated for by a decrease in the volume of one of the other components.

As a first response to an increase in the volume of any of these components, the CSF is shunted or displaced from the

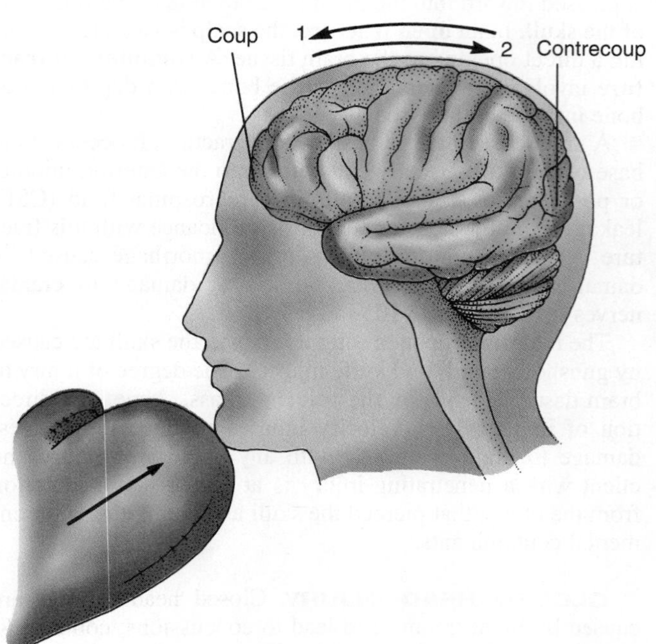

Figure 45-8 ● Coup (site of impact) injury to frontal area of brain, and contrecoup injury to frontal and temporal areas of the brain.

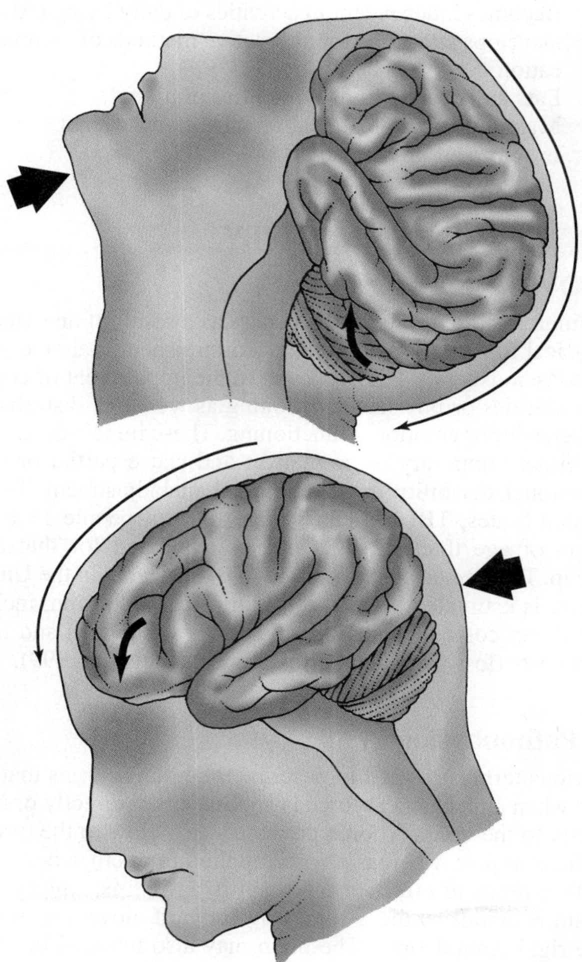

Figure 45-9 ● Head movement during acceleration-deceleration injury, which is typically seen in motor vehicle accidents.

cranial compartment to the spinal subarachnoid space, or the rate of CSF absorption is increased. An additional response, if needed, is a decrease in cerebral blood volume by the displacement of cerebral venous blood into the sinuses. As long as the brain is able to compensate for the increase in volume and remain compliant, there are minimal increases in ICP.

Increased ICP is the leading cause of death from head trauma in clients who reach the hospital alive. It occurs when compliance no longer takes place and the brain cannot accommodate further volume changes. As ICP increases, cerebral blood flow decreases, leading to tissue hypoxia, a decrease in serum pH level, and an increase in carbon dioxide level. This process causes cerebral vasodilation, edema, and a further increase in ICP, and the cycle continues. If the condition remains untreated, the brain herniates downward toward the brainstem, causing irreversible brain damage and possibly death **(uncal herniation).**

Two types of edema may cause increased ICP: vasogenic edema and cytotoxic edema. A third type (interstitial edema) occurs in the presence of acute brain swelling. Vasogenic edema is seen most often as a cause of increased ICP in the adult. It is characterized by an increase in brain tissue volume caused by an abnormal permeability of the walls of the cerebral vessels, which allows protein-rich plasma infiltrate to leak into the extracellular space of the brain. The fluid collects primarily in the white matter.

Cytotoxic, or cellular, edema may occur as a result of a hypoxic insult, which causes a disturbance in cellular metabolism, the sodium pump, and active ion transport. The brain is quickly depleted of available oxygen, glucose, and glycogen and converts to anaerobic metabolism. The sodium pump fails, and sodium enters the cells and pulls water from the extracellular space. A concomitant decrease in serum sodium level to less than 120 mEq/L occurs. As a result, there is an abnormal accumulation of fluid in the brain cells and a decrease in the extracellular fluid space. Cytotoxic edema may lead to vasogenic edema and a further in increase ICP.

Interstitial edema occurs in the presence of acute brain swelling and is associated with elevated blood pressure or increased CSF pressure. Edema develops rapidly in the perivascular and periventricular white space and can be controlled through measures to reduce blood pressure, decrease CSF pressures, or increase the cerebral perfusion pressure. Cerebral perfusion pressure (CPP) is the amount of pressure needed to deliver oxygen and nutrients to brain tissue. CPP is influenced by oxygenation, cerebral blood volume, blood pressure, cerebral edema, and intracranial pressure. Maintenance of a CPP above 70 mm Hg provides adequate metabolic needs.

HEMORRHAGE. Hemorrhages, which cause hematomas (clots), are classified as secondary injury and are caused by vascular damage from the shearing force of the trauma. All hematomas are potentially life threatening because they act as space-occupying lesions and are surrounded by edema. Three types of hemorrhages include epidural hematoma, subdural hematoma, and intracerebral hemorrhage.

EPIDURAL HEMATOMA. An **epidural hematoma** results from arterial bleeding into the space between the dura and the inner table of the skull (Figure 45-10). It is often caused by a fracture of the temporal bone, which houses the middle meningeal artery. Epidural hematomas are characterized by the presence of a "lucid interval" that lasts for minutes, during which time the client is awake and talking. This follows a momentary unconsciousness that occurred within

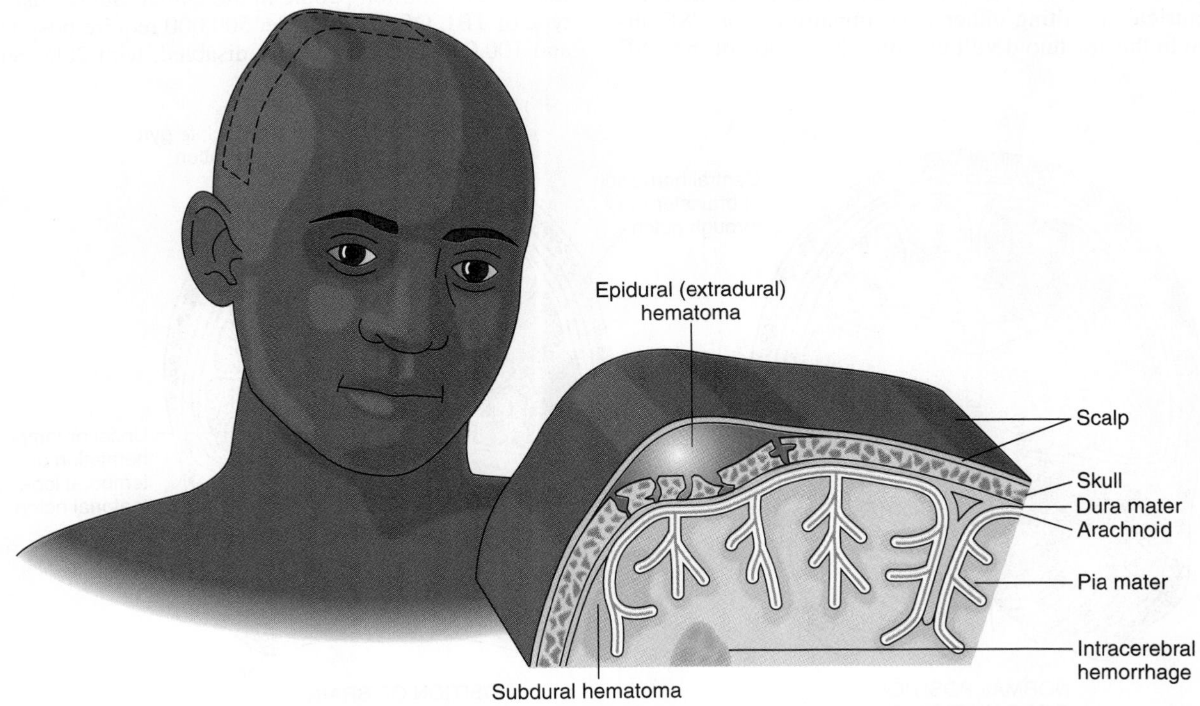

Figure 45-10 ● Epidural hematoma (outside the dura mater of the brain), subdural hematoma (under the dura mater), and intracerebral hemorrhage (within the brain tissue).

minutes of the injury. The client becomes increasingly symptomatic and may progress to coma.

SUBDURAL HEMATOMA. A **subdural hematoma (SDH)** results from venous bleeding into the space beneath the dura and above the arachnoid (see Figure 45-10). It results most often from a tearing of the bridging veins within the cerebral hemispheres or from a laceration of brain tissue. Bleeding from this injury occurs more slowly than from an epidural hematoma. SDHs are subdivided into acute, subacute, and chronic. An acute SDH presents within 48 hours after impact; the subacute SDH, between 48 hours and 2 weeks; and the chronic SDH, from 2 weeks to several months following injury. SDHs have the highest mortality rate.

INTRACEREBRAL HEMORRHAGE. An intracerebral hemorrhage is the accumulation of blood within the brain tissue caused by the tearing of small arteries and veins in the subcortical white matter (see Figure 45-10). A brainstem hemorrhage occurs as a result of direct trauma, fractures, or torsion injuries to the brainstem.

LOSS OF AUTOREGULATION. Through the process of cerebral autoregulation, blood flow to the brain remains relatively constant despite variations in systemic blood pressure. A loss of autoregulation causes the cerebral blood flow to fluctuate passively with the systemic blood pressure. Systemic hypertension may cause an increase in ICP (from an increase in cerebral blood flow) and the potential for vasogenic edema. Hypoxemia and hypercapnia cause marked cerebral vasodilation and therefore an increase in cerebral blood flow, which contributes to increased ICP.

HYDROCEPHALUS. Hydrocephalus is an abnormal increase in CSF volume. It is caused by dilation of the cerebral ventricles resulting either from impairment of CSF absorption in the arachnoid villi or from obstruction of the CSF circulation pathway. This increase in CSF volume may lead to increased ICP.

HERNIATION. In the presence of increased ICP, the brain tissue may shift and herniate downward. Of the several types of herniation syndromes (Figure 45-11), uncal (transtentorial) herniation is the most clinically significant because it is life threatening. It is caused by a shift of one or both areas of the temporal lobe, known as the uncus. This shift creates pressure on the third cranial nerve and results in dilated and nonreactive pupils, ptosis, and a rapidly deteriorating level of consciousness. Central herniation is caused by a downward shift of the brainstem and the diencephalon from a supratentorial lesion. It is clinically manifested by Cheyne-Stokes respirations and pinpoint, nonreactive pupils.

A shift of the cingulate gyrus below the falx cerebri is known as cingulate herniation. A type of infratentorial herniation, cerebellar tonsillar herniation, occurs when the cerebellar tonsils shift and compress the medulla. This may lead to respiratory and cardiovascular compromise or arrest. All herniation syndromes are potentially life threatening, and the physician must be notified immediately when they are suspected.

Etiology

The most common causes of traumatic brain injury (TBI) in the United States are accidents involving motor vehicles, including both automobiles and motorcycles. All too often, alcohol and drugs are contributing factors to the accident. Falls, acts of violence, and sports-related injuries are the next most common causes.

Incidence/Prevalence

Each year 7 million people in the United States sustain some type of TBI. Of these people, 500,000 require hospitalization and 100,000 are permanently disabled, with 2000 remaining

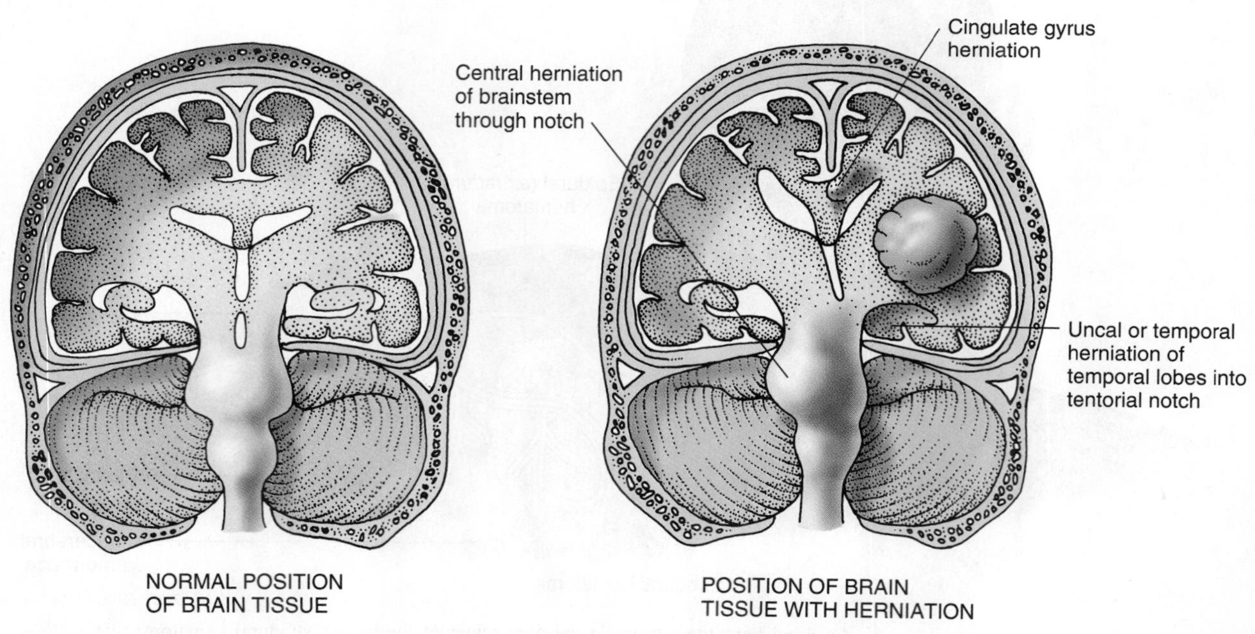

Figure 45-11 ● Herniation syndromes.

in a persistent vegetative state. Studies indicate that the summer and spring months, evenings, nights, and weekends are associated with a high number of injuries (McNair, 1999).

Head injuries occur three times more often in males than in females. More than 70% of these injuries occur in people between 10 and 39 years of age, with a peak incidence between 15 and 24 years of age (McNair, 1999).

CONSIDERATIONS FOR OLDER ADULTS
Clients older than 60 years of age have a higher mortality rate because they are at higher risk for developing secondary injury related to the initial TBI (Chart 45-7).

COLLABORATIVE MANAGEMENT

Assessment

HISTORY

Obtaining an accurate history from a client who has sustained craniocerebral trauma may be difficult because of either the seriousness of the injury or the presence of amnesia. It is not unusual for the client to experience **amnesia** (loss of memory) for the events before or after the injury. The client with a serious head injury is often admitted to the hospital unconscious or in a confused and combative state. If the client is unable to provide information, the history can be obtained from rescue workers or witnesses to the injury. The nurse should ask when, where, and how the injury occurred. Did the client lose consciousness? If so, for how long? Has there been a change in the level of consciousness?

The nurse obtains information about the events immediately after the injury. Clients with a severe injury may have several different reactions. The client may be completely unresponsive after the injury; alternatively, the client may initially be responsive and deteriorate rapidly within a few minutes to several hours. In another typical presentation, the client is initially unconscious for a few minutes as a result of the primary brain injury, returns to a normal level of consciousness, and then rapidly deteriorates as a consequence of secondary insult to the brain.

The nurse determines whether the client experienced any seizure activity before or after the injury or if there is a history of a seizure disorder. It is important to obtain precise information about the circumstances of falls, particularly in the older client. Other pertinent information includes hand dominance, any diseases of or injuries to the eyes, and any allergies to medications or food, particularly seafood. People allergic to seafood are often allergic to the contrast media used in diagnostic tests. The nurse obtains a history of alcohol or drug use and abuse, because drugs or alcohol may mask the symptoms of increased ICP.

CHART 45-7

NURSING FOCUS *on the* OLDER ADULT
Head Injury

- Head injury is the fifth leading cause of death in older adults
- The 65- to 75-year age-group has second highest incidence of head injury of all age-groups.
- Falls and motor vehicle accidents are the most common cause of head injury.
- The following factors contribute to high mortality:
  - Falls causing subdural hematomas (closed-head injuries), especially chronic subdural hematomas
  - Poorly tolerated systemic stress, which is increased by admission to a high-stimuli environment
  - Medical complications, such as hypotension, hypertension, and cardiac problems
  - Decreased protective mechanisms, which make clients susceptible to infections (especially pneumonia)
  - Decreased immunologic competence, which is further diminished by head injury

PHYSICAL ASSESSMENT/CLINICAL MANIFESTATIONS

No two injuries are alike. The client with a TBI may have a variety of signs and symptoms depending on the severity of injury and the resulting increase in intracranial pressure (ICP) (see Chart 45-5). The goals of the nursing assessment are the establishment of baseline data and the early detection of and prevention of increased ICP, systemic hypotension, hypoxia, or hypercapnia (increased blood levels of carbon dioxide). The early detection of subtle changes in the client's neurologic status enables the health care team to prevent or treat potentially life-threatening complications.

Because it is estimated that 5% to 20% of clients with TBI have associated cervical spinal cord injuries, all clients with head trauma are treated as though they have spinal cord injury until radiographic studies prove otherwise. The nurse assesses for indicators of spinal cord injury, such as loss of motor and sensory function, tenderness along the spine, and abnormal head tilt. The client may experience respiratory problems and diaphragmatic breathing, and his or her reflexes may be diminished or absent.

AIRWAY AND BREATHING PATTERN ASSESSMENT. The first priority is the assessment of the client's airway and breathing pattern. Hypoxia and hypercapnia are best detected through arterial blood gas analysis, but the nursing assessment is vital to identify the client at risk for respiration-related complications. Injuries to the brainstem may cause a change in the client's breathing pattern, such as Cheyne-Stokes respirations, central neurogenic hyperventilation, and apneustic, cluster, or ataxic breathing. Table 45-4 describes the common respiratory patterns of comatose clients.

VITAL SIGNS ASSESSMENT. The mechanisms of autoregulation are often impaired as the result of craniocerebral trauma. The more serious the injury, the more severe the impact on autoregulation. The nurse or assistive nursing personnel monitors the client's blood pressure and pulse to detect possible changes in cerebral blood flow caused by impaired autoregulation as a result of hypotension or hypertension. The **Cushing reflex,** a classic yet late sign of increased ICP, is manifested by severe hypertension with a widened pulse pressure and bradycardia. As ICP increases, the pulse becomes thready, irregular, and rapid. Cerebral blood flow increases in response to hypertension, and vasogenic edema may occur, further increasing ICP. In contrast, hypotension and tachycardia are symptomatic of hypovolemic shock. This decrease in blood volume may lead to decreased cerebral perfusion pressure and eventually to ischemia and infarct of the brain tissue.

Hypovolemic shock is usually due to intra-abdominal bleeding or bleeding into the soft tissue around major fractures—not

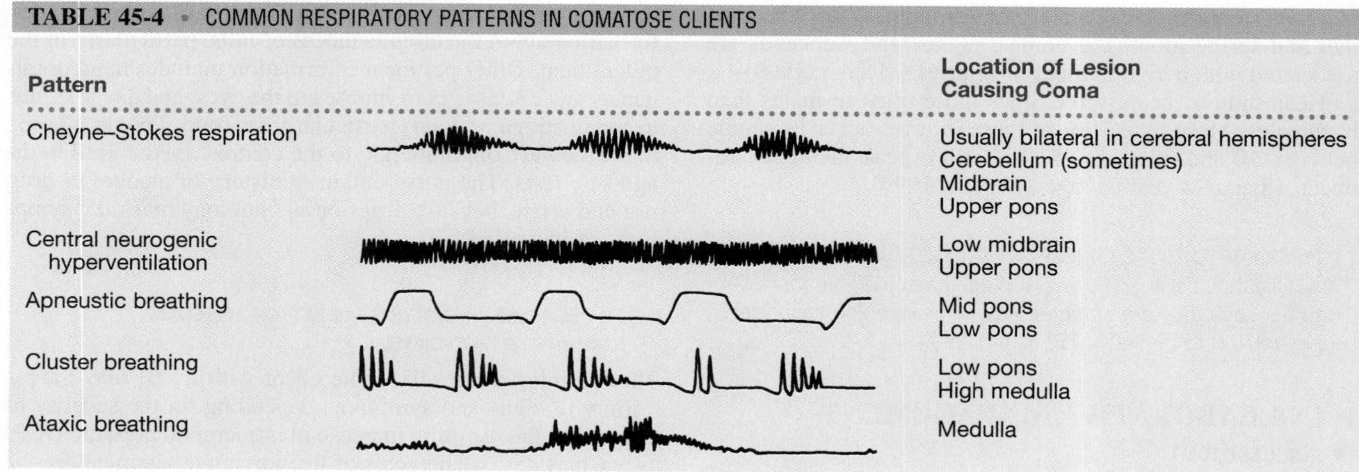

TABLE 45-4 • COMMON RESPIRATORY PATTERNS IN COMATOSE CLIENTS

Pattern	Location of Lesion Causing Coma
Cheyne–Stokes respiration	Usually bilateral in cerebral hemispheres Cerebellum (sometimes) Midbrain Upper pons
Central neurogenic hyperventilation	Low midbrain Upper pons
Apneustic breathing	Mid pons Low pons
Cluster breathing	Low pons High medulla
Ataxic breathing	Medulla

to intracranial bleeding. Cardiac dysrhythmias may result from chest trauma, bruising of the heart, or interference with the autonomic nervous system.

NEUROLOGIC ASSESSMENT. Many hospitals use the Glasgow Coma Scale to assess neurologic status (see Chapter 41). The most important variable to assess is level of consciousness. A decrease or change in level of consciousness is typically the first sign of a deterioration in neurologic status. Changes in the content of consciousness or orientation are due to injury to the cerebral cortex. A decrease in arousal or increased sleepiness and coma are caused by pressure on the reticular activating system within the brainstem. Early indicators of a change in level of consciousness include behavior changes (e.g., restlessness or irritability), which are often subtle in nature.

EYE ASSESSMENT. The nurse elicits a history of previous eye injury or medications that affect pupillary dilation and constriction, such as anticholinergics and adrenergics. The nurse also checks the pupils for size and reaction to light. Any changes in pupil size, shape, and reactivity must be reported to the health care provider immediately, because such changes indicate an increase in ICP. Pupillary changes or eye signs differ depending on which areas of the brain are damaged. Pinpoint and nonresponsive pupils are indicative of brainstem dysfunction at the level of the pons. Of particular importance is the ovoid pupil, which is regarded as the midstage between a normal-sized pupil and a dilated pupil. This finding indicates the development of increased ICP.

The nurse may check gross vision if the client's condition permits. The nurse can have the client read any printed material (e.g., the nurse's name tag) or count the number of fingers that the nurse holds within the visual field. Loss of vision is usually caused by injury to the occipital lobe, which produces temporary cortical blindness.

If the client is able to cooperate, the health care provider or neurosurgical nurse tests cranial nerves III, IV, and VI. Extraocular movements may be diminished due to the presence of increased ICP and hydrocephalus. Damage to the optic chiasm, optic tract, or optic radii may cause visual field deficits or diplopia. In the unconscious client, the oculocephalic and oculovestibular tests are performed to test the integrity of the brainstem and of cranial nerves III, VI, and VII. Chapter 41 describes these techniques in detail.

MOTOR ASSESSMENT. The nurse also assesses for bilateral motor responses to avoid missing lateralizing signs. The client's motor loss or dysfunction usually appears contralateral to the site of the lesion. For example, a left-sided hemiparesis is indicative of an injury to the right cerebral hemisphere. A deterioration in motor function or the development of abnormal posturing (decerebrate or decorticate posturing) or flaccidity is another indicator of increased ICP. These changes are attributable to dysfunction within the pyramidal system or cerebral peduncles. Brainstem or cerebellar injury may cause ataxia, decreased or increased muscle tone, and weakness.

ADDITIONAL NEUROLOGIC ASSESSMENT. If the client is able to cooperate, a full neurologic assessment is completed as outlined in Chapter 41. Particular attention is given to cranial nerves I, V, VII, IX, and X. The first cranial nerve is often damaged where the frontal lobe passes over the irregularly shaped bones of the anterior and middle fossa; this results in the loss of smell (anosmia). Cranial nerves V, VII, IX, and X are important for chewing and swallowing abilities and phonation. The client's ability to speak must be assessed, with particular attention directed toward differentiating aphasias (caused by injury to the cerebral cortex) from communication impairments (caused by damage to the cranial nerves and cerebellum). Damage to the cranial nerves occurs from disruption of the nerve trunk, either intracranially or along its extracranial course in the skull or face. Cranial nerve damage may result from direct trauma or compression associated with pressure or hemorrhage.

The nurse assesses for other signs of increased ICP (see Chart 45-5). These include severe headache, nausea, vomiting, seizures, and papilledema (seen by ophthalmoscopic examination). **Papilledema,** also known as a **choked disk,** is edema and hyperemia of the optic disk. It is always a sign of increased ICP. Headache and seizures are a response to the injury and may or may not be associated with increased ICP. In general, a single neurologic finding is not indicative of increased ICP. However, the nurse must remember that the client can have a marked increase in ICP yet be relatively asymptomatic.

The nurse carefully assesses the client's ears and nose for any signs of cerebrospinal fluid (CSF) leaks that result from a basilar skull fracture. CSF placed on a white absorbent background can be distinguished from other fluids by the "halo" sign, a yellowish stain surrounded by bloody drainage. CSF tests positively for glucose when a strip testing method (Dipstix) is used, but this method of determining a CSF leak is not always reliable. If there is a CSF leak, the client should be assessed for any signs of nuchal rigidity (stiff neck), which may indicate infection or blood in the CSF. Nuchal rigidity is not checked until a spinal cord injury has been ruled out.

The client's head is palpated to detect the presence of fractures or hematomas. The nurse looks for areas of ecchymosis (bruising), tender areas of the scalp, and lacerations.

Clients with a *minor* head injury should be assessed for signs and symptoms of postconcussion syndrome. Symptoms include a wide array of physical and cognitive problems that range from persistent headache, weakness, and dizziness to personality and behavior changes, loss of memory, and problems with perception, reasoning abilities, and concept formation. The symptoms may persist for a few days or weeks to several months after the injury. For some clients, severe physical and cognitive problems remain despite a relatively benign initial clinical presentation and normal diagnostic test findings.

PSYCHOSOCIAL ASSESSMENT

The person who has had a moderate or severe head injury is never the same as before the injury. Most often, the client with a major head injury has personality changes manifested by temper outbursts, depression, risk-taking behavior, and denial of disability. The client may become talkative and develop a very outgoing personality. Memory, especially recent or short-term memory, is affected and should not be confused with problems of aphasia. The ability to learn new information and concentration may be affected. Finally, the client may exhibit problems with insight and planning. All of these problems may lead to difficulties within the family structure and with social and work-related interactions. Coping strategies that have been used in the past must be assessed to determine the client's ability to adapt to the changes in physical and cognitive abilities. Although they have no focal signs, clients with a mild head injury may still have symptoms of disability 1 year after injury.

The nurse assesses family dynamics, particularly if the client is discharged to the family's care directly from the acute care hospital. The family or significant others must also cope with changes in the client's physical appearance and cognitive abilities. Many families are angry at the client for being injured, especially when his or her behavior or their own behavior resulted in an injury that could have been prevented. They may feel guilty that they did not or were not able to prevent the injury. The family or significant others may feel overwhelmed by the complexity of care required and the long recovery period. Both the family and the client need to develop coping strategies to deal with the potential role reversals and role changes caused by the injury.

LABORATORY ASSESSMENT

There are no laboratory tests to diagnose a primary brain injury; however, several laboratory tests are used to diagnose or indicate measures to prevent secondary brain insult. Arterial blood gases (ABGs) are analyzed, with particular attention given to oxygen and carbon dioxide levels. The health care provider also orders a complete blood count (CBC) and determination of serum glucose and electrolyte levels and osmolality. These tests are performed to monitor hemodynamic status or to identify electrolyte imbalance or the presence of infection.

RADIOGRAPHIC ASSESSMENT

The health care provider orders computed tomography (CT) scanning to identify the extent and scope of injury to the brain. This diagnostic test can identify the presence of a lesion that requires surgical intervention, such as epidural or subdural hematoma. Radiography of the cervical spine and the skull is done to rule out fractures and dislocations. A chest x-ray study is done to identify fractured ribs or other chest injuries. A flat plate of the abdomen may be obtained to assist in the diagnosis of abdominal bleeding or bowel laceration.

OTHER DIAGNOSTIC ASSESSMENT

Magnetic resonance imaging (MRI) is particularly useful in the diagnosis of diffuse axonal injury but is not recommended for clients with ICP monitoring devices or other invasive monitoring devices. As the client's condition stabilizes, the physician may order other diagnostic tests to identify the extent of injury to the brain. For example, the integrity of the cerebral vessels is measured through the use of Doppler flow studies or an arteriogram; cerebral perfusion is measured by cerebral blood flow studies. Evoked potentials provide information on the functioning sensory pathways and may be useful in predicting outcome.

Interventions

The client with a *severe* head injury is admitted to the critical care unit or a trauma center. Clients with moderate head injuries are either admitted to the general nursing unit or the critical care unit, where they are closely observed for at least 24 hours. Clients with mild TBI are sent home from the emergency department with instructions (Chart 45-8).

NONSURGICAL MANAGEMENT. Nursing interventions for all clients with a head injury are directed toward preventing or detecting increased ICP, promoting fluid and electrolyte balance, and monitoring the effects of treatments and medications.

ASSESSMENT OF VITAL SIGNS. The nurse or assistive nursing personnel takes and records the client's vital signs every 1 to 2 hours. The health care provider may order medications to prevent severe hypertension or hypotension. The client in the critical care unit is connected to a cardiac monitor to detect any cardiac dysrhythmias. Nonspecific ST-segment or T-wave changes may occur, possibly in response to stimulation of the autonomic nervous system or an increase in the level of circulating catecholamines. The nurse documents and reports cardiac irregularities to the health care provider.

The client with a head injury is often admitted with a fever—a defense mechanism in the presence of trauma. Fever

CHART 45-8

CLIENT EDUCATION GUIDE
Minor Head Injury

- If the person is sleeping, wake him or her every 3 to 4 hours for the first 2 days, asking his or her name, where he or she is, and the name of the caregiver.
- Expect the person to complain of headache, nausea, or dizziness for at least 24 hours. If these symptoms are severe or do not improve, contact the physician immediately or take the person back to the emergency department.
- For a headache, give acetaminophen (Tylenol) every 4 hours as needed.
- Avoid giving the person sedatives, sleeping pills, or alcoholic beverages for at least 24 hours unless the physician instructs otherwise.
- Do not allow the person to engage in strenuous activity for at least 48 hours.
- Do not allow nose blowing or ear cleaning for 48 hours.
- If any of the following symptoms occur, take the person back to the emergency department immediately:
  - Blurred vision
  - Drainage from the ear or nose
  - Weakness
  - Slurred speech
  - Progressive sleepiness
  - Vomiting
  - Worsening headache
  - Unequal pupil size
- Keep follow-up appointments with the health care provider.

as a consequence of infection may develop later in the course of the disease. A third cause of fever is a central fever caused by hypothalamic damage. It is manifested by an absence of sweating and no diurnal (daily) variation; this type of fever is high and lasts several days to weeks. In addition, this type of fever responds better to cooling (hypothermia blanket, sponge bath) than to the administration of antipyretic drugs such as acetaminophen (Tylenol, Ace-Tabs✤).

POSITIONING. The nurse positions the client to avoid extreme flexion or extension of the neck and to maintain the head in the midline, neutral position. The nurse logrolls the client during turning to avoid extreme hip flexion and keeps the head of the bed elevated 30 degrees. All of these measures enhance venous drainage, which helps prevent increased intracranial pressure (ICP).

HYPERVENTILATION. Prophylactic hyperventilation during the first 20 hours after injury is usually avoided, because it may produce ischemia by causing cerebral vasoconstriction with a resulting decrease in cerebral blood volume and ICP. In acute neurologic deterioration, however, hyperventilation may be used for brief periods. Intracranial hypertension that does not respond to standard treatment may also require hyperventilation for longer periods of time (American Association of Neurological Surgeons, 1997).

The client who requires mechanical ventilation is hyperventilated to maintain a partial pressure of arterial carbon dioxide ($Paco_2$) of 27 to 35 mm Hg. Carbon dioxide is a very potent vasodilator that can contribute to increases in ICP. The $Paco_2$ must not be allowed to fall to less than 20 mm Hg, which may result in hypoxia caused by *severe* vasoconstriction. Arterial oxygen levels (Pao_2) are maintained between 80 and 100 mm Hg to prevent cerebral vasodilation resulting from hypoxemia. Arterial blood gas values are monitored at least twice per day and after each change in the ventilator setting.

INDUCTION OF BARBITURATE COMA. Clinical trails in the use of barbiturate coma have been disappointing yet remain an option for clients whose ICP cannot be controlled by other means. Pentobarbital sodium (Nembutal, Novopentobarb✤) is the drug of choice. This drug works by decreasing the metabolic demands of the brain and cerebral blood flow, stabilizing cell membranes, decreasing the formation of vasogenic edema, and producing a more uniform blood supply. The provider adjusts the dosage to maintain complete unresponsiveness. As a consequence, it is difficult for the nurse to recognize subtle or unsubtle neurologic changes. The client requires mechanical ventilation, sophisticated hemodynamic monitoring, and ICP monitoring. Complications of barbiturate coma include cardiac dysrhythmias, hypotension, and fluid and electrolyte disturbances.

DRUG THERAPY. Glucocorticoids (dexamethasone [Decadron, Dexasone]) and methylprednisolone sodium succinate [Solu-Medrol, Medrol]) have no demonstrated benefit in the management of increased ICP as a result of head injury or cerebral infarction. Mannitol (Osmitrol), an osmotic diuretic, is used to treat cerebral edema by pulling water out of the extracellular space of the edematous brain tissue, but it does not cross the blood-brain barrier. It is most effective when given in boluses rather than as a continuous infusion. Furosemide (Lasix), a loop diuretic, is often used as adjunctive therapy to reduce the incidence of rebound from mannitol and also enhances its therapeutic action. Furosemide also reduces edema and blood volume, decreases sodium uptake by the brain, and decreases the production of CSF at the choroid plexus.

The nurse administers mannitol through a filter in the IV tubing or, if given by IV push, draws it up through a filtered needle to eliminate microscopic crystals. The client receiving either osmotic or loop diuretics is monitored for intake and output and severe dehydration, as well as for indications of acute renal failure, weakness, edema, and changes in urinary output. A Foley catheter must be inserted to maintain strict measurement of output. The client's serum and urine osmolality are checked daily.

Codeine or fentanyl (Sublimaze) may be used with ventilated clients to decrease agitation and control restlessness. These agents can be easily reversed with naloxone (Narcan). Neuromuscular blocking agents (NMBAs), such as pancuronium bromide (Pavulon), have no analgesic effect but when used with sedation help to decrease the cerebral metabolic rate associated with agitation. Neuromuscular muscular blocking agents *must never be used without sedation.*

Anticonvulsants, such as phenytoin (Dilantin), are given to prevent seizures. Acetaminophen (Tylenol, Ace-Tabs✤) and aspirin (Ancasal✤) are given to clients who are febrile (temperature greater than 101° F [39° C]) to reduce fever.

FLUID AND ELECTROLYTE MANAGEMENT. The client with craniocerebral trauma is at risk for diabetes insipidus and the syndrome of inappropriate antidiuretic hormone (SIADH) because the pituitary gland may be injured or compressed from cerebral edema (see Fluid and Electrolyte

Imbalances, p. 1005). Fluid overload can occur in the client with multiple trauma from the rapid administration of IV fluids, plasma expanders, or corticosteroids. Fluids may be restricted to 2 L/day initially to decrease increased ICP and swelling, but this practice is less common today. The amount of fluid restriction is also influenced by the response to diuretic therapy and an evaluation of laboratory values. Serum osmolality should be maintained below 310 mOsm. Urine specific gravity is checked every 1 to 4 hours. Serum and urine osmolality and electrolytes are monitored frequently.

STRATEGIES FOR SENSORY/PERCEPTUAL ALTERATIONS. The client with a *major* head injury may exhibit changes in the following areas: sense of smell; ability to taste, swallow, or feel the presence of food within the oral cavity; and vision, pain, and temperature sensation. As a result, the client is at risk for nutritional deficits, which may interfere with the healing process. The client may be injured from falling over objects outside the field of vision, or burn injuries could occur because of the inability to perceive variations in water temperatures.

The nurse ensures that mealtime and the surrounding environment is a pleasant experience and positions the client to maximize swallowing ability. The speech-language pathologist identifies strategies to prevent food from accumulating in the cheek of the affected side. In general, clients who have swallowing problems are able to tolerate or swallow soft or semisoft foods and liquids (mechanical soft or dental diet, junior baby foods, custards, scrambled eggs) better than thin liquids (water, juice, or milk). Powdered thickener (Thick-It) may be added to thicken foods to a more manageable consistency. The nurse collaborates with the dietitian to find a diet appropriate for the client with dysphagia.

If there is a large lesion of the parietal lobe, the client may experience a loss of sensation for pain, temperature, touch, and proprioception, which prevents the client from responding appropriately to environmental stimuli. A hazard-free environment is necessary to prevent injury (e.g., from burns, if the client's coffee is too hot; or from falls, if the siderails on the bed are not kept up). A sensory stimulation program should be integrated into the comatose or stuporous client's routine care activities. Sensory stimulation is done to facilitate a meaningful response to the environment. The nurse presents visual, auditory, or tactile stimuli one at a time and explains the purpose and the type of stimulus presented. For example, the nurse shows a picture of the client's mother and says, "This is a picture of your mother." The picture is shown several times, and the same words are used to describe the picture. If auditory tapes are used, they should not be longer than 10 to 15 minutes. If the stimulus is presented for a longer period, it simply becomes "white" noise, or meaningless background noise.

The client may be disoriented and experience a short-term memory loss. The nurse always introduces himself or herself to the client before any interaction. Explanations of procedures and activities should be short and simple and given immediately before and throughout the procedure. A sleep-wake cycle must be maintained, with scheduled rest periods. The nurse orients the client to time (day, month, and year) and place and explains the reason for the hospitalization. The client is reassured that he or she is safe and that family members know where he or she is. The nurse should ask the family to bring in familiar objects, such as pictures. Orientation cues within the environment, such as a large clock with numbers or a single-date calendar, should be provided.

PULMONARY MANAGEMENT. Pulmonary secretions tend to pool as the result of a decreased level of consciousness, an ineffective cough, or an altered breathing pattern. The secretions may be thick because of the fluid intake restriction used to prevent cerebral edema. Chest physiotherapy and frequent turning may be needed as indicated by the results of the respiratory assessment.

The client with increased intracranial pressure (ICP) should be carefully observed when suctioned. If the client is intubated, he or she should be manually hyperventilated (preoxygenated) with 100% oxygen for 60 seconds between each pass of the catheter. The client should be allowed a rest period of a few minutes after suctioning to prevent increased ICP. Lidocaine given intravenously or endotracheally may be used to suppress the cough reflex, which would increase ICP.

BEHAVIORAL MANAGEMENT. The client is at risk for seizure activity, and actions are taken as outlined in the discussion of epilepsy (see Chapter 42). The nurse or assistive nursing personnel keeps the bed in a low position with the siderails up. Hand mittens may be applied if the client attempts to pull out the IV line or nasogastric tube. Restraining any extremity increases agitation and fear. The client's behavior is observed and documented at least every hour. Alternatives to restraints should be attempted according to hospital policy. For example, covering the client's IV site with the I.V. House or other device may prevent dislodgement (see Chapter 14). Keeping the client's hands busy with activity pillows or puzzles accomplishes the same goal.

The nurse or assistive nursing personnel orients the client to the surroundings as needed and provide a quiet environment. The nurse closely monitors the client's response to television programs or the radio. Often, he or she is unable to differentiate these situations or programs from what is happening within his or her own environment.

STRATEGIES FOR PREVENTING COMPLICATIONS OF IMMOBILITY. Chapter 10 discusses mobility and ADL skills in detail as well as ways to prevent complications of immobility. Several additional interventions are provided in this section.

Until the client is fully mobile, he or she should wear pneumatic compression boots or sequential compression stockings to prevent venous stasis, which could lead to either a pulmonary embolus or deep vein thrombosis. Administration of prophylactic anticoagulants such as heparin, aspirin, or low–molecular weight heparinoids may be ordered.

In collaboration with the physical therapist and occupational therapist, a program of exercises to maintain function, prevent complications of immobility, and accomplish activities of daily living (ADLs) is implemented. The nurse, assistive nursing personnel, or significant other provides passive or active-assistive range-of-motion exercises at least once every 2 to 3 hours, with particular attention given to the joints of the fingers and the wrist. Splints for the affected limbs should be custom-fitted by physical or occupational therapists. The client whose feet are flaccid may wear high-topped tennis shoes to prevent footdrop. Such shoes may be used for the client who is spastic, but only after consultation with the occupational or physical therapist. The nurse or assistive nursing personnel applies and removes splints and supportive shoes and inspects the skin for signs of irritation several times each day.

NUTRITION MANAGEMENT. The client who is moderately to severely injured usually has a decreased level of consciousness, at least temporarily. As a result, the client is unable to chew or swallow and must receive nutrition and fluids by an alternative method. The client initially receives IV fluids until stabilized. If there is no improvement in level of consciousness, long-term nutritional support via enteral feeding is usually instituted. A small-lumen nasogastric or nasoduodenal tube or percutaneous endoscopic gastrostomy (PEG) tube is used for continuous or intermittent feeding. Small-bore tubes decrease the risk for aspiration in a client who is at high risk. Care of the client receiving enteral feeding is described in Chapter 61.

With the use of either type of tube, the nurse weighs the client daily, collaborates with the dietitian to determine if caloric needs are being met, and monitors serum albumin, prealbumin, and transferrin levels to ensure adequate protein intake. The client is assessed daily for signs of dehydration, such as dry mucous membranes and poor skin turgor. Supplements such as milkshakes and Ensure may be needed to meet the client's caloric and protein requirements if he or she is not receiving total enteral nutrition.

SURGICAL MANAGEMENT. The physician may elect to insert an ICP monitoring device to evaluate the client's pressure more closely. All devices are inserted through a burr hole that is placed in the skull using a twist drill. Each device is connected to a transducer that is connected to a monitor. The monitor is able to record the pressure waves and provide a digital readout of the pressure.

INTRACRANIAL PRESSURE MONITORING. Various types of devices for monitoring ICP are used. An *intraventricular catheter (IVC)* is a small tube that is inserted into the anterior horn of the lateral ventricle of the nondominant cerebral hemisphere. The advantage of this system is that cerebrospinal fluid (CSF) can be drained to decrease ICP, and specimens can be obtained for laboratory analysis. The *subarachnoid screw* or *bolt* is a hollow device placed into the subarachnoid space for direct pressure measurement. A disadvantage of the system is that CSF cannot be drained to treat increased ICP; however, it is less invasive, which lowers the risk of infection (Table 45-5).

An *epidural catheter* or *sensor* is a transducer that is placed between the skull and the dura, leaving the dura intact. A similar device is the *subdural catheter,* which is placed under the dura mater. Its major advantage is the decreased risk of infection from an open dural space. The *fiberoptic transducer tipped pressure sensor* is the most common device for ICP monitoring. It is easily transported and can be placed in the subdural or subarachnoid space, in the ventricle, or directly into brain tissue. The nurse follows the agency's protocols for the management of these devices.

CRANIOTOMY. In extreme cases in which the client's ICP cannot be controlled, the physician may elect to perform a craniotomy to remove ischemic tissue or the tips of the temporal lobes. The removal of nonvital brain tissue allows expansion of brain tissue without further compromise of ICP. A craniotomy may also be performed to remove epidural or subdural

TABLE 45-5 • ADVANTAGES AND DISADVANTAGES OF INTRACRANIAL PRESSURE MONITORING DEVICES

Monitoring Device	Advantages	Disadvantages
Intraventricular catheter (IVC)	Allows accurate measurement of intracranial pressure (ICP) Allows drainage or sampling of cerebrospinal fluid (CSF) Allows instillation of contrast media Provides reliable evaluation of cerebral compliance	Provides additional site for potential infection Most invasive method for monitoring ICP Must be balanced and recalibrated frequently Catheter can become occluded by blood or tissue Insertion can be difficult with small or collapsed ventricles CSF leakage can occur around insertion site Associated with increased infection rate
Subarachnoid bolt or screw	Lower infection rates than with IVC Quickly and easily placed Can be used with small or collapsed ventricles Does not penetrate brain parenchyma	Tendency for dampened waveform Less accurate at high ICP May become occluded by blood or tissue Must be balanced and recalibrated frequently (i.e., every 4 hours and whenever client is repositioned) Baseline drift and tendency for dampened waveform Does not provide for CSF sampling
Subdural/epidural catheter or sensor	Least invasive Decreased risk for infection Easily and quickly placed	Increasing baseline drift over time; therefore accuracy and reliability are questionable Does not provide for CSF sampling or drainage
Fiberoptic transducer tipped catheter	Can be placed in subdural or subarachnoid space, in ventricle, or into brain tissue Easily transported Requires zeroing only once (during insertion) Baseline drift to 1 mm Hg/day Decreased risk of infection Less waveform artifact No need to adjust transducer to client's position Easy to insert	Does not provide for CSF sampling or drainage Cannot be recalibrated after placement Probe needs periodic replacement Fragile fiberoptic cable easily damaged and broken

hematomas. Care of the client with a craniotomy is discussed under Postoperative Assessment (Brain Tumor), p. 1003.

Community-Based Care

The client with a *major* head injury requires case management and ongoing rehabilitation following hospitalization. Information on the selection of a head injury rehabilitation facility can be obtained from the National Head Injury Foundation (NHIF). Other preparation includes the development of a detailed client care plan to be given to the rehabilitation facility. This enables the provision of consistent care and decreases the initial anxiety related to the changes that the client may experience. The discharge summary states medications, including dosage, possible reactions, and special preparation; the current client care plan; techniques used to motivate or calm the client; and strategies to assist the family to adapt to the situation.

The goal of rehabilitation after head injury is to maximize the client's ability to return to his or her highest level of functioning. Rehabilitation activities such as occupational therapy (OT), physical therapy (PT), and speech therapy may continue in the home after discharge from the rehabilitation facility. Adaptation of the home environment to safely accommodate the client may be needed. The family may require assistance in obtaining adaptive devices needed for ADLs and ambulation.

HEALTH TEACHING

The staff nurse or case manager provides the client and family with both written and verbal instructions. The teaching plan for the client with craniocerebral trauma includes a review of seizure precautions and strategies to adapt to sensory dysfunction and to cope with the personality or behavior problems that may arise. The nurse explains the purpose, dosage, schedule, and route of administration of any medications. The client is encouraged to participate in activities as tolerated. Demonstrations and return demonstrations of care activities may facilitate the competence of family members in skill performance. The nurse stresses the importance of regular follow-up visits with therapists and health care providers.

With the family and the client, the nurse reinforces the same strategies used in the hospital to treat sensory or perceptual changes. In addition, the family or significant others are taught about the importance of not moving furniture or other objects in the home to a different place, because this can lead to an injury in the client with visual problems or might confuse the client with cognitive impairments.

Clients with personality and behavior problems respond best to a structured and consistent environment. The nurse instructs the family to develop a home routine that provides structure, repetition, and consistency. The family must also be instructed on the importance of reinforcing positive behaviors and not reinforcing negative behaviors.

The nurse teaches the client who has sustained a *minor* head injury (e.g., a concussion) that postconcussion syndrome may occur. This syndrome is a group of clinical manifestations including, but not limited to, the following:

- Personality changes
- Irritability
- Headaches
- Dizziness
- Restlessness
- Nervousness
- Insomnia
- Memory loss

Many clients with head injuries experience some of these manifestations during recovery. However, some clients have these problems for weeks, months, or even years to the extent that they interfere with daily activities such as employment. The prolonged pattern is classified as post-trauma syndrome. The exact cause of the phenomenon is not known, but physiologic and psychologic theories have been espoused. Support groups and professional counseling are the most effective interventions.

Most clients with moderate-to-severe craniocerebral trauma are discharged with physical and cognitive disabilities. Changes in personality and behavior are not unusual. The family must learn to cope with the client's increased fatigue, irritability, temper outbursts, depression, and memory problems. These clients often require constant supervision at home, and eventually the families feel socially isolated. The nurse instructs the family to plan for regular respite care, either in a structured day-care respite program or through relief provided by a friend or neighbor. Family members, particularly the primary caretaker, may become depressed and experience feelings of loneliness. They may also experience isolation, increased responsibilities, and role reversals. In addition, the family may feel angry at the client because of the additional responsibilities (financial or emotional) that his or her care has placed on them. To help the family cope with these problems, the nurse suggests that they join and actively participate in a local head injury support group.

The client needs assistance in identifying realistic expectations for discharge. Because of cognitive deficits, it may not be possible for the client to return to his or her previous employment or educational pursuits. The client may experience a sense of isolation and loneliness, because personality and behavior changes make it difficult to resume or maintain the social contacts he or she had before the injury.

HOME CARE MANAGEMENT

Little home care preparation is needed for the client with a concussion unless he or she is experiencing symptoms of post-traumatic sequelae. The nurse or discharge planner assesses the client's home for potential hazards before discharge from the hospital. There must be functioning smoke and fire alarms, because the client with a head injury often loses the sense of smell. This information can be obtained from the admission data or by a home visit. Home adaptations and referrals to outside agencies should be completed before discharge.

HEALTH CARE RESOURCES

The nurse or case manager refers families and significant others and clients to the National Head Injury Foundation (NHIF), as well as to the local or state group, for information and support. The NHIF and its state chapters maintain lists of rehabilitation facilities for clients with head injuries. The NHIF will send family members and other interested persons guidelines for selecting a rehabilitation facility. Families should inquire about the facility's experience in caring for the person with a head injury, how many admissions the facility has had in the previous 2 to 3 years, and the results or outcome statistics on those clients (e.g., how many went home and at what functional recovery level—poor, fair, or good). Other helpful groups include the National Easter Seal Society and the National Institute of Handicapped Research.

BRAIN TUMORS

OVERVIEW

Brain tumors can arise anywhere within the brain structures and are named according to the cell or tissue from which they originate. Primary tumors originate within the central nervous system (CNS) and rarely metastasize outside this area. Secondary brain tumors result from metastasis from other areas of the body, such as the lungs, breast, kidney, and gastrointestinal tract.

Pathophysiology

Primary brain tumors occur as a rapid proliferation or abnormal growth of cells normally found within the CNS. Secondary brain tumors occur as malignant cells from other tumors outside the CNS that metastasize to the brain. Regardless of origin, the tumor expands in an irregular fashion and invades, infiltrates, or compresses normal brain tissue. This leads to the following:

- Cerebral edema
- Increased intracranial pressure (ICP)
- Focal neurologic deficits
- Obstruction of the flow of cerebrospinal fluid (CSF)
- Pituitary dysfunction

COMPLICATIONS OF TUMORS

Cerebral edema, or more specifically vasogenic edema, results from changes in capillary endothelial tissue permeability, which allows plasma to seep into the extracellular spaces. This leads to increased ICP, and herniation of the brain tissue may occur. A variety of focal neurologic deficits result from edema, infiltration, and compression of surrounding brain tissue. The cerebral blood vessels may become compressed because of edema and increased ICP. This compression leads to ischemia of the area supplied by the vessel. In addition, the tumor may infiltrate the walls of the vessel, causing it to rupture and hemorrhage into the tumor bed or adjacent brain tissue. Approximately 33% of clients who have brain tumors experience seizure activity attributable to interference with the brain's normal conduction pathways.

Increased ICP may also result from obstruction of the flow of CSF or displacement of the lateral ventricles by the expanding lesion. Typically, a tumor obstructs the aqueduct of Sylvius or one of the ventricles or encroaches on the subarachnoid space. Posterior fossa tumors may obstruct the flow of CSF from the fourth ventricle to the foramen of Luschka or Magendie. With any brain tumor, the obstruction of normal CSF flow causes hydrocephalus and eventually leads to increased ICP.

Pituitary dysfunction may occur as the tumor compresses the pituitary gland and causes the syndrome of inappropriate antidiuretic hormone (SIADH) or diabetes insipidus (DI). These disorders result in severe fluid and electrolyte imbalances and can be life threatening (see Chapter 63 for a complete description).

CLASSIFICATION OF TUMORS

Brain tumors are usually classified as either malignant or benign (Table 45-6). Benign tumors are generally associated with a favorable outcome, which is often not the case with malignant tumors. However, benign tumors may be malignant by virtue of their location. If the tumor cannot be completely removed or treated, it continues to grow. As it invades other brain tissue, cerebral edema, focal neurologic deficits, and increased ICP occur. Herniation of brain tissue eventually leads to death. Benign tumors also may undergo histologic changes and become malignant.

A second classification system is based on location. Supratentorial tumors, which occur most often in adults, are located in the area above the tentorium, the tentlike fold of dura that surrounds the cerebellar hemisphere and supports the occipital lobe. In other words, supratentorial tumors are located within the cerebral hemispheres. Located beneath the tentorium is the infratentorial area, the area of the brainstem structures and cerebellum.

A third classification system depends on the cellular, histologic, or anatomic origins of the tumor. The nervous system is composed of two types of cells: (1) neurons, which are responsible for nerve impulse conduction; and (2) neuroglial cells, which provide support, nourishment, and protection for neurons. Four specific types of cells are neuroglial cells: astrocytes, oligodendroglia, ependymal cells, and microglia. When classifying tumors according to this system, tumors are named by their cell type. For example, an astrocytoma is a tumor of astrocytes.

GLIOMAS. Gliomas are malignant tumors. They account for 60% of all brain tumors in adults and arise from the neuroglial cells of the brain and brainstem. Malignant gliomas have a peak incidence in people 40 to 60 years of age. They infiltrate and invade surrounding brain tissue. The most common type of glioma is the astrocytoma, which may be found anywhere within the cerebral hemispheres. It is usually treated by surgery, followed by radiation and chemotherapy. Oligodendrogliomas, another type of glioma, are generally located within the frontal lobes of the brain. These tumors are slow-growing and are usually calcified. Surgical removal is possible, and the long-term prognosis is good. A glioblastoma is a highly malignant, grade III or higher, rapidly growing, in-

TABLE 45-6 • CLASSIFICATION OF BRAIN TUMORS

BENIGN	MALIGNANT
• Acoustic neuroma	• Astrocytoma
• Meningioma	Grade 2
• Pituitary adenoma	Grade 3
• Astrocytoma	Grade 4 (also known as glioblastoma multiforme)
Grade 1 (may undergo changes and become malignant)	• Oligodendroglioma
	• Ependymoma
	• Medulloblastoma
• Chondroma	• Chondrosarcoma
• Craniopharyngioma	• Glioma
• Hemangioblastoma	• Lymphoma

vasive astrocytoma. Although improved surgical techniques and advanced treatment have improved the outlook and quality of life for a client with this type of tumor, fewer than 15% of affected clients survive 18 months after diagnosis. Ependymomas arise from the lining of the ventricles and are difficult to treat surgically because of their location. The treatment of choice involves radiation and shunting procedures to control the hydrocephalus caused by the blocking of normal CSF flow by the tumor. Chemotherapy may also be used for these tumors.

Gliomas are graded according to their cellular differentiation or how closely the tumor cells resemble normal cells. Grade I tumors are well differentiated, grade II tumors are moderately differentiated, and grade III tumors are poorly differentiated. Grade III tumors may rapidly change to grade IV tumors, which are poorly differentiated. A grade III or IV astrocytoma is referred to as glioblastoma multiforme and is associated with a poor outcome. Grade I and II tumors often undergo cellular changes and become grade III or IV tumors.

MENINGIOMAS. **Meningiomas** arise from the coverings of the brain (the meninges). They are the most common benign tumor, with a peak incidence at age 50 years. Females are affected more than males by a 2:1 ratio. This tumor is encapsulated, globular, and well demarcated and causes compression and displacement of surrounding brain tissue. Although complete removal of the tumor is possible, it tends to recur. It tends to occur in areas where the meninges predominate.

PITUITARY TUMORS. Pituitary tumors that occur in the anterior lobe account for 10% to 25% of brain tumors and may cause endocrine dysfunction. The most common type of pituitary tumor is the adenoma, which is subdivided into chromophobe, secretory, and nonsecretory adenomas. These tumors are benign and often occur in young and middle-aged adults. The presenting symptoms are often visual disturbances. These tumors also produce hypopituitary signs, such as loss of body hair, diabetes insipidus, sterility, visual field defects, and headaches.

ACOUSTIC NEUROMAS. Acoustic neuromas arise from the sheath of Schwann cells in the peripheral portion of cranial nerve VIII. They are also referred to as cerebellar pontine angle (CPA) tumors to describe their anatomic location. Acoustic neuromas compress brain tissue and tend to surround adjacent cranial nerves (VII, V, IX, X), making surgical removal difficult without causing permanent cranial nerve dysfunction. Females are twice as likely as males to have acoustic neuromas. Common symptoms include hearing loss, **tinnitus** (ringing in the ears), and dizziness.

Metastatic, or secondary tumors, account for nearly 30% of brain tumors. Metastatic cells from the lungs, breast, colon, pancreas, and kidney can travel to the brain via the blood and the lymphatic system. Multiple metastatic lesions are not uncommon.

Etiology

The exact cause of brain tumors is unknown. Several areas under investigation include genetic changes, heredity, errors in fetal development, ionizing radiation, electromagnetic fields, environmental hazards, diet, viruses, and injury. Recently, the use of cellular phones has been i development of brain tumors.

Incidence/Prevalence

Brain tumors account for 1.8% of all cancer deat dence rate for all primary brain tumors is 11.8 per 100,0 persons; the incidence rate for malignant tumors is 6.4 per 100,000 persons. In 1999, 16,800 new cases were diagnosed, and there were 13,100 deaths (Landis et al., 1999). Brain tumors in the adult population are seen primarily in clients 40 to 60 years of age.

CONSIDERATIONS FOR OLDER ADULTS

The incidence rate of brain tumors is higher in men and in Caucasians. Meningiomas are seen more often in middle-aged women and in older women, whereas gliomas are seen slightly more often in older men. The incidence of malignant tumors increases with age, with the greatest increases in those over 70 years of age (Prados, Berger, & Wilson, 1998).

COLLABORATIVE MANAGEMENT

Assessment

The clinical manifestations of brain tumors vary with the site of the tumor (Chart 45-9). In general, symptoms of a brain tumor include the following:

- Headaches that are usually more severe upon awakening in the morning
- Nausea and vomiting
- Visual symptoms
- Seizures
- Changes in mentation or personality
- Papilledema (swelling of the optic disk)

Neurologic deficits result from the destruction, distortion, or compression of brain tissue. Supratentorial tumors usually result in paralysis, seizures, memory loss, cognitive impairment, language impairment, or vision problems. Infratentorial

CHART 45-9

KEY FEATURES *of* Common Brain Tumors

Cerebral Tumors
- Headache (most common feature)
- Vomiting unrelated to food intake
- Changes in visual acuity and visual fields; diplopia (visual changes caused by papilledema)
- Hemiparesis or hemiplegia
- Hypokinesia
- Hyperesthesia, paresthesia, decreased tactile discrimination
- Seizures
- Aphasia
- Changes in personality and/or behavior

Brainstem Tumors
- Hearing loss (acoustic neuroma)
- Facial pain and weakness
- Dysphagia, decreased gag reflex
- Nystagmus
- Hoarseness
- Ataxia and dysarthria (cerebellar tumors)

tors produce ataxia, autonomic nervous system dysfunction, vomiting, drooling, hearing loss, and vision impairment. As the tumor grows, intracranial pressure increases, and the symptoms become progressively more severe.

Diagnosis is based on the history, neurologic assessment, clinical examination, and results of neurodiagnostic testing. Noninvasive diagnostic studies such as computed tomography (CT), magnetic resonance imaging (MRI), and skull films are conducted first. The CT and MRI identify the size, location, and extent of the tumor. The MRI may be used for initial diagnostic evaluation, whereas the CT is often used for follow-up during the hospital course.

Cerebral angiography is usually not indicated to diagnose a brain tumor but may be used to provide additional information about vascular supply to the tumor. Electroencephalography (EEG), lumbar puncture (LP), myelogram, brain scan, and positron emission tomography (PET) may be indicated to provide further information about the size, location, and characteristics of the tumor. Laboratory tests may also be ordered to evaluate endocrine function, renal status, and electrolyte balance.

Interventions

When possible, the nurse obtains a history from both the client and the family, including current signs and symptoms. A complete neurologic assessment is needed to establish baseline data and to determine the nature and extent of neurologic deficits.

NONSURGICAL MANAGEMENT. The goal of treatment of brain tumors is to decrease tumor size, improve quality of life, and improve survival time. The type of treatment selected depends on the tumor size and location, client symptoms and general condition, and whether the tumor is recurrent. The treatment of brain tumors may include radiation, chemotherapy, and surgery. A number of experimental treatment modalities are being investigated, including blood-brain barrier disruption, recombinant deoxyribonucleic acid (DNA), monoclonal antibodies, new antineoplastic drugs, immunotherapy, and hyperthermia. Gliadel wafers have recently been approved by the Food and Drug Administration (FDA) for use as adjunct therapy in clients with recurrent glioblastoma multiforme. These wafers are placed in the resection cavity of the tumor (Rhone-Poulenc, 1996).

DRUG THERAPY. The health care provider may prescribe a variety of medications to treat the client's symptoms and to prevent complications. Analgesics, such as codeine and acetaminophen (Tylenol, Ace-Tabs♣), are given for headache. Dexamethasone (Decadron) is usually given to control cerebral edema. Research supports the efficacy of administering glucocorticoids for the treatment of edema resulting from brain tumors. Phenytoin (Dilantin) is used to prevent seizure activity. Histamine blockers such as ranitidine hydrochloride (Zantac, Apo-Ranitidine♣) or nizatidine (Axid, Axid AR) are given to decrease gastric acid secretion and prevent the development of stress ulcers. Prochlorperazine dimaleate (Compazine) and other antiemetics are used to treat nausea and vomiting.

RADIATION THERAPY AND CHEMOTHERAPY. Radiation therapy may be used alone, after surgery, or in combination with chemotherapy and surgery. Chapter 25 discusses radiation treatment for cancer in detail. Chemotherapy may be given alone, in combination with radiation and surgery, and with tumor progression. Although these drugs may control tumor growth or decrease tumor burden, the benefit usually is very short-lived. Chemotherapy usually involves more than one agent and may be given intravenously, intra-arterially, or intrathecally through an Ommaya reservoir.

RADIOSURGICAL PROCEDURES. Radiosurgical procedures are an alternative to surgery. These techniques include the modified linear accelerator using accelerated x-rays, a particle accelerator using beams of protons (cyclotron), isotope seeds implanted in the tumor (brachytherapy), and the gamma knife (Figure 45-12).

The gamma knife is a type of stereotactic radiosurgical procedure that uses a single high dose of ionized radiation to focus 201 beams of cobalt-60 radiation to selectively destroy intracranial lesions without damaging surrounding healthy tissue. Combining neurodiagnostic imaging tools—including magnetic resonance imaging (MRI), computed tomography (CT), magnetic resonance angiography (MRA), and angiography—with the gamma knife allows for precise localization of deep-seated or anatomically difficult lesions and the delivery of a customized dose of cobalt-60 radiation to the desired area only. Treatment usually takes less than an hour, and clients require only overnight hospitalization. Advantages of this technique include its noninvasive nature, a lower risk than the traditional craniotomy, surgical precision, and decreased cost, morbidity, length of hospital stay, and recovery time.

The gamma knife is used primarily for brain tumors or arteriovenous malformations (AVMs) that are in an inaccessible location and therefore unresectable by craniotomy. Tumors typically treated in this manner are acoustic neuromas, meningiomas, and metastatic tumors. The gamma knife may also be used with clients who refuse conventional surgery, for clients whose age and physical condition precludes general anesthesia, as an adjunct to radiation therapy, and for recurrent or residual AVM or tumors after embolization or craniotomy.

SURGICAL MANAGEMENT. The most important modality in the treatment of brain tumors is a biopsy to determine the specific pathology. A craniotomy is the most common sur-

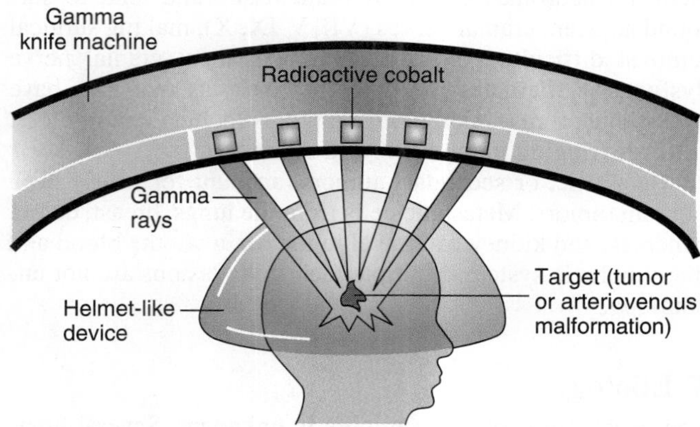

Figure 45-12 ● A gamma knife treatment. The radiation beams are widely dispersed over the surface of the head to prevent damage to healthy brain tissue. The beams are intense only at the point of the target.

gical treatment and may be done to improve symptoms related to the lesion or to decrease pressure effects. The challenge for the surgeon is to remove the tumor as completely as possible without damaging normal tissue. Complete removal is possible with some benign tumors, which results in a "surgical cure." Postoperatively, the client is usually admitted to the critical care unit.

POSTOPERATIVE ASSESSMENT. The Client Care Plan on p. 1004 highlights the major aspects of postoperative nursing care following a craniotomy. The focus of postoperative care is to monitor the client to detect changes in status and to prevent or minimize complications, especially increased ICP. The nurse assesses neurologic and vital signs every 30 minutes for the first 4 to 6 hours after surgery and then every hour. If the client is stable for 24 hours, the frequency of these checks may be decreased to every 2 to 4 hours, depending on the agency's policy. Potential neurologic deficits include a decreased level of consciousness, motor weakness or paralysis, aphasia, visual changes, and personality changes. Periorbital edema and ecchymosis of one or both eyes is not unusual and is treated with cold compresses to decrease swelling. The nurse irrigates the affected eye with warm saline solution or artificial tears to improve client comfort.

The client in the critical care unit is routinely connected to the cardiac monitor. Dysrhythmias may occur after posterior fossa surgery or result from fluid and electrolyte imbalance. Other nursing interventions include strict recording of the client's intake and output and a fluid restriction to 1500 mL/day. Range-of-motion exercises to all extremities are performed at least every 2 to 3 hours. The nurse or assistive nursing personnel assists the client to turn, cough, and breathe deeply every 2 hours. To prevent the development of deep vein thrombosis, sequential compression stockings or pneumatic compression boots are kept in place until the client is ambulating.

Positioning. Clients who have undergone supratentorial surgery should have the head of the bed elevated 30 degrees to promote venous drainage from the head. The nurse positions the client to avoid extreme hip or neck flexion and maintains the head in a midline, neutral position. The client may be turned side-to-side or remain supine. If a large tumor has been removed, it is recommended that the client be placed on the nonoperative side to prevent displacement of the cranial contents by gravity. The client with an infratentorial craniotomy should be kept flat and positioned on either side for 24 to 48 hours. This prevents pressure on the neck-area incision site. It also prevents pressure on the internal tumor excision site from higher cerebral structures. The client should receive nothing by mouth (NPO status) for 24 hours, because edema around the medulla and lower cranial nerves may place the client at risk for vomiting and aspiration.

Monitoring the Dressing. The nurse checks the head dressing every 1 to 2 hours for signs of drainage. The area of drainage is marked once during each shift for baseline comparison. A small or moderate amount of drainage is expected. Some clients may have a Hemovac, Jackson-Pratt, or other surgical drain in place for 24 hours after surgery. The nurse measures the drainage every 8 hours and records the amount and color; a typical amount of drainage is 30 to 50 mL per shift (8 hours). The nurse follows the manufacturer's and physician's instructions to maintain suction within the drain. Excessive amounts of drainage (a saturated head dressing or drainage greater than 50 mL/8 hr) should be reported immediately to the physician.

Monitoring Laboratory Values. The laboratory studies monitored postoperatively include complete blood count (CBC), serum electrolyte levels and osmolality, coagulation studies, and arterial blood gas (ABG) measurements.

The client's hematocrit and hemoglobin concentration may be abnormally low from blood loss during surgery or perhaps elevated if the blood was replaced. Hyponatremia may occur as a result of fluid volume overload, syndrome of inappropriate antidiuretic hormone (SIADH), or steroid administration. Hypokalemia may cause cardiac irritability. Weakness, a change in level of consciousness, and confusion are symptoms of hyponatremia and hypokalemia. Hypernatremia may be caused by meningitis, dehydration, or diabetes insipidus (DI). It is manifested by muscle weakness, restlessness, extreme thirst, and dry mouth. Untreated hypernatremia may lead to seizure activity. ABG values are monitored to ensure adequate cerebral oxygenation.

Ventilating the Client. Often the client is electively mechanically ventilated and hyperventilated for the first 24 to 48 hours after surgery to prevent increased intracranial pressure (ICP). The goal of hyperventilation is to keep the partial pressure of arterial carbon dioxide at 27 to 35 mm Hg, with normal arterial oxygen levels. This produces cerebral vasoconstriction, which decreases ICP. If the client is awake or attempting to breathe at a rate other than that set on the ventilator, medications such as fentanyl citrate (Sublimaze) are given. The client who is intubated is suctioned if indicated by the findings of frequent respiratory assessments. The nurse must remember to hyperoxygenate the client before suctioning.

DRUG THERAPY. Medications routinely given postoperatively include anticonvulsants, histamine blockers, and corticosteroids, such as dexamethasone (Decadron). Analgesics such as codeine are given for pain, and acetaminophen is given for fever or mild pain. Some physicians may elect to administer prophylactic antibiotics to prevent infection.

PREVENTING POSTOPERATIVE COMPLICATIONS. Postoperative complications are listed in Table 45-7.

Increased Intracranial Pressure. The major postoperative complication of supratentorial surgery is increased ICP from cerebral edema, hemorrhage, or obstruction of the normal flow of cerebrospinal fluid (CSF). Symptoms of increased ICP include severe headache, deteriorating level of consciousness, restlessness, irritability, and dilated or pinpoint pupils that are slow to react or are nonreactive to light.

Treatment of increased ICP includes placing the client supine with the head of the bed elevated 30 degrees unless contraindicated. The head should be maintained in a midline, neutral position to facilitate venous drainage from the brain. Osmotic diuretics such as mannitol (Osmitrol), glucocorticoids, or loop diuretics may be given to decrease cerebral edema. After computed tomography or other diagnostic tests determine the exact cause of increased ICP, the client may be connected to a ventilator and hyperventilated. A monitoring device may be inserted to measure ICP more accurately. Surgery may be needed to correct the problem (e.g., hematoma) or to relieve pressure. Treatment of increased ICP is discussed more fully under Ineffective Tissue Perfusion (Stroke), p. 983.

Client Care Plan • THE CLIENT REQUIRING A CRANIOTOMY

NURSING DIAGNOSIS NO. 1 • Deficient Knowledge related to the surgical procedure

Expected Outcomes	Nursing Interventions	Rationale
The client will verbalize preoperative and postoperative routines. The client will be free of postoperative complications.	Provide preoperative teaching: • Answer questions. • Reinforce information provided by the surgeon. Explain preoperative preparation, such as laboratory work, chest x-ray studies, electrocardiogram. Explain anesthesia procedures.	An informed client is less anxious and fearful.
	Explain the procedure for preparing the client's head for surgery. Tell the client and the family how long the procedure will take and where the client will go after surgery (perianesthesia care unit or critical care unit).	The client's hair is shaved in the surgical site.
	Discuss how the client will look after surgery. Tell the family where to wait while the client is in surgery. [D] Ensure that all permits are signed. If possible, arrange a visit to the critical care unit so the client and family can meet the staff. Explain routine postoperative care—head dressing, urinary catheter, endotracheal tube, IVs, incentive spirometry, pain management.	The client will have a head dressing, may have periorbital edema and bruising, and may be intubated and on a ventilator.

NURSING DIAGNOSIS NO. 2 • Ineffective Tissue Perfusion (Cerebral) related to the surgical procedure

Expected Outcomes	Nursing Interventions	Rationale
The client's level of consciousness and neurologic status will improve or remain the same.	Check vital signs and neurologic signs every hour postoperatively or more often as clinically indicated. Report changes to the physician. Monitor for signs of increased ICP. Implement nursing measures to prevent increased ICP: • Elevate the head of the bed 30 degrees. [D] • Position the client in bed to avoid extreme hip and neck flexion. [D] • Maintain the client's head in a midline, neutral position. [D] • Avoid clustering nursing activities. [D] • Avoid talking about the client at the bedside. [D] • Provide a quiet environment. [D]	The client is at risk for increased intracranial pressure (ICP).
	Record strict measurement of intake and output. [D] Monitor serum electrolyte levels, serum and urine osmolality, and urine specific gravity. Administer medications as ordered if ICP increases.	Fluid intake is generally restricted postoperatively. The client is at risk for dehydration and fluid and electrolyte imbalance.
	Check the head dressing for drainage: • Circle and date the area of drainage. • Notify the physician of a significant increase in drainage. • Notify the physician of cerebrospinal fluid (CSF) drainage immediately.	A small amount of bloody drainage is not unusual; CSF drainage is not normal.

NURSING DIAGNOSIS NO. 3 • Acute Pain related to the surgical procedure

Expected Outcomes	Nursing Interventions	Rationale
The client's pain will be alleviated or reduced.	Assess level and extent of pain. Give pain medication as ordered; document the client's response. Assess the effectiveness of pain relief, and collaborate with the physician for an effective pain management protocol. Use nonpharmaceutical pain relief measures, such as imagery, relaxation, distraction, or music, as needed. Organize a plan of care to allow the client uninterrupted periods of rest.	Pain management enables the client to participate fully in the plan of care.
	Apply an ice pack to the eyes as needed. [D] Provide comfort measures: • Provide a back rub. [D] • Apply cool compress to forehead. [D]	The client may have periorbital edema.
	Provide frequent mouth care: [D] • Apply moisturizer to the lips. [D] • Provide ice chips. [D]	The client's mouth may be dry because of the fluid restriction.

TABLE 45-7 • POSTOPERATIVE COMPLICATIONS OF CRANIOTOMY

Increased intracranial pressure (ICP) Hematomas • Subdural hematoma • Epidural hematoma • Subarachnoid hemorrhage Hypovolemic shock Hydrocephalus Respiratory complications • Atelectasis • Hypoxia • Pneumonia • Neurogenic pulmonary edema	Wound infection Meningitis Fluid and electrolyte imbalances • Dehydration • Hyponatremia • Hypernatremia Seizures Cerebrospinal fluid (CSF) leak Cerebral edema

Cerebral edema is often present before surgery and may be further increased by tissue manipulation during the surgical procedure. Edema usually reaches a peak within 72 hours after surgery and, if no further complications occur, gradually subsides during the next few weeks. Cerebral edema is manifested by a change in the level of consciousness and other symptoms of increased ICP.

Hematomas. Subdural and epidural hematomas and intracranial hemorrhage are manifested by severe headache, a change in level of consciousness, progressive neurologic deficits, and herniation syndromes. Bleeding into the posterior fossa may lead to sudden cardiovascular and respiratory arrest. Treatment of a hematoma necessitates surgical removal, whereas an intracranial hemorrhage is treated with aggressive medical management (e.g., osmotic diuretics and ICP monitoring).

Hydrocephalus. Hydrocephalus is caused by obstruction of the normal CSF pathway from edema, an expanding lesion such as a hematoma, or blood in the subarachnoid space. Rapidly progressive hydrocephalus produces the classic symptoms of increased ICP. Slowly progressive hydrocephalus is manifested by headache, decreased level of consciousness, irritability, blurred vision, and urinary incontinence. This condition is often self-limiting and resolves without any treatment or with daily lumbar punctures to remove CSF. If treatment is required, a surgical shunt is inserted to drain CSF to another area of the body. A ventriculoperitoneal or, less often, a ventriculoatrial or lumbar peritoneal shunt procedure is usually performed. A major complication of the shunting procedure is a subdural hematoma from the tearing of bridging veins. An external lumbar drain may also be used temporarily. Additional information about shunts may be found in neuroscience nursing textbooks.

Respiratory Problems. Respiratory complications include atelectasis, pneumonia, and neurogenic pulmonary edema. Atelectasis and pneumonia can be prevented by providing appropriate pulmonary hygiene, turning the client frequently, and encouraging the client to take frequent deep breaths to expand the lungs each hour. The provision of humidified air and incentive spirometry are useful techniques to prevent these complications. Other treatment modalities include endotracheal or oral tracheal suctioning and chest physiotherapy. These measures may cause an increase in ICP. However, close monitoring of the client's status and ICP waveforms allows him or her to receive the benefits of aggressive pulmonary hygiene despite the potential risk.

Neurogenic pulmonary edema is an infrequent but life-threatening complication of neurologic insult such as TBI, brain tumors, or surgery. Its symptoms are the same as those of acute pulmonary edema, but there are no associated cardiac problems. In spite of aggressive treatment, most clients with neurogenic pulmonary edema do not survive the insult.

Wound Infection. Wound infections occur more often in older and debilitated clients and in clients with a history of diabetes, long-term steroid use, obesity, and previous infections. The client may contribute to the problem by rubbing or scratching the wound. If infection is present, the wound appears reddened and puffy. It may begin to separate, is sensitive to touch, and feels warm. The client may or may not be febrile. Treatment is based on the degree and extent of the infection. The nurse may treat a localized infection by simply cleaning it with alcohol or by applying local antibiotics. For more severe infections, systemic antibiotic administration may be required. If the underlying bone is involved, it may need to be removed.

Meningitis. Meningitis is an inflammation of the meninges and may occur as a result of surgery or wound infection, a cerebrospinal fluid (CSF) leak, or contamination during surgery. (See the discussion of meningitis in Chapter 44 for a more complete explanation of this complication.)

Fluid and Electrolyte Imbalances. Complications related to fluid and electrolyte imbalance include diabetes insipidus (DI), syndrome of inappropriate antidiuretic hormone (SIADH), and cerebral salt wasting (CSW). DI is seen most often after supratentorial surgery, especially procedures involving the pituitary gland or hypothalamus. Failure of the posterior pituitary gland to secrete antidiuretic hormone (ADH) leads to failure of the renal tubules to reabsorb water. The client's urine output increases dramatically (it may be up to 10 L/day), and the urine specific gravity drops to below 1.005. Urine osmolality decreases, whereas serum osmolality increases. The client may become dehydrated, with hypovolemic shock developing if this condition is left untreated. Fluid replacement to replace urinary losses and prevent dehydration may be accomplished by having the client increase oral intake or use IV fluids if he or she can do so. Hormonal replacement may also be necessary, especially if fluid loss is greater than 6 L/24 hr.

Aqueous vasopressin is short-acting, lasting only 6 to 8 hours. Desmopressin acetate (DDAVP) may be administered for long-term replacement therapy.

SIADH occurs when the posterior pituitary gland secretes too much ADH, causing water retention. The client becomes anuric, with a urinary output of less than 20 mL/hr. Sodium concentration in the urine is normal or elevated, whereas the serum sodium level falls. Other indications of SIADH are loss of thirst, irritability, muscle weakness, and decreased level of consciousness. SIADH is treated by fluid restriction, which is usually sufficient to correct the hyponatremia. Slow IV infusion of 3% hypertonic sodium may be needed for severe hyponatremia (<118 mEq/L).

CSW is thought to result from the extra renal influence of atrial natriuretic factor (ANF). ANF cells are located in the hypothalamus and the right atrium and regulate fluid volume. CSW is believed to be the primary cause of hyponatremia in the neurosurgical population. It is characterized by hyponatremia, decreased serum osmolality, and decreased blood volume. Serum vasopressin and ANF levels can differentiate CSW and SIADH. CSW is treated with the replacement of sodium and isotonic fluid volume.

Clients with complications related to fluid and electrolyte imbalance undergo strict measurement of their intake and output. An accurate daily weight measurement is an essential aspect of nursing care. The nurse assesses carefully for indications of fluid overload or dehydration during treatment. Serum electrolyte levels and osmolality are measured daily (or more often if clinically indicated). Chapter 12 and 13 provide additional information on fluid and electrolyte imbalances, and Chapter 63 provides further discussion of SIADH and DI.

CRITICAL THINKING CHALLENGE

You are a nurse in the neurosurgical step-down unit of a large tertiary care center. Today you receive a client transferred from the neurosurgical intensive care unit who had a craniotomy 3 days ago to remove a malignant brain tumor. He has had an uneventful postoperative course and is planning to undergo radiation and chemotherapy after he recovers from surgery. His prognosis is guarded at this time.

- What postoperative complications should you monitor for?
- With what members of the interdisciplinary team might you need to collaborate?
- What health teaching will he need before he is discharged from the hospital?

For suggested answer guidelines, go to SIMON http://www.wbsaunders.com/SIMON/Iggy/.

Community-Based Care

The client with a brain tumor is managed at home if possible. The nurse or case manager mobilizes health resources to support the client and family at home. Maintaining a reasonable quality of life is an important goal for recovery and rehabilitation (see the Evidence Based Practice for Nursing box at right).

HEALTH TEACHING

It is important that the client and family fully understand the importance of any recommended follow-up health care appointments. The nurse writes the date, time, and place on a card and gives it to the client or family member, significant other, or other caregiver. The discharge summary should state the name of the person who has given the follow-up information.

Information given to the client and the family or significant others includes the name of the medications, the dosage, the timing of administration, the number of days to take the medication, and any side effects. The nurse explains what to do or whom to call if any adverse reactions occur. The client is taught to refrain from taking any over-the-counter medications unless authorized by the health care provider.

The nurse instructs the client to maintain a program of regular physical exercise within the limits of any disabilities. Referral to the dietitian may be necessary to ensure adequate caloric intake for the client receiving radiation or chemotherapy.

Seizures are a potential complication that can occur at any time for as long as 1 year or more postoperatively. The nurse provides the client and the family with information about seizure precautions and what to do if a seizure occurs.

If long-term changes or disability is expected, the client needs to be prepared for major lifestyle changes. Chapter 10 discusses coping with disability in more detail.

EVIDENCE-BASED PRACTICE FOR NURSING

How do clients with brain tumors view their quality of life?

Fox, S., & Lantz, C. (1998). The brain tumor experience and quality of life: A qualitative study. *Journal of Neuroscience Nursing, 30*(4), 245-252.

The purpose of this qualitative study was to explore the quality of life (QOL) experienced by clients with brain tumors and their families to more clearly define QOL in brain tumor clients and to contribute to gaps in the existing QOL literature.

Semistructured interviews were conducted with 23 adults with brain tumors and 21 significant others. Data were organized into five conceptual themes: the stigma of a mind-body illness, an invasive disease of the self, my family has a brain tumor, dealing with medical diplomats, and QOL—no substitute for living. It was difficult for the researchers to separate QOL from the context of the brain tumor experience, because many participants commented that no experience had prepared them to deal with the brain tumor. Many equated QOL with dying because it had not been mentioned until no other treatment options existed. Two significant themes—invasive disease of the self and associated stigma of a mind-body illness—were revealed as unique to the brain tumor population.

Critique. Despite the small convenience sample, this study provides valuable information about QOL in clients with brain tumors and in their families. There was no attempt to control for tumor type or grade, and the presence of significant others during the interview process may have influenced clients' responses. Therefore it is not possible to extrapolate the study's results to the general brain tumor population.

Implications for Nursing. This study helps nurses understand what is important to clients with brain tumors and their families in order to cope with the diagnosis. The experience of having a brain tumor is devastating and has a catastrophic impact on the family. Although most nurses would expect physical care to be of the highest priority, study participants point out that their need for information and guidance about to what to expect during the course of the tumor, especially the changes to expect, are paramount in planning care. The authors note that QOL in clients with brain tumors is "uncharted water." This study is an important beginning in charting this course.

HOME CARE MANAGEMENT

Unless the client has a permanent disability, no special home care preparation is needed. Clients with hemiparesis need assistance to ensure that their home is accessible according to their method of mobility (e.g., cane, walker, or wheelchair). The environment should be made safe to prevent falls. For example, scatter rugs should be removed and grab bars placed in the bathroom.

Information about the selection of rehabilitation or chronic care facility, if needed, can be obtained from the social worker or discharge planner. The selected facility should have experience in providing care for neurologically impaired clients. A psychologist should be available to provide input in the evaluation of the cognitive disabilities often exhibited by the client.

HEALTH CARE RESOURCES

The nurse refers the client and the family or significant others to the American Brain Tumor Association or the National Brain Tumor Foundation. The American Cancer Society is also an appropriate community resource for clients with malignant tumors. Home care agencies are available to provide both the physical and rehabilitative care that the client may need at home. Hospice services and palliative care may be needed for the terminally ill client. Brain tumor support groups may also be a valuable asset to the client and family.

BRAIN ABSCESS

OVERVIEW

A brain abscess is a purulent infection of the brain in which pus forms in the extradural, subdural, or intracerebral area of the brain. The causative organisms are most often bacteria, which invade the brain directly or indirectly.

In general, organisms from the ear, sinus, or mastoid area enter the brain by traveling along the wall of the cerebral veins, and therefore they may spread to any area of the brain. At times, the organisms (especially those from the ear) erode the bone, form a tract, and enter the brain directly. Septic emboli from the heart, the lungs, or a dental or peritonsillar abscess may break off and enter the systemic circulation. These organisms may become lodged in a cerebral vessel and produce a localized infection. Penetrating trauma, open head injuries, and neurosurgical procedures provide a potential means for the direct entry of an organism into the brain. In the past 15 years, the number of clients with a brain abscess as a consequence of immunosuppression, organ transplantation, and acquired immunodeficiency syndrome (AIDS) has increased rapidly.

The organisms cause a local infection, and acute inflammation surrounds the involved area. Within a few days, necrosis of the tissue takes place, and pus formation and liquefaction of the tissue occur. This is followed by the development of cerebral edema owing to localized vascular congestion in response to inflammation. During the subsequent 2 weeks, the area becomes encapsulated, first by fibrous granulation tissue and later by collagenous connective tissue. The abscess usually occurs deep within the cerebral hemisphere and involves the white matter of the brain. Occasionally, the abscess does not become encapsulated but instead spreads through the brain tissue to the subarachnoid space and ventricular system.

The organism varies with the source of the abscess. *Streptococci* are the most common organisms and are often found with other anaerobes such as *Bacteroides*. *Enterobacteriaceae* such as *Escherichia coli* and *Proteus* organisms may also be combined with *Streptococcus*. Yeast and fungi are now implicated in 9% to 17% of cases of cerebral abscess formation, particularly in clients who are immunosuppressed. *Toxoplasma gondii* is the most commonly seen central nervous system (CNS) opportunistic infection in the AIDS population.

Most brain abscesses occur in the frontal and temporal lobes. It is estimated that 5% to 20% of affected clients have more than one abscess. Mortality rates vary from 30% to 60%; abscesses that occur in immunosuppressed clients are associated with a higher mortality rate.

COLLABORATIVE MANAGEMENT

Assessment

PHYSICAL ASSESSMENT/CLINICAL MANIFESTATIONS

The clinical manifestations of a brain abscess are insidious. The client may present with headache, fever, and focal neurologic deficits or nonspecific signs and symptoms. The nurse begins the examination by performing a complete neurologic assessment. The client is usually mildly lethargic and somewhat confused. The pupillary response to light is normal in the early stages. As increased intracranial pressure (ICP) progresses, the pupils dilate and become nonresponsive. Examination of the client's visual fields often reveals a temporal field blindness (decrease in peripheral vision). If the abscess affects the cerebral hemispheres, nystagmus and a dysconjugate gaze may be noted. Motor examination reveals a generalized weakness. More significant motor problems, such as hemiplegia, may be apparent in the presence of a frontal lobe abscess. An ataxic gait is seen with a cerebellar abscess. Sensory impairment varies, although the client often exhibits no sensory deficits. The client may have varying degrees of aphasia in the presence of a frontal or temporal lobe abscess. Seizure activity may occur because of irritation of the cortical tissue. Late in the disease process, more severe symptoms of increased ICP occur and include severe headache, coma, a widened pulse pressure, bradycardia, and irregular respirations. The client with AIDS often presents with systemic infection, central nervous system involvement, and lymphoma.

DIAGNOSTIC TESTS

A complete blood count and erythrocyte sedimentation rate (ESR) are typically performed. The white blood cell count and ESR are usually elevated, indicating the presence of infection. If the abscess is encapsulated, the white blood cell count may be normal. The nurse obtains specimens for aerobic and, when possible, anaerobic cultures of the blood, ear, nose, and throat to determine the primary source of infection.

The health care provider orders a computed tomography (CT) scan to determine the presence of cerebritis, hydrocephalus, or a midline shift. Magnetic resonance imaging (MRI) is also useful in detecting the presence of an abscess early in the course of the disease. An electroencephalogram can localize the lesion in most cases and shows high-voltage, slow-wave activity; electrical silence may be noted in the area of the abscess. Radiography of the sinuses and the mastoid is often indicated. A lumbar puncture is not usually performed because of the risks of cerebral herniation.

The nurse assesses the client using the Glasgow Coma Scale (GCS) (see Chapter 41) at least every 2 hours or more often if clinically indicated. Included in this assessment are the client's vital signs. The client is at risk for increased ICP, which may initially be manifested by a change in level of consciousness. Late signs of increased ICP include seizures, pupillary changes, and a widened pulse pressure and bradycardia. The nurse elevates the head of the bed 30 degrees to promote venous drainage from the head. Other interventions for the treatment of increased ICP are discussed earlier under Preventing Postoperative Complications (Brain Tumors), p. 1003.

Interventions

The nurse gives the medications ordered by the physician to treat the abscess. Typically used antibiotics include penicillin G benzathine (Bicillin) and nafcillin sodium (Nafcil, Unipen). Metronidazole (Flagyl, Novonidazol🍁) may be used if an anaerobic organism is the causative agent. These agents are particularly useful in the early stages (cerebritis) of abscess formation. A combination of antibiotics is used, particularly if the abscess resulted from septic emboli. Anticonvulsants, such as phenytoin (Dilantin), may be used prophylactically to prevent seizures. The nurse strictly adheres to the medication schedule to maintain therapeutic blood levels. Analgesics may be ordered to treat headache.

The physician may surgically drain an encapsulated abscess via a bur hole to reduce the mass effect of the lesion. In certain cases a craniotomy may be performed to remove the abscess. The decision to perform surgery is based on the client's general condition, the stage of abscess development, and the site of the abscess. The nurse provides routine preoperative and postoperative care for the client undergoing a craniotomy, as discussed earlier under Postoperative Assessment (Brain Tumor), p. 1003.

The client with a brain abscess is discharged to home if few or no neurologic deficits are present. Clients with severe dysfunction are usually transferred to long-term care or a rehabilitation facility. Thirty percent of surviving clients have neurologic deficits.

ONLINE RESOURCES

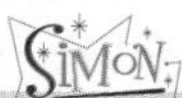

For suggested readings and Internet resources, go to http://www.wbsaunders.com/SIMON/Iggy/.

SELECTED BIBLIOGRAPHY

Asterisk indicates a classic or definitive work on this subject.

*Adams, H.P., et al. (1996). Guidelines for thrombolytic therapy for acute stroke: A supplement to the guidelines for the management of patients with acute ischemic stroke. *Circulation, 94*(1), 167-171, 174.

Adams, R.D., Victor, M., & Ropper, A.H. (1997). *Principles of neurology* (6th ed.). New York: McGraw-Hill.

Allen, K.M., & Phillips, J.M. (1997). *Women's health across the lifespan: A comprehensive perspective.* Philadelphia: J.B. Lippincott.

American Association of Neurological Surgeons. (1997). *Guidelines for the management of severe head injuries.* Chicago: Author.

American Association of Neuroscience Nurses. (1997). *Clinical guidelines series: Intracranial pressure monitoring.* Chicago: Author.

American Association of Neuroscience Nurses. (1997). *Clinical guideline series: Epilepsy.* Chicago: Author.

*American Brain Tumor Association. (1996). *A primer of brain tumors.* Des Plaines, IL: American Brain Tumor Association.

*Blank-Reid, C. (1996). How to have a stroke at an early age: The effects of crack, cocaine, and other illicit drugs. *Journal of Neuroscience Nursing, 28*(1), 19-27.

Bohan, E.M., & Weingart, J. (1998). Neurosurgical management of primary brain tumors: Diagnosis, treatment and future trends. *Journal of Neuroscience Nursing, 30*(6), 361-362.

Bohan, E.M. (1998). Neurosurgical management of patients with central nervous system malignancies. *Seminars in Oncology Nursing, 14*(1), 8-17.

Bonnono, C., et al. (2000). Emergi-paths and stroke teams: An emergency department approach to acute ischemic stroke. *Journal of Neuroscience Nursing, 32*(6), 298-305.

Cawley, M., Marberger, R., & Earl. G. (1998). Investigational neuroprotective drugs in traumatic brain injury. *Journal of Neuroscience Nursing, 30*(6), 369-374.

Doolittle, N., et al. (1998). Blood-brain barrier disruption for the treatment of malignant brain tumors: The national program. *Journal of Neuroscience Nursing, 30*(2), 81-90.

Fox, S., & Lantz, C. (1998). The brain tumor experience and quality of life: A qualitative study. *Journal of Neuroscience Nursing, 30*(4), 245-252.

*Gershman, G.E., et al. (1995). *Post stroke rehabilitation: Assessment, referral and patient management. Clinical practice guidelines and quick reference guide for clinicians No. 16.* AHCPR Pub. No. 95-0663. Rockville, MD. Agency for Health Care Policy and Research, Public Health Service, U.S. Department of Health and Human Services.

*Gershman, G.E., et al. (1995). *Post stroke rehabilitation: Clinical practice guidelines and quick reference guide for clinicians No. 16.* AHCPR Pub. No. 95-0662. Rockville, MD. Agency for Health Care Policy and Research, Public Health Service, U.S. Department of Health and Human Services.

Gonzaga-Camfield, R. (1999). Developing an emergency department team for treatment of stroke with recombinant tissue plasminogen activator. *Critical Care Nursing Clinics of North America, 11*(2), 261-268.

Hall, P. (1998). Acute ischemic stroke. *Journal of the American Academy of Nurse Practitioners, 10*(12), 559-570.

Hickey, J.V. (1997). *The clinical practice of neurological and neurosurgical nursing* (4th ed.). Philadelphia: J.B. Lippincott.

Hickman, J.L. (1998). Outcomes management for stroke patients using thrombolytics. *Critical Care Nursing Clinics of North America, 10*(1),101-115.

Hinkle, J.L. (1997). New developments in managing transient ischemic attacks and acute stroke. *AACN Clinical Issues: Advanced Practice in Acute and Critical Care, 8*(2), 205-213.

Hock, N. (1998). Neuroprotective and thrombolytic agents: Advances in stroke treatment. *Journal of Neuroscience Nursing, 30*(3), 175-184.

Hock, N. (1999). Brain attack: The stroke continuum. *Nursing Clinics of North America, 34*(3), 689-724.

Landis, S.H., et al. (1999). Cancer statistics, 1999. *CA Cancer Journal for Clinicians, 49*(1), 8-31.

Marion, D.W. (1999). *Traumatic brain injury.* New York: Thieme.

Marler, J.R., Jones, D.W., & Emr, M. (1997). *Proceedings of a national symposium on rapid identification and treatment of acute stroke.* National Institute of Neurological Disorders and Stroke, National Institutes of Health.

McNair, N. (1999). Traumatic brain injury. *Nursing Clinics of North America, 34(*3), 637-659.

Mitchell, A., Steffenson, N., & Davenport, K. (1997). Hypopituitarism due to traumatic brain injury: A case study. *Critical Care Nurse, 17*(4), 34-51.

Murphy, M.P., et al. (1998). Discharge planning for individuals with neurocognitive barriers. *The Journal of Care Management, 4*(4), 28-35.

NIH Consensus Development Panel on rehabilitation of Persons with Traumatic Brain Injury (2000). Rehabilitation of persons with traumatic brain injury. *Journal of the American Medical Association, 282*(10), 974-986.

NINDS rt-PA Stroke Study Group (1997). rt-PA stroke treatment (Special issue). *Journal of Neuroscience Nursing, 29*(6), 349-396.

Prados, M.D., Berger, M.S., & Wilson, C.B. (1998). Primary central nervous system tumors: Advances in knowledge and treatment. *CA: Cancer Journal for Clinicians, 48*(6), 331-360.

*Rhone-Polenc Rorer Pharmaceuticals. (1996). Gliadel package insert.

Shapiro, W.R. (1998). The therapy of primary brain tumors. *BNI Quarterly, 14*(2), 4-14.

Shapiro, W.R., & Shapiro, J.R. (1998). Biology and treatment of malignant glioma. *Oncology, 12*(2), 233-246.

*Shpritz, D.W. (1996). *Rapid nursing intervention: Neurologic.* Albany, NY: Delmar.

Smillova, A., & Walker, E. (2000). Meningococcemia: A critical care emergency. *Critical Care Nurse, 20*(5), 28-38.

Thompson, H.J. (2000). Managing patients with lumbar drainage devices. *Critical Care Nurse, 20*(5), 59-68.

Wong, F.W.H. (2000). Prevention of secondary brain injury. *Critical Care Nurse, 20*(5), 18-27.

UNIT 10

PROBLEMS OF SENSATION

Management of Clients with Problems of the Sensory System

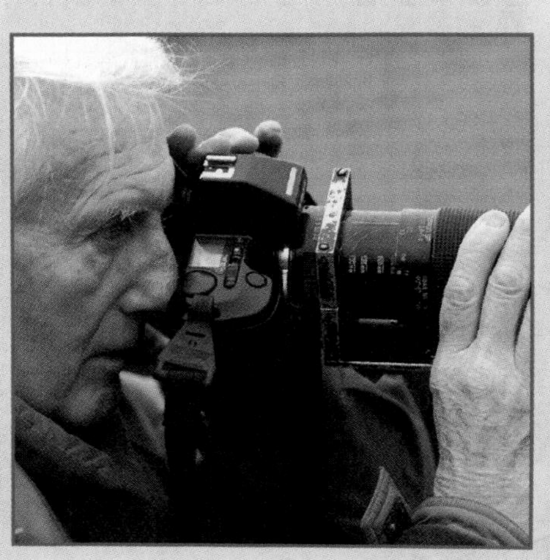

Problems of Sensation: Eyes and Ears ■ Core Concepts Grid

Anatomy	Physiology	Pathophysiology	History	Physical Exam	Diagnostic Tests	Interventions	Pharmacology
• **Cranial nerves** Optic (II) Oculomotor (III) Trochlear (IV) Trigeminal (V) Abducens (VI) Facial (VII) Vestibulocochlear (VIII) • **Ears** External canal Tympanic membrane Middle ear Ossicles Eustachian tube Inner ear Semicircular canals Cochlea Endolymph Perilymph Organ of Corti • **Eyes** Eyelids/eyeballs Conjunctiva Lacrimal glands Cornea Uvea Iris/lens/retina Canal of Schlemm Aqueous/vitreous humor	• **Sound transmission** • **Light transmission** • **Color discrimination** • **Refraction** • **Accommodation** • **Coordination**	• **Inflammation** • **Obstruction** • **Tinnitus** • **Vertigo** • **Dizziness** • **Hearing loss** • **Hyperopia** • **Myopia** • **Astigmatism** • **Increased intraocular pressure (IOP)** • **Opacity of lens** • **Retinal detachment** • **Hemorrhage** • **Vision loss**	• **Client past medical history** Systemic medical conditions Past injuries • **Family history** • **Social history** Medications Occupation Gender Diet history Leisure activities Age	• **Ear** Otoscopic examination Light reflex Voice test Watch test Tuning fork Rinne test Weber test • **Eye** Exophthalmos Ptosis Scleral color Anisocoria Pupillary reaction Snellen chart Visual fields Jaeger card Six cardinal positions of gaze Corneal light reflex Cover/uncover test	• **Cultures** • **Computed tomography (CT)** • **Audiometry** Bone conduction Pure tone Speech • **Tympanometry** • **Slit-lamp examination** • **Corneal staining** • **Tonometry** • **Ophthalmoscopy** • **Gonioscopy**	• **Ear medication installations** • **Removal of cerumen** • **Removal of foreign objects from ear canal** • **Ear medication installation** • **Care for the deaf** • **Communication with the deaf** Signing Speech reading • **Eye care** Eye glasses Artificial eyes Contact lenses • **Care for the blind** • **Communication with the blind** Clock TTY Braille	• **Systemic antibiotics** • **Ear medications** Antibiotic Antifungal Anti-inflammatory • **Antivertigo agents** • **Antiemetics** • **Artificial tears** • **Eye medications** Antibiotic Antifungal Anti-inflammatory • **Midriatics** • **Miotics** Beta blockers Pilocarpine Carbonic anhydrase inhibitors

CHAPTER 46

Assessment of the Eye and Vision

M. LINDA WORKMAN

Learning Objectives

After studying this chapter, you should be able to:

1. Explain the concept of refraction in relation to how the cornea, lens, aqueous humor, and vitreous humor contribute to vision.
2. Describe age-related changes in the eye, eyelids, and vision.
3. List five systemic disorders that have an impact on the eye and vision.
4. Discuss which elements of a client's history might predict visual impairment later in life.
5. Discuss the educational needs of a client undergoing fluorescein angiography.
6. Explain the relationship between intraocular pressure and eye health.
7. Use proper technique to instill eyedrops.

SIMON

Go to http://www.wbsaunders.com/SIMON/Iggy/ for self-assessment questions related to these Learning Objectives.

Many people consider vision to be their most important sense and the major way to communicate with the world. Vision begins with the eye and is fully perceived in the brain. Many conditions can affect the eye and alter vision temporarily or permanently. Changes in the eye and vision can provide important data regarding the client's general health status and the problems that might be encountered in self-care.

ANATOMY AND PHYSIOLOGY REVIEW

Structure

The eyeball, a ball-shaped or spherical organ about 2.5 cm in length and 2.3 cm in diameter, is located in the anterior portion of the orbit. The **orbit** is the bony socket of the skull that surrounds and protects the eye and the attached muscles, nerves, vessels, and tear-producing glands.

LAYERS OF THE EYEBALL

The eye has three layers, or coats (Figure 46-1). The external layer is the **sclera** (the opaque tissue making up the "whites" of the eye) and the transparent cornea on the front of the eye.

The middle layer, or **uvea,** is heavily pigmented. This layer consists of the choroid, the ciliary body, and the iris. The **choroid,** a dark brown membrane between the sclera and the retina, lines most of the sclera. The choroid has many blood vessels that supply nutrients to the retina.

The **ciliary body** connects the choroid with the iris and secretes **aqueous humor.** The **iris** is the colored portion of the external eye; its center opening is the **pupil.** The muscles of the iris contract and relax to control pupil size and the amount of light entering the eye.

The innermost layer is the **retina,** a thin, delicate structure through which the sensory fibers that transmit impulses to the optic nerve are distributed. The retina contains blood vessels and two types of photoreceptors called **rods** and **cones.** The rods work at low levels of light and provide peripheral vision. The cones are active at bright levels of light and provide color and central vision.

The **optic fundus** is the area at the inside back of the eye that can be seen with an ophthalmoscope. This area contains the **optic disk,** a creamy pink to white depressed area in the retina (Figure 46-2). The optic nerve enters the eyeball at this point. The optic disk is sometimes called the **blind spot** because it contains only nerve fibers and no photoreceptor cells. To one side of the optic disk is a small, yellowish-pink area called the **macula lutea.** The center of the macula is the **fovea centralis,** where vision is the most acute.

REFRACTIVE STRUCTURES AND MEDIA

Light waves pass through the following structures on the way to the retina: cornea, aqueous humor, lens, and vitreous humor. Each of these structures has a different density, which causes the light waves to bend, or **refract,** to some degree and focus images on the retina. These structures are the **refracting media** of the eye.

The **cornea** is the clear layer that forms the external coat on the front of the eye (see Figure 46-1). The **aqueous humor** is a clear, watery fluid that fills the anterior and posterior chambers of the eye. Aqueous humor is continually produced

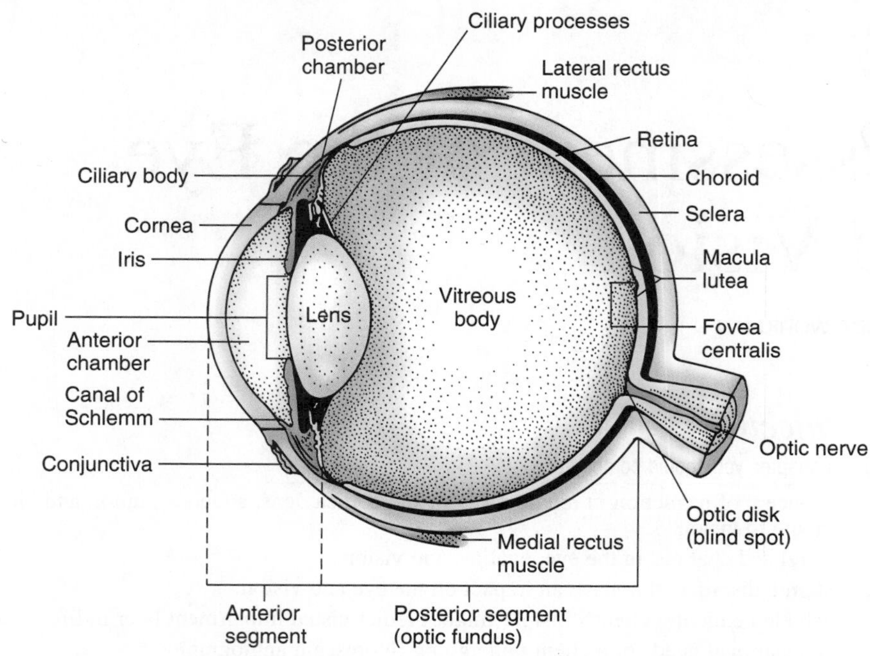

Figure 46-1 ● Anatomic features of the eye.

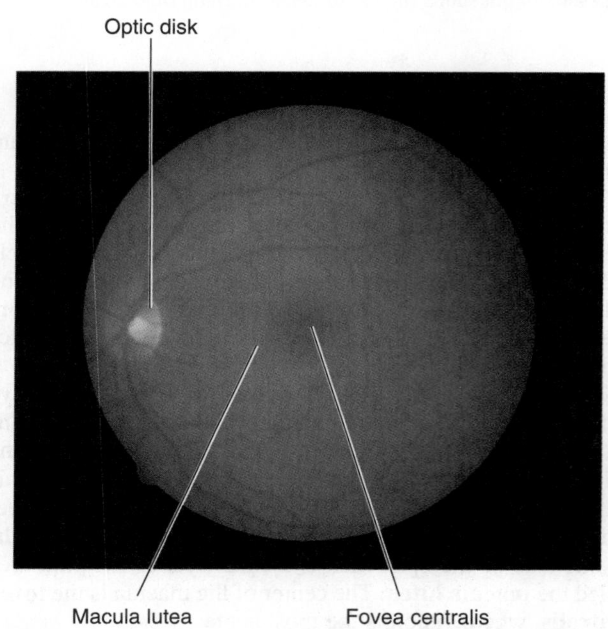

Figure 46-2 ● A normal optic fundus.

by the ciliary processes and passes from the posterior chamber, through the pupil, and into the anterior chamber. This fluid drains through the **canal of Schlemm** into the blood to maintain a balanced intraocular pressure (IOP, or the pressure within the eye).

The **lens** is a circular, convex structure that lies behind the iris and in front of the vitreous body. It is normally transparent. The lens bends the rays of light entering through the pupil so they focus properly on the retina. The curve of the lens changes to focus on near or distant objects.

The **vitreous body** is a gelatinous substance that fills the vitreous chamber (the space between the lens and the retina). This gelatin-like body transmits light and shapes the eye.

EXTERNAL STRUCTURES

The eyelids are thin, movable folds of skin that protect the eyes, shut out light during sleep, and keep the cornea moist. The upper eyelid is larger than the lower one. The **canthus** is the place at which the two eyelids meet at the corner of the eye.

The **conjunctivae** are the mucous membranes of the eye. The **palpebral conjunctiva** is a thick, vascular membrane that lines the under surface of each eyelid. Located over the sclera is the thin, transparent **bulbar conjunctiva.**

Tears are produced by a small **lacrimal gland,** which is located in the upper outer part of each orbit (Figure 46-3). Tears flow across the front of the eye, toward the nose, and into the inner canthus. They drain out through the **punctum** (found at the nasal side of the lid edges), into the **lacrimal duct** and **sac,** and then into the nose through the nasolacrimal duct.

MUSCLES

Six voluntary muscles rotate the eye and coordinate eye movements (Figure 46-4). Table 46-1 summarizes the functions of these muscles. Coordinated eye movements ensure that the retina of each eye receives an image at the same time so only a single image is seen.

NERVES

The extraocular muscles are innervated by the following cranial nerves: oculomotor (cranial nerve III), trochlear (cranial nerve IV), and abducens (cranial nerve VI). The **optic nerve** (cranial nerve II) is the nerve of sight, connecting the optic

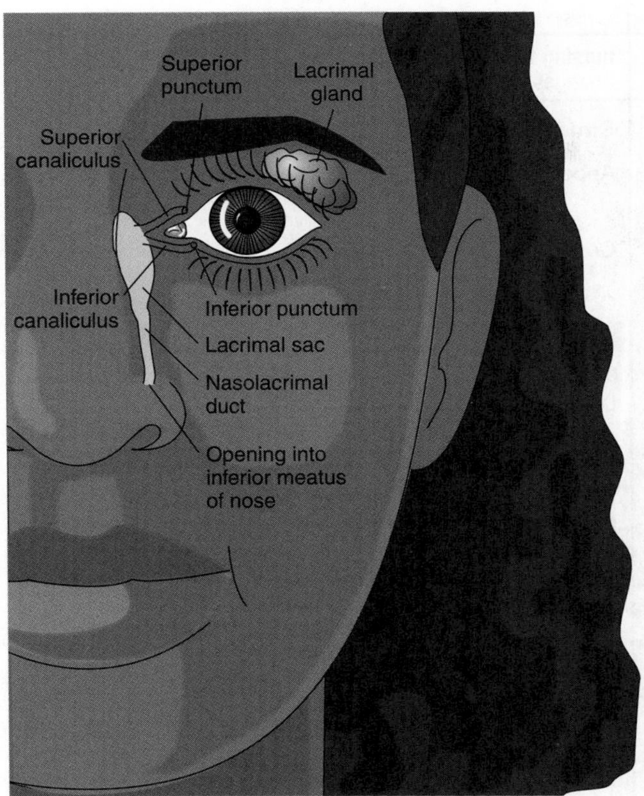

Figure 46-3 ● Anterior view of the eye and adjacent struc-

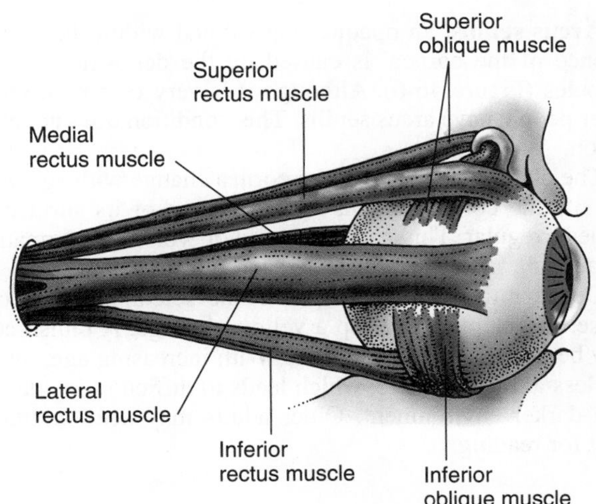

Figure 46-4 ● The extraocular muscles.

disk to the brain. Part of the trigeminal nerve (cranial nerve V) causes the sensory portion of the blink reflex and is stimulated when the cornea is touched. The facial nerve (cranial nerve VII) innervates the lacrimal glands and muscles controlling lid closure.

BLOOD VESSELS

The ophthalmic artery brings oxygenated blood to the structures in the orbit. This artery branches to supply blood to the

TABLE 46-1 • FUNCTIONS OF OCULAR MUSCLES

SUPERIOR RECTUS MUSCLE
- Together with the lateral rectus, this muscle moves the eye diagonally upward toward the side of the head.
- Together with the medial rectus, this muscle moves the eye diagonally upward toward the middle of the head.

LATERAL RECTUS MUSCLE
- Together with the medial rectus, contraction of this muscle holds the eye in a straight position.
- Contracting alone, this muscle turns the eye toward the side of the head.

MEDIAL RECTUS MUSCLE
- Contracting alone, this muscle turns the eye toward the nose.

INFERIOR RECTUS MUSCLE
- Together with the lateral rectus, this muscle moves the eye diagonally downward toward the side of the head.
- Together with the medial rectus, this muscle moves the eye diagonally downward toward the middle of the head.

SUPERIOR OBLIQUE MUSCLE
- Contraction pulls the eye downward.

INFERIOR OBLIQUE MUSCLE
- Contraction pulls the eye upward.

retina. The ciliary arteries supply the sclera, choroid, ciliary body, and iris. Venous drainage is through the two ophthalmic veins.

Function

Three functions of the eye provide clear images of near and far objects: refraction, pupillary constriction, and accommodation.

REFRACTION

The different curved surfaces and refractive media of the eye allow light to pass through to the retina. Each surface and media bends (refracts) light differently to focus an image on the retina. **Emmetropia** is the ideal refraction of the eye: with the lens at rest, light rays from a distant source (6 m or more) are focused into a sharp image on the retina. Figure 46-5 shows the normal refraction of light within the eye. Images fall on the retina inverted and reversed left to right. For example, an object in the lower nasal visual field strikes the upper outer area of the retina.

Errors of refraction are common. **Hyperopia** (also called hypermetropia or farsightedness) is a condition in which the eye does not refract light enough. As a result, images actually fall (converge) behind the retina (see Figure 46-5). Vision beyond 20 feet is normal, but near vision is poor. Hyperopia is corrected with a convex lens in eyeglasses or contact lenses.

Myopia (nearsightedness) is a condition in which the eye overrefracts or overbends the light. As a result, images are focused in front of the retina (see Figure 46-5). Near vision is normal, but distance vision is poor. Myopia is corrected with a biconcave lens in eyeglasses or contact lenses.

Astigmatism is a refractive error caused by unevenly curved surfaces on or in the eye, which results in visual distortion. Astigmatism is usually caused by uneven corneal surfaces.

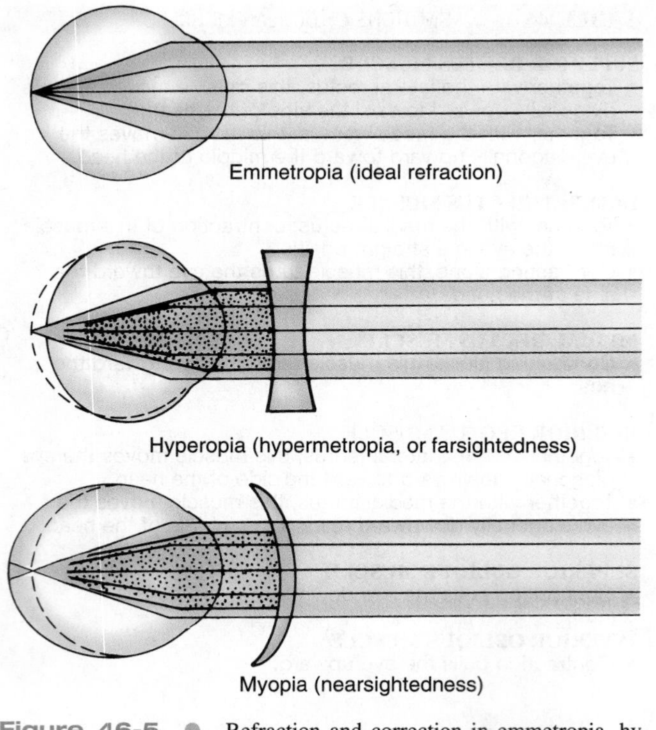

Figure 46-5 ● Refraction and correction in emmetropia, hyperopia, and myopia.

PUPILLARY CONSTRICTION

The pupil controls the amount of light that enters the eye. If the level of light to one or both eyes is increased, both pupils constrict (become smaller). The amount of constriction depends on how much light is available and how well the retina can adapt to light changes. Pupillary constriction is called **miosis,** and pupillary dilation is called **mydriasis.** Medications can alter pupillary constriction.

ACCOMMODATION

The healthy eye can focus sharp images on the retina whether the image is close to the eye or more distant. The process of maintaining a clear visual image when the gaze is shifted from a distant to a near object is known as **accommodation.** The eye is able to adjust its focus by changing the curve of the lens.

Eye Changes Associated with Aging

Changes directly within the eye cause visual acuity to decrease with age. Age-related changes within the nervous system and in the structures supporting the eye also contribute to decreasing visual function (Chart 46-1).

AGE-ASSOCIATED STRUCTURAL CHANGES

In the older adult, decreased eye muscle tone reduces the ability to maintain an upward gaze and to keep focused on a single object. The lower eyelid may relax and fall away from the eye **(ectropion),** exposing more of the eye and leading to dry eye symptoms.

CHART 46-1

nursing focus *on the* Older adult
Changes in the Eye Related to Aging

Structure/Function	Change
Appearance	Eyes appear to be sunken. Arcus senilis forms. Sclera yellows.
Cornea	Cornea flattens, which causes blurring of vision.
Ocular muscles	Muscle strength is reduced, which results in a diminished capacity to maintain an upward gaze and to maintain a single image.
Lens	Elasticity is lost, which increases the near point of vision. Lens hardens and becomes compact. Cataracts form.
Iris	Decrease in ability to dilate results in small pupil size and poor adaptation to darkness.
Pupil	Pupil size is smaller. Aperture size takes longer to change, which reduces ability to see in dim light.
Color vision	Discrimination among colors of short wavelength (green, blue, violet) decreases.
Tears	Diminished tear production results in dry eyes, increasing discomfort and risk for infection.

Arcus senilis, an opaque ring formed within the circumference of the cornea, is caused by the deposition of fatty globules (Figure 46-6). Although it is very common, not all older people have arcus senilis. This condition does not affect vision.

The clarity and shape of the cornea change with age. After age 65, the cornea flattens and the curve of its surface becomes irregular. This change causes or worsens astigmatism. As a result, images are distorted and blurred.

Degenerative changes occur in the sclera; fatty deposits cause the sclera to develop a yellowish tinge. A bluish color may be noted as the sclera thins. With increasing age, the iris has less ability to dilate, which leads to difficulty in adapting to a darker environment. Older adults may need additional light for reading.

AGE-ASSOCIATED FUNCTIONAL CHANGES

The lens yellows with aging, which affects the ability of the eye to transmit and focus light. The aging lens hardens, shrinks, and loses elasticity. As the lens loses elasticity, the ability of the eye to accommodate is gradually lost. The **near point of vision** (the closest distance at which the eye can see an object clearly) increases. Near objects (especially reading material) must be placed farther from the eye to be seen clearly. This age-related change is called **presbyopia.** In addition, the **far point** (farthest point at which an object can be distinguished) decreases. Thus the older person has a narrower visual field.

As a person ages, general color sensitivity decreases, as does discrimination among the colors of green, blue, and vio-

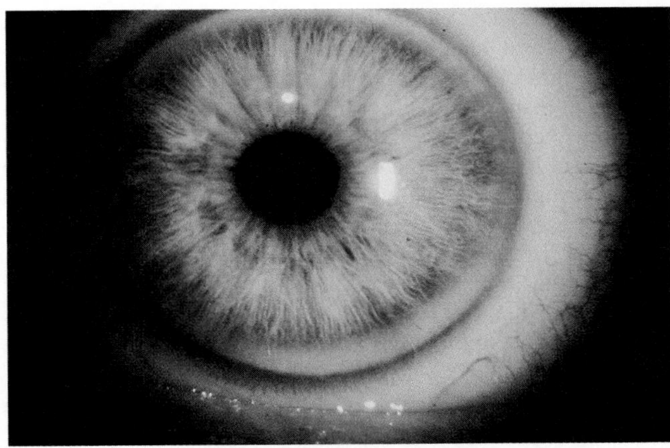

Figure 46-6 ● Arcus senilis of the iris.

let. More light is needed to stimulate the visual receptors. Intraocular pressure (IOP) is slightly higher in older than in younger adults.

CHART 46-2

eye and vision Assessment Using Gordon's Functional Health Patterns

Cognition Perceptual Pattern

Do you have any difficulty seeing objects at a distance?
Do you have any difficulty reading fine print or doing close work?
Do you wear eyeglasses or contact lenses?
What type of light do you use for reading?
Do you wear sunglasses or a hat when outdoors?
Do you have frequent headaches?
Have you noticed any change in your ability to see things at night?
When did you last have your eyes examined?
Do you go to an ophthalmologist or an optometrist?
When were you last tested for glaucoma?

Based on Gordon, M. (2000). *Manual of nursing diagnosis* (9th ed.). St. Louis: Mosby.

TABLE 46-2 • EXTRAOCULAR CONDITIONS AFFECTING THE EYE AND VISION

SYSTEMIC DISORDERS	DRUGS
• Diabetes mellitus	• Antihistamines
• Hypertension	• Decongestants
• Lupus erythematosus	• Antibiotics
• Sarcoidosis	• Opioids
• Thyroid dysfunction	• Anticholinergics
• Acquired immunodeficiency syndrome	• Cholinergic agonists
	• Sympathomimetics
• Cardiac disease	• Oral contraceptives
• Multiple sclerosis	• Antineoplastic agents
	• Corticosteroids
	• Carbonic anhydrase inhibitors
	• Beta blockers

ASSESSMENT TECHNIQUES

History

The nurse collects subjective information from the client to determine whether problems with the eye or vision have an impact on daily functioning. Chart 46-2 suggests some questions to ask when assessing eye and vision history.

DEMOGRAPHIC DATA

Age is an important factor to consider when assessing the visual processes and eye structure. The incidence of glaucoma and cataract formation increases with aging. Presbyopia commonly begins in the 40s.

Gender also may be important. For example, retinal detachments are more common in men, and dry eye symptoms are more common in women.

PERSONAL AND FAMILY HISTORY

The nurse asks the client about a family history of eye problems. Some conditions, such as a refractive error, show a familial tendency. The nurse also asks about any systemic medical conditions that could have ocular involvement or cause complications (Table 46-2).

The client is asked about past accidents, injuries, surgeries, or blows to the head that may have led to the present problem. The nurse asks specifically about previous laser surgeries, because clients often do not classify laser treatment as surgery. The nurse asks about the types of sports the client plays; some injuries are more common to specific sports.

The client is asked about medications, particularly decongestants and antihistamines. The ocular effects of these drugs are well documented. Many clients do not consider over-the-counter eyedrops to be medication. The name, strength, dose, and scheduling for all ophthalmic medications are recorded. Many systemic drugs can cause eye disturbances (see Table 46-2). Clinical manifestations of ocular drug effects include **pruritus** (itching), foreign body sensation, redness, tearing, sensitivity to light **(photophobia),** and the development of cataracts or glaucoma.

DIET HISTORY

Because some ocular problems are caused by or made worse with vitamin deficiencies, the nurse asks the client about his or her food choices. For example, vitamin A deficiency can cause conjunctival dryness, keratomalacia, and blindness.

SOCIOECONOMIC STATUS

The nurse asks the client about his or her work and specifically how the eyes are used. In some occupations, such as computer programming, constant exposure to monitor screens may lead to eyestrain and the need for eyeglasses. Machine operators are at risk for eye injury because of the high speeds at which particles can be thrown at the eye. The client who works in industrial settings is asked about the use of protective eyewear, such as goggles. Chronic exposure to infrared or ultraviolet light may cause photophobia and cataract formation.

CURRENT HEALTH PROBLEMS

The nurse asks the client about the onset of visual changes. Has the change occurred rapidly or slowly? *A client with a sudden or persistent loss of vision within the past 48 hours should be seen immediately by an ophthalmologist, as should the client experiencing trauma, a foreign body in the eye, sudden ocular pain, or sudden redness.* The client is asked whether the same symptoms are present to the same degree in both eyes.

The following questions are asked if ocular injury or eye trauma is involved:

- How long ago did the injury occur?
- What was the client doing when it happened?
- If a foreign body was involved, what was its source?
- Was any first aid administered at the scene? If so, what actions were taken?

Physical Assessment

INSPECTION

The nurse looks for head tilting, squinting, or other noticeable actions that offer clues to compensatory stances for attaining clear vision. For example, clients with double vision may cock the head to the side in an attempt to focus the two images into one, or they may close one eye to see more clearly.

The nurse observes for symmetry in the appearance of the eyes. The eyes are checked to determine if they are an equal distance from each other, of the same size, and of the same degree of prominence. The eyes also are assessed for their placement in the orbits and for symmetry of movement. **Exophthalmos** (proptosis) is a condition in which the eyes protrude; in **enophthalmos,** the eyeballs are sunken.

The nurse assesses the eyebrows and eyelashes for hair distribution. The direction of the eyelashes is determined. Eyelashes normally point outward and away from the eyelid. The eyelids are assessed for **ptosis** (drooping), redness, lesions, or swelling. The lids normally close completely, with the upper and lower lid edges touching. When the eyes are open, the upper lid covers a small portion of the iris. The edge of the lower lid lies below the line between the cornea and sclera. No sclera should be visible between the eyelid and the iris.

Scleral and Corneal Assessment

The sclera is examined for color; it is usually white. A yellow color may indicate jaundice or systemic problems. In dark-skinned people the normal sclera may appear yellow, and small, pigmented dots may be visible (Jarvis, 2000).

The nurse can best observe the cornea by directing a light at it from the side using several angles. The cornea should be transparent, smooth, shiny, and bright. Any cloudy areas or specks may be the result of accidents or injuries.

The blink reflex is assessed by bringing a fist quickly toward the client's face; clients with vision will blink. Alternatively, a syringe full of air can be expelled toward the eyes. The client blinks if the reflex is intact.

Pupillary Assessment

The pupils are usually round and of equal size. Approximately 5% of people normally have a slight but noticeable difference in the size of their pupils **(anisocoria).** Pupil size varies in people exposed to the same amount of light. Pupils are smaller in older adults. People with myopia have larger pupils; people with hyperopia have smaller pupils. The normal pupil diameter is between 3 and 5 mm.

The nurse observes the pupils for their response to light. Increasing light causes pupillary constriction, whereas decreasing light causes dilation. Constriction of both pupils is the normal response to direct light. Pupils also constrict in response to accommodation. The nurse assesses pupillary reaction to light by asking the client to look straight ahead while quickly bringing the beam of a penlight in from the side and directing it at the right **(oculus dexter [OD])** pupil. Constriction of the right pupil is a direct response to shining the penlight into that eye. Constriction of the left **(oculus sinister [OS])** pupil when light is shined at the right pupil is known as a **consensual response.** Direct and consensual responses are assessed for each eye.

Each pupil is evaluated for speed of reaction. The pupil should immediately constrict when a light is directed at it. This rapid response is termed **brisk.** If the pupil takes more than 1 second to constrict, the response is termed **sluggish.** Pupils that fail to react are termed **nonreactive** or **fixed.** The reactivity speed of right and left pupils is compared, and any discrepancy is noted.

In assessing for accommodation, the nurse holds the index finger about 18 cm from the client's nose and moves it toward the nose. The client's eyes normally converge during this movement, and the pupils constrict equally. When accommodation stops, the pupils begin to enlarge and return to their normal size.

MEASUREMENT OF VISION

Vision is measured by various tests. Each eye is tested separately, and then both eyes are tested together. Clients who routinely wear corrective lenses are tested both without and with their corrective lenses.

Acuity

Visual acuity tests measure both distance and near vision. The Snellen chart, or "eye chart," is a simple tool to measure distance vision. This chart has letters, numbers, pictures, or a single letter presented in various positions (Figure 46-7). The client stands 20 feet from the chart, covers one eye, and uses the other eye to read the line that appears most clear. If the client can do this accurately, he or she is asked to read the next lower line. This sequence is repeated to the last line on which the client can correctly identify most characters. The procedure is repeated for the other eye. Findings are recorded as a comparison between what the client can read at 20 feet and the distance at which a person with normal vision can read the same line. For example, 20/50 means that the client is able to see at 20 feet from the chart what a "healthy eye" can see at 50 feet.

For clients who are in a confined space that does not permit a 20-foot distance to the eye chart or who cannot see the 20/400 character, visual acuity is assessed by holding fingers in front of their eyes and asking them to count (Figure 46-8). This procedure is repeated five times. Acuity is recorded as "count fingers vision at 5 feet," or the farthest distance at which the client can count the fingers correctly.

Clients who cannot count fingers are tested for **hand motion (HM) acuity.** The nurse stands about 2 to 3 feet in front of the client. The eye not being tested is covered. A light is directed onto the hand from behind the client. The nurse demonstrates the three possible directions in which the hand can move during the test (stationary, left-right, or up-down).

LETTER CHART FOR 20 FEET
Snellen Scale

E 200 ft

H N 100 ft

D F N 70 ft

P T X Z 50 ft

U Z D T F 40 ft

D F N P T H 30 ft

P H U N T D Z 20 ft

N P X T Z F H 15 ft

Figure 46-7 ● A typical Snellen chart. (Courtesy National Society to Prevent Blindness, Schaumburg, IL.)

The nurse moves the hand slowly (1 second per motion) and asks the client, "What is my hand doing now?" This procedure is repeated at least five times. Visual acuity is recorded as HM at the farthest distance at which the client correctly identifies most of the hand motions.

If the client cannot detect hand movement, the nurse tests acuity by measuring **light perception (LP).** The client is first asked to cover the left eye (OS). In a darkened room, the beam of a penlight is directed at the right eye (OD) from a distance of 2 to 3 feet for 1 to 2 seconds. Clients are instructed to say "on" when the beam of light is perceived and "off" when it is no longer detected. This procedure is repeated five times. If the client identifies the presence or absence of light three times correctly, acuity is recorded as LP.

Near-Vision Testing

Near vision is tested for clients who have difficulty reading and in clients older than 40 years of age. The nurse uses a small, handheld Snellen chart called a Jaeger card (Figure 46-9) or a Rosenbaum Pocket Vision Screener. The client holds the card

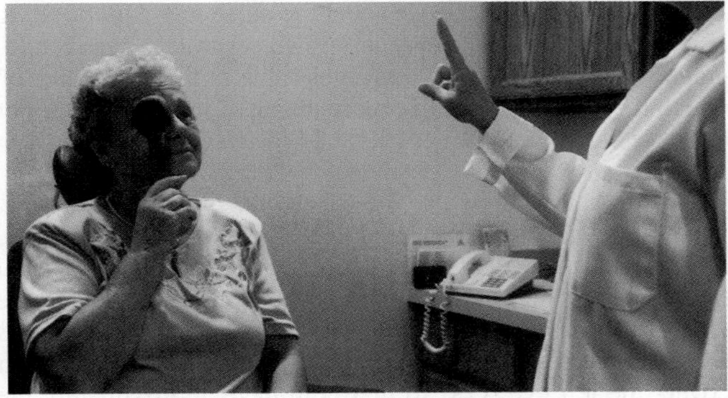

Figure 46-8 ● Client counting fingers during determination of visual acuity.

ROSENBAUM POCKET VISION SCREENER

	Point	Jaeger	distance equivalent
95			20/800
874			20/400
2843	26	16	20/200
638 E Ш Ǝ X O O	14	10	20/100
8 7 4 5 Ǝ m Ш O X O	10	7	20/70
6 3 9 2 5 m E Ǝ X O X	8	5	20/50
4 2 8 3 6 5 Ш E m O X O	6	3	20/40
3 7 4 2 5 8 Ǝ Ш Ǝ X X O	5	2	20/30
9 3 7 8 2 6 Ш m E X O O	4	1	20/25
4 2 8 7 3 9 E Ш m O O X	3	1+	20/20

Card is held in good light 14 inches from eye. Record vision for each eye separately with and without glasses. Presbyopic patients should read thru bifocal segment. Check myopes with glasses only.

DESIGN COURTESY J. G. ROSENBAUM, M.D., CLEVELAND, OHIO

PUPIL GAUGE (mm.)

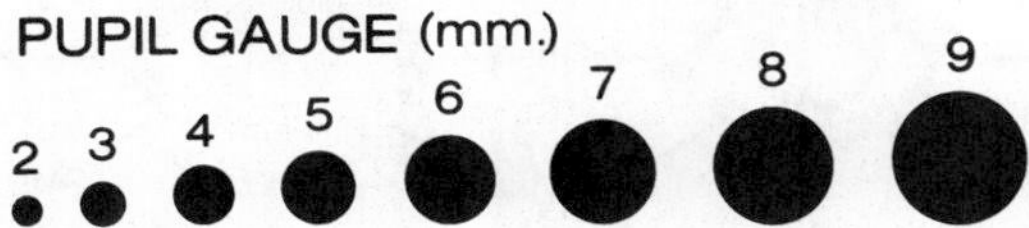

Figure 46-9 ● A typical Jaeger card. (Courtesy of SMP Division, Cooper Laboratories [P.R.], San German, Puerto Rico.)

14 inches away from the eyes, and the nurse asks him or her to read the characters. The eyes are tested separately and then together. The nurse records the Jaeger value of the lowest line on which the client can identify more than half the characters. For example, acuity might read "J2 at 14 inches."

Assessment of Visual Fields

A **confrontation test** is used to examine the client's visual fields, or peripheral vision. During the test, the nurse and the client sit facing each other and look directly into each other's eyes. The nurse covers his or her right eye (OD) and the client covers the left eye (OS) so that both have approximately the same visual field. The nurse moves a finger or an object from a nonvisible area into the client's line of vision.

This test provides only a crude estimate of the client's visual fields but can reveal large-field defects such as **hemianopia** (blindness in one half of the field of vision), **quadrantanopia** (blindness in one fourth of the field of vision), or large **scotomas** (blind spots in the visual field).

Assessment of Extraocular Muscle Function

Assessment of extraocular muscle function includes three components: the corneal light reflex, the six cardinal positions of gaze, and the cover-uncover test. The nurse also observes for parallelism of the eyes and smoothness of ocular movements.

The corneal light reflex determines alignment of the two eyes. After asking the client to stare straight ahead, the nurse shines a penlight at both corneas from a distance of 12 to 15 inches. The bright dot of light reflected from the shiny surface of the cornea should be in a symmetric position (e.g., at the 1 o'clock position in the right eye and at the 11 o'clock position in the left eye). An asymmetric reflex indicates a deviating eye and possible muscle imbalance.

The six cardinal positions of gaze are used to assess muscle function (Figure 46-10). The eye will not turn to a particular position if the muscle is weak or if the controlling nerve is affected. The nurse asks the client to hold his or her head still and to move the eyes to follow a small object such as a pen. The nurse moves the object to the client's right (lateral), upward and right (temporal), down and right, left (lateral), upward and left (temporal), and down and left (see Figure 46-10). While the client moves the eyes to these positions, the nurse observes for parallel eye movements and any deviation of movement. **Nystagmus,** an involuntary, rhythmic, and rapid twitching of the eyeball, is a normal finding for the far lateral gaze. It may also be caused by abnormal innervation or prolonged reduced vision.

A different method of assessing muscle function is the cover-uncover test. The nurse asks the client to use both eyes to look at a specific fixed point, such as the nurse's nose. One of the client's eyes is covered with a card. The nurse observes the uncovered eye to see if it moves to fix on the object; if the eye moves, it was not focused on the fixed point before the other eye was covered. The nurse then removes the cover and observes for any movement in the eye just uncovered. The presence and direction of any deviations of eye movement are recorded.

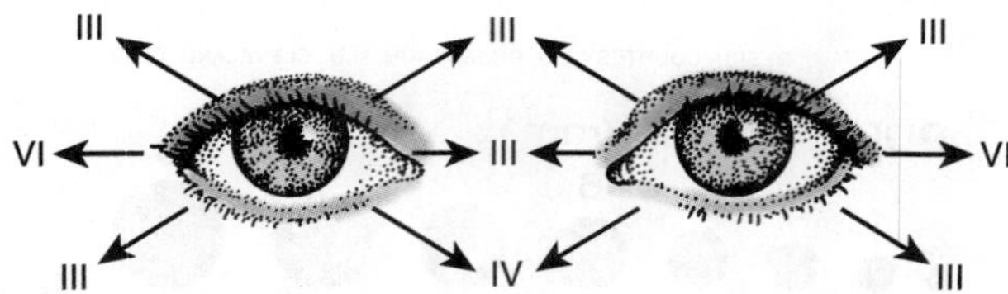

Figure 46-10 ● Checking extraocular movements in the six cardinal positions indicates the functioning of cranial nerves III, IV, and VI.

Assessment of Color Vision

Several methods are available for testing color vision. The most commonly used tool is the **Ishihara chart,** which shows numbers composed of dots of one color within a circle of dots of a different color (Figure 46-11). Testing each eye separately, the examiner asks the client what numbers he or she sees on the chart. The ability to read the numbers correctly depends on the normal functioning of color vision.

Psychosocial Assessment

Clients undergoing changes in visual perception may be anxious or fearful about a possible loss of vision. Clients with severe visual defects may be unable to perform normal activities of daily living and may need to change their leisure activities. The sense of dependency resulting from reduced vision can affect self-esteem. The nurse investigates the client's feelings about the visual disturbances and assesses the effectiveness of his or her coping techniques. The nurse also discusses the client's concerns with family members or significant others to determine whether support is available. The client's current knowledge and use of available services for the visually impaired are assessed.

Diagnostic Assessment

LABORATORY TESTS

Cultures and smears of corneal or conjunctival swabs and scrapings aid in the diagnosis of infections. A sample of the exudate is obtained for culture before antibiotics or topical

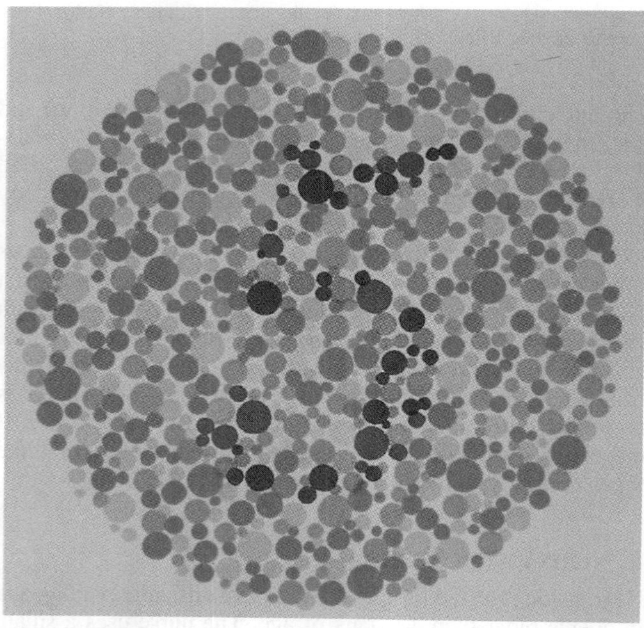

Figure 46-11 ● An Ishihara chart for testing color vision.

anesthetics are instilled. Swabs are taken from the conjunctivae and any ulcerated or inflamed areas.

RADIOGRAPHIC EXAMINATIONS

Computed Tomography

Computed tomography (CT) is a radiographic diagnostic method in which computers form a cross-sectional image. It is valuable in visualizing the eyes, extraocular muscles, and optic nerves. It is a sensitive method for detecting tumors in the orbital space. Data are obtained by scanning the skull and orbits with beams of low-intensity x-rays. Because contrast material is not usually administered, no special client preparation or follow-up care is required. The nurse informs the client that this test is not painful. However, the client must be positioned in a confined space and keep the head still during the procedure.

Radioisotopic Scanning

Radioisotopes are used to locate tumors and lesions in various body organs. Isotope studies differentiate an intraocular tumor from a hemorrhage, especially in the choroid layer.

CLIENT PREPARATION. After the informed consent process, the client receives a tracer dose of the radioactive isotope, either orally or by injection.

PROCEDURE. The client is asked to lie still and breathe normally. The scanner measures the radioactivity emitted by the radioactive atoms concentrated in the area being studied. Clients who are restless, anxious, or agitated may require sedation.

FOLLOW-UP CARE. The nurse assures the client that the amount of radioisotope used as a tracer is extremely small and that he or she is not radioactive. No other special follow-up care is required.

OTHER DIAGNOSTIC TESTS

A variety of techniques are used to examine specific eye structures. Such techniques are not necessary in the routine visual assessment of all people but may be indicated for those with special risks, symptoms, or exposures. Such techniques require special skill and are used only by physicians, optometrists, or advanced practice nurses.

Slit-Lamp Examination

The slit lamp permits the examination of anterior ocular structures under microscopic magnification (Figure 46-12). The client leans on a chin rest to stabilize the head. A narrow beam (slit) of light is aimed so that it brightly illuminates only a narrow segment of the eye. This technique allows the examiner to locate accurately the position of any abnormality in the cornea, lens, or anterior vitreous humor. The slit beam also may help identify the abnormal presence of cells in the aqueous humor.

Corneal Staining

Corneal staining consists of placing fluorescein or other topical dye into the conjunctival sac. The dye outlines irregularities of the corneal surface that are not easily visible. Corneal staining is indicated in cases of corneal trauma, problems caused by a contact lens, or the presence of foreign bodies, abrasions, ulcers, or other corneal disorders.

This procedure is noninvasive and is performed under aseptic conditions. The dye is applied topically to the eye, and the eye is then viewed through a blue filter. Nonintact areas of the cornea stain a bright green color.

Tonometry

A **tonometer** is an instrument for measuring **intraocular pressure (IOP).** Normal IOP readings are 10 to 21 mm Hg. About 5% of clients with healthy eyes have a slightly higher pressure. Tonometer readings are indicated for all clients older than 40 years of age. Adults with a family history of glaucoma should have their IOP measured once or twice a year.

IOP varies throughout the day. It tends to be highest in the morning but may peak at any time of the day, depending on the individual. Therefore the time of IOP measurement is always documented.

Several methods and instruments are available to measure IOP (Figure 46-13). Some involve direct contact with the eye, whereas others use a noncontact technique. Table 46-3 compares the advantages and disadvantages of each method.

Ophthalmoscopy

The direct ophthalmoscope allows viewing of the eye's external structures and interior. It is easiest to examine the fundus when the room is dark because the pupil will dilate. When performing direct ophthalmoscopy, the nurse holds the instrument with the right hand when examining the right eye and with the left hand when examining the left eye. The nurse stands on the same side as the eye being examined. The client is instructed to look straight ahead at an object on the wall behind the nurse. A thumb can be placed on the client's eyebrow to assist in knowing the distance from the ophthalmoscope to the client. The ophthalmoscope is held firmly against the examiner's face and is aligned so that the examiner's eye sees through the sight hole (Figure 46-14).

When using the ophthalmoscope, the nurse comes toward the client's eye from about 12 to 15 inches away and about

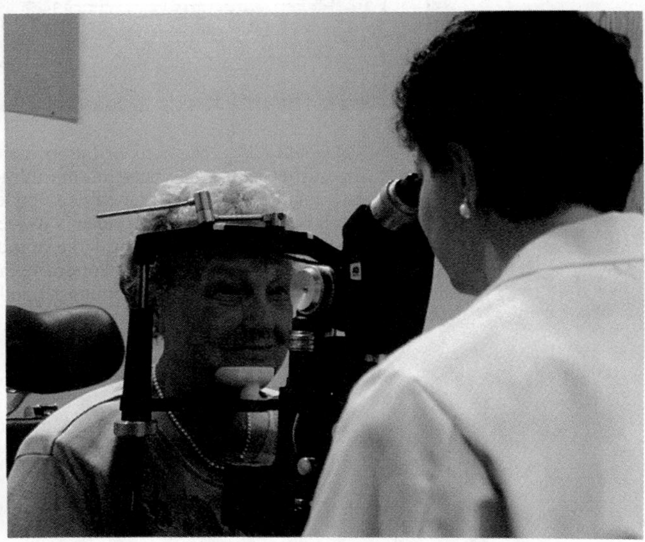

Figure 46-12 ● Slit-lamp ocular examination.

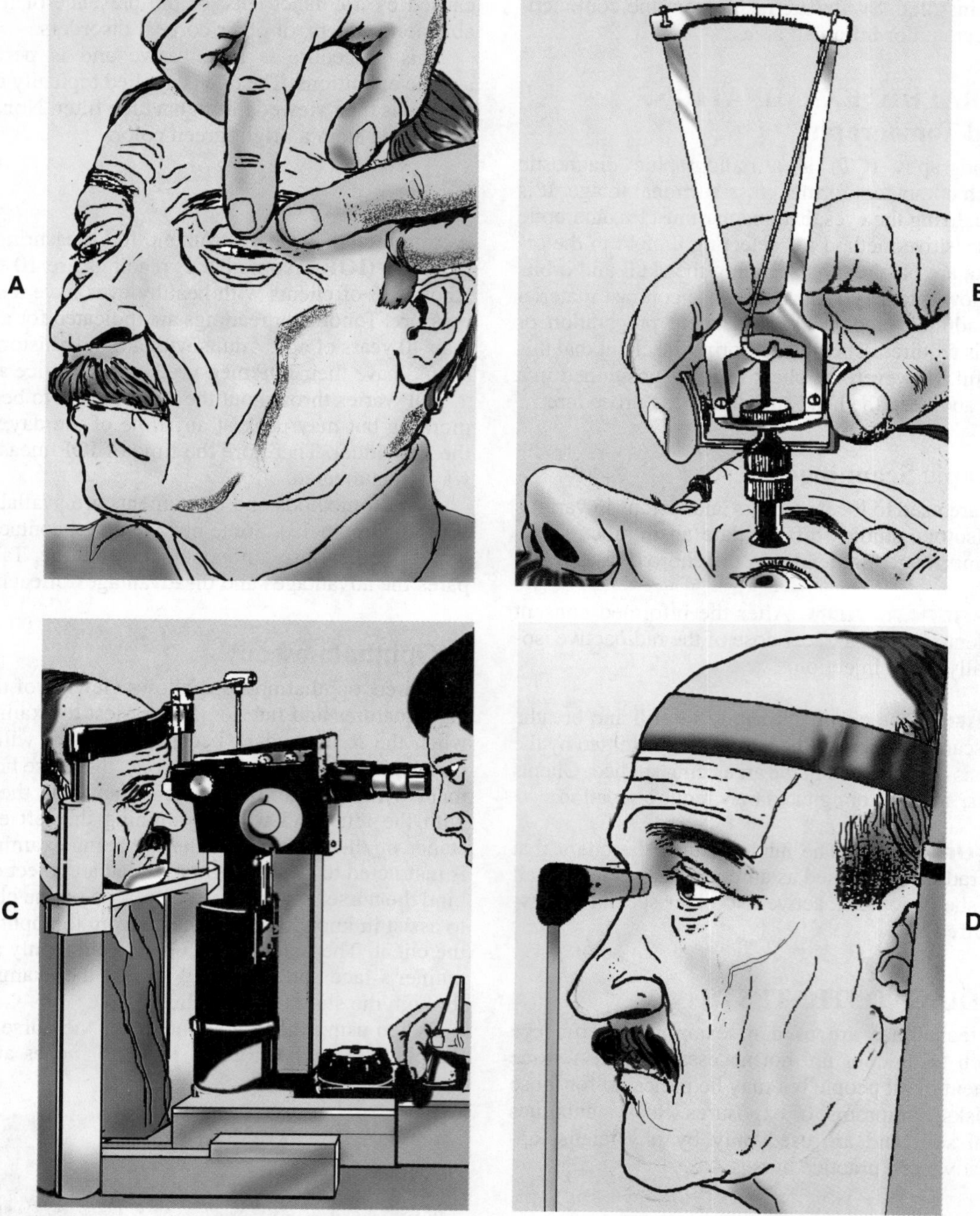

Figure 46-13 ● Methods of intraocular pressure estimation. **A,** Finger palpation is useful only when a large difference exists between the intraocular pressure of the two eyes, as in unilateral angle-closure glaucoma. **B,** Schiötz tonometry can be learned readily. Because the tonometer is relatively inexpensive, it can be used in every physician's office to screen for chronic simple glaucoma. **C,** The air-puff tonometer can be used for screening large numbers of clients but is far more expensive than Schiötz's tonometer. **D,** Goldman's applanation tonometer, used with a slit lamp, is the standard instrument for glaucoma diagnosis and management for most ophthalmologists. It is expensive and requires considerable skill.

TABLE 46-3 • TYPES OF TONOMETRY

Type of Tonometry	Advantages	Disadvantages
Noncontact (air-puff) tonometer A puff of air indents the cornea	No direct contact with the client's cornea No anesthesia needed Very rapid	Less accurate than direct contact methods The puff of air is unpleasant and may startle the client
Schiötz tonometer A small pressure gauge is placed on the cornea, and a weighted plunger is depressed	Reliable readings Portable Low cost	Touches the client's cornea Requires topical anesthetic May abrade or infect the cornea
Goldman's applanation tonometer The machine exerts a force against the cornea	Highly accurate Rapid	Touches the client's cornea Requires topical anesthetic Danger of infection Machine is expensive
Tono-Pen XL A penlight-sized appliance is placed against the cornea and exerts a force against the cornea	Rapid Portable Accurate Uses a sleeve to prevent infection	Touches the client's cornea Requires topical anesthetic

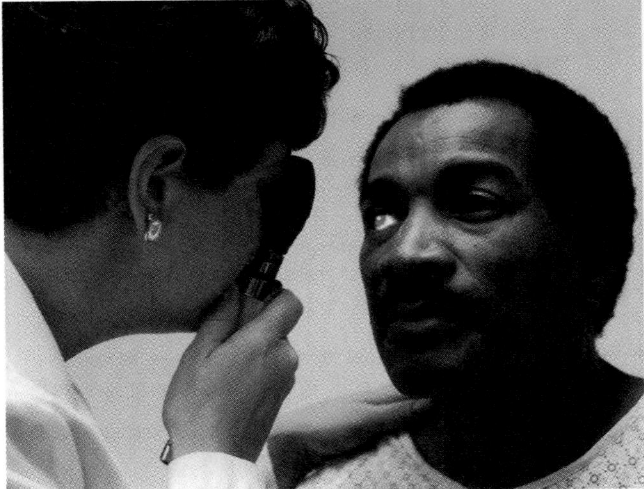

Figure 46-14 ● Proper technique for direct ophthalmoscopic visualization of the retina.

15 degrees lateral to the client's line of vision. As the ophthalmoscope is directed at the pupil, a red glare **(red reflex)** is seen in the pupil. The red reflex is a reflection of the light on the retina. An absent red reflex may indicate an opacity in the lens or cloudiness of the vitreous. The nurse, who has both eyes open, moves toward the client's pupil while following the red reflex. The retina should then be visible through the ophthalmoscope. Structures examined with the ophthalmoscope include the optic disk, optic vessels, fundus, and macula. Table 46-4 lists the features that should be observed in each structure.

Ultrasonography

Ultrasonography is used to examine the orbit and eye with high-frequency sound waves. This noninvasive test aids in the diagnosis of trauma, intraorbital tumors, proptosis, and choroidal or retinal detachments. It is also used to determine gross outline changes in the eye and the orbit in clients with cloudy corneas or lenses, which prevents examination of the fundus. Ultrasonography helps calculate the length of the eye, one of the measurements used to determine the strength of the intraocular lens implant needed after cataract surgery.

TABLE 46-4 • STRUCTURES TO ASSESS BY DIRECT OPHTHALMOSCOPY

RED REFLEX
- Presence or absence

OPTIC DISK
- Color
- Margins (sharp or blurred)
- Cup size
- Presence of rings or crescents

OPTIC BLOOD VESSELS
- Size
- Color
- Kinks or tangles
- Light reflection
- Narrowing
- Nicking at arteriovenous crossings

FUNDUS
- Color
- Tears or holes
- Lesions
- Bleeding

MACULA
- Presence of blood vessels
- Color
- Lesions
- Bleeding

CLIENT PREPARATION. The nurse explains the test to the client and instills anesthetic drops into the lower lid. The client is cautioned to avoid rubbing the eye. Clients are seated upright with the chin in the chin rest.

PROCEDURE. The probe is touched against the client's anesthetized cornea, and sound waves are bounced through the eye. The sound waves return to the transducer when they strike a non–fluid-filled structure. The anatomic structures that reflect sound waves are the cornea, anterior and posterior lens capsule, and retina. When these reflected sound waves return to the transducer, a characteristic "spike" pattern appears on the screen.

FOLLOW-UP CARE. The nurse reminds the client not to rub or bump the eye until the effects of the anesthetic drops have worn off.

Magnetic Resonance Imaging

Magnetic resonance imaging (MRI) has many ophthalmic uses and avoids exposing the client to radiation. *It is not used with an actual or suspected metallic foreign body, because the magnetic pull can move the metal fragment and damage the eye.*

The nurse explains to the client that the MRI study may be performed in an enclosed space (although MRI units with open sides are becoming more available). Sedation may be necessary. If the client is sedated, pulse oximetry is performed during the procedure because direct observation of respiratory status is not possible. All metallic jewelry is removed until the procedure is completed.

Fluorescein Angiography

Fluorescein angiography provides a detailed image and permanent record of eye circulation. Photographs are taken in rapid succession after the intravenous (IV) administration of dye. This test is useful for the diagnosis of conditions affecting the circulation of the retina (e.g., diabetic retinopathy and macular degeneration) or for the diagnosis of intraocular tumors.

CLIENT PREPARATION. The nurse explains the procedure to the client, asks about allergies and previous reactions to dyes, and instills mydriatic eyedrops (cause pupil dilation) approximately 1 hour before the test. Chart 46-3 describes the best practice patterns for the correct instillation of eyedrops. The nurse checks that the informed consent has been signed by the client or responsible person. The nurse warns that the dye may cause the skin to appear yellow for several hours after the test. The stain is gradually eliminated through the urine, which changes color.

PROCEDURE. IV access must be obtained. After the catheter is in the vein, 5 mL of a 10% solution of fluorescein is injected into the client's peripheral vein. A camera is set up with ophthalmologic equipment to photograph retinal and choroidal blood vessels as the dye passes through them. The procedure takes only minutes because the vessels fill quickly.

FOLLOW-UP CARE. After the test, the client may feel weak and nauseated. After the nausea resolves, clients are encouraged to drink fluids to help eliminate the dye. The nurse encourages rest and emphasizes that any yellow staining of the skin will disappear in a few hours. After the test, the urine will be bright green until the dye is excreted. The client is instructed to avoid direct sunlight until pupil dilation returns to normal.

CHART 46-3

BEST PRACTICE *for* Instillation of Ophthalmic Drops

- Wash your hands.
- Don gloves if secretions are present.
- Explain the procedure to the client.
- Check the name, strength, and expiration date of the solution.
- Stand behind the client.
- Instruct the client to tilt the head backward, open the eyes, and look up.
- Have the client's head rest against your body.
- Pull the lower lid downward against the cheekbone.
- Hold the medication bottle like a pencil, with the tip down.
- Rest the wrist holding the bottle on the client's cheek.
- Without touching the tip of the bottle to the client's conjunctiva, squeeze the bottle gently and release the correct number of drops into the conjunctival pocket.
- Gently release the lower eyelid.
- Instruct the client to close the eyes gently, without squeezing the lids together.

Electroretinography

Electroretinography is the process of graphing the retina's response to light stimulation. An electroretinogram is obtained by placing a contact lens electrode on an anesthetized cornea. Lights at varying speeds and intensities are flashed, and the neural response is graphed. The measurement from the cornea is identical to the response that would be obtained if electrodes were placed directly on the retina.

Preparation includes instilling an anesthetic into the eye. Afterward, the client is reminded to avoid rubbing the eye until the effects of the anesthetic have disappeared.

This procedure is especially helpful in detecting and evaluating retinal blood vessel changes such as diabetic or hypertensive retinopathy; trauma to the retinal blood supply, such as with retinal detachment; toxic changes from the use of drugs; and systemic disorders, such as vitamin A deficiency.

CRITICAL THINKING CHALLENGE

The client is a 60-year-old Hispanic woman who speaks no English. She is scheduled to have a slit-lamp evaluation and measurement of intraocular pressure by the Schiötz method. As she comes into the examination area, she begins to cry and cover her eyes. There is no one who can speak Spanish in the clinic.

- What is your first priority?
- How will you explain what is involved in these tests?
- How will you reduce her concerns about pain or eye damage?

For suggested answer guidelines, go to SIMON http://www.wbsaunders.com/SIMON/Iggy/.

ONLINE RESOURCES

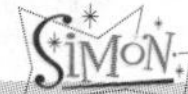

For suggested readings and Internet resources, go to http://www.wbsaunders.com/SIMON/Iggy/.

SELECTED BIBLIOGRAPHY

Asterisk indicates a classic or definitive work on this subject.

Bron, A. (2001). The architecture of the corneal stroma. *British Journal of Ophthalmology, 85*(4), 379-381.

Cleary, B. (1997). Age-related changes in the special senses. In M. Matteson, E. McConnell, & A. Linton (Eds.), *Gerontological nursing: Concepts and practice* (2nd ed., pp. 384 405). Philadelphia: W.B. Saunders.

*Cleary, M. (1995). Helping the person who is visually impaired: Concerns, questions, remedies, and sources. *Journal of Ophthalmic Nursing and Technology, 14*(5), 205-211.

Cohen, S., & Kawasaki, A. (1999). Introduction to formal visual field testing: Goldman and Humphrey perimeter. *Journal of Ophthalmic Nursing and Technology, 18*(1), 7-11.

Cotran, R., Kumar, V., & Collins, T. (1999). *Robbins pathologic basis of disease* (5th ed.). Philadelphia: W.B. Saunders.

Garber, N. (1999). Applanation tonometry. *Journal of Ophthalmic Nursing and Technology, 18*(6), 270-279.

Garber, N. (1999). Iris and pupil evaluation: Key considerations. *Journal of Ophthalmic Nursing and Technology, 18*(5), 207-218.

Garber, N. (2000). A guide to performing basic manifest refractometry. *Journal of Ophthalmic Nursing and Technology, 19*(2), 84-95.

Garber, N. (2000). Performing direct ophthalmoscopy. *Journal of Ophthalmic Nursing and Technology, 19*(3), 120-133.

Gordon, M. (2000). *Manual of nursing diagnosis* (9th ed.). St. Louis: Mosby.

Guyton, A., & Hall, J. (2000). *Textbook of medical physiology* (10th ed.). Philadelphia: W.B. Saunders.

Jarvis, C. (2000). *Physical examination and health assessment* (3rd ed.). Philadelphia: W.B. Saunders.

Ramos, M. (1999). Prevention of work-related injuries: A look at eye protection use and suggested prevention strategies. *Journal of Ophthalmic Nursing and Technology, 18*(3), 117-119.

Segal, W., et al. (2001). Disinfection of Goldman tonometers after contamination with hepatitis C virus. *American Journal of Ophthalmology, 131*(2), 184-187.

Shoemaker, J. (1997). Adult vision screening by nonphysicians. *Journal of Ophthalmic Nursing & Technology, 16*(5), 244-250.

*Sullivan, N. (1983). Vision in the elderly. *Journal of Gerontological Nursing, 9*(4), 228-235.

*Vaughan, D., Asbury, T., & Riordan-Eva, P. (Eds.). (1995). *General ophthalmology* (14th ed.). Norwalk, CT: Appleton & Lange.

CHAPTER 47

Interventions for Clients with Eye and Vision Problems

M. LINDA WORKMAN

Learning Objectives

After studying this chapter, you should be able to:

1. Describe how to correctly instill ophthalmic drops and ointment into the eye.
2. Explain the consequences of increased intraocular pressure (IOP).
3. Identify common practices that increase IOP.
4. Prioritize educational needs for the client after cataract surgery with and without lens replacement.
5. Compare and contrast myopia and hyperopia and the correction needed for each.
6. Describe the pathologic bases, symptoms, and nursing care priorities for primary open-angle glaucoma and acute angle-closure glaucoma.
7. Identify the nursing care priorities for the donor when corneal donation is planned.
8. Explain how diabetes mellitus and hypertension affect vision.
9. Prioritize educational needs for the client after corneal transplantation.
10. Describe the common visual deficits for the client with dry macular degeneration.
11. Identify nursing interventions to promote home safety for the client with impaired vision.

SIMON

Go to http://www.wbsaunders.com/SIMON/Iggy/ for self-assessment questions related to these Learning Objectives.

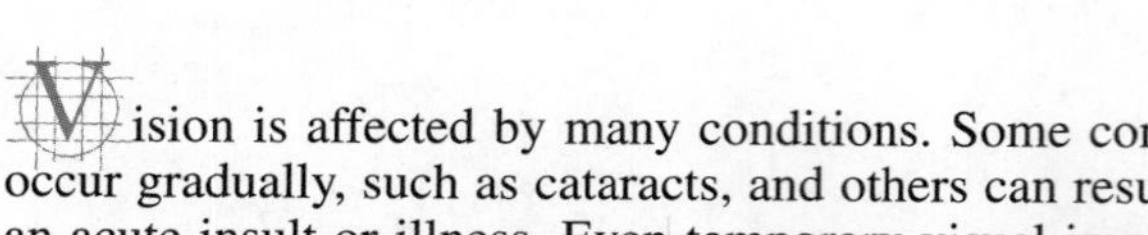

Vision is affected by many conditions. Some conditions occur gradually, such as cataracts, and others can result from an acute insult or illness. Even temporary visual impairment causes the client distress and necessitates some changes in function or lifestyle.

EXTERNAL EYE DISORDERS: EYELID DISORDERS

The eyelid is composed of small muscles and thin skin. The eyelid protects the external eye surface and is responsible for the spread of tears. Disorders can be related to changes in the structure, function, or position of the eyelid. Lid structure may also be altered by age (Figures 47-1 and 47-2).

Blepharitis

OVERVIEW

Blepharitis, an inflammation of the eyelid edges, is most common in the older adult and is often associated with *dry eye syndrome* (see Keratoconjunctivitis Sicca, p. 1027). The lack of sufficient tears with this disorder may lead to bacterial invasion of the eye structures, because tears are bacteriostatic.

➤ COLLABORATIVE MANAGEMENT

Clients usually have itchy, red, and burning eyes. **Seborrhea** (greasy, itchy scaling) of the eyebrows and eyelids is often present. On slit-lamp examination, greasy scales and mattering may be seen on the eyelid-eyelash margin.

Blepharitis is best controlled by a regimen of eyelid care using warm, moist compresses followed by gentle scrubbing with dilute baby shampoo. The nurse instructs the client to avoid rubbing the eyes, because this action can spread the infection to other eye structures.

Entropion

OVERVIEW

An **entropion** is an inversion of the eyelid causing the eyelashes to rub against the eye. The condition usually develops after age 40 years. Entropion can be caused by eyelid muscle spasms or by scarring and deformity of the eyelid itself as a result of trauma. Older clients are susceptible to entropion because of a loss of tissue support with aging.

➤ COLLABORATIVE MANAGEMENT

The client usually reports "feeling something in my eye." Pain and tearing may also be present. On inspection, the eyelid is turned inward, and the conjunctiva appears inflamed. Corneal abrasion may result from constant irritation.

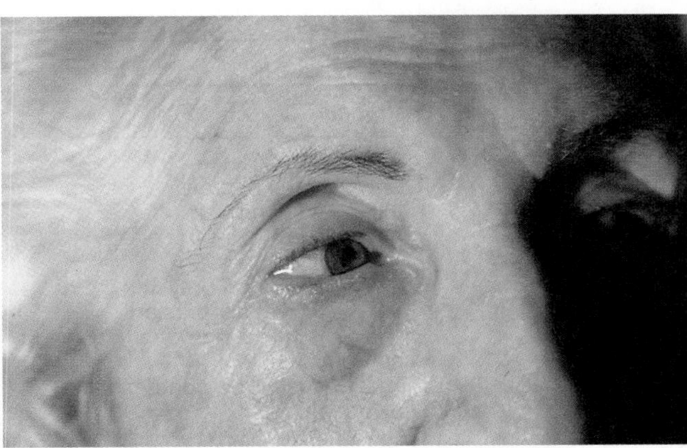

Figure 47-1 ● Eyelid eversion (ectropion).

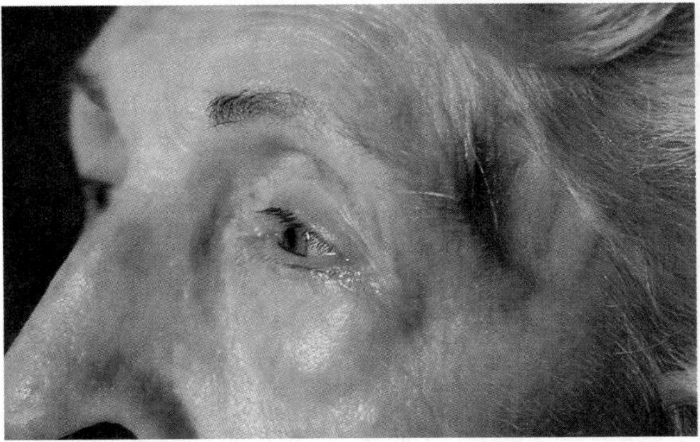

Figure 47-2 ● "Bags" under the eyes.

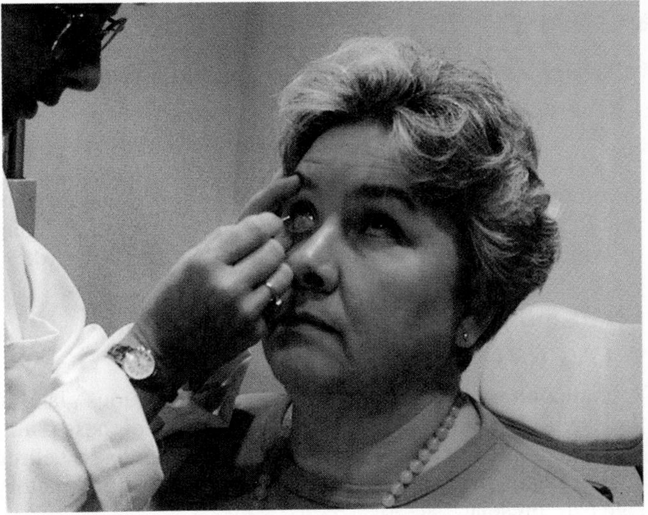

Figure 47-3 ● Application of ophthalmic ointment.

Surgery may correct the position of the eyelid by either tightening the orbicular muscle (thus moving the eyelid to a normal position) or directly preventing inward rotation of the eyelid margin. After surgery, the eye is usually covered with a patch, and the client is discharged a few hours later.

CHART 47-1

BEST PRACTICE *for*
Instillation of Ophthalmic Ointments

- Wash your hands.
- Wear gloves.
- Explain the procedure to the client.
- Check the name, strength, and expiration date of the medication.
- Instruct the client to tilt the head backward, open the eyes, and look up.
- Pull the client's lower lid downward, toward the cheekbone, creating a "pocket" in the lower lid.
- Hold the tube like a pencil, with the tip downward.
- Rest the wrist holding the tube on the client's cheek.
- Do not touch the tip of the tube to the conjunctiva.
- Squeeze the tube gently until a small amount of ointment is in the pocket.
- Release the lower eyelid.
- Instruct the client to close the eye gently.
- Tell the client that vision may be blurred by the ointment.
- Instruct the client to remove the ointment before driving or operating equipment.
- Remove ointment by closing the eye and wiping the closed lid from the inner canthus outward with a clean tissue.

The nurse demonstrates instillation of eyedrops and evaluates the client's ability to instill the drops. The client is instructed to leave the patch in place until he or she is seen by the ophthalmologist and to inform the ophthalmologist of any pain or drainage under the patch. The nurse teaches the client or significant other how to clean the suture line with a cotton swab and the prescribed solution. A small amount of antibiotic ointment may be applied (Figure 47-3). Chart 47-1 describes best practices for applying ophthalmic ointment; Chart 47-2 summarizes important information on ophthalmic drugs.

Ectropion

OVERVIEW

An **ectropion** is the outward sagging and eversion of the eyelid (see Figure 47-1) that is usually associated with aging. Ectropion is caused by relaxation of the orbicular muscle. This lid position does not permit tears to wash adequately over the anterior surface of the eye, leading to corneal drying and ulceration.

COLLABORATIVE MANAGEMENT

Clients frequently have complaints of constant tearing and outward deviation of the eyelid. Surgery is required to restore proper lid alignment. After surgery, the eye is covered with a patch and the client is discharged. Nursing interventions are the same as those for an entropion.

Hordeolum

OVERVIEW

A **hordeolum,** or **stye,** can be external or internal. An external hordeolum is an infection of the sweat glands in the eyelid, occurring near the emergence of the eyelashes from the eyelid (called the **eyelid-eyelash margin**). A red, swollen, tender area is noted on the skin surface side of the eyelid. An internal hordeolum is caused by an infection of the eyelid sebaceous glands. The most common causative organisms are *Staphylo-*

CHART 47-2

DRUG THERAPY *for* Eye Problems

Drug	Nursing Interventions	Rationale
TOPICAL ANESTHETICS		
Proparacaine HCl, or proxymetacaine (AK-Taine, Alcaine, Ocu-Caine, Ophthetic)	Use nasal punctal occlusion.	This technique decreases systemic absorption and side effects.
Tetracaine HCl, cocaine HCl (Pontocaine)	Remind the client not to rub or touch the eye while it is anesthetized.	Touching may injure the eye.
	Patch the eye if the client leaves the facility before the anesthetic wears off.	The use of a patch prevents injury, such as corneal abrasion.
	Do not use discolored solution.	Discoloration is a sign of altered drug composition.
	Store the bottle tightly closed.	Air may cause drug contamination and oxidation.
TOPICAL STEROIDS		
Prednisolone acetate (Ocu-Pred, Ophtho-Tate✤) Prednisolone phosphate (Inflamase)	Shake vigorously before use.	Medication is a suspension; shaking is required to distribute the medication evenly in the solution.
Dexamethasone (Dexair, Dexotic, Maxidex) Betamethasone (Betnesol)	Monitor the client for signs of corneal ulceration.	Steroid use predisposes the client to local infection.
Fluorometholone (Fluor-Op, Liquifilm)	Advise the client not to share eyedrops with others.	Disease transmission is possible when sharing eyedrops.
ANTI-INFECTIVE AGENTS		
Gentamicin (Alcomicin✤, Garamycin, Genoptic) Tobramycin (Tobrex)	Be sure to obtain a specimen for culture before use.	Use of an antibiotic before a culture specimen is obtained may alter culture results.
Ciprofloxacin (Ciloxan) Erythromycin (Ilotycin) Chlortetracycline (Aureomycin) Sulfisoxazole (Gantrisin)	Clean exudate from the eyes before administering drops.	Cleansing decreases the risk of contaminating the medication and increases contact of the conjunctiva with the medication.
Ofloxacin (Ocuflox)	Reinforce the importance of completing the prescribed medication regimen.	Compliance is critical to maintain a therapeutic level of medication.
ANTIBIOTIC-STEROID COMBINATIONS		
Tobramycin with dexamethasone (TobraDex) Neomycin sulfate with polymyxin B sulfate and dexamethasone (Maxitrol)	This is the same as for each component alone.	This is the same as for each component alone.
TOPICAL ANTIVIRAL AGENTS		
Idoxuridine (Herplex, Stoxil) Trifluridine (Viroptic)	Refrigerate and protect from light.	Cool temperatures and absence of light ensures medication stability.
Vidarabine (Vira-A)	Monitor the client for itching lids and burning eyes.	Sensitivity to this drug is common.

coccus aureus, Staphylococcus epidermidis, and *Streptococcus.* The hordeolum usually affects only one eyelid at a time. Vision is not affected.

➤ COLLABORATIVE MANAGEMENT

Small, beady, edematous areas may be seen on the skin side of the eyelid or on the conjunctival side of the eyelid-eyelash margin. As the hordeolum forms, it fills with purulent material, causing pain.

Treatment includes the use of warm compresses four times a day and an antibacterial ointment. When the lesion opens, either spontaneously or after application of the warm compresses, the purulent material drains and the pain subsides.

Nursing interventions include applying a clean washcloth compress and instructing the client in this application. Chart 47-3 describes the proper technique for applying ocular compresses.

After the compresses have been applied for the prescribed time, the nurse instills antibiotic ointment. The client is advised that ointments may cause blurred vision and is taught to remove the ointment from the eyes before driving or operating machinery. To remove the ointment, the client closes the eye and gently wipes the closed eyelid from the inner canthus outward.

Chalazion

OVERVIEW

A **chalazion** is a sterile inflammation of a sebaceous gland in the eyelid. It begins with inflammation and tenderness (similar to the hordeolum), followed by a gradual painless swelling at the gland. In its fully developed state, no inflammatory signs are present.

➤ COLLABORATIVE MANAGEMENT

Most chalazia protrude on the conjunctival side of the eyelid. The client has eye fatigue, sensitivity to light, and possibly excessive tearing **(epiphora).**

Treatment includes the use of warm compresses for 15 minutes four times a day, followed by instillation of ophthalmic ointment. The physician excises the chalazion if it is

CHART 47-2

DRUG THERAPY *for* Eye Problems—cont'd

Drug	Nursing Interventions	Rationale
ADRENERGICS		
Dipivefrin HCl (Propine)	Instruct the client to use nasal punctal occlusion during administration.	Nasal punctal occlusion decreases systemic absorption and side effects.
	Monitor the client's heart rate and blood pressure.	Systemic absorption increases the heart rate and blood pressure.
BETA BLOCKERS		
Carteolol (Ocupress) Levobunolol (Betagan) Timolol (Timoptic, Apo-Timop✤)	Instruct the client to use nasal punctal occlusion during administration.	Nasal punctal occlusion decreases systemic absorption and side effects.
	Monitor the client's heart rate and blood pressure.	Systemic absorption slows the heart rate and may decrease blood pressure, causing orthostatic hypotension.
MIOTICS		
Carbachol (Isopto Carbachol, Miostat) Pilocarpine HCl (Isopto Carpine, Miocarpine✤, Pilocar, Spersacarpine✤)	Warn the client that visual acuity is decreased in low-light environments.	This drug causes severe pupillary constriction.
	Use with caution in clients who have urinary tract obstruction.	This drug mimics the parasympathetic system and can cause urinary retention.
MYDRIATICS AND CYCLOPLEGICS		
Atropine (Atropair, Minims Atropine✤, Ocu-Tropine) Cyclopentolate (Cyclogyl, Minims Cyclopentate✤) Phenylephrine (Minims Phenylephrine✤, Neo-Synephrine, Ocu-Phrin, Spersaphrine✤) Tropicamide (Minims Tropicamide✤, Mydriacyl, Tropicacyl)	Instruct the client to wear sunglasses until the drug wears off.	This drug causes photophobia.
	Instruct the client to avoid driving or operating hazardous machinery until the drug wears off.	This drug causes blurred vision.
	Instruct the client to use nasal punctal occlusion during administration.	This technique decreases systemic absorption and side effects.
NONSTEROIDAL ANTI-INFLAMMATORY AGENTS		
Flurbiprofen (Ocufen) Diclofenac (Voltaren) Ketorolac (Acular)	Monitor the client for bleeding in the eye.	These drugs disrupt platelet aggregation.
	Instruct the client not to wear soft contact lenses during therapy with these drugs.	These drugs interact with contact lens materials and increase the risk for infection.

CHART 47-3

CLIENT EDUCATION GUIDE
Application of an Ocular Compress

1. Wash your hands.
2. Fold a clean washcloth into fourths.
3. Soak the washcloth with running tap water that is warm to your inner wrist. (If cool compresses are needed, follow the same steps using cold running tap water.)
4. Place the cloth over your *closed* eye.
5. Keep the cloth in place with minimal pressure until the cloth cools.
6. Refold the washcloth so that a different "fourth" will be held against the eye.
7. Resoak the cloth with running tap water.
8. Repeat applications three times for as many times each day as are ordered by your physician.

large enough to affect vision, is cosmetically displeasing to the client, or recurs frequently.

After excision, antibiotic ointment is instilled and the eye is covered with a patch. Best practices for proper application of a nonpressure eyepatch are described in Chart 47-4.

The client is instructed to leave the eyepatch intact for 4 to 6 hours and then remove the patch and begin applying warm, moist compresses. Antibiotic eyedrops are instilled after use of the compresses. The nurse instructs the client to report any evidence of infection, increasing redness, purulent drainage, or reduced vision to the ophthalmologist immediately.

LACRIMAL APPARATUS DISORDERS: KERATOCONJUNCTIVITIS SICCA

OVERVIEW

The lacrimal system moistens the external eye with tears and removes tears from the external surface of the eye. Problems can arise from insufficient tear production or from infection or inflammation in any part of the lacrimal system.

Keratoconjunctivitis sicca, or dry eye syndrome, results from changes in the composition of tears, lacrimal gland malfunction, or altered tear distribution. Decreased tear production can also occur during antihistamine, beta-adrenergic blocking agent, or anticholinergic drug therapy. Diseases associated with decreased tear production include rheumatoid arthritis, leukemia, sarcoidosis, multiple sclerosis, mumps, and lymphoma. Radiation or chemical burns can also decrease lacrimal system function. Injury to the facial nerve (cranial nerve VII) can inhibit tearing. Eye dryness may follow vision-enhancing surgery.

CHART 47-4

BEST PRACTICE *for* Application of an Eyepatch

Nonpressure Eyepatch

1. Assemble the equipment:
   - Eyepatch
   - Skin preparation
   - Nonallergenic paper tape
2. Explain the procedure to the client.
3. Wash your hands.
4. Apply a skin preparation to the client's forehead and cheek.
5. Instruct the client to close both eyes gently.
6. Place a patch over the closed eyelid.

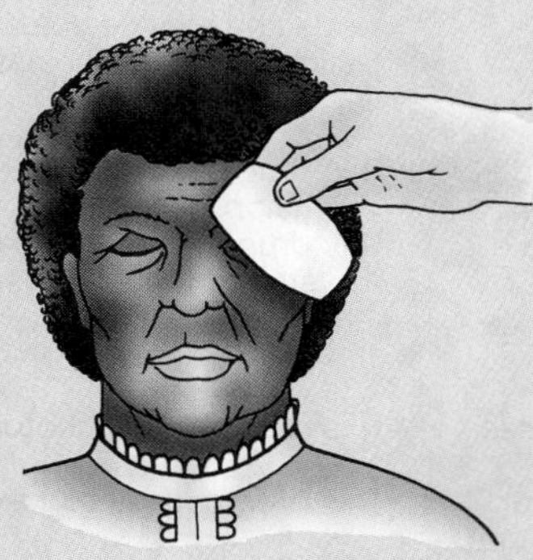

7. Apply tape from the cheek to the middle of the forehead in a diagonal line.

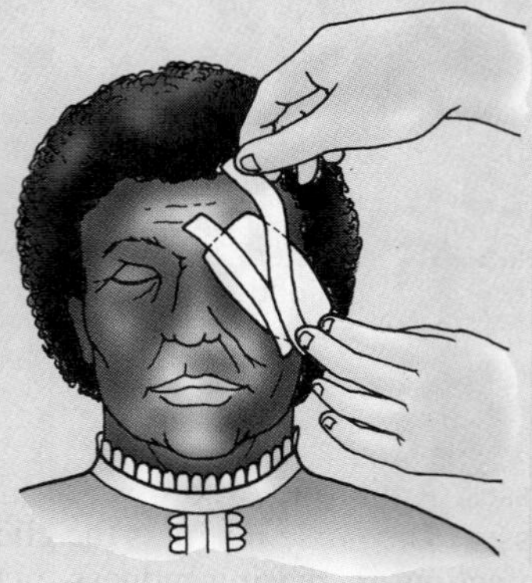

8. Cover the patch with overlapping pieces of tape.

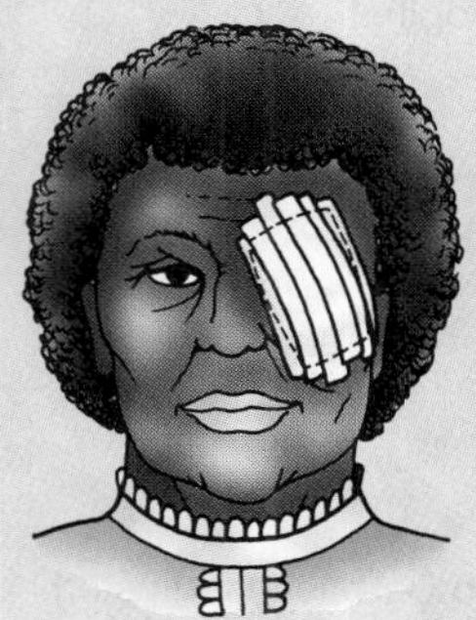

Pressure Eyepatch

1. Assemble the equipment:
   - Two eyepatches for each eye requiring treatment
   - Skin preparation pad
   - Nonallergenic paper tape

2-5. Follow corresponding steps under Nonpressure Eyepatch.

6. Fold one eyepatch in half, place it over the closed eyelid, and apply a second eyepatch (unfolded) over the folded one.

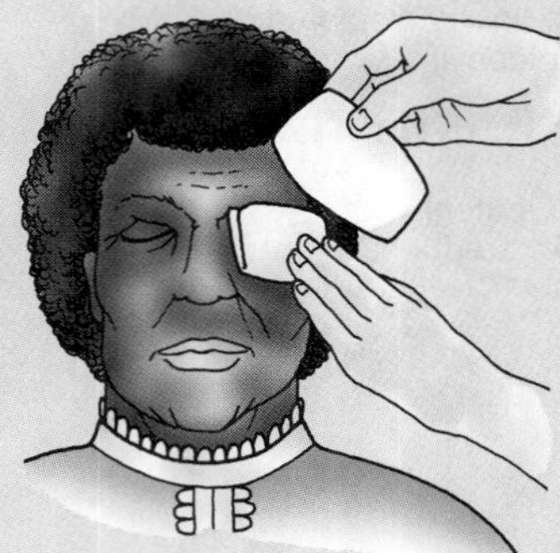

7, 8. Follow corresponding steps under Nonpressure Eyepatch.

▶ COLLABORATIVE MANAGEMENT

The client has the sensation of a foreign body in the eye, burning and itching eyes, and photophobia (increased sensitivity to light). The corneal light reflex is dulled or distorted. The tear film may contain strands of mucus.

Treatment depends on the severity of the symptoms. Artificial tears (HypoTears, Refresh) are prescribed for daytime use to reduce dryness and can be used as often as necessary. A lubricating ointment (Lacri-Lube S.O.P., Refresh P.M.) is used at night. If the dry eye syndrome is caused by an abnormal eyelid position or function, surgery may be required.

CONJUNCTIVAL DISORDERS

The conjunctiva is a thin mucous membrane that covers and protects the eye. Because of its location, the conjunctiva is subject to trauma and exposure to noxious gases; it is also susceptible to infection.

Subconjunctival Hemorrhage

OVERVIEW

Subconjunctival blood vessels are fragile and can break after increased pressure resulting from sneezing, coughing, or vomiting. These hemorrhages may also be associated with hypertension, trauma, or blood dyscrasias.

▶ COLLABORATIVE MANAGEMENT

The small, well-defined area of hemorrhage is bright red under the conjunctiva. The client is usually quite concerned about its appearance. No pain or visual impairment accompanies the hemorrhage, and it resolves gradually within 10 to 14 days without treatment.

Conjunctivitis

OVERVIEW

Conjunctivitis is an inflammation or infection of the conjunctiva. Inflammatory conjunctivitis results from exposure to allergens or irritants and is not contagious. Infectious conjunctivitis occurs as a result of bacterial or viral infection and is readily transmitted from person to person.

COLLABORATIVE MANAGEMENT

Symptoms of allergic conjunctivitis include conjunctival edema, a sensation of burning, **vascular injection** (engorgement of blood vessels—"bloodshot" appearance), excessive tearing, and itching.

Treatment includes the instillation of vasoconstrictors and corticosteroid eyedrops. The client is instructed to avoid using makeup until all symptoms of conjunctivitis subside.

Bacterial conjunctivitis, or "pink eye," is caused by *Staphylococcus aureus, Haemophilus influenzae,* or *Pseudomonas aeruginosa.* Symptoms include blood vessel dilation, mild conjunctival edema, tearing, and discharge. The discharge is watery at first and then gradually becomes thicker, with shreds of mucus.

Cultures of the drainage are obtained to identify the causative microorganism. Treatment is aimed at controlling the infection. Appropriate topical antibiotics are administered.

Nursing interventions focus on preventing the spread of the disease. For example, cross-contamination may spread the infection to the other eye. The amount, color, and type of drainage are noted. The nurse reviews hygienic principles with the client, including handwashing after touching the eye and before instilling eyedrops. The client is warned not to touch the unaffected eye without first washing the hands and to avoid sharing washcloths and towels with others.

Trachoma

OVERVIEW

Trachoma is a chronic, bilateral scarring form of conjunctivitis caused by *Chlamydia trachomatis.* Trachoma is the chief cause of blindness in the world. The incidence is highest in warm, moist climates where hygienic practices are substandard.

COLLABORATIVE MANAGEMENT

The incubation period is 5 to 14 days. Initially, trachoma resembles bacterial conjunctivitis. Symptoms include tearing, photophobia, edema of the eyelids, and conjunctival edema. Follicles form on the upper eyelid conjunctiva. As the disease progresses, the eyelid scars and turns inward, causing the eyelashes to damage the cornea.

Specimens are obtained for culture to identify the causative organism. A 4-week course of oral tetracycline (Achromycin, Apo-Tetra✱) or erythromycin (Apo-Erythro-EC✱, E-Mycin, E.E.S.) is given. These drugs may be applied topically if the systemic forms are unavailable.

Nursing interventions focus on infection control. The client is instructed to wash the hands before and after touching the eyes. The nurse advises the client to keep washcloths separate from those of unaffected people and to launder them separately. The nurse also emphasizes the importance of completing the prescribed course of antibiotics.

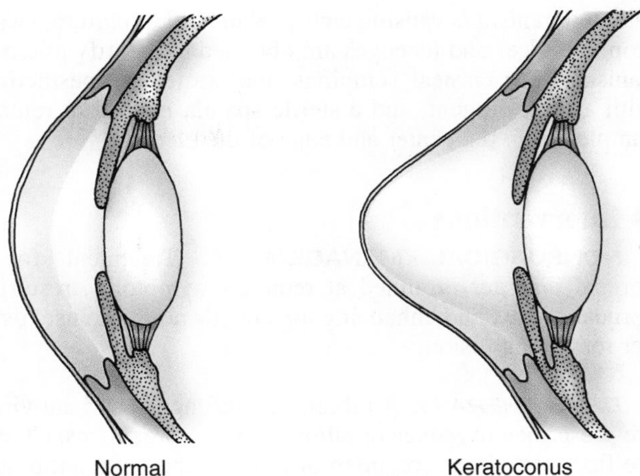

Figure 47-4 ● Profiles of a normal eyeball and one with keratoconus.

TABLE 47-1 • COMMON CAUSES OF CORNEAL DISORDERS

KERATOCONUS • Autosomal recessive trait • Down syndrome • Aniridia • Marfan syndrome • Atopic allergy • Retinitis pigmentosa	**KERATITIS (*ACANTHAMOEBA*)** • Protozoal infection
KERATITIS (EXPOSURE) • Ectropion/entropion • Exophthalmos • Neurologic deficits	**CORNEAL ULCERS** • Mechanical injury • Chemical injury • Drying • Infection

CORNEAL DISORDERS

OVERVIEW

For a sharp image to be focused on the retina, the cornea must be transparent and intact. Corneal problems are the leading cause of visual impairment in the United States and Canada. Corneal disorders may be caused by degeneration of the cornea (keratoconus) (Figure 47-4); deposition of substances in the cornea, altering its refracting power (dystrophies); inflammation from either irritation or infection (keratitis); or ulceration of the corneal surface. Table 47-1 lists common causes of corneal disorders.

COLLABORATIVE MANAGEMENT

Assessment

The client with a corneal disorder usually has pain, reduced vision, photophobia, and eye secretions. Cloudy or purulent (pus-filled) fluid may be present on the eyelids or eyelashes. Gloves are worn during the examination when secretions are noted.

The cornea may look hazy or cloudy. An altered corneal light reflex may be noted. The cornea may no longer be intact, and patchy areas may be visible on examination. When fluorescein is used, these areas appear green.

No definitive tests confirm corneal disease, although microbial culture and corneal scrapings can help determine which organism is causing a corneal ulcer. For culture, swabs from the ulcer and its edges are obtained to identify microorganisms. For corneal scrapings, the cornea is anesthetized with a topical agent, and a sterile spatula is used to remove samples from the center and edge of the ulcer.

Interventions

NONSURGICAL MANAGEMENT. Treatment for a corneal disorder is aimed at reducing symptoms, restoring corneal clarity, and enhancing the client's ability to use his or her remaining vision.

DRUG THERAPY. Antibiotics, antifungals, and antivirals are prescribed to reduce or eliminate microorganisms. Clients are first started on a regimen of a broad-spectrum antibiotic, which may be changed when the results of the culture are known. Steroids may be used with antibiotics to reduce the inflammatory response in the eye. Drugs can be administered topically as eyedrops, injected subconjunctivally, or administered intravenously. Chart 47-5 describes best practices for eyedrop administration.

CHART 47-5

BEST PRACTICE *for* Eyedrop Administration

- Administer drugs at frequent, precise intervals. *The timing of administration is critical.* Clients with eye problems are often given several broad-spectrum antibiotics. If each drug is administered every hour, create separate dosage schedules. For example, give antibiotic A at 7:00, 8:00, 9:00, and 10:00. Then give antibiotic B at 7:30, 8:30, 9:30, and 10:30.
- If two medications must be administered *at the same time, separate the instillation by 5 minutes.* For example, a client with glaucoma and a bacterial ulcer receives timolol (Apo-Timop✱, Timoptic) at 7:00 and tobramycin (Tobrex) at 7:05.
- If the same medication is required for both eyes and one eye is infected, use *separate* bottles of medication.
- Clearly label each bottle for the appropriate eye (OS for the left eye, OD for the right eye).
- Wear gloves when ocular drainage is present.
- Wash your hands before and after administering eyedrops.

VISION ENHANCEMENT. The nurse assists clients in using their functional vision, suggesting sunglasses and indirect lighting if glare creates difficulties. The nurse also informs clients about assistive devices, such as magnifiers and special light fixtures.

SURGICAL MANAGEMENT. Keratoplasty, or corneal transplant, is the surgical removal of diseased corneal tissue and replacement with tissue from a human donor cornea. Transplantation restores vision by removing corneal deformities and replacing them with healthy corneal tissue.

PREOPERATIVE CARE. Corneal transplantation is performed as a scheduled surgical procedure or when donor tissue becomes available. Usually the client is quite anxious. The nurse's calm approach is helpful during discussions. The nurse assesses the client's knowledge of the surgery and of preoperative and postoperative routines, providing information as needed.

The client's eyes are examined for signs of infection, and any redness, drainage, or edema around the eye is reported to the ophthalmologist. Antibiotic drops are instilled into the eye to reduce the risk for infection. Intravenous (IV) access is placed before surgery.

OPERATIVE PROCEDURE. The surgeon removes the center 7 to 8 mm of the diseased cornea (Figure 47-5) with a **trephine,** a circular knife that operates much like a cookie cutter. The same trephine is used to cut the tissue graft from

The diseased cornea is removed with a trephine.

A button, or graft, of donor cornea is removed with the same trephine so that the cuts are identical.

The donor cornea is placed on the eye and stitched into place with suture material that is finer than a human hair.

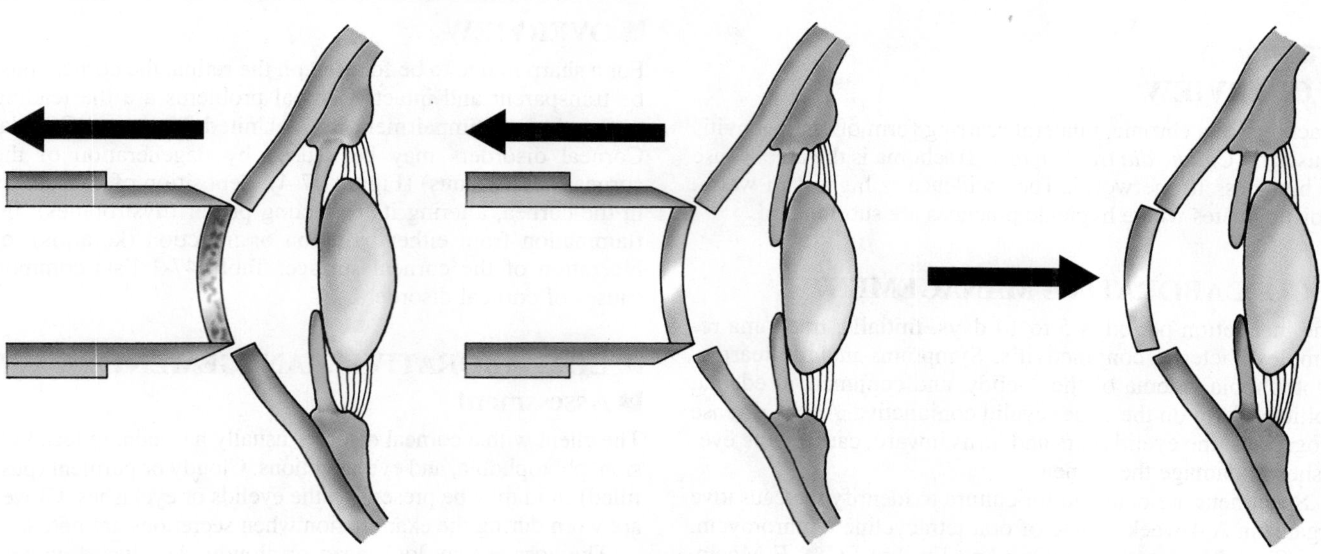

Figure 47-5 ● The steps involved in corneal transplantation (penetrating keratoplasty).

the donor cornea. The donor corneal graft is positioned on the eye and sutured into place. Figure 47-6 shows the eye after corneal transplantation.

During a keratoplasty, the client is usually under regional anesthesia. The nerves around and behind the eye are numbed so that the client cannot move or see out of the eye.

POSTOPERATIVE CARE. After the procedure is completed, a subconjunctival antibiotic injection is given and an antibiotic ointment instilled. The eye is covered with a pressure patch and a protective shield. This initial dressing is left in place until the next day. The nurse does not remove or change the dressing without a specific order from the ophthalmologist.

The nurse notifies the ophthalmologist of changes in vital signs or of drainage on the dressing. The client is instructed to lie on the nonoperative side to reduce intraocular pressure (IOP). During the immediate postoperative period, he or she cannot see out of the affected eye because of the eyepatch and shield.

If the client is to maintain the patches after discharge, the nurse shows him or her how to apply a patch and obtains a return demonstration. For the first postoperative month, the client is instructed to wear the shield at night and whenever he or she is around small children or pets. Complications after corneal transplant surgery include bleeding, wound leakage, infection, and graft rejection.

Although the cornea has no blood supply, graft rejection is possible. The inflammatory process starts in the donor cornea near the graft edge and moves centrally. Vision is reduced, and the cornea becomes cloudy. The client is treated with frequent applications of topical corticosteroids. If the rejection process continues, the graft becomes opaque, and blood vessels may begin to branch into the opaque tissue.

EYE DONATION. Tissue for a keratoplasty is obtained from a local eye or tissue bank. An eye bank obtains its supply of corneal tissue from volunteer donors. These donors must be free of infectious disease or cancer at the time of death.

If a deceased client is a potential eye donor, the nurse:

- Raises the head of the bed 30 degrees
- Instills antibiotic eyedrops, such as Neosporin or tobramycin
- Closes the eyes and applies a *small* ice pack to the closed eyes
- Contacts the family and physician to discuss eye donation

INTRAOCULAR DISORDERS: LENS DISORDERS

Cataract

OVERVIEW

The lens is a biconvex, transparent, refractive elastic structure suspended behind the iris. A cataract is an opacity of the lens that distorts the image projected onto the retina (Figure 47-7). The degree of reduced vision created by the cataract is determined by the location and density of the opacification. Intervention is indicated when visual acuity has been reduced to a level that the client finds unacceptable or that adversely affects lifestyle.

Pathophysiology

With aging, the lens gradually loses water and increases in density. This increased density results from the compression of older lens fibers and the production of new fibers in the outer layers. Opacities can develop in any part of the lens or capsule. A cataract forms as compaction of fibers reduces lens water content, causing lens proteins to precipitate and form crystals. Over time, a progressive and painless loss of lens transparency occurs. Both eyes may have cataracts; however, the rate of progression in each eye is usually different.

Etiology

Cataracts are classified by nature or by onset. They may be present at birth or develop at any time. Cataracts may be age related or result from trauma or exposure to toxic substances. Cataract formation is also associated with specific diseases and other ocular disorders (Table 47-2).

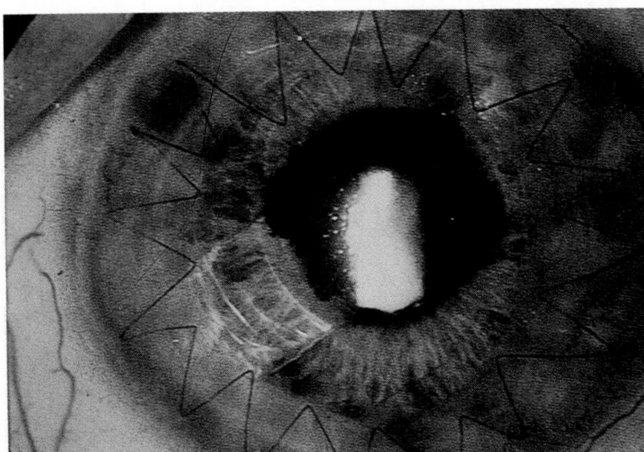

Figure 47-6 ● The appearance of the eye with sutures in place after corneal transplantation. (Courtesy John A. Costin, MD.)

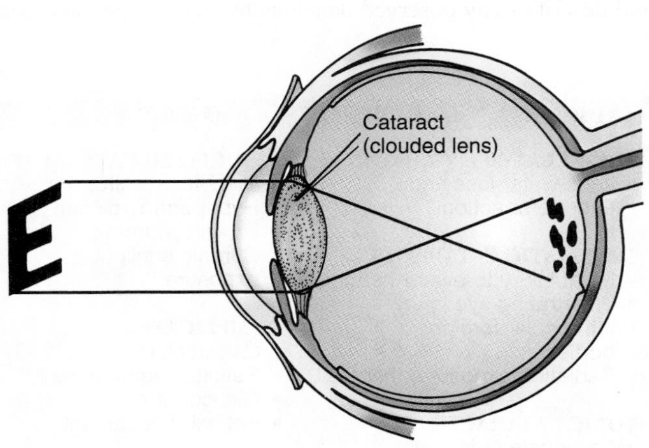

Figure 47-7 ● The visual impairment produced by the presence of a cataract.

Incidence/Prevalence

Cataracts develop in approximately 5 to 10 million people worldwide every year. The age-related cataract is the most common type. Some degree of cataract formation is expected in all people older than 70 years of age (Vaughan, Asbury, & Riordan-Eva, 1995).

COLLABORATIVE MANAGEMENT

SIMON Activity Link

Assessment

HISTORY

When taking a history from a client with cataracts, the nurse notes his or her age, because cataracts are most prevalent in the older adult. The nurse asks about other predisposing factors, including the following:

- Recent or past trauma to the eye
- Exposure to radioactive materials or x-rays
- Systemic disease (such as diabetes mellitus, hypoparathyroidism, Down syndrome, or atopic dermatitis)
- Use of medications (such as corticosteroids, chlorpromazine, or miotic drugs)
- Intraocular disease (such as recurrent uveitis)

The nurse asks the client to describe his or her vision. For example, the nurse might say, "Tell me what you can see well and what you have difficulty seeing." This technique helps the nurse determine the impact of visual deficits on the client.

PHYSICAL ASSESSMENT/CLINICAL MANIFESTATIONS

Early manifestations of cataract development include slightly blurred vision and decreased color perception (Chart 47-6). As lens cloudiness continues, the client may complain of a decrease in vision adversely affecting daily activities. Blurred and double vision may occur. Without surgical intervention, visual impairment can progress to blindness. *No pain or eye redness is associated with age-related cataract formation.*

Visual acuity is significantly reduced. Vision is tested using a Snellen chart and brightness acuity testing (see Chapter 46). The nurse evaluates the client's acuity under various lighting conditions, which can help determine the degree of visual disability.

The nurse examines the lens with the direct ophthalmoscope and describes any observed densities by size, shape, and location. As the cataract matures, the opacity makes visualization of the retina increasingly difficult. Eventually, the red reflex is absent. When this occurs, the pupil is white (Figure 47-8); this is the most easily detected symptom of a cataract.

TABLE 47-2 • COMMON CAUSES OF CATARACTS

AGE-RELATED CATARACTS • Lens water loss and fiber compaction **TRAUMATIC CATARACTS** • Blunt injury to eye or head • Penetrating eye injury • Intraocular foreign bodies • Radiation exposure, therapy **TOXIC CATARACTS** • Corticosteroids • Phenothiazine derivatives • Miotic agents	**ASSOCIATED CATARACTS** • Diabetes mellitus • Hypoparathyroidism • Down syndrome • Chronic sunlight exposure **COMPLICATED CATARACTS** • Retinitis pigmentosa • Glaucoma • Retinal detachment

PSYCHOSOCIAL ASSESSMENT

Loss of vision is gradual, and the client may not be aware of the change until activities such as reading, meal preparation, and driving are affected. Fear of losing one's eyesight can be overwhelming, and the client may exhibit great anxiety during an ocular evaluation.

Analysis

COMMON NURSING DIAGNOSES AND COLLABORATIVE PROBLEMS

The most common nursing diagnosis for clients with cataracts is Disturbed Sensory Perception (Visual) related to ocular lens opacity.

ADDITIONAL NURSING DIAGNOSES AND COLLABORATIVE PROBLEMS

In addition to the most common nursing diagnosis, clients with cataracts may have one or more of the following:

- Fear related to loss of eyesight, scheduled surgery, or inability to regain eyesight
- Risk for Injury related to decreased vision, age, or presence in an unfamiliar environment

CHART 47-6

KEY FEATURES *of* Cataracts

Early
- Blurred vision
- Decreased color perception

Late
- Diplopia
- Reduced visual acuity progressing to blindness
- Absence of red reflex
- Presence of white pupil

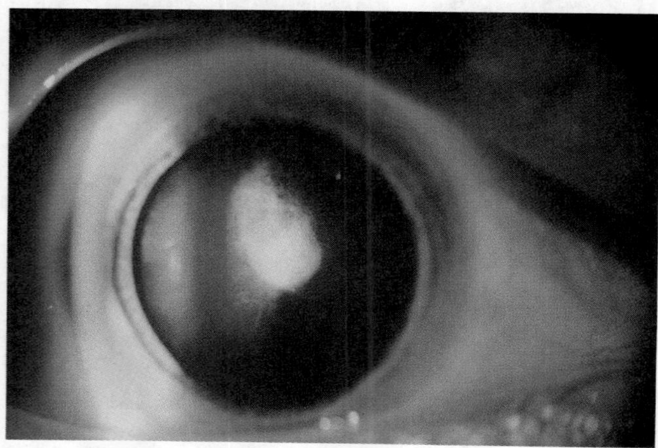

Figure 47-8 ● The appearance of an eye with a mature cataract. (Courtesy John A. Costin, MD.)

- Social Isolation related to reduced visual acuity, fear of injury, decreased ability to navigate in the community, or fear of embarrassment
- Self-Care Deficit related to visual impairment
- Deficient Knowledge (Cataract Pathophysiology and Treatment) related to lack of information or misinterpretation of previously acquired information
- Impaired Home Maintenance related to age, limited vision, or activity restrictions imposed by surgery

CRITICAL THINKING CHALLENGE

The client is a 75-year-old woman with changes in vision that have taken place over the past 3 years. She tells you that her glasses always seem dirty; she can no longer tell blue, green, and purple apart; she cannot distinguish shapes at night; and when car headlights approach, she sees "sparklers." You suspect that she has cataracts.

- What additional assessment questions should you ask to distinguish cataracts from glaucoma?
- What physical findings would you expect?
- How would cataracts affect her visual fields?

For suggested answer guidelines, go to SIMON http://www.wbsaunders.com/SIMON/Iggy/.

Planning and Implementation

DISTURBED SENSORY PERCEPTION (VISUAL)

PLANNING: EXPECTED OUTCOMES. The client with cataracts is expected to have improved vision.

INTERVENTIONS. Surgery and a variety of nursing interventions facilitate the client's recovery of vision.

PREOPERATIVE CARE. The health care provider gives the client accurate information so that he or she can make informed decisions about treatment. The nurse teaches about the nature of cataracts, their progression, and their treatment.

Because cataract surgery is usually an outpatient procedure and most clients are older, adequate preoperative teaching is problematic. The nurse assesses how the client's vision affects the activities of daily living, especially dressing, eating, and ambulating.

An IV infusion is usually started in the operating room. A sedative is given preoperatively, and oral acetazolamide (Acetazolam✤, Diamox) may be given on the morning of surgery to reduce intraocular pressure (IOP). The nurse instills a series of sympathomimetic drugs, such as phenylephrine (Neo-Synephrine, Spersaphrine✤), preoperatively to achieve mydriasis and vasoconstriction. Parasympatholytic drops, such as tropicamide (Minims Tropicamide✤, Mydriacyl) or cyclopentolate hydrochloride (Cyclogyl, Minims Cyclopentolate✤), are also administered to induce paralysis to prevent lens movement.

After the client is in the surgical area, a local anesthetic is administered into the muscle cone behind the eye to achieve anesthesia and ensure eye paralysis. The client may receive an IV injection of midazolam (Versed) to create a few minutes of light anesthesia during the administration of local anesthesia.

CRITICAL THINKING CHALLENGE

Your 75-year-old client has been diagnosed with cataracts and is scheduled to have surgery for removal of one cataract, to be followed immediately with an intraocular lens implant.

- What is your teaching priority for this client?

For suggested answer guidelines, go to SIMON http://www.wbsaunders.com/SIMON/Iggy/.

OPERATIVE PROCEDURE. Extraction of the cataractous lens can be extracapsular or intracapsular (Figure 47-9). The most common procedure is extracapsular cataract extraction (ECCE). The anterior portion of the capsule is opened and removed. The ophthalmologist then removes the lens cortex and nucleus. Any remaining lens material is carefully removed from the eye. The posterior lens capsule is left inside the eye.

In intracapsular cataract extraction, the ophthalmologist removes the lens and capsule completely. A disadvantage of this approach is that the protective posterior capsule is removed, placing the eye at greater risk for retinal detachment and resulting in the loss of a supportive structure for the intraocular lens (IOL) implant.

After the lens with the cataract is removed, the eye has no accommodative power and has lost most of its refractive ability **(aphakia).** A replacement lens is required to focus light rays in the retina. Most often, a small, clear, high-density plastic lens is implanted at the same time that the cataract is removed. Replacement lenses can be selected to allow correction of a specific refractive error. Some clients have distant vision restored to 20/20 and may need glasses only for reading or close work. A newer replacement lens with multiple focal planes may correct all vision for a client to the extent that glasses or contact lenses are either no longer needed or are only minimally needed.

POSTOPERATIVE CARE. Immediately after surgery, the nurse administers an antibiotic subconjunctivally and instills an antibiotic plus steroid ointment. The eye may or may not be covered with a patch and a protective shield. The client is positioned in semi-Fowler's position or on the nonoperative

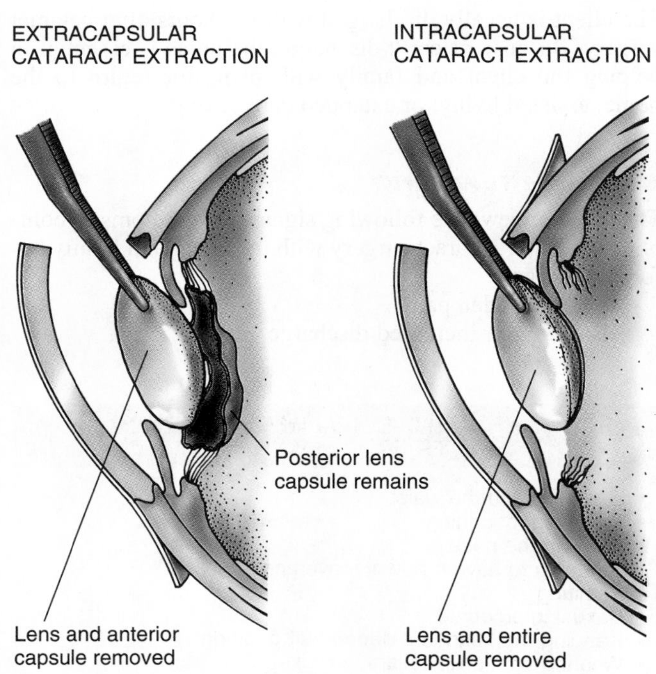

Figure 47-9 ● Surgical approaches to lens removal for cataracts.

side. The nurse observes the dressing for evidence of drainage and reports any drainage to the surgeon.

If a dressing is used, the ophthalmologist usually performs the first dressing change and examines the eye with a slit-lamp microscope the next day. Antibiotic-steroid eyedrops, such as tobramycin combined with dexamethasone (TobraDex), are instilled.

Mild itching caused by the small stitches used to close the incision is normal. Cool compresses may be beneficial. Discomfort at the site is controlled by a mild analgesic such as acetaminophen (Abenol✱, Tylenol) or acetaminophen with oxycodone (Endocet✱, Percocet, Tylox). Aspirin is avoided because of its effects on blood coagulation.

Pain in the early postoperative period may indicate a serious complication, such as increased IOP or hemorrhage. The nurse instructs the client to contact the ophthalmologist if pain accompanied by nausea or vomiting is present.

To minimize increases in IOP (the major complication during the postoperative period), the nurse enforces and teaches the client and family about activity restrictions. Activities that can cause a sudden rise in IOP are listed in Table 47-3.

Another major complication is infection. The client is instructed to observe for increasing redness of the eye, a change in visual acuity, tearing, and photophobia. Creamy white, dry, crusty drainage on the eyelids and lashes is normal. Yellow or green drainage must be reported, however.

Bleeding into the anterior chamber of the eye also may occur, usually several days after surgery. Blood may come from the incision, iris, or ciliary body. The client is instructed to report any change in vision immediately to the ophthalmologist.

Most clients experience a dramatic improvement in vision as early as the day of surgery. The nurse cautions, however, that final best vision will not be present until 4 to 6 weeks after surgery.

Community-Based Care

The client is usually discharged within 2 hours after cataract surgery. Because of early discharge, the nurse is essential in helping the client and family with plans for return to the home, assisted living, or extended care setting.

HEALTH TEACHING

The nurse reviews the following signs and symptoms of complications after cataract surgery with the client and family before discharge:

- Sharp, sudden pain
- Bleeding or increased discharge
- Lid swelling
- Decreased vision
- Flashes of light or floating shapes

The nurse also tells the client to avoid activities that might increase IOP (see Table 47-3). The client may wash his or her hair a day or two after surgery, but only with the head tilted back, such as in a beauty salon or barber shop, to avoid getting water in the eye. For the immediate postoperative period, the client is advised to stand in the shower with the face held away from the shower head.

Cooking and light housekeeping are permitted, but vacuuming should be avoided for several weeks because of the forward flexion involved and the rapid, jerky movements required. The client is also advised to refrain from driving, operating machinery, and participating in certain sports, such as golf, until given specific permission from the ophthalmologist.

TABLE 47-3 • ACTIVITIES THAT INCREASE INTRAOCULAR PRESSURE

- Bending from the waist
- Sneezing, coughing
- Blowing the nose
- Straining to have a bowel movement
- Vomiting
- Sexual intercourse
- Keeping the head in a dependent position
- Wearing tight shirt collars

CRITICAL THINKING CHALLENGE

Your 75-year-old client, who just underwent cataract surgery with intraocular lens replacement, cleans her own house, does her own shopping, eats lunch out with her friends once each week, volunteers in a soup kitchen one day per week, plays cards once each week, plays golf once each week, and plays bingo three times each week. She also drinks one glass of wine with dinner each day and bakes her own bread.

- Which activities may she continue, and which activities should she avoid for the first week following surgery?

For suggested answer guidelines, go to SIMON http://www.wbsaunders.com/SIMON/Iggy/.

NIC MEDICATION ADMINISTRATION: EYE. The nurse reviews the procedure for instilling eyedrops with the client or caretaker. If the client is concerned that the drops may not be correctly instilled, the nurse may advise him or her to refrigerate the eyedrops. Then, when the eyedrop falls into the conjunctival sac, the client will experience a cool feeling. Eyedrops are typically prescribed for 4 to 6 weeks after cataract surgery (Chart 47-7).

CHART 47-7

NIC INTERVENTION ACTIVITIES *for* The Client Requiring Topical Eye Medication

Medication Administration: Eye: *Preparing and instilling ophthalmic medications*

- Wash hands before preparing or administering medication.
- Follow the five rights of medication administration.
- Note client's medical history and history of allergies.
- Determine client's knowledge of medication and understanding of method of administration.
- Position client supine with neck slightly hyperextended; ask client to look at ceiling.
- Instill medication into the conjunctival sac using aseptic technique.
- Apply gentle pressure to nasolacrimal sac if medication has systemic effects.
- Instruct client to close eye gently to help distribute medication.
- Wash hands after eye medication administration.

NIC intervention activities selected from McCloskey, J.C., & Bulechek, G.M. (2000). *Nursing interventions classification (NIC)* (3rd ed.). St. Louis: Mosby.

HOME CARE MANAGEMENT

If the client has difficulty instilling eyedrops, a supportive neighbor, friend, or family member can be taught the procedure. Adaptive equipment that positions the bottle of eyedrops directly over the eye can also be purchased. Chart 47-8 lists items to cover in the focused assessment of a client in the home environment after cataract surgery.

HEALTH CARE RESOURCES

If the client lives alone and has no family or significant others, the nurse arranges for a home care nurse to assess the client and the home situation. If the client is unable to instill eyedrops independently, a friend, neighbor, or family member can be taught this technique.

CRITICAL THINKING CHALLENGE

About 8 hours after cataract surgery and intraocular lens replacement, your 75-year-old client calls and tells you that her pupil on the operative side is twice as large as the pupil in the nonoperative eye and that the operative eye itches.

- What additional information should you obtain?
- Should this client be seen tonight, or should she keep her morning appointment?

For suggested answer guidelines, go to SIMON http://www.wbsaunders.com/SIMON/Iggy/.

Evaluation: Outcomes

The nurse evaluates the care of the client with cataracts on the basis of the identified nursing diagnoses and collaborative problems. The expected outcomes include that the client will:

- Have improved vision
- Recognize signs and symptoms of complications
- Instill eyedrops correctly
- State activities that might increase IOP
- Remain free from injury

Glaucoma

OVERVIEW

Glaucoma is a group of ocular diseases resulting in increased IOP. When IOP is greater than the tissues can tolerate, the cells of the retina and the optic nerve are damaged. If the condition progresses, blindness results. In most common forms of glaucoma, vision is lost gradually and painlessly, without the person's awareness.

Pathophysiology

Intraocular pressure (IOP) is the fluid (aqueous humor) pressure within the eye. A normal IOP of 10 to 21 mm Hg is maintained when there is a balance between production and outflow of aqueous humor. IOP can be raised by decreasing the outflow of aqueous fluid through the anterior chamber or by overproducing aqueous humor. In people with glaucoma, aqueous humor builds up inside the eye, and the increased pressure reduces blood flow to the optic nerve and retina. The sensitive nerve tissue becomes ischemic and dies. Tissue damage usually starts in the periphery and moves inward toward the fovea centralis. Left untreated, glaucoma can result in blindness.

There are several causes and types of glaucoma (Table 47-4). Glaucoma is classified as primary, secondary, or associated. In primary glaucoma, the most common form, the structures involved in circulation and reabsorption of the aqueous humor undergo direct pathologic change.

Primary open-angle glaucoma (POAG), the most common form of primary glaucoma, is usually bilateral and asymptomatic in the early stages. There is reduced outflow of aqueous humor through the chamber angle. Because the fluid cannot leave the eye at the same rate at which it is produced, IOP gradually increases.

Angle-closure glaucoma (also called closed-angle glaucoma, narrow-angle glaucoma, or acute glaucoma) is much less common, has a sudden onset, and is treated as an emergency. The basic problems are a narrowed angle and forward displacement of the iris. Displacement of the iris against the cornea narrows or closes the chamber angle, obstructing the

CHART 47-8

FOCUSED ASSESSMENT *of* Home Care Clients After Cataract Surgery

Assess the eye and vision, including:
- Visual acuity in both eyes using a Jaeger card
- Visual fields of both eyes
- Compare operative eye with nonoperative eye for presence or absence of:
  - Redness
  - Tearing
  - Drainage

Ask the client about:
- Pain in or around the operative eye
- Any change in visual acuity (decreased or improved) in the operative eye
- Whether any of the following has been noticed in the operative eye:
  - Dark spots
  - Increase in the number of floaters
  - Bright flashes of light

Assess the home environment for:
- Safety hazards (especially tripping and falling hazards)
- Kitchen hazards
- Level of room lighting

Assess client compliance with and understanding of treatment and limitations, including:
- Signs and symptoms to report
- Medication regimen
- Activity restrictions

Assess functional ability, including:
- Activities of daily living
- Compliance with medication regimen

TABLE 47-4 • COMMON CAUSES OF GLAUCOMA

PRIMARY GLAUCOMA
- Aging
- Heredity
- Central retinal vein occlusion

SECONDARY GLAUCOMA
- Uveitis
- Iritis
- Neovascular disorders
- Trauma
- Ocular tumors
- Degenerative disease
- Eye surgery

ASSOCIATED GLAUCOMA
- Diabetes mellitus
- Hypertension
- Severe myopia
- Retinal detachment

outflow of aqueous humor. This can happen suddenly and without warning.

Secondary glaucoma results from ocular diseases that cause a narrowed angle or an increased volume of fluid within the eye. These diseases or conditions indirectly disrupt the activity of the structures involved in circulation and reabsorption of aqueous humor. This can happen suddenly and without warning.

Incidence/Prevalence

Glaucoma is a common cause of blindness in industrialized countries. Incidence is age related, with as many as 10% of people older than 80 years of age affected (Vaughan, Asbury, & Riordan-Eva, 1995).

COLLABORATIVE MANAGEMENT

Primary open-angle glaucoma develops slowly, usually without symptoms. The gradual loss of visual fields associated with this disease may go unnoticed because central vision is unaffected. At times, the client may have foggy vision, reduced accommodation, mild aching in the eyes, or headaches and may require frequent changes in eyeglass prescriptions. Late symptoms of glaucoma occur after irreversible damage to optic nerve function and include visual field losses, decreased visual acuity not correctable with eyeglasses, and the appearance of halos around lights. Chart 47-9 lists common clinical manifestations of glaucoma.

Assessment

PHYSICAL ASSESSMENT/CLINICAL MANIFESTATIONS

Ophthalmoscopic examination of the client with glaucoma reveals cupping and atrophy of the optic disk. The disk becomes wider and deeper and turns white or gray (Figure 47-10).

To determine the extent of peripheral field losses, visual fields are measured. A visual field examination (to detect blind spots) maps the areas seen by the eye while it fixates on a central point. In chronic open-angle glaucoma, the visual fields initially show a small crescent-shaped defect that gradually progresses to a larger field defect. In acute angle-closure glaucoma, the visual fields can quickly decrease.

The clinical manifestations of acute angle-closure glaucoma differ from those of open-angle glaucoma. The onset of symptoms is acute, and the client complains of sudden, excruciating pain around the eyes that radiates over the sensory distribution of the fifth cranial nerve. Headache or brow ache, nausea, vomiting, and abdominal discomfort also may occur. Other symptoms may include seeing colored halos around lights and sudden blurred vision with decreased light perception.

On examination, the sclera may appear reddened and the cornea foggy. Ophthalmoscopic examination reveals a shallow anterior chamber, cloudy aqueous humor, and a moderately dilated, nonreactive pupil.

CHART 47-9

KEY FEATURES *of* Glaucoma

Early
- Increased intraocular pressure
- Diminished accommodation

Late
- Diminished visual fields (loss of peripheral vision)
- Decreased visual acuity not correctable with glasses
- Halos around lights
- Headache or eye pain (acute closed-angle glaucoma)
- Increased cup-disk ratio
- Pale optic disk

OTHER DIAGNOSTIC ASSESSMENT

TONOMETRY. Intraocular pressure (IOP), as measured by tonometry, is elevated in glaucoma. If an elevated reading is found during routine screening examination, the nurse takes several readings over a period of time at various times of the day to determine a pattern, because IOP varies during the day. In open-angle glaucoma, the tonometry reading is between 22 and 32 mm Hg (normal is 10 to 21 mm Hg). In angle-closure glaucoma, the tonometry reading may be 30 mm Hg or higher.

TONOGRAPHY. Tonography combines the use of an electronic indentation tonometer with a recording device. The outflow of aqueous humor from the eye is measured while a weight rests on the globe. The slope of the graph is significant. A flat tracing indicates a reduced rate of outflow, as in glaucoma. A steep downhill tracing indicates adequate drainage.

GONIOSCOPY. A special lens that eliminates the corneal curve facilitates the view of the drainage angle in the anterior chamber of the eye. The entire 360-degree circumference of the iridocorneal angle is examined. Adhesions, abnormal blood vessels, sites of trauma, and other data are noted as possible causes of secondary glaucoma.

Interventions

NONSURGICAL MANAGEMENT. Blindness from glaucoma can be prevented by early detection, lifelong treatment, and a commitment to close monitoring and follow-up care. Usually some degree of vision loss is experienced. Chart 47-10 provides information that the nurse can use to help the older client with impaired vision to remain as independent as possible.

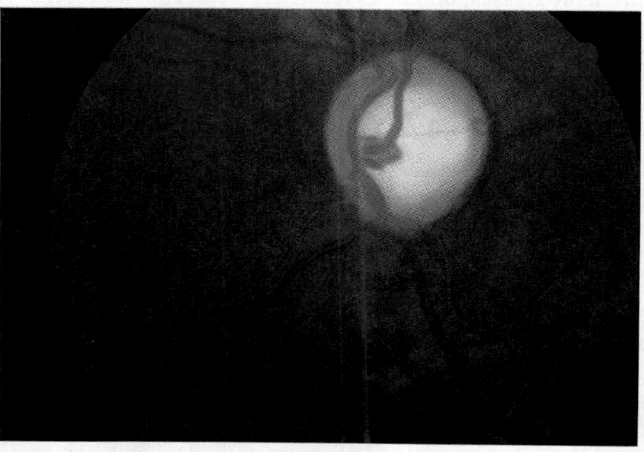

Figure 47-10 ● The optic fundus of a client with glaucoma.

DRUG THERAPY. Drug therapy for glaucoma focuses on reducing IOP through two mechanisms:

- Physically constricting the pupil so that the ciliary muscle is contracted, which allows better circulation of the aqueous humor to the site of absorption
- Inhibiting the production of aqueous humor

Pupillary Constriction. Drugs that constrict the pupil and contract the ciliary muscle **(miotics),** such as pilocarpine hydrochloride (Isopto Carpine, Pilocar, Spersacarpine✱), are commonly used to treat glaucoma. In acute angle-closure glaucoma, constriction of pupil size is also desired, because it stretches the iridocorneal angle and enhances aqueous outflow. Carbachol (Isopto Carbachol, Miostat) may be used with or in place of pilocarpine. Echothiophate iodide (Phospholine Iodide) produces miosis and increases outflow. The nurse reminds the client that miotics may cause blurred vision for 1 to 2 hours after use and that adaptation to dark environments is difficult because of the pupillary constriction.

Inhibition of Aqueous Humor. Beta blockers such as timolol (Apo-Timop✱, Timoptic) and levobunolol (Betagan) are the drug of choice for decreasing IOP. When used as eyedrops, beta blockers reduce aqueous humor production without causing pupillary constriction.

Carbonic anhydrase inhibitors, such as acetazolamide (Acetazolam✱, Diamox) and methazolamide (Neptazane), reduce aqueous humor production to help maintain a lowered IOP. Epinephrine 0.5% to 2% and dipivefrin hydrochloride (Propine) also reduce aqueous humor production. Epinephrine-containing agents are not used in angle-closure glaucoma because of the pupillary dilation caused by their sympathomimetic action.

Osmotic agents may be administered systemically for a client with angle-closure glaucoma as part of emergency treatment to rapidly reduce IOP. Such agents include oral glycerin (Osmoglyn) and IV mannitol (Osmitrol).

SURGICAL MANAGEMENT

LASER SURGERY. When a medical regimen for the client with open-angle glaucoma has been ineffective at controlling IOP, laser surgery is indicated.

Preoperative Care. Nursing interventions include informing the client about laser technology, expected sights and

CHART 47-10

NURSING FOCUS *on the* OLDER ADULT

Promote Independent Living in Clients with Impaired Vision

MEDICATIONS

- Having a neighbor, relative, friend, or visiting nurse visit once a week to measure the proper medications for each day may be helpful.
  - If the client is to take medications more than once each day, it is helpful to use a container of a different shape (with a lid) each time. For example, if the client is to take medication at 9 AM, 1 PM, and 9 PM, the 9 AM medications would be placed in a round container, the 1 PM medications in a square container, and the 9 PM medications in a triangular container.
  - It is helpful to place each day's medication containers in a separate box with raised letters on the side of the box spelling out the day.
- "Talking clocks" are available for the client with low vision.

COMMUNICATION

- Telephones with large, raised block numbers may be helpful. The best models are those with black numbers on a white phone or white numbers on a black phone.
- Telephones that have a programmable, automatic dialing feature are very helpful. Programmed numbers should include those for the fire department, police, relatives, friends, neighbors, and 911.

SAFETY

- It is best to leave furniture the way the client wants it and not move it.
- Throw rugs are best eliminated.
- Appliance cords should be short and kept out of walkways.
- Lounge-style chairs with built-in footrests are preferable to footstools.
- Nonbreakable dishes, cups, and glasses are preferable to breakable ones.
- Cleansers and other toxic agents should be labeled with large, raised letters.
- Hook-and-loop (Velcro) strips at hand level may help to mark the locations of switches and electrical outlets.

FOOD PREPARATION

- Meals on Wheels is a service that many older adults find helpful. This service brings meals at mealtime, cooked and ready to eat. The cost of this service varies, depending on the client's ability to pay.
- Many grocery stores offer a "shop by telephone" service. The client can either complete a computer booklet indicating types, amounts, and brands of items desired, or the store will complete this booklet over the telephone by asking the client specific information. The store then delivers groceries to the client's door (many stores also offer a "put away" service) and charges the client's bank card.
- A microwave oven is a safer means of cooking than a standard stove, although many older clients are afraid of microwave ovens. If the client has and will use a microwave oven, others can prepare meals ahead of time, label them, and freeze them for later use. Also, many complete, microwavable frozen dinners that comply with a variety of dietary restrictions are available.
- Friends or relatives may be able to help with food preparation. Often relatives do not know what to give an older person for birthdays or other gift-giving occasions. One suggestion is a homemade prepackaged frozen dinner that the client enjoys.

PERSONAL CARE

- Handgrips should be installed in bathrooms.
- The tub floor should have a nonskid surface.
- Male clients should use an electric shaver rather than a razor.
- Choosing a hairstyle that is becoming but easy to care for (avoiding parts) will help in independent living.
- Home hair care services may be available.

DIVERSIONAL ACTIVITY

- Some clients are able to use large-print books, newspapers, and magazines (available through local libraries and vision services).
- Books, magazines, and some newspapers are available on audiotape.
- Clients experienced in knitting or crocheting may be able to create items fashioned from straight pieces, such as afghans.
- Card games, dominoes, and some board games that are available in large, high-contrast print may be helpful for clients with low vision.

sounds commonly heard during this procedure, and expected outcomes.

Operative Procedure. A laser **trabeculoplasty** burns the trabecular meshwork, scarring it and causing the meshwork fibers to tighten. This tightening of the fibers increases the size of the spaces between the fibers, allowing outflow of aqueous humor and a reduction in IOP. Topical or local anesthesia is used. Clients commonly experience a temporary increase in IOP immediately after this procedure.

Laser surgery is also indicated for clients with angle-closure glaucoma. The laser makes a hole near the edge of the iris, allowing aqueous humor to flow from the posterior chamber to the anterior chamber and then into the trabecular meshwork.

Postoperative Care. The client is instructed to arrange for transportation home because driving is prohibited immediately after the surgery. Because laser procedures can sometimes increase IOP, the pressure should be re-evaluated 1 hour after surgery and before discharge. The ophthalmologist may prescribe an ocular steroid, such as prednisolone acetate (Ocu-Pred, Ophtho-Tate♣).

STANDARD SURGICAL THERAPY. In open-angle glaucoma that fails to respond to drug and laser therapy and in selected cases of angle-closure glaucoma, surgical intervention is required. This surgery either creates a new drainage channel for aqueous humor or destroys the structures responsible for its production.

Glaucoma surgery is performed either in a hospital or on an outpatient basis. The usual length of stay is several hours to several days.

After surgery, the ophthalmologist administers an antibiotic subconjunctivally. The eye is covered with a patch after an antibiotic-steroid ointment is inserted, and a protective shield is applied over it. The client is instructed to avoid taking aspirin, to avoid lying on the operative side, and to report any brow pain, severe eye pain, or nausea.

The most serious complication after glaucoma surgery is choroidal hemorrhage. If IOP is too low, fluid may enter the suprachoroid space and cause a choroidal detachment. The accumulation of fluid in this space may break blood vessels located there. Symptoms of choroidal hemorrhage include the following:

- Acute pain deep in the eye
- Decreased vision
- Vital sign changes

OCULAR CHAMBER DISORDERS: VITREOUS HEMORRHAGE

OVERVIEW

The vitreous is the gelatinous body that makes up the posterior two thirds of the eye and provides the eye's shape. Vitreous hemorrhage (bleeding into the vitreous cavity) may result from aging, systemic diseases, or trauma, or it may occur spontaneously. With aging, the vitreous may spontaneously detach from the retina. If blood vessels are torn, bleeding into the vitreous results. Diseases that disrupt the retinal blood vessels, such as hypertensive retinopathy and proliferative diabetic retinopathy, also may cause blood leakage into the vitreous.

COLLABORATIVE MANAGEMENT

The primary symptom of vitreous hemorrhage is reduced visual acuity; the degree of reduction varies with the severity of the hemorrhage. A mild hemorrhage may cause the client to see a red haze or series of vitreous "floaters." The client experiencing a moderate hemorrhage may graphically describe seeing "black streaks" or "tiny black dots." Severe hemorrhage may cause visual acuity to be reduced to hand motion. Eye examination shows a reduced red reflex because light rays are blocked from reaching the retina. Ultrasonography is used to determine the location and extent of the hemorrhage.

A vitreous hemorrhage may absorb slowly with no treatment. If the hemorrhage is still present several weeks to months later, a **vitrectomy** (surgical removal of the vitreous) is indicated.

UVEAL TRACT DISORDERS: UVEITIS

OVERVIEW

The uveal tract is composed of three distinct but related parts: the iris, the ciliary body, and the choroid. The most common problem associated with these structures is inflammation, or **uveitis.** Uveitis may occur in the anterior or posterior portion of the eye.

Anterior uveitis can include inflammation of the iris, inflammation of the ciliary body, or both. The cause of anterior uveitis is unknown, but the condition is associated with exposure to allergens, infectious agents, trauma, or systemic disease (rheumatoid arthritis, ankylosing spondylitis, herpes simplex, herpes zoster). It can follow any local or systemic bacterial infection. Symptoms include aching around the eye; tearing; blurred vision; photophobia; a small, irregular, nonreactive pupil; and a "bloodshot" appearance of the sclera.

Posterior uveitis is the common term for **retinitis** (inflammation of the retina) and **chorioretinitis** (inflammation of both the choroid and the retina). Posterior uveitis is associated with tuberculosis, syphilis, and toxoplasmosis.

The onset of symptoms is slow and insidious. Visual impairment in the affected eye, the primary symptom, results from protein-rich fluid, fibrin, and cells leaking into the vitreous cavity. The pupil is small, nonreactive, and irregularly shaped. Black dots are visible against the red background of the fundus. Chorioretinal lesions appear as grayish yellow patches on the retinal surface.

COLLABORATIVE MANAGEMENT

Treatment of the client with anterior or posterior uveitis includes resting the ciliary body with a cycloplegic agent. The pupil is dilated to prevent adhesions between the iris and the lens. Steroid drops are administered every hour to decrease the inflammatory response of the eye and to prevent adhesions of the iris to the cornea and lens. Subconjunctival injections of steroids may be used in posterior uveitis or when topical steroids have been ineffective. Analgesics that contain neither aspirin nor opioids are ordered for pain. Antibiotic therapy may be started for the client with posterior uveitis or when infection is present with anterior uveitis.

Cool or warm compresses are applied for ocular pain. Darkening the room and wearing sunglasses reduce the discomfort of photophobia. Because of blurred vision from the cycloplegic drops, the nurse instructs the client not to drive or operate machinery. The nurse reviews the signs and symptoms of bacterial and fungal ulcers and the indications of increased intraocular pressure (IOP).

RETINAL DISORDERS

Hypertensive Retinopathy

OVERVIEW

Many Americans have hypertension. Hypertension causes blood vessel changes in the eyes that lead to retinal damage and decreased vision.

Hypertensive retinopathy is classified by grades. With each increasing grade, progressive changes are noted in the retina. A direct relationship exists between narrowing of the retinal arterioles and elevation of the diastolic blood pressure.

COLLABORATIVE MANAGEMENT

As blood pressure increases, retinal arterioles narrow and take on a characteristic "copper wire" appearance (Figure 47-11). Nicking, or narrowing, of the vessel at arteriovenous crossings is apparent. If blood pressure remains elevated, areas of localized ischemia, known as soft exudates or "cotton wool" spots, develop as a result of occlusion of the arteriole. Small hemorrhages may be noted. The client may also have headaches and vertigo. Left untreated, hypertensive retinopathy can cause retinal detachment.

Treatment focuses primarily on management of the systemic hypertension (see Chapter 36) and controlling IOP.

Diabetic Retinopathy

OVERVIEW

Diabetic retinopathy is the vascular complication of diabetes in the retina. The longer the person has diabetes, the greater is the incidence and severity of retinopathy (Cotran, Kumar, & Collins, 1999). Another factor influencing the severity of retinopathy is blood glucose control. Good control lessens the severity of the disease. There are two types of diabetic retinopathy: background diabetic retinopathy and proliferative diabetic retinopathy.

In **background diabetic retinopathy,** the supporting cells of the retinal vessels die, and the capillary walls of the retina allow fluid to leak. As this fluid is absorbed, thick yellow-white deposits, or hard exudates, are formed. The retinal capillaries become diseased and lose their ability to transport needed oxygen and nutrients. Outpouches in the walls of capillaries **(microaneurysms)** are formed. These fragile capillaries bleed easily and cause intraretinal hemorrhages in the nerve fiber layer of the retina (Figure 47-12). Visual acuity is diminished by reduction of the capillary blood supply to the retina or by macular edema.

In clients with **proliferative diabetic retinopathy,** a network of fragile new blood vessels develops, leaking blood and protein into the surrounding tissue. Development of these blood vessels is stimulated by the hypoxic state of the retina that results from poor capillary perfusion of retinal tissues. New blood vessels grow in the retina, encroach onto the iris, and grow into the posterior face of the vitreous. The vitreous contracts and pulls away from the retina, causing blood vessels to break and bleed into the vitreous.

COLLABORATIVE MANAGEMENT

Treatment of the client with diabetic retinopathy depends on the degree of retinal involvement. Laser therapy can be used to seal microaneurysms, resulting in decreased bleeding. Scattering of laser burns across the retina can also decrease the retina's need for oxygen and control the growth of new blood vessels.

A vitrectomy is performed if frequent bleeding into the vitreous occurs and the body is unable to reabsorb it or if fibrin bands threaten to detach the retina. Fibrin bands within the vitreous are severed and removed. An endolaser may be used in the eye during surgery to seal leaking or bleeding blood vessels.

Macular Degeneration

OVERVIEW

Macular degeneration (deterioration of the macula, the area of central vision) can be atrophic (age related, or *dry*) or exudative *(wet)*. Atrophic degeneration is characterized by scle-

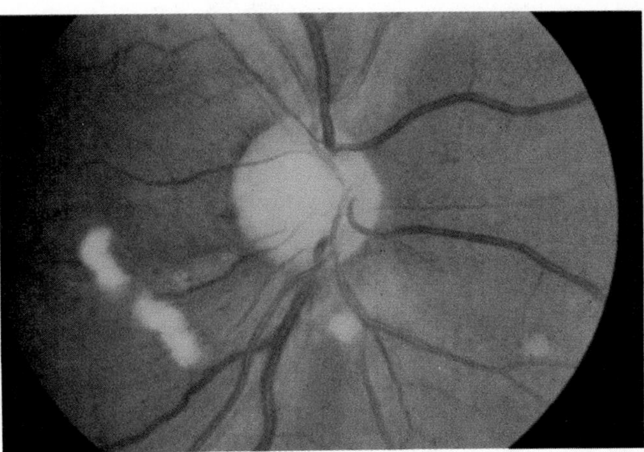

Figure 47-11 ● The optic fundus of a client with hypertension.

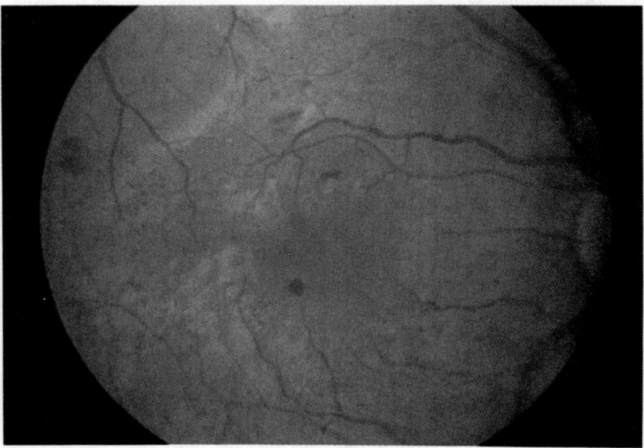

Figure 47-12 ● The optic fundus of a client with diabetes.

rosing of retinal capillaries, causing macular cells to become ischemic and necrotic. Rod and cone photoreceptors die. Central vision declines, and clients describe "mild blurring and distortion." This type of degeneration is more common and progresses at a faster rate among smokers than among nonsmokers. Current research into nutrition therapy suggests that the risk for atrophic macular degeneration can be reduced by increasing long-term dietary intake of antioxidants and the carotenoids lutein and zeaxanthin (see the Evidence-Based Practice for Nursing box below).

Clients with exudative degeneration experience a sudden decrease in vision after a serous detachment of pigment epithelium in the macula. Blood vessels invade this injured area and cause fluid and blood to accumulate under the macula (like a blister), resulting in scar formation and progressive distortion of vision.

COLLABORATIVE MANAGEMENT

Treatment of atrophic macular degeneration aims to help the client maximize remaining vision. The associated loss of central vision may interfere with the ability to read, write, recognize safety hazards, and drive. The nurse suggests alternative strategies (such as large-print books and public transportation) and referrals to community organizations that provide a wide range of adaptive equipment.

Management of clients with exudative macular degeneration is geared toward slowing the process and identifying further changes in visual perception. Fluid and blood may resorb in a small percentage of clients with exudative degeneration. Laser therapy to seal the leaking blood vessels in or near the macula can limit the extent of the damage.

EVIDENCE-BASED PRACTICE FOR NURSING

Prevention of age-related macular degeneration starts early

Pratt, S. (1999). Dietary prevention of age-related macular degeneration. *Journal of the American Optometric Association, 70*(1), 39-47.

This study represents a meta-analysis of research for the past 20 years regarding modifiable factors associated with the development of age-related macular degeneration (ARMD). The analysis includes studies of different types with variable sample sizes and different degrees of rigor. Data were obtained from multiple sites using different methodologies. Although some conflicting data were found, there was agreement regarding two modifiable risk factors. Smoking was strongly correlated to the development of ARMD, with heavier smokers at greater risk than nonsmokers. Long-term ingestion of diets high in the carotenoids lutein and zeaxanthin, found in dark green, leafy vegetables, appeared to have a protective effect against the development of ARMD. It was not known whether vitamin supplements containing synthetic carotenoids could induce the same degree of protection.

Critique. This review analyzed data from studies that were not consistent in design, size, or rigor. Data obtained were largely retrospective in nature. The information derived in this study was trend oriented. Large, prospective clinical trials are needed to demonstrate whether dietary modification can significantly protect against the development of ARMD.

Implications for Nursing. ARMD is a leading cause of visual impairment in older adults, and the lost vision is permanent, interfering with independent living. The link between smoking and the eventual development of ARMD is stronger than the link between dietary ingestion of specific carotenoids and protection against ARMD. Lifestyle modification, however, has no known harmful side effects and does have many benefits for decreasing cardiovascular and cancer risks. Therefore nurses can support recommendations for the suggested lifestyle modifications.

Retinal Holes, Tears, and Detachments

OVERVIEW

A retinal hole is a break in the integrity of the peripheral sensory retina. Retinal holes can be caused by trauma or can occur with aging.

A retinal tear is a more jagged and irregularly shaped break in the retina. It can result from traction on the retina.

A retinal detachment is the separation of the sensory retina from the pigmented epithelium. Retinal detachments are classified by the nature of their development.

Rhegmatogenous detachments occur following a hole or tear in the retina caused by mechanical force, creating an opening for the vitreous to filter into the subretinal space. When sufficient fluid collects in this space, the retina detaches.

Traction detachments are created when the retina is pulled away from the epithelium by bands of fibrous tissue in the vitreous.

Exudative detachments are caused by fluid accumulation in the subretinal space; they occur in association with a systemic disease or with ocular tumors. No retinal break occurs.

COLLABORATIVE MANAGEMENT

The onset of a retinal detachment is usually sudden and painless because no pain fibers are located in the retina. Clients may suddenly see bright flashes of light (**photopsia**) or floating dark spots in the affected eye. During the initial phase of the detachment or if the detachment is partial, the client may describe the sensation of a curtain being pulled over part of the visual field. The visual field loss corresponds to the area of detachment.

Assessment

On ophthalmoscopic examination, detachments appear as gray bulges or folds in the retina that quiver with movement. This appearance is in marked contrast to the flat pink-orange color of the choroid as it shows through the transparent retina. Depending on the cause of the detachment, a hole or tear also may be seen at the edge of the detachment.

Interventions

If a retinal hole or tear is discovered before it causes a detachment, the ophthalmologist may elect to close or seal the break. Closure prevents the accumulation of fluid under the retina, reducing the likelihood of a detachment. Treatment aims to create an inflammatory response that will bind the retina and choroid together around the break. This inflammatory response can be created through external application of **cryotherapy** (a freezing probe), **photocoagulation** (laser), or **diathermy** (high-frequency current).

Spontaneous reattachment of the retina is rare. Surgical repair is required to place the retina in contact with the underlying structures. A common repair procedure is scleral buckling.

PREOPERATIVE CARE. Clients requiring retinal surgery are anxious and fearful about a possible permanent loss of vision. The nurse provides information and reassurance to allay fears.

Depending on the location and size of the retinal break, activity restrictions may be necessary immediately to prevent further tearing or detachment and to promote drainage of any subretinal fluid.

The nurse places an eyepatch over the client's affected eye to reduce eye movement. Topical medications to inhibit accommodation and constriction of the pupil are administered before surgery.

OPERATIVE PROCEDURE. The surgery is performed with the client under general anesthesia. In scleral buckling, the ophthalmologist repairs wrinkles or folds in the retina so that the retina can assume its normal smooth position, and the sclera flattens against the retina. To promote reattachment, a small piece of silicone is placed against the sclera and held in place by an encircling band (Figure 47-13). These devices keep the retina in contact with the choroid and sclera to promote attachment. Any subretinal fluid present is drained.

To further encourage retinal reattachment, a gas such as sulfahexafluoride (SF6) or silicone oil can be used. These agents float up against the retina to hold it in place until healing occurs.

POSTOPERATIVE CARE. After retinal reattachment surgery, an eyepatch and shield are applied. The nurse monitors the client's vital signs and checks the eyepatch and shield for any drainage.

Activity status varies. If gas or oil has been used, the nurse positions the client on his or her abdomen to allow the gas to float against the retina. The client lies with the head turned so that the operative eye is facing up, for several days or until the gas has been absorbed. As an alternative, he or she can sit on the side of the bed and place the head on an over-the-bed table. Bathroom privileges are allowed once the client is fully awake.

The client may experience nausea and pain postoperatively. The nurse administers analgesics and antiemetics as prescribed. Any complaint of a sudden increase in pain or pain accompanied by nausea is reported to the ophthalmologist because these symptoms may indicate the development of complications. The nurse also instructs the client to avoid activities that increase intraocular pressure (IOP) (see Table 47-3).

In the first week after retinal detachment surgery, the client must avoid reading, writing, and close work, such as sewing, because these activities cause rapid eye movements. The nurse teaches the client about the signs and symptoms associated with infection and detachment. The client is instructed to notify the nurse or physician if any signs or symptoms occur.

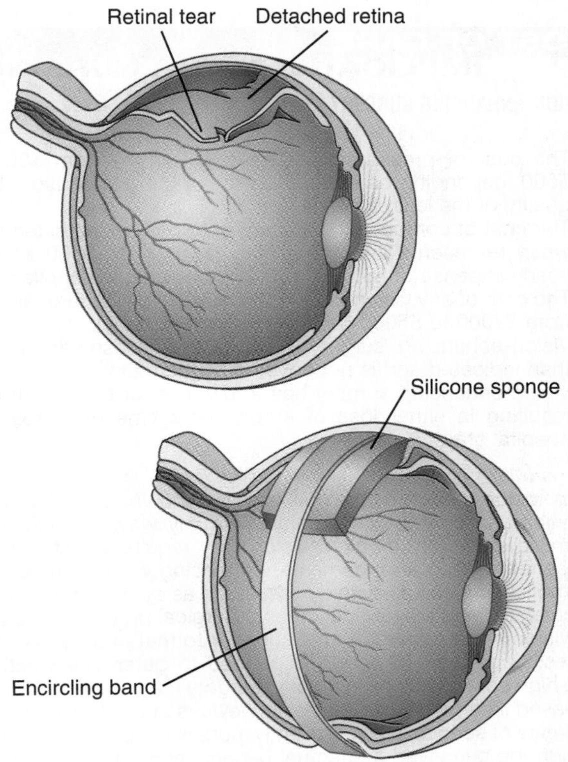

Figure 47-13 ● The scleral buckling procedure for repair of retinal detachment.

Retinitis Pigmentosa

OVERVIEW

Several types of bilateral retinal disorders with progressive degeneration of the retina and a loss of visual receptors lead to blindness. Retinitis pigmentosa is a condition in which retinal nerve cells degenerate and the pigmented cells of the retina grow and move into the sensory areas of the retina, causing further degeneration. Different forms of this disorder can be inherited as an autosomal dominant trait, an autosomal recessive trait, or an X-linked recessive trait (Cotran, Kumar, & Collins, 1999).

COLLABORATIVE MANAGEMENT

The most common early clinical manifestation experienced by a person with retinitis pigmentosa is night blindness. Over time, decreased visual acuity progresses to total blindness. Ophthalmoscopic examination of the retina shows excessive pigmentation in a lattice-like pattern. Cataracts may accompany this disorder.

No current therapy has proved effective in preventing or slowing the degenerative process. Because some retinal destruction resembles that seen with vitamin A deficiency, a regimen of vitamin A, along with decreased exposure of the retina to bright light, is being tried.

REFRACTIVE ERRORS

OVERVIEW

The ability of the eye to focus images on the retina depends on the length of the eye from front to back and the refractive power of the lens system. **Refraction** is the bending of light rays. Problems in either eye length or refraction can result in refractive errors.

Myopia

In **myopia** (nearsightedness), the refractive ability of the eye is too strong for the eye length. Images are bent and fall in front of, not on, the retina.

Hyperopia

In **hyperopia,** or **hypermetropia** (farsightedness), the refractive ability of the eye is too weak, causing images to be focused behind the retina. A shorter length of the eye may contribute to the development of hyperopia.

Presbyopia

As people age, the crystalline lens loses its elasticity and is less able to alter its shape to focus the eye for close work **(presbyopia).** As a result, images fall behind the retina. Presbyopia usually occurs in people in their 30s and 40s.

Astigmatism

Astigmatism occurs when the curve of the cornea is uneven. Because light rays are not refracted equally in all directions, a focus point on the retina is not achieved.

COLLABORATIVE MANAGEMENT

Assessment

Refractive errors are diagnosed through a process known as **refraction.** The client is asked to view an eye chart while lenses of different strengths are systematically placed in front of the eye, and is then asked whether the lenses sharpen or worsen vision. The power or strength of the lens necessary to permit focusing of the image on the retina is expressed in measurements called **diopters.**

Interventions

NONSURGICAL MANAGEMENT. Errors of refraction must be corrected through the use of a lens to permit light rays to focus on the retina (see Figure 46-5). Myopic vision is corrected to bring the image forward onto the retina with a concave lens. Hyperopic vision is corrected with a convex lens to move the focused image back to the retina.

EYEGLASSES. Eyeglasses commonly correct errors of refraction. Advantages of eyeglasses, when compared with other refractive error corrections, include ease of use, durability, availability, and low cost. Disadvantages include a change in physical appearance, the weight of the frame on the nose, and reduced peripheral vision (vision is corrected only when the client looks through the center of the lens).

CONTACT LENSES. Contact lenses can also correct refractive errors. Round plastic disks rest against the cornea and fit under the eyelid.

Hard Lenses. Hard contact lenses correct refractive errors by changing the shape of the cornea, which increases its refracting ability, and by placing the specific refractive power and shape needed in front of the eye so that light rays can be correctly focused onto the retina.

Complications of hard contact lens wear include corneal edema, which occurs when the lenses are worn for an extended period. Corneal abrasions can result from overwear, which dries the epithelium and causes minute breaks, or from the irritation of the contact lens against the cornea.

Soft Lenses. Soft contact lenses are larger but better tolerated than hard contact lenses. They resemble the thickness of plastic wrap and can be worn for longer periods because the lenses' hydrophilic character allows greater corneal access to moisture and oxygen. Most problems with wearing soft lenses are related to lens deterioration, deposits in the lens, and lack of compliance with lens care practices.

There are two types of soft contact lenses: daily-wear lenses (worn during waking hours) and extended-wear lenses. Extended-wear contact lenses can be worn continuously for several days to several weeks, depending on the client's environment, activities, and tolerance of the lenses.

SURGICAL MANAGEMENT. Surgery is becoming a popular alternative for the treatment of refractive errors. Such vision-enhancing surgeries include radial keratotomy, photorefractive keratectomy, laser in-situ keratomileusis, and placement of Intacs corneal ring segments. All surgical procedures are much more expensive than eyeglasses or any type of contact lens. These procedures are rarely covered by insurance (see the Cost of Care box below).

RADIAL KERATOTOMY. **Radial keratotomy (RK)** is an outpatient surgical procedure for the treatment of mild to moderate myopia. Eight to 16 diagonal incisions are made through 90% of the peripheral cornea. Because the central cornea is not incised, vision is not diminished. These incisions flatten the cornea, which decreases the length of the eye and allows the image to be focused closer to the retina.

Slight overcorrection or undercorrection of the refractive error is possible, in which case the client still must wear some form of visual correction after the surgery. Other complications include corneal scarring and chronic dry eyes.

COST OF CARE IMPLICATIONS FOR NURSING

VISION-ENHANCING SURGERY

Cost of Care

- The cost of prescription eyeglasses ranges from $50 to $500, depending on the complexity of the prescription, the quality of the lens, and the frames.
- The cost of contact lenses (hard, soft, daily wear, extended wear) represents an initial outlay of $100 to $300 and a yearly expense of $80 to $150 for consumable supplies.
- The cost of any vision-enhancing surgical procedure ranges from $2000 to $5000 per eye (varies regionally).
- Vision-enhancing surgery is considered cosmetic rather than indicated and is not covered by insurance.
- Vision-enhancing surgery has a low level of complications resulting in either loss of employment time or increased hospital stay.

Implications for Nursing

Poor vision decreases the quality of life and vocational opportunities and contributes to injury in many ways. In addition, some clients with impaired vision may require assistance or dependent living arrangements. Enhancing vision can be accomplished with assistive devices such as eyeglasses or contact lenses and by surgical means. Surgical procedures result in vision enhancement that is superior to that of assistive devices. Long-term follow-up is needed to determine whether the high cost of vision-enhancing surgery may be offset by decreased lifetime costs of assistive devices or by decreased incidence of serious injury. Currently, nurses need to help clients weigh the perceived and actual benefits against the costs related to different types of vision enhancement.

PHOTOREFRACTIVE KERATECTOMY. **Photorefractive keratectomy (PRK)** is an alternative for people with mild to moderate stable myopia and low astigmatism. PRK is not a laser version of radial keratotomy but a completely different procedure. An excimer laser pulses a brief but powerful beam of ultraviolet light on the central superficial cornea. This beam removes small portions of the tissue surface, reshaping the cornea to properly focus an image on the retina.

Photorefractive keratectomy is performed as an outpatient procedure with the client under local anesthesia. One eye is treated at a time, usually at least 3 months apart. The eye is patched after surgery. Complete healing to best vision may take up to 6 months.

Most people do not need corrective lenses for distance vision after PRK but may still need reading glasses. Expected side effects of PRK in the postoperative period include pain, hazy vision, light sensitivity, tearing, and pupil enlargement. Possible complications include difficulty with night vision, corneal clouding, undercorrection, far-sightedness, increased intraocular pressure (IOP), chronic dry eyes, and glare.

LASER IN-SITU KERATOMILEUSIS. **Laser-in-situ keratomileusis (LASIK)** is a newer procedure for correcting near-sightedness, far-sightedness, and astigmatism using the excimer laser. With this procedure, the superficial layers of the cornea are lifted temporarily as a flap and brief but powerful laser pulses reshape the deeper corneal layers. After reshaping the deeper layers, the superficial cornea is placed back into its original position.

LASIK is performed as an outpatient procedure with the client under local anesthesia. Usually both eyes are treated at the same time, although some clients prefer separate surgeries. Most clients have improved functional vision within an hour after surgery; complete healing to best vision may take up to 4 weeks.

This procedure is thought to be superior to PRK because the outer corneal layer is not damaged. Pain is reportedly less than for PRK, and the time to best vision is reduced. Most clients require less postoperative medication, and a wider variety of refractive errors can be treated with LASIK than with PRK.

After LASIK correction of refractive errors, many clients no longer require eyeglasses or contact lenses. Overcorrection or undercorrection is possible, however, and some clients may need a mild prescription for a refractive error. The risk for complications is reportedly less than for other types of vision-enhancing surgery and includes corneal clouding and chronic dry eyes.

INTACS CORNEAL RING. Intacs corneal ring placement is the most recent vision-enhancing procedure for near-sightedness. This surgery does not involve the use of a laser and has the advantage of being reversible. With this procedure, the shape of the cornea is changed by placing a polymeric ring in the outer edges of the cornea (outside of the optical zone).

Intacs ring placement is performed as an outpatient procedure with the client under local anesthesia. Healing to best vision is immediate. Overcorrection or undercorrection of refraction is possible; however, removal, replacement, or adjustment of ring tightness can enhance satisfaction. In addition, replacements can be made if the client's vision changes further as a result of aging. Because the ring is applied to the cornea outside of the optical zone, the risk for corneal clouding or scarring is lower than with other surgical procedures.

TRAUMATIC DISORDERS

Trauma to the eye or periorbital area can result from almost any activity. Care varies depending on the area of the eye affected and whether the globe of the eye has been penetrated.

Hyphema

OVERVIEW

A **hyphema** is a hemorrhage in the anterior chamber. It occurs when a force is applied to the eye and breaks the blood vessels.

COLLABORATIVE MANAGEMENT

If the hyphema is large, it may block the pupil and reduce vision, possibly causing pain and photophobia. Hemolysis of the blood occurs, and the blood is filtered out of the eye through the trabecular meshwork. If the hemolyzed blood obstructs the trabecular meshwork, increased intraocular pressure (IOP) results.

The client with a hyphema is treated by bedrest in semi-Fowler's position to use gravity as an aid in keeping the hyphema away from the optical center of the cornea. Minimal or no sudden eye movements are permitted for 3 to 5 days to decrease the risk for rebleeding. Cycloplegic eyedrops may be ordered to place the eye at rest, and the eye is protected by a patch and shield. Television and reading are restricted. A hyphema usually resolves in 5 to 7 days.

Contusion

OVERVIEW

A contusion of the eyeball and surrounding tissue is caused by traumatic contact with a blunt object. The force of the blow pushes the eye back in the socket. The globe is compressed, and stretching of the ocular soft tissues occurs, which can produce damage and possibly rupture the globe.

Results of the injury may not be seen immediately. These results include edema of the eyelids, subconjunctival hemorrhage, corneal edema, and hyphema.

COLLABORATIVE MANAGEMENT

Periorbital ecchymosis, or "black eye," a common contusion injury, is usually caused by blunt trauma. Bleeding into the soft tissue occurs, creating the characteristic purple bruise. The color fades gradually and disappears in approximately 10 days. Visual acuity is usually not affected, although orbital pain, photophobia, eyelid edema, and diplopia may be present.

Treatment begins at the time of injury. Ice is applied immediately. The client should receive a thorough eye examination to rule out any other eye injuries.

Foreign Bodies

OVERVIEW

Eyelashes, dust, fingernails, dirt, and airborne particles can come in contact with the conjunctiva or cornea and irritate or abrade the surface. If nothing is seen on the cornea or conjunctiva, the eyelids are everted to examine the palpebral and bulbar conjunctivae.

➤ COLLABORATIVE MANAGEMENT

The client complains of "feeling something in my eye" or of blurry vision. Pain is a common symptom if the corneal epithelium is injured. Tearing and photophobia may be present.

Evaluation of vision is done before treatment. The nurse examines the eye of any client with a suspected or known corneal abrasion with fluorescein, followed by ocular irrigation with normal saline (0.9%) to gently remove the particles. Best practices for ocular irrigation are described in Chart 47-11.

After the foreign body is removed and the eyepatch applied, the nurse tells the client how long the patch must be left in place (usually overnight). The client is reminded to seek follow-up care to have the patch removed and the eye examined.

Lacerations

OVERVIEW

Lacerations are wounds caused by sharp objects and projectiles. Lacerations can occur to any part of the eye, but the most common areas of involvement are the eyelids and the cornea.

➤ COLLABORATIVE MANAGEMENT

Initially, the eye is closed and a small ice pack is applied to decrease bleeding. The client receives medical attention as soon as possible.

CHART 47-11

BEST PRACTICE *for* Ocular Irrigation

1. Assemble equipment:
   - Normal saline IV (1000-mL bag)
   - Macrodrip IV tubing
   - IV pole
   - Eyelid speculum
   - Topical anesthetic (proparacaine hydrochloride)
   - Gloves
   - Collection receptacle (emesis basin works well)
   - Towels
   - pH paper
2. Quickly obtain a history from the client while flushing the tubing with normal saline:
   - Nature and time of the injury
   - Type of irritant or chemical (if known)
   - Type of first aid administered at the scene
   - Any allergies to the "caine" family of medications
3. Evaluate the client's visual acuity *before* treatment:
   - Ask the client to read your name tag with the affected eye while covering the good eye.
   - Ask the client to "count fingers" with the affected eye while covering the good eye.
4. Put on gloves.
5. Place a strip of pH paper in the cul-de-sac of the client's affected eye.
6. Instill proparacaine hydrochloride eyedrops as ordered.
7. Place the client in a supine position with the head turned slightly toward the affected eye.
8. Have the client hold the affected eye open, or position an eyelid speculum.
9. Direct the flow of normal saline across the affected eye from the nasal corner of the eye toward the outer corner of the eye.
10. Assess the client's comfort during the procedure.
11. If both eyes are affected, irrigate them simultaneously using separate personnel and equipment.

If the client can open the eye, the nurse checks visual acuity and cleans the eyelids. Minor lacerations of the eyelid can be sutured in an emergency department, an urgent care center, or an ophthalmologist's office. A microscope is necessary in the operating room if the client has a laceration that involves the eyelid margin, affects the lacrimal system, involves a large area, or has jagged edges.

Corneal lacerations are considered an ocular emergency because ocular contents may prolapse through the laceration. Symptoms include severe eye pain, photophobia, tearing, decreased visual acuity, and inability to open the eyelid. If the laceration is the result of a penetrating injury, an object may be noted protruding from the eye. *This object must never be removed except by the ophthalmologist, because it may be holding ocular structures in place.*

Antibiotics are initiated to reduce the likelihood of an infection. Depending on the depth of the laceration, scarring may develop. If the scar alters vision, a corneal transplant may be needed later. If the ocular contents have prolapsed through the laceration or if the injury is severe, enucleation (surgical eye removal) may be indicated.

Penetrating Injuries

OVERVIEW

Clients with penetrating ocular injuries have the poorest chance of retaining vision in the injured eye. Glass, high-speed metallic or wood particles, BB pellets, and bullets are common causes of penetrating injuries. The particles can enter the eye through the eyelid, sclera, or cornea and can lodge in or behind the eyeball.

➤ COLLABORATIVE MANAGEMENT

The client usually complains of some eye pain and relates a history of "suddenly feeling hit in the eye." An entrance wound may be visible. Depending on the location of the entrance and the resting place of the projectile, vision may be affected.

X-ray studies and computed tomography (CT) scans of the orbit are obtained. Ultrasonography of the globe and orbit may also be performed. *Magnetic resonance imaging (MRI) is contraindicated because the procedure may move any metal-containing projectile and cause more injury.*

Surgery is usually required to remove the foreign object. In some cases, foreign bodies need to be removed by a vitrectomy. IV antibiotics are started before surgery to reduce the chance of an infection or endophthalmitis. A tetanus booster is administered if necessary.

Visual acuity is assessed and documented. If the client cannot see print, the nurse determines whether he or she can count fingers or see directional movement of the nurse's hand. If the client cannot see movement, the nurse assesses his or her ability to see light.

OCULAR MELANOMA

OVERVIEW

Melanoma is the most common intraocular malignant tumor in adults. This tumor occurs most often in the uveal tract among people in their 30s and 40s.

Because of its rich blood supply, an ocular melanoma can spread easily. Common pathways for metastatic spread are extension through the sclera or through invasion of other intraocular structures into surrounding tissue and the brain.

COLLABORATIVE MANAGEMENT

Assessment

Symptoms of malignant melanoma may not be readily apparent; the tumor may be discovered during a routine examination. Blurring of vision may occur if the macular area is invaded. Visual acuity is reduced if the tumor grows inward toward the center of the eye from the choroid and alters the visual pathway. Increased intraocular pressure (IOP) can result if the tumor invades the canal of Schlemm and obstructs outflow of aqueous humor. A change in iris color may occur if the tumor infiltrates the iris. Sudden loss of a portion of the visual field may result from tumor invasion of the subretinal space, producing retinal detachment.

Diagnostic tests for a malignant melanoma depend on the size and growth rate of the tumor. Ultrasonography is performed to determine the tumor's location and size.

Interventions

Treatment also depends on the tumor's size and growth rate, as well as the condition of the other eye. Small lesions of the iris not affecting the iris root are monitored until growth is observed. Tumors of the choroid can be treated by surgical enucleation or by radiation therapy with a radioactive cobalt plaque.

SURGERY. **Enucleation** (surgical removal of the entire eyeball) is performed with the client under general anesthesia. After the eye is removed, a ball implant is inserted to provide a base for the socket prosthesis and to ensure the best cosmetic result.

The implant is covered with surrounding tissue, muscles, and conjunctiva. A plastic conformer is placed over the conjunctiva to maintain the shape of the eyelids until a prosthesis can be fitted. After the dressing is removed, a pressure patch is placed over the eye for 24 hours.

Until the prosthesis is fitted (usually 1 month after surgery), an antibiotic-steroid ointment is inserted into the cul-de-sac once a day. Best practices for the insertion and removal of the prosthesis are presented in Chart 47-12.

RADIATION THERAPY. Radiation therapy can reduce the size and thickness of malignant melanomas. The radioactive plaque, a round, flat disk about the size of a dime and containing a radioactive material, such as cobalt-60 or iodine-125, is sutured to the sclera overlying the tumor site. The length of time the plaque remains sutured to the sclera depends on the size of the tumor and the dose of radiation to be delivered.

Complications of radiation therapy include vascular changes, retinopathy, glaucoma, necrosis of the sclera, and cataract formation. Vitreous hemorrhage may develop as the tumor becomes smaller and pulls or breaks blood vessels.

While the plaque is in place, the eye may or may not be covered with a patch. Cycloplegic eyedrops and an antibiotic-steroid combination are administered. The nurse teaches the client how to instill eyedrops.

BLINDNESS

OVERVIEW

Different forms of blindness exist and may affect any or all aspects of vision, including color, light, image, movement, and acuity. Clients are classified as legally blind if their best visual acuity with corrective lenses is 20/200 or less in the better eye or if the widest diameter of the visual field in that eye is no greater than 20 degrees.

Blindness can occur in one or both eyes. When one eye is affected, the field of vision is narrowed and depth perception is impaired.

Central vision can be impaired by diseases involving the macula, such as macular edema or macular degeneration. Loss of peripheral vision is associated with glaucoma. The loss of side vision affects the client's ability to drive and his or her awareness of hazards in the periphery.

COLLABORATIVE MANAGEMENT

The nurse teaches the client techniques to make better use of existing vision. Moving the head slightly up and down can enhance a three-dimensional effect. When shaking hands or pouring water, the client can line up the object and move toward it. He or she should choose a position that favors the good eye; for example, people with vision in the right eye should position people and items on their right.

Nursing interventions for the client with reduced sight fall into four areas: orientation, ambulation, self-care, and support.

ORIENTATION. Most clients seen in health care settings have varied degrees of sight. Most clients categorized as "blind" had sight at some time and thus have a background knowledge regarding size and shape on which the nurse can rely when providing information. When talking with a client who has limited sight or is blind, the nurse always uses a normal tone of voice.

The nurse first orients the client to the immediate environment, including the approximate size of the room. One object in the room, such as an examination chair or hospital bed, serves as the focal point during the nurse's description. The nurse guides the client to the focal point and orients him or her to the environment from that point. For example, the nurse might say, "To the left of the bed is a chair." The nurse then describes all other objects in relation to the focal point. The nurse accompanies the client to other important areas, such as the bathroom, so that the client can learn their locations. The nurse highlights the location of the toilet, sink, and toilet paper holder. The client with limited sight is never left in the center of an unfamiliar room.

Clients with limited sight prefer to establish the location of important objects, such as the call bell, water pitcher, and clock. Once their location has been fixed, these items are not moved without the client's consent. The location of movable items, such as chairs, stools, and wastebaskets, are not disturbed without consulting him or her.

At mealtime, the nurse or assistive nursing personnel sets up food on the tray using clock placement. For example, "There is sliced ham at 6 o'clock; peas are located at 3 o'clock; to the right of the plate is coffee; salt and pepper are next to the coffee."

CHART 47-12

BEST PRACTICE *for* Insertion and Removal of an Ocular Prosthesis

Insertion

1. Assemble equipment:
   - Prosthesis
   - Gloves
   - Towel
2. Explain the procedure to the client.
3. Wash your hands.
4. Cover the work area with a cloth or towel.
5. Don gloves.
6. Remove the prosthesis from its container and rinse it with tepid water.
7. Lift the client's upper lid using your nondominant hand.

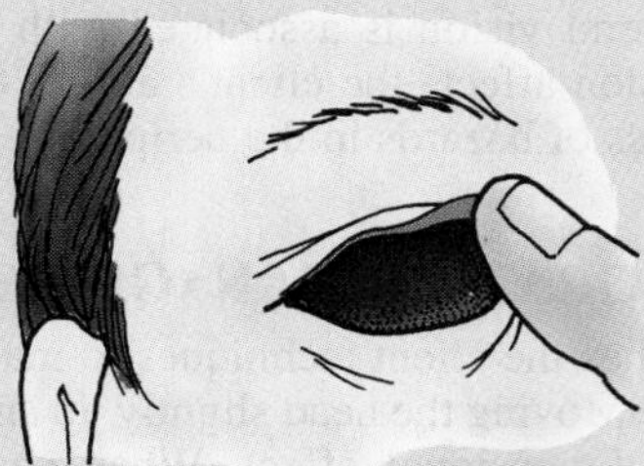

8. Place the prosthesis between the thumb and forefinger of your dominant hand. The notched end of the prosthesis should be closest to the client's nose.

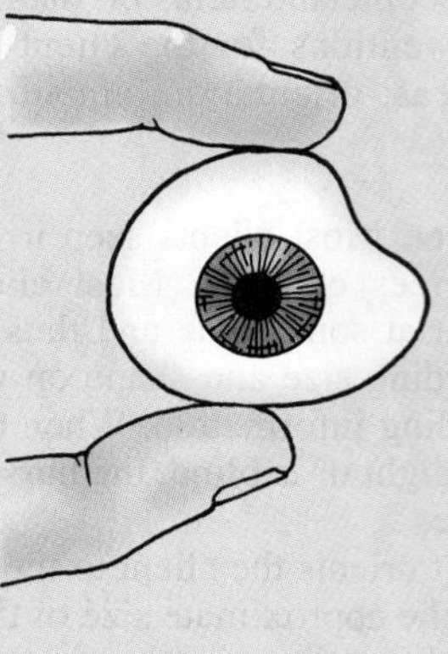

9. Insert the prosthesis with the top edge slipping under the upper lid. Continue until most of the iris is covered by the upper lid.

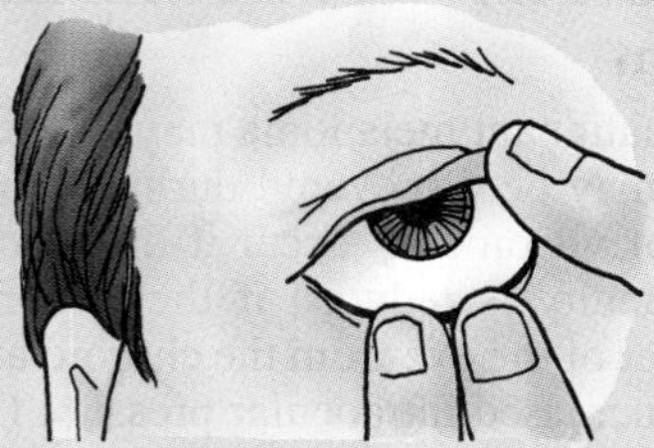

10. Gently release the upper eyelid.
11. Retract the lower lid slightly until the bottom edge of the prosthesis slips behind it.

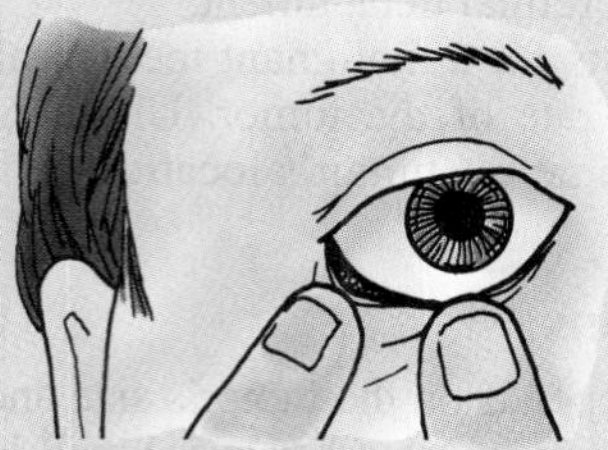

12. Release your hands slowly.

Removal

1. Assemble equipment:
   - Normal saline-filled labeled container
   - Gloves
2. Explain the procedure to the client.
3. Wash your hands.
4. Don gloves.
5. Instruct the client to sit up and tilt the head slightly downward.
6. Place your hand against the client's cheek, palm side up.
7. Pull the lower lid slightly down and laterally.
8. Allow the prosthesis to slide out onto your hand, or pull gently if necessary.
9. Place the prosthesis in a container filled with normal saline labeled with the client's name. Cover the container.

AMBULATION. When helping a client with limited sight to ambulate, the nurse allows him or her to grasp the nurse's arm at the elbow. The arm is kept close to the nurse's body so that the client can detect the direction of movement. When obstacles are noted in the path ahead, the nurse alerts the client.

Clients may use a cane to detect obstacles, such as furniture, walls, or curbs. The cane is held in the dominant hand several inches off the floor and sweeps the ground where the client's foot will be placed next. The laser cane sends out signals to help a blind client detect obstacles.

SELF-CARE. The ability to control the environment is important to the client with a visual impairment. The nurse knocks on the door before entering the hospital room or any other environment of a client with limited sight. The nurse states his or her name and reason for visiting when entering the room.

SUPPORT. Clients' reaction to the loss of sight is similar to the reaction to loss of a body part. Newly blind clients may experience a period of physical or psychologic immobility. A period of grieving is needed for the "dead" (nonseeing) eye. Clients often experience hopelessness and denial. With time, anger usually gives way to acceptance. The ability to cope may begin within days, but some clients mourn for months or years.

Clients benefit from the honest, empathetic support that nurses can provide. They need to hear that it is normal to mourn, to cry, and to feel the loss. Nurses help clients move toward acceptance by encouraging the mastery of one task at a time and by providing positive reinforcement for each success.

ONLINE RESOURCES

For suggested readings and Internet resources, go to http://www.wbsaunders.com/SIMON/Iggy/.

SELECTED BIBLIOGRAPHY

Asterisk indicates a classic or definitive work on this subject.

*Bass, S., & Giovinazzo, V. (1996). Laser treatment of macular disease. *Optometry Clinics, 5*(1), 161-173.

*Cleary, M. (1995). Helping the person who is visually impaired: Concerns, questions, remedies, and sources. *Journal of Ophthalmic Nursing and Technology, 14*(5), 205-211.

Cohen, S., & Kawasaki, A. (1999). Introduction to formal visual field testing: Goldman and Humphrey perimeter. *Journal of Ophthalmic Nursing and Technology, 18*(1), 7-11.

Collins, M., et al. (2001). Effect of laser in situ keratomileusis (LASIK) on the corneal endothelium three years postoperatively. *American Journal of Ophthalmology, 131*(1), 1-6.

Cotran, R., Kumar, V., & Collins, T. (1999). *Robbins pathologic basis of disease* (5th ed.). Philadelphia: W.B. Saunders.

DuBosar, R. (1999). Age-related macular degeneration: New treatments show promise. *Journal of Ophthalmic Nursing and Technology, 18*(2), 60-70.

Gilbard, J. (1999). Dry eye, blepharitis, and chronic eye irritation: Divide and conquer. *Journal of Ophthalmic Nursing and Technology, 18*(3), 109-115.

Jarvis, C. (2000). *Physical examination and health assessment* (3rd ed.). Philadelphia: W.B. Saunders.

Kearney, K. (1997). Emergency! Retinal detachment. *American Journal of Nursing, 97*(8), 50.

McCloskey, J.C, & Bulechek, G.M. (2000). *Nursing interventions classification (NIC)* (3rd ed.). St. Louis: Mosby.

Moore, L. (2000). Severe visual impairment in older women. *Western Journal of Nursing Research, 22*(5), 571-595.

Noecker, R., & Golightly, S. (1999). Pharmacology of ocular surgery. *Journal of Ophthalmic Nursing and Technology, 18*(3), 101-108.

Pratt, S. (1999). Dietary prevention of age-related macular degeneration. *Journal of the American Optometric Association, 70*(1), 39-47.

Rakow, P. (1999). Making miracles with prosthetic soft lenses. *Journal of Ophthalmic Nursing and Technology, 18*(3), 120-122.

Ramos, M. (1999). Prevention of work related injuries: A look at eye protection use and suggested prevention strategies. *Journal of Ophthalmic Nursing and Technology, 18*(3), 117-119.

Ramponi, D. (2000). Go with the flow during an eye emergency. *Nursing2000, 30*(8), 54-56.

Rapaport, M. (2000). Eyelid dermatitis. *Dermatology Nursing, 12*(5), 352-354.

Shoemaker, J. (1997). Adult vision screening by nonphysicians. *Journal of Ophthalmic Nursing and Technology, 16*(5), 244-250.

Smith, S. (1999). The role of antioxidants in AMD: Ongoing research. *Journal of Ophthalmic Nursing and Technology, 18*(2), 68-70.

*Sullivan, N. (1983). Vision in the elderly. *Journal of Gerontological Nursing, 9*(4), 228-235.

United States Pharmacopeia Dispensing Information (USP DI): Vol. I. Drug information for the health care professional (20th ed.). (2000). Englewood, CO: Micromedix.

*Vader, L. (1992). Vision and vision loss. *Nursing Clinics of North America, 27*(3), 705-714.

*Vaughan, D., Asbury, T., & Riordan-Eva, P. (Eds.). (1995). *General ophthalmology* (14th ed.). Norwalk, CT: Appleton & Lange.

Whitaker, R., Whitaker, V., & Dill, C. (1999). Glaucoma: What the ophthalmic nurse should know. *Insight: The Journal of the American Society of Ophthalmic Registered Nurses, 24*(3), 86- 91.

CHAPTER 48

Assessment of the Ear and Hearing

JUDY MALKIEWICZ

Learning Objectives

After studying this chapter, you should be able to:

1. Describe the key elements to inspect when performing assessment of the external ear.
2. Describe age-related changes in the structure of the ear and hearing.
3. Identify 10 drugs that have an impact on hearing.
4. Demonstrate the correct use of an otoscope.
5. Describe the landmarks of the tympanic membrane.
6. Compare and contrast air conduction and bone conduction of sound.
7. Demonstrate the correct use of a tuning fork in performing the Weber and Rinne tests for hearing.
8. Prioritize educational needs for the client about to undergo pure tone audiometry and electronystagmography.

SIMON

Go to http://www.wbsaunders.com/SIMON/Iggy/ for self-assessment questions related to these Learning Objectives.

Ear and hearing assessment are important skills for nurses caring for clients of all ages. Many difficulties with the ear and hearing develop over a long period of time, and hearing may also be affected by several medications. An understanding of the anatomy and physiology of the ear is essential. Table 48-1 defines terms commonly used in assessing the ear and hearing.

ANATOMY AND PHYSIOLOGY REVIEW

Structure

The ear consists of three structural parts: the external ear, the middle ear, and the inner ear; each is important to the hearing process.

EXTERNAL EAR

The external ear develops in the embryo at the same time as the kidneys and urinary tract. Therefore any person with a defect of the external ear must also be examined for possible problems or defects of the renal and urinary systems.

The external ear **(pinna),** which is composed of cartilage covered by skin, is embedded in the temporal bone bilaterally at the level of the eyes, attached to the head by skin and cartilage at approximately a 10-degree angle. The external ear extends from the pinna through the external canal to the **tympanic membrane,** or eardrum (Figure 48-1). The external ear canal is slightly S-shaped and lined with **cerumen** (wax)–producing glands (which help protect and lubricate the ear canal), sebaceous glands, and hair follicles. The hair follicles and cerumen protect the tympanic membrane and the middle ear. In the adult, the distance from the opening of the external canal to the tympanic membrane is approximately 1 to 1½ inches (2.5 to 3.75 cm). The external ear includes the **mastoid process,** the bony ridge located over the temporal bone behind the pinna.

MIDDLE EAR

The middle ear begins at the medial side of the tympanic membrane. It consists of the **epitympanum,** a compartment containing the three bony **ossicles** (Figure 48-2): the malleus, the incus, and the stapes. The proximal end of the eustachian tube also opens in the middle ear.

The tympanic membrane is a thick, transparent sheet of tissue providing a barrier between the external ear and the middle ear. The landmarks on the tympanic membrane include the annulus, the pars flaccida, and the pars tensa. The tympanic membrane is attached to the first bony ossicle, the **malleus** (hammer), at the **umbo** (Figure 48-3). The bony ossicles behind the tympanic membrane are joined, although not rigidly, allowing vibratory movement.

The pars flaccida and pars tensa are parts of the tympanic membrane. The pars flaccida is that portion of the tympanic membrane above the short process of the malleus; the pars tensa is that portion surrounding the long process of the malleus. It is usually transparent, opaque, or pearly gray and moves when air is injected into the external canal. The umbo is seen through the tympanic membrane as a white dot at the end of the long process of the malleus. The short process of the malleus, the long process of the malleus, and the umbo are structures seen through the transparent tympanic membrane.

The middle ear is separated from the inner ear by the round window and the oval window. The eustachian tube originates from the floor of the middle ear at the proximal end and opens at the distal end in the nasopharynx. The distal opening in the nasopharynx is surrounded by adenoid lymphatic tissue (Figure 48-4). The eustachian tube allows equalization of pressure on both sides of the tympanic membrane. Secretions from the middle ear drain through it.

TABLE 48-1 • TERMINOLOGY COMMONLY USED IN EAR AND HEARING ASSESSMENT

cerumen Waxlike secretion of the external ear canal
conductive hearing loss Hearing loss resulting from a physical disruption in the transmission of sound waves
decibel A unit of sound for expressing loudness
masking The process of hiding a specific sound from one ear while the other ear is tested for its ability to hear that sound
Meniere's disease An intermittent but progressive deterioration of hearing and balance
otitis media Inflammation/infection of the middle ear
otosclerosis Formation of spongy bone around structures of the middle and inner ear, leading to low-tone hearing impairment
ototoxic Damaging to the structures important for hearing
presbycusis Age-related degenerative changes in the ear, leading to decreased hearing acuity
sensorineural Hearing loss resulting from neural defects
spondee Words of two syllables on which equal stress is placed during pronunciation
vestibular hearing loss Relating to the functions of the ear for the sense of balance and position

INNER EAR

The inner ear, lying on the other side of the oval window, contains the semicircular canals, the cochlea, and the distal end of the eighth cranial nerve (see Figure 48-2). The **semicircular canals** contain fluid and hair cells connected to the sensory nerve fibers of the vestibular portion of the eighth cranial nerve; fluid and hair cells help to maintain the sense of balance.

The **cochlea,** the spiral organ of hearing, is divided into the scala tympani and the scala vestibuli. Reissner's membrane stretches across the scala vestibuli and forms the duct of the cochlea, or the scala media. The scala media is filled with **endolymph,** a fluid similar to intracellular fluid. The scala tympani and scala vestibuli are filled with **perilymph.** Endolymph and perilymph are fluids that protect the cochlea and the semicircular canals; these structures literally float in the fluids and are thus cushioned against abrupt movements of the head.

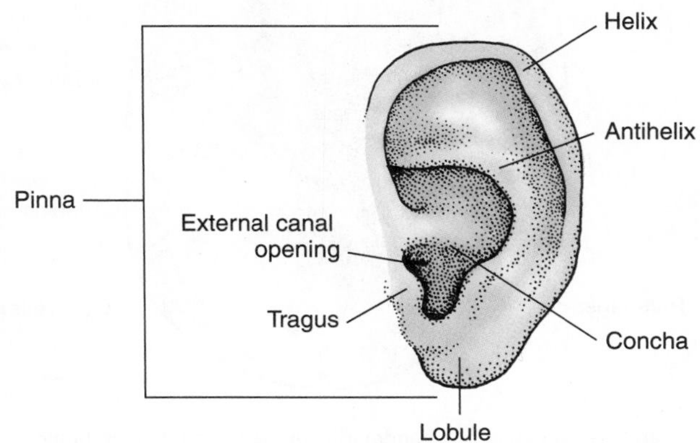

Figure 48-1 ● Anatomic features of the external ear.

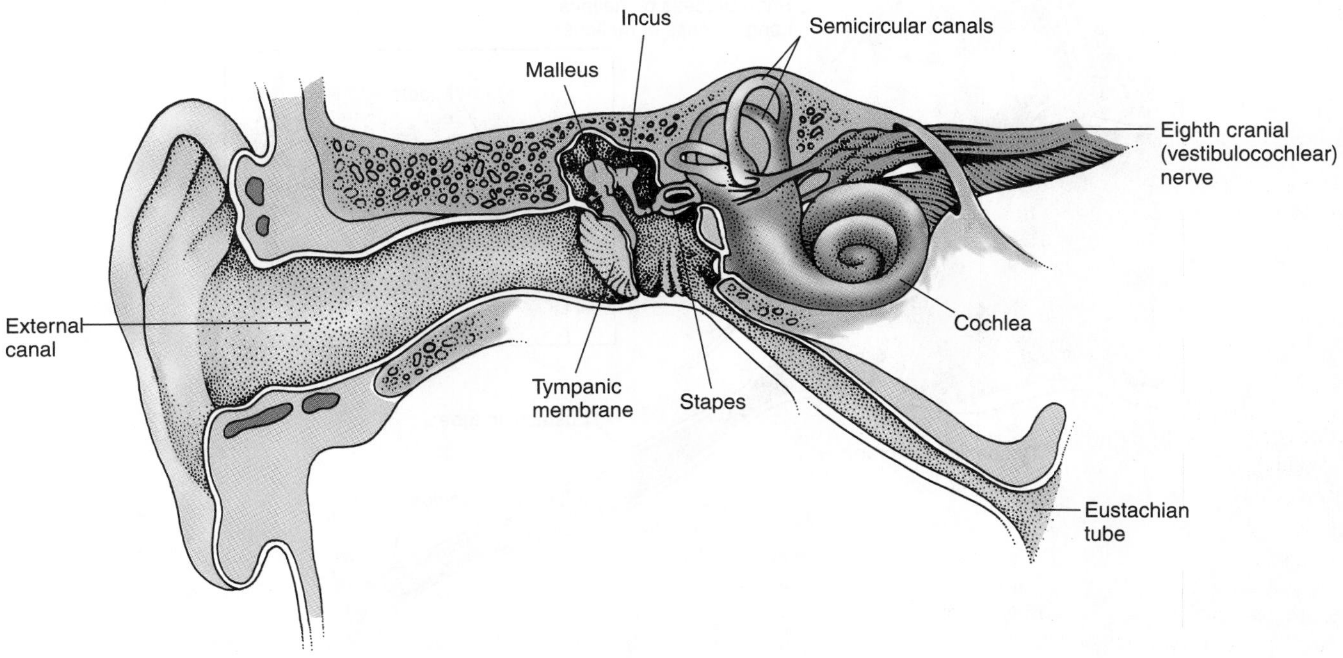

Figure 48-2 ● Anatomic features of the internal ear.

The **organ of Corti** is the receptor end-organ of hearing located on the basilar membrane of the cochlea. The cochlea contains hair cells that detect vibration from sound and stimulate the eighth cranial nerve.

Function

The ear's main function is hearing, which is accomplished when sound is delivered through the air to the external ear canal and the temporal bone covering the mastoid air cells. The sound waves strike the mastoid and the movable tympanic membrane, which is connected to the first bony ossicle, the malleus, at the umbo. The sound wave vibrations are transferred from the tympanic membrane to the malleus, the incus, and the stapes. From the stapes the vibrations are transmitted to the cochlea. Receptors there **transduce** (change) the vibrations into action potentials, conducted to the brain as neural impulses by the cochlear portion of the eighth cranial (or auditory) nerve. Sound is processed and interpreted by the brain.

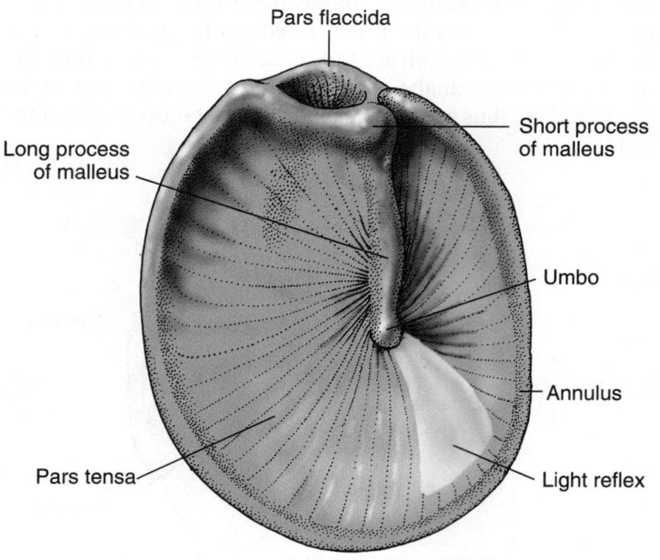

Figure 48-3 ● Landmarks on the tympanic membrane.

Ear and Hearing Changes Associated with Aging

Ear and hearing changes related to aging are summarized in Chart 48-1. Some of these changes are harmless (see the Evidence-Based Practice for Nursing box on p. 1052); others pose serious threats to the hearing ability of older clients and call for nursing interventions.

ASSESSMENT TECHNIQUES

History

The nurse obtains a thorough history from the client. Informal hearing assessment begins as the nurse observes the client listening to and answering questions. The client's posture and appropriateness of responses provide additional information about his or her hearing acuity.

During the interview, the nurse sits in adequate light, facing the client, which allows the client to see the nurse speaking. The nurse is careful to use ordinary language. The nurse also assesses demographic data, personal and family history, socioeconomic status, and current health problems. Chart

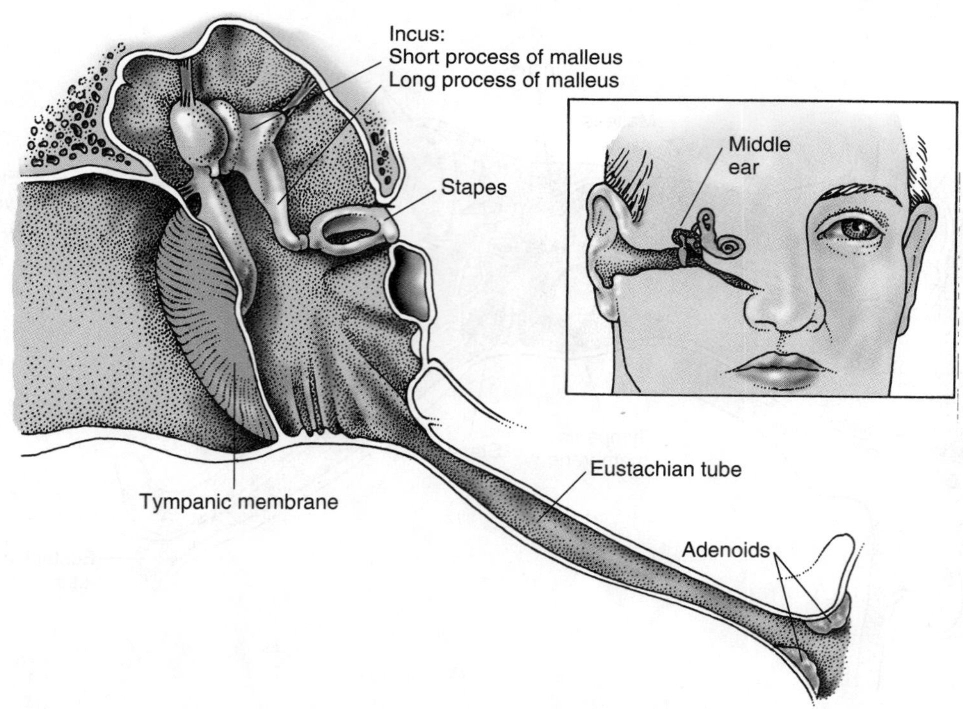

Figure 48-4 ● Anatomic features and attached structures of the middle ear.

48-2 lists important questions to ask regarding ear and hearing assessment.

DEMOGRAPHIC DATA

The gender of the client is important. Some auditory disorders, such as otosclerosis, are more common in women; others, such as Meniere's disease, are more common in men. Age is also a significant factor in hearing loss.

PERSONAL AND FAMILY HISTORY

Personal history includes information on past or current signs and symptoms of ear pain, ear discharge, vertigo, tinnitus, decreased hearing, and difficulty understanding people when they talk or difficulty hearing environmental noises. The nurse asks the client about the following:

- Ear trauma
- Ear surgery
- Past infections
- Excessive cerumen
- Ear itch
- Any invasive instruments routinely used to clean the ear
- Type and pattern of ear hygiene
- Exposure to loud noise or music
- Air travel (especially in unpressurized aircraft)
- Swimming habits and the use of protective ear devices for swimming
- History of hereditary factors and health conditions causing changes in the blood supply to the ear (heart disease, hypertension, diabetes)
- History of vitiligo (a pigment disorder in which there may be a loss of melanin-containing cells [and their protective function] in the inner ear, resulting in hearing loss)
- History of smoking (nicotine increases the carboxyhemoglobin in the blood, resulting in a decreased oxygen supply to the cochlea, possibly increasing sensory cell damage)
- History of vitamin B_{12} and folate deficiency (appears to be associated with age-related hearing loss)

CHART 48-1

NURSING FOCUS *on the* OLDER ADULT
The Ear and Hearing

Physiologic Change	Nursing Implications	Rationale
The pinna becomes elongated because of normal loss of subcutaneous tissue and decreased tissue elasticity.		
Hair becomes coarser and longer, especially in men.		
Cerumen-producing glands decrease in number and function.	Irrigate ear canal weekly.	Irrigation removes excess cerumen, preventing impaction and enhancing transmission of sound waves.
Cerumen tends to be drier in older clients; it becomes impacted, which causes hearing loss.	Place 1-2 drops of oil into ear canal 8 hr before irrigation.	Oil softens impacted cerumen, facilitating removal.
The tympanic membrane loses elasticity; it may normally appear dull and retracted.		
Bony ossicles have decreased movement.		
The cochlea undergoes degenerative changes.		
Disturbed vestibular function results in occasional dizziness, vertigo, and sensations of unsteadiness in 50%–60% of older clients.	Assist the client with standing and initial ambulation.	The nurse provides a stable point of reference. Assistance decreases the risk of falling as a result of vestibular disorientation.
Hearing acuity diminishes with advancing age.	Establish that a hearing deficiency exists.	Determine whether interventions are needed. Not all older clients have diminished hearing acuity.
The ability to hear high-frequency sounds is nearly gone by age 60, which affects speech reception and increases auditory reaction time greatly. Clients have particular difficulty with the *f, s, sh,* and *pa* sounds. Some older clients hear a persistent noise (tinnitus). Presbycusis (a sensorineural type of hearing loss) is common in older adults.	When speaking to an older client with a hearing deficiency: • Provide a quiet environment. • Face the client. • Speak slowly in a deeper voice.	This makes it easier for the client to hear and communicate. • Extraneous noise may interfere with the client's auditory perception. • The client can benefit by being able to see lip movement. • The client may be able to discern lower frequencies more easily.

EVIDENCE-BASED PRACTICE FOR NURSING

Ear size as a predictor of chronologic age

Tan, R., Osman, V., & Tan, G. (1997). Ear size as a predictor of chronological age. *Archives of Gerontology and Geriatrics, 25*(2), 187-191.

This study examined the external ear circumference in 100 Caucasian men (n=79) and women (n=21) between the ages of 21 and 98 years. It was found that the external ear circumference increased in size an average of 0.51 mm/year.

Critique. External ear circumference was found to be predictive of chronologic age in the population studied. Since the external ear is composed of elastic cartilage covered by skin, it was thought that the increases in external ear circumference with age were due to changes in collagen.

Implications for Nursing. Older clients can be reassured that increasing external ear circumference is common.

CHART 48-2

EAR AND HEARING ASSESSMENT
Using Gordon's Functional Health Patterns

Cognitive-Perceptual Pattern

- Do you notice that you have the volume of the television or radio set at an increased level?
- Are you sitting closer to the television or radio in order to hear more clearly?
- Do you have difficulty in your ability to hear or follow conversations in a noisy environment, such as a restaurant?
- Do you have difficulty hearing high-pitched sounds like the doorbell?

Health Perception/Health Management Pattern

- Have you had your hearing checked?
- If you are or were exposed to environmental noise, have you consistently used appropriate hearing protection?
- Do you avoid cleaning your ear canals with foreign objects such as toothpicks or paper clips?
- Have you discussed with your health care provider the side effects of any drugs you may be taking that might affect your ear and hearing?

Based on Gordon, M. (2000). *Manual of nursing diagnosis* (9th ed.). St. Louis: Mosby.

If the client uses a hearing aid, the nurse determines how well it works, the date of the last hearing test, the type of test given, and the results. The client is asked about other conditions that may impair hearing, such as allergies, upper respiratory tract infection, hypothyroidism, arteriosclerosis, head trauma, and recent head, facial, or dental surgery.

A thorough medication history is crucial because many drugs are ototoxic (Table 48-2).

The client is asked about his or her occupation and any hobbies involving exposure to excessive environmental noise or music. The nurse also investigates the use of protective ear devices or any devices inserted into the ear, such as a telephone operator headset or a stethoscope. Information about hearing loss among family members is important because some types of hearing loss are hereditary or have a genetic component.

SOCIOECONOMIC STATUS

The nurse assesses the client's socioeconomic status to determine the availability of health care. Clients of lower socioeconomic status often do not seek health care for ear-related problems until hearing damage is extensive. Clients at any socioeconomic level, however, might hesitate to have their hearing loss diagnosed because of the fear of wearing a hearing amplification device.

TABLE 48-2 • IMPACT OF OTOTOXIC SUBSTANCES ON AUDITORY FUNCTION

Drug	Auditory Effects
ANTIBIOTICS	
Amikacin (Amikin)	++
Chloramphenicol (Chloromycetin, Novochlorocap✤)	+ to ++
Erythromycin (Apo-Erythro E-C✤, E.E.S., E-Mycin, Novorythro✤)	+ to ++
Gentamicin (Cidomycin✤, Garamycin)	++
Kanamycin (Kantrex)	++
Neomycin	++
Streptomycin	++
Tobramycin (Nebcin)	++
Vancomycin (Lyphocin, Vancocin)	++
DIURETICS	
Acetazolamide (Apo-Acetazolamide✤, Diamox)	++
Ethacrynic acid (Edecrin)	++
Furosemide (Apo-Furosemide✤, Lasix, Furoside✤)	++
NONSTEROIDAL ANTI-INFLAMMATORY AGENTS	
Ibuprofen (Advil, Amersol✤, Motrin, Novoprofen✤)	+
Indomethacin (Indocid✤, Indocin)	+
Naproxen (Anaprox, Apo-Napro-Na✤, Naprosyn, Novonaprox✤)	+
Salicylates (Apo-ASA✤, Ascriptin, Bufferin, Entrophen✤)	++
MISCELLANEOUS	
Carbamazepine (Tegretol)	++
Cisplatin (Abiplatin✤, Platinol)	++
Mechlorethamine (Mustargen)	+
Quinine (Legatrin, NovoQuinine✤, Quinamm)	+
Quinidine (Apo-Quinidine✤, Cardioquin, Quinidex)	+

+, Slight impact; ++, significant impact.

CURRENT HEALTH PROBLEMS

The nurse assesses current ear-related health problems, asking whether the client has noticed any "trouble with" his or her ears, ear pain, or discharge, including any earwax. The client is asked about any change in hearing, such as an intolerance for sound levels that do not bother other people (hyperacusis), or associated problems, such as ringing in the ears. If a change in hearing is reported, the nurse asks whether one or both ears are involved and whether the change was sudden or gradual. The client is also asked about any problems with dizziness (an off-balance feeling or lightheadedness) or **vertigo** (spinning sense of movement).

Physical Assessment

Inspection and palpation are the only examination techniques used to assess the ear. The nurse begins the examination by placing the client in either a sitting or a supine position. Uncooperative clients are carefully restrained to prevent injury to the external canal. Any hearing aids should be removed during the examination. After the otoscopic examination, the nurse inspects the hearing aid for cracks, debris, and a proper fit. Ear examination is divided into external ear and mastoid assessment, otoscopic assessment, and auditory assessment.

EXTERNAL EAR AND MASTOID ASSESSMENT

The mastoid process is inspected for redness and swelling, which indicate inflammation. To assess for tenderness, the nurse gently taps with one finger over the mastoid process, compresses the tragus with one finger, and gently manipulates the pinna forward and backward. Any tenderness suggests an inflammatory process in either the external ear or the mastoid.

The entire external ear is inspected for shape, location of attachment to the head, and condition of the visible external canal. The normal pinna is uniformly shaped without additional skin tags or deformity. The pinna should be attached vertically to the side of the head at a posterior angle of no greater than 10 degrees. It should fall within or touch the eye-occiput line, an imaginary line drawn from the greatest protuberance on the occiput to the lateral canthus of the eye. Any variation from the normal ear shape and attachment is recorded.

Abnormalities of the pinna include swelling, nodules, and lesions. In chronic gout, accumulations of uric acid crystals result in hard, irregular, painless nodules called tophi on the helix and antihelix portions of the pinna. Other painless nodules on the pinna might be due to basal cell carcinoma or rheumatoid arthritis. Small, crusted, ulcerated, or indurated lesions on the pinna that fail to heal could be squamous cell carcinoma.

The normal external canal is free from lesions, dry, clean, and not reddened. The nurse assesses for the following abnormalities:

- Furuncles
- Large accumulations of cerumen
- Scaliness
- Redness
- Swelling of or drainage from the ear associated with a foreign object (insects or inanimate substances), trauma, or infection

The nurse also notes any other drainage (blood, cerebrospinal fluid, pus, or serous fluid) and its character.

OTOSCOPIC ASSESSMENT

An instrument called an otoscope is used to examine the ear. Many types are available. An otoscope (Figure 48-5) consists of a light, a handle, a magnifying lens, and a pneumatic attachment for injecting air into the external canal to test mobility of the tympanic membrane.

Specula of various diameters attach to the head of the otoscope; the largest that most comfortably fits the client's external canal is selected for the examination. *The speculum is never blindly introduced into the external canal because of the risk of perforating the tympanic membrane.*

If the client experiences any pain during external ear examination, the nurse attempts a cautious otoscopic examination. (The speculum will cause extreme pain if it comes in contact with inflamed tissue in the external canal.) The nurse must become familiar with and memorize all of the structures of the tympanic membrane and middle ear before attempting to visualize them with an otoscope.

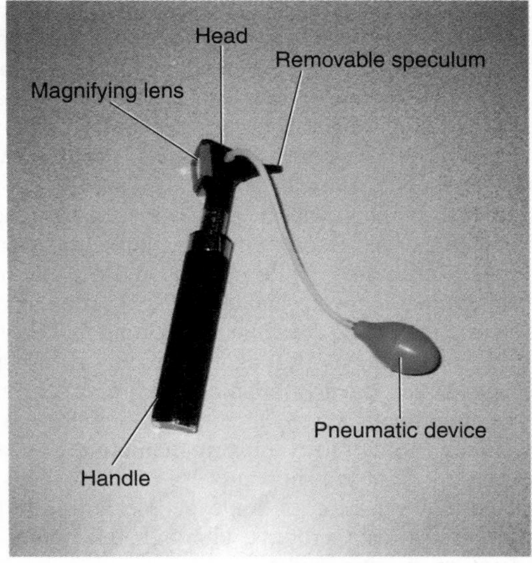

Figure 48-5 ● Functional components of an otoscope.

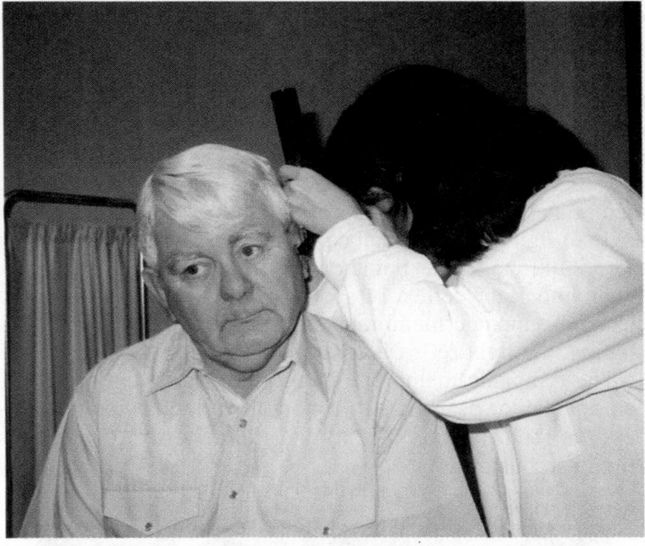

Figure 48-6 ● Proper technique for an otoscopic examination.

When performing an otoscopic examination, the nurse tilts the client's head slightly away and holds the otoscope upside down, like a large pen (Figure 48-6). This position permits the nurse's hand to lie against the client's head for support. If the client moves, both the nurse's hand and the otoscope move as well, preventing damage to the external canal or tympanic membrane. The nurse holds the otoscope in the dominant hand and gently pulls the pinna up and back with the non-dominant hand. The external canal is visualized while the speculum is slowly inserted. The examiner uses caution and avoids jamming the speculum into the walls of the external canal, which causes pain.

After the pinna is correctly displaced and the otoscope is comfortably introduced in the external canal, the tympanic membrane is observed for color, intactness, and shape. The nurse further assesses for lesions and the amount and consistency of cerumen and hair. The normal external canal is skin colored, intact, and without lesions; it contains various amounts of soft cerumen and has small, fine hairs.

Next, the tympanic membranes are assessed for intactness, normal structures seen through the tympanic membrane (the long and short processes of the malleus and the umbo), portions of the tympanic membrane itself (light reflex, pars flaccida, and pars tensa), and the color, shape, and mobility of the membrane, as well as any lesions. Figure 48-7 shows an otoscopic view of a normal tympanic membrane. The normal tympanic membrane is always intact. The long process of the malleus is seen through the tympanic membrane as a whitish streak extending from the short process of the malleus to the umbo. A normal variation in some people with allergies is vascularity of the long process, although this might be an early indication of otitis media.

The short process of the malleus is seen through the tympanic membrane as a white structure that seems more three-dimensional (projecting out toward the otoscope) than the other structures on the tympanic membrane. The umbo appears as a round, white dot.

The long and short processes of the malleus, in addition to the umbo, are always easily identified in the normal ear. Abnormal variations are caused by serous otitis and otitis media, among other disorders.

Reflection of the otoscope's light off of the tympanic membrane reveals the **light reflex,** a clearly demarcated triangle of light in the normal ear. The base of the triangle is on the annulus, and the point of the triangle is on the umbo. When the light reflex is spotty or multiple because of a changed tympanic membrane shape from either retraction or bulging, the light reflex is termed **diffuse.**

The tympanic membrane is normally shiny and transparent, opaque, or pearly gray. Abnormal variations include redness (as seen in otitis media) and dullness or retraction (as seen in serous otitis).

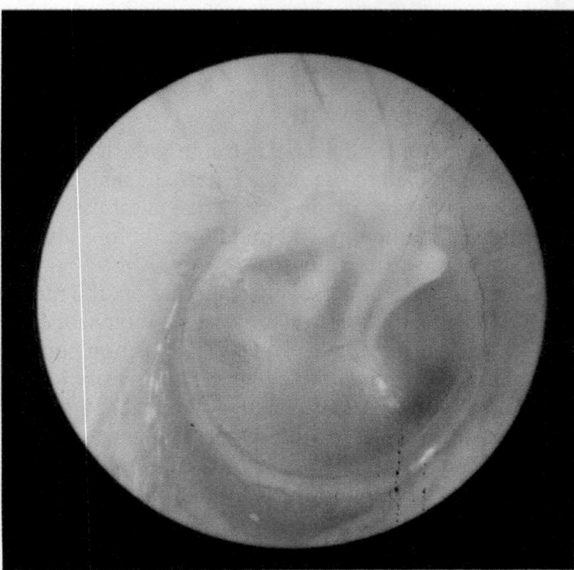

Figure 48-7 • Otoscopic view of a normal tympanic membrane.

The normal tympanic membrane is slightly concave, allowing the pars tensa portion to move gently on testing with a puff of air from the pneumatic device on the otoscope.

The normal tympanic membrane is free of lesions. The most common lesion is scarring caused by previous ear infection and perforation. A scar thickens the tympanic membrane, which makes it difficult or impossible to see through the membrane at the point of the scar and reduces the mobility of the tympanic membrane.

The nurse tests the mobility of the tympanic membrane by gently injecting a small puff of air through the pneumatic device into the external canal and watching the pars tensa portion for movement. The normal tympanic membrane moves gently. Decreased or absent mobility results from scarring, retraction, bulging, the presence of fluid in the middle ear, and decreased mobility of the ossicles associated with aging.

CULTURAL CONSIDERATIONS

Cerumen is generally moist and tan or brown in Caucasian and African-American clients. It is dry and light brown to gray in Asians and Native Americans. The color of the lining of the external ear canal varies with the client's skin tone.

CRITICAL THINKING CHALLENGE

The client is an older nursing home resident who speaks no English. The staff, who do not understand her native language, have noticed that her right external ear is red with peeling skin on the inner aspect. You are to perform an external and otoscopic examination on her.

- How will you explain these procedures to the client (you also do not speak her native language)?
- Describe how you will proceed with the inspection of the external ear.
- How will you select the proper-size speculum for the otoscopic examination?

For suggested answer guidelines, go to SIMON http://www.wbsaunders.com/SIMON/Iggy/.

AUDITORY ASSESSMENT

After completing bilateral external ear and otoscopic examinations, the nurse assesses the client's hearing acuity. Sound is transmitted by air conduction and bone conduction. Air conduction of sound is normally more sensitive than bone conduction. If hearing acuity is decreased, the hearing loss is categorized as follows:

- **Conductive hearing loss,** resulting from any physical obstruction of sound wave transmission (such as a foreign body in the external canal, a retracted or bulging tympanic membrane, or fused bony ossicles)
- **Sensorineural hearing loss,** resulting from a defect in the cochlea, the eighth cranial nerve, or the brain itself
- **Mixed conductive-sensorineural hearing loss,** a profound hearing loss

Each of the auditory function tests determines the degree of hearing loss and differentiates the type of loss.

Voice Test

A simple hearing acuity test can be conducted by asking the client to block one external ear canal while standing 1 to 2 feet (30 to 60 cm) away. The examiner quietly whispers a statement and asks the client to repeat it. Each ear is tested separately. If the client does not respond correctly, a louder whisper is used. If the client is suspected of lip-reading, the examiner's hand can be used to block his or her view of the examiner's mouth.

Watch Test

A ticking watch is used to test hearing acuity for high-frequency sounds. The nurse holds a ticking watch about 5 inches (12.7 cm) from each of the ears and asks whether the ticking is heard. The client with normal hearing should be able to hear it.

Audioscopy

The lightweight audioscope allows the examiner to visualize the external ear and tympanic membrane. Hearing can be measured at a 40-decibel (dB) intensity at frequencies of 500, 1000, 2000, and 4000 cycles per second (cps), or hertz (Hz). The audioscope is larger than a conventional otoscope, and nurses can easily use it to assess hearing.

Tuning Fork Tests

Hearing acuity can be tested by the Weber and Rinne tuning fork tests. Tuning fork tests are useful, although limited, in differentiating between conductive and sensorineural hearing losses. The frequency range of the tuning fork used for these tests corresponds to that of normal speech: 512 or 1024 Hz. To perform this assessment, the nurse stands in front of the sitting client.

WEBER TUNING FORK TEST

To perform the Weber tuning fork test, the nurse places the vibrating tuning fork on the middle of the client's head, at the midline of the forehead, or above the upper lip over the teeth. Many clients object to the vibration over the upper lip, so the preferred site is the midline of the skull (Figure 48-8). The nurse takes care to hold the vibrating tuning fork by the stem only, not by the vibrating fork. The nurse asks the client in which ear the sound is louder. The normal test result is sound heard equally in both ears. If the client hears the sound louder in one ear, the term *lateralization* describes the side on which the sound is the loudest.

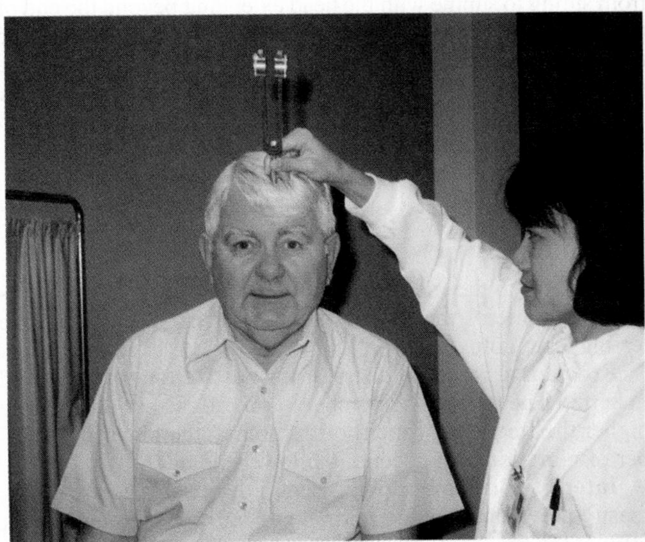

Figure 48-8 ● Correct placement of the tuning fork for the Weber test.

RINNE TUNING FORK TEST

The Rinne tuning fork test compares hearing by air conduction with hearing by bone conduction. Sound is normally heard two to three times longer by air conduction than by bone conduction. The nurse performs the Rinne tuning fork test by placing the vibrating tuning fork stem on the client's mastoid process. The client indicates when he or she no longer hears the sound, and the nurse quickly brings the tuning fork in front of the pinna without touching the client, asking whether he or she still hears the sound (Figure 48-9). The nurse records the duration of both phases, bone conduction followed by air conduction, and compares the times. The client normally continues to hear the sound two times longer in front of the pinna after not hearing it with the tuning fork touching the mastoid process.

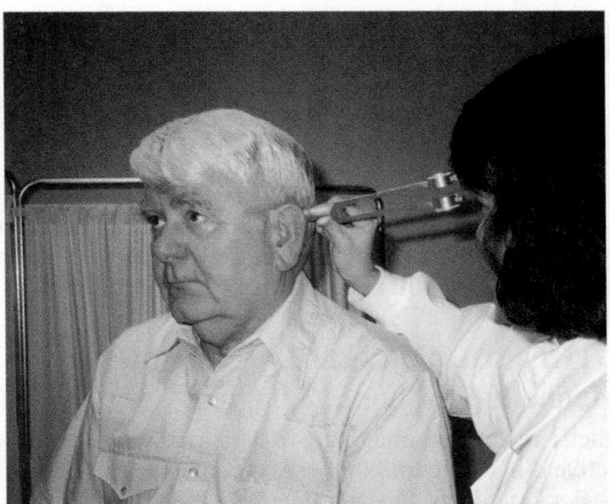

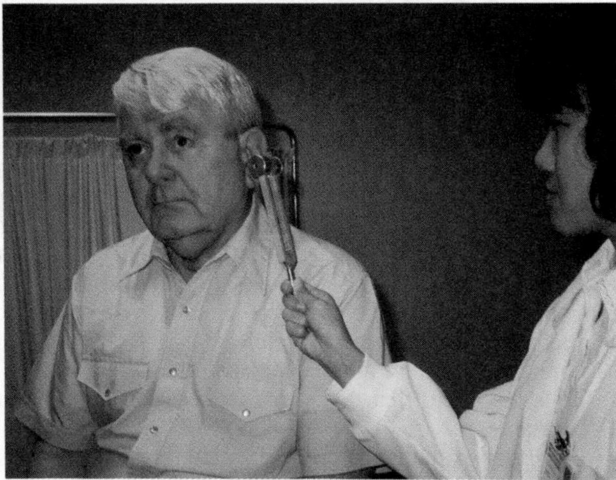

Figure 48-9 ● Correct placement of the tuning fork for the Rinne test.

Psychosocial Assessment

The client may become irritable, frustrated, and depressed by an inability to hear and respond appropriately. The inability to hear results in frustrating experiences and often isolates the client from the world. Depression may result from the sensory isolation of hearing loss. The nurse is sensitive to the client and conducts the interview at a pace appropriate for that individual.

The nurse investigates the social and work relationships to determine whether the client experiences isolation because of hearing problems. In addition, the client is encouraged to express feelings related to hearing loss and discuss changes in daily living activities for coping. The nurse also obtains information from family members, especially if the client denies having a hearing problem. Throughout the assessment, the nurse remains patient and empathetic.

Diagnostic Assessment

LABORATORY TESTS

Laboratory tests are not of value in determining hearing acuity except for determinations of cholesterol (low-density liprotein–high-density lipoprotein [LDL/HDL]) ratios in older women. Women with high LDL/HDL ratios have better hearing (by 5 dB) than women with low LDL/HDL ratios. For an external ear infection, microbial culture and antibiotic sensitivity tests can determine the causative organism and the most appropriate antibiotic.

RADIOGRAPHIC EXAMINATIONS: COMPUTED TOMOGRAPHY

Computed tomography (CT), with or without contrast enhancement, reveals the structures of the ear in great detail by multiple x-ray scans of the head, which are then averaged by a computer. CT is especially helpful in diagnosing acoustic tumors.

OTHER DIAGNOSTIC ASSESSMENT

Magnetic Resonance Imaging

Magnetic resonance imaging (MRI) is a noninvasive, nonradioactive diagnostic tool that uses a computer to generate images. Because of its superior contrast resolution, no bony artifacts can obscure tissue. Therefore MRI has great sensitivity to soft-tissue changes. Clients with internal metal vascular clips cannot have MRI.

Auditory Brainstem-Evoked Response

Auditory brainstem-evoked response (ABR) is done to assess hearing in clients who are unable to indicate, or are unreliable in indicating, recognition of sound stimuli during hearing testing. This test helps diagnose both conductive and sensorineural hearing losses. Electrodes are placed on the scalp during the test. After the test, the client's hair should be cleansed to remove the electrode gel.

To prepare the client for ABR testing, the nurse:

- Tells the client that no fasting or sedation is necessary for the test
- Carefully explains the procedure and its purpose
- Informs the client that the procedure usually takes about 30 minutes

Electronystagmography

Electronystagmography (ENG) is a cost-effective test that is sensitive in detecting both central and peripheral disease of the vestibular system in the ear. The ENG detects **nystagmus** (involuntary eye movements) that can be recorded. Electrodes are taped to the skin near the eyes, and one or more procedures (caloric testing, changing gaze position, or changing head position) are done to stimulate nystagmus. Failure of nystagmus to occur with cerebral stimulation suggests an abnormality in the vestibulocochlear apparatus, the cerebral cortex, the auditory nerve, or the brainstem.

To prepare the client for ENG, the nurse:

- Carefully explains the procedure and its purpose
- Tells the client to fast for several hours before the test and to avoid caffeine-containing beverages for 24 to 48 hours before the test
- Tells clients with pacemakers that they should not have the test
- Carefully introduces fluids after the test to prevent nausea and vomiting

Caloric Testing

Caloric testing is performed to evaluate the vestibular (inner-ear) portion of the auditory nerve. Water warmer or cooler than body temperature is infused into the ear. A normal response is demonstrated by the onset of **vertigo** (spinning sensation) and nystagmus (involuntary eye movements) within 20 to 30 seconds. To prepare the client for caloric testing, the nurse:

- Carefully explains the procedure and its purpose
- Tells the client to fast for several hours before the test
- Tells the client that the affected side will be tested first
- Explains that the client will be maintained on bedrest after the procedure with careful introduction of fluids to prevent nausea and vomiting

Dix-Hallpike Test for Vertigo

The Dix-Hallpike test for vertigo is performed by assisting the client to a sitting position on an examination table. The nurse stands to the side of the client and quickly repositions him or her from sitting to supine with the head extending beyond the end of the table. This change of position is done first to one side and then to the other side. A client with benign positional vertigo will have a burst of nystagmus after a delay of 5 to 10 seconds.

To prepare the client for the Dix-Hallpike test, the nurse:

- Carefully explains the procedure and its purpose
- Explains that double vision may occur during the test

Audiometry

Audiometry is the measurement of hearing acuity. To understand audiometry, the nurse must first understand audiometric testing terminology.

Frequency is the highness or lowness of tones (expressed in hertz). The greater the number of vibrations per second, the higher the frequency (pitch) of the sound; the fewer the number of vibrations per second, the lower the pitch.

Intensity of sound is expressed in decibels. The lowest intensity at which a young, normal ear can detect sound (about 50% of the time) is 0 dB. Sound at 110 dB is so intense (loud) that it is painful for most people with normal hearing. Conversational speech is generally around 60 dB, and a soft whisper is around 20 dB (Table 48-3). A hearing loss of 45 to 50 dB renders the person unable to hear speech without a hearing aid. A person with a hearing loss of 90 dB may not be able to hear speech even with a hearing aid.

Threshold is the lowest level of intensity at which pure tones and speech are heard by a client (about 50% of the time). **Pure tones** are generated by an **audiometer** (Figure 48-10) to determine hearing acuity. There are two types of audiometry: pure tone audiometry and speech audiometry.

PURE TONE AUDIOMETRY

Tones generated by an audiometer are presented to the client at frequencies for hearing speech, music, and other common sounds. Pure tone audiometry is performed by air conduction testing or bone conduction testing. The results of pure tone audiometry are plotted on an **audiogram** (Figure 48-11). For some clients, the hearing of one ear is "masked" while the hearing of the other ear is tested.

AIR CONDUCTION TEST. Pure tone air conduction testing determines whether a client hears normally or has a hearing loss. It is designed to test air conduction hearing sensitivity (through earphones) at frequencies of 125, 250, 500, 750, 1000, 1500, 2000, 3000, 4000, 6000, and 8000 Hz, but thresholds are usually confined to the frequencies of 250, 500, 1000, 2000, 4000, and 8000 Hz. The intensities for the pure tones generally range from 10 to 110 dB.

CLIENT PREPARATION. The client is placed in a sound-isolated room in which ambient noise does not exceed American National Standards Institute noise standards. The nurse sits facing the client because his or her facial expressions are frequently helpful in evaluating responses. Hearing-impaired clients may benefit from lip-reading the nurse's instructions. The nurse instructs the client as follows:

"I am going to test your hearing. The object of the test is to find the point at which you can just barely hear the tones. The tones will sound like soft bells or tuning forks. Every time you hear one, no matter how soft, signal by raising your hand (or pushing the button) on the side you hear the tone." (If the client cannot raise a hand or push a button because of physical or motor disabilities, a yes-no verbal response is appropriate.)

"When you no longer hear the tone, lower your hand (or release the button). This lets me know when you hear the tone and when it goes away."

TABLE 48-3 • DECIBEL INTENSITY AND SAFE EXPOSURE TIME FOR COMMON SOUNDS

Sound	Decibel Intensity (dB)	Safe Exposure Time*
Threshold of hearing	0	
Whispering	20	
Average residence or office	40	
Conversational speech	60	
Car traffic	70	>8 hr
Motorcycle	90	8 hr
Chain saw	100	2 hr
Rock concert, front row	120	3 min
Jet engine	140	Immediate danger
Rocket launching pad	180	Immediate danger

*For every 5-dB increase in intensity, the safe exposure time is cut in half.

PROCEDURE. The ear with the better hearing is tested first. Before beginning the test, the nurse adjusts the audiometric equipment by:

1. Setting the frequency control at 1000 Hz and the hearing level control at 40 dB

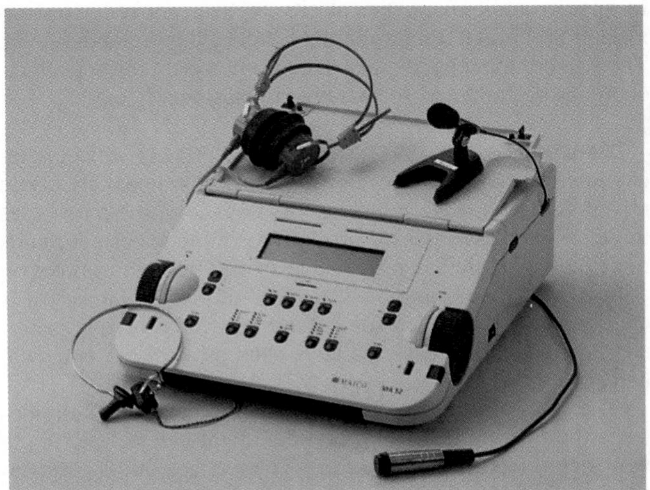

Figure 48-10 • A pure tone audiometer. (Courtesy Maico, Inc., Minneapolis, MN.)

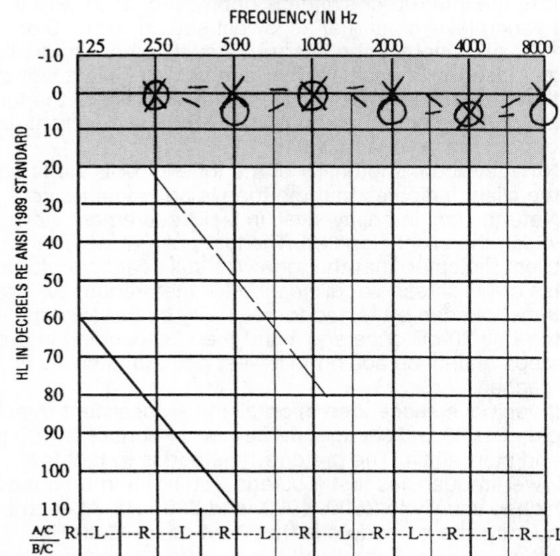

Figure 48-11 • Audiogram pattern depicting normal hearing. (Courtesy Cleveland Hearing and Speech Center, Cleveland, OH.)

2. Putting on the earphones and listening to the tone while switching from one ear to the other
3. In each earphone, listening to the tone while gradually turning the hearing level control toward 0 dB
4. Testing the signal cord and light to make sure they are working

Best practices for conduction audiometry to obtain a profile of the client's hearing for pure tones across the frequencies tested, from low to high frequencies, are presented in Chart 48-3. No special follow-up care is needed.

BONE CONDUCTION TEST. Pure tone bone conduction testing determines whether the hearing loss detected by air conduction testing is due to conductive or sensorineural factors, or to a combination of the two. It is used only when the results of air conduction testing are abnormal. There are restrictions on both the frequency and the intensity of the sound produced by the device. The frequencies are usually restricted to those between 250 and 4000 Hz. Because a bone conduction oscillator requires great power to vibrate the skull, maximal outputs for bone conduction are also lower.

CHART 48-3

BEST PRACTICE *for* Pure Tone Air Conduction Audiometry

1. After explaining the procedure to the client, place the earphones on the client. Make sure that the side marked *left* is on the left ear and the side marked *right* is on the right ear. The earphones must cover the ears.
2. If the client reports a hearing difference between the two ears, test the ear with better hearing first.
3. Begin the testing at 1000 Hz. This frequency is near the middle of the ear's sensitivity spectrum, and it has been demonstrated to have good test-retest reliability.
4. Adjust the audiometer so that the tone is inaudible unless the interrupter switch is depressed. Start with the hearing level control at its lowest setting, either 0 or −10 dB. Depress the interrupter switch, and gradually increase the intensity of the tone until the client signals that the tone is heard. Increase the intensity of the tone beyond this point by about 20 dB to give the client an opportunity to hear it well.
5. Now reduce the intensity of the tone in 5-dB steps until the client indicates that the tone is no longer heard. Note the last intensity level, in 5-dB decrement steps, at which the client signaled. The last point at which the client indicated that the tone was still heard should be his or her threshold for hearing for that frequency. The threshold can be tested for reliability by increasing the tone by 20 dB once again and then descending in 5-dB steps until once again the lowest point in intensity is reached.
6. If you have succeeded in obtaining a consistent threshold at 1000 Hz, change the frequency control to 500 Hz and start again. The preferred method is to test the lower frequencies first (500 and 250 Hz) and then move higher, usually to 2000, 4000, and 8000 Hz. At each frequency, the procedure is the same as for 1000 Hz.
7. After you have completed the threshold measurements on the first ear, switch the output selector to the opposite earphone. Proceed in the same manner to obtain thresholds for the other ear, also beginning at 1000 Hz.
8. If the thresholds of the second ear seem to differ by 40 dB or more from those of the first ear, masking of the better-hearing ear is indicated to rule out its participation in the test.
9. In operating the interrupter switch, make sure that you do not fall into rhythmic patterns that the client can follow. The pattern of tonal presentations should be irregular so that the client cannot predict when the tone will be presented.

CLIENT PREPARATION. The nurse explains that hearing sensitivity for bone conduction is going to be checked. The sounds and how the client should respond are the same as those for the air conduction test.

PROCEDURE. The ear with greater acuity is tested first. If neither ear is "better," it makes no difference which is tested first.

The bone conduction vibrator is placed behind the pinna, firmly on the mastoid process. The nurse then follows steps 4 through 9 of Chart 48-3. Remember that restrictions are placed on both the intensity and the frequency used in bone conduction testing. Restrictions are usually described on the face of the audiometer. No special follow-up care is needed.

INTERPRETATION OF RESULTS. Audiometric evaluation determines whether the client's hearing is within normal limits or, with a hearing impairment, whether the hearing loss is conductive, sensorineural, or mixed. The type of loss can be determined by the configuration of the audiogram after completion of pure tone air and bone conduction audiometry.

In the hands of an experienced clinician, the audiometer is a useful tool for evaluating the extent and type of hearing loss. For interpreting the results of a hearing test, the expertise of the person who performed the test and the reliability of the client's responses must be considered. In reality, the audiogram is the diagnostician's best estimate of hearing, based on observations of the client's auditory behavior in the testing situation.

Figure 48-11 is an audiogram showing normal results of air and bone conduction tests. Hearing is generally considered normal when the pure tone thresholds are at 10 dB or better. The line at 0 dB on the audiogram represents the hearing thresholds of a young person with normal hearing. Figure 48-12 depicts audiogram representations of various types of hearing loss.

SPEECH AUDIOMETRY

In speech audiometry, the ability to hear spoken words is measured through a microphone connected to an audiometer. The two components of speech audiometry are the speech reception threshold and speech discrimination.

SPEECH RECEPTION THRESHOLD. Speech reception threshold is the level of intensity at which a client can repeat simple words. In testing this threshold, the nurse tries to determine how intense (or loud) a simple speech stimulus must be before the client can hear it well enough to repeat it correctly. In one common test, lists of two-syllable words called **spondee** are used (i.e., words in which there is generally equal stress on each syllable, such as *airplane, railroad,* and *cowboy*).

The speech reception threshold measured by the audiometer is the hearing level at which the client can repeat simple words correctly 50% of the time. The test is administered essentially in the same manner as for the pure tone tests, but the microphone is activated through the audiometer. The intensity dial on the audiometer regulates word level intensity.

SPEECH DISCRIMINATION. Speech discrimination testing establishes the ability to discriminate among similar sounds or among words that contain similar sounds. The ability to understand speech is considered the most important measurable aspect of human auditory function. Speech discrimination testing assesses understanding of speech. A hearing loss may not only decrease sensitivity to sound but also impair understanding of what is being said.

A standard format contains lists of 25 to 50 **monosyllabic** (one-syllable) words, such as *carve, day, toe,* and *ran,* phonemically balanced (designed to include the phonemes of American English in the proper proportion) and with equal word difficulty between lists. The lists are presented to the client through earphones at a selected loudness level, generally about 30 to 40 dB above the speech reception threshold, or at the client's most comfortable listening level. A percentage score is derived from the number of words repeated correctly.

Tympanometry

Tympanometry assesses compliance (mobility) of the tympanic membrane and structures of the middle ear as a function

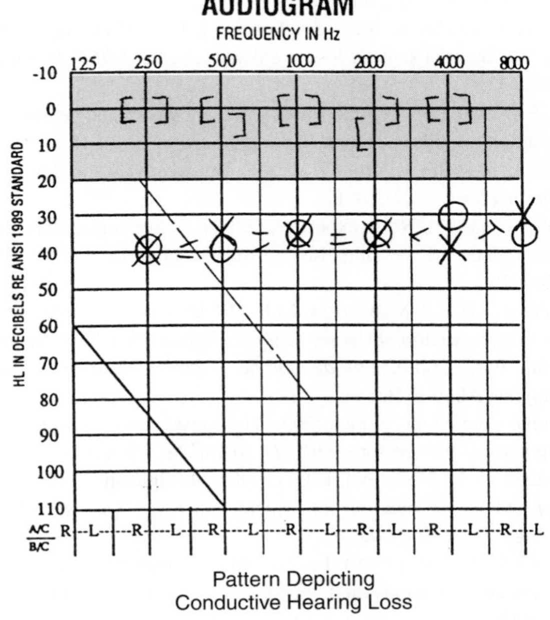

Pattern Depicting Conductive Hearing Loss

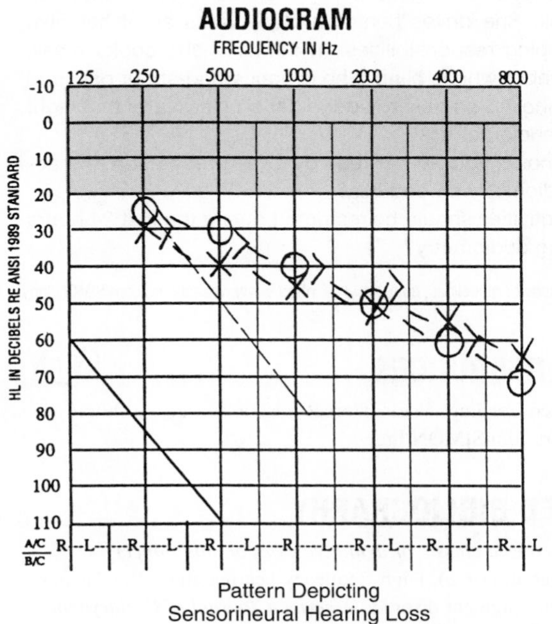

Pattern Depicting Sensorineural Hearing Loss

AUDIOGRAM

FREQUENCY IN Hz

Pattern Depicting Conductive and Sensorineural Hearing Loss

Audiogram Key	Left	Right		Left	Right
AC Unmasked	x	o	AC Masked	□	Δ
BC Unmasked	>	<	BC Masked	]	[
No Response	↘	↙	SF		S

Figure 48-12 ● Audiogram patterns depicting various types of hearing loss. (Courtesy Cleveland Hearing and Speech Center, Cleveland, OH.)

of systematically varied air pressure in the external auditory canal. The progression or resolution of serous otitis and otitis media can be accurately monitored with this procedure.

Tympanometry is helpful in distinguishing middle-ear pathologic conditions, such as otosclerosis, ossicular disarticulation, otitis media, and perforation of the tympanic membrane. It is also valuable for assessing patency of the eustachian tube and for observing postsurgical recovery of middle-ear function.

CRITICAL THINKING CHALLENGE

Your client is an 86-year-old woman who lives at home and is scheduled to have pure tone audiometry performed next week. She drives herself and performs all of her own housekeeping responsibilities. In addition, she cooks meals for a neighbor who is blind. She is concerned about pain and whether she will be able to attend her art class later that night after the audiometry.

- What should you tell her regarding the preparation and actual audiometry procedures?
- What activities should be restricted during the first 24 hours following audiometry?

For suggested answer guidelines, go to 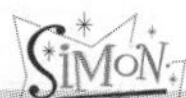 http://www.wbsaunders.com/SIMON/Iggy/.

ONLINE RESOURCES

For suggested readings and Internet resources, go to http://www.wbsaunders.com/SIMON/Iggy/.

SELECTED BIBLIOGRAPHY

Asterisk indicates a classic or definitive work on this subject.

Ardic, F.N., et al. (1998). High-frequency hearing and reflex latency in patients with pigment disorder. *American Journal of Otolaryngology, 19*(6), 365-369.

Bagley, M. (1998). Helping older adults to live better with hearing and vision losses. *Journal of Case Management, 7*(4), 147-152.

Baloh, R.W. (1998). Decision making in medicine: Dizzy patients: The varieties of vertigo. *Hospital Practice, 33*(6), 55-58, 61-63, 67-68.

*Benjamin, B., et al. (1994). *A color atlas of otorhinolarynogology.* Philadelphia: Lippincott-Raven.

*Bess, F.H., & Humes, L.E. (1995). *Audiology: The fundamentals.* Baltimore: Williams & Wilkins.

Cavendish, R. (1998). Clinical snapshot: Adult hearing loss. *American Journal of Nursing, 98*(8), 50-51.

Chaimoff, M., et al. (1999). Sudden hearing loss as a presenting symptom of acoustic neuroma. *American Journal of Otolaryngology, 20*(3), 157-160.

de la Cruz, M., & Bance, M. (1999). Carbamazepine-induced sensorineural hearing loss. *Archives of Otolaryngology–Head and Neck Surgery, 125*(2), 225-227.

Friedman, E.M., et al. (1997). When and how to retrieve foreign bodies. *Patient Care, 31*(13), 186-190, 193-194, 197-200.

Gates, G.A., Couropmitree, N.N., & Myers, R.H. (1999). Genetic associations in age-related hearing thresholds. *Archives of Otolaryngology–Head and Neck Surgery, 125*(6), 654-659.

Guyton, A., & Hall, J. (2000). *Textbook of medical physiology* (10th ed.). Philadelphia: W.B. Saunders.

Houston, D.K., et al. (1999). Age-related hearing loss, vitamin B-12, and folate in elderly women. *American Journal of Clinical Nutrition, 69*(3), 564-571.

Hsu, R., & Levine, S.C. (1998). Sudden hearing loss: How to identify the cause promptly. *Consultant, 38*(1), 23-26, 31-32.

Hull, R.H. (1997). *Aural rehabilitation: Serving children and adults* (3rd ed.). San Diego: Singular Publishing.

Jarvis, C. (2000). *Physical examination and health assessment* (3rd ed.). Philadelphia: W.B. Saunders.

Larson, P.D., Hazen, S.E.; & Martin, J.L.H. (1997). Assessment and management of sensory loss in elderly patients. *AORN Journal, 65*(2), 432-437.

Lee, F.S., et al. (1998). Analysis of blood chemistry and hearing levels in a sample of older persons. *Ear and Hearing, 19*(3), 180-190.

Lucas, L. & Matthews-Flint, L. (2001). Sound advice about hearing aids. *Nursing2001, 31*(2), 59-61.

Lusk, S.L. (1997). Noise exposures: Effects of hearing and prevention of noise induced hearing loss. *AAOHN Journal, 45*(8), 397-405, 409-410.

Malarkey, L.M., & McMorrow, M.E. (1999). *Nurse's manual of laboratory tests and diagnostic procedures.* Philadelphia: W.B. Saunders.

Martin, F.N. (2000). *Introduction to audiology* (7th ed.). Needham Heights: Allyn & Bacon.

National Council on Aging. (2000). The consequences of untreated hearing loss in older persons. *ORL–Head and Neck Nursing, 18*(1), 12-16.

Noorhassim, I., & Rampal, K.G. (1998). Multiplicative effect of smoking and age on hearing impairment. *American Journal of Otolaryngology, 19*(4), 240-243.

Ota, Y., & Oda, M. (1999). Lesion site in sudden deafness: Study with electrocochleography and transiently evoked otoacoustic emission. *Acta Oto-Laryngologica, 119*(1), 33-41.

Pagana, K.D., & Pagana, T.J. (1999a). *Diagnostic testing and nursing implications: A case study approach* (5th ed.). St. Louis: Mosby.

Pagana, K.D., & Pagana, T.J. (1999b). *Mosby's diagnostic and laboratory test reference* (4th ed.). St. Louis: Mosby.

Shaw, L. (1997). Protocol for detection and follow-up of hearing loss. *Clinical Nurse Specialist, 11*(6), 240-247.

Sheehan, J. (2000). Caring for the deaf: Do you do enough? *RN, 63*(3), 69-72.

Stewart, M.G., et al. (1999). Cost-effectiveness of the diagnostic evaluation of vertigo. *Laryngoscope, 109*(4), 600-605.

Stone, C.M. (1999). Clinical outlook: Preventing cerumen impaction in nursing facility residents. *Journal of Gerontological Nursing, 25*(5), 43-45.

Tan, R., Osman, V., & Tan, G. (1997). Ear size as a predictor of chronological age. *Archives of Gerontology and Geriatrics, 25*(2), 187-191.

Thobaden, M. (1998). Helping clients with presbycusis. *Home Care Provider, 3*(4), 186-188.

CHAPTER 49

Interventions for Clients with Ear and Hearing Problems

JAN HOOT MARTIN

Learning Objectives

After studying this chapter, you should be able to:

1. Compare and contrast the clinical manifestations and interventions for external otitis and otitis media.
2. Describe how to correctly instill medications into the ear.
3. Explain the procedures to safely remove impacted cerumen from the ear canal of an older client.
4. Prioritize educational needs for the client with Meniere's disease.
5. Compare and contrast the causes and interventions for conductive versus sensorineural hearing loss.
6. Prioritize nursing care needs for the client after tympanoplasty.
7. Prioritize educational needs for the client after stapedectomy.
8. Identify an appropriate method for communicating with a client who has recently become hearing impaired.
9. Develop a teaching plan for a client who is learning to use a hearing aid.

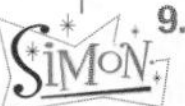
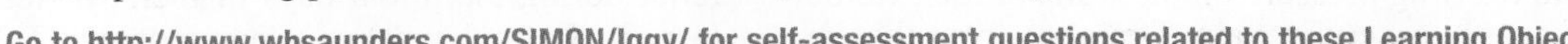

Go to http://www.wbsaunders.com/SIMON/Iggy/ for self-assessment questions related to these Learning Objectives.

Although often underappreciated, the ears play an important role in daily functioning. Disorders of the ears can cause a variety of problems ranging from hearing difficulties to problems of balance and functional ability. Hearing difficulties can lead to confusion, mistrust, social isolation, and the inability to give and receive accurate information. When a person is unable to maintain adequate balance, functional ability and the ability to provide adequate self-care needs become questionable. Disorders of the ear and of hearing are often easily treated with proper diagnosis; however, early recognition and intervention are necessary to prevent additional damage and to promote a maximal level of wellness.

CONDITIONS AFFECTING THE EXTERNAL EAR

The external ear is the outermost part of the ear structures and, as such, is subject to outside forces that can cause problems. Disorders of the external ear include **congenital malformation** (birth defects), trauma, and infectious or noninfectious lesions of the pinna, auricle, or auditory canal. Ear structures (external, middle, and inner ear) develop at different times during fetal development; thus the presence of birth defects in one area does not necessarily mean that other areas will be affected similarly. Abnormalities of the external ear range from crumpling or falling forward of the pinna to absence **(atresia)** of the auditory canal. In addition, trauma can damage or destroy the auricle and external canal. Surgical reconstruction, generally completed in phases, can reform the pinna with skin grafts and plastic prostheses. Trauma to the auricle resulting in a hematoma necessitates the removal of blood via needle aspiration to prevent calcification and hardening, which is often referred to as a **cauliflower** or **boxer's ear.**

Benign cysts or polyps of the auricle or external canal are surgically removed if they grow large enough to block the canal and affect hearing. Malignant cells, most commonly basal cell carcinoma, can also be found on the pinna. In general, treatment consists of simple excision. As the lesion becomes larger, its proximity to the skull and facial nerve makes treatment more difficult.

External Otitis

OVERVIEW

External otitis is a painful condition caused when irritating or infective agents come into contact with the skin of the external ear. The result to the external auditory canal or auricle is either an allergic response or inflammation with or without infection. Affected skin becomes red, swollen, and tender to touch or movement. Swelling of the auditory canal can lead to hearing loss due to canal obstruction. Allergic external otitis is commonly caused by contact with cosmetics, hair sprays, earphones, earrings, or hearing aids. The most common infectious organisms, usually bacterial or fungal, are *Pseudomonas aeruginosa,*

Streptococcus, Staphylococcus, and *Aspergillus.* Table 49-1 compares external otitis and otitis media.

External otitis occurs more often in hot, humid environments, especially in the summer, and is commonly referred to as **swimmer's ear** because of the high incidence in people involved in water sports. In addition, clients who have traumatized and opened lesions in their external auditory canal with sharp or small objects (such as hairpins or cotton-tipped applicators) or through headphones are more susceptible to external otitis.

Necrotizing or **malignant external otitis** is the most virulent form of external otitis; the organism spreads beyond the external auditory canal into the adjacent structures of the ear and skull. The high mortality rate seen with malignant external otitis results from complicating disorders such as meningitis, brain abscess, and destruction of cranial nerves, especially the facial nerve (cranial nerve VII).

COLLABORATIVE MANAGEMENT

Assessment

Clinical manifestations of external otitis include a variety of complaints, ranging from mild itching to pain with movement of the pinna or tragus. Clients have pain with physical manipulation of the pinna and tragus or when upward pressure is applied to the external canal. They report feeling as though the ear is plugged and hearing is reduced.

The nurse uses extreme caution during otoscopic examination to avoid exerting pressure on the walls of the external canal, which causes excessive pain. Drainage from the ear, when present, is often greenish white. To prevent cross-contamination, the nurse is careful to dispose of the otoscope tip and wash his or her hands thoroughly before examining the opposite ear. Hearing loss can be severe on the affected side when inflammation causes obstruction of the auditory canal and reduces access of sounds to the tympanic membrane.

TABLE 49-1 • COMPARISON OF FEATURES BETWEEN EXTERNAL OTITIS AND OTITIS MEDIA

Etiology	Clinical Manifestations	Treatment
EXTERNAL OTITIS		
Allergic reactions Bacterial or fungal infection Swimming Local trauma	Pain Itching Hearing loss Plugged feeling in ear Redness and edema Exudate	Topical antibiotics Corticosteroids Oral analgesics Local heat
OTITIS MEDIA		
Bacterial or viral infection Accumulation of fluid	Pain Pressure in ear Hearing loss Tinnitus Fever Malaise Nausea or vomiting Bulging tympanic membrane Fluid behind tympanic membrane	Systemic antibiotics Analgesics Local heat Antipyretics Antihistamines Decongestants Myringotomy

Interventions

Treatment of external otitis focuses on reducing local inflammation, edema, and pain. The nurse or assistive nursing personnel applies heat locally for 20 minutes three times a day, using towels warmed with water and then wrapped in a plastic bag, or heating pads placed on a low setting. Bedrest is often helpful in limiting head movements, thereby reducing pain.

Topical antibiotic and steroid therapies are the most effective means of decreasing inflammation and pain. The nurse reviews best practices for instilling eardrops with the client, as shown in Chart 49-1. The nurse observes the client to make sure that he or she uses proper technique. If edema has caused an obstruction of the external canal, an earwick is inserted past the blockage, with medicated drops applied to the outside end (Figure 49-1). A long piece of gauze dressing serves as an earwick, which the physician or nurse practitioner inserts using forceps to push carefully through the blocked external auditory canal to the tympanic membrane. The earwick may be removed when medication can flow freely into the canal. Thorough handwashing is strictly enforced. Systemic oral or intravenous antibiotics are used in severe cases, especially when cellulitis is present or the auricular lymph nodes are enlarged.

Analgesics, including opioids, may be necessary for pain relief during the initial days of therapy. Acetylsalicylic acid (aspirin, Entrophen✤) or acetaminophen (Tylenol, Abenol✤) can be given to relieve less severe pain.

After the inflammation has subsided, diluted alcohol may be dropped into the ear to keep it clean and dry and to prevent recurrence. The nurse teaches the client not to use cotton-tipped applicators to dry the ears, because use could lead to trauma to the canal and increase the risk for infection or inflammation. The use of ear plugs when engaging in water sports is recommended for clients with recurrent episodes of external otitis after swimming.

Furuncle

OVERVIEW

Often called localized external otitis, a **furuncle** is caused by bacterial infection, usually *Staphylococcus,* of a hair follicle. A furuncle is located on the outer half of the external canal.

CHART 49-1

BEST PRACTICE *for* Instillation of Eardrops

1. Gather the solutions to be administered.
2. Check the labels to ensure correct dosage and time.
3. Remove and discard any ear packing.
4. Irrigate the ear if the tympanic membrane is intact.
5. Place the bottle of eardrops (with the top on tightly) in a bowl of warm water for 5 minutes.
6. Tilt the client's head in the opposite direction of the affected ear and place the drops in the ear.
7. With the head tilted, gently move the head back and forth five times.
8. Insert a cotton ball into the opening of the ear canal to act as packing.

COLLABORATIVE MANAGEMENT

The clinical manifestations of a furuncle include intense local pain to light touch. The area is swollen and red, with tight skin covering the area, possibly with a purulent head. No drainage is noted unless the furuncle has ruptured. Hearing is impaired if the lesion occludes the canal.

Treatment is similar to that of other types of external otitis: local and systemic antibiotic administration and localized heat application. An earwick may be used with one-half strength Burow's solution to relieve pain. The furuncle might need to be incised and drained if it does not resolve with the use of antibiotics.

Cerumen or Foreign Bodies

OVERVIEW

Many objects can enter or be placed in the external auditory canal. Cerumen, or wax, is the most common cause of an impacted canal. Vegetables, beads, pencil erasers, and insects are other common items that may also enter the ear, with or without the client's help. Although uncomfortable, these are rarely true emergencies, and the nurse takes care when removing cerumen or foreign bodies.

COLLABORATIVE MANAGEMENT

Assessment

Clients have a sensation of fullness in the ear, with or without associated hearing loss, and may have ear pain, itching, and/or bleeding from the ear. The object may or may not be visible with direct inspection.

Interventions

When the occluding material is cerumen, the nurse irrigates the canal with a mixture of water and hydrogen peroxide at body temperature (Figure 49-2), following best practices for proper irrigation (Chart 49-2). Removal of wax by irrigation is a slow process and may take more than one sitting. When cerumen obstruction is the cause of hearing loss, however, removal results in increased hearing. Between 50 and 70 mL of solution is the maximum amount that the client can tolerate at one sitting. Irrigation is contraindicated in clients who have tympanic membrane perforation or otitis media.

If the cerumen is thick and dry or cannot be removed easily, the health care provider may prescribe a ceruminolytic product such as Cerumenex to soften the wax before trying to remove it. Another way to soften cerumen is to add 3 drops of glycerin or mineral oil to the ear at bedtime and 3 drops of hydrogen peroxide twice a day. After several days of this treatment, the cerumen is more easily removed through irrigation. In some cases, a small curette or cerumen spoon may be used to scoop out the wax. Only trained health care providers should use this method, because damage to the canal or the tympanic membrane is likely with improper technique. Refer to Chart 49-3 for nursing care considerations of older adult clients with cerumen impaction.

Irrigation is *not* used when the foreign object is vegetable matter, because this material expands with hydration, worsening the impaction. The object needs to be physically removed by an experienced health care provider.

Insects are killed before removal unless they can be coaxed out by a flashlight or a humming noise. Mineral oil or diluted alcohol is instilled into the ear to suffocate the insect, which is then removed with ear forceps.

If the client has local irritation, an antibiotic or steroid ointment may be applied to prevent infection and reduce local irritation. Hearing acuity is tested if hearing loss is not resolved by removal of the object.

In rare cases, surgical removal of the foreign object is necessary. The object is removed through the transcanal route using a wire bent at a 90-degree angle. The wire is looped around the object, and the object is pulled out. Because this procedure is painful, general anesthesia is necessary.

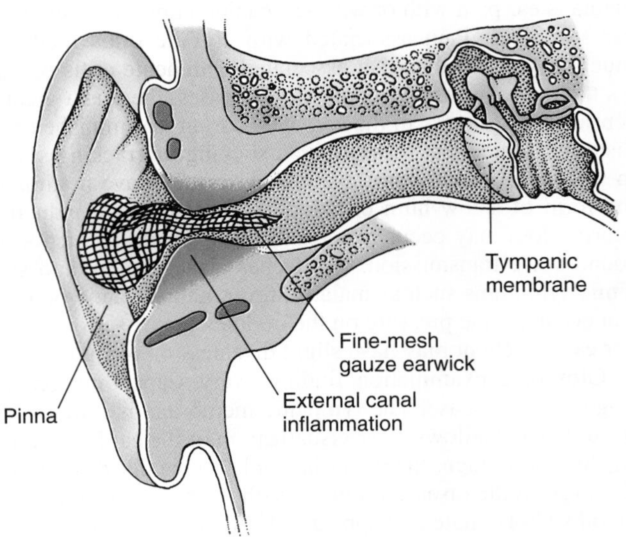

Figure 49-1 ● Earwick for instillation of antibiotics into the external canal. When edema occludes the external auditory canal, it is difficult for antibiotic solutions to enter the canal adequately. An earwick is placed through the meatus. Solutions placed on the external portion of the earwick are absorbed through the canal.

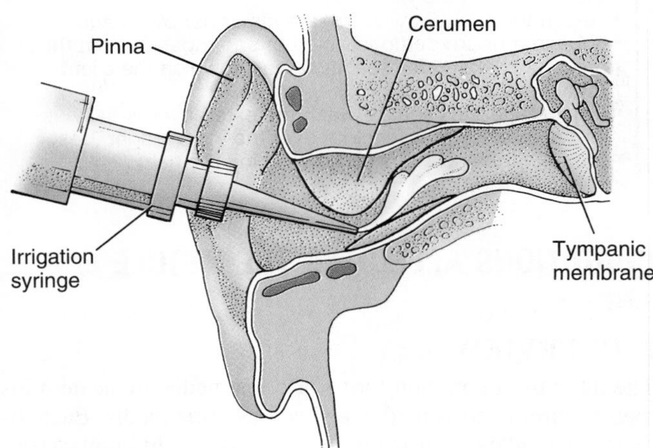

Figure 49-2 ● Irrigation of the external canal. Cerumen and debris can be removed from the ear by irrigation with warm water. The stream of water is aimed above or below the impaction to allow back-pressure to push it out rather than further down the canal.

CHART 49-2

BEST PRACTICE *for* Ear Irrigation

1. Gather the proper equipment: basin, syringe, otoscope, towel.
2. Warm tap water to body temperature.
3. Fill a syringe with warm water.
4. Place a towel around the client's neck.
5. Place a basin under the ear to be irrigated.
6. Use an otoscope to check the location of the impacted cerumen; ascertain that the tympanic membrane is intact and that the client does not have otitis media.
7. Place the tip of the syringe at an angle so that the fluid pushes on one side and not directly on the impaction (this helps to loosen the impaction instead of forcing it further into the canal).
8. Watch the fluid return for signs of cerumen plug removal.
9. Continue to irrigate the ear with approximately 70 mL of fluid.
10. If the cerumen does not drain out, wait 10 minutes and repeat the irrigation procedure.
11. Monitor the client for signs of nausea.
12. If the client becomes nauseated, stop the procedure.
13. If the cerumen cannot be removed by irrigation, the client may place mineral oil into the ear three times a day for 2 days to soften dry, impacted cerumen, after which irrigation may be repeated.

CHART 49-3

NURSING FOCUS *on the* OLDER ADULT
Cerumen Impaction

- Assess the hearing of all older clients using simple voice tests (see Chapter 48).
- Perform a gentle otoscopic inspection of the external canal and tympanic membrane of any older client who has a problem with hearing acuity, especially the client who wears a hearing aid.
- Use ear irrigation to remove any impacted cerumen.
- Make certain that the irrigating fluid is approximately 98° F (37° C) to reduce the chance of stimulating the vestibular sense.
- Use no more than 5 to 10 mL of irrigating fluid at a time.
- If nausea, vomiting, or dizziness develops, stop the irrigation immediately.
- Teach the client how to irrigate his or her own ears.
- Obtain a return demonstration of ear irrigation from the client, observing for specific areas in which the client may need assistance.
- Encourage the client to wash the external ears daily using a soapy, wet washcloth over the index finger (best done in the shower or while washing the hair).

CONDITIONS AFFECTING THE MIDDLE EAR

Otitis Media

OVERVIEW

The three most common forms of otitis media are acute otitis media, chronic otitis media, and serous otitis media. Each affects the middle-ear structures but has slightly different causes, incidences, and pathologic changes. If otitis progresses or remains untreated, permanent conductive hearing loss may occur. Otitis media is less common in adults than in children but does occur.

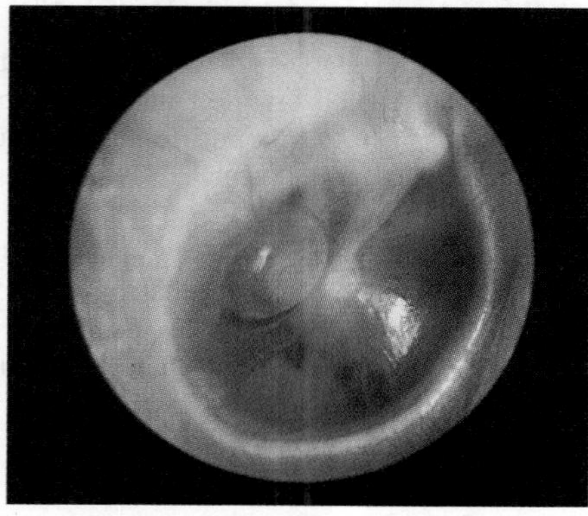

Figure 49-3 ● Otoscopic view of otitis media.

Acute otitis media and chronic otitis media, also known as suppurant or purulent otitis media, are similar in pathophysiology. An infecting agent introduced into the middle ear causes an inflammation within the mucosa, leading to swelling and irritation of the ossicles within the middle ear. This process is followed by a purulent inflammatory exudate. Acute disease has a sudden onset and a relatively short duration of 3 weeks or less. Chronic otitis media usually follows repeated acute episodes, has a longer duration, and can be associated with greater morbidity or injury to the middle ear.

The eustachian tube and mastoid, connected to the middle ear by a continuation of cells, are also affected by the infection. If the tympanic membrane perforates and infective materials spill into the external ear, external otitis also develops, which, untreated, thickens and scars the middle ear. Necrosis of the ossicles leads to destruction of the middle-ear structures.

COLLABORATIVE MANAGEMENT

Assessment

The chief complaint of the client with acute or chronic otitis media is ear pain with or without manipulation of the external ear structures. Pain associated with chronic otitis media is much less severe than that associated with acute otitis media. As the pressure in the middle ear increases, there is a greater sensation of fullness in the ear, and hearing is diminished and distorted. The client may notice a sticking or cracking sound in the ear on yawning or swallowing or may have tinnitus in the form of a low hum or a low-pitched sound. Conductive hearing loss may occur as a result of physical obstruction in sound wave transmission. Headaches are common, and systemic symptoms such as malaise, fever, nausea, and vomiting can occur. As the pressure on the middle ear presses on the inner ear, the client may have slight dizziness or vertigo.

Otoscopic examination findings vary, depending on the stage of the disease. The tympanic membrane is initially retracted, which allows clear visualization of the ear landmarks. At this early stage, the client has only vague ear discomfort; however, as the disease progresses, the tympanic membrane's blood vessels dilate and appear red (Figure 49-3). In the third stage, the tympanic membrane becomes red, thickened, and bulging, with loss of landmarks. Decreased membrane mobility is evident on inspection with a pneumatic otoscope. Exudate behind the membrane may be visible.

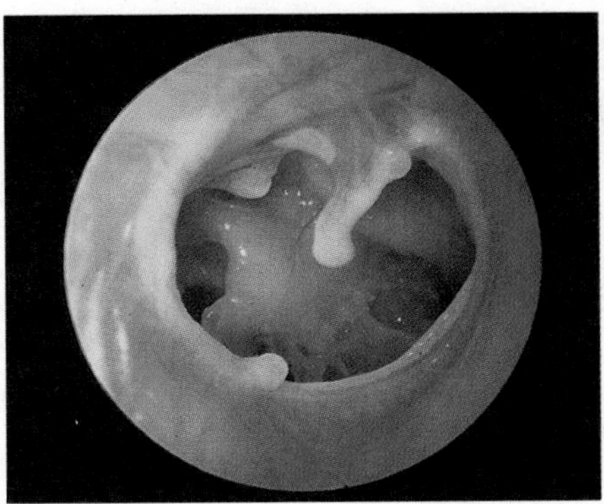

Figure 49-4 ● Otoscopic view of a perforated tympanic membrane.

If the disease progresses, the tympanic membrane spontaneously **perforates** (breaks open) and pus or blood drains from the ear (Figure 49-4). This discharge may be pulsating when viewed through the otoscope. When the membrane ruptures, the client notices a marked decrease in pain as the pressure on middle-ear structures is relieved (Figure 49-5). Tympanic perforations from any cause may heal if the underlying problem is controlled. The membrane covering initially appears thinner over the healed perforation. A simple central perforation does not interfere with hearing unless the ossicles of the middle ear are damaged or the perforation is large. However, repeated perforations with extensive scarring can cause hearing loss.

Cultures of drainage after a perforation from uncontrolled otitis media may reveal the infecting agent. Cultures are rarely taken unless previous treatment has been ineffective. When the tympanic membrane is not perforated, a needle aspiration or myringotomy draws fluid for culture.

Interventions

NONSURGICAL MANAGEMENT. Treatment can be as simple as putting the client in a quiet environment without distractions. Bedrest limits head movements that intensify the pain. Localized heat may be applied by using a heating pad adjusted to a low setting. Application of cold may occasionally relieve pain.

Systemic antibiotic therapy can decrease pain by reducing inflammation. Topical antibiotics are not used to treat otitis media. Analgesics such as acetylsalicylic acid (aspirin, Entrophen♣) and acetaminophen (Tylenol, Abenol♣) aid in pain relief, and their antipyretic effects help the client feel better by relieving an elevated temperature. When the client has severe pain, opioid analgesics such as codeine and meperidine hydrochloride (Demerol) also may be used.

Antihistamines and decongestants are prescribed to decrease mucus production in the nasopharynx and to decrease fluid in the middle ear. The body can then reabsorb the fluid, reducing pressure and pain.

SURGICAL MANAGEMENT. If the pain persists after initial antibiotic therapy and the tympanic membrane continues to bulge, a **myringotomy** (surgical opening of the pars tensa of the tympanic membrane) is performed. Myringotomies drain middle-ear fluids and almost immediately relieve pain.

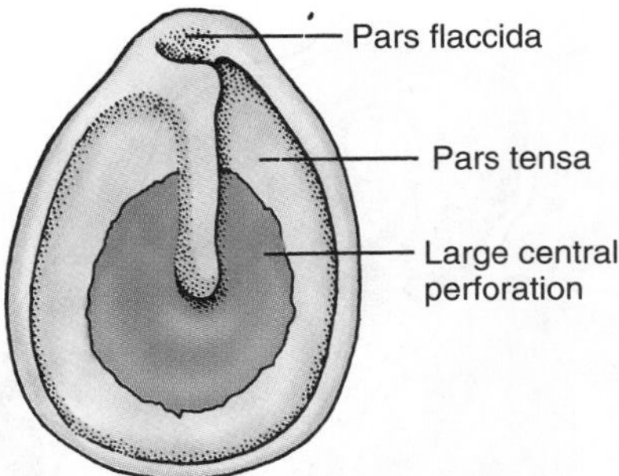

With a **large central perforation,** clients complain of significant hearing loss.

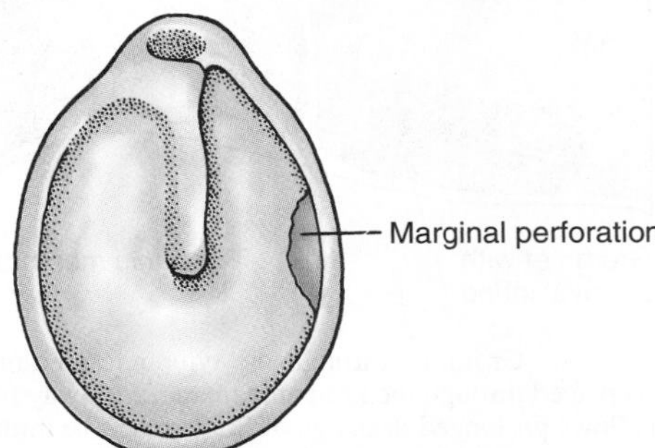

With a **marginal perforation,** clients might complain of significant hearing loss.

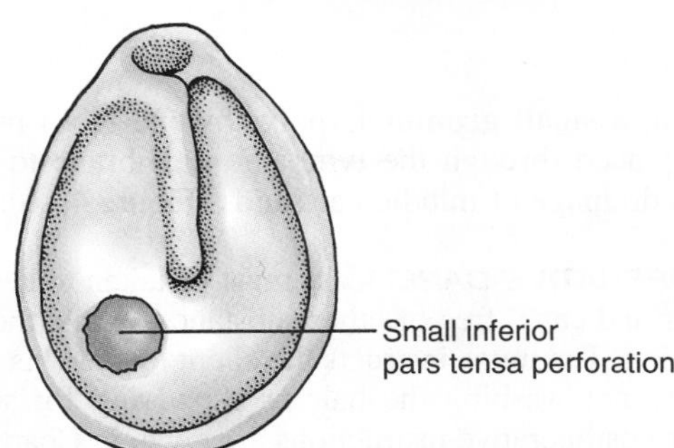

With a **small inferior pars tensa perforation,** clients do not complain of much interference with hearing.

Figure 49-5 ● Perforations of the tympanic membrane. Central perforations heal more quickly than marginal perforations. Marginal perforations that do not heal allow cholesteatoma formation.

PREOPERATIVE CARE. The nurse reassures the client that the myringotomy will relieve pain and is usually performed without anesthesia. Many people are apprehensive about a perforation and its effect on hearing. To relieve some of this anxiety, the nurse discusses the reasons for the procedure with the client and encourages relaxation techniques such as deep breathing before and during the procedure. Systemic antibiotic therapy continues before and after this procedure. The nurse cleans the external canal with a bacteriostatic solution such as povidone-iodine (Betadine) before the myringotomy.

OPERATIVE PROCEDURE. The small surgical incision can be performed in an office or clinic setting and heals rapidly. An alternative is the removal of fluid from the middle ear via needle aspiration. For relief of pressure caused by serous

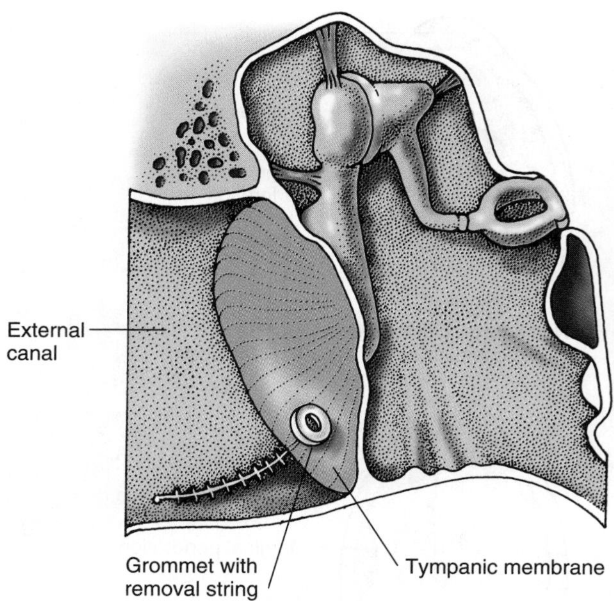

Figure 49-6 ● Grommet through the tympanic membrane. A small grommet is placed through the tympanic membrane away from the margins, which allows prolonged drainage of fluids from the middle ear. The grommet can be removed later, and the tympanic membrane can be allowed to heal naturally or be patched with a small piece of homogenous tissue.

otitis media, a small **grommet** (polyethylene tube) may be surgically placed through the tympanic membrane to allow continuous drainage of middle-ear fluids (Figure 49-6).

POSTOPERATIVE CARE. Care must be taken to keep the external ear and canal free of other substances while the incision is healing. The nurse instructs the client to keep his or her head dry by not washing the hair or showering for several days. Other postoperative instructions are given in Chart 49-4.

CRITICAL THINKING CHALLENGE

You are assigned to care for a 28-year-old man who has been admitted with diabetic ketoacidosis. During the course of his hospitalization, he tells you that he thinks he has an ear infection.

- What assessment information will you need before notifying the health care provider?
- What nursing interventions would you perform regardless of the location of the infection?
- If otitis media is diagnosed, what is the proper route for antibiotic therapy, and why?

For suggested answer guidelines, go to SIMON http://www.wbsaunders.com/SIMON/Iggy/.

Mastoiditis

OVERVIEW

The epithelial lining of the middle ear is continuous with the epithelial lining of the mastoid air cells, which are embedded in the temporal bone. **Mastoiditis** is a secondary disorder resulting from untreated or inadequately treated otitis media and can be acute or chronic. Before antibiotic therapy, mastoiditis

CHART 49-4

CLIENT EDUCATION GUIDE
Recovery from Ear Surgery

- Avoid straining when you have a bowel movement.
- Do not drink through a straw for 2 to 3 weeks.
- Avoid air travel for 2 to 3 weeks.
- Avoid excessive coughing for 2 to 3 weeks.
- Stay away from people with colds.
- If you need to blow your nose, blow gently, one side at a time, with your mouth open.
- Avoid getting your head wet, washing your hair, and showering for 1 week.
- Keep your ear dry for 6 weeks by placing a ball of cotton coated with petroleum jelly (such as Vaseline) in your ear. Change the cotton ball daily.
- Avoid rapidly moving the head, bouncing, and bending over for 3 weeks.
- Change your ear dressing every 24 hours as directed.
- Report excessive drainage immediately to your physician.

was a leading cause of death in children and of hearing loss in adults. Today, antibiotic therapy is aimed at treating the middle-ear infection before it progresses to mastoiditis.

COLLABORATIVE MANAGEMENT

Assessment

The clinical manifestations of mastoiditis include swelling behind the ear and pain with minimal movement of the tragus, the pinna, or the head. Pain is not relieved by myringotomy. **Cellulitis** (infection spreading laterally through the tissues of the skin) develops on the skin or external scalp over the mastoid process. Otoscopic examination reveals a red, dull, thick, immobile tympanic membrane with or without perforation. Postauricular lymph nodes are tender and enlarged. Clients with mastoiditis also have low-grade fever, malaise, and anorexia.

Interventions

NONSURGICAL MANAGEMENT. Antibiotic therapy aims to prevent the continued spread of infection from the otitis media or mastoiditis but has limited use in actual mastoiditis treatment because of the difficulty of achieving effective antibiotic levels within the bony structure of the mastoid. Cultures obtained from the ear drainage or myringotomy determine the sensitivities of infecting organisms to specific antibiotics.

SURGICAL MANAGEMENT. Surgical removal of the infected tissue is necessary if the client does not respond to antibiotic administration within a few days. A simple or modified radical mastoidectomy with tympanoplasty is the most common treatment. All infected tissue must be removed so that the infection does not spread to other structures. A tympanoplasty is then performed to reconstruct the ossicles and the tympanic membrane to restore hearing. Client preparation, the operative procedure, and follow-up care for tympanoplasty are discussed on pp. 1073 and 1074.

Complications arise when infective material has not been removed completely or when other structures outside the mastoid and middle ear are contaminated. Complications of mastoiditis include damage to the abducens and facial cranial nerves (cranial nerves VI and VII), decreasing the client's ability to look laterally (cranial nerve VI) and causing a drooping of the mouth on the affected side (cranial nerve VII). Other complications include vertigo, meningitis, brain abscess, chronic purulent otitis media, and wound infection.

Trauma

OVERVIEW

Trauma and damage may occur to the tympanic membrane and ossicles by infection, by direct damage to the structures, or through rapid changes in the middle-ear cavity pressure. Foreign objects placed in the external canal may exert pressure on the tympanic membrane and cause perforation. If the objects continue through the canal, the bony structure of the stapes, incus, and malleus may be damaged. Blunt injury to the basal skull and ears can also damage middle-ear structures through fractures extending to the middle ear. Slapping of the external ear increases the pressure in the external auditory canal, tearing the eardrum when the pressure is great enough. The tympanic membrane has a limited stretching ability and gives way under high pressure. Excessive nose blowing and rapid changes of pressure that occur with nonpressurized air flight **(barotrauma)** can cause an increase in pressure within the middle ear. High pressure damages the ossicles and can cause outward perforation of the eardrum.

COLLABORATIVE MANAGEMENT

Tympanic membrane perforations usually heal within 24 hours. Repeated perforations, especially from chronic otitis media, heal slower, with tympanic scarring. Depending on the amount of damage to the ossicles, hearing may or may not return. Hearing aids can improve hearing in this type of hearing loss. Surgical reconstruction of the ossicles and tympanic membrane through a tympanoplasty or a myringoplasty may also improve hearing (see later discussion of nursing care under Tympanoplasty, pp. 1073-1074).

Preventive measures should be taken to avoid trauma. The nurse instructs clients to avoid inserting objects into the external canal. Ear protectors can be used when blunt trauma is likely, especially in sports such as boxing.

Neoplasms

OVERVIEW

Tumors of the middle ear are rare. The most common type of tumor is the glomus jugulare, a highly vascular benign lesion arising from the jugular vein. Extremely rare malignant tumors include primary adenocarcinoma, adenoid cystic carcinoma, and mucoepidermoid carcinoma. The growth of any lesion within the middle-ear fossa disrupts conductive hearing, erodes the ossicles, and has the potential to involve the inner ear and adjacent cranial nerves.

COLLABORATIVE MANAGEMENT

Clients experience progressive hearing loss and tinnitus. Infection and pain are rarely associated with glomus jugulare tumors. A physical examination reveals bulging of the tympanic membrane or a mass extending to the external auditory canal. The highly vascular nature of the glomus jugulare tumor gives it a reddish color and a visible pulsation when seen through the eardrum.

Diagnosis is made by physical examination, tomography, and angiography. Neoplasms are removed by surgery, which generally sacrifices hearing in the affected ear. If all of the margins of the tumor can be seen clearly through the tympanic membrane, a transcanal approach is used to remove the lesion. When the tumor margins extend past the tympanic membrane, further diagnostic tests are necessary to determine the extent of growth and vascular involvement. Radiation therapy is used to decrease the vascularity of the glomus jugulare tumor but is not the preferred method of treatment. Benign lesions are removed because, with continued growth of the neoplasm, cranial structures other than the middle ear can be affected, further damaging the facial or trigeminal nerve. When possible, reconstructive surgery of the middle ear structures is performed later to restore conductive hearing.

CONDITIONS AFFECTING THE INNER EAR

Tinnitus

OVERVIEW

Tinnitus (continuous ringing or noise perception in the ear) is one of the most common complaints of clients with ear or hearing disorders. The health care provider cannot use diagnostic testing to confirm tinnitus, nor does the disorder have observable characteristics, but tinnitus can lead to particularly disturbing emotional consequences for the person afflicted with this disorder.

COLLABORATIVE MANAGEMENT

Symptoms of tinnitus range from mild ringing, which can go unnoticed during the day, to a loud roaring in the ear, which can interfere with thinking and attention span. When clients report tinnitus, the nurse is alert to the wide variety of pathologic disorders and other factors that cause tinnitus: presbycusis, **otosclerosis** (irregular bone growth around ossicles), Meniere's disease, certain drugs, exposure to loud noise, and other inner-ear abnormalities.

The exact pathophysiology and treatment of tinnitus vary with the underlying cause. When no underlying cause can be found or the disorder is untreatable, therapy focuses on ways to mask the tinnitus with background sound, noisemakers, and music during sleeping hours. Ear mold hearing aids can amplify sounds to drown out the tinnitus during the day. The American Tinnitus Association assists clients in coping with tinnitus when other therapy is unsuccessful.

Vertigo and Dizziness

OVERVIEW

Vertigo and dizziness are common clinical manifestations of many ear disorders. Dizziness is a disturbed sense of a person's proper relationship to space. Clients vary greatly in defining dizziness. Vertigo is often used interchangeably with dizziness, but the definition, as well as the cause, is somewhat different. True **vertigo** is a real sense of whirling or turning in space.

The visual system, the vestibular system (cochlea, semicircular canals), and the proprioceptive system (muscles and nerve endings) combine to give input to the cerebellum about balance. Dysfunction in any of these areas leads to a disturbed sense of balance or motion. Common factors affecting the ear that cause vertigo include Meniere's disease, labyrinthitis, acoustic neuromas, benign paroxysmal vertigo, trauma, motion sickness, and drug or alcohol ingestion.

➤ COLLABORATIVE MANAGEMENT

Associated symptoms of vertigo include nausea, vomiting, falling, nystagmus, hearing loss, and tinnitus. Until the underlying cause of the vertigo can be treated, each clinical manifestation is treated. Clients are advised to:

- Restrict head motions and move more slowly
- Maintain adequate hydration, especially after vomiting
- Take medications with antivertiginous effects, such as dimenhydrinate (Dramamine, Gravol♣), diazepam (Valium, Apo-Diazepam♣), and scopolamine (Transderm Scop, Transderm-V♣).

Many clients are dissatisfied with treatment because side effects of the medications, especially drowsiness, can be worse than the vertigo. The nurse cautions clients to maintain a safe, uncluttered environment to prevent accidents during periods of vertigo and to use a cane or walker to maintain balance. The nurse further instructs clients not to drive or operate machinery when taking antivertiginous drugs.

Labyrinthitis

OVERVIEW

Labyrinthitis is an infection of the labyrinth, which occasionally occurs as a complication of acute or chronic otitis media. Infection results from an erosion of the bony capsule, allowing infective materials to invade the inner ear. Labyrinthitis often results from the growth of a **cholesteatoma** (benign overgrowth of squamous cell epithelium) from the middle ear into the lateral semicircular canal. Labyrinthitis may follow middle-ear or inner-ear surgery when infection is present. When the infecting organism is viral, the labyrinthitis may be part of a systemic viral infection such as an upper respiratory tract infection or infectious mononucleosis.

➤ COLLABORATIVE MANAGEMENT

Clinical manifestations include hearing loss, tinnitus, spontaneous nystagmus to the affected side, and vertigo with associated nausea and vomiting. **Meningitis** (infection of the brain covering) is the most common complication of labyrinthitis.

Treatment of labyrinthitis includes the use of systemic antibiotics such as ampicillin (Omnipen, Apo-Ampi♣). Clients are advised to stay in bed in a darkened room until clinical manifestations have diminished. Antiemetics, such as chlorpromazine hydrochloride (Thorazine, Novo-Chlorpromazine♣), and antivertiginous medications, such as dimenhydrinate (Dramamine, Gravol♣), relieve symptoms.

The client also needs psychosocial support. Hearing loss on the affected side may be permanent, although vertigo subsides as the inflammation resolves. Persistent balance problems may improve with gait training and physical therapy.

Meniere's Disease

OVERVIEW

Meniere's disease has three distinct characteristics—tinnitus, unilateral sensorineural hearing loss, and vertigo—occurring in attacks that can last for several days. Clients are almost totally incapacitated during an attack, and several days are needed for full recovery. The pathologic changes of Meniere's disease are either overproduction or decreased reabsorption of endolymphatic fluid, causing a distortion of the entire inner-canal system. This distortion leads to decreased hearing from dilation of the cochlear duct, vertigo because of damage to the vestibular system, and tinnitus from unknown cause. Involvement is generally unilateral. The initial hearing loss is reversible, but repeated damage to the cochlea, caused by increased fluid pressure, leads to permanent hearing loss.

The cause of Meniere's disease is unknown but is associated with viral or bacterial infections, allergic reactions, and biochemical disturbances that increase fluid imbalances. Mild long-term stress also seems to be associated with Meniere's disease.

➤ COLLABORATIVE MANAGEMENT

Assessment

The onset of Meniere's disease symptoms usually occurs in people between the ages of 20 and 50 years, with a greater prevalence in men and Caucasians. Times of severe, debilitating attacks alternate with almost symptom-free periods. Clients often have certain clinical manifestations before an attack of vertigo, such as headaches, increasing tinnitus, and a feeling of fullness in the affected ear. Clinical manifestations are unilateral in 60% to 70% of the cases.

Clients describe the tinnitus as a continuous, low-pitched roar or a humming sound, which worsens just before and during a severe attack. Hearing loss is initially of the low-frequency tones but worsens to include all levels after repeated episodes. Hearing loss is worse during an attack. In the early stages of Meniere's disease, periods of remission are marked by normal or nearly normal hearing, but permanent hearing loss develops as the attacks increase.

Clients describe the vertigo as periods of whirling, which might even cause them to fall. The vertigo is so intense that even while lying down, clients hold the bed or ground to prevent the whirling. The severe vertigo usually lasts 3 to 4 hours, but clients continue to feel dizzy long after the attack. Nausea and vomiting are common. Other clinical manifestations include rapid eye movements and severe headaches.

Interventions

NONSURGICAL MANAGEMENT. The nurse instructs clients to make slow head movements to prevent worsening of the vertigo. Dietary and lifestyle changes, such as salt and fluid restrictions that reduce the amount of endolymphatic fluid, are recommended. Clients are advised to stop smoking because of the vasoconstrictive effects.

Drug therapy aims to control the vertigo and vomiting and restore normal balance. Mild diuretics are prescribed to decrease endolymph volume. Nicotinic acid has been found to be useful because of its vasodilatory effect. Antihistamines such as diphenhydramine hydrochloride (Benadryl, Allerdryl♣) and dimenhydrinate (Dramamine, Gravol♣) help reduce the severity of or stop an acute attack. Antiemetics such as chlorpromazine hydrochloride (Thorazine, Novo-Chlorpromazine♣), droperidol (Inapsine), and trimethobenzamide hydrochloride (Arrestin, Tigan) help control the nausea and vomiting. Diazepam (Valium, Apo-Diazepam♣) calms the anxious client; controls vertigo, nausea, and vomiting; and allows the client to rest quietly during an attack.

SURGICAL MANAGEMENT. Surgical treatment of Meniere's disease remains controversial because the hearing in the affected ear is often sacrificed. When medical therapy is ineffective and the client's functional hearing level has decreased significantly, surgery is performed. The most radical procedure involves resection of the vestibular nerve or total removal of the labyrinth **(labyrinthectomy),** performed via the transcanal route. The footplate of the stapes is moved aside, and the labyrinth is removed through the oval window with fine forceps.

Another procedure performed early in the course of the disease is **endolymphatic decompression** with drainage and a shunt. The endolymphatic sac is drained, and a small tube is inserted to enhance fluid drainage. Some clients report relief of vertigo and preservation of their hearing.

If an endolymphatic decompression has been performed, manipulation of the vestibular structures of the inner ear causes postoperative vertigo. The nurse reassures the client that the vertigo is temporary as a result of the surgical procedure, not the disease.

Acoustic Neuroma

OVERVIEW

An **acoustic neuroma** is a benign tumor of cranial nerve VIII. The location makes it destructive because of the frequent involvement of the cerebellum. Depending on the size and exact location of the tumor, damage to hearing, facial movements, and sensation can occur. Also, other neurologic-pathologic disorders associated with a lesion occupying intracranial space may result.

COLLABORATIVE MANAGEMENT

Clinical manifestations begin with tinnitus and progress to gradual sensorineural hearing loss in more than 90% of clients. Later, clients experience constant mild vertigo. As the tumor enlarges, adjacent cranial nerves are damaged.

Acoustic neuromas are diagnosed with computed tomography (CT) scanning and magnetic resonance imaging (MRI). Audiograms diagnose sensorineural hearing loss. Cerebrospinal fluid assays show increased pressure and positive results for protein.

Surgical removal via a craniotomy is necessary, and the remaining hearing is sacrificed. Extreme care is taken to preserve the function of the facial nerve (cranial nerve VII). Routine postcraniotomy care is discussed in Chapter 45. Acoustic neuromas rarely recur after surgical removal.

HEARING LOSS

OVERVIEW

Pathophysiology

Hearing loss is one of the most common physical handicaps in North America. Hearing loss may be conductive, sensorineural, or a combination of the two (Figure 49-7). Conductive hearing loss occurs when sound waves are blocked from contact with inner-ear nerve fibers because of external-ear or middle-ear disorders. If the inner-ear nerve, or sensory, fibers that lead to the cerebral cortex are damaged, the hearing loss is termed sensorineural. Combination hearing loss is known as mixed conductive-sensorineural.

The differences in conductive and sensorineural hearing loss are summarized in Table 49-2. Disorders that lead to conductive hearing loss can often be corrected with no or minimal permanent damage. Sensorineural hearing loss is often permanent, and measures must be taken to prevent further damage or to amplify sounds as a means to improve hearing.

Etiology

COMMON CAUSES OF CONDUCTIVE HEARING LOSS

Any inflammatory process or obstruction of the external or middle ear by cerumen or foreign objects leads to conductive hearing loss. Changes in the tympanic membrane such as bulges, retractions, and perforations may indicate damage to middle-ear structures, which leads to conductive hearing loss. Tumors, scar tissue buildup, and overgrowth of soft bony tissue (otosclerosis) on the ossicles from previous middle-ear surgery also lead to conductive hearing loss.

COMMON CAUSES OF SENSORINEURAL HEARING LOSS

When the inner ear or auditory nerve (cranial nerve VIII) is damaged, sensorineural hearing loss develops. Prolonged exposure to loud noise can damage the hair cells of the cochlea. Many drugs are toxic **(ototoxic)** to the inner-ear structures, and their effects on hearing can be transient or permanent, unilateral or bilateral, dose related, or non–dose related. When ototoxic drugs (such as those listed in Table 48-2) are given to clients with reduced renal function, increased ototoxicity can result because drug elimination takes longer. Older clients are especially susceptible to ototoxicity because of reduced kidney function.

Presbycusis is a common cause of sensorineural hearing loss associated with the process of aging. This hearing loss is commonly caused by degeneration or atrophy of the ganglion cells in the cochlea, loss of elasticity of the basilar membrane, or a decreased vascular supply to the inner ear. Recent research findings suggest that deficiencies of vitamin B_{12} and folic acid may play a role in presbycusis (see the Evidence-Based Practice for Nursing box on p. 1071). Other causes of sensorineural hearing loss include inherited disorders, circulatory disorders (such as arteriosclerosis and hypertension), bacterial or viral infections, prolonged fever, Meniere's disease, diabetes mellitus, and ear surgery. Each is thought to accelerate degenerative changes of the cochlea. Trauma to the ear or the head also contributes to sensorineural hearing loss.

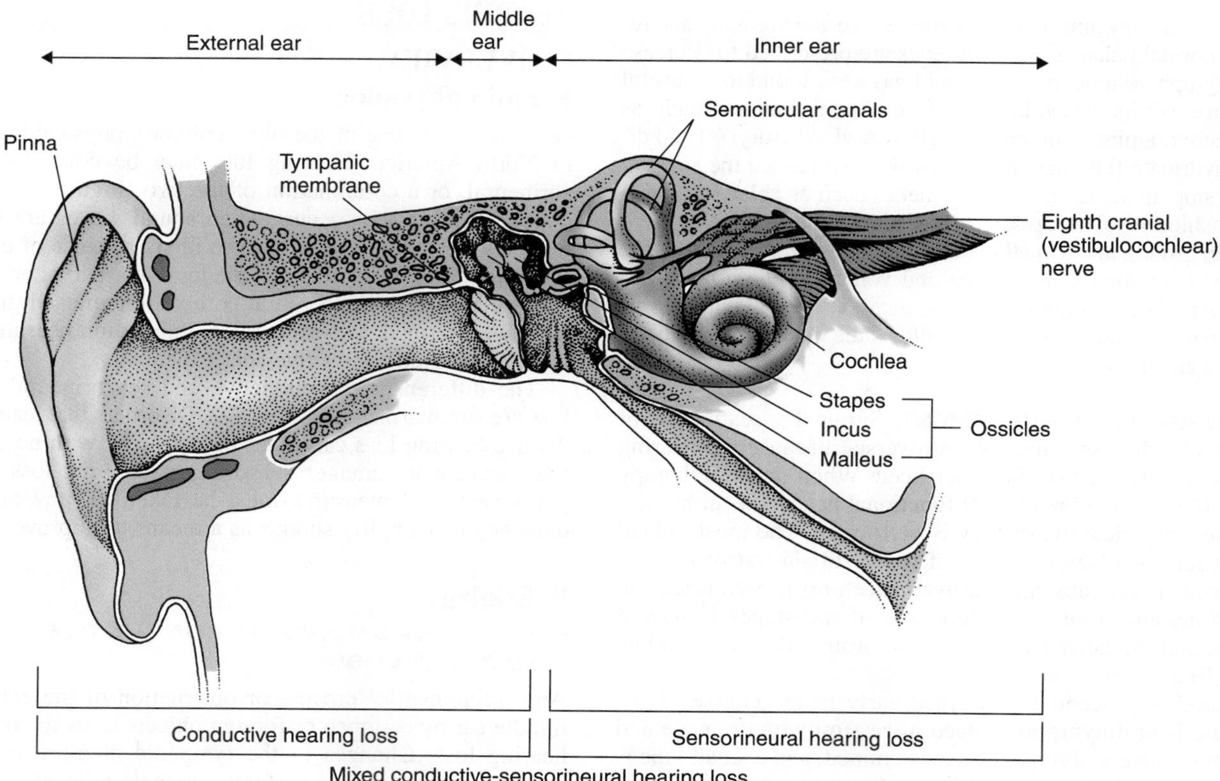

Figure 49-7 • Anatomy of hearing loss. Hearing loss can be divided into three types: (1) conductive loss (difficulty in the external or the middle ear), (2) sensorineural loss (difficulty in the inner ear or the acoustic nerve), and (3) mixed conductive-sensorineural loss (a combination of the two).

TABLE 49-2 • DIFFERENTIAL FEATURES OF CONDUCTIVE AND SENSORINEURAL HEARING LOSS

Conductive Hearing Loss	Sensorineural Hearing Loss
CAUSES	
Cerumen Foreign body Perforation of the tympanic membrane Edema Infection of the external or middle ear Tumors Otosclerosis	Prolonged exposure to noise Presbycusis Ototoxic substances Meniere's disease Acoustic neuroma Diabetes mellitus Labyrinthitis Infection Myxedema
ASSESSMENT FINDINGS	
Evidence of obstruction with otoscope Abnormality in tympanic membrane Speaking softly Hearing best in a noisy environment Rinne test: air conduction greater than bone conduction Weber test: lateralization to affected ear	Normal appearance of external canal and tympanic membrane Tinnitus common Occasional dizziness Speaking loudly Hearing poorly in loud environment Rinne test: air conduction less than bone conduction Weber test: lateralization to unaffected ear

Incidence/Prevalence

Because hearing loss may be gradual and affect only some aspects of hearing, many adults are unaware that their hearing is impaired. The actual incidence of hearing loss is not known exactly; however, approximately 30% to 35% of people ages 65 to 75 years have a hearing loss, and as many as half of the people older than 85 years of age have some degree of hearing loss (National Institute on Deafness and Other Communications Disorders).

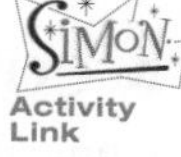

➤ COLLABORATIVE MANAGEMENT

• Assessment

HISTORY

The nurse asks clients how long they have noticed a difference in their hearing and whether the changes occurred suddenly or gradually. Age is an important factor, because some ear and hearing changes occur with advanced age; also, chronic otitis media is diagnosed more often in the older adult. The nurse notes occupational exposure to loud or continuous noises, as well as current or previous use of ototoxic drugs. Clients are also asked about any history of external-ear or middle-ear infection and whether tympanic membrane perforation accompanied the infection. The nurse questions clients about any history of direct trauma to the ears. Because some types of hearing loss have a genetic predisposi-

EVIDENCE-BASED PRACTICE FOR NURSING

Can dietary modification reduce age-related hearing loss?

Houston, D., et al. (1999). Age-related hearing loss, vitamin B-12, and folate in elderly women. *American Journal of Clinical Nutrition, 69*(3), 564-571.

The authors undertook this study to examine possible causes of presbycusis, or age-related hearing loss. As the title suggests, the hypothesis was that deficiencies in vitamin B_{12} and folate might play a role in the hearing loss so common in older adults. For analysis, subjects were recruited and included or excluded depending on criteria that suggested they either had or could have hearing loss due to specific causes such as infections, ototoxicity, trauma, or conductive hearing loss. Data collections included blood counts, hematologic measures, and serum tests for hepatic, renal, and thyroid function. In addition, serum vitamin B_{12}, red blood cell folate, and serum folate levels were determined. Auditory examinations were conducted, and hearing function was categorized using criteria similar to those of the National Health and Nutrition Examination Survey. Correlation coefficients and chi-square analysis were used for analysis demonstrating poor vitamin B_{12} and folate status associated with greater hearing loss.

Critique. The investigators used a very complex methodology to examine this question. Much was done to ensure close control over the variables. This study was conducted with a larger study examining bone health and auditory functioning and included only white women ages 60-71 years. These demographics limit generalization of the findings, but the notion of a vitamin deficiency leading to age-related hearing loss is unique.

Implications for Nursing. Nurses are educated to pay attention to the nutritional status of clients. This study suggests an additional reason for the importance of proper nutrition. Although serum vitamin and red blood cell folate levels are not measured often in general practice, the nurse can become an advocate for instituting supportive nutrition when necessary.

tion, the nurse asks whether any family members are hearing impaired.

When pain accompanies acute-onset hearing loss, the nurse asks about recent upper respiratory tract infection and possible allergies affecting the upper respiratory system.

PHYSICAL ASSESSMENT/CLINICAL MANIFESTATIONS

Chart 49-5 presents focused assessment techniques for clients with suspected hearing loss. Hearing loss may be sudden or gradual and is often bilateral. The ability to hear high-frequency soft, discriminating consonants—especially *s, sh, f, th,* and *ch* sounds—is lost first. Clients often state that they have no problem with hearing but cannot understand specific words. They might think that the speaker is mumbling. They often experience high-pitched, continuous bilateral tinnitus. Vertigo may be present, depending on the extent of inner-ear involvement.

TUNING FORK TESTS. Tuning fork tests help diagnose hearing loss (see Chapter 48). With the Weber test, the client can usually hear sounds well in the ear with a suspected conductive hearing loss because of the preserved bone conduction. With the Rinne test, the client reports that sound transmitted by bone conduction is louder and more sustained than that transmitted by air conduction.

OTOSCOPIC EXAMINATION. The nurse performs an otoscopic examination to assess the external auditory canal,

CHART 49-5

FOCUSED ASSESSMENT *of* The Client with Suspected Hearing Loss

Assess whether the client has any of the following ear complaints:
- Pain
- Feeling of fullness or congestion
- Dizziness or vertigo
- Tinnitus
- Difficulty understanding conversations, especially in a noisy room
- Difficulty hearing sounds
- Needing to strain to hear
- Needing to turn the head to favor one ear or needing to lean forward to hear

Assess visible ear structures, particularly the external canal and tympanic membrane:
- Position and size of the pinna
- Patency of the external canal; presence of cerumen or foreign bodies, edema, or inflammation
- Condition of the tympanic membrane: intact, edema, fluid, inflammation

Assess functional ability, including:
- Frequency of asking people to repeat statements
- Withdrawal from social interactions or large groups
- Shouting in conversation
- Failing to respond when not looking in the direction of the sound
- Answering questions incorrectly

the tympanic membrane, and structures of the middle ear visible through the tympanic membrane (see Chapter 48). Physical findings from examination vary, depending on the cause of the hearing loss.

Obstruction of the external auditory canal can result in hearing loss. The nurse inspects the canal and notes the following:
- Whether the canal is open
- The amount and character of cerumen present
- The integrity of the skin lining the canal
- The presence of redness, exudates, lesions, or foreign objects

Middle-ear infections can also diminish hearing. In infection or inflammation, the tympanic membrane appears red, thickened, and bulging, with a loss of landmarks. Loss of mobility of the membrane is evident with inspection through a pneumatic otoscope. The nurse notes the presence of any scars or perforations on the tympanic membrane. With close observation, the nurse may be able to see exudate behind the membrane.

PSYCHOSOCIAL ASSESSMENT

For persons with a hearing loss, communication can become a struggle, and they may isolate themselves because of the difficulty in talking and listening. Social isolation can lead to depression, fear, and despair. The nurse is sensitive to emotional changes that may be related to reduced hearing and a decline in conversational skills.

LABORATORY ASSESSMENT

No laboratory tests can definitively diagnose hearing loss. However, some laboratory findings can indicate pathologic problems that might affect hearing.

White blood cell counts are elevated in the client with acute or chronic otitis media. Microbial culture and antibiotic sensitivity tests can determine the causative organism and the most appropriate antibiotic therapy when infection causes hearing loss.

The client with hearing loss associated with peripheral neuropathy may have other systemic diseases, including poorly controlled diabetes mellitus. The fasting blood glucose level may be elevated, and the blood, even when diluted, may be positive for serum acetone.

RADIOGRAPHIC ASSESSMENT

Radiographic assessment can determine nonauditory problems affecting hearing ability. Some auditory problems can be diagnosed using radiographic techniques: skull x-ray films to determine bony involvement in otitis media and the location of otosclerotic lesions, and computed tomography (CT) and magnetic resonance imaging (MRI) to determine soft-tissue involvement and the presence and location of tumors.

OTHER DIAGNOSTIC ASSESSMENT

Audiometry can assist in the diagnosis and determine the extent and type of hearing loss. An audiogram shows whether hearing loss is only conductive or whether it has a sensorineural component. This is important in determining possible causes of the hearing loss and in planning appropriate interventions.

CRITICAL THINKING CHALLENGE

You are assigned treatment of an 85-year-old woman who is admitted for congestive heart failure, hypertension, type 2 diabetes mellitus, and degenerative joint disease with a history of bilateral hip replacements. She reports that she has been losing some of her hearing for the past few years, but that since being admitted to the hospital her hearing has become much worse.

- What physical assessment findings are needed to gain additional information?
- Considering the woman's admitting diagnoses, what factors associated with treatment of these other disorders may play a role in her hearing loss?

For suggested answer guidelines, go to SIMON http://www.wbsaunders.com/SIMON/Iggy/.

Analysis

COMMON NURSING DIAGNOSES AND COLLABORATIVE PROBLEMS

The following are common nursing diagnoses for clients with any degree of hearing impairment:

1. Disturbed Sensory Perception (Auditory) related to obstruction, infection, damage to the middle ear, or damage to the auditory nerve
2. Anxiety related to an inability to communicate

ADDITIONAL NURSING DIAGNOSES AND COLLABORATIVE PROBLEMS

In addition to the common nursing diagnoses, clients with hearing loss or impairment may have one or more of the following:

- Deficient Knowledge related to treatment and prevention
- Activity Intolerance related to pain
- Social Isolation related to pain and decreased hearing
- Risk for Injury related to altered auditory perception and infection
- Acute Pain related to an inflammatory process and fluid in the middle ear
- Impaired Physical Mobility related to vertigo

Planning and Implementation

DISTURBED SENSORY PERCEPTION (AUDITORY)

PLANNING: EXPECTED OUTCOMES. The client with hearing loss or impairment is expected to either experience an increase in auditory sensory perception to a functional level or maintain existing levels of hearing.

INTERVENTIONS. Interventions aim at identifying the problem, halting the pathologic processes, and improving auditory sensory perception.

NIC **EAR CARE.** For most people, hearing is accepted as an important factor in social interactions and to gain knowledge. With special care to the ears, hearing can be preserved at maximal levels (Chart 49-6).

NONSURGICAL MANAGEMENT. Nonsurgical interventions include early detection of hearing impairment, use of drug therapy and comfort measures, and use of assistive devices to amplify or augment the client's auditory perception.

CHART 49-6

NIC INTERVENTION ACTIVITIES *for* Care of the Ears

Ear Care: *Prevention or minimization of threats to ear or hearing*

- Monitor for drainage from ears, as appropriate.
- Irrigate the ear, as appropriate.
- Avoid placing sharp objects in the ear.
- Administer eardrops, as appropriate.
- Explain the relationship between balance and the inner ear, as appropriate.
- Monitor for episodes of dizziness associated with ear problems, as appropriate.
- Determine if cerumen in the ear canal is causing pain or hearing loss.
- Instill mineral oil in the ear to soften impacted cerumen before irrigation.
- Irrigate the ear canal with a Water Pik (or similar device) on low setting using warm water (80° to 90° F), as appropriate.
- Demonstrate proper technique for ear irrigation to caregiver, as appropriate.
- Monitor frequency of ear infections.
- Instruct how to monitor and regulate high-volume noise exposure.
- Instruct client to wear hearing protection for exposure to high-intensity noise.
- Instruct client concerning the potential danger of exposure to high-volume music, especially with headphones.
- Instruct client with pierced ears how to avoid infection at the insertion site.
- Encourage use of earplugs for swimming, if client is susceptible to ear infections.

NIC intervention activities selected from McCloskey, J.C., & Bulechek, G.M. (Eds.). (2000). *Nursing interventions classification (NIC)* (3rd ed.). St. Louis: Mosby.

EARLY DETECTION. Early detection helps correct the problem causing the hearing loss. When hearing loss is gradual, the client can compensate. The nurse assesses for indications of hearing loss, as listed in Chart 49-6.

DRUG THERAPY. Drug therapy is aimed at either correcting the underlying pathologic change or reducing the side effects of disorders associated with hearing loss. Local (topical) antibiotics are administered to clients with external otitis. Systemic antibiotics are necessary when clients have other auditory infections. By treating the infection, antibiotics resolve local edema and improve hearing. When pain accompanies hearing disorders, local or systemic analgesics are often used, depending on the type and location of the pain. Many ear disorders disturb equilibrium, causing vertigo and dizziness with nausea and vomiting. Antiemetic, antihistamine, antivertiginous, and benzodiazepine drugs can help correct nausea, vertigo, and dizziness.

ASSISTIVE DEVICES. Many devices are useful for clients with permanent, progressive hearing loss. Telephone amplifiers increase telephone volume, allowing the caller to speak in a normal voice. Flashing lights activated by the ringing telephone or doorbell alert clients visually. In some cases, clients may be referred for the use of a specially trained dog to help them be aware of sounds (ringing telephones or doorbells, cries of other people, and potential dangers), in much the same way that a seeing eye dog assists a blind person.

Small, portable audio amplifiers can assist the nurse in communicating with clients experiencing hearing loss but who have chosen not to use a hearing aid. The use of audio amplifiers or allowing clients to use a stethoscope helps nurses to communicate with elders and others who require additional volume to hear speech.

Hearing Aids. A hearing aid is a miniature electronic amplifier that is usually used for clients with conductive hearing loss. Hearing aids are less effective for sensorineural hearing loss and may make functional hearing worse by amplifying background noise. The amplifier can be worn in one or both ears. Local agencies offer special rehabilitation classes for the hearing impaired that will help the wearer obtain the most benefit from this device.

The nurse offers some special tips to help the client adjust to the hearing aid. Hearing with a hearing aid can be different from natural hearing. The client is encouraged to start using the hearing aid slowly, initially wearing it only at home and only during part of the day. Listening to television and the radio and reading aloud can help the client get used to new sounds. The tone or volume of the hearing aid can be adjusted. The most important and difficult aspect of a hearing aid is the amplification of background noise, as well as voices. The client must learn to concentrate and filter out background noises.

The client must also learn to care for the hearing aid (Chart 49-7). Hearing aids are delicate electronic devices that should be handled only by people who know how to care for them properly. The cost of the aids varies greatly but represents a significant investment.

Cochlear Implants. Cochlear implantation may help clients with sensorineural hearing loss. A small computer converts sound waves into electronic impulses. Electrodes are placed by the internal ear, with the computer attached to the external ear. The electronic impulses then directly stimulate nerve fibers. Some clients have a 50% return of their hearing with this method.

SURGICAL MANAGEMENT. Many surgical interventions are available for clients with specific disorders leading to hearing loss.

TYMPANOPLASTY. Tympanoplasty reconstructs the middle ear to improve hearing caused by conductive hearing loss. The procedures vary from simple reconstruction of the tympanic membrane **(myringoplasty)** to replacement of the ossicles within the middle ear. A type I tympanoplasty is used for a myringoplasty; a type II tympanoplasty is used in cases of greater damage and to provide more extensive reconstruction (Figure 49-8).

Preoperative Care. The nurse gives specific instructions to the client scheduled for a tympanoplasty. Systemic antibiotics reduce the numbers of infecting organisms. Before surgery, the nurse irrigates the ear with a solution of equal parts of vinegar and sterile water to restore normal ear pH. The client follows other measures to decrease the chances of postoperative infection, such as avoiding people with upper respiratory tract infections, getting adequate rest, eating a balanced diet, and maintaining an adequate fluid intake.

The nurse assures the client that initial hearing loss after surgery is normal because of the packing in the canal, and that hearing will improve on packing removal. The nurse explains the importance of deep breathing and coughing postoperatively but emphasizes that forceful coughing increases pressure in the middle ear and must be avoided.

Operative Procedure. Surgical treatment is performed only if the middle ear is free of infection and if the condition of the eustachian tube does not promote continued infection. If an infection is present, the graft is more likely to become infected and not heal properly. Surgery of the tympanic membrane and

CHART 49-7

CLIENT EDUCATION GUIDE
Hearing Aid Care

- Keep the hearing aid dry.
- Clean the ear mold with mild soap and water while avoiding excessive wetting.
- Clean debris from the hole in the middle of the part that goes into your ear with a toothpick or a pipe cleaner.
- Turn off the hearing aid and remove the battery when not in use.
- Check and replace the battery frequently.
- Keep extra batteries on hand.
- Keep the hearing aid in a safe place.
- Avoid dropping the hearing aid or exposing it to temperature extremes.
- Adjust the volume to the lowest setting that allows you to hear, to prevent feedback squeaking.
- Avoid using hair spray, cosmetics, oils, or other hair and face products that might come into contact with the receiver.
- If the hearing aid does not work:
  - Change the battery.
  - Check the connection between the ear mold and the receiver.
  - Check the on/off switch.
  - Clean the sound hole.
  - Adjust the volume.
  - Take the hearing aid to an authorized service center for repair.

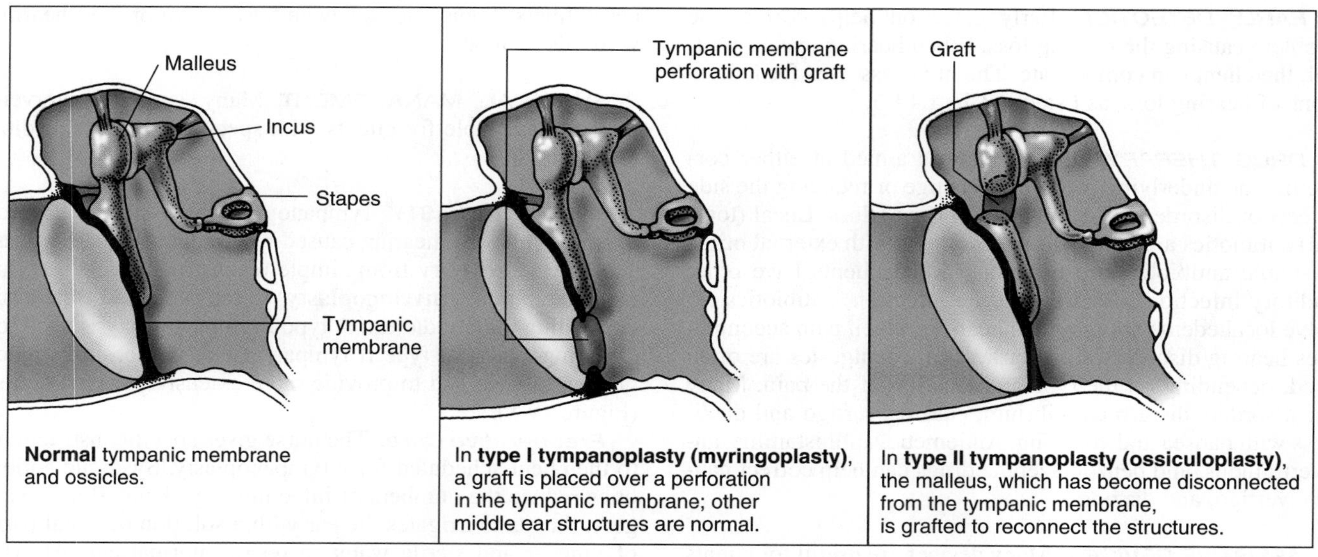

Normal tympanic membrane and ossicles.

In **type I tympanoplasty (myringoplasty)**, a graft is placed over a perforation in the tympanic membrane; other middle ear structures are normal.

In **type II tympanoplasty (ossiculoplasty)**, the malleus, which has become disconnected from the tympanic membrane, is grafted to reconnect the structures.

Figure 49-8 ● A normal tympanic membrane and two types of tympanoplasties.

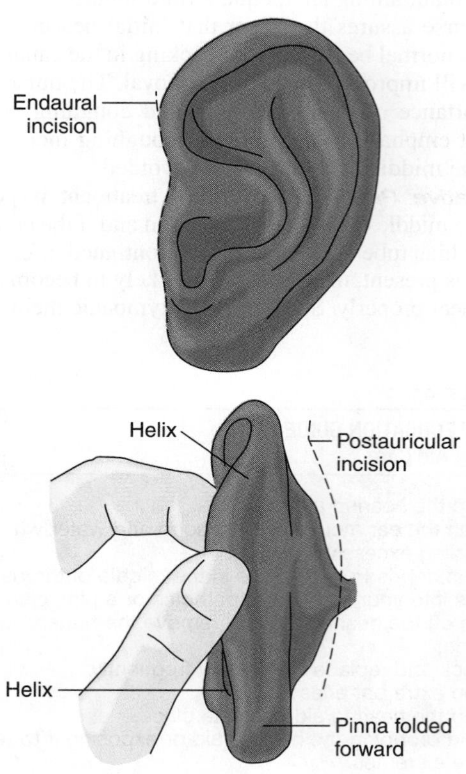

Figure 49-9 ● Surgical approaches for the ear. The endaural approach is used when the external canal is too small to use for a transcanal approach (not shown because no external incision is used). The postauricular approach is used for more extensive repair of the middle-ear and inner-ear structures.

ossicles requires the use of a microscope and is a delicate procedure. Local anesthesia can be used, although general anesthesia is often chosen to prevent the client from moving.

The surgeon can repair the tympanic membrane with a variety of materials, including temporal muscle fascia, a split-thickness skin graft, and venous tissue. If the ossicles are damaged, more extensive measures must be taken to repair or replace them. The surgeon reaches the ossicles via a transcanal approach, an endaural incision, or the postauricular route with a mastoidectomy (Figure 49-9).

The surgeon then removes diseased tissue and cleans the middle-ear cavity. The ossicles are assessed for damage and the extent to which repair or replacement is necessary. The surgeon uses autogenous cartilage or bone, cadaver ossicles, stainless steel wire, or polytetrafluoroethylene (Teflon) to repair or replace the ossicles.

Postoperative Care. An antiseptic-soaked gauze, such as iodoform gauze (Nu Gauze), is packed in the auditory canal. If the postauricular or endaural incision is used, an external dressing is placed over the operative site. Dressings are kept clean and dry, and the nurse uses sterile technique when changing them. The client is kept flat, with the head turned to the side and the operative ear facing up for at least 12 hours postoperatively. Antibiotic therapy is used to prevent infections from recurring.

Clients generally report hearing improvement after the canal packing is removed. Until that time, the nurse communicates as with a hearing-impaired client, directing conversation to the unaffected ear. The nurse also instructs the client in postoperative care and activity restrictions (see Chart 49-4).

STAPEDECTOMY. A partial or complete stapedectomy with a prosthesis effectively corrects hearing loss. This procedure is most effective for clients with hearing loss related to otosclerosis.

Preoperative Care. To prevent the introduction of infective material to the middle-ear structures, no signs or symptoms of external otitis can be present at surgery. The nurse instructs the client to follow measures that prevent middle-ear or external-ear infections (Chart 49-8).

The nurse reviews the expected outcomes and possible complications of the surgery. Hearing is initially worse after a stapedectomy. The success rate of this procedure is high; however, as with all ear procedures, it carries a risk of failure

CHART 49-8

CLIENT EDUCATION GUIDE
Prevention of Ear Infection or Trauma

- Do not use small objects, such as cotton-tipped applicators, matches, toothpicks, or hairpins, to clean your external ear canal.
- Wash your external ear and canal daily in the shower or while washing your hair.
- Blow your nose gently.
- Do not occlude one nostril while blowing your nose.
- Sneeze with your mouth open.
- Wear sound protection around loud or continuous noises.
- Avoid activities with high risk for head or ear trauma, such as wrestling, boxing, motorcycle riding, and skateboarding.
- Wear head and ear protection when engaging in these activities.
- Keep the volume on head receivers at the lowest setting that allows you to hear.
- Frequently clean objects that come into contact with your ear (headphones, telephone receivers, and so on).
- Avoid environmental conditions with rapid changes in air pressure.

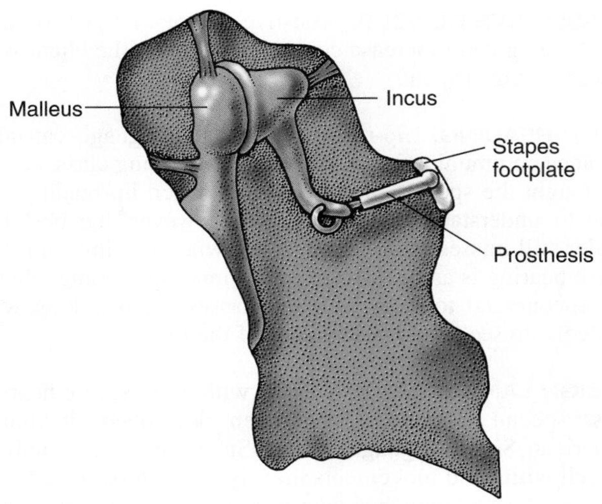

Figure 49-10 ● Prosthesis used with stapedectomy. The stapes is removed, leaving the footplate. After a hole is drilled in the footplate, a metal or plastic prosthesis is connected to the incus and inserted through the hole to act as a vibration device, much as the stapes worked before the development of otosclerosis.

that might lead to total deafness on the affected side. Other possible complications include prolonged vertigo, infection, and facial nerve damage. A decision to proceed with surgery should be made with the client's full knowledge and understanding of these complications.

Operative Procedure. A stapedectomy is usually performed through the external auditory canal with the client under local anesthesia. The head and neck of the stapes and, less often, the footplate are removed. After removal of the immobile bone, a small hole is drilled in the footplate; a metal or plastic prosthesis in the shape of a piston is connected between the incus and the footplate (Figure 49-10). Sounds cause the prosthesis to vibrate as the stapes did. After stapedectomy, up to 90% of clients experience restoration of practical hearing.

Postoperative Care. The nurse informs the client that noticeable improvement in hearing may not occur until 6 weeks after surgery. Initially, the ear packing interferes with hearing. Postoperative swelling in the ear continues to affect hearing until the edema has resolved. Medications for pain help reduce discomfort, and antibiotics are given to reduce the risk for infection at the surgical site. The nurse instructs the client to follow the postoperative procedures in Chart 49-4.

The surgical procedure is performed in an area where cranial nerves VII, VIII, and X might be damaged by direct trauma or by postoperative swelling. The nurse observes for complications of surgery by assessing for facial nerve damage or muscle weakness and changes in tactile sensation or taste. Vertigo, nausea, and vomiting are common complaints because of the proximity to inner-ear structures.

Antivertiginous drugs, such as meclizine hydrochloride (Antivert, Bonamine♣), and antiemetic medications, such as droperidol (Inapsine), are given. Care is taken to prevent injury, especially during times of increased vertigo. The nurse assists the client with ambulating during the first 1 to 2 days after surgery. Siderails on the bed are kept up, and the nurse reminds the client to move the head slowly when changing position, to avoid vertigo.

CHART 49-9

BEST PRACTICE *for*
Communicating with a Hearing-Impaired Client

- Position yourself directly in front of the client.
- Make sure that the room is well lighted.
- Get the client's attention before you begin to speak.
- Move closer to the better-hearing ear.
- Speak clearly and slowly.
- Do not shout (shouting raises the frequency of the sound and often makes understanding more difficult).
- Keep hands and other objects away from your mouth when talking to the client.
- Attempt to have conversations in a quiet room with minimal distractions.
- Have the client repeat your statements rather than just indicating assent.
- Rephrase sentences and repeat information to aid in understanding.
- Use appropriate hand motions.
- Write messages on paper if the client is able to read.

ANXIETY

PLANNING: EXPECTED OUTCOMES. The client with hearing loss or impairment is expected to state that anxiety about communication is reduced and become proficient in alternative communication techniques.

INTERVENTIONS. Interventions focus on facilitating communication and reducing anxiety.

Best practices for communicating with a hearing-impaired client are listed in Chart 49-9. Shouting to the client is of little benefit, because the sound may be projected at a higher frequency, making him or her less able to understand. The most obvious means of communicating with such a client is by the written word (if he or she is able to see, read, and write) or with pictures of familiar phrases and objects. Many television programs are now closed captioned (subtitled) for the hearing impaired.

ASSISTIVE DEVICES. Assistive devices, described on p. 1073, can greatly increase communication for the client with a hearing impairment.

LIP-READING. Lip-reading and sign language can also enhance communication. In a formal lip-reading class, clients are taught the special cues to look for when lip-reading and how to understand body language. However, the best lip-reader still misses more than 50% of what is being said. Because hearing is assisted by even minimal lip-reading, clients are encouraged to wear their eyeglasses when talking with someone to see subtle movements of the lips.

SIGN LANGUAGE. For clients with more severe hearing loss, special languages have been developed, including American Sign Language (ASL). Such languages combine speech with hand movements that signify letters, words, and phrases. These languages take time and effort to learn, and many people are unable to learn them, just as many people cannot learn foreign languages. However, as the hearing-impaired person become less able to function, motivation to learn may increase.

MANAGING ANXIETY. A major source of anxiety is the possibility of permanent hearing loss. The nurse provides honest and accurate information about the likelihood of hearing returning. When the hearing impairment is likely to be permanent or become more profound, the nurse reassures clients that communication and social interaction can be maintained.

To reduce anxiety and prevent social isolation, clients use remaining resources to make social contact satisfying. The most obvious way to decrease social isolation is by improving communication (as previously described). The nurse asks about past or present diversional activities to identify the client's most satisfying activities and social interactions and determine the amount of effort necessary to continue them. Activities can be altered to maximize client satisfaction. Someone accustomed to large gatherings might choose smaller groups instead. A quiet evening meal at home with friends might substitute for dinner in a noisy restaurant.

Community-Based Care

Lengthy hospitalization is rare for most clients with ear and hearing disorders. If surgical repair is necessary and the procedure is completed without complications, the procedure may be completed as an outpatient or the hospital stay is usually only a day.

HEALTH TEACHING

The nurse gives clients written instructions about how to take medications and when to return for follow-up care. If the client cannot read, the nurse gives these instructions to a family member who may assist with care. The nurse teaches clients how to instill eardrops (see Chart 49-1) and irrigate the ears (see Chart 49-2), and asks for a return demonstration.

To promote health and prevent late postoperative infections, clients are instructed to follow the suggestions in Chart 49-8. For clients who use a hearing aid, the nurse teaches them how to use it effectively.

COST OF CARE IMPLICATIONS FOR NURSING

HEARING LOSS

Cost of Care

- The cost of assistive devices for hearing-impaired individuals can be staggering.
- Hearing aids are available in a variety of styles and vary greatly, depending on the style and circuitry options available. Prices for hearing aids range from $700 to $2400 for one device, with the cost doubling if two devices are needed.
- Batteries for hearing aids must be changed as often as every few days to once a week, depending on the volume settings. Batteries cost about $1 to $2 per battery, depending on how many are purchased at the same time.
- Telephone devices for the deaf (TDD) also vary in cost and options. These devices cost from $300 to $600 per unit. Portable amplifiers cost approximately $25.
- In addition to the cost of hearing aids and telephone devices, there are a variety of devices that are needed to either improve the quality of life for hearing-impaired individuals or aid in their safety needs. Examples include alert systems, doorbells, baby alarms, fire alarms, and alarm clocks. A special alarm clock called the Sonic Boom cost $90. Complete security systems for hearing-impaired individuals range from $377 to $775.

Implications for Nursing

People with severe hearing loss require devices that people with normal hearing would never need. Hearing aids are generally used by the individual at all times when he or she is awake. However, they are removed at night for sleeping, and given their small size, these devices can be easily misplaced or broken if care is not taken to secure them in the institutional setting. Nurses need to familiarize themselves with how to replace batteries and how to turn hearing aids on and off to preserve battery life.

Data from Department of Speech and Communication Disorders, Audiology Section, University of Northern Colorado, Greeley, CO.

HOME CARE MANAGEMENT

Clients who experience persistent vertigo, either in association with the disorder or as a side effect of surgery, remain in danger of falling. The home must therefore be assessed for potential hazards and to determine whether family members or significant others are available to assist with meal preparation and other activities of daily living. A nurse case manager can, in collaboration with the home care nurse, assist clients and their families in determining the best ways to maintain adequate self-care abilities, maintain a safe environment, decide about assistance needs, and provide needed care.

HEALTH CARE RESOURCES

If clients do not have family or friends to help during the postoperative period, a referral to a home care agency is necessary. Assistance with meal preparation, cleaning, and personal hygiene can be contracted for with the hospital discharge planners.

Follow-up hearing tests are scheduled for clients when the lesions are well healed, in about 6 to 8 weeks. Audiograms done before and after treatment are compared, and evaluation for further intervention to improve hearing begins. A complication of an unsuccessful surgery is continued disability or complete loss of hearing in the affected ear. Surgery is performed on the ear with the greatest hearing loss. If the surgery does not improve hearing, clients

TABLE 49-3 • AGENCIES OFFERING SERVICES FOR EAR AND HEARING DISORDERS

HOUSE EAR INSTITUTE
2100 West Third Street, Fifth Floor
Los Angeles, CA 90057
Voice: (800) 352-8888
TTY: (213) 484-2642
Internet: http://www.hei.org

NATIONAL INFORMATION CENTER ON DEAFNESS
Gallaudet University
800 Florida Avenue NE
Washington, DC 20002
Voice: (202) 651-5051
TTY: (202) 651-5000
E-mail: nidc@gallux.gallaudet.edu
Internet: http://www.gallaudet.edu

AMERICAN ACADEMY OF OTOLARYNGOLOGY/HEAD AND NECK SURGERY
One Prince Street
Alexandria, VA 22314
Voice: (703) 519-1589
TTY: (703) 836-4444
Internet: http://www.entnet.org

AMERICAN SPEECH-LANGUAGE-HEARING ASSOCIATION
10801 Rockville Pike
Rockville, MD 20852
Voice/TTY: (301) 897-5700
Voice: (800) 638-8255
Internet: http://www.asha.org

SELF HELP FOR HARD OF HEARING PEOPLE, INC. (SHHH)
7910 Woodmont Avenue, Suite 1200
Bethesda, MD 20814
Voice: (301) 657-2248
TTY: (301) 657-2249
Fax: (301) 913-9413
Internet: http://www.shhh.org

must decide to either attempt surgical correction of the other ear or continue to use an amplification device. When the underlying disorder causing the hearing impairment is progressive, this decision is difficult. The nurse supports clients by listening to their concerns and giving additional information when needed.

Costs to the individual with a hearing impairment can be extensive (see the Cost of Care box on p. 1076). Information and support can come from several organizations that publish informative articles to help clients reduce hearing loss (Table 49-3). Many public and private institutions offer hearing evaluations, as well as supplying information and counseling for clients with hearing disorders.

Evaluation: Outcomes

NOC The nurse evaluates the care of the client with hearing loss or impairment on the basis of the identified nursing diagnoses and collaborative problems. The expected outcomes include that the client will:

- State that the hearing is at least partially improved
- State that anxiety is reduced
- Demonstrate proper technique for using assistive devices
- Identify potential postoperative hazards
- State the importance of follow-up hearing assessments
- Be able to communicate effectively with family, friends, co-workers, and health care professionals
- Have receptive ability for communication
- Acknowledge messages received
- Maintain satisfactory social contacts
- State that the pain is reduced or alleviated
- Describe the proper use of antibiotic therapy
- Demonstrate proper techniques when using eardrops, ointments, powders, or irrigation liquids
- Identify and avoid potential causes of otitis media
- Seek assistance with activities of daily living until vertigo and dizziness have subsided

ONLINE RESOURCES

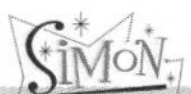

For suggested readings and Internet resources, go to http://www.wbsaunders.com/SIMON/Iggy/.

SELECTED BIBLIOGRAPHY

Asterisk indicates a classic or definitive work on this subject.

Bagley, M. (1998). Helping older adults to live better with hearing and vision losses. *Journal of Case Management, 7*(4), 147-152.

Baloh, R. (1998a). *Dizziness, hearing loss, and tinnitus.* Philadelphia: F.A. Davis.

Baloh, R. (1998b). Dizzy patients: The varieties of vertigo. *Hospital Practice, 33*(6), 55-63.

Barry, B., et al. (1999). Otogenic intracranial infections in adults. *Laryngoscope, 109*(3), 483-487.

Bellenir, K., & Shin, L. (1998). *Ear, nose, and throat disorders sourcebook.* Detroit: Omnigraphics.

Berger, M. (Ed.). (1998). *Ear, nose and throat disorders.* Philadelphia: W.B. Saunders.

Billue, J. (1998). Subjective idiopathic tinnitus. *Clinical Excellence for Nurse Practitioners, 2*(2), 73-82.

Bumby, A., & Stephens, S. (1997). Clonazepam in the treatment of tinnitus—A pilot study. *Journal of Audiological Medicine, 6*(2), 98-104.

Cavendish, R. (1998). Clinical snapshot: Adult hearing loss. *American Journal of Nursing, 98*(8), 50-51.

Chaimoff, M., et al. (1999). Sudden hearing loss as a presenting symptom of acoustic neuroma. *American Journal of Otolaryngology, 20*(3), 157-160.

*Clinical guidelines: Adult screening for hearing. (1996). *Nurse Practitioner, 21*(6), 106, 108, 115.

Cook, R. (1998). Ear syringing. *Nursing Standard, 13*(13-15), 56-61.

de la Cruz, M., & Bance, M. (1999). Carbamazepine-induced sensorineural hearing loss. *Archives of Otolaryngology–Head and Neck Surgery, 125*(2), 225-227.

Dhillon, R., & East, C. (1999). *Ear, nose, and throat, and head and neck surgery: An illustrated colour text.* New York: Churchill Livingstone.

Doyle, W., et al. (1999). Illness and otological changes during upper respiratory virus infection. *Laryngoscopy, 109*(2), 324-328.

Erber, N., Holland, J., & Osborn, R. (1998). Communicating with elders: Effects of speaker-listener distance. *British Society of Audiology, 32*(3), 135-138.

Flatau, E., et al. (1998). Hearing impairment in residents of a long-term care facility: Prevalence and relationship to cognitive dysfunction. *Annals of Long Term Care, 6*(13), 410-413.

Garstecki, D., & Erler, S. (1998). Hearing and aging. *Topics in Geriatric Rehabilitation, 14*(2), 1-17.

Gates, G., Couropmitree, N, & Myers, R. (1999). Genetic association in age-related hearing thresholds. *Archives in Otolaryngology–Head and Neck Surgery, 125*(6), 654-659.

Gelfand, S. (1998). *Hearing: An introduction to psychological and physiological acoustics* (3rd ed.). New York : Marcel Dekker.

Hagnebo, C., et al. (1997). The influence of vertigo, hearing impairment and tinnitus on the daily life of Meniere's patients. *Scandinavian Audiology, 26*(2), 69-76.

Heath, H. (1997). Sensory function in older people. *Community Nurse, 3*(11), 13-14.

Herdman, S. (1997). Advances in the treatment of vestibular disorders. *Physical Therapy, 77*(6), 602-618.

Hope, B. (1999). Create sensitivity to the elderly's sensory changes. *Homecare Education Management, 2*, 26-27.

Houston, D., et al. (1999). Age-related hearing loss, vitamin B-12, and folate in elderly women. *American Journal of Clinical Nutrition, 69*(3), 564-571.

Hsu, R., & Levine, S. (1998). Sudden hearing loss: How to identify the cause promptly. *Consultant, 38*(1), 23-26.

Kaufman, G. (1998). Ear problems: Care and prevention. *Practice Nurse, 15*(6), 338-342.

Kendrick, J. (1997). New strategies for hearing protection. *Occupational Health and Safety, 66*(10), 134-138.

Kujdychy, N. (1999). Prescribing trends in the treatment of acute otitis media. *ADVANCE for Nurse Practitioners, 7*(8), 30-35.

LaRosa, S. (1998). Primary care management of otitis externa. *Nurse Practitioner, 23*(6), 125-128.

Larsen, P., Hazen, S., & Martin, J. (1997). Assessment and management of sensory loss in elderly patients. *AORN Journal, 65*(2), 432-437.

Leblanc, A. (1999). *Atlas of hearing and balance organs : a practical guide for otolaryngologists.* New York: Springer.

Lorentine, M., et al. (1998). On the behavioral characteristics of loud-music listening. *Ear and Hearing, 19*(6), 420-428.

Lucas, L., & Matthews-Flint, L. (2001). Sound advice about hearing aids. *Nursing2001, 31*(2), 59-61.

Lucente, F., & Har-El, G. (1999). *Essentials of otolaryngology* (4th ed.). Philadelphia: Lippincott, Williams, & Wilkins.

Ludman, H., & Wright, T. (1998). *Diseases of the ear* (3rd ed.). New York: Oxford University Press.

Lusk, S. (1997). Noise exposures. *AAOHN Journal, 45*(8), 397-409.

Luxon, L. (1998). Disorders of hearing and balance. *Reviews in Clinical Gerontology, 8*(1), 31-43.

Martin, R. (1998). Nuts and bolts: What to do when the patient "can't understand the words." *Hearing Journal, 51*(6), 70-72.

Mostafapour, S., Lahargoue, K., & Gates, G. (1998). Noise-induced hearing loss in young adults: The role of personal listening devices and other sources of leisure noise. *Laryngoscope, 108*(12), 1832-1839.

National Council on the Aging. (2000). The consequences of untreated hearing loss in older persons. *ORL–Head and Neck Nursing, 18*(1), 12-16.

National Institute on Deafness and Other Communication Disorders. (1999). What is presbycusis? NIH Pub. No. 97-4233; http://www.nidcd.nih.gov/.

Noorhassin, I., & Rampal, K. (1998). Multiplicative effect of smoking and age on hearing impairment. *American Journal of Otolaryngology, 19*(4), 240-243.

Nusbaum, N. (1999). Aging and sensory senescence. *Southern Medical Journal, 92*(3), 267-275. Also available at http://www.medscape.com/SMA/SMJ/1999/v92.n03/smj9203.02.nusb/smj9203.02.nusb-01.html.

Ramsay, H., Karkainen, J., & Palva, T. (1997). Success in surgery for otosclerosis: Hearing improvement and other indicators. *American Journal of Otolaryngology, 18*(1), 23-28.

*Ross, V., Echevarria, K., & Robinson, B. (1991). Geriatric tinnitus: Causes, clinical treatment, and prevention. *Journal of Gerontological Nursing, 17*(10), 6-11.

Sanna, M. (1999). *Color atlas of otoscopy: From diagnosis to surgery.* New York: Thieme.

Shaw, L. (1997). Protocol for detection and follow-up of hearing loss. *Clinical Nurse Specialist, 11*(6), 240-247.

Sheehan, J. (2000). Caring for the deaf: Do you do enough? *RN, 63*(3), 69-72.

Silverstein, H., et al. (1999). Direct round window membrane application of gentamicin in the treatment of Meniere's disease. *Archives of Otolaryngology–Head and Neck Surgery, 120*(5), 649-655.

Simpson, J., Donaldson, I., & Davies, W. (1998). Use of homeopathy in the treatment of tinnitus. *British Journal of Audiology, 32*(4), 227-233.

Singhal, S., et al. (1999). Genetic correlation in otosclerosis. *American Journal of Otolaryngology, 20*(2), 102-105.

Stone, C. (1999). Preventing cerumen impaction in nursing facility residents. *Journal of Gerontological Nursing, 25*(5), 43-45.

Thobaben, M. (1998). Helping clients with presbycusis. *Home Care Provider, 3*(4), 186-188.

Tolson, D. (1997). Age-related hearing loss: A case for nursing intervention. *Journal of Advanced Nursing, 26*(6), 1150-1157.

Tolson, D., & Stephens, D. (1997). Age-related hearing loss in the dependent elderly population: A model for nursing care. *International Journal of Nursing Practice, 3*(4), 224-230.

Vilholm, O., Moller, K., & Jorgensen, K. (1998). Effect of traditional Chinese acupuncture on severe tinnitus: A double-blind placebo-controlled, clinical investigation with open therapeutic control. *British Journal of Audiology, 32*(3), 197-204.

Waddinton, C., McKennis, A., & Goodlett, A. (1997). Treatment of conductive hearing loss with ossicular chain construction procedures. *AORN Journal, 65*(3), 511-518.

Walker, J., & Barnes, B. (1998). Dizziness. *Emergency Medicine Clinics of North America, 16*(4), 845-875.

Wazen, J., et al. (1998). Long-term hearing results following vestibular surgery in Meniere's disease. *Laryngoscope, 108*(10), 1470-1473.

Weimert, T. (1997). The acute ear. *Emergency Medicine, 29*(12), 34-45.

*Winslow, E.H. (1994). Hearing loss? Check for impacted cerumen. *American Journal of Nursing, 94*(10), 55.

UNIT 11

PROBLEMS OF MOBILITY

Management of Clients with Problems of the Musculoskeletal System

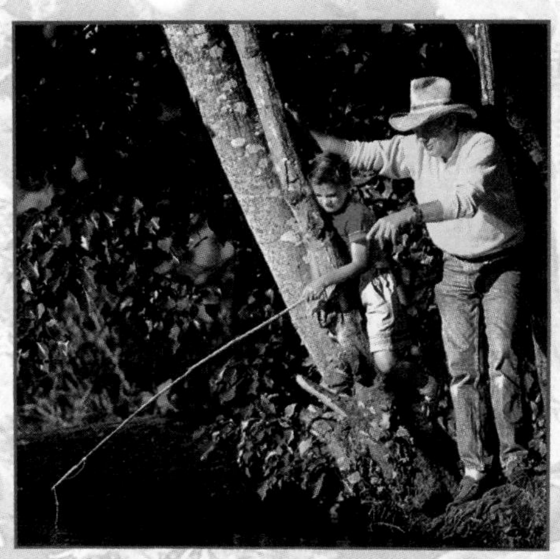

UNIT 11

PROBLEMS OF MOBILITY: MUSCULOSKELETAL SYSTEM ■ Core Concepts Grid

Anatomy	Physiology	Pathophysiology	History	Physical Exam	Diagnostic Tests	Interventions	Pharmacology
• **Skeletal system** Bones Cartilage Tendons Ligaments Joints • **Muscular system**	• **Calcium storage** • **Hematopoesis** • **Protection** • **Form/framework** • **Motion** • **Joint articulation**	• **Fracture** • **Sprain** • **Contusion** • **Trauma** • **Osteoporosis** • **Infection**	• **Client medical history** Injury Illness Musculo-skeletal Systemic • **Family history** Congenital problems • **Social history** Occupation Sports Nutrition Age Race Gender • **Risk factors** Diet Exercise	• **Joint appearance** • **Gait** • **Range of motion** • **Flexion** • **Extension** • **Hyperextension** • **Abduction** • **Adduction** • **Pronation** • **Supination** • **Circumduction** • **Rotation** • **Inversion** • **Eversion** • **Alignment** • **Bruising/skin trauma** • **Kyphosis**	• **Radiologic studies** • **Arthroscopy** • **Magnetic resonance imaging (MRI)** • **Bone scan** • **Serum calcium** • **Serum phosphorus**	• **Cast care** • **Traction** • **Neurovascular checks** • **Braces/splints** • **Pin tract care** • **Skin assessment** • **Positioning** • **Logroll turning** • **Range-of-motion exercises** • **Body alignment** • **Lifestyle modifications** Diet Exercise • **Rest** • **Physical rehabilitation** • **Preventing immobility complications**	• **Analgesics** • **Muscle relaxants** • **Nonsteroidal anti-inflammatory drugs (NSAIDs)** • **Antibiotics** • **Calcium** • **Vitamin D** • **Selective estrogen receptor modulators** • **Anticoagulants**

CHAPTER 50

Assessment of the Musculoskeletal System

DONNA D. IGNATAVICIUS

Learning Objectives

After studying this chapter, you should be able to:

1. Recall the anatomy and physiology of the musculoskeletal system.
2. Perform a musculoskeletal assessment using Gordon's Functional Health Patterns.
3. Evaluate important assessment findings in a client with a musculoskeletal health problem.
4. Explain the use of laboratory testing for a client with a musculoskeletal health problem.
5. Identify the use of radiography in diagnosing musculoskeletal health problems.
6. Plan follow-up care for clients undergoing musculoskeletal diagnostic testing.

SIMON **Go to http://www.wbsaunders.com/SIMON/Iggy/ for self-assessment questions related to these Learning Objectives.**

The musculoskeletal system is the second largest body system; it includes the bones, joints, and skeletal muscles, as well as their supporting structures. Disease, surgery, and trauma often affect one or more parts of this system, yet its assessment is often overlooked by nurses. This chapter does not include diagnostic testing related to arthritis or specific tests for osteoporosis. Descriptions of those tests are found in Chapters 21 and 51 under discussions of those diseases.

ANATOMY AND PHYSIOLOGY REVIEW

Skeletal System

The skeletal system consists of 206 bones and multiple joints. The growth and development of these structures occur during childhood and adolescence and are not discussed in this text.

BONES

Types

Bones may be classified by their shape. *Long bones,* such as the femur, are cylindric with rounded ends; they often bear weight. *Short bones,* such as the phalanges, are small and bear little or no weight. *Flat bones,* such as the scapula, protect vital organs and often contain blood-forming cells. Bones that have unique shapes are known as *irregular bones* (e.g., the carpal bones in the wrist). The *sesamoid bone* is the least common type and develops within a tendon; the patella is a typical example.

Structure

As shown in Figure 50-1, the outer layer of bone, or cortex, is composed of dense, compact bone tissue. The inner layer, in the medulla, contains spongy, cancellous tissue. Almost every bone has both tissue types but in varying quantities. The long bone typically has a shaft, or diaphysis, and two knoblike ends, or epiphyses.

The structural unit of the cortical, compact bone is the haversian system, as detailed in Figure 50-1. The haversian system is a complex canal network containing microscopic blood vessels, which supply nutrients and oxygen to bone, and lacunae, which are small cavities that house osteocytes (bone cells). The canals run longitudinally within the hard, cortical bone tissue.

The softer, cancellous tissue contains large spaces, or trabeculae, which are filled with red and yellow marrow. Hematopoiesis (production of blood cells) occurs in the red marrow. The yellow marrow contains fat cells, which can be dislodged and enter the bloodstream to cause fat embolism syndrome (FES), a life-threatening complication. Volkmann's canals connect bone marrow vessels with the haversian system and periosteum, the outermost covering of the bone. Osteogenic cells, which later differentiate into **osteoblasts** (bone-forming cells) and **osteoclasts** (bone-destroying cells), are found in the deepest layer of the periosteum.

Bone also contains a matrix (also called *osteoid*) consisting chiefly of collagen, mucopolysaccharides, and lipids. Deposits of inorganic calcium salts (carbonate and phosphate) in the matrix provide the hardness of bone.

Bone is a very vascular tissue; its estimated total blood flow is between 200 and 400 mL/min. Each bone has a principal nutrient artery, which enters near the middle of the shaft and branches into ascending and descending vessels. These vessels supply the cortex, the marrow, and the haversian system. Sympathetic and afferent (sensory) fibers constitute the sparse nerve supply to bone. Dilation of blood vessels is controlled by the sympathetic nerves. The afferent fibers transmit

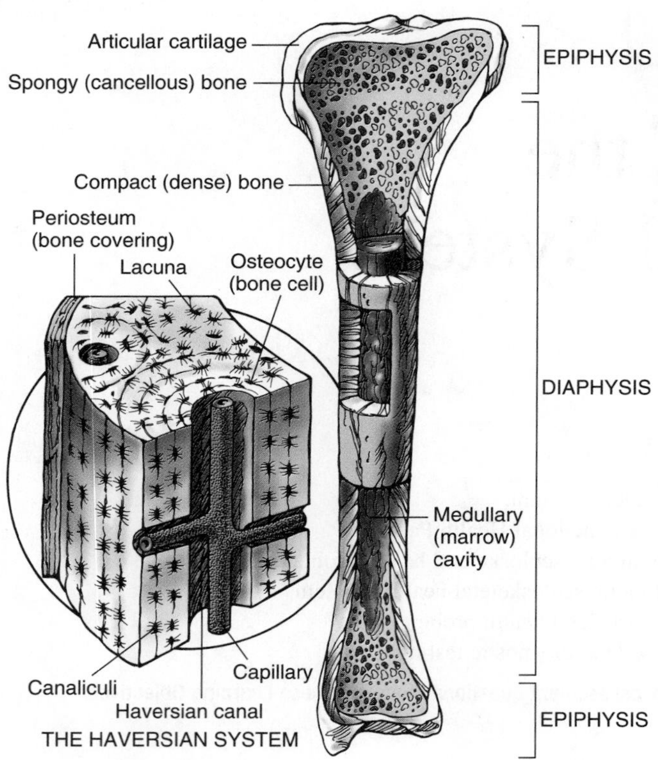

Figure 50-1 ● The structure of a typical long bone. The cortex, or outer layer, is composed of dense, compact tissue. The microscopic structure of this compact cortical tissue is the haversian system.

the pain experienced by clients who have primary lesions of the bone.

Growth and Metabolism

After puberty, bone reaches its maturity and maximal growth. Bone is a dynamic tissue, however, that undergoes a continuous process of formation and resorption, or destruction, at equal rates until the age of 35 years. In later years, bone resorption accelerates, decreasing bone mass and predisposing clients to injury. (See Chapter 51 for a discussion of the effects of aging on bone metabolism.)

Bone growth and metabolism are affected by numerous minerals and hormones, including the following:

- Calcium
- Phosphorus
- Calcitonin
- Vitamin D
- Parathyroid hormone (PTH)
- Growth hormone
- Glucocorticoids
- Estrogens and androgens
- Thyroxine
- Insulin

CALCIUM AND PHOSPHORUS

Bone accounts for approximately 99% of the calcium in the body and 90% of the phosphorus. The serum concentrations of calcium and phosphorus maintain an inverse relationship; for example, when calcium levels rise, phosphorus levels decrease. When serum levels of calcium and phosphorus are altered, calcitonin and PTH work to maintain equilibrium. If the calcium level of the blood is decreased, for example, the bone (which stores calcium) releases calcium into the vascular system in response to PTH stimulation.

CALCITONIN

Calcitonin is produced by the thyroid gland and *decreases* the serum calcium concentration if it is increased above its normal level. Calcitonin inhibits bone resorption and increases renal excretion of calcium and phosphorus as needed.

VITAMIN D

Vitamin D and its metabolites are produced in the body and transported in the blood to promote the absorption of calcium and phosphorus from the small intestine. They also seem to enhance PTH activity in the release of calcium from the bone. A decrease in the body's vitamin D level can result in osteomalacia in the adult. An external source of vitamin D may be given to clients at risk for or diagnosed with osteomalacia. Vitamin D metabolism and osteomalacia are detailed in Chapter 51.

PARATHYROID HORMONE

When serum calcium levels are lowered, parathyroid hormone (PTH, or parathormone) secretion increases and stimulates bone to promote osteoclastic activity and *donate* calcium to the blood. PTH reduces the renal excretion of calcium and facilitates its absorption from the intestine. Conversely, when serum calcium levels increase, PTH secretion diminishes to preserve the bone calcium supply; this is an example of the feedback loop system of the endocrine system.

GROWTH HORMONE

Growth hormone secreted by the anterior lobe of the pituitary gland is responsible for increasing bone length and determining the amount of bone matrix formed before puberty. During childhood, an increased secretion results in gigantism, and a decreased secretion results in dwarfism. In the adult, an increase causes acromegaly, which is characterized by bone and soft-tissue deformities (see Chapter 63).

GLUCOCORTICOIDS

Adrenal glucocorticoids regulate protein metabolism, either increasing or decreasing catabolism to reduce or intensify the organic matrix of bone. They also aid in regulating intestinal calcium and phosphorus absorption.

ESTROGENS AND ANDROGENS

Estrogens stimulate osteoblastic activity and inhibit PTH. When estrogen levels decline at menopause, women are susceptible to low serum calcium levels with subsequent bone loss (osteoporosis). Androgens, such as testosterone, promote anabolism and increase bone mass. External sources of estrogen and testosterone may be prescribed for clients at risk for or diagnosed with osteoporosis.

THYROXINE

Thyroxine is one of the principal hormones secreted by the thyroid gland. Its primary function is to increase the rate of protein synthesis in all types of tissue, including bone.

INSULIN

Insulin works together with growth hormone to build and maintain healthy bone tissue.

Function

The skeletal system:

- Provides a framework for the body
- Supports the surrounding tissues (e.g., muscle and tendons)
- Assists in movement through muscle attachment and joint formation
- Protects vital organs, such as the heart and lungs
- Manufactures blood cells in red bone marrow
- Provides storage for mineral salts (e.g., calcium and phosphorus)

JOINTS

A **joint** is a space in which two or more bones come together. The primary function of a joint is to provide movement and flexibility in the body.

Types

There are three types of joints in the body:

- Synarthrodial, or completely immovable, joints (e.g., in the cranium)
- Amphiarthrodial, or slightly movable, joints (e.g., in the pelvis)
- Diarthrodial (synovial), or freely movable, joints (e.g., the elbow and knee)

Although any of these joints can be affected by disease or injury, the diarthrodial joints are most commonly involved.

Structure and Function

The **diarthrodial,** or **synovial, joint** is the most common type of joint in the body. Synovial joints are so named because they are the only type lined with synovium, a membrane that secretes synovial fluid for lubrication and shock absorption. As illustrated in Figure 50-2, the synovium lines the internal portion of the joint capsule but does not normally extend onto the surface of the cartilage at the spongy bone ends. Articular cartilage consists of a collagen fiber matrix impregnated with a complex ground substance. Bursae, small sacs located at joints to prevent friction, are also lined with synovial membrane.

Synovial joints are subtyped by their anatomic structures. *Ball-and-socket* joints (shoulder, hip) permit movement in any direction. *Hinge* joints (elbow) allow motion in one plane, flexion, and extension. The knee is often classified as a hinge

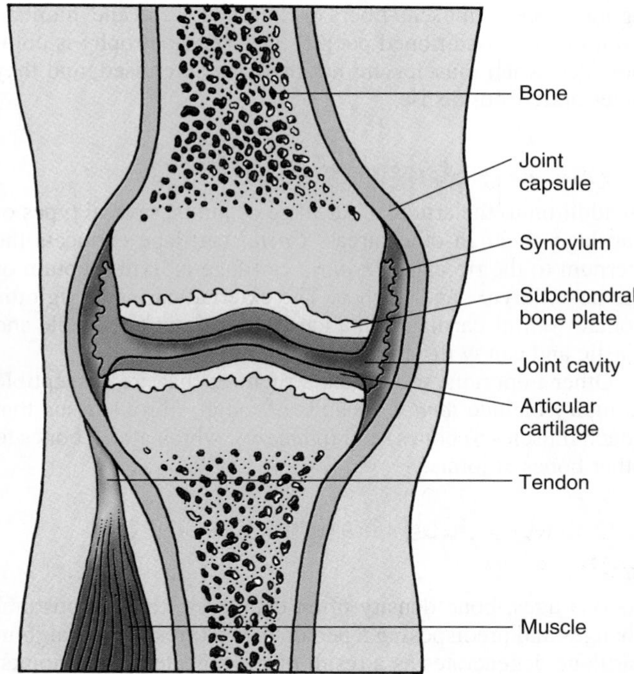

Figure 50-2 ● The structure of a diarthrodial joint. Synovium lines the joint capsule but does not extend into the articular cartilage.

joint, but it rotates slightly, as well as flexes and extends. It is best described as a *condylar* type of synovial joint. The gliding movement of the wrist is characteristic of the *biaxial* joint. *Pivot* joints permit rotation only, as in the radioulnar area.

Muscular System

There are three types of muscle in the body: smooth muscle, cardiac muscle, and skeletal muscle. Smooth, or nonstriated, involuntary muscle is responsible for contractions of organs and blood vessels and is controlled by the autonomic nervous system. Cardiac muscle, or the myocardium, is also controlled by the autonomic nervous system. The smooth and cardiac muscles are discussed with the body systems to which they belong in the assessment chapters.

Structure

In contrast to smooth and cardiac muscle, skeletal muscle is voluntarily controlled by the central and peripheral nervous systems. The junction of a peripheral motor nerve and the muscle cells that it supplies is sometimes referred to as a motor end plate. Muscle fibers are held in place by connective tissue in bundles, or fasciculi. The entire muscle is surrounded by dense, fibrous tissue (fascia) containing the muscle's blood, lymph, and nerve supply.

Function

The primary function of skeletal muscle is movement of the body and its parts. When bones, joints, and supporting structures are adversely affected by injury or disease, the adjacent muscle tissue is often involved, limiting mobility. During the aging process, muscle fibers decrease in size and number, even in well-conditioned people. This senile atrophy is compounded when muscles are not regularly exercised, and they deteriorate from disuse.

Supporting Structures

In addition to the articular cartilage of joints, several types of cartilage occur in other areas. *Costal* cartilage connects the sternum to the rib cage. *Hyaline* cartilage is in the septum of the nose, larynx, and trachea. The external ear and epiglottis contain *yellow* cartilage. In all areas, the tissue is flexible and elastic and can withstand enormous tension.

Other important supporting structures that are susceptible to injury include *tendons* (bands of tough, fibrous tissue that attach muscles to bones) and *ligaments,* which attach bones to other bones at joints.

Musculoskeletal Changes Associated with Aging

As one ages, bone density often decreases, causing postural changes and predisposing a person to fractures. Synovial joint cartilage degenerates as a result of the repeated use of joints, especially weight-bearing joints such as the hips and knees. The result is often degenerative joint disease. Muscle tissue atrophy occurs, but its rate may be slowed by increased activity and exercise. Collectively, these changes cause decreased coordination, gait changes, and predisposition to falls with injury. Chart 50-1 lists the major anatomic and physiologic changes and suggested nursing interventions.

ASSESSMENT TECHNIQUES

History

In the assessment of a client with an actual or potential musculoskeletal problem, a detailed history aids the nurse in identifying diagnoses and subsequent interventions (Chart 50-2).

DEMOGRAPHIC DATA

Young men are at the greatest risk for trauma related to motor vehicle crashes. Older adults are at the greatest risk for falls that result in fractures and soft-tissue injury (see Chapter 5).

WOMEN'S HEALTH CONSIDERATIONS

The age and sex of the client are important indicators in musculoskeletal disorders. Older women, for example, are most likely to have metabolic bone disease, such as osteoporosis. Women of any age are at the highest risk for most types of arthritis.

PERSONAL AND FAMILY HISTORY

Accidents, illnesses, and medications may relate to a client's current problem. When taking a personal health history, the nurse questions the client about all traumatic incidents, regardless of the date of occurrence. An injury to the lumbar spine 30 years previously may contribute to a client's current complaint of low back pain. A motor vehicle crash can be the cause of traumatic arthritis years after the event.

Previous or concurrent diseases may affect musculoskeletal status. For example, a client with diabetes who is treated for a foot ulcer is at high risk for acute or chronic osteomyelitis (bone infection). In addition, diabetes slows the healing process. Certain disorders have a familial or genetic tendency. Osteoporosis (age-related bone loss), for instance, often occurs in several generations of a family, and bone cancer tends to be genetically linked. It is also important for the nurse to determine a history of previous hospitalizations and illnesses or complications.

The nurse also asks about previous and current use of medications. Some drugs, such as steroids, can affect calcium metabolism and promote bone loss. Other drugs may be taken to relieve musculoskeletal pain. The client should also be asked about herbal or biologic compounds that may be used for arthritis, such as chondroitin. Complementary and alternative therapies are commonly employed by clients with various types of arthritis (see Chapter 21).

CHART 50-1

NURSING FOCUS *on the* OLDER ADULT

Changes in the Musculoskeletal System Related to Aging

Physiologic Change	Nursing Implications	Rationale
Decreased bone density	Teach safety tips to prevent falls. Reinforce need to exercise, especially weight-bearing exercise.	Porous bones are more likely to fracture. Exercise slows bone loss.
Increased bone prominence	Prevent pressure on bone prominences.	There is less soft tissue to prevent skin breakdown.
Kyphotic posture: widened gait, shift in the center of gravity	Teach proper body mechanics; instruct the client to sit in supportive chairs with arms.	Correction of posture problems prevents further deformity; the client should have support for bony structures.
Cartilage degeneration	Provide moist heat, such as a shower or warm, moist compresses.	Moist heat increases blood flow to the area.
Decreased ROM	Assess the client's ability to perform ADLs and mobility.	The client may need assistance with self-care skills.
Muscle atrophy, decreased strength	Teach isometric exercises.	Exercises increase muscle strength.
Slowed movement	Do not rush the client; be patient.	The client may become frustrated if hurried.

ROM, Range of motion; *ADLs,* activities of daily living.

DIET HISTORY

An evaluation of the client's diet history helps determine the cause of inadequate nutrition. For example, most people, especially women, do not consume adequate amounts of calcium. People who cannot afford to buy food are especially at risk for undernutrition.

CONSIDERATIONS FOR OLDER ADULTS

An inadequate intake of calcium or protein or insufficient exposure to sunlight predisposes the older adult to loss of bone and lean muscle. Homebound or institutionalized older clients are particularly at risk if they are not exposed to sunlight.

Inadequate protein or insufficient vitamin C in the diet inhibits healing of bone and tissue. Obesity places excess stress and strain on bones and joints, with resultant fractures and degeneration of cartilage. In addition, obesity inhibits mobility in clients with musculoskeletal problems, which predisposes them to complications such as respiratory and circulatory problems.

SOCIOECONOMIC STATUS

When assessing a client with a possible musculoskeletal alteration, the nurse inquires about lifestyle. A person's occupation can cause or contribute to an injury. For instance, fractures are not uncommon in clients whose jobs require manual labor, such as carpenters and mechanics. Certain occupations, such as computer-related jobs, may predispose a person to carpal tunnel syndrome (entrapment of the median nerve in the wrist). Construction workers may experience back injury from prolonged standing and excessive lifting. Amateur and professional athletes often experience acute musculoskeletal injuries, such as joint dislocations and fractures, or chronic disorders, such as degenerative joint disease.

CHART 50-2

MUSCULOSKELETAL ASSESSMENT
Using Gordon's Functional Health Patterns

Activity-Exercise Pattern

Do you have sufficient energy for desired/required activities?
What is your exercise pattern? Type of exercise? Regularity?
What spare time (leisure) activities do you engage in?
What is your perceived ability for (code for level according to key below):

Feeding?	Level 0: Full self-care
Bathing?	Level I: Requires use of equipment or device
Toileting?	
Bed mobility?	Level II: Requires assistance or supervision of another person
Dressing?	
Grooming?	Level III: Requires assistance or supervision of another person and equipment or device
General mobility?	
Cooking?	
Home maintenance?	Level IV: Is dependent and does not participate
Shopping?	

Cognitive-Perceptual Pattern

Do you experience any discomfort?
Do you have pain? If so, how do you manage it?
What is the easiest way for you to learn things?
Do you have any difficulty learning?

Based on Gordon, M. (2000). *Manual of nursing diagnosis* (9th ed.). St. Louis: Mosby.

Socioeconomic status may be related to the client's occupation and therefore affect the likelihood of musculoskeletal problems. For example, an executive working in an office is less likely to sustain a musculoskeletal injury than is a painter or roofer engaged in manual labor and activities such as climbing ladders.

CULTURAL CONSIDERATIONS

The body proportions of African Americans differ from those of Caucasians, Asian Americans, and Native Americans. African Americans have shorter trunks and longer legs than do other groups. Their long bones are significantly longer and narrower than those of Caucasians. All bones are denser, and African-American men have denser bones than do African-American women. Caucasian women have the least amount of bone density of any group, which makes them the most susceptible to osteoporosis and fractures (Ignatavicius, 1998).

Many African Americans also have a lactose intolerance (i.e., an inability to convert lactose to glucose and galactose). Because milk and dairy products are good sources of calcium for bone building but are rich in lactose, African Americans may need to obtain their calcium from other food sources, such as dark green, leafy vegetables. Inuits also have a low tolerance for milk, and the adult diet is low in calcium.

A client's ethnic and cultural background may also be helpful in ascertaining his or her tolerance to pain. There may be differences in reactions to pain among cultural populations, as discussed in Chapter 7. The nurse uses this information to aid in pain assessment.

CURRENT HEALTH PROBLEM

The nurse gathers data pertinent to the client's presenting complaint as follows:

- Date and time of onset
- Factors that cause or exacerbate (worsen) the problem
- Course of the problem (e.g., intermittent or continuous)
- Clinical manifestations (as expressed by the client) and the pattern of their occurrence
- Measures that improve clinical manifestations (e.g., heat)

The most common complaint of people with musculoskeletal problems is pain. The pain may be acute or chronic, depending on its onset and duration. The nurse may use the PQRST model to elicit a complete assessment of the client's pain:

P Provoking incident? (Was there a certain incident or event that precipitated the pain or caused an exacerbation of the pain?)

Q Quality of pain? (What does the pain feel like in descriptive terms? Is it burning, throbbing, stabbing?)

R Region, radiation, and relief? (Exactly where is the pain located? Does the pain travel or radiate? Does anything help relieve the pain?)

S Severity of the pain? (How severe is the pain? The client may use a pain scale [see Chapter 7] or describe how the pain has interfered with his or her ability to function.)

T Time? (How long does the pain last? When does it occur? Is it worse at night or during the day? If the pain awakens a person at night, the source of the pain is most likely inflammatory, not degenerative.)

With any pain assessment, it is always best if the client describes the pain in his or her own words and points to its location, if possible.

Physical Assessment

Although bones, joints, and muscles are usually assessed simultaneously in a head-to-toe approach, each subsystem is described separately for emphasis and understanding. For physical assessment of the musculoskeletal system, the nurse incorporates inspection, palpation, active range of motion (ROM), and special techniques for specific problems. A general assessment is described in this chapter. More specific assessment techniques are discussed in the interventions chapters that follow for each musculoskeletal problem.

ASSESSMENT OF THE SKELETAL SYSTEM

General Inspection

The nurse observes the client's posture, gait, and mobility for gross deformities and impairment.

POSTURE

Posture includes the person's body build and alignment when standing and walking. The nurse observes the curvature of the spine and the length, shape, and symmetry of extremities. Figure 50-3 illustrates some common spinal deformities. Muscle mass is also inspected for size and symmetry.

GAIT

Most clients with musculoskeletal problems eventually have a problem with gait. The two phases of normal, automatic gait (Figure 50-4) are the stance phase and the swing phase.

The nurse or therapist evaluates the client's balance, steadiness, and ease and length of stride; any limp or other asymmetric leg movement or deformity is noted. An abnormality in the stance phase of gait is called an *antalgic* gait. When part of one leg is painful, the person shortens the stance phase on the affected side. An abnormality in the swing phase is called a *lurch.* This abnormal gait occurs when the muscles in the buttocks and/or legs are too weak to allow the person to change weight from one foot to the other. In this case, the shoulders are moved either side to side or front to back for help in shifting the weight from one leg to the other. Some clients, such as those with chronic hip pain and muscle atrophy from arthritic disorders, have a combination of an antalgic gait and lurch.

MOBILITY

In collaboration with the physical or occupational therapist, the nurse observes the client's need for or use of ambulatory devices, such as canes and walkers, during transfer from bed to chair and while walking and climbing stairs. The nurse also assesses mobility by asking the client to perform activities of daily living (ADLs) such as dressing and bathing. Pain and deformity may limit physical mobility and function. A complete discussion of functional assessment is found in Chapter 10.

After performing a functional assessment, the nurse assesses major bones, joints, and muscles by inspection, palpation, and determination of ROM. A goniometer (used by physical therapists and clinical specialists) provides an exact measurement of ROM, but the degree of joint mobility can be estimated by having the client put each joint through its ROM. The nurse uses the movements shown in Figure 50-5. As long as the client can function to meet personal needs, a limitation in ROM may not be significant. For each anatomic location, the skin is observed for color, elasticity, and lesions that may relate to musculoskeletal dysfunction.

Assessment of the Head and Neck

The nurse inspects and palpates the skull for shape, symmetry, tenderness, and masses. The temporomandibular joints (TMJs) are best evaluated by palpation. The client is asked to open his or her mouth while the nurse palpates the TMJs. Common abnormal findings are tenderness or pain, crepitus (a grating sound), and a spongy swelling caused by excess synovium and fluid.

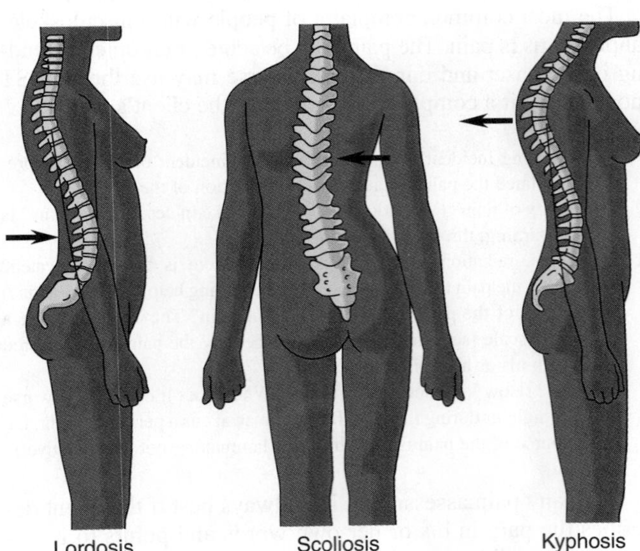

Figure 50-3 ● Common spinal deformities.

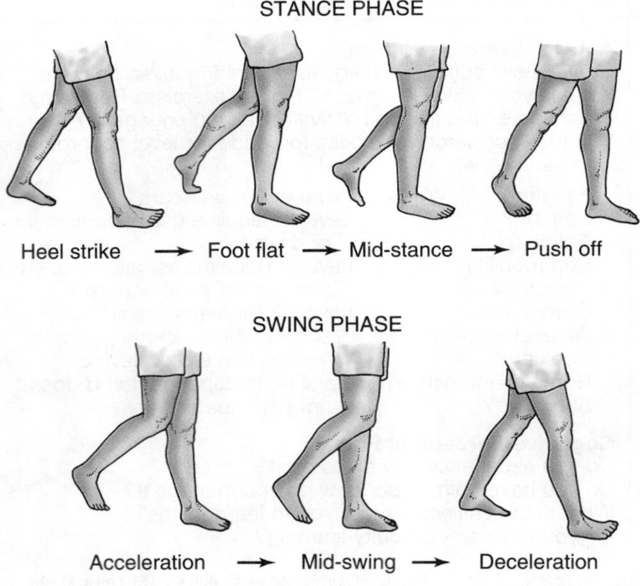

Figure 50-4 ● The phases of gait.

The nurse then inspects and palpates each vertebra of the spine in the neck. Clinical findings may include malalignment; tenderness; or inability to flex, extend, and rotate the neck as expected.

Assessment of the Spine

The thoracic spine, lumbar spine, and sacral spine are evaluated in the same manner as the neck. Spinal alignment problems are common (see Figure 50-3). In addition, the nurse places both hands over the lumbosacral area and applies pressure with the thumbs to elicit tenderness. Many clients do not complain of discomfort until the area is palpated.

Assessment of the Upper Extremities

The nurse assesses both extremities concurrently. For example, both shoulders are inspected and palpated for size, swelling, deformity, malalignment, tenderness or pain, and mobility. A shoulder injury may prevent the client from combing his or her hair with the affected arm, but severe arthritis may inhibit movement in both arms. The elbows and wrists are assessed in a similar way.

Because the hand has multiple joints in a single digit, assessment of hand function is perhaps the most critical part of the examination. The nurse inspects and palpates the metacarpophalangeal (MCP), proximal interphalangeal (PIP), and distal interphalangeal (DIP) joints. The same digits are compared on the right and left hands (Figure 50-6). The nurse also determines range of motion (ROM) for each joint by observing active movement, if such movement is possible. For a quick and easy assessment of ROM, the client is asked to make a fist and then appose each finger to the thumb. If he or she can perform these maneuvers, ROM of the hand is not seriously restricted.

Assessment of the Lower Extremities

Evaluation of the hip joint relies primarily on determination of its degree of mobility, because the joint is deep and difficult to inspect or palpate. The client with hip pain usually experiences pain in the *groin* area, or the pain may radiate to the knee. The knee is readily accessible for nursing assessment, particularly when the client is sitting and the knee is flexed. Fluid accumulation, or effusion, is easily detected in the knee joint; limitations in movement with accompanying pain are common findings. The knees may be malaligned, as in genu valgum ("knock-knee") or genu varum ("bowlegged") deformities.

The ankles and feet are often neglected in the physical examination; however, they contain multiple bones and joints that can be affected by disease and injury. The nurse observes and palpates each joint and tests for ROM.

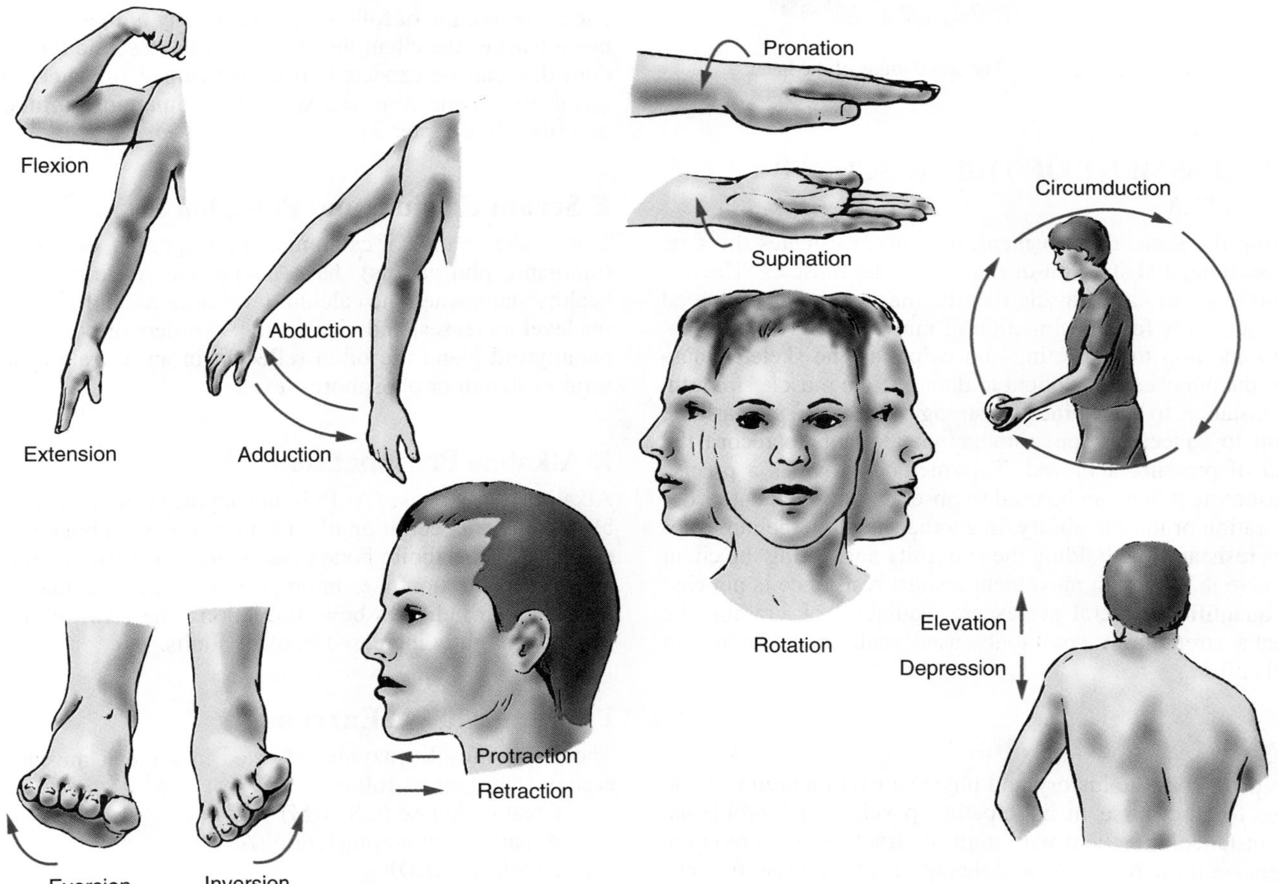

Figure 50-5 ● Movements of the skeletal muscles. (Modified from Jarvis, C. [2000]. *Physical examination and health assessment* [3rd ed.]. Philadelphia: W.B. Saunders.)

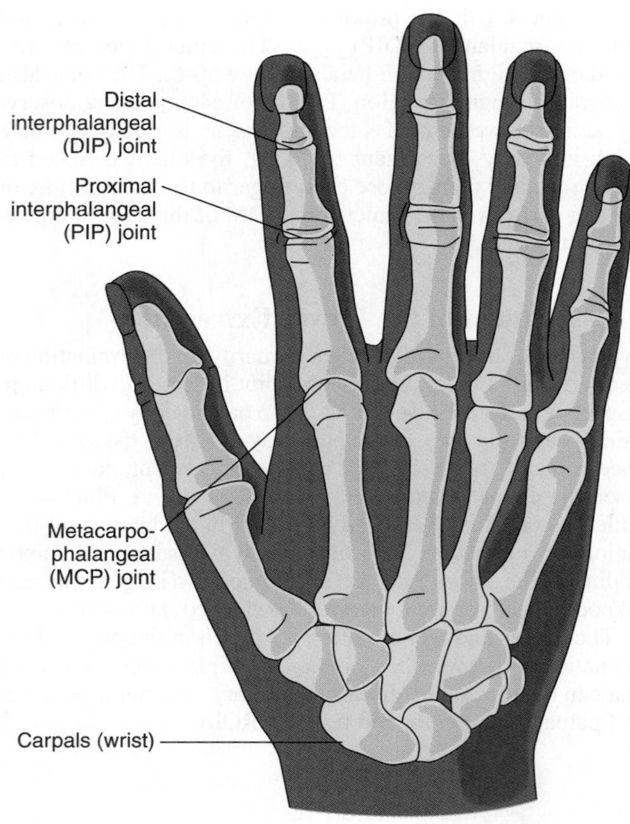

Figure 50-6 ● The small joints of the hand.

ASSESSMENT OF THE MUSCULAR SYSTEM

During the skeletal assessment, the nurse evaluates the size, shape, tone, and strength of major skeletal muscles. The circumference of each muscle may be measured and compared symmetrically for an estimation of muscle mass.

In addition to inspecting and palpating the skeletal muscles, the nurse asks the client to demonstrate muscle strength. For instance, to determine grip strength, the nurse may ask the client to squeeze a sphygmomanometer bulb to record the level of pressure achieved. This method provides a precise measurement that can be used to observe improvement or deterioration of muscle ability. In another method, the nurse applies resistance by holding the extremity and asking the client to move it. Although movement against resistance is not easily quantified, several scales are available for grading the client's strength. A commonly used scale is delineated in Table 50-1.

TABLE 50-1 • LOVETT'S SCALE FOR GRADING MUSCLE STRENGTH

Rating	Description
5	Normal: ROM unimpaired against gravity with full resistance
4	Good: can complete ROM against gravity with some resistance
3	Fair: can complete ROM against gravity
2	Poor: can complete ROM with gravity eliminated
1	Trace: no joint motion and slight evidence of muscle contractility
0	Zero: no evidence of muscle contractility

ROM, Range of motion.

Psychosocial Assessment

The data from the history and physical examination provide clues for the nurse in anticipating psychosocial problems. For instance, the client with multiple fractures who requires extensive immobilization and therapy is at high risk for sensory deprivation. Prolonged absence from employment or permanent disability may cause the client to lose his or her job or occupation. Further stress may be experienced if chronic pain ensues and he or she cannot cope with numerous stressors simultaneously. Deformities resulting from musculoskeletal disease or injury can affect a person's body image and self-concept.

Diagnostic Assessment

LABORATORY TESTS

Chart 50-3 lists the major laboratory tests used in assessing clients with musculoskeletal disorders. There is no special client preparation or follow-up care for any of these tests. The nurse teaches the client the purpose of the test and the procedure that can be expected. Tests performed for clients with connective tissue diseases, such as rheumatoid arthritis, are described in Chapter 21.

Serum Calcium and Phosphorus

The concentrations of calcium and phosphorus, or phosphate (inorganic phosphorus), have an inverse relationship. In a healthy state, when the calcium level decreases, the phosphorus level increases, and vice versa. Disorders of bone and the parathyroid gland are often reflected in an alteration of the serum calcium or phosphorus level.

Alkaline Phosphatase

Alkaline phosphatase (ALP) is an enzyme normally present in blood. The concentration of ALP increases with bone or liver damage. In metabolic bone disease and bone cancer, the enzyme concentration rises in proportion to the osteoblastic activity, which indicates bone formation. The level of ALP is normally slightly increased in older adults.

Serum Muscle Enzymes

The major muscle enzymes affected in skeletal muscle disease or injury are as follows:

- Creatine kinase (CK-MM)
- Aspartate aminotransferase (AST)
- Aldolase (ALD)
- Lactate dehydrogenase (LDH)

As a result of damage, the muscle tissue releases additional amounts of these enzymes, which increases serum levels.

CHART 50-3

LABORATORY PROFILE

Musculoskeletal Assessment

Test	Normal Range for Adults	Significance of Abnormal Findings
Serum calcium	8.6-10.0 mg/dL (2.15-2.50 mmol/L) >60 yr: Slightly lower >90 yr: 8.2-9.6 mg/dL	*Hypercalcemia* (increased calcium) • Metastatic cancers of the bone • Paget's disease • Bone fractures in healing stage *Hypocalcemia* (decreased calcium) • Osteoporosis • Osteomalacia
Serum phosphorus	2.7-4.5 mg/dL (0.87-1.45 mmol/L) >60 yr: 2.3-3.7 mg/dL (M) 2.8-4.1 mg/dL (F)	*Hyperphosphatemia* (increased phosphorus) • Bone fractures in healing stage • Bone tumors • Acromegaly *Hypophosphatemia* (decreased phosphorus) • Osteomalacia
Alkaline phosphatase (ALP)	25-100 units/L	*Elevations* may indicate: • Metastatic cancers of the bone • Paget's disease • Osteomalacia
Serum muscle enzymes		
Creatine kinase (CK_3)	Total CK: • Men: 38-174 units/L • Women: 26-140 units/L >90 yr: 21-203 (M) 22-99 (F)	*Elevations* may indicate: • Muscle trauma • Progressive muscular dystrophy • Effects of electromyography
Lactate dehydrogenase (LDH)	Total LDH: 140-280 units/L 60-90 yr: 110-210 units/L >90 yr: 99-284 units/L LDH_5: 0%-5%	*Elevations* may indicate: • Skeletal muscle necrosis • Extensive cancer • Progressive muscular dystrophy
Aspartate aminotransferase (AST)	8-10 units/L (slightly lower in women) >60 yr: 11-26 units/L (M) 10-20 units/L (F)	*Elevations* may indicate: • Skeletal muscle trauma • Progressive muscular dystrophy
Aldolase (ALD)	1.0-7.5 units/L	*Elevations* may indicate: • Polymyositis and dermatomyositis • Muscular dystrophy

M, Males; *F*, females.

The serum CK level begins to rise 2 to 4 hours after muscle injury and is elevated early in muscle disease, such as muscular dystrophy. The CK molecule has two subunits: M (muscle) and B (brain). Three isoenzymes have been identified. Skeletal muscle CK (CK-MM, or CK_3) is the only isoenzyme that rises in concentration with damage to skeletal muscle.

AST is moderately elevated (three to five times normal) in certain muscle diseases, such as muscular dystrophy and dermatomyositis. The levels of the isoenzymes aldolase A (ALD-A) and LDH_5 also increase in clients with these disorders.

RADIOGRAPHIC EXAMINATIONS

Standard Radiography

The skeleton is readily visible on standard x-ray films. Anteroposterior and lateral projections are the initial screening views. Other approaches, such as oblique or stress views, depend on the part of the skeleton to be evaluated and the necessity of the x-ray study.

Observations of bone density, alignment, swelling, and intactness are made. The conditions of joints can be determined, including the size of the joint space, the smoothness of articular cartilage, and synovial swelling. Soft-tissue involvement may be evident but not clearly differentiated.

The nurse informs the client that the x-ray table is hard and cold and instructs him or her to remain still during the filming process.

Tomography and Xeroradiography

Whereas standard x-ray studies superimpose one structure on another, tomography produces planes, or slices, for focus and blurs the images of other structures. This procedure is helpful in detailing the musculoskeletal system, because the many close structures make visualization difficult.

Xeroradiography highlights the contrast between structures. Margins and edges can be clearly seen (edge enhancement). Disadvantages of xeroradiography are the higher radiation dose to the client and inability of xeroradiography to determine tissue densities.

Myelography

Myelography involves the injection of contrast medium, or dye, into the subarachnoid space of the spine, usually by spinal puncture. The vertebral column, intervertebral disks, spinal nerve roots, and blood vessels can be visualized. Although this test is still performed, it is far less popular; computed tomography (CT) and magnetic resonance imaging

(MRI) have often replaced such invasive, and potentially painful, diagnostic techniques. Further discussion of myelography is found in Chapter 43.

Arthrography

An arthrogram is an x-ray study of a joint after contrast medium (air or solution) has been injected to enhance its visualization. Double-contrast arthrography, which uses both air and contrast, may be performed when a traumatic injury is suspected. The physician can often determine bone chips, torn ligaments, or other loose bodies within the joint.

CLIENT PREPARATION. The most common joints studied are the knee and the shoulder. The client is questioned about allergy to shellfish or iodine.

The radiology nurse or technician informs the client that the test may be uncomfortable because of pressure at the needle insertion site. The joint may be swollen for several days after the test, and strenuous physical activity should be avoided for 12 to 24 hours. The joint may be wrapped, and ice may be applied at intervals for the first few hours after the test to decrease swelling.

PROCEDURE. If the knee is examined, the client is supine while the knee is flexed. After a local anesthetic is applied, the physician injects an iodine-based contrast medium directly into the joint through a medial or lateral approach. The client feels pressure but should not experience pain. X-ray images are then taken of the joint, which may be put through range of motion (ROM) during the test.

FOLLOW-UP CARE. Because the contrast medium mixes with synovial fluid, it is not withdrawn after the procedure. As a result, the client's joint is enlarged and slightly uncomfortable. Some clients state that they feel the solution moving in the joint and hear "swishing" noises for several days until the solution is absorbed by the body. If these sensations continue, the health care provider should be contacted.

In most cases, the client can resume usual activities but should avoid strenuous exercise, such as participating in contact sports, for at least 12 hours after the test. If the client has an identified joint injury, he or she may require a longer period of immobilization. An elastic support bandage may be worn around the joint for several days. The application of ice may reduce some of the swelling.

Computed Tomography

Computed tomography (CT) has gained wide acceptance for the detection of musculoskeletal problems, particularly those of the vertebral column. It may be used with or without a contrast medium, which is given orally or intravenously. If the administration of a contrast agent is planned, the radiology nurse or technician checks that the client has been allowed nothing by mouth (NPO) for at least 4 hours and is not allergic to iodine.

As a noninvasive procedure, the CT scan requires minimal nursing intervention except for client education. During the procedure, the client must remain still for 30 to 60 minutes on a hard table while the affected part is encased in the machine. Complaints of claustrophobia and annoyance from the clicking sounds made by the scanner on rotation are common, but the client is reassured that there is no danger from the machine.

OTHER DIAGNOSTIC TESTS

Bone Biopsy

In a bone biopsy, the physician extracts a specimen of bone for microscopic examination. This invasive test may confirm the presence of infection or neoplasm. One of two techniques may be used to retrieve the specimen: needle (closed) biopsy or incisional (open) biopsy.

CLIENT PREPARATION. The nurse teaches the client about the procedure and post-test care. The open technique is more invasive and requires more care.

PROCEDURE. The health care provider may perform bone biopsy in the client's room, in a special procedures room in the radiology department, or in the operating room with the use of local or general anesthesia. If the client is not given a general anesthetic, this procedure is quite painful. After anesthesia is induced, the health care provider inserts a long needle into the bone cortex or makes a small incision to reveal the bone tissue. A sterile dressing is applied after extraction of the osseous tissue. If an incision is made, a pressure dressing is applied.

FOLLOW-UP CARE. The nurse inspects the biopsy site for bleeding, swelling, and hematoma formation, which are the most common complications of bone biopsy during the first 24 hours after the procedure. Because the pressure dressing inhibits observation, the nurse monitors the client's level of pain. If internal bleeding or marked swelling occurs, the client complains of severe pain instead of the mild to moderate discomfort usually associated with the procedure. For decreasing the likelihood of bleeding, he or she is taught to immobilize the affected extremity for 12 to 24 hours. If bone infection occurs as a complication of bone biopsy, the client's temperature may be elevated 1 to 3 days after the procedure.

A mild analgesic often relieves the discomfort resulting from the procedure. After an open biopsy, the nurse teaches the client to reapply the dressing daily over the incision site while inspecting the wound for signs of inflammation or infection, such as redness, warmth, and tissue swelling.

Muscle Biopsy

Muscle biopsy is done for the diagnosis of atrophy (as in muscular dystrophy) and inflammation (as in polymyositis). The procedure and care for clients undergoing muscle biopsy are the same as those for clients undergoing bone biopsy.

Electromyography

Electromyography (EMG) is usually accompanied by nerve conduction studies for determining the electrical potential generated in an individual muscle. EMG helps in the diagnosis of neuromuscular, lower motor neuron, and peripheral nerve disorders.

CLIENT PREPARATION. The nurse informs the client that EMG may cause temporary discomfort, especially when the client is subjected to episodes of electrical current. For selected clients, mild sedation is ordered. The physician may also order a temporary discontinuation of skeletal muscle relaxants several days before the procedure to prevent medication from having effects on the test results.

PROCEDURE. The test may be performed at the bedside or in an EMG laboratory. When both EMG and nerve conduction studies are done, nerve conduction is usually tested first. Flat electrodes are placed along the nerve to be evaluated, and low electrical currents are passed through the electrodes to the nerve and muscle innervated. If nerve conduction is accomplished, the muscle contracts.

For testing muscle potential, multiple needle electrodes varying from ½ to 3 inches (1.3 to 7.5 cm) are inserted. The client may be asked to perform activities for measurement of muscle potential during minimal and maximal contraction. The degree of nerve and muscle activity is recorded on an oscilloscope, which provides a graphic readout for later interpretation.

FOLLOW-UP CARE. A few medical complications are associated with EMG. The nurse provides comfort measures and inspects the needle sites for hematoma formation. The application of ice can prevent this complication. The client may also complain of increased pain and anxiety after the test.

Arthroscopy

An arthroscope is a fiberoptic tube inserted into a joint for direct visualization; the knee and shoulder are most commonly evaluated. In addition, synovial biopsy and surgical procedures to repair traumatic injury can be accomplished through the arthroscope.

CLIENT PREPARATION. Because the knee is most commonly "scoped," the care described for the client undergoing arthroscopy relates to that joint. Arthroscopy is performed on an ambulatory basis or as same-day surgery. Clients who cannot flex their knees at least 40 degrees or who have infected knees are not candidates for the procedure. The client must be able to flex the knee, and joint infection may worsen from the mechanical trauma of arthroscope insertion.

If possible, the client should have a physical therapy consultation before arthroscopy to learn the leg exercises that are necessary after the test, especially if the procedure will be surgical. Straight-leg raises (SLRs) and quadriceps setting exercises (isometrics with the leg extended) are practiced in sets of 10 each. Range-of-motion (ROM) exercises are also taught but may not be allowed immediately after arthroscopic surgery. The nurse in the surgeon's office or at the surgical center can teach these exercises or reinforce the information provided by the physical therapist. The nurse also explains the procedure and post-test care.

PROCEDURE. The client is usually given local, light general, or epidural anesthesia, depending on the purpose of the procedure. In some settings, a large pneumatic tourniquet is used around the thigh to minimize bleeding during the procedure. Medications promoting vasoconstriction for control of bleeding may be used alone or in conjunction with the tourniquet.

The knee is flexed to at least 40 degrees, and saline or lactated Ringer's solution is used to irrigate the knee. As shown in Figure 50-7, the arthroscope is inserted through a small incision less than ¼ inch (0.6 cm) long. Multiple incisions may be required to allow inspection at a variety of angles. After the procedure, a bulky pressure dressing and an elastic bandage may be applied, depending on the amount of manipulation during the test or surgery.

FOLLOW-UP CARE. The nurse evaluates the neurovascular status of the client's affected limb frequently, in accordance with the nursing standard of care. Initially, the typical protocol is every hour. The technique for this assessment is described in detail in Chapter 52 and includes monitoring distal pulses, warmth, color, capillary refill, pain, movement, and sensation of the affected extremity.

The nurse encourages the client to perform exercises as taught before the examination. For the mild discomfort experienced after the diagnostic arthroscopy, the physician prescribes a mild analgesic, such as acetaminophen (Tylenol, Ace-Tabs♣). The client has short-term activity restrictions, depending on the musculoskeletal problem. Ice is often used for 24 hours, and the extremity should be elevated for 24 to 48 hours. When arthroscopic surgery is performed, the health care provider usually prescribes an opioid-analgesic combination, such as oxycodone and acetaminophen (Percocet, Tylox).

Although complications are not common, the nurse monitors and teaches the client to monitor for the following:

- Swelling
- Hypothermia (decreased body temperature) resulting from the use of the tourniquet during the procedure
- Increased joint pain attributable to mechanical injury
- Thrombophlebitis
- Infection

Severe joint or limb pain after discharge may indicate a possible complication and warrants that the client contact the

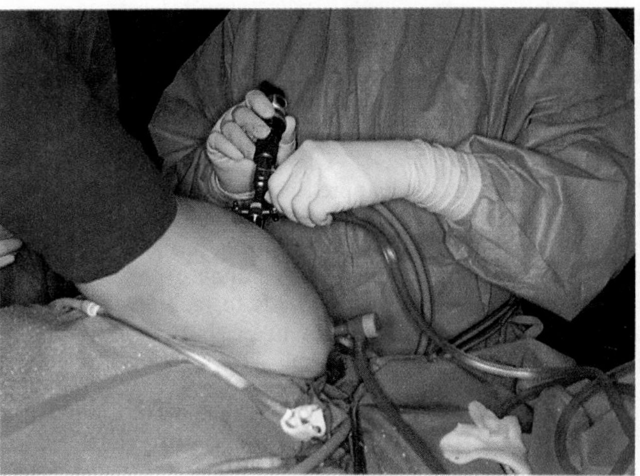

Figure 50-7 ● An arthroscope is used in the diagnosis of pathologic changes in the joints. This client is undergoing arthroscopy of the shoulder.

physician immediately. The health care provider may see the client about 1 week after the test to check for complications.

CRITICAL THINKING CHALLENGE

A young male client complains of severe left knee pain following a ski trip last weekend. The orthopedic surgeon suspects damage to the meniscus and schedules the client for an arthroscopy.

- As his office nurse, what health teaching will you need to provide to prepare the client for this procedure?
- What immediate post-test care will the client require? What discharge instructions will the postanesthesia care unit (PACU) nurse need to review?

For suggested answer guidelines, go to SIMON http://www.wbsaunders.com/SIMON/Iggy/.

Bone Scan

The bone scan is a radionuclide test in which radioactive material is injected for visualization of the entire skeleton. It is used primarily to detect tumors, arthritis, osteomyelitis, osteoporosis, vertebral compression fractures, and unexplained bone pain.

CLIENT PREPARATION. A nuclear medicine physician or technician injects the client intravenously with the radioactive isotope of technetium (^{99m}Tc) several hours before the scanning procedure. As a bone-seeking substance, the isotope migrates to bone. The nurse assures the client that the dose is minimal and that no complications will result from receipt of the material. He or she is asked to void immediately before the scan to prevent an obliterated view of the pelvis by the urinary bladder.

PROCEDURE. The client is taken to the nuclear medicine department and placed on the scanning table. For an accurate image, the client must be able to lie still for 30 to 60 minutes during scanning. Clients who are older, restless, or in pain may find this test uncomfortable and may need mild sedation. The examiner looks for areas of bone in which there is increased uptake, or concentration, of the isotope. These hot lesions indicate abnormal bone metabolism, a sign of bone disease. Cold lesions, in which there is decreased uptake, indicate poor blood flow to bone, as in severe arteriosclerosis.

FOLLOW-UP CARE. The amount of radioactivity in the isotope is minimal and presents no hazard to the client or the nurse. The substance is excreted in urine and stool. Because the substance rapidly deteriorates in the body, no special precautions are required for handling excreta. The nurse encourages the client to push fluids to facilitate urinary excretion. Repeated scans may be taken, but no additional injection of the radioisotope is required.

Gallium/Thallium Scans

The gallium or thallium scan is similar to the bone scan but is more specific and sensitive in detecting bone problems. Gallium citrate (^{67}Ga) is the radioisotope most commonly used. This substance also migrates to brain, liver, and breast tissue and therefore is used in examination of these structures when disease is suspected.

For clients with osteosarcoma, thallium (^{201}Tl) is better than gallium or technetium for diagnosing the extent of the disease. Thallium has traditionally been used for the diagnosis of myocardial infarctions but is now also used for evaluation of cancers of the bone.

CLIENT PREPARATION. Because bone takes up gallium slowly, the nuclear medicine physician or technician administers the isotope 1 to 2 days before scanning. Other tests that require contrast media or other isotopes cannot be given during this time.

The nurse instructs the client that the radioactive material poses no threat because it readily deteriorates in the body. Because gallium is excreted through the intestinal tract, it tends to collect in feces before the scanning procedure.

PROCEDURE. Depending on the tissue to be examined, the client is taken to the nuclear medicine department 1 to 2 days after injection. The procedure takes 30 to 60 minutes, during which time the client must lie still for accurate test results to be achieved. Mild sedation may be necessary to facilitate relaxation and cooperation during the procedure for confused older clients or those in severe pain.

FOLLOW-UP CARE. No special care is required after the test. The radioisotope is excreted in stool and urine, but no precautions are taken in handling the excreta. The nurse encourages the client to push fluids to facilitate urinary excretion.

Magnetic Resonance Imaging

Magnetic resonance imaging (MRI), with or without the use of contrast media, can be used to diagnose musculoskeletal disorders. Its use is expanding and replacing some of the more traditional tests, such as bone scans. The MRI is more accurate than computed tomography (CT) and myelography for many spinal and knee problems (Patel & Lauerman, 1997).

The image is produced through the interaction of magnetic fields, radio waves, and atomic nuclei showing hydrogen density. Simply put, the radio waves "bounce" off the body tissues being examined. Because each tissue has its own density, the computer image clearly distinguishes normal and abnormal tissues. For some tissues, the cross-sectional image is better than that produced by radiography or CT. The lack of hydrogen ions in cortical bone makes it easily distinguishable from soft tissues. The test is particularly useful in identifying problems with muscles, tendons, and ligaments.

The nurse ensures that the client removes all metal objects and checks for clothing zippers and metal fasteners. Although joint implants made of titanium or stainless steel are safe, pacemakers and surgical clips are not. Chart 50-4 lists questions that the nurse or technician should consider in preparing the client for MRI. Open MRIs prevent the claustrophobia that occurs with the older, encased machines.

Gadolinium-DTPA (diethylenetriamine-pentaacetic acid) is the only contrast agent approved for MRI. It is most commonly used to diagnose degenerative vertebral disease and recurrent disk herniation—sometimes referred to as the failed back surgery syndrome (Patel & Lauerman, 1997).

CHART 50-4

BEST PRACTICE *for*
The Client Preparing for Magnetic Resonance Imaging

- Is the client pregnant?
- Does the client have magnetic metal fragments or implants, such as an aneurysm clip?
- If the client has an IV catheter, can it be converted to a heparin lock temporarily?
- Does the client have a pacemaker or electronic implant?
- Can the client be without supplemental oxygen for an hour?
- Can the client tolerate the supine position for 20 to 30 minutes?
- Can the client lie still for 20 to 30 minutes?
- Does the client need life support equipment?
- Can the client communicate clearly and understand verbal communication?

Ultrasonography

Sound waves produce an image of the tissue in ultrasonography. An ultrasound procedure may be used to visualize the following:

- Soft-tissue disorders, such as masses and fluid accumulation
- Traumatic joint injuries
- Osteomyelitis
- Surgical hardware placement

A jelly-like substance applied to the skin over the site to be examined promotes the movement of a metal probe. No special preparation or post-test care is necessary. A quantitative ultrasound (QUS) may be done for determining fractures or bone density.

ONLINE RESOURCES

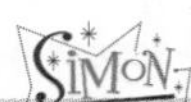

For suggested readings and Internet resources, go to http://www.wbsaunders.com/SIMON/Iggy/.

SELECTED BIBLIOGRAPHY

Asterisk indicates a classic or definitive work on this subject.

Burke, M.M., & Walsh, M.B. (1997). *Gerontologic nursing: Wholistic care of the older adult* (2nd ed.). St. Louis: Mosby.

Corbett, J.V. (1998). Laboratory tests and diagnostic procedures in orthopaedic nursing practice. *Nursing Clinics of North America, 33*(4), 685-700.

Eliopoulos, C. (1997). *Gerontological nursing* (4th ed.). Philadelphia: J.B. Lippincott.

*Guyton, A.C. (1995). *Textbook of medical physiology.* Philadelphia: W.B. Saunders.

Ignatavicius, D.D. (1998). *Introduction to long-term care.* Philadelphia: F.A. Davis.

Jarvis, C. (2000). *Physical examination and health assessment* (3rd ed.). Philadelphia: W.B. Saunders.

Mangini, M. (1998). Physical assessment of the musculoskeletal system. *Nursing Clinics of North America, 33*(4), 643-652.

Martsolf, D.S. (1999). Cultural aspects of orthopaedic nursing. *Orthopaedic Nursing, 18*(2), 65-71.

Matteson, M.A., McConnell, E.S., & Linton, A.D. (1997). *Gerontological nursing: Concepts and practice* (2nd ed.). Philadelphia: W.B. Saunders.

Neal, L. (1997). Basic musculoskeletal assessment: Tips for the home health nurse. *Home Healthcare Nurse, 15*(4), 227-235.

O'Hanlon-Nichols, T. (1998). Basic assessment series: A review of the adult musculoskeletal system. *American Journal of Nursing, 98*(6), 48-52.

Pagana, K.D., & Pagana, T.J. (1999). *Mosby's diagnostic and laboratory test reference* (4th ed.). St. Louis: Mosby.

Patel, P.R., & Lauerman, W.C. (1997). The use of magnetic resonance imaging in the diagnosis of lumbar disc disease. *Orthopaedic Nursing, 16*(1), 59-65.

Scura, K.W., & Whipple, B. (1997). How to provide better care for the postmenopausal woman. *American Journal of Nursing, 97*(4), 36-44.

CHAPTER 51

Interventions for Clients with Musculoskeletal Problems

DONNA D. IGNATAVICIUS

Learning Objectives

After studying this chapter, you should be able to:

1. Explain the risk factors for primary and secondary osteoporosis.
2. Describe ways to decrease the risk for osteoporosis.
3. Discuss the role of drug therapy in the prevention and management of osteoporosis.
4. Compare and contrast osteoporosis and osteomalacia.
5. Identify common assessment findings in clients with Paget's disease of the bone.
6. Differentiate acute and chronic osteomyelitis.
7. Analyze assessment data to determine common nursing diagnoses and collaborative problems for the client with a malignant bone tumor.
8. Discuss the psychosocial aspects associated with a diagnosis of bone cancer.
9. Develop a community-based plan of care for a client with a malignant bone tumor.
10. Evaluate the nursing care of a client with a bone tumor using expected outcome criteria.
11. Explain the pathophysiology and risk factors for carpal tunnel syndrome.
12. Discuss treatment options for the client diagnosed with carpal tunnel syndrome.
13. Describe common disorders of the foot, including hallux valgus and plantar fasciitis.
14. Explain the role of the nurse when caring for a client with muscular dystrophy.

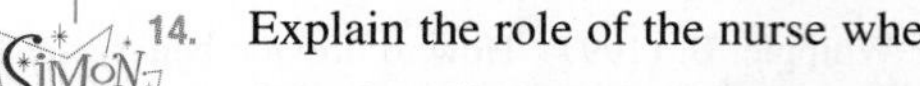

Go to http://www.wbsaunders.com/SIMON/Iggy/ for self-assessment questions related to these Learning Objectives.

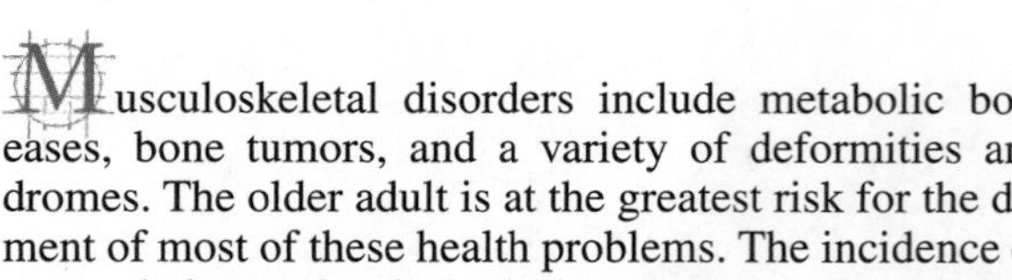

Musculoskeletal disorders include metabolic bone diseases, bone tumors, and a variety of deformities and syndromes. The older adult is at the greatest risk for the development of most of these health problems. The incidence of bone cancer is increasing in both the young and the older population. As technologic advances occur and clients survive longer with primary lesions, metastatic cancer becomes more prevalent. This chapter focuses on selected disorders not covered in Chapter 21 on connective tissue diseases.

METABOLIC BONE DISEASES

Osteoporosis

OVERVIEW

Osteoporosis is a metabolic disease in which bone demineralization results in decreased density and subsequent fractures. The wrist, hip, and vertebral column are most often affected.

The World Health Organization (WHO) has developed a standard for osteoporosis diagnosis based on **bone mineral density (BMD)** values using T-scores. A T-score is the number of standard deviations above or below the average BMD. Low bone mass **(osteopenia)** is present when the T-score is between −1 and −2.5. Osteoporosis in postmenopausal women is defined as a BMD T-score at or below −2.5 (Ott, 1999).

Osteoporosis is a major health problem in many countries. Therefore a World Congress on Osteoporosis was convened in 2000 to explore how to best prevent and treat this costly health problem. The estimated cost for osteoporosis-related health care in the United States alone is more than $14 billion each year (Cutson & Meuleman, 2000).

Pathophysiology

Bone is a dynamic tissue. Throughout a person's life span, new bone is formed by osteoblastic activity, whereas old bone is resorbed through osteoclastic activity; this process is known as bone modeling. BMD determines bone strength and peaks between 30 and 35 years of age. After the peak years, bone resorption activity exceeds bone-building activity, and bone density decreases. Trabecular, or cancellous (spongy), bone is lost first, followed by loss of cortical (compact) bone.

BMD decreases rapidly in postmenopausal women as serum estrogen levels diminish. Approximately 40% to 45% of a woman's bone mass is lost during her life span. It is estimated that 50% of all women older than 65 years of age have symptomatic osteoporosis.

More than half of all Caucasian women have at least one osteoporotic fracture during their lifetime. Men also develop osteoporosis and resulting fractures. Studies have shown that although men are less likely than women to experience a fracture, the lifetime risk of fracture in men is 13% to 25% (Bilezikian, 1999).

CLASSIFICATION OF OSTEOPOROSIS

Osteoporosis is an irreversible osteopenia. There are two major types: primary osteoporosis and secondary osteoporosis. **Primary osteoporosis** is more common and is not associated with an underlying pathologic condition. It occurs in both genders at any age but most often affects women after menopause and men in their later years. **Secondary osteoporosis** results from an associated medical condition, such as hyperparathyroidism; long-term drug therapy, such as with corticosteroids; or prolonged immobility, such as that seen with spinal cord injury (Table 51-1). Treatment of the secondary type is directed toward the cause of the osteoporosis when possible.

Primary osteoporosis can be divided into two subtypes. *Type I* (postmenopausal) osteoporosis occurs in women between the ages of 55 and 65 years. Estrogen presumably prevents or decreases the rate of bone resorption in women and is unavailable in sufficient quantities after menopause. Vertebral and wrist fractures are common in postmenopausal women because the predominant bone type in the vertebrae and wrists is cancellous.

Type II (senile) osteoporosis occurs in those older than 65 years of age and affects women twice as often as men. Hip and vertebral fractures are often seen in clients with type II disease.

THEORIES OF OSTEOPOROSIS DEVELOPMENT

The exact pathophysiology of osteoporosis is unclear, but two theories of disease development have been advocated. First, osteoporosis may result from decreased osteoblastic activity. The osteoblasts, or bone-forming cells, may have a shortened life span or may be less efficient in the client with osteoporosis. The second, and more popular, theory suggests an increase in osteoclastic (bone resorption) activity. The latter theory has gained increased recognition over the past decade and has resulted in treatment directed toward measures to prevent rapid bone resorption.

TABLE 51-1 • CAUSES OF SECONDARY OSTEOPOROSIS

DISEASES/CONDITIONS
- Diabetes mellitus
- Hyperthyroidism
- Hyperparathyroidism
- Cushing's syndrome
- Growth hormone deficiency
- Metabolic acidosis
- Female hypogonadism
- Paget's disease
- Osteogenesis imperfecta
- Rheumatoid arthritis
- Prolonged immobilization
- Marfan's syndrome
- Bone cancer
- Cirrhosis
- Chronic airway limitation

DRUGS (CHRONIC USE)
- Corticosteroids
- Heparin
- Anticonvulsants
- Ethanol (alcohol)
- Drugs that induce hypogonadism (decreased levels of sex hormones)
- High levels of exogenous (external) thyroid hormone

Etiology

The exact cause of primary osteoporosis is unknown; however, numerous risk factors have been identified (Chart 51-1). In view of the high cost of osteoporosis in both health care dollars and quality of life, young women need to be aware of appropriate health and lifestyle practices that can prevent this potentially disabling disease (see the Meeting Healthy People 2010 Objectives box on p. 1096). A nursing study by Berarducci et al. (2000) found that most health care providers focus on the risk of osteoporosis in women over 50 years of age and do not assess risk as often in women age 49 years and younger (see the Evidence-Based Practice for Nursing box on p. 1096).

Primary osteoporosis most often occurs in women after menopause as a result of decreased estrogen levels. Women lose approximately 2% of their bone mass every year in the first 5 years after menopause. For women who cannot take estrogen replacement, such as breast cancer survivors, the risk of osteoporosis increases.

In addition, body build seems to predict the occurrence of the disease. Osteoporosis occurs more often in thin, lean-built Caucasian and Asian women, particularly those who do not exercise regularly. Obese women can store estrogen in their tissues for use as necessary to maintain a normal level of serum calcium. Exercise decreases bone resorption and stimulates bone formation. Immobilization, such as prolonged bedrest, produces rapid bone loss.

The relationship of osteoporosis to dietary factors is not as well established. A diet deficient in calcium and vitamin D stimulates the parathyroid gland to produce parathyroid hormone (PTH). PTH triggers the release of calcium from the bony matrix. Malabsorption, caused by disease or drugs, also contributes to low serum calcium levels. Institutionalized or homebound people who are not exposed to sunlight may be at a higher risk because they do not receive adequate vitamin D for the metabolism of calcium.

Protein deficiency may contribute to the incidence of bone demineralization, although this theory is controversial. Be-

CHART 51-1

BEST PRACTICE *for*
Assessing Risk Factors for Primary Osteoporosis

Assess for the following:
- Client's age greater than 60
- Family history of osteoporosis
- Caucasian or Asian race
- Thin, lean body build
- Low, lifetime calcium intake
- Estrogen deficiency
- Androgen deficiency
- Smoking history
- High alcohol intake
- Lack of physical exercise or prolonged immobility

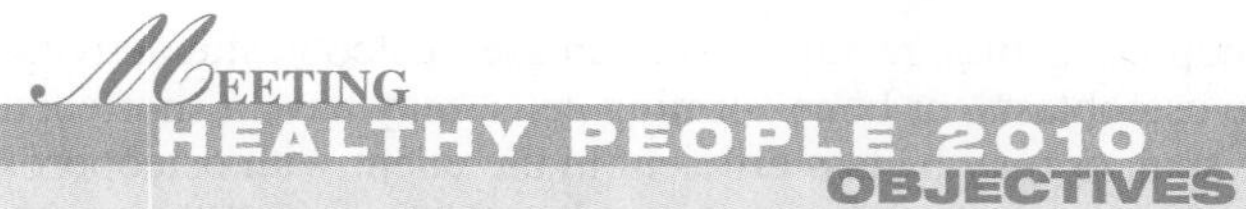

OSTEOPOROSIS

Objective 2.10: Reduce the proportion of adults who are hospitalized for vertebral fractures associated with osteoporosis.

- Teach women of all ages about osteoporosis as a disease and cause of potentially life-threatening fractures.
- Teach young and middle-aged women the need to practice a lifestyle that reduces the risk factors for osteoporosis (e.g., no smoking, increased exercise, increased calcium intake).
- Teach middle-aged and older adults to have bone mineral density screening tests to determine their bone loss percentage (often available at no or minimal cost at local health fairs or pharmacies).
- Remind clients to use proper body mechanics, such as using large leg muscles rather than back muscles for lifting.
- If clients are at high risk for osteoporosis, tell them to avoid jarring activities such as jogging or horseback riding.
- If clients are at high risk for osteoporosis, tell them to consult with a health care provider and comply with preventive treatment.

EVIDENCE-BASED PRACTICE FOR NURSING

Do health care providers assess knowledge of osteoporosis in young women?

Berarducci, A., et al. (2000). Health-promoting educational practices related to osteoporosis. *Applied Nursing Research, 13*(4), 173-180.

This descriptive study was designed to determine if health care providers educate women of all ages about osteoporosis, including assessing risk factors for the disease. The researchers surveyed 90 health care providers in southwest Florida. Forty-nine surveys were returned, and 47 were usable. The responses of the providers showed significant differences between women 49 years of age and younger and women over 50 years of age. Health care providers routinely assessed risk factors in older women and educated these women, but they did not identify risk factors or provide education for younger women.

Critique. Although the sample size was small and the subjects constituted a convenience sample, this research is one of the few studies that address the issue of health promotion to prevent osteoporosis in young women. The study cannot be generalized and needs to be repeated using a larger sample in a larger geographic area.

Implications for Nursing. Nurses and other health care professionals in any setting have a responsibility to educate all women, regardless of age, about the risk factors for osteoporosis and how to reduce them. Other studies have supported the belief that lifestyle changes in young adulthood can prevent or minimize the risk for osteoporosis as women age.

cause 50% of serum calcium is protein bound, protein is needed for calcium utilization; however, excessive protein intake may increase calcium loss in the urine. Protein is needed, however, for bone healing when a fracture occurs.

Alcohol consumption and cigarette smoking are other possible risk factors. Although the exact mechanisms are not known, these substances may promote acidosis, which in turn increases bone loss. Alcohol also has a direct toxic effect on bone tissue, resulting in decreased bone formation and increased bone resorption (Leslie, 2000). Excessive caffeine intake can increase calcium loss in the urine.

Hereditary factors may play a role for both men and women, but this hypothesis has not been confirmed (Orwell, 2000). Several of the suspected risk factors, such as body build, are determined in part by heredity; however, heredity or a genetic influence alone probably is not predictive for osteoporosis.

CONSIDERATIONS FOR OLDER ADULTS

Aging is a major risk factor for osteoporosis. As aging occurs, serum concentrations of 1,25-dihydroxycholecalciferol, a vitamin D metabolite, decrease. Osteoporosis is often accompanied by low levels of serum calcitonin, a hormone secreted by the thyroid gland that helps maintain a normal serum calcium level. In addition, some older adults living at home or in health care settings are undernourished and deficient in calcium and protein.

Incidence/Prevalence

Between 25 and 35 million Americans, 80% of whom are women, have osteoporosis. The incidence of the disease is greater in women than in men (at least 5:1) because men usually have larger bones and protection provided by bone-building testosterone. Ninety percent of men and women over age 75 suffer from osteoporosis.

Osteoporosis results in more than 1.5 million fractures each year, 300,000 of which are hip fractures. In people older than 90 years of age, one third of women and one fifth of men experience at least one hip fracture. The mortality for older clients with hip fractures is very high, especially within the first 6 months, and the debilitating effects can be devastating (McClung, 2000).

CULTURAL CONSIDERATIONS

Caucasian women are affected more often than African-American women. It is well documented that African-American women have 10% more bone mass than Caucasian women. Northern European and Asian-American women are at a higher risk than Caucasian women (McClung, 2000).

COLLABORATIVE MANAGEMENT

Assessment

Typically, a diagnosis of osteoporosis is made after the client sustains a vertebral, wrist, or hip fracture. The client may be asymptomatic before admission with one or more bone fractures. When taking a history, the nurse determines the risk factors for osteoporosis, as described under Etiology, p. 1095.

PHYSICAL ASSESSMENT/CLINICAL MANIFESTATIONS

When performing a musculoskeletal assessment, the nurse inspects and palpates the vertebral column. The classic "dowager's hump," or kyphosis of the dorsal spine, is usually present (Figure 51-1). The client often states that height has been shortened, perhaps as much as 2 to 3 inches (5 to 7 cm) within the previous 20 years. Height and weight should be measured and compared with previous measurements if they are available.

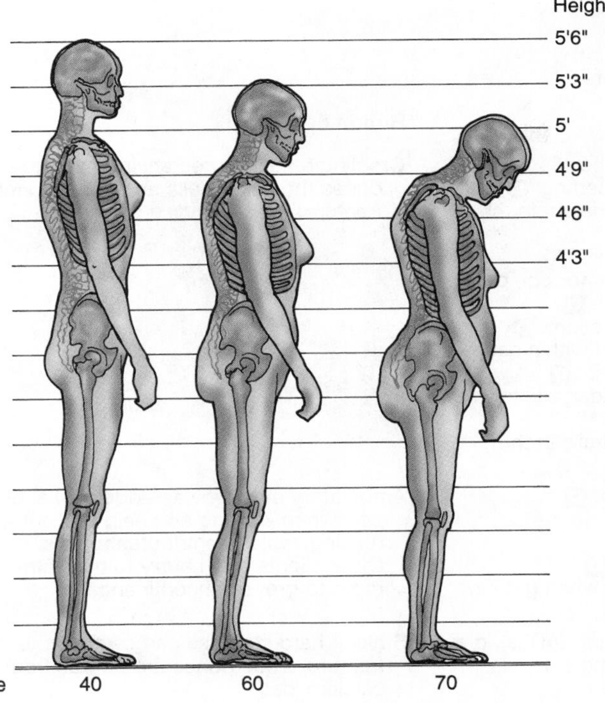

Figure 51-1 ● A normal spine at age 40 years and osteoporotic changes at ages 60 and 70 years. These changes can cause a loss of as much as 6 inches in height and can result in the so-called dowager's hump *(far right)* in the upper thoracic vertebrae.

Accompanying the spinal deformity is the complaint of back pain, which often occurs after lifting, bending, or stooping. The pain may be sharp and acute in onset. Pain is worse with activity and is relieved by rest. Palpation of the vertebrae, particularly the lower thoracic and lumbar vertebrae, usually increases the client's discomfort. Therefore palpation should be gentle.

Back pain accompanied by tenderness and voluntary restriction of spinal movement suggests one or more compression vertebral fractures, the most common type of osteoporotic fracture. Movement restriction and spinal deformity may result in constipation, abdominal distention, reflux esophagitis, and respiratory compromise in severe cases. The most likely area for fracture occurrence is between T8 and L3.

Fractures are also common in the distal end of the radius and the upper third of the femur (hip). The nurse directs special attention to these areas as part of the physical assessment.

PSYCHOSOCIAL ASSESSMENT

Women often associate osteoporosis with menopause, getting older, and becoming less independent. The disease can result in suffering, deformity, and disability that can affect the client's well-being and life satisfaction. The quality of life may be further impacted by pain, insomnia, depression, and **fallophobia** (fear of falling).

The nurse assesses the client's concept of body image, especially if the client is severely kyphotic. For example, the client may have difficulty finding clothes that fit properly. Social interactions may be curtailed because of a change in appearance or the physical limitations of being unable to sit in chairs in restaurants, movie theaters, and other places. Alterations in sexuality may occur as a result of poor self-esteem or the discomfort imposed by positioning during intercourse.

Because osteoporosis readily predisposes a client to fractures, the client must be extremely cautious about activities. As a result, the threat of fracture can create anxiety and fear and result in further limitation of social or physical activities. The nurse assesses for the presence of these feelings because they may affect the response to health care. For instance, the client may be anxious to the point that he or she will not exercise as prescribed for fear that a fracture will occur.

LABORATORY ASSESSMENT

There are no definitive laboratory tests that confirm a diagnosis of primary osteoporosis; however, a number of biochemical markers can provide information about bone modeling. A battery of tests can be performed to rule out secondary osteoporosis or other metabolic bone diseases, such as osteomalacia and Paget's disease. These include determination of serum calcium, vitamin D, phosphorus, and alkaline phosphatase levels.

Urinary calcium levels may also be assessed. Serum protein measurements and thyroid function tests are performed to exclude hyperthyroidism.

A simple, more specific and sensitive test to evaluate bone resorption is being used with clients with spinal cord injury and others at risk. The Upyr Crosslinks assay measures urinary concentrations of pyridinium, a collagen substance found in bone and cartilage. An increase in urinary levels indicates increased bone resorption (loss). The advantage of this test is its ability to detect bone loss early. In addition, no special client preparation is required. The disadvantage of the test is its cost, which is high because the test is relatively new. However, pyridinium and other biochemical markers of bone modeling may be used in the future as a routine screening test (Hunt, Civitelli, & Halstead, 1995).

RADIOGRAPHIC ASSESSMENT

X-ray studies of the spine and long bones show loss of bone density and the presence of fractures. However, radiographic findings of bone density changes are evident only after a 25% to 40% bone loss has occurred.

In the search for a more sensitive diagnostic test to detect early bone changes, computed tomography (CT) has been used extensively, particularly for the spine. CT allows better visualization of changes in the cancellous bone than in the cortical bone. Because the vertebral column consists primarily of cancellous bone, the test is helpful in the early diagnosis of osteoporosis. Quantitative CT (QCT) measures the bone density of vertebral bone.

In the past decade, technologic advances have enabled the detection of early changes in bone density. One of the newer diagnostic tools is dual photon absorptiometry, sometimes called **dual energy x-ray absorptiometry (DEXA).** DEXA is a painless scan that measures bone mineral density (BMD) in the hip, wrist, or vertebral column. It is the best tool currently available for diagnosis. In July 1998, Medicare began covering the cost of bone density studies for high-risk clients. No special client preparation or follow-up care is required.

CLIENT CARE PLAN • THE CLIENT WITH OSTEOPOROSIS

NURSING DIAGNOSIS NO. 1 • Risk for Falls related to trivial accidents

Expected Outcomes	Nursing Interventions	Rationale
The client will not experience falls or fractures resulting from falls.	Create a hazard-free environment for the client while he or she is in the hospital or other setting. [D] Get the client out of bed with the bed height in the lowest position. [D] Teach the client to wear nonskid slippers. [D] Inspect the floor for spills and the room for equipment that may cause tripping or stumbling. [D] Provide additional lighting for an older client. [D] Place necessary items close to the bed within easy reach (e.g., water pitcher and call bell). [D] Keep two siderails up, especially for older adults who are confused. [D] Teach the importance and use of handrails in the bathroom. [D]	Creating a hazard-free environment reduces the risk of falls and subsequent fracture.
	Provide ambulatory support as needed. [D] Assess the need for a cane or a walker. Consult with a physical therapist. Teach the client to call for assistance. [D] Teach the client to take his or her time when getting out of bed and walking. [D]	Ambulatory aids provide additional support when walking and help prevent rushing, which contributes to falls. Older clients often hurry to the bathroom to prevent incontinence.
	When helping with activities of daily living (ADLs), prevent the client from accidentally hitting siderails, door frames, and so on. [D]	Striking hard surfaces can cause bone fracture, since bones are porous from calcium loss.
	Teach the client to bend or stoop slowly and not to lift or move heavy objects, such as hospital furniture.	Quick body movements can easily lead to vertebral compression fractures in the client with osteoporosis.
	Monitor side effects for any drugs the client may be taking for concurrent medical conditions.	Diuretics, phenothiazines, and tranquilizers can cause dizziness, drowsiness, and weakness, predisposing the client to falls.
	Teach the importance of diet in preventing further osteoporosis. Refer to dietary consultation. Teach the client which foods are high in calcium content. Teach the need to decrease caffeine and alcohol intake.	Dietary calcium is needed to maintain the serum level, thus preventing additional loss from bone. Caffeine excess can increase calcium loss in urine; alcohol excess can promote acidosis, which increases bone resorption.
	Teach the effect of cigarette smoking on bone remodeling (if the client is a smoker).	Cigarette smoking can promote acidosis.

[D] Indicates tasks that can be delegated to assistive nursing personnel.

OTHER DIAGNOSTIC ASSESSMENT

Magnetic resonance imaging (MRI) is sometimes used instead of the CT scan to detect the presence of bone density changes, especially in the spine. Ultrasound has recently been approved to detect osteoporotic bone changes. Although not as precise as DEXA, it is less expensive and more available, making it a good screening tool for the disorder.

Interventions

Because the client is predisposed to fractures, drugs and diet therapy are used to retard bone resorption and form new bony tissue. Exercise and education can prevent osteoporosis or slow its progress. These measures help to reduce the chance of fracture and subsequent complications (see the Client Care Plan above).

DRUG THERAPY. The health care provider may prescribe estrogen, calcium supplements, vitamin D, biphosphonates (BPs), selective estrogen receptor modulators, calcitonin, or a combination of several drugs to treat osteoporosis, as well as to prevent it (Chart 51-2). Other agents have been given, but with limited success. Estrogen is the least expensive of the drugs used for osteoporosis.

ESTROGEN. Estrogen blocks bone resorption by inhibiting cytokines, which are chemicals that stimulate osteoclastic activity. Therefore estrogen replacement (ERT) is effective in slowing bone loss and treating established disease. Studies have shown a remarkable reduction of fractures in women undergoing estrogen therapy (Capriotti, 2000). It is recommended, however, that the drug be initiated shortly after menopause and continued on a long-term basis.

The health care provider may prescribe low doses, such as 0.625 mg, of conjugated estrogens (Premarin, C.E.S.♣) because the side effects of the drug, such as endometrial or breast cancer, are potentially serious. Some providers do not use the drug for preventive purposes. Others believe that the

CLIENT CARE PLAN • THE CLIENT WITH OSTEOPOROSIS—cont'd

NURSING DIAGNOSIS NO. 2 • Impaired Physical Mobility related to decreased muscle tone, dysfunction secondary to previous fractures, or pain secondary to recent fractures

Expected Outcomes	Nursing Interventions	Rationale
The client will increase mobility to the level of ADL independence.	Consult with the physical therapist regarding an exercise program to include strengthening and weight-bearing exercises. Assist the client as necessary with exercises [D] Teach the client that ADLs do not replace prescribed exercises. Teach the importance of exercises.	Strengthening exercises increase joint movement, increase muscle tone, and stimulate blood circulation to bone and muscle tissue. Weight-bearing exercises decrease the rate of bone loss and increase bone formation.
	Assist with ADLs as necessary, allowing the client to be as independent as possible. [D]	Pain and poor muscle tone may limit the client's ability to be independent, especially after a fracture.
	Assess the need for assistive and adaptive devices in order to perform ADLs; consult with the occupational therapist to obtain appropriate equipment.	Devices may be needed for the client to be independent in ADLs. Overuse and reliance, however, should be discouraged.

NURSING DIAGNOSIS NO. 3 • Acute Pain and Chronic Pain related to effects of vertebral fracture

Expected Outcomes	Nursing Interventions	Rationale
The client will experience alleviation or reduction of pain so that he or she can be independent in care.	Assess the need for pain medication: opioid or non-opioid analgesics, muscle relaxants, or anti-inflammatory drugs.	Clients usually receive pain medication on a prn schedule. Older clients often do not request pain medication even if needed; therefore the nurse must anticipate this need.
	Maintain orthotic devices for vertebral fracture. Check that the brace or corset fits properly. Inspect the skin where the device causes pressure. [D] Apply the device for use when the client gets out of bed. [D]	Orthotic devices maintain spine alignment and provide spinal column support.
	Apply moist heat to the back (heat packs or hot compresses) as needed to reduce pain. (The physical therapist may do this.) (See also Chapter 7.)	Heat increases blood circulation to affected areas, thus relieving muscle spasms, which cause pain.

[D] Indicates tasks that can be delegated to assistive nursing personnel.

benefit of estrogen in preventing potentially debilitating and life-threatening fractures outweighs its risks. The health care provider often prescribes progesterone along with the estrogen (hormone replacement therapy [HRT]) to minimize cancer occurrence. For middle-aged women, especially those in their 40s and early 50s (sometimes referred to as the "transition years"), birth control pills may be used to provide these supplements. However, some clients do not want to have uterine bleeding and breast tenderness.

A newer form of estrogen, the estrogen patch (Estraderm, Estrace, Femogex♣), delivers an even, continuous amount of estrogen when applied several times each week. These patches are available in several doses, from 4 mg/10 cm (0.05 mg/24 hr) to 8 mg/10 cm (0.1 mg/24 hr).

CALCIUM. If a person cannot ingest sufficient quantities of calcium in the diet, calcium supplements are used. Natural calcium sources, such as oyster shells, are preferable. Supplements should be started in the high-risk population in young adulthood, because bone resorption accelerates after age 30 to 35 years. Calcium carbonate, found in over-the-counter (OTC) drugs such as Tums, is one of the most cost-effective and is best taken with food, since gastric acid is needed to absorb it. Calcium citrate does not require gastric acid for absorption and is therefore most often recommended as a calcium supplement (Capriotti, 2000). Forty percent of calcium carbonate is elemental calcium that can be used by the body. For example, a 600-mg tablet contains about 240 mg of elemental calcium.

The client should take calcium supplements under the supervision of a health care provider. **Hypercalcemia** (excess serum calcium) can cause serious damage to the urinary system. The amount of calcium prescribed is affected by the addition of estrogen therapy and the presence of risk factors for osteoporosis.

In the United States the typical daily intake of dietary calcium is between 450 and 550 mg. The recommended daily allowance (RDA) of calcium is 1200 mg. Many clinicians and researchers believe that the RDA is insufficient to meet the calcium requirements of postmenopausal women, who may require as much as 1500 mg or more daily to prevent osteoporosis. An increased calcium intake may prevent bone loss in men as well. The nurse teaches the client to consume foods rich in calcium, such as milk and dairy products and dark green, leafy vegetables (see Chapter 11 for a list of foods high in calcium).

VITAMIN D. Vitamin D supplementation may be necessary for the institutionalized or homebound client or for those

CHART 51-2

DRUG THERAPY *for* Osteoporosis

Drug	Usual Dosage	Nursing Interventions	Rationale
Calcium (e.g., Os-Cal, Tums, Caltrate-600, Citracal)	1.0-1.5 g in divided doses PO	Give a third of daily dose at bedtime. Push fluids.	Calcium is most readily utilized by the body when the client is fasting and immobile. Increased fluid intake aids in preventing the formation of calcium-based urinary stones.
		Assess for a history of urinary stones.	Calcium supplements are not given to clients who are susceptible to urinary stone formation.
		Monitor serum calcium level.	Hypercalcemia, or calcium excess, is a side effect of calcium supplementation.
		Monitor urinary calcium level (no more than 4 mg/kg in 24 hr).	The kidneys attempt to excrete excess calcium.
		Observe for signs of hypercalcemia.	Hypercalcemia can result in urinary stones, cardiac arrhythmias, and an increase or decrease in skeletal muscle tone.
Estrogen (e.g., Premarin, Estinyl, Estrace C.E.S.✤, Transderm) may be given with progesterone on days 16-25	0.425-1.25 mg PO for 25 days/mo 0.05 mg/24 hr or 0.1 mg/24 hr transdermally	Assess for history of tumors, hypertension, thromboembolytic disease, or liver or gallbladder disease.	Estrogen therapy is withheld from clients with susceptibility to an exacerbation of one or more of these problems.
		Teach the importance of gynecologic examinations every 6 months.	Endometrial and breast cancer can result from estrogen therapy.
		Teach breast self-examination.	Clients can detect potentially malignant lesions early so that treatment can begin immediately.
		Observe for vaginal bleeding.	Vaginal bleeding is a side effect of estrogen therapy and a sign of possible endometrial cancer.
		Monitor blood pressure.	Hypertension and other cardiovascular complications may result from combined estrogen-progesterone therapy.
		Observe for thrombus formation.	Deep vein thrombosis is a complication of combined estrogen-progesterone therapy.
		Monitor serum liver enzyme and cholesterol levels.	An elevation of liver enzyme levels may be indicative of liver involvement resulting from estrogen. An elevated cholesterol level can result in hypertension and thrombus formation.
Alendronate (Fosamax)	5 mg/day PO	Take early in AM with 8 oz water; do not lie down until after breakfast.	Although not common, esophagitis or esophageal ulcers may result from alendronate therapy.
Raloxifene (Evista)	60 mg qd	Teach client to monitor weight and BP frequently.	Drug causes increased water and sodium retention.
		Monitor liver function tests (LFTs) in collaboration with health care provider.	Raloxifene can cause increased LFTs or worsen hepatic disease (should not be given to client who has liver disease).
Calcitonin (e.g., Calcimar [salmon], Cibacalcin [human], Miacalcin [salmon; nasal spray])	100 IU/day SC or IM 200 IU/day intranasally, alternating nostrils	Rotate injection sites for parenteral administration.	Injection sites become irritated and reddened.
		Monitor for flushing, headache, nausea, and vomiting.	These are common side effects of calcitonin.
		Monitor renal function, calcium, and vitamin D levels.	Toxicity from calcitonin can cause renal problems.

who do not meet daily requirements. An adequate level of vitamin D is needed for optimal calcium absorption in the intestines. The prescribed dosage is usually 400 to 800 international units (IU)/day. Higher doses can produce toxic effects, such as hypercalcemia and hyperphosphatemia.

BIPHOSPHONATES. Biphosphonates (BPs) inhibit bone resorption by binding with crystal elements in bone, especially spongy, trabecular bone tissue. Two BPs, alendronate (Fosamax) and etidronate (Didronel) have been approved for the prevention and management of osteoporosis, Paget's disease, and hypercalcemia associated with cancer.

Although side effects are not common, when they do occur, they tend to be serious. Esophagitis and esophageal ulcers have been reported with the use of Fosamax, especially when the pill is not completely swallowed. The nurse teaches clients taking this drug to take it early in the morning with 8 ounces of water. They should not lie down until after breakfast. If chest pain occurs, a symptom of esophageal irritation, they should discontinue the drug and contact their health care provider. Clients with poor renal function, hypocalcemia, or gastrointestinal reflux disease (GERD) should not take BPs.

Other BPs, such as risedronate, are being investigated. Because of poor gastrointestinal absorption of most BPs, parenteral administration is also being studied. Clodronate may be given every 2 weeks intramuscularly to enhance bone mineral density (BMD), but the injection is very painful. Ibandronate, given intravenously every 3 months, has shown increases in vertebral bone mass (Capriotti, 2000).

SELECTIVE ESTROGEN RECEPTOR MODULATORS. Selective estrogen receptor modulators (SERMs), a newer class of drugs, are designed to mimic estrogen in some parts of the body while blocking its effect elsewhere. Raloxifene (Evista) is used for prevention and management of osteoporosis in postmenopausal women. It increases BMD, reduces bone resorption, and lowers serum cholesterol. The recommended dose is 60 mg/day. The drug should not be given to women who have a history of thromboembolitic disease (Leslie, 2000).

CALCITONIN. Calcitonin is a thyroid hormone that inhibits osteoclastic activity, thus decreasing bone loss. It is used for the treatment of osteoporosis, Paget's disease, and hypercalcemia associated with cancer. The drug also has an analgesic effect after vertebral fracture, thereby promoting early recovery.

Calcitonin (salmon) can be given intramuscularly, subcutaneously, or intranasally (Miacalcin). Nasal administration is preferred because it improves compliance, minimizes side effects, and is convenient. The nurse teaches the client to alternate nostrils to prevent nasal mucosal irritation, a common side effect.

OTHER AGENTS. Androgens, such as testosterone propionate (Testex, Malogen🍁), have been successful in decreasing bone resorption and increasing bone growth. When given to postmenopausal women, however, androgens cause masculine traits and may lead to liver disease. Androgens may decrease bone resorption in men, however, particularly older men.

DIET THERAPY. The dietary considerations for the treatment of a client with a diagnosis of osteoporosis are the same as those for preventing the disease. Adequate amounts of protein, magnesium, vitamin K, and trace minerals are needed for bone formation. Calcium and vitamin D intake needs to be increased, and alcohol and caffeine consumption should be discouraged. For the client who has sustained a fracture, intake of protein, vitamin C, and iron is increased to promote bone healing.

PREVENTION OF FALLS. The client must be careful to prevent falls and other activities that can cause a fracture. A hazard-free environment is necessary to meet this goal, and the nurse must teach the client about its importance.

Many hospitals and long-term care facilities have risk management programs in which clients are assessed for their risk for falls. For those at high risk, programs such as the Falling Star protocol have reduced falls by making the staff aware of the client's high risk. In this program, a star is placed at the head of the bed to designate a person at high risk. Chapter 5 discusses fall prevention in health care agencies and at home in more detail.

Hip protectors are inexpensive devices that can prevent hip fracture if the client experiences a fall. A hip protector is a pad that is worn while ambulating. If the client falls onto his or her trochanter, the probability of hip fracture is lessened.

EXERCISE. Exercise is important in the prevention and management of osteoporosis. It also plays a vital role in pain management, cardiovascular function, and an improved sense of well-being.

In collaboration with the health care provider, the physical therapist prescribes exercises for strengthening the abdominal and back muscles. These exercises improve posture and provide an improved support for the spine. Abdominal isometrics, deep breathing, and pectoral stretching are stressed in order to increase pulmonary capacity. Exercises for the extremity muscles include isometric, resistive, and range-of-motion (ROM) exercises. The nurse encourages active ROM exercises, which improve joint mobility and increase muscle tone.

In addition to exercises for muscle strengthening, a general weight-bearing exercise program is implemented. Walking for 30 minutes three times a week, swimming, or bicycling are recommended activities. The nurse teaches the client that certain high-impact recreational activities, such as bowling and horseback riding, may cause vertebral compression and should be avoided.

PAIN MANAGEMENT. The pain management program depends on the intensity and duration of the pain. With treatment, pain from spinal fractures often resolves 6 to 8 weeks after injury; treatment usually includes drug therapy and orthotic devices. The health care provider prescribes analgesics (opioid and nonopioid) during the acute phase of the pain (i.e., from the time of injury to as long as several weeks afterward). Muscle relaxants, which ease the discomfort associated with muscle spasms, are often used for spinal fractures. Nonsteroidal anti-inflammatory drugs (NSAIDs) are beneficial for pain relief and for decreasing spinal nerve root inflammation from crushed vertebrae. The nurse is alert to the problems associated with NSAIDs, such as gastrointestinal bleeding and congestive heart failure, particularly in older adults.

ORTHOTIC DEVICES. Known as dorsolumbar orthoses, orthotic devices immobilize the spine during the acute pain phase and provide spinal column support (Figure 51-2). The physical therapist or orthotist custom fits the client for this lightweight device. The client is taught to inspect the skin for irritation and report tolerance to the device.

CRITICAL THINKING CHALLENGE

You are working in a nursing home where one of your older female residents has fallen three times this week. When you review her chart, you note that she has been diagnosed with osteoporosis for about 10 years but has not been treated. The resident ambulates independently without an assistive device.

- What assessments will you want to perform on this resident?
- What options might the resident have for medical management of her osteoporosis?
- What health teaching should you plan for her?

For suggested answer guidelines, go to SIMON: http://www.wbsaunders.com/SIMON/Iggy/.

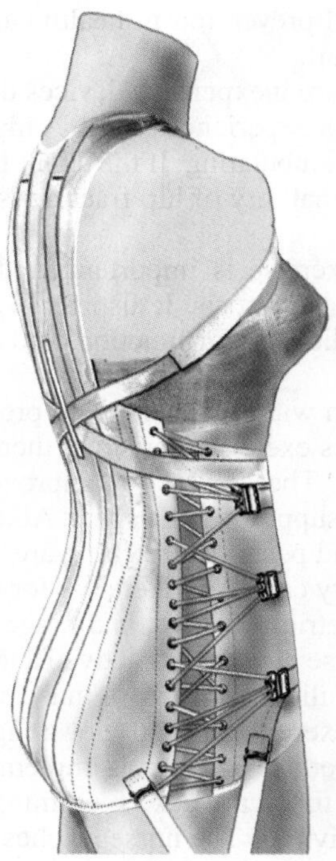

Figure 51-2 ● A dorsolumbar orthosis. (Courtesy Truform Orthotics and Prosthetics, Cincinnati, OH.)

Community-Based Care

Clients with osteoporosis are usually managed at home. However, some experience fractures that may require hospitalization.

The client with osteoporosis who has one or more fractures can be discharged to the home setting. In some instances, the client is discharged to a long-term care facility for rehabilitation or permanent residence when support systems are not available.

HOME CARE MANAGEMENT

If the client is discharged to the home setting, the nurse must assess the environment for potential hazards before discharge. The nurse uses the database completed by the nurse or occupational therapist at the time of admission to ascertain whether alterations in the home environment are necessary. For example, if scatter rugs are used in the home, the client is advised to have these removed to reduce the chance of falling.

A two-story house or apartment may be a problem if physical mobility is limited or if an adequate support railing is not available to assist with stair climbing. The social worker, discharge planner, or case manager, in conjunction with the nurse, helps the client identify adaptations that may have to be made to create as hazard free an environment as possible.

Assistive or adaptive devices for personal use may be needed, if only for a short time. Devices to assist with activities of daily living (ADLs), such as a dressing stick to put on pants, are helpful in maintaining the client's independence. The occupational therapist works with the nurse to determine the need for assistive devices. Chapter 10 describes the promotion of ADL independence in detail.

The nurse and physical therapist assess the need for ambulatory aids in the home. A walker or cane may provide the additional support necessary to prevent falls.

HEALTH TEACHING

The teaching plan for the client with osteoporosis includes prevention of falls (see the Meeting Healthy People 2010 Objectives box on p. 1096), exercise, diet therapy, and drug therapy. Psychosocial support is also important to help the client maintain the highest quality of life possible.

PREVENTION OF FALLS. Clients must be extremely careful to prevent falls. Ambulatory aids should be used for additional support, although some clients refuse to be seen in public with a cane or walker. Similarly, clients may not want to wear orthotic devices because of embarrassment or discomfort. The nurse and physical therapist provide a thorough explanation of the necessity and the proper method for using these devices.

EXERCISE. The physical therapist prescribes a structured exercise program, which the nurse reinforces. Strengthening, ROM, and weight-bearing exercises are taught. Follow-up physical therapy visits ensure that clients have learned the exercises and are compliant.

DIET THERAPY. The nurse emphasizes the importance of a diet rich in calcium-containing foods. A diet consultation before discharge can help clients select foods they like and that are high in the essential nutrients. If a fracture has occurred, the nurse encourages clients to eat foods rich in vitamin C, protein, and iron. The nurse also instructs them to decrease caffeine and alcohol consumption and to stop smoking.

DRUG THERAPY. For clients who will be homebound or institutionalized, sunlight exposure should be promoted as an essential source of vitamin D. The importance of sunlight should be stressed to the long-term care facility where the client may be transferred. The nurse teaches about the therapeutic and adverse effects associated with drug therapy for osteoporosis (see Chart 51-2).

PSYCHOSOCIAL SUPPORT. Because clients are often afraid that they will sustain a fracture, it is extremely important to allay their fears to the extent possible. The degree of osteoporosis determines the likelihood of injury. The more severe the osteoporosis, the more limited the activities should be. For example, a woman with severe osteoporosis may sustain vertebral compression fractures from stooping or bending. For most clients, an aggressive treatment plan prevents fractures from trivial trauma.

Explaining the importance of orthotic and ambulatory aids in the prevention of injury increases compliance and decreases reluctance to use the devices. A supportive spouse, family member, or significant other can encourage clients to adhere to the treatment plan.

CONSIDERATIONS FOR OLDER ADULTS

Because most clients with osteoporosis are older, they may not comply with the diet or exercise. Often the older adult is used to eating less than the required daily nutrients. Consumption of milk and dairy products is usually minimal. As a result, the health care provider prescribes calcium supplements for long-term maintenance. The nurse instructs clients to take only the prescribed amount; too much calcium can lead to hypercalcemia. Exercise compliance may also be a problem for older adults.

Clients who are receiving estrogen therapy need to have frequent gynecologic checkups to detect early signs of endometrial cancer. The nurse teaches clients how to monitor for side effects. Follow-up visits to the health care provider are scheduled frequently to monitor calcium blood levels and determine further progression of osteoporosis.

HEALTH CARE RESOURCES

If the client cannot return home after a fracture, placement in a nursing home may be necessary, at least for a short time. The hospital nurse or case manager documents the client's needs on the transfer record and communicates the special considerations required.

If returning to a home environment, the client may need equipment for ADLs and ambulation. Financial resources are assessed before equipment is obtained. If the client's insurance or other third-party payer will not reimburse him or her, other sources are explored. Religious and support organizations are possible resources for free materials. Items are often donated to these groups for use as needed in the community. Rental of equipment is also an option. The hospital or local medical supplier can provide cost estimates of renting versus purchasing the needed equipment. The equipment should be accessible before the client returns home.

A home care nurse may be needed for follow-up in the home environment. The nurse in this setting can be contacted to assist in the discharge planning for the client, to assess potential environmental hazards, and to obtain equipment and supplies. The home care nurse determines the need for physical or occupational therapy, social work, and homemaking personnel in the home.

In addition to home care resources, the Osteoporosis Foundation provides information to clients and health care professionals regarding the disease and its treatment. Large metropolitan hospitals often have osteoporosis specialty clinics and support groups for clients with osteoporosis.

Osteomalacia

OVERVIEW

Osteomalacia is a reversible metabolic disease in which there is a defect in the mineralization of bone. Unlike in osteoporotic tissue, the amount and quality of bone matrix (osteoid) in osteomalacia are normal but mineralization is delayed or inadequate (Table 51-2).

Pathophysiology

Osteomalacia is the adult equivalent of rickets, or vitamin D deficiency, in children. In its natural form, vitamin D is obtained from the ultraviolet radiation of the sun and from certain foods. In combination with calcium and phosphorus, the vitamin is necessary for bone formation.

Vitamin D is actually a group of vitamins, including vitamins D_2 and D_3. The naturally occurring substance is D_3 (cholecalciferol), which is manufactured by photochemical activation in the skin, which is triggered by the sun's ultraviolet light. As illustrated in Figure 51-3, the D_3 from either the skin or food is carried to the liver bound to an alpha globulin as transcalciferin. There, part of the substance is converted to 25-hydroxycholecalciferol, or calcidiol.

TABLE 51-2 • DIFFERENTIAL FEATURES OF OSTEOPOROSIS AND OSTEOMALACIA

Characteristic	Osteoporosis	Osteomalacia
Definition	Decreased bone mass	Demineralized bone
Pathophysiology	Lack of calcium	Lack of vitamin D
Radiographic findings	Osteopenia, fractures	Pseudofractures, Looser's zones, fractures
Calcium level	Normal	Low or normal
Phosphate level	Normal	Low or normal
Parathyroid hormone	Normal	High or normal
Alkaline phosphatase	Normal	High

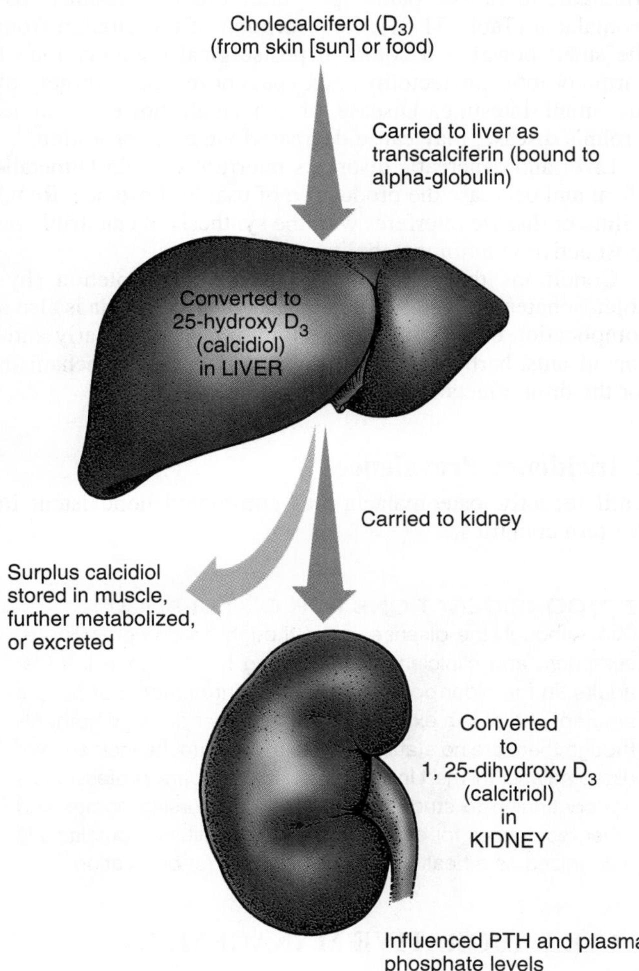

Figure 51-3 • Process of vitamin D metabolism in the body. (*PTH,* Parathyroid hormone.)

Calcidiol is then transported to the kidney for transformation into the major active vitamin D metabolite, 1,25-dihydroxycholecalciferol, or calcitriol. The amount of calcitriol produced is regulated by parathyroid hormone (PTH) and the blood level of phosphate, the inorganic form of phosphorus. Calcitriol production increases when there is an increase in PTH or a decrease in serum phosphate levels.

Calcitriol is needed for optimal intestinal absorption of calcium and works in combination with PTH for the release of calcium from bone to assist in serum calcium regulation. Consequently, calcitriol or vitamin D deficiency results in decreased calcium absorption from the gut, which in turn leads to PTH stimulation and a decrease in both serum phosphate and calcium levels.

In osteomalacia, a primary or secondary vitamin D deficiency causes insufficient bone mineralization. Nonmineralized or poorly mineralized osteoid accumulates over the surfaces of both cortical and cancellous bone.

Etiology

In addition to primary vitamin D deficiency related to lack of sunlight exposure or dietary intake, vitamin D deficiency attributable to various pathologic conditions may result in osteomalacia (Table 51-3). Malabsorption of the vitamin from the small bowel is a common postsurgical complication of partial or total gastrectomy and bypass or resection surgery of the small intestine. Disease of the small bowel, such as Crohn's disease, may cause decreased vitamin absorption.

Liver and pancreatic disorders interrupt vitamin D metabolism and decrease the production of usable substance. Renal failure or disease interferes with the synthesis of calcitriol, the most active vitamin metabolite.

Conditions that contribute to phosphate depletion (hypophosphatemia) lead to osteomalacia. Osteomalacia is also a complication of the intake of certain drugs, particularly anticonvulsants, barbiturates, and fluoride. The exact mechanism for the drug effects is not known.

Incidence/Prevalence

Until recently, osteomalacia was considered nonexistent in Western countries.

CONSIDERATIONS FOR OLDER ADULTS

Although the disease is not thought to be common, researchers and clinicians are exploring its incidence in older adults. In the older population, significant numbers of people are deprived of sun exposure, maintain poor diets, or both. Although there are no statistical data to indicate the incidence of osteomalacia in the United States, health care professionals are continuing to study its occurrence in nursing homes and other residences for older adults. As a result, osteomalacia is recognized as a health problem for the older population.

COLLABORATIVE MANAGEMENT

Assessment

The important data for the nurse to obtain for a client with osteomalacia or suspected osteomalacia include age, exposure to sunlight, and skin pigmentation. The older adult who has been homebound or chronically institutionalized is at the greatest risk. People who have dark skin and consume minimal protein are more at risk than light-skinned people with the same dietary habits. The nurse also takes a thorough diet history to determine the intake of foods containing vitamin D and calcium.

PHYSICAL ASSESSMENT/CLINICAL MANIFESTATIONS

Osteomalacia is easily confused with osteoporosis. Many of the clinical manifestations are similar, and both disorders may occur at the same time.

In the early stages of osteomalacia, the manifestations are nonspecific. Muscle weakness and bone pain are often misdiagnosed as arthritis or rheumatism. In some cases, proximal muscle weakness in the shoulder and pelvic girdle areas is the only complaint.

Muscle weakness in the lower extremities may cause a waddling and unsteady gait, which contributes to falls and subsequent fractures. Hypophosphatemia leads to an inadequate production of muscle cell adenosine triphosphate, thus resulting in a decrease in muscle cell energy. If hypocalcemia is present, muscle cramping may accompany the weakness.

The nurse assesses muscle strength and observes the client's gait. The nurse records complaints of muscle cramps and bone pain. The skeletal discomfort is often vague and generalized. The spine, ribs, pelvis, and lower extremities are most often affected. The client usually describes the pain as aggravated by activity and worse at night.

In addition to the client's subjective complaint of pain, the nurse palpates the affected bones for tenderness. Bone tenderness can be elicited by pressure on the tibia or rib cage. The nurse observes skeletal malalignment as long-bone bowing or spinal deformity, similar to that seen in osteoporosis. In extreme cases, the pelvis narrows, so that vaginal childbirth is difficult.

If osteomalacia is untreated, vertebral, rib, and long-bone fractures may occur. The client may be misdiagnosed as having bone cancer or osteoporosis.

DIAGNOSTIC ASSESSMENT

Table 51-2 shows the changes in laboratory values that help to support the diagnosis of osteomalacia. X-ray studies of bone tissue with osteomalacia show a decrease in the trabeculae of cancellous bone and lack of osteoid sharpness. The classic diagnostic finding specific to the disease, however, is the presence of radiolucent bands (Looser's lines or zones). Looser's zones are pseudofractures; they represent stress fractures that have not mineralized. They often appear symmetrically in the inner femora, ribs, and inferior pubic rami and may progress to complete fractures with minimal trauma.

TABLE 51-3 • CAUSES OF OSTEOMALACIA

VITAMIN D DISTURBANCE	KIDNEY DISEASE
Inadequate production	Chronic renal failure
Lack of sunlight exposure	Renal tubular disorders
Dietary deficiency	• Acidosis
Abnormal metabolism	• Hypophosphatemia
Drug therapy	
• Phenytoin (Dilantin)	**FAMILIAL METABOLIC ERROR**
• Fluoride	Hypophosphatemia
• Barbiturates	
Liver disease	
Renal disease	
Inadequate absorption	
• Postgastrectomy	
• Malabsorption syndrome	
Inflammatory bowel disease	

Interventions

Because the nursing diagnoses for osteomalacia are the same as those for osteoporosis, the client goals are also similar. An increase in vitamin D through dietary intake, sun exposure, and drug supplementation is promoted. The nurse teaches about foods high in vitamin D and the importance of frequent sun exposure for the manufacture of the vitamin.

The recommended daily allowance (RDA) of vitamin D is 10 μg, or 400 international units (IU). Because older adults are at risk for bone demineralization from aging, as well as for osteomalacia, a safe and adequate daily requirement may be as high as 15 to 20 g, or 600 to 800 IU. Chart 51-3 lists interventions for helping older clients meet the daily requirement of vitamin D.

Paget's Disease of the Bone

OVERVIEW

Paget's disease, or osteitis deformans, is a metabolic disorder of bone remodeling, or turnover, in which increased resorption or loss results in bone deposits that are weak, enlarged, and disorganized. First described in 1876 by Sir James Paget, an English surgeon, the disease was thought to be an inflammatory process, infectious in origin. Until the 1960s, Paget's disease was considered a medical curiosity and given little attention. With the growing number of affected older adults in Western countries, interest in the disease has increased and treatment has improved.

Three pathophysiologic phases of the disorder have been described: active, mixed, and inactive. In the first phase (the active phase), a prolific increase in osteoclasts (cells that break down bone) causes massive bone destruction and deformity. The osteoclasts of pagetic bone are large and multinuclear, unlike the osteoclasts of normal bone tissue.

In the mixed phase, the osteoblasts (bone-forming cells) react in a compensatory manner to form new bone. The result is bone that is disorganized and chaotic in structure. The new trabecular bone has a mosaic pattern with a volume twice that of normal bone.

When the osteoblastic activity exceeds the osteoclastic activity, the inactive phase occurs. The newly formed bone becomes sclerotic and Ivory hard. The number of osteoclasts begins to return toward normal.

As a result of the metabolic bone process, the vascularity of the newly formed bone tissue is increased. The arterial capillaries of pagetic bone become hypertrophied, causing marrow sinus and venous system distention. Paget's disease occurs in one bone or in multiple sites. The most common areas of involvement are the vertebrae, the femur, the skull, the sternum, and the pelvis.

The exact cause of Paget's disease is unknown, but it may be the result of a latent viral infection contracted in young adulthood and manifesting as a disease 20 to 40 years later. Bone biopsy specimens have revealed an antigen from a respiratory virus and measles. Because the disorder is present in monozygotic twins, a familial autosomal dominant pattern has been suggested. The disease has been noted in up to 30% of people with a positive family history for Paget's disease.

CHART 51-3

NURSING FOCUS *on the* OLDER ADULT
Meeting the Daily Requirement for Vitamin D

- Advise clients to get sun exposure for at least 5 minutes weekly, even in the summer and winter.
- Recommend that clients eat food high in calcium to promote vitamin D absorption and utilization in the small intestines.
- Suggest that clients eat natural and fortified foods containing vitamin D, including milk and dairy products, such as ice cream (or ice milk), yogurt, and cheese.
- Recommend that clients exercise on a regular basis (at least three times a week for 20 to 30 minutes) to prevent bone loss.

CONSIDERATIONS FOR OLDER ADULTS

Approximately 1 to 3 million people in the United States suffer from Paget's disease. It is primarily a disease of the older age-group. It occurs in a very small percentage of people younger than 40 years of age.

CULTURAL CONSIDERATIONS

Because Paget's disease occurs more often in Europe and less often in Asia and Scandinavia, there may be a possible link between the disease and ethnic origin.

COLLABORATIVE MANAGEMENT

Assessment

PHYSICAL ASSESSMENT/CLINICAL MANIFESTATIONS

Of clients with Paget's disease, 80% are asymptomatic. The disease may be confined to one bone. The disease is often accidentally discovered during a routine laboratory or radiographic examination. In more severe disease, the manifestations are diverse and potentially fatal (Chart 51-4).

MUSCULOSKELETAL AND NEUROLOGIC ASSESSMENT. Bone pain causes the client to seek medical attention. The pain is aching, poorly described, deep, and worsened by pressure and weight bearing. It is most noticeable at night or when the client is resting, and the pain is typically mild to moderate. Back pain and headache are common complaints.

CHART 51-4

KEY FEATURES *of* Paget's Disease of the Bone

Musculoskeletal Manifestations
- Bone and joint pain (may be in a single bone) that is aching, poorly described, and aggravated by walking
- Low back and sciatic nerve pain
- Bowing of long bones
- Loss of normal spinal curvature
- Enlarged, thick skull
- Pathologic fractures
- Osteogenic sarcoma

Skin Manifestations
- Flushed, warm skin

Other Manifestations
- Apathy, lethargy, fatigue
- Hyperparathyroidism
- Gout
- Urinary or renal stones
- Heart failure from fluid overload

The pain associated with the disorder may result from metabolic bone activity, secondary arthritis, impending fracture, or nerve impingement. Arthritis occurs at the joints of the affected bones, but its relationship to Paget's disease is unclear. Nerve impingement is particularly common in the lumbosacral area of the vertebral column, presenting as back pain that radiates along one or both lower extremities.

The nurse assesses the location and extent of the client's pain to determine the areas involved. Posture, stance, and gait are also observed to identify gross bony deformities. Because of the enlargement of the vertebrae, loss of normal spinal curvature, and lower extremity malalignment, the client is usually short. Long-bone bowing in the arms and legs with subsequent varus deformity of the elbows and knees is often symmetric. Flexion contractures of the hips are often present.

When performing a musculoskeletal assessment in a client with Paget's disease, the nurse pays particular attention to the size and shape of the skull, which is typically soft, thick, and enlarged. Involvement of the temporal bone may lead to deafness and vertigo, whereas basilar complications can compress any of the cranial nerves and result in neurologic compromise. Platybasia, or basilar invagination, causes brainstem manifestations that threaten life. In some cases, the bony enlargement of the skull blocks cerebrospinal fluid (CSF), resulting in hydrocephalus.

Pathologic fractures may be the presenting clinical manifestation of the disorder. As many as 30% of clients with Paget's disease sustain at least one incomplete or complete fracture. The femur and the tibia are most often affected, and fracture of these bones can result from minimal trauma. The fracture line is usually perpendicular to the long axis of the bone, and healing is unpredictable because of abnormal metabolic activity within the bone.

The most dreaded complication of Paget's disease is neoplasm, most commonly osteogenic sarcoma (see the discussion under Malignant Bone Tumors, p. 1112). Sarcomas occur in about 1% of clients with pagetic bone. They appear primarily in the pelvis, the femur, and the humerus and carry a grave prognosis because of early metastasis to the lung or extensive local invasion. They are often multifocal, and they occur more often in men. When severe bone pain is present in a client with Paget's disease, neoplasm is suspected.

SKIN ASSESSMENT. The nurse assesses the skin for its color and temperature. In people with Paget's disease, the skin is typically flushed and warm because of increased vascularity. In addition, the nurse assesses the client's energy level. The client usually complains of apathy, lethargy, and fatigue.

OTHER MANIFESTATIONS. Other, less common manifestations of Paget's disease include hyperparathyroidism and gout. Secondary hyperparathyroidism leads to an increase in serum and urinary calcium levels. In severe cases, calcium excess results from prolonged immobilization. Calcium deposits occur in joint spaces or as stones in the urinary tract. Hyperuricemia (serum uric acid excess) and gout occur because the increased metabolic activity of bone creates an increase in nucleic acid catabolism.

In a few cases, increased vascularity causes an increase in cardiac output, resulting in congestive heart failure. Cardiac complications tend to occur only when more than a third of the skeleton is involved.

LABORATORY ASSESSMENT

Increases in serum alkaline phosphatase (ALP) and urinary hydroxyproline levels are the primary laboratory findings indicating the probability of Paget's disease. Overactive osteoblasts cause the alteration in ALP level. An evaluation of the 24-hour urinary hydroxyproline level reflects an increase in bone collagen turnover and indicates the degree of the disease process. The higher the value of hydroxyproline, the greater the severity of Paget's disease.

The calcium levels in blood and urine are normal or elevated. The immobilized client is more likely to have an increase in calcium levels as a result of calcium moving from bone into the blood.

Paget's disease often causes an elevation of uric acid because nucleic acid from overactive bone metabolism increases. This finding may be misinterpreted as primary gout.

RADIOGRAPHIC ASSESSMENT

X-ray studies of pagetic bone reveal radiolucent, or punched-out, areas indicative of increased bone resorption. Depending on the phase of the disease, the overall bone mass is enlarged and the cortices are thickened. Malalignment deformities, fractures, and secondary arthritic changes may be present.

Computed tomography (CT) is useful in the detection of sarcomas, changes in the skull, and spinal cord or nerve compression.

OTHER DIAGNOSTIC ASSESSMENT

Bone scans using radioactive isotopes are only slightly more sensitive than routine x-ray studies in delineating the bone changes of Paget's disease. When the diagnosis is difficult, the physician may perform a bone biopsy. Magnetic resonance imaging (MRI) may also be used for the same purpose as the CT scan.

Interventions

Nonsurgical or surgical management may be necessary to reduce pain. Nonsurgical interventions are used initially.

NONSURGICAL MANAGEMENT. Drug therapy is the primary intervention used for pain relief. Not only can drugs relieve pain, but also they may cause the disease to go into remission for a period of time by reducing pagetic bone resorption. Other pain relief measures are also used.

DRUG THERAPY. The purpose of drug therapy in Paget's disease is to relieve pain and to decrease bone resorption. Mild to moderate pain may be alleviated by aspirin or nonsteroidal anti-inflammatory drugs (NSAIDs), such as ibuprofen (Motrin, Apo-Ibuprofen✤). When the calcium level is more than twice the normal value and multisystem disease is present, the physician usually prescribes more potent drugs, such as calcitonin, etidronate disodium (EHDP), mithramycin, or one of the new biphosphonates (BPs).

Calcitonin. Calcitonin is a thyroid hormone that is 75% effective in initiating a remission of Paget's disease. It seems to retard bone resorption and, subsequently, relieve pain. The drug often causes a dramatic decrease in the alkaline phosphatase level in a few weeks. Given intramuscularly, subcutaneously, or intranasally (Miacalcin), calcitonin (salmon) is a fairly safe medication but has side effects, including nausea, flushing, and rash. Intranasal administration can cause nasal mucosal irritation. Most of these effects occur within 1 hour of drug administration. The usual duration of therapy is 6 months, followed by a 6-month course of etidronate.

Etidronate. Etidronate (Didronel), an older BP, is prescribed orally in a dosage range of 5 to 20 mg/kg/day and tends to have a longer-lasting effect on Paget's disease as compared with calcitonin. The dosage is kept to a minimum because high dosages may cause osteomalacia or vitamin D deficiency. Its major disadvantage is that the drug is poorly absorbed from the small intestine. Therefore etidronate should be taken on an empty stomach 1 to 2 hours after breakfast or at bedtime with water or juice. Milk or milk products inhibit the drug's absorption as well. Diarrhea may occur in a few clients, but this problem is treated with an antidiarrheal medication.

Calcitonin and Didronel are often the first drugs prescribed and are often used in combination. If repeated courses of these drugs are not effective, mithramycin or other BPs may be added to the drug regimen.

Mithramycin. Mithramycin (plicamycin, Mithracin) is a potent antineoplastic and antibiotic with many side effects. It is reserved for clients with marked hypercalcemia or severe disease with neurologic compromise. By suppressing both osteoblast and osteoclast activity, the drug can relieve bone pain in 4 to 5 days. The usual dosage range is 10 to 25 μg/kg/day IV, with 15 μg/kg being the most commonly administered dosage. The nurse observes for signs of toxicity to the liver, gastrointestinal tract, and kidneys. Liver and kidney function test results and intake and output are monitored daily. Because mithramycin also suppresses platelets, daily platelet counts and bleeding precautions are taken. When liver enzyme levels become extremely high, drug therapy is interrupted temporarily.

Biphosphonates. Calcitonin and etidronate typically reduce pain and achieve a 50% reduction in bone resorption. Newer and more potent biphosphonates (BPs) achieve a greater reduction and promote disease remission. The duration of remission may exceed 1 year or more after a single course of drug therapy (Siris, 1999).

BPs work by binding with crystal elements in the bone to inhibit bone resorption. A number of BPs have been established in many countries as effective treatment for Paget's disease of the bone, myeloma, and bone metastases. Examples include tiludronate, alendronate, and risedronate. Short-term therapy with oral olpadronate has been successful for treatment of clients with Paget's disease in countries other than the United States.

The nurse and health care provider monitor the client's alanine phosphatase levels periodically to determine drug effectiveness. Periodic x-ray studies may also be ordered to assess bone changes during and after drug therapy.

OTHER PAIN RELIEF INTERVENTIONS. In addition to administering medication, the nurse uses physical measures to reduce pain. These measures may include application of heat, massage, and institution of an exercise program, and they are performed in conjunction with a physical therapist. The client may be fitted for an orthotic device to immobilize and provide support for the vertebrae or long bones. Additional interventions for pain relief, such as relaxation techniques, are discussed in Chapter 7.

The nurse provides the client with the address for the Paget's Disease Foundation and the local chapter of the Arthritis Foundation. These resources provide information and support for the client and family or significant others.

SURGICAL MANAGEMENT. When a client with Paget's disease has secondary arthritis and pain relief is not achieved, he or she may undergo a partial or total joint replacement (see Chapter 21).

OSTEOMYELITIS

OVERVIEW

Osteomyelitis is the term used to describe any infection of the bone. Even with current antibiotic treatment options, osteomyelitis continues to be a common problem and a difficult challenge for the health care team.

Pathophysiology

Osteomyelitis is divided into two major types: acute osteomyelitis and chronic osteomyelitis. An infection lasting less than 4 weeks is acute; an infection lasting longer than that time is chronic.

Regardless of the type of osteomyelitis, the pathophysiologic process is the same. On invasion by one or more pathogenic microorganisms, the bone, and often the surrounding soft tissues, becomes inflamed. The resulting increased vascularity promotes edema. Within several days, vessel thromboses develop, causing ischemia (decreased blood flow) to the involved bone, which consequently dies. The presence of necrotic bone (sequestrum) retards bone healing and causes superimposed infection, often in the form of bone abscess. As shown in Figure 51-4, the cycle repeats itself as the superimposed infection

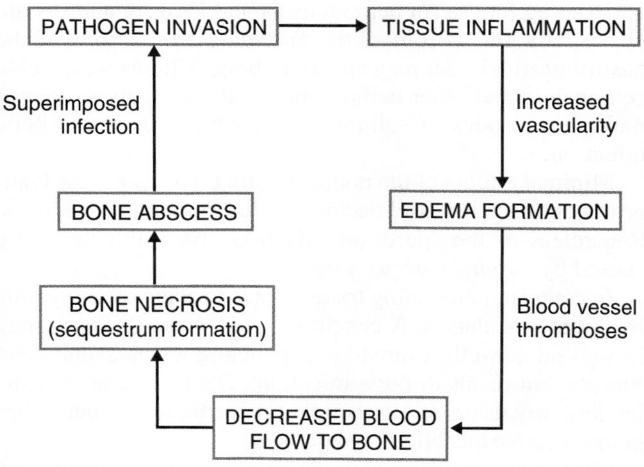

Figure 51-4 ● Infection cycle of osteomyelitis.

leads to further inflammation, vessel thromboses, and necrosis. Increased attention has been given to the mechanisms by which pathogens invade bone tissue: hematogenous spread, direct inoculation, or contiguous spread.

ACUTE OSTEOMYELITIS

Acute hematogenous osteomyelitis occurs more often in children, but it is becoming increasingly common in adults, particularly older adults. An infection occurring in another part of the body moves to and invades bone tissue, particularly the long bones (such as the femur) and the vertebrae. Pathogenic microbes favor bone that has a rich vascular supply and a marrow cavity.

Osteomyelitis resulting from direct inoculation often occurs in adults. The client experiences penetrating trauma, which allows the offending organism direct access to bone tissue. The microbe may originate from the client's skin or from a penetrating object, such as a nail.

Contiguous spread of microorganisms occurs when surrounding soft tissue becomes infected. This mechanism is common in adults who have vascular compromise, as in those with diabetes or peripheral vascular disease. The client with vascular insufficiency is typically older than 50 years of age and has soft-tissue infections of the small bones in the feet or hands. Many different types of microbes invade the adjacent bone simultaneously.

CHRONIC OSTEOMYELITIS

Chronic osteomyelitis may result from any of the acute types. The adult with a compromised vascular supply is at greatest risk for chronic infection. Advanced age and concurrent disease may prolong the course of the infection for as long as a year or more.

Etiology

Each type of bone infection has its own causative factors. Acute hematogenous spread results from bacteremia, underlying disease, or nonpenetrating trauma. Urinary tract infections, particularly in older men, tend to spread to the lower vertebrae. Long-term intravenous (IV) catheters, such as Hickman catheters, are primary sources of infection. Clients undergoing long-term hemodialysis and IV drug abusers are also at risk for osteomyelitis. *Salmonella* infections of the gastrointestinal tract may spread to bone. Clients with sickle cell anemia and other hemoglobinopathies often experience multiple episodes of salmonellosis, which can cause bone infection.

Minimal trauma of the nonpenetrating type can cause hemorrhages or small-vessel occlusions, leading to bone necrosis. Regardless of the source of infection, many infections are caused by *Staphylococcus aureus.*

In contrast, penetrating trauma leads to acute osteomyelitis by direct inoculation. A concurrent soft-tissue infection may be present as well. Animal bites, puncture wounds, and bone surgery can result in bone infection. The most common offending organism is *Pseudomonas aeruginosa,* but other gram-negative bacteria may be found.

Contiguous spread occurs when adjacent soft tissues are infected. Poor dental hygiene and radiation therapy can predispose the mandible to infection.

> **CONSIDERATIONS FOR OLDER ADULTS**
> Malignant external otitis media involving the base of the skull and mastoid bones is seen in older clients with diabetes. The most common case of contiguous spread is found in the client with diabetes or peripheral vascular disease who has a slow-healing foot ulcer. Multiple organisms are responsible for the subsequent osteomyelitis.

If bone infection is misdiagnosed or inadequately treated, chronic osteomyelitis occurs. Inadequate treatment results when the treatment period is too short or when the treatment is delayed or inappropriate. Gram-negative bacteria alone or mixed with gram-positive organisms account for nearly 50% of all chronic bone infections.

COLLABORATIVE MANAGEMENT

Assessment

The client with acute osteomyelitis manifests fever, usually above 101° F (38° C). The area around the infected bone swells and is tender when palpated. Erythema (redness) and heat may also be present.

When vascular insufficiency is suspected, the nurse assesses circulation in the distal extremities. Draining ulcers may be present on the feet or hands, indicating inadequate healing ability as a result of poor circulation.

Bone pain, with or without other manifestations, is a common complaint of clients with bone infection. The pain is described as a constant, localized, pulsating sensation that intensifies with movement. When there is severe vascular compromise, clients may not feel discomfort because of nerve damage from lack of blood supply.

Fever, swelling, and erythema are less common in those with chronic osteomyelitis. Ulceration resulting in sinus tract formation, localized pain, and drainage are more characteristic of chronic infection (Chart 51-5).

The client with osteomyelitis usually has an elevated white blood cell (leukocyte) count, often double the normal value. In chronic infection, normal or slight elevations are not uncommon.

The erythrocyte sedimentation rate (ESR) may be normal early in the course of the disease but rises as the condition progresses. The rate may remain elevated for as long as 3 months after drug therapy is discontinued.

If bacteremia is present, a blood culture identifies the offending organisms to determine which antibiotics should be

CHART 51-5

KEY FEATURES *of* Acute and Chronic Osteomyelitis

Acute Osteomyelitis
- Fever, temperature usually above 101° F (38° C)
- Swelling around the affected area
- Erythema of the affected area
- Tenderness of the affected area
- Bone pain that is constant, localized, and pulsating; intensifies with movement

Chronic Osteomyelitis
- Ulceration of the skin
- Sinus tract formation
- Localized pain
- Drainage from the affected area

used in treatment. Approximately 50% of clients with acute hematogenous infection have positive blood cultures.

Although bone changes cannot be detected early with standard x-ray studies, changes in blood flow can be seen early in the course of the disease by radionuclide scanning. A bone scan, using technetium or gallium, is extremely helpful in the diagnosis of osteomyelitis and identifies most cases. In some cases, magnetic resonance imaging (MRI) may be more sensitive than traditional bone scanning in the diagnosis of osteomyelitis.

The definitive diagnosis of osteomyelitis may be made by bone biopsy. A culture of soft tissue or of the sinus tract may not identify the offending microbes invading the bone. Often the organisms affecting soft tissue and bone are different, and each must be treated.

Interventions

The specific treatment protocol depends on the type and number of microbes present in the infected tissue. If other measures fail to resolve the infectious process, surgical management may be needed.

NONSURGICAL MANAGEMENT. To reverse osteomyelitis, the health care provider initiates antibiotic therapy as soon as possible. Contact precautions prevent the spread of the offending organism to other clients and health care personnel (see Chapter 26 for a discussion of contact precautions).

DRUG THERAPY. IV antibiotic therapy is usually prescribed for several weeks for acute osteomyelitis. More than one antibiotic may be needed to combat the presence of multiple types of organisms. The hospital or home care nurse gives the drugs at specifically ordered times so that therapeutic serum levels are achieved. The nurse must become familiar with the drugs' actions, side effects, toxicity, interactions, and precautions for administration. Family members in the home setting are taught how to administer the antibiotics.

The optimal drug regimen for clients with chronic osteomyelitis is not well established. Prolonged therapy for more than 3 months may be needed to eliminate the infection. Because of the cost of lengthy hospital stays, clients are typically discharged to the home setting with central IV catheters, such as the Hickman catheter, for medication administration. After discontinuation of IV drugs, oral antibiotic therapy may be needed for weeks or months. A cost-saving alternative to IV drug therapy is the use of newer and more potent oral antibiotics, such as fleroxacin (Megalone).

In addition to parenteral or oral drug administration, the wound may be irrigated, either continuously or intermittently, with one or more antibiotic solutions. The nurse is responsible for drug administration and uses sterile technique at all times. A technique in which beads are impregnated with an antibiotic and packed into the wound provides direct contact of the antibiotic with the offending organism.

INFECTION CONTROL. If an open wound or ulcer is present in the hospital or long-term care setting, the client's treatment usually includes standard precautions for limited infections in which the wound is covered, but this practice varies according to health care agency policy. Contact precautions are reserved for more severe infections, particularly when the purulent material cannot be adequately contained by a dressing. The open area is covered, and strict aseptic technique is used when dressings are changed to prevent further contamination. Wounds may be managed through the window of a cast, which must remain dry during dressing or irrigation procedures.

HYPERBARIC OXYGEN THERAPY. One fairly new treatment to increase tissue perfusion for clients with chronic, unremitting osteomyelitis is the use of a hyperbaric chamber or portable device to administer hyperbaric oxygen (HBO) therapy. These devices are usually available in large teaching hospitals and may not be accessible to all clients who might benefit from them. With HBO therapy, the affected area is exposed to a high concentration of oxygen that diffuses into the tissues to promote healing. In conjunction with high-dose antibiotic therapy and surgical debridement, HBO has proved very useful in treating a number of anaerobic infections.

SURGICAL MANAGEMENT. Antibiotic therapy alone may not be sufficient to meet the goals of treatment. Surgical techniques are used to minimize the disfigurement that heretofore has been a devastating result of severe osteomyelitis. Most often, surgery is reserved for clients with chronic osteomyelitis.

SEQUESTRECTOMY. Because bone cannot heal in the presence of necrotic tissue, a sequestrectomy is performed to debride the infected bone and allow revascularization of tissue.

BONE GRAFTS. The excision of devitalized and infected bone often results in a sizable cavity, or bone defect. The use of cancellous bone grafts to obliterate bone defects began in the 1940s and is still widely used today. One of the most popular surgical techniques is the Papineau procedure, or open cancellous bone graft, which is used primarily with large bone and soft-tissue defects.

As a three-step procedure, the surgeon excises necrotic bone, grafts the bone, and covers the skin, if necessary (Figure 51-5). The donor bone is most often taken from the client's posterior ileum. The surgeon tightly packs small chips of bone into the cavity and applies a pressure dressing. In 4 or 5 days, the first postoperative dressing is applied in the operating room under sterile conditions. Daily sterile dressings are applied until about 2 weeks later, when the graft stabilizes. If needed, the surgeon performs a skin graft, usually a simple split-thickness graft, between 8 and 16 weeks after the bone graft.

BONE SEGMENT TRANSFERS. When infected bone is extensively resected, reconstruction with microvascular bone transfers may be useful. In general, a bone transfer is reserved for larger skeletal defects.

The most common donor sites are the client's fibula and iliac crest. The bone graft may have an attached muscle or skin flap, if necessary. The steps of the procedure are similar to those of cancellous grafting in that debridement precedes bone transfer.

MUSCLE FLAPS. If the bony defect is relatively small, a muscle flap may be the only surgery required. Local muscle flaps are used in the treatment of chronic osteomyelitis when soft tissue does not obliterate the dead space, or cavity, resulting from bone debridement. The flap provides wound coverage and enhances blood flow to promote healing. A split-thickness skin graft is often applied several days after the muscle flap.

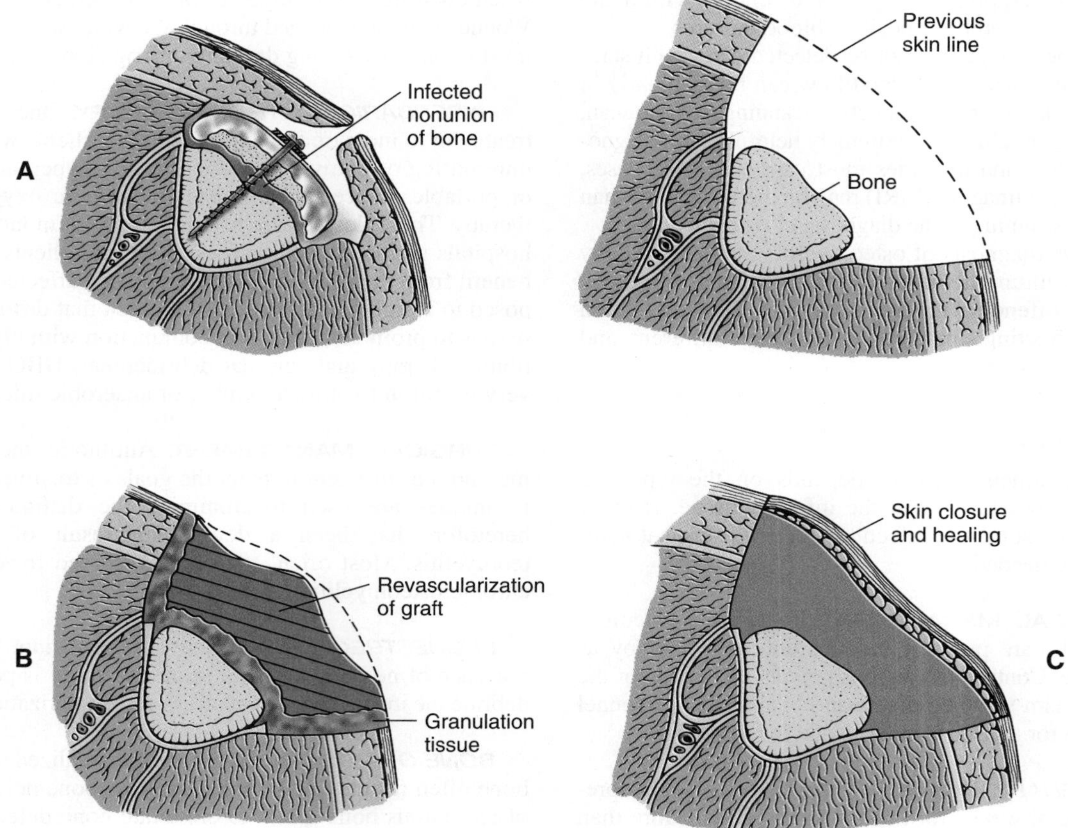

Figure 51-5 ● The three stages of the Papineau procedure. **A,** Stage 1: excision and stabilization, allowing tissue to granulate. **B,** Stage 2: open cancellous bone graft showing vascularization. **C,** Stage 3: skin coverage if not spontaneous.

AMPUTATION. When the previously described surgical procedures are not appropriate or successful, the affected limb may need to be amputated. The physical and psychologic care for a client who has undergone an amputation is discussed in Chapter 52.

For all of the surgical procedures and their recovery phases, long-term antibiotic treatment is necessary. The preoperative and postoperative nursing care is similar to that for repair of musculoskeletal trauma.

CRITICAL THINKING CHALLENGE

A 58-year-old man with a history of diabetes mellitus, coronary artery disease, hypertension, and pulmonary emphysema comes with a foot wound to the clinic where you work. He states that he attempted to cut out an ingrown toenail last week, but his "little knife" slipped and entered the soft tissue around the nail. On inspection, the area is red, warm, and slightly tender. He has a temperature of 101.8° F (39° C).

- What other physical assessment should be performed at this time?
- What laboratory tests will the nurse practitioner most likely order?
- Based on his probable diagnosis, what treatments may the client have?

For suggested answer guidelines, go to SIMON http://www.wbsaunders.com/SIMON/Iggy/.

BONE TUMORS

Benign Bone Tumors

OVERVIEW

Benign bone tumors are often asymptomatic and may be discovered on routine x-ray examination or as the cause of pathologic fractures. The cause of benign bone tumors is not known.

Tumors may arise from several types of tissue. The major classifications include chondrogenic tumors (from cartilage), osteogenic tumors (from bone), and fibrogenic tumors (from fibrous tissue and found most often in children) (Table 51-4). The cause of bone tumors, like other neoplasms, is unknown. Although many specific benign tumors have been identified, only the common ones are described here.

Chondrogenic Tumors

OSTEOCHONDROMA

PATHOPHYSIOLOGY/ETIOLOGY. The most common benign bone tumor is the osteochondroma. Although its onset is usually in childhood, the tumor grows until skeletal maturity and may not be diagnosed until adulthood. The tumor may be a single growth or multiple growths and can occur in any bone. The femur and the tibia are most often involved.

TABLE 51-4 • CLASSIFICATION OF PRIMARY BONE TUMORS

BENIGN	MALIGNANT
Chondrogenic	***Chondrogenic***
Osteochondroma	Chondrosarcoma
Chondroma	
	Osteogenic
Osteogenic	Osteosarcoma
Osteoid osteoma	
Osteoblastoma	***Fibrogenic***
Giant cell tumor	Fibrosarcoma
	Unknown Origin
	Ewing's sarcoma

On gross appearance, the tumor has a large cartilaginous cap with a bony stalk protruding from the bone. As the cap grows, the tumor ossifies and may become malignant. About 10% of osteochondromas change into sarcomas.

INCIDENCE/PREVALENCE. Osteochondromas account for about 40% of all benign bone tumors and typically affect males more often than females.

CHONDROMA

PATHOPHYSIOLOGY/ETIOLOGY. The chondroma, or endochondroma, is closely related to the osteochondroma in histologic (cellular) presentation. Unlike the osteochondroma, however, the chondroma is a lesion of mature hyaline cartilage affecting primarily the hands and the feet. The ribs, the sternum, the spine, and the long bones may also be involved. Chondromas are slow growing and often cause pathologic fractures after trivial injury.

INCIDENCE/PREVALENCE. Chondromas are found in people of all ages, occur in both males and females, and can affect any bone.

Osteogenic Tumors

OSTEOID OSTEOMA

PATHOPHYSIOLOGY/ETIOLOGY. The osteoid osteoma is distinguished by its pinkish, granular appearance, resulting from the proliferation of osteoblasts. Unlike other tumors, a single lesion is usually less than 0.4 inch (1 cm) in diameter. Any bone can be affected, but the femur and the tibia are most often involved. When the osteoid osteoma occurs in the spinal column and sacrum, the clinical manifestations resemble those of the lumbar disk syndrome. The client complains of unremitting bone pain, probably attributable to the increase in prostaglandin levels associated with the tumor.

INCIDENCE/PREVALENCE. Approximately 10% of all benign bone tumors are osteoid osteomas. The lesion occurs in children and young adults, with a predominance among males.

OSTEOBLASTOMA

PATHOPHYSIOLOGY/ETIOLOGY. Often called *giant osteoid osteoma,* the osteoblastoma affects the vertebrae and long bones. The tumor is larger than the osteoid osteoma and lies in cancellous bone. Its reddish, granular appearance facilitates diagnosis.

INCIDENCE/PREVALENCE. The lesion accounts for fewer than 1% of primary bone tumors and affects adolescent boys and young adults of both sexes.

GIANT CELL TUMOR

PATHOPHYSIOLOGY/ETIOLOGY. The origin of the giant cell tumor remains uncertain. This lesion is aggressive and can be extensive. On gross examination, the lesions are gray to reddish brown and may involve surrounding soft tissue. Although classified as benign, giant cell tumors can metastasize to the lung.

INCIDENCE/PREVALENCE. Unlike most other benign bone tumors, giant cell tumors affect women older than 20 years of age; the peak incidence occurs in clients in their 30s. Approximately 18% of all benign bone tumors are giant cell tumors.

➤ COLLABORATIVE MANAGEMENT

Assessment

PHYSICAL ASSESSMENT/CLINICAL MANIFESTATIONS

If a client experiences clinical manifestations of a benign bone tumor, pain is the most frequent complaint. The pain can range from mild to moderate, as seen with chondromas, to unremitting and intense, as is typical with osteoid osteomas. Pain can be caused by direct tumor invasion into soft tissue, compressing peripheral nerves, or by a resulting pathologic fracture.

In addition to collecting information regarding the nature of the client's pain, the nurse observes and palpates the suspected involved area. When the tumor affects the lower extremities or the small bones of the hands and feet, local swelling may be detected as the neoplasm enlarges. In some cases, muscle atrophy or muscle spasm may be present. The nurse palpates the bone and muscle to detect these changes and elicit tenderness.

DIAGNOSTIC ASSESSMENT

Routine radiography and conventional tomography are extremely beneficial in localizing and visualizing neoplasms of the bone. Benign tumors are characterized by sharp margins, intact cortices, and smooth, uniform periosteal bone.

Computed tomography (CT) is less useful, except in complex anatomic areas, such as the spinal column and sacrum. The test is helpful in evaluating the extent of soft-tissue involvement.

When the diagnosis of a benign tumor is uncertain, an open or needle biopsy of the bone is performed. The open, surgical method is preferred in order to obtain a sufficient amount of tissue.

A bone scan is not specific in distinguishing a benign tumor from a malignant one, but it allows the extent of the lesions to be better visualized as compared with most radiographic examinations.

Magnetic resonance imaging (MRI) may be helpful in viewing problems of the spinal column.

Interventions

NONSURGICAL MANAGEMENT. The physician uses drug therapy and surgery in combination when possible. Nondrug pain relief measures are also used. Depending on the client's preference and tolerance, measures such as application of heat or cold may be helpful to relieve pain.

In addition to ordering analgesics to reduce pain, the health care provider usually prescribes one or more nonsteroidal anti-inflammatory drugs (NSAIDs) to inhibit prostaglandin synthesis and thus relieve pain in the client with an osteoid osteoma. The nurse observes for drug actions and side effects, administering the drug after meals or with milk and crackers.

SURGICAL MANAGEMENT. The most common surgical procedure used for clients with benign bone tumors is curettage, or simple excision of the tumor tissue. If the tumor is small, surgery may not be indicated. When the lesion is extremely extensive, as in a giant cell tumor, the neoplasm is removed with care to restore or maintain the function of the adjacent joint, most often the knee. In some cases, the knee is replaced with a prosthetic device or is fused (arthrodesis). Bone grafting may be needed. The nursing care for clients undergoing these surgical procedures is discussed in Chapter 21.

Malignant Bone Tumors

OVERVIEW

Malignant bone tumors may be primary (those that originate in bone; see Table 51-4) or secondary (those that originate in other tissues and metastasize to bone). Primary tumors occur most often in people between 10 and 30 years of age and make up a small percentage of bone cancers. As for other forms of cancer, the exact cause of bone cancer is unknown. Metastatic lesions most often occur in the older age-group and account for most bone cancers.

Primary Tumors

OSTEOSARCOMA

PATHOPHYSIOLOGY/ETIOLOGY. Osteosarcoma, or osteogenic sarcoma, is the most common type of primary malignant bone tumor. More than 50% occur in the distal femur, followed, in decreasing order of occurrence, by the proximal tibia and humerus. Flat-bone and long-bone incidence is about equal in people older than 25 years of age.

The lesion is relatively large, causing pain and swelling of short duration. The involved area is usually warm, since the vascularity to the site increases. The central portion of the mass is sclerotic from increased osteoblastic activity; the periphery is soft, extending through the bone cortex in the classic sunburst appearance associated with the neoplasm. An inward expansion into the medullary canal is also common.

Osteosarcoma may be osteoblastic, chondroblastic, or fibroblastic, depending on the tissue of origin. Regardless of its source, the lesion typically metastasizes to the periphery of the lung within 2 years of treatment; metastasis usually results in death.

INCIDENCE/PREVALENCE. Osteosarcoma occurs more often in males than in females (2:1), between ages 10 and 30 years, and in older clients with Paget's disease. Clients who have received radiation for other forms of cancer or who have benign lesions are also at high risk.

EWING'S SARCOMA

PATHOPHYSIOLOGY/ETIOLOGY. Although Ewing's sarcoma is not as common as other tumors, it is the most malignant. Like other primary tumors, it causes pain and swelling. In addition, systemic manifestations, particularly low-grade fever, leukocytosis, and anemia, characterize the lesions. The pelvis and the lower extremity are most often affected. Pelvic involvement is a poor prognostic sign.

On a cellular level the tumor is similar to bone lymphoma. On x-ray examination the characteristic mottled destructive pattern and "onion skin" appearance of the bone surface distinguish the neoplasm as Ewing's sarcoma. Like other malignant tumors, it is not encapsulated and often extends into soft tissue. Death results from metastasis to the lungs and other bones.

INCIDENCE/PREVALENCE. Five percent of all malignant bone tumors are Ewing's sarcoma. Although the tumor can be seen in clients of any age, it usually occurs in children and young adults in their 20s. Men are affected more often than women.

CHONDROSARCOMA

PATHOPHYSIOLOGY/ETIOLOGY. In contrast to the client with osteosarcoma, the client with chondrosarcoma experiences dull pain and swelling for a long period. The tumor typically affects the pelvis and proximal femur near the diaphysis. Arising from cartilaginous tissue, the lesion destroys bone and often calcifies. The client with chondrosarcoma has a better prognosis than the client with osteogenic sarcoma.

INCIDENCE/PREVALENCE. Chondrosarcoma occurs in middle-aged and older people, with a slight predominance in men, and accounts for fewer than 10% of all malignant bone tumors.

FIBROSARCOMA

PATHOPHYSIOLOGY/ETIOLOGY. Arising from fibrous tissue, fibrosarcomas can be divided into subtypes, of which malignant fibrous histiocytoma (MFH) is the most malignant. Most often, the clinical presentation of MFH is slow and insidious, without specific manifestations. Local tenderness, with or without a palpable mass, occurs in the long bones of the lower extremity. Like other bone cancers, the lesion can metastasize to the lungs.

INCIDENCE/PREVALENCE. Although MFH affects people of all ages, it typically occurs in middle-aged men. Fortunately, the lesion is not common.

Metastatic Bone Disease

PATHOPHYSIOLOGY/ETIOLOGY. Primary tumors of the prostate, breast, kidney, thyroid, and lung are called *bone-seeking* cancers; they metastasize to the bone more often than other primary tumors. The vertebrae, pelvis, femur, and ribs are the bone sites commonly affected. Simply stated, primary tumor cells, or seeds, are carried to bone through the bloodstream. Almost all metastatic lesions are of epithelial origin and begin in the bone marrow.

Pathologic fractures, which occur in 10% to 15% of cases, are a major concern in management. The most commonly affected areas for fracture are the acetabulum and the proximal femur.

INCIDENCE/PREVALENCE. Metastatic bone tumors greatly outnumber primary malignant neoplasms. Metastatic bone disease primarily affects people older than 40 years of age. In clients with a history of cancer and local pain, metastasis is suspected. The incidence of bone metastasis ranges from 20% to 70%, depending on the statistical reporting source. It is suspected that the reported incidence of metastasis is grossly understated.

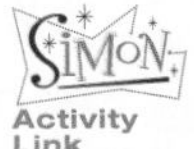

COLLABORATIVE MANAGEMENT

Assessment

HISTORY

The data collected for the client suspected of having a malignant tumor are similar to the data required for the client with a benign growth. In addition, the nurse asks whether the client has had previous radiation therapy for cancer and elicits information about the client's general health.

PHYSICAL ASSESSMENT/CLINICAL MANIFESTATIONS

The clinical manifestations seen in the client with a primary malignant tumor or metastatic disease vary, depending on the specific type of lesion. Most often, the client has a group of nonspecific complaints, including pain, local swelling, and a tender, palpable mass. Marked disability may be present in advanced metastatic bone disease.

In a client with Ewing's sarcoma, a low-grade fever may occur because of the systemic features of the neoplasm. For this reason, Ewing's sarcoma is often confused with osteomyelitis. Fatigue and pallor resulting from anemia are also common.

In performing a musculoskeletal assessment, the nurse inspects the involved area and palpates the mass for size characteristics and tenderness. The client's ability to perform mobility tasks and activities of daily living (ADLs) is also determined. The nurse observes the client performing mobility tasks and may record the results on a functional assessment tool (see Chapter 10). The degree of disability can then be determined for comparison with later measurements after medical and nursing intervention.

PSYCHOSOCIAL ASSESSMENT

Often, clients with malignant bone tumors are young adults whose socially productive lives are just beginning. They need support systems to help cope with the diagnosis and its treatment. Family, significant others, and health care professionals are major components of the needed support. The nurse assesses the systems available to clients.

Clients often experience a loss of control over their lives when a diagnosis of malignancy is made. As a result, they become anxious and fearful about the outcome of their illness. Coping with the diagnosis becomes a challenge. They go through the grieving process; initially, there is denial. The nurse identifies the anxiety level and assesses the stage or stages of the grieving process. The nurse also identifies any maladaptive behavior, indicating ineffective coping mechanisms. Chapter 25 further elaborates on the psychosocial assessment for clients with malignancy.

LABORATORY ASSESSMENT

The client with a primary malignant or metastatic bone tumor typically shows elevated serum alkaline phosphatase (ALP) levels, indicating the body's attempt to form new bone by increasing osteoblastic activity.

The client with Ewing's sarcoma or metastatic bone lesions often has normocytic anemia. In addition, leukocytosis is common with Ewing's sarcoma.

In some clients with bone metastasis from the breast, kidney, or lung, the serum calcium level is elevated. Massive bone destruction stimulates release of the mineral into the bloodstream.

In clients with Ewing's sarcoma and bone metastasis, often the erythrocyte sedimentation rate (ESR) is elevated, which is probably attributable to secondary tissue inflammation.

RADIOGRAPHIC ASSESSMENT

As with benign bone tumors, routine x-ray studies and computed tomography (CT) allow for adequate visualization of malignant lesions. Although each tumor type has its own characteristic radiographic pattern, certain findings are common to all. Malignant tumors typically show poor margination, bone destruction, irregular periosteal new bone, and cortical breakthrough.

Metastatic lesions may increase or decrease bone density, depending on the amount of osteoblastic and osteoclastic activity. CT is helpful in determining the extent of soft-tissue damage.

OTHER DIAGNOSTIC ASSESSMENT

BONE BIOPSY. A bone biopsy may be performed to diagnose the tumor type. A needle biopsy is usually done when metastasis to the bone is suspected. An open method, through a surgical incision, is preferred for primary lesions. The surgeon keeps the incision as small as possible. The biopsy scar is removed during bone cancer surgery to eliminate a possible source of tumor seeds.

After biopsy, the cancer is staged according to the grade of the tumor. One popular method is the TNM staging system, which uses determinations of *t*umor size, *n*odal involvement, and evidence of *m*etastasis.

Another surgical staging method is to correlate the tumor grade (high or low), tumor site (intracompartmental or extracompartmental), and presence of metastatic disease (positive or negative). Staging guides the health care team in their decision regarding treatment.

BONE SCAN. Although a bone scan is not helpful in determining the type of tumor, it allows the extent of the cancer to be visualized. A scan is almost always ordered when bone metastasis is suspected.

Analysis

COMMON NURSING DIAGNOSES AND COLLABORATIVE PROBLEMS

The following are common nursing diagnoses for clients with malignant bone tumors:

1. Acute Pain and Chronic Pain related to direct tumor invasion into soft tissue
2. Anticipatory Grieving related to a change in body image or impending death
3. Disturbed Body Image related to the effects of chemotherapy, radiation therapy, or surgery

A common collaborative problem is Potential for Fractures.

ADDITIONAL NURSING DIAGNOSES AND COLLABORATIVE PROBLEMS

In addition to the common nursing diagnoses and collaborative problems, clients with malignant bone tumors may have one or more of the following:

- Fear and Anxiety related to the medical diagnosis, possible disfiguring surgery, or impending death
- Ineffective Coping related to nonacceptance of the medical diagnosis
- Compromised Family Coping related to nonacceptance of the medical diagnosis
- Dysfunctional Grieving related to an inability to cope with the medical diagnosis
- Impaired Physical Mobility related to the size and extent of the tumor, weakness, and/or the effects of terminal metastatic disease
- Imbalanced Nutrition: Less Than Body Requirements related to an increased metabolic process secondary to cancer
- Disturbed Sleep Pattern related to pain
- Self-Care Deficit (Total) related to impaired physical mobility and weakness
- Ineffective Role Performance related to a temporary or permanent inability to maintain the family or community role
- Spiritual Distress related to fear of death

Planning and Implementation

ACUTE PAIN; CHRONIC PAIN

NOC **PLANNING: EXPECTED OUTCOMES.** The client with a malignant bone tumor is expected to experience a reduction or alleviation of pain associated with the bone lesion as indicated by self-report.

INTERVENTIONS. Because the pain is often due to direct tumor invasion, treatment is aimed at reducing the size of or removing the tumor. A combination of nonsurgical and surgical management is often used to promote client comfort and eliminate the complications of bone cancer.

NONSURGICAL MANAGEMENT. In addition to analgesics for local pain relief, chemotherapeutic agents and radiation therapy are often administered in an attempt to cause tumor regression. In clients with vertebral metastatic disease, bracing and immobilization with cervical traction reduce back pain.

DRUG THERAPY. The physician may prescribe chemotherapy to be given alone or in combination with radiation or surgery. Certain proliferating tumors, such as Ewing's sarcoma, are sensitive to cytotoxic medications. Others, such as chondrosarcomas, are often totally drug resistant. Chemotherapy seems to work best for small, metastatic lesions and may be administered before or after surgery. For most tumors, the physician orders a combination of agents. At present, there is no universally accepted protocol of chemotherapeutic agents. The drugs selected are determined in part by the primary source of the cancer in metastatic disease. For example, when metastasis occurs from breast cancer, estrogens and progesterones may be used.

The nurse observes the client carefully for side and toxic effects and monitors laboratory tests diligently. Chapter 25 discusses the nursing care associated with the administration of cytotoxic agents.

RADIATION THERAPY. Radiation is used for selected types of malignant tumors. For clients with Ewing's sarcoma and early osteosarcoma, radiation may be the treatment of choice in reducing tumor size and thus pain.

For clients with metastatic disease, radiation is given primarily for palliation. The therapy is directed toward the painful sites in an attempt to provide a more comfortable life span. One or more treatments are given, depending on the extent of disease. With precise planning, radiation therapy can be used with minimal complications. The nursing care for clients receiving radiation therapy is described in Chapter 25.

SURGICAL MANAGEMENT. The treatment of primary bone tumors is surgery, often combined with radiation or chemotherapy.

PREOPERATIVE CARE. Preoperatively, the nurse thoroughly evaluates the client to assist the physician in the selection of the surgical procedure to be performed. In addition to the nature, progression, and extent of the tumor, the client's age and general health state are taken into consideration. Chemotherapy may be administered preoperatively.

As for any client preparing for cancer surgery, the client with bone cancer needs psychologic support from the nurse and other members of the health care team. The nurse assesses the level of understanding of the client and the family or significant others. As a client advocate, the nurse encourages the expression of concerns and questions and provides information regarding hospital routines and procedures. Spiritual support is important to some clients, who may prefer to contact their own clergy, rabbi, or spiritual leader or talk with the clergy affiliated with the hospital. The nurse helps to arrange for spiritual assistance if needed.

Postoperative needs are anticipated and planned for as much as possible before the client undergoes surgery. The nurse informs the client what to expect postoperatively and how to help ensure adequate recovery.

OPERATIVE PROCEDURES. Wide or radical resection procedures are commonly performed for clients with bone sarcomas. Wide excision is removal of the lesion surrounded by an intact cuff of normal tissue and leads to cure of low-grade tumors only. A radical resection includes removal of the lesion, the entire muscle, bone, and other tissues directly involved. It is the only procedure adequate for high-grade tumors.

In the past, limb amputation was commonly performed for bone tumors, with or without disarticulation (joint removal). Today, advances in reconstructive surgery allow for resection of the tumor and repair of the resulting bony defect to salvage the limb. The following are used to correct bone defects:

- Total joint replacements with prosthetic implants, either whole or partial
- Custom metallic implants
- Allografts from the iliac crest, rib, or fibula

In a few cases, arthrodesis (joint fusion) may be the procedure of choice. Total joint replacements are discussed in Chapter 21.

As an alternative to total replacement, an allograft may be implanted with internal fixation for those clients who do not have metastases. This is a common procedure for sarcomas of the proximal femur. Allograft procedures for the knee are also performed, particularly in young adults. Preoperative chemotherapy is given to enhance the likelihood of success. Allografts with adjacent tendons and ligaments are harvested from cadavers and can be frozen or freeze-dried for a prolonged period. The graft is fixed with a series of bolts, screws, or plates. The nurse observes for signs of hemorrhage, infection, or fracture.

For clients with metastatic disease, intractable pain is surgically treated with percutaneous cordotomy (cutting of the spinal nerve roots). Cryosurgery (cold application) may reduce pain and tumor size.

POSTOPERATIVE CARE. The surgical incision for a limb salvage procedure is often extensive. A pressure dressing with wound suction is typically maintained for up to 5 days.

The client who has undergone a limb salvage procedure has resulting impaired physical mobility and a self-care deficit. The nature and extent of the alterations depend on the location and extent of the surgery.

Promotion of Physical Mobility. Usually, muscle strengthening and range-of-motion (ROM) exercises begin immediately postoperatively and continue for at least a year. After upper extremity surgery, the client can engage in active-assistive exercises by using the opposite hand to help achieve motions such as forward flexion and abduction of the shoulder. Continuous passive motion (CPM) using a CPM machine may be initiated as early as the first postoperative day for either upper extremity or lower extremity procedures.

After lower extremity surgery, the emphasis is on strengthening the quadriceps muscles by using passive and active motion when possible. Maintaining muscle tone is an important prerequisite to weight bearing, which progresses from toe touch or partial weight bearing to full weight bearing by 3 months postoperatively.

The client who has had a bone graft has a plaster cast that remains in place for several months. Weight bearing is prohibited until there is evidence that the graft is incorporated into the adjacent bone tissue.

During the recovery phase, the client also needs assistance with activities of daily living (ADLs), particularly if the surgery involves the upper extremity. The nurse assists if needed, but at the same time tries to encourage the client to do as much as possible unaided.

Neurovascular Assessment. Surrounding tissues, including nerves and blood vessels, may be sacrificed during surgery. Vascular grafting is common, but the lost nerve is usually not replaced. The nurse assesses the neurovascular status of the affected extremity and its digits thoroughly and frequently. Splinting or casting of the limb may also cause neurovascular compromise and needs to be checked for proper placement.

Pelvic lesions, although not commonly seen, are also excised. Reconstruction generally entails bone fusion with muscle and nerve preservation. A hip spica cast or brace may be necessary until graft incorporation has occurred. The client may need a cane for ambulation.

The major complications peculiar to reconstructive surgery for which the nurse should observe are superficial and deep wound infection, dislocation or loosening of the implants, and rapid neurovascular compromise.

An increase in pain or temperature or a rapid deterioration in circulatory status alerts the nurse to notify the physician promptly.

Psychologic Support. In addition to needing psychologic help in coping with physical disabilities, the client may need help coping with the surgery and its effects postoperatively. Having identified the available support systems preoperatively, the nurse helps to mobilize them for use after surgery.

As a result of most of the surgical procedures, the client experiences an alteration in body image. The nurse can suggest ways to minimize cosmetic changes. For example, a shoulder droop can be covered by a custom-made pad worn under clothing. The client can cover lower extremity defects with pants.

ANTICIPATORY GRIEVING

NOC **PLANNING: EXPECTED OUTCOMES.** The client with a malignant bone tumor is expected to work through the grieving process by taking action to manage stressors and accept the prognosis.

INTERVENTIONS. The nurse's most important role is to be an active listener and to encourage the client and family or significant others to verbalize their feelings. Counselors and members of the clergy or spiritual leaders may provide additional assistance in promoting acceptance of the diagnosis, treatment, or possibly, impending death. Chapter 9 provides information about death and dying.

NIC **GRIEF WORK FACILITATION.** Regardless of the prognosis, a diagnosis of bone cancer is a major stressor that causes the client and family or significant others to grieve. The nurse helps the client and others to cope with the loss and resolve the grief (Chart 51-6).

ADVOCACY. The nurse also acts as an advocate for the client and the family and often promotes the physician-client relationship. For instance, the client may not completely understand the medical or surgical treatment plan but may be hesitant to question the physician. The nurse's intervention increases communication, which is essential in successful management of the client with cancer.

DISTURBED BODY IMAGE

NOC **PLANNING: EXPECTED OUTCOMES.** The client with a malignant bone tumor is expected to experience a positive perception of, and adjust to changes in, his or her body appearance.

CHART 51-6

NIC INTERVENTION ACTIVITIES *for* The Client with Bone Cancer (Psychosocial Care)

Grief Work Facilitation: *Assistance with the resolution of a significant loss*
- Identify the loss.
- Assist the client to identify the nature of the attachment to the lost object or person.
- Assist the client to identify the initial reaction to the loss.
- Encourage expression of feelings about the loss.
- Instruct in phases of the grieving process, as appropriate.
- Support progression through personal grieving stages.
- Identify significant others in discussion and decisions, as appropriate.
- Assist to identify personal coping strategies.
- Communicate acceptance of discussing loss.
- Identify sources of community support.
- Reinforce progress made in the grieving process.
- Assist in identifying modifications needed in lifestyle.

Body Image Enhancement: *Improving a client's conscious and unconscious perceptions and attitudes toward his/her body*
- Assist client to discuss changes caused by illness or surgery, as appropriate.
- Help client determine the extent of actual changes in the body or its level of functioning.
- Assist to determine the influence of a peer group on the client's perception of present body image.
- Identify the significance of the client's culture, religion, race, sex, and age on body image.
- Monitor whether client can look at the changed body part.
- Determine if a change in body image has contributed to increased social isolation.
- Assist client to identify actions that will enhance appearance.
- Identify support groups available to client.

NIC intervention activities selected from McCloskey, J.C., & Bulechek, G.M. (2000). *Nursing interventions classification (NIC)* (3rd ed.). St. Louis: Mosby. No part of this work is to be altered without prior written permission from the Publisher.

INTERVENTIONS. The client's self-perception of body image is closely associated with his or her ability to accept the illness. The nurse recognizes and accepts the client's view about the body image alteration. A trusting nurse-client relationship allows the client freedom to verbalize negative feelings. The client's strengths and remaining capabilities are emphasized. Realistic mutual goals regarding lifestyle are established (see Chart 51-6).

POTENTIAL FOR FRACTURES

PLANNING: EXPECTED OUTCOMES. As with other bone diseases in which pathologic fracture is a possible complication (e.g., osteoporosis), the client with a malignant bone tumor is expected to avoid falls and minimize trauma to prevent fractures. In people with metastatic bone disease, fractures occur more readily and are not as preventable because of resulting destructive bone changes. A more realistic outcome for people with metastatic disease, then, may be that the client's pain will be minimized through treatment of the fracture.

INTERVENTIONS. Radiation or surgery may be required to reinforce or replace the diseased bone to prevent fracture. In recent years, surgical techniques have also been improved for fracture fixation.

NONSURGICAL MANAGEMENT. Newer techniques in radiation therapy have improved the incidence of bone healing for actual and impending pathologic fractures. To improve muscle tone and, consequently, to reduce the risk for fracture, the client performs strengthening exercises. Physical therapy on an ambulatory basis is commonly prescribed.

SURGICAL MANAGEMENT. The principles of surgery for metastatic fractures include the following:
- Replacing as much defective bone as possible
- Being thorough in technique to avoid a second procedure
- Aiming to return the client to a functional state with a minimum of hospitalization and immobilization

Fractures of the proximal femur are very common. Prosthetic replacement reinforced with polymethylmethacrylate is preferred over open reduction with internal fixation (ORIF) when feasible. The surgeon uses intramedullary rods and compression screws for more distal fractures. Prophylactic fixation may be indicated for microscopic fractures that cause chronic pain. Chapter 52 discusses the nursing management for clients undergoing repair of a fractured hip.

CRITICAL THINKING CHALLENGE

You are caring for a young adult who has had reconstructive surgery for tibial bone carcinoma. Before his diagnosis, he had been very active in sports, especially skiing and snowmobiling. He tells you that he is very concerned that the cancer diagnosis and surgery will markedly change his life, particularly his relationship with his long-time girl friend.
- What questions might you ask the client as part of a psychosocial assessment?
- What nursing diagnoses might you anticipate?
- What realistic outcomes should he expect to achieve?
- What health teaching will you need to provide?

For suggested answer guidelines, go to SIMON http://www.wbsaunders.com/SIMON/Iggy/.

Community-Based Care

After medical treatment for a primary malignant tumor, the client is usually managed at home with follow-up care. The client with metastatic disease may remain in the home or, when home support is not available, may be admitted to a long-term care facility for extended or hospice care. His or her care may be managed by a case manager.

HEALTH TEACHING

For the client receiving intermittent chemotherapy on an ambulatory basis, the nurse emphasizes the importance of keeping appointments. The nurse reviews the side effects and toxic effects of the medications. The client is taught how to treat minor side effects and when to alert the health care provider. If the drugs are administered at home via long-term IV catheter, the nurse explains the care involved with daily dressing changes and potential catheter complications. Chapter 14 describes the health teaching required for a client receiving infusion therapy at home.

The client receiving radiation therapy is also taught the importance of keeping appointments and recognizing the complications of treatment. The nurse reviews interventions that can be used at home for minor complications.

If the client has undergone surgery, he or she has a wound and limited mobility. The nurse teaches how to care for the wound and perform activities of daily living (ADLs) and mobility activities independently. Physical and occupational therapists assist in ADL teaching and provide or recommend assistive and adaptive devices if necessary. The physical therapist also teaches the proper use of ambulatory aids, such as crutches, and exercises.

Pain management can be a major problem, particularly in the client with metastatic bone disease. The nurse reviews nondrug pain relief measures, including relaxation and music therapy. The nurse emphasizes those techniques that worked during hospitalization.

The client with bone cancer typically fears that the malignancy will return. The nurse acknowledges this possibility but reinforces confidence in the health care team and medical treatment chosen.

Realistic goals regarding return to work, recreational activities, and so forth are mutually established. The nurse encourages the client to resume a functional lifestyle but cautions that it should be gradual. Certain activities, such as participating in sports, may be prohibited.

The client with advanced metastatic bone disease needs to prepare for death. The nurse and other support personnel assist the client through the stages of death and dying and identify resources that can help the client write a will, visit with distant family members, or do whatever he or she thinks is needed to die in peace.

HOME CARE MANAGEMENT

In collaboration with the occupational therapist, the nurse evaluates the client's home environment for structural barriers that may hinder mobility. The client may be discharged with a cast, crutches, or a wheelchair.

Accessibility to eating and toileting facilities is essential to promote independence. Because the client with metastatic disease is susceptible to pathologic fractures, potential hazards that may contribute to falls or injury should be removed.

HEALTH CARE RESOURCES

In addition to family and significant others, cancer support groups are helpful to the client with bone cancer. Some organizations, such as I Can Cope, provide information and emotional support; others, such as CanSurmount, are geared more toward client and family education.

The hospital staff nurse, discharge planner, or case manager also ensures that follow-up care, including nursing care and physical or occupational therapy, is available in the home. The client with terminal cancer may choose to become part of a hospice program (see Chapter 9).

Evaluation: Outcomes

NOC The nurse evaluates the care of the client with a malignant bone tumor on the basis of the identified nursing diagnoses and collaborative problems. The expected outcomes may include that the client will:

- State that pain is reduced or alleviated
- Perform ADLs and ambulation activities independently
- Seek health care resources as needed, including cancer support groups
- State that body image perception is improved

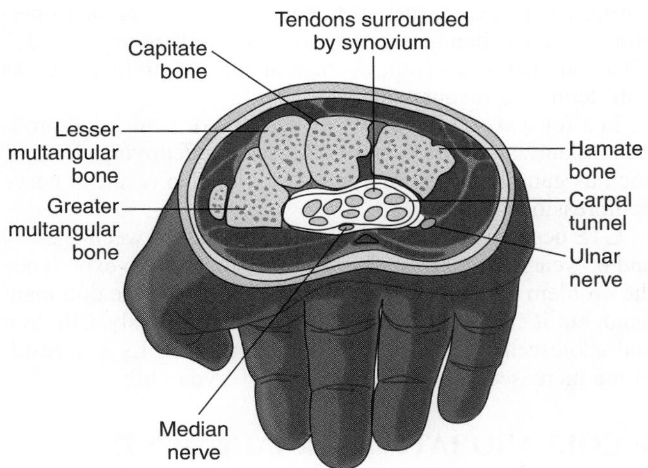

Figure 51-6 ● Anatomy of the carpal tunnel.

- Return to a functional lifestyle (or accept impending death in the case of advanced metastasis)
- State that anxiety regarding medical diagnosis and treatment is decreased

DISORDERS OF THE HAND

Carpal Tunnel Syndrome

OVERVIEW

Carpal tunnel syndrome (CTS) is a common condition in which the median nerve in the wrist becomes compressed, causing pain and numbness. The carpal tunnel is a rigid canal lying between the carpal bones and a fibrous tissue sheet called the flexor retinaculum. As seen in Figure 51-6, a group of nine tendons enveloped by synovium share space with the median nerve in the carpal tunnel. When the synovium becomes swollen or thickened, the nerve is compressed.

The median nerve supplies the motor, sensory, and autonomic function for the first three digits of the hand and the palmar aspect of the fourth digit. Because of the median nerve's proximity to other structures, wrist flexion causes nerve impingement against the flexor retinaculum; extension causes increased pressure in the distal portion of the carpal tunnel.

CTS usually manifests as a chronic problem; acute cases are rare. Excessive hand exercise, edema or hemorrhage into the carpal tunnel, or thrombosis of the median artery can lead to acute CTS. Clients with a Colles' fracture of the wrist or hand burns are particularly at risk for rapid CTS development.

In most cases, however, the causative factors may not result in neurologic deficit for years. CTS is a common complication of certain metabolic and connective tissue diseases. For example, synovitis (inflammation of the synovium) occurs in clients with rheumatoid arthritis. The hypertrophied synovium compresses the median nerve. In other chronic disorders such as diabetes mellitus, inadequate blood supply can cause median nerve neuropathy, or dysfunction, resulting in CTS.

CTS is the most common repetitive strain injury (RSI)—the fastest growing type of occupational injury. People whose jobs require repetitive hand activities involving pinch or grasp during wrist flexion, such as factory workers, computer operators, and jackhammer operators, are predisposed to CTS. CTS can also result from overuse in sports activities such as golf, tennis, or racquetball.

In a few cases, CTS may be a familial or congenital problem, manifesting in adulthood. Space-occupying lesions, such as ganglia, tophi, and lipomas, can also result in nerve compression.

CTS occurs in adults of all ages but peaks between ages 30 and 60 years. Women are five times more likely to experience the problem than men. Most often, CTS affects the dominant hand, but it can occur in both hands simultaneously. Children and adolescents are beginning to experience CTS as a result of the increased use of computers in everyday life.

COLLABORATIVE MANAGEMENT

Assessment

On the basis of the client's history and complaint of hand pain and numbness, a medical diagnosis is often made without further assessment. The nurse questions clients regarding the nature, intensity, and location of the pain. Clients often state that the pain is worse at night as a result of flexion or direct pressure during sleep. The pain may radiate to the arm, the shoulder and neck, or the chest.

In addition to the complaint of numbness, clients with carpal tunnel syndrome (CTS) may also experience paresthesia (painful tingling). Sensory changes usually precede motor manifestations by weeks or months.

PHYSICAL ASSESSMENT/CLINICAL MANIFESTATIONS

The health care provider performs several tests to elicit abnormal sensory findings. Phalen's wrist test, sometimes called **Phalen's maneuver,** produces paresthesia in the median nerve distribution within 60 seconds. The client is asked to relax the wrist into flexion or place the backs of the hands together and flex both wrists simultaneously (Figure 51-7). Of clients with CTS, 80% have a positive Phalen's test result.

The same sensation can be elicited by tapping lightly over the area of the median nerve in the wrist **(Tinel's sign).** If the test is unsuccessful, a blood pressure cuff can be placed on the upper arm and inflated to the client's systolic pressure. The result is often pain and tingling.

Motor changes begin with a weak pinch, clumsiness, and difficulty with fine movements and then progress to muscle weakness and wasting. The nurse may test for pinching ability and ask the client to perform a fine-movement task, such as threading a needle. Strenuous hand activity worsens the subjective complaints.

In addition to inspecting for muscle atrophy and task performance, the nurse observes the wrist for swelling. The area is palpated, and characteristics are described. Autonomic changes may be evidenced by skin discoloration; nail changes, such as brittleness; and increased or decreased palmar sweating.

DIAGNOSTIC ASSESSMENT

Routine x-ray studies are ordered to visualize bone changes, space-occupying lesions, and synovitis. If these causative factors are not suspected, a client with CTS may not have x-ray studies done.

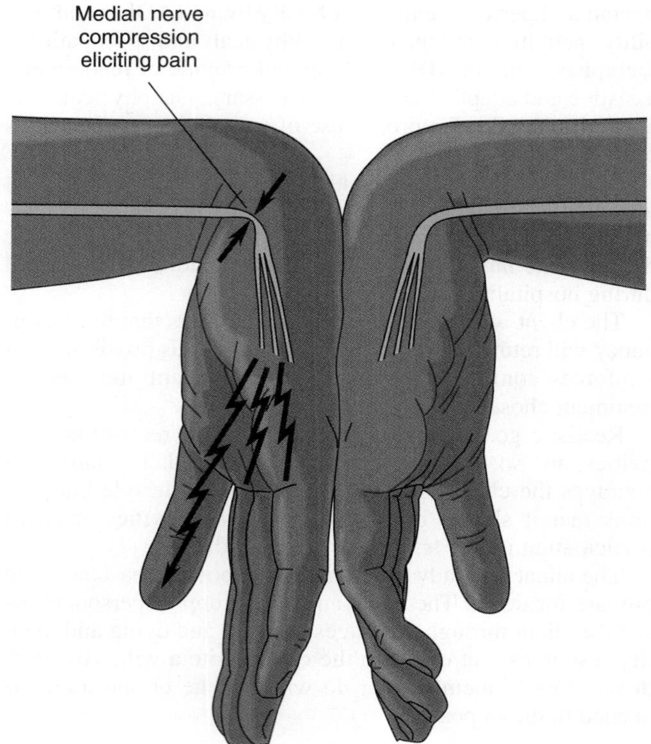

Figure 51-7 ● Phalen's maneuver for detection of carpal tunnel syndrome.

The health care provider may order electromyography (EMG), magnetic resonance imaging (MRI), or ultrasonography when a definitive diagnosis is uncertain. Problems of the cervical spine and spinal nerves can mimic the clinical manifestations of CTS. EMG testing reveals nerve dysfunction before muscle atrophy is observed. More recently, MRI has been used to help diagnose CTS. The most common finding is an enlarged median nerve within the carpal tunnel. The newest technique for diagnosis is the use of ultrasound.

Interventions

The health care provider uses conservative measures before surgical intervention. With either type of treatment, however, CTS can recur.

NONSURGICAL MANAGEMENT. Drug therapy and immobilization of the wrist are the major components of nonsurgical management. The nurse teaches the client the importance of these modalities in the hope of preventing surgical intervention.

DRUG THERAPY. The most commonly prescribed drugs for the relief of pain and inflammation, if present, are aspirin and other nonsteroidal anti-inflammatory drugs (NSAIDs).

In addition to or instead of systemic medications, the physician may inject corticosteroids directly into the carpal tunnel. If the client responds to the medication, several additional weekly or monthly injections are given.

As with any medication, the nurse monitors the effects of drug therapy. Aspirin and NSAIDs are given with or after meals to reduce gastric irritation.

IMMOBILIZATION. A splint may be used to immobilize the wrist during the day, during the night, or both. Many clients experience temporary relief with splinting. The occupational therapist places the wrist in the neutral position or in slight extension. Even when a splint is not used, the nurse instructs the client to minimize hand activities, at least temporarily.

PREVENTION OF CARPAL TUNNEL SYNDROME. Many businesses have recognized the hazards of repetitive motion as a primary cause of occupational injury and disability. Young men and women in the labor force are experiencing increasing numbers of repetitive strain injuries (RSIs). Occupational health nurses have played an important role in the development of ergonomically appropriate furniture and other aids to decrease CTS and other musculoskeletal injuries. Federal and state legislation has been passed to ensure that businesses provide ergonomically appropriate workstations for their employees.

SURGICAL MANAGEMENT. Surgery is necessary in about 50% of clients with CTS. Surgery can relieve the pressure on the median nerve by providing nerve decompression.

PREOPERATIVE CARE. The nurse in the physician's office or same-day surgical center reinforces the teaching provided by the surgeon regarding the nature of the surgery. Postoperative care is reviewed so that the client knows what to expect.

OPERATIVE PROCEDURES. The two most common surgeries are the open carpal tunnel release (OCTR) and the newer endoscopic carpal tunnel release (ECTR). When CTS is a complication of rheumatoid arthritis, a synovectomy (removal of excess synovium via incision) through an inner-wrist incision may resolve the problem. Removal of a space-occupying lesion, if present, also decompresses the nerve. Whatever the cause of nerve compression, the physician removes it either by cutting or by the newer laser technique. In some cases, CTS recurs months to years after surgery.

An alternative to OCTR is the endoscopic release. The surgeon makes a very small incision (less than ½ inch [1.2 cm]) through which the endoscope is inserted. The surgeon then uses special instruments, which may include a laser, to free the trapped median nerve.

POSTOPERATIVE CARE. Although ECTR is less invasive and costs less than the open procedure, the client may experience pain and numbness for a longer time postoperatively as compared with recovery from OCTR. Major surgical complications are rare following CTS surgery.

In addition to monitoring vital signs, the nurse checks the pressure dressing carefully for drainage and tightness. If the endoscopic procedure has been performed, the dressing is very small. The surgeon may require that the client's hand and arm be elevated above heart level for 1 or 2 days to reduce swelling from surgery. The nurse checks the neurovascular status of the digits every hour during the immediate postoperative period, encouraging the client to move all fingers of the affected hand frequently. The nurse offers pain medication and assures the client that he or she will be given a prescription for analgesics for use at home during recovery.

After surgery, the client's wrist is placed in a splint that allows thumb and finger movements. The splint is usually applied after the sutures have been removed and may be used for up to 2 weeks.

Hand movements, including lifting heavy objects, may be restricted for 4 to 6 weeks. The client can expect weakness and discomfort for weeks or perhaps months. The nurse teaches how to assess for neurovascular status.

The client must realize that the surgical procedure might not be a cure. For instance, synovitis may recur in the client with rheumatoid arthritis and may recompress the median nerve. Multiple operations and other treatments are not uncommon with CTS.

The client may need assistance with routine daily tasks or even self-care activities during recovery. The nurse ensures that assistance in the home is available; this is usually provided by the family or significant others.

Dupuytren's Contracture

Dupuytren's contracture, or deformity, is a slowly progressive contracture of the palmar fascia, resulting in flexion of the fourth or fifth digit of the hand. The third digit is occasionally affected. Although Dupuytren's contracture is a fairly common problem, the cause is unknown. It usually occurs in older men, tends to be familial, and can be bilateral.

When function becomes impaired, surgical release is required. A partial or selective fasciectomy (removal of fascia) is performed. After removal of the dressing and drain, a splint may be used. Nursing care is similar to that for the client with carpal tunnel repair.

Ganglion

A **ganglion** is a round, cystlike lesion, often overlying a wrist joint or tendon. The synovium surrounding the tendon degenerates, allowing the tendon sheath tissue to become weak and distended. Ganglia are painless on palpation, but they can cause joint discomfort after prolonged joint use or minor trauma, such as a strain. The lesion can disappear and then recur. Ganglia are most likely to develop in people between 15 and 50 years of age.

Although the fluid within the lesion can be aspirated, total excision is preferred. The postoperative care is the same as that for the client undergoing other hand surgery.

DISORDERS OF THE FOOT

Hallux Valgus

The **hallux valgus** deformity, sometimes referred to as a bunion, is a common foot problem. The great toe deviates laterally at the metatarsophalangeal (MTP) joint (Figure 51-8). Although hallux valgus is often congenital, it can occur as a result of arthritis or poorly fitted shoes. As the deviation worsens, the bony prominence enlarges and causes pain, particularly when shoes are worn. Women are affected more often than men.

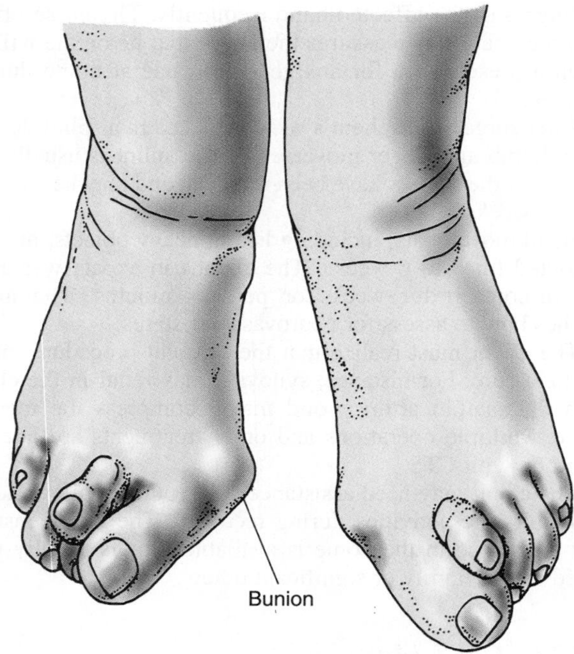

Figure 51-8 ● Appearance of hallux valgus with a bunion.

The surgical procedure, a simple bunionectomy, involves removal of the bony overgrowth and bursa. When other toe deformities accompany the condition or if the bony overgrowth is large, several osteotomies, or bone resections, may be performed. In this case, Kirschner wires are inserted vertically through the toes until healing occurs (Figure 51-9). If both feet are affected, one foot is treated at a time.

Hammertoe

Often clients have hammertoes and hallux valgus deformities simultaneously. As shown in Figure 51-10, a **hammertoe** is the dorsiflexion of any MTP joint with plantar flexion of the adjacent proximal interphalangeal (PIP) joint. The second toe is most often affected. As the deformity worsens, corns may develop on the dorsal side of the toe and calluses may appear on the plantar surface. Clients are uncomfortable when wearing shoes and walking.

Hammertoe is treated by surgical correction of the deformity with osteotomies and the insertion of Kirschner wires for fixation (see Figure 51-9). The postoperative course is similar to that for the client with hallux valgus repair. The client uses crutches until full weight bearing is allowed 3 to 4 weeks postoperatively.

Morton's Neuroma

In the client with **Morton's neuroma,** or plantar digital neuritis, a small tumor grows in a digital nerve of the foot. The client usually describes the pain as an acute, burning sensation in the web space. The pain involves the entire surface of the third and fourth toes.

Treatment involves surgical removal of the neuroma and application of a pressure dressing. Ambulation is usually permitted immediately after surgery.

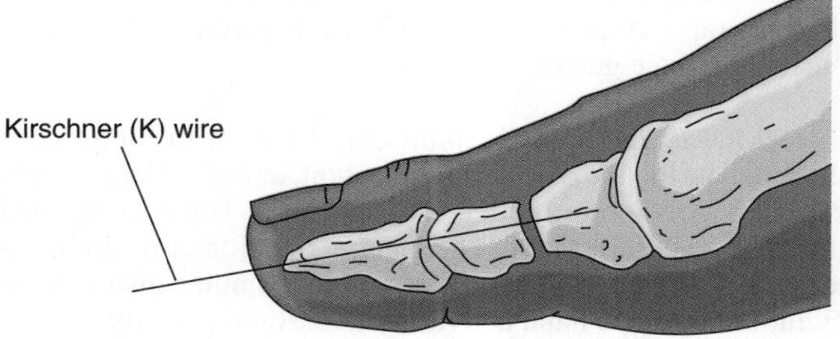

Figure 51-9 ● Use of Kirschner wires to repair hallux valgus and other toe deformities.

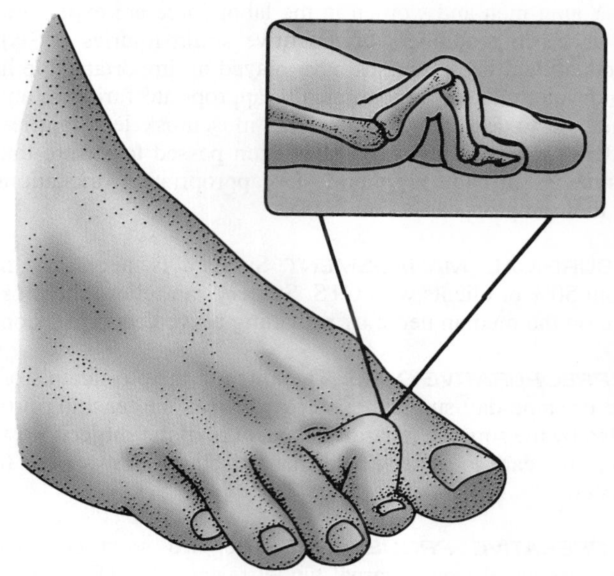

Figure 51-10 ● Hammertoe of the second metatarsophalangeal joint.

Tarsal Tunnel Syndrome

Tarsal tunnel syndrome is the ankle version of carpal tunnel syndrome (CTS). The posterior tibial nerve in the ankle becomes compressed, resulting in loss of sensation and pain in a portion of the foot. Typically, the median and lateral plantar branches, which supply the sole of the foot and the distal phalanges, are affected by the nerve compression. Diagnosis and treatment are similar to those for CTS.

Plantar Fasciitis

Plantar fasciitis is an inflammation of the plantar fascia, which is located in the area of the arch of the foot. It is often seen in middle-aged and older adults, as well as athletes, especially runners. In ambulatory care settings, plantar fasciitis accounts for 10% of running injuries. Obesity is also a contributing factor.

Clients complain of pain in the arch of the foot, especially when getting out of bed. The pain is worsened with weight bearing. Although most clients experience unilateral plantar fasciitis, the problem can affect both feet.

More than 90% of clients respond to conservative management, which includes rest, ice, stretching exercises, strapping of the foot to maintain the arch, shoes with good support, and or-

TABLE 51-5 • TREATMENT OF COMMON FOOT PROBLEMS

Description/Cause	Treatment
CORN	
Induration and thickening of the skin caused by friction and pressure, painful conical mass	Surgical removal by podiatrist
CALLUS	
Flat, poorly defined mass on the sole over a bony prominence caused by pressure	Padding and lanolin cremes; overall good skin hygiene
INGROWN NAIL	
Nail sliver penetration of the skin, causing inflammation	Removal of sliver by podiatrist; warm soaks; antibiotic ointment
HYPERTROPHIC UNGUAL LABIUM	
Chronic hypertrophy of nail lip caused by improper nail trimming; results from untreated ingrown nail	Surgical removal of necrotic nail and skin; treatment of secondary infection

thotics. Nonsteroidal anti-inflammatory drugs (NSAIDs) or steroids may be needed to control pain and inflammation. If conservative measures are unsuccessful, endoscopic surgery to remove the inflamed tissue may be required.

Nursing care involves teaching the client about the importance of complying with the treatment plan and coordinating care with the physical therapist for instruction in exercise.

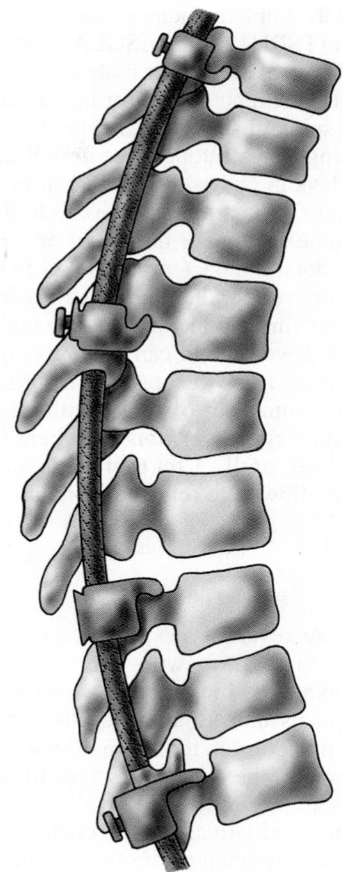

Figure 51-11 • Correction of the lateral spine contour with Cotrel-Dubousset instrumentation and spinal fusion.

Other Problems of the Foot

Table 51-5 cites other common foot problems. Although clients are usually not hospitalized for these conditions, the nurse may recognize a foot disorder and alert the physician.

OTHER DISORDERS OF THE SKELETON

Scoliosis

OVERVIEW

Scoliosis is a C- or S-shaped lateral curvature of the vertebral spine (see Figure 50-3). Many individuals with scoliosis are diagnosed and treated before adolescence. Children are typically screened for scoliosis during their middle school years. Information about caring for children with scoliosis is presented in most pediatric nursing texts.

➤ COLLABORATIVE MANAGEMENT

Assessment

In the adult with scoliosis, the impairment is usually cosmetic, although severe deviations of more than 50 degrees can compromise cardiopulmonary function. The abnormal curvature can cause low back pain, for which treatment is initiated. Women are affected more often than men.

Methods of treating adult scoliosis differ from those used for children. The adult spinal column is less flexible and therefore less likely to respond to exercises, weight reduction, bracing, and casting for correction of the deformity. In the adult, the disorder is progressive and can result in an additional 1 degree of deviation each year.

Clients who underwent scoliosis surgery 20 to 25 years previously are returning with progressive, debilitating back pain from degenerative disk disease below the fusion and with "flat back" syndrome (loss of lumbar curvature). In some of these clients, fusion was not accomplished with instrumentation, and surgery may be necessary to resolve the pain.

Interventions

Surgical intervention is the most common treatment for adults. The procedure consists of surgical fusion and insertion of instrumentation. The surgeon performs one or more spinal fusions by packing cancellous bone chips, usually from the iliac crest, between the affected vertebrae for support and stabilization. Both an anterior and a posterior approach may be needed. If so, the surgeon may perform both procedures during the same operative day or may stage them 7 to 10 days apart.

The metal instrumentation straightens the spine and immobilizes the fused area during healing (Figure 51-11). The earlier instrumentation systems include those by Harrington, Dwyer, and Luque. In the 1980s, Cotrel-Dubousset (CD) implants became popular and are still used today. Other systems similar to the CD implant include the Texas Scottish Rite Hospital system (TSRH) and the ISOLA system.

The nursing care of the client undergoing corrective surgery for scoliosis is similar to that for the client undergoing a laminectomy or spinal fusion (see Chapter 43). The major difference is the length of postoperative immobilization, which can be several days in bed with Harrington or Dwyer procedures. Luque and CD instrumentation allow the client to be out of bed the same evening or the day after surgery. A thoracolumbosacral (dorsolumbar) orthosis (TLSO) is typically used to support the vertebral column (see Figure 51-2).

With the newer surgical techniques, the client may return to work in about 3 weeks and can resume activities such as swimming and bicycling. Recreational sports, such as tennis, are usually resumed in 6 weeks with CD implant surgery, but other surgery may prevent the client from performing these activities until 3 to 6 months postoperatively. Many clients are allowed to return to contact sports within a year or less.

Osteogenesis Imperfecta

Although there are several types of osteogenesis imperfecta (OI), the milder tarda form with autosomal inheritance is more prevalent in adults. In this rare hereditary disease, a defect of connective tissue formation results in fragile and deformed bones. In addition to multiple fractures and poor skeletal development, the client may have blue sclerae; soft, brownish teeth; and presenile deafness.

The treatment is palliative, and the client's life span is often shortened. The physician prescribes steroids, calcium, vitamin C, and sodium fluoride. Physical therapy, casting or bracing, and intramedullary rodding are used to maintain mobility and promote ambulation if possible. The nurse refers the client to the Osteogenesis Foundation in the United States or to the "Brittle Bones" society in other countries for information and support.

MUSCULAR DISEASES

Progressive Muscular Dystrophies

OVERVIEW

At least nine types of **muscular dystrophy (MD)** have been clinically identified. They can be broadly categorized as slowly progressive or rapidly progressive. The slowly progressive types are most commonly seen in adults.

Five forms of MD are often seen in adults. Each type has its own distinct characteristics and causes, but all are progressive (Table 51-6).

The exact pathophysiologic mechanisms are unknown, but three theories have been advocated. The vascular theory suggests that a lack of blood flow causes the typical degeneration of muscle tissue seen in MD. Microscopic necrotic areas in dystrophied muscle tissue support this hypothesis, although this finding does not explain the marked degree of degeneration often seen in the disease.

The neurogenic theory proposes a disturbance in nerve-muscle interaction. Research has failed, however, to locate the nature of the disturbance.

The most popular belief is the membrane theory. This theory suggests that cell membranes are genetically altered,

TABLE 51-6 • DIFFERENTIAL FEATURES OF COMMON MUSCULAR DYSTROPHIES

Onset	Genetics	Clinical Manifestations	Progression
DUCHENNE (SEVERE X-LINKED) DYSTROPHY			
18 mo-4 yr	Sex-linked recessive, expression in males	Symmetric pelvic and shoulder girdle muscle weakness; waddling gait; cardiac involvement common; mental retardation in one third	Severely progressive, leading to inability to walk between 7 and 11 yr of age; death from cardiac or respiratory failure in 20s or 30s
BECKER (BENIGN X-LINKED) DYSTROPHY			
5-25 yr	Sex-linked recessive, expression in males	Wasting of pelvic and shoulder muscles; normal cardiac and mental function	Gradual progression; inability to walk 25 yr after onset; usually normal life span
LIMB-GIRDLE DYSTROPHY			
Usually 20s or 30s	Usually autosomal dominant, expression in either sex	Upper extremity and neck muscles and lower extremity and hip muscle weakness	Extremely variable; severe disability within 10-20 yr after onset; life span shortened by 10-20 yr
FACIOSCAPULOHUMERAL (LANDOUZY-DEJERINE) DYSTROPHY			
Usually in 20s	Autosomal dominant, expression in either sex	Facial and shoulder girdle muscle involvement	Usually benign; normal life span
MYOTONIC (STEINERT) DYSTROPHY			
Birth to 40s	Autosomal dominant, expression in either sex	Muscle atrophy with multiple organ involvement (e.g., heart, lungs, smooth muscle, and endocrine system)	Usually gradual if onset in adulthood

causing a compromise in cell integrity. An increase in the activity of muscle proteolytic enzymes may accompany the membrane alteration, leaving the muscle cell vulnerable to degeneration. Increased enzyme activity has been documented in the client with dystrophied muscles.

The cause of MD is unknown, but there may be a genetic influence for most of the major types. Some forms of MD are transmitted as autosomal dominant or recessive traits, whereas others are sex linked.

The most commonly occurring type of MD is the severe X-linked recessive variety initially described by Guillaume Duchenne in 1868. Each year, 20 to 33 cases are reported per 100,000 live male births. In an X-linked recessive disorder, one half of the male children of an unaffected mother, or carrier, manifest the disease. Becker's dystrophy is also inherited in an X-linked recessive manner, but it is less common than Duchenne's dystrophy. The other types of MD seen in adults can occur in either sex.

➤ COLLABORATIVE MANAGEMENT

Diagnosis of MD is often difficult because the clinical manifestations are similar to those of other muscular disorders. Muscle biopsy often confirms the diagnosis. Muscle weakness and trophic changes are characteristic of all types of MD. Serum muscle enzyme values may be elevated, and electromyographic (EMG) findings are often abnormal.

Management of the client with MD is supportive and involves the entire health care team. Physical and occupational therapy helps the client maintain as much function and independence as possible. Major organ or body system involvement is medically managed, but the life span is often shortened from these manifestations of the disease. With the exception of prednisone, no drug has been found to slow the progression of the disorder, although immunosuppressive agents, anabolic steroids, and growth factors have been tried.

An experimental treatment called myoblast transfer therapy (MTT) has been supported by the Food and Drug Administration (FDA). MTT involves injections of healthy muscle cells (myoblasts) taken from a donor and multiplied in a laboratory. The cells are then given to the client with MD, where they theoretically fuse with each other and the recipient's unhealthy muscle cells. Effective gene therapy may also be an option for curing MD in the future.

Nursing interventions focus on making the client as comfortable as possible and reinforcing techniques and exercises taught in the physical therapy program. The nurse's role in caring for a client with cardiac or other organ involvement is the same as for any client with dysfunction of these areas.

Other Muscular Disorders

Most muscular disorders are classified as neuromuscular disorders, such as myasthenia gravis, or as connective tissue diseases, such as polymyositis. Therefore these disorders are discussed in Chapters 44 and 21, respectively.

ONLINE RESOURCES

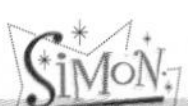

For suggested readings and Internet resources, go to http://www.wbsaunders.com/SIMON/Iggy/.

SELECTED BIBLIOGRAPHY

Asterisk indicates a classic or definitive work on this subject.

Ailinger, R.L., & Emerson, J. (1998). Women's knowledge of osteoporosis. *Applied Nursing Research, 11*(3), 111-114.

Ashworth, L. (1997). Can alendronate help my osteoporosis? *Home Care Provider, 2*(1), 37-39.

Bayles, C.M., Cochran, K., & Anderson, C. (2000). The psychosocial aspects of osteoporosis in women. *Nursing Clinics of North America, 35*(1), 279-286.

Berarducci, A., et al. (2000). Health-promoting educational practices related to osteoporosis. *Applied Nursing Research, 13*(4), 173-180.

Bilezikian, J.P. (1999). Osteoporosis in men. *Journal of Endocrinology and Metabolism, 84*(10), 3431-3434.

Capriotti, T. (2000). Pharmacologic prevention and treatment of osteoporosis in women. *MEDSURG Nursing, 9*(2), 86-90.

Cutson, T.M., & Meuleman, E. (2000). Managing menopause. *American Family Physician, 61*(5), 1391-1400.

Dowd, R., & Cavalieri, R.J. (1999). Help your patient live with osteoporosis. *American Journal of Nursing, 99*(4), 55, 57-60.

Hall, J., & Riley, R.E. (1999). Nutritional strategies to reduce the risk of osteoporosis. *MEDSURG Nursing, 8*(5), 281-293.

*Hunt, A.H. (1996). The relationship between height change and bone mineral density. *Orthopaedic Nursing, 15*(3), 57-71.

*Hunt, A.H., Civitelli, R., & Halstead, L. (1995). Evaluation of bone resorption: A common problem during impaired mobility. *SCI Nursing, 12*(3), 90-94.

*Kessenich, C.R., & Rosen, C.J. (1996). Vitamin D and bone status in elderly women. *Orthopaedic Nursing, 15*(3), 67-71.

LeBoff, M.S. (1997). Metabolic bone disease. In W.N. Kelley et al. (Eds.), *Textbook of rheumatology* (5th ed., pp. 1563-1580). Philadelphia: W.B. Saunders.

Leslie, M. (2000). Issues in the nursing management of osteoporosis. *Nursing Clinics of North America, 35*(1), 189-197.

Lewis, T., et al. (1999). Caring for the patient with Paget's disease of the bone. *Nurse Practitioner, 24*(7), 53, 57-58.

Maher, A.B., Salmond, S.W., & Pellino, T.A. (1999). *Orthopaedic nursing* (2nd ed.). Philadelphia: W.B. Saunders.

Mahon, S.M. (1998). Osteoporosis: A concern for cancer survivors. *Oncology Nursing Forum, 25*(5), 843-851.

Marchigiano, G. (1997). Osteoporosis: Primary prevention and intervention strategies for women at risk. *Home Care Provider, 2*(2), 76-82.

Matteson, M.A., McConnell, E.S., & Linton, A.D. (1997). *Gerontological nursing: Concepts and practice* (2nd ed.). Philadelphia: W.B. Saunders.

McClung, B.L. (2000). *Nursing practice guideline: Clinical management of patients at risk for or diagnosed with osteoporosis.* New York: Medical Information Services.

*National Osteoporosis Foundation. (1995). *Position paper: Current perspective on diagnosis, prevention, and treatment of osteoporosis.* Washington, DC: Author.

Orwell, E. (2000). Men with osteoporosis. Presented at the World Congress on Osteoporosis 2000, June 17, 2000, Chicago.

Ott, S.M. (1999). Osteoporosis and osteomalacia. In W.R. Hazzard et al. (Eds.), *Principles of geriatric medicine and gerontology* (4th ed., pp. 1057-1084). New York: McGraw-Hill.

Peterson, J.A. (2001). Osteoporosis overview. *Geriatric Nursing, 22*(1), 17-23.

*Piasecki, P.A. (1996). Nursing care of the patient with metastatic bone disease. *Orthopaedic Nursing, 15*(4), 25-33.

*Quaschnick, M.S. (1996). The diagnosis and management of plantar fasciitis. *Nurse Practitioner, 21*(4), 50-63.

Sedlak, C.A., et al. (1998). Osteoporosis prevention in young women. *Orthopaedic Nursing, 17*(3), 53-60.

Siris, E.S. (1999). Goals of treatment for Paget's disease of bone. *Journal of Bone and Mineral Research, 14*(Suppl. 2), 49-52.

Solomon, J. (1998). Osteoporosis: When support weakens. *RN, 61*(5), 37-40.

Tawil, R. (1999). Outlook for therapy in the muscular dystrophies. *Seminars in Neurology, 19*(1), 81-86.

Vanderford, V. (1999). Using bone density measurements in the detection and treatment of osteoporosis. *Geriatric Nursing, 20*(4), 211.

Wright, A. (1998). Nursing interventions with advanced osteoporosis. *Home Healthcare Nurse, 16*(3), 145-151.

CHAPTER 52

Interventions for Clients with Musculoskeletal Trauma

ANN BUTLER MAHER

Learning Objectives

After studying this chapter, you should be able to:

1. Compare and contrast common types of fractures.
2. Discuss the usual healing process for bone.
3. Identify common complications of fractures.
4. Explain the typical clinical manifestations that are seen in clients with one or more fractures.
5. Analyze common nursing diagnoses for the client with a fracture.
6. Describe the nursing care of the client with a cast, including client education.
7. Describe the nursing care of the client in traction.
8. Discuss pain management for the client with a fracture.
9. Prioritize nursing care for the postoperative client who has undergone open reduction with internal fixation of the hip.
10. Evaluate the nursing care of a client with a fracture.
11. Identify common types of amputations.
12. Explain the psychosocial aspects related to amputations.
13. Develop a community-based teaching plan for a client who has undergone an elective amputation.
14. Describe the collaborative management for the client with complex regional pain syndrome.
15. Identify the common types of sports-related injuries and their management.

SIMON

Go to http://www.wbsaunders.com/SIMON/Iggy/ for self-assessment questions related to these Learning Objectives.

Musculoskeletal injury is one of the primary causes of disability in the United States. Trauma to the musculoskeletal system ranges from simple muscle strain to multiple bone fractures with severe soft-tissue damage. With advancing age, a person is more likely to develop decreased bone mass (osteoporosis), which causes fractures. Hip, wrist, vertebral, and pelvic fractures are common in late adulthood.

FRACTURES

OVERVIEW

A **fracture** is a break or disruption in the continuity of a bone. Fractures can occur anywhere in the body and at any age. All fractures have the same basic pathophysiologic mechanism and nursing management, regardless of fracture type or location.

Pathophysiology

CLASSIFICATION OF FRACTURES

A fracture is classified by the extent of the break as follows:

- *Complete fracture.* The break is across the entire width of the bone in such a way that the bone is divided into two distinct sections.
- *Incomplete fracture.* The fracture does not divide the bone into two portions, because the break is through only part of the bone.

A fracture is described by the extent of associated soft-tissue damage as **open** (or **compound**) or **closed** (or **simple**). The skin surface over the broken bone is disrupted in a compound fracture, which causes an external wound. These fractures are often graded to define the extent of tissue damage. Grade I is the least severe injury, and skin damage is minimal. In grade II, an open fracture is accompanied by skin and muscle contusions. The most severe injury is grade III, in which there is damage to skin, muscle, nerve tissue, and blood vessels; the wound is more than 2.4 to 3.2 inches (6 to 8 cm) in diameter. A closed (simple) fracture does not extend through the skin. Therefore there is no visible wound.

Figure 52-1 illustrates common types of fractures. The nurse needs to be familiar with the differences in these types because they often dictate the specific nursing care required for the client.

In addition to being identified by type, fractures are characterized by their cause. A **pathologic (spontaneous) fracture** occurs after minimal trauma to a bone that has been weakened by disease. For example, a client with bone cancer or osteoporosis can easily sustain a pathologic fracture. A **fatigue or**

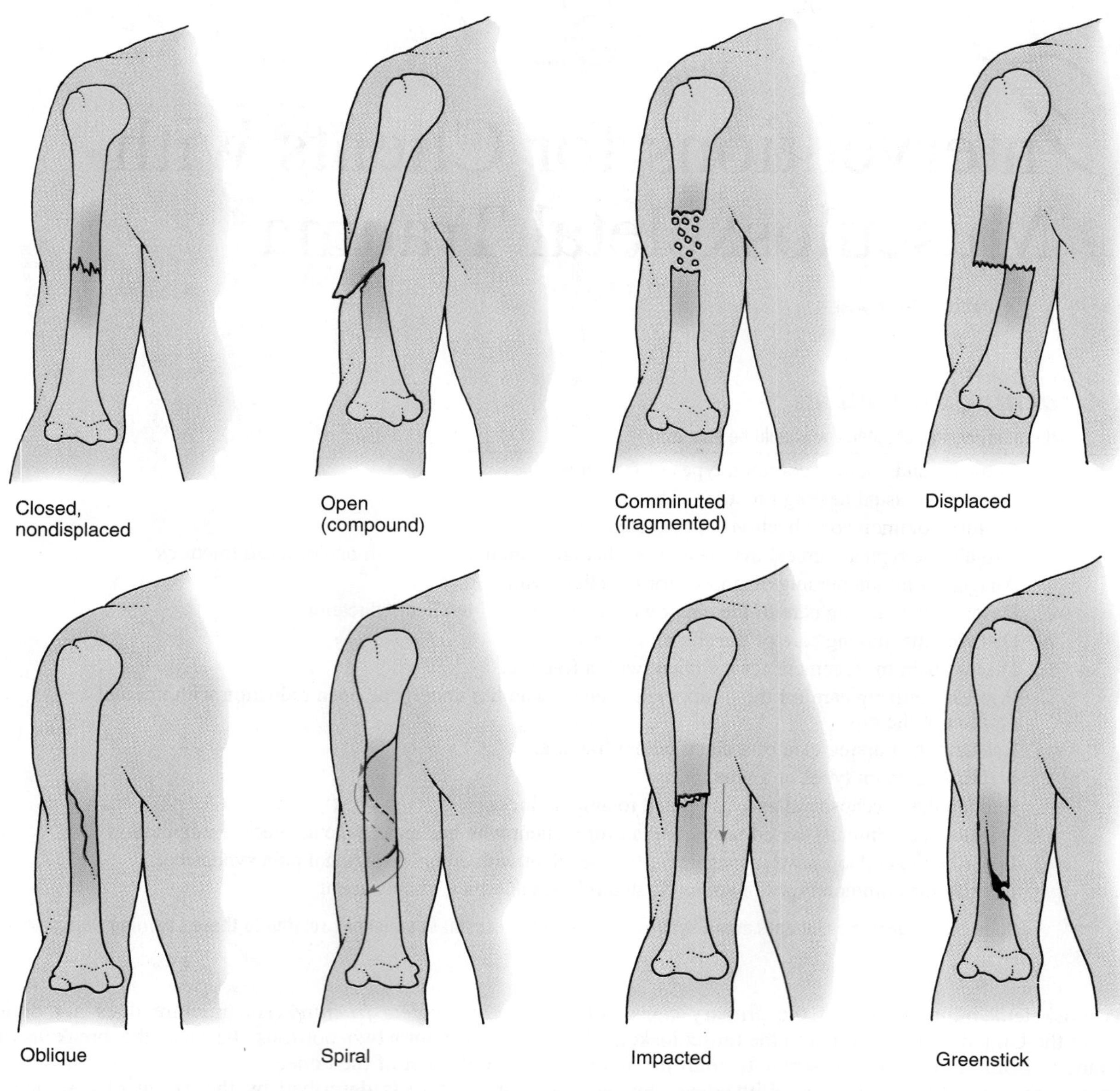

Figure 52-1 ● Common types of fractures.

stress fracture results from excessive strain and stress on the bone. **Compression fractures** are produced by a loading force applied to the long axis of cancellous bone. They commonly occur in the vertebrae of clients with osteoporosis.

STAGES OF BONE HEALING

When a bone is broken, the body immediately begins the healing process to repair the injury and restore the body's equilibrium. Within 48 to 72 hours after the injury, a hematoma forms at the site of the fracture because bone is extremely vascular. Blood supply to and within the bone usually diminishes because of the injury, which causes an area of bone necrosis. The dead cells prompt migration of fibroblasts and osteoblasts to the fracture site as part of the inflammatory process. This prompts the formation of fibrocartilage, providing the foundation for bone healing (within 3 days to 2 weeks).

As a result of vascular and cellular proliferation, the fracture site is surrounded by new vascular tissue known as a callus (within 2 to 6 weeks). Callus formation is the beginning of a nonbony union. As healing continues, the callus is transformed from a loose, fibrous tissue into bone (within 3 weeks to 6 months). Excess callus is resorbed. During the final phase of healing, consolidation, and remodeling, bone continues to be resorbed and deposited in response to stress, reshaping to meet mechanical demands. This process may start as early as 6 weeks after fracture and can continue for up to 1 year. Figure 52-2 summarizes the stages of bone healing.

In young, healthy adult bone, healing takes about 6 weeks. In the older person who has reduced bone mass, healing time is lengthened; complete healing often takes 3 to 6 months. Other factors that affect healing include the severity of the trauma, the type of bone injured, inadequate immobilization, infections at the fracture site, and avascular necrosis (AVN).

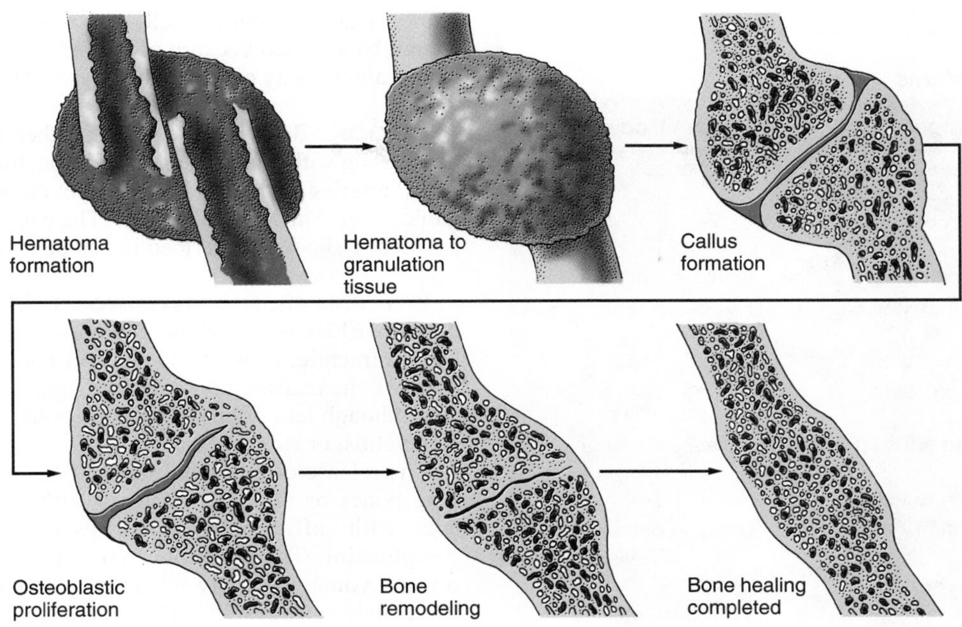

Figure 52-2 ● The stages of bone healing.

CONSIDERATIONS FOR OLDER ADULTS

Healing can be affected by a number of factors in addition to the aging process. Bone formation and strength rely on adequate nutrition. Calcium, phosphorus, vitamin D, and protein are necessary for the production of new bone (see Chapter 53). For women, the loss of estrogen after menopause is detrimental to the body's ability to form new bone tissue. Concurrent diseases can also affect the rate at which bone heals. For instance, peripheral vascular diseases, such as arteriosclerosis, reduce arterial circulation to bone; thus the bone receives less oxygen and lesser amounts of nutrients, both of which are needed for repair.

COMPLICATIONS OF FRACTURES

Regardless of the type or location of the fracture, several limb and life-threatening complications can result from the injury. The nurse must be able to recognize the clinical manifestations of impending complications so that treatment can be started immediately. In some cases, careful monitoring and assessment can prevent these complications.

ACUTE COMPARTMENT SYNDROME. Compartments are sheaths of inelastic fascia that support and partition muscles, blood vessels, and nerves in the body. **Acute compartment syndrome (ACS)** is a serious condition in which increased pressure within one or more compartments causes massive compromise of circulation to the area. The most common sites for ACS are the compartments in the lower leg and the dorsal and volar compartments of the forearm.

The pressure to the compartment can be from an external or internal source. Tight, bulky dressings and casts are examples of external pressure. Blood or fluid accumulation is a common source of internal pressure. ACS is not limited to clients with musculoskeletal problems; clients with severe burns, extensive insect bites, or massive infiltration of intravenous (IV) fluids are also susceptible to compartment syndrome. In these situations, edema increases pressure in one or more compartments.

PATHOPHYSIOLOGIC CHANGES. The primary pathophysiologic changes of increased compartment pressure are sometimes referred to as the ischemia-edema cycle. Capillaries within the viable muscle dilate, which raises capillary pressure. Capillaries become more permeable because of the release of histamine by the ischemic muscle tissue. As a result, plasma proteins leak into the interstitial fluid space, and edema occurs. Edema causes pressure on nerve endings and subsequent pain. Blood flow to the area is reduced, and further ischemia results. Sensory deficits (e.g., paresthesia) generally appear before changes in vascular or motor signs. The color of the tissue pales, and pulses begin to weaken but rarely disappear; the affected area is usually palpably tense, and pain can be elicited with passive motion of the extremity. If the condition is not treated, cyanosis, tingling, numbness, paresis, and severe pain occur. Chart 52-1 summarizes the sequence of pathophysiologic events in compartment syndrome and the associated clinical assessment findings.

ACS is not common, but it creates an emergency situation when it does occur. Within 4 to 6 hours after the onset of compartment syndrome, neuromuscular damage is irreversible. The limb can become useless in 24 to 48 hours.

In some cases, clients at especially high risk for ACS are monitored by an invasive procedure. Compartment pressures can be monitored on a one-time basis with a handheld device with a digital display, or they can be monitored continuously. Continuous monitoring requires placement of a wick or slit-tip catheter connected to a transducer and is recommended for comatose or unresponsive at-risk clients.

If ACS is verified, the surgeon may perform a **fasciotomy** by making an incision through the skin and subcutaneous tissues into the fascia of the affected compartment. This proce-

CHART 52-1

KEY FEATURES *of* Compartment Syndrome

Physiologic Change	Clinical Findings
Increased compartment pressure	No change
Increased capillary permeability	Edema
Release of histamine	Increased edema
Increased blood flow to area	Pulses present Pink tissue
Pressure on nerve endings	Pain
Increased tissue pressure	Referred pain to compartment
Decreased tissue perfusion	Increased edema
Decreased oxygen to tissues	Pallor
Increased production of lactic acid	Unequal pulses Flexed posture
Anaerobic metabolism	Cyanosis
Vasodilation	Increased edema
Increased blood flow	Tense muscle swelling
Increased tissue pressure	Tingling Numbness
Increased edema	Paresthesia
Muscle ischemia	Severe pain unrelieved by medication
Tissue necrosis	Paresis/paralysis

dure relieves the pressure in order to restore circulation to the affected area. No consensus exists on what pressure requires fasciotomy (normal = 0 to 8 mm Hg); compartment pressures must be considered in relation to the client's hemodynamic status. After fasciotomy, the nurse packs and dresses the open wound on a regular basis until secondary closure occurs, usually in 4 to 5 days. At that time, the surgeon usually debrides the wound and may apply a skin graft to promote healing.

POSSIBLE RESULTS OF COMPARTMENT SYNDROME. Specific problems resulting from compartment syndrome include infection, persistent motor weakness in the affected extremity, contracture, and myoglobinuric renal failure. In extreme cases, amputation may be necessary.

Infection from the necrotic tissue may become severe enough that amputation of the limb is warranted. *Motor weakness* from injured nerves is not reversible, and the client may require braces or other orthotic devices for assistance in movement. Volkmann's *contractures,* which can begin within 12 hours of the pressure increase, result from shortening of the ischemic muscle and from nerve involvement.

Myoglobinuric renal failure (rhabdomyolysis) is a potentially fatal complication of compartment syndrome. It commonly occurs when large or multiple compartments are involved. Injured muscle tissues release myoglobulin (muscle protein) into the circulation, where it can occlude the distal convoluted tubule and precipitate acute renal failure. Although the exact pathophysiologic mechanisms are unknown, it is suspected that myoglobulin has a direct toxic effect on the kidney. Damaged muscle cells also release potassium, which cannot be excreted because of the renal failure. The resulting hyperkalemia may cause cardiac dysrhythmias.

SHOCK. Bone is quite vascular; therefore there is a risk of bleeding with bone injury. In addition, trauma can sever adjacent arteries and cause hemorrhage; consequently, hypovolemic shock can develop rapidly. (The pathophysiology of hypovolemic shock is described in Chapter 37.)

FAT EMBOLISM SYNDROME. Fat embolism syndrome (FES) is a serious complication, usually resulting from a fracture, in which fat globules are released from the yellow bone marrow into the bloodstream. FES may also occur, although less often, with pancreatitis, diabetic coma, osteomyelitis, or sickle cell anemia.

The release of fat emboli is most likely with fractures of long bones or multiple fractures, although a break in any bone with sufficient bone marrow content can cause the complication. The problem can occur at any age or in either sex, but young men between ages 20 and 40 years and older adults between ages 70 and 80 years are at the greatest risk. The older client with a fractured hip has the highest risk, but FES is also common in clients with fractures of the pelvis.

Several theories have been offered to explain how fat is released from the bone marrow. The metabolic theory proposes that the elevated concentration of catecholamines as a result of trauma causes mobilization of free fatty acids, which leads to platelet aggregation and the formation of fat globules. The mechanical theory suggests that the pressure within yellow bone marrow is greater than capillary pressure, and therefore fats are released directly from the bone. In either case, the fat globules are deposited in small blood vessels that supply the major organs of the body, most commonly the lungs.

The *earliest* manifestation of FES is altered mental status, which is caused by a low arterial oxygen level. The client then typically experiences respiratory distress, tachycardia, tachypnea, fever, and petechiae (a macular, measles-like rash over the neck, upper arms, and/or chest and abdomen). Petechiae are characteristic of fat emboli, but the physiologic basis for their development is not known.

Laboratory findings in FES include the following:

- Increased erythrocyte sedimentation rate (ESR)
- Decreased serum calcium levels
- Decreased red blood cell and platelet counts
- Increased serum lipase level

These changes in blood values are poorly understood, but they aid in diagnosis of the condition.

Fat embolism usually occurs within 48 hours of the fracture and can result in respiratory failure or death, often from pulmonary edema. When the lungs are affected, the complication may be misdiagnosed as a pulmonary embolism from a blood clot (Chart 52-2).

THROMBOEMBOLITIC COMPLICATIONS. Deep vein thrombosis (DVT) often develops in people who are immobile because of trauma, surgery, or disability. It is the most common complication of lower extremity surgery or trauma and the most often fatal complication of musculoskeletal surgery. A person who smokes, is obese, has heart disease, or has

CHART 52-2

KEY FEATURES *of* Pulmonary Emboli: Fat Embolism Versus Blood Clot Embolism

Fat Embolism	Blood Clot Embolism
Definition	
Obstruction of the pulmonary vascular bed by fat globules	Obstruction of the pulmonary artery by a blood clot or clots
Origin	
95% from fractures of the long bones; occurs usually within 48 hr	85% from deep vein thrombosis in the legs or pelvis; can occur anytime
Assessment Findings	
Altered mental status (earliest sign) Increased respirations, pulse, temperature Chest pain Dyspnea Crackles Decreased Sa_{O_2} Petechiae (50%-60%) Retinal hemorrhage (not common) Mild thrombocytopenia	Same as for fat embolism, except no petechiae
Treatment	
Bedrest Gentle handling Oxygen Hydration (IV fluids) Possibly steroid therapy Fracture immobilization	Preventive measures (e.g., leg exercises, antiembolism stockings, SCDs) Bedrest Oxygen Possibly mechanical ventilation Anticoagulants Thrombolytics Possible surgery: pulmonary embolectomy, vena cava umbrella

Sa_{O_2}, Arterial oxgen saturation; SCD, Sequential compression device.

a history of thromboembolitic complications is at an increased risk for DVT. The incidence of life-threatening embolic conditions is highest in older adults, particularly during the first 2 to 3 days after musculoskeletal surgery.

Certain fracture sites are more often associated with life-threatening thrombi. For example, DVT that leads to pulmonary embolism is more likely to develop in clients with fractures of the lower extremities and pelvis. Local venous stasis secondary to trauma or surgical procedures (e.g., use of tourniquets in lower extremity injuries) increases the chance of DVT in clients with musculoskeletal trauma. A further discussion of DVT is found in Chapter 36.

INFECTION. Any time there is trauma to tissues, the body's defense system is disrupted. Wound infections are the most common type of infection resulting from orthopedic trauma; they range from superficial skin infections to deep wound abscesses. Infection can also be caused by implanted hardware used to repair a fracture surgically, such as pins, plates, or rods. Clostridial infections can result in gas gangrene or tetanus and can prevent the bone from healing properly.

Bone infection, or osteomyelitis, is most common with open fractures in which skin integrity is lost and after surgical repair of a fracture (see Chapter 53). For clients experiencing this type of trauma, the risk of hospital-acquired (nosocomial) infections is increased.

AVASCULAR NECROSIS. Avascular necrosis (AVN) is sometimes referred to as aseptic or ischemic necrosis or osteonecrosis. Blood supply to the bone is disrupted, which results in the death of bone tissue. AVN is most often a complication of hip fractures, or any fracture in which there is displacement of bone. Surgical repair of fractures also can lead to AVN because the hardware can interfere with circulation.

FRACTURE BLISTERS. Fracture blisters are associated most commonly with high-energy fractures and twisting injuries in the lower extremities. Extensive tissue edema allows fluid to move into the weakened space between the epidermis and the dermis. The increased colloidal osmotic pressure then pulls more fluid into the space. Fracture blisters can lead to wound infection and delayed fracture treatment, which may then contribute to potential nonunion. Nursing measures that can assist in preventing or minimizing fracture blisters include maintaining proper immobilization before definitive treatment, and elevation to limit edema.

DELAYED UNION, NONUNION, AND MALUNION. Delayed union describes a fracture that has not healed within 6 months of injury. Some fractures never achieve union; that is, they never completely heal (nonunion); others heal incorrectly (malunion). These problems are most common in clients with tibial fractures, fractures for which a number of different treatment techniques have been used (e.g., cast, traction), and pathologic fractures. Union may also be delayed or not achieved in the older client. If bone does not heal, the client typically experiences pain and immobility from deformity.

Etiology

The primary cause of a fracture is trauma from a motor vehicle accident or fall. The trauma experienced may be a direct blow to the bone or an indirect force from muscle contractions or pulling forces on the bone. Sports, vigorous exercise, and malnutrition are contributing factors. Bone diseases, such as osteoporosis, increase the risk of a fracture in older adults.

Incidence/Prevalence

The incidence of fractures depends on the location of the injury. Rib fractures are the most common type in the adult population. Femoral shaft fractures occur most often in young and middle-aged adults. The incidence of proximal femur (hip) fractures is highest in older adults. Humeral fractures are common in adults; the older the person, usually the more proximal the fracture. Wrist (Colles') fractures are typically seen in middle and late adulthood.

WOMEN'S HEALTH CONSIDERATIONS

It is estimated that more than 1 million fractures occur annually in the United States as a result of osteoporosis, and most occur in middle-aged and older women. By age 80, 1 in 5 women has suffered a hip fracture.

CULTURAL CONSIDERATIONS

Hip fractures occur less often in African Americans or in men of any race than in Caucasian and Asian women because of a lower incidence of osteoporosis. This is due in some degree to the denser bone mass in African Americans and in men of any race.

SIMON Activity Link

COLLABORATIVE MANAGEMENT

Assessment

HISTORY

The nurse collects data to determine the cause of the fracture, which helps in developing an individualized plan of care for the client.

PRECEDING EVENTS. The nurse asks the client to recall the specific events up to the time of the injury. Some type of force, such as incisional, crush, acceleration or deceleration, shearing, or friction, leads to most musculoskeletal injuries. As a result, several body systems are often affected.

Incisional (as from a knife wound) and crush injuries cause hemorrhage and disrupt blood flow to major organs. Acceleration or deceleration injuries cause direct trauma to the spleen, brain, and kidneys when these organs are moved from their fixed locations in the body. Shearing and friction damage the skin and cause a high level of wound contamination.

By asking about the events leading to the injury, the nurse can determine which forces have been experienced and therefore which body systems or parts of the body to assess. For example, a forward fall often results in Colles' fracture of the wrist because the person tries to catch himself or herself with an outstretched hand. Knowing the mechanism of injury also helps the nurse determine whether other types of injury, such as head and spinal cord injury, may be present.

OTHER HISTORY. A medication history, including substance abuse (recreational drug use), is important regardless of age. For example, a young adult may have had an excessive amount of alcohol, which contributed to a motor vehicle accident or to a fall at the work site. Many older adults also consume alcohol and an assortment of prescribed and over-the-counter drugs, which can cause dizziness and loss of balance.

A medical history elicits possible causes of the fracture and gives clues as to how long it will take for the bone to heal. Certain diseases, such as bone cancer and Paget's disease, cause pathologic fractures that often do not achieve union.

The nurse asks about the client's occupation and recreational activities. Some occupations are more hazardous than others; for instance, construction work is potentially more physically dangerous than office work. Certain hobbies and recreational activities are also extremely hazardous (e.g., skiing and in-line skating). Contact sports, such as football and ice hockey, often result in musculoskeletal injuries, including fractures. Other activities do not have such an obvious potential for injury but can cause fractures nonetheless. For instance, daily jogging and frequent marching in a band can lead to fatigue fractures.

Because inadequate nutrition contributes to fractures and can inhibit bone healing, the nurse takes a complete diet history. Health promotion counseling is a major focus for comprehensive health care today.

CONSIDERATIONS FOR OLDER ADULTS

A diet history is especially important for older adults. For example, some older clients eat poorly because of loss of companionship and poor finances. They may be unable to prepare meals and thus rely on others for proper nutrition. Inadequate exposure to sunlight in many older adults may contribute to vitamin D deficiency.

PHYSICAL ASSESSMENT/CLINICAL MANIFESTATIONS

BODY SYSTEM ASSESSMENT. The client with a fracture often sustains trauma to other body systems. Consequently, the nurse assesses all major body systems *first* for life-threatening complications, including head, thoracic, and abdominal injuries. The assessment of these areas is described elsewhere in this text.

MUSCULOSKELETAL ASSESSMENT. When inspecting the site of a possible fracture, the nurse observes for a change in bone alignment. The bone may appear deformed, or a limb may be internally or externally rotated. Accompanying these deviations may be an alteration in the length of the extremity (usually a shortening) or a change in bone shape. The nurse asks the client to move the involved body part. If pain is elicited, the movement is stopped immediately. Range of motion (ROM) is typically decreased. When the affected part is moved, the nurse may hear **crepitation,** a continuous grating sound created by bone fragments.

The nurse also observes the skin for integrity. If the skin is intact (closed fracture), the area over the fracture may be ecchymotic (bruised) from bleeding into the underlying soft tissues. Subcutaneous emphysema, the appearance of bubbles under the skin because of air trapping, is not uncommon but is seen later.

Swelling at the fracture site is rapid and can result in marked neurovascular compromise. Therefore the nurse performs a thorough neurovascular assessment and compares the injured area with its symmetric counterpart. Skin color and temperature, sensation, mobility, pain, and pulses are assessed distal to the fracture site. If the fracture involves an extremity, the nurse checks the nails for capillary refill by applying pressure to the nail and observing for the speed of blood return. If nails are brittle or thick, the skin adjacent to the nail is assessed. Chart 52-3 describes the procedure for a neurovascular assessment, which evaluates circulation, movement, and sensation.

For an open fracture, the nurse determines the degree of soft-tissue damage and the amount of overt bleeding. The area may be lightly palpated for tenderness, but a sterile glove is worn if the skin is disrupted.

Clients often complain of moderate to severe pain at the site of the fracture or in an adjacent or distal area. For example, clients with a fractured hip may have groin pain or pain referred to the back of the knee. Pain is usually due to muscle spasm and edema, which result from the fracture. In clients with one or more fractured ribs, severe pain occurs when deep

CHART 52-3

BEST PRACTICE *for* Assessment of Neurovascular Status in Clients with Musculoskeletal Injury

ASSESSMENT TECHNIQUE	NORMAL FINDINGS
Skin Color	
Inspect the area distal to the injury.	No change in pigmentation compared with other parts of the body.
Skin Temperature	
Palpate the area distal to the injury (the dorsum of the hands is most sensitive to temperature).	The skin is warm.
Movement	
Ask the client to move the affected area or the area distal to the injury (active motion).	The client can move without discomfort.
Move the area distal to the injury (passive motion).	No difference in comfort compared with active movement.
Sensation	
Ask the client if numbness or tingling is present (paresthesia).	No numbness or tingling.
Palpate with a paper clip (especially the web space between the first and second toes or the web space between the thumb and forefinger).	No difference in sensation in the affected and unaffected extremities. (Loss of sensation in these areas indicates perineal nerve or median nerve damage.)
Pulses	
Palpate the pulses distal to the injury.	Pulses are strong and easily palpated; no difference in the affected and unaffected extremities.
Capillary Refill	
Press the nail beds distal to the injury until blanching occurs (or the skin near the nail if nails are thick and brittle).	Blood returns (return to usual color) within 3 seconds (5 seconds for older clients).
Pain	
Ask the client about the location, nature, and frequency of the pain.	Pain is usually localized and is often described as stabbing or throbbing. (Pain out of proportion to the injury and unrelieved by analgesics might indicate compartment syndrome.)

breaths are taken. The nurse assesses respiratory status, which may be severely compromised from pain or pneumothorax (air in the pleural cavity).

SPECIAL ASSESSMENT CONSIDERATIONS. For fractures of the shoulder and upper arm, the physical assessment is best done with the client in a sitting or standing position, if possible, so that shoulder drooping or other abnormal positioning can be seen. The nurse supports the affected arm and flexes the elbow to promote comfort during the assessment. For more distal areas of the arm, the assessment is done with the client in a supine position so that the extremity can be elevated to reduce swelling.

The nurse places the client in a supine position for assessment of the lower extremities and pelvis. A client with an impacted hip fracture may be able to walk for a short time after injury, although this is not recommended. The client with any type of hip fracture has pain and decreased ROM in the hip.

Some fractures can cause internal organ damage, resulting in hemorrhage. When a pelvic fracture is suspected, the nurse assesses vital signs, skin color, and the level of consciousness for indications of possible hypovolemic shock. The urine is checked for blood, which indicates damage to the urinary system, often the bladder. If the client is unable to void, the nurse suspects damage to the urethra.

PSYCHOSOCIAL ASSESSMENT

The psychosocial status of a client with a fracture depends on the extent of the injury and other complications. Hospitalization is usually not required for a single, uncomplicated fracture, and the client may return to usual daily activities within a few days. Healing is usually complete in a young adult in 4 to 6 weeks.

In contrast, a client suffering multiple trauma can be hospitalized for weeks and may undergo many surgical procedures and other treatments. For these clients, disruptions in lifestyle can create a high level of stress.

The stresses that result from a chronic condition affect relationships between the client and family members or significant others. The nurse assesses the client's feelings about himself or herself as a person and asks about how he or she coped with previously experienced stressful events. Body image and sexuality may be altered by deformity, treatment modalities for fracture repair, and/or long-term immobilization.

LABORATORY ASSESSMENT

No special laboratory tests are available for assessment of fractures. The client's hemoglobin level and hematocrit are often low because of bleeding caused by the injury. If extensive soft-tissue damage accompanies the fracture, the erythrocyte sedimentation rate (ESR) may be elevated, which indicates the expected inflammatory response. If the ESR increases during fracture healing, the client may have a bone infection. During the healing stages, serum calcium and phosphorus levels are often increased as the bone releases these elements into the blood.

RADIOGRAPHIC ASSESSMENT

The health care provider orders standard x-ray studies and tomograms to confirm a diagnosis of fracture. These reveal the bone disruption, malalignment, or deformity. If the x-ray film does not show a fracture but the client is symptomatic, the x-ray study is usually repeated with additional views.

The computed tomography (CT) scan is useful in detecting fractures of complex structures, such as the hip and pelvis. It also identifies compression fractures of the spine.

OTHER DIAGNOSTIC ASSESSMENT

The health care provider may order a bone scan (with technetium or gallium) for help in detecting certain types of fractures, particularly pathologic fractures. It is impossible for fractures of small bones or occult fractures to be visualized by conventional x-ray studies as early as by a bone scan. In addition, the bone scan can better determine fracture complications, such as delayed bone healing, nonunion, infection, and avascular necrosis (AVN).

Magnetic resonance imaging (MRI) is useful in determining the amount of soft-tissue damage that may have occurred with the fracture. It is also helpful in visualizing vertebral and skull fractures.

Analysis

COMMON NURSING DIAGNOSES AND COLLABORATIVE PROBLEMS

The following are common nursing diagnoses for clients with fractures:

1. Risk for Peripheral Neurovascular Dysfunction related to bone and soft-tissue trauma and immobility
2. Acute Pain related to bone disruption, soft-tissue damage, muscle spasm, and edema
3. Risk for Infection related to bone trauma and soft-tissue damage
4. Impaired Physical Mobility related to pain
5. Imbalanced Nutrition: Less Than Body Requirements related to additional metabolic need for healing of bone and soft tissues

ADDITIONAL NURSING DIAGNOSES AND COLLABORATIVE PROBLEMS

In addition to the common nursing diagnoses, clients with fractures may have one or more of the following:

- Activity Intolerance related to pain and impaired mobility
- Constipation related to prolonged immobility (particularly in older adults)
- Ineffective Coping related to prolonged immobility, hospitalization, and/or lifestyle changes
- Compromised Family Coping related to prolonged hospitalization and/or lifestyle changes
- Deficient Diversional Activity related to prolonged hospitalization and rehabilitation
- Anticipatory Grieving related to altered lifestyle
- Self-Care Deficit related to pain and immobility
- Disturbed Body Image related to deformity and/or treatment modality
- Sexual Dysfunction related to pain and immobility
- Disturbed Sleep Pattern related to chronic pain and/or prolonged hospitalization
- Fear related to possible nursing home placement and/or death (particularly in older adults)
- Impaired Skin Integrity and Impaired Tissue Integrity related to bone injury

The following collaborative problems may be appropriate for clients with severe fractures:

- Potential for Acute Compartment Syndrome
- Potential for Hypovolemic Shock
- Potential for Fat Embolism Syndrome
- Potential for Thromboembolitic Complications
- Potential for Avascular Necrosis
- Potential for Delayed Healing, Malunion, or Nonunion

Planning and Implementation

RISK FOR PERIPHERAL NEUROVASCULAR DYSFUNCTION

NOC **PLANNING: EXPECTED OUTCOMES.** The client with a fracture is expected to have sufficient blood flow for adequate oxygen and nutrient delivery to tissues, especially distal to the fracture site, as indicated by strong distal peripheral pulses, brisk capillary refill, normal skin color, and intact muscle function.

INTERVENTIONS. A fracture can occur anywhere. The nurse provides emergency interventions until medical treatment in a hospital is available.

EMERGENCY CARE. A fracture may be accompanied by multiple injuries to vital organs. Therefore the nurse *first* assesses the client for respiratory distress, bleeding, and head injury. If any of these is present, the nurse provides lifesaving care before being concerned about the fracture.

The fracture injury is then assessed (Chart 52-4). If the person is clothed, the nurse or another person trained in first aid cuts away clothing from the fracture site for best visualization. Bleeding is controlled by direct pressure on the area and digital pressure over the proximal artery nearest the fracture. At the same time, to prevent shock, the nurse checks vital signs, places the client in a supine position, and keeps him or her warm with coverings.

The nurse also:

- Inspects the fracture site for intactness of skin, swelling, and deformity (e.g., shortening and rotation)
- Palpates the area *lightly* to determine temperature (coolness), decreased sensation, and blanching
- Assesses distal pulses by comparing affected and unaffected extremities, if applicable
- Assesses for motor function by asking the client to move an area distal to the fracture (e.g., if a femoral fracture is suspected, he or she is asked to move the ankle and foot on the affected side; the upper portion of the leg remains immobilized)

To prevent further damage, reduce pain, and increase circulation, the nurse immobilizes the area of the fracture by splinting. Any object or device that extends to the joints above and below the fracture can be used as a splint. At the scene of an accident, the nurse may need to improvise by using avail-

CHART 52-4

BEST PRACTICE *for* Emergency Care of the Client with an Extremity Fracture

1. Remove the client's clothing (cut, if necessary) to inspect the affected area while supporting the injured area above and below the injury. Do not remove shoes, since this can cause increased trauma.
2. Apply direct pressure on the area if there is bleeding and pressure over the proximal artery nearest the fracture.
3. Keep the client warm and in a supine position.
4. Check the neurovascular status of the area distal to the extremity: temperature, color, sensation, movement, and capillary refill. Compare affected and unaffected limbs.
5. Immobilize the extremity by splinting; include joints above and below the fracture site. Recheck circulation after splinting.
6. Cover the affected area with a dressing (preferably sterile).

able materials, such as a board. If the skin is broken, the nurse loosely applies a clean (preferably sterile) cloth to prevent further contamination of the wound. Neurovascular assessment is rechecked following splinting.

In the emergency department, physician's office, or clinic, fracture management begins with reduction and immobilization of the fracture:

- Reduction, or realignment of the bone ends for proper healing, is accomplished by a closed method (e.g., traction) or an open (surgical) procedure.
- Immobilization is achieved by the use of bandages, casts, traction, internal fixation, or external fixation.

The health care provider selects the treatment method on the basis of the type, location, and extent of the fracture. These interventions prevent further injury and reduce discomfort. The nurse is responsible for maintaining these devices and for assessing, preventing, and intervening for complications that can result from their use.

> **CRITICAL THINKING CHALLENGE**
>
> A 30-year-old man arrives at your emergency department via ambulance. He was the driver of a motorcycle involved in a collision with a sport utility vehicle (SUV). Paramedics report that the client was hit from the side; the bike fell on him, and he was trapped underneath the SUV. Initial reports from the ambulance en route describe an individual in shock with a mangled left leg below the knee and a left wrist fracture. The client was wearing a helmet at the time of the crash.
>
> - What information given above is helpful in predicting other injuries this client may have sustained?
> - What are the priority assessments you should perform when he arrives at the hospital?
> - What assessments of the leg injury will determine the type and grade of the fracture?
> - What initial assessments of the injured leg should you perform?

For suggested answer guidelines, go to SIMON http://www.wbsaunders.com/SIMON/Iggy/.

NIC **NEUROVASCULAR MONITORING.** The nurse performs a neurovascular assessment (Chart 52-5) at frequent intervals if the client is admitted to the hospital, depending on the severity and extent of the fracture and agency policy. The nurse pays particular attention to *early* signs and symptoms of acute compartment syndrome (ACS) by doing a thorough pain assessment. The client with early ACS typically complains of severe, diffuse pain that is not relieved by analgesics; pain during passive motion is greater than pain during active motion. If the client presents with this complaint, the nurse notifies the health care provider *immediately.*

NONSURGICAL MANAGEMENT. Nonsurgical management typically involves closed reduction and immobilization with a bandage, splint, cast, or traction. For each modality, the nurse's primary concern is assessment and prevention of neurovascular dysfunction or compromise.

CLOSED REDUCTION. **Closed reduction** is the most common nonsurgical method for managing a simple fracture. While applying a manual pull, or traction, on the bone, the health care provider manipulates the bone ends so that they realign. Anesthesia or analgesia may be used during this procedure to minimize pain. An x-ray verifies that the bone ends are approximated before the bone is immobilized.

Bandages and Splints. For certain areas of the body, such as the scapula and clavicle, an elastic bandage or commercial mobilizer may be used to immobilize the bone during healing. Because upper extremity bones do not bear weight, splints may be sufficient to keep bone fragments in place. Figure 52-3 illustrates the use of a wrist splint for fracture immobilization. Thermoplast, a durable, flexible material for splinting, allows custom fitting to the client's body part.

The nurse's primary responsibility is to assess the area distal to the bandage or splint for neurovascular compromise. The client usually complains of increased discomfort that is not relieved by analgesics if the splint or bandage is too tight. The nurse reinforces the need for elevation as appropriate and teaches how to assess for circulatory changes. The client is reminded to keep the device as dry and clean as possible to prevent skin breakdown and infection.

Casts. For more complex fractures or fractures of the lower extremity, the physician or orthopedic technician ap-

CHART 52-5

NIC INTERVENTION ACTIVITIES *for* The Client at Risk for Peripheral Neurovascular Dysfunction

Circulatory Care (Arterial Insufficiency/Venous Insufficiency): *Promotion of arterial and venous circulation.*

- Perform a comprehensive appraisal of peripheral circulations (e.g., check peripheral pulses, edema, capillary refill, color, and temperature).
- Monitor degree of discomfort or pain.
- Palpate limb with caution.
- Place extremity in a dependent position, as appropriate.

Peripheral Sensation Management: *Prevention or minimization of injury or discomfort in the client with altered sensation.*

- Monitor for paresthesia: numbness, tingling, hyperesthesia, and hypoesthesia.
- Monitor fit of bracing devices, prosthesis, shoes, and clothing.
- Administer analgesics, as necessary.
- Discuss or identify causes of abnormal sensations or sensation changes.

NIC intervention activities selected from McCloskey, J.C., & Bulechek, G.M. (2000). *Nursing interventions classification (NIC)* (3rd ed.). St. Louis: Mosby.

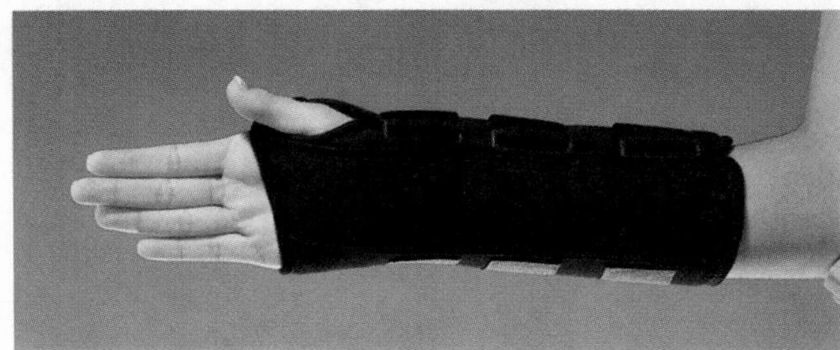

Figure 52-3 ● A universal wrist and forearm splint used for immobilization. (Courtesy Smith & Nephew, Inc., Orthopaedics Division, Memphis, TN.)

plies a cast to hold bone fragments in place after reduction. A **cast** is a rigid device that immobilizes the affected body part while allowing other body parts to move. A cast also allows early mobility and reduces pain. Although its most common use is for fractures, a cast may be applied for correction of deformities (such as clubfoot) or for prevention of deformities (such as those seen in some clients with rheumatoid arthritis).

Cast Materials. Several types of materials are used to make casts. The traditional plaster of Paris (anhydrous calcium sulfate) cast requires application of a well-fitted stockinette under the material. If the stockinette is too tight, it may impair circulation; if it is too loose, wrinkles can lead to the development of pressure ulcers and subsequent skin breakdown. Padding is applied over the stockinette, followed by wet plaster rolls wrapped around the extremity or other body part. The cast feels hot because an immediate chemical reaction occurs, but it soon becomes damp and cool. This type of cast takes 24 to 72 hours to dry, depending on the size and location of the cast. A wet cast feels cold, smells musty, and is grayish. The cast is dry when it feels hard and firm, is odorless, and has a shiny white appearance.

On occasion, the plaster cast may have rough edges, which can crumble and cause skin irritation. To resolve this problem, the nurse petals the cast if the underlying stockinette does not cover the edges of the cast. Small strips of tape are placed over the rough edges to protect the skin. If the skin under the cast was disrupted, the health care provider, orthopedic technician, or specially trained nurse cuts a window into the cast so that the wound can be observed and cared for. A window is also an access for taking pulses, removing wound drains, or relieving abdominal distention when the client is in a body or spica cast.

If the cast is too tight, it may be cut with a cast cutter to relieve pressure or allow tissue swelling. The physician may choose to bivalve the cast (cut it lengthwise into two equal pieces) if bone healing is almost complete. The nurse can remove either half of the cast for inspection or for provision of care. The two pieces are then reunited by an elastic bandage wrap.

Synthetic materials for casts include fiberglass and polyester–cotton knit (Figure 52-4). These materials are lighter than plaster and require minimal drying time. Fiberglass casts are dry in 10 to 15 minutes and can bear weight 30 minutes after application. Polyester–cotton knit casts take 7 minutes to dry and can withstand weight bearing in approximately 20 minutes. Some health care providers use synthetic casts for upper extremities and plaster of Paris casts for lower extremities because plaster casts can bear more weight for a longer time.

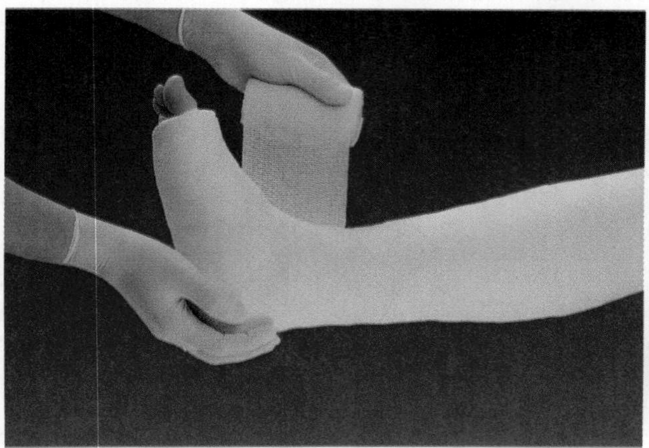

Figure 52-4 ● Application of a fiberglass synthetic cast. (Courtesy Smith & Nephew, Inc., Orthopaedics Division, Memphis, TN.)

Types of Casts. Casts can be generally divided into four main groups: arm casts, leg casts, cast braces, and body or spica casts. Table 52-1 describes specific casts that are used for various parts of the body.

When a client is in bed with an *arm cast,* a sling is used to elevate the arm above the heart to reduce swelling. The hand should be higher than the elbow. Ice may be ordered for the first 24 to 48 hours. When the client is out of bed, the arm is supported with a sling placed around the neck to alleviate fatigue caused by the weight of the cast. The sling should distribute the weight over a large area of the shoulders and trunk, not just the neck. Some health care providers prefer that after the first few days in an arm cast, particularly a short-arm cast, the client not use a sling, to encourage normal movement of the mobile joints and enhance bone healing.

A *leg cast* permits mobility and requires the client to use ambulatory aids, such as crutches. A cast shoe, sandal, or boot that attaches to the foot or a rubber walking pad attached to the sole of the cast assists in ambulation (if weight bearing is allowed) and helps prevent damage to the cast. The affected leg is elevated on several pillows to reduce swelling, and ice is applied for the first 24 hours or as ordered.

A *cast brace* enables the client to bend unaffected joints while the fracture is healing. The fracture must show signs of healing and minimal tissue edema before application of this cast. Two cylindric casts are made and connected by a hinge to allow joint movement. As healing occurs, the casts may be removed and replaced with a soft brace. Commercial immobilizers, which serve the same function as a cast brace, are available and may be used in some cases.

A *body cast* encircles the trunk of the body; a *spica cast* encases a portion of the trunk and one or two extremities. A client with either of these casts presents a special challenge for nursing care. Potential complications related to severe impairment in mobility include the following:

- Skin breakdown
- Respiratory dysfunction, such as pneumonia and atelectasis
- Constipation
- Joint contractures

Cast syndrome (superior mesenteric artery syndrome), an uncommon but serious complication, is most often seen in orthopedic clients who have been placed in a hip spica or body cast. Partial or complete upper intestinal obstruction results in classic symptoms: abdominal distention, epigastric pain, nausea, and vomiting. The vomiting often occurs after meals, and clients may have normal bowel sounds. Partial obstruction occurs initially from compression of the third portion of the duodenum between the superior mesenteric artery and the aorta. This progresses to complete obstruction from duodenal edema caused by continued vomiting and distention. Placing a window in the abdominal portion of the cast or bivalving the cast may be sufficient to relieve pressure on the duodenum. Management of intestinal obstruction is the same as for any client with this complication (see Chapter 57).

Cast Care. Before the cast is applied, the nurse explains the purpose of the cast and the procedure for its application.

With a plaster cast, it is particularly important for the nurse to warn the client about the heat that will be felt immediately after the wet cast is applied. The new cast is not covered; this facilitates air-drying.

When a client with a wet plaster cast is moved and turned, the nurse handles the cast with the palms of the hands to prevent indentations and resultant areas of pressure on the skin. The client is turned every 1 to 2 hours to allow air to circulate and dry all parts of the cast. If the client is hospitalized, the nurse or assistive nursing personnel places a sign at the head of the bed as a reminder that the cast is wet and requires special handling. If the health care provider orders that the cast be elevated to reduce swelling, a cloth-covered pillow is used instead of one encased in plastic, which could cause the cast to retain heat and prevent drying. Elevation of the casted extremity reduces edema but may impair arterial circulation to the affected limb. Uniform support is needed while the cast is drying to prevent development of pressure points.

For preventing contamination by urine or feces, the perineal area of a dry long leg or body cast is encased in a plastic, protective covering. Fracture pans are preferred over traditional bedpans because they are smaller and more comfortable for the client. Care is taken to prevent spillage onto the cast.

The nurse checks to ensure that the cast is not too tight and frequently monitors the client's neurovascular status, usually every hour for the first 24 hours after application (see Chart 52-3 for a description of the procedure and normal findings). The nurse should be able to insert a finger between the cast and the skin. Ice may be applied for the first 24 to 36 hours to reduce swelling and inflammation.

Once the plaster cast is dry, it is inspected at least once every 8 hours for drainage, cracking, crumbling, alignment, and fit. Areas of drainage on the cast should be measured and documented, although there is no direct relationship between the amount of cast drainage and the amount of drainage from the wound. Plaster casts act like sponges and absorb drainage, whereas synthetic casts act like a wick, pulling drainage away from the drainage site. Padding can also absorb wound drainage. Drainage on any cast should always be measured and documented in the client record; however, sources disagree on whether drainage should be circled on the cast, because it may increase anxiety. The nurse immediately reports sudden increases in the amount of drainage or a change in the integrity of the cast to the health care provider. After swelling decreases, it is not uncommon for the cast to become too loose and need replacement. If the client is not admitted to the hospital, he or she is given instructions regarding cast care, as discussed later under Community-Based Care, p. 1141.

Cast Complications. During hospitalization, the nurse assesses for other complications resulting from casting that can

TABLE 52-1 • TYPES OF CASTS USED FOR MUSCULOSKELETAL TRAUMA

Type and Characteristics of Cast	Use
UPPER EXTREMITY CASTS	
Short-arm cast (SAC) (extends from below the elbow to and including part of the hand)	Stable fractures of the wrist (metacarpals, carpals, or distal radius)
Long-arm cast (LAC) (includes the upper arm to and including part of the hand)	Unstable fractures of the wrist, distal humerus, radius, or ulna
Hanging-arm cast (same as LAC but heavier, with added loop at the mid-forearm)	Fractures of the humerus that cannot be aligned by LAC (Light traction is possible while the client is in bed or by an attached strap that extends around the neck.)
Thumb spica (gauntlet) cast (similar to SAC with the thumb casted in abduction)	Fractures of the thumb
Shoulder spica cast (the shoulder is casted in abduction with the elbow flexed)	Unstable fractures of the shoulder girdle or humerus; dislocations of the shoulder
LOWER EXTREMITY CASTS	
Short-leg cast (SLC) (from below the knee to the base of the toes)	Fractures of the ankle, metatarsals, or foot
Long-leg cast (LLC) (from the mid-upper thigh to the base of the toes)	Unstable fractures of the tibia, fibula, or ankle
Walking cast (a walking device on the bottom of SLC or LLC)	Same as for SLC or LLC
Leg cylinder (similar to SLC, but the ankle and foot are not casted)	Stable fractures of the tibia, fibula, or knee
Long-leg cylinder (similar to LLC, but the ankle and foot are not casted)	Stable fractures of the distal femur, proximal tibia, or knee
CAST BRACES (OR BRACE CASTS)	
Patellar weight-bearing cast (similar to SLC or leg cylinder)	Midshaft or distal shaft fractures of the femur
External polycentric knee hinge cast (a hinge connects the lower and upper leg and allows 90 degrees of knee flexion)	Same as for the patellar weight-bearing cast
BODY CASTS	
Hip spica (extends from below the nipple line down the affected leg [single], down the leg and half of the unaffected leg [1½], or down both legs [double])	Dislocation of the hip; pelvic or hip injuries
Risser's cast (the body jacket extends from the shoulders to beyond the iliac crests and hips, with a large opening over the anterior chest)	Scoliosis; thoracic spinal fractures
Halo cast (the body jacket contains a halo brace)	Fractures of the cervical spine

be serious and life threatening, such as infection, circulation impairment, and peripheral nerve damage. If the client returns home after cast application, the client and family are taught how to monitor for these complications and when to notify the health care provider.

Infection most often results from the breakdown of skin under the cast (pressure necrosis). If pressure necrosis occurs, the client typically complains of a very painful "hot spot" under the cast, and the cast may feel warmer in the affected area. The nurse smells the area for mustiness or an unpleasant odor that would indicate infected material. If the infection progresses, a fever may develop.

Circulation impairment and peripheral nerve damage can result from constriction of the cast. The nurse performs frequent neurovascular assessments, as described in Chart 52-3. A client with a new cast may require hourly assessments. A client with a cast that is 3 or 4 days old usually requires assessments every 4 to 8 hours.

The client with a cast may be immobilized for a prolonged period, depending on the extent of the fracture and the type of cast. The nurse assesses for complications of immobility, such as skin breakdown, pneumonia, atelectasis, thromboembolism, and constipation. Before the cast is removed, the nurse informs the client that the cast cutter will not injure the skin but that heat may be felt during the procedure.

Because of prolonged immobilization, a joint may become contracted, usually in a fixed state of flexion, or degenerative arthritis may develop from lack of weight bearing, which is necessary for cartilage viability. Muscle can also atrophy from lack of exercise during prolonged immobilization of the affected body part, usually an extremity.

CRITICAL THINKING CHALLENGE

Following initial assessment in the emergency department, your client who was injured in the motorcycle accident has a closed reduction of the wrist fracture and application of a long-arm cast. He is alert and oriented when he arrives on the orthopedic unit.

- What assessment should you perform to evaluate the neurovascular status of the client's injured arm?
- What is a potential cause of compartment syndrome in this client's fractured arm?
- What symptoms would raise suspicion of compartment syndrome?

For suggested answer guidelines, go to SIMON http://www.wbsaunders.com/SIMON/Iggy/.

Traction. **Traction** is the application of a pulling force to a part of the body to provide reduction, alignment, and rest. Traction can also decrease muscle spasm (thus relieving pain) and prevent or correct deformity and tissue damage. A client in traction is usually hospitalized longer, but in some cases home care is possible even for skeletal traction.

Mechanical traction can be either of the following:

- Continuous, as in fracture treatment
- Intermittent, for relief of muscle spasm in other types of musculoskeletal/neurologic trauma, such as cervical nerve root compression

Traction may also be classified as running traction or balanced suspension. In running traction, the pulling force is in one direction and the client's body acts as countertraction. Moving the body or bed position can alter the countertraction force. Balanced suspension provides the countertraction, so that the pulling force of the traction is not altered when the bed or client is moved. This allows for increased client movement and facilitates care.

Types of Traction. Traction is typically one of five types: skin traction, skeletal traction, plaster traction, brace traction, or circumferential traction. Skin traction involves the use of a Velcro boot (Buck's traction) (Figure 52-5), belt, or halter, which is secured around a body part. The primary purpose of skin traction is to decrease painful muscle spasms that accompany fractures. The weight used as a pulling force is limited (5 to 10 pounds [2.3 to 4.5 kg]) to prevent injury to the skin.

In skeletal traction, pins (e.g., Steinmann), wires (e.g., Kirschner), tongs (e.g., Crutchfield), or screws are surgically inserted directly into bone. These allow the use of longer traction time and heavier weights (usually 15 to 30 pounds [6.8 to 13.6 kg]). Skeletal traction aids in bone realignment.

Plaster traction combines skeletal traction and a plaster cast. A brace traction device exerts a pull for correction of alignment deformities. Circumferential traction uses a belt around the body, such as pelvic traction for low back problems. Table 52-2 describes commonly used types of traction for various parts of the body.

Traction Care. The nurse may set up or assist in the setup of traction. In larger or specialty hospitals or units, orthopedic technicians may set up traction. Once traction is applied, the nurse is responsible for maintaining the correct balance between traction pull and countertraction force. Weights are not usually removed without an order; they are not usually lifted manually or allowed to sit on the floor. Weights should be freely hanging at all times. The nurse teaches this important point to staff members on the unit and to other personnel, such as in the radiology department.

The skin should be inspected at least every 8 hours for signs of irritation or inflammation. When possible, the nurse removes the belt or boot that is used for skin traction every 8 hours to inspect under the device.

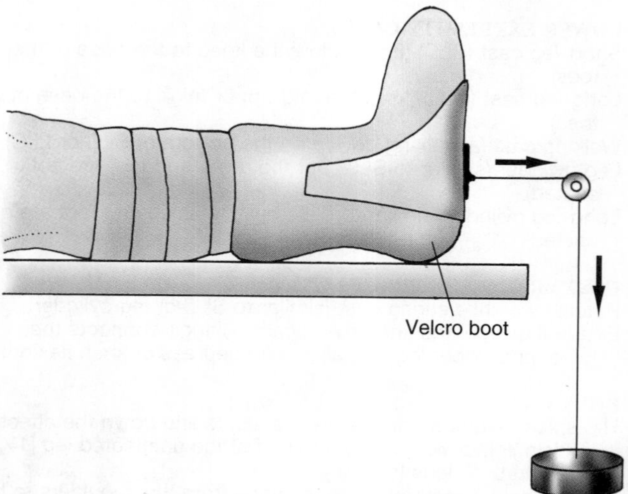

Figure 52-5 ● Buck's traction with a hook-and-loop fastener (Velcro) boot, commonly used for hip fractures.

When skeletal traction is used, the nurse pays particular attention to the points of entry of pins, wires, or screws for signs of inflammation or infection. A small amount of clear fluid drainage ("weeping") is expected. Most health care providers prefer that the nurse perform pin care every day. No standardized method or protocol for pin care has been established throughout the United States. Some health care providers and nurse specialists believe that cleaning the pins disrupts the skin's natural barrier to infection and advise against this practice. In any case, the nurse observes pin sites at least every 8 hours for drainage, color, odor, and severe redness, which indicate inflammation and possible infection. Infection of the pin tract may result in osteomyelitis.

The nurse is responsible for checking traction equipment to ensure its proper functioning. All ropes, knots, and pulleys are inspected at least every 8 hours for loosening, fraying, and positioning. The nurse checks the weight for consistency with the health care provider's order. At times, the health care provider or qualified technician changes the weight without notifying the nurse or modifying the written order; the nurse contacts the person responsible for a new order for confirmation of the change. Sometimes one of the weights is accidentally displaced by a staff member or visitor who bumps into it. The nurse replaces the weights if they are not correct and notifies the health care provider or orthopedic technician.

If the client complains of severe pain from muscle spasm, the weights may be too heavy or the client may need realignment. The nurse reports the pain to the health care provider if body realignment fails to reduce the discomfort. The nurse also assesses the neurovascular status of the affected body part to detect circulatory compromise and subsequent tissue damage. For clients with casts, circulation is usually monitored every hour for the first 24 hours after traction is applied and every 4 hours thereafter (see Chart 52-3).

CONSIDERATIONS FOR OLDER ADULTS

Older clients often have peripheral vascular disease, connective tissue disease, and/or diabetes. Therefore they are at high risk for problems caused by skin or skeletal traction because of inadequate circulation and sensation. Traction of any type is not the ideal treatment for the older client, because it necessitates a prolonged period of immobilization; serious complications can result, such as pneumonia and pulmonary emboli. Abrasions, ulcers, and other skin problems should be reported to the health care provider. Care must be taken to avoid pressure on the bony prominences and superficial nerves. Pressure on the peroneal nerve at the point where it passes around the neck of the fibula must also be avoided, or footdrop could occur.

SURGICAL MANAGEMENT. For some types of fractures, casts and traction are not appropriate or sufficient treatment techniques. Surgical intervention may be needed to realign the bone for the healing process.

PREOPERATIVE CARE. For stabilizing the fracture, the client may be placed in traction before surgery. This procedure is typical for managing a fractured hip when Buck's traction may be used preoperatively (see Figure 52-5). The nurse teaches the client and family or significant others what to expect during and after the surgery. The preoperative care for a client undergoing musculoskeletal surgery is similar to that for any client preparing for surgery with general or epidural anesthesia. (See Chapter 17 for a thorough discussion of preoperative nursing care.)

TABLE 52-2 • TYPES OF TRACTION USED FOR MUSCULOSKELETAL TRAUMA

Type and Characteristics of Traction	Use
UPPER EXTREMITY TRACTION	
Sidearm skin or skeletal traction (the forearm is flexed and extended 90 degrees from the upper part of the body)	Fractures of the humerus with or without involvement of the shoulder and clavicle
Overhead or 90-90 traction, skin or skeletal (the elbow is flexed and the arm is at a right angle to the body over the upper chest)	Same as above (depends on the physician's preference)
Plaster traction (pins inserted through the bone are fixed in the cast)	Fractures of the wrist
LOWER EXTREMITY TRACTION	
Buck's extension traction (skin) (the affected leg is in extension)	Fractures of the hip or femur preoperatively Prevention of hip flexion contractures Hip dislocation
Russell's traction (similar to Buck's traction, but a sling under the knee suspends the leg)	Fractures of the hip or end of the femur
Balanced skin or skeletal traction (the limb is usually elevated in a Thomas splint with Pearson's attachment, or a Böhler-Braun splint is used)	Fractures of the femur or pelvis (acetabulum)
SPINAL COLUMN AND PELVIC TRACTION	
Cervical halter (a strap under the chin)	Cervical muscle spasms, strain/sprain, or arthritis
Cervical skeletal (e.g., halo brace, Crutchfield tongs)	Cervical fractures of the spine Muscle spasms
Pelvic belt (a strap around the hips at the iliac crests is attached to weights at the foot of the bed)	Pain, strain, sprain, or muscle spasms, in the lower back
Pelvic sling (a wide strap around the hips is attached to an overhead bar to keep the pelvis off the bed)	Pelvic fractures; other pelvic injuries

OPERATIVE PROCEDURES. **Open reduction with internal fixation (ORIF)** is a common method of reducing and immobilizing a fracture. When this method is not feasible, **external fixation with closed reduction** is used. Although the nurse does not decide which surgical technique is used, the nurse's understanding of the procedures enhances client teaching and care.

Open Reduction with Internal Fixation. ORIF permits early mobilization. Consequently, it is often the preferred surgical method for an older adult who is susceptible to the complications of immobility.

Open reduction allows the surgeon direct visualization of the fracture site. Internal fixation uses pins, screws, rods, plates, and/or prostheses to immobilize the fracture during healing. The surgeon makes an incision to gain access to the broken bone and implants the device. After the bone achieves union, the hardware may be removed, depending on the location and type of fracture (e.g., fractured ankle). Specific types of internal fixation devices are discussed later under Fractures of Specific Sites, p. 1142.

External Fixation. An alternative modality for the initial management of fractures is the external fixation apparatus, as shown in Figure 52-6. After fracture reduction, the physician makes small percutaneous incisions so that pins may be implanted into the bone. All pins are self-drilling. The pins are held in place by an external metal frame to prevent bone movement.

Advantages and Disadvantages. External fixation has several advantages over other immobilization techniques:

- There is minimal blood loss in comparison with internal fixation.
- The device allows early ambulation and exercise of the affected body part while relieving pain.
- The device maintains alignment in closed fractures that will not maintain position in a cast and stabilizes comminuted fractures that require bone grafting.
- In open fractures, in which skin and tissue trauma accompanies the fracture, the device permits easy access to the wound and promotes healing. This method is often preferred over the use of a window in a cast for wound care.

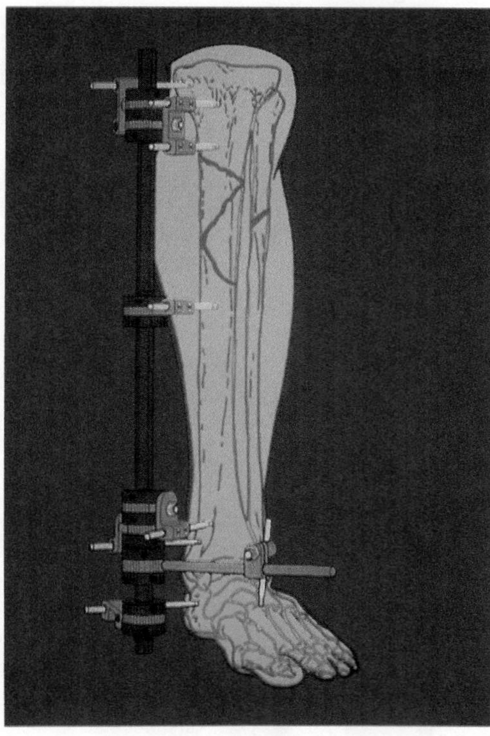

Figure 52-6 ● The Hex-Fix external fixation system for tibial fractures. (Courtesy Smith & Nephew, Inc., Orthopaedics Division, Memphis, TN.)

A disadvantage of external fixation is pin tract infection. Pin tract infections can lead to osteomyelitis, which is serious and difficult to treat (see Chapter 51). For prevention of these infections, some agencies have a pin care procedure that is performed several times a day. The procedure is similar to that described earlier for skeletal traction pins (see Traction Care, p. 1136). As with skeletal traction, the need for special cleaning of the pins and the area around the pins is controversial. Regardless of whether pin care is done, the nurse inspects the pin sites at least daily for severe redness, swelling, and purulent drainage.

Care of the Client with an External Fixator. As with any fracture treatment, the nurse assesses the neurovascular status of the extremity distal to the fracture. External fixators may be used for an extremity or for fractures of the pelvis. External fixation is not definitive treatment for fractures. After a fixator is removed, the client may be placed in a cast until healing is complete.

The client with an external fixator may experience a disturbed body image. The frame may be large and bulky, and the affected area may have massive tissue damage with dressings. The nurse is sensitive to this possibility in planning care.

CRITICAL THINKING CHALLENGE

Following evaluation in the emergency department, the client injured in the motorcycle accident is sent to the operating room for removal of his ruptured spleen, ORIF of an unstable pelvic fracture, and application of an external fixator to the grade III comminuted fracture of his left tibia and fibula.

- What are the advantages of external fixation for treating fractures of the tibia and fibula?
- What assessments of the external fixator should you perform frequently?
- Your client tells you that when the fixator is removed, his leg will be completely healed and he will be able to bear weight completely. What does this statement indicate about the client's understanding of the role of external fixation in fracture management?

For suggested answer guidelines, go to SIMON http://www.wbsaunders.com/SIMON/Iggy/.

Circular External Fixation. The Ilizarov technique of circular external fixation is sometimes used to treat new fractures (closed, comminuted fractures and open fractures with bone loss), as well as malunion or nonunion of fractures. It may also be used to treat congenital bone deformities, especially in children. This procedure originated in Russia about 50 years ago and was introduced in the United States in 1986.

A circular external fixation device stimulates bone growth. Unlike the traditional fixator, the Ilizarov external fixator promotes rotation, angulation, shortening, lengthening, and/or widening of bone while allowing healing of the soft-tissue defect. The nursing care of the client with this device is similar to the care of the client with other external fixation systems except in one major regard: if the device is being used for filling bone gaps, using bone transport or distraction, the client must be taught how to manually turn the four-sided nuts (clickers), usually four times a day, unless he or she has an automated device. Daily distraction rates vary among clients, but 1 mm/day is common. Screening and teaching are particularly important because the client adjusts and cares for the apparatus for a prolonged time.

POSTOPERATIVE CARE. The postoperative care for a client undergoing ORIF or external fixation is similar to that provided for any client undergoing surgery (see Chapter 19). However, because bone is a vascular, dynamic body tissue, the client is at risk for certain complications specific to fractures and musculoskeletal surgery. These problems (e.g., fat embolism and deep vein thrombosis [DVT]) are discussed earlier under Complications of Fractures, pp. 1127-1129.

PROCEDURES FOR NONUNION. Some surgical repairs are not successful, because the bone does not heal. Several additional options are available to the surgeon to promote bone union, such as electrical bone stimulation, bone grafting, and the newest therapy, ultrasound fracture treatment.

For selected clients, electrical bone stimulation may be successful. This procedure is based on research showing that bone has inherent electrical properties that are used in healing. The exact mechanism of action is unknown. Several types of devices have been developed. A noninvasive system uses magnetic coils applied on the skin or over a cast to deliver a pulsed magnetic field. There are no known risks with this system, although clients with pacemakers cannot use this device on an upper extremity. Implanted direct-current stimulators are placed directly in the fracture site and have no external apparatus. Both systems require about 6 months of treatment, and weight bearing is at the discretion of the health care provider.

Another method of treating nonunion is bone grafting. A bone graft may also replace diseased bone or increase bone tissue for joint replacement. In most cases, chips of bone are taken from the client's iliac crest or other site and are packed or wired between the bone ends to facilitate union. Allografts from cadavers may also be used. These grafts are frozen or freeze-dried and stored under sterile conditions in a bone bank, usually in a hospital.

Bone banking from living donors is becoming increasingly popular. If qualified, clients undergoing total hip replacement may donate their femoral heads to the bank for later use as bone grafts for other clients. Careful screening ensures that the bone is healthy and that the donor has no communicable disease. The bone cannot be donated without the client's written consent.

One of the newest modalities for fracture healing is low-intensity pulsed ultrasound (also called Exogen therapy). Used for slow-healing fractures or for new fractures as an alternative to surgery, ultrasound treatment has yielded excellent results. The client applies the treatment for about 20 minutes each day. It has no contraindications or adverse effects.

ACUTE PAIN

NOC **PLANNING: EXPECTED OUTCOMES.** The client with a fracture is expected to experience a reduction or alleviation of pain as indicated by the absence of or a decrease in reported pain, no changes in vital signs, and no facial expressions of pain.

INTERVENTIONS. The nonsurgical or surgical management of fractures through reduction and immobilization helps reduce pain and prevents neurovascular injury. The client often requires drug therapy and other pain relief measures.

DRUG THERAPY. Musculoskeletal pain related to soft-tissue damage, bone disruption, and muscle spasm is one of the most severe types of pain that can be experienced. The client often has the pain for a prolonged time, which makes pain management difficult. The health care provider commonly prescribes opioid analgesics, anti-inflammatory drugs, and muscle relaxants.

For clients with chronic, severe pain, opioid and nonopioid drugs are alternated or given together to manage pain both centrally and peripherally. The nurse and client mutually decide on the best times for the strong pain relievers to be administered (e.g., before a complex dressing change and at bedtime). The nurse observes the client carefully for the effectiveness of the medication and its side effects. An early sign of acute compartment syndrome (ACS) is often the sudden inability of pain medication to relieve pain. Chapter 7 discusses the various methods of pain management, including epidural analgesia and patient-controlled analgesia.

COMPLEMENTARY AND ALTERNATIVE THERAPIES. With chronic, severe pain, the client cannot depend solely on drugs for relief. The nurse uses temporary pain relief measures, such as ice or heat, depending on the cause of the pain. If swelling causes pressure on the affected area, ice and elevation of the affected body part may be appropriate. Muscle spasms are best relieved by application of heat and massage. Other physical measures include a warm, soothing bath, a back rub, and the use of therapeutic touch.

If these measures are not effective in reducing pain, the nurse may use distraction, imagery, or music therapy as alternatives. The nurse teaches relaxation techniques, such as deep breathing, for use during periods of severe pain. Chapters 4 and 7 discuss these techniques in detail.

RISK FOR INFECTION

PLANNING: EXPECTED OUTCOMES. The client with a fracture is expected to be free of a wound or bone infection.

INTERVENTIONS. When caring for a client with a fracture, particularly an open fracture, the nurse uses strict aseptic technique for dressing changes and wound irrigations. Signs and symptoms of local inflammation with purulent drainage are reported immediately to the physician. Other infections, such as pneumonia and urinary tract infection, may occur days after the fracture. The nurse or assistive nursing personnel monitors the client's vital signs every 4 to 8 hours; increases in temperature and pulse often indicate systemic infection.

For most clients with an open fracture, the health care provider prescribes one or more broad-spectrum antibiotics prophylactically. This treatment is especially important for fractures requiring surgical repair.

IMPAIRED PHYSICAL MOBILITY

NOC **PLANNING: EXPECTED OUTCOMES.** The client with a fracture is expected to be free of consequences of impaired mobility and independent in ambulation and mobility, such as transferring from bed to chair.

INTERVENTIONS. The interventions necessary for this diagnosis can be grouped into two types: those that help prevent complications of impaired mobility and those that help increase mobility.

PREVENTION OF COMPLICATIONS. The nurse plays a vital role in preventing and assessing complications in immobilized clients with fractures. Additional information about nursing care for preventing problems associated with immobility is found in Chapter 10 and earlier in this chapter in the discussion of specific complications under Complications of Fractures, pp. 1127-1129.

CONSIDERATIONS FOR OLDER ADULTS
The risk of each complication related to impaired mobility is dramatically increased if surgery is performed. Older clients are at the greatest risk; physiologic changes and prolonged immobility predispose them to these complications.

PROMOTION OF MOBILITY. The use of crutches or a walker increases mobility and assists in ambulation. The client may progress to use of a cane.

CRUTCHES. Crutches are the most commonly used ambulatory aid for many types of musculoskeletal trauma (e.g., fractures, sprains, and amputations). In most agencies, the physical therapist fits the client for crutches and teaches him or her how to ambulate with them on flat surfaces and stairs. The nurse's role may be to reinforce the instructions and evaluate whether the client is using the crutches correctly. However, in emergency department and ambulatory settings nurses routinely teach clients how to use crutches.

Walking with crutches requires strong upper extremities, balance, and coordination. For this reason, crutches are not used as often for older adults.

The therapist pads the tips and axillary bars of the crutches; padding prevents the tips from slipping and the bars from damaging the axillae. To prevent pressure on the axillary nerve, there should be two to three finger breadths between the axilla and the top of the crutch when the crutch tip is at least 6 inches (15 cm) diagonally in front of the foot. The crutch is adjusted by the therapist so that the elbow is flexed no more than 30 degrees when the palm is on the handle (Figure 52-7).

There are several types of gaits for walking with crutches. The most common one for musculoskeletal injury is the three-point gait, which allows minimal weight bearing on the affected leg.

WALKER. A walker is most often used by the older client who needs additional support for balance. The physical therapist assesses the strength of the upper extremities and the unaffected leg. Strength is improved with exercise as needed.

CANE. A cane is sometimes used if the client needs only minimal support for an affected leg. The straight cane offers the least support. A hemi-cane or quad-cane provides a broader base for the cane and therefore more support. The cane is placed on the *unaffected* side and should create no more than 30 degrees of flexion of the elbow. The top of the cane should be parallel to the greater trochanter of the femur.

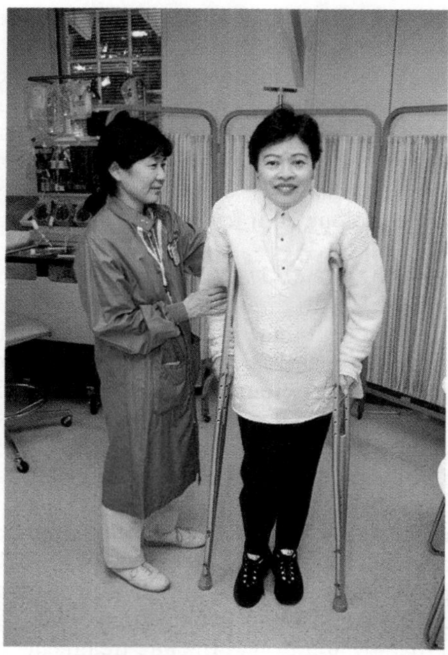

Figure 52-7 ● Assisting the client with crutch walking. Note how the therapist guards the client and how the client's elbows are at no more than 30 degrees of flexion.

IMBALANCED NUTRITION: LESS THAN BODY REQUIREMENTS

PLANNING: EXPECTED OUTCOMES. The client with a fracture is expected to maintain an adequate dietary intake to promote healing and prevent complications.

INTERVENTIONS. Nursing interventions focus on meeting the client's nutritional needs. The dietitian assesses the client's food likes and dislikes and collaborates with him or her to plan meals that are both appealing and nutritional. For promotion of bone and tissue healing, the client needs a high-protein, high-calorie diet. Supplements of vitamins B and C are also required for tissue nutrition. Clients with fractures may be immobilized for extended periods; thus they are predisposed to hypocalcemia, which results in loss of calcium from bone and in subsequent bone fragility. The nurse teaches the client to increase intake of foods high in calcium, particularly milk and milk products if they are tolerated.

A negative nitrogen balance can develop 7 to 10 days after injury in an immobilized client because of an increase in catabolism without compensatory protein intake. The nurse offers frequent small feedings and supplements of high-protein liquids, such as Ensure or Carnation Instant Breakfast preparations. Milk shakes are an excellent protein and calorie supplement, as well as a source of calcium.

Because of less weight bearing on long bones, the immobilized client with a fracture often becomes anemic. Blood loss from the injury or reparative surgery contributes to the anemic state. The nurse encourages intake of foods high in iron content. The health care provider may prescribe an oral iron supplement. It is not uncommon for the client to receive a daily multivitamin with iron.

Community-Based Care

The client with an uncomplicated fracture is usually discharged to home from the emergency department. Older adults with hip or other fractures or clients with multiple trauma are hospitalized and then often transferred to a rehabilitation setting or to a long-term care facility for rehabilitation or permanent residence. To ensure continuity of care, the case manager or the discharge planner in the hospital communicates the plan of care to the health care agency receiving the client.

HEALTH TEACHING

The client with a fracture may be discharged from the hospital, emergency department, office, or clinic with a bandage, splint, cast, or external fixator. The nurse provides verbal and written instructions on the care of these devices. Chart 52-6 describes care of the affected extremity after removal of the cast.

The client may also need to continue wound care at home. The nurse teaches the client and caregiver how to assess and dress the wound to promote healing and prevent infection. The client is taught how to recognize complications (see Complications of Fractures, p. 1127) and when and where to seek professional health care should complications occur.

Additional educational needs depend on the type of fracture and fracture repair. Care of external fixators and casts is discussed earlier under Cast Care (p. 1134) and External Fixation (p. 1138).

HOME CARE MANAGEMENT

If the client is discharged to home, the nurse or case manager assesses the home environment for structural barriers to mobility, such as stairs.

CONSIDERATIONS FOR OLDER ADULTS

A home assessment is particularly important for older clients. A cast is bulky and requires room for maneuvering and ambulating. In collaboration with the therapy team, the nurse instructs the client and family or significant others to remove scatter rugs and other items that can contribute to falls. The rooms should not be cluttered with furniture, so that the client can maneuver with crutches, a walker, or a cane. An elevated toilet seat or shower chair may be needed to promote independence in toileting.

HEALTH CARE RESOURCES

The nurse identifies potential or actual problems in the hospital and arranges for follow-up care at home. For example, professional counseling for depression may need to continue after discharge from the hospital. A social worker may need to help the client apply for funds to pay medical bills. If there is severe bone and tissue damage, the nurse must be realistic and help the client understand the long-term nature of the recovery period, particularly if he or she experiences a major complication, such as infection, while in the hospital. Multiple treatment techniques and surgical procedures required for complications can be mentally and emotionally draining for the client and family. A vocational counselor may be needed to help the client seek a different type of job, depending on the nature of the fracture.

CHART 52-6

CLIENT EDUCATION GUIDE
Care of the Extremity After Cast Removal

- Remove scaly, dead skin carefully by soaking—do not scrub.
- Move the extremity carefully. Expect discomfort, weakness, and decreased range of motion.
- Support the extremity with pillows or your orthotic device until strength and movement return.
- Exercise slowly as instructed by your physical therapist.
- Wear support stockings or elastic bandages to prevent swelling (for lower extremity).

The client with a severe injury and multiple treatment modalities may need follow-up care in the home by a home care nurse. An older or incapacitated client may need assistance with activities of daily living (ADLs), which is provided by home care aides. The nurse in the hospital anticipates the client's needs and arranges for these services, usually with the assistance of the case worker or discharge planner.

It is extremely important for the hospital nurse to communicate the client's needs to the nurse or aide who will care for the client at home. A physical therapist may come to the home, or the client may go to a clinic, hospital, or private office for follow-up physical therapy after discharge from the hospital. An occupational therapist assists with retraining in the home environment for ADLs; adaptations in the home enable the client to be independent.

In addition to individual follow-up, it is the nurse's responsibility to participate in community education about injury prevention. Injury ranked fifth as the leading cause of death in 1996 and since 1980 has remained the leading cause of death between ages 1 and 44.

The cost to individuals and society at large is enormous (see the Cost of Care box on p. 1142). For every death due to injury, there are 16 hospitalizations and 400 outpatient visits. Each year, about 90,000 people sustain injuries serious enough to cause long-term disability. Injury is a definable, correctable event with specific identifiable risks. It is imperative that nurses be active in educating the public on prevention of injury through programs that highlight the major risk factors: alcohol, illicit drugs, and firearms among the young, and falls in older adults (see also Chapter 51).

Evaluation: Outcomes

NOC The nurse evaluates the care of the client with a fracture on the basis of the identified nursing diagnoses and collaborative problems. The expected outcomes include that the client:

- Maintains adequate tissue perfusion as indicated by strong distal peripheral pulses, brisk capillary refill, normal skin color, and intact muscle formation
- Reports that pain is reduced or alleviated
- Does not acquire an infection of the bone or soft tissues

COST OF CARE IMPLICATIONS FOR NURSING

MUSCULOSKELETAL TRAUMA

Cost of Care

- The cost of fractures due to osteoporosis could escalate to approximately $62 billion by the year 2020.
- The cost of hip fracture includes not only the cost of the fracture during hospitalization but also the cost of associated morbidities and posthospital care. Annual costs in the year following hip fracture have been estimated at $37,250 per person.
- Estimates place the lifetime cost of injury at more than $250 billion. The majority of this sum is related to the indirect cost of productivity—loss from death or disability. The direct cost of medical services accounts for approximately 30%.

Implications for Nursing

Injuries are the primary cause of musculoskeletal trauma. Injuries are not accidents; injuries have identifiable risk factors and patterns. Nurses can play a major role in injury prevention by educating the community about these risks. Prevention is a key factor in reducing costs related to musculoskeletal trauma.

Data from American College of Surgeons, Committee on Trauma. (1999). Injury prevention slide presentation; Anderson, E.G. (1997). Osteoporosis: Epidemic of the 21st century? *Geriatrics, 52*(6), 76-78; and Brainsky, A., et al. (1997). The economic cost of hip fractures in community-dwelling older adults: A prospective study. *Journal of the American Geriatrics Society, 45*(3), 281-287.

- Independently ambulates with or without ambulatory aids and provides self-care
- Does not experience consequences of immobility
- Maintains an adequate nutritional intake, as evidenced by bone and soft-tissue healing

Fractures of Specific Sites

UPPER EXTREMITY FRACTURES

Fractures of the Clavicle

Fractures of the clavicle typically result from a fall on an outstretched hand, a fall on the shoulder, or a direct injury. Most clavicular fractures are self-healing; a splint or bandage is used for immobilization. Complicated fractures, although uncommon, may require open reduction with internal fixation (ORIF) by pins, wires, or screws.

Fractures of the Scapula

Scapular fractures are not common and are usually caused by direct impact to the area. Serious internal trauma, including pneumothorax, pulmonary contusion, and fractured ribs, can accompany these fractures.

The shoulder is immobilized with a sling and swathe or a shoulder immobilizer until the fracture heals, usually in 2 to 4 weeks. Intra-articular neck and glenoid fractures may require surgical intervention with plate and screw fixation.

Fractures of the Humerus

Fractures of the proximal humerus, particularly impacted or displaced fractures, are common in the older adult. An impacted injury is usually treated conservatively, with a sling for immobilization. A displaced fracture often requires ORIF with pins or a prosthetic device.

Humeral shaft fractures are generally corrected by closed reduction and application of a hanging-arm cast or splint. If necessary, the fracture is repaired surgically (with an intramedullary rod or metal plate and screws) or with external fixation. Nonunion of the bone and radial nerve palsy are frequent complications of this fracture. Bone grafting facilitates union; prolonged splinting is necessary while the radial nerve regenerates.

A direct blow to the condyles of the distal humerus can cause either or both condyles to fracture, usually in a T- or Y-shaped configuration. The most serious complication is damage to the brachial or median nerve. Condylar fracture is usually treated by ORIF with a series of screws, although skeletal traction and casting can be used.

Fractures of the Olecranon

Fractures of the olecranon are relatively common in adults and typically result from a fall on the elbow. Many are successfully treated by closed reduction and application of a cast. The healing process usually takes more than 2 months, and several additional months may be needed before full use of the elbow is achieved. ORIF is performed for displaced fractures, and a splint is worn during the healing phase.

Fractures of the Radius and Ulna

Forearm fractures of the ulna without accompanying injury to the radius are rare. As with other fractures of long bones, closed reduction with casting may be the appropriate treatment. If the fracture is displaced, ORIF with intramedullary rods or plates and screws is required.

WOMEN'S HEALTH CONSIDERATIONS

Colles' fracture, or distal radius fracture, is common among older adults (particularly women); it results most often from a fall on an open hand. The distal radius has a large percentage of cancellous bone, the type that is initially affected by osteoporosis. Chapter 51 describes osteoporosis, or loss of bone mass, in detail. The options for reduction and immobilization include splinting, casting, plaster-and-pin fixation, or external fixation with a frame. External fixation may be used even with soft tissue damage.

Fractures of the Wrist and Hand

One or more of the bones in the wrist and hand can break, but the most common fracture is of the carpal scaphoid bone in young adult men. This is also one of the most misdiagnosed fractures because it is poorly visualized on an x-ray film. Closed reduction and casting for 6 to 12 weeks is the treatment of choice. If the bone does not heal, open reduction and bone grafting are performed.

Fractures of the metacarpals and phalanges are usually not displaced, which makes their treatment less difficult than that of other fractures. Metacarpal fractures are immobilized for 3 to 4 weeks. Phalangeal fractures are immobilized in finger splints for 10 to 14 days.

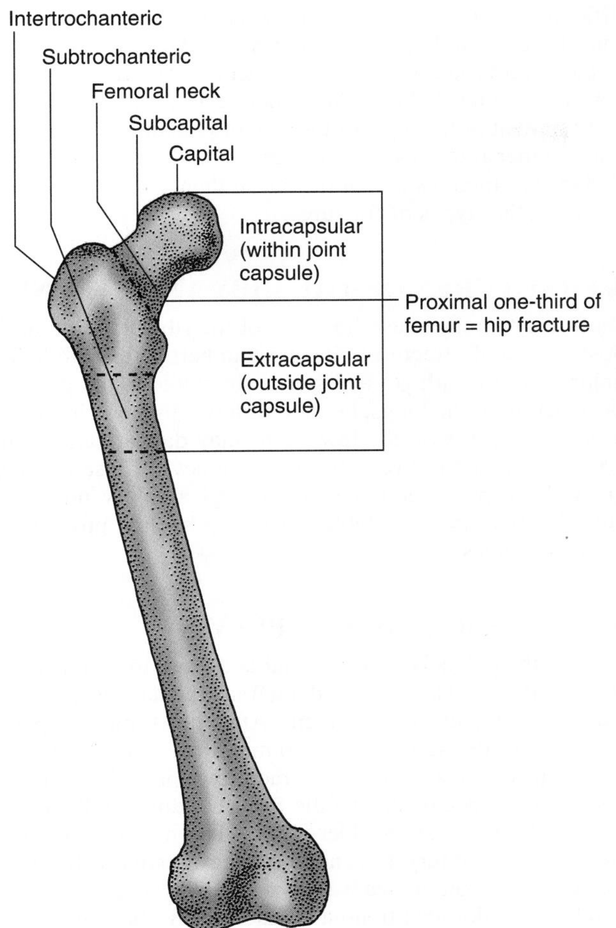

Figure 52-8 ● The types of hip fractures.

LOWER EXTREMITY FRACTURES

Fractures of the Hip

Hip fractures include those involving the upper third of the femur and are classified as intracapsular (within the joint capsule) or extracapsular (outside the joint capsule). These types are further divided according to fracture location (Figure 52-8).

CONSIDERATIONS FOR OLDER ADULTS

Hip fractures occur most often in older persons, particularly women who have osteoporosis. Repair of hip fracture is rapidly becoming the most common surgical procedure for people older than 85 years of age. As many as one third of older clients who sustain a hip fracture die within 1 year of injury from medical complications caused by the fracture or by immobility that occurs after the fracture. Approximately 50% cannot return home or live independently after the fracture (Lappe, 1998). Because of the poor prognosis of clients experiencing hip fractures, public education on osteoporosis and fracture prevention is crucial. Studies suggest that older, thin, Caucasian women are at the most risk for hip fracture (see the Evidence-Based Practice for Nursing box above).

EVIDENCE-BASED PRACTICE FOR NURSING

Preventing hip fractures due to osteoporosis

Turner, L.W., Faile, P.A., & Tomlinson, R., Jr. (1999). Osteoporosis diagnosis and fracture. *Orthopaedic Nursing, 18*(5), 21-27.

This study examined correlates for osteoporosis diagnosis and hip fracture among a national sample of women over 50 years of age using data extracted from the Third National Health and Nutrition Examination Survey (NHANES III). Correlates for screening and diagnosis of osteoporosis included advancing age and race. Risk factors predicting hip fracture included age, race, low body mass index, and inactivity.

Critique. Randomly selected data from a large sample (n = 2336) confirmed prior research results. The NHANES III survey from which the data were derived included an oversampling of African Americans, Hispanics, and individuals over 60 years of age.

Implications for Nursing. Results of the present study combined with information from prior research can be used to formulate nursing guidelines for prevention of osteoporosis and related fractures among older women. Nurses should (1) screen and target high-risk women: those who are older, Caucasian, and underweight; (2) focus on helping clients to achieve and maintain a healthy body weight; (3) encourage safe physical activity two or more times per week consistent with the client's lifestyle and health status; and (4) promote public education regarding osteoporosis.

Falls cause most hip fractures; impaction or displacement, especially of the femoral neck, often results. If the degree of osteoporosis is so severe that it prevents surgical intervention, the client may be incapacitated for the remainder of his or her life.

The treatment of choice is surgical repair, when possible, to allow the older client to get out of bed. Buck's traction may be applied before surgery, which should be scheduled within 24 hours of injury if at all possible. Depending on the exact location of the fracture, open reduction with internal fixation (ORIF) may include an intramedullary rod, pins, a prosthesis, or a fixed sliding plate (such as a compression screw). The client with a compression screw can usually ambulate a few days after surgery and has a decreased chance of infection and nonunion, in comparison with clients for whom other procedures are used. If the femoral neck or head is fractured, a prosthetic device is implanted. Depending on the age of the client and prior mobility status, the surgeon replaces the femoral head only (Moore prosthesis) or performs a total hip replacement. Figures 52-9 and 52-10 illustrate examples of these devices used for ORIF of the hip. Nonsurgical options are Buck's traction and skeletal traction, followed by use of a cast brace (Taggart, 1999).

Hip fractures are common. Nurses in all health care settings need to know how to care for the special needs of the older adult with a hip fracture (see the Client Care Plan on p. 1145). The care is similar to that needed by older clients undergoing total hip replacement (see Chapter 21).

Fractures of the Femur

Fractures of the lower two thirds of the femur usually result from trauma (often from a motor vehicle accident). A femoral fracture is seldom immobilized by casting, because the powerful muscles of the thigh become spastic, which causes displacement of bone ends. Extensive hemorrhage is associated with femoral fracture.

Skeletal traction, followed by a cast brace or hip spica cast, is the typical nonsurgical treatment. Surgical treatment is ORIF with nails, rods, or a compression screw. In a few cases, external fixation may be employed. Healing time for a femoral fracture may be 6 months or longer.

Fractures of the Patella

Like most other fractures, patellar fractures result from direct impact. The surgeon typically repairs the fracture by closed reduction and casting or internal fixation with screws.

Fractures of the Tibia and Fibula

Trauma to the lower leg most often causes fractures of both the tibia and the fibula, particularly the lower third ("tib-fib" fractures). The three basic treatment techniques are closed reduction with casting, internal fixation, and external fixation. If closed reduction is used, the client wears a cast for at least 8 to 10 weeks. Delayed union is not unusual with this type of fracture. Internal fixation with nails or a plate and screws, followed by a long leg cast for 4 to 6 weeks, is another option. When the fractures cause extensive skin and soft-tissue damage, the initial treatment may be external fixation, often for 6 to 10 weeks. This is usually followed by application of a cast until the fracture is completely healed.

Fractures of the Ankle and Foot

Ankle fractures are described by their anatomic place of injury. For example, a bimalleolar (Pott's) fracture involves the medial malleolus of the tibia and the lateral malleolus of the fibula. Because of the instability of the ankle joint, the fracture can result from supination and eversion, pronation and abduction, or pronation and eversion. These forces generally create spiral, transverse, or oblique breaks, which are often difficult to treat and present problems in healing. A combination of closed and open techniques may be used, depending on the severity and extent of the fracture. An arthrodesis (fusion) may be needed if the bone does not heal.

Treatment of fractures of the foot or phalanges is similar to that of other fractures, with either closed or open reduction. Phalangeal fractures are more painful than, but not as serious as, most other types of fractures.

FRACTURES OF THE RIBS AND STERNUM

Chest trauma may cause fractures of the ribs or sternum; the most commonly fractured ribs are numbers 4 through 8. The major concern with rib and sternal fractures is the potential for puncture of the lungs, heart, or arteries by bone fragments or ends. Fractures of the lower ribs may damage underlying organs, such as the liver, spleen, or kidneys. These fractures tend to heal spontaneously without surgical intervention. The client is often uncomfortable during the healing process and requires analgesia.

FRACTURES OF THE PELVIS

Because the pelvis is very vascular and close to major organs and blood vessels, associated internal damage is the chief concern in fracture management. After head injuries, pelvic fractures are the second most common cause of death from trauma. In young adults, pelvic fractures typically result from motor vehicle accidents or falls from buildings; falls are the most common cause in older adults. The major concern related to pelvic injury is venous oozing or arterial bleeding. Loss of blood volume leads to hypovolemic shock.

Internal abdominal trauma is assessed by checking for the presence of blood in the urine and stool and by watching the

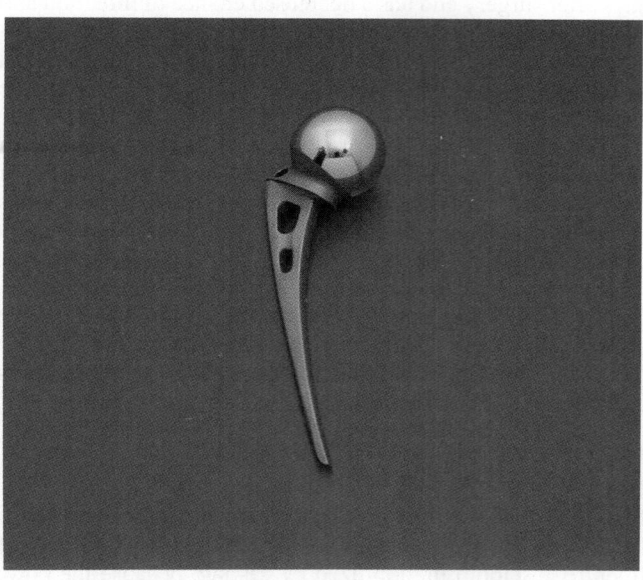

Figure 52-9 ● The Moore prosthesis, which is used for hip fractures. (Courtesy Smith & Nephew, Inc., Orthopaedics Division, Memphis, TN.)

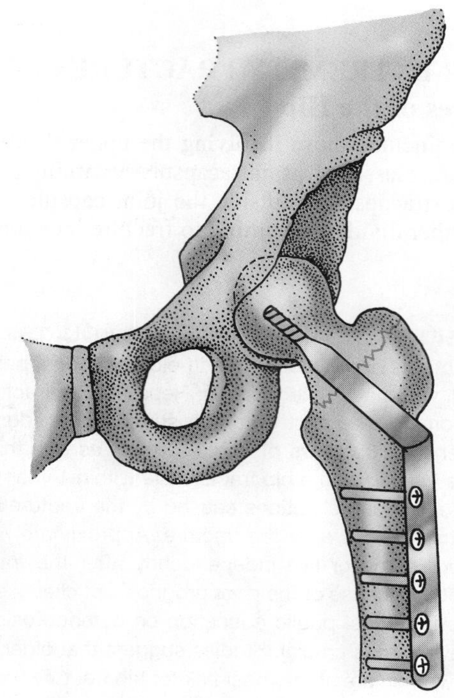

Figure 52-10 ● A compression hip screw used for open reduction with internal fixation (ORIF) of the hip.

CLIENT CARE PLAN • THE CLIENT UNDERGOING OPEN REDUCTION WITH INTERNAL FIXATION FOR A FRACTURED HIP

NURSING DIAGNOSIS NO. 1 • Risk for Injury related to subluxation or dislocation

Expected Outcomes	Nursing Interventions	Rationale
The client will not experience subluxation or dislocation of the operative hip during the hospital stay.	Place an abduction pillow, a splint, or a bed pillow between the client's legs in bed. [D]	Adduction of the affected leg beyond the body's midline can cause dislocation of the hip.
	Use a leg cradle or similar device to align the affected leg. [D]	These devices help prevent internal or external rotation of the affected hip, which could result in dislocation.
	Turn the client carefully toward either side to prevent adduction (check the physician's order). [D]	Adduction of the leg can cause dislocation of the hip.
	Do not flex the operative hip beyond 90 degrees. [D] Use an elevated toilet seat. [D] Have the client sit in a supporting chair with a straight back and seat. [D]	Hyperflexion of the operative hip can cause dislocation.
	Teach the client not to cross the legs.	Crossing the legs causes adduction.

NURSING DIAGNOSIS NO. 2 • Acute Pain related to surgical incision

Expected Outcomes	Nursing Interventions	Rationale
The client will experience alleviation or reduction of surgical pain.	Give pain medication as needed; anticipate the client's need if the client cannot verbalize (epidural or patient-controlled analgesia [PCA] may be used).	Relieving the client's pain helps the client to participate more fully in the plan of care.
	Give pain medication before the physical therapy session (if it does not cloud the client's sensorium) or other periods of increased activity.	
	Use a fracture pan instead of a traditional bedpan. [D]	A fracture pan does not require as much lifting by the client; lifting increases pain.
	Use nondrug pain relief measures, such as distraction, music, and relaxation exercises as needed.	These measures work synergistically with medications; they may reduce the use of opioids and their side effects.

NURSING DIAGNOSIS NO. 3 • Risk for Infection related to impaired skin integrity

Expected Outcomes	Nursing Interventions	Rationale
The client will not experience surgical wound infection.	Inspect the surgical dressing for drainage, and document the type and amount.	Purulent drainage indicates wound infection.
	Monitor and measure the drainage collected in a surgical drain, such as a Hemovac. Empty and compress only if there is an order (opening to remove drainage increases the risk of contaminating the surgical site).	Drains allow the removal of exudate, which can be a medium for bacterial growth.
	After removal of the surgical dressing, inspect the incision for redness, swelling, and warmth, as well as approximation of wound edges.	Signs of inflammation may indicate an infectious process.
	If a dressing is used, change the dressing by using sterile technique.	Sterile conditions reduce the chance of infection.
	Monitor vital signs every 4 hr for 1-3 days. [D]	Elevated pulse and temperature may indicate wound infection.

NURSING DIAGNOSIS NO. 4 • Impaired Physical Mobility related to hip precautions and surgical pain

Expected Outcomes	Nursing Interventions	Rationale
The client will experience increased physical mobility.	Reinforce transfer and ambulation techniques (walker or crutches) as taught by the physical therapist. Have the trapeze and overhead frame on the bed before surgery and teach the client to use the device. Teach the client to bear weight to tolerance (or to bear weight partially for at least 6 wk postoperatively). Assess the client's need for assistive/adaptive devices to perform activities of daily living (ADLs) independently; consult with an occupational therapist.	Increasing mobility promotes the client's independence and return to society as a functional member.
	Assess for and prevent complications of prolonged immobility, such as deep vein thrombosis, skin breakdown, or hypostatic pneumonia. (See Chapter 10 and earlier portions of this chapter for nursing assessment and prevention of complications.)	Complications of immobility cause the client discomfort and prolonged hospitalization.

[D] Indicates tasks that can be delegated to assistive nursing personnel.

abdomen for the development of rigidity or swelling. The trauma team may use peritoneal lavage, computed tomography (CT) scanning, or ultrasound (the newest diagnostic modality) for assessment of hemorrhage. Ultrasound is noninvasive, rapid, reliable, and cost-effective, and it can be done at the bedside in real time.

There are many classification systems for pelvic fractures. A system that is particularly useful for nurses divides fractures of the pelvis into two broad categories: non–weight-bearing fractures and weight-bearing fractures.

When a non–weight-bearing part of the pelvis is fractured, such as one of the pubic rami or the iliac crest, treatment can be as minimal as bedrest on a firm mattress or bed board. This type of fracture can be quite painful, and the client may need stool softeners to facilitate defecation because of hesitancy to move. Well-stabilized fractures usually heal in 2 months.

A weight-bearing fracture, such as multiple fractures of the pelvic ring creating instability or a fractured acetabulum, necessitate external fixation and/or open reduction with internal fixation (ORIF). Less commonly used now are skeletal traction or double-hip spica casts. Progress to weight bearing depends on the stability of the fracture following fixation. Some clients may fully bear weight within days of surgery, whereas others managed with traction may not bear weight for as long as 12 weeks.

FRACTURES AT OTHER SITES

Because the skull and vertebral column protect the brain and spinal cord, these fractures are described in Chapter 43. The nurse must be aware of the special care required for these clients because of possible neurologic damage resulting from these fractures. Fractures of the mandible or nose and other facial trauma are discussed elsewhere in the text.

AMPUTATIONS

OVERVIEW

An **amputation** is the removal of a part of the body. The nurse recognizes that the psychosocial ramifications of the procedure are often more devastating than the physical impairment that results. The loss experienced is complete and permanent and causes a change in body image and often in self-esteem. As with other types of loss, the client can be expected to progress through phases of the grieving process.

Pathophysiology

SURGICAL AMPUTATION

Amputations range from removal of part of a digit to removal of nearly half the entire body. The surgeon performs an amputation by one of two methods: open (or guillotine) method or closed (or flap) method.

The open method is used for clients who have, or are likely to develop, an infection. The wound remains open, and drains allow exudate to escape from the site until the infection clears. The surgeon may suture the skin flaps over the wound at a later time. In the closed technique, the surgeon pulls the skin flaps over the bone end and sutures them in place as part of the amputation procedure. One or more drains are typically inserted.

In either the closed or open method, the surgeon attempts to preserve as much of the part as possible and to keep major joints intact for maximal postoperative mobility.

TRAUMATIC AMPUTATION

Not all amputations are surgically planned. Some, classified as traumatic amputations, occur when a body part is severed unexpectedly (e.g., by a chain saw). Because the amputated part in these clients is usually healthy, attempts to replant it may be made.

One of the most likely replantations involves one or more digits. The current recommendation for prehospital care is that the severed digit be wrapped in a cool, dry cloth and moistened with normal saline, if possible, or bottled water. The digit should then be placed in a sealed plastic bag. The bag is placed in ice water, never directly on ice. Contact between the digit and the water is avoided to prevent tissue damage. Any semi-detached parts of the digit should not be removed.

LEVELS OF AMPUTATION

LOWER EXTREMITY. Lower extremity amputations are performed much more frequently than upper extremity amputations. Five types of lower extremity amputations may be performed (Figure 52-11).

The loss of any or all of the small toes presents a minor disability. Loss of the great toe is significant because it affects balance, gait, and "push off" ability during walking. Midfoot amputations (e.g., the Lisfranc amputation and the Chopart amputation) and the Syme amputation are common procedures for peripheral vascular disease. In the Syme amputation, most of the foot is removed but the ankle remains. The

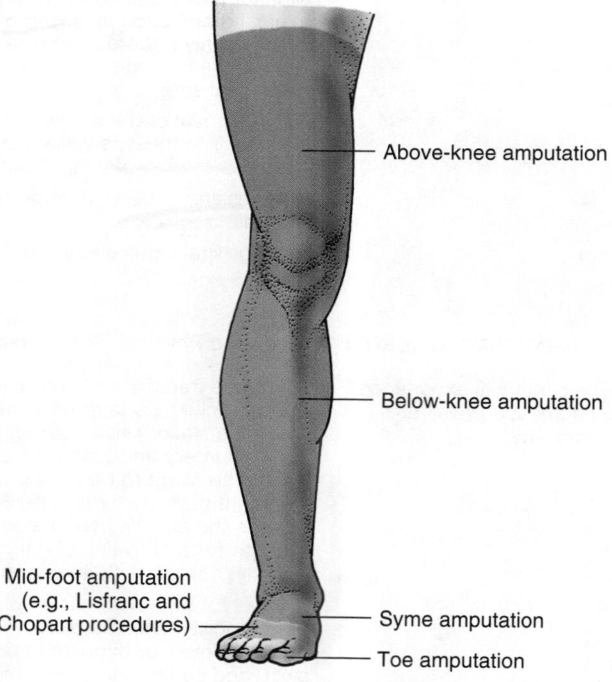

Figure 52-11 ● Common levels of lower extremity amputation.

advantage of this surgery over traditional amputations below the knee is that weight bearing can be accomplished without use of a prosthesis and without pain.

An intense effort is made to preserve knee joints with below-knee amputation (BKA) rather than above-knee amputation (AKA). When the cause for the amputation extends beyond the knee, however, above-knee or higher amputations are performed. Hip disarticulation, or removal of the hip joint, and hemipelvectomy procedures are more common in younger clients than in older clients, who cannot easily handle the cumbersome prostheses required for ambulation. The higher the level of amputation, the more energy is required for ambulation. These higher-level procedures are typically done for cancer of the bone, osteomyelitis, or trauma. Hemicorporectomy (hemipelvectomy and translumbar amputation) is a rare radical procedure performed as a last resort for cancer.

UPPER EXTREMITY. Fewer than 10% of all amputations are upper extremity amputations. An amputation of any part of the upper extremity is generally more incapacitating than one of the leg. The arms and hands are necessary for activities of daily living (ADLs), such as feeding, bathing, dressing, and driving a car. As much length as possible is saved to maintain function. Early replacement with a prosthetic device is vital for the client with this type of amputation.

COMPLICATIONS OF AMPUTATIONS

The following are common complications of elective or traumatic amputations:

- Hemorrhage
- Infection
- Phantom limb pain
- Problems associated with immobility
- Neuroma
- Flexion contractures

HEMORRHAGE. When a person loses part or all of an extremity either by surgery or by trauma, major blood vessels are severed, which causes bleeding. If the bleeding is uncontrolled, the client is at risk for hypovolemic shock and possibly death.

INFECTION. As with any surgical procedure or trauma, infection can occur in the wound or the bone (osteomyelitis). The older adult who is debilitated and confused is at the greatest risk because excreta may soil the wound, or the client may remove the dressing and pick at the incision.

PHANTOM LIMB PAIN. **Phantom limb pain (PLP)** is a frequent complication of amputation. Most clients experience phantom limb sensation in the early postoperative period. Sensation is perceived in the phantom foot or hand and diminishes over time. When phantom limb sensation persists and is unpleasant or painful, it is referred to as PLP. PLP is more common in clients who have experienced chronic limb pain before surgery and rare in those who experience traumatic amputations.

No one theory explains or predicts PLP. Three theories are being researched:

- Peripheral nervous system theory
- Central nervous system theory
- Psychologic theory

The peripheral nervous system theory implies that sensations remain as a result of severing peripheral nerves during the amputation. The central nervous system theory states that PLP results from a loss of inhibitory signals that are usually generated through afferent impulses from the amputated limb. When many sensory fibers are destroyed by amputation, the loss of inhibitory influences allows repetitive neural activity, which results in pain. Neither of these physiologic theories completely explains PLP. Most likely, a psychologic component helps predict and explain this phenomenon. Stress, anxiety, and depression often worsen or trigger an episode of PLP but are not likely to be the causative factors.

When experiencing PLP, the client complains of pain in the removed body part, most often shortly after surgery. The pain is often described either as an intense burning or crushing sensation or as cramping. Some clients say they feel as if the removed part is in a distorted, uncomfortable position; they experience numbness and tingling (sometimes called phantom limb sensation), as well as pain.

Some clients report that the most distal area of the removed part feels as if it is retracted into the residual limb end. For most clients, the pain is triggered by touching the residual limb, by temperature or barometric pressure changes, by concurrent illness, by fatigue, or by emotional stress. Routine activities, such as urination, can trigger the pain in other clients. If pain is long-standing, especially if it existed before the amputation, any stimulus can cause it, including touching any part of the body.

PROBLEMS ASSOCIATED WITH IMMOBILITY. Because the client experiences reduced mobility as a result of surgery, the complications of atelectasis, pneumonia, thromboembolism, and skin breakdown can readily occur. These problems are discussed earlier under Complications of Fractures, p. 1127.

NEUROMA. Neuroma—a sensitive tumor consisting of nerve cells found at severed nerve endings—forms most often in amputations of the upper extremity but can occur anywhere.

FLEXION CONTRACTURES. Flexion contractures of the hip or knee are seen in clients with amputations of the lower extremity. This complication must be avoided so that the client can ambulate with a prosthesis.

Etiology

Most knowledge about amputations was obtained during World War II, when trauma often necessitated a loss of one or more body parts. Today, with highly sophisticated microsurgery for revascularization of tissues, amputations related to trauma are less likely to be needed. Limb salvage procedures, such as those described in Chapter 51 (under Surgical Management in the section on malignant bone tumors), have reduced the need for amputation.

Traumatic amputations most often result from accidents. A person may be cleaning lawn mower blades or a snow blower without disconnecting the machine. A motor vehicle or industrial machine accident may also cause an amputation.

CONSIDERATIONS FOR OLDER ADULTS

The primary indication for surgical amputation is *ischemia* from peripheral vascular disease in the older client (see Chapter 36). The rate of lower extremity amputation, for example, is much greater among clients with diabetes than among other clients because of peripheral neuropathy and peripheral vascular disease (Spollett, 1998). In addition, these older diabetic clients have visual, cardiac, and kidney problems. A client with an amputation of one leg because of poor circulation will often have an amputation of the other leg within 5 years. Older adults of advanced age may not be candidates for prostheses because of the energy required for ambulation. The more proximal the amputation in the lower extremity, the more energy required for ambulation.

Incidence/Prevalence

Surgical amputations are not as common as they were in the past, because the success rates of revascularization and limb salvage techniques have improved over the last 30 years. However, more than 100,000 amputations are performed yearly in the United States, about half of these in clients with coexisting diabetes.

The typical client undergoing the procedure is a middle-aged or older man with diabetes and a lengthy history of smoking. The client most likely has failed to care for his feet properly, which has resulted in a nonhealing, infected foot ulcer and possibly gangrene.

The second largest group with amputations consists of young men who experience motorcycle or other vehicular accidents or who are injured at work by industrial equipment. These men may either experience a traumatic amputation or undergo a surgical amputation because of a severe crushing injury and massive soft-tissue damage.

CULTURAL CONSIDERATIONS

The incidence of lower extremity amputations is greater in the African-American and Hispanic populations because the incidence of major diseases leading to amputation, such as diabetes and arteriosclerosis, is greater in this population. Limited access to care for these minority groups may also play a major role in limb loss (Spollett, 1998).

COLLABORATIVE MANAGEMENT

Assessment

PHYSICAL ASSESSMENT/CLINICAL MANIFESTATIONS

When the client has peripheral vascular disease, the nurse's primary concern preoperatively is to assess circulation in other parts of the body The nurse assesses skin color, temperature, sensation, and pulses in both affected and unaffected extremities. Capillary refill is evaluated by applying pressure to the nail bed and waiting for the brisk return of normal color. In the older adult, however, this test may be difficult to do because the nails may be thick and opaque. In this situation, the skin near the nail bed can be assessed (see Chart 52-3).

PSYCHOSOCIAL ASSESSMENT

People react differently to the loss of a body part. The nurse needs to be aware that an amputation of a portion of one finger can be traumatic to the client; therefore the loss must not be underestimated. The client undergoing an amputation faces a complete, permanent loss. The nurse assesses the client's psychologic preparation for a planned amputation and expects him or her to experience the grieving process. Adjustment to a traumatic, unexpected amputation is often more difficult than accepting a planned one. The young client may be bitter, hostile, and uncooperative. In addition to loss of a body part, the client may lose a job, the ability to participate in favorite recreational activities, or a social relationship if the other person cannot accept the body change. Chapter 9 discusses the nursing assessment for a client experiencing loss.

The client is faced with an altered self-concept. The physical alteration that results from an amputation affects body image and self-esteem. For example, a client may think that an intimate relationship with a mate is no longer possible. An older adult may feel a loss of independence. The nurse assesses the client's feelings about himself or herself to identify areas in which he or she needs emotional support.

The nurse tries to determine the client's willingness and motivation to withstand prolonged rehabilitation after the amputation. Asking questions about how the client has dealt with previous life crises can provide clues. The client's willingness to change careers or other activities is also determined. Adjustment to the amputation and rehabilitation is less difficult if the client is willing to make necessary changes.

In addition to assessing the client's psychosocial status, the nurse assesses the family's or significant others' reaction to the surgery. The family's response usually correlates directly with the client's progress during recovery and rehabilitation. The family can be expected to grieve for the loss and must be allowed to adjust to the change in the client.

The nurse also assesses the client's coping abilities and helps him or her to identify personal strengths and weaknesses. The nurse ascertains that the client's religious or spiritual beliefs have been determined, because certain groups require that the amputated body part be stored for later burial with the rest of the body or be buried now.

DIAGNOSTIC ASSESSMENT

Routine preoperative x-ray studies, such as a chest x-ray, are done as appropriate for any client undergoing surgery. The surgeon determines which tests are performed to assess for viability of the limb. A large number of noninvasive techniques are available to assist the physician in this evaluation. For complete accuracy, the health care provider does not rely on any single test.

One procedure is measurement of segmental limb blood pressures, which can also be used by the nurse at the bedside. In this test, an ankle-brachial index (ABI) is calculated by dividing ankle systolic pressure by brachial systolic pressure. A normal ABI is greater than or equal to 1.

Blood flow in an extremity can also be assessed by many other noninvasive tests, including Doppler ultrasonography, laser Doppler flowmetry, and transcutaneous oxygen pressure ($TcPO_2$). The ultrasonography measures the velocity of blood flow in the limb. The $TcPO_2$ measures oxygen pressure to indicate blood flow in the limb. Angiography is the most commonly used invasive method; however, it is not helpful in predicting healing of amputations. Transcutaneous oxygen pressure has proved reliable for predicting healing.

Interventions

Clients undergoing amputation today are not confined to a wheelchair. Advancements in the design of prosthetics have enabled clients to become independent in ambulation. Therefore complications from extended bedrest are not common, even for older adults.

ASSESSMENT OF TISSUE PERFUSION. The nurse's primary focus is to monitor for signs indicating that there is sufficient tissue perfusion but no hemorrhage. The skin flap at the end of the residual limb should be pink in a light-skinned person and not discolored (lighter or darker than other skin pigmentation) in a dark-skinned client. The area should be warm but not hot. The nurse assesses the closest proximal pulse for strength and compares it with that in the other extremity. If the client has bilateral vascular disease, however, comparison of limbs is not an accurate way of measuring blood flow.

MANAGEMENT OF PAIN. Phantom limb pain (PLP) must be distinguished from stump pain, since they are managed differently. Pain management related to stump pain is not unlike that for any client in pain (see Chapter 7). If the client complains of PLP, the nurse recognizes that the pain is real. It is not therapeutic for the nurse to remind the client that the limb cannot be hurting, because it is missing. To prevent increased pain, the nurse handles the residual limb carefully when assessing the site or changing the dressing.

DRUG THERAPY. Some studies have shown that opioids are not as effective for PLP as they are for residual limb pain. The health care provider prescribes medication on the basis of the type of PLP the client experiences. For instance, beta-blocking agents such as propranolol (Inderal, Apo-Propranolol✱, Detensol✱) are used for constant, dull burning. Anticonvulsants, such as phenytoin (Dilantin) and carbamazepine (Tegretol), may be used for knifelike pain; antispasmodics such as baclofen may be prescribed for muscle spasms or cramping.

COMPLEMENTARY AND ALTERNATIVE THERAPIES. More than 50 treatments for PLP have been used worldwide. Transcutaneous electrical nerve stimulation (TENS) has had the most consistent pain relief rates. Other treatment measures include the following:

- Ultrasound therapy
- Massage
- Exercises
- Biofeedback
- Distraction therapy
- Hypnosis
- Psychotherapy

PREVENTION OF INFECTION. The surgeon typically prescribes broad-spectrum prophylactic antibiotics for several days postoperatively. The initial pressure dressing and drains are usually removed by the surgeon 48 to 72 hours after surgery. The nurse:

- Inspects the wound site for signs of inflammation (e.g., redness and swelling)
- Monitors the healing process
- Records the characteristics of drainage, if present
- Changes the soft dressing every day until the sutures are removed

The below-the-knee limb may be casted in the operating room for protection, prevention of edema, and prevention of knee contractures. On the third postoperative day, a window is opened in the distal end of the cast to inspect the suture line.

PROMOTION OF AMBULATION. The nurse or health care provider consults with a physical therapist to initiate exercises as soon as possible after surgery. If the amputation is a planned one, the therapist often works with the client before surgery to start muscle strengthening exercises and to evaluate the need for aids, such as crutches. If the client can be instructed preoperatively in the use of these devices, learning how to ambulate after surgery is facilitated.

EXERCISE. For clients with above-knee amputations (AKAs) or below-knee amputations (BKAs), the nurse teaches range-of-motion (ROM) exercises for prevention of flexion contractures, particularly of the hip and knee. A trapeze and an overhead frame, as shown in Figure 52-12, aid in strengthening the upper extremities and allow the client to move independently in bed.

A firm mattress is essential for preventing contractures with a lower extremity amputation. The nurse assists the client into a prone position every 3 to 4 hours for 20- to 30-minute periods. This position may be uncomfortable initially, but it is necessary to prevent hip flexion contractures. The nurse instructs the prone client to pull the residual limb close to the other leg and contract the gluteal muscles of the buttocks. For BKAs, the nurse also teaches the client to push the residual limb down toward the bed while supporting it on a pillow. After the sutures are removed, the physical therapist may begin resistive exercises with a "sling-and-spring" apparatus, which can also be used at home.

Elevation of a lower leg residual limb on a pillow while the client is in a supine position is controversial. Some practitioners advocate avoiding this procedure at all times because it promotes hip or knee flexion contracture. Others allow ele-

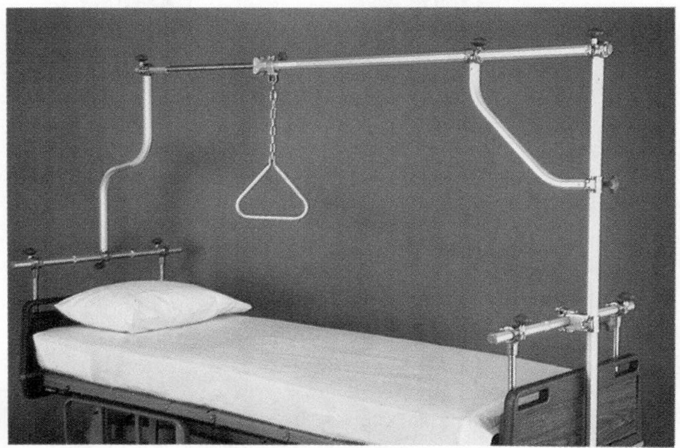

Figure 52-12 • The placement of an overhead frame and trapeze on a bed.

vation for the first 24 hours to reduce swelling and subsequent discomfort. The nurse inspects the residual limb daily to ensure that it lies completely flat on the bed.

PROSTHESES. For an elective amputation, the nurse arranges for the client to see a certified prosthetist-orthotist (CPO) so that planning can begin for the client's postoperative needs. Arrangements for replacing an upper extremity are especially important so that the client can provide self-care. Some clients are fitted with a temporary prosthesis at the time of surgery. Other clients, particularly older clients with vascular disease, are fitted after the residual limb has healed.

The client being fitted with a lower extremity prosthesis should bring a sturdy pair of shoes to the fitting. The prosthesis will be adjusted to that heel height.

PREPROSTHETIC CARE. Several devices help shape and shrink the residual limb in preparation for the prosthesis. Rigid, removable dressings are preferred because they decrease edema, protect and shape the limb, and allow easy access to the wound for inspection. The Jobst air splint, a plastic inflatable device, is sometimes used for this purpose. This device is usually inflated to 20 mm Hg for 22 out of every 24 hours. One of its disadvantages is air leakage.

Wrapping with elastic bandages can be effective in reducing edema, shrinking the limb, and holding the wound dressing in place. Most surgeons prefer elastic bandages over a shrinker sock, although it is easier for the client to apply a sock than to wrap elastic bandages.

For wrapping to be effective, the nurse reapplies the bandages every 4 to 6 hours or more often if they become loose. Figure-eight wrapping prevents restriction of blood flow. The nurse decreases the tightness of the bandages while wrapping in a distal-to-proximal direction. After wrapping, the nurse anchors the bandages to the most proximal joint, such as above the knee for BKAs (Figure 52-13).

PROSTHESIS APPLICATION. The design of and materials for prostheses have improved dramatically over the years. Computer-assisted design and manufacturing (CAD-CAM) is now available for a custom fit. One of the biggest developments in lower extremity prosthetics is the ankle-foot prosthesis. The Flex-Foot is used by more active amputees.

PROMOTION OF BODY IMAGE. The client often experiences feelings of inadequacy as a result of losing a body part, especially the older adult who was in poor health before surgery. If possible, the nurse arranges for the client to meet with a rehabilitated amputee. If the client is older, an older amputee is the ideal person with whom the client should interact.

Use of the word *stump* for referring to the remaining portion of the limb is controversial. Clients have reported feeling as if they were part of a tree when the term was used. However, some rehabilitation specialists who routinely work with amputees believe the term is appropriate because it forces the client to realize what has happened and enhances adjustment to the amputation. This discussion uses *residual limb* instead.

The nurse assesses the client's verbal and nonverbal references to the affected area. Some clients behave euphorically and seem to have accepted the loss. The nurse should not jump to the conclusion that acceptance has occurred. The client is asked to describe his or her feelings about changes in body image and self-esteem. The client may verbalize acceptance but refuse to look at the area during a dressing change.

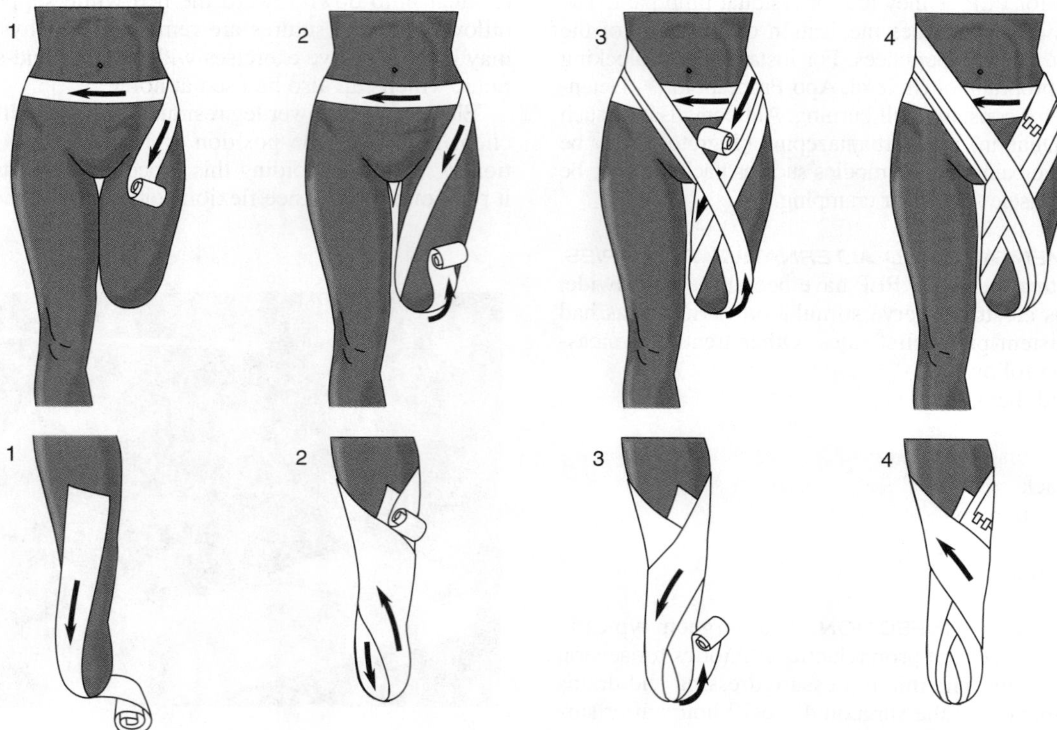

Figure 52-13 ● A common method of wrapping an amputation stump. *Top,* Wrapping for above-knee amputation. *Bottom,* Wrapping for below-knee amputation.

This inconsistent behavior is not unusual and should be noted by the nurse.

PROMOTION OF LIFESTYLE ADAPTATIONS. The client may believe that it will be impossible to return to a previous lifestyle, including intimate relationships, his or her job, and recreational activities. With advancements in prostheses, many clients can return to their jobs and other activities. Professional athletes who use prostheses are quite successful in sports. Clients with amputations ski, hike, bowl, and participate in other physically demanding activities. More than 20,000 amputees in the United States currently participate actively in sports; about a fourth of these individuals are engaged in organized competition.

If a job or career change is necessary, the nurse consults with a social worker for evaluation of the client's other skills that could be used in another capacity. A supportive family or significant other is important for the client's adjustment to this change. The client may also think that an intimate relationship is no longer possible because of physical changes. The nurse works with the sexual partner to help in the client's adjustment to the amputation. Professional assistance from a sex counselor or psychologist may be needed.

The nurse helps the client to set realistic goals and to take one day at a time. He or she is helped to recognize personal strengths, which are emphasized and taken into account in setting goals. If the goals are not realistic, frustration and disappointment may dampen the client's motivation during rehabilitation. Basic principles of rehabilitation are discussed in Chapter 10.

Community-Based Care

The client is discharged directly to home or to a rehabilitation facility, depending on the extent of the amputation. In the few cases in which rehabilitation is not feasible (e.g., for a debilitated, confused older client), he or she may be discharged to a long-term care facility. The case manager or discharge planner coordinates this transfer.

HEALTH TEACHING

After the sutures are removed (several weeks after surgery), the client begins residual limb care. The home care nurse teaches the client how to care for the residual limb and how to care for the prosthesis if it is available. The limb should be rewrapped three times a day with an elastic bandage applied in a figure-eight manner (see Figure 52-13) by the client or family member. After the residual limb is healed, it is cleaned each day with the rest of the body during bathing with soap and water, and it is inspected for signs of inflammation or skin breakdown.

Prostheses require special care for ensuring their reliability and proper function, and the prosthetist plays an important role in the rehabilitation team effort. Prostheses are custom made, taking into account the client's level of amputation, lifestyle, and occupation. Proper teaching regarding correct cleansing of the socket and inserts, wearing the correct liners, assessing shoe wear, and a schedule of follow-up care is essential before discharge.

A client who seemed to adjust to the amputation during hospitalization may realize that it is difficult to cope with the loss after discharge from the hospital. The nurse in the hospital setting should tell the client that this can happen. During the hospital stay, the nurse helps the client to identify strong support systems on which he or she can rely after discharge. The home care or rehabilitation nurse reinforces this supporting information.

HOME CARE MANAGEMENT

The client with a lower extremity amputation needs to have enough room at home to maneuver a wheelchair if the leg prosthesis is not yet available. He or she must be able to use toileting facilities and have access to areas necessary for self-care, such as the kitchen. Structural changes may be required before the client goes home.

HEALTH CARE RESOURCES

For the older adult or for the client with an extensive amputation, such as a hemipelvectomy, the case manager or discharge planner arranges for follow-up care in the home by a home care nurse (Chart 52-7). Physical therapy may continue in the home or on an ambulatory care basis.

The client with an upper extremity amputation may need occupational therapy to relearn activities of daily living (ADLs). The nurse or case manager also makes arrangements for vocational or family counseling, as needed. Some clients are discharged to a rehabilitation facility for 2 to 3 weeks for these services. Chapter 10 describes the rehabilitation phase of health care in detail. The nurse teaches the client to explore support groups for amputees that may be available in the client's community.

CRUSH SYNDROME

When multiple compartments in the leg or arm are injured, crush syndrome (CS) can occur. CS is a potentially life-threatening, systemic complication after a severe crush injury. Its pathophysiologic mechanism is similar to that of acute compartment syndrome (see p. 1127).

Specific causes of CS include the following:

- Prolonged use of a pneumatic antishock garment (PASG) or military antishock trousers (MAST) (For this reason, these devices are seldom used today.)
- Wringer-type injuries
- Natural disasters, such as earthquakes
- Work-related injuries, such as being trapped under heavy equipment or material

CHART 52-7

FOCUSED ASSESSMENT *of*
The Client with a Lower Extremity Amputation in the Home

Assess the residual limb for:
- Adequate circulation
- Infection
- Healing
- Flexion contracture
- Dressing/elastic wrap

Assess the client's ability to perform activities of daily living (ADLs) in the home.
Evaluate the client's ability to use ambulatory aids and care for the prosthetic device (if available).
Assess the client's nutritional status.
Assess the client's ability to cope with body image change.

- Drug/alcohol overdose, when one or more limbs may be compressed by body weight for a prolonged time

Regardless of the cause, CS is characterized by the following:

- Acute compartment syndrome
- Hypovolemia
- Hyperkalemia
- Rhabdomyolysis (myoglobulin release from skeletal muscle into the bloodstream)
- Acute tubular necrosis (ATN) resulting from hypovolemia and rhabdomyolysis

Nursing assessments include signs and symptoms of hypovolemia, hyperkalemia, and compartment syndrome. Treatments focus on preventing acute tubular necrosis secondary to myoglobin release and cardiac dysrhythmias related to hyperkalemia. Adequate IV fluids, diuretics, and low-dose dopamine to enhance renal perfusion may be ordered. An output of 100 to 200 ml/hr is the goal. Sodium bicarbonate is given to treat acidosis. Kayexalate may reduce serum potassium adequately, but hemodialysis may be required if potassium levels remain high or renal failure occurs.

COMPLEX REGIONAL PAIN SYNDROME

Complex regional pain syndrome (CRPS) (less commonly called **reflex sympathetic dystrophy syndrome [RSDS]**) is a poorly understood complex disorder that includes pain, trophic changes, autonomic dysfunction, and motor impairment (most notably muscle paresis). It is probably caused by an abnormally hyperactive sympathetic nervous system. It most often results from traumatic injury and commonly occurs in the feet and hands (Aprile, 1998).

The syndrome tends to progress through three classic stages. In stage 1, which lasts 1 to 3 months, the client complains of locally severe, burning pain; edema; vasospasm; and muscle spasm. Over the next 3 months, clients in stage 2 have more severe, diffuse pain and edema, muscle atrophy, and spotty osteoporosis, as shown on x-ray examination. In stage 3, the final stage, the client presents with marked muscle atrophy, intractable (unrelenting) pain, severely limited mobility of the affected area, contractures, and marked, diffuse osteoporosis. Timing of diagnosis is important, since the syndrome is more difficult to treat when diagnosed in the later stages.

The first priority of management is pain relief. Nurses play an important role in pain management, which includes drug therapy and an array of nonpharmacologic modalities. Chapter 7 discusses pain management in detail.

In collaboration with the physical and occupational therapist, the nurse also assists in maintaining adequate range of motion (ROM). The skin of a client with CRPS tends to alternate between warm, swollen, and red to cool, clammy, and bluish. Skin care needs to be gentle, with minimal stimulation.

The nurse assists the client in coping with CRPS. Psychotherapy may be indicated. The RSDS Association is available to help clients organize or locate support groups and other resources for clients with this syndrome.

SPORTS-RELATED INJURIES

In addition to the bone and muscle problems already discussed, trauma can cause cartilage, ligament, and tendon injury. Many musculoskeletal injuries are the result of participation in sports or other strenuous physical activities. These injuries have become so common that large metropolitan hospitals have sports medicine clinics and physicians who specialize in this field.

Although the specific types of injury are numerous, this chapter includes only the most common ones seen by the nurse in a hospital or ambulatory care setting. The principles of injury to one part of the body are analogous to those of similar injuries in other parts. For example, a tendon rupture in a knee is cared for in the same manner as a tendon rupture in the wrist. Chart 52-8 lists general emergency measures for sports-related injuries.

Because the knee is most often injured, it is discussed as a typical example of other areas of the body. Trauma to the knee results in internal derangement, a broad term for disturbances of an injured knee joint. When surgery is required to resolve the problem, most surgeons prefer to perform the procedure through an arthroscope when possible. A general description of arthroscopy is presented in Chapter 50.

Knee Injuries: Meniscus

OVERVIEW

There are two semilunar cartilaginous structures, or menisci, in the knee joint: the medial meniscus and the lateral meniscus. These pads act as shock absorbers, but they can tear. Tearing is usually a result of twisting the leg when the knee is flexed and the foot is placed firmly on the ground. The medial meniscus is much more likely to tear than the lateral meniscus because it is less mobile. Internal rotation causes a tear in the medial meniscus; external rotation causes a tear in the lateral meniscus.

Tears can be anterior or posterior, longitudinal or transverse. In the medial meniscus, a longitudinal tear, or "bucket handle" injury, often causes the knee to lock; that is, the torn cartilage jams between the femur and the tibia and prevents extension of the knee. Surgery is often required for this type of injury. In transverse tears, the knee does not lock, and surgery may not be required.

COLLABORATIVE MANAGEMENT

The client with a torn meniscus typically has pain, swelling, and tenderness in the knee. A clicking or snapping sound can often be heard when the knee is moved.

A common diagnostic technique is the **McMurray test.** The examiner flexes and rotates the knee and then presses on

CHART 52-8

BEST PRACTICE *for*
Emergency Care of Sports-Related Injuries

- Do not move the victim until spinal cord injury is ascertained (see Chapter 45 for assessment of spinal cord injury).
- Immobilize the injured part; immobilize the joint above and below the injury by applying a splint.
- Apply ice intermittently for the first 24-48 hours (heat may be used thereafter).
- Elevate the affected limb to decrease swelling.
- Always assume the area is fractured until x-ray studies are done.
- Assess neurovascular status in the area distal to the injury.

the medial aspect while slowly extending the leg. The test result is positive if clicking is palpated or heard. A negative finding, however, does not rule out a tear.

For a locked knee, the treatment may be manipulation followed by casting for 3 to 6 weeks. If the problem recurs, a partial or total **meniscectomy** is performed. An open meniscectomy requires a surgical incision for removal of all or part of the meniscus and is rarely performed. Most surgeons prefer to remove only the affected portion, which can be accomplished through an arthroscope during a closed meniscectomy as a same-day surgical procedure. As described in Chapter 50, an arthroscope is a metal tubular instrument used for examination or surgery of joints. One or more small incisions (less than ¼ inch [0.6 cm] long) are made in the knee for insertion of the arthroscope. The surgeon threads a cutting device through the arthroscope for removal of the torn cartilage while the knee is irrigated with saline or lactated Ringer's solution, depending on the type of equipment used. The surgeon may use a laser during the procedure, depending on the type and severity of the injury. A bulky pressure dressing is applied after the procedure, and the affected leg is wrapped in elastic bandages.

As for any postoperative client, the nurse checks the surgical dressing for bleeding and monitors vital signs after the client is readmitted to the unit. The nurse performs circulation checks, as outlined in Chart 52-3, usually every hour for the first few hours and then every 4 hours.

The client begins leg exercises immediately after surgery to strengthen the leg, prevent thrombophlebitis, and reduce swelling. Quadriceps setting, in which the client straightens the leg while pushing the knee against the bed, is done in sets of 10 or more. Straight-leg raises are also performed as soon as the client awakens from anesthesia. Range-of-motion (ROM) exercises are usually not started for several days.

To prevent the client from bending the affected knee, the physician may order a knee immobilizer, such as the one shown in Figure 52-14. The nurse elevates the leg on one or two pillows according to the physician's preference and applies ice to reduce postoperative swelling. Full weight bearing is restricted for several weeks, depending on the amount of cartilage removed. The client is usually discharged from the hospital with crutches in less than 23 hours.

Knee Injuries: Ligaments

OVERVIEW

The cruciate and collateral ligaments in the knee are predisposed to injury, often from sports or vehicular accidents. The anterior cruciate ligament (ACL) is the most commonly torn ligament in the knee. Athletes often experience ACL injuries during skiing or gymnastics.

When the ACL is torn, the person feels a snap; the knee gives way because of ACL laxity. Within hours, the knee is swollen, stiff, and painful.

COLLABORATIVE MANAGEMENT

Physical examination by the health care provider shows positive ligamentous laxity. The diagnosis of ACL deficiency is confirmed by x-ray studies, magnetic resonance imaging (MRI), or assessment with an arthrometer (an instrument for measuring the amount of tibial displacement).

Treatment may be nonsurgical or surgical, depending on the severity of the injury and the anticipated activity of the client. Exercises, bracing, and limits on activities while the ligament heals may be sufficient. If medical management is not effective, surgery may be needed.

The surgeon repairs the tear by reattaching the torn portions of the ligament, and the leg is placed in a cast. If the ligament cannot be repaired, reconstructive surgery may be performed with the use of autologous grafts. Since the early 1980s, the Food and Drug Administration (FDA) has approved several artificial knee ligaments. The Gore-Tex ligament is a permanent implant. A ligament augmentation device is used temporarily while the autograft heals. Both of these materials can be implanted through an arthroscope.

Complete healing of knee ligaments after surgery can take 6 to 9 months or longer. Nursing management is similar to the care of any client in a cast, which is described earlier in this chapter under Cast Care, p. 1134.

Tendon Ruptures

Rupture of the Achilles tendon is common in adults who participate in strenuous sports. In the older adult, quadriceps tendon rupture may occur from a fall down several steps. For severe damage, the tendon is surgically repaired and the leg is immobilized in a cast for 6 to 8 weeks. If the tendon is beyond repair, a tendon transplant (also known as tendon reconstruction) is performed. A tendon is removed from one part of the body and transplanted to the affected area. The nursing care for these clients is similar to that discussed earlier for a client with a cast (see Cast Care, p. 1134).

Dislocations and Subluxations

Dislocation of a joint occurs when the articulating surfaces are no longer in proximity. If the dislocation is not complete,

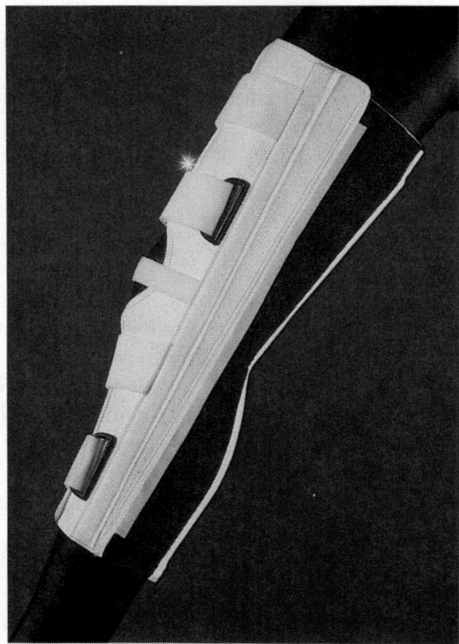

Figure 52-14 ● A knee immobilizer. (Courtesy Zimmer, Inc., Warsaw, IN.)

the joint is partially dislocated, or subluxed. Dislocation can occur in any diarthrodial (synovial) joint but is common in the shoulder, hip, knee, and fingers. This injury is most often the result of trauma but can be congenital or pathologic (resulting from joint disease, such as arthritis).

The typical manifestations of dislocation are as follows:

- Pain
- Immobility
- Alteration in contour of the joint
- Deviation in length of the extremity
- Rotation of the extremity

The health care provider performs a closed manipulation, or reduction, of the joint and forces it back into its original position while the client is anesthetized or under conscious sedation. The joint is immobilized by a cast or immobilizer until healing occurs.

Recurrent dislocations are common in the knee and shoulder. For this problem, the joint is fixed with wires to prevent further displacement; a cast, splint, or traction is applied for 3 to 6 weeks.

Strains

A strain is excessive stretching of a muscle or tendon when it is weak or unstable. Strains are sometimes referred to as muscle pulls. Falls, lifting of heavy items, and exercise often cause this injury.

Strains are classified according to their severity:

- A first-degree (mild) strain causes mild inflammation but little bleeding. Swelling, ecchymosis, and tenderness are usually present.
- A second-degree (moderate) strain involves tearing of the muscle or tendon fibers without complete disruption. Muscle function may be impaired.
- A third-degree (severe) strain involves a ruptured muscle or tendon with separation of muscle from muscle, tendon from muscle, or tendon from bone. Severe pain and disability result from severe strains.

Management usually involves cold and heat applications, exercise, and activity limitations. The health care provider may prescribe anti-inflammatory drugs to decrease inflammation and pain. Muscle relaxants may also be used. In third-degree strains, surgical repair of the ruptured muscle or tendon may be necessary.

Sprains

A sprain is excessive stretching of a ligament. Twisting motions from a fall or sports activity typically precipitate the injury. Sprains are classified according to severity:

- A first-degree (mild) sprain involves tearing of a few fibers of a ligament. Function of the joint is not impaired.
- In a second-degree (moderate) sprain, more fibers are torn, but stability of the joint remains intact.
- A third-degree (severe) sprain causes marked instability of the joint.

Pain and swelling characterize ligament injuries. The treatment for mild (first-degree) sprains is minimal:

- Rest
- Use of ice for the first 24 to 48 hours
- Application of a compression bandage for a few days to reduce swelling and provide joint support
- Elevation

Second-degree sprains require immobilization (elastic bandage and Air Stirrup ankle brace, splint, or cast) and partial weight bearing while the tear heals. For severe ligament damage (third-degree sprain), immobilization for 4 to 6 weeks is necessary. Surgery may be recommended, particularly for chronic instability, as discussed earlier under Knee Injuries: Ligaments, p. 1153.

For more specific client education, refer to the Clinical Pathway on p. 1833.

Rotator Cuff Injuries

The musculotendinous, or rotator, cuff of the shoulder functions to stabilize the head of the humerus in the glenoid cavity during shoulder abduction. The rotator cuff typically undergoes degenerative changes as one gets older. Young adults usually sustain a tear of the cuff by substantial trauma, such as may occur during a fall, while throwing a ball, or with heavy lifting. Older adults tend to have small tears related to aging, repetitive motions, or falls.

Clients with a torn rotator cuff have shoulder pain and cannot initiate or maintain abduction of the arm at the shoulder. When the arm is abducted, the client usually drops the arm because abduction cannot be maintained (drop arm test).

The health care provider usually treats the client conservatively with nonsteroidal anti-inflammatory drugs (NSAIDs), physical therapy, sling support, and ice/heat applications while the tear heals.

For clients who do not respond to conservative treatment or for those who have a complete tear, the surgeon repairs the cuff. After surgery, the affected arm is usually immobilized in a sling for several weeks. Pendulum exercises are started on the third or fourth postoperative day and progress to active exercises in about 2 weeks. If the surgery is extensive, the client's arm may be immobilized for a longer time before exercises begin.

ONLINE RESOURCES

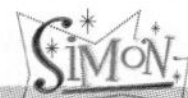

For suggested readings and Internet resources, go to http://www.wbsaunders.com/SIMON/Iggy/.

SELECTED BIBLIOGRAPHY

Aprile, A.E. (1998). Complex regional pain syndrome. *Journal of the American Association of Nurse Anesthetists, 65*(6), 557-560.

Boulanger, B.R., Rozycki, G.S., & Rodriquez, A. (1999). Sonographic assessment of traumatic injury. *Surgical Clinics of North America, 79*(6), 1297-1316.

Browner, B.D., Alberta, F.G., & Mastrella, D.J. (1999). A new era in orthopedic trauma care. *Surgical Clinics of North America, 79*(6), 1431-1448.

Byrne, T. (1999). The set-up and care of a patient in Buck's traction. *Orthopaedic Nursing, 18*(2), 79-83.

Childs, S.G. (Ed.). (1999). *The upper extremity: Traumatic injuries and conditions.* Pitman, NJ: National Association of Orthopaedic Nurses.

Childs, S.G., & Holmes, S.B. (1998). *Guidelines for orthopaedic nursing: Adult trauma.* Pitman, NJ: National Association of Orthopaedic Nurses.

Church, V. (2000). Staying on guard for DVT and PE. *Nursing2000, 30*(2), 35-42.

Hager, C.A., & Brncick, N. (1998). Fat embolism syndrome. *Orthopaedic Nursing, 17*(2), 41-46, 58.

Hoover, T.J., & Seifert, J.A. (2000). Soft tissue complications of orthopedic emergencies. *Emergency Medicine Clinics of North America, 18*(1), 115-139.

Lappe, J.M. (1998). Prevention of hip fractures: A nursing imperative. *Orthopaedic Nursing, 17*(3), 15-26.

Ludwick, R., Dieckman, B., & Snelson, C.M. (1999). Assessment of geriatric orthopaedic trauma. *Orthopaedic Nursing, 18*(6), 13-20.

Maher, A.B. (2001). Trauma. In D.C. Schoen (Ed.), *Core curriculum for orthopaedic nursing* (4th ed.) Pitman, NJ: National Association of Orthopaedic Nurses.

Maher, A.B., Salmond, S.W., & Pellino, T.A. (Eds.). (1998). *Orthopaedic nursing.* Philadelphia: W.B. Saunders.

McCann, S., & Gruen, G. (1997). Fracture blisters: A review of the literature. *Orthopaedic Nursing, 16*(2), 17-23.

Plociak, B.J., Lato, A., & Palumbo, M. (1999). Case study: Fractured ankle. *Orthopaedic Nursing, 18*(4), 21-26.

Roberts, D. (1999). Introduction to bone: Structure and function, fractures, and osteoporosis. In C.M. Ceccio, J.A. Deuschle, D.R. Eckhouse-Ekeberg (Eds.), *An introduction to orthopaedic nursing* (2nd ed., pp. 3-16). Pitman, NJ: National Association of Orthopaedic Nurses.

Rudman, N., & McIlmail, D. (2000). Emergency department evaluation and treatment of hip and thigh injuries. *Emergency Medicine Clinics of North America, 18*(1), 29-66.

Spollett, G.R. (1998). Preventing amputations in the diabetic population. *Nursing Clinics of North America, 33*(4), 629-641.

Sprague, J. (1998). Cast syndrome: The superior mesenteric artery syndrome. *Orthopaedic Nursing, 17*(4), 12-15.

Taggart, H. (1999). Caring for the elderly hip fracture patient. In C.M. Ceccio, J.A. Deuschle, D.R. Eckhouse-Ekeberg (Eds.), *An introduction to orthopaedic nursing* (2nd ed., pp. 113-122). Pitman, NJ: National Association of Orthopaedic Nurses.

Turner, L.W., Faile, P.A., & Tomlinson, R., Jr. (1999). Osteoporosis diagnosis and fracture. *Orthopaedic Nursing, 18*(5), 21-27.

Williamson, V.C. (Ed.). (1998). *Management of lower extremity fractures.* Pitman, NJ: National Association of Orthopaedic Nurses.

UNIT

12

PROBLEMS OF DIGESTION, NUTRITION, AND ELIMINATION

Management of Clients with Problems of the Gastrointestinal System

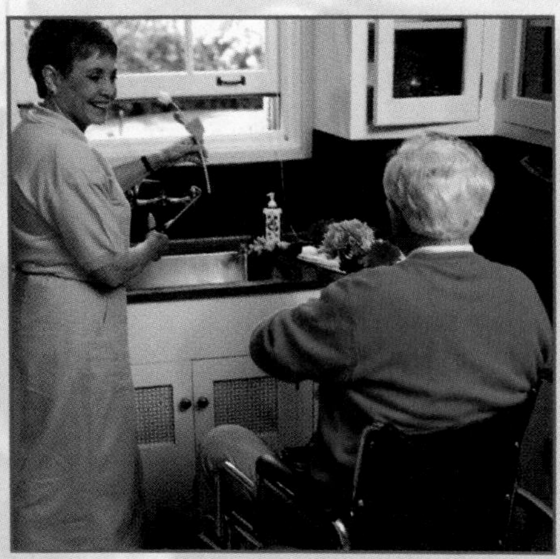

Problems of Digestion, Nutrition, and Elimination: GI System ■ Core Concepts Grid

Anatomy	Physiology	Pathophysiology	History	Physical Exam	Diagnostic Tests	Interventions	Pharmacology
• **Oropharynx** • **Esophagus** • **Stomach** • **Small intestine** • **Large intestine** • **Liver** • **Gallbladder** • **Pancreas** • **Rectum** • **Anus**	• **Absorption** • **Specialized secretions** • **Digestion** Hydrochloric acid Lipase Amylase • **Phagocytosis** • **Coagulation** • **Synthesis of** Proteins Carbohydrates Fats Vitamins • **Detoxification**	• **Inflammation** • **Infection** • **Obstruction** • **Hemorrhage** • **Perforation** • **Dumping syndrome** • **Erosion** • **Ascites**	• **Client history of** Past problems Pain • **Family history of digestive system problems** • **Social history** Alcohol Drugs Stress management Occupation Age Race Gender • **Bowel habits** • **Diet**	• **Mouth** • **Skin** Striae Cullen's sign Grey-Turner's sign Color • **Peristalsis** • **Bowel sounds** • **Bruits** • **Tympany** • **Masses** • **Abdominal distention** • **Swallowing** • **Intake** • **Vital signs**	• **Upper/lower GI series** • **Endoscopy** • **Esophagastroduodenoscopy (EGD)** • **Endoscopic retrograde cholangiopancreatography (ERCP)** • **Ultrasonography** • **CAT scan** • **Liver biopsy** • **Gastric analysis** • **Fecal analysis** • **Serum bilirubin** • **Aspartate aminotransferase (AST)** • **Alanine aminotransferase (ALT)** • **Lactate dehydrogenase (LDH)** • **Amylase** • **Lipase** • **Culture *Helicobacter pylori***	• **Therapeutic diets** • **Saline lavage** • **Sclerotherapy** • **Tamponade** • **Extracorporeal shock wave lithotripsy (ESWL)** • **Rest** • **Tube** Blakemore Nasogastric Nasoenteric Gastrostomy • **Ostomies** Colostomy Ileostomy • **Postoperative care** • **Rest** • **Fluid replacement** • **Blood transfusion** • **Health teaching**	• **Antacids** • **Histamine blockers** • **Vasocontrictors** • **Corticosteroids** • **Anticholinergics** • **Chenodeoxycholic acid** • **Urodeoxycholic acid** • **Immune serum globulin** • **Hepatitis A vaccine (HAV)** • **Hepatitis B vaccine (HBV)** • **Bowel stimulants** • **Antidiarrheals** • **Antibiotics** • **Lactulose** • **Chemotherapeutic agents**

CHAPTER 53

Assessment of the Gastrointestinal System

CONSTANCE VISOVSKY

Learning Objectives

After studying this chapter, you should be able to:

1. Recall the anatomy and physiology of the gastrointestinal (GI) system.
2. Perform a GI assessment using Gordon's Functional Health Patterns.
3. Evaluate important assessment findings in a client with a GI health problem.
4. Explain the use of laboratory testing for a client with a GI health problem.
5. Identify the use of radiography in diagnosing GI health problems.
6. Plan follow-up care for clients having endoscopic procedures.

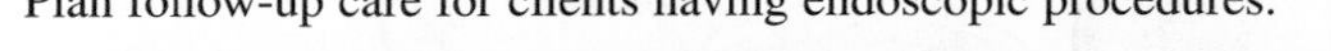

Go to http://www.wbsaunders.com/SIMON/Iggy/ for self-assessment questions related to these Learning Objectives.

The gastrointestinal (GI) system includes the GI tract, consisting of the mouth, esophagus, stomach, small and large intestines, and rectum. The salivary glands, liver, gallbladder, and pancreas secrete substances into the GI tract by connecting ducts (Figure 53-1). The adult GI tract is approximately 15 feet long. The main function of the GI tract, with the aid of organs such as the pancreas and the liver, is the digestion of food. Nutritional assessment is discussed in Chapter 61. The GI tract is susceptible to many pathologic conditions, including structural problems, impairments in motility, infection, and cancer.

ANATOMY AND PHYSIOLOGY REVIEW

Overview of the Gastrointestinal Tract

Structure

The GI tract consists of a hollow tube—the lumen—surrounded by a layer of surface and epithelial cells called the mucosa. The mucosa includes a thin layer of smooth muscle and some exocrine gland cells. This layer is surrounded by the submucosa, which is made up of connective tissue. The outermost layer is composed of both circular and longitudinal smooth muscles, which work to keep contents moving through the tract. Although the GI tract is continuous from the mouth to the anus, it is divided into specialized regions. The mouth, pharynx, esophagus, stomach, and small and large intestines each perform a specific function. In addition, the secretions of the salivary, gastric, and intestinal glands; liver; and pancreas empty into the GI tract to aid digestion.

Function

The functions of the GI tract include secretion, digestion, absorption, and motility. Food and fluids are ingested, swallowed, and propelled along the lumen to be eliminated. Contractions of the smooth muscles in the GI tract move food from the mouth to the anus. Before food can be absorbed, it must be dissolved and broken down. Digestion is a mechanical and chemical process whereby complex foodstuffs are broken down into simpler forms that can be used by the body. During digestion, the stomach secretes hydrochloric acid, the liver secretes bile, and digestive enzymes are released, aiding in food breakdown. After the digestive process is complete, absorption takes place. Absorption is carried out as the nutrients produced by digestion move from the lumen of the GI tract into the body's circulatory system for uptake by individual cells (Figure 53-2).

Nerve Supply

Innervation of the GI tract occurs in two ways. First, intrinsic contractile stimulation is provided by two internal nerve plexuses: the *myenteric* plexus (an outer plexus found in the longitudinal and circular smooth muscle) and the *submucosal* plexus (an inner nerve plexus in the submucosa). These nerve plexuses connect with each other along the entire length of the GI tract to maintain the tone of the smooth muscle and to stimulate movements.

The second type of innervation is provided by the autonomic nervous system, which connects with nerve fibers from the intrinsic nerve plexuses. Parasympathetic stimulation is provided primarily by the vagus nerve (cranial nerve X), which innervates the esophagus, the stomach, and to a lesser extent, the small intestine, the gallbladder, and part of the large intestine. This stimulation causes increased motor and secretory activity and relaxation of sphincters. Sympathetic stimulation via the thoracic and lumbar splanchnic nerves is provided to all parts of the GI tract; it slows movement, inhibits secretions, and contracts sphincters.

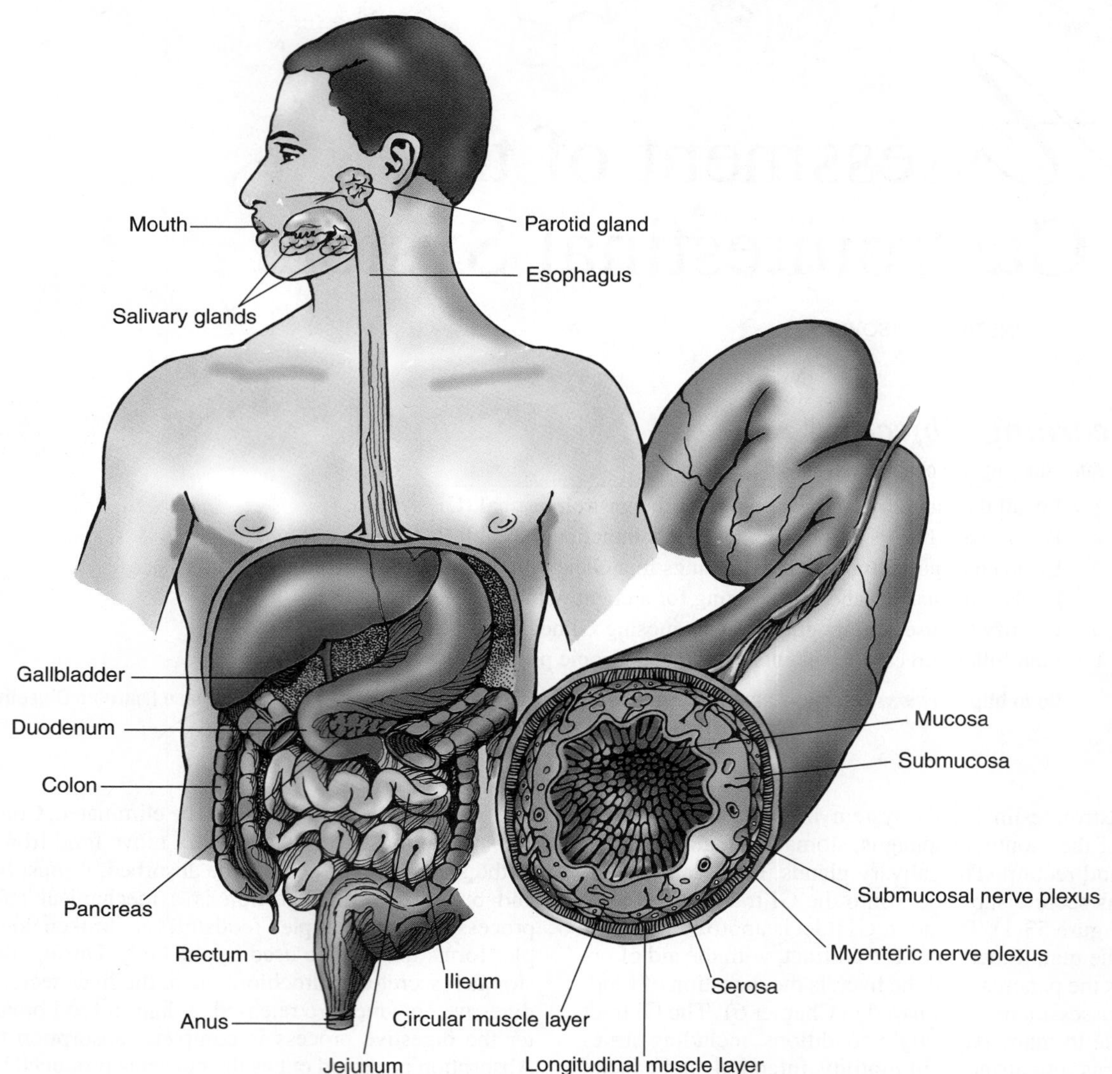

Figure 53-1 ● The gastrointestinal system (GI tract) can be thought of as a tube (with accessory structures) extending from the mouth to the anus for a 25-foot length. The structure of this tube (shown enlarged) is basically the same throughout its length.

Blood Supply

The blood supply to the GI tract originates from the aorta and branches to the many arteries throughout the length of the tract: the celiac, gastric, splenic, common hepatic, internal and external iliac, and superior and inferior mesenteric arteries. The venous system that carries absorbed nutrients away from the lumen of the GI tract consists of the gastric vein, the splenic vein, and other veins that drain into the portal vein of the liver. This blood circulates through the liver to the hepatic vein and returns to the heart via the inferior vena cava.

Oral Cavity

Structure

The oral cavity includes the buccal mucosa, lips, tongue, hard palate, soft palate, teeth, and salivary glands. The buccal mucosa is the mucous membrane lining the inside of the oral cavity. The lips are external to the oral cavity and are pink-red. The tongue lies on the floor of the mouth, anchored to the hyoid bone. The tongue is involved in speech, taste, and **mastication** (chewing). The mucous membrane covering the tongue consists of small projections, called papillae, that house the taste buds and provide a roughened surface, permitting the movement of food in the mouth during chewing. The hard palate and the soft palate together form the roof of the mouth.

Adults have 32 permanent teeth: 16 in each arch. The teeth are composed of a hard, calcified substance called dentin, which is then covered by enamel. There are four types of teeth: incisors, canines, premolars, and molars. The oral cavity contains three major salivary glands: the parotid glands, the submandibular glands, and the sublingual glands. These glands produce 1 to 1.5 L of saliva per day to assist in digestion by moistening food, thus enabling it to be formed into a bolus for swallowing.

The pharynx (throat) extends from the soft palate to the esophagus. It is lined with mucous membrane and contains three pairs of organs: the adenoids, the lingual tonsils (at the base of the tongue), and the tonsils.

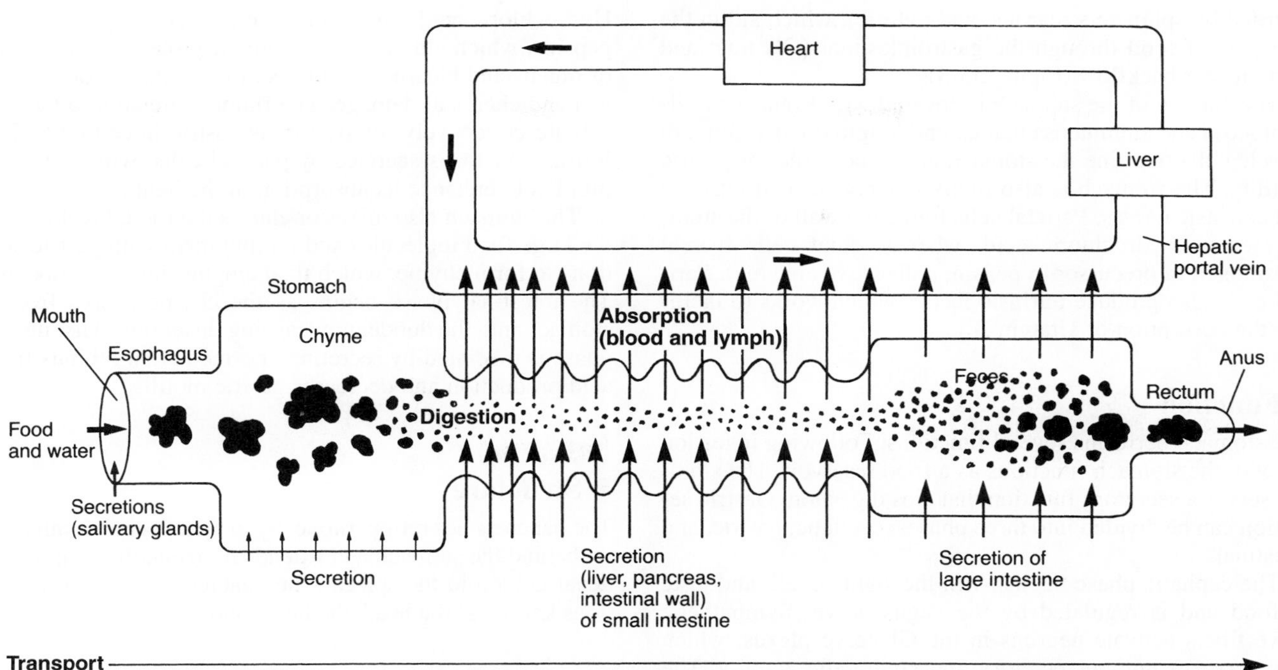

Figure 53-2 ● A conceptual view of the gastrointestinal system. (From Vander, A.J., Sherman, J.H., & Luciano, D.S. [1990]. *Human physiology* [5th ed.]. New York: McGraw-Hill. Used with permission.)

Function

The different types of teeth function to prepare food for digestion by cutting, tearing, crushing, or grinding the food. Swallowing begins after food is taken into the mouth and chewed. Saliva is secreted in response to the presence of food in the mouth and begins to soften the food. Saliva contains mucin and an enzyme, salivary amylase (also known as ptyalin), which begins the breakdown of carbohydrates.

The four phases of swallowing are oral preparatory, oral, pharyngeal, and esophageal. The *oral preparatory* phase begins with the intake of food into the mouth. The mandible, teeth, and tongue work to soften the food and form a bolus. The tongue acts to move the bolus toward the back of the mouth. The *oral* phase begins with the movement of the bolus toward the back of the mouth. The tongue presses the bolus against the hard palate, toward the anterior faucial arches, triggering the swallowing reflex.

The *pharyngeal* phase begins as the swallowing reflex is triggered. As the bolus is forced into the pharynx, the soft palate elevates, which seals the nasal cavity. At this time, the swallowing reflex also inhibits respiration and allows the opening of the esophagus so that the food can enter. The oral and pharyngeal phases are extremely rapid, usually taking less than 1 second.

The *esophageal* phase begins when the bolus enters the esophagus at the cricopharyngeal juncture. A peristaltic wave passes the food to the stomach, which takes about 9 seconds.

Esophagus

Structure

The esophagus is a muscular canal approximately 10 inches (24 cm) long; it extends from the pharynx to the stomach and passes through the hiatus in the center of the diaphragm. The wall of the esophagus consists of mucosa, submucosa, and muscularis propria. The mucosal layer is composed of squamous epithelial cells. The submucosa is composed of loose connective tissue containing blood vessels, lymphatics, and nerve fibers. The muscularis propria consists of smooth and striated muscle fibers. The portion of the esophagus proximal to the gastroesophageal junction is referred to as the lower esophageal sphincter (LES).

Function

The primary function of the esophagus is to propel food and fluids from the pharynx to the stomach and to prevent reflux of gastric contents into the esophagus. The propulsive function is the result of coordinated contractions of the muscular layers of the esophagus. The esophageal walls secrete mucus to lubricate the food and aid in the transport of the bolus to the stomach. As peristalsis pushes the bolus along the esophagus, the cardiac sphincter relaxes to allow the bolus to enter the stomach. The activity of the LES is regulated by smooth muscle, as well as neural and hormonal influences.

Stomach

Structure

The stomach is a glandular digestive and endocrine organ located in the midline and left upper quadrant (LUQ) of the abdomen. The stomach has four anatomic regions. The *cardia* is the narrow portion of the stomach that is distal to the gastroesophageal junction. The *fundus* is the area to the left above the gastroesophageal junction. The main area of the stomach is referred to as the *body* or *corpus.* The *antrum* is the distal portion of the stomach and is separated from the duodenum by the pyloric sphincter. Both ends of the stomach are guarded by sphincters (cardiac and pyloric), which aid in the transport of food through the gastrointestinal (GI) tract and also prevent backflow (Figure 53-3).

The surface of the stomach is covered with *rugae,* or folds of mucosa and submucosa that extend longitudinally. Smooth muscle cells that line the stomach are responsible for gastric motility. The stomach is also richly innervated with intrinsic and extrinsic nerves. Parietal cells lining the wall of the stomach secrete hydrochloric acid, whereas chief cells secrete pepsinogen (a precursor to pepsin, a digestive enzyme). Parietal cells also produce intrinsic factor, which works to facilitate the absorption of vitamin B_{12}.

Function

The stomach performs several functions. Following ingestion of food, the stomach functions as a food reservoir. The stomach serves a secretory function that aids digestion. Gastric secretion can be divided into three phases: cephalic, gastric, and intestinal.

The cephalic phase begins with the sight, smell, and taste of food and is regulated by the vagus nerve. Sympathetic nerve fibers activate neurons in the GI nerve plexus, which then serve to initiate secretory and contractile activity. The gastric phase begins with the presence of food in the stomach. The G-cells in the antrum secrete the hormone gastrin, which promotes the secretion of hydrochloric acid and pepsinogen.

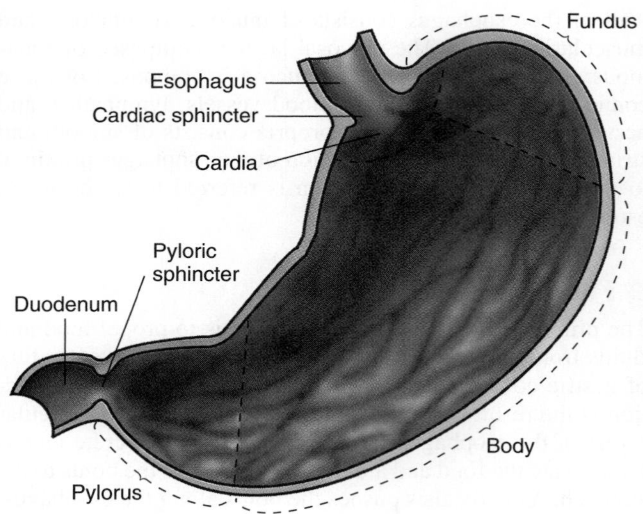

Figure 53-3 ● The anatomy of the stomach.

Hydrochloric acid transforms inactive pepsinogen into active pepsins, which aid in the digestion of proteins. The secretion of mucus and bicarbonate protect the stomach from mechanical and chemical damage. The fluids secreted into the stomach are collectively referred to as gastric juice (Table 53-1). Intrinsic factor is secreted by parietal cells, which bind vitamin B_{12} to enhance its absorption in the ileum.

The stomach also mixes or churns the food, breaking apart the large food molecules and mixing them with gastric secretions to form chyme, which then empties into the duodenum. The intestinal phase begins as the chyme passes from the stomach into the duodenum, causing distention. The intestinal phase is mediated by secretin, a hormone that inhibits further acid production and decreases gastric motility.

Pancreas

Structure

The pancreas lies retroperitoneally in the upper abdominal cavity behind the stomach and extends horizontally from the duodenal C-loop to the spleen. The pancreas is divided into portions known as the head, the body, and the tail (Figure 53-4).

Function

Two major cellular bodies within the pancreas have separate functions: exocrine and endocrine. The *exocrine* part of the pancreas constitutes approximately 80% of the organ and consists of acinar cells, which secrete the enzymes that are necessary for the digestion of carbohydrates, fats, and proteins (trypsin, chymotrypsin, amylase, and lipase) (Table 53-2). The *endocrine* part of the pancreas is made up of the islets of Langerhans, with alpha cells producing glucagon and beta cells producing insulin. Although the islet cells account for less than 2% of the volume of the pancreas, the hormones produced are essential in the regulation of metabolism. Chapter 62 describes the endocrine function of the pancreas.

Liver

Structure

The liver is the largest organ in the body and is mainly located in the right upper quadrant (RUQ) of the abdomen. The liver is divided into two major regions: a larger right lobe and a smaller left lobe. The lobes are divided by the falciform ligament, which attaches the liver to the diaphragm. The liver is made up of functioning units called lobules (Figure 53-5). The organ has a connective tissue covering, called the Glisson capsule, which protects it. Hepatocytes, or liver cells, are arranged

TABLE 53-1 • GASTROINTESTINAL HORMONES

Hormone	Source	Effect
Gastrin	Secreted by the gastric mucosa in the presence of peptides	Stimulates gastric motility and secretion of hydrochloric acid
Secretin	Secreted by the duodenum in the presence of hydrochloric acid	Stimulates the secretion of pancreatic juice and bile from the liver
Pancreozymin	Secreted by the duodenum in the presence of hydrochloric acid and peptides	Stimulates the secretion of pancreatic juice
Cholecystokinin	Secreted by the duodenum in the presence of amino acids and fatty acids	Stimulates the secretion of pancreatic enzymes and bile from the gallbladder

into cellular plates, which radiate from a central vein. Small bile channels fit between the plates and empty into terminal bile ducts. The right and left hepatic ducts transport bile from the liver. The liver receives its blood supply from the hepatic artery and the hepatic portal vein. Approximately 1500 mL of blood flows through the liver every minute.

Function

The liver performs more than 400 functions in three major categories: storage, protection, and metabolism. The liver stores several minerals and vitamins: copper, iron, magnesium, vitamin B_{12}, folic acid, vitamin B_6, niacin, and the fat-soluble vitamins A, D, E, and K.

The protective function of the liver involves phagocytic Kupffer's cells, which are part of the body's reticuloendothelial system. They engulf harmful bacteria and anemic red blood cells. The liver also detoxifies potentially harmful compounds (such as drugs, chemicals, and alcohol) that are ingested.

The liver functions in the metabolism of proteins considered vital for human survival. It breaks down amino acids to remove ammonia, which is then converted to urea and is excreted via the kidneys. In addition, the liver synthesizes several plasma proteins, including albumin, prothrombin, and fibrinogen. The liver's role in carbohydrate metabolism involves storing and releasing glycogen as the body's energy requirements change. The liver synthesizes, breaks down, and temporarily stores fatty acids and triglycerides.

TABLE 53-2 • MAJOR DIGESTIVE ENZYMES AND BILE

Substance	Source	Substrate	End Product
Salivary amylase (ptyalin)	Salivary glands	Starch	Dextrins, maltose
Gastric pepsin (protease)	Stomach	Proteins	Polypeptides
Gastric lipase	Stomach	Emulsified fats	Fatty acids* and glycerol*
Bile (contains no enzymes)	Liver; stored and released from the gallbladder	Unemulsified fats	Emulsified fats
Trypsin	Pancreas	Proteins and polypeptides	Polypeptides and amino acids*
Chymotrypsin	Pancreas	Proteins and polypeptides	Polypeptides and amino acids*
Carboxypeptidase	Pancreas	Polypeptides	Smaller polypeptides
Amylase	Pancreas	Starch	Maltose, lactose, and sucrose
Lipase	Pancreas	Bile and emulsified fats	Glycerol* and fatty acids*
Enterokinase	Duodenal mucosa	Trypsinogen	Trypsin
Peptidases	Intestine	Peptides	Amino acids*
Lactase	Intestine	Lactose (milk sugar)	Glucose* and galactose*
Maltase	Intestine	Maltose (malt sugar)	Glucose*
Sucrase	Intestine	Sucrose (cane sugar)	Glucose* and fructose*

*End product ready for digestion.

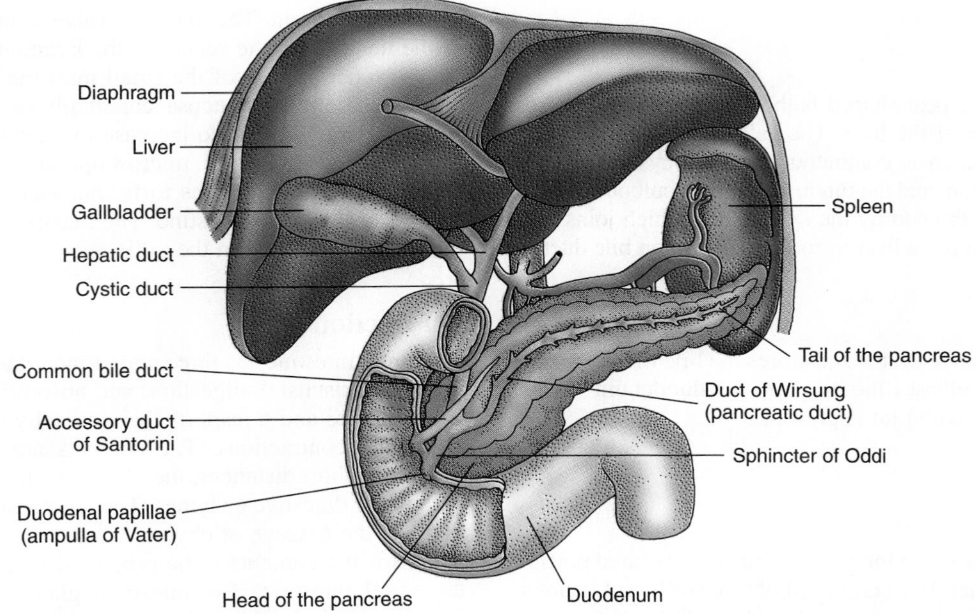

Figure 53-4 • The anatomy of the pancreas, the liver, and the gallbladder.

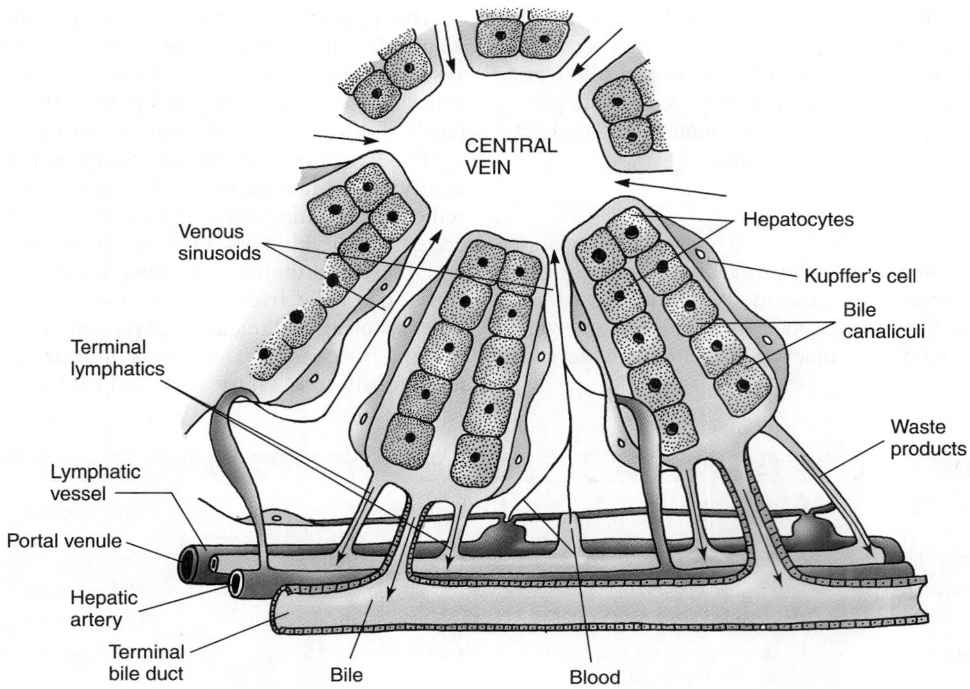

Figure 53-5 ● The anatomy and physiology of the liver lobule. Blood flows from the portal vein and hepatic artery to the central vein. As blood passes through the sinusoids, waste products are removed from the blood and excreted via the lymphatics. Bile is manufactured by the hepatocytes (liver cells) and is secreted into the bile canaliculi. From there, it flows into the bile ducts and then to the gallbladder.

The liver forms and continually secretes bile. Bile is essential for the emulsification of fat. The constituents of bile are bile salts, cholesterol, phospholipids (lecithin), water, electrolytes, and bile pigments (bilirubin). The secretion of bile increases in response to gastrin, secretin, and cholecystokinin. Bile is secreted into small ducts that empty into the common bile duct and into the duodenum at the sphincter of Oddi. However, if the sphincter is closed, the bile goes to the gallbladder for storage.

Gallbladder

Structure

The gallbladder is a pear-shaped bulbous sac that is located on the inferior surface of the liver. The gallbladder has three portions: the neck, which is continuous with the cystic duct; the body, or main portion; and the fundus, the lower bulbous section. The gallbladder is drained by the cystic duct, which joins with the hepatic duct from the liver to form the common bile duct.

Function

The gallbladder concentrates and stores the bile that has come from the liver. It releases the bile into the duodenum via the common bile duct when fat is present.

Small Intestine

Structure

The small intestine is the longest and most convoluted portion of the digestive tract. It is composed of three different regions: the duodenum, the jejunum, and the ileum. The duodenum is the first 10 inches (25 cm) of the small intestine and is attached to the distal end of the pylorus. It is C-shaped, curving left around the head of the pancreas and bending behind the transverse portion of the large intestine. The common bile duct and pancreatic duct join to form the ampulla of Vater, emptying into the duodenum at the duodenal papilla. This papillary opening is surrounded by sphincter muscle known as the sphincter of Oddi. The 8-foot (2.5-m) portion of the small intestine that follows the sphincter of Oddi is the jejunum. The last 8 to 12 feet (2.5 to 4 m) of the small intestine is called the ileum. The ileocecal valve separates the entrance of the ileum from the cecum of the large intestine.

The inner surface of the small intestine has circular folds of mucosa and submucosa called plicae circulares, which project into the lumen to increase the surface area for digestion and absorption. Villi, microscopic finger-like projections, cover the plicae circulares to further increase the absorptive surface of the small intestine. The mucosa contains intestinal glands located between the villi.

Function

The small intestine has three main functions: movement (mixing and peristalsis), digestion, and absorption. The small intestine mixes and transports the chyme by movements called segmental contractions. The contents are moved back and forth over short distances, thereby allowing the chyme to mix with many digestive enzymes. The ileocecal valve opens only to allow the passage of chyme. It takes an average of 3 to 10 hours for the contents to be propelled by peristalsis through the small intestine. The intestinal glands secrete intestinal juice containing epithelial cells that are used to replace surface epithelial cells of the villi as they are lost. The intestinal

CHART 53-1

NURSING FOCUS *on the* OLDER ADULT
Changes in the Gastrointestinal System Related to Aging

Physiologic Change	Disorders Related to Change	Nursing Implications	Rationale
STOMACH			
Atrophy of the gastric mucosa is characterized by a decrease in the ratio of gastrin-secreting cells to somatostatin-secreting cells. This change leads to decreased hydrochloric acid levels (hypochlorhydria).	Decreased hydrochloric acid levels lead to decreased absorption of iron and vitamin B_{12} and to proliferation of bacteria. Atrophic gastritis occurs as a consequence of bacterial overgrowth.	Encourage frequent feedings of bland foods high in vitamins and iron. Assess for epigastric pain.	Frequent feedings help prevent gastritis. Assessment helps detect gastritis.
LARGE INTESTINE			
Peristalsis decreases, and nerve impulses are dulled.	Decreased sensation to defecate can result in postponement of bowel movements, which leads to constipation and impaction.	Encourage a high-fiber diet and 1500 mL of fluid intake daily (if not contraindicated). Encourage as much activity as tolerated.	These interventions increase the sensation of needing to defecate.
PANCREAS			
Distention and dilation of pancreatic ducts change. Calcification of pancreatic vessels occurs with a decrease in lipase production.	Decreased lipase level results in decreased fat absorption and digestion. Steatorrhea, or excess fat in the feces, occurs because of decreased fat digestion.	Encourage small, frequent feedings. Assess for diarrhea.	Small, frequent feedings help prevent steatorrhea. Diarrhea may be steatorrhea.
LIVER			
A decrease in the number and size of hepatic cells leads to decreased liver weight and mass. This change and an increase in fibrous tissue lead to decreased protein synthesis and changes in liver enzymes. Enzyme activity and cholesterol synthesis are diminished.	Decreased enzyme activity depresses drug metabolism, which leads to accumulation of drugs—possibly to toxic levels.	Assess all clients for adverse effects of all drugs, even those administered in normal doses.	Assessment detects drug toxicity.

cells also produce cells that contain enzymes aiding in the digestion of proteins, carbohydrates, and lipids.

Many digestive hormones and enzymes aid in the digestion of the chyme, each having a specific function (see Tables 53-1 and 53-2). Carbohydrates, fats, proteins, vitamins, water, and electrolytes are absorbed by both diffusion and active transport.

Large Intestine

Structure

The large intestine extends approximately 5 to 6 feet in length from the ileocecal valve to the anus and is lined with columnar epithelium that has absorptive and mucous cells. It begins with the cecum, with the appendix forming a narrow tube extending down from the cecum. The large intestine then extends upward from the cecum as the colon. The colon consists of four divisions: the ascending colon, the transverse colon, the descending colon, and the sigmoid colon. The sigmoid colon empties into the rectum.

Following the sigmoid colon, the large intestine bends downward to form the rectum. The last 3 to 4 cm of the large intestine is called the anal canal, which opens to the exterior of the body through the anus. The anal canal is surrounded by sphincter muscles.

Function

The large intestine's functions are movement, absorption, and elimination. Movement in the large intestine consists mainly of segmental contractions, like those in the small intestine, to allow enough time for the absorption of water. In addition, three or four strong peristaltic contractions per day are triggered by colonic distention in the proximal large intestine to propel the contents toward the rectum, where the material is stored until the urge to defecate occurs.

Absorption of water and some electrolytes occurs in the large intestine to reduce the fluid volume of the chyme, which creates a more solid material, the feces, for elimination. GI changes associated with aging are summarized in Chart 53-1.

ASSESSMENT TECHNIQUES

History

One method of assessing gastrointestinal (GI) functioning is to use the nutritional-metabolic and elimination patterns found in Gordon's Functional Health Patterns (Chart 53-2). The goal of the health history is to determine the events related to the current health problem.

CHART 53-2

GASTROINTESTINAL ASSESSMENT
Using Gordon's Functional Health Patterns

Nutritional-Metabolic Pattern

What is your typical daily food intake? Describe a day's meals, snacks, and vitamins.
How much salt do you typically add to your food? Do you use salt substitutes?
How is your appetite? Any recent change?
Do you have any difficulty chewing or swallowing?
Do you wear dentures? How well do they fit?
Do you ever experience indigestion or "heartburn"? How often? What seems to cause it? What helps it?
Do you have pain, diarrhea, gas, or any other problems? Do any specific foods cause this for you?
What is your typical daily fluid intake? What types of fluids (water, juices, soft drinks, coffee, tea)? How much?
Have you had any recent change in your weight? Weight gain? Weight loss? How much?
Have you noticed a change in the tightness of your rings or shoes? Tighter? Looser?
Have you noticed any difference in the size of your abdomen?

Elimination Pattern

What is your usual bowel elimination pattern? Frequency? Character? Discomfort? Laxatives?
Do you have any pain or bleeding associated with bowel movements?
Have you experienced any changes in your usual bowel pattern?
When was your last rectal examination?
Have you ever had an endoscopy or a colonoscopy?
What is your usual urinary elimination pattern? Frequency? Amount? Color? Odor? Control?
Have you noticed a change in the amount of urine?

Based on Gordon, M. (2000). *Manual of nursing diagnosis* (9th ed). St. Louis: Mosby.

DEMOGRAPHIC DATA

The nurse or assistive nursing personnel collects demographic data about the client, such as age, gender, culture, and occupation. This information can provide information regarding predispositions to particular GI tract disorders. For example, familial adenomatous polyposis (FAP) is an inherited autosomal dominant disorder that predisposes the client to colon cancer.

CONSIDERATIONS FOR OLDER ADULTS

The majority of GI tract cancers occur in adults age 50 and older. In addition, the incidence of hiatal hernia increases with each decade of life. Diverticulosis and gallstones are also seen increasingly in people older than 40 years of age.

CULTURAL CONSIDERATIONS

Inflammatory bowel diseases are more common in Caucasians than in African Americans or Asians. Ulcerative colitis is three to six times more prevalent among people of Jewish descent (Glickman, 1998). The incidence of GI cancers also varies among ethnic groups. For example, gastric cancer is prevalent in Japan, Korea, and southern China. Colon cancer is more prevalent among African-American men (Garlick Roll, 1999; Hawkins, 1999).

PERSONAL AND FAMILY HISTORY

A thorough review of the client's overall health status is an important part of every history. The nurse questions the client about previous GI disorders or abdominal surgery.

The client is asked about prescription medications being taken, including how much, when the drugs are administered, and why they have been prescribed. The nurse also explores whether the client takes over-the-counter medications, which he or she may use independently. In particular, the nurse asks whether aspirin, nonsteroidal anti-inflammatory drugs (NSAIDs) (such as ibuprofen), laxatives, or enemas are routinely taken. Large amounts of aspirin or NSAIDs can predispose the client to peptic ulcer disease and GI bleeding. Long-term use of laxatives or enemas can cause dependence on such stimulation and result in constipation.

Finally, the nurse investigates the client's travel history. The nurse asks the client whether he or she has traveled outside of the country recently. This information may provide clues as to the origin of symptoms such as diarrhea.

DIET HISTORY

A diet history is important when assessing GI tract function. Many conditions of the GI tract manifest themselves as a result of alterations in dietary intake and absorption of nutrients. The goals of a nutritional assessment are to gather information about ingestion, digestion, absorption, and metabolism (Hammond, 1999). The nurse inquires about any special diet and whether there are any known food allergies. The nurse also asks the client to describe the usual foods that are eaten daily and the times meals are taken.

The nurse explores with the client any changes that have occurred in eating habits as a result of illness. Anorexia (loss of appetite for food) can occur with GI disease. The nurse also asks about changes in taste and any difficulty or pain with swallowing (dysphagia) that could be associated with esophageal disorders. The nurse ascertains if abdominal pain or discomfort accompanies eating, and if the client has experienced any nausea, vomiting, or dyspepsia (indigestion or heartburn). Unknown food allergies often cause these symptoms. The nurse inquires about any unintentional weight loss, since some cancers of the GI tract may present in this manner. It is also important to assess alcohol and caffeine consumption, because both substances are associated with many GI disorders, such as gastritis and peptic ulcer disease.

CULTURAL CONSIDERATIONS

Cultural and religious patterns are important in obtaining a complete diet history. The nurse determines if culturally based foods pose a problem for the client. For example, the spices or hot pepper used in cooking in many cultures can aggravate or precipitate GI tract complaints, such as indigestion. The nurse should also note religious patterns such as fasting or abstinence.

Approximately 80% to 90% of African Americans are lactose intolerant (Greenberger & Isselbacher, 1998). A much smaller percentage of Caucasians also have this problem. Lactose intolerance causes bloating, cramping, and diarrhea as a result of lack of the enzyme lactase. Lactase is needed to convert lactose in milk and other dairy products to glucose and galactose.

SOCIOECONOMIC STATUS

Knowledge of the client's socioeconomic status can give the nurse valuable clues for determining his or her ability to obtain food, medications, and medical care. People who have limited budgets, such as elders or the unemployed, may not be able to purchase foods required for a balanced diet. In addition, they may substitute less expensive, and perhaps less effective, over-the-counter medications for prescription medications. Necessary medical care may be delayed, and clients may not seek health care until conditions are well advanced. Clients who are financially restricted may benefit from suggestions for managing nutrition while on a budget.

CURRENT HEALTH PROBLEMS

GI tract clinical manifestations are often vague and difficult for the client to describe. The nurse obtains a chronologic account of the current problem, symptoms, and any treatments taken. Furthermore, the nurse explores the characteristics associated with each symptom, including the location, quality, quantity, timing (onset, duration), and factors that may aggravate or alleviate the symptom (see Chart 53-2). The following examples are topics to explore with clients about specific GI tract symptoms.

A change in bowel habits is a significant complaint. The nurse explores the following with the client:

- Pattern of bowel movements
- Color and consistency of the feces
- Occurrence of diarrhea or constipation
- Effective action taken to relieve diarrhea or constipation
- Presence of frank blood or tarry stools
- Presence of abdominal distention or gas

An unintentional weight gain or loss is a symptom that warrants further investigation. The nurse assesses the client concerning the following:

- Normal weight
- Weight gain or loss
- Period of time for weight change
- Changes in appetite or oral intake

Smoking predisposes the client to several types of cancer, especially oral cancer, because nicotine is a GI irritant. The nurse obtains a smoking history, including the number of packs of cigarettes smoked per day per number of years. The nurse also asks about any history or current use of cigars, pipe tobacco, or chewing tobacco.

Pain is a common complaint in clients with GI tract disorders. The nurse asks about pain in relation to the following:

- Presence
- Location
- Radiation to another site
- Factors that make the pain better or worse
- Intensity

Abdominal pain is often vague and difficult to evaluate. Asking the client to apply descriptors to the type of pain, such as burning, gnawing, or stabbing, is often helpful. The location of the pain can be determined by asking the client to point to the involved site. The nurse also asks about the relationship of food intake to the onset or worsening of pain. For example, a high-fat meal often triggers gallbladder pain.

Changes in the skin can result from several GI tract disorders, such as liver and biliary system obstruction. The nurse asks the client about the following:

- Skin discolorations or rashes
- Itching
- Jaundice
- Increased susceptibility to bruising
- Increased tendency to bleed

Physical Assessment

Physical assessment of the gastrointestinal (GI) system involves a comprehensive examination of the client's nutritional status, the mouth and pharynx, the abdomen, and the extremities. Nutritional assessment is discussed in detail in Chapter 61.

MOUTH AND PHARYNX

Assessment of the mouth involves inspection and palpation. To begin the examination of the mouth, the nurse puts on gloves, faces the client, and inspects the lips for color, moisture, cracking, or lesions. To continue, the nurse needs a penlight and a tongue depressor. The medical-surgical nurse inspects the inner surfaces of the lips and the oral mucosa, starting on the client's left side and moving in a clockwise fashion. The advanced-practice nurse (APN) carefully palpates the U-shaped area under the tongue for nodules, since oral malignancies are most likely to develop in this area. The tongue is inspected for color, coating, ulcers, and variations in size and shape.

The nurse examines the teeth for evidence of dental caries and notes the absence of teeth. Tooth discoloration may be the result of excessive tobacco use. Referral to a dentist is appropriate if the nurse detects abnormalities or decay.

The gums should be pink, moist, and smooth. African-American clients may have a dark line on the margins of the gingiva. If the client wears dentures, they are removed. Throughout this examination, the nurse is alert to any significant mouth odors that suggest disease. For instance, a fruity smell may indicate uncontrolled diabetes mellitus.

Oral lesions or nodules are noted. For example, lesions from Kaposi's sarcoma may be seen in clients with acquired immunodeficiency syndrome (AIDS).

ABDOMEN

In preparation for examination of the abdomen, the client is instructed to empty his or her bladder and then to lie in a supine position with the knees bent, keeping the arms at the sides to prevent inadvertent tensing of the abdominal muscles.

During the abdominal examination, the nurse usually begins at the client's right side and proceeds in a systematic fashion (Figure 53-6):

- Right upper quadrant (RUQ)
- Left upper quadrant (LUQ)
- Left lower quadrant (LLQ)
- Right lower quadrant (RLQ)

Table 53-3 lists the organs that lie in each of these topographic areas.

If areas of pain or discomfort are noted from the history, the nurse places this area last in the examination sequence. This

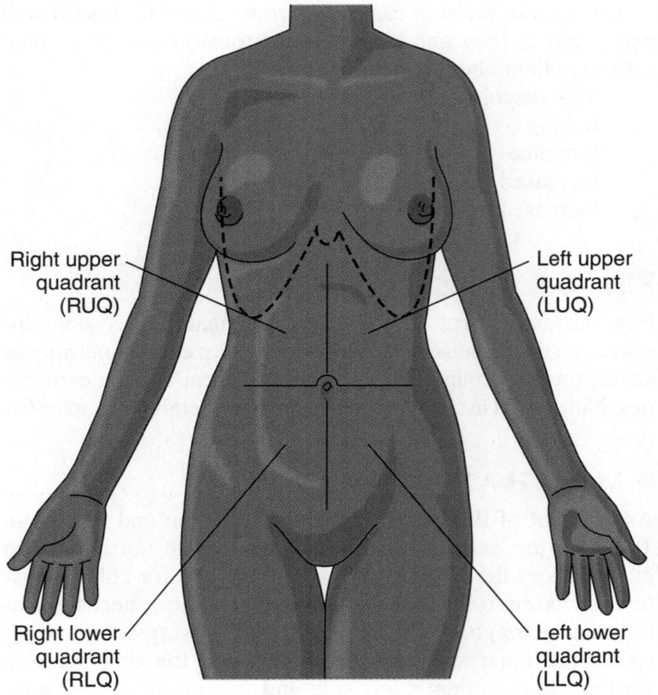

Right upper quadrant (RUQ)
Left upper quadrant (LUQ)
Right lower quadrant (RLQ)
Left lower quadrant (LLQ)

Figure 53-6 ● A topographic division of the abdomen into quadrants.

TABLE 53-3 • LOCATION OF BODY STRUCTURES IN EACH ABDOMINAL QUADRANT

RIGHT UPPER QUADRANT (RUQ) • Most of the liver • Gallbladder • Duodenum • Head of the pancreas • Hepatic flexure of the colon • Part of the ascending and transverse colon	**LEFT LOWER QUADRANT (LLQ)** • Part of the descending colon • Sigmoid colon • Left ureter • Left ovary and fallopian tube • Left spermatic cord
LEFT UPPER QUADRANT (LUQ) • Left lobe of the liver • Stomach • Spleen • Body and tail of the pancreas • Splenic flexure of the colon • Part of the transverse and descending colon	**RIGHT LOWER QUADRANT (RLQ)** • Cecum • Appendix • Right ureter • Right ovary and fallopian tube • Right spermatic cord **MIDLINE** • Abdominal aorta • Uterus (if enlarged) • Bladder (if distended)

sequence should prevent the client from tensing abdominal muscles because of the pain, which would make the examination difficult. The nurse examines any area of tenderness cautiously and instructs the client to state whether it is too painful. His or her face is observed for signs of distress or pain.

The nurse assesses the abdomen by using the four techniques of examination, but in a sequence different from that used for other body systems: inspection, auscultation, percussion, and then palpation. This sequence is preferred so that palpation and percussion do not increase intestinal activity and hence increase bowel sounds. Palpation is not performed if appendicitis or an abdominal aneurysm is suspected.

Inspection

The nurse inspects the skin and notes the following:

- Overall symmetry of the abdomen
- Presence of discolorations (rashes, lesions, striae, petechiae, scars, distended superficial veins, jaundice, and any other pigmentation changes)
- Abdominal distention
- Bulging flanks
- Taut, glistening skin

The nurse assesses the architecture of the abdomen by observing its contour and symmetry. The contour of the abdomen is the abdominal profile and can be rounded, flat, concave, or distended. The contour is best seen if one stands at the side of the bed. The nurse notes whether the contour is symmetric or asymmetric. Asymmetry in the upper quadrants can be indicative of a tumor, pancreatic cyst, or gastric dilation. Asymmetry in the lower quadrants can be caused by ovarian tumors, fibroid tumors, pregnancy, or bladder distention (O'Hanlon-Nichols, 1998). The nurse inspects the shape and position of the umbilicus for any deviations. The presence of ecchymosis around the umbilicus (Cullen's sign) is also noted as an indication of intraperitoneal hemorrhage (Wrobleski, Barth, & Oyen, 1999).

Finally, the nurse inspects the client's abdominal movements, including the normal rising and falling with inspiration and expiration, and notes any distress during movement. Occasionally, pulsations may be visible, particularly in the area of the abdominal aorta. Peristaltic movements are rarely seen on inspection unless the client is thin and has markedly increased peristalsis. If such movements are observed, the nurse notes the quadrant of origin and the direction of peristaltic flow. This finding is reported to the health care provider, since it may indicate an intestinal obstruction.

Auscultation

The nurse performs auscultation of the abdomen with the diaphragm of the stethoscope, since bowel sounds are usually high pitched. The stethoscope is placed lightly on the abdominal wall while the nurse listens for bowel sounds in all four quadrants, beginning in the RLQ at the ileocecal valve area.

Bowel sounds are created as air and fluid move through the GI tract. They are normally heard as relatively high pitched gurgles every 5 to 15 seconds, with a normal frequency range of 5 to 30 per minute. Bowel sounds are characterized as normal, hypoactive, or hyperactive. The nurse listens for the character and frequency of the sounds. Bowel sounds may be irregular, so the nurse must listen for *at least* 1 full minute in each quadrant to confirm the absence of bowel sounds. Bowel sounds are diminished or absent after abdominal surgery or in the client with peritonitis or paralytic ileus. Increased bowel sounds, especially loud gurgling sounds, result from hypermotility of the bowel (borborygmus). These sounds are usually heard in the client with diarrhea or gastroenteritis or above a complete intestinal obstruction.

The nurse also auscultates the abdomen for vascular sounds or bruits ("swooshing" sounds) over the abdominal aorta, the renal arteries, and the iliac arteries. A bruit heard over the aorta usually indicates the presence of an aneurysm. If this sound is heard, the nurse discontinues the examination and notifies the health care provider immediately.

The nurse may auscultate for two other abnormal circulatory sounds: friction rubs and venous hums. A friction rub, which sounds like two pieces of leather rubbing together, can be heard over the spleen or the liver and indicates the presence of a splenic infarct or a hepatic tumor. A continuous venous hum is heard in the periumbilical region in the presence of engorged liver circulation, as in hepatic cirrhosis.

Percussion

Percussion may be used during the abdominal assessment to determine the size of solid organs; to detect the presence of masses, fluid, and air; and to estimate the size of the liver and spleen. This part of the physical assessment is usually performed by a physician or advanced-practice nurse (APN). The examiner elicits percussion notes by placing the middle finger of the nondominant hand over the abdominal area to be percussed, striking his or her finger lightly with the tip of the middle finger of the dominant hand several times. Each quadrant is systematically assessed by comparing sounds over different areas. The **percussion notes** normally heard in the abdomen are termed **tympanic** (the high-pitched, loud, musical sound of an air-filled intestine) or **dull** (the medium-pitched, softer, thudlike sound over a solid organ, such as the liver).

To percuss the size of the liver span, the physician or APN begins from below the right nipple in the midclavicular line and is careful to percuss between ribs. The percussion note should change from resonance of the lung tissue to dullness of the liver when the upper liver border is reached. The examiner marks the area where percussion tones change, then percusses up from the iliac crest in the midclavicular line until the percussion note changes from tympany of the bowel to dullness of the liver at the lower border. Again, this area is marked. The distance between the two marks is the approximate liver span, which is normally 2.4 to 5 inches (6 to 12 cm). An enlarged liver span indicates **hepatomegaly** (liver enlargement).

The examiner may use percussion techniques to determine the size and position of the spleen at the tenth intercostal space in the left midaxillary line. Dullness heard forward of the midaxillary line or in the left anterior axillary line indicates enlargement of the spleen (splenomegaly). Mild to moderate splenomegaly can be detected before the spleen becomes palpable. Percussion can also be used to detect a distended bladder.

Palpation

The purpose of palpation is to determine the size and location of abdominal organs and to assess for the presence of masses or tenderness. Palpation of the abdomen consists of two types: light palpation and deep palpation. Only physicians and APNs, such as clinical nurse specialists and nurse practitioners, should perform deep palpation.

LIGHT PALPATION

The technique of light palpation is used to detect large masses and areas of tenderness and to help the client achieve muscular relaxation. The nurse places the first four fingers of the palpating hand close together and then places them lightly on the abdomen and proceeds smoothly and systematically from quadrant to quadrant. The abdomen is depressed to a depth of 0.5 to 1 inch (1.25 to 2.5 cm), and the assessment proceeds with a rotational movement of the palpating hand. Any areas of tenderness or guarding are noted, because these areas are examined last and cautiously during deep palpation. While performing light palpation, the nurse is alert to signs of rigidity, which, unlike voluntary guarding, is a sign of peritoneal inflammation. Areas of pain should be evaluated for rebound tenderness (Blumberg's sign). With fingers placed at a 90-degree angle in relation to the abdomen, the examiner pushes slowly and deeply, releasing quickly. Pain felt on release is a positive sign for rebound tenderness and should be reported to the health care provider.

DEEP PALPATION

Deep palpation is used to further determine the size and shape of abdominal organs and masses. The APN uses the palm and fingers of one or both hands and proceeds deliberately around the abdominal wall to a maximal depth. If both hands are used (bimanual palpation), one hand is placed on top of the other for palpation of a deep organ. This technique may be required in order to overcome the resistance felt by a large, obese abdomen.

There are two techniques that can be used for palpating the liver. For the first technique, the examiner stands at the client's right side and places the left hand under the client's back parallel to the eleventh and twelfth ribs. The right hand is placed in the right upper quadrant (RUQ) parallel to the midline. The client is then instructed to take a deep breath as the examiner presses the hand inward and upward under the rib cage until a maximal depth is reached. The liver may or may not be palpable, but the edge of the liver may be felt over the fingertips of the palpating hand as the client breathes.

The second technique for palpating the liver is the *hooking technique.* The examiner stands at the client's right side behind the shoulder and places both hands, next to one another, below the lower border of the liver. The client is instructed to take a deep breath while the nurse presses in with the fingers of both hands at the costal margin. The examiner attempts to feel the lower border of the liver as it descends.

Palpation is also used to detect an enlarged spleen; however, the spleen must be three times its original size before it is palpable. The same two techniques for palpating the liver are used for the spleen, but on the left side. The pancreas, the gallbladder, and the left kidney are not usually palpable in most healthy adults.

Psychosocial Assessment

Psychosocial assessment focuses on how the current complaint affects the client's lifestyle. The nurse asks whether there has been any interruption of, or disturbance to, usual activities, including employment. The nurse questions about recent stressful events experienced. Emotional stress has been associated with the development or exacerbation of irritable bowel syndrome (IBS).

CRITICAL THINKING CHALLENGE

A male client has been admitted to your unit complaining of RUQ pain and fever for the last 2 days. His usual dietary pattern consists of eating at restaurants several times weekly. The symptoms began 2 hours after eating a dinner of fried foods at a local restaurant.

- What specific areas of the history should you seek further information or clarification about?
- What physical assessment findings would you be most likely to find during the abdominal examination?

For suggested answer guidelines, go to SIMON http://www.wbsaunders.com/SIMON/Iggy/.

Diagnostic Assessment

LABORATORY ASSESSMENT

To make an accurate assessment of the many possible causes of gastrointestinal (GI) tract abnormalities, laboratory testing of blood, urine, and stool specimens can be performed.

Blood Tests

COMPLETE BLOOD COUNT

A complete blood count (CBC) aids in the diagnosis of anemia and infection; it also detects changes in the blood's formed elements. In adults, GI bleeding is the most frequent cause of anemia.

CLOTTING FACTORS

Because the liver is the main site of all proteins involved in coagulation, the prothrombin time is useful in evaluating the levels of these clotting factors. Prothrombin time measures the rate at which prothrombin is converted to thrombin, a process that is dependent on most of the vitamin K–associated clotting factors. Severe acute or chronic liver damage leads to prolongation of the prothrombin time secondary to impaired synthesis of clotting proteins.

SERUM ELECTROLYTES

Many electrolytes are altered in GI tract dysfunction. For example, calcium is absorbed in the GI tract and may be measured to detect malabsorption. Excessive vomiting or diarrhea causes electrolyte depletion, requiring replacement.

SERUM ENZYME ASSAYS AND LIVER FUNCTION TESTS

Assays of serum enzymes are important in the evaluation of liver damage. **Aspartate aminotransferase (AST)** and **alanine aminotransferase (ALT)** are two enzymes found in the liver and other organs. These enzymes are elevated in most liver disorders, but they are highest in conditions that cause necrosis, such as severe viral hepatitis.

Elevations in serum **amylase** and **lipase** are indicative of acute pancreatitis. In acute pancreatitis, serum amylase levels begin to elevate within 24 hours of onset and remain elevated for up to 5 days unless extensive pancreatic necrosis, obstruction, or a pseudocyst is present. Serum amylase and lipase measurements are the best indicators of the presence of acute pancreatitis, with elevations corresponding to pancreatitis in 75% to 80% of cases (Toskes & Greenberger, 1998; Wrobleski, Barth, & Oyen, 1999).

Bilirubin is the primary pigment in bile, which is normally conjugated and excreted by the liver and biliary system. It is measured as total serum bilirubin, conjugated (direct) bilirubin, and unconjugated (indirect) bilirubin. These measurements are important in the evaluation of jaundice and in the evaluation of liver and biliary tract functioning (Hass, 1999). Elevations in direct and indirect bilirubin levels can indicate impaired secretion or conjugation.

The serum level of ammonia is also measured to evaluate hepatic function. Ammonia is normally used to rebuild amino acids or is converted to urea for excretion. Elevated ammonia levels are seen in conditions that cause hepatocellular injury, such as cirrhosis of the liver.

TUMOR MARKERS

Two **oncofetal antigens**—CA19-9 and CEA—are evaluated to monitor the success of cancer therapy and to assess for the recurrence of cancer in the GI tract. These antigens may also be increased in benign GI conditions. Chart 53-3 lists blood tests commonly used by the health care provider in the diagnosis of GI disorders.

URINE TESTS

The presence of amylase can be detected in the urine. In acute pancreatitis, there is increased renal clearance of amylase. Amylase levels in the urine remain high even after serum levels return to normal; therefore there may be false-positive findings associated with this particular test.

Urine urobilinogen is a form of bilirubin that is converted by the intestinal flora and excreted in the urine. Its measurement is useful in the evaluation of hepatic and biliary obstruction, since the presence of bilirubin in the urine often precedes the development of jaundice (Chart 53-4).

STOOL TESTS

Several stool examinations are used in the evaluation of GI tract dysfunction (see Chart 53-4). Stool testing for occult blood is called the **fecal occult blood test (FOBT).** The FOBT measures the presence of blood in the stool from GI bleeding, a common finding associated with colorectal cancer.

Stool samples are collected to test for ova and parasites to aid in the diagnosis of parasitic infection. Stool samples tested for fecal fats are evaluated for steatorrhea and malabsorption. Fat is normally absorbed in the small intestine in the presence of biliary and pancreatic secretions. In malabsorption, fat is abnormally excreted in the stool.

WOMEN'S HEALTH CONSIDERATIONS

Compared with women of lower socioeconomic status, women of higher socioeconomic status are more likely to have regular physical examinations that include an annual FOBT and a proctosigmoidoscopy every 3 to 5 years after the age of 50. An annual FOBT reduces mortality from colorectal cancer in women (Allen & Phillips, 1997).

CHART 53-3

LABORATORY PROFILE
Gastrointestinal Assessment

Test	Normal Range for Adults	Significance of Abnormal Findings
Calcium (total)	*18-60 yr:* 8.6-10.0 mg/dL or 2.15-2.50 mmol/L *60-90 yr:* 8.8-10.2 mg/dL or 2.20-2.55 mmol/L *>90 yr:* 8.2-9.6 mg/dL or 2.15-2.40 mmol/L	*Decreased* values indicate possible: Malabsorption Renal failure Acute pancreatitis
Potassium	*Male:* 3.5-4.5 mEq/L or 3.5-4.5 mmol/L *Female:* 3.4-4.4 mEq/L or 3.4-4.4 mmol/L	*Decreased* values indicate possible: Vomiting Gastric suctioning Diarrhea Drainage from intestinal fistulas
Albumin	*18-60 yr:* 3.4-4.8 g/dL *60-90 yr:* 3.2-4.6 g/dL	*Decreased* values indicate possible: Hepatic disease
Alanine aminotransferase (ALT)	*18-60 yr, male:* 10-40 units/L *female:* 7-35 units/L *60-90 yr, male:* 13-40 units/L *female:* 10-28 units/L *>90 yr, male:* 6-38 units/L *female:* 5-24 units/L	*Increased* values indicate possible: Liver disease Hepatitis Cirrhosis
Aspartate aminotransferase (AST)	*18-60 yr:* 8-20 units/L *>60 yr, male:* 11-26 units/L *female:* 10-20 units/L	*Increased* values indicate possible: Liver disease Hepatitis Cirrhosis
Lactate dehydrogenase (LDH)	140-280 units/L	*Increased* values indicate possible damaged liver caused by hepatitis and other hepatocellular disorders
Alkaline phosphatase	25-100 units/L or 0.43-1.70 μKat/L	*Increased* values indicate possible: Hepatic disease Biliary obstruction
Bilirubin		
Total serum	*18-60 yr:* 0.3-1.2 mg/dL or 5-21 μmol/L *60-90 yr:* 0.2-1.1 mg/dL or 3-19 μmol/L *>90 yr:* 0.2-0.9 mg/dL or 3-15 μmol/L	*Increased* values indicate possible: Hemolysis Biliary obstruction Hepatic damage
Conjugated (direct)	<0.2 mg/dL or 3.4 μmol/L	*Increased* values indicate possible biliary obstruction
Unconjugated (indirect)	<1.1 mg/dL or 19 μmol/L	*Increased* values indicate possible: Hemolysis Hepatic damage
Ammonia	19-60 μg/dL or 11-35 μmol/L	*Increased* values indicate possible hepatic disease such as cirrhosis
Xylose absorption	*5-g dose in 2 hr:* >20 mg/dL or >1.3 mmol/L *25-g dose in 2 hr:* >25 mg/dL or >1.7 mmol/L	*Decreased* values in blood and urine indicate possible malabsorption in the small intestine
Serum amylase	*18-60 yr:* 27-131 IU/L or 0.46-2.23 μKat /L *60-90 yr:* 24-151 IU/L or 0.41-2.57 μKat /L	*Increased* values indicate possible acute pancreatitis
Serum lipase	13-141 units/L or 0.22-2.40 μKat/L *>60 yr:* 0-302 units/L or 0.0-5.13 μKat /L	*Increased* values indicate possible acute pancreatitis
Cholesterol	<200 mg/dL or 5.18 mmol/L	*Increased* values indicate possible: Pancreatitis Biliary obstruction *Decreased* values indicate possible liver cell damage
Carbohydrate antigen 19-9 (CA19-9)	<37 units/mL	*Increased* values indicate possible: Cancer of the pancreas, stomach, colon Acute pancreatitis Inflammatory bowel disease
Carcinoembryonic antigen (CEA)	*Nonsmoker:* <2.5 ng/mL *Smoker:* up to 5 ng/mL	*Increased* values indicate possible: Colorectal, stomach, pancreatic cancer Ulcerative colitis Crohn's disease Hepatitis Cirrhosis

CHART 53-4

LABORATORY PROFILE

Common Urine and Stool Tests Used in Gastrointestinal Assessment

Test	Normal Range for Adults	Significance of Abnormal Findings
Urine bilirubin	Negative	*Increased* values indicate possible: Biliary obstruction Cirrhosis Hepatitis
Urobilinogen	Urine: 0.1-1.0 Ehrlich unit/mL	*Increased* values indicate possible: Hepatitis Cirrhosis *Absence* indicates possible obstructive jaundice
Urine amylase	Various levels, depending on unit of measure	*Increased* values indicate possible: Acute pancreatitis Pancreatic obstruction
Stool for occult blood	Negative	*Presence* indicates possible: Carcinoma Peptic ulcer Ulcerative colitis
Ova and parasites	Negative	*Presence* is diagnostic of infection
Fecal fat	<7 g/24 hr with normal diet	*Increased* values indicate possible: Crohn's disease Malabsorption syndrome Pancreatic disease

RADIOGRAPHIC EXAMINATIONS

Radiographic examinations and similar diagnostic procedures are useful in detecting structural and functional disorders of the gastrointestinal (GI) tract. The role of the nurse is to properly prepare the client for the examination, to provide an explanation of the procedure, and to provide the necessary post-procedure care. As with most invasive procedures, many of the diagnostic tests outlined here require a witnessed and signed informed consent.

Flat-Plate Film of the Abdomen

A flat-plate film of the abdomen is generally the first x-ray study that the health care provider orders when diagnosing a GI problem. A flat-plate film visualizes organs in the abdomen. This simple film has the ability to reveal abnormalities such as masses, tumors, and strictures or obstructions to normal movement. Patterns of bowel gas appear light on the abdominal film and can be useful in detecting ileus from obstruction. There is no required client preparation except to wear a hospital gown and remove any jewelry or belts, which may interfere with the film.

Upper Gastrointestinal Series and Small-Bowel Series

An upper GI radiographic series is an x-ray visualization from the oral part of the pharynx to the duodenojejunal junction. The upper GI series is used to detect disorders of structure or function of the esophagus (barium swallow), stomach, or duodenum. An extension of the upper GI series, the small-bowel follow-through (SBFT), continues the tracing of the barium through the small intestine up to and including the ileocecal junction to detect disorders of the jejunum or ileum.

CLIENT PREPARATION. The client is instructed to abstain from foods or liquids for 8 hours before the test. If possible, opioid analgesics and anticholinergic medications are withheld for 24 hours before the test, since they decrease intestinal tract motility.

The client is instructed about the barium preparation and the need to drink approximately 16 ounces of the barium. The radiology nurse or technician explains that a rotating examination table will be used to assist the client in assuming the vertical, supine, prone, and lateral positions required for this test.

PROCEDURE. The client drinks a mixture of barium sulfate, and fluoroscopy is used to trace the barium through the esophagus and stomach. The client stands against the x-ray table for this part of the test. The table then moves the client to a lying position for more views of the stomach and duodenum. Lying in a prone position, the client drinks more barium as quickly as possible while x-ray films are taken. To attempt to make the client as comfortable as possible, a pillow for the head and a sheet to prevent chilling are supplied whenever possible. The position changes help to coat the mucosa and identify gastroesophageal reflux and hiatal hernia.

If a small-bowel radiographic series is included, the client drinks additional barium, and more x-ray films are taken at intervals. This series can take several hours, depending on how long it takes the barium to reach the cecum.

FOLLOW-UP CARE. After either of these series, the nurse teaches the client to drink plenty of fluids to help eliminate the barium. The client may be given a mild laxative or stool softener to assist in elimination of the barium. The radiology nurse or technician instructs the client that stools may be chalky white for 24 to 72 hours as barium is excreted. The client is informed that when all barium is passed, brown stools return. If the client is at home, he or she is instructed to report abdominal fullness, pain, or a delay in return to brown stools.

Barium Enema

A barium enema examination, also known as a lower GI series, is a radiographic visualization of the large intestine. This test is usually ordered for a client with a complaint of blood or mucus in the stool or a change in bowel pattern, such as diarrhea or constipation. A barium enema can also detect bowel obstruction from volvulus (Korsten & Abittan, 1999). This test is usually contraindicated in clients when colon perforation or fistula is suspected, since there is the potential for barium to enter the venous circulation, causing cardiac arrest.

CLIENT PREPARATION. Adequate client preparation for a barium enema study is very important. The client consumes clear liquids 12 to 24 hours before the examination to reduce the amount of fecal matter in the bowel. The client is allowed nothing by mouth (NPO) after midnight on the night before the test. In addition, the health care provider orders a potent laxative, such as magnesium citrate, and possibly an oral liquid preparation, such as GoLYTELY, for cleaning the bowel the evening before the examination. In some cases, a cleansing enema is needed or required according to the agency's procedure.

PROCEDURE. To begin the barium enema examination, a rectal catheter with an inflatable balloon is inserted. Approximately 500 to 1500 mL of barium is instilled slowly by gravity, and the client is instructed to hold the barium. Films are taken with the client in supine, prone, and lateral positions. He or she may experience abdominal cramps and the urge to defecate as the barium enema is given. This procedure can be extremely uncomfortable, especially for older adults. The client is instructed to take slow, deep breaths and to hold the anal sphincter as tightly closed as possible. The test takes about 45 minutes to 1 hour. In some cases, a double-contrast study is ordered. In this study, air is instilled to enhance the contrast and outline small lesions.

FOLLOW-UP CARE. After the study is completed, the client is allowed to expel the barium. The radiology nurse or technician teaches the client to drink plenty of fluids to assist in eliminating the barium. A laxative is given to help remove the barium from the intestinal tract. The client is informed that the stools will be chalky white for about 24 to 72 hours, until all barium is expelled.

Percutaneous Transhepatic Cholangiography

Percutaneous transhepatic cholangiography is an x-ray study of the biliary duct system using an iodinated dye instilled via a percutaneous needle inserted into the hepatic ducts of the liver. This procedure is usually performed when a client has jaundice or persistent upper abdominal pain even after cholecystectomy.

CLIENT PREPARATION. A laxative is usually given to the client the evening before the procedure. He or she is on NPO status for 12 hours before the test, and the nurse asks about allergies to iodine or seafood. If the client has either of these allergies, the nurse informs the health care provider. Coagulation tests are monitored, since impaired clotting is a contraindication to this procedure. Before the procedure begins, an intravenous (IV) infusion is started for the administration of sedatives.

PROCEDURE. The client is placed in a supine position on the fluoroscopy table. The site is prepared and draped, and a local anesthetic is injected into the skin. During the test, the client is instructed to hold his or her breath on expiration while a needle is inserted into the liver under x-ray visualization. The dye is injected slowly until the biliary tree is filled. X-ray images are taken as the dye reaches the biliary duct system. A tilt table may be used to place the client in various positions to visualize the entire biliary tree. At the end of the test, the biliary ducts are aspirated of contrast medium. The procedure usually takes 30 minutes to 1 hour.

FOLLOW-UP CARE. After a percutaneous transhepatic cholangiography, the client is confined to bed for 6 hours. The nurse checks vital signs frequently, since there is a risk of hemorrhage and sepsis. The client is placed on the right side with a firm pillow or sandbag placed against the lower ribs and abdomen. The nurse inspects the lower right rib cage area for signs of bleeding, hematoma, ecchymosis, or bile leakage.

Gallbladder Series

A gallbladder radiographic series, or oral cholecystography, is an x-ray visualization of the gallbladder after oral ingestion of radiopaque, iodine-based contrast medium. It is not commonly performed today because of the availability and accuracy of gallbladder ultrasound. After the contrast medium is ingested, it is eventually cleared from the blood by the liver, and it is then deposited into the hepatic and biliary ducts and gallbladder. The test may be performed to identify causes of obstruction, such as stones, but gallbladder ultrasonography is more commonly done for this purpose. A gallbladder radiographic series should be done before any barium studies.

CLIENT PREPARATION. Before the gallbladder radiographic series, the nurse checks with the client about any allergies to iodine or seafood. On the day before the test, the client eats a fat-free or low-fat diet and takes 6 radiopaque iodine tablets (iopanoic acid [Telepaque]) approximately 2 hours after the evening meal. One tablet is taken with water every 5 minutes until all 6 tablets are consumed. The nurse instructs the client that the tablets can cause diarrhea. The client is on NPO status from midnight on the night before the test until after the test is completed.

PROCEDURE. The client is usually in the radiology department for about 60 minutes while several views of the gallbladder are taken. These films will identify any stones present in the gallbladder. The client is then given a fatty meal, or synthetic substitute, to cause contraction of the gallbladder within 10 to 30 minutes. A second series of films helps to confirm the presence of contrast material in the cystic duct, common duct, and duodenum.

FOLLOW-UP CARE. The nurse remains alert for allergic reaction to the contrast material.

Intravenous Cholangiography

Intravenous cholangiography (IVC) is an x-ray study of the gallbladder and biliary ducts. This test may be performed if the gallbladder is not visualized by a gallbladder radiographic series or gallbladder ultrasonography, or if biliary symptoms occur in a client who has had a cholecystectomy. It may also be done during surgery.

CLIENT PREPARATION. Before the test, the nurse checks with the client about any allergies to iodine or seafood and reports allergies to the physician. The client is on NPO status after midnight on the night before the test. Some agencies may require a bowel preparation. The nurse notifies the client that a sensation of warmth or flushing may be felt with the injection of the contrast medium.

PROCEDURE. The client may be in the radiology department for 2 to 4 hours for IVC. The client is given an IV injection of a contrast material, and x-ray films are taken at 20-minute intervals for 1 hour, or until the biliary ducts are visualized. The gallbladder should be visualized in 1 to 2 hours.

FOLLOW-UP CARE. The radiology personnel and nurse monitor the client for allergic reaction to the contrast material so that emergency measures can be instituted if necessary.

Computed Tomography of the Gastrointestinal Tract

Computed tomography (CT), also referred to as a CT scan, is a cross-sectional x-ray visualization that can detect tissue densities and abnormalities in the abdomen, liver, pancreas, spleen, and biliary tract. CT may be performed with or without contrast media.

CLIENT PREPARATION. The client is instructed that he or she will need to lie still in a rather enclosed space of the machine. The client is instructed to remove jewelry or metal from the x-ray field. If the use of a contrast medium is scheduled, the nurse asks about allergies to seafood and iodine. The client is on NPO status for 4 to 8 hours before the test if a contrast medium is to be used. IV access will be required for injection of the contrast medium. The client is advised that a warm, flushing feeling may be felt on injection.

PROCEDURE. The radiologic technician instructs the client to lie still and to hold his or her breath when asked. The client is placed on the examining table, and a series of x-ray images are taken. The contrast medium may be given by IV injection for a second set of images. The test takes approximately 1 to 2 hours to complete.

FOLLOW-UP CARE. No particular follow-up care is needed after a CT scan unless sedatives were administered. If the client was sedated, the nurse monitors vital signs until the client is alert and fully awake.

CRITICAL THINKING CHALLENGE

The health care provider suspects that your client may have an inflammation of the gallbladder as a result of gallstones.

- What diagnostic procedure will probably be ordered for this client to confirm the diagnosis?
- What information should the nurse ask the client about before the test is scheduled?

For suggested answer guidelines, go to SIMON http://www.wbsaunders.com/SIMON/Iggy/.

OTHER DIAGNOSTIC TESTS

Endoscopy

Endoscopy is direct visualization of the gastrointestinal (GI) tract by means of a flexible fiberoptic endoscope. Endoscopes of various sizes are used for different areas of the GI tract. Visualization of the esophagus, stomach, biliary system, and bowel is possible. Endoscopy is usually ordered to evaluate bleeding, ulceration, inflammation, masses, tumors, and cancerous lesions. Obtaining specimens for biopsy and cytologic studies is also possible through the endoscope. There are several types of endoscopic examinations.

ESOPHAGOGASTRODUODENOSCOPY

Esophagogastroduodenoscopy (EGD), a visual examination of the esophagus, stomach, and duodenum, is accomplished using a fiberoptic endoscope. The distal end of the endoscope is flexible, allowing visualization of the entire area.

CLIENT PREPARATION. The client preparing for an upper GI endoscopic examination is usually on NPO status after midnight on the night before the test, or 8 to 12 hours before the procedure. The nurse explains that during the test a flexible tube is passed down the esophagus with the client under conscious sedation. The physician usually orders medication, such as midazolam hydrochloride (Versed), meperidine (Demerol), or diazepam (Valium, E-Pam✤), to sedate the client. Atropine may be administered to dry secretions. In addition, a local anesthetic is sprayed to inactivate the gag reflex and facilitate passage of the tube. The nurse explains that this anesthetic will calm the gag reflex and that swallowing will be difficult. If the client has dentures, they are removed.

PROCEDURE. After the medications are administered, the client is usually placed in the left lateral decubitus (Sims') position with a towel or basin at the mouth for secretions. The physician passes the tube through the mouth and into the esophagus (Figure 53-7). The procedure takes approximately 30 minutes.

FOLLOW-UP CARE. The nurse checks vital signs frequently as ordered (usually every 30 minutes) until the sedation wears off. The siderails of the bed are raised during this time. The client remains on NPO status until the gag reflex returns (usually in 2 to 4 hours). The nurse monitors for signs of perforation, such as pain, bleeding, or fever. The client is instructed not to drive for 12 hours following the test. He or she is informed that a hoarse voice or sore throat may persist for several days following the test. Throat lozenges can be used to relieve throat discomfort.

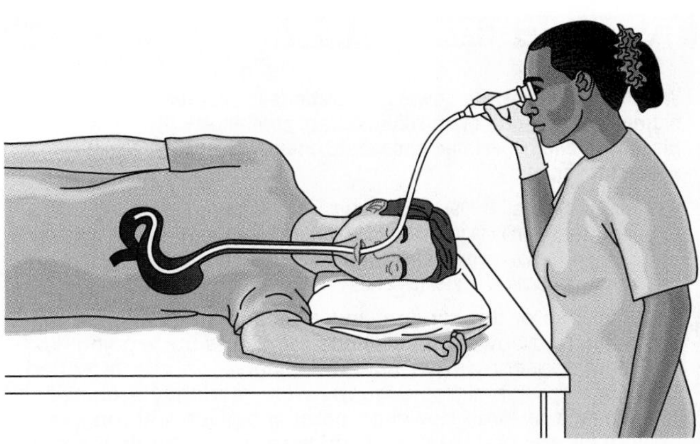

Figure 53-7 ● Esophagogastroduodenoscopy allows visualization of the esophagus, the stomach, and the duodenum. If the esophagus is the focus of the examination, the procedure is called esophagoscopy. If the stomach is the focus, the procedure is called gastroscopy.

ENDOSCOPIC RETROGRADE CHOLANGIOPANCREATOGRAPHY

Endoscopic retrograde cholangiopancreatography (ERCP) includes visual and radiographic examination of the liver, gallbladder, and pancreas to identify the cause and location of obstruction. After the cannula is inserted into the main duct, a radiopaque dye is inserted, followed by several x-ray images. The physician may perform a papillotomy, a small incision in the sphincter around the ampulla of Vater, to remove gallstones.

CLIENT PREPARATION. The client is prepared in the same manner as for an EGD, including being on NPO status after midnight on the night before the test. The client will require IV access for the administration of sedation. The nurse asks about prior exposure to x-ray dye and any sensitivities or allergies.

PROCEDURE. The endoscopic portion of an ERCP is similar to that of an EGD, except that the endoscope is advanced farther, to the duodenum and into the biliary tract. Once the cannula is in the common duct, the radiologist or the radiologic technician injects contrast medium, and x-ray films are taken to evaluate the biliary tract. A tilt table assists in distributing the contrast medium to all branches of the biliary tree. Following examination of the biliary tree, the cannula is directed into the pancreatic duct for examination. The ERCP lasts from 30 minutes to 2 hours.

FOLLOW-UP CARE. The nurse assesses vital signs frequently, usually every 15 minutes, until the client is stable. The nurse observes for several postprocedure complications, including cholangitis, perforation, sepsis, and pancreatitis. These problems do not occur immediately after the procedure but may take several hours to 2 days to develop. Colicky abdominal pain can occur secondary to the air instilled during the procedure. The client is instructed to report abdominal pain, fever, nausea, or vomiting that fails to resolve. He or she remains on NPO status until the gag reflex returns. Once the gag reflex is intact, the client can begin taking clear fluids.

COLONOSCOPY

Colonoscopy is an endoscopic examination of the entire large bowel. The physician may also obtain tissue biopsy specimens or remove polyps through the colonoscope. A colonoscopy is also used to evaluate the cause of chronic diarrhea or locate the source of GI bleeding.

CLIENT PREPARATION. The client should have a liquid diet for at least 24 hours before a colonoscopy and is usually on NPO status after midnight on the night before the procedure.

CONSIDERATIONS FOR OLDER ADULTS

A complete bowel preparation ("prep") is necessary to enable the physician to visualize the entire colon. For many clients, especially older adults, the "prep" is the worst part of the procedure, resulting in weakness and fatigue.

An oral liquid preparation for cleaning the bowel (e.g., polyethylene glycol electrolyte solution [GoLYTELY]) is given to the client the evening before the examination. The solution should be chilled to make it more palatable. Even though it has a salty taste, the solution should not be diluted with water or ice. The nurse instructs the client to drink the preparation quickly—8 ounces (240 mL) every 10 minutes until all 4 L are consumed. This solution produces a watery diarrhea that begins in approximately 1 hour. The bowel clears in 4 to 5 hours. In some cases, the client may require laxatives, suppositories (e.g., bisacodyl [Dulcolax]), or one or more cleansing enemas. IV access is necessary for the administration of conscious sedation.

PROCEDURE. The physician orders medication to aid in relaxation, usually midazolam hydrochloride (Versed) or meperidine (Demerol). Initially, the client is placed on the left side with the knees drawn up while the endoscope is passed into the rectum to the cecum. Air may be instilled for better visualization. The entire procedure lasts approximately 60 minutes. Atropine sulfate is kept available in case of bradycardia resulting from vasovagal response.

FOLLOW-UP CARE. The nurse checks vital signs every 15 minutes until the client is stable. Siderails are kept up until sedation wears off. The client is observed for signs of perforation and hemorrhage. The nurse instructs the client that a feeling of fullness, cramping, and passage of flatus are expected for several hours after the test. If a polypectomy or tissue biopsy was performed, there may be a small amount of blood in the first stool after the colonoscopy. Excessive bleeding should be reported immediately to the health care provider (Chart 53-5). If the procedure was performed in an ambulatory care setting, the client will need another person to provide transportation home. The client should avoid driving for 8 to 12 hours after the procedure because of the effects of sedation.

PROCTOSIGMOIDOSCOPY

Proctosigmoidoscopy is an endoscopic examination of the rectum and sigmoid colon using a flexible or rigid scope. The

CHART 53-5

BEST PRACTICE *for* Care of the Client After a Colonoscopy

- Do not allow the client to take anything by mouth until sedation wears off and the client is alert.
- Take vital signs every 15 to 30 minutes until the client is alert.
- Keep the siderails up until the client is alert.
- Assess for rectal bleeding or blood clots.
- Remind the client that fullness and mild abdominal cramping are expected for several hours.
- Assess for manifestations of bowel perforation, including *severe* abdominal pain and guarding. Fever may occur later.
- Assess for manifestations of hypovolemic shock, including dizziness, lightheadedness, decreased blood pressure, tachycardia, pallor, and altered mental status (may be the first sign).
- If the procedure is performed in an ambulatory care setting, arrange for another person to drive the client home.

purpose of this test is to screen for colon cancer, investigate the source of GI bleeding, or diagnose or monitor inflammatory bowel disease. If proctosigmoidoscopy is used as an alternative to colonoscopy for colorectal cancer screening, it is recommended that screening begin at 50 to 55 years of age (Levin et al., 1999).

CLIENT PREPARATION. The client should have a liquid diet for at least 24 hours before a sigmoidoscopy; a cleansing enema or sodium biphosphate (Fleet's) enema is usually given the morning of the procedure. A laxative may also be ordered the evening before the test (see the Evidence-Based Practice for Nursing box at right).

PROCEDURE. For a proctosigmoidoscopy, the client is placed on the left side in the knee-chest position or on a special table in the proctoscopic position. No sedation is required. The scope is lubricated and inserted into the anus to the required depth for visualization. Tissue biopsy may be performed during this procedure. The examination usually lasts about 30 minutes.

FOLLOW-UP CARE. The client is informed that mild gas pain and flatulence may be experienced from air instilled into the rectum during the examination. If a biopsy was obtained, a small amount of bleeding may be observed.

Gastric Analysis

Gastric analysis measures the hydrochloric acid and pepsin content for evaluation of gastric and duodenal disorders. There are two tests in gastric analysis: basal gastric secretion and gastric acid stimulation. Basal gastric secretion measures the secretion of hydrochloric acid between meals. If only small amounts of secretion are collected, a follow-up gastric stimulation test is given.

CLIENT PREPARATION. The client is on NPO status for at least 12 hours before the test. Alcohol, tobacco, and medications that may affect gastric secretion are avoided for 24 hours before the test. The nurse inserts a nasogastric (NG) tube and removes and discards the residual contents of the stomach.

EVIDENCE-BASED PRACTICE FOR NURSING

Which of the following bowel preparations is best for flexible sigmoidoscopy: oral magnesium citrate combined with oral bisacodyl, one hypertonic phosphate enema, or two hypertonic phosphate enemas?

Fincher, R., et al. (1999). A comparison of bowel preparations for flexible sigmoidoscopy: Oral magnesium citrate combined with oral bisacodyl, one hypertonic phosphate enema, or two hypertonic phosphate enemas. *American Journal of Gastroenterology, 94*(8), 2122-2127.

The purpose of this randomized clinical trial was to compare three differing bowel preparations for clients undergoing flexible sigmoidoscopy. Two hundred ninety-one clients scheduled for a routine sigmoidoscopy were randomly assigned to receive one of three bowel preparations given with oral magnesium citrate: oral bisacodyl and magnesium citrate the night before the procedure, one hypertonic phosphate enema 1 hour before the procedure, or two hypertonic enemas given at 2 hours and 1 hour before the procedure. The physicians performing the endoscopy were blinded to the type of preparation the client received and were asked to rate the quality of the preparation. Clients were asked to rate their comfort and overall satisfaction.

There was no statistical difference in the bowel preparation quality between the three methods, and clients preferred the oral regimen, even though it was associated with more diarrhea.

Critique. Despite the lack of statistical differences in bowel preparations, this study builds on previous work by the same authors examining routine practices for their scientific basis and application to clinical practice. The rating scale of bowel preparation by the physicians may not have been clear enough to differ between excellent and good ratings.

Implications for Nursing. Proper bowel preparation is critical to an accurate procedure. No previous studies have identified a superior means of providing bowel preparation. An oral bowel preparation that is well tolerated may have implications for decreasing the number of repeat procedures needed because of lack of visualization, thereby decreasing test-associated costs. A completely oral regimen could reduce nursing time associated with administering enemas.

PROCEDURE. The NG tube is attached to suctioning equipment for collecting the contents at 15-minute intervals for 1 hour. The nurse collects each sample and labels the time and volume of each specimen.

For the gastric acid stimulation test, the NG tube is left in place, and a drug that stimulates gastric acid secretion (e.g., pentagastrin or betazole dihydrochloride [Histalog]) is given subcutaneously. Fifteen minutes after injection of the drug, specimens are again collected at 15-minute intervals for 1 hour. The nurse collects, labels, and measures the specimens.

Depressed levels of gastric secretion suggest the presence of gastric carcinoma. Increased levels of gastric secretion indicate Zollinger-Ellison syndrome and duodenal ulcers (see Chapter 56).

FOLLOW-UP CARE. After the test is completed, the NG tube is removed and the client can resume normal eating patterns. No other follow-up is necessary.

Ultrasonography

Ultrasonography is a technique in which high-frequency, inaudible vibratory sound waves are passed through the body via a transducer; the echoes of the sound waves created are then recorded. The echoes are then converted into images and photographed for analysis. Ultrasound testing is commonly used to image soft tissues, such as the liver, the spleen, the pancreas, the gallbladder, and the biliary system.

CLIENT PREPARATION. The client is usually on NPO status for 8 to 12 hours before ultrasonography of the abdomen. The nurse informs the client that it will be necessary to lie still during the study. He or she instructed to drink 1 to 2 L of fluid just before the test, because a full bladder is necessary for accurate visualization.

PROCEDURE. The client is placed in a prone or supine position. The technician applies insulating gel to the end of the transducer and on the area of the abdomen under study. This gel allows airtight contact of the transducer with the skin. The technician moves the transducer back and forth over the skin until the desired images are obtained. The study takes about 15 to 30 minutes.

FOLLOW-UP CARE. No follow-up care is necessary after ultrasonography.

Endoscopic Ultrasonography

Endoscopic ultrasonography (EUS) provides images of the gastrointestinal (GI) wall and high-resolution images of the digestive organs. The ultrasonography is performed through the endoscope. This procedure is useful in diagnosing the presence of lymph node tumors, mucosal tumors, and tumors of the pancreas, stomach, and rectum. The client preparation and follow-up care are similar to the preparation and follow-up care for both endoscopy and ultrasonography.

Liver-Spleen Scan

A liver-spleen scan uses IV injection of a radioactive colloid that is taken up primarily by the liver and secondarily by the spleen. The scan evaluates the liver and the spleen for tumors or abscesses, organ size and location, and vascularity. This scan is useful in evaluating hepatocellular disease.

CLIENT PREPARATION. The nurse instructs the client about the need to lie still during the scanning. The client is assured that the colloid injection has only small amounts of radioactivity and is not dangerous. The nurse should ask female clients of childbearing age if they may be pregnant or are currently breastfeeding. The radionuclide can be found in breast milk, and radiation from x-ray studies should be avoided in pregnancy.

PROCEDURE. The technician or the physician gives the radioactive injection through an IV line, and a wait of about 15 minutes is necessary for uptake. The client is placed in many different positions while the scanning takes place. No follow-up care is necessary after a liver scan.

FOLLOW-UP CARE. The client should be instructed that the radionuclide is eliminated from the body through the urine in 24 hours. Careful handwashing following toileting will decrease the exposure to any radiation present in the urine.

ONLINE RESOURCES

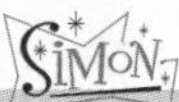

For suggested readings and Internet resources, go to http://www.wbsaunders.com/SIMON/Iggy/.

SELECTED BIBLIOGRAPHY

Allen, K.M., & Phillips, J.M. (1997). *Women's health across the lifespan.* Philadelphia: Lippincott-Raven.

Berne, R.M., & Levy, M.N. (1998). *Physiology* (4th ed.). St. Louis: Mosby.

Chai, C., & Blackington, E. (2000). Colorectal cancer. *ADVANCE for Nurse Practitioners, 8*(4), 34-39.

Dammel, T. (1997). Fecal occult blood testing: Looking for hidden danger. *Nursing97, 27*(7), 44-45.

Fincher, R., et al. (1999). A comparison of bowel preparations for flexible sigmoidoscopy: Oral magnesium citrate combined with oral bisacodyl, one hypertonic phosphate enema, or two hypertonic phosphate enemas. *American Journal of Gastroenterology, 94*(8), 2122-2127.

Garlick Roll, M. (1999). Colon cancer. In C. Miaskowski & P. Buchsel (Eds.), *Oncology nursing: Assessment and clinical care* (pp. 863-887). St. Louis: Mosby.

Glickman, R. (1998). Inflammatory bowel disease: Ulcerative colitis and Crohn's disease. In A.S. Fauci, E. Braunwald, & K.J. Isselbacher (Eds.), *Harrison's principles of internal medicine* (14th ed., pp. 1633-1648). New York: McGraw-Hill.

Gordon, M. (2000). *Manual of nursing diagnosis* (9th ed.). St. Louis: Mosby.

Greenberger, N., & Isselbacher, K. (1998). Disorders of absorption. In A.S. Fauci, E. Braunwald, & K.J. Isselbacher (Eds.), *Harrison's principles of internal medicine* (14th ed., pp. 1616-1633). New York: McGraw-Hill.

Hammond, K. (1999). Nutrition-focused physical assessment. *Home Healthcare Nurse, 17*(6), 354-355.

Hass, P. (1999). Differentiation and diagnosis of jaundice. *AACN Clinical Issues: Advanced Practice in Acute and Critical Care, 10*(4), 433-441.

Hawkins, B. (1999). Stomach cancer. In C. Miaskowski & P. Buchsel (Eds.), *Oncology nursing: Assessment and clinical care* (pp. 863-887). St. Louis: Mosby.

Korsten, M., & Abittan, C. (1999). Obstipation and lower abdominal pain. *The Clinical Advisor, 2*(6), 68-70.

Levin, T.R., et al. (1999). Predicting advanced proximal colonic neoplasia with screening sigmoidoscopy. *Journal of the American Medical Association, 281*(17), 1611-1617.

Linton, A.D. (1997). Age-related changes in the gastrointestinal system. In M.A. Matteson, E.S. McConnell, & A.D. Linton (Eds.), *Gerontological nursing: Concepts and practice* (2nd ed., pp. 317-335). Philadelphia: W.B. Saunders.

Malarkey, L.M., & McMorrow, M.E. (1998). *Nurse's manual of laboratory tests and diagnostic procedures.* Philadelphia: W.B. Saunders.

O'Hanlon-Nichols, T. (1998). Basic assessment series: Gastrointestinal system. *American Journal of Nursing, 98*(4), 48-53.

Toskes, P., & Greenberger, N. (1998). Disorders of the pancreas. In A.S. Fauci, E. Braunwald, & K.J. Isselbacher (Eds.), *Harrison's principles of internal medicine* (14th ed., pp. 1737-1740). New York: McGraw-Hill.

Wellman, N. (1997) A case manager's guide to nutrition screening and intervention. *The Journal of Care Management, 3*(2), 12-27.

Wrobleski, D., Barth, M. & Oyen, L. (1999). Necrotizing pancreatitis: Pathophysiology, diagnosis, and acute care management. *AACN Clinical Issues: Advanced Practice in Acute and Critical Care, 10*(4), 464-477.

CHAPTER 54

Interventions for Clients with Oral Cavity Problems

CONSTANCE VISOVSKY

Learning Objectives

After studying this chapter, you should be able to:

1. Develop a teaching plan for clients who have stomatitis.
2. Explain the common causes of malignant oral tumors.
3. Identify common nursing diagnoses for clients with oral cancer.
4. Prioritize postoperative care for clients undergoing surgery for oral cancer.
5. Develop a teaching plan for community-based care of clients with oral cancer.

SIMON Go to http://www.wbsaunders.com/SIMON/Iggy/ for self-assessment questions related to these Learning Objectives.

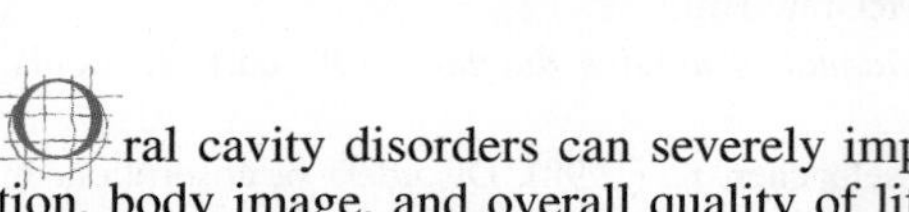

Oral cavity disorders can severely impact speech, nutrition, body image, and overall quality of life. Nurses play an important role in maintaining and restoring oral cavity health in their clients through nursing interventions and client education. Chart 54-1 lists ways for clients to maintain a healthy oral cavity.

STOMATITIS

OVERVIEW

Stomatitis is characterized by painful, single or multiple ulcerations of the oral mucosa that appear as inflammation and denudation of the oral mucosa, impairing the protective lining of the mouth. These ulcerations are commonly referred to as canker sores. Although the terms *stomatitis* and *mucositis* may be used interchangeably, stomatitis is contained in the oral cavity, and mucositis may be more generalized throughout the mucous membranes. The ulceration causes pain, and open areas predispose the individual to bleeding and infection. Although infection remains the most life-threatening complication of stomatitis, pain is the most common complaint (Eilers, 1997). Mild erythema (redness) may respond to topical treatments, whereas extensive stomatitis may require treatment with opioid analgesics.

Stomatitis is classified according to the cause of the inflammation. *Primary* stomatitis includes aphthous stomatitis, herpes simplex stomatitis, and traumatic ulcers. *Secondary* stomatitis generally results from infection by opportunistic viruses or bacteria, particularly in clients with immunosuppressive disorders.

Pathophysiology

The oral mucosa is a protective lining of stratified, squamous, and nonkeratinizing epithelium that extends from the mouth at the junction of the lips to the oropharynx (throat). Inflammatory processes induced by infectious agents, allergy, vitamin deficiency, systemic disease, or antineoplastic drugs cause injury to oral cavity membranes. Cells that are damaged by the inflammatory process slough off, leading to an ulcerated oral mucosa. The ulcerations formed are painful, and bleeding results secondary to erosion of oral mucous membranes (Eilers, 1997).

Etiology

Stomatitis can result from infection, allergy, vitamin deficiency, systemic disease, chemotherapy, or radiation. Infectious agents, such as bacteria and viruses, may have a role in the development of recurrent aphthous stomatitis. L-forms of streptococcus bacteria have been isolated from aphthous ulcers. Although viruses have not been successfully cultured from aphthous lesions, recurrent lesions have been associated with latent zoster or cytomegalovirus (CMV).

The implication that certain foods trigger allergic responses that result in the formation of aphthous ulcers remains controversial. Foods such as coffee, potatoes, cheese, nuts, citrus fruits, and gluten may be precipitating factors. In some cases, strict elimination diets have resulted in the improvement of ulcers. Deficiencies in vitamin B_{12}, folate, and iron associated with malnutrition can contribute to the formation of stomatitis.

Systemic diseases such as human immunodeficiency virus (HIV) infection and chronic renal failure can also predispose a person to stomatitis. Approximately 50% of first-degree relatives of individuals with aphthous ulcers also have the disease, suggesting a genetic link to stomatitis (Woo & Sonis, 1996). Treatment of disease states such as cancer can predispose an individual to the development of painful stomatitis or mucositis. Thirty-nine to fifty percent of clients undergoing chemotherapy or radiation to the head and neck for cancer re-

CHART 54-1

CLIENT EDUCATION GUIDE
Maintaining a Healthy Oral Cavity

- Perform a self-examination of your mouth every month; report any unusual finding.
- Be sure to eat a balanced diet.
- Brush and floss your teeth every day. Set a routine and keep to it.
- Manage your stress as much as possible; learn how to maintain your emotional health.
- Avoid contact with agents that may cause inflammation of the mouth, such as mouthwashes that contain alcohol.
- If possible, avoid medications that may cause inflammation of the mouth or reduce the flow of saliva.
- Be aware of any changes in the occlusion of your teeth, mouth pain, or swelling; seek medical attention promptly.
- See your dentist regularly; have problems attended to promptly.
- If you wear dentures, make sure they are in good repair and fit properly.

port experiencing stomatitis (Hyland, 1997). The severity of stomatitis is related to the type and dose of therapy, as well as to client-related factors, such as pretreatment oral health (Eilers, 1997). (See Chapter 25 for nursing care of the client undergoing radiation and chemotherapy.)

The symptoms of stomatitis range in severity from a dry, painful mouth to open ulcerations, predisposing the client to infection. Mouth ulcerations can alter nutritional status as a result of difficulty with food ingestion or swallowing. When severe, stomatitis and the edema that can accompany it have the potential to impact airway integrity.

Incidence/Prevalence

Aphthous stomatitis is the most common oral lesion treated by primary care providers. It has been found to affect more than 50% of the population and is especially common in North America (Peterson & Baughman, 1996). The incidence of stomatitis in clients undergoing cancer chemotherapy is approximately 40% (Beck, 1996).

WOMEN'S HEALTH CONSIDERATIONS

A hormonal influence has been suggested in relation to women and aphthous stomatitis. Women generally have a higher prevalence of the disorder, with an increased incidence of oral ulceration during the luteal phase of the menstrual cycle. A moderation or absence of lesions during pregnancy has been attributed to increased steroid levels (Peterson & Baughman, 1996).

Primary Stomatitis

APHTHOUS STOMATITIS

Aphthous stomatitis is a noninfectious inflammatory condition of the oral mucosa. Aphthous ulcers are categorized as minor, major, or herpetiform. Eighty percent of aphthous lesions are minor ulcers, measuring less than 0.4 inch (1 cm) in diameter and occurring in groups of up to five lesions. These lesions appear most commonly on the buccal mucosa, soft palate, oropharyngeal mucosa, and lateral and ventral areas of the tongue. The lesions appear as shallow, painful ulcerations covered by a yellow-gray pseudomembrane and exterior erythematous ring. Major aphthous ulcers make up 7% to 20% of aphthous ulcers, are larger than 1 cm, persist for months, and may heal with scarring. Herpetiform ulcers make up 7% to 10% of aphthous ulcers, occur in groups of 10 or more, and are usually located in the posterior part of the mouth (Woo & Sonis, 1996).

HERPES SIMPLEX STOMATITIS

The herpes simplex virus (HSV) is responsible for the development of primary herpes simplex stomatitis, also called acute herpetic stomatitis. The uniformly sized vesicles occur most often on the tongue, palate, and buccal and labial mucosae. The vesicles rupture soon after appearing, leaving painful, ulcerated areas surrounded by erythematous margins. The lesions at this stage are similar to aphthous ulcers. The ulcerated areas heal in 10 to 14 days. The mucosal vesicles are generally accompanied by acute inflammation of the gingiva, occasionally with herpetic lesions. The tongue has a characteristic white coating, and the client complains of a foul breath. Primary HSV infection is characterized by symptoms of generalized infection, including malaise, fever, and lymphadenopathy.

HSV enters injured oral mucosal tissue, where it replicates in the cells of the dermis and epidermis, resulting in primary HSV infection. Although stomatitis caused by HSV can occur as either a primary or secondary (recurrent) infection, secondary infections are more common. Two types of HSV have been identified: HSV type 2, which causes genital lesions (discussed in Chapter 77), and HSV type 1, which is responsible for nongenital lesions.

HSV infection is extremely common. Primary herpetic stomatitis is usually contracted in childhood but may be seen in adults. Immunocompromised clients tend to experience more severe and extensive HSV infections.

VINCENT'S STOMATITIS

Vincent's stomatitis, or acute necrotizing stomatitis, is an acute bacterial infection of the gingiva characterized by erythema, ulceration, and necrosis of the gingival margins. The gingival papillae between the teeth appear worn away and raw. The gingivae often bleed spontaneously or from mild irritation, such as chewing. Clients complain of severe pain; foul breath; thick, ropy secretions; and increased salivation. Systemic clinical manifestations can include malaise, poor appetite, and occasionally, enlargement of cervical lymph nodes.

The disease has a sudden onset and is related to a decreased resistance of tissues to normal oral bacterial flora. Systemic etiologic factors that decrease tissue resistance include poor nutrition, leukemia, and severe infections such as pyelonephritis. Poor oral hygiene and extreme emotional stress have been suggested as contributing factors.

Necrotizing gingivitis occurs primarily in adults, and the incidence seems to increase with aging. Older adults have an increased susceptibility to infections because of decreased immunocompetence.

TRAUMATIC ULCERS

Oral trauma is thought to be the most common precipitating factor in the development of recurrent aphthous stomatitis

(Peterson & Baughman, 1996). Traumatic ulcers can develop at the site of an injury. Traumatic insults, such as injuries from dental procedures, cheek biting, and hot foods, can lead to ulceration. Such injuries can also allow the entry of bacteria, resulting in secondary infection.

Traumatic ulcers are commonly found in clients with malocclusion, ill-fitting dentures, or broken teeth and in those who habitually bite their oral mucosa. In addition, individuals with recurrent aphthous stomatitis are predisposed to developing additional ulcers at the site of a traumatic injury.

Secondary Stomatitis

LICHEN PLANUS

Lichen planus is an inflammatory mucocutaneous disease involving both the skin and the oral mucous membranes. The lesions may be active or in remission, with external lesions affecting the extremities and the genitalia. Symmetric white oral lesions of various patterns appear on the tongue and buccal and labial mucosae. Eighty percent of all lichen planus lesions are bilateral, appearing on the buccal mucosa (Burkhart, Burkes, & Burker, 1997). The remaining 20% are localized to the tongue or lips.

The etiology of the disease is unknown, but recent developments indicate that there may be a cell-mediated immune response involved in the progression of the lesions. Disease states such as diabetes and hypertension may invoke lichenoid reactions from the medications used to treat these conditions. Oral lichen planus may also be associated with hepatitis C infection (Bagan et al., 1998). Local irritants and trauma are contributing factors associated with the progression of lichenoid lesions. There has been conflicting evidence suggesting stress as a mediator of lichen planus. In addition, the chronic inflammatory nature of lichen planus may prove to be a risk factor for oral cancer.

Lichen planus affects 1% to 2% of the population, occurring more often in women than in men and occurring most often in clients ages 40 to 50 years (Burkhart, Burkes, & Burker, 1997). It occurs in all races, with variations in severity among the racial groups. Although the oral lesions themselves are often asymptomatic, an erosive form of the disorder can cause pain that interferes with speech and swallowing. The diagnosis of lichen planus is confirmed through tissue biopsy.

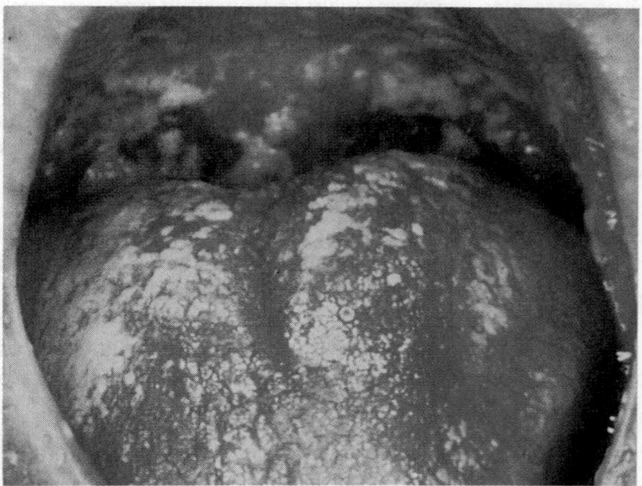

Figure 54-1 • Oral candidiasis. (From Radford, J., & Thatcher, N. [1988]. The toxicity of cancer chemotherapy in adults. *Cancer Care, 5,* 4-7.)

CANDIDIASIS (MONILIASIS)

In oral candidiasis, white plaquelike lesions appear on the tongue, palate, pharynx, and buccal mucosa (Figure 54-1). When these patches are wiped away, the underlying surface appears red and sore (Sheff, 1999). Clients rarely complain of actual pain but describe the lesions as dry or hot.

Candida albicans is part of the normal flora of the oral cavity. **Candidiasis,** also called moniliasis, is a fungal infection resulting from an overgrowth of this normal flora. With recurrent candidiasis, as with all secondary stomatitis, a causative systemic disorder should be sought. Antibiotic therapy destroys the normal flora that usually prevent fungal infections; thus candidiasis can occur in clients receiving long-term antibiotic therapy. Candidiasis of the oral cavity is common in clients undergoing immunosuppressive therapy (chemotherapy, radiation, steroid therapy, or antirejection medication). For example, chemotherapy affects the rapidly dividing cells of the oral mucosa, leading to ulcerations that have a propensity to become infected secondary to a decreased immune response. Candidiasis is also very common among HIV-infected individuals, becoming increasingly likely as CD4+ cell counts fall (Klaus & Grodesky, 1998).

CONSIDERATIONS FOR OLDER ADULTS

Older adults are especially at high risk for candidiasis because aging causes a decrease in immune function. The risk increases for clients who are diabetic, malnourished, or under emotional stress. Older adults who wear dentures may use soft denture liners that provide comfort but can also be colonized by *C. albicans,* contributing to denture stomatitis (Dixon, Breeding, & Faler, 1999).

COLLABORATIVE MANAGEMENT

Assessment

HISTORY

The nurse collects information concerning possible etiologic factors, such as recent infections, a history of stomatitis, nutritional compromise, oral hygiene habits, oral trauma, stress, or immunocompromise. A medication history should also be collected. The nurse records the course of the current outbreak and ascertains if episodes of stomatitis are recurrent. The client is asked if the lesions interfere with swallowing or eating.

PHYSICAL ASSESSMENT/CLINICAL MANIFESTATIONS

While examining the oral cavity, the nurse wears nonsterile gloves for protection against infection. Adequate lighting, including a flashlight or penlight, and a tongue blade facilitate the examination. The nurse assesses the oral cavity for lesions, coating, cracking, and fissures. Characteristics of the lesions are described in terms of location, size, shape, color, and drainage. Any odors that may be present are noted and described.

If lesions are noted along the pharynx, and if the client reports dysphagia or pain on swallowing, the nurse should suspect that the lesions may extend farther down the esophagus. Additional diagnostic testing may be required.

The physical examination may also include examination of the cervical and submandibular lymph nodes for swelling. Any elevation in temperature is noted.

LABORATORY ASSESSMENT

Laboratory tests are usually not needed. However, serum albumin, vitamin B_{12}, folate, and iron levels may be obtained if nutritional status appears to be compromised. A complete blood count may reveal the presence of infection, neutropenia, or anemia. A Tzank smear can assist in distinguishing between herpatic and aphthous ulcers. Fluid from herpetic vesicles in herpes simplex stomatitis may be obtained for viral culture. Bacterial culture of exudate from the oral mucosa validates Vincent's stomatitis or secondary infection. A potassium hydroxide slide preparation or a routine culture and Gram stain can help identify *Candida* organisms.

Interventions

Interventions for stomatitis are aimed toward the promotion of oral health through scrupulous oral hygiene and careful food selection.

ORAL HYGIENE. The nurse or assistive nursing personnel uses a soft-bristled toothbrush or disposable foam swabs (toothettes) to stimulate gums and clean the oral cavity. The nurse encourages frequent rinsing of the mouth with any of the following: sodium bicarbonate solution, warm saline, or hydrogen peroxide solution. The client should avoid commercial mouthwashes because they have a high alcohol content, causing a burning sensation in irritated or ulcerated oral mucosa.

The nurse instructs the client to increase mouth care to every 2 hours and twice at night if the stomatitis is not controlled. Frequent gentle mouth care enhances debridement of ulcerated lesions and can prevent superinfections. Frequent oral care also promotes a general feeling of well-being. Chart 54-2 lists measures for special oral care.

CHART 54-2

BEST PRACTICE *for* Care of Clients with Problems of the Oral Cavity

- Remove dentures if the client has severe stomatitis or oral pain.
- Encourage the client to perform oral hygiene, or provide it after each meal and as often as needed.
- Increase mouth care to every 2 hours or more often if stomatitis is not controlled.
- Use a soft toothbrush, toothette, or gauze for oral care.
- Encourage frequent rinsing of the mouth with hydrogen peroxide, warm saline, sodium bicarbonate (baking soda) solution, or a combination of these solutions.
- Teach the client to avoid commercial mouthwashes and lemon-glycerin swabs.
- Assist the client in selecting soft, bland, and nonacidic foods.
- Apply topical analgesics or anesthetics as ordered by the physician and monitor their effectiveness.

DRUG THERAPY. Anti-infective agents, including antibiotics and antifungals, may be necessary for control of infection in the client with stomatitis. The nurse administers anti-infectives as ordered and provides instruction on how to take them. The health care provider prescribes systemic antibiotics severe recurrent or Vincent's stomatitis. Investigations have linked recurrent aphthous stomatitis to strains of L-streptococci. Tetracycline syrup 250 mg/10 mL four times a day for 10 days may be prescribed. The client rinses for 2 minutes and swallows the syrup, thus obtaining both topical and systemic therapy. Chlorhexidine, an oral rinse, can be beneficial in preventing infection, since it is active against numerous bacteria and fungi. However, chlorhexidine prepared in the United States is 9.6% alcohol and therefore may cause stinging and burning on administration. Chlorhexidine causes a brown discoloration of the teeth that can be removed with oxidizing agents and abrasives.

Antibiotics are of little value in viral or fungal stomatitis unless a secondary infection is present. Systemic antibiotics are ineffective for lichen planus and are not recommended.

A regimen of intravenous (IV) acyclovir (Zovirax) is usually prescribed for immunocompromised clients who contract herpes simplex stomatitis. Acyclovir is typically administered to clients with normal renal function at a dose of 5 mg/kg, infused at a constant rate over a 1-hour period every 8 hours for 7 days. Clients with competent immune systems may be given acyclovir in oral or topical form.

For clients with oral candidal infection, an antifungal agent is prescribed, such as nystatin (Mycostatin, Nadostine) oral suspension 600,000 units four times daily for 7 to 10 days. The nurse teaches the client to swish the solution around in the mouth before swallowing. Oral troches (lozenges) may also be effective. Clients who are taking inhaled steroids should be advised to use a spacer to decrease the amount of medication left in the mouth. In addition, the client should rinse the mouth with warm water after using inhalers, to rinse away any deposited drug (Shuster, 1998). Systemic steroids can be of benefit in long-standing lichen planus.

ANALGESICS. Interventions for clients with stomatitis should include pain control, because pain is consistently present during an outbreak. The nurse performs a comprehensive assessment of pain that includes the following: location, characteristics, onset and duration, frequency, quality, intensity, severity, and precipitating factors.

Topically applied agents or oral analgesics temporarily relieve severe oral pain (Table 54-1). Agents containing 20% benzocaine provide temporary pain relief and can be applied

TABLE 54-1 • DRUGS COMMONLY USED FOR ORAL PAIN RELIEF

ORAL AGENTS
- Lidocaine 2%, viscous
- Diphenhydramine elixir
- Opioids such as acetaminophen with codeine (codeine phosphate 12 mg, acetaminophen 120 mg/5 mL) and morphine sulfate

TOPICAL AGENTS
- Dyclonine (Dyclone) 0.5%
- Benzocaine 20%
- Lidocaine protective gel (Zilactin-L)

to the affected areas three to four times daily. Fifteen milliliters of 2% viscous lidocaine every 3 hours (maximum of 8 doses per day) can be used as a gargle or mouthwash.

The health care provider often prescribes topical swishes for herpes simplex stomatitis and lichen planus. These suspensions can be offered in frozen form; the numbing effects of the cold provide longer analgesia. Topical corticosteroids are indicated for aphthous ulcers, lichen planus, and the lesions of primary herpes simplex virus (HSV) infection. Triamcinolone cream is applied with the finger or a cotton-tipped applicator, or the corticosteroid can be injected directly into the lesion.

Occasionally, systemic approaches to pain relief need to be employed. For moderate to severe stomatitis, around-the-clock administration of combinations of opioid and nonopioid analgesics, such as acetaminophen and codeine, is recommended. If the pain is unrelieved, or if the stomatitis is severe, morphine may be used until healing occurs. Any time a client receives an intervention for pain, the nurse monitors the effectiveness of the pain control measures through an ongoing assessment of the pain experience.

TUMORS

OVERVIEW

Oral cavity tumors can be benign, premalignant, or malignant. Whether benign or malignant, tumors of the oral cavity impact many daily functions. Activities such as swallowing, chewing, and speaking can be affected. Pain accompanying the tumor can also impose limitations on daily activities and self-care. Oral cavity tumors affect body image, especially if treatment involves removal of the tongue or part of the mandible, or requires a tracheostomy.

Premalignant Lesions

LEUKOPLAKIA

Leukoplakia presents as slowly developing changes in the oral mucous membranes that are characterized by thickened, white, firmly attached patches. These patches appear slightly raised and sharply circumscribed. Leukoplakial lesions undergo malignant transformation in approximately 3% to 6% of cases (Olsen, 1999). Although leukoplakia can be found anywhere on the oral mucosa, lesions on the lips or tongue are more likely to progress to malignancy. Leukoplakia results from mechanical factors that cause long-term oral mucous membrane irritation, such as poorly fitting dentures, chronic cheek nibbling, or broken or poorly repaired teeth. In addition, oral hairy leukoplakia can be found in clients with HIV infection. The use of tobacco products has also been implicated in the development of leukoplakia, which is sometimes referred to as "smoker's patch." Oral leukoplakia can be confused with oral candidal infection. However, unlike candidal infection, leukoplakia cannot be removed by scraping.

Leukoplakia is the most common oral lesion among adults; it affects 3% of the population and accounts for 18% of all oral lesions (Shugars & Patton, 1997). Oral hairy leukoplakia is an early manifestation of HIV infection and is highly correlated with progression from HIV infection to acquired immunodeficiency syndrome (AIDS). Leukoplakia not associated with HIV infection is more often seen in people over age 40. Men have twice the incidence of leukoplakia that women have, but this ratio is changing because increasing numbers of women are smoking.

ERYTHROPLAKIA

Erythroplakia presents as a red, velvety mucosal lesion on the surface of the oral mucosa. There is a higher degree of malignant transformation in erythroplakia than in leukoplakia. As such, these lesions should be regarded with suspicion and analyzed by biopsy. Erythroplakia is most commonly found on the floor of the mouth, tongue, palate, and mandibular mucosa. Erythroplakia can be difficult to distinguish from inflammatory or immune reactions.

Malignant Tumors

SQUAMOUS CELL CARCINOMA

PATHOPHYSIOLOGY. More than 90% of oral cancers are squamous cell carcinomas that begin on the surface of the epithelium. Over a period of many years, premalignant (or dysplastic) changes begin. Cells begin to vary in size and shape; alterations in the thickness of the lining of the epithelium develop, resulting in atrophy. These tumors usually grow slowly, and the lesions may be large before the onset of symptoms unless ulceration is present. Mucosal erythroplasia is the earliest sign of oral carcinoma. Oral lesions that appear as red, raised, eroded areas are suspicious for carcinoma.

The American Joint Committee on Cancer has devised the TNM classification system for tumors of the lip and oral cavity (Table 54-2). Each lesion is defined by the following:

T—the size or degree of penetration of the tumor
N—the presence, size, number, and location of involved cervical lymph nodes
M—the presence of distant metastasis (spread)

ETIOLOGY. Squamous cell carcinoma is the most common oral malignancy. Squamous cell carcinomas can be found on the lips, tongue, buccal mucosa, and oropharynx. The major risk factors in the development of oral cancers are increasing age, tobacco use, and alcohol ingestion. Ninety-five percent of all oral cancers occur in people over 40 years of age. Tobacco use in any form (e.g., smoking or chewing tobacco) can increase the risk of cancer by 5% to 25%. The use of smokeless tobacco has nearly tripled in the last 20 years. This form of tobacco contains carcinogens and large quantities of nicotine, which can lead to nicotine addiction. Alcohol ingestion can potentate the carcinogenic effects of tobacco.

An increased rate of oral carcinoma is found in individuals with certain occupations, such as textile workers, plumbers, and coal and metal workers. Additional factors, such as sun exposure, poor dietary habits, poor oral hygiene, and infection with the human papillomavirus (HPV), require further research.

Common signs and symptoms of oral carcinoma include unusual lumps or thickening of the buccal mucosa, or red or white patches appearing on the gums, tongue, or oral mucous membranes. Cancers of the lip are strongly associated with chronic exposure to the sun and often present as a sore that fails to heal. Soreness, pain, or a burning sensation may also be present. In later stages, the client may experience difficulty chewing or swallowing. Advanced cancers of the tongue can cause

TABLE 54-2 • TNM CLASSIFICATION FOR TUMORS OF THE LIP AND ORAL CAVITY

PRIMARY TUMOR (T)
- T_X Primary tumor cannot be assessed
- T_0 No evidence of primary tumor
- T_{is} Carcinoma in situ
- T_1 Tumor 2 cm or less in greatest dimension
- T_2 Tumor more than 2 cm but not more than 4 cm in greatest dimension
- T_3 Tumor more than 4 cm in greatest dimension
- T_4 (Lip) Tumor invades adjacent structures (e.g., through the cortical bone, the tongue, and the skin of the neck)
- T_4 (Oral cavity) Tumor invades adjacent structures (e.g., through the cortical bone, into the deep [extrinsic] muscle of the tongue, the maxillary sinus, and the skin)

LYMPH NODE (N)
- N_X Regional lymph nodes cannot be assessed
- N_0 No regional lymph node metastasis
- N_1 Metastasis in a single ipsilateral lymph node, 3 cm or less in greatest dimension
- N_2 Metastasis in a single ipsilateral lymph node, more than 3 cm but not more than 6 cm in greatest dimension; or multiple ipsilateral lymph nodes, none more than 6 cm in greatest dimension; or bilateral or contralateral lymph nodes, none more than 6 cm in greatest dimension
  - N_{2a} Metastasis in a single ipsilateral lymph node more than 3 cm but not more than 6 cm in greatest dimension
  - N_{2b} Metastasis in multiple ipsilateral lymph nodes, none more than 6 cm in greatest dimension
  - N_{2c} Metastasis in bilateral or contralateral lymph nodes, none more than 6 cm in greatest dimension
- N_3 Metastasis in a lymph node more than 6 cm in greatest dimension

DISTANT METASTASIS (M)
- M_X The presence of distant metastasis cannot be assessed
- M_0 No distant metastasis
- M_1 Distant metastasis

STAGE GROUPING

Stage	T	N	M
0	T_{is}	N_0	M_0
I	T_1	N_0	M_0
II	T_2	N_0	M_0
III	T_3	N_0	M_0
	T_1	N_1	M_0
	T_2	N_1	M_0
	T_3	N_1	M_0
IV	T_4	N_0	M_0
	T_4	N_1	M_0
	Any T	N_2	M_0
	Any T	N_3	M_0
	Any T	Any N	M_1

From American Joint Committee on Cancer. O.H. Beahrs, et al. (Eds.). (1998). *Manual for staging of cancer* (3rd ed.). Philadelphia: J.B. Lippincott.

pain that radiates to the ear. Cervical lymph nodes may become enlarged, hardened, and fixed secondary to metastatic invasion.

INCIDENCE/PREVALENCE. Carcinomas of the oral cavity account for approximately 6% of all cancers diagnosed each year in the United States. In 1999 in the United States, approximately 30,000 cases of oral cancer were diagnosed, and 8000 deaths were attributed to the disease (Greenlee et al., 2000). Worldwide, cancers of the mouth and pharynx account for 363,000 new cases and 200,000 deaths annually (Parkin, Pisani, & Ferlay, 1999).

CONSIDERATIONS FOR OLDER ADULTS

The incidence of oral cancer is expected to increase as the population of older adults increases. Carcinoma of the oral cavity is primarily a disease of older adults that is prevalent in the sixth and seventh decades of life.

WOMEN'S HEALTH CONSIDERATIONS

Along with an increase in tobacco use among women, there has been an increase in oral cancer rates among women. The estimated incidence for women in the United States is 6.4 per 100,000 (Parkin, Pisani, & Ferlay, 1999).

CULTURAL CONSIDERATIONS

African Americans have a higher rate of oral carcinoma than Caucasians (Shugars & Patton, 1997). The relative 5-year survival rate for Caucasians with cancer of the oral cavity or pharynx is 55%, compared with a relative 5-year survival rate of 32% for African Americans with oral cancer (National Cancer Institute, 1999). Higher mortality rates from oral cancer have been associated with limited access to health care.

BASAL CELL CARCINOMA

Basal cell carcinoma of the oral cavity occurs primarily on the lips. The lesion is asymptomatic and resembles a raised scab. With time, the lesion evolves into a characteristic ulcer with a raised pearly border. Basal cell carcinomas do not metastasize but can aggressively involve the skin of the face. The major etiologic factor in basal cell carcinoma is exposure to sunlight.

Basal cell carcinoma occurs as a result of the failure of basal cells to mature into keratinocytes. It is the second most common type of oral cancer but is much less common than squamous cell carcinoma.

CULTURAL CONSIDERATIONS

Clients who work outdoors or who sunbathe excessively, especially Caucasians with fair skin, are more likely to have basal cell carcinomas.

KAPOSI'S SARCOMA

Kaposi's sarcoma is a malignant lesion arising in blood vessels. Kaposi's sarcoma is usually painless and appears as a raised purple nodule or plaque. In the mouth the hard palate is the most common site of Kaposi's sarcoma, but it can also be found on the gums, tongue, or tonsils. It is most often associated with AIDS. (See Chapter 22 for a complete discussion of Kaposi's sarcoma.)

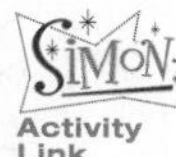

COLLABORATIVE MANAGEMENT

Assessment

HISTORY

A priority for nurses in the prevention and detection of oral cancers is the identification of high-risk groups. Individuals at high risk for developing oral cancer tend to use large amounts of alcohol and tobacco and are over 40 years of age. The nurse asks about occupation and exposure to known oral carcinogens or irritants, such as sunlight or other source of ultraviolet radiation. A family history of cancer and a history of previous oral cancer alert health care providers to be especially observant for signs of cancer.

The nurse assesses the client's routine oral hygiene regimen and use of dentures or oral appliances, which might add to discomfort or mechanically irritate the mucosa. The client should be asked about bleeding, which might indicate an ulcerative lesion. The nurse determines the status of the client's past and current appetite and nutritional state, including difficulty with chewing or swallowing. A continuing trend of weight loss may be related to metastasis, heavy alcohol intake, difficulty in eating or chewing, or an underlying disorder.

PHYSICAL ASSESSMENT/CLINICAL MANIFESTATIONS

An examination of the oral cavity requires adequate lighting for proper visualization. The nurse thoroughly inspects the oral cavity for any lesions, evidence of pain, or restriction of movement. Using a tongue blade, the nurse can visually examine all areas of the oral cavity. The nurse notes any alteration in speech attributable to tongue restriction. Following inspection, the advanced-practice nurse uses bimanual palpation of any visible nodules to determine size and fixation. The cervical lymph nodes should also be palpated (Figure 54-2).

PSYCHOSOCIAL ASSESSMENT

The functioning and appearance of the oral cavity are strongly linked with body image and quality of life. Therefore the nurse assesses the impact of oral lesions on the client's self-concept. In addition, the nurse assesses the client for any educational or cultural needs regarding instruction or therapy and evaluates the client's support system and past mechanisms of coping.

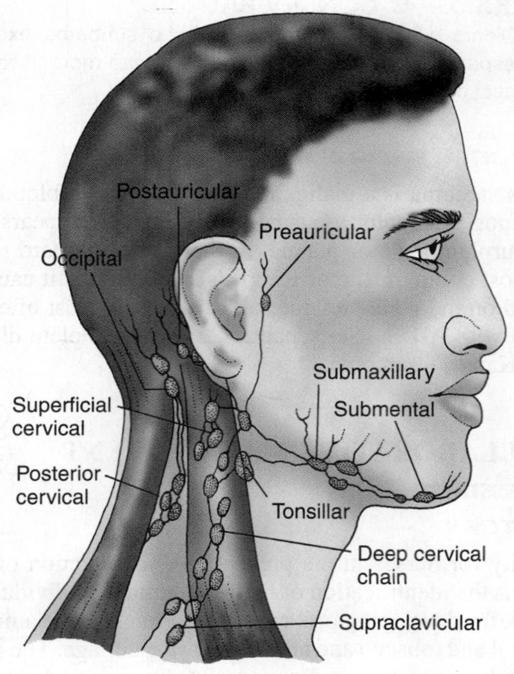

Figure 54-2 ● The lymph nodes of the cervical region.

RADIOGRAPHIC ASSESSMENT

The purpose of radiologic diagnostic tests for cancer of the oral cavity is to assess the extent and spread of the tumor. Computed tomography (CT) scans are helpful in determining the extent of the tumor and lymphatic or bone involvement.

OTHER DIAGNOSTIC ASSESSMENT

Biopsy is the definitive method for diagnosis of oral cancer; therefore the physician obtains a biopsy specimen of the oral tissue to assess for malignant or premalignant changes. Incisional biopsies allow for collection of normal and abnormal tissue. An intraoral biopsy can be done with the client under local anesthesia. In very small lesions, an excisional biopsy can permit complete tumor removal. Magnetic resonance imaging (MRI) is useful in detecting perineural involvement and in evaluating thickness in cancers of the tongue. Both CT and MRI can be used to determine metastatic spread to the liver or lungs if further staging of the disease is warranted.

An aqueous solution of toluidine blue 1% can be applied to oral lesions to determine if they are malignant. This preparation stains malignant lesions, leaving normal tissue unaffected. However, a lesion that is the result of an inflammatory process may also pick up the stain, leading to a false-positive result. Although a biopsy is still needed to confirm a cancer diagnosis, toluidine blue may be useful for screening high-risk individuals.

> **CRITICAL THINKING CHALLENGE**
>
> You are a nurse in a busy family practice clinic. A 67-year-old woman comes in for her annual physical examination. In the course of providing her recent health history, she tells you that she has developed several white patches on her tongue "that won't go away, no matter what I do."
>
> - What questions would be appropriate for the nurse to ask this client in gathering more of her health history?
> - What aspects of the oral cavity assessment should the nurse pay particular attention to?

For suggested answer guidelines, go to SIMON http://www.wbsaunders.com/SIMON/Iggy/.

Analysis

COMMON NURSING DIAGNOSES AND COLLABORATIVE PROBLEMS

The following are priority nursing diagnoses for clients with malignant tumors of the oral cavity:

1. Risk for Ineffective Airway Clearance related to obstruction by the tumor, edema, or secretions
2. Impaired Oral Mucous Membrane related to effects of the tumor

ADDITIONAL NURSING DIAGNOSES AND COLLABORATIVE PROBLEMS

In addition to the common nursing diagnoses, clients with tumors of the oral cavity may have one or more of the following:

- Impaired Verbal Communication related to the tumor or surgery
- Disturbed Body Image related to impaired oral mucous membrane, surgery, chemotherapy, or radiation therapy
- Acute Pain related to impaired oral mucous membrane
- Risk for Infection related to impaired oral mucous membrane

- Impaired Swallowing related to presence of the oral tumor, surgery, or radiation
- Imbalanced Nutrition: Less Than Body Requirements related to pain and/or edema

Planning and Implementation

RISK FOR INEFFECTIVE AIRWAY CLEARANCE

NOC **PLANNING: EXPECTED OUTCOMES.** The client with a malignant tumor of the oral cavity is expected to maintain a patent airway as evidenced by effective coughing, increased air exchange, and the absence of aspiration.

INTERVENTIONS. Extensive tumor involvement and tenacious secretions can impede airway patency. Nursing measures for maintaining airway patency center on assessment for dyspnea, inability to cough effectively, or inability to swallow.

NONSURGICAL MANAGEMENT. The nurse assesses for difficulty breathing and/or decreased air exchange and dysphagia. Measures to increase air exchange, remove secretions, and prevent aspiration are instituted (Chart 54-3).

NIC ***AIRWAY MANAGEMENT.*** The nurse assesses for dyspnea resulting from the obstructive presence of the tumor or from excessive secretions. The nurse assesses the quality, rate, and depth of respirations and auscultates the lungs for decreased or absent ventilation, or for the presence of adventitious sounds. If oral secretions are excessive or thick, the nurse attempts to aid the client in expectorating secretions. To increase air exchange, the client is placed in a semi-Fowler's or high Fowler's position to maximize ventilation potential. Secretions can be mobilized by encouraging fluids to help liquefy secretions, by chest physiotherapy, and by measures to encourage effective coughing. If oral secretions remain problematic, oral suction equipment with a dental tip or a tonsil tip (Yankauer catheter) can be employed.

If edema is associated with oral cavity lesions, the client may receive steroids for reducing inflammation. Antibiotics may be ordered if infection is present, since infection can increase inflammation and edema in the lesion. A cool mist supplied by a face tent may assist with oxygen transport and control of edema.

NIC ***COUGH ENHANCEMENT.*** Measures that promote deep inhalation generate high intrathoracic pressure, which assists the client in producing an effective cough to mobilize secretions. The nurse assists the client to a sitting position with the head slightly flexed and the knees flexed. The nurse then instructs him or her to take several deep breaths, hold the breath for 2 seconds, and then cough two to three times in succession. He or she is instructed to follow coughing with several maximal inhalation breaths. The client can also be instructed to enhance coughing by inhaling deeply several times and coughing at the end of exhalation.

NIC ***ASPIRATION PRECAUTIONS.*** Aspiration precautions prevent or minimize the risk factors associated with aspiration. The nurse assesses the client's level of consciousness, gag reflex, and ability to swallow. To prevent aspiration, the client is placed upright at 90 degrees (high Fowler's position). As a precaution, suction equipment should be kept nearby. Clients at risk of aspiration should be fed in small amounts; thickened liquids can be used to prevent gagging.

SURGICAL MANAGEMENT. The client with an oral lesion may require a tracheostomy preoperatively. This may be due to the extent of surgical excision required to remove the tumor, or it may be due to excessive edema. A tracheostomy re-establishes a patent airway and can be performed by the physician with the client under local or general anesthesia. The tracheostomy tube is usually left in place until edema resolves and the airway is patent. If the tumor is the major cause of the oral airway blockage, however, the tracheostomy may be maintained through the perioperative period until oral healing begins, and in some cases it may be permanent. After postoperative edema resolves, the client is decannulated (the tracheostomy tube is removed). (Refer to Chapter 28 for nursing care of the client with a tracheostomy.)

CHART 54-3

NIC INTERVENTION ACTIVITIES *for* The Client with Oral Cancer

Airway Management: *Facilitation of patency of air passages*
- Position the client to maximize ventilation potential.
- Remove secretions by encouraging coughing or suctioning.
- Instruct how to cough effectively.
- Auscultate breath sounds, noting areas of decreased or absent ventilation and presence of adventitious sounds.
- Administer humidified air or oxygen, as appropriate.
- Position to alleviate dyspnea.
- Monitor respiratory and oxygenation status, as appropriate.

Cough Enhancement: *Promotion of deep inhalation by the client with subsequent generation of high intrathoracic pressures and compression of underlying lung parenchyma for the forceful expulsion of air*
- Assist the client to a sitting position with the head slightly flexed, shoulders relaxed, and knees flexed.
- Encourage client to take several deep breaths.
- Encourage client to take a deep breath, hold it for 2 seconds, and cough two or three times in succession.
- Instruct client to inhale deeply, bend forward slightly, and perform three or four huffs (against an open glottis).
- Instruct client to inhale deeply several times, to exhale slowly, and to cough at the end of exhalation.
- Instruct client to follow coughing with several maximal inhalation breaths.
- Promote systemic fluid hydration, as appropriate.

Aspiration Precautions: *Prevention or minimization of risk factors in the client at risk for aspiration*
- Monitor level of consciousness, cough reflex, gag reflex, and swallowing ability.
- Monitor pulmonary status.
- Maintain an airway.
- Position upright 90 degrees or as far as possible.
- Feed in small amounts.
- Avoid liquids or use thickening agent.
- Offer foods or liquids that can be formed into a bolus before swallowing.
- Cut food into small pieces.
- Request medication in elixir form.
- Break or crush pills before administration.
- Keep head of bed elevated 30 to 45 minutes after eating.

NIC intervention activities selected from McCloskey, J.C., & Bulechek, G.M. (2000). *Nursing interventions classification (NIC)* (3rd ed.). St. Louis: Mosby.

IMPAIRED ORAL MUCOUS MEMBRANE

PLANNING: EXPECTED OUTCOMES. The client with a malignant tumor of the oral cavity is expected to maintain or re-establish oral mucosal integrity.

INTERVENTIONS. Both the presence of tumors of the oral cavity and the effects of treatment of oral tumors pose threats to the integrity of the oral mucosa. Oral cavity lesions can be treated by surgical excision, by nonsurgical treatments such as radiation or chemotherapy, or by a combination of treatments (referred to as multimodal therapy), which is the most expensive treatment option (see the Cost of Care box below). Nursing interventions focus primarily on the restoration and maintenance oral health.

NONSURGICAL MANAGEMENT. The purpose of nonsurgical management is to promote tissue healing and to maintain and promote oral hygiene for the client with oral lesions.

ORAL CARE. The nurse works with the client to establish an oral hygiene routine. Ideally, oral hygiene is performed every 2 hours for ulcerated lesions or infection, or in the immediate postoperative period. Modifications might be needed because of oral discomfort, bleeding, or edema. Oral care with a soft-bristled toothbrush is preferred. In the event of a fall in the platelet count below 40,000/mm^3, the client should be switched to an ultrasoft "chemobrush." The use of toothettes or a disposable foam brush is discouraged because these products may not adequately control bacteremia-promoting plaque (Toth et al., 1995)(see the Evidence-Based Practice for Nursing box at right). Lubricant can be applied to moisten the lips and oral mucosa as needed.

Clients with ulcerative or bleeding lesions should avoid using commercial mouthwashes and lemon-glycerin swabs. Commercial mouthwashes contain alcohol, and lemon-glycerin swabs are acidic. These substances can cause a burning sensation and contribute to drying of the oral mucous membranes. The nurse encourages frequent rinsing of the mouth with sodium bicarbonate solution, warm saline, or hydrogen peroxide solution (see also Chart 54-2).

RADIATION THERAPY. Radiation therapy has been used alone, as well as in conjunction with surgery and chemotherapy, in the treatment of cancer of the oral cavity. The goal of radiation therapy is tumor eradication while preserving function and appearance. There are several ways to apply radiotherapy. In collaboration with the client, the physician chooses the best mode on the basis of the tumor site and staging.

Radiation therapy for oral cancers can be given by external beam or interstitial implantation. External beam radiation passes through the skin or mucous membrane to the tumor site. Typically, treatments are given as five daily treatments per week over a 6- to 9-week period. Special precautions are taken to minimize the dose of radiation to the brain or spinal cord. Another option is the implantation of radioactive substances (interstitial radiation therapy) to either boost the dosage or deliver a radiation dose close to the tumor bed. This form of implant therapy can be curative in early-stage lesions in the floor of the mouth or anterior tongue, or to add an ad-

COST OF CARE IMPLICATIONS FOR NURSING

ORAL CAVITY PROBLEMS

Cost of Care

- The cost of medical-surgical care for clients with oral cancer in the United States is thought to be approximately $3.7 billion.
- The variables identified as being significantly associated with treatment costs are TNM stage, single-modality treatment versus multimodality treatment, and comorbidity grade.
- The majority of costs are incurred during the treatment phase.

Implications for Nursing

The majority of the costs associated with oral cavity cancer care are incurred during treatment, especially if treatment involves a combination of surgery, chemotherapy, and radiation. Measures to permit early identification and treatment of the disease at a stage where single-modality treatment can be used more effectively would yield substantial decreases in management costs. Client education about the risk factors for oral cancer plus rigorous assessment of those with high-risk profiles (e.g., heavy alcohol and tobacco use) would be cost-effective in reducing the incidence and permitting early diagnosis and treatment of the disease.

Data from Funk, G.F., et al. (1998). Cost-identification analysis in oral cavity cancer management. *Otolaryngology–Head and Neck Surgery, 118*(2), 211-220.

EVIDENCE-BASED PRACTICE FOR NURSING

Do foam swabs work as well as toothbrushes to remove dental plaque?

Pearson, L. (1996). A comparison of the ability of foam swabs and toothbrushes to remove dental plaque: Implications for nursing practice. *Journal of Advanced Nursing, 23,* 62-69.

The purpose of this study was to compare the effectiveness of a toothbrush and a foam swab in the removal of dental plaque over a 6-day period. Three experiments were conducted using the mouth of the author and a volunteer. A plaque scoring system was used to quantify the amount of plaque left on teeth adjacent to periodontal tissue. Plaque amounts were measured at the gum-tooth margin (gingival crevice plaque) and between teeth (approximal plaque).

At the end of 6 days, the ability of the toothbrush to remove plaque was noted to be superior to that of the foam swab; the toothbrush usually achieved complete removal of all visible plaque from the sites examined. The sites cleansed by the foam swabs revealed remaining plaque after using the "scrubbing" or "swabbing" technique outlined. When plaque was allowed to accumulate over a 6-day period, similar results were obtained. This study suggests that toothbrush use is more effective than foam swabs in removing plaque, but results could be impacted by user technique.

Critique. The very small sample size (2), as well as the use of the researcher as a study subject, may have permitted bias to be introduced into this study. It is also unclear who assigned the plaque scores to the study subjects. However, as nursing builds knowledge for evidence-based practice, the efficiency and utility of using these two mouth cleansing modalities need further examination.

Implications for Nursing. Nurses need to consider the aim of the intervention in selecting an instrument for mouth care. If the aim is to hydrate oral mucosa, a foam swab will deliver moisture to the tissues in an adequate fashion. Also, if damage to fragile oral mucosal tissue is a concern, a foam swab causes minimal damage. However, if removal of dental debris is the aim of mouth care, then the selection of a toothbrush appears to be more appropriate. This becomes important, since controlling plaque is a concern for those clients who may be immunocompromised (the overgrowth and invasion of organisms from plaque can be of concern).

ditional boost of radiation to a tumor that received external beam radiation.

Interstitial radiation is used for smaller lesions that do not infiltrate surrounding tissues. The following can be radioactive materials:

- Seeds, which are permanently implanted into the tissue (usually for tumors unable to be completely excised, or in neck nodes)
- Needles or wires, which are extracted at the end of therapy
- Radiation catheters or holders, which are loaded with radioactive materials
- A "mold" of radioactive material placed directly over the lesion for a specific time

The dose of interstitial therapy is often difficult to calculate. With the exception of radioactive seeds, which have a low level of activity, clients receiving interstitial radiation are usually hospitalized for the duration of treatment. Radiation isolation precautions must be instituted while the materials are active or in place. A tracheostomy may be required with interstitial implants because of edema and increased oral secretions. (See Chapter 25 for nursing care of clients undergoing radiation therapy.)

CRITICAL THINKING CHALLENGE

The white patches on your client's tongue have been diagnosed as leukoplakia. In addition, a biopsy performed on a nodule located on the floor of the mouth was determined to be squamous cell carcinoma. The client is preparing to undergo surgical excision and adjunctive treatment with radiation.

- What should the nurse include in the preoperative teaching for this client?
- What complications from the treatment is this client at risk for?
- What measures should the nurse include in the oral hygiene care for this client?

For suggested answer guidelines, go to SIMON http://www.wbsaunders.com/SIMON/Iggy/.

CHEMOTHERAPY. The client may receive one or more chemotherapeutic agents (Table 54-3). The advantages of chemotherapy instead of, or as an adjunct to, surgery or radiation for cancer of the oral cavity continue to be evaluated.

Recent trials have been conducted on the use of two individual agents—mitomycin and cisplatin—to prevent local recurrence and improve survival. Response rates have varied from 0% to 30% (Vikram, 1998; Witt, 1998). The nurse instructs the client undergoing chemotherapy about the anticipated side effects of the medication, which vary with each agent. The nurse administers antiemetic medications as prescribed and provides other comfort measures as needed.

SURGICAL MANAGEMENT. The physician can often excise small, noninvasive lesions of the oral cavity in an ambulatory setting with local anesthesia. The surgical defect is usually small enough to be closed by sutures. These smaller lesions are also responsive to carbon dioxide laser therapy or *cryotherapy* (extreme cold application), which can be performed as an ambulatory care procedure in a surgical center (but may require general anesthesia).

Small oral cancers are equally responsive to radiation therapy and to surgery. More invasive lesions (stage III and IV) require more extensive surgical excision and result in a greater loss of function and disfigurement. Not all lesions can be excised by the peroral approach (through the mouth). The goal of surgical resection is the removal of the tumor with a surgical margin that is free of tumor involvement.

PREOPERATIVE CARE. Before excision of a lesion of the oral cavity, the nurse assesses and documents the client's level of understanding of the disease process, the rationale for the surgery, and the planned intervention. Information is reinforced as needed. The nurse identifies family members or other caregivers and includes them in health teaching.

For small, local excisions, postoperative restrictions include a liquid diet for a day, then soft foods. There are no activity limitations, and postoperative analgesics are prescribed.

The nurse instructs the client undergoing large surgical resections about the following:

- The placement of a temporary tracheostomy for approximately 10 days and the concomitant nursing care (oxygen therapy and suctioning)
- Temporary loss of speech due to the tracheostomy
- The need for vital signs to be taken frequently postoperatively
- The need to take nothing by mouth (remain on NPO status) for 10 to 14 days until intraoral suture lines are healed
- The need to have IV lines in place for medication delivery and hydration
- Postoperative medications and activity (out of bed on the first postoperative day)
- Any surgical drains

The nurse also assesses the client's ability to read and write. The client and nurse select the method of communication to use postoperatively with staff and family members (e.g., Magic Slate, picture board, or pad and pencil).

OPERATIVE PROCEDURES. Three factors influence the type of surgery performed for oral cancers: the size and location of the tumor, tumor invasion into the bone, and the presence of metastasis to neck lymph nodes (Olsen, 1999). Small tumors (2 cm or less) located near the mouth opening can be excised perorally (inside the mouth). Otherwise, an external approach may be used. The surgeon may approach the oral cavity from under the mandible or may split the lower lip and retract the lips and cheek for exposure. The mandible is occasionally split as well and pushed aside for oral access; it is wired at the end of the operation. The most extensive oral operations are composite resections, which combine partial or total **glossectomy** (tongue removal) and partial mandibulectomy. In the *commando* (co-mandible) *procedure,* the surgeon excises a segment of the mandible with the oral lesion, usually in conjunction with a radical neck dissection (see Chapter 29). If the anterior mandible is resected to treat tumor invasion in that area, the mandible is reconstructed after the

TABLE 54-3 • COMMON CHEMOTHERAPEUTIC DRUGS USED IN CLIENTS WITH SQUAMOUS CELL CARCINOMA OF THE HEAD AND NECK

• Methotrexate	• Doxorubicin
• Bleomycin	• Vincristine
• Cisplatin (*cis*-platinum)	• 5-Fluorouracil
• Cyclophosphamide	• Hydroxyurea

resection to decrease speech and swallowing problems postoperatively and improve appearance. For clients undergoing a complete glossectomy, a prosthesis will be necessary to aid in swallowing and speech.

Metastasis to cervical lymph nodes usually indicates a poor prognosis for clients with cancer of the oral cavity. In clients with cervical node metastasis, a neck dissection may also be performed. A radical neck dissection involves the removal of submental; submandibular; upper, mid, and lower jugular; and posterior triangular levels of the cervical lymph nodes, along with cranial nerve XI, the internal jugular vein, and the sternocleidomastoid muscle. Modified and selective neck dissections may be done in individuals with minimal lymph node involvement.

POSTOPERATIVE CARE. Postoperative care of the client with cancer of the oral cavity focuses on airway management as a priority. The client will have a temporary tracheostomy placed, requiring intensive nursing care to promote airway clearance. In addition, care must be taken to protect the surgical incision site from mechanical damage and infection. Nursing interventions to relieve pain or discomfort and promote nutrition are also important.

Maintaining Airway Patency. After extensive excision or resection, the most important nursing intervention is maintaining airway patency. The client may not recall on awakening from anesthesia that a tracheostomy tube is in place and may initially panic because of the inability to speak. The nurse reminds the client why he or she cannot speak and provides reassurance that the vocal cords are intact (unless a total laryngectomy has been performed, then the loss of voice is permanent). The nurse provides the client with the predetermined method of communication.

Nursing interventions are aimed at keeping the temporary tracheostomy patent. Frequent suctioning, using sterile technique, may be required for excessive secretions. Humidified oxygen may be ordered to help liquefy secretions in the early postoperative phase. After the immediate postoperative phase, the client may be able to cough effectively enough to decrease the need for suctioning. After oral edema has decreased and the tracheostomy tube has been changed to a noncuffed type, the client can speak by plugging the stoma with the fingertip. The nurse and physician determine the appropriateness of instructing the client in this technique. (See Chapter 28 for care of the client with a tracheostomy.)

When the client has been determined to have an adequate airway through the areodigestive tract and can effectively clear secretions by coughing, the tracheostomy tube is removed. An airtight dressing is placed over the tracheostomy site, and the incision heals without the need for sutures. The client is instructed to press fingers over the dressing to prevent the incision from separating during coughing (Reese, 1996).

Clients who have undergone extensive resection may have slurred speech or difficulty in speaking. The nurse assesses the need for consultation with a speech/language pathologist.

Protecting the Operative Area. The surgical incision site requires careful attention to avoid infection. The nurse or assistive nursing personnel provides gentle mouth care for cleaning away thick secretions and stimulating the flow of saliva. The delivery of oral care depends on the nature and extent of the surgical procedure. Oral care should be provided every 4 hours in the early postoperative phase. The presence of unusual odors from the mouth can indicate infection. In the early postoperative phase, care must be taken to avoid disruption of the suture line during oral hygiene.

The nurse elevates the head of the bed to at least 30 degrees to assist in decreasing edema by gravity. If skin grafting was done, the nurse inspects the donor site (generally on the anterior thigh) during every nursing shift for bleeding or manifestations of infection. (See Chapter 29 for specific nursing care of the client with a radical neck dissection.)

Relieving Pain. To provide optimal pain relief in the postoperative period, the nurse relies on subjective and objective data to assess the need for analgesics and the effectiveness of the medications given. The goal of pain medication during this period is relief of pain while allowing the client to function at an optimal level. Clients who have undergone surgery for oral carcinomas describe their pain as throbbing or pounding. IV morphine is usually the initial postoperative pain medication given. Oral acetaminophen combined with codeine (Tylenol with Codeine) may be used for systemic relief of moderate pain.

Promoting Nutrition. Clients who have undergone extensive resections of the oral cavity remain on NPO status for 5 to 7 days or longer. This allows healing in the oral cavity before food contacts the incision. Nasogastric feeding or total parenteral nutrition is needed during this time (see Chapter 61). The tubes are usually inserted in the operating room.

When oral fluid intake is begun, the nurse assesses for and documents difficulty in swallowing, aspiration, or leakage of saliva or fluids from the suture line. Nursing care should also include the monitoring of weight and hydration. Nutritional supplementation may be used to improve the client's quality of life (see the Legal/Ethical Issues in Health Care box below). Clients experiencing weight loss or having difficulty maintaining hydration may be candidates for gastrostomy tube placement.

A speech/language pathologist is often consulted to assist with swallowing techniques. A swallowing impairment may be temporary or permanent. The client is encouraged to perform swallowing exercises.

Legal/Ethical Issues in Health Care

NUTRITIONAL SUPPLEMENTATION IN CLIENTS UNDERGOING RADIATION TREATMENTS

Maintaining optimal nutritional status for individuals with oral carcinoma is a difficult task, considering the many aspects of digestion impacted by the disease and treatment. Radiation therapy can pose additional challenges to nutrition because of the decreased saliva flow and alterations in taste that can result. Not only does increasing evidence point to nutritional status as a predictor of overall survival, but the ability to eat and enjoy food is an important component of quality of life.

The purpose of the study by McCarthy and Weihofen (1999) was to describe the effect of nutritional supplements on the food intake of clients undergoing radiotherapy. Forty clients beginning external beam radiation therapy were given weekly dietary counseling. The daily food intake was recorded 3 days per week for 4 weeks. One half of the subjects were assigned to ingest a nutritional supplement between meals and at bedtime. Findings suggested that those who ingested the nutritional supplements significantly increased their total caloric and protein intake while not reducing their food-derived caloric and protein intake. Based on this study, the addition of nutritional supplements to the normal food intake for clients undergoing radiotherapy for the treatment of oral cancer may be a viable option in helping to maintain adequate nutrition.

From McCarthy, D. & Weihofen, D. (1999). The effect of nutritional supplements on food intake in patients undergoing radiotherapy. *Oncology Nursing Forum, 26*(5), 897-900.

Community-Based Care

Continuing care for the client with an oral tumor depends on the severity of the tumor, the treatment for the tumor, and available support systems. Most clients are maintained at home during follow-up care. Ongoing nutritional management remains a vital part of the treatment plan. In addition, the short- and long-term effects of the treatment for cancers of the oral cavity must be monitored once the client is discharged home.

HOME CARE MANAGEMENT

If radiation therapy is part of the client's treatment plan, home care considerations include preparatory information and management strategies. Complications due to radiation to the head or neck can be acute or delayed. Acute effects include treatment-related mucositis, stomatitis, and alterations in taste. Long-term effects such as xerostomia (excessive mouth dryness) and dental decay require ongoing oral care, the use of saliva substitutes, and follow-up dental visits. Although ongoing dental care is important, the possible adverse effects that radiation has on the cellular elements of the bone make elective oral surgical procedures, such as tooth extraction, impossible in the area of the radiation. Fatigue, which can be either short or long term, is a common side effect of radiation and chemotherapy.

The client whose tracheostomy has been removed is often taking a soft diet by mouth before discharge. Occasionally, however, clients are discharged from the hospital while still requiring tracheostomy suction, oral suction, and nasogastric feedings. Suction equipment, nutritional supplies, and nursing care can be provided by home care companies. (See Chapter 61 for home care preparation for the client receiving home parenteral nutrition and Chapter 28 for home care preparation for the client with a tracheostomy.)

HEALTH TEACHING

The nurse instructs the client and family about medications, diet or feedings, any treatments (such as tracheostomy care, suture line care, and dressing changes), and early symptoms of infection.

Alterations in taste and dysphagia make maintaining adequate nutritional status a challenge. Alterations in taste occur when the taste buds are included in the radiation treatment field. Taste sensation begins to return several weeks after the completion of treatment. Changes in taste include aversions for meat, such as beef or pork, and metallic tastes in the mouth. Clients can be taught to add seasonings to foods, to use gravies or sauces to make foods more palatable, and to use high-protein foods such as cheeses, milk, eggs, puddings, and legumes in place of meat. Clients with dysphagia are instructed in swallowing exercises. Thickened liquids are recommended, since thin liquids, such as water, are difficult to control during swallowing. In collaboration with the dietitian, the nurse instructs the client and family on how to assess the nutritional intake of the client who is just beginning to eat. Liquid dietary supplements are usually recommended at this time. If bleeding is a problem, or if mucositis is present, a diet of soft foods that will not cause injury to the mucous membranes is preferred.

The nurse instructs the client and/or family members to inspect the oral cavity daily for areas of redness, indicating the onset of mucositis, or for lesions indicative of stomatitis. Meticulous oral hygiene should be continued in the postoperative phase, especially if adjuvant chemotherapy or radiation is planned or underway. The nurse reinforces the oral hygiene routine, putting particular emphasis on the need for frequent rinsing of the oral cavity to reduce the number of microorganisms and maintain hydration. The client should use a chemobrush, should rinse the chemobrush with hydrogen peroxide and water following each use, and should change chemobrushes weekly.

If the salivary glands were part of the radiation field, the client is instructed in the daily use of a fluoride gel to prevent dental caries. A 1% sodium fluoride gel is placed in a customized applicator that completely covers the tooth surface. This applicator is worn for 10 minutes daily. Saliva production is greatly reduced as a consequence of radiation. The resulting xerostomia results in the inability to eat dry foods. The nurse instructs the client in the use of saliva substitutes.

Skin reactions are also a common side effect of radiation. The nurse should instruct the client to avoid sun exposure, to avoid perfumed lotions or powders, and to cleanse the face or neck area with a gentle, nondeodorant soap.

To increase retention of the information, the client and the family demonstrate the skills they are taught. The nurse evaluates and documents their understanding of the treatments.

> **CONSIDERATIONS FOR OLDER ADULTS**
>
> For the older client with metastatic or invasive oral cancer, skilled home care or nursing home services are required for pain management, nutrition maintenance, and emotional support. Older adults often take subtherapeutic doses of analgesics for fear of becoming addicted. The home care nurse teaches the client about the need to promote comfort to improve nutrition and prevent depression. Chart 54-4 summarizes the focused nursing assessment for the older adult with oral cancer. (See Chapter 7 for further information on pain management in older adults.)

HEALTH CARE RESOURCES

Clients who have undergone composite resection often require community services, because they have both physical and psychosocial needs. Clients who have undergone surgical excision experience depression related to a change in body image. Excision of a portion of the mandible can leave a facial defect that may be difficult to hide. A social worker or other health care professional may be needed for client and family counseling. Clients who have undergone a total glossectomy may be able to speak with special training and the use of an intraoral prosthesis fashioned by a maxillofacial prosthodontist. The prosthesis is similar to dentures, with augmentation to approximate the oral articulating surfaces.

CHART 54-4

FOCUSED ASSESSMENT *of* The Older Adult with Oral Cancer

- Assess the mouth and surrounding tissues for candidiasis, mucositis, pain, and loss of appetite and taste.
- Monitor the client's weight.
- Monitor nutritional and fluid intake.
- Assess for difficulty in eating or speech.
- Assess pain status and measures used to control pain.
- Monitor the client's response to medications.
- Identify psychosocial problems, such as depression, anxiety, and fear.

The nurse consults the social worker or case manager for assistance in obtaining special equipment or nutritional resources required by the client at home. The case manager assesses the financial needs of the client and makes referrals to government, community, and religious organizations as needed.

Evaluation: Outcomes

NOC The nurse evaluates the care of the client with a malignant tumor of the oral cavity on the basis of the identified nursing diagnoses and collaborative problems. The expected outcomes include that the client:

- Maintains a patent oral airway through removal of oral secretions
- Maintains nutritional status by eating foods that are well tolerated and nutritious
- Communicates thoughts and feelings to family members, friends, and health care personnel
- Maintains the integrity of the oral mucous membrane

DISORDERS OF THE SALIVARY GLANDS

Acute Sialadenitis

OVERVIEW

Acute sialadenitis, the inflammation of a salivary gland, can be caused by infectious agents, irradiation, or immunologic disorders. Salivary gland inflammation can have a bacterial or viral etiology. Acute sialadenitis can be caused by infection with cytomegalovirus (CMV). The most common bacterial organisms are *Staphylococcus aureus, Staphylococcus pyogenes, Streptococcus pneumoniae,* and *Escherichia coli.* This disorder most commonly affects the parotid or submandibular gland in adults.

A decrease in the production of saliva (as in dehydrated or debilitated clients or in those who are on NPO status postoperatively for an extended time) usually precipitates acute sialadenitis. The bacteria or viruses enter the gland through the ductal opening in the oral cavity. Systemic medications, such as phenothiazines, chloramphenicol, and oxytetracycline, can also precipitate an episode of acute sialadenitis. Untreated infections of the salivary glands can evolve into abscesses, which can rupture and spread infection into the tissues of the neck and the mediastinum.

Clients who receive radiation for the treatment of cancers of the head and neck or thyroid may develop decreased salivary flow, predisposing them to acute or persistent sialadenitis. The effect of radiation on the salivary glands is rapid and dose related (Mandel & Mandel, 1999; McEwen & Sanchez, 1997). Immunologic disorders such as HIV infection can cause enlargement of the parotid gland that can be due to secondary infection. Sjögren's syndrome, an autoimmune disorder, is characterized by chronic salivary gland enlargement and inflammation (see Chapter 21).

COLLABORATIVE MANAGEMENT

Assessment

During the initial interview, the nurse assesses for any predisposing factors for sialadenitis, such as ionizing radiation to the head or neck area. The nurse asks about systemic illnesses such as HIV infection and collects a thorough medication history.

The presence of dehydration can be noted by assessing the oral cavity and the skin for turgor. Other assessment findings include pain and swelling of the face over the affected gland. Cranial nerve function is tested, since the branches of the facial nerve lie close to the salivary glands. Fever and general malaise also occur, and purulent drainage can often be massaged from the affected duct in the oral cavity (Chart 54-5).

Interventions

Collaborative management includes the administration of IV fluids and measures such as the following to treat the underlying cause and increase the flow of saliva:

- Hydration
- Application of warm compresses
- Massage of the gland
- Use of a saliva substitute
- Use of **sialagogues** (substances that stimulate the flow of saliva)

Sialagogues include lemon slices and fruit- or citrus-flavored candy. Massage is accomplished by milking the edematous gland with the fingertips toward the ductal opening. Elevation of the head of the bed promotes gravity drainage of the edematous gland.

Acute sialadenitis is best prevented by adherence to routine oral hygiene. This practice prohibits infections from ascending to the salivary glands from the oral cavity.

Postirradiation Sialadenitis

The salivary glands are sensitive to ionizing radiation, such as from radiation therapy or radioactive iodine treatment of thyroid cancers. Exposure of the glands to radiation produces **xerostomia** (very dry mouth caused by severe reduction in the flow of saliva) within 24 hours. Radiation to the salivary glands can also produce pain and edema, which generally abate after several days.

Xerostomia may be temporary or permanent, depending on the dose of radiation and the percentage of total salivary gland tissue irradiated. Little can be done to relieve the client's dry mouth during the course of radiation therapy. Frequent sips of water and frequent mouth care, especially before meals, are the most effective interventions. After the course of radiation therapy has been completed, saliva substitutes may provide moisture for 2 to 4 hours at a time. Over-the-counter solutions are available, or solutions may be mixed with methylcellulose (Cologel), glycerin, and saline.

Salivary Gland Tumors

OVERVIEW

Tumors of the salivary glands are relatively rare; they constitute 5% of all oral tumors. Initially they present as slow-growing, painless masses (McEwen & Sanchez, 1997). Malignant tumors are characterized by more rapid growth than that of be-

CHART 54-5

KEY FEATURES *of* Sialadenitis

- Swelling on the sides of the face or under the tongue, which increases when the client eats
- Alteration in the quantity or appearance of saliva
- Pain, especially during eating
- Purulent drainage from the affected duct

nign tumors and are generally associated with pain. Involvement of the facial nerve, more common with malignant tumors, results in facial weakness or paralysis (partial or total) on the affected side. Needle aspiration biopsy and open biopsy are useful procedures in establishing a diagnosis.

COLLABORATIVE MANAGEMENT

Assessment

The nurse collects information concerning prior radiation exposure, since radiation to the head and neck areas is associated with the occurrence of salivary gland tumors. Salivary gland malignancies present as localized, firm masses. In advanced stages of salivary gland tumors, the nurse may note a large preauricular mass accompanied by facial nerve paralysis. Submandibular and minor salivary gland tumors may be tender or painful. Tumor invasion of the hypoglossal nerve causes impaired movement of the tongue, and a loss of sensation can follow. The nurse pays particular attention to assessment of the facial nerve because of its close proximity to the salivary glands. The nurse assesses the client's ability to:

- Wrinkle the brow
- Raise the eyebrows
- Squeeze the eyes shut
- Wrinkle the nose
- Pucker the lips
- Puff out the cheeks
- Grimace or smile

Interventions

The treatment of choice for both benign and malignant tumors of the salivary glands is surgical excision. However, radiation therapy is often used for salivary gland cancers that are large, have recurred, show evidence of residual disease after excision, or are highly malignant.

Clients who have undergone **parotidectomy** (surgical removal of the parotid glands) or submandibular gland surgery are at risk for weakness or loss of function of the facial nerve because the nerve courses directly through the gland. Facial nerve repair with autogenous nerve grafting can be done at the time of surgery. The majority of studies support combining surgery with postoperative radiation for advanced disease.

ONLINE RESOURCES

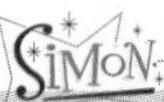

For suggested readings and Internet resources, go to http://www.wbsaunders.com/SIMON/Iggy/.

SELECTED BIBLIOGRAPHY

Asterisk indicates a classic or definitive work on this subject.

Aubertin, M.A. (1997). Home care of the elderly oral cancer patient. *Home Healthcare Nurse, 15*(6), 381-390.

Bagan, J., et al. (1998). Preliminary investigation of the association of oral lichen planus and hepatitis C. *Oral Surgery, Oral Medicine, Oral Pathology, Oral Radiology, and Endodontics 85*(5), 532-535.

*Barnes, L., et al. (1996). Basaloid squamous cell carcinoma of the head and neck: Clinicopathological features and differential diagnosis. *Annals of Otology, Rhinology, and Laryngology, 105,* 75-82.

*Beck, S. (1996). Mucositis. In S. Groenwald et al. (Eds.), *Cancer symptom management* (pp. 308-323). Boston: Jones & Bartlett.

Burkhart, N.W., Burkes, E.J., & Burker, E.J. (1997). Meeting the educational needs of patients with oral lichen planus. *General Dentistry,* 126-131.

Dixon, D., Breeding, L., & Faler, T. (1999). Microwave disinfection of denture base materials colonized with *Candida albicans. Journal of Prosthetic Dentistry, 81*(2), 207-214.

*Dose, A. (1995). The symptom experience of mucositis, stomatitis, and xerostomia. *Seminars in Oncology Nursing, 11*(4), 248-255.

Eilers, J. (1997). Stomatitis as a side effect of cancer treatment. *Quality of Life: A Nursing Challenge, 5*(3), 68-74.

Freer, S.K. (2000). Use of an oral assessment tool to improve practice. *Professional Nurse, 15*(10), 635-639.

Greenlee, R., et al. (2000). Cancer statistics, 2000. *Ca: A Cancer Journal for Clinicians, 50*(1), 7-33.

Hyland, S. (1997). Assessing the oral cavity. In M. Frank-Stromborg & S. Olsen (Eds.), *Instruments for clinical health care research* (2nd ed.). Boston: Jones & Bartlett.

Klaus, B., & Grodesky, M. (1998). Common oral manifestations seen in patients with HIV/AIDS. *Nurse Practitioner, 23*(6), 134-139.

Mandel, S., & Mandel, R. (1999). Persistent sialadenitis after radioactive iodine therapy: Report of two cases. *Journal of Oral Maxillofacial Surgery, 57*(7), 738-741.

McCarthy, D., & Weihofen, D. (1999). The effect of nutritional supplements on food intake in patients undergoing radiotherapy. *Oncology Nursing Forum, 26*(5), 897-900.

McEwen, D., & Sanchez, M. (1997). A guide to salivary gland disorders. *AORN Journal, 65*(3), 554-566.

National Cancer Institute. (1999). *SEER cancer incidence public-use database CD-ROM, 1973-1999,* Bethesda, MD: Public Health Service, U.S. Department of Health and Human Services.

Olsen, M. (1999). Oral cavity cancer. In C. Miaskowski & P. Buchsel (Eds.), *Oncology nursing: Assessment and clinical care* (pp. 1177-1201). St. Louis: Mosby.

Parkin, D., Pisani, P., & Ferlay, J. (1999). Global cancer statistics. *CA: A Cancer Journal for Clinicians, 49*(1), 33-64.

*Pearson, L. (1996). A comparison of the ability of foam swabs and toothbrushes to remove dental plaque: Implications for nursing practice. *Journal of Advanced Nursing, 23,* 62-69.

*Peterson, M.J., & Baughman, R. (1996). Recurrent aphthous stomatitis: Primary care management. *Nurse Practitioner, 21*(5), 36-47.

*Ransier, A., et al. (1995). A combined analysis of a toothbrush, foam brush, and a chlorhexidine-soaked foam brush in maintaining oral hygiene. *Cancer Nursing, 18*(5), 393-396.

*Reese, J. (1996). Head and neck cancers. In R. McCorkle et al. (Eds.), *Cancer nursing: A comprehensive textbook* (2nd ed., pp. 773-795). Philadelphia: W.B. Saunders.

Sheff, B. (1999). Oral *Candida albicans. Nursing99, 29*(7), 25.

Shugars, D., & Patton, L. (1997). Detecting, diagnosing, and preventing oral cancer. *Nurse Practitioner, 22*(6), 105-129.

Shuster, J. (1998). Inhaled steroids and oral candidiasis. *Nursing98,* May, p.25.

*Toth, B., et al. (1995). Minimizing oral complications of cancer treatment. *Oncology, 9*(9), 851-858.

Vikram, B., (1998). Adjuvant therapy in head and neck cancer. *Ca: A Cancer Journal for Clinicians, 48*(4): 199-209.

Walton, J.C., Miller, J., & Tordecilla, L. (2001). Elder oral assessment and care. *MEDSURG Nursing, 10*(1), 37-44.

Witt, M.E. (1998). Radiation and chemotherapy as combined treatment for advanced head and neck cancer. *MEDSURG Nursing, 7*(3), 159-164.

*Woo, S., & Sonis, S. (1996). Recurrent aphthous ulcers: A review of diagnosis and management. *Journal of the American Dental Association, 127,* 1202-1211.

CHAPTER

55

Interventions for Clients with Esophageal Problems

CONSTANCE VISOVSKY

Learning Objectives

After studying this chapter, you should be able to:

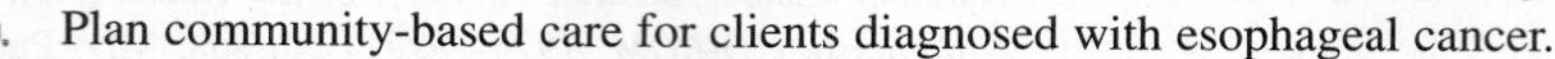

1. Explain the pathophysiology of gastroesophageal reflux disease (GERD).
2. Assess the client who is experiencing GERD.
3. Plan the nursing care for clients with GERD.
4. Develop a postoperative teaching plan for the client having a hiatal hernia repair.
5. Identify the differences in the incidence of esophageal cancer among cultural groups.
6. Describe the risk factors for esophageal cancer.
7. Analyze assessment data to determine common nursing diagnoses for the client with esophageal cancer.
8. Discuss the priorities for postoperative care of the client undergoing surgery for esophageal cancer.
9. Plan community-based care for clients diagnosed with esophageal cancer.

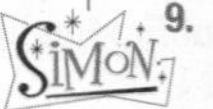

Go to http://www.wbsaunders.com/SIMON/Iggy/ for self-assessment questions related to these Learning Objectives.

Esophageal disorders affect approximately 546,000 people in the United States. One third of the population experiences symptoms associated with the reflux of stomach acid into the esophagus. Impaired gastroesophageal motility resulting from achalasia or diverticula is responsible for 400,000 visits to health care providers annually (see the Cost of Care Box on p. 1193).

The esophagus is a hollow, distensible muscular tube located behind the trachea that acts primarily as a conduit for food from the mouth to the stomach. It passes through the diaphragm at the esophageal hiatus and extends to the gastroesophageal junction. The esophagus is susceptible to a variety of inflammatory, structural, motor, and neoplastic disorders. Collaborative management involves medical and surgical therapies in addition to diet and lifestyle modifications. Nurses have a significant role in assisting clients in making the lifestyle changes necessary for the successful prevention and management of esophageal disorders.

GASTROESOPHAGEAL REFLUX DISEASE

OVERVIEW

Esophageal reflux is defined as the backward flow of gastrointestinal contents into the esophagus. Reflux produces its characteristic symptoms by exposing the esophageal mucosa to the irritating effects of gastric and/or duodenal contents, resulting in inflammatory changes of the esophageal mucosa. A person with acute symptoms of inflammation is often described as having **reflux esophagitis,** a hallmark of gastroesophageal reflux disease (GERD). Reflux esophagitis is graded according the extent and severity of the lesions.

Pathophysiology

The following physiologic factors are implicated in the development of GERD (Tucker & Schumann, 1999):

- An incompetent lower esophageal sphincter
- Irritation from the refluxate
- Abnormal esophageal clearance
- Delayed gastric emptying

The reflux of gastric contents into the esophagus is normally prevented by the presence of two high-pressure areas that remain relatively contracted in the resting phase. A 3-cm (1.2-inch) segment at the proximal end of the esophagus is called the upper esophageal sphincter (UES). Another 2- to 4-cm (0.8- to 1.6-inch) portion just proximal to the gastroesophageal junction is called the lower esophageal sphincter (LES). The function of the LES is supported by its anatomic placement in the abdomen, where the surrounding pressure is significantly higher than in the low-pressure thorax. Sphincter function is also supported by the acute angle (angle of His) that is formed as the esophagus enters the stomach. Esophageal reflux can occur when gastric volume or intra-abdominal pressure is elevated, when the sphincter tone of the LES is decreased, or when the LES undergoes inappropriate relaxation.

COST OF CARE IMPLICATIONS FOR NURSING

ESOPHAGEAL PROBLEMS

Cost of Care

- Ambulatory care for clients with Barrett's esophagus costs approximately $103 per month, or $1241 per year.
- Clients with low-grade dysplasia (tissue changes) are three times as likely to have more than 3 endoscopies per year as compared to clients who do not have dysplasia.
- Endoscopies and clinic visits account for 31% and 5.9%, respectively, of the monthly medical costs.
- The medication costs per month for clients with Barrett's esophagus is $65.
- Proton-pump inhibitors account for 64.6% of the total medication cost.
- Medications account for more than 50% of the total cost of care.

Implications for Nursing

Prolonged gastrointestinal reflux leading to Barrett's esophagus or disease results in a relatively high cost of care in terms of the need for health care services. Clients require ongoing monitoring by endoscopy for dysplastic changes in the mucosa, long-term medication adherence to control reflux, and primary care provider visits. Nurses can play an integral role in the prevention of gastrointestinal reflux by educating their clients about the risk factors for developing reflux, strategies for managing reflux, and the necessity of making lifestyle adjustments that prevent esophageal damage.

Data from Eloubeidi, M., et al. (1999). A cost analysis of outpatient care for patients with Barrett's esophagus in a managed care setting. *The American Journal of Gastroenterology, 94*(8), 2033-2036.

An individual experiencing reflux may be asymptomatic and relatively unaware that reflux is occurring. However, the esophagus has only a limited resistance to the damaging effects of the acidic gastrointestinal (GI) contents. The pH of acid secreted by the stomach ranges from 1.5 to 2.0, whereas the pH of the distal esophagus is normally neutral (6.0 to 7.0). Repeated exposure of the esophageal mucosa to highly acid gastric secretions is associated with the development of erosive esophagitis.

Refluxed material is returned to the stomach by a combination of gravity, saliva, and peristalsis. The effectiveness of the clearance mechanism is very important. An inflamed esophagus cannot eliminate the refluxed material as quickly or efficiently as a healthy one, and therefore the duration of exposure increases with each reflux episode.

Hyperemia (increased blood flow) and erosion occur in the esophagus in response to the chronic inflammation. Gastric acid and pepsin are responsible for the tissue injury. Minor capillary bleeding often accompanies the erosion, but frank hemorrhage is rare. During the process of healing, the body may substitute a columnar epithelium (Barrett's epithelium) for the normal squamous cell epithelium of the lower esophagus. Although this new tissue is more resistant to acid and therefore supports esophageal healing, it is considered premalignant and is associated with an increased risk of cancer in 10% to 15% of clients with prolonged GERD (Sharma, 1999). The fibrosis and scarring that accompanies the healing process can produce esophageal stricture, resulting in a narrowing of the esophageal lumen. The stricture leads to progressive difficulty in swallowing. Uncontrolled esophageal reflux also creates a risk for other serious complications such as esophageal ulceration, hemorrhage, and aspiration pneumonia. GERD has been implicated as one of the causes of adult-onset asthma, laryngitis, and dental deterioration.

TABLE 55-1 • FACTORS CONTRIBUTING TO DECREASED LOWER ESOPHAGEAL SPHINCTER PRESSURE

- Fatty foods
- Caffeinated beverages, such as coffee, tea, and cola
- Chocolate
- Nicotine in cigarette smoke
- Calcium channel blockers
- Nitrates
- Peppermint, spearmint
- Alcohol
- Anticholinergic drugs
- High levels of estrogen and progesterone
- Nasogastric tube placement

Etiology

Current evidence suggests that GERD is a result of impaired LES function, which permits the reflux of gastric contents into the esophagus and the subsequent exposure of the esophageal mucosa to gastric contents from impaired esophageal clearance (Claussen, 1999). Currently, the role that hiatal hernia (see p. 1198) plays in the development of GERD is controversial, because each of these disorders often present independently of one another. Nighttime reflux tends to result in prolonged exposure of the esophagus to acid because recumbency tends to impair peristalsis and gravity clearance mechanisms.

Gastric distention caused by the ingestion of large meals or by conditions associated with delayed gastric emptying predispose the client to reflux. A number of individual factors, including certain foods and medications, have been identified as influencing the tone and contractility of the LES (Table 55-1). Clients who have a nasogastric tube often experience compromised esophageal sphincter function. The tube keeps the cardiac sphincter open and allows acidic contents from the stomach to enter the esophagus. Other factors that increase intra-abdominal and intragastric pressure (e.g., wearing tight belts, obesity, bending over, and ascites) overcome the gastroesophageal pressure gradient maintained by the LES and allow reflux to occur.

Incidence/Prevalence

The incidence of GERD is approximately 2% to 3% per year and affects 25% to 35% of the population. Ten percent of the population reports experiencing symptoms of reflux daily, and 44% report experiencing symptoms once a month (Scott & Gelhot, 1999). Gastroesophageal reflux disease (GERD) can occur at any age but is more common in people over 45 years of age. The incidence of GERD may be underestimated because many people with mild disease relate the symptoms to episodes of stress or dietary indiscretion.

CULTURAL CONSIDERATIONS

The prevalence of GERD is higher in females than in males and is found more often in Caucasians than in other ethnic groups. Severe esophagitis is more common in males than in females and is more prevalent in Caucasians than in African Americans.

COLLABORATIVE MANAGEMENT

Assessment

HISTORY

The nurse assesses the client for a history of heartburn or atypical chest pain associated with the reflux of gastrointestinal contents. The client is assessed for dysphagia (difficulty swallowing) or odynophagia (painful swallowing), either of which can indicate the development of a stricture. The nurse further investigates whether the client has a history of newly diagnosed asthma, morning hoarseness, or pneumonia, which are suggestive of severe reflux reaching the pharynx or mouth and/or pulmonary aspiration.

PHYSICAL ASSESSMENT/CLINICAL MANIFESTATIONS

The clinical manifestations of reflux may vary substantially in severity (Chart 55-1).

DYSPEPSIA. A diagnosis of GERD is made principally by a history of **dyspepsia** (also called pyrosis or heartburn), which is the characteristic symptom. Clients often describe this pain as a substernal or retrosternal burning sensation that tends to move up and down the chest in a wavelike fashion. If severe, the pain may radiate to the neck or jaw or may be referred to the back. The pain typically worsens when the client bends over, strains, or is in a recumbent position.

With severe GERD, the pain occurs after each meal and persists for 20 minutes to 2 hours. Clients usually experience prompt relief by ingesting fluids or antacids or by maintaining an upright posture. Some clients experience *atypical chest pain,* which mimics angina and needs to be carefully differentiated from cardiac disease.

REGURGITATION. Regurgitation, which is associated with neither belching nor nausea, is another common symptom. The client reports the occurrence of warm fluid traveling up the throat. If the fluid reaches the level of the pharynx, the client notes a sour or bitter taste in the mouth. This effortless regurgitation can even occur when the client is in an upright position. The danger of aspiration is increased if regurgitation occurs when the client is in a recumbent position.

If the client experiences regurgitation, the nurse carefully auscultates the chest for crackles, which is an indication of associated aspiration. The nurse assesses for coughing, hoarseness, or wheezing at night, which may be related to recumbent regurgitation. Assessment for bronchitis may be necessary in clients experiencing long-term regurgitation.

CHART 55-1

KEY FEATURES *of* Gastroesophageal Reflux Disease

- Dyspepsia (heartburn or pyrosis)
- Regurgitation (may lead to aspiration or bronchitis)
- Coughing, hoarseness, or wheezing at night
- Water brash
- Dysphagia
- Odynophagia (painful swallowing)
- Chest pain
- Belching
- Flatulence

HYPERSALIVATION. A reflex salivary hypersecretion known as **water brash** occurs in response to reflux. Water brash must be carefully distinguished from regurgitation. The client reports a sensation of fluid in the throat, but unlike with regurgitation, there is no bitter or sour taste.

DYSPHAGIA AND ODYNOPHAGIA. Chronic GERD can involve **dysphagia** (difficulty in swallowing). Dysphagia may be the presenting symptom in 33% of clients with GERD. This symptom is usually fairly mild; it is not progressive and occurs with the first swallow of each meal. Dysphagia does not interfere with oral nutrition and does not produce weight loss. Careful assessment is required if a client reports progressive or persistent dysphagia, because this usually indicates the development of a stricture or cancer. The nurse assesses the following:

- The degree of dysphagia
- Whether dysphagia occurs with the ingestion of solids, liquids, or both
- Whether dysphagia is intermittent or occurs with each swallowing effort

Odynophagia (painful swallowing) is a possible symptom of GERD but is relatively rare in people with uncomplicated reflux disease. Severe and long-lasting chest pain may be present if spasms occurring in the esophagus cause the muscle to contract with excess force. The resulting pain can be agonizing and last for hours.

OTHER CLINICAL MANIFESTATIONS. Eructation (belching), flatulence (gas), or bloating after eating are other common complaints. Nausea and vomiting occur infrequently, and unplanned weight loss is rare.

RADIOGRAPHIC ASSESSMENT

No single test is considered to be a gold standard for diagnosing GERD. A barium swallow can be used to rule out complications associated with GERD or to evaluate dysphagia, but it is not sensitive enough to be diagnostic. The most accurate method of diagnosing gastroesophageal reflux disease (GERD) is 24-hour pH monitoring; this involves placing pH probes 2 inches (5 cm) above the lower esophageal sphincter (LES). A barium swallow with fluoroscopy then outlines the structure of the esophagus and its peristaltic patterns. Twenty-four hour ambulatory pH monitoring is widely used but is helpful only in evaluating acid reflux. Endoscopy is useful in diagnosing or evaluating reflux esophagitis or in monitoring complications such as Barrett's esophagus. During endoscopy, tissue samples can be obtained for biopsy, and strictures can be dilated (see Chapter 53).

OTHER DIAGNOSTIC ASSESSMENT

The health care provider orders esophageal manometry, or motility testing, when the diagnosis is uncertain. Water-filled catheters are inserted via the client's nose or mouth and are connected to transducers that record pressures from various sites in the esophagus as the catheters are withdrawn. Manometry quantifies the resting pressure of the LES and helps to evaluate sphincter competence, but when used alone it is not sensitive or specific enough to establish a diagnosis of GERD.

In Bernstein's test, an acidic solution is infused via a tube inserted into the distal esophagus. Clients with normal esophageal mucosa experience no symptoms when acid is infused, but clients with esophagitis experience immediate heartburn.

Scintigraphy involves preloading the stomach with a liquid radioisotope via the mouth or a tube. Scintillation counts are performed over the lower esophagus and are compared with counts obtained over the stomach. If a client is experiencing frequent reflux, the radioisotope will be refluxed back into the esophagus, which significantly elevates the scintillation counts over the lower esophageal region. Scintigraphy may be used in conjunction with pH monitoring.

Interventions

Interventions begin with thorough teaching that GERD is a chronic condition that warrants ongoing management. This knowledge base is essential for a client's understanding of and adherence to the prescribed regimen of drugs, diet therapy, and lifestyle modifications.

NONSURGICAL MANAGEMENT. The goals of treatment for GERD are the relief of symptoms, treatment of esophagitis, and prevention of complications such as strictures or Barrett's esophagus. Although GERD can be controlled by diet therapy, education, lifestyle changes, and drug therapy, it is important to note that, even after the esophagitis is healed, 40% to 80% of clients relapse in 6 months after their medication is discontinued.

DIET THERAPY. Diet therapy is used to relieve symptoms in clients with relatively mild GERD. In collaboration with the dietitian, the nurse explores the client's basic meal patterns and food preferences. The nurse and dietitian work with both the client and the family to plan modifications that may decrease reflux symptoms. For adherence at home to be successful, it is essential that family members who do the shopping and cooking be included in this discussion.

In conjunction with the dietitian, the nurse counsels the client to limit or eliminate foods that decrease LES pressure. The client should also restrict spicy and acidic foods (e.g., orange juice, tomatoes) until esophageal healing can occur, because these foods irritate the inflamed tissue and cause heartburn (Goldsmith, 1998).

Because large meals increase the volume of and pressure in the stomach and delay gastric emptying, the nurse or dietitian instructs the client to eat four to six small meals each day rather than three large ones. Carbonated beverages should also be avoided because they increase pressure in the stomach. Clients are encouraged to avoid evening snacks and to eat no food for at least 3 hours before going to bed, because reflux episodes are most damaging at night. Clients may have the most difficulty adhering to the restriction of evening snacks. The nurse also advises the client to eat slowly and chew thoroughly to facilitate digestion and prevent eructation (belching). The client is encouraged to investigate which particular diet changes best reduce the frequency and severity of symptoms.

CLIENT EDUCATION. The nurse educates the client about the risk factors for the development of reflux, including contributing lifestyle factors. Lifestyle factors that can exacerbate the disease are reviewed, and the client is counseled on ways to eliminate them. The nurse also educates the client regarding the need for ongoing monitoring, particularly if the client has developed strictures, ulcerations, or Barrett's esophagus.

LIFESTYLE CHANGES. The control of GERD involves some lifestyle adjustments on the part of the client. For example, he or she is instructed to elevate the head of the bed by 8 to 12 inches for sleep to prevent nighttime reflux. In addition, he or she is instructed to sleep in the left lateral decubitus position to minimize the effects of nighttime episodes of reflux (see the Evidence-Based Practice for Nursing box below). Nighttime reflux is extremely common, and infrequent swallowing in combination with a recumbent position significantly impairs esophageal clearance. Although wooden blocks have traditionally been recommended to elevate the head of the bed, foam wedges may also achieve satisfactory results. The client or the client's spouse or partner may find elevation of the bed unacceptable at first. The nurse emphasizes the importance of this intervention and investigates all possible approaches for achieving compliance (Chart 55-2).

For clients with a history of smoking, the nurse explores the possibility and means of smoking cessation and makes the appropriate referrals. The nurse explains that smoking causes a prompt and significant drop in LES pressure and optimally should be stopped. The nurse also explores the client's normal pattern and amount of alcoholic beverage use. The client is taught about the effects of alcohol on LES sphincter pressure. The nurse can assist the client in finding appropriate alcohol cessation programs if needed.

EVIDENCE-BASED PRACTICE FOR NURSING

What sleeping position would be most beneficial for clients with gastroesophageal reflux disease?

Khoury, R., et al. (1999). Influence of spontaneous sleep positions on nighttime recumbent reflux in patients with gastroesophageal reflux disease. *The American Journal of Gastroenterology, 94*(8), 2069-2073.

The purpose of this study was to investigate the influence of body position during sleep on recumbent reflux in 10 clients with gastroesophageal reflux disease. The 10 subjects (3 female, 7 male) were fed a standardized, high-fat dinner and bedtime snack. A single-channel pH probe was placed 5 cm above the lower esophageal sphincter (LES) in each client to measure the percentage of reflux episodes (pH <4) that occurred during four sleeping positions. A body position sensor taped to the client's sternum recorded spontaneous changes in posture during sleep.

The right lateral position was associated with the greatest percentage of time the pH remained under 4 and longer esophageal acid clearance when compared to the left, supine, and prone positions. The supine position resulted in a greater overall number of gastroesophageal reflux episodes that occurred within 1 minute of assuming this position. This study determined that the preferred sleeping position for clients with gastroesophageal reflux is the left lateral position.

Critique. Although the sample size was small, this was the first study to examine the effects of sleeping positions on recumbent reflux in clients with gastroesophageal reflux.

Implications for Nursing. Previous research supports the theory that body position influences gastroesophageal reflux. Nurses can incorporate information concerning sleeping position into their teaching plan for clients faced with damaging nighttime reflux. In addition to elevating the head of the bed, clients can be instructed to lie in the left lateral position for sleep to reduce the number of reflux episodes and the length of time the esophageal mucosa is exposed to acidic contents.

CHART 55-2

CLIENT EDUCATION GUIDE
Lifestyle Modifications to Control Reflux

- Eat four to six small meals a day.
- Limit or eliminate fatty foods, coffee, tea, cola, and chocolate.
- Reduce or eliminate from your diet any food or spice that causes pain.
- Limit or eliminate alcohol and tobacco.
- Do not snack in the evening, and take no food for 2 to 3 hours before you go to bed.
- Eat slowly, and chew your food thoroughly to reduce belching.
- Remain upright for 1 to 2 hours after meals, if possible.
- Elevate the head of your bed 8 to 12 inches using wooden blocks or a foam wedge. Never sleep flat in bed.
- If you are overweight, lose weight.
- Do not wear constrictive clothing.
- Avoid heavy lifting, straining, and working in a bent-over position.

If the client is obese, the nurse collaborates with the dietitian to examine approaches to weight reduction. Decreasing intra-abdominal pressure often reduces reflux symptoms.

Other lifestyle factors cause increased abdominal pressure, and the nurse explores these with the client. Wearing constrictive clothing, lifting heavy objects or straining, and working in a bent-over or stooped position should be avoided. The nurse emphasizes that these general adaptations are an essential and effective component of disease management and can produce prompt results in uncomplicated cases.

DRUG THERAPY. Some medications can cause reflux. Therefore the nurse, in conjunction with the primary health care provider, explores the possibility of eliminating from the client's regimen those medications implicated in reflux. Three principles guide drug therapy for gastroesophageal reflux: (1) to inhibit gastric acid secretion, (2) to accelerate gastric emptying, and (3) to protect the gastric mucosa (Chart 55-3).

Antacids. In uncomplicated cases of GERD, antacids are effective for occasional episodes of heartburn. Antacids act by elevating the pH level of the gastric contents, thereby deactivating pepsin. They are inadequate for the control of frequent symptoms because their duration of action is too short and their nighttime effectiveness is minimal.

Antacids containing aluminum hydroxide or magnesium hydroxide may be used. Maalox and Mylanta consist of a combination of these two agents, and clients often tolerate them better because they produce fewer side effects such as constipation and diarrhea. The nurse instructs the client to take the antacid 1 hour before and 2 to 3 hours after each meal. Some antacids are prepared as double-strength (DS) suspensions or tablets. The advantage of DS preparations is that the client can take a smaller amount of the drug. For example, 30 mL of regular Mylanta equals 15 mL of Mylanta-II (DS preparation).

Gaviscon, a combination of aluminum hydroxide and magnesium carbonate, is a commonly used and very effective medication for GERD. It forms a viscous foam that floats on top of the gastric contents and theoretically decreases the incidence of reflux. If reflux occurs, the foam enters the esophagus first and buffers the acid in the refluxed material. The nurse reminds the client to take this drug when food is in the stomach.

Histamine Receptor Antagonists. Histamine blockers, such as famotidine (Pepcid), ranitidine (Zantac), cimetidine (Tagamet), and nizatidine (Axid) are the main pharmacologic means of inhibiting gastric acid secretion. With histamine receptor antagonists available over the counter (OTC) and widely advertised for heartburn, many clients self-medicate before seeking professional assistance from their health care provider. When clients who have self-medicated with OTC preparations experience uncontrolled symptoms, the health care provider usually prescribes a *higher* dose of a histamine receptor antagonist.

Cimetidine (Tagamet) is not used as often as the longer-acting preparations. It has an inhibitory effect on the elimination of certain other medications, and therefore significant drug interactions can occur in clients taking warfarin, theophylline, phenytoin, nifedipine, or propranolol. Ranitidine and the other preparations are longer acting, and less frequent dosing is necessary. They also appear to produce fewer side effects and are safe for long-term administration. Although these drugs do not affect the occurrence of reflux directly, they do reduce gastric acid secretion, provide symptomatic improvement, and support healing of the inflamed esophageal tissue.

The proton pump inhibitors, such as omeprazole (Prilosec), lansoprazole (Prevacid), and rabeprazole (Aciphex), demonstrate effective, long-acting inhibition of gastric acid secretion. They are typically reserved for the treatment of severe GERD that is refractory to treatment with histamine blockers, and they play an important role in maintaining the remission of both GERD and Barrett's esophagus. These potent drugs can reduce gastric acid secretion by about 90% over a 24-hour period and can be given in a single daily dose. If once-a-day dosing fails to control symptoms, twice-a-day dosing is appropriate (Sharma, 1999). For example, omeprazole (Prilosec) is usually prescribed as a 20-mg oral dose once a day for 4 to 8 weeks. Complete healing of esophagitis is seen in 80% to 97% of clients (Tucker & Schumann, 1999). Proton pump inhibitors promote rapid tissue healing, but recurrence is common when the drug is stopped.

Other Drugs. Prokinetic drugs are used to accelerate gastric emptying and improve lower esophageal sphincter (LES) pressure and esophageal peristalsis. The health care provider may add bethanechol (Urecholine) or metoclopramide (Reglan) to the drug regimen for clients who experience severe and ongoing symptoms of reflux.

Bethanechol is a cholinergic drug; it increases the secretion of gastric acid and usually requires the simultaneous administration of a histamine receptor antagonist and antacids. Bethanechol is usually prescribed in 25-mg doses four times a day. The nurse teaches the client to take bethanechol 30 to 60 minutes before meals and warns the client about the typical side effects, which include abdominal cramping, diarrhea, increased salivation, and urinary urgency.

The primary action of metoclopramide is to increase the rate of gastric emptying. It does not affect gastric acid secretion or directly heal esophageal tissue. Its use is also associated with a high incidence of neurologic and psychotropic side effects such as fatigue, anxiety, ataxia, and hallucinations. Long-term use is not recommended.

SURGICAL MANAGEMENT. Antireflux surgery is usually indicated for otherwise healthy clients who have failed to respond to medical treatment or to demonstrate complications related to GERD or for whom the cost of long-term drug ther-

CHART 55-3

DRUG THERAPY *for* Gastroesophageal Reflux Disease (GERD)

Drug	Usual Dosage	Nursing Interventions	Rationale
Antacids, either aluminum or magnesium salts	30 mL PO between meals and as needed (PRN) throughout the day and at bedtime	Give 1 hr before meals, 2-3 hr after meals, and at bedtime. Give prn as instructed by physician.	Antacids neutralize acid and produce prompt relief of heartburn.
		Observe the client for constipation or diarrhea.	Aluminum products produce constipation, and magnesium products induce diarrhea.
		Suggest the use of combination mixtures or alternating use of aluminum and magnesium products.	Balancing their effects is important for client adherence.
Gaviscon, antacid plus alginic acid	1 tablet or 10-20 mL PO throughout the day and at bedtime	Give after meals and at bedtime.	Alginic acid forms a viscous foam that floats on top of the gastric contents, impeding reflux or buffering its effects when it occurs.
Histamine receptor antagonists		Instruct the client to take the drug with meals.	These drugs dramatically suppress gastric acid secretion and promote healing.
Cimetidine (Tagamet)	300 mg qid PO or 900-1200 mg PO at bedtime	Observe the client for side effects; fatigue, headache, and diarrhea are common. Instruct client about potential toxicity with some medications.	
Ranitidine (Zantac)	150 mg bid PO	Administer with meals and at bedtime.	Ranitidine and famotidine are more potent, longer-acting drugs, yet they produce fewer side effects.
Famotidine (Pepcid)	40 mg PO daily or 20 mg bid PO		
Nizatidine (Axid)	150 mg bid PO	Use cautiously and in reduced dosages in clients with renal disease.	Clients need an adequate creatinine clearance to prevent drug toxicity.
		Observe for dysrhythmias.	Dysrhythmias are common adverse effects of the drug.
		Do not mix with tomato-based, mixed-vegetable juices; apple juice is the preferred choice.	This drug may be less potent when mixed with tomato-based, mixed-vegetable juices.
Bethanechol (Urecholine)	25 mg qid PO	Instruct the client to take the drug 30-60 min before meals. Continue with antacids and histamine receptor antagonists as ordered.	This drug increases lower esophageal sphincter (LES) pressure and increases the rate of esophageal clearance.
		Observe the client for typical side effects: abdominal cramping, diarrhea, urinary urgency, and increased salivation.	Bethanecol has cholinergic effects and increases the secretion of gastric acid.
		Counsel the client about the control of side effects.	Typical associated cholinergic effects occur with the use of bethanechol.
Metoclopramide (Reglan)	10 mg tid or qid PO	Instruct the client to take the drug before meals.	This drug increases the rate of gastric emptying.
		Teach the client to report any neurologic or psychotropic side effects, such as restlessness, anxiety, ataxia, or hallucinations.	Long-term drug use produces adverse effects in up to one third of clients.
Omeprazole (Prilosec, Losec♣)	20-30 mg PO daily	Instruct the client to take the drug before meals. Observe the client for typical side effects: abdominal cramping, diarrhea, headache.	Gastric acid suppression is greater than 90%. Action is prolonged, but gastrointestinal effects are severe in some clients.
Lansoprazole (Prevacid)	15 mg PO daily for gastroesophageal reflux disease (GERD) Up to 60 mg PO for gastrointestinal ulcers or Zollinger-Ellison syndrome	Instruct the client to take the drug before meals.	Same as above.
		For the client who has difficulty swallowing or has a nasogastric tube, open the capsule and mix granules in apple juice (or applesauce if not tube fed).	The drug is safe to administer by opening (not crushing) the capsule.

apy is prohibitive. Various surgical procedures may be used. The three major surgical procedures are Nissen fundoplication, the Hill repair, and the Belsey repair (Figure 55-1).

In each of these procedures, the surgeon wraps and sutures the gastric fundus around the esophagus, which anchors the LES area below the diaphragm and reinforces the high-pressure area. For a more complete description of the three major procedures, see Operative Procedures (Hiatal Hernia), p. 1202.

The Client Care Plan on pp. 1199 and 1200 outlines the nursing care of clients undergoing esophageal surgery. Clients who have surgery are encouraged to continue following the basic antireflux regimen of antacids and diet therapy, because the rate of recurrence is significant.

Placement of the synthetic Angelchik prosthesis is also used for clients with severe reflux. This surgical procedure is associated with fewer long-term problems with achalasia (failure of the lower esophageal muscles and sphincter to relax properly). The surgeon performs a laparotomy and ties a C-shaped silicone prosthesis filled with gel around the distal esophagus (Figure 55-2). The prosthesis anchors the LES in the abdomen and reinforces sphincter pressure. Dysphagia is the primary complication of this procedure.

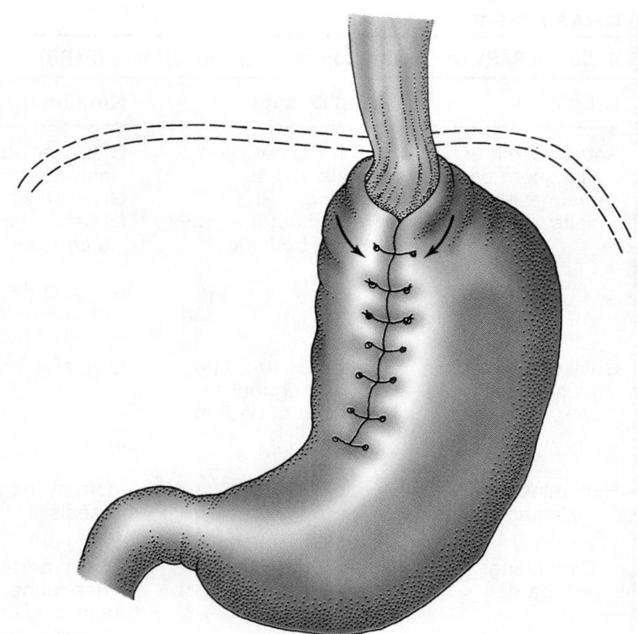

Figure 55-1 ● Nissen fundoplication for gastroesophageal reflux disease or hiatal hernia repair.

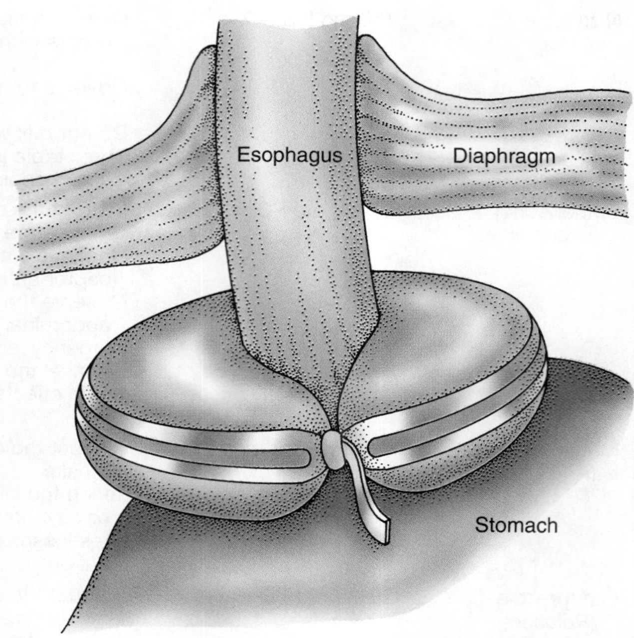

Figure 55-2 ● Placement of the Angelchik antireflux prosthesis.

HIATAL HERNIA

OVERVIEW

The esophageal hiatus is the opening in the diaphragm through which the esophagus passes from the thorax to the abdomen. **Hiatal hernias,** also called diaphragmatic hernias, involve the protrusion of the stomach through the esophageal hiatus of the diaphragm into the thorax. Clients with hiatal hernias may be completely asymptomatic or may experience daily symptoms similar to those of clients with GERD.

Pathophysiology

The two major types of hiatal hernias are sliding hernias and paraesophageal (rolling) hernias.

SLIDING HERNIA

Sliding hernias are the most common type of hernia and account for 90% of the total number of hiatal hernias. The esophagogastric junction and a portion of the fundus of the stomach slide upward through the esophageal hiatus into the thorax (Figure 55-3). The hernia generally moves freely and slides into and out of the thorax during changes in position or intra-abdominal pressure. Although volvulus (twisting) and obstruction do occur rarely, the major concern in a client with a sliding hernia is the development of esophageal reflux and its complications. The development of reflux appears to be related to chronic exposure of the lower esophageal sphincter (LES) to the low pressure of the thorax, which significantly reduces the effectiveness of the LES. Symptoms associated with LES pressure are worsened by positions that favor reflux, such as bending or lying supine.

ROLLING HERNIA

With paraesophageal hernias, the gastroesophageal junction remains in its normal intra-abdominal location, but the fundus (and possibly portions of the stomach's greater curvature) roll through the esophageal hiatus and into the thorax beside the esophagus (see Figure 55-3). The herniated portion of the stomach may be small or quite large; in rare cases, the stomach completely inverts into the thorax. Reflux is rarely a concern because the LES remains anchored below the diaphragm, but the risks of volvulus, obstruction, and strangulation are high. The development of iron deficiency anemia is common, because slow bleeding secondary to venous obstruction causes the gastric mucosa

Client Care Plan • THE CLIENT UNDERGOING TRADITIONAL OPEN ESOPHAGEAL SURGERY

NURSING DIAGNOSIS NO. 1 • Risk for Infection related to surgical incision

Expected Outcomes	Nursing Interventions	Rationale
The client will manifest no signs or symptoms of infection.	Do not reposition or replace the nasogastric tube. Do not perform endotracheal suctioning on a client with esophageal anastomosis or repair.	Moving the tube can cause trauma, which could puncture or irritate the incision; trauma to the area might open a potential route of infection.
	Encourage the client to suction or expectorate oral secretions rather than swallow them.	Clients are kept on nothing by mouth (NPO) status to avoid active peristalsis.
	Assess the cutaneous suture line for redness, drainage, and other signs of infection. Observe the dressing for bleeding; document and report any findings to the physician.	Monitor the client to detect complications and early signs of infection as soon as possible.
	Clean sutures once each shift with half-strength peroxide; dry the area and apply a small amount of antibacterial ointment.	Cleaning removes crusts and secretions, which could be an ideal media for bacterial growth.
	Monitor vital signs per the physician's orders. [D] Document and report any significant changes to the physician.	Monitoring provides early detection of and intervention for hemorrhage or infection.

NURSING DIAGNOSIS NO. 2 • Risk for Imbalanced Nutrition: Less than Body Requirements related to NPO status and surgical disruption of the esophagus

Expected Outcomes	Nursing Interventions	Rationale
The client will maintain adequate nutritional intake by nasogastric tube until oral feedings are begun.	Remind the client of NPO status when he or she is alert. [D]	Older clients may demonstrate memory deficit; clients are often on NPO status until the intraoral incision is healed.
	Monitor IV hydration while the client is on NPO status and before tube feedings are begun; monitor and record intake and output every shift.	Monitor hydration status for overload or retention; older clients are often susceptible to overload of fluids.
	Assess and document bowel sounds every shift until tube feedings are well tolerated.	Establish a baseline for bowel sounds; the return of bowel sounds postoperatively is often an indication to begin tube feedings.
	Measure and record the client's weight daily. [D]	Weight gives information on fluid status.
	Maintain proper functioning of the nasogastric tube; while it is attached to suction, measure and record drainage every shift. When tube feedings are begun, flush the tube carefully with water after each feeding or medication administration.	Monitor and maintain patency to permit drainage and to allow a route for the administration of medications and nutrition.
	Elevate the head of the bed 30 degrees at rest and 90 degrees for feeding and for ½ hr after feeding.	Raising the head helps prevent reflux; the incidence of reflux is greatest during and ½ hr after tube feedings.
	Provide the client with written and oral instructions regarding tube feedings.	Written and oral instructions provide the client with resources when the nurse is not available.
	Include the family/significant other in all teaching.	Including loved ones ensures support for the client to perform the procedures.
	Have the client give a return demonstration of the procedure.	A return demonstration aids in retention of the learned procedure and provides a means of evaluation for the nurse.
	When oral fluids are begun, assess and document swallowing difficulties, aspiration, or leakage, including signs of increased pulse rate, increased temperature, increased respiratory rate, subcutaneous emphysema, or a change in chest tube drainage indicating contamination from the gastrointestinal tract.	Clients occasionally have difficulty swallowing after esophageal surgery; assessment provides documentation of a real or perceived difficulty. The nurse observes carefully for signs of leakage from the esophageal anastomosis site or from a perforation.
	If the client is experiencing difficulty in swallowing, consult a speech-language pathologist for assessment or assistance in swallowing.	Speech-language pathologists are often experts at evaluating swallowing disorders; providing the client with techniques of head positioning, breath holding, or oral exercises can help overcome minor swallowing difficulties.
	Collaborate with the dietitian as appropriate.	A change in food consistency often eases swallowing difficulties.
	Observe the client for any epigastric burning, retrosternal or back pain, or pain radiating to the chin or shoulder indicative of esophageal reflux; document any findings.	Esophageal reflux, once documented, can be treated by positioning the client or dietary changes; analgesics may be required before mealtimes.

[D] Indicates tasks that can be delegated to assistive nursing personnel.

Continued

CLIENT CARE PLAN • THE CLIENT UNDERGOING TRADITIONAL OPEN ESOPHAGEAL SURGERY—cont'd

NURSING DIAGNOSIS NO. 3 • Acute Pain related to incision; Chronic Pain related to reflux

Expected Outcomes	Nursing Interventions	Rationale
The client will verbalize control of pain, facilitating adequate nutritional intake and participation in activities of daily living.	Assess and document the level of pain, relying on subjective and objective symptoms of pain and pain relief. Assess and document the relief obtained from the analgesic regimen.	Clients are often unwilling to demonstrate evidence of pain and often are unwilling to use analgesics, particularly opioids, as often as prescribed.
	Assess the client for pain related to esophageal reflux or perforation: epigastric burning; pain radiating to the shoulder, chin, or back; change in vital signs; change in character of chest tube drainage (if present); subcutaneous emphysema. Document and report all findings to the physician.	Early detection of esophageal perforation is imperative to begin effective treatment; documentation of reflux communicates to other health care workers the need to prevent reflux aspiration.
	Instruct the client to keep the head of the bed raised 30 degrees at all times and 90 degrees at meals and for ½ hr after meals. **D**	Raising the head of the bed not only reduces edema by facilitating gravity drainage but also facilitates food passage and prevents esophageal reflux.
	Explore dietary modifications with the client to alleviate discomfort related to reflux.	Smaller, more frequent meals with a change in food consistency can reduce the discomfort associated with reflux.
	Explore various positioning changes to facilitate food passage and alleviate symptoms of reflux.	Varying the positions assumed while eating and after eating can reduce the discomfort associated with reflux or dysphagia.
	Instruct the client to use analgesic medication ½ hr before meals, chest physiotherapy, and other treatments as needed.	Ensuring a peak analgesic effect during activities that the client reports as being most uncomfortable can increase compliance with those activities and efforts to obtain adequate nutritional intake.
	Instruct the client and family/significant other about the timing, side effects, and restrictions of the prescribed medications; provide written and oral instructions.	Written and oral instructions are given because the client may have memory loss.
	Instruct the client to monitor his or her own comfort.	The client gains a feeling of control concerning discomfort.

D Indicates tasks that can be delegated to assistive nursing personnel.

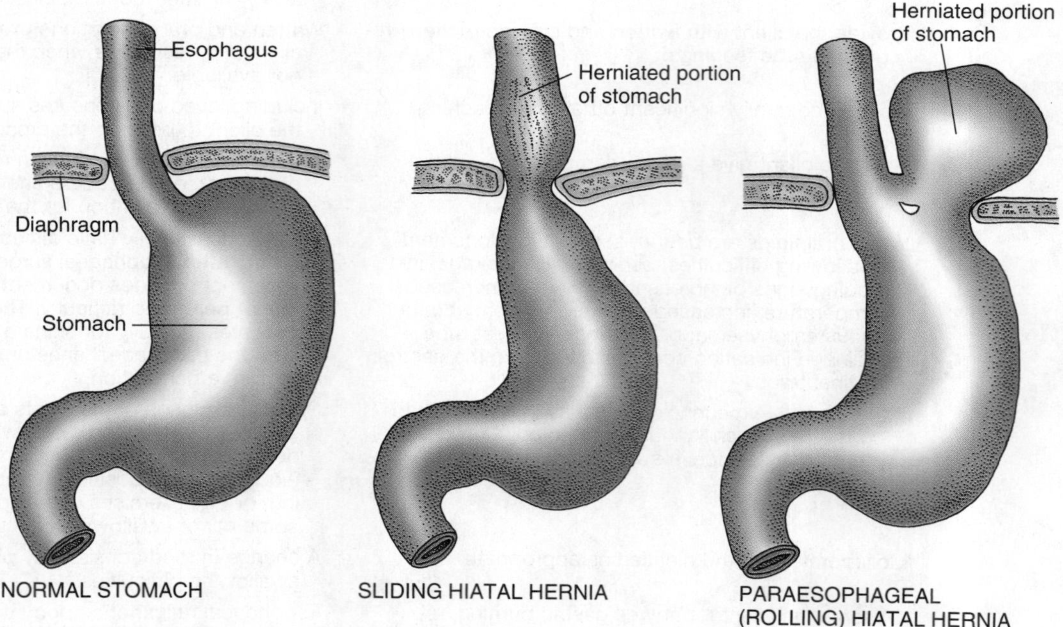

Figure 55-3 • A comparison of the normal stomach and sliding and paraesophageal (rolling) hiatal hernias.

to become engorged and ooze. Significant bleeding or hemorrhage is rare.

Etiology

Sliding hiatal hernias are believed to develop from muscle weakening in the esophageal hiatus, which loosens the esophageal supports and permits the lower portion of the esophagus to rise into the thorax. Congenital weaknesses, trauma, obesity, or surgery may also play a significant role. The development of the hernia is the result of the combined effects of weakened support structures and prolonged increases in abdominal pressure.

Muscle weakening does not appear to cause paraesophageal hernias. Instead, it is theorized that the stomach is not properly anchored below the diaphragm, and the hernia results from an anatomic defect rather than a structural weakness. Paraesophageal hernias can also be caused by previous esophageal surgeries, including sliding hernia repair.

Incidence/Prevalence

Hiatal hernia is one of the more common disorders that affect the upper gastrointestinal tract, and it affects women more often than men. Hiatal hernias have been reported in up to 20% of adults (Crawford, 1999).

CONSIDERATIONS FOR OLDER ADULTS
The incidence of sliding hiatal hernias increases with age in both genders and reaches a prevalence of approximately 60% in the sixth decade of life. As many as 80% of clients with hiatal hernias are asymptomatic or experience only mild, transient symptoms associated with reflux.

COLLABORATIVE MANAGEMENT

Assessment

The nurse carefully assesses for heartburn, regurgitation, pain, dysphagia, and belching. An assessment of the client's general physical appearance and nutritional status is also included. The nurse notes the location, onset, duration, quality, and aggravating and alleviating factors associated with the presence of pain. The primary symptoms of sliding hiatal hernias are associated with reflux. The nurse auscultates the thorax and lungs, as pulmonary symptoms similar to asthma may be triggered by episodes of aspiration, particularly at night. A detailed history is crucial in attempting to differentiate angina from noncardiac chest pain due to gastroesophageal reflux. Symptoms resulting from hiatal hernia typically worsen after a meal or when the client is in a recumbent position (Chart 55-4).

In clients with paraesophageal (rolling) hernias, the nurse assesses for symptoms related to the stretching or displacement of thoracic contents by the hernia. Clients may report a feeling of fullness after eating and may even experience breathlessness or a feeling of suffocation if the hernia interferes with breathing. Some clients experience chest pain associated with reflux that mimics angina.

The barium swallow study with fluoroscopy is the most specific diagnostic test for identifying hiatal hernia. Paraesophageal hernias are usually clearly visible, and sliding hernias can often be observed as the client is moved through a series of positions that increase intra-abdominal pressure.

CHART 55-4

KEY FEATURES *of* Hernias

Sliding Hiatal Hernias
- Heartburn
- Regurgitation
- Chest pain
- Dysphagia
- Belching

Paraesophageal Hernias
- Feeling of fullness after eating
- Breathlessness after eating
- Feeling of suffocation
- Chest pain that mimics angina
- Worsening of manifestations in a recumbent position

Clients with sliding hernias usually experience symptoms of reflux. Therefore any or all of the diagnostic tests used for gastroesophageal reflux disease (GERD) may be used to fully evaluate the extent of reflux and the degree of esophageal damage (see Other Diagnostic Assessment [GERD], p. 1194).

Interventions

Clients with hiatal hernias may be managed either medically or surgically. The health care provider's choice of management is based on the severity of the client's symptoms and the risk of serious complications. Sliding hiatal hernias are most commonly treated medically. Large paraesophageal hernias can become strangulated or obstructed; therefore early surgical repair is encouraged.

NONSURGICAL MANAGEMENT. The interventions for clients with hiatal hernia closely follow those outlined for clients with GERD and include drug therapy, diet therapy, lifestyle modifications, and client education. The health care provider typically prescribes antacids and histamine receptor antagonists, such as ranitidine (Zantac), in an attempt to control reflux and its symptoms.

Diet therapy is also an integral part of the conservative management of hiatal hernia and follows the guidelines discussed earlier for GERD, p. 1195. The client is encouraged to avoid eating in the late evening and to avoid foods associated with reflux. In collaboration with the dietitian, the nurse works with the client to modify the diet to reduce body weight (if appropriate), because obesity increases intra-abdominal pressure and worsens both the hernia and the symptoms of reflux.

The nurse carefully explains the underlying condition to increase the client's understanding of the disorder and increase adherence to the treatment regimen. Teaching about positioning, as described earlier for GERD (p. 1195) is also extremely important. It is essential that clients:

- Sleep at night with the head of the bed elevated 8 to 12 inches
- Remain upright for several hours after eating
- Avoid straining or excessive vigorous exercise
- Refrain from wearing clothing that is tight or constrictive around the abdomen

SURGICAL MANAGEMENT. The physician usually schedules surgery when the risk of complications is high or when damage from chronic reflux becomes severe.

PREOPERATIVE CARE. If the surgery is not urgent, the surgeon encourages clients who are overweight to lose weight before surgery. Clients are advised to quit or significantly reduce smoking. As part of preoperative teaching, the nurse reinforces the surgeon's instructions and prepares the client for the postoperative course.

Before developing the teaching plan, the nurse must know which surgical approach is planned. For the thoracic surgical approach, for example, the client is taught about chest tubes. The nurse also informs the client that a nasogastric tube will be inserted during surgery and will remain in place for several days. Oral intake is started gradually with clear liquids after peristalsis is re-established, or to stimulate peristalsis. The nurse also instructs the client about techniques for effective deep breathing and use of the incentive spirometer. These measures are essential to prevent postoperative respiratory complications. The high incision makes deep breathing extremely painful for the client. The nurse educates the client concerning the aspects of postoperative pain and assures the client that adequate postoperative analgesia will be administered.

OPERATIVE PROCEDURES. Although several hiatal hernia repair procedures are in use, each involves reinforcement of the lower esophageal sphincter (LES) through some degree of fundoplication. The surgeon wraps a portion of the stomach fundus around the distal esophagus to anchor it and reinforce the LES. The eventual recurrence for either type of hernia following surgical repair is 10% to 15% over 5 years (Ferguson, 1997).

The **Nissen repair** is the most commonly used procedure (see Figure 55-1) for hiatal hernia repair. An abdominal approach is usually chosen. The surgeon wraps the fundus a full 360 degrees around the lower esophagus. The sphincter reinforcement is tight and usually controls reflux effectively. Laparoscopic Nissen fundoplication (LNF) is a relatively new surgical technique that involves the creation of an antireflux valve or fundoplication laparoscopically through 5 ½-inch incisions in the abdomen. The fundus is then wrapped 360 degrees around the LES to strengthen it (Vaca et al., 1998).

In the Hill repair, an abdominal approach is also used, but the fundoplication is wrapped 180 degrees around the esophagus. The angle of His is restructured to accentuate the angle at which the esophagus enters the stomach. The Belsey repair usually involves a 280-degree esophageal wrap and uses a thoracic approach.

Surgeons do not agree about which surgical repair is most appropriate or effective, because each procedure has unique advantages and disadvantages. For example, the laparoscopic Nissen fundoplication is associated with all the risks of a major surgery; pneumonia, myocardial infarction, wound infection, and bleeding (Vaca et al., 1998).

POSTOPERATIVE CARE. Postoperative care following hiatal hernia repair closely follows that required after any esophageal surgery (see the Client Care Plan on pp. 1199 and 1200). The nurse carefully assesses for complications of fundoplication surgery and reports their occurrence to the physician (Chart 55-5).

Respiratory Care. The primary focus of postoperative care is the prevention of respiratory complications. The nurse or assistive nursing personnel elevates the head of the client's bed at least 30 degrees to lower the diaphragm and facilitate lung expansion. The client is assisted out of bed and is ambulated as soon as possible. The incision must be supported during coughing to reduce pain and to prevent excessive strain on the suture line, especially with obese clients.

CHART 55-5

BEST PRACTICE *for*
Assessment of Postoperative Complications Related to Fundoplication Procedures

COMPLICATION	ASSESSMENT FINDINGS
Temporary dysphagia	The client has difficulty swallowing when oral feeding begins.
Gas bloat syndrome	The client has difficulty belching to relieve distention.
Atelectasis, pneumonia	The client experiences dyspnea, chest pain, and/or fever.
Obstructed nasogastric tube	The client experiences nausea, vomiting, and/or abdominal distention. The nasogastric tube does not drain.

Incentive spirometry and deep breathing are routinely used after surgery to maintain patency of the airways. Adequate analgesia is essential for client compliance and should be administered as needed. Clients with a smoking history or chronic airway limitation (chronic obstructive pulmonary disease, asthma) require more aggressive respiratory management by the respiratory therapist to prevent atelectasis and pneumonia. Clients with large hiatal hernias are at high risk for developing respiratory complications.

Nasogastric Tube Management. Postoperative management also involves the care of the nasogastric (NG) tube. Inserting a large-diameter NG tube during surgery prevents the fundoplication wrap from becoming too tight around the esophagus. The nasogastric drainage is initially dark brown with old blood but should become normal yellowish green within the first 8 hours after surgery. The nurse checks every 4 to 8 hours for proper placement of the tube in the stomach. The NG tube should be properly anchored so it cannot be displaced, because it cannot be safely reinserted without risking perforation of the incision.

Frequent assessment of the patency of the tube is essential to keep the stomach decompressed; this prevents retching or vomiting, which can strain or rupture the stomach sutures. Because the tube is irritating, the nurse or assistive nursing personnel provides frequent oral hygiene. The nurse also assesses the client's hydration status regularly, including accurate measures of intake and output. Adequate fluid replacement helps to thin respiratory secretions.

Nutritional Care. The client may begin oral intake with clear fluids after peristalsis is re-established or in an effort to stimulate peristalsis. Some surgeons create a temporary gastrostomy for feeding to allow for undisturbed healing of the repair. The client gradually progresses to a near-normal diet during the first 6 weeks. A few foods, such as caffeinated or carbonated beverages and alcohol, are either restricted or eliminated. The food storage area of the stomach is reduced by the surgery, and meals need to be both smaller and more frequent.

The nurse carefully supervises the first oral feedings, because temporary dysphagia is common. Persistent dysphagia usually indicates that the fundoplication is too tight, and dilation may be required.

Another common complication of fundoplication surgery is the gas bloat syndrome, in which clients are unable to voluntarily eructate (belch). The syndrome is usually temporary but may persist. The nurse teaches the client to avoid drinking carbonated beverages, eating gas-producing foods (especially high-fat foods), chewing gum, and drinking with a straw.

Many clients acquire the habit of aerophagia (air swallowing) from attempting to reverse or clear acid reflux. The nurse teaches these clients to consciously relax before and after meals, eat and drink slowly, and chew all food thoroughly.

Air in the stomach that cannot be removed by belching can be extremely uncomfortable. Frequent position changes and ambulation are effective interventions for eliminating air from the gastrointestinal tract.

Community-Based Care

Clients undergoing one of the three major surgical repairs require activity restrictions during the 4- to 6-week postoperative recovery period. For laparoscopic surgery, activity is typically restricted for a shorter time, and the client can return to his or her usual lifestyle more quickly. For long-term management, the nurse teaches the client and family about appropriate diet modifications, but the use of stool softeners or bulk laxatives is recommended for the first postoperative weeks until healing is complete. The nurse instructs the client to avoid straining and prevent constipation.

The client is taught to inspect the healing incision daily and to notify the physician or health care provider if swelling, redness, tenderness, discharge, or fever occurs. The nurse advises the client to avoid contact with people with respiratory infections and to contact the physician if symptoms of a cold or influenza develop. Persistent coughing can cause the incision or the fundoplication to dehisce. The client is also advised to avoid smoking.

The nurse and dietitian educate the entire family or significant other about diet. Full support is essential for the client to successfully modify the size and timing of meals. Relatively few ongoing diet restrictions are needed, but overeating or eating the wrong types of foods can produce discomfort if the client cannot belch. The client avoids foods that produce discomfort, and the nurse encourages cautious experimentation with new foods. The nurse instructs the client to report the recurrence of reflux symptoms to the health care provider.

Although severe surgical complications are relatively rare, conditions such as gas bloat syndrome and dysphagia are common and may persist. The nurse helps the client prepare for these problems and for the potential that reflux may not be completely controlled or may occur again. Although surgery controls the condition, a cure is rare, and lifestyle modifications need to be ongoing.

ACHALASIA

OVERVIEW

Achalasia is an esophageal motility disorder in which the lower esophageal sphincter (LES) fails to relax properly with swallowing and in which the normal peristalsis of the esophagus is replaced with abnormal contractions. It is characterized by chronic and progressive dysphagia. Regurgitation of ingested food may also occur, especially at night, resulting in aspiration. If left untreated, progressive dysphagia can result in weight loss. Chest pain is experienced by one third of clients with the disorder.

Achalasia is thought to result from esophageal denervation (loss of nerve impulse passage). The exact cause of denervation is unknown. A genetic basis to the disorder has been proposed as suggested by occasional familial clustering and phenotype (observable characteristics) association.

Over time, peristaltic failure plus spasm can produce a massively dilated esophagus, which further slows food passage. Achalasia is an uncommon disorder that usually manifests itself in young adulthood. Both genders appear to be equally affected. Approximately 5% to 10% of individuals with this disorder develop esophageal squamous cell carcinoma (Crawford, 1999). Complications of achalasia also include esophageal candidiasis, lower esophageal diverticula, airway obstruction, and aspiration pneumonia.

COLLABORATIVE MANAGEMENT

Assessment

The nurse assesses for the primary symptoms of achalasia, such as dysphagia and regurgitation of solids, liquids, or both. The client is asked about the presence of chest pain associated with these symptoms.

Achalasia is often a chronic condition. The symptoms worsen over time, which poses an increased threat to health and functioning as the disorder progresses. The nurse questions the client about factors that aggravate the symptoms (e.g., body position or diet changes) as well as medications or home treatments that relieve the symptoms. The client is asked about a history of previous esophageal surgery or trauma, which compound the progressive dysphagia. Respiratory history and current respiratory-associated symptoms are particularly important with regard to their direct relationship to reflux, regurgitation, and aspiration.

To determine the effect of the esophageal symptoms, the nurse obtains a nutritional history, including dietary habits, food tolerances, and weight loss. The nurse also notes the presence of halitosis (foul mouth odor), which can be caused by the regurgitation of previously ingested food. The nurse auscultates the lungs for adventitious sounds secondary to pulmonary aspiration of retained saliva and food. The nurse or assistive nursing personnel weighs the client and compares this weight with the client's usual weight.

A chest x-ray study reveals a distorted and dilated tubular esophagus, the absence of a gastric air bubble and, occasionally, a tubular mediastinal mass next to the aorta. A barium swallow reveals esophageal dilation with a persistent beaklike narrowing at the terminal esophagus—the hallmark of a nonrelaxing LES. Esophageal manometry typically reveals an elevated resting LES pressure and incomplete sphincter relaxation when the client swallows. Endoscopy is used to evaluate the appearance of the esophageal mucosa, especially for changes associated with cancer or the presence of candida.

Interventions

The symptoms associated with achalasia can be treated with a variety of approaches. A combination of dietary measures, pharmacologic agents, esophageal dilation and surgery are used.

DRUG AND DIET THERAPY. Mild cases of achalasia can be managed with calcium channel blockers or nitrates to reduce LES pressure. Drug therapy is given for symptom relief and is not recommended as an alternative to more definitive therapy.

The nurse advises the client to experiment with changes in diet because they can often ease the pressure and reflux associated with achalasia. The nurse discusses with the client any food habits he or she has noted that aggravate or relieve the symptoms. Semisoft foods are often better tolerated, as are warm foods and liquids. Eating four to six smaller meals rather than three large meals during the day facilitates the passage of food. The nurse collaborates with the dietitian for additional suggestions about diet changes and nutritional balance.

Nocturnal reflux of foods and liquids from the dilated esophagus into the hypopharynx and oral cavity often can be prevented if the client sleeps with the head of the bed elevated or in a semisitting position. The nurse also advises the client to experiment with various changes in position while eating, because such changes can reduce pressure sensations during meals. Some clients benefit from arching the back while swallowing. The nurse cautions the client to avoid wearing restrictive clothing, which can increase esophageal pressure and regurgitation.

ESOPHAGEAL DILATION. More severe cases of achalasia require dilation of the LES. The traditional treatment involves the passage of progressively larger sizes of esophageal bougies (dilators). Balloon dilation of the esophagus (using polyurethane balloons on a catheter) is considered the most effective treatment for achalasia. The procedure is performed on an ambulatory care basis. Typically, pneumatic dilators are positioned across the esophageal junction with fluoroscopy and local anesthesia. The balloon, which is filled with air or water, is inflated to a predetermined level for 30 to 60 seconds (Figure 55-4). This method lowers the basal LES pressure by tearing the esophageal sphincter muscle fibers.

After the procedure, the nurse monitors the client for bleeding and signs of perforation, such as chest and shoulder pain, elevated temperature, subcutaneous emphysema (air under the skin), or hemoptysis (coughing up blood). The client is taught to expectorate rather than swallow any secretions that may be produced. The client is also instructed to take nothing by mouth (NPO) for 1 hour and is instructed to limit dietary intake to liquids for 24 hours. The procedure may be repeated in 2 to 3 months if needed. Most clients report improvement in swallowing.

ESOPHAGOMYOTOMY. Surgical procedures for clients with achalasia are aimed at facilitating the passage of food. **Esophagomyotomy,** in which the LES is incised, has been used successfully for decades. Both thoracic and abdominal approaches can be used. An antireflux wrap **(fundoplication)** may or may not be part of the procedure.

Esophagomyotomy is a more complex surgical treatment for achalasia. General anesthesia is required, and the client is hospitalized for several days. A thoracotomy approach permits exposure of the esophagus. The surgeon cuts muscle fibers around the LES to open the sphincter and thereby provide less obstruction to food passage.

For long-term refractory achalasia, the surgeon may attempt excision of the affected portion of the esophagus, with or without replacement by a segment of colon or jejunum (partial esophagectomy).

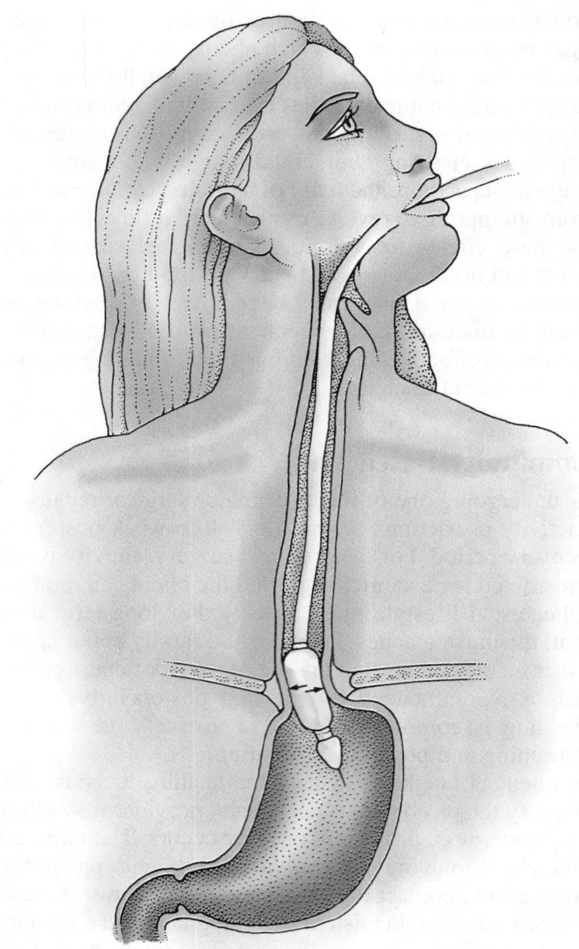

Figure 55-4 ● Balloon (pneumatic) dilation of the lower esophagus.

Postoperative care for clients undergoing esophagomyotomy or esophagectomy includes managing chest tubes and drains, assessing healing of the thoracotomy or abdominal incision, pain control, and managing nasogastric feedings. (See Chapter 19 for general postoperative care and Chapter 30 for care of the client with a thoracotomy.)

ESOPHAGEAL TUMORS

OVERVIEW

Tumors occurring in the esophagus can be benign or malignant. Benign tumors, usually in the form of leiomyomas, are extremely uncommon and are usually asymptomatic. No specific treatment is required unless they produce symptoms, and then they are generally removed.

Worldwide, esophageal cancer is the third most common gastrointestinal (GI) cancer and the eighth most common cancer (Parkin, Pisani, & Ferlay, 1999). A relatively uncommon cancer in the United States, it represents about 6% of all cancers of the GI tract, and mortality from the disease remains very high (Landis et al., 1999).

Pathophysiology

Most malignant esophageal tumors arise from the epithelium. Fifteen percent of all esophageal cancers are located in the upper esophagus and are primarily squamous cell in origin. Thirty-five percent of tumors appear in the mid-thoracic region and can be either squamous cell or adenocarcinomas. The lower esophagus is the site of approximately 50% of all esophageal cancers, primarily adenocarcinomas. The local and regional lymphatic spread of the disease differs according to the site of the original tumor. It has been proposed that esophageal cancers result from mutations in suppressor genes and proto-oncogenes (see Chapter 24 for a more complete discussion).

Esophageal tumors exhibit rapid local growth because there is no serosal layer to limit their extension. Because the esophageal mucosa is richly supplied with lymphatics, there is early spread of tumors to lymph nodes. Esophageal tumors can protrude into the esophageal lumen and either take on a flattened and infiltrative form to cause thickening of the lumen or manifest as a necrotic ulceration that invades deeply into surrounding tissue. In rare cases the lesion may be confined to the epithelial layer (in situ). In the majority of cases, the tumor is relatively large and well established on diagnosis.

Etiology

In the United States, the two primary risk factors associated with the development of squamous cell carcinoma of the esophagus are tobacco use and alcohol ingestion. The compounds in tobacco smoke may be responsible for the genetic mutations seen in one half of esophageal tumors. A smoker has two to six times the risk of eventually developing esophageal cancer than does a nonsmoker. Some alcoholic beverages contain potent carcinogens that may be responsible for the development of esophageal tumors. Smoking and alcohol ingestion act synergistically in the development of esophageal cancer.

Long-term exposure to gastric contents, such as that caused by gastroesophageal reflux disease (GERD), also plays a role in esophageal cancer development. Exposure to acid and pepsin leads to the replacement of normal distal squamous mucosa with columnar epithelium as a response to tissue injury, causing Barrett's disease or esophagus. This tissue undergoes dysplasia and, ultimately, malignant transformation.

In other parts of the world where esophageal cancer is common, the incidence of squamous cell carcinoma appears to be linked to high levels of nitrosamines (which are found in pickled and fermented foods) and foods high in nitrate. Diets that are chronically deficient in fresh fruits and vegetables have been implicated in the development of squamous cell carcinoma.

Certain genetic factors may have a role in the development of esophageal cancer. Overexpression and/or mutations of the p53 tumor suppressor gene have been found in esophageal cancer. In addition, the presence of the p53 gene may be an indication of advanced disease. Tumor cells with a mutated p53 gene have demonstrated resistance to chemotherapy.

Incidence/Prevalence

In the United States, cancer of the esophagus accounts for fewer than 1% of all newly diagnosed cancers and 6% of all tumors involving the gastrointestinal tract. In 1999 there was an estimated 316,000 new cases of esophageal cancer and 286,000 deaths worldwide (Parkin, Pisani, & Ferley, 1999). Although squamous cell cancer accounts for most cases, the rate of adenocarcinoma of the esophagus is also rapidly increasing. It is usually found at the gastroesophageal junction and the distal portion of the esophagus. The greatest incidence of adenocarcinoma can be found in Caucasian males of middle to upper socioeconomic status (Quinn & Reedy, 1999).

Esophageal cancer is extremely virulent and has a 5-year survival rate of less than 5%.

CULTURAL CONSIDERATIONS

Over the past several decades there have been statistically significant annual increases in the incidence of squamous cell cancer of the esophagus in the United States, particularly in African Americans. Mortality rates for esophageal cancer are now second only to those for cancer of the lung.

The incidence of esophageal cancer is extremely high in areas of northwest China, the Caspian Sea (around Russia and Iran), Japan, and the Transkei region of southern Africa. In these groups, the disease is found primarily in the upper to middle esophageal area. Residents of some provinces in China have a 30% to 40% probability of dying from esophageal cancer. The causes of these extreme variations are being researched but have not been satisfactorily explained.

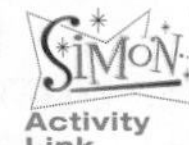

COLLABORATIVE MANAGEMENT

Assessment

HISTORY

The nurse assesses the client's racial and cultural background, age, sex, and any pertinent history of alcohol consumption, tobacco use, dietary habits, and other esophageal problems (e.g., dysphagia, stricture, or reflux). In collaboration with the dietitian, the nurse also collects a nutrition history, including the ingestion of pickled foods, changes in appetite, changes in taste, or a decline in weight. The degree of weight loss over time is also an important consideration.

Cancer of the esophagus is a silent tumor in its early stages, with few signs to identify on assessment. By the time the tumor causes symptoms, it usually has spread rather extensively.

PHYSICAL ASSESSMENT/CLINICAL MANIFESTATIONS

The primary clinical manifestations of esophageal cancer are dysphagia (most common) and weight loss (Brooks-Brunn, 2000). The nurse carefully assesses the degree and severity of dysphagia. Tumor-induced dysphagia is both persistent and progressive. It is initially associated with swallowing solids, particularly meat, and then progresses rapidly over a period of weeks or months to difficulty in swallowing soft foods and liquids. Late in the disease, even saliva can induce choking. Clients usually report a sensation that food is sticking in the throat or in the substernal area. Careful assessment of the dysphagia is an important part of the diagnosis because the dysphagia associated with other esophageal disorders is not usually continuous. Dysphagia does not usually appear until at least 60% of the esophageal diameter is narrowed by the tumor.

Odynophagia (painful swallowing) is present in most clients and is reported as a steady, dull, substernal pain that may radiate. The presence of severe or persistent pain often indicates tumor invasion of the mediastinal structures. The nurse also assesses for the occurrence of regurgitation, vomiting, foul breath, and chronic hiccups, which often accompany advanced disease. In most clients, pulmonary complications develop at some point, and the nurse assesses for the presence of chronic cough, increased secretions, and a history of recent infections.

Tumors in the upper esophagus may involve the larynx and thus cause hoarseness. Chart 55-6 summarizes the clinical manifestations of esophageal tumors.

PSYCHOSOCIAL ASSESSMENT

The symptoms and diagnosis of esophageal cancer can affect a client in profound ways. The disease produces significant daily symptoms, requires major modifications in basic eating patterns, and is terminal. The fear of choking can transform normal mealtimes into frightening experiences that the client may wish to avoid. The nurse carefully assesses the client's response to the diagnosis and prognosis and explores his or her coping strengths and resources. The impact of the disease on the usual pattern of activities is also assessed. The nurse also assesses the availability of support systems and the potential financial impact of the disease and its treatment.

RADIOGRAPHIC ASSESSMENT

To arrive at a diagnosis of esophageal cancer, the physician first uses a barium swallow study with fluoroscopy. The tumor margins of large masses can often be outlined during this test. A definitive diagnosis of cancer necessitates histologic evidence by means of a tissue biopsy.

OTHER DIAGNOSTIC ASSESSMENT

The definitive diagnosis of esophageal cancer is made by esophagogastroduodenoscopy (EGD) with biopsies of the esophagus and tumor. The physician performs an endoscopic examination to inspect the esophagus and to obtain specimens for cytologic studies and staging. Multiple tissue samples may be required when the suspected tumor is in the distal esophagus, because clear tissue samples are difficult to obtain.

A complete staging workup is performed to determine the extent of the disease. A computed tomography (CT) scan assists in identifying metastatic disease that can be present in the chest or abdomen. Positron emission tomography (PET) is a newer technology that may identify metastatic disease with more accuracy than a CT scan. Metastasis can also be diagnosed by bone and brain scans or exploratory laparoscopy. An endoscopic ultrasound (EUS) is a staging technique that can help determine the size and depth of tumor invasion. (These tests are described elsewhere in this text.)

CHART 55-6

KEY FEATURES *of* Esophageal Tumors

- Persistent and progressive dysphagia (most common feature)
- Feeling of food sticking in the throat
- Odynophagia (painful swallowing)
- Severe, persistent chest or abdominal pain or discomfort
- Regurgitation
- Chronic cough with increasing secretions
- Hoarseness
- Anorexia
- Nausea and vomiting
- Weight loss (often >20 pounds)
- Changes in bowel habits (diarrhea, constipation, bleeding)

CRITICAL THINKING CHALLENGE

You are gathering the initial history on a 65-year-old female Asian client admitted with dysphagia and a recent weight loss of 20 pounds over 3 months. The client states she used to smoke 2 packs of cigarettes per day for 30 years but quit 15 years ago. The client also admits to a 5-year history of gastrointestinal reflux, especially after eating in the late evening.

- What lifestyle and cultural factors place this client at risk for esophageal cancer?
- What specific questions would you ask concerning her swallowing difficulties?
- What additional clinical manifestations should you inquire about?

For suggested answer guidelines, go to SIMON http://www.wbsaunders.com/SIMON/Iggy/.

Analysis

COMMON NURSING DIAGNOSES AND COLLABORATIVE PROBLEMS

The priority nursing diagnosis for clients with cancer of the esophagus is Imbalanced Nutrition: Less than Body Requirements related to impaired swallowing.

ADDITIONAL NURSING DIAGNOSES AND COLLABORATIVE PROBLEMS

In addition to the common nursing diagnosis, the client with esophageal cancer may develop any of the following due to the impact of the disease and/or treatment:

- Risk for Aspiration related to impaired swallowing secondary to esophageal strictures
- Impaired Swallowing related to obstruction by the tumor or the effects of radiotherapy
- Acute Pain or Chronic Pain related to the pressure of the tumor mass in the esophagus or mediastinum
- Ineffective Coping and Compromised Family Coping related to the effects of the disease and to the terminal prognosis
- Anticipatory Grieving related to declining physical status and terminal prognosis
- Spiritual Distress related to impending death

The additional collaborative problem is Potential for Metastasis due to the close proximity of the esophagus to other body structures.

Planning and Implementation

IMBALANCED NUTRITION: LESS THAN BODY REQUIREMENTS

NOC **PLANNING: EXPECTED OUTCOMES.** The major concern for a client with esophageal cancer is weight loss secondary to dysphagia. Therefore the client is expected to ingest a sufficient quantity of balanced nutrients to meet the body's needs and to maintain a stable weight.

INTERVENTIONS. Interventions to maintain or improve the nutritional status of the client must focus on treatments to remove or shrink the obstructive tumor and on ameliorating the effects of treatment that can impact nutritional status.

Treatment options for cancer of the esophagus that can assist in both disease and nutrition management include the following:

- Nutritional support
- Radiotherapy
- Photodynamic therapy
- Dilation of strictures
- Prosthesis insertion
- Chemotherapy
- Surgical removal of the tumor

Much has been done over the last decade to try to improve the outcome for clients diagnosed with esophageal cancer. The typical treatment plan uses a combination of the above approaches. The current trend includes chemotherapy with or without surgery in an effort to improve the odds of obtaining a cure. Clients with cancer of the esophagus can experience many problems, and relieving symptoms becomes an essential consideration.

NIC **NUTRITION THERAPY.** The purpose of nutrition therapy is the administration of food and fluids to support the metabolic processes of a client who is malnourished or at high risk for becoming malnourished. A thorough nutritional assessment provides members of the health care team with baseline information concerning the client's nutritional status. The dietitian determines the caloric needs of the client to meet nutritional requirements. The nurse or assistive nursing personnel weighs the client daily. Careful positioning is essential for a client who is experiencing frequent regurgitation or who has prosthetic tubes to keep the esophagus patent. The nurse teaches the client to remain upright for several hours after meals and to avoid lying completely flat. The head of the bed is always elevated 30 degrees or more to prevent reflux.

Semisoft foods and thickened liquids are preferred because they are easier to swallow. Caloric intake and the amount of fluids ingested are monitored daily to monitor progress toward nutritional goals. In addition, liquid nutritional supplements can be used between feedings to increase caloric intake. Ongoing efforts are made to preserve the ability to swallow, but feeding tubes may be needed temporarily when dysphagia is severe. In clients with complete obstruction or life-threatening fistula formation, it may be necessary to create a gastrostomy or jejunostomy. The nurse monitors laboratory and clinical indicators of nutritional status. The client may also benefit from diet teaching and planning.

NIC **SWALLOWING THERAPY.** The nurse consults with the speech-language pathologist to assist with oral exercises to improve swallowing. A lollipop given to the client to suck on can enhance tongue strength. The client is instructed to reach for food particles on the lips or chin using the tongue. In preparation for swallowing, the nurse assists the client to position the head in forward flexion (chin tuck). The client is instructed to place food at the back of the mouth. The nurse monitors for the sealing of lips and for tongue movements while eating and also checks for pocketing of food after swallowing. It is important the nurse monitor for signs of aspiration. Family members and/or caregivers are taught how to feed the client, monitor for aspiration, and institute appropriate measures should choking occur. Chart 55-7 provides a summary of NIC interventions.

NONSURGICAL MANAGEMENT. Treatment decisions are based on the location and size of the tumor, the presence of metastasis, the client's concurrent health status, and the client's ability to withstand radical surgery.

The focus of nonsurgical treatment is palliative care. The outcomes of palliative care are the relief of symptoms and improved duration of survival. A combination of chemotherapy, radiation, pain control, and nutritional support measures can be used. The physician selects nonsurgical management when a client is either unable or unwilling to undergo extensive surgery.

RADIATION THERAPY. Radiation therapy to manage esophageal cancer is only moderately effective and can be used alone or in combination with other modalities. Used alone, radiation has been effective in the palliation of advanced esophageal cancer, with improvement in symptoms in 50% to 76% of cases (Behrend, 1999). Radiation therapy is contraindicated for clients with tracheoesophageal fistula,

CHART 55-7

NIC INTERVENTION ACTIVITIES *for* The Client with Esophageal Problems

Nutrition Therapy: *Administration of food and fluids to support metabolic processes of a client who is malnourished or at high risk for becoming malnourished*

- Determine—in collaboration with the dietitian, as appropriate—number of calories and type of nutrients needed to meet nutrition requirements.
- Assist the client to a sitting position before eating or feeding.
- Encourage the client to select semisoft food, if lack of saliva hinders swallowing.
- Select malts, shakes, and ice cream to supplement nutrition
- Monitor food/fluid ingested and calculate daily caloric intake, as appropriate
- Determine need for nasogastric tube feedings

Swallowing Therapy: *Facilitating swallowing and preventing complications of impaired swallowing*

- Collaborate with speech therapist to instruct client/family about swallowing exercise regimen.
- Explain the rationale of the swallowing regimen to client/family.
- Provide a lollipop for client to suck on to enhance tongue strength, if appropriate.
- Assist client to position head in forward flexion in preparation for swallowing ("chin tuck").
- Assist client to place food at back of mouth and on unaffected side.
- Monitor for signs and symptoms of aspiration.
- Instruct family/caregiver how to position, feed, and monitor client.
- Instruct client/caregiver on emergency measures for choking.

NIC intervention activities selected from McCloskey, J.C., & Bulechek, G.M. (Eds.). (2000). *Nursing interventions classification (NIC)* (3rd ed.). St. Louis: Mosby.

mediastinitis, mediastinal hemorrhage, or infiltration of the cancer to the trachea or bronchus (Gregoire & Fitzpatrick, 1998). Radiation reduces tumor size and offers clients consistent short-term relief. Although higher doses of radiation demonstrate better results, esophageal stricture or stenosis can result in 30% to 50% of clients requiring esophageal dilation. Normal esophageal tissue is very sensitive to the effects of radiation. The treatment is typically administered in twenty episodes over 4 weeks.

In the first weeks of treatment, radiation produces edema and epithelial desquamation, which often create acute esophagitis and odynophagia (painful swallowing). Profound anorexia, nausea, and vomiting may also result. Symptoms persist until treatment is completed. The nurse assesses the client frequently to determine the incidence and severity of symptoms. Systemic analgesics are often required to control discomfort, and the nurse administers topical lidocaine (Viscous Xylocaine) before each attempt at oral feeding.

The nurse works with the client to modify the diet to meet nutritional needs and maintain comfort. Small, frequent, soft or semiliquid meals are offered. Sweet, light foods are often tolerated best, and protein powder may be used to supplement the nutritional content of the diet. The nurse maintains accurate records of calorie counts, intake and output, and daily weights and also assesses skin turgor and mucous membranes regularly. In collaboration with the physician and dietitian, the nurse assesses the need for enteral nutrition if oral intake is insufficient.

For clients receiving radiation therapy, frequent gentle mouth care is important. Clients are at risk for monilial esophagitis, and the nurse is alert to any abrupt worsening of symptoms. Chapter 25 describes additional nursing interventions for the client undergoing radiation therapy.

PHOTODYNAMIC THERAPY. Photodynamic therapy (PDT) was originally used for the treatment of skin cancer. In 1995 it was approved for use as a palliative treatment for individuals with advanced esophageal cancer, who are not candidates for surgery. The client is injected with porfimer sodium (Sanofi Pharmaceuticals, New York), a light-sensitive drug that acts to amass cancer cells. Two days after the injection, a fiberoptic probe with a light at the tip is threaded into the esophagus. The light activates the Photofrin, destroying only cancer cells. PDT is far less invasive than surgery and is performed on an ambulatory care basis under conscious sedation.

The side effects of Photofrin are rare but include nausea, fever, and constipation. After the procedure, the client is given written guidelines concerning photosensitivity measures. The client is instructed to avoid exposure to sunlight for 1 month. Sunglasses and protective clothing that covers all exposed body areas are essential. The client may experience chest pain secondary to tissue damage and will require pain relief with opioids for a short time. The client is instructed to follow a clear liquid diet for 3 to 5 days after the procedure and advance to full liquids as tolerated (Durkin, 1999).

ESOPHAGEAL DILATION. Esophageal dilation may be performed as necessary throughout the course of the disease to achieve temporary but immediate relief of dysphagia. Esophageal dilation can be performed on an ambulatory care basis. The physician uses dilators to tear soft tissue, widening the esophageal lumen. In most cases, malignant tumors may be dilated safely, but perforation remains a significant risk. Bacteremia can also occur. To reduce the risk of endocarditis, the American Heart Association recommends prophylaxis with antibiotics (Behrend, 1999). The treatment is repeated as often as needed to preserve the client's ability to swallow (see p. 1204).

PROSTHESIS INSERTION. The physician may insert a semirigid prosthesis to bypass disabling dysphagia and to prevent aspiration in clients who have advanced disease or tracheoesophageal (TE) or esophagobronchial (EB) fistulas. Prosthesis insertion can maintain an open esophagus and preserve the client's ability to receive oral nourishment and thus palliate the symptoms related to obstruction. The procedure is not without risk, and acute complication rates have been reported to occur in 16% to 18% of clients (Raltz & Kozarek, 1999). The prosthesis can become dislodged, migrate, or perforate the esophagus as tumor bulk increases.

The nurse's primary care emphasis is the prevention of aspiration. The prosthesis interrupts the function of the lower esophageal sphincter (LES) and permits the free reflux of gastric contents. The nurse supervises the client closely, offers small oral feedings, and ensures that the client does not lie flat in bed.

CHEMOTHERAPY. The use of chemotherapy in the treatment of esophageal cancer has been only moderately effective. The two chemotherapeutic agents used to treat squamous cell carcinoma are 5-fluorouracil (5-FU) and cisplatin. Currently, there is no standard treatment for adenocarcinoma of the esophagus. Chemotherapy can be given before surgery to decrease tumor size, thereby facilitating surgical resection (Quinn & Reedy, 1999). Chemotherapy appears to be more effective when given in combination with radiation. Cisplatin and 5-FU make the tumor cells more sensitive to the effects of radiation. Chemotherapy can be administered concurrently with radiotherapy before surgery. This treatment is thought to provide the client with the best chance of cure.

CRITICAL THINKING CHALLENGE

Your client has been diagnosed with esophageal cancer and is undergoing preoperative radiation for tumor reduction before surgical resection.

- What possible complications related to this treatment should the nurse assess for?
- What nursing interventions could be instituted to assist the client in maintaining adequate nutritional intake?
- What should the nurse include in the teaching plan for this client?

For suggested answer guidelines, go to SIMON http://www.wbsaunders.com/SIMON/Iggy/.

SURGICAL MANAGEMENT. Radical surgery represents the only definitive treatment for esophageal cancer and is the preferred treatment for clients with no evidence of advanced disease. The goals of surgical resection vary from palliation to cure. Esophagectomy is an extensive surgical procedure and is associated with significant morbidity and mortality. Mortality from the surgical procedure ranges from 10% to 20%. Complications from surgery (e.g., fistula formation, abscess, and respiratory complications) occur in 20% to 50% of individuals (Behrend, 1999; Mayer, 1998).

PREOPERATIVE CARE. Preoperative preparation for clients undergoing esophagectomy or esophagogastrostomy can be quite extensive. Clients are advised to stop smoking 2 to 4 weeks before surgery to enhance their pulmonary functioning. Client preparation for surgery may include 5 days to 2 to 3 weeks of nutritional support in an effort to improve their nutritional status and decrease postoperative morbidity. Ideally, this supplementation is given orally, but most clients usually require tube feeding or parenteral nutrition. The role of parenteral nutritional support in these clients remains controversial (Sikora et al., 1998). The nurse carefully monitors the client's weight, intake and output, and fluid and electrolyte balance. A preoperative dental evaluation may be required to remove pre-existing dental caries. Meticulous oral care is performed four times daily to decrease the risk of postoperative infection.

Preoperative nursing care also focuses on teaching and on psychologic support. The nurse ensures that the client is knowledgeable about the surgery and its outcomes. The physician's instructions are clarified and reinforced as needed. The nurse explains the following:

- The number and sites of all incisions and drains
- The placement of a jejunostomy tube for initial enteral feedings
- The need for chest tubes if the pleural space is entered
- The purpose of the nasogastric tube
- The need for intravenous (IV) infusion

The client visits the critical care unit, if possible, and initiates contacts with unit staff.

The nurse instructs the client about routines for turning, coughing, deep breathing, and chest physiotherapy. The crucial nature of postoperative respiratory care is emphasized. The nurse addresses the probable need for ventilator support, because respiratory management is a major focus of postoperative care. If colon interposition is planned, the client also undergoes a complete bowel preparation with laxatives and enemas before surgery.

The client facing a serious illness and extensive surgery can be expected to display feelings of grief and anxiety. The nurse encourages the client to talk about personal feelings and fears and involves the family or significant others in all preoperative teaching and discussions. A primary nurse or case manager can be extremely helpful in providing continuity of care and support to the entire family.

OPERATIVE PROCEDURES. A subtotal or total *esophagectomy* is usually required because tumors are often quite large and involve distant lymph nodes. Several procedures have been used, but the preferred surgical procedure is an **esophagogastrostomy.** The diseased portion of the esophagus is removed, and the cervical portion is anastomosed (connected) to the stomach. The cervical portion of the stomach is then brought up into the thorax through the esophageal hiatus (Figure 55-5). A vagotomy is also usually performed with this type of resection, resulting in hypertonicity of the pylorus. A pyloromyotomy is created to prevent gastric motility disturbances. Lastly, a jejunostomy tube is placed for postoperative enteral feeding.

For a client with early stage tumors of the lower third of the esophagus, a transhiatal esophagectomy is the preferred surgical approach. The surgery is performed through an upper midline cervical incision. With this approach there is no entry into the pleural space, thereby minimizing respiratory complications.

For a client with tumors in the upper esophagus, radical neck dissection and laryngectomy may also be required because of the spread of disease to the larynx. The surgeon may perform a colon interposition when the tumor involves the stomach or the stomach is otherwise unsuitable for anastomosis. A section of right or left colon is removed and brought up into the thorax to substitute for the esophagus (see Figure 55-5).

These surgical procedures pose cardiovascular risks for the client. Intraoperative hypotension can result from pressure on the posterior heart. Decreased lymphatic pulmonary clearance can predispose the client to pulmonary edema when mediastinal lymph nodes and lymphatics are resected. The stress placed on the heart by extensive surgery can increase the risk of myocardial ischemia and dysrhythmias, especially if the client has underlying coronary disease.

The client with compromised nutritional status or prior radiation or chemotherapy is predisposed to an increased risk of infection. For clients who undergo more radical surgical procedures, there is a serious risk of leakage at the anastomosis site. This situation is especially true with colon interpositions because several anastomosis sites are vulnerable to the effects of tension, poor blood supply, and delayed healing. Mediastinitis resulting from an anastomotic leak can lead to fatal sepsis.

POSTOPERATIVE CARE. The client requires meticulous postoperative care and is at risk for multiple serious complications. The Client Care Plan on pp. 1199 and 1200 outlines client interventions for esophageal surgery.

Respiratory Care. Respiratory care is the *highest* postoperative priority, and the client is usually intubated and mechanically ventilated for at least the first 24 hours. Postoperative pulmonary complications include atelectasis and pneumonia. The risk of postoperative pulmonary complications is increased in the client who has received preoperative radiation. Once the client is extubated, the nurse begins deep breathing, turning, and coughing routines. Chest physiotherapy is initiated as ordered, usually every 2 to 4 hours. The nurse assesses the client for decreased breath sounds and shortness of breath every 1 to 2 hours. Incisional support and adequate analgesia are essential for effective coughing and should be administered regularly if the client's vital signs remain stable. The nurse keeps the client in a semi-Fowler's or high Fowler's position to support ventilation and prevent reflux. The physician prescribes prophylactic antibiotics and supplemental oxygen; blood gases are ordered regularly. The nurse ensures the patency of the water seal drainage system for chest tubes and monitors for changes in the volume or color of the drainage.

Cardiovascular Care. Hypotension can occur secondary to pressure placed on the posterior heart and may respond well to vigorous IV fluid administration. The nurse also monitors for signs and symptoms of fluid volume overload, particularly in clients who have undergone lymph node dissection. The nurse assesses for edema, crackles in the lungs, and increased jugular venous pressure. In the immediate postoperative phase, the client may be admitted to the intensive care unit. Critical care nurses assess hemodynamic parameters such as cardiac output, cardiac index, and systemic vascular resistance every 2 hours to monitor for myocardial ischemia.

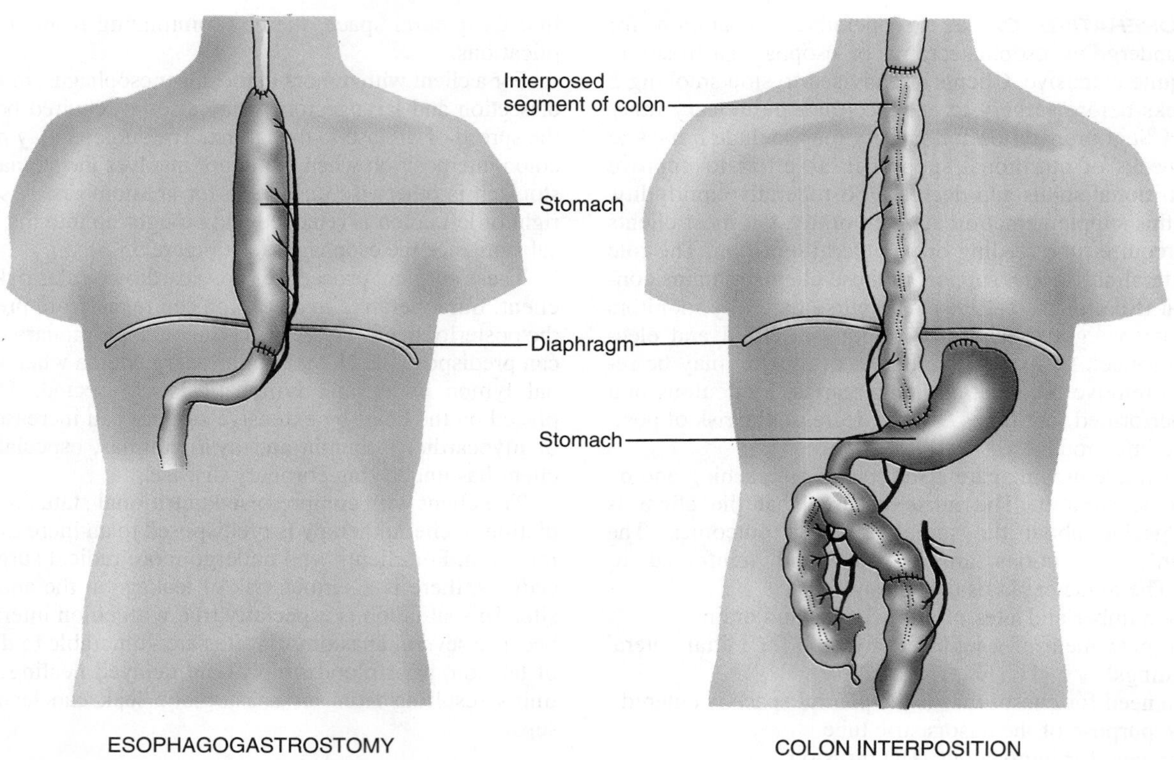

Figure 55-5 ● Surgical approaches to the treatment of esophageal cancer.

Atrial fibrillation is a dysrhythmia that results from irritation of the vagus nerve during surgery. Management of atrial fibrillation can include digitalization, beta blockers, or cardioversion. (See Chapter 34 for more information on atrial fibrillation.)

Wound Management. Wound management is another significant postoperative concern because the client typically has multiple incisions and drains. The nurse provides incisional support during turning and coughing to prevent dehiscence. Wound infection usually occurs 4 to 5 days after surgery. Postoperative leakage from the site of anastomosis is a dreaded complication that can appear 2 to 10 days after surgery. If an anastomic leak occurs, all oral intake is discontinued and is not resumed until the leak has healed. Nutrition may be given through the jejunostomy tube during the healing process. The nurse carefully assesses for fever, fluid accumulation, general signs of inflammation, and symptoms of early shock (e.g., tachycardia, tachypnea) and reports these findings to the health care provider immediately.

Nasogastric Tube Management. A nasogastric (NG) tube is placed intraoperatively to decompress the suture line. The nurse monitors the NG tube for patency and carefully secures the tube to prevent dislodgment, which can disrupt the sutures at the anastomosis. The nurse *does not* independently irrigate or reposition the NG tube in clients who have undergone esophageal surgery. The initial nasogastric drainage is bloody but should change to a greenish yellow color by the end of the first postoperative day. The continued presence of blood may indicate bleeding at the suture line. The nurse provides oral hygiene every 2 to 4 hours while the tube is in place (Chart 55-8).

CHART 55-8

BEST PRACTICE *for*
Managing the Client with a Nasogastric Tube After Esophageal Surgery

- Check for tube placement every 4 to 8 hours.
- Ensure that the tube is patent (open) and draining; drainage should turn from bloody to yellowish green by the end of the first postoperative day.
- Secure the tube well to prevent dislodgment.
- Do not irrigate or reposition the tube without a physician's order.
- Provide meticulous oral and nasal hygiene every 2 to 4 hours.
- Keep the head of the bed elevated to at least 30 degrees.
- When the client is permitted to have a small amount of water, place the client in an upright position and observe for dysphagia (difficulty swallowing).
- Observe for leakage from the anastomosis site, as indicated by fever, fluid accumulation, and manifestations of early shock (tachycardia, tachypnea, altered mental status).

Nutritional Care. The nutritional management of the client who has undergone an esophageal surgery is an early postoperative concern. On the second postoperative day, initial feedings begin through the jejunostomy tube. The feedings are slowly increased over the next several days. Feeding by this method can be discontinued once the client is taking adequate oral nutrition. However, some clients may require jejunostomy feedings for approximately 1 month if small amounts of aspiration are detected.

Before beginning oral feedings, a cine-esophagram study is performed to detect the presence of anastomotic leaks, strictures, or signs of aspiration. If no leaks are detected, an esophageal diet is begun, starting with liquids. If liquids are well tolerated, the client's diet is advanced to include semisolid foods and then solid foods. The nurse supervises the client during all initial swallowing efforts and ensures that he or she is in an upright position. The food storage area of the stomach has been radically decreased, and gravity is the client's only real defense against reflux. The nurse continues to assess for signs of leakage.

The client is instructed to consume 6 to 8 meals per day and to ingest fluids between, rather than with, meals to prevent diarrhea. Diarrhea can occur 20 minutes to 2 hours after eating and can be symptomatically managed with loperamide before meals. The diarrhea is thought to be the result of **vagotomy syndrome,** which develops as a result of the interruption of vagal fibers to the abdominal viscera during surgery. This syndrome is diminished by pyloroplasty.

CRITICAL THINKING CHALLENGE

Your client has completed a course of preoperative radiation therapy, and has undergone an esophagogastrostomy as part of her esophageal cancer treatment.

- What postoperative complications should you assess for and why?
- What nursing interventions would be most appropriate for preventing postoperative complications?

For suggested answer guidelines, go to SIMON http://www.wbsaunders.com/SIMON/Iggy/.

Community-Based Care

Clients with esophageal cancer have many challenges to face once they are discharged home. The combination treatment regimens cause long-lasting side effects, such as fatigue and weakness. These complex treatments also require the client to be knowledgeable about symptom management and to know when to report issues of concern to the health care provider. (See Chapter 25 for care of the client undergoing radiation therapy and chemotherapy.)

HOME CARE MANAGEMENT

The care given in the hospital is continued after discharge to the community. Ongoing respiratory care is a priority, and family members are instructed to assist with ambulation, splinting incisions, and use of the incentive spirometer. The nurse teaches the family to protect the client from infection and to contact the physician immediately if signs of respiratory infection develop. The client is encouraged to be as active as possible and to avoid excessive bedrest and its complications at all costs.

HEALTH TEACHING

Wound healing is also an ongoing concern. The nurse teaches the client and family to inspect the incisions daily for redness, tenderness, swelling, odor, and discharge. The client and family are instructed to report a temperature greater than 101° F (38.3° C).

The nurse prepares written instructions about the signs of anastomosis leakage and the importance of reporting them to the physician or other health care provider immediately. The client and family members are instructed to report the presence of fever and a swollen, painful neck incision, which indicates a cervical anastomotic leak (Gregoire & Fitzpatrick, 1998).

Nutritional support also remains a concern. The nurse encourages the client to continue increasing oral feedings as tolerated. The client is reminded to eat a high-calorie, high-protein diet that contains soft and easily swallowed foods. Meals should be small and frequent, and nutritionally empty foods are avoided. Eggnogs and milkshakes may be easily prepared and enriched to supplement meals. The client needs to learn what foods can be tolerated and needs to adjust his or her eating pattern to ingest food more slowly than before. Individuals who have undergone esophageal resection can lose up to 10% of their body weight. The client is taught to monitor his or her weight at home and to report a weight loss of 5 pounds or more. If sufficient oral intake is not possible, the family may need instruction about tube feedings or parenteral nutrition at home. (See the Legal/Ethical Issues in Health Care box above.)

The nurse emphasizes the importance of keeping the client upright after meals and elevating the head of the bed on blocks. Families are counseled that dysphagia or odynophagia may recur because of stricture, reflux, or cancer recurrence. These symptoms should be promptly reported to the health care provider.

Despite radical surgery, the client with cancer of the esophagus still has a terminal illness and a relatively short life expectancy. Emphasis is placed on maximizing quality of life. Realistic planning is important as the client's condition eventually worsens, and the client and family are assisted to plan for the future together. The nurse assists family members in exploring formal and informal sources of support. When

LEGAL/ETHICAL ISSUES IN HEALTH CARE

WITHHOLDING FOOD AND FLUIDS

Providing nutrition and hydration by means of IV catheters or gastric intubation raises many issues. Societal norms surround the provision of food and fluids to individuals who are deemed vulnerable, and this act is viewed differently than complex medical interventions. In addition, there is concern that withholding food and fluids may cause discomfort or suffering. Although there is agreement that ethical principles should be used to guide decision making in the provision or withdrawal of food and fluids, there is evidence to suggest that there are few potential benefits to providing nutrition to those with terminal or protracted illnesses.

Although there are no easy answers to this dilemma, a guide to decision making is suggested. The first consideration should be the previous wishes and evidence of current sensation of the individual involved. Second, the benefits and burdens of nutrition and hydration need to be evaluated in terms of long- and short-term goals. Finally, the interests of all parties involved should be represented. Clinicians should focus on reaching a consensus by incorporating an existing knowledge of feeding and hydration with consideration based on the wishes of the individual. The views of all stakeholders, and the given benefits and burdens of each case should also weigh in the decision.

From Daly, B. (2000) The special challenges of withholding food and fluids. *Gerontological Nursing, 26*(9), 25-31.

needed, the nurse helps the family or significant others arrange for hospice care.

HEALTH CARE RESOURCES

The nurse initiates referrals to community or home care organizations to assist the family in providing the needed home care. The client may need transportation to the radiation treatment center 5 times per week for up to 6 weeks. Oncology nursing care may be needed to monitor and evaluate the client who is receiving chemotherapy at home through venous access devices or portable infusion pumps. In addition, the nurse informs the family about the services available through the American Cancer Society. The nurse may also acquaint the family with area hospice services for future planning.

Evaluation: Outcomes

NOC The nurse evaluates the care of the client with esophageal cancer on the basis of the identified nursing diagnoses and collaborative problems. The expected outcomes are that the client:

- Maintains hemodynamic stability free of cardiovascular complications
- Maintains a patent airway free of respiratory complications
- Is free of infection
- Is able to consume adequate nutrition and maintain a stable weight
- Is able to swallow comfortably
- States that pain is controlled through pharmacologic and nonpharmacologic pain control measures
- Successfully adapts to the stresses surrounding the diagnosis and treatment with meaningful support from family or significant others

DIVERTICULA

OVERVIEW

Diverticula are sacs resulting from the herniation of esophageal mucosa and submucosa into surrounding tissue. Clients complain of dysphagia, regurgitation, nocturnal cough, and halitosis (bad breath).

Diverticula may develop anywhere along the length of the esophagus. No environmental risk factors are known to be involved in the development of esophageal diverticula. The incomplete or late opening of the cricopharyngeal muscle during swallowing leads to high pressures in the hypopharynx and leads to *Zenker's diverticulum,* the most common form. Zenker's diverticulum occurs most often in older adults. Clients with esophageal diverticula can be at risk for esophageal perforation because the mucosa is without the protection of the normal esophageal muscle layer.

COLLABORATIVE MANAGEMENT

The diagnosis of esophageal diverticula is made by x-ray examination and barium swallow. Endoscopy must be performed with strict care in these clients, because perforation can occur.

Diet therapy and positioning are the major interventions for controlling symptoms related to diverticula. The dietitian assists the client in exploring variations in the size and frequency of meals and in food texture and consistency. Semisoft foods and smaller meals are often best tolerated and may reduce or relieve the symptoms of pressure and reflux. Individual food tolerances and intolerances are explored with the client.

As with other forms of reflux, nocturnal problems associated with diverticula are best managed by sleeping with the head of the bed elevated and avoiding the recumbent position for at least 2 hours after eating. The client is also counseled to avoid vigorous exercise after meals. The nurse advises the client to avoid restrictive clothing and frequent stooping or bending.

Surgical management is aimed at excising the diverticula and reapproximating the mucosa. Most physicians use the cervical surgical approach above the clavicle. Postoperatively, the client takes nothing by mouth for several days to promote healing and receives IV fluids for hydration, tube feedings, and then oral fluid and food. The nurse provides pain relief measures and monitors for complications such as bleeding or perforation. A nasogastric (NG) tube is placed during surgery for decompression and is *not* irrigated or repositioned unless specifically ordered by the surgeon. This tube may be used later for feeding.

Community-based care includes teaching the client and family about the following:

- Tube feeding and resuming an oral diet
- Positioning guidelines to prevent reflux
- Warning signs of complications

Community resources are usually not needed for uncomplicated cases.

TRAUMA

OVERVIEW

Trauma to the esophagus can result from blunt injuries, chemical burns, surgery or endoscopy, or the stress of protracted severe vomiting (Table 55-2). Trauma may affect the esophagus directly, impairing swallowing and nutrition, or it may create problems and complications in related structures such as the lungs or mediastinum. The incidence of most forms of esophageal trauma is low in adults.

When excessive force is exerted on the esophageal mucosa, it may perforate or rupture, allowing the caustic acid secretions to enter the mediastinal cavity. These tears are associated with a high mortality rate related to shock, respiratory impairment, or sepsis.

Chemical injury is usually a result of the accidental or intentional ingestion of caustic substances. The oral cavity is also usually damaged, and the damage is rapid and severe. Acid burns tend to affect the superficial layers of the esophagus, whereas alkaline substances cause deeper penetrating injuries.

TABLE 55-2 • CAUSES OF ESOPHAGEAL PERFORATION

- Straining
- Seizures
- Trauma
- Foreign objects
- Instruments or tubes
- Chemical injury
- Complications of esophageal surgery
- Ulcers

Strong alkalis can cause full perforation of the esophagus within 1 minute. Additional problems may include aspiration pneumonia and hemorrhage. Strictures may develop as scar tissue forms. Table 55-3 lists caustic substances commonly found in the home.

➤ COLLABORATIVE MANAGEMENT

Most clients with esophageal trauma are initially evaluated and treated in the emergency department. Assessment focuses on the nature of the injury and the circumstances surrounding it. The nurse assesses for the presence of an airway, chest pain, dysphagia, vomiting, and bleeding.

If the risk of extending the damage is not excessive, the physician may order an x-ray or endoscopic study to evaluate tears or perforation. A computed tomography (CT) scan of the chest reveals the presence of mediastinal air.

After the injury, the client is allowed nothing by mouth to prevent further leakage of esophageal secretions. Esophageal and gastric suction is used for drainage and to rest the esophagus. Esophageal rest is maintained for at least 10 days after injury to allow for initial healing of the mucosa. The physician orders total parenteral nutrition (TPN) to provide calories and protein for wound healing while the client is not eating.

To prevent sepsis, the physician prescribes broad-spectrum antibiotics. High-dose corticosteroids may be administered to suppress inflammation and prevent strictures. The physician may prescribe opioid and nonopioid analgesics for pain management. When caustic burns involve the oral cavity, topical agents, such as 50/50 diphenhydramine hydrochloride (Benadryl) and kaolin with pectin (Ka-Pectolin) or topical lidocaine (Viscous Xylocaine), may be used for topical analgesia and local anti-inflammatory action.

If nonsurgical management is not effective in healing traumatized esophageal tissue, the client may need surgery to remove the damaged tissue. The client with severe injuries may require resection of part of the esophagus with a gastric pull-through and repositioning or replacement by a bowel segment. (See Surgical Management [Esophageal Tumors], pp. 1208 and 1209.)

TABLE 55-3 • ACTIVE INGREDIENTS OF COMMON HOUSEHOLD CORROSIVES

Types	Corrosive	Active Ingredient
Acids		
Liquid	Mister Plumber	Sulfuric acid 8.5%
	Lysol Toilet Bowl Cleaner	Hydrochloric acid
	Sno-Bol Toilet Bowl Cleaner	Hydrochloric acid 15%
Granular	ZUD Rust and Stain Remover	Oxalic acid
	Sani-Flush Toilet Bowl Cleaner	Sodium bisulfite 75%
	Vanish Toilet Bowl Cleaner	Sodium acid sulfate 62%
Alkalis	Liquid Drāno	Sodium hydroxide 9.5%
	Crystal Drāno	Sodium hydroxide 80%
	Liquid Plumr	Sodium hypochlorite and hydroxide 8%
	Easy-Off Liquid Oven Cleaner	Sodium hydroxide
	Mr. Muscle Oven Cleaner	Sodium hydroxide
	Industrial/Professional Drāno	Sodium hydroxide 32%
	Ammonia	Ammonium hydroxide
Bleaches	Clorox	
	Peroxide	
Thermal agents	Dry ice	
	Hot water	
Detergents	Cascade (dish)	Sodium tripolyphosphate
	Amway (dish)	Sodium tripolyphosphate

ONLINE RESOURCES

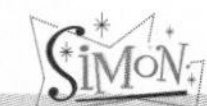

For suggested readings and Internet resources, go to http://www.wbsaunders.com/SIMON/Iggy/.

SELECTED BIBLIOGRAPHY

Behrend, S.W. (1999). Esophageal cancer. In Miaskowski, C. & Buchsel, P. (Eds.), *Oncology nursing: Assessment and clinical care* (pp. 889-917). St. Louis: Mosby.

Brooks-Brunn, J.A. (2000). Esophageal cancer: An overview. *MEDSURG Nursing, 9*(5), 248-254.

Cameron, A. (1999). Barrett's esophagus: Prevalence and size of hiatal hernia. *The American Journal of Gastroenterology, 94*(8), 2054-2059.

Claussen, J. (1999). Gastroesophageal reflux disease: A rational approach to management. *Clinician Reviews, 9*(6), 69-82.

Crawford, J. (1999). The gastrointestinal tract. In R.S. Cotran et al. (Eds.), *Robbins pathologic basis of disease* (6th ed., pp. 775-787). Philadelphia: W.B. Saunders.

Daly, B. (2000). The special challenges of withholding artificial nutrition and hydration. *Journal of Gerontological Nursing, 26*(9), 25-31.

Durkin, S. (1999). Photodynamic therapy: A cancer treatment for the 21st century. *Gastroenterology Nursing, 22*(3), 115-120.

Eloubeidi, M., et al. (1999). A cost analysis of outpatient care for patients with Barrett's esophagus in a managed care setting. *The American Journal of Gastroenterology, 94*(8), 2033-2036.

Fackeer, W.K., & Richter, J.E., (2000). Refractory GERD: What next? *Consultant,* May, pp. 973-983.

Ferguson, M.K. (1997). Pitfalls and complications of antireflux surgery: Nissen and Collis-Nissen techniques. In Fell & Bains (Eds.), *Chest surgery clinics of North America* (pp. 489-509). Philadelphia: W.B. Saunders.

Goldsmith, C. (1998). Gastroesophageal reflux disease. *American Journal of Nursing, 98*(9), 44-45.

Gregoire, A.S., & Fitzpatrick, E. (1998). Esophageal cancer: Multisystem nursing management. *Dimensions of Critical Care Nursing, 17*(1), 28-36.

Kessenich, C. (1999). Differential diagnosis of chest pain: A case report. *Gastroenterology Nursing, 22*(1), 10-13.

Khoury, R., et al. (1999). Influence of spontaneous sleep positions on nighttime recumbent reflux in patients with gastroesophageal reflux disease. *The American Journal of Gastroenterology, 94*(8), 2069-2073.

Landis, S.H., et al. (1999). Cancer statistics 1999. *CA: A Cancer Journal for Clinicians, 49*(1), 8-31.

Mayer, R. (1998). Gastrointestinal tract cancer. In A.S. Fauci, E. Braunwald, & K.J. Isselbacher (Eds.), *Harrison's principles of internal medicine* (14th ed., pp. 568-577). New York: McGraw-Hill.

O'Connor, J., Falk, G., & Richter, J. (1999). The incidence of adenocarcinoma and dysplasia in Barrett's esophagus. *The American Journal of Gastroenterology, 94*(8), 2037-2042.

Parkin, D.M., Pisani, P., & Ferlay, J. (1999). Global cancer statistics. *CA: A Cancer Journal for Clinicians, 49*(1), 33-64.

Quinn, K., & Reedy, A. (1999). Esophageal cancer: Therapeutic approaches and nursing care. *Seminars in Oncology Nursing, 15*(1), 17-25.

Raltz, S., & Kozarek, R. (1999). Do age, gender, or tumor location affect outcomes when using metallic stents in the palliative treatment of esophageal carcinoma? *Gastroenterology Nursing, 22*(6), 249-253.

Scott, M., & Gelhot, A.R. (1999). Gastroesophageal reflux disease: Diagnosis and management. *American Family Physician,* 59(5), 1161-1169.

Sharma, P. (1999). Barrett's esophagus: Put guidelines into practice. *Patient Care for the Nurse Practitioner, 2*(9), 23-26.

Sikora, S., et al. (1998). Role of nutrition support during induction chemoradiation therapy in esophageal cancer. *Journal of Parenteral and Enteral Nutrition, 22*(1), 18-21.

Tucker, K., & Schumann, L. (1999). Gastroesophageal reflux disease. *The Clinical Advisor,* April, pp. 52-58.

Vaca, K., et al. (1998). The role of laparoscopic Nissen fundoplication in gastroesophageal reflux disease. *MEDSURG Nursing, 7*(6), 364-370.

CHAPTER 56

Interventions for Clients with Stomach Disorders

CONSTANCE VISOVSKY

Learning Objectives

After studying this chapter, you should be able to:

1. Compare etiologies and assessment findings of acute and chronic gastritis.
2. Describe the key components of collaborative management for clients with gastritis.
3. Compare and contrast assessment findings associated with gastric and duodenal ulcers.
4. Identify the most common medical complications that can result from peptic ulcer disease (PUD).
5. Analyze assessment data to determine common nursing diagnoses associated with PUD.
6. Develop a teaching plan related to drug therapy for clients experiencing PUD.
7. Prioritize interventions for clients with upper gastrointestinal bleeding.
8. Plan preoperative and postoperative care for the client undergoing gastric surgery.
9. Develop a community-based plan of care for clients who have undergone gastric surgery.
10. Evaluate outcomes for clients with PUD.
11. Explain Zollinger-Ellison syndrome and its associated clinical manifestations.
12. Analyze risk factors for gastric carcinoma, including cultural considerations.
13. Plan postoperative care for clients who have undergone surgery for gastric cancer.
14. Discuss the psychologic and emotional concerns of clients with gastric cancer.

SIMON **Go to http://www.wbsaunders.com/SIMON/Iggy/ for self-assessment questions related to these Learning Objectives.**

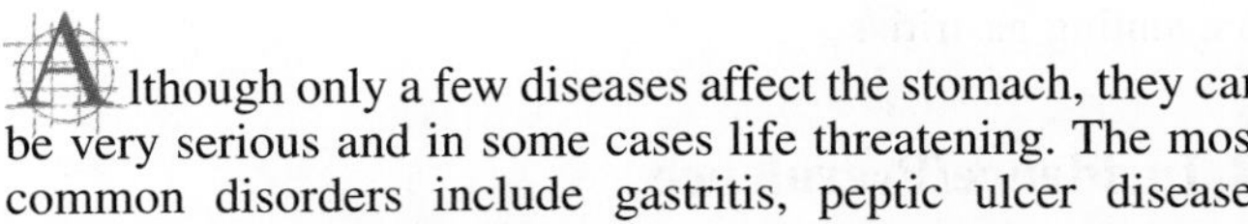

Although only a few diseases affect the stomach, they can be very serious and in some cases life threatening. The most common disorders include gastritis, peptic ulcer disease, Zollinger-Ellison syndrome, and gastric carcinoma (cancer).

GASTRITIS

OVERVIEW

Gastritis is defined as inflammation of the gastric mucosa (stomach lining). It can be diffuse or localized and can be classified according to cause, cellular changes, or distribution of the lesions. Gastritis can be designated as erosive (acute gastritis, stress ulcers) or nonerosive (chronic gastritis). Although the mucosal changes accompanying acute gastritis typically resolve after several months, this is not true for chronic gastritis.

Pathophysiology

Prostaglandins provide a protective mucosal barrier that prevents the stomach from digesting itself by a process called acid autodigestion. If there is a break in the protective barrier, mucosal injury occurs. The resulting injury is compounded by histamine release and vagal nerve stimulation. Hydrochloric acid can then diffuse back into the mucosa and injure small vessels. This back-diffusion results in edema, hemorrhage, and erosion of the stomach's lining. The pathologic changes of gastritis include vascular congestion, edema, acute inflammatory cell infiltration, and degenerative changes in the superficial epithelium of the stomach lining.

The early pathologic manifestation of gastritis is a thickened, reddened mucous membrane with prominent rugae, or folds. As the disease progresses, the walls and lining of the stomach thin and atrophy. With progressive gastric atrophy from chronic mucosal injury, the function of the parietal (acid-secreting) cells decreases and the source of intrinsic factor is lost. The intrinsic factor is critical for absorption of vitamin B_{12}. When body stores of vitamin B_{12} are eventually depleted, pernicious anemia results. The amount and concentration of acid in stomach secretions gradually decrease until the secretions consist of only mucus and water.

Chronic gastritis is associated with an increased risk of gastric cancer as the persistent inflammation extends deep into the mucosa, causing destruction of the gastric glands and cellular changes. Hemorrhage may occur after an episode of acute gastritis or with ulceration caused by chronic gastritis.

ACUTE GASTRITIS

Inflammation of the gastric mucosa or submucosa after exposure to local irritants can result in acute gastritis. Various degrees of mucosal necrosis and inflammatory reaction occur in acute disease. The diagnosis cannot be based solely on clinical symptoms without an endoscopic examination. Complete regeneration and healing usually occur within a few days. If the stomach muscle is not involved, complete recovery usually occurs with no residual evidence of gastric inflammatory reaction.

CHRONIC GASTRITIS

Chronic gastritis appears as a patchy, diffuse (spread out) inflammation of the mucosal lining of the stomach. Chronic gastritis usually heals without scarring, but it can progress to hemorrhage and the formation of an ulcer.

Chronic gastritis may be categorized as type A, type B, or atrophic. Type A (nonerosive) chronic gastritis refers to an inflammation of the glands, as well as the fundus and body of the stomach. Type B chronic gastritis usually affects the glands of the antrum but may involve the entire stomach. In atrophic chronic gastritis, diffuse inflammation and destruction of deeply located glands accompany the condition. Chronic atrophic gastritis affects all layers of the stomach, thus decreasing the number of cells. The muscle becomes thickened, and inflammation is present. Chronic atrophic gastritis is characterized by total loss of fundal glands, minimal inflammation, thinning of the gastric mucosa, and intestinal metaplasia (abnormal tissue development).

Etiology

ACUTE GASTRITIS

The onset of infection with *Helicobacter pylori* can result in acute gastritis. *H. pylori* is a gram-negative, spiral-shaped organism that penetrates the mucosal gel layer of the gastric epithelium. Although it is uncommon, other forms of bacterial gastritis from organisms such as staphylococci, streptococci, *Escherichia coli,* or salmonella can cause life-threatening consequences such as sepsis and extensive tissue necrosis (Friedman & Peterson, 1998). Other infectious causes of acute gastritis can be found in clients with immunosuppressive disorders. In clients with acquired immunodeficiency syndrome (AIDS), for example, gastric erosions can be found with herpes simplex viral infection and disseminated cytomegalovirus (CMV) infection.

Nonsteroidal anti-inflammatory drug (NSAID) use poses a risk for the development of acute gastritis. Gastritis occurs in 5% to 25% of NSAID users, but the exact mechanism of the role of NSAIDs in the development of gastritis is not well understood. Other drugs, including alcohol, cytotoxic agents, caffeine, and corticosteroids, have also been implicated; however, scientific evidence is lacking. Acute gastritis is also caused by local irritation from radiation therapy and accidental or intentional ingestion of corrosive substances, including acids or alkalis (such as lye and drain cleaners [Mister Plumber, Drano]). In the client who is allowed nothing by mouth (NPO), gastritis may result from lack of stimulation of normal secretions. Acute stress-induced gastritis, characterized by multiple shallow erosions of the proximal stomach, may be present in 80% to 100% of critically ill clients.

CHRONIC GASTRITIS

Type A gastritis has been associated with the presence of antibodies to parietal cells and intrinsic factor; therefore an autoimmune pathogenesis for this type of gastritis has been proposed. Parietal cell antibodies have been found in 90% of clients with pernicious anemia and in more than one half of individuals with type A gastritis. A genetic link to this disease, with an autosomal dominant pattern of inheritance, has been noted in the relatives of clients with pernicious anemia (Centanni et al., 1999).

The most common form of the disease is type B gastritis, caused by *H. pylori* infection. There is a direct correlation between the number of organisms and the degree of cellular abnormality present. Although serum antibodies have been isolated in some clients, it is believed that these antibodies are not representative of an autoimmune process but are the result of prolonged inflammation. Fifty percent of clients who have gastric ulcers have associated chronic gastritis.

Chronic local irritation and toxic effects caused by alcohol ingestion, radiation therapy, and smoking have been implicated in the development of chronic gastritis. Surgical procedures that involve the pyloric sphincter, such as the Billroth II procedure, can lead to gastritis by causing reflux of alkaline secretions into the stomach. Other systemic disorders such as Crohn's disease, graft-versus-host disease, and uremia can also precipitate the development of chronic gastritis.

CHRONIC ATROPHIC GASTRITIS. Atrophic gastritis is a type of chronic gastritis that is seen most often in older adults. It can occur after exposure to toxic substances in the workplace (e.g., benzene, lead, and nickel) or *H. pylori* infection, or it can be related to autoimmune factors.

Although atrophic gastritis is often present in people with gastric cancer, it is not always considered a precancerous lesion. Gastric carcinoma develops in fewer than 10% of clients who have atrophic gastritis. Chart 56-1 lists guidelines for preventing gastritis.

Incidence/Prevalence

Approximately 2.7 million people in the United States have been diagnosed with gastritis. The incidence of gastritis is higher in men than in women; however, it has been suggested that more women have chronic atrophic gastritis. Acute and

CHART 56-1

CLIENT EDUCATION GUIDE
Gastritis Prevention

- Avoid drinking excessive amounts of alcoholic beverages.
- Use caution in taking large doses of aspirin, nonsteroidal anti-inflammatory drugs (such as ibuprofen), and corticosteroids. Prolonged use of small doses of corticosteroids may also cause gastritis.
- Avoid excessive intake of caffeine-containing beverages.
- Avoid eating contaminated foods or drinking contaminated water.
- Stop smoking.
- Protect yourself against exposure to toxic substances in the workplace, such as lead and nickel.
- Seek medical treatment if you are experiencing symptoms of esophageal reflux (see Chapter 55).

chronic forms of the disease are more prevalent in heavy smokers and persons who abuse alcohol. The incidence of chronic gastritis increases with age.

COLLABORATIVE MANAGEMENT

Assessment

PHYSICAL ASSESSMENT/CLINICAL MANIFESTATIONS

Physical assessment findings may include abdominal tenderness and bloating, **hematemesis** (vomiting blood), or **melena** (traces of blood in the stool). In stress-induced gastritis, symptoms of intravascular volume depletion and shock may be present.

ACUTE GASTRITIS. Symptoms of acute gastritis can range from mild to severe. Epigastric discomfort, anorexia, cramping, nausea, and vomiting may be present. In some cases, gastric hemorrhage is the presenting symptom (Chart 56-2). The symptoms last only a few hours or days and vary with the cause. Aspirin-related gastritis may result in dyspepsia (heartburn). Gastritis from alcohol abuse may cause vomiting and hematemesis. Gastritis or food poisoning caused by endotoxins, such as staphylococcal endotoxin, has an abrupt onset; severe nausea and vomiting often occur within 5 hours of ingestion of the contaminated food.

CHRONIC GASTRITIS. Chronic gastritis causes few symptoms. Clients may complain of nausea, vomiting, or upper abdominal discomfort. Periodic epigastric pain may simulate ulcer-like distress, which is relieved on ingestion of food. Some clients may have anorexia, and pain may be exacerbated by eating fatty or spicy foods (see Chart 56-2).

DIAGNOSTIC ASSESSMENT

Esophagogastroduodenoscopy (EGD) via an endoscope with biopsy is the gold standard for diagnosing gastritis, as well as detecting the presence of *H. pylori.* The health care provider uses biopsy to establish a definitive diagnosis of the type of gastritis. If lesions are patchy and diffuse, biopsy of several suspicious areas may be necessary to avoid misdiagnosis. A cytologic examination of the biopsy specimen is performed to confirm or rule out gastric cancer.

CHART 56-2

KEY FEATURES *of* Gastritis

Acute Gastritis
- Rapid onset of epigastric pain or discomfort
- Nausea and vomiting
- Hematemesis (vomiting blood)
- Gastric hemorrhage
- Dyspepsia (heartburn)
- Anorexia

Chronic Gastritis
- Vague complaint of epigastric pain that is relieved by food
- Anorexia
- Nausea or vomiting
- Intolerance of fatty and spicy foods
- Pernicious anemia

Interventions

Clients with gastritis are not often seen in the acute care setting unless they have an exacerbation of acute or chronic gastritis that results in fluid and electrolyte imbalance or bleeding. Management is directed toward supportive care for relieving the symptoms and removing the cause of discomfort.

Acute gastritis is treated symptomatically and supportively because the healing process is spontaneous, usually occurring within a few days. When the cause is removed, pain and discomfort usually subside. If hemorrhage is severe, a blood transfusion may be necessary. Fluid replacement is indicated in clients with severe fluid loss. Surgery, such as partial gastrectomy, pyloroplasty, and/or vagotomy, may be indicated for clients with major bleeding or ulceration. Treatment of chronic gastritis varies with the cause. General treatment goals include the eradication of causative agents, treatment of any underlying disease (e.g., uremia, Crohn's disease), and avoidance of toxic substances (e.g., alcohol, tobacco, nonsteroidal anti-inflammatory drugs [NSAIDs]).

NONSURGICAL MANAGEMENT. The identification and elimination of the causative factors, such as eradication of *H. pylori* infection, is the primary treatment modality. Drugs and diet therapy are also used in the treatment of gastritis.

DRUG THERAPY. In the acute phase, the nurse directs actions toward relief of pain and discomfort. The health care provider may order medications that block and buffer gastric acid secretions to relieve pain.

H_2-receptor antagonists are commonly used to block gastric secretions. These agents include ranitidine (Zantac), famotidine (Pepcid), and nizatidine (Axid). Sucralfate (Carafate, Sulcrate♣), a mucosal barrier fortifier, may also be prescribed. Antacids used as buffering agents include aluminum hydroxide combined with magnesium hydroxide (Maalox) and aluminum hydroxide combined with simethicone and magnesium hydroxide (Mylanta) (Chart 56-3). The nurse monitors for symptom relief and side effects of these medications and notifies the health care provider of any untoward effects or worsening of gastric distress.

Clients with chronic gastritis may require vitamin B_{12} for prevention or treatment of pernicious anemia. If *H. pylori* is found in biopsy specimens, the health care provider may treat the infection and reverse or prevent impairment of mucosal defenses. A common drug regimen for *H. pylori* infection is bismuth subsalicylates (Pepto-Bismol), metronidazole (Flagyl, Novonidazol♣), and tetracycline or ampicillin (Amcill, Ampicin♣).

The nurse, health care provider, or pharmacist instructs clients about the medications associated with gastric irritation. These medications include chemotherapeutic agents, corticosteroids, erythromycin (E-Mycin, Erythromid♣), and NSAIDs, such as aspirin, indomethacin (Indocin, Novomethacin♣) and ibuprofen (Motrin, Advil, Amersol♣, Novo-Profen♣).

The health care provider may change the dose, frequency, or type of medication if symptoms of gastric irritation appear or persist. The nurse instructs clients to avoid stomach-irritating over-the-counter (OTC) medications, such as aspirin and ibuprofen.

DIET THERAPY. The nurse or dietitian instructs the client with gastric disease to limit intake of any foods and spices

CHART 56-3

DRUG THERAPY *for* Peptic Ulcer Disease

Drug	Usual Dosage	Nursing Interventions	Rationale
ANTACIDS			
Magnesium hydroxide with aluminum hydroxide (Maalox, Mylanta)	50-80 mEq 1 hr + 3 hr pc (after meals) + hs (at bedtime)	Give 2 hr after meals and at bedtime.	Hydrogen ion load is high after ingestion of foods.
		Use liquid rather than tablets.	Suspensions are more effective than chewable tablets.
		Do not give other drugs within 1-2 hr of antacids.	Antacids interfere with absorption of other drugs.
		Assess the client for a history of renal disease.	Hypermagnesemia may result.
		Assess the client for a history of congestive heart failure.	These antacids have a high sodium content.
		Observe the client for the side effect of diarrhea.	Magnesium often causes diarrhea.
Aluminum hydroxide (Amphojel)	50-80 mEq 1 hr + 3 hr pc + hs	Give 1 hr after meals and at bedtime.	Hydrogen ion load is high after ingestion of food.
		Use liquid rather than tablets if palatable.	Suspensions are more effective than chewable tablets.
		Do not give other drugs within 1-2 hr of antacids.	Antacids interfere with absorption of other drugs.
		Observe the client for the side effect of constipation. If constipation occurs, consider alternating with magnesium antacid.	Aluminum causes constipation, and magnesium has a laxative effect.
		Use for clients with renal failure.	Aluminum binds with phosphates in the gastrointestinal (GI) tract.
H_2 ANTAGONISTS			
Ranitidine (Zantac)	150 mg bid or 300 mg hs PO; 50 mg q6h IV or 8 mg/hr IV (continuous)	Give single dose at bedtime.	Bedtime administration suppresses nocturnal acid production.
Famotidine (Pepcid)	40 mg once daily or in two divided doses PO; 20 mg q12h IV	Give single dose at bedtime.	Bedtime administration suppresses nocturnal acid production. Compliance may improve with less frequent administration.
Nizatidine (Axid)	150 mg bid or 300 mg hs PO	Give single dose at bedtime.	Bedtime administration suppresses nocturnal acid production. Compliance may improve with less frequent administration.
Sucralfate (Carafate, Sulcrate♣)	1 g qid or 2 g bid PO	Give 1 hr before and 2 hr after meals, and at bedtime.	Food may interfere with drug's adherence to mucosa.
		Do not give within 30 min of giving antacids or other drugs.	Antacids may interfere with effect.

that cause distress. Tea, coffee, cola, chocolate, mustard, paprika, cloves, pepper, and hot spices may increase discomfort. Alcohol and tobacco should also be avoided.

After the client has an acute episode of gastritis, the nurse helps him or her to identify foods that aggravate discomfort. New foods should be introduced one at a time. Avoidance of substances that cause symptoms is important. Most clients seem to progress better with a soft, bland diet and smaller, more frequent meals.

STRESS REDUCTION. The nurse may assist the client with various techniques that reduce stress and discomfort, such as progressive relaxation, cutaneous stimulation, guided imagery, and distraction. (See Chapter 4 for a discussion of these therapies.)

SURGICAL MANAGEMENT. Partial gastrectomy, pyloroplasty, vagotomy, or even total gastrectomy may be indicated for clients who have major bleeding caused by severe erosive gastritis. Such surgery is necessary only if more conservative measures have not controlled the bleeding. Surgical interventions are discussed under Surgical Management (Peptic Ulcer Disease), p. 1228.

PEPTIC ULCER DISEASE

OVERVIEW

A **peptic ulcer** is a mucosal lesion of the stomach or duodenum. The term *peptic ulcer* is used to describe both gastric and duodenal ulcers. **Peptic ulcer disease (PUD)** results

CHART 56-3

DRUG THERAPY *for* Peptic Ulcer Disease—cont'd

Drug	Usual Dosage	Nursing Interventions	Rationale
ANTISECRETORY AGENTS			
Omeprazole (Prilosec, Losec✽)	20 mg bid or 40 mg hs PO	Have the client take capsule whole; do not crush.	Delayed-release capsules allow absorption after granules leave the stomach.
		Give single dose at bedtime for ulcer disease.	Bedtime administration suppresses nocturnal acid production.
Lansoprazole (Prevacid)	15 or 30 mg hs PO	Give single dose at bedtime for ulcer disease; do not crush.	Bedtime administration suppresses nocturnal acid production.
Rabeprazole (AcipHex)	20 mg once daily PO	Take following the morning meal.	Drug promotes healing and symptom relief of duodenal ulcers.
		Do not crush capsule.	Drug is a sustained-release capsule.
PROSTAGLANDIN ANALOGS			
Misoprostol (Cytotec)	200 μg qid PO	Take with food.	Drug protects against nonsteroidal anti-inflammatory drug (NSAID)–induced ulcers.
		Avoid magnesium-containing antacids.	Both misoprostol and magnesium-containing antacids can cause diarrhea.
ANTIMICROBIALS			
Clarithromycin (Biaxin)	500 mg tid PO	Antimicrobials should be given as part of therapy to eradicate *Helicobacter pylori* infection.	*H. pylori* is a gram-negative bacterium implicated in the development of peptic ulcer disease (PUD).
Amoxicillin (Amoxil)	1 g bid PO	The selection of the specific drug depends on its effectiveness, side effects, and drug interactions.	
Tetracycline	500 mg qid PO		
Metronidazole (Flagyl)	250 mg tid and hs PO		

when gastric mucosal defenses become impaired and no longer protect the epithelium from the effects of acid and pepsin (Figure 56-1).

Pathophysiology

GASTRIC ULCERS

Acid, pepsin, and *Helicobacter pylori* infection play an important role in the development of gastric ulcers. The gastric mucosal barrier overlies the epithelium. The secretion of mucus and bicarbonate provides a first line of defense in maintaining a near-normal pH on the gastric epithelium and protects the mucosal barrier against acid. Gastromucosal prostaglandins increase the barrier's resistance to ulceration. The integrity of the barrier is enhanced by the rich blood supply of the mucosa of the stomach and duodenum.

When a break in the mucosal barrier occurs, hydrochloric acid injures the epithelium. Gastric ulcers may then result from back-diffusion of acid or dysfunction of the pyloric sphincter (see Figure 56-1). Without normal functioning and competence of the pyloric sphincter, bile refluxes into the stomach. This reflux of bile acids may break the integrity of the mucosal barrier and produce hydrogen ion back-diffusion, which leads to mucosal inflammation. Toxic agents and bile then destroy the lipid plasma membrane of the gastric mucosa.

Gastric emptying is often delayed in clients with gastric ulceration; this causes regurgitation of duodenal contents, which compounds the gastric mucosal injury. A decreased blood flow to the gastric mucosa may also alter the defense barrier and thereby allow ulceration to occur. Characteristically, gastric ulcers are deep and penetrating, and they usually occur on the lesser curvature of the stomach, near the pylorus (Figure 56-2).

DUODENAL ULCERS

Ninety-five percent of duodenal ulcers occur in the first portion of the duodenum. Duodenal ulcers present as deep, sharply demarcated lesions that penetrate through the mucosa and submucosa into the muscularis propria (muscle layer). The floor of the ulcer consists of a necrotic area residing on granulation tissue and surrounded by areas of fibrosis.

The characteristic feature of a duodenal ulcer is high gastric acid secretion, although a wide range of secretory levels is found. In clients with duodenal ulcers, pH levels are low in the duodenum for long periods. Protein-rich meals, calcium, and vagal excitation stimulate acid secretion. Combined with

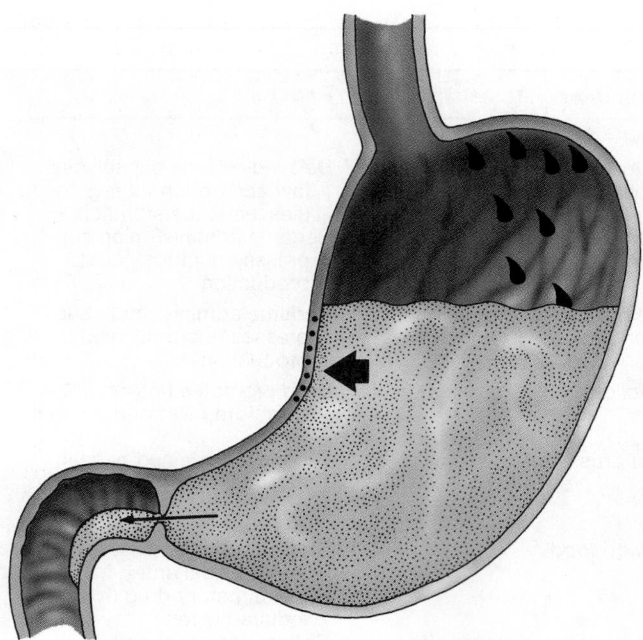

Conditions favoring the development of **gastric ulcers** are normal gastric acid secretion and delayed stomach emptying with *increased diffusion of gastric acid back into the stomach tissues.*

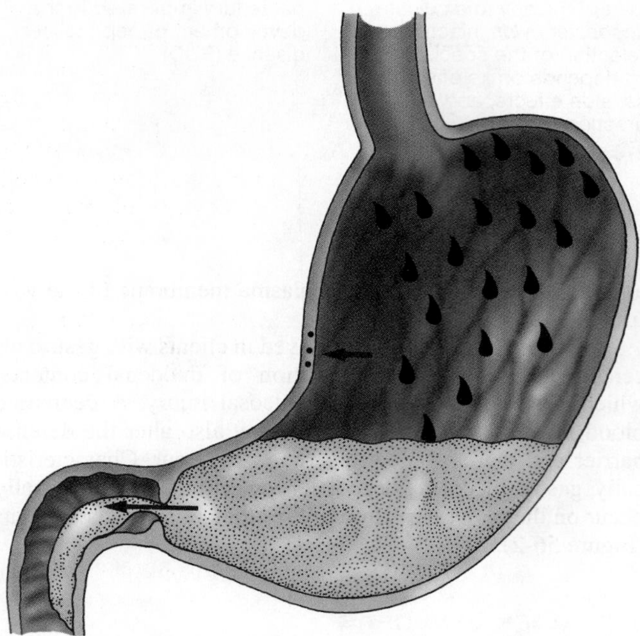

Conditions favoring the development of **duodenal ulcers** are normal diffusion of acid back into stomach tissues with *increased secretion of gastric acid* and *increased stomach emptying.*

Figure 56-1 ● The pathophysiology of peptic ulcer.

hypersecretion, a rapid emptying of food from the stomach reduces the buffering effect of food and delivers a large acid bolus to the duodenum (see Figure 56-1). Inhibitory secretory mechanisms and pancreatic secretion may be insufficient to control the acid load.

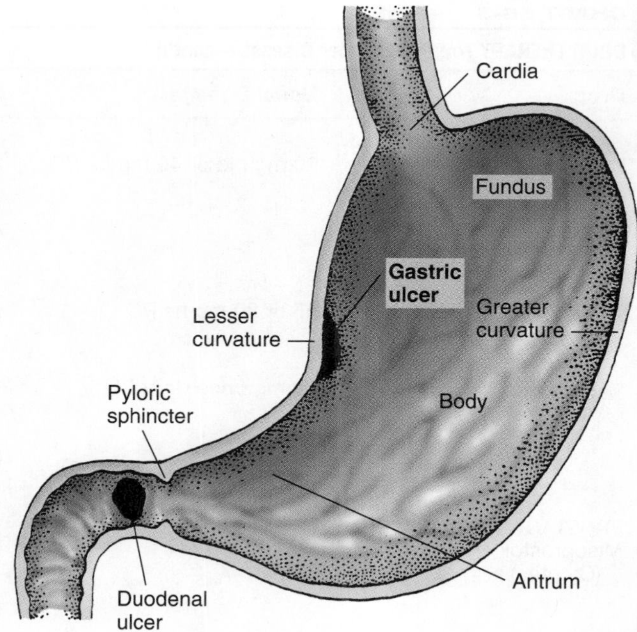

Figure 56-2 ● The most common sites for peptic ulcers.

Up to 95% to 100% of clients with duodenal ulcer disease have confirmed *H. pylori* infection (Friedman & Peterson, 1998). *H. pylori* produces substances that damage the gastric mucosa. Urease produced by *H. pylori* catalyzes the hydrolysis of urea to ammonia. Hydrogen ions are then released in response to the presence of ammonia and contribute further to gastric mucosal damage.

STRESS ULCERS

Stress ulcers are acute gastric mucosal lesions occurring after an acute medical crisis or trauma. Stress ulcers have been associated with head injury, burns, respiratory failure, shock, and sepsis. Bleeding caused by gastric erosion is the principal manifestation of acute stress ulcers.

Multifocal lesions associated with stress ulcers occur in the proximal portion of the stomach and duodenum. These lesions begin as focal areas of ischemia and evolve into erosions and ulcerations that may progress to massive hemorrhage. Little is known of the exact etiology of stress ulcers; however, in the presence of elevated levels of hydrochloric acid, ischemic areas can progress to erosive gastritis and subsequent ulcerations.

COMPLICATIONS OF ULCERS

The most common complications of PUD are hemorrhage, perforation, pyloric obstruction, and intractable disease.

HEMORRHAGE. Hemorrhage occurs in approximately 15% to 25% of clients with PUD and is the most serious complication (Figure 56-3). It tends to occur more often in clients with gastric ulcers and in older adults. Of those with an initial bleed, 40% experience a recurrence of bleeding if underlying infection with *H. pylori* remains untreated or if therapy does not include an H_2 antagonist. With massive bleeding, the client

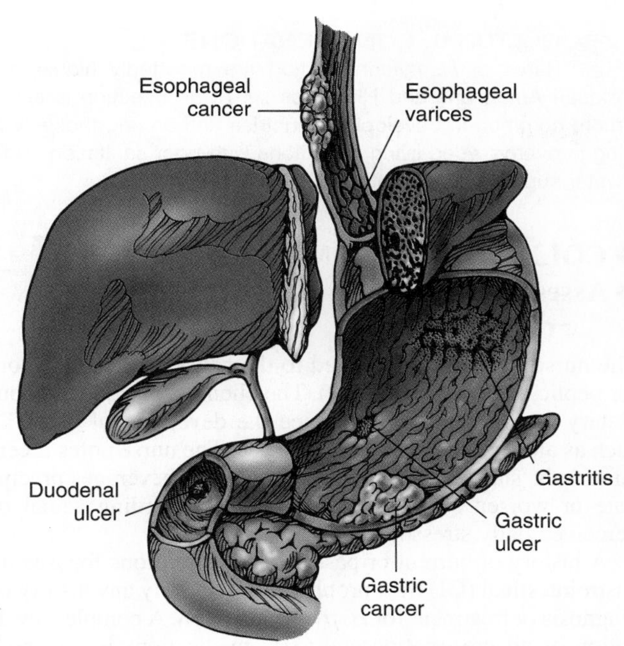

Figure 56-3 ● Common causes of upper gastrointestinal bleeding.

vomits bright red or coffee-ground blood (hematemesis). Hematemesis usually indicates bleeding at or above the duodenojejunal junction (upper gastrointestinal [GI] bleeding).

Minimal bleeding from ulcers is manifested by occult blood in a tarry stool (melena). Melena may occur in clients with gastric ulcers but is more common in those with duodenal ulcers. Gastric acid digestion of blood typically results in a granular dark vomitus (coffee-ground appearance); the digestion of blood within the duodenum and small intestine may result in a black stool.

PERFORATION. Perforation into the peritoneal cavity occurs in approximately 2% to 3% of clients with duodenal ulceration. Simultaneous hemorrhage accompanies perforation in 10% of clients and carries a 6% to 7% mortality rate (Blackington, 1999). In clients with perforation, the gastroduodenal contents (acid peptic juice, bile, and pancreatic juice) empty through the anterior wall of the stomach or duodenum into the peritoneal cavity. Sudden, sharp pain begins in the mid-epigastric region and spreads over the entire abdomen. The amount of pain correlates with the amount and type of GI contents spilled. The characteristic pain causes the client to be apprehensive. The abdomen is tender, rigid, and boardlike, and the client assumes the knee-chest position in an attempt to decrease the tension on the abdominal muscles. The client may become desperately ill within hours. Chemical peritonitis soon occurs; bacterial septicemia and hypovolemic shock follow. Peristalsis diminishes, and paralytic ileus develops. Peptic ulcer perforation is considered a surgical emergency.

PYLORIC OBSTRUCTION. Pyloric obstruction occurs in 2% to 4% of clients and is manifested by vomiting caused by stasis and gastric dilation. Obstruction occurs at the pylorus (the gastric outlet) and is caused by scarring, edema, inflammation, or a combination of these factors.

Symptoms of gastric outlet obstruction include abdominal bloating, nausea, and vomiting. When vomiting persists, the client may experience hypochloremic (metabolic) alkalosis from loss of large quantities of acid gastric juice (hydrogen and chloride ions) in the vomitus. Hypokalemia may also result from the vomiting or metabolic alkalosis. The health care provider typically hospitalizes the client so he or she may receive intravenous (IV) fluid and electrolyte replacement.

INTRACTABLE DISEASE. One third of all clients with ulcers have a single episode with no recurrence. Intractability may develop from complications of ulcers, excessive stressors in the client's life, or an inability to adhere to long-term therapy. The client no longer responds to conservative management, or recurrences of symptoms interfere with activities of daily living (ADLs). In general, the client continues to have recurrent pain and discomfort despite treatment. Clients who fail to respond to traditional treatments or who have a relapse following discontinuation of therapy should be referred to a gastroenterologist.

Etiology

Peptic ulcer development is primarily associated with nonsteroidal anti-inflammatory drug (NSAID) use and bacterial infection with *H. pylori.* NSAIDs (such as aspirin or ibuprofen) break down the mucosal barrier and disrupt the mucosal protection mediated systemically by cyclooxygenase (COX) inhibition. In addition, NSAIDs cause the depletion of endogenous prostaglandins, resulting in local gastric mucosal injury. The risk of developing PUD is 5 to 20 times higher in individuals who use NSAIDs than in the general population (Graham et al., 1999c). GI complications from NSAID use can occur at any time, even after long-term uncomplicated use. NSAID-related ulcers are difficult to treat, even with long-term therapy, since these ulcers have a high rate of recurrence.

Certain drugs may contribute to gastroduodenal ulceration by altering gastric secretion, producing localized damage to mucosa and interfering with the healing process. Theophylline (Theo-Dur) and caffeine stimulate hydrochloric acid production. Caffeine may contribute to vascular stasis and mucosal anoxia. The use of corticosteroids is also associated with an increased incidence of peptic ulceration.

H. pylori infection is transmitted from person to person, but exactly how this transmission takes place remains unknown. In one study, *H. pylori* was successfully cultivated from vomitus and occasionally from stool and saliva, indicating that the organism may be transmissible during GI tract illness, particularly if the person is vomiting (see the Evidence-Based Practice for Nursing box on p. 1222).

Incidence/Prevalence

In the United States, there are 450,000 new cases of PUD diagnosed each year, and a total of 4 million people see a health care provider for health issues related to peptic ulcers. The prevalence of peptic ulcers has risen from a rate of 19.9 per 1000 persons to a rate of 23 per 1000 (Astarita, 1999). The prevalence of duodenal ulcers ranges from 6% to 15%, and they occur with equal frequency in men and women. Sixty percent of duodenal ulcers recur within 1 year, and 90% recur

EVIDENCE-BASED PRACTICE FOR NURSING

Fecal and oral shedding of *Helicobacter pylori* from healthy infected adults

Parsonnet, J., Shmuely, H. & Haggerty, T. (1999). Fecal and oral shedding of *Helicobacter pylori* from healthy adults. *Journal of the American Medical Association, 282*(23), 2240-2245.

The purpose of this study was to determine how humans shed the organism *Helicobacter pylori* into the environment. A controlled clinical experiment involving healthy volunteers recruited through advertisement was conducted from February through December 1998. All subjects meeting eligibility criteria underwent serum immunoglobulin G (IgG) and 13C breath testing for *H. pylori* infection. A total of 16 asymptomatic *H. pylori*–infected adults and 10 uninfected adults participated in the study.

The *H. pylori*–infected subjects were given a cathartic (sodium phosphate) and an emetic (ipecac). One uninfected control subject also underwent the emesis portion of the experiment. Stool samples were collected during the 8 hours following cathartic administration. Following an overnight fast, subjects were administered 5 mL of ipecac followed by 480 mL of water. A saliva sample was obtained before and following emesis. Air samples were tested throughout the emesis period by using agar plates with a Fluoropore filter covering half of the plate's diameter. A new plate was replaced every 30 minutes. Ten subjects had a second air sampler placed 1.2 m away to determine the radius of bacterial aerosolization. The 10 uninfected subjects provided normal stool and saliva samples.

All vomitus samples from infected subjects grew *H. pylori,* often in high quantities. Air samples taken during vomiting episodes grew *H. pylori* in 37.5% of infected subjects. Saliva tested before and after vomiting grew small quantities of *H. pylori.* Only 22 (21.8%) of 101 stools from infected subjects grew the organism, and no stools or other samples from uninfected subjects contained *H. pylori.*

Critique. Although the sample in this case control study is relatively small, this study provides intriguing evidence of the presence and possible routes of transmission of *H. pylori.*

Implications for Nursing. Since *H. pylori* can be cultured from both vomitus and stools of healthy *H. pylori*–infected individuals, there may be implications for modifications in nursing practice and client education. Since much of the culture grew from vomitus, episodes of emesis could be a mechanism for the spread of *H. pylori* into the environment by means of gastric-oral transmission. Organisms are also dispersed into the air during periods of emesis. *H. pylori* was also cultured from saliva of infected individuals, inferring an oral-oral transmission. Since transmission of *H. pylori* has been demonstrated to occur under conditions that induce vomiting, further research is needed to determine the extent of nursing interventions necessary during episodes of gastrointestinal illness to prevent spread of the organism. Furthermore, as more is learned about *H. pylori* transmission, client education initiatives to prevent spread within households may also be necessary.

within 2 years. The incidence of gastric ulcers is not really known, since some afflicted individuals are asymptomatic (Friedman & Peterson, 1998).

CONSIDERATIONS FOR OLDER ADULTS

Both duodenal and gastric ulcers occur more often following the sixth decade of life. Older adults tend to use over-the-counter (OTC) remedies, often delaying appropriate treatment for symptoms of PUD. In addition, they often suffer from one or more chronic illnesses that require the use of medications that can precipitate or worsen PUD. There is also evidence that older adults may be at increased risk for complications and death following acute peptic ulcer bleeding.

CULTURAL CONSIDERATIONS

Rates of *H. pylori* infection are reportedly higher in African Americans and Hispanics. *H. pylori* infection is also more common in developing countries and among those living in overcrowded living conditions with poor sanitation and water supplies (Blackington, 1999).

COLLABORATIVE MANAGEMENT

SIMON Activity Link

Assessment

HISTORY

The nurse collects data related to the causes and risk factors for peptic ulcer disease (PUD). The client is questioned about dietary factors that can influence the development of PUD, such as alcohol intake and tobacco use. The nurse notes if certain foods, such as tomatoes, or caffeinated beverages precipitate or worsen symptoms. Information regarding actual or perceived daily stressors is also elicited.

A history of current or past medical conditions focuses on gastrointestinal (GI) tract problems, particularly any history of diagnosis or treatment for *H. pylori* infection. A complete evaluation of all prescription and OTC medications is obtained. The nurse specifically inquires if the client is taking corticosteroids, aspirin, or other nonsteroidal anti-inflammatory drugs (NSAIDs). The nurse also asks whether the client has ever undergone radiation treatments.

A history of GI upset, pain and its relationship to eating and sleep patterns, and actions taken to relieve pain is also important. The nurse inquires about any changes in the character of the pain, since this may signal the development of complications. For example, if pain that was once intermittent and relieved by food and antacids becomes constant and radiates to the back or upper quadrant, this may indicate impending ulcer perforation. It is important to note that many individuals with active duodenal or gastric ulcers report having no ulcer symptoms.

PHYSICAL ASSESSMENT/CLINICAL MANIFESTATIONS

Physical assessment findings may reveal epigastric tenderness, usually located at the midline between the umbilicus and the xiphoid process. If perforation into the peritoneal cavity is present, the client will exhibit a rigid, boardlike abdomen accompanied by rebound tenderness. Initially, auscultation of the abdomen may reveal hyperactive bowel sounds, but these may diminish with progression of the disorder.

Dyspepsia (indigestion), which is defined as discomfort centered around the epigastrium or upper abdomen, is the most commonly reported symptom associated with PUD. This pain or discomfort is described as sharp, burning, or gnawing. Some clients may perceive discomfort as a sensation of abdominal pressure or of fullness or hunger. Pain is less often the initial complaint in the older client. In this age-group, melena is often the presenting sign.

Gastric ulcer pain often occurs in the upper epigastrium with localization to the left of the midline and may be accentuated by food. *Duodenal* ulcer pain is usually located to the right of the epigastrium (Table 56-1). The pain associated with a duodenal ulcer occurs 90 minutes to 3 hours after eating and often awakens the client at night. Pain may also be exacerbated by certain foods (such as tomatoes, hot spices, fried

TABLE 56-1 • DIFFERENTIAL FEATURES OF GASTRIC AND DUODENAL ULCERS

Feature	Gastric Ulcer	Duodenal Ulcer
Age	Usually 50 yr or older	Usually 40-50 yr
Gender	Male/female ratio of 1.1:1	Equal male/female ratio
Blood group	No differentiation	Most often type O
General nourishment	May be malnourished	Usually well nourished
Stomach acid production	Normal secretion or hyposecretion	Hypersecretion
Occurrence	Mucosa exposed to acid-pepsin secretion	Mucosa exposed to acid-pepsin secretion
Clinical course	Healing and recurrence	Healing and recurrence
Pain	Occurs ½-1 hr after a meal; at night: rarely	Occurs 90 min-3 hr after a meal; at night: often awakens client between 1 and 2 AM
	Accentuated by ingestion of food	Relieved by ingestion of food
Response to treatment	Healing with appropriate therapy	Healing with appropriate therapy
Hemorrhage	Hematemesis more common than melena	Melena more common than hematemesis
Malignant change	Perhaps in less than 10%	Rare
Recurrence	Tends to heal and recurs often in the same location	60% recur within 1 yr; 90% recur within 2 yr
Surrounding mucosa	Atrophic gastritis	No gastritis

foods, onions, alcohol, or caffeine drinks) and certain medications (such as aspirin, NSAIDs, or corticosteroids).

Vomiting may be a symptom accompanying ulcer disease, most commonly in conjunction with pyloric sphincter dysfunction. It results from gastric stasis associated with pyloric obstruction. Appetite is generally maintained in clients with a peptic ulcer unless pyloric obstruction is present.

To assess for fluid volume deficit, which can occur secondary to bleeding, the nurse takes orthostatic vital signs of all clients suspected of PUD. Orthostatic changes are characterized by a decrease of more than 20 mm Hg in systolic blood pressure, a decrease of 10 mm Hg in diastolic blood pressure, and/or an increase in pulse when the client rises from a lying to an erect (sitting or, if possible, standing) position. The nurse also assesses for dizziness, especially when the client is upright, since this is another symptom of fluid volume deficit.

CRITICAL THINKING CHALLENGE

A client with a long-standing history of rheumatoid arthritis comes to the clinic where you work with complaints of vague, episodic epigastric abdominal discomfort over the last month.

- During the initial interview, what pertinent questions should you ask regarding this client's symptoms?
- How might the treatment for arthritis relate to the client's symptoms?
- What might you expect to find when assessing this client?

For suggested answer guidelines, go to SIMON http://www.wbsaunders.com/SIMON/Iggy/.

PSYCHOSOCIAL ASSESSMENT

The nurse assesses the impact of ulcer disease on the client's lifestyle, occupation, family, and social and leisure activities. Questions about lifestyle, occupation, and leisure can yield important information. The nurse evaluates the impact that lifestyle changes will have on the client. This assessment determines the client's ability to comply with the prescribed treatment regimen and to obtain the needed social support to alter his or her lifestyle.

LABORATORY ASSESSMENT

Hemoglobin and hematocrit values may be low, indicating bleeding. The stool specimen may be positive for occult blood if bleeding is present.

RADIOGRAPHIC ASSESSMENT

A barium examination of the GI tract can be used to establish a duodenal ulcer. A duodenal ulcer appears as a discrete crater in the duodenal bulb. This is often the initial test for a client who does not have severe symptoms. If perforation is suspected, the health care provider usually first orders a flat-plate film of the abdomen to identify the presence of free air.

OTHER DIAGNOSTIC ASSESSMENT

The major diagnostic test for PUD is esophagogastroduodenoscopy (EGD), which is the most accurate means of establishing a diagnosis. Visualization of the ulcer crater by EGD allows the health care provider to take specimens for *H. pylori* testing and for biopsy and cytologic studies for ruling out gastric cancer (see the Legal/Ethical Issues in Health Care box on p. 1224). EGD may be repeated at 4- to 6-week intervals while the health care provider evaluates the progress of healing in response to therapy.

Urea breath testing has been employed to detect *H. pylori* when endoscopy is not clinically indicated. To perform this test, the client must be on NPO status after midnight on the night before the test. The client drinks a carbon-enriched urea solution. The presence of *H. pylori* will cause the bacteria to break down the solution and release carbon dioxide, which the client inhales in a collection container for analysis. The carbon dioxide excreted in the breath is then measured and compared with a baseline measurement to determine the presence of *H. pylori.* In addition to its noninvasive nature, this test assesses the entire stomach and may prove especially helpful after the client has been treated to determine if treatment was successful (Blackington, 1999).

A second noninvasive test for *H. pylori* involves IgG serologic testing. Infection with *H. pylori* causes immunoglobulin

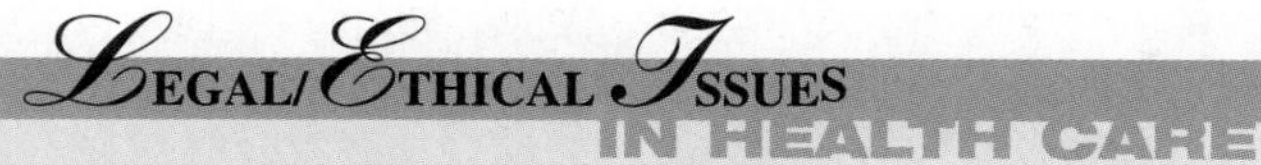

QUALITY OF CARE FOR MEDICARE CLIENTS WITH PEPTIC ULCER DISEASE

Economic constraints on the health care system have resulted in efforts to provide cost-effective, high-quality care. In an effort to improve the quality of care delivered to Medicare beneficiaries with peptic ulcer disease (PUD), a chart review of 2644 Medicare beneficiaries was conducted to measure compliance with National Institute of Health (NIH) guidelines for the detection and treatment of *Helicobacter pylori* in PUD.

In this particular study, only 57% of hospitalized Medicare recipients with PUD were tested for *H. pylori.* In addition, only 74% of clients with known *H. pylori* infection were treated with appropriate antimicrobial therapy. Medical record review also noted that 74% of clients were screened for nonsteroidal anti-inflammatory drug (NSAID) use. Only 24% had documented counseling regarding the risks associated with NSAID use, and only 2% had documented education of the ulcer-associated risks of NSAID use.

Although limited documented education may be in part to blame for the poor quality of care regarding *H. pylori*–related ulcers, NIH clinical practice guidelines for the diagnosis and treatment of peptic ulcer disease are clearly underutilized. Quality improvement initiatives are needed to improve the care delivered to Medicare beneficiaries with PUD. *H. pylori* screening and treatment guidelines need to be enforced to ensure that appropriate treatment is received, especially by older adults.

Data from Offman, J., et al. (2000). The quality of care for Medicare patients with peptic ulcer disease. *American Journal of Gastroenterology* 95(1), 106-113.

antibodies to form. Although antibody assays have a high sensitivity and specificity (>95%) for detecting *H. pylori,* antibody assays cannot be used to document eradication of the organism, since antibody levels can remain elevated despite successful treatment.

A complete medication history needs to be obtained before diagnostic testing is done for *H. pylori.* False-negative results could be obtained if the client has received antibiotic treatment, used a bismuth preparation (Pepto-Bismol), or used a proton-pump inhibitor within the 4-week period before testing for *H. pylori.* Other medications, such as misoprostol, sucralfate, or an H_2 blocker administered within the week before the test may also yield a false-negative result. Use of over-the-counter medications (OTC), such as Pepcid AC, Tagamet, and Zantac, can also affect test results.

Analysis

COMMON NURSING DIAGNOSES AND COLLABORATIVE PROBLEMS

The following are priority nursing diagnoses for clients with peptic ulcer disease (PUD):

1. Acute Pain or Chronic Pain related to gastric and/or duodenal mucosal injury
2. Risk for Deficient Fluid Volume related to hemorrhage or vomiting

ADDITIONAL NURSING DIAGNOSES AND COLLABORATIVE PROBLEMS

In addition to the common nursing diagnoses, clients with PUD may have one or more of the following:

- Ineffective Therapeutic Regimen Management related to long-term treatment and lifestyle changes
- Ineffective Coping related to intractable progressive disease
- Imbalanced Nutrition: Less Than Body Requirements related to anorexia, nausea, or diet constraints
- Disturbed Sleep Pattern related to discomfort
- Risk for Falls related to orthostatic hypotension
- A collaborative problem that could occur is Potential for Metabolic Alkalosis.

Planning and Implementation

ACUTE PAIN; CHRONIC PAIN

NOC **PLANNING: EXPECTED OUTCOMES.** PUD causes significant discomfort that impacts many aspects of daily living. The client with PUD is expected to experience reduction or alleviation of pain as indicated by self-report.

INTERVENTIONS. Interventions to manage pain related to PUD are accomplished with specific ulcer therapy and dietary modifications. One of the primary purposes for employing drug therapy in the management of PUD is to reduce or eliminate pain. Analgesics are not the mainstay of pain relief for PUD. Instead, the ulcer drug regimen itself promotes relief of pain by eradicating *H. pylori* infection and promoting healing of gastric mucosa.

The nurse performs a comprehensive pain assessment that includes the following aspects of pain:

- Location
- Characteristics
- Onset/duration
- Frequency
- Quality
- Severity
- Precipitating and alleviating factors

Any changes in the characteristics or location of peptic ulcer pain are carefully assessed, since such changes often accompany the development of complications. The nurse teaches the client to eliminate factors (such as spicy foods) that can precipitate or increase pain from ulcer disease.

Measures to promote adequate rest and sleep may be necessary, since ulcer pain can cause the client to awaken. The nurse assists the client in achieving compliance with the medication regimen, since adherence to the drug regimen will promote relief of pain and discomfort. The client's satisfaction with the level of pain relief achieved is monitored.

DRUG THERAPY. The primary goals of drug therapy in the treatment of PUD are (1) to provide pain relief, (2) to eradicate *H. pylori* infection, (3) to heal ulcerations, and (4) to prevent recurrence (see Chart 56-3). Several different regimens can be used to achieve these goals. In selecting a therapeutic drug regimen, the health care provider must consider the efficacy of the treatment, the anticipated side effects, the ability of the client to comply with the regimen, and the cost of the treatment (Astarita, 1999).

Although numerous drugs have been evaluated for the treatment of *H. pylori* infection, no single agent has been used successfully against the organism. Current practice involves using a combination of agents to achieve treatment goals. The most successful regimen used is a triple therapy consisting of a bismuth compound, metronidazole, and either amoxicillin or tetracycline. Triple therapy is supple-

COST OF CARE IMPLICATIONS FOR NURSING

PEPTIC ULCER DISEASE

Cost of Care

- The cost of selected 2-week regimens for the treatment of *Helicobacter pylori*–associated peptic ulcer disease (PUD) ranges from $75 to $215, depending on the extent and combination of drugs used.
- Treatment of *H. pylori*–associated PUD decreases the need for hospitalization secondary to bleeding episodes. This reduces the economic burden to the health care system.
- The direct and indirect costs of diagnosis and treatment account for $5 billion to $6 billion annually.
- Treatment of *H. pylori*–related PUD provides substantial savings in terms of direct costs (e.g., medications, office visits) and indirect costs (lost workdays due to the illness).

Implications for Nursing

The treatment of *H. pylori*–associated PUD reduces recurrence from 80% to less than 10% in 1 year. However, in clinical practice, appropriate antimicrobial therapy is underutilized. Nurses need to understand the pathogenesis of PUD in order to advocate for appropriate treatment for their clients. In addition, nurses need to educate their clients concerning the role of *H. pylori* infection in ulcer disease in order to assist them in effective management of this disorder.

Data from Lane, L., & Fendrick, A.M. (1998). *Helicobacter pylori* and peptic ulcer disease. *Postgraduate Medicine, 103*(3), 231-243; and Graham, D., et al. (1999). Recognizing peptic ulcer disease: Keys to clinical and laboratory diagnosis. *Postgraduate Medicine, 105*(3), 113-128.

CHART 56-4

NURSING FOCUS *on the* OLDER ADULT

Giving Ulcer Medications Safely

- Assess the client's complete drug regimen. Older adults are more susceptible to adverse side effects from multiple drugs.
- Monitor the client carefully for signs of adverse effects.
- Keep dosage schedules simple when a client is at home.
- Assess the client's understanding of instructions related to medications. Provide a written list and instructions for each medication.

mented by the addition of an H_2-receptor antagonist to facilitate ulcer healing and prevent recurrence (see the Cost of Care box above). Although this regimen is the most effective and least expensive, adherence to the regimen is difficult for most clients. A client must consume medications four times daily, and adverse effects occur in 20% to 30% of individuals, especially older adults (Chart 56-4). Recently, some strains of *H. pylori* have begun to demonstrate metronidazole resistance, raising concerns about long-term treatment with this regimen.

HYPOSECRETORY DRUGS. Hyposecretory drugs produce a reduction in gastric acid secretions. These drugs include antisecretory agents, H_2-receptor antagonists, and prostaglandin analogs (see Chart 56-3).

ANTISECRETORY AGENTS. Omeprazole (Prilosec), lansoprazole (Prevacid), and the newest proton pump inhibitor, rabeprazole (Aciphex) suppress the H^+,K^+-ATPase enzyme system of gastric acid production. These medications are available as sustained-release tablets; therefore they must not be crushed before administration.

H_2-RECEPTOR ANTAGONISTS. Drugs that block histamine-stimulated gastric secretions are effective in the management of ulcer disease. These medications may be used for indigestion and heartburn, and lower-dose forms are available in over-the-counter (OTC) products. H_2-receptor antagonists block the action of the H_2 receptors of the parietal cells, thus inhibiting gastric acid secretion. The most common drugs are ranitidine (Zantac), famotidine (Pepcid), and nizatidine (Axid). These drugs are typically administered in a single dose at bedtime and are used for 4 to 6 weeks in combination with triple therapy.

PROSTAGLANDIN ANALOGS. Prostaglandins are naturally abundant in the gastrointestinal (GI) tract and have been shown to be effective in clinical trials in the treatment of duodenal ulcers. Prostaglandin analogs reduce gastric acid secretion and enhance gastric mucosal resistance to tissue injury. Misoprostol (Cytotec), the most commonly used drug in this category, *prevents* NSAID-induced ulcers. Some NSAIDs are being manufactured in combination with misoprostol. A significant adverse effect of this drug is uterine contraction; therefore its use is contraindicated in pregnant women.

ANTACIDS. Antacids buffer gastric acid and prevent the formation of pepsin. Antacids have demonstrated effectiveness in accelerating the healing of duodenal ulcers. Liquid suspensions are the most therapeutic form, but tablets may be more convenient and enhance compliance. The most widely used preparations are mixtures of aluminum hydroxide and magnesium hydroxide, since this combination overcomes the unpleasant GI side effects of either of these preparations when used alone. Mylanta and Maalox are examples of this type of combination antacid formulation. The aluminum and magnesium hydroxide combination products neutralize well at small doses. Aluminum and magnesium-based products must also be administered cautiously to those with renal impairment, since these substances cannot be eliminated adequately by the kidneys and are consequently retained in excessive amounts in the body.

The nurse instructs the client that to achieve a therapeutic effect, sufficient antacid must be ingested to neutralize the hourly production of acid. For optimal effect, antacids are given about 2 hours after meals to reduce the hydrogen ion load in the duodenum. Antacids may be effective from 30 minutes to 3 hours after ingestion. Antacids taken with an empty stomach are quickly evacuated; thus the neutralizing effect is reduced. Calcium carbonate (Tums) is a potent antacid, but it triggers gastrin release, causing a rebound acid secretion. Therefore its use in acid inhibition is not recommended.

Antacids can interact with certain drugs, such as phenytoin (Dilantin), tetracycline, and ketoconazole, and interfere with their effectiveness. The nurse determines what other drugs the client is using before recommending a specific antacid. Medications are administered 1 to 2 hours before or after the antacid. The nurse informs the client that flavored antacids, especially wintergreen, should be avoided. The flavoring increases the emptying time of the stomach; thus the desired effect of the antacid is negated.

The nurse teaches the client with past or present heart failure to avoid antacids containing a high sodium content, such as aluminum hydroxide, magnesium hydroxide, sodium bicarbonate, and simethicone combination products (Gelusil and Mylanta). Magaldrate (Riopan) has the lowest sodium concentration.

MUCOSAL BARRIER FORTIFIERS. Sucralfate (Carafate) is sulfonated disaccharide that forms complexes with proteins at the base of a peptic ulcer. This protective coat prevents further digestive action of both acid and pepsin.

Sucralfate does not inhibit acid secretion. Rather, it binds bile acids and pepsins, reducing injury from these substances. Sucralfate may be used in conjunction with H_2-receptor antagonists and antacids but should not be administered within 1 hour of the antacid. Sucralfate is given on an empty stomach 1 hour before each meal and at bedtime. The main side effect of this drug is constipation.

DIET THERAPY. The value of diet in the management of ulcer disease is highly controversial. There is no evidence that dietary restriction reduces gastric acid secretion or promotes tissue healing, although a bland diet may assist in relieving symptoms. Food itself acts as an antacid by neutralizing gastric acid for 30 to 60 minutes. An increased rate of gastric acid secretion, called rebound, may follow. If diet therapy is used, it may be directed toward neutralizing acid and reducing hypermotility, which may alleviate symptoms.

The nurse instructs the client to avoid substances that increase gastric acid secretion. This includes caffeine-containing beverages (coffee, tea, and cola). Both caffeinated and decaffeinated coffees should be avoided, since coffee contains peptides that stimulate gastrin release.

In collaboration, the nurse and dietitian teach the client to exclude any foods that cause discomfort. A bland, nonirritating diet is recommended during the acute symptomatic phase. Bedtime snacks are avoided because they may stimulate gastric acid secretion. Eating six smaller daily meals may help, but this regimen is no longer a regular part of therapy. There is no evidence to support the theory that eating six daily meals promotes healing of the ulcer, and this practice actually stimulates gastric acid secretion. Clients should avoid alcohol and tobacco because of their stimulatory effects on gastric acid secretion.

RISK FOR DEFICIENT FLUID VOLUME

PLANNING: EXPECTED OUTCOMES. Fluid volume loss secondary to the development of complications is a risk associated with PUD. Blood loss due to hemorrhage can carry significant morbidity and mortality. Fluid volume loss secondary to vomiting can lead to dehydration and electrolyte imbalances. The client with peptic ulcer disease (PUD) is expected to benefit from prevention or early detection of disease complications.

INTERVENTIONS. Monitoring and early recognition of complications are critical to the successful management of PUD. Interventions aimed at managing complications associated with PUD include prevention and/or management of bleeding, perforation, and gastric outlet obstruction. In some cases, surgical treatment of complications becomes necessary.

NIC **HYPOVOLEMIA MANAGEMENT.** The purpose of managing hypovolemia is to expand intravascular fluid in a client who is volume depleted. The nurse or assistive nursing personnel monitors vital signs and observes for fluid loss from bleeding or vomiting. The nurse carefully monitors the client's fluid status, including intake and output. Fluid replacement in older adults should be closely monitored to prevent fluid overload. An infusion pump is used to ensure accurate delivery of the desired volume. Serum electrolytes are also monitored, since depletions from vomiting or nasogastric suctioning must be replaced. The nurse should ensure that two large-bore peripheral IV catheters are inserted so that both fluids and blood lost to vomiting or hemorrhage can be replaced. Volume replacement with isotonic crystalloid solutions (0.9 normal saline solution, or lactated Ringer's solution) should be started immediately, since adequate fluid volume replacement is essential. The health care provider may order blood products, such as packed red blood cells, to expand volume and correct abnormalities in the complete blood count (CBC). For clients with active bleeding, fresh frozen plasma may be given if the prothrombin time is 1.5 times higher than the midrange control value. To prevent injury from falls secondary to orthostatic hypotension, the client is assisted with ambulation.

NIC **BLEEDING REDUCTION: GASTROINTESTINAL.** The purpose of interventions to reduce bleeding is to limit the amount of blood loss from the upper and lower gastrointestinal (GI) tract resulting from complications related to PUD. The nurse monitors the client for signs and symptoms indicating GI bleeding. All excretions are observed for the presence of frank or occult bleeding. With GI bleeding, the presence of frank blood or coffee-ground vomitus may be observed. Stools can contain frank blood or appear black and tarry. Occult blood loss may be detected by stool examination and may be accompanied by progressive iron deficiency anemia.

The nurse monitors the client's hematocrit, hemoglobin, and coagulation studies for changes from the baseline measurements. The nurse or assistive nursing personnel monitors vital signs. With mild bleeding (less than 500 mL), slight feelings of weakness and mild perspiration may be present. When blood loss exceeds 1 L/24 hr, signs and symptoms of shock may be manifested, such as hypotension, chills, palpitations, diaphoresis, and a weak, thready pulse. (See Chapter 38 for the treatment of shock.)

The nurse immediately notifies the health care provider of major bleeding. Transfusion therapy may be required to replace blood loss. (See Chapter 40 for nursing interventions for clients undergoing blood transfusion.) The health care provider may order H_2 blockers to avoid extremes in gastric pH levels. If appropriate and as ordered, the nurse inserts a nasogastric (NG) tube, monitors secretions, and performs nasogastric lavage to decompress the stomach and alleviate bleeding. In addition, the client and family are instructed to avoid the use of anti-inflammatory medications that can precipitate or worsen GI bleeding.

NIC interventions are summarized in Chart 56-5.

NONSURGICAL MANAGEMENT. Because prevention or early detection of complications is critical in obtaining a satisfactory outcome, the nurse monitors the client carefully and immediately reports changes to the health care provider. The type of nonsurgical intervention selected will depend on the type and severity of the complication.

The goals of therapeutic interventions for bleeding secondary to PUD are as follows:

- Cessation of the acute bleeding episode
- Prevention of rebleeding

CHART 56-5

NIC INTERVENTION ACTIVITIES *for* The Client with Stomach Disorders

Hypovolemia Management: *The expansion of intravascular fluid volume in a client who is volume depleted*
- Monitor vital signs, as appropriate.
- Monitor fluid status, including intake and output, as appropriate.
- Monitor for fluid loss (e.g., bleeding, vomiting, diarrhea, perspiration, and tachypnea).
- Arrange availability of blood products for transfusion, if necessary.
- Administer blood products (e.g., platelets and fresh frozen plasma), as appropriate.
- Monitor for blood reaction, if appropriate.

Bleeding Reduction: Gastrointestinal: *The limitation of the amount of blood loss from the upper and lower gastrointestinal tract and related complications*
- Monitor for signs and symptoms of persistent bleeding (e.g., check all secretions for frank or occult blood).
- Hematest all excretions and observe for blood loss in emesis, sputum, feces, urine, nasogastric drainage, and wound drainage, as appropriate.
- Document color, amount, and character of stools.
- Monitor coagulation studies and complete blood count (CBC) with WBC differential.
- Insert nasogastric tube to suction and monitor secretions, if appropriate
- Perform nasogastric lavage, as appropriate.
- Avoid extremes in gastric pH level by administration of appropriate medication (e.g., antacids or histamine-2 blocking agent).
- Instruct the client and/or family on the need for blood replacement, as appropriate.
- Instruct the client and/or family to avoid the use of anti-inflammatory medications (e.g., aspirin and ibuprofen).

NIC intervention activities selected from McCloskey, J.C., & Bulechek, G.M. (2000). *Nursing interventions classification (NIC)* (3rd ed.). St. Louis: Mosby. No part of this work is to be altered without prior written permission from the Publisher.
WBC, White blood cell.

A combination of several different therapeutic interventions, including endoscopic therapy, acid suppression, NG tube placement, and saline lavage, can be used to control acute bleeding and prevent rebleeding. Therapeutic trials have been conducted to determine the optimal treatment for bleeding due to peptic ulcers. Endoscopic therapy and suppression of gastric acid are the primary therapies used to control active bleeding caused by PUD. H_2-receptor antagonists, proton pump inhibitors, and antacids are the primary medications used to treat this bleeding.

ENDOSCOPIC THERAPY. Endoscopic therapy via an esophagogastroduodenoscopy (EGD) can assist in achieving homeostasis during an acute bleeding episode. The three primary methods of endoscopic therapy are (1) thermal contact using a heater probe or multi-electrocoagulation, (2) injection of the bleeding site with diluted epinephrine or a sclerosing agent (alcohol), and (3) laser therapy. All three methods are effective in achieving blood clot formation. Thermal contact and injection are most commonly used. Laser therapy is costly and therefore is used less often. Endoscopic therapy is most beneficial for clients with active bleeding; however, persistent or re-bleeding despite endoscopic therapy continues to be problematic. No consensus has been reached on the appropriate management of re-bleeding.

ACID SUPPRESSION. Aggressive acid suppression is used to prevent re-bleeding. When acute bleeding is stopped and clot formation has taken place within the ulcer crater, the clot remains in contact with gastric contents. Acid-suppressive agents are used to stabilize the clot by raising the pH level of gastric contents. Several drugs are used to achieve acid suppression in clients with a bleeding episode. H_2-receptor antagonists prevent acid from being produced by parietal cells. Proton pump inhibitors prevent the transport of acid across the parietal cell membrane, whereas antacids buffer acid produced in the stomach.

NASOGASTRIC TUBE PLACEMENT. Upper GI bleeding may require the health care provider or nurse to insert a nasogastric (NG) tube to:
- Ascertain the presence or absence of blood in the stomach
- Assess the rate of bleeding
- Prevent gastric dilation
- Administer saline lavage

Nasogastric aspiration is an important part of diagnostic and prognostic evaluation of the client. The presence of red blood in emesis, nasogastric aspirate, or stools is correlated with a poor outcome (Terdiman, 1998).

Once the NG tube is placed, confirmation of proper positioning of the tube is determined by x-ray examination. The nurse irrigates the NG tube to maintain its patency and prevent obstruction with clotted blood.

SALINE LAVAGE. Saline lavage requires the insertion of a large-bore NG tube with instillation of saline in volumes of 50 to 200 mL. The saline and blood are repeatedly withdrawn until returns are clear or light pink and without clots. For protection against exposure to blood, practitioners may use the following procedure with a closed system for irrigation and suction. A Y-connector is attached to the NG tube, and an IV bag of normal saline is attached to tubing at one end of the Y-connector. The opposite connector is attached to tubing connected to wall suction. After the stomach is initially drained by suctioning, the tubing attached to the wall suction is clamped off, and up to 200 mL of normal saline is allowed to drain into the client through the NG tube. After the saline is instilled, the tube connecting the saline to the NG tube is clamped off, and the clamp to suction is released. The nurse instructs the client to lie on the left side during this procedure to limit the flow of saline out of the stomach and prevent aspiration.

NONSURGICAL MANAGEMENT OF PERFORATION. To prevent peritonitis from GI contents that have entered the peritoneum, perforation is managed by the immediate replacement of fluid, blood, and electrolytes and the administration of antibiotics. The nurse maintains nasogastric suction to drain gastric secretions and thus prevent further peritoneal spillage. The client remains on NPO status, and the nurse carefully monitors intake and output. The nurse or assistive nursing personnel checks vital signs at least hourly and monitors the client for clinical manifestations of septic shock, such as fever, pain, tachycardia, lethargy, or anxiety.

NONSURGICAL MANAGEMENT OF PYLORIC OBSTRUCTION. Pyloric obstruction is caused by edema, spasm, or scar tissue. Symptoms of obstruction related to difficulty in emptying the stomach include feelings of fullness, distention, or nausea after eating, as well as vomiting of copious amounts of undigested food.

Treatment of obstruction is directed toward restoration of fluid and electrolyte balance and decompression of the dilated stomach. Obstruction related to edema and spasm generally responds to medical therapy. First, the stomach must be decompressed with nasogastric suction; next, interventions are directed at correcting metabolic alkalosis and dehydration. The NG tube is clamped after about 72 hours, and the client is checked for retention of gastric contents. If the amount retained is not more than 350 mL in 30 minutes, the health care provider may allow oral fluids. In some cases, surgical intervention may be required.

CRITICAL THINKING CHALLENGE

Your client has been diagnosed with a nonsteroidal anti-inflammatory drug (NSAID)–induced duodenal ulcer, and the presence of *H. pylori* infection has been confirmed.

- What complications of peptic ulcer disease (PUD) is this client most at risk for?
- What dietary instructions should you give to this client?
- What should you teach this client about the medical treatment for PUD?

For suggested answer guidelines, go to SIMON http://www.wbsaunders.com/SIMON/Iggy/.

SURGICAL MANAGEMENT. New guidelines for the treatment of PUD that include *H. pylori* eradication and the development of nonsurgical means of controlling bleeding have led to a decline in the need for surgical intervention. In PUD, surgical intervention is used to:

- Reduce the acid-secreting ability of the stomach
- Treat clients who do not respond to medical therapy
- Treat a surgical emergency that develops as a complication of PUD

PREOPERATIVE CARE. Before surgery, an NG tube is inserted and connected to suction to remove secretions and empty the stomach. This allows surgery to take place without contamination of the peritoneal cavity by gastric secretions. Chart 56-6 describes the procedure for inserting the NG tube and nursing care associated with NG tube maintenance. The NG tube remains in place postoperatively to prevent the accumulation of secretions, which may lead to vomiting or gastrointestinal (GI) distention and pressure on the suture line.

Other preoperative nursing measures for the client undergoing gastric surgery are the same as those for any client undergoing abdominal surgery and general anesthesia (see Chapter 17).

CHART 56-6

BEST PRACTICE *for* Nasogastric Tubes

1. Inform the client about the procedure and its potential discomfort.
2. Seat the client with pillows behind the shoulders.
3. Lubricate the tube with a water-soluble lubricant.
4. Measure the length of the tube to be passed.
   a. Measure from the bridge of the nose to the earlobe to the xiphoid process.
   b. Indicate this length with a piece of tape on the tube.

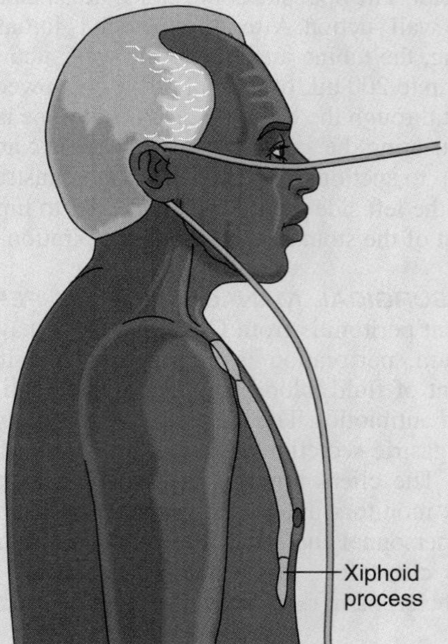

5. Determine which nostril is more patent.
6. Encourage the client to swallow or drink water if the level of consciousness and treatment plan permit.
7. Insert the tube.
   a. Pass the tube gently into the nasopharynx. Ask the client to swallow repeatedly while the tube is advanced.
   b. If resistance is met, rotate the tube slowly, aiming downward and toward the closer ear.
   c. In the intubated or semiconscious client, flex the client's head toward the chest while passing the tube.
8. Withdraw the tube immediately if any change is noted in the client's respiratory status.
9. Test for tube placement by using one or more of the following techniques:
   a. Obtain a sample of the gastric contents by aspirating with a 50-mL catheter-tipped syringe.
   b. Test the pH of the gastric contents (should be between 1 and 3.5).
   c. Obtain an order for an x-ray study to confirm placement.
10. Connect the tube to suction at low pressure.
    a. The Levin tube is connected to intermittent low suction.
    b. The Salem sump or Anderson tube is connected to continuous low suction.
11. Secure the tube to the client's nose with adhesive tape and to the client's gown.
    a. Tie a slipknot around the tube with a rubber band.
    b. Pin a rubber band to the client's gown.
12. Check the client's intake and output every 4 hr or more often, as indicated.
13. Observe the client for nausea, vomiting, abdominal fullness, or distention.
14. If irrigation is indicated, use only a normal saline solution.
15. Observe the client for alterations in fluid and electrolyte balance.
16. If indicated, instruct the client about movement that will not dislodge the tube and cause nasal irritation.
17. Remove the adhesive tape securing the tube to the nose daily and prn to clean skin; reapply tape.

OPERATIVE PROCEDURES. There is no definitive single procedure for PUD. The most commonly performed surgical procedures are gastroenterostomy, vagotomy and pyloroplasty.

Gastroenterostomy. A simple **gastroenterostomy** permits neutralization of gastric acid by regurgitation of alkaline duodenal contents into the stomach. The surgeon creates a passage between the body of the stomach and the small bowel, often the jejunum (Figure 56-4). The benefit may be offset by interference with acid inhibition of gastrin release, which results in a net increase in acid secretion.

If the gastroenterostomy drains the stomach, it reduces motor activity in the pyloroduodenal area. Drainage of the gastric contents diverts acid from the ulcerated area and facilitates healing. However, the secretory capacity of the parietal cell mass of the stomach has not been reduced, and the gastrin mechanism continues to function. For this reason, a vagotomy is usually combined with gastroenterostomy for reduction of the vagal influences.

Vagotomy. Three types of **vagotomy** have been used in the treatment of duodenal ulcers: truncal vagotomy, selective vagotomy, and proximal gastric vagotomy (Figure 56-5). Vagotomy eliminates the acid-secreting stimulus to gastric cells and decreases the responsiveness of parietal cells. In a truncal vagotomy, the vagal trunks are transected and the antrum is removed. The remaining stomach is anastomosed to the proximal duodenum (Billroth I) or to a loop of jejunum (Billroth II) (Figures 56-6 and 56-7).

With selective vagotomy, only the branches of the vagus nerve that supply the stomach are transected; the remaining abdominal viscera still has intact vagal innervation. Selective vagotomy results in a more complete response, reduced ulcer recurrence, and fewer postoperative complications.

Proximal gastric vagotomy interrupts the nerve supply to only the acid-secreting portion of the stomach; it spares the branches of the vagus nerve that innervate the antrum, making pyloroplasty unnecessary.

Pyloroplasty. The surgeon often performs **pyloroplasty** in conjunction with a vagotomy to widen the exit of the pylorus. This facilitates emptying of stomach contents. The most common procedure is the Heineke-Mikulicz pyloroplasty (Figure 56-8). In this procedure the surgeon enlarges the pyloric stricture by incising the pylorus longitudinally and sutures the incision transversely.

POSTOPERATIVE CARE. The postoperative care is similar for all of the surgical procedures (see the Client Care Plan on p. 1231). The nurse provides the usual postoperative care for clients who have had general anesthesia (see Chapter 19).

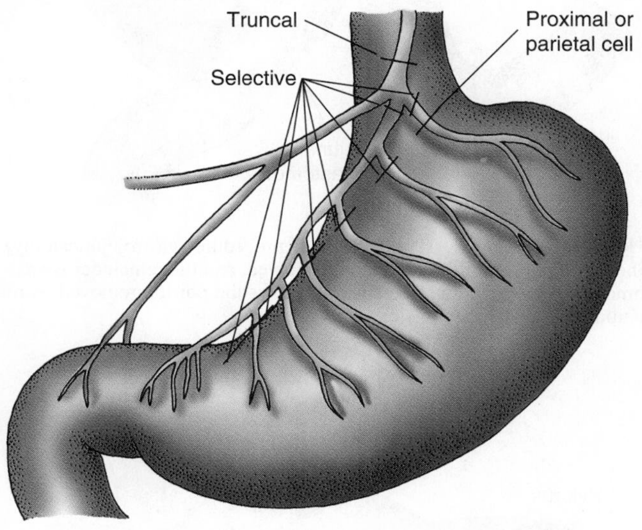

Figure 56-5 ● The types of vagotomies.

Figure 56-4 ● Gastroenterostomy (the creation of a passage between the body of the stomach and the jejunum).

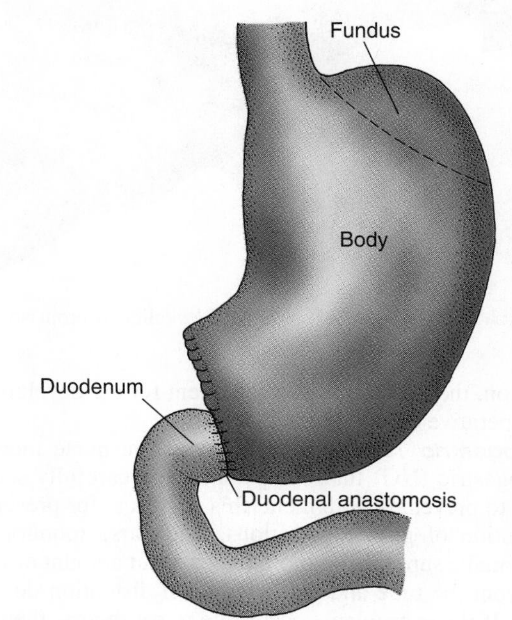

Figure 56-6 ● The Billroth I procedure (gastroduodenostomy). The distal portion of the stomach is removed, and the remainder is anastomosed to the duodenum. The shading shows the portion removed.

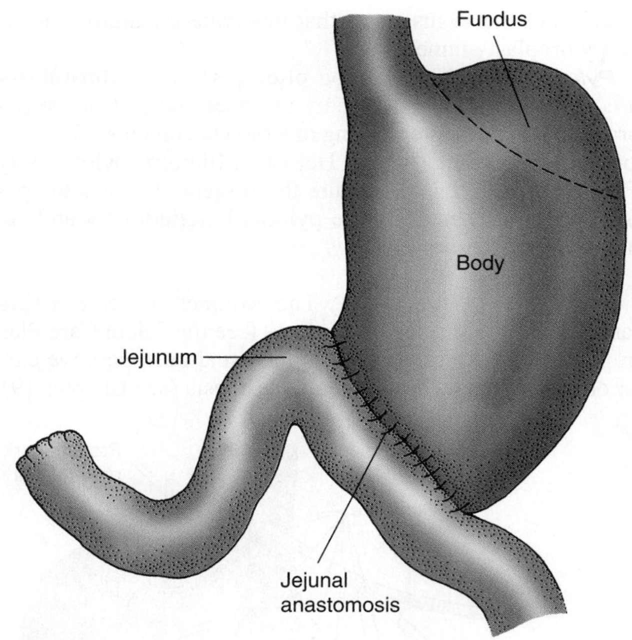

Figure 56-7 ● The Billroth II procedure (gastrojejunostomy). The lower portion of the stomach is removed, and the remainder is anastomosed to the jejunum. The shading shows the portion removed. A remaining duodenal stump is closed.

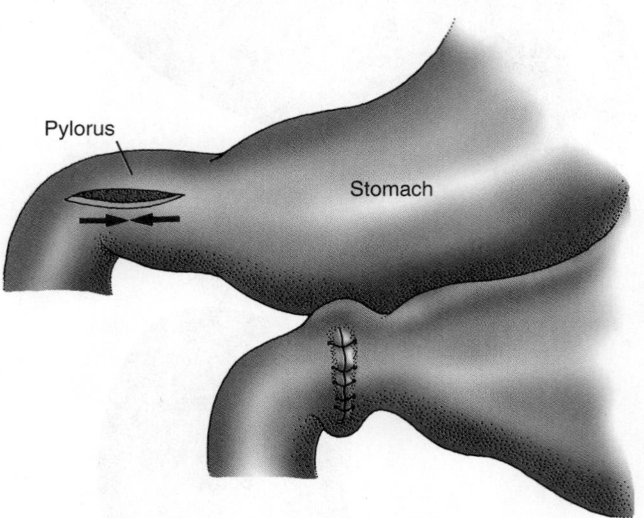

Figure 56-8 ● The Heineke-Mikulicz pyloroplasty.

In addition, the nurse monitors the client for the development of postoperative complications.

Nasogastric Tube Management. The nurse monitors the nasogastric (NG) tube for patency and carefully secures the tube to prevent dislodgment; this is critical for preventing the retention of gastric secretions. The nurse monitors the client to make sure that no more than a scant amount of blood drains from the tube and that abdominal distention does not develop. If these problems occur, the nurse reports them immediately to the surgeon. Irrigation or repositioning of the NG tube is not done after gastric surgery unless specifically ordered by the surgeon.

Monitoring for Postoperative Complications. The nurse observes the client carefully for possible complications and reports them immediately to the health care provider. In the immediate postoperative period, many complications may occur. Table 56-2 summarizes surgical procedures and potential complications.

A disruption in the patency of the NG tube can result in *acute gastric dilation* postoperatively; this is manifested by epigastric pain and a feeling of fullness, hiccups, tachycardia, and hypotension. Irrigation or replacement of the NG tube by order of the surgeon can relieve these symptoms.

Dumping syndrome is a term that refers to a constellation of vasomotor symptoms after eating, especially following a Billroth II procedure. This syndrome is believed to occur as a result of the rapid emptying of gastric contents into the small intestine, which shifts fluid into the gut, causing abdominal distension. The nurse observes for *early* manifestations of this syndrome, which typically occurs within 30 minutes of eating. Symptoms include vertigo, tachycardia, syncope, sweating, pallor, palpitations, and the desire to lie down.

Late dumping syndrome, which occurs 90 minutes to 3 hours after eating, is caused by a release of an excessive amount of insulin. The insulin release follows a rapid rise in the blood glucose level that results from the rapid entry of high-carbohydrate food into the jejunum. The nurse observes for intestinal manifestations, including dizziness, lightheadedness, palpitations, diaphoresis, and confusion.

Dumping syndrome is managed by dietary measures that include decreasing the amount of food taken at one time and eliminating liquids ingested with meals. In collaboration with the dietitian, the nurse instructs the client to consume a high-protein, high-fat, low-carbohydrate diet (Table 56-3). Pectin administered in the form of a dry powder may *prevent* the syndrome. A somatostatin analog, octreotide, may be ordered in severe cases.

Alkaline *reflux gastropathy,* also known as *bile reflux gastropathy,* is a complication of gastric surgery in which the pylorus is bypassed or removed (e.g., pyloroplasty, gastric resection with gastroduodenostomy [Billroth I procedure], and gastrojejunostomy [Billroth II procedure]). Endoscopic examination reveals regurgitated bile in the stomach and mucosal hyperemia. Symptoms include early satiety, abdominal discomfort, and vomiting.

Delayed gastric emptying is often present after gastric surgery and usually resolves within 1 week. Edema at the anastomosis or adhesions obstructing the distal loop may be mechanical causes. Metabolic causes (such as hypokalemia, hypoproteinemia, or hyponatremia) should be considered. The edema is resolved with nasogastric suction, maintenance of fluid and electrolyte balance, and proper nutrition.

Afferent loop syndrome may occur when the duodenal loop is partially obstructed after a Billroth II resection. Pancreatic and biliary secretions fill the intestinal loop, which becomes distended. Painful contractions attempt to propel these secretions from the loop. The nurse monitors for clients reporting abdominal bloating and pain 20 to 60 minutes after eating, often followed by nausea and vomiting. Treatment consists of surgical correction of the incomplete loop obstruction.

Recurrent ulceration occurs in approximately 5% of clients who have undergone gastric surgery for PUD. Recurrent ulcers can be due to incomplete vagotomy or persistent *H. pylori* in-

CLIENT CARE PLAN • THE CLIENT RECOVERING FROM GASTRIC SURGERY

NURSING DIAGNOSIS NO. 1 • Acute Pain or Chronic Pain related to gastric or mucosal injury or gastric surgery

Expected Outcomes	Nursing Interventions	Rationale
The client is expected to experience reduced pain as evidenced by verbalization of pain reduction or alleviation.	Teach the client what to expect regarding the postoperative pain experience. Explain possible effects of fatigue and anxiety. Instill a sense of control of the situation in relation to the temporary nature of the problem.	These interventions reduce the client's anxiety level and fatigue. Increased anxiety and fatigue ultimately intensify the pain experience by reducing the body's or mind's adaptive capacity to deal with uncomfortable stimuli or situations.
	Assess the client's sleep patterns and the influence of pain on sleep. D	Sleep disturbances are common with ulcer disease, and pain may exacerbate this problem.
	Encourage rest and provide an opportunity for rest during the day. D	Fatigue can intensify the pain experience.
	Administer appropriate analgesics as ordered for postoperative pain. Administer antiulcer therapy as ordered.	Analgesics are used in conjunction with comfort measures to reduce or alleviate postoperative pain. Pain control secondary to gastric mucosal injury is treated with agents to decrease gastric acid secretion, promote healing, and eradicate *H. pylori* infection.
	Teach nonpharmacologic techniques used in conjunction with medications to promote comfort, such as relaxation, cutaneous stimulation, and massage.	Nonpharmacologic pain relief measures provide an additional means of managing pain and discomfort.
	Encourage positioning to improve chest expansion (i.e., semi-Fowler's position or reclining). Demonstrate techniques to splint the incision during coughing. D	Proper positioning and incision splinting can lessen pain associated with movement and encourage deep breathing and coughing to prevent postoperative respiratory problems.
	Avoid, or use with caution, drugs that decrease mucosal resistance (aspirin, nonsteroidal anti-inflammatory drugs [NSAIDs], steroids) or drugs that alter gastric acid production. Discourage the use of stimulants (e.g., caffeine and nicotine) or spices (e.g., mustard, paprika, pepper, and Tabasco sauce) that are known to cause pain or discomfort.	Identification of factors that can exacerbate pain or discomfort can assist the client in eliminating individualized pain triggers. Certain substances are known gastric irritants and should be avoided.
	Eliminate the use of alcohol. Avoid the concurrent use of alcohol and aspirin.	Alcohol irritates the mucosal lining and may provoke gastritis. Alcohol and aspirin together greatly irritate the mucosal lining.
	Identify increases in pain or changes in pain characteristics. Instruct the client to report signs of complications, a feeling of fullness, weakness, or hematemesis.	Increasing pain or discomfort may indicate the development of complications.
	Gradually increase food until the client is able to eat three to six meals a day. D	Return of function of the stomach and intestines is evaluated postoperatively.
	If discomfort recurs, decrease the size of meals and the amount of fluids. D	Small enteral feedings are better tolerated than three large meals per day. Fluids should be offered between meals.

NURSING DIAGNOSIS NO. 2 • Risk for Deficient Fluid Volume related to vomiting, hemorrhage, or perforation

Expected Outcomes	Nursing Interventions	Rationale
The client is expected to maintain vascular, cellular, and intracellular perfusion as evidenced by: • Intact mental status • Stable blood pressure • Warm, dry skin • Urine output of at least 30 mL/hr	Assess for nausea, vomiting, tarry stools, occult or frank blood in stools, thirst, diaphoresis, pain, tachycardia, and hypotension.	Assessment detects fluid volume deficit and evaluates its severity.
	Assess urine output and hemoglobin and hematocrit values.	Early detection of hypovolemia secondary to fluid volume depletion or hemorrhage can prevent excessive losses.
	Monitor client's fluid status, including intake and output. D Replace fluids and administer blood products as ordered by the health care provider.	If fluid volume deficit occurs, these same interventions assess the effectiveness of treatment.

D Indicates tasks that can be delegated to assistive nursing personnel.

TABLE 56-2 • SURGICAL MANAGEMENT OF PEPTIC ULCER DISEASE AND POTENTIAL COMPLICATIONS OF PEPTIC ULCER DISEASE

Surgery	Description	Possible Adverse Effects
Vagotomy Truncal (total abdominal vagotomy)	Cuts the vagus nerve at the esophageal level; severs both anterior and posterior trunks; destroys vagal and abdominal innervation; destroys gastrointestinal (GI) motility	Gastric emptying is inhibited; pyloroplasty or antrectomy must be performed to prevent gastric stasis. Some clients experience a feeling of fullness after eating (33%), dumping syndrome (10%), or diarrhea (10%).
Selective	Cuts the vagus nerve to the stomach, but other abdominal innervation remains; acid production stops	Gastric emptying is inhibited; pyloroplasty or antrectomy must be performed to prevent gastric stasis.
Proximal, or parietal cell (can be done without pyloroplasty or antrectomy)	Cuts the parietal branches of the vagus nerve; alters innervation to acid-producing cells but does not alter GI motility	Few negative consequences because innervation of the antrum and the pyloric sphincter remains.
Vagotomy with antrectomy	Cuts the vagus nerve and removes the antrum (lower half) of the stomach; removes the source of gastrin secretion	Some clients may have a feeling of fullness after eating, dumping syndrome, diarrhea, anemia, malabsorption, or recurrent ulceration.
Pyloroplasty	Enlarges the pylorus by surgically enlarging the pyloric sphincter	The stomach may empty too rapidly; alkaline reflux gastropathy can occur.
Vagotomy and pyloroplasty	Cuts the right and left branches of the vagus nerve; widens the existing pyloric sphincter to prevent stasis and to enhance emptying of the stomach	The stomach may empty too rapidly; alkaline reflux gastropathy can occur.
Subtotal gastrectomy Billroth I (gastroduodenostomy after resection) hemigastrectomy	Removes the distal one third to one half of the stomach and anastomoses with the duodenum; removes the antral portion of the stomach and the pylorus	Dumping syndrome, anemia, malabsorption, weight loss, or alkaline reflux may occur.
Billroth II (gastrojejunostomy after resection)	Removes the distal segment of the stomach and antrum and anastomoses with the jejunum; retains the duodenum; secretions of the liver and pancreas flow to the jejunum; preferred procedure	Afferent loop syndrome, malabsorption-related weight loss, vitamin B_{12} deficiency, alkaline reflux, or dumping syndrome may occur.
Total gastrectomy (esophagojejunostomy)	Removes the stomach from the level of the lower esophageal sphincter to the duodenum and anastomoses the duodenum to the esophagus	Gastric function is altered. Dumping syndrome and anemia may occur.

fection. Recurrence is most common following vagotomy with antrectomy, and ulcerations tend to occur at the site of anastomosis (stomal or marginal ulcer) or immediately distal in the small intestine. Abdominal pain, usually located in the epigastrium, is the most commonly reported symptom of recurrent peptic ulcer. The health care provider may order H_2-receptor antagonists and proton pump inhibitors to assist with the healing process. The eradication of *H. pylori* in the case of recurrent stomal ulcerations is controversial.

NUTRITIONAL MANAGEMENT. Several problems related to nutrition develop as a result of partial removal of the stomach, including deficiencies of vitamin B_{12}, folic acid, and iron; impaired calcium metabolism; and reduced absorption of calcium and vitamin D. These problems are caused by a shortage of intrinsic factor. The shortage results from the resection and from inadequate absorption because of rapid entry of food into the bowel. In the absence of intrinsic factor, clinical manifestations of pernicious anemia occur. The nurse should assess for the development of atrophic glossitis secondary to vitamin B_{12} deficiency. In atrophic glossitis, the tongue takes on a shiny and "beefy" appearance. The client may also have signs of anemia secondary to folic acid and iron deficiency. The nurse monitors the complete blood count (CBC) for signs of megaloblastic anemia and leukopenia. These manifestations are corrected by the administration of vitamin B_{12}. The health care provider may also prescribe folic acid or iron preparations.

Community-Based Care

Clients may be discharged from the hospital as long as there is no evidence of ongoing bleeding, orthostatic changes, or cardiopulmonary distress or compromise. Clients discharged following treatment for peptic ulcer disease (PUD) and/or complications secondary to the disease must face several challenges in order to manage the disease successfully. Long-term adherence to medication regimens requires the client to take many oral medications on a daily basis. Permanent lifestyle alterations in dietary habits must also be made. Clients must be knowledgeable about complications related to PUD and know when to report symptoms to the health care provider.

HOME CARE MANAGEMENT

Clients are discharged to the home, subacute unit, or skilled nursing facility to continue recuperation. Clients who have undergone surgery or have had complications, such as hemor-

TABLE 56-3 • DIET FOR DUMPING SYNDROME

Food Group	Foods Allowed or Encouraged	Foods to Use with Caution	Foods That Must Be Excluded
Soups		Fluids 1 hr before and after meals	Spicy soups
Meat and meat substitutes	8 oz or more per day: fish poultry, beef, pork, veal, lamb, eggs, cheese, and peanut butter		Spicy meats or meat substitutes
Potato and substitutes	Potato, rice, pasta, starchy vegetables	Foods made with milk	Highly spiced potatoes or substitutes
Bread and cereal	White bread, rolls, muffins, crackers, and cereals	Whole-grain bread, rolls, crackers, and cereals	Breads with frosting or jelly, sweet rolls, and coffee cake
Vegetables	Two or more cooked vegetables	Gas-producing vegetables, such as cabbage, onions, broccoli, or raw vegetables	
Fruits	Limit three per day: unsweetened cooked or canned fruits	Unsweetened juice or fruit drinks 30-45 min after meals; fresh fruit	Sweetened fruit or juice
Beverages	Dietetic drinks	Limit to 1 hr after meals; caffeine-containing beverages, such as coffee, tea, and cola; if tolerated, diet carbonated beverages	Milk shakes, malts, and other sweet drinks; regular carbonated beverages and alcohol
Fats	Margarine, oils, shortening, butter, bacon, and salad dressings	Mayonnaise	Any fats with milk products
Desserts	Fruit (see Fruits)	Sugar-free gelatin, pudding, and custard	All sweets, cakes, pies, cookies, candy, ice cream, and sherbet
Seasonings and miscellaneous	Diet jelly, diet syrups, sugar substitutes	Excessive amounts of salt	Excessive amounts of spices, sugar, jelly, honey, syrup, or molasses

GENERAL PRINCIPLES
- Five to six small meals daily
- Relatively high fat and protein content
- Low roughage
- Relatively low carbohydrate content
- No milk, sweets, or sugars
- Liquid between meals *only*

rhage, may require visits from a home care nurse to assess clinical progress.

HEALTH TEACHING

The primary focus of home care preparation is client teaching regarding risk factors for the recurrence of PUD; clients are also taught to recognize and report the development of complications related to the disease process or surgical intervention.

The nurse instructs the client and family or significant others about factors related to the development of an ulcer. A risk assessment assists in identifying gastric irritants and lifestyle stressors that may be contributory to ulcer formation. Strategies for lifestyle changes are developed together with the client. The nurse teaches about symptoms that should be brought to the attention of the health care provider after discharge from the hospital, such as abdominal pain; nausea and vomiting; black, tarry stools; and weakness or dizziness. To demonstrate understanding, the client describes the symptoms back to the nurse.

The nurse also teaches the client about diets to be used for avoiding postprandial distention or dumping syndrome. For postsurgical clients, especially those who have undergone partial stomach removal, a smaller meal may be required. In collaboration with the dietitian, the nurse instructs the client to:

- Eat small, frequent meals
- Avoid drinking liquids with meals
- Abstain from foods that contribute to discomfort
- Eliminate caffeine and alcohol consumption
- Begin a smoking cessation program
- Receive B_{12} injections, as appropriate

The client is also taught to avoid any over-the-counter (OTC) product containing aspirin or ibuprofen. The nurse emphasizes the importance of adhering to the treatment regimen. Long-term medication compliance is critical for eradicating *H. pylori* infection and achieving healing of the ulcer. The importance of keeping all follow-up appointments is also emphasized, since early detection of recurrence or the development of complications is desirable.

The nurse helps the client to identify situations that cause stress, describe feelings during stressful situations, and develop a plan for coping with stressors (Chart 56-7). The nurse encourages the client to learn and use relaxation techniques, such as exercise, biofeedback, humor, and imagery (see Chapter 4). Psychotherapy may be indicated to help some clients cope with excessive anxiety or stress. Ulcer disease is difficult to eradicate, so it is essential for the client and family to understand how modifying living, working, and eating habits minimizes the risk of ulcer recurrence.

HEALTH CARE RESOURCES

Following discharge, home care nursing visits may be indicated if clients and family members or significant others require instruction or assistance with follow-up care, such as dressing changes, monitoring of potential complications, and continued nutritional problems.

Evaluation: Outcomes

NOC The nurse evaluates the care of the client with peptic ulcer disease (PUD) on the basis of the identified nursing diagnoses and collaborative problems. The expected outcomes are that the client:

- Maintains hemodynamic stability, free of disease or surgical complications
- States that pain is reduced or alleviated by prescribed interventions
- Identifies potential causes and risks of disease recurrence
- Avoids the intake of irritating foods and beverages
- Avoids smoking
- Avoids over-the-counter medications containing aspirin or ibuprofen
- Identifies early symptoms of recurrence or complications
- Identifies and copes successfully with stressful situations
- Adheres to long-term medication regimen and appropriate follow-up with the health care provider

CHART 56-7

FOCUSED ASSESSMENT *of* Ambulatory Care with Ulcer Disease

Assess gastrointestinal and cardiovascular status, including:
- Vital signs, including orthostatic vital signs
- Skin color
- Presence of abdominal pain (location, severity, character, duration, precipitating factors, and relief measures)
- Character, color, and consistency of stools
- Changes in bowel elimination pattern
- Hemoglobin and hematocrit
- Bowel sounds; palpate for areas of tenderness

Assess nutritional status, including:
- Dietary patterns and habits
- Intake of caffeine and alcohol
- Relationship of food to symptoms

Assess medication history.
- Use of steroids
- Use of nonsteroidal anti-inflammatory drugs (NSAIDs)
- Use of over-the-counter medications

Assess client's coping style
- Recent stressors
- Past coping style

Assess client's understanding of illness and ability to comply with therapeutic regimen.
- Symptoms to report to health care provider
- Expected and side effects of medications
- Food and drug interactions
- Need for smoking cessation

ZOLLINGER-ELLISON SYNDROME

OVERVIEW

Zollinger-Ellison syndrome (ZES) is manifested by upper gastrointestinal (GI) tract ulceration, increased gastric acid secretion, and the presence of a non–beta cell islet tumor of the pancreas, called a gastrinoma. Affected individuals may have more than one gastrinoma. Approximately two thirds of gastrinomas are malignant. Recent developments indicate that a benign but aggressive form of the disease may exist (Yu et al., 1999). Although most gastrinomas grow slowly, a small portion of them develop rapidly and metastasize widely. Metastasis occurs mainly in the liver and regional lymph nodes. Gastrinoma remains a relatively uncommon disease, with an incidence of 1 to 3 new cases per year per million people.

In 20% to 60% of clients with ZES, the gastrinoma results from an autosomal dominant disorder called multiple endocrine neoplasia type 1 (MEN-1) syndrome. Gastrinomas contain multiple hormones, but adrenocorticotropic hormone (ACTH) is most commonly found. As a result, Cushing's syndrome with increased ACTH levels is reported in approximately 8% of clients with ZES.

In the early course of the disease, symptoms resemble those of peptic ulcer disease (PUD). However, these symptoms tend to progress, and they respond poorly to traditional ulcer therapy. Diarrhea may be a manifestation of this disorder, occurring in 40% of clients. The diarrhea may be associated with large amounts of hydrochloric acid secreted into the proximal duodenum. **Steatorrhea** (an excessive amount of fat in the feces) results from the inactivation of pancreatic lipase secondary to the large concentrations of acid and decreased amounts of bile acids.

COLLABORATIVE MANAGEMENT

Assessment

Radiographic and endoscopic findings for ZES are similar to those for PUD. However, infection with *Helicobacter pylori* is usually absent. The diagnosis is usually made by radioimmunoassay studies that reveal increased serum gastrin levels in conjunction with the clinical features of the disease.

Interventions

The aim of therapy is to suppress acid secretion in order to control the client's symptoms. The H^+,K^+-ATPase inhibitors, such as lansoprazole and omeprazole (given as 60 mg/day in a single dose) are the drugs of choice to reduce gastric acid secretion and heal ulcers in clients with ZES. However, long-term treatment with these drugs can lead to significant decreases in vitamin B_{12} levels (Termanini et al., 1998). High doses of H_2-receptor antagonists, such as ranitidine (Zantac), are also effective in reducing gastric acid and providing symptom relief.

If medical therapy fails, the health care provider may choose to perform a vagotomy and pyloroplasty to supplement pharmacologic means of controlling hypersecretion. A total gastrectomy is the surgical approach of choice for this disorder if vagotomy, pyloroplasty, and medical therapy are inadequate. (See the earlier discussion of these surgeries under Surgical Management [Peptic Ulcer Disease], p. 1228.)

The consequences of the malignant properties of the tumor are now being more widely recognized, and complete surgical resection of the tumor appears to be the optimal treatment. Clients with aggressive disease can also be treated with chemotherapeutic agents such as 5-fluorouracil and doxorubicin to reduce the tumor and control symptoms.

GASTRIC CARCINOMA

OVERVIEW

Gastric carcinoma refers to malignant neoplasms in the stomach. Adenocarcinomas account for 85% to 95% of all gastric cancers (Mayer, 1998, O'Connor, 1999). The remaining 15% are due to non-Hodgkin's lymphoma and leiomyosarcomas. In the United States, 30% of gastric cancers are in the distal stomach, 20% are in the midsection of the stomach, and 37% arise in the proximal third of the stomach. The remaining cases of gastric carcinoma involve the entire stomach. The onset is insidious, and the disease is often advanced when detected.

Pathophysiology

Gastric adenocarcinoma can be characterized as *intestinal* or *diffuse.* Intestinal adenocarcinomas result from atrophic gastritis or intestinal metaplasia, both of which are considered precancerous conditions. The diffuse form of the disease is found primarily in areas where gastric cancer is endemic. Early, superficial gastric cancers produce no notable symptoms. On microscopic examination, the cells resemble intestinal metaplasia (abnormal tissue development).

Gastric cancers spread by direct extension through the gastric wall and into regional lymphatics. The intramural lymphatics readily allow horizontal spread within the gastric wall. Extramural lymphatics carry tumor deposits to lymph nodes in more than 50% of operable cases. Direct invasion of and adherence to adjacent organs (e.g., the liver, pancreas, and transverse colon) may also result. Hematogenous spread via the portal vein to the liver and via the systemic circulation to the lungs and bones is the most common mode of metastasis. Peritoneal seeding of cancer cells from the involved gastric serosa to the omentum, peritoneum, ovary, and pelvic cul-de-sac can also occur.

In people with advanced gastric cancer, there is invasion of the muscularis (stomach muscle) or beyond. These lesions are not amenable to curative resection. Most clients in the United States have advanced (stage III or stage IV) disease when diagnosed. The 5-year survival rate following surgical resection is 20% to 25% for tumors located in the distal stomach, 10% for proximal tumors, and 5% when the entire stomach is involved (Hawkins, 1999).

Etiology

Recent evidence has provided a strong link between infection with *H. pylori* and the subsequent development of gastric cancer. Metabolic products produced by the organism transform the gastric mucosa while producing a state of chronic inflammation. Such chronic inflammatory states can induce cancer by increasing cell proliferation and free radical formation.

Clients with pernicious anemia, gastric polyps, chronic atrophic gastritis, and achlorhydria (absence of secretion of hydrochloric acid) are two to three times more likely to develop gastric cancer.

Gastric cancer seems to be positively correlated with the ingestion of pickled foods, salted fish, salted meat, and nitrates from processed foods, as well as a high consumption of salt. The ingestion of these foods over a long period of time can lead to atrophic gastritis, a precancerous condition.

The role of cigarette smoking and alcohol consumption in the development of gastric carcinoma is controversial, although some studies support the conclusion that smokers are 1.5 to 3 times more likely to develop gastric cancer as compared with nonsmokers (O'Connor, 1999).

Genetic factors may play a role in the development of gastric cancer; an increased incidence of the disease has been noted among direct relatives of clients with gastric cancer. First-degree relatives of individuals with gastric cancer are two to three times more likely to develop the disease themselves. In addition, individuals with type A blood appear to have a slight risk of gastric cancer.

Gastric surgery, especially a Billroth II procedure, seems to increase the risk for gastric cancer because of the eventual development of atrophic gastritis, which results in changes to the mucosa. Clients with Barrett's esophagus have an increased risk of adenocarcinoma of the gastric cardia.

Incidence/Prevalence

Although the incidence of gastric cancer is decreasing in the United States, it is the fourteenth most common cause of all cancer-related deaths, and it is one of the top five causes of cancer-related deaths for minority populations (O'Connor, 1999). Men appear to have a greater incidence of developing the disease than women, and the average age of onset is from 50 to 70 years of age.

CULTURAL CONSIDERATIONS

Japan, Chile, and Costa Rica have the highest incidence of gastric cancer. In some Nordic countries, such as Scandinavia, an increased incidence and prevalence of the disease has been noted over the last several decades. Native Americans, African Americans, and Hispanics are two times as likely to develop gastric cancer as compared with Caucasians (O'Connor, 1999).

COLLABORATIVE MANAGEMENT

Assessment

HISTORY

The nurse questions the client regarding the known risk factors for the development of gastric cancer. The nurse elicits information regarding preferred foods, especially pickled, salted, or smoked foods. Information regarding tobacco use and alcohol ingestion is also gathered. The nurse inquires if the client has ever been diagnosed or treated for *H. pylori* infection, gastritis, or pernicious anemia. The nurse notes if the client has a history of gastric surgery or polyps. The nurse also inquires if any of the client's immediate relatives have been diagnosed with gastric cancer. If known, the nurse makes a notation of the client's blood type.

PHYSICAL ASSESSMENT/CLINICAL MANIFESTATIONS

Although clients with *early* gastric cancer may be asymptomatic, indigestion (heartburn) and abdominal discomfort are the *most* common symptoms (Chart 56-8). These symptoms are often ignored, however, or a change in diet or use of antacids relieves them. As the tumor grows, these symptoms become more severe and do not respond to diet changes or antacids. Epigastric, back, or retrosternal pain is also an early symptom that may go unrecognized. Two thirds of clients will complain of epigastric pain following eating. This pain is described as a vague feeling of fullness or discomfort (Hawkins, 1999).

In *advanced* gastric carcinoma, progressive weight loss, nausea, and vomiting can occur. Vomiting represents pronounced dilation, thickening of the stomach wall, or pyloric obstruction. Obstructive symptoms appear earlier with tumors located near the pylorus than with fundic lesions. Clients with advanced disease may have weakness, fatigue, and anemia.

Physical assessment findings in advanced disease may be absent, or a palpable epigastric mass may suggest hepatomegaly from metastatic disease. Hard, enlarged lymph nodes in the left supraclavicular chain, left axilla, or umbilicus may be the result of metastasis from gastric cancer. Masses on the right suggest metastasis in the perigastric lymph nodes or liver. Signs of distant metastasis include the following:

- Virchow's (sentinel or signal) nodes (enlarged supraclavicular lymph nodes, especially on the left)
- Blumer's shelf, resulting from peritoneal seeding that produces a firm mass palpable on rectal or vaginal examination
- "Sister Mary Joseph nodes" (subcutaneous periumbilical deposits)
- Krukenberg's tumor (metastatic ovarian nodules)

LABORATORY ASSESSMENT

In clients with advanced disease, anemia is evidenced by low hematocrit and hemoglobin values. Clients may have macrocytic or microcytic anemia associated with decreased iron or vitamin B_{12} absorption. The stool may be positive for occult blood.

Hypoalbuminemia and abnormal results of liver tests (such as bilirubin and alkaline phosphatase) occur with advanced disease and with hepatic metastasis. The level of carcinoembryonic antigen (CEA) is elevated in *advanced* cancer of the stomach.

CHART 56-8

KEY FEATURES *of* Early Versus Advanced Gastric Cancer

Early Gastric Cancer
- Indigestion
- Abdominal discomfort initially relieved with antacids
- Feeling of fullness
- Epigastric, back, or retrosternal pain

(NOTE: Many clients with early gastric cancer have no clinical manifestations.)

Advanced Gastric Cancer
- Nausea and vomiting
- Obstructive symptoms
- Iron deficiency anemia
- Palpable epigastric mass
- Enlarged lymph nodes
- Weakness and fatigue
- Progressive weight loss
- Signs of distant metastasis
  - Virchow's nodes
  - Blumer's shelf
  - "Sister Mary Joseph nodes"
  - Krukenberg's tumor

RADIOGRAPHIC ASSESSMENT

A double-contrast upper gastrointestinal (GI) series is usually the first diagnostic test. The use of a double-contrast medium assists in the detection of small lesions. A polypoid mass, ulcer crater, or thickened fibrotic gastric wall may suggest gastric cancer.

A computed tomography (CT) scan is used to evaluate gastric malignancies. CT scans of the chest, abdomen, and pelvis are used in determining the extent of the disease.

OTHER DIAGNOSTIC ASSESSMENT

The health care provider uses esophagogastroduodenoscopy (EGD) for definitive diagnosis of gastric cancer. The lesion can be visualized directly, and biopsies of all visible lesions can be obtained to determine the presence of cancer cells. During the endoscopy, an endoscopic ultrasound (EUS) of the gastric mucosa can also be performed. This technology allows the health care provider to evaluate the depth of the tumor and the presence of lymph node involvement that permits more accurate staging of the disease.

Interventions

Management of gastric cancer includes drug therapy, radiation, and/or surgery.

NONSURGICAL MANAGEMENT. The treatment of gastric cancer is highly dependent on the stage of the disease. Surgical resection of the tumor is usually combined with chemotherapy and/or radiation. Radiation and chemotherapy commonly prolong survival of clients with advanced gastric disease.

DRUG THERAPY. The role of chemotherapy in gastric cancer remains uncertain. No specific chemotherapeutic protocol has had a positive effect on survival. Chemotherapy with single agents such as fluorouracil (5-FU), doxorubicin, mitomycin-C, cisplatin, and etoposide have been used, but the use of a combination of agents appears to have superior results. Bone marrow suppression, nausea, and vomiting are common side effects. Chapter 25 discusses chemotherapy in detail.

RADIATION THERAPY. Although gastric cancers are somewhat sensitive to the effects of radiation, the use of this treatment is limited, since the disease is often widely disseminated to other abdominal organs on diagnosis. Organs such as the liver and kidneys, as well as the spinal cord, have limits as to the amount of radiation they can endure. Postoperative radiation has not significantly increased survival. Intraoperative radiotherapy (IORT) is available at only a few institutions in the United States, since special operative suites, equipment, and personnel are required.

The most common side effects experienced by clients undergoing radiation include impaired skin integrity, fatigue, and anorexia. Nausea, vomiting, and diarrhea may occur approximately 1 week after treatment is initiated and diminish a month or more after treatment ends. (See Chapter 25 for more information on radiation therapy.) The most common potential problems of IORT are hemorrhage and fistula development.

SURGICAL MANAGEMENT. Surgical resection is the preferred method for treating gastric cancer. The primary surgical procedures for the treatment of gastric cancer are total gastrectomy and subtotal gastrectomy. In early stages, surgery plus adjuvant chemotherapy or radiation may be curative. Most clients with advanced disease are candidates for palliative surgical treatment. Metastasis in the supraclavicular lymph nodes (Virchow's nodes), inguinal lymph nodes, liver, umbilicus, or perirectal wall indicates that the opportunity for cure by resection has been lost. Palliative resection may significantly improve the quality of life for a client suffering from obstruction, hemorrhage, or pain.

PREOPERATIVE CARE. The health care provider gives the client and family an explanation of the disease and the available treatment options (potentially curative or palliative). The nurse reinforces and clarifies the information given. Preoperative care is similar to that provided for the client undergoing general anesthesia and abdominal surgery (see Chapter 17).

OPERATIVE PROCEDURES. When the tumor is located in the mid or distal (lower) portions of the stomach, a subtotal gastrectomy is typically performed. The surgeon uses a Billroth I or Billroth II procedure (discussed earlier under Operative Procedures [Peptic Ulcer Disease], p. 1229). The omentum, spleen, and relevant nodes are also removed.

For the client with a resectable growth in the upper third of the stomach, a total gastrectomy is performed (Figure 56-9). In this procedure the surgeon removes the entire stomach along with en bloc removal of the lymph nodes and omentum. The surgeon sutures the esophagus to the duodenum or jejunum to re-establish continuity of the GI tract. More radical surgery involving removal of the spleen and distal pancreas is controversial. The overall mortality rate for clients undergoing total gastrectomy surgery is 10% to 15% (Hawkins, 1999). For clients with advanced disease, total gastrectomy is performed only when gastric bleeding or obstruction is present.

Clients with tumors at the gastric outlet who are not candidates for subtotal or total gastrectomy may undergo gastroenterostomy for palliation. The surgeon creates a passage between the body of the stomach and the small bowel, often the duodenum (see Figure 56-4).

POSTOPERATIVE CARE. Clients require the standard postoperative care that is given to those who have had general anesthesia (see Chapter 19). Complications after gastric surgery may include the following:

- Pneumonia
- Anastomotic leak
- Hemorrhage
- Reflux aspiration
- Sepsis
- Reflux (acute) gastritis (discussed earlier under Acute Gastritis, p. 1216)
- Paralytic ileus
- Bowel obstruction
- Wound infection
- Dumping syndrome (discussed earlier under Monitoring for Postoperative Complications [Peptic Ulcer Disease], p. 1230).

The nurse monitors the client for the development of postoperative complications. The nurse auscultates the lungs for adventitious sounds and monitors for the return of bowel sounds. Monitoring vital signs is performed as appropriate to detect signs of infection or bleeding. Aggressive pulmonary exercises and early ambulation can help prevent respiratory complications and deep vein thrombosis. The nurse also inspects the operative site every 8 hours for the presence of redness, swelling, or drainage, which indicates wound infection. The nurse also ensures proper positioning of the client to prevent aspiration from reflux.

Since weight loss is problematic for clients with gastric cancer, nutrition therapy is a vital aspect of preoperative and postoperative management. Preoperatively, compression by the tumor can impede adequate nutritional intake. To correct malnutrition before surgery, the health care provider may prescribe supplements to the diet and/or total parenteral nutrition (TPN). Vitamin, mineral, iron, and protein supplements are essential for correction of nutritional deficits.

Postoperatively, the client's inability to ingest normal-size meals, along with poor nutrient absorption due to decreased stomach size, can prevent the client from taking in adequate nutrition. Therefore the surgeon may place an enteral feeding tube during surgery for continued nutritional support. When feasible, oral intake should begin with fluids and progress to solids as tolerated. For clients who have undergone gastric surgery, regurgitation may result from overeating or from eating too quickly.

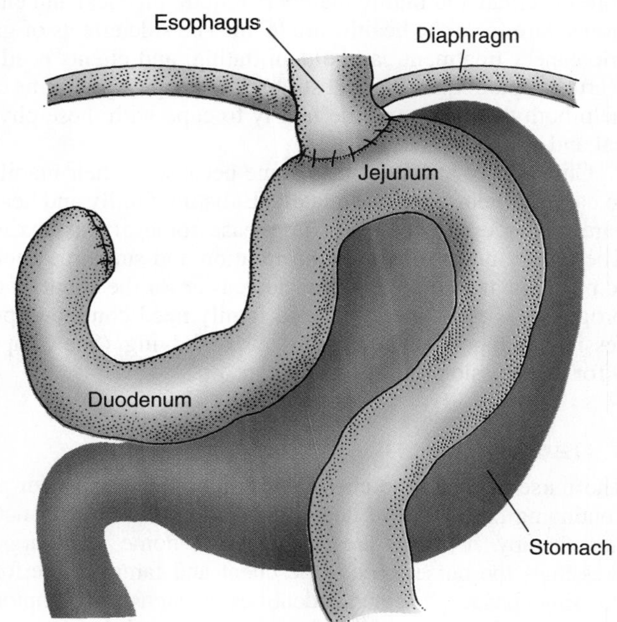

Figure 56-9 ● Total gastrectomy, with anastomosis of the esophagus to the jejunum (esophagojejunostomy), is the principal medical intervention for extensive gastric cancer.

After oral feedings are restarted, the nurse observes the client for signs and symptoms of dumping syndrome and teaches the manifestations and management of this syndrome. The client is advised to eat six small meals per day and to consume a diet high in protein and fat but low in carbohydrate-rich foods (see Table 56-3). Liquids should not be taken with meals. Milk and dairy products are usually eliminated because many clients are lactose-intolerant and have symptoms after the ingestion of milk-containing products.

In collaboration with the dietitian, the nurse guides the client and family in providing the most nutrients and calories. Counseling about methods of preparation and types of foods that increase caloric and protein intake is essential. The nurse maintains intake, output, and calorie counts on a daily basis and records weights at least weekly. Anemia, as well as vitamin B_{12} and folate deficiency, can result following gastrectomy. Oral folate and iron replacement and vitamin B_{12} injections can help correct these deficiencies.

Community-Based Care

Clients who have undergone total gastrectomy and those who are debilitated with advanced gastric cancer are discharged to home with maximal assistance or to a subacute unit or skilled nursing facility. Clients who have undergone subtotal gastrectomy and are not debilitated may be discharged to home with partial assistance for activities of daily living (ADLs). Recurrence of the cancer is common, and clients will need regular follow-up examinations and radiographic assessments. A case manager may be assigned to ensure continuity of care and thorough follow-up with diagnostic testing.

HOME CARE MANAGEMENT

Gastric cancer is considered a life-threatening illness; therefore the client and family members require physical and emotional care from the health care team. The side effects of gastric cancer treatment can be debilitating, and clients need to learn symptom management strategies. Hospice programs can help both the client and the family to cope with these physical and emotional needs.

Clients may fear returning home because of their inability to care for themselves adequately. Enlisting family and health care resources for the client may ease some of this anxiety. The family needs adequate information and support systems to make the transition to home care easier for the client. If the prognosis is poor, the client and family need continued professional support to cope with death and dying. (See Chapter 9 for a discussion of end-of-life care.)

HEALTH TEACHING

The nurse instructs the client and family members about any continuing postoperative needs, adjuvant treatment, and nutrition therapy. If clients are discharged to home with surgical dressings, the nurse teaches the client and family to perform dressing changes. The nurse identifies the signs and symptoms of incisional infection (e.g., fever, redness, and drainage) that are to be reported.

Clients who will be receiving radiation therapy or chemotherapy require instructions related to the side effects of these treatments. Nausea and vomiting are common side effects of chemotherapy, and instruction in the use of prescribed antiemetics may be needed. (See Chapter 25 for education for clients receiving chemotherapy or radiation therapy.)

The nurse, in conjunction with the dietitian, educates the client and family concerning the type and quantity of foods that will provide optimal nutritional value. Interventions to minimize dumping syndrome are also emphasized (see Table 56-3).

HEALTH CARE RESOURCES

A home care referral provides ongoing assessment, assistance, and encouragement to the client and family or significant others at home. A home care nurse can help with physical care procedures and can also provide valuable psychologic support. Additional referrals to a dietitian, professional counselor, or clergy may be necessary. Referral to a hospice agency can be of great assistance. Hospice care may be delivered in the home or in an institutional setting. Appropriate support groups (such as I Can Cope, provided by the American Cancer Society) can be a major resource.

ONLINE RESOURCES

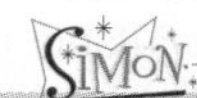

For suggested readings and Internet resources, go to http://www.wbsaunders.com/SIMON/Iggy/.

SELECTED BIBLIOGRAPHY

Aronson, B. (1998). Update on peptic ulcer drugs. *American Journal of Nursing, 98*(1), 41-46.

Astarita, T. (1999). Update on peptic ulcer disease management. *Patient Care for the Nurse Practitioner, 2*(12), 39-51.

Blackington, E. (1999). The gastric demon. *ADVANCE for Nurse Practitioners, 7*(8), 37-44.

Centanni, M., et al. (1999). Atrophic body gastritis in patients with autoimmune thyroid disease: An underdiagnosed association. *Archives of Internal Medicine, 159*(15), 1726-1730.

Cromwell, D., et al. (1999). Can restrictions on reimbursement for antiulcer drugs decrease Medicaid pharmacy costs without increasing hospitalizations? *Health Services Research, 33*(6), 1593-1608.

Curtas, S. (1999). Diagnosing gastrointestinal malignancies. *Seminars in Oncology Nursing, 15*(1), 10-16.

Friedman, L., & Peterson, W. (1998). Peptic ulcer and related disorders. In A.S. Fauci, E. Braunwald, & K.J. Isselbacher (Eds.), *Harrison's principles of internal medicine* (14th ed., pp. 1596-1616). New York: McGraw-Hill.

Graham, D., et al. (1999a). Practical advice on eradicating *Helicobacter pylori* infection. *Postgraduate Medicine, 105*(3), 137-148.

Graham, D., et al. (1999b). Recognizing peptic ulcer disease: Keys to clinical and laboratory diagnosis. *Postgraduate Medicine, 105*(3), 113-128.

Graham, D., et al. (1999c). Scope and consequences of peptic ulcer disease: How important is asymptomatic *Helicobacter pylori* infection? *Postgraduate Medicine, 105*(3), 100-108.

Hawkins, B. (1999). Stomach cancer. In C. Miaskowski & P. Buchsel (Eds.), *Oncology nursing: Assessment and clinical care* (pp. 1015-1030). St. Louis: Mosby.

Heslin, J.M. (1997). Peptic ulcer disease. *Nursing97, 27*(1), 34-40.

Lane, L., & Fendrick, A.M. (1998). *Helicobacter pylori* and peptic ulcer disease. *Postgraduate Medicine, 103*(3), 231-243.

Levy, R., & Feld, A. (1999). Increasing patient adherence to gastroenterology treatment and prevention regimens. *American Journal of Gastroenterology, 94*(7), 1734-1742.

Marshall, J., Collins, S., & Gafni, A. (2000). Prediction of resource utilization and case cost for acute nonvariceal upper gastrointestinal hemorrhage at a Canadian community hospital. *American Journal of Gastroenterology, 94*(7), 1841-1846.

Mayer, R. (1998). Gastrointestinal tract cancer. In A.S. Fauci, E. Braunwald, & K.J. Isselbacher (Eds.), *Harrison's principles of internal medicine* (14th ed., pp. 568-578). New York: McGraw-Hill.

Navuluri, R., & Yue, S. (1999). Understanding peptic ulcer disease pharmacotherapeutics. *Nurse Practitioner, 24*(3), 128-132.

Norton, J.A., Fraker, D.L., & Alexander, H.R. (1999). Surgery to cure Zollinger-Ellison syndrome. *New England Journal of Medicine, 341*(9), 635-644.

O'Connor, K. (1999). Gastric cancer. *Seminars in Oncology Nursing, 15*(1), 26-35.

Offman, J., et al. (2000). The quality of care for Medicare patients with peptic ulcer disease. *American Journal of Gastroenterology 95*(1), 106-113.

Parkman, H., MacMillan Rodney, W., & Rogers, H. (2001). Empiric therapy for nonulcer dyspepsia. *Patient Care for the Nurse Practitioner, 3*(1), 23-24.

Parsonnet, J., Shmuely, H., & Haggerty, T. (1999). Fecal and oral shedding of *Helicobacter pylori* from healthy adults. *Journal of the American Medical Association, 282*(23), 2240-2245.

Ridenour, K. (1998). Medication history and *Helicobacter pylori* testing. *Gastroenterology Nursing, 21*(1), 24-25.

Saddler, D. (1999). Education for the gastroenterology cancer patient. *Gastroenterology Nursing, 22*(3), 121-126.

Schwartz, R., Karpeh, M., & Brennan, M. (1999). In J.M. Daly, T.P.J. Hennessy, & J.V. Reynolds (Eds.), *Management of upper gastrointestinal cancer* (pp. 83-101). Philadelphia: W.B. Saunders.

Terdiman, J. (1998). Update on upper gastrointestinal bleeding: Basing treatment decisions on patient's risk level. *Postgraduate Medicine, 103*(6), 43-63.

Termanini, B., et al. (1998). Effect of long-term gastric acid suppressive therapy on serum vitamin B_{12} levels in patients with Zollinger-Ellison syndrome. *American Journal of Medicine, 104*(5), 422-430.

Weber, H.C., et al. (1997). Studies on the interrelation between Zollinger-Ellison syndrome, *Helicobacter pylori,* and proton pump inhibitor therapy. *Gastroenterology, 112*(1), 84-91.

Yu, F., et al. (1999). Prospective study of the clinical course, prognostic factors, causes of death and survival in patients with long-standing Zollinger Ellison syndrome. *Journal of Clinical Oncology, 17*(2), 615-630.

CHAPTER 57

Interventions for Clients with Noninflammatory Intestinal Disorders

CONSTANCE VISOVSKY

Learning Objectives

After studying this chapter, you should be able to:

1. Explain the risk factors for irritable bowel syndrome (IBS) and cancer of the colon.
2. Develop a teaching-learning plan for clients with IBS.
3. Differentiate the most common types of hernias.
4. Develop a plan of care for a client undergoing a hernia repair.
5. Interpret diagnostic assessments for clients with colorectal cancer.
6. Discuss the psychosocial aspects associated with colorectal cancer and related surgeries.
7. Explain the role of the nurse in managing the client with colorectal cancer.
8. Develop a perioperative plan of care for a client undergoing a colon resection and colostomy.
9. Construct a community-based teaching-learning plan for clients requiring colostomy care.
10. Identify community-based resources for clients with colorectal cancer.
11. Analyze the differences between small-bowel and large-bowel obstructions.
12. Describe assessment findings associated with mechanical and nonmechanical obstructions.
13. Explain the role of the nurse when caring for clients with nasogastric tubes.
14. Develop a plan of care for a client experiencing intestinal obstruction.
15. Prioritize nursing care for the client with abdominal trauma.

SIMON

Go to http://www.wbsaunders.com/SIMON/Iggy/ for self-assessment questions related to these Learning Objectives.

The most common presenting symptoms associated with noninflammatory intestinal disorders include alterations in bowel patterns, abdominal pain, and rectal bleeding (Figure 57-1). Symptoms of this type require investigation, since they can be associated with serious illnesses, such as intestinal obstruction or colorectal cancer.

IRRITABLE BOWEL SYNDROME

OVERVIEW

Irritable bowel syndrome (IBS) is the most common digestive disorder seen in clinical practice. IBS is a functional gastrointestinal (GI) disorder, characterized by the presence of chronic or recurrent diarrhea, constipation, and/or abdominal pain and bloating (Alderman, 1999). IBS is estimated to occur in 10% to 22% of the population of the United States. It is believed to be due to impairment in the motor or sensory function of the GI tract. Motility changes result in changes in the normal bowel elimination pattern to a pattern of diarrhea, constipation, or alternating diarrhea and constipation. Symptoms of IBS typically begin to appear in young adulthood. The exact cause is unknown, since no structural or infectious etiology has been identified. Physical factors, such as diverticular disease, ingestion of coffee or other gastric stimulants, or lactose intolerance may contribute to IBS. IBS follows a pattern of intermittent remissions and exacerbations.

The diagnosis of IBS is made by careful history taking, documenting the presence of characteristic symptoms; laboratory tests; and any other diagnostic tests to exclude a more serious condition. There are no specific biomarkers for IBS, but characteristic symptoms known collectively as the Manning criteria are typically present in clients with IBS. The Manning criteria include abdominal pain relieved by defecation or associated with changes in stool frequency or consistency, abdominal distention, the sensation of incomplete evacuation of stool, and the presence of mucus with stool passage. Bowel function changes progressively and eventually forms the characteristic pattern.

Recent studies have demonstrated that clients with IBS experience alteration in rectal visceral sensation. Balloon distention in the rectum or sigmoid colon resulted in abdominal

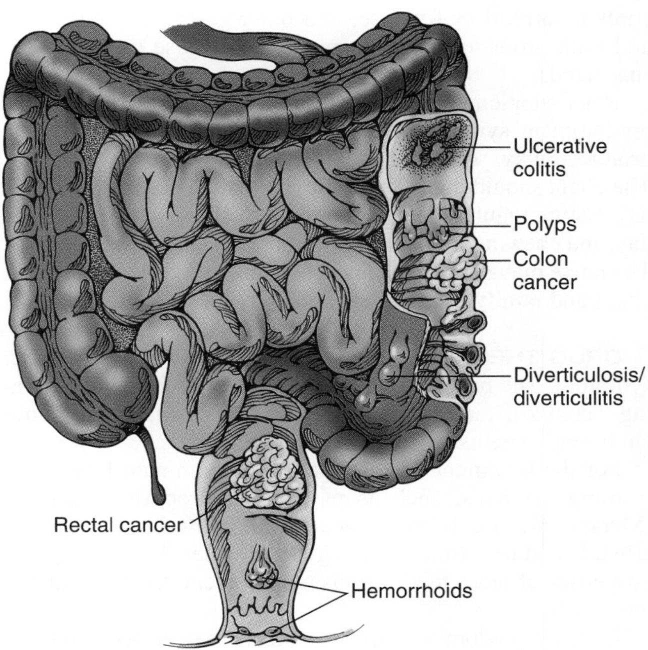

Figure 57-1 ● Common causes of lower gastrointestinal bleeding.

pain at levels higher in clients with IBS than in those without IBS (Schmulson et al., 2000).

The course of the illness is generally specific to the client, and most clients can identify factors that precipitate exacerbations, such as diet, stress, or anxiety. There are no changes in the bowel mucosa and therefore no serious health consequences. However, the irregular bowel patterns and associated cramps often wreak havoc on the person's lifestyle. Psychosocial factors have been thought to play a significant role in IBS. However, the evidence is often contradictory (Carlson, 1998). Food intolerance may be associated with IBS. Dairy products and grains can contribute to bloating, flatulence, and distention. In one study, individuals who reported intolerances to multiple foods were more likely to report IBS (Locke et al., 2000). Finally, IBS symptoms have also been associated with analgesic use (see the Evidence-Based Practice for Nursing box at right).

WOMEN'S HEALTH CONSIDERATIONS

The prevalence of IBS in women is 2:1 as compared with men. Furthermore, several studies indicate that there may be a link between a history of physical, sexual, or emotional abuse and the subsequent development of IBS in women (Toner & Akman, 2000).

EVIDENCE-BASED PRACTICE FOR NURSING

What are the possible risk factors for irritable bowel syndrome?

Locke, G.R., et al. (2000). Risk factors for irritable bowel syndrome: Role of analgesics and food sensitivities. *American Journal of Gastroenterology, 95*(1), 157-164.

The purpose of this study was to identify additional risk factors for the development of irritable bowel syndrome (IBS), since previous evaluations of traditional risk factors have not led to insight into the pathogenesis of this disorder. Questionnaires were mailed to an age (30 to 64 years) and gender–stratified sample of 892 individuals residing in Olmsted County, Minnesota. Six hundred forty-three individuals returned the surveys. A self-report questionnaire listing gastrointestinal symptoms required for a diagnosis of IBS, measures of potential risk factors, and a psychosomatic symptom checklist were used. Logistic regression was used in the analysis. Age, gender, and psychosomatic symptoms were controlled for.

Results showed that 12% of respondents reported IBS symptoms. IBS was significantly associated with the use of analgesics, particularly aspirin. IBS was also correlated with reports of food allergies and ratings of somatic symptoms. The odds of having IBS were higher among subjects taking analgesics and among those reporting multiple food sensitivities.

Critique. Although this study provides early insight into possible risk factors not before associated with IBS, the results must be interpreted with caution. Although the sample size is adequate, the self-selection and cross-sectional design, and limited geographic area lend bias and an inability to generalize the results to the study. Moreover, the self-report methodology and the fact that the subjects were not necessarily medically evaluated for their symptoms limits the interpretation of the findings.

Implications for Nursing. Although the study results cannot be generalized to the population, nurses collecting history information can include questions concerning analgesic use and food allergies in individuals suspected of having IBS. Individuals who identify themselves as having food sensitivities may also have symptoms of IBS that require investigation. Although analgesics in themselves may not be causative, it is possible that clients with IBS present with other forms of pain induced by the disorder. Careful questioning during the intake history can provide more information into the pathogenesis of IBS.

COLLABORATIVE MANAGEMENT

Assessment

The client is asked about a history of abdominal pain, changes in the bowel pattern or consistency of stools, and the passage of mucus. The nurse collects information on all medications the client is taking, since many medications cause GI symptoms similar to those of IBS. A careful dietary history, including the use of caffeinated beverages or beverages sweetened with sorbitol or fructose, which can cause bloating or diarrhea, should be elicited.

A flare-up consisting of worsening cramps, abdominal pain, and diarrhea or constipation usually brings the client to the health care provider. The most common symptom of IBS is pain in the left lower quadrant of the abdomen. The client reports increased pain after eating and relief after a bowel movement. Nausea may be associated with mealtime and defecation. The crampy abdominal patterns are accompanied by constipation or diarrhea. The constipated stools are small and hard and are generally followed by several softer stools. The diarrheal stools are soft and watery, and mucus is often present in the stools. Clients with IBS often complain of belching, gas, anorexia, and bloating.

The client generally appears well, with a stable weight, and nutritional and fluid levels are within normal ranges. The nurse inspects and auscultates the abdomen. Bowel sounds are generally within normal range and may be somewhat quiet with constipation. On percussion of the abdomen, tympanic sounds may be heard over loops of filled bowel. On palpation, there may be diffuse (widespread) tenderness, which is generally worse if the sigmoid colon is palpable. The rectal examination may reveal hard or soft stool.

Routine laboratory work (including a complete blood count [CBC], serologic tests, serum albumin, erythrocyte sedimentation rate, and stools for occult blood) is normal in IBS. The health care provider typically orders a barium enema examination for clients suspected of having IBS. Colonic spasm is often noted during the procedure; however, this finding is not diagnostic. In the absence of other diagnostic findings, colonic spasm supports the diagnosis (Figure 57-2).

The evaluation of IBS is not complete without flexible sigmoidoscopy in adults younger than 40 years of age or colonoscopy in adults older than 40 years of age. A colonoscopy often demonstrates intense spastic contractions, which often stimulate painful sensations. Otherwise, the bowel mucosa appears continuous, smooth, and pink.

Interventions

The client with IBS is most often cared for on an ambulatory basis. Interventions are directed at education, dietary modification, drug therapy, and stress management.

CLIENT EDUCATION. The nurse educates the client regarding the chronic nature of the disorder. Education is also directed at identifying food intolerances and needed dietary modifications. Information regarding what constitutes normal bowel function and laxative abuse is provided. The client must be alert to the urge to defecate and evacuate promptly to avoid straining and should plan to allow time and privacy in the bathroom.

DIET THERAPY. The initial treatment of IBS focuses on dietary modifications. The nurse assists the client in identifying and eliminating offending or upsetting foods. He or she is advised to limit caffeine and to avoid alcohol, beverages that contain sorbitol or fructose, and other gastric irritants. Milk and milk products are to be avoided if lactose intolerance is suspected.

Fiber supplements are usually recommended whatever the predominant symptom may be. Dietary fiber and bulk help produce bulky, soft stools and establish regular bowel habits. The client should ingest approximately 30 to 40 g of fiber each day. Eating regular meals, drinking 8 to 10 cups of liquid each day, and chewing food slowly promote normal bowel function. The nurse may need to collaborate with the dietitian to help the client and family or significant others with meal planning.

DRUG THERAPY. Drug therapy is directed at the major symptom. The health care provider may prescribe bulk-forming laxatives, antidiarrheal agents, $5HT_3$ antagonists, anticholinergic agents, or tricyclic antidepressants.

For the treatment of constipation-predominant IBS, bulk-forming laxatives, such as psyllium hydrophilic mucilloid (Metamucil) or calcium polycarbophil (Mitrolan), are generally taken at mealtimes with a glass of water. The hydrophilic properties of these medications help prevent dry, hard, or liquid stools.

Diarrhea-predominant IBS is typically treated with antidiarrheal agents, such as diphenoxylate hydrochloride with atropine sulfate (Lomotil) or loperamide (Imodium) (Chart 57-1).

For IBS where pain is the predominant symptom, anticholinergics or antispasmodics, such as dicyclomine hydrochloride (Bentyl) and propantheline bromide (Pro-Banthine), help relieve abdominal cramping and intestinal spasm. Tricyclic antidepressants have also been successfully used in this form of IBS. It is unclear whether their effectiveness is due to the antidepressant or anticholinergic effects of the drugs. If clients experience postprandial discomfort (discomfort after eating), they should take these medications 30 to 45 minutes before mealtime.

STRESS MANAGEMENT. Stress management is based on the client's current and ongoing stressors and available resources. After the nurse completes a detailed psychosocial assessment, the nurse and the client set expected outcomes and plan appropriate interventions. Relaxation techniques can help the client learn skills for managing the illness. Understanding the illness empowers the client to take certain actions (e.g., diet modification and exercise) that can significantly affect the course of the illness.

If the client is in a stressful work or family situation, personal counseling may be helpful. The nurse may need to make appropriate referrals or assist in making appointments. The opportunity to discuss problems and attempt creative problem solving is often helpful. The nurse teaches the client that regular exercise is important for managing stress and promoting regular bowel elimination.

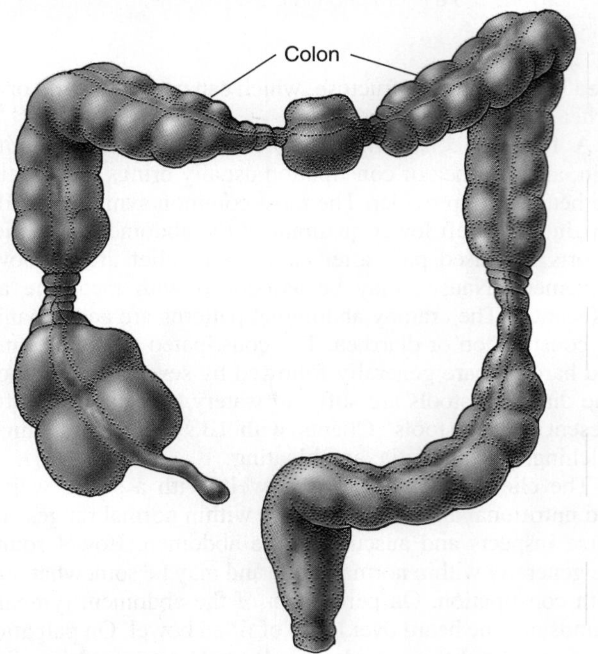

Figure 57-2 ● Spastic contractions of the colon as they occur with irritable bowel syndrome.

HERNIATION

OVERVIEW

A **hernia** is a weakness in the abdominal muscle wall through which a segment of the bowel or other abdominal structure protrudes. Hernias can also penetrate through any other defect in the abdominal wall, through the diaphragm, or through other structures in the abdominal cavity.

Defects in the muscle wall result from weakened collagen or widened spaces at the inguinal ligament. These muscle weaknesses can be inherited or acquired as part of the aging process. Increases in intra-abdominal pressure as a result of pregnancy, obesity, abdominal distention, ascites, heavy lifting, or coughing can contribute to their occurrence.

The most common types of abdominal hernias (Figure 57-3) are indirect, direct, femoral, umbilical, and incisional. An *indirect* inguinal hernia is a sac formed from the peritoneum that contains a portion of the intestine or omentum. The hernia pushes downward at an angle into the inguinal canal. In males, indirect inguinal hernias can become large and often descend into the scrotum. *Direct* inguinal hernias, in contrast, pass through a weak point in the abdominal wall.

Femoral hernias protrude through the femoral ring. A plug of fat in the femoral canal enlarges and eventually pulls the peritoneum and often the urinary bladder into the sac. *Umbilical* hernias are congenital or acquired. Congenital umbilical hernias appear in infancy. Acquired umbilical hernias directly result from increased intra-abdominal pressure. They are most commonly seen in obese individuals.

Incisional, or ventral, hernias occur at the site of a previous surgical incision. These hernias result from inadequate healing of the incision, which is most often caused by postoperative wound infections, inadequate nutrition, and obesity.

Hernias may also be classified as **reducible,** irreducible (incarcerated), or strangulated. A hernia is reducible when the contents of the hernial sac can be placed back into the abdominal cavity by gentle pressure. An **irreducible** (incarcerated) hernia cannot be reduced or placed back into the abdominal cavity. Any hernia that is not reducible requires immediate surgical evaluation.

A hernia is **strangulated** when the blood supply to the herniated segment of the bowel is cut off by pressure from the hernial ring (the band of muscle around the hernia). If a hernia is strangulated, there is ischemia and obstruction of the bowel loop. This can lead to necrosis of the bowel and possibly bowel perforation. Signs of strangulation are abdominal distention, nausea, vomiting, pain, fever, and tachycardia.

The most important elements in the development of a hernia are congenital or acquired muscle weakness and increased intra-abdominal pressure. The most significant factors contributing to increased intra-abdominal pressure are obesity, pregnancy, and lifting of heavy objects.

Indirect inguinal hernias, the most common type, are most frequent in men because they follow the tract that develops when the testes descend into the scrotum before birth. Direct

CHART 57-1

DRUG THERAPY *for* the Treatment of Diarrhea-Predominant Irritable Bowel Syndrome

Drug	Usual Dosage	Nursing Interventions	Rationale
Diphenoxylate hydrochloride and atropine sulfate (Lomotil)	1 tablet 6 times/day; no more than 6 tablets in 24 hr	Assess for abdominal distention, pain, and fever.	These symptoms may indicate a bacterial organism in the gastrointestinal (GI) tract. Diarrhea should not be suppressed in the presence of GI infection.
		Assess for sedation, dry mouth, urinary retention, and rash.	These are common side effects.
Loperamide (Imodium)	2 mg after each loose stool; maximum of 16 mg/day	Assess for abdominal distention, pain, and fever.	These symptoms may indicate a bacterial organism in the GI tract. Diarrhea should not be suppressed if GI infection is present.

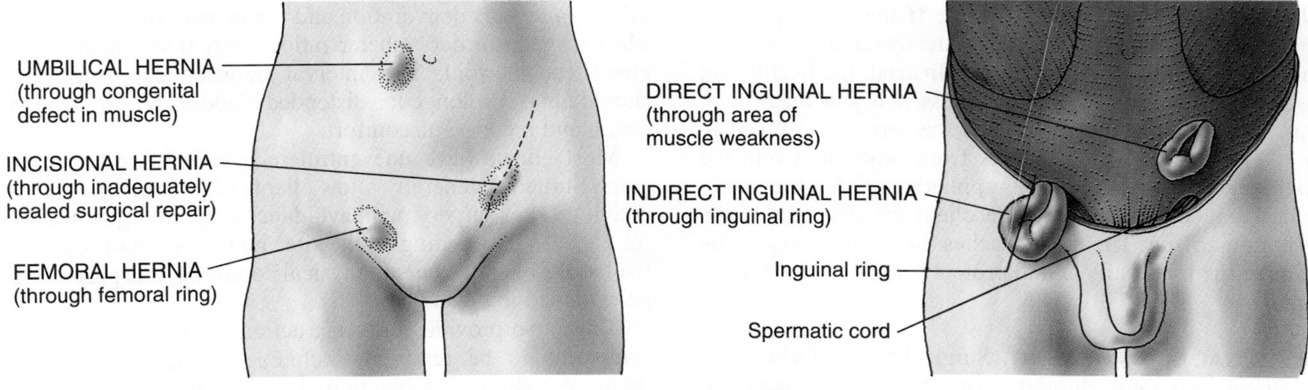

Figure 57-3 ● The types of abdominal hernia.

hernias occur more often in older adults. Femoral and adult umbilical hernias are most common in obese or pregnant women. Incisional hernias can occur in people who have undergone abdominal surgery.

CONSIDERATIONS FOR OLDER ADULTS

The older adult with a strangulated hernia may not complain of pain but instead may present with nausea and vomiting. The nurse must carefully evaluate the client complaining of any of these symptoms, since they may require immediate medical and eventually surgical intervention.

COLLABORATIVE MANAGEMENT

Assessment

The client with a hernia typically comes to the health care provider's office or the emergency department with a complaint of a "lump" or protrusion felt at the involved site. The development of the hernia may be associated with straining or lifting.

To perform an abdominal assessment, the nurse inspects the abdomen when the client is lying and again when he or she is standing. If the hernia is reducible, it may disappear when the client is lying flat. The examiner asks the client to strain or perform the Valsalva maneuver and observes for bulging. The abdomen is auscultated for active bowel sounds. Absent bowel sounds may indicate obstruction and strangulation.

To palpate the hernia, the health care provider gently examines the ring and its contents by inserting a finger in the ring and noting any changes when the client coughs. The nurse never forces the hernia to reduce; that maneuver could cause strangulated intestine to rupture.

If a male client suspects a hernia in his groin, the health care provider has him stand for the examination. Using the right hand for the client's right side and the left hand for the client's left side, the health care provider invaginates the loose scrotal skin with the index finger, following the spermatic cord upward to the external inguinal cord. At this point, the client is asked to cough, and the health care provider notes any palpable herniation.

Interventions

The type of treatment selected will depend on client factors, as well as the type of hernia.

NONSURGICAL MANAGEMENT. If the client is not a surgical candidate and the hernia is incarcerated, no attempt should be made to reduce the hernia. Instead, the health care provider may prescribe a truss. A truss is a pad made with firm material; it is held in place over the hernia with a belt to help keep the abdominal contents from protruding into the hernial sac. If a truss is used, it is applied only after the physician has reduced the hernia. The client usually applies the truss before arising. The nurse teaches the client to assess the skin under the truss daily and to protect it with a light layer of powder.

SURGICAL MANAGEMENT. Surgical repair of a hernia is the treatment of choice. Surgery is often performed on an ambulatory care basis for adult clients who have no pre-existing health conditions that would complicate the operative course. In same-day surgery centers, anesthesia may be local, regional, or general, and the surgery may be laparoscopic. More extensive surgery, such as a bowel resection or temporary colostomy, may be necessary if strangulation results in a gangrenous section of bowel. Clients undergoing extensive surgery are hospitalized for a longer period of time.

Herniorrhaphy is the surgery of choice for hernia repair. Hernioplasty is performed less often but can be performed in conjunction with a herniorrhaphy.

PREOPERATIVE CARE. The nurse prepares the client for surgery (see Chapter 17). He or she may be instructed to have one or two enemas the night before or the morning of surgery, depending on the surgeon's preference. If outpatient surgery is planned, the nurse assists the client in making appropriate arrangements for travel to home and for home care.

OPERATIVE PROCEDURES. During a **herniorrhaphy,** the surgeon makes an abdominal incision and places the contents of the hernial sac back into the abdominal cavity before closing the opening. When a **hernioplasty** is performed, the surgeon reinforces the weakened muscle wall with mesh, fascia, or wire. The surgeon may opt to perform the surgery through a laparoscope instead of using the open surgical method.

POSTOPERATIVE CARE. Postoperative care of the client is the same as that described in Chapter 19, except that clients who have undergone surgery for hernias are told to avoid coughing. To promote lung expansion, the nurse encourages deep breathing and frequent turning. With repair of an indirect inguinal hernia, the physician often orders a scrotal support and ice bags to be applied to the scrotum to prevent swelling, which often contributes to pain. Elevation of the scrotum with a soft pillow helps prevent and control swelling. The nurse encourages early ambulation on the day of surgery if it is not contraindicated by scrotal swelling or pre-existing conditions. Ambulation helps promote comfort and a feeling of well-being and decreases the risk of postoperative complications.

In the immediate postoperative period, the client may experience difficulty voiding. The nurse allows the male client to stand to allow a more natural position for gravity to facilitate voiding and bladder emptying. Techniques to stimulate voiding, such as allowing water to run, may also be used. Careful monitoring of intake and output alerts the nurse to voiding problems early. The nurse carefully palpates the abdomen for distention. A fluid intake of at least 1500 to 2500 mL/day prevents dehydration and maintains urinary function. Most surgeons order catheterization every 6 to 8 hours if the client cannot void. The interval between catheterizations should not be prolonged; a distended bladder can stress the incision and increase discomfort.

Most clients have uneventful recoveries after hernia repairs. Surgeons generally allow clients to return to their usual activities after surgery, with avoidance of straining and lifting for 2 weeks. Depending on the site and the extent of repair, as well as the client's general physical condition, this period may be extended to 6 weeks.

The nurse provides oral instructions and a written list of symptoms to be reported, including fever, chills, wound drainage, redness or separation of the incision, and increasing incisional pain.

The client is also instructed to keep the wound dry and clean and to replace the sterile dressing daily if indicated. Showering is permitted if allowed by the surgeon.

COLORECTAL CANCER

OVERVIEW

Cancer of the colon and rectum is the third most common cancer in the United States and occurs equally in men and women. Cancer of the colon ranks third in estimates for cancer deaths in the United States (Greenlee et al., 2000). Colorectal cancer can occur at any age but is most prevalent in individuals over the age of 50. Although the death rate from large-bowel cancer may be decreasing slightly, this disease is lethal in a significant number of cases because it is often not detected until an advanced stage, when metastasis has occurred.

Pathophysiology

Ninety-five percent of colorectal cancers are adenocarcinomas. Adenocarcinomas are tumors that arise from the glandular epithelial tissue of the colon. Colorectal cancer develops as a multistep process, resulting in a number of molecular changes, such as loss of key tumor suppressor genes and activation of certain oncogenes that alter colonic mucosa cell division. The increased proliferation of the colonic mucosa forms polyps that can be transformed into malignant tumors. The majority of colorectal cancers are believed to arise from adenomatous polyps that present as a visible protrusion from the mucosal surface of the bowel.

Tumors occur in different areas of the colon, with 70% occurring on the right side of the proximal colon. The percentages in Figure 57-4 indicate an increased incidence of cancer in the proximal sections of the large intestine in the last 20 years.

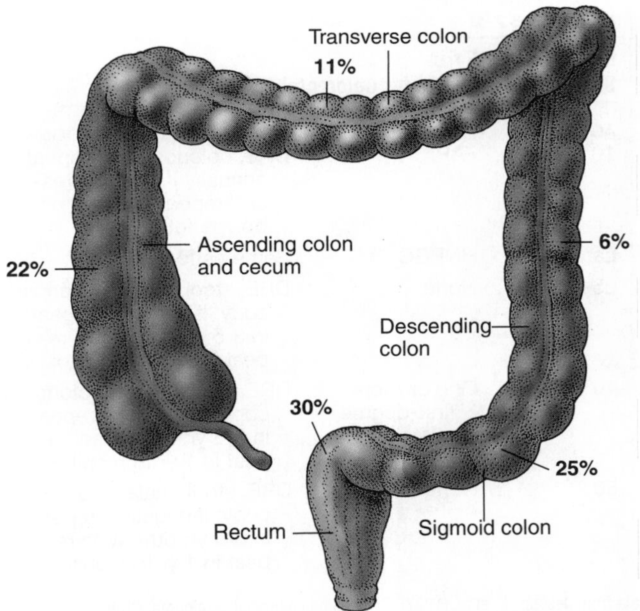

Figure 57-4 ● The incidence of cancer in relation to colorectal anatomy.

Colorectal cancer can metastasize by means of direct extension or by spreading through the blood or lymph. The tumor may spread locally into the four layers of the bowel wall and into neighboring organs. The tumor may enlarge into the lumen of the bowel or spread through the lymphatics or the circulatory system. The circulatory system is entered directly from the primary tumor through blood vessels in the bowel or via the lymphatics. The liver is the most frequent site of metastasis from circulatory spread. Of clients with colorectal cancer, 15% to 30% will develop metastasis to the liver in spite of surgical resection of the tumor. Metastasis to the lungs, brain, bones, and adrenal glands may also be found. Colon tumors can also spread by peritoneal seeding during surgical resection of the tumor. Seeding occurs when a tumor is excised and cancer cells break off from the tumor into the peritoneal cavity.

Complications related to the increasing growth of the tumor locally or through metastatic spread include bowel obstruction or perforation with resultant peritonitis, abscess formation, and fistula formation to the urinary bladder or the vagina. The tumor may invade neighboring blood vessels and cause frank bleeding. A tumor growing into the bowel lumen can gradually obstruct the intestine and eventually block it completely. Tumor extending beyond the bowel wall may place pressure on neighboring organs (uterus, urinary bladder, and ureters) and cause symptoms that mask those of the cancer. Twenty percent of clients diagnosed with colorectal cancer are diagnosed at the time of an emergency hospitalization for bowel obstruction or other life-threatening complication (Hardcastle, 1997).

Etiology

Risk factors for the development of colorectal cancer include genetic predisposition, personal and dietary factors, and inflammatory bowel disease.

GENETIC PREDISPOSITION

Individuals with a first-degree relative diagnosed with colorectal cancer have a threefold to fourfold risk of developing the disease. An autosomal dominant inherited genetic disorder known as familial adenomatous polyposis (FAP) accounts for 1% of colorectal cancers. In these individuals, thousands of adenomatous polyps develop over the course of 10 to 15 years and have a 100% chance of becoming malignant. By the age of 20, most individuals require surgical intervention to prevent cancer. Hereditary nonpolyposis colorectal cancer (HNPCC) is another autosomal dominant disorder and accounts for 10% of all colorectal cancers. This disorder is characterized by the development of colorectal cancer at an average age of 45 years (Cavalieri & Franklin, 1998; Saddler & Ellis, 1999). Clients with this type of genetic disorder may also have a higher incidence of endometrial, ovarian, and ureteral cancers.

PERSONAL FACTORS

Approximately 75% of all colorectal cancers have no known predisposing cause. Age is considered a risk factor in the development of colorectal cancer, since 95% of cases are diagnosed in persons over 50 years of age. Individuals who have been diagnosed and treated for colorectal cancers have an increased risk of developing a second primary colorectal cancer, often at the site of the surgical anastomosis. Individuals with adenomatous polyps are at an increased risk of developing colorectal cancer. Such individuals need regular follow-up with colonoscopy to visualize and remove polyps.

DIETARY FACTORS

It is theorized that decreased bowel transit time and certain foods containing chemical mutagens may place individuals at risk for colorectal cancer (Table 57-1). These foods also aid in decreasing bowel transit time, which would increase the time that the bowel is exposed to carcinogens (cancer-causing substances). A high-fat diet, particularly animal fat from red meats, increases bile acid secretion and anaerobic bacteria, which are thought to be carcinogenic within the bowel. Fried and broiled meats and fish are also thought to contain chemical mutagens that are carcinogenic. Diets with large amounts of refined carbohydrates that lack fiber decrease bowel transit time.

INFLAMMATORY BOWEL DISEASE

Inflammatory bowel diseases, such as ulcerative colitis and Crohn's disease, pose an increased risk of colorectal cancer, especially if the disease has had a long, severe course.

Incidence/Prevalence

Americans have a 6% lifetime risk of developing colorectal cancer. Approximately 130,000 people in the United States were diagnosed with colorectal cancer in 1999, with an estimated 55,000 deaths (Landis et al., 1999). Most clients with colorectal cancer are older than 50 years of age; only 2% to 6% are younger than 40 years of age. The peak incidence of colorectal cancer occurs in the sixth decade of life. The overall incidence of colorectal cancer is equivalent in men and women, with cancer of the rectum being more common in men. Anal cancers account for approximately 4% of colorectal cancers.

CULTURAL CONSIDERATIONS

Both male and female African Americans have an increased frequency of colorectal cancer in advanced stages at the time of diagnosis, and consequently an increase in death rates from colorectal cancer, as opposed to male and female Caucasian Americans (Saddler & Ellis, 1999). The incidence of colorectal cancer is higher in industrialized regions of the world, with the highest rates found in North America and Australia.

TABLE 57-1 • FOODS THAT AFFECT A PERSON'S RISK FOR COLORECTAL CANCER

FOODS TO AVOID
- Red meat
- Animal fat
- Fatty foods
- Fried or broiled meats and fish
- Refined carbohydrates (e.g., concentrated sweets)

FOODS TO CONSUME
- Fruits and vegetables, especially cruciferous vegetables from the cabbage family (e.g., broccoli, cabbage, cauliflower, brussels sprouts)
- Whole-grain products
- Adequate fluids, especially water

COLLABORATIVE MANAGEMENT

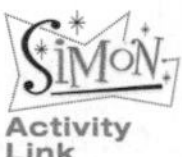

Assessment

HISTORY

In taking a history from a client with colorectal cancer, the nurse obtains the client's diet history and asks about major risk factors, such as a personal history of breast, ovarian, or endometrial cancer; ulcerative colitis; Crohn's disease; familial polyposis; or adenomas; or a family history of colorectal cancer. The nurse also assesses the client's participation in age-specific screening guidelines for colorectal cancer (Chart 57-2).

The nurse also asks about changes in bowel habits, such as diarrhea or constipation, with or without blood in the stool. The client may also report fatigue (related to anemias), abdominal fullness, pain, or weight loss, which, unfortunately, are signs of advanced disease.

PHYSICAL ASSESSMENT/CLINICAL MANIFESTATIONS

The signs of colorectal cancer depend on the location of the tumor. However, the most common signs are rectal bleeding, anemia, and a change in the stool. Stools may contain microscopic amounts of blood that are not noticeably visible, or the client may have mahogany-colored or bright red stools. Gross blood is not usually detected with tumors of the right side of the colon but is common (but not massive) with tumors of the left side of the colon and the rectum.

Tumors arising in the transverse and descending colon result in symptoms of obstruction as growth of the tumor impedes the passage of stool. The client may complain of "gas pains," cramping, or incomplete evacuation. Tumors arising in the rectosigmoid colon are associated with hematochezia (the passage of red blood via the rectum), straining to pass stools, and narrowing of stools. Clients may complain of dull

CHART 57-2

BEST PRACTICE *for* Screening Guidelines for Colorectal Cancer

AGE	FAMILY HISTORY	DIAGNOSTIC EXAMINATIONS
10	FAP	DRE, colonoscopy; repeat annually if polyps present; repeat in 3 yr if no polyps found
Late teens	HNPCC	Same as for FAP
25	None	DRE, stool guaiac, colonoscopy; if negative, repeat in 3-5 yr; otherwise, repeat in 1 yr to monitor
40	One or more first-degree relatives	DRE, stool guaiac, colonoscopy; if negative, repeat in 3-5 yr; otherwise, repeat in 1 yr to monitor
50	None	DRE, stool guaiac, colonoscopy; if negative, repeat in 3-5 yr; otherwise repeat in 1 yr to monitor

Data from Jessup, J., et al. (1997). Diagnosing colorectal carcinoma: Clinical and molecular approaches. *CA: A Cancer Journal for Clinicians, 47*(2), 70-92.

DRE, Digital rectal examination; *FAP,* familial adenomatous polyposis; *HNPCC,* hereditary nonpolyposis colorectal cancer.

pain. Right-sided tumors can grow quite large without disrupting bowel patterns or appearance, since the stool consistency is more liquid in this part of the colon. These tumors ulcerate and bleed intermittently, so stools can contain dark or mahogany-colored blood. A mass may be palpated in the lower right quadrant, and the client often has anemia secondary to blood loss.

Examination of the abdomen begins with assessment for obvious distention or masses. Visible peristaltic waves accompanied by high-pitched or tingling bowel sounds may indicate a partial bowel obstruction from the tumor. Total absence of bowel sounds after listening for 5 full minutes indicates a complete bowel obstruction. Palpation and percussion are performed to evaluate the liver and spleen for enlargement and to evaluate for masses along the colon. The health care provider may perform a digital rectal examination to palpate the rectum and lower sigmoid colon for masses.

PSYCHOSOCIAL ASSESSMENT

The psychologic consequences associated with a diagnosis of colorectal cancer are many. Clients must cope with a diagnosis that inspires fear and anxiety about treatment, pain, possible disfigurement, and a shortened life span. In addition, if the cancer is believed to have a genetic origin, there is anxiety concerning implications for the client's immediate family members. Possible loss of health insurance and excessive costs of genetic testing are also sources of fear and anxiety.

LABORATORY ASSESSMENT

COMPLETE BLOOD COUNT AND BLOOD CHEMISTRIES. Hemoglobin and hematocrit values are usually decreased as a result of the intermittent bleeding associated with the tumor. Colorectal cancer that has metastasized to the liver will cause liver function tests to be elevated.

FECAL OCCULT BLOOD TESTS. A positive test result for occult blood in the stool **(fecal occult blood test [FOBT])** confirms bleeding in the gastrointestinal (GI) tract. False-positive reactions can be caused by a number of foods and medications. The client avoids meat, peroxidase-containing foods (horseradish and beets), aspirin, and vitamin C for 48 hours before giving a stool specimen. The nurse assesses whether the client is taking anti-inflammatory drugs (such as ibuprofen, corticosteroids, or salicylates). These medications may be discontinued for a period before the test to reduce the risk of a false-positive result (Held-Warmkessel, 1998). Two separate stool samples should be tested on 3 consecutive days. Negative results do not completely rule out the possibility of colorectal cancer.

ONCOFETAL ANTIGEN TESTING. Carcinoembryonic antigen (CEA) may be elevated in 70% of people with colorectal cancer. There is no relationship between the CEA level and the cancer stage. CEA is not specifically associated with the colorectal cancer, and it may be elevated in the presence of other benign or malignant diseases and in smokers. CEA is often used to monitor the effectiveness of treatment and identify disease recurrence.

RADIOGRAPHIC ASSESSMENT

BARIUM ENEMA. A double-contrast barium enema (air and barium are instilled into the colon) provides better visualization of polyps and small lesions than barium alone. This test may demonstrate an occlusion in the bowel, where the tumor is decreasing the size of the lumen.

COMPUTED TOMOGRAPHY. Computed tomography (CT) of the abdomen, pelvis, lungs, or liver helps confirm the existence of a mass and the extent of disease.

CHEST X-RAY STUDY. A chest x-ray study and liver scan may locate distant sites of metastasis.

> **CRITICAL THINKING CHALLENGE**
>
> You are gathering the initial history for a 44-year-old woman admitted to your unit with intermittent rectal bleeding over the last 3 months. The client states that her maternal uncle died of colorectal cancer at the age of 52.
>
> - What personal factors place this client at risk for colorectal cancer?
> - What specific questions would you ask concerning the rectal bleeding she reports?
> - What abnormalities in laboratory values would you suspect?

For suggested answer guidelines, go to SIMON http://www.wbsaunders.com/SIMON/Iggy/.

OTHER DIAGNOSTIC ASSESSMENT

SIGMOIDOSCOPY. A sigmoidoscopy provides visualization of the lower colon using a fiberoptic scope. Polyps can be visualized, and samples can be taken for biopsy.

COLONOSCOPY. A colonoscopy provides visualization of the entire large bowel from the rectum to the ileocecal valve. As with sigmoidoscopy, polyps can be visualized and removed, and tissue samples can be taken for biopsy. Colonoscopy is the definitive test for the diagnosis of colorectal cancer.

LIVER SCAN. A liver scan may locate distant sites of metastasis.

Analysis

COMMON NURSING DIAGNOSES AND COLLABORATIVE PROBLEMS

The priority nursing diagnosis for clients with colorectal cancer is Anticipatory Grieving related to the diagnosis of a potentially terminal illness, a disturbance in body image, and the possible loss of fecal continence. The priority collaborative problem is Potential for Metastasis.

ADDITIONAL NURSING DIAGNOSES AND COLLABORATIVE PROBLEMS

In addition to the common nursing diagnoses and collaborative problems, clients with colorectal cancer may develop one or more of the following:

- Acute Pain or Chronic Pain related to tumor obstruction of the intestine, with possible pressure on other organs
- Disturbed Body Image related to the creation of a stoma or fear of incontinence

- Compromised Family Coping related to alteration in roles, lifestyle changes, and fear of the client's death
- Imbalanced Nutrition: Less Than Body Requirements related to the diagnostic workup
- Fear related to the disease process
- Powerlessness related to the presence of a life-threatening illness and its treatment

Planning and Implementation

ANTICIPATORY GRIEVING

NOC **PLANNING: EXPECTED OUTCOMES.** A client faced with a diagnosis of colorectal cancer experiences feelings and anxieties that can tax his or her ability to cope with present and future issues related to the disease and treatment. The client with colorectal cancer is expected to identify, develop, and use effective coping methods in dealing with the perceived changes and losses experienced.

INTERVENTIONS. The client and family are faced with a possible loss of or alteration in body functions. Medical and surgical interventions for the treatment of colorectal cancer may result in cure, disease control, or palliation. Interventions are designed to assist the client in formulating effective strategies for expressing feelings of grief and developing coping skills.

The nurse observes and identifies the following:

- The client's and family's current methods of coping
- Effective sources of support used in past crises
- The client's and family's present perceptions of the health problem
- Signs of anticipatory grief, such as crying, anger, and withdrawal from usual relationships

The nurse encourages the client to verbalize feelings about the diagnosis, treatment, and anticipated alteration in body functions if a colostomy is planned (see later discussion of the operative procedure under Surgical Management, p. 1249). Sadness, anger, feelings of loss, and depression are normal responses to this change in body functions.

If a colostomy is planned, the nurse teaches the client what to expect about the appearance and care of the colostomy. Postoperatively, the client is encouraged to look at and touch the stoma. When the client is physically able, the nurse asks him or her to participate in colostomy care. Participation helps to restore the client's sense of control over his or her lifestyle and thus facilitates improved self-esteem.

NIC **GRIEF WORK FACILITATION.** The purpose of grief work is to assist the client with the resolution of a significant loss. The nurse assists in identifying the nature of and reaction to the loss. Encouraging the client to verbalize feelings and identify fears helps to move him or her through the appropriate phases of the grief process. The nurse establishes a trusting, ongoing relationship with the client and provides support through the personal grieving stages.

The nurse, in collaboration with the psychologist when appropriate, assists the client in identifying personal coping strategies. The client is encouraged to implement cultural, religious, and social customs associated with the loss and to identify sources of community support available to the client and family. Modifications in lifestyle can be anticipated in clients with a diagnosis of colorectal cancer. The nurse assists in identifying the necessary modifications in lifestyle that may be necessary. The chaplain, social worker, and/or family assists in discussions and decisions concerning treatment, the prognosis, and end-of-life decisions, as appropriate.

NIC **GENETIC COUNSELING.** Genetic counseling entails the use of an interactive helping process focusing on the prevention of a genetic disorder or on the ability to cope with a family member who has a genetically based disorder. The nurse may be asked to provide a referral to a genetics center by clients who are believed to have familial colorectal cancers. Specially trained nurses can discuss the purposes and goals of genetic testing. Privacy and confidentiality need to be ensured. A review of the family history may provide important information concerning the pattern of colorectal cancer inheritance. To make an informed decision, the client and family need information about the advantages, risks, and costs of appropriate genetic tests. The nurse will need to carefully monitor the client's response on learning of his or her genetic risk factors.

NIC interventions are summarized in Chart 57-3.

POTENTIAL FOR METASTASIS

PLANNING: EXPECTED OUTCOMES. The client with colorectal cancer is expected to not have the cancer spread to vital organs; thus the client's life expectancy will be increased and the quality of life will be improved.

INTERVENTIONS. Although surgical resection is the primary means used to control the disease, several adjuvant

CHART 57-3

NIC INTERVENTION ACTIVITIES *for* The Client with Noninflammatory Intestinal Disorders

Grief Work Facilitation: *Assistance with the resolution of a significant loss*

- Assist the client to identify the nature of the attachment to the lost object or person.
- Assist the patient to identify the initial reaction to the loss.
- Encourage expression of feelings about the loss.
- Instruct in phases of the grieving process, as appropriate.
- Support progression through personal grieving stages.
- Include significant others in discussions and decisions, as appropriate.
- Assist to identify personal coping strategies.
- Encourage client to implement cultural, religious, and social customs associated with the loss.
- Identify sources of community support.
- Assist in identifying modifications needed in lifestyle.

Genetic Counseling: *Use of an interactive helping process focusing on assisting an individual, family, or group, manifesting or at risk for developing or transmitting a birth defect or genetic condition, to cope.*

- Provide privacy and ensure confidentiality.
- Discuss the client's purpose, goals, and agenda for the genetic counseling session.
- Discuss the advantages, risks, and costs of genetic tests.
- Monitor response when patient learns about own genetic risk factors.
- Provide referral to genetic health care specialists, as necessary.

NIC intervention activities selected from McCloskey, J.C., & Bulechek, G.M. (2000). *Nursing interventions classification (NIC)* (3rd ed.). St. Louis: Mosby.

therapies are employed as well. Adjuvant therapies are administered before or after surgery to affect a cure and to prevent recurrence.

NONSURGICAL MANAGEMENT. The type of therapy used is based on the pathologic staging of the disease. Dukes' staging classification is most often used. This method classifies colorectal tumors by designating them as either A, B, C, or D according to the depth of invasion into the mucosa and distant spread.

Dukes' stage A indicates that the tumor has penetrated into, but not through, the bowel wall. Stage B indicates that the tumor has penetrated through the bowel wall. Stage C indicates that the tumor has penetrated through the bowel wall and that there is lymph node involvement. Stage D indicates that the tumor has metastasized to any of a number of distant sites.

RADIATION THERAPY. The administration of preoperative radiation therapy has not improved overall survival from colorectal cancer but has been effective in providing local or regional control of the disease. Postoperative radiation has not demonstrated any consistent improvement in survival or recurrence. As a palliative measure, radiation therapy may be used to control pain, hemorrhage, bowel obstruction, or metastasis to the lung in advanced disease. Unlike the case with colorectal cancer, radiation therapy is almost always a part of the treatment plan for rectal cancer. The nurse explains the radiation therapy procedure to the client and family and monitors for possible side effects (e.g., diarrhea and fatigue). (See Chapter 25 for care of clients undergoing radiation therapy.)

CHEMOTHERAPY. Adjuvant chemotherapy after primary surgery is recommended for clients with stage II (Dukes' stage B_2) or stage III (Dukes' stage C) disease to improve survival. The drug of choice is intravenous (IV) 5-fluorouracil (5-FU) with or without levamisole or leucovorin. The side effects of 5-FU and levamisole or leucovorin are diarrhea, mucositis, and skin effects. Oxaliplatin is a relatively new platinum analog chemotherapeutic agent. It has been used with 5-FU and levamisole or leucovorin with good results in clients with metastatic disease. The dose-limiting toxicity for this agent is peripheral sensory neuropathy.

In 1997 irinotecan (Camptosar) was approved as second-line treatment for metastatic disease if disease has recurred or progressed after treatment with 5-FU. With this drug, myelosuppression (bone marrow suppression) and diarrhea are the most frequent dose-limiting toxicities. Current clinical trials using a 17-1A monoclonal antibody and a colorectal tumor vaccine are in progress. In addition, new oral agents consisting of a fluorinated pyrimidine and leucovorin are being tested. Intrahepatic arterial chemotherapy, often with 5-FU, may be administered to clients with liver metastasis.

SURGICAL MANAGEMENT. Surgical removal of the tumor with margins free of disease is the best method of ensuring removal of colorectal cancer. The size of the tumor, its location, the extent of metastasis, the integrity of the bowel, and the condition of the client determine which surgical procedure is performed for colorectal cancer (Table 57-2). Because the majority of colorectal cancers are diagnosed when the cancer has extended beyond the tumor, the three most common surgeries performed are *hemicolectomy* (resection of the tumor and regional lymph nodes) with reanastomosis, *colon resection* with *colostomy (temporary or permanent),* and *abdominoperineal resection* (Saddler & Ellis, 1999).

Small tumors indicate an early stage of cancer and are well differentiated without evidence of vascular or lymphatic invasion. They can be removed with clean margins and may be treated with local excision and close follow-up. A transanal approach without an abdominal incision is the technique most commonly used; this approach decreases the risk for postoperative complications and shortens the hospital stay. Only 5% of clients with colorectal cancer, however, meet the criteria of early-stage cancer. Currently, clinical trials are being conducted to evaluate the use of laparoscopic techniques in the treatment of colorectal cancer.

HEMICOLECTOMY AND COLON RESECTION. A **hemicolectomy** involves excision of the involved area of the colon, leaving an area of clean margins. If the integrity of the intestine is optimal (e.g., without inflammation, as with bowel obstruction or perforation), and if the rectal sphincter can be left intact, reanastomosis can usually be accomplished and an ostomy can be avoided. If healing of a reanastomosed bowel is thought to be in jeopardy, a temporary or permanent colostomy will be performed. A **colostomy** is the surgical creation of an opening of the colon onto the surface of the abdomen.

Preoperative Care. The nurse helps the client to prepare for colon resection by reinforcing the physician's explanation of the planned surgical procedure. The client is told as accurately as possible what anatomic and physiologic changes will occur with surgery. The location and number of incision sites and drains are also discussed.

Before evaluating the tumor and colon during surgery, the physician may not be able to determine whether a colostomy will be necessary. If this is the case, the physician informs the client that a colostomy is a possibility. If the surgeon informs

TABLE 57-2 • SURGICAL PROCEDURES FOR COLORECTAL CANCERS IN VARIOUS LOCATIONS

RIGHT-SIDED COLON TUMORS
- Right hemicolectomy for smaller lesions
- Right ascending colostomy or ileostomy for large, widespread lesions
- Cecostomy (opening into the cecum with intubation to decompress the bowel)

LEFT-SIDED COLON TUMORS
- Left hemicolectomy for smaller lesions
- Left descending colostomy for larger lesions (e.g., the Hartmann procedure)

SIGMOID COLON TUMORS
- Sigmoid colectomy for smaller lesions
- Sigmoid colostomy for larger lesions (e.g., the Hartmann procedure)
- Abdominoperineal resection for large, low sigmoid tumors (near the anus) with colostomy (the rectum and the anus are completely removed, leaving a perineal wound)

RECTAL TUMORS
- Resection with anastomosis or pull-through procedure (preserves anal sphincter and normal elimination pattern)
- Colon resection with permanent colostomy
- Abdominoperineal resection with colostomy

the client that a colostomy is inevitable, the nurse consults an enterostomal therapist (ET) to advise on optimal placement of the ostomy and instructs the client about the rationale and general principles of ostomy care. An ET is a registered nurse who has completed specialized training and is certified in ostomy nursing care. Some are also certified in wound and incontinence care.

The client who requires low rectal surgery is faced with the risk of postoperative sexual dysfunction and urinary incontinence as a result of nerve damage during surgery. The physician discusses the risk for these problems with the client before surgery and allows him or her to verbalize concerns and questions related to this risk. The nurse reinforces teaching about abdominal surgery performed with the client under general anesthesia and reviews the routines for turning and deep breathing (see Chapter 17).

If the bowel is not obstructed or perforated, elective surgery is planned. The client receives a thorough cleaning of the bowel, or "bowel prep," to minimize bacterial growth and prevent complications. In preparation for the bowel prep, the client is usually instructed to restrict the diet to clear liquids for 1 to 2 days before surgery. Mechanical cleaning is accomplished with laxatives and enemas or with "whole-gut lavage." For whole-gut lavage, the client usually ingests large quantities of a sodium sulfate and polyethylene glycol solution (e.g., GoLYTELY). This solution overwhelms the absorptive capacity of the small bowel and clears feces from the colon.

To reduce the risk of infection, the surgeon may prescribe oral or IV antibiotics to be given the day before surgery (Held-Warmkessel, 1998). Before surgery, a nasogastric (NG) tube is placed for decompression of the stomach following surgery. A peripheral IV line is also placed for fluid and electrolyte replacement while the client is taking nothing by mouth (NPO).

The client with colorectal cancer faces a serious illness with long-term consequences of the disease and treatment. A case manager can be very helpful in identifying client and family needs, as well as continuity of care and support.

Operative Procedure. The surgeon makes an incision in the abdomen and explores the abdominal cavity to determine if the tumor can be removed. The portion of the colon with the tumor is excised, and the two open ends of the bowel are irrigated before **anastomosis** (reattachment) of the colon. If an anastomosis is not feasible because of the location of the tumor or the bowel is inflamed, a colostomy is created.

A colostomy may be created in the ascending, transverse, descending, or sigmoid colon (Figure 57-5). One of three basic techniques is used to construct a colostomy. A loop **stoma** (surgical opening) is made by bringing a loop of colon to the skin surface, severing and everting the anterior wall, and suturing it to the abdominal wall. Loop colostomies are usually performed in the transverse colon and are usually temporary (Bradley & Pupiales, 1997). An external rod is used to support the loop until the intestinal tissue adheres to the abdominal wall. Care must be taken to avoid displacing the rod, especially during appliance changes.

An end stoma is often constructed, most often in the descending or sigmoid colon, when a colostomy is intended to

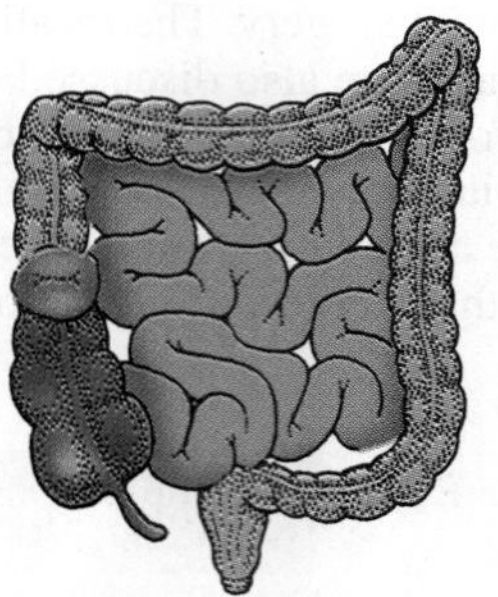

The **ascending colostomy** is done for right-sided tumors.

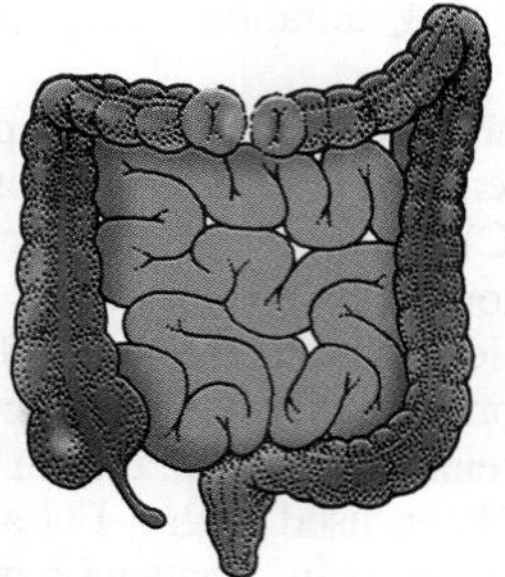

The **transverse (double-barreled) colostomy** is often used in such emergencies as intestinal obstruction or perforation because it can be created quickly. There are two stomas. The proximal one, closest to the small intestine, drains feces. The distal stoma drains mucus.

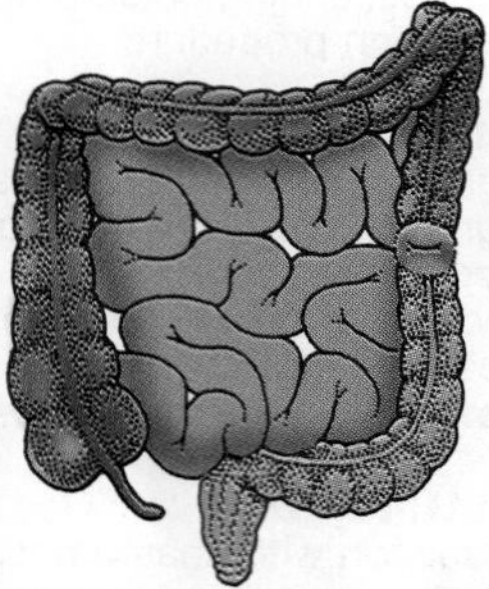

Descending colostomy

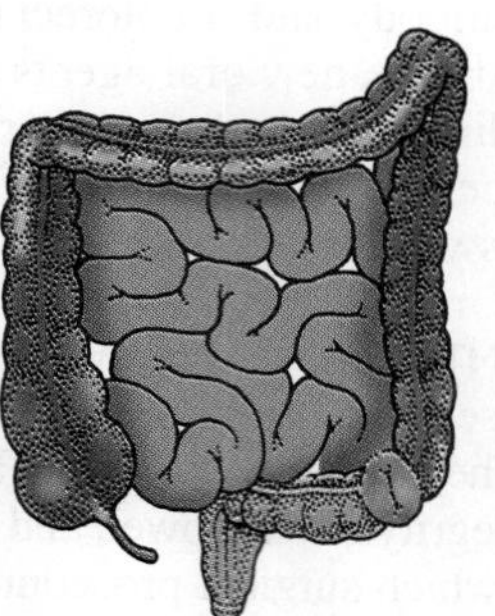

Sigmoid colostomy

Figure 57-5 ● Different locations of colostomies in the colon.

be permanent. It may also be done in conjunction with a Hartmann procedure, when the surgeon oversews the distal stump of the colon and places it in the abdominal cavity, preserving it for future reattachment. An end stoma is constructed by severing the end of the proximal portion of the bowel and bringing it out through the abdominal wall.

The least common colostomy is the double-barrel stoma, which is created by dividing the bowel and bringing both the proximal and distal portions to the abdominal surface to create two stomas. The proximal stoma (closest to the client's head) is the functioning stoma and eliminates stool; the distal stoma (farthest from the head) is considered nonfunctioning, although it may secrete some mucus. The distal stoma is sometimes referred to as a mucous fistula.

Postoperative Care. Clients who have undergone a colon resection without a colostomy receive care similar to that of clients undergoing any abdominal surgery (see Chapter 19).

Colostomy Management. The client who has a colostomy created may return from surgery with an ostomy pouch system in place. If there is no pouch system in place, a petrolatum gauze dressing is usually placed over the stoma to keep it moist, and this is covered with a dry, sterile dressing. In collaboration with the enterostomal therapist (ET), the nurse places a pouch system as soon as possible. The colostomy pouch system allows more convenient and acceptable collection of stool than a dressing does.

The nurse assesses the color and integrity of the stoma. A healthy stoma should be reddish pink and moist and will protrude about ¾ inch (2 cm) from the abdominal wall. A small amount of bleeding at the stoma is common.

The nurse reports any of the following problems related to the colostomy to the surgeon:

- Signs of ischemia and necrosis (dark red, purplish, or black color; dry, firm, or flaccid)
- Unusual bleeding
- Mucocutaneous separation (breakdown of the suture line securing the stoma to the abdominal wall)

The nurse also assesses the condition of the peristomal skin and frequently checks the pouch system for proper fit and signs of leakage. The peristomal skin should be intact, smooth, and without redness or excoriation.

The colostomy should start functioning 2 to 4 days postoperatively. When the colostomy begins to function, the pouch may need to be emptied frequently because of excess gas collection. It should be emptied when it is one-third to one-half full of stool. Stool is liquid immediately postoperatively but becomes more solid, depending on where in the colon the stoma was placed. For example, the stool from a colostomy in the ascending colon is liquid, the stool from a colostomy in the transverse colon is pasty, and the stool from a colostomy in the descending colon is more solid (similar to usual stool expelled from the rectum).

ABDOMINOPERINEAL RESECTION. When rectal tumors are present, the rectum and rectal support structure may need to be removed. An abdominoperineal resection usually requires a permanent colostomy for evacuation. However, with improvements in surgical techniques, more clients can undergo a colon resection with the rectal sphincter left intact; thus the need for a colostomy is avoided.

Preoperative Care. The preoperative care for the client undergoing an abdominoperineal resection is similar to that provided for the client undergoing a colon resection.

Operative Procedure. The surgeon removes the distal sigmoid colon, the rectosigmoid colon, the rectum, and the anus through combined abdominal and perineal incisions. A permanent end-sigmoid colostomy is created.

Postoperative Care. Postoperative care after an abdominoperineal resection is similar to that given after a colon resection with the creation of a sigmoid colostomy. The nurse collaborates with the ET to provide colostomy care and client and family education. In addition, the nurse monitors for postoperative complications, including pneumonia, dehydration, anastomotic leakage, and wound infection.

Wound Management. The perineal wound is generally surgically closed, and two bulb suction drains, such as Jackson-Pratt drains, are placed in the wound or through stab wounds near the wound. The drains help prevent drainage from collecting within the wound and are usually left in place for several days, depending on the character and amount of drainage.

Monitoring drainage from the perineal wound and cavity is important because of the possibility of infection and abscess formation. Serosanguineous drainage from the perineal wound may be observed for 1 to 2 months after surgery. Complete healing of the perineal wound may take 6 to 8 months. This wound can be a greater source of discomfort than the abdominal incision and ostomy, and more care may be required. The client may experience phantom rectal sensations because sympathetic innervation for rectal control has not been interrupted. Rectal pain and itching may occasionally occur after healing; however, there is no known physiologic explanation for these sensations. Interventions may include use of antipruritic medications, such as benzocaine, and sitz baths. The nurse continually assesses for signs of infection, abscess, or other complications and implements methods for promoting wound drainage and comfort (Chart 57-4).

Colostomy Management. The care of the permanent colostomy created as a result of the abdominal-perineal re-

CHART 57-4

BEST PRACTICE *for* Perineal Wound Care

Wound Care

- Place an absorbent dressing (Kerlix or abdominal pad) over the wound.
- Instruct the client that he or she may:
  - Use a feminine napkin as a dressing
  - Wear jockey-type shorts rather than boxers

Comfort Measures

- If ordered, soak the wound area in a sitz bath for 10 to 20 minutes three or four times per day.
- Administer pain medication as ordered and assess its effectiveness.
- Instruct the client about permissible activities. The client should:
  - Assume a side-lying position in bed; avoid sitting for long periods
  - Use foam pads or a soft pillow to sit on whenever in a sitting position
  - Avoid the use of air rings or rubber doughnut devices

Prevention of Complications

- Maintain fluid and electrolyte balance by monitoring intake and output and by monitoring output from the perineal wound.
- Observe suture line integrity and monitor wound drains; watch for erythema, edema, bleeding, purulent drainage, unusual odor, and excessive or constant pain.

section is similar to that of a hemicolectomy with a colostomy (see Surgical Management, p. 1249).

CRITICAL THINKING CHALLENGE

Your client is about to undergo a colon resection with the creation of a temporary colostomy for colorectal cancer.

- What preoperative teaching should be included for this client?
- What physical parameters should you assess the stoma for in the early postoperative period?
- What postoperative complications should you monitor for?

For suggested answer guidelines, go to SIMON http://www.wbsaunders.com/SIMON/Iggy/.

Community-Based Care

Clients undergoing an uncomplicated colon resection are typically hospitalized for 5 to 7 days. Discharge planning with the assistance of a discharge planner or case manager assists clients and their families in coping with the immediate postoperative phase of recovery. Following hospitalization for surgery, the client with colorectal cancer is usually managed at home. Radiation therapy or chemotherapy is typically done on an ambulatory (outpatient) basis. For the client with advanced cancer, hospice care is an option (see Chapter 9).

HOME CARE MANAGEMENT

The nurse assesses all clients for their ability to perform incision care and activities of daily living (ADLs) within limitations. For clients requiring assistance with these activities, home care visits by nurses or assistive nursing personnel can be provided.

For the client who has undergone a colostomy, the nurse or case manager reviews the home situation to aid the client in arranging for care. Ostomy products should be kept in an area (preferably the bathroom) where the temperature is neither hot nor cold (skin barriers may become stiff or melt in extreme temperatures) to ensure proper functioning. The enterostomal therapist (ET) may serve as a consultant after the client is discharged home to ensure continuity of care.

No changes are needed in sleeping accommodations. A rubber covering may initially be placed over the bed mattress if clients feel insecure about the pouch system. The client may consume his or her usual diet on discharge.

HEALTH TEACHING

Before discharge, clients are instructed to avoid lifting heavy objects or straining on defecation to prevent tension on the anastomosis site. The client is advised to avoid driving for 4 to 6 weeks while the incision heals. A stool softener may be prescribed to keep stools at a soft consistency for ease of passage. Clients are instructed to note the frequency, amount, and character of the stools. In addition to this information, the nurse teaches all clients with colon resections to watch for and report clinical manifestations of intestinal obstruction and perforation (e.g., cramping, abdominal pain, nausea, and vomiting). A normal diet may be resumed; however, the client is advised to avoid gas-producing foods and carbonated beverages. Four to six weeks may be required to establish the effects of certain foods on bowel patterns.

COLOSTOMY CARE. Rehabilitation after ostomy surgery requires that clients and family members learn the principles of colostomy care and the psychomotor skills needed to facilitate this care. Providing information is important, but the nurse must also allow adequate opportunity for clients to learn the psychomotor skills involved in ostomy care before discharge. Sufficient practice time is planned for clients and family or significant others so that they can handle, assemble, and apply all ostomy equipment. The nurse teaches clients and family or other caregiver about the following:

- The normal appearance of the stoma
- Signs and symptoms of complications
- Measurement of the stoma
- The choice, use, care, and application of the appropriate appliance to cover the stoma
- Measures to protect the skin adjacent to the stoma
- Dietary measures to control gas and odor
- Resumption of normal activities, including work, travel, and sexual intercourse

The appropriate pouch system must be selected and fitted to the stoma. Clients with flat, firm abdomens may use either flexible (bordered with paper tape) or nonflexible (full skin barrier wafer) pouch systems. A firm abdomen with lateral creases or folds requires a flexible system. Clients with deep creases, flabby abdomens, a retracted stoma, or a stoma that is flush or concave to the abdominal surface benefit from a convex appliance with a stoma belt (Bradley & Pupiales, 1997). This type of system presses into the skin around the stoma, causing the stoma to protrude. This protrusion helps tighten the skin and prevents leaks around the stoma opening onto the peristomal skin.

Measurement of the stoma is necessary to determine the correct size of the stomal opening on the appliance. The opening should be large enough not only to cover the peristomal skin but also to avoid stomal trauma. The stoma will shrink within 6 to 8 weeks of surgery; therefore it needs to be measured at least once weekly during this time and as needed if the client gains or loses weight. The client and family caregiver should be taught to trace the pattern of the stomal area on the wafer portion of the appliance and to cut an opening about $\frac{1}{8}$ to $\frac{1}{16}$ inch larger than the stomal pattern to ensure that stomal tissue will not be constricted (Catanzaro & Serembus, 1998).

Skin preparation may include clipping peristomal hair or shaving the area to achieve a smooth surface, prevent unnecessary discomfort when the wafer is removed, and minimize the risk of infected hair follicles. The client is advised to avoid using moisturizing soaps to clean the area because the lubricants can interfere with adhesion of the appliance. The client and family caregiver are taught to apply a skin sealant and allow it dry before application of the appliance (colostomy bag) to facilitate less painful removal of the tape or adhesive. If peristomal skin becomes raw, the client or caregiver checks to see whether the sealant contains alcohol and, if so, reconsiders using it to avoid causing a burning sensation to the skin. Stoma powder or paste, or a combination, may also be used for erythematous peristomal skin. The paste is also used to fill in crevices and creases to create a flat surface for the faceplate of the colostomy bag. If the client develops a fungal rash, an antifungal cream or powder is used, as ordered.

Control of gas and odor from the colostomy is often a significant goal for clients with new ostomies. Although a leaking or inadequately closed pouch is the usual cause of odor, flatus can also contribute to the odor. The nurse teaches the client and family caregiver that although there are generally no forbidden foods for ostomates, certain foods and habits can cause flatus or contribute to odor when the pouch is open. Broccoli, brussels sprouts, cabbage, cauliflower, cucumbers, mushrooms, and peas often cause flatus, as does chewing gum, smoking, drinking beer, and skipping meals. Crackers, toast, and yogurt can help prevent gas. Asparagus, broccoli, cabbage, turnips, eggs, fish, and garlic contribute to odor when the pouch is open. Buttermilk, cranberry juice, parsley, and yogurt will help prevent odor; charcoal filters, pouch deodorizers, or placement of a breath mint in the pouch will eliminate odors. The client should be cautioned not to put aspirin tablets in the pouch because they may cause ulceration of the stoma (Table 57-3).

The client with a sigmoid colostomy may benefit from colostomy irrigation to regulate elimination. However, most clients with a sigmoid colostomy can become regulated through diet. An irrigation is similar to an enema but is administered through the stoma rather than the rectum.

In addition to instructing the client about the clinical manifestations of obstruction and perforation, the nurse also advises the client with a colostomy to report any fever or sudden onset of pain or swelling around the stoma. Other assessments performed by the home care nurse are listed in Chart 57-5.

PSYCHOSOCIAL PREPARATION. The diagnosis of cancer can be emotionally immobilizing for the client and family or significant others, but treatment may be welcomed because it may provide hope for control of the disease. The nurse explores the client's reactions to the illness and perceptions of planned interventions.

The client's reaction to ostomy surgery, which may include disfigurement, may involve the following:

- Fear of not being accepted by others
- Feelings of grief related to disturbance in body image
- Concerns about sexuality

The nurse allows the client to verbalize his or her feelings. By teaching how to physically manage the ostomy, the nurse can help the client begin to restore self-esteem and improve body image. Inclusion of family and significant others in the rehabilitation process may help maintain relationships and raise the client's self-esteem. Anticipatory instruction includes information on leakage accidents, odor control measures, and adjustments to resuming normal sexual relationships.

HEALTH CARE RESOURCES

Several resources are available to complement nursing care, maintain continuity of care in the home environment, and provide for client needs that the nurse is not able to meet. The nurse makes a referral to the case manager or social worker, who can provide further emotional counseling to the client and family or significant others, aid in managing the financial concerns that the client and family may have, or arrange home care or extended care (e.g., in a nursing home, group home, or hospice) as needed.

The nurse makes a referral to the enterostomal therapist (ET) to aid in preoperative stoma teaching, evaluate and mark the stoma site, and provide consultation for problems in care. The enterostomal therapist (ET) may also conduct an ambulatory care clinic for ongoing client needs.

Information about the United Ostomy Association, a self-help group of people who have ostomies, is provided. Literature, such as the organization's publication *(Ostomy Quarterly),* and information about a local chapter are given to the client. This organization conducts a visitor program that sends specially trained visitors (who have an ostomy) to talk with clients. After obtaining the client's consent, the nurse makes a referral to the visitor program so that the visitor can see the client both preoperatively and postoperatively. A physician's consent for visitation is generally necessary.

The local division or unit of the American Cancer Society (ACS) can help provide necessary medical equipment and supplies, home care services, travel accommodations, and other resources for the client who is undergoing cancer treatment or ostomy surgery. The nurse informs the client and family of the programs available through the local division or unit.

Because of short hospital stays, clients with new ostomies receive most of their instruction on colostomy care from nurses working for home care agencies. This resource also facilitates provision for physical care needs, medication management, and emotional support for clients with or without colostomies. If the client has advanced colorectal cancer, a referral for hospice services in the home, nursing home, or other long-term care setting may be appropriate. The home care nurse informs the client and family about what ostomy supplies are needed and where they can be purchased. Price and location are considered before recommendations are made.

Evaluation: Outcomes

NOC The nurse evaluates the care of the client with colorectal cancer on the basis of the identified nursing diagnoses and collaborative problems. The expected outcomes are that the client:

- Maintains hemodynamic stability following surgery
- Is free of infection and postoperative complications
- Demonstrates appropriate incision care and, if applicable, appropriate colostomy care with minimal assistance
- Acquires or maintains effective coping patterns throughout the diagnosis, treatment, and rehabilitative phases of recovery

INTESTINAL OBSTRUCTION

OVERVIEW

Intestinal obstruction is defined as "a partial or complete obstruction of the small or large bowel that impedes the natural progression of digestive processing" (Shelton, 1999, p. 478). Intestinal obstruction is a common and serious disorder caused by a variety of conditions and is associated with significant morbidity. Bowel obstruction accounts for up to 20% of emergency admissions to a surgical service. It can occur anywhere in the intestinal tract, although the ileum in the small intestine (the narrowest part of the intestinal tract) is the most common site. The nurse assesses for clinical manifestations of obstruction in all clients with gastrointestinal (GI) disorders, since obstruction occurs fairly often and is associated with a variety of conditions.

Pathophysiology

Intestinal obstructions can be partial or complete and are classified as mechanical or nonmechanical. In **mechanical ob-**

TABLE 57-3 • SOLUTIONS TO SPECIAL PROBLEMS IN OSTOMY USE

Problems	Solutions
ODOR	
Foods Dairy products (boiled milk, eggs, and some cheese), fish, onion, garlic, coffee, alcohol, nuts, prunes, beans, cabbage, cucumbers, asparagus, radishes, broccoli, turnips, peas, highly seasoned foods	Spinach, cranberry juice, yogurt, buttermilk, dark green vegetables (parsley is particularly helpful), increased vitamin C in food or vitamin preparations
Drugs Antibiotics, vitamins, iron	***Oral Medications*** Chlorophyll tablets (Derifil) for fecal odors (absorb gas) Charcoal tablets Bismuth bicarbonate (0.6 g tid with meals) Bismuth subgallate (Devrom or Biscaps) 1 or 2 tablets with meals and 1 tablet at bedtime ***Pouch Preparations*** Odor-proof pouch or pouch with odor-control mechanism Manufactured preparations (place small amounts in pouch): Banish II or Superbanish (United), Odor-Guard (Marlan), Ostobon (Pettibone Labs), activated charcoal, ostomy deodorant (Sween), Nilodor, Devko tablets (Parthenon), D-Odor, M-9 (Mason Lab) Sodium bicarbonate solution (soaked cotton balls in pouch) Vanilla, peppermint, lemon, or almond extracts (put 10 drops into pouch or soak cotton balls) Favorite spice, cloves, or cinnamon (place $^{1}/_{4}$ tsp in pouch) Mouthwash (e.g., Cēpacol, Listerine) (several drops in pouch or soaked cotton balls in pouch) ***Cleaning Reusable Pouches*** Wisk and water (1:1 solution) Baking soda and water (1:1 solution) Household white vinegar and water (1:1 solution) Manufactured products: Uri-Kleen, Uni-Wash (United), Peri-Wash (Sween), Skin Care cleaner (Bard) Baking soda (after drying the pouch, powder inside with baking soda)
FLATULENCE	
Activities Eating fast and talking at same time, gum chewing, smoking, snoring, skipping meals, emotional upset	Avoid these activities; eat solids before taking liquids
Foods Mushrooms, onions, beans, cabbage, brussels sprouts, spinach, cheese, eggs, beer, carbonated beverages, fish, highly seasoned foods, some fruit drinks, corn, pork, peas, coffee, high-fat foods	***Pouch Adaptation*** Use pouches with gas or odor filters
SKIN IRRITATION	
Allergy Erythema, erosion, edema, weeping, bleeding, itching, burning, stinging, irritation the same shape as the allergic material	Creams: Sween cream, Unicare cream, or Hollister Skin Conditioning Cream (use small amount and rub in; tapes will adhere when dry)
Chemical Exposure Stool, urine, glues, solvents, soaps, detergents, proteolytic digestive enzymes	Powders (karaya gum, Stomahesive, cornstarch) used with skin gel (Skin Prep, Skin Gel) Antacids: aluminum hydroxide (Amphojel, Maalox) used with skin sealant (Skin Prep, Skin Gel)
Epidermal Hyperplasia Increased formation of epidermal cells causing a generalized thickening of the outer layer of the skin	Skin sealant alone (for slightly reddened skin) Skin barriers: one application left on for 24 hr or longer may clear irritations quickly Pastes (Hollister Premium, Stomahesive) used to fill in creases and spaces
Mechanical Trauma Pressure, friction, or stripping of the skin (e.g., adhesives, tape, belts)	Hair dryer on cool setting to decrease moisture Do not patch or tape leaks; correct the leakage problem immediately
Infection *Candida albicans* infection indicated by pustular, reddened, weepy, white spots	***For Candidiasis*** Use nystatin (Mycostatin) powder; cover with skin sealant (Skin Prep or Skin Gel)
Radiation Therapy Erythema, weeping	Use drying agent (e.g., acroflavin) Place skin barrier (Stomahesive) over site

CHART 57-5

FOCUSED ASSESSMENT *of* The Home Care Client with a Colostomy

Assess gastrointestinal status, including:
- Dietary and fluid intake and habits
- Presence or absence of nausea and vomiting
- Weight gain or loss
- Bowel elimination pattern and characteristics and amount of effluent (stool)
- Bowel sounds

Assess condition of stoma, including:
- Location, size, protrusion, color, and integrity
- Signs of ischemia, such as dull coloring or dark or purplish bruising

Assess periostomal skin for:
- Presence or absence of excoriated skin, leakage underneath drainage system
- Fit of appliance and effectiveness of skin barrier and appliance

Assess client's and family's coping skills, including:
- Self-care abilities in the home
- Acknowledgment of changes in body image and function
- Sense of loss

struction, the bowel is physically obstructed by disorders outside the intestine (e.g., adhesions or hernias) or by blockages in the lumen of the intestine (e.g., tumors, inflammation, strictures, or fecal impactions). **Nonmechanical obstruction** (also known as paralytic ileus or adynamic ileus because it is a result of neuromuscular disturbance) does not involve a physical obstruction in or outside the intestine. Instead, peristalsis is decreased or absent, resulting in a slowing of the movement or a backup of intestinal contents.

Intestinal contents are composed of ingested fluid and saliva; gastric, pancreatic, and biliary secretions; and swallowed air. In both mechanical and nonmechanical obstructions, the intestinal contents accumulate at and above the area of obstruction. Intestinal distention results from the intestine's inability to absorb the contents and mobilize them down the intestinal tract. To compensate for the lag, peristalsis increases in an effort to move the intestinal contents forward. The increase in peristalsis stimulates more secretions, which leads to additional distention. This causes edema of the bowel with increased capillary permeability. Plasma leaking into the peritoneal cavity and fluid trapped in the intestinal lumen markedly decrease the absorption of fluid and electrolytes into the vascular space. Reduced circulatory blood volume and electrolyte imbalances typically occur. Hypovolemia ranges from mild to extreme (hypovolemic shock).

Specific fluid and electrolyte problems result, depending on the part of the intestine that is blocked. An obstruction high in the small intestine causes a loss of gastric hydrochloride, which can lead to *metabolic alkalosis.* Obstruction below the duodenum but above the large bowel results in loss of both acids and bases, so that acid-base imbalance is usually not compromised. Obstruction at the end of the small intestine and lower in the intestinal tract causes loss of alkaline fluids, which can lead to *metabolic acidosis.*

If the resultant hypovolemia is severe, renal insufficiency or even death can occur. Bacterial peritonitis with or without actual perforation can also result. Bacteria in the intestinal contents lie stagnant in the obstructed intestine. This is not a problem unless the blood flow to the intestine is compromised. However, with so-called closed-loop obstruction (blockage in two different areas) or a **strangulated obstruction** (obstruction with compromised blood flow), the risk for peritonitis is greatly increased. Bacteria without blood supply can form an endotoxin, and release of the endotoxin into the peritoneal or systemic circulation results in septic shock. With a strangulated obstruction, major blood loss into the intestine and the peritoneum can result. Current mortality rates for bowel obstruction range from 3.5% to 6% but may be as high as 14% in older adults.

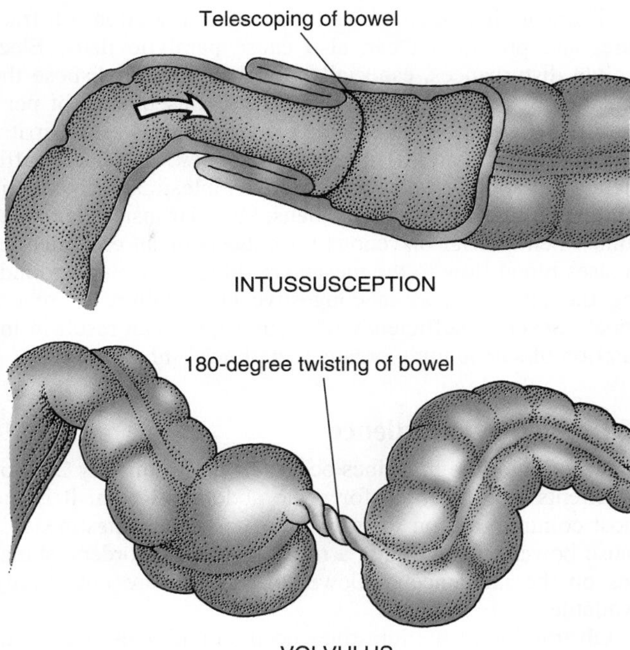

Figure 57-6 ● Two types of mechanical obstruction.

Etiology

Mechanical obstruction can result from adhesions, tumors, hernias, fecal impactions, strictures due to Crohn's disease or radiation, intussusception (telescoping of a segment of the intestine within itself), volvulus (twisting of the intestine), fibrosis due to disorders such as endometriosis, and vascular disorders (e.g., emboli and arteriosclerotic narrowing of mesenteric vessels) (Figure 57-6). In individuals age 65 or older, diverticulitis and tumors are the most common causes of obstruction.

Regardless of age, adhesions are the most common cause of mechanical obstruction, accounting for 45% to 60% of cases. Adhesions are bands of granulation and scar tissue that develop as a result of an inflammatory response, encircling the intestine and constricting its lumen.

Paralytic, or **adynamic, ileus** is a nonmechanical obstruction caused by physiologic, neurogenic, or chemical imbalances associated with decreased peristalsis from trauma or the effect of a toxin on autonomic intestinal control. Adynamic ileus occurs to some degree following abdominal surgery or trauma. Paralytic ileus can be caused by handling of the intestines during abdominal surgery; intestinal function is lost for a few hours to several days.

Thoracic diseases such as myocardial infarction, rib fracture, and pneumonia can also cause paralytic ileus. Electrolyte disturbances, especially hypokalemia, predispose the client to ileus. Paralytic ileus can be a consequence of peritonitis, since leakage of colonic contents causes severe irritation and triggers an inflammatory response. Vascular insufficiency to the bowel, also referred to as intestinal ischemia, is a potential cause of adynamic ileus. Vascular insufficiency results when arterial or venous thrombosis or an embolus decreases blood flow to the mesenteric blood vessels surrounding the intestines, as in congestive heart failure or severe shock. Severe insufficiency of blood supply can result in infarction of surrounding organs (e.g., bowel infarction).

Incidence/Prevalence

Obstruction of the intestines occurs in approximately 20% of all clients who are seen for acute abdominal pain. It is the most common reason for surgery of the small intestine. Because bowel obstruction is a result of other disorders, statistics on the incidence of bowel obstruction are not readily available.

Obstruction of the intestines occurs in all age-groups, but the incidence differs with age. In adults, 75% of all obstructions occur in the small intestine and 15% occur in the large intestine. In order of occurrence, adhesions, hernias, and tumors are the most common causes of small-bowel obstruction; cancer of the colon, diverticulitis, and volvulus cause most large-bowel obstructions in adults.

CONSIDERATIONS FOR OLDER ADULTS

The physiologic changes associated with aging, such as decreased peristalsis and decreased mobility, contribute to fecal impactions in older adults. Fecal impactions can lead to partial or complete bowel obstruction.

COLLABORATIVE MANAGEMENT

Assessment

HISTORY

The nurse collects information concerning the following:

- Past or recent abdominal surgery
- Radiation therapy
- History of inflammatory bowel disease
- Gallstones
- Hernias
- Trauma
- Peritonitis
- Cancer

The client is asked about recent occurrence of nausea or vomiting. The nurse also asks about the passage of flatus and the time, character, and consistency of the last bowel movement. Singultus (hiccups) is common with all types of intestinal obstruction.

The nurse assesses for a family history of colorectal cancer and asks the client about blood in the stool or a change in bowel pattern. The body temperature with obstruction is rarely higher than 100° F (37.8° C). A temperature higher than this, with or without guarding and tenderness, and a sustained elevation in pulse indicate a strangulated obstruction or peritonitis.

PHYSICAL ASSESSMENT/CLINICAL MANIFESTATIONS

MECHANICAL OBSTRUCTION. The client with mechanical obstruction in the small intestine often has mid-abdominal pain or cramping. The pain can be sporadic, and the client may feel comfortable between episodes. If strangulation is present, the pain becomes more localized and steady. Vomiting often accompanies obstruction and is more profuse with obstructions in the proximal small intestine. The vomitus may contain bile and mucus or be orange-brown and foul smelling as a result of bacterial overgrowth with low ileal obstruction. Obstipation (no passage of stool) and failure to pass flatus accompany complete obstruction. Diarrhea may be present in partial obstruction.

Mechanical colonic obstruction causes a milder, more intermittent colicky abdominal pain than is seen with small-bowel obstruction. Lower abdominal distention may be present, as well as obstipation, or ribbon-like stools if obstruction is partial. Alterations in bowel patterns and blood in the stools accompany the obstruction if colorectal cancer or diverticulitis is the cause.

On examination of the abdomen, the nurse may observe abdominal distention, which is common in all forms of intestinal obstruction. Peristaltic waves may also be visible. The nurse auscultates for proximal high-pitched bowel sounds **(borborygmi),** which are associated with cramping early in the obstructive process as the intestine tries to push the mechanical obstruction forward. In later stages of mechanical obstruction, the bowel sounds are absent, especially distal to the obstruction. Abdominal tenderness and rigidity are usually minimal. The presence of a tense, fluid-filled bowel loop mimicking a palpable abdominal mass may signal a closed-loop, strangulating small-bowel obstruction.

NONMECHANICAL OBSTRUCTION. In most types of nonmechanical obstruction (paralytic, or adynamic, ileus), the pain is described as a constant, diffuse discomfort. Colicky cramping is not characteristic of this type of obstruction. Pain associated with obstruction attributable to vascular insufficiency or infarction is usually severe and constant. On inspection, abdominal distention is typically present. On aus-

CHART 57-6

KEY FEATURES *of* Small-Bowel and Large-Bowel Obstructions

Small-Bowel Obstructions	Large-Bowel Obstructions
Abdominal discomfort/pain, possibly accompanied by visible peristaltic waves in upper and mid abdomen	Intermittent lower abdominal cramping
Upper or epigastric abdominal distention	Lower abdominal distention
Nausea and early, profuse vomiting	Minimal or no vomiting (may contain fecal material)
Obstipation	Obstipation or ribbon-like stools
Severe fluid and electrolyte imbalances	No major fluid and electrolyte imbalances
Metabolic alkalosis	Metabolic acidosis

cultation of the abdomen, the nurse notes decreased bowel sounds in early obstruction and absent bowel sounds in later stages. Vomiting of gastric contents and bile is frequent, but the vomitus rarely has a foul odor and is rarely profuse. Obstipation may or may not be present. Chart 57-6 compares small-bowel and large-bowel obstructions.

LABORATORY ASSESSMENT

There is no definitive laboratory test to confirm a diagnosis of mechanical or nonmechanical obstruction. White blood cell (WBC) counts may be normal unless there is a strangulated obstruction, in which case there may be leukocytosis (increased WBCs). Hemoglobin, hematocrit, creatinine, and blood urea nitrogen (BUN) values are often elevated, indicating dehydration. Serum sodium, chloride, and potassium concentrations are reduced because of loss of fluid and electrolytes. Elevations in serum amylase levels may be found with strangulating obstructions, which can damage the pancreas.

High obstruction in the small intestine is likely to show an elevated serum venous carbon dioxide concentration and other values indicative of metabolic alkalosis. Obstruction in the large intestine is likely to show a low serum venous carbon dioxide concentration and other values suggestive of metabolic acidosis.

RADIOGRAPHIC ASSESSMENT

The health care provider obtains flat-plate and upright abdominal x-ray films as soon as an obstruction is suspected. Distention of loops of intestine with fluid and gas in the small intestine, in conjunction with the absence of gas in the colon, indicates an obstruction in the small intestine. However, x-ray findings are often normal when a strangulated obstruction actually exists in the small intestine. Therefore obstruction cannot be ruled out on the basis of x-ray findings.

Obstruction of the large intestine often shows gas distention of the colon on abdominal x-ray studies. A finding of free air under the diaphragm on abdominal x-ray examination indicates a perforated intestine.

OTHER DIAGNOSTIC ASSESSMENT

The diagnostic examination chosen depends on the suspected location of the obstruction. The physician may perform endoscopy (sigmoidoscopy or colonoscopy) or a barium enema study to determine the cause of the obstruction, except in cases where perforation is suspected. A computed tomography (CT) scan is useful in uncovering the cause and location of the obstruction and may be the diagnostic tool of choice when symptoms are severe (see the Cost of Care Box at right).

Interventions

Interventions are aimed at uncovering the cause and relieving the obstruction. Intestinal obstructions can be relieved by nonsurgical or surgical means. If the obstruction is partial and there is no evidence of strangulation, nonsurgical management is the treatment of choice. Decompression of the intestinal tract is initiated along with fluid and electrolyte replacement.

NONSURGICAL MANAGEMENT. Paralytic ileus responds well to nonsurgical methods of relieving obstruction. Nonsurgical approaches are also preferred in the treatment of clients with terminal disease associated with bowel obstruction. In addition to being on NPO status, clients with intestinal obstruction typically have a nasogastric or, more rarely, nasointestinal tube inserted. These tubes provide decompression of the bowel by draining fluid and air and are attached to suction; the type of suction depends on the type of tube inserted.

NASOINTESTINAL TUBES. The physician *occasionally* inserts nasointestinal (NI) tubes (such as the Miller-Abbott, Cantor, and Harris tubes) for obstruction of the small intestine. These longer tubes extend into the small intestine. Mercury-filled balloons at the end of a lumen act as a bolus of food, stimulating peristalsis and advancing down the intestinal tract. The Cantor and Harris tubes are single-lumen tubes with mercury-filled balloons at the tips and suction ports within the same lumen, proximal to the tip. The Miller-Abbott tube has two separate lumens for mercury and drainage.

The nurse assists with progression of the tube by helping the client change position every 2 hours and, if ordered, by advancing the tube 3 to 4 inches at specified times. These tubes are never taped to the nose until they reach a specified position in the intestine. As the tube is being inserted and advanced, it drains by gravity. The nurse monitors the drainage; if drainage stops, the nurse obtains a physician's order to inject 10 mL of air. The nurse does not irrigate the NI tube with fluid without an order by the health care provider. If ordered, the nurse attaches low intermittent suction to the suction lumen when the tube has stopped advancing.

COST OF CARE IMPLICATIONS FOR NURSING

INTESTINAL OBSTRUCTION

Cost of Care

- The cost of plain abdominal films in the diagnosis of intestinal obstruction is approximately $200 to $300 and provides an overall accuracy of 57%.
- A barium swallow or enema can cost $300 to $500, with an overall accuracy of 78%.
- Computed tomography (CT) can cost $500 to $800. The overall accuracy of CT in diagnosing intestinal obstruction ranges from 91% to 97%.
- The use of ultrasound in the diagnosis of intestinal obstruction is gaining popularity. The cost of this procedure is $300 to $600, with an overall accuracy of 81% to 96%.
- Laparoscopy is indicated to evaluate the need for laparotomy. The cost of this procedure can range from $1000 to $2000, with an overall accuracy of 94%.

Implications for Nursing

There are a variety of diagnostic tests that can be used in confirming the diagnosis of intestinal obstruction. Excessive costs to the health care system occur when an inappropriate diagnostic test is chosen, or if because of inadequate preparation, the examination needs to be repeated. Advanced-practice nurses require a working knowledge of diagnostic testing in order to ensure that their clients undergo the appropriate examination. Nurses responsible for preparing clients to undergo diagnostic procedures should ensure that proper preparation for the examination has been carried out (e.g., bowel prep, maintaining NPO status) to avoid inaccurate or incomplete results requiring the client to undergo additional testing that could add to the client burden and health care costs.

Data from Shelton, B. (1999). Intestinal obstruction. *AACN Clinical Issues: Advanced Practice in Acute and Critical Care, 10*(4), 478-491.

Most health care providers avoid the use of NI tubes because insertion of the mercury-filled lumen is often difficult; the time it takes to insert the tube also delays treatment. Insertion of this tube can be uncomfortable for clients.

NASOGASTRIC TUBES. Most clients with an obstruction have at least a **nasogastric (NG) tube** in place unless the obstruction is mild. Salem sump and Anderson tubes are examples of NG tubes that sit distally in the stomach and are attached to *low continuous* suction. Levin tubes are connected to *low intermittent* suction.

At least every 4 hours, the nurse assesses the client with an NG tube for proper placement of the tube, tube patency, and output. The nasal skin is also monitored daily for integrity. The nurse assesses for peristalsis by auscultating for bowel sounds with the suction disconnected (suction will mask peristaltic sounds).

The nurse questions the client regarding the passage of flatus and records the passage, amount, and character of bowel movements daily. Abdominal girth is measured at the same point each day. The client is also assessed for nausea and asked to report this manifestation.

NG tubes must be monitored for proper functioning. Occasionally, NG tubes move out of optimal drainage position or become plugged. In this case, the nurse notes a decrease in gastric output or stasis of the tube's contents. The client is assessed for nausea, vomiting, increased abdominal distention, and placement of the tube. If the NG tube is repositioned or replaced, confirmation of proper placement is obtained by x-ray examination before use. After appropriate placement is established, the contents are aspirated and the tube is irrigated with 30 mL of normal saline every 4 hours or as needed to maintain patency.

OTHER NONSURGICAL TECHNIQUES. Most types of nonmechanical obstruction respond to nasogastric decompression in conjunction with medical treatment of the primary disorder. Incomplete mechanical obstruction can sometimes be successfully treated without surgery. Obstruction caused by fecal impaction usually resolves after disimpaction and enema administration. Intussusception may respond to hydrostatic pressure changes during a barium enema.

FLUID AND ELECTROLYTE REPLACEMENT. IV fluid replacement and maintenance are indicated for all clients with intestinal obstruction, since the client is on NPO status and fluid and electrolyte loss (particularly potassium) through vomiting and nasogastric suction is great. On the basis of serum electrolytes and blood urea nitrogen (BUN) levels, the health care provider orders aggressive fluid replacement with 2 to 4 L of normal saline or lactated Ringer's solution with potassium added. Care must be taken with clients who are prone to fluid overload (e.g., the client with a history of congestive heart failure). The nurse carefully monitors lung sounds, weight, and intake and output parameters. Blood replacement may be indicated in strangulated obstruction because of blood loss into the bowel or peritoneal cavity.

The nurse or assistive nursing personnel monitors the client's vital signs and other measures of fluid status (e.g., urine output, skin turgor, and mucous membranes). Edema from third spacing is assessed because fluid is lost, mostly from the vascular space, into surrounding spaces (e.g., the peritoneal cavity). In collaboration with the dietitian, the physician may order total parenteral nutrition (TPN) to improve the nutritional status of the client, especially if he or she has had chronic nutritional problems and has been on NPO status for an extended period. Chapter 61 discusses the nursing care of clients receiving TPN.

Because of fluid losses, the client with intestinal obstruction is characteristically thirsty. The nurse provides frequent mouth care to help maintain moist mucous membranes. Lemon-glycerin swabs are avoided because they can increase mouth dryness. A small amount of ice chips may be allowed if the client is not having surgery; however, the health care provider should be consulted first. Ice chips can provide more free water than electrolytes; thus potassium and hydrochloric acid are washed out of the NG tube. The nurse monitors intake and output carefully to avoid electrolyte imbalance and false interpretation of gastric output measurements.

PAIN MANAGEMENT. The abdominal distention commonly noted with intestinal obstruction can cause a great deal of discomfort, especially when distention is severe. The colicky, crampy pain that comes and goes with mechanical obstruction and the nausea, vomiting, dry mucous membranes, and thirst contribute to the client's discomfort. The nurse continually assesses the character and location of the pain and immediately reports any pain that significantly increases or changes from a colicky, intermittent type to a constant discomfort. Such changes can indicate perforation of the intestine or peritonitis.

Opioid analgesics are normally withheld in the diagnostic period so that clinical manifestations of perforation or peritonitis are not masked. The nurse explains to the client and family the rationale for not giving analgesics. In addition, if analgesics such as morphine or meperidine are given, they slow intestinal motility and can cause vomiting. The nurse must be alert to this side effect, because nausea and vomiting are also signs of NG tube obstruction or worsening bowel obstruction.

The nurse helps the client obtain a position of comfort with frequent position changes to promote increased peristalsis. A semi-Fowler's position helps alleviate the pressure of abdominal distention on the chest. Not only is this a good comfort technique, but it also facilitates adequate thoracic excursion and normal breathing patterns.

Discomfort is generally less with nonmechanical obstruction than with mechanical obstruction. With both types of obstruction, discomfort is aggravated by ingestion of food or fluids.

DRUG THERAPY. If strangulation is thought to be likely, the health care provider prescribes IV broad-spectrum antibiotics. In addition, in cases of partial obstruction or paralytic ileus, medications that enhance gastric motility, such as octreotide acetate (Sandostatin), may be used.

SURGICAL MANAGEMENT. In all cases of complete mechanical obstruction and in many cases of incomplete mechanical obstruction, surgical intervention is necessary to relieve the obstruction. A strangulated obstruction is inevitably complete, and surgical intervention is always required. An **exploratory laparotomy** (a surgical opening of the abdominal cavity to investigate the cause of the obstruction) is initially performed for most clients with obstruction. More specific surgical procedures depend on the cause of the obstruction.

PREOPERATIVE CARE. The nurse provides preoperative teaching as discussed in Chapter 17. If time permits, all clients who require surgery for obstruction undergo nasogastric intubation and suction before surgery. However, in cases of complete obstruction, surgery should proceed without delay.

OPERATIVE PROCEDURES. The surgeon enters the abdominal cavity and explores for obstruction. If adhesions are found to be the cause of the obstruction, the adhesions are lysed (cut and released). Obstruction caused by a tumor or diverticulitis requires a colon resection with primary anastomosis or a temporary or permanent colostomy. If obstruction is caused by intestinal infarction, an embolectomy, thrombectomy, or colon resection (partial removal) may be necessary, particularly if the intestine is gangrenous.

POSTOPERATIVE CARE. Postoperative care for the client undergoing an exploratory laparotomy with lysis of adhesions, colon resection, thrombectomy, or embolectomy is similar to that described in Chapter 19. All clients have an NG tube in place until peristalsis (as characterized by the return of bowel sounds) resumes. The NG tube is removed slowly by first discontinuing suction and then clamping the tube for a scheduled amount of time. Residual drainage is checked at each stage to assess peristalsis without decompression before removing the NG tube entirely.

Community-Based Care

All clients with intestinal obstruction are hospitalized for monitoring and treatment. The length of stay varies according to the type of obstruction, the treatment, and the presence of complications. Clients who have complicated obstruction, such as strangulation or incarceration, are at greater risk for peritonitis, sepsis, and shock. The hospital stay may be up to several weeks, depending on the severity of complications.

Clients with nonmechanical (adynamic) intestinal obstruction are less likely to require a lengthy hospitalization because of the obstruction alone. Adynamic obstruction generally responds to NG intubation and suction within a few days.

HOME CARE MANAGEMENT

For the client who has had an intestinal obstruction, preparation for home care depends on the cause of the obstruction and the treatment required. Clients who have resolution of obstruction without surgical intervention are assessed for their knowledge of strategies to avoid recurrent obstruction. For example, if fecal impaction was the cause of the obstruction, the nurse assesses the client's ability to carry out a bowel regimen independently. For clients who have undergone surgery, the nurse evaluates their ability to function at home with the added tasks of incision care and possibly colostomy care.

HEALTH TEACHING

The nurse instructs the client to report any abdominal pain or distention, nausea, or vomiting, with or without constipation, since these symptoms might indicate recurrent obstruction. The client should be reassured, however, that recurrent paralytic ileus is not usually a problem. The client who has had mechanical obstruction as a result of fecal impaction (often the older adult) needs to have a structured bowel regimen to prevent recurrence (Chart 57-7). The nurse instructs this client to adhere to high-fiber diets, to exercise, and to drink at least 24 ounces of water daily, unless contraindicated. The physician may also order bulk-forming laxatives to help maintain a consistent elimination pattern.

The nurse teaches the client who has had surgery about incision care, drug therapy, and activity limitations. Drug therapy consists of an oral opioid analgesic, such as oxycodone hydrochloride with acetaminophen (Tylox, Percocet, Endocet✤), to be taken as needed for incisional discomfort. As with any opioid therapy, a stool softener is added to the medication regimen to prevent constipation and possible recurrent obstruction.

With resolution of obstruction, educational efforts by the nurse are aimed at prevention of obstruction by examining the cause of the obstruction and how to prevent recurrence. The nurse also reinforces important signs and symptoms to report to the health care provider. The client who had curative treatment of the underlying cause most likely requires less support than the client who underwent treatment of obstruction related to a serious disease that will require further treatment. The client is encouraged to express fears and concerns about the future. The nurse assesses the client's understanding and needs with regard to treatment plans.

HEALTH CARE RESOURCES

The need for follow-up appointments depends on the cause of the obstruction and the treatment required. If the client is at risk for fecal impaction, the nurse can arrange for a home care nurse to assess the gastrointestinal (GI) function and dietary habits of the client on an ongoing basis. Arrangements should also be made for the services of a home care nurse if the client needs help with incision or colostomy care. Medicare guidelines or insurance precertification requirements must be met before approval is given for home care visits. The discharge planner or case manager assist in setting up home care follow-up.

CHART 57-7

NURSING FOCUS *on the* OLDER ADULT
Fecal Impaction

- Teach the client to eat high-fiber foods, including plenty of raw fruits and vegetables and whole-grain products.
- Encourage the client to drink adequate amounts of fluids, especially water.
- Do not routinely administer a laxative; teach the client that laxative abuse decreases abdominal muscle tone and contributes to an atonic colon.
- Encourage the client to exercise regularly, if possible. Walking every day is an excellent exercise for promoting intestinal motility.
- Use natural foods to stimulate peristalsis, such as warm beverages and prune juice.
- Take bulk-forming products, such as Metamucil, to provide fiber.
- Check the client's stool for amount and frequency; oozing of soft or diarrheal stool often indicates a fecal impaction.
- Have the client sit on a toilet or bedside commode, rather than on a bedpan, for elimination.

ABDOMINAL TRAUMA

OVERVIEW

Abdominal trauma is defined as injury to the structures located between the diaphragm and the pelvis, which occurs when the abdomen is subjected to blunt or penetrating forces. Organs injured may include the large or small bowel, liver, spleen, duodenum, pancreas, kidneys, and urinary bladder.

At least one half of all blunt abdominal trauma occurs from motor vehicle accidents (MVAs) (Sommers & Johnson, 1997). Other causes of blunt trauma include falls, aggravated assaults, and contact sports. *Penetrating abdominal trauma* is caused by gunshot wounds, stabbing, or impalement with an object. The liver is the most commonly injured organ in blunt and penetrating trauma. The spleen is the most commonly injured organ in blunt abdominal trauma. The small intestine is the third most commonly injured organ in abdominal trauma; 80% of injuries are caused by gunshot wounds (GSWs).

> **CULTURAL CONSIDERATIONS**
> MVAs are three times more common in males than in females in the 15- to 24-year age-group. In the 15- to 34-year age-group, European Americans (Caucasians) have a death rate from MVAs that is 40% higher than that of African Americans (Sommers & Johnson, 1997). Penetrating injuries from GSWs and stab wounds are more common in preteen and young adults than in older adults and are more common in African Americans than in European Americans.

COLLABORATIVE MANAGEMENT

Assessment

In the emergency phase of treatment, health care providers focus on the risks of hemorrhage, shock, and peritonitis. Mental status and skin perfusion are *priority* nursing assessments, with skin perfusion being the most reliable clinical guide in assessing hypovolemic shock:

- In a person with mild shock, the skin is pale, cool, and moist.
- With moderate shock, diaphoresis is more marked and urine output ceases.
- With severe shock, changes in mental status are manifested by agitation, disorientation, and recent memory loss.

The nurse assesses for abdominal trauma by asking the client about the presence, location, and quality of pain. The abdomen, flanks, back, genitalia, and rectum are inspected for contusions, abrasions, lacerations, ecchymosis, penetrating injuries, and symmetry. All of the client's clothes must be removed. If pneumatic garments such as antishock trousers are in place, they are usually not removed unless aggressive fluid replacement has been given to the client, a surgical team is available to immediately intervene, and the attending physician orders it to be done. After pneumatic garments are removed, uncontrolled hemorrhage can occur. Antishock trousers have a constrictive effect on hemorrhage in the trunk and facilitate circulatory return to the heart. However, they can cause compartment syndrome to the lower extremities; consequently, their use is controversial.

Inspection of the abdomen may reveal distention. To perform an adequate inspection, the nurse turns the client while maintaining spinal immobilization. Ecchymosis may signify internal bleeding. Ecchymosis present in the distribution of a lap seat belt should be reported to the health care provider immediately, since investigation for occult injury to the bowel is necessary. Ecchymosis around the umbilicus is known as **Cullen's sign,** and ecchymosis on either flank (known as **Turner's sign**) may indicate retroperitoneal bleeding into the abdominal wall.

The nurse auscultates the abdomen for bowel sounds. Absent or diminished bowel sounds may be caused by the presence of blood, bacteria, or a chemical irritant in the abdominal cavity. The nurse also auscultates for bruits in the abdomen, which indicate renal artery injury.

During percussion, an abnormal sign associated with abdominal trauma is resonance over the right flank with the client lying on the left side. This is known as **Ballance's sign** and is found with a ruptured spleen. Resonance over the normally dull liver is due to free air, which is pathologic. Palpation for lower rib fractures should increase suspicion of liver or spleen injuries. Injury to the spleen is present in 20% of individuals with left lower rib fractures. Liver injury is present in 10% of individuals with right lower rib fractures. The presence of **Kehr's sign,** left shoulder pain resulting from diaphragmatic irritation, may be present in splenic injury.

Dullness over hollow organs that normally contain gas, such as the stomach and the large and small intestines, may indicate blood or fluid. Light abdominal palpation identifies areas of tenderness, rebound tenderness, guarding, rigidity, and spasm. If the nurse palpates a mass, it may be blood or a fluid collection.

The client without obvious significant bleeding or definite signs of peritoneal irritation undergoes abdominal radiography, diagnostic peritoneal lavage (DPL), and computed tomography (CT). For peritoneal lavage, the physician inserts a large-bore catheter into the abdomen and allows fluid to enter the abdominal cavity. If the return drainage from the abdomen is pink or grossly bloody, the health care team prepares the client for surgery. Abdominal ultrasound has recently been used successfully in diagnosing blunt abdominal trauma and may replace CT and DPL for diagnosis (Levins, 2000). Clients with hemodynamic instability or peritonitis are candidates for immediate laparotomy.

Interventions

Nonsurgical and surgical interventions are aimed at preserving or restoring hemodynamic stability, preventing or decreasing blood loss, and preventing complications.

NONSURGICAL MANAGEMENT. Nursing interventions include placement of at least two large-bore IV catheters in the upper extremities. IV catheters are not used in the lower extremities; if the vasculature has been injured, fluid can pool in the abdomen. The health care provider may insert a central venous catheter to assist with rapid fluid volume infusion. IV fluid consists of a balanced saline solution, crystalloids, and possibly blood.

The following physiologic parameters are monitored:

- Arterial blood gases
- Complete blood count (CBC)
- Serum electrolyte, glucose and amylase, and blood urea nitrogen (BUN) determinations
- Liver function tests
- Clotting studies

Measuring arterial blood gases may be of assistance in determining the severity of shock. Hemoglobin and hematocrit values do not initially reflect true blood loss; values can be skewed because of hemoconcentration from volume loss or the dilutional effects of IV fluids. Serial hemoglobin and hematocrit measurements may be more accurate in determining true blood loss. An elevated white blood cell (WBC) count may indicate a ruptured spleen or intestinal injury. Elevated levels of serum transaminases may indicate liver injury. Elevation of serum amylase activity may signal injury to the pancreas or the bowel. All laboratory work is compiled so that values can be compared and subtle changes noted.

Continuous cardiac monitoring is begun in the emergency department. The nurse inserts an indwelling urinary (Foley) catheter unless there is blood at the urinary meatus. Initially and hourly thereafter, the nurse evaluates urine output for bleeding and specific gravity. Laboratory tests indicate the amount of blood and protein in the urine. If there is an open abdominal wound or evisceration, the nurse covers it with a sterile dry dressing unless the physician orders otherwise. Unless it is contraindicated, as in the case of a concomitant skull fracture, the physician or nurse inserts a nasogastric (NG) tube, which is kept in place to identify bleeding and to minimize the risk of vomiting and aspiration. Antibiotics are administered as ordered to reduce the risk of peritonitis.

If the client with known abdominal trauma has no definite clinical manifestations of active bleeding or abdominal injury, he or she is admitted to the hospital for observation. Blunt trauma can cause active, but often not obvious, damage. The nurse assesses for abdominal or referred pain and nausea. Every 15 to 30 minutes in the early postinjury period and then hourly, the nurse evaluates the client's:

- Mental status
- Vital signs
- Clinical findings, such as vomiting, guarding, rigidity, or rebound tenderness
- Skin temperature
- Bowel sounds
- Urine output

The nurse reports any change immediately to the health care provider. It is more important for the nurse to recognize the high risk of an active abdominal injury and assess for general signs of abdominal injury (e.g., hemorrhage and peritonitis) than to identify the exact nature of the abdominal injury. Analgesics for pain are not prescribed at this time so that clinical manifestations are not masked or overlooked. The nurse explains the rationale for withholding analgesics to the client and family or significant others.

SURGICAL MANAGEMENT. For the client with severe abdominal trauma, the surgeon performs an exploratory laparotomy and repairs abdominal injuries immediately if there are definite signs of peritoneal irritation. These signs include rebound tenderness, significant blood loss, evisceration, or a gunshot wound (GSW) with possible peritoneal involvement.

Most stab wounds require exploratory laparotomy, but as many as 25% are superficial and do not involve the peritoneum. Using local anesthesia, the surgeon explores and cleans superficial stab wounds; the client does not require an exploratory laparotomy.

Before discharge from the hospital, the client who has experienced abdominal trauma is taught the signs and symptoms of abdominal bleeding whether or not surgery has been performed. The nurse instructs the client to report abdominal pain, nausea, vomiting, bloody or black stools, fever, weakness, and dizziness.

Hemorrhage can occasionally occur weeks after blunt abdominal trauma, despite medical evaluation. For the client who undergoes surgery or exploration of wounds, the nurse provides instructions on wound care before discharge from the hospital.

POLYPS

OVERVIEW

Polyps in the intestinal tract are small growths covered with mucosa and attached to the surface of the intestine. Although most are benign, polyps are significant in that some have the potential to become malignant.

Polyps are identified by their tissue type. The presence of adenomas always necessitates medical consultation because of their malignant potential. Although only 2% to 5% of adenomas progress to cancer, almost all colorectal cancers develop from an adenoma (Markowitz & Winawer, 1997). Adenomas are further classified as villous or tubular. Of these, villous adenomas pose a greater cancer risk.

Familial adenomatous polyposis (FAP) and hereditary nonpolyposis colorectal cancer (HNPCC) are inherited syndromes characterized by progressive development of colorectal adenomas. Unless these syndromes are treated, colorectal cancer inevitably occurs by the fourth to fifth decade of life (Markowitz & Winawer, 1997).

Other types of polyps include hyperplastic and hamartomatous polyps. Hyperplastic polyps, which include mucosal and inflammatory varieties, are entirely benign with no malignant potential. Hamartomatous polyps include juvenile and Peutz-Jeghers syndrome polyps. Although both types are generally benign, rare reports of malignant changes have been reported in juvenile polyps.

In addition to being classified by their tissue type, polyps are described according to their appearance (Figure 57-7). Pedunculated polyps are stalklike; a thin stem attaches them to the intestinal wall. They become elongated as peristalsis pulls them into the lumen of the intestine. Polyps attached to the intestinal walls by a broad base are described as sessile. A malignant polyp may be pedunculated or sessile.

COLLABORATIVE MANAGEMENT

Polyps are usually asymptomatic and are discovered during routine diagnostic testing, including tests for blood in the stool. However, they can cause gross rectal bleeding, intestinal

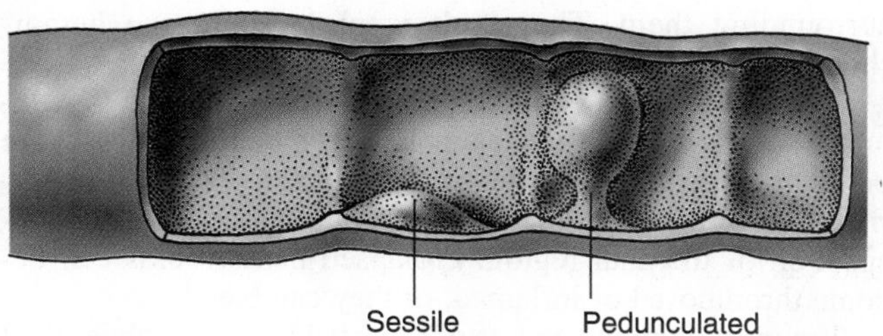

Figure 57-7 ● Pedunculated and sessile polyps. Pedunculated polyps, such as tubular adenomas, are stalklike. Sessile polyps, such as villous adenomas, are broad based.

obstruction, or intussusception (telescoping of the bowel). Diagnostic studies involve a barium enema examination and proctosigmoidoscopy or colonoscopy for ruling out cancer. Biopsy specimens of polyps can be obtained, or the entire polyp can be removed (polypectomy) with the use of an electrocautery snare that fits through the sigmoidoscope or colonoscope. This often eliminates the need for abdominal surgery to remove a suspicious or definitely malignant polyp. The client with FAP often requires a total colectomy (colon removal) to prevent the development of cancer.

Nursing care focuses on client education. The nurse instructs the client about the following:

- The nature of the polyp
- Clinical manifestations to report to the health care provider
- The need for regular, routine monitoring

The client with a known benign polyp that does not need to be removed has frequent sigmoidoscopic or colonoscopic examinations to monitor for any growth or change in the polyp or for an increase in the number of polyps. If the client has undergone a polypectomy, follow-up sigmoidoscopic or colonoscopic examinations are needed, because there is an increased risk of multiple polyps in the client who has had at least one polyp.

Nursing care of the client who has undergone a polypectomy of the colorectal area includes monitoring for abdominal distention and pain, rectal bleeding, mucopurulent rectal drainage, and fever.

A small amount of blood might appear in the stool after a polypectomy, but this should be temporary. Nursing care of the client who has undergone a total colectomy is described in Chapter 58 under Crohn's Disease.

HEMORRHOIDS

OVERVIEW

Hemorrhoids are unnaturally swollen or distended veins in the anorectal region. Hemorrhoids are common and not significant unless they cause pain or bleeding. The veins involved in the development of hemorrhoids are part of the normal structure in the anal region. With limited distention, the veins function as a valve overlying the anal sphincter that assists in continence. Increased intra-abdominal pressure causes elevated systemic and portal venous pressure, which is transmitted to the anorectal veins. Arterioles in the anorectal region shunt blood directly to the distended anorectal veins, which increases the pressure. With repeated elevations in pressure from increased intra-abdominal pressure and engorgement from arteriolar shunting of blood, the distended veins eventually separate from the smooth muscle surrounding them. The result is prolapse of the hemorrhoidal vessels.

Hemorrhoids can be internal or external (Figure 57-8). Internal hemorrhoids, which cannot be seen on inspection of the perineal area, lie above the anal sphincter. External hemorrhoids lie below the anal sphincter and can be seen on inspection of the anal region. Prolapsed hemorrhoids can become thrombosed or inflamed, or they can bleed.

The most common causes of repeated increased abdominal pressure resulting in hemorrhoids are straining at stool, pregnancy, portal hypertension, and colorectal cancer.

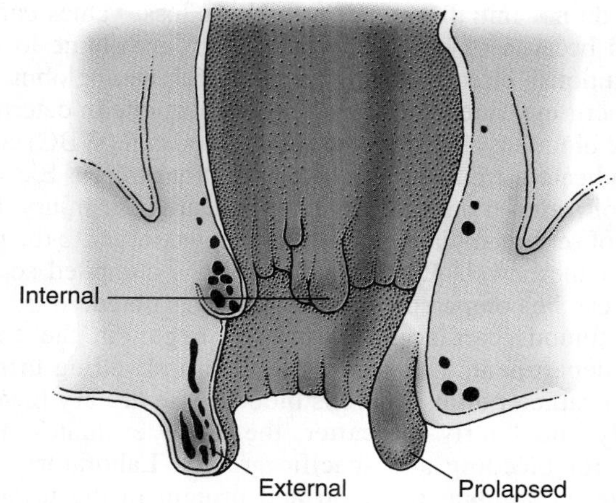

Figure 57-8 ● Internal, external, and prolapsed hemorrhoids. Internal hemorrhoids lie above the anal sphincter and cannot be seen on inspection of the anal area. External hemorrhoids lie below the anal sphincter and can be seen on inspection of the anal region. Hemorrhoids that enlarge, fall down, and protrude through the anus are called prolapsed hemorrhoids.

➤ COLLABORATIVE MANAGEMENT

Assessment

The most common symptoms of hemorrhoids are bleeding and prolapse. Blood is characteristically bright red and is present on toilet tissue or outside the stool. Pain is a common symptom and is often associated with thrombosis, especially if thrombosis occurs suddenly. Other symptoms include itching and a mucous discharge. Diagnosis is made by inspection, digital examination, proctoscopy, or proctoscopic ultrasonography.

Interventions

Interventions are typically conservative and are aimed at reducing symptoms with a minimum of discomfort, cost, and time lost from usual activities.

NONSURGICAL MANAGEMENT. Local treatment and diet therapy are initiated when symptoms begin. Cold packs applied to the anorectal region for a few minutes at a time beginning with the onset of pain and hot sitz baths three or four times a day are often enough to relieve discomfort, even if the hemorrhoids are thrombosed.

Witch hazel soaks (e.g., Tucks) are also effective for pain. Topical anesthetics, such as lidocaine (Xylocaine), are useful for severe pain. Dibucaine (Nupercainal) ointment, an over-the-counter remedy, may be applied for mild to moderate pain. This ointment should be used only temporarily, however, because it can mask worsening symptoms and delay diagnosis of a severe disorder. If itching or inflammation is present, the health care provider prescribes a steroid preparation, such as hydrocortisone. Cleansing the anal area with moistened cleansing tissues rather than standard toilet tissue helps to avoid irritation. The anal area should be cleansed gently by dabbing, rather than by wiping.

Diets high in fiber and fluids are recommended to promote regular bowel movements without straining. Stool softeners, such as docusate sodium (Colace), can be used temporarily. Irritating laxatives are avoided, as well as foods and beverages that can make hemorrhoids worse. Spicy foods, nuts, coffee, and alcohol can be irritating. Clients are encouraged to avoid sitting for long periods of time. The health care provider may prescribe oral analgesics for pain if the hemorrhoids are thrombosed.

Conservative treatment should alleviate symptoms in 3 to 5 days. If symptoms continue or recur frequently, the client may require surgical intervention.

SURGICAL MANAGEMENT. The surgeon can perform several procedures for symptomatic hemorrhoids. The type of surgery depends on the degree of prolapse, whether there is thrombosis, and the overall condition of the client. Surgical methods include sclerotherapy, elastic band ligation, cryosurgery, and hemorrhoidectomy.

In **sclerotherapy,** the surgeon injects a sclerosing agent into the tissues around the hemorrhoids to obliterate the vessels. Sclerotherapy can be done on an outpatient basis without long-term pain. However, it can be done only for low-grade hemorrhoids.

Elastic band ligation is considered a better method because of its success rate. One or two rubber bands are put on at one ambulatory care visit, and repeated visits may be needed for ligation of all hemorrhoids. Local pain after ligation does occur, and hemorrhage may also occur.

Cryosurgery, which can be done on an ambulatory care basis, involves freezing the hemorrhoid with a probe to cause necrosis. Because of its many disadvantages (e.g., profuse and foul drainage lasting up to 6 weeks; hemorrhage; large, painful skin tags; and incomplete destruction), cryosurgery is no longer a widely accepted method.

Hemorrhoidectomy, the standard treatment, can now be performed in an ambulatory care/same-day surgical setting. Approximately 10% of clients with symptomatic hemorrhoids undergo hemorrhoidectomies. The most common problem following a hemorrhoidectomy is pain, which is severe for 1 to 2 days after surgery. Urinary retention can also occur because of rectal spasms and anorectal tenderness. Hemorrhage, which may be internal and not visible or external, is a rare but potential complication.

The nurse teaches clients with hemorrhoids about the need for adhering to high-fiber, high-fluid diets to promote regular bowel patterns. The nurse advises clients to avoid stimulant laxatives, which are habit forming.

For clients who undergo any type of surgical intervention, the nurse monitors for hemorrhage and pain postoperatively. These clients, in particular, require ongoing interventions for pain because of its severity. Appropriate nursing interventions include the following:

- Assisting clients to a side-lying position
- Keeping fresh ice packs over the dressing until the packing is removed
- Use of moist heat (as in sitz baths) three or four times a day after the first 12 hours postoperatively

Vasodilation from the sitz bath redirects blood to the rectal area, which might cause the client to feel faint. The nurse may place an ice bag on the client's head during the sitz bath to prevent feelings of faintness. A flotation pad can be used under the buttocks for sitting.

The first postoperative bowel movement may be very painful. The physician usually prescribes stool softeners, such as docusate sodium, to begin on the first postoperative day. Opioid analgesics are administered before the client attempts to defecate, and the caregiver should stay nearby during the first defecation. All clients who have undergone a hemorrhoidectomy are monitored for urinary retention.

MALABSORPTION SYNDROME

OVERVIEW

Malabsorption is a syndrome associated with a variety of disorders and intestinal surgical procedures. Malabsorption interferes with the ability to absorb nutrients and is a result of a generalized flattening of the mucosa of the small intestine. With various disorders, physiologic mechanisms limit absorption of nutrients because of one or more of the following abnormalities:

- Bile salt deficiencies
- Enzyme deficiencies
- Presence of bacteria
- Disruption of the mucosal lining of the small intestine
- Altered lymphatic and vascular circulation
- Decrease in the gastric or intestinal surface area

The nutrient involved in malabsorption depends on the type and location of the abnormality in the intestinal tract.

Deficiencies of bile salts can lead to malabsorption of fats and fat-soluble vitamins. Bile salt deficiencies can result from decreased synthesis of bile in the liver, bile obstruction, or alteration of bile salt absorption in the small intestine.

Enzymes normally found in the intestine split disaccharides (complex sugars) to monosaccharides (simple sugars). Examples of these enzymes are lactase, sucrase, maltase, and isomaltase. Lactase deficiency is the most common disaccharide enzyme deficiency. Without sufficient amounts of this enzyme, the body is not able to break down lactose. Lactase deficiency can be due to genetic transmission, injury to intestinal mucosa from viral hepatitis, bacterial proliferation in the intestine, or sprue. Deficiencies of the other disaccharide enzymes are rare.

Pancreatic enzymes are also necessary for absorption of vitamin B_{12}. With destruction or obstruction of the pancreas or insufficient pancreatic stimulation, these nutrients are malabsorbed. Chronic pancreatitis, pancreatic carcinoma, resection of the pancreas, and cystic fibrosis can cause these malabsorption problems.

Loops of bowel can accumulate intestinal contents, resulting in bacterial overgrowth, when there is a decrease in peristalsis. Bacteria at these sites break down bile salts, and fewer salts are available for fat absorption. These bacteria can also ingest vitamin B_{12}, which contributes to vitamin B_{12} deficiency. This phenomenon can occur after a gastrectomy or with progressive systemic sclerosis and diabetic enteropathy.

Disruption of the mucosal lining of the intestine is responsible for the malabsorption that occurs with celiac (nontropical) sprue, tropical sprue, Crohn's disease, and ulcerative colitis.

In celiac (nontropical) sprue, the absorptive surface area in the small intestine is lost; there is malabsorption of most nutrients. Celiac sprue is thought to be due to a genetic immune hypersensitivity response to gluten or its breakdown products or to result from the accumulation of gluten in the diet with peptidase deficiency.

Tropical sprue is caused by an infectious agent that has not been identified but is thought to be bacterial. Mucosal changes occur in a more widespread manner than in celiac sprue. However, the changes are not as severe as in celiac sprue. Tropical sprue results in malabsorption of fat, folic acid, and vitamin B_{12} in later stages of the disease.

The inflammation in Crohn's disease interferes with the surface of cells absorbing bile salts and therefore leads to fat malabsorption. In ulcerative colitis, protein loss may occur.

Obstruction to lymphatic flow in the intestine can lead to loss of plasma proteins along with loss of minerals (such as iron, copper, and calcium), vitamin B_{12}, folic acid, and lipids. Lymphatic obstruction can be caused by many conditions. Certain cancers, such as lymphoma, inflammatory states, radiation enteritis, Crohn's disease, Whipple's disease, congestive heart failure, and constrictive pericarditis, are causes of lymphatic obstruction.

Interference with blood flow to the intestinal mucosa, which occurs in celiac and superior mesenteric artery disease, results in malabsorption. With intestinal surgery, there is loss of the surface area needed to facilitate absorption. Resection of the ileum results in vitamin B_{12}, bile salt, and other nutrient deficiencies. Gastric surgery is one of the most common causes of malabsorption and maldigestion. Other conditions associated with maldigestion and malabsorption include small-bowel ischemia and radiation enteritis.

➤ COLLABORATIVE MANAGEMENT

Assessment

Diarrhea is the classic symptom of malabsorption. It occurs secondary to unabsorbed nutrients, which add to the bulk of the stool, and unabsorbed fat. Steatorrhea (greater than normal amounts of fat in the feces) is a common sign. Steatorrhea is a result of bile salt deconjugation, nonabsorbed fats, or bacteria in the intestine. Not all clients with malabsorption will have diarrhea; instead, many clients manifest an increased stool mass. Other clinical manifestations include the following:

- Weight loss
- Bloating and flatus (carbohydrate malabsorption)
- Decreased libido
- Easy bruising (purpura)
- Anemia (with iron and folic acid or vitamin B_{12} deficiencies)
- Bone pain (with calcium and vitamin D deficiencies)
- Edema (caused by hypoproteinemia)

Laboratory studies reveal a decrease in mean corpuscular volume (MCV), mean corpuscular hemoglobin (MCH), and mean corpuscular hemoglobin concentration (MCHC). These decreases indicate hypochromic microcytic anemia resulting from iron deficiency. Increased MCV and variable MCH and MCHC values indicate macrocytic anemia resulting from vitamin B_{12} and folic acid deficiencies. Serum iron levels are low in protein malabsorption because of insufficient gastric acid for use of iron. Serum cholesterol levels may be low from decreased absorption and digestion of fat. Low serum calcium levels may indicate malabsorption of vitamin D and amino acids. Low levels of serum vitamin A (retinol) and carotene, its precursor, indicate a bile salt deficiency and malabsorption of fat. Serum albumin and total protein levels are low if protein loss occurs. A quantitative fecal fat analysis is elevated in either malabsorption or maldigestion.

A lactose tolerance test result that shows less than a 20% rise in the blood glucose level over the fasting blood glucose level indicates lactose intolerance. A monosaccharide test validates or rules out lactase deficiency. The xylose absorption test can reveal low urine and serum D-xylose levels if malabsorption in the small intestine is present, a common finding in celiac sprue. An abnormal D-xylose test can indicate bacterial overgrowth in the small intestine.

The Schilling test measures urinary excretion of vitamin B_{12} for diagnosis of pernicious anemia and a variety of other malabsorption syndromes. The bile acid breath test assesses the absorption of bile salt. If the client has bacterial overgrowth, the bile salts will become deconjugated, and the carbon dioxide level in the breath will peak earlier than expected.

Biopsy of the small intestine is performed via an oral endoscopic procedure for diagnosis of tropical sprue or celiac sprue. Ultrasonography is used to diagnose pancreatic tumors and tumors in the small intestine that are causing malabsorption. X-ray studies of the gastrointestinal (GI) tract reveal pancreatic calcifications, tumors, or other abnormalities that cause malabsorption. Barium enema examination shows mucosal changes representative of celiac sprue or other abnormalities.

Interventions

Interventions for most malabsorption syndromes focus on avoidance of dietary substances that aggravate malabsorption and supplementation of nutrients. Surgical or nonsurgical management of the primary disease may be indicated. Drug therapy may also improve or resolve malabsorption.

Dietary management includes a low-fat diet for clients who have gallbladder disease, severe steatorrhea, cystic fibrosis, and progressive systemic sclerosis. A low-fat diet may or may not be indicated for pancreatic insufficiency, because this disorder improves with enzyme replacement. Some clinicians believe that limitation of fat intake is not necessary with enzyme replacement. Dietary intake of fat is actually beneficial to the client because it has a high amount of calories. After a total gastrectomy, a high-protein, high-calorie diet and small, frequent meals are recommended. Lactose-free or lactose-restricted diets are available for clients with lactase deficiency, and gluten-free diets are available for clients with celiac sprue.

The physician orders nutritional supplements according to the specific deficiency. Common supplements include the following:

- Water-soluble vitamins, such as folic acid, vitamin B_{12}, and vitamin B complex
- Fat-soluble vitamins, such as vitamin A, vitamin D, and vitamin K
- Minerals, such as calcium, iron, and magnesium
- Pancreatic enzymes, such as pancrelipase (Pancrease, Viokase)

Antibiotics are used to treat tropical sprue, Whipple's disease, and other disorders involving bacterial overgrowth. Tropical sprue is treated with trimethoprim/sulfamethoxazole (Bactrim, Septra). Bacterial overgrowth can be caused by a variety of disorders but is often treated with tetracycline and metronidazole (Flagyl, Novonidazol🍁). Steroids are sometimes given in celiac disease to decrease inflammation.

Drug therapy is used to control the clinical manifestations of malabsorption. Antidiarrheal agents, such as diphenoxylate hydrochloride and atropine sulfate (Lomotil) or kaolin with pectin (Kaopectate, Kao-Con), are often used to control diar-

CHART 57-8

BEST PRACTICE *for*
Special Skin Care for Clients with Chronic Diarrhea

- Use medicated wipes or premoistened disposable wipes rather than toilet tissue to clean the perineal area.
- Clean the perineal area well with mild soap and warm water after each stool; rinse soap from the area well.
- If the physician allows, provide a sitz bath several times a day.
- Apply a thin coat of vitamin A & D ointment or other medicated protective covering, such as aloe products, after each stool.
- Keep the client off the affected buttock area.
- For open areas, cover with thin DuoDerm or Tegaderm occlusive dressing to promote rapid healing.
- Observe for fungal or yeast infections, which appear as dark red rashes. Obtain an order for medication if this problem occurs.

rhea and steatorrhea (see Chart 57-1). Anticholinergics, such as dicyclomine hydrochloride (Bentyl, Bentylol✤), are often given before meals to inhibit gastric motility. IV fluids may be necessary to replenish fluid losses associated with diarrhea.

The nurse provides special measures to protect the skin when diarrhea occurs (Chart 57-8). The nurse conducts an ongoing assessment for clinical manifestations of malabsorption and relates these to activities and dietary intake. For example, clients with steatorrhea are monitored for fluid and electrolyte imbalances and are encouraged to ingest electrolyte-rich liquids liberally. The nurse teaches clients the rationale for dietary, drug, and surgical management of nutritional deficiencies and evaluates interventions on the basis of changes in or resolution of clinical manifestations.

ONLINE RESOURCES

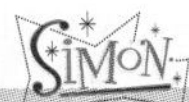

For suggested readings and Internet resources, go to http://www.wbsaunders.com/SIMON/Iggy/.

SELECTED BIBLIOGRAPHY

Alderman, J. (1999). Managing irritable bowel syndrome. *ADVANCE for Nurse Practitioners, 7*(1), 40-46.

American Cancer Society. (1997). Colorectal cancer. *CA: A Cancer Journal for Clinicians, 47*(2), 66-128.

Beackington, E. (2000). Irritable bowel syndrome: An update on treatment options. *Advance for Nurse Practitioners,* October, pp. 32-36.

Bonci, L., et al. (1998). Is malabsorption causing your patient's GI symptoms? *Patient Care,* March, pp. 93-116.

Bradley, M., & Pupiales, M. (1997). Essential elements of ostomy care. *American Journal of Nursing, 97*(7), 38-46.

Cantanzaro, J., & Serembus, J. (1998). High tech wound and ostomy care in the home setting. *Critical Care Nursing Clinics of North America, 10*(3), 327-338.

Carlson, E. (1998). Irritable bowel syndrome. *Nurse Practitioner, 23*(1), 82-93.

Cavalieri, J., & Franklin, B. (1998). Hereditary nonpolyposis colon cancer. *American Journal of Nursing, 98*(10), 42-43.

Clevenger, F., & Tepas, J. (1997). Perioperative management of patients with major trauma injuries. *AORN Journal, 65*(3), 583-594.

Greenlee, R., et al. (2000). Cancer statistics 2000. *CA: A Cancer Journal for Clinicians, 50*(1), 16.

Hardcastle, J.D. (1997). Colorectal cancer. *CA: A Cancer Journal for Clinicians, 47*(2), 66-68.

Harris, H., et al. (1999). Leukocytosis and free fluid are important indicators of isolated intestinal injury after blunt trauma. *Journal of Trauma, Injury, Infection, and Critical Care, 46*(4), 656-659.

Held-Warmkessel, J. (1998). Colon cancer: Prevention and detection strategies. *ADVANCE for Nurse Practitioners, 6*(7), 42-45.

Jenks, J.M., Morin, K.H., & Tomaselli, N. (1997). The influence of ostomy surgery on body image in patients with cancer. *Applied Nursing Research, 10*(4), 174-180.

Jeppesen, P., et al. (1997). Essential fatty acid deficiency in patients with severe fat malabsorption. *American Journal of Clinical Nutrition, 65,* 837-843.

Jessup, J.M., et al. (1997). Diagnosing colorectal carcinoma: Clinical and molecular approaches. *CA: A Cancer Journal for Clinicians, 47*(2), 70-92.

Koloski, N., Talley, N., & Boyce, P. (2000). The impact of functional gastrointestinal disorders on quality of life. *American Journal of Gastroenterology, 95*(1), 67-71.

Korsten, M., & Abittan, C. (1999). Obstipation and lower abdominal pain. *Clinical Advisor, 2*(6), 68-70.

Landis, S.H., et al. (1999). Cancer statistics, 1999. *Ca: A Cancer Journal for Clinicians, 49*(1), 8-32.

Lerman, C., et al. (1999). Genetic testing in families with hereditary nonpolyposis colon cancer. *Journal of the American Medical Association, 281*(17), 1618-1622.

Levins, T.T. (2000). Using ultrasound to assess blunt abdominal trauma. *Nursing2000, 30*(5), 32cc14-32cc15.

Locke, G.R., et al. (2000). Risk factors for irritable bowel syndrome: Role of analgesics and food sensitivities. *American Journal of Gastroenterology, 95*(1), 157-164.

Markowitz, A.J., & Winawer, S.J. (1997). Management of colorectal polyps. *CA: A Cancer Journal for Clinicians, 47*(2), 93-112.

O'Brien, B. (1999). Coming of age with an ostomy. *American Journal of Nursing, 99*(8), 71-74.

Pharmacia & Upjohn Company. (1997). Data on file. Kalamazoo, MI: Author.

Pontieri-Lewis, V. (2000). Colorectal cancer: Prevention and screening. *MEDSURG Nursing, 9*(1), 9-13.

Saddler, D., & Ellis, C. (1999). Colorectal cancer. *Seminars in Oncology Nursing, 15*(1), 58-69.

Schmulson, M., et al. (2000). Correlation of symptom criteria with perception thresholds during rectosigmoid distension in irritable bowel syndrome patients. *American Journal of Gastroenterology, 95*(1), 152-155.

Shelton, B. (1999). Intestinal obstruction. *AACN Clinical Issues: Advanced Practice in Acute and Critical Care, 10*(4), 478-491.

Sommers, M.S., & Johnson, S.A. (1997). *Davis's manual of nursing therapeutics for diseases and disorders.* Philadelphia: F.A. Davis.

Toner, B., & Akman, D. (2000). Gender role and irritable bowel syndrome: Literature review and hypothesis. *American Journal of Gastroenterology, 95*(1), 11-16.

Town, J. (1997). Bringing acute abdomen into focus. *Nursing97, 27*(5), 52-57.

Weber, T., et al. (1999). Novel hMLH1 and hMSH2 germline mutations in African-Americans with colorectal cancer. *Journal of the American Medical Association, 281*(24), 2316-2320.

Yoshii, H., et al. (1998). Usefulness and limitations of ultrasonography in the initial evaluation of blunt abdominal trauma. *Journal of Trauma, Injury, Infection and Critical Care, 45*(1), 45-51.

CHAPTER 58

Interventions for Clients with Inflammatory Intestinal Disorders

CONSTANCE VISOVSKY

Learning Objectives

After studying this chapter, you should be able to:

1. Compare and contrast the typical physical assessment findings associated with appendicitis and peritonitis.
2. Prioritize nursing care for the client who has peritonitis.
3. Discuss the common causes of gastroenteritis.
4. Compare and contrast the pathophysiology and clinical manifestations of ulcerative colitis and Crohn's disease.
5. Analyze priority nursing diagnoses and collaborative problems for clients with chronic inflammatory bowel disease (IBD).
6. Explain the purpose of and nursing implications related to drug therapy for clients with IBD.
7. Formulate a postoperative plan of care for a client undergoing a colon resection/colectomy and colostomy or ileostomy.
8. Develop a teaching plan for a client needing community-based care for a new ostomy.
9. Identify expected outcomes for clients with chronic IBD.
10. Explain the role of diet therapy in managing the client with diverticular disease.
11. Describe the comfort measures that the nurse can use for the client with an anal abscess, fissure, or fistula.
12. Discuss ways that helminthic infestation, parasitic infection, and food poisoning can be prevented.

SIMON

Go to http://www.wbsaunders.com/SIMON/Iggy/ for self-assessment questions related to these Learning Objectives.

Inflammatory bowel disease (IBD) is a condition of the small and/or large intestine involving inflammation that can be acute or chronic in duration. Chronic forms of IBD are characterized by periods of exacerbation and remission. Inflammatory and infectious intestinal disorders are often difficult to differentiate, since many of the characteristics of infectious processes mimic those of more chronic conditions. The nurse's involvement in assessing and managing intestinal disorders is essential to early diagnosis and successful treatment.

ACUTE INFLAMMATORY BOWEL DISORDERS

Appendicitis, peritonitis, and gastroenteritis are the most common acute inflammatory bowel problems. These disorders are potentially life threatening, and can have major systemic complications if not treated promptly.

Appendicitis

OVERVIEW

Appendicitis is acute inflammation of the vermiform appendix—the blind pouch attached to the cecum of the colon that is usually located in the right iliac region, just below the ileocecal valve. The appendix has no known function. As part of the cecum, it fills with food and empties on a regular basis. Inflammation of the appendix can occur when the lumen (opening) of the appendix is obstructed. Inflammation leads to infection as bacteria invade the wall of the appendix.

When the lumen is blocked, the mucosa continues to secrete fluid until the pressure within the lumen exceeds venous pressure. Blood flow to the appendix is restricted, and infection causes more swelling, which further impedes blood flow. Gangrene from hypoxia or perforation can occur within 24 to 36 hours. If this process occurs slowly, adjacent organs may wall off the area, and a localized abscess develops. If the infectious process occurs rapidly, peritonitis (inflammation of the peritoneum) may result. All complications of peritonitis are serious. Acute appendicitis is the most common cause of acute inflammation in the right lower quadrant. Consequently, it is one of the most common indications for emergency abdominal surgery.

When obstruction is present, calculi composed of fecal material (fecaliths), calcium phosphate–rich mucus, and inorganic salts may be the most common cause of the initial obstruction. Other causes of obstruction include tumors, viral infections, and worms. However, recent evidence points to ulceration of the mucosa as the primary cause of appendicitis (Silen, 1998). Infection by viral or fungal pathogens has been suggested as the cause of ulceration. Although appendicitis affects a person at any age, the peak incidence is between the ages of 20 and 30 years. Appendicitis affects men and women equally, except before 25 years of age, when males are affected more often than females at a 3:2 ratio (Silen, 1998).

It is thought that chronic infection of the appendix can occur, but this is not usually the cause of abdominal pain that lasts for weeks or months. Recurrent acute appendicitis does sometimes occur, often with complete remission of inflammation between acute attacks. In rare instances, acute appendicitis may be the first manifestation of Crohn's disease.

CONSIDERATIONS FOR OLDER ADULTS

Appendicitis is relatively rare at extremes in age; however, perforation is more common in older people, causing a higher mortality rate. The diagnosis of appendicitis is difficult to establish in older adults, as symptoms of pain and tenderness are not as pronounced in this age-group. As a result, 30% of older clients with appendicitis develop perforation due to a delay in diagnosis. The development of peritonitis is associated with a 15% mortality rate in older adults (Silen, 1998).

COLLABORATIVE MANAGEMENT

Assessment

The history obtained from the client outlining the sequence of events provides the most important assessment of appendicitis. The most common symptom is abdominal pain, which results from contractions of the appendix or distention of its lumen. With *classic* appendicitis, abdominal pain in the epigastric or periumbilical area is the initial symptom. Pain may not be localized, however, and can exist anywhere in the abdomen or flanks. The pain at this time is described as mild or cramping. Nausea and vomiting follow in 50% to 60% of cases. As the inflammation spreads to the peritoneal surface, the pain becomes more steady and severe and the location shifts to the right lower quadrant. Abdominal pain that increases with cough or movement and is relieved by flexion of the right hip or the knees suggests a perforated appendix with peritonitis. Anorexia is a frequent finding associated with acute appendicitis.

Abdominal tenderness on palpation is the most common, important, and reliable symptom. In later stages of inflammation, tenderness becomes more localized and is noted with palpation of the right lower quadrant. This area is referred to as **McBurney's point;** it is located midway between the anterior iliac crest and the umbilicus in the right lower quadrant (Figure 58-1). The nurse may feel tenseness of the muscles (muscle rigidity) over the tender area. Rigidity over the whole abdomen, accompanied by tense positioning and guarding, indicates a perforated appendix with peritonitis. Perforation rarely occurs within 24 hours of the onset of symptoms, but the incidence of peritonitis rises to as high as 80% after 48 hours. Rebound tenderness is a term used to describe a sensation of severe pain that occurs after deep pressure is applied and released. This maneuver involves pressing a finger into the abdomen at a point away from the pain and is performed by the physician or advanced-practice nurse.

The client's temperature is usually normal or slightly elevated at 99° to 100.5° F (37.2° to 38° C). A temperature of 101° F (38.2° C) or higher suggests the presence of peritonitis. As the temperature rises, a corresponding rise in pulse rate will be noted.

Because the clinical manifestations associated with many other medical conditions are similar to those of acute appendicitis, arriving at a diagnosis is often difficult. It is important for the nurse to determine the sequence of symptoms. For example, nausea and vomiting that precede abdominal pain often indicate gastroenteritis.

Clinical manifestations that do not follow the classic pattern can occur as a result of variations in the anatomic location of the appendix. The appendix can be located deep in the pelvis, in the right upper quadrant, or even in the left lower quadrant.

Laboratory findings do not establish the diagnosis, but there is often a moderate elevation of the white blood cell (WBC) count (leukocytosis) to 10,000 to 18,000/mm³ with a "shift to the left" (an increased number of immature WBCs). A WBC elevation greater than 20,000/mm³ may indicate a perforated appendix. An ultrasound study may show the presence of an enlarged appendix. If symptoms are recurrent or prolonged, a barium enema or computed tomography (CT) scan may reveal the presence of a fecalith.

Interventions

All clients with suspected or confirmed appendicitis are hospitalized and examined by a surgeon. If the diagnosis is questionable, the health care team observes the client before surgical exploration.

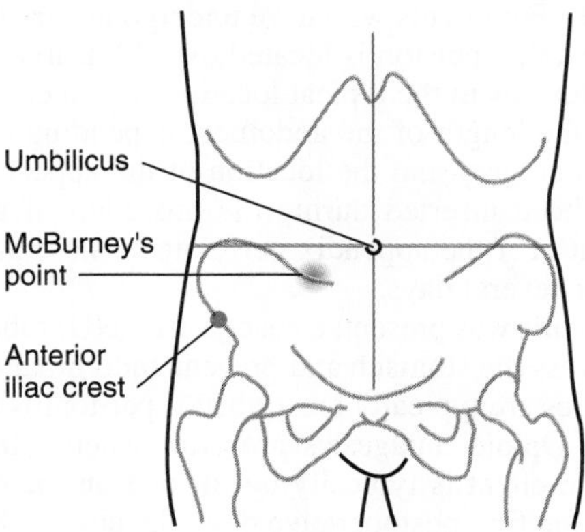

Figure 58-1 ● McBurney's point is located midway between the anterior iliac crest and the umbilicus in the right lower quadrant. This is the classic area for localized tenderness during the later stages of appendicitis.

NONSURGICAL MANAGEMENT. After admission to the hospital, the physician keeps the client with suspected or known appendicitis on nothing by mouth (NPO) status to prepare for the possibility of emergency surgery and to avoid aggravating the inflammatory process. The nurse administers intravenous (IV) fluids, as ordered, to prevent fluid and electrolyte imbalance and to replenish fluid volume. If the semi-Fowler's position can be tolerated, the nurse advises the client to maintain this position so that abdominal drainage, if any, can be contained in the lower abdomen.

Once the diagnosis of appendicitis is confirmed, the surgeon schedules surgery. The nurse may administer opioid analgesics, as ordered, while the client is being prepared for surgery. The client with suspected appendicitis should not receive laxatives or enemas, which can cause perforation of the appendix. Heat should never be applied to the abdomen because this may increase circulation to the appendix and result in increased inflammation and perforation.

SURGICAL MANAGEMENT. Surgery is required as soon as possible. If the diagnosis is not definitive but the client is at high risk for complications from suspected appendicitis, the surgeon may perform an exploratory laparotomy to rule out appendicitis.

PREOPERATIVE CARE. Preoperative teaching is often limited because the client is in pain or may be transferred to the operating suite for emergency surgery. The nurse prepares the client for general anesthesia and surgery (see Chapter 17).

OPERATIVE PROCEDURES. An **appendectomy** is the removal of the inflamed appendix. In a *traditional,* uncomplicated appendectomy, the surgeon removes the appendix through an incision approximately 3 inches (7.5 cm) long in the right lower quadrant. The incision is larger if the appendix is in an atypical position or if peritonitis is present.

An appendectomy is often done via **laparoscopy.** The surgeon makes several small incisions through which an endoscope is inserted. A cutting instrument is threaded through the endoscope, and the appendix is removed.

POSTOPERATIVE CARE. Postoperative care of the client who has undergone an appendectomy includes the care required for any client who has received general anesthesia (see Chapter 19). For clients who have undergone a traditional appendectomy, the incision is located over McBurney's point if the appendix was in the typical location. The incision may be as long as the length of the abdomen, depending on the area explored in surgery and the location of the appendix. Drains may have been inserted during the procedure if an abscess was present or if the appendix perforated. The drains are left in place for several days.

If peritonitis was present, a nasogastric (NG) tube is placed to decompress the stomach and prevent abdominal distention. IV antibiotics are typically prescribed if peritonitis or abscess is present. Opioid analgesics are administered for pain as needed. The client is typically out of bed on the evening of surgery or the first postoperative day. The client who has had an uncomplicated appendectomy via laparoscopy may stay overnight or may be discharged on the day of surgery. In this case, no NG tubes or drains are needed.

The client who has undergone an uncomplicated appendectomy usually recovers rapidly. After a traditional surgical procedure, he or she can resume normal activity in 2 to 4 weeks. If surgery has been complicated by perforation or peritonitis, he or she is hospitalized for 5 to 7 days or longer.

If the client is discharged to a home setting, the nurse assesses his or her ability to function with the added tasks of incision care, drug therapy, and some activity restrictions. The nurse assesses the home environment and the need for support to meet physical needs.

Peritonitis

OVERVIEW

Peritonitis is an acute inflammation of the endothelial lining of the abdominal cavity, or peritoneum. Peritonitis can be classified as primary or secondary, localized or generalized. Peritonitis is a life-threatening illness and is associated with several abdominal disorders.

Pathophysiology

PATHOLOGIC CHANGES

Normally, the peritoneal cavity contains approximately 50 mL of sterile fluid (transudate), which serves to prevent friction in the abdominal cavity during peristalsis (Hirsch & Caswell, 1999). When the peritoneal cavity is contaminated by bacteria, the body initially produces an inflammatory reaction that walls off a localized area to fight the infection. This local reaction involves vascular dilation and increased capillary permeability, allowing for transport of leukocytes and subsequent phagocytosis of the offending organisms. If this walling off process fails, the inflammation spreads and contamination becomes massive, resulting in diffuse peritonitis.

COMPLICATIONS

Vascular dilation continues, along with hyperemia (increased blood flow) and a fluid shift. The body responds to the infectious process by shunting extra blood to the area of inflammation. Fluid is shifted from the extracellular fluid (ECF) compartment into the peritoneal cavity, connective tissues, and gastrointestinal (GI) tract ("third spacing"). This shift of fluid out of the vascular space can result in a significant decrease in circulatory volume. The rate of decreasing circulatory volume is proportional to the degree of peritoneal involvement. Severely decreased circulatory volume can result in insufficient perfusion of the kidneys, leading to renal failure with electrolyte imbalance.

Peristalsis slows or stops in response to severe peritoneal infection, and the lumen of the bowel becomes distended with gas and fluid. Fluid that normally flows to the small bowel and the colon for reabsorption accumulates in the intestine in volumes of 7 to 8 L daily. The toxins or bacteria responsible for the peritonitis can also enter the bloodstream from the peritoneal area, leading to bacteremia or septicemia (bacterial invasion of the blood).

Respiratory problems can occur as a result of increased abdominal pressure against the diaphragm from intestinal distention and fluid shifts to the peritoneal cavity. Pain can interfere with ventilatory efforts when the client has an increased oxygen demand because of the infectious process.

TYPES OF PERITONITIS

Primary peritonitis is an acute bacterial infection that develops as a result of contamination of the peritoneum through the vascular system. Tuberculous peritonitis that arises from a tuberculin infection originating elsewhere in the body is a type of primary peritonitis. Clients with alcoholic cirrhosis and ascites, in the absence of a perforated organ, often manifest peritonitis, which may be due to leakage of bacteria through the wall of the intestine.

Secondary peritonitis is usually caused by bacterial invasion as a result of an acute abdominal disorder. Secondary peritonitis can develop as a result of a gangrenous bowel, perforation of the viscera by blunt or penetrating trauma, or bile leakage.

Etiology

Peritonitis is caused by contamination of the peritoneal cavity by bacteria or chemicals. Bacteria gain entry into the peritoneum by perforation or from an external penetrating wound. The most common causes of bacterial peritonitis are appendicitis and perforations associated with peptic ulcer disease, diverticulitis, a gangrenous gallbladder, or bowel obstruction. Bacterial invasion can also occur from an ascending infection through the reproductive tract, as in salpingitis or a septic abortion. Other causes of peritonitis include perforating tumors, ulcerative colitis, foreign bodies (from trauma), leakage or contamination during a surgical procedure, and infection by skin pathogens in clients undergoing continuous ambulatory peritoneal dialysis (CAPD). Bacteria responsible for peritonitis include *Escherichia coli, Streptococcus, Staphylococcus, Pneumococcus,* and *Gonococcus.* Chemical peritonitis arises from leakage of bile, pancreatic enzymes, and gastric acid.

Incidence/Prevalence

Primary peritonitis accounts for only a small percentage of the cases of peritonitis. The incidence of secondary peritonitis is difficult to determine because data usually relate to the underlying cause, such as appendicitis or peptic ulcer.

COLLABORATIVE MANAGEMENT

Assessment

HISTORY

The nurse questions the client regarding a history of abdominal pain and determines if the pain is localized or generalized. The nurse also asks about a history of a low-grade fever or recent spikes in temperature.

PHYSICAL ASSESSMENT/CLINICAL MANIFESTATIONS

Physical findings of peritonitis (Chart 58-1) depend on several factors: the stage of the disease, the ability of the body to localize the process by walling off the infection, and whether the inflammation has progressed to generalized peritonitis. The client typically appears acutely ill, lying still, possibly with the knees flexed. Movement is guarded, and the client may report and show signs of pain (e.g., facial grimacing) with coughing or movement of any type. During inspection, the nurse may observe progressive abdominal distention if the inflammation markedly reduces intestinal motility. The nurse may auscultate for bowel sounds, but these usually disappear with progression of the inflammation.

The cardinal signs of peritonitis are abdominal pain and tenderness. In the client with localized peritonitis, the abdomen is tender on palpation in a well-defined area of the abdomen with rebound tenderness in this area. With generalized peritonitis, tenderness is widespread. Abdominal wall rigidity is a common finding. The client may have a high fever because of the infectious process, with tachycardia occurring in response to the fever. The nurse assesses whether the client has dry mucous membranes with poor tissue turgor and a low urine output. A low urine output occurs because fluid accumulates in the peritoneal cavity, the GI tract, and connective tissues, resulting in a fluid deficit in the vascular space. Nausea and vomiting may also be present. Hiccups may occur as a result of diaphragmatic irritation. Depending on the severity of the peritonitis, the nurse may find that the client has a compromised respiratory status.

DIAGNOSTIC ASSESSMENT

White blood cell (WBC) counts are commonly elevated to 20,000/mm^3 with a high neutrophil count. A series of blood culture studies may be done to determine whether septicemia has occurred and to identify the causative organism to enable appropriate therapy.

The health care provider orders laboratory tests to assess fluid and electrolyte balance and renal status, including the following:

- Electrolytes
- Blood urea nitrogen (BUN)
- Creatinine
- Hemoglobin
- Hematocrit

Arterial blood gas values are obtained to assess respiratory function and acid-base balance.

CHART 58-1

KEY FEATURES *of* Peritonitis

- Abdominal pain (localized, poorly localized, or referred to the shoulder or thorax)
- Rigid, boardlike abdomen
- Distended abdomen
- Nausea, anorexia, vomiting
- Diminishing bowel sounds
- Inability to pass flatus or feces
- Rebound tenderness in the abdomen
- High fever
- Tachycardia
- Dehydration from high fever (poor skin turgor)
- Decreased urine output
- Hiccups
- Possible compromise in respiratory status

Abdominal x-ray films are obtained to assess for free air or fluid in the abdominal cavity, which indicates perforation. The x-ray films may also show dilation, edema, and inflammation of the small and large intestines.

The physician may perform a diagnostic peritoneal lavage by instilling 1 L of fluid through a peritoneal dialysis catheter. Lavage fluid positive for peritonitis is characterized by the following: more than 500 WBCs/mL^3 of fluid, more than 50,000 red blood cells (RBCs)/mL, or the presence of bacteria on a Gram stain. Bile-stained green fluid may indicate a ruptured gallbladder or perforated intestine, which can lead to chemical peritonitis.

Interventions

All clients with peritonitis are hospitalized because of the severe nature of the illness. If complications are extensive, the client may be admitted to a critical care unit. Nursing interventions focus on the early identification of complications.

NONSURGICAL MANAGEMENT. The physician prescribes IV fluids and broad-spectrum antibiotics immediately after establishing the diagnosis of peritonitis. IV fluids are necessary to replace fluids collected in the peritoneum and bowel. Daily weight and intake and output are monitored to assess fluid status. A nasogastric (NG) tube is inserted to decompress the stomach and the intestine, and the client is on NPO status. The nurse administers oxygen, as ordered, according to the client's respiratory status. The health care provider will most likely institute pain management with IV analgesics, such as morphine sulfate administered via a patient-controlled analgesia (PCA) pump. Even with nonsurgical management of peritonitis, the nurse can expect the health care provider to order a surgical consultation in the event that surgery becomes necessary.

SURGICAL MANAGEMENT. Abdominal surgery is the optimal treatment for identifying and repairing the cause of the peritonitis. If the client is so critically ill that surgery would be life threatening, it may be delayed. Surgery focuses on controlling the contamination, removing foreign material from the peritoneal cavity, and draining collected fluid.

The surgeon performs an **exploratory laparotomy** to remove or repair the inflamed or perforated organ. The abdominal cavity is opened surgically and explored for inflamed and perforated organs or other abnormalities.

PREOPERATIVE CARE. The preoperative care for the client undergoing an exploratory laparotomy is similar to that described in Chapter 17 for the client receiving general anesthesia.

OPERATIVE PROCEDURES. For an exploratory laparotomy, the surgeon makes an incision through the abdominal wall and explores the abdominal cavity. Part or all of a perforated or inflamed organ may be removed, depending on that organ's function. For example, an appendectomy is performed for an inflamed appendix; a colon resection, with or without a colostomy, is indicated for a perforated diverticulum or perforated colon secondary to a tumor. Before the abdominal cavity is closed, the surgeon irrigates the peritoneum with antibiotic solutions. Two to four catheters may also be inserted to drain the cavity and provide a route for irrigation postoperatively.

POSTOPERATIVE CARE. Postoperative care is similar to that for other clients undergoing surgery (see Chapter 19). Clients with peritonitis may have actual or potential multisystem complications. Therefore the nurse initially monitors level of consciousness, vital signs, respiratory status (respiratory rate and breath sounds), and fluid and electrolyte status (intake and output and laboratory values) at least hourly.

Positioning. The nurse maintains the client in a semi-Fowler's position to promote drainage of peritoneal contents in the inferior region of the abdominal cavity. This position also facilitates adequate respiratory excursion in that the diaphragm and abdominal contents are impinging on respiratory muscles.

Wound Care. The client is likely to have multiple incisions and drains. Because contamination at the time of surgery impedes healing of an incision with edges well approximated (by first intention), incisions are allowed to heal by second or third intention. These incisions necessitate meticulous care involving manual irrigation or packing, as ordered by the surgeon. If the surgeon orders peritoneal irrigation through a drain, the nurse maintains sterile technique during manual irrigation, usually by using a catheter-tipped syringe. The nurse determines that the client is not retaining irrigant by ensuring the absence of abdominal distention or pain and by monitoring irrigant intake and output.

As a result of the loss of fluids from the extracellular space to the peritoneal cavity, IV fluid replacement and maintenance are indicated for all clients with peritonitis. Fluid volume deficit also occurs as a result of nasogastric suctioning and NPO status. Normal saline or a balanced saline solution with potassium is administered intravenously according to electrolyte, BUN, and serum creatinine values. To assess fluid volume, the nurse monitors the client's vital signs, urine output, skin turgor, integrity of mucous membranes, and most important, weight. The nurse also assesses for edema from third spacing.

CONSIDERATIONS FOR OLDER ADULTS

The older adult often does not have characteristic signs and symptoms of dehydration. A change in mental status may be an early sign of fluid deficit. The nurse assesses skin turgor on an older client using the skin over the forehead or sternum. The nurse provides frequent mouth care to help maintain moist mucous membranes. The use of lemon-glycerin swabs is avoided because they can increase dryness.

Community-Based Care

The length of hospitalization depends on the extent and severity of the infectious process. Clients who have a localized abscess drained and who respond to antibiotics and IV fluids without respiratory, renal, or cardiac complications are discharged in about a week. Clients who experience complications of peritonitis, along with sepsis or shock, may require mechanical ventilation or hemodialysis, with hospital stays lasting for several weeks. Discharge planning varies with the degree of involvement of all body systems. Some clients may be transferred to a subacute unit to complete their antibiotic therapy and recovery.

If the client is being discharged to home, the nurse assesses his or her ability to function at home with the added task of incision care and a diminished activity tolerance. The nurse provides the client with written and oral instructions to report the following:

- Unusual or foul-smelling drainage
- Swelling, redness, or warmth or bleeding from the incision site
- A temperature higher than 101° F (38.2° C)
- The presence of abdominal pain

The nurse also instructs the client in proper handwashing and dressing change techniques, which include directions to dress wounds separately to avoid cross-contamination.

The physician prescribes an oral opioid analgesic and possibly an antibiotic. The nurse reviews information about these medications with the client and caregiver. For clients taking opioid analgesics for any length of time, a stool softener should be prescribed.

The nurse also explains diet and activity limitations. Diet depends on the type of surgery performed and the client's specific food tolerances at the time of discharge. All clients are told to refrain from any lifting for *at least* 6 weeks. Other activity limitations are made on an individual basis with the physician's recommendation.

Peritonitis is a life-threatening and consequently frightening illness. Incisional care can be demanding, and activity intolerance can be overwhelming. If complications have resolved, the nurse reassures clients that they can realistically expect to resume their previous lifestyle. Convalescence is often longer than that required for other types of surgery, however, because of the multisystemic involvement.

Clients with an incision healing by second or third intention may require dressings, solution, and catheter-tipped syringes to irrigate the wound. The nurse may arrange for a home care nurse to assess, irrigate, or pack the wound and change the dressing as needed. If a client needs assistance with activities of daily living, a home care aide or temporary placement in a skilled care facility may be indicated. The case manager collaborates with the health care team to determine the most appropriate setting for community-based care.

Gastroenteritis

OVERVIEW

Acute diarrheal illnesses cause significant morbidity among young children and adults, especially in less-developed nations of the world. **Gastroenteritis** is an increase in the frequency and water content of stools and/or vomiting as a result of inflammation of the mucous membranes of the stomach and intestinal tract. Gastroenteritis primarily affects the small bowel and can be of either viral or bacterial origin. Both forms have similar manifestations and are considered self-limiting in their course unless complications occur. All organisms that are implicated in gastroenteritis cause diarrhea; however, the organisms discussed in this section have distinguishing characteristics.

Authors disagree on classification of the infectious diseases described as gastroenteritis. Some investigators include shigellosis when discussing gastroenteritis; others consider shigellosis separately as a dysentery type of illness. Dysenteries affect the *large* bowel; gastroenteritis affects the *small* bowel. Other authors classify infectious disease of the intestine as bacterial, viral, or parasitic, without using the term *gastroenteritis.*

Food poisoning is sometimes described in conjunction with gastroenteritis, with specific reference to the organism causing the food poisoning. Gastroenteritis, however, differs from food poisoning with regard to transmission in the body, incubation time, and effect on immunity.

The following discussion of gastroenteritis includes the viral forms (epidemic viral, rotavirus) and the bacterial forms (*Campylobacter, Escherichia coli,* and shigellosis) (Table 58-1). Organisms associated with food poisoning and parasitic infections are discussed under Food Poisoning, p. 1295.

Pathophysiology/Etiology

Infection with viral and bacterial organisms can produce gastrointestinal (GI) illnesses in which watery diarrhea is the primary feature. These disorders can be caused by noninflammatory, inflammatory, or penetrating mechanisms. The infecting organism (e.g., enterotoxigenic *E. coli*) can release enterotoxin

TABLE 58-1 • COMMON TYPES OF GASTROENTERITIS AND THEIR CHARACTERISTICS

Type	Characteristics
VIRAL GASTROENTERITIS	
Epidemic viral	Caused by many parvovirus-type organisms Transmitted by the fecal-oral route in food and water Incubation period 10-51 hr Communicable during acute illness
Rotarvirus and Norwalk virus	Transmitted by the fecal-oral route and possibly the respiratory route Incubation in 48 hr Rotavirus is most common in infants and young children Norwalk virus affects young children and adults
BACTERIAL GASTROENTERITIS	
Campylobacter enteritis	Transmitted by the fecal-oral route or by contact with infected animals or infants Incubation period 1-10 days Communicable for 2-7 weeks
Escherichia coli diarrhea	Transmitted by fecally contaminated food, water, or fomites
Shigellosis	Transmitted by direct and indirect fecal-oral routes Incubation period 1-7 days Communicable during the acute illness to 4 weeks after the illness Humans possibly carriers for months

(a noninflammatory toxic substance specific to the intestinal mucosa), which results in diarrhea. The organism (e.g., *Shigella* or *Campylobacter*) can also attach itself to mucosal epithelium without penetrating it. Cells of the intestinal villi are then destroyed, and malabsorption results. Infections that are mediated by bacterial toxins cause the absorptive capacity of the distal small bowel and proximal colon to be overcome, resulting in diarrhea. Finally, the organism (e.g., rotavirus) can penetrate the intestine, causing cellular destruction, necrosis, and a potential for ulceration. Diarrhea occurs often with white blood cells (WBCs) or red blood cells (RBCs) present in the stool.

All of these situations result in *increased* GI motility, with fluids and electrolytes being secreted into the intestine at rapid rates. Invading organisms have increased capabilities of attaching to the intestinal mucosa if the normal intestinal flora is altered. This can occur in clients who are receiving antibiotics, are malnourished, or are debilitated. Two groups of viruses, the rotaviruses and Norwalk virus, as well as bacterial pathogens, are primary etiologic agents involved in the development of gastroenteritis.

TYPES OF GASTROENTERITIS

VIRAL GASTROENTERITIS. Many types of rotaviruses cause rotavirus gastroenteritis. The reservoir of these viruses is in humans. The viruses are transmitted via the fecal-oral route and possibly via the respiratory tract. Incubation is 48 hours. The period of communicability is during the acute stage and shortly after. Rotavirus infection is generally limited to infants and young children; by age 2 years, most children have acquired antibodies against most types of these viruses.

Norwalk virus infection can occur year-round and affects adults and children alike. This virus is spread by the oral-fecal route and is responsible for one third of all epidemics of viral gastroenteritis in developed countries. The virus is also a common cause of waterborne epidemics of gastroenteritis.

BACTERIAL GASTROENTERITIS. There are three general types of bacterial gastroenteritis:

- *E. coli* diarrhea ("traveler's diarrhea")
- *Campylobacter enteritis* ("traveler's diarrhea")
- *Shigellosis* (bacillary dysentery)

E. coli is the most common organism implicated in traveler's diarrhea. The reservoirs of *E. coli* are humans, who are often asymptomatic. The organism is transmitted through fecally contaminated food, water, or fomites (any other substance that transmits infection).

The etiologic feature of *Campylobacter* enteritis is the bacterium *Campylobacter jejuni;* reservoirs are domestic or wild animals and birds. *C. jejuni* is transmitted through the fecal-oral route by ingestion of water or food contaminated with feces or by direct contact with infected animals or infants. Incubation ranges from 1 to 10 days. The organism is communicable for several days to weeks throughout the course of the infection (usually 2 to 7 weeks).

Shigellosis is caused by infection with *Shigella* bacteria. Direct or indirect fecal-oral transmission can occur from an infected person or carrier. The incubation period before the illness is 1 to 7 days. The illness can be communicated during the acute phase and for up to 4 weeks after the onset of the illness. A person may be a carrier of this illness for months after the acute illness.

Incidence/Prevalence

Acute GI illnesses are the second most common disease worldwide. Acute diarrheal illnesses are the most common cause of morbidity and mortality among children and older adults in Asia, Africa, and Latin America. Gastroenteritis often occurs in epidemic outbreaks among groups of people.

Campylobacter enteritis occurs worldwide, commonly in epidemic outbreaks. Its incidence is highest during warm months. Diarrhea caused by *E. coli* also occurs worldwide, commonly in epidemics. The highest incidence is in areas of poor sanitation during warm months. Shigellosis occurs worldwide in every age-group but is most frequent in children under the age of 10 years. Children and older adults are more susceptible to *Shigella* because of their immature or depressed immune systems. Outbreaks of shigellosis are common in areas with crowded living conditions.

COLLABORATIVE MANAGEMENT

Assessment

The history elicited from the client can provide information related to the potential cause of the illness. The nurse questions the client regarding a recent history of travel, especially to tropical regions of Asia, Africa, or Central or South America. Traveler's diarrhea can begin 3 days to 2 weeks following the client's arrival.

The client who has gastroenteritis usually appears ill. Nausea and vomiting can occur with all types of gastroenteritis but are usually limited to the first 1 or 2 days of the illness. All clients with gastroenteritis classically have diarrhea, which varies in consistency and amount with the causative organism.

In clients with epidemic viral gastroenteritis, myalgia (muscle aches), headache, and malaise are often reported. The nurse notes slight abdominal distention. The nurse auscultates hyperactive bowel sounds and finds diffuse tenderness on palpation. However, there should be *no* rebound tenderness, which might indicate peritonitis. Depending on the amount of fluids lost through diarrhea and vomiting, the client may have varying degrees of dehydration manifested by the following:

- Poor skin turgor
- Dry mucous membranes
- Orthostatic blood pressure changes
- Hypotension
- Oliguria

In some cases, dehydration may be severe, and shock may occur if diarrhea is prolonged. Dehydration occurs rapidly in older adults.

Diarrhea associated with epidemic viral gastroenteritis is typically limited to 24 to 48 hours. In rotavirus gastroenteritis, there is an elevated temperature and watery diarrhea lasting 2 to 6 days. Mucus may be present in the stools of individuals infected with rotavirus. Infection with the Norwalk virus is characterized by the rapid onset of nausea, abdominal cramps, vomiting, and diarrhea. The illness is usually mild, lasting 24 to 48 hours (Greenberg, 1998). *Campylobacter* enteritis is a more severe disease with foul-smelling stools that contain blood and that can number 20 to 30 per day for up to

7 days. *E. coli* gastroenteritis may or may not involve blood or mucus in the stool; diarrhea can last for up to 10 days. *Shigella* causes stools containing blood and mucus, which can continue for up to 5 days.

As part of the laboratory assessment, Gram stain of stool is usually done before culture. Many white blood cells (WBCs) on Gram stain suggest shigellosis. The presence of WBCs and red blood cells (RBCs) in the stool indicates *Campylobacter* gastroenteritis.

A stool culture that is positive for enterotoxigenic *E. coli* is diagnostic of *E. coli* diarrhea. Culture of stool that is positive for *Shigella* when there are pus cells or WBCs present in the stool is diagnostic of shigellosis.

Sophisticated electron microscopy and immunoassay procedures can identify epidemic viral gastroenteritis or rotavirus gastroenteritis; however, such examinations are rarely done because they are expensive and tedious to perform.

Interventions

For clients with most types of gastroenteritis, supportive treatment is instituted. Therapy is focused on fluid replacement, and the amount and route of fluid administration are determined by fluid status.

FLUID REPLACEMENT. For mild cases of gastroenteritis, the client is treated on an ambulatory care basis or in the nursing home if he or she is a resident there. If the fluid volume is severely depleted, the client is admitted to the hospital for administration of IV fluids. For older clients at home or in a long-term care setting, oral rehydration therapy (ORT) with commercially prepared rehydration products, such as Resol, may prevent hospitalization.

The nurse obtains weight, orthostatic blood pressure, and other vital sign measurements at the time of admission. Hypotonic IV fluids, such as half-strength normal saline (0.45% sodium chloride), are infused as ordered. The nurse monitors the client's vital signs, intake and output, and weight. A rapid gain or loss of 1 kg (2.2 pounds) of body weight is equivalent to the gain or loss of 1 L of fluid. Standard precautions are consistently observed when handling vomitus and stool.

The health care provider may order a potassium supplement to be added to IV fluids if the serum potassium level is low. To help assess renal function and prevent hyperkalemia, the nurse verifies that the client is voiding before and during potassium replacement. The client is advised to rest in bed, especially during periods of nausea or vomiting.

Depending on the type of gastroenteritis, the local health department may need to be notified. It is mandatory that every case of shigellosis be reported. In some endemic areas, *Campylobacter* enteritis needs to be reported on a case-by-case basis. Other types of gastroenteritis must be reported only if they occur in epidemic proportions. The nurse or case manager investigates state and local health department guidelines for reporting requirements.

DIET THERAPY. Diet therapy is the same for the client who remains at home as for the client in the hospital. If the client is not actively vomiting, the nurse recommends small volumes of clear liquids with electrolytes (e.g., Gatorade) for 24 hours. The frequency and amount of oral intake can be increased if nausea and vomiting are *not* present. If nausea and vomiting continue, the nurse withholds food and fluids until these symptoms subside. The nurse advises the client *not* to drink water, because it does not contain any electrolytes to replace those lost. After 24 hours, the diet for all clients can be advanced to include saltine crackers, toast, and jelly. When the client can tolerate this diet, bland foods (e.g., nonfat soup, custard, yogurt, cottage cheese, mashed or baked potatoes, and cooked vegetables) may be added. Caffeine is avoided, since it can increase intestinal motility. The client may progress to a regular diet as tolerated.

DRUG THERAPY. Drugs that suppress intestinal motility, such as anticholinergics and antiemetics, are *not* routinely given for bacterial or viral gastroenteritis. Use of these drugs can prevent the infecting organisms from being eliminated from the body. If the health care provider determines that antiperistaltic agents are necessary, an initial dose of loperamide 4 mg may be administered orally, followed by 2 mg after each loose stool, up to 16 mg/day. Bismuth subsalicylate (Pepto-Bismol) 30 mL or 2 tablets every 30 minutes for a maximum of 8 doses may be given to reduce the watery volume of the stool.

Treatment with antibiotics may be warranted if the gastroenteritis is due to bacterial infection with fever and severe diarrhea. The health care provider may order norfloxacin (Chibroxin, Noroxin) 400 mg twice a day PO or ciprofloxacin (Cipro) 500 mg twice a day PO for 3 days. If the gastroenteritis is due to shigellosis, anti-infective agents, such as trimethoprim/sulfamethoxazole (Septra, Bactrim), are administered.

For relatively short-term diarrhea of 24 to 48 hours' duration, the diagnosis is based primarily on the client's history and clinical manifestations without validation by a stool examination. When diarrhea is severe or persists for long periods, the stool is examined in an effort to determine the causative organism and to begin specific treatment. It should be determined if the diarrhea is caused by *Salmonella* or parasites, because these organisms respond to specific medications (see Parasitic Infection, p. 1292). Diarrhea that continues longer than 10 days is probably *not* due to gastroenteritis, and a thorough investigation for the cause is warranted.

SKIN CARE. Frequent stools that are rich in electrolytes and enzymes, as well as frequent wiping and washing of the anal region, can irritate the skin. The nurse teaches the client to avoid toilet paper and harsh soaps. Ideally, the client can gently clean the area with warm water or absorbent cotton, followed by thorough drying with absorbent cotton. Cream, oil, or gel can be applied to a damp, warm washcloth to remove excrement adhering to excoriated skin. Hydrocortisone cream or protective barrier cream should be applied to the skin between stools. Witch hazel compresses (e.g., Tucks) and sitz baths for 10 minutes, two to three times daily, can also relieve discomfort.

If leakage of stool is a problem, the client can put absorbent cotton next to the anal orifice and keep it in place with snug underwear. For clients who are incontinent, the nurse keeps the perineal and buttock areas clean and dry. The use of incontinent pads instead of briefs allows air to circulate to the skin and prevents irritation.

HEALTH TEACHING. During the acute phase of the illness, the nurse teaches about the importance of fluid replacement measures. The nurse teaches the client to follow the diet described earlier under Diet Therapy, p. 1273, and about any necessary medications. The nurse also teaches the client and family about the importance of minimizing the risk of transmission of gastroenteritis. Clients are advised to:

- Wash their hands meticulously with an antibacterial soap, especially after bowel movements, and maintain good personal hygiene
- Restrict the use of glasses, dishes, eating utensils, and tubes of toothpaste to themselves only
- Maintain clean bathroom facilities to avoid exposure to stool
- Inform the health care provider if symptoms persist beyond 3 days

Clients adhere to these precautions for up to 7 weeks after the illness or up to several months if *Shigella* was the offending organism. If the client is employed as a food handler, the public health department should be consulted for recommendations about the return to work (Chart 58-2).

CHRONIC INFLAMMATORY BOWEL DISEASE

Chronic inflammatory bowel disease (chronic IBD) refers to several inflammatory disorders of the gastrointestinal (GI) tract with no known etiology. Chronic IBDs may be divided into two major groups: ulcerative colitis and Crohn's disease (Table 58-2).

Ulcerative Colitis

OVERVIEW

Ulcerative colitis is a chronic inflammatory process affecting the mucosal lining of the colon or rectum. This chronic inflammatory process can result in loose stools containing blood and mucus, poor absorption of vital nutrients, and thickening of the colon wall. Over time, the client experiences episodes of abdominal discomfort and extraintestinal manifestations of the disease that cause disruption of lifestyle. The affected client may have only minor periodic health problems, necessitating only ambulatory care, or serious problems, such as malnutrition and physical debilitation, requiring multiple hospitalizations.

CHART 58-2

CLIENT EDUCATION GUIDE
Measures to Prevent the Transmission of Gastroenteritis

- Wash your hands meticulously with an antibacterial soap, especially after having a bowel movement.
- Do not share your dishes, glasses, or toothpaste.
- Keep the commode clean to prevent exposure to your stool.
- Do not prepare or handle food that will be consumed by others.

Pathophysiology

Ulcerative colitis is characterized by diffuse inflammation of the intestinal mucosa; the result is a loss of surface epithelium with ulceration and possibly abscess formation. Generally, the disease begins in the rectum and proceeds in a uniform, continuous manner proximally toward the cecum. The inflammatory process progresses to epithelial cell damage and loss, leaving areas of ulceration. The colon appears ulcerated, reddened, and hemorrhagic. Ulcerative colitis is characterized by periods of remission and exacerbation.

Clients with *acute* ulcerative colitis may have vascular congestion, hemorrhage, edema, and ulceration of the bowel mucosa. As the disease course progresses, *chronic* changes in the colon occur. Fibrosis and retraction of the bowel result in muscle hypertrophy, deposition of fat and fibrous tissue, and a narrower and shorter colon. With long-term disease, dysplastic changes to the surface epithelium occur. These changes are associated with an increased risk of colon cancer.

Complications of ulcerative colitis include the following:

- Intestinal perforation with resultant peritonitis and fistula formation
- **Toxic megacolon**
- Hemorrhage
- Increased risk of colon cancer
- Abscess formation
- Malabsorption
- Bowel obstruction
- Extraintestinal clinical manifestations, such as arthritis

Table 58-3 describes these common complications.

Etiology

The exact cause of ulcerative colitis is unknown. A genetic basis of the disease has been proposed because of the increased incidence seen in families, certain ethnic groups, and twins. Immunologic theories, including autoimmune dysfunction, have been explored because of the extraintestinal manifestations of the disease. One hypothesis suggests that

TABLE 58-2 • DIFFERENTIAL FEATURES OF ULCERATIVE COLITIS AND CROHN'S DISEASE

Feature	Ulcerative Colitis	Crohn's Disease
Location	Begins in the rectum and proceeds in a continuous manner toward the cecum	Most often in the terminal ileum, with patchy involvement through all layers of the bowel
Etiology	Unknown	Unknown
Peak incidence at age	15-25 yr and 55-65 yr	15-40 yr
Stools	10-20 liquid, bloody stools per day	5-6 soft, loose stools per day, rarely bloody
Complications	Hemorrhage Perforation Fistulas Nutritional deficiencies	Fistulas Nutritional deficiencies

IBD results from an abnormal response to normal flora present in the intestines; another possibility is that there may be a defect in intestinal permeability that permits antigens to leak through the mucosa, stimulating an inflammatory response. Psychologic factors have also been implicated, since stress often results in a flare-up of the disease. However, there is little evidence to relate psychologic factors to the cause of the disease.

Incidence/Prevalence

There is a higher geographic distribution of the disease in northern Europe and North America. The annual incidence of ulcerative colitis is approximately 2 to 10 new cases per 100,000 persons. The prevalence is 40 to 100 cases per 100,000 people in the United States. There is a tenfold risk of the disease if an individual has a first-degree relative with the disease.

Peak incidence is between the ages of 15 and 25 years, with another peak occurring between ages of 55 and 65 years. Females are more often affected than men. Jewish Caucasians of European or Ashkenazic origin are at highest risk compared with other Caucasian groups (Rubin, 1998).

CULTURAL CONSIDERATIONS

Ulcerative colitis is four to five times more common among people of Jewish origin and commonly affects Caucasians in developed Western society. It is seen more often in individuals of Jewish European or Ashkenazic origin, but not in those of Sephardic origin. Although the disease is more common in Caucasians, the incidence in African Americans is increasing.

TABLE 58-3 • COMPLICATIONS OF ULCERATIVE COLITIS AND CROHN'S DISEASE

Complication	Description
Hemorrhage/perforation	Lower gastrointestinal bleeding results from erosion of the bowel wall.
Abscess formation	Localized pockets of infection develop in the ulcerated bowel lining.
Toxic megacolon	Paralysis of the colon causes dilation and subsequent bowel obstruction.
Malabsorption	Essential nutrients cannot be absorbed through the diseased intestinal wall, causing anemia and malnutrition (most common in Crohn's disease).
Bowel obstruction	Obstruction results from toxic megacolon or cancer.
Fistulas	Fistulas can occur anywhere, but usually track between the bowel and bladder. Pyuria and fecaluria result.
Colorectal cancer	Clients with ulcerative colitis for 7-10 yr or longer have a high risk for colorectal cancer. This complication accounts for about one third of all deaths related to ulcerative colitis.
Extraintestinal complications	Complications include arthritis, hepatic and biliary disease (especially cholelithiasis), oral and skin lesions, and ocular disorders, such as iritis. The cause is unknown.

COLLABORATIVE MANAGEMENT

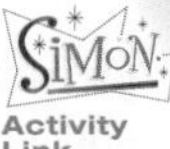

Assessment

HISTORY

The nurse collects data on any family history of inflammatory bowel disease (IBD) and previous and current therapy for the illness, as well as dates and types of surgery. Obtaining a diet history is essential. The history should include the client's usual dietary patterns and the relationship of elimination patterns to intolerance of milk and milk products and greasy, fried, spicy, or hot foods. A history of weight loss may be seen in clients with severe disease.

The nurse asks about the symptoms of acute ulcerative colitis, which often include abdominal pain, cramping, urgency, and diarrhea with up to 10 to 20 liquid, bloody stools per day, as well as anorexia and fatigue. The client is questioned regarding his or her usual bowel elimination pattern; the color, consistency, and character of stools; and the presence or absence of blood in all stools. The nurse notes the relationship between the occurrence of diarrhea and the timing of meals, pain, emotional distress, and activity. The client is questioned regarding extraintestinal symptoms such as arthritis, mouth sores, vision problems, and skin disorders.

PHYSICAL ASSESSMENT/CLINICAL MANIFESTATIONS

The client with ulcerative colitis may have symptoms that vary with the acuteness of onset and with complications of the disease process. The client may complain of abdominal pain, bloody diarrhea, and **tenesmus** (uncontrollable straining). Vital signs are usually within normal limits in mild disease. In more severe cases, the client may have a low-grade fever (99° to 100° F [37.2° to 37.8° C]). The physical assessment findings are typically nonspecific, and in milder cases the physical examination may be normal.

The nurse may note some mild abdominal distention along the colon. Palpation may reveal areas of increased or localized tenderness. Rebound tenderness may suggest peritonitis. The nurse may note localized areas of abdominal pain or cramping over areas of diseased bowel. The client may be febrile and tachycardic, indicating possible complications, such as peritonitis, dehydration, and bowel perforation.

PSYCHOSOCIAL ASSESSMENT

The intestinal and extraintestinal symptoms associated with ulcerative colitis can be taxing. The nurse evaluates the client's understanding of the illness and its impact on his or her lifestyle. The client is encouraged and supported while the following are explored:

- The relationship of life events to disease exacerbations
- Stress factors that produce symptoms
- Family and social support systems
- Concerns regarding the possible genetic basis and associated cancer risks of the disease

Many clients are very apprehensive regarding the frequency of stools and the presence of blood. The uncontrollability of the disease symptoms, particularly diarrhea, can be disruptive and stress producing. More severe illness may limit the client's activities outside the home. As a result of the excessive diarrhea, the client may become dependent on the proximity of a bathroom. Eating may be associated with pain and cramping, as well as an increased frequency of stools. Mealtimes may become unpleasant experiences. Frequent visits to health care providers and vigilant monitoring of the colonic mucosa for dysplastic (irregular) changes can be anxiety provoking.

LABORATORY ASSESSMENT

As a result of chronic blood loss, hematocrit and hemoglobin levels may be low, reflecting anemia and a chronic disease state. An increased white blood cell (WBC) count and elevated erythrocyte sedimentation rate (ESR) are consistent with inflammatory disease. Sodium, potassium, and chloride concentrations may be depleted secondary to frequent diarrheal stools and malabsorption resulting from the diseased bowel. Hypoalbuminemia is found in clients with extensive disease.

Viral and bacterial dysenteries can cause symptoms similar to those of ulcerative colitis. Before an invasive diagnostic workup, the stools are examined for occult blood, ova (eggs), and parasites, and specimens for culture are obtained. Other problems must be ruled out before a definitive diagnosis of ulcerative colitis is made.

RADIOGRAPHIC ASSESSMENT

Barium enemas with air contrast demonstrate differences between Crohn's disease and ulcerative colitis and identify complications, mucosal patterns, and the distribution and depth of disease involvement. In early disease, the barium enema will show incomplete filling as a result of inflammation and fine ulcerations along the bowel contour. These ulcerations appear deeper in more advanced disease.

OTHER DIAGNOSTIC ASSESSMENT

The sigmoidoscopic examination is probably the most definitive diagnostic procedure for ulcerative colitis. The physician can directly visualize the sigmoid and transverse colon. Common findings include an edematous, friable bowel mucosa with a loss of vascular pattern and frequent ulcerations. Biopsy specimens can also be taken to determine if inflammation or dysplastic changes are present.

> **CRITICAL THINKING CHALLENGE**
>
> A 65-year-old female client is admitted to your unit with a 10-year history of mild to moderate ulcerative colitis. Recently she has noted an increasing amount of abdominal pain and cramping following meals. She has also experienced an increase in stools from 1 to 3 per day to 8 to 12 per day. She reports that the stools contain blood and mucus. Her vital signs are normal except for a slight increase in temperature to 100° F (37.8° C).
>
> - What additional information in the history should you elicit from the client?
> - What actions should you take considering this client's increase in temperature and gastrointestinal (GI) symptoms?
> - What long-term consequences of the disease is this client most at risk for?

For suggested answer guidelines, go to SIMON http://www.wbsaunders.com/SIMON/Iggy/.

Analysis

COMMON NURSING DIAGNOSES AND COLLABORATIVE PROBLEMS

The following are common nursing diagnoses for clients with ulcerative colitis:

1. Diarrhea related to inflammation of the bowel mucosa
2. Acute and Chronic Pain related to inflammation and ulceration of the bowel mucosa and accompanying skin irritation

The most common collaborative problem is Potential for Gastrointestinal Bleeding.

ADDITIONAL NURSING DIAGNOSES AND COLLABORATIVE PROBLEMS

In addition to the common nursing diagnoses and collaborative problems, clients with ulcerative colitis may have one or more of the following:

- Imbalanced Nutrition: Less Than Body Requirements related to diarrhea and malabsorption
- Disturbed Body Image related to increased bowel elimination or surgical intervention
- Activity Intolerance related to fatigue and anemia
- Ineffective Coping related to chronic physical illness and repeated hospitalizations
- Risk for Deficient Fluid Volume related to diarrhea
- Impaired Oral Mucous Membrane related to extraintestinal oral disease
- Anxiety related to increased risk of colon cancer and lifestyle interruptions

Planning and Implementation

DIARRHEA

NOC **PLANNING: EXPECTED OUTCOMES.** A major concern for a client with ulcerative colitis is the occurrence of frequent, bloody diarrhea. The client with ulcerative colitis is expected to experience decreased diarrhea through measures to reduce the inflammation of the intestinal lining.

INTERVENTIONS. Many measures are used to relieve symptoms and to reduce intestinal motility, decrease inflammation, and promote intestinal healing. Medical management of ulcerative colitis is the preferred and initial treatment option.

NONSURGICAL MANAGEMENT. Nonsurgical management includes drug and diet therapy. The provision of physical and emotional rest are also important considerations.

NIC ***DIARRHEA MANAGEMENT.*** The purpose of diarrhea management (Chart 58-3) is the prevention and alleviation of diarrhea. It is important to instruct the client with exacerbations of diarrhea to record the color, volume, frequency, and consistency of stools to determine the severity of the problem. The nurse, in collaboration with the dietitian, assists in identifying factors that may cause or contribute to diarrhea.

The nurse monitors the skin in the perianal area for irritation and ulceration due to loose, frequent stools. Stool cultures may be sent if diarrhea continues. The client and family members are instructed in the appropriate use of antidiarrheal medications. The nurse or assistive nursing personnel weighs the client regularly. In severe exacerbations of the disease, the

CHART 58-3

NIC INTERVENTION ACTIVITIES *for* The Client with Inflammatory Bowel Disease

Diarrhea Management: *Management and alleviation of diarrhea*
- Instruct client/family members to record color, volume, frequency, and consistency of stools.
- Identify factors (e.g., medications, bacteria, tube feedings) that may cause or contribute to diarrhea.
- Teach the client to eliminate gas-forming and spicy foods from diet.
- Suggest trial elimination of foods containing lactose.
- Instruct in low-fiber, high-protein, high-calorie diet, as appropriate.
- Teach client appropriate use of antidiarrheal medications.
- Monitor the skin in perianal area for irritation and ulceration.
- Weigh the client regularly.
- Perform actions to rest the bowel (NPO liquid diet).

Pain Management: *Alleviation of pain or a reduction in pain to a level of comfort that is acceptable to the client*
- Perform a comprehensive pain assessment to include location, characteristics, onset/duration, frequency, quality, intensity or severity of pain, and precipitating factors.
- Evaluate, with the client and the health care team, the effectiveness of past pain control measures that have been used.
- Reduce or eliminate factors that can precipitate or increase the pain experience (e.g., fear, fatigue, monotony, and lack of knowledge).
- Teach the use of nonpharmacologic measures (e.g., biofeedback, TENS, hypnosis, relaxation, guided imagery, music therapy, distraction, activity therapy, acupressure, hot/cold application, and massage) before, after and, if possible, during painful activities; before pain occurs or increases; and along with other pain relief measures.

NIC intervention activities selected from McCloskey, J.C., & Bulechek, G.M. (2000). *Nursing interventions classification (NIC)* (3rd ed.). St. Louis: Mosby. No part of this work is to be altered without prior written permission from the Publisher.
TENS, Transcutaneous electrical nerve stimulation.

nurse, in collaboration with the health care provider, performs actions to rest the bowel.

DRUG THERAPY. The health care provider prescribes a combination of drugs, including salicylate compounds, corticosteroids, immunosuppressants, and antidiarrheals.

Salicylate Compounds. Sulfasalazine (Azulfidine, PMS-Sulfasalazine✹) is one of the primary treatments for ulcerative colitis. It is thought to act by inhibiting prostaglandin synthesis. These compounds may be administered orally or rectally to reduce inflammation. Sulfasalazine is used to prevent recurrences of the disease, as well as to treat acute exacerbations of mild to moderate severity (Glickman, 1998). The usual dose of sulfasalazine is 2 to 4 g/day. The nurse teaches the client to take the drug with a full glass of water and to increase fluids throughout the day. The drug should be taken after meals to prevent GI discomfort. Blood dyscrasias, such as leukopenia and anemia, may occur.

Oral mesalamine (Asacol, Pentasa, Salofalk✹) is used for its anti-inflammatory effect in the acute phase of the illness. The recommended dose of Asacol is 800 mg three times a day or Pentasa 4 g daily in divided doses. Tablets should not be crushed, broken, or chewed. The drug is also available for rectal administration.

Olsalazine (Dipentum) 1 g daily is a salicylate used for maintenance therapy. Side effects of oral mesalamine include occasional flare-ups of colitis.

Clients with mild to moderate colitis of the distal bowel may be treated with mesalamine suppositories given two or three times daily or with retention enemas (Rowasa enema) given once daily at bedtime.

Corticosteroids. Oral or IV corticosteroid therapy may be prescribed during exacerbations of the disease. Prednisone (Deltasone, Winpred) 40 to 65 mg daily is usually given orally. For a severely ill client, prednisolone (Delta-Cortef) 45 to 60 mg daily may be given intravenously. Once clinical improvement has been established, the corticosteroids are tapered over a 2- to 3-month period following discharge because of the long-term adverse effects that commonly occur with steroid therapy. Examples include hyperglycemia (increased blood glucose), osteoporosis, peptic ulcer disease, and increased risk for infection. For clients with rectal symptoms, topical steroids in the form of small-retention enemas may be prescribed. Hydrocortisone rectal foam (Cortifoam) is ordered one to two times daily for 2 to 3 weeks, then every other day. Hydrocortisone enemas (Cortenema) are given at bedtime for 21 days, then tapered and discontinued.

Immunosuppressive Drugs. As single agents, immunosuppressive drugs are not effective in the treatment of ulcerative colitis. However, when given in combination with steroids, they may help to reduce the amount of steroids necessary to obtain a response. Cyclosporine given at 4 mg/kg/day can be beneficial in severely ill clients who might otherwise require a colectomy. Oral mercaptopurine (Purinethol) may be given at a dose of 1.5 to 2.5 mg/kg/day. The nurse observes for side effects of this medication, which include thrombocytopenia (decreased platelets), leukopenia (decreased white blood cells [WBCs]), anemia, renal failure, infection, headache, GI ulceration, stomatitis (oral cavity inflammation), and hepatotoxicity. Therefore it is important to monitor blood counts and note signs of infection.

Antidiarrheal Drugs. To provide symptomatic management of diarrhea, antidiarrheal drugs may be ordered. These drugs are given very cautiously, however, since they can precipitate colonic dilation and toxic megacolon. Common antidiarrheal drugs include diphenoxylate hydrochloride and atropine sulfate (Lomotil) and loperamide (Imodium).

DIET THERAPY. The severity of the client's ulcerative colitis determines the type of diet required. Clients may begin with one form of diet therapy and progress to a more advanced diet as symptoms diminish, with the goal of preventing hyperactive bowel activity.

Clients with severe symptoms are kept on NPO status to ensure bowel rest. The physician often orders total parenteral nutrition (TPN) for these clients (see Chapter 61). Clients with slightly less severe symptoms may be given elemental formulas, such as Vivonex or Ensure, which are absorbed in the upper bowel, thus minimizing bowel stimulation. Clients with significant but less severe symptoms may be restricted to a low-fiber (low-residue) diet. Clients following a low-fiber diet should avoid foods such as whole-wheat grains, nuts, and fresh fruits or fresh vegetables (Table 58-4). There is controversy whether fiber needs to be restricted during the chronic phase of the illness. If fiber intake does not induce symptoms, the intake of fiber need not be limited. However, because the role of diet in inflammatory bowel disease (IBD) is not well defined, and because individual tolerance to foods vary, clients with controlled symptoms may only need to limit or omit those foods that cause them discomfort or diarrhea.

Typically, lactose-containing foods are poorly tolerated and should be reduced or eliminated. All clients should be cautioned that caffeinated beverages, pepper, alcohol, and smoking are common GI stimulants that could cause discomfort.

REST. At the onset of treatment, activity is generally restricted because rest can reduce intestinal activity, provide comfort, and promote healing. The nurse ensures that the client has easy access to a bedpan, commode, or bathroom in case of urgency or tenesmus.

CRITICAL THINKING CHALLENGE

Your older client with ulcerative colitis has developed mouth ulcers and is complaining of stiffness in her joints. Her abdominal pain and diarrhea have improved with aggressive treatment, including immunosuppressives.

- What relationship does the client's mouth sores and joint pain have to her disease process?
- What possible complications of immunosuppressive therapy should you be alert for?
- What laboratory values would be most important for you to monitor for in this client?

For suggested answer guidelines, go to SIMON http://www.wbsaunders.com/SIMON/Iggy/.

TABLE 58-4 • GUIDELINES FOR A LOW-FIBER DIET

Foods Allowed	Foods Not Allowed
BEVERAGES	
Only 2 glasses of milk, if allowed, boiled or evaporated; strained fruit juices, coffee, tea, and carbonated beverages	Alcohol
EGGS	
Prepared in any manner, except fried	Fried
CHEESE	
Cottage, cream, milk, American, and Tillamook (use in small amounts)	Highly flavored
MEATS OR POULTRY	
Roasted, baked, or broiled tender beef, lamb, liver, veal, fish, chicken, or turkey	Tough meats, pork; fried or highly spiced meats
SOUPS	
Bouillon, broth, and strained cream soups from foods allowed	Any others
FATS	
Butter, margarine, oils, 30 mL (1 oz) of cream daily	None
VEGETABLES	
Canned or cooked vegetables, such as asparagus, beets, carrots, peas, potatoes, pumpkin, squash, spinach, and young string beans; tomato juice	Raw or whole cooked vegetables (e.g., potato with skin)
FRUITS	
Strained fruit juices; cooked or canned apples, apricots, Royal Ann cherries, peaches, pears, dried fruit purée, and ripe banana and avocado; all of the above *without skins or seeds*	All other raw or cooked fruits
BREAD AND CRACKERS	
Refined bread, toast, rolls, and crackers	Pancakes, waffles, and whole-grain bread or rolls
CEREALS	
Cooked cereal, such as Cream of Wheat, Malt-O Meal, strained oatmeal, cornmeal, cornflakes, puffed rice, Rice Krispies, and puffed wheat	Whole-grain cereals; other prepared cereals
POTATOES/RICE/PASTA	
White rice, macaroni, noodles, and spaghetti	Fried potato, potato chips, and brown rice
DESSERTS	
Gelatin desserts, tapioca, angel food or sponge cake, plain custards, water ice or ice cream without fruit or nuts, and rennet or simple puddings	Rich pastries, pies, and anything with nuts or dried fruit
SWEETS	
Sugar, jelly, honey, syrups, gumdrops, hard candy, plain creams, milk chocolate	Other candy; jam, marmalade
MISCELLANEOUS FOODS	
Cream sauce and plain gravy	Nuts, olives, popcorn, rich gravies, pepper, spices, and vinegar

Modified from Williams, S. R. (1998). *Nutrition and diet therapy* (8th ed.). St. Louis: Mosby.

SURGICAL MANAGEMENT. Approximately 20% to 25% of individuals with ulcerative colitis require a colectomy (Glickman, 1998). Indications for surgery include bowel perforation, toxic megacolon, hemorrhage, colon cancer, and conventional treatment failure. The surgeon may choose one of several surgical procedures to alleviate these problems.

TOTAL PROCTOCOLECTOMY WITH A PERMANENT ILEOSTOMY. Total proctocolectomy (or colectomy) with a permanent ileostomy has traditionally been the standard surgical procedure for clients undergoing a colectomy.

Preoperative Care. When an ileostomy is indicated, the nurse provides extensive explanations to the client and family or significant other. Preoperative teaching includes aspects that relate to abdominal surgery (see Chapter 17) and those that relate to ileostomy. The surgeon consults with the enterostomal therapist (ET) preoperatively for recommendations on the location of the ostomy (stoma). (An ET is a nurse specializing and certified in skin and ostomy care.) A visit from an ostomate (a client with an ostomy) may be appropriate before surgery if the client agrees to this. The surgeon orders oral or parenteral antibiotics, such as neomycin sulfate (Mycifradin, Neo-fradin), as a bowel antiseptic. Mechanical cleansing of the bowel with enemas or laxatives may also be required.

Operative Procedure. During a total proctocolectomy with a traditional permanent ileostomy, the colon, rectum, and anus are removed, followed by closure of the anus. The surgeon brings the end of the terminal ileum out through the abdominal wall and forms a stoma, or ostomy. The stoma is usually placed in the right lower quadrant of the abdomen, below the belt line (Figure 58-2). The surgeon makes a perineal incision to remove the rectum and supporting tissues.

Postoperative Care. Initially after surgery, the output from the ileostomy is a loose, dark green liquid that may contain some blood. Over time, a process called ileostomy adaptation occurs. The small intestine begins to absorb increased amounts of sodium and water (a former function of the large intestine, which was removed by surgery). Stool volume decreases, becomes thicker (pastelike), and turns yellow-green or yellow-brown. The effluent (fluid material) usually has little odor or a sweet odor. Any foul or unpleasant odor may be a symptom of some underlying problem (e.g., blockage or infection).

Depending on the frequency and irritation of stool drainage, the client must wear a pouch system at all times. Disposable systems are most often used.

Prevention of skin problems (irritation, excoriation, ulceration) is critical for the client with an ileostomy. The output from the small intestine is rich in proteolytic enzymes and bile salts, which can quickly irritate and injure the skin. A pouch system that has some type of skin barrier (gelatin or pectin) provides sufficient protection for most clients. Other products are also available.

Most clients undergoing surgical intervention for ulcerative colitis have lived with chronic illness for some time. They may view surgery positively as a relief from the multiple problems caused by the disease. Initially, however, they may not perceive life with an ileostomy as a positive alternative.

Total proctocolectomy with a permanent ileostomy results in an alteration in appearance and body function. The goals for a client undergoing this procedure are to become proficient in self-care, to adapt his or her lifestyle to include care of an ostomy, and to successfully resume presurgery activities.

TOTAL COLECTOMY WITH A CONTINENT ILEOSTOMY. As an alternative to the traditional ileostomy with an external pouch, the surgeon may create an internal system—a Kock's ileostomy or ileal reservoir. This procedure is sometimes referred to as a continent ileostomy. The surgeon constructs an intra-abdominal pouch or reservoir from the terminal ileum (Figure 58-3), where stool is stored in the pouch until it is drained by the client using a soft rubber catheter. The care of a Kock's ileostomy involves the connection of the pouch to the stoma, which is constructed with a nipple-like valve made from an intussuscepted portion of the ileum. The stoma is flush with the skin.

The nursing care of the client undergoing this procedure is similar to the care of the client undergoing a proctocolectomy with a permanent ileostomy (see the previous section). Immediately postoperatively, an indwelling Foley catheter is placed in the pouch, which is connected to low intermittent suction and irrigated as ordered.

The nurse monitors the character and quality of effluent (drainage). Approximately 2 weeks after surgery, the nurse teaches the client to drain the stoma. Initially, the pouch holds only 50 to 75 mL; over time, the pouch capacity reaches 500 to 700 mL. When the pouch needs to be emptied, the client experiences a sensation of fullness. The client drains the pouch several times a day and wears a small dressing over the stoma to keep it moist and to protect clothing from the moist stoma. This procedure has several advantages. The client does not need to wear an external pouch for collection of stool and experiences minimal skin problems. Unfortunately, the need

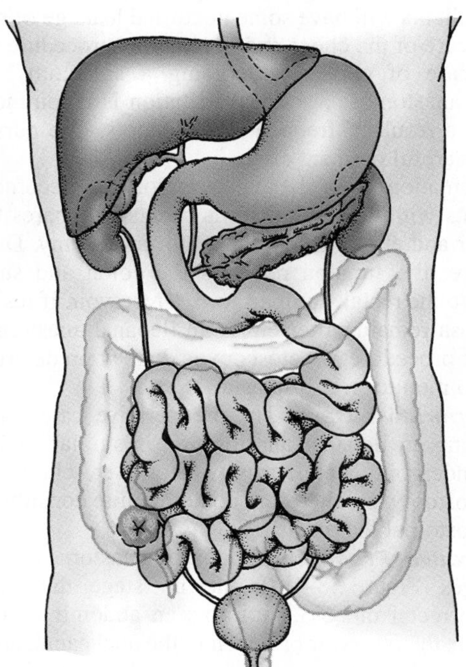

Figure 58-2 ● Total proctocolectomy with a permanent ileostomy. This involved removal of the colon, the rectum, and the anus with closure of the anus. Note the missing colon, rectum, and anus with the resultant stoma in the right lower quadrant.

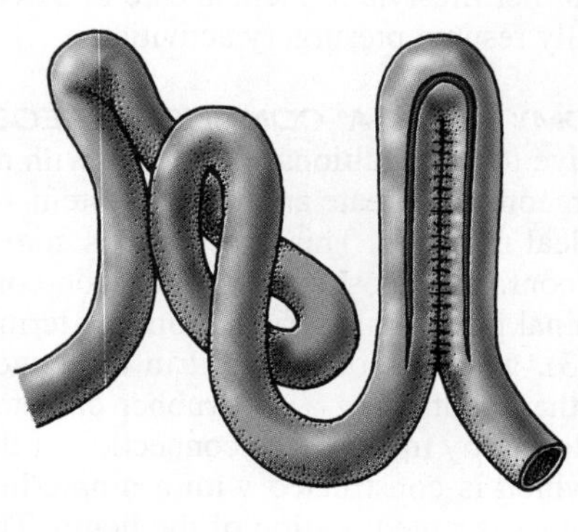

1. A reservoir, in which the client will retain stool until draining it, is constructed from a loop of ileum folded and sutured together, then cut.

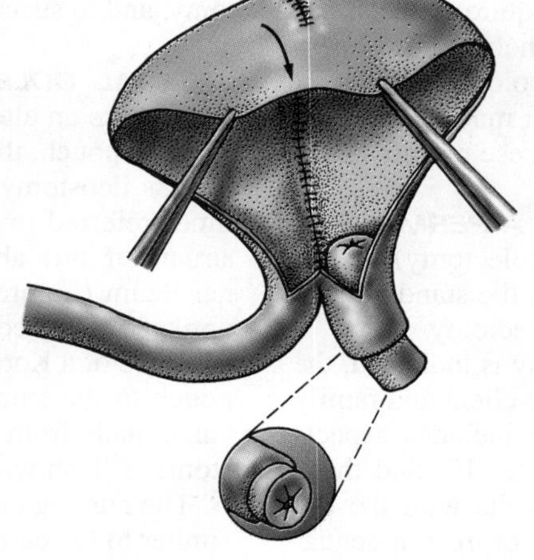

2. A portion of the ileum is intussuscepted to form a nipple valve, and the upper part of the stitched and cut ileum is pulled down and sutured to form a pouch.

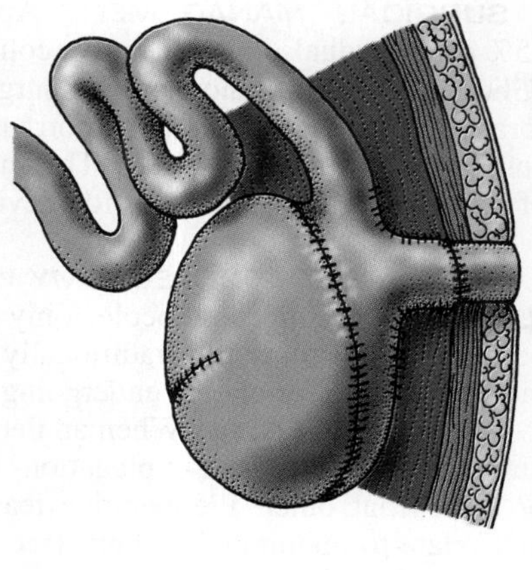

3. The nipple valve, which shuts tight against pressure from a filled pouch, is pulled through the stoma and sutured flush with the abdomen.

Figure 58-3 ● The creation of a Kock's (continent) ileostomy.

for frequent revisions and problems with leakage have made this procedure less desirable.

TOTAL COLECTOMY WITH ILEOANAL ANASTOMOSIS; ILEOANAL RESERVOIR. During a total colectomy with ileoanal anastomosis, the surgeon removes the colon and the rectum and sutures the ileum into the anal canal. Usually continence is excellent following this procedure, but up to 20% of clients will have some nocturnal leakage of stool. The nursing care of the client undergoing this procedure is similar to the care of clients undergoing a colectomy. With an ileoanal anastomosis, perineal irritation is a common occurrence as a result of frequent, loose stools. The nurse should provide careful perineal care.

The creation of an ileoanal reservoir has become popular for clients with ulcerative colitis because it spares the rectal sphincter and eliminates the need for an ostomy. During this procedure, the surgeon removes the colon and sutures the ileum into the rectal stump to form a reservoir. If residual rectal mucosa remains after either an ileoanal anastomosis or a reservoir procedure, proctoscopy is done at predetermined intervals to monitor for dysplasia.

Preoperative Care. The preoperative care for a client undergoing an ileoanal anastomosis is similar to that for a client undergoing an ileostomy. However, clients will not have an ostomy and therefore do not require consultation with an enterostomal therapist (ET).

Operative Procedure. Ileoanal anastomosis occurs in two stages (Figure 58-4). In the first stage, the surgeon excises the rectal mucosa, performs an abdominal colectomy, constructs the reservoir or pouch to the anal canal, and creates a temporary loop ileostomy. The loop ileostomy is necessary to allow adequate healing of the internal pouch and all anastomosis sites and to allow for an increase in the capacity of the internal reservoir through fluid instillations. After 3 to 4 months the client returns to have the loop ileostomy closed. Stool formation resembles that in clients who have undergone a traditional ileostomy.

Postoperative Care. The nurse provides the usual postoperative interventions for clients who have undergone abdominal surgery. All clients requiring surgical intervention for ulcerative colitis have an abdominal incision. Initially, most clients are maintained on NPO status and a nasogastric (NG) tube is used for suction.

ACUTE PAIN; CHRONIC PAIN

NOC **PLANNING: EXPECTED OUTCOMES.** The client with ulcerative colitis is expected to experience relief from painful abdominal cramping and skin irritation as indicated by self-report.

INTERVENTIONS. Pain control may be accomplished through pharmacologic and nonpharmacologic measures. The client's symptoms can cause physical discomfort, which can also contribute to emotional discomfort. The use of a variety of symptom-reducing interventions and supportive measures can provide increased comfort.

NIC **PAIN MANAGEMENT.** The purpose of pain management is the alleviation of pain or a reduction in pain to a level of comfort that is acceptable to the client (see Chart 58-3). The client with ulcerative colitis experiences abdominal pain and cramping, particularly with exacerbations of the disease. Increases in pain may also signal the development of complications such as peritonitis. Frequent bowel movements can cause skin irritation and increase the client's discomfort. The nurse performs a comprehensive pain assessment. With the client and the health care team, the nurse evaluates the effectiveness of past pain control measures used.

The nurse assists the client in reducing or eliminating factors that can precipitate or increase the pain experience. An-

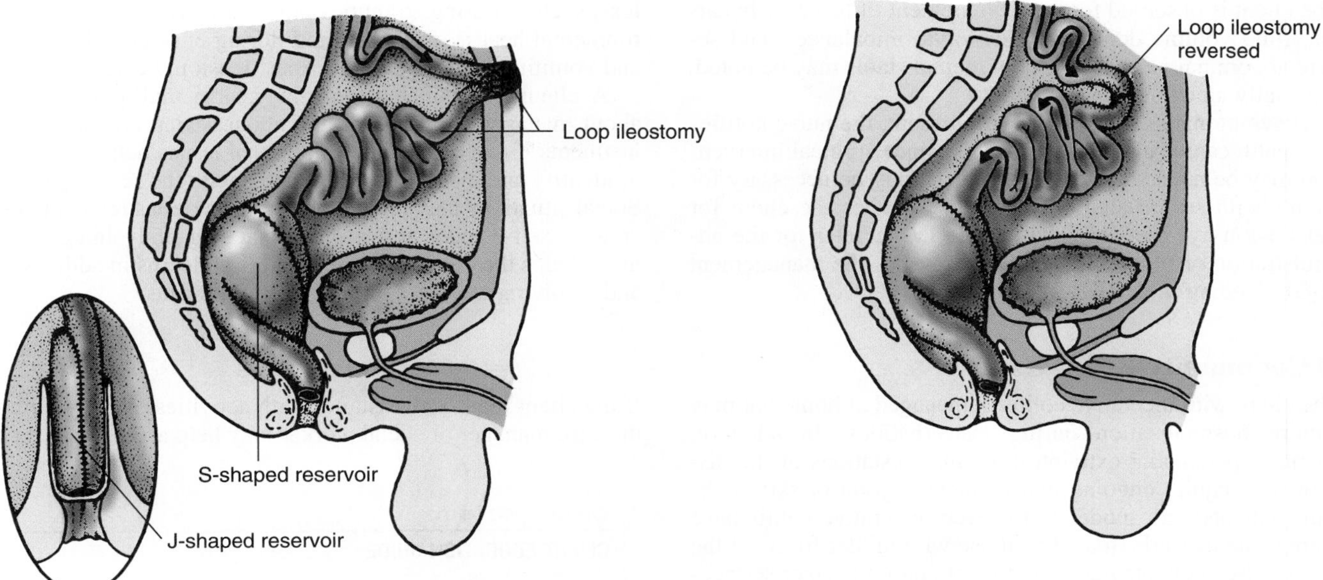

Stage 1.
After removal of the colon, a temporary loop ileostomy is created and an ileoanal reservoir is formed. The reservoir is created in an S-shaped reservoir (using three loops of ileum) or a J-shaped reservoir (suturing a portion of ileum to the rectal cuff, with an upward loop).

Stage 2.
After the reservoir has had time to heal–usually several months–the temporary loop ileostomy is reversed, and stool is allowed to drain into the reservoir.

Figure 58-4 ● The creation of an ileoanal reservoir.

tidiarrheal medications may be prescribed to control diarrhea but must be used cautiously, since they can precipitate toxic megacolon. The client may benefit from diet teaching and meal planning as a means of decreasing abdominal discomfort related to cramping and bloating. Excoriated skin can contribute to pain and discomfort. Scrupulous skin care prevents painful excoriation of the skin. The nurse can also teach the client to use nonpharmacologic measures (e.g., biofeedback, music therapy, guided imagery) as a means of pain modification.

DRUG THERAPY. Antidiarrheal medications are used to control diarrhea and thereby reduce the resulting discomfort. These must be used with caution, since toxic megacolon can develop. The physician may prescribe anticholinergics, such as propantheline bromide (Pro-Banthine), before meals to provide relief from the pain and cramping that may occur with diarrhea. Opioids are used sparingly and cautiously, since these drugs can mask symptoms of life-threatening complications.

DIET THERAPY. Dietary measures help to control symptoms and thereby promote relief from discomfort. The nurse assesses the client's needs for diet teaching and evaluates the effects of implemented dietary measures on an ongoing basis.

PERINEAL SKIN CARE. Perineal skin can be irritated by frequent contact with loose stools and frequent cleaning. This irritation can be a major contributor to the client's discomfort. The nurse explains special measures for skin care. For example, cleaning the perineal area with mild soap and warm water after each bowel movement keeps the skin free of any stool. Frequent sitz baths may be helpful, particularly after a bowel movement. The application of a thin coat of mineral oil, petroleum jelly, vitamin A and D ointment, aloe creams, or medicated foam applications may provide relief. Use of medicated wipes with witch hazel (e.g., Tucks) is soothing if the rectal area is tender or sensitive from the use of toilet tissue.

Various manufacturers of ostomies (e.g., Hollister and Convatec) produce a three-product system for skin care that may help prevent and heal perineal skin irritation, thus relieving discomfort. Such systems include a skin-cleaning solution, a moisturizing and healing cream, and a petroleum jelly–like ointment that prevents contact of moisture and stool with the skin.

POTENTIAL FOR GASTROINTESTINAL BLEEDING

PLANNING: EXPECTED OUTCOMES. The client with ulcerative colitis is expected to experience a reduction in or cessation of the gastrointestinal (GI) bleeding that accompanies chronic ulcerative colitis. The client is also expected to remain free of complications of the disease that can cause bleeding, such as perforation.

INTERVENTIONS. The nurse's primary responsibility is to monitor the client closely for signs and symptoms of GI bleeding resulting from acute disease or complications. All stools are monitored for blood, using both gross and occult examination. The nurse monitors the client's hematocrit, hemoglobin, and electrolyte values for abnormalities. The nurse or assistive nursing personnel monitors the client's vital signs.

The client is observed for the development of fever, tachycardia, fluid volume depletion, electrolyte imbalances, and severe abdominal pain. Changes in mental status may be noted, especially among older adults.

If symptoms of GI bleeding are present, the nurse notifies the health care provider immediately, since surgical intervention may be necessary. Blood products may be necessary for clients with severe anemia. The nurse readies the client for transfusion by inserting a large-bore IV catheter for the administration of blood. Chapter 56 describes the management of GI bleeding in detail.

Community-Based Care

The client with ulcerative colitis is managed at home but may require hospitalization during exacerbations. In addition, clients experiencing extraintestinal manifestations of the disease will require ongoing management of joint or skin problems. Clients with moderate to severe ulcerative colitis have more acute exacerbations than those with milder forms of the disease. Such clients may benefit from case manager services to coordinate and facilitate quality care in a cost-effective way.

HOME CARE MANAGEMENT

For clients with ulcerative colitis, home care management focuses on managing symptoms and monitoring for complications. The nurse instructs the client in measures to reduce or control abdominal pain, cramping, and diarrhea. The nurse also instructs the client and family members regarding symptoms that should be reported immediately to the health care provider. For clients returning home or transferring to nursing home or subacute care following surgery, ongoing respiratory care, incision care, ostomy care, and pain management are additional concerns.

HEALTH TEACHING

The nurse educates the client about the nature of ulcerative colitis with regard to its acute episodes, remissions, and symptom management. The nurse emphasizes that even though the cause is unknown, relapses can be resolved with proper health care.

The nurse teaches the client dietary measures to reduce bloating and cramping. The client needs to learn what foods are best tolerated and adjust his or her diet accordingly. The nurse teaches about prescribed medications and medication side effects to remain alert for. Clients taking immunosuppressive drugs should be taught to report signs of infection, such as sore throat, to the health care provider. The nurse prepares written instructions for the client and family members about the signs of colonic dilation and perforation and reiterates the importance of notifying the health care provider if these signs occur.

If the client has undergone a surgical diversion to manage colon effluent, the nurse or enterostomal therapist (ET) explains and demonstrates the required care. The client is encouraged to demonstrate self-care of the ileostomy. The nurse also teaches clients with an ileostomy to include adequate amounts of salt and water in their diets because the ileostomy promotes the loss of these elements. They are taught to be cautious in situations that promote profuse sweating or fluid loss, such as during strenuous physical activities, when environmental heat is excessive, and during episodes of diarrhea and vomiting. Chart 58-4 describes ileostomy care in detail.

A client with an ileostomy may have multiple concerns about management at home and about sexual and social adjustments. Considering possible sexual issues helps the client to identify and discuss these concerns with the sexual partner. Social situations may precipitate some anxieties related to decreased self-esteem and a disturbance in body image. The nurse helps the client explore possible concerns in addressing and resolving these potentially stressful events.

HEALTH CARE RESOURCES

If the client requires assistance with activities of daily living, the case manager or social worker may help arrange the serv-

CHART 58-4

CLIENT EDUCATION GUIDE
Ileostomy Care

Pouch Care
- Empty your pouch when it is one-third to one-half full.
- Change the pouch during inactive times, such as before meals, before retiring at night, on waking in the morning, and 2 to 4 hours after eating.
- Change the entire pouch system every 3 to 7 days.

Skin Protection
- Use a pectin-based skin barrier (not karaya gum) to protect your skin from contact with contents from the ostomy.
- Use skin care products, such as skin sealants and ostomy skin creams, if your skin continues to come into contact with ostomy contents.
- Watch your skin for any irritation or redness.

Diet
- Chew food thoroughly.
- Be cautious of high-fiber and high-cellulose foods. You may need to eliminate these from the diet if they cause severe problems (diarrhea, constipation, or blockage). Examples include popcorn, peanuts, coconut, Chinese vegetables, string beans, tough-fiber meats, shrimp and lobster, rice, bran, and skinned vegetables (tomatoes, corn, and peas).

Medications
- Avoid taking enteric-coated and capsule medications.
- Inform any health care provider who is prescribing medications for you that you have an ostomy. Before having prescriptions filled, inform your pharmacist that you have an ostomy.
- Do not take any laxatives or enemas. You should usually have loose stool and should contact a physician if no stool has passed in 6 to 12 hours.

Symptoms to Watch for
- Report any drastic increase or decrease in drainage to your health care provider.
- If stomal swelling, abdominal cramping, or distention occurs, or if ileostomy contents stop draining, do the following:
  - Remove the pouch with faceplate.
  - Lie down, assuming a knee-chest position.
  - Begin abdominal massage.
  - Apply moist towels to the abdomen.
  - Drink hot tea.
  - If none of these maneuvers is effective in resuming ileostomy flow, or if abdominal pain is severe, call your health care provider right away.

ices of a home care aide. If the client is discharged from the hospital with an ileostomy, the case manager makes a referral to a home care agency. A home care nurse can provide assessment and guidance in integrating ostomy care into the client's lifestyle and possibly provide wound care, including the monitoring of wound healing (Chart 58-5). The client needs to know where to purchase ostomy supplies, along with the name, size, and manufacturer's order number. The ET or case manager contacts local and regional supply companies for prices and availability of supplies.

The nurse or ET can identify the local ostomy support group by contacting the United Ostomy Association. A support group or the Crohn's and Colitis Foundation of America may be of assistance in obtaining supplies, as well as providing education for ostomates. The nurse also informs the client and family or significant others of available ostomy outpatient clinics and ETs. If the client agrees, a visit from an ostomate can be initiated or continued on an outpatient basis.

Evaluation: Outcomes

NOC The nurse evaluates the care of the client with ulcerative colitis on the basis of the identified nursing diagnoses and collaborative problems. Expected outcomes may include that the client will:

- Be free of diarrhea, rectal bleeding, and cramping
- Maintain adequate hydration
- Understand the factors that can influence exacerbations of the disease
- Maintain ideal body weight
- Understand and adhere to the prescribed drug regimen
- Remain free of complications of the disease
- Identify and seek care for extraintestinal manifestations of the disease

In addition, the client with an ileostomy can be expected to:

- Engage in self-care of the ileostomy
- Maintain peristomal skin integrity
- Demonstrate behaviors that integrate ostomy care into his or her lifestyle
- Verbalize signs and symptoms of stoma complications

Crohn's Disease

OVERVIEW

Crohn's disease, also known as *regional enteritis* or *granulomatous colitis,* is a chronic inflammatory bowel disease (IBD) that can affect any part of the gastrointestinal (GI) tract, from the mouth to the anus. Approximately one million people in the United States have the disease (Klonowski & Masoodi, 1999). The peak incidence is between 15 and 40 years of age. The cause of Crohn's disease is uncertain; however, infectious, genetic, and immune etiologies have been proposed.

Mycobacterium paratuberculosis has been proposed as an environmental stimulus that could be implicated in the development of Crohn's disease, since granulomas similar to those seen in individuals with pulmonary tuberculosis have been found on biopsy of the intestines of people with the disease. A genetic predisposition to the disease has also been proposed, since the disease tends to cluster in families and appears equally in identical twins. However, the most widely accepted cause is believed to be a defect in the immunoregulation of inflammation in the presence of bacteria or viruses in the intestinal tract, along with a genetic predisposition for the disease (Norton, 1998).

Chronic, nonspecific inflammation of the entire intestinal tract characterizes the disease, with the terminal ileum being the site most often affected. Eventually, deep fissures and ulcerations develop and often extend through all bowel layers, predisposing the individual to the development of bowel fistulas. The result is severe diarrhea and malabsorption of vital nutrients. Chronic pathologic changes include thickening of the bowel wall, resulting in narrowing of the bowel lumen and strictures. In advanced disease, the bowel mucosa demonstrates nodular swelling (granulomas) intermingled with deep ulcerations.

The complications associated with Crohn's disease are similar to those of ulcerative colitis. As shown in Table 58-3, hemorrhage is more common in ulcerative colitis but can occur in Crohn's disease as well (see the Evidence-Based Practice for Nursing box on p. 1284). Severe malabsorption by the small intestine is more common in clients with Crohn's disease. Cancer of the small bowel and colon may develop in the client with Crohn's disease but usually occurs after the disease has been present for 15 to 20 years. Fistula formation is a common complication of Crohn's disease. Fistulas can occur between segments of the intestine or present as cutaneous fistulas or perirectal abscesses. Fistulas can also extend from the bowel to other organs and body cavities, such as the bladder or vagina (Figure 58-5). Twenty to thirty percent of individuals with the disease will develop intestinal obstruction. Initially, obstruction results from inflammation and edema. Over time, fibrosis develops and obstruction results secondary to a narrowing of the bowel (Glickman, 1998).

CHART 58-5

FOCUSED ASSESSMENT *of* Home Care of Clients with Inflammatory Bowel Disease

Assess gastrointestinal function and nutritional status, including:
- Abdominal cramping or pain
- Bowel elimination pattern; specifically frequency, characteristics and amount of stools, presence or absence of blood in stools
- Dietary and fluid intake and habits (include relationship of specific foods to cramping and stools)
- Weight gain or loss
- Signs and symptoms of dehydration
- Presence or absence of fever, rectal tenesmus, or urgency
- Bowel sounds
- Condition of perianal skin, including presence or absence of perianal fistula or abscess

Assess client's and family's coping skills, including:
- Current and ongoing stress level and coping style
- Availability of support system

Assess home environment, including:
- Adequacy and availability of bathroom facilities
- Opportunity for rest and relaxation

Assess ability to manage therapeutic regimen, including:
- Knowledge of medications
- Signs and symptoms to report
- Dietary management
- Availability of community resources
- Importance of follow-up care

EVIDENCE-BASED PRACTICE FOR NURSING

What are the characteristics of clients with acute lower gastrointestinal bleeding related to Crohn's disease?

Belaiche, J., et al. (1999). Acute lower gastrointestinal bleeding in Crohn's disease: Characteristics of a unique series of 34 patients. *American Journal of Gastroenterology, 94*(8), 2177-2181.

The purpose of this study was to assess the characteristics of clients with lower gastrointestinal (GI) bleeding related to Crohn's disease. In this study, 34 clients presenting to the hospital with lower GI bleeding were identified and data concerning the following characteristics were analyzed: client characteristics, blood transfusion requirements, site of bleeding, treatment, and follow-up.

In eight clients, the first manifestation of Crohn's disease was an episode of severe bleeding. Clients received 1 to 5 units of blood. The hemorrhage was found to be more frequent in clients with colonic disease than in those with disease confined to the small bowel. In 95% of cases, bleeding was caused by an area of ulceration, usually found in the sigmoid colon. Treatment consisted of blood transfusions and supportive measures such as corticosteroids, immunosuppressants, or endoscopy to identify the lesion and to apply either laser coagulation or adrenaline to stop bleeding from the lesion. Treatment was successful in 80% of clients with a first-time bleed. Bleeding was not significantly associated with steroid therapy in this study. In follow-up, 12 clients experienced recurrent bleeding episodes.

Critique. The relatively small sample size and convenience sampling method limits the generalizability of the findings. The definition and severity of GI bleeding may vary across the several medical centers used for subject recruitment, although the authors attempted to standardize this by recruiting subjects who received 2 or more units of blood.

Implications for Nursing. Although the results of the study cannot be generalized to all clients with Crohn's disease, new data about the presentation of the disease and its course were presented. The characteristics of hemorrhagic forms of Crohn's disease are not well described in the literature. This study can serve to make nurses more aware of bleeding as a complication more often associated with the disease than was previously thought. Nurses who care for individuals with disease in the colon can monitor their clients more closely for GI bleeding. Also, the study finding that more conservative treatments were successful in treating 80% of first-time hemorrhages can be shared with clients. Finally, although steroids were not associated with the development of bleeding in this study, other medications can increase the risk of GI bleeding. Clients need to be taught to avoid nonsteroidal anti-inflammatory drugs or aspirin-containing products while taking steroids, since the risk of bleeding increases. In addition, concomitant warfarin treatment may also increase the risk of bleeding.

CULTURAL CONSIDERATIONS

Crohn's disease is more common among people of Jewish descent, Caucasians of Western cultures, and those of middle European origin. The incidence of Crohn's disease is 20% greater in women than in men.

COLLABORATIVE MANAGEMENT

Assessment

HISTORY

A detailed history will assist in uncovering signs and symptoms specific to Crohn's disease. A history of fever, abdominal pain, and loose stools is commonly seen in a client with Crohn's disease. He or she is asked about recent unintentional loss of weight. The nurse should ask about the frequency, consistency, and presence of blood in the stool. The nurse also ascertains if the client has any first-degree relatives with the disease.

PHYSICAL ASSESSMENT/CLINICAL MANIFESTATIONS

The nurse performs a thorough abdominal examination, assesses for clinical manifestations of the disease, and evaluates the client's nutritional and hydration status. When performing an abdominal assessment, the nurse often notes findings that are consistent with those in acute appendicitis (e.g., tenderness, guarded movement, and a palpable mass in the right lower quadrant).

On inspection of the abdomen, the nurse assesses for distention, masses, or visible peristalsis. Inspection of the perianal area may reveal ulcerations or fissures. During auscultation, bowel sounds may be decreased or absent in the client with severe inflammation or obstruction. An increase in high-pitched or rushing sounds may be present over areas of narrowed bowel loops. Muscle guarding, masses, rigidity, or tenderness may be noted on palpation.

The clinical presentation of Crohn's disease can vary greatly from client to client. Depending on the parts of the bowel involved, the nurse may identify several clinical manifestations. Most clients report diarrhea, abdominal pain, and low-grade fever. Fever is also commonly present with complications such as fistulas and severe inflammation. If the disease occurs only in the ileum, diarrhea occurs five or six times per day, often with a soft, loose stool. Steatorrhea (fatty diarrheal stools) is common. The stool may contain bright red blood, but this is a rare finding.

Abdominal pain from the inflammatory process is usually constant and is located in the right lower quadrant. Clients also experience periumbilical pain before and after bowel movements. If the lower colon is diseased, pain is often experienced in both lower abdominal quadrants.

Weight loss is experienced by approximately 80% of individuals with Crohn's disease. Clients often experience nutritional problems as a result of increased catabolism secondary to chronic inflammation, anorexia, malabsorption, or self-imposed dietary restrictions. The result is fluid and electrolyte imbalances, as well as protein, iron, vitamin, and mineral deficiencies.

The marked inflammatory bowel changes decrease the small bowel's ability to absorb nutrients, which may be worsened by surgery and fistulas. The nurse is acutely aware of how important it is to detect clinical manifestations of peritonitis, bowel obstruction, and nutritional and fluid imbalances. The early detection of a change in the client's status helps to minimize these life-threatening complications.

PSYCHOSOCIAL ASSESSMENT

The client experiencing Crohn's disease needs a complete psychosocial assessment. The chronicity of the problem and the troublesome complications can greatly affect clients and their families. The assessment should be ongoing and should continuously reflect the client's status, as well as the family's.

DIAGNOSTIC ASSESSMENT

The health care provider may order a number of laboratory studies for clients with Crohn's disease; however, no disease-specific tests are available to confirm the diagnosis. The re-

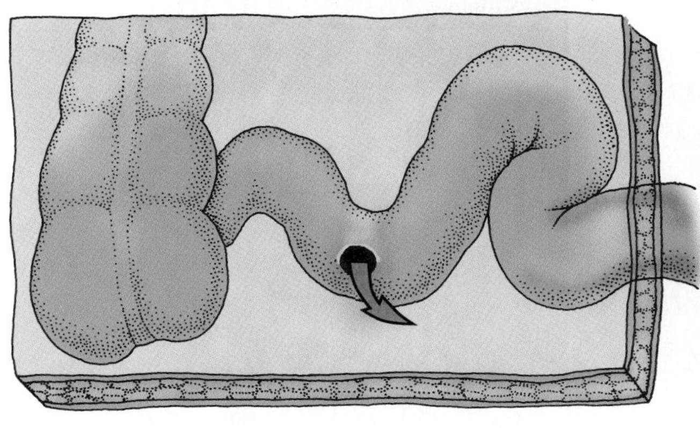

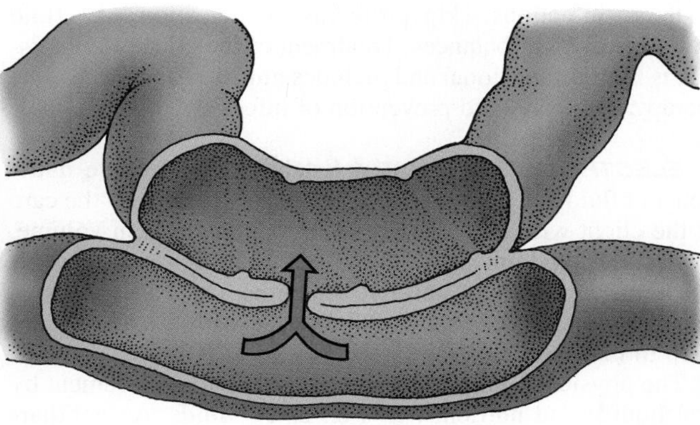

Figure 58-5 ● The types of fistulas that are complications of Crohn's disease.

sults of laboratory tests often indicate the extent and severity of inflammation associated with the disease.

If bleeding is present, the client may experience anemia. The nurse may note decreased hemoglobin and hematocrit values as a result of slow blood loss. Serum levels of folic acid and cobalamin (vitamin B_{12} group) are generally low because of malabsorption, further contributing to anemia. Amino acid malabsorption may result in decreased albumin levels. An elevated erythrocyte sedimentation rate (ESR) is consistent with the presence of inflammation. White blood cells (WBCs) in the urine may indicate infection (pyuria), which may be caused by ureteral obstruction or an enterovesical (bowel to bladder) fistula. If significant diarrhea is present, the client will experience electrolyte losses, particularly potassium and magnesium.

The results of the contrast barium enema and upper gastrointestinal (GI) series often provide more specific diagnostic information. X-ray studies show narrowing, ulcerations, strictures, and fistulas consistent with Crohn's disease. In the acute illness, these tests are often deferred until the risk of perforation lessens.

Depending on which areas of the bowel are diseased, the sigmoidoscopic examination may not be diagnostic. If the rectosigmoid colon is involved, the physician may see ulcerations and inflamed mucosa, areas of fissure, fistula, and abscess formation of the perianal and perirectal areas.

Colonoscopy is used when other tests, especially the barium enema examination, have not led to a specific diagnosis.

Interventions

Treatment of Crohn's disease is similar to that described earlier under Nonsurgical Management (Ulcerative Colitis), p. 1276.

NONSURGICAL MANAGEMENT. Specific interventions vary with the severity of disease and complications present.

DRUG THERAPY. The drugs used to manage Crohn's disease are similar to those used in the treatment of ulcerative colitis (see Drug Therapy [Ulcerative Colitis], p. 1277). Sulfasalazine (Asulfidine, PMS-Sulfasalazine♣) 1.5 to 2 g twice a day PO has been shown to be effective in treating exacerbations of Crohn's disease. Although glucocorticoids can be effective, sepsis can result from abscesses or fistulas that may be present. These medications mask the symptoms of infection; therefore they must be used with caution and require vigilant monitoring by the nurse for signs of infection.

Metronidazole (Flagyl, Novonidazol♣) 250 to 500 mg three times a day PO has been helpful in clients with fistulas. Immunosuppressive therapy has been effective in clients with refractory disease or fistulas. Azathioprine (Imuran), an immunosuppressive agent, 50 mg/day for 12 months may be instituted. After that time the health care provider may attempt to withdraw the drug, but long-term therapy may be needed in some cases.

Since a defect in immunoregulation of inflammation may be implicated in the development of Crohn's disease, neutralization of a cytokine (specifically, tumor necrosis factor) may prove useful in decreasing bowel inflammation. A relatively new drug, infliximab (Remicade) a chimeric monoclonal antibody form of antitumor necrosis factor alpha, has been approved for use. The usual dose of 5 mg/kg has demonstrated efficacy in the treatment of active Crohn's disease and fistulas. Further investigation is needed to determine the long-term safety and efficacy of the drug (Mikula, 1999).

NUTRITIONAL MANAGEMENT. Long-standing nutritional deficits can have severe consequences for the client with Crohn's disease. Malnutrition can result in poor fistula and wound healing, loss of lean muscle mass, decreased immune system response, and increased morbidity and mortality. With severe exacerbations of the disease, the health care provider may order hospitalization to provide bowel rest and nutritional enhancement with total parenteral nutrition (TPN). For less severe exacerbations, the health care provider may prescribe an elemental diet using products such as Vivonex to induce remission. Elemental diets are absorbed in the jejunum and therefore permit rest of the distal small intestine and colon. Once remission is achieved, the health care provider will usually prescribe a low-residue diet. Nutritional supplements, such as Ensure or Sustacal, can be added to provide nutrients and added calories.

COMPLICATION MANAGEMENT. **Fistulas** (abnormal tract from intestine to skin or intestine to intestine) are common occurrences with acute exacerbations of Crohn's disease. Clients with fistulas often experience complications, such as systemic infections, skin problems, malnutrition, and fluid and electrolyte imbalances. Treatment of the client with a fistula is multidimensional and includes nutrition and electrolyte therapy, skin care, and prevention of infection.

ELECTROLYTE THERAPY. Establishing adequate nutrition and fluid and electrolyte balance takes priority in the care of the client with a fistula. GI secretions are high in volume, electrolytes, and enzymes. The client is at high risk for malnutrition, dehydration, and hypokalemia. The nurse assesses for these complications and collaborates with the health care team to manage them.

The physician orders fluids and electrolyte replacement by oral liquids and nutrients, as well as IV fluids. An antidiarrheal agent, such as diphenoxylate hydrochloride or atropine sulfate (Lomotil), may be prescribed to decrease fluid loss from diarrhea, but these drugs are not commonly used and must be given with caution.

When a fistula begins to develop, the client's nutritional status is usually compromised. After the fistula has developed, nutritional status worsens. The client requires at least 3000 calories/day to promote healing of the fistula. If the client cannot take adequate oral fluids and nutrients, the physician may order TPN. In collaboration with the dietitian, the nurse:

- Carefully monitors the client's tolerance to diet
- Assists the client in selecting high-calorie, high-protein, high-vitamin, low-fiber meals
- Offers enteral supplements, such as Ensure and Vivonex
- Records food intake for accurate calorie counts

SKIN CARE. Proteolytic enzymes and bile contribute to the problem of skin irritation and excoriation. Skin irritation needs to be prevented; this is usually accomplished through the use of skin barriers, application of pouches, and insertion of drains (Figure 58-6). By applying a pouch to the draining fistula, the nurse prevents skin irritation and can measure the effluent (drainage).

In one approach to drainage management, the nurse covers the area surrounding the fistula with barriers, such as Stomahesive or DuoDerm, and then applies a wound drainage system over the fistula, securing it to the protective dressing. The skin adjacent to the fistula is cleaned with normal saline solution and gently patted dry.

The nurse collaborates with the enterostomal therapist (ET) to provide wound management. Wound drainage must *never* be allowed to be in direct contact with skin without prompt cleaning, because intestinal fluid enzymes are caustic.

PREVENTION OF INFECTION. Clients with fistulas are at extremely high risk for intra-abdominal abscesses and sepsis. Intra-abdominal fistulas are treated with careful nursing interventions, containment of wound drainage, and antibiotic therapy. The nurse observes for subtle signs of infection or sepsis, such as fever, abdominal pain, or change in mental status.

SURGICAL MANAGEMENT. Surgery to remove diseased portions of intestine is controversial for clients with Crohn's disease because risk for recurrence is considerable. However, those who continue to have symptoms after long-term medical treatment and those with complications such as fistulas may undergo a small-bowel resection and anastomosis with or without a colon resection to improve quality of life (see the Legal/Ethical Issues in Health Care box on p. 1287).

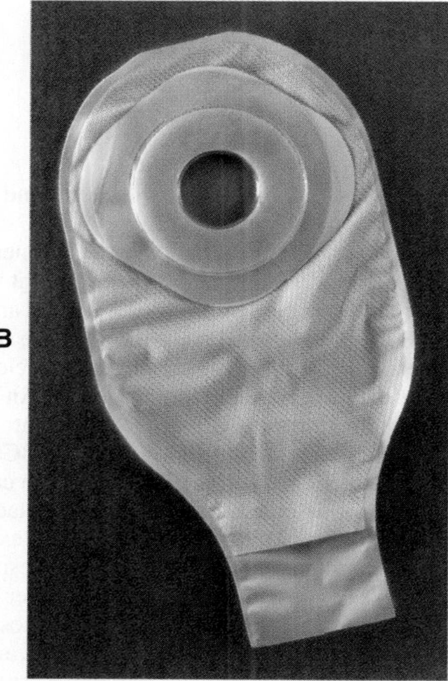

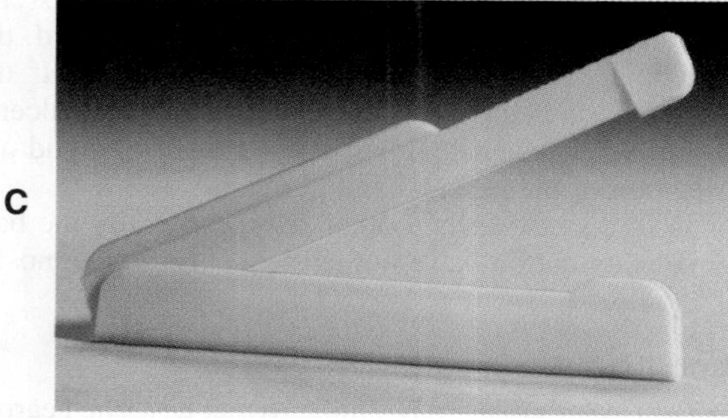

Figure 58-6 ● Skin barriers, such as wafers **(A),** are cut to fit ⅛ inch around fistula. A drainable pouch **(B)** is applied over the wafer and clamped **(C)** until the pouch is to be emptied. Effluent should drain into the bag and not contact the skin. (Courtesy ConvaTec, A Bristol-Myers Squibb Company, Skillman, NJ.)

Strictureplasty may be performed for bowel strictures related to Crohn's disease. This procedure, which involves incising along the length of the stricture and suturing the incised area on the horizontal plane, allows for an increase in the bowel diameter. Preoperative and postoperative care for each

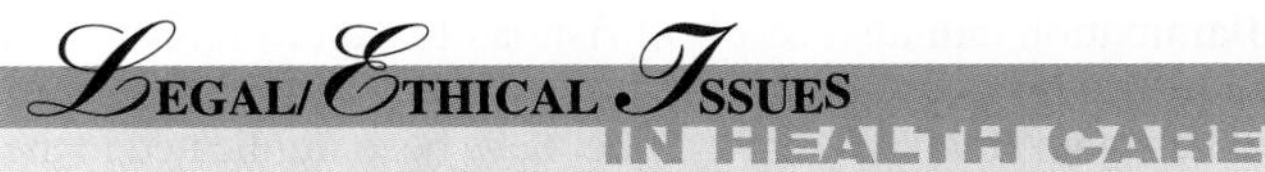

THE IMPACT OF SURGERY FOR CROHN'S DISEASE ON HEALTH-RELATED QUALITY OF LIFE

When clients are questioned regarding their concerns relative to the disease process, surgery appears to be one of their greatest worries, particularly if the surgery will require them to have an ostomy. This study examined whether surgical treatment of Crohn's disease modified health-related quality of life (QOL) as compared with inactive Crohn's disease, active disease, or healthy controls.

Clients with active Crohn's disease reported the lowest health-related QOL. The most important factor in determining health-related QOL is the severity of the disease and accompanying symptoms. It is apparent that the severe symptoms accompanying active disease seriously impair perceived QOL. QOL improves during disease remission, regardless of whether the remission was achieved by medical or surgical means. To improve QOL, it is more important to achieve remission, regardless of the approach used.

Data from Casellas, F., et al. (2000). Impact of surgery for Crohn's disease on health-related quality of life. *American Journal of Gastroenterology, 95*(1), 177-181.

of these surgical procedures is similar to care for clients undergoing other types of abdominal surgery.

Community-Based Care

The discharge care plan for the client with Crohn's disease is similar to that for the client with ulcerative colitis (see Community-Based Care [Ulcerative Colitis], p. 1282). The nurse or case manager helps the client with a draining fistula plan for care of the fistula at home.

HOME CARE MANAGEMENT

The interventions begun in the hospital to manage the disease need to be carried out to some extent in the home. Measures to control the disease and related symptoms and manage nutrition need to be reinforced. Supplies for wound and/or fistula care may be required. The client's home should be arranged so that the client has easy access to the bathroom, as well as privacy to perform fistula care. To ensure adequate nutrition, the client should have easy access to a well-supplied kitchen of readily prepared foods.

HEALTH TEACHING

The teaching plan for the client with Crohn's disease is similar to that for the client with ulcerative colitis. He or she is taught the usual course of the disease, symptoms of complications, and when to notify the health care provider. Medication teaching, including purpose, dose, and side effects, is incorporated into the teaching plan. The nurse, in collaboration with the dietitian, teaches the client to follow a low-residue, high-calorie diet and to avoid foods that cause discomfort.

The nurse teaches the client to provide for rest periods, especially during exacerbations of the disease. If stress appears to increase symptoms of the disease, the nurse may teach the client stress management techniques or recommend counseling. For long-term follow-up, the client is educated regarding the increased risk of bowel cancer and the advisability of having a colonoscopy yearly as a means of early detection of changes in the mucosa (Hirsch & Caswell, 1999).

COST OF CARE
IMPLICATIONS FOR NURSING

INFLAMMATORY BOWEL DISEASE

Cost of Care

- The average cost of hospitalization for Crohn's disease is $12,528 excluding physician's fees.
- The mean cost per admission for all cases of ulcerative colitis is $3726.
- Surgical treatment for Crohn's disease accounts for 49.8% of all admissions and accounts for 60% to 55% of all costs.
- Clients treated surgically for Crohn's disease had more costly hospitalizations than those treated medically.
- Total parenteral nutrition accounts for 63% of all pharmacy costs when clients are admitted for exacerbations of Crohn's disease.
- Admissions for Crohn's disease that include surgical interventions are the most costly.

Implications for Nursing

Chronic diseases such as Crohn's disease are characterized by periods of remission and exacerbation. Vigilant monitoring of the client's status by home care nurses could significantly reduce costs by identifying complications so that treatment is initiated in the early phases. Nurses play an important role in the education of their clients and families. Teaching initiatives that assist clients with symptom management and recognition of complications could possibly avoid more costly hospital admissions and subsequent invasive treatments. Therapies that decrease the number of surgical hospitalizations should reduce the cost of inpatient care associated with Crohn's disease.

Data from Cohen, R., et al. (2000). The cost of hospitalization for Crohn's disease. *American Journal of Gastroenterology, 95*(2), 524-530.

If a client has developed a fistula, the nurse explains and demonstrates fistula care. The client needs opportunities to practice the care in the hospital. Ideally, the client should be independent in fistula care before leaving the hospital. However, because of the perirectal or vaginal location of the fistula or an obese abdomen, the client may need assistance in this care. If this is the case, a family member or a caregiver must learn and practice the care, or the nurse or case manager can arrange for home care services.

HEALTH CARE RESOURCES

The client discharged to home following resection and anastomosis may require visits from a home care nurse to assess the surgical wound and monitor for complications. The nurse assesses the client's and family's ability to monitor the progress of fistula healing and to watch for signs and symptoms of infection and sepsis. Home care nursing visits may also be appropriate for this purpose. A home care aide might be considered for clients who cannot meet their nutritional needs, who need help with meal preparation, and who need help in purchasing groceries.

If the client needs equipment for fistula care, such as skin barriers and wound drainage bags, the nurse or case manager contacts medical supply companies or local pharmacies to ascertain their availability and price (see the Cost of Care box above). A support group sponsored by the United Ostomy Association or a local hospital in the community may also be available to assist the client and family with physical, as well as psychosocial, needs.

Diverticular Disease

OVERVIEW

Diverticula are congenital or acquired pouchlike herniations of the mucosa through the muscular wall of the small intestine or colon. **Diverticulosis** is the presence of many abnormal pouchlike herniations (diverticula) in the wall of the intestine. **Diverticulitis** is the term used to describe an inflammation of one or more diverticula.

Pathophysiology

Diverticula can occur in any part of the small or large intestine, but they occur most commonly in the sigmoid colon (Figure 58-7). The musculature of the colon hypertrophies, thickens, and becomes rigid, and herniation of the mucosa and submucosa through the colon wall is seen. Diverticula seem to occur at points of weakness in the intestinal wall, often at areas where blood vessels interrupt muscular continuity. The muscle weakness develops as part of the aging process.

In and of themselves, diverticula cause few problems. If undigested food or bacteria become trapped in a diverticulum, however, blood supply to that area diminishes and bacteria invade the diverticulum. Diverticulitis results when the diverticulum perforates and a local abscess forms. The perforated diverticulum can also progress to an intra-abdominal perforation with generalized peritonitis.

Bleeding from diverticula can range from minor, localized bleeding to massive hemorrhage. Minor bleeding is often due to localized inflammation in areas of vascular granulation tissue at the base of the diverticulum. Hemorrhage can result when a blood vessel is eroded within a diverticulum. Inflammation secondary to recurrent diverticulitis can lead to narrowing of the bowel lumen, which may result in obstruction. Inflammation can also result in fistulas to other organs, such as the bladder and the vagina.

Diets with small amounts of fiber have been implicated in the development of diverticula in that they cause less bulky stool and possibly constipation. For diverticulosis and diverticulitis to occur, there must be an increase in intraluminal pressure and muscle contractions to move fecal material through the colon.

The etiologic factor in diverticulitis may be retained undigested food in diverticula, which compromises the blood supply to that area and facilitates bacterial invasion of the sac.

Incidence/Prevalence

The incidence of diverticulosis is difficult to determine, but it is estimated that millions of people are affected. Diverticular disease affects one third of adults over age 60 years. Although diverticulosis is common, only 1 out of 5 people with this disease displays symptoms. Diverticular disease occurs more often in men than in women (Isselbacher & Epstein, 1998).

CONSIDERATIONS FOR OLDER ADULTS

The incidence of diverticula increases with age. There is a reported incidence of 20% to 50% in Western populations over the age of 50 (Isselbacher & Epstein, 1998).

COLLABORATIVE MANAGEMENT

Assessment

HISTORY

Clients with diverticulosis are usually asymptomatic, and unless pain and/or bleeding develops, the condition may go undiagnosed or be found incidentally on routine colonoscopy. Occasionally, diverticulosis causes symptoms. For clients

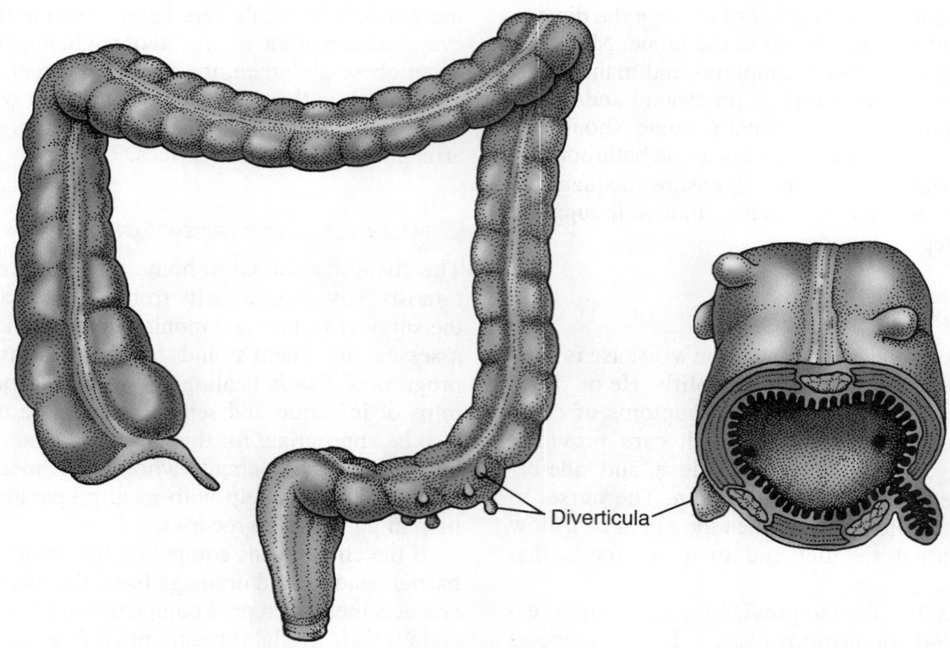

Figure 58-7 ● Several abnormal outpouchings, or herniations, in the wall of the intestine, which are diverticula. These can occur anywhere in the small or large intestine but are found most often in the sigmoid as shown in this figure. Diverticulitis is the inflammation of a diverticulum that occurs when undigested food or bacteria become trapped in the diverticulum.

with uncomplicated diverticulosis, the nurse asks about a history of intermittent pain in the left lower quadrant and a history of constipation. If diverticulitis is suspected, the client is asked about a history of fever and abdominal pain. The nurse inquires about recent bowel elimination patterns, since constipation may develop as a result of intestinal inflammation. The client is also questioned about the presence of bleeding from the rectum.

PHYSICAL ASSESSMENT/CLINICAL MANIFESTATIONS

On physical examination of the client with uncomplicated diverticulosis, no clinical manifestations of the disorder may be present. Occasionally the nurse may elicit tenderness on abdominal palpation.

The client with diverticulitis has abdominal pain, most often localized to the left lower quadrant. The pain may be intermittent at first but becomes progressively steady. Occasionally pain may be suprapubic or may occur on one side. Abdominal pain is generalized if peritonitis has occurred. The client's temperature is elevated, ranging from a low-grade fever to 101° F (38.2° C), and may be accompanied by chills. The nurse may note the presence of tachycardia secondary to fever. Nausea and vomiting are also commonly present.

On examination of the abdomen, the nurse may observe distention. Tenderness on palpation may be noted over the area involved (usually the left lower quadrant). The colon may be palpable. If localized peritoneal irritation is present, localized muscle spasm, guarded movement, and rebound tenderness are usually present. If generalized peritonitis is present, abdominal muscle spasm, guarding, and rebound tenderness are more diffuse.

If the perforated diverticulum is close to the rectum, the health care provider may palpate a tender mass during the rectal examination. Blood pressure checks may show orthostatic changes. If bleeding is massive, the client may have hypotension and dehydration that result in shock. If generalized peritonitis has occurred, sepsis and manifestations of hypotension and septic or hypovolemic shock can occur.

DIAGNOSTIC ASSESSMENT

For the client with uncomplicated diverticulosis, laboratory studies are not indicated. The client with diverticulitis, however, has an elevated white blood cell (WBC) count. Decreased hematocrit and hemoglobin values are noted if chronic or severe bleeding is present. In stool tests for occult blood, results are positive in 20% of clients (also called a positive guaiac). Urinalysis may show a few red blood cells (RBCs) if the left ureter is in proximity to a perforated diverticulum.

X-ray studies of the intestinal tract with barium contrast show diverticula. An upper gastrointestinal (GI) series shows diverticula of the small intestine, and barium enema examination shows diverticula of the large intestine. X-ray studies are not indicated in clients with uncomplicated diverticulosis, because symptoms are usually minimal or nonexistent.

The client with diverticulitis usually does *not* undergo a barium enema examination in the acute phase of the illness because of the risk of rupture of the inflamed diverticulum. A barium enema examination may be completed after the client has been treated with antibiotics and the inflammation has resolved. A flat-plate film of the abdomen may reveal free air and fluid in the left lower quadrant, suggesting an abscess or free air under the diaphragm, indicating perforation. The health care provider may also order a computed tomography (CT) scan to diagnose an abscess or thickening of the bowel related to diverticulitis.

Ultrasonography, a noninvasive test, may reveal bowel thickening or an abscess. The physician may perform a sigmoidoscopy or colonoscopy *after the acute phase* of the illness, usually to rule out the presence of a tumor in the large intestine, particularly if the client has rectal bleeding. If the sigmoidoscope or colonoscope enters a diverticulum, however, the chances of perforating the diverticulum are high.

Interventions

Clients may be treated on an ambulatory care basis when symptoms are mild, with a temperature lower than 101° F (38.2° C) and a WBC count ranging from 13,000 to 15,000/mm^3. The client who is an outpatient should be monitored for any prolonged or increased fever, abdominal pain, or blood in the stool.

Clients with moderate to severe diverticulitis require hospitalization. Clinical manifestations that suggest the need for admission are a temperature higher than 101° F (38.2° C), persistent abdominal pain for more than 3 days, or evidence of lower GI bleeding.

NONSURGICAL MANAGEMENT. For the client with diverticulitis, a combination of drug and diet therapy with rest to decrease inflammation and improve tissue perfusion is indicated. This plan is preferred for older adults and others with mild to moderate disease (Chart 58-6).

DRUG THERAPY. For clients with mild diverticulitis, the health care provider prescribes broad-spectrum antibiotics, such as metronidazole (Flagyl) plus trimethoprim/sulfamethoxazole (Bactrim, Septra) or ciprofloxacin (Cipro). A mild analgesic may be given for pain.

The health care provider admits clients with more severe pain to the hospital and orders IV fluids to correct dehydration, as well as IV antibiotics such as cefoxitin plus metro-

CHART 58-6

NURSING FOCUS *on the* OLDER ADULT
Diverticulitis

- Provide antibiotics, analgesics, and anticholinergics as ordered. Observe older clients carefully for side effects of these drugs, especially confusion (or increased confusion), urinary retention or failure, and orthostatic hypotension.
- Do not give laxatives or enemas. Teach the client and the family about the importance of avoiding these measures.
- Encourage the client to rest and to avoid activities that may increase intra-abdominal pressure, such as straining and bending.
- While diverticulitis is active, provide a *low*-fiber diet (see Table 58-4). When the inflammation resolves, provide a *high*-fiber diet. Teach the client and family about these diets and when they are appropriate.
- Because older clients do not always experience the typical pain or fever expected, observe carefully for signs of active disease.
- Perform frequent abdominal assessments to determine distention and tenderness on palpation.
- Check stools for occult or frank bleeding.

nidazole. Anticholinergics, such as propantheline bromide (Pro-Banthine), may reduce intestinal hypermotility. For clients with moderate to severe diverticulitis, an opioid analgesic, such as meperidine hydrochloride (Demerol) or morphine sulfate, can alleviate pain.

Laxatives are avoided because they increase intestinal motility. Enemas are avoided because they increase intraluminal pressure. The nurse assesses the client for clinical manifestations of fluid and electrolyte imbalance on an ongoing basis.

REST. The nurse instructs the client to remain in bed during the acute phase of illness. He or she is advised to refrain from lifting, straining, coughing, or bending to avoid an increase in intra-abdominal pressure, which can result in perforation of the diverticulum.

DIET THERAPY. During the acute phase of the illness, the client's diet is restricted to clear liquids. Clients who have more severe symptoms are admitted to the hospital and are kept on NPO status. A nasogastric (NG) tube is inserted if nausea, vomiting, or abdominal distention is severe. The nurse administers IV fluids, as ordered, for hydration. In collaboration with the dietitian, the client increases dietary intake slowly as symptoms subside. When inflammation has resolved and bowel function returns to normal, a fiber-containing diet is introduced gradually. If active diverticulitis recurs, fiber intake is stopped for the acute phase of the illness.

SURGICAL MANAGEMENT. The client with diverticulitis may need to undergo surgery for any of the following conditions:

- Rupture of the diverticulum with subsequent peritonitis
- Pelvic abscess
- Bowel obstruction
- Fistula
- Persistent fever or pain after 4 days of medical treatment
- Uncontrolled bleeding

The surgeon performs emergency surgery if peritonitis, bowel obstruction, or pelvic abscess is present. Colon resection, with or without a colostomy, is the most common surgical procedure for clients with diverticular disease.

PREOPERATIVE CARE. Preparation of the client for surgery depends on the severity of the condition. The surgery might be performed on an emergency basis, or it might be done with a few weeks' notice. The surgeon informs the client whether a temporary or permanent colostomy might be required.

If the client is *not* in the acute stage of diverticulitis, a thorough bowel preparation *may* be given, consisting of enemas and laxatives daily for 2 to 3 days before surgery. Because of the risk of perforation, however, the surgeon may forgo an aggressive bowel preparation. If the client has an acutely inflamed diverticulum or persistent fever and abdominal pain, the bowel preparation is most likely withheld.

The client who is to undergo emergency surgery or who has not responded to medical intervention is maintained on NPO status with an NG tube in place. He or she receives IV fluids with appropriate electrolyte replacements.

For clients without acute inflammation, a well-structured preoperative diet is ordered. The client usually has a low-fiber diet for 4 to 5 days, followed by a full-liquid diet for 2 days, then a clear-liquid diet the evening before surgery.

Preoperative teaching may include information about the possible need for a colostomy. If a colostomy is a possible outcome, the enterostomal therapist (ET) or office nurse describes its function and purpose. The nurse need not discuss colostomy care in detail unless the client wishes this information at this time.

OPERATIVE PROCEDURES. In a resection of the colon, the surgeon excises the portion that is inflamed or diseased and, if possible, creates an anastomosis of the colon to restore patency. Inflammation and infection, however, may preclude the feasibility of an anastomosis. If this is the case, the surgeon may perform a colostomy. Select clients may be candidates for colostomy closure and anastomosis after the bowel has been allowed to rest for 3 to 6 months.

POSTOPERATIVE CARE. The immediate physical care for clients undergoing a colon resection for diverticulitis is the same as that for clients undergoing abdominal surgery (see Chapter 19).

Wound Care. The client has a drain in place at the abdominal incision site for 2 to 3 days. If a colostomy has been performed, the stoma may be covered with petroleum gauze dressing because the colostomy does not drain for approximately 2 days, or a colostomy bag may be placed over the stoma. If the stoma is visible, the nurse monitors its color and integrity. The stoma should be pinkish to cherry red without retraction or prolapse into the abdomen.

Diet Therapy. The client is maintained on NPO status with an NG tube in place for 2 to 3 days after a colon resection with or without a colostomy. When peristalsis returns, the nurse removes the NG tube, according to the health care provider's order, and introduces clear liquids *slowly. Gradually,* the diet is advanced to solids, depending on the return of peristalsis and bowel function.

If the client has had a colostomy created, it should begin functioning in 2 to 4 days. Most clients who undergo surgery and colostomy formation for diverticulitis have a sigmoid colostomy because the sigmoid colon is the most common site of diverticulitis. Drainage from a sigmoid colostomy initially consists of loose stool, but eventually the stool becomes formed. A tight seal around the stoma is essential to avoid contact of feces with the skin. Colostomy care is detailed in Chapter 57.

Emotional Support. If a colostomy has been performed, the nurse gives the client an opportunity to express feelings about the ostomy. The nurse discusses these feelings with the client, acknowledging that anger and depression are normal responses. When the client is physically able, the nurse encourages him or her to look at the stoma and touch the apparatus.

Community-Based Care

The length of hospitalization for clients with diverticulitis ranges from 4 to 10 days, depending on the response to medical treatment and the need for surgery. Discharge plans vary according to the treatment.

HOME CARE MANAGEMENT

For the client with diverticulitis who has responded to medical treatment, home care focuses on proper diet. The nurse assesses the client's ability to obtain and prepare the recommended high-fiber foods. The client who has required surgical intervention has the added responsibilities of incision care and possibly colostomy care, with some temporary limitations placed on activities.

HEALTH TEACHING

DIET THERAPY. All clients with diverticular disease require education regarding a high-fiber diet. For clients with diverticulosis, an increase in dietary fiber can regulate bowel function and bring about partial relief of symptoms. The nurse and dietitian encourage the client with diverticulosis to eat a diet high in cellulose and hemicellulose types of fiber. These substances can be found in wheat bran, whole-grain breads, and cereals. The client should ingest at least 25 to 35 g of fiber per day. This requirement can be derived from four slices of 100% whole-wheat bread and a 3-ounce serving of all-bran cereal. The nurse also teaches the client to eat fresh fruits and vegetables with high-fiber content to add bulk to stools.

The client who is not accustomed to eating high-fiber foods should add them to the diet gradually to avoid flatulence and abdominal cramping. If the client cannot tolerate the recommended fiber requirement, a bulk-forming laxative, such as psyllium hydrophilic mucilloid (Metamucil), can be taken to increase fecal size and consistency. An adequate intake of fluids will help to prevent the bloating that may accompany a high-fiber diet. The client should also avoid alcohol because it irritates the bowel. Clients are instructed to avoid foods containing seeds or indigestible material that may block a diverticulum, such as nuts, corn, popcorn, cucumbers, tomatoes, figs, strawberries, and caraway seeds. In collaboration with the dietitian, the nurse teaches the client that dietary fat intake should not exceed 30% of the total daily caloric intake.

Clients should *avoid all fiber* when they have symptoms of *diverticulitis* because high-fiber foods are irritating. As diverticulitis resolves, fiber can gradually be added until progression to a high-fiber diet is once again obtained. The client who has undergone surgery is usually taking solid food by the time of discharge from the hospital.

The nurse explains the usual disease course and factors that can exacerbate the disease to the client. Follow-up with the health care provider approximately 1 month following resolution of symptoms is recommended, and a repeat flexible sigmoidoscopy or barium enema may be preformed at that time.

SURGICAL FOLLOW-UP. Clients who have had abdominal surgery need oral and written instructions on incision care and the signs and symptoms to report to the health care provider. These are similar to the instructions given to clients after other types of abdominal surgery. The nurse provides instructions on colostomy care for clients who have a temporary or permanent colostomy.

GENERAL INSTRUCTIONS. The nurse instructs clients *with any type of diverticular disease,* orally and in writing, about signs and symptoms of acute diverticulitis, including fever, abdominal pain, and bloody, mahogany, or tarry stools. The client should be advised to avoid the use of laxatives (other than bulk-forming types) and enemas. All clients can also benefit from avoiding the activities that increase intra-abdominal pressure, such as straining at stool, bending, or lifting heavy objects.

The nurse reassures clients with diverticulosis that this disorder need not cause problems if a proper diet is followed. The client is informed that this illness does not commonly recur and that with proper diet and elimination patterns, recurring episodes and potential complications can be avoided.

The client with a colostomy has special needs with regard to the alteration in body image and loss of body function. The nurse encourages the client to verbalize concerns about body image.

Clients who have undergone surgery may need assistance with incision and colostomy care. The nurse or case manager arranges for a home care nurse to assess wound healing and proper functioning of the ostomy and the appliance. If the client is interested, the nurse can arrange for a visit from an ostomy volunteer or an enterostomal therapist (ET). For information about other ostomy resources, the nurse or the client can contact the United Ostomy Association.

ANORECTAL ABSCESS

OVERVIEW

Anorectal abscesses most often result from obstruction of the ducts of glands in the anorectal region by feces, foreign bodies, or trauma. Stasis of obstructing contents occurs and causes infection that spreads into adjacent tissue. Most abscesses begin as cryptitis (a pocket of infection in an anal crypt).

The client may experience diarrhea or rectal pain as the first symptom. There may be no clinical manifestations at the time of the first physical assessment, but local swelling, erythema, and tenderness on palpation are apparent within a few days after the onset of pain. If the abscess becomes chronic, discharge, bleeding, and pruritus (itching) may exist. Fever occurs if larger abscesses are present.

COLLABORATIVE MANAGEMENT

Anorectal abscesses are managed by surgical incision and drainage. The physician can often incise simple perianal and ischiorectal abscesses using a local anesthetic. For clients with more extensive abscesses, a regional or general anesthetic may be needed. Systemic antibiotics are given only for clients who are immunocompromised, are diabetic, have valvular disease or a prosthetic valve, or have extensive subcutaneous fat. Incision and drainage in these clients is performed after antibiotic therapy.

Nursing interventions are focused on helping the client to maintain comfort and optimal perineal hygiene (Chart 58-7). The nurse encourages the use of sitz baths, analgesics, bulk-producing agents, and stool softeners during the perioperative period until healing occurs. The nurse also emphasizes the importance of ongoing perineal hygiene after all bowel movements and the maintenance of a regular bowel pattern with a high-fiber diet.

ANAL FISSURE

OVERVIEW

An anal fissure is a superficial erosion of the anal canal. Fissures can be primary or secondary, acute or chronic. *Primary* fissures are idiopathic with no known cause. *Secondary* fis-

CHART 58-7

BEST PRACTICE *for* Promoting Perineal Comfort

- Keep the perineal area clean with mild soap.
- Pat the perineal area dry instead of rubbing it.
- Provide warm sitz baths or apply warm compresses to the area.
- If the area is acutely inflamed, apply cold packs.
- Provide a chair cushion or a soft, inflatable ring for the seated client. For the older or debilitated client, monitor the skin carefully to prevent pressure sores.
- Use absorbent pads for drainage, if any, and change them often.
- Use premoistened wipes for cleaning the perineal area after a bowel movement.
- Use witch hazel wipes (e.g., Tucks) to relieve pain.
- Give bulk-forming agents, such as psyllium mucilloid (Metamucil), as ordered, to reduce pain associated with defecation.
- Apply a topical anesthetic cream to the perineal area, as ordered.
- Give oral analgesics, as prescribed, for pain relief.
- Do not administer enemas or give potent laxatives.

sures are associated with another disorder (e.g., Crohn's disease, tuberculosis, or leukemia) or with trauma (e.g., from a foreign body, childbirth, or perirectal surgery). Constipated stool, diarrhea, or spasm of the anal sphincter is another possible cause.

➤ COLLABORATIVE MANAGEMENT

An acute anal fissure is superficial and resolves spontaneously or heals quickly with conservative treatment. Chronic fissures recur, and surgical treatment may be needed. Pain during and after defecation and bleeding noted outside the stool are the most common symptoms. Other clinical manifestations associated with chronic fissures are pruritus, urinary frequency or retention, dysuria, and dyspareunia (painful intercourse).

The health care provider makes the diagnosis by inspecting and stretching the perianal skin. If the client is having pain at the time of the examination, diagnostic testing is usually limited to inspection. If the client is not in severe pain, a digital examination and possibly a sigmoidoscopy are performed. When painless or multiple fissures are present, the physician may perform a barium enema and sigmoidoscopy to rule out an associated inflammatory bowel disorder.

Management of an acute fissure is nonsurgical, with interventions aimed at local, symptomatic pain relief and softening of stools to reduce trauma to the area. Warm sitz baths and analgesia are recommended along with the use of bulk-producing agents, such as psyllium hydrophilic mucilloid (Metamucil), which help minimize pain associated with defecation. If fissures do not respond to medical management within several days to weeks, surgical excision of the fissure with a local anesthetic may be necessary.

The nurse explains the appropriate pain control measures to the client. When nonsurgical management is initiated, the nurse instructs clients to notify the health care provider if pain is not relieved within a few days. The nurse instructs the client who undergoes surgery to continue with the same pain management and bowel regimen, including sitz baths, analgesics, and bulk-forming agents. He or she is reminded to report any drainage or bleeding from the rectum to the health care provider.

ANAL FISTULA

OVERVIEW

An anal fistula, or *fistula in ano,* is an abnormal tract leading from the anal canal to the perianal skin. Most anal fistulas result from anorectal abscesses, which are caused by obstruction of anal glands (see Anorectal Abscess, p. 1291). Fistulas can also be associated with tuberculosis, Crohn's disease, or cancer.

➤ COLLABORATIVE MANAGEMENT

The client with an anal fistula has pruritus (itching), purulent discharge, and tenderness or pain that is worsened by bowel movements. The physician uses a proctoscope to identify the source of symptoms and to locate the fistula. Because fistulas do not heal spontaneously, surgery is necessary. To perform a fistulotomy, the surgeon incises the tissue overlying the tract and performs curettage (scraping) of the base. The incision site heals by secondary intention. In a client with a high fistula, a special surgical technique is necessary because important sphincters are often affected. Postoperatively, the nurse instructs the client about sitz baths, analgesics, and the use of bulk-producing agents or stool softeners to minimize pain.

PARASITIC INFECTION

OVERVIEW

Parasites can enter and invade the gastrointestinal (GI) tract and cause infections leading to varying degrees of illness. Parasites commonly enter through the mouth by means of fecal-oral transmission from the following:

- Contaminated food or water
- Oral-anal sexual practices
- Contact with feces from a contaminated person

Common parasites that cause infection in humans are *Entamoeba histolytica,* which causes amebiasis (amebic dysentery), *Giardia lamblia,* which causes giardiasis, and *Cryptosporidium.*

Infection with *Entamoeba histolytica*

Humans are the only known hosts for *E. histolytica* (also known as amebiasis). This organism occurs in cysts and trophozoites (sporozoan parasites). Trophozoites die rapidly after they leave the body in stool. Cysts, however, can remain viable in the right type of environment for weeks or months. Humans who eliminate cysts are infectious. Flies have been found to be vectors for transmission of the cysts, and transmission is increased in areas that use human excrement for fertilizer. Transmission occurs by the fecal-oral route.

Amebiasis occurs worldwide, but it is most prevalent and most severe in tropical areas. Prevalence rates are as high as 40% in areas with poor sanitation, crowding, and poor nutrition. Amebiasis causes 40,000 to 100,000 deaths annually worldwide. The disease causes less severe symptoms and often goes undiagnosed in temperate climates. The organism may occur in 2% to 5% of some populations in the United States.

E. histolytica either feeds on bacteria in the intestine or invades and ulcerates the mucosa of the large intestine. The parasite can be limited to the GI tract (intestinal amebiasis), or it can extend outside the intestines (extraintestinal amebiasis). People can have intestinal amebiasis without having any symptoms, or symptoms can range from mild to severe.

Infection with *Giardia lamblia*

G. lamblia is a protozoal parasite that causes superficial invasion, destruction, and inflammation of the mucosa in the small intestine. Like *E. histolytica, G. lamblia* has a trophozoite and cyst form, and cysts can transmit the organism. Humans are hosts to this organism, but beavers and dogs may be reservoirs for infection. *G. lamblia* is transmitted by the fecal-oral route. Giardiasis is a well-recognized problem in travelers, campers, male homosexuals, and immunosuppressed people.

Modes of transmission are similar to those for amebiasis; in the United States, however, giardiasis is much more prevalent and is the most common parasitic infection. Giardiasis affects only the intestinal system, causing acute diarrhea, chronic diarrhea, or malabsorption syndrome. The acute phase usually is self-limiting, lasting days or weeks. The chronic phase can last for years. Diarrhea is usually mild in both forms, but it can be severe. As stools increase in frequency, they become more watery, greasy, frothy, and malodorous with mucus. Weight loss and weakness are also common. Malabsorption can occur with diarrhea that continues for longer than 3 weeks. Manifestations result from malabsorption of fat, protein, vitamin B_{12}, and lactase deficiency.

Infection with *Cryptosporidium*

Cryptosporidium is another parasitic infestation transmitted by the fecal-oral route that is manifested by diarrhea. This infection commonly occurs in immunosuppressed clients, particularly those with human immunodeficiency virus (HIV). (See Chapter 22 for a discussion of HIV infection.)

COLLABORATIVE MANAGEMENT

Assessment

A thorough history can provide information about potential sources of exposure to parasitic infection. A history of travel to parts of the world where such infections are prevalent increases suspicion for infection with parasites. GI symptoms related to travel may be delayed as long as 1 to 2 weeks following the return home. A diet history is especially helpful if several people become ill. Common water supplies may be infected with *Giardia* or *Cryptosporidium.* Trichinosis should be considered if the client has ingested pork products.

Mild to moderate *E. histolytica* infestation causes clinical manifestations, including the daily passage of several strongly odoriferous stools, possibly with mucus but without blood, accompanied by abdominal cramping, flatulence, fatigue, and weight loss.

Clients experience characteristic remissions and recurrences. Severe amebic dysentery is manifested by frequent, more liquid, and odoriferous stools with mucus *and* blood. Fever up to 105° F (40° C), tenesmus (ineffectual and painful straining to defecate), generalized abdominal tenderness, and vomiting can also occur. The ulcerations characteristic of invading amebiasis that occur in the colon can cause pain, bleeding, and obstruction. Ulcerations can also be localized in the rectum, resulting in formed stool with blood. Complications are rare but include appendicitis and bowel perforation.

Extraintestinal amebiasis can occur without symptoms of intestinal infection. The most common form is amebic liver abscess, which causes symptoms of fever, pain, and an enlarged liver. The abscess can rupture, and death can result if the infection is not treated and complications occur.

The diagnosis of amebiasis is made by examination of stool for parasites. Because *E. histolytica* is difficult to detect, serial stool examinations are needed if the disease is suspected. The use of sigmoidoscopy may detect ulcerations in the rectum or colon. Exudate obtained during sigmoidoscopic examination is studied for the parasite. The white blood cell (WBC) count can be as high as 20,000/mm^3 when severe dysentery is present.

The diagnosis of giardiasis is also confirmed by stool examination for parasites. Because organisms may not be detected for at least 1 week after symptoms appear, multiple stool samples should be examined. Duodenal aspirate can also be examined for the parasite.

Infection with *Cryptosporidium* is usually self-limiting in individuals who are not immunocompromised. Drug therapy for clients with immunosuppression may consist of paromomycin 500 to 750 mg four times daily.

Interventions

INTERVENTIONS FOR AMEBIASIS. Treatment for all types of amebiasis mandate the use of amebicide drugs. The physician commonly prescribes metronidazole (Flagyl, Novonidazol✤) and diloxanide furoate (Entamide), or diloxanide furoate and tetracycline hydrochloride (Sumycin) followed by chloroquine. Clients with severe dysentery require IV fluids for replacement and maintenance of fluid volume and possibly opiates, such as diphenoxylate hydrochloride and atropine sulfate (Lomotil), to control bowel motility. Clients with extraintestinal amebiasis or severe dehydration are hospitalized. Clients with asymptomatic, mild, or moderate disease are treated as outpatients with drug therapy. For all clients, at least three stools are examined for parasites at 2- to 3-day intervals, starting 2 to 4 weeks after drug therapy has been completed.

INTERVENTIONS FOR GIARDIASIS. Treatment for giardiasis is drug therapy. Metronidazole is the drug of choice, and the usual dose is 250 mg three times a day PO for 5 days. Tinidazole (Fasigyn) can be used as an alternative. Stools are examined 2 weeks after treatment is begun to assess for eradication.

The nurse explains modes of transmission and means to avoid the spread of infection and recurrent contact with parasitic organisms. Clients are taught that they can transmit the infection to others until amebicides effectively kill the parasites. The nurse instructs clients to:

- Avoid contact with stool
- Keep toilet areas clean
- Wash their hands meticulously with an antimicrobial soap after bowel movements
- Maintain personal hygiene
- Avoid stool from dogs and beavers

The client is also advised to avoid sexual practices that allow rectal contact until drug therapy is completed. The nurse informs the client that all household and sexual contacts should undergo stool examinations for parasites. If the water supply is suspected as the source, a sample is obtained and sent for analysis. Multiple infections are common in households, often as a result of contaminated water supplies. Well water and water from areas with inadequate or no filtration equipment can be sources of contamination.

HELMINTHIC INFESTATION

Helminths are wormlike animals; they are often parasitic and capable of causing infectious disease in humans. There are many species of helminths, which, for purposes of classification, are divided into three general categories:

- Roundworms (nematodes)
- Flukes (trematodes)
- Tapeworms (cestodes)

Helminths can cause various degrees of gastrointestinal (GI) symptoms in humans. Most often, they enter the human body through the skin or via the oral route with ingestion of food, water, or other substances contaminated with worms. Some helminths gain access to the human body via insects, such as flies and mosquitoes. Helminths that are typically transmitted via insects are limited to tropical areas, however, and are not discussed here. Flukes (trematodes), which are passed to humans via snail-contaminated water, are also limited to tropical and subtropical areas outside the United States and are not discussed here.

Roundworms

Roundworms are commonly the cause of helminthic infections in the United States and worldwide. These infections include enterobiasis, trichinosis, and hookworm.

Enterobiasis

Enterobiasis ("pinworm infection") is caused by *Enterobius vermicularis* and is the most common helminthic infection in the United States. It is transmitted by oral ingestion of contaminated food, drink, or fomites. The most common clinical manifestations of infection include nocturnal perianal pruritus, vaginitis, insomnia, and restlessness.

The client may have vague GI symptoms, such as abdominal pain, nausea, vomiting, and diarrhea. However, many infected clients have no symptoms. Diagnosis is made when eggs of the helminth are found on the perianal skin or on cellulose tape that has been applied to the perianal skin.

Treatment of enterobiasis includes meticulous handwashing techniques after defecation and before meals to prevent spread of the worms to others. Drug therapy is indicated for all clients with symptoms and in some clients who are infected but are not symptomatic. Household cohabitants of an infected client may be treated with drug therapy even if they are asymptomatic. Pyrantel pamoate (Antiminth, Combantrin🍁) or mebendazole (Vermox, Nemasol🍁) is given orally in one dose, which is repeated at 2 and 4 weeks.

Infection with pinworms is curable and is not usually associated with complications; however, recurrences are common.

Trichinosis

Trichinosis is another helminthic disease caused by roundworms. The incidence in the United States is 50 to 100 cases annually, but many mild or asymptomatic cases are not diagnosed, since the person is usually asymptomatic. *Trichinella spiralis,* which lives in the intestine of humans, pigs, bears, and rats, causes trichinosis. The organism is usually transmitted to people who ingest undercooked pork or pork products. Ingestion of other meats, such as ground beef, can also promote transmission if a meat grinder has been used for both beef and pork. Following ingestion, the larvae, encased in cysts, are released by the digestive action of acid and pepsin. Incubation is 12 hours to 28 days after ingestion. Clinical manifestations range from none to severe; death rarely results.

During the first week following infection, diarrhea results from the invasion of the gut by large numbers of the parasite. Abdominal pain, nausea, and vomiting may follow. During the second week, the larvae begin to invade the muscle, instigating a hypersensitivity reaction characterized by fever, periorbital and facial edema, and subconjunctival hemorrhage. Occasionally a rash or dyspnea develops. Two to three weeks after infection, symptoms of myositis, myalgia, and muscle weakness develop, particularly in the lower back, neck, jaw, biceps, and extraocular muscles. Vague muscle pain and malaise characterize the convalescence phase, which can last for several months.

A diagnosis of trichinosis is confirmed by a history of ingestion of raw or undercooked meat. White blood cell (WBC) and eosinophil counts are elevated for 2 weeks after meat is ingested. Biopsy of skeletal muscle shows larvae of the *Trichinella* organism. Worms are rarely seen in feces.

During the first week after infection, the client is treated with oral mebendazole. During the stage of muscle invasion, he or she must be hospitalized to receive high doses of corticosteroids.

Hookworms

Hookworms are also roundworms. They differ from pinworms and *Trichinella* in that they initially enter the human body through the skin. Hookworm disease is caused by either *Ancylostoma duodenale* or *Necator americanus.*

Hookworms infect a quarter of the world's population, but the disease is rare in areas outside the tropics or in areas with little rain. Worms are infective outside the body in warm, moist soil for up to 1 week. Transmission occurs when larvae penetrate through the skin. The organism can migrate to pulmonary capillaries via the bloodstream and enter alveoli. Cilia carry the organisms up the respiratory tree to the pharynx and the mouth, where they are swallowed and enter the GI tract. Hookworms probably also enter the GI tract when a person ingests contaminated food.

Early symptoms of hookworm disease include a pruritic, erythematous, raised vesicular inflammation of the skin. Infection in the GI tract may produce no symptoms, or it may cause anorexia, diarrhea, or mild abdominal and epigastric discomfort. Bleeding and anemia may occur when worms suck blood at sites of attachment in the GI tract. If blood loss is severe, the client may have symptoms of iron deficiency anemia, such as pallor, hair thinning, deformed nails, pica, and shortness of breath.

Diagnosis of hookworm infection is based on the presence of ova (eggs) in the feces. Occult blood is often present in the stool. There may be a low hemoglobin concentration and hematocrit value or a low serum iron level and high iron-binding capacity, indicating hypochromic microcytic anemia. The WBC counts and eosinophil counts are elevated.

All clients with symptoms receive iron therapy and a diet high in protein and vitamins for at least 3 months after anemia is corrected. Pyrantel pamoate (Antiminth) or mebendazole (Vermox) is given for a complete recovery. Severe hookworm disease can cause malabsorption and protein loss, necessitating nutritional support in addition to other treatments.

Tapeworms

Five types of tapeworms (cestodes) may infect humans: tapeworms found in cattle, fish, dogs pigs, and rodents. Tapeworm infections generally cause either no symptoms or only occasional GI upset, such as nausea, diarrhea, or abdominal pain.

Transmission of tapeworms occurs when a person ingests undercooked beef, raw fish, or other contaminated food or water or accidentally swallows infected lice or fleas from dogs. People can also accidentally ingest arthropods, such as cockroaches, in stored foods or cereals.

The diagnosis of tapeworm infestation is made by laboratory examination of eggs found in the stool (test of stool for ova and parasites). Clients are treated with medications for this type of infection.

• • •

When caring for clients with helminths, the nurse follows standard precautions or body substance precautions when in contact with any stool. All clients are taught to wash their hands after defecating and before eating. They should avoid ingesting undercooked beef, fish, or pork, as well as drinking water that may be contaminated. After petting dogs, clients should take care to keep their mouth closed and wash their hands. All stored foods should be kept tightly closed to avoid contamination by cockroaches and other insects.

FOOD POISONING

Foodborne illnesses are a common problem, with 6.5 cases occurring in the United States every year (Van Benden et al., 1999). Food poisoning has been linked to as many as 9000 deaths per year in the United States (Shewmake & Dillon, 1998). Food poisoning results when a person ingests infectious organisms in food. Unlike gastroenteritis, food poisoning is not directly communicable from person to person, and incubation periods are shorter. Like gastroenteritis, it causes diarrhea, nausea, and vomiting. The nurse can differentiate food poisoning from gastroenteritis by obtaining a thorough history of common food intake in clients who have common symptoms of acute diarrhea, nausea, and vomiting.

The common types of food poisoning are caused by pathogens and include the following (Table 58-5):

- Gram-negative Salmonella
- *Staphylococcal aureus*
- *Escherichia coli*
- Botulism

TABLE 58-5 • COMMON TYPES OF FOOD POISONING

STAPHYLOCOCCAL INFECTION
- Caused by contaminated meats and dairy products
- Can be transmitted by human carriers
- Causes abrupt onset of vomiting and diarrhea without fever

***ESCHERICHIA COLI* INFECTION**
- Caused by meat contaminated with animal feces
- Causes abrupt vomiting, diarrhea, abdominal cramping, and fever

BOTULISM
- Commonly associated with improperly canned foods, especially fruits and vegetables
- Nausea, vomiting, diarrhea, and weakness progressing to paralysis
- Diplopia, dysphagia, and dysarthria

SALMONELLOSIS
- Caused by contaminated food or drink but can be transmitted by the fecal-oral route
- Fever, nausea, vomiting, abdominal cramping, and diarrhea lasting for 3 to 5 days

All cases of botulism and salmonellosis need to be reported to the local health department. Cases of staphylococcal and *E. coli* food poisoning are reported if epidemic outbreaks occur.

Salmonellosis

Salmonellosis is a bacterial infection caused by the *Salmonella* organism. It can be transmitted by the "five Fs": flies, fingers, food, feces, and fomites.

Incubation is 8 to 48 hours after the person has ingested the contaminated food or liquid. Symptoms usually last for 3 to 5 days and include fever with or without chills, nausea, vomiting, cramping abdominal pain, and diarrhea, which may be bloody.

Salmonellosis is usually self-limiting, but bacteremia with localization in joints or bone may occur. The definitive diagnosis is made by stool culture. Treatment is symptomatic, and drug therapy is not usually indicated unless bacteremia occurs; in that case, the physician prescribes antibiotics.

Clients may be carriers of the bacterium for up to 1 year. The nurse instructs all clients with *Salmonella* gastroenteritis and their contacts to wash their hands before meals and after defecating to avoid transmission of the organism. The treatment for *Salmonella* infection is controversial, since antibiotics tend not to shorten the illness. In some studies, quinolones have been shown to be effective, but these are usually reserved for individuals with severe manifestations of the illness.

Staphylococcal Infection

Staphylococcus is associated with 25% of reported food poisoning outbreaks. *Staphylococcus* is found in meats and dairy products and can be transmitted by carriers of the organism. For staphylococcal food poisoning to occur, there must be contamination of food and a period of time (hours) during which the organisms multiply. This can take place during the slow cooling of food after it is cooked.

Symptoms of staphylococcal food poisoning include an abrupt onset of vomiting, abdominal cramping, and diarrhea. The person usually has symptoms 2 to 4 hours after ingesting the contaminated food. There is no fever, but the client is weak.

A diagnosis can be made when stool culture yields 100,000 enterotoxin-producing staphylococci; however, symptoms rarely last more than 24 hours, and people do not always seek medical attention. Antimicrobial drug therapy is not usually indicated unless an agent produces progressive systemic involvement. Parenteral fluids may be necessary if fluid volume is grossly depleted.

Escherichia coli Infection

E. coli is not usually associated with food poisoning. Since 1992, however, there have been several outbreaks of *E. coli* food poisoning in the United States. Enterohemorrhagic strains of *E. coli* produce cytotoxins that cause outbreaks of hemorrhagic colitis and hemolytic-uremic syndrome. Treatment of the client with *E. coli* food poisoning includes IV fluids and antibiotic therapy.

Botulism

Botulism is a paralytic disease resulting from ingestion of a toxin in food contaminated with *Clostridium botulinum.* Botulism is most commonly associated with home-canned foods, particularly vegetables, fruits, condiments, and less commonly, meat and fish. It can be associated with commercially prepared products and with products not adequately heated to destroy toxins before they are eaten.

Incubation is usually 18 to 36 hours. After this time, symptoms occur; illness may be mild or severe, with paralysis, respiratory failure, and death. Initial symptoms include diplopia, dysphagia, and dysarthria.

Weakness can progress rapidly from the neck to the arms, thorax, and legs. Paralytic ileus, severe constipation, and urinary retention can also occur. Nausea, vomiting, and abdominal pain may occur before or after the onset of paralysis.

The diagnosis is made on the basis of the client's history and a stool culture of *C. botulinum.* The serum may be positive for toxins.

Treatment with trivalent botulism antitoxin (ABE) is given as soon as the diagnosis is made if the client is not hypersensitive to it. The physician may lavage the stomach to stop absorption of toxin. All clients are hospitalized to observe for and treat respiratory paralysis. Nothing is given orally until swallowing and respiratory difficulties pass. The physician orders IV fluids as needed. If respiratory paralysis occurs, tracheostomy and mechanical ventilation are implemented. If ventilation can be maintained, the client can survive with no neurologic deficits after the illness.

To prevent botulism, the nurse teaches clients the importance of discarding cans of food that are punctured or swollen or that have defective seals. Containers for home-canned foods must be sterilized by boiling for 20 minutes to destroy *C. botulinum* spores before canning.

ONLINE RESOURCES

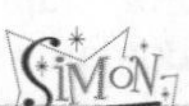

For suggested readings and Internet resources, go to http://www.wbsaunders.com/SIMON/Iggy/.

SELECTED BIBLIOGRAPHY

Belaiche, J., et al. (1999). Acute lower gastrointestinal bleeding in Crohn's disease: Characteristics of a unique series of 34 patients. *American Journal of Gastroenterology, 94*(8), 2177-2181.

Bernstein, C., et al. (2000). Direct hospital costs for patients with inflammatory bowel disease in a Canadian tertiary care university hospital. *American Journal of Gastroenterology, 95*(3), 677-683.

Borwell, B. (1997). The psychosexual needs of stoma patients. *Professional Nurse, 12*(4), 250-255.

Butterton, J., & Calderwood, S. (1998). Acute infectious diarrheal diseases and bacterial food poisoning. In A.S. Fauci, E. Braunwald, & K.J. Isselbacher (Eds.), *Harrison's principles of internal medicine* (14th ed., pp. 796-801). New York: McGraw-Hill.

Casellas, F., et al. (2000). Impact of surgery for Crohn's disease on health-related quality of life. *American Journal of Gastroenterology, 95*(1), 177-181.

Cohen, R., et al. (2000). The cost of hospitalization for Crohn's disease. *American Journal of Gastroenterology, 95*(2), 524-530.

Delco, F., & Sonnenberg, A. (1999). Commonalities in the time trends of Crohn's disease and ulcerative colitis. *American Journal of Gastroenterology, 94*(8), 2172-2176.

Eckes, L.M., & Norton, B.A. (1997). Ulcerative colitis: From medical management to ileal pouch anal anastomosis—A patient's perspective. *Gastroenterology Nursing, 20*(3), 91-100.

Glickman, R. (1998). Inflammatory bowel disease: Ulcerative colitis and Crohn's disease. In A.S. Fauci, E. Braunwald, & K.J. Isselbacher (Eds.), *Harrison's principles of internal medicine* (14th ed., pp. 1633-1645). New York: McGraw-Hill.

Greenberg, H. (1998). Viral gastroenteritis. In A.S. Fauci, E. Braunwald, & K.J. Isselbacher (Eds.), *Harrison's principles of internal medicine* (14th ed., pp. 1116-1118). New York: McGraw-Hill.

Hirsch, C., & Caswell, D. (1999). Gastrointestinal disorders. In American Association of Critical-Care Nurses—A. Gawlinski & D. Hamwi (Eds.), *Acute care nurse practitioner clinical curriculum and certification review* (pp. 618-722). Philadelphia: W.B. Saunders.

Isselbacher, K., & Epstein, A. (1998). Diverticular, vascular, and other disorders of the intestine and peritoneum. In A.S. Fauci, E. Braunwald, & K.J. Isselbacher (Eds.), *Harrison's principles of internal medicine* (14th ed., pp. 1648-1656). New York: McGraw-Hill.

Klonowski, E., & Masoodi, J. (1999). The patient with Crohn's disease. *RN, 62*(3), 32-37.

Lynn, R., & Friedman, L. (1998). Irritable bowel syndrome. In A.S. Fauci, E. Braunwald, & K.J. Isselbacher (Eds.), *Harrison's principles of internal medicine* (14th ed., pp. 1646-1648). New York: McGraw-Hill.

Martin, F. (1997). Ulcerative colitis. *American Journal of Nursing 97*(8), 38-39.

Mikula, C. (1999). Anti-TNF alpha: New therapy for Crohn's disease. *Gastroenterology Nursing, 22*(6), 245-248.

Mishkin, S. (1997). Dairy sensitivity, lactose malabsorption, and elimination diets in inflammatory bowel disease. *American Journal of Clinical Nutrition, 65*(2), 564-567.

Moore, S., et al. (1998). Nurse perceptions of ostomy patients and their ostomy care competence. *Home Care Provider, 3*(4), 214-220.

Northouse, L.L., et al. (1999). The concerns of patients and spouses after the diagnosis of colon cancer: A qualitative analysis. *Journal of Wound, Ostomy, and Incontinence Nursing, 26*(1), 8-17.

Norton, B. (1998). Crohn's disease: A review of medical, surgical and nutritional management. *ADVANCE for Nurse Practitioners, 6*(9), 42-50.

Olmstead, J. (1998). Evaluation and management of the patient with ulcerative colitis. *Gastroenterology Nursing, 21*(4), 176-180.

Rayhorn, N. (1999). Understanding inflammatory bowel disease. *Nursing99, 29*(12), 57-61.

Rubin, D. (1998). Small and large bowel dysfunction. In Jameson, J.L. (Ed.), *Principles of molecular medicine.* New Jersey: Humana Press.

Shewmake, R., & Dillon, B. (1998). Food poisoning. *Postgraduate Medicine, 103*(6), 125-131.

Silen, W. (1998). Acute appendicitis. In A.S. Fauci et al. (Eds.), *Harrison's principles of internal medicine* (14th ed., pp. 1658-1660). New York: McGraw-Hill.

Van Benden, C., et al. (1999). Multiple outbreak of Salmonella enterica serotype Newport infections due to contaminated alfalfa sprouts. *Journal of the American Medical Association, 281*(2), 158-162.

Worley, J. (1999). Diagnosis and management of inflammatory bowel disease. *Journal of the American Academy of Nurse Practitioners, 11*(1), 23-31.

CHAPTER 59

Interventions for Clients with Liver Problems

JANICE TAZBIR

Learning Objectives

After studying this chapter, you should be able to:

1. Describe the pathophysiology and complications associated with cirrhosis of the liver.
2. Interpret laboratory test findings commonly seen in clients with cirrhosis.
3. Analyze assessment data from clients with cirrhosis to determine priority nursing diagnoses and collaborative problems.
4. Formulate a collaborative plan of care for the client with severe late-stage cirrhosis.
5. Identify emergency interventions for the client with bleeding esophageal varices.
6. Evaluate care for clients with cirrhosis.
7. Develop a community-based teaching plan for the client with cirrhosis of the liver.
8. Compare and contrast the transmission of hepatitis A, B, and C viral infections.
9. Explain ways in which each type of hepatitis can be prevented.
10. Discuss the primary concerns about the increasing incidence of hepatitis C in the United States.
11. Identify treatment options for clients with cancer of the liver.
12. Describe the typical complications that result from liver transplantation.

SIMON Go to http://www.wbsaunders.com/SIMON/Iggy/ for self-assessment questions related to these Learning Objectives.

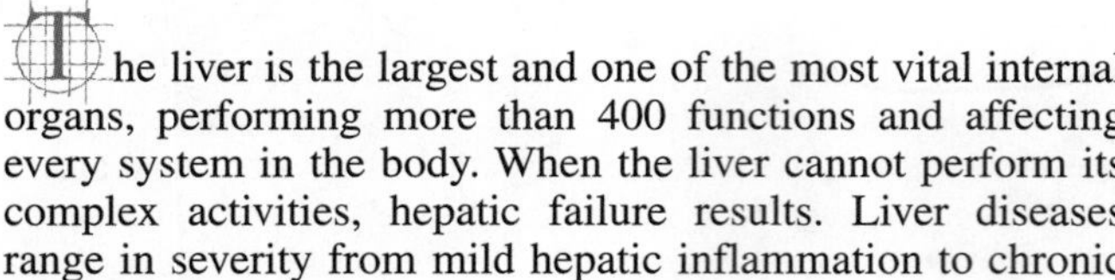

The liver is the largest and one of the most vital internal organs, performing more than 400 functions and affecting every system in the body. When the liver cannot perform its complex activities, hepatic failure results. Liver diseases range in severity from mild hepatic inflammation to chronic end-stage cirrhosis.

CIRRHOSIS

OVERVIEW

Cirrhosis is a chronic, progressive liver condition. It usually develops insidiously and has a prolonged, destructive course. As an end-stage process, it is essentially an irreversible reaction to hepatic inflammation and necrosis.

Pathophysiology

Cirrhosis is characterized by diffuse fibrotic bands of connective tissue that distort the liver's normal architecture. Extensive degeneration and destruction of hepatocytes (hepatic [liver] cells) occur. In attempts to regenerate with new nodule formation, a disorganized lobular pattern develops. Flow alterations in the vascular system and lymphatic bile duct channels result from compression caused by the proliferation of fibrous tissue.

TYPES OF CIRRHOSIS

There are four major types of cirrhosis (Table 59-1):

1. Laënnec's, or alcoholic cirrhosis
2. Postnecrotic cirrhosis
3. Biliary cirrhosis
4. Cardiac cirrhosis

LAËNNEC'S CIRRHOSIS. Laënnec's cirrhosis, or alcoholic cirrhosis, is also called nutritional, or portal, cirrhosis. Alcohol has a direct toxic effect on the liver cells (hepatocytes) and causes liver inflammation (alcoholic hepatitis), which usually precedes the onset of alcoholic cirrhosis. Metabolic changes in the liver that are induced by alcohol lead to fatty infiltration of the hepatocytes and scarring between the lobules. The liver becomes enlarged, with cellular degeneration and infiltration by fat, leukocytes, and lymphocytes (white blood cells). As the inflammatory process decreases, the destructive phase increases. Early scar formation is caused by fibroblast infiltration and collagen formation. Damage to the hepatic parenchyma progresses as a result of malnutrition and repeated exposure to the hepatotoxin (alcohol). If alcohol is withheld, the fatty infiltration is reversible. If alcohol abuse continues, widespread scar tissue formation and fibrosis infiltrate the liver as a result of cellular necrosis.

TABLE 59-1 • MAJOR TYPES OF CIRRHOSIS OF THE LIVER

LAËNNEC'S CIRRHOSIS
- Most common type
- Caused by long-term use of alcohol
- Liver becomes enlarged, firm, and hard in early disease, and smaller and nodular in end-stage disease

POSTNECROTIC CIRRHOSIS
- Caused by massive hepatic cell necrosis, usually from acute viral hepatitis or exposure to certain hepatotoxins, such as industrial chemicals

BILIARY CIRRHOSIS
- Caused by chronic biliary obstruction, bile stasis, and inflammation
- Liver becomes fibrotic; hepatic cells are destroyed

CARDIAC CIRRHOSIS
- Caused by severe or chronic heart failure (also called vascular cirrhosis).
- Liver becomes enlarged and congested with venous blood, resulting in cell necrosis from anoxia

In early cirrhosis, the liver capsule is enlarged, firm, and hard. The regenerated nodules give the capsule a hobnailed, or bumpy, appearance. As the pathologic process of cirrhosis progresses, the liver shrinks in size. The capsule is covered with fine nodules surrounded by gray connective tissue.

POSTNECROTIC CIRRHOSIS. Postnecrotic cirrhosis occurs after massive liver cell necrosis. Broad bands of scar tissue cause the destruction of liver lobules and entire lobes. The liver enlarges and then becomes shrunken with large nodules, representing macronodular structural changes throughout the organ. Postnecrotic cirrhosis occurs most often as a complication of acute viral hepatitis or after exposure to industrial or chemical hepatotoxins (e.g., carbon tetrachloride). This type of cirrhosis is suspected in clients who exhibit signs of chronic liver disease and do not have a history of excessive alcohol intake.

BILIARY CIRRHOSIS. Biliary cirrhosis develops as a result of chronic biliary obstruction, bile stasis, inflammation, or diffuse hepatic fibrosis. *Primary* biliary cirrhosis results from intrahepatic bile stasis. *Secondary* biliary cirrhosis is caused by obstruction of the hepatic or common bile ducts, which produces bile stasis in the liver. The accumulation of excessive hepatic bile leads to progressive fibrosis, hepatocellular destruction, and regenerated nodules. Severe obstructive jaundice is a key clinical manifestation in both types of biliary cirrhosis.

CARDIAC CIRRHOSIS. Cardiac cirrhosis, or vascular cirrhosis, is associated with severe right-sided heart failure. It develops in clients with long-standing heart failure after cor pulmonale, constrictive pericarditis, and valvular insufficiency (see Chapter 35). The liver becomes enlarged, is congested with venous blood, and appears edematous and dark in color. The liver serves as a reservoir for large amounts of venous blood that the failing heart cannot pump back into the systemic circulation. The increase in hepatic volume and pressure causes severe venous congestion. The liver becomes anoxic, which results in hepatic cell necrosis and fibrosis.

COMPLICATIONS OF CIRRHOSIS

Common problems and complications associated with hepatic cirrhosis depend on the amount of damage sustained by the liver. The loss of hepatic function contributes to the development of metabolic abnormalities. Hepatic cell degeneration may lead to the following:

- Portal hypertension
- Ascites (accumulation of abdominal fluid)
- Bleeding esophageal varices
- Coagulation defects
- Jaundice
- Portal-systemic encephalopathy (PSE) with hepatic coma
- Hepatorenal syndrome

PORTAL HYPERTENSION. **Portal hypertension,** a persistent increase in pressure within the portal vein, is a major complication of cirrhosis. It results from increased resistance to or obstruction of the flow of blood through the portal vein and its tributaries. The blood meets resistance to flow and seeks collateral venous channels around the high-pressure area.

Blood flow backs into the spleen, causing splenomegaly. Veins in the esophagus, stomach, intestines, abdomen, and rectum become dilated. Portal hypertension can result in ascites, esophageal varices, prominent abdominal veins (caput medusae), and hemorrhoids.

ASCITES. **Ascites** is the accumulation of free fluid containing almost pure plasma within the peritoneal cavity. Increased hydrostatic pressure from portal hypertension causes plasma to leak into the peritoneal cavity. The accumulation of plasma protein, primarily albumin, in the peritoneal fluid reduces the amount of circulating plasma protein in the blood. When this decrease is combined with the inability of the liver to synthesize albumin because of impaired hepatocyte functioning, the effective serum colloid osmotic pressure is decreased in the circulatory system.

Increased hepatic lymph formation also contributes to ascites formation. The lymphatic system is unable to channel the increased amounts of lymph, and weeping of liver plasma ("liver sweat") occurs as a result. The decrease of effective intravascular circulation from massive ascites may cause renal vasoconstriction, triggering the renin-angiotensin system. This results in sodium and water retention, which increases hydrostatic pressure and lymph formation, and the vicious circle of ascites formation continues.

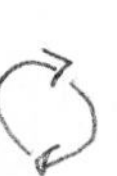

BLEEDING ESOPHAGEAL VARICES. As the blood backs up away from the liver, it enters the esophageal and gastric vessels that carry it into the systemic circulation. **Bleeding esophageal varices** occur when these fragile, thin-walled esophageal veins become distended or irritated and rupture. Variceal bleeding may be caused by the following:

- Any chemical irritant, such as alcohol, medications, and refluxed gastric acid
- Mechanical trauma from abrasions by poorly chewed food, vomiting, or nasogastric (NG) tube insertion
- Increased pressure in the esophagus caused by vigorous physical exercise, coughing, or retching and vomiting

Varices occur most often in the distal end of the esophagus but are also noted in the proximal esophagus and stomach. Gastric ulceration or erosion also puts the client at risk for hemorrhage from the stomach. Endoscopy, if possible, can differentiate between gastrointestinal and esophageal bleeding.

The client with bleeding esophageal varices loses large volumes of blood from hematemesis and may go into shock from hypovolemia. This condition is a medical emergency and needs immediate medical intervention (see Potential for Hemorrhage, p. 1308).

COAGULATION DEFECTS. With cirrhosis, there is a decrease in the synthesis of bile fats in the liver; this prevents the absorption of fat-soluble vitamins (e.g., vitamin K). Without vitamin K, clotting factors II, VII, IX, and X are not produced in sufficient quantities, and the client is susceptible to bleeding and easy bruising. Therefore when a client has bleeding esophageal varices, the blood does not clot and hemorrhage occurs.

CRITICAL THINKING CHALLENGE

You are the nurse for a client with Laënnec's cirrhosis. You go into the client's room and find the client in the bathroom vomiting what appears to be hematemesis (blood in the vomitus).

- What actions will you take?
- In what order of priority should you implement these interventions?
- How can you differentiate if this is a gastrointestinal bleed or an esophageal bleed?

For suggested answer guidelines, go to SIMON http://www.wbsaunders.com/SIMON/Iggy/.

JAUNDICE. Jaundice in clients with hepatic cirrhosis is caused by one of two mechanisms (Table 59-2): hepatocellular disease or intrahepatic obstruction. Hepatocellular jaundice develops because the liver cannot metabolize bilirubin. The liver's normal uptake of bilirubin from the blood is thus impaired. This decreased excretion results in excessive circulating bilirubin levels. Intrahepatic obstructive jaundice results from edema, fibrosis, or scarring of the hepatic bile channels and bile ducts, which interferes with normal bile and bilirubin excretion.

PORTAL-SYSTEMIC ENCEPHALOPATHY. Portal-systemic encephalopathy (PSE) is also known as **hepatic encephalopathy** and **hepatic coma** in the later stages. It is a clinical disorder seen in end-stage hepatic failure and cirrhosis. PSE is manifested by neurologic symptoms and is characterized by an altered level of consciousness, impaired thinking processes, and neuromuscular disturbances.

PSE may develop insidiously in clients with chronic liver disease and go undetected until the late stages. Symptoms develop rapidly in acute liver dysfunction. Four stages of development have been identified: prodromal, impending, stuporous, and comatose (Table 59-3). The client's symptoms may gradually progress to coma or fluctuate among the four stages.

The exact mechanisms of PSE have not been identified. The most probable cause is impaired ammonia metabolism. Most of the ammonia in the body is found in the gastrointestinal (GI) tract. Protein provided by the diet is transported to the liver by the portal vein. The liver breaks down protein by a series of enzymatic reactions. Protein is initially broken down into glutamine (a nontoxic substance) and ammonia. Ammonia is further broken down into urea. Urea diffuses into the body fluids and is eventually excreted in the urine by the kidneys.

Some ammonia is normally formed in the GI tract by the action of intestinal bacteria on protein products. Gastric juices are also a source of ammonia, and peripheral tissue metabolism produces some ammonia. The kidney may be a source of endogenous ammonia if hypokalemia is present.

TABLE 59-2 • LABORATORY DIAGNOSTIC DIFFERENTIATION OF JAUNDICE

Test	Hepatocellular Jaundice	Obstructive Jaundice	Hemolytic Jaundice
Serum bilirubin			
Indirect (unconjugated)	Increased	Slightly increased	Increased
Direct (conjugated)	Increased	Moderately increased	Normal
Urine bilirubin	Increased	Increased	None
Urobilinogen			
Stool	Normal to decreased	None	Increased
Urine	Normal to increased	None	Increased

TABLE 59-3 • STAGES OF PORTAL-SYSTEMIC ENCEPHALOPATHY

STAGE I: PRODROMAL
- Subtle manifestations that may not be recognized immediately
- Personality changes
- Behavior changes (agitation, belligerence)
- Emotional lability (euphoria, depression)
- Impaired thinking
- Inability to concentrate
- Fatigue, drowsiness
- Slurred or slowed speech
- Sleep pattern disturbances

STAGE II: IMPENDING
- Continuing mental changes
- Mental confusion
- Disorientation to time, place, or person
- Asterixis (see Figure 59-3)

STAGE III: STUPOROUS
- Progressive deterioration
- Marked mental confusion
- Stuporous, drowsy, but arousable
- Abnormal electroencephalogram tracing
- Muscle twitching
- Hyperreflexia
- Asterixis

STAGE IV: COMATOSE
- Unresponsiveness, leading to death in 85% of clients progressing to this stage
- Unarousable, obtunded
- Response to painful stimulus
- No asterixis
- Positive Babinski's sign
- Muscle rigidity
- Fetor hepaticus (characteristic liver breath—musty, sweet odor)
- Seizures

If the liver is incapable of adequate protein degradation and cannot convert ammonia to urea, an excessive amount of circulating ammonia develops. Elevated ammonia levels are toxic to central nervous system tissue (glial and nerve cells), interfering with normal cerebral metabolism and function.

Factors that may precipitate PSE include the following:

- High-protein diet
- Infections
- Hypovolemia (deficient fluid volume)
- Hypokalemia (deficient serum potassium)
- Constipation
- GI bleeding (causes a large protein load in the intestines)
- Drugs (e.g., hypnotics, opioids, sedatives, analgesics, diuretics)

PSE may also occur after paracentesis or shunting procedures. The prognosis for a client with PSE depends on the severity of the underlying cause, the precipitating factors, and the degree of liver dysfunction.

HEPATORENAL SYNDROME. The development of **hepatorenal syndrome** indicates a poor prognosis for the client with hepatic failure. It is one of the primary causes of death in end-stage cirrhosis. Progressive oliguric renal failure associated with hepatic failure results in functional impairment of kidneys with normal anatomic and morphologic features. This syndrome is manifested by the following:

- A sudden decrease in urinary flow
- Elevated blood urea nitrogen and creatinine levels, with abnormally decreased urine sodium excretion
- Increased urine osmolarity

Hepatorenal syndrome often occurs after clinical deterioration from GI bleeding or the onset of PSE. Drugs such as indomethacin (Indocin) and possibly acetaminophen (Tylenol, Exdol✤) and aspirin (acetylsalicylic acid [ASA]) may precipitate renal failure when administered to the client with cirrhosis. Hepatorenal syndrome is generally accompanied by elevated serum ammonia levels with an increase in jaundice and serum bilirubin levels. The kidneys cannot excrete these products in the urine. Hepatorenal syndrome may also complicate other liver diseases, including acute hepatitis and hepatic malignancy.

Etiology

The exact factors contributing to cirrhosis have not been clearly defined. There is a genetic component, with a familial tendency to develop cirrhosis and a familial hypersensitivity to alcohol in some people. Many alcoholics do not experience cirrhosis, whereas others have cirrhosis even when adequate nutrition is maintained.

The cause of cirrhosis varies with the type. Chronic infection with the hepatitis B virus is the number-one cause of cirrhosis in the world (Rollier et al., 1999). Laënnec's (alcoholic) cirrhosis results from the hepatotoxic effect of alcohol. Poor nutritional intake compounds the problem of a malnourished liver in most adults. Postnecrotic cirrhosis usually occurs after acute viral hepatitis, which may result from blood transfusions. It is seen after exposure to industrial or chemical hepatotoxins (e.g., carbon tetrachloride, arsenic, and phosphorus). Biliary cirrhosis results from chronic biliary obstruction and inflammation. Cardiac cirrhosis is associated with prolonged hepatic venous congestion. Cirrhosis often develops as an idiopathic process.

Incidence/Prevalence

Cirrhosis may develop at any age. Cirrhosis and chronic liver disease was the tenth leading cause of death in 1997, accounting for 25,175 deaths (Centers for Disease Control and Prevention [CDC], 1999). Of all cases of cirrhosis, 10% to 30% are postnecrotic and 5% to 10% are primary biliary. Laënnec's cirrhosis is the most common type of cirrhosis in industrialized countries. Most cases of cirrhosis could be prevented by eliminating alcohol intake. The death rate for cirrhosis in men is two times the rate for females, regardless race or ethnicity (National Institutes of Health [NIH], 1999).

CULTURAL CONSIDERATIONS

In the United States, mortality from cirrhosis is higher in African Americans and Hispanics (CDC, 1999). The cause is unknown.

COLLABORATIVE MANAGEMENT

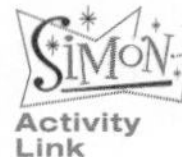

Assessment

HISTORY

The nurse obtains historical data from clients with suspected cirrhosis, including age, sex, race, history of or present substance use, and employment history, especially exposure to harmful chemical toxins. The nurse determines whether there is a history of alcoholism in the family. The client is asked to describe his or her alcohol intake, including the amount consumed during a given period of time. The nurse also asks the client about previous medical conditions, such as acute viral hepatitis, biliary tract disorders, viral infections, blood transfusions, and a history of heart failure or respiratory disorders.

PHYSICAL ASSESSMENT/CLINICAL MANIFESTATIONS

Because cirrhosis has an insidious onset, many of the early signs and symptoms are vague and nonspecific. The client may report the following:

- Generalized weakness
- Weight loss
- GI symptoms (loss of appetite, early morning nausea and vomiting, dyspepsia, flatulence, and changes in bowel habits, with constipation and bouts of diarrhea)
- Abdominal pain and liver tenderness (both of which are often ignored by the client)

Hepatic function abnormalities are often detected when a physical examination or laboratory tests are completed for an unrelated illness or problem. The development of late signs of advanced cirrhosis may cause the client to seek medical treatment. GI bleeding, jaundice, ascites, and spontaneous bruising indicate deteriorating hepatic function and represent complications of cirrhosis.

The nurse thoroughly assesses the client with liver dysfunction or hepatic failure, because it affects every body system (Figure 59-1). The clinical picture and course vary from client to client depending on the severity of hepatic failure. An inspection may reveal the following:

- Obvious yellowing of the skin (jaundice) and the sclerae (icterus)
- Dry skin

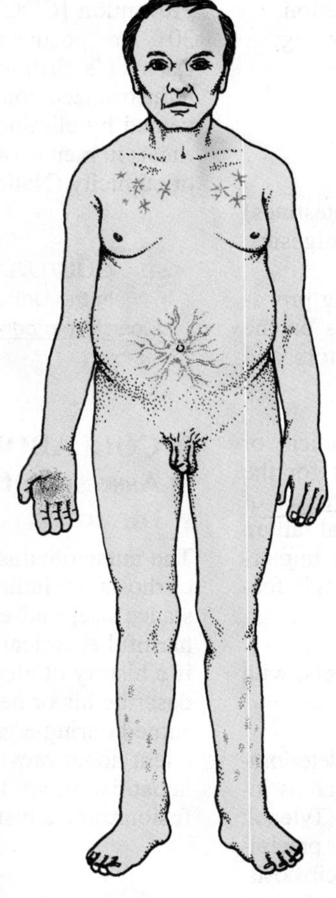

Figure 59-1 ● The clinical picture of a client with liver dysfunction. Signs and symptoms vary according to the progression of the disease. Early signs and symptoms are noted in color.

- Rashes
- Purpuric lesions, such as petechiae (round, pinpoint, red-purple lesions) or ecchymosis (large purple, blue, or yellow bruises)
- Warm and bright red palms of the hands (palmar erythema)
- Vascular lesions with a red center and radiating branches, known as "spider angiomas" (telangiectasias, spider nevi, or vascular spiders), on the nose, cheeks, upper thorax, and shoulders
- Peripheral dependent edema of the extremities and sacrum

ABDOMINAL ASSESSMENT. The nurse may readily detect *massive* ascites as a distended abdomen with bulging flanks. The umbilicus may protrude, and dilated abdominal veins (caput medusae) may radiate from the umbilicus. Ascites can cause physical problems; for example, orthopnea and dyspnea from increased abdominal distention can interfere with lung expansion. The client may have difficulty maintaining an erect body posture, and problems with balance may affect walking. The nurse inspects and palpates for the presence of inguinal or umbilical hernias, which are likely to develop in clients with ascites because of increased intra-abdominal pressure.

Minimal ascites is often more difficult to detect. Advanced assessment techniques, such as the percussion test for shifting dullness and the presence of a fluid wave, may be performed by the health care provider.

When performing an assessment of the abdomen, the nurse keeps in mind that hepatomegaly occurs in 60% of all cases of early cirrhosis. The advanced practice nurse or other health care provider palpates the right upper quadrant for **hepatomegaly** (enlarged liver) below the costal (rib cage) border. The presence of hepatomegaly may be determined by percussing for dullness over the enlarged liver.

The nurse measures the client's abdominal girth to evaluate the progression of ascites (Figure 59-2). To measure abdominal girth, the client lies flat while the nurse pulls a tape measure around the largest diameter of the abdomen. The girth is measured at the end of exhalation. The abdominal skin

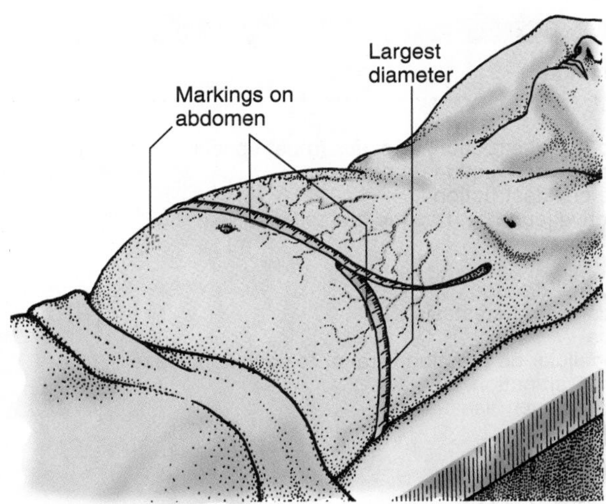

Figure 59-2 ● How to measure abdominal girth. With the client supine, the nurse brings the tape measure around the client and takes a measurement at the level of the umbilicus. Before removing the tape, the nurse marks the client's abdomen along the sides of the tape on the client's flanks (sides) and midline to ensure that later measurements are taken in the same place.

and flanks should be marked to ensure the same tape measure placement on subsequent readings.

OTHER PHYSICAL ASSESSMENT. The nurse assesses nasogastric (NG) tube drainage (if present), vomitus, and stool for the presence of blood. This may be indicated by frank blood in the excrement or by a positive result of an *o*-toluidine test for occult blood content (Hema-Check, Hematest). Gastritis, stomach ulceration, or oozing esophageal varices may be responsible for the presence of blood **(melena).**

The nurse may note fetor hepaticus, which is the distinctive breath odor of chronic liver disease and portal-systemic encephalopathy (PSE). It is characterized by a fruity or musty odor. Fetor hepaticus results from the inability of the damaged liver to metabolize and detoxify mercaptan, which is produced by bacterial degradation of methionine, a sulfurous amino acid.

Amenorrhea may occur in women, and men may exhibit testicular atrophy, **gynecomastia** (enlarged breasts), and impotence as a result of inactive hormones. Clients with problems of the hematologic system caused by hepatic failure may have bruising, **petechiae** (small, purplish hemorrhagic spots on the skin), and an enlarged spleen.

The nurse continually assesses the client's neurologic functioning. Subtle changes in mentation and personality often progress to coma, a late complication of PSE. The nurse also assesses for **asterixis** (liver flap or flapping tremor), a coarse tremor characterized by rapid, nonrhythmic extensions and flexions in the wrists and fingers. Asterixis also appears in the ankles, corners of the mouth, eyelids, and tongue. Figure 59-3 illustrates the technique used to elicit asterixis during physical assessment.

PSYCHOSOCIAL ASSESSMENT

The client with hepatic cirrhosis may undergo subtle or obvious personality, cognitive, and behavior changes, such as agitation and belligerence. He or she may experience sleep pattern disturbances or may exhibit signs of emotional lability, euphoria, or depression. The nurse performs a psychosocial assessment to identify needs and help guide client care. For reasons unknown, individuals living in poorer, inner city communities experience a disproportionate percentage of liver disease (Frieden et al., 1999)

Repeated hospitalizations are common for clients with alcohol-induced cirrhosis who do not adhere to treatment plans. The nurse assesses the impact of the hospitalizations on the client's lifestyle and self-esteem. Social workers assess the client's financial capabilities to help determine whether assistance is needed.

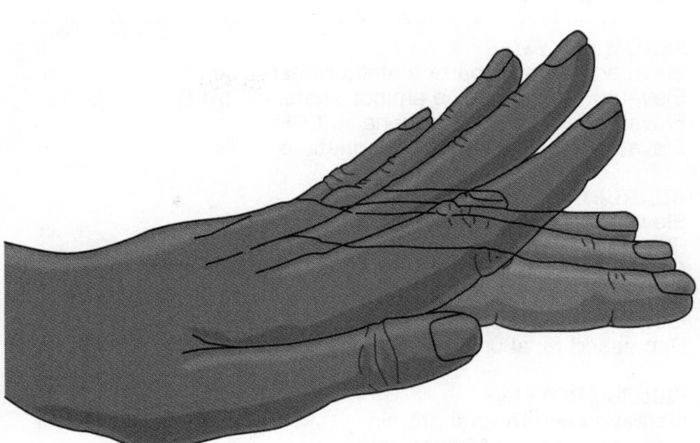

Figure 59-3 ● To elicit asterixis (flapping tremor), have the client extend the arm, dorsiflex the wrist, and extend the fingers. Observe for rapid, nonrhythmic extensions and flexions.

LABORATORY ASSESSMENT

Characteristic abnormalities are common in laboratory studies of clients with liver disease (Table 59-4). Serum levels of aspartate aminotransferase (AST), alanine aminotransferase (ALT), and lactate dehydrogenase (LDH) are elevated because these enzymes are released into the blood with the destruction of hepatic cells. Alkaline phosphatase levels are sensitive to mild extrahepatic or intrahepatic biliary obstruction and therefore increase in clients with cirrhosis.

Total serum bilirubin levels also rise. Indirect bilirubin levels rise in clients with cirrhosis because of the inability of the failing liver to conjugate bilirubin. Therefore bilirubin is present in the urine (urobilinogen) in increased amounts. Fecal urobilinogen concentration is decreased in clients with biliary tract obstruction, which occurs in biliary cirrhosis. These clients exhibit light- or clay-colored stools.

Total serum protein and albumin levels are decreased in clients with severe or chronic liver disease as a result of decreased synthesis by the liver. Serum levels of globulins (alpha, beta, and gamma) are elevated because of their increased synthesis by the reticuloendothelial system of the liver, which indicates an immune response to hepatic disease.

Prothrombin time (PT) is prolonged because the liver decreases the synthesis of prothrombin, reflecting hepatocellular

TABLE 59-4 • ASSESSMENT OF ABNORMAL LABORATORY FINDINGS IN LIVER DISEASE

Abnormal Finding	Significance
SERUM ENZYMES	
Elevated serum aspartate aminotransferase (AST)	Hepatic cell destruction, hepatitis (most specific indicator)
Elevated serum alanine aminotransferase (ALT)	Hepatic cell destruction, hepatitis
Elevated lactate dehydrogenase (LDH)	Hepatic cell destruction
Elevated serum alkaline phosphatase	Obstructive jaundice, hepatic metastasis
BILIRUBIN	
Elevated serum total bilirubin	Hepatic cell disease
Elevated serum direct conjugated bilirubin	Hepatitis, liver metastasis
Elevated serum indirect unconjugated bilirubin	Cirrhosis
Elevated urine bilirubin	Hepatocellular obstruction, viral or toxic liver disease
Elevated urine urobilinogen	Hepatic dysfunction
Decreased fecal urobilinogen	Obstructive liver disease
SERUM PROTEINS	
Increased serum total protein	Acute liver disease
Decreased serum total protein	Chronic liver disease
Decreased serum albumin	Severe liver disease
Elevated serum globulin	Immune response to liver disease
OTHER TESTS	
Elevated serum ammonia	Advanced liver disease or portal-systemic encephalopathy (PSE)
Prolonged prothrombin time (PT) or INR	Hepatic cell damage and synthesis of prothrombin

INR, International Normalized Ratio.

or obstructive biliary tract disease. Anemia may be reflected by an altered complete blood count (CBC), with decreased hemoglobin and hematocrit values. The white blood cell (WBC) count may also be decreased. Increased toxins in the blood lead to premature cell death. Ammonia levels are elevated in the presence of advanced liver disease and PSE because the conversion of ammonia to urea for excretion is decreased.

RADIOGRAPHIC ASSESSMENT

Abdominal x-ray studies may reveal an enlarged liver, gas or cysts within the liver and biliary tract, calcification of the liver, and massive ascites.

The upper gastrointestinal (GI) radiographic series is an examination of the esophagus, stomach, and small bowel. It may show the presence of esophageal varices or gastric or duodenal ulceration, all of which complicate the care of a client with cirrhosis.

The physician may order angiographic studies to identify actual arterial bleeding sites within the stomach. A computed tomography (CT) scan is helpful in detecting minimal ascites and provides information about the volume and character of fluid collections.

OTHER DIAGNOSTIC ASSESSMENT

The physician may perform an esophagogastroduodenoscopy (EGD) to directly visualize the upper GI tract and to detect the presence of bleeding or oozing esophageal varices, stomach irritation and ulceration, or duodenal ulceration and bleeding. Injection sclerotherapy may be performed as a palliative measure during the endoscopic procedure to halt variceal bleeding (see Potential for Hemorrhage, p. 1308).

Radioisotope liver scans show abnormal hepatic thickening and identify liver masses. The physician may use liver biopsy as the definitive test for cirrhosis. A hepatic tissue biopsy reveals destruction and fibrosis of the hepatic cells, which is indicative of the disease.

Analysis

COMMON NURSING DIAGNOSES AND COLLABORATIVE PROBLEMS

The most common nursing diagnosis for clients with cirrhosis is Excess Fluid Volume related to portal hypertension (causing ascites) and decreased serum colloid osmotic pressure.

The following are the primary collaborative problems for clients with cirrhosis:

1. Potential for Hemorrhage
2. Potential for Portal-Systemic Encephalopathy (PSE)

ADDITIONAL NURSING DIAGNOSES AND COLLABORATIVE PROBLEMS

In addition to the common nursing diagnoses and collaborative problems, clients with cirrhosis may have one or more of the following:

- Imbalanced Nutrition: Less than Body Requirements related to anorexia, nausea, and faulty absorption, metabolism, and storage of nutrients and vitamins
- Ineffective Breathing Pattern related to ascites and decreased diaphragmatic excursion and pressure on the diaphragm from ascites
- Impaired Comfort related to abdominal pressure
- Risk for Infection related to a decreased number of white blood cells
- Risk for Impaired Skin Integrity related to pruritus secondary to jaundice, edema, and ascites
- Ineffective Coping related to a chronic and potentially fatal disease process
- Sexual Dysfunction related to altered hormonal function and decreased libido

- Disturbed Body Image related to distended abdomen and skin lesions

Additional collaborative problems include the following:

- Potential for Drug Toxicity
- Potential for Hypokalemia

Planning and Implementation

EXCESS FLUID VOLUME

NOC **PLANNING: EXPECTED OUTCOMES.** The client with cirrhosis is expected to experience a decrease in extravascular and intra-abdominal fluid as indicated by (1) a decrease or absence of ascites, (2) serum electrolytes within normal limits (WNL), and (3) blood pressure in expected range (IER).

INTERVENTIONS. Fluid accumulations are minimal during the early stages of ascites, and therefore interventions are aimed at preventing the accumulation of additional fluid and mobilizing the existing fluid collection. Nonsurgical treatment measures usually control ascites. If respiratory or abdominal functioning is compromised, surgical measures may be necessary. (See the Concept Map for chronic liver failure on p. 1306.)

NONSURGICAL MANAGEMENT. Supportive measures to control abdominal ascites include diet therapy, drugs, paracentesis, and comfort measures. The nurse also carefully monitors fluid and electrolyte status.

DIET THERAPY. The health care provider usually places the client with abdominal ascites on a low sodium diet as an initial means of controlling fluid accumulation in the abdominal cavity. The amount of daily sodium intake restriction typically varies from 500 mg to 2 g. In collaboration with the dietitian, the nurse explains the purpose of the diet and advises the client to eliminate table salt and salty foods. (See Chapter 13 for a list of high-sodium foods.) The absence of salt in low-sodium diets is distasteful to most people, so the dietitian suggests alternative flavoring additives such as lemon, vinegar, parsley, oregano, and pepper.

The health care provider may limit the client's fluid intake if serum sodium levels fall. The kidneys retain sodium, and dilutional hyponatremia results, primarily from excessive fluid volume. Intravenous (IV) and oral fluids are restricted to 1000 to 1500 mL/day in an effort to reverse the fluid overload and raise the serum sodium level. The nurse calculates the permitted amount of oral fluids on the basis of the ordered IV intake.

In general, clients with cirrhosis are malnourished and have multiple dietary deficiencies. Vitamin supplements, such as thiamine, folate, and multivitamin preparations, are typically added to the IV fluids because of the inability of the liver to store vitamins. Oral vitamins are given when IV fluid administration is discontinued.

DRUG THERAPY. The health care provider usually orders a diuretic to reduce fluid accumulation and to prevent cardiac and respiratory impairment.

The nurse monitors the effect of diuretic therapy by assessing intake and output, weighing the client daily, measuring abdominal girth, and monitoring electrolyte levels. Serious electrolyte imbalances, such as hypokalemia (decreased potassium) and hyponatremia (decreased sodium), may accompany diuretic therapy. (See Chapter 13 for discussion of electrolyte imbalances.) Depending on the diuretic selected, the provider may order an oral or IV potassium supplement.

Clients with cirrhosis often require antacid therapy for GI symptoms. Because most antacids are high in sodium, the physician prescribes a low-sodium antacid such as magaldrate (Riopan).

PARACENTESIS. Abdominal **paracentesis** may be indicated if dietary restrictions and drug administration fail to control ascites (Chart 59-1). The procedure is performed at the bedside. The physician inserts a trocar catheter into the abdomen to remove and drain ascitic fluid from the peritoneal cavity.

Once a primary treatment modality for ascites, paracentesis is more commonly used as a diagnostic tool to examine ascitic fluid. It is also used as a palliative measure to relieve abdominal pressure, because ascites may cause severe respiratory and abdominal distress. To relieve acute symptoms, the physician slowly drains the ascitic fluid (usually 1 to 3 L). Hypovolemia with a fluid volume deficit may occur with rapid fluid removal, because these clients have adjusted to the excessive fluid volume in the abdomen. Rapid, drastic removal of ascitic fluid leads to decreased abdominal pressure, which may contribute to vasodilation and shock. The nurse observes for impending signs of shock from fluid shifts during and immediately after the procedure.

Repeated paracentesis procedures are contraindicated because of the increased incidence of protein depletion, hypovolemia, and electrolyte imbalances (hypokalemic alkalosis), which can contribute to the development of portal-systemic encephalopathy in the client with cirrhosis.

COMFORT MEASURES. Excessive ascitic fluid volume in the abdomen may cause the client to experience respiratory difficulty. Dyspnea may develop as a result of increased intra-abdominal pressure, which limits thoracic expansion and diaphragmatic excursion. The nurse or assistive nursing personnel elevates the head of the bed to at least 30 degrees or as high as the client wishes in an effort to minimize shortness of breath. The client is encouraged to sit in a chair. This upright position, with his or her feet elevated to discourage dependent ankle edema, often relieves dyspnea.

To weigh the client, the nurse or assistive nursing personnel uses a standard upright bedside scale (if the client can stand). Weighing on a bed scale necessitates that the client lie flat; this supine position can cause the client to feel increasingly short of breath and can increase anxiety.

NIC ***FLUID/ELECTROLYTE MANAGEMENT.*** The nurse monitors the client for fluid and electrolyte imbalances as a result of the disease or treatment. Laboratory tests, such as blood urea nitrogen (BUN), serum protein, hematocrit, and electrolytes help to determine fluid and electrolyte status. Nursing activities are listed in Chart 59-2.

SURGICAL MANAGEMENT. When medical management fails to control ascites, the physician may choose surgical intervention to divert ascites into the venous system by creating a shunt. However, the shunt has limited use as an effective treatment for ascites. Clients with ascites are poor sur-

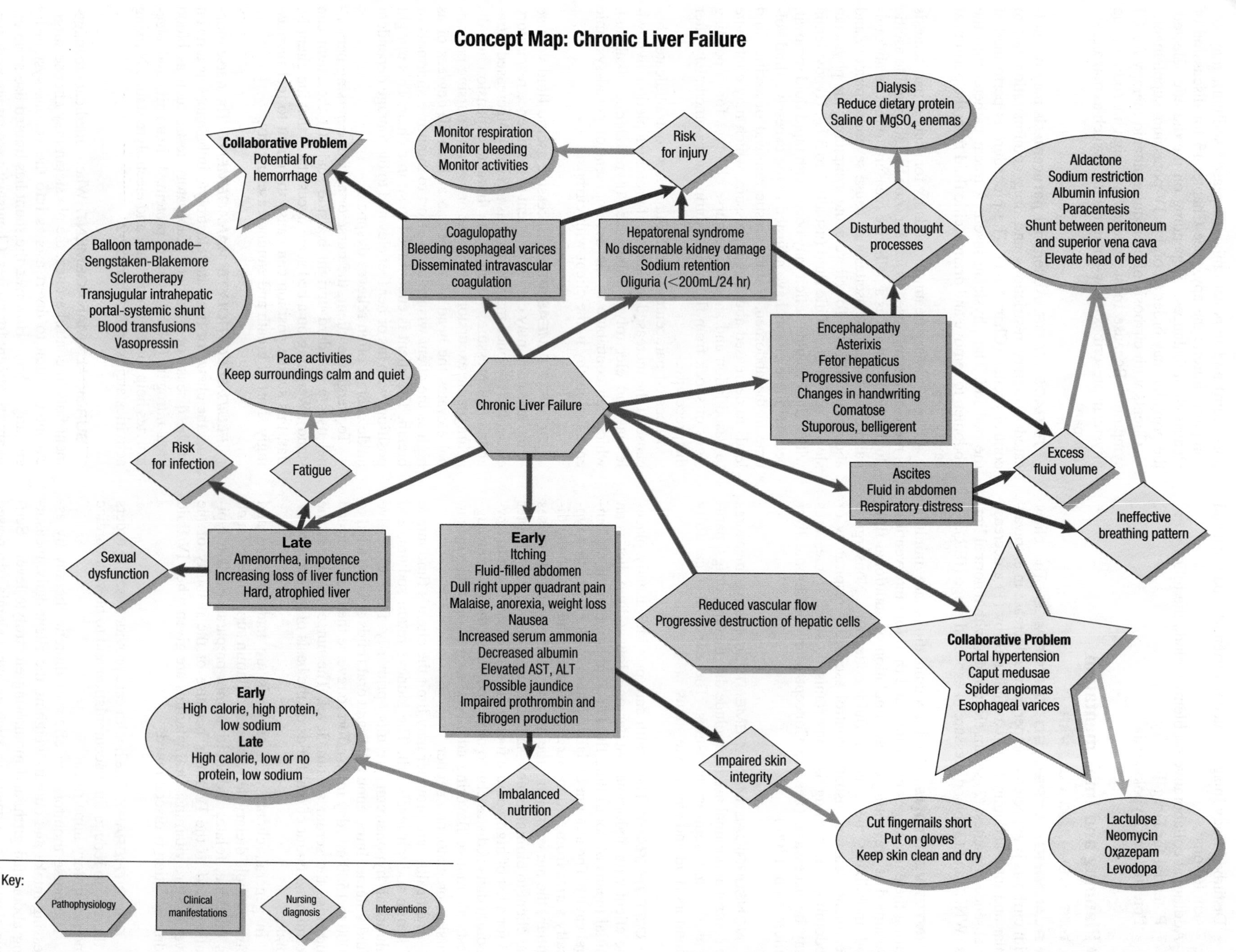
Concept Map: Chronic Liver Failure
Collaborative Problem
Potential for hemorrhage
Monitor respiration
Monitor bleeding
Monitor activities
Risk for injury
Dialysis
Reduce dietary protein
Saline or $MgSO_4$ enemas
Balloon tamponade–Sengstaken-Blakemore
Sclerotherapy
Transjugular intrahepatic portal-systemic shunt
Blood transfusions
Vasopressin
Coagulopathy
Bleeding esophageal varices
Disseminated intravascular coagulation
Hepatorenal syndrome
No discernable kidney damage
Sodium retention
Oliguria (<200mL/24 hr)
Disturbed thought processes
Aldactone
Sodium restriction
Albumin infusion
Paracentesis
Shunt between peritoneum and superior vena cava
Elevate head of bed
Pace activities
Keep surroundings calm and quiet
Chronic Liver Failure
Encephalopathy
Asterixis
Fetor hepaticus
Progressive confusion
Changes in handwriting
Comatose
Stuporous, belligerent
Risk for infection
Fatigue
Excess fluid volume
Ascites
Fluid in abdomen
Respiratory distress
Ineffective breathing pattern
Sexual dysfunction
Late
Amenorrhea, impotence
Increasing loss of liver function
Hard, atrophied liver
Early
Itching
Fluid-filled abdomen
Dull right upper quadrant pain
Malaise, anorexia, weight loss
Nausea
Increased serum ammonia
Decreased albumin
Elevated AST, ALT
Possible jaundice
Impaired prothrombin and fibrogen production
Reduced vascular flow
Progressive destruction of hepatic cells
Collaborative Problem
Portal hypertension
Caput medusae
Spider angiomas
Esophageal varices
Early
High calorie, high protein, low sodium
Late
High calorie, low or no protein, low sodium
Imbalanced nutrition
Impaired skin integrity
Cut fingernails short
Put on gloves
Keep skin clean and dry
Lactulose
Neomycin
Oxazepam
Levodopa
Key:
Pathophysiology
Clinical manifestations
Nursing diagnosis
Interventions

CHART 59-1

BEST PRACTICE *for*
Care of the Client Having a Paracentesis

- Explain the procedure, and answer the client's questions.
- Obtain vital signs, measure the client's abdominal girth, and weigh the client.
- Ask the client to void completely or drain the Foley catheter.
- Position the client. Assist him or her to sit in an upright position at the side of the bed with the feet propped on a stool. Support the client to maintain this position during the procedure.
- Monitor vital signs every 15 minutes during the procedure.
- Measure the drainage and record on the intake and output record.
- Describe the collected fluid (e.g., clear, straw-colored, hazy, or cloudy). Send specimens for laboratory analysis.
- After the physician removes the trocar catheter, apply a dressing to the puncture site. Assess for fluid leakage.
- Position the client in bed and maintain bedrest until vital signs are stable and return to baseline.

gical risks because of their susceptibility to infection, as evidenced by the following:

- A decreased WBC count
- Disseminated intravascular coagulation (DIC)
- Bleeding esophageal varices
- Anesthesia reactions

Mortality in these clients having shunt procedures can be as great as 11% perioperatively; complication rates are approximately 30% (Ziser et al., 1999).

PREOPERATIVE CARE. Because the client with cirrhosis has many underlying medical problems, an optimal physical state is desired before surgery is performed. Electrolyte imbalances are corrected, and abnormal coagulation is treated with the administration of fresh frozen plasma and vitamin K. Packed red blood cells are made available for transfusion, because these clients have bleeding tendencies.

OPERATIVE PROCEDURES. One of several types of shunts may be created, such as the peritoneovenous and Denver shunts.

Peritoneovenous Shunt. A peritoneovenous shunt, also known as a peritoneojugular or LeVeen shunt (Figure 59-4), drains ascites through a one-way valve into a silicone rubber tube that terminates in the superior vena cava. A pressure gradient develops between the peritoneal cavity and the vena cava, facilitating the flow of ascitic fluid through the valve into the venous system. During inspiration, the diaphragm descends, which increases peritoneal fluid (ascites) pressure; pressure in the superior vena cava also increases, which creates the needed gradient. A pressure difference of greater than 3 cm H_2O is necessary to open the valve. The valve closes when the pressure is decreased.

After the shunt has been inserted, the client is expected to lose weight, show a decrease in abdominal girth, have increased urinary output, and exhibit an increased renal excretion of sodium. These clinical improvements result from restored adequate peripheral circulation.

Denver Shunt. The Denver shunt has a subcutaneous pump that can be manually compressed. It is often preferred for clients whose ascites contains large particles (common in neoplastic ascites). These particles can cause the flow to become sluggish and result in a clotted shunt. Compressing the pump of the Denver shunt helps to irrigate the tubing to maintain patency.

CHART 59-2

NIC INTERVENTION ACTIVITIES *for*
The Client with Cirrhosis

Fluid/Electrolyte Management: *Regulation and prevention of complications from altered fluid and/or electrolyte levels*

- Obtain laboratory specimens for monitoring of altered fluid and electrolyte levels (i.e. hematocrit, BUN, protein, sodium and potassium levels) as appropriate.
- Keep an accurate record of intake and output.
- Weigh daily and monitor trends.
- Monitor for signs and symptoms of fluid retention.
- Monitor vital signs, as appropriate.
- Administer prescribed supplemental electrolytes, as appropriate.

Bleeding Precautions: *Reduction of stimuli that may induce bleeding or hemorrhage in at-risk clients*

- Monitor the client closely for hemorrhage.
- Monitor for signs and symptoms of persistent bleeding (e.g., check all secretions for frank or occult blood)
- Monitor coagulation studies, including prothrombin time (PT), partial prothrombin time (PTT), fibrinogen, fibrin degradation/split products, and platelet counts, as appropriate
- Monitor orthostatic vital signs, including blood pressure.
- Use electric razor, instead of straight-edge, for shaving
- Use soft toothbrush or toothettes for oral care.
- Avoid injections (IV, IM, or SQ), as appropriate.
- Protect the client from trauma, which may cause bleeding.

Neurologic Monitoring: *Collection and analysis of client data to prevent or minimize neurologic complications*

- Monitor level of consciousness.
- Monitor level of orientation.
- Monitor recent memory, attention span, past memory, mood, affect, and behaviors.
- Monitor vital signs: temperature, blood pressure, pulse, and respirations.

NIC intervention activities selected from McCloskey, J.C., & Bulechek, G.M. (Eds.). (2000). *Nursing interventions classification (NIC)* (3rd ed.) St. Louis: Mosby.
BUN, Blood urea nitrogen.

POSTOPERATIVE CARE. The nurse provides the usual postoperative care for a client undergoing abdominal surgery (see Chapter 19). The nurse remains aware that the ascitic fluid is routed into the venous system, resulting in vascular volume expansion and hemodilution. The vital signs are monitored carefully; an increase in blood pressure reflects an increase in vascular volume. If the client has a central venous or pulmonary artery catheter in place, the nurse determines whether pressure is elevated. Breath sounds are auscultated for the presence of crackles, which indicates excessive lung fluid. A diuretic, such as furosemide (Lasix), is usually ordered to rid the body of excessive fluid.

The nurse notes any abnormal results of coagulation studies (prothrombin time [PT] and partial thromboplastin time [PTT]). Reabsorption of clotting factors in ascitic fluid may further inhibit an already altered clotting mechanism and lead to DIC and bleeding abnormalities.

The nurse or assistive nursing personnel measures the client's weight, abdominal girth, and urinary output each shift to determine the effectiveness of the shunting procedure.

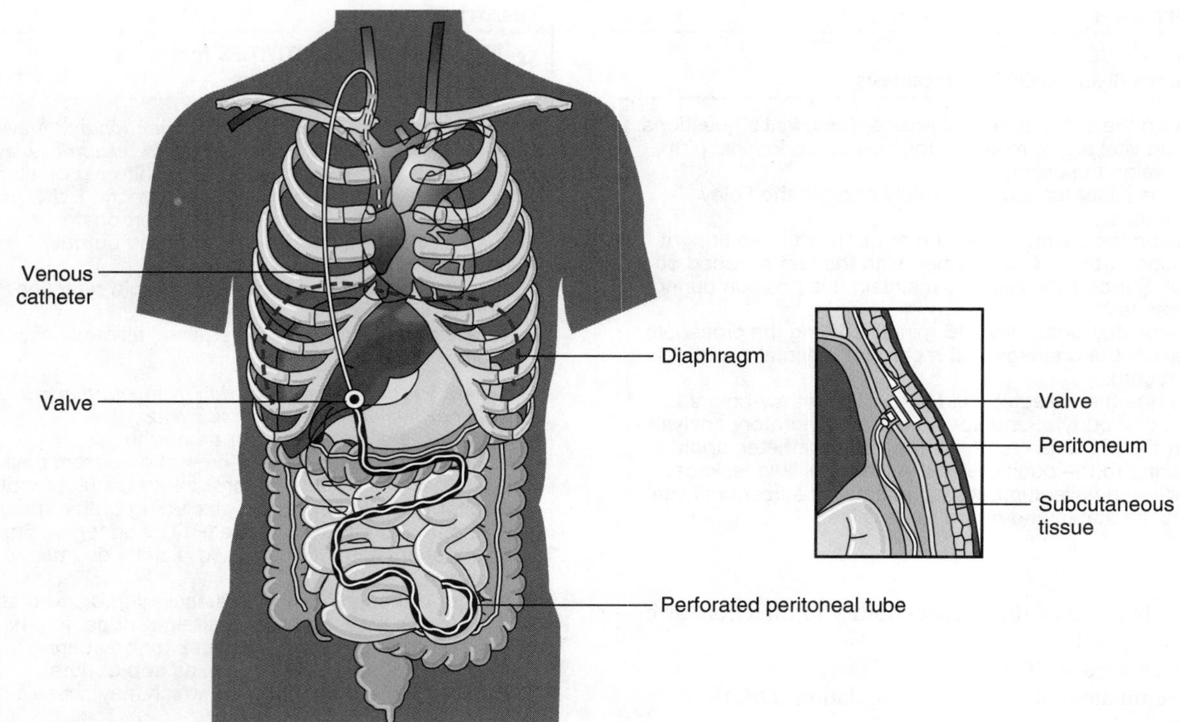

Figure 59-4 ● Peritoneovenous (LeVeen) shunting for treatment of ascites.

POTENTIAL FOR HEMORRHAGE

PLANNING: EXPECTED OUTCOMES. If the client experiences hemorrhage, it is expected to be controlled through medical and nursing interventions.

INTERVENTIONS. During the acute phase of bleeding, early interventions are based on identifying the source of bleeding and initiating treatment to halt it. Because massive esophageal bleeding can cause rapid blood loss, emergency interventions are initiated. If the client is a known alcoholic with a history of variceal bleeding, measures to treat the esophageal varices are initiated and therefore valuable time is not wasted looking for another source of bleeding.

NONSURGICAL MANAGEMENT. The health care team intervenes quickly to control bleeding by providing gastric intubation, balloon tamponade, drug therapy, replacement of blood products, injection sclerotherapy, or transjugular intrahepatic portal-systemic shunt (TIPS). The client is managed in the critical care unit. After the acute bleeding episode has been controlled, the client may require surgical intervention to decrease portal hypertension, thereby decreasing the risk of further variceal bleeding.

GASTRIC INTUBATION. Early in the hospitalization, the client's reports of hematemesis should be investigated. The physician usually inserts an 18-gauge Salem sump tube and lavages the stomach until the fluid returned is clear. The introduction of saline or water lavage may be used to achieve vasoconstriction of the bleeding gastric ulceration or varices. The physician may add norepinephrine (Levophed) to the solution to produce further constriction.

If endoscopy identifies the bleeding site as a gastric ulcer, the physician initiates medical treatment with drug therapy (antacids and histamine receptor antagonists) and blood product replacement. If bleeding continues from the ulcer, surgical intervention is necessary.

ESOPHAGOGASTRIC BALLOON TAMPONADE. If the physician suspects that hematemesis has occurred because of bleeding esophageal varices, he or she inserts an esophagogastric tamponade tube. Bleeding varices are a medical emergency and necessitate immediate intervention. The primary nursing intervention is maintaining a patent airway. Vomiting and the accumulation of blood in the oropharynx may result in aspiration, occlusion of the airway, and respiratory compromise. The nurse attempts to keep the client's oropharynx clear by suctioning secretions, turning the client's head, and keeping the head of the bed elevated during vomiting episodes to prevent aspiration.

Types of Esophagogastric Tubes. The classic method of treating bleeding esophageal varices is by compressing the bleeding vessels with an esophagogastric tube, such as the Sengstaken-Blakemore tube (Blakemore tube), which has two balloons. This type of tube is also referred to as a **tamponade tube.** When inflated, the large esophageal balloon compresses the esophagus. The smaller gastric balloon helps anchor the tube and exerts pressure against bleeding varices in the distal esophagus and the cardia of the stomach. A third lumen terminates in the stomach and is connected to suction, allowing the aspiration of gastric contents and blood. A Salem sump tube is used in conjunction with the Sengstaken-Blakemore tube and is placed in the proximal esophagus to enable clearing of collected esophageal secretions, saliva, and blood.

Insertion of an Esophagogastric Tube. Before the physician inserts the tube, the nurse inspects it and inflates and deflates the balloons to check for integrity and leaks. Each lumen is identified and labeled to prevent errors in adding or removing pressure and air volume.

The physician usually anesthetizes the client's nose and oropharynx, introduces the tube through the nares, and gently inserts it into the stomach. After tube placement is verified, the stomach is aspirated and irrigated. The gastric balloon is inflated with up to 300 mL of air. The nurse assists the physician in securing the tube and applying traction, which provides additional tamponading pressure. This is accomplished by taping the tube to the face guard of a football helmet or by securing it to an overbed traction apparatus and applying a 1-pound (0.45-kg) traction weight.

Care of the Client with an Esophagogastric Tube. Inflation of the esophageal balloon is measured with a sphygmomanometer. Pressure should be maintained between 20 and 25 mm Hg. The nurse periodically checks the balloon pressures and volumes to prevent loss of pressure (with further bleeding or erosion) or rupture of the esophagus caused by overinflation (Chart 59-3). The esophagogastric balloon is usually removed after 48 hours. The nurse attaches the esophageal and gastric drainage lumina to low intermittent suction and monitors the amount and type of drainage.

Placement of the tamponade tube should halt variceal bleeding. After bleeding is controlled, the traction is released, and esophageal pressure is gradually decreased. The gastric balloon is deflated, and the tube is removed. Another tube should be kept at the bedside for potential reinsertion if bleeding recurs.

The nurse and assistive nursing personnel should be alert for sudden respiratory compromise with acute distress caused by airway obstruction from upward displacement of the esophageal balloon. A pair of scissors is *always* kept at the bedside. If the tube becomes dislodged, the nurse cuts both balloon ports to rapidly deflate the balloon and quickly removes the tube.

BLOOD TRANSFUSIONS. Massive hemorrhage necessitates replacement by blood products. Blood is drawn to identify the client's blood type. Until the blood is available, the nurse administers large crystalloid (IV fluids) or colloid (plasma) volumes, as ordered, into large-bore IV access routes to maintain blood pressure.

The nurse administers packed red blood cells and fresh frozen plasma (per physician order and agency policy) to replace blood volume and clotting factors. The physician and the nurse monitor trends in hemoglobin and hematocrit levels, and additional blood products are transfused as indicated.

DRUG THERAPY. To prevent the incidence of esophageal hemorrhage, the client may be placed on propranolol (Inderal, Apo-Propranolol♣) therapy. By decreasing heart rate and systemic blood pressure, the chance of bleeding may be reduced.

In a client who is actively bleeding, the physician may use a vasoconstrictor (e.g., vasopressin [Pitressin]), to temporarily control hemorrhage by lowering pressure within the portal blood flow system. This drug causes contraction of smooth muscle in the vascular bed. By constricting preportal splanchnic arterioles, blood flow is decreased to the abdominal organs, which reduces portal pressure and portal blood flow.

Vasopressin is administered by infusion pump intravenously or through a catheter placed in the superior mesenteric artery. The IV route is indicated initially because it allows easy, rapid access. The insertion of a superior mesenteric artery catheter is an invasive procedure performed by the physician or radiologist through fluoroscopy. Both infusion methods have demonstrated effective short-term control of variceal bleeding, but recurrent hemorrhage is common. An initial bolus dose of 20 to 40 units of vasopressin in 100 to 200 mL of 5% dextrose in water (D_5W) is typically given, followed by a continuous infusion of 200 units in 500 mL of D_5W at 0.2 to 0.4 units/min.

CHART 59-3

BEST PRACTICE *for*
Care of Clients with Esophageal Tamponade Tubes

- Assist the physician with tube placement. Before the gastric balloon is inflated, make sure that a chest x-ray film is obtained and is available *immediately* on tube insertion.
- Elevate the head of the bed when the tube is in place.
- Clearly label all lumina of the tamponade tube.
- Keep a pair of scissors at the bedside. Cut the tube and remove it immediately if signs of respiratory distress or airway obstruction occur.
- Apply gentle tension to the tube by securing it to the face guard of a football helmet or by applying an overhead traction setup with a 1-pound (0.45-kg) traction weight.
- Apply a cut gauze sponge around the tube under the client's nose.
- Insert a drainage tube into the esophagus, above the inflated balloon, if the tamponade tube does not have an esophageal drainage port. If an esophageal drainage port is available, maintain drain patency.
- Provide the client with frequent mouth care.
- Restrain the client's hands loosely *if necessary* to prevent dislodgement of the tube.
- Maintain the specified balloon pressures and volumes. (Esophageal balloon pressure is measured in millimeters of mercury; gastric balloon volume is measured in milliliters or cubic centimeters.) Release the pressure at specified intervals. (The client may experience substernal pressure when the esophageal balloon is inflated. This is an expected feeling.)
- Assess the client's sudden report of back and upper abdominal pain. Monitor vital signs for a drop in blood pressure and an increase in the heart rate. Report these signs immediately.

The nurse closely monitors the pulse, blood pressure, and intake and output ratio of the client receiving vasopressin. The occurrence of abdominal cramping, chest pain, and cardiac dysrhythmias is noted and reported immediately to the health care provider. Vasopressin may precipitate acute angina or myocardial infarction in clients with coronary artery disease. The nurse immediately reports any abnormal assessment findings to the physician. Concurrent IV administration of nitroglycerin, a vasodilator, may help prevent vasoconstriction of the coronary arteries during vasopressin therapy.

INJECTION SCLEROTHERAPY. The use of endoscopic injection sclerotherapy in clients with bleeding esophageal varices is a treatment reserved for clients who have repeated hemorrhagic episodes despite conservative medical management. Before the endoscopy, the nurse obtains baseline vital signs values. The physician usually administers the first dose of sedative, usually diazepam (Valium) or midazolam hydrochloride (Versed). The physician sprays the client's throat with a topical anesthetic, such as benzocaine (Cetacaine).

Injection sclerotherapy is performed in conjunction with esophagogastroduodenoscopy. During the endoscopic examination, the physician introduces a sclerosing agent, or sclerosant, through a flexible injector (Figure 59-5).

Bleeding from the varices should stop within 2 to 5 minutes. If it continues, the physician makes a second injection attempt below the bleeding site. Prophylactic injection sclerotherapy may be performed on other distended, nonbleeding varices. Because the procedure is usually done during an acute bleeding episode, the nurse or assistive nursing personnel closely monitors the client's vital signs during this hour-long procedure, which is done at the bedside or in an endoscopy clinic.

The client may report noncardiac chest discomfort for 24 to 72 hours after the injection; this discomfort is relieved by analgesia. The nurse assesses the complaint of chest pain and administers pain medication. Esophageal perforation and ulceration are other complications of injection sclerotherapy and cause severe chest pain. The nurse immediately reports acute changes to the physician.

Because aspiration may occur and cause pneumonia and pleural effusion, the nurse assesses lung sounds for decreased aeration and adventitious sounds. After injection sclerotherapy, caution is necessary when nasogastric (NG) tubes are used and inserted. Some physicians prefer not to reinsert NG tubes to decrease the risk of injury to the sclerosed esophagus.

ENDOSCOPIC LIGATION. Endoscopic variceal ligation uses bands to ligate the bleeding varices and can be used to prevent esophageal varices from bleeding. This procedure is similar to sclerotherapy except that the varices are ligated with bands instead of injected. This procedure is thought to be safer and more cost-effective than propranolol therapy in preventing esophageal varices from bleeding (Sarin et al., 1999).

TRANSJUGULAR INTRAHEPATIC PORTAL-SYSTEMIC SHUNT. Insertion of a **transjugular intrahepatic portal-systemic shunt (TIPS)** is a nonsurgical procedure performed in the radiology department in a special procedures room or an interventional radiology suite. This procedure is usually reserved for clients who have not responded to any other nonsurgical management. With the client under IV conscious sedation, the physician passes a shunt through a catheter and implants it between the portal vein and the hepatic vein. This technique reduces portal venous pressures and therefore controls bleeding.

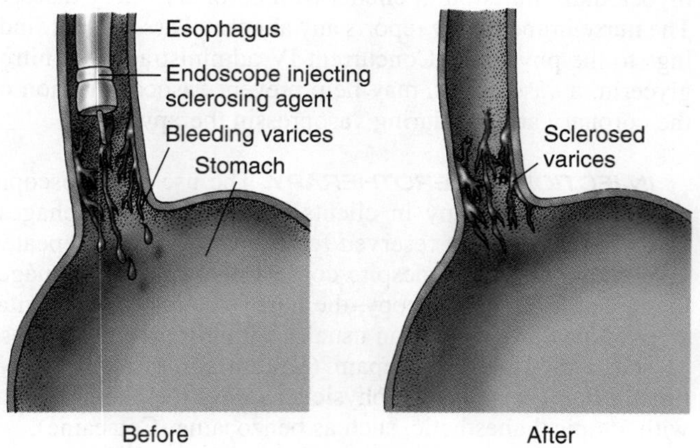

Figure 59-5 ● Injection sclerotherapy.

Before the procedure, the physician obtains informed consent from the client. The client should know that the procedure is painful even though droperidol (Inapsine), meperidine hydrochloride (Demerol), or midazolam hydrochloride (Versed) is given in high doses for IV conscious sedation. Complications may include stenosis and thrombosis. After TIPS, the client can usually go home within 2 to 4 days.

SURGICAL MANAGEMENT. Portal-systemic shunts are considered a last-resort intervention for clients with portal hypertension and esophageal varices. The high mortality rate associated with shunting procedures occurs because clients with end-stage liver disease have coagulation abnormalities, are susceptible to infection, tolerate anesthesia poorly, and have ascites. In recent years, liver transplantation has also been commonly performed for end-stage cirrhosis (see Liver Transplantation, p. 1324).

Surgical bypass shunting procedures decrease portal hypertension by diverting a portion of the portal vein blood flow from the liver. The goal is to decrease the incidence of variceal bleeding while maintaining sufficient blood flow to the liver, thereby preserving hepatocellular function.

PREOPERATIVE CARE. The client with hepatic cirrhosis has multiple underlying problems. The client with esophageal bleeding must be transfused before surgery with packed red blood cells and fresh frozen plasma to correct clotting deficiencies.

OPERATIVE PROCEDURES. The shunting procedures most commonly used are the portacaval and splenorenal shunts (Figure 59-6).

The portacaval shunt diverts the portal venous blood flow into the inferior vena cava to decrease portal pressure. The portal vein is anastomosed to the inferior vena cava. Splenorenal shunting involves splenectomy with anastomosis of the splenic vein and left renal vein. There are several variations of these procedures. With the *mesocaval* shunt, the superior mesenteric vein is anastomosed to the inferior vena cava.

Portal-systemic decompression shunting procedures are not as common as they once were because of complications such as bleeding, portal-systemic encephalopathy (PSE), shunt thrombosis, and infection, as well as the increase in number of liver transplants. A shunt may decrease the occurrence of variceal bleeding, but survival time is usually not prolonged.

POSTOPERATIVE CARE. The client is usually admitted to the critical care unit immediately after surgery. The extent of care needed depends on the client's preoperative health status, extent of hepatic disease, and magnitude of the procedure.

The nurse provides constant observation and careful monitoring, including a frequent assessment of vital signs, central venous pressure, and pulmonary artery pressure (if indicated), as well as an hourly intake and urinary output measurements. In collaboration with the physician and the respiratory therapist, the nurse monitors respiratory status if the client is intubated, protects the client's artificial airway (endotracheal tube), and checks the ventilator for correct settings. The usual postoperative care measures to prevent atelectasis and pneumonia are instituted.

Although the intubated client has an increased need for sedatives, the nurse exercises discretion in providing opioid analgesics for pain relief and sedation during the postoperative period. These drugs are contraindicated in clients with chronic hepatic failure, because most drugs are metabolized in the liver.

After these shunting procedures, clients are susceptible to oliguria. They are often hypovolemic as a result of the following:

- Uncompensated blood loss
- Excessive fluid loss from prolonged exposure of the peritoneal space during surgery, resulting in fluid evaporation
- The recurrence of ascites
- Preoperative fluid restriction
- Diuretic therapy

The nurse administers the ordered fluid volume and assesses the effects of the volume by monitoring for increased blood pressure, decreased heart rate, and increased urinary output. Excessive increases in the central venous pressure or pulmonary artery pressure after fluid challenge are reported. Volume replacement may be given as fresh frozen plasma (to correct postoperative coagulopathy), IV solution boluses, and packed red blood cells.

Recurrent esophageal variceal bleeding after a portal-systemic shunt is not uncommon and may indicate the return of elevated portal pressures caused by a thrombosed (clotted) shunt. A rapid reaccumulation of abdominal fluid may also suggest a failed shunt or excessive sodium administration. The physician may need to reinstitute diuretic therapy. The nurse continues to measure the client's abdominal girth and reports sudden girth increases to the physician.

The nurse should be alert for the development of postshunt encephalopathy, because it is common in these clients (see care measures for portal-systemic encephalopathy [PSE] in the next section).

Clients requiring portal-systemic shunts have increased nutritional requirements and are often given total parenteral nutrition (TPN) to provide the needed calories, vitamins, and minerals. The nurse also administers albumin intravenously several times per day to replace the albumin lost in ascites. (See Chapter 61 for care associated with TPN administration.)

NIC ***Bleeding Precautions.*** The nurse monitors the client closely for hemorrhage. Coagulation studies, including prothrombin time (PT), partial thromboplastin time (PTT), platelet count, and International Normalized Ratio (INR), are also monitored carefully. Chart 59-2 lists additional interventions for clients at risk for bleeding.

POTENTIAL FOR PORTAL-SYSTEMIC ENCEPHALOPATHY

PLANNING: EXPECTED OUTCOMES. It is expected that the nurse report and document findings for clients who exhibit signs of portal-systemic encephalopathy (PSE).

INTERVENTIONS. During the early stages of PSE in clients with hepatic cirrhosis, interventions are focused on decreasing ammonia formation in an effort to decrease progressive cerebral dysfunction. The diseased liver cannot convert ammonia to a less toxic form, and ammonia is carried by the circulatory system to the brain, where high levels of ammonia are toxic to normal cerebral function. The aim of PSE management is to halt this process.

Because ammonia is formed in the gastrointestinal (GI) tract by the action of bacteria on protein, nonsurgical treatment measures to decrease ammonia production include dietary limitations and drug therapy to reduce bacterial breakdown. The nurse collaborates with the dietitian and physician to plan and implement these treatment measures.

DIET THERAPY. The client with cirrhosis has increased nutritional requirements. The client needs high-carbohydrate, moderate-fat, and high-protein foods. The diet is often modified for clients who have elevated serum ammonia levels and exhibit the signs of PSE. The client's intake of dietary protein is typically limited in an effort to reduce the

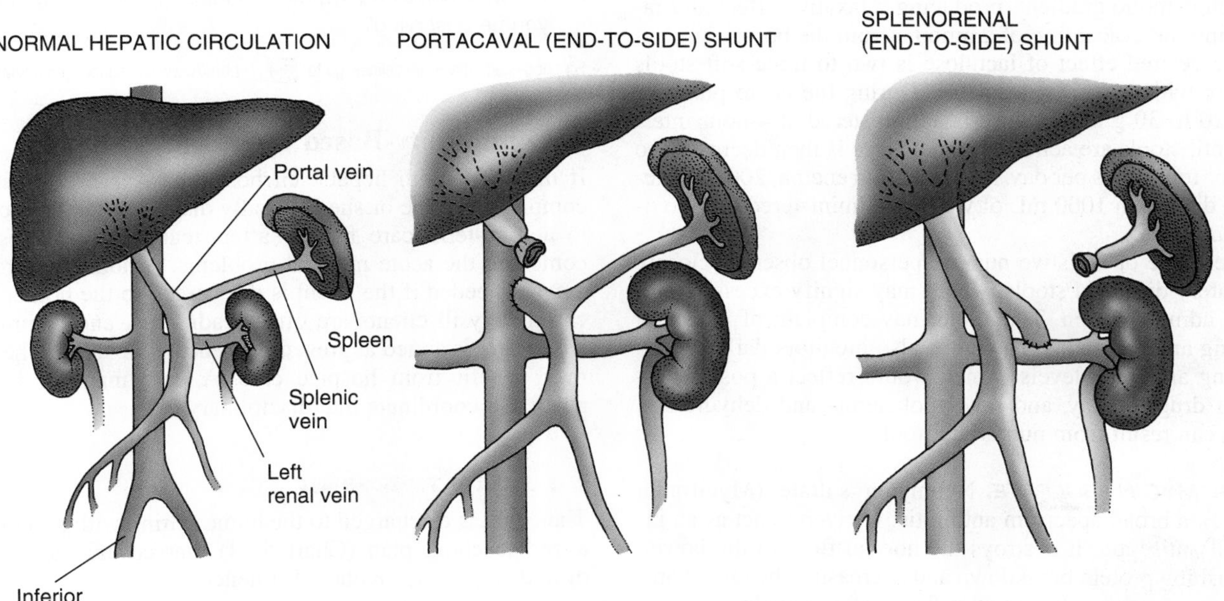

Figure 59-6 ● Surgical shunting diverts portal venous blood flow from the liver to decrease portal and esophageal pressure.

excessive breakdown of protein into ammonia by intestinal bacteria.

The diet for a client with PSE or elevated ammonia levels usually includes low-protein foods and simple carbohydrates, such as fruit juice. As the client's mental status deteriorates, proteins may be totally eliminated from the diet. When PSE fluctuates among the four stages, the nurse avoids giving foods high in protein content, such as meat, fish, poultry, eggs, and dairy products.

Clients with cirrhosis often experience GI bleeding, which results in the formation of increased amounts of ammonia as intestinal bacteria attempt to metabolize the blood cells. GI bleeding may precipitate hepatic coma (stage IV of PSE). These clients are maintained on nothing by mouth (NPO) status with a nasogastric (NG) tube or an esophageal tamponade tube, depending on the source of the bleeding. Nutritional maintenance with IV total parenteral nutrition is often necessary.

DRUG THERAPY. Several types of drugs can eliminate or reduce ammonia levels in the body.

LACTULOSE. The health care provider orders the administration of lactulose (Cephulac) to promote the excretion of ammonia in the stool. Lactulose, a disaccharide with high molecular weight, is a viscous, sticky, sweet-tasting liquid that the nurse administers either orally or by NG tube. When giving the drug orally, the nurse dilutes the lactulose with fruit juice to help the client tolerate the sweet taste. Lactulose retention enemas are often necessary when the client cannot tolerate oral administration or when liquids are contraindicated in the upper GI tract.

Lactulose creates an acidic environment in the bowel by keeping ammonia in its ionized state; this decreases the colon's pH from 7 to 5. This causes ammonia to leave the circulatory system and move into the colon, which reverses the normal passage of ammonia from the colon to the bloodstream. The acidic environment also discourages the growth of bacteria. Lactulose draws water into the bowel because of its high osmotic gradient, producing a laxative effect and facilitating the evacuation of ammonia from the bowel.

The desired effect of lactulose is two to three soft stools per day with an acidic fecal pH. During the acute phase of PSE, 20 to 30 g of lactulose is administered at 4-hour intervals until stools are achieved; the dosage is then decreased to three or four times per day. As a retention enema, 200 g of lactulose diluted in 1000 mL of water is administered at 4- to 6-hour intervals.

The nurse or assistive nursing personnel observes closely for watery diarrheal stools, which may signify excessive lactulose administration. The client may complain of intestinal bloating and cramping. The nurse also monitors daily for decreasing ammonia levels, which would reflect a positive effect of drug therapy, and for hypokalemia and dehydration, which can result from numerous stools.

NEOMYCIN SULFATE. Neomycin sulfate (Mycifradin Sulfate), a broad-spectrum antibiotic, is given to act as an intestinal antiseptic. It destroys the normal flora in the bowel, diminishing protein breakdown and decreasing the rate of ammonia production. Maintenance doses of neomycin are given orally but may also be administered as a retention enema.

Because constipation may lead to increased bacterial action on retained stool, with a resulting increase in ammonia levels, stool softeners should be included in the long-term treatment plan. The administration of medications that are potentially toxic to the liver, such as opioid analgesics, sedatives, and barbiturates, must be restricted.

OTHER DRUGS. Because the client with PSE exhibits progressive neurologic changes and is often confused, combative, uncooperative, or belligerent, the nurse may need to give sedatives to prevent him or her from self-harm or harm of others. In such cases, the judicious use of drugs such as oxazepam (Serax) is warranted.

Levodopa (Dopar, Larodopa) has been used with some success in the treatment of chronic PSE. The use of levodopa (a precursor of dopamine and norepinephrine) is based on the theory that encephalopathy involves defective neurotransmitters. Deficient dopamine and norepinephrine are replaced by false transmitters—amine products from the breakdown of dietary protein. Synthetic levodopa provides the pathway for normal transmission.

NIC **NEUROLOGIC MONITORING.** The nurse or assistive nursing personnel continually assesses for changes in level of consciousness and orientation (see Chart 59-2). An individualized neurologic assessment is developed for each client and includes the assessment of simple tasks such as name writing, bilateral handgrasping, and serial subtractions and additions.

The nurse also continually assesses for the presence of asterixis (liver flap) and fetor hepaticus (liver breath). These signs suggest worsening encephalopathy.

CRITICAL THINKING CHALLENGE

You are caring for a client in the prodromal stage of PSE.

- In planning care, which common medications are hepatotoxic and should be avoided?
- What type of dietary restrictions might be ordered?
- How will you maintain the client's safety?
- For what signs and symptoms indicating worsening PSE will you be observing?

For suggested answer guidelines, go to SIMON http://www.wbsaunders.com/SIMON/Iggy/.

Community-Based Care

If the client with hepatic cirrhosis survives life-threatening complications, he or she is usually discharged to the home or to a long-term care facility after treatment measures have combated the acute medical problems. A home care referral may be needed if the client is discharged to the home. These chronically ill clients are often readmitted, and community-based care is aimed at preventing rehospitalization. The client may benefit from hospice care. A case manager is often needed to coordinate interdisciplinary care.

HEALTH TEACHING

The client is discharged to the home setting with an individualized teaching plan (Chart 59-4) that covers diet therapy, drug therapy, and alcohol abstinence.

DIET THERAPY. In collaboration with the dietitian, the nurse provides strict dietary instructions. Most clients need a diet high in calories, protein, and vitamins. Depending on the

CHART 59-4

CLIENT EDUCATION GUIDE
Cirrhosis

Diet Therapy
- Consume a diet high in calories, protein, and vitamins unless your health care provider has told you to avoid high-protein foods.
- If you have excessive fluid in the abdomen, follow the low-sodium diet prescribed for you.
- Eat small, frequent meals that are nutritionally well balanced.
- Include in your diet daily supplemental liquids (e.g., Ensure or Ensure Plus) and a multivitamin. Low-protein supplements are available if needed.

Drug Therapy
- Take the diuretics prescribed for you. If you experience weakness or cardiac irregularities, report these symptoms to your health care provider.
- Take the H_2-receptor antagonist prescribed for you to prevent gastrointestinal bleeding.
- Do *not* take any other medication unless specifically ordered by your health care provider.

Alcohol Abstinence
- Do not consume any alcohol.
- Seek support services for help.

presence or absence of ascites, the client may require a diet low in sodium. The dietitian plans meals and menus with the client's favorite foods and provides lists of foods high in calories, protein, and vitamins.

The client with portal-systemic encephalopathy (PSE) must avoid high-protein foods at home in an effort to decrease the incidence of progressive neurologic dysfunction. If the client's nutritional intake is decreased after discharge, multivitamin supplements and supplemental liquid feedings (e.g., Ensure) are usually needed.

DRUG THERAPY. The client is often discharged while receiving diuretics. The nurse provides written instructions and the health care provider's prescription for the diuretic. Written information about the signs and symptoms of potential electrolyte imbalances that may result from diuretic therapy (e.g., hypokalemia) is also essential. The client may need to take a potassium supplement.

If the client has had problems with bleeding from gastric ulcers, the provider prescribes antacids or an H_2-receptor antagonist agent, such as ranitidine hydrochloride (Zantac). The nurse provides written guidelines and administration schedules for all medications to be taken at home.

The nurse advises the client to avoid all over-the-counter medications and to consult the physician for follow-up medical care. The client is instructed to notify the physician immediately if any gastrointestinal (GI) bleeding is noted so that re-evaluation can be initiated quickly.

ALCOHOL ABSTINENCE. One of the most important aspects of ongoing care for the nurse to stress is the need for alcohol abstinence (see Chapter 8). Avoiding alcohol can do the following:
- Prevent further fibrosis of the liver from scarring
- Allow the liver to regenerate
- Prevent gastric and esophageal irritation
- Reduce the incidence of bleeding
- Prevent other life-threatening complications

HOME CARE MANAGEMENT

The nurse, case manager, client, and family or significant other should identify any physical adaptations needed to prepare the client's home for convalescence. The client's rest area should be close to a bathroom, because diuretic therapy increases the frequency of urination. If the client has difficulty reaching the toilet, additional equipment (e.g., urinals, bedpans, and bedside commodes) is necessary. Special, adult-sized incontinence pads or briefs may be helpful if the client has an altered mental status and has urinary incontinence.

Initial home activity may be limited for the client who has undergone surgical intervention. If the client experiences shortness of breath from massive ascites, elevating the head of the bed and maintaining the client in a semi-Fowler's to high Fowler's position may help alleviate respiratory distress. Alternatively, a reclining chair with a foot elevator may be used.

HEALTH CARE RESOURCES

The client with chronic cirrhosis may require a home care nurse to assess the client's tolerance of dietary restrictions. The home care nurse can also monitor the effectiveness of drug therapy or the surgical shunt in controlling ascites. Individual and group therapy sessions may be arranged to assist the client in dealing with alcohol abstinence. The nurse may refer the client and family to self-help groups, such as Alcoholics Anonymous and Al-Anon. The client may also desire spiritual support. Other possible resources include hospice and long-term care in a nursing home.

Evaluation: Outcomes

NOC The nurse evaluates the care of the client with cirrhosis on the basis of the identified nursing diagnoses and collaborative problems. The expected outcomes include that the client will:
- Experience a decrease in or no ascites
- Have electrolytes within normal limits (WNL)
- Have blood pressure WNL
- Not experience hemorrhage, or be managed immediately if bleeding occurs
- Not experience PSE, or be managed immediately if PSE occurs
- Have the optimal quality of life possible

HEPATITIS

OVERVIEW

Hepatitis is the widespread inflammation of liver cells. *Viral* hepatitis is the most prevalent type and can be either acute or chronic. **Viral hepatitis** results from an infection caused by one of five major categories of viruses:
- Hepatitis A virus (HAV)
- Hepatitis B virus (HBV)
- Hepatitis C virus (HCV)
- Hepatitis D virus (HDV)
- Hepatitis E virus (HEV)

Hepatitis F and G have also been identified but are uncommon.

Liver injury with inflammation can also develop after exposure to a number of pharmacologic and chemical agents by inhalation, ingestion, or parenteral (IV) administration. *Toxic* and *drug-induced hepatitis* can result from exposure to hepatotoxins (e.g., industrial toxins, alcohol, and medications).

Hepatitis may also occur as a secondary infection during the course of infections with other viruses, such as Epstein-Barr, herpes simplex, varicella-zoster, and cytomegalovirus.

Clients usually recover from hepatitis but may have residual liver damage. Mortality from hepatitis is relatively low, but severe hepatitis may be fatal. With increasing numbers of people developing chronic hepatitis, the mortality is rising.

Pathophysiology

After the liver has been exposed to causative agents (e.g., a virus), it becomes enlarged and congested with inflammatory cells, lymphocytes, and fluid, resulting in right upper quadrant pain and discomfort. As the disease process continues and progresses, the liver's normal lobular pattern becomes distorted as a result of widespread inflammation, necrosis, and hepatocellular regeneration. This distortion increases pressure within the portal circulation, interfering with the blood flow into the hepatic lobules. Edema of the liver's bile channels results in intrahepatic obstructive jaundice.

Specific data on the pathogenesis of hepatitis A, C, D, and E are limited. Clinical manifestations of acute HBV inflammation are determined by an immunologic response of the host (client). Immune complex–mediated tissue damage may contribute to the extrahepatic manifestations of acute hepatitis B. Clinical responses include an urticarial rash (hives) and arthritic joint pain.

There are three phases of hepatitis. The **preicteric** or prodromal phase begins with the infection and the start of signs and symptoms and generally lasts a week. The **icteric** phase starts with the onset of jaundice and lasts approximately 4 to 6 weeks. The **posticteric** or recovery phase of hepatitis is marked by active phagocytosis and enzyme activity; damaged hepatic cells are removed, allowing for regeneration of the cells. This phase may last up to 4 months. Unless serious complications develop, most clients recover normal hepatic function after a viral hepatic insult.

CLASSIFICATION OF HEPATITIS AND ETIOLOGIES

VIRAL HEPATITIS. The five types of acute viral hepatitis vary by mode of transmission, manner of onset, and incubation periods (Table 59-5). These viruses are classified as enteral or parenteral in reference to the mechanism of transmission.

Enteral forms (hepatitis A and E) are transmitted by the fecal-oral route. Parenteral forms (hepatitis B, C, and D) are primarily transmitted via venous blood transfer or through intimate sexual contact. Vaccines to prevent hepatitis A and B are currently available.

HEPATITIS A. The causative agent of hepatitis A, hepatitis A virus (HAV), is a ribonucleic acid (RNA) virus of the enterovirus family. HAV is characterized by a mild course similar to that of a typical viral syndrome and often goes unrecognized. It is spread via the fecal-oral route by the oral ingestion of fecal contaminants. Sources of infection include contaminated water, shellfish caught in contaminated water, and food contaminated by food handlers infected with HAV. The virus may also be spread by oral-anal sexual activity. The incubation period of hepatitis A is usually 15 to 50 days. The disease is usually not life threatening. Individuals exposed to the virus should be given immune globulin immediately and not later than 2 weeks after the exposure.

HEPATITIS B. Hepatitis B is caused by a double-shelled particle containing deoxyribonucleic acid (DNA) composed of a core antigen (HBcAg), a surface antigen (HBsAg), and an independent protein (HBeAg) that circulates in the blood.

The primary mode of transmission of hepatitis B virus (HBV) is via the skin and mucous membrane route by contamination with blood and serous fluid. Lower concentrations of HBV are also found in semen, vaginal fluid, and saliva. Although transmission can occur through bites, there are no documented cases of transmission through kissing. Hepatitis B may be spread through the following modes of transmission:

- Sexual contact with multiple partners (heterosexual and homosexual)
- Sharing needles
- Accidental needle sticks or injuries from sharp instruments in health care workers
- Blood transfusion
- Hemodialysis
- Acupuncture, tattooing, ear or body piercing
- Maternal-fetal route

The clinical course of hepatitis B may be varied. It may have an insidious onset with mild signs and symptoms, or it may result in serious complications such as fulminant hepatitis, chronic hepatitis, cirrhosis, and hepatocellular carcinoma, a rare but increasing problem in the United States. The incubation period is generally 45 to 180 days, but hepatitis B commonly develops 60 to 90 days after exposure. Chronic HBV infection develops in about 1% to 10% of adult clients with acute HBV infection (CDC, 1999).

HEPATITIS C. The causative virus of hepatitis C (HCV) is an enveloped, single-stranded RNA virus. It is transmitted by exposure of the skin and mucous membrane to blood and plasma; it is rarely transmitted sexually or from mother to fetus.

HCV is spread by contaminated items such as the following:

- Illicit IV drug needles (highest incidence)
- Tattoo, ear, or body piercing needles
- Razors, nail clippers, and scissors
- Toothbrushes and Water Piks
- Tampons or sanitary napkins
- Blood, blood products, or organ transplants received before 1992

Health care workers, such as nurses and phlebotomists, are also at risk for HCV infection following a needle stick injury with HCV-contaminated blood. HCV infection is also common in hemodialysis centers.

The incubation period for HCV is 21 to 140 days, with an average incubation period of 7 weeks. Approximately 85% of infected individuals develop chronic hepatitis (Hoofnagle, 1999). Approximately 2.7 million Americans are chronically infected with HCV, with 65% between 30 and 49 years of age (Alter, 1999). This suggests that the health care system may be burdened as infected individuals age and develop worsening liver damage (see the Cost of Care box on p. 1316).

Hepatitis C is a leading cause of cirrhosis and hepatocellular carcinoma worldwide. Approximately half of the liver transplants performed in the United States are for end-stage hepatitis C (Hepatitis Foundation International, 1999). Unfor-

TABLE 59-5 • DIFFERENTIAL FEATURES OF THE FIVE TYPES OF VIRAL HEPATITIS*

Hepatitis A	Hepatitis B	Hepatitis C	Hepatitis D	Hepatitis E
SYNONYMS				
Infectious hepatitis	Serum hepatitis	Post-transfusion hepatitis		Epidemic non-A, non-B hepatitis or enterically transmitted hepatitis
DIAGNOSIS OF ACUTE DISEASE				
Anti-HAV IgM in serum	HBsAg in serum	Anti-HCV in serum	Anti-HDV in serum	Anti-HEV in serum
INCUBATION PERIOD				
15-50 days	48-180 days	14-180 days	14-56 days	15-64 days
HIGH-RISK GROUPS				
More common in young children and institutional settings	All age-groups affected, especially drug addicts and health care personnel	All ages of drug users Persons with hemophilia	Drug addicts Persons with hepatitis B	Persons living in underdeveloped countries
SEASON				
Fall and early winter	All year	All year	All year	All year
TRANSMISSION				
Usually by oral-fecal route among persons living in close contact; ingestion of contaminated water or contaminated shellfish	Primarily blood; drug abuse, sexual contact, mother to child at birth	Primarily blood; drug abuse, sexual contact (rarely), mother to child at birth	Co-infects with hepatitis B; nonpercutaneous; close personal contact	Oral-fecal route; transmitted principally by contaminated water
CLINICAL FINDINGS				
Majority of type A infections (mild and anicteric); symptoms similar to those of influenza	Changes similar to those of hepatitis A	Changes similar to those of hepatitis A	Changes similar to those of hepatitis A, but symptoms often more severe than those in hepatitis A and hepatitis B	Resembles hepatitis A
	Fatigue, anorexia, low-grade fever, abdominal discomfort, arthralgias, rashes, enlarged and tender liver, light stools, dark urine, jaundice Elevated serum AST and ALT levels (early), hyperbilirubinemia, abnormal liver function test results	Tends to have more severe symptoms; sometimes necessitates hospitalization for extended periods	Often asymptomatic	
VIRUS IN FECES?				
Yes	Not infectious	Not identified	Not identified	Possible
VIRUS IN SERUM?				
Anti-HAV in serum during acute phase and incubation period is rare	HBsAg is in serum throughout the clinical course	Anti-HVC test is approximately 95% reliable; often takes up to 8 weeks to show antibody	Anti-HDV in serum	
NOSOCOMIAL PROBLEM?				
No	Yes	Yes	Yes	No
MORTALITY				
Less frequent	More frequent, chronic form can be fatal	More frequent, chronic form can be fatal	Increased	Unknown

Anti-HAV, antibody to HAV; IgM, immunoglobulin M; *HBsAg,* hepatitis B surface antigen; *anti-HCV,* antibodies to HCV; *anti-HDV,* antibodies to HDV; *anti-HEV,* antibodies to HEV; *AST,* aspartate aminotransferase; *ALT,* alanine aminotransferase; *HBIG,* hepatitis B immune globulin; *anti-HBs,* hepatitis B surface antibody; *anti-HBc,* hepatitis B core antibody; *anti-HBe,* hepatitis Be antibody.

Continued

TABLE 59-5 • DIFFERENTIAL FEATURES OF THE FIVE TYPES OF VIRAL HEPATITIS*—cont'd

Hepatitis A	Hepatitis B	Hepatitis C	Hepatitis D	Hepatitis E
INCIDENCE OF CHRONIC ACTIVE HEPATITIS AS A COMPLICATION				
Low	Approximately 15% will develop chronic form	Approximately 85% will develop chronic form	Yes	No
IMMUNE GLOBULIN (IG) (PROPHYLAXIS)				
IG	HBIG or IG	No		None; recommended IG
VACCINE				
Yes	Yes	No	Prevention of hepatitis B with vaccine prevents hepatitis D	No
ANTIBODY				
Anti-HAV	Anti-HBs, anti-HBc, anti-HBe	Anti-HCV	Anti-HDV	Anti-HEV

Anti-HAV, antibody to HAV; IgM, immunoglobulin M; *HBsAg,* hepatitis B surface antigen; *anti-HCV,* antibodies to HCV; *anti-HDV,* antibodies to HDV; *anti-HEV,* antibodies to HEV; *AST,* aspartate aminotransferase; *ALT,* alanine aminotransferase; *HBIG,* hepatitis B immune globulin; *anti-HBs,* hepatitis B surface antibody; *anti-HBc,* hepatitis B core antibody; *anti-HBe,* hepatitis Be antibody.

COST OF CARE IMPLICATIONS FOR NURSING

HEPATITIS C

Cost of Care

- An estimated 3.9 million Americans, nearly 2% of the population, are chronically infected with hepatitis C.
- The cost of hepatitis C infections and related diseases is more than $600 million dollars per year.
- More than half of the liver transplants performed in the United States are for hepatitis C. The average first-year cost for a liver transplant exceeds $200,000.
- From the year 2010 through 2019, the projected cost in direct medical expenses is $10.7 billion, with 165,900 deaths due to chronic liver disease and 27,200 deaths due to hepatocellular carcinoma.

Implications for Nursing

Nurses are at high risk for getting hepatitis C and becoming part of these statistics. As these costs rise, health care will be impacted further from this disease. Nurses must strive to disseminate information about this disease to prevent others from obtaining it and to help reduce costs.

Data from Wong, J.B., et al. (2000). Estimating future hepatitis C morbidity, mortality, and costs in the United States. *American Journal of Public Health, 90*(10), 1562-1569.

LEGAL/ETHICAL ISSUES IN HEALTH CARE

LIVER TRANSPLANTATION FOR CLIENTS WITH HEPATITIS C

More than half of the transplants performed in the United States are for clients with end-stage liver disease related to hepatitis B and hepatitis C. When these individuals receive a transplant, many "new livers" become reinfected with the hepatitis. As a result, another transplantation is required.

As of October 1999 more than 14,000 people are awaiting a transplant, and approximately 4500 transplants are performed each year. Is it ethical to provide transplants for individuals with hepatitis? Is it a lifesaving or life-prolonging procedure for these individuals? Is it an appropriate use of a scarce resource? Should the diagnosis come into consideration with transplantation, given that the clients often choose to participate in high-risk behaviors that make them susceptible to hepatitis C?

tunately, the newly transplanted liver often becomes reinfected with the virus (see the Legal/Ethical Issues box below, left).

HEPATITIS D. Hepatitis D (delta hepatitis, or HDV) is caused by a defective RNA virus that needs the helper function of HBV. HDV co-infects with HBV and needs its presence for viral replication. Hepatitis D can co-infect a client with HBV or can occur as a superinfection in a client with chronic HBV. Superinfection usually develops into chronic HDV. The incubation period is approximately 14 to 56 days. As with HBV, the disease is transmitted primarily by parenteral routes.

CULTURAL CONSIDERATIONS

In the United States, Canada, and northern Europe, hepatitis D (delta infection) is most prevalent in people exposed to blood and blood products (e.g., drug addicts and hemophiliacs).

The prevalence of hepatitis D usually corresponds to the prevalence of hepatitis B. Southern Italy, Africa, South America, and parts of Russia and Romania have a high prevalence, whereas northern Italy, Spain, Turkey, and Egypt have a moderate prevalence (CDC [Hepatitis Branch], 1997).

HEPATITIS E. The hepatitis E virus (HEV) was originally identified by its association with waterborne epidemics of hepatitis in the Indian subcontinent. Since then, it has occurred in epidemics in Asia, Africa, the Middle East, Mexico, and Central and South America. Many large outbreaks have occurred after heavy rains and flooding.

In the United States, hepatitis E has been found only in travelers returning from these endemic areas. The nonenveloped, single-stranded RNA virus is transmitted via the fecal-oral route, and the clinical course resembles that of hepatitis A. HEV has an incubation period of 15 to 64 days. There is no evidence at this time of a chronic form of HEV.

TOXIC AND DRUG-INDUCED (CHEMICAL) HEPATITIS. Two major types of toxic hepatitis have been recognized—direct toxic hepatitis and idiosyncratic toxic hepatitis.

DIRECT TOXIC HEPATITIS. Direct toxic hepatitis (DTH) results in necrosis and fatty infiltration of the liver. Agents causing toxic hepatitis are generally systemic poisons or are converted in the liver to toxic metabolites. People with repeated, regular exposure to an offending agent (e.g., alcohol [alcoholic hepatitis]) or with a dose-related toxicity range can have direct toxic hepatitis. For example, acetaminophen (Tylenol), a commonly used over-the-counter (OTC) analgesic, can cause severe hepatic necrosis when taken in large amounts, such as in suicide attempts or accidental ingestion by children.

Industrial toxins such as carbon tetrachloride, trichloroethylene, and yellow phosphorus also have a direct toxic effect on the liver.

IDIOSYNCRATIC TOXIC HEPATITIS. Idiosyncratic toxic hepatitis (ITH) results in morphologic changes to the liver that are similar to those found in viral hepatitis. In idiosyncratic drug reactions, the occurrence of hepatitis is unpredictable and uncommon. It may occur at any time during or shortly after exposure to the drug. Examples of agents that result in idiosyncratic toxic hepatitis are isoniazid (INH, Isotamine♣), an antituberculosis drug, and phenytoin (Dilantin), an anticonvulsant.

Treatment of toxic and drug-induced hepatitis is supportive. Transplantation may be considered if fulminating liver failure is present. Withdrawal of the suspected agent is indicated at the first sign of a reaction. Chemical exposure of the liver to drugs and toxins has resulted in the development of chronic active hepatitis and cirrhosis.

COMPLICATIONS OF HEPATITIS

Failure of the liver cells to regenerate, with progression of the necrotic process, results in a severe and often fatal form of hepatitis known as **fulminant hepatitis.** This form of massive hepatic necrosis is rare.

Hepatitis is considered to be chronic when liver inflammation lasts longer than several months (usually defined as 6 months). **Chronic hepatitis** usually occurs as a result of hepatitis B or hepatitis C. Superimposed infection with hepatitis D (HDV) in clients with chronic HBV may also result in chronic hepatitis.

With **chronic active hepatitis (CAH),** liver damage is progressive and is characterized by hepatic necrosis, acute inflammation, and progressive fibrosis. The client may be asymptomatic for long periods of the hepatic disease process, or the continued fibrosis may lead to liver failure, cirrhosis, and death. Chronic active hepatitis may be manifested by the following:

- Persistent clinical symptoms and hepatomegaly
- The continual presence of HBsAg (hepatitis B surface antigen) or anti-HCV (HCV antibodies)
- Elevated, fluctuating serum levels of aspartate aminotransferase (AST), bilirubin, and alkaline phosphatase for 6 months or longer after the acute hepatitis episode

Liver biopsy is necessary to establish the diagnosis of chronic hepatitis.

In people with *chronic persistent* hepatitis and *chronic lobar* hepatitis, liver damage does not progress after the initial insult. These types of hepatitis result from infections with hepatitis B and C viruses. Most clients with chronic persistent hepatitis are asymptomatic, and physical findings are normal. Laboratory data may reveal a mild elevation of serum AST and alkaline phosphatase levels that may persist for up to 1 year. Routine screening of blood donors and the elimination of commercial blood sources have virtually eliminated the incidence of hepatitis B or C caused by blood transfusion. Case reporting to local health departments for all types of *viral* hepatitis is mandatory. Measures to prevent viral hepatitis for health care workers and others in contact with infected clients are listed in Charts 59-5 and 59-6.

CHART 59-5

BEST PRACTICE *for*
Prevention of Viral Hepatitis in Health Care Workers

- Use standard precautions to prevent the transmission of disease between clients or between clients and health care staff (see Chapter 26).
- Eliminate needles and other sharps by substituting needleless systems. (Needle sticks are the major source of hepatitis B transmission in health care workers.)
- Take the hepatitis B vaccine (Hepatovax-B, Recombivax HB), which is given in a series of three injections. This vaccine also prevents hepatitis D. (See Chapter 26 for more information on this requirement of the United States Occupational Safety and Health Administration [OSHA].)
- For postexposure prevention of hepatitis A or B, seek medical attention immediately for immunoglobulin (IG) administration.
- Report all cases of hepatitis to the local health department.

CHART 59-6

CLIENT EDUCATION GUIDE
Prevention of Viral Hepatitis

- Maintain adequate sanitation and personal hygiene. Wash your hands before eating and after using the toilet.
- Drink water treated by a water purification system.
- If traveling in underdeveloped or nonindustrialized countries, drink only bottled water. Avoid food washed or prepared with tapwater, such as raw vegetables, fruits, and soups.
- Use adequate sanitation practices to prevent the spread of the disease between family members.
- Do not share bed linens, towels, eating utensils, or drinking glasses.
- Do not share needles for injection, body piercing, or tattooing.
- Do not share razors, nail clippers, toothbrushes, or Water Piks.
- Use a condom during sexual intercourse.

Etiology

In addition to the hepatitis A, B, C, D, and E viruses, other causes of hepatitis include the following:

- Drugs, chemicals, and toxins
- Blood transfusion reactions from exposure to the hepatitis virus
- Hyperthyroidism
- Ingestion of ethyl alcohol (ETOH), resulting in alcoholic hepatitis
- Wilson's disease (increased serum copper)
- Other viruses, such as Epstein-Barr, cytomegalovirus, and yellow fever

Incidence/Prevalence

There are an estimated 125,000 to 200,000 infections of hepatitis A every year. Approximately one third of Americans have evidence of past infection, but many are not aware that they were infected (CDC, 1999).

Hepatitis B occurs primarily in young adults between 20 and 39 years of age. The incidence of hepatitis B is between 140,000 to 320,000 infections each year. There has been a decrease during the first half of the 1990s, most likely as a result of the hepatitis B vaccine. Approximately 10% of clients with hepatitis B develop chronic hepatitis.

The prevalence of hepatitis C is highest in individuals with high-risk drug behaviors, such as sharing needles. The incidence is approximately 36,000 new infections per year. It is estimated that 4 million of the U.S. population has been infected. The chronic form develops in approximately 85% of those infected.

COLLABORATIVE MANAGEMENT

Assessment

HISTORY

If viral hepatitis is suspected, the nurse asks the client whether he or she has had known exposure to a person with hepatitis. The nurse determines whether the client has had recent blood transfusions or undergoes hemodialysis for renal failure. The client should be asked about the following:

- Sexual activities
- Social activities
- Injectable drug use
- Recent ear or body piercing and/or tattooing
- Close living accommodations, such as military barracks, correctional institutions, overcrowded apartments, long-term care facilities
- Receiving blood, blood products, or a transplant before 1992

The client's employment history is obtained. The nurse specifically asks about employment as a health care worker. The client is asked about recent travel to a foreign country or to an area with inadequate environmental sanitation. The client is also questioned about the ingestion of water from a possibly contaminated source or the recent ingestion of shellfish.

PHYSICAL ASSESSMENT/CLINICAL MANIFESTATIONS

VIRAL HEPATITIS. The courses and clinical manifestations of all five types of viral hepatitis are somewhat similar (see Table 59-5). The nurse assesses the client's general subjective complaints, determining whether symptoms occurred acutely (hepatitis A and E) or insidiously (hepatitis B and C).

The client may verbalize feelings of fatigue and loss of appetite. The nurse explores further to assess whether the client is experiencing the following:

- Abdominal pain
- Arthralgia (joint pain)
- Myalgia (muscle pain)
- Diarrhea/constipation
- Fever
- Irritability
- Lethargy
- Malaise
- Nausea/vomiting

The nurse lightly palpates the right upper abdominal quadrant to assess for liver tenderness. The client may report right upper quadrant pain with jarring movements. The skin, sclerae, and mucous membranes are inspected for the presence of jaundice. The client may present for medical treatment only after jaundice appears, believing that other vague symptoms are related to an influenza-like syndrome.

Jaundice in hepatitis results from intrahepatic obstruction and is caused by edema of the liver's bile channels. Dark urine and clay-colored stools are often reported by the client. The nurse obtains a urine and stool specimen for visual inspection and laboratory analysis. The skin is inspected for the presence of rashes in clients with suspected hepatitis B and hepatitis C. Irregular patches of redness or urticaria (hives) may occur. The client often reports pruritus (itching) and may have skin abrasions from scratching.

The client with hepatitis A usually has a fever, and the temperature may range from 100° to 104° F (38° to 40° C). Fever may be low-grade or absent with hepatitis B and hepatitis C.

TOXIC AND DRUG-INDUCED HEPATITIS. The clinical picture in toxic and drug-induced hepatitis depends on the causative agent. Idiosyncratic reactions may result in clinical manifestations that are indistinguishable from those of viral hepatitis or may simulate extrahepatic bile duct obstruction symptoms such as severe jaundice, rash, arthralgia, and fever.

PSYCHOSOCIAL ASSESSMENT

Viral hepatitis usually occurs as an acute illness. Its symptoms may be mild and abate rapidly or go undetected. Emotional problems for affected clients often center on their anger about being sick and being fatigued. General malaise, inactivity, and vague complaints contribute to depression and despondency. These clients worry about the long-term effects and complications.

Clients with viral hepatitis often feel guilty about having exposed others to the virus. Infectious diseases such as hepatitis continue to have a social stigma. The client may feel embarrassed by the isolation and hygiene precautions that are imposed in the hospital and continue to be necessary at home. This embarrassment may cause the client to limit social interactions. Self-imposed visitor restrictions may be instituted by the client out of fear of spreading the virus to family and friends.

Family members are sometimes afraid of contracting the disease and may distance themselves from the client. The nurse allows the client and family to verbalize these feelings and explores the reasons for these fears. Precautionary isolation measures evoke anxiety for the client and the family.

Clients are unable to return to work until the results of blood tests for serologic markers are negative. The loss of wages and the cost of hospitalization for a client without insurance coverage may produce great anxiety and financial burden for the client and the family.

> **CRITICAL THINKING CHALLENGE**
>
> You are the nurse caring for a 52-year old man recently diagnosed with chronic hepatitis C. He denies any high-risk behavior but admits to getting a tattoo in Vietnam. How will you reply to his following questions?
>
> - Could I have gotten this by a tattoo?
> - Could my wife and children have hepatitis?
> - How could I not have known I had hepatitis?
> - What is the cure?

For suggested answer guidelines, go to SIMON http://www.wbsaunders.com/SIMON/Iggy/.

LABORATORY ASSESSMENT

The presence of hepatitis A, B, and C is usually indicated by acute elevations in levels of liver enzymes, indicating liver cellular damage, and by specific serologic markers.

SERUM LIVER ENZYMES. Levels of alanine aminotransferase (ALT) may be elevated to more than 1000 mU/mL and may rise to as high as 4000 mU/mL in severe cases of viral hepatitis. Aspartate aminotransferase (AST) levels may rise to 1000 to 2000 mU/mL. Alkaline phosphatase levels may be normal (30 to 90 IU/L) or mildly elevated. Serum total bilirubin levels are elevated to greater than 2.5 mg/dL and are consistent with the clinical appearance of jaundice. Elevated levels of bilirubin are also present in the urine.

SEROLOGIC MARKERS/ENZYME ASSAYS. The presence of *hepatitis A* is established when hepatitis A virus (HAV) antibodies (anti-HAV) are identified in the blood. Ongoing inflammation of the liver by HAV is evidenced by the presence of immunoglobulin M (IgM) antibodies, which persist in the blood for 4 to 6 weeks. Previous infection is indicated by the presence of immunoglobulin G (IgG) antibodies. These antibodies persist in the serum and provide permanent immunity to HAV.

The presence of the *hepatitis B* virus (HBV) is established if serologic testing confirms the presence of hepatitis B antigen-antibody systems in the blood. HBV is a double-shelled DNA virus consisting of an inner core and an outer shell. Antigens located on the surface (shell) of the virus (HBsAg) and IgM antibodies to hepatitis B core antigen (anti-HBc IgM) are the most significant serologic markers. The presence of these markers establishes the diagnosis of hepatitis B. The client is considered infectious as long as HBsAg is present in the blood. Persistence of this serologic marker after 6 months or longer indicates a carrier state or chronic hepatitis. HBsAg levels normally decline and disappear after the acute hepatitis B episode. The presence of antibodies to HBsAg (anti-HBs) in the blood indicates recovery and immunity to hepatitis B.

Enzyme-linked immunosorbent assay (ELISA) is the initial screening test for clients suspected of being infected with *hepatitis C* virus (HCV), and it is the most commonly used enzyme test for HCV antibodies (anti-HCV). False-positive results can occur in clients with normal ALT levels and no risk factors. In these cases, a more specific assay called the recombinant immunoblot assay (RIBA) is used. Because HCV can often be detected within 2 to 3 weeks of exposure, the virus may be measured directly using the reverse transcription polymerase chain reaction (RT-PCR) test.

The presence of *hepatitis D* virus (HDV) can be confirmed by the identification of intrahepatic delta antigen or, more often, by a rise in the hepatitis D virus antibodies (anti-HDV) titer.

Hepatitis E virus (HEV) testing is usually reserved for travelers in whom hepatitis is present, but the viruses cannot be detected. The presence of the hepatitis E antibodies (anti-HEV) is found in individuals infected with the virus.

OTHER DIAGNOSTIC ASSESSMENT

Chronic hepatitis is diagnosed by percutaneous liver biopsy. The biopsy distinguishes between chronic active and chronic persistent hepatitis. It is also the gold standard test for assessing the extent of injury and prognosis of HCV disease. The finding of fatty infiltrates in liver biopsy specimens and inflammation with neutrophils is consistent with Laënnec's (alcohol-induced) hepatitis.

Interventions

The client with viral hepatitis can be mildly or acutely ill depending on the severity of the inflammation. Most clients are not hospitalized. The plan of care for all clients with viral hepatitis is based on measures to rest the liver, promote cellular regeneration, and prevent complications (see the Client Care Plan on pp. 1320 and 1321).

NONSURGICAL MANAGEMENT. During the acute stage of viral hepatitis, interventions are aimed at resting the inflamed liver to promote hepatic cell regeneration. Rest is an essential intervention to reduce the liver's metabolic demands and increase its blood supply. Treatment is generally supportive.

PHYSICAL REST. The nurse and assistive nursing personnel assess the client's response to activity and rest periods. Strict bedrest may be indicated during the early icteric phase of hepatitis. The client is usually tired and expresses feelings of general malaise. Complete bedrest is usually not required, but rest periods alternating with periods of activity are indicated and are often sufficient to promote hepatic healing.

The nurse individualizes the client's plan of care and changes it as needed to reflect the severity of symptoms, fatigue, and the results of liver function tests and enzyme determinations. The client and nursing staff should adhere to scheduled rest periods. Activities such as self-care and ambulating are gradually added to the activity schedule as tolerated.

PSYCHOLOGIC REST. Emotional and psychologic rest is essential for the client. Because bedrest and inactivity can produce anxiety, the nurse includes diversional activities in the plan of care. The nurse asks the hospitalized client's family to bring in small craft projects, reading materials (e.g., magazines, books, newspapers), or a portable radio. Staff and family members are encouraged to spend time in the client's room.

DIET THERAPY. A special diet is usually not required. The diet should be high in carbohydrates and calories with moderate amounts of fat and protein. Small, frequent meals are often preferable to three standard meals. The nurse asks the client about food preferences, because favorite foods are tolerated better than randomly selected foods. The nurse or assistive nursing personnel encourages the client to select foods that are appealing. High-calorie snacks may be needed.

The health care provider typically orders supplemental vitamins. If caloric intake is low, the nurse may need to provide supplemental commercial feedings, such as Ensure.

DRUG THERAPY. An antiemetic to relieve nausea, such as trimethobenzamide hydrochloride (Tigan) and dimenhydrinate (Dramamine), may be prescribed. Prochlorperazine maleate (Compazine), a phenothiazine, is avoided because of its potential hepatotoxic effects.

There are no drugs specific for hepatitis A management. Interferon, a biologic response modifier given by injection over several months, has been approved for the treatment of *hepatitis B*. However, interferon has a number of side effects that often are so severe the client cannot continue the therapy. Side effects include flu-like symptoms of headaches, fever,

CLIENT CARE PLAN • THE CLIENT WITH VIRAL HEPATITIS

NURSING DIAGNOSIS NO. 1 • Activity Intolerance related to decreased metabolic energy production secondary to liver dysfunction.

Expected Outcomes	Nursing Interventions	Rationale
The client will gradually increase activity to the level experienced before hepatitis occurred.	Provide several periods of rest during the day. D Organize care so the client is not fatigued. D Reinforce the need for bedrest in the immediate recovery period. D Gradually add activities to the client's daily schedule. For example, self-care activities are allowed before ambulation. D	Rest promotes healing of the liver; inflammation of hepatic cells decreases.
	Provide or encourage diversional activities on the basis of the client's interests, such as reading, watching television, or doing small crafts. D Encourage family members and significant others to visit the client for short periods. D Place frequently used items close within reach. D	Diversions such as visits and independent activities decrease anxiety, which can prevent rest. The nurse needs to caution against excessive visitation, because the client may become more fatigued.

NURSING DIAGNOSIS NO. 2 • Imbalanced Nutrition: Less than Body Requirements related to anorexia, nausea, and vomiting

Expected Outcomes	Nursing Interventions	Rationale
The client will achieve an optimal intake of nutrients and calories to promote liver tissue healing.	Provide a diet high in carbohydrates and calories; in collaboration with the dietitian, provide moderate amounts of fat and protein.	A diet high in carbohydrates and calories provides energy. Protein is needed for hepatic cell regeneration.
	Provide small, frequent meals that are attractively presented.	The appearance of a large meal can cause anorexia. Eating a large quantity of food can cause abdominal distention and nausea or vomiting.
	Obtain a diet history to determine food preferences. Encourage significant others to bring in foods, if permitted. Allow the client to select meals from the menu. D Offer high-calorie, high-protein snacks such as milkshakes. D Provide supplemental vitamins and liquid feedings, such as Ensure or Ensure Plus, as ordered. Avoid fried and fatty foods, which can increase nausea.	
	Administer antiemetic medication, such as trimethobenzamide hydrochloride (Tigan), as ordered. Administer acid suppression therapy as ordered.	Antiemetics and acid suppression therapy minimize gastric distress, which allows the client to consume adequate oral nutrition.
	Remove noxious odors or move unpleasant objects or substances away from the client. D	Noxious odors or substances, such as a full bedside commode, can contribute to nausea.

D indicates tasks that can be delegated to assistive nursing personnel.

INR, International Normalized Ratio.

fatigue, loss of appetite, nausea, and vomiting. Other side effects include hair loss, depression, and bone marrow suppression that decreases white blood cell and platelet production.

Two antiviral drugs have recently been used to treat acute HBV: ribavirin (Virazole, Rebetol) and lamivudine (Epivir). Lamivudine is also used after liver and heart transplantation. Both of these drugs can cause sudden, severe anemia and cardiac arrest.

Hepatitis C can be treated with interferon (usually alfa), ribavirin (Virazole, Rebetol), or the more effective combination of Rebetol and interferon alfa-2b, a recombinant called Rebetron. Long-term results are better with the combination drug, which is now considered the first-line drug for HCV (Dougherty & Dreher, 2001).

COMFORT MEASURES. Some foods and smells may stimulate nausea. If possible, the nurse or assistive nursing personnel removes the stimulus causing the nausea. In an effort to stimulate appetite, the nurse or assistive nursing personnel provides mouth care or instructs the client to perform mouth care before meals. The meal may be more palatable when the client is sitting up in a chair. The nurse empties bedpans, urinals, and bedside commodes promptly and provides an air freshener for the room if the client can tolerate it.

SURGICAL MANAGEMENT. Liver transplantation may be performed for clients with chronic hepatitis, especially for hepatitis C, but many become reinfected (see the later discussion of liver transplantation, p. 1324).

Client Care Plan • THE CLIENT WITH VIRAL HEPATITIS—cont'd

NURSING DIAGNOSIS NO. 3 • Deficient Knowledge related to causes of hepatitis and modes of transmission

Expected Outcomes	Nursing Interventions	Rationale
The client will verbalize knowledge about the causes of hepatitis and the modes of transmission.	Assess client's knowledge about disease and modes of transmission, and educate as necessary.	A baseline for the client's level of knowledge must be obtained.
	Instruct the client with hepatitis B or C that a chronic form of the disease may develop and that he or she will need monitoring once discharged.	If the client does not realize the risk for a chronic form, he or she may continue risk behaviors and accidentally infect others.
	If it is identified that the client has a drug or alcohol problem, refer to appropriate persons.	Abstaining from risk behaviors will help reduce transmission.
	Instruct clients that they should not donate blood.	The blood would be wasted because it is contaminated.
	Teach clients to modify sexual practices as directed by health care providers.	Depending on sexual practices, all types of viral hepatitis may be transmitted sexually.
	Use direct, nonjudgmental questions to identify risk behaviors.	Clients may not understand why they are being questioned about sexual and drug behaviors.

NURSING DIAGNOSIS NO. 4 • Risk for Impaired Skin integrity related to pruritus secondary to hepatic dysfunction

Expected Outcomes	Nursing Interventions	Rationale
The skin will remain intact.	Keep the client's skin hydrated with proper moisture. Avoid hot baths, and use emollients. D	Dry skin can lead to more pruritus and make the skin more at risk to breakdown.
	Keep client's fingernails short, and encourage using knuckles if client must scratch. D	Fingernails may scratch and tear the skin.
	Administer antihistamines as prescribed, closely observing for sedation.	Antihistamines may relieve pruritus but may cause excessive sedation.

NURSING DIAGNOSIS NO. 5 • Ineffective Protection related to increased risk of bleeding secondary to decreased vitamin K absorption and possible thrombocytopenia

Expected Outcomes	Nursing Interventions	Rationale
The client is free from bleeding.	Monitor prothrombin time, INR, and platelet levels.	Increased levels for prothrombin time and INR and decreased platelet levels indicate that the client is at greater risk for bleeding.
	Observe for signs of overt and occult bleeding (e.g., bleeding gums, gastrointestinal bleeding, tarry stools). D	If any type of bleeding occurs, the health care provider must be notified immediately.
	Avoid intramuscular injections whenever possible; use small-gauge needles if injection is necessary.	Intramuscular injections may cause bleeding.
	Administer vitamin K as ordered.	Vitamin K helps decrease the chance for bleeding.
	Teach client to use a soft toothbrush and an electric razor.	Less harsh objects help minimize injury to the mucosa and face.

D indicates tasks that can be delegated to assistive nursing personnel.

INR, International Normalized Ratio.

Community-Based Care

HEALTH TEACHING

The nurse teaches the client and the family to observe measures to prevent infection transmission (see Chart 59-6). In addition, the nurse instructs the client with viral hepatitis to avoid alcohol and any nonprescription, over-the-counter medications, particularly acetaminophen (Tylenol, Exdol♣) and sedatives, for 3 to 12 months because of the hepatotoxic effects (Chart 59-7). Clients who develop chronic hepatitis should always avoid these products.

The client must determine patterns for rest on the basis of physical tolerance of increased activity. The nurse encourages the client to increase activity gradually to prevent fatigue. The client should eat small, frequent meals of high-carbohydrate and low-fat foods. In collaboration with the dietitian, the nurse provides diet teaching and menu planning. The nurse teaches the client to follow precautionary measures and avoid sexual activity until the results of hepatitis B surface antigen (HBsAg) tests are negative.

HOME CARE MANAGEMENT

Home care management varies according to the type of hepatitis. A primary focus is preventing the spread of the infec-

CHART 59-7

CLIENT EDUCATION GUIDE
Viral Hepatitis

- Avoid all medications, including over-the-counter drugs, such as acetaminophen (Tylenol, Exdol♣), unless prescribed by your physician.
- Avoid all alcohol.
- Rest frequently throughout the day, and get adequate sleep at night.
- Eat small, frequent meals with a high-carbohydrate, low-fat content.
- Avoid sexual intercourse until antibody testing results are negative.
- Follow the guidelines for preventing transmission of the disease (see Chart 59-6).

tion. For hepatitis transmitted by the fecal-oral route, careful handwashing and sanitary disposal of feces are important. Standard precautions are used for hepatitis transmitted percutaneously and permucosally. Education is therefore very important.

HEALTH CARE RESOURCES

Clients with viral hepatitis and their families may contact the local health department for further information on infection control and prevention. Clients discharged home with limited activity tolerance or minimal family support may need the assistance of a home care aide in performing activities of daily living, particularly meal preparation.

FATTY LIVER

A fatty liver is caused by the accumulation of triglycerides and other fats in the hepatic cells. In severe cases, fat may constitute as much as 40% of the liver's weight and cause changes in liver function. Minimal, temporary fatty changes are usually reversible by eliminating the cause. The most common cause of fatty liver is chronic alcoholism. Other causes include the following:

- Malnutrition
- Diabetes mellitus
- Obesity
- Pregnancy
- Prolonged total parenteral nutrition (TPN)
- Exposure to large doses of drugs toxic to the liver

Fatty infiltration of the liver may result from faulty fat metabolism in the liver and the mobilization of fatty acids from adipose tissue.

Many clients with a fatty liver are asymptomatic. The most common and typical finding is hepatomegaly. Other symptoms include the following:

- Right upper abdominal pain
- Ascites
- Edema
- Jaundice
- Fever
- Signs of late cirrhosis, depending on the severity of the fat infiltration and the longevity of the occurrence

A liver biopsy confirms excessive fat in the liver. Interventions are aimed at removing the underlying cause of the infiltration and providing dietary restrictions.

HEPATIC ABSCESS

OVERVIEW

Although hepatic abscesses are uncommon, they carry a high mortality rate. Liver abscesses occur when the liver is invaded by bacteria or protozoa. These organisms destroy the liver tissue, producing a necrotic cavity filled with infective agents, liquefied liver cells and tissue, and leukocytes. The infectious necrotic tissue walls off the abscess from the healthy liver.

A *pyogenic* liver abscess occurs when bacteria invade the liver. Infecting organisms include *Escherichia coli* and *Klebsiella, Enterobacter, Salmonella, Staphylococcus,* and *Enterococcus* species. A pyogenic abscess is generally solitary and confined to the right lobe, but occasionally they are multiple in nature. The usual cause is acute cholangitis, which occurs as a complication of cholelithiasis. Pyogenic liver abscesses may also result from liver trauma, abdominal peritonitis, and sepsis, or an abscess can extend to the liver after pneumonia or bacterial endocarditis.

The protozoan *Entamoeba histolytica* causes an *amebic* hepatic abscess, which may occur after amebic dysentery. These abscesses usually occur in the form of a single abscess in the right hepatic lobe.

COLLABORATIVE MANAGEMENT

Clients with hepatic abscesses are generally ill. On occasion, an abscess is not diagnosed until autopsy. In clients with a pyogenic liver abscess, the onset of symptoms is usually sudden. Amebic abscesses cause a more insidious onset of symptoms. Common complaints include the following:

- Right upper abdominal pain with a palpable, tender liver
- Anorexia
- Weight loss
- Nausea and vomiting
- Fever and chills
- Shoulder pain
- Dyspnea
- Pleural pain if the diaphragm is involved

A hepatic abscess is usually diagnosed by liver scan. Hepatic arteriography differentiates an abscess from a malignancy. Blood cultures assist in identifying the causative organism in pyogenic abscesses, and stool cultures may identify *E. histolytica.* With ultrasonographic guidance, a liver abscess may be aspirated percutaneously. Surgical drainage is indicated only for a single pyogenic abscess or for an amebic abscess that fails to respond to long-term antibiotic treatment.

LIVER TRAUMA

OVERVIEW

The liver is the most common organ to be injured in clients with penetrating trauma of the abdomen (e.g., gunshot wounds, stab wounds, and rib fractures) and is the second most commonly injured organ in clients who have blunt abdominal trauma. Liver damage or injury should be suspected whenever any upper abdominal or lower chest trauma is sustained. The liver is often injured by steering wheels in vehicular accidents. Common injuries to the liver include simple lacerations, multiple lacerations, avulsions (tears), and crush injuries.

The liver is a highly vascular organ and receives approximately 29% of the body's cardiac output. When hepatic trauma occurs, blood loss can be massive. The client may exhibit signs of hemorrhagic shock, such as the following:

- Hypotension
- Tachycardia
- Tachypnea
- Pallor
- Diaphoresis
- Cool, clammy skin
- Confusion

A decreased hematocrit may confirm suspected blood loss. Clinical manifestations include right upper quadrant pain with abdominal tenderness, distention, guarding, and rigidity. Abdominal pain exaggerated by deep breathing and referred to the right shoulder (Kehr's sign) may indicate diaphragmatic irritation (Chart 59-8).

CHART 59-8

KEY FEATURES *of* Liver Trauma

- Right upper quadrant pain with abdominal tenderness
- Abdominal distention and rigidity
- Guarding of the abdomen
- Increased abdominal pain exaggerated by deep breathing and referred to the right shoulder (Kehr's sign)
- Indicators of hemorrhage and hypovolemic shock:
  - Tachycardia
  - Tachypnea
  - Pallor
  - Diaphoresis
  - Cool, clammy skin
  - Confusion or other change in mental state

COLLABORATIVE MANAGEMENT

When hepatic and other abdominal organ trauma is suspected, the physician performs an emergency peritoneal lavage to confirm injury. If trauma is present, the lavage reveals gross blood or a high red blood cell count.

The physician then performs an exploratory laparotomy to identify and control the source and type of bleeding. Minor surgical interventions, such as suture placement, wound packing, decompression, or a combination of these procedures, are often performed to halt bleeding. Liver lobe resection is required in some extensive liver injuries.

Clients with hepatic trauma require the administration of multiple blood products, packed red blood cells, and fresh frozen plasma, as well as massive volume infusion to maintain adequate hydration. Postoperatively, the client with hepatic trauma is admitted to a critical care unit. The nurse monitors the client for persistent bleeding. Complete blood count and coagulation studies must be closely monitored for trends in changes.

CANCER OF THE LIVER

OVERVIEW

Primary hepatic cancer, or **hepatocellular carcinoma** (cancer originating in the liver), is one of the leading causes of death in the world. The incidence is higher in African-American males and is increasing in people age 40 to 60 years of age (El-Serag & Mason, 1999). Possible reasons for this trend include the increase in people with hepatitis B and hepatitis C infections, which often lead to cancer of the liver.

CULTURAL CONSIDERATIONS

Hepatocellular carcinoma (HCC) is rare in the United States but is one of the most common malignancies in other parts of the world (e.g., Africa). The geographic variation probably reflects the prevalence of chronic hepatitis B and chronic hepatitis C infection in other countries. Hepatitis B or C virus is thought to be the primary carcinogen in as many as 80% of clients with HCC worldwide. Men are affected three times more than women, and blacks worldwide are affected twice as often as Caucasians (El-Serag & Mason, 1999).

Carcinoma of the liver most often develops as a metastatic process. Because of the increased vascularity of the liver, the organ is a common site for metastasis from (1) primary cancers of the esophagus, stomach, colon, rectum, breasts, and lungs; or (2) a malignant melanoma.

Between 30% and 70% of clients with primary hepatic cancer also have cirrhosis, and the risk is 40 times greater in clients with cirrhosis. Men with cirrhosis are more likely than women to develop HCC. Increased testosterone and decreased estrogens may promote the development of HCC in men with cirrhosis (Tanaka et al., 2000).

Primary hepatic cancer has also been associated with trauma, nutritional deficiencies, and exposure to carcinogens and hepatotoxins, such as aflatoxin, thorium dioxide, *Senecio* alkaloids, and the fungus *Aspergillus.*

COLLABORATIVE MANAGEMENT

Clients with liver metastasis initially complain of epigastric or right upper quadrant abdominal pain, fatigue, anorexia, and weight loss. Later they typically experience the same manifestations of HCC, such as jaundice, ascites, bleeding, and encephalopathy. A nuclear radioisotope liver scan detects metastasis in many cases, but ultrasonography with needle biopsy may be required to confirm the metastasis.

Liver cancer is usually fatal within 6 months of diagnosis. Surgical management may be indicated for clients with a single metastatic lesion confined to one liver lobe. Liver lobe resection for surgical excision of metastasis has been successful in achieving survival rates of up to 5 years.

Unfortunately, 75% of clients are not candidates for surgical excision because their tumors are unresectable. A newer procedure, cryosurgical ablation of the liver, has produced remissions that offer hope for long-term survival (Leininger, 1997). In this procedure, the surgeon makes a subcostal or midline abdominal incision and selects which tumors are appropriate for either resection or cryoablation. The cryotherapy probes circulate liquid nitrogen and freeze the tumors. Postoperatively, the client is admitted to the critical care unit for monitoring of complications, including hypothermia, renal failure, and bleeding.

Other standard treatments for liver cancer include high-dose chemotherapy, usually with fluorouracil (5-FU) and hepatic artery ligation to deprive the metastatic lesion of oxygen. Both treatments can be accomplished without systemic effect because of the unique portal vein circulation in the liver. Hepatic chemotherapy is administered by a surgically implanted infusion pump, which enables controlled infusion for up to 14 days at a time. (See Chapter 25 for a discussion of intra-arterial chemotherapy.) Transplantation may also be used to treat liver cancer.

LIVER TRANSPLANTATION

OVERVIEW

The first liver transplantation was performed in 1963, and in 1983 it was decided that liver transplantation no longer be considered experimental. In 1998, 4487 liver transplants were performed, and 1-year survival rates are now approximately 84% (United Network for Organ Sharing (UNOS), 1998).The client with end-stage liver disease who has not responded to conventional medical or surgical intervention is a potential candidate for liver transplantation. In the adult, diseases treated by liver transplantation include the following:

- Primary or secondary biliary cirrhosis
- Chronic active hepatitis with cirrhosis
- Hepatic metabolic diseases, such as protoporphyria and Wilson's disease
- Budd-Chiari syndrome (hepatic vein thrombosis)
- Primary sclerosing cholangitis
- Lannëac's cirrhosis, if the person has abstained from alcohol

Liver transplantation is not commonly performed for clients with malignant neoplasms. Because the tumor is likely to recur in immunosuppressed clients, the procedure remains controversial.

The client for potential transplantation undergoes extensive physiologic and psychologic assessment and evaluation by physicians and transplant coordinators to identify contraindications to the procedure.

Clients who are not considered candidates for transplantation are those with severe end-stage liver disease with life-threatening complications, such as the following:

- Repeated episodes of esophageal variceal bleeding
- Sepsis
- Severe cardiovascular instability with advanced cardiac disease
- Acquired immunodeficiency syndrome (AIDS)
- Diabetes mellitus
- Severe respiratory disease

Additional identified risk factors include the existence of the following:

- Portal vein thrombosis
- Advanced catabolic state
- Active alcoholism
- Age older than 60 years
- Primary and metastatic malignant disease
- A lack of knowledge and understanding of the procedure and necessary postoperative care measures
- A poor psychosocial support system
- Psychologic instability

Liver transplantation has become the most effective treatment for clients with an increasing number of acute and chronic liver diseases, although they are more common in children than in adults. Indications and contraindications continue to vary among transplantation centers and are continually revised as treatment options change and surgical techniques improve.

Donor livers are obtained primarily from head trauma victims and in the United States. They are distributed through a nationwide program, the United Network of Organ Sharing (UNOS). This system distributes donor livers on the basis of regional considerations and recipient acuity. A new program for living donors has also been established. Recipients with the highest level of acuity receive highest priority.

Acute Graft Rejection

The success of all transplantations has greatly improved since the introduction in 1980 of cyclosporine (cyclosporin A), an immunosuppressant drug. Cyclosporine has been the primary agent to prevent rejection of the donor organ graft, but azathioprine (Imuran) and prednisone (Deltasone) are also used. Most recipients receive a combination of cyclosporine, steroids, and azathioprine.

A newer immunosuppressant agent discovered in 1984, tacrolimus (FK 506), is more potent than cyclosporine. FK 506 has been shown to be effective as a form of rescue therapy for clients who continue to reject a liver graft. Mycophenolate mofetil (CellCept) is the one of the newest approved immunosuppressants for the treatment of rejection in liver transplants and for those who are unable to tolerate cyclosporin or FK 506.

A majority of clients still experience a rejection response after liver transplantation beginning 1 to 2 weeks after surgery. Clinical manifestations of acute rejection include tachycardia, fever, right upper quadrant or flank pain, decreased bile pigment and volume, and increasing jaundice. Laboratory findings include elevated serum bilirubin, alkaline phosphatase levels, and increased prothrombin time and aminotransferase levels.

Transplant rejection is treated with IV doses of methylprednisolone (Solu-Medrol). If this drug is not effective, antibodies to lymphocytes such as muromonab-CD3 (OKT3) may also be used. OKT3 is T-cell specific and is more potent, but it increases the client's risk of infection. Mycophenolate mofetil may also be used against rejection. As with all rejection treatments, the client is at a greater risk for infection. If none of these drugs is effective, a rapid deterioration of liver function occurs. Multisystem organ failure, including respiratory and renal involvement, develops along with diffuse coagulopathies and portal-systemic encephalopathy. The only alternative for treatment is emergency transplantation.

Infection

Infection is another potential threat to the transplanted graft and the client's survival. Immunosuppressant therapy, which must be used to prevent and treat organ rejection, significantly increases the client's susceptibility to and risk for infection. Other risk factors include the presence of multiple tubes and intravascular lines, immobility, and prolonged anesthesia.

The average liver transplant client acquires at least one bacterial infection and has a 40% to 50% chance of developing a viral or fungal infection. In the early post-transplantation period, common infections include pneumonia, wound infections, and urinary tract infections. Opportunistic infections usually develop after the first postoperative month and include cytomegalovirus, mycobacterial infections, and parasitic infections. Latent infections such as tuberculosis and herpes simplex are often reactivated.

Transplant complications cause clients to be very anxious. The nurse and other members of the health care team assure the client that these problems are common and usually successfully treated (see the Evidence-Based Practice for Nursing on box at right).

The physician prescribes broad-spectrum antibiotics for prophylaxis during and after surgery. The nurse obtains culture specimens from all lines and tubes and collects specimens for culture at predetermined time intervals as dictated by the agency's policy. If an infection is detected, the physician prescribes organism-specific anti-infective agents.

Other Complications

The biliary anastomosis is susceptible to breakdown, obstruction, and infection. If leakage occurs or if the site becomes necrotic or obstructed, an abscess can form or peritonitis, bacteremia, and cirrhosis may develop. Other potential complications include the following:

- Hemorrhage
- Hepatic artery thrombosis
- Fluid and electrolyte imbalances

EVIDENCE-BASED PRACTICE FOR NURSING

How much anxiety is experienced by clients undergoing a liver transplant?

Chappell, S., & Case, P. (1997). Anxiety in liver transplant patients. *MEDSURG Nursing, 6*(2), 98-103.

The purpose of this study was to describe the anxiety of adult liver transplant recipients during their hospitalization. Speilberg's model of state and trait anxiety was the framework for the study. Speilberg's State Trait Anxiety Inventory (STAI) and a visual analog scale (VAS) were completed at the following stages: admission for transplantation, transfer to the nursing floor, first liver biopsy, first signs of infection, first signs of a rejection episode, immediately after the first teaching session with the transplant coordinator, and discharge from the hospital. The highest mean anxiety scores occurred at the first liver biopsy, the first episode of rejection, and the first infection.

Critique. Although the sample size for this study was small, the researchers aimed to explore the psychosocial aspects of this major surgery and life-changing event. Data from this study can help nurses better care for their clients by addressing both their psychosocial needs and their physical needs.

Implications for Nursing. Nurses should anticipate that clients will be extremely anxious during the first liver biopsy and during episodes of rejection or infection. Nurses caring for clients during these procedures and times should exercise additional support. Other people on the health care team, as well as the clients' families, should also be made aware that clients will experience anxiety at these times; they should be taught to be as supportive and understanding as possible.

TABLE 59-6 • ASSESSMENT AND PREVENTION OF COMMON POSTOPERATIVE COMPLICATIONS ASSOCIATED WITH LIVER TRANSPLANTATION

Assessment	Prevention
ACUTE GRAFT REJECTION	
Occurs from the fourth to tenth postoperative day Manifested by tachycardia, fever, right upper quadrant (RUQ) or flank pain, diminished bile drainage or change in bile color, or increased jaundice Laboratory changes include increased levels of serum bilirubin, transaminases, and alkaline phosphatase, as well as prolonged prothrombin time.	Prophylaxis with immunosuppressant agents, such as cyclosporine Early diagnosis to treat with more potent antirejection drugs, such as muromonab-CD3 (OKT3)
INFECTION	
Can occur at any time during recovery Frequent cultures of tubes, lines, and drainage Manifested by fever or excessive, foul-smelling drainage (urine, wound, or bile); other indicators depend on location and type of infection Early removal of invasive lines Good handwashing	Antibiotic prophylaxis Early diagnosis and treatment with organism-specific anti-infective agents
HEPATIC COMPLICATIONS (BILE LEAKAGE, ABSCESS FORMATION, HEPATIC THROMBOSIS)	
Manifested by decreased bile drainage, increased RUQ abdominal pain with distention and guarding, nausea or vomiting, increased jaundice, and clay-colored stools Laboratory changes include increased levels of serum bilirubin and transaminases	Keep T-tube in dependent position and secure to client; empty frequently, recording quality and quantity of drainage Report manifestations to physician immediately May necessitate surgical intervention
ACUTE RENAL FAILURE	
Caused by hypotension, antibiotics, cyclosporine, acute liver failure, or hypothermia Indicators of hypothermia include shivering, hyperventilation, increased cardiac output, vasoconstriction, and alkalemia Early indicators of renal failure include changes in urine output, increased BUN and creatinine levels, and electrolyte imbalance	Monitor all drug levels with nephrotoxic side effects Prevent hypotension Observe for early signs of renal failure and report them immediately to the physician

**BUN,* Blood urea nitrogen

- Pulmonary atelectasis
- Acute renal failure
- Chronic graft rejection
- Psychologic maladjustment

➤ COLLABORATIVE MANAGEMENT

Care of the client undergoing liver transplantation requires an interdisciplinary team approach. Case managers are an important part of the team. After the client is identified as a candidate and a donor organ is procured, the actual liver transplantation surgical procedure usually takes 8 hours. The length of the procedure can vary greatly. The procedure involves five anastomoses between recipient and donor organs, including the following vascular anastomosis sites:

- Suprahepatic inferior vena cava
- Infrahepatic vena cava
- Portal vein
- Hepatic artery
- Biliary tract

The biliary anastomosis site varies depending on the client's extrahepatic biliary tract. Two common sites are end-to-end anastomosis between the donor and the recipient common bile duct and anastomosis between the donor common bile duct and the recipient jejunum.

In the immediate postoperative period, the client who has undergone liver transplantation is managed in the critical care unit and requires aggressive monitoring and care. The nurse assesses for signs and symptoms of complications of surgery and immediately reports their occurrence to the physician (Table 59-6).

The nurse monitors the client's temperature and reports temperatures greater than 100° F (38° C) and increased abdominal pain, distention, and rigidity, which are indicators of peritonitis. Nursing assessment also includes monitoring for a change in neurologic status that could indicate encephalopathy from a nonfunctioning liver. Signs of coagulopathy (e.g., continuous bloody oozing from a catheter, a drain, and incision sites; petechiae; or ecchymosis) are reported to the physician immediately because they can indicate impaired function of the transplanted liver.

ONLINE RESOURCES

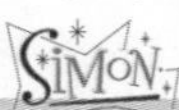

For suggested readings and Internet resources, go to http://www.wbsaunders.com/SIMON/Iggy/.

SELECTED BIBLIOGRAPHY

Alter, M. (1999). *Epidemiology of hepatitis C.* NIH Consensus Development Conference on Management of Hepatitis C; http://gi.ucsf.edu/ALF/CC/CCMAlter.html.

Bockhold, K.M. (2000). Who's afraid of hepatitis C? *American Journal of Nursing, 100*(5), 26-31.

Centers for Disease Control and Prevention (Hepatitis Branch) (April 28, 1997). *Epidemiology and prevention of viral hepatitis A to E: An overview;* http://www.cdc.gov/ncidod/diseases/hepatitis/slideset/httoc.htm.

Centers for Disease Control and Prevention. (1999). *Hepatitis fact sheet;* http://www.cdc.gov/ncidod/diseases/hepatitis.htm.

Chappell, S., Case, P. (1997). Anxiety in liver transplant patients. *MEDSURG Nursing, 6*(2), 98-103.

Dougherty, A.S., & Dreher, H.M. (2001). Hepatitis C: Current treatment strategies for an emerging epidemic. *MEDSURG Nursing, 10*(1), 9-13.

El-Sarag, H., & Mason, A. (1999). Rising incidence of hepatocellular carcinoma in the United States. *New England Journal of Medicine, 340*(10), 745-750.

Frieden, T., et al. (1999). Chronic liver disease in central Harlem: The role of alcohol and viral hepatitis. *Hepatology, 29*(3), 883-888.

Groen, K.A. (1999). Primary and metastatic liver cancer. *Seminars in Oncology Nursing, 15*(1), 48-57.

Hepatitis Foundation International. (September 1999). *Hepatitis fact sheet;* http://hepfi.org/Hepinfo/FACT%201-99.htm.

Hoofnagle, J. (1999). Hepatitis C: *The clinical spectrum of disease.* NIH Consensus Development Conference on Management of Hepatitis C; http://www.hepnet.com/hepc/hoofnagl.html.

Leininger, S.M. (1997). Managing patients with cryosurgical ablation of the prostate and liver. *MEDSURG Nursing, 6*(6), 359-363, 386.

LoBiondo-Wood, G., et al. (1997). Impact of liver transplantation on quality of life: A longitudinal perspective. *Applied Nursing Research, 10*(1), 27-32.

National Institutes of Health (Hepatitis Branch). (September 1999). *Program and abstracts.* NIH Consensus Development Conference on Management of Hepatitis C; http://odp.od.nih.gov/consensus/cons/105/105_abstract.pdf.

Neuman, A., et al. (1998). Hepatitis C viral dynamics in vivo and the antiviral efficacy of interferon-alpha therapy. *Science, 282,* 103-107.

Rollier, C., et al. (1999). Protective and therapeutic effect of DNA-based immunization against Hepadnavirsus large envelope protein. *Gastroentereology, 116*(3), 658-665.

Sarin, S., et al. (1999). Comparison of endoscopic ligation and propranolol for the primary prevention of variceal bleeding. *New England Journal of Medicine, 340,* 988-993.

Shovein, J.T., et al. (2000). Hepatitis A: How benign is it? *American Journal of Nursing, 100*(3), 43-47.

Starzl, T., et al. (1997). Liver transplantation. *Gastroenterology, 112*(1), 288-291.

Tanaka, K, et al. (2000). Serum testosterone: Estradiol ration and the development of hepatocellular carcinoma among male cirrhotic patients. *Cancer Research, 60*(18), 5106-5110.

United Network for Organ Sharing. (1998). *1998 Annual Report;* http://www.unos.org.

Wiley, T., et al. (1998). Impact of alcohol on the histological and clinical progression of hepatitis C infection. *Hepatology, 28*(3), 805-809.

Wong, J.B., et al. (2000). Estimating future hepatitis C morbidity, mortality, and costs in the United States. *American Journal of Public Health, 90*(10), 1562-1569.

Ziser, A., et al. (1999). Morbidity and mortality in cirrhotic patients undergoing anesthesia and surgery. *Anesthesiology, 90*(1),42-53.

CHAPTER 60

Interventions for Clients with Problems of the Gallbladder and Pancreas

E. JEAN HAYES

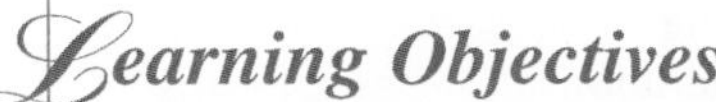

After studying this chapter, you should be able to:

1. Identify the common causes of cholecystitis and cholelithiasis (gallbladder disease).
2. Explain the role of testing in diagnosis of gallbladder disease.
3. Compare postoperative care of clients undergoing a traditional cholecystectomy with that of clients undergoing a laparoscopic cholecystectomy.
4. Develop a community-based teaching plan for clients with gallbladder disease, including care of a T-tube.
5. Compare and contrast the pathophysiology of acute and chronic pancreatitis.
6. Interpret common assessment findings associated with acute pancreatitis and those associated with chronic pancreatitis.
7. Prioritize nursing care for clients with acute pancreatitis and clients with chronic pancreatitis.
8. Explain the use and adverse effects of drug therapy for clients with chronic pancreatitis.
9. Develop a postoperative plan of care for clients undergoing a Whipple procedure.
10. Construct a discharge plan for care of clients with pancreatic cancer in the community.
11. Discuss the psychosocial needs of the client with pancreatic cancer and associated nursing interventions.

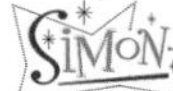

Go to http://www.wbsaunders.com/SIMON/Iggy/ for self-assessment questions related to these Learning Objectives.

Disorders of the gallbladder and pancreas begin as single-organ processes, but the inflammatory response may extend to other organs if the primary disorder is not treated. This occurs because of the anatomic proximity of the liver, gallbladder, and pancreas and because the flow of bile from the liver through the biliary (gallbladder) ductal system may be impeded. Inflammation of the gallbladder, liver, or pancreas is caused by obstruction in the biliary system from gallstones, edema, stricture, or tumors. For example, gallstones impacted in the cystic duct cause cholecystitis; gallstones lodged in the ampulla of Vater impede the flow of bile and pancreatic secretions, which can result in pancreatitis.

BILIARY DISORDERS

Cholecystitis

OVERVIEW

The two most common problems that occur within the biliary tree are stone formation (cholelithiasis) and associated chronic inflammation (cholecystitis). Cholecystitis may occur as an acute or chronic inflammation of the gallbladder wall (Table 60-1). Chronic inflammation may be complicated by an acute attack if an obstruction is present.

Pathophysiology

ACUTE CHOLECYSTITIS

Acute **cholecystitis** (inflammation of the gallbladder) usually develops in association with **cholelithiasis** (gallstones). Either condition may occur singly, but they frequently occur together. Cholelithiasis is discussed in detail later in this chapter (p. 1333).

Acalculous cholecystitis (inflammation occurring in the absence of gallstones) is believed to be due to bacterial invasion via the lymphatic or vascular route. *Escherichia coli* is the most common causative bacterium found, but group D *Streptococcus, Salmonella,* and *Staphylococcus* may also be found.

Acute cholecystitis usually follows obstruction of the cystic duct by a stone, which evokes the inflammatory response. This response may be the result of a mechanical, chemical, or

TABLE 60-1 • COMPARISON OF ACUTE AND CHRONIC CHOLECYSTITIS

Acute Cholecystitis	Chronic Cholecystitis
Inflammation present	Inflammation followed by fibrosis
Most commonly occurs as a result of cholelithiasis (gallstones) but can occur from bacterial invasion or biliary spasm	Most commonly occurs as a result of cholelithiasis
Bile obstruction *not* common	Bile obstruction common; may result in cholangitis and pancreatitis
Jaundice *not* common	Jaundice very common

bacterial process (Greenberger & Isselbacher, 1998). When the gallbladder is inflamed, trapped bile is reabsorbed and acts as a chemical irritant to the gallbladder wall; that is, the bile has a toxic effect. The presence of bile, in combination with impaired circulation, edema, and distention of the gallbladder, causes ischemia of the gallbladder wall. The result is tissue sloughing with necrosis and gangrene. Perforation (rupture) of the gallbladder wall may occur. If the perforation is small and localized, an abscess may form. Peritonitis may result if the perforation is large.

In some cases, painful episodes of cholecystitis may be the result of organ or bile duct spasticity. The spasticity temporarily prevents the release of an adequate amount of bile for fat digestion.

CHRONIC CHOLECYSTITIS

Chronic cholecystitis results, possibly from repeated bouts of acute or subacute cholecystitis, when gallbladder muscle wall disease and inefficient emptying of bile by the gallbladder persist. Gallstones are almost always present. In chronic cholecystitis, the gallbladder becomes fibrotic and contracted, which results in decreased motility and deficient absorption.

Pancreatitis and **cholangitis** (inflammation of the common bile duct) can occur as complications of cholecystitis. Pancreatitis and cholangitis result from the backup of bile throughout the biliary tract. Bile obstruction leads to jaundice.

Jaundice (yellow discoloration of the skin and mucous membranes) and **icterus** (yellow discoloration of the sclerae) can occur in clients with acute cholecystitis but is most commonly seen in clients with chronic gallbladder inflammation. Impeded or obstructed bile flow caused by edema of the ducts or gallstones contributes to *extrahepatic obstructive* jaundice. Jaundice in cholecystitis may also be caused by direct liver involvement. Inflammation of the liver's bile channels or bile ducts may cause *intrahepatic* obstructive jaundice, resulting in an increase in circulating levels of bilirubin, the principal pigment of bile.

When the concentration of bilirubin in the blood increases to greater than 2.5 mg/dL, jaundice occurs (Pagana & Pagana, 1998). In a person with obstructive jaundice, the normal flow of bile into the duodenum is blocked, allowing excessive bile salts to accumulate in the skin. This accumulation of bile salts leads to pruritus (itching) or a burning sensation. The bile flow blockage also prevents bilirubin from reaching the large intestine, where it is converted to urobilinogen. Because urobilinogen accounts for the normal brown color of feces, clay-colored stools result. Water-soluble bilirubin is normally excreted by the kidneys in the urine. When an excess of circulating bilirubin occurs, the urine becomes dark and foamy because of the kidneys' effort to clear the bilirubin.

Etiology

The exact etiology of cholecystitis is unknown. In addition to the formation of gallbladder calculi, causes of acute cholecystitis include the following:

- Trauma
- Inadequate blood supply
- Prolonged anesthesia and surgery
- Adhesions
- Edema
- Neoplasms (tumors)
- Long-term fasting
- Prolonged dehydration
- Gallbladder trauma
- Prolonged immobility
- Excessive opioid use

Any condition that affects the regular filling or emptying of the gallbladder or causes "gallbladder shock" (a decrease in blood flow to the gallbladder) can result in acute cholecystitis. Cholecystitis has also been attributed to anatomic problems such as twisting or kinking of the gallbladder neck or cystic duct resulting in pancreatic enzyme reflux into the gallbladder.

Incidence/Prevalence

More than 20 million persons in the United States have gallbladder disease, which causes more than 800,000 hospitalizations each year (see the Cost of Care Box on p. 1329). Gallstones are very common in the United States, with approximately 20% of the population being affected. Native Americans, particularly the Pima Indians of Arizona, have an unusually high incidence of gallstones, with Mexican Americans and Caucasians following (Everhart et al., 1999; Price & Wilson, 1997). A high incidence of biliary tract disease and cholecystitis occurs in people with a sedentary lifestyle, a familial tendency to biliary disease, obesity, or diabetes mellitus.

WOMEN'S HEALTH CONSIDERATIONS

The incidence of gallbladder disease is higher in women, especially Caucasian women. By age 60 years, nearly one third of obese women develop biliary disease (Allen & Phillips, 1997).

COLLABORATIVE MANAGEMENT

Assessment

PHYSICAL ASSESSMENT/CLINICAL MANIFESTATIONS

Clients with acute cholecystitis frequently present with pain, although clinical manifestations vary in intensity and frequency (Chart 60-1).

The nurse or assistive nursing personnel obtains the client's height and weight and determines his or her sex, age, race, and ethnic group. The nurse asks about food preferences and determines whether excessive fat and cholesterol are included in the diet. The client is asked whether any foods are

COST OF CARE IMPLICATIONS FOR NURSING

GALLBLADDER DISORDERS

Cost of Care

- Approximately 800,000 hospitalizations occur each year for gallstone disease at a cost exceeding $2 billion annually.
- The cost of medical care for the client with a biliary disorder varies according to the type of problem present and the medical/surgical management needed to resolve the problem.
- Obesity is a major contributing factor to the formation of gallstones, a major cause of cholecystitis.
- The health-related economic cost of obesity to U.S. business represents approximately 5% of the total medical costs.
- Surgical management of gallbladder disease, without complications, can cost from a low of approximately $4000 to a high of around $12,000. Complications will increase the cost expenditure.
- Laparoscopic cholecystectomy has reduced the length of stay and the cost of treatment of gallbladder disease.

Implications for Nursing

Because of the high cost of obesity, and the significance of obesity to gallbladder disorders, nurses need to become familiar with the management of obesity. The nurse will want to consult with a nutritionist or dietitian to develop a dietary plan for the client. The plan needs to allow the client to reduce weight in a slow, safe manner, since rapid weight loss is a causative factor in gallstone formation. Preventing the formation of gallstones will decrease the number of surgeries needed each year.

Nurses need to continue to be proficient in providing care for the client undergoing an outpatient laparoscopic procedure, including preoperative and postoperative teaching to prevent complications. The prevention of complications will reduce the cost factor by decreasing the number of days the client will need to stay in the hospital and lowering the number of interventions such as antibiotic therapy.

Data from Thompson, D., et al. (1998). Estimated economic costs of obesity to U.S. business, *American Journal of Health Promotion, 13*(2), 120-127; and Howard, D.E., & Fromm, H. (1999). Nonsurgical management of gallstone disease, *Gastroenterology Clinics of North America, 28*(1), 133-141.

not tolerated. The nurse asks whether any of the following gastrointestinal (GI) symptoms occur in relation to the intake of fatty food: flatulence, dyspepsia (indigestion), eructation (belching), anorexia, nausea, vomiting, and abdominal pain or discomfort.

The client is asked to describe the pain, including its intensity and duration, precipitating factors, and any measures that relieve it. The pain may be described as indigestion of varying intensity, ranging from a mild, persistent ache to a steady, constant pain in the right upper abdominal quadrant. The pain may radiate to the right shoulder or scapula. The abdominal pain of chronic cholecystitis may be vague and nonspecific. The usual pattern of more acute pain is episodic. Clients often refer to these episodes as "gallbladder attacks."

The nurse also asks the client to describe his or her daily activity or exercise routines to determine whether his or her lifestyle is sedentary. The client is questioned whether there is a family history of gallbladder disease, since there is a familial tendency for biliary tract diseases. If the client is female, the nurse also determines whether estrogen replacement therapy (ERT) is being taken, because this therapy may contribute to biliary disorders.

Because of gallbladder tenderness, it is difficult to use abdominal palpation and percussion in assessment of the client with acute cholecystitis. With right subcostal palpation, pain

CHART 60-1

KEY FEATURES *of* Cholecystitis

- Episodic or vague abdominal pain or discomfort that can radiate to the right shoulder
- Pain triggered by a high-fat or high-volume meal
- Anorexia
- Nausea or vomiting
- Dyspepsia
- Eructation
- Flatulence
- Feeling of abdominal fullness
- Rebound tenderness (Blumberg's sign)
- Fever
- Jaundice, clay-colored stools, dark urine, steatorrhea (most common with chronic cholecystitis)

increases with deep inspiration (Murphy's sign). Guarding and rigidity, as well as rebound tenderness (Blumberg's sign), are reliable indicators of peritoneal irritation.

Assessment for rebound tenderness and deep palpation are reserved for physicians and advanced-practice nurses. To elicit rebound tenderness, the nurse pushes his or her fingers deeply and steadily into the client's abdomen, then quickly releases the pressure. Pain that results from the rebound of the palpated tissue indicates peritoneal inflammation. Deep palpation below the liver border in the right upper quadrant may reveal a sausage-shaped mass, representing the distended, inflamed gallbladder. Percussion over the posterior rib cage intensifies localized abdominal pain.

In *chronic* cholecystitis, clients may have insidious symptoms and may not seek medical treatment until late symptoms such as jaundice, clay-colored stools, and dark urine result from an obstructive process. Steatorrhea (fatty stools) occurs because fat absorption is decreased owing to the lack of bile. Bile is needed for the absorption of fats and fat-soluble vitamins in the intestine. As with any inflammatory process, the client may have an elevated temperature of 99° to 102° F (37° to 39° C), tachycardia, and dehydration from fever and vomiting.

DIAGNOSTIC ASSESSMENT

There are no laboratory tests specific for gallbladder disease. A differential diagnosis must rule out other diseases that may cause similar symptoms, such as peptic ulcer disease, gastroesophageal reflux disorder, and pancreatitis. Serum levels of alkaline phosphatase, aspartate aminotransferase (AST), and lactate dehydrogenase (LDH) may be elevated, indicating abnormalities in liver function. The direct (conjugated) and indirect (unconjugated) serum bilirubin levels are elevated if an obstructive process is present. An increased white blood cell (WBC) count with a left shift on the differential count indicates inflammation. If there is pancreatic involvement, serum and urine amylase levels are elevated.

Ultrasonography of the right upper quadrant is the best diagnostic test for cholecystitis and has largely replaced the older cholecystogram. It is safe, accurate, and painless. Acute cholecystitis is evidenced by edema of the gallbladder wall and pericholecystic fluid, both of which are determined by the ultrasound (Nahrwold, 1997). The health care provider may also order an upper GI radiographic series to rule out other causes of abdominal pain, such as gastritis and peptic ulcer disease. A cholecystogram may be ordered if other diagnostic tests are inconclusive.

A hepatobiliary scan with cholecystokinin using technetium ^{99m}Tc disofenin or mebrofenen can be performed to visualize the gallbladder and determine patency of the biliary system. The pretest fasting period for this scan can be as short as 4 hours, making it preferable to a diagnostic study that would require a longer fasting time. Visualization of the gallbladder excludes the diagnosis of acute cholecystitis with a high degree of certainty (Fischbach, 2000).

Interventions

Nonsurgical treatment measures prescribed during the acute phase of cholecystitis are directed at resting the inflamed gallbladder in an effort to reduce the inflammatory process and relieve the pain. Because of the risk of sepsis and perforation, however, acute cholecystitis is generally managed surgically.

NONSURGICAL MANAGEMENT. Nonsurgical measures to relieve pain include diet and drug therapy. The physician, nurse, and dietitian often collaborate when implementing these interventions.

DIET THERAPY. For clients with acute cholecystitis, the health care provider may recommend withholding food and fluids or modifying the diet by avoiding high-fat or high-volume meals. These dietary measures decrease stimulation of the gallbladder and help prevent pain, nausea, and vomiting. For clients with severe nausea and vomiting, decompression of the stomach may be necessary. A nasogastric tube is inserted to empty the stomach contents. (The nurse's role in caring for a client with a nasogastric [NG] tube is described in Chapter 58.)

The nurse encourages the client with chronic cholecystitis to consume a low-fat diet to decrease stimulation of the gallbladder. Smaller, more frequent meals assist some clients in tolerating food better.

CRITICAL THINKING CHALLENGE

Your client with chronic cholecystitis tells you that she has been avoiding fried foods and eating a low-fat diet but is still having problems with pain and nausea after meals. You want to determine what she considers to be "low fat."

- Using a daily caloric intake of 1800 calories, determine how many grams of fat your client can consume to remain at a 20% total dietary fat intake.
- What questions might you ask her to evaluate whether she can determine the percentage of fat in a food item by reading the label?
- Who else might you involve in this client's care to assist with nutritional needs?

For suggested answer guidelines, go to SIMON http://www.wbsaunders.com/SIMON/Iggy/.

DRUG THERAPY. For clients in severe pain, the health care provider may order opioid analgesics, such as meperidine hydrochloride (Demerol), to relieve abdominal pain and spasm. Traditionally, morphine has not been given, because it can cause spasms of the sphincter of Oddi and increase pain. Meperidine, like all opioids, can increase smooth muscle tone in the biliary tract as well, causing biliary and pancreatic secretions to decrease and bile duct pressure to increase. This can also result in spasms of the sphincter of Oddi (Pasero, 1998). Antispasmodic agents, such as anticholinergics (e.g., dicyclomine hydrochloride [Bentyl, Lomine♣), may be used to relax the smooth muscles, preventing biliary contraction. Decreased muscle contraction minimizes secretions and assists in the reduction of pain. The health care provider usually prescribes antiemetics, such as trimethobenzamide hydrochloride (Tigan), to relieve nausea and vomiting.

SURGICAL MANAGEMENT. The usual surgical treatment of clients with acute and chronic cholecystitis is cholecystectomy, the removal of the gallbladder. Two operative procedures are available to the surgeon for performing a cholecystectomy: the traditional open approach and laparoscopic laser cholecystectomy.

TRADITIONAL CHOLECYSTECTOMY. Use of the traditional surgical approach has markedly declined during the past decade. The client undergoing this surgery is usually hospitalized for several days following the procedure.

Preoperative Care. The nurse provides the usual preoperative care in the operating suite on the day of surgery (see Chapter 17). The nurse reinforces teaching of aggressive measures to prevent respiratory complications. To minimize abdominal/incisional jarring during coughing, deep breathing, and turning, the nurse demonstrates splinting methods using a pillow or folded blanket. These clients, especially older adults and smokers, are also susceptible to postoperative atelectasis. The nurse instructs the client in the use of sustained maximal inspiration (SMI) devices, such as an incentive spirometer.

The importance of early mobilization in preventing complications is also emphasized. The nurse informs the client to expect to get out of bed the evening of surgery.

Operative Procedure. The surgeon not only removes the gallbladder through a right subcostal incision but also often explores the biliary ducts for the presence of stones. If the common bile duct is explored, the surgeon typically inserts a T-tube drain to ensure patency of the duct (Figure 60-1). Trauma to the common bile duct stimulates inflammation, which can impede bile flow and contribute to bile stasis. In addition, the surgeon usually inserts a drainage tube, such as a Jackson-Pratt (JP) drain. This drainage tube is positioned in the gallbladder bed to prevent fluid accumulation. The drainage is usually serosanguinous (serous fluid mixed with blood) and is bile stained in the first 24 hours postoperatively.

Postoperative Care. Postoperative incisional pain relief after a traditional cholecystectomy is usually achieved with meperidine hydrochloride (Demerol) using a patient-controlled analgesia (PCA) pump. The client participates in coughing and deep breathing exercises more readily when pain is minimized. Therefore the nurse plans for the coughing and deep breathing exercises to be performed when pain relief is optimal.

Antiemetics may be necessary for clients with episodes of postoperative nausea and vomiting. The nurse administers the antiemetic early, as ordered, to prevent retching associated with vomiting and thus decrease the incidence of pain related to muscle straining.

The nurse cares for the incision, the surgical drain, and the T-tube. The surgeon typically removes the surgical dressing and drain within 24 to 48 hours after surgery. The T-tube,

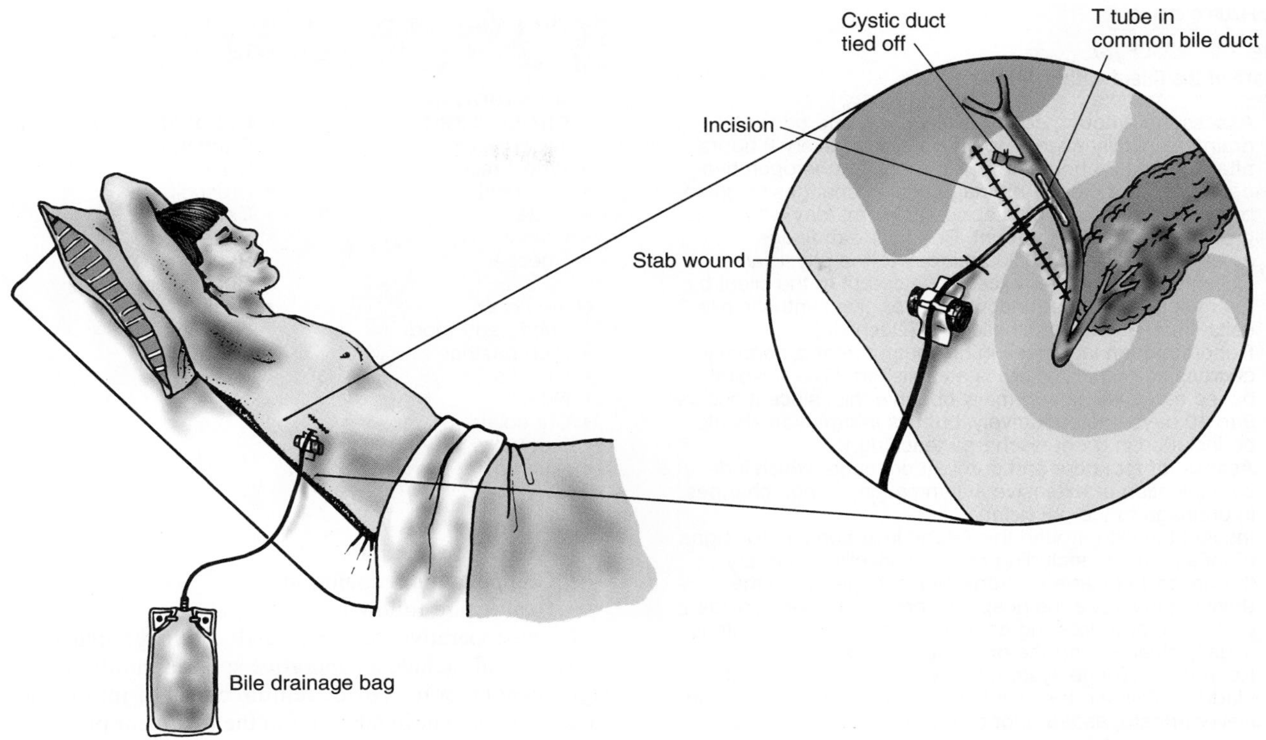

Figure 60-1 ● Placement of a T-tube.

however, may remain in place for 6 weeks or longer. Chart 60-2 highlights the important nursing care activities associated with the T-tube system.

The client usually receives nothing by mouth (NPO) for about 8 to 24 hours postoperatively. If gallbladder disease is severe, a nasogastric (NG) tube provides stomach decompression during this period. When peristalsis returns, the nurse removes the NG tube as ordered. The physician places the client on a clear liquid diet. The nurse gradually advances the diet from clear liquids to solid foods as tolerated. Within a day or two, the client resumes the ingestion of solid foods and is discharged to home.

The amount of fat allowed in the client's diet after a cholecystectomy depends on his or her tolerance of fat. In the early postoperative period, if bile flow is reduced, a low-fat diet may reduce discomfort and prevent nausea. For most clients, a special diet is not required. The nurse advises the client to eat nutritious meals and avoid excessive intake of fat. If the client is obese, the nurse recommends a weight reduction program. The nurse collaborates with the physician and the dietitian in planning the appropriate diet.

LAPAROSCOPIC CHOLECYSTECTOMY. Laparoscopic cholecystectomy, introduced in 1988, has quickly gained in popularity (see the Clinical Pathway on p. 1852). It is now considered the treatment of choice by many surgeons and is performed more often than the traditional open cholecystectomy. From studies involving 4000 clients undergoing a laparoscopic cholecystectomy, data show very positive results, including the following:

- Complications are very uncommon.
- Conversion to open cholecystectomy is about 5%.
- The death rate is very low (i.e., <0.1%).
- Bile duct injuries are rare.

These data indicate why the laparoscopic approach to gallbladder removal is now considered the "gold standard" (Greenberger & Isselbacher, 1998).

Preoperative Care. The laparoscopic procedure is commonly done on an ambulatory care basis in a same-day surgery suite. The surgeon explains the procedure; the nurse answers questions and reinforces the physician's instructions. There is no special preoperative preparation for the client. However, the physician typically orders the usual preoperative laboratory tests and requires the client to be on NPO status before the surgery. Chapter 17 describes general preoperative care for the client undergoing anesthesia.

Operative Procedure. The surgeon makes a 10-mm midline puncture at the umbilicus. The abdominal cavity is insufflated with 3 to 4 L of carbon dioxide. Gasless laparoscopic cholecystectomy using abdominal wall lifting devices is a more recent innovation. This technique results in improved pulmonary and cardiac function (Strasberg, 1999). A trocar catheter is inserted, through which a laparoscope is introduced. The laparoscope is attached to a video camera, and the abdominal organs are viewed on a monitor. The surgeon makes three small punctures through which to introduce laparoscopic forceps to manipulate the gallbladder. A laser is used to dissect the gallbladder away from the liver bed and to close off the cystic artery and the duct. The surgeon mobilizes the gallbladder, aspirates the bile and crushes any large stones, and then extracts the gallbladder through the umbilical port.

Postoperative Care. Removing the gallbladder with the laparoscopic technique reduces the risk of wound complications. Some clients have a problem with "free air pain" from

CHART 60-2

BEST PRACTICE *for* Care of the Client with a T-Tube

- Assess the amount, color, consistency, and odor of drainage initially every 2 to 4 hours, then every 8 hours after the first 24 hours. In the immediate postoperative period, expect bloody drainage, which changes to green-brown bile. Bile output is about 400+ mL/day with a gradual decrease in amount. Report bile drainage amounts in excess of 1000 mL/day to the physician.
- Collect and administer excess bile output to the client by the nasogastric tube (uncommon), or give synthetic bile salts, such as dehydrocholic acid (Decholin).
- Report sudden increases in bile output after a normally decreasing output pattern is established. (The hospital-based nurse will not normally observe this, since it occurs 9 to 10 days postoperatively, but this information should be included in client discharge teaching.)
- Assess for foul odor and purulent drainage, which indicate infection or extensive inflammation. Report changes in drainage to the physician.
- Inspect the skin around the T-tube insertion site for signs of inflammation, including redness, swelling, and erythema, and observe for frank bile leakage. Keep the dressing dry. (Use the hospital's procedure and provide drain care and dressing change per protocol. The site is usually cleaned and the dressing changed daily.)
- Keep the drainage system below the level of the gallbladder. Maintain the client in the semi-Fowler's position.
- *Never* irrigate, aspirate, or clamp a T-tube without a physician's order.
- Assess the drainage system for pulling, kinking, or tangling of tubing, especially when the client is positioned toward the right side. Assist the client with early turning and ambulation. Drape and secure the section of the T-tube emerging from the stab wound over a small roll of gauze taped to the client's skin to help prevent its lumen from occluding as a result of pressure.
- When ordered by the physician, raise the drainage bag to the level of the abdomen (usually on the fourth or fifth postoperative day). Then assess the client for feelings of fullness, nausea, or pain.
- When the client is allowed to eat, clamp the T-tube for 1 to 2 hours (per physician's orders) before and after meals. Assess the client's response to determine tolerance of food.
- Observe stools for return of brown color 7 to 10 days postoperatively.

carbon dioxide retention in the abdomen. The nurse teaches about the importance of early ambulation to promote absorption of the carbon dioxide. Far less opioid analgesia is necessary after the laparoscopic procedure than following the open cholecystectomy procedure.

The client is usually discharged from the hospital or surgery center within 1 day. Following laparoscopic surgery, the client can return to usual activities, including work, much sooner than if an open cholecystectomy had been done. Most clients are able to resume usual activities within 1 to 3 weeks.

Community-Based Care

HEALTH TEACHING

With a cholecystectomy, discharge teaching for the client and the family may include the following:

- Pain management
- Diet therapy
- Wound, drain, and incision care
- Activity restrictions
- Complication recognition
- Health care follow-up

TABLE 60-2 • FOODS FOR CLIENTS WITH CHOLECYSTITIS OR CHOLELITHIASIS TO AVOID

FOODS HIGH IN CHOLESTEROL	GAS-FORMING VEGETABLES
Dairy Products	• Cabbage
• Whole milk	• Onions
• Ice cream	• Broccoli
• Butter	• Cauliflower
• Cream	• Sauerkraut
• Cheese	• Radishes
	• Cucumbers
Other Foods	• Beans
• Fried, fatty foods	
• Rich pastries	
• Gravies	
• Nuts	
• Chocolate	
• Egg yolks	
• Avocado	

In postoperative teaching and discharge planning, the nurse should include a supportive spouse, family member, or significant other to provide reinforcement of information and to assist the client in adhering to the treatment plan.

Diet therapy for the client who has undergone a cholecystectomy is based on his or her tolerance of fats. The nurse or dietitian consults with the client to develop a nutrition program that includes nutritious, well-balanced meals that include the client's preferences, when possible. If the client has a poor tolerance of fats, a low-fat diet is developed and a list of foods to avoid is provided (Table 60-2). The dietitian may provide printed menu-planning guidelines. Some clients need to maintain a low-fat diet for 6 months or longer. They are advised to add fatty foods to the diet slowly and as tolerated.

If the client has problems tolerating three large meals a day, the nurse advises him or her to try smaller, more frequent meals. If the client is obese, a weight reduction diet is recommended and teaching is tailored to provide appropriate dietary guidelines.

Clients are leaving the hospital sooner after traditional open gallbladder surgery than in the past. Since a T-tube is usually left in place for several weeks, clients are sent home with the drainage systems intact. The nurse instructs the client and one or more family members to inspect the incision wound and the T-tube drainage site for signs and symptoms of inflammation. These signs and symptoms include redness, swelling, warmth, extreme tenderness, excessive drainage, and increased incisional pain. Any of these findings should be reported to the health care provider. The nurse provides oral and written instructions for drainage tube care (Chart 60-3).

The client with cholecystitis who either refuses or postpones surgery must be instructed on the signs of potential complications of chronic cholecystitis, including fever, recurrent abdominal pain, and jaundice. If these signs occur, the client should notify the health care provider for prompt medical care.

HOME CARE MANAGEMENT

After a traditional cholecystectomy, clients usually need short-term assistance with procuring foods, preparing meals,

CHART 60-3

CLIENT EDUCATION GUIDE
Home Care for the Client with a T-Tube

- Wear loose-fitting clothes.
- Wear older clothes to prevent ruining good-quality clothes.
- If staining occurs, soak the garment in a solution of detergent, baking soda, and bleach.
- Take showers instead of baths.
- Avoid heavy lifting and strenuous activity.
- Remove the dressing around the T-tube every day. Hold the tube in place and use an alcohol wipe to clean the skin around the tube. Apply a precut dressing around the catheter and tape it in place.
- Empty the drainage bag at the same time each day. Allow the bile to flow from the bag's spout; do not disconnect the system.
- The physician may advise you to clamp the T-tube for 1 to 2 hours before and after meals. Otherwise, you should keep the T-tube unclamped.
- Observe the amount, color, and odor of the drainage. Report any change in drainage, abdominal pain, nausea, or vomiting to your physician.
- Coil the drainage tubing and secure it to your abdomen by taping or using a belt with Velcro fasteners. Keep the drainage bag below the level of the T-tube.
- Inspect the wound for signs of infection, including redness, swelling, warmth, abdominal firmness, pain, and purulent drainage at the tube site. Take your temperature, and report a temperature of 100° F (37° C) or greater to your physician.
- Return to the hospital as scheduled for a cholangiogram.

performing dressing changes, and caring for the T-tube. Clients who have undergone traditional gallbladder surgery may also need transportation to follow-up appointments with the health care provider. The surgeon typically allows these clients to return to their usual activities 4 to 6 weeks after surgery.

HEALTH CARE RESOURCES

For clients at home with a T-tube or for those older adults who cannot manage self-care, a home care nurse may be needed to provide support and follow-up nursing care and teaching. The home care nurse assesses the client's adaptation to the treatment plan and evaluates wound healing and the integrity of the T-tube drainage system. The home care nurse also determines the need for further wound and skin care interventions and implements these interventions as needed.

Cholelithiasis

OVERVIEW

Cholelithiasis, the presence of one or more gallstones, is the most common disorder of the biliary tract. It is estimated that 16 to 20 million persons in the United States have gallstones, with approximately 1 million new cases developing each year (Greenberger & Isselbacher, 1998). Gallstones form when bile, stored in the gallbladder, hardens into stonelike material. In more than 90% of clients with cholecystitis, the cause of inflammation is bile stasis resulting from impaction of the cystic duct by gallstones. Chronic cholecystitis occurs when repeated episodes of cystic duct obstruction result in chronic inflammation.

Pathophysiology

PATHOLOGIC CHANGES

The exact pathophysiology of gallstone formation is not clearly understood, but abnormal metabolism of cholesterol and bile salts plays an important role in their formation. Contributing factors may include the following:

- Supersaturation of bile with cholesterol
- Excessive bile salt losses
- Decreased gallbladder-emptying rates
- Changes in bile concentration or bile stasis within the gallbladder

Gallstones may lie dormant within the gallbladder or may move to other areas of the biliary tree as the gallbladder empties and refills with bile. Stones may migrate and lodge within the gallbladder neck, cystic duct, or common bile duct, causing obstruction (Figure 60-2). Common bile duct stones are seen in 20% of clients age 65 years or older who undergo a cholecystectomy (Howard & Fromm, 1999). Gallstones interfere with or totally obstruct normal bile flow from the gallbladder to the duodenum, causing vascular congestion as a result of impeded venous return. Edema and congestion occur and contribute to the initial inflammatory process. When bile cannot flow from the gallbladder, the stasis of bile and local irritation from the gallstones lead to cholecystitis (see Acute Cholecystitis, p. 1327).

Cholangitis, usually associated with choledocholithiasis (common bile duct stones), involves infection of the bile ducts. *Ascending* cholangitis (inflammation of the biliary tree) occurs after bacterial invasion of the ducts. Bacterial invasion can lead to life-threatening *suppurative* cholangitis when symptoms are not recognized quickly and pus accumulates in the ductal system.

TYPES OF GALLSTONES

The gallbladder provides an excellent environment for the production of gallstones. In particular, the gallbladder only occasionally mixes its normally abundant mucus with its highly viscous, concentrated bile. The constant temperature within the gallbladder also contributes to stone formation by delaying bile emptying, causing biliary stasis.

Gallstones are composed of substances normally found in bile, such as cholesterol, bilirubin, bile salts, calcium, and various proteins. Stones are classified as either cholesterol stones or pigment stones.

Cholesterol stones form as a result of metabolic imbalances of cholesterol and bile salts. They are the most common type found in people in the United States, accounting for 90% of all gallstones, and generally originate from the gallbladder (Howard & Fromm, 1999).

Etiology

There appears to be a familial tendency in the development of cholelithiasis, but this may be related to familial dietary habits (excessive dietary cholesterol intake) and familial sedentary lifestyles. Gallstones are seen more frequently in obese clients, probably as a result of impaired fat metabolism or increased cholesterol. Cholesterol-lowering drugs, which lower cholesterol levels in the blood, actually increase the amount of cholesterol secreted in bile. Age is also a factor, with people over 60 years of age more likely to develop stones than

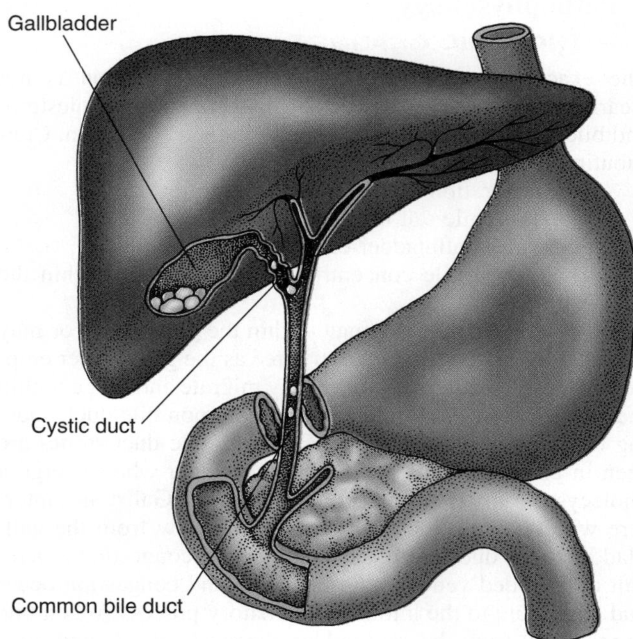

Figure 60-2 ● Gallstones within the gallbladder and obstructing the common bile and cystic ducts.

younger people. Persons with type 1 diabetes are also at increased risk for the development of gallstones and cholecystitis because of the higher levels of fatty acids (triglycerides) they generally have.

Cholesterol is increased following rapid weight loss, when the liver excretes extra cholesterol into bile (National Institutes of Health [NIH], 1999). The ingestion of low-calorie or liquid protein diets also increases the susceptibility to gallstone development. These diets cause the liberation of cholesterol from tissues; the cholesterol is excreted as crystals in bile. Alcohol abuse may contribute to the formation of pigment stones, but alcohol in moderate amounts appears to reduce the formation of cholesterol stones (Howard & Fromm, 1999). Cholelithiasis is seen with hemolytic blood disorders, with bowel disease such as Crohn's disease, and after jejunoileal bypass surgery as a treatment of morbid obesity.

WOMEN'S HEALTH CONSIDERATIONS

Women who are between 20 and 60 years of age are twice as likely to develop gallstones as men. Obesity is a major risk factor for gallstone formation, especially in women (NIH, 1999). Pregnancy tends to worsen gallstone formation. Pregnancy, as well as drugs such as estrogen and birth control pills, especially the older oral contraceptives, alter hormone levels and delay muscular contraction of the gallbladder, causing a decreased rate of bile emptying. The incidence of gallstones is higher in women who have had multiple pregnancies. Combinations of causative factors increase the incidence of stone formation, especially in women. For example, an obese pregnant woman or an obese woman taking birth control pills may be at higher risk.

Incidence/Prevalence

Cholelithiasis is common and a major source of morbidity in the United States, accounting for 800,000 hospitalizations each year for both men and women at a cost exceeding $2 billion annually (Howard & Fromm, 1999). Because gallstones are so prevalent, with up to 20 million persons having the disorder, several thousand deaths are attributed to them each year. This places gallstone disorder among the most common causes of death due to nonmalignant digestive disease (Everhart et al., 1999). The incidence of gallstone disease increases with age: 50% of women and 16% of men in their 70s and 80% of men and women in their 80s have the disorder (Howard & Fromm, 1999). Male clients who have cholelithiasis are usually 50 years of age or older. Two thirds of people with gallstones also experience chronic cholecystitis (Greenberger & Isselbacher, 1998).

CULTURAL CONSIDERATIONS

Gallstones are more prevalent among Native Americans and less prevalent among African Americans and Asians (Howard & Fromm, 1999). There is a lower prevalence of gallbladder disease among both non-Hispanic black men and women than among non-Hispanic whites. Age-standardized prevalence is similar for non-Hispanic white and Mexican-American men, with both having a higher prevalence than non-Hispanic black men. Among women, the age-adjusted prevalence is highest for Mexican Americans, followed by non-Hispanic whites and non-Hispanic blacks (Everhart et al., 1999).

COLLABORATIVE MANAGEMENT

Assessment

The same historical database may be obtained for clients with cholecystitis and clients with cholelithiasis (see Assessment [Cholecystitis], p. 1328).

PHYSICAL ASSESSMENT/CLINICAL MANIFESTATIONS

The severity of pain and presentation of symptoms in the client with cholelithiasis depend on the following:

- Whether the stone is stationary or mobile
- The size and location of the stone
- The degree of obstruction
- The presence and extent of inflammation

Initially, the pain of cholelithiasis is usually a steady, mild ache located in the mid-epigastric area. It may increase in intensity and duration and may radiate to the right shoulder or back.

The severe pain of **biliary colic** is produced by obstruction of the cystic duct of the gallbladder. When a stone is moving through or is lodged within the duct, tissue spasm occurs in an effort to mobilize the stone through the small duct. This intense pain may be so severe that it is accompanied by tachycardia, pallor, diaphoresis, and prostration (extreme exhaustion).

Any of the clinical manifestations seen in acute or chronic cholecystitis may occur in cholelithiasis (see Chart 60-1). Clients with chronic cholecystitis and acute ductal obstruction may experience the excruciating pain of biliary colic as well. On inspection, the nurse may observe jaundice of the skin, the sclerae, the upper palate, and the oral mucous membranes. If gallstones occlude the common bile duct, prolonged severe inflammation and hepatic damage may also occur.

LABORATORY ASSESSMENT

There are no specific laboratory tests for cholelithiasis. As in cholecystitis, the serum alkaline phosphatase, lactate dehydrogenase, aspartate aminotransferase, and direct and indirect bilirubin levels may be elevated. Examination of a random stool specimen may reveal absent or low levels of urobilinogen in the feces, indicating an obstructive process. If pancreatic involvement accompanies gallstone impaction, serum and urine amylase levels are elevated.

RADIOGRAPHIC ASSESSMENT

Calcified gallstones are easily visualized on abdominal x-ray examination. An oral cholecystogram is diagnostic when the stones are radiopaque. The physician may order intravenous (IV) cholecystography (or cholangiography) for clients who are unable to absorb oral contrast agents.

Percutaneous transhepatic cholangiography is a fluoroscopic examination of the biliary ducts and may be used to diagnose obstructive jaundice and visualize stones located in the ducts. Another procedure that permits radiographic visualization of the common bile duct, pancreas, pancreatic ducts, and biliary tree is endoscopic retrograde cholangiopancreatography (ERCP). This procedure permits the gastroenterologist to precisely pinpoint the nature of a biliary obstruction (see Chapter 53).

OTHER DIAGNOSTIC ASSESSMENT

Ultrasound of the gallbladder is most commonly used procedure to determine the presence of stones within the biliary system. It is the test of choice to confirm the diagnosis of cholelithiasis and to distinguish between obstructive and nonobstructive jaundice. Ultrasound of the gallbladder is reported to be 95% accurate in detecting gallstones. The exception is a stone found in the common bile duct, which rarely visualizes on ultrasound (McCormick, 1999).

CRITICAL THINKING CHALLENGE

Your client is scheduled to have an ERCP performed in the morning. She asks you how this test can determine what is causing her jaundice and expresses concern about the safety of the procedure.

- What answers will you give this client?
- How does jaundice develop in the biliary tree?
- What does an ERCP detect that other procedures might not?
- What are the risks and benefits of an ERCP?
- What postprocedure assessments and interventions will you need to provide for this client?

For suggested answer guidelines, go to SIMON http://www.wbsaunders.com/SIMON/Iggy/.

Interventions

The health care provider may institute supportive medical treatment for clients with cholelithiasis as an alternative to or before surgical removal of the gallbladder and gallstones.

NONSURGICAL MANAGEMENT. Two thirds of gallstones are asymptomatic, or silent (Howard & Fromm, 1999). Asymptomatic stones are usually managed conservatively with no medical or surgical intervention. Acute pain occurs when the gallstones partially or totally obstruct the cystic or common bile duct. Measures aimed at resting the inflamed gallbladder are the same as those discussed earlier for cholecystitis, p. 1330. Symptomatic clients require treatment, and laparoscopic cholecystectomy is the accepted first-line therapy (Strasberg, 1999).

DIET THERAPY. In general, the client must adhere to a low-fat diet to prevent further pain of biliary colic. If gallstones are causing an obstruction of bile flow, the health care provider may order replacement of fat-soluble vitamins (such as vitamins A, D, E, and K) and the administration of bile salts to facilitate digestion and vitamin absorption. Food and fluids are withheld if nausea and vomiting occur.

DRUG THERAPY. Pain caused by acute obstruction with gallstones necessitates opioid analgesia with meperidine hydrochloride (Demerol). Older clients should not be given Demerol, since it can cause acute confusion and nausea (see Chapter 7). Morphine is usually not used, because it is thought to cause biliary spasm and constrict the sphincter of Oddi. Antispasmodic or anticholinergic drugs, such as dicyclomine hydrochloride (Bentyl, Lomine🍁), may be given to relax smooth muscles and decrease ductal tone and spasm. The health care provider orders antiemetics to control nausea and vomiting.

Bile acid therapy has been effective in dissolving gallstones, depending on the type of stones. Chenodeoxycholic acid (CDCA; chenodiol; Chenix) and ursodeoxycholic acid (UDCA; ursodiol; Actigall) reduce cholesterol stones by unsaturating bile. They do this by decreasing coupling of cholesterol to bile acids during bile secretion. Adverse effects of chenodiol are lessened when it is used in conjunction with ursodiol. Ursodiol has also been shown to be effective in preventing gallstone formation after rapid weight loss (Howard & Fromm, 1997).

Chenodiol may be effective in dissolving small stones (less than 5 mm). This treatment is generally reserved for older adults who have mild or asymptomatic gallstone disease and those who are poor surgical risks. Unfortunately, it may take up to 2 years to dissolve gallstones, and compliance with taking medications over an extended length of time can be a problem. These drugs are expensive, and stones can recur if the client is not maintained on low drug dosages for even more prolonged periods. The nurse observes for and reports diarrhea, the common side effect of chenodiol therapy.

Ursodiol has been approved in the United States as an anticholelithic agent since 1988. This drug dissolves small (less than 20-mm) cholesterol gallstones. As is the case for chenodiol, ursodiol may take up to 1 year to dissolve the stone or stones. Moreover, in up to 50% of treated clients, the stones recur within 5 years. Therefore this treatment is best for clients who have mild or infrequent clinical manifestations, those who refuse surgery, or those who are poor surgical risks.

Obstructive jaundice in cholelithiasis is caused by impeded bile flow through the common bile duct as a result of gallstone obstruction. It may lead to excessive accumulation of bile salts in the skin. As a result, severe pruritus may occur. Cholestyramine resin (Questran) binds with bile acids in the intestine, forming an insoluble compound that is excreted in the feces. As a result, excessive bile salts are removed and itching is decreased. The nurse mixes the powder form of the drug with fruit juices or milk. It should be given before meals and at bedtime.

EXTRACORPOREAL SHOCK WAVE LITHOTRIPSY. Extracorporeal shock wave lithotripsy is a noninvasive procedure that is used for ambulatory treatment of clients with gallstones in some settings. A machine–a lithotriptor–generates powerful shock waves to shatter the gallstones (Figure 60-3). Clients who are eligible for this procedure must have three or fewer cholesterol stones (measuring between 5 and 30 mm), have a functioning gallbladder, and have no history of liver or pancreatic disease. Clients who have pacemakers or who are pregnant are not candidates for lithotripsy.

During the hour-long procedure, up to 1500 shocks are repeated until the gallstone is completely fragmented. The minute particles are then able to travel through the biliary ductal system to be excreted via the intestines. Because some clients experience mild pain as gallbladder spasms occur in an effort to expel the tiny stone fragments, the physician may use IV conscious sedation with fentanyl citrate (Alfenta, Sublimaze) or midazolam hydrochloride (Versed).

Eating and drinking are permitted almost immediately after the procedure. The nurse informs the client that right upper quadrant discomfort after the procedure is not uncommon and usually resolves within 2 days. Acetaminophen (Tylenol, Exdol✱) often provides enough analgesia to relieve this pain.

PERCUTANEOUS TRANSHEPATIC BILIARY CATHETER INSERTION. The physician may insert a percutaneous transhepatic biliary catheter under fluoroscopic guidance. This procedure decompresses obstructed extrahepatic ducts so that bile can flow (Figure 60-4). It is primarily used for inoperable hepatic, pancreatic, or bile duct carcinoma. It may be a nonsurgical alternative for the treatment of biliary obstruction caused by gallstones and hepatic dysfunction associated with obstructive jaundice and biliary sepsis in high-risk candidates. Nursing care associated with this treatment is outlined in Chart 60-4.

SURGICAL MANAGEMENT. One of several procedures may be indicated in the surgical treatment of cholelithiasis (Table 60-3). **Cholecystotomy** (an opening into the gallbladder) may be an emergency procedure to remove gallstones. This procedure is often performed for older adults or critically ill clients with life-threatening multisystem problems who may not withstand a prolonged surgical procedure. If the stones are located in the common bile duct, a **choledocholithotomy** (an incision into the common bile duct to remove stones) is necessary. If the common bile duct is explored, the surgeon inserts a T-tube drain into the duct to ensure patency until edema subsides and to allow collection of excessive bile drainage.

A simple, traditional **cholecystectomy** or laparoscopic cholecystectomy is performed when stones are confined to the gallbladder. The common bile duct and adjacent ducts are explored for the presence of additional stones or stone fragments and crystals in this traditional surgical procedure (see Surgical Management [Cholecystitis], p. 1330).

After a cholecystectomy with T-tube placement, the surgeon may prescribe drugs to stimulate bile production and bile flow from the liver. Bile flow promotes the digestion and absorption of fat, fat-soluble vitamins, and cholesterol in the duodenum. Hydrocholeretic drugs, such as dehydrocholic acid (Decholin, Cholan), which are synthetic bile salts, increase the solubility of cholesterol. Increased solubility prevents the accumulation of cholesterol in bile, thereby decreasing the recurrence of biliary calculi and promoting drainage of (potentially infected) bile through the T-tube drainage system.

A postoperative T-tube cholangiogram can identify retained stones. Direct visualization of the biliary tract with an endoscope **(choledochoscopy)** enables the removal of calculi retained in the common bile duct. Choledochoscopy is performed through a T-tube or an incision into the common bile duct. An instrument with a small, basket-like attachment is used to snare the stone (Figure 60-5). If this method fails, a fiberoptic endoscope is introduced into the duodenum. An incision into the papillae (papillotomy) allows the stone to pass into the duodenum.

The preoperative and postoperative nursing care measures for the client undergoing gallbladder surgical procedures are

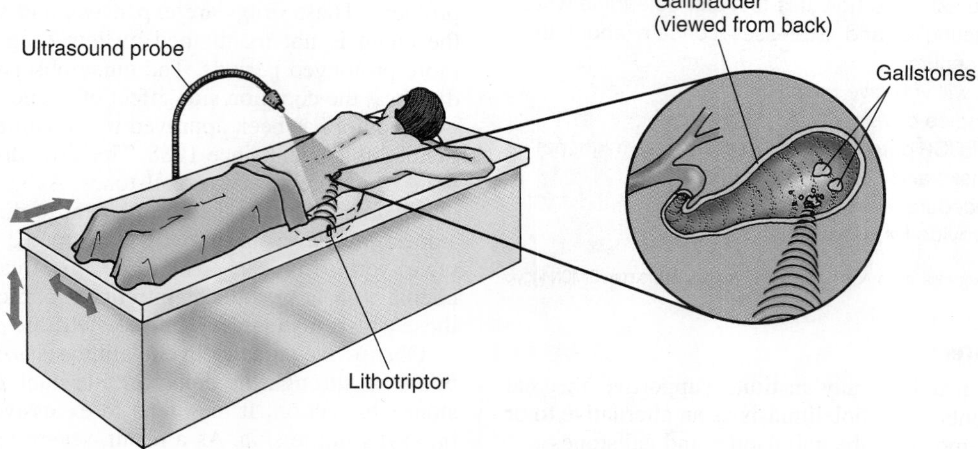

Figure 60-3 ● Biliary lithotripsy. With the assistance of a computer and an ultrasound monitor, the physician positions the client over a shock wave generator (lithotriptor) by means of a table that moves upward and downward, forward and backward, and from side to side. When the client is positioned properly, the physician fires the lithotriptor. Particles slough off the gallstones until they are completely fragmented, and the fragments pass through the biliary ductal system.

the same as those for cholecystectomy (see Surgical Management [Cholecystitis], p. 1330).

An additional therapeutic intervention, used in conjunction with or as an alternative to surgery, is endoscopic retrograde cholangiopancreatography (ERCP). This procedure allows the physician radiographic visualization of the common bile duct, gallbladder, pancreatic ducts, and biliary tree. Since about 10% of clients with gallstone disease also have common duct stones, this can be significant (Nahrwold, 1997). If gallstones are present in the bile ducts, the surgeon may use ERCP in removing them, either before or during gallbladder surgery.

Community-Based Care

Most often, the client with cholelithiasis has surgery and is discharged to home postoperatively (see Community-Based Care [Cholecystitis], p. 1332). The client may be discharged with a T-tube drainage system intact (see Chart 60-3) and will need instructions as to care of the tube.

The nurse provides information to the client and family about the potential for **postcholecystectomy syndrome,** in which the clinical manifestations of biliary tract disease occur following cholecystectomy in a small percentage of clients. Postcholecystectomy syndrome is caused by residual or recurring calculi, inflammation, or stricture of the common bile duct.

The nurse instructs the client to report symptoms of biliary tract disease, including jaundice of the skin or sclera, darkened urine, light-colored stools, pain, fever, or chills, to the physician or nurse practitioner.

Cancer of the Gallbladder

OVERVIEW

Primary cancer of the gallbladder is rare and is more common in women than in men (NIH, 1999). Adenocarcinoma and squamous cell carcinoma of the gallbladder account for the majority of gallbladder cancers. They typically infiltrate the liver and ducts, as well as the gallbladder. These rare gallbladder carcinomas appear more frequently in clients with pre-existing chronic cholecystitis and cholelithiasis.

The diagnosis of gallbladder cancer is difficult. Early symptoms, when present, are insidious in onset and similar to those of chronic cholecystitis and cholelithiasis. Characteristic signs and symptoms include the following:

- Anorexia
- Weight loss

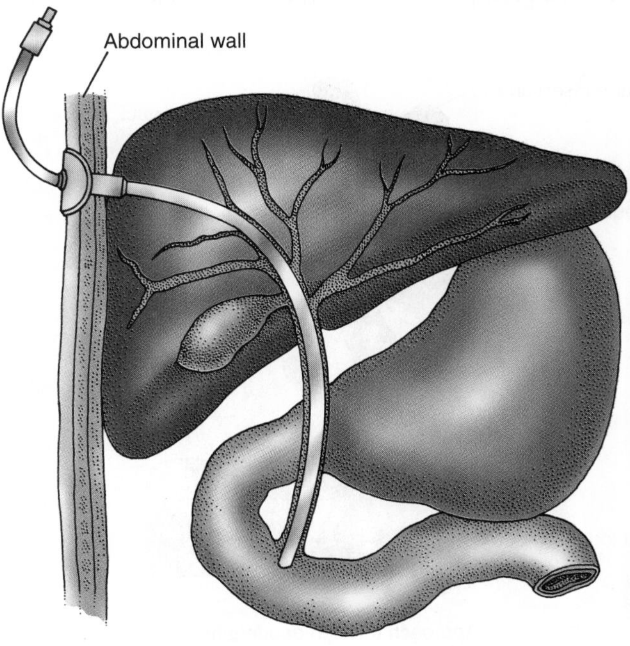

Figure 60-4 ● Transhepatic biliary catheterization.

CHART 60-4

BEST PRACTICE *for* The Client with a Transhepatic Biliary Catheter

- Change the catheter insertion site dressing daily, according to the hospital's policy. Recommended care includes cleaning the skin with hydrogen peroxide and applying antibiotic ointment and a small sterile dressing to the site.
- During the first several days after catheter insertion, unclamp the catheter and allow it to drain into an external drainage system (per physician's order).
- Using a three-way stopcock system located between the catheter and the drainage bag, irrigate the catheter twice daily with 5 to 20 mL of bacteriostatic (preservative-free) saline. Check the physician's orders for the amount of solution and the frequency of irrigation. Flush the tubing to the client and to the bag to ensure that the tubing is patent. (Occlude the stopcock with a sterile cap when the irrigation procedure is complete.)
- Instruct the client that he or she may experience discomfort during irrigation. Observe for abdominal cramping or excessive pain, and notify the physician if any occurs.
- If pain is severe and abdominal rigidity develops, notify the physician immediately.
- Assess the client for decreasing jaundice. Stools should change from clay color to normal brown, and urine should change from dark to straw color. Monitor serum bilirubin test results for decreasing levels.
- Assess the client for fever, chills, and hypotension, and report these findings to the physician.
- Inspect the catheter for the presence of blood, and notify the physician immediately if any occurs.
- Inspect the catheter for patency.
- The drainage bag should remain in a dependent position. Do not place the bag on the bed or above the level of the client.
- Affix the bag to the client's gown (not to the bed).
- Provide discharge instructions to the client or a family member, including:
  - Dressing care
  - Signs of catheter malfunction, infection, and dislodgment
  - Outpatient and cholangiography appointments

TABLE 60-3 ● COMMON GALLBLADDER SURGICAL PROCEDURES

Surgical Procedure	Description
Traditional cholecystectomy	Removal of the gallbladder through a high (subcostal) abdominal incision
Laparoscopic laser cholecystectomy	Removal of the gallbladder by laser through a laparoscope
Cholecystotomy	Incision into the gallbladder to remove gallstones
Choledochotomy	Incision into the common bile duct
Choledocholithotomy	Incision into the common bile duct to remove gallstones

- Nausea
- Vomiting
- General malaise
- Jaundice
- Hepatosplenomegaly
- Chronic, progressively severe epigastric or right upper quadrant pain

A moderately tender, irregularly shaped mass may be palpated. Often, gallbladder carcinoma is discovered during other procedures for diagnosis of suspected cholecystitis or during cholecystectomy.

COLLABORATIVE MANAGEMENT

The prognosis for the client with cancer of the gallbladder is poor. Three treatments are used: surgery, radiation therapy, and chemotherapy. Surgical intervention, when performed, is usually extensive. A bile drainage tube (transhepatic biliary catheter) may be inserted to relieve symptoms such as jaundice and itching (see Chart 60-4).

PANCREATIC DISORDERS

Acute Pancreatitis

OVERVIEW

Acute pancreatitis is a serious and, at times, life-threatening inflammatory process of the pancreas. This inflammatory process is brought on by a premature activation of pancreatic enzymes that destroy ductal tissue and pancreatic cells, resulting in autodigestion and fibrosis of the pancreas. The pathologic changes occur in variable degrees. The severity of pancreatitis depends on the extent of inflammation and tissue destruction. Pancreatitis can range from mild involvement evidenced by edema and inflammation to necrotizing hemorrhagic pancreatitis (NHP). NHP affects approximately 20% of clients diagnosed with pancreatitis and is characterized by diffusely bleeding pancreatic tissue with fibrosis and tissue death.

Pathophysiology

The pancreas is unusual in that it functions as both an exocrine gland and an endocrine gland. The primary endocrine disorder is diabetes and is discussed in Chapter 65. The exocrine function of the pancreas is responsible for secreting enzymes that assist in the breakdown of starches, proteins, and fats. These enzymes are normally secreted in the inactive form and become activated once they enter the intestine. Early activation (i.e., activation within the pancreas rather than the intestinal lumen) results in the inflammatory process of pancreatitis. Direct toxic injury to the pancreatic cells and the production and release of pancreatic enzymes (trypsin, elastase, phospholipase A, lipase, and kallikrein) result from the obstructive damage. Following pancreatic duct obstruction, increased pressure within the pancreas and the pancreatic ducts may contribute to ductal rupture, allowing spillage of trypsin and other enzymes into the pancreatic parenchymal tissue. In acute pancreatitis, four major pathophysiologic processes occur: lipolysis, proteolysis, necrosis of blood vessels, and inflammation.

LIPOLYSIS

The hallmark of pancreatic necrosis is enzymatic fat necrosis of the endocrine and exocrine cells of the pancreas caused by the enzyme lipase. Fatty acids are released during this lipolytic process and combine with ionized calcium to form a soaplike product. The initial rapid lowering of serum calcium levels is not readily compensated for by the parathyroid gland. Because the body needs ionized calcium and cannot use bound calcium, hypocalcemia occurs.

PROTEOLYSIS

The pathogenesis of pancreatitis involves **autodigestion** of the pancreatic parenchyma by the enzymes normally produced by the pancreas (Figure 60-6). Trypsin is the key element that activates all other proteolytic enzymes involved in autodigestion.

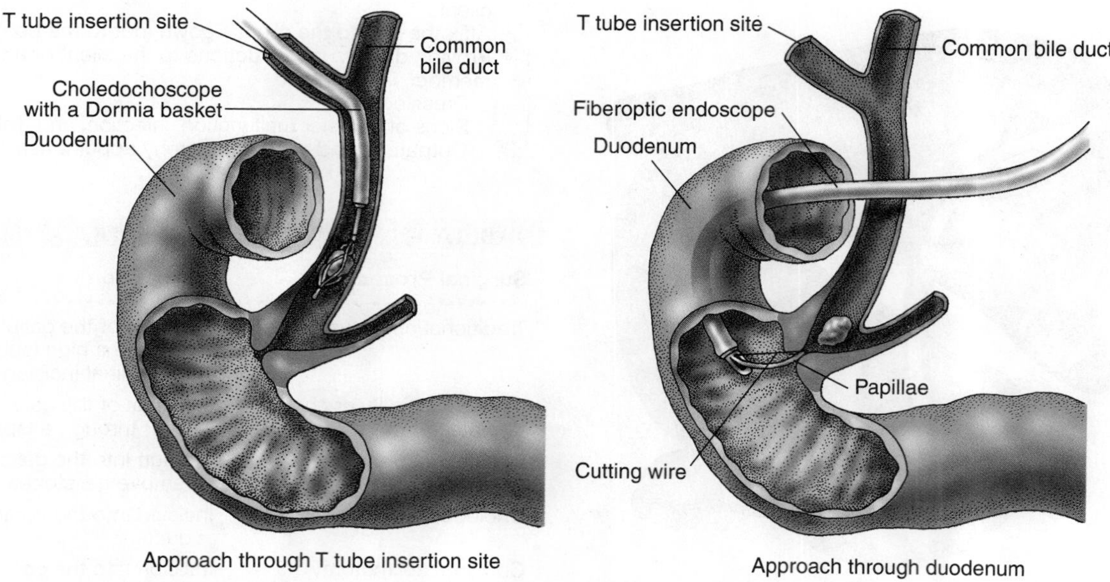

Figure 60-5 ● Choledochoscopic removal of gallstones.

The agent that triggers the premature activation of trypsin to trypsinogen has not been identified and is being investigated. Proteolysis involves the splitting of proteins by hydrolysis of the peptide bonds, resulting in the formation of smaller polypeptides. Proteolytic activity may lead to thrombosis and gangrene of the pancreas. Pancreatic destruction may be localized and confined to one area or may involve the entire organ.

NECROSIS OF BLOOD VESSELS

Elastase is activated by trypsin and causes elastic fibers of the blood vessels and ducts to dissolve. The necrosis of blood vessels results in bleeding, ranging from minor bleeding to massive hemorrhage of pancreatic tissue. Another pancreatic enzyme, kallikrein, causes the release of vasoactive peptides, bradykinin, and a plasma kinin known as kallidin. These substances contribute to vasodilation and increased vascular permeability, further compounding the hemorrhagic process. This massive destruction of blood vessels by necrosis may lead to generalized hemorrhage with blood escaping into the retroperitoneal tissues. The client with hemorrhagic pancreatitis is critically ill, and extensive pancreatic destruction and shock may lead to death. The majority of deaths in clients with acute pancreatitis result from irreversible shock.

INFLAMMATION

The inflammatory stage occurs when leukocytes cluster around the hemorrhagic and necrotic areas of the pancreas. A secondary bacterial process may lead to suppuration (pus formation) of the pancreatic parenchyma or the formation of an abscess (see later discussion under Pancreatic Abscess, p. 1348). Infected lesions that are mild may be absorbed. When infected lesions are severe, calcification and fibrosis occur. If the infected fluid becomes walled off by fibrous tissue, a pancreatic pseudocyst is formed (see Pancreatic Pseudocyst, p. 1349).

THEORIES OF ENZYME ACTIVATION

Several theories explain the triggering mechanisms leading to enzyme activation in acute pancreatitis. The *bile reflux* ("common channel") theory proposes that an obstruction of the common channel (the common bile duct and the main pancreatic duct channel) causes reflux of the bile into the pancreatic tissue, resulting in activation of the enzymes. Not all biliary tracts have this common channel. If the common channel is absent, the common bile and pancreatic ducts merge into the duodenum separately.

According to the *hypersecretion-obstruction* theory, the pancreatic duct ruptures and the resulting disruption or tearing of the cell membrane allows pancreatic secretions and enzymes to leak back into the parenchymal tissue.

The exact mechanism of *alcohol-induced* changes in pancreatitis is unclear. Alcohol appears to have a direct metabolic effect on the pancreas by stimulating hydrochloric acid and secretin production, which in turn stimulates exocrine functions of the pancreas. Alcohol also causes edema of the duodenum and the ampulla of Vater, obstructing the flow of pancreatic se-

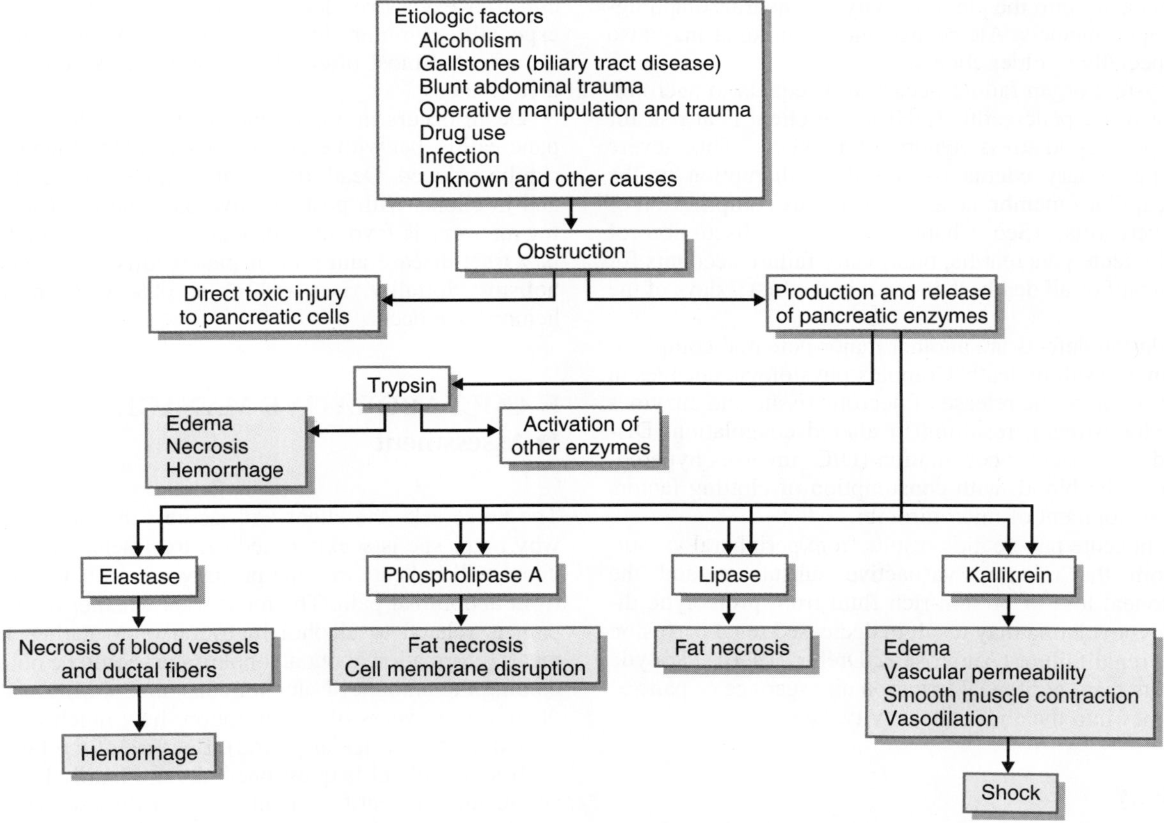

Figure 60-6 ● The process of autodigestion in acute pancreatitis.

cretions. Alcohol may decrease the tone of the sphincter of Oddi and cause sphincter spasm and duodenal reflux.

According to the fourth theory, reflux of duodenal contents can occur from biliary tract disease, gallstones in the bile duct (causing the sphincter of Oddi to dilate), or a generalized loss of tone caused by alcohol ingestion. Duodenal contents can enter the pancreatic duct through the weakened sphincter, activating the pancreatic enzymes.

The generalized abdominal pain of acute pancreatitis is related to peritoneal irritation. Ductal release of digested proteins and lipids into the peripancreatic tissues, along with stretching of the pancreatic tissue, causes the seepage of these substances into the mesentery. The resultant peritonitis stimulates the sensory nerves, contributing to intense pain in the back and flanks.

COMPLICATIONS OF ACUTE PANCREATITIS

Acute pancreatitis may result in severe, life-threatening complications. Jaundice occurs from swelling of the head of the pancreas, which impedes bile flow through the common bile duct. The bile duct may also be compressed by calculi or a pancreatic pseudocyst. The resulting total bile flow obstruction causes severe jaundice. Transient hyperglycemia occurs as a result of the release of glucagon, as well as the decreased release of insulin due to damage to the pancreatic islet cells. Total destruction of the pancreas may occur, leading to type 1 diabetes.

Left lung pleural effusions frequently develop in the client with acute pancreatitis. Amylase effusions probably occur when exudate containing pancreatic enzymes passes from the peritoneal cavity into the pleural cavity via the transdiaphragmatic lymph channels. Atelectasis and pneumonia may also occur, especially in older clients.

Multisystem organ failure occurs as a sequela to necrotizing hemorrhagic pancreatitis (NHP). The client is at risk for acute respiratory distress syndrome (ARDS). This severe form of pulmonary edema is caused by disruption of the alveolar-capillary membrane and is a serious complication of acute pancreatitis. (See Chapter 32 for a discussion of ARDS.) In acute pancreatitis, pulmonary failure accounts for more than half of all deaths that occur in the first 7 days of the disease.

Coagulation defects are another major potential complication and may result in death. Complex physiologic changes in the pancreas cause the release of necrotic tissue and enzymes into the bloodstream, resulting in altered coagulation. Disseminated intravascular coagulation (DIC) involves hypercoagulation of the blood, with consumption of clotting factors and the development of microthrombi.

Shock in acute pancreatitis results from peripheral vasodilation from the released vasoactive substances and the retroperitoneal loss of protein-rich fluid from proteolytic digestion. Hypovolemia may result in decreased renal perfusion and acute renal failure (Ambrose & Dreher, 1996). Paralytic ileus results from peritoneal irritation and seepage of pancreatic enzymes into the abdominal cavity.

Etiology

In many cases, the cause of pancreatitis is not known. Many factors can produce injury to the pancreas. The most commonly cited factor is biliary tract disease, with gallstones accounting for 45% of the cases of obstructive pancreatitis. Excessive alcohol ingestion is the second leading cause of pancreatitis. Iatrogenic acute pancreatitis may occur as a result of trauma from surgical manipulation after biliary tract, pancreatic, gastric, and duodenal procedures, such as cholecystectomy, the Whipple procedure, and partial gastrectomy. The trauma may also originate as a complication of the diagnostic procedure endoscopic retrograde cholangiopancreatography (ERCP).

Other etiologic factors include the following:

- Trauma: external (blunt trauma) or operative
- Pancreatic obstruction: tumors, cysts, or abscesses; abnormal organ structure
- Metabolic disturbances: hyperlipidemia, hyperparathyroidism, or hypercalcemia
- Renal disturbances: failure or transplantation
- Familial, inherited conditions
- Penetrating gastric or duodenal ulcers, resulting in peritonitis
- Viral infections, such as coxsackievirus B infection
- Toxicities of drugs, including opiates, sulfonamides, thiazides, steroids, and oral contraceptives (The exact mechanism by which these and other drugs cause pancreatitis is unknown.)

Incidence/Prevalence

Steady, heavy alcohol intake for 5 to 10 years is likely to be the causative mechanism for pancreatitis in the middle-aged male population. Episodes of acute pancreatitis usually occur after excessive alcohol consumption. These attacks are especially common during holidays and vacations. Women are affected most often after cholelithiasis and biliary tract disturbances.

Death occurs in approximately 10% of clients with acute pancreatitis, but with early diagnosis and treatment, mortality can be reduced. Death occurs at a higher rate in older adults and in clients with postoperative pancreatitis. The prognosis for recovery is favorable for pancreatitis associated with biliary tract disease and poor if pancreatitis accompanies alcoholism. Mortality rises as high as 60% when necrosis and hemorrhage occur.

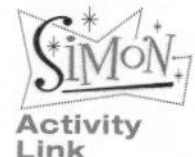

COLLABORATIVE MANAGEMENT

Assessment

HISTORY

The nurse asks the client with acute pancreatitis to indicate why he or she is seeking medical treatment. Most often, the client will indicate that the primary reason is to obtain relief from abdominal pain. The nurse asks whether the abdominal pain is related to alcohol ingestion or to eating a high-fat meal. Information about alcohol usage should be obtained, including the amount of alcohol consumed during what period of time (i.e., years of consumption, how much usually consumed over a particular period). Because of the familial connection, the client is questioned about a family history of alcoholism, pancreatitis, or biliary tract disease. The client is questioned concerning a personal history of any biliary tract problems, such as gallstones. The nurse further determines whether any abdominal surgical interventions, such as cholecystectomy, or diagnostic procedures, such as ERCP, have been performed recently.

The nurse assesses for the presence of other medical problems known to cause pancreatitis, including peptic ulcer disease, renal failure, vascular disorders, hyperparathyroidism, and hyperlipidemia. The client is also asked whether any recent viral infections have been experienced and to list all prescription and over-the-counter (OTC) drugs taken recently.

PHYSICAL ASSESSMENT/CLINICAL MANIFESTATIONS

Diagnosis of pancreatitis is made on the basis of the clinical presentation combined with the results of diagnostic studies—both laboratory and radiologic. Clinical manifestations of acute pancreatitis vary widely and depend on the severity of the inflammation. Typically, a client is diagnosed after presenting with abdominal pain that localizes in the epigastrium; this is the most frequent symptom. The nurse obtains in-depth data about the pain. The client often states that the pain had a sudden onset, is located in the mid-epigastric area or the left upper quadrant, and radiates to the back, left flank, or left shoulder. The pain is described as intense and continuous, and it is worsened by lying in the supine position. Often the client finds relief by assuming the fetal position (with the knees drawn up to the chest and the spine flexed) or when sitting upright and bending forward. The client may report weight loss resulting from nausea and vomiting.

When performing an abdominal assessment, the nurse may find the following on inspection:

- Generalized jaundice
- Gray-blue discoloration of the abdomen and periumbilical area **(Cullen's sign)**
- Gray-blue discoloration of the flanks **(Turner's sign),** caused by pancreatic enzyme leakage to cutaneous tissue from the peritoneal cavity

The nurse listens for bowel sounds; absent or decreased bowel sounds usually indicate paralytic (adynamic) ileus. On light palpation, the nurse notes abdominal tenderness, rigidity, and guarding as a result of peritonitis. A palpable mass may be found if a pancreatic pseudocyst is present. Pancreatic ascites creates a dull sound on percussion.

The nurse or assistive nursing personnel takes and records vital signs frequently to assess for elevated temperature, tachycardia, and decreased blood pressure. The nurse uses these data to determine whether complications are occurring. Respiratory complications, such as left lung pleural effusions, atelectasis, and pneumonia, are common in clients with acute pancreatitis. The nurse auscultates the lung fields for adventitious sounds or decreased aeration and observes respirations for dyspnea or orthopnea.

Changes in vital signs may indicate the life-threatening complication of shock. Hypotension and tachycardia may result from pancreatic hemorrhage, excessive fluid volume shifting, or the toxic effects of abdominal sepsis from enzyme damage. The nurse also observes the client for changes in behavior and sensorium that may be related to alcohol withdrawal, hypoxia, or impending sepsis with shock (see Chapter 8).

PSYCHOSOCIAL ASSESSMENT

Excessive alcohol intake, particularly in men, is the most frequent cause of acute pancreatitis. Thus the nurse tactfully explores the client's alcohol intake history. The nurse and the client should discuss the intake of alcohol and the reasons for overindulging. The nurse asks him or her when increased drinking episodes occur, in particular, whether binges occur during holidays, vacations, or weekends or revolve around particular activities, such as card playing or television viewing. The client is also questioned about any recent traumatic event that may have contributed to increased alcohol consumption, such as the death of a family member or a job loss.

LABORATORY ASSESSMENT

Diagnostic laboratory abnormalities are found in clients with acute pancreatitis (Table 60-4). Elevated serum amylase and lipase levels provide the most reliable and direct evidence of pancreatitis and are considered the cardinal diagnostic signs. Serum amylase levels usually increase within 12 to 24 hours and remain elevated for 3 to 4 days. A level of serum amylase three times greater than normal is considered diagnostic (Greenberger, Toskes, & Isselbacher, 1998). Persistent elevations of amylase levels may be an indicator of pancreatic abscess or pseudocyst (Lillemoe & Yeo, 1998). Lipase is considered more specific in the diagnosis of acute pancreatitis, and serum levels remain elevated for up to 2 weeks. Because serum lipase levels stay elevated for such a long time, the physician may find this test useful in diagnosing clients who are not examined until several days after the initial onset of symptoms (Hoerner, 1998). Amylase levels in 24-hour urine collections are also elevated as a result of the inflammatory process and remain elevated for up to 2 weeks. However, testing the urine for amylase is no more sensitive than testing serum amylase, yet it costs more. Testing the urine is sometimes useful several days after the onset of symptoms, when serum amylase levels may be normal.

If pancreatitis is accompanied by biliary dysfunction (biliary pancreatitis), serum bilirubin and alkaline phosphatase

TABLE 60-4 • CAUSES OF LABORATORY DIAGNOSTIC ABNORMALITIES IN ACUTE PANCREATITIS

Abnormal Finding	Cause
CARDINAL DIAGNOSTIC TESTS	
Increased *serum* amylase	Pancreatic cell injury
Elevated *serum* lipase	Pancreatic cell injury
Elevated *urine* amylase	Pancreatic cell injury
OTHER DIAGNOSTIC TESTS	
Elevated serum glucose	Pancreatic cell injury, resulting in impaired carbohydrate metabolism; decreased insulin release
Decreased serum calcium	Fatty acids combined with calcium; seen in fat necrosis
Elevated bilirubin	Hepatobiliary obstructive process
Elevated aspartate transaminase (AST)	Hepatobiliary involvement
Elevated white blood cell count	Inflammatory response

levels are usually elevated. A sensitive indicator of biliary obstruction in acute pancreatitis is serum alanine aminotransferase (ALT). A threefold or greater rise in concentration offers a 95% probability that the diagnosis of acute biliary pancreatitis is correct (Baillie, 1997). Elevated white blood cell (WBC) count and serum glucose levels are also common in acute pancreatitis (Ambrose & Dreher, 1996).

Decreased serum calcium and magnesium levels are seen with fat necrosis. Calcium levels may fall and remain decreased for 7 to 10 days. Calcium levels that consistently remain below 8 mg/dL are associated with a poor prognosis.

RADIOGRAPHIC ASSESSMENT

Computed tomography (CT) provides a reliable diagnosis of acute pancreatitis. This noninvasive technique may be used to rule out pancreatic pseudocyst or ductal calculi. A chest x-ray film may reveal elevation of the left side of the diaphragm or pleural effusion.

OTHER DIAGNOSTIC ASSESSMENT

In the client with severe pancreatitis, ultrasonography and magnetic resonance imaging (MRI) of the pancreas help confirm an initial clinical impression, assess for the degree of inflammatory resolution, and reveal common bile duct dilation from obstruction or gallstones. The MRI study provides information similar to that of a CT scan but is much more costly and offers no real advantage over the less expensive CT scan. Endoscopic retrograde cholangiopancreatography (ERCP) is the definitive test to locate and assist in removing gallstones, which can cause biliary pancreatitis.

Analysis

COMMON NURSING DIAGNOSES AND COLLABORATIVE PROBLEMS

The following are priority nursing diagnoses for clients with acute pancreatitis:

1. Acute Pain related to the effects of pancreatic inflammation and enzyme leakage
2. Imbalanced Nutrition: Less Than Body Requirements related to the effects of pancreatic dysfunction, nausea, vomiting, and anorexia

ADDITIONAL NURSING DIAGNOSES AND COLLABORATIVE PROBLEMS

In addition to the common nursing diagnoses, clients with acute pancreatitis may have one or more of the following:

- Deficient Fluid Volume related to pancreatic hemorrhage, fluid loss into the abdominal cavity, nausea and vomiting, and nasogastric suctioning
- Ineffective Breathing Pattern related to the complications of pleural effusion or acute respiratory distress syndrome (ARDS)
- Risk for Activity Intolerance related to debilitation
- Anxiety related to severe illness and a possibly chronic condition
- Disturbed Sleep Pattern related to pain
- Impaired Health Maintenance related to insufficient knowledge about the illness, its causative factors, and the treatment plan

The client with pancreatitis is also likely to have the following collaborative problems:

- Potential for Hyperglycemia
- Potential for Hemorrhage
- Potential for Fluid and Electrolyte Imbalances

Planning and Implementation

ACUTE PAIN

NOC **PLANNING: EXPECTED OUTCOMES.** The client with acute pancreatitis is expected to verbalize a decrease in or absence of abdominal pain, as evidenced by a pain scale measurement.

INTERVENTIONS. Abdominal pain is the prominent symptom of pancreatitis. The main focus of nursing care is aimed at reducing discomfort and pain by the use of interventions that decrease gastrointestinal (GI) tract activity, thus decreasing pancreatic stimulation. Pain assessment to measure the effectiveness of these interventions is a vital nursing activity (see Chapter 7).

NONSURGICAL MANAGEMENT. The health care team initially attempts to achieve pain relief with nonsurgical interventions, which include fasting, drug therapy, and comfort measures.

FASTING. In an effort to rest the pancreas and reduce pancreatic enzyme secretion, food and fluids are withheld in the acute period. The health care provider orders IV fluid administration to maintain hydration. IV replacement of calcium and magnesium may also be needed.

Nasogastric drainage and suction may be necessary to decrease gastric distention and to suppress pancreatic secretion. Gastric decompression prevents gastric digestive juices from flowing into the duodenum. Because paralytic (adynamic) ileus is a common complication of acute pancreatitis, prolonged nasogastric intubation may be necessary. The nurse assesses for the presence of bowel sounds before the nasogastric (NG) tube is removed.

NIC ***ANALGESIC ADMINISTRATION*** (Chart 60-5). Pain management for acute pancreatitis should begin with titration of opioids by means of patient-controlled analgesia (PCA). Meperidine hydrochloride (Demerol) is the traditional drug of choice for relieving abdominal pain associated with acute pancreatitis (Pasero, 1998). It has been thought that meperidine hydrochloride causes less incidence of spasm of the smooth musculature of the pancreatic ducts and the sphincter of Oddi than do other analgesics such as morphine. In mild pancreatitis, the pain usually subsides in 3 to 4 days; however, with severe acute pancreatitis, the abdominal pain and tenderness may persist for up to 2 weeks. The nurse individualizes dosages and intervals of medication administration, as ordered, according to the severity of the disease and the symptoms.

CRITICAL THINKING CHALLENGE

Your client with acute pancreatitis tells you that he is not getting much relief from the pain with the shots you are giving him every 4 hours.

- What should you include in this client's comprehensive pain assessment?

CHART 60-5

NIC INTERVENTION ACTIVITIES *for* The Client with Acute Pancreatitis

Analgesic Administration: *Use of pharmacologic agents to reduce or eliminate pain*

- Determine pain location, characteristics, quality, and severity before medicating client.
- Check medical order for drug, dose, and frequency of analgesic prescribed.
- Choose the appropriate analgesic or combination of analgesics when more than one is prescribed.
- Choose the IV route, rather than IM, for frequent pain medication injections, when possible.
- Attend to comfort needs and other activities that assist relaxation to facilitate response to analgesia.
- Administer analgesics around-the-clock to prevent peaks and troughs of analgesia, especially with severe pain.
- Administer adjuvant analgesics and/or medications when needed to potentiate analgesia.
- Consider use of continuous infusion, whether alone or in conjunction with bolus opioids, to maintain serum levels.
- Institute safety precautions for those receiving narcotic analgesics, as appropriate.
- Correct misconceptions/myths client or family members may hold regarding analgesics, particularly opioids (e.g., addiction and risks of overdose).
- Evaluate the effectiveness of analgesic at regular frequent intervals after each administration, but especially after the initial doses, also observing for any signs and symptoms of untoward effects (e.g., respiratory depression, nausea and vomiting, dry mouth, and constipation).
- Document response to analgesic and any untoward effects.
- Implement actions to decrease untoward effects of analgesics (e.g., constipation and gastric irritation).
- Collaborate with the health care provider if drug, dose, route of administration, or interval changes are indicated, making specific recommendations based on equianalgesic principles.

Pain Management: *Alleviation of pain or a reduction in pain to a level of comfort that is acceptable to the client*

- Perform a comprehensive assessment of pain to include location, characteristics, onset/duration, frequency, quality, intensity or severity of pain, and precipitating factors.
- Observe for nonverbal cues of discomfort, especially in those unable to communicate effectively.
- Ensure that client receives attentive analgesic care.
- Consider cultural influences on pain response.
- Determine the impact of the pain experience on quality of life (e.g., sleep, appetite, activity, cognition, mood, relationships, performance of job, and role responsibilities).
- Evaluate, with the client and the health care team, the effectiveness of past pain control measures that have been used.
- Control environmental factors that may influence the client's response to discomfort (e.g., room temperature, lighting, and noise).
- Reduce or eliminate factors that precipitate or increase the pain experience (e.g., fear, fatigue, monotony, and lack of knowledge).
- Consider the client's willingness to participate, ability to participate, preference, support of significant others for method, and contraindications when selecting a pain relief strategy.
- Select and implement a variety of measures (e.g., pharmacologic, nonpharmacologic, interpersonal) to facilitate pain relief, as appropriate).
- Provide the person optimal pain relief with prescribed analgesics.
- Implement the use of patient-controlled analgesia (PCA), if appropriate.
- Use pain control measures before pain becomes severe.
- Verify level of discomfort with client, note changes in the medical record, and inform other health professionals working with the client.
- Evaluate the effectiveness of the pain control measures used through ongoing assessment of the pain experience.
- Institute and modify pain control measures on the basis of the client's response.
- Promote adequate rest/sleep to facilitate pain relief.
- Notify the health care provider if measures are unsuccessful or if current complaint is a significant change from client's past experience of pain.
- Inform other health care professionals/family members of nonpharmacologic strategies being used by the client to encourage preventive approaches to pain management.
- Use a multidisciplinary approach to pain management, when appropriate.
- Consider referrals for client, family, and significant others to support groups and other resources, as appropriate.
- Provide accurate information to promote family's knowledge of and response to the pain experience.
- Incorporate the family in the pain relief modality, if possible.
- Monitor client satisfaction with pain management at specified intervals.

Patient-Controlled Analgesia (PCA) Assistance: *Facilitating client control of analgesic administration and regulation*

- Collaborate with health care providers, client, and family members in selecting the type of narcotic to be used.
- Ensure that the client is not allergic to the analgesic to be administered.
- Teach the client and family to monitor pain intensity, quality, and duration.
- Teach the client and family to monitor respiratory rate and blood pressure.
- Teach the client and family members how to use the PCA device.
- Teach the client and family members the action and side effects of pain-relieving agents.
- Document client's pain, amount and frequency of drug dosing, and response to pain treatment in a pain flow sheet.
- Recommend a bowel regimen to avoid constipation.
- Consult with clinical pain experts for a client who is having difficulty achieving pain control.

NIC intervention activities selected from McCloskey, J.C., & Bulechek, G.M. (2000). *Nursing interventions classification (NIC)* (3rd ed.). St. Louis: Mosby.

- What medication is he probably receiving, and why?
- What actions should you take in regard to his statement about lack of adequate pain relief?
- What options does the health care team have for pain management?

For suggested answer guidelines, go to SIMON http://www.wbsaunders.com/SIMON/Iggy/.

DRUG THERAPY. Decreasing the release of secretin reduces pancreatic stimulation. Secretin is an intestinal hormone that stimulates the release of enzymes and bicarbonate from the pancreas when acidic chyme is present in the duodenum. Antacids administered orally or via an NG tube that is clamped for 20 minutes after administration neutralize gastric secretions. The health care provider orders histamine receptor antagonists, such as ranitidine hydrochloride (Zantac), to decrease hydrochloric acid production so that pancreatic enzymes are not activated by an acidic pH. These interventions are also useful in reducing the occurrence of GI erosion and bleeding. Anticholinergics, such as dicyclomine hydrochloride (Bentyl, Lomine✤), are indicated to decrease vagal stimulation, decrease GI motility, and inhibit pancreatic enzyme and bicarbonate volume and concentration. However, these drugs can cause unwanted side effects for older adults, such as dry mouth, urinary retention, constipation, and acute confusion.

An additional drug that the care provider might prescribe is somatostatin or its synthetic analog, octreotide. This is used in an attempt to decrease pancreatic activity, but the research is still inconclusive about the value of the therapy (Uhl et al., 1999).

COMFORT MEASURES. Helping the client to assume the fetal position (with the legs drawn up to the chest) may decrease the abdominal pain of pancreatitis.

If the client has an NG tube in place, the nurse provides frequent oral hygiene measures to keep mucous membranes moist and free of inflammation or crusting. Because of the drying effect of anticholinergic drugs and the absence of oral fluids, the mouth and oral cavity may be extremely dry, resulting in considerable discomfort.

Lowering the client's anxiety level may also substantially reduce pain. The nurse provides thorough explanations of procedures. The client is encouraged to express the emotions and responses he or she is experiencing. The nurse also provides reassurance and diversional activities, such as television, music, and reading material, and encourages visitors to direct attention away from the pain.

SURGICAL MANAGEMENT. Surgical intervention for acute pancreatitis is usually not indicated. However, complications of pancreatitis, such as pancreatic pseudocyst and abscess, may necessitate surgical drainage. If pancreatitis is caused by biliary tract obstruction, the physician may perform a laparotomy (abdominal exploration) for common bile duct exploration and the release of obstruction.

PREOPERATIVE CARE. In addition to general preoperative care measures, the client usually has an NG tube inserted and begins receiving IV fluids. The client is frequently in pain, a factor that inhibits the learning process, so the nurse provides preoperative teaching in a manner that takes the client's comfort level into account. Postoperative reminders may be needed to reinforce the preoperative learning. The nurse teaches the client to expect a pancreatic drainage tube and explains its care during the postoperative period. The nurse needs to be certain that the client knows how to promote respiratory function by turning, coughing, deep breathing, and splinting the incision, because the client with an NG tube is at increased risk for postoperative pulmonary complications.

OPERATIVE PROCEDURE. When an abscess or pseudocyst is incised and drained with the client under general anesthesia, drainage tubes are inserted, sutured in place, and connected to low suction (80 mm Hg or less) to prevent further tissue erosion.

POSTOPERATIVE CARE. Postoperatively, the nurse monitors drainage tubes for patency by assessing for kinks in the tubes and maintaining the ordered drain suction pressure and system integrity. The nurse records the output amount from the drain and describes the character of the drainage. A sump type of drain is usually inserted. The nurse ascertains that the drain is functioning, as indicated by a hissing noise from the sump lumen.

The nurse provides meticulous skin care and dressing changes. The client is monitored for the first signs of redness or skin irritation because pancreatic enzyme drainage is particularly excoriating to the skin. Skin barriers, such as a Stomahesive wafer around the drainage tube, are applied to repel drainage from the skin. The nurse continually assesses for further deterioration of the tissue. The nurse should also collaborate with an enterostomal therapist (ET) for measures to promote skin integrity, such as the use of individualized ostomy appliances and the application of topical ointments.

IMBALANCED NUTRITION: LESS THAN BODY REQUIREMENTS

NOC **PLANNING: EXPECTED OUTCOMES.** The client with acute pancreatitis is expected to have sufficient nutritional intake to maintain body weight and a decrease in pancreatic stimulation.

INTERVENTIONS. The client is maintained on NPO status in the early stages of pancreatitis. Clients who have severe pancreatitis and are unable to eat for 7 to 10 days should receive nutritional support in the form of total parenteral nutrition (TPN) (see Chapter 61) or total enteral nutrition (TEN) (see the Evidence-Based Practice for Nursing box on p. 1345). If TPN is used for nutritional support, the nurse assesses for glucose intolerance by monitoring for elevated blood glucose levels. This is extremely important in clients with pancreatitis because pancreatic dysfunction affects the release of insulin. Some clients require insulin administration during an acute episode of the disease. TEN has been shown to produce fewer episodes of glucose elevation and other complications associated with the use of TPN yet has been shown to be as effective in maintaining nutritional status (Scolapio et al., 1999).

When food is tolerated during the recovery phase, the health care provider generally orders small, frequent, moderate- to high-carbohydrate, high-protein, low-fat meals. Foods should be bland with little spice; caffeine-containing foods (tea, coffee, cola, and chocolate), as well as alcohol, should be avoided.

To boost caloric intake, commercial liquid nutritional preparations, such as Ensure and Isocal, supplement the diet. If caloric intake is less than desired, an NG tube may be required for additional nutrition via enteral feedings. The health care provider may also prescribe fat-soluble and other vitamin and mineral replacement supplements.

Community-Based Care

HEALTH TEACHING

Education needs to be started early in the hospitalization period—as soon as the acute episodes of pain have subsided. The nurse assesses the client's and family members' or significant others' knowledge of the disease.

The goals of discharge planning and education are to avoid further episodes of pancreatitis and prevent progression to a chronic disease. The nurse instructs the client to abstain from

EVIDENCE-BASED PRACTICE FOR NURSING

What is the best method for ensuring optimal nutrition in clients with acute pancreatitis? Is early total enteral nutrition (TEN) or total parenteral nutrition (TPN) going to provide the client with mild acute pancreatitis the best nutrition?

McClave, S., et al. (1997). Comparison of the safety of early enteral vs parenteral nutrition in mild acute pancreatitis. *Journal of Parenteral and Enteral Nutrition, 21*(1), 14-20.

Acute pancreatitis creates a catabolic stress state that promotes, among other things, nutritional deterioration. Total parenteral nutrition (TPN) has been the standard of practice for providing exogenous nutrients while avoiding pancreatic stimulation. Based on evaluation of other studies conducted, the authors determined that more information was needed to determine if the widespread use of TPN was warranted. Clients admitted to the hospital with acute pancreatitis were prospectively randomized to receive either total enteral nutrition (TEN) (nasojejunal route) or TPN. There were no differences on admission in mean age, Ranson criteria, multiple organ failure score (MOF), or APACHE III score between the TEN and TPN groups. Both groups were studied, and the authors found that TEN was as safe and effective as TPN and had some advantages over TPN: less costly, more rapid resolution of the toxicity, and less stress-induced hyperglycemia.

Critique. Because of the small sample size of 32 (16 per group), the cost of nutrition was the only study end point to reach statistical significance. The study was performed in clients with mild acute pancreatitis, predominantly alcoholic related, so results may not be directly applied to persons with severe acute pancreatitis.

Implications for Nursing. The nurse caring for a client with acute pancreatitis needs to recognize the impact the illness has on the nutritional well-being of the individual. The traditional method of treatment includes avoiding pancreatic stimulation by having the client remain on NPO status (receiving nothing by mouth) and using alternative nutritional support. The nurse needs to familiarize himself or herself with the unique needs of the client with jejunal feeding. Traditional complications associated with TPN may also be decreased, such as fewer episodes of hyperglycemia and fewer nosocomial infections.

alcohol to prevent further pain attacks and extension of inflammation and pancreatic insufficiency. The client is told that if alcohol is consumed, pain will be experienced, and further autodigestion of the pancreas will lead to chronic pancreatitis and chronic pain.

The nurse also teaches the client to notify the health care provider after discharge to home if acute abdominal pain or biliary tract disease (as evidenced by jaundice, clay-colored stools, or darkened urine) occurs. These signs and symptoms are possible indicators of complications or disease progression.

HOME CARE MANAGEMENT

Home care preparation will need to be individualized for each client's circumstances. Some clients with acute pancreatitis may be severely weakened from their acute illness and need to confine activity to one floor, limiting stair climbing and other strenuous activities until they regain their strength.

HEALTH CARE RESOURCES

Clients with acute pancreatitis require visits by a home care nurse if the hospital course was complicated. In these cases, home care may be needed for wound care and assistance with activities of daily living (ADLs). The client requires medical follow-up with the primary care physician or nurse practitioner for monitoring of the disease process. For clients with alcoholism, the nurse provides information about groups such as Alcoholics Anonymous (AA). Family members may attend support groups such as Al-Anon and Al-Ateen.

Evaluation: Outcomes

NOC The nurse evaluates the care of the client with acute pancreatitis on the basis of the identified nursing diagnoses and collaborative problems. The expected outcomes include that the client will:

- Experience an alleviation of or reduction in abdominal pain, as indicated by self-report
- Maintain adequate nutritional intake with a decrease in pancreatic stimulation as evidenced by weight maintenance
- Not experience a recurrence of pancreatitis

Chronic Pancreatitis

OVERVIEW

Chronic pancreatitis is a progressive, destructive disease of the pancreas, characterized by remissions and exacerbations (recurrence). Inflammation and fibrosis of the tissue contribute to pancreatic insufficiency and diminished function of the organ. Chronic pancreatitis usually develops after repeated episodes of alcohol-induced acute pancreatitis. It may also be associated with chronic obstruction of the common bile duct. Chronic pancreatitis may develop in the absence of a known acute disorder. Relief of pain, prevention of recurrence of attacks, prevention of complications, and nutritional support are the principal interventions.

Pathophysiology

TYPES OF CHRONIC PANCREATITIS

Alcohol-induced chronic pancreatitis is also known as *chronic calcifying pancreatitis (CCP).* Protein precipitates that plug the ducts and lead to ductal obstruction, atrophy, and dilation characterize CCP. As the protein plugging becomes diffuse, the epithelium of the ducts undergoes histologic changes, resulting in metaplasia (cell replacement) and ulceration. This inflammatory process causes fibrosis of the pancreatic tissue. Intraductal calcification and marked pancreatic parenchymal destruction develop in the late stages. Cystic sacs containing pancreatic secretions and enzymes form on the pancreas. The organ becomes hard and firm as a result of acinar cell atrophy and pancreatic insufficiency.

Chronic obstructive pancreatitis develops from inflammation, spasm, and obstruction of the sphincter of Oddi. Inflammatory and sclerotic lesions occur in the head of the pancreas and around the ducts, causing an obstruction and backflow of pancreatic secretions (see Complications of Acute Pancreatitis, p. 1340).

PATHOLOGIC CHANGES

Pancreatic insufficiency in chronic pancreatitis is characterized by the loss of exocrine function. Pancreatic exocrine secretion is divided into two components: aqueous bicarbonate and enzymes.

The aqueous component neutralizes the duodenal contents and pancreatic enzymes that are essential to normal digestion and absorption. Most clients with chronic pancreatitis have a decreased output of pancreatic secretion and bicarbonate. Pancreatic enzyme secretion must be reduced by more than 80% to produce steatorrhea resulting from severe malabsorption of fats. These characteristic stools are pale, bulky, and frothy and have an offensive odor. The action of colonic bacteria on unabsorbed lipids and proteins is responsible for the foul odor. On inspection of the stools, the fat content is visible. In severe chronic pancreatitis, stool fat output may exceed 40 g/day.

Fat malabsorption also contributes to weight loss and muscle wasting (a decrease in muscle mass) and leads to general debilitation of the client. Protein malabsorption results in a "starvation" edema of the feet, legs, and hands caused by decreased levels of circulating albumin.

The loss of pancreatic endocrine function is responsible for the development of frank diabetes mellitus in clients with chronic pancreatic insufficiency. (See Chapter 65 for a complete discussion of diabetes mellitus.)

The client with chronic pancreatitis may have pulmonary complications, such as pleuritic pain, pleural effusions, and pulmonary infiltrates. Pancreatic ascites may impede diaphragmatic excursion and decrease lung expansion, resulting in impaired ventilation. In the ill client with chronic pancreatitis, acute respiratory distress syndrome (ARDS) may develop.

Etiology

The cause of chronic calcifying pancreatitis is persistent excessive alcohol intake that results in repeated episodes of acute pancreatitis. The most common cause of chronic obstructive pancreatitis is cholelithiasis and biliary tract disease, which results in persistent inflammation. Other etiologic factors include pancreatic pseudocyst, postoperative ductal scarring, and cancer of the pancreas or duodenum. All of these factors can produce obstruction of the pancreatic duct. Prolonged starvation and prolonged use of parenteral feedings for nutritional support can result in pancreatic atrophy, causing pancreatic insufficiency.

Incidence/Prevalence

Approximately 75% of clients with chronic pancreatitis are alcoholics (Price & Wilson, 1997). Alcohol-induced pancreatitis is predominantly found in men, but the incidence in women is increasing. In women, chronic pancreatitis occurs more commonly among those with biliary tract disease (cholecystitis and cholelithiasis). The age at occurrence of chronic pancreatitis is variable but is usually between 45 and 60 years.

COLLABORATIVE MANAGEMENT

Assessment

Clinical manifestations of chronic pancreatitis differ from those of an acute inflammation, although, as with acute pancreatitis, abdominal pain is the major clinical manifestation (Chart 60-6). The client with chronic pancreatitis typically describes the pain as a continuous burning or gnawing dullness with periods of acute exacerbation. The pain is intense and relentless. The frequency of acute exacerbations may increase as the pancreatic fibrosis develops.

CHART 60-6

KEY FEATURES *of* Chronic Pancreatitis

- Intense abdominal pain (major clinical manifestation) that is continuous and burning or gnawing
- Abdominal tenderness
- Ascites
- Possible left upper quadrant mass (if pseudocyst or abscess is present)
- Respiratory compromise manifested by adventitious or diminished breath sounds, dyspnea, or orthopnea
- Steatorrhea; clay-colored stools
- Weight loss
- Jaundice
- Dark urine
- Polyuria, polydipsia, polyphagia (diabetes mellitus)

The nurse performs the same abdominal assessment as for clients with acute pancreatitis, but the findings may not be as significant. Abdominal tenderness is less intense. A mass may be palpated in the left upper quadrant, which is indicative of a pancreatic pseudocyst or abscess (see Pancreatic Pseudocyst, p. 1349). Massive pancreatic ascites may be present, producing dullness on abdominal percussion. Because respiratory complications can accompany the condition, the nurse auscultates the lung fields for adventitious sounds or decreased aeration and observes for dyspnea or orthopnea.

The client is asked to collect a random stool specimen, if able, or is asked to describe the stools. The nurse or assistive nursing personnel collects the stool specimen for diagnostic studies. The specimen may show the presence of steatorrhea (foul-smelling fatty stools that may increase in volume as pancreatic insufficiency progresses and lipase production decreases). The nurse observes the client's anal area for excoriation resulting from frequent defecation.

The client may also experience weight loss, muscle wasting, jaundice, dark urine, and the signs and symptoms of diabetes mellitus, such as polyuria, polydipsia, and polyphagia.

In chronic pancreatitis, significant laboratory findings include normal or moderately elevated serum amylase and lipase levels. Obstruction of the intrahepatic bile duct can cause elevated serum bilirubin and alkaline phosphatase levels. Transient elevations in serum glucose levels are common and can be detected by blood glucose monitoring, both fasting and nonfasting.

The only definitive diagnostic test for chronic pancreatitis is the identification of calcification of pancreatic tissue in a biopsy specimen. If direct evidence of chronic pancreatitis is needed, the health care provider may order a secretin test. This test is the most sensitive and specific for chronic pancreatitis, other than histology (Amann, DiMagno, & Rubin, 1997). Secretin is an intestinal hormone that stimulates hepatic and pancreatic secretion. In this test, the client swallows a double-lumen gastrointestinal (GI) tube. The tip should reach the duodenum, with the proximal lumen port located in the stomach. Gastric and duodenal contents are aspirated before and after IV administration of secretin. An abnormal volume of enzymes and bicarbonate in the GI contents may indicate chronic pancreatitis.

Abdominal ultrasonography is also a helpful diagnostic tool, especially to reveal pseudocysts. Endoscopic retrograde cholangiopancreatography (ERCP) may reveal ductal system abnormalities, such as calcification and strictures, or it may delineate the presence of pancreatic pseudocyst.

Interventions

The focus of caring for the client with chronic pancreatitis is to manage pain, assist in maintaining a sufficient nutritional intake, and prevent recurrence.

NONSURGICAL MANAGEMENT. Nonsurgical interventions primarily include drug and diet therapy.

DRUG THERAPY. The major intervention for the pain of chronic pancreatitis is drug therapy. In addition, the nurse teaches the client to avoid ingesting irritating substances that can precipitate pain.

NIC ***Analgesic Administration*** (see Chart 60-5). The nurse medicates the client, as ordered, according to the assessment of the level and intensity of pain and evaluates the effectiveness of the drug intervention. Opioid analgesia with meperidine hydrochloride (Demerol) is most frequently used, but opioid dependency may become a problem. Nonopioid analgesics may be tried to relieve pain. (See Chapter 7 for other interventions for chronic pain.)

If drug dependency becomes a problem, behavior modification programs and drug and alcohol counseling will be necessary. The health care provider may need to admit these clients to drug and alcohol dependency programs.

Enzyme Replacement. Pancreatic enzymes (non–enteric-coated preparations) are essential dietary supplements (Chart 60-7). These are given with meals or snacks to aid in digestion and absorption of fat and protein. Drugs such as pancreatin (Donnazyme) and pancrelipase (Cotazym, Viokase, or Pancrease) are prescribed in capsule, tablet, or powder form and contain amylase, lipase, and protease. Cotazym also contains calcium carbonate to increase depleted calcium levels. The nurse mixes the powder form in applesauce or fruit juice to make it more palatable. Enzyme preparations should not be mixed with foods containing proteins, because the enzymatic action dissolves the food into a watery substance. The nurse advises the client to wipe his or her lips with a wet towel to prevent the skin irritation and breakdown that residual enzymes can cause.

The dosage of pancreatic enzymes depends on the severity of the malabsorption and maldigestion. The nurse records the number and consistency of stools per day to monitor the effectiveness of enzyme therapy. If pancreatic enzyme treatment is effective, the stools should become less frequent and less fatty.

Insulin Therapy. If the client has diabetes, the health care provider prescribes insulin or oral hypoglycemic agents for glucose control. Clients maintained on total parenteral nutrition (TPN) are particularly susceptible to labile glucose levels and may require regular insulin additives to the solution. The nurse closely monitors blood glucose levels so that hyperglycemia is controlled and insulin or diabetic shock is prevented. The use of glucometers allows frequent assessment of glucose levels during the critical insulin dosage adjustment period. The nurse, laboratory technician, or assistive nursing personnel checks glucose levels every 2 to 4 hours.

CHART 60-7

CLIENT EDUCATION GUIDE
Enzyme Replacement for the Client with Chronic Pancreatitis

- Give pancreatic enzymes with meals and snacks.
- Administer pancreatin after antacid or H_2 blockers; decreased pH inactivates drug.
- Tell the client to swallow the tablets without chewing to minimize oral irritation.
- Mix the powder form in applesauce or fruit juice.
- Do not mix enzyme preparations in protein-containing foods.
- Have the client wipe his or her lips after taking enzymes to avoid skin irritation.
- Do not crush enteric-coated preparations.
- Monitor serum uric acid levels (pancrelipase can cause an increase in uric acid levels).

Other Drugs. The health care provider may also prescribe histamine receptor antagonists, such as ranitidine hydrochloride (Zantac), to decrease gastric acid. Gastric acid destroys the lipase needed to break down fats. Controlling the acidity of the stomach with H_2 blockers or proton pump inhibitors or neutralizing stomach acid with oral sodium bicarbonate may enhance the effectiveness of the non–enteric-coated enzyme therapy. Subcutaneous octreotide (Sandostatin), a growth hormone similar to somatostatin, is ordered by some physicians if pain and diarrhea persist (Amann, DiMagno, & Rubin, 1997).

DIET THERAPY. Protein and fat malabsorption results in significant weight loss and decreased muscle mass in the client with chronic pancreatitis. Therefore the nutritional interventions for acute pancreatitis are also relevant for the chronic phase of pancreatitis. The client often limits food intake to avoid the recurrent pain, which is exacerbated by eating. For this reason, nutrition maintenance is often difficult to achieve, and clients are provided with TPN or total enteral nutrition (TEN), including vitamin and mineral replacement.

For long-term dietary management, the client needs an increased number of calories, up to 4000 to 6000 calories/day, to maintain weight. Foods high in carbohydrates and protein also assist in the healing process. Foods high in fat are avoided because they cause or increase diarrhea.

SURGICAL MANAGEMENT. Surgery is not a primary intervention for the treatment of chronic pancreatitis. However, it may be indicated for intractable abdominal pain, incapacitating relapses of pain, or complications such as abscesses and pseudocysts.

The underlying pathologic changes determine the procedure indicated. The surgeon incises and drains an abscess or pseudocyst. Cholecystectomy or choledochotomy (incision of the common bile duct) may be indicated if biliary tract disease is an underlying cause of pancreatitis. If the pancreatic duct sphincter is fibrotic, the surgeon performs a sphincterotomy (incision of the sphincter) to enlarge it.

In pancreaticojejunostomy, the pancreatic duct is opened and anastomosed to the jejunum to relieve obstruction. This procedure relieves pain and preserves pancreatic tissue and function. The preoperative and postoperative care is similar to that for clients undergoing the Whipple procedure (discussed under Surgical Management [Pancreatic Carcinoma], p. 1352). A partial pancreatectomy (resection of the pancreas) may be performed for clients with advanced pancreatitis or disabling pain. Vagotomy with gastric antrectomy is done to alter nerve stimulation and decrease pancreatic secretion. (See Chapter 56 for a discussion of nursing care.)

In a few cases, pancreas transplantation may be done. However, this procedure is performed most often for clients with severe, uncontrolled diabetes. Chapter 65 discusses pancreas transplantation.

Community-Based Care

The care of the client with pancreatitis usually involves a case manager or discharge planner. A community-based case manager may continue to follow the client while he or she requires health care in the home or other community-based setting.

HEALTH TEACHING

Because there is no known cure for chronic pancreatitis, client and family education is aimed at preventing further acute exacerbations of this chronic disease, providing long-term care, and promoting health maintenance (Chart 60-8).

DIET THERAPY. The nurse instructs the client to avoid known precipitating factors, such as the ingestion of caffeinated beverages and alcohol. The dietitian elicits the participation of the family or significant other in diet planning and food preparation. Diet teaching focuses on eating bland, low-fat, frequent meals and avoiding rich, fatty foods. The nurse and dietitian stress the importance of dietary compliance and the need for increased nutritional intake to prevent acute exacerbations of this chronic illness. Written instructions on diet and pancreatic enzyme replacement therapy are essential.

The nurse instructs the client and family members or significant others on the importance of adhering to the pancreatic enzyme replacement treatment. The client must take the prescribed enzymes with meals and snacks to aid in the digestion of food and promote the absorption of fats and proteins. The nurse teaches the client to take the enzymes at the beginning of the meal and to report to the health care provider any increase in the occurrence of foul-smelling, frothy, fatty stools; abdominal distention; and cramping so that pancreatic enzyme replacement may be increased as needed. The client should report any skin excoriation or breakdown so that therapeutic interventions to promote skin integrity can be instituted.

CHART 60-8

CLIENT EDUCATION GUIDE
Prevention of Exacerbations of Chronic Pancreatitis

- Avoid things that make your symptoms worse, such as drinking caffeinated beverages.
- Avoid alcohol ingestion; refer to self-help group for assistance.
- Avoid nicotine.
- Eat bland, low-fat, high-protein, moderate-carbohydrate meals; avoid gastric stimulants, such as spices.
- Eat small meals and snacks high in calories.
- Take the pancreatic enzymes that have been prescribed for you with meals.
- Rest frequently; restrict your activity to one floor until you regain your strength.

SKIN CARE. The frequency of defecation (whether continent or incontinent) poses challenging skin care problems. The nurse instructs the client to keep his or her skin dry and free of the abrasive fatty stools, which are excoriating to the skin. The skin should be cleaned thoroughly after each stool and a soothing emollient, such as Sween, applied. To prevent breakdown and maintain skin integrity, a skin barrier may be needed. Many products on the market, such as zinc oxide cream, actively repel stool from the skin.

DRUG THERAPY. The client and family members must be able to state the desired effect of the prescribed drugs, the schedule for drug administration, and potential side effects. The nurse provides written guidelines as reinforcement.

If the client develops diabetes mellitus as a result of chronic pancreatitis from endocrine dysfunction, management of elevated glucose levels after discharge from the hospital may necessitate oral hypoglycemic agents or insulin injections. If this is the case, the client and the family require in-depth teaching concerning diabetes, its signs and symptoms, medical management, insulin administration, dietary management, urine and blood glucose monitoring, and general care information. (See Chapter 65 for a discussion of diabetes.)

HOME CARE MANAGEMENT

Client with chronic pancreatitis are usually discharged to home, but some may require care in a long-term care setting. If the client is discharged to home, the activity area should be limited to one floor until he or she regains strength and can increase activity. Toilet facilities must be easily accessible because of chronic steatorrhea and frequent defecation. If toilet facilities are not available in the immediate rest area, a bedpan or bedside commode is obtained for the home.

HEALTH CARE RESOURCES

Chronic illnesses are devastating for families. The high costs of medical insurance, medical treatment, and drug therapy cause serious financial problems. Often the client with chronic pancreatitis is unable or unwilling to work. Case management to coordinate care and manage resources should be instituted during hospitalization and continue throughout the course of the illness.

The client may require home visits by nurses and a dietitian, depending on the severity of the chronic health problems and home maintenance and support needs. The home care nurse assesses the client for pain management, compliance with dietary guidelines and alcohol abstinence, the effectiveness of pancreatic enzyme therapy, and psychosocial adaptation to a chronic illness.

The nurse or case manager refers the client to a counselor or a self-help group, such as Alcoholics Anonymous, if appropriate.

Pancreatic Abscess

OVERVIEW

Pancreatic abscesses are the most serious complication of pancreatitis. If untreated, they are always fatal. After surgery, the recurrence rate is higher than 30%. The abscesses form from collections of purulent liquefaction of the necrotic pancreas.

Pancreatic abscesses occur after severe acute pancreatitis, exacerbations of chronic pancreatitis, or biliary tract surgery. The development of either a single abscess or multiple abscesses results from extensive inflammatory necrosis of the pancreas that is readily invaded by infectious organisms such as *Escherichia coli, Klebsiella, Bacteroides, Staphylococcus,* and *Proteus.* They can erode through the retroperitoneum into the bowel mesentery, the mediastinum, the pleural space, or the pelvis.

➤ COLLABORATIVE MANAGEMENT

Clients with pancreatic abscesses often appear more seriously ill than clients with pseudocysts. Clinical manifestations are similar; however, the temperature in clients with abscesses may spike to as high as 104° F (40° C). Blood cultures are helpful in revealing the infective organism. Pleural effusions commonly accompany these abscesses. Ultrasonography and computed tomography (CT) cannot differentiate between pancreatic pseudocysts and abscesses.

Pancreatic abscesses that are not surgically drained carry 100% mortality. Drainage should be performed as soon as possible to prevent sepsis. Antibiotic treatment alone does not resolve the abscess. Mortality remains as high as 60%, even after surgical drainage. Many clients require multiple drainage procedures for recurrent abscesses.

CRITICAL THINKING CHALLENGE

Your client has indicated that he does not intend to alter his alcohol consumption after he is discharged; in fact, he plans to stop for a drink at his favorite bar on the way home after his release later today.

- What is the connection between alcohol consumption and chronic pancreatitis?
- What questions should you ask to determine if the client fully understands the connection between alcohol consumption and recurrence of pancreatitis?
- What resources are available to him to assist with his alcohol problem?
- What nursing diagnoses are appropriate for this client?

For suggested answer guidelines, go to SIMON http://www.wbsaunders.com/SIMON/Iggy/.

Pancreatic Pseudocyst

OVERVIEW

Pancreatic pseudocysts develop as a complication of acute or chronic pancreatitis. **Pseudocysts** occur in pancreatitis caused by alcoholism, biliary tract disease, or abdominal or surgical trauma. Pseudocysts develop in 10% to 20% of all people with pancreatitis, and mortality is reported at approximately 10%.

Pancreatic pseudocysts, or false cysts, are so named because, unlike true cysts, they do not have an epithelial lining. Pseudocysts are encapsulated saclike structures that form on or surround the pancreas. The pseudocyst wall is inflamed, vascular, and fibrotic. It may contain up to several liters of straw-colored or dark-brown viscous fluid, the enzymatic exudate of the pancreas.

➤ COLLABORATIVE MANAGEMENT

A pseudocyst can be palpated as an epigastric mass in approximately 50% of cases. The primary presenting symptom is epigastric pain radiating to the back. Other common clinical manifestations include abdominal fullness, nausea, vomiting, and jaundice.

Pseudocysts are diagnosed, and their growth and resolution monitored, by serial abdominal ultrasonographic examination or CT.

Complications of pseudocyst formation include the following:

- Hemorrhage
- Infection
- Obstruction of the bowel, biliary tract, or splenic vein
- Abscess
- Fistula formation
- Pancreatic ascites

Pseudocysts may spontaneously resolve, or they may rupture and produce hemorrhage. Surgical intervention is necessary if the pseudocyst does not resolve within 6 weeks or if complications develop. To accomplish internal drainage, the surgeon creates an opening (ostomy) between the pseudocyst and the stomach (cystogastrostomy), the jejunum (cystojejunostomy), or the duodenum (cystoduodenostomy). To provide external drainage, the surgeon inserts a sump drainage tube to remove pancreatic secretions and exudate. Pseudocysts recur in almost 10% of cases. Pancreatic fistulas are common after surgery, and skin breakdown from corrosive pancreatic enzymes presents a major nursing care challenge (see earlier discussion under Postoperative Care [Acute Pancreatitis], p. 1344).

Pancreatic Carcinoma

OVERVIEW

Cancer of the pancreas is one of the leading causes of cancer-related mortality, accounting for 2% to 3% of the new cancer cases each year and for high costs of care (see the Cost of Care Box on p. 1350) (Sauter & Coleman, 1999).

Pathophysiology

Pancreatic tumors usually originate from epithelial cells of the pancreatic ductal system. If the tumor is discovered in the early stages, the tumor cells may be localized within the glandular organ; however, this is highly unlikely. Most often, the tumor is discovered in the late stages of development and may be a well-defined mass or is diffusely spread throughout the pancreas.

The tumor may be a primary cancer, or it may result from metastasis from cancers of the lung, breast, thyroid, or kidney or from skin melanoma. Primary pancreatic tumors are generally adenocarcinomas and grow in well-differentiated glandular patterns. Pancreatic adenocarcinoma grows rapidly and spreads to surrounding organs (stomach, duodenum, gallbladder, and intestine) by direct extension and invasion of lymphatic and vascular systems. This highly metastatic lesion may eventually invade the lung, peritoneum, liver, spleen, and lymph nodes.

Clinical manifestations depend on the site of origin or metastasis. The head of the pancreas is the most common site of pancreatic carcinoma. Pancreatic tumors are usually small lesions with poorly defined margins. Jaundice results from tumor compression and obstruction of the common bile duct and from gallbladder dilation, causing the organ to enlarge.

Carcinomas of the body and tail of the pancreas are usually large and invade the entire tail and body. These tumors may

COST OF CARE IMPLICATIONS FOR NURSING

PANCREATIC CANCER

Cost of Care

- Pancreatic cancer ranks eleventh in incidence and fifth in cancer deaths.
- Total annual costs are $4.9 billion (men: $3.0 billion; women: $1.9 billion).
- Total direct costs are $881.3 million.
  Seventy-one percent of total direct costs ($627.1 million/$881.3 million) are for those over 65 years of age.
  Total hospital costs are 77% ($679.5 million/$881.3 million) of total direct costs.
- Total indirect costs are $4 billion.
  Sixty-three percent of total indirect costs ($2518.43 million/$4018 million) are for those ages 45 to 64 years.
  Mortality costs are $3.7 billion—93% ($3739 million/$4018 million) of indirect costs.

Implications for Nursing

Pancreatic cancer has a very low 5-year survival rate, with fewer than 20% of those diagnosed with the disease living longer than 1 year after diagnosis.

Because of the cost of pancreatic cancer, it is important that nurses recognize the role they might play in the disease process. This role might include education about the risk factors and prevention, the signs and symptoms, and the treatment of this cancer.

Currently there is no known diagnostic test to predict the individual's susceptibility to this type of cancer, nor is the exact cause of the cancer known.

Nurses need to identify who might be at higher risk to develop pancreatic cancer: some possible links have been shown with alcohol and caffeine consumption and with a diet high in fat and protein. Smoking is known to be the single most significant risk factor for the development of pancreatic cancer. These actual and potential risk factors are modifiable.

Data from Wilson, L., & Lightwood, J. (1999). Pancreatic cancer: Total costs and utilization of health services, *Journal of Surgical Oncology, 71*(3), 171-181; and Sauter, P.L., & Coleman, J. (1999). Pancreatic cancer: A continuum of care. *Seminars in Oncology Nursing, 15*(1), 36-47.

be palpable abdominal masses, especially in the thin client. Through metastatic spread via the splenic vein, metastasis to the liver may cause hepatomegaly (enlargement of the liver up to two to three times its normal size). Carcinomas of the body and tail spread more extensively than do pancreatic head carcinomas, with invasion of the retroperitoneum, vertebral column, spleen, adrenal glands, colon, or stomach. Regardless of where it originates, pancreatic cancer spreads rapidly through the lymphatic and venous systems to other organs.

Thrombophlebitis is a common complication of pancreatic carcinoma. It is attributed to an increase in the levels of thromboplastic factors in the blood. Necrotic products of the pancreatic tumor are believed to have thromboplastic properties, resulting in the blood's hypercoagulable state. Thrombophlebitis is due to the client's confinement to bed and extensive surgical manipulation.

Etiology

The exact cause of pancreatic carcinoma is unknown. The single most prevalent risk factor for pancreatic cancer is smoking. A diet high in protein and fat, and high coffee or alcohol consumption have also been investigated for possible linkage to the disease, but current studies do not show a substantial direct association (Sauter & Coleman, 1999). Research does support the theory that there might be a genetic link in the development of pancreatic cancer (McEwen et al., 1996).

Incidence/Prevalence

Approximately 28,000 people develop pancreatic cancer each year, and an equal number of people die from the disease each year. Fewer than 20% of persons diagnosed with pancreatic cancer survive longer than 1 year after diagnosis (Sauter & Coleman, 1999).

CONSIDERATIONS FOR OLDER ADULTS

The incidence of pancreatic cancer increases with age. The highest rates of incidence are in people between 60 and 70 years of age, and pancreatic cancer rarely develops before the age of 50. The disease appears to be somewhat more common in men than in women, but the difference is slight (Mayer, 1999; Sauter & Coleman, 1999).

CULTURAL CONSIDERATIONS

Cancer of the pancreas occurs in developed countries. A slightly higher incidence among African Americans has been reported (Sauter & Coleman, 1999).

COLLABORATIVE MANAGEMENT

Assessment

Pancreatic cancer often presents in an insidious manner. The presenting symptoms depend somewhat on the location of the tumor. The first clue to the presence of pancreatic carcinoma may be the appearance of jaundice, which is a late sign (Chart 60-9). Jaundice appears as the initial sign in two thirds of all cases because the gallbladder and liver are commonly involved. As the tumor spreads, the green-gold skin color associated with obstructive jaundice progressively worsens. On noting the jaundice, the nurse asks the client whether the color of the stool and urine has changed. As a result of the obstructive process, the stool is clay colored and the urine is dark and frothy. The nurse inspects the skin for dryness and scratch marks, indicating pruritus from jaundice. The nurse also assesses the sclerae for icterus and the mucous membranes for signs of jaundice.

By the time jaundice appears, the pancreatic carcinoma is usually in an advanced stage. The nurse may be able to palpate the enlarged gallbladder and liver. In advanced cases of pancreatic carcinoma, the tumor may be palpated as a firm, fixed mass in the left upper abdominal quadrant or epigastric region.

The most common complaint, often misinterpreted by even the client, is fatigue. This fatigue is described as a diminished energy level and an increased need for rest disproportionate to the level of activity. The client notices an inability to perform usual physical or intellectual activities (Sauter & Coleman, 1999).

The nurse questions the client about abdominal pain, which may be described as a vague, constant dullness in the upper abdomen and nonspecific in nature. Pain, a common early complaint in clients with pancreatic carcinoma, is also present in the advanced stages of the disease. Pain may be related to eating or activity.

CHART 60-9

KEY FEATURES *of*
Presenting Signs and Symptoms of Pancreatic Carcinoma

- Jaundice (lesions of pancreatic head only)
- Clay-colored stools
- Dark urine
- Abdominal pain: usually vague, dull, or nonspecific
- Weight loss
- Anorexia
- Nausea or vomiting
- Glucose intolerance
- Splenomegaly
- Flatulence
- Gastrointestinal bleeding
- Ascites
- Leg or calf pain (from thrombophlebitis)
- Weakness

In addition, the nurse asks the client whether he or she is experiencing pain in other areas of the body. Referred back pain may be caused by pressure on the nerve plexus. Some clients have leg or calf pain with swelling and redness as a result of thrombophlebitis, a complication of pancreatic carcinoma.

The nurse or assistive nursing personnel weighs the client and determines the extent of weight loss and whether it has occurred rapidly. The client is questioned about food intake and intolerances. Anorexia accompanied by early satiety, nausea, flatulence, and vomiting is common. Gastrointestinal (GI) bleeding may develop from esophageal or gastric varices caused by the tumor pressing on the portal vein. A new diagnosis of diabetes is found in some clients.

The nurse performs a general abdominal assessment. In particular, the nurse percusses the abdomen for dullness, which may indicate the presence of ascites. Pancreatic ascites occurs in the advanced stages of the disease process.

There are no specific blood tests to diagnose pancreatic carcinoma. Serum amylase and lipase levels, as well as alkaline phosphatase and bilirubin levels, are elevated. The degree of elevation depends on the acuteness or chronicity of the pancreatic and biliary damage. Elevated carcinoembryonic antigen (CEA) levels occur in 80% to 90% of clients with pancreatic carcinoma. This test may provide early information about the presence of tumor cells. CA 19-9, another tumor marker, has been found to be the most useful serologic test for monitoring a proven diagnosis and for continuing surveillance of the cancer for potential spread or recurrence (Sauter & Coleman, 1999).

Computed tomography (CT) can confirm the presence of a tumor and can differentiate the tumor from a cyst. Biopsy of pancreatic tissue by needle aspiration reveals malignant cells. Ultrasonographic examinations do not distinguish pancreatic carcinoma from other pancreatic disorders. Endoscopic retrograde cholangiopancreatography (ERCP) visualization and cytologic study of aspirate provide the most definitive diagnostic data. An alternative to ERCP is a percutaneous transhepatic biliary cholangiogram with placement of a percutaneous transhepatic biliary drain (PTBD). This drain decompresses the blocked biliary system by draining bile, either internally or externally (Sauter & Coleman, 1999). Aspiration of pancreatic ascitic fluid by abdominal paracentesis may reveal malignant cells and elevated amylase levels. When the secretin test is performed (see Assessment [Chronic Pancreatitis], p. 1346), duodenal or gastric aspirate may reveal malignant cells.

EVIDENCE-BASED PRACTICE FOR NURSING

Improving the quality of life for clients with pancreatic cancer: A cooperative team approach by a diverse group of health care providers can improve the life experiences of persons with pancreatic cancer

Sauter, P.K., & Coleman, J. (1999). Pancreatic cancer: A continuum of care. *Seminars in Oncology Nursing, 15*(1), 36-47.

A diagnosis of pancreatic cancer leads a person to consider both quality and quantity of life, since cancer of the pancreas is a disease with a poor prognosis. Many physical symptoms are associated with advanced disease—symptoms that are sometimes feared more that the cancer itself. Fewer than 20% of clients diagnosed with pancreatic cancer live longer than 1 year after diagnosis, and only 3% survive for 5 years. The authors' objectives were to provide information about the etiology, manifestations, treatment, and symptom management of pancreatic cancer. To this end, information was gathered from textbooks, research studies, and review articles. The course of the disease was tracked, from diagnosis to medical management, with appropriate nursing interventions identified for all aspects of care. It was recommended that the nurse place emphasis on empowering the client and caregivers in the management of the disease, when possible.

Critique. Although the authors presented detailed information on the medical management of the disease, they did not provide the same detailed information on ways to involve or empower the client. An excellent research suggestion was given: develop an accurate marker for pancreatic cancer that can be easily detected in a screening test for persons at risk for the disease. Research needs to make progress in the identification of a genetic marker to identify familial links to pancreatic cancer.

Implications for Nursing. Providing care for the client with pancreatic cancer presents many nursing challenges. The nurse needs to understand the disease progression and its multiple treatments in order to provide knowledgeable care to the client. Caring for the client with pancreatic cancer needs to be rendered in a manner that empowers both the client and the caregivers. To accomplish this, the nurse needs to become an integral part of the health care team, which can address treatment, symptom management, and meeting the psychologic, social, and spiritual needs of the client and family as the disease progresses.

Interventions

Management of the client with pancreatic carcinoma is geared toward preventing tumor spread and decreasing pain. These measures are not curative, only palliative (see the Evidence-Based Practice for Nursing box above). The cancers are often multifocal and recur despite treatment.

NONSURGICAL MANAGEMENT. As in other types of cancer, chemotherapy or radiation is used to relieve pain. (See Chapter 25 for nursing interventions associated with these treatment modalities.)

DRUG THERAPY. In an effort to keep the pain under control, the nurse medicates the client, as ordered, with opioid analgesics (usually morphine) and provides comfort measures before the pain escalates and reaches a peak. Because of the poor prognosis, drug dependency is not a consideration. High doses of opioid analgesics may be needed for the intense abdominal and back pain that occurs in the late stages of the disease.

Chemotherapeutic interventions for pancreatic carcinoma have had limited success. Combining agents such as fluorouracil (5-fluorouracil [5-FU]) and carmustine (BCNU) has been more successful than single-agent chemotherapy. 5-FU is an antimetabolite that interferes with deoxyribonucleic acid (DNA) synthesis in rapidly dividing cells. Two other drugs prescribed are mitomycin (Mutamycin), an antitumor antibiotic that inhibits synthesis of ribonucleic acid (RNA), and streptozocin (Zanosar), a nitrosourea that interferes with the replication of DNA. The nurse provides the client with symptomatic relief and comfort measures for the adverse effects of chemotherapeutic agents, such as nausea and vomiting. Gemcitabine, a new cytotoxic agent, is now standard therapy for the treatment of clients whose cancer is nonresectable or whose cancer has metastasized. The major benefit to the client is pain management, with shrinkage of tumor size and prolonged survival a secondary benefit (Sauter & Coleman, 1999).

RADIATION THERAPY. Intensive external beam radiation therapy to the pancreas may offer pain relief by shrinking tumor cells, alleviating obstruction, and improving food absorption; it does not improve survival rates. Implantation of radioactive iodine (^{125}I) seeds, in combination with systemic or intra-arterial administration of floxuridine (FUDR), has also been used. The client may experience discomfort during and after the radiation treatments. Supportive nursing interventions for the relief of symptoms are indicated.

SURGICAL MANAGEMENT. Complete surgical resection of the pancreatic tumor offers the individual with pancreatic cancer the only effective treatment, but the surgery is only possible in a small percentage of cases. The mean survival rate for clients with nonresectable pancreatic cancer is 6 months after diagnosis (Mayer, 1999). Clients with tumors confined to the head of the pancreas are candidates for curative resection. Clients with tumors of the body and tail generally are not candidates for surgery, because in most cases their tumors have spread to other organs. The surgeon may perform either a total pancreatectomy or the Whipple procedure (pancreaticoduodenectomy).

PREOPERATIVE CARE. The client with pancreatic carcinoma is a poor surgical risk because of malnutrition and debilitation. A nasogastric (NG) tube for decompression is inserted, and the administration of IV fluids or total parenteral nutrition (TPN) is typically started before surgery.

The client experiences anorexia with early satiety and often experiences nausea and vomiting, making the oral intake of nutrition difficult to maintain. Management is geared toward providing optimal nutrition preoperatively and postoperatively.

Tube Feedings. As long as intestinal function is adequate, the client may be maintained nutritionally with enteral tube feedings. When tube feedings are tolerated, a small-lumen silicone feeding tube, such as a Dobbhoff tube, is inserted to avoid the complications of larger-lumen tubes, such as sinusitis and nasal irritation. Commercially prepared products chosen by the health care provider or dietitian provide specific nutrients. Feedings are given by bolus or continuous infusion, depending on the client's tolerance and residual volumes.

Often, in the late stages of pancreatic carcinoma or during the Whipple procedure, the physician inserts a small catheter into the jejunum (jejunostomy) so that enteral feedings may be given. This feeding method is preferred to prevent reflux and to facilitate absorption. Feedings are initiated in low concentrations and volumes and are gradually increased as tolerated. The nurse delivers feedings by means of a tube-feeding pump to maintain a constant volume and assesses for diarrhea frequency as a means of measuring tolerance (see Chapter 61).

Total Parenteral Nutrition. For optimal nutrition, hyperalimentation by TPN may be necessary in addition to tube feedings or as a single measure to provide nutrition. When central venous access is required, a Hickman catheter or other type of catheter may be necessary. Meticulous IV line care is an important nursing measure to prevent catheter sepsis. Sterile dressing changes and site observation are extremely important (see Chapter 14). The nurse also performs finger sticks to obtain blood for glucose measurements. These measurements help to monitor the client's pancreatic function and tolerance of dextrose in the solution. Additional nursing care measures for the client receiving TPN are given in Chapter 61.

OPERATIVE PROCEDURES. The Whipple procedure (radical pancreaticoduodenectomy) involves extensive surgical manipulation and is used to treat cancer of the head of the pancreas. The procedure entails removal of the proximal head of the pancreas, the duodenum, a portion of the jejunum, the stomach (partial or total gastrectomy), and the gallbladder, with anastomosis of the pancreatic duct (pancreaticojejunostomy), the common bile duct (choledochojejunostomy), and the stomach (gastrojejunostomy) to the jejunum (Figure 60-7). In addition, the surgeon may remove the spleen (splenectomy).

As a palliative measure to relieve biliary obstruction in the likelihood of extensive tumor invasion, a cholecystojejunostomy may be done as a bypass procedure.

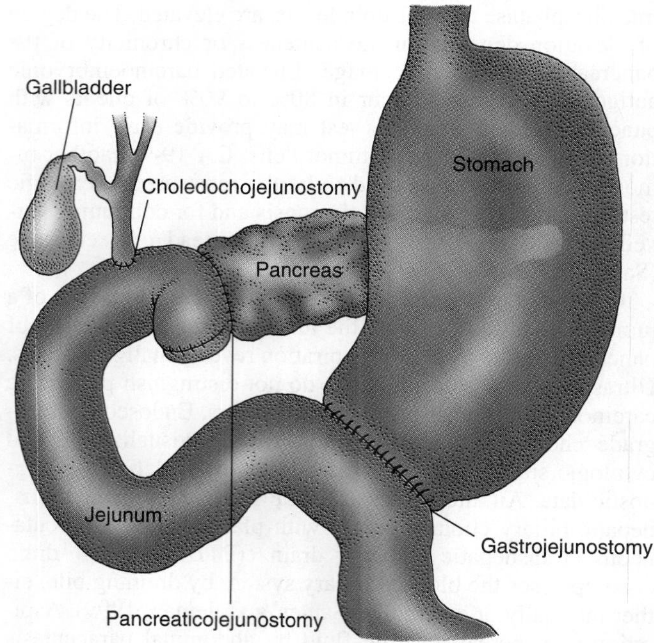

Figure 60-7 ● The three anastomoses that constitute the Whipple procedure: choledochojejunostomy, pancreaticojejunostomy, and gastrojejunostomy.

POSTOPERATIVE CARE. In addition to routine postoperative care measures, the client who has undergone a radical pancreaticoduodenectomy requires intensive nursing care and is usually admitted to a surgical critical care unit. The nurse assesses for potential complications of the Whipple procedure (Table 60-5).

Gastrointestinal Drainage Monitoring. The monitoring of gastrointestinal (GI) drainage and NG tube patency is an important aspect of postoperative nursing care. Drainage tubes are strategically placed during surgery to remove drainage and secretions from the area and to prevent stress on the anastomosis sites. The nurse assesses the tubes and drainage devices for undue stress or kinking and maintains the drainage tubes in a dependent position. The suction pressure gauge is checked frequently to maintain the desired suction level. Most often, Salem sump tubes are used and connected to low continuous suction (80 mm Hg or less) to maintain drain patency.

The nurse monitors the drainage for color, consistency, and amount. The drainage should be serosanguineous; the appearance of clear, colorless, bile-tinged drainage or frank blood with an increase in output may indicate disruption or leakage of an anastomosis site. Most of the disruptions of the anastomosis site occur within a week to 10 days after surgery. Hemorrhage can occur as an early or late complication.

If the NG tube is obstructed, the nurse instills air first. If this method does not keep the drainage lumen open, irrigation with 10 to 20 mL of normal saline is gently performed. If the problem continues, the nurse may need to notify the physician for additional interventions.

The development of a fistula (an abnormal passageway) is the most common and most serious postoperative complication. Biliary, pancreatic, or gastric fistulas result from partial or total breakdown of an anastomosis site. The secretions that drain from the fistula contain bile, pancreatic enzymes, or gastric secretions, depending on which anastomosis site is ruptured. These secretions, particularly pancreatic fluid, are corrosive and irritating to the skin, and internal leakage causes a chemical peritonitis. Peritonitis (inflammation and infection of the peritoneum) necessitates treatment with multiple antibiotics.

TABLE 60-5 • POTENTIAL COMPLICATIONS OF THE WHIPPLE PROCEDURE

CARDIOVASCULAR COMPLICATIONS
- Hemorrhage at anastomosis sites with hypovolemia
- Myocardial infarction
- Heart failure
- Thrombophlebitis

PULMONARY COMPLICATIONS
- Atelectasis
- Pneumonia
- Pulmonary embolism
- Acute respiratory distress syndrome
- Pulmonary edema

GASTROINTESTINAL COMPLICATIONS
- Adynamic (paralytic) ileus
- Gastric retention
- Gastric ulceration
- Bowel obstruction from peritonitis
- Pancreatitis
- Hepatic failure
- Thrombosis to mesentery

WOUND COMPLICATIONS
- Infection
- Dehiscence
- Fistulas: pancreatic, gastric, and biliary

METABOLIC COMPLICATIONS
- Unstable diabetes mellitus
- Renal failure

Positioning. The nurse places the client in the semi-Fowler's position to reduce stress on the suture line and anastomosis site, as well as to optimize lung expansion. Stress on the gastric suture line can be minimized by maintaining NG tube drainage at a low suction level to keep the remaining stomach (if a partial gastrectomy is done) or the jejunum (if a total gastrectomy is done) free of excessive fluid buildup and pressure. The NG tube is also used to reduce stimulation of the remaining pancreatic tissue.

Assessment of Fluids and Electrolytes. Because the Whipple procedure is extensive and can take 6 to 10 hours to complete, maintaining fluid and electrolyte balance can be difficult. Clients tend to experience significant intraoperative blood loss and postoperative bleeding. The intestine is exposed to air for long periods, and evaporation of fluid occurs. Significant losses of fluid and electrolytes occur from NG and other drainage tubes. In addition, these clients are usually malnourished and have low serum levels of protein and albumin, which maintain colloid osmotic pressure within the circulating system. Reduction in the serum osmotic pressure makes the client susceptible to third spacing of body fluids, with fluid moving from the intravascular to the interstitial space, resulting in shock.

For these reasons, the nurse closely monitors vital signs for decreased blood pressure and increased heart rate, decreased vascular pressures with a central venous line or pulmonary artery catheter (Swan-Ganz catheter), and decreased urine output to detect early signs of hypovolemia and prevent shock. The nurse is also alert for pitting edema of the extremities, dependent edema in the sacrum and back, and an intake that far exceeds output. Nutritional repletion via hyperalimentation and the administration of albumin promote the shift of fluid from the interstitial space back into the intravascular space.

Maintenance of ordered IV fluid volume replacement is important. The nurse monitors hemoglobin and hematocrit values to assess for blood loss and the need for blood transfusions. Electrolyte values are reviewed for decreased serum levels of sodium, potassium, chloride, and calcium. IV fluid concentrations must be altered to correct these electrolyte imbalances. The physician orders replacement of electrolytes as needed.

CRITICAL THINKING CHALLENGE

Your client had a Whipple procedure performed 3 days ago, and he has come to your unit from the surgical intensive care unit. He still has an NG tube to low suction and a wound drain in place.

- What physical assessments need to be made initially on placement in your care unit?
- Which postoperative complications would you assess the client for at this point?
- What changes in nasogastric output might signify a complication? What should the normal output look like?

For suggested answer guidelines, go to SIMON http://www.wbsaunders.com/SIMON/Iggy/.

Glucose Monitoring. Immediately after the Whipple procedure, the client may have transient hyperglycemia or hypoglycemia as a result of stress and surgical manipulation of the pancreas. Most of the endocrine cells (islets of Langerhans, responsible for insulin and glucose secretion) are located in the body and tail of the pancreas. In most clients, up to half of the gland remains, and diabetes does not develop; however, a large number of clients are diabetic before surgery. The nurse monitors glucose levels frequently during the early postoperative period and administers insulin injections, as prescribed.

Community-Based Care

The client with pancreatic cancer is usually followed by a case manager, both in the hospital and in the home or other community-based setting. The role of the case manager is to ensure that the client receives cost-effective treatment and that his or her biopsychosocial needs are met.

HEALTH TEACHING

When the client is discharged to home, many of the care measures are palliative and aimed at providing relief of symptoms such as pain. Care measures and teaching information are similar to those for clients with chronic pancreatitis.

In many cases, the diagnosis of pancreatic cancer is made a few months before death occurs. The client needs time to adjust to the diagnosis, which is usually made too late for cure or prolonged survival. The nurse helps the client identify what needs to be done to prepare for death. For example, the client may want to write a will or see family members and friends whom he or she has not seen recently. The client needs to make specific requests for the funeral or memorial service known to family members or significant others. These actions help the client prepare for death in a dignified manner. Chapter 9 discusses anticipatory grieving and preparation for death in detail.

HOME CARE MANAGEMENT

The stage of progression of pancreatic carcinoma and available home care resources dictate whether the client can be discharged to home or whether additional care is needed in a skilled nursing facility or hospice. Home care preparations depend on the client's physical and activity limitations and should be tailored to his or her needs. The nurse needs to coordinate care with the client and whoever will be used as the care provider after discharge from the hospital—home care provider, hospice care provider, or extended care provider.

The client and family need emotional support to deal with issues related to this illness. The nurse assists family members in ascertaining realistically and objectively the amount of physical care required for the client. The family members must be told that their own physical and emotional health is at risk during this stressful period and that supportive counseling is indicated. If the family does not have a religious affiliation or a spiritual leader (e.g., a minister or a rabbi) to provide support, the nurse suggests alternative counseling options. It is appropriate for the nurse to make the initial contact or appointment according to the client's or family's wishes.

HEALTH CARE RESOURCES

Regular home care nursing and assistive nursing personnel visits are scheduled to assist the client and family by providing physical, psychologic, and supportive care. The nurse supplies information about local hospice care (see Chapter 9) and cancer support groups.

ONLINE RESOURCES

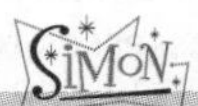

For suggested readings and Internet resources, go to http://www.wbsaunders.com/SIMON/Iggy/.

SELECTED BIBLIOGRAPHY

Asterisk indicates a classic or definitive work on this subject.

Allen, K.M., & Phillips, J.M. (1997). *Women's health across the lifespan: A comprehensive perspective.* Philadelphia: J.B. Lippincott.

Amann, S.T., DiMagno, E., & Rubin, W. (1997). Pancreatitis: Diagnostic and therapeutic interventions. *Patient Care, 31*(11), 200-202, 205-212, 215-216.

*Ambrose, M.S., & Dreher, H.M. (1996). Pancreatitis: Managing a flare-up. *Nursing, 26*(4), 33-39.

American Cancer Society. (2000). *Cancer facts and figures—2000.* Report No. 00-300M-No.5008.00 Atlanta: Author.

*Bagg, A. (1988). Whipple's procedure: Nursing guidelines. *Critical Care Nurse 8*(5), 34-45.

Baillie, J. (1997). Treatment of acute biliary pancreatitis. *New England Journal of Medicine, 336*(4), 286-287.

Banks, P. (1997). Practice guidelines in acute pancreatitis. *American Journal of Gastroenterology, 92*(3), 377-386.

Barton-Burke, M. (1999). Gemcitabine: A pharmacologic and clinical overview. *Cancer Nursing, 22*(2), 176-183.

*Carson, C., Seidel, S., & Bushmiaer, M. (1996). Recovery from laparoscopic cholecystectomy procedures. *AORN Journal, 63*(6), 1099-1113.

*Conner, M., & Deane, D. (1995). Patterns of patient controlled analgesia and intramuscular analgesia. *Applied Nursing Research, 8*(2), 67-72.

Cooper, A.D. (1999). Bile salts: Metabolic, pathologic, and therapeutic considerations. *Gastroenterology Clinics of North America, 28*(1), xi, 1-245.

Coyne, P.J. (1998a). Pain control: Assessing and treating the pain of pancreatitis. *American Journal of Nursing, 98*(11), 14, 16.

Coyne, P.J. (1998b.) *Pancreatitis.* In M. McCaffery & C. Passero. (Eds.), *Pain: Clinical manual* (2nd ed.). St. Louis: Mosby.

Everhart, J.E., et al. (1999). Prevalence and ethnic differences in gallbladder disease in the United States. *Gastroenterology, 177*(3), 632-639.

*Fain, J.A., & Amato-Vealey, E. (1988). Acute pancreatitis: A gastrointestinal emergency. *Critical Care Nurse, 8*(6), 47-63.

Fischbach, F. (2000). *A manual of laboratory and diagnostic tests* (6th ed.). Philadelphia: J.B. Lippincott.

Greenberger, N., Isselbacher, K. (1998). Diseases of the gallbladder and bile ducts. In A.S. Fauci, C. Braunwald, & K.J. Isselbacher (Eds.), *Harrison's principles of internal medicine* (14th ed., p. 1504). New York: McGraw-Hill.

Greenberger, N., Toskes, P.P., & Isselbacher, K.J. (1998). Acute and chronic pancreatitis. In A.S. Fauci, C. Braunwald, & K.J. Isselbacher (Eds.), *Harrison's principles of internal medicine* (14th ed., pp. 1741-1752). New York: McGraw-Hill.

Held-Warmkessel, J., Volpe, H., & Waldman, A.R. (1998). Symptom management for patients with pancreatic cancer. *Clinical Journal of Oncology Nursing, 2*(4), 135-139.

Hoerner, M. (1998). Continuing education forum: Diagnosis and management of acute pancreatitis. *Journal of the American Academy of Nurse Practitioners, 10*(10), 471-477.

Howard, D.E., & Fromm, H. (1999). Nonsurgical management of gallstone Disease. *Gastroenterology Clinics of North America, 28*(1), 133-144.

Izbicki, J.R., et al. (1999). Surgical treatment of chronic pancreatitis and quality of life after operation. *Surgical Clinics of North America, 79*(4), 913-944.

Katz, J. (1997). Back to basics: Providing effective patient teaching. *American Journal of Nursing, 97*(5), 33-36.

*Kowdley, K. (1996). Update on therapy for hepatobiliary diseases. *Nurse Practitioner, 21*(7), 78-88.

Krumberger, J. (1999). Ask the experts: What is the most current recommendation for analgesic agents and pain management in patients with pancreatitis and other obstructive gastrointestinal disorders? *Critical Care Nurse, 19*(2), 110-111.

Levin, B. (1999). Gallbladder carcinoma. *Annals of Oncology, 10* (Suppl. 4), 129-130.

Lillemoe, K. (1998). Palliative therapy for pancreatic cancer. *Surgical Oncology Clinics of North America, 7*(1), 199-216.

Lillemoe, K., & Yeo, C. (1998). Management of the complications of pancreatitis. *Current problems in Surgery, 35,* 3-98.

Mayer, R. (1999). *Pancreatic cancer;* http://www.harrisononline.com.

McClave, S.A., et al. (1997). Comparison of the safety of early enteral vs parenteral nutrition in mild acute pancreatitis. *Journal of Parenteral and Enteral Nutrition, 21*(1), 14-20.

McCormick, M.E. (1999). Endoscopic retrograde cholangiopancreatography. *American Journal of Nursing, 99*(2), 24HH-JJ.

*McEwen, D., et al. (1996). Managing patients with pancreatic cancer. *AORN Journal, 64*(5), 716-734.

*McGrath, P., Sloan, D., & Kenady, D. (1996). Surgical management of pancreatic carcinoma. *Seminars in Oncology, 23*(2), 200-212.

Meissner, J.E. (1997). Disease review: Caring for patients with pancreatitis. *Nursing, 27*(10), 50-51.

Nahrwold, D.L. (1997). Gallstone disease: Update on diagnostic and therapeutic options. *Consultant, 37*(8), 2049-2052, 2057-2058.

National Institutes of Health. (1999). Gallstones; http://www.niddk.nih.gov/health/digest/pubs/gallstns/gallstns.htm.

Norton, I.D., & Petersen, B.T. (1999). Interventional treatment of acute and chronic pancreatitis: Endoscopic procedures. *Surgical Clinics of North America, 79*(4), 895-911, xii.

Nowazek, V. (1996). Nursing management of the patient with acute pancreatitis. In S.D. Ruppert, J.G. Kernicki, & J.T. Dolan (Eds.), *Dolan's critical care nursing* (2nd ed., pp. 832-847). Philadelphia: F.A. Davis.

Pagana, K.D., & Pagana, T.J. (1998). *Mosby's manual of diagnostic and laboratory tests,* St. Louis: Mosby.

Pasero, C. (1998). Assessing and treating the pain of pancreatitis. *American Journal of Nursing, 98*(11), 14, 16.

Peterson, A. (1997). Analgesics. *RN, 60*(4), 45-50.

*Pinto, K. (1996). Acalculous cholecystitis: A case report. *Nurse Practitioner, 21*(10), 120-122.

Price, S.A., & Wilson, L. (1997). *Pathophysiology: Clinical concepts of disease processes* (5th ed., pp. 376-383, 396-400). St. Louis: Mosby.

Runzi, M., & Layer, P. (1999). Nonsurgical management of acute pancreatitis: Use of antibiotics. *Surgical Clinics of North America, 79*(4), 759-765, xii.

Rutecki, G.W., & Whittier, F.C. (1998). Decision points in hypocalcemia: Is emergent therapy required? Complications may include tetany, seizures, and arrhythmias. *Journal of Critical Illness, 13*(2), 84-86, 89-90.

Sauter, P.K., & Coleman, J. (1999). Pancreatic cancer: A continuum of care. *Seminars in Oncology Nursing, 15*(1), 36-47.

Scolapio, J.S., Mahli-Chowla, N., & Ukleja, A. (1999). Nutrition supplementation in patients with acute and chronic pancreatitis. *Gastroenterology Clinics of North America, 28*(3), 695-707.

Simon, J.A. & Hudes, E.S. (1998). Serum ascorbic acid and other correlates of gallbladder disease among U.S. adults. *American Journal of Public Health, 88*(8), 1208-1212.

Simpson, J.P., Savarise, M.T., & Moore, J. (1999). Outpatient laparoscopic cholecystectomy: What predicts the need for admission? *American Surgeon, 65*(6), 525-528.

Snow, L.L., et al. (1999). Management of bile duct stones in 1527 patients undergoing laparoscopic cholecystectomy. *American Surgeon, 65*(6), 530-545.

*Steer, M.L., Waxman, I., & Freedman, S. (1995). Chronic pancreatitis. *New England Journal of Medicine, 332*(22), 1482-1490.

Strasberg, S. (1999). Laparoscopic biliary surgery. *Gastroenterology Clinics of North America, 28*(1), 117-130.

Thompson, D., et al. (1998). Estimated economic costs of obesity to U.S. business. *American Journal of Health Promotion, 13*(2), 120-127.

*Tierney, L.M., McPhee, S.J., & Papadakis, M.A. (1996). *Current medical diagnosis and treatment* (35th ed.). Stamford, CN: Appleton & Lange.

Tseng, M., Everhart, J.E., & Sandler, R.S. (1999). Dietary intake and gallbladder disease: A review. *Public Health Nutrition, 2*(2), 161-172.

Uhl, W., et al. (1999). The role of Octreotide and Somatostatin in acute and chronic pancreatitis. *Digestion, 60* (Suppl. 2), 22-30.

Understanding gallstone formation. (1999). *Nursing, 29*(4), 14.

CHAPTER 61

Interventions for Clients with Malnutrition and Obesity

DONNA D. IGNATAVICIUS

Learning Objectives

After studying this chapter, you should be able to:

1. Identify three anthropometric measurements that the nurse can use to evaluate a client's nutritional status.
2. Explain the potential consequences and complications associated with malnutrition.
3. Describe the risk factors for malnutrition, especially for older adults.
4. Discuss the role of laboratory testing in the diagnosis of malnutrition.
5. Analyze assessment data to determine common nursing diagnoses for the client with malnutrition.
6. Identify expected outcomes for clients who are malnourished.
7. Describe the nursing care of clients receiving total enteral nutrition (TEN).
8. Prioritize nursing care for clients receiving total parenteral nutrition (TPN).
9. Identify complications associated with TPN.
10. Explain the potential consequences and complications associated with obesity.
11. Discuss the role of culture and gender as factors in the prevalence of obesity.
12. Identify the role of drug therapy in the management of obesity.
13. Develop a postoperative teaching plan for clients having a gastroplasty or intestinal bypass.

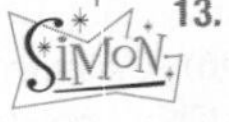

Go to http://www.wbsaunders.com/SIMON/Iggy/ for self-assessment questions related to these Learning Objectives.

Nutrition plays a major role in promoting and maintaining health. Nutritional health not only contributes to positive care outcomes but also saves health care dollars. As part of a comprehensive health assessment, the nurse should include nutritional screening to identify clients who have nutritional deficits or are at risk for developing nutritional deficits. Nurses may also conduct a complete nutritional assessment (Grindel & Costello, 1996).

NUTRITION STANDARDS

Dietary Planning

Several national standards are available for planning and evaluating nutrition. The standard most widely accepted in the United States is the Recommended Dietary Allowance (RDA), established in 1943 by the Food and Nutrition Board (FNB) of the National Research Council/National Academy of Sciences. The most current revision in 1989 establishes recommendations for energy intake, protein, vitamins, and minerals for a healthy population. Healthy adults require approximately 1800 calories/day and 0.8 g of protein/kg of body weight to meet basal energy needs.

The RDA can be used to estimate the adequacy of nutrient intake over time. If a client does not meet 100% of the RDA, it is incorrect to assume that he or she is nutritionally deficient. The risk of inadequate intake for any nutrient is not presumed to be increased until less than 70% of the RDA is consumed. It is also incorrect to assume that all clients in a specific population who meet 100% of the RDA are not at risk for malnutrition.

The FNB, with the involvement of Health Canada, has recommended Dietary Reference Intakes (DRI) replace the RDA. The first DRI released recommended the intake of nutrients related to bone health (Food and Nutrition Board, 1997). The established standard of Canada, the Recommended Nutrient Intake (RNI), is similar to that of the United States.

Disease Prevention and Health Promotion

The role of diet and nutrition in disease has been a subject of interest for many years. The current focus is on health promotion and the prevention of disease. In 1995, the Dietary Guidelines for Americans were revised by the U.S. Department of Agriculture (USDA) and the U.S. Department of Health and Human Services (DHHS). These seven guidelines emphasize the importance of selecting foods to maintain a healthful diet with balance, moderation, and variety (Figure 61-1). One of the most noticeable changes from previous editions occurs in the weight guideline. For the first time, diet and physical activity are emphasized in the second guideline with the goal of maintaining or improving body weight (Kennedy, Meyers, & Layden, 1996).

The Nutrition Recommendations for Canadians (Table 61-1) are similar to the Dietary Guidelines for Americans. In addition, they recommend limiting the caffeine content of the diet to no more than the equivalent of four cups of coffee per day, as well as adding fluoride to community water supplies to a level of 1 mg/L.

The USDA developed the Food Guide Pyramid in 1992 to translate food recommendations into a practical graphic format (Figure 61-2). A pyramid format was chosen to communicate three key dietary principles: variety, moderation, and proportionality. The pyramid design emphasizes building the diet on a base of grains, fruits, and vegetables. Moderate quantities of lean meats, protein sources, and dairy products are added, and the intake of fats and sweets is limited. This guide to daily food choices has replaced the basic four food groups as the standard for evaluating the nutritional adequacy of dietary intake. Table 61-2 suggests the daily servings of each food group and clarifies the size of a serving. Adhering to this pattern results in a nutritionally adequate intake if a variety of foods is chosen.

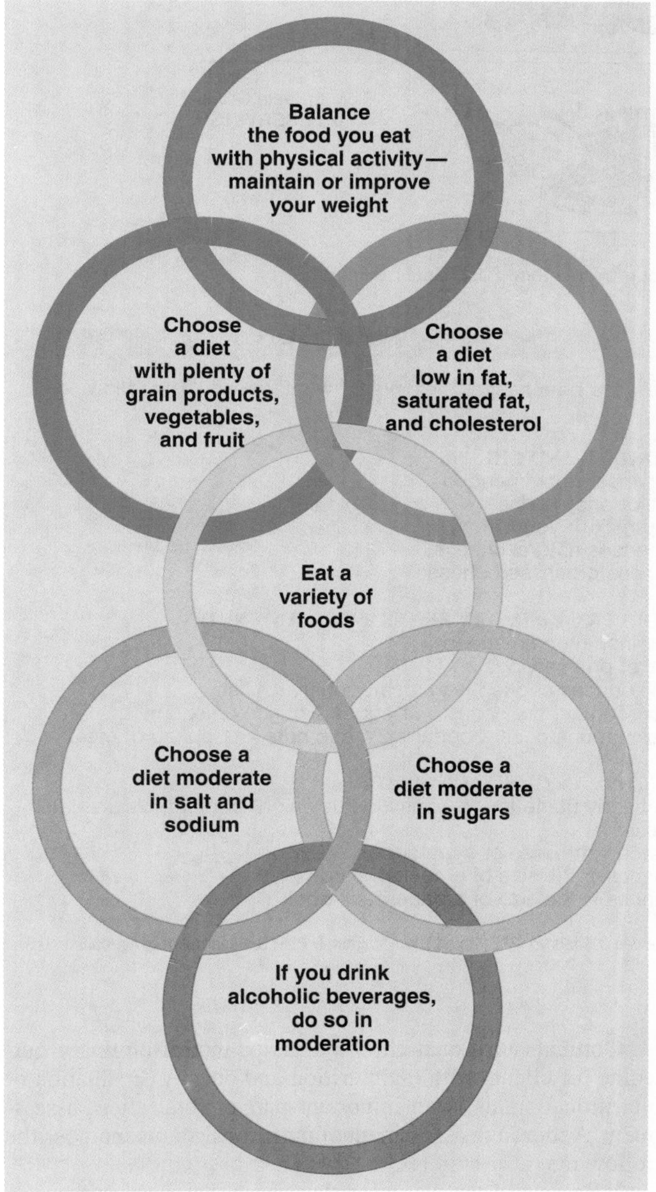

Figure 61-1 ● Dietary guidelines developed by the U.S. Department of Agriculture and the U.S. Department of Health and Human Services.

A variety of vegetarian diet patterns are being adopted by increasing numbers of people for health, environmental, and moral reasons. The **lacto-vegetarian** eats milk, cheese, and dairy foods but avoids meat, fish, poultry, and eggs. The **lacto-ovo-vegetarian** also includes eggs. The **vegan** eats only foods of plant origin. Vegans can develop megaloblastic anemia as a result of vitamin B_{12} deficiency. Vegans should include a daily source of vitamin B_{12} in their diets, such as a fortified breakfast cereal, fortified soy beverage, or meat analog (Messina & Burke, 1997). All vegetarians should ensure that they get adequate amounts of calcium, iron, zinc, and vitamins D and B_{12}. Well-planned vegetarian diets can provide adequate nutrition. The Vegetarian Food Pyramid, endorsed by the Vegetarian Resource Group, can assist vegetarians with daily food choices (Figure 61-3).

NUTRITIONAL ASSESSMENT

Malnutrition and obesity are common nutrition problems that occur as progressive changes within the client. When nutritional deficiencies or excesses develop, the body adapts through the use of homeostatic mechanisms. As the intake moves farther away from the accepted range, however, the body accommodates by reducing functional levels or changing the status or size of the affected body compartments. The nutritional status of a client can be determined by the presence or absence of these adaptations.

Nutritional status reflects the balance between nutrient requirements and nutrient intake. Factors affecting nutrient requirements include disease, infection, and psychologic stress. Nutrient intake is influenced by disease, eating behavior, economic factors, emotional stability, medication, and cultural factors.

TABLE 61-1 • NUTRITION RECOMMENDATIONS FOR CANADIANS

- The sodium content of the Canadian diet should be reduced.
- The Canadian diet should include no more than 5% of total energy as alcohol, or two drinks daily, whichever is less.
- The Canadian diet should contain no more caffeine than the equivalent of four cups of regular coffee per day.
- Community water supplies containing less than 1 mg/L of fluoride should be fluoridated to that level.
- The Canadian diet should provide energy consistent with the maintenance of body weight within the recommended range.
- The Canadian diet should include essential nutrients in amounts specified in the Recommended Nutrient Intake.
- The Canadian diet should include no more than 30% of energy as fat (33 g/1000 kcal or 39 g/5000 kJ) and no more than 10% as saturated fat (11 g/1000 kcal or 13 g/5000 kJ).
- The Canadian diet should provide 55% of energy as carbohydrates (138 g/1000 kcal or 165 g/5000 kJ) from a variety of sources.

From Communications/Implementation Committee, Minister of National Health and Welfare. (1990). *Action towards healthy eating: Canada's guidelines for healthy eating and recommended strategies for implementation.* Cat. No. H39-166/1990E. Ottawa: Branch Publications Unit.

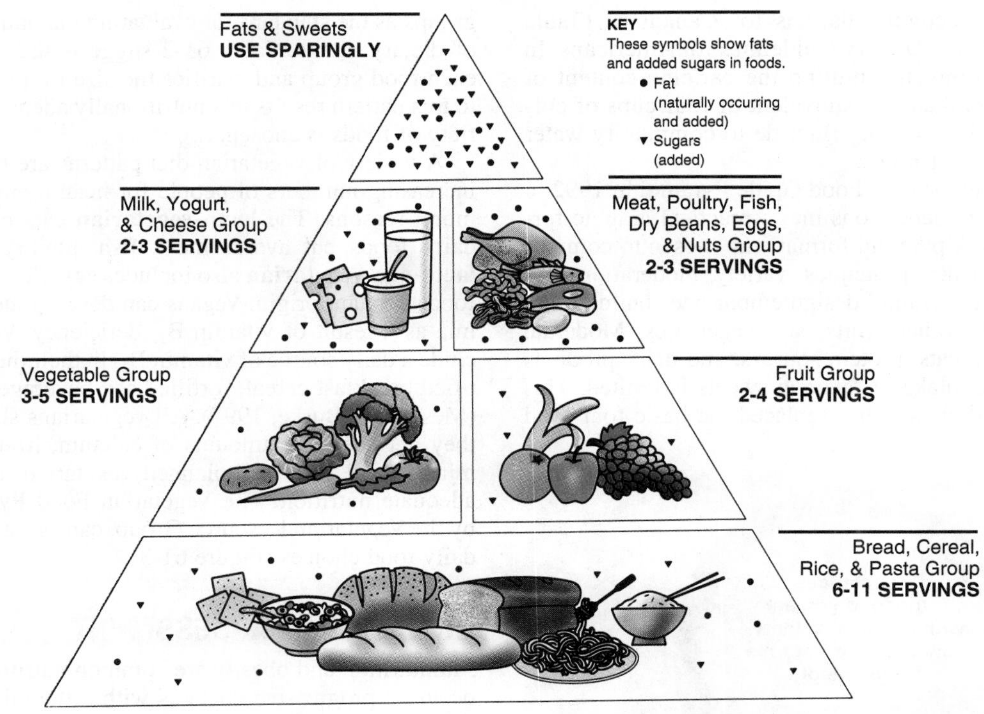

Figure 61-2 ● The U.S. Department of Agriculture Food Guide Pyramid.

TABLE 61-2 • SERVING SIZES FOR EACH FOOD GROUP

With the Food Guide Pyramid, what counts as a "serving" may not always be a typical "helping" of what you eat. The following are some examples of servings.

BREAD, CEREAL, RICE, AND PASTA
6 to 11 servings recommended
Examples of one serving:
- 1 slice of bread
- 1 ounce ready-to-eat cereal
- ½ cup cooked cereal, rice, or pasta

VEGETABLES
3 to 5 servings recommended
Examples of one serving:
- 1 cup raw leafy vegetables
- ½ cup other vegetables, cooked or chopped raw
- ¾ cup vegetable juice

FRUITS
2 to 4 servings recommended
Examples of one serving:
- 1 medium apple, banana, or orange
- ½ cup chopped, cooked, or canned fruit
- ¾ cup fruit juice

MILK, YOGURT, AND CHEESE
2 to 3 servings recommended
Examples of one serving:
- 1 cup milk or yogurt
- 1½ ounces natural cheese
- 2 ounces processed cheese

MEAT, POULTRY, FISH, DRY BEANS, EGGS, AND NUTS
2 to 3 servings recommended
Examples of one serving:
- 2 to 3 ounces cooked lean meat, poultry, or fish
- ½ cup cooked dry beans or 1 egg = 1 ounce of lean meat
- 2 tablespoons peanut butter or ⅓ cup nuts = 1 ounce of meat

HOW MUCH IS AN OUNCE OF MEAT?
Here is a handy guide for determining the weight of meat, chicken, fish, or cheese:
- 1 ounce = the size of a matchbox
- 3 ounces = the size of a deck of cards
- 8 ounces = the size of a paperback book

Modified from Nutrition and your health: Dietary guidelines for Americans. (1995). *Home and Garden Bulletin No. 232* (4th ed.). Washington, D.C.: U.S. Department of Agriculture, U.S. Department of Health and Human Services.

CULTURAL CONSIDERATIONS

Lactose intolerance (inability to tolerate milk and milk products) is a relatively common condition that occurs in a number of ethnic groups. It is found in more than 66% of Mexican Americans and 79% of African Americans, as well as in some Native American tribes, Asian Americans, and Ashkenazic Jews (Giger & Davidhizar, 1999). A small percentage of Caucasians are also lactose intolerant. The cause of lactose intolerance is an insufficient amount of the lactase enzyme, which converts lactose into absorbable glucose.

Optimal nutritional care is a major interdisciplinary outcome for clients with malnutrition and obesity. Evaluation of nutritional status is an important part of total client assessment. A thorough assessment of nutritional status includes the following:

- Review of the diet history
- Food and fluid intake record
- Laboratory data
- Food-medication interactions
- Physical examination and health history

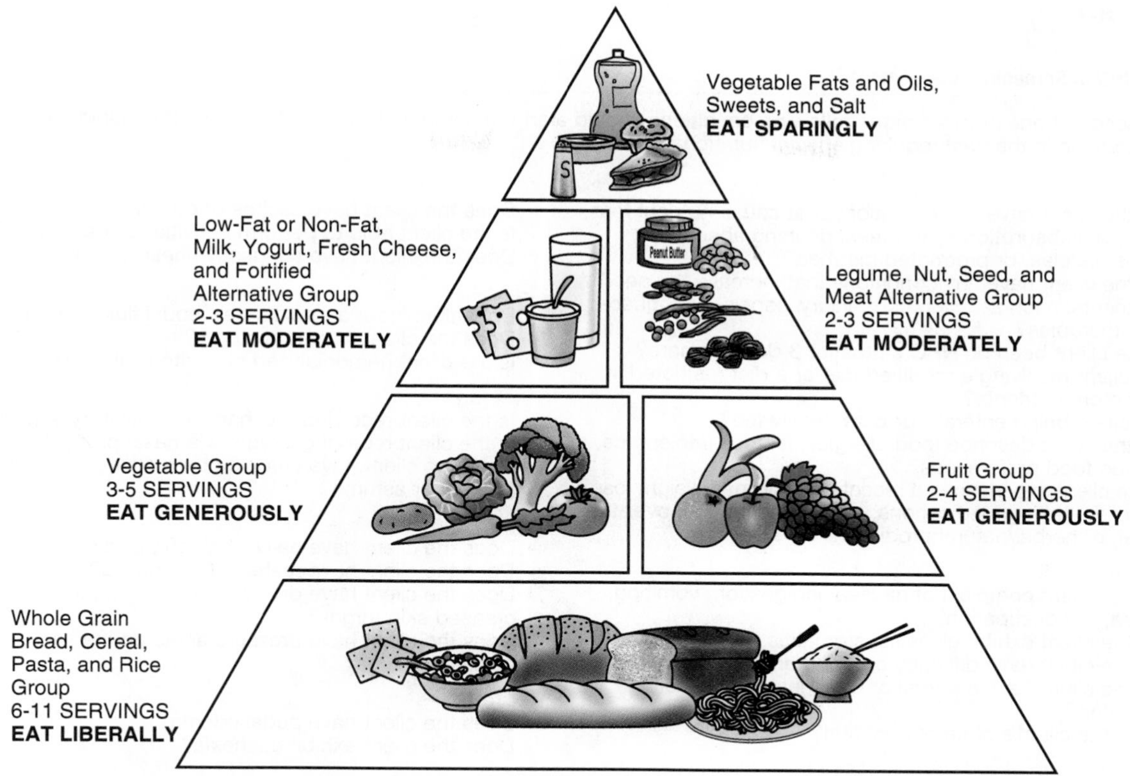

Figure 61-3 ● Food pyramid for a vegetarian diet. (Courtesy The Health Connection.)

- Anthropometric measurements
- Psychosocial assessment

Monitoring the nutritional care of a client is as important as the initial assessment. The health care provider, nurse, and dietitian collaborate to identify clients at risk for nutritional problems.

Initial Nutritional Screening

Not every client needs a complete nutritional assessment, but it is important to identify clients at risk for nutritional problems through screening. An initial nutritional screening provides the nurse with an inexpensive, quick way of determining which clients need more extensive nutritional assessment by the health care provider and dietitian.

The initial nutritional screening includes visual inspection, measured height and weight, weight history, usual eating habits, ability to chew and swallow, and any recent changes in appetite or food intake. Questions that may alert the nurse to clients at risk for nutritional problems can be incorporated into the history and physical assessment (Chart 61-1).

CONSIDERATIONS FOR OLDER ADULTS

Nutritional screening can take place in the home, ambulatory care setting, hospital, or nursing home. The Nutrition Screening Manual for Professionals Caring for Older Americans (1991) is a multidisciplinary project of the American Dietetic Association, the American Academy of Family Physicians, and the National Council on the Aging. The goal of this 5-year initiative was to use a collaboration of health care professionals to promote routine nutrition screening to older Americans in all community health and medical care settings. Risk factors for malnutrition in older adults include inappropriate intake, poverty, social isolation, dependency or disability, acute or chronic diseases or conditions, and chronic medication use. The Nutrition Screening initiative developed a three-tiered approach to nutrition screening:

1. The *DETERMINE* Your Nutritional Health Checklist to alert older adults about the warning signs for poor nutritional health (Figure 61-4)
2. The Level I screen developed for use by professionals in health or social service settings, such as adult day-care centers, congregate meal programs, and assisted-living facilities
3. The Level II screen developed for use in medical settings such as acute care hospitals, physicians' offices, and long-term care facilities.

Another nutritional assessment tool, the Mini Nutritional Assessment (MNA), has recently been designed and tested worldwide to provide a single, rapid assessment of older adults in ambulatory care, hospitals, and nursing homes (Vellas et al., 1999). The MNA can be completed in about 10 minutes; a low score indicates malnutrition or a risk for malnutrition.

Anthropometric Measurements

Anthropometric measurements are noninvasive methods of evaluating nutritional status. These measurements include height and weight and assessment of body fat.

CHART 61-1

BEST PRACTICE *for*
Initial Nutrition Screening Assessment

The presence of one or more of the following conditions should alert the nurse that the client is at risk for malnutrition or has had a condition in the past requiring special nutritional care.

General
- Does the client have any conditions that cause nutrient loss, such as malabsorption syndromes, draining abscesses, wounds, fistulas, or protracted diarrhea?
- Does the client have any conditions that increase the need for nutrients, such as fever, burn, injury, sepsis, or antineoplastic therapies?
- Has the client been on NPO status for 3 days or more?
- Is the client receiving a modified diet or a diet restricted in one or more nutrients?
- Is the client being enterally or parenterally fed?
- Does the client describe food allergies, lactose intolerance, or limited food preferences?
- Has the client experienced a recent, unexplained weight loss?
- Is the client taking medications, either prescription, over-the-counter, or herbal/natural products?

Gastrointestinal
- Does the client complain of nausea, indigestion, vomiting, diarrhea, or constipation?
- Does the client exhibit glossitis, stomatitis, or esophagitis?
- Does the client have difficulty chewing or swallowing?
- Does the client have a partial or total gastrointestinal obstruction?
- What is the client's state of dentition?

Cardiovascular
- Does the client have ascites or edema?
- Is the client able to perform activities of daily living?
- Does the client have congestive heart failure?

Genitourinary
- Does fluid input approximately equal fluid output?
- Does the client have an ostomy?
- Is the client hemodialyzed or peritoneally dialyzed?

Respiratory
- Is the client receiving mechanical ventilatory support?
- Is the client receiving oxygen via nasal prongs?
- Does the client have chronic obstructive pulmonary disease (COPD) or asthma?

Integumentary
- Does the client have nail or hair changes?
- Does the client have rashes or dermatitis?
- Does the client have dry or pale mucous membranes or decreased skin turgor?
- Does the client have pressure areas on the sacrum, hips, or ankles?

Extremities
- Does the client have pedal edema?
- Does the client exhibit cachexia?

Modified with permission of Ross Products Division, Abbott Laboratories, Columbus, OH.
NPO, Nothing by mouth.

MEASUREMENT OF HEIGHT AND WEIGHT

Height and weight provide a baseline determination of nutritional status. The nurse or assistive nursing personnel obtains accurate measurements, because clients who report their own measurements tend to overestimate height and underestimate weight. Subsequent measurements may indicate an early change in nutritional status.

Height

Clients should be measured and weighed while wearing minimal clothing and no shoes. The nurse or assistive nursing personnel determines the client's height in inches or centimeters with the measuring stick of a weight scale. The client should stand erect and look straight ahead, with the heels together and the arms at the sides.

CONSIDERATIONS FOR OLDER ADULTS
Some older adults may have difficulty standing erect, and their actual height may be less than their height on recall. If height cannot be measured directly, it should be estimated by arm span or with use of a knee-height caliper, which provides a more precise height estimate.

Weight

The nurse or assistive nursing personnel weighs ambulatory clients with an upright balance beam scale. Nonambulatory clients can be weighed with a movable wheelchair balance beam scale or a bed scale. The manufacturer should calibrate weight scales twice yearly to ensure accurate readings. For daily or sequential weights, the nurse or assistive nursing personnel notes the time and obtains the weight at the same time each day, if possible. Conditions such as heart failure and renal disease affect fluid balance and, therefore, weight.

Normal weights for adult men and women are shown in the Metropolitan Life tables (Table 61-3). The latest U.S. Department of Agriculture (USDA) and U.S. Department of Health and Human Services (DHHS) Dietary Guidelines contain weight guidelines that emphasize both weight maintenance and weight loss. The same healthy weight guideline applies to all adults. Older adults are no longer permitted a higher weight standard. The weight range appears in the guidelines as a chart with three categories: healthy weight, moderate overweight, and severe overweight (Figure 61-5). Either the Metropolitan Life tables or the New Weight Guidelines from the USDA and the DHHS may be used for comparison with a client's height and weight. Some health care professionals prefer the Metropolitan Life tables because they consider body build differences by gender.

Changes in body weight can be expressed by three different formulas:

1. Weight as a percentage of ideal body weight (IBW):

$$\%\text{IBW} = \frac{\text{Current weight} \times 100}{\text{Ideal weight}}$$

2. Current weight as a percentage of usual body weight (UBW):

$$\%\text{UBW} = \frac{\text{Current weight} \times 100}{\text{Usual weight}}$$

3. Change in weight:

$$\text{Weight change} = \frac{\text{Usual weight} - \text{Current weight}}{\text{Usual weight}} \times 100$$

The Warning Signs of poor nutritional health are often overlooked. Use this checklist to find out if you or someone you know is at nutritional risk.

DETERMINE YOUR NUTRITIONAL HEALTH

Read the statements below. Circle the number in the yes column for those that apply to you or someone you know. For each yes answer, score the number in the box. Total your nutritional score.

	YES
I have an illness or condition that made me change the kind and/or amount of food I eat.	2
I eat fewer than 2 meals per day.	3
I eat few fruits or vegetables, or milk products.	2
I have 3 or more drinks of beer, liquor or wine almost every day.	2
I have tooth or mouth problems that make it hard for me to eat.	2
I don't always have enough money to buy the food I need.	4
I eat alone most of the time.	1
I take 3 or more different prescribed or over-the-counter drugs a day.	1
Without wanting to, I have lost or gained 10 pounds in the last 6 months.	2
I am not always physically able to shop, cook and/or feed myself.	2
TOTAL	

Total Your Nutritional Score. If it's —

0-2 **Good!** Recheck your nutritional score in 6 months.

3-5 **You are at moderate nutritional risk.** See what can be done to improve your eating habits and lifestyle. Your office on aging, senior nutrition program, senior citizens center or health department can help. Recheck your nutritional score in 3 months.

6 or more **You are at high nutritional risk.** Bring this checklist the next time you see your doctor, dietitian or other qualified health or social service professional. Talk with them about any problems you may have. Ask for help to improve your nutritional health.

Remember that warning signs suggest risk, but do not represent diagnosis of any condition. Turn the page to learn more about the Warning Signs of poor nutritional health.

These materials developed and distributed by the Nutrition Screening Initiative, a project of:

AMERICAN ACADEMY OF FAMILY PHYSICIANS

THE AMERICAN DIETETIC ASSOCIATION

NATIONAL COUNCIL ON THE AGING, INC.

Figure 61-4 ● "DETERMINE Your Nutritional Health" checklist used to alert older adults to the warning signs of poor nutritional health. (Courtesy The Nutrition Screening Initiative, Washington, D.C.)

Continued

The Nutrition Checklist is based on the Warning Signs described below. Use the word DETERMINE to remind you of the Warning Signs.

DISEASE

Any disease, illness or chronic condition which causes you to change the way you eat, or makes it hard for you to eat, puts your nutritional health at risk. Four out of five adults have chronic diseases that are affected by diet. Confusion or memory loss that keeps getting worse is estimated to affect one out of five or more of older adults. This can make it hard to remember what, when or if you've eaten. Feeling sad or depressed, which happens to about one in eight older adults, can cause big changes in appetite, digestion, energy level, weight and well-being.

EATING POORLY

Eating too little and eating too much both lead to poor health. Eating the same foods day after day or not eating fruit, vegetables, and milk products daily will also cause poor nutritional health. One in five adults skip meals daily. Only 13% of adults eat the minimum amount of fruit and vegetables needed. One in four older adults drink too much alcohol. Many health problems become worse if you drink more than one or two alcoholic beverages per day.

TOOTH LOSS/ MOUTH PAIN

A healthy mouth, teeth and gums are needed to eat. Missing, loose or rotten teeth or dentures which don't fit well or cause mouth sores make it hard to eat.

ECONOMIC HARDSHIP

As many as 40% of older Americans have incomes of less than $6,000 per year. Having less—or choosing to spend less—than $25-30 per week for food makes it very hard to get the foods you need to stay healthy.

REDUCED SOCIAL CONTACT

One third of all older people live alone. Being with people daily has a positive effect on morale, well-being and eating.

MULTIPLE MEDICINES

Many older Americans must take medicines for health problems. Almost half of older Americans take multiple medicines daily. Growing old may change the way we respond to drugs. The more medicines you take, the greater the chance for side effects such as increased or decreased appetite, change in taste, constipation, weakness, drowsiness, diarrhea, nausea, and others. Vitamins or minerals when taken in large doses act like drugs and can cause harm. Alert your doctor to everything you take.

INVOLUNTARY WEIGHT LOSS/GAIN

Losing or gaining a lot of weight when you are not trying to do so is an important warning sign that must not be ignored. Being overweight or underweight also increases your chance of poor health.

NEEDS ASSISTANCE IN SELF CARE

Although most older people are able to eat, one of every five have trouble walking, shopping, buying and cooking food, especially as they get older.

ELDER YEARS ABOVE AGE 80

Most older people lead full and productive lives. But as age increases, risk of frailty and health problems increase. Checking your nutritional health regularly makes good sense.

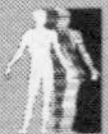

The Nutrition Screening Initiative • 1010 Wisconsin Avenue, NW • Suite 800 • Washington, DC 20007
The Nutrition Screening Initiative is funded in part by a grant from Ross Laboratories, a division of Abbott Laboratories.

Figure 61-4, cont'd • "DETERMINE Your Nutritional Health" checklist used to alert older adults to the warning signs of poor nutritional health. (Courtesy The Nutrition Screening Initiative, Washington, D.C.)

TABLE 61-3 • METROPOLITAN LIFE HEIGHT AND WEIGHT TABLES

Height*		Weight†			Height*		Weight†		
Feet	Inches	Small Frame	Medium Frame	Large Frame	Feet	Inches	Small Frame	Medium Frame	Large Frame
MEN					**WOMEN**				
5	2	128-134	131-134	138-150	4	10	102-111	109-121	118-131
5	3	130-136	133-143	140-153	4	11	103-113	111-123	120-134
5	4	132-138	135-145	142-156	5	0	104-115	113-126	122-137
5	5	134-140	137-148	144-160	5	1	106-118	115-129	125-140
5	6	136-142	139-151	146-164	5	2	108-121	118-132	128-143
5	7	138-145	142-154	149-168	5	3	111-124	121-135	131-147
5	8	140-148	145-157	152-172	5	4	114-127	124-138	134-151
5	9	142-151	148-160	155-176	5	5	117-130	127-141	137-155
5	10	144-154	151-163	158-180	5	6	120-133	130-144	140-159
5	11	146-157	154-166	161-184	5	7	123-136	133-147	143-163
6	0	149-160	157-170	164-188	5	8	126-139	136-150	146-167
6	1	152-164	160-174	168-192	5	9	129-142	139-153	149-170
6	2	155-168	164-178	172-197	5	10	132-145	142-156	152-173
6	3	158-172	167-182	176-202	5	11	135-148	145-159	155-176
6	4	162-176	171-187	181-207	6	0	138-151	148-162	158-179

Reprinted courtesy of Metropolitan Life Insurance Company, 1983.
*Shoes with 1-inch heels.
†Weight in pounds. Men: allow 5 pounds of clothing. Women: allow 3 pounds of clothing

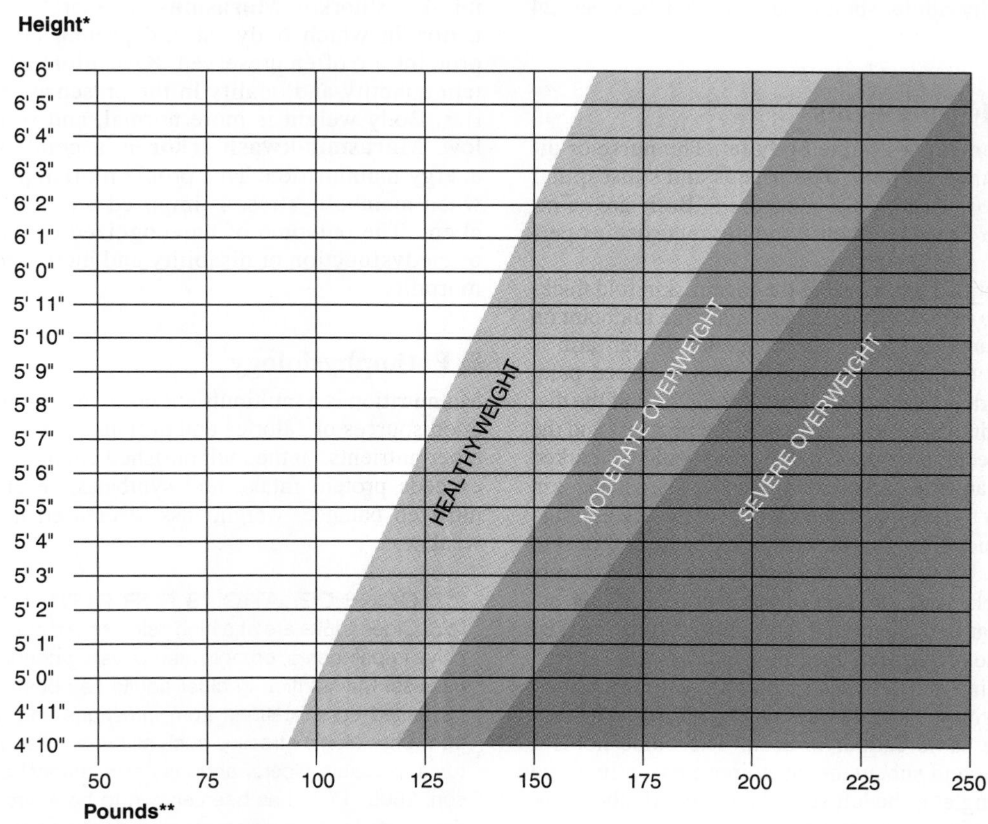

* Without shoes.
** Without clothes. The higher weights apply to people with more muscle and bone, such as many men.

Figure 61-5 ● The U.S Department of Agriculture and the U.S. Department of Health and Human Services guidelines for determining proper weight or degree of obesity. (Redrawn from http://www.nalusda.gov/fnic/Dietary/9dietgui.htm.)

An involuntary weight loss of 10% at any time significantly affects nutritional status. Weights may need to be taken daily, several times a week, or weekly for monitoring status and the effectiveness of nutritional support.

ASSESSMENT OF BODY FAT

Body Mass Index

The body mass index (BMI), or Quetelet index, is a measure of nutritional status that does not depend on frame size. The BMI indirectly estimates total fat stores within the body by the relationship of weight to height:

$$\text{BMI} = \frac{\text{Weight (kg)}}{\text{Height}^2\ (\text{m}^2)}$$

A simpler calculation for estimating BMI can be programmed into handheld computers:

$$\text{BMI} = \frac{\text{Weight (lb)}}{\text{Height}^2\ (\text{inches}^2)} \times 705$$

BMI can also be determined using a nomogram. The least risk of death from malnutrition is associated with scores between 20 and 25 (Mahan & Escot-Stump, 1996). BMIs above and below these values are associated with increased health risks. Older, healthy adults should have a BMI between 24 and 27.

Skin Fold Measurements

Skin fold measurements estimate body fat. The nurse or dietitian may measure the client. The triceps and subscapular skin folds are most commonly measured. Both are compared with standard measurements and are recorded as percentiles.

The nurse or dietitian can measure the triceps skin fold thickness by using a tape measure to locate and mark the midpoint on the client's upper arm. To obtain the midpoint, the left arm is bent 90 degrees at the elbow, and the forearm is placed palm down across the middle of the body. The midpoint is half the distance between the tip of the shoulder (acromion process) and the tip of the elbow (olecranon process). The skin should be marked at this point before any measurements are made. The triceps skin fold is measured on the back of the left arm over the triceps muscle at the marked midpoint. The nurse holds a double fold of skin and subcutaneous adipose tissue between the fingers and thumb. The skin fold is held until the jaws of the skin fold caliper are placed perpendicular to the length of the skin fold at the marked midpoint. The nurse records this measurement.

Subscapular skin fold thickness indirectly estimates body fat. The body position is the same as for triceps skin fold thickness, and the same caliper is used. The nurse holds a double fold of skin and subcutaneous adipose tissue in a line from the inferior angle of the left scapula to the left elbow, applies the calipers, and records the measurement.

Arm Circumference

The midarm circumference (MAC) can be obtained to measure muscle mass and subcutaneous fat. To measure MAC, the nurse or dietitian places a flexible tape around the arm at the same marked midpoint used to measure skin fold thickness, taking care to hold the tape firmly but gently to avoid compressing the tissue. This measurement is recorded in centimeters. The midarm muscle mass (MAMM) measures the amount of muscle in the body and is a more sensitive indicator of protein reserves. It can be computed from the MAC and the triceps skin fold measure.

MALNUTRITION

OVERVIEW

Carbohydrates, protein, and fat supply the body with energy. Under healthy conditions, the majority of this energy undergoes digestion and is absorbed from the gastrointestinal tract. Food energy is used to maintain body temperature, respiration, cardiac output, muscle function, protein synthesis, and the storage and metabolism of food sources.

Energy balance refers to the relationship between energy expended and energy stored. When energy expended exceeds energy intake, energy stores are used to supply the deficit; this results in weight loss. Body proteins are used for energy when calorie intake is insufficient. The body attempts to meet its calorie requirements even if it is at the expense of protein needs.

Many severely ill or traumatized hospitalized clients are at risk for **protein-calorie malnutrition (PCM),** also known as protein-energy malnutrition (PEM). PCM may present in three forms: marasmus, kwashiorkor, and marasmic-kwashiorkor. **Marasmus** is generally a calorie malnutrition in which body fat and protein are wasted. Serum proteins are often preserved. **Kwashiorkor** is a lack of protein quantity and quality in the presence of adequate calories. Body weight is more normal, and serum proteins are low. **Marasmic-kwashiorkor** is a combined protein and energy malnutrition. This problem often presents clinically when metabolic stress is imposed on a chronically starved client. The outcome of unrecognized or untreated PCM is often dysfunction or disability and increased morbidity and mortality.

Pathophysiology

Malnutrition is a multinutrient problem because foods that are good sources of calories and protein are also good sources of other nutrients. In the malnourished client, protein catabolism exceeds protein intake and synthesis, resulting in negative nitrogen balance, weight loss, decreased muscle mass, and weakness.

> **CONSIDERATIONS FOR OLDER ADULTS**
> Older adults are at a high risk for poor nutrition due to cognitive impairments, complicated physical conditions, or chronic disease. Malnutrition in older adults has been associated with increased complications from infections and slower recovery from physiologic stresses such as surgical wounds, bone fractures, pressure ulcers, and loss of functional capacity (Anderson, 2000). PCM has been shown to be a strong independent risk factor for 1-year posthospital discharge mortality.

The functional ability of the liver, heart, lungs, gastrointestinal tract, and immune system diminishes in the client with malnutrition. A decrease in serum proteins **(hypoproteinemia)** occurs as protein synthesis in the liver decreases. Vital capacity is also reduced as a result of respiratory muscle atrophy; cardiac output diminishes. Malabsorption occurs because of atrophy of gastrointestinal mucosa and the loss of intestinal villi.

Other complications of severe malnutrition in adults include the following:

- Leanness and cachexia (muscle wasting)
- Decreased effort tolerance
- Lethargy
- Intolerance to cold
- Edema
- Dry, flaking skin and various types of dermatitis
- Poor wound healing and a higher than usual number of infections, particularly postoperative infection

Etiology

Malnutrition results from inadequate nutrient intake, increased nutrient losses, and increased nutrient requirements. Inadequate nutrient intake can be linked to poverty, lack of education, substance abuse, decreased appetite, and a decline in functional ability to eat independently. Infectious diseases, such as tuberculosis and human immunodeficiency virus (HIV) infection, are also precipitating factors in PCM. Diseases that produce diarrhea and respiratory and other infections leading to anorexia result in negative calorie and protein balance; anorexia then leads to poor food intake. Vomiting leads to decreased absorption with increased nutrient losses. Medical treatments such as chemotherapy can also cause malnutrition. In addition, catabolic processes increase nutrient requirements and metabolic losses.

Inadequate nutrient intake can also result when a person is admitted to the hospital or nursing home (Dudek, 2000). Decreased staffing may not allow time for clients who need to be fed, especially older adults who may eat slowly (Anderson, 2000). Many diagnostic tests and surgery require a period of having nothing by mouth (NPO).

Unrecognized dysphagia is a common problem in nursing homes and can cause malnutrition, dehydration, and aspiration pneumonia. A study by Kayser-Jones and Pengilly (1999) found that 45 of 82 residents in one nursing home had some degree of dysphagia (difficulty swallowing) ranging from mild to profound. Only 10 of the 45 residents had been referred for dysphagia evaluation by a speech-language pathologist.

Eating disorders, such as anorexia nervosa and bulimia nervosa, also lead to malnutrition. **Anorexia nervosa** is a self-induced starvation resulting from a fear of fatness, even though the client is underweight. **Bulimia nervosa** is characterized by episodes of binge eating in which the client ingests a large amount of food in a short time. The binge eating is followed by some form of purging behavior, such as self-induced vomiting and/or an excessive use of laxatives and diuretics. If not treated, death can result from starvation, infection, or suicide. Information about eating disorders can be found in textbooks on mental health nursing.

Incidence/Prevalence

Malnutrition is present in many hospitalized clients (Dudek, 2000). In a review of eight studies with more than 1347 hospitalized adults, 40% to 55% were determined to be malnourished or at risk for malnutrition, and up to 12% were severely malnourished. Malnourished clients heal more slowly, suffer more complications, and have a higher mortality rate. Surgical clients with a likelihood of malnutrition were two to three times more likely to experience minor and major complications and excess mortality. Length of hospitalization in malnourished medical-surgical clients can be extended by as much as 90%, which clearly increases health care costs (Gallagher-Allred et al., 1996).

The prevalence of PCM in long-term care facilities has been reported to range from 10% to 85% (Anderson, 2000). In one study, the prevalence of malnutrition in 100 clients admitted consecutively to a skilled nursing facility was 39%. The highest prevalence of malnutrition was found in clients admitted from acute care hospitals (Nelson et al., 1993).

Acute PCM may develop in clients who were adequately nourished before hospitalization if they experience starvation while in a catabolic state from infection, stress, or injury. *Chronic* PCM can occur in clients who have cancer, end-stage renal or hepatic disease, or chronic neurologic disease.

WOMEN'S HEALTH CONSIDERATIONS

As many as 25% of the general older adult population may be malnourished, most of them women (Wellman, 1997). Older women are particularly at risk for PCM (Chart 61-2) because of the following:

- Acute and chronic disease
- Processes that lead to a reduction of food intake
- Malabsorption and maldigestion
- Decreased efficiency of nutrient use
- Multiple medication therapy
- Poverty
- Social isolation
- Dependency/disability

Women, especially adolescents and young adults, are more likely than men to have eating disorders. Caucasian women are at the highest risk for these health problems.

CULTURAL CONSIDERATIONS

In Western countries, cultural factors do not seem to have a major influence on the development of malnutrition. However, newly arriving immigrants from developing countries may be at risk for malnutrition because of limited food supplies, poverty, and eating habits.

In the Native American population of the United States, poor nutrition has also been directly related to several leading causes of death, including heart disease and cirrhosis of the liver. The diets of many Native American tribes continue to be inadequate in protein, calcium, and vitamins A and C. These deficiencies may result from an unavailability of or a lack of money to purchase foods that are high in these nutrients (Giger & Davidhizar, 1999).

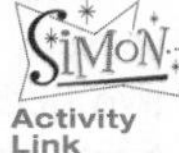

COLLABORATIVE MANAGEMENT

Assessment

HISTORY

The nurse reviews the medical history to determine the diagnosis, possibility of increased metabolic needs or nutritional losses, chronic disease, recent surgery of the gastrointestinal tract, drug and alcohol abuse, and recent, significant weight loss. Each of these conditions can contribute to malnutrition. For older adults, the nurse also explores mental status deterioration, poor eyesight or hearing, diseases affecting major organs, constipation or incontinence, slowed reactions, a review of prescription and over-the-counter medications (including herbal and natural supplements), and physical disabilities.

CHART 61-2

NURSING FOCUS *on the* OLDER ADULT
Risk Assessment for Malnutrition

- Recognize that clinical manifestations of malnutrition may not be apparent because they are similar to physiologic changes associated with aging (e.g., dry skin, decreased muscle tone, dry hair).
- Assess body weight and compare it with the usual body weight or ideal body weight.
- Be aware that multiple chronic diseases, especially gastrointestinal disorders such as malabsorption syndromes, predispose the client to malnutrition.
- Assess the client's financial ability to buy healthy food.
- Assess the client's physical and mental ability to prepare food.
- Inspect the client's oral cavity for the presence of teeth or dentures, gum disease, or oral lesions that could affect food intake.
- Review the client's medications, including prescription and over-the-counter (OTC) drugs. Many drugs interact with food or cause anorexia or nausea.
- Use the DETERMINE checklist and Level I or II screen, if appropriate.

For clients who live independently, the nurse or occupational therapist assesses the performance of instrumental activities of daily living (IADLs). Functional status can best be evaluated for institutionalized clients by assessing their performance of activities of daily living (ADLs). An inability to perform any of the eight IADLs or any of the six ADLs indicates a high level of dependence and the potential for disease and poor nutritional status (*Nutrition Screening Manual,* 1991). When functional status is evaluated with nutritional status, there appears to be a strong predictability of infections and complications among institutionalized adults. Chapter 10 describes functional assessment in detail.

The nurse interviews the client to obtain information about his or her usual daily food intake, eating behaviors, change in appetite, and recent weight changes. The client is asked to describe the usual foods eaten daily and the times of meals and snacks. This information is then compared with the Food Guide Pyramid for gross deficiencies. The dietitian can more thoroughly analyze the diet, if necessary.

The nurse explores with the client any changes in eating habits as a result of illness. Any change in appetite, taste, and weight loss is recorded. A weight loss of 5% or more in 30 days, a weight loss of 10% in 6 months, or a weight that is below ideal body weight is significant for malnutrition.

Difficulty or pain in chewing or swallowing is also assessed. The nurse asks the client whether any foods are avoided and why. The occurrence of nausea, vomiting, heartburn, or any other symptoms of discomfort with eating is also recorded. Finally, the client is asked about dental health problems, including the presence of dentures. Dentures or partial plates that do not fit well interfere with food intake.

TABLE 61-4 • SIGNS AND SYMPTOMS OF NUTRIENT DEFICIENCIES

Sign/Symptom	Potential Nutrient Deficiency
HAIR	
Alopecia	Zinc, essential fatty acids
Easy pluckability	Protein, essential fatty acids
Lackluster hair	Protein, zinc
"Corkscrew" hair	Vitamin C, vitamin A
Decreased pigmentation	Protein, copper
EYES	
Xerosis of conjunctiva	Vitamin A
Corneal vascularization	Riboflavin
Keratomalacia	Vitamin A
Bitot's spots	Vitamin A
GASTROINTESTINAL TRACT	
Nausea, vomiting	Pyridoxine
Diarrhea	Zinc, niacin
Stomatitis	Pyridoxine, riboflavin, iron
Cheilosis	Pyridoxine, iron
Glossitis	Pyridoxine, zinc, niacin, folic acid, vitamin B_{12}
Magenta tongue	Riboflavin
Swollen, bleeding gums	Vitamin C
Fissured tongue	Niacin
Hepatomegaly	Protein
SKIN	
Dry and scaling	Vitamin A, essential fatty acids, zinc
Petechiae/ecchymoses	Vitamin C, vitamin K
Follicular hyperkeratosis	Vitamin A, essential fatty acids
Nasolabial seborrhea	Niacin, pyridoxine, riboflavin
Bilateral dermatitis	Niacin, zinc
EXTREMITIES	
Subcutaneous fat loss	Calories
Muscle wastage	Calories, protein
Edema	Protein
Osteomalacia, bone pain, rickets	Vitamin D
Arthralgia	Vitamin C
HEMATOLOGIC	
Anemia	Vitamin B_{12}, iron, folic acid, copper, vitamin E
Leukopenia, neutropenia	Copper
Low prothrombin time, prolonged clotting time	Vitamin K, manganese
NEUROLOGIC	
Disorientation	Niacin, thiamine
Confabulation	Thiamine
Neuropathy	Thiamine, pyridoxine, chromium
Paresthesia	Thiamine, pyridoxine, vitamin B_{12}
CARDIOVASCULAR	
Congestive heart failure, cardiomegaly, tachycardia	Thiamine
Cardiomyopathy	Selenium

PHYSICAL ASSESSMENT/CLINICAL MANIFESTATIONS

The nurse assesses for signs and symptoms of various nutrient deficiencies (Table 61-4). The nurse inspects the client's hair, eyes, oral cavity, nails, and musculoskeletal and neurologic systems. The condition of the skin, including any reddened or open areas, is observed. The anthropometric measurements previously described may also be obtained. The nurse or assistive nursing personnel monitors all food and fluid intake, observes the client at mealtime, and notes any mouth pain or difficulty in chewing or swallowing.

PSYCHOSOCIAL ASSESSMENT

The psychosocial history provides information about the client's economic status, occupation, educational level, living and cooking arrangements, and mental status. The nurse determines whether financial resources are adequate for providing the necessary food. If resources are inadequate, the social worker may refer the client to available community services.

LABORATORY ASSESSMENT

Routine laboratory tests provide additional information about nutritional status. These tests supply objective data that can support subjective data and identify preclinical deficiencies. Laboratory tests must be carefully interpreted with regard to the total client; an isolated value may yield an inaccurate conclusion.

HEMATOLOGY. Hemoglobin is measured to detect iron deficiency anemia. A low hemoglobin level may indicate anemia, recent hemorrhage, or hemodilution caused by fluid retention. Hemoglobin may be low secondary to conditions such as low serum albumin, infection, catabolism, or cancer. High hemoglobin levels may indicate hemoconcentration or dehydration, or they may be secondary to liver disease.

Hematocrit, a measure of cell volume, indicates iron status. Low hematocrit levels may reflect anemia, hemorrhage, excessive fluid, renal disease, or cirrhosis. High hematocrit levels may indicate dehydration or hemoconcentration.

PROTEIN STUDIES. Serum albumin, transferrin, and thyroxine-binding prealbumin can be measured in the laboratory. Serum albumin indicates the body's protein status but is not sensitive enough to detect early changes in nutritional status. The normal serum albumin level for men and women is greater than 3.5 g/dL. Table 61-5 indicates the level of protein depletion based on the serum albumin level.

Serum **transferrin,** an iron-transport protein, can be measured directly or calculated as an indirect measurement of total iron-binding capacity (TIBC) as follows:

$$\text{Calculated transferrin} = (0.68 \times \text{TIBC}) + 21$$

Serum transferrin has a shorter half-life of 8 to 10 days and therefore is a more sensitive indicator of protein status than is albumin. Table 61-6 indicates the level of protein depletion based on serum transferrin level.

Thyroxine-binding **prealbumin (PAB)** provides a more sensitive indicator of protein deficiency because of its short half-life of 2 days. Depending on the laboratory test used, the normal PAB range is 17 to 40 mg/dL. PAB can also assess improvement in nutritional status with refeeding; levels can increase by 1 mg/dL/day with adequate nutritional support. However, this test is expensive, and its cost may be prohibitive except at large facilities.

SERUM CHOLESTEROL. Cholesterol levels normally range between 160 and 200 mg/dL in adult men and women. Values are typically low with malabsorption, liver disease, pernicious anemia, terminal stages of cancer, sepsis, or stress. A cholesterol level below 160 mg/dL has been identified as a possible indicator of malnutrition.

TABLE 61-5 • METHOD OF ASSESSING VISCERAL PROTEIN MASS FROM SERUM ALBUMIN LEVELS

When Serum Albumin (mg/dL) Is	The Level of Visceral Protein Depletion Is
>3.5	None
2.8-3.5	Mild
2.1-2.7	Moderate
<2.1	Severe

Modified with permission of Ross Products Division, Abbott Laboratories, Columbus, OH.
NOTE: Because the half-life of serum albumin is relatively long (about 20 days), albumin indicates initial visceral protein status but is not sensitive enough for detecting early changes in nutritional status.

TABLE 61-6 • METHOD OF ASSESSING VISCERAL PROTEIN MASS FROM SERUM TRANSFERRIN LEVELS

Serum transferrin is measured or calculated from total iron-binding capacity (TIBC) by the following equation:

$$\text{Calculated transferrin} = (0.68\ \text{TIBC}) + 21$$

When Serum Transferrin (mg/dL) Is	The Level of Visceral Protein Depletion Is
>200	None
151-200	Mild
100-150	Moderate
<100	Severe

Modified with permission of Ross Products Division, Abbott Laboratories, Columbus, OH.
NOTE: Serum transferrin has a half-life of approximately 8 days and therefore reflects acute changes in visceral protein status. The disadvantage of measuring serum transferrin is that the test is not routinely available in many clinical laboratories. Several formulas have been derived to calculate serum transferrin from TIBC, a measurement that is more readily available. However, measured transferrin is more accurate and is preferable when possible.

OTHER LABORATORY TESTS. Total lymphocyte count (TLC) can be used to assess immune function. Malnutrition suppresses the immune system and leaves the client more vulnerable to infection. When a client is malnourished, the TLC is usually decreased below 1500 mm^3 (Bender et al., 2000).

Analysis

COMMON NURSING DIAGNOSES AND COLLABORATIVE PROBLEMS

The most common diagnosis for the client with malnutrition is Imbalanced Nutrition: Less Than Body Requirements related to inadequate food intake or increased nutrient requirements.

ADDITIONAL NURSING DIAGNOSES AND COLLABORATIVE PROBLEMS

In addition to the common nursing diagnosis, clients with malnutrition may have one or more of the following:

- Risk for Impaired Skin Integrity related to depleted protein stores
- Risk for Infection related to suppressed immune system
- Risk for Disturbed Body Image related to physical changes from weight loss

Some clients with malnutrition are at risk for collaborative problems such as the following:

- Anemia
- Immunocompromised state

Planning and Implementation

IMBALANCED NUTRITION: LESS THAN BODY REQUIREMENTS

NOC **PLANNING: EXPECTED OUTCOMES.** The client with malnutrition is expected to (1) demonstrate an adequate nutrient intake, (2) maintain body mass and weight within normal limits (WNL), and (3) maintain laboratory values WNL (e.g., albumin).

INTERVENTIONS. The preferred route for feeding is through the gastrointestinal tract because it enhances the immune system and is safer, easier, less expensive, and more physiologically sound (Chart 61-3).

NIC **NUTRITION MANAGEMENT.** In collaboration with the health care provider and dietitian, the nurse provides high-calorie, high-protein foods (e.g., milkshakes, cheese and crackers). A feeding schedule of six small meals benefits many clients. If the client has difficulty chewing or is edentulous (toothless), a pureed or dental soft diet may facilitate food intake.

Malnourished ill clients often need to be encouraged to eat. The nurse provides a quiet environment, which is conducive to eating. Some clients, especially older adults, may take a long time to eat even small quantities of food.

Restorative feeding programs help nursing home residents who need special assistance. These residents eat in a separate dining area so that time and attention can be given to them. Chart 61-4 offers additional interventions to increase nutritional intake for older adults in any setting.

DRUG THERAPY. Medications may be given to some clients to stimulate appetite. For example, cyproheptadine (Periactin), an antihistamine, may be ordered for clients who are underweight, especially those with eating disorders. Megestrol acetate (Megace), an antineoplastic drug, may be used to increase appetite in clients who have cachexia, acquired immunodeficiency syndrome (AIDS), or unexplained weight loss. The mechanism for how these drugs work to increase appetite is unknown.

PARTIAL ENTERAL NUTRITION. The dietitian calculates the nutrients required daily and translates these requirements into meals for the client. If the client cannot ingest sufficient nutrients as food, **partial enteral nutrition** with fortified medical nutritional supplements (MNSs) (e.g., Ensure or Carnation Instant Breakfast) may be given, especially for older adults. Many commercial enteral products are available. For clients with medical diagnoses such as liver and renal disease, special products that meet their needs are also available. The client must enjoy the taste of the product for acceptability and optimal intake.

CONSIDERATIONS FOR OLDER ADULTS

Supplements used in acute care, long-term care, and home care are costly. In addition, older adults may refuse them, and the supplements are then wasted. Bender at al. (2000) found that a more successful alternative to having the MNS distributed by food service or nursing assistant staff in the nursing home was to have the supplements delivered by nurses during their usual medication passes. In this study, the nurses gave 60 mL or more of the MNS at least four times a day with the clients' medications. The subjects increased weight and had fewer pressure ulcers, thus making the program very cost-effective.

Nutritional supplements are supplied as liquid formulas, powders, bars, and puddings in a variety of flavors. They come in different degrees of sweetness and are also available as modular supplements that provide single nutrients. Examples of modular supplements are Polycose for carbohydrates and ProPac for protein. Carbohydrate modulars are useful only if additional calories are needed. Protein modulars are indicated when metabolic stress causes a need for higher protein intake.

The nurse bases adequate daily fluid intake on 30 mL of fluid per kilogram of body weight. This recommendation is

CHART 61-3

NIC INTERVENTION ACTIVITIES *for* The Client with Malnutrition

Nutrition Management: *Assisting with or providing a balanced dietary intake of foods and fluids*

- Ascertain client's food preferences.
- Determine, in collaboration with the dietitian, as appropriate, number of calories and type of nutrients needed to meet nutrition requirements.
- Encourage increased intake of protein, iron, and vitamin C, as appropriate.
- Offer snacks (e.g., frequent drinks, fresh fruits/fruit juice), as appropriate.
- Adjust diet to client's lifestyle, as appropriate.
- Weigh client at appropriate intervals.
- Encourage client to wear properly fitted dentures and/or acquire dental care.
- Assist client in receiving help from appropriate community nutritional programs, as needed.

NIC intervention activities selected from McCloskey, J.C., & Bulechek, G.M. (Eds.). (2000). *Nursing intervention classification (NIC)* (3rd ed.). St. Louis: Mosby. No part of this work is to be altered without prior written permission from the Publisher.

CHART 61-4

NURSING FOCUS *on the* OLDER ADULT
Promoting Nutritional Intake

- Observe the client during meals for food intake.
- Ask the client about food likes and dislikes.
- Encourage self-feeding, or feed the client slowly.
- Create an environment that is conducive to eating and socialization and relaxation, if possible.
- Serve snacks with activities, especially in long-term care settings.
- Document the percentage of food eaten at each meal and snack.
- Ensure that meals are visually appealing, appetizing, and properly prepared.
- Review the client's medication profile and discuss with the health care provider the use of drugs that may be suppressing appetite.
- If the client is depressed, be sure that the depression is treated by the health care provider.

not for clients with severe cardiac problems or fluid restrictions. The health care provider may also prescribe vitamin and mineral supplements.

The nurse or assistive nursing personnel maintains a daily calorie count and fluid intake to assess whether the client can meet the goals of nutritional therapy. The dietitian usually asks the nursing staff to keep the food intake record for at least 3 consecutive days. Accurate daily or weekly weights are also essential depending on the amount of depletion.

TOTAL ENTERAL NUTRITION. Clients often cannot meet the goals of nutritional therapy through their usual oral intake because of increased metabolic demands or a decreased ability to eat. In such cases, enteral tube feeding may be necessary to supplement oral intake or to provide total nutritional support.

CANDIDATES FOR TOTAL ENTERAL NUTRITION. Clients likely to receive **total enteral nutrition (TEN)** can be divided into three groups:

- Clients who can eat but cannot maintain adequate nutrition by oral intake of food alone
- Clients who have permanent neuromuscular impairment and cannot swallow
- Clients who do not have permanent neuromuscular impairment but are critically ill and cannot eat because of their condition

Clients in the first group are often older adults or clients receiving cancer treatment who cannot meet their calorie and protein needs (see the Legal/Ethical Issues in Health Care box below). Clients in the second group usually have permanent swallowing problems and require some type of feeding tube for delivery of the enteral product on a long-term basis. Examples of conditions that can cause permanent swallowing problems are strokes, severe head trauma, and advanced multiple sclerosis. Clients in the third group receive enteral nutrition for as long as their illness lasts. The feeding is discontinued when the client improves and can eat again. Total enteral nutrition is contraindicated for clients with diffuse peritonitis, severe pancreatitis, intestinal obstruction, intractable vomiting or diarrhea, and paralytic ileus (Bowers, 1996).

TYPES OF ENTERAL PRODUCTS. Many commercially prepared enteral products are available. An appropriate combination of carbohydrates, fat, vitamins, minerals, and trace elements is available in liquid form. Differences among products allow the dietitian to select the right formula for each client. An order from the health care provider is required for enteral nutrition, but the dietitian usually makes the recommendation and computes the amount and type of product needed for each client.

METHODS OF ADMINISTRATION OF TOTAL ENTERAL NUTRITION. TEN is administered as "tube feedings" through one of the available gastrointestinal tubes, either via a **nasoenteric tube (NET)** or an **enterostomal tube.**

Types of Tubes. A nasoenteric tube is any feeding tube inserted nasally and then advanced into the gastrointestinal tract. Commonly used NETs include the **nasogastric (NG) tube** and the **nasoduodenal tube (NDT).** A nasojejunal tube (NJT) is also available but is used less often than the other NETs. NDTs and NJTs are usually indicated for critically ill clients at risk for aspiration or delayed stomach emptying.

NETs are used for delivering short-term enteral feedings because they are easy to use and are safer for the client at risk for aspiration *if* the tip of the tube is placed below the pyloric sphincter of the stomach. Small-bore polyurethane or silicone tubes from 8 to 12 French external diameter are preferred over large-bore plastic or latex tubes. The smaller tubes are more comfortable and are less likely to cause complications such as nasal irritation, sinusitis, tissue erosion, and pulmonary compromise.

Enterostomal feeding tubes are used for clients who need long-term enteral feeding. The most common types are gastrostomies and jejunostomies. The physician directly accesses the gastrointestinal tract using various surgical, endoscopic, and laparoscopic techniques.

A **gastrostomy** is a stoma created from the abdominal wall into the stomach through which a short feeding tube is inserted by the physician. The gastrostomy may require a small abdominal incision or may be placed endoscopically; these tubes are called **percutaneous endoscopic gastrostomy (PEG)** or dual access gastrostomy-jejunostomy (PEG/J) tubes. The PEG does not require general anesthesia and is more secure and more durable than traditional gastrostomies. An alternative to either device is the **low-profile gastrostomy device (LPGD).** The LPGD is available with a firm or balloon-style internal bumper or retention disk. An antireflux valve keeps gastrointestinal contents from leaking onto the skin. This device is less irritating to the skin, longer lasting, and more cosmetically pleasing, and it allows greater client independence. However, skin-level devices do not allow easy access for checking residuals.

Jejunostomies are used less often than gastrostomies. A **jejunostomy** is used for long-term feedings when it is desirable to bypass the stomach, such as with gastric disease, upper gastrointestinal obstruction, and abnormal gastric or duodenal emptying.

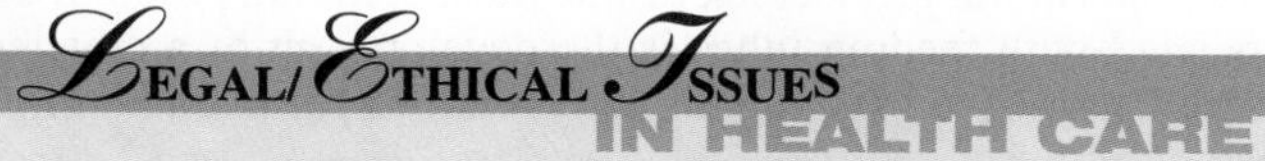

TOTAL ENTERAL NUTRITION FOR OLDER ADULTS

Total enteral nutrition provides a client's total daily nutrient and fluid requirements. In some cases, this artificial nutrition and hydration may not be desired by the older adult. For example, some clients have advance directives that state they do not want to be kept alive by artificial nutrition and hydration if certain conditions exist. However, questions arise when clients are not able to make their wishes known.

For many years it was believed that withholding food and fluids would cause discomfort. Recent cancer research indicates that clients who do not eat and drink do not suffer and in fact may be more comfortable if food and fluids are withheld. The decision to feed is complex, and there is no clear right or wrong answer. To compound this dilemma, medical complications (e.g., aspiration, pressure ulcers) are common in older adults who are tube fed.

When clinicians are making decisions about the desirability of tube feedings in these cases, the focus should be on achieving consensus by:

- Reviewing what is known about tube feedings, especially their risks and benefits
- Reviewing the medical facts about the client
- Investigating any available evidence that would help understand the client's wishes
- Obtaining the opinions of all stakeholders in the situation
- Delaying any action until consensus is achieved

Data from Daly, B.J. (2000). Special challenges of withholding artificial nutrition and hydration. *Journal of Gerontological Nursing. 26*(9), 25–31.

Types of Feedings. Tube feedings are administered by bolus feeding, continuous feeding, and cyclic feeding. **Bolus feeding** is an intermittent feeding of a specified amount of enteral product at specified times during a 24-hour period—typically every 4 hours. This method can be accomplished manually or by infusion through a mechanical pump or controller device. A more popular method of tube feeding is continuous enteral feeding. **Continuous feeding** is similar to IV therapy in that small amounts are continuously infused (by gravity drip or by a pump or controller device) over a specified time. **Cyclic feeding** is the same as continuous feeding except that the infusion is stopped for a specified time in each 24-hour period, usually 6 to 10 or more hours ("down time"). Down time typically occurs in the morning to allow bathing, bed making, and other treatments.

Infusion rates for continuous and cyclic feedings (and to some extent for intermittent bolus feeding) vary with the total amount of solution to be infused, the specific composition of the product, and the response of the client to the procedure.

The health care provider and dietitian usually decide the type, rate, and method of tube feeding, as well as the amount of additional water needed. If the client can swallow small amounts of food, he or she may also eat orally while the tube is in place.

The nurse is responsible for the care and maintenance of the feeding tube and the enteral feeding. Chart 61-5 lists the major nursing interventions for the client receiving an enteral feeding.

COMPLICATIONS OF TOTAL ENTERAL NUTRITION. The nurse is responsible for the prevention, assessment, and management of complications associated with tube feeding. Some complications of therapy result from the type of tube used to administer the feeding, and other complications result from the enteral product itself. The most common problem associated with feeding tubes is the development of a clogged tube. Chart 61-6 lists nursing interventions for maintaining a patent tube.

A less common but more serious complication is dislodgement of the tube. Several techniques should be used to confirm proper placement. An x-ray study is the most accurate confirmation method and should always be done on initial tube insertion. After the initial placement is confirmed, the nurse checks the placement before each intermittent feeding or at least every 8 hours during continuous or cyclic feeding.

The traditional auscultatory method is not reliable, especially for clients with small-bore tubes (see the Evidence-Based Practice for Nursing box on p. 1371). In this method, the nurse instills 20 to 30 mL of air into the tube while listening over the stomach with a stethoscope. The whooshing sound that results does not guarantee correct tube placement. The nurse should instead aspirate a sample of the gastrointestinal content, observe its color, and test its pH. When aspirating fluid, the nurse waits at least 1 hour following medication administration, then flushes the tube with 20 mL of air to clear it. The aspirate is collected and tested with pH paper. The pH of gastric fluid ranges from 0 to 4.0. If the tube has migrated down into the intestines, the pH will be between 7.0 and 8.0. If the tube is in the lungs, the pH will be greater than 6.0 (Metheney at al., 1998). The pH may also be as high as 6 if the client takes certain medications, such as H_2 blockers (e.g., ranitidine [Zantac] and famotidine [Pepcid]).

CHART 61-5

BEST PRACTICE *for*
Tube Feeding Care and Maintenance

- If nasogastric or nasoduodenal feeding is ordered, use a soft, flexible, small-bore feeding tube (smaller than 12 French). The initial placement of the tube should be confirmed by x-ray study. Secure the tube with tape or a commercial attachment device after applying a skin protectant; change the tape regularly.
- Check tube placement by x-ray study when the correct position of the tube is in question; an x-ray study is the only reliable method. Checking the pH of the aspirant is a useful adjunct. Other traditional methods for determining tube placement have not proved to be reliable (see the Evidence-Based Practice for Nursing box on p. 1371).
- If a gastrostomy or jejunostomy tube is used, assess the insertion site for signs of infection or excoriation (e.g., excessive redness and drainage). Rotate the tube 360 degrees each day and check for in-and-out play of about ¼ in (0.5 cm). If the tube cannot be moved, notify the health care provider immediately, because the retention disk may be embedded in the tissue. Cover the site with a dry sterile dressing, and change the dressing at least once a day.
- Check and record the residual volume every 4 hours by aspirating stomach contents into a syringe. If residual feeding is obtained, check the physician's order for the appropriate intervention (usually to slow or stop the feeding for a time).
- Check the feeding pump or controller device (if used) to ensure proper mechanical operation.
- Ensure that the prescribed enteral product is infused at the ordered rate (mL/hr).
- Change the feeding bag and tubing every 24 hours; label the bag with the date and time of the change. Use an irrigation set for no more than 24 hours.
- For continuous or cyclic feeding, add only 4 hours of product to the bag each time to prevent bacterial growth; a closed system may be used for 24 hours.
- To prevent aspiration, keep the head of the bed elevated at least 30 degrees during the feeding and for 1 hour after the feeding.
- Monitor laboratory values, especially blood urea nitrogen (BUN), serum electrolytes, hematocrit, albumin, prealbumin, and glucose.
- Monitor for complications of tube feeding, especially diarrhea.
- Monitor and carefully record the client's weight and intake and output.

CHART 61-6

BEST PRACTICE *for*
Maintaining a Patent Feeding Tube

- Flush the tube with 30 to 60 mL of water (amount usually ordered by the health care provider or dietitian):
  - At least every 4 hours during a continuous tube feeding
  - Before and after each intermittent tube feeding
  - Before and after medication administration (use warm water)
  - After checking residual volume
- If the tube becomes clogged, use 30 mL of water for flushing, applying gentle pressure with a 50-mL piston syringe.
- Avoid the use of carbonated beverage, except for existing clogs *when water is not effective.* Do not use cranberry juice.
- Whenever possible, use liquid medications instead of crushed tablets.
- Do not mix medications with the feeding product. Crush tablets as finely as possible and dissolve in warm water.
- Consider use of automatic flush feeding pump such as Flexiflo, Quantum, or Kangaroo.

EVIDENCE-BASED PRACTICE FOR NURSING

What is the best way to determine whether a nasogastric tube is in the right place?

Metheney, N., et al. (1998). pH, color, and feeding tubes. *RN, 61*(1), 25-27.

Next to x-ray studies, pH testing of aspirate is the most dependable method of confirming tube placement. In this study, the researchers aspirated gastrointestinal fluid from more than 1000 feeding tubes in acutely ill clients with new tubes. The pH of gastric contents ranged between 0 and 4. When the tube was in the small intestine, the pH increased to 7. The researchers also found that the color of gastric contents was different from aspirates from the pulmonary system or intestines. Gastric fluid was green, tan, off-white, bloody, or brown, whereas duodenal samples were a medium to golden yellow. Aspirates from the tracheobronchial tree in clients whose tubes were malpositioned were off-white in color and heavily tinged with mucus.

Critique. For more than 10 years the primary author of this study has been researching the most reliable methods for confirming proper placement of nasogastric tubes. This study replicated previous findings and added the assessment of color as another tool. A large sample of homogeneous clients was used to help generalize conclusions.

Implications for Nursing. The researchers clearly demonstrated that pH and color are more reliable indicators for ensuring proper placement of nasoenteric tubes than the auscultatory method, although the latter is common practice in clinical agencies. Nurses should use all of these methods to prevent enteral feeding into the lungs.

Fluid Imbalances. Clients receiving enteral nutrition therapy are at an increased risk for fluid imbalances. Clients who receive this therapy are often older or debilitated and may also have cardiac or renal problems. Fluid imbalances associated with enteral nutrition are usually related to the body's response to increased serum osmolarity.

Increased Osmolarity. Osmolarity is the amount or concentration of particles dissolved in solution. This concentration exerts a specific osmotic pressure within the solution. Normal osmolarity of extracellular fluid (ECF) ranges between 270 and 300 mOsm. Enteral feeding products range in osmolarity from isotonic (about 300 mOsm) to extremely hypertonic (600 mOsm). Electrolytes (including sodium) contribute to this hypertonicity, but more of the osmolarity is determined by the concentration of proteins and sugar molecules in the enteral product. Even when the product is isotonic, the ECF can become hyperosmolar unless some hypotonic fluids are also administered to the client. This situation is most likely to develop in clients who are unconscious, unable to respond to the thirst reflex, on fluid restrictions, or receiving hyperosmotic enteral preparations.

An increase in the osmolarity of the plasma increases the osmotic pressure of the plasma. Because this increased osmolarity is largely a result of extra glucose and proteins (which tend to remain in the plasma rather than move to interstitial spaces), the plasma osmotic pressure (water-pulling pressure) is increased. In this situation, intracellular and interstitial water move into and expand the plasma volume. This volume expansion results in an increased renal excretion of water (among clients with normal renal function) and leads to osmotic dehydration. If clients do not have normal renal and cardiac function, the expansion of the plasma volume can lead to circulatory overload and the formation of pulmonary edema, especially in older adults. The nurse assesses for signs and symptoms of circulatory overload and collaborates with the dietitian and physician in planning the correct amount of fluid to be provided to the client.

Dehydration. Excessive diarrhea may develop when hyperosmolar enteral preparations are delivered quickly. This situation can also lead to dehydration through excessive water loss. The nurse consults with the health care provider and dietitian for recommendations to prevent diarrhea.

First, the dietitian usually changes the feeding to a more iso-osmolar formula. Most of these formulas can be started full-strength but slowly at 15 to 20 mL/hr. The rate is gradually increased as the client tolerates and as the expected nutritional outcome is achieved. If diarrhea continues, the client should be evaluated for *Clostridium difficile* and its toxins.

In some cases, diarrhea may be the result of liquid medications, such as elixirs and suspensions that have a very high osmolality. Examples include acetaminophen, digoxin, furosemide, phenytoin, and potassium chloride. Clients receiving multiple liquid medications need to be evaluated to determine if their drug regimen can be changed to prevent diarrhea. Diluting these liquids may also be an option.

Another cause of diarrhea-related fluid imbalance among clients receiving enteral feeding preparations is lactose intolerance. Clients receiving milk-based enteral feeding preparations may become lactose intolerant. Most commercial enteral products, such as Ensure, are lactose free.

Vines et al. (1992) conducted a comprehensive review of research on diarrhea related to tube feeding. They concluded that diarrhea often results from bacterial contamination, and they implemented interventions for decreasing this risk.

Electrolyte Imbalances. Depending on the client's state of health, certain electrolyte imbalances can be avoided. This is achieved by the use of enteral preparations containing lower concentrations of the electrolytes that the client cannot handle well.

In addition to the client's specific electrolyte imbalances, the two most common electrolyte imbalances associated with enteral nutrition therapy are hyperkalemia and hypernatremia. Both of these conditions may be related to hyperglycemia-induced hyperosmolarity of the plasma and the resultant osmotic diuresis. Electrolyte imbalances are discussed in detail in Chapter 13.

CRITICAL THINKING CHALLENGE

An older adult in your nursing home has been eating less than 50% of her meals since admission the previous week. She has lost 3 pounds in 5 days. The nursing assistant reports to you today that the resident has a reddened area on her sacrum that does not blanch. When you speak to this client, she tells you that she is upset about being "put in a home."

- What other assessments should you perform at this time?
- What are her priority nursing diagnoses?
- What interventions are appropriate for her now?

For suggested answer guidelines, go to SIMON http://www.wbsaunders.com/SIMON/Iggy/.

PARENTERAL NUTRITION. When a client cannot effectively use the gastrointestinal tract for nutrition, parenteral nutrition therapy may maintain or improve his or her nutritional status. This form of IV therapy differs from standard IV therapy in that *all* nutrients (carbohydrates, proteins, fats, vitamins, minerals, and trace elements) are delivered to the client.

One liter of fluid containing 5% dextrose, which is often used as standard IV therapy, provides only 170 kcal. A hospitalized client typically receives 3 or 4 L a day for a total number of calories ranging between 500 and 700 a day. This calorie intake is not sufficient when the client requires IV therapy for a prolonged period and cannot eat an adequate diet or has increased calorie needs for tissue repair and building.

Parenteral nutrition (**hyperalimentation,** or "hyperal") is subdivided into two categories:

- Partial parenteral nutrition, or peripheral parenteral nutrition
- Total parenteral nutrition, or central parenteral nutrition

As suggested by the names, these categories differ by the site of administration and the content of the solutions.

PARTIAL PARENTERAL NUTRITION. **Partial parenteral nutrition (PPN)** provides nutritional support to clients who are unable or unwilling to take a feeding via the gastrointestinal tract. PPN is typically used when a client has a prolonged postoperative ileus or when placement of a central IV line is not advised. It is used when nutritional support is needed less than 14 days. The client should be able to tolerate large fluid volumes and have readily accessible peripheral veins.

PPN is usually delivered through a cannula or catheter in a large distal vein of the arm. Two types of solutions are commonly used in various combinations for PPN: lipid (fat) emulsions and amino acid dextrose solutions.

Most lipid emulsions (20%) are isotonic, but the tonicity of commercially prepared amino acid dextrose solutions ranges from 300 mOsm to nearly 1200 mOsm. Amino acid dextrose solutions are considered more stable than the lipid emulsions, and therefore additives (e.g., vitamins, minerals, electrolytes, and trace elements) tend to be mixed with the amino acid dextrose solutions. The amino acid dextrose solution must be delivered through an in-line filter. Lipids and amino acid dextrose solutions are administered by a pump or controller device for accuracy and constancy in delivery rate.

A newer product for PPN is a *mixture* of lipids (10% or 20% fat emulsion) and an amino acid dextrose (usually 10%) solution. This mixture of three types of nutrients is referred to as a 3:1, total nutrient admixture (TNA), or triple-mix solution; it is available in 3-L bags.

TOTAL PARENTERAL NUTRITION. When the client requires intensive nutritional support for an extended time, the health care provider prescribes centrally administered **total parenteral nutrition (TPN).** TPN is delivered through access to central veins, usually the subclavian or internal jugular veins. Central venous catheters and associated nursing care are described in detail in Chapter 14.

TPN solutions contain higher concentrations of dextrose and proteins, usually in the form of synthetic amino acids or protein hydrolysates (3% to 5%). These solutions are hyperosmotic (three to six times the osmolarity of normal blood). The base solutions are available as commercially prepared solutions. The hospital or community pharmacist adds components (specific electrolytes, minerals, trace elements, and insulin) according to the client's nutritional needs. This therapy provides needed calories and spares body proteins from catabolism for energy requirements.

TPN solutions are administered with a pump or an infusion controller device. The osmolarity of the fluid and the concentrations of the specific components make controlled delivery essential.

COMPLICATIONS OF PARENTERAL NUTRITION. Clients receiving PPN or TPN are at risk for a wide variety of serious and potentially life-threatening complications. Complications may result from the PPN and TPN solutions or from the central venous catheter. The following discussion is limited to the complications of PPN and TPN that involve fluid or electrolyte balance. Complications of IV cannulas and central venous catheters are discussed in Chapter 14.

Fluid Imbalances. Clients receiving PPN or TPN are at increased risk for fluid imbalance. Not only is fluid delivered directly into the venous system, but the extreme hyperosmolarity of the solutions stimulates fluid shifts between body fluid compartments.

The hyperosmolarity of parenteral nutrition solutions is caused by their amino acid and dextrose concentrations. Increased dextrose causes hyperglycemia. As a result, some of the dextrose moves into the interstitial and intracellular spaces, where it is metabolized. However, dextrose remains in the plasma volume when the solutions are administered too rapidly, without enough insulin coverage, or in the presence of hyponatremia and hypokalemia. The result is a shift of water from the interstitial and intracellular spaces into the plasma. Expansion of the plasma volume together with hyperglycemia can cause osmotic diuresis and lead to serious dehydration and hypovolemic shock. If the client has an accompanying cardiac or renal dysfunction, the situation can lead to overhydration, congestive heart failure, and pulmonary edema.

The nurse monitors for these complications by taking daily weights and by recording accurate intake and output while the client is receiving parenteral nutrition. Serum glucose and electrolyte values are also monitored (Chart 61-7). Any major changes or abnormalities are reported to the health care provider.

CHART 61-7

BEST PRACTICE *for*
Care and Maintenance of Total Parenteral Nutrition

- Check each bag of total parenteral nutrition (TPN) solution for accuracy by comparing it with the physician's order.
- Monitor the IV pump for accuracy in delivering the prescribed hourly rate.
- If the TPN solution is temporarily unavailable, give 10% dextrose/water (D/W) or 20% D/W until the TPN solution can be obtained.
- If the TPN administration is not on time ("behind"), do not attempt to "catch up" by increasing the rate.
- Monitor the client's weight daily or according to agency protocol.
- Monitor serum electrolytes and glucose daily or per agency protocol. (Some agencies require finger stick blood sugars [FSBSs] every 4 hours, especially if the client is receiving insulin. Urine testing for ketones may also be ordered.)
- Monitor and carefully record the client's intake and output.
- Assess the client's IV site for signs of infection or infiltration (see Chapter 14).
- Change the IV tubing every 24 hours or per agency protocol.
- Change the dressing around the IV site every 48 to 72 hours or per agency protocol.

Electrolyte Imbalances. Clients receiving either PPN or TPN are at an increased risk for many different electrolyte imbalances, depending on the electrolyte composition of the solution and whether a fluid imbalance occurs. The health care provider usually orders daily determinations of serum electrolyte levels to detect these imbalances. The risk of metabolic and electrolyte complications is reduced when the rate of administration is carefully controlled and clients are closely monitored for response to treatment. Potassium and sodium imbalances are common among clients receiving PPN and TPN, especially when insulin is also administered as part of the therapy. Calcium imbalances, especially hypercalcemia, are associated with PPN and TPN, although immobility may play more of a role than the actual parenteral therapy in the development of this imbalance.

EFFECTS OF MEDICATION. There is no specific drug therapy for malnutrition, although multivitamins and an iron preparation may be prescribed to treat or prevent anemia. The nurse carefully reviews the client's medications because of food-medication interactions. Medications can affect nutritional status, and the foods ingested can affect the efficacy of medications.

Community-Based Care

Malnourished clients can be cared for in a variety of settings, including the acute care hospital, subacute unit, nursing home, or their own home. Malnutrition is often diagnosed when the client is admitted to the acute care hospital or as a consequence of events that occur after hospitalization, such as poor wound healing or sepsis. If the client is severely compromised, he or she may require admission to a subacute unit or traditional nursing home for either transitional or long-term care and be followed by a case manager. If adequate home support is available, the client may be discharged to home in the care of a family member, significant other, or other caregiver. Home care nurses may be needed to monitor and direct the care.

HEALTH TEACHING

The dietitian instructs the malnourished client and the family about high-calorie, high-protein diet and nutritional supplements. The pharmacist reviews any parenteral solutions with the client and family or significant others.

The nurse reinforces the importance of adhering to the diet and reviews any medications the client may be taking. If the client takes an iron preparation, the nurse teaches the importance of taking the medication immediately before or during meals. The nurse also cautions the client that iron tends to cause constipation. For the older adult already susceptible to constipation, the nurse stresses measures for prevention, including adequate fiber intake, adequate fluids, and exercise.

HOME CARE MANAGEMENT

The malnourished client needs a variety of resources at home to continue aggressive nutrition support. If the client can consume food by the oral route, the case manager or other discharge planner determines whether his or her financial resources are adequate for providing the necessary food and nutrition supplements. If the hospital provides ambulatory nutrition counseling services, the client is scheduled for follow-up after discharge for assessment of weight gain. The nurse assesses the ability of the client and family to understand and comply with instructions.

The malnourished client discharged to home on enteral or parenteral nutrition support needs the specialized services of a home nutrition therapy team. This team generally consists of the physician, nurse, dietitian, pharmacist, and social worker. Several commercial companies supply these services to clients in addition to the feeding supplies and formulas.

HEALTH CARE RESOURCES

The malnourished client may need help from community resources. Once nutrition therapy has progressed, the client may be discharged to the home setting or to a long-term care facility. The nurse collaborates with the case manager or discharge planner to find the best placement for each client. If the client is discharged to home, a home care nurse may visit until the client is stable.

Whether the client is discharged to home or to another facility, the dietitian provides written instructions about the diet and nutritional supplements. Communication with the new care provider is essential for continuity of care.

Evaluation: Outcomes

NOC The nurse evaluates the care of the malnourished client on the basis of the identified nursing diagnoses and collaborative problems. Expected outcomes include that the client:

- Has an adequate intake of all required nutrients on a daily basis
- Experiences no further weight loss or has a weight increase
- Has laboratory values within normal limits (WNL)

OBESITY

OVERVIEW

The terms **obesity** and **overweight** are often used interchangeably, but they refer to different conditions. Overweight is an increase in body weight for height compared with a reference standard, such as the Metropolitan Life height and weight tables (see Table 61-3) or 10% greater than ideal body weight. However, this weight may not reflect excess body fat. It is possible for well-developed athletes to appear overweight because of increased muscle mass; in such cases the proportion of muscle to fat is greater than average.

An obese person weighs at least 20% above the upper limit of the normal range for ideal body weight. **Morbid obesity** refers to a weight that has a negative effect on health—usually more than 100% above ideal body weight.

Pathophysiology

Obesity refers to an excess amount of body fat. It is possible to be obese at a weight that is within normal range according to a reference standard. The normal amount of body fat in *men* is between 15% and 20% of body weight. Obese young men have body fat greater than 22%, and older obese men have body fat greater than 25%. For *women,* the normal amount of body fat is 18% to 32%. Obese young women have body fat greater than 35% (Bray, 1994). Body fat can be measured in several ways. Height and weight are the easiest and most practical measurements for determining the degree of overweight.

OBESITY INDICES

To establish the percentage of ideal body weight (IBW), the height and weight of the client are compared with the midpoint of the desirable weight for a medium frame of the client's height and sex in the Metropolitan Life height and weight tables (see Table 61-3). The body mass index (BMI), as described previously on p. 1363, is a measure of heaviness and is only an indirect indicator of body fat. It reflects the combined effects of body build, proportions, lean body mass, and body fat. However, BMI has exhibited substantial correlations with fat mass for adult men and women and has been validated as a risk factor for cardiovascular disease. As a general rule, a BMI of 27 indicates obesity and an increased risk for health problems. Arm circumference and skin fold measurements more completely define body composition and adiposity.

The distribution of excess body fat rather than the degree of obesity has been used to predict increased health risks. The waist-to-hip ratio (WHR) or abdominal/gluteal ratio (AGR) differentiates a predominantly peripheral (gynecoid) lower body obesity from a central (android) upper body obesity. A WHR of 0.95 or greater in men (0.8 or greater in women) indicates android obesity with excess fat at the waist and abdomen; this pattern carries the greatest health risk. Two risk groups have been identified by location of abdominal fat: one with subcutaneous fat and one with intra-abdominal fat. The group with subcutaneous fat had fewer complications than did the group with excess intra-abdominal fat. Cross-sectional studies have shown that increased abdominal fat has been related to stroke, insulin resistance, hyperinsulinemia, and frank diabetes mellitus. Excessive abdominal fat may also enhance the risk for gallbladder disease (Pi-Sunyer, 1993).

COMPLICATIONS OF OBESITY

Obesity is a major public health problem and is associated with many complications, including death. As a result of this increasing problem, the Healthy People 2010 agenda addresses the need to reduce the proportion of children, adolescents, and adults who are obese. Nurses can help meet this goal through education and role modeling (see the Meeting Healthy People 2010 Objectives box above).

Complications of obesity that improve with weight loss include the following:

- Diabetes mellitus
- Hypertension
- Hyperlipidemia (increased serum lipids)
- Cardiac disease
- Sleep apnea
- Cholelithiasis
- Chronic back pain
- Early degenerative arthritis
- Certain types of cancer

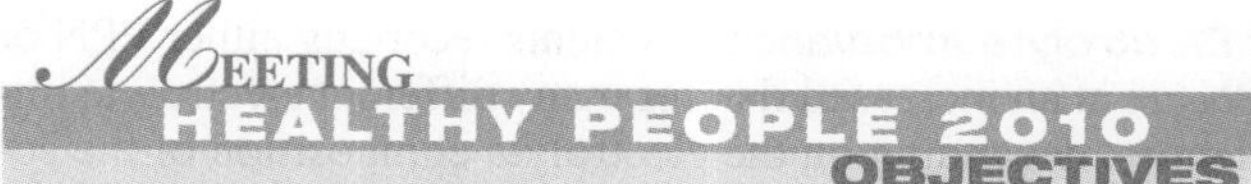

NUTRITION AND OVERWEIGHT

Objective 19.2: Reduce the proportion of adults who are obese.

- Teach the client the potential consequences and complications of obesity.
- Teach the client the importance of eating a healthy diet, including a variety of foods, especially grain products, vegetables, and fruits. The diet should be moderate in salt and sugar and low in fats and cholesterol.
- Remind the client that foods eaten away from home tend to be higher in fat, cholesterol, and salt and are lower in calcium than foods prepared at home.
- Reinforce the need to engage regularly in moderate physical activity for at least 30 minutes each day.
- Begin education regarding diet and physical activity for children and adolescents, and continue throughout adulthood. (Once an adolescent becomes overweight, he or she is likely to remain overweight.)

TABLE 61-7 • CLASSIFICATION OF OBESITY BASED ON BODY MASS INDEX

Body Mass Index	Class	Risk for Disease Associated with Obesity
20-25	0	Low (not obese)
25-30	1	Low
30-35	2	Moderate
35-40	3	High
40+	4	Very high risk

Data from Bray, G.A. (1994). Etiology and prevalence of obesity. In C. Bouchard (Ed.). *The genetics of obesity* (pp. 17-33): Boca Raton, FL: CRC Press.

Obese people are also more susceptible to infectious diseases than are thinner people.

CLASSIFICATION

Bray (1994) has developed a classification of obesity based on BMI and the corresponding risk for disease (Table 61-7). This classification system eliminates describing obesity in unflattering and prejudicial terms such as *morbid* or *gross.*

Etiology

The cause of obesity involves complex interrelationships of many factors, including the following:

- Genetic
- Environmental
- Psychologic
- Social
- Cultural
- Pathologic
- Physiologic

Five major causes of both human and animal obesity have been identified (Bray, 1994). The first, neuroendocrine causes, include injury to the hypothalamus, Cushing's disease, polycystic ovary failure, hypogonadism, and growth hormone deficiency and insulinoma.

A second cause is dietary obesity associated with high-fat diets. Data suggest that obesity associated with a high-fat diet is more pronounced when the diet contains a significant amount of saturated fat.

Genetic factors are being studied as a third cause. They are found in clinically uncommon states, such as Prader-Willi syndrome. Genetic composition may predispose some people but not others to obesity. Researchers have recently identified the *ob* gene in mice, which helps to regulate energy balance. Leptin, the hormone encoded by the *ob* gene, appears to send a message to the brain that the body has stored enough fat; this serves as a signal to stop eating. For obese humans, a variant in this gene may mean that the body does not receive the signal to stop eating. More recent evidence suggests that energy balance and adiposity are regulated not only by the hormonal action of leptin and its receptors but also by the interaction of leptin and insulin with the hypothalamic neuropeptide Y system (Schwartz & Seeley, 1997).

The fourth cause of obesity is drug treatment. Drugs that promote obesity include the following:

- Corticosteroids
- Estrogens
- Nonsteroidal anti-inflammatory drugs
- Antihypertensives
- Antidepressants
- Antiepileptics
- Phenothiazines

Physical inactivity has been identified as the fifth cause. The major identified barriers to increasing physical activity include a lack of time and a lack of safe environments in which to be active. Regular exercise is associated with lower death rates for adults of any age. It also increases lean muscle, decreases body fat, aids in weight control, and enhances psychologic well-being. Regular exercise can also decrease the risk of falling in older adults.

Incidence/Prevalence

The number of overweight children, adolescents, and adults has continued to rise over the past four decades. In the United States, the total cost (medical cost and lost productivity) of obesity is more than $100 billion each year. Phase 1 of the third National Health and Nutrition Examination Survey (NHANES III) was conducted between 1988 and 1991 and concluded that 58 million adults in the United States were overweight. This figure represents 33.4% of Americans. "Overweight" in this study was a BMI equal to or greater than 27.8 for men (approximately 124% of IBW) and a BMI equal to or greater than 27.3 for women (approximately 120% of IBW) (Kuczmarski et al., 1994). In 2000, an estimated 107 million adults in the United States were overweight or obese.

Familial and genetic factors play an important role in obesity. When both parents are overweight, approximately 80% of their children will be overweight. If neither parent is overweight, fewer than 10% of the children will be overweight. In studies of identical twins, nonidentical twins, and parent-sibling relationships, about 50% of the difference in body fatness is transmitted to children, and approximately 50% of this amount is genetically controlled. A combination of improper diet and lack of physical activity produces obesity in genetically predisposed people.

CULTURAL CONSIDERATIONS

Culture seems to be a factor in the prevalence of obesity. The prevalence of obesity among ethnic minorities, including African Americans, Hispanic Americans, Asian Americans and Pacific Islanders, Native Americans, Native Alaskans, and Native Hawaiians, is substantially higher than in Caucasians, especially among women (Kumanyika, 1993). A study by Harrell and Gore (1998) found that African-American women of low and middle socioeconomic status (SES) were much more likely to be obese and inactive than were African-American women of high SES. Among Caucasian women, those with low SES had the greatest prevalence of obesity and inactivity. After controlling for income and education, African-American women were twice as likely as Caucasian women to be obese and inactive.

Further research by Gore (1999) found that African Americans' frame of reference for "normal" body weight is much larger that the standard indicator for weight. Another factor contributing to larger body size in African-American women is that Caucasian women engage in weight loss methods for significantly longer periods of time than do African-American women (Tyler, Allan, & Alcozer, 1997).

A descriptive study of Hispanic women and their daughters demonstrated that daughters ate more fat than did their mothers (Garcia-Maas, 1999). The greater the fat intake, the more negatively women seemed to perceive their health status.

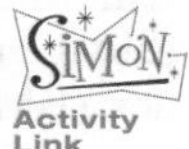

COLLABORATIVE MANAGEMENT

Assessment

HISTORY

The nurse or dietitian collects the following information about the client:

- Economic status
- Usual food intake
- Eating behavior
- Cultural background
- Attitude toward food
- Appetite
- Chronic diseases
- Medications
- Physical activity

A diet history usually incorporates a 24-hour recall of food intake and the frequency with which foods are consumed. The nurse or dietitian is objective but understands the personal nature of these questions. The adequacy of the diet can be rapidly evaluated by comparing the amount and types of foods consumed daily with the Dietary Guidelines for Americans (see Figure 61-1). Gross inadequacies for specific nutrients can be identified with this approach. The dietitian can provide a more detailed analysis of dietary intake.

WOMEN'S HEALTH CONSIDERATIONS

Women have a unique risk for nutrition-related diseases and conditions and weight-related problems due to biologic, social, and political factors. The American Dietetic Association (ADA) and the Canadian Dietetic Association (CDA) issued a joint position paper on women's health and nutrition (ADA, 1995). Five of the leading causes of morbidity and mortality in North American women are cardiovascular disease, cancer, osteoporosis, diabetes, and overweight. Women are vulnerable to several weight-related health risks associated with being overweight. Recent estimates of North American women who are overweight range from 25% to 33%, with certain native and ethnic populations reporting even higher percentages.

Being overweight adds many risks for women, especially if the fat stores are located in the abdominal or truncal areas of the body. A waist/hip ratio of 0.85 puts women at higher risk for coronary heart disease, hypertension, dyslipidemia, diabetes, gallstone formation, and cancer of the reproductive organs. In addition to these medical risks, women are vulnerable to the social, economic, and emotional pressures associated with being overweight. Overweight women may find it difficult to feel good about themselves when challenged by society's discrimination against the overweight. The constant struggle for many women to lose weight often ends in failure and leads to patterns of weight cycling or disordered eating. Prevention and early intervention programs for overweight women and their families remain a critical need. The ADA and CDA will continue their efforts to include nutrition in clinical and preventive services for women because it is such a critical component of both risk reduction and treatment for weight-associated conditions.

PHYSICAL ASSESSMENT/CLINICAL MANIFESTATIONS

In collaboration with the dietitian, the nurse accurately obtains the client's height and weight and calculates the percentage of ideal body weight (% IBW) and the body mass index (BMI). The dietitian may:

- Calculate the waist/hip ratio
- Make the necessary skin fold measurements and record them in the chart

The nurse also examines the skin of the obese client for reddened or open areas; these may not be easily visible because of excess fat.

PSYCHOSOCIAL ASSESSMENT

The nurse obtains a psychosocial history to determine the client's circumstances and emotional factors that might prevent success of therapy or be worsened by it. The nurse or social worker interviews the client to determine his or her perception of current weight. The client may or may not view weight as a problem, which will affect treatment and outcome.

The nurse explores the client's past history to assess the following:

- Cause and duration of weight gain
- Family history of obesity
- Past attempts at weight reduction and outcomes

The nurse asks about the following:

- Current reasons for wanting to lose weight
- Stressors (e.g., home, employment, personal, financial, or community) that might prevent success
- Exercise patterns
- Current medications
- Perceptions of self-worth

The diet history provides a detailed analysis of the client's eating habits. As a member of the health care team, the nurse can evaluate the data to coordinate an interdisciplinary approach that incorporates diet, exercise, behavior modification, and psychologic support. The client may be referred to a community support group if one is available.

LABORATORY ASSESSMENT

There are no significant laboratory tests for obesity. However, the nurse should review all laboratory test results to assess the nutritional status of the client.

Analysis

COMMON NURSING DIAGNOSES AND COLLABORATIVE PROBLEMS

The following are the most common nursing diagnoses for clients with obesity or overweight:

1. Imbalanced Nutrition: More Than Body Requirements related to a dysfunctional eating pattern or neuroendocrine disorder
2. Activity Intolerance related to a sedentary lifestyle

ADDITIONAL NURSING DIAGNOSES AND COLLABORATIVE PROBLEMS

In addition to the common nursing diagnoses, clients may have one or more secondary problems associated with obesity and overweight, which include the following:

- Situational Low Self-Esteem or Chronic Low Self-Esteem related to guilt associated with eating style
- Disturbed Body Image related to physical appearance
- Disturbed Thought Processes related to depression
- Ineffective Sexuality Patterns related to body image perception, rejection by partner, or difficulty assuming sexual positions
- Impaired Social Interaction related to poor self-esteem and rejection by others
- Impaired Physical Mobility related to decreased strength and endurance

Some clients with obesity are at risk for collaborative problems, which include the following:

- Diabetes mellitus
- Cardiovascular disease
- Hypertension

Planning and Implementation

IMBALANCED NUTRITION: MORE THAN BODY REQUIREMENTS

NOC **PLANNING: EXPECTED OUTCOMES.** The client with obesity or overweight is expected to (1) participate in a structured weight loss program, (2) approach ideal body weight, and (3) establish a lasting, healthful dietary pattern that will result in permanent, sustained weight loss.

INTERVENTIONS. Weight is lost only when energy expended is greater than intake. Weight loss may be accomplished by dietary restriction with or without the aid of drugs. Clients who are candidates for surgical treatment:

- Repeatedly fail at nonsurgical techniques
- Have a body mass index (BMI) equal to or greater than 40 (class IV)
- Weigh more than 100% above ideal body weight (IBW)
- Have medically significant obesity

NONSURGICAL MANAGEMENT. The first clinical practice *Guidelines for Treatment of Adult Obesity* outlines treatment decisions based on risk assessment. Recommendations for appropriate weight reduction strategies or weight maintenance to prevent further weight gain are also included (Shape Up America and American Obesity Association, 1996). Various diet programs and medications have attempted to help obese clients achieve permanent weight loss.

DIET PROGRAMS. Modalities for helping people lose weight include fasting, very-low-calorie diets, balanced and unbalanced low-energy diets, and novelty diets.

Fasting. Short-term fasting programs have not been successful in treating morbidly obese clients, and prolonged fasting does not produce permanent benefits. Most clients regain the weight that was lost by this method. In addition, the risks associated with fasting (e.g., severe ketosis) require close medical supervision.

Very-Low-Calorie Diets. Very-low-calorie diets generally provide 200 to 800 calories/day. Two types of very-low-calorie diets are the *protein-sparing modified fast* and the *liquid formula diet.*

The protein-sparing modified fast provides protein of high biologic value (1.5 g/kg of desirable body weight/day) within a limited number of calories. The diet produces rapid weight loss while preserving lean body mass. The liquid formula diet provides between 33 and 70 g of protein daily.

Both diets require an initial cardiac evaluation, supervision by an interdisciplinary health team with monitoring by a physician, nutrition counseling by a registered dietitian, and supplementation with vitamins and minerals. These diets are only one part of a weight reduction program. Clients who are following these diets should receive nutrition education, psychologic counseling, exercise, and behavior therapy. Comparable weight losses have been achieved with both diets, but most clients do not sustain the weight loss and regain the weight.

Balanced and Unbalanced Low-Energy Diets. Nutritionally balanced diets generally provide 1200 calories/day with a conventional distribution of carbohydrate, protein, and fat. Vitamin and mineral supplements may be necessary if energy intakes fall below 1200 calories for women and 1800 calories for men. This diet provides conventional foods that are economical and easy to obtain; thus the goal of weight loss is facilitated, and that loss is maintained.

Unbalanced low-energy diets, such as the low-carbohydrate diet (e.g., Atkins diet), restrict one or more nutrients. No evidence supports the claim that the restricted nutrient increases or decreases weight loss beyond the calorie deficit it produces.

Novelty Diets. Novelty diets, such as the grapefruit diet, are often nutritionally *inadequate.* This type of diet implies that a certain food increases metabolic rate or accelerates the oxidation of body fat. Weight loss is achieved because energy is restricted by food choice, but clients do not sustain weight loss after terminating the diet.

DIET THERAPY. Diet recommendations for each client should be developed through close interaction between the client, physician, and dietitian. The diet should meet the client's needs and habits and should be realistic.

The dietitian develops a diet plan and instructs the client. At a minimum, the diet should:

- Have a scientific rationale
- Be nutritionally adequate for all nutrients except energy
- Have a low risk/benefit ratio
- Be practical and conducive to long-term success

Calorie estimates are easily calculated. Resting metabolic rate is determined using a gender-specific formula that incorporates the appropriate activity factor. This figure reflects the total calories needed daily for maintaining current weight. To encourage a weight loss of 1 pound (2.2 kg) a week, the dietitian subtracts 500 calories/day. To encourage a weight loss of 2 pounds (4.4 kg) a week, the dietitian subtracts 1000 calories/day. The amount of weight lost varies with the client's food intake, level of physical activity, and water losses. Carbohydrate, protein, and fat can be calculated as in Table 61-8. A reasonable goal of 5% to 10% loss of body weight has been shown to improve glycemic control and reduce cholesterol and blood pressure, and these benefits continue if the weight loss is sustained (Wing & Jeffery, 1995).

DRUG THERAPY. A BMI of 30, or a BMI of 27 with co-morbidities, is one indicator for the use of drug therapy (Shape Up America and American Obesity Association, 1996). Anorectic drugs suppress appetite, which reduces food intake and over time may result in weight loss. These drugs play a valuable role in a comprehensive weight reduction program but should be used only as part of such a program. Currently available drugs to treat obesity act on either the noradrenergic or serotonergic systems in the central nervous system. The most commonly used anorectic drug for the treatment of obesity is sibutramine (Meridia). Sibutramine is an anorectic drug that inhibits the re-uptake of serotonin (which enhances satiety [feeling full when eating]) and norepinephrine (which raises metabolic rate). Adverse effects include dry mouth, constipation, and insomnia.

Orlistat (Xenical) is a different type of drug that inhibits lipase and leads to partial hydrolysis of triglycerides. Because fats are only partially digested and absorbed, calorie intake is decreased. Most clients taking orlistat experience gastrointestinal symptoms that include loose stools, abdominal cramps, and nausea.

TABLE 61-8 • NUTRIENT NEEDS DURING WEIGHT REDUCTION

Calorie Level	Protein	Carbohydrate	Fat	Multivitamin and Mineral Supplement
<600	1.5 g/kg/day*	50 g/day minimum	3-6 g/day linoleic acid minimum	Yes 100% of RDA or RNI
600-1200	1-1.5 g/kg/day	≥55% of calories	≤30% of calories	Yes 100% of RDA or RNI
1200	0.8-1.5 g/kg/day	≥55% of calories	≤30% of calories	Optional

Minimum at all calorie levels: Sodium, 500 mg/day; potassium, 2000 mg/day; calcium, 800 mg/day; iron, 15 mg/day; noncaloric fluids, 2 L/day.

Modified from Dwyer, J. T. (1991). Nutrient needs in weight management. *Contemporary Management of the Overweight Patient, 3,* 1-8.
*This requirement may necessitate more than 600 calories/day. Protein needs are based on ideal body weight.
RDA, Recommended Dietary Allowance; *RNI,* Recommended Nutrient Intake (Canada).

BEHAVIORAL TREATMENT. Behavioral treatment of obesity consists of various strategies to change daily eating habits to achieve weight loss. This ongoing process should produce a change in behavior. Self-monitoring techniques include keeping a record of foods eaten (food diary), exercise patterns, and emotional and situational factors. Stimulus control involves controlling the external cues that promote overeating. Reinforcement techniques are used to self-reward the behavior change. Cognitive restructuring involves modifying negative beliefs by learning positive coping self-statements.

Fairburn and Cooper (1996) have developed a cognitive behavioral approach to the acquisition of weight maintenance behavior skills. Clients are encouraged to accept modest weight loss goals and are further discouraged from losing more weight. The treatment focuses on the acquisition of weight maintenance skills and on cognitive factors and any tendency to evaluate self-worth in terms of body size. The client's focus is shifted from physical appearance to a concern for health.

CRITICAL THINKING CHALLENGE

You are caring for a 42-year-old female hospitalized client who is preparing to have bilateral knee replacements. She tells you that she has been obese her entire life and now has severe arthritis in both knees. She has tried every novelty diet available but regains the weight shortly after completing the diet. Her husband left her last year because he was embarrassed to be with her.

- What are the priority nursing diagnoses related to her obesity?
- What other options does she have for managing her nutritional problem?
- What is the psychologic impact of being obese?

For suggested answer guidelines, go to SIMON http://www.wbsaunders.com/SIMON/Iggy/.

SURGICAL MANAGEMENT. Clients who do not respond to traditional dietary intervention may be considered for a surgical procedure aimed at producing permanent weight loss. All clients with a body mass index (BMI) ≥40, or a BMI ≥35 with additional risk factors, should be considered for surgery (Shape Up America and American Obesity Association, 1996). Most surgical procedures fall into three categories:

1. Mechanical or physical (adipose tissue removal or intake restriction)
2. Malabsorptive (bypass of the gastrointestinal tract)
3. Regulatory (directly affecting hunger or thirst)

PREOPERATIVE CARE. The nurse reinforces health teaching before the client has surgery. Preoperative care is similar to that for any client undergoing abdominal surgery (see Chapter 17).

OPERATIVE PROCEDURES. Surgical procedures that physically restrict the intake of food include the following:

- Maxillomandibular fixation (jaw wiring)
- Esophageal banding
- Gastroplasty (banding or stapling the stomach)
- Intestinal bypass, in which the stomach and jejunum are connected

One of the most common procedures is gastroplasty, which decreases the size of the stomach. Stapling horizontally across the top of the stomach leaves only a small opening (0.8 to 1 cm) into the distal stomach. However, the fundic pouch created is often stretched too much, which inhibits weight loss. The vertical banded gastroplasty evolved from earlier forms of gastroplasty. It is designed with a less distensible vertical pouch that reduces the capacity for a meal by 100-fold. The small pouch outlet delays emptying and provides an internal cue for satiety.

Gastric restrictive operations sometimes produce maladaptive eating behaviors, such as the following:

- "Soft calorie syndrome" (consumption of excessive amounts of soft or liquid, calorically dense foods)
- Vomiting from inadequate chewing
- Inappropriate consumption of liquids after solids

An intestinal bypass reduces the size of the stomach with stainless steel staples but connects a small opening in the upper portion of the stomach to the small intestine by means of an intestinal loop (Figure 61-6). Complications of the intestinal bypass include bloating of the pouch. The incidence of nausea and vomiting is similar to that with gastroplasty. Intestinal bypass usually leads to greater weight loss that does gastroplasty, in part because of dumping syndrome as the use of the lower part of the stomach is omitted. Intestinal bypass operations have been modified to avoid blind loop bacterial overgrowth syndromes and are now performed as a biliointestinal bypass, jejunoileal bypass with ileogastrostomy, or duodenoileal bypass.

Surgical treatment of clinically severe obesity by either vertical banded gastroplasty or Roux-en-Y gastric bypass is a viable option for selected clients (NIH Consensus Development Conference Panel, 1991). Maximum weight loss from these procedures generally occurs 18 to 24 months after surgery. Two years after surgery, Roux-en-Y clients lost 60% to 70% of their weight, whereas gastroplasty clients lost 40% to 60%.

POSTOPERATIVE CARE. The client has a nasogastric (NG) tube put in place immediately after gastroplasty or intestinal bypass. In gastroplasty, the NG tube drains both the proximal pouch and the distal stomach. The nurse closely monitors the tube for patency. The tube is never repositioned because its movement can disrupt the suture line.

The NG tube is removed on the third day if the client has bowel sounds and is passing flatus. The nurse gives the client 1 ounce (30 mL) of water in a 1-ounce medicine cup and instructs the client to sip it slowly over 1 hour. Clear liquids are given if the client can tolerate water, and 1-ounce cups are used for each serving. Pureed foods, juice, and soups thinned with broth, water, or milk are added to the diet 24 to 48 hours after clear liquids are tolerated. Typically, the client can increase the volume to 1 ounce over 5 minutes or until satisfied, but the diet is limited to liquids or pureed foods for 6 weeks. The client then progresses to three meals a day, with an emphasis on nutrient-dense foods. Nausea, vomiting, or discomfort occurs if too much liquid is ingested.

Before discharge from the hospital, the nurse instructs the client to take liquid or chewable multivitamins daily and to consume adequate protein to promote wound healing. To avoid blockage of the pouch opening, clients are encouraged to eat slowly, chew foods well, and avoid swallowing chunks of food that cannot be liquefied completely.

ACTIVITY INTOLERANCE

PLANNING: EXPECTED OUTCOMES. The client with obesity or overweight is expected to (1) tolerate usual activity as evidenced by endurance, energy conservation, and self-care; and (2) incorporate daily exercise into his or her lifestyle.

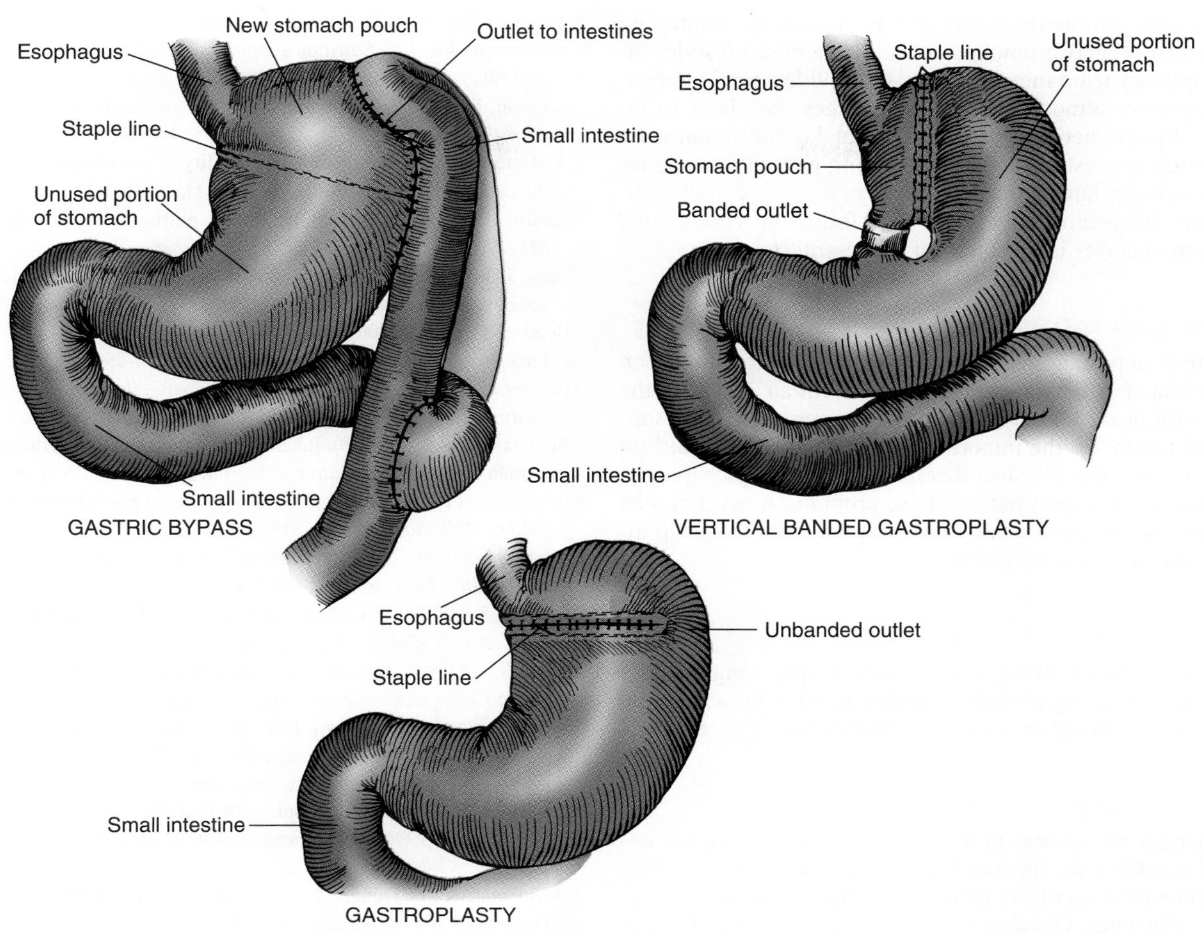

Figure 61-6 ● Surgical procedures for obesity. (Redrawn from Mahan, L.K., & Escott-Stump, S. [1996], *Krause's food, nutrition, & diet therapy* [9th ed.]. Philadelphia: W.B. Saunders.)

INTERVENTIONS. Management of the overweight or obese client is an interdisciplinary effort. The nurse collaborates with the physician, dietitian, and physical therapist or exercise physiologist to meet the goal of improving the client's physical activity tolerance. The major intervention is to increase the type and amount of daily exercise to create a calorie deficit along with modification of eating habits. Adding exercise to a diet intervention produces more weight loss than just dieting alone. More of the weight lost is fat, which preserves lean body mass. An increase in exercise produces a reduction in the waist/hip ratio.

Increasing and maintaining physical activity levels is important in maintaining weight loss. Many overweight or obese clients are so unfit that it may take several months of conditioning before they can exercise sufficiently to achieve weight loss.

The nurse or physical therapist or exercise physiologist first obtains a clinical exercise history. It is important to determine the client's current exercise pattern and exercise habits over a lifetime. The client should understand the importance of an exercise component in a weight loss program. The nurse also ascertains the client's desire to participate in an exercise program and his or her preferred types of exercise.

The health care provider evaluates the client by an exercise stress test. Not all clients need a stress test, but those with chronic disease may need a stress test and more specific exercise recommendations. The nurse counsels clients about unusual signs and symptoms during exercise (e.g., chest pain) and what to do if they occur. The physical therapist or exercise physiologist first emphasizes the importance of exercising consistently and then stresses duration, intensity, and frequency.

A minimal-level workout should be developed for the client so that consistency can be achieved. The goal for the client is to maintain a lifetime of increased physical activity. The client is apt to be less fatigued and discouraged with a low-intensity, short-duration program. Sedentary clients are encouraged to increase their activity by walking 30 to 40 minutes daily (15 to 20 minutes/mile) or the equivalent. The activity may be performed all at once or divided over the course of the day. The nurse teaches the client to exercise only under the supervision of the physician. All members of the interdisciplinary team should provide encouragement and support for any increase in physical activity.

Community-Based Care

Obese clients can be cared for in a variety of settings, including the acute care hospital and subacute unit (particularly following surgical treatment for obesity) or in their own home. Obesity is a chronic, lifelong problem. Diets, drug therapy, exercise, and behavior modification can produce short-term weight losses with reasonable safety. However, most clients who do lose weight often regain the weight. Treatment of obesity should focus on the long-term reduction of health risks and medical problems associated with obesity, improving quality of life, and promoting a health-oriented lifestyle. Interdisciplinary team members need to provide a nonjudgmental, supportive atmosphere that encourages the client to increase physical activity, decrease fat intake and reliance on medication use, establish a normal eating pattern in response to physiologic hunger, and address psychologic problems. Frequent, long-term ambulatory care follow-up coordinated by a case manager is essential for successful treatment.

HEALTH TEACHING

The most important features of client education focus on health-related behavior patterns. The dietitian counsels the client on a healthful eating pattern. The nurse provides support and reinforces the importance of maintaining a healthful eating pattern. The physical therapist or exercise physiologist recommends an appropriate exercise program. A psychologist recommends cognitive restructuring approaches that help alter dysfunctional eating patterns.

HOME CARE MANAGEMENT

The overweight or obese client needs proper weighing devices and measuring utensils to follow the diet prescribed by the physician. No other home care preparation is needed.

HEALTH CARE RESOURCES

The chances for success in a weight control program are enhanced if additional support is available. The nurse provides the client with a list of available community resources, such as Weight Watchers, Overeaters Anonymous, Take Off Pounds Sensibly (TOPS), comprehensive interdisciplinary treatment programs, and a list of professionals that includes a registered dietitian, psychologist, and exercise physiologist who may provide frequent follow-up in an ambulatory care setting.

Evaluation: Outcomes

NOC The nurse evaluates the care of the client with obesity or overweight on the basis of the identified nursing diagnoses and collaborative problems. Expected outcomes include that the client:

- Establishes a lasting, healthful dietary pattern that results in permanent, sustained weight loss
- Slowly increases the amount of physical exercise to aid in promoting weight loss
- Incorporates daily exercise into lifestyle
- Participates in usual daily activities

ONLINE RESOURCES

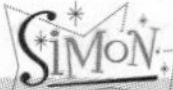

For suggested readings and Internet resources, go to http://www.wbsaunders.com/SIMON/Iggy/.

SELECTED BIBLIOGRAPHY

Asterisk indicates a classic or definitive work on this subject.

*American Dietetic Association. (1995). Position of the American Dietetic Association and the Canadian Dietetic Association: Women's health and nutrition. *Journal of the American Dietetic Association, 95*(3), 362-366.

*American Society of Parenteral and Enteral Nutrition. (1993). Section II: Rationale for adult nutrition support guidelines. *Journal of Parenteral and Enteral Nutrition, 17*(4), 5SA-6SA.

Ammon, P.K. (1999). Individualizing the approach to treating obesity. *Nurse Practitioner, 24*(2), 27-31, 36-38, 41-43.

Anderson, E.B. (2000). Facilitating quality of life through nutrition. *Advance for Nurses (DC/Baltimore), 2*(11), 17-18, 30.

Andris, D.A. (1998). Total parenteral nutrition in surgical patients. *MEDSURG Nursing, 7*(2), 76-83.

*Bass, J.D., et al. (1996). The effect of dietary fiber on tube-fed elderly patients. *Journal of Gerontology Nursing, 22*(10), 37-44.

Bender, S., et al. (2000). Malnutrition: Role of the TwoCal® HN Med Pass Program. *MEDSURG Nursing, 9*(6), 284-296.

*Booker, M., & Ignatavicius, D. (1996). *Infusion therapy: Techniques and medications.* Philadelphia: W.B. Saunders.

*Bouchard, C., et al. (1988). Inheritance of the amount and distribution of human body fat. *International Journal of Obesity, 12*(3), 205-215.

*Bowers, S. (1996). Tubes: A nurse's guide to enteral feeding devices. *MEDSURG Nursing, 5*(5), 313-324.

Bowers, S. (1999). Nutrition support for malnourished, acutely ill adults. *MEDSURG Nursing, 8*(3), 145-166.

Bowers, S. (2000). All about tubes: Your guide to enteral feeding devices. *Nursing2000, 30*(12), 41-48.

*Bray, G.A. (1994). Etiology and prevalence of obesity. In C. Bouchard (Ed.), *The genetics of obesity* (pp. 17-33). Boca Raton, FL: CRC Press.

Cammon, S.A., & Hackshaw, H.S. (2000). Are we starving our patients? *American Journal of Nursing, 100*(5), 43-47.

*Conway, J.M. (1995). Ethnicity and energy stores. *American Journal of Clinical Nutrition, 62*(5 Suppl.), 1067S-1071S.

*Costello, M.C. (1996). Home health nutrition. *MEDSURG Nursing, 5*(4), 229-239.

*Davidhizar, R., & Dunn, C. (1996). Malnutrition in the elderly. *Home Healthcare Nurse, 14*(12), 948-956.

Dudek, S.G. (2000). Malnutrition in hospitals: Who's assessing what patients eat? *American Journal of Nursing, 100*(4), 36-43.

Edwards, S.J., & Metheney, N.A. (2000). Measurement of gastric residual volume: State of the science. *MEDSURG Nursing, 9*(3), 125-128.

Epley, D. (1999). Nutritional assessment in home care patients. *Home Care Provider, 4*(3), 102-105.

*Fairburn, C.G., & Cooper, Z. (1996). New perspectives on dieting and behavioural treatments for obesity. *International Journal of Obesity, 20*(Suppl. 1), S9-S13.

Fellows, L.S., et al. (2000). Evidence-based practice for enteral feedings: Aspiration prevention strategies, bedside detection, and practice change. *MEDSURG Nursing, 9*(1), 27-32.

Food and Nutrition Board, Institute of Medicine, National Academy of Sciences. (1997). *Dietary reference intakes: Calcium, phosphorus, magnesium, vitamin D, and fluoride.* Washington, D.C.: National Academy Press.

*Food and Nutrition Board, National Research Council/National Academy of Sciences. (1989). *Recommended dietary allowances* (10th ed.). Washington, D.C.: National Academy Press.

*Gallagher-Allred, C.R., et al. (1996). Malnutrition and clinical outcomes: The case for medical nutrition therapy. *Journal of the American Dietetic Association, 96,* 366-369.

Garcia-Maas, L.D. (1999). Intergenerational analysis of dietary practices and health perceptions of Hispanic women and their adult daughters. *Journal of Transcultural Nursing, 10*(3), 213-219.

Giger, J.N., & Davidhizar, R.E. (1999). *Transcultural nursing: Assessment and intervention* (3rd ed.). St. Louis: Mosby.

Goff, K.L. (1997). The nuts and bolts of enteral infusion pumps. *MEDSURG Nursing, 6*(1), 9-16.

*Goldstein, D.J., & Potvin, J.H. (1994). Long-term weight loss: The effect of pharmacologic agents. *American Journal of Clinical Nutrition, 60*(5), 647-657.

Gore, S.V. (1999). African-American women's perceptions of weight: Paradigm shift for advanced practice. *Holistic Nursing Practice, 13*(4), 71-79.

*Grindel, C.G., & Costello, M.C. (1996). Nutrition screening: An essential assessment parameter. *MEDSURG Nursing, 5*(3), 145-156.

Harrell, J.S., & Gore, S.V. (1998). Cardiovascular risk factors and socioeconomic status in African American and Caucasian women. *Research in Nursing and Health, 21*(4), 285-295.

Jones, S.A., & Guenter, P. (1997). Automatic flush feeding pumps. *Nursing97, 27*(2), 56-59.

Kayser-Jones, J., & Pengilly, K. (1999). Dysphagia among nursing home residents. *Geriatric Nursing, 20*(2), 77-84.

*Kennedy, E., Meyers, L., & Layden, W. (1996). The 1995 dietary guidelines for Americans: An overview. *Journal of the American Dietetic Association, 96*(3), 234-237.

Kohn-Keeth, C. (2000). How to keep feeding tubes flowing freely. *Nursing2000, 30*(3), 58-59.

*Kuczmarski, R. J., et al. (1994). Increasing prevalence of overweight among U.S. adults: The National Health and Nutrition Examination Surveys, 1960-1991. *Journal of the American Medical Association, 272*(3), 205-211.

*Kumanyika, S. (1993). Special issues regarding obesity in minority populations. *Annals of Internal Medicine, 119*(7 Pt. 2), 650-654.

*Lord, L.M., Lipp, J., & Stull, S. (1996). Adult tube feeding formulas. *MEDSURG Nursing, 5*(6), 407-420.

Lyman, B., & Marquardt, P. (1997). Nutrition screening tool development and utilization for home care patients. *Home Healthcare Nurse, 15*(12), 835-842.

Messina, V.K., & Burke, K.I. (1997). Position of the American Dietetic Association: Vegetarian diets. *Journal of the American Dietetic Association, 97*(11), 1317-1321.

*Metheney, N., et al. (1990). Effectiveness of the auscultatory method in predicting feeding tube location. *Nursing Research, 39,* 262-267.

Metheney, N., et al. (1998). pH, color, and feeding tubes. *RN, 61*(1), 25-27.

Metheney, N., et al. (1998). Testing feeding tube placement: Auscultation vs. pH method. *American Journal of Nursing, 98*(5), 37-43.

Miller, D. (2000). To crush or not to crush? *Nursing2000, 30*(2), 50-52.

*Nelson, K.J., et al. (1993). Prevalence of malnutrition in the elderly admitted to long-term care facilities. *Journal of the American Dietetic Association, 93*(4), 459-461.

*NIH Consensus Development Conference Panel. (1991). Gastrointestinal surgery for severe obesity. *Annals of Internal Medicine, 115*(12), 956-961.

*Nutrition and your health: Dietary guidelines for Americans. (1995). *Home and Garden Bulletin No. 232* (4th ed.). Washington, D.C.: U.S. Department of Agriculture and U.S. Department of Health and Human Services.

**Nutrition Screening Manual for Professionals Caring for Older Americans: Nutrition Screening Initiative.* (1991). Washington, D.C.: Greer, Margois, Mitchell, Grunwald & Associates. (Available from The Nutrition Screening Initiative, 2626 Pennsylvania Ave., N.W., Suite 301, Washington, D.C. 20037.)

*Pi-Sunyer, F.X. (1993). Medical hazards of obesity. *Annals of Internal Medicine, 119,*(7 Pt. 2), 655-660.

Pontieri-Lewis, V. (1997). The role of nutrition in wound healing. *MEDSURG Nursing, 6*(4), 187-192.

Rotkoff, N. (1999). Care of the morbidly obese patient in a long-term care facility. *Geriatric Nursing, 20*(6), 309-313.

Schwartz, M.W., & Seeley, R.J. (1997). The new biology of body weight regulation. *Journal of the American Dietetic Association, 97,* 54-58.

*Shape Up America and American Obesity Association. (1996). *Guidelines for treatment of adult obesity.* Bethesda, MD: Shape Up America.

Tyler, D.O., Allan, J.D., & Alcozer, F.R. (1997). Weight loss used by African American and Euro-American women. *Research in Nursing and Health, 20*(5), 413-423.

*Vegetarian food pyramid. (1994). *Vegetarian Journal, 13,* 21.

Vellas, B., et al. (1999). The Mini Nutritional Assessment (MNA) and its use in grading the nutritional state of elderly patients. *Nutrition, 15*(2), 159-161.

*Viall, C.D. (1996). Location, location, location. *Nursing96, 26*(9), 43-45.

*Vines, S.W., et al. (1992). Research utilization: An evaluation of the research related to causes of diarrhea in tube-fed patients. *Applied Nursing Research, 5,* 164-173.

*Webber-Jones, J., et al. (1992). How to declog a feeding tube. *Nursing, 22*(4), 62-64.

Wellman, N.S. (1997). A case manager's guide to nutrition screening and intervention. *The Journal of Care Management, 3*(2), 12-27.

*Wing, R.R. & Jeffery, R.W. (1995). Effect of modest weight loss on changes in cardiovascular risk factors: Are there differences between men and women or between weight loss and maintenance? *International Journal of Obesity, 19,* 67-73.

Yen, P.K. (1999). Cancer treatment compromises nutrition. *Geriatric Nursing, 20*(5), 278-279.

UNIT

13

PROBLEMS OF REGULATION AND METABOLISM

Management of Clients with Problems of the Endocrine System

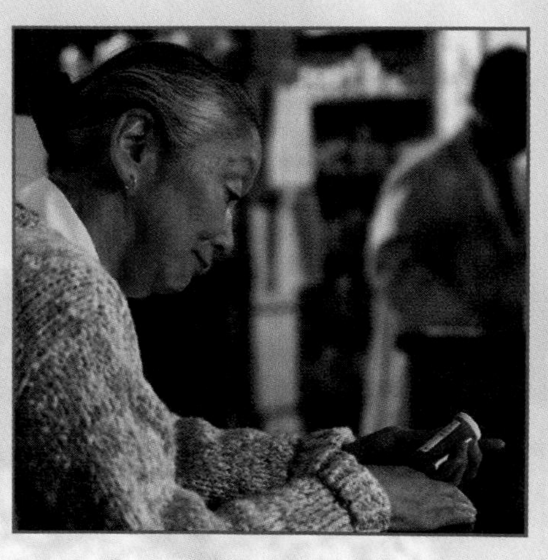

UNIT 13 PROBLEMS OF REGULATION AND METABOLISM: ENDOCRINE SYSTEM ■ Core Concepts Grid

Anatomy	Physiology	Pathophysiology	History	Physical Exam	Diagnostic Tests	Interventions	Pharmacology
• **Glands** Anterior pituitary Posterior pituitary Thyroid Parathyroid Pancreas Adrenal • **Hormones** Antidiuretic hormone (ADH) Thyroid-stimulating hormone (TSH) Adrenocorticotropic hormone (ACTH) Growth hormone (GH) Mineralocorticoids Glucocorticoids Androgens Epinephrine Norepinephrine Thyroxine Thyrocalcitonin Parathormone Insulin Glucagon	• **Neuroregulation** • **Hypothalamus** • **Regulation** Metabolism Fluids/electrolytes Glucose levels Stress response	• **Inflammation** • **Hypersecretion** • **Hyposecretion** • **Infection** • **Diabetic ketoacidosis** • **Hyperglycemic hyperosmolar nonketotic syndrome (HHNKS)** • **Adrenal crisis**	• **Client history** Energy level Elimination pattern Nutrition Reproductive function Libido • **Family history** Endocrine disease • **Social history** Drug/alcohol use Coping skills Age Gender • **Weight change**	• **Appearance** Skin Hair Body fat distribution Muscle mass Bruising Petechiae Edema Face Genitalia • **Size of thyroid** • **Vital signs** • **Weight**	• **Adrenocorticotropic hormone (ACTH) levels** • **Aldosterone assay** • **Antidiuretic hormone (ADH)** • **Blood glucose** • **Catecholamines** Vanillylmandelic acid (VMA) • **Cortisol** • **Glycosolated hemoglobin A_{lc}** • **17-hydroxycorticosteroids** • **Ketones** • **Parathyroid hormone level** • **T_3/T_4** • **Thyroid scan**	• **Hormone replacement** • **Nutrition** • **Fluid management** • **Stress management** • **Client education** Diet Exercise Hormone replacement regimen Overdose Underdose Foot care Signs of complications Need for carrying emergency medical information • **Postoperative care/monitoring for complications** Thyroidectomy Adrenalectomy Pancreas transplantation • **Monitoring for hypoglycemia and hyperglycemia**	• **Glucagon** • **Insulin** • **Oral hypoglycemic agents** • **Thyroid replacement** • **Thyroid inhibitors** • **Pituitary hormone replacements** • **Pituitary hormone inhibitors** • **Parathyroid hormone replacement** • **Parathyroid hormone inhibitors** • **Calcium** • **Adrenal hormone replacements** • **Adrenal hormone inhibitors**

CHAPTER 62

Assessment of the Endocrine System

M. LINDA WORKMAN

Learning Objectives

After studying this chapter, you should be able to:

1. Describe the relationship between hormones and receptor sites.
2. Explain negative feedback as a control mechanism for hormone secretion.
3. Discuss the structure and function of the hypothalamus.
4. Discuss the structure and function of the anterior and posterior pituitary glands.
5. Discuss the structure and function of the adrenal glands.
6. Discuss the structure and function of the thyroid and parathyroid glands.
7. Discuss the structure and function of the pancreas.
8. Describe changes in the endocrine system associated with aging.
9. Identify laboratory tests that aid in determining endocrine function and dysfunction.

SIMON

Go to http://www.wbsaunders.com/SIMON/Iggy/ for self-assessment questions related to these Learning Objectives.

The endocrine system is composed of glands in many tissues and organs in a variety of body areas (Figure 62-1). A key feature of all endocrine glands is the secretion of hormones. **Hormones** are biochemicals that exert their effects on specific tissues known as **target tissues.** Target tissues are usually located some distance from the endocrine gland, with no direct physical connection between the endocrine gland and its target tissue. For this reason endocrine glands are called "ductless" glands and must use the circulatory system to transport secreted hormones to the target tissues. Endocrine glands include the following:

- Pituitary gland
- Adrenal glands
- Thyroid gland
- Islet cells of the pancreas
- Parathyroid glands
- Gonads

The endocrine system works with the nervous system to regulate overall physiologic function. Such control is called **neuroendocrine regulation.** Many interactions must occur between the endocrine system and all other body systems to ensure that each system maintains a constant normal balance **(homeostasis)** in response to environmental changes. For example, neuroendocrine control of other body systems keeps the internal body temperature at or near 98.6° F (37° C), even when environmental temperatures are lower or higher. Other neuroendocrine actions help keep the serum sodium level between 136 and 145 mEq/L (mmol/L), regardless of whether a person eats 2 g or 12 g of sodium per day.

Table 62-1 lists the specific hormones secreted by various endocrine glands. Hormones usually travel through the bloodstream to all body areas but exert their actions only on target tissues. Hormones recognize their target tissues and exert their actions by binding to receptor sites on or within the target tissue cells. In general, each receptor site type is specific for only one hormone. Hormone-receptor interactions work in a "lock and key" manner in that only the correct hormone (key) can bind to and activate the receptor site (lock) (Figure 62-2). Binding a hormone to its receptor causes the target tissue to change its activity. In this way, hormones produce specific responses even though they circulate throughout the body. Table 62-2 lists the key features of hormones.

Disorders of the endocrine system are related to either an excess or a deficiency of a specific hormone or to a defect at its receptor site. The onset of these disorders can be either slow and insidious or abrupt and life threatening.

The nurse's observation and interviewing skills are especially important in assessing the endocrine system. Except for the thyroid gland and the testicles, the endocrine glands cannot be examined directly. A knowledge of the anatomy and physiology of the endocrine system together with data obtained from the history and laboratory diagnostic tests is essential in assessing the endocrine system.

ANATOMY AND PHYSIOLOGY REVIEW

The control of cellular function by any hormone depends on a series of reactions working through **negative feedback control mechanisms.** Hormone secretion is dependent on the need of the body for the final action of that hormone. When a body condition starts to move away from the normal range and a specific action or response is needed to correct this change,

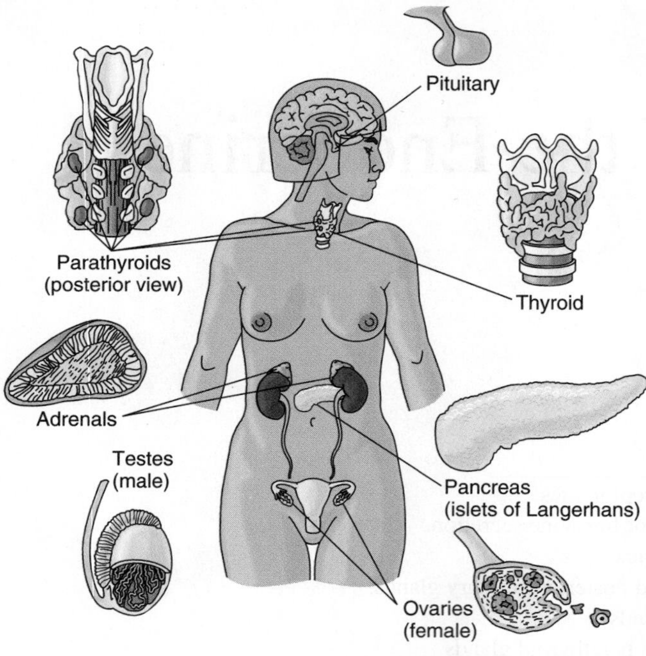

Figure 62-1 ● The endocrine system.

TABLE 62-1 ● PRINCIPAL HORMONES OF THE ENDOCRINE GLANDS

Gland	Hormones
Anterior pituitary	Thyroid-stimulating hormone (TSH) Adrenocorticotropic hormone (ACTH, corticotropin) Luteinizing hormone (LH) Follicle-stimulating hormone (FSH) Prolactin (PRL) Growth hormone (GH) Melanocyte-stimulating hormone (MSH)
Posterior pituitary	Vasopressin (antidiuretic hormone [ADH]) Oxytocin
Thyroid	Triiodothyronine (T_3) Thyroxine (T_4) Calcitonin
Parathyroids	Parathyroid hormone
Adrenal cortex	Glucocorticoids (cortisol) Mineralocorticoids (aldosterone)
Ovary	Estrogen Progesterone
Testes	Testosterone
Pancreas	Insulin Glucagon Somatostatin

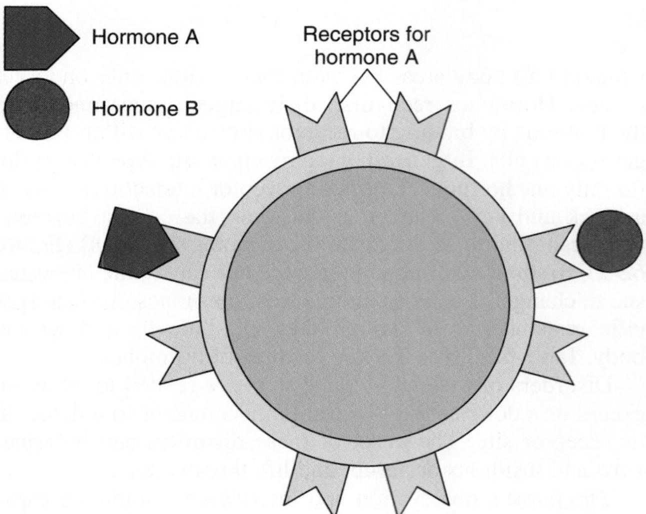

Figure 62-2 ● "Lock and key" hormone-receptor binding. Hormone A fits and binds to receptor sites, causing a change in cell action. Hormone B does not fit or bind to receptor sites, and therefore no change in cell action results.

TABLE 62-2 ● COMMON KEY FEATURES OF HORMONES

- All hormones exert their effects at low blood concentrations.
- Receptors on or within target tissues are needed for *all* hormones to exert an effect.
- Most hormones (except for thyroid and adrenal medullary hormones) are not stored to any great extent and must be produced as needed.
- Hormones in the blood are bound to plasma proteins.
- Only free hormones (those not bound to plasma proteins) can bind to their receptor sites.
- Most hormones cause target tissues to increase or decrease their activity by changing gene activity either directly or indirectly. Exceptions are hormones that alter membrane permeability.
- The activity of most hormones is of short duration.
- Continued hormone activity requires continued production and secretion.
- The clearance of secreted hormones occurs through cellular uptake, enzymatic breakdown, gastrointestinal excretion, or urinary excretion.

secretion of the hormone capable of causing the correcting action or response is stimulated until the need (demand) is met. As the correction occurs, hormone secretion decreases (and may halt). This type of control for hormone synthesis is considered negative feedback because the hormone causes the opposite action of the initial condition change.

An example of a simple negative feedback hormone response is the control of insulin secretion. When blood glucose levels start to rise above normal, the hormone insulin is secreted. Insulin causes glucose to be taken up by the cells, causing a decrease in blood glucose levels. Thus the action of insulin (decreasing blood glucose levels) is opposite of the condition that stimulated insulin secretion (elevated blood glucose levels).

Some hormones that use negative feedback mechanisms have more complex interactions. These interactions involve a series of reactions in which more than one endocrine gland is stimulated as well as the final target tissues. In such a situation, the first hormone in the series may have another endocrine gland as its target tissue. For this type of mechanism to maintain homeostasis, the following series of interactions must occur:

- The central nervous system receives and reacts to various stimuli transmitted to the hypothalamus.

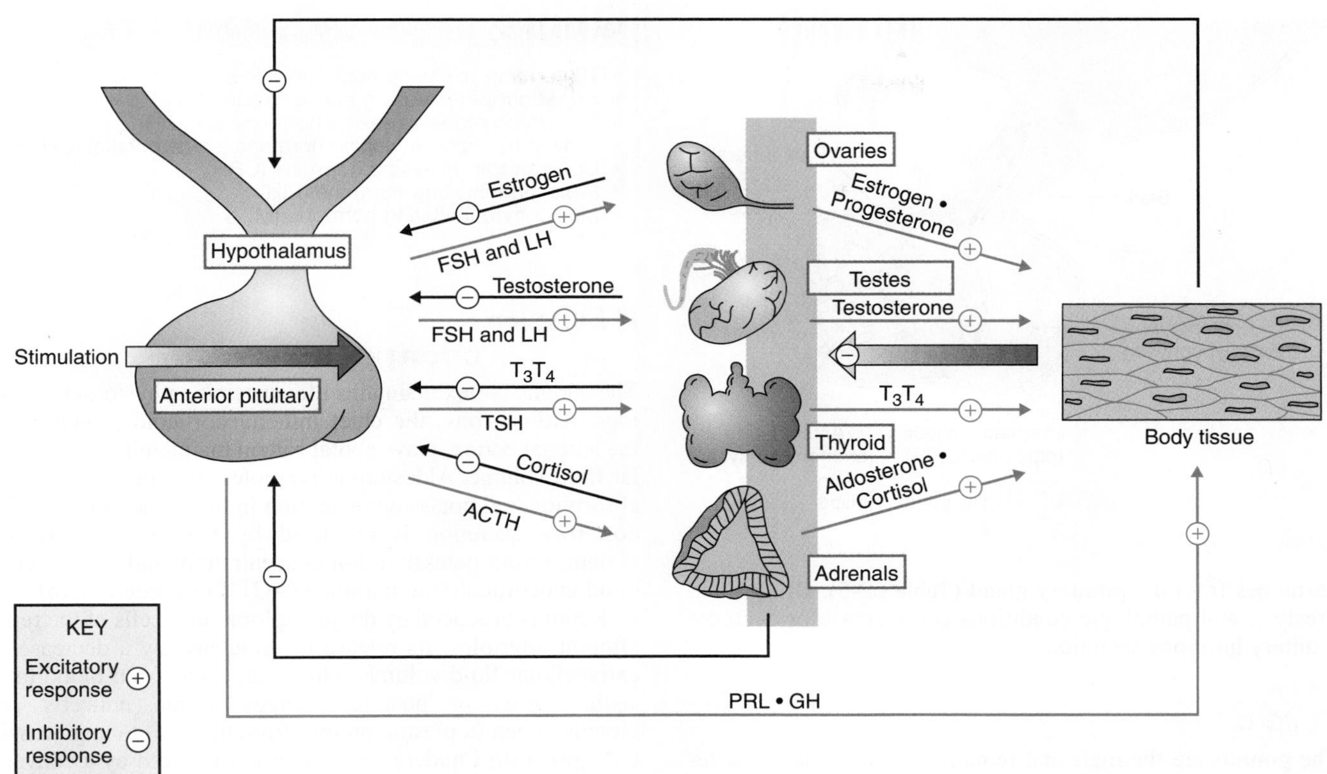

Figure 62-3 ● The feedback system of the hypothalamic-pituitary-target gland axis. (*ACTH,* Adrenocorticotropic hormone; *TSH,* thyroid-stimulating hormone; T_3, triiodothyronine; T_4, thyroxine; *FSH,* follicle-stimulating hormone; *LH,* luteinizing hormone; *PRL,* prolactin; *GH,* growth hormone.)

- The hypothalamus responds to the stimuli with the production and release of either releasing or inhibiting factors, which are transported to the pituitary.
- In the pituitary gland, the releasing or inhibiting factors either stimulate or inhibit the release of specific hormones.
- The anterior pituitary responds to these hormones by controlling the secretion of hormones from target organs or tissue.

This type of complex control is demonstrated by the interaction of the hypothalamus and the anterior pituitary with a target tissue (e.g., thyroid, adrenal cortex, or gonads) (Figure 62-3). The normal blood level range of each hormone is well defined. Excesses or deficiencies of hormone secretion can lead to pathologic conditions.

Hypothalamus and Pituitary Glands

Structure

The hypothalamus plays a major role in regulating endocrine function. The hypothalamus consists of nervous tissue located beneath the cerebral hemispheres and thalamus on each side of the third ventricle in the brain. Nerve fibers connect the hypothalamus to the rest of the central nervous system. The hypothalamus shares a miniature circulatory system with the anterior pituitary gland. This system is known as the **hypothalamic-hypophysial portal system** and allows hormones produced in the hypothalamus to travel directly to the anterior pituitary gland.

The pituitary gland is located at the base of the brain in an indentation of the sphenoid bone called the sella turcica (see Figure 62-1). The oval pituitary gland is about 1 cm in diameter and is divided into three lobes (Figure 62-4). The anterior lobe, or **adenohypophysis,** makes up about 70% of the gland. The posterior lobe, or **neurohypophysis,** stores hormones produced in the hypothalamus. Nerve fibers in the hypophysial stalk, a structure extending from the hypothalamus, connect the hypothalamus to the posterior pituitary. The area between the anterior and posterior lobes is the intermediate lobe **(pars intermedia).**

Function

The hypothalamus has both endocrine and nonendocrine functions. The endocrine function is to produce regulatory hormones (Table 62-3). Some of these hormones are released into the bloodstream and travel to the anterior pituitary, where they either stimulate or inhibit the release of anterior pituitary hormones.

In response to the releasing hormones of the hypothalamus, the anterior pituitary secretes **tropic hormones,** which stimulate various glands. Other anterior pituitary hormones, such as growth hormone (somatotropin) and prolactin, produce their primary effect directly on final target tissues (Table 62-4).

The hormones of the posterior pituitary, vasopressin (antidiuretic hormone [ADH]) and oxytocin, are produced in the hypothalamus and transported by the nerve tracts that connect the hypothalamus with the posterior pituitary. These hormones are stored in the nerve endings of the posterior pituitary and are released into the blood vessels when needed.

Other conditions or substances can affect the release of

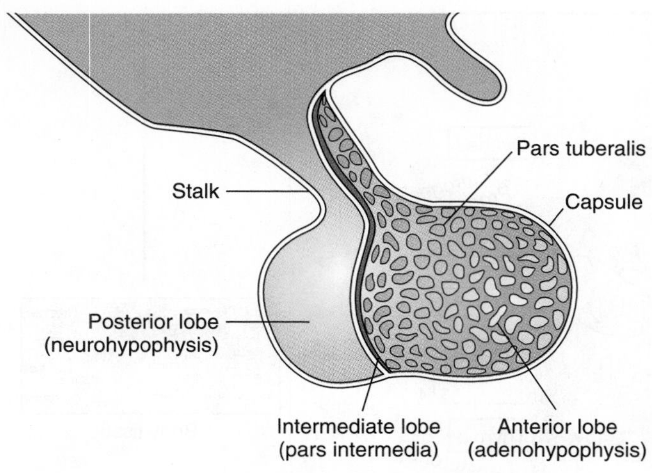

Figure 62-4 ● The pituitary gland.

hormones from the pituitary gland (Table 62-5). Drugs, diet, lifestyle, and pathologic conditions can increase or decrease pituitary hormone secretion.

Gonads

The **gonads** are the male and female endocrine glands of reproduction. Male gonads are the testes, and female gonads are the ovaries. Although these glands are formed prenatally and are present at birth, their function does not begin until puberty.

During puberty in the male, the increased secretion of gonadotropins (luteinizing hormone [LH] and follicle-stimulating hormone [FSH]) from the anterior pituitary gland stimulates maturation of the testes, production of testosterone, and maturation of the external genitalia. During puberty in the female, increased secretion of the same gonadotropins stimulates ovarian maturation, estrogen production, ovulation, and maturation of the external genitalia. The structure and function of the testes and ovaries are detailed in Chapter 73.

Adrenal Glands

The adrenal glands are highly vascular, tent-shaped organs located at the top of each kidney (see Figure 62-1). Each gland is about 3.3 cm long and weighs $\frac{1}{16}$ to $\frac{1}{8}$ ounce (1.8 to 3.5 g).

The adrenal gland consists of an outer portion **(cortex)** and an inner portion **(medulla);** each has independent functions. The hormones of the adrenal glands have physiologic effects throughout the body.

ADRENAL CORTEX

Structure

The adrenal cortex makes up about 90% of the adrenal gland and consists of cells divided into three zones or layers (Figure 62-5). **Mineralocorticoids** are produced in the zona glomerulosa and help control the body's mineral content, especially sodium and potassium. Glucocorticoids, androgens, and estrogens are produced in the zona fasciculata and zona reticularis. The hormones produced and secreted by the cortex are often called **adrenal steroids** or **corticosteroids.**

TABLE 62-3 • HYPOTHALAMIC HORMONES

- Thyrotropin-releasing hormone (TRH)
- Gonadotropin-releasing hormone (Gn-RH)
- Growth hormone–releasing hormone (GH-RH)
- Growth hormone–inhibiting hormone (somatostatin) (GH-IH)
- Corticotropin-releasing hormone (CRH)
- Prolactin-inhibiting hormone (PIH)
- Melanocyte-inhibiting hormone (MIH)

Function

MINERALOCORTICOIDS

The adrenal cortex maintains life-sustaining physiologic activities. **Aldosterone,** the chief mineralocorticoid produced by the adrenal cortex, plays a vital role in maintaining extracellular fluid volume. Aldosterone promotes sodium and water reabsorption and potassium excretion in the kidney tubules. Aldosterone secretion is regulated by the renin-angiotensin system, serum potassium ion concentration, and the presence of adrenocorticotropic hormone (ACTH or corticotropin).

Renin is produced by the juxtaglomerular cells of the renal afferent arterioles. Its release is stimulated by a decrease in extracellular fluid volume, which can occur from blood loss, sodium loss, or posture changes. Renin converts angiotensinogen (a plasma protein from the live) to angiotensin I. Angiotensin I undergoes a reaction catalyzed by a converting enzyme to form angiotensin II, the active form of angiotensin. In turn, angiotensin II stimulates the secretion of aldosterone. Chapters 11 (Figure 11-8), 12 (Figure 12-2), and 69 further describe the renin-angiotensin system. Aldosterone causes kidney reabsorption of sodium and water to bring the plasma volume and concentration back to normal.

Serum potassium ion concentration also has a regulatory effect on aldosterone secretion. The adrenal cortex secretes aldosterone when the serum potassium concentration increases above normal by as little as 0.1 mEq/L (Orth & Kovacs, 1998).

ACTH has a weak stimulatory effect on aldosterone secretion. When ACTH is administered, aldosterone secretion rapidly rises during the first hour then decreases rapidly to basal levels.

GLUCOCORTICOIDS

The principal glucocorticoid secreted by the adrenal cortex is **cortisol.** Cortisol affects the following:

- Carbohydrate, protein, and fat metabolism
- The body's response to stress
- Emotional stability
- Immune function

Cortisol has a permissive effect on other physiologic processes. It must be present for other physiologic processes to occur, such as catecholamine action and the maintenance of normal excitability of the myocardium. Glucocorticoid functions are summarized in Table 62-6.

The release of glucocorticoids is regulated directly by the anterior pituitary hormone ACTH and indirectly by the hypothalamic corticotropin-releasing hormone (CRH). The release of CRH and ACTH is affected by the serum concentration of free cortisol, the diurnal sleep-wake cycle, and stress.

TABLE 62-4 • PITUITARY HORMONES: TARGET TISSUES AND SUBSEQUENT ACTIONS

Hormone	Target Tissue	Actions
ANTERIOR PITUITARY		
TSH (thyroid-stimulating hormone)	Thyroid	Stimulates synthesis and release of thyroid hormone
ACTH (adrenocorticotropic hormone, corticotropin)	Adrenal cortex	Stimulates synthesis and release of corticosteroids and adrenocortical growth
LH (luteinizing hormone)	Ovary Testes	Stimulates ovulation and progesterone secretion Stimulates testosterone secretion
FSH (follicle-stimulating hormone)	Ovary Testes	Stimulates estrogen secretion and follicle maturation Stimulates spermatogenesis
PRL (prolactin)	Mammary glands	Stimulates breast milk production
GH (growth hormone)	Bone and soft tissue	Promotes growth through lipolysis, protein anabolism, and insulin antagonism
MSH (melanocyte-stimulating hormone)	Melanocytes	Promotes pigmentation
POSTERIOR PITUITARY*		
Vasopressin (antidiuretic hormone [ADH])	Kidney	Promotes water reabsorption
Oxytocin	Uterus and mammary glands	Stimulates uterine contractions and ejection of breast milk

*These hormones are synthesized in the hypothalamus and are stored in the posterior pituitary gland. They are transported from the hypothalamus to the posterior pituitary while bound to neurophysins.

When levels of serum cortisol are low, the hypothalamus secretes CRH, which stimulates the pituitary to release ACTH. ACTH then stimulates the adrenal cortex to secrete cortisol. Conversely, adequate or elevated levels of circulating free cortisol *inhibit* the release of CRH and ACTH. This inhibitory effect is an example of a negative feedback system.

Glucocorticoid release peaks in the morning and reaches its lowest level 12 hours before and after each peak. Emotional, chemical, or physical stress results in an increased release of glucocorticoids.

SEX HORMONES

Small amounts of androgens and estrogens are secreted by the adrenal cortex in both genders. Adrenal secretion of these hormones is usually not significant because the **gonads** (ovaries and testes) secrete much larger amounts of estrogens and androgens. In women, however, the adrenal gland is the major source of androgens. Women who have adrenal insufficiency or who have undergone surgical removal of the adrenals may need a small amount of testosterone replacement.

ADRENAL MEDULLA

Structure

The adrenal medulla is actually a sympathetic nerve ganglion with glandular secretory cells. Stimulation of the sympathetic nervous system results in the release of adrenal medullary hormones, the **catecholamines.** Catecholamines travel to all areas of the body through the bloodstream and exert their effects on target cells. The adrenal medullary hormones are not essential for life but play a role in the physiologic stress response.

Function

The adrenal medulla secretes two catecholamines, **norepinephrine (NE)** and **epinephrine,** in proportions of 15% and

TABLE 62-5 • FACTORS AFFECTING SECRETION/RELEASE OF SELECTED PITUITARY HORMONES

VASOPRESSIN

Potential Causes of Increased Secretion
- Congestive heart failure
- Hemorrhage
- Diuretics
- Opioids
- Chlorpropamide
  - Diabinese
  - Novo-Propamide♣
- Cyclophosphamide
- Vincristine
- Nicotine
- Stress
- Hypoxia

Potential Causes of Decreased Secretion
- Alcohol consumption
- Phenytoin

GROWTH HORMONE

Potential Causes of Increased Secretion
- High-protein diet
- Deep sleep
- Hypoglycemia
- Fasting
- Estrogen
- Glucagon
- Dopamine

Potential Causes of Decreased Secretion
- REM sleep
- Hyperglycemia
- Obesity
- Hypothyroidism

PROLACTIN

Potential Causes of Increased Secretion
- Stress
- Nipple manipulation
- Estrogen
- Dopamine antagonists
- Chlorpromazine
  - Thorazine
  - Chlorpromanyl♣

Potential Causes of Decreased Secretion
- Dopamine
- Hyperthyroidism

OXYTOCIN

Potential Causes of Increased Secretion
- Nipple manipulation
- Orgasm
- Extracellular fluid hypertonicity

Potential Causes of Decreased Secretion
- Stress
- Opioids

Data from Wilson, J., et al. (Eds.). (1998). *William's textbook of endocrinology* (9th ed.). Philadelphia: W.B. Saunders.

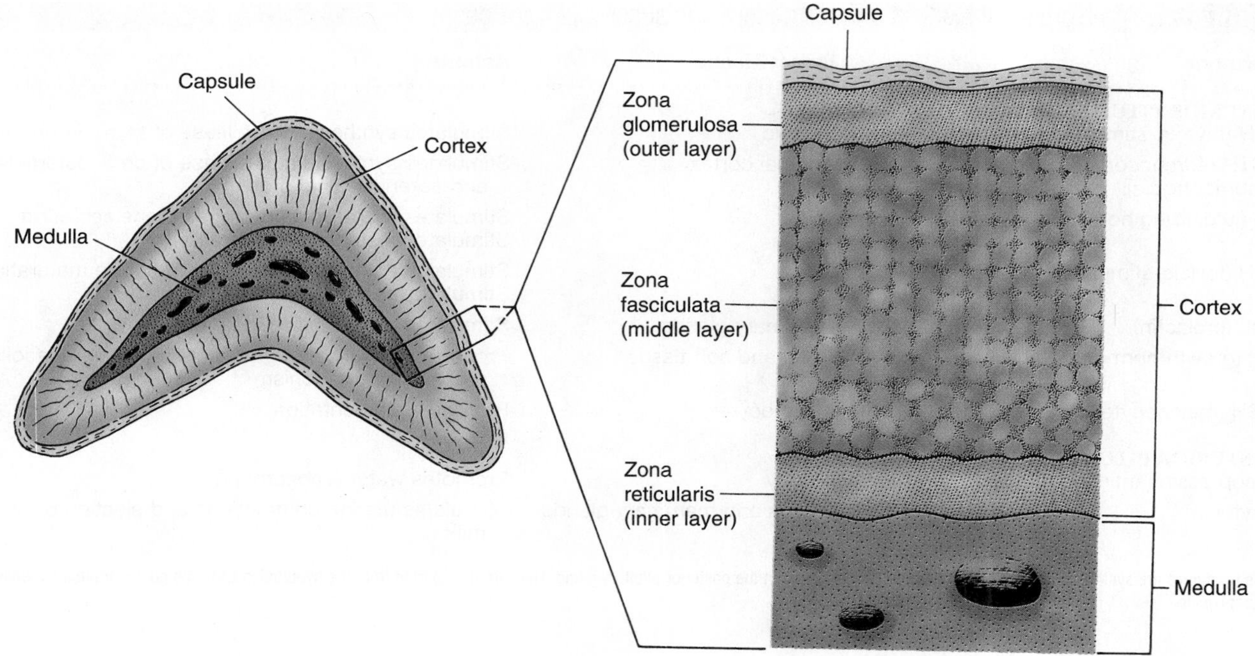

Figure 62-5 • The structural detail of the adrenal gland.

TABLE 62-6 • FUNCTIONS OF GLUCOCORTICOID HORMONES

- Maintain blood glucose level by increasing hepatic gluconeogenesis and inhibiting peripheral glucose use
- Increase lipolysis, releasing glycerol and free fatty acids
- Increase protein catabolism
- Degrade collagen and connective tissue
- Increase the number of polymorphonuclear leukocytes released from bone marrow
- Exert anti-inflammatory effects that decrease the migration of inflammatory cells to sites of injury
- Maintain behavior and cognitive functions

85%, respectively. The effects of catecholamines vary according to the specific receptor in the cell membranes of the target tissue.

These receptors are of two types: alpha adrenergic and beta adrenergic. Both types of receptors are further classified as alpha$_1$- and alpha$_2$-receptors and beta$_1$-, beta$_2$-, and beta$_3$-receptors. NE acts primarily on alpha-adrenergic receptors, whereas epinephrine most often stimulates beta-adrenergic receptors.

Catecholamines exert their actions on many target organs. Table 62-7 summarizes the effects of adrenal medullary hormone stimulation on body tissues and organs.

Activation of the sympathetic nervous system, with the subsequent release of adrenal medullary catecholamines, is an important component of the body's response to stress. Catecholamines are secreted in small amounts at all times to maintain homeostasis. Severe physical or psychologic stress triggers the increased secretion of catecholamines. This sympathetic activation results in the "fight-or-flight" response, a state of heightened physical and emotional awareness. (See Chapter 41 for more information on the sympathetic [adrenergic] nervous system.)

TABLE 62-7 • CATECHOLAMINE RECEPTORS AND EFFECTS OF ADRENAL MEDULLARY HORMONE STIMULATION ON SELECTED ORGANS AND TISSUES

Organ or Tissue	Receptors	Effects
Heart	Beta$_1$	Chronotropic action Inotropic action
Blood vessels	Alpha Beta$_2$	Vasoconstriction Vasodilation
Gastrointestinal tract	Alpha Beta	Increased sphincter tone Decreased motility
Kidney	Beta$_2$	Increased renin release
Bronchioles	Beta$_2$	Relaxation; dilation
Bladder	Alpha Beta$_2$	Sphincter contractions Relaxation of detrusor muscle
Skin	Alpha	Increased sweating
Fat cells	Beta	Increased lipolysis
Liver	Alpha	Increased gluconeogenesis and glycogenolysis
Pancreas	Alpha Beta	Decreased glucagon and insulin release Increased glucagon and insulin release
Eyes	Alpha	Dilation of pupils

Thyroid Gland

Structure

The thyroid gland is located anteriorly in the neck, directly below the cricoid cartilage (Figure 62-6). In the average adult, the thyroid weighs approximately $\frac{3}{5}$ of an ounce (18 g). It has

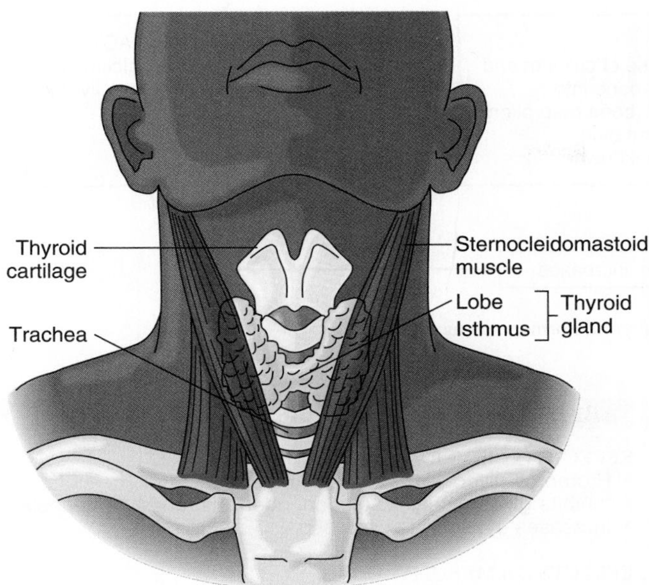

Figure 62-6 ● Anatomic location of the thyroid gland.

two lobes joined by a thin **isthmus** that lies in front of the trachea.

The thyroid gland has a rich blood supply. The right lobe has a greater blood supply and is often larger than the left lobe. The thyroid is composed of follicular and parafollicular cells. Follicular cells produce and secrete the thyroid hormones **thyroxine (T_4)** and **triiodothyronine (T_3).** Parafollicular cells produce and secrete **thyrocalcitonin** (calcitonin), which plays a role in calcium regulation.

Function

REGULATION OF BASAL METABOLIC RATE

Both T_3 and T_4 increase the basal metabolic rate, which causes an increase in oxygen consumption and heat production. The two hormones differ not in function but rather in structure. Approximately 99.5% of circulating T_4 and T_3 is bound to plasma proteins, including prealbumin, albumin, and thyroid-binding globulin, but the proportion of bound hormone is in equilibrium with the free hormone. The free hormone is transported into the cell, where it binds to a specific receptor in the cell nucleus. Once in the cell, T_4 is converted to T_3—the most active form of the hormone. The cellular conversion of T_4 to T_3 is impaired by a number of factors that include stress, starvation, radiopaque dyes, beta blockers, and propylthiouracil (PTU); cold temperatures seem to increase conversion. Table 62-8 summarizes thyroid hormone function.

The secretion of T_3 and T_4 is regulated by a hypothalamic-pituitary-thyroid gland axis, or feedback mechanism. The anterior pituitary secretes thyroid-stimulating hormone (TSH), which stimulates the thyroid gland to release thyroid hormone. The circulating level of thyroid hormone is the major factor regulating the release of TSH: if thyroid hormone levels are high, TSH release is inhibited; if low, TSH release is increased. This is a classic example of a negative feedback system. Secretion of TSH is also affected by the hypothalamic secretion of thyrotropin-releasing hormone (TRH). Cold and stress are two factors that cause the hypothalamus to secrete TRH, which then stimulates the anterior pituitary to secrete TSH.

TABLE 62-8 • FUNCTIONS OF THYROID HORMONES

- Fetal development, particularly neural and skeletal systems
- Control metabolic rate of all cells
- Promote sufficient pituitary secretion of GH and gonadotropins
- Regulate protein, carbohydrate, and fat metabolism
- Exert chronotropic and inotropic cardiac effects
- Increase red blood cell production
- Affect respiratory rate and drive
- Increase bone formation and decrease bone resorption of calcium
- Act as insulin antagonists

GH, Growth hormone.

The synthesis of thyroid hormones involves a series of steps. A sufficient dietary intake of protein and iodine in food and water is essential to produce thyroid hormones. Iodine is absorbed from the gastrointestinal tract as iodide. The thyroid gland withdraws iodide from the circulation and concentrates it. After its transport in the thyroid, iodide enters into a series of reactions that result in the formation of T_4 or T_3. The hormones are bound to thyroglobulin and are stored in the follicular cells of the thyroid gland. With stimulation, T_4 and T_3 break off from thyroglobulin and are released into the circulation.

CALCIUM AND PHOSPHATE REGULATION

Calcitonin is another thyroid hormone produced in the medullary portion of the thyroid. Calcitonin lowers serum calcium and serum phosphate levels by inhibiting bone resorption (breakdown). It works in opposition to parathyroid hormone (PTH).

The primary factor influencing calcitonin secretion is the serum calcium level. Low serum calcium levels suppress the release of calcitonin; elevated serum calcium levels increase its secretion. Additional factors that cause an increased release of calcitonin are pregnancy, a high-calcium diet, and an increased secretion of gastrin.

Parathyroid Glands

Structure

The parathyroid glands consist of four small glands located close to, embedded in, or attached to the posterior surface of the thyroid gland (see Figure 62-1). The parathyroid glands are composed of two types of cells: chief and oxyphil. Only the chief cells, which produce and secrete PTH, have endocrine function.

Function

PTH regulates calcium and phosphate metabolism as a result of its effect on three target organs: bone, kidney, and the gastrointestinal (GI) tract (Figure 62-7). Bone is the primary storage site of calcium in the body. PTH promotes increased bone resorption, thus increasing serum calcium. In the kidney

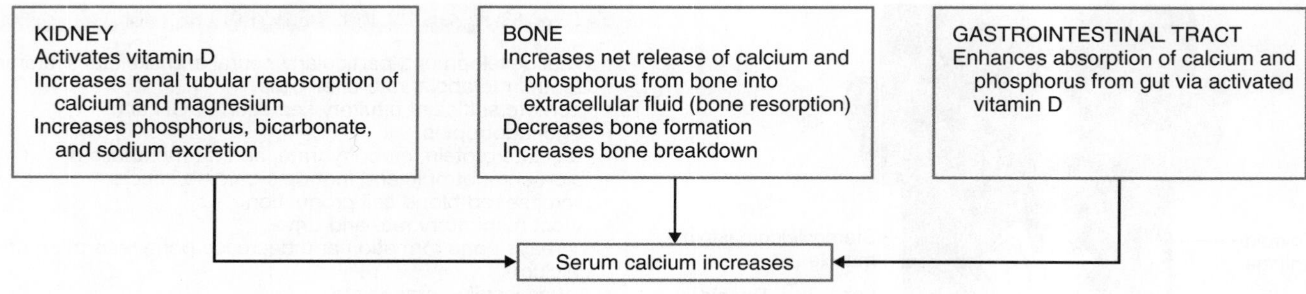

Figure 62-7 ● Effects of parathyroid hormone on target organs.

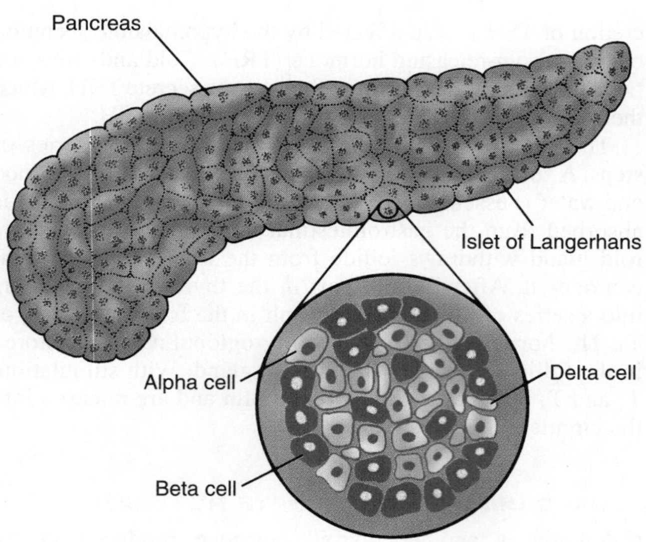

Figure 62-8 ● The islets of Langerhans of the pancreas.

tubules, PTH activates vitamin D, which increases the absorption of calcium and phosphate from the GI tract.

Calcium is the major controlling factor of PTH secretion. PTH secretion decreases when serum calcium levels are elevated, and it increases when serum calcium levels are low. Serum phosphate levels also affect PTH secretion, most likely because of its effect on serum calcium levels. PTH and calcitonin work together to maintain a normal level of ionic calcium in the extracellular fluid.

Pancreas

Structure

The pancreas lies behind the stomach and has endocrine and exocrine functions. The **islets of Langerhans** perform the endocrine functions of the pancreas (Figure 62-8). There are about 1 million islet cells throughout the pancreas.

The islets of Langerhans are composed of three distinct cell types: alpha cells, which secrete **glucagon;** beta cells, which secrete **insulin;** and delta cells, which secrete **somatostatin.** Glucagon and insulin affect carbohydrate, protein, and fat metabolism. Somatostatin, which is secreted not only in the pancreas but also in the gut and the brain, inhibits the release and action of glucagon and insulin from the pancreas. It also inhibits the release and action of gastrin, secretin, and other peptides in the gut.

TABLE 62-9 • ANABOLIC EFFECTS OF INSULIN

EFFECTS ON LIVER
- Promotes glycogen synthesis and storage
- Inhibits glycogenolysis, gluconeogenesis, and ketogenesis
- Increases triglyceride synthesis

EFFECTS ON MUSCLE
- Promotes protein synthesis
- Increases amino acid transport
- Promotes glycogenesis

EFFECTS ON FAT
- Increases fatty acid synthesis
- Promotes triglyceride storage
- Decreases lipolysis

Function

The exocrine function of the pancreas involves the secretion of digestive enzymes through ducts that empty into the duodenum (see Chapter 53). The primary endocrine function of the pancreas is to regulate blood glucose (sugar).

Glucagon increases blood glucose levels. Glucagon is stimulated by a decrease in blood glucose levels and an increase in blood amino acid levels. In conjunction with epinephrine, growth hormone (GH), and the glucocorticoids, glucagon maintains blood glucose levels. In the liver, the primary target organ of glucagon, glucagon causes **glycogenolysis** (the conversion of glycogen to glucose). In addition, glucagon enhances amino acid transport from muscle and promotes **gluconeogenesis** (the conversion of amino acids to glucose). In fat metabolism, glucagon enhances **lipolysis** (fat breakdown) and subsequent ketone formation.

Insulin, an **anabolic** hormone (one that stimulates growth), promotes the synthesis and storage of carbohydrate (CHO), protein, and fat (Table 62-9). Insulin lowers blood glucose levels by enhancing glucose diffusion across cell membranes in many tissues. Basal levels of insulin are secreted continuously in the fasting state to control metabolism. Insulin secretion rises in response to an increase in blood glucose levels. CHO is the major stimulus for insulin secretion; amino acids may produce an effect that is similar but not as potent. More information on insulin is presented in Chapter 65.

Endocrine Changes Associated with Aging

The effects of aging on the endocrine system vary considerably. It is difficult to distinguish normal from abnormal en-

CHART 62-1

NURSING FOCUS *on the* OLDER ADULT

Changes in the Endocrine System Related to Aging

Physiologic Change	Nursing Actions	Rationale
Increased antidiuretic hormone (ADH)	Assess for diluted urine and polyuria.	Ongoing assessment helps to detect early signs of complications.
	Monitor fluid intake and output. Encourage fluid intake unless contraindicated.	A sufficient fluid intake may help prevent dehydration.
Decreased ovarian function	Teach the client the signs and symptoms of estrogen deficiency.	The client's ability to cope with changes may be enhanced with knowledge.
	Promote exercise and calcium intake.	Sufficient exercise and calcium intake delay bone loss and prevent osteoporosis.
Decreased glucose tolerance	Identify at risk clients by obtaining a family history of diabetes mellitus and obesity. Assess for greater-than-ideal body weight or body mass index, little physical exercise, frequent yeast infections, polydipsia, polyuria.	Identification of at-risk clients helps in early detection of complications and conditions such as diabetes.
	Teach the client the signs and symptoms of hyperglycemia.	Knowledge helps improve the client's ability to recognize hyperglycemia.
Decreased peripheral metabolism	Assess for signs and symptoms of hypothyroidism, especially constipation, lethargy, dry skin, and mental deterioration.	Ongoing assessment helps differentiate hypothyroidism from the clinical features of aging.

docrine activity because of age-related variables such as the following:

- Acute and chronic illnesses
- Alterations in diet, activity, and lean body mass/fat ratio
- Disturbances in sleep patterns
- Decreased metabolic clearance rate of hormones
- Increased use of multiple drugs that may affect hormone function

The nurse considers these variables when assessing the client with endocrine dysfunction.

The nurse encourages the older adult client to participate in regular screening examinations, including fasting and postprandial blood glucose checks, calcium level determinations, and thyroid function testing. Chart 62-1 summarizes the endocrine changes that occur in the older adult and lists related nursing interventions.

ASSESSMENT TECHNIQUES

History

A systems approach is used for obtaining the history of clients with a suspected endocrine problem. This approach can be difficult because of the variety and combination of clinical symptoms. The information gathered from the history provides a basis for physical assessment and for planning care. The nurse identifies the client's response to actual or perceived changes and discusses the potential diagnostic and treatment plan. Chart 62-2 presents some assessment questions based on Gordon's Functional Health Patterns. Although endocrine problems can disturb any health pattern, the patterns most commonly affected are Nutritional-Metabolic, Activity, Elimination, Sleep-Rest, and Sexuality-Reproductive. These data are combined with physical, psychosocial, and laboratory findings for a complete assessment of endocrine function.

DEMOGRAPHIC DATA

The age and gender of the client provide essential baseline assessment data. Certain disorders are more common in older than in younger clients, such as hyperosmolar states, loss of ovarian function, and decreased thyroid and parathyroid function. In particular, decreased glucose tolerance is common among older adults.

Manifestations of endocrine disorders can be gender related, such as the sexual effects of hyperpituitarism and hypopituitarism (see Chapter 63).

PERSONAL AND FAMILY HISTORY

The client is asked about any family history of obesity, growth or development difficulties, diabetes mellitus, infertility, or thyroid disorders. The nurse further assesses the client for a history of the following:

- Endocrine dysfunction
- Signs or symptoms that could indicate an endocrine disorder
- Hospitalizations

The client is asked about past and current medications, such as hydrocortisone, levothyroxine, oral contraceptives, and antihypertensive drugs.

DIET HISTORY

Nutritional changes or gastrointestinal (GI) tract disturbances may reflect a variety of endocrine problems. The nurse as-

CHART 62-2

ENDOCRINE ASSESSMENT
Using Gordon's Functional Health Patterns

Nutritional-Metabolic Pattern
What is your typical daily food intake? Describe a day's meals, snacks, and vitamins.
How much salt do you typically add to your food? Do you use salt substitutes?
How is your appetite?
Do you have any difficulty chewing or swallowing?
What is your typical daily fluid intake? What types of fluids (water, juices, soft drinks, coffee, tea)? How much?
Have you had any recent change in your weight? Weight gain? Weight loss? How much?
Have you noticed a change in the tightness of your rings or shoes? Tighter? Looser?

Elimination Pattern
What is your usual bowel elimination pattern? Frequency? Character? Discomfort? Laxatives?
What is your usual urinary elimination pattern? Frequency? Amount? Color? Odor? Control?
Have you noticed a change in the amount of urine?
Do you have any problem with excessive perspiration?
Do you have any other type of drainage?

Sleep-Rest Pattern
Do you have any difficulty falling asleep when you go to bed?
Is there a change in the number of hours you sleep per night?
Do you take any medication to help you sleep?
About how many times to you wake up during the night?
Do you have any difficulty getting back to sleep?
Are you bothered by nightmares or vivid dreams?
Do you have difficulty waking up in the morning?
Do you feel generally rested and ready for daily activities after sleep?
Do you take scheduled naps or rest periods during the day?
Do you find yourself falling asleep at work or at home while reading or watching television?

Sexuality-Reproductive Pattern
Are you sexually active?
Are you satisfied with your level of sexual activity?
Do you participate in sex as often as you would like?
Do you participate in sex as often as your partner would like?
Have you noticed a change in your interest in having sex over the past year?
Female:
At what age did menstruation start?
How regular are your periods?
Do you have any pain, cramping, or clotting during your periods?
Have you ever been pregnant? What was the outcome of the pregnancy(ies)?
Do you use contraceptives? What type? Have you had any problems with your chosen method of contraception?

Activity-Exercise Pattern
Do you feel you have sufficient energy to perform tasks or routines that are required of you?
Do you feel you have sufficient energy to do what you would like to do?
Do you exercise? How often? For how long each time? What type(s) of exercise do you perform?
What activities do you perform in your spare time?
What is your ability to perform the following tasks?

Feeding _____	Grooming _____
Bathing _____	General Mobility _____
Toileting _____	Cooking _____
Bed Mobility _____	Home Maintenance _____
Dressing _____	Shopping _____

Functional Levels Code
Level 0: Full self-care
Level I: Requires use of equipment or device
Level II: Requires assistance or supervision of another person
Level III: Requires assistance or supervision of another person and use of equipment or device
Level IV: Is dependent and does not participate

Based on Gordon, M. (2000). *Manual of nursing diagnosis* (9th ed.). St. Louis: Mosby.

sesses for a history of nausea, vomiting, and abdominal pain. An increase or decrease in food or fluid intake may also indicate specific disorders. For example, diabetes insipidus is characterized by excessive thirst, and primary adrenal hypofunction is characterized by salt craving. Hunger and thirst may also be increased in diabetes mellitus. Rapid changes in weight without accompanying changes in diet can signal the onset of a number of endocrine disorders, including diabetes mellitus and thyroid dysfunction.

SOCIOECONOMIC STATUS

Because the client's socioeconomic status can be a sensitive issue, the nurse explores with the client whether his or her resources are adequate to maintain a healthy diet, purchase needed medications, and seek consistent health care follow-up. This initial determination of socioeconomic status allows the nurse to involve social service and home care agencies at an early stage.

CURRENT HEALTH PROBLEMS

The nurse focuses on the client's reason for seeking health care, asking questions such as the following:

- Did the client's symptoms occur gradually, or was the onset sudden?
- Has the client been treated for this problem in the past?
- How have the current symptoms interfered with activities of daily living?

Such questioning provides clues to specific endocrine disorders. The nurse also explores changes in energy levels, elimination patterns, sexual and reproductive functions, and physical characteristics.

Energy Levels

Changes in energy levels are associated with a number of endocrine problems, particularly of the thyroid (see Chapter 64) and adrenal glands (see Chapter 63). The nurse asks the client about any change in ability to perform daily activities and assesses the client's current energy level. For instance, has the client been sleeping longer or experiencing fatigue or generalized weakness?

Elimination

Elimination patterns are also affected by the endocrine system. The nurse identifies the client's past pattern of elimination to determine deviations from the normal routine. The client is asked about urine amount and frequency. Does he or she urinate frequently in large amounts? Does the client wake during the night to urinate **(nocturia),** or does he or she experience pain on urination **(dysuria)**? Information about the frequency of bowel movements and their consistency and color may provide clues to problems in fluid balance or metabolic rate (i.e., thyroid function).

Sex and Reproduction

Sexual and reproductive functions are greatly affected by disturbances in the endocrine system. Women are asked about any changes in the menstrual cycle such as increased flow, duration, and frequency of menses; pain or excessive cramping; or a recent change in the regularity of menses. Men are asked whether they have experienced impotence. The nurse questions both men and women about a change in libido or any fertility problems.

Physical Appearance

The nurse discusses any changes in physical characteristics that the client perceives. Overt changes are identified during the physical assessment, but clients may be able to describe subtle changes that the nurse might miss. The client is asked about changes in the following:

- Hair texture or distribution
- Facial contours
- Voice quality
- Body proportions
- Secondary sexual characteristics

For example, the nurse might ask a man if he is shaving less often or a woman if she has noticed an increase in facial hair. These changes may be associated with pituitary, thyroid, parathyroid, or adrenal dysfunction.

CRITICAL THINKING CHALLENGE

The client is a 27-year-old woman who stopped having menstrual periods 6 months ago. She is not pregnant. At the beginning of the interview, the client shouts at you because she had to wait 15 minutes beyond her assigned appointment time. After the shouting, the client suddenly bursts into tears and apologizes to you.

- Given the client's age, gender, and initial presentation, are there any endocrine glands that do not need to be assessed? If so, which ones and why?
- What would be an appropriate response to this client's expressed anger and apology?
- What specific questions regarding her menstrual cycle should you ask?

For suggested answer guidelines, go to SIMON http://www.wbsaunders.com/SIMON/Iggy/.

Physical Assessment

INSPECTION

An endocrine problem can result in characteristic physical changes because of its effect on growth and development, regulation of sex hormone levels, fluid and electrolyte balance, and the body's use of nutrients. The nurse should be cautious, however, because many different clinical findings can be associated with multiple endocrine disorders or with nonendocrine pathologic processes.

Inspection of the client using a head-to-toe approach is often effective. The client's general appearance is observed, and height, weight, fat distribution, and muscle mass are assessed in relation to age. It is important to remember that heredity and age rather than a pathologic condition may be responsible for significant deviations (e.g., short stature).

When examining the head, the nurse focuses on abnormalities of facial structure, features, and expression, such as the following:

- Prominent forehead or jaw
- Round or puffy face
- Dull or flat expression
- Exophthalmos (protruding eyeballs and retracted upper lids)

The lower half of the neck is observed for a visible enlargement of the thyroid gland. In most instances the thyroid tissue cannot be observed. The isthmus may be noticeable when the client swallows. Jugular vein distention may be noted on inspection of the neck and can indicate fluid overload (see Chapter 12).

Skin abnormalities may reflect a dysfunction of specific endocrine glands. The nurse observes skin color and notes areas of hypopigmentation or hyperpigmentation. Fungal skin infections, slow wound healing, bruising, and petechiae are often seen in clients with adrenocortical hyperfunction. Skin infections, foot ulcers, and slow wound healing are common among clients with diabetes mellitus. In secondary hypofunction of the adrenal glands, the skin over the finger joints, elbows, and knees, as well as any scar tissue, may show increased pigmentation due to increased levels of ACTH and melanocyte-stimulating hormone.

Vitiligo (patchy areas of depigmentation with increased pigmentation at the edges) is seen with primary hypofunction of the adrenal glands and is due to autoimmune destruction of melanocytes in the skin. Areas of decreased pigmentation most often occur on the face, neck, and extremities. Mucous membranes can exhibit large areas of pigmentation. The nurse documents the location, distribution, color, and size of all skin discolorations and lesions.

The nurse inspects the client's fingernails for malformation, thickness, or brittleness, all of which may suggest thyroid gland difficulties. The extremities and the base of the spine are examined for edema, which suggests a disturbance in fluid and electrolyte balance.

Visual examination of the trunk can show signs of specific endocrine dysfunction. The nurse notes any abnormalities in chest size and symmetry. Truncal obesity, supraclavicular fat pads, and a "buffalo hump" may indicate adrenocortical excess. Hormonal imbalance may also change secondary sexual characteristics. The nurse inspects the breasts of both men and women for size, symmetry, pigmentation, and discharge. **Striae** (usually reddish purple "stretch marks") on the breasts or abdomen are often seen with adrenocortical excess.

The nurse assesses the client's hair distribution for indications of endocrine gland dysfunction, including **hirsutism** (abnormal growth of body hair, especially on the face, chest, and the linea alba of the abdomen of women), excessive hair loss, or changes in hair texture.

Examination of the genitalia may reveal a dysfunction in hormone secretion. The nurse notes the size of the scrotum and penis or of the labia and clitoris in relation to standards for the client's age. The distribution and quantity of pubic hair are often affected in hypogonadism.

PALPATION

The thyroid gland and the testes can be examined by palpation. Chapters 69 and 73 discuss examination of the testes. During the initial assessment, a specially trained nurse palpates the thyroid gland for size, symmetry, general shape, and the presence of nodules or other irregularities.

The nurse palpates the thyroid gland by standing either behind or in front of the client (Figure 62-9); the posterior approach may be easier. Offering the client sips of water to promote swallowing during the examination helps the clinician palpate the thyroid gland.

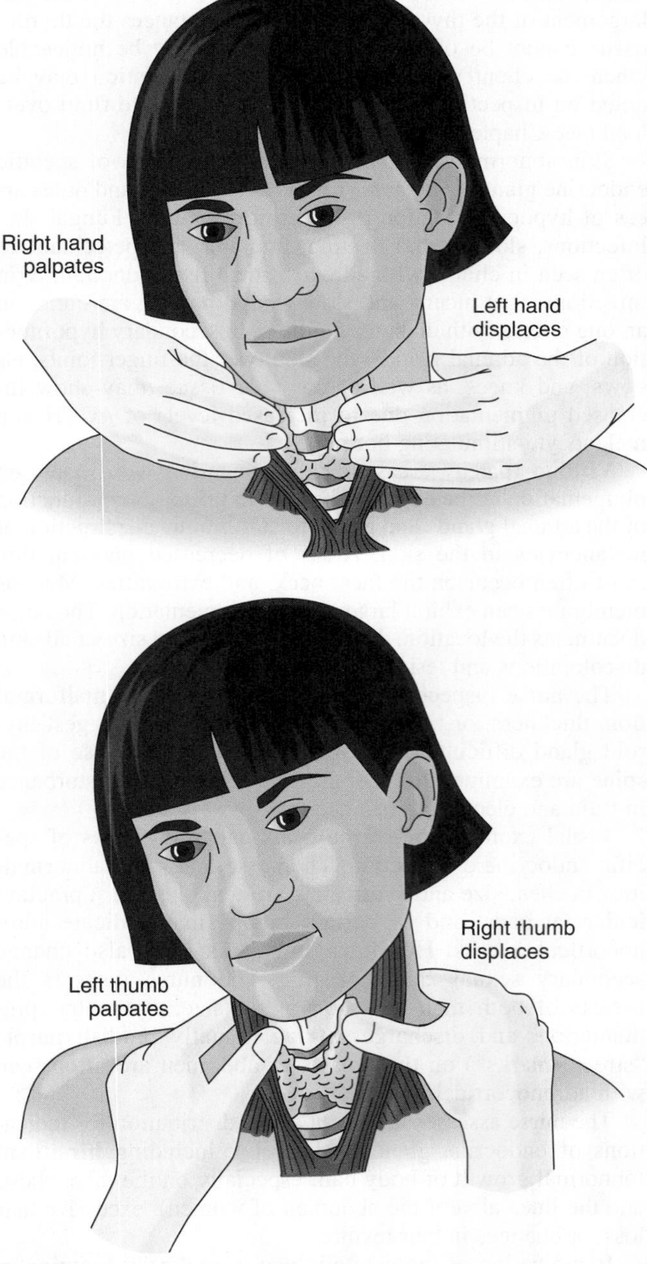

Figure 62-9 ● Palpation of the thyroid gland.

The client is asked to sit and to lower the chin. Using the posterior approach, the thumbs of both hands are placed on the back of the client's neck, with the fingers curved around to the front of the neck on either side of the trachea. The client is asked to swallow, and the nurse locates the isthmus of the thyroid and feels it rising. The anterior surface of the thyroid lobe is also identified. To examine the right lobe, the nurse:

- Turns the client's head to the right
- Displaces the thyroid cartilage to the right with the fingers of the left hand
- Palpates the right lobe with the right hand

This procedure is reversed for examination of the left lobe.

AUSCULTATION

The nurse auscultates the client's chest to establish baseline vital signs and to determine irregularities in cardiac rate and rhythm. A variety of endocrine disturbances can cause dehydration and volume depletion. Therefore the nurse documents any difference in the client's blood pressure and pulse in the lying, standing, or sitting positions (orthostatic vital signs).

If an enlarged thyroid gland is palpated, the area of enlargement is auscultated for bruits. Hypertrophy of the thyroid gland causes an increase in vascular flow, which may result in bruits.

Psychosocial Assessment

Information obtained from the history and physical examination aids the nurse in identifying potential or actual psychosocial problems. The nurse assesses the client's coping skills, support systems, and health-related beliefs.

A number of endocrine disorders seriously affect the client's perception of self. For example, body characteristics can change significantly in disorders of the pituitary, adrenal, and thyroid glands. Infertility, impotence, and other changes in sexual functioning may result from endocrine dysfunction. The nurse addresses any difficulty in coping with such changes. Additional support from social or counseling services may be appropriate when planning care.

Clients with endocrine problems may require lifelong medication and follow-up care. The nurse assesses the client's readiness to learn and his or her ability to carry out specific self-management skills. Clients may also face financial difficulties resulting from a prolonged medical regimen or interruption of employment. A referral to social service agencies may be necessary.

Diagnostic Assessment

LABORATORY TESTS

For the client with suspected endocrine dysfunction, laboratory tests are an essential part of the diagnostic process. The highly specialized testing for specific disorders is described in Chapters 63 to 65. Some generalizations can be made. Best practices for the collection of specimens for endocrine testing are listed in Chart 62-3.

CHART 62-3

BEST PRACTICE *for* Endocrine Testing

- Explain the procedure to the client.
- Emphasize the importance of taking a medication prescribed for the test on *time.* Tell the client to set an alarm if the medication is to be taken during the night.
- Instruct the client to begin the urine collection (whether for 2, 4, 8, 12, or 24 hours) by emptying his or her bladder. Tell the client *not* to save the urine specimen that begins the collection. The timing for the urine collection begins after this specimen. To end the collection, the client empties his or her bladder at the end of the timed period and adds that urine to the collection.
- Make sure that the preservative has been added to the collection container at the beginning of the collection, if necessary. Tell the client of its presence in the container.
- Check your laboratory's method of handling hormone test samples. Blood samples drawn for certain hormones (e.g., catecholamines) must be placed on ice and taken to the laboratory immediately.
- If you are drawing blood samples from a line, clear the IV line thoroughly. Do not use a double- or triple-lumen line to obtain samples; contamination or dilution from another port is possible.

Stimulation/Suppression Tests

Measurement of specific hormone levels does not always distinguish between the normal and the abnormal. The wide normal range for some hormones makes it necessary to elicit responses by stimulation or suppression tests.

In the client with suspected underactivity of an endocrine gland, a stimulus may be provided to determine whether the gland is capable of normal hormone production. This method is called *stimulation testing.* Measured amounts of selected hormones are given to stimulate the target gland to maximal production. Hormone levels are then measured and interpreted against a given norm. Failure of the hormone level to rise with stimulation denotes hypofunction.

Suppression tests are used when hormone levels are high or in the upper range of normal. Failure of hormone production to be suppressed during standardized testing indicates hyperfunction. (See the specific tests in Chapters 63 and 64.)

Radioimmunoassay

Radioimmunoassay is a competitive binding assay in which radioactively labeled amounts of hormone (antigen) compete with unlabeled hormones from the plasma or serum for antibody binding sites. Various techniques measure the amount of unbound and bound hormone. The unbound hormone is the active hormone.

Urine Tests

In addition to the measurement of hormones in the blood, hormone levels and the metabolites of specific hormones in the urine are often measured. Because many of the endocrine hormones are secreted in a pulsatile fashion, measurement of a specific hormone in a 24-hour urine collection better reflects the overall function of certain glands, such as the adrenal gland. The nurse teaches the client how to collect a 24-hour urine sample (see also Chart 62-3).

Certain hormones require additives in the container at the beginning of the collection. The nurse instructs the client not to discard the preservative from the container and to use caution when handling it, because some solutions are caustic. The client is also reminded that this collection is timed for *exactly* 24 hours. The nurse instructs the client to avoid taking any unnecessary medications during endocrine testing; drugs may interfere with the laboratory assays.

Tests for Glucose

Tests for functions of the islet cells of the pancreas are indirect; they measure the *result* of pancreatic islet cell function. Blood glucose values and the oral glucose tolerance test help the physician or nurse practitioner make a diagnosis of diabetes mellitus. The glycosylated hemoglobin (HbA_{1C}) value reveals the *average* blood glucose level over a period of 2 to 3 months. Its primary use is in assessing overall control of glucose level in diabetes mellitus. (See Chapter 65 for a full discussion of diabetes mellitus.)

RADIOGRAPHIC EXAMINATIONS

Anterior, posterior, and lateral skull x-ray studies may be used to visualize the sella turcica. Erosion of the sella turcica indicates invasion of the wall from an abnormal growth.

Computed tomography (CT) and magnetic resonance imaging (MRI) scans can show the extent of growth or locate a tumor buried within the pituitary. CT and MRI scans, sometimes using contrast media, also reveal the size and shape of other glands and nearby structures.

Angiography and venography may reveal structural abnormalities, such as aberrant blood vessels. Ultrasonography, especially of the thyroid gland, can indicate whether nodules or masses are solid or cystic.

OTHER DIAGNOSTIC TESTS

Needle biopsy is a relatively safe and quick outpatient procedure and can be used to indicate the composition of thyroid nodules. It is primarily used to determine whether surgical intervention is necessary.

CRITICAL THINKING CHALLENGE

The 27-year-old client with an absence of menses is scheduled to have blood drawn for follicle-stimulating hormone (FSH) levels, an ultrasound of the ovaries, a 24-hour urine collection for estradiol beta-17 levels, and a CT scan of the head. She is very anxious about the tests and the results.

- How should you prepare her physically for each test?
- What special instructions should you provide for the 24-hour urine test?
- The client is very concerned about pain and modesty.
- What reassurances can you provide for the level of pain expected?
- Is the client's modesty at risk with any of these procedures? If so, how? What precautions can be taken to reduce exposure?

For suggested answer guidelines, go to SIMON http://www.wbsaunders.com/SIMON/Iggy/.

ONLINE RESOURCES

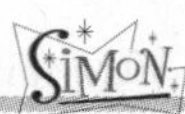

For suggested readings and Internet resources, go to http://www.wbsaunders.com/SIMON/Iggy/.

SELECTED BIBLIOGRAPHY

Asterisk indicates a classic or definitive work on this subject.

Cook, L. (1999). The value of lab values. *American Journal of Nursing, 99*(5), 66-75.

Gordon, M. (2000). *Manual of nursing diagnosis* (9th ed.). St. Louis: Mosby.

Guyton, A., & Hall, J. (2001). *Textbook of medical physiology* (9th ed.). Philadelphia: W.B. Saunders.

Kelley, W. (Ed.). (1997). *Textbook of internal medicine* (3rd ed.). Philadelphia: Lippincott-Raven.

*Kokko, J., & Tannen, R. (1996). *Fluids and electrolytes* (3rd ed.). Philadelphia: W.B. Saunders.

Larsen, P.R., Davies, T., & Hay, I. (1998). In J. Wilson et al. (Eds.). *William's textbook of endocrinology* (9th ed., pp. 389-515). Philadelphia: W.B. Saunders.

*Mooradian, A. (1995). Normal age-related changes in thyroid hormone economy. *Clinics in Geriatric Medicine, 11*(2), 159-169.

Orth, D., & Kovacs, W. (1998). The adrenal cortex. In J. Wilson et al. (Eds.). *William's textbook of endocrinology* (9th ed., pp. 517-664). Philadelphia: W.B. Saunders.

Pagana, K., & Pagana, T. (1999). *Diagnostic testing and nursing implications: A case study approach.* St. Louis: Mosby.

Reeves, W.B., Bichet, D., & Andreoli, T. (1998). In J. Wilson et al. (Eds.). *William's textbook of endocrinology* (9th ed., pp. 341-387). Philadelphia: W.B. Saunders.

Sagre, G., & Brown, E. (1998). Measurement of hormones. In J. Wilson et al. (Eds.). *William's textbook of endocrinology* (9th ed., pp. 43-54). Philadelphia: W.B. Saunders.

Thorner, M., et al. (1998). The anterior pituitary. In J. Wilson et al. (Eds.). *William's textbook of endocrinology* (9th ed., pp. 249-340). Philadelphia: W.B. Saunders.

Wilson, J., et al. (Eds.). (1998). *William's textbook of endocrinology* (9th ed.). Philadelphia: W.B. Saunders.

*Winger, J., & Hornick, T. (1996). Age-associated changes in the endocrine system. *Nursing Clinics of North America, 31*(4), 827-844.

CHAPTER 63

Interventions for Clients with Pituitary and Adrenal Gland Problems

M. LINDA WORKMAN

Learning Objectives

After studying this chapter, you should be able to:

1. Compare and contrast the common clinical manifestations associated with pituitary hypofunction and pituitary hyperfunction.
2. Use clinical changes and laboratory data to determine the effectiveness of interventions for pituitary hypofunction.
3. Identify the teaching priorities for the client taking hormone replacement therapy for pituitary hypofunction.
4. Prioritize nursing care for the client immediately after a transsphenoidal hypophysectomy.
5. Use clinical changes and laboratory data to determine the effectiveness of interventions for pituitary hyperfunction.
6. Compare and contrast the problems associated with oversecretion and undersecretion of antidiuretic hormone.
7. Explain the effect of diabetes insipidus on blood and urine volumes and blood and urine osmolarity.
8. Explain the effects of the syndrome of inappropriate antidiuretic hormone (SIADH) on blood and urine volumes and blood and urine osmolarity.
9. Use clinical changes and laboratory data to determine the effectiveness of interventions for diabetes insipidus.
10. Identify teaching priorities for the client with diabetes insipidus.
11. Use clinical changes and laboratory data to determine the effectiveness of interventions for SIADH.
12. Identify teaching priorities for the client with SIADH.
13. Compare and contrast the clinical manifestations of Cushing's syndrome and Addison's disease.
14. Use clinical changes and laboratory data to determine the effectiveness of interventions for Cushing's syndrome.
15. Identify teaching priorities for the client with Cushing's syndrome.
16. Use clinical changes and laboratory data to determine the effectiveness of interventions for Addison's disease.
17. Identify teaching priorities for the client with Addison's disease.

SIMON

Go to http://www.wbsaunders.com/SIMON/Iggy/ for self-assessment questions related to these Learning Objectives.

Pituitary and adrenal gland problems can be caused by, or can cause, oversecretion or undersecretion of one or more hormones. At times, the correct amount of hormone may be produced but cannot be used because of receptor site failure.

Hormones secreted from the anterior pituitary gland regulate growth, metabolism, and sexual development. These functions are affected when the pituitary gland secretes too much or too little of one or more hormones. The posterior pituitary gland secretes **vasopressin** (antidiuretic hormone [ADH]). Dysfunction of the posterior pituitary gland results in fluid and electrolyte imbalance. The adrenal gland produces and secretes hormones that influence homeostasis and are life sustaining.

The effects of endocrine problems occur throughout the body and may induce psychologic, as well as physical, changes. Nursing care for the client with pituitary or adrenal gland disorders includes the following:

- Performing a careful assessment
- Educating clients
- Evaluating responses to therapy
- Providing psychosocial support

A complete history and physical examination are performed during the assessment to detect specific clinical findings. The client also often undergoes a variety of diagnostic tests and relies on the nurse for specific instructions and explanations. Surgical intervention may be indicated. The client often needs hormone replacement therapy for the rest of his or her life. Physical and emotional support are critical.

DISORDERS OF THE PITUITARY GLAND

DISORDERS OF THE ANTERIOR PITUITARY GLAND

The anterior pituitary gland **(adenohypophysis)** controls growth, metabolic activity, and sexual development through the actions of the following hormones:

- Growth hormone (GH; somatotropin)
- Prolactin (PRL)
- Thyrotropin (thyroid-stimulating hormone [TSH])
- Corticotropin (adrenocorticotropic hormone [ACTH])
- Follicle-stimulating hormone (FSH)
- Luteinizing hormone (LH)
- Melanocyte-stimulating hormone (MSH)

Disorders of hormones secreted by the anterior pituitary gland can result from problems arising within the anterior pituitary gland itself **(primary pituitary dysfunction)** or from problems in the hypothalamus that change anterior pituitary function **(secondary pituitary dysfunction).** In either case, one or more hormones may be undersecreted **(pituitary hypofunction)** or oversecreted **(pituitary hyperfunction).**

Hypopituitarism

OVERVIEW

Pathophysiology

A person with hypopituitarism has a deficiency of one or more anterior pituitary hormones, resulting in metabolic abnormalities and sexual dysfunction. Decreased production of *all* of the anterior pituitary hormones is an extremely rare condition known as **panhypopituitarism.**

More commonly, there is a marked decrease in the secretion of one hormone and a lesser decrease in the other hormones. Deficiencies of adrenocorticotropic hormone (ACTH) and thyroid-stimulating hormone (TSH) are the *most* life threatening because they result in a corresponding decrease in the secretion of vital hormones from the adrenal and thyroid glands. Adrenal hypofunction is discussed on pp. 1412-1415; hypothyroidism is discussed in Chapter 64.

Deficiency of the **gonadotropins** (luteinizing hormone [LH] and follicle-stimulating hormone [FSH]—hormones that stimulate the ovaries and testes to produce sex hormones) changes sexual function in both men and women. In males, gonadotropin deficiency results in testicular failure, with decreased testosterone production from the Leydig cells and decreased or absent spermatogenesis from the seminiferous tubules. Decreased testosterone levels in males cause delayed onset of puberty and sterility. In females, gonadotropin deficiency results in ovarian failure, amenorrhea, and infertility.

Growth hormone (GH) deficiency changes tissue growth patterns indirectly. GH itself has little effect on tissues and cells. Rather, the presence of GH stimulates the liver to produce substances known as **somatomedins** (Guyton & Hall, 2000). These somatomedins, especially somatomedin C (insulin-like growth factor-1 [IGF-1]), then enhance growth activities in cells and tissues. Somatomedin C is responsible for bone and cartilage growth and maintenance.

GH deficiency may be a result of insufficient production of GH, failure of the liver to produce somatomedins, or a failure of the cells or tissues to respond to the presence of the somatomedins. GH deficiency in children leads to short stature and other manifestations of growth retardation. GH deficiency in adults produces no obvious anatomic changes but does increase the rate of bone destructive activity, leading to thinner, more fragile bones.

Etiology

The cause of hypopituitarism varies. Benign or malignant pituitary tumors can compress and destroy pituitary tissue. Pituitary function can be impaired by severe malnutrition or rapid loss of body fat, such as in people with **anorexia nervosa** (a disorder in which people see themselves as overweight and eat so little that excessive weight loss and starvation result). Poor circulation to the pituitary gland can cause hypoxia and infarction. Other causes of hypopituitarism are listed in Table 63-1. **Idiopathic hypopituitarism** may result in an isolated hormone deficiency, and often the cause is unknown.

Postpartum hemorrhage is the most common cause of pituitary infarction, which results in decreased hormone secretion. This clinical problem is known as **Sheehan's syndrome.** The pituitary gland normally enlarges during pregnancy, and when hypotension results from hemorrhage, ischemia and necrosis of the gland occur. Usually this condition develops immediately postpartum, although some cases have occurred several years after delivery.

COLLABORATIVE MANAGEMENT

Assessment

Some changes in physical appearance and target organ function are associated with deficiencies of specific pituitary hormones (Chart 63-1). Gonadotropin (LH and FSH) deficiency results in the loss of or change in secondary sex characteristics in men and women. While assessing the male client, the nurse notes the key signs and symptoms of facial and body hair loss. The nurse asks about episodes of impotence and decreased **libido** (sex drive). Female clients may report **amen-**

TABLE 63-1 • CAUSES OF HYPOPITUITARISM

CAUSES OF PRIMARY HYPOPITUITARISM
- Pituitary tumor (craniopharyngioma)
- Partial or total surgical hypophysectomy
- Radiation
- Infarction
- Metastatic disease
- Granulomatous process
- Trauma

CAUSES OF SECONDARY HYPOPITUITARISM
- Infection
- Trauma
- Brain tumor
- Congenital defects

orrhea (absence of menstrual periods), **dyspareunia** (painful intercourse), **infertility** (difficulty in achieving pregnancy), and decreased libido. While examining the female client, the nurse checks for dry skin, breast atrophy, and a decreased amount or absence of axillary and pubic hair.

Neurologic manifestations of hypopituitarism due to tumor growth often first occur as changes in visual perception. The nurse evaluates the client's visual acuity, particularly peripheral vision, for changes or loss. Bilateral temporal headaches are a common finding. Other manifestations may include **diplopia** (double vision) and ocular muscle paralysis, limiting eye movement.

Laboratory findings vary widely in people with hypopituitarism. Some pituitary hormone levels may be measured directly. Often, however, the *effects* of the hormones, rather than their actual levels, are assessed. Basal levels of triiodothyronine (T_3) and thyroxine (T_4) from the thyroid, as well as testosterone and estradiol from the gonads, are measured easily. If levels of one or all of these hormones are low or in the low-normal range, hypopituitarism is a possibility and further evaluation is necessary. Levels of pituitary gonadotropins (LH and FSH) and TSH are sufficient if function of the target organ is apparent. Function of LH and FSH is assessed by observing for the presence of secondary sexual characteristics; function of TSH is assessed by measuring circulating levels of thyroid hormones. ACTH levels may be normal or low, and prolactin (PRL) levels are low to high.

Some tests for pituitary function involve administering agents that are known to stimulate secretion of specific pituitary hormones and then measuring the response. Such tests are called **stimulation tests.** For example, the presence of insulin in people with normal pituitary function causes an increased release of GH and ACTH. The stimulation test for either GH or ACTH assessment involves injecting the client with regular insulin (0.05 to 1 units/kg of body weight) and checking the circulating levels of GH and ACTH. The stimulation test for TSH involves injecting thyrotropin-releasing hormone (TRH) and measuring the blood levels of thyroid hormones. The stimulation test for LH and FSH involves administering gonadotropin-releasing hormone (GnRH). In people with no pituitary problems, this injection results in a peak release of LH and FSH within 15 to 45 minutes after the injection. The stimulation test for PRL is the same as that for TSH.

Pituitary abnormalities may cause changes in the **sella turcica** (the bony nest where the pituitary gland rests) that can be seen with skull x-ray studies. Such changes may include enlargement, erosion, and calcifications in the area of the sella turcica as a result of pituitary tumors. Computed tomography (CT) and magnetic resonance imaging (MRI) can more distinctly define bone or soft-tissue lesions. An angiogram may be indicated to rule out the presence of an aneurysm or congenital vascular malformations, especially before any surgical intervention.

CHART 63-1

KEY FEATURES *of* Pituitary Hypofunction

Deficient Hormone	Clinical Manifestations
Anterior Pituitary Hormones	
Growth hormone (GH)	Decreased bone density Pathologic fractures Decreased muscle strength Increased serum cholesterol levels
Gonadotropins (luteinizing hormone [LH], follicle-stimulating hormone [FSH])	Women: • Amenorrhea • Anovulation • Low circulating estrogen levels • Breast atrophy • Loss of bone density • Decreased axillary and pubic hair • Decreased libido • Fine facial wrinkles Men: • Decreased facial hair • Decreased ejaculate volume • Reduced muscle mass • Loss of bone density • Decreased body hair • Decreased libido • Impotence • Fine facial wrinkles
Thyrotropin (Thyroid-stimulating hormone [TSH])	Decreased circulating TSH levels Decreased circulating thyroid hormone levels Weight gain Intolerance to cold Scalp alopecia Hirsuitism Menstrual abnormalities Decreased libido Slowed cognition Lethargy
Adrenocorticotropic hormone (ACTH)	Decreased serum cortisol levels Pale, sallow complexion Malaise and lethargy Anorexia Postural hypotension Headache Hypoglycemia Hyponatremia Decreased axillary and pubic hair (women)
Posterior Pituitary Hormones	

Vasopressin (antidiuretic hormone [ADH])	Diabetes insipidus
	• Greatly increased urine output
	• Low urine specific gravity (<1.005)
	• Hypovolemia
	  Hypotension
	  Dehydration
	• Increased plasma osmolarity
	• Increased thirst
	• Output does not decrease when fluid intake decreases

Data from Thorner, M., et al. (1998). The anterior pituitary. In J. D. Wilson et al. (Eds.), *Williams textbook of endocrinology* (9th ed., pp. 249-340). Philadelphia: W.B. Saunders; and Reeves, W.B., Bichet, D., & Andreoli, T. (1998). Posterior pituitary and water metabolism. In J.D. Wilson et al. (Eds.), *Williams textbook of endocrinology* (9th ed., pp. 341-387). Philadelphia: W.B. Saunders.

Interventions

Management of the adult with hypopituitarism focuses on replacement of deficient hormones. Older clients or those with a chronic disease often require a lower amount of hormone replacement. Men who have gonadotropin deficiency are treated with **androgens** (testosterone). The most widely used and most effective route of administration is intramuscular (IM), although use of transdermal testosterone patches is increasing. The nurse instructs the client in self-administration. Therapy is usually initiated with high-dose testosterone and is continued until **virilization** (presence of male secondary sex characteristics) is achieved. Maximal effects of treatment include increases in penis size, libido, muscle mass, bone size, and bone strength. Chest, facial, pubic, and axillary hair growth also increase, and the voice deepens. Clients usually report improved self-esteem and body image after therapy is initiated. The dose may then be decreased, but therapy continues throughout life.

Androgen therapy is avoided in men with prostate cancer. Side effects of testosterone therapy include **gynecomastia** (the development of breast tissue in men), baldness, and prostatic hypertrophy.

Achieving fertility in these clients is difficult and requires additional parenteral testosterone therapy. The nurse educates the client about the course of additional therapy and supports the client and family members emotionally because the outcome of fertility treatment is uncertain.

Women who have gonadotropin deficiency receive hormone replacement with a combination of estrogen and progesterone administered at their menstrual cycle, which causes withdrawal bleeding. The risk for hypertension or **thrombosis** (formation of blood clots in deep veins) is increased with estrogen therapy, especially among women who smoke. The nurse emphasizes measures to reduce risk and the need for regular health visits. For women who wish to become pregnant, clomiphene citrate (Clomid) may be given to induce ovulation. Menotropins in conjunction with human chorionic gonadotropin (hCG) are used to stimulate ovulation when therapy with clomiphene citrate has failed.

Adult clients who have GH deficiency may be treated with injections of GH, although this treatment is rare.

Hyperpituitarism

OVERVIEW

Hyperpituitarism is a condition of hormone oversecretion that occurs when a client has pituitary tumors or hyperplasias. Tumors usually arise from the somatotropic cells (growth hormone [GH]), the lactotropic cells (prolactin [PRL]), and the corticotropic cells (adrenocorticotropic hormone [ACTH[) of the anterior pituitary gland **(adenohypophysis).** An exception is the overproduction of PRL, which may occur in response to tumors that overproduce GH and ACTH. Hypersecretion of ACTH is sometimes associated with increased secretion of melanocyte-stimulating hormone (MSH).

Pathophysiology

A common reason for hyperpituitarism is the presence of a pituitary adenoma, a benign epithelial tumor. Adenomas are classified by size, the degree of invasiveness, and the hormone secreted. An invasive pituitary adenoma involves a portion or all of the sella turcica. When the sella turcica is not involved, the adenoma is "enclosed."

As an adenoma gets larger and compresses brain tissue, neurologic symptoms, as well as endocrine symptoms, may occur. Such symptoms may include visual changes, headache, and increased intracranial pressure.

PRL-secreting tumors are the most common of the pituitary adenomas. Excessive PRL secretion inhibits the secretion of gonadal steroids and gonadotropins in men and women, resulting in **galactorrhea** (production of breast milk), amenorrhea, and infertility.

Overproduction of GH results in **gigantism** (Figure 63-1) or **acromegaly** (Figure 63-2). The onset of the disease may be gradual with slow progression, and changes may remain unnoticed for years before diagnosis of the disorder. Early detection and treatment are essential to prevent irreversible changes in the soft tissues, such as those of the face, hands, feet, and skin. These changes are, to a certain extent, reversible after treatment, but skeletal changes are permanent.

In the client with gigantism, the onset of GH hypersecretion occurs *before* puberty, which causes rapid proportional growth in the length of all bones. In the client with acromegaly, excessive GH secretion occurs *after* puberty and produces increased skeletal thickness, hypertrophy of the skin,

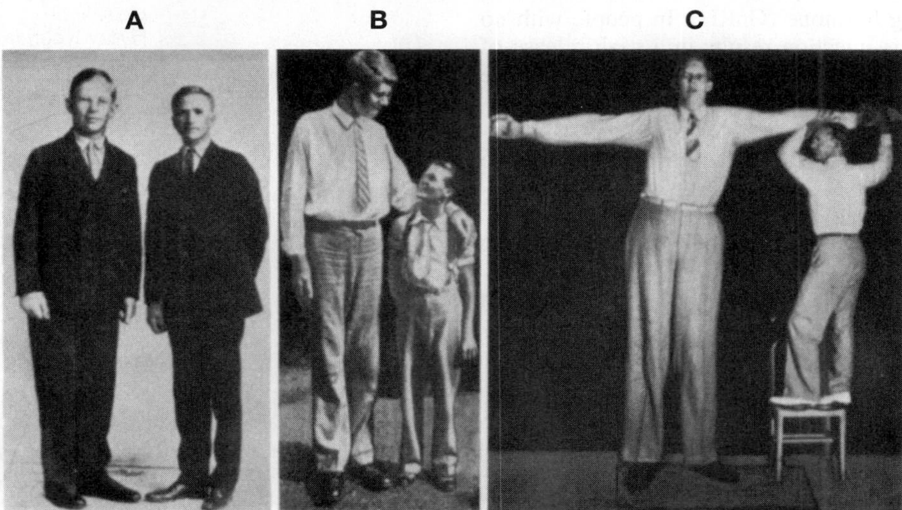

Figure 63-1 ● The clinical features of GH excess. Robert Wadlow, the "Alton giant," weighed 9 pounds at birth but grew to 30 pounds by the time he was 6 months old. By his first birthday, he had reached 62 pounds. At the time of his death at age 22 from cellulitis of the feet, he was 8 feet 11 inches tall and weighed 457 pounds. (**A** and **B** from Fadner, F. [1944]. *Biography of Robert Wadlow.* Courtesy Bruce Humphries, Publishers. **C** courtesy C.M. Charles and C.M. MacBryde.)

and enlargement of many visceral organs, such as the liver and heart.

Bony changes related to excessive GH occur slowly and include thickening, tufting of terminal phalanges (arrowhead fingertips), and bone cell overgrowth. Degeneration of joint cartilage and hypertrophy of ligaments, vocal cords, and eustachian tube mucosa are common. Nerve entrapment occurs because of tissue overgrowth with demyelinization of peripheral nerves. Because GH is an insulin **antagonist** (blocks the action of insulin), **hyperglycemia** (elevated blood glucose levels) is also common.

Hypersecretion of ACTH results in overstimulation of the adrenal cortex. This stimulation produces excessive amounts of glucocorticoids, mineralocorticoids, and androgens, which lead to the development of Cushing's disease (see Hypercortisolism [Cushing's Syndrome], p. 1416).

Etiology

Most cases of hyperpituitarism result from hormone-secreting adenomas arising from one pituitary cell type. Hyperpituitarism can also be caused by hypothalamic dysfunction in which excessive amounts of releasing hormones are produced and then overstimulate the normal pituitary gland.

Adenomas can develop in clients without a family history or as part of a syndrome known as **multiple endocrine neo-**

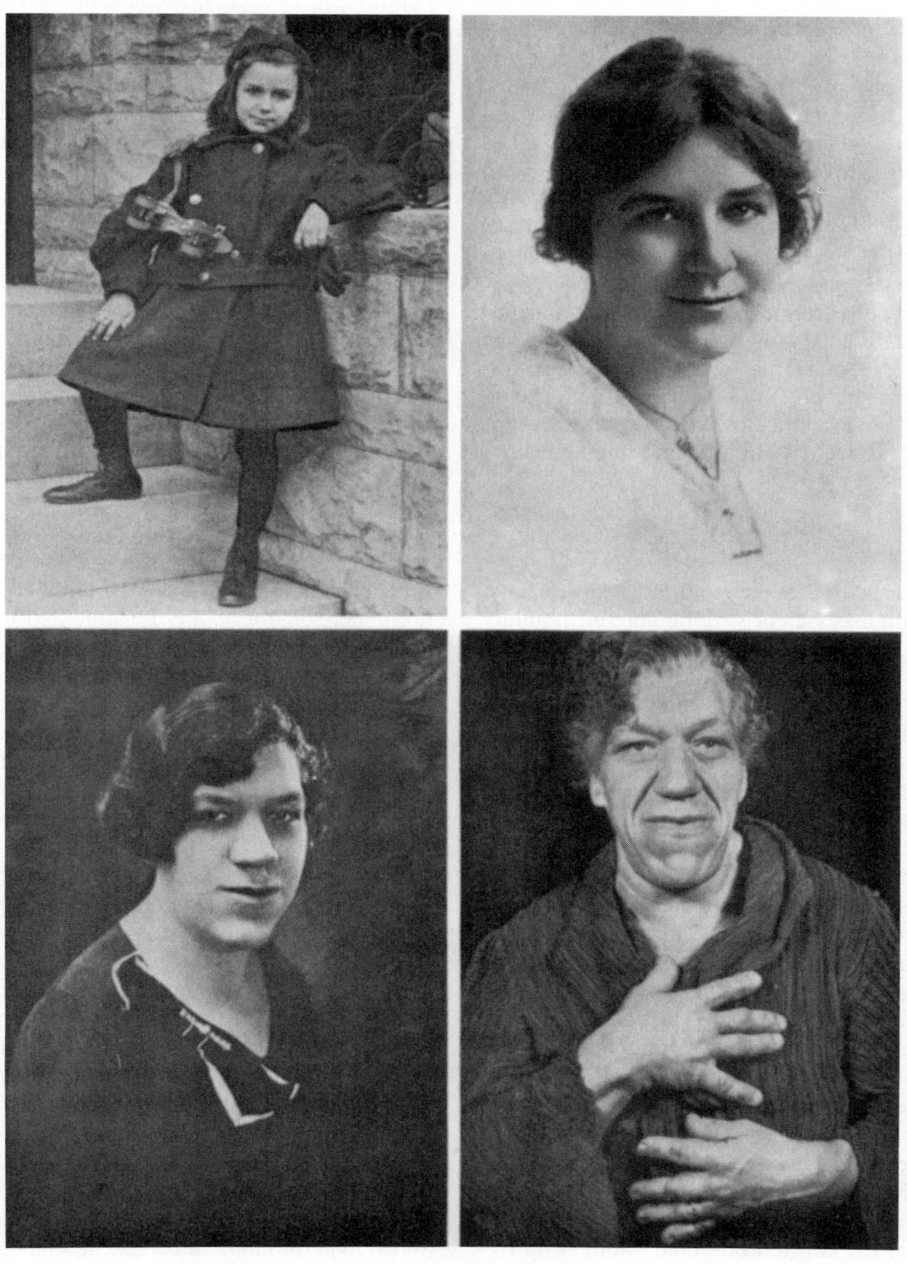

Figure 63-2 ● The progression of acromegaly. (From Mendelhoff, A., & Smith, D.E., [Eds.]. [1956]. Acromegaly, diabetes, hypermetabolism, proteinuria, and heart failure. Clinical Pathological Conference. *American Journal of Medicine, 20,* 133.)

plasia. This familial disorder, inherited as an autosomal dominant trait, may include parathyroid and pancreatic tumors.

Incidence/Prevalence

Hyperpituitarism is a rare disorder. The most common secretory tumors are prolactinomas, followed by GH-producing adenomas. Tumors secreting gonadotropin or thyroid-stimulating hormone (TSH) are the least common. Of all pituitary tumors for which surgery is performed, approximately 70% secrete one or more hormones.

COLLABORATIVE MANAGEMENT

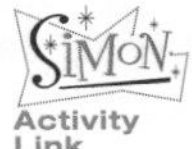

Assessment

HISTORY

The symptoms of hyperpituitarism vary, depending on which hormone is produced in excess. The nurse obtains data about the client's age, gender, and family history. The client is asked about any change in hat, glove, ring, or shoe size. Fatigue and lethargy are common. The client with excessively high GH levels may have backache and **arthralgias** (joint pain) in response to bone changes. He or she is asked specifically about the presence of headaches and changes in vision.

The client with hypersecretion of PRL (hyperprolactinemia) often reports difficulties in sexual functioning. The nurse asks women about menstrual changes (e.g., amenorrhea, irregular menses, and difficulty in achieving pregnancy) and about decreased libido or **dyspareunia** (painful intercourse). Men may report decreased libido and impotence.

PHYSICAL ASSESSMENT/CLINICAL MANIFESTATIONS

Some changes in physical appearance and target organ function are associated with excesses of specific anterior pituitary hormones (Chart 63-2). Initial manifestations of GH hypersecretion are changes in the facial features, including increases in lip and nose sizes; increases in head, hand, and foot sizes; and a prominent supraorbital ridge. **Prognathism,** a projection of the jaw beyond the facial features, becomes marked. The client is assessed for difficulty in chewing and for dentures that no longer fit. Arthritic changes causing joint pain and decreased mobility may also be noted. Fingers and toes may have an "arrowhead" or tufted shape on x-ray films and a thickened appearance. At onset, acromegaly is characterized by increased metabolism and strength. As the disease progresses, these manifestations are replaced with lethargy and weakness.

The nurse assesses the client's vision for any changes related to compression of the optic nerves. The nurse also notes any increased perspiration and oil secretion on the skin. Other prominent features include the following:

- Organomegaly (cardiac or hepatic)
- Hypertension
- Dysphagia caused by an enlarged tongue
- Deepening of the voice caused by hypertrophy of the larynx

Hypersecretion of PRL is often observed, along with hypogonadism and galactorrhea (fluid leakage from the breast). Galactorrhea may be present in either gender but is predominant in females.

PSYCHOSOCIAL ASSESSMENT

The client with hyperpituitarism often seeks health care because of dramatic changes in physical appearance. The nurse assesses the impact of these physical changes on the client's interpersonal relationships.

In clients who are disturbed by an inability to conceive, the nurse identifies symptoms of emotional distress, such as crying, reports of depression, irritability, and hostility. They may express fear of the diagnosis, subsequent surgery, and prognosis, especially when a tumor is suspected.

LABORATORY ASSESSMENT

In a person with hyperpituitarism, usually only one hormone is produced in excess, because the cell types within the pituitary gland are so discretely organized. The most common hormones produced in excess are PRL, ACTH, and GH. Tumors producing TSH, luteinizing hormone (LH), or follicle-stimulating hormone (FSH) are extremely rare. Elevated levels of any of these hormones usually warrant further investigation. Elevations of LH and FSH, however, are normal in the postmenopausal woman.

RADIOGRAPHIC ASSESSMENT

Radiographic evaluation of the client with hyperpituitarism is identical to that for a client with hypopituitarism. Conventional skull x-ray films are made to identify abnormalities of the sella turcica. Computed tomography (CT) and magnetic resonance imaging (MRI) can define soft-tissue lesions, and angiography can rule out an aneurysm or congenital vascular malformations.

OTHER DIAGNOSTIC ASSESSMENT

Rather than just measuring the circulating level of a specific hormone, some tests are dynamic and measure how well the endocrine gland responds to stimulation changes. Suppression tests are a type of dynamic endocrine testing that can help in the diagnosis of hyperpituitarism. These tests involve administering agents that induce a suppressive response from the pituitary gland, and they can determine whether the normal negative feedback control mechanisms for hormonal regulation are intact. For example, high circulating levels of glucose have a suppressive effect on the release of GH. In a suppression test, 100 g of oral glucose or 0.5 g/kg of body weight is given intravenously. GH levels are measured serially for up to 120 minutes. GH levels that do not fall below 5 ng/mL indicate a positive (abnormal) result.

Another example of a suppression test is the administration of intravenous (IV) cortisol in the form of dexamethasone (Decadron). This agent should result in suppression of ACTH. When ACTH production continues in the presence of dexamethasone administration, the client may have pituitary Cushing's disease.

Analysis

When hyperpituitarism is present, one or more of the anterior pituitary hormones are overproduced. The nursing diagnoses focus on the client's responses to excesses of prolactin (PRL) and growth hormone (GH).

CHART 63-2

KEY FEATURES *of* Pituitary Hyperfunction

Excess Hormone	Clinical Manifestations
Anterior Pituitary Hormones	
Prolactin (PRL)	Hypogonadism (loss of secondary sexual characteristics) Decreased gonadotropin levels Galactorrhea Increased body fat Increased serum prolactin levels
Growth hormone (GH)	Acromegaly • Thickened, oily skin (facial) • Thickened lips • Folding of the scalp skin • Deepening of the voice • Enlarged hands and feet • Increasing head size • Protrusion of the lower jaw • Joint enlargement and pain (knees, hips, and shoulders) • Kyphosis and backache • "Barrel chest" • Excessive sweating (especially of the hands, feet, head, and face) • Coarse facial features • Tufting of the fingertips • Hyperglycemia • Airway narrowing, sleep apnea • Enlarged heart, lungs, and liver
Adrenocorticotropic hormone (ACTH)	Cushing's syndrome • Elevated plasma cortisol levels • Weight gain • Truncal obesity • "Moon face" • Extremity muscle wasting • Loss of bone density • Hypertension • Hyperglycemia • Purple striae • Acne • Thin, easily damaged skin • Hyperpigmentation
Thyrotropin (thyroid-stimulating hormone [TSH])	Elevated plasma TSH levels Elevated plasma thyroid hormone levels Weight loss Tachycardia Heat intolerance Increased gastrointestinal (GI) motility Fine tremors
Gonadotropins (luteinizing hormone [LH], follicle-stimulating hormone [FSH])	Men: • Elevated LH and FSH levels • Hypogonadism or hypergonadism Women: • Normal LH and FSH levels (The most common clinical manifestations in men and women are related to the physical presence of a tumor rather than to excessive hormone secretion.)
Posterior Pituitary Hormones	
Vasopressin (antidiuretic hormone [ADH])	Syndrome of inappropriate antidiuretic hormone (SIADH) • Decreased urine output • Increased urine osmolarity • Increased plasma volume • Decreased plasma osmolarity • Weight gain • Hyponatremia • Nonpitting edema • Central nervous system (CNS) changes (confusion, seizures)

Data from Thorner, M., et al. (1998). The anterior pituitary. In J.D. Wilson et al. (Eds.), *Williams textbook of endocrinology* (9th ed., pp. 249-340). Philadelphia: W.B. Saunders; and Reeves, W.B., Bichet, D., & Andreoli, T. (1998). Posterior pituitary and water metabolism. In J.D. Wilson et al. (Eds.), *Williams textbook of endocrinology* (9th ed., pp. 341-387). Philadelphia: W.B. Saunders.

COMMON NURSING DIAGNOSES AND COLLABORATIVE PROBLEMS

The following are common nursing diagnoses for clients with hyperpituitarism:

1. Disturbed Body Image related to altered physical appearance
2. Sexual Dysfunction related to actual limitation imposed by disease (e.g., loss of libido, infertility, impotence)

ADDITIONAL NURSING DIAGNOSES AND COLLABORATIVE PROBLEMS

In addition to the common nursing diagnoses, clients with hyperpituitarism may have one or more of the following:

- Acute Pain and Chronic Pain related to compression of tissues by tumor (e.g., discomfort, headache), backache, or arthralgia secondary to the effects of excessive GH levels; or to dyspareunia secondary to excessive PRL levels
- Fear related to a perceived threat of death from an intracranial tumor
- Anxiety related to a threat of or change in health status
- Ineffective Coping related to impaired self-concept and loss of control over the body
- Activity Intolerance related to the effects of excessive GH levels (e.g., pain or discomfort, lethargy, and weakness)
- Disturbed Sensory Perception (Visual) related to altered nerve transmission as a consequence of nerve compression from tumor or surrounding structures
- Deficient Knowledge (diagnosis and treatment regimen) related to unfamiliarity with information

Planning and Implementation

DISTURBED BODY IMAGE

NOC **PLANNING: EXPECTED OUTCOMES.** The client with hyperpituitarism is expected to experience a sense of congruence between body reality, body ideal, and body presentation.

INTERVENTIONS. The goals of therapy for the client who has hyperpituitarism are to return hormone levels to normal or near normal, correct the problems of headache and visual disturbances, prevent complications, reverse as many of the body changes as possible, and preserve as much normal pituitary function as possible. The client who has excessive GH levels may have skeletal changes that cannot be reversed with treatment.

NONSURGICAL MANAGEMENT. The client is encouraged to verbalize concerns and fears about his or her altered physical appearance. The nurse helps the client identify personal strengths and positive characteristics, reinforcing each client's uniqueness and importance.

Galactorrhea, gynecomastia, and difficulties in sexual functioning can cause disturbances in body image and personal identity. The nurse reassures the client that treatment may alleviate some of these symptoms and encourages him or her to discuss his or her feelings.

DRUG THERAPY. Drug therapy may be used alone or in combination with surgery and/or radiation. The most common drugs used are dopamine agonists, especially bromocriptine mesylate (Parlodel). This drug group stimulates dopamine receptors in the brain and inhibits the release of many pituitary hormones, most specifically GH and PRL. In most cases, small tumors **(microadenomas)** decrease until the pituitary gland is of normal size, and large pituitary tumors **(macroadenomas)** decrease to some extent. In clients with acromegaly, bromocriptine has reduced GH levels and decreased tumor size, especially when GH levels remain high after surgery or before the full effect of radiation therapy has occurred.

Side effects of bromocriptine include **orthostatic** (postural) hypotension, gastric irritation, nausea, headaches, abdominal cramps, and constipation. Bromocriptine is given with a meal or a snack to reduce some of these side effects. Treatment is usually initiated with a low dose and is gradually increased until the desired level (usually 7.5 mg/day) is reached. *If pregnancy occurs, the drug is stopped immediately.*

Other agents used for acromegaly are the somatostatin analogs, especially octreotide (Sandostatin). This drug group inhibits GH release through negative feedback. Although this therapy is effective in reducing GH levels, a disadvantage is the fact that it must be administered daily as a subcutaneous injection. A major side effect is gallbladder disease.

RADIATION THERAPY. Radiation therapy is not useful in the management of acute hyperpituitarism. Radiation therapy regimens take a long time to complete, and several years may pass before a therapeutic effect is evident. Side effects of radiation therapy include hypopituitarism, optic nerve damage, reduced coordinated eye movement, and visual field defects.

SURGICAL MANAGEMENT. Surgical removal of a microadenoma of the pituitary gland **(hypophysectomy)** is often indicated for clients with hyperpituitarism.

PREOPERATIVE CARE. The nurse explains that hypophysectomy decreases hormone levels, relieves headaches, and may reverse changes in sexual functioning. Body changes, visceral enlargement, and visual changes are not usually reversible. The nurse explains that because nasal packing is present for 2 to 3 days postoperatively, it will be necessary to breathe through the mouth, and a "mustache" dressing ("drip" pad) will be placed under the nose. The client is instructed not to brush teeth, cough, sneeze, blow the nose, or bend forward after surgery. These activities can open the muscle graft, increase intracranial pressure, and hinder healing of the incision. Nasal and oral mucous membrane swab specimens for bacterial culture and sensitivity are obtained preoperatively because surgery, especially the transsphenoidal approach, can cause infectious organisms from these areas to spread systemically.

OPERATIVE PROCEDURE. A transsphenoidal approach to the pituitary gland is most commonly used (Figure 63-3). Transsphenoidal hypophysectomy is microscopic surgery performed with the client under general anesthesia and in a semisitting position. The surgeon makes the initial incision just above the upper lip and reaches the pituitary gland through the sphenoid sinus. After the gland is removed, a muscle graft is taken, often from the anterior thigh, to support the area and prevent leakage of cerebrospinal fluid (CSF). The surgeon inserts nasal packing after the incision is closed and applies a mustache dressing. If the tumor cannot be reached by this approach, a craniotomy may be indicated (see Chapter 45).

POSTOPERATIVE CARE. The nurse monitors the client's neurologic response and documents any changes in vision, mental status, altered level of consciousness, or decreased strength of the extremities. The client is observed for postoperative complications (e.g., transient diabetes insipidus).

In a client with diabetes insipidus, urine specific gravity measurements are low and urine output is excessive. The nurse monitors the intake of IV fluid, encourages fluid intake in response to thirst, and administers vasopressin as indicated. A Foley catheter may be inserted for accurate measuring of urine output, and daily weights are taken.

The client is instructed to report any postnasal drip, which might indicate leakage of CSF. The head of the bed is elevated postoperatively. The nurse assesses nasal drainage for quantity, quality, and the presence of glucose (which indicates that the fluid is CSF). A light yellow color at the edge of the clear drainage on the dressing is called the "halo sign" and indicates CSF. If the client complains of persistent, severe headaches, CSF fluid may have leaked into the sinus area. Most CSF leaks resolve with bedrest. If the CSF leak persists, the physician may perform a spinal tap to reduce CSF pressure. Surgical intervention is rarely necessary.

Coughing is avoided postoperatively because it increases pressure in the incisional area and may lead to a CSF leak. The nurse reminds the client to perform deep breathing exercises frequently to prevent pulmonary complications. Clients may also have mouth dryness as a result of mouth breathing. The nurse or assistive nursing personnel performs frequent oral rinses and applies petroleum jelly to dry lips.

Infection can occur postoperatively as well. The nurse is particularly alert for symptoms of meningitis, such as headache, fever, and **nuchal** (neck) rigidity. The surgeon may prescribe antibiotics, analgesics, and antipyretics.

If the entire pituitary gland has been removed, thyroid hormones and glucocorticoids must be replaced. (Gonadotropin deficiency is also noted in both male and female clients.) Best practices for postoperative care are reviewed in Chart 63-3.

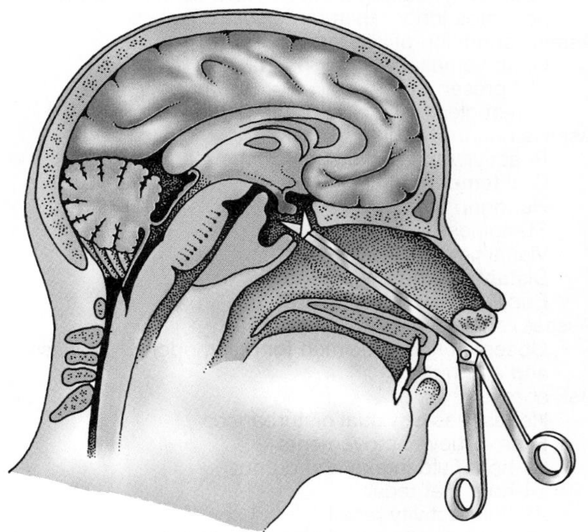

Figure 63-3 ● The transsphenoidal surgical approach to the pituitary gland. Selective adenomectomy leaves normal pituitary tissues undisturbed.

SEXUAL DYSFUNCTION

PLANNING: EXPECTED OUTCOMES. The client with hyperpituitarism is expected to achieve a personal desired level of sexual functioning.

INTERVENTIONS. The nurse identifies the specific problems that the client is experiencing and encourages him or her to discuss any effect that sexual dysfunction has had on his or her sexual partner. Drug therapy with bromocriptine can decrease prolactin (PRL) levels in clients with PRL-secreting tumors. After PRL levels are decreased, gonadotropin function often returns to normal. Clients requiring hypophysectomy may experience sexual dysfunction as a result of postsurgical gonadotropin deficiency and require hormone replacement (discussed earlier under Interventions [Hypopituitarism], p. 1401).

CRITICAL THINKING CHALLENGE

The client is 24 hours postoperative from a transsphenoidal hypophysectomy. Her IV has been discontinued even though she still feels nauseated and does not want to eat or drink. She tells you that she would like to get up to use the bathroom because it seems like she has to use the bedpan every 15 minutes to urinate. She also asks you to change her moustache dressing because it is very wet and is irritating her skin.

- What additional assessment data should you obtain?
- Is it safe to let the client get up out of bed?
- What information should you relay to the surgeon?

For suggested answer guidelines, go to SIMON http://www.wbsaunders.com/SIMON/Iggy/.

Community-Based Care

Clients who have advanced acromegaly may experience arthritic changes. The nurse assesses the degree of mobility impairment and identifies appropriate adaptations, such as the

CHART 63-3

BEST PRACTICE *for* The Client After Hypophysectomy

- Monitor the client's neurologic status.
- Monitor fluid balance, especially for output greater than intake, because transient diabetes insipidus can occur.
- Encourage the client to maintain pulmonary hygiene through deep breathing exercises.
- Instruct the client *not* to cough, blow the nose, or sneeze.
- Instruct the client to use dental floss and oral mouth rinses because brushing the teeth is not permitted until the incision heals sufficiently.
- Instruct the client to avoid bending at the waist for any reason, because this position increases intracranial pressure.
- Monitor the nasal drip pad for the type and amount of drainage. The presence of the halo sign may indicate a CSF leak.
- Monitor bowel movements to prevent constipation and subsequent "straining."
- Teach the client self-administration of the prescribed hormones.

CSF, Cerebrospinal fluid.

use of ambulatory aids (cane or walker) and the accessibility of bathroom facilities.

HEALTH TEACHING

After a transsphenoidal hypophysectomy, the nurse advises the client to avoid activities that might interfere with healing. Bending over from the waist to pick up objects or tie shoes must be avoided because doing so increases intracranial pressure. The client is instructed to bend the knees and then lower the body to retrieve fallen objects. Intracranial pressure also increases when the client strains to have a bowel movement. The nurse suggests techniques to prevent constipation, such as eating high-fiber foods, drinking additional fluids, and using stool softeners or laxatives. Both bending and straining with bowel movements should be avoided for up to 2 months after surgery.

The client must avoid toothbrushing for about 2 weeks after surgery until the incision has undergone significant healing. Frequent mouth care (every 4 to 6 hours) with mouthwash and daily flossing during this period provides adequate oral hygiene. Transient numbness in the area of the incision and a decreased sense of smell are expected after surgery and usually last 3 to 4 months. The nurse advises the client to use a mirror to check the gums for bleeding, because reduced sensation increases the risk for injury.

After a hypophysectomy, hormone replacement with vasopressin may be necessary to maintain fluid balance (see later discussion under Interventions [Diabetes Insipidus], p. 1410). If the anterior portion of the pituitary gland is removed, the client may require instruction in cortisol, thyroid, and gonadal hormone replacement. The nurse instructs the client to report the return of any symptoms of hyperpituitarism immediately to the primary health care provider.

HOME CARE MANAGEMENT

After treatment, the client who has hyperpituitarism may require daily self-management regimens and frequent checkups. The client may also need to develop strategies to minimize stress to prevent alterations of hormone production. The nurse performs a focused assessment during the first several home visits to a client who has undergone a hypophysectomy (Chart 63-4). Medication regimens, signs and symptoms of infection, and cerebral edema are reviewed with the family.

HEALTH CARE RESOURCES

The client with decreased mobility related to acromegaly or who has had recent surgery may require a home care aide or nurse to help maintain activities of daily living (ADLs). In addition, the client with hyperpituitarism must continue to have hormone levels monitored at regular intervals to detect any recurrence of tumor. Regularly scheduled follow-up with the health care team is essential.

Evaluation: Outcomes

NOC The nurse evaluates the care of the client with hyperpituitarism on the basis of the identified nursing diagnoses and collaborative problems. The expected outcomes include that the client will:

- Experience an improvement in body image
- Achieve a personal desired level of sexual functioning
- Demonstrate adjustment to physical appearance
- Be willing to use strategies to enhance appearance and function

DISORDERS OF THE POSTERIOR PITUITARY GLAND

Disorders of the posterior pituitary (**neurohypophysis**) are directly related to a deficiency or excess of the hormone vasopressin **(antidiuretic hormone [ADH]).** Two disorders associated with ADH deficiency or excess are diabetes insipidus and the syndrome of inappropriate antidiuretic hormone (SIADH).

Diabetes Insipidus

OVERVIEW

Diabetes insipidus is a disorder of water metabolism caused by a deficiency of ADH—either a decrease in ADH synthesis or an inability of the kidneys to respond appropriately to ADH. ADH deficiency results in the excretion of large volumes of dilute urine. Without the presence of ADH, the distal tubules and collecting ducts of the kidney remain impermeable to water. Thus water is excreted as urine rather than being absorbed in these areas, which leads to **polyuria** (excessive urination with loss of free water).

Dehydration caused by this massive diuresis results in an increase in plasma osmolality, which stimulates the osmore-

CHART 63-4

FOCUSED ASSESSMENT *of* Home Care Clients Who Have Undergone Transsphenoidal Hypophysectomy for Hyperpituitarism

Assess cardiovascular status.
- Vital signs, including apical pulse, pulse pressure, presence or absence of orthostatic hypotension, and the quality/rhythm of peripheral pulses.

Assess cognition and mental status.
- Level of consciousness
- Orientation to time, place, and person
- Accurately reading a seven-word sentence containing no words longer than three syllables

Assess condition of operative site.
- Observe nasal area for drainage
  - If present, note color, clarity, and odor
  - Test clear drainage for the presence of glucose

Assess neuromuscular status.
- Reactivity of patellar and biceps reflexes
- Oral temperature
- Handgrip strength
- Steadiness of gait
- Visual fields
- Distant and near visual acuity
- Pupillary responses to light

Assess renal system.
- Observe urine specimen for color, odor, cloudiness, and amount

Ask about:
- Headaches or visual disturbances
- Ease of bowel movements
- 24-hour fluid intake and output
- 24-hour diet recall
- 24-hour activity recall
- Over-the-counter and prescribed medications taken

Assess client's understanding of illness and compliance with treatment.
- Signs and symptoms to report to health care provider
- Medication plan (correct timing and dose)

ceptors to relay a sensation of thirst to the cerebral cortex. Normally, thirst promotes increased fluid intake and aids in maintaining water homeostasis. If the thirst mechanism is inadequate or absent, or if the person is unable to obtain water, dehydration becomes more severe.

ADH deficiency can be classified as nephrogenic, drug-related, primary, or secondary, depending on whether the problem is caused by insufficient production of ADH or an inability of the kidney to respond to the presence of ADH.

Nephrogenic diabetes insipidus is an inherited disorder. The renal tubules do not respond to the actions of ADH, which results in inadequate water reabsorption by the kidney. The actual amount of hormone produced is not deficient.

Primary diabetes insipidus is caused by a defect in the hypothalamus or pituitary gland, resulting in a lack of ADH production or release. Secondary diabetes insipidus results from tumors within or adjacent to the hypothalamus or pituitary gland, head trauma, infectious processes, surgical procedures (hypophysectomy), or metastatic tumors, usually from the lung or the breast. Less commonly, it is caused by brain hemorrhage, brain disease, or cerebral aneurysm. All of these problems can reduce the production of ADH.

Drug-related diabetes insipidus is caused by the administration of lithium carbonate (Eskalith, Lithobid, Carbolith♣) and demeclocycline (Declomycin). These drugs can interfere with the kidneys' response to ADH.

➤ COLLABORATIVE MANAGEMENT

● Assessment

Most of the clinical manifestations of diabetes insipidus are related to dehydration (Chart 63-5). The nurse notes the key symptoms of an increase in the frequency of urination and excessive thirst. The client is asked about a history of any known etiologic factors, such as recent surgery, head trauma, or medication use (e.g., lithium). Although increased fluid intake usually prevents serious dehydration and volume depletion, the client who is deprived of fluids or who cannot increase oral fluid intake may experience shock caused by fluid loss and plasma hyperosmolality. Signs of dehydration, such as poor skin turgor and dry or cracked mucous membranes or skin, may be present in varying degrees. (See Chapter 12 for further discussion of clients with dehydration.)

Loss of free water produces expected changes in blood and urine tests. The initial step in diagnosis is to measure a 24-hour fluid intake and output. The amount of the client's food and fluid is not restricted during this measurement. Urine output must be more than 4 L during this period for diabetes insipidus to be diagnosed. The amount of urine excreted in 24 hours may vary from 4 to 30 L/day. Urine is dilute and therefore has a low specific gravity (less than 1.005) and low osmolality (50 to 200 mOsm/kg). Fluid deprivation and hypertonic saline tests are also used for diagnosis of the disorder (Table 63-2).

CHART 63-5

KEY FEATURES *of* Diabetes Insipidus

Cardiovascular Manifestations
- Hypotension
- Decreased pulse pressure
- Tachycardia
- Peripheral pulses weak, easily obliterated
- Hemoconcentration
  - Increased hemoglobin
  - Increased hematocrit

Renal/Urinary Manifestations
- Increased urine output
  - Dilute, low specific gravity
  - Hypo-osmolar

Integumentary Manifestations
- Poor turgor
- Dry mucous membranes

Neurologic Manifestations
- Increased sensation of thirst
  - Irritability*
  - Decreased cognition*
  - Hyperthermia*
  - Lethargy to coma*
  - Ataxia*

*Occurs when access to water is limited and rapid dehydration results.

TABLE 63-2 • CARE OF THE CLIENT UNDERGOING SPECIAL TESTS FOR DIABETES INSIPIDUS

Nursing Interventions	Rationale
FLUID DEPRIVATION TEST (TO IDENTIFY THE CAUSE OF POLYURIA)	
Obtain baseline vital signs; then check them hourly.	Assessment permits the nurse to detect changes, especially postural hypotension and tachycardia.
Deprive the client of fluid. Observe the client for compliance with fluid restriction.	Fluid restriction must be maintained for test results to be of diagnostic importance.
Measure urine output, specific gravity, and osmolality hourly.	Urine testing results determine whether testing can proceed.
Weigh the client hourly.	Testing can proceed if urine osmolality stabilizes for three samples and 3% weight loss is noted.
Give 5 units of aqueous vasopressin (subcutaneously), as ordered. Continue hourly urine measurements.	Vasopressin triggers—and ongoing assessment detects—changes in urine specific gravity and osmolality. Specific gravity and osmolality decrease with primary and secondary diabetes insipidus. No response is seen with nephrogenic diabetes insipidus.
HYPERTONIC SALINE TEST (TO STIMULATE RELEASE OF ADH)	
Administer a normal water load to the client, followed by infusion of hypertonic saline. Measure urine output hourly.	The procedure detects ADH release. A sudden decrease in urine output is a sign of ADH release.

ADH, Antidiuretic hormone.

Interventions

Medical management is aimed at controlling the symptoms of the disease through drug therapy (Chart 63-6). If only a partial deficit of ADH is present, effective control can be achieved with oral chlorpropamide (Diabinese, Novo-Propamide✤) or clofibrate (Atromid-S, Claripex✤). These drugs increase the action of existing ADH and possibly have a direct stimulating effect on the production of ADH in the hypothalamus. They have some undesirable side effects, however, and are not used as often as synthetic vasopressin.

When ADH deficiency is severe, ADH is replaced in amounts sufficient to maintain water balance. Desmopressin acetate (DDAVP) is a synthetic form of vasopressin administered intranasally in a metered spray and is the drug of choice. The frequency of administration varies in different clients. Each metered spray delivers 10 g, and the client with mild diabetes insipidus may require only 1 to 2 doses in 24 hours. For the client with more severe diabetes insipidus, 1 to 2 metered doses two to three times per day may be needed. Lypressin (Diapid) is an older form of the drug and is given by nasal spray or subcutaneously when short-acting therapy is indicated. Subcutaneous injections last only 3 to 6 hours. During an acute exacerbation or severe dehydration, ADH may be given intravenously or intramuscularly. Ulceration of the mucous membranes, allergy, a sensation of chest tightness, and pulmonary inhalation of the spray may occur with use of the intranasal preparations. If side effects occur, or if the client has an upper respiratory tract infection, subcutaneous vasopressin is used.

Nursing management is aimed at the early detection of dehydration and the maintenance of adequate hydration. Interventions include accurately measuring fluid intake and output, checking urine specific gravity, and recording the client's weight daily.

The nurse encourages the client to consume amounts of oral fluids approximately equal to urine output. If fluids are administered intravenously, the nurse ensures the patency of the access catheter and pays meticulous attention to the amount infused each hour.

The client with permanent diabetes insipidus requires lifelong vasopressin therapy. The nurse must assess the client's ability to follow instructions and willingness to participate in health care. The client using vasopressin preparations is instructed to recognize polyuria and polydipsia as signals for the need for another dose of medication. *All clients taking vasopressin need to record daily weight measurements to identify weight gain.* The nurse emphasizes the importance of using the same scale and weighing at the same time of day while wearing a similar amount of clothing. If weight gain occurs, the client is instructed to notify the health care provider. Clients with diabetes insipidus should also wear a medical alert bracelet identifying the disorder and current medication.

Syndrome of Inappropriate Antidiuretic Hormone

OVERVIEW

The **syndrome of inappropriate antidiuretic hormone (SIADH)** occurs when vasopressin (antidiuretic hormone [ADH]) is secreted even when plasma osmolality is low or normal. A decrease in plasma osmolality normally inhibits

CHART 63-6

DRUG THERAPY *for* Diabetes Insipidus

Drug	Usual Dosage	Nursing Interventions	Rationale
Lypressin (Diapid)	4-8 sprays (5-10 pressor units) (nasal spray) in divided doses	Monitor for upper respiratory tract infections or allergy.	The effectiveness of nasal sprays is affected by upper respiratory tract infections.
Desmopressin (DDAVP)	0.1-0.4 mL in single or divided dose (nasal spray)	Teach the client the proper method of administration.	Some clients may have difficulty with measuring and inhaling.
Aqueous vasopressin (Pitressin)	5-20 units in divided doses (SC, IM, or nasal spray)	Instruct the client to sit upright when spraying.	An upright position promotes effective absorption in the nasal mucosa.
		Instruct the client to hold his or her breath when using nasal spray.	Holding one's breath prevents nasal spray from entering the lungs and potentially causing pneumonia.
		Monitor the client's intake and output.	Intake and output measurement helps to guide dosage regulation.
		Have the client space fluid intake during waking hours.	Extra fluid intake at night can cause nocturia.
		Monitor the client frequently (every 3-4 hr) for a recurrence of symptoms.	Monitoring detects the need for additional doses of these short-acting medications.
		Monitor the client's weight.	Water retention can be detected by weight gain.
Clofibrate (Atromid-S, Claripex✤)	6-8 g in 4 doses qod PO	Watch for signs of SIADH.	The drug can potentiate the action of vasopressin.
Chlorpropamide (Diabinese, Novo-Propamide✤)	125-250 mg qod PO *Older adults:* 100-125 mg qod PO	Monitor the client for signs and symptoms of hypoglycemia.	Hypoglycemia is a potentially severe side effect.

SIADH, Syndrome of inappropriate antidiuretic hormone.

ADH production and secretion. SIADH is also known as the Schwartz-Bartter syndrome. SIADH is also discussed in Chapter 25 as a complication of cancer and cancer therapy.

In SIADH, the feedback mechanisms that regulate ADH do not function properly. ADH continues to be released even when plasma is hyposmolar. Water is *retained,* which results in dilutional **hyponatremia** (a decreased serum sodium level due to dilution) and expansion of the extracellular fluid volume. The increase in plasma volume causes an increase in the glomerular filtration rate and inhibits the release of renin and aldosterone. The combined effect is an increased sodium loss in urine, further contributing to hyponatremia.

SIADH is associated with a variety of pathologic conditions and specific drugs. Table 63-3 lists common causes of SIADH.

COLLABORATIVE MANAGEMENT

Assessment

HISTORY

The client is asked about his or her medical history, which may reveal conditions associated with the development of SIADH. The nurse pays particular attention to a history of the following:

- Recent trauma
- Cerebrovascular disease
- Tuberculosis or other pulmonary disease
- Cancer
- All past and current medication use

PHYSICAL ASSESSMENT/CLINICAL MANIFESTATIONS

Initially, the symptoms of SIADH are related to water retention. Gastrointestinal (GI) disturbances, such as loss of appetite, nausea, and vomiting, may occur first. The nurse weighs the client and documents any recent weight gain. In clients with SIADH, free water (not salt) is retained and dependent edema is not usually present, even though water is retained.

Water retention, hyponatremia, and fluid shifts affect central nervous system function, especially when the serum sodium level drops below 115 mEq/L. The client may experience lethargy, headaches, hostility, and disorientation. A change in level of consciousness is an early sign of SIADH. Neurologic symptoms can progress from lethargy and headaches to decreased responsiveness, seizures, and coma. The nurse assesses deep tendon reflexes, which are often decreased or sluggish.

Vital sign changes include tachycardia (caused by the increased fluid volume) and hypothermia (caused by central nervous system disturbance). Chapter 13 presents other findings associated with hyponatremia.

TABLE 63-3 • CONDITIONS CAUSING THE SYNDROME OF INAPPROPRIATE ANTIDIURETIC HORMONES

MALIGNANCIES	CNS DISORDERS
• Small cell carcinoma of the lung	• Trauma
• Pancreatic, duodenal, and GU carcinomas	• Infection
• Thymoma	• Tumors (primary or metastatic)
• Ewing's sarcoma	• Strokes
• Hodgkin's lymphoma	• Porphyria
• Non-Hodgkin's lymphoma	• Systemic lupus erythematosus
PULMONARY DISORDERS	**DRUGS**
• Viral and bacterial pneumonia	• Exogenous ADH
• Lung abscesses	• Chlorpropamide
• Active tuberculosis	• Vincristine
• Pneumothorax	• Cyclophosphamide
• Chronic lung diseases	• Carbamazepine
• Mycoses	• Opioids
• Positive-pressure ventilation	• Tricyclic antidepressants
	• General anesthetics

GU, Genitourinary; *CNS,* central nervous system; *ADH,* antidiuretic hormone.

DIAGNOSTIC ASSESSMENT

Water retention changes both plasma and urine osmolality. Urine volume decreases, and urine osmolarity increases. Plasma volume increases, and plasma osmolarity decreases. Elevated urine sodium levels and elevated specific gravity reflect increased urine concentration. Serum sodium levels are decreased, often as low as 110 mEq/L, because of volume expansion and sodium excretion.

Radioimmunoassay of ADH can diagnose SIADH when ADH levels are inappropriately elevated in relation to plasma osmolality. (When plasma osmolality is normal or decreased, ADH levels should be low.)

Interventions

Interventions to treat SIADH focus on restricting fluid intake, promoting the excretion of water, replacing lost sodium, interfering with the action of ADH, and preventing injury if the client experiences increased cranial pressure or seizures.

FLUID RESTRICTION. Fluid restriction is essential in the management of the client with SIADH because fluid intake further dilutes the plasma sodium concentration. In some cases, fluid intake may be kept as low as 500 to 600 mL/24 hr. Tube feedings are diluted with a solution other than plain water, and saline is used to irrigate GI tubes. The nurse mixes any medications for GI tube administration with saline.

Measurement of intake, output, and daily weights determines the degree of fluid restriction necessary. A weight gain of 2 pounds (1 kg) or more per day or a gradual increase over several days is cause for concern. A 1-kg weight increase is equal to a 1000-mL fluid retention (1 kg = 1 L). The client is often uncomfortable during fluid restriction, and the nurse keeps mucous membranes moist by offering frequent oral rinsing (reminding the client not to swallow these rinses).

DRUG THERAPY. Diuretics are sometimes used to treat SIADH, particularly if congestive heart failure results from fluid overload. The nurse must be aware of the potential effect of electrolyte losses; sodium loss can be potentiated, further contributing to the problems caused by SIADH.

Hypertonic saline (i.e., 3% sodium chloride [3% NaCl]) is often used to treat SIADH. IV saline is given cautiously because it may add to existing fluid overload and promote congestive heart failure. If the client needs routine IV fluids, the physician orders a saline solution rather than a water solution.

The administration of drugs such as lithium carbonate (Eskalith, Lithobid, Carbolith✱) and demeclocycline (Declomycin) is associated with the development of diabetes insipidus. Their use has therefore been explored in the treatment of SIADH. Lithium is seldom used because of its toxicity; demeclocycline is more common.

PROVIDING A SAFE ENVIRONMENT. The nurse observes for and documents changes in the client's neurologic status. The nurse assesses for subtle changes, such as muscle twitching, before they progress to seizures or coma. Orientation to time, place, and person is checked every 2 hours because disorientation or confusion may be present. Environmental noise and lighting are reduced to prevent overstimulation.

Flow sheets with continuing information about the level of consciousness, motor and sensory neurologic assessments, and pertinent laboratory data are helpful in detecting neurologic trends. The frequency of neurologic checks depends on the status of the client: for the client with SIADH who is hyponatremic but alert, awake, and oriented, neurologic checks every 4 hours are sufficient. For the client who has had a change in level of consciousness, neurologic checks take place at least every hour. The nurse also inspects the environment at regular intervals, making sure that basic safety measures, such as siderails securely in place, are observed.

CRITICAL THINKING CHALLENGE

The client is a 63-year-old man with late-stage lung cancer who is being cared for at home by his wife. He has SIADH and is on a fluid restriction of 800 mL/day. During a home visit, the client seems to be more confused than when you last saw him. His wife tells you that his mouth is always dry and he does not want to eat. She also tells that you he would eat ice cream but that she has not given it to him because of the fluid restriction.

- What additional assessment data should you obtain?
- What comfort measures could you suggest?
- Should this client be permitted to have a serving of ice cream? Why or why not?

For suggested answer guidelines, go to SIMON http://www.wbsaunders.com/SIMON/Iggy/.

DISORDERS OF THE ADRENAL GLAND

ADRENAL GLAND HYPOFUNCTION

OVERVIEW

Production of adrenocortical steroids may decrease as a result of inadequate secretion of adrenocorticotropic hormone (ACTH), dysfunction of the hypothalamic-pituitary control mechanism, and complete or partial destruction of the adrenal glands. Manifestations may develop gradually or occur quickly with stress. In acute adrenocortical insufficiency **(adrenal crisis),** life-threatening manifestations may appear without warning. Figure 63-4 outlines the normal pathway for adrenocortical hormone synthesis.

Loss of the adrenal medulla, which produces **catecholamines** (dopamine, norepinephrine, and epinephrine), does not upset the maintenance of homeostasis. This is because catecholamines are also synthesized and released from other areas in the sympathetic nervous system.

Pathophysiology

Insufficiency of adrenocortical steroids causes problems through the loss of mineralocorticoid **(aldosterone)** and glucocorticoid **(cortisol)** action. Impaired secretion of cortisol results in decreased **gluconeogenesis** (making glucose from proteins) along with depletion of liver and muscle glycogen, leading to **hypoglycemia** (low blood glucose levels). The glomerular filtration rate and gastric acid production decrease, leading to a reduction in urea nitrogen excretion, causing anorexia and weight loss.

Reduced aldosterone secretion causes potassium, sodium, and water imbalances. Potassium excretion is decreased, causing hyperkalemia; sodium and water excretion is increased, causing hyponatremia and hypovolemia. Potassium retention also promotes reabsorption of hydrogen ions, which can ultimately lead to acidosis.

Lower adrenal androgen levels result in the decrease or loss of body, axillary, and pubic hair, especially in women, because the adrenals produce most of the androgens in fe-

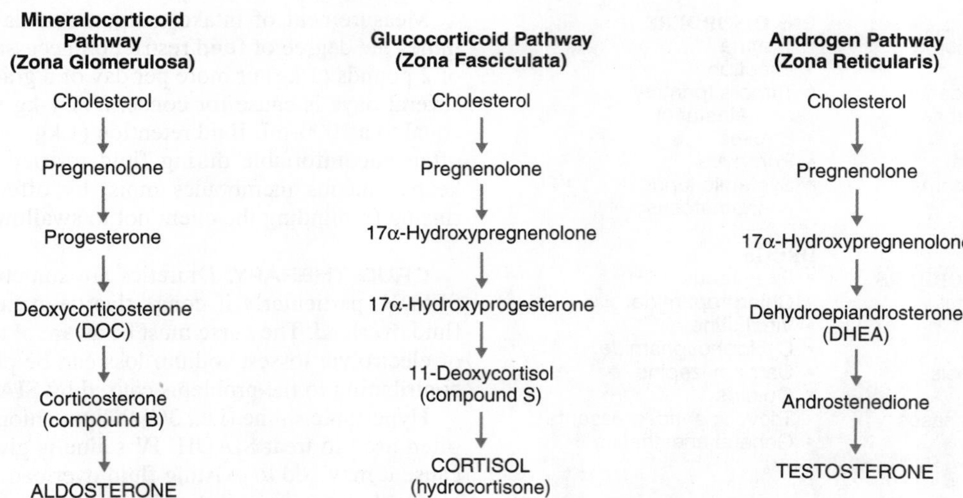

Figure 63-4 ● A simplified explanation of the major pathways of adrenal steroidal synthesis from the adrenal cortex.

males. The severity of symptoms is related to the degree of deficiency in hormone secretion.

Acute adrenal insufficiency, or **Addisonian crisis,** is a life-threatening event in which the physiologic need for glucocorticoid and mineralocorticoid hormones is greater than the available supply. In most cases, acute adrenal insufficiency occurs in response to a stressful event (e.g., surgery, trauma, or severe infection), especially when the adrenal hormone output is already compromised. The pathophysiology of acute adrenal crisis is almost the same as that of chronic insufficiency; the one difference occurs in clients with acute adrenal crisis related to bilateral adrenal hemorrhage. These clients may have normal sodium and potassium levels because the time between the initial incident and the presentation may be too short for a change in electrolyte composition to occur. Unless intervention is initiated promptly, however, sodium levels fall and potassium levels rise rapidly. More severe hypotension results from the blood volume depletion that occurs with the loss of aldosterone. Best practices for emergency care of clients with acute adrenal insufficiency (Addisonian crisis) are outlined in Chart 63-7.

Etiology

Adrenal insufficiency may be classified as primary or secondary. Causes of primary and secondary adrenal insufficiency are listed in Table 63-4. One of the most frequent causes of secondary adrenal insufficiency is the sudden cessation of long-term, high-dose glucocorticoid therapy. This therapy suppresses production of glucocorticoids through negative feedback. Glucocorticoid drugs must be withdrawn gradually to allow for pituitary production of ACTH and adrenal production of cortisol.

COLLABORATIVE MANAGEMENT

Assessment

HISTORY

While taking a history from the client with suspected adrenal hypofunction, the nurse asks questions about symptoms and factors contributing to adrenal hypofunction. The client is also asked about any change in activity level, because lethargy, fatigue, and muscle weakness are often present. Questions about salt intake are included because salt craving is often a symptom of adrenal hypofunction.

Gastrointestinal (GI) problems, such as anorexia, nausea, vomiting, diarrhea, and abdominal pain, often occur. The nurse asks about weight loss during the past weeks or months. Female clients report menstrual changes related to weight loss, and male clients may report impotence.

The medical history identifies potential causes of adrenal hypofunction. The nurse asks whether the client has had radiation to the abdomen or head. Significant medical problems (e.g., tuberculosis or previous intracranial surgery) and all past and current medications, especially steroids, anticoagulants, or cytotoxic drugs, are documented.

PHYSICAL ASSESSMENT/CLINICAL MANIFESTATIONS

The clinical manifestations of adrenal hypofunction vary, and the severity of symptoms is related to the degree of hormone deficiency (Chart 63-8). In clients with primary adrenal hypofunction, plasma ACTH and melanocyte-stimulating hormone (MSH) levels are elevated because of the loss of the adrenal-hypothalamic-pituitary feedback system. Elevated MSH levels result in areas of increased pigmentation (Figure 63-5). In primary autoimmune disease, areas of decreased pigmentation may occur because of destruction of pigment-producing cells in the skin (melanocytes). Body hair may also be decreased. In secondary disease, there is no increase in skin pigmentation.

CHART 63-7

BEST PRACTICE *for* Nursing Care of the Client with Acute Adrenal Insufficiency

- Before initiating treatment, obtain a complete blood count and electrolyte, blood urea nitrogen, and plasma cortisol levels, as ordered by the physician.
- Give an initial dose of hydrocortisone sodium succinate (Solu-Cortef) 100 to 300 mg intravenously; then infuse 100 mg over an 8-hour period, as ordered by the physician.
- Give concomitant doses of hydrocortisone 50 mg intramuscularly every 12 hours, as ordered by the physician.
- After resolution of the crisis, adjust the dosage of medications, as ordered by the physician:
  - Give oral glucocorticoids (e.g., hydrocortisone).
  - Decrease the dosage of oral glucocorticoids during several days as maintenance levels are reached.
  - Give supplemental mineralocorticoids, such as fludrocortisone (Florinef), as the glucocorticoid dosage is tapered.

TABLE 63-4 • CAUSES OF PRIMARY AND SECONDARY ADRENAL INSUFFICIENCY

PRIMARY CAUSES	SECONDARY CAUSES
• Idiopathic (autoimmune) disease* • Tuberculosis • Metastatic cancer • Fungal lesions • AIDS • Hemorrhage • Gram-negative sepsis (Waterhouse-Friderichsen syndrome) • Adrenalectomy • Abdominal radiation therapy • Drugs (mitotane) and toxins	• Pituitary tumors • Postpartum pituitary necrosis (Sheehan's syndrome) • Hypophysectomy • High-dose pituitary radiation • High-dose whole-brain radiation

*Most common cause.

CHART 63-8

KEY FEATURES *of* Adrenal Insufficiency

Neuromuscular Manifestations
- Muscle weakness
- Fatigue
- Joint/muscle pain

Gastrointestinal Manifestations
- Anorexia
- Nausea, vomiting
- Abdominal pain
- Bowel changes (constipation/diarrhea)
- Weight loss
- Salt craving

Integumentary Manifestations
- Vitiligo
- Hyperpigmentation

Cardiovascular Manifestations
- Anemia
- Hypotension
- Hyponatremia
- Hyperkalemia
- Hypercalcemia

The nurse assesses the client for symptoms of hypoglycemia (e.g., sweating, headaches, tachycardia, and tremors) and volume depletion (postural hypotension and dehydration). **Hyperkalemia** (elevated blood levels of potassium) can cause dysrhythmias with an irregular heart rate and result in cardiac arrest.

PSYCHOSOCIAL ASSESSMENT

Depending on the degree of metabolic imbalance, clients may appear lethargic, apathetic, depressed, confused, and even psychotic. The nurse observes the client and checks his or her orientation to person, place, and time. Families may report that the client has a decreased energy level, experiences wide mood swings, and is forgetful.

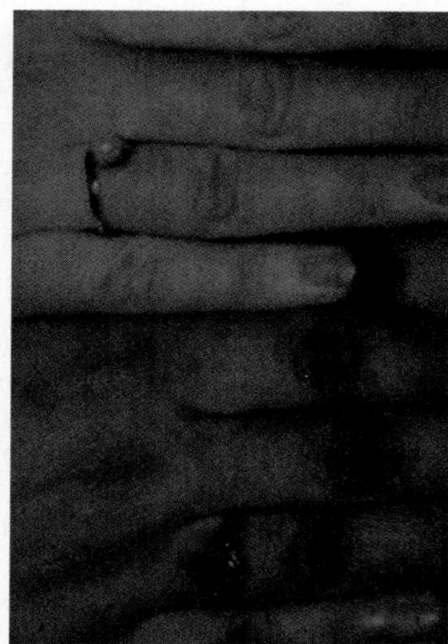

Figure 63-5 ● Hand of a client with hyperpigmentation related to adrenocortical insufficiency *(bottom),* shown alongside the hand of an unaffected person. Note the deep hyperpigmentation of the knuckles. (From Wilson, J.D, et al. (1998). *Williams textbook of endocrinology* (9th ed.). Philadelphia: W.B. Saunders. Courtesy Dr. H. Patrick Higgins.)

DIAGNOSTIC ASSESSMENT

Laboratory findings usually include low serum cortisol, decreased fasting blood glucose, low sodium, elevated potassium, and increased serum blood urea nitrogen (BUN) levels (Chart 63-9). In primary disease, the eosinophil count and ACTH level are elevated. Plasma cortisol levels fail to rise during stimulation tests.

Urinary 17-hydroxycorticosteroids are the glucocorticoid metabolites, and 17-ketosteroid levels reflect the adrenal androgen metabolites. Both levels are in the low or low-normal range in adrenal hypofunction. Table 63-5 lists drugs that can interfere with test results.

Skull x-ray films, computed tomography (CT), magnetic resonance imaging (MRI), and arteriography may aid in the search for a cause of pituitary problems leading to adrenal insufficiency.

Noninvasive procedures of the adrenal gland, such as CT scans without dye, may occasionally show atrophy of the gland. CT scans may help determine adrenal hypofunction.

An ACTH (cosyntropin [Cortrosyn], synthetic ACTH) stimulation test is the most definitive test for adrenal insufficiency. A rapid ACTH stimulation test may be administered on an outpatient basis. Cosyntropin 0.25 to 1 mg is given intramuscularly or intravenously, and plasma cortisol levels are obtained at 30-minute and 1-hour intervals after the baseline value is established. In primary insufficiency, the cortisol response is absent or markedly decreased; in secondary insufficiency, it is decreased.

A longer ACTH stimulation test uses a continuous infusion of 50 units of ACTH in saline for 24 hours or an 8-hour

CHART 63-9

LABORATORY PROFILE
Adrenal Gland Assessment

Test	Normal Range for Adults	Significance of Abnormal Findings: Hypofunction of the Adrenal Gland	Significance of Abnormal Findings: Hyperfunction of the Adrenal Gland
Sodium	136-145 mEq/L	Decreased	Increased
Potassium	3.4-4.5 mEq/L	Increased	Decreased
Glucose	74-106 mg/dL *Older adults:* slightly increased	Normal to decreased	Normal to increased
Calcium	8.6-10.0 mg/dL (total) 4.6-5.08 mg/dL (ionized) *Older adults:* slightly decreased	Increased	Decreased
Leukocytes	20%-40%	Normal	Increased
Eosinophils	1%-4%	Increased	Decreased
Bicarbonate	22-29 mEq/L	Increased	Decreased
BUN	6-20 mg/dL *Older adults:* may be slightly higher	Increased	Normal
Cortisol	6 AM-8 AM 5-23 μg/dL or 138-635 SI units (nmol/L) 4 PM-6 PM 3-16 μg/dL or 83-441 SI units (nmol/L)	Decreased	Increased

BUN, Blood urea nitrogen; *SI,* System Internationale.

infusion daily for 4 to 5 days, with simultaneously collected 24-hour urine samples. Levels of urinary 17-hydroxycorticosteroids and urinary free cortisol are also measured. In clients with primary adrenal insufficiency, the response is low or absent; in those with secondary insufficiency, the value for 17-hydroxycorticosteroids fails to rise above 20 mg per total volume.

Interventions

Nursing interventions are aimed at promoting fluid balance and monitoring for fluid deficit (Chart 63-10). The nurse or assistive nursing personnel weighs the client daily and records intake and output. Vital signs are assessed every 1 to 4 hours, depending on the client's condition and the occurrence of dysrhythmias or postural hypotension. Laboratory values are monitored to identify hemoconcentrations (e.g., increased hematocrit or BUN). Chapter 12 discusses fluid volume deficit in detail.

Glucocorticoid and mineralocorticoid deficiencies are completely corrected by replacement therapy. Hydrocortisone corrects glucocorticoid deficiency (Chart 63-11). Glucocorticoid replacement regimens vary. Generally, divided doses are given, with two thirds given in the morning and one third in the late afternoon to mimic the normal adrenal hormone secretion rhythm. Although most clients do well on this regimen, some may not tolerate the dosage or may need more.

An additional mineralocorticoid hormone, such as fludrocortisone (Florinef), may be needed to maintain correct electrolyte balance (especially sodium and potassium). Adjustments in dosage may be necessary in hot weather, when additional sodium is lost because of excessive perspiration. *Salt restriction or diuretic therapy should not be started without considering whether it might precipitate an adrenal crisis.*

TABLE 63-5 • SOME DRUGS THAT INTERFERE WITH TESTS FOR URINARY 17-HYDROXYCORTICOSTEROIDS AND URINARY 17-KETOSTEROIDS

- Acetaminophen
- Acetazolamide
- Acetylsalicylic acid
- Amphetamines
- Ascorbic acid
- Barbiturates
- Calcium gluconate
- Carbon disulfide
- Chloral hydrate
- Chlordiazepoxide
- Chlormerodrin
- Chlorothiazide
- Chlorpromazine
- Chlorthalidone
- Colchicine
- Corticotropin
- Cortisone
- Dexamethasone
- Diazepam
- Digitoxin
- Digoxin
- Diphenhydramine
- Diphenylhydantoin
- Erythromycin
- Estrogens
- Fructose
- Glutethimide
- Hydralazine
- Iodides
- Medroxyprogesterone
- Meperidine
- Meprobamate
- Metyrapone
- Mitotane
- Morphine
- Nalidixic acid
- Oral contraceptives
- Paraldehyde
- Penicillin
- Pentazocine
- Perphenazine
- Phenobarbital
- Phenothiazines
- Phenylbutazone
- Promazine
- Propoxyphene
- Quinidine
- Quinine
- Reserpine
- Secobarbital
- Spironolactone
- Testosterone
- Vitamin K

ADRENAL GLAND HYPERFUNCTION

Unlike adrenal gland hypofunction, which results in a generalized deficiency of all adrenal hormones, the adrenal gland may oversecrete just one or all hormones. Hypersecretion by the adrenal cortex may result in excessive amounts of glucocorticoids, leading to **hypercortisolism** (e.g., **Cushing's syndrome**), **hyperaldosteronism** (excessive mineralocorticoid production), or excessive androgen production.

Hypersecretion of the adrenal medulla caused by a tumor **(pheochromocytoma)** results in excessive secretion of catecholamines, of which 80% is epinephrine and the remainder is norepinephrine.

CHART 63-10

NIC INTERVENTION ACTIVITIES *for* Clients with Adrenal Insufficiency

Electrolyte Management: Hyperkalemia: *Promotion of potassium balance and prevention of complications resulting from serum potassium levels higher than desired*
- Administer electrolyte-binding and electrolyte-excreting resins (e.g., Kayexalate) as prescribed, if appropriate.
- Monitor lab values for changes in oxygenation or acid-base balance, as appropriate.
- Administer prescribed medications to shift potassium into the cell (e.g., 50% dextrose and insulin, sodium bicarbonate, calcium chloride, and calcium gluconate), as appropriate.
- Avoid potassium-sparing medications (e.g., spironolactone [Aldactone] and triamterene [Dyrenium]), as appropriate.
- Maintain potassium restrictions.
- Administer prescribed diuretics, as appropriate.
- Monitor fluid status, including intake and output, as appropriate.
- Monitor potassium levels after diuresis.
- Monitor cardiac manifestations of hyperkalemia (e.g., decreased cardiac output, heart blocks, peaked T waves, fibrillation, or asystole).
- Respond to cardiac arrest.

Hypoglycemia Management: *Preventing and treating low blood glucose levels*
- Determine recognition of hypoglycemia signs and symptoms.
- Monitor blood glucose levels, as indicated.
- Monitor for signs and symptoms of hypoglycemia (e.g., shakiness, tremor, sweating, nervousness, anxiety, irritability, impatience, tachycardia, palpitations, chills, clamminess, lightheadedness, pallor, hunger, nausea, headache, tiredness, drowsiness, weakness, warmth, dizziness, faintness, blurred vision, nightmares, crying out in sleep, paresthesias, difficulty concentrating, difficulty speaking, incoordination, behavior change, confusion, coma, seizure).
- Provide simple carbohydrate, as indicated.
- Administer glucagon, as indicated.
- Maintain IV access, as appropriate.
- Instruct client and significant others on signs and symptoms, risk factors, and treatment of hypoglycemia.
- Instruct client to have simple carbohydrate available at all times.
- Instruct client to obtain and carry/wear appropriate emergency identification.

NIC intervention activities selected from McCloskey, J.C., & Bulechek, G.M. (2000). *Nursing interventions classification (NIC)* (3rd ed.). St. Louis: Mosby.

Hypercortisolism (Cushing's Syndrome)

OVERVIEW

Pathophysiology

Cushing's syndrome exaggerates the normal actions of glucocorticoids, causing widespread problems. Excessive stimulation of adrenocorticotropic hormone (ACTH) of either pituitary or ectopic origin causes adrenocortical hyperplasia, which results in loss of normal hormone secretion rhythms. The client's endocrine tissues have decreased responsiveness to releasing hormones, especially prolactin (PRL), thyrotropin, and gonadotropin. Many clients also experience abnormal sleep patterns. Most of these changes are due to excessive amounts of glucocorticoids.

The client with Cushing's syndrome has alterations of nitrogen, carbohydrate, and mineral metabolism. An increase in total body fat results from slow turnover of plasma fatty acids, and a redistribution of fat produces the typical body pattern of truncal obesity, "buffalo hump," and "moon face" (Figure 63-6). Increases in the breakdown of tissue protein and an increase in urine nitrogen excretion also occur, resulting in decreased muscle mass, **atrophic** (thin) skin, and bone density loss.

High levels of corticosteroids kill lymphocytes and shrink organs containing lymphocytes, such as the liver, the spleen, and the lymph nodes. Thus protection of the inflammatory and immune responses is reduced.

In most cases, increased androgen production causes acne, **hirsutism** (increased hair growth), and occasionally, clitoral hypertrophy. Increased androgen production can also interrupt the normal hormone feedback mechanism for the ovary, decreasing the ovary's production of estrogens and progesterone. **Oligomenorrhea** (scant or infrequent menses) occurs as a result.

Etiology

Cushing's syndrome is a group of clinical problems caused by an excess of cortisol, secreted by the adrenal cortex **(endogenous)** or administered for another clinical disorder (**exogenous** or **iatrogenic**). Table 63-6 lists causes of cortisol excess. Women are affected eight times more often than men.

COLLABORATIVE MANAGEMENT

Assessment

A thorough history and physical assessment aid in detecting clinical features of hypercortisolism, which result from glucocorticoid excess.

HISTORY

The client who has hypercortisolism has varied changes because of the widespread effect of excessive cortisol levels in the body. The nurse asks about changes in activity or sleep patterns, fatigue, and muscle weakness. Osteoporosis is common in hypercortisolism, and the client is asked about bone pain or a history of fractures. The nurse also questions the client about a history of frequent infections and easy bruising, which suggest hypercortisolism. Women may report a cessation of menses. Gastrointestinal (GI) complaints may indicate ulcer formation from increased hydrochloric acid secretion.

The nurse also refers to the client's medical history. Steroid or alcohol abuse can produce the clinical and biochemical features of Cushing's syndrome.

PHYSICAL ASSESSMENT/CLINICAL MANIFESTATIONS

The client with hypercortisolism has characteristic physical changes (see Figure 63-6). The general appearance of the client is observed. Changes in fat distribution may result in fat pads on the neck, back, and shoulders ("buffalo hump"); an enlarged trunk with thin arms and legs; and a round face ("moon face"). Other characteristics include generalized muscle wasting and weakness.

The nurse also inspects the client for skin changes resulting from increased blood vessel fragility, such as bruises, thin or translucent skin, and wounds that have not healed properly. Reddish purple **striae** ("stretch marks") are often present on

CHART 63-11

MAINTENANCE DRUG THERAPY *for* Hypofunction of the Adrenal Gland

Drug	Usual Dosage	Nursing Interventions	Rationale
Cortisone	25-50 mg PO either once daily in AM or daily in divided doses	Instruct the client to take the drug with meals or a snack.	Gastrointestinal irritation can occur
Hydrocortisone (Cortef, Hycort♣)	20-50 mg PO either once daily in AM or daily in divided doses	Instruct the client to report the following signs or symptoms of excessive drug therapy: • Rapid weight gain • Round face • Fluid retention	Cushing's syndrome, which indicates a need for dosage adjustment, can occur.
Prednisone (Winpred♣)	5-10 mg PO either once daily in AM or daily in divided doses	Instruct the client to report illness, such as: • Severe diarrhea • Vomiting • Fever	Other conditions may indicate a need for dosage change. The usual daily dosage may not be adequate during periods of illness or severe stress
Fludrocortisone (Florinef)	0.05-0.2 mg PO daily	Monitor the client's blood pressure.	Hypertension is a potential side effect.
		Instruct the client to report weight gain or edema.	Sodium-related fluid retention is possible.

the abdomen, upper thighs, and upper arms because of the degradative effect of cortisol on collagen.

Excessive cortisol secretion may result in a fine coating of hair over the face and body and in acne. In the female client, the nurse looks for the presence of hirsutism, clitoral hypertrophy, and male pattern balding related to androgen excess.

Elevations in blood glucose levels are also a frequent finding. Hypertension from water and sodium retention is common.

PSYCHOSOCIAL ASSESSMENT

Hypercortisolism can result in emotional lability, and the nurse asks about mood swings, irritability, confusion, or depression. The client may become neurotic or psychotic as a result of changes in blood cortisol levels.

DIAGNOSTIC ASSESSMENT

Plasma cortisol levels are elevated in clients with hypercortisolism. Blood for cortisol assays is obtained at the same time of day because levels vary throughout the day. Further diagnostic testing is performed to confirm the diagnosis of hypercortisolism, because an increase in cortisol levels is also seen in acute illness and trauma. Plasma ACTH levels vary, depending on the cause of hypercortisolism. In ectopic (ACTH-producing) syndromes, ACTH levels are elevated. In Cushing's syndrome (primary disease of the adrenal gland), ACTH levels are low to immeasurable. Additional laboratory findings may include the following:

- Increased blood glucose level
- Elevated white blood cell count
- Elevated lymphocyte count
- Increased sodium level
- Decreased serum calcium level
- Decreased serum potassium level

Urine is tested to measure levels of free cortisol and the adrenal metabolites of cortisol and androgens (17-hydroxycorticosteroids and 17-ketosteroids). The client is instructed to save *all* urine for 24 hours. In Cushing's disease, basal levels of urinary free cortisol, 17-ketosteroids, and 17-hydroxycorticosteroids are all elevated, as are urine levels of calcium, potassium, and glucose.

Radiographic studies, computed tomography (CT) scans, magnetic resonance imaging (MRI), and arteriography may identify lesions of the adrenal or pituitary glands, lung, GI tract, or pancreas in a client with clinical manifestations of cortisol hypersecretion.

The *overnight dexamethasone suppression test* is an initial screening test for Cushing's syndrome. The client is instructed not to take medications, especially phenytoin (Dilantin) or phenobarbital, for at least 2 days before the test. Normally, plasma cortisol levels are lower than 5 μg/dL. Higher levels indicate that further, definitive testing is necessary.

For the *3-day, low-dose* dexamethasone suppression test, the client must take no medications for at least 2 days before the test (if possible) and have no stressful procedures (e.g., barium enema, myelogram, or an intense physical therapy session) performed during the test. Table 63-5 lists drugs that interfere with testing. A baseline 24-hour urine sample is collected on day 1. Dexamethasone 0.5 mg is administered every 6 hours on days 2 and 3, during which time 24-hour urine collections are taken. The 24-hour urine collections are tested for 17-ketosteroids, 17-hydroxycorticosteroids, creatinine, and urinary free cortisol. Normally, urinary 17-hydroxycorticosteroid excretion and free cortisol levels are suppressed by dexamethasone, and Cushing's syndrome is ruled out. If these levels are not suppressed, a higher-dose dexamethasone test is performed.

The *high-dose* (8-mg) dexamethasone suppression test distinguishes between bilateral adrenocortical hyperplasia (e.g., Cushing's syndrome) and an adrenocortical neoplasm as the cause of hypercortisolism. This test can be performed as an overnight test or a 2-day test and is similar to the tests previously discussed but uses higher doses of dexamethasone. In the overnight high-dose test, the client with Cushing's disease will have a reduced plasma cortisol level that is less than 50% of baseline. This test is more reliable than the 2-day high-dose test.

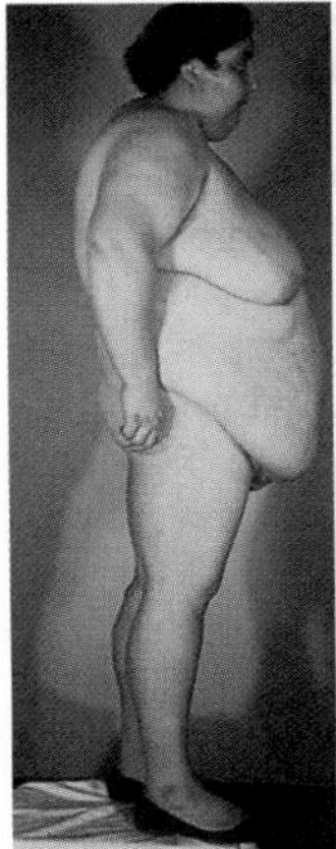
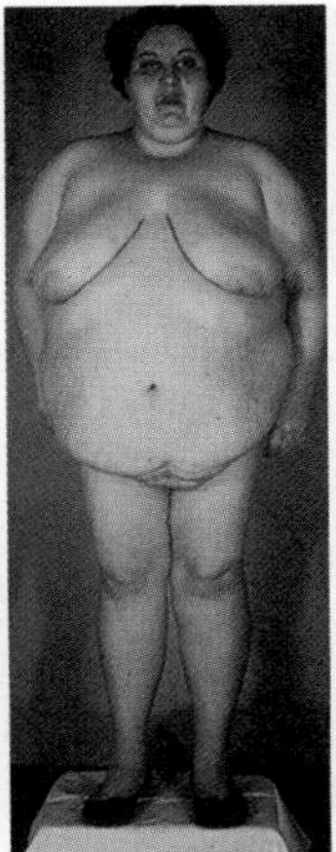
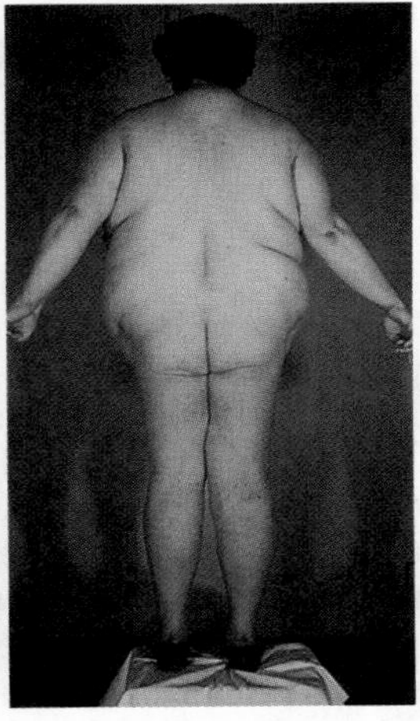

Figure 63-6 • The typical appearance of a client with Cushing's disease or syndrome. Note truncal obesity, "moon face," "buffalo hump," thinner arms and legs, and abdominal striae. (From Wenig B.M., Heffess, C.S., & Adair, C.F. (1997). *Atlas of endocrine pathology.* Philadelphia: W.B. Saunders.

TABLE 63-6 • CONDITIONS CAUSING INCREASED CORTISOL SECRETION

ENDOGENOUS SECRETION
- Bilateral adrenal hyperplasia*
- Pituitary adenoma increasing the production of ACTH (pituitary Cushing's syndrome)
- Malignancies: carcinomas of the lung, gastrointestinal tract, pancreas
- Adrenal adenomas or carcinomas

EXOGENOUS ADMINISTRATION
- Therapeutic use of ACTH or glucocorticoids—most commonly for treatment of:
  - Asthma
  - Autoimmune disorders
  - Organ transplantation
  - Cancer chemotherapy
  - Allergic responses
  - Chronic fibrosis

ACTH, Adrenocorticotropic hormone.
*Most common cause.

Interventions

Goals of treatment for hypercortisolism include reduction of plasma cortisol levels, removal of tumors, prevention of complications, and restoration of normal or acceptable body appearance. Specific nursing interventions and drug therapy address the problems of clients who have hypercortisolism. Preoperative and postoperative nursing care is an integral part of the management of the client with endogenous hypercortisolism because surgical intervention is usually necessary for the relief of symptoms.

NONSURGICAL MANAGEMENT. The nurse weighs the client daily and monitors intake and output to assess hydration status. Restriction of fluid intake is sometimes necessary to maintain fluid balance.

DRUG THERAPY. Most clients with endogenous hypercortisolism undergo surgery. Drugs that interfere with adrenocorticotropic hormone (ACTH) production or adrenal hormone synthesis, however, may be used for palliation. Mitotane (Lysodren) is an adrenal cytotoxic agent used for inoperable adrenal tumors. Aminoglutethimide (Elipten, Cytadren) is an adrenal enzyme inhibitor that decreases cortisol production. Trilostane (Modrastane), also an enzyme inhibitor, has not always been effective. Cyproheptadine (Periactin) is less commonly used to treat clients with adrenal hyperfunction resulting from pituitary-related Cushing's disease because it interferes with ACTH production. During all drug therapy, the nurse assesses the client for therapy effectiveness and side effects or symptoms of toxicity.

RADIATION THERAPY. Radiation, applied internally or externally, may be used to treat hypercortisolism caused by pituitary adenomas. However, radiation is not always effective and also may destroy normal tissue. The nurse observes for any changes in the client's neurologic status, such as headache, elevated blood pressure or pulse, disorientation, or changes in pupil size or reaction. The client may experience skin dryness, redness, flushing, or alopecia at the radiation site. The nurse reviews these possible side effects with the client. Chapter 45 specifically discusses radiation therapy to the head.

SURGICAL MANAGEMENT. The surgical treatment of adrenocortical hypersecretion depends on the cause of the disease. When adrenal hyperfunction is due to increased pituitary secretion of ACTH, transsphenoidal removal of an adenoma may be attempted. In many instances, small adenomas cannot be localized and **hypophysectomy** (surgical removal of the pituitary gland) is needed. Hypophysectomy is performed via the transsphenoidal or transfrontal craniotomy route. (See earlier discussion of hypophysectomy on pp. 1406 and 1407; see also Chapter 45 for nursing care of clients undergoing a craniotomy.)

If hypercortisolism is caused by adrenal adenomas or carcinomas, a partial or complete **adrenalectomy** (removal of the adrenal gland) may be needed.

PREOPERATIVE CARE. Electrolyte imbalances are corrected before surgery, and the nurse monitors potassium, sodium, and chloride values. Dysrhythmias from potassium imbalance may occur, and cardiac monitoring may be indicated. Hyperglycemia, if present, is controlled before surgery, and the nurse monitors blood glucose levels.

The client with hypercortisolism is susceptible to complications such as infections and fractures. The nurse and assistive nursing personnel attempt to prevent infection with handwashing and aseptic technique. The risk for falls is decreased by raising the siderails of the bed and encouraging the client to ask for assistance when getting out of bed. The physician orders a high-calorie, high-protein diet before surgery.

Glucocorticoid preparations are administered preoperatively as ordered. The client continues to receive glucocorticoids throughout the operative procedure to prevent adrenal crisis. The removal of the tumor results in a sudden drop in cortisol levels. The nurse discusses postoperative care and long-term medication therapy during preoperative teaching.

OPERATIVE PROCEDURES. A **unilateral adrenalectomy** is performed when one gland is involved. A **bilateral adrenalectomy** is necessary when ectopic ACTH-producing tumors cannot be treated by other means or when both adrenal glands are diseased.

Surgery can be abdominal or through the lateral flank. Abdominal surgery causes a higher degree of illness and risk. In the flank approach (the preferred approach), the abdominal cavity is not entered, and the morbidity and mortality rates are reduced. A new approach, laparoscopic adrenalectomy, may reduce the incidence of some postoperative complications.

POSTOPERATIVE CARE. After an adrenalectomy, the client is usually sent to a critical care unit. In the immediate postoperative period, the nurse assesses the client every 15 minutes to identify symptoms of cardiovascular collapse or shock (e.g., hypotension, a rapid, weak pulse, and a decreasing urine output) due to possible insufficient glucocorticoid replacement. The nurse monitors ongoing vital signs and other hemodynamic variables (central venous pressure, pulmonary wedge pressure), intake and output, daily weights, and serum electrolyte levels.

After a bilateral adrenalectomy, clients require lifelong glucocorticoid and mineralocorticoid replacement. The nurse administers glucocorticoid preparations as ordered. In unilateral adrenalectomy, glucocorticoid replacement continues until the remaining gland increases hormone production. This therapy may be required for up to 2 years after surgery.

PREVENTING COMPLICATIONS. The client who has hypercortisolism is prone to injury from skin breakdown, pathologic bone fractures, and gastrointestinal (GI) bleeding. Prevention of such injuries is a major nursing care focus.

Skin Breakdown. The nurse assesses the client's skin to detect reddened areas, excoriation, breakdown, and edema. If mobility is decreased, the client is turned frequently and bony prominences are padded to prevent skin breakdown.

The nurse instructs the client to avoid activities that can result in skin trauma. To minimize tissue injury, the client may use a soft toothbrush and electric razor. Proper hygiene is important, and clients are instructed to keep the skin clean and to dry it thoroughly after washing. Excessive dryness can be prevented by using a moisturizing lotion.

Adhesive tape frequently causes breakdown of the skin. This tape is used sparingly, and extreme caution is used when removing it. After venipuncture or arterial puncture, the client may experience an increase in bleeding because of blood vessel fragility. Pressure over the site is exerted for longer than normal to prevent excessive bleeding and **ecchymosis** (bruising).

Pathologic Fractures. Hypercortisolism results in demineralization of bone, which, if it persists, may lead to osteoporosis. The nurse instructs the client about safety issues and dietary needs. The client with osteoporosis is susceptible to fractures as a result of accidental falls or bumps. When helping the client to move in bed, the nurse uses a lift sheet instead of grasping him or her. The nurse instructs the client to call for assistance when ambulating. The nurse also reviews the use of ambulatory aids (walkers or canes), if needed. Rooms should be kept free of extraneous objects that might cause a fall. When assisting with daily activities, the nurse prevents the client from bumping into hard objects.

A dietitian is consulted to counsel the client about diet therapy. A high-calorie diet is ordered that includes items from all of the major food groups and increased amounts of calcium and vitamin D. Generous amounts of milk, cheese, yogurt, and green leafy and root vegetables add considerable amounts of calcium to the diet. The client is advised to avoid substances containing caffeine and alcohol.

Gastrointestinal Bleeding. Interventions are aimed at minimizing gastric irritation, usually through drug therapy. Drug therapy involves two different types of agents: those that protect the GI mucosa and those that decrease the secretion of hydrochloric acid.

Agents Protecting the Gastrointestinal Mucosa. Antacids are prescribed to buffer stomach acids and to protect the GI mucosa. The nurse teaches the client that these drugs should be taken on a regular schedule, rather than on a prn (as-needed) basis.

Agents Inhibiting the Secretion of Hydrochloric Acid. The most effective agents are those that block the H_2-receptor site in the gastric mucosa. When histamine binds to this receptor site, a series of membrane actions occur that result in the release of hydrochloric acid. Drugs that block the H_2-receptor site include cimetidine (Tagamet, Peptol♣, Novo-Cimetine♣), ranitidine (Zantac, Apo-Ranitidine♣), famotidine (Pepcid), and nizatidine (Axid). Omeprazole (Losec♣, Prilosec) inhibits the gastric proton pump and prevents the formation of hydrochloric acid.

Prevention of Irritation. The client is encouraged to reduce or eliminate habits that contribute to gastric irritation, such as consuming alcohol or caffeine, smoking, and fasting. The nurse discusses other prescribed and over-the-counter medications that the client may be taking. Nonsteroidal anti-inflammatory drugs (NSAIDs) and drugs that contain aspirin or other salicylates can cause gastritis and intensify any bleeding episode.

HEALTH TEACHING. Lifelong hormone replacement is required after bilateral adrenalectomy. The nurse educates the client and family members about compliance with the medication regimen and its side effects. Wearing a medical alert bracelet is essential. Education of clients after bilateral adrenalectomy and hypophysectomy is the same as that for those who have undergone cortisol replacement (Chart 63-12).

CHART 63-12

CLIENT EDUCATION GUIDE
Cortisol Replacement Therapy

- Take your medication in divided doses, the first dose in the morning and the second dose between 4 and 6 PM.
- Take your medication with meals or snacks.
- Weigh yourself daily.
- Increase your dosage as directed for increased physical stress or severe emotional stress, including surgery, dental work, influenza, fever, pregnancy, and family problems.
- Never skip a dose of medication. If you have persistent vomiting or severe diarrhea and cannot take your medication by mouth for 24 to 36 hours, call your physician. If you cannot reach your physician, go to the nearest emergency department. You may need an injection to take the place of your usual oral medication.
- Always wear your medical alert bracelet or necklace.
- Make regular visits for health care follow-up.
- Learn how to give yourself an intramuscular injection of hydrocortisone.

CRITICAL THINKING CHALLENGE

The client is a 76-year-old woman who has been taking 25 mg of prednisone daily for 2 years to treat a chronic inflammatory lung disease. She is now in an extended care facility recovering from a hip-pinning procedure following a fracture. The staff does not like working with her, because she claims she is hungry all the time and she has frequent spells of shouting at people that are intermixed with periods of weeping. She has many bruises, and her family is asking whether she is being physically abused.

- How should you approach the assistive nursing personnel about this "problem" client?
- What will you tell the family about the bruising?
- What interventions can you institute to reduce this client's risk for injury?
- How can her appetite be managed?

For suggested answer guidelines, go to SIMON http://www.wbsaunders.com/SIMON/Iggy/.

Hyperaldosteronism

OVERVIEW

In clients with hyperaldosteronism, increased secretion of aldosterone results in mineralocorticoid excess. **Primary hyperaldosteronism (Conn's syndrome)** is due to excessive secretion of aldosterone from one or both adrenal glands, which is most commonly caused by an adenoma. In a person with **secondary hyperaldosteronism,** the continuous excessive secretion of aldosterone is caused by high levels of angiotensin II that are due to high plasma renin activity. Causes of this renin activation include renal hypoxemia and the use of thiazide diuretics.

Increased aldosterone levels affect the renal tubules and cause sodium retention with potassium and hydrogen ion excretion. Hypernatremia, hypokalemia, and metabolic alkalosis result. Sodium retention increases blood and interstitial fluid volume, which elevates blood pressure and suppresses renin production. The elevated blood pressure may cause strokes and renal damage. Peripheral edema rarely occurs because of the "renal escape mechanism," in which the proximal tubule decreases sodium reabsorption. However, no compensatory mechanism exists to stop or reverse the loss of potassium. (See Chapter 13 for further discussion of electrolyte imbalances.)

Hyperaldosteronism occurs three times more frequently in women than in men and is most prevalent in clients between 30 and 60 years of age.

COLLABORATIVE MANAGEMENT

Assessment

Symptoms related to hypokalemia and elevated blood pressure are the most common problems of the client with hyperaldosteronism. The history may reveal nonspecific findings, such as headache, fatigue, muscle weakness, **nocturia** (excessive urination at night), and loss of stamina. **Polydipsia** (excessive fluid intake) and **polyuria** (excessive urine output) occur less frequently. **Paresthesias** (sensations of numbness and tingling) may occur if potassium depletion is severe. The client may have visual changes related to hypertension.

The diagnosis of primary hyperaldosteronism is made on the basis of laboratory studies and x-ray findings. Serum potassium levels are decreased, and sodium levels are elevated. Plasma renin levels are low; aldosterone levels are elevated. Increased hydrogen ion secretion results in metabolic alkalemia (elevated blood pH). Urine studies show low specific gravity and elevated aldosterone levels. Computed tomography (CT) scans reveal the presence and location of adrenal adenomas.

Interventions

Surgery is the treatment of choice for hyperaldosteronism if the problem is identified in its early stages. Adrenalectomy may be unilateral or bilateral. Surgery is not performed, however, until the client's potassium levels are normal. The physician orders spironolactone (Aldactone, Novospiroton✦, Sincomen✦), a potassium-sparing diuretic and aldosterone antagonist, to promote fluid balance. Potassium supplements may be ordered to increase potassium levels before surgery. The client may also benefit from a low-sodium preoperative diet, but no dietary restrictions are needed after surgery because aldosterone levels should return to normal.

The client who has undergone a unilateral adrenalectomy may require temporary glucocorticoid replacement, and the client who has undergone a bilateral adrenalectomy needs lifelong replacement. Glucocorticoids are administered before surgery to prevent adrenal hypofunction. The client receiving long-term replacement therapy should wear a medical alert bracelet. (See the discussion of adrenalectomy under Hypercortisolism [Cushing's syndrome], pp. 1418 and 1419, for further postoperative care and client education.)

When surgery is inadvisable, spironolactone therapy is continued to control the symptoms of hypokalemia and hypertension. Because spironolactone is a potassium-sparing diuretic, hyperkalemia can occur in clients who have impaired renal function or excessive potassium intake. The nurse advises the client to avoid potassium supplements and foods rich in potassium (see Chart 13-6). Because hyponatremia can occur with spironolactone therapy, the client may require increased dietary sodium. He or she is instructed to report symptoms of hyponatremia, such as dryness of the mouth, thirst, lethargy, or drowsiness. The nurse alerts clients to report any additional side effects of spironolactone therapy, including gynecomastia, diarrhea, drowsiness, headache, rash, **urticaria** (hives), confusion, inability to maintain an erection, hirsutism, and amenorrhea.

Pheochromocytoma

OVERVIEW

Pheochromocytoma is a catecholamine-producing tumor that arises in chromaffin cells. Pheochromocytomas usually occur as single, unilateral tumors on the right side; approximately 10% are bilateral tumors, and another 10% are found in the abdomen. Pheochromocytomas are most often benign, but about 10% are malignant. The tumors produce and store catecholamines.

Pheochromocytomas release the catecholamines epinephrine and norepinephrine (NE). Excessive epinephrine and NE stimulate alpha receptors and beta receptors and can have wide-ranging adverse effects mimicking stimulation of the sympathetic division of the autonomic nervous system.

Causes are unknown, but some are associated with inherited disorders such as neurofibromatosis and multiple endocrine neoplasia type II syndrome. Pheochromocytomas are rare and occur slightly more frequently in women. The tumors can occur at any age but appear most commonly in clients between 40 and 60 years of age.

COLLABORATIVE MANAGEMENT

Assessment

The history may include intermittent hypertensive episodes or attacks that vary in length from a few minutes to several hours. During these episodes, the client experiences severe headaches, palpitations, profuse diaphoresis, flushing, apprehension, or a feeling of impending doom. Pain in the chest or abdomen, with nausea and vomiting, can also occur. Certain stimuli, such as increased abdominal pressure, urination, and vigorous abdominal palpation, can provoke a hypertensive crisis. The client may also report heat intolerance, weight loss, and tremors.

Diagnostic tests include 24-hour urine collections for vanillylmandelic acid (VMA) (a product of catecholamine metabolism), metanephrine, and free catecholamines, all of which are elevated in the presence of a pheochromocytoma. Best practices for VMA testing are listed in Chart 63-13. Basal plasma catecholamine levels are elevated after the client has been at rest for at least 30 minutes. The clonidine suppression test is used in the diagnosis of a pheochromocytoma. When oral clonidine hydrochloride (Catapres, Dixarit✦) is given to a person who does not have a pheochromocytoma, the clonidine suppresses catecholamine release and reduces the serum catecholamine levels. The response is not seen in the client who has a pheochromocytoma.

When the client suspected of having a pheochromocytoma has severe hypertension, testing for the disorder may include alpha-adrenergic blockade with phentolamine. Phentolamine (Regitine, Rogitine✦) is administered intravenously at a dose of 5 mg, and blood pressure is measured every 30 seconds for 3 minutes, then every minute for 7 minutes. When a rapid drop of at least 35 mm Hg systolic pressure and 25 mm Hg diastolic pressure results, the test is considered positive.

CHART 63-13

BEST PRACTICE *for* Vanillylmandelic Acid Testing

- Describe the test to the client and explain that his or her participation is needed for accurate test results.
- Instruct the client on the special vanillylmandelic acid (VMA)–restricted diet that starts 2 or 3 days before the 24-hour urine collection.
- Restricted foods include those containing caffeine (coffee, tea, cola, and chocolate or cocoa), certain fruits (citrus fruits and bananas), vanilla-containing foods, and licorice. Check your laboratory for a more inclusive food list.
- Confer with the physician about which medications should not be given during the 3- or 4-day test. Medications usually withheld include aspirin and antihypertensive agents.
- Be aware that strenuous physical activity, stress, and starvation can increase VMA levels; monitor, intervene, and teach the client as appropriate.
- Instruct the client about how to collect an accurate 24-hour urine sample: the collection is started with an empty bladder, and then all urine formed over the next 24 hours is collected in one container. At the end of the 24-hour period, the client voids and adds that urine to the collection.
- Obtain a urine collection container with preservative from the laboratory. Check with the laboratory about keeping the collection on ice.
- When the collection is complete, send the urine to the laboratory promptly.
- Help the client understand the test results; normal VMA excretion in 24 hours is 2 to 7 mg, or 10 to 35 μmol.

Catecholamine stimulation tests can be useful in the diagnosis of a pheochromocytoma; however, the danger of uncontrolled hypertension and effects on the heart limit the usefulness of this test. These tests involve the administration of histamine, glucagon, or tyramine to stimulate catecholamine release. Blood and urine catecholamine levels are measured. Catecholamine stimulation of **glycogenolysis** (breakdown of glycogen) and suppression of insulin may cause **hyperglycemia** (elevated blood glucose levels) and **glycosuria** (presence of glucose in the urine).

After diagnosis, computed tomography (CT) scans of the adrenal glands locate intra-adrenal tumors. Chest x-ray films and tomograms can locate tumors in the thoracic area; arteriograms can locate intra-abdominal tumors.

Interventions

Surgery is the treatment of choice for a pheochromocytoma. One or both adrenal glands are removed (depending on whether the tumor is bilateral). Preoperatively, the nurse focuses on adequate tissue perfusion, nutritional needs, and comfort measures.

Hypertension is the hallmark of the disease. The nurse monitors the blood pressure regularly and places the cuff consistently on the same arm, with the client in lying and standing positions. The nurse also identifies stressors that may precede a hypertensive crisis and attempts to minimize them. The client is instructed not to smoke, drink caffeine-containing beverages, or change position suddenly. The abdomen *should not be palpated.* A diet rich in calories, vitamins, and minerals is provided.

The client often benefits from preoperative hydration therapy because inadequate blood volume increases the risk for intraoperative and postoperative hypotension. The nurse assesses the client's hydration status and notes symptoms of dehydration or fluid overload.

A calm, restful environment is provided because the client with a pheochromocytoma may experience incapacitating headaches. The client is instructed to limit activity. A private, darkened room helps to promote rest. If the client is sleeping, interruptions are avoided if possible.

The physician stabilizes the client with alpha-adrenergic blocking agents before surgery because of the increased risk for hypertension during surgery. Anesthetic agents and manipulation of the tumor during surgery can produce a release of catecholamines. The physician orders the short-acting alpha-adrenergic blocker phentolamine via IV bolus or drip for a hypertensive crisis. Oral phenoxybenzamine hydrochloride (Dibenzyline) produces long-acting alpha-adrenergic blockade and is used most frequently for preoperative management of hypertension and prevention of hypertensive crisis. It is also a drug of choice for long-term management of the client who is not a candidate for surgery.

The physician adjusts drug dosages for 2 to 3 weeks before surgery until blood pressure is controlled and no further hypertensive attacks occur. The blood volume expands, and blood pressure with the client in the supine position returns to normal.

The physician avoids using beta-adrenergic blocking agents in clients with a suspected or confirmed pheochromocytoma until after alpha-adrenergic blockade has been initiated, because these drugs may cause blood pressure to rise. After alpha-adrenergic blockade, low doses of propranolol hydrochloride (Inderal, Detensol✤) may be used to treat tachycardia and dysrhythmias.

Postoperative nursing care is similar to that for the client who has undergone an adrenalectomy (see Hypercortisolism [Cushing's Syndrome], pp. 1418 and 1419). The nurse closely monitors the client for hypotension related to the sudden decrease in catecholamine level and for hypovolemia, especially when the client was inadequately prepared for surgery. Hemorrhage and shock are possible, and the nurse administers plasma expanders and fluids as prescribed. Vital signs, as well as fluid intake and output, are monitored. If opioids are administered, the nurse observes their effect on blood pressure.

Tumors may be inoperable because of the client's other medical conditions. Treatment in these cases is medical, with alpha-adrenergic and beta-adrenergic blocking agents, because these tumors do not respond well to chemotherapy or radiation therapy. For clients who are medically managed, self-measurement of blood pressure with home monitoring equipment is essential.

ONLINE RESOURCES

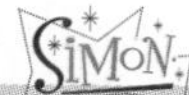

For suggested readings and Internet resources, go to http://www.wbsaunders.com/SIMON/Iggy/.

SELECTED BIBLIOGRAPHY

Ahern-Gould, K., & Stark, J. (1998). Quick resource for electrolyte imbalance. *Critical Care Nursing Clinics of North America, 10*(4), 477-490.

Carson, P. (2000). Emergency: Adrenal crisis. *American Journal of Nursing, 100*(7), 49-50.

Castiglione, V. (2000). Emergency: Hyperkalemia. *American Journal of Nursing, 100*(1), 55-56.

Chmielewski, C. (1998). Hyperkalemic emergencies: Mechanisms, manifestations, and management. *Critical Care Clinics of North America, 10*(4), 449-457.

Clayton, L., & Dilley, K. (1998). Cushing's syndrome. *American Journal of Nursing, 98*(7), 40-41.

Cotran, RS., Kumar, V., & Collins, T. (1999). *Robbins' pathologic basis of disease* (6th ed.). Philadelphia: W.B. Saunders.

Eisenberg, A., & Redick, E. (1999). Caring for a patient after resection of pituitary adenoma. *Nursing99, 29*(12), 32cc1-32cc2, 32cc4-32cc6.

Ezzone, S. (1999). Clinical focus: SIADH. *Clinical Journal of Oncology Nursing, 3*(4), 187-188.

Fabius, D. (1998). How to recognize electrolyte imbalances on an ECG. *Nursing98, 28*(2), 32hn1-32hn6.

Goldberg, M. (2000). The diagnostic challenge—Hyperaldosteronism caused by bilateral adrenal hyperplasia. *Emergency Medicine, 32*(3), 55-56.

Guyton, A.C., & Hall, J.E. (2000). *Textbook of medical physiology* (10th ed.). Philadelphia: W.B. Saunders.

Heater, D. (1999a). If ADH goes out of balance: Diabetes insipidus. *RN, 62*(7), 44-46.

Heater, D. (1999b). If ADH goes out of balance: SIADH. *RN, 62*(7), 47-49.

Kearney, K. (2000). Emergency: Adrenal crisis. *American Journal of Nursing, 100*(7), 49-50.

Luken, K. (1999). Clinical manifestations and management of Addison's disease. *Journal of the American Academy of Nurse Practitioners, 11*(4), 151-154.

McCloskey, J.C, & Bulechek, G.M (2000). *Nursing interventions classification (NIC)* (3rd ed.). St. Louis: Mosby.

Nayback, A. (2000). Hyponatremia as a consequence of acute adrenal insufficiency and hypothyroidism. *Journal of Emergency Nursing, 26*(2), 130-133.

O'Donnell, M. (1997). Addisonian crisis. *American Journal of Nursing, 97*(3), 41.

Orth, D., & Kovacs, W. (1998). The adrenal cortex. In J.D. Wilson et al. (Eds.), *Williams textbook of endocrinology* (9th ed., pp. 517-664). Philadelphia: W.B. Saunders.

Reeves, W.B., Bichet, D., & Andreoli, T. (1998). Posterior pituitary and water metabolism. In J.D. Wilson et al. (Eds.), *Williams textbook of endocrinology* (9th ed., pp. 341-387). Philadelphia: W.B. Saunders.

Reincke, M. (2000). Subclinical Cushing's syndrome. *Endocrinology and Metabolism Clinics of North America, 29*(1), 43-56.

Thorner, M., et al. (1998). The anterior pituitary. In J.D. Wilson et al. (Eds.), *Williams textbook of endocrinology* (9th ed., pp. 249-340). Philadelphia: W.B. Saunders.

United States Pharmacopeia Dispensing Information (USP DI): Vol. I. Drug information for the health care professional. (20th ed.). (2000). Englewood, CO: Micromedix.

CHAPTER 64

Interventions for Clients with Problems of the Thyroid and Parathyroid Glands

M. LINDA WORKMAN

Learning Objectives

After studying this chapter, you should be able to:

1. Compare and contrast the common clinical manifestations associated with hyperthyroidism and hypothyroidism.
2. Explain the pathophysiology of Graves' disease.
3. Use clinical changes and laboratory data to determine the effectiveness of interventions for hyperthyroidism.
4. Prioritize nursing care for the client during the first 24 hours following a total thyroidectomy.
5. Explain the pathophysiology of Hashimoto's thyroiditis.
6. Identify teaching priorities for the client taking thyroid hormone replacement therapy.
7. Use clinical changes and laboratory data to determine the effectiveness of interventions for hypothyroidism.
8. Compare and contrast the clinical manifestations associated with hyperparathyroidism and hypoparathyroidism.
9. Prioritize nursing care for the client during the first 24 hours following a parathyroidectomy.
10. Use clinical changes and laboratory data to determine the effectiveness of interventions for parathyroid problems.

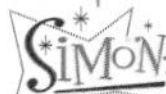

Go to http://www.wbsaunders.com/SIMON/Iggy/ for self-assessment questions related to these Learning Objectives.

Hormones from the thyroid and parathyroid glands affect general metabolism, electrolyte balance, and excitable membrane activity. Therefore a disturbance in either thyroid or parathyroid function usually has widespread clinical manifestations. With mild disturbances, the problems are subtle. With more severe disturbances, the problems may be life threatening.

THYROID DISORDERS

Hyperthyroidism

OVERVIEW

Excessive thyroid hormone secretion results in **hyperthyroidism.** The clinical manifestations of hyperthyroidism are referred to as **thyrotoxicosis.** Thyroid hormones affect all metabolic processes in all body organs and therefore produce numerous and varied clinical manifestations. Hyperthyroidism can be temporary or permanent depending on the cause.

Pathophysiology

In hyperthyroidism, the normal feedback control over thyroid hormone secretion fails. Because thyroid hormones stimulate most body systems, excessive thyroid hormones produce a state of **hypermetabolism** with increased sympathetic nervous system activity. Many of the clinical manifestations of hyperthyroidism are caused by the body's response to the demands of hypermetabolism (Chart 64-1).

Thyroid hormones directly stimulate the heart. The increased heart rate and stroke volume in hyperthyroidism cause an increase in cardiac output and peripheral blood flow. This excessive or **hyperdynamic** circulatory state results from an increase in the number of adrenergic receptors on the heart muscle.

Elevated levels of thyroid hormones affect protein, carbohydrate, and lipid metabolism. Protein **synthesis** (buildup) and **degradation** (breakdown) are increased. Breakdown exceeds buildup, causing a net loss of protein known as a **negative nitrogen balance.** Glucose tolerance is decreased, and

CHART 64-1

KEY FEATURES *of* Hyperthyroidism

Integumentary Manifestations
- Diaphoresis (excessive sweating)
- Fine, soft, silky hair (body)
- Smooth, warm, moist skin
- Thinning of scalp hair

Pulmonary Manifestations
- Shortness of breath with or without exertion

Cardiovascular Manifestations
- Palpitations
- Chest pain
- Increased systolic blood pressure
- Widened pulse pressure
- Tachycardia
- Dysrhythmias

Gastrointestinal Manifestations
- Weight loss
- Increased appetite
- Diarrhea

Musculoskeletal Manifestations
- Muscle weakness

Neurologic Manifestations
- Blurred or double vision
- Eye fatigue
- Corneal ulcers or infections
- Increased tears
- Injected (red) conjunctiva
- Photophobia
- Eyelid retraction, eyelid lag*
- Globe lag*
- Hyperactive deep tendon reflexes
- Tremors
- Insomnia

Metabolic Manifestations
- Increased basal metabolic rate
- Heat intolerance
- Low-grade fever

Psychologic/Emotional Manifestations
- Decreased attention span
- Restlessness
- Irritability
- Emotional lability
- Manic behavior

Reproductive Manifestations
- Amenorrhea
- Decreased menstrual flow
- Increased libido

Other Manifestations
- Goiter
- Wide-eyed (startled) appearance*
- Weakness, fatigue

*Present in Graves' disease only

TABLE 64-1 • CAUSES OF HYPERTHYROIDISM

Cause	Mechanism
Graves' disease (toxic diffuse goiter)	Autoimmune in nature. Antibodies (TSHAb) bind to TSH receptors and keep them activated, increasing the size of the gland and increasing the production of thyroid hormones.
Toxic multinodular goiter	Multiple thyroid nodules, resulting in thyroid hyperfunction.
Thyroid adenoma	Independent and inappropriate functioning of adenoma of follicular cells.
Pituitary hyperthyroidism	Pituitary adenoma resulting in excessive TSH secretion.
Thyroiditis (radiation-induced)	T_3 and T_4 secretion increased before destruction of gland. Hyperthyroid state usually transient.
T_3 thyrotoxicosis	Increase in thyroid secretion of T_3. Cause unknown.
Factitious hyperthyroidism	Ingestion of excessive amounts of thyroid hormone.
Jod-Basedow phenomenon (iodine induced)	Administration of iodine to an individual with endemic goiter, resulting in excessive production of thyroid hormone.
Struma ovarii	Dermoid tumor of the ovary that secretes thyroid hormone.
Thyroid carcinoma	Uncommon, usually occurs with large follicular carcinomas.
Trophoblastic tumors	Choriocarcinoma, hydatidiform mole, and embryonal carcinoma with high concentrations of chorionic gonadotropins that stimulate T_3 and T_4 secretion.

T_3, Triiodothyronine; *T_4*, thyroxine; *TSH*, thyroid-stimulating hormone.

the client has **hyperglycemia** (elevated blood glucose levels). Fat metabolism is increased, which results in decreased body fat stores. Although the client has an increased appetite, food intake does not meet energy demands, and the client loses weight. With prolonged hyperthyroidism, the client is in a state of chronic nutritional deficiency.

Thyroid hormones are produced in response to the stimulation hormones secreted by the hypothalamus and anterior pituitary glands. Thus oversecretion of thyroid hormones changes the secretion of hormones from the hypothalamus and anterior pituitary gland. In addition, thyroid hormones have some influence over sex hormone production in both men and women. If hyperthyroidism is present before puberty, sexual development is delayed. If hyperthyroidism develops after puberty, women experience menstrual irregularities and decreased fertility. Both men and women with hyperthyroidism experience an increased **libido** (sexual urge or interest).

Etiology

The causes of hyperthyroidism are numerous (Table 64-1). The most common cause is **Graves' disease,** also called toxic diffuse goiter. The client with Graves' disease usually has hyperthyroidism, a **goiter** (enlargement of the thyroid gland), **exophthalmos** (abnormal protrusion of the eyes), and **pretibial myxedema** (dry, waxy swelling of the front surfaces of the lower legs). *Not all clients with a goiter have hyperthyroidism.*

Graves' disease is an autoimmune disorder in which antibodies **(immunoglobulins)** are made and attach to the thyroid stimulating hormone (TSH) receptor sites on the thyroid tissue. When these antibodies, known as thyroid-stimulating immunoglobulins (TSIs), bind to the thyroid gland, the gland increases in size and overproduces thyroid hormones. In addition to the manifestations caused by hypermetabolism, the client with Graves' disease also has exophthalmos and pretibial edema.

Hyperthyroidism caused by multiple thyroid nodules is termed **toxic multinodular goiter.** Affected clients usually have had this goiter for years. The overproduction of thyroid hormone is usually milder than that seen in Graves' disease, and the client does not have exophthalmos or pretibial edema.

Hyperthyroidism also can be caused by overmedication with thyroid hormone **(exogenous hyperthyroidism).** Thyroid hormone has been abused by people trying to control weight or to increase their energy levels.

A condition called thyroid storm or thyroid crisis can occur when hyperthyroidism is untreated or poorly controlled or when the client is severely stressed. This condition is an extreme state of hyperthyroidism in which all clinical manifestations are more severe and life threatening.

Incidence/Prevalence

Hyperthyroidism is a common endocrine disorder. Graves' disease can occur at any age but is diagnosed most often in women between 20 and 40 years of age. Toxic multinodular goiter usually occurs after the age of 50 and affects women four times as often as men.

COLLABORATIVE MANAGEMENT

Assessment

HISTORY

The client may have noticed many changes and problems, because hyperthyroidism can affect nearly all body systems. Age, gender, and usual weight are recorded. The client may report a recent weight loss and an increased appetite. Diarrhea is common.

A hallmark of hyperthyroidism is heat intolerance. The client may have **diaphoresis** (increased sweating) even when environmental temperatures are comfortable for others. The client often wears lighter clothing in cold weather. The client may also report palpitations or chest pain as a result of the cardiovascular effects. The nurse asks about changes in breathing patterns, because dyspnea (with or without exertion) is common.

Visual changes may be the earliest problem noted in the client with hyperthyroidism, especially ophthalmopathy with Graves' disease (Figure 64-1). The client is asked about changes in vision, such as blurring or double vision and tiring of the eyes.

The nurse inquires whether the client has noticed a change in energy level or his or her ability to perform activities of daily living (ADLs). Fatigue, weakness, and insomnia are common. Family and friends may report that the client has become more irritable or depressed.

Women are asked about changes in menses, because amenorrhea or a decreased menstrual flow is common. Initially, both men and women may experience an increase in libido.

The nurse explores the client's medical history. A history of thyroid surgery or radiation therapy to the neck is important, because some people remain hyperthyroid after surgery or are resistant to radiation therapy. The client is asked about past and current medications, especially the use of thyroid hormone replacement or antithyroid drugs.

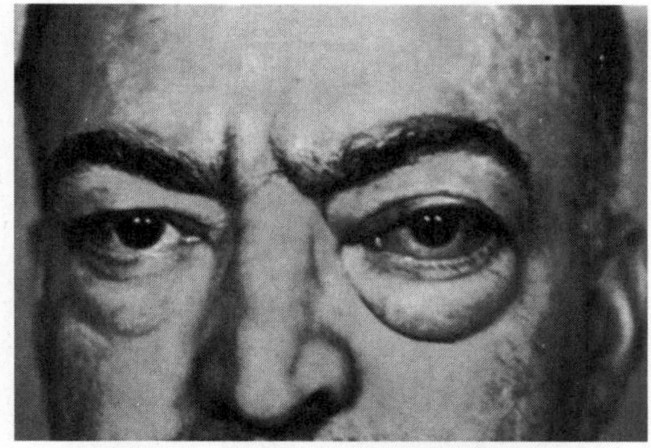

Figure 64-1 ● Ophthalmopathy. The client has proptosis.

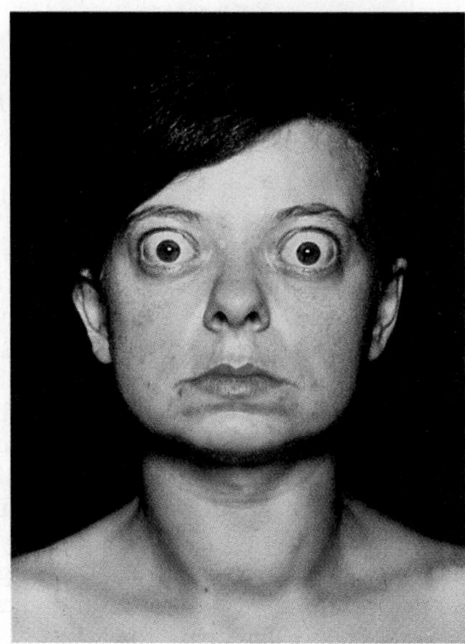

Figure 64-2 ● Exophthalmos. (From Seidel, H.M., et al. [1999]. *Mosby's guide to physical examination* [4th ed.]. St. Louis: Mosby.)

PHYSICAL ASSESSMENT/CLINICAL MANIFESTATIONS

The nurse notes the client's general appearance. Two types of **ophthalmopathy** (abnormal eye appearance or function) are common with hyperthyroidism: eyelid retraction (eyelid lag) and globe (eyeball) lag. In eyelid lag, which occurs in all forms of thyrotoxicosis, the upper eyelid fails to descend when the client gazes slowly downward. In globe lag, the upper eyelid pulls back faster than the eyeball when the client gazes upward. During assessment, the client is asked to look down and then up, and the response is documented.

Infiltrative ophthalmopathy, which leads to exophthalmos, is common in clients with Graves' disease (Figure 64-2). The wide-eyed or "startled" look is due to edema in the extraocular muscles and increased fatty tissue behind the eye, which

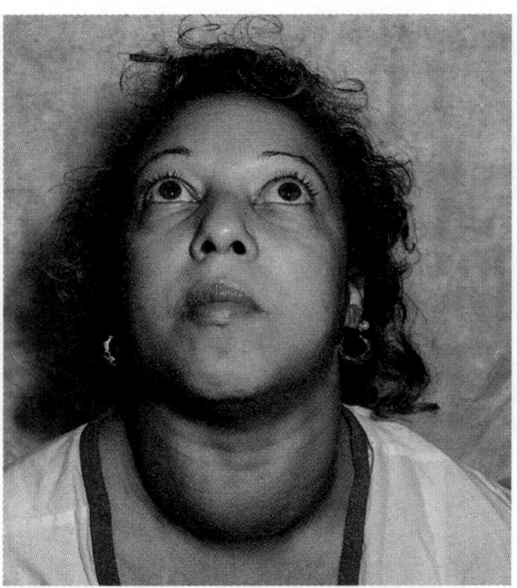

Figure 64-3 ● Goiter. (From Schwartz, M.H. [1998]. *Textbook of physical diagnosis: History and examination* [3rd ed.]. Philadelphia: W.B. Saunders.)

pushes the globe forward. Pressure on the optic nerve may impair vision. Swelling and shortening of the muscles may cause problems with focusing. If the eyelid fails to close completely and the eye is unprotected, the eye may become overdry and prone to corneal ulceration or infection. The nurse observes the client's eyes for excessive tearing and a bloodshot appearance and asks about sensitivity to light **(photophobia).**

The nurse palpates the thyroid gland to determine the presence of a mass or general enlargement, observing the size and symmetry of the gland. In goiter, a generalized thyroid enlargement in people with Graves' disease, the thyroid gland may increase to four times its normal size (Figure 64-3). **Bruits** (turbulence from increased blood flow) may be heard with a stethoscope. (See Chapter 62 for a full discussion of thyroid palpation and auscultation.)

The nurse inspects the client's hair and skin. Fine, soft, silky hair and smooth, moist skin are common with hyperthyroidism. The client may have extremity muscle weakness, hyperactive deep tendon reflexes, or tremors. Gross motor movements are observed for tremors, especially of the hands. Reflexes may be hyperactive. The client may appear extremely restless, irritable, and fatigued.

PSYCHOSOCIAL ASSESSMENT

The client with hyperthyroidism often experiences emotional **lability** (mood instability), irritability, decreased attention span, and manic behavior. Mild to severe hyperactivity often leads to a state of fatigue because of the inability to sleep well. The nurse asks the client whether he or she has been crying or laughing inappropriately or has had difficulty concentrating. The client's family members or significant other often report these changes in mental or emotional status.

LABORATORY ASSESSMENT

The diagnostic workup for hyperthyroidism includes measurement of the following serum values: triiodothyronine (T_3), thyroxine (T_4), T_3 resin uptake (T_3RU), and thyroid-stimulating hormone (TSH). Antibodies to TSH (TSHRAb) are measured to determine the presence of Graves' disease. Laboratory findings in clients with hyperthyroidism are summarized in Chart 64-2.

OTHER DIAGNOSTIC ASSESSMENT

THYROID SCAN. The thyroid scan evaluates the position, size, and functioning of the thyroid gland. Radioactive iodine (RAI [^{123}I]) is given by mouth, and the uptake of iodine by the thyroid gland (RAIU) is measured. The half-life of ^{123}I is short, and radiation precautions are not necessary. Pregnancy, however, should be ruled out before the scan is performed.

Normally the thyroid has an uptake of 5% to 35% of the administered dose when measured at 24 hours. RAIU is increased in clients with hyperthyroidism. RAI not used by the thyroid is excreted by the kidney.

The nurse assesses whether the client has undergone procedures or has taken medications that might affect the results of the scan. Procedures that use iodine-containing dye (e.g., intravenous pyelogram [IVP]) should not be performed for at least 4 weeks before a thyroid scan. Any medication that contains iodine should be discontinued for 1 week before the scan.

ULTRASONOGRAPHY. Ultrasonography of the thyroid gland can be used to determine its size and the composition of any masses or nodules. This procedure takes approximately 30 minutes to perform, and the nurse reassures the client that it is painless.

ELECTROCARDIOGRAPHY. An electrocardiogram (ECG) usually shows tachycardia. Other ECG changes with hyperthyroidism include atrial fibrillation and alterations in P and T waveforms.

CRITICAL THINKING CHALLENGE

The client is a 53-year-old woman who is brought to the emergency department after collapsing at her daughter's wedding rehearsal. She is 5' 8" tall and weighs 125 pounds. Her vital signs are as follows: blood pressure, 186/122; pulse, 104; respirations, 28. She has fine tremors of her hands.

The client is crying and yelling because the wedding rehearsal has been interrupted. Her daughter tells you that the client has not slept at all for the last three nights while finishing the dresses for the bridesmaids. The client insists that she is okay, only a little hungry after skipping lunch today. She says she has no health problems and is not being treated for any disorder. The health care team suspects hyperthyroidism and thyroid storm.

- What additional questions should you ask related to her weight?
- What diagnostic tests do you anticipate will be requested?
- What are your care priorities given the client's current clinical manifestations?
- The client insists that she must get back to the wedding rehearsal and threatens to leave immediately.
- How will you prevent her from leaving?

For suggested answer guidelines, go to SIMON http://www.wbsaunders.com/SIMON/Iggy/.

Interventions

Because Graves' disease is the most common form of hyperthyroidism, the interventions discussed in the following sections include those specific for the problems associated with Graves' disease as well as with other types of hyperthyroidism.

CHART 64-2

LABORATORY PROFILE
Thyroid Function

Test	Normal Range for Adults	Significance of Abnormal Findings	
		Hyperthyroidism	Hypothyroidism
Serum T_3	110-230 ng/dL, or 1.2-1.5 SI units	Increased	Decreased
Serum T_4	4.6-11 μg/dL, or 59-142 SI units	Increased	Decreased
Free T_4 index	0.8-2.8 ng/dL, or 10-30 SI units	Increased	Decreased
T_3 resin uptake	25%-35% (varies with different laboratories)	Increased	Decreased
TRH stimulation test	Doubling of baseline TSH 30 min after IV injection of 500 μg TRH (women have greater response)	Little or no TSH response	Delayed or poor TSH response in secondary hypothyroidism (pituitary failure) Elevated two or more times the normal in primary hypothyroidism (thyroid gland failure)
Thyroid suppression test	N/A	Fails to suppress RAIU or T_4 levels	No change in RAIU or T_4 levels
TSH stimulation test (thyroid stimulation test)	>10% in RAIU or >1.5 μg/dL	N/A (test differentiates primary from secondary hypothyroidism)	No response in primary hypothyroidism Normal response in secondary hypothyroidism
Thyroid antibodies (antithyroglobulin antibody)	Titer <1:100	High titer of antithyroglobulin antibodies	Increased titers
Thyrotropin receptor antibodies (TSH-RAb)	Titer <130% of basal activity	High titers indicate Graves' disease	No response

TSH, thyroid-stimulating hormone; *RAIU,* radioactive iodine uptake; *N/A,* not applicable; T_3, triiodothyronine; T_4, thyroxine; *TRH,* thyrotropin-releasing hormone, *SI,* System Internationale.

The cardiac problems of hyperthyroidism include increased systolic blood pressure, a widened pulse pressure, tachycardia, and other dysrhythmias. The goals of nonsurgical management are to decrease the effect of thyroid hormone on cardiac function and to reduce thyroid hormone secretion. Surgery may be necessary when nonsurgical interventions are unsuccessful.

NONSURGICAL MANAGEMENT. The nurse monitors the client's apical pulse, blood pressure, and temperature at least every 4 hours. The client is instructed to report any palpitations, dyspnea, vertigo, or chest pain immediately.

The nurse and other assistive nursing personnel minimize the client's discomfort from the clinical effects of hyperthyroidism. Fatigue is common, and the client is encouraged to rest. The environment is kept as quiet as possible. Frequent bed linen changes, sponge baths, and a cool environment decrease discomfort caused by diaphoresis and heat intolerance.

DRUG THERAPY. The most commonly ordered antithyroid drugs are the thioamides, including propylthiouracil (PTU) and methimazole (Tapazole), which block thyroid hormone production (Chart 64-3). The response to these drugs is delayed because the client may have large amounts of thyroid hormone stored that continues to be released. Other drugs are needed to control the manifestations (especially cardiac) of hyperthyroidism until hormone production and release are reduced.

Iodine preparations decrease blood flow through the thyroid gland. This action reduces the production and release of thyroid hormone. Improvement usually occurs within 2 weeks, but weeks may be needed before metabolism returns to normal. This treatment can result in hypothyroidism, and the client must be closely monitored for the need for medication changes.

Lithium carbonate also inhibits thyroid hormone release. However, its use is limited because of certain side effects such as depression, nephrogenic diabetes insipidus, tremors, nausea, and vomiting. Lithium may be prescribed when a client cannot tolerate other antithyroid drugs.

Beta-adrenergic blocking drugs, such as propranolol (Inderal, Detensol✤) and atenolol (Tenormin), relieve diaphoresis, anxiety, tachycardia, and palpitations.

RADIOACTIVE IODINE THERAPY. *Radioactive iodine (RAI) therapy is contraindicated in pregnant women because ^{131}I crosses the placenta and can adversely affect the fetal thyroid gland.* The client with hyperthyroidism may receive RAI in the form of oral ^{131}I. The dosage depends on the thyroid gland's size and sensitivity to radiation. The thyroid gland picks up the RAI, and some of the cells that produce thyroid hormone are destroyed by the local radiation. Because the thyroid gland stores thyroid hormone to some degree, the client may not experience complete symptom relief until 6 to 8 weeks after RAI therapy. The client usually needs drug therapy for hyperthyroidism during the first few weeks after RAI treatment.

RAI therapy usually involves one dose and can be performed on an outpatient basis. Occasionally a client needs a second or third dose. The radiation dose is usually low enough that radiation precautions are not required. The nurse reassures the client that the radioactivity is quickly eliminated. The de-

CHART 64-3

DRUG THERAPY *for* Hyperthyroidism

Drug	Usual Dosage	Nursing Interventions	Rationale
Propylthiouracil (PTU, Propyl-Thyracil✱)	100-150 mg tid PO	Give at 8-hr intervals around-the-clock	Spreading out dosage helps maintain suppression of hormone.
Methimazole (Tapazole)	5-15 mg tid PO	Monitor vital signs. Weigh the client weekly. Observe for sore throat, fever, headache, and skin eruptions.	Changes in vital signs or weight and appearance or other signs and symptoms may indicate adverse reactions, which may necessitate discontinuation of drug use.
Iodine products Strong iodine (Lugol's) solution Saturated solution of potassium iodide (SSKI) Potassium iodide tablets, solution, and syrup	Dosage varies, depending on the type of iodine prescribed, the manufacturer, and the form supplied (tablet, solution, or syrup)	Give in fruit juice or water. Observe for fever, rash, metallic taste, sore mouth, severe GI distress, and burning mouth and throat. Instruct the client to take tablets after meals.	Giving in fruit juice or water improves taste. Signs of iodism may necessitate discontinuation of drug use. Taking after meals enhances absorption.
Lithium carbonate (Lithobid, Carbolith✱, Lithizine✱)	Individualized 900-1200 mg/day PO in divided doses	Observe for signs of hypothyroidism. Instruct the client to drink 10-12 glassfuls of fluid a day Instruct the client to maintain normal sodium intake.	Signs of hypothyroidism may indicate drug-induced thyroid enlargement. Extra fluid intake helps to prevent dehydration. Reduced sodium intake can cause retention of the drug.
Propranolol (Inderal, Detensol✱) Atenolol (Tenormin)	20 mg/day qid in divided doses 25-50 mg PO qd	Weigh the client daily. Measure intake and output. Instruct the client to take the drug with food. Instruct the client to avoid smoking. Monitor the client's pulse.	Increased weight and decreased output may indicate congestive heart failure. Taking the drug with food enhances absorption. The drug's effect is reduced by smoking. Tachycardia is a sign of hyperthyroidism.

GI, Gastrointestinal.

gree of thyroid destruction is variable. Some clients become hypothyroid as a result of treatment. This complication may occur within a few weeks or may take several years to develop. The client then needs lifelong thyroid hormone replacement. All clients who have undergone RAI therapy should be monitored regularly for changes in thyroid function.

SURGICAL MANAGEMENT. Antithyroid drugs and RAI therapy are now the most common treatments for clients with hyperthyroidism. Surgery to remove all or part of the thyroid gland may be necessary for clients who have a large goiter causing tracheal or esophageal compression or who are unresponsive to antithyroid drugs. Removal of all **(total thyroidectomy)** or part **(subtotal thyroidectomy)** of the thyroid tissue decreases the production of thyroid hormones. Clients undergoing a total thyroidectomy must take lifelong thyroid hormone replacement. This surgery is also indicated in certain types of thyroid cancer.

PREOPERATIVE CARE. If possible, the client is treated with drug therapy first and experiences near-normal thyroid function **(euthyroid)** before thyroid surgery. The euthyroid state is achieved with antithyroid drugs that decrease the secretion of thyroid hormone. Iodine preparations are also used to decrease the size and vascularity of the gland, thereby reducing the risk for hemorrhage and the potential for thyroid storm during surgery.

Cardiac problems of hypertension, dysrhythmias, and tachycardia must be controlled before surgery. The client with hyperthyroidism is often not at an optimal weight and may need to follow a high-protein, high-carbohydrate diet for days or weeks before surgery.

The nurse instructs the client to perform coughing and deep-breathing exercises. Teaching the client how to support the neck when coughing or moving is critical. Placing both hands behind the neck when moving reduces the strain on the suture line. The nurse explains that hoarseness may be present for a few days as a result of endotracheal tube placement during surgery.

Clients often fear thyroid surgery, perhaps because the incision is in the neck area. The nurse reassures the client by calmly explaining the surgery and postoperative care and by answering any questions the client and family may have.

OPERATIVE PROCEDURES. A thyroidectomy is performed with the client under general anesthesia. During surgery, the client's neck is extended and the surgeon makes a "collar" incision 1 to 2 cm above the clavicle. The surgeon identifies and avoids the parathyroid glands and recurrent laryngeal nerves to minimize complications and injury.

With a *subtotal thyroidectomy,* the remaining thyroid tissues are sutured to the trachea. With a *total thyroidectomy,* the surgeon leaves the parathyroid glands with an intact blood supply and removes the entire thyroid gland.

POSTOPERATIVE CARE. Vital signs are monitored every 15 minutes until the client is stable and are then monitored every 30 minutes. Monitoring of vital signs is increased or decreased depending on changes in the client's condition and on the physician's orders.

The nurse assesses the client's level of discomfort. Sandbags or pillows are used to support the head and neck. The client is placed in a semi-Fowler's position when awake. When positioning the client, the nurse decreases tension on the suture line by avoiding neck extension. Pain medications are administered as needed and as ordered.

Humidification of the air promotes easier respiration and thins respiratory secretions. The nurse assists the client in coughing and deep breathing every 30 minutes to 1 hour and also suctions oral and tracheal secretions when necessary.

Thyroid surgery can cause several complications, including hemorrhage, respiratory distress, parathyroid gland injury (resulting in **hypocalcemia** [low serum calcium levels] and **tetany** [hyperexcitability of nerves and muscles]), damage to the laryngeal nerves, and thyroid storm. The nurse is alert to the potential for complications and identifies manifestations early.

Hemorrhage. Hemorrhage is most likely to occur during the first 24 hours after surgery. After surgery, the nurse inspects the neck dressing and behind the client's neck for blood. A drain may be present with a moderate amount of serosanguineous drainage. Hemorrhage may also be seen as bleeding at the incision site or as respiratory distress caused by tracheal compression.

Respiratory Distress. Respiratory distress can also result from swelling or tetany. Laryngeal **stridor** (harsh, high-pitched respiratory sounds) is heard in acute respiratory obstruction. Emergency tracheostomy equipment is kept in the client's room. The nurse checks that oxygen and suctioning equipment are nearby and in working order. In some instances, nurses are instructed to remove clips or sutures when medical assistance is not immediately available.

Hypocalcemia and Tetany. The parathyroid glands can be damaged or their blood supply impaired during thyroid surgery. Hypocalcemia and tetany result when parathyroid hormone (PTH) levels decrease. The nurse assesses the client for symptoms of tingling around the mouth or of the toes and fingers and muscular twitching as signs of calcium deficiency. Calcium gluconate or calcium chloride for intravenous (IV) administration must be available in an emergency situation. (For information on the later signs of hypocalcemia, see Postoperative Care [Hyperparathyroidism], p. 1438, and Assessment [Hypoparathyroidism], p. 1438. The care of clients with hypocalcemia is discussed in Chapter 13.)

Laryngeal Nerve Damage. Hoarseness and a weak voice can result if the laryngeal nerve is injured during surgery. The nurse assesses the client's voice at 2-hour intervals and documents any changes. The client is reassured that hoarseness is usually temporary.

Thyroid Storm. Thyroid storm or **thyroid crisis** is a life-threatening event that occurs in clients with uncontrolled hyperthyroidism and is usually caused by Graves' disease. Signs and symptoms of crisis develop quickly. Thyroid storm is usually triggered by a major stressor such as trauma or infection. Other conditions that can lead to thyroid storm include vigorous palpation of the goiter, exposure to iodine, and radioactive iodine (RAI) therapy. In the past, thyroid storm often occurred in the postoperative period when clients were not pretreated with antithyroid drugs and supportive drugs. Today postoperative thyroid storm is rare because clients receive antithyroid drugs, beta blockers, steroids, and iodides before thyroid surgery to prevent thyroid crisis.

CHART 64-4

BEST PRACTICE *for*
Emergency Care of the Client During Thyroid Storm

- Maintain a patent airway and adequate ventilation.
- Give antithyroid drugs as ordered: propylthiouracil (PTU, Propyl-Thyracil✱), 300 to 900 mg/day; methimazole (Tapazole), up to 60 mg/day.
- Administer sodium iodide solution, 2 g/day IV as ordered.
- Give propranolol (Inderal, Detensol✱), 1 to 3 mg IV as ordered. Give slowly over 3 minutes; the client should be connected to a cardiac monitor, and a central venous pressure catheter should be in place.
- Give glucocorticoids as ordered: hydrocortisone, 100 to 500 mg/day IV; prednisone, 4 to 60 mg/day IV or IM.
- Monitor continually for cardiac dysrhythmias.
- Monitor vital signs every 30 minutes.
- Provide comfort measures, including a cooling blanket.
- Give nonsalicylate antipyretics as ordered.

The signs and symptoms of thyroid storm are caused by excessive thyroid hormone release that leads to a large increase in the metabolic rate. Symptoms include the following:

- Fever
- Tachycardia
- Systolic hypertension

The client may have gastrointestinal symptoms such as abdominal pain, nausea, vomiting, and diarrhea. Typically, the client with thyroid storm is agitated and anxious and has tremors. As the crisis progresses, he or she may become restless, confused, and psychotic and may have seizures, leading to coma. *Even with treatment, thyroid storm has a mortality rate of 25%.*

Emergency measures to prevent death vary with the intensity and type of specific symptoms. After the causative event has been identified, the following are primary concerns:

- Maintaining airway patency
- Providing adequate ventilation
- Stabilizing the hemodynamic status

Chart 64-4 outlines the best practices for the management of thyroid storm.

INFILTRATIVE OPHTHALMOPATHY. Treatment for hyperthyroidism does not affect the eye and vision problems of Graves' disease. Treatment of the client with infiltrative ophthalmopathy is symptomatic. The nurse instructs the client with mild symptoms to elevate the head of the bed at night and use an eye lubricant (artificial tears). If photophobia (sensitivity to light) is present, dark glasses or eye patches are often helpful. For the client who cannot close the eyelids completely, the nurse recommends gently taping the lids closed with nonallergenic tape. These actions prevent irritation and injury. If pressure behind the eye continues and forces the eye forward, blood supply to the eye can be compromised, leading to ischemia and blindness. (See Chapter 46 for more discussion regarding eye protection.)

In severe cases the physician prescribes short-term steroid therapy to reduce swelling and halt the infiltrative process. Prednisone (Deltasone, Winpred✦) is often administered in high doses (often 120 mg/day) initially and then tapered down according to the client's response. The nurse explains the need to gradually reduce the prednisone and reviews its side effects with the client.

The physician may prescribe diuretics to decrease edema around the eye. Surgical intervention (orbital decompression) may be necessary if loss of sight or damage to the eyeball is possible.

HEALTH TEACHING. The signs and symptoms of hyperthyroidism are reviewed and the client is instructed to report an increase or recurrence of symptoms. The symptoms of hypothyroidism (discussed in the next section) and the need for thyroid hormone replacement are reviewed. The nurse reinforces the need for regular follow-up, because hypothyroidism can occur several years after radioactive iodine therapy.

If the client has had surgery, the surgeon usually removes the sutures on the third or fourth postoperative day. The client is instructed to inspect the incision area and to report redness, tenderness, drainage, or swelling to a member of the health care team.

The discharged client may continue to experience mood changes as a result of hyperthyroidism. The nurse explains the reason for emotional lability to the client and family and reassures them that it will decrease with continued treatment.

Hypothyroidism

OVERVIEW

The clinical manifestations of hypothyroidism (Chart 64-5) are the result of decreased metabolism from low levels of thyroid hormones. Hypothyroidism can occur at any time throughout the life span.

Pathophysiology

Thyroid cells may fail to produce sufficient levels of thyroid hormones for several reasons. Sometimes the cells themselves are damaged and no longer function normally. Other times the thyroid cells are functional but the person does not ingest enough of the substances needed to make thyroid hormones, especially iodide and tyrosine. When the production of thyroid hormones (THs) is too low or absent, the blood levels of TH are very low and the client has a decreased metabolic rate. This lowered metabolism causes the hypothalamus and anterior pituitary gland to make stimulatory hormones, especially thyroid-stimulating hormone (TSH), as compensation. The TSH binds to thyroid cells and causes the thyroid gland to enlarge, forming a **goiter.**

Most tissues and organs are affected by the low metabolic rate caused by hypothyroidism. Cellular energy production is decreased, and many metabolites build up. The metabolites are compounds of proteins and sugars called **glycosaminoglycans.** These compounds build up inside cells, which increases the mucous and water, forms cellular edema, and changes organ texture. The cellular edema is mucinous edema (called **myxedema**) rather than edema caused by water alone (Figure 64-4). This edema changes the appearance of the

CHART 64-5

KEY FEATURES *of* Hypothyroidism

Integumentary Manifestations
- Cool, pale or yellowish, dry, coarse, scaly skin
- Thick, brittle nails
- Dry, coarse, brittle hair
- Decreased hair growth, with loss of eyebrow hair

Pulmonary Manifestations
- Hypoventilation
- Pleural effusion
- Dyspnea

Cardiovascular Manifestations
- Bradycardia
- Dysrhythmias
- Enlarged heart
- Decreased activity tolerance
- Hypotension

Metabolic Manifestations
- Decreased basal metabolic rate
- Decreased body temperature
- Cold intolerance

Musculoskeletal Manifestations
- Muscle aches and pains
- Delayed contraction and relaxation of muscles

Neurologic Manifestations
- Slowing of intellectual functions
  - Slowness or slurring of speech
  - Impaired memory
  - Inattentiveness
- Lethargy or somnolence
- Confusion
- Hearing loss
- Paresthesia (numbness and tingling) of the extremities
- Decreased tendon reflexes

Psychologic/Emotional Manifestations
- Apathy
- Agitation
- Depression
- Paranoia
- Withdrawal

Gastrointestinal Manifestations
- Anorexia
- Weight gain
- Constipation
- Abdominal distention

Reproductive Manifestations

Women
- Changes in menses (amenorrhea or prolonged menstrual periods)
- Infertility
- Anovulation
- Decreased libido

Men
- Decreased libido
- Impotence

Other Manifestations
- Periorbital edema
- Facial puffiness
- Facial coarseness
- Nonpitting edema of the hands and feet
- Hoarseness
- Goiter (enlarged thyroid gland)
- Thick tongue
- Increased sensitivity to opioids and tranquilizers
- Blank expression
- Weakness, fatigue
- Decreased urine output
- Anemia
- Easy bruising
- Iron deficiency
- Folate deficiency
- Vitamin B_{12} deficiency

client with full-blown hypothyroidism. Nonpitting edema forms everywhere and is especially evident around the eyes, in the hands and feet, and between the shoulder blades. These same compounds cause the tongue to thicken and edema to form in the larynx, making the voice more husky. It is likely that these metabolites build up in other tissues and organs, decreasing general physiologic function.

Myxedema coma is a rare but serious complication of untreated or inadequately treated hypothyroidism. The decrease in metabolism in cardiac tissue causes the heart muscle to become flabby and the chamber size to increase. The result is decreased cardiac output and decreased perfusion to the brain and other vital organs. The decreased perfusion makes the already slowed cellular metabolism worse, resulting in tissue and organ failure. *The mortality rate for myxedema coma is extremely high, and this condition is considered a life-threatening emergency.* Myxedema coma can be caused by a variety of events or conditions (Table 64-2).

Etiology

Most cases of hypothyroidism in the United States occur as a result of thyroid surgery and radioactive iodine (RAI) treatment of hyperthyroidism. Worldwide, hypothyroidism is common in areas where the soil and water have little natural iodide, causing **endemic goiter.** (This problem was common in the midwest region of the country before iodide was added to table salt and before fresh saltwater fish was widely available.) Hypothyroidism is also caused by a variety of other conditions and factors (Table 64-3).

Incidence/Prevalence

Hypothyroidism occurs most often in women between 30 and 60 years of age. Women are affected 7 to 10 times more often than men (Larsen, Davis, & Hay, 1998). A link between diabetes mellitus and the development of hypothyroidism has been established. This link is supported by the finding of an increased incidence of hypothyroidism among minority populations at high risk for diabetes mellitus, such as Native Americans (see the Evidence-Based Practice for Nursing box on p. 1432).

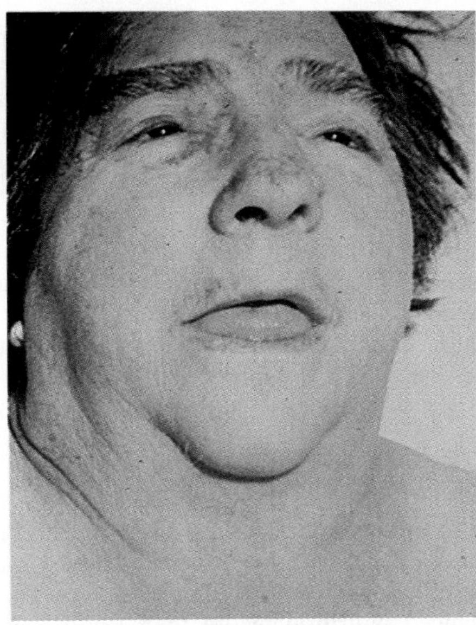

Figure 64-4 ● Myxedema. (From Seidel H.M., et al. [1999]. Mosby's guide to physical examination [4th ed.]. St. Louis: Mosby.)

COLLABORATIVE MANAGEMENT

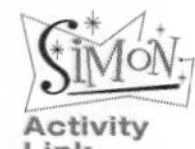

Assessment

HISTORY

A decrease in thyroid hormone produces a variety of signs and symptoms related to decreased metabolic activity. The client often reports an increase in time spent sleeping, sometimes up to 14 to 16 hr/day. The client may also have generalized weakness, anorexia, muscle aches, and paresthesias. Constipation is common. The client often has cold intolerance, and the nurse asks if more blankets at night or sweaters and extra clothing in warm weather have been needed.

Both male and female clients may identify a decrease in libido. In addition, women with hypothyroidism may have had difficulty becoming pregnant or experienced changes in menses (heavy, prolonged bleeding or amenorrhea). Men can have problems with impotence and fertility.

TABLE 64-2 • CONDITIONS OR EVENTS PRECIPITATING MYXEDEMA COMA

- Acute illness
- Anesthesia
- Surgery
- Hypothermia
- Chemotherapy
- Sedatives/opioids
- Rapid withdrawal of thyroid medications
- Untreated hypothyroidism
- Inadequately treated hypothyroidism

TABLE 64-3 • CAUSES OF HYPOTHYROIDISM

PRIMARY CAUSES

Decreased Thyroid Tissue

- Surgical removal of the thyroid
- Radiation-induced thyroid destruction
- Autoimmune thyroid destruction
- Congenital thyroid agenesis
- Congenital thyroid hypoplasia
- Congenital thyroid dysgenesis
- Cancer (thyroidal or metastatic)

Decreased Synthesis of Thyroid Hormone

- Endemic iodine deficiency
- Excessive exposure to iodine
- Medications
  - Lithium
  - Phenylbutazone
  - Propylthiouracil
  - Sodium or potassium perchlorate
  - Aminoglutethimide

SECONDARY CAUSES

Inadequate Production of Thyroid-Stimulating Hormone

- Pituitary tumors, trauma, infections, or infarcts
- Congenital pituitary defects
- Hypothalamic tumors, trauma, infections, or infarcts

EVIDENCE-BASED PRACTICE FOR NURSING

Native American diabetics more at risk for hypothyroidism

Michalek, A., Mahoney, M., & Calebaugh, D. (2000). Hypothyroidism and diabetes mellitus in an American Indian population, *Journal of Family Practice, 49*(7), 638-640.

A clinical relationship between the presence of diabetes mellitus and the development of hypothyroidism among the general population is beginning to be recognized, although the exact cause of this link is only speculated. Few minority populations have been examined for this phenomenon. During the past 30 years, the incidence and prevalence of both type I and type II diabetes mellitus among Native Americans has increased well beyond that of the general population. The incidence of hypothyroidism among this group is not known. The purpose of this study was to determine the incidence of hypothyroidism among members of a northeastern Native American nation who were also diabetic.

The researchers performed a chart review of 892 northeastern Native Americans living in an isolated area. All charts were from one clinic setting. Of the 892 charts reviewed, 156 clients were identified as having diabetes mellitus, and 25 of these clients also had hypothyroidism. Of particular interest was the fact that many more women than men had either or both of these disorders, especially women over the age of 60.

Critique. This descriptive survey included a large sample size, strengthening the validity of the findings. The retrospective nature of the design and the fact that data was obtained only from medical records clouds the issue of the true incidence and prevalence rates for either diabetes mellitus or hypothyroidism (many people with type II diabetes are unaware that they have the disease). It is likely that the actual incidence and prevalence for these disorders is even higher than the reported results. Nonetheless, the results of this study represent an important beginning for prevention and early detection strategies.

Implications for Nursing. When taking a history from any client, nurses need to obtain more specific racial/ethnic information to determine if a client has any degree of Native American heritage. Even more important, when a client is known to be Native American, the nurse needs to ask specific questions related to the clinical manifestations of both diabetes mellitus and hypothyroidism. The development of educational materials targeted to Native American populations regarding risk factors, early detection methods, and clinical manifestations can be a nursing priority.

The client is asked about his or her current or previous use of medications, such as lithium, aminoglutethimide, sodium or potassium perchlorate, thiocyanates, or cobalt. All of these drugs can impair the production of thyroid hormone. The client is asked whether he or she is taking any tranquilizers or opioids (hypothyroidism increases the sensitivity to these drugs as a result of decreased metabolism).

PHYSICAL ASSESSMENT/CLINICAL MANIFESTATIONS

The client's overall appearance is observed. Figure 64-4 shows the typical appearance of an adult with hypothyroidism. Common changes in appearance include coarse features, edema around the eyes and face, a blank expression, and a thick tongue. The client's overall muscle movement is slow.

PSYCHOSOCIAL ASSESSMENT

Hypothyroidism causes many problems in psychosocial functioning. Depression is the most common reason for seeking medical attention. Family members often bring the client for the initial evaluation. The client may be too lethargic, apathetic, or drowsy to recognize changes in his or her condition. Families may report that the client is withdrawn.

The nurse assesses the client's attention span and memory, both of which can be impaired by hypothyroidism. Paranoia and agitation may be additional findings.

LABORATORY ASSESSMENT

In general, laboratory findings for hypothyroidism are the opposite of those for hyperthyroidism. Triiodothyronine (T_3) and thyroxine (T_4) serum levels are decreased. TSH levels are elevated in primary hypothyroidism but can be decreased or near-normal in clients with secondary and tertiary hypothyroidism. More information is presented in Chart 64-2.

CRITICAL THINKING CHALLENGE

The client is a 22-year-old college senior nursing student who has been brought to the student health service by her friends, who say she is not "acting right." This former straight-A student has been oversleeping and missing classes. Her grades have dropped to Bs and Cs. She has gained 40 pounds during the past semester and has not had a period for 5 months. Today she did not recognize her roommate's brother. She is not taking any prescribed or over-the-counter medications. She is wearing two sweaters and asking for a blanket even though the room is quite warm. The health care team suspects hypothyroidism.

- What assessment data should you obtain first?
- What comfort measures will you provide to this client?
- What questions will you ask the client, and what questions will you ask her friends?

For suggested answer guidelines, go to SIMON http://www.wbsaunders.com/SIMON/Iggy/.

Analysis

COMMON NURSING DIAGNOSES AND COLLABORATIVE PROBLEMS

The following are common nursing diagnoses for clients with hypothyroidism:

1. Decreased Cardiac Output related to decreased stroke volume as a result of electrical or mechanical malfunction from bradycardia and arteriosclerotic coronary artery disease
2. Ineffective Breathing Pattern related to decreased energy, obesity, fatigue, and inactivity
3. Disturbed Thought Processes related to increased interstitial edema and water retention

The major collaborative problem is the Potential for Myxedema Coma.

ADDITIONAL NURSING DIAGNOSES AND COLLABORATIVE PROBLEMS

In addition to the common nursing diagnoses and collaborative problems, clients with hypothyroidism may have one or more of the following:

- Imbalanced Nutrition: More than Body Requirements related to decreased metabolic need
- Hypothermia related to decreased metabolic rate
- Constipation related to decreased gastrointestinal motility

- Impaired Physical Mobility related to fatigue, decreased strength and endurance, depression, obesity, and pain
- Disturbed Body Image related to changes in physical appearance
- Deficient Knowledge of condition, diagnosis, and treatment related to low energy level and fatigue

Additional collaborative problems for clients with hypothyroidism are Potential for Paralytic Ileus and Potential for Cardiomyopathy.

Planning and Implementation

DECREASED CARDIAC OUTPUT

NOC **PLANNING: EXPECTED OUTCOMES.** The client with hypothyroidism is expected to maintain normal cardiovascular function.

INTERVENTIONS. NIC interventions for the client with hypothyroidism are outlined in Chart 64-6. The client with hypothyroidism can have decreased blood pressure, bradycardia, and dysrhythmias. The nurse monitors blood pressure, heart rate, and rhythm and observes closely for signs of shock, such as hypotension, decreasing urine output, and mental status changes.

If hypothyroidism has been chronic, the client may have cardiovascular disease. The client is instructed to report episodes of chest pain or discomfort immediately.

The client with hypothyroidism requires lifelong thyroid hormone replacement. Synthetic hormone preparations are usually prescribed; the most common is levothyroxine sodium (Synthroid, T_4, Eltroxin✤). Therapy is started with low doses and gradually increased over a period of weeks. *The client with more severe symptoms of hypothyroidism is started on the lowest dose of thyroid hormone replacement.* This caution is especially important when the client has known cardiac problems. Starting at too high a dose or increasing the dose too rapidly can cause severe hypertension, heart failure, and myocardial infarction.

The nurse assesses the client for chest pain and dyspnea during initiation of therapy. The final dosage is determined by blood levels of TSH and the client's physical responses. The dosage and time required for symptom relief vary with each client. The nurse monitors for and teaches the client the signs and symptoms of hyperthyroidism, which can occur with replacement therapy.

CHART 64-6

NIC INTERVENTION ACTIVITIES *for* The Client with Hypothyroidism

Respiratory Monitoring: *Collection and analysis of client data to ensure airway patency and adequate gas exchange*
- Monitor rate, rhythm, depth, and effort of respirations.
- Note chest movement, watching for symmetry.
- Monitor breathing patterns for bradypnea.
- Monitor for diaphragmatic muscle fatigue (paradoxical motion).
- Note changes in Sao_2 and Svo_2.
- Monitor client's ability to cough effectively.
- Monitor for dyspnea and events that improve and worsen it.

Shock Prevention: *Detecting and treating a client at risk for impending shock.*
- Monitor circulatory status: BP, skin color, skin temperature, heart sounds, heart rate and rhythm, presence and quality of peripheral pulses, and capillary refill.
- Monitor for signs of inadequate tissue oxygenation.
- Monitor for apprehension, increased anxiety, and changes in mental status.
- Monitor intake and output.
- Administer oxygen and/or mechanical ventilation, as appropriate.

Hypothermia Treatment: *Rewarming and surveillance of a client whose core body temperature is below 35° C.*
- Monitor client's temperature, using a low-recording thermometer if necessary.
- Place on a cardiac monitor, as appropriate.
- Cover with warmed blankets, as appropriate.
- Administer heated oxygen, as appropriate.
- Monitor vital signs, as appropriate.
- Monitor skin color and temperature.
- Monitor intake and output.
- Avoid giving IM or subcutaneous medications during the hypothermic state.
- Give client warm oral fluids, if alert and able to swallow.
- Teach client to consume a caloric intake sufficient to maintain a normal body temperature.
- Emphasize the importance of wearing warm, protective clothing when going into a cold environment.

NIC intervention activities selected from McCloskey, J.C., & Bulechek, G.M. (Eds.). (2000). *Nursing interventions classification (NIC)* (3rd ed.). St. Louis: Mosby. No part of this work is to be altered without prior written permission from the Publisher.
Sao_2, Arterial oxygen saturation; Svo_2, venous oxygen saturation.

INEFFECTIVE BREATHING PATTERN

NOC **PLANNING: EXPECTED OUTCOMES.** The client with hypothyroidism is expected to have normal respiratory function as evidenced by respiratory rate and depth within normal limits (WNL) and pulse oximetry in expected range (IER).

INTERVENTIONS. The nurse observes and records the rate and depth of respirations. The lungs are auscultated for any abnormalities, such as a decrease in breath sounds. If hypothyroidism is severe, the client may have such severe respiratory distress that ventilatory support is required. Severe respiratory distress is usually associated with myxedema coma.

Sedating a client with hypothyroidism can make respiratory difficulties worse and is avoided, if possible. When a tranquilizer or sedative is needed, the dosage is reduced because hypothyroidism increases sensitivity to these drugs. The nurse assesses the client for signs of respiratory difficulty.

ALTERED THOUGHT PROCESSES

PLANNING: EXPECTED OUTCOMES. The client with hypothyroidism is expected to have improved thought processes with correction of the hypothyroidism.

INTERVENTIONS. The nurse notes the presence and severity of symptoms, including lethargy, drowsiness, memory deficit, inattentiveness, and difficulty communicating. Symptoms should decrease with thyroid hormone treatment, and mental awareness usually returns to normal levels in adults within 2 weeks. The nurse orients the client to person, place, and time, explains all procedures slowly and carefully, and provides a safe environment.

Family members or significant others may have difficulty coping with the client's symptoms. The nurse encourages them to accept the mood changes and mental slowness as manifestations of the disease, which should improve with therapy.

MYXEDEMA COMA

Any client with hypothyroidism who has any other health problem or who is newly diagnosed is at risk for myxedema coma. Factors leading to myxedema coma are listed in Table 64-2. The following problems are associated with this condition:

- Coma
- Respiratory failure
- Hypotension
- Hyponatremia
- Hypothermia
- Hypoglycemia

Untreated myxedema coma leads to shock, organ damage, and death. The nurse assesses the client with hypothyroidism every shift for changes that indicate increasing severity of hypothyroid symptoms, especially changes in mental status.

The physician institutes treatment quickly according to the client's clinical presentation and history and without waiting for laboratory confirmation. Best practices for emergency care of the client with myxedema coma are outlined in Chart 64-7.

CONSIDERATIONS FOR OLDER ADULTS

Metabolic rate and thyroid hormone production decrease with advancing age, particularly among people older than 80 years (Chart 64-8). Until recently, however, data regarding normal levels of T_3 and T_4 were established only for adults between 20 and 30 years of age. By such criteria, older people with T_3 and T_4 levels 15% to 20% below the "normal levels" established for a younger population were considered to have hypothyroidism, and therapy with thyroid hormone was initiated. However, many of these clients were not truly hypothyroid, and therapy caused **pseudohyperthyroidism**, stressing many tissues and organs (Wallace & Hofmann, 1998). In addition, daily thyroid hormone therapy decreases the activity of the anterior pituitary gland and the thyroid gland, creating actual hypothyroidism. Health care providers need to assess more than just laboratory data to determine hypothyroidism in the older adult.

Community-Based Care

Hypothyroidism is usually a chronic condition. Clients with hypothyroidism are managed on an outpatient basis and may reside in the home, in an assisted-living environment, or in a long-term care facility. Clients in acute care settings, subacute care settings, and rehabilitation centers may have long-standing hypothyroidism in addition to other acute or chronic health problems. The nurse needs to ensure that whoever is responsible for overseeing daily care is aware of the condition and understands its treatment.

HEALTH TEACHING

Most of the education needed by the client with hypothyroidism concerns hormone replacement therapy. The nurse emphasizes the need for lifelong medication and reviews the signs and symptoms of both hyperthyroidism and hypothyroidism. This information helps the client and family know when to seek medical interventions for dosage adjustment. All aspects of medication information are reviewed, including side effects. The client is instructed not to take any over-the-counter (OTC) medication because thyroid hormone preparations interact with many other drugs. The older adult client may need additional information about the effects of aging on the thyroid gland (see Chart 64-8).

The nurse advises the client to maintain a well-balanced diet with adequate fiber and fluid intake to prevent constipation. Excessive dietary fiber or fiber supplements may interfere with the absorption of thyroid hormone. The client is reminded of the importance of adequate rest periods before resuming a full schedule of daily activities. Family members are encouraged to voice their concerns to the health care provider.

The nurse discusses the necessity for follow-up care. All clients with hypothyroidism should wear a MedicAlert identification bracelet.

The time required for resolution of hypothyroidism symptoms varies; the nurse focuses on educating the family to be tolerant of any mental dullness or slowness in their loved one. Family members are instructed to orient the client frequently and to explain everything clearly and simply.

HOME CARE MANAGEMENT

The client with hypothyroidism does not usually require changes in the home unless cognition has decreased to the point that he or she poses a danger to self. Activity intolerance and fatigue may necessitate one-floor living for a short time. If symptoms have not cleared before discharge from the hospital, the nurse discusses the need for extra heat or clothing because of cold intolerance. The client who continues to have a decreased attention span may need assistance with the med-

CHART 64-7

BEST PRACTICE *for*
Emergency Care of the Client During Myxedema Coma

- Maintain a patent airway.
- Replace fluids as ordered.
- Give levothyroxine sodium IV as ordered.
- Administer glucose IV as ordered.
- Administer corticosteroids as ordered.
- Check the client's temperature frequently.
- Monitor blood pressure.
- Cover the client with warm blankets.
- Monitor for changes in mental status.

CHART 64-8

NURSING FOCUS *on the* OLDER ADULT
Thyroid Problems

Teach the client the following facts about changes in the thyroid gland related to aging:

- The thyroid gland decreases in size with increasing age.
- Thyroid hormone secretion decreases with age, but the hormone level remains stable because cellular clearance of the hormone also decreases with age.
- The basal metabolic rate decreases with age, usually as a result of decreased activity. This decrease changes the body composition from predominantly muscular to predominantly fatty.
- Older clients require lower doses of replacement thyroid hormone. Too large a dose may adversely affect the heart muscle.

ication regimen. The nurse discusses this issue with the family and client and develops a plan for medication administration. One person should be clearly designated as responsible for medication preparation and administration so that doses are neither missed nor duplicated.

HEALTH CARE RESOURCES

Immediately after returning home, the client may require a support person to stay and provide more attention than could be given by a visiting nurse or home care aide. Contact with the health care team is necessary for follow-up and identification of potential problems. The client taking thyroid medication may have symptoms of hypothyroidism if the dosage is inadequate or symptoms of hyperthyroidism if the dose is too high. The nurse performs a focused assessment at every home visit to the client under treatment for thyroid dysfunction (Chart 64-9).

CRITICAL THINKING CHALLENGE

The 22-year-old nursing student is started on oral levothyroxine (Synthroid). She tells you that she is scheduled to take the NCLEX exam in 10 days.

- What teaching priorities for her medication regimen will you establish?
- How will she be able to tell whether or not the medication is effective?
- Should she take the NCLEX as currently scheduled? Why or why not?

For suggested answer guidelines, go to SIMON http://www.wbsaunders.com/SIMON/Iggy/.

CHART 64-9

FOCUSED ASSESSMENT *for* Home Care Clients with Thyroid Dysfunction

Assess cardiovascular status.
- Vital signs, including apical pulse, pulse pressure, presence or absence of orthostatic hypotension, and the quality and rhythm of peripheral pulses
- Presence or absence of peripheral edema
- Weight gain or loss

Assess cognition and mental status.
- Level of consciousness
- Orientation to time, place, and person
- Accurately reading a seven-word sentence containing no words greater than three syllables
- Can the client count backward from 100 by 3s?

Assess condition of skin and mucous membranes.
- Moistness of skin, most reliable on chest and back
- Skin temperature and color

Assess neuromuscular status.
- Reactivity of patellar and biceps reflexes
- Oral temperature
- Handgrip strength
- Steadiness of gait
- Presence or absence of fine tremors in the hand

Ask about the following:
- Sleep in the past 24 hours
- Client warm enough or too warm indoors
- 24-hour diet recall
- 24-hour activity recall
- Over-the-counter and prescribed medications taken
- Last bowel movement

Assess client's understanding of illness and compliance with treatment.
- Signs and symptoms to report to health care provider
- Medication plan (correct timing and dose)

Evaluation: Outcomes

NOC The nurse evaluates the care of the client with hypothyroidism on the basis of the identified nursing diagnoses and collaborative problems. The expected outcome is that the client will:

- Maintain normal cardiovascular function
- Maintain adequate respiratory function as evidenced by respiratory rate and depth WNL and pulse oximetry IER
- Experience improvement in thought processes

Thyroiditis

OVERVIEW

Thyroiditis is an inflammation of the thyroid gland. There are three types: acute, subacute, and chronic. Chronic thyroiditis (Hashimoto's disease) is the most common type.

Acute Thyroiditis

Acute thyroiditis, which is caused by bacterial invasion of the thyroid gland, is uncommon. Signs and symptoms include pain, neck tenderness, malaise, elevated temperature, and **dysphagia** (difficulty swallowing). This condition is treated symptomatically and usually responds to antibiotic therapy.

Subacute Thyroiditis

Subacute or granulomatous thyroiditis results from a viral infection of the thyroid gland, occasionally after a cold or other upper respiratory tract infection. Manifestations include fever, chills, dysphagia, and muscle and joint pain. Pain can radiate to the ears and the jaw. The thyroid gland feels hard and moderately enlarged on palpation. Thyroid function can remain normal, although hyperthyroidism or hypothyroidism may develop.

The client with mild subacute thyroiditis is managed with rest, fluids, and acetylsalicylic acid (aspirin). In more severe cases, corticosteroids are given to reduce inflammation.

Chronic Thyroiditis

Chronic thyroiditis (Hashimoto's disease) is a type of hypothyroidism that affects women more often than men, most commonly clients in their 30s to 50s. Hashimoto's disease is an autoimmune disorder. The thyroid becomes invaded with antithyroid antibodies and lymphocytes, causing thyroid tissue destruction. When large amounts of the gland are destroyed, serum thyroid hormone levels are low and secretion of thyroid-stimulating hormone is increased.

COLLABORATIVE MANAGEMENT

The clinical manifestations of Hashimoto's disease include dysphagia and painless enlargement of the gland. Diagnosis is based on the presence of circulating antithyroid antibodies and needle biopsy findings of the thyroid gland. Serum thyroid hormone levels, TSH levels, and radioactive iodine uptake (RAIU) vary depending on the stage of the disease.

The client is treated with thyroid hormone to prevent hypothyroidism and to suppress TSH secretion, thereby decreasing the size of the thyroid gland. Surgery (subtotal thyroidectomy) is necessary if the goiter does not respond to thyroid hormone, is disfiguring, or compresses other structures.

Nursing interventions focus on promoting client comfort and educating the client about hypothyroidism, medications, and surgery (see Surgical Management [Hyperthyroidism], p. 1428.)

Thyroid Cancer

OVERVIEW

There are four distinct types of thyroid cancer: papillary, follicular, medullary, and anaplastic. The initial clinical manifestation of thyroid cancer is a solitary, painless lump or nodule in the thyroid gland. Additional signs and symptoms depend on the presence and location of **metastasis** (spread of cancer cells).

Papillary Carcinoma

Papillary carcinoma, the most common type of thyroid cancer, is found more often in women and in clients younger than 40 years of age. It is a slow-growing tumor and can be present for years before spreading to nearby lymph nodes. When the tumor is confined to the thyroid gland, the chance for cure is good with a partial or total thyroidectomy.

Follicular Carcinoma

About 25% of all thyroid cancers are follicular carcinomas. This tumor primarily affects clients older than 50 years of age. The cancer invades blood vessels and spreads to bone and lung tissue. It rarely spreads to lymph nodes but can adhere to the trachea, neck muscles, great vessels, and skin, resulting in **dyspnea** (difficulty breathing) and **dysphagia** (difficulty swallowing). When the tumor involves the recurrent laryngeal nerves, the client may have a hoarse voice. The prognosis is fair when metastasis is minimal at the time of diagnosis.

Medullary Carcinoma

Medullary carcinoma accounts for 5% to 10% of all thyroid cancers and is more common in clients older than 50 years of age. Metastasis occurs through lymph nodes and invasion of surrounding structures. This tumor often occurs as part of multiple endocrine neoplasia (MEN) type II, a familial endocrine disorder. There is excessive secretion of calcitonin, adrenocorticotropic hormone (ACTH), prostaglandins, and serotonin.

Anaplastic Carcinoma

Anaplastic carcinoma is a rapid-growing, extremely aggressive tumor that directly invades nearby structures to cause symptoms of **stridor** (harsh, high-pitched respiratory sounds), hoarseness, and dysphagia. The prognosis is poor, and most clients die within a year after diagnosis. The client with anaplastic carcinoma may be treated with palliative surgery, radiation, or chemotherapy.

COLLABORATIVE MANAGEMENT

Surgery is the treatment of choice for papillary, follicular, and medullary carcinomas. A total thyroidectomy is usually performed with a nodal neck dissection if regional lymph nodes are involved. The physician prescribes postoperative suppressive doses of thyroid hormone for 3 months. A radioactive iodine uptake (RAIU) study is performed after medication is withdrawn. If there is RAI uptake, the client is treated with **ablative** (enough to destroy the tissue) amounts of RAI. If thyroid cancer does not respond to RAI, a course of chemotherapy is initiated.

PARATHYROID DISORDERS

Hyperparathyroidism

OVERVIEW

The parathyroid glands maintain calcium and phosphate balance (Figure 64-5). Serum calcium concentration is normally maintained within a narrow range; phosphate levels vary more widely. Increased levels of parathyroid hormone (PTH) act directly on the kidney, causing increased kidney reabsorption of calcium and increased phosphate excretion. These processes cause **hypercalcemia** (excessive calcium) and **hypophosphatemia** (inadequate phosphate) in the client with hyperparathyroidism.

In the bone, excessive PTH levels increase bone **resorption** (bone loss of calcium) by decreasing **osteoblastic** (bone production) activity and increasing **osteoclastic** (bone destruction) activity. This process releases calcium and phosphate into the circulation and demineralizes bone. When the normal solubility of calcium in the serum is exceeded, as in long-standing hypercalcemia, calcium is deposited in soft tissues.

Although the exact triggering mechanisms are unknown, *primary* hyperparathyroidism results when one or more parathyroid glands does not respond to the normal feedback of serum calcium. In 80% to 85% of the cases, the cause is a benign tumor in one parathyroid gland. Table 64-4 lists other causes of hyperparathyroidism.

COLLABORATIVE MANAGEMENT

Assessment

The nurse asks about the client's symptoms and any bone fractures, recent weight loss, arthritis, or psychologic distress. Any history of radiation treatment to the head or neck is also

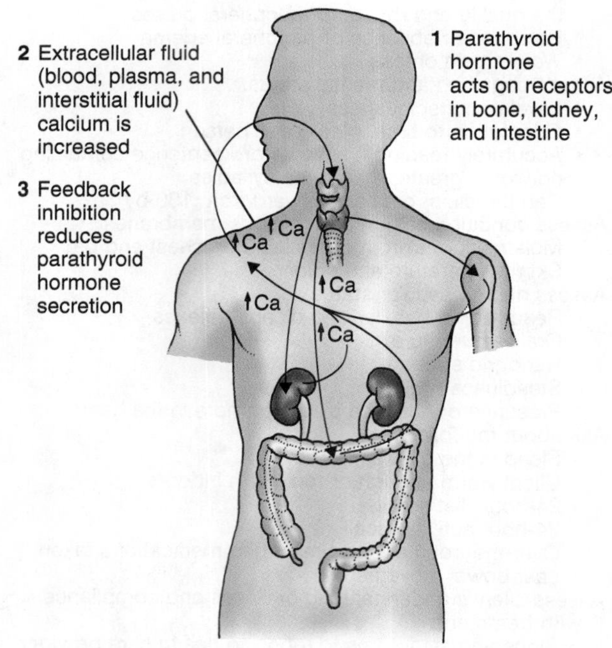

Figure 64-5 ● The physiologic actions of parathyroid hormone.

obtained. The client with long-standing disease may have a waxy pallor of the skin and bone deformities in the extremities and back.

The clinical features of hyperparathyroidism may be related either to the effects of excessive PTH or to the effects of the accompanying hypercalcemia.

High levels of PTH cause **renal calculi** (kidney stones) and **nephrocalcinosis** (deposits of calcium in the soft tissue of the kidney). Bone lesions are due to an increased rate of bone destruction and result in pathologic fractures, bone cysts, and osteoporosis in advanced cases.

Gastrointestinal manifestations (e.g., anorexia, nausea, vomiting, epigastric pain, constipation, and weight loss) are common, particularly when serum calcium levels are high. **Hypergastrinemia** (elevated serum gastrin levels) is caused by hypercalcemia and leads to peptic ulcer disease. Fatigue and lethargy may be present and become more severe as the serum calcium levels increase. When serum calcium levels are greater than 12 mg/dL, the client may have psychosis with mental confusion, which leads to coma and death if left untreated. (See Chapter 13 for more information on the effects of hypercalcemia.)

Serum PTH, calcium, and phosphate levels and urine cyclic adenosine monophosphate (cAMP) are the most commonly used laboratory tests to detect hyperparathyroidism (Chart 64-10). X-rays may show kidney stones, calcium deposits, and bone lesions, such as cysts or fractures. Generalized bone demineralization and resorption in the long bones occur in the client with chronic hyperparathyroidism. Other diagnostic tests include arteriography, computed tomography (CT), venous catheterization of the thyroid veins with sampling of the blood for PTH levels, and ultrasonography. The nurse explains the procedures and cares for the client undergoing diagnostic tests.

TABLE 64-4 • CAUSES OF PARATHYROID DYSFUNCTION

CAUSES OF HYPERPARATHYROIDISM
- Parathyroid adenoma
- Parathyroid carcinoma
- Congenital hyperplasia
- Neck trauma or radiation
- Vitamin D deficiency
- Chronic renal failure with hypocalcemia
- Parathyroid hormone-secreting carcinomas of the lung, kidney, or gastrointestinal tract

CAUSES OF HYPOPARATHYROIDISM
- Surgical or radiation-induced thyroid ablation
- Parathyroidectomy
- Congenital dysgenesis
- Idiopathic (autoimmune) hypoparathyroidism
- Hypomagnesemia

Interventions

NONSURGICAL MANAGEMENT

DIURETIC AND FLUID THERAPY. The most common therapy for reducing serum calcium levels in clients who are not candidates for surgery is hydration and furosemide (Lasix, Uritol♣), a diuretic that increases kidney excretion of calcium. IV saline in large volumes also promotes renal calcium excretion.

The nurse monitors cardiac function and intake and output every 2 to 4 hours during hydration therapy. Continuous cardiac monitoring may be required. The nurse closely monitors serum calcium levels and immediately reports any precipitous drop to the physician. Sudden drops in calcium levels may cause tingling and numbness in the muscles.

DRUG THERAPY. When hydration and furosemide cannot reduce hypercalcemia, or if it becomes necessary to discontinue IV fluids, additional medications can help to reduce the clinical manifestations of hyperparathyroidism, especially those related to hypercalcemia.

Phosphates. Oral phosphates inhibit bone resorption and interfere with calcium absorption. IV phosphates are used only when serum calcium levels must be lowered rapidly.

Calcitonin. Calcitonin decreases skeletal calcium release and increases the kidney excretion of calcium. Calcitonin is not effective when used alone because of its short duration of action. Its therapeutic effects are greatly enhanced if given in conjunction with glucocorticoids.

Calcium Chelators. Some drugs lower calcium levels by binding **(chelating)** calcium, which reduces the levels of free calcium. Mithramycin, a cytotoxic agent, is the most effective and potent calcium chelator used to lower serum calcium levels. In most clients a single IV dose of 10 to 15 mg/kg of body weight by slow infusion can lower serum calcium levels within 48 hours. However, the toxic effects limit its use to two or three doses. **Thrombocytopenia** (decreased circulating platelets and an increased tendency to bleed) and kidney and

CHART 64-10

LABORATORY PROFILE
Parathyroid Function

Test	Normal Range for Adults	Significance of Abnormal Findings: Hyperthyroidism	Hypothyroidism
Serum calcium	Total: 8.6-10.0 mg/dL, or 2.20-2.55 SI units Ionized (active): 4.64-5.28 mg/dL, or 1.16-1.32 SI units	Increased in primary hyperparathyroidism	Decreased
Serum phosphate	2.7-4.5 mg/dL, or 0.87-1.45 SI units *Older adults:* May be slightly lower	Decreased	Increased
Serum parathyroid hormone	<2000 pg/mL	Increased	Decreased
Urinary cAMP	1-11.5 μmol/dL	Increased	Decreased

cAMP, Cyclic adenosine monophosphate; *SI,* System Internationale.

liver toxicity can result after only one dose. Liver function studies, blood urea nitrogen and creatinine, complete blood count (CBC), and serum calcium levels are closely monitored in the client receiving mithramycin. Another calcium chelator is penicillamine (Cuprimine, Pendramine).

SURGICAL MANAGEMENT. Surgical management of hyperparathyroidism involves a parathyroidectomy.

PREOPERATIVE CARE. Before parathyroidectomy, the client is stabilized and calcium levels are decreased to near-normal. If mithramycin has been used to lower serum calcium levels, the physician orders studies to determine bleeding and clotting times and orders a CBC to determine bone marrow function.

The nurse advises the client that coughing and deep-breathing exercises should be performed postoperatively and that talking may be painful for the first day or two after surgery. The nurse demonstrates neck support by having the client place both hands behind the neck to assist in elevating the head.

OPERATIVE PROCEDURES. Using general anesthesia and with the client's neck hyperextended, the surgeon makes a transverse incision in the lower neck. After the muscles are retracted, both sides of the neck are examined to evaluate all four parathyroid glands. Starting on one side, the surgeon examines the glands for enlargement. If only one gland on that side is enlarged, a frozen section is done on both glands. If a tumor is present on one side but the other side is normal, the surgeon removes the tumor and leaves the remaining gland intact.

POSTOPERATIVE CARE. The nurse observes the client for signs of respiratory distress, which may be due to compression of the trachea by hemorrhage or swelling of neck tissues. The nurse ensures that emergency equipment, including suction, oxygen, and tracheostomy equipment, is at the bedside. If severe swelling occurs, the surgeon may need to remove clips from the incision to preserve the airway. The nurse monitors vital signs, identifies any change in status, and checks the neck dressing for abnormal amounts of drainage or bleeding. A small amount (1 to 5 mL) of drainage is normal.

The remaining glands, which may be nonfunctional as a result of PTH overproduction, require several days to several weeks to return to normal function. A hypocalcemic crisis can occur during this critical period. Serum calcium levels are determined immediately after surgery and are monitored every 4 hours until calcium levels stabilize. The nurse monitors for signs and symptoms of hypocalcemia, such as tingling and twitching in the extremities and face. The nurse checks for Trousseau's and Chvostek's signs, either of which signal potential tetany (see Chapter 13).

Damage to the recurrent laryngeal nerve is rare, but the nurse assesses the client for persistent changes in voice patterns and hoarseness.

When hyperparathyroidism is due to **hyperplasia** (tissue overgrowth), three glands plus half of the fourth gland are usually removed; the remaining portion of the fourth gland is tagged to make it easy to find if future surgery is necessary. If all four glands are removed, a small portion of a gland may be implanted in the forearm, where it produces PTH and maintains calcium homeostasis. If all of these maneuvers fail, the client will need lifelong treatment with calcium and vitamin D because the resulting hypoparathyroidism is permanent.

Hypoparathyroidism

OVERVIEW

Hypoparathyroidism is an uncommon endocrine disorder in which parathyroid function is decreased. Problems are directly related to a lack of parathyroid hormone (PTH) secretion or to decreased effectiveness of PTH on target tissue. Whether the problem is a lack of PTH secretion or an ineffectiveness of PTH on tissues, the result is the same—hypocalcemia.

Iatrogenic hypoparathyroidism, the most common form, is caused by the removal of all parathyroid tissue during total thyroidectomy or by deliberate surgical removal of the parathyroid glands.

Idiopathic hypoparathyroidism is a rare condition that can occur spontaneously. The exact cause is unknown, but an autoimmune basis is suspected because antiparathyroid antibodies are present in many affected clients. In addition, hypoparathyroidism is often associated with the following autoimmune disorders: adrenal insufficiency, hypothyroidism, diabetes mellitus, pernicious anemia, gonadal failure, and vitiligo.

Hypomagnesemia (decreased serum magnesium levels) may also cause hypoparathyroidism. Hypomagnesemia is seen in alcoholics and in clients with malabsorption syndromes, chronic renal disease, and malnutrition. It causes impairment of PTH secretion and may interfere with PTH effects on the bones and kidneys.

COLLABORATIVE MANAGEMENT

Assessment

The nurse begins assessment of the client with suspected hypoparathyroidism by asking about any head or neck surgery or radiation therapy, because these treatments may cause hypoparathyroidism. The client is asked about the signs and symptoms of hypoparathyroidism, which may range from mild tingling and numbness to tetany. Tingling and numbness around the mouth or in the hands and feet reflect mild to moderate hypocalcemia. Severe muscle cramps, carpopedal spasms, and seizures (with no loss of consciousness or incontinence) reflect a more severe hypocalcemia. The client or caregiver may notice mental changes ranging from irritability to psychosis.

The physical assessment may show excessive or inappropriate muscle contractions that cause finger, hand, and elbow flexion; this can signal an impending attack of tetany. The nurse checks for Chvostek's sign and Trousseau's sign; positive responses indicate potential tetany. A parkinsonian-like syndrome may be evident. The presence of cataracts denotes chronic hypocalcemia. Bands or pits may encircle the crowns of the teeth, which indicates a loss of calcium from the teeth and causes enamel loss. The roots of the client's teeth may be defective.

Diagnostic tests for hypoparathyroidism include electroencephalography (EEG), blood tests, and computed tomography (CT). EEG changes are nonspecific and revert to normal with correction of hypocalcemia. Serum calcium, phosphate, magnesium, vitamin D, and urine cyclic adenosine monophosphate (cAMP) levels may be used in the diagnostic workup for hypoparathyroidism (see Chart 64-9). The CT scan can show brain calcifications, which indicate chronic hypocalcemia.

Interventions

Management of hypoparathyroidism focuses on correcting hypocalcemia, vitamin D deficiency, and hypomagnesemia. For clients with acute and severe hypocalcemia, IV calcium is administered as a 10% solution of calcium chloride or calcium gluconate over 10 to 15 minutes. Acute vitamin D deficiency is treated with calcitriol (Rocaltrol), 0.5 to 2.0 mg/day. Acute hypomagnesemia is corrected with 50% magnesium sulfate in 2-mL doses (up to 4 g/day) either intramuscularly or intravenously. Long-term oral therapy for hypocalcemia involves the administration of calcium, 0.5 to 2.0 g/day in divided doses.

Long-term therapy for vitamin D deficiency is 50,000 to 400,000 units of ergocalciferol daily. The dosage is adjusted to keep the client's calcium level in the low-normal range (slightly hypocalcemic), enough to prevent symptoms of hypocalcemia. It must also be low enough to prevent increased urine calcium concentrations, which can lead to stone formation.

Nursing management includes teaching about the medication regimen and interventions to reduce anxiety. The client is instructed to eat foods high in calcium but low in phosphorus. Milk, yogurt, and processed cheeses are avoided because of their high phosphorus content. *The nurse stresses that therapy for hypocalcemia is lifelong.* The client is advised to use some form of identification, such as a MedicAlert bracelet or a wallet card. With adherence to the prescribed drug and diet regimen, the calcium level usually remains high enough to prevent a hypocalcemic crisis.

ONLINE RESOURCES

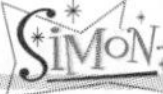

For suggested readings and Internet resources, go to http://www.wbsaunders.com/SIMON/Iggy/.

SELECTED BIBLIOGRAPHY

Asterisk indicates a classic or definitive work on this subject.

American Cancer Society. (2001). *Cancer facts and figures 2001.* Atlanta: Author; 01-300M-No. 5008.01.

Assessing thyroid disorder in women. (1998). *AWHONN Lifelines, 2*(5), 14.

Braverman, L., Dworkin, H., & Macindoe, J. (1997). Thyroid disease: When to screen, when to treat. *Patient Care, 31*(6), 18-20, 29, 34.

Clement, B. (1998). Parathyroid pathophysiology. *Seminars in Perioperative Nursing, 7*(3), 186-192.

Cotran, R., Kumar, V., & Collins, T. (1999). *Robbins' pathologic basis of disease* (6th ed.). Philadelphia: W.B. Saunders.

Elliott, B. (2000). Diagnosing and treating hypothyroidism. *The Nurse Practitioner, 25*(3), 92-105.

Goldsmith, C. (1999). Hypothyroidism. *American Journal of Nursing, 99*(6), 42-43.

Guyton, A., & Hall, J. (2000). *Textbook of medical physiology* (10th ed.). Philadelphia: W.B. Saunders.

*Kennedy, L.W., & Caro, J.F. (1996). The ABCs of managing hyperthyroidism in the older patient. *Geriatrics, 51*(5), 22-24, 27, 31, 32.

Klein, I., & Ojamaa, K. (2001). Thyroid hormone and the cardiovascular system. *New England Journal of Medicine, 344*(7), 501-509.

Larsen, P.R., Davies, T., & Hay, I. (1998). The thyroid gland. In J. Wilson et al. (Eds.). *William's textbook of endocrinology* (9th ed., pp. 389-515). Philadelphia: W.B. Saunders.

McCloskey, J.C., & Bulechek, G.M. (2000). *Nursing interventions classification (NIC)* (3rd ed.). St. Louis: Mosby.

Mead, M. (2000). Thyroid function tests. *Practice Nurse, 19*(6), 283.

Michalek, A., Mahoney, M., & Calebaugh, D. (2000). Hypothyroidism and diabetes mellitus in an American Indian population. *Journal of Family Practice, 49*(7), 638-640.

Mitchell, S. (1997). Thyroid eye disease: A patient's point of view. *Ophthalmic Nursing: International Journal of Ophthalmic Nursing, 1*(3), 14-16.

Payton, R., Gardner, R., & Reynolds, D. (1997). Pharmacologic considerations and management of common endocrine disorders in women. *Journal of Nurse-Midwifery, 42*(3), 186-206.

Sagre, G., & Brown, E. (1998). Measurement of hormones. In J. Wilson et al. (Eds.). *William's textbook of endocrinology* (9th ed.). (pp. 43-54). Philadelphia: W.B. Saunders.

Screening for thyroid disease: The latest guidelines. (1998). *Consultant, 38*(10), 2447-2448.

The thyroid "neck check": Thyroid blues. (1998). *ORL: Head and Neck Nursing, 16*(2), 31.

Trotto, N. (1999). Hypothyroidism, hyperthyroidism, hyperparathyroidism. *Patient Care, 33*(14), 186-188, 191, 195-200.

United States Pharmacopeia Dispensing Information (USP DI): Vol. I. Drug information for the health care professional (2000). (20th ed.). Englewood, CO: Micromedix.

Wallace, K., & Hofmann, M. (1998). Thyroid dysfunction: How to manage overt and subclinical disease in older patients. *Geriatrics, 53*(4), 32-41.

Walpert, N. (1998). The highs and lows of autoimmune thyroid disease. *Nursing98, 28*(12), 58-60.

Young, J. (1999). Myxedema coma. *Nursing99, 29*(1), 64.

CHAPTER 65

Interventions for Clients with Diabetes Mellitus

M. ELAINE McLEOD

Learning Objectives

After studying this chapter, you should be able to:

1. Compare and contrast the age of onset, clinical manifestations, and pathologic mechanisms of type 1 and type 2 diabetes mellitus.
2. Identify clients at risk for developing type 2 diabetes mellitus.
3. Explain the effects of insulin on carbohydrate, protein, and fat metabolism.
4. Evaluate laboratory data to determine whether the client is using the prescribed dietary, medication, and exercise interventions for diabetes.
5. Explain the effect of aerobic exercise on blood glucose levels.
6. Describe the significance of the presence of ketone bodies in the urine of a diabetic client.
7. Use the exchange system to plan a menu for a client with diabetes who is prescribed to eat 1800 calories per day, divided into three meals and a snack, with 15% of calories from fat, 20% of calories from protein, and the remaining calories from carbohydrate sources.
8. Compare the mechanisms of action of the sulfonylureas, biguanides, alpha-glucosidase inhibitors, meglitinides, thiazolidinediones, and D-phenylalanine derivatives as antidiabetic agents.
9. Explain the effect of hypertension on the development of diabetic nephropathy and diabetic retinopathy.
10. Identify clients at risk for the development of hypoglycemia.
11. Prioritize nursing interventions for the client with mild to moderate hypoglycemia and moderate to severe hypoglycemia.
12. Identify clients at risk for developing diabetic ketoacidosis (DKA).
13. Prioritize nursing interventions for clients with DKA.
14. Identify clients at risk for developing hyperglycemic-hyperosmolar nonketotic syndrome (HHNS).
15. Prioritize nursing interventions for clients with HHNS.
16. Use laboratory data and clinical manifestations to determine the effectiveness of the interventions for DKA and HHNS.
17. Describe the steps required for subcutaneous insulin administration.
18. Describe the correct technique to use when mixing different types of insulin within the same syringe.
19. Compare and contrast the clinical manifestations of hyperglycemia and hypoglycemia.
20. Perform foot assessment and foot care for the client with diabetes.

SIMON

Go to http://www.wbsaunders.com/SIMON/Iggy/ for self-assessment questions related to these Learning Objectives.

Diabetes mellitus is a common chronic disease requiring lifelong behavioral and lifestyle changes. Diabetes is best managed with an interdisciplinary team approach that helps empower the client to successfully manage his or her disease. As part of the team, the nurse plans, organizes, and coordinates care among the various health disciplines involved; provides care and education; and promotes the client's health and well-being. The Evidence-Based Practice for Nursing box on p. 1441 provides an example of the effects of team intervention on diabetes management.

OVERVIEW

Diabetes is a major public health problem worldwide. The complications of the disease cause many devastating health problems. The financial cost of diabetes is discussed in the Cost of Care box on p. 1441. In the United States, diabetes is the leading cause of new cases of blindness, end-stage renal disease requiring dialysis or transplantation, and lower limb amputations. A large percentage of the U.S. population with diabetes is undiagnosed, and many of those who are diagnosed have unacceptably high blood glucose levels. Studies

EVIDENCE-BASED PRACTICE FOR NURSING

Teamwork for diabetes treatment pays off!

Koproski, J., Pretto, Z., & Poretsky, L. (1997). Effect of an intervention by a diabetes team in hospitalized patients with diabetes. *Diabetes Care, 20*(10): 1553-1555.

A randomized controlled trial was conducted to determine the effects of a diabetes team on length of hospital stay, glucose control, and readmission rates in hospitalized clients with diabetes. The study was conducted at a 492-bed community teaching hospital in New York City. Clients with concurrent or new-onset diabetes from November 1993 through November 1994 were selected for the study. There were 85 clients in the intervention group and 94 in the control group. A diabetes nurse educator and an endocrinologist visited clients in the intervention group daily. The client's plan of care was discussed with the primary care physician, and consultations were requested with a dietitian and social worker as needed. The control group received care in the "usual manner." Measures were obtained for length of stay, blood glucose control, insulin administration and blood glucose monitoring instructions, nutrition and social service consults, and readmission rates.

Clients in the intervention group received more education about diabetes. Documented instructions for blood glucose monitoring were present in 89% of cases in the intervention group as opposed to 57% in the control group. Documented instructions for insulin administration were present in 69% of the charts of the intervention group as opposed to 25% of the charts in the control group. Eighty-seven percent of clients had documentation of education of any kind in the intervention group as compared with 37% in the control group. Seventy-six percent of clients in the intervention group had nutrition consultation as compared with 40% in the control group. There was no difference in the amount of social worker contact.

Clients treated by the diabetes team had shorter lengths of stay, achieved better glycemic control early in the study, and demonstrated a significant reduction in readmission rates. Clients with a primary diagnosis of diabetes had a median length of stay of 5.5 days in the intervention group as compared with 7.5 days in the control group. The percentage of clients with "good" blood glucose control (75% of capillary blood glucose readings between 80 and 180 mg/dL) was 75% for the intervention group as compared with 46% in the control group during the first month of the program. In the intervention group 15% were readmitted within 3 months after discharge as compared with 32% in the control group.

Critique. Characteristics of the client population may have biased results of the study. There was a significant difference between the initial blood glucose levels between the two groups. The admission blood glucose levels were significantly higher in the intervention group, indicating that initial glycemic control was worse. Clients in the intervention group were younger. Younger diabetic clients tend to have acute illness that resolves quickly with treatment. They also tend not to have the number of chronic complications of diabetes. It is also difficult to prevent readmission of an older diabetic client with multiple chronic complications of diabetes.

Implications for Nursing. Clients in the intervention group clearly had more education documented and had more nutrition consultation than did the control group. Improved statistics for the implementation group are due in part to education provided by a multidisciplinary team. The nurse is an integral part of that team.

confirm that **glycemic** (blood glucose) control reduces complications of diabetes.

Today, interventions exist to reduce the incidence of blindness, drug therapy can reduce the incidence of kidney and coronary artery disease, and regular evaluation of the feet can reduce the incidence of amputation. The challenge for the nurse is to assist the client with diabetes in achieving and maintaining tight glycemic control so that long-term chronic complications are prevented.

COST OF CARE IMPLICATIONS FOR NURSING

DIABETES MELLITUS

Cost of Care

- The economic burden of diabetes mellitus in the United States is enormous. Direct medical expenses attributed to diabetes in 1997 totaled $44.1 billion. This figure includes $7.7 billion for diabetes and acute glycemic care, $11.8 billion for high prevalence of related chronic conditions, and $24.6 billion for high prevalence of general medical conditions (American Diabetes Association, 1999b).
- Medical care for diabetic clients accounts for 10% to 15% of all health care costs in the United States and 25% of all Medicare costs (Roman & Harris, 1997).
- The cost of diabetes is shared by all citizens, not just those with diabetes. In the United States, 60% of the medical costs for diabetic care are paid for with public money through agencies such as Medicare, Medicaid, and the Veterans Administration (Harris, 1998).
- Adults with diabetes are hospitalized more frequently and have longer hospital stays than nondiabetic individuals. Results of the National Medical Expenditure Survey indicated that the average per capita cost each year was over $11,000 for people with diabetes as compared with $2,600 for those without diabetes, with about 64% of the cost being due to inpatient hospitalization (Harris, 1998).

Implications for Nursing

If costs related to diabetes are to be reduced, attention must be directed to the prevention and treatment of chronic complications of diabetes. Therapies are available to reduce the incidence of blindness, medications are available to reduce the incidence of kidney and coronary artery disease, and regular sensory evaluation of the foot will reduce the incidence of amputation. The challenge for the nurse is to assist the diabetic client in achieving and maintaining meticulous glycemic control so that long-term chronic complications are prevented.

Data from American Diabetes Association. (1999). Reviews: Economic consequences of diabetes mellitus in the U.S. *Diabetes Care,* 22(2), 296-309; Harris, M. I. (1998). Diabetes in America: Epidemiology and scope of the problem. *Diabetes Care,* 21(suppl 3), 11-14; and Roman, S. H. & Harris, M. I. (1997). Management of diabetes mellitus from a public health perspective. *Endocrinology and Metabolism Clinics for North America,* 26(3), 443-474.

Pathophysiology

CLASSIFICATION OF DIABETES

For all types of diabetes mellitus, the main feature is chronic **hyperglycemia** (high blood glucose level) resulting from problems with insulin secretion, insulin action, or both. The disease is classified by age of onset, the underlying problem causing a lack of insulin, and the severity of the deficiency. Table 65-1 outlines the different types of diabetes.

THE ENDOCRINE PANCREAS

The endocrine portion of the pancreas consists of about 1 million small glands, the **islets of Langerhans,** scattered throughout the gland. The islet cells compose only a small portion of the gland, with most of the gland having exocrine functions for digestive processes. Four types of islet cells have been identified: alpha, beta, D, and F. Glucagon is produced by alpha cells, insulin is produced by beta cells, somatostatin is produced by D cells, and pancreatic polypeptide

TABLE 65-1 • CLASSIFICATION OF DIABETES MELLITUS

TYPE 1 DIABETES
- Primary beta-cell destruction leading to absolute insulin deficiency
  - Autoimmune process
  - Idiopathic

TYPE 2 DIABETES
- Ranges from insulin resistance with an insulin deficiency to secretory deficit with insulin resistance

OTHER SPECIFIC TYPES (CONDITIONS RESULTING IN HYPERGLYCEMIA)
- Genetic defects of beta-cell function
- Genetic defects in insulin action
- Diseases of the exocrine pancreas: pancreatitis, trauma, neoplasia, cystic fibrosis, hemochromatosis
- Endocrinopathies: acromegaly, Cushing's disease, glucagonoma, pheochromocytoma, hyperthyroidism, aldosteronoma
- Drug- or chemical-induced conditions (from use of pentamidine, nicotinic acid, glucocorticoids, thyroid hormone, diazoxide, beta-adrenergic agonists, thiazides, Dilantin, interferon-alpha, other drugs)
- Infections: congenital rubella, cytomegalovirus
- Uncommon forms of immune-related diabetes
- Other genetic syndromes associated with diabetes: Down syndrome, Klinefelter's syndrome, Turner's syndrome, Huntington's chorea, and others

GESTATIONAL DIABETES MELLITUS (GDM)
- Carbohydrate intolerance is first recognized during pregnancy.
- Children of mothers with GDM are at greater risk for neonatal mortality, congenital malformation, and macrosomia (large body size).
- Studies indicate that children of mothers with GDM have an increased risk of obesity and impaired glucose tolerance later in life.
- Clients with GDM are at high risk for developing diabetes after pregnancy.
- Diagnosis is based on the results of a 100-g oral glucose tolerance test during pregnancy.

Data from American Diabetes Association. (2000). Committee Report: Report of the Expert Committee on the Diagnosis and Classification of Diabetes Mellitus. *Diabetes Care,* 23(Suppl. 1), 4-19; and American Diabetes Association. (2000). Position statement: Gestational diabetes mellitus. *Diabetes Care, 23*(Suppl. 1), 77-79.

is produced by F cells. This chapter focuses on the activity of glucagon and insulin. **Glucagon** is a major "counterregulatory" hormone that has actions opposite those of insulin and releases glucose from cell storage sites whenever blood glucose levels are low. **Insulin** plays a key role in allowing body cells to store and use carbohydrate, fat, and protein.

INSULIN PHYSIOLOGY

Insulin is a protein made up of 51 amino acids contained within two peptide chains: an alpha chain with 21 amino acids and a beta chain with 30 amino acids. **Preproinsulin** is produced initially. This protein is known as a **precursor molecule** because it is inactive and must be modified and made smaller to eventually become the active hormone insulin. Preproinsulin is cut by enzymes to proinsulin (a precursor that includes the alpha and beta chains of the insulin molecule) and an additional fragment called the C-peptide chain. In the islet cells, proinsulin is converted into equal amounts of insulin and C-peptide (Figure 65-1). C-peptide is not active and can

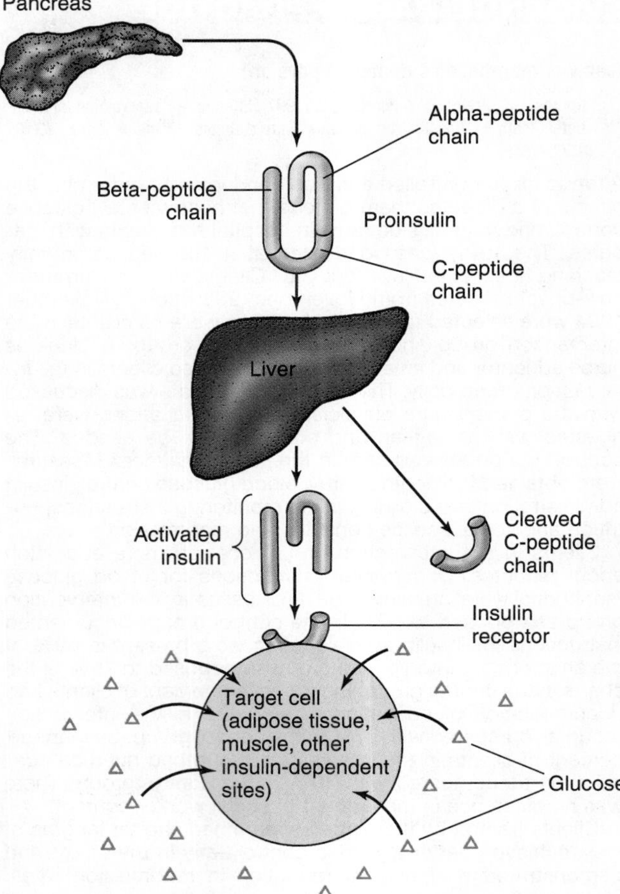

Figure 65-1 ● Proinsulin, secreted by and stored in the beta cells of the islets of Langerhans in the pancreas, is transformed by the liver into activated insulin. Insulin attaches to receptors on target cells, where it promotes glucose transport into the cells through the cell membranes.

be used to measure the rate that pancreatic beta cells are secreting insulin.

The action of insulin allows glucose in the blood to move into cells to make energy. Thus insulin is like a key to unlock cell membrane entryways for glucose. Insulin action starts by binding to insulin receptors on the membranes of target cells. The liver is the first major organ to be reached by insulin in the blood. In the liver, insulin promotes tissue-building metabolism **(anabolism)** by causing both the production and storage of glycogen **(glycogenesis)** at the same time that it inhibits glycogen breakdown into glucose **(glycogenolysis).** Insulin increases protein and **lipid** (fat) synthesis and very-low-density lipoprotein (VLDL) formation. Insulin inhibits tissue-degrading metabolism **(catabolism)** by inhibiting liver glycogenolysis, **ketogenesis** (conversion of fats to acids), and **gluconeogenesis** (conversion of proteins to glucose). In muscle, insulin promotes protein and glycogen synthesis. In fat cells, insulin promotes the storage of triglycerides. Overall, insulin keeps blood glucose levels from becoming too high and also helps maintain blood lipid levels in the normal range.

The pancreas secretes about 40 to 50 units of insulin per day. Insulin is secreted directly into liver circulation in a **biphasic** (two-step) manner. Insulin is secreted at low levels during the fasting state **(basal insulin secretion)** and at increased levels after eating **(prandial).** There is an early burst of insulin secretion within 10 minutes of eating, followed by a progressively increasing phase of insulin release that lasts as long as hyperglycemia is present.

GLUCOSE HOMEOSTASIS

Glucose is the primary fuel for the central nervous system (CNS). Because the brain cannot produce or store much glucose, a continuous supply from the body's circulation is needed. Outside the CNS, fatty acids can be used as fuel for energy formation (Halperin & Goldstein, 1999). The circulating fuels of glucose and free fatty acids are stored inside cells as glycogen in the liver and muscles and as triglyceride in fat cells. Fat, in the form of triglyceride, is the most efficient means of storing energy. Fat has 9 calories of stored energy per gram, whereas protein and carbohydrate have only 4 calories per gram. Although protein can be degraded for fuel use during starvation, protein is not used for fuel under normal conditions.

The combined actions of insulin and counterregulatory hormones (discussed in the next section) keep blood glucose within the range of 65 to 105 mg/dL (3.6 to 5.8 mmol/L) to supply glucose for CNS functions. When glucose levels fall, insulin secretion stops and glucagon release is stimulated. Glucagon causes the release of glucose from the liver. Liver glucose is made available through **glycogenolysis** (breakdown of glycogen to glucose) and gluconeogenesis. When glucose is unavailable, **lipolysis** (breakdown of fat) and **proteolysis** (breakdown of amino acids) occur to provide fuel for energy.

Counterregulatory hormones increase blood levels of glucose by actions opposite those of insulin when more energy is needed. Glucagon is the main counterregulatory hormone. Other hormones that increase blood glucose levels are epinephrine, norepinephrine, growth hormone, and cortisol. In type 1 diabetes, glucagon secretion in response to hypoglycemia is lost, increasing the risk for severe hypoglycemic reactions.

ABSENCE OF INSULIN

The lack of insulin in diabetes, either from lack of insulin production or from a problem with the use of insulin at its cell receptor, prevents some cells from using glucose as an energy source. Insulin is needed to supply glucose to most of the body's tissues. Without insulin, the body enters a serious state of breaking down body fat and protein. Levels of counterregulatory hormones increase in an attempt to increase the availability of glucose from other sources. Table 65-2 outlines the body's response to insufficient insulin.

Without insulin, glucose builds up in the blood, causing **hyperglycemia** (high blood glucose levels). Hyperglycemia causes fluid and electrolyte imbalances, leading to the classic symptoms of diabetes: *polyuria, polydipsia,* and *polyphagia.*

Polyuria (frequent and excessive urination) results from an osmotic diuresis caused by excess glucose in the urine. As a result of diuresis, sodium, chloride, and potassium are excreted in the urine in large amounts, accompanied by severe water loss. The resulting dehydration stimulates the thirst mechanism, and **polydipsia** (excessive thirst) occurs. Because the cells are not receiving any food (glucose), the sense of cell starvation results in **polyphagia** (excessive eating). In spite of eating vast amounts of food, the person remains in a state of starvation until insulin is available to move glucose into the cells.

TABLE 65-2 • PHYSIOLOGIC RESPONSE TO INSUFFICIENT INSULIN

- Decreased glycogenesis (conversion of glucose to glycogen)
- Increased glycogenolysis (conversion of glycogen to glucose)
- Increased gluconeogenesis (formation of glucose from non-carbohydrate sources, such as amino acids and lactate)
- Increased lipolysis (breakdown of triglycerides to glycerol and free fatty acids)
- Increased ketogenesis (formation of ketones from free fatty acids)
- Proteolysis (breakdown of protein with amino acid release in muscles)

With insulin deficiency, fats break down **(lipolysis),** releasing free fatty acids. Conversion of free fatty acids to **ketone bodies** (small acids) provides a backup energy source. Because ketone bodies, or "ketones," are incomplete and abnormal degradation products of free fatty acids, they are not further metabolized and may accumulate in the blood when insulin is not available. This accumulation causes metabolic acidosis.

Because of the dehydration associated with diabetes mellitus, **hemoconcentration** (increased blood concentration) and **hypovolemia** (decreased blood volume) develop, leading to **hyperviscosity** (thick, concentrated blood) and **hypoperfusion** (decreased circulation) of tissues and poor tissue oxygenation **(hypoxia).** Hypoxic cells are unable to metabolize glucose efficiently, the Kreb's cycle is blocked, and lactic acid accumulates, causing more acidosis. Restoring tissue perfusion and oxygenation by treating the lack of insulin is the key to halting lactic acid production.

The excess acids present during a lack of insulin increase the hydrogen ion (H^+) and carbon dioxide (CO_2) concentrations of the blood and other extracellular fluids. These products stimulate the respiratory control areas of the brain to increase the rate and depth of respiration in an attempt to excrete more carbon dioxide and acid. This type of breathing is known as **Kussmaul respiration.** Acetone is exhaled, giving the breath a "fruity" odor. When the lungs can no longer offset acidosis, the pH drops. Arterial blood gas studies show a primary **metabolic acidosis** (decreased pH accompanied by decreased arterial bicarbonate [HCO_3] levels) and **compensatory respiratory alkalosis** (decreased partial pressure of arterial carbon dioxide [$Paco_2$]) (see Chapter 16).

The absence of insulin causes total-body potassium depletion. Because of the increased fluid loss with hyperglycemia, excessive potassium is excreted in the urine, leading to *low* serum potassium levels. However, *high* serum potassium levels may occur in acidosis because of the shift of potassium from inside the cells to the blood and other extracellular fluids. Serum potassium levels in diabetes, then, may be low **(hypokalemia),** elevated **(hyperkalemia),** or even normal, depending on hydration, the severity of the acidosis, and the client's response to treatment. Chapters 15 and 16 discuss acid-base balance and acidosis in more detail.

ACUTE COMPLICATIONS OF DIABETES

Three emergencies related to abnormal blood glucose levels can occur in clients who have diabetes: **diabetic ketoacidosis**

(DKA) caused by lack of insulin and ketosis; **hyperglycemic-hyperosmolar nonketotic syndrome (HHNS)** associated with insulin deficiency, profound dehydration, and the absence of ketosis; and **hypoglycemia** occurring when too much insulin or too little glucose is present. *All three conditions require emergency treatment and can result in death if inappropriately treated or not treated at all.* The bases for these complications, along with the appropriate interventions, are described in the next section.

CHRONIC COMPLICATIONS OF DIABETES

Diabetes mellitus is a major risk factor for morbidity and mortality because of changes in the larger or generalized body blood vessels **(macrovascular),** as well as changes in small blood vessels **(microvascular)** within tissues and organs. These blood vessel changes lead to many complications as a result of poor tissue circulation and cell death. *Macrovascular* complications, including coronary heart disease, cerebrovascular disease, and peripheral vascular disease, are responsible for increased early death among diabetic clients as compared with the general population. *Microvascular* complications involve abnormalities of blood vessel wall structure and function, leading to nephropathy (kidney dysfunction), neuropathy (nerve dysfunction), and retinopathy (vision problems). Three theories have been used to explain the cause and progression of diabetic vascular complications:

- Chronic hyperglycemia causes irreversible structural changes resulting in basement membrane thickening and organ damage.
- Glucose toxicity directly or indirectly affects functional cell integrity.
- Chronic ischemia in microcirculatory branches results in connective tissue hypoxia and microischemia.

Strong evidence supports the association between chronic high blood glucose levels and the development of microvascular complications. The association between poor blood glucose control and the development of macrovascular complications is less clear. The development of macrovascular complications in people with type 2 diabetes seems to be more related to hypertension, a sedentary lifestyle, high blood lipid levels, and smoking than it does to hyperglycemia. The additional risk factor of obesity is important for people with type 2 diabetes. About 80% of clients with type 2 diabetes are obese, and cardiovascular events account for most of their deaths.

The National Diabetes Data Group of the National Institutes of Health estimates that the onset of type 2 diabetes may occur 9 to 12 years before the disorder is diagnosed. During the time that diabetes is not being treated, complications are developing. Up to 21% of clients are found to have retinopathy at the time of diagnosis (American Diabetes Association [ADA], 2000f). Many older diabetic clients do not develop classic signs of high blood glucose levels, and the diagnosis is made when the person seeks treatment for an acute illness or for complications caused by diabetes.

The Diabetes Control and Complications Trial (DCCT), an ongoing study involving 29 medical centers and more than 1400 people with type 1 diabetes, provides evidence that hyperglycemia is a critical factor in the development of long-term diabetic complications. Intensive therapy with good glucose control (maintaining blood glucose levels within identified ranges) delayed the onset and slowed the progression of retinopathy, nephropathy, and neuropathy. Clients in the group receiving intensive treatment had a mean blood glucose level of less than 155 mg/dL (8.6 mmol/L) and a glycosylated hemoglobin (hemoglobin A_{1c} [HbA_{1c}]) concentration of 7.2% (ADA, 2000j).

The United Kingdom Prospective Diabetes Study (UKPDS) established that intensive therapy with lowered blood glucose levels reduced the onset of retinopathy, nephropathy, and possibly neuropathy in clients with type 2 diabetes. Analysis of UKPDS data showed a strong relationship between risks for microvascular complications and the blood glucose level. For every percentage point decrease in HbA_{1c}, there was a 35% reduction in the risk for kidney and eye complications. Lowering the blood glucose level was not shown to have an effect on cardiovascular complications (ADA, 2000k).

MACROVASCULAR COMPLICATIONS

CARDIOVASCULAR DISEASE. Cardiovascular disease is the major cause of death in clients with diabetes mellitus; it accounts for about 80% of all deaths in these clients. Three fourths of these deaths are from coronary artery disease (Herlitz & Malmberg, 1999). Death from coronary artery disease is about 3 to 10 times higher in clients with type 1 diabetes, and 2 to 4 times higher in clients with type 2 diabetes, than in people who do not have diabetes.

Diabetic clients have a greater incidence of acute myocardial infarction and a higher death rate from this complication than nondiabetic individuals (Herlitz & Malmberg, 1999). Several factors account for this difference. Diabetic clients tend to have extensive coronary artery disease, diabetic cardiomyopathy, and abnormal blood clotting. In addition, after myocardial infarction, complications of left ventricular dysfunction with cardiac failure and fatal cardiac dysrhythmias are more common in the diabetic population.

Complications from atherosclerosis in clients with diabetes are very common. Diabetic clients also have more extensive disease. Although clients with diabetes do not develop larger infarcts, they have a higher incidence of pump failure. Heart failure is increased 600% in men with diabetes and 900% in women with diabetes (Garber, 1998).

Risk factors for cardiovascular disease include hyperglycemia, hypertension, **hyperinsulinemia** (excessive blood insulin levels), **hyperlipidemia** (excessive blood levels of cholesterol and other fats), clotting abnormalities, and blood vessel problems (Sowers & Lester, 1999). In addition to being an early indication of nephropathy, **albuminuria** (presence of albumin in the urine) is associated with greater cardiovascular disease in both type 1 and type 2 diabetes. The finding of even microscopic amounts of albumin in the urine is used as an indication for further screening for vascular disease and aggressive intervention to reduce cardiovascular risk factors (ADA, 2000e).

Data from the DCCT strongly indicate that tight blood glucose control by strict insulin treatment is critical for prevention of cardiovascular disease in clients with diabetes. Studies indicate that cardiovascular disease complication rates with diabetes can be reduced through aggressive treatment of hypertension and hyperlipidemia. The American Diabetes Association (ADA) recommends that blood pressure be maintained at levels lower than 130/85 mm Hg and that low-density lipoprotein (LDL) cholesterol be lowered to less than 100 mg/dL (<2.60 mmol/L) (ADA, 2000t).

CEREBROVASCULAR DISEASE. Diabetes is a risk factor for cerebral infarction and stroke. The presence of other risk factors, such as hyperlipidemia, hypertension, coronary artery disease, nephropathy, peripheral vascular disease, and excessive alcohol and tobacco use, along with diabetes, greatly increases the risk for stroke (Davis et al., 1999).

Elevated blood glucose levels at the time of the stroke are associated with greater brain injury. In addition, some studies have shown that hyperglycemia worsens cerebral damage after a stroke.

MICROVASCULAR COMPLICATIONS

EYE AND VISION COMPLICATIONS. Legal blindness, defined as a corrected visual acuity of 20/200 or less, is 25 times more common in diabetic individuals than in nondiabetic individuals. In the United States, diabetic retinopathy is the most frequent cause of new cases of blindness among adults ages 20 to 74 years. Retinopathy is strongly related to the duration of diabetes. After 20 years of diabetes, nearly all clients with type 1 diabetes and 60% of those with type 2 diabetes have some degree of retinopathy.

The cause and progression of diabetic retinopathy are related to problems with retinal blood vessels that cause leakage and blockage of blood flow, leading to retinal hypoxia. **Nonproliferative diabetic retinopathy (NPDR)** (Figure 65-2) is characterized by structural abnormalities of retinal blood vessels, but growth of new blood vessels is not stimulated. With this problem, there are areas of poor retinal circulation, edema, hard fatty deposits in the eye, and retinal hemorrhages. **Microaneurysms** (small capillary wall dilations seen as red dots with an ophthalmoscope) form throughout the eye. They leak fluid and blood into the retina, causing retinal edema and hard exudates. Other abnormal retinal findings include intraretinal hemorrhages, nerve fiber atrophy from hypoxia, and venous beading. **Venous beading** is the abnormal appearance of retinal veins in which areas of swelling and constriction along a segment of vein resemble links of sausage. Venous beading occurs in areas of retinal ischemia and is a predictor of progression to proliferative diabetic retinopathy. NPDR develops slowly *over time* and rarely causes blindness. Clients with severe NPDR have a 50% chance of developing proliferative diabetic retinopathy (Neeley et al., 1998).

Proliferative diabetic retinopathy (PDR) is the growth of new retinal blood vessels **(neovascularization).** When circulation to the retina is poor and hypoxia develops, retinal cells secrete a "growth factor" that stimulates the formation of new blood vessels within the eye. These new vessels are thin, fragile, and prone to bleeding, resulting in eye hemorrhage and more vision loss (Figure 65-3). Reddish black particles floating across the field of vision indicate bleeding into vitreous fluid. Fibrous tissue bands, developing along with new blood vessels, cause retinal detachment and irreversible vision loss. Chapter 47 discusses treatment of retinal problems.

The incidence of retinopathy is associated with fasting blood glucose levels higher than 129 mg/dL. Hyperglycemia and hypertension have been found to predict progression of retinopathy in clients with type 1 diabetes (Cohen et al., 1999). A 1% increase in total glycosylated hemoglobin (HbA_{1c}) was associated with a 10% increase in risk for progression of retinopathy. The Diabetes Control and Complications Trial (DCCT) established that intensive diabetes management to obtain **near-euglycemic** (near-normal blood glucose levels) control could prevent or delay the progression of diabetic retinopathy (ADA, 2000f).

Vision loss can also occur from macular degeneration, corneal scarring, and changes in lens shape or clarity. Hyperglycemia may cause blurred vision, even through prescription eyeglasses. The diabetic client may report double vision during periods of hypoglycemia. Cataracts occur in diabetic clients at a younger age, progress at a faster rate, and occur with greater frequency than in nondiabetic individuals. Open-angle glaucoma is more common in clients with diabetes. The management and treatment of cataracts and glaucoma are the same as for nondiabetic clients (see Chapter 47).

> **CONSIDERATIONS FOR OLDER ADULTS**
> The older client with diabetic retinopathy has the additional effect of visual changes that occur with aging. As a result, the older diabetic client's ability to perform self-care activities may be more seriously affected than that of a younger person with diabetes (see Chapter 47). The ability to discriminate among blues, greens, and violets decreases with normal aging. This deterioration of color perception makes performing visual blood glucose monitoring more difficult.

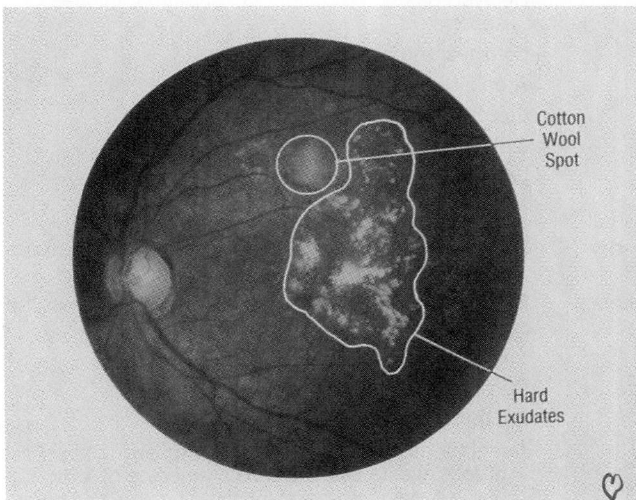

Figure 65-2 ● Select ophthalmic changes seen in nonproliferative diabetic retinopathy.

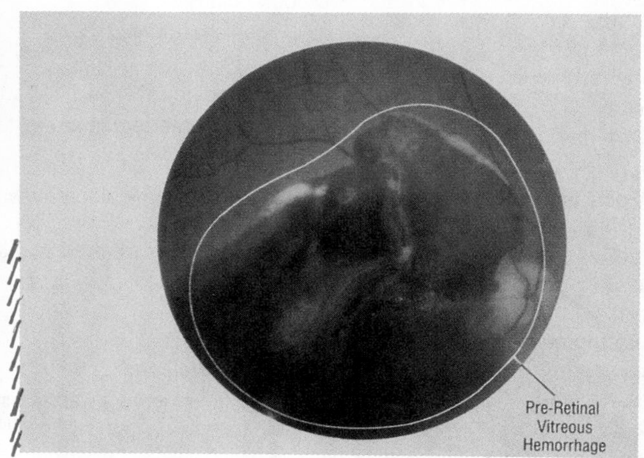

Figure 65-3 ● Ophthalmic hemorrhage that is possible with proliferative diabetic retinopathy.

DIABETIC NEUROPATHY. **Neuropathy** is a progressive deterioration of the nerves that results in loss of nerve function. Neuropathy is a common complication of diabetes and often involves all parts of the body. Damage to sensory nerve fibers results in either pain or loss of sensation. Damage to motor nerve fibers results in muscle weakness. Damage to nerve fibers in the autonomic nervous system results in widespread loss of many functions.

Diabetic neuropathy can be focal or diffuse, with each type having different causes, rates of progression, and treatments. The most common neuropathies among clients with diabetes are the diffuse neuropathies. **Diffuse neuropathies** involve generalized or widespread nerve function loss. These neuropathies have a slow onset, affect both sides of the body, involve motor and sensory nerves, progress slowly, and are usually irreversible. Diffuse neuropathies include autonomic nerve dysfunction. Late complications of diffuse neuropathies include foot ulcers and deformities.

Focal neuropathies are limited to a single nerve or nerve group. They are usually caused by a specific acute, ischemic event (ischemic neuropathy) or by the physical trapping of a nerve (entrapment neuropathy) within other tissues. Both types lead to nerve damage or nerve death. Ischemic neuropathies occur when the blood supply to a nerve or group of nerves is disrupted. The symptoms are sudden in onset, affect only one side of the body or body area, and are self-limiting in duration. Recovery time varies from nerve to nerve. Entrapment neuropathies occur because of compression of a nerve within a body compartment or between tissues. Symptoms are gradual in onset and can occur anywhere. They may be bilateral, having a waxing and waning course without spontaneous recovery. An example of focal entrapment neuropathy is carpal tunnel syndrome.

Insulin deficiency and hyperglycemia are thought to lead to neuropathy through blood vessel changes that cause inadequate oxygenation (hypoxia) to nerves. Both the axon and its myelin sheath are damaged by reduced blood flow, resulting in blocked nerve impulse transmission. Excessive glucose is converted to sorbitol, which accumulates in nerves. The increased sorbitol also slows motor nerve conduction. Commonly seen diabetic neuropathies are listed in Table 65-3. Neuropathy in the autonomic nervous system can lead to problems in cardiovascular, gastrointestinal (GI), and urinary function. Maintaining blood glucose levels within the normal range delays the onset and reduces the severity of diabetic neuropathies.

The cardiovascular problems of **orthostatic** (postural) hypotension and **syncope** (brief loss of consciousness), place the client with diabetes at risk for injury by falling. Common GI symptoms from diabetic neuropathy are **dysphagia** (difficulty swallowing), heartburn, nausea and vomiting, and bowel elimination problems. Diarrhea caused by diabetes is chronic, may be severe, often occurs at night, and may be associated with anal incontinence. Constipation, the most common GI symptom, is intermittent and may alternate with bouts of diarrhea. **Gastroparesis** (delay in gastric emptying) is a frequent cause of hypoglycemia. Loss of nerve input to the blad-

TABLE 65-3 • FEATURES OF DIABETIC NEUROPATHY

	Complication	Manifestation
DIFFUSE NEUROPATHIES		
Distal symmetric polyneuropathy	Sensory alterations	Paresthesias: burning/tingling sensations, starting in toes and moving up legs Dysthesias: burning, stinging, or stabbing pain Anesthesia: loss of sensation
	Motor alterations in intrinsic muscles of foot	Foot deformities: high arch, claw toes, hammertoes; shift of weight bearing to metatarsal heads and tips of toes
Autonomic neuropathy	Anhidrosis	Drying, cracking of skin
	Gastroparesis	Delayed gastric emptying, constipation, nausea, anorexia
	Diabetic diarrhea	Diarrhea and bowel incontinence
	Neurogenic bladder	Atonic bladder, urinary retention
	Impotence	Erectile dysfunction
	Loss of cardiac reflexes	Orthostatic hypotension, resting tachycardia
	Defective counterregulation	Loss of warning signs of hypoglycemia
FOCAL NEUROPATHIES		
Focal ischemia	Thoracolumbar radiculopathy with sensory and reflex loss	Pain radiating across back, side, and front of chest or abdomen
	Cranial nerve palsies, third and sixth nerves	Sudden diplopia or ptosis; eye pain
	Amyotrophy	Pain; asymmetric weakness; wasting of iliopsoas, quadriceps, and adductor muscles
Entrapment neuropathies	Median nerve	Carpal tunnel syndrome
	Popliteal nerve/knee	Footdrop
	Posterior tibial nerve at tarsal tunnel	Tarsal tunnel syndrome: sensory impairment in sole of foot; weakness of intrinsic muscles of foot; burning pain and paresthesias at ankle and plantar surface

der results in incomplete emptying, which leads to urinary infection and kidney problems.

DIABETIC NEPHROPATHY. Nephropathy is the development of pathologic changes in the kidney that reduce kidney function and may lead to renal failure. Diabetes mellitus is the leading cause of end-stage renal disease (ESRD) and renal failure in the United States. Diabetic nephropathy develops in 40% of individuals with type 1 diabetes and in 50% of individuals with type 2 diabetes (Bell & Alele, 1999). Native Americans, Hispanics (especially Mexican Americans), and African Americans have much higher risks of developing ESRD than non-Hispanic whites. Renal failure is a common cause of death in clients with type 1 diabetes. Maintaining blood glucose levels within the normal range can delay the onset of diabetic nephropathy and, in some cases, may prevent it.

In addition to hyperglycemia, a genetic predisposition to kidney problems in a person with diabetes increases the risk for developing diabetic nephropathy. Examples of known or suspected genetic predisposition to kidney disease include a mutation of the gene for angiotensin-converting enzyme (ACE), polycystic kidney disease (see Chapter 71), and a family history of hypertension (Ravid, 1997). In addition, clients with diabetes who also produce excess collagen (such as people who form keloid scars) are at greater risk for developing diabetic nephropathy.

The earliest clinical sign of nephropathy is **microalbuminuria** (presence of very small amounts of albumin in the urine). The American Diabetes Association (ADA) recommends a test for microalbuminuria in clients who have had type 1 diabetes for at least 5 years and in all clients with type 2 diabetes.

Chronic high blood glucose levels cause hypertension in kidney blood vessels and excess kidney perfusion. The increased pressure damages the kidney in many ways. The blood vessels become more leaky, especially in the glomerulus. This leakiness allows filtration of larger particles (including albumin and other proteins), which then form deposits in the kidney tissue and blood vessels. Deposits narrow the vessels, decreasing kidney oxygenation and leading to kidney cell hypoxia and cell death. These processes worsen with the duration of diabetes. The blood vessels in the glomerulus become scarred and are unable to filter urine from the blood, leading to renal failure. After protein is found in the urine **(proteinuria),** progression to ESRD and renal failure is inevitable within the next 7 to 15 years.

Renal damage is also related to the mean arterial blood pressure increases seen as part of cardiovascular disease in diabetic clients. Both systolic and diastolic hypertension greatly accelerates the progression of diabetic nephropathy.

MALE ERECTILE DYSFUNCTION. Erectile dysfunction (ED) is defined as inability to achieve or maintain an erection sufficient for satisfactory sexual performance. ED occurs at a higher rate and at an earlier age among men with diabetes as compared with the general population. About half of diabetic men have ED. This occurs 10 to 15 years earlier than in the general population (Korenman, 1998). In diabetes, ED is related to poor blood glucose control, obesity, medically treated hypertension, heavy cigarette smoking, and the presence of other chronic microvascular and macrovascular complications of diabetes.

ED may be caused by neuropathy, vascular disease, psychologic factors, or accompanying endocrine disorders. Autonomic neuropathy and/or vascular changes are responsible for persistent ED in diabetes. Chapter 76 discusses erectile function problems in depth.

Etiology

TYPE 1 DIABETES

Type 1 diabetes is an autoimmune disorder in which beta-cell destruction in the pancreas occurs in a genetically susceptible individual (Table 65-4). In autoimmune disease, the immune

TABLE 65-4 • DIFFERENTIATION OF TYPE 1 AND TYPE 2 DIABETES

Features	Type 1	Type 2
Former names	Juvenile-onset diabetes Ketosis-prone diabetes Insulin-dependent diabetes mellitus (IDDM)	Maturity-onset diabetes Ketosis-resistant diabetes Non–insulin-dependent diabetes mellitus (NIDDM)
Age at onset	Usually under age 30 yr, occurs at any age	Peaks in 50s; may occur earlier
Symptoms	Abrupt onset, thirst, weight loss	Frequently none; thirst, fatigue, visual blurring, vascular or neural complications
Etiology	Viral infection	Not known
Pathology	Pancreatic beta-cell destruction	Insulin resistance Dysfunctional pancreatic beta cell
Antigen patterns	HLA-DR4, HLA-DR3	None
Antibodies	ICAs present at diagnosis	None
Endogenous insulin and C-peptide	None	Low, normal, or high
Inheritance	Recessive	Unknown
Nutritional status	Usually nonobese	60%-80% obese
Insulin	All dependent on insulin	Required for 20%-30%
Sulfonylurea therapy	None	Effective for most clients
Medical nutrition therapy	Mandatory	Mandatory

ICAs, Islet cell antibodies.

system fails to recognize normal body cells as "self" and takes destructive actions against them. In type 1 diabetes, immune system cells and cell products attack and destroy insulin-secreting cells within the islets. Although the exact cause or why a person's immune system would begin to attack normal body cells is not known, people with certain tissue types are more likely to develop autoimmune diseases, including type 1 diabetes. Specifically, people who have the tissue types HLA-DR3 and/or HLA-DR4 are at an increased risk for the development of type 1 diabetes. Certain viral infections, such as mumps, congenital rubella, and coxsackievirus infection, appear to be able to trigger autoimmune destruction of pancreatic beta cells.

Indicators, or **markers,** of immune damage to insulin-producing cells (a key feature of type 1 diabetes) are the presence of antibodies in the blood directed against the beta cells themselves or against substances made by the beta cells. Most clients with type 1 diabetes have islet cell antibodies (ICAs), autoantibodies to insulin (IAAs), autoantibodies to glutamic acid decarboxylase (GAD), and/or autoantibodies to tyrosine phosphates. Circulating ICA and IAA may be present before clinical manifestations of type 1 diabetes develop.

Risk for developing type 1 diabetes is determined by inheritance of the HLA-DR3 and HLA-DR4 genes. *It is important to remember, however, that although inheritance of these genes increases the risk, most people with these genes do not develop type 1 diabetes.* Development of the disease appears to be an interactive effect of genetic predisposition and exposure to the right environmental factors. In addition, it appears that the exposure must occur within a sensitive time period for it to enhance the predisposition. It is thought that the environmental exposure(s) insults or damages the beta cells of the pancreas, although time may be needed before the damage has the result of decreasing insulin production (Ilonen & Akerblom, 1999). The risk for developing type 1 diabetes in the general population ranges from 1 in 400 to 1 in 1000. The risk greatly increases for those people who have at least one parent with diabetes (from 1 in 20 to 1 in 50) (Funnell et al., 1998). It is unclear why some genetically susceptible people develop diabetes and others do not.

TYPE 2 DIABETES

Clients with type 2 diabetes have a reduction in the ability of most cells to respond to insulin **(insulin resistance),** poor control of liver glucose output, and decreased beta-cell function, eventually leading to beta-cell failure. Most people with type 2 diabetes are obese adults older than 40 years of age. The specific causes of type 2 diabetes are not known. Both insulin resistance and beta-cell failure have many genetic and nongenetic

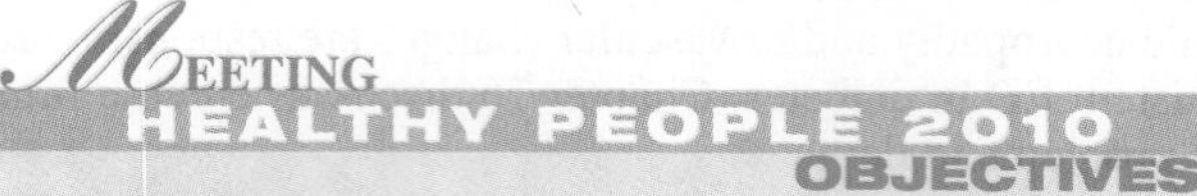

DIABETES MELLITUS

Objective 18.4: Reduce the diabetes death rates (diabetes as the underlying cause) to no more than 12.0 per 100,000 persons.

- Encourage all people to have a yearly screening physical examination that includes blood testing for diabetes.
- Inform all clients who have a sedentary lifestyle and who are overweight about the risk factors for and complications of diabetes.
- Assist diabetic clients who smoke to reduce or quit smoking.
- Instruct clients with diabetes mellitus to achieve and maintain body weight within 5 pounds of identified ideal weight for age and body size.
- Provide one-to-one education sessions, group education sessions, and printed and videotape information on diabetes treatment and care to clients diagnosed with diabetes.
- Educate clients about the specific medications prescribed to manage their disease.
- Demonstrate the use of the diet strategy individually planned for the client with diabetes.
- Encourage all clients with diabetes to participate in an individualized exercise program at least 3 days per week.
- Assist those clients with diabetes who also have hypertension to understand the importance of adhering to the prescribed drug therapies for both health problems.
- Instruct clients with diabetes to obtain annual vaccinations against influenza.
- Teach clients with type 2 diabetes to maintain adequate hydration, especially when any other illness is also present.
- Participate in mass screenings to identify people with undiagnosed type 2 diabetes among the general population.
- Develop culturally sensitive and literacy-appropriate education materials targeted to high-risk minority populations.

Objective 18.9: Reduce the frequency of foot ulcers in persons with diabetes.

- Include foot assessment whenever caring for a client with diabetes.
- Include sensory testing of the feet for all clients with diabetes.
- Instruct the client with diabetes about proper foot care.
- Teach the client with diabetes the importance of always wearing protective footwear whenever the client is out of bed.
- Show the client the proper type of footwear to prevent foot injury.
- Find resources for those diabetic clients who are unable to afford properly fitting shoes.
- Teach the client how to monitor the circulatory status of his or her feet.
- Encourage the client to see a podiatrist twice a year.
- Refer the client with foot lesions to a wound management specialist.
- Encourage the client with diabetes who smokes to reduce or quit smoking.

Objective 18.23: Increase to 52% the proportion of persons with diabetes who have received formal diabetes education.

- Evaluate the diabetes education materials and programs currently in place at your institution for currency, literacy, cultural sensitivity, and adequacy.
- Identify resources within your agency and community for diabetes education and support.
- Meet with the diabetes educator at your agency and establish means for collaboration and referral.
- If a diabetes educator is not available at your agency, work with existing personnel to enhance diabetes knowledge and awareness.
- Assist in policy-making decisions within your agency to develop a formalized teaching plan for all clients with diabetes, regardless of whether the clients are newly diagnosed or have had diabetes for a long time.
- Develop and offer diabetes education programs within your community in a variety of settings.

causes. Heredity plays a major role in the development of type 2 diabetes. Offspring of clients with type 2 diabetes have a 15% chance of developing the actual disease and a 30% risk of having impaired glucose tolerance. Specific gene defects have been identified in certain groups with high prevalence rates of type 2 diabetes. Pima Indians have a 50% prevalence of type 2 diabetes, with insulin resistance and hyperinsulinemia identified as a dominant trait (Funnell et al., 1998).

Incidence/Prevalence

Diabetes has become one of the most common chronic diseases in the United States. Diagnosed and undiagnosed diabetes affects 7% of all adults over the age of 20, with rates reaching 18.8% by age 60 (Harris et al., 1998).

The prevalence of diabetes has increased steadily over the past 40 years. In 1998 an estimated 10.5 million people had diabetes. About 90% of these individuals have type 2 diabetes. Diagnosed diabetes is most prevalent in middle-aged and older adult populations, affecting about 6% of people 45 to 64 years of age and 11% of those older than 65 years of age. Approximately 10% of clients diagnosed with diabetes are over 70 years of age. After the age of 40, new-onset diabetes is almost always non–insulin dependent. The prevalence of diabetes is similar for men and women.

Prevention

The fact that diabetes is a common disorder and causes many preventable but devastating complications makes the disease a major public health problem. The U.S. government has identified control of diabetes and its complications as a major focus for health promotion activities (see the Meeting Healthy People 2010 box on p. 1448).

Specific immune studies can accurately detect individuals who will develop immune-related type 1 diabetes. Measurement of ICA levels in relatives of clients with type 1 diabetes identifies those at risk for developing the disease. ICA measurement can predict 35% of relatives who will develop type 1 diabetes within 5 years and 60% to 70% of relatives likely to develop type 1 diabetes within 10 years (Dahlquist, 1999).

Treatment of increased blood glucose levels in clients who have glucose intolerance may help delay the onset of diabetes. Insulin therapy given to susceptible individuals appears to slow destruction of pancreatic beta cells. Sulfonylurea drugs decrease hyperglycemia and stimulate both insulin secretion and insulin action. Metformin (Glucophage), which inhibits intestinal absorption of glucose and improves insulin action, has been shown to be effective in preventing type 2 diabetes. Other interventions that prevent or delay diabetes include drug therapy to reduce the immune response and promote repair of deoxyribonucleic acid (DNA) damage. Immunosuppressive therapy can prolong the person's ability to secrete insulin. Nicotinamide (niacin) decreases the likelihood of diabetes caused by DNA damage.

Risk factors of obesity, physical inactivity, and a high-fat diet can be modified by behavioral changes. Weight reduction prevents type 2 diabetes. Reduced caloric intake improves insulin sensitivity, and weight reduction further improves insulin action. Low-fat diets, coupled with weight loss and increased exercise, have been shown to delay progression to type 2 diabetes in susceptible individuals. Studies are being conducted to determine if diabetes can be prevented or delayed through intervention with insulin during the "prediabetic" phase of the disease in high-risk relatives (ADA, 2000p).

CULTURAL CONSIDERATIONS

Certain ethnic groups have an increased risk of developing type 2 diabetes when compared with the U.S. population as a whole. African Americans have twice the risk of Caucasians for developing type 2 diabetes. The risk in Hispanics, especially those of Puerto Rican or Mexican origin, is approximately 2.5 times higher than the risk in Caucasians, whereas Native Americans show a fivefold increase in risk (Haffner, 1998a). Groups at high risk for type 2 diabetes are presented in Table 65-5.

The incidence and prevalence of type 2 diabetes have increased dramatically among Native Americans as a result of changes in physical activity and dietary habits. Obesity is a major risk factor for diabetes in Pima Indian tribes.

Harris et al. (1999) found racial and ethnic differences in glycemic control among U.S. adults with type 2 diabetes. Non-Hispanic black women and Mexican-American men were disproportionately represented among those with poor glycemic control. Minorities have a higher risk for complications even after adjusting for differences in blood glucose control.

CRITICAL THINKING CHALLENGE

You are caring for a 62-year-old woman who has had type 2 diabetes for more than 20 years. She is blind and has renal failure. Her 28-year-old daughter asks you what her own chances are for developing diabetes. The daughter reports that her 38-year-old sister has just been diagnosed with type 2 diabetes. You note that the daughter is 5 feet 8 inches tall and weighs about 140 pounds. She is a physical education teacher at a local high school and has a 1-year-old son.

- What personal questions should you ask the daughter to help determine her risk?
- Explain the genetics of type 2 diabetes.
- What tests (if any) might be helpful in determining this person's risk?
- How could the daughter reduce her risk or delay the development of the disease?

For suggested answer guidelines, go to SIMON http://www.wbsaunders.com/SIMON/Iggy/.

TABLE 65-5 • MAJOR RISK FACTORS FOR TYPE 2 DIABETES

- Family history of diabetes (parents or siblings)
- Obesity (more than 20% above a person's ideal body weight)
- Origin (African-American, Hispanic, Native American, or Asian-American)
- Age older than 45 years plus any of the preceding factors
- Previously identified impaired glucose tolerance or use of certain prescription drugs
- Hypertension (>140/90 mm Hg)
- High-density lipoprotein cholesterol levels <35 mg/dL (0.90 mmol/L) and triglyceride levels >250 mg/dL (2.82 mmol/L)
- History of gestational diabetes or delivery of infants weighing more than 9 pounds

Data from American Diabetes Association (2000). Position statement: Screening for type 2 diabetes. *Diabetes Care, 23*(Suppl. 1), 20-23.

➤ COLLABORATIVE MANAGEMENT

Assessment

HISTORY

The nurse asks questions and collects data about risk factors, as well as symptoms related to diabetes. The client's age is important because type 2 diabetes is more common in older people, especially among African-American and Mexican-American clients. Women are asked how large their children were at birth because many women who develop type 2 diabetes had gestational diabetes or were glucose intolerant during pregnancy. These women often give birth to infants that weigh 9 pounds or more.

Assessing weight and weight change is important because excess weight and obesity are risk factors for type 2 diabetes. The client with type 1 diabetes often experiences weight loss with increased appetite during the weeks before diagnosis. For both types of diabetes, clients usually experience fatigue, polyuria, and polydipsia. They are asked about recent major or minor infections. In particular, women are asked about frequent vaginal yeast infections. All clients are asked if they have noticed whether small skin injuries become infected more easily or seem to take a longer time to heal.

The family history is explored for parents and siblings with diabetes. If the client has one or more relatives with diabetes, it is important to determine whether these relatives use insulin or control their disease with diet, exercise, and/or oral antidiabetic medications.

LABORATORY ASSESSMENT

BLOOD TESTS. The health care provider uses blood glucose values to diagnose diabetes. The nurse, the client, or a family member monitors the ongoing status of the disease by performing capillary blood glucose testing using a blood glucose meter. The physician and the nurse assess the overall result of treatment through review of glycosylated hemoglobin (hemoglobin A_{1c} [HbA_{1c}]) and fructosamine levels.

Instructions for blood glucose testing are presented in Chart 65-1. The American Diabetes Association (ADA) defines normal blood glucose values in Chart 65-2. ADA criteria for the diagnosis of adult diabetes mellitus are outlined in Table 65-6.

FASTING BLOOD GLUCOSE TEST. The results of the fasting blood glucose test are most accurate when the test is performed on blood obtained by venipuncture. The client should be fasting for at least 8 hours (water is permitted). The blood needs to be obtained before insulin or oral antidiabetic agents have been administered. A diagnosis of diabetes is made with two separate test results greater than 126 mg/dL (7 mmol/L) (ADA, 2000a).

ORAL GLUCOSE TOLERANCE TEST. The oral glucose tolerance test (OGTT) is the most sensitive test for the diagnosis of diabetes, although it is not routinely used, except in diagnosis of gestational diabetes. The test is inconvenient to clients, costly, and time consuming compared with the fasting plasma glucose measure. Before the test, the nurse reviews instructions from Chart 65-1 with the client. Carbohydrate intake restriction or bedrest before the test alters glucose tolerance. The client drinks a beverage containing a glucose load of 75 g, and blood samples are collected at 30-minute intervals for 2 hours. A diagnosis of diabetes is made if the venous blood glucose is greater than 200 mg/dL (11.1 mmol/L) at 120 minutes.

CHART 65-1

CLIENT EDUCATION GUIDE
Blood Glucose Testing

Fasting Plasma Blood Glucose
- Do not eat any food or drink any liquid for at least 8 hours.

Oral Glucose Tolerance Test
- Eat a balanced diet with carbohydrate intake of at least 150 g for a minimum of 3 days while maintaining normal physical activity.
- Carbohydrate restriction, bedrest, acute illness, and certain drugs interfere with the test. Phenytoin (Dilantin), anovulatory drugs, diuretics, nicotinic acid, and glucocorticoids adversely affect results.
- The test is performed in the morning after a 10- to 12-hour fast.
- A fasting blood sample is obtained.
- You will be asked to drink 300 mL (75 g) of a flavored beverage within 5 minutes of the fasting blood sample.
- Blood samples are drawn at 30-minute intervals for 2 hours.
- During the test, you will remain at rest and not be able to smoke or drink liquids.
- Report any signs suggesting hypoglycemia, such as weakness, dizziness, nervousness, and confusion.

CHART 65-2

LABORATORY PROFILE
Blood Glucose Values

Test	Normal Range for Adults	Significance of Abnormal Results
Fasting blood glucose test	<110 mg/dL (6.1 mmol/L) *Older Adults:* Levels rise 1 mg/dL per decade with age.	Levels >126 mg/dL (7.0 mmol/L) obtained on at least two occasions are diagnostic of diabetes, even in older adults.
Glucose tolerance test (2-hour post-load result)	<140 mg/dL (7.8 mmol/L)	Levels >140 mg/dL (7.8 mmol/L) and <200 mg/dL (11.1 mmol/L) indicate impaired glucose tolerance. Levels >200 mg/dL (11.1 mmol/L) indicate provisional diagnosis of diabetes.
Glycosylated hemoglobin (hemoglobin A_{1c} [HbA_{1c}]) test	4% to 6%	Levels over 8% indicate poor diabetic control with need for adherence to regimen or changes in therapy.

Data from American Diabetes Association. (2000). Committee report: Report of the Expert Committee on the Diagnosis and Classification of Diabetes Mellitus. *Diabetes Care, 23*(Suppl. 1), 4-19, and American Diabetes Association. (2000). Position statement: Tests for glycemia in diabetes. *Diabetes Care, 23*(Suppl. 1), 80-82.

GLYCOSYLATED HEMOGLOBIN ASSAYS. Glycosylated hemoglobin (HbA_{1c}) is the best indicator of the average blood glucose level. Because glucose attaches to the hemoglobin molecule, measurement of HbA_{1c} indicates the average blood glucose level during the previous 120 days—the life span of the average red blood cell. HbA_{1c} testing can be used

TABLE 65-6 • CRITERIA FOR THE DIAGNOSIS OF TYPE 2 DIABETES

Symptoms of diabetes plus casual blood glucose concentration greater than 200 mg/dL (11.1 mmol/L). Casual is defined as any time of day without regard to time since last meal. The classic symptoms of diabetes include polyuria, polydipsia, and unexplained weight loss.

Or

Fasting plasma glucose greater than 126 mg/dL (7.0 mmol/L). Fasting is defined as no caloric intake for at least 8 hours.

Or

2-hour plasma glucose greater than 200 mg/dL during an oral glucose tolerance test. The test should be performed using a glucose load containing the equivalent of 75 g glucose dissolved in water.

NOTE: Each test must be confirmed, on a subsequent day, under similar circumstances.

Data from American Diabetes Association. (2000). Committee report: Report of the Expert Committee on the Diagnosis and Classification of Diabetes Mellitus. *Diabetes Care, 23*(Suppl. 1), 4-19.

to assess long-term glycemic control, as well as to predict risk for the development of chronic complications. Unlike results of the fasting blood glucose test, HbA_{1c} test results are not influenced by changing one's eating habits the day before the test. It is recommended that HbA_{1c} testing be performed at the time of initial diagnosis and at intervals frequent enough to permit evaluation of the therapeutic plan. Hemolysis, blood loss, and pregnancy all increase red blood cell turnover and reduce HbA_{1c} levels. Triglycerides and bilirubin interfere with the assay, leading to overestimation of HbA_{1c} levels in clients with hypertriglyceridemia. The ADA recommends HbA_{1c} testing at least twice a year in clients who are meeting treatment goals and have stable blood glucose control, and quarterly assessments in clients whose therapy has changed and who are not meeting glycemic goals (ADA, 2000t).

GLYCOSYLATED SERUM PROTEINS AND ALBUMIN. Serum proteins and albumin become increasingly glycosylated with elevated blood glucose levels in the same way that HbA_{1c} does. However, because serum proteins and albumin turn over in 14 days, compared with the 120 days of red blood cells, glycosylated serum albumin (GSA) and glycosylated serum proteins (GSP) can be used to indicate blood glucose control over a shorter period. These measures are useful in conditions in which tight control of blood glucose levels is necessary (e.g., pregnancy) or in short-term follow up of treatment changes (ADA, 2000u).

URINE TESTS

URINE TESTING FOR KETONE BODIES. Ketones are a waste product of fat metabolism. The presence of urine ketones may indicate impending ketoacidosis. The ADA recommends testing urine for ketones during acute illness or stress, when blood glucose levels are consistently greater than 300 mg/dL (>16.7 mmol/L), during pregnancy, or when any symptoms of ketoacidosis are present (ADA, 2000u). Ketone testing is recommended for diabetic clients participating in a weight loss program.

TESTS FOR RENAL FUNCTION. The presence of urine protein when no symptoms of renal problems are present may indicate microvascular changes in the kidney. Urine albumin excretion rates of 20 to 200 g/min (30 to 300 mg/hr) indicate microalbuminuria. Even minor elevations of albumin excretion are associated with increased mortality.

Once clinical proteinuria has been detected, kidney function (e.g., glomerular filtration rate) is assessed by creatinine clearance tests (see Chapter 69). In clients with known nephropathy, a rise in serum creatinine levels is related to both poor blood glucose control and hypertension.

URINE TESTING FOR GLUCOSE. Indirect measures of blood glucose may be obtained through urine testing for glucose, although this method is less precise than blood glucose testing. Fluid intake, urine concentration, time interval since last voiding, and certain drugs affect the results (ADA, 2000u).

OTHER DIAGNOSTIC ASSESSMENTS

The presence of certain autoantibodies can accurately indicate if a person will develop type 1 diabetes. Measurement of islet cell antibody (ICA) levels of relatives of clients with type 1 diabetes identifies those at high risk for diabetes development (Dahlquist, 1999). Insulin autoantibody (IAA) levels correlate with the rate of progression to diabetes and the age at which type 1 diabetes develops (the younger the age at which diabetes develops and/or the faster the progression to diabetes, the higher the level of IAA). Measurement of C-peptide levels indicates beta secretory function of the pancreas. C-peptide levels correlate well with insulin levels.

Analysis

COMMON NURSING DIAGNOSES AND COLLABORATIVE PROBLEMS

The following are common nursing diagnoses for clients with diabetes:

1. Risk for Injury related to hyperglycemia
2. Risk for Injury related to stress of surgery
3. Risk for Injury related to sensory alterations (diabetic neuropathy)
4. Chronic Pain related to peripheral nerve dysfunction (diabetic neuropathy)
5. Risk for Injury related to visual sensory-perceptual alterations (diabetic retinopathy)
6. Ineffective Renal Tissue Perfusion related to the renal effects of vascular abnormalities (diabetic nephropathy)

The following are primary collaborative problems:

1. Potential for Hypoglycemia
2. Potential for Diabetic Ketoacidosis
3. Potential for Hyperglycemic-Hyperosmolar Nonketotic Syndrome

ADDITIONAL NURSING DIAGNOSES AND COLLABORATIVE PROBLEMS

In addition to the common nursing diagnoses and collaborative problems, clients with diabetes may have one or more of the following:

- Imbalanced Nutrition: More Than Body Requirements related to an imbalance of food intake and physical activity, lack of knowledge, and ineffective coping skills

- Risk for Deficient Fluid Volume related to fluid shifts, failure of regulatory mechanisms, hyperglycemic osmotic diuresis, polyuria, vomiting, diarrhea, decreased oral intake, and dehydration
- Acute Pain related to insulin injections or capillary blood glucose testing
- Impaired Oral Mucous Membrane related to microvascular circulatory changes and uncontrolled blood glucose levels
- Deficient Knowledge related to a lack of familiarity with information resources about the disease process, diet, exercise, medications, weight control, and mouth care
- Impaired Urinary Elimination and Urinary Retention (with Overflow Incontinence) related to diabetic neuropathy
- Constipation related to diabetic neuropathy
- Diarrhea related to diabetic neuropathy
- Risk for Impaired Skin Integrity related to decreased circulation, increased blood glucose levels, decreased mobility, and decreased sensation
- Risk for Infection related to increased blood glucose levels, decreased tissue perfusion, inadequate primary defenses (e.g., breaks in skin integrity), and the effects of chronic disease
- Risk for Infection related to wounds, urinary tract infection, intravenous (IV) access site, or oral mucous membranes
- Risk for Ineffective Sexuality Patterns (Male) related to autonomic neuropathy, decreased circulation, or psychologic problems
- Risk for Ineffective Sexuality Patterns (Female) related to the physical and psychologic stressors of diabetes
- Sexual Dysfunction related to impotence, impaired lubrication, painful intercourse with the changes in neurologic control of the genitalia, the effects of actual or perceived limitations imposed by the disease or therapy, and altered self-concept
- Situational Low Self-Esteem related to an inability to deal with the self-care demands of the diabetic regimen
- Anxiety related to the diagnosis of diabetes, potential complications of diabetes, and self-care regimens
- Fear related to the diagnosis of diabetes, potential complications of diabetes, and self-care regimens
- Ineffective Coping and Compromised Family Coping related to a chronic disease, a complex self-care regimen, and decreased social support
- Powerlessness related to the complications of diabetes (blindness, amputations, renal failure, and neuropathy)
- Social Isolation related to visual impairment or blindness
- Noncompliance with self-care related to the complexity and chronicity of the prescribed regimen
- Ineffective Health Maintenance related to insufficient knowledge of ADA exchange diet, weight control, weight maintenance, benefits and risks of exercise, self-monitoring of blood glucose, medications, sick-day care, foot care, hypoglycemia, and available resources

Planning and Implementation

The management of diabetes mellitus is complicated and involves considerable client cooperation and education. The Concept Map on p. 1453 highlights care issues for the client with type 2 diabetes mellitus.

RISK FOR INJURY RELATED TO HYPERGLYCEMIA

NOC **PLANNING: EXPECTED OUTCOMES.** The client with diabetes is expected to maintain blood glucose levels in the expected range and avoid acute and chronic complications of diabetes.

INTERVENTIONS. The treatment of diabetes uses nonsurgical and surgical interventions.

NONSURGICAL MANAGEMENT. Nonsurgical management of diabetes mellitus involves dietary interventions, monitoring of blood glucose levels, a planned exercise program, and in some instances, medications to lower blood glucose levels. The nurse, in collaboration with the client, physician, dietitian, pharmacist, and in some cases, physical therapist, plans, organizes, and delivers care.

The American Diabetes Association (ADA) has proposed the following treatment goals in relation to glycosylated hemoglobin (HbA_{1c}) and blood glucose levels (ADA, 2000t):

- HbA_{1c} levels should be maintained at 7% or below.
- The majority of premeal blood glucose levels should be 80 to 120 mg/dL (4.4 to 6.7 mmol/L).
- Blood glucose values at bedtime should be between 100 and 140 mg/dL (5.6 to 7.8 mmol/L).

CONSIDERATIONS FOR OLDER ADULTS

The primary aim of therapy in the older diabetic client is to maintain quality of life by maintaining blood glucose levels in the range that avoids both hypoglycemia and hyperglycemia. This precaution may require an aggressive therapy program with insulin in cases where the effects of uncontrolled hyperglycemia are greater than the risk of hypoglycemia occurring as a result of the therapy.

DRUG THERAPY. Medication administration is indicated when a client with type 2 diabetes does not have blood glucose control with dietary modification, regular exercise, and stress management. See Table 65-7 for the cost of diabetes medications.

Oral Therapy. Oral agents are prescribed only after dietary control has been shown to be insufficient.

Sulfonylurea Agents. Sulfonylurea agents are appropriate only for clients with some remaining pancreatic beta-cell function. These drugs stimulate insulin secretion (which reduces liver glucose output and increases cell uptake of glucose) and enhance the number or sensitivity of receptor sites on the cell for interaction with insulin. These drugs differ in strength, overall effects, metabolism, and risk for complications (Chart 65-3).

Hypoglycemia is the most serious complication of sulfonylurea therapy. Hypoglycemic episodes are more likely to occur with chlorpropamide (Diabinese, Novopropamide) because of its long duration of action. Underweight older clients with cardiovascular, liver, or kidney impairment are more susceptible to hypoglycemia.

Other, less common side effects include hematologic reactions (leukopenia, thrombocytopenia, hemolytic anemia), allergic skin reactions, and gastrointestinal (GI) effects (nausea, epigastric fullness, heartburn). In addition, many drugs can potentiate or interfere with the actions of sulfonylurea agents (Table 65-8).

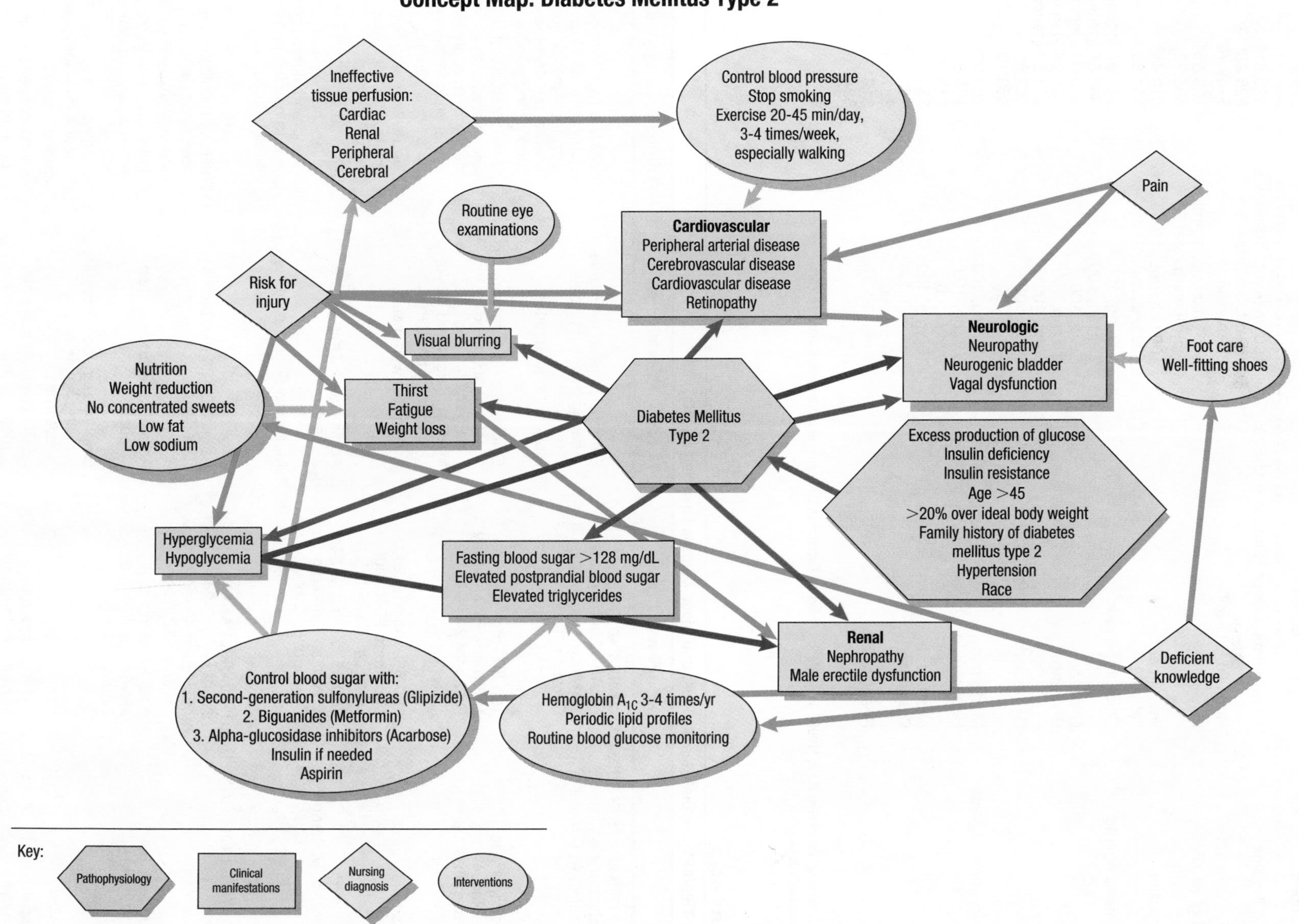
Concept Map: Diabetes Mellitus Type 2
Ineffective tissue perfusion: Cardiac Renal Peripheral Cerebral
Control blood pressure
Stop smoking
Exercise 20-45 min/day, 3-4 times/week, especially walking
Pain
Routine eye examinations
Cardiovascular
Peripheral arterial disease
Cerebrovascular disease
Cardiovascular disease
Retinopathy
Risk for injury
Visual blurring
Neurologic
Neuropathy
Neurogenic bladder
Vagal dysfunction
Foot care
Well-fitting shoes
Nutrition
Weight reduction
No concentrated sweets
Low fat
Low sodium
Thirst
Fatigue
Weight loss
Diabetes Mellitus Type 2
Excess production of glucose
Insulin deficiency
Insulin resistance
Age >45
>20% over ideal body weight
Family history of diabetes mellitus type 2
Hypertension
Race
Hyperglycemia
Hypoglycemia
Fasting blood sugar >128 mg/dL
Elevated postprandial blood sugar
Elevated triglycerides
Renal
Nephropathy
Male erectile dysfunction
Deficient knowledge
Control blood sugar with:
1. Second-generation sulfonylureas (Glipizide)
2. Biguanides (Metformin)
3. Alpha-glucosidase inhibitors (Acarbose)
Insulin if needed
Aspirin
Hemoglobin A1C 3-4 times/yr
Periodic lipid profiles
Routine blood glucose monitoring
Key:
Pathophysiology
Clinical manifestations
Nursing diagnosis
Interventions

TABLE 65-7 • COST OF DIABETES MEDICATIONS

Medications	Specific Product	Size	Price
Humulin insulins	All products except Humulin R U-500:	100 units/mL, 10-mL vial	$20.81*
		1.5-mL cartridge, 5	$25.28*
	Humulin R U-500:	20-mL vial	$149.72*
Humalog insulin	Insulin lispro	100 units/mL, 10-mL vial	$28.55
		1.5-mL cartridge, 5	$35.32
Iletin insulins	Iletin I beef	100 units/mL, 10-mL vial	$19.44*
	Iletin II pork	100 units/mL 10-mL vial	$34.88*
Sulfonylurea agents	Chlorpropamide	100 mg, 100	$21.97 (generic brand)
		250 mg, 100	$35.37 (generic brand)
	Glipizide	5 mg, 100	$15.64 (generic brand)
	Glyburide	1.5 mg, 100	$24.96 (generic brand)
		3 mg, 100	$31.37 (generic brand)
	Glimepiride	1 mg, 100	$22.60
		4 mg, 100	$69.10
Nonsulfonylurea agents	Metformin	500 mg, 100	$54.82
	Repaglinide	0.5 mg, 100	$55.83
		2 mg, 100	$79.03
	Acarbose	100 mg, 100	$64.42
	Pioglitazone	15 mg, 90	$236.24
		30 mg, 90	$372.01
	Rosiglitazone	4 mg, 90	$191.75
		8 mg, 90	$348.08

Data from *1998 Drug Topics Red Book.* (1998). Montvale, NJ: Medical Economics Company; and http://www.planetrx. com.
*Average wholesale price.

CHART 65-3

DRUG THERAPY *for* Diabetes Mellitus: Oral Blood Glucose Lowering Agents

Drug	Dosage and Duration	Nursing Interventions	Rationale
FIRST-GENERATION SULFONYLUREA AGENTS			
Acetohexamide (Dymelor♣, Dimelor♣)	*Usual:* 0.25-1.5 g/day *Maximum:* 1.5 g/day *Duration:* 12-24 hr	Emphasize need for regular eating habits and patterns. Monitor renal function.	There is a high incidence of hypoglycemia in diabetic clients with renal impairment. Older clients can develop exaggerated hypoglycemia responses.
Chlorpropamide (Diabinese, Novo-propamide♣)	100-500 mg q24h *Maximum:* 500 mg/day *Duration:* 24-60 hr	Emphasize need for regular eating habits and patterns.	The long half-life of the drug is associated with a high incidence of hypoglycemia.
		Monitor weight and intake and output patterns.	There is an increased potential for severe hyponatremia.
Tolazamide (Tolinase)	100-500 mg q12-24h *Maximum:* 2000 mg/day *Duration:* 12-24 hr	Administer with meals.	Taking with meals helps to avoid gastrointestinal upset.
Tolbutamide (Orinase, Mobenol♣)	750-1500 mg q12-24h *Maximum:* 3000 mg/day *Duration:* 6-10 hr	Administer 30 min before meals.	Taking 30 min before meals gives the best reduction in postprandial hyperglycemia.
		Monitor weight and intake and output patterns.	Use with caution in patients with renal failure.
SECOND-GENERATION SULFONYLUREA AGENTS			
Glipizide (Glucotrol)	2.5-5 mg q12-24h *Maximum:* 40 mg/day *Duration:* 12-24 hr	Administer 30 min before meals.	The long half-life of the drug is associated with a high incidence of hypoglycemia.
Glyburide (DiaBeta♣)	1.25 to 20 mg/day *Maximum:* 20 mg/day *Duration:* 24 hr	Administer with first main meal.	Administration with food helps reduce gastrointestinal side effects.
		Emphasize need for regular eating habits and patterns.	Hypoglycemia is more likely to occur with insufficient caloric intake.
Glimepiride (Amaryl)	1-4 mg once daily *Maximum:* 8 mg/day *Duration:* 24 hr	Administer with first main meal. Emphasize need for regular eating habits and patterns.	Individuals with impaired renal function are more sensitive to blood glucose–lowering effects of glimepiride.

CHART 65-3

DRUG THERAPY *for* Diabetes Mellitus: Oral Blood Glucose Lowering Agents—cont'd

Drug	Dosage and Duration	Nursing Interventions	Rationale
NONSULFONYLUREA AGENTS			
Metformin (Glucophage)	500 mg bid or 850 mg once a day *Maximum:* 2550 mg/day *Duration:* 12 hr	Administer with food.	Primary side effects are nausea, diarrhea, and abdominal discomfort.
		Monitor weight and intake and output patterns.	Use with caution in patients with renal failure. Lactic acidosis occurs with greater frequency in patients with impaired renal function.
Repaglinide (Prandin)	0.5-2 mg *Maximum:* 16 mg/day *Duration:* 2-3 hr	Administer 30 min before meals.	Taking 30 min before meals gives the best reduction in postprandial hyperglycemia.
ALPHA-GLUCOSIDASE INHIBITORS			
Acarbose (Precose)	Individualized *Maximum:* 100 mg tid *Duration:* 2-4 hr	Instruct client to take with the first bite of each main meal.	Acarbose must be taken at the beginning of a meal to be fully effective.
Miglitol (Glyset)	Individualized Usual dose: 50 mg tid *Maximum:* 100 mg tid *Duration:* ≈1 hr	Instruct client to take with the first bite of each main meal.	Glyset must be taken at the beginning of a meal to be fully effective.
		Monitor renal function.	Drug may accumulate in clients with renal dysfunction; not recommended for clients with serum creatinine greater than 2 mg/dL.
THIAZOLIDINEDIONES			
Pioglitazone (Actos)	15-30 mg once a day *Maximum:* 45 mg daily	Emphasize need for liver function tests as recommended.	Rare cases of liver failure have occurred with pioglitazone. Liver function tests are measured at start of therapy and at regular times thereafter.
		Emphasize need to report symptoms of unexplained nausea, vomiting, abdominal pain, fatigue, anorexia, or dark urine.	
		Advise women of childbearing age to use adequate contraception.	Administration of troglitazone with certain oral contraceptives may reduce the plasma concentration of the oral contraceptive.
Rosiglitazone (Advandia)	4 mg daily *Maximum:* 8 mg	Emphasize need for liver function tests as recommended.	Rare cases of liver failure have occurred with rosiglitazone. Liver function tests are measured at start of therapy and at regular times thereafter.
		Instruct client to report signs and symptoms of nausea, vomiting, abdominal pain, fatigue, anorexia, or dark urine.	
		Advise women of childbearing age to use adequate contraception.	Improved insulin sensitivity may allow ovulation to resume, increasing the chance of pregnancy.
D-PHENYLALANINE DERIVATIVES			
Nateglinide (Starlix)	*Usual:* 60-120 mg tid before meals *Maximum:* Optimal dose has not been defined *Duration:* 4 hr	Administer 1-30 min before meals.	Stimulates rapid secretion of insulin to reduce increases in blood glucose levels that occur soon after eating.
		Instruct client to omit medication when skipping a meal.	Reduces the risk of hypoglycemia.

TABLE 65-8 • DRUG INTERACTIONS WITH SULFONYLUREA AGENTS

POTENTIATE HYPOGLYCEMIA	WORSEN HYPERGLYCEMIA
Allopurinol (Zyloprim)	Amphetamines
Ammonium chloride	Asparaginase (Elspar)
Androgens (testosterone [Testoderm])	Bumetanide (Bumex)
Angiotensin-converting agents (captopril [Capoten], enalapril [Vasotec])	Calcium channel blockers (diltiazem, nifedipine)
Anticoagulants, oral (dicumarol)	Cholestyramine (Questran)
Antifungal azoles, systemic (fluconazole [Diflucan], miconazole [Monistat])	Chlorthalidone (Hygroton)
Barbiturates	Clonidine (Catapres)
Beta-adrenergic blocking agents (atenolol, propranolol)	Corticosteroids (prednisone)
Bromocriptine	Corticotropin (ACTH)
Calcium channel blockers (verapamil)	Danazol (Danocrine)
Clofibrate (Atromid-S)	Diazoxide, parenteral (Hyperstat)
Disopyramide (Norpace)	Dextrothyroxine (Choloxin)
Ethanol	Diuretics, thiazide (hydrochlorothiazide)
Fenfluramine (Pondimin)	Estrogen (Estrace, Premarin)
Fluoroquinolone anti-infectives (ciprofloxacin)	Estrogen-progesterone–containing oral contraceptives (Brevicon, Depo-Provera, Estrostep)
Guanethidine (Ismelin)	Furosemide (Lasix)
Histamine H_2 antagonists (cimetidine [Tagamet], ranitidine [Zantac])	Gemfibrozil (Lopid)
MAO inhibitors (phenelzine [Nardil])	Glucagon
Methyldopa (Aldomet)	Isoniazid (INH)
NSAIDs (indomethacin [Indocin], ibuprofen [Advil])	Lithium (Lithobid)
Octreotide (Sandostatin)	Morphine (morphine sulfate)
Probenecid (Benemid, Probalan)	Nicotinic acid (Nicolar)
Pyridoxine (vitamin B_6)	Pentamadine (pentamadine isethionate)
Quinidine (quinidine gluconate)	Phenothiazines (prochlorperazine [Compazine], trifluoperazine [Stelazine])
Quinine (quinine sulfate)	Phenytoin (Dilantin)
Sulfinpyrazone (Anturane)	Rifampin (Rifadin)
Sulfonamides (trimethoprim/sulfamethoxazole [Bactrim], sulfisoxazole [Gantrisin])	Salicylates (large doses)
Tetracycline	Thyroid hormones (liothyronine [Cytomel], levothyroxine [Levothroid, Synthroid])

Meglitinides. Repaglinide (Prandin) is an agent that has actions and adverse effects similar to those of sulfonylureas, although it binds to a different receptor site. The drug is taken before meals, has a rapid onset, and has a limited duration of action. Adverse effects associated with Repaglinide (Prandin) include hypoglycemia, GI disturbances, upper respiratory tract infection, arthralgia or back pain, and headache.

Biguanides. Metformin (Glucophage) lowers glucose by decreasing liver glucose release and by decreasing cellular insulin resistance. This drug does not stimulate insulin release, and when given alone, it does not cause hypoglycemia. Its major route of excretion is through the kidney and should not be given to anyone with renal disease (creatinine ≥1.5 in males, ≥1.4 in females). The drug should be withheld for 48 hours after administration of contrast material (Mahler & Adler, 1999).

Metformin can cause lactic acidosis in diabetic clients with renal insufficiency and should not be used with conditions that decrease oxygenation or decrease drug clearance, such as renal insufficiency, liver disease, alcoholism, severe congestive heart failure, severe peripheral vascular disease, or severe chronic obstructive pulmonary disease (Samos & Roos, 1998). The symptoms of lactic acidosis are often subtle and nonspecific. The nurse teaches the client to report symptoms of fatigue, unusual muscle pain, difficulty breathing, unusual or unexpected stomach discomfort, dizziness, lightheadedness, or irregular heartbeats to the primary care provider. Clients are instructed to take metformin with meals to reduce GI effects. The nurse cautions against alcohol intake because alcohol potentiates the effects of metformin on lactate metabolism.

Alpha-Glucosidase Inhibitors. Alpha-glucosidase inhibitors reduce postprandial hyperglycemia by slowing digestion and absorption of carbohydrate within the intestine. These agents inhibit enzymes in the intestinal tract, delaying the digestion of carbohydrate. The prolonged digestion time reduces the rate of glucose absorption and lowers postprandial blood glucose levels. The most frequent side effects are flatulence, diarrhea, and abdominal discomfort. There are two drugs in this class. Acarbose (Precose) is well tolerated when dosing is started at a low range (25 mg once daily to three times daily with meals) and increased slowly. At higher doses, symptoms of carbohydrate malabsorption are common. Miglitol (Glyset) should be taken three times daily at the start (with the first bite) of each main meal. Clients using alpha-glucosidase inhibitors as combination therapy may experience hypoglycemia secondary to insulin or sulfonylureas. Because these drugs interfere with the conversion of complex sugars to glucose during digestion, only simple sugars or milk is used for oral correction of hypoglycemia.

Thiazolidinedione Antidiabetic Agents. Thiazolidinediones enhance insulin action, thus promoting glucose utilization in peripheral tissues. They are known as "insulin sensitizers" and include rosiglitazone (Avandia) and pioglitazone (Actos). These drugs improve sensitivity to insulin in muscle and fat tissue and inhibit gluconeogenesis. They can be used in combination with a sulfonylurea agent or insulin to improve blood glucose control because their mechanisms of action are different. Clients taking any drug of this class should have liver function studies performed at the start of therapy and regularly thereafter because of potential liver damage. Clients with liver enzyme values more than 2.5 times higher than normal should not start therapy, and those with values more than 3 times higher should have the drug discontinued (Rosiglitazone, 1999). All drugs in this class have effects on serum lipids.

Other side effects of this drug class include infection, headache, and pain. Administration of thiazolidinediones can reduce the effectiveness of oral contraceptives.

D-Phenylalanine Derivatives. Nateglinide (Starlix) lowers blood glucose by stimulating insulin secretion via interaction with the ATP-sensitive potassium channel on pancreatic beta cells. This action is dependent on functioning beta cells in the pancreatic islet cells. Nateglinide (Starlix) is rapidly absorbed and stimulates insulin secretion within 20 minutes of oral administration. It is taken just before meals to control mealtime hyperglycemia, resulting in improved overall glycemic control in clients with type 2 diabetes. Adverse effects include hypoglycemia, upper respiratory infection, and diarrhea. Clients who skip meals should also skip their scheduled dose of Starlix to reduce the risk of hypoglycemia.

Combination Agents. Newer oral agents combine drugs from two different classes. Glucovance, for example, combines the second-generation sulfonylurea glyburide with metformin. This combination of drugs is more efficient than either drug alone and decreases blood glucose levels at lower doses because these agents have different mechanisms of action.

Drug Administration. Drugs are started initially at the lowest effective dosage, and increases in dosage are made every 1 to 2 weeks until acceptable blood glucose control or maximal dosage is reached. If the maximal dosage does not control blood glucose levels, a different oral agent is used.

Antidiabetic drugs are not a substitute for dietary modification and exercise. The client is taught about the need for continuing dietary restrictions and regular exercise while taking antidiabetic medication. To avoid adverse drug interactions, the nurse teaches the client to consult with the primary care provider before using any over-the-counter drugs.

Drug Selection. The choice of oral antidiabetic drug is based on cost, the client's ability to manage multiple drug doses, and the client's age and response to the drugs. Sulfonylureas are less expensive than other oral antidiabetic agents, can be taken once daily, and are associated with few side effects. Metformin (Glucophage) is more expensive than sulfonylurea agents and is associated with GI side effects. Acarbose must be taken before each meal.

Beta-cell function often declines over time, reducing the effectiveness of oral antidiabetic drugs. The treatment regimen for the client with type 2 diabetes may eventually require insulin therapy either alone or in combination with oral agents.

Insulin Therapy. Insulin therapy is needed for type 1 diabetes and for moderate to severe type 2 diabetes. The safety of insulin therapy in older clients may be affected by decreasing vision, mobility and coordination problems, and decreased memory. There are many types of insulin and regimens, all aimed at achieving normal blood glucose levels.

Types of Insulin. Insulin is obtained from animal sources (beef or pork pancreas), combinations of animal sources and semisynthetic human insulin, and synthetic human insulin (made through recombinant DNA technology). There are differences in strength and onset of action between human insulin and animal-source insulin. Thus dose and timing adjustments are needed when a client changes from one type of insulin to the other. Human insulin tends to have a more rapid onset of action, a shorter peak action, and a shorter duration of action than animal-source insulin. Human insulin is preferred for pregnant women or women considering pregnancy, clients with allergies or resistance to animal-source insulins, clients beginning insulin therapy, and clients expected to use insulin only intermittently (ADA, 2000l).

Rapid-, short-, intermediate-, and long-acting forms of insulin can be injected separately or mixed in the same syringe. Insulin is available in concentrations of 100 units/mL (U-100) and 500 units/mL (U-500). U-500 is used only in rare cases of insulin resistance. U-500 and insulin lispro are the only insulins that require a prescription. Velosulin BR and Velosulin Human (both U-100 insulins) contain phosphate buffers for use with external insulin pumps. U-400 is being used in some implantable pumps on an experimental basis.

The nurse teaches the client that the insulin type and species, the injection technique, the site of injection, and the individual response can all affect the absorption, onset, degree, and duration of insulin activity. The nurse reinforces the information that changing insulins may affect blood glucose control and should be done only under careful supervision (ADA, 2000l). Table 65-9 reviews the types and sources of available insulin preparations, and Table 65-10 outlines the time activity of subcutaneous human insulin.

Insulin Regimens. Insulin regimens try to duplicate the normal release pattern of insulin from the pancreas. The pancreas produces a constant *(basal)* amount of insulin that balances liver glucose production with glucose use and maintains normal blood glucose levels between meals. The pancreas also produces additional *(prandial)* insulin, stimulated by food, that prevents postmeal blood glucose elevations. The insulin dose required for acceptable blood glucose control varies considerably among clients. A usual starting dose is between 0.5 and 1 units/kg of body weight per day. For multiple-dose regimens or continuous subcutaneous insulin infusion (CSII), basal insulin makes up about 40% to 50% of the total daily dosage, with the remainder divided into premeal doses of regular insulin. Dosage adjustments are based on the results of blood glucose monitoring. Because the rate of absorption is slowed by increasing the dosage, adjustments in dosage should be made no more often than every 3 to 4 days (Hirsh, 1998).

Most of the insulin regimens use NPH insulin for basal insulin coverage. Humulin U Ultralente insulin provides a lower basal rate and may be used instead of NPH insulin when frequent hypoglycemic episodes occur. Insulin glargine (Lantus), a long-acting insulin analog, is available for once-daily subcutaneous injection at bedtime to provide basal insulin coverage. The client determines the effect of long-acting insulin by monitoring fasting blood glucose values. Different insulin protocols (regimens or programs) are shown in Figure 65-4.

Single Daily Injection Protocol. Many clients inject insulin only once daily. This protocol may include only intermediate-acting insulin or a combination of short- and intermediate-

TABLE 65-9 • INSULIN PREPARATIONS

Type	Source
INSULIN ANALOG	
• Humalog (Lilly)	DNA technology
• Insulin aspart (Novo Nordisk)	DNA technology
SHORT-ACTING INSULINS	
Insulin injection (regular crystalline insulin):	
• Iletin II R (Lilly)	Pork (purified)
• Regular (Novo Nordisk)	Pork (purified)
Insulin human injection (regular human insulin):	
• Humulin R (Lilly)	DNA technology
• Novolin R (Novo Nordisk)	DNA technology
• Velosulin BR (Novo Nordisk)	Semisynthetic
• Velosulin BR (Novo Nordisk)	DNA technology
CONCENTRATED INSULIN	
Insulin injection (regular crystalline insulin):	
• Iletin II U-500 (Lilly)	Pork (purified)
INTERMEDIATE-ACTING INSULINS	
Isophane insulin suspension (NPH insulin):	
• Iletin II (Lilly)	Pork (purified)
• NPH pork (Novo Nordisk)	Pork (purified)
• Humulin N (Lilly)	DNA technology
• Novolin N (Novo Nordisk)	DNA technology
Insulin zinc suspension (Lente insulin):	
• Iletin II (Lilly)	Pork (purified)
• Lente L (Novo Nordisk)	Pork (purified)
• Humulin L (Lilly)	DNA technology
• Novolin L (Novo Nordisk)	DNA technology
FIXED-COMBINATION INSULINS	
• Humulin 50/50 (Lilly)	DNA technology
• Humulin 70/30 (Lilly)	DNA technology
• Novolin 70/30 (Novo Nordisk)	DNA technology
LONG-ACTING INSULINS	
• Humulin U (Lilly)	DNA technology
• Insulin Glargine (Aventis)	DNA technology
BUFFERED INSULINS FOR USE IN EXTERNAL PUMPS	
• Humulin BR (Lilly)	DNA technology
• Velosulin BR (Novo Nordisk)	Semisynthetic
• Velosulin BR (Novo Nordisk)	DNA technology

acting insulin. A single dose of intermediate-acting insulin may not match the blood insulin level with food intake. When fasting glucose levels become elevated, a multiple-injection protocol should be considered.

Two-Dose Protocol. Combinations of short- and intermediate-acting insulin are injected twice daily. Two thirds of the daily dose is given before breakfast, and one third is given before the evening meal. Initially, intermediate-acting and regular insulin are usually given in a 2:1 ratio, and the evening (or bedtime) dose is given in a 1:1 ratio. Changes in these ratios are then based on results of blood glucose monitoring. Disadvantages of this schedule are that nighttime hypoglycemia is common and the blood glucose value in the morning is higher than desired (Hirsh, 1998).

TABLE 65-10 • TIME ACTIVITY OF SUBCUTANEOUS HUMULIN INSULIN

Insulin	Onset	Peak	Duration
Rapid-acting (lispro insulin)	15-30 min	1-2 hr	3-4 hr
Short-acting (regular)	0.5-1 hr	2-4 hr	6-8 hr
Intermediate-acting (NPH, Lente)	1-4 hr	4-12 hr	18-24 hr
Long-acting (Ultralente)	4-8 hr	18 hr	24-36 hr

Three-Dose Protocol. A combination of short- and intermediate-acting insulin is given before breakfast, short-acting insulin is given before the evening meal, and intermediate-acting insulin is given at bedtime. Giving intermediate-acting insulin at bedtime results in lower fasting and after-breakfast blood glucose levels. This schedule avoids nighttime hypoglycemia but may not provide enough coverage for the noon meal (Funnell et al., 1998).

Four-Dose Protocol. Giving short-acting insulin 30 minutes before meals allows the greatest amount of insulin to be present during the greatest insulin need. Basal insulin is provided by twice-daily injection of intermediate-acting insulin or a bedtime injection of long-acting insulin. Injection of premeal short-acting insulin based on anticipated carbohydrate intake allows some highly motivated clients with type 1 diabetes to have more flexibility in meal timing and size. Insulin lispro should be given within 15 minutes of eating a meal; peak action usually occurs within 30 to 90 minutes. Because this insulin duration of action is short, the client taking insulin lispro also requires longer-acting insulin for basal insulin requirements.

Combination Therapy. A combination of oral agents and intermediate-acting insulin is given to clients with type 2 diabetes who do not have reasonable control of blood glucose levels with oral agents alone. Obese diabetic clients with higher fasting C-peptide levels may be more likely to respond to combination therapy than to single therapy.

Intensified Therapy Regimens. Intensified regimens are composed of a basal dose of intermediate-acting insulin and a bolus dose of short-acting insulin designed to bring the next blood glucose value into the target range. The client's blood glucose patterns determine insulin dosage. The frequency of blood glucose monitoring is based on the timed action of short- and intermediate-acting insulins and may be required as often as eight times daily. Blood glucose testing 1 hour after meals and within 10 minutes before the next meal helps determine the adequacy of the bolus dose. The client determines the effects of basal insulin by monitoring pre-evening meal and fasting blood glucose values. Blood glucose values at 3 AM can detect nighttime hypoglycemia and indicate adequacy of both short- and intermediate-acting insulin doses.

Clients on intensified insulin regimens need extensive education to achieve target blood glucose values. The client needs to understand clearly how to self-adjust insulin doses and must understand nutrition therapy so that dietary flexibility can be maintained within target blood glucose values.

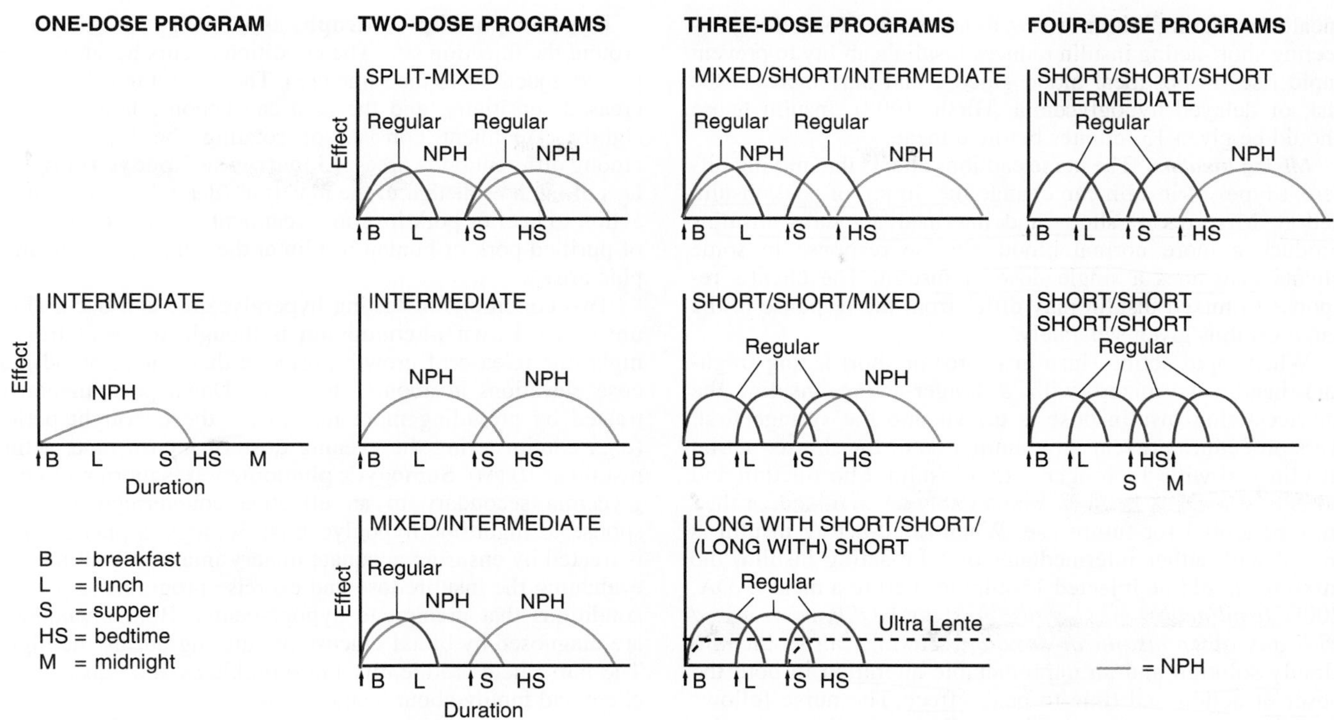

Figure 65-4 ● Insulin regimens. One injection a day of short-acting or intermediate-acting insulin may be enough to control blood glucose levels. However, split doses (two, three, or four injections of the daily dose) or split mixed doses (a mixture of short-acting and longer-acting insulins) may give better control.

Clients must also be able to perform blood glucose monitoring with precision so that therapy decisions can be based on accurate data.

Pharmacokinetics of Insulin. The action of insulin to move glucose into the cells after insulin injection depends on various factors, including physical factors and injection techniques.

Injection Site. Figure 65-5 shows common insulin injection sites. The site of injection affects the speed of insulin absorption. Absorption is fastest in the abdomen, followed by the deltoid, thigh, and buttocks. Rotating injection sites, either within one body area or between body areas, prevents **lipohypertrophy** (increased fat deposits in the skin) or **lipoatrophy** (loss of fatty tissue, leaving an uneven appearance). Rotation *within* one anatomic site is preferred to rotation from one site to another to prevent day-to-day changes in absorption. The abdomen (except for a 2-inch radius around the navel) is the preferred site of injection because it provides the most rapid insulin absorption.

Absorption Rate. Characteristics of insulin affect its absorption. The longer the duration of insulin action, the more unpredictable its absorption. Ultralente provides less consistent absorption than shorter-acting insulin preparations. The larger the dose of insulin, the more prolonged the absorption (Hirsh, 1998). Factors that increase blood flow from the injection site, such as local application of heat, massage of the area, and exercise of the injected area, increase insulin absorption. Scarred sites often become favorite injection sites because they are less sensitive to pain, but injection into scar tissue may delay absorption. Lipodystrophy does not affect the rate of insulin absorption (Burge & Schade, 1997).

Injection Depth. Injections are usually made into the subcutaneous tissue. Most individuals are able to lightly grasp a fold of skin and inject at a 90-degree angle. Aspiration for blood is not necessary. Thin individuals may need to pinch the skin and inject at a 45-degree angle to avoid intramuscular (IM) injection. IM injection produces a slightly faster absorption than does subcutaneous injection but is not recommended for routine insulin administration because of the risk for hypoglycemia (ADA, 2000l). The nurse assesses the older client's ability to administer insulin and arranges for assistance when self-care is no longer possible.

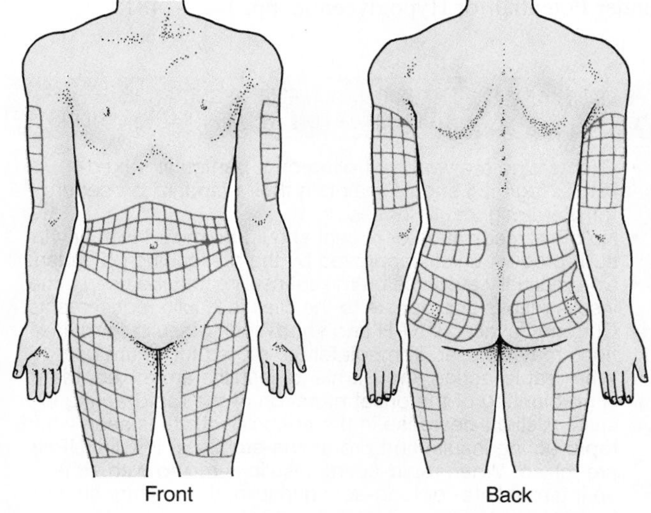

Figure 65-5 ● Common insulin injection sites.

Time of Injection. Injecting regular insulin 30 minutes before meals provides a greater amount of plasma free-insulin at mealtime. Eating within a few minutes after (or before) injecting short-acting insulin reduces insulin's ability to prevent rapid rises in postmeal blood glucose and may increase the risk of delayed hypoglycemia (Hirsh, 1998). Insulin lispro should be given 15 minutes before a meal.

Mixing Insulins. The nurse cautions clients that mixing different types of insulin can change the timing of peak insulin action. Mixtures of short- and intermediate-acting insulins produce a more normal blood glucose response in some clients than does a single dose of insulin. The client's response to mixed insulin may differ from the response to the same insulins given separately.

When rapid-acting (insulin lispro) or short-acting (regular) insulin is mixed with a longer-acting insulin, the shorter-acting insulin dose is drawn into the syringe first. This procedure prevents contamination of the shorter-acting insulin vial with the longer-acting insulin. Short-acting and NPH insulins may be used immediately when mixed, or they may be stored for future use. When rapid-acting insulin is mixed with either intermediate- or long-acting insulin, the mixture should be injected 15 minutes before a meal (ADA, 2001). *Insulin glargine (Lantus) must not be diluted or mixed with any other insulin or solution.* Mixing can result in a cloudy solution and an unpredictable alteration in both the onset of action and time to peak effect. The nurse follows American Diabetes Association (ADA) guidelines for mixing insulins (Table 65-11).

Complications of Insulin Therapy. Hypoglycemia, the result of excessive insulin levels, has a variety of causes. Manifestations and treatment of hypoglycemia are discussed later under Potential for Hypoglycemia, pp. 1478-1481.

TABLE 65-11 • AMERICAN DIABETES ASSOCIATION GUIDELINES FOR THE MIXING OF INSULINS

- Clients who are well controlled on a particular mixed-insulin regimen should maintain their standard procedure for preparing insulin doses.
- No other medication or diluent should be mixed with any insulin product unless approved by the prescribing physician.
- Commercially available premixed insulins may be used if the insulin ratio is appropriate to the client's insulin requirements.
- Currently available NPH and short-acting insulin formulations may be used immediately or stored for future use.
- When rapid-acting and Ultralente insulins are mixed, there is no blunting of the onset of action of the rapid-acting insulin. A slight decrease in the absorption rate is seen when rapid-acting insulin and protamine-stabilized insulin (NPH) are mixed. When rapid-acting insulin is mixed with either an intermediate- or long-acting insulin, the mixture should be injected 15 minutes before a meal.
- Mixing of short-acting and Lente insulin is not recommended, except for a few clients already controlled on this mixture.
- On mixing, zinc present in Lente preparations binds with the regular insulin and delays its onset of action.
- Clients using Lente mixed with regular insulin should standardize the interval between mixing and injecting.
- Phosphate-buffered insulins (NPH) should not be mixed with Lente insulins. Zinc phosphate, present in NPH insulin, may precipitate and convert the longer-acting insulin to a short-acting insulin, with unpredictable results.
- There is no rationale for mixing animal insulins with human insulins.

Data from American Diabetes Association. (2000). Position statement: Insulin administration. *Diabetes Care, 23*(Suppl. 1), 86-89.

Hypertrophic lipodystrophy is a spongy swelling at or around the injection site. The condition occurs because of repeated injections in the same area. The overlying skin has decreased sensitivity, and the area can become large and unsightly. Treatment consists of rotating the injection site among different body areas. **Lipoatrophic lipodystrophy** is a loss of fat at or distant to the injection site and occurs as a reaction to beef or pork insulin. Treatment consists of injection of purified pork or human insulin at the edge of the lipoatrophic area.

Two conditions of fasting hyperglycemia can occur (Figure 65-6). **Dawn phenomenon** is thought to result from a nighttime release of growth hormone that causes blood glucose elevations at about 5 to 6 AM. Dawn phenomenon is treated by providing more insulin for the overnight period (e.g., administering the evening dose of intermediate-acting insulin at 10 PM). **Somogyi's phenomenon** is morning hyperglycemia secondary to an effective counterregulatory response to nighttime hypoglycemia. Somogyi's phenomenon is treated by ensuring adequate dietary intake at bedtime and evaluating the insulin dose and exercise programs to prevent conditions that precipitate hypoglycemia. Both phenomena are diagnosed by blood glucose monitoring during the night. The nurse helps to identify these problems and educates the client and family about management.

Alternative Methods of Insulin Administration. Many methods of insulin delivery are available in addition to traditional intermittent subcutaneous injections.

Continuous Subcutaneous Infusion of Insulin. Continuous subcutaneous infusion of a basal dose of insulin (CSII) with increases in insulin at mealtimes seems to be more effective in controlling blood glucose levels than a multiple-injection schedule. CSII allows for total flexibility in meal timing, because if a meal is skipped, the mealtime dose of insulin is not administered. CSII is administered by an externally worn pump containing a syringe and reservoir with rapid- or short-acting insulin and connected to the client by an infusion set. The nurse teaches the client to adjust the amount of insulin received on the basis of data from blood glucose monitoring.

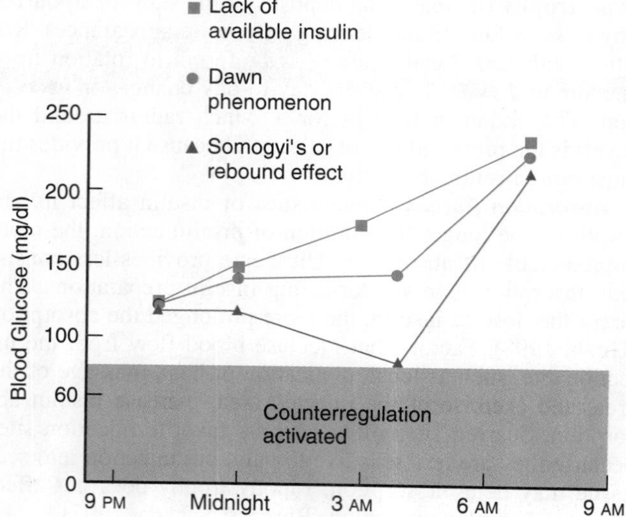

Figure 65-6 • Three blood glucose phenomena in diabetic clients.

Lispro is an appropriate insulin for insulin infusion pumps. The stability of this insulin in both MiniMed and Disetronic pumps has been confirmed (Figure 65-7). Lispro is not approved for use in pregnancy (ADA, 2000c).

Skin infections may occur when the infusion site is not cleaned or the needle placement is not changed every 3 days. When the client is receiving rapid-acting insulin and has normal blood glucose levels, cessation of insulin administration quickly results in hyperglycemia. The use of CSII is associated with more frequent and more severe ketoacidosis than with other methods of insulin administration. Ketoacidosis is related to inexperience in using the pump, infection, accidental cessation of insulin infusion, infusion set obstruction, or mechanical problems related to the pump. Buffered insulin may be used to prevent the precipitation of insulin crystals within the catheter. The nurse stresses the importance of regular testing for the presence of ketones.

Intensive education for clients using CSII is necessary. Because of the potential for hypoglycemia, as well as hyperglycemia, the client must perform all necessary functions to ensure accurate insulin administration. The nurse teaches the client to operate the pump, make adjustments in settings, and respond appropriately to alarms. Removal of the pump for any length of time can result in hyperglycemia. The nurse provides supplemental insulin schedules for times when the pump is not operational. CSII is expensive, compared with traditional insulin injections, and not all costs are covered by insurance.

Implanted Insulin Pumps. Insulin pumps are implanted in the peritoneal cavity, where insulin can be absorbed by blood vessels in the peritoneum in a manner similar to that of natural insulin release (Figure 65-8). Absorption of insulin into the portal circulation is believed to reduce peripheral hyperinsulinemia. The pump is surgically implanted in a subcutaneous pocket in the lower abdomen. The pump reservoir is refilled with U-400 insulin every 1 or 2 months. The major complications of implanted insulin pumps (IIPs) have been catheter blockage, inflammation in the subcutaneous pocket, and pump mechanical failure. Because mechanical problems associated with the pump, catheter, and insulin delivery have not been solved, the implantable pump is not widely available.

Injection Devices. In addition to traditional insulin syringes, injection devices include a needleless system and a pen-type injector. With a needleless device, the needle is replaced by an ultrathin liquid stream of insulin forced through the skin under high pressure. Insulin administered by jet injection is absorbed at a faster rate, with a resulting shorter duration of insulin action. How these changes affect overall metabolic control is yet to be determined. Cost is a primary drawback to this system.

Pen-type injectors hold small, lightweight, prefilled insulin cartridges. The injectors are easy to carry and make intensive insulin therapy with multiple injections easier to accomplish. These devices allow greater accuracy than traditional insulin syringes, especially when measuring doses lower than 5 units (Robertson, Glazer, & Campbell, 2000). The nurse discusses methods of maintaining the insulin cartridges at an appropriate temperature when using this device away from home. The nurse is cautious when recommending pen-type injectors for visually or neurologically impaired individuals. The packaging for all insulin pens includes a statement that they are not meant for independent use by visually impaired people (Williams, 1999b).

New Technology. Insulin absorption across the nasal mucosa is rapid, making nasal insulin delivery a possible alternative to parenteral injection. However only a small amount of insulin is actually absorbed through the mucosa, making blood glucose control inconsistent. A nasal spray, administered via nebulizer, is one new means of insulin administration. Studies are also underway to evaluate the effects of aerosolized insulin given by nebulized inhaler. Regular insulin (U-500) is delivered in an inhaler during inspiration (the lungs provide a large surface for absorption of insulin). Routine use of inhalers is imprecise and dependent on how the client times the dose with inhalation. Newer inhaler systems are being developed that trigger a precise dose of medication

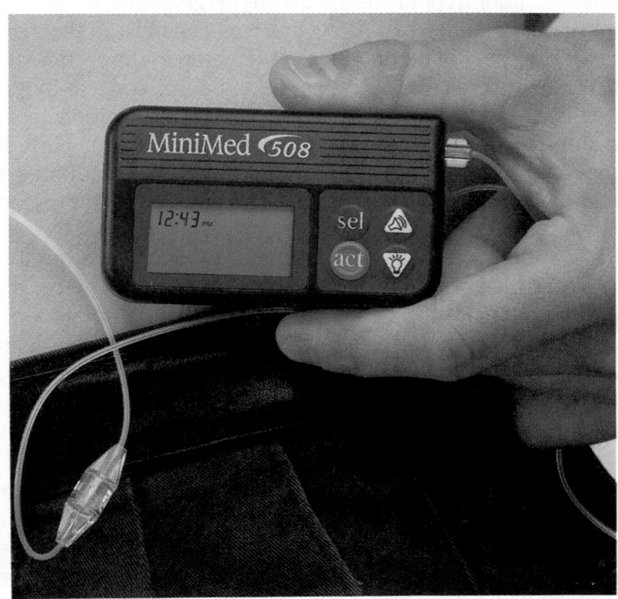

Figure 65-7 ● External insulin pump. (Courtesy MiniMed, Inc., Northridge, CA.)

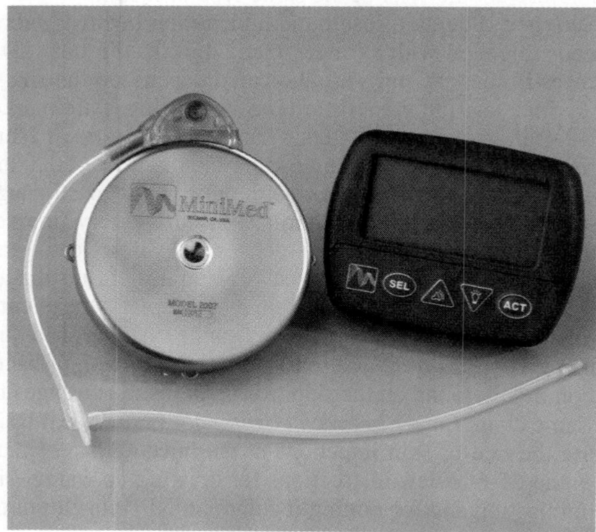

Figure 65-8 ● Internal insulin pump. (Courtesy MiniMed, Inc., Northridge, CA.)

at the time when airflow from inhalation reaches a certain rate (Saudek, 1997).

Transdermal (through the skin) delivery of insulin is being tested. This method of drug delivery appears to be predictable but slower than delivery with traditional injections (Robertson, Glazer, & Campbell, 2000).

NIC **Client Education: Prescribed Medication.** The nurse provides specific instructions to the client undergoing insulin therapy. Chart 65-4 lists NIC intervention activities for assisting with self-medication.

Storage. Insulin not in use should be refrigerated; refrigeration maintains potency, prevents exposure to sunlight, and inhibits bacterial growth. Insulin in use may be kept at room temperature to limit local irritation at the injection site, which may occur when cold insulin is used.

To prevent loss of drug potency, the client is taught to avoid subjecting insulin to temperatures less than 36° F (2.2° C) or greater than 86° F (30° C) or to excessive agitation. Ideally, insulin lispro is refrigerated but not frozen. The vial or cartridge of insulin lispro can be unrefrigerated for up to 28 days, as long as it is kept as cool as possible (not greater than 86° F [30° C]) and away from direct heat and light.

The client is instructed to always have a spare bottle of each type of insulin used. A slight loss in potency may occur after the bottle has been in use for more than 30 days even when the expiration date has not been passed. When refrigerated, prefilled syringes are stable up to 30 days. If possible, the syringes are stored in the vertical (upright) position, with the needle pointing upward, so that insulin particles do not clog the needle. The predrawn syringe should be rolled between the hands before administration. The primary care provider assesses the effect of premixing insulins on blood glucose control by examining blood glucose levels (ADA, 2000l).

Dose Preparation. The person administering the insulin inspects the bottle before each use for changes (e.g., clumping, frosting, precipitation, or change in clarity or color) that may signify loss in potency. Rapid- and short-acting insulins should be clear, and all other types of insulin should be uniformly cloudy after gently rolling the vial between the hands. If the potency of an insulin vial is questionable, the person should use another vial of the same type of insulin.

Syringes. Standard insulin administration involves subcutaneous injection with syringes marked in insulin units. Differences in the way units are indicated depend on the size of the syringe and the manufacturer. Some syringes are marked in 1-unit increments, and other syringes are marked in 2-unit increments. Syringes are manufactured in 0.25-, 0.3-, 0.5- and 1-mL capacity. The needle sizes range from 27 to 30 gauge. Needle lengths may be standard (12.7 mm), a very fine version (15.9 mm), or a short version (8 mm). Short needles are not used for obese clients because of variability of insulin absorption. To ensure accurate insulin measurement, the client is instructed to always buy the same type of syringes. Most insulin preparations have additives that inhibit growth of bacteria commonly found on the skin. Reuse of insulin syringes for the same client *(never between clients)* does not appear to increase the rate of skin infections at the injection site. Charts 65-5 and 65-6 review instructions for drawing up a single insulin injection and for mixing regular and NPH insulin in the same syringe (ADA, 2000l).

Client Education: Blood Glucose Monitoring. Self-monitoring of blood glucose levels (SMBG) provides information that allows the client to adjust therapy. The nurse teaches the client to use the physician's prescribed formulas to (1) self-adjust diet, exercise, or pharmacologic therapy; (2) identify and properly treat hyperglycemia and hypoglycemia; and (3) improve decision making and problem solving. See Table 65-12 for costs of blood glucose monitors and strips.

The American Diabetes Association (ADA) recommends SMBG for clients taking insulin or oral agent therapy. Ongoing knowledge of blood glucose levels is especially important for the following clients:

- Any diabetic client attempting to maintain glucose levels in the near-normal range
- Pregnant clients
- Clients with a tendency to develop severe ketosis or hypoglycemia
- Clients with hypoglycemic unawareness
- Clients undergoing intensive treatment programs, especially those using portable infusion devices, or taking multiple daily insulin injections

The operating principles of most self-monitoring systems are the same. The finger is pricked, and a drop of blood is made to flow over a reagent pad on a testing strip. Meters measure blood glucose by using color reflectance or sensor technology. With reflectance meters, the glucose in a drop of blood reacts with an enzyme in the strip, changing the color of the strip. The meter reads the color of the strip and gives a number for the blood glucose value. Meters that use sensor technology measure small electrical currents produced by the interaction between the glucose in the blood and the chemicals on the strip (Peragallo-Dittko, 1999). The client can also perform visual blood glucose monitoring by comparing the color on a test strip with the strip on the test strip vial.

There is some variation between glucose concentration in whole blood by SMBG systems and that measured by clinical laboratory procedures. The ADA has set the performance goal to be a total error of no more than 10% at glucose concentrations ranging between 30 and 400 mg/dL (1.6 and 22.2 mmol/L) (ADA, 1996). The accuracy of SMBG systems decreases at both hypoglycemic and hyperglycemic levels. The overall performance of SMBG systems depends on the accuracy of the specific blood glucose meter, operator proficiency, and test strip quality. Results may be influenced by the amount of blood on the strip; the meter's calibration to the strip currently in use; environmental conditions of altitude, temperature, and moisture; and client-specific conditions of hematocrit level, triglyceride concentration, and the presence of hypotension.

Most meters indicate blood glucose results as a number, but some have voice readouts, memories that can be displayed, or capabilities for graphic displays on a computer. A client's visual impairments, including color blindness, determine the method of SMBG selected. Some models have large, bold display screens and simple, user-friendly procedures. Other models use voice modules to announce the display messages.

The client and nurse follow Centers for Disease Control and Prevention (CDC) guidelines for infection control during SMBG. The chance of becoming infected from blood glucose monitoring processes can be reduced by handwashing before monitoring and not reusing lancets. Clients are instructed not to share their blood glucose monitoring equipment. Hepatitis B virus can survive in a dried state for at least 1 week. Infec-

CHART 65-4

NIC INTERVENTION ACTIVITIES *for* The Diabetic Client with Hyperglycemia

Hyperglycemia Management: *Preventing and treating above-normal blood glucose levels*
- Monitor blood glucose levels, as indicated.
- Monitor for signs and symptoms of hyperglycemia: polyuria, polydipsia, polyphagia, weakness, lethargy, malaise, blurring of vision, or headache.
- Monitor urine ketones, as indicated.
- Monitor ABG, electrolyte, and β-hydroxybutyrate levels, as available.
- Monitor orthostatic blood pressure and pulse, as indicated.
- Administer insulin, as prescribed.
- Encourage oral fluid intake.
- Monitor fluid status (including I&O), as appropriate.
- Maintain IV access, as appropriate.
- Administer IV fluids, as needed.
- Administer potassium, as prescribed.
- Consult physician if signs and symptoms of hyperglycemia persist or worsen.
- Identify possible causes of hyperglycemia.
- Anticipate situations in which insulin requirements will increase (e.g., intercurrent illness).
- Restrict exercise when blood glucose levels are >250 mg/dL, especially if urine ketones are present.
- Instruct client and significant others on prevention, recognition, and management of hyperglycemia.
- Encourage self-monitoring of blood glucose levels.
- Instruct on urine ketone testing, as appropriate.
- Instruct client and significant others on diabetes management during illness, including use of insulin and/or oral agents, monitoring fluid intake, carbohydrate replacement, and when to seek health professional assistance, as appropriate.
- Provide assistance in adjusting regimen to prevent and treat hyperglycemia (e.g., increasing insulin or oral agent), as indicated.

Teaching: Prescribed Medication: *Preparing a client to safely take prescribed medications and monitor for their effects*
- Instruct the client to recognize distinctive characteristics of the medication(s), as appropriate.
- Inform the client of both the generic and brand names of each medication.
- Instruct the client on the purpose and action of each medication.
- Instruct the client on the dosage, route, and duration of each medication.
- Instruct the client on the proper administration/application of each medication.
- Evaluate the client's ability to self-administer medications.
- Instruct the client to perform needed procedures before taking a medication (e.g., check pulse, glucose), as appropriate.
- Inform the client what to do if a dose of medication is missed.
- Inform the client of consequences of not taking or abruptly discontinuing medication(s), as appropriate.
- Instruct the client on which criteria to use when deciding to alter the medication/dosage schedule, as appropriate.
- Instruct the client on possible adverse side effects of each medication.
- Instruct the client on how to relieve and/or prevent certain side effects, as appropriate.
- Instruct the client on appropriate actions to take if side effects occur.
- Instruct the client on the signs and symptoms of overdosage or underdosage.
- Inform the client of possible drug/food interactions, as appropriate.
- Instruct the client how to properly store the medication(s).
- Instruct the client on the proper care of devices used for administration.
- Instruct the client on proper disposal of needles and syringes at home, as appropriate, and where to dispose of the sharps container in their community.
- Provide the client with written information about the medication action, purpose, side effects, and so on.
- Assist the client to develop a written medication schedule.
- Instruct the client to carry documentation of his or her prescribed medication regimen.
- Instruct the client how to fill his or her prescription(s), as appropriate.
- Inform the client of possible changes in appearance and/or dosage when filling generic medication prescriptions.
- Warn the client of the risks associated with taking expired medications.
- Determine the client's ability to obtain required medications.
- Provide information on medication reimbursement, as appropriate.
- Provide information on cost savings programs/organizations to obtain medications and devices, as appropriate.
- Provide information on medication alert devices and how to obtain them.
- Reinforce information provided by other health care team members, as appropriate.
- Include the family/significant others, as appropriate.

Teaching: Prescribed Diet: *Preparing a client to correctly follow a prescribed diet*
- Appraise the client's current level of knowledge about prescribed diet.
- Determine the client's/significant other's feelings/attitude toward prescribed diet and expected degree of dietary compliance.
- Instruct the client on the proper name of the prescribed diet.
- Explain the purpose of the diet.
- Instruct the client about how to keep a food diary, as appropriate.
- Instruct the client on allowed and prohibited foods.
- Inform the client of possible drug/food interactions, as appropriate.
- Assist the client to accommodate food preferences into the prescribed diet.
- Assist the client in substituting ingredients to conform favorite recipes to the prescribed diet.
- Instruct the client about how to read labels and select appropriate foods.
- Observe the client's selection of foods appropriate to prescribed diet.
- Instruct the client about how to plan appropriate meals.
- Provide written meal plans, as appropriate.
- Reinforce information provided by other health care team members, as appropriate.
- Refer client to dietitian/nutritionist, as appropriate.
- Include the family/significant others, as appropriate.

NIC intervention activities selected from McCloskey J.C., & Bulechek, G.M. (2000). *Nursing interventions classification (NIC)* (3rd ed.). St. Louis: Mosby.

ABG, Arterial blood gas; *I&O,* intake and output.

tion can be spread in the lancet holder even when the lancet itself has been changed. Small particles of blood can stick to the device and infect multiple users. Regular cleaning of the meter is important in infection control. Health care personnel who perform blood glucose testing and family members who assist with testing should wear gloves to provide protection from infection (American Association of Diabetes Educators, 1997).

Interpretation of Results. Accuracy of blood glucose measurements may be reduced by errors in technique, equipment failure, or misrepresentation. The data obtained from SMBG are evaluated together with other measures of blood glucose levels (e.g., glycosylated hemoglobin, or hemoglobin A_{1c} [HbA_{1c}], values) or periodic laboratory blood glucose tests. Even when SMBG is performed correctly, the results are affected by hematocrit values (anemia falsely elevates hematocrit values; polycythemia falsely depresses them) and may be unreliable in the hypoglycemic or severe hyperglycemic ranges. Accuracy of the meter itself is also an issue. Even when highly trained personnel tested meters under optimal conditions, there was wide variation in accuracy and precision between capillary blood glucose monitoring devices approved for the clinical market. Laboratory glucose determinations are more accurate than SMBG.

Frequency of Testing. The frequency of monitoring varies with the complexity of the medication schedules and the goals of therapy. Diabetic clients with unstable blood glucose levels, as well as those undergoing intensive treatment regimens

CHART 65-5

CLIENT EDUCATION GUIDE
Subcutaneous Insulin Administration

- Wash your hands.
- Inspect the bottle for the type of insulin and the expiration date.
- Gently roll the bottle of intermediate-acting insulin in the palms of your hands to mix the insulin.
- Clean the rubber stopper with an alcohol swab.
- Remove the needle cover and pull back the plunger to draw air into the syringe. The amount of air should be equal to the insulin dose. Push the needle through the rubber stopper and inject the air into the insulin bottle.
- Turn the bottle upside down and draw the insulin dose into the syringe.
- Remove air bubbles in the syringe by tapping on the syringe or injecting air back into the bottle. Redraw the correct amount.
- Make certain the tip of the plunger is on the line for your dose of insulin. Magnifiers are available to assist in measuring accurate doses of insulin.
- Remove the needle from the bottle. Recap the needle if the insulin is not to be given immediately.
- Select a site within your injection area that has not been used in the past month.
- Clean your skin with an alcohol swab. Lightly grasp an area of skin and insert the needle at a 90-degree angle.
- Push the plunger all the way down. This will push the insulin into your body. Release the pinched skin.
- Pull the needle straight out quickly. Do not rub the place where you gave the shot.
- Dispose of the syringe and needle without recapping in a puncture-proof container.

Data from American Diabetes Association. (2000). Position statement: Insulin administration. *Diabetes Care, 23*(Suppl. 1), 86-89.

CHART 65-6

CLIENT EDUCATION GUIDE
How to Mix a Prescribed Dose of 10 Units of Regular Insulin and 20 Units of NPH Insulin

- Wash your hands.
- Inspect the bottles for the type of insulin and the expiration date.
- Gently roll the bottle of intermediate insulin in the palms of your hands to mix the insulin.
- Clean the rubber stopper with an alcohol swab.
- Inject 20 units of air into the NPH insulin bottle. The amount of air should be equal to the dose of insulin needed. Always inject air into the intermediate-acting insulin first. Withdraw the syringe.
- Inject 10 units of air into the regular insulin bottle. The amount of air is equal to the dose of insulin desired.
- Withdraw 10 units of regular insulin. Be sure that the syringe is free of air bubbles. Always withdraw the shorter-acting insulin first.
- Withdraw 20 units of NPH insulin with the same syringe, being careful not to inject any short-acting insulin into the bottle. (A total of 30 units should be in the syringe.)

Data from American Diabetes Association. (2001). Position statement: Insulin administration. *Diabetes Care, 23*(Suppl. 1), 86-89.

TABLE 65-12 • COST OF BLOOD GLUCOSE MONITORS AND STRIPS

Meter	Cost of Meter	Test Strips (50)	Test Strips (100)
Accu Chek Advantage:	Complete Care Kit: $97.99 (Rebate: $25.00, trade-in: $50.00)	Comfort Curve: $33.95	Comfort Curve: $59.44
One Touch Profile	One Touch Profile System: $97.99 (Rebate: $25.00, trade-in: $50.00)	$34.75	$61.29
Glucometer	Encore Diabetes Kit: $74.95 (Rebate: $30.00, trade-in: $10.00)	$31.99	
	Glucometer Elite XL Diabetes Care System: $49.95 (Rebate: $25.00, trade-in: $25.00)	$32.97	$59.99
Precision QID	QID: $54.99 (Rebate: $35.00, trade-in: $20.00)	$35.77	$56.95
Sure Step	Sure Step Blood Glucose System: $59.99 (Rebate: $40.00, trade-in: $20.00)	$33.95	$59.44
Exact Tech	R.S.G. Meter: $29.99 (Rebate: $20.00, Trade-in: $10.00)	$24.97	$43.99

Data from http://www.diabeteswebsite.com.

(continuous subcutaneous insulin infusions with pumps or more than three injections daily) require frequent blood glucose monitoring. Clients undergoing minimal treatment regimens designed to prevent symptomatic hyperglycemia or clients with type 2 diabetes receiving oral agents require less frequent monitoring.

Blood Glucose Therapy Goals. The nurse works with the client to reach set goals for blood glucose therapy. Target blood glucose levels are set individually for each client. On the basis of the Diabetes Control and Complications Trial (DCCT) results, a diabetes policy group recommends that clients with type 1 diabetes aim for premeal glucose levels of 80 to 120 mg/dL (4.4 to 6.7 mmol/L) and a bedtime level of 100 to 140 mg/dL (6.1 to 7.8 mmol/L) (Goldstein & Little, 1997).

Accuracy of Self-Monitoring of Blood Glucose Levels. All meters currently available are reasonably accurate when the manufacturer's directions are followed. Results are technique dependent regardless of whether test strips are read visually or with a meter. The nurse helps the client select a meter on the basis of the cost of the meter and strips, ease of use, availability of repair and maintenance service, and ability to discriminate color. The nurse provides training, including an explanation and demonstration of the procedures, assesses visual acuity, tests for color blindness as indicated, and checks the learner's ability to accurately perform the procedure through a return demonstration. Assessment of the diabetic client's ability to discriminate between colors is vital for those who do not use a blood glucose meter.

The most common error in SMBG is failure to follow instructions about properly applying blood on the test strip, timing, and removing blood samples from the monitor. Because performance accuracy deteriorates over time, continued retraining of clients performing SMBG is necessary to ensure that results are accurate.

CONSIDERATIONS FOR OLDER ADULTS

Visual interpretation of blood glucose values is affected by the normal changes of aging. The ability to discriminate shades of blue, violet, and green becomes less accurate. Older clients require three times as much light to see things as they did at age 20. It is more effective to place high-intensity light on the object or surface than to increase light for the entire room.

New Technology. Blood glucose measurements can be obtained "continuously" by means of a glucose sensor placed under the skin of the abdomen. The sensor measures glucose in interstitial fluid every 5 minutes. The information shows blood glucose fluctuations over the course of the day and allows adjustments in intensive insulin therapy to be made more accurately.

Several noninvasive monitoring systems that measure glucose in interstitial fluid are under development. The GlucoWatch received approval from the Advisory Panel of the Food and Drug Administration (FDA) in December 1999. The device sends a tiny electrical current through the skin and measures glucose from interstitial fluid just beneath the surface of the skin. Glucose measurements can be obtained every 20 minutes. The GlucoWatch is meant to supplement, not replace, finger stick tests. Because the reliability of this device has not yet been determined, the FDA recommends that insulin be given only after confirming the results of the GlucoWatch with a finger stick test (Trecroci, 1999) (Table 65-13).

Systems for obtaining blood without finger sticks are also being developed. The Professional Lancette uses a laser beam to vaporize a pinpoint of skin on the user's finger to get a drop of blood.

DIET THERAPY. Effective self-management of diabetes requires that the meal plan, education, and counseling program be individualized for each client (see Chart 65-4). Because of the complexity of nutrition issues, a registered dietitian should be a member of the treatment team. The nurse, dietitian, client, and family work together on all aspects of the meal plan. The meal plan must be realistic and as flexible as possible.

Goals of Diet Therapy. Diet therapy for clients with diabetes focuses on the following goals:

- Maintenance of as near-normal blood glucose levels as possible
- Achievement of optimal serum lipid levels: low-density lipoprotein (LDL) cholesterol less than 100 mg/dL (2.60 mmol/L) and triglyceride levels less than 200 mg/dL (<2.30 mmol/L) (ADA, 2000m, 2000t)
- Achievement of optimal blood pressure goals, usually less than 130/85 mm Hg (ADA, 2000t)
- Ensuring adequate calories for achieving reasonable weight for adults, meeting increased metabolic needs during pregnancy and lactation, or promoting recovery from illness
- Prevention and treatment of the acute complications of hypoglycemic medications, short-term illness, and exercise-related problems
- Prevention and treatment of complications of diabetes, such as renal disease, neuropathy, and cardiovascular disease
- Improvement of overall health through optimal nutrition (ADA, 2000n)

Principles of Nutrition in Diabetes. The dietitian formulates a meal plan based on the client's usual food intake. Day-to-day consistency in the timing and amount of food consumed helps control blood glucose. Clients receiving insulin therapy need to eat at consistent times that are coordinated with the timed action of insulin. Clients receiving in-

TABLE 65-13 • COST OF BLOOD GLUCOSE MONITORING PRODUCTS

Product	Cost	Cost of Supplies	Comments
Lasette	$995	Disposable cartridge: $30 for a two-pack ($0.12 per test)	Cartridge is good for 120 uses. Battery is rechargeable, with 50 uses per charge.
GlucoWatch	$250-$350	Disposable pads: $4 to $5	Pads must be changed every 12 hours. Watch should last 2-3 yr.

Data from http://www.cellrobotics.com/perslasette.html; and http://www.glucowatch.com.

tense insulin therapy can be taught to adjust premeal insulin to allow for timing and quantity changes in their meal plan (ADA, 2000n).

Protein. The recommended protein intake for the client with diabetes is the same as that for the general population, with 10% to 20% of total caloric intake coming from protein. A dietary protein intake of 10% of calories (0.8 g/kg of body weight) is recommended for clients with nephropathy (ADA, 2000n).

Fat and Carbohydrate. The amount of calories from fat and carbohydrates is based on individualized nutritional goals. Of the remaining 80% to 90% of caloric intake, less than 10% should be from saturated fat and up to 10% should be from polyunsaturated fat. The remaining 60% to 70% of caloric intake is obtained from monounsaturated fat and carbohydrates (ADA, 2000n).

Further dietary fat restrictions for clients with diabetes are determined by a dietitian on the basis of specific lipid abnormalities. Adults with diabetes should be tested annually for lipid abnormalities. These tests include fasting serum cholesterol, triglyceride, high-density lipoprotein (HDL) cholesterol, and calculated LDL cholesterol levels (ADA, 2000m).

The percentage of calories obtained from carbohydrate sources is also individualized for each client. Various starches have different blood glucose responses. Emphasis is placed on the total amount of carbohydrate consumed each day rather than the source of the carbohydrate. Little scientific evidence supports the assumption that sugars are more rapidly absorbed than starches and cause blood glucose values to increase more rapidly.

Fiber. High-fiber diets seem to improve carbohydrate metabolism and lower cholesterol levels. The client is taught to select foods with moderate to high amounts of dietary fiber (e.g., legumes, lentils, roots, green leafy vegetables, all types of whole-grain cereals, and fruits). An intake of 20 to 35 g of dietary fiber per day is ideal.

The nurse teaches the client that incorporating high-fiber foods into the diet gradually can minimize abdominal cramping, discomfort, loose stools, and flatulence. An increase in fluid intake should accompany increased fiber intake. The nurse and the client pay careful attention to blood glucose levels because hypoglycemia can result when dietary fiber intake increases significantly.

Nonnutritive Sweeteners. The use of products to enhance the taste of food while not disturbing blood glucose control is desirable. The FDA has approved four nonnutritive sweeteners for use: saccharin, aspartame, acesulfame K, and sucralose.

Fat Replacers. Fat replacers are introduced into food processing to create good-tasting, lower-fat foods but may increase carbohydrate content. The dietitian and the nurse provide training to clients with diabetes on how to incorporate fat replacers into their meal plan. General guidelines regarding the use of fat replacers are as follows (ADA, 2000r):

- Fat replacer should be less than 20 calories or less than 5 g of carbohydrate per serving if it is a "free food."
- Limit fat replacer to three servings per day.
- From 6 to 10 g of carbohydrate per serving is one half of a carbohydrate choice.
- From 11 to 20 g of carbohydrate per serving is one carbohydrate choice.

Alcohol. Blood glucose levels will not be affected by *moderate* use of alcohol when diabetes is well controlled. The nurse teaches clients using insulin that two alcoholic beverages for men and one for women can be ingested with, and in addition to, the usual meal plan. (One alcoholic beverage = 12 ounces of beer, 5 ounces of wine, or 1.5 ounces of distilled spirits.) Because of the potential for alcohol-induced hypoglycemia, the client is instructed to ingest alcohol only with or shortly after meals. Because alcohol elevates plasma triglycerides, reducing or abstaining from alcohol may be recommended for diabetic clients with hyperlipidemia, a history of alcohol abuse, or during pregnancy. One alcoholic beverage is substituted for two fat exchanges when calculating caloric intake (ADA, 2000n).

Food Labeling. Nutrient and ingredient information help clients make appropriate food choices and select appropriate portions. For clients with diabetes, foods containing sucrose or other sugars are not restricted. These foods should be used sparingly and substituted for other carbohydrates in the individual meal plan. The client is instructed to use the food label to determine food carbohydrate content to aid in blood glucose control (ADA, 2000g).

Client Education: Prescribed Diet. The 1994 Nutrition Recommendations for Diabetes recognized that no one single meal plan is appropriate for all clients with diabetes. Each client's nutrition recommendations are based on blood glucose monitoring results, total blood lipid levels, and glycosylated hemoglobin. Results from self-monitoring of blood glucose levels (SMBG) help to determine whether current patterns of meals and exercise need adjustment or whether present habits need reinforcement. A specific dietary prescription is developed for each client.

The nurse supports and reinforces nutrition information provided by the dietitian. The diabetic client needs to understand how to make adjustments in nutritional intake during illness, planned exercise, and social occasions (such as restaurant meals) where the usual time of eating is delayed. The client may be unable to follow the prescribed diet because of an inability to see, read, or understand printed materials. Dietary information is shared with the person who prepares the meals. The dietitian sees each client at least yearly to note subtle changes in lifestyle and make appropriate diet therapy changes. The dietitian also sees those clients assessed by the case manager to be at *high risk* for nutritional problems. Some clients, such as those with weight control problems or low incomes, may require more frequent evaluation and counseling.

Meal Planning Strategies. A variety of meal planning approaches are available. Each approach emphasizes different aspects of nutrition.

Exchange System. The exchange system is based on three food groups: carbohydrates, meat and meat substitutes, and fat. The client's prescription identifies how many items from each food group are to be eaten at a meal or snack. Table 65-14 provides an example of the exchange system of diet therapy. The exchange list for meal planning assumes that foods with similar nutrient content affect blood glucose concentrations similarly. Diets based on the exchange system have been shown to produce predictable blood glucose responses.

Carbohydrate Counting. Carbohydrate (CHO) counting provides a simple approach to meal planning and is helped by the fact that the nutritional content of most packaged food items is listed on the label. Because fat and protein have little effect on postmeal blood glucose levels, CHO counting emphasizes the nutrient that has the greatest impact on these levels. CHO counting uses total grams of carbohydrate, regardless of the food source. The dietitian determines the number of grams of carbohydrate to be eaten at each meal and snack

TABLE 65-14 • EXCHANGE SYSTEM OF MEDICAL NUTRITION THERAPY

	Nutrient Content				
Food Content	**Carbohydrate (g)**	**Protein (g)**	**Fat (g)**	**Calories**	**Examples**
Carbohydrates	15	3	1 or less	80	1 slice bread, 1/2 bagel, 1/2 hamburger bun, 1/2 cup corn, 1/2 cup mashed potato
Fruit	15			60	1 apple, 1/2 banana, 1/2 grapefruit
Milk					
Skim	12	8	0-3	90	1 cup skim milk
Low-fat	12	8	5	120	1 cup 2% milk
Whole	12	8	5	150	1 cup whole milk
Other carbohydrates	Varies	Varies	Varies	Varies	1 glazed donut, 1 granola bar, 1 sweet roll
Vegetables	5	2		25	Carrots, green beans, spinach, 1/2 cup cooked, 1 cup raw; 1 large tomato
Meat or meat substitutes					
Very lean		7	0.1	35	1 oz chicken (white meat, skinless), 1 oz fat-free cheese
Lean		7	3	55	1 oz lean beef, chicken (skinless), or fish; 1/4 cup cottage cheese
Medium-fat		7	5	75	1 oz most beef, pork, lamb, or chicken with skin; 1/4 cup tuna fish
High-fat		7	8	100	1 oz pork sausage, 1 tbsp peanut butter, 1 oz regular cheese
Fat			5	45	1 tsp butter or margarine, 1 strip bacon

Courtesy of Carole Colebanks.

and assists the client in making appropriate food choices. CHO counting is effective in achieving overall blood glucose control. Blood glucose control requires a consistent carbohydrate intake from day to day.

Clients who are receiving intensive insulin or pump therapies can use CHO counting to determine insulin coverage. After the amount of insulin needed to cover the usual meal is determined, insulin may be added or subtracted for changes in carbohydrate intake. The usual formula of 1 unit of short-acting insulin for each 15 g of carbohydrate provides flexibility to meal plans.

Special Considerations for Type 1 Diabetes. A meal plan based on the client's usual food intake is developed, and insulin therapy is integrated into the usual eating and exercises patterns. To prevent wide swings in blood glucose levels, day-to-day consistency in the timing and amount of food is important for a client using standard insulin therapy (one to two daily insulin injections). To match the effects of insulin, the daily caloric intake is distributed among three main meals, a bedtime snack, and one or more between-meal snacks. Clients receiving intensified insulin therapy with multiple daily injections of insulin or an insulin pump have more flexibility in the choice and timing of meals and snacks.

In addition to maintaining blood glucose levels within a target range, a second goal for the treatment of clients with type 1 diabetes is to avoid gaining weight. **Hyperinsulinemia** (chronic high blood insulin levels), which can occur with intensive treatment schedules, may result in weight gain. These clients may need to treat hyperglycemia by caloric restriction rather than by increases in insulin dosage. Weight gain can be minimized by adhering to the prescribed meal plan, consistently eating an evening snack, and avoiding overtreatment of hypoglycemia (Franz, 1997).

Special Considerations for Type 2 Diabetes. With type 2 diabetes, diet therapy is directed toward weight reduction and improvement in blood glucose and lipid levels in the obese person. For clients in whom caloric reduction and exercise has not been successful in achieving long-term weight loss, emphasis is on reducing blood glucose and lipid levels. A moderate caloric restriction (250 to 500 calories less than the average daily intake) and an increase in physical activity improves diabetes control and weight control. Losing only as much as 10 to 20 pounds improves blood glucose control (Franz, 1997). Decreasing high dietary intake of cholesterol-raising fatty acids is important in reducing the risk for cardiovascular disease (ADA, 2000m).

CONSIDERATIONS FOR OLDER ADULTS

Older diabetic clients are at increased risk for malnutrition and hypoglycemia and are particularly prone to developing dehydration, a factor in the development of hyperglycemic-hyperosmolar nonketotic syndrome (HHNS). Many factors contribute to malnutrition. Older clients who prepare their own food or have tooth loss or poorly fitting dentures may not eat enough food. Neuropathy with gastric retention or diarrhea compounds poor food intake. Impaired cognition and depression may disrupt self-management. Older clients may have a marginal food supply because of inadequate income, may have poor understanding of meal planning goals, or may live alone and have reduced incentive to prepare or eat proper meals. They may eat in restaurants or live in situations where they have little control over meal preparation. Regular visits by home care nurses can assist the older client in following a diabetic meal plan.

A realistic approach to diet therapy is essential. Changing eating habits of 60 to 70 years' duration is very difficult. The nurse, the dietitian, and the client assess the usual eating patterns. The older client taking antidiabetic drugs is taught about the importance of eating meals and snacks at the same time every day, eating the same amount of food from day to day, and eating all food allowed on the diet.

EXERCISE THERAPY. Regular physical exercise is an essential part of a total diabetic treatment plan. Regular exercise has beneficial effects on carbohydrate metabolism and insulin sensitivity. In addition, exercise improves the client's sense of well-being and reduces the risk for atherosclerosis (ADA, 2000d).

In the person without diabetes, glucose use during exercise is matched by glucose production by the liver; thus exercise does not induce hyperglycemia or hypoglycemia. The client with type 1 diabetes is unable to make these hormonal adaptations. In the diabetic client without an adequate insulin supply, cells are unable to use glucose. Low insulin levels stimulate release of glucagon and epinephrine to increase hepatic glucose production, further raising blood glucose levels. In the absence of insulin, free fatty acids become the source of energy. Exercise in the client with uncontrolled diabetes results in further hyperglycemia and the formation of ketone bodies.

Exercise in the person with diabetes can cause hypoglycemia because of increased muscle glucose uptake and the inhibition of glucose release from the liver. Hypoglycemia can occur during exercise and for up to 24 hours after exercise. Replacement of muscle and liver glycogen stores, along with increased insulin sensitivity following exercise, causes insulin requirements to drop (Franz, 1997).

Diabetic clients may have prolonged elevated blood glucose levels after vigorous exercise periods. Liver glucose production increases to provide the energy needs for exercise. In nondiabetic clients, this increased glucose production is balanced by an increase in plasma insulin secretion so that fluctuations in blood glucose levels are avoided. The client with type 1 diabetes is unable to increase plasma insulin levels, and postexercise hyperglycemia develops.

Benefits of Exercise. Regular exercise of moderate intensity helps regulate blood glucose levels and results in lowered insulin requirements for clients with type 1 diabetes. Regular exercise improves diabetic control by increasing insulin sensitivity, improving cell uptake of glucose, and promoting weight loss.

Regular exercise decreases risk factors for cardiovascular disease. In response to training, clients with type 1 diabetes have decreases in most blood lipid levels and an increase in high-density lipoproteins (HDLs). Exercise decreases blood pressure and improves cardiovascular function. Regular vigorous physical activity appears to have an important role in the prevention of type 2 diabetes by reducing body weight, insulin resistance, and glucose intolerance.

Risks Related to Exercise. The client with diabetes is assessed for potential risk for injury related to exercise. Prolonged hypoglycemia or hyperglycemia can occur, particularly after sustained high-intensity exercise.

Several complications of diabetes can be made worse by exercise. The client with proliferative retinopathy is advised to avoid the **Valsalva maneuver** (breath holding while bearing down) and activities that increase blood pressure. Heavy lifting, rapid head motion, or jarring activities can cause vitreous hemorrhage or retinal detachment. Exercise may increase proteinuria in clients with diabetic nephropathy. The risk for foot and joint injury is increased for clients with peripheral neuropathy. Autonomic neuropathy can cause postexercise orthostatic hypotension (ADA, 2000d).

Screening Before Initiating an Exercise Program. The diabetic client is advised to have a complete history and physical examination before beginning a physical activity program. Regular physical activity increases the risk of both musculoskeletal injury and life-threatening cardiovascular events. The ability of the heart to respond to increasing levels of exercise on a treadmill, as well as the presence of other risk factors, forms the basis of the exercise prescription. For clients who are unable to perform vigorous exercise, the heart's ability to tolerate exercise is tested with cardiac stressor drugs (e.g., coronary vasodilators, dipyridamole thallium scans). The client needs to be carefully evaluated for the presence of macrovascular and microvascular complications that may be worsened by exercise (ADA, 2000d).

Guidelines for Exercise. The client determines blood glucose levels before exercise. When levels are greater than 250 mg/dL (13.8 mmol/L), the client tests the urine for ketones. The absence of urine ketones indicates that enough insulin is available to promote glucose transport and use, and that exercise should be effective in lowering blood glucose levels. The presence of ketones contraindicates exercise. Ketones indicate that current insulin levels are not adequate and that exercise would elevate blood glucose levels.

Low-intensity aerobic exercise for longer durations is most effective in achieving desired health effects for clients with diabetes. Such exercises are those that require slow, submaximal effort, continue for greater than 12 to 15 minutes, are rhythmic in nature, and result in a moderately elevated heart rate (above 50% of maximal heart rate). Examples of appropriate aerobic activities include walking briskly, running, jogging, stationary or regular bicycling, swimming, dancing, rowing, and cross-country skiing. These activities improve cardiac output.

For individuals with type 1 diabetes, the aerobic exercise should endure for 20 to 40 minutes and be performed 4 to 7 days per week. A 5- to 10-minute warm-up period with stretching and low-intensity exercise before aerobic exercise and a 5- to 10-minute cool-down period after aerobic exercise reduce the risk for dysrhythmias. Daily exercise increases total energy expenditure, facilitates weight loss, and improves blood glucose control.

NIC ***Client Education: Exercise Promotion.*** Chart 65-7 lists NIC intervention activities for exercise. The client is instructed to wear shoes with good traction and cushioning and to examine the feet daily and after exercise. Exercise in extreme heat or cold or during periods of poor control of diabetes is avoided. The client is advised to maintain hydration, especially during and after exercise in a warm environment.

Exercise is not performed within 1 hour of insulin injection or at the peak time of insulin action, because this activity can increase absorption of insulin from the injection site, causing an increase in blood insulin levels. The risk for hypoglycemia increases when insulin is injected into an area that is exercised.

The nurse makes certain that all diabetic clients engaging in exercise know the risks for hypoglycemia and teaches preventive measures. Clients taking oral medications or insulin should perform self-monitoring of blood glucose levels (SMBG) to determine the effects of their exercise program. The client is taught that supplemental snacks containing rapidly absorbable carbohydrate may be taken before and during exercise to maintain blood glucose levels within normal ranges. Additional carbohydrate may be taken for up to 24 hours after exercise to prevent postexercise hypoglycemia. The amount of additional carbohydrate intake is directed by

CHART 65-7

NIC INTERVENTION ACTIVITIES *for* The Diabetic Client Needing to Increase Physical Activity

Exercise Promotion: *Facilitation of regular physical exercise to maintain or advance to a higher level of fitness and health*

- Appraise client's health beliefs about physical exercise.
- Encourage verbalization of feelings about exercise or need for exercise.
- Include client's family/caregivers in planning and maintaining the exercise program.
- Inform client about health beliefs and physiologic effects of exercise.
- Instruct client about appropriate type of exercise for level of health, in collaboration with physician and/or exercise physiologist.
- Instruct client about desired frequency, duration, and intensity of the exercise program.
- Instruct client about conditions warranting cessation of or alteration in the exercise program.
- Instruct client on proper warm-up and cool-down exercises.
- Instruct the client in techniques to avoid injury while exercising.
- Assist client to develop an appropriate exercise program to meet needs.
- Assist client to set short-term and long-term goals for the exercise program.
- Assist client to schedule regular periods for the exercise program into weekly routine.
- Monitor client's response to exercise program.
- Provide positive feedback for client's efforts.

Vital Signs Monitoring: *Collection and analysis of cardiovascular, respiratory, and body temperature data to determine and prevent complications*

- Monitor blood pressure, pulse, temperature, and respiratory response, as appropriate.
- Monitor for and report signs and symptoms of hypothermia and hyperthermia.
- Monitor presence and quality of pulses.
- Monitor cardiac rhythm and rate.
- Monitor heart tones.
- Monitor respiratory rate and rhythm (e.g., depth and symmetry).
- Monitor for abnormal respiratory patterns (e.g., Cheyne-Stokes, Kussmaul, Biot, apneustic, ataxic, and excessive sighing).
- Monitor skin color, temperature, and moistness.
- Identify possible causes of changes in vital signs.

NIC intervention activities selected from McCloskey J.C., & Bulechek, G.M. (2000). *Nursing interventions classification (NIC)* (3rd ed.). St. Louis: Mosby. No part of this work is to be altered without prior written permission from the Publisher.

the results of blood glucose monitoring. The nurse instructs the client to adjust insulin dosage before planned exercise as directed.

Clients with type 1 diabetes should perform vigorous exercise only if blood glucose levels are in the range of 80 to 250 mg/dL (4.4 to 13.8 mmol/L) and if there are no ketones present in the urine. In the nonobese client who is taking insulin, the nurse recommends a carbohydrate-containing snack before exercise if at least 1 hour has elapsed since the last food was eaten or if high-intensity exercise is planned. There is no need for additional carbohydrate intake when the blood glucose level is greater than 100 mg/dL (5.6 mmol/L) before exercise and the planned activity is of low intensity and short duration. When vigorous activity of long duration is planned, the client should eat an additional 15 to 30 g of carbohydrate for every 30 to 60 minutes of exercise. Snacks such as fruit, fruit juice, bread products, and whole milk are effective in preventing hypoglycemia. The client is instructed to carry a simple sugar (hard candy) to eat if symptoms of hypoglycemia occur. The nurse also instructs the client to carry identifying information about having diabetes.

CONSIDERATIONS FOR OLDER ADULTS

With age, the ability of the heart and lungs to deliver oxygen to tissues and organs declines. These changes may be due more to a decline in muscle mass than to changes in cardiac output. Aerobic activities are thought to be important in maintaining muscle mass. Healthy older clients are able to maintain cardiac output by increasing stroke volume during exercise.

Specific exercise programs are beneficial for *frail older adults* who, because of weak muscles and poor balance, are at greater risk for falls and fractures. Clients who are limited to low-intensity programs can achieve benefits when exercise is performed at least three times per week. Some level of exercise is beneficial even to severely debilitated clients (Samos & Roos, 1998).

SURGICAL MANAGEMENT. Surgical interventions for diabetes mellitus include transplantation of all or part of the pancreas. Successful pancreas and islet cell transplantations are the only therapies that achieve blood glucose control by providing normal insulin secretion that responds to feedback regulation (Robertson et al., 2000). Clients' quality of life is improved when they no longer have to take insulin injections and are free of diabetic dietary restrictions.

WHOLE-PANCREAS TRANSPLANTATION. Improved surgical techniques and newer immunosuppressive therapies have improved outcomes in pancreatic transplantation. Simultaneous pancreas and kidney transplantation shows a 1-year client survival rate of greater than 90% and a 1-year **graft** (transplanted organ) survival rate of 82%. Pancreatic graft survival is defined as not needing insulin injections. The degree of tissue-type matching affects the results. Both graft and client survival are improved when a living related donor kidney is available (Manske, 1999). Pancreatic transplantation is performed in one of three situations: transplantation of the pancreas alone (PTA), transplantation of the pancreas after successful kidney transplantation (PAK), and simultaneous pancreas and kidney transplantation (SPK). The ideal procedure for diabetic clients with uremia is SPK. These clients are generally poor surgical candidates because of the presence of complications from the diabetes. The problems of diabetes must be severe enough to balance the expected toxicity of immunosuppressive drugs. Pancreatic transplantation is only partially successful in reversing the long-term complications of diabetes (ADA, 2000o).

Operative Procedure. The majority of pancreas transplants have been performed using the technique of **systemic venous delivery of insulin and bladder drainage of exocrine secretions (systemic-bladder).** This procedure involves attaching the donated pancreas to the client's urinary bladder. Because this procedure results in hyperinsulinemia and has urologic complications, techniques were developed to allow systemic venous delivery of insulin to the intestinal tract (systemic-enteric) and bladder drainage of pancreatic enzymes. Complications of this procedure include blood clot formation, duodenal leak, wound infections, and urologic problems.

Rejection Management. Transplant rejection accounts for 32% of graft failures in the first year after a pancreas transplant (Stratta, 1999). Most transplant centers use a combination of four drug and antibody types to reverse rejection. (See Chapter 20 for a listing of agents used to prevent or treat transplant rejection.) Clients undergoing immunosuppressive therapy initially receive drug therapy to prevent viral, bacterial, and fungal infection because of the risk of opportunistic infections.

Pancreatic transplantation is considered successful when the client is independent from insulin therapy, blood glucose levels are normal, and glycosylated hemoglobin values are normal. In nearly 90% of rejection episodes, kidney problems occur earlier than pancreatic problems. An increase in serum creatinine is an indication of rejection of both the transplanted kidney and the pancreas. In diabetic clients with urinary drained pancreas transplants, a decrease in the urine amylase level by 25% is used as an indication to treat rejection. High blood glucose levels are a later marker of rejection and usually indicate irreversible graft failure.

Long-Term Effects. Long-term immunosuppressive therapy is associated with increased risk for infections, cancer, and atherosclerosis. The transplanted pancreas does not duplicate all of the functions of a normal pancreas. Because the pancreas is transplanted into the peritoneal cavity, insulin drains into the systemic rather than the portal circulation, causing elevations in blood insulin levels **(hyperinsulinemia).** Hyperinsulinemia is a risk factor for both hypertension and macrovascular disease.

Complications. Complications are common in clients receiving organ transplants and requiring long-term immunosuppressive therapy. Major complications of a pancreas transplant include venous thrombosis, rejection, and infection. Careful monitoring of laboratory values, fluid and electrolyte status, physical signs and symptoms, and changes in vital signs can alert the nurse to possible complications and the need to notify the physician for therapy. Early removal of IV and intra-arterial lines, use of sterile technique with dressing changes and catheter irrigations, strict handwashing by health care personnel, and good pulmonary hygiene all help to prevent infection.

Thrombosis of blood vessels to the pancreas occurs in as many as 30% of clients who have had pancreas transplants. Changes in surgical technique have reduced the incidence of this complication. The nurse observes for, and reports to the physician, any sharp and sudden drop in urine amylase levels, rapid increases in blood glucose, gross hematuria **(bloody urine),** and tenderness or pain in the graft area (iliac fossa).

The nurse assesses the client for signs and symptoms of rejection. In acute rejection, decreased kidney function is indicated by increased serum creatinine of 0.3 mg/dL or greater (Stratta, 1999), decreased urine output, hypertension, increased weight, graft tenderness, and fever. Proteinuria is often the first indicator of chronic graft rejection. The nurse observes for signs and symptoms of rejection, including elevations of serum amylase, lipase, or glucose; decreased urine amylase; graft tenderness; hyperglycemia; and fever. It is especially important to assess for signs and symptoms of infection and initiate appropriate treatment. Fever can be a sign of both infection and rejection.

The nurse monitors for side effects of the various immunosuppressive drugs. Cyclosporine (Neoral) is **nephrotoxic** (toxic to the kidney). Symptoms of nephrotoxicity include a rise in creatinine and a decrease in urine output. White blood cell counts are monitored daily, since azathioprine (Imuran) is associated with bone marrow suppression. Prednisone has multiple side effects, including elevated blood glucose levels. Common side effects of tacrolimus (Prograf) are nephrotoxicity, neurotoxicity, gastrointestinal (GI) toxicity, and glucose intolerance. Hypertension is a common adverse effect of tacrolimus.

The client's quality of life improves as a result of freedom from the need for insulin, a less restricted lifestyle, and a return to a normal diet. The nurse must stress, however, the potential for the need for insulin injections to treat hyperglycemia caused by immunosuppressive drugs.

ISLET CELL TRANSPLANTATION. Islet cell transplantation in rats and dogs successfully eliminates the requirement for insulin administration and provides protection from the complications of diabetes. Human transplantation of islet cells is limited by the technical inability to obtain a sufficient number of islet cells. Tissue type (HLA)–matched pancreas glands from cadavers are used, and isolated islet cells are injected into the portal vein or implanted beneath the kidney capsule or into the spleen. Successful transplantation has occurred in a small number of clients. Islet cell transplantation is currently considered an experimental procedure (ADA, 2000o).

RISK FOR INJURY RELATED TO STRESS OF SURGERY

PLANNING: EXPECTED OUTCOMES. The client with diabetes undergoing a surgical procedure is expected to have a satisfactory and complete postoperative recovery without complications.

INTERVENTIONS. Surgery is a physical and emotional stressor, and the diabetic client has a higher than average risk for complications. Acute stress increases the supply of glucose through the action of the counterregulatory hormones. These hormones suppress the action of insulin, increasing the risk for ketoacidosis and metabolic acidosis. Fasting contributes to the development of ketoacidosis. Diuresis from hyperglycemia can cause severe dehydration and loss of electrolytes.

Coronary artery disease, diabetic nephropathy, and autonomic neuropathy further increase the risk of surgical complications. Diabetic nephropathy makes fluid management more difficult. Cardiac dysrhythmias may result from the combined effect of anesthesia and autonomic neuropathy on the cardiovascular system. Autonomic neuropathy may cause paralytic ileus and urinary retention postoperatively.

Blood glucose must be controlled to prevent acute complications of hypoglycemia, diabetic ketoacidosis (DKA), and hyperglycemic-hyperosmolar nonketotic syndrome (HNNS). Blood glucose control is also necessary to reduce infection and promote wound healing. Keeping perioperative blood glucose levels between 120 and 200 mg/dL (6.7 and 11.1 mmol/L) has been found to prevent complications and promote wound healing (Hirsh & Paauw, 1997).

PREOPERATIVE CARE. Chlorpropamide (Diabinese) is discontinued for at least 36 hours before surgery. Metformin (Glucophage) is discontinued 48 hours before the surgical procedure and restarted only after renal function is normal. All other oral agents are discontinued the day of surgery. Adjustments in insulin therapy are based on preoperative blood glucose levels. When the client is admitted, the nurse starts IV fluids as ordered to maintain hydration, monitors blood glucose results, and administers insulin as ordered.

Operative procedures for clients with type 1 diabetes are performed early in the day to cause the least disruption in blood glucose control. Stable blood glucose levels can be achieved by administration of IV insulin when surgery is scheduled later in the day. Withholding normal insulin doses can cause hyperglycemia, ketosis, and electrolyte abnormalities. Moreover, giving a portion of the normal subcutaneous insulin dose involves guesswork and may cause a large, unpredictable release of insulin after surgery is underway (Hirsh & Paauw, 1997). The nurse performs frequent blood glucose monitoring throughout the perioperative period to determine the need for additional insulin.

Plans for postoperative pain control need to be made in the preoperative period. Pain, a stressor, stimulates the release of counterregulatory hormones, causing high blood glucose levels and increasing insulin needs. The older client who receives opioid analgesic drugs is more at risk for confusion, paralytic ileus, hypoventilation, and hypotension. The effects of opioid analgesics on slowing GI motility and the effects on blood glucose levels need to be considered. Many clients with long-standing diabetes have delayed gastric emptying. Compared with IM injections of opioids, patient-controlled analgesia (PCA) systems have fewer respiratory complications and a lower incidence of confusion. (See Chapter 7 for interventions related to pain and Chapter 17 for general preoperative care.)

INTRAOPERATIVE CARE. The frequency of blood glucose assessment depends in part on the type of anesthetic agent used. Epidural anesthesia minimally affects glucose metabolism. During general anesthesia, glucose levels increase early and remain elevated throughout the operative period. Surgery lasting 3 to 5 hours or longer leads to greater hyperglycemia, with these clients needing supplemental short-acting insulin.

IV administration of short-acting insulin in 5% to 10% glucose is recommended for all insulin-treated clients, as well as for clients with poorly controlled type 2 diabetes who are undergoing general anesthesia. Blood glucose levels less than 200 mg/dL during surgery reduce the incidence of wound infection during the postoperative period. Larger than normal doses of insulin may be needed during surgery because of stress-induced release of glucagon and epinephrine. The physician orders insulin/glucose infusion rates based on results of hourly capillary blood glucose tests.

NIC intervention activities for monitoring of vital signs are presented in Chart 65-7. The nurse monitors the client's temperature because body temperature is deliberately lowered in some operative procedures and inadvertently in others. Low operating room temperatures and large surgical incisions lower body temperature. Hypothermia decreases metabolic needs, depresses heart rate and contractility, causes vasoconstriction, and impairs insulin release, resulting in high blood glucose levels. The arterial blood gas values are monitored for acidosis.

POSTOPERATIVE CARE. The nurse continues glucose and insulin infusions, as ordered, until the client is stable and able to tolerate oral feedings. Supplemental short-acting insulin, with the dosage based on blood glucose monitoring, may be needed to control blood glucose levels until the client's usual medication regimen can be restarted. Short-term insulin therapy may be needed postoperatively for the client who usually uses oral agents alone. For the client receiving insulin therapy, changes in the usual insulin dosage may be needed until the stress of surgery subsides. To prevent the potential development of insulin allergy, only human insulin should be used for short-term therapy.

MONITORING. Clients with autonomic neuropathy or vascular disease require careful monitoring to avoid hypotension or respiratory arrest. Clients whose hypertension is well controlled with beta-blocking drugs must be monitored carefully for hypoglycemia (beta blocking agents mask hypoglycemia). Clients with **azotemia** (increased nitrogen waste products in the blood) may have problems with fluid management. The nurse monitors central venous pressure or pulmonary artery pressure as necessary.

Hyperkalemia (elevated blood potassium level) is often seen in clients with mild to moderate kidney failure and can lead to an acute cardiac dysrhythmia. In other clients, **hypokalemia** (low blood potassium levels) may be present and is made worse by insulin and glucose therapy given during surgical treatment. The nurse monitors the client's cardiac rhythm and serum potassium values as ordered.

Cardiovascular Monitoring. Serial electrocardiograms (ECGs) are recommended for older diabetic clients, those with long-standing type 1 diabetes, and those with known heart disease. Diabetic clients have a high incidence of postoperative myocardial infarctions that are associated with a high mortality rate. Alterations in ECGs or in potassium levels may indicate a silent myocardial infarction.

Renal Monitoring. Careful monitoring of fluid balance helps detect acute kidney failure. Diagnosis of renal impairment may require the use of x-ray studies using dyes, which may be nephrotoxic. Treatment of infections may require the use of nephrotoxic antibiotics. The physician and nurse ensure adequate hydration of the client when these drugs are used. The nurse monitors for impending renal failure through careful assessment of the client's fluid and electrolyte status.

NUTRITIONAL CARE. The use of **total parenteral nutrition (TPN)** in diabetic clients can result in severe metabolic changes. Frequent capillary blood glucose monitoring is used to determine the need for supplemental short-acting insulin. After a stable dose of insulin is reached, insulin can be added to the TPN solution and the frequency of capillary blood glucose monitoring decreased.

Returning to a normal meal plan as soon as possible after surgery promotes healing and re-establishes homeostasis. When oral foods are tolerated, the nurse ensures that the client takes at least 150 to 200 g of carbohydrate daily to prevent hypoglycemia.

RISK FOR INJURY RELATED TO SENSORY ALTERATIONS

NOC **PLANNING: EXPECTED OUTCOMES.** The client with diabetes is expected to identify factors that increase the potential for injury, practice proper foot care to prevent injury (as evidenced by cleansing and inspecting the feet for cleanliness and healthy skin), and maintain intact skin on the feet.

INTERVENTIONS. Foot injury is the most common complication of diabetes leading to hospitalization. Diabetes is the leading cause of amputation worldwide. The overall risk of amputation is 15 times greater in diabetic clients than in nondiabetic clients. For clients who have had a previous amputation, the risk of amputation in the second leg is 10 to 20 times greater than the risk of amputation in the general population. The 5-year mortality rate after lower extremity amputation ranges from 39% to 68%.

Intensive education about foot care is needed for clients with diabetes. Low levels of high-density lipoprotein (HDL) cholesterol, high levels of plasma glucose and glycosylated hemoglobin (hemoglobin A_{1c} [HbA_{1c}]), and long duration of diabetes are associated with increased risk for amputation.

Sensory neuropathy, ischemia, and infection are the leading causes of foot disease associated with diabetes. Peripheral neuropathy is present in more than 80% of diabetic clients with foot ulcers (Abbott et al., 1998). Loss of pain, pressure and temperature sensation in the foot increases the chance of injury and development of ulcerations. Impaired blood flow to the foot limits healing of the wound.

Up to half of all people with diabetes have a hammertoe or claw toe deformity created by motor neuropathy (Mayfield et al., 1998). Toes become hyperextended, which increases pressure on the **metatarsal heads** ("ball" of the foot), resulting in ulceration. Thinning or shifting of the fat pad under the metatarsal heads decreases the cushioning and increases areas of pressure. These changes predispose the client to callus formation, ulceration, and infection. Figure 65-9 shows **hallux valgus** (turning of the great toe), and Figure 65-10 shows a hammertoe.

The **Charcot foot** is an example of a diabetic foot deformity. The Charcot foot is warm, swollen, and painful. Continued ambulation collapses the arch, shortens the foot, and gives the foot a "rocker bottom" shape.

Although sensory neuropathy may manifest as tingling or burning, it is more often evident as numbness and reduced sensation. Neuropathy causes loss of normal sweating and skin temperature regulation, resulting in dry and atrophic skin. Cracks and fissures in the skin increase the risk for infection.

The loss of sensation allows painless trauma to cause major foot problems. Because sensation is absent, the client does not notice physical, thermal, or chemical injuries to the foot. Thus the client does not take measures to treat these injuries. Foot injuries can be caused by walking barefoot, wearing ill-fitting shoes, sustaining thermal injuries from hot water (e.g., hot water bottles, heating pads, and baths), or receiving caustic burns caused by over-the-counter medications to treat corns. Because the blood supply to the diabetic foot is poor, these injuries sometimes lead to amputation.

Ulcers result from continued pressure. **Plantar** ulcers (ulcers on the bottom of the foot) are due to standing or walking, whereas ulcers on the top or sides of the foot are usually due to shoe pressure. The foot responds to increased pressure by callus formation. Most diabetic plantar ulcers are located under the metatarsal heads. Ulcerations usually occur over or around the great toe, under the metatarsal heads, and on the tops of claw toes.

The risk for infection increases whenever there is a break in the skin. Skin breaks tend to occur in areas of excessive or repetitive pressure. Infection is common in diabetic foot ulcers and, once present, is difficult to treat. Decreased immune function in diabetic clients increases the risk for infection. Infection also impairs glucose control, leading to higher blood glucose levels and reduced immune defense mechanisms.

PREVENTION OF HIGH-RISK CONDITIONS. Neuropathy of the lower extremities can be delayed by keeping blood glucose levels as near normal as possible. Poor blood glucose control increases the risk of neuropathy and amputation. Intensive therapy reduces the risk of development of peripheral

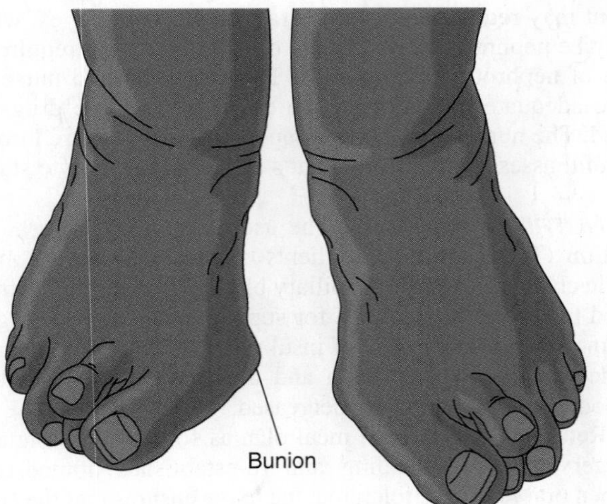

Figure 65-9 ● The appearance of hallux valgus with a bunion.

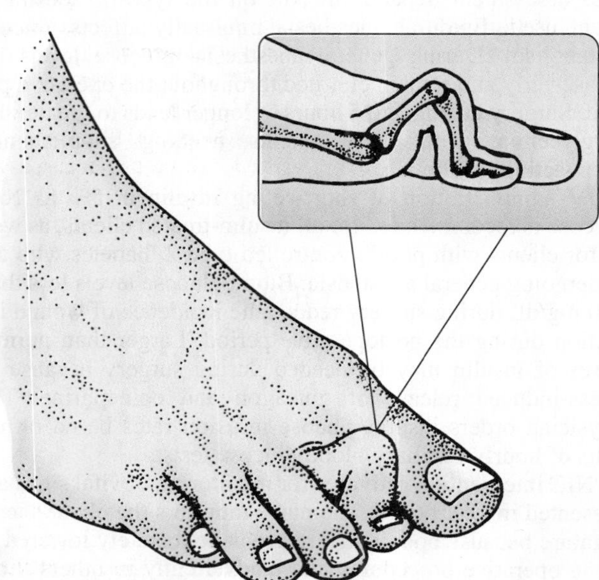

Figure 65-10 ● Hammertoe of the second metatarsophalangeal joint.

sensory neuropathy by 60%. Smoking cessation is encouraged to reduce the risk of vascular complications (ADA, 2000q).

The risk of ulcers or amputation is increased in clients who have had diabetes more than 10 years, are male, have poor glucose control, or have cardiovascular, retinal, or renal complications. Foot-related risks include poor gait and stepping mechanics, peripheral neuropathy, evidence of increased pressure (callus, erythema, hemorrhage under a callus, limited joint mobility, foot deformities, or severe nail pathology), peripheral vascular disease, and a history of ulcers or amputation (ADA, 2000q).

NIC PERIPHERAL SENSATION MANAGEMENT. An in-depth circulatory, sensory, musculoskeletal, and skin evaluation of the feet should be done at least annually (ADA, 2000q). Chart 65-8 lists NIC intervention activities for peripheral sensation management and foot care, and Table 65-15 outlines foot risk categories. Sensory examination with Semmes-Weinstein monofilaments remains the single most practical measure of the risk for foot ulcers. The monofilaments are nylon wires of varying calibrated thickness. The threads are rigid but bend when pressure is applied. More pressure is needed to bend the thicker filaments. The client is asked to close his or her eyes. The nurse presses the tip of the thinnest filament to a defined area on the sole of the foot. The filament is pressed against the skin until either it bends or the client announces that he or she feels the pressure. If the filament bends before the client feels the sensation, the next-thicker filament is applied. Inability to feel the medium-size monofilament indicates high risk for injury. The nurse completes a full assessment of the diabetic foot as outlined in Chart 65-9.

NIC FOOT CARE. All clients with diabetes need to wear shoes that protect the feet from injury. Shoes need to be fitted to the client by an experienced shoe fitter, such as a certified podiatrist. The shoe should be ½ to ⅝ inch longer than the longest toe. Heels should be less than 2 inches in height to avoid shifting the body weight onto the metatarsal heads, increasing the risk for foot ulcerations. Pressure from shoes that are too tight causes tissue damage when the shoes are worn for 4 hours or more with no relief. The nurse teaches the client to change his or her shoes by midday and again in the evening. Socks or stockings need to fit properly and be appropriate for the planned activity. Stockings should feel soft and not have thick seams, creases, or holes that can irritate the skin. Stockings should provide padding for the foot and be able to absorb excess moisture. Stockings that are tight or have constricting bands are to be avoided. Clients with toe deformities need to buy custom shoes with high, wide toeboxes and extra depth. Clients with severely deformed feet, such as Charcot feet, need specially molded shoes. All new shoes should have a slow break-in period, with periodic self-inspection of both feet for signs of irritation or blistering.

All clients with diabetes require education about preventive foot care and an examination of the feet and legs at each visit to a health care provider. The nurse or case manager identifies clients with *high-risk* foot conditions and provides education about foot care. Clients at risk are taught about the problems of the loss of protective sensation, the importance of monitoring their feet on a daily basis, the proper care of the feet (including nail and skin care), and how to select appropriate footwear. The client with neuropathy is advised to break in new shoes slowly to reduce blister formation (ADA, 2000q).

The nurse assesses the client's ability to inspect all areas of the foot and to perform appropriate care. Family members are taught principles of foot care for those clients with visual difficulties, physical limitations, or cognitive problems that prevent complete inspection of their feet (ADA, 2000q). Clients with diabetes are taught to inspect their feet daily. Chart 65-10 outlines foot care instructions.

CHART 65-8

NIC INTERVENTION ACTIVITIES *for* The Diabetic Client with Reduced Sensation in the Lower Extremities

Peripheral Sensation Management: *Prevention or minimization of injury or discomfort in the client with altered sensation*
- Monitor for sharp/dull and/or hot/cold discrimination.
- Monitor for paresthesia: numbness, tingling, hyperesthesia, and hypoesthesia.
- Encourage client to use the unaffected body part to determine temperature of foods, liquids, bathwater, and so on.
- Instruct client or family to monitor position of body parts while bathing, sitting, lying, or changing position.
- Instruct client or family to examine skin daily for alteration in skin integrity.
- Monitor fit of bracing devices, prosthesis, shoes, and clothing.
- Instruct client or family to use thermometer to test water temperature.
- Encourage use of gloves or other protective clothing over affected body part when body part is in contact with objects that—because of their thermal, textural, or other characteristics—may be potentially hazardous.
- Avoid or carefully monitor use of heat or cold, such as heating pads, hot water bottles, and ice packs.
- Encourage client to wear well-fitting, low-heeled, soft shoes.
- Check shoes, pockets, and clothing for wrinkles or foreign objects.
- Instruct client to use timed intervals, rather than presence of discomfort, as a signal to alter position.
- Protect body parts from extreme temperature changes.
- Discuss or identify causes of abnormal sensation or sensation changes.
- Instruct client to visually monitor position of body parts, if proprioception is impaired.

Foot Care: *Cleansing and inspecting the feet for the purposes of relaxation, cleanliness, and healthy skin*
- Inspect skin for irritation, cracking, lesions, corns, calluses, deformities, or edema.
- Inspect client's shoes for proper fit.
- Dry carefully between toes.
- Apply lotion.
- Clean nails.
- Apply moisture-absorbing powder, as indicated.
- Discuss with client usual foot care routine.
- Instruct client/family on the importance of foot care.
- Offer positive feedback about self-care foot activities.
- Monitor client's gait and weight distribution on feet.
- Monitor cleanliness and general condition of shoes and stockings.
- Instruct client to inspect inside of shoes for rough areas.
- Monitor hydration level of feet.
- Monitor for arterial insufficiency in lower legs.
- Monitor legs and feet for edema.
- Instruct client to monitor temperature of feet using the back of the hand.
- Instruct client in the importance of inspection, especially when sensation is diminished.
- Cut normal-thickness toenails when soft, using a toenail clipper and using the curve of the toe as a guide.
- Refer to podiatrist for trimming of thickened nails, as appropriate.

NIC intervention activities selected from McCloskey J.C., & Bulechek, G.M. (2000). *Nursing interventions classification (NIC)* (3rd ed.). St. Louis: Mosby.

TABLE 65-15 • FOOT RISK CATEGORIES

RISK CATEGORIES	MANAGEMENT CATEGORIES
Risk Category 0 • Has disease that leads to insensitivity • Has protective sensation • Has not had a plantar ulcer	*Management Category 0* • Examine feet at each visit, at least 4 times per year • Foot clinic once a year • Client education
Risk Category 1 • Does not have protective sensation • Has not had a plantar ulcer • Does not have a foot deformity	*Management Category 1* • Examine feet at each visit, at least 4 times per year • Foot clinic visit every 6 months • Soft insoles • Client education
Risk Category 2 • Does not have protective sensation • Has not had a plantar ulcer • Does have a foot deformity	*Management Category 2* • Examine feet at each visit, at least 4 times per year • Foot clinic visit every 3-4 months • Custom-molded insoles • Prescription footwear • Client education
Risk Category 3 • Does not have protective sensation • Has history of plantar ulcer	*Management Category 3* • Examine feet at each visit, at least 4 times per year • Foot clinic visit every 1-2 months • Custom-molded insoles • Prescription footwear • Client education

From Gillis W. Long Hansen's Disease Center Rehabilitation Branch (1992). *Foot screening: Care of the foot in diabetes: The Carville approach.* Carville, LA: Department of Health and Human Services.

CHART 65-9

FOCUSED ASSESSMENT *of* The Diabetic Foot

Assess the client for risk of diabetic foot problems:
- History of previous ulcer
- History of previous amputation

Assess the foot for abnormal skin/nail conditions:
- Dry, cracked, fissured skin
- Ulcers
- Toenails: thickened, long nails; ingrown nails
- Tinea pedis; onychomycosis (mycotic nails)

Assess the foot for status of circulation:
- Symptoms of claudication
- Presence or absence of dorsalis pedis or posterior tibial pulse
- Prolonged capillary filling time (>25 seconds)
- Presence or absence of hair growth on the top of the foot

Assess the foot for evidence of deformity:
- Calluses, corns
- Prominent metatarsal heads (metatarsal head is easily felt under the skin)
- Toe contractures: clawed toes, hammertoes
- Hallux valgus or bunions
- Charcot foot ("rocker bottom")

Assess the foot for loss of strength:
- Limited ankle joint range of motion
- Limited motion of great toe

Assess the foot for loss of protective sensation:
- Numbness, burning, tingling
- Semmes-Weinstein monofilament testing at 10 points on each foot

CHART 65-10

CLIENT EDUCATION GUIDE
Foot Care Instructions

- Inspect your feet daily, especially the area between the toes.
- Wash your feet daily with lukewarm water and soap. Dry thoroughly.
- Apply moisturizing cream to your feet after bathing. Do not apply to the area between your toes.
- Change into clean cotton socks every day.
- Do not wear the same pair of shoes 2 days in a row, and wear only leather shoes.
- Check your shoes for foreign objects (nails, pebbles) before putting them on. Check inside the shoes for cracks or tears in the lining.
- Purchase shoes that have plenty of room for your toes. Buy shoes later in the day, when feet are normally larger. Break in new shoes gradually.
- Wear socks to keep your feet warm.
- Trim your nails straight across with a nail clipper. Smooth the nails with an emery board.
- See your physician or nurse immediately if you have blisters, sores, or infections. Protect area with a dry, sterile dressing. Do not use adhesive tape to secure dressing.
- Do not treat blisters, sores, or infections with home remedies.
- Do not smoke.
- Do not step into the bathtub without checking the temperature of the water with your wrist. Optimal temperature is 95° F (29.4° to 35° C).
- Do not use very hot or cold water. Never use hot water bottles, heating pads, or portable heaters to warm your feet.
- Do not treat corns, blisters, bunions, calluses, or ingrown toenails yourself.
- Do not go barefooted.
- Do not wear sandals with open toes or straps between the toes.
- Do not cross your legs or wear garters or tight stockings that constrict blood flow.
- Do not soak your feet.

WOUND CARE. The Wound Healing Society's standards of care for diabetic ulcers are a moist wound environment, debridement of necrotic tissue, and off-loading (Eaglstein & Falagna, 1997).

WOUND ENVIRONMENT. Dressings are used to reduce or prevent infection, allow painless debridement, reduce wound pain, and stimulate development of granulation tissue. Many commercial products achieve these purposes. Antiseptics such as povidone iodine, hydrogen peroxide, and chlorhexidine tend to be toxic to skin cells and interfere with wound healing. Research has not provided convincing evidence of their effectiveness (Lipsky, 1998). Dressings that keep the wound moist are essential.

DEBRIDEMENT. The value of debridement lies in removal of dead tissues that support bacterial growth. This is accomplished through surgical procedures, topically applied debriding agents, and dressing materials. Placing a wet dressing, letting it dry, and then tearing out the adherent tissue debrides the wound; however, this technique also delays wound repair (Hunt & Hopf, 1997).

ELIMINATION OF PRESSURE. The elimination of pressure on an infected area is essential to wound healing. Pressure is reduced through specialized orthotic devices; custom-molded shoe inserts, or shoe modifications that redistribute weight. Clients with foot ulcers are instructed not to wear a shoe on the affected foot while the ulcer is healing. Even the most ideally fitting prescription shoes will not take the pressure off a wound or ulcer nearly as well as a total-contact cast or removable cast walker (Armstrong & Lavery, 1998). Total-contact casts are used to aid in healing of ulcers. Casting material is molded to the foot and leg, allowing weight-bearing forces to be spread out along the entire surface of contact, thereby reducing vertical force. The almost complete elimination of motion of the total-contact cast reduces plantar shear forces. The cast is removed 24 to 48 hours after application and weekly thereafter until the ulcer is healed. The client must understand that unless measures are taken to redistribute weight on a permanent basis, foot ulcers will recur.

GROWTH FACTORS. Growth factors applied directly to wounds can increase the rate of healing by stimulating granulation tissue formation and enhancing cell growth (Steed, 1997). Diabetic foot ulcers that have been present for many months or even years are being healed with this treatment. Because treatment with growth factors is expensive and based on having other aspects of diabetes controlled, this treatment is generally performed in specialized treatment centers.

CHRONIC PAIN

NOC **PLANNING: EXPECTED OUTCOMES.** The client with diabetes who has neuropathic pain is expected to experience relief of pain, use preventive measures, and use available resources to increase comfort.

INTERVENTIONS. NIC intervention activities to manage pain are listed in Chart 65-11. Achieving and maintaining normal blood glucose levels may prevent neuropathy and relieve symptoms of acute nerve dysfunction. Anticonvulsant drugs are commonly used in the treatment of pain caused by diabetic neuropathy. Agents such as gabapentin (Neurontin) have been shown to reduce mean pain scores and improve the perceived quality of life in diabetic clients with neuropathic pain (Vinik, 1999). Tricyclic antidepressants, particularly amitriptyline hydrochloride (Elavil, Levate✱) and nortriptyline (Pamelor), also are beneficial in treating pain caused by neuropathy. These drugs have an analgesic effect, and smaller doses are required for analgesia than for antidepressant effects.

The burning typical of C-fiber neuropathy may respond to capsaicin cream 0.075% (Axsain✱, Zostrix-HP). This drug promotes depletion of neuropeptide substance P, which is involved in pain transmission (see Chapter 7). The nurse instructs the client in the application of capsaicin. Topical applications four times daily are needed for several weeks before relief is achieved. Neuropathic pain may often worsen for several days after therapy is initiated before improving.

RISK FOR INJURY RELATED TO VISUAL SENSORY-PERCEPTUAL ALTERATIONS

NOC **PLANNING: EXPECTED OUTCOMES.** The client with diabetes is expected to maintain optimal vision and be free of injury related to decreased visual acuity.

CHART 65-11

NIC INTERVENTION ACTIVITIES *for* The Diabetic Client Experiencing Pain

Analgesic Administration: *Use of pharmacologic agents to reduce or eliminate pain*
- Determine pain location, characteristics, quality, and severity before medicating client.
- Check medical order for drug, dose, and frequency of analgesic prescribed.
- Attend to comfort needs and other activities that assist relaxation to facilitate response to analgesia.
- Set positive expectations regarding the effectiveness of analgesics to optimize client response.
- Document response to analgesic and any untoward effects.
- Teach about the use of analgesics, strategies to decrease side effects, and expectations for involvement in decisions about pain relief.

Teaching: Individual: *Planning, implementation, and evaluation of a teaching program designed to address a client's particular needs*
- Establish rapport.
- Determine the client's learning needs.
- Appraise the client's current level of knowledge and understanding of content.
- Appraise the client's educational level.
- Appraise the client's cognitive, psychomotor, and affective abilities/disabilities.
- Determine the client's ability to learn specific information (i.e., developmental level, physiologic status, orientation, pain, fatigue, unfulfilled basic needs, emotional state, and adaptation to illness).
- Set mutual, realistic learning goals with the client.
- Identify learning objectives necessary to reach goals.
- Determine the sequence for presenting the information.
- Appraise the client's learning style.
- Select appropriate teaching methods/strategies.
- Select appropriate educational materials.
- Tailor the content to the client's cognitive, psychomotor, and/or affective abilities/disabilities.
- Adjust instruction to facilitate learning, as appropriate.
- Provide an environment conducive to learning.
- Instruct the client, when appropriate.
- Evaluate the client's achievement of the stated objectives.
- Reinforce behavior, as appropriate.
- Correct information misinterpretations, as appropriate.
- Provide time for the client to ask questions and discuss concerns.
- Select new teaching methods/strategies, if previous ones were ineffective.
- Refer the client to other specialists/agencies to meet the learning objectives as appropriate.
- Document the content presented, the written materials provided, and the client's understanding of the information or client behaviors that indicate learning on the permanent medical record.
- Include the family/significant others, as appropriate.

NIC intervention activities selected from McCloskey J.C., & Bulechek, G.M. (2000). *Nursing interventions classification (NIC)* (3rd ed.). St. Louis: Mosby.

INTERVENTIONS

BLOOD GLUCOSE CONTROL. Poor blood glucose control, proteinuria, diastolic hypertension, and long duration of diabetes are associated with the development of diabetic retinopathy. Retinopathy and vision loss can be markedly reduced with good control of blood glucose. Surgical intervention for retinal hemorrhage or new retinal blood vessel growth can also reduce vision loss.

Only about 10% of all clients with visual impairment are totally blind. The rest have reduced vision. In addition to regular eye examinations to evaluate retinopathy, the nurse encourages the client with diabetes and visual impairment to be examined by an optometrist or ophthalmologist for assessment of remaining vision and prescription of appropriate eyewear. A functional vision assessment, performed by a low-vision technician, rehabilitation teacher, or diabetes educator, is a task-specific evaluation that determines the client's use of lighting, contrast, nonoptical and low-vision devices, and large-print options. Included in the functional vision assessment is whether the client uses central or peripheral vision. Diabetic clients with macular edema have loss of central vision. This process causes difficulties with detail discrimination, reading printed materials, preparing insulin syringes for injection, and performing self-monitoring of blood glucose levels (SMBG).

ENVIRONMENTAL MANAGEMENT. Not all diabetic clients with visual impairment require the use of special devices. Adjustments in lighting, contrast, color, distance, type size of printed materials, and eye movement often improve visual abilities. The nurse recommends that the client supplement overhead fluorescent lighting with an incandescent lamp directed toward the workspace. Placing dark equipment against a white or yellow background (or vice versa) provides contrast to enhance vision. Coding objects such as vials of insulin with bright colors or with felt-tipped markers will aid in identification of the correct bottle to be used. Bringing the blood glucose lancet or insulin syringe close to the eye makes it easier to see. The nurse directs the client to sources of materials printed with a large type size or bold print to enhance ease of reading. The client is instructed to use peripheral fields of vision by learning how to move the eye to maximize vision.

Visually adapted devices make it possible for the client to self-administer insulin doses independently. Preset dose gauges (used to measure the space between the end of the syringe barrel and the plunger) allow a client to draw up the correct amount of insulin by feeling this distance. Variable dose gauges draw insulin in variable and mixed doses of 1-, 2-, and 10-unit increments. The client sets the desired dose by pressing a lever or turning a screw on the device. Critical points to stress when teaching the client to use an adaptive device include the following:

- Differentiating between bottles of fast-acting and slower-acting insulin (One commonly used method is to wrap a rubber band around the fast-acting insulin bottle.)
- Ensuring proper placement of the device on the syringe for correct measurements
- Holding the insulin bottle upright when measuring insulin
- Avoiding air bubbles in the syringe by pulling a small amount of insulin into the syringe, moving the plunger in and out three times, and measuring insulin on the fourth draw

A system to determine how many doses can be drawn from a bottle of insulin needs to be established so that the client does not inject air from an empty bottle rather than insulin (Williams, 1997, 1999b).

The nurse assists the diabetic client with visual impairment in maintaining blood glucose control to limit the amount of functional vision change that normally occurs with hypoglycemia and hyperglycemia.

CRITICAL THINKING CHALLENGE

The client has had diabetes mellitus for several years. He takes 30 units of NPH with 10 units of regular insulin in the morning before breakfast and 20 units of NPH insulin before the evening meal. He has recently undergone laser therapy for treatment of diabetic retinopathy. He wants to be independent in insulin administration, and your assessment indicates that he has the intellectual ability to learn the needed skills.

- List three methods for preventing both hypoglycemia and hyperglycemia that you would stress during your teaching sessions.
- Discuss four ways of altering the environment to aid in measurement of accurate insulin doses.
- List five critical points that would be included in a teaching session on adaptive devices for use with insulin syringes.

For suggested answer guidelines, go to SIMON http://www.wbsaunders.com/SIMON/Iggy/.

INEFFECTIVE RENAL TISSUE PERFUSION

PLANNING: EXPECTED OUTCOMES. The client with diabetes is expected to maintain a urine elimination pattern in the expected range and urine protein levels within normal limits.

INTERVENTIONS

PREVENTION. Tight control of blood glucose levels may reverse microalbuminuria and reduce the progression of renal disease in clients with type 1 diabetes. Control of hypertension also has been demonstrated to reduce the rate of progression of diabetic nephropathy and to reduce the complications of hypertensive nephropathy (ADA, 2000t).

The nurse stresses the need for yearly evaluation of kidney function according to American Diabetes Association (ADA) Standards of Care. Screening is performed by three methods: (1) measurement of the albumin-creatinine ratio in a random, spot urine collection; (2) 24-hour urine collection with creatinine, allowing for the simultaneous measurement of creatinine clearance; and (3) timed urine collection (e.g., 4 hours or overnight) (ADA, 2000t). The nurse explains the implications of the test and helps the client collect the specimen if necessary.

Aggressive control of blood glucose and hypertension in diabetic clients without microalbuminuria has been shown to avoid nephropathy. However, once microalbuminuria develops, end-stage renal disease is inevitable. Measures are then directed toward preventing progression of the disease. This is accomplished by treating hypertension, avoiding nephrotoxic agents, promptly treating urinary tract infections (UTIs), and preventing dehydration.

Control of blood pressure and blood glucose levels depends on the participation and cooperation of the client. Prescribed medications must be taken according to schedules, and dietary restriction must be maintained. All clients with diabetes must be aware of the roles of blood pressure and blood glucose levels in the development of renal disease. Nursing measures are directed toward assisting the client in maintaining normal blood glucose levels and blood pressure levels below 130/85 mm Hg (ADA, 2000e). In addition, the nurse stresses the need for yearly screening for microalbuminuria.

Any UTI has the potential to cause kidney infection and further irreversible decline in renal function. The nurse educates the client about the signs and symptoms of UTI. The client is instructed to take medications exactly as prescribed, making certain that the course of treatment is completed. The client needs to see the physician or nurse for follow-up urine cultures to reduce the risk of renal damage. Indwelling urinary catheters are avoided when possible.

Drugs can affect renal function either through toxic effects on the kidney or by an acute but reversible reduction in function. The most common nephrotoxic drugs are aminoglycoside antibiotics such as amikacin (Amikin), streptomycin, kanamycin (Kantrex), gentamicin (Garamycin), and tobramycin (Tobrex). Anticancer agents, such as cisplatin (Platinol); acetaminophen (Tylenol); other nonsteroidal anti-inflammatory drugs such as ibuprofen (Advil) or naproxen (Aleve); and antifungal agents (amphotericin B) should be avoided (Bell & Alele, 1999). Radiocontrast dyes and materials can also affect renal function. To prevent accidental ingestion of nephrotoxic drugs; the nurse cautions the client to check with his or her health care provider before taking any over-the-counter or prescription medication.

DIET THERAPY. Restriction of dietary protein to 0.8 g/kg of body weight per day is recommended for individuals with overt nephropathy. Once the glomerular filtration rate (GFR) begins to fall, further restriction to 0.6 g/kg may slow the decline in renal function (ADA, 2000e). Because of the difficulty in maintaining lifelong dietary restrictions, the nurse provides ongoing education to assist with dietary compliance.

NIC **FLUID/ELECTROLYTE MANAGEMENT.** The nurse institutes fluid and electrolyte management measures to prevent deterioration of renal status. NIC intervention activities for fluid and electrolyte management are listed in Chart 65-12. Avoiding dehydration is important in maintaining renal function. Any acute illness that causes dehydration is treated aggressively with IV fluids (Bell & Alele, 1999). The nurse assesses the status of fluid balance in the diabetic client and institutes measures to prevent dehydration. The most common cause of dehydration in clients with diabetic neuropathy is the overuse of diuretics. Clients are instructed to report edema or symptoms of orthostatic hypotension to their health care

CHART 65-12

NIC INTERVENTION ACTIVITIES *for* The Diabetic Client Experiencing Fluid and Electrolyte and Acid-Base Imbalances

Fluid/Electrolyte Management: *Regulation and prevention of complications from altered fluid and/or electrolyte levels*

- Monitor for abnormal serum electrolyte levels, as available.
- Obtain laboratory specimens for monitoring of altered fluid or electrolyte levels (e.g., hematocrit, BUN, protein, sodium, and potassium levels), as appropriate.
- Weigh daily and monitor trends.
- Promote oral intake (e.g., provide oral fluids that are the client's preference, place in easy reach, provide a straw, and provide fresh water) as appropriate.
- Set an appropriate intravenous infusion (or blood transfusion) flow rate.
- Monitor laboratory results relevant to fluid balance (e.g., hematocrit, BUN, albumin, total protein, serum osmolality, and urine specific gravity levels).
- Monitor hemodynamic status, including CVP, MAP, PAP, and PCWP levels, if available.
- Keep an accurate record of intake and output.
- Monitor for signs and symptoms of fluid retention.
- Monitor vital signs, as appropriate.
- Maintain intravenous solution containing electrolyte(s) at a constant flow rate, as appropriate.
- Monitor client's response to prescribed electrolyte therapy.
- Monitor for manifestations of electrolyte imbalance.
- Assess client's buccal membranes, sclera, and skin for indications of altered fluid and electrolyte balance (e.g., dryness, cyanosis, and jaundice).
- Consult physician if signs and symptoms of fluid and/or electrolyte imbalance persist or worsen.
- Administer prescribed supplemental electrolytes, as appropriate.
- Monitor for fluid loss (e.g., bleeding, vomiting, diarrhea, perspiration, and tachypnea).

Acid-Base Management: Metabolic Acidosis: *Promotion of acid-base balance and prevention of complications resulting from serum HCO_3 levels lower than desired.*

- Obtain ordered specimens for laboratory analysis (e.g., ABG, urine, and serum levels), as appropriate.
- Monitor ABG levels for decreasing pH level, as appropriate.
- Maintain patent IV access.
- Monitor intake and output.
- Monitor determinants of tissue oxygen delivery (e.g., Pao_2, Sao_2, and hemoglobin levels and cardiac output), if available.
- Monitor for electrolyte imbalances associated with metabolic acidosis (e.g., hyponatremia, hyperkalemia or hypokalemia, hypocalcemia, hypophosphatemia, and hypomagnesemia), as appropriate.
- Monitor for decreasing bicarbonate from excessive nonvolatile acids (e.g., renal failure, diabetic ketoacidosis, tissue hypoxia, and starvation), as appropriate.
- Administer prescribed alkaline medications (e.g., sodium bicarbonate), as appropriate, based on ABG results.
- Prevent complications from excessive $NaHCO_3$ administration (e.g., metabolic alkalosis, hypernatremia, volume overload, decreased oxygen delivery, decreased cardiac contractility, and enhanced lactic acid production).
- Administer fluids as prescribed.
- Administer insulin and fluid hydration (isotonic and hypotonic) for diabetic ketoacidosis, causing metabolic acidosis, as appropriate.
- Institute seizure precautions.
- Monitor for CNS manifestations of metabolic acidosis (e.g., headache, drowsiness, decreased mentation, seizures, and coma), as appropriate.
- Monitor for cardiopulmonary manifestations of metabolic acidosis (e.g., hypotension, hypoxia, arrhythmias, and Kussmaul respiration), as appropriate.
- Monitor for GI manifestations of metabolic acidosis (e.g., anorexia, nausea, and vomiting), as appropriate.
- Provide comfort measures to deal with the GI effects of metabolic acidosis.
- Instruct the client and/or family on actions instituted to treat the metabolic acidosis.

NIC intervention activities selected from McCloskey J.C., & Bulechek, G.M. (2000). *Nursing interventions classification (NIC)* (3rd ed.). St. Louis: Mosby. No part of this work is to be altered without prior written permission from the Publisher.

BUN, Blood urea nitrogen; *CVP,* central venous pressure; *MAP,* mean arterial pressure; *PAP,* pulmonary artery pressure; *PCWP,* pulmonary capillary wedge pressure; *ABG,* arterial blood gas; *Pao_2,* partial pressure of arterial oxygen; Sao_2, arterial oxygen saturation; *$NaHCO_3$,* sodium bicarbonate; *CNS,* central nervous system; *GI,* gastrointestinal.

provider. The nurse also provides ongoing education to assist with dietary compliance.

Dialysis treatment for diabetic clients with renal failure is the same as for clients without diabetes (see Chapter 72). The dosage of insulin needs to be adjusted when dialysis is started.

POTENTIAL FOR HYPOGLYCEMIA

Proper central nervous system (CNS) function depends on a continuous supply of glucose in the blood. The brain cannot make glucose and stores only a few minutes' supply as glycogen. This needed continuous supply of glucose cannot be maintained when blood glucose concentration falls below critical levels.

The first defense against falling blood glucose levels in the nondiabetic client is decreased insulin secretion, decreased glucose use, and increased glucose production. Decreased insulin secretion normally occurs when blood glucose levels drop to about 83 mg/dL (4.5 mmol/L). Critical glucose counterregulatory hormones are activated at about 68 mg/dL (3.8 mmol/L), a blood glucose threshold well above the level for symptoms of hypoglycemia. The primary counterregulatory hormone is glucagon; epinephrine also becomes important in diabetic clients who have deficient glucagon levels. Both glucagon and epinephrine raise blood glucose levels by stimulating liver glycogenolysis and gluconeogenesis. In addition, epinephrine limits secretion of insulin.

Type 1 diabetes mellitus causes severe problems in the body's response to hypoglycemia. These changes are evident within 1 to 5 years of diagnosis. Regulation of circulating insulin levels is lost in clients with type 1 diabetes because the source of insulin is an injection rather than the pancreas. As blood glucose levels fall, insulin levels do not decrease. The ability of the pancreas to secrete glucagon in response to hypoglycemia is lost in clients with long-standing diabetes. After a few more years of type 1 diabetes, epinephrine response to falling blood glucose levels is also reduced. Epinephrine responses will occur but will require a lower blood glucose level to become active. These problems dramatically increase the risk for severe hypoglycemia.

A second problem found in clients with long-standing type 1 diabetes is **hypoglycemic unawareness.** These clients no longer have the warning symptoms of impending hypoglycemia that prompt them to take appropriate preventive action. Hypoglycemic unawareness is reported to occur in 50% of all clients with very-long-standing (>30 years) type 1 diabetes and in an estimated 25% of clients overall.

Symptoms of hypoglycemia are divided into two categories. **Neuroglycopenic** symptoms result directly from brain glucose deprivation and are associated with a more gradual decline in blood glucose. **Neurogenic** symptoms result from autonomic nervous system activation triggered by hypoglycemia and occur when there is a rapid decline in blood glucose (Table 65-16). Awareness of hypoglycemia is largely the result of perception of neurogenic symptoms (Cryer, 1999).

Blood glucose levels that cause symptoms of hypoglycemia vary among individuals. Many clients with diabetes have hypoglycemic symptoms when blood glucose levels are well above 50 mg/dL (2.8 mmol/L), especially if the level has dropped rapidly or if they are accustomed to sustained hyperglycemia. Thus clinical criteria are used to categorize hypoglycemic severity. In mild hypoglycemia, the client remains totally alert and is able to treat symptoms. In severe hypoglycemia, neurologic function is so impaired that the assistance of another person is needed for treatment.

TABLE 65-16 • SYMPTOMS OF HYPOGLYCEMIA

NEUROGLYCOPENIC SYMPTOMS	NEUROGENIC SYMPTOMS
• Headache • Confusion • Slurred speech • Behavior changes • Coma • Warm • Weak • Faint • Dizzy • Blurred vision	• Adrenergic: Shaky/tremulous Heart pounding Nervous/anxious • Cholinergic: Sweaty Hungry Tingling

Data from Towler, D.A., et al. (1993). Mechanism of awareness of hypoglycemia. Perception of neurogenic (predominantly cholinergic) rather than neuroglycopenic symptoms. *Diabetes, 42,* 1791.

PLANNING: EXPECTED OUTCOMES. The client with diabetes is expected to have an optimal level of mental status functioning (e.g., alert and oriented to person, place, and time, with a Glasgow Coma Scale score greater than 7) and have decreased episodes of hypoglycemia.

INTERVENTIONS. Many diabetic clients have symptoms of hypoglycemia at levels above 50 mg/dL. A blood glucose level below 70 mg/dL alerts the nurse to assess for signs and symptoms of hypoglycemia (Funnell et al., 1998) (Table 65-17; see also Table 65-16).

NIC **HYPOGLYCEMIA MANAGEMENT.** NIC intervention activities for hypoglycemia are listed in Chart 65-13. The nurse monitors blood glucose levels before administering antidiabetic agents, before meals, and before the hour of sleep, or when the client is symptomatic. All clients who take insulin or sulfonylurea agents to lower blood glucose levels are at risk for hypoglycemia, especially if they are older, have liver or kidney impairment, or are taking medications that potentiate the effects of oral antidiabetic drugs. Recognition of sulfonylurea-induced hypoglycemia is often delayed because the usual neurologic symptoms are often absent (Marks & Teale, 1999).

DIET THERAPY. When the client is hypoglycemic, the nurse starts treatment with carbohydrate replacement per physician orders or standing protocols. When the client can swallow, a liquid form of carbohydrate is administered, although virtually any low-fat source of carbohydrate can be used to treat hypoglycemia. Specific treatment recommendations are listed in Chart 65-14. The level of blood glucose being treated may determine the form of glucose to be used. Fluid is absorbed much more quickly from the gastrointestinal (GI) tract than solids. Highly concentrated sweetened fluids, such as juice with several spoonfuls of sugar added or a soft drink, may retard absorption. Commercially available products provide predictable amounts of glucose.

DRUG THERAPY. Glucagon administered subcutaneously or intramuscularly and 50% dextrose administered intravenously are given to diabetic clients who are unable to swal-

TABLE 65-17 • DIFFERENTIATION OF HYPOGLYCEMIA AND HYPERGLYCEMIA

Feature	Hypoglycemia	Hyperglycemia
Skin	Cool, clammy	Hot, dry*
Dehydration	Absent	Present
Perspiration	Profuse*	Absent
Respirations		Rapid, deep*; Kussmaul type; acetone odor to breath
Mental status	Anxious, nervous,* irritable, mental confusion,* seizures, coma	Varies from alert to stuporous, obtunded, or frank coma
Symptoms	Weakness,* double vision, blurred vision, hunger, tachycardia, palpitations	No specific symptoms for DKA Acidosis: hypercapnea; abdominal cramps, nausea and vomiting Dehydration: decreased neck vein filling, orthostatic hypotension, tachycardia, poor skin turgor
Glucose	50 mg/dL (2.8 mmol/L)	>250 mg/dL (13.8 mmol/L)
Ketones	Negative	Positive

DKA, Diabetic ketoacidosis.
*Classic symptoms.

CHART 65-13

NIC INTERVENTION ACTIVITIES *for* The Diabetic Client Experiencing or at Risk for Hypoglycemia

Hypoglycemia Management: *Preventing and treating low blood glucose levels*

- Identify clients at risk for hypoglycemia.
- Monitor blood glucose levels, as indicated.
- Monitor for signs and symptoms of hypoglycemia (e.g., shakiness, tremor, sweating, nervousness, anxiety, irritability, impatience, tachycardia, palpitations, chills, clamminess, lightheadedness, pallor, hunger, nausea, headache, tiredness, drowsiness, weakness, warmth, dizziness, faintness, blurred vision, nightmares, crying out in sleep, paresthesias, difficulty concentrating, difficulty speaking, incoordination, behavior change, confusion, coma, seizure).
- Provide simple carbohydrate, as indicated.
- Provide complex carbohydrate and protein, as indicated.
- Administer glucagon, as indicated.
- Contact emergency medical services, as necessary.
- Administer intravenous glucose, as indicated.
- Maintain patent airway, as necessary.
- Maintain IV access, as appropriate.
- Protect from injury, as necessary.
- Review events prior to hypoglycemia to determine probable cause.
- Provide feedback regarding appropriateness of self-care management of hypoglycemia.
- Instruct client and significant others on signs and symptoms, risk factors, and treatment of hypoglycemia.
- Instruct client to have simple carbohydrates available at all times.
- Instruct client to obtain and carry/wear appropriate emergency identification.
- Instruct significant others on the use and administration of glucagon, as appropriate.
- Instruct on interaction of diet, insulin/oral agents, and exercise.
- Provide assistance in making self-care decisions to prevent hypoglycemia (e.g., reducing insulin/oral agents and/or increasing food intake for exercise).
- Encourage self-monitoring of blood glucose levels.
- Encourage ongoing telephone contact with diabetes care team for consultation regarding adjustments in treatment regimen.

NIC intervention activities selected from McCloskey J.C., & Bulechek, G.M. (2000). *Nursing interventions classification (NIC)* (3rd ed.). St. Louis: Mosby. No part of this work is to be altered without prior written permission from the Publisher.

CHART 65-14

CLIENT EDUCATION GUIDE
Treatment of Hypoglycemia at Home

For *mild* hypoglycemia (hungry, irritable, shaky, weak, headache, fully conscious; blood glucose usually less than 60 mg/dL [3.4 mmol/L]):
- Treat the symptoms of hypoglycemia with 10 to 15 g of carbohydrate. You may use one of the following:
  - Glucose tablets or glucose gel (dosage is printed on the package)
  - 1/2 cup of fruit juice
  - 1/2 cup of regular (nondiet) soft drink
  - 8 ounces of skim milk
  - 6 to 10 hard candies
  - 4 cubes of sugar
  - 4 teaspoons of sugar
  - 6 saltines
  - 3 graham crackers
  - 1 tablespoon of honey or syrup
- Retest blood glucose in 15 minutes.
- Repeat this treatment if symptoms do not resolve.
- Eat a small snack of carbohydrate and protein if your next meal is more than an hour away.

For *moderate* hypoglycemia (cold and clammy skin; pale; rapid pulse; rapid, shallow respirations; marked change in mood; drowsiness; blood glucose usually less than 40 mg/dL [2.2 mmol/L]):
- Treat the symptoms of hypoglycemia with 15 to 30 g of rapidly absorbed carbohydrate.
- Take additional food, such as low-fat milk or cheese, after 10 to 15 minutes.

For *severe* hypoglycemia (unable to swallow; unconsciousness or convulsions; blood glucose usually less than 20 mg/dL [1.0 mmol/L]):

Treatment administered by family members:
- Administer 1 mg of glucagon as intramuscular or subcutaneous injection.
- Administer a second dose in 10 minutes if the person remains unconscious.
- Notify a primary care provider immediately, and follow instructions.
- If still unconscious, transport the person to the emergency department.
- Give a small meal when the person wakes up and is no longer nauseated.

low. Glucagon converts liver glycogen to glucose and is not effective in severely starved clients. The nurse takes care to prevent aspiration in clients receiving glucagon, since it often causes vomiting. The nurse gives 50% dextrose carefully to avoid extravasation. The effects of glucagon and dextrose are temporary, and after the client responds, the nurse administers a simple sugar followed by a small snack or meal. IV glucose may be ordered to maintain mild hyperglycemia. Diazoxide (Proglycem), a specific antidote to sulfonylurea-induced hypoglycemia, or octreotide (Sandostatin), which inhibits sulfonylurea-induced insulin release, may be required if there is difficulty keeping blood glucose levels up by infusion alone (Marks & Teale, 1999).

The nurse evaluates the results of treatment by monitoring blood glucose levels for several hours. Symptoms may persist for an hour or more after treatment of hypoglycemia. A target blood glucose level is 70 to 110 mg/dL (3.9 to 6.2 mmol/L).

PREVENTION STRATEGIES. The nurse teaches the diabetic client how to prevent future episodes of hypoglycemia. Four common causes of hypoglycemia are (1) excess insulin, (2) deficient intake or absorption of food, (3) exercise, and (4) alcohol.

INSULIN EXCESS. Even when insulin is injected in a consistent manner in a nonexercised body area, variations in absorption can cause hypoglycemia. Excess insulin can be caused by lowered insulin resistance, which occurs with termination of pregnancy or resolution of an infection. Increased insulin sensitivity can occur with weight loss or exercise programs and also leads to excess insulin. The nurse instructs the individual taking insulin not to change brands or change from animal-source to human insulin without medical supervision. Differences in formulation of insulin can result in hypoglycemia.

DEFICIENT FOOD INTAKE. Inadequate or incorrectly timed dietary intake can result in hypoglycemia. Irregularities in gastric absorption sometimes cause hypoglycemia in clients with delayed gastric emptying. This problem is more common in clients with diabetes of long duration, is more severe with solid than with liquid meals, and is made worse by illness or poor metabolic control. The nurse instructs the client about the importance of regularity in timing and quantity of food eaten.

EXERCISE. Blood glucose levels commonly decline during exercise in a client with type 1 diabetes. Severe and/or prolonged exercise can increase the rates of cellular glucose uptake and use for several hours after the exercise has been completed. The nurse instructs the client in blood glucose monitoring and carbohydrate supplementation during exercise.

ALCOHOL. The cause of alcohol-induced hypoglycemia is the inhibition of liver gluconeogenesis. Alcohol produces hypoglycemia only when fasting is prolonged and when glycogen stores are depleted before drinking begins (Marks & Teale, 1999). Alcohol cannot be converted to glucose and interferes with the counterregulatory response to hypoglycemia (Funnell et al., 1998). Alcohol may also impair glycogen breakdown and makes exercise-induced hypoglycemia more severe. Alcohol also potentiates the effects of insulin and sulfonylurea-induced hypoglycemia. The nurse instructs the diabetic individual to ingest alcohol according to ADA guidelines—only with or shortly after eating a meal with enough carbohydrate to prevent hypoglycemia (ADA, 2000n). The client is cautioned about avoiding excess alcohol at bedtime to prevent nighttime hypoglycemia.

CLIENT EDUCATION. The cause of hypoglycemia may be subtle. At the onset of menses, a fall in progesterone level may decrease insulin requirements and contribute to hypoglycemia. When clients switch to a new bottle of insulin, hypoglycemia may be noted because the old bottle of insulin had lost its potency. Some clients report hypoglycemia when they change injection sites. Drugs such as propranolol (Inderal, Detensol✤) or other beta blockers mask the early warning signs and thus predispose clients to severe hypoglycemia. Some episodes of hypoglycemia occur without an obvious cause, and many are due to the erratic absorption of insulin, a problem that is not eliminated even in the most careful client.

The nurse can help each diabetic client to develop a personal treatment plan for hypoglycemia. Routine administration of 10 to 15 g of carbohydrate results in overtreatment of hypoglycemic episodes in some individuals and undertreatment in others. The exact glucose rise produced by a given amount of carbohydrate varies. Using the estimate that each 5 g of carbohydrate raises blood glucose about 20 mg/dL, a personal treatment plan can be developed that will provide direction for treatment of specific blood glucose levels. As an example, the client may be directed to take the following Farkas-Hirsh, 2000):

- 20 to 30 g of carbohydrate for a blood glucose level of 50 mg/dL (2.8 mmol/L) or less
- 10 to 15 g of carbohydrate for a blood glucose level of 51 to 70 mg/dL (2.9 to 3.9 mmol/L)

This treatment plan is revised or reinforced by blood glucose monitoring results.

The client is instructed to wear a medical alert bracelet to advise others of the diabetic status. This bracelet is helpful if clients become hypoglycemic and are unable to provide self-care. The nurse assists the client in obtaining the medical alert bracelet.

The nurse teaches the client and family about the signs and symptoms of hypoglycemia. Clients and family members must know that delaying a meal for more than 30 minutes increases the risk for hypoglycemia. The client should have a carbohydrate source with him or her at all times.

The cause of any episodes of hypoglycemia should be determined, and measures taken to prevent recurrence. Hypoglycemia is a major risk associated with exercise programs for clients receiving intensive insulin protocols. Nightmares or headaches on days after prolonged or severe exercise are associated with hypoglycemia, and this possibility should be understood by the client and his or her family.

ESTABLISHING TREATMENT PLANS. Blood glucose monitoring provides information on successful treatment of hypoglycemia. Treatment is continued until blood glucose target ranges have been achieved and maintained. Once treatment is successful and blood glucose control are regained, the specific cause of each hypoglycemic episode must be determined and measures taken to prevent further recurrences.

POTENTIAL FOR DIABETIC KETOACIDOSIS

Metabolic problems of diabetic ketoacidosis (DKA) are caused by a total or partial lack of insulin combined with the action of counterregulatory hormones (Figure 65-11). Laboratory diagnosis of DKA is shown in Table 65-18. DKA occurs in 2% to 5% of all clients with type 1 diabetes mellitus and is most often started by infection. *Death occurs in 1% to 10% of these clients even with appropriate treatment.* Mortality is highest for clients over 60 years of age. Most deaths in older clients occur when there are additional health problems, such as infection, stroke, myocardial infarction, vascular thrombosis, intestinal obstruction, or pneumonia, along with DKA.

Polyuria, polydipsia, and polyphagia start before the actual DKA. Central nervous system (CNS) depression results in changes in consciousness varying from lethargy to coma. The client is dehydrated and has signs and symptoms of severe fluid loss. Kussmaul respiration, abdominal pain, nausea, and vomiting are associated with the metabolic acidosis. Initial serum sodium levels may be low or normal. Initial potassium levels depend on how long DKA has existed before treatment. After therapy is initiated, serum potassium levels begin to drop quickly. Serum white blood cell counts of 20,000 cells/mm indicate dehydration; counts greater than 30,000 cells/mm^3 usually indicate infection.

PLANNING: EXPECTED OUTCOMES. The client with diabetes is expected to maintain a normal blood glucose level and have minimized episodes of hyperglycemia.

INTERVENTIONS

HYPERGLYCEMIA MANAGEMENT. The nurse monitors for signs and symptoms of DKA (see Table 65-18 and Figure 65-11). In the initial phases of treatment, the nurse checks the client's blood pressure, pulse, and respirations every 15 minutes until stable. The nurse records urine output, temperature, and mental status every hour. When a central venous catheter has been placed, the nurse assesses central venous pressure as ordered, usually every 30 minutes. Assessing the client's airway patency, level of consciousness, hydration status, status of fluid and electrolyte replacement, and levels of blood glucose are primary nursing measures. After treatment is underway and these variables are stable, monitoring vital signs and recording values every 4 hours is acceptable. Blood glucose values can be measured either by laboratory or bedside glucose monitoring. Results indicate the adequacy of insulin replacement and establish when to switch from saline to dextrose-containing solutions.

FLUID AND ELECTROLYTE MANAGEMENT. Close assessment of the *fluid status* of the diabetic client is essential. The kidneys are less able to respond to changes in pH or fluid and electrolyte balance, to concentrate urine, or to regulate blood osmolarity. The risk for kidney failure also rises with age. Impaired bicarbonate reabsorption and acid excretion in poorly functioning renal tubules can progress to acidosis. Car-

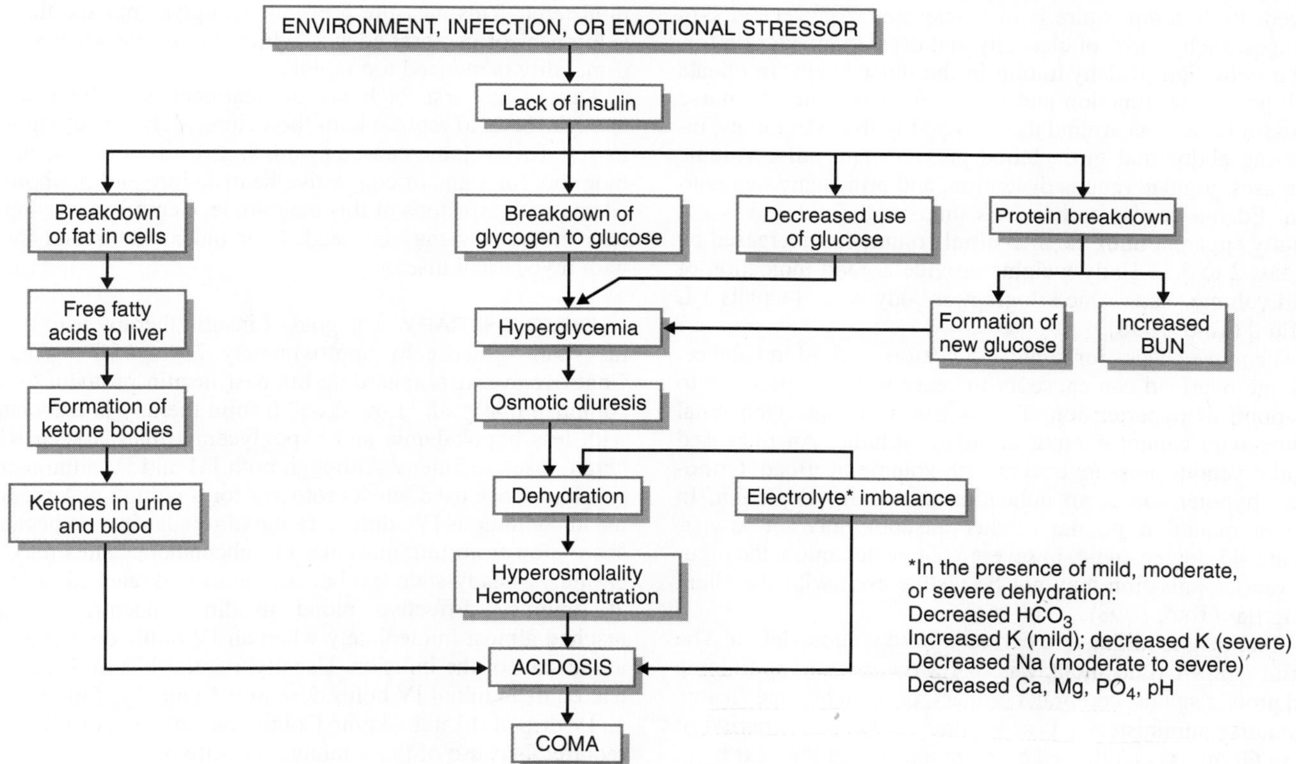

Figure 65-11 ● The pathophysiologic mechanism of diabetic ketoacidosis.

TABLE 65-18 • DIFFERENCES BETWEEN DIABETIC KETOACIDOSIS AND HYPERGLYCEMIC-HYPEROSMOLAR NONKETOTIC SYNDROME

	Diabetic Ketoacidosis (DKA)	Hyperglycemic-Hyperosmolar Nonketotic Syndrome (HHNS)
Onset	Sudden	Gradual
Precipitating factors	Infection Other stressors Inadequate insulin dose	Infection Other stressors Poor fluid intake
Manifestations	Ketosis: Kussmaul respiration, "fruity" breath, nausea, abdominal pain Dehydration or electrolyte loss: polyuria, polydipsia, weight loss, dry skin, sunken eyes, soft eyeballs, lethargy, coma	Altered central nervous system function with neurologic symptoms Dehydration or electrolyte loss: same as for DKA
LABORATORY FINDINGS		
Serum glucose	>300 mg/dL (16.7 mmol/L)	>800 mg/dL (44.5 mmol/L)
Osmolality	Variable	>350 mOsm/L
Serum ketones	Positive at 1:2 dilutions	Negative
Serum pH	<7.35	>7.4
Serum HCO_3	<15 mEq/L	>20 mEq/L
Serum Na	Low, normal, or high	Normal or low
Serum K	Normal; elevated with acidosis, low following dehydration	Normal or low
BUN	>20 mg/dL; elevated because of dehydration	Elevated
Creatinine	>1.5 mg/dL; elevated because of dehydration	Elevated
Urine ketones	Positive	Negative

HCO_3, Bicarbonate.

diovascular disease can cause fluid retention. The dehydrated client's lips and mouth may appear dry, and the tongue furrowed. Body temperature is often elevated. Age-related skin changes, such as loss of elasticity and dryness, make skin turgor a poor sign of dehydration in the older client. In clients with poor renal function and excess fluid volume, the nurse assesses for edema around the eyes and in the extremities, increasing abdominal girth, blood pressure and pulse volume increases, jugular venous distention, and orthostatic hypotension. Edema occurs with excess interstitial fluid and is not usually apparent until the interstitial volume has increased by at least 2 to 3 L. Daily weights provide a good indication of fluid volume status. One kilogram of body weight equals 1 L of fluid (Toto, 1998).

The nurse checks for clinical indicators of fluid imbalance. Volume overload can cause an increase in blood pressure to the point of hypertension. This is true in clients with renal failure who cannot excrete the extra volume. An increased jugular venous pressure occurs with volume overload. Orthostatic hypotension is an indication of volume depletion. In volume depletion, jugular venous pulsation may not be visible at a 45-degree angle. In severe volume depletion, the jugular venous pulsation may not be visible even with the client lying flat (Toto, 1998).

Treatment is initiated to correct a fluid volume deficit. The initial goal of fluid therapy is to restore circulating volume and protect against cerebral, coronary, or renal hypoperfusion. The nurse administers 1 L of isotonic saline over a period of 30 to 60 minutes, followed by a second liter in the next hour, or as ordered.

The second objective of fluid therapy, which is to replace total body and intracellular losses, is achieved more slowly, usually using 0.45% saline. When blood glucose levels reach 250 mg/dL (13.8 mmol/L), 5% dextrose in 0.45% saline is administered. This measure prevents hypoglycemia and the development of cerebral edema, which can occur when serum osmolality is reduced too rapidly.

During the first 24 hours of treatment, the client needs enough fluids to replace both the volume deficit and ongoing losses. This volume can be as much as 6 to 10 L. The nurse monitors for signs of congestive heart failure and pulmonary edema with infusions of this magnitude. Central venous pressure monitoring may be needed for older clients and those with myocardial disease.

DRUG THERAPY. The goal of insulin therapy is to lower the serum glucose by approximately 75 to 150 mg/dL/hr. Controversy exists regarding the best insulin protocol to accomplish this goal. "Low-dose" insulin therapy is associated with less hypokalemia and hypoglycemia than is seen with "high-dose" regimens. Although both IM and IV administration have been used, most protocols for treating DKA recommend continuous IV administration of regular insulin because absorption from intramuscular or subcutaneous sites may be erratic. A steady-state level of insulin can be reached in 25 to 30 minutes. Effective blood insulin concentrations are reached almost immediately when an IV bolus dose is given at the start of the infusion. Usually, regular insulin is administered in an initial IV bolus dose of 0.1 units/kg, followed by an IV drip of 0.1 units/kg/hr. Continuous infusion of insulin is required because of the 4-minute half-life of IV insulin. Subcutaneous insulin is started when the client can take oral nourishment and ketosis has stopped. The effects of insulin therapy are assessed by hourly blood glucose measurements.

ACIDOSIS MANAGEMENT. Regardless of the initial potassium value, there is a large total-body potassium deficit. With insulin therapy, the serum potassium level falls rapidly as potassium shifts into the cells. The nurse monitors the client for signs of hypokalemia, including fatigue, malaise, confusion, muscle weakness, shallow respirations, abdominal distention or paralytic ileus, hypotension, and weak pulse. An electrocardiogram (ECG) shows cardiac conduction changes related to potassium. Hypokalemia is a significant cause of death in the treatment of DKA. Before administering IV potassium, the nurse ensures that the client's urine output is at least 30 mL/hr.

Bicarbonate therapy is indicated only for *severe* acidosis. Inappropriate use of bicarbonate may reverse acidosis too rapidly and result in severe hypokalemia, which can cause fatal cardiac dysrhythmias. Rapid correction of acidosis can worsen the client's mental status. Metabolic acidosis is corrected with fluid replacement and insulin therapy. Sodium bicarbonate, administered by slow IV infusion over several hours, is indicated when the arterial pH is 7.0 or less or the serum bicarbonate level is less than 5 mEq/L (5 mmol/L).

After acid-base disturbances have been corrected, the health team's efforts are directed toward determining the cause of DKA. Infection is the most common precipitating cause (see Table 65-18).

CLIENT EDUCATION: PREVENTION. Investigation of the factors leading to DKA helps the nurse plan specific educational efforts. The nurse teaches the client to perform self-monitoring of blood glucose levels (SMBG) every 4 to 6 hours as long as symptoms such as anorexia, nausea, and vomiting are present and as long as SMBG results are greater than 250 mg/dL (13.8 mmol/L). The client checks urine ketone levels when blood glucose levels exceed 300 mg/dL (>16.7 mmol/L).

The client is taught to minimize the risk for dehydration by maintaining food and fluid intake. When nausea is present, the client is instructed to take liquids containing both glucose and electrolytes (e.g., soda pop, diluted fruit juice, and sports drinks [Gatorade]). Small amounts of fluid may be tolerated even when vomiting is present. The client should take 8 to 12 ounces (240 to 360 mL) of calorie-free and caffeine-free liquids every hour while awake.

Liquids containing carbohydrate can be taken when the diabetic client is unable to eat solid food. The risk of starvation ketosis is reduced by a minimum daily carbohydrate intake of 150 g. After consulting with the primary care provider, the nurse may instruct the client to take additional rapid-acting (lispro) or short-acting (regular) insulin on the basis of SMBG results.

The nurse instructs the client to consult the primary care provider when the following occur:

- SMBG results are greater than 250 mg/dL (13.8 mmol/L).
- Ketonuria is present for more than 24 hours.
- The client is unable to take food or fluids.
- Illness persists for more than 1 to 2 days.

The nurse also instructs the client or the primary caregiver to detect hyperglycemia by performing SMBG whenever the client is ill. Significant illness can result in dehydration with DKA, hyperglycemic-hyperosmolar nonketotic syndrome, or both. The sooner the client seeks treatment, the less severe is the degree of metabolic alteration. Chart 65-15 reviews guidelines for the ill client to follow.

CHART 65-15

CLIENT EDUCATION GUIDE
Sick-Day Rules

- Notify your health care provider that you are ill.
- Monitor your blood glucose at least every 4 hours.
- Test your urine for ketones when your blood glucose level is greater than 240 mg/dL (13.8 mmol/L).
- Continue to take insulin or oral antidiabetic agents.
- To prevent dehydration, drink 8 to 12 ounces of sugar-free liquids every hour that you are awake.
- Continue to eat meals at regular times.
- If unable to tolerate solid food because of nausea, consume more easily tolerated foods or liquids equal to the carbohydrate content of your usual meal.
- Call your primary care provider for any of the following danger signals:
  - Persistent nausea and vomiting
  - Moderate or large ketones
  - Blood glucose elevation after 2 supplemental doses of insulin
  - High (101.5° F [38.6° C]) or rising fever; fever for more than 24 hours.
- Treat your symptoms (e.g., diarrhea, nausea, vomiting, and fever) as directed by your primary care provider.
- Get plenty of rest.

POTENTIAL FOR HYPERGLYCEMIC-HYPEROSMOLAR NONKETOTIC SYNDROME AND COMA

Hyperglycemic-hyperosmolar nonketotic syndrome (HHNS) is a **hyperosmolar** (increased blood osmolarity) state caused by hyperglycemia of any origin. The pathophysiologic processes associated with HHNS are outlined in Figure 65-12. Although both HHNS and diabetic ketoacidosis (DKA) are associated with hyperglycemia, HHNS is different from DKA because of the absence of ketosis and the much higher than average blood glucose levels and osmolality. Often blood glucose levels are greater than 800 mg/dL (44.5 mmol/L) and blood osmolality is greater than 350 mOsL when HHNS is present. Other biochemical problems with HHNS tend to be more severe than those with DKA. Table 65-18 outlines the differences between DKA and HHNS.

CONSIDERATIONS FOR OLDER ADULTS

HHNS occurs most often in older clients and almost exclusively in people with type 2 diabetes mellitus, many of whom were previously undiagnosed. Mortality rates in older clients have been as high as 40% to 70%. The onset of HHNS is slow and may not be recognized. The older client typically seeks medical attention later and is sicker than the younger client. *HHNS does not occur in adequately hydrated individuals.* Older clients with diabetes are at greater risk for dehydration and HHNS because of age-related changes in thirst perception and poor urine-concentrating abilities.

Conditions such as myocardial infarction, sepsis, pancreatitis, and stroke, and drugs such as glucocorticoids, diuretics, phenytoin sodium (Dilantin), propranolol (Inderal), and calcium channel blockers also may precipitate HHNS. Central nervous system (CNS) changes range from confusion to complete coma. In contrast to clients with DKA, those with HHNS may have generalized seizures, myoclonic jerking, and reversible paralysis.

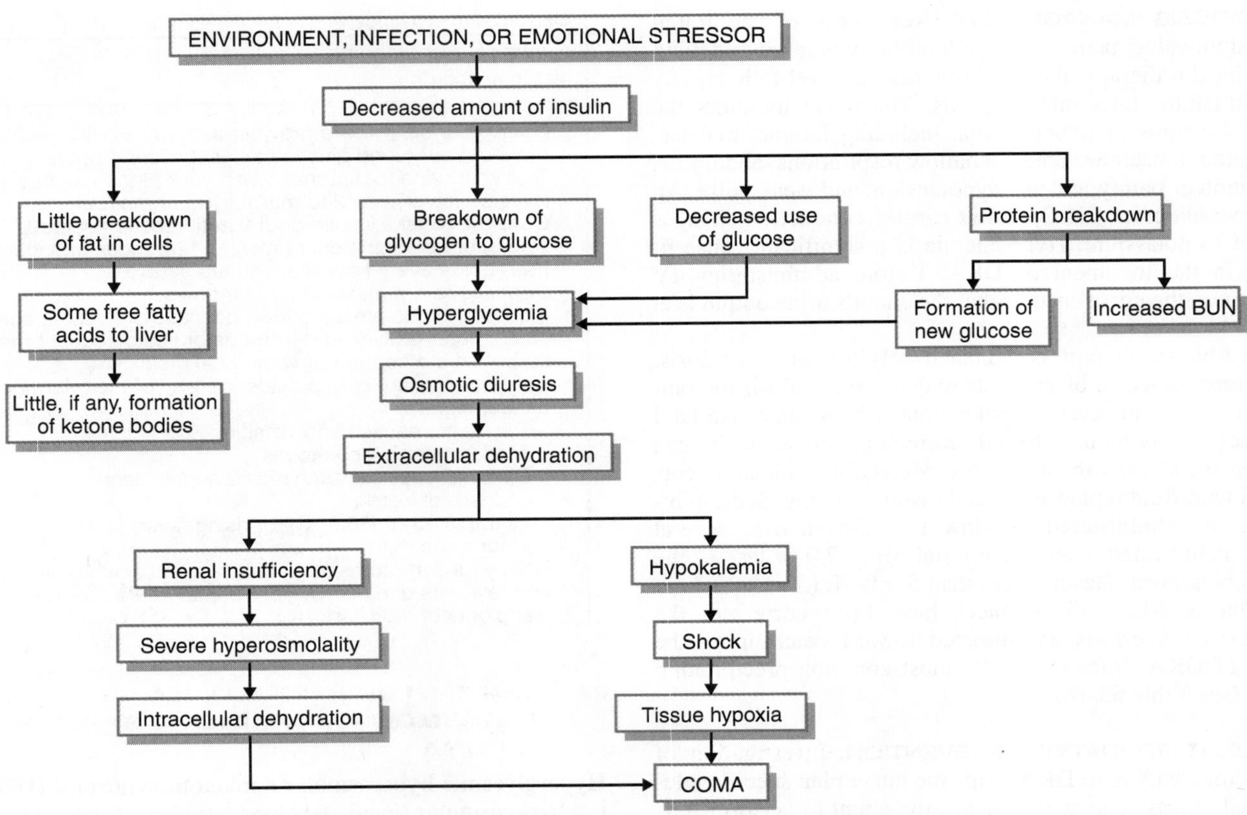

Figure 65-12 ● The pathophysiologic mechanism of hyperglycemic-hyperosmolar nonketotic syndrome.

The development of HHNS rather than DKA in any client is related to residual insulin secretion. In HHNS, the client secretes just enough insulin to prevent ketosis but not enough to prevent hyperglycemia. The hyperglycemia of HHNS is more severe than that of DKA, greatly increasing the blood osmolality and causing profound osmotic diuresis. Severe dehydration and electrolyte loss occur, and the client may lose 15% to 25% of body fluid. When dehydration is severe, glucose is not filtered into the urine, causing even greater hyperglycemia and hyperosmolality. Impairment of the thirst center in the brain occurs, making it impossible for the client to drink enough fluid to prevent dehydration.

PLANNING: EXPECTED OUTCOMES. The client with diabetes is expected to maintain a normal blood glucose level and have minimized episodes of hyperglycemia.

INTERVENTIONS

MONITORING. The nurse monitors for signs and symptoms of HHNS (see Tables 65-17 and 65-18 for symptoms of hyperglycemia). The nurse performs ongoing assessment of fluid status.

FLUID THERAPY. The goal of therapy is to complete rehydration and obtain normal blood glucose levels within 36 to 72 hours. The choice of fluid replacement and the rate of administration are critical in the management of HHNS. The severity of the CNS problems is related to the level of blood hyperosmolarity and cellular dehydration. Re-establishing fluid balance in brain cells is a difficult and slow process, and many clients do not recover baseline CNS function until several hours after blood glucose levels have returned to normal.

As with DKA, the *initial* objective for fluid replacement in HHNS is to increase circulating blood volume. If shock or severe hypotension is present, normal saline is given initially. Otherwise, half-normal saline is preferable because it more rapidly corrects the free-water deficit (Samos & Roos, 1998). The fluids are infused at a rate of 1 L/hr until central venous pressure or pulmonary capillary wedge pressure begins to rise or until the blood pressure and urine output are adequate. The rate is then reduced to 100 to 200 mL/hr. Half of the estimated water deficit is replaced in the first 12 hours, and the remainder is given during the next 36 hours. Body weight, urine output, kidney function, and the presence or absence of pulmonary congestion and jugular venous distention determine the rate of fluid administration. In clients with known congestive heart failure, renal insufficiency, or acute kidney failure, central venous pressure monitoring is indicated. The nurse assesses the client hourly for signs of cerebral edema. *Changes in the level of consciousness; changes in pupil size, shape or reaction; or seizures are reported immediately to the physician* (Konick-McMahan, 1999). Lack of any improvement in level of consciousness may indicate inadequate rates of fluid replacement or reduction in plasma osmolarity. Regression after initial improvement may indicate too rapid a reduction in plasma osmolarity. A slow but steady improvement in CNS function is the best evidence that fluid management is satisfactory.

CONTINUING THERAPY. IV insulin given at a rate of 10 units/hr is usually required to reduce blood glucose levels. Although fluid replacement reduces hyperglycemia, it cannot by itself return blood glucose levels to normal. A reduction of 10% per hour in the blood glucose level is a reasonable goal (Samos & Roos, 1998). Potassium loss occurs in HHNS, although not to the degree that it does in DKA. Because of the initial low urine output **(oliguria)** or absent urine output **(anuria),** potassium replacement may not be needed at the onset of therapy. Client education and interventions to minimize dehydration are similar to those for ketoacidosis.

Community-Based Care

HEALTH TEACHING

Education to attain blood glucose control must begin at the time of diagnosis of diabetes. Education is conducted in a hospital or outpatient setting, clinic, or primary care provider's office and involves the coordinated efforts of physicians, dietitians, nurses, pharmacists, social workers, and psychologists (see Chart 65-11).

ASSESSING LEARNING NEEDS. Although some education can be conducted in group settings, most will need to be done on a one-to-one basis. Continuing education will need to take place over time to master the knowledge, skills, and flexibility required to maintain long-term blood glucose control. The nurse or case manager assesses educational needs of the client and assures that education is provided by the appropriate disciplines.

The client's awareness of diabetes and the needs of the person and his or her family must be assessed before initiating teaching (Brink et al., 1995). This assessment includes the following:

- Age, occupation
- Likes, dislikes, fears
- Current lifestyle
- Evaluation of general health, attitudes about health, self-care behaviors
- Learning ability and style, willingness to learn
- Acceptance of diabetes, current knowledge of diabetes
- Skills needed, attitudes, goals
- Ethnic background, language
- Home situation

Before beginning actual diabetic education, the nurse assesses the client's baseline knowledge of diabetes and its treatment, determining what concerns the client the most about having diabetes. Adult learners are interested in information that applies directly to their situation. It is appropriate to ask what the client wants to learn. Starting with what he or she already knows and building on that base is a good way to increase knowledge and correct any errors in information that the client may have. To capture interest and motivate clients for further learning, the nurse presents material relevant to their first questions. Because they will be required to manage their own care after discharge, clients tend to focus on issues most important to them. Teaching about treatment measures that need to be started soon after diagnosis may be of more interest to the client than long-term control.

The client's physical condition dictates the timing of teaching efforts. When blood glucose levels are fluctuating, the client does not have the energy to learn complex information. Telling the client that good control of blood glucose levels improves the sense of well-being can help him or her accept the recommended therapy. An informal teaching program is started until the client feels able to attend a formal class. The nurse teaches and observes the client's technique for injections and blood glucose monitoring.

Individual clients learn in individual ways. A successful diabetic education program combines several different teaching methods. Some clients learn better when they read pamphlets; others learn better when they watch videotapes. Learning is enhanced when the equipment is handled, techniques are practiced, success is rewarded, and errors are corrected immediately.

ASSESSING PHYSICAL, COGNITIVE, AND EMOTIONAL LIMITATIONS. The nurse assesses the educational and reading levels of the client to determine what level of information to present. The client's visual ability to read printed information is assessed. In addition, the client taking insulin needs to be able to read the labels and markings on syringes and equipment. Many clients with type 2 diabetes have **presbyopia** (age-related far-sightedness) and baseline visual difficulties that are made worse by blurred vision caused by fluctuating blood glucose levels. The client must be able to understand the printed material that is presented. Even highly educated clients do not want to read complicated information when they are sick. Much of the printed material from drug companies is printed at the sixth- or seventh-grade level. The International Diabetes Center prepares printed diabetic education material at the second- and third-grade levels. The nurse develops creative teaching strategies for the client who cannot read.

The nurse also assesses the client's ability to conceptualize. The adjustment of insulin dosage on the basis of blood glucose monitoring is a difficult concept to understand and may not be appropriate for some clients who are unable to understand these concepts. Self-management of medication, exercise, and diet requires complex interpretation and behavior.

The nurse assesses manual dexterity and any physical limitations that may alter the teaching plan. A history of hand injury, the presence of hand tremors, or severe arthritis requires modification in insulin preparation instruction.

Information is best learned when the client is ready. Clients with newly diagnosed diabetes are facing a life crisis. Some may be more motivated to learn information that will be beneficial and are willing to change lifelong behaviors. Others may grieve the loss of their previous lifestyle and use denial as a means of coping with the diagnosis. In this instance, the client may not be able to learn needed information at this time.

EXPLAINING SURVIVAL SKILLS. The initial phase of diabetic education involves basic survival skills. The basic pathologic changes of diabetes and the relationship of diet, medication, and exercise to overall metabolic control are important.

A dietitian provides the initial diet instruction. The diabetic client needs to understand what food is to be eaten, how much food is to be eaten, and when the food is to be eaten. The nurse stresses the importance of eating meals on time, as well as the dangers of skipping meals. The client must be able to explain how to maintain food intake during illness. The nurse reinforces dietary instruction, answers questions, and refers questions to the dietitian or physician as indicated.

After the nurse provides medication instruction, the client should be able to identify the specific medication needed for control of blood glucose levels. When insulin administration is needed, the client must be able to prepare and administer the ordered dose accurately using sterile technique. The client must also be able to verbalize when insulin injections are to be taken, where insulin is to be injected, and how insulin is to be stored. The nurse stresses the dangers of skipping insulin doses. Possible drug interactions must be carefully reviewed with the client, particularly older individuals taking oral antidiabetic agents.

The diabetic client should be able to state a plan for regular physical activity. The client must be able to verbalize the relationship between exercise and blood glucose control and identify situations when activity is not appropriate. The nurse provides guidelines for additional carbohydrate intake to prevent hypoglycemia as a result of excessive exercise.

The diabetic client also must be able to verbalize the plan for monitoring blood glucose. The person performing self-monitoring of blood glucose levels (SMBG) must be able to do the procedure with accuracy and understanding of the results. The nurse provides guidelines for when SMBG is to be performed, acceptable ranges, and actions to be taken when results are out of these ranges. When the client is unable to perform SMBG, the nurse or case manager ensures that a resource (e.g., home care agency, health clinic, or primary care provider's office) will be available to do monitoring during times of illness).

The client must understand the significance, symptoms, causes, and treatment of hypoglycemia. It is essential for the diabetic client to verbalize the causes of hypoglycemia and the activities needed to prevent recurrence. He or she must be able to describe appropriate carbohydrate resources to have available and the intent to notify the physician regarding hypoglycemic episodes.

The client also must understand the significance of hyperglycemia and its relationship to illness. The client must describe actions to take during illness and when to communicate with the primary care provider.

Most of this survival information is retained when the client is ready to learn. Client education is a challenge to nurses because clients tend to be hospitalized for shorter periods. All of the diabetic education may be provided in an outpatient setting, where contact with the client is limited. It becomes necessary to squeeze important information into the time frames available. Many clients, regardless of the duration of their disease, do not progress in self-management beyond the survival level because of psychologic barriers.

COUNSELING. The major goal of in-depth counseling is to assist the client in becoming self-sufficient in diabetes management. Educational sessions with the client and family members are necessary in order to individualize the diabetes regimen to their particular needs, skills, and abilities. Education is often provided through the team efforts of a physician, a nurse educator, a dietitian, a social worker, a pharmacist, a psychologist, and other health care professionals as needed, and it occurs in a variety of outpatient settings.

In addition to knowledge gained at the survival level, the diabetic client should be able to discuss the action of insulin in the body and the effects of insulin deficiency on various body systems. The client should also be able to explain the effects of diet, medication, and activity on control of blood glucose levels. He or she should be able to relate the metabolic goals of maintaining normal blood glucose levels to the prevention of complications. This aspect involves being able to relate variations in SMBG results to the possible need for a change in insulin dosage.

The client must be able to describe the meal plan and explain what adjustments in dietary intake are needed to meet diabetic diet requirements. He or she should state how food intake needs to be altered when increased physical activity is planned and when he or she eats in restaurants or at family gatherings. It is essential that the client be able to list appropriate foods to be eaten to prevent and treat hypoglycemia, as well as adjustments to make when feeling ill.

The diabetic client must be able to demonstrate accuracy in insulin preparation and administration. He or she should be able to discuss the onset, peak, and duration of the specific insulin preparation. In reviewing insulin administration practices, the nurse stresses the importance of injection site selection and site rotation. The nurse carefully reviews guidelines for adjustment in insulin dosage on the basis of SMBG results (when permitted by the physician) and explains that follow-up SMBG results are needed to evaluate the effects of additional insulin. The client should explain the method of protecting insulin when traveling. For clients with the potential for severe hypoglycemia, the nurse observes a family member's ability to inject glucagon. When the client is taking oral diabetic medications, the nurse asks him or her to identify the medication and describe its schedule of administration. Because of the potential for drug interactions, the client must identify over-the-counter drugs with the potential to cause adverse drug interactions and the need to inform the primary care provider of the drug regimen.

Within the physical limitations imposed by the baseline health status, the client should be able to perform any desired physical activities. The diabetic client must state the SMBG levels that are safe for exercise, the frequency of performing SMBG during exercise, the food intake required before exercise, and what food to have available during exercise if symptoms of hypoglycemia occur. He or she should be aware of the potential for injury during exercise and explain the importance of protective footwear.

The goals of in-depth education are for the nurse to assist the diabetic client in solving problems of blood glucose fluctuation through the use of SMBG. The client should be able to identify practices, such as travel (Chart 65-16), that result in blood glucose fluctuations and to treat these problems with supplemental insulin administration, changes in physical activity levels, or changes in diet. The nurse asks the client to demonstrate urine ketone testing techniques and identify the conditions during which urine ketones should be measured.

The diabetic client must be able to describe a plan for periodic evaluation of the control of blood glucose levels by the primary care provider, as well as periodic dental and eye examinations. He or she must be able to demonstrate appropriate foot care, wear properly fitting shoes, and describe hazards related to foot care. The client must be able to relate plans to reduce specific risk factors, such as cigarette smoking and hypertension.

The client must verbalize that diabetes is a lifelong disease that necessitates lifestyle changes, describe the changes in progress, and indicate those that need to be made. He or she should be able to identify stress-producing situations and discuss methods for stress reduction.

PSYCHOSOCIAL PREPARATION

The diagnosis of diabetes may represent a loss of control. All but a few clients lose flexibility in routines. Life becomes ordered; time schedules and routines must be followed. Certain events surrounding diabetes are predictable. Taking an insulin injection and not eating for several hours causes hypoglycemia. Poorly controlled diabetes leads to complications and premature death. Tight control of blood glucose levels prevent these complications.

The stress of diabetes is in addition to the demands of normal daily life. The client must be able to integrate the demands of diabetes into daily and recreational schedules so as not to cause blood glucose alterations.

The nurse can assist in healthy psychologic adaptation to diabetes by providing successful educational experiences. The mastery of blood glucose monitoring assists the client in feeling that he or she has control over the disease. Knowledge of the effects of extra activities or extra food, as well as the result of taking additional insulin, is helpful in making future adjustments in regimens.

The client's feeling a sense of control over the condition does much to provide a positive psychologic attitude about diabetes. Success in self-injection of insulin provides concrete evidence that he or she is able to master the disease. The nurse breaks a task into small, achievable units to ensure mastery of techniques; for example, a client may begin learning how to administer an injection by first obtaining an accurate dose of insulin.

It is appropriate to devote as much time as possible to insulin injection and blood glucose monitoring techniques. Clients with newly diagnosed diabetes are often fearful of giving themselves injections. After insulin injection technique has been mastered, clients become less anxious and are able to attend to other tasks.

CRITICAL THINKING CHALLENGE

The client is a 60-year-old business man recently diagnosed with type 2 diabetes after developing hyperglycemic-hyperosmolar nonketotic syndrome (HHNS) following 2 days of vomiting and diarrhea. He has been started on a second-generation sulfonyl urea oral antidiabetic drug. Last week he attended a group class for clients with newly diagnosed diabetes. He tells you that he feels fortunate that his diabetes can be cured with oral medication instead of insulin injections. He also explains that eating in restaurants and having alcoholic cocktails with his customers are a major part of his occupation, and he wonders if the "pills will interfere with his drinking habits."

- How will you identify this client's most urgent educational needs?
- What, if any, referrals are most appropriate for this client?
- Do you have any suggestions for how this client could manage social contact with his customers without increasing his risk for diet- and alcohol-related changes in blood glucose levels?

For suggested answer guidelines, go to SIMON http://www.wbsaunders.com/SIMON/Iggy/.

CHART 65-16

CLIENT EDUCATION GUIDE
Travel Tips for Diabetic Clients

Before traveling visit your primary care provider and diabetes educator.
- See your physician to make certain you do not have any other health problems.
- Obtain a letter from your physician (typed on office letterhead) that indicates you have diabetes and lists the medications you are taking.
- Obtain any needed immunizations or inoculations.
- Obtain prescriptions from your physician for your medications, including glucagon if you take insulin, and prescriptions for motion sickness, nausea and vomiting, and traveler's diarrhea.
- Develop a plan for changing strengths of insulin if you are traveling to a country that does not carry the type of insulin you use. Learn how to use a U-100 syringe to draw up U-40 insulin.
- Develop a plan for meal and medication adjustment across time zones. Eastbound travel will shorten the day, requiring a reduction in the amount of medication needed. Westbound travel may add an extra meal to the day and require additional medication.
- Obtain a list of foods from your diabetes educator that you can substitute for food served in restaurants or airplanes.

If you are traveling by air, train, or boat, call ahead and request special meals for individuals with diabetes.
- Plan for delays in eating.
- Eat something every 4 hours.
- Drink a glass of water every 2 hours to prevent dehydration.
- Do not assume that special meals will be available; substitute items you cannot eat with foods you have in your travel kit.

Notify airline and hotel personnel that you have diabetes.
- Always wear medical alert identification and keep your medical alert card in your wallet.

While traveling:
- Check your blood glucose level frequently.
- Do not engage in activities when blood glucose levels are lower than 65 mg/dL.
- Stretch and walk around every 2 hours to help your circulation.
- Check your feet frequently for blisters and sores. You may be doing more walking than usual.
- Take extra shoes with you, and plan to change shoes often when walking more than normal.
- Protect your skin against exposure to the sun. Drug-induced photosensitivity can occur with some oral hypoglycemic agents.

Always have your travel kit with you; do not check your kit along with the rest of your luggage. Include these items in your travel kit:
- Twice as much medication and twice as many supplies as you think you will need (Pack medications separately from checked luggage.)
- Insulin stored in an insulated carrying case that will maintain temperatures according to the manufacturer's directions
- The letter from your physician (typed on office letterhead) that indicates you have diabetes and lists the medications you are taking
- A supply of fast-acting sugar (such as glucose tablets or gel, hard candy, and sugar cubes), as well as longer-acting foods (such as cheese and crackers and peanut butter and crackers)
- A self-monitoring diary

CHART 65-17

FOCUSED ASSESSMENT *of* The Insulin-Dependent Diabetic Client During a Home or Clinic Visit

Assess overall mental status, wakefulness, ability to converse.
Take vital signs and weight:
- Fever could indicate infection.
- Are blood pressure and weight within target range? Why or why not?

Question client regarding any change in visual acuity; check current visual acuity.
Inspect oral mucous membranes, gums, and teeth.
Question client about injection areas used; inspect areas being used; assess whether client is utilizing areas and sites appropriately.
Inspect skin for intactness, wounds that have not healed, new sores, ulcers, bruises, or burns; assess any previously known wounds for infection, progression of healing.
Question client regarding foot care.
Assess lower extremities and feet for peripheral pulses, lack of or decreased sensation, abnormal sensations, breaks in skin integrity, condition of toes and nails.
Question client regarding color and consistency of stools and frequency of bowel movements; assess abdomen for bowel sounds.
Review client's home health diary:
- Is blood glucose within targeted range? Why or why not?
- Is glucose monitoring being recorded often enough?
- Is the client's food intake adequate and appropriate? Why or why not?
- Is exercise occurring regularly? Why or why not?

Assess client's ability to perform self-monitoring of blood glucose.
Assess client's procedures for obtaining and storing insulin and syringes, cleaning equipment, disposing of syringes and needles.
Assess client's insulin preparation and injection technique.

HOME CARE MANAGEMENT

Maintaining blood glucose control depends on the client's self-management skills. The primary role of the health care professional is to provide ongoing support and education and to empower the client to make informed decisions. Diabetes education aims to help the client acquire knowledge regarding the management of diabetes, behavior change skills, and communication skills to participate effectively as part of the health care team (Childs, 1998).

The nurse provides information about resources. The client must know whom to contact in case of an emergency. Older adults who live alone must have daily telephone contact with a friend or neighbor. The client may also need assistance with grocery shopping and meal preparation. He or she may have limited access to transportation out of the home and may not have sufficient supplies of food, particularly in bad weather. Because of the high frequency of visual problems in older clients, they may need assistance in preparing insulin syringes for injection or in performing blood glucose monitoring. The nurse or case manager initiates referrals to home care or public health agencies as appropriate. Such referral is especially important for older women with diabetes who are insulin dependent. Studies have reported that these women have greater cognitive decline with memory loss than do men with diabetes or women of the same age who do not have diabetes (Gregg et al., 2000). Chart 65-17 identifies areas for assessment during a home or clinic visit.

TABLE 65-19 • OUTCOME CRITERIA FOR DIABETIC TEACHING

Before being discharged to home, the diabetic client or the significant other should be able to:
- Tell why insulin or an oral hypoglycemic agent is being prescribed
- Name which insulin or oral hypoglycemic agent is being prescribed, and name the dosage and frequency of administration
- Discuss the relationship between mealtime and the action of insulin or the oral hypoglycemic agent
- Discuss plans to follow diabetic diet instructions
- Prepare and administer insulin accurately
- Test blood for glucose, or state plans for having blood glucose levels monitored
- Test urine for ketones, and state when this test should be done
- Verbalize how to store insulin
- List symptoms that indicate a hypoglycemic reaction
- Tell what carbohydrate sources are used to treat hypoglycemic reactions
- Tell what symptoms indicate hyperglycemia
- Tell what dietary changes are needed during illness
- Verbalize when to call the physician or the nurse (frequent episodes of hypoglycemia, symptoms of hyperglycemia)
- Verbalize the procedures for proper foot care

HEALTH CARE RESOURCES

A wide array of diabetic education material is available from drug companies. The American Diabetes Association (ADA) will refer a diabetic client to the appropriate agencies or resources (phone [800] 232-3472 in the United States; [703] 549-1500 in Canada). The American Association of Diabetes Educators can refer a diabetic client to a certified diabetes educator in his or her area for information about diabetes (phone [800] TEAM-UP-4). Additional resources are listed in the Selected Bibliography.

Evaluation: Outcomes

NOC The nurse evaluates the care of the client with diabetes on the basis of the identified nursing diagnoses and collaborative problems. The ultimate evaluation of the success of survival-level and in-depth diabetic education is the ability of the client to maintain blood glucose levels within the normal range. Specific outcome criteria for client education are listed below and in Table 65-19. The expected outcomes include that the client will:
- Achieve blood glucose control as evidenced by maintaining blood glucose levels in the expected range
- Avoid acute and chronic complications of diabetes
- Have a satisfactory and complete postoperative recovery without complications
- Identify factors that increase the potential for injury
- Modify lifestyle to reduce the risk for injury
- Monitor health status changes
- Practice proper foot care to prevent injury, as evidenced by cleansing and inspecting the feet for cleanliness and healthy skin
- Maintain intact skin on the feet
- Experience relief of pain
- Recognize causal factors of pain
- Use preventive measures to avoid pain
- Use available resources to increase comfort
- Maintain optimal vision

- Be free of injury related to decreased visual acuity
- Maintain a urine elimination pattern in the expected range
- Maintain urine proteins within normal limits
- Have an optimal level of mental status functioning
- Have decreased episodes of hypoglycemia
- Have decreased episodes of hyperglycemia

ONLINE RESOURCES

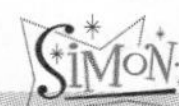

For suggested readings and Internet resources, go to http://www.wbsaunders.com/SIMON/Iggy/.

SELECTED BIBLIOGRAPHY

Asterisk indicates a classic or definitive work on this subject.

Abbott, C.A., et al. (1998). Multicenter study of the incidence of and predictive risk factors for diabetic neuropathic foot ulceration. Diabetes Care, 21(12), 1071-1075.

Ahern-Gould, K. (1998). Quick resource for electrolyte imbalance. *Critical Care Nursing Clinics of North America, 10*(4), 477-490.

Aiello, L.P., Gardner, T.W., & King, G.L. (1998). Technical review: Diabetic retinopathy. *Diabetes Care, 21*(1), 143-156.

Alberts, M.J. (1999). Diagnosis and treatment of ischemic stroke. *American Journal of Medicine, 106*(2), 211-221.

Amanti, M., & Schumann, L. (1998). Coronary artery disease: A link between hypertension, diabetes, hyperlipidemia and obesity. *Journal of the American Academy of Nurse Practitioners, 10*(2), 77-81.

American Association of Diabetes Educators. (1997). Position statement: Blood glucose monitoring, http://www.aadenet.org.

*American Diabetes Association. (1996). Consensus statement: Self-monitoring of blood glucose. *Diabetes Care, 19*(Suppl. 1), 62-66.

American Diabetes Association. (1998). Consensus development conference on the diagnosis of coronary heart disease in people with diabetes. *Diabetes Care, 21*(9), 1551-1559.

American Diabetes Association. (1999a). Consensus development conference on diabetic foot wound care. *Diabetes Care, 22*(8), 1354-1399.

American Diabetes Association. (1999b). Reviews: Economic consequences of diabetes mellitus in the U.S. *Diabetes Care, 22*(2), 296-309.

American Diabetes Association. (2000a). Committee report: Report of the Expert Committee on the Diagnosis and Classification of Diabetes Mellitus. *Diabetes Care, 23*(Suppl. 1), 4-19

American Diabetes Association. (2000b). Position statement: Aspirin therapy in diabetes. *Diabetes Care, 23*(Suppl. 1), 61-62.

American Diabetes Association. (2000c). Position statement: Continuous subcutaneous insulin infusion. *Diabetes Care, 23*(Suppl. 1), 90.

American Diabetes Association. (2000d). Position statement: Diabetes mellitus and exercise. *Diabetes Care, 23*(Suppl. 1), 50-54.

American Diabetes Association. (2000e). Position statement: Diabetic nephropathy. *Diabetes Care, 23*(Suppl. 1), 69-72.

American Diabetes Association. (2000f). Position statement: Diabetic retinopathy. *Diabetes Care, 23*(Suppl. 1), 73-76.

American Diabetes Association. (2000g). Position statement: Food labeling, *Diabetes Care, 23*(Suppl. 1), 94-95.

American Diabetes Association. (2000h). Position statement: Gestational diabetes mellitus. *Diabetes Care, 23*(Suppl. 1), 77-79.

American Diabetes Association. (2000i). Position statement: Hospital admission guidelines for diabetes mellitus. *Diabetes Care, 23*(Suppl. 1), 83.

American Diabetes Association. (2000j). Position statement: Implications of the diabetes control and complications trial. *Diabetes Care, 23*(Suppl. 1), 24-26.

American Diabetes Association. (2000k). Position statement: Implications of the United Kingdom prospective diabetes study. *Diabetes Care, 23*(Suppl. 1), 27-31.

American Diabetes Association. (2000l). Position statement: Insulin administration. *Diabetes Care, 23*(Suppl. 1), 86-89.

American Diabetes Association. (2000m). Position statement: Management of dyslipidemia in adults with diabetes. *Diabetes Care, 23*(Suppl. 1), 57-60.

American Diabetes Association. (2000n). Position statement: Nutritional recommendations and principles for individuals with diabetes. *Diabetes Care, 23*(Suppl. 1), 43-46.

American Diabetes Association. (2000o). Position statement: Pancreas transplantation for patients with diabetes mellitus. *Diabetes Care, 23*(Suppl. 1), 85.

American Diabetes Association. (2000p). Position statement: Prevention of type 1 diabetes mellitus. *Diabetes Care, 23*(Suppl. 1), 108.

American Diabetes Association. (2000q). Position statement: Preventive foot care in people with diabetes. *Diabetes Care, 23*(Suppl. 1), 55-56.

American Diabetes Association. (2000r). Position statement: Role of fat replacers in diabetes medical nutrition therapy. *Diabetes Care, 23*(Suppl. 1), 96-97.

American Diabetes Association. (2000s). Position statement: Screening for type 2 diabetes. *Diabetes Care, 23*(Suppl. 1), 20-23.

American Diabetes Association. (2000t). Position statement: Standards of medical care for patients with diabetes mellitus. *Diabetes Care, 23*(Suppl. 1), 32-42.

American Diabetes Association. (2000u). Position statement: Tests for glycemia in diabetes. *Diabetes Care, 23*(Suppl. 1), 80-82.

Apfel, S.C. (1999). Neurotrophic factors in the therapy of diabetic neuropathy. *American Journal of Medicine, 107*(2B), 34-42.

Arezzo, J.C. (1999). New developments in the diagnosis of diabetic neuropathy. *American Journal of Medicine, 107*(2B), 9-16.

Armstrong, D., & Lavery, L.A. (1998). Shoes and the diabetic foot. *Practical Diabetology, 17*(1), 23-26.

Armstrong, D., Lavery, L.A., & Bushman, T.R. (1998). Peak foot pressures influence the healing time of diabetic foot ulcers treated with total contact casts. *Journal of Rehabilitation Research and Development, 35*(1), 1-5.

Armstrong, D., et al. (1998). Choosing a practical screening instrument to identify patients at risk for diabetic foot ulceration. *Archives of Internal Medicine, 158*(3), 289-292.

Bagley, M. (1998). Helping older adults to live better with hearing and vision loss. *Journal of Case Management, 7*(4), 147-152.

Bell, D.S., & Alele, J. (1999). Dealing with diabetic nephropathy. *Postgraduate Medicine, 105*(2), 83-94.

Bell, P.M., & Hadden, D.S. (1997). Metformin. *Endocrinology and Metabolism Clinics of North America, 26*(3), 523-537.

Bennett, G.A. (1998). Neuropathic pain: New insights, new interventions. *Hospital Practice, 33*(10), 95-114.

Bichler, L.M. (1999). Foot ulcers in diabetes. *ADVANCE for Nurse Practitioners, 7*(1), 49-52.

Bloomgarden, Z.T. (1999). New approaches to insulin treatment and glucose monitoring. *Diabetes Care, 22*(12), 2078-2082.

Bohannon, N.N.V. (1997). Benefits of lispro insulin. *Postgraduate Medicine, 101*(2), 73-80.

Bolli, G.B., & Fanelli, C.G. (1999). Physiology of glucose counterregulation to hypoglycemia. *Endocrinology and Metabolism Clinics of North America, 28*(3), 467-493.

Boulton, A.J.M., & Malik, R.A. (1998). Diabetic neuropathy. *Medical Clinics of North America, 82*(4), 909-929.

Brenner, Z.R. (1999). Preventing postoperative complications. *Nursing99, 29*(10), 34-39.

*Brink, S., et al. (1995). *Diabetes education goals.* Alexandria, VA: American Diabetes Association.

Brown, J.B., Pedula, K., & Bakst, A.W. (1999). The progressive cost of complications in type 2 diabetes mellitus. *Archives of Internal Medicine, 159*(16), 1873-1880.

Browne, A.C., & Sibbald, R.G. (1999). The diabetic neuropathic ulcer: An overview. *Ostomy/Wound Management, 45*(1A), 6-22.

Brunner, G., et al. (1998). Validation of home blood glucose meters with respect to clinical and analytical approaches. *Diabetes Care, 21*(4), 585-590.

Burge, M.R., & Schade, D.S. (1997). Insulins. *Endocrinology and Metabolism Clinics of North America, 26*(3), 575-598.

Burke, J., et al. (1999). Rapid rise in the incidence of type 2 diabetes from 1987 to 1996. *Archives of Internal Medicine, 159*(13), 1450-1456.

Capriotti, T., & McLeughlin. (1998). A revitalized battle against diabetes mellitus for the new millennium. *MEDSURG Nursing, 7*(6), 323-342.

Caspi, A. (1998). Sildenafil: A new drug treatment for male erectile dysfunction. *Pharmacy and Therapeutics, 23*(5), 233-240.

Childs, B.P. (1998). Diabetes care: Compliance versus empowerment. *Case Review, 4*(3), 14-20.

Clark, C.M. (1998). The burden of chronic hyperglycemia. *Diabetes Care, 21*(Suppl. 3), 32-34.

*Cleary, M.E. (Ed.). (1994). *Diabetes and visual impairment: An educator's resource guide.* Chicago: American Association of Diabetes Educators.

Cohen, R.A., et al. (1999). Determinants of retinopathy progression in type 1 diabetes. *American Journal of Medicine, 107*(1), 45-51.

Consensus development conference on diabetic foot wound care. (1999). *Ostomy/Wound Management, 45*(9), 32-47.

Culleton, J.L. (1999). Preventing diabetic foot complications. *Postgraduate Medicine, 106*(1), 74-83.

Cryer, P.E. (1997). *Hypoglycemia: Pathophysiology, diagnosis and treatment.* New York: Oxford University Press.

Cryer, P.E. (1999). Symptoms of hypoglycemia, thresholds for their occurrence and hypoglycemic unawareness. *Endocrinology and Metabolism Clinics of North America, 28*(3), 495-499.

Dagogo-Jack, S., & Santiago, J.V. (1997). Pathophysiology of type 2 diabetes and modes of action of therapeutic interventions. *Archives of Internal Medicine, 157*(16), 1802-1817.

Dahlquist, G. (1999). Primary and secondary prevention strategies of pre-type 1 diabetes. *Diabetes Care, 22*(Suppl. 2), 4-6.

Dahn, M.S. (1998). The role of growth factors in wound management of diabetic foot ulcers. *Federal Practitioner, 15*(Suppl. 7), 14-19.

Davidson, M.B. (1998). *Diabetes mellitus: Diagnosis and treatment.* Philadelphia: W.B. Saunders.

Davis, T.M.E., et al. (1999). Risk factors for stroke in type 2 diabetes mellitus. *Archives of Internal Medicine, 159*(10), 1097-1103.

Declair, V. (1999). The importance of growth factors in wound healing. *Ostomy/Wound Management, 45*(4), 64-80.

DePree, P.A. (1998). Lispro insulin. *Nursing98, 28*(11), 54-55.

Despres, J.P. (1999). Insulin resistance and hyperglycemic associated risk factors. *Diabetes Care, 22*(Suppl. 2), 38-40.

Dewey, C.M., & Riley, W.J. (1999). Have diabetes, will travel. *Postgraduate Medicine, 101*(2), 111-126.

Diabetes Prevention Program Research Group. (1999). The diabetes prevention program: Design and methods for a clinical trial in the prevention of type 2 diabetes. *Diabetes Care, 22*(4), 623-634.

Dinneen, S.F., & Gerstein, H.C. (1997). The association of albuminuria and mortality in non–insulin dependent diabetes mellitus. *Archives of Internal Medicine, 157*(13), 1413-1418.

Dinsmoor, R. (1999). Tools of the trade: New insulins, drugs and devices. *Diabetes Self-Management, 16*(6), 46-54.

Eaglstein, W.H., & Falanga, V. (1997). Chronic wounds. *Surgical Clinics of North America, 77*(3), 689-700.

Fagan, T., & Sowers, J. (1999). Type 2 diabetes mellitus: Greater cardiovascular risk factors and greater benefits of therapy. *Archives of Internal Medicine, 159*(10), 1033-1034.

Farkas-Hirsh, R. (Ed.). (2000). All about hypoglycemia. *Diabetes Self-Management, 17*(1), 21-27.

Feinglos, M.N., & Bethel, M.A. (1998). Treatment of type 2 diabetes. *Medical Clinics of North America, 82*(4), 757-790.

Fishman, L.M. (1999). The normal pathophysiology of aging. *Journal of Long-Term Home Health Care, 1*(2), 114-124.

Fleming, D.R. (1999). Challenging traditional insulin injection practices. *American Journal of Nursing, 99*(2), 72-73.

Franz, M.J. (1997). Lifestyle modifications for diabetes management. *Endocrinology and Metabolism Clinics of North America, 26*(3), 499-510.

Funnell, M., & Barlage, D. (2000). Saying a mouthful about oral diabetes drugs. *Nursing2000, 30*(11), 34-39.

Funnell, M.M., et al. (1998). *A core curriculum for diabetes education.* Chicago: American Association of Diabetes Educators.

Garber, A.J. (1998). Vascular disease and lipids in diabetes. *Medical Clinics of North America, 82*(4), 931-948.

Garg, S.K., et al. (1999). Correlation of fingerstick blood glucose measurements with GlucoWatch Biographer Glucose results in young subjects with type 1 diabetes. *Diabetes Care, 22*(10), 1708-1714.

Gaster, B., & Hirsh, I.B. (1998). The effects of improved glycemic control on complications of type 2 diabetes. *Archives of Internal Medicine, 158*(2), 134-140.

*Gillis W. Long Hansen's Disease Center Rehabilitation Branch. (1992). *Foot screening: Care of the foot in diabetes: The Carville approach.* (1992). Carville, LA: Department of Health and Human Services.

Goldberg, R.B. (1998). Prevention of type 2 diabetes. *Medical Clinics of North America, 82*(4), 805-821.

Goldstein, D.E., & Little, R.R. (1997). Monitoring glycemia in diabetes: Short term assessment. *Endocrinology and Metabolism Clinics of North America, 26*(3), 475-486.

Green, K., & Lydon, S. (1998). The continuum of patient care. *American Journal of Nursing, 98*(10), 16BBB-DDD.

Greene, D.A., Stevens, M.J., & Feldman, E.L. (1999). Diabetic neuropathy: The scope of the problem. *American Journal of Medicine, 107*(2B), 2-8.

Greenspan, F.S., & Strewler, G.J. (1997). *Basic and clinical endocrinology.* Stamford, CT: Appleton & Lange.

Gregg, E., et al. (2000). Is diabetes associated with cognitive impairment and cognitive decline among older women? *Archives of Internal Medicine, 160*(2), 174-180.

Grinslade, S., & Buck, E.A. (1999). Diabetic ketoacidosis: Implications for the medical-surgical nurse. *MEDSURG Nursing, 8*(1), 37-45.

Guerrero-Romero, F., & Rodriguez-Moran, M. (1999). Proteinuria is an independent risk factor for ischemic stroke in non–insulin dependent diabetes mellitus. *Stroke, 30*(9), 1787-1791.

Haffner, S.M. (1998a). Epidemiology of type 2 diabetes: Risk Factors. *Diabetes Care, 21*(Suppl. 3), 3-6.

Haffner, S.M. (1998b). Technical review: Management of dyslipidemia in adults with diabetes. *Diabetes Care, 21*(1), 160-178.

Halperin, M.L., & Goldstein, M.B. (1999). *Fluid, electrolyte and acid-base physiology.* Philadelphia, W.B. Saunders.

Halpin-Landry, J.E., & Goldsmith, S. (1999). Feet first: Diabetes care. *American Journal of Nursing, 99*(2), 26-33.

Harris, M.I. (1998). Diabetes in America: Epidemiology and scope of the problem. *Diabetes Care, 21*(Suppl. 3), 11-14.

Harris, M.I., Flegal, K.M., & Cowie, C.C. (1998). Prevalence of diabetes, impaired fasting glucose, and impaired glucose tolerance in U.S. adults. *Diabetes Care, 21*(4), 518-524.

Harris, M.I., et al. (1999). Racial and ethnic differences in glycemic control of adults with type 2 diabetes. *Diabetes Care, 22*(3), 403-408.

Hazlewood, F.J., Rodriguez, D.J. & Cypress, M. (1999). Exploring the roles of case managers in diabetes care. *Case Manager, 9*(2), 57-63.

Henry, R.R. (1997). Thiazolidinediones. *Endocrinology and Metabolism Clinics of North America, 26*(3), 553-573.

Herlitz, J., & Malmberg, K. (1999). How to improve the cardiac prognosis for diabetes. *Diabetes Care, 22*(Suppl. 3), 89-96.

Hernandez, D. (1998). Microvascular complications of diabetes: Nursing assessment and intervention. *American Journal of Nursing, 98*(6), 26-32.

Hirsh, I.B. (1998). Intensive treatment of type 1 diabetes. *Medical Clinics of North America, 82*(4), 689-719.

Hirsh, I.B., & Paauw, D.S. (1997). Diabetes management in special situations. *Endocrinology and Metabolism Clinics of North America, 26*(3), 631-645.

Hunt, T.K., & Hopf, H.W. (1997). Wound healing and wound infection. *Surgical Clinics of North America, 77*(3), 587-606.

Hunter, S.J., & Garvey, T. (1998). Insulin action and insulin resistance: Diseases involving defects in insulin receptors, signal transduction, and the glucose transport effector system. *American Journal of Medicine, 105*(4), 331-345.

Hussar, D.A. (2000). New drugs 2000. *Nursing2000, 30*(1), 55-56.

Ilonen, J., & Akerblom, H. (1999). New technologies and genetics of type 1 diabetes. *Diabetes Technology and Therapeutics, 1*(2), 205-207.

Inlow, S., Kalla, T. P., & Rahman, J. (1999). Downloading plantar foot pressures in the diabetic patient. *Ostomy/Wound Management, 45*(10), 28-38.

Jacober, S., & Sowers, J. (1999). An update on perioperative management of diabetes. *Archives of Internal Medicine, 159*(20), 2405-2411.

Janisse, D.J. (1998). Picking the shoe to fit the occasion. *Diabetes Self-Management, 15,* 30-33.

Jaremko, J., & Rorstad, O. (1998). Advances toward the implantable artificial pancreas for treatment of diabetes. *Diabetes Care, 21*(3), 444-450.

Joseph, S.E., Hopkins, D., & Korzon-Burokowska, A. (1998). The action profile of lispro is not blunted by mixing in the syringe with NPH insulin. *Diabetes Care, 21*(12), 2098-2102.

Kendall, D.M., & Robertson, R.P. (1997). Pancreas and islet transplantation. *Endocrinology and Metabolism Clinics of North America, 26*(3), 611-630.

Keown, P.A. (1999). Therapeutic strategies for optimal use of novel immunosuppressants. *Transplantation Proceedings, 31*(4), 1790-1793.

Kong, M.F., et al. (1999). Natural history of diabetic gastroparesis. *Diabetes Care, 22*(3), 503-507.

Konick-McMahan, J. (1999). Riding out a diabetic emergency. *Nursing99, 29*(9), 34-40.

Koproski, J., Pretto, Z., & Poretsky, L. (1997). Effect of an intervention by a diabetes team in hospitalized patients with diabetes. *Diabetes Care, 20*(10), 1553-1555.

Korenman, S.G. (1998). New insights into erectile dysfunction: A practical approach. *American Journal of Medicine, 105*(2), 135-144.

Kumar, A., et al. (1999). Combined kidney and pancreatic transplantation. *British Medical Journal, 318*(7188), 886-887.

Larsen, J. (1998). Dyslipidemia in diabetes. *ADVANCE for Nurse Practitioners, 6*(4), 36-43.

Lavery, L. (1998). Practical criteria for screening patients at high risk for diabetic foot ulceration. *Archives of Internal Medicine, 158*(2), 157-162.

Lebovitz, H.E. (1997). Alpha-glucosidase inhibitors. *Endocrinology and Metabolism Clinics of North America, 26*(3), 539-551.

LeRoith, D., Taylor, S., & Olefsky, J. (1997). *Diabetes mellitus.* Philadelphia: Lippincott-Raven.

*Letho, S., et al. (1996). Risk factors predicting lower extremity amputation in patients with NIDDM. *Diabetes Care, 19*(6), 607-612.

Lipsky, B.A. (1998). Overview of the diabetic foot: Epidemiology, pathophysiology and the role of infection. *Federal Practitioner, 15*(Suppl. 7), 2-7.

Lougheed, W.D., et al. (1997). Stability of insulin lispro in insulin infusion systems. *Diabetes Care, 20*(7), 1061-1065.

Mahler, R.J., & Adler, M.L. (1999). Type 2 diabetes mellitus: Update on diagnosis, pathophysiology and treatment. *Journal of Endocrinology and Metabolism, 84*(4), 1165-1171.

Malmberg, K. (1997). Intensive glucose control produced better long-term outcomes after myocardial infarction. *British Medical Journal, 314*(7093), 1512-1515.

Manske, C.L. (1999). Risks and benefits of kidney and pancreas transplantation for diabetic patients. *Diabetes Care, 22*(Suppl. 2), 114-120.

Marks, J.B., & Raskin, P. (1998). Nephropathy and hypertension in diabetes. *Medical Clinics of North America, 82*(4), 877-907.

Marks, V., & Teale, J.D. (1999). Drug-induced hypoglycemia. *Endocrinology and Metabolism Clinics of North America, 28*(3), 555-577.

Mayfield, J.A., et al. (1998). Technical review: Preventive foot care in people with diabetes. *Diabetes Care, 21*(12), 2161-2177.

Miettinen, H., et al. (1998). Impact of diabetes on mortality after first myocardial infarction. *Diabetes Care, 21*(1), 69-75.

Moss, S.E., Klein, R., & Klein, B. (1999). Risk factors for hospitalization in people with diabetes. *Archives of Internal Medicine, 159*(17), 2053-2057.

Muha, J. (1999). Local wound care in diabetic foot complications. *Postgraduate Medicine, 106*(1), 97-102.

*National Institute of Diabetes and Digestive and Kidney Diseases. (1995). *Diabetes in America.* NIH Pub. No. 95-1468, Bethesda, MD: National Institutes of Health.

Neeley, K.A., et al. (1998). Diabetic retinopathy. *Medical Clinics of North America, 82*(4), 847-876.

Nehra, A., Barrett, D.M., & Moreland, R.B. (1999). Pharmacologic advances in the treatment of erectile dysfunction. *Mayo Clinic Proceedings, 74*(7), 709-721.

O'Brien, T., Nguyen, T.T., & Zimmerman, B.R. (1998). Hyperlipidemia and diabetes mellitus. *Mayo Clinic Proceedings, 73*(10), 969-976.

O'Hanlon-Nichols. (1999). Neurologic assessment: The basis of a comprehensive examination. *American Journal of Nursing, 99*(6), 44-50.

O'Neill, K., & Ross-Kerr, J.C. (1999). Impact of an instructional program on nurse's accuracy in capillary blood glucose monitoring. *Clinical Nursing Research, 8*(2), 166-179.

Parry, G.J. (1999). Management of diabetic neuropathy. *American Journal of Medicine, 107*(2B), 27-33.

Peragallo-Dittko, V. (1999). Blood glucose meter roundup. *Diabetes Self-Management, 16*(2), 7-16.

Peters, S. (1998). Diabetic foot ulcers: Prevention is the key to successful management. *ADVANCE for Nurse Practitioners, 6*(6), 59-62.

Petronic, V., & Bhisitkul, R. (1999). Lasers and diabetic retinopathy: The art of gentle destruction. *Diabetes Technology and Therapeutics, 1*(2), 177-187.

Pieber, T., et al. (2000). Efficacy and safety of HOE 901 versus NPH insulin in patients with type 1 diabetes. *Diabetes Care, 23*(2), 157-162.

Pinzur, M.S. (1999). The American Orthopaedic and Foot and Ankle Society guidelines. *Practical Diabetology, 18*(1), 6-13.

Rabinovitch, A., & Skyler, J.S. (1998). Prevention of type 1 diabetes. *Medical Clinics of North America, 82*(4), 739-755.

Rassam, A., et al. (1999). Optimal administration of lispro insulin in hyperglycemic type 1 diabetes. *Diabetes Care, 22*(1), 133-136.

Ravid, M., et al. (1997). Main risk factors for nephropathy in type 2 diabetes mellitus are plasma cholesterol levels, mean blood pressure and hyperglycemia. *Archives of Internal Medicine, 158*(9), 998-1004.

Reddy, K.S., et al. (1999). Surgical complications after pancreas transplantation with portal-enteric drainage. *Transplantation Proceedings, 31*(1-2), 617-618.

Riddle, M.C. (1997). Tactics for type 2 diabetes. *Endocrinology and Metabolism Clinics of North America, 26*(3), 659-677.

Robbins, J. (1998). Foot ulcerations: Causes, therapy, prevention and care. *Federal Practitioner, 15*(Suppl. 7), 9-13.

Robertson, K., Glazer, N., & Campbell, R. (2000). The latest development in insulin injection devices. *Diabetes Educator, 26*(1), 135-152.

Robertson, R.P, et al. (2000). Technical review: Pancreas and islet transplantation for patients with diabetes. *Diabetes Care, 23*(1), 112-116.

Roman, S.H., Harris, M.I. (1997). Management of diabetes mellitus from a public health perspective. *Endocrinology and Metabolism Clinics of North America, 26*(3), 443-474.

Rosenbloom, A.L., et al. (1999). Emerging epidemic of type 2 diabetes in youth. *Diabetes Care, 22*(2), 345-354.

Rosiglitazone for type 2 diabetes mellitus. (1999) *Medical Letter, 41*(1059), 71-73.

Rosscamp, R.H., & Park, G. (1999). Long-acting insulin analogs. *Diabetes Care, 22*(Suppl. 2), 109-113.

*Ruderman, N., & Devlin, J.T. (Eds). (1995). *The health professional's guide to diabetes and exercise.* Alexandria, VA: American Diabetes Association.

Ryan, A., et al. (2001). Insulin action after resistive training in insulin-resistant older men and women. *Journal of the American Geriatrics Society, 49*(3), 254-262.

Samos, L.F., & Roos, B.A. (1998). Diabetes mellitus in older persons. *Medical Clinics of North America, 82*(4), 791-803.

Saudek, C. (1997). Novel forms of insulin delivery. *Endocrinology and Metabolism Clinics of North America, 26*(3), 599-610.

Scheen, A.J., & Lefebvre, P.J. (1999). Troglitazone: Antihyperglycemic activity and potential role in the treatment of type 2 diabetes. *Diabetes Care, 22*(9), 1568-1577.

Schrier, R.W. (1997). *Renal and electrolyte disorders.* Philadelphia: Lippincott-Raven.

Service, F.J. (1999). Classification of hypoglycemic disorders. *Endocrinology and Metabolism Clinics of North America, 28*(3), 501-517.

Setter, S.M, Baker, D.E., & Campbell, R.K. (1999). Sildenafil (Viagra) for the treatment of erectile dysfunction in men with diabetes. *Diabetes Educator, 25*(1), 79-89.

Shorr, R.I., et al. (1997). Incidence and risk factors for serious hypoglycemia in older persons using insulin or sulfonylureas. *Archives of Internal Medicine, 157*(15), 1681-1686.

Simon, R.R., Aminoff, M.J., & Greenberg, D.A. (1999). *Clinical neurology.* Stamford, CT: Appleton & Lange.

Skyler, J.S. (1997a). Insulin therapy in type 11 diabetes. *Postgraduate Medicine, 101*(2), 85-96.

Skyler, J.S. (1997b). Tactics for type 1 diabetes. *Endocrinology and Metabolism Clinics of North America, 26*(3), 647-657.

Slovenkai, M.P. (1998). Foot problems in diabetes. *Medical Clinics of North America, 82*(3), 949-972.

Sollinger, H.W., et al. (1998). Experience with 500 simultaneous pancreas-kidney transplants. *Annals of Surgery, 228*(3), 284-293

Sowers, J.R., & Lester, M.A. (1999). Diabetes and cardiovascular disease. *Diabetes Care, 22*(Suppl. 3), 14-20.

Spollett, G.R. (1999). Assessment and management of erectile dysfunction in men with diabetes. *Diabetes Educator, 25*(1), 65-75.

Steed, D.L. (1997). The role of growth factors in wound healing. *Surgical Clinics of North America, 77*(3), 575-586.

Steiner, G. (1999). Risk factors for macrovascular disease in type 2 diabetes: Classic lipid abnormalities. *Diabetes Care, 22*(Suppl. 3), 6-9.

Stratta, R.J. (1999). Optimal immunosuppression in pancreas transplantation. *Transplantation Proceedings, 31*(1/2), 619-621.

Stratta, R.J., et al. (1999). Evolution in pancreas transplantation techniques: Simultaneous kidney-pancreas transplantation using portal-enteric drainage without antilymphocyte induction. *Annals of Surgery, 229*(5), 701-708.

Sutherland, D.E.R., Cecka, M., & Gruessner, A. (1999). Report from the International Transplant Registry—1998. *Transplantation Proceedings, 27*(1/2), 597-601.

Taub, L.F. (1998). The ADA's clinical practice recommendations in action. *American Journal of Nursing, 98*(10), 16B-16D.

Taylor, H.R. (1997). Diabetic retinopathy: A public health challenge. *American Journal of Ophthalmology, 123*(4), 543-545.

Tomky, D. (1997). Diabetes: Taking a new look at an old adversary. *American Journal of Nursing, 97*(11), 41-45.

Toto, K.H. (1998). Fluid balance assessment. *Critical Care Clinics of North America, 10*(4), 383-400.

Trecroci, D. (1999). FDA panel backs GlucoWatch monitor. *Diabetes Interview, 9*(1), 15.

Troglitazone for non-insulin dependent diabetes mellitus. (1997). *Medical Letter, 39*(1001), 49-51.

Vinik, A.I. (1999). Diabetic neuropathy: Pathogenesis and therapy. *American Journal of Medicine, 107*(2B), 17-26.

Ward, J.D. (1999). Improving prognosis in type 2 diabetes. *Diabetes Care, 22*(Suppl. 2), 84-87.

Wei, M., et al. (1998). Effects of diabetes and level of glycemia on all-cause and cardiovascular mortality. *Diabetes Care, 21*(7), 1167-1172.

White, J.R., Campbell, R.K., & Hirsh, I. (1997). Insulin analogues. *Postgraduate Medicine, 101*(2), 58-70.

Wierman, M.E. (1998). Erectile dysfunction: A multifaceted disorder. *Hospital Practice, 33*(10), 65-90.

Williams, A.S. (1997). Teaching nonvisual diabetes self-care: Choosing appropriate tools and techniques for visually impaired individuals. *Diabetes Spectrum, 10*(2), 128-134.

Williams, A.S. (1999a). Adjusting to vision loss. *Diabetes Self-Management, 16*(2), 45-51.

Williams, A.S. (1999b). Independent insulin management. *Diabetes Self-Management, 16*(5), 33-41.

Zimmerman, B.R. (1997). Sulfonylureas. *Endocrinology and Metabolism Clinics of North America, 26*(3), 511-522.

Zinman, B., et al. (1997). Insulin lispro in CSII. *Diabetes, 46*(3), 440-443.

UNIT 14

PROBLEMS OF PROTECTION

Management of Clients with Problems of the Skin, Hair, and Nails

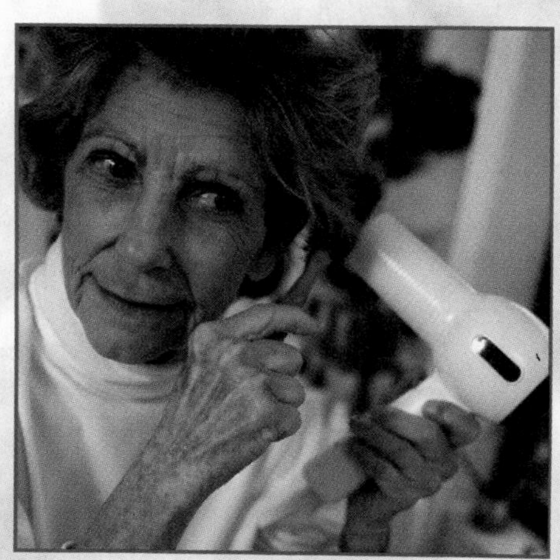

UNIT 14

Problems of Protection: Skin, Hair, and Nails ■ Core Concepts Grid

Anatomy	Physiology	Pathophysiology	History	Physical Exam	Diagnostic Tests	Interventions	Pharmacology
• **Skin** Subcutaneous fat Epidermis Dermis • **Hair** • **Nails** • **Glands**	• **Protection** • **Regulation** Fluid balance Electrolyte balance Temperature • **Vitamin synthesis**	• **Inflammation** • **Infection** • **Tumors** • **Burns** Thermal Chemical Electrical	• **Client history** Dermatologic problems Medications Liver, gallbladder, renal disease • **Family history** Chronic skin problems • **Social history** Occupation Nutritional status Sun exposure Age Race • **Risk for pressure ulcers**	• **Skin** Color Lesions Moisture Vascular markings Edema Intactness Tattoos Temperature Texture Turgor Depth (stage) of wound Drainage • **Hair/nails** Shape Distribution Texture	• **Cultures** • **Skin tests** Patch Scratch • **Biopsy**	• **Burn wound assessment** Depth Area Rule of Nines • **Burn fluid replacement formulas** • **Graft care** • **Care of burn wounds** • **Hypertrophy** • **Precautions for itching** • **Emotional support** • **Debridement** • **Wound dressings** • **Nutrition** • **Prevention of pressure ulcers** • **Skin/wound ongoing assessment**	• **Topical antibiotics** • **Topical antiinflammatories** • **Keratolytic agents** • **Antipsoriasis agents** • **Debriding agents** • **Systemic antibiotics**

CHAPTER 66

Assessment of the Skin, Hair, and Nails

JANICE CUZZELL

Learning Objectives

After studying this chapter, you should be able to:

1. Compare the structures and function of the dermis with those of the epidermis.
2. Describe the integumentary changes associated with aging.
3. Use proper terminology to describe different skin lesions.
4. Describe techniques to assess skin changes in clients with dark skin.
5. Distinguish between normal variations and abnormal skin manifestations with regard to skin color, texture, warmth, and moisture.
6. Explain the role of melanocytes in determining skin color.
7. Describe the ABCD method of assessing skin lesions for cancer.
8. Prioritize educational needs for the client undergoing an excisional biopsy for a skin lesion.

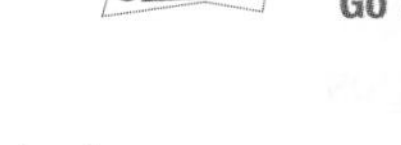

Go to http://www.wbsaunders.com/SIMON/Iggy/ for self-assessment questions related to these Learning Objectives.

The integumentary system is composed of the skin, hair, and nails. This system is the first line of defense in protecting the inner organs from the external environment. The skin is the largest organ of the body and plays a major role in homeostasis. Not only is it a barrier to microorganisms, it also helps to regulate body temperature and maintains fluid and electrolyte balance. Changes in the skin can communicate information about a person's health and well-being.

Emotional stress, systemic disease, and skin injury or disease can alter the function, appearance, and texture of the skin. Therefore the nurse examines the skin for important clues about the client's health. Because the skin has many sensory receptors, the client can report subjective skin sensations that may indicate specific health problems. The sensory function of the skin allows the nurse to use touch as a therapeutic intervention to provide comfort, relieve pain, and communicate caring.

ANATOMY AND PHYSIOLOGY REVIEW

Structure of the Skin

As shown in Figure 66-1, the skin has three distinct layers: fat, dermis, and epidermis. Each layer has unique properties that contribute to the skin's ability to maintain its complex functions.

SUBCUTANEOUS FAT (ADIPOSE TISSUE)

The innermost layer of the skin, which lies over muscle and bone, is the site for fat formation and storage. Fat cells act as heat insulators for the body. They absorb shock and protect against mechanical injury by padding internal structures. The distribution of fat varies with anatomic area, age, and gender. Many blood vessels perforate the fatty layer and extend into the dermal layer, forming capillary networks that supply nutrients and remove waste products.

DERMIS (CORIUM)

Above the subcutaneous fat lies the **dermis,** a layer of connective tissue that contains no cells. The dermis is composed of collagen and elastic fibers that are interwoven to give the skin both flexibility and mechanical strength.

Collagen, the main component of dermal tissue, is a protein formed by dermal cells called fibroblasts. The production of collagen increases in areas of tissue injury and helps form scar tissue. Fibroblasts also produce **ground substance,** a lubricating material composed of protein and sugar groups that surrounds the dermal cells and fibers and contributes to the skin's normal suppleness and turgor.

The elasticity of the skin depends on both the quantity and quality of the elastic fibers, which are scattered among the collagen fibers. The major component of the elastic fiber is **elastin.**

The dermis houses a network of capillaries and lymph vessels in which the exchange of oxygen and heat occurs. The dermis is also rich in sensory nerves that transmit the sensations of touch, pressure, temperature, pain, and itch.

EPIDERMIS

Anchored to the dermis by fingerlike projections of dermal tissue **(dermal papillae)** is the outermost layer of skin: the

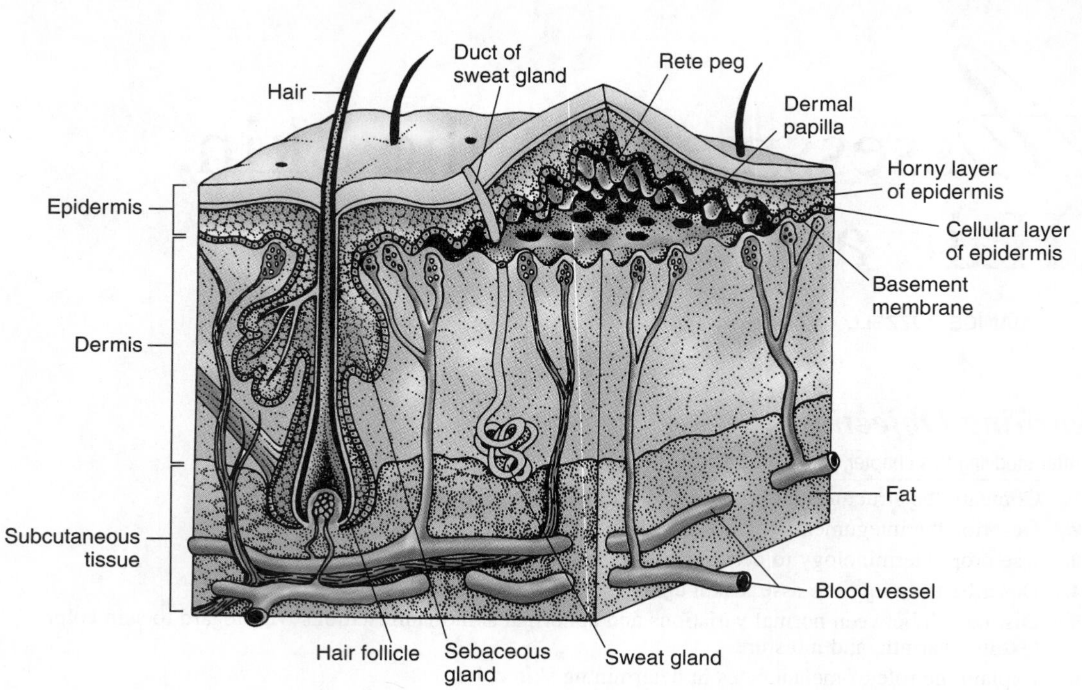

Figure 66-1 ● Anatomy of the skin.

epidermis. The fingers of epidermal tissue that project into the dermis are called **rete pegs.** The epidermis is less than 1 mm thick, but it is the protective barrier between the body and noxious stimuli in the environment.

The epidermis does not have a separate blood supply. It receives its nutrients by diffusion from the many blood vessels in the dermal layer through a porous basement membrane at the dermal-epidermal junction. Attached to the basement membrane are the keratinocytes. The basal cells (those keratinocytes capable of cell division and located closest to the basement membrane) continuously divide to form new cells. Older keratinocytes are pushed upward to form the stratified layers of the epithelium **(malpighian layers).** As keratinocytes move toward the surface, they flatten and eventually die. The outermost skin layer, the **stratum corneum** (horny layer), is composed of these dead cells. **Keratin,** the protein produced by keratinocytes, makes the horny layer relatively waterproof. A keratinocyte takes about 28 to 45 days to move from the basement membrane to the skin surface, where it is shed **(exfoliated).**

The final synthesis of vitamin D occurs primarily within the epidermis. Vitamin D is activated by ultraviolet (UV) light.

Melanocytes are found at the level of the basement membrane in a ratio of about 1 melanocyte for every 10 keratinocytes. These pigment-producing cells give color to the skin and account for the racial differences in skin tone. Darker skin tones are not caused by increased numbers of melanocytes; it is the size of the pigment granules (melanin) contained in each cell that determines the color. UV light stimulates the production of melanin, which protects against the harmful effects of sun exposure. Melanin production increases locally in response to endocrine changes or inflammation.

Structure of the Skin Appendages

HAIR

Hair, a remnant of the thick protective pelt worn by most mammals, is mainly a cosmetic feature for modern humans. Hair growth varies with race, gender, age, and genetic predisposition. Individual hairs can differ in both structure and rate of growth, depending on body location.

Hair follicles are located in the dermal layer of the skin but are actually extensions of the epidermal layer (see Figure 66-1). Within each hair follicle, a round column of keratin forms the mature hair shaft. The increased sulfur content of hair keratin (in contrast to that of keratin found in the cells of the stratum corneum) toughens the hair shaft as it forms. Hair color is genetically determined by a person's rate of melanin production.

Hair growth occurs in cycles; a growth phase **(anagen)** is followed by a resting phase **(telogen).** Local and systemic stressors can alter the growth cycle and result in temporary hair loss. Permanent baldness, such as common male pattern baldness, is genetic in origin and is seldom influenced by personal or environmental factors.

NAILS

Well-groomed fingernails and toenails have cosmetic value and serve as useful tools with which to scrape and grasp. Like hair follicles, the nails are extensions of the keratin-producing epidermal layers of the skin.

The white, crescent-shaped portion of the nail at the lower end of the nail plate **(lunula)** reflects the underlying nail matrix, where nail keratin is formed and nail growth begins (Figure 66-2). Unlike hair growth, which is cyclic, nail growth is a continuous but slow process. Total replacement of a fingernail

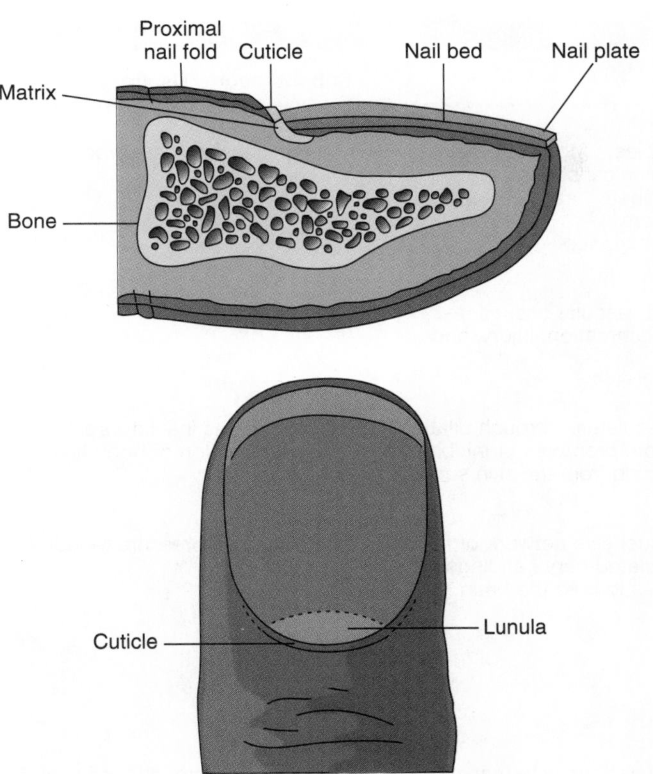

Figure 66-2 ● Anatomy of the nail.

from the matrix to the end of the finger requires 3 to 4 months. Total replacement of a toenail may take up to 12 months.

The **cuticle,** a layer of keratin produced by the epithelial cells of the proximal nail fold, attaches the nail plate to the soft tissue of the nail fold. The nail body is largely translucent; the pinkish hue reflects a rich capillary blood supply beneath the nail surface. Nail growth and appearance are often altered during systemic disease or serious illness.

GLANDS

SEBACEOUS GLANDS. The sebaceous glands are distributed over the entire skin surface, except for the palms of the hand and soles of the feet. Most sebaceous glands are directly connected to the hair follicles (Figure 66-3). The sebaceous glands of the eyelids, nipple areolae, and genitalia are freestanding.

Sebaceous glands continuously produce **sebum,** a mildly bacteriostatic, fat-containing substance. Sebum lubricates the skin and reduces water loss from the skin surface.

SWEAT GLANDS. The skin has two types of sweat glands: eccrine and apocrine. **Eccrine sweat glands** originate from the epithelial cells. They are found over the entire skin surface and are not associated with the hair follicle. The odorless, colorless, isotonic secretions of the eccrine glands are the single most important factor in the regulation of body temperature. Stimulation of the eccrine sweat glands and the resultant evaporative water loss enable the body to lose as much as 10 to 12 L of fluid in a single day.

Apocrine sweat glands are in direct contact with the hair follicle. They occur primarily in the areas of the axillae, perineum, nipple areolae, and periumbilicus. The interaction of skin bacteria with the secretions of the apocrine glands causes the characteristic body odor.

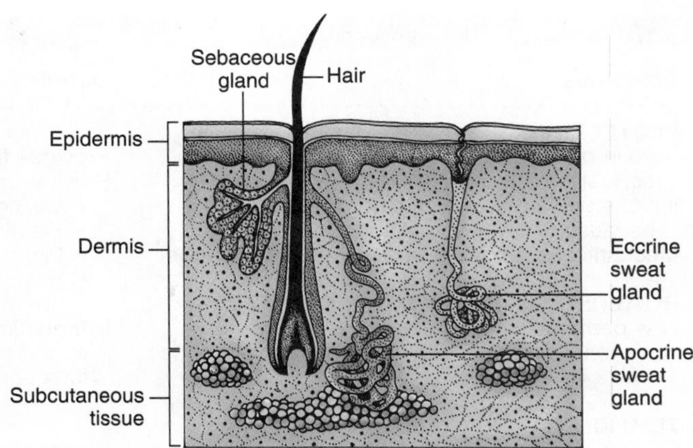

Figure 66-3 ● Anatomy of the hair follicle and sebaceous and sweat glands.

Functions of the Skin

The skin is a complex organ responsible for the regulation of many body functions throughout the life span (Table 66-1). Although the skin has mainly protective and regulatory functions, the dynamic relationship between the skin and the outside world makes it an important way to communicate a client's state of health and body image.

Skin Changes Associated with Aging

The process of aging begins at birth. As changes in physiology progress with aging, the skin undergoes age-related alterations in both structure and function (Chart 66-1). Figures 66-4 through 66-15 show some common age-related skin changes.

There are individual differences in how quickly and to what degree the skin ages. Although genetic background, hormonal changes, and systemic disease may change the appearance of the skin over time, chronic sun exposure is the single most important factor leading to degeneration of the skin components (Figure 66-16).

ASSESSMENT TECHNIQUES

History

Before examining the skin, the nurse obtains an accurate history from the client so that actual and potential skin problems can be readily identified. Chart 66-2 summarizes the best practices for obtaining a history from a client with a skin problem. The nurse begins by gathering information about integumentary changes and current skin care practices.

DEMOGRAPHIC DATA

The nurse obtains demographic data from clients with actual or potential skin disorders. Age is important because many changes in the integumentary system are normal manifestations of the aging process.

TABLE 66-1 • FUNCTIONS OF THE SKIN

Epidermis	Dermis	Subcutaneous Tissue
PROTECTION		
Keratin provides protection from injury by corrosive materials Inhibits proliferation of microorganisms because of dry external surface Mechanical strength through intracellular bonds	Provides fibroblasts for wound healing Provides mechanical strength • Collagen fibers • Elastic fibers • Ground substance	Mechanical shock absorber
HOMEOSTASIS (WATER BALANCE)		
Low permeability to water and electrolytes prevents systemic dehydration and electrolyte loss	Lymphatic and vascular tissues respond to inflammation, injury, and infection	
TEMPERATURE REGULATION		
Eccrine sweat glands allow dissipation of heat through evaporation of sweat secreted onto the skin surface	Cutaneous vasculature, through dilation or constriction, promotes or inhibits heat conduction from the skin surface	Fat cells act as insulators and assist in retention of body heat
SENSORY ORGAN		
Transmits a variety of sensations through the neuroreceptor system	Encloses an extensive network of free and encapsulated nerve endings for relaying sensations to the brain	Contains large pressure receptors
VITAMIN SYNTHESIS		
7-Dehydrocholesterol is present in large concentrations in malpighian cells; photoconversion to vitamin D takes place	No function	No function
PSYCHOSOCIAL		
Body image alterations with many epidermal diseases, such as generalized psoriasis	Body image alterations with many dermal diseases, such as scleroderma	Body image alterations may result from increases, decreases, and redistribution of body fat stores

Race and nationality can also be important. Some variations in skin appearance are normal among clients of specific races and nationalities but are abnormal for clients of other races or nationalities.

Information regarding the client's occupation and hobbies can provide clues to chronic skin exposure to chemicals, irritants, abrasive substances, and other environmental factors that may contribute to skin problems.

PERSONAL AND FAMILY HISTORY

The nurse obtains the client's medical history, including previous or current illnesses and surgical procedures. This information helps to determine whether skin changes are a manifestation of an underlying systemic disorder.

Because a predisposition to many skin diseases can be inherited, the nurse explores any family tendency toward chronic skin problems. An examination of the immediate family's current health status may identify a communicable disease that has been transferred between family members.

MEDICATION HISTORY

Because skin reactions to systemic medications are common, the client is asked about any recent use of prescription and over-the-counter (OTC) preparations (e.g., laxatives, antacids, and cold remedies). Information is obtained regarding when each medication was started, the dose and frequency of the medication, and the time the last dose was taken. A medication history also helps identify skin changes that result from the treatment of other medical problems, such as the changes that occur with long-term steroid or anticoagulant therapy.

DIET HISTORY

The client's weight, height, body build, and food preferences are noted. Poor nutrition, especially protein deficiencies, vitamin deficiencies, and obesity, can predispose a client to skin lesions and delay wound healing. Fat-free diets and chronic alcoholism can lead to vitamin deficiencies and related skin changes. Some skin diseases, such as chronic urticaria and acne, may be worsened by certain foods or food additives.

SOCIOECONOMIC STATUS

The nurse asks the client about his or her social and economic background to identify environmental factors that might contribute to skin disease. Recent travel may be a source of skin infections or unusual lesions.

If the client is well tanned, the nurse asks about the amount of time spent in the sun and tanning booths and whether he or she has experienced any skin problems associated with sun exposure.

Skin problems related to poor hygiene are common. The client is asked about living conditions, bathing practices, and the availability of running water.

CHART 66-1

NURSING FOCUS *on the* OLDER ADULT

Changes in the Integumentary System Related to Aging

Physical Changes	Clinical Findings	Changes in Functional Ability
EPIDERMIS		
Decreased thickness in epidermal layer	Increased skin transparency and fragility	
Decreased epidermal mitotic activity	Delayed wound healing	Decreased cell replacement
Decreased epidermal mitotic homeostasis	Skin hyperplasia, such as hyperkeratoses and skin cancers (especially in sun-exposed areas)	
Increased epidermal permeability	Increased susceptibility to irritant reactions	Decreased barrier function
Decreased number of Langerhans cells	Decreased cutaneous inflammatory response	Decreased injury response
Decreased number of active melanocytes	Increased sensitivity to sun exposure	
Hyperplasia of melanocytes at the dermal-epidermal junction (especially in sun-exposed areas)	Mottled hyperpigmentation and hypopigmentation (e.g., liver spots and age spots)	
Decreased vitamin D production	Increased susceptibility to osteomalacia	Decreased vitamin D production
Flattening of the dermal-epidermal junction	Increased susceptibility to shearing forces, with resultant blisters, purpura, skin tears, and pressure-related skin problems	
DERMIS		
Decreased dermal blood flow	Increased susceptibility to dry skin (xerosis)	Decreased chemical clearance
Decreased vasomotor responsiveness	Increased thermoregulatory alterations (predisposition to heat stroke and hypothermia)	Decreased vascular responsiveness
Decreased dermal thickness	Paper-thin, transparent skin with an increased susceptibility to trauma	Decreased injury response
Degeneration of elastic fibers	Decreased tone and elasticity (wrinkles)	Body image alterations
Benign proliferation of capillaries	Cherry hemangiomas	
Abnormal nerve endings	Alterations in sensory perception	Decreased sensory perception
SUBCUTANEOUS LAYER		
Redistribution of adipose tissue	"Bags," cellulite, double chin, abdominal apron	Body image alterations
Thinning of subcutaneous fat layer	Increased susceptibility to hypothermia Decreased resistance to mechanical injury (especially pressure necrosis)	Decreased thermoregulation Decreased injury response
HAIR		
Decreased number of hair follicles and rate of growth	Increased hair thinning	Decreased cell replacement
Decreased number of active melanocytes in follicle	Gradual loss of hair color (graying)	Body image alterations
NAILS		
Decreased rate of growth	Increased susceptibility to fungal infections	Decreased cell replacement
Decreased blood flow beneath the nail bed	Longitudinal nail ridges	
GLANDS		
Decreased sebum production despite sebaceous gland hyperplasia	Increased size of pores (especially on nose); large comedones in malar region	Decreased sebum production
Decreased eccrine and apocrine gland activity	Increased susceptibility to dry skin Decreased perspiration, leading to decreased cooling effect Decreased need for antiperspirants	Decreased sweat production Decreased thermoregulation

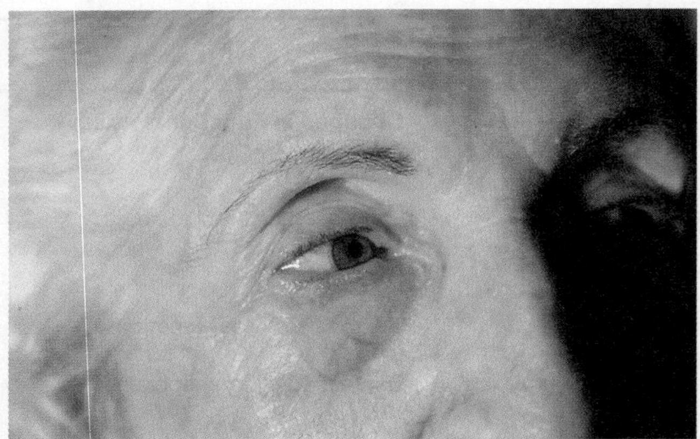

Figure 66-4 ● Eyelid eversion.

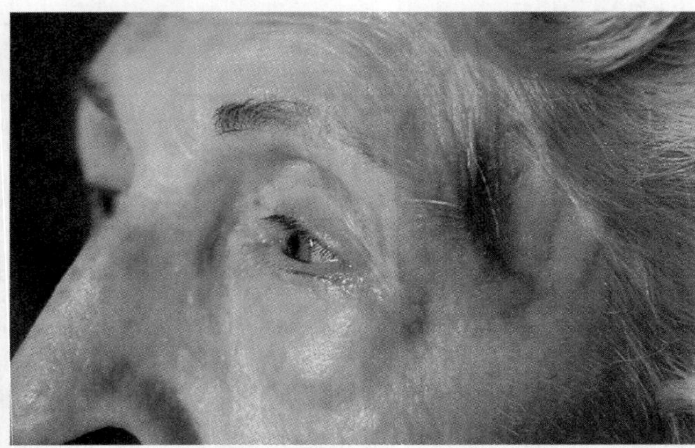

Figure 66-7 ● Changes in the body contour: "bags" under the eyes.

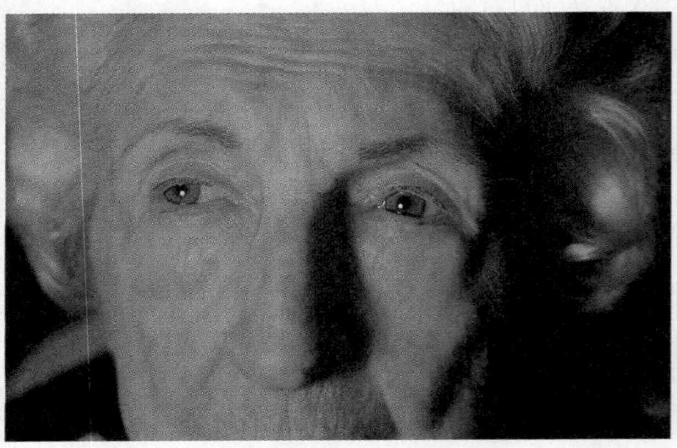

Figure 66-5 ● Deepening of the orbit.

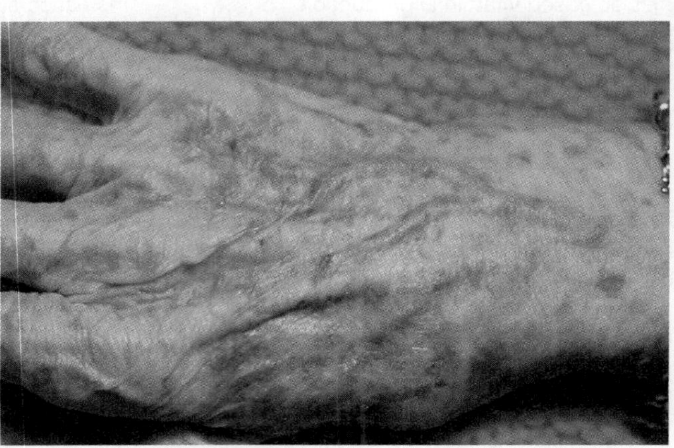

Figure 66-8 ● Paper-thin, transparent skin.

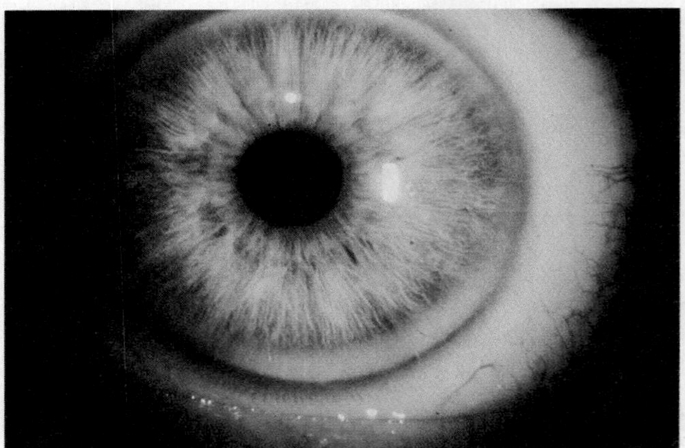

Figure 66-6 ● Arcus senilis of the iris.

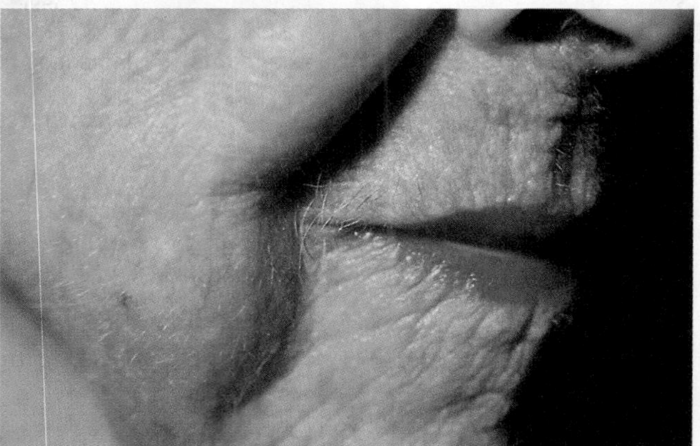

Figure 66-9 ● Wrinkles.

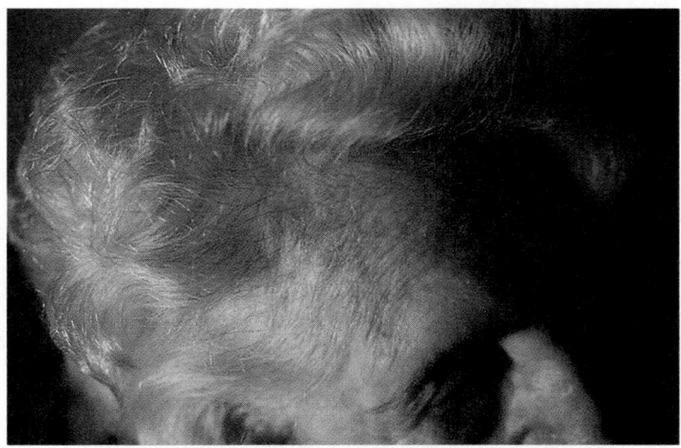

Figure 66-10 ● Graying and thinning of the hair.

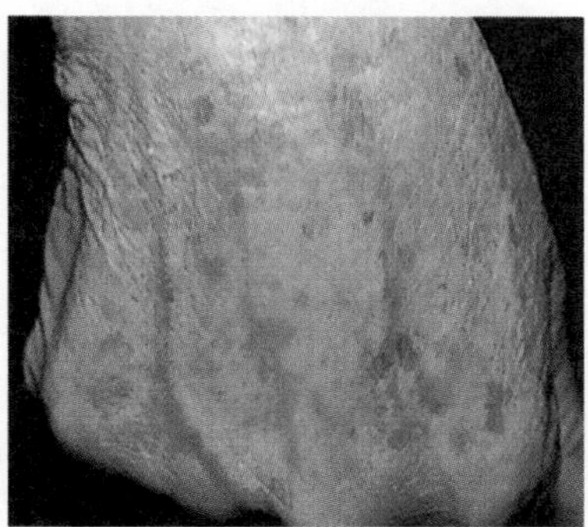

Figure 66-13 ● Actinic lentigo (liver spots).

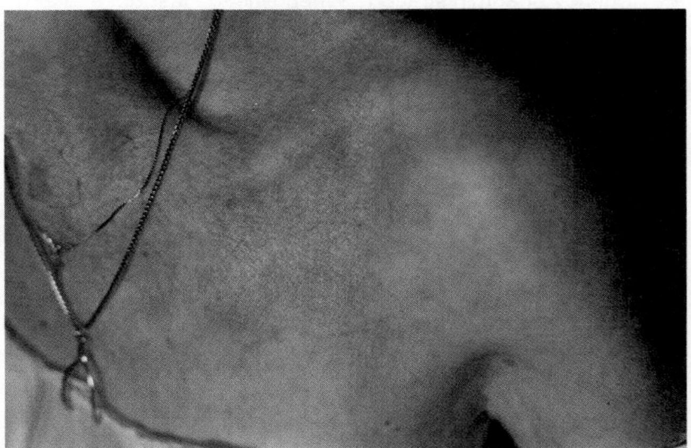

Figure 66-11 ● Xerosis (dry skin).

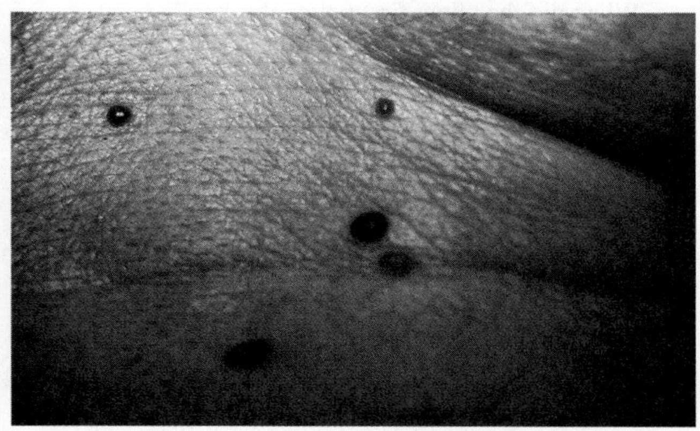

Figure 66-14 ● Senile (cherry) angiomas.

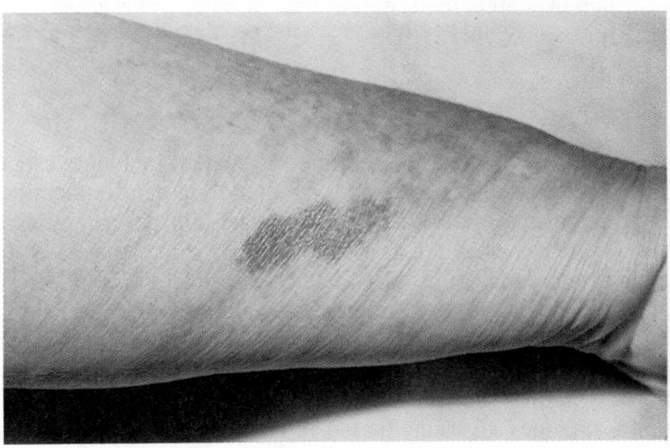

Figure 66-12 ● Actinic purpura.

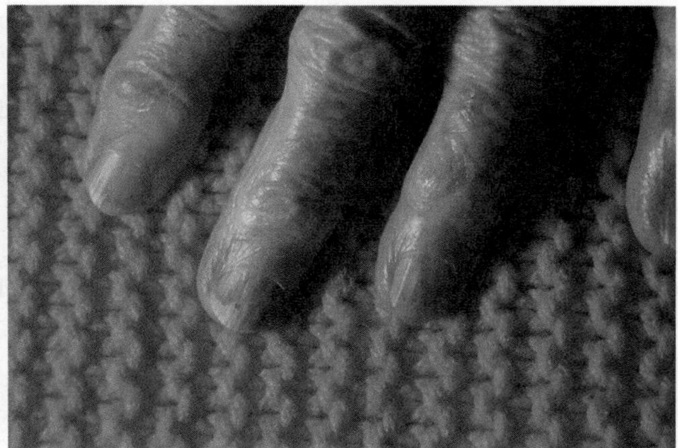

Figure 66-15 ● Nail changes, longitudinal ridges and thickening.

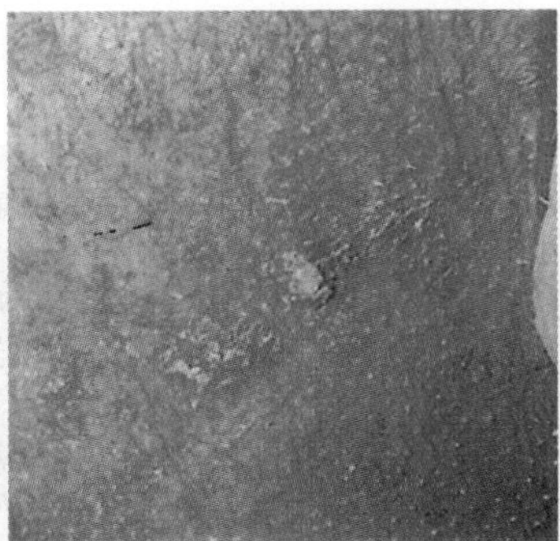

Figure 66-16 ● Actinic (solar) keratosis.

CURRENT HEALTH PROBLEM

If a skin problem is identified, the nurse obtains more information about the specific problem, such as the following:

- When did the client first notice the rash?
- Where on the body did the rash begin?
- Has the problem improved or become worse?

If a similar problem has occurred before, the client is asked to describe the course of the skin lesion and how it was treated. The nurse tries to link the problem with specific symptoms, such as itching, burning, numbness, pain, fever, sore throat, stiff neck, or nausea and vomiting. The client is asked to identify anything that seems to make the problem better or worse.

Physical Assessment

SKIN ASSESSMENT

Inspection

Skin changes may be related to specific skin diseases and may also reflect an underlying systemic disorder. By using skin assessment skills, the nurse is in a unique position to identify obvious and subtle clues about a client's state of wellness.

A thorough assessment of the skin is best accomplished with the client partially or completely disrobed. Skin examination for actual or potential impairments is incorporated as a routine part of daily care while bathing or assisting the client.

The nurse inspects the client's skin surfaces in a well-lighted room; natural or bright fluorescent lighting enhances the visibility of subtle skin changes. Although no special equipment is needed, a penlight is often helpful for close inspection of lesions and for illumination of the oral cavity.

Each skin surface is assessed systematically, including the scalp, hair, nails, and mucous membranes. Particular attention is given to the skin fold areas. The moist, warm environment of skin folds can harbor opportunistic microorganisms, such as yeast or bacteria. The following features are noted and documented:

- Obvious changes in color and vascularity
- The presence or absence of moisture
- Edema
- Skin lesions
- Skin integrity

In addition, the cleanliness of the various body areas may indicate a need for further evaluation of self-care activities.

CHART 66-2

BEST PRACTICE *for* Obtaining an Accurate Nursing History of the Client with a Skin Problem

Medical-Surgical History

- Does the client have any current or previous medical problems?
- Has the client undergone any recent or previous surgical procedures?

Family History

- Is there any family tendency toward chronic skin problems?
- Do any members of the immediate family have recent skin complaints?

Medication History

- Is the client allergic to any systemic or topical medication? If so, have the client describe the reaction.
- What prescription drugs has the client taken recently? When was the drug started? What is the dose or frequency of administration? When was the last dose taken?
- What over-the-counter drugs has the client taken recently? When was the drug started? What is the dose or frequency of administration? When was the last dose taken?

Social History

- What is the client's occupation?
- What recreational activities does the client enjoy?
- Has the client traveled recently?
- What is the client's nutritional status?

Current Health Problem

- When did the client first notice the skin problem?
- Where on the body did the problem begin?
- Has the problem gotten better or worse?
- Has a similar skin condition ever occurred before? If so, have the client describe the typical course and how it was treated.
- Is the problem associated with any of the following: itching, burning, stinging, numbness, pain, fever, nausea and vomiting, diarrhea, sore throat, cold, stiff neck, new foods, new soaps or cosmetics, new clothing or bed linens, or stressful situations?
- Does anything seem to make the problem worse (e.g., sun exposure, medications, heat or cold, and menses)?
- Does anything seem to make the problem better?

COLOR

Skin color is affected by a number of factors, including blood flow, oxygenation, body temperature, and pigment production. In addition to these factors, the wide variability in natural skin tones often makes color assessment difficult, especially in clients with darker skin. (See Cultural Considerations, pp. 1510 and 1511, for suggestions for assessing clients with darker skin.)

Changes in skin color are described by their appearance (Table 66-2). The nurse documents alterations in color and notes whether the distribution is generalized or localized. Color changes are accentuated in the areas of least pigmentation, such as the buccal mucosa, sclera, nail beds, and the palms and soles. Therefore an inspection of these areas may help confirm more subtle color alterations of general body areas.

LESIONS

Skin disease is clinically described in terms of primary and secondary lesions (Figure 66-17). **Primary lesions** represent an initial reaction to an underlying problem that alters one of

TABLE 66-2 • COMMON ALTERATIONS IN SKIN COLOR

Alteration	Underlying Cause	Location	Significance
White (pallor)	Decreased hemoglobin level Decreased blood flow to the skin (vasoconstriction)	Conjunctivae Mucous membranes Nail beds Palms and soles Lips	Anemia Shock or blood loss Chronic vascular compromise Sudden emotional upset Edema
	Genetically determined defect of the melanocyte (decreased pigmentation)	Generalized	Albinism
	Acquired patchy loss of pigmentation	Localized	Vitiligo; tinea versicolor
Yellow-orange	Increased total serum bilirubin level (jaundice)	Generalized Mucous membranes Sclera	Increased hemolysis of red blood cells Liver disorders
	Increased serum carotene level (carotenemia)	Perioral Palms and soles Absent in sclera and mucous membranes	Increased ingestion of carotene-containing foods (carrots) Pregnancy Thyroid deficiency Diabetes
	Increased urochrome level	Generalized Absent in sclera and mucous membranes	Chronic renal failure (uremia)
Red (erythema)	Increased blood flow to the skin (vasodilation)	Generalized	Generalized inflammation (e.g., erythroderma)
		Localized (to area of involvement)	Localized inflammation (e.g., sunburn, cellulitis, trauma, and rashes)
		Face, cheeks, nose, and upper chest	Fever, increased alcohol intake
		Area of exposure	Exposure to cold
Blue	Increase in deoxygenated blood (cyanosis)	Nail beds Mucous membranes Generalized	Cardiopulmonary disease Methemoglobinemia
	Bleeding from vessels into tissue: • Petechiae (1-3 mm) • Ecchymosis (>3 mm)	Localized	Thrombocytopenia Increased blood vessel fragility
Reddish blue	Increased overall amount of hemoglobin	Generalized	Polycythemia vera
	Decreased peripheral circulation	Distal extremities, nose	Inadequate tissue perfusion
Brown	Increased melanin production	Localized (to area of involvement) Pressure points, areolae, palmar creases, and genitalia Face, areolae, vulva, and linea nigra	Chronic inflammation Exposure to sunlight Addison's disease Pregnancy; oral contraceptives (melasma)
	Café au lait spots (tan-brown patches)		
	• <6 spots	Localized	Nonpathogenic
	• >6 spots	Generalized	Neurofibromatosis
	Melanin and hemosiderin deposits (bronze or grayish tan color)	Distal lower extremities Exposed areas or generalized	Chronic venous stasis Hemochromatosis

the structural components of the skin. **Secondary lesions** are changes in the appearance of the primary lesion. These changes occur with normal progression of the underlying disease or in response to therapeutic intervention in the form of a topical or systemic treatment.

For example, acute dermatitis often occurs as primary vesicles with associated **pruritus** (itching). Secondary lesions in the form of crusts occur as the client scratches, the vesicles are opened, and the exudate dries. With chronic dermatitis, the skin often becomes **lichenified** (thickened) because of the client's continual rubbing of the epidermis to relieve itching.

Lesions are described in terms of their color, size, location, and configuration. The nurse notes whether the lesions occur as isolated changes or are grouped to form a distinct pattern. Table 66-3 defines terms commonly used to describe lesions.

The nurse assesses each lesion for the following ABCD characteristics associated with skin cancer:

A Asymmetry of shape
B Border irregularity
C Color variation within one lesion
D Diameter greater than 5 mm

A dermatologist or surgeon evaluates any lesion with one or more of the ABCD characteristics.

In describing the location of lesions, the nurse notes whether they are generalized or localized. If the lesions are localized, the specific body regions involved are identified. This information is important because some diseases are associated with a specific pattern of skin lesions. Involvement of only the sun-exposed areas of the body is important information when a possible cause is being considered. Rashes limited to the skin fold areas (e.g., on the axillae, beneath the

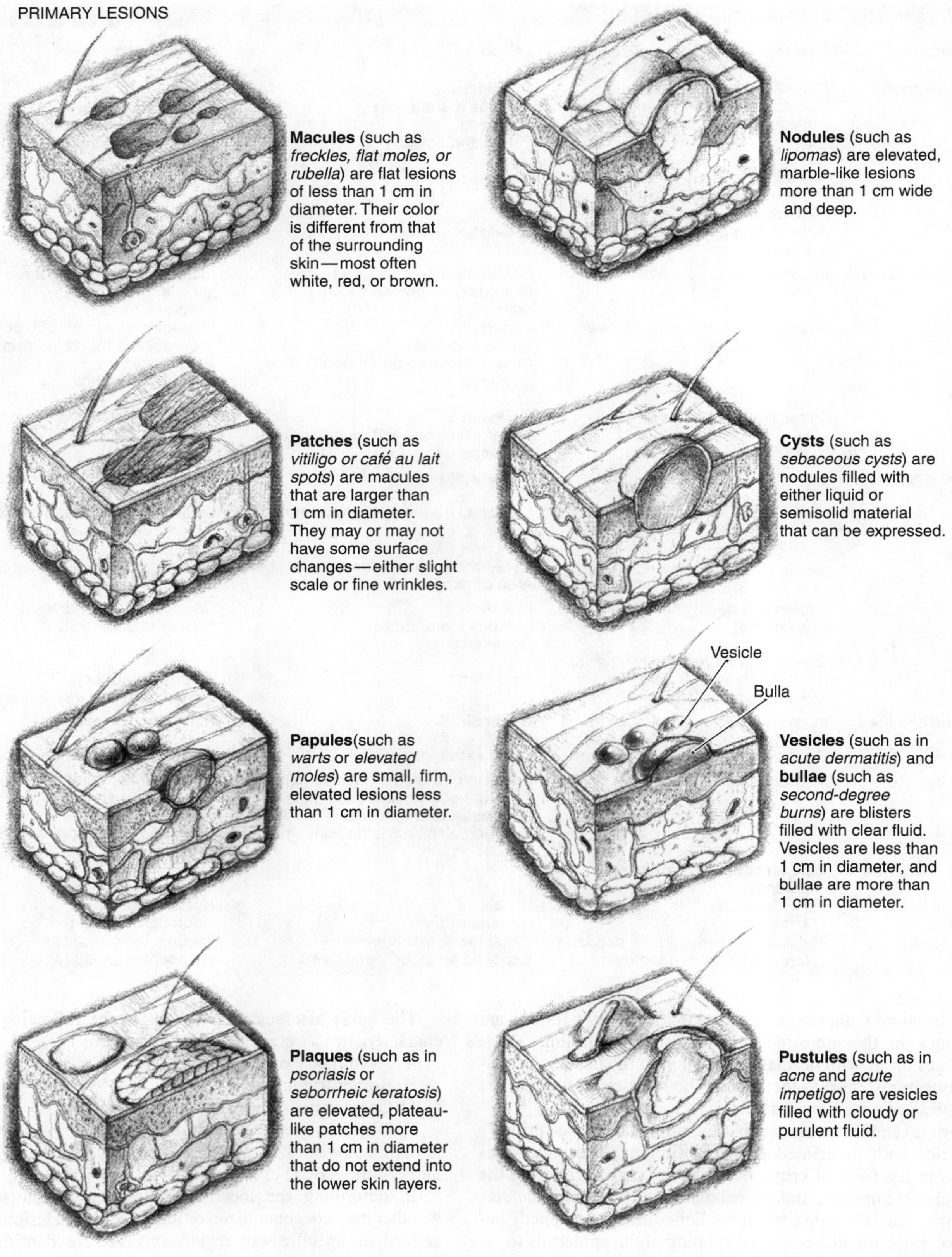

PRIMARY LESIONS

Macules (such as *freckles, flat moles, or rubella*) are flat lesions of less than 1 cm in diameter. Their color is different from that of the surrounding skin—most often white, red, or brown.

Patches (such as *vitiligo or café au lait spots*) are macules that are larger than 1 cm in diameter. They may or may not have some surface changes—either slight scale or fine wrinkles.

Papules(such as *warts* or *elevated moles*) are small, firm, elevated lesions less than 1 cm in diameter.

Plaques (such as in *psoriasis* or *seborrheic keratosis*) are elevated, plateau-like patches more than 1 cm in diameter that do not extend into the lower skin layers.

Nodules (such as *lipomas*) are elevated, marble-like lesions more than 1 cm wide and deep.

Cysts (such as *sebaceous cysts*) are nodules filled with either liquid or semisolid material that can be expressed.

Vesicle

Bulla

Vesicles (such as in *acute dermatitis*) and **bullae** (such as *second-degree burns*) are blisters filled with clear fluid. Vesicles are less than 1 cm in diameter, and bullae are more than 1 cm in diameter.

Pustules (such as in *acne* and *acute impetigo*) are vesicles filled with cloudy or purulent fluid.

Figure 66-17 ● Classification of skin lesions.

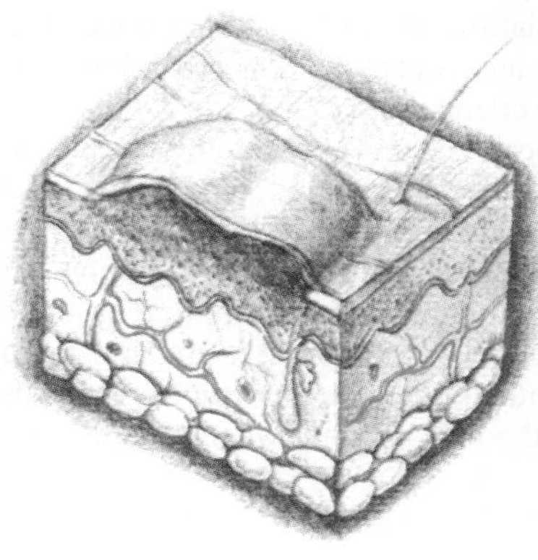

Wheals (such as *urticaria* and *insect bites*) are elevated, irregularly shaped, transient areas of dermal edema.

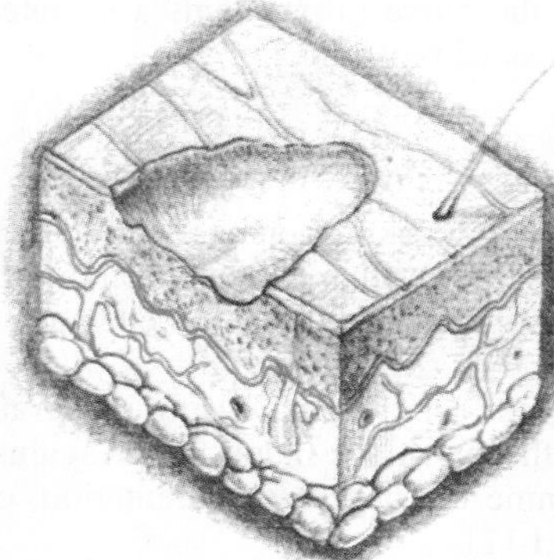

Erosions (such as in *varicella*) are wider than fissures but involve only the epidermis. They are often associated with vesicles, bullae, or pustules.

SECONDARY LESIONS

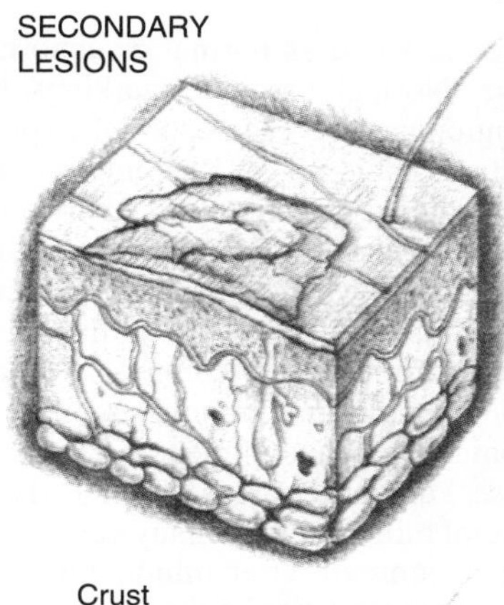

Scales (such as in *exfoliative dermatitis* and *psoriasis*) are visibly thickened stratum corneum. They appear dry and are usually whitish. They are seen most often with papules and plaques.

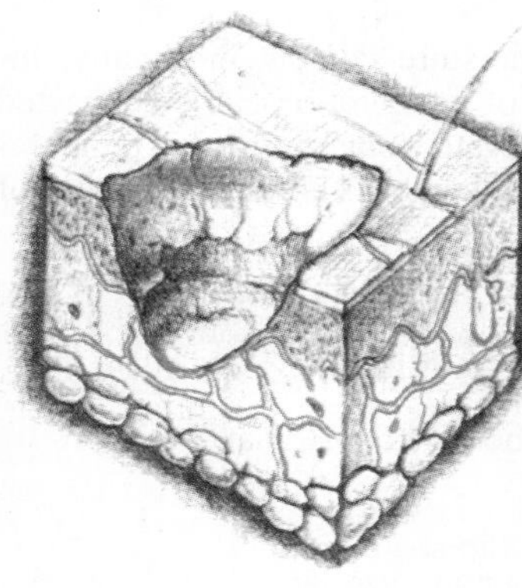

Ulcers (such as *stage 3 pressure sores*) are deep erosions that extend beneath the epidermis and involve the dermis and sometimes the subcutaneous fat.

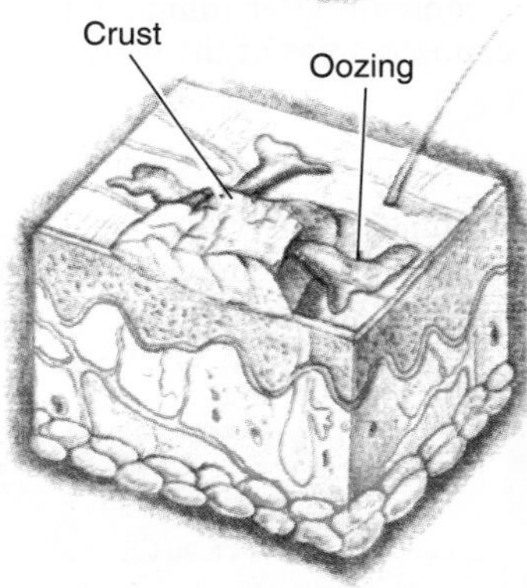

Crusts and oozing (such as in *eczema* and *late-stage impetigo*) are composed of dried serum or pus on the surface of the skin, beneath which liquid debris may accumulate. Crusts frequently result from broken vesicles, bullae, or pustules.

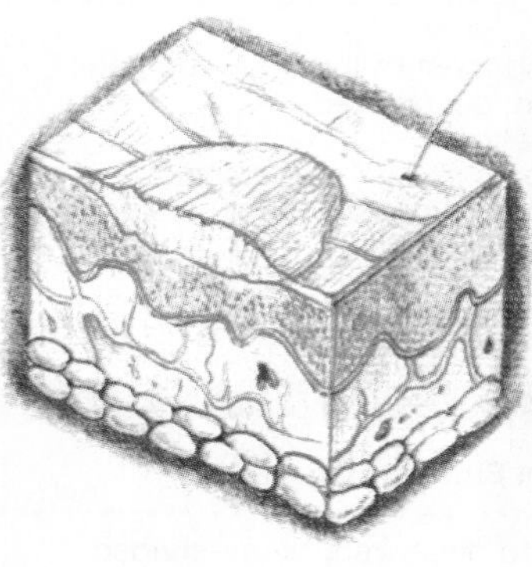

Lichenifications (such as in *chronic dermatitis*) are palpably thickened areas of epidermis with accentuated skin markings. They are caused by chronic rubbing and scratching.

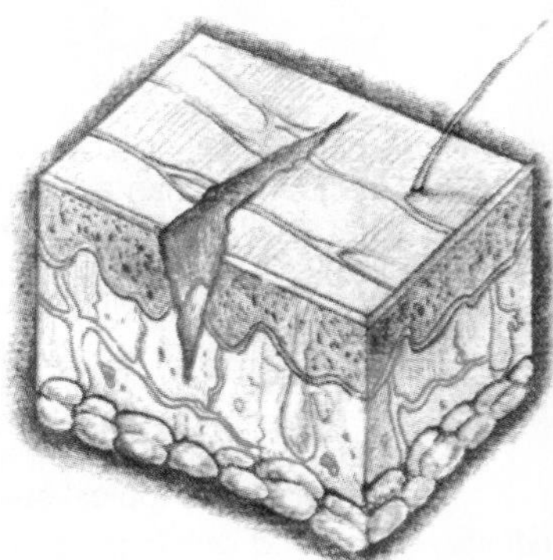

Fissures (such as in *athlete's foot*) are linear cracks in the epidermis, which often extend into the dermis.

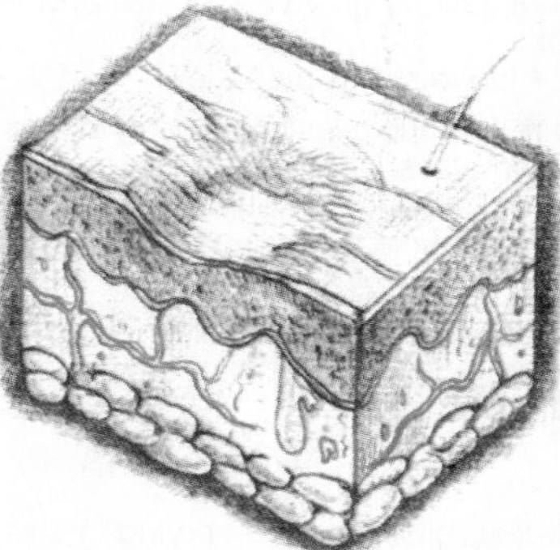

Atrophy (such as *striae* [stretch marks] and *aged skin*) is characterized by thinning of the skin surface with loss of skin markings. The skin is translucent and paper-like. Atrophy involving the dermal layer results in skin depression.

Figure 66-17, cont'd ● Classification of skin lesions.

breasts, in the groin) alert the nurse to problems associated with friction, heat, and excessive moisture.

EDEMA

The presence of edema causes the skin to appear shiny, taut, and paler than uninvolved skin. During skin inspection, the location, distribution, and color of any areas of edema are documented.

Skin elasticity is also affected by edema. Using moderate pressure, the nurse places the tip of the index finger against edematous tissue to determine the degree of indentation, or pitting (see Chapters 11 and 12).

MOISTURE

The skin is examined for moisture content. Normally, increased moisture in the form of perspiration can be expected with increased activity or elevated environmental temperatures. Dampness of the skin fold areas is common because of decreased air circulation where the skin surfaces touch. Excess moisture can cause eventual skin breakdown in bedridden and debilitated clients.

Overly dry skin can be caused by factors such as a dry environment, improper skin lubrication, inadequate fluid intake, and the normal processes of aging. Dry skin usually has scaling of the stratum corneum. Dry skin may be especially marked in areas of limited circulation, such as the feet and lower legs. Dry skin becomes a problem for most adults during the winter months, when the air contains less moisture, and in the hospital environment, where humidity is often poorly controlled.

TABLE 66-3 • TERMS COMMONLY USED TO DESCRIBE SKIN LESION CONFIGURATIONS

annular Ringlike with raised borders around flat, clear centers of normal skin
circinate Circular
circumscribed Well defined with sharp borders
clustered Several lesions grouped together
coalesced Lesions that merge with one another and appear confluent
diffuse Widespread, involving most of the body with intervening areas of normal skin; generalized
linear Occurring in a straight line
serpiginous With wavy borders, resembling a snake
universal All areas of the body involved, with no areas of normal-appearing skin

VASCULAR MARKINGS

Vascular changes are classified as normal or abnormal depending on the cause. Normal vascular markings include birthmarks, cherry angiomas (see Figure 66-14), spider angiomas, and venous stars (Table 66-4). Bleeding into the tissue results in purpuric lesions: petechiae and ecchymosis.

Petechiae are small vascular lesions (<0.5 mm in diameter) that do not fade or blanch when pressure is applied (Figure 66-18). They often indicate increased capillary fragility. Petechiae of the lower extremities are commonly associated with stasis dermatitis, a condition commonly seen in clients with a history of chronic venous insufficiency.

Ecchymoses (bruises) are larger areas of hemorrhage that range in size from several millimeters to many centimeters. In older adults, bruising is common after minor trauma to the skin, especially on sun-exposed areas of the body.

INTEGRITY

The nurse thoroughly examines areas with actual breaks in skin integrity. For example, skin tears are a common finding in older people as a result of a flattening of the dermal-

TABLE 66-4 • COMMON VASCULAR SKIN LESIONS

Lesion	Clinical Findings	Location	Significance
Cherry angioma (senile angioma)	Bright to dusky red, dome-shaped papule 2-5 mm in diameter Adjacent lesions may vary in size and color Partial blanching on palpation	Chest and back	Normal skin change with aging
Spider angioma	Bright red, starlike lesion varying in size from small to 2 cm Center of "star" is sometimes raised and may pulsate when palpated	Face, neck, and upper trunk	Associated with liver disease, pregnancy (change in estrogen level), and vitamin B deficiency May be normal finding
Telangiectasia	Reddish blue linear or star-like lesion caused by enlargement of the superficial blood vessels	Face and trunk	Associated with sun exposure and prolonged alcohol intake May be seen in systemic scleroderma and after continued use of potent topical steroids
Venous star	Spider-like, blue marking varying in size from small to several inches May have a "cascading" appearance Does not blanch with pressure	Legs (near veins) and anterior chest Face, scalp, and groin	Associated with increased pressure in superficial veins (varicose veins)
Port-wine stain	Large, dark red to purple area of discoloration Does not blanch with pressure		Congenital abnormality If on the face, may be associated with neurologic disorders and ocular abnormalities

epidermal junction with aging. The thin, fragile skin is easily disrupted by friction or shearing forces, especially if areas of ecchymosis are already present. The nurse looks for skin tears in the following areas:

- In areas where constricting clothing rubs against the skin surface
- On the upper extremities, where the skin is grasped when assisting a client to ambulate
- In areas where adhesive tapes or dressings have been applied and removed

The nurse remains alert to the presence of multiple abrasions or early pressure-related skin changes. These may signal previously unrecognized impairments in physical mobility or alterations in sensory perception.

Breaks in skin integrity are described by their location, size, color, and distribution, as well as by the presence of drainage or any signs of infection. The evaluation of partial-thickness and full-thickness wounds, including objective criteria that describe progress toward healing, is discussed in Chapter 68.

CLEANLINESS

The nurse evaluates the cleanliness of the skin to gain information about self-care needs. The hair, nails, and skin are inspected closely for excessive soiling and offensive odor. Depending on a client's degree of self-care deficit, hard-to-reach areas (e.g., perirectal and inguinal skin folds, axillae, feet) may be less clean than other skin surface areas.

Palpation

Because skin inspection alone can be misleading, palpation is performed to gather additional information about skin lesions, moisture, temperature, texture, and turgor (Table 66-5).

Palpation confirms the size of the lesions and determines whether they are flat or slightly raised. The consistency of larger lesions can vary from soft and pliable to firm and solid. With eyes closed, the nurse can detect more subtle changes, such as the difference between a fine **macular** (flat) rash and a **papular** (raised) rash. The client is asked whether he or she experiences pain or tenderness during palpation of the skin.

The nurse touches areas of excess moisture to determine the thickness and consistency of secretions. In areas of excess dryness, a finger is rubbed against the skin surface to determine the degree of flaking or scaling.

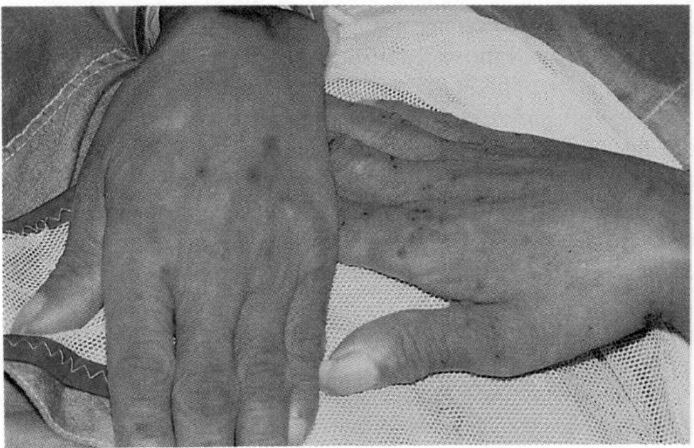

Figure 66-18 ● Petechiae.

Both generalized and localized changes in skin temperature can be detected by placing the back of a hand on the skin surface. Before assessing for changes in skin temperature, the nurse makes certain to have warm hands. Cold hands interfere with accurate assessment and are uncomfortable for the client.

The skin surfaces are palpated to assess texture, which differs according to body region and exposure to environmental irritants. For example, areas of long-term sun exposure have a rougher texture than that of protected skin surfaces. The client whose occupation requires repeated exposure to harsh soaps or chemicals may show skin changes related to this exposure. Increased skin thickness from scarring, lichenification, or edema usually decreases elasticity.

Turgor indicates the amount of skin elasticity. The turgor of the skin can be altered by a number of factors, including water content and age. The skin is gently pinched between the thumb and forefinger and released. If skin turgor is normal, the skin immediately returns to its original state when released. Poor skin turgor is evidenced by "tenting" of the skin, with a gradual return to the original state (see Chapter 11). A normal loss of elasticity with aging makes the assessment of skin turgor difficult in an older client. If the client is in a supine position, the forehead or chest tissue gives the best indication of skin hydration.

HAIR ASSESSMENT

During the skin assessment, the hair is inspected and palpated for cleanliness, distribution, quantity, and quality. Hair is normally found in an even distribution over most of the body surfaces, with the hair on the scalp, in the pubic region, and in the axillary folds thicker and coarser than hair on the trunk and extremities. Although color and growth patterns vary widely, sudden or marked changes in hair characteristics may reflect an underlying disease process. As with skin changes, the nurse investigates any abnormal findings by obtaining an in-depth history of the circumstances surrounding any change.

How well the hair is groomed, including the cleanliness of areas of thicker hair growth, can confirm information already gathered about a client's social history and health care needs. If the client has intense itching or scratches continually, the scalp and pubis are examined for lice and **nits** (lice eggs). The scalp is inspected for excessive scaling, redness, lesions, excoriation, crusting, and tenderness.

Dandruff, an accumulation of patchy or diffuse white or gray scales that appear on the surface of the scalp, is common. Dandruff is mainly a cosmetic problem, but an excessively oily scalp can result in inflammatory changes with erythema and pruritus. Severe inflammatory dandruff can extend to involve the eyebrows and the skin of the face and neck. *If severe dandruff is not treated, hair loss can occur.*

Although gradual hair loss is associated with aging, sudden asymmetric or patchy hair loss at any age is of concern. The nurse assesses the scalp for distribution and thickness of the hair and notes variations.

Hirsutism is excessive body hair growth or hair growth in abnormal body areas. Increased hair growth across the face and anterior chest in women is a sign of hirsutism. Hirsutism is one manifestation of hormonal imbalance. If hirsutism is apparent, the nurse looks for changes in fat distribution and

TABLE 66-5 • COMMON CLINICAL FINDINGS IN SKIN PALPATION

Clinical Findings	Cause	Location	Examples of Predisposing Conditions
EDEMA			
Localized	Inflammatory response	Area of injury or involvement	Trauma
Dependent or pitting	Fluid and electrolyte imbalance Venous and cardiac insufficiency	Ambulatory: dorsum of foot and medial ankle Bedridden: buttocks, sacrum, and lower back	Congestive heart failure Renal disease Hepatic cirrhosis Venous thrombosis or stasis
Nonpitting	Endocrine imbalance	Generalized, but more easily seen over the tibia	Hypothyroidism (myxedema)
MOISTURE			
Increased	Autonomic nervous system stimulation	Face, axillae, skin folds, palms, and soles	Fever, anxiety, activity Hyperthyroidism
Decreased	Dehydration Endocrine imbalance	Buccal mucous membranes with progressive involvement of other skin surfaces	Fluid loss Postmenopausal status Hypothyroidism Normal aging
TEMPERATURE			
Increased	Increased blood flow to the skin	Generalized Localized	Fever, hypermetabolic states Inflammation
Decreased	Decreased blood flow to the skin	Generalized Localized	Impending shock, sepsis, anxiety Hypothyroidism Interference with vascular flow
TURGOR			
Decreased	Decreased elasticity of the dermis (tenting when pinched)	Abdomen, forehead, or radial aspect of the wrist	Severe dehydration Sudden, severe weight loss Normal aging
TEXTURE			
Roughness or thickness	Irritation, friction	Pressure points (e.g., soles, palms, and elbows)	Calluses Chronic eczema Atopic skin diseases
	Sun damage	Areas of sun exposure	Normal aging
	Excessive collagen production	Localized or generalized	Scleroderma Keloids
Softness or smoothness	Endocrine disturbances	Generalized	Hyperthyroidism

capillary fragility, which can occur in Cushing's disease; and for clitoral enlargement and deepening of the voice, which may indicate ovarian dysfunction.

NAIL ASSESSMENT

Dystrophic (abnormal) nails often reflect a serious systemic illness or local skin disease involving the epidermal keratinocytes. The fingernails and toenails are evaluated for color, shape, thickness, texture, and the presence of lesions.

Many variations in color, texture, and grooming of the nails are influenced by factors unrelated to disease, such as occupation. When assessing the older adult, the nurse notes minor variations associated with the aging process (see Figure 66-15), such as a gradual thickening of the nail plate, the presence of longitudinal ridges, or a yellowish-gray discoloration.

COLOR

The color of the nail plate depends on many factors, including thickness and transparency of the nail, blood composition, adequacy of arterial blood flow, and pigment deposits (Table 66-6). Figure 66-19 shows normal variations in nail color. Changes in color can be attributed to external factors, such as the chemical damage encountered in some occupations and in the long-term use of nail polish.

During examination, the client's fingers and toes should be free of any surface pressure that might interfere with local blood flow or alter the appearance of the digits. To differentiate between color changes attributable to the underlying vascular supply and those resulting from pigment deposition, the nail bed is blanched to see whether a significant color change occurs with pressure. This technique involves gently squeezing the end of the finger or toe, exerting downward pressure on the nail bed, and then releasing the pressure. Color caused by vascular alterations changes as pressure is applied and returns to the original state when pressure is released. Color caused by pigment deposition remains unchanged.

SHAPE

Nail shape may indicate early or late changes consistent with systemic disease. For example, fingernail clubbing is diagnostic for impaired gas exchange.

TABLE 66-6 • COMMON ALTERATIONS IN NAIL COLOR

Alteration	Clinical Findings	Significance
White	Horizontal white banding or areas of opacity Generalized pallor of nail beds	Chronic hepatic or renal disease (hypoalbuminemia) Shock Anemia Early arteriosclerotic changes (toenails) Myocardial infarction
Yellow-brown	Diffuse yellow to brown discoloration	Jaundice Peripheral lymphedema Bacterial or fungal infections of the nail Psoriasis Diabetes Cardiac failure Staining from tobacco, nail polish, or dyes Long-term tetracycline therapy Normal aging (yellow-gray color)
	Vertical brown banding extending from the proximal nail fold distally	Normal finding in African-American clients Nevus or melanoma of nail matrix in Caucasian clients
Red	Thin, dark red vertical lines 1-3 mm in length (splinter hemorrhages)	Bacterial endocarditis Trichinosis Trauma to the nail bed Normal finding in some clients
	Red discoloration of the lunula	Cardiac insufficiency
	Dark red nail beds	Polycythemia vera
Blue	Diffuse blue discoloration that blanches with pressure	Respiratory failure Methemoglobinuria Venous stasis disease (toenails)

The nail shape is evaluated by examining the curve of the nail plate and surrounding soft tissue from all angles. The fingertips are palpated to define areas of sponginess, tenderness, or marked edema. Table 66-7 describes common variations in nail shape.

THICKNESS

The nail plate can thicken as a result of trauma, chronic dermatologic disease, or decreased arterial blood flow. In older clients, the nurse looks for a "heaped-up" appearance of the toenails, which is commonly associated with fungal infection **(onychomycosis).**

CONSISTENCY

Nail consistency is described as hard, soft, or brittle. Nail plates may become hard, with increased thickening. A warm-water soak or lubrication with petroleum jelly is required to soften the nail plates before they can be trimmed.

Soft nail plates, which are thin and bend easily with pressure, have been associated with malnutrition, chronic arthritis, myxedema, and peripheral neuritis.

Brittle nails can split, as in the client with onychomycosis or advanced psoriasis. Splitting of the nail plate is also caused by repeated exposure to water and detergents, which damage the plate over time.

LESIONS

Separation of the nail plate from the nail bed **(onycholysis)** creates an air pocket beneath the nail plate. The pocket first appears as a grayish white opacity. The color may change as

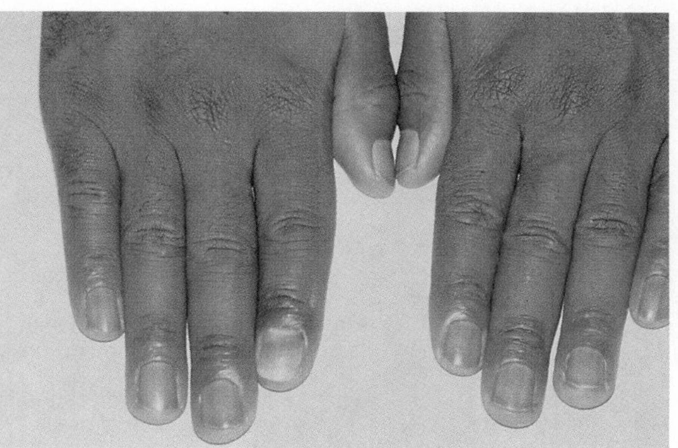

A

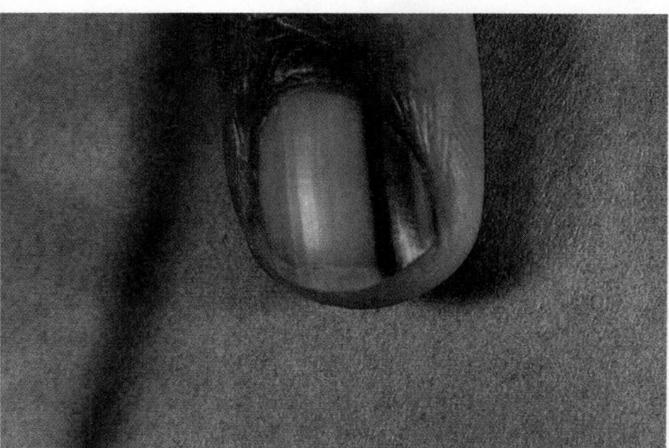

B

Figure 66-19 • **A,** Diffuse nail pigmentation. **B,** Linear nail pigmentation.

TABLE 66-7 • COMMON VARIATIONS IN NAIL SHAPE

Nail Shape	Clinical Findings	Significance
Normal	Angle of 160 degrees between the nail plate and the proximal nail fold • Nail surface slightly convex • Nail base firm when palpated	Normal finding
Clubbing		
Early clubbing	Straightening of angle between the nail plate and the proximal nail fold to 180 degrees • Nail base spongy when palpated	Hypoxia Lung cancer
Late clubbing	Angle between the nail plate and the proximal nail fold exceeds 180 degrees • Nail base visibly edematous and spongy when palpated • Enlargement of the soft tissue of the fingertips gives a "drumstick" appearance when viewed from above	Prolonged hypoxia Advanced lung cancer
Spoon nails (koilonychia)		
Early koilonychia	Flattening of the nail plate with an increased smoothness of the nail surface	Iron deficiency (with or without anemia) Poorly controlled diabetes >15 yr in duration
Late koilonychia	Concave curvature of the nail plate	Local injury Psoriasis Chemical irritants Developmental abnormality
Beau's grooves	1-mm wide horizontal depressions in the nail plates caused by growth arrest (involves all nails)	Acute, severe illness Prolonged febrile state Isolated periods of severe malnutrition
Pitting	Small, multiple pits in the nail plate • May be associated with plate thickening and onycholysis • Most often involves the fingernails (several or all)	Psoriasis Alopecia areata

dirt and keratin collect in the pocket, and the area begins to have a bad odor. Onycholysis is common with fungal infections and after trauma. Separation of the nail plate may also occur with psoriasis or as a result of prolonged contact with chemicals.

The nurse inspects the soft-tissue folds around the nail plate for localized redness, heat, swelling, and tenderness. Inflammation of the skin around the nail **(acute paronychia)** is usually associated with a torn cuticle or an ingrown toenail. If acute paronychia occurs in an immunocompromised client, an opportunistic infection caused by the *Staphylococcus* organism is probable.

Chronic paronychia is more common and is characterized by inflammation that persists for months. People at risk for chronic paronychia are men and women with frequent exposure to water, such as homemakers, bartenders, and laundry workers.

CULTURAL CONSIDERATIONS

Pallor, erythema, cyanosis, and other color changes reflective of the physical state are more difficult to recognize in clients with naturally dark skin tones. Although physiologic processes are the same for both light-skinned and dark-skinned clients, the amount of skin pigmentation greatly alters how the skin appears in response to physiologic alterations. Consequently, the nurse develops assessment skills to detect the more subtle color changes. He or she becomes familiar with the normal appearance of a dark-skinned client's mucous membranes, nail beds, and skin tone so that variations from normal can be identified.

Assessment of Pallor in Dark-Skinned Clients

To detect generalized pallor, the nurse inspects the mucous membranes for an ash gray color. If the lips and the nail beds are not heavily pigmented, they appear paler than normal for that client. The skin is examined under appropriate lighting for the absence of the underlying red tones that normally give heavily pigmented skin a healthy glow. With generalized decreased blood flow to the skin, brown skin appears yellow-brown, and very dark brown skin is ash gray.

Assessment of Cyanosis in Dark-Skinned Clients

Cyanosis is even more difficult to detect in a client with dark skin. If impaired gas exchange is suspected, the nurse examines the lips, tongue, nail beds, conjunctivae, and palms and soles at regular intervals for subtle color changes. In a client with cyanosis, the lips and tongue are gray, and the palms, soles, conjunctivae, and nail beds have a bluish tinge. To support these observations, the nurse assesses for the more obvious manifestations of hypoxia, including tachycardia, hypotension, changes in respiratory rate or rhythm, decreased breath sounds, changes in level of consciousness, and any increase in the amount or viscosity of secretions.

Assessment of Inflammation in Dark-Skinned Clients

If areas of acute inflammation are suspected, the back of the examiner's hand is used to palpate for the increased warmth that occurs when blood flow to the skin increases. With the fingertips, the nurse palpates for hardened areas deep in the tissue, which may give the skin a "woody" feeling. Inflamed skin is tender and edematous. If edema is extensive, the skin is taut and shiny.

Areas of the body where inflammation (e.g., inflammatory rash or cellulitis) has recently resolved appear darker than the normal skin tone. This is due to stimulation of the melanocytes during the inflammatory process and to the increased pigment production that continues after inflammation subsides. More extensive injury to the skin with destruction of melanocytes (e.g., deep ulcer, full-thickness burn) may heal with color changes that are lighter than the normal skin tone. Unlike acute changes, chronic inflammatory changes seldom produce tenderness on palpation. If scar tissue is present, the skin may feel less supple, especially over the joints. If chronic inflammatory changes are suspected, the nurse asks the client about a history of skin problems in that area of the body.

Assessment of Jaundice in Dark-Skinned Clients

Jaundice in a client with dark skin is best assessed by inspecting the oral mucosa, especially the hard palate, for yellow discoloration. Inspection of the conjunctivae and adjacent sclera may be misleading, because normal deposits of subconjunctival fat produce a yellowish hue that is visible in contrast to the dark periorbital skin. Therefore the nurse examines the sclera closest to the cornea for a more accurate determination of jaundice. The palms and soles of dark-skinned clients may appear yellow if they are callused; a callus should not be mistaken for jaundice.

Assessment of Skin Bleeding in Dark-Skinned Clients

Purpuric lesions may be difficult to detect depending on the degree of skin pigmentation. Areas of ecchymosis appear darker than normal skin; they may be tender and easily palpable, depending on whether hematoma is present. In most cases, the client relates a history of trauma to the area that confirms the assessment. Petechiae are rarely visible in dark skin and may be seen only in the oral mucosa and conjunctiva.

Psychosocial Assessment

Actual impairments in skin integrity are commonly associated with altered perceptions in body image, especially when more visible skin surfaces (e.g., face, hair, hands) are involved. The nurse assesses the client's body language for clues indicating a disturbance in self-concept. For example, the avoidance of eye contact or the use of garments to cover the affected areas communicates concern about physical appearance. Clients with chronic skin diseases often relate a history of social isolation that is attributable to a fear of rejection by others or a belief that the skin problem is contagious.

Skin changes linked to poor hygiene are common in clients from low socioeconomic backgrounds. The nurse assesses the client's overall appearance for excessive soiling, matted hair, body odor, or other self-care deficits. The nurse confirms unsanitary living conditions by obtaining a social history. Clients may relate similar skin problems among family members, friends, and sexual contacts.

If skin problems related to poor hygiene are identified in older clients, the nurse also evaluates any physical limitations that may be contributing to poor health maintenance. For example, visual problems or limited mobility can make it difficult for clients to see or reach skin surfaces to clean them.

> **CRITICAL THINKING CHALLENGE**
>
> The client is a 75-year-old Caucasian woman who shows you an area on the left side of her chest—over her ribs and under the arm—that has numerous small red lesions. The lesions are macular and do not blanche with pressure.
>
> - What additional physical assessment techniques should you use?
> - What specific questions should you ask this client?

For suggested answer guidelines, go to SIMON http://www.wbsaunders.com/SIMON/Iggy/.

Diagnostic Assessment

LABORATORY TESTS

When a fungal, bacterial, or viral pathogen is suspected as the cause of certain skin changes, confirmation by microscopic examination is necessary.

Cultures for Fungal Infections

When superficial fungal **(dermatophyte)** infections are suspected, scales are gently scraped from the skin lesions into a Petri dish or a similar clean container and taken to the laboratory for culture. Fingernail clippings and hair are collected in a similar manner. Unfortunately, waiting for culture results can delay treatment of a superficial fungal infection. For this reason, the specimen is also treated with a potassium hydroxide (KOH) preparation and examined microscopically. Fungal infections show branched hyphae when viewed under a microscope after treatment with KOH. A positive KOH test often eliminates the need for a culture.

For deeper fungal infections, a piece of tissue is obtained for culture. The physician obtains the specimen by punch biopsy (see Skin Biopsy, below). The biopsy specimen may be sent for cell analysis and special fungal stains; the tissue specimen is bisected, or two separate biopsy specimens are obtained.

Cultures for Bacterial Infections

Specimens for bacterial culture are obtained from intact primary lesions (bullae, vesicles, or pustules), if possible. Material is expressed from the lesion, collected with a cotton-tipped applicator, and placed in a bacterial culture medium. For intact lesions, **unroofing** (lifting or puncturing of the outer surface) may be required with a sterile small-gauge needle before the material can be easily expressed. If secondary lesions in the form of crusts are present, the nurse removes the crusts and swabs the underlying exudate.

A biopsy of deep bacterial infections may be required to obtain a specimen for culture. If bacterial cellulitis is suspected, nonbacteriostatic saline can be injected deep into the tissue and aspirated; the aspirant is sent for culture.

Cultures for Viral Infections

Viral cultures are indicated if a herpes virus infection is suspected. The physician uses a cotton-tipped applicator to obtain vesicle fluid from intact lesions. Unlike bacterial and fungal specimens, which can remain at room temperature until being transported to the laboratory, viral culture tubes are placed on ice immediately after the specimen is obtained and are transported to the laboratory as soon as possible.

OTHER DIAGNOSTIC TESTS

Skin Biopsy

To establish an accurate diagnosis or assess the effectiveness of an intervention, the physician must often obtain a small piece of skin tissue for histopathologic study. Before preparing the client, the nurse checks with the physician to determine the number, location, and type of skin biopsies to be performed.

TYPES OF BIOPSIES. Depending on the size, depth, and location of the skin changes, the physician may perform a punch biopsy, shave biopsy, or scalpel excision (excisional biopsy).

PUNCH BIOPSY. The punch biopsy is the most basic technique. A small circular cutting instrument, or punch, ranges in diameter from 2 to 6 mm. After the site is injected with a local anesthetic, a small plug of tissue is cut to the depth of the subcutaneous fat and removed with forceps and scissors. The biopsy site may be closed with one or two sutures if it is on the face or lower extremity. Some physicians allow the biopsy site to heal without suturing.

SHAVE BIOPSY. A shave biopsy removes only that portion of the skin elevated above the surrounding tissue by injection of the local anesthetic. A scalpel or razor blade is moved parallel to the skin surface to remove the tissue specimen. Shave biopsies are usually indicated for superficial or raised lesions. Suturing is not necessary.

EXCISIONAL BIOPSY. In rare instances, larger or deeper specimens are obtained by excision with a scalpel. Deep incisions are made and then sutured after the specimen is removed. In contrast to punch and shave biopsies, excisional biopsies usually involve more discomfort for the client while the site is healing.

CLIENT PREPARATION. As with any invasive procedure, the nurse prepares the client for a biopsy by briefly explaining what to expect. The nurse emphasizes that a biopsy is a minor procedure with few, if any, complications. If a punch or shave biopsy is planned, the client is reassured that scarring is minimal because of the small size of the tissue removed. If an excisional biopsy is planned, the nurse tells the client to expect a cosmetic result similar to that of a healed surgical incision.

PROCEDURE. The nurse establishes a sterile field and assembles all necessary supplies and instruments. A syringe with the physician's choice of local anesthetic is available. A small-gauge needle (No. 25) is attached to the syringe to minimize discomfort during injection. Although preparation of the biopsy site differs according to the physician's preference, the skin is simply wiped with alcohol in most cases.

The most uncomfortable time for the client is during the injection of a local anesthetic agent, which produces a burning or stinging sensation. The nurse reassures the client that the discomfort will subside as the anesthetic takes effect. Talking the client through the procedure with a quiet voice, in combination with a gentle touch, has a calming effect.

After removal, tissue specimens for routine pathologic study are placed directly in 10% formalin for fixation. Specimens for culture are placed in sterile saline solution. Bleeding of the biopsy site is sometimes controlled with Monsel's solution, a topical hemostatic agent. If topical treatment does not stop the bleeding, suturing is considered.

FOLLOW-UP CARE. After bleeding is under control and any sutures have been placed, the site is covered with an adhesive bandage or a dry gauze dressing. The nurse instructs the client to keep the dressing dry and in place for a minimum of 8 hours. After the dressing is removed, the site is cleaned once a day with tap water or saline to remove any dried blood or crusts. The physician may also prescribe an antibiotic ointment to minimize local bacterial colonization. The biopsy site may be left open unless a covering is preferred for cosmetic reasons or because the site is an area often soiled. The nurse instructs the client to report any erythema or excessive drainage at the site. Sutures are usually removed 7 to 10 days after biopsy.

Wood's Light Examination

A handheld, long-wave length ultraviolet (black) light or Wood's light is sometimes used during physical examination. Areas of blue-green or red fluorescence are associated with certain skin infections. Hypopigmented skin becomes more prominent when it is viewed under black light, which greatly facilitates the evaluation of pigment changes in fair-skinned clients.

Examination of the skin under a Wood's light is always carried out in a darkened room. The nurse reassures the client that no discomfort is associated with a Wood's light examination.

Diascopy

Diascopy is a noninvasive and painless technique that eliminates erythema caused by increased blood flow to the skin, thereby facilitating the inspection of skin lesions. A glass slide or lens is pressed down over the area to be examined, blanching the skin and revealing the shape of the underlying lesions.

Skin Testing

If a client's rash is thought to be an allergic contact dermatitis, patch testing may identify the responsible allergen. The technique for allergy testing of the skin is described in Chapter 23.

CRITICAL THINKING CHALLENGE

The client is a 45-year-old Asian woman who speaks no English. She has a large, black, papular lesion with irregular borders on her left cheek. Her daughter is serving as the interpreter. You are concerned that this lesion may be a melanoma. The daughter tells you that this mark has been on her mother's face for at least 20 years and that her mother considers it a "mark of beauty."

- Should this lesion be examined by a surgeon or dermatologist? Why or why not?
- What additional information should you obtain from the mother (with the daughter's assistance)?
- What additional physical assessment data should you obtain regarding this lesion?

For suggested answer guidelines, go to SIMON http://www.wbsaunders.com/SIMON/Iggy/.

ONLINE RESOURCES

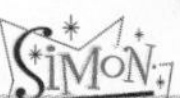

For suggested readings and Internet resources, go to http://www.wbsaunders.com/SIMON/Iggy/.

SELECTED BIBLIOGRAPHY

Asterisk indicates a classic or definitive work on this subject.

Ebersole, P., & Hess, P. (1998). *Toward healthy aging* (5th ed.). St. Louis: Mosby.

*Gaskin, F.C. (1986). Detection of cyanosis in the person with dark skin. *Journal of the National Black Nurses Association, 1*(1), 52-60.

Guyton, A., & Hall, J. (2000). *Textbook of medical physiology* (10th ed.). Philadelphia: W.B. Saunders.

Jarvis, C. (2000). *Physical examination and health assessment* (3rd ed.). Philadelphia: W.B. Saunders.

Lookingbill, D.P., & Marks, J.G., Jr. (2000). *Principles of dermatology* (3rd ed.). Philadelphia: W.B. Saunders.

Matteson, M. (1997). Age-related changes in the integument. In M.A. Matteson, E.S. McConnell, & A.D. Linton (Eds.), *Gerontological nursing: Concepts and practice* (2nd ed., pp. 174-195). Philadelphia: W.B. Saunders.

CHAPTER

67

Interventions for Clients with Skin Problems

JANICE CUZZELL

Learning Objectives

After studying this chapter, you should be able to:

1. Prioritize nursing care for a client with dry skin.
2. Compare and contrast wound healing by first, second, and third intention.
3. Identify clients at risk for pressure ulcer development.
4. Plan an individualized strategy for pressure ulcer prevention for a specific client at increased risk.
5. Differentiate the clinical manifestations for stage I through stage IV pressure ulcers.
6. Prioritize the nursing interventions for a client with a stage III pressure ulcer.
7. Evaluate the effectiveness of interventions for pressure ulcer management.
8. Compare the clinical manifestations and modes of transmission for bacterial, viral, and fungal skin infections.
9. Prioritize nursing care and educational needs for clients who have parasitic skin infections.
10. Explain the rationale for drug therapy for psoriasis.
11. Explain the rationale for ultraviolet therapy for psoriasis.
12. Identify interventions for prevention of skin cancer.
13. Describe the clinical manifestations of melanoma.

SIMON **Go to http://www.wbsaunders.com/SIMON/Iggy/ for self-assessment questions related to these Learning Objectives.**

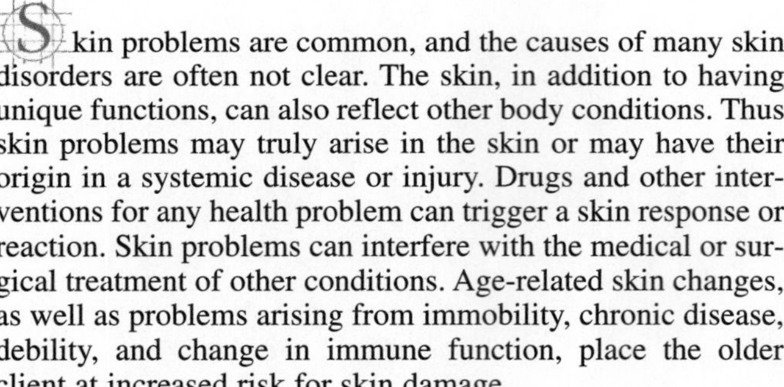

Skin problems are common, and the causes of many skin disorders are often not clear. The skin, in addition to having unique functions, can also reflect other body conditions. Thus skin problems may truly arise in the skin or may have their origin in a systemic disease or injury. Drugs and other interventions for any health problem can trigger a skin response or reaction. Skin problems can interfere with the medical or surgical treatment of other conditions. Age-related skin changes, as well as problems arising from immobility, chronic disease, debility, and change in immune function, place the older client at increased risk for skin damage.

MINOR IRRITATIONS

Dryness

OVERVIEW

Dry skin is a common problem, especially in older clients. Dry skin is a fine flaking of the **stratum corneum** (outermost skin layer), which is more pronounced over the distal lower extremities. Dehydration of the stratum corneum **(xerosis)** is often accompanied by a generalized **pruritus** (itching). In clients with chronic skin conditions, unrelieved pruritus may result in secondary skin lesions, excoriations, **lichenification** (thickening), and infection as they scratch and rub the skin in an attempt to relieve the intense itching.

Xerosis is worse in dry climates. Central heating and air-conditioning reduce the humidity in the air and increase skin dryness. Wind, cold, and sunlight also contribute to the problem. Frequent bathing with harsh soap and hot water and poor application of moisturizers further dries the skin; however, frequent bathing with moisturizing soaps, oils, and lotions may reduce dryness.

COLLABORATIVE MANAGEMENT

Immediate nursing intervention is aimed at rehydration of the skin and relief of itching. A 20-minute soak in a mildly warm bath, followed by application of an emollient cream or lotion, can rehydrate the skin and promote comfort. If the client is bedridden or if tub baths are contraindicated, the trunk and extremities can be wrapped in warm, moist towels covered by plastic sheeting and additional blankets to prevent chilling. Skin creams or lotions are always applied to slightly damp skin after these procedures or within 2 to 3 minutes after routine bathing.

Contrary to popular belief, the cream or lotion is *not* what makes the skin soft and supple. Water is the agent that softens the outer skin layers. Lubricating creams and lotions seal in the moisture provided by water, promoting suppleness and preventing flaking. Some skin lotions are **hydrophilic** (water seeking) and actually draw moisture from the skin, making the dryness worse if they are not applied directly to damp skin.

The nurse educates clients and family members or significant others in measures to maintain healthy skin. Chart 67-1 lists practical ways to avoid drying the skin.

Pruritus

OVERVIEW

Pruritus, or itching, is a distressing symptom that may or may not be associated with skin disease. Pruritus is caused by stimulation of itch-specific nerve fibers at the dermal-epidermal junction. Physical or chemical agents either act directly on these nerve fibers or activate chemical mediators, such as histamine, which then act on the itch receptors.

As a subjective sensation similar to pain, pruritus varies among clients in location and severity. Regardless of the underlying cause, clients usually report that pruritus is worse at night. Pruritus can be made worse by poor skin hydration, increased skin temperature, perspiration, and emotional stress.

CHART 67-1

CLIENT EDUCATION GUIDE
Prevention of Dry Skin

- Use a room humidifier during the winter months or whenever the furnace is in use.
- Take a complete bath or shower only every other day (wash face, axillae, perineum, and any soiled areas daily).
- Use tepid water.
- Use a superfatted, nonalkaline soap instead of deodorant soap.
- Rinse the soap thoroughly from your skin.
- If you like bath oil, add the oil to the water at the end of the bath.
- Pat rather than rub skin surfaces dry.
- Avoid clothing that continuously rubs the skin, such as tight belts, nylon stockings, or pantyhose.
- Maintain a daily fluid intake of 3000 mL unless contraindicated for another medical condition.
- Do not apply rubbing alcohol, astringents, or other drying agents to the skin.
- Avoid caffeine and alcohol ingestion.

COLLABORATIVE MANAGEMENT

Clients usually seek relief from pruritus by scratching or rubbing the skin, a response that further stimulates the itch receptors and causes a pattern referred to as the **"itch-scratch-itch" cycle.** When the pruritus is associated with skin lesions, relief can usually be obtained by treatment of the underlying dermatologic disorder with appropriate topical and systemic medications. Systemic diseases, such as liver and venous disorders, can also cause pruritus without skin lesions.

The nurse plans care to promote comfort and prevent alterations in skin integrity that can result from vigorous scratching. Because dry skin is often a contributing factor, proper bathing and skin lubrication techniques are emphasized (see Chart 67-1). Clients are encouraged to keep the fingernails trimmed short, with rough edges filed, to minimize skin excoriation. They may wear mittens or splints at night to prevent inadvertent scratching during sleep.

A cool sleeping environment combined with a larger dose of sedating antihistamines at bedtime (when the side effect of drowsiness is welcome) may provide an uninterrupted night's sleep. Therapeutic baths **(balneotherapy)** containing colloidal oatmeal preparations or tar extracts may provide temporary relief (Table 67-1).

If antihistamines are ordered, the nurse closely monitors the client's response to therapy so that the dosage can be adjusted as needed. The anti-inflammatory properties of many topical steroid preparations can be maximized if the ointment or cream is applied to slightly damp skin.

Sunburn

OVERVIEW

Sunburn is a first-degree or superficial burn and one of the most common skin injuries. Excessive exposure to ultraviolet (UV) light injures the superficial dermis, with subsequent di-

TABLE 67-1 • USES OF THERAPEUTIC BATHS

Agents	Disease	Purpose
ANTIBACTERIAL BATHS		
Potassium permangenate (1:32,000; 1:64,000)	Infected eczema Pemphigus Multiple infected ulcerations	To lower skin bacterial load
COLLOIDAL BATHS		
Starch and baking soda (1 cup each per tub) Aveeno colloidal oatmeal (1 cup per tub) Aveeno oilated colloidal oatmeal	Atopic eczema Psoriasis Chickenpox	To relieve itching To soothe To lubricate
EMOLLIENT BATHS*		
Bath oils; Alpha Keri Lubath Mineral oil	Any dry skin condition	To clean and hydrate the skin
TAR BATHS*		
Bath oils with tar: Balnetar, Zetar, Polytar Coal tar concentrate (liquor carbonis, detergents)	Scaly dermatosis Psoriasis Eczema	To loosen scale To relieve itching To potentiate ultraviolet A or ultraviolet B light therapy

Modified from Rosen, T., Lanning, M.B., & Hill, M.J. (1983). *The nurse's atlas of dermatology.* Boston: Little, Brown & Co. ©1983 by Theodore Rosen and Marilyn B. Lanning.
*For emollient and tar baths, add 3 to 6 capfuls of therapeutic agent per standard bathtub.

lation of the capillaries, erythema, tenderness, edema, and occasional blister formation. Involvement of large areas of the body may also produce systemic symptoms, such as headache, nausea, and fever.

COLLABORATIVE MANAGEMENT

Redness (erythema) and pain begin within a few hours after sunburn has occurred and gradually increase in intensity for 1 to 2 days before subsiding. Treatment is directed toward symptomatic relief and includes cool baths and soothing lotions, such as bland lubricants or refrigerated moisturizing lotions. Antibiotic ointments are used only if blistering of the skin causes secondary infection. If pain is severe, topical corticosteroids may decrease the inflammation temporarily.

Urticaria

OVERVIEW

Urticaria (hives) is the presence of white or red edematous papules or plaques of varying sizes. Urticaria is usually caused by exposure to a specific noxious stimulus, which releases histamine in the dermal tissue, causing vasodilation and leakage of plasma protein to form lesions or wheals. Unfortunately, the exact cause of urticaria is identified in only a small number of cases. The following factors are thought to cause urticaria: drugs, foods, infections, autoimmune diseases, malignancies, physical stimuli, and psychogenic responses.

COLLABORATIVE MANAGEMENT

Treatment is aimed at removal of the potential stimulus and relief of symptoms. Because the skin reaction is caused by histamine release, antihistamines are the drugs of choice. The nurse instructs the client to avoid overexertion, alcohol consumption, and warm environments, which contribute to vasodilation and make the symptoms worse.

TRAUMA

OVERVIEW

Skin trauma can vary from a neat, aseptic surgical incision performed in a controlled environment to a grossly infected, draining pressure ulcer with tissue destruction. Injury to the skin stimulates a series of events for repair and re-establishment of the body's protective barrier.

Phases of Wound Healing

Wound healing occurs in three phases: the inflammatory, or "lag," phase; the fibroblastic, or connective tissue repair phase; and the maturation, or remodeling, phase. Table 67-2 summarizes the key events of normal wound healing. The length of each phase depends on the type of injury and whether the wound is allowed to heal by first, second, or third intention (Figure 67-1).

A wound without tissue loss, such as a clean laceration or a surgical incision, can be closed with sutures or staples. The wound edges are brought together, with the skin layers approximated and held in place until healing is complete. Because the wound can be easily corrected and dead space eliminated, healing by **first intention** shortens the phases of tissue repair. Inflammation resolves quickly, and connective tissue repair is minimal, resulting in a thin scar.

TABLE 67-2 • NORMAL WOUND HEALING

INFLAMMATORY PHASE
- Begins at the time of injury or cell death and lasts 3-5 days.
- Immediate responses are vasoconstriction and clot formation.
- After 10 minutes, vasodilation with increased capillary permeability and leakage of plasma (and plasma proteins) into the surrounding tissue.
- Migration of white blood cells (especially macrophages) into the wound.
- Clinical manifestations of local edema, pain, erythema, and warmth.

FIBROBLASTIC PHASE
- Begins about the fourth day after injury and lasts 2-4 weeks.
- Fibrin strands form a scaffold or framework.
- Mitotic fibroblast cells migrate into the wound, attach to the framework, divide, and stimulate the secretion of collagen.
- Collagen, together with ground substance, builds tough and inflexible scar tissue.
- Capillaries in areas surrounding the wound form "buds" that grow into new blood vessels.
- Capillary buds and collagen deposits form the "granulation" tissue in the wound, and the wound contracts.
- Epithelial cells grow over the granulation tissue bed.

MATURATION PHASE
- Begins as early as 3 weeks after injury and may continue for a year.
- Collagen is reorganized to provide greater tensile strength.
- Scar tissue gradually becomes thinner and paler in color.
- The mature scar is firm and inelastic when palpated.

Deeper tissue injuries or wounds with tissue loss, such as a chronic pressure ulcer or venous stasis ulcer, result in a cavity-like defect that requires gradual filling in of the dead space with connective tissue. Consequently, healing by **second intention** prolongs the repair process.

Wounds with a high potential for infection, such as surgical incisions that enter a nonsterile body cavity or traumatic wounds that occur under unclean conditions, may be intentionally left open for several days. After debris and exudate have been removed and inflammation has subsided, the wound is closed by first intention. Healing by delayed primary closure, or **third intention,** results in a scar similar to that found in wounds that heal by first intention. As shown in Table 67-3, healing can be impaired by a number of factors.

Mechanisms of Wound Healing

The body restores skin integrity through the processes of epithelialization and contraction. The degree to which these processes can close the wound depends on the depth of injury and the extent of tissue loss. The mechanisms of epithelialization and contraction can be easily understood if two categories of injury are considered: partial-thickness wounds and full-thickness wounds.

PARTIAL-THICKNESS WOUNDS

Partial-thickness, or superficial, wounds heal by **epithelialization,** the production of new skin cells by epithelial cells re-

The Process of Wound Healing

▶ Healing by First Intention

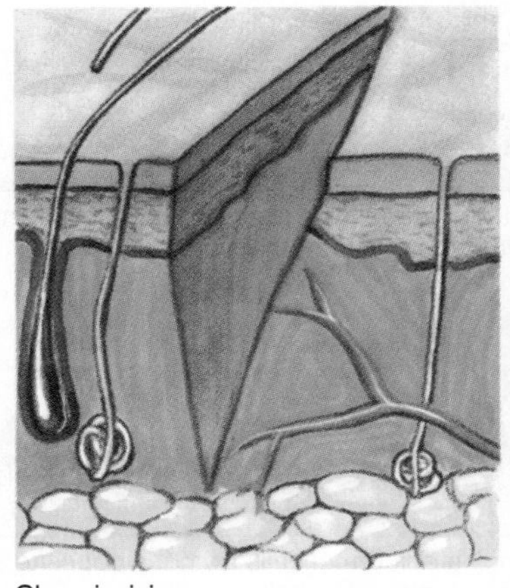

Clean incision

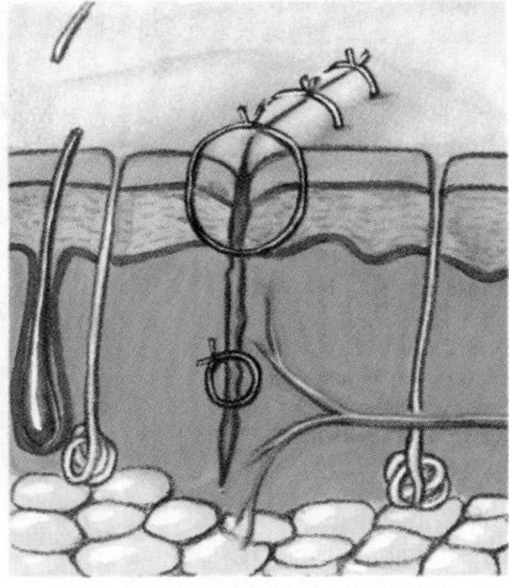

Early suture

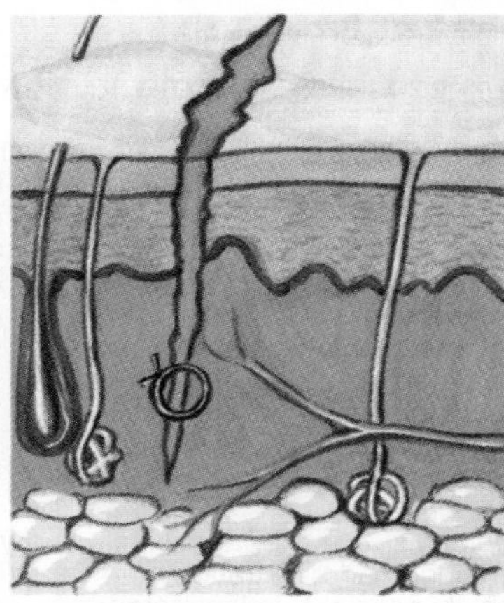

"Hairline" scar

An aseptically made wound with minimal tissue destruction and minimal tissue reaction begins to heal as the edges are approximated by close sutures or staples. No open areas or dead spaces are left to serve as potential sites of infection.

▶ Healing by Second Intention (Granulation) and Contraction

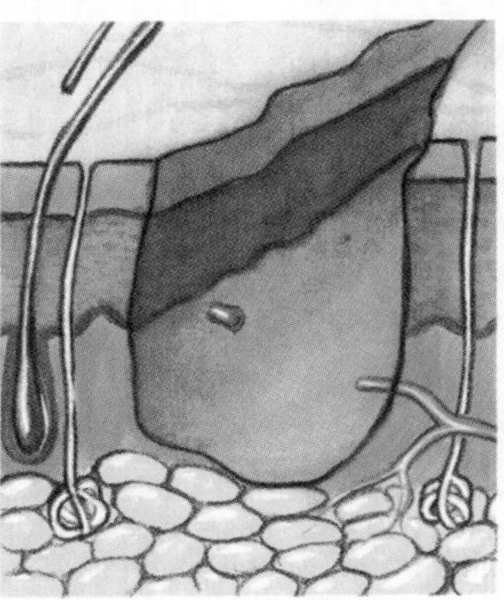

Gaping, irregular wound

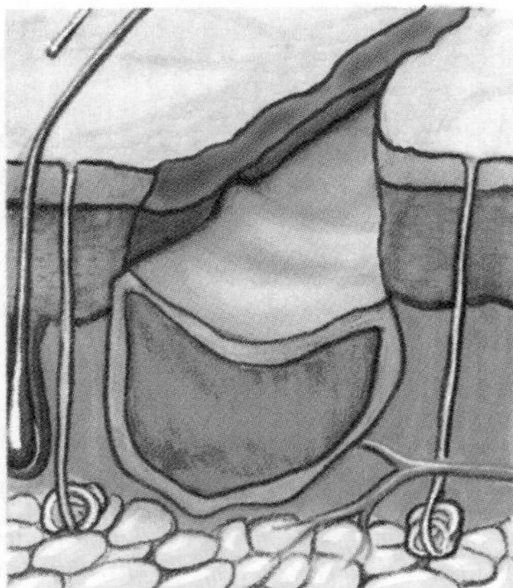

Granulation and contraction

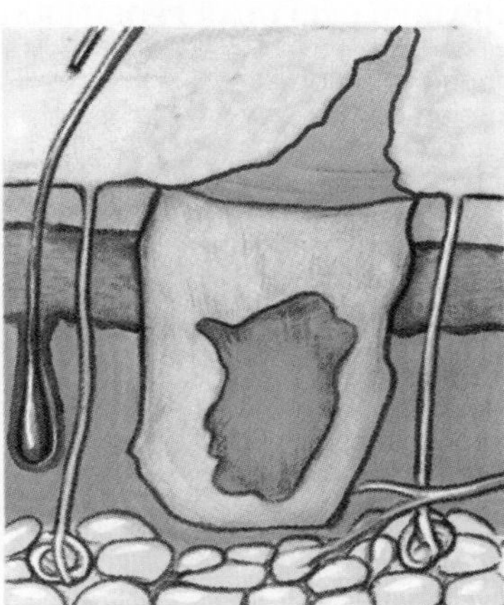

Growth of epithelium over scar

An infected or chronic wound or one with tissue damage so extensive that the edges cannot be smoothly approximated is usually left open and allowed to heal from the inside out. The nurse periodically cleans and assesses the wound for healthy tissue production. Scar tissue is extensive, and healing is prolonged.

▶ Healing by Third Intention (Delayed Closure)

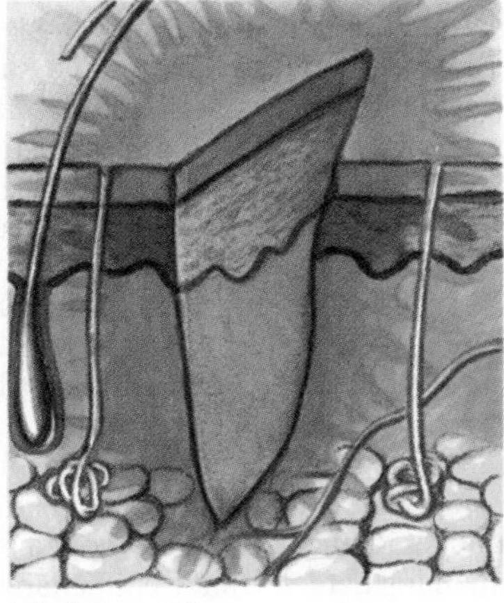

Infected wound

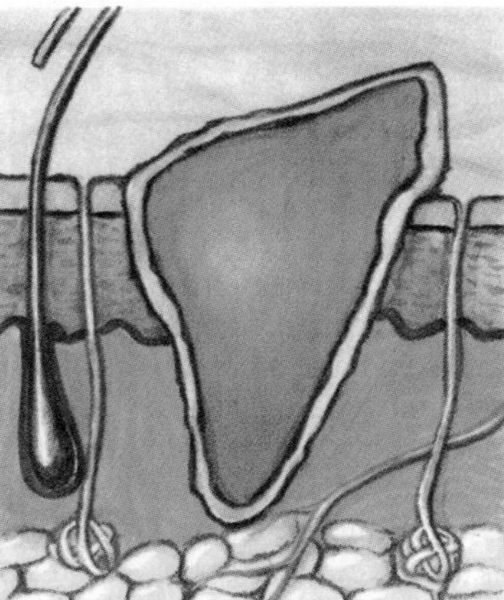

Granulation

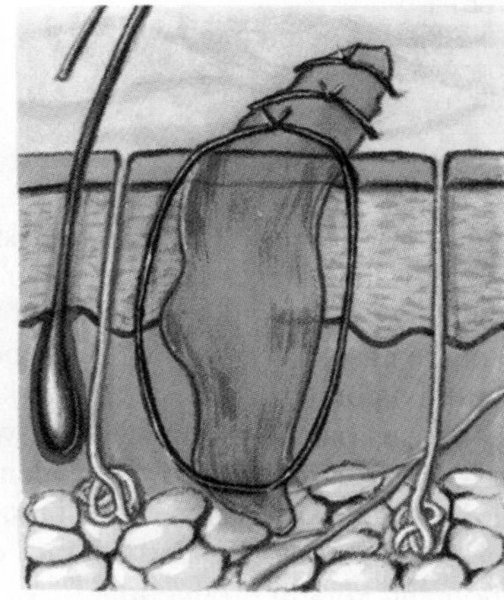

Closure with wide scar

A potentially infected surgical wound may be left open for several days. If no clinical signs of infection occur, the wound is then closed surgically.

Figure 67-1 ● The process of wound healing.

TABLE 67-3 • CAUSES OF IMPAIRED WOUND HEALING

Cause	Mechanism
ALTERED INFLAMMATORY RESPONSE	
Local	
Arteriosclerosis Diabetes Vasculitis Thrombosis Venous insufficiency Lymphedema Pharmacologic vasoconstriction Irradiated tissue Crush injuries Primary closure under tension	Altered local tissue circulation, resulting in ischemia, impaired leukocytic response to wounding, and increased probability of wound infection
Systemic	
Leukemia Prolonged administration of high-dose anti-inflammatory drugs • Corticosteroids • Aspirin	Systemic inhibition of leukocytic response, resulting in impaired host resistance to infection
IMPAIRED CELLULAR PROLIFERATION	
Local	
Wound infection Foreign body Necrotic tissue Repeated injury or irritation Movement of wound (e.g., across a joint) Wound desiccation or maceration	Prolonged inflammatory response, which can result in low tissue oxygen tension and further tissue destruction
Systemic	
Aging Chronic stress Nutritional deficiencies • Calories • Protein • Vitamins • Minerals • Water Impaired oxygenation • Pulmonary insufficiency • Heat failure • Hypovolemia Cirrhosis Uremia Prolonged hypothermia Coagulation disorders Cytotoxic drugs	Impaired cellular proliferation and collagen synthesis Decreased wound contraction

maining in the dermal layer of the skin and at the base of the epidermal appendages (Figure 67-2). On injury, a fibrin clot forms. Undamaged epithelial cells at the basement membrane and at the base of the hair follicles and glands undergo a burst of cell division (mitosis). The new skin cells move into "cell-free" spaces on the wound surface, where the fibrin clot acts as a frame. Regrowth across the open area **(resurfacing),** initially only one cell layer thick, proceeds with thickening or layering of the new epidermis and, eventually, rete peg formation and keratin production.

In a healthy client, healing of a partial-thickness wound by epithelialization takes 5 to 7 days. Epithelialization occurs best in tissue that is well hydrated, is well oxygenated, and has few microorganisms.

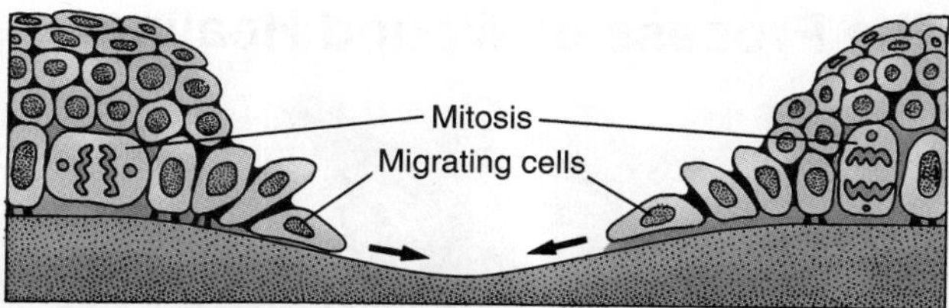

Skin cells at the edge of the wound begin multiplying and migrate toward the center of the wound.

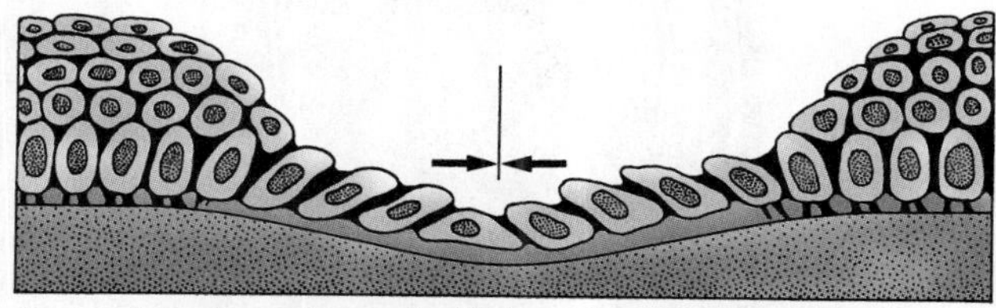
Once advancing epidermal cells from the opposite sides of the wound meet, migration halts.

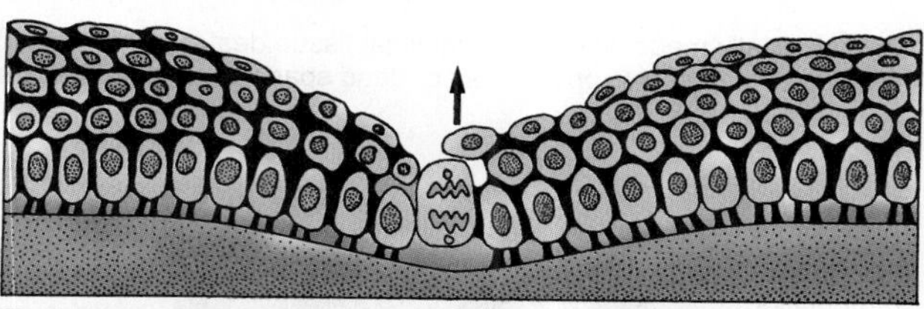
Epithelial cells continue to divide until the thickness of the new skin layer approaches normal.

Figure 67-2 • Epithelialization. (Modified from Swaim, S.F. (1980). *Surgery of traumatized skin.* Philadelphia: W.B. Saunders.)

FULL-THICKNESS WOUNDS

In a client with a deeper, or full-thickness, wound, most if not all of the epithelial remnants have been destroyed, except those remaining at the wound margins. For a full-thickness wound to heal, the **nonviable** (dead) tissue must be removed so that gradual filling in of the defect with granulation tissue can progress.

Drawing together of the wound edges occurs at the same time as collagen synthesis and wound revascularization. This type of healing is known as **contraction** (see Figure 67-1). Unlike epithelialization, in which new tissue is formed, wound contraction decreases the surface area of a full-thickness wound by stretching and thinning the existing tissue surrounding the wound. Fibroblastic cells in the wound bed exert a mechanical force on the wound edges, causing the wound to decrease in size at a uniform rate of about 0.6 to 0.75 mm/day. Complete closure of a wound by contraction depends on the mobility of the surrounding skin as tension is applied to it. Necrotic tissue provides a physical obstacle to wound contraction and must be removed for healing to occur.

If tension in the surrounding skin exceeds the force of contraction, wound closure does not occur, and the wound remains open until epithelial cells at the wound edges eventually bridge the remaining defect. Unlike epithelialization in partial-thickness wounds, in which the skin integrity soon returns to normal, the movement of epithelial cells from wound edges over fibrous connective tissue results in an unstable epithelial surface that is poorly attached to the underlying tissue and thus is susceptible to reinjury. A venous stasis leg ulcer is one example of a skin defect in an area where effective movement of the surrounding skin is usually not sufficient to allow wound healing by contraction. As a result, the thin epithelial covering cannot withstand environmental hazards and abrades easily.

Epithelialization and contraction do not continue indefinitely. Natural healing processes can slow down or even be halted by the presence of infection, pressure, or mechanical obstacles, such as a poorly applied dressing. In the case of chronic wounds, healing can cease spontaneously and without a clearly defined cause.

➤ COLLABORATIVE MANAGEMENT

Specific treatment of skin trauma varies with the depth and circumstances of the injury. The focus of all treatment for any type of skin trauma is to enhance wound healing, prevent infection, and restore function to the area. Management for pressure ulcers presents common interventions, as does treatment for burns (see Chapter 68).

PRESSURE ULCERS

OVERVIEW

A **pressure ulcer** is any lesion caused by unrelieved pressure resulting in damage of underlying tissue or a lesion that is a clearly localized area of cellular necrosis due to vascular insufficiency in an area of tissue under pressure. This type of injury most commonly occurs over bony prominences. These skin lesions are a specific type of skin trauma that occurs almost exclusively in people with limited mobility. Once formed, pressure ulcers are slow to heal, requiring weeks to years, and result in increased morbidity and health care costs. The term *pressure ulcer* matches the guidelines provided by the Agency for Healthcare Research and Quality (formerly the Agency for Health Care Policy and Research) of the U.S. Department of Health and Human Services.

Pathophysiology

Mechanical forces exerted to or on the skin lead to the formation of pressure ulcers. These forces—pressure, friction, and shear—lead to direct and ischemic tissue damage. Although injury occurs more often to skin over bony prominences, pressure ulcers may occur anywhere. Excessive skin moisture increases the susceptibility of the skin to damage when mechanical forces are exerted.

PRESSURE

Pressure occurs as a result of gravity. Dependent tissues in contact with a fixed surface experience varying degrees of pressure. Pressure is determined by the amount of weight exerted at the point of contact, the distribution of weight at the point of contact, and the density of the contacting surface. Excessive or prolonged pressure can compress blood vessels at the point of contact, leading to ischemia, inflammation, and tissue necrosis. Pressure occurs when the client is positioned on a hard, unyielding surface that does not diffuse the weight or when he or she remains in the same position too long.

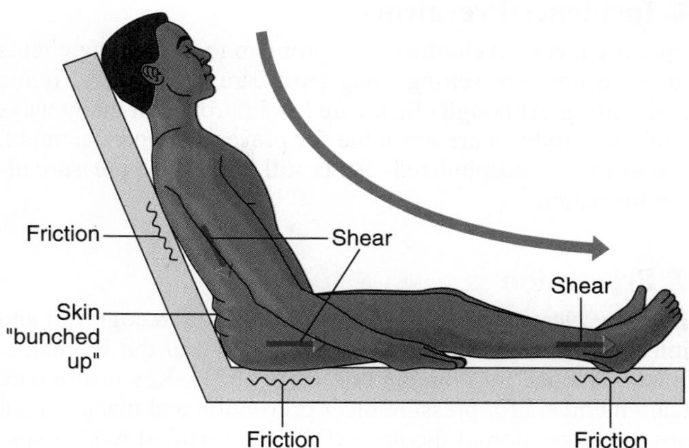

Figure 67-3 ● Shearing forces pulling skin layers away from deeper tissue. The skin is "bunched up" against the back of the mattress while the rest of the bone and muscle in the area press downward on the lower part of the mattress. Blood vessels become kinked, obstructing circulation and leading to tissue death.

FRICTION

Friction occurs when surfaces rub the skin and irritate or directly pull off epithelial tissue. Such forces are generated when the client is dragged or pulled across bed linen.

SHEAR

Shear or shearing forces are generated when the skin itself remains stationary and the tissues below the skin (such as fat and muscle) shift or move (Figure 67-3). The movement of the deeper tissue layers reduces the blood supply to the skin, leading to skin hypoxia, anoxia, ischemia, inflammation, and necrosis.

Gravity plays a role in the development of shearing forces. A shear injury commonly occurs when a client is in bed in a semisitting position and gradually slides downward. Often, the skin over the sacrum does not slide down at the same pace as the deeper tissues; thus the skin is mechanically "sheared," causing blood vessels to stretch and leading to soft-tissue ischemia, although no break in external skin integrity is observed.

Etiology

Pressure ulcers occur as a result of mechanical trauma and tissue anoxia.

CONSIDERATIONS FOR OLDER ADULTS

Older adults are at particular risk for pressure ulcers because of the presence of age-related skin changes. Progressive flattening of the dermal-epidermal junction predisposes older people to skin tears from mechanical shearing forces, such as the removal of adhesive tape and friction from tightly applied restraints. In addition, skin moisture and irritation from incontinence and friction over bony prominences can lead to partial-thickness skin destruction and early pressure ulcer formation. *If pressure is unrelieved, tissue destruction progresses to full-thickness injury.*

Incidence/Prevalence

Pressure ulcer development is a problem found among clients in the acute care setting, long-term care facility, and home care setting. Although client care has improved in many ways and new products are available for prevention and treatment, 3% to 14% of hospitalized clients still experience pressure ulcer formation.

Prevention

Pressure ulcers can be prevented if the risk is recognized and intervention begins early (see Chart 67-2 and the Evidence-Based Practice for Nursing box on p. 1521). Key health care team members for pressure ulcer prevention and management are the enterostomal therapist (ET), the certified wound specialist, and the registered dietitian (RD).

A pressure ulcer prevention program consists of two steps: (1) identification of high-risk clients and (2) implementation of aggressive intervention for prevention with the use of pressure relief/reduction devices. Many facilities do not recognize the value of preventing pressure ulcers with appropriate consultation, use of pressure relief/reduction products, and ensuring adequate nutrition. The costs of implementing such prevention strategies is more than justified by the savings seen in comparison with the costs of interventions for care when actual ulceration is present (see the Cost of Care box on p. 1521).

Risk identification and prevention measures must include education of the client and the caregiver. Documentation of risk assessment, prevention measures implemented, and education of all individuals involved in the care of the client at risk for pressure ulcer formation is key to the plan's success. Periodic reassessment of risk and continuing evaluation of the implemented plan are necessary as client conditions change.

IDENTIFICATION OF HIGH-RISK CLIENTS

All clients admitted to a health care facility or home care agency should be assessed for pressure ulcer risk, as recommended by the Agency for Healthcare Research and Quality (AHRQ). The use of a risk assessment tool increases the chances of identifying those clients at greater risk for skin breakdown. The two risk assessment tools recommended by the AHRQ guidelines are the Norton Scale and the Braden Scale (Figure 67-4).

Other factors to consider when determining the risk category for pressure ulcer formation are mental status, activity/mobility, nutritional status, and incontinence.

MENTAL STATUS. The client's mental status determines whether he or she is a partner in the prevention of pres-

CHART 67-2

NIC INTERVENTION ACTIVITIES *for* The Client at Risk for or with Pressure Ulcers

Pressure Ulcer Prevention: *Prevention of pressure ulcers for a client at high risk for developing them*
- Use an established risk assessment tool to monitor client's risk factors (e.g., Braden scale).
- Document skin status on admission and daily.
- Monitor any reddened areas closely.
- Remove excessive moisture on the skin resulting from perspiration, wound drainage, and fecal or urinary incontinence.
- Apply protective barriers, such as creams or moisture-absorbing pads, to remove excess moisture, as appropriate.
- Turn every 1 to 2 hours, as appropriate.
- Turn with care to prevent injury to fragile skin.
- Post a turning schedule at the bedside, as appropriate.
- Inspect skin over bony prominences and other pressure points when repositioning at least daily.
- Avoid massaging over bony prominences.
- Position with pillows to elevate pressure points off the bed.
- Keep bed linens clean, dry, and wrinkle free.
- Utilize specialty beds and mattresses, as appropriate.
- Use devices on the bed (e.g., sheepskin) that protect the client.
- Moisturize dry, unbroken skin.
- Avoid hot water and use mild soap when bathing.
- Apply elbow and heel protectors, as appropriate.
- Facilitate small shifts of body weight frequently.
- Ensure adequate dietary intake, especially protein, vitamins B and C, iron, and calories, using supplements, as appropriate.
- Instruct family member/caregiver about signs of skin breakdown, as appropriate.

Pressure Ulcer Care: *Facilitation of healing in pressure ulcers*
- Describe characteristics of pressure ulcers at regular intervals, including size (L × W × D), stage (I to IV), location, exudate, granulation or necrotic tissue, and epithelialization.
- Monitor color, temperature, edema, moisture, and appearance of surrounding skin.
- Keep ulcer moist to aid in healing.
- Cleanse the skin around the ulcer with mild soap and water.
- Debride ulcer, as needed.
- Cleanse the ulcer with the appropriate nontoxic solution, working in a circular motion from the center.
- Note characteristics of any drainage.
- Apply dressings, as appropriate.
- Monitor for signs and symptoms of infection in the wound.
- Position every 1 to 2 hours to avoid prolonged pressure.
- Use specialty beds and mattresses, as appropriate.
- Ensure adequate dietary intake.
- Monitor nutritional status.
- Teach client/family member(s) wound care procedures.
- Initiate consultation services of the enterostomal therapy nurse, as needed.

Pressure Management: *Minimizing pressure to body parts*
- Place on appropriate therapeutic mattress/bed.
- Place on a polyurethane foam pad, as appropriate.
- Refrain from applying pressure to the affected body part.
- Elevate injured extremity.
- Turn the immobilized client at least every 2 hours, according to a specific schedule.
- Facilitate small shifts of body weight.
- Monitor skin for areas of redness and breakdown.
- Use an established risk assessment tool to monitor client's risk factors (e.g., Braden scale).
- Monitor the client's nutritional status.
- Monitor for sources of pressure and friction.

NIC intervention activities selected from McCloskey J.C., & Bulechek, G.M. (2000). *Nursing interventions classification (NIC)* (3rd ed.). St. Louis: Mosby.

sure. When the client understands that turning and shifting of weight prevents tissue damage, the risk for pressure ulcer formation decreases. When he or she has a mental status problem because of stroke, head injury, organic brain disease, Alzheimer's disease, or other problem with cognition, the risk for pressure ulcer formation increases.

ACTIVITY/MOBILITY. The level of the client's independent mobility is a direct factor in the risk for pressure ulcer formation. Those clients who have unimpaired mobility and can respond to physical sensation changes are at low risk for pressure ulcer formation. Any client, regardless of age, who requires assistance with turning and positioning or who is less aware of physical sensation changes is at high risk for pressure ulcer formation. A client who must be confined to bed or a chair is at higher risk than a client who requires assistance with ambulation.

NUTRITIONAL STATUS. Nutritional status is a critical risk factor for the development of pressure ulcers. Maintenance of skin integrity and wound healing are dependent on a positive nitrogen balance and adequate serum protein levels. The client in a negative nitrogen balance not only heals more slowly but also is at greater risk for tissue destruction. In addition, draining wounds are a route of protein loss.

Attaining and maintaining adequate nutrition is as important as pressure reduction in the prevention of pressure ulcer formation. A dietitian or other nutrition specialist should be a part of the pressure reduction team or program.

Nutritional status assessment includes laboratory studies, evaluation of weight and weight change, ability of the client to consume an adequate diet, and the need for vitamin, mineral, or protein supplementation. Nutrition is considered inadequate when the client's serum albumin level is lower than 3.5 mg/dL or the lymphocyte count is less than 1800/mm^3. Other indicators of inadequate nutrition include a weight loss of 15% of total body weight or greater.

A positive nitrogen balance requires an intake of 30 to 35 calories/kg of body weight per day with a protein intake of 1.25 to 1.5 g/kg/day. Up to 2 g/kg/day of protein may be required when nutritional deficits are severe or protein loss is ongoing. Vitamin supplementation is individualized according to the client's nutritional status.

INCONTINENCE. Incontinence results in prolonged contact of the skin with such substances as urea, bacteria, yeast, and enzymes carried in urine and feces. These substances are irritants and lead to skin breakdown. The excessive moisture associated with incontinence macerates intact skin, increasing the risk for breakdown. Daily inspection of the skin for any areas of redness or skin breakdown is a major part of pressure ulcer prevention. Maintenance of clean, intact skin also assists in the prevention process. The skin should be washed with a pH-balanced soap to maintain the normal acid level. Creams or lotions are used to lubricate and moisturize the skin. Barrier ointment protection is needed

EVIDENCE-BASED PRACTICE FOR NURSING

Assess and reassess for accurate predictability

Bergstrom, N., et al. (1998). Predicting pressure ulcer risk. *Nursing Research, 47*(5), 261-269.

This prospective, investigator-controlled/coordinated study of 843 randomly selected subjects conducted at multiple sites sought to test the Braden Scale for predictive validity and established cutoff points in assessing pressure ulcer risk. Sites of the study included two tertiary care hospitals, two Veterans Administration Medical Centers, and two skilled nursing facilities. Subjects ranged in age from 19 to 102 years, with a mean age of 63 years. Research staff were trained in scoring the Braden Scale, staging ulcers, and recording data on the skin assessment tool. Videotapes were used in initial and refresher training. The inter-rater reliability was established at .95 and maintained throughout the study. The Braden Scale has six subscale items for rating with a possible score ranging from 6 to 23 points. The critical cutoff point in previous studies was established at 16. Subjects were assessed on admission and every 48 to 72 hours until discharge for a maximum of 4 weeks.

None of the subjects had observable pressure ulcers on admission. One hundred eight subjects (12.8%) developed one or more pressure ulcers during their stay at the facility. The critical cutoff score in this study was higher than that of previous studies: 18 rather than 16. The Braden Scale was determined to be predictive on admission but even more predictive for the assessments completed at 48 to 72 hours after admission. The subjects who developed pressure ulcers had a mean age 10 years greater than those who did not develop pressure ulcers. Women were more likely to develop pressure ulcers than men.

Critique. This clinical study was well designed and well controlled. The methods of study were appropriate for the questions asked.

Implications for Nursing. The Braden Scale has demonstrated reliability, validity, sensitivity, and specificity in predicting pressure ulcer risk. The study underscores the importance of risk reassessment beyond admission, when client conditions can change and risk increases. This scale should be used for ongoing evaluation of pressure ulcer risk throughout the client's stay in the facility.

COST OF CARE IMPLICATIONS FOR NURSING

PRESSURE ULCER PREVENTION

Cost of Care

- Medicare reimbursement for medically complex residents of long-term care decreased from an average of $408 to $231 per day, beginning in 1997.
- Most residents with complex wounds and stage III or IV pressure ulcers fall into the category of medically complex.
- Pressure relief/reduction devices and appropriate dressing materials cost more than the available reimbursement.
- Many long-term care facilities made product choices based on cost alone.
- Use of pressure relief/reduction devices for prevention of pressure ulcers was limited.
- The number and severity of pressure ulcers among residents of long-term care facilities increased during this budget reduction period.

Implications for Nursing

An ounce of prevention may be worth tons rather than pounds of cure. Although on the surface, pressure relief/reduction devices, high-protein diets, and appropriate dressing materials appear expensive, the actual cost in nursing hours, equipment, devices, and consumable supplies when caring for a client with even one pressure ulcer is far greater. New legislation, signed in late 1999, will allow prevention costs, as well as care costs, to be justly reimbursed. Nurses need to consider pressure ulcer prevention in the care setting as a number one priority of care.

Data from Motta, G. (2000). Reimbursement relief. *Continuing Care, 19*(4), 14-16.

Client's name ______	Evaluator's name ______				Date of assessment	
Sensory perception Ability to respond meaningfully to pressure-related discomfort	**1. Completely limited** Unresponsive to painful stimuli (does not moan, flinch, or grasp) because of diminished level of consciousness or sedation OR limited ability to feel pain over most of body surface	**2. Very limited** Responds only to painful stimuli; cannot communicate discomfort except by moaning or restlessness OR has a sensory impairment that limits the ability to feel pain or discomfort over half of the body	**3. Slightly limited** Responds to verbal commands but cannot always communicate discomfort or need to be turned OR has some sensory impairment that limits ability to feel pain or discomfort in one or two extremities	**4. No impairment** Responds to verbal commands; has no sensory deficit that would limit ability to feel or voice pain or discomfort		
Moisture Degree to which skin is exposed to moisture	**1. Constantly moist** Skin is kept moist almost constantly by perspiration, urine; dampness is detected every time the client is moved or turned	**2. Very Moist** Skin is often but not always moist; linen must be changed at least once a shift	**3. Occasionally moist** Skin is occasionally moist, requiring an extra linen change approximately once a day	**4. Rarely moist** Skin is usually dry; linen requires changing only at routine intervals		
Activity Degree of physical activity	**1. Bedfast** Confined to bed	**2. Chairfast** Ability to walk severely limited or nonexistent; cannot bear own weight and must be assisted into chair or wheelchair	**3. Walks occasionally** Walks occasionally during the day but for very short distances, with or without assistance; spends the majority of each shift in bed or chair	**4. Walks frequently** Walks outside the room at least twice a day and inside the room at least once every 2 hours during waking hours		
Mobility Ability to change or control body position	**1. Completely immobile** Does not make even slight changes in body or extremity position without assistance	**2. Very limited** Makes occasional slight changes in body or extremity position but unable to make frequent or significant changes independently	**3. Slightly limited** Makes frequent though slight changes in body or extremity position independently	**4. No limitations** Makes major and frequent changes in position without assistance		
Nutrition Usual food intake pattern	**1. Very poor** Never eats a complete meal; rarely eats more than a third of any food offered; eats two servings or less of protein (meat or dairy products) per day; takes fluids poorly; does not take a liquid dietary supplement OR is NPO or maintained on clear liquids or IV for more than 5 days	**2. Probably inadequate** Rarely eats a complete meal and generally eats only about half of any food offered; protein intake includes only three servings of meat or dairy products per day; occasionally will take a dietary supplement OR receives less than optimal amount of liquid diet or tube feeding	**3. Adequate** Eats over half of most meals; eats a total of four servings of protein (meat, dairy products) each day; occasionally will refuse a meal, but will usually take a supplement if offered OR is receiving tube feeding or total parenteral nutrition, which probably meets most nutritional needs	**4. Excellent** Eats most of every meal; never refuses a meal; usually eats a total of four or more servings of meat and dairy products; occasionally eats between meals; does not require supplementation		
Friction and shear	**1. Problem** Requires moderate to maximum assistance in moving; complete lifting without sliding against sheets is impossible; frequently slides down in bed or chair, requiring frequent repositioning with maximum assistance; spasticity, contractures, or agitation leads to almost constant friction	**2. Potential problem** Moves feebly or requires minimum assistance during a move; skin probably slides to some extent against sheets, chair, restraints, or other devices; maintains relatively good position in chair or bed most of the time but occasionally slides down	**3. No apparent problem** Moves in bed and in chair independently and has sufficient muscle strength to lift up completely during move; maintains good position in bed or chair at all times			
Scoring system: 15-16 = mild risk, 12-14 = moderate risk, <11 = severe risk				Total score		

Figure 67-4 ● The Braden Scale for predicting pressure ulcer risk. (From Barbara Braden and Nancy Bergstrom. Copyright 1988. Reprinted with permission.)

whenever incontinence is present. Absorbent pads or garments must be changed quickly with each incontinence episode to avoid prolonged skin contact with urine and/or feces. Reddened areas are *never* massaged, since this action can damage capillary beds and increase tissue necrosis.

PRESSURE RELIEVING TECHNIQUES

The cornerstone in the prevention (and treatment) of pressure ulcers is the provision of adequate pressure relief. A consideration in pressure relief is the **capillary closing pressure,** the amount of pressure needed to occlude skin capillary blood flow, in the area at risk. The normal capillary closing pressure ranges from 12 to 32 mm Hg. Any device used must provide pressure relief below the capillary closing pressure in order to prevent tissue ischemia. *Most devices have a standardized guaranteed pressure relief reading; however, these readings do not ensure that capillary blood flow for any given client is adequate. Therefore the nurse must use observation of skin color, integrity, and temperature to determine capillary flow adequacy.*

Devices are categorized according to whether they relieve pressure or merely reduce pressure. In addition, devices are further categorized as dynamic or static. Dynamic systems alternate air inflation and deflation of the device through the use of electricity. Static devices, made of gel, water, foam, or air, are in a constant state of inflation that distributes the client pressure load over a larger area, thus reducing the pressure any one area experiences.

Pressure relief/reduction products come in many forms, such as specialty beds, mattress replacements, overlays, and assistive devices. Choosing the correct product is important in the success of the prevention or management plan. The product selected is re-evaluated daily for effectiveness in reducing pressure, comfort, and elimination of "bottoming out," wherein the client's bony prominences sink into the mattress or cushion, causing him or her to have pressure even with the product in place.

PRESSURE RELIEF DEVICES. Pressure relief devices consistently reduce pressure below capillary closing pressure. These devices are recommended for clients who:

- Need prevention of skin breakdown because they cannot turn
- Need prevention of extension of skin breakdown that has already occurred
- Need promotion of healing of breakdown present on several turning surfaces

PRESSURE REDUCTION DEVICES. Pressure reduction devices lower pressure below that provided by a standard hospital mattress or chair surface but do not consistently reduce pressure below the capillary closing pressure. Such devices must be used in conjunction with an individualized turning schedule.

POSITIONING. A good plan for positioning is the 30-degree rule. This rule involves ensuring that the client is positioned and propped so that whatever part of the body is elevated is tilted back at least 30 degrees to the mattress, rather than resting directly on a dependent bony prominence. This rule applies to side-lying, as well as head-of-bed elevation, positions. The client who must be elevated to a full 90 degrees because of respiratory difficulties should be tilted forward even more than 90 degrees, with pillows behind the back to keep pressure off of the sacral/coccyx area.

The client at risk for pressure ulcer formation in bed is also at risk while sitting. Careful assessment for proper wheelchair or regular chair cushioning is essential for pressure ulcer prevention. Physical therapists and rehabilitation specialists may be consulted for selection of these products.

Even with an appropriate mattress or cushion, the client must change or be assisted in changing positions periodically. Many facilities require turning and positioning every 2 hours. *However, pressure can occur in less time, and the actual turning/repositioning schedule for each client should be individualized.*

Pillows and other positioning/padding devices are used to keep heels pressure free at all times for high-risk clients. Frequent assessment of heel positioning is needed to ensure that pressure is not redistributed to another high-risk area, such as the sides of the feet. Assessment is needed even more frequently when devices that hide the feet, such as boots, are used, especially if the client has a peripheral vascular problem.

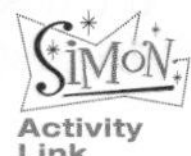

COLLABORATIVE MANAGEMENT

Assessment

HISTORY

When taking a history from the client with a pressure ulcer, the nurse identifies the underlying cause of skin loss, as well as factors that may impair healing. The specific circumstances of the skin loss are investigated. In general, clients with chronic pressure ulcerations usually have a history of delayed healing or recurrence of the ulcer after healing has occurred. Because pressure-related skin loss is common among the severely debilitated, the nurse remains alert to the following contributing factors:

- Prolonged bedrest
- Immobility
- Incontinence
- Inadequate nutrition or hydration
- Altered mental status (decreased sensory perception)

PHYSICAL ASSESSMENT/CLINICAL MANIFESTATIONS

The nurse inspects the entire body, including the back of the head, for areas of skin injury or pressure. Special attention is given to bony prominences (such as the heels, sacrum, elbows, trochanter, and posterior and anterior iliac spines) and areas that are vulnerable to excessive moisture. In addition, the nurse assesses the client's general appearance for issues related to skin health. Such issues include body weight and the proportion of weight to height, because obese persons, as well as thin persons, are at increased risk for pressure ulcer formation. Overall cleanliness of the skin, hair, and nails is noted, as is any alteration in mobility or range of joint motion.

WOUND ASSESSMENT

The appearance of pressure ulcers changes with the depth of the injury. Chart 67-3 lists the characteristics of the four stages of pressure ulceration, and Figures 67-5 to 67-8 show examples.

Wounds are assessed for location, size, color, extent of tissue involvement, cell types in the wound base and margins, exudate, condition of surrounding tissue, and presence of foreign bodies. This initial assessment is documented to serve as a starting point for determining the nature of the intervention plan and its effectiveness. How often a wound is assessed is determined by the written policies and procedures at the facility or agency. Weekly documented assessment is the standard in many facilities. *However, the wound should be assessed at each dressing change, with the existing parameters compared with previous documentation to determine the current state of healing or deterioration.*

The location and size of the wound are the first two clinical parameters recorded. Wounds are sized by length, width, and depth, using millimeters or centimeters. In standardizing the wound size for documentation and communication purposes, the wound is assessed as a clock face with 12 o'clock in the direction of the client's head and 6 o'clock in the direction of the client's feet. The length is always measured from 12 o'clock to 6 o'clock, and the width is measured at 9 o'clock and 3 o'clock. The depth is the distance from the deepest portion of the wound base to skin level. When all caregivers use this format, measurement is accurate and wound progress can be determined.

The nurse inspects the wound margins for **cellulitis** (inflammation of the skin cells) extending beyond the area of injury. Progressive tissue destruction, as reflected by an increase in the size or depth of the ulcer and accompanied by increased wound drainage, usually indicates an impairment in the client's ability to resist infection if proper measures have been taken to relieve pressure.

CHART 67-3

KEY FEATURES *of* Pressure Ulcers

Stage I
- Skin is intact.
- Area is red and does not blanch with external pressure.
- For clients with darker skin that does not blanch†:

Observable pressure-related alteration of intact skin—changes are compared with an adjacent or opposite area and include one or more of the following:
- Skin temperature (warmth or coolness)
- Tissue consistency (firm or boggy)
- Sensation (pain, itching)

The ulcer appears as a defined area of persistent redness in lightly pigmented skin, whereas in darker skin tones, the ulcer may appear with persistent red, blue, or purple hues.

Stage II
- Skin is not intact.
- There is partial-thickness skin loss of the epidermis or dermis.
- Ulcer is superficial and may be characterized as an abrasion, a blister, or a shallow crater.

Stage III
- Skin loss is full thickness.
- Subcutaneous tissues may be damaged or necrotic.
- Damage extends down to but not through the underlying fascia.
- There is a deep crater-like appearance or eschar present.
- Undermining may or may not be present.

Stage IV
- Skin loss is full thickness with extensive destruction, tissue necrosis, or damage to muscle, bone, or supporting structures.
- Undermining is present.
- Sinus tracts may develop.

Data from U.S. Department of Health and Human Services. (1992). *Pressure ulcers in adults: Prediction and prevention, Clinical Practice Guideline, No. 3.* Rockville, MD: Agency for Health Care Policy and Research, Public Health Service, U.S. Department of Health and Human Services.

†Data from Henderson, C., et al. (1997). Draft definition of stage I pressure ulcers: Inclusion of persons with darkly pigmented skin. *Advances in Wound Care, 10*(5), 16-19.

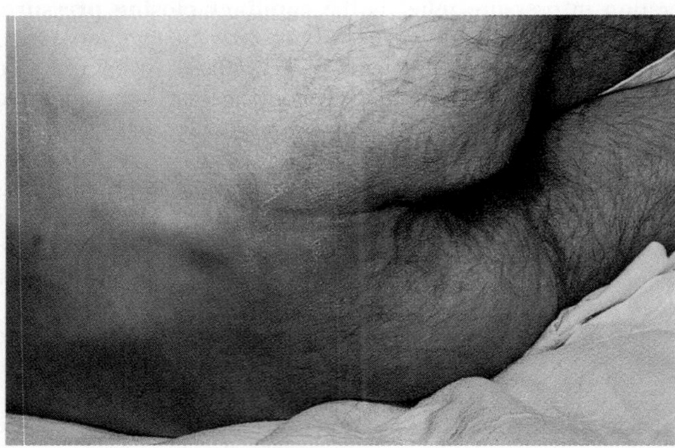

Figure 67-5 ● A stage I pressure ulcer.

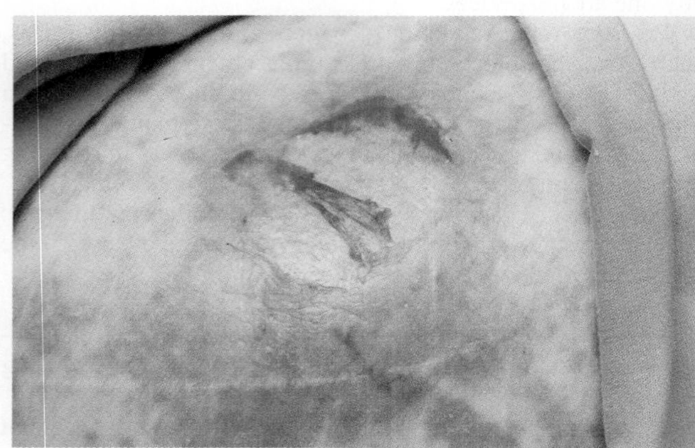

Figure 67-6 ● A stage II pressure ulcer.

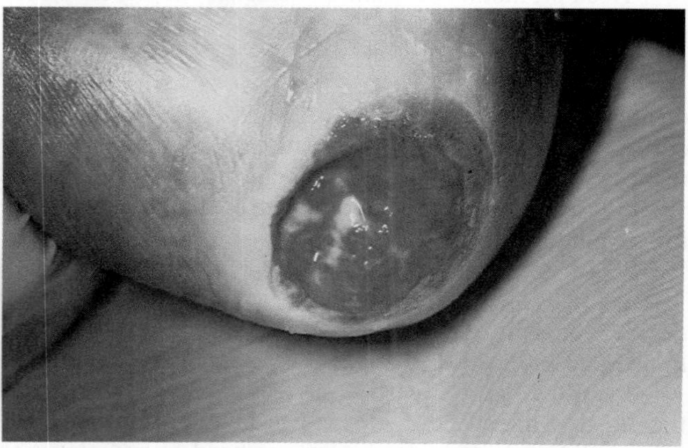

Figure 67-7 ● A stage III pressure ulcer.

The nurse inspects the wound for the presence or absence of necrotic tissue. Because of the depth of tissue destruction, a full-thickness pressure ulcer is initially covered by a layer of black, gray, or brown, nonviable, denatured collagen called wound **eschar.**

In the early stages of wound healing, the eschar is dry, leathery, and firmly attached to the wound surface. As the inflammatory phase of wound healing begins and removal of wound debris progresses, the eschar starts to lift up and separate from the tissue beneath. When disrupted, this nonviable eschar is an excellent breeding ground for bacteria normally found on the skin surface, as well as those inadvertently introduced by other means. As bacteria increase in number, they release enzymes, which increase the liquefaction of necrotic tissue. This tissue becomes softer and more yellow. In the presence of bacterial colonization, wound exudate increases substantially; the color and odor of wound exudate indicate the predominant microorganism present. The characteristics of wound exudate are presented in Table 67-4.

Beneath the separating dead tissue, granulation tissue appears. Early granulation is pale pink, progressing to a beefy red color as it grows and fills the wound. A wound with poor local arterial blood supply appears dry, with pale immature granulation tissue present. Venous obstruction causes an excessively moist ulcer surface with a deep red color (reflective of the deoxygenated blood beneath the ulcer surface).

The nurse palpates the ulcerated area or wound to determine the texture of the granulations. Healthy granulations have a slightly spongy texture. Pressure ulcers may involve more extensive tissue destruction than is first evident on inspection. Separation of the skin layers at the wound margins from the underlying granulation tissue is known as **undermining.** The nurse inspects undermined areas for gradual filling with healthy granulations and for wound healing progress. The nurse palpates the bony prominences for deep hardening of the surrounding soft tissue, which often suggests tissue ischemia well beneath the surface of the skin.

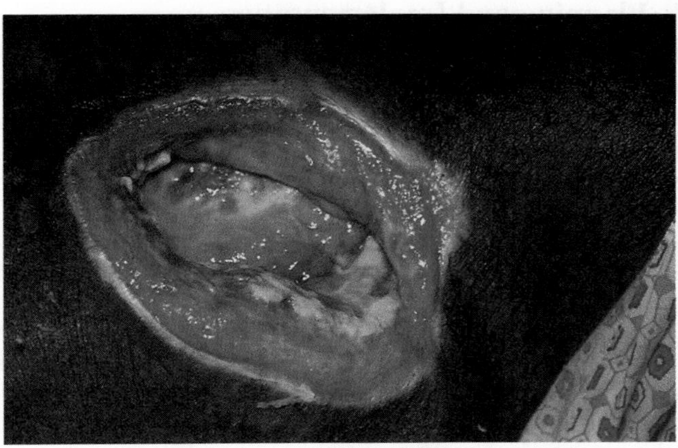

Figure 67-8 ● A stage IV pressure ulcer.

After ischemia has occurred, continued pressure over the area of injury results in the progression of tissue destruction from the deep tissue layers toward the surface. This "hidden" wound may first appear as a small opening in the skin through which purulent drainage exudes. If such an opening is observed, the nurse uses a cotton-tipped applicator to probe gently for a much larger pocket of necrotic tissue beneath the opening.

PSYCHOSOCIAL ASSESSMENT

The client with one or more pressure ulcers may have an altered body image. Ineffective coping patterns emerge as the client and family or significant others strive to comply with changes in lifestyle that are necessary to facilitate healing. In addition, chronic, slow-healing ulcers are often painful and costly to treat.

The nurse assesses the client's and family's or significant others' knowledge of the treatment goals at each stage of the healing process, as well as compliance with the prescribed treatment regimen. The client's skills in cleaning the wound and applying a dressing are assessed as well. Noncompliance with pressure ulcer care procedures may reflect an inability to accept the diagnosis or to cope with the pain, cost, or potential scarring associated with prolonged healing. Depending on his or her activity level and the location of the ulcer, the client may need the assistance of a family member or home care nurse to care adequately for the pressure ulcer at home.

The nurse explores with the client specific changes in activities of daily living (ADLs) that are needed to relieve pressure and promote healing. Increased activity is promoted whenever possible to enhance circulation to the affected tissue. Frequent bedrest with elevation of the legs may be necessary for healing when ulcers occur on the lower legs, particularly in the client with venous insufficiency and lower leg edema. When the client is bedridden, frequent repositioning to relieve pressure (every 2 hours in bed; every 1 hour in a chair) can be labor intensive. In the home environment, repositioning, incontinence management, and dressing changes are often required around the clock, disrupting family routines and contributing to stress.

TABLE 67-4 • TYPES OF WOUND EXUDATE

Characteristics	Significance
SEROSANGUINEOUS EXUDATE	
Blood-tinged amber fluid consisting of serum and red blood cells	Normal for first 48 hr after injury Sudden increase in amount precedes wound dehiscence in wounds closed by first intention
PURULENT EXUDATE	
Creamy yellow pus	Colonization with *Staphylococcus*
Greenish-blue pus, causing staining of dressings and accompanied by a "fruity" odor	Colonization with *Pseudomonas*
Beige pus with a "fishy" odor	Colonization with *Proteus*
Brownish pus with a "fecal" odor	Colonization with aerobic coliform and *Bacteroides* (usually occurs after intestinal surgery)

LABORATORY ASSESSMENT

A wound that is exposed is always *contaminated* but not always *infected.* **Contamination** is the presence of microorganisms without any clinical manifestation of infection. The normal body immune defenses keep the number of bacteria to a minimum and prevent infection. **Wound infection** is contamination with pathogenic microorganisms to the degree that growth and spread cannot be controlled by the body's immune defenses. Wounds that exhibit inflammation, induration, odor, erythema, and moderate to heavy exudate should be evaluated by culture and sensitivity studies for infection to identify the causative microorganism. The presence of pus as exudate alone does not indicate an infection, since pus formation occurs when necrotic tissue debrides and liquifies through autolysis.

If wounds are extensive, if the client is severely immunocompromised, or if local blood supply to the wound is impaired, bacterial growth may exceed the body's ability to defend against invasion into deeper tissue layers. The result is deep wound infection and, eventually, bacteremia and sepsis (systemic infection).

Swab cultures are helpful only in identifying the types of bacteria present on the ulcer surface and may be misleading when trying to identify or quantify bacteria in the underlying tissues. Tests such as quantitative wound biopsies allow the numbers of bacteria to be analyzed. Unfortunately, these tests are time consuming, costly, and unavailable in many medical laboratories. Therefore the clinical indicators of infection—cellulitis, progressive increase in ulcer size or depth, changes in the quantity and quality of exudate, and systemic signs of bacteremia—are important criteria in the diagnosis and subsequent treatment of an infection.

OTHER DIAGNOSTIC ASSESSMENT

Any additional laboratory studies are performed on the basis of the suspected cause of the wound. For pressure ulcers to show progress toward healing, the underlying factors contributing to delayed healing must be diagnosed and treated. For example, noninvasive and invasive arterial blood flow studies are indicated if arterial occlusion is suspected in delayed healing of a pressure ulcer on the heel or ankle. Similarly, blood tests to establish specific nutritional deficiencies are helpful in treating the debilitated, malnourished client with a pressure ulcer.

> **CRITICAL THINKING CHALLENGE**
>
> The client is a 78-year-old woman admitted preoperatively for a total right hip replacement. She has been donating her own blood for several weeks before the surgery to reduce the need for an unknown donor blood transfusion. This woman is 5 feet tall and weighs 98 pounds. She has some degenerative joint disease in her left hip as well.
>
> - What risk factors does this client have for pressure ulcer development?
> - What additional assessment data should you obtain?
> - What (if any) preoperative interventions could be made to reduce her risk for pressure ulcer formation?
>
> For suggested answer guidelines, go to SIMON http://www.wbsaunders.com/SIMON/Iggy/.

Analysis

COMMON NURSING DIAGNOSES AND COLLABORATIVE PROBLEMS

The most common nursing diagnosis for clients with pressure ulcers is Impaired Skin Integrity related to vascular insufficiency and traumatic circumstances. The most common collaborative problem is Risk for Infection and Wound Extension related to disruption of the skin's protective barrier and impaired local blood supply.

ADDITIONAL NURSING DIAGNOSES AND COLLABORATIVE PROBLEMS

In addition to the common nursing diagnoses and collaborative problems, clients with pressure ulcers may have one or more of the following:

- Acute Pain or Chronic Pain related to skin trauma, wound infection, and wound treatment
- Disturbed Body Image related to loss of skin and altered appearance
- Ineffective Coping related to the chronicity of the ulcer, alteration in body image, and changes in lifestyle required to promote healing
- Imbalanced Nutrition: Less Than Body Requirements related to inadequate intake of calories, protein, vitamins, and minerals
- Ineffective (Peripheral) Tissue Perfusion related to vascular disease and prolonged alterations in fluid volume
- Deficient Knowledge related to lack of information about or unclear explanation of the treatment regimen

Planning and Implementation

IMPAIRED SKIN INTEGRITY

NOC **PLANNING: EXPECTED OUTCOMES.** The client with a pressure ulcer is expected to (1) protect the viable cells on the wound surface until healing is completed; (2) experience complete ulcer healing by second intention as evidenced by granulation, epithelialization, and resolution of wound size; (3) have skin thickness in the expected range in the pressure ulcer area; and (4) not experience the formation of other pressure ulcers.

INTERVENTIONS. Wound care techniques for pressure ulcers vary according to each client's needs and the physician's preference. Although aggressive removal of necrotic tissue by surgical excision may be indicated in a severely immunosuppressed client who is susceptible to a life-threatening wound infection, a nonsurgical approach to ulcer debridement is preferred for an older client who has adequate host defenses but is too ill or debilitated to undergo surgery.

NONSURGICAL MANAGEMENT. NIC interventions for pressure ulcer prevention and management are listed in Chart 67-2. Nonsurgical intervention of pressure ulcers is often left to the discretion of the nurse, who collaborates with the physician to select a method of wound dressing on the basis of the identified goal of wound management.

DRESSINGS. A properly designed dressing can expedite healing by removing unwanted debris from the ulcer surface, protecting exposed viable tissues, and re-establishing a temporary barrier between the body and the environment until ulcer closure is complete. For a client with a draining, necrotic ulcer, the dressing must be designed to remove excessive exudate and loose debris without damaging migrating epithelial cells or newly formed granulation tissue. If necrosis is extensive and the eschar is thick, nonviable (dead) tissue must be surgically or chemically removed before further debridement with dressings will be effective. Depending on the dressing material used, dressings help to remove debris either through mechanical entrapment and detachment of dead tissue or by creating an environment that promotes self-digestion of necrotic material by the bacterial enzymes (Table 67-5).

After all of the nonviable tissue has been removed, protection of any exposed vital structures, such as tendon, bone, and newly formed collagen, becomes a primary objective of pressure ulcer care. The ideal environment for healing by epithelialization and contraction is a clean, *slightly* moist ulcer surface with minimal bacterial colonization. Heavy moisture from an excessively secreting ulcer or a dressing that is too wet can interfere with healing by promoting the growth of microorganisms and causing maceration of healthy tissue. Likewise, if a clean ulcer surface is exposed to air or if highly absorbent dressing materials are used for prolonged periods, the subsequent drying effect can lead to dehydration of viable surface cells, scab formation, or conversion to a deeper injury.

The nurse assesses the ulcer for the presence or absence of nonviable tissue and the quantity of exudate. A dressing material with properties that promote an optimal environment for healing is selected (Table 67-6). For example, a material that does not stick to the wound surface and does not remove fragile epithelial cells when it is changed is the dressing of choice for protecting new tissue. Depending on the amount of drainage, the nurse selects either a hydrophobic or a hydrophilic material:

- A **hydrophobic** (nonabsorbent, waterproof) material is beneficial when the wound is relatively free of drainage and the objective is to protect the ulcer from external contamination, such as urine or feces.
- A **hydrophilic** (absorbent) material draws excessive drainage away from the ulcer surface, preventing maceration.

A variety of synthetic materials with hydrophilic and hydrophobic properties are available. Unlike cotton gauze dressings, these may be left intact for extended periods. Some biologic skin substitutes can also prevent tissue dehydration and promote healing (see Chapter 68). These substances include **homograft** (human cadaver skin), **heterograft** (pigskin), collagen material, amniotic membrane, and cultured human skin cells (epithelium).

The frequency of dressing changes depends on the amount of necrotic material or exudate. Dry gauze dressings are changed when "strike through" occurs or when the outer layer of the dressing first becomes saturated with exudate. Gauze dressings used for debridement, such as those placed on a wound wet, allowed to dry, and then removed, are changed frequently enough to take off any loose debris or exudate, usually every 4 to 6 hours. Synthetic dressings are changed when accumulation of exudate causes the adhesive seal to break and leakage to occur.

Before reapplying any dressing, the nurse gently cleans the ulcer surface with saline or a nontoxic wound cleanser as prescribed. If an antibacterial cleanser is ordered, the nurse dilutes the agent to minimize tissue toxicity and then rinses and dries the surface thoroughly before applying the dressing.

PHYSICAL THERAPY. As an adjunct to the use of dressings for ulcer debridement, the use of daily whirlpool treatments can facilitate mechanical removal of dead tissue. The ulcerated area is immersed in warm tap water to which an antibacterial cleansing agent has been added. Continuous agitation of the water mechanically loosens the debris and washes away exudate and particulate matter. During treatment, the ulcer surface is cleaned with a gauze pad. After treatment, the therapist or certified wound specialists often uses instruments to trim away any obvious bits of dead tissue that are still loosely attached to the ulcer surface.

DRUG THERAPY. Clean, healthy granulation tissue is vascular and capable of providing white blood cells and antibodies to the ulcer surface to combat infection. However, if extensive necrosis is present or local tissue defenses are impaired, topical antibacterial agents are often needed to control bacterial growth. (Chapter 68 details the advantages and uses of topical antimicrobial agents.) In the absence of established ulcer infection, prophylactic antibiotics are usually avoided because of the danger of the development of resistant strains of bacteria.

DIET THERAPY. Successful healing of pressure ulcers depends on adequate nutritional stores of calories, protein, vitamins, minerals, and water. Nutritional deficiencies are common among older adults and chronically ill clients. Such deficiencies contribute to an increased risk of skin breakdown

TABLE 67-5 • COMMON DRESSING TECHNIQUES FOR WOUND DEBRIDEMENT

Technique	Mechanism of Action
Wet-to-dry saline-moistened gauze	Dry, necrotic debris is softened by the saline, allowing it to become more effectively entrapped in the interstices as the gauze dries and shrinks. Dressing may also entrap healing tissue.
Wet-to-damp saline-moistened gauze	As with the wet-to-dry technique, necrotic debris is mechanically removed, but with less trauma to healing tissue.
Continuous wet gauze	The wound surface is continually bathed with a wetting agent of choice, promoting dilution of viscous exudate and softening of dry eschar.
Topical enzyme preparations	Proteolytic action on thick, adherent eschar causes breakdown of denatured protein and more rapid separation of necrotic tissue.
Moisture-retentive dressing	Spontaneous separation of necrotic tissue is promoted by autolysis.

TABLE 67-6 • COMMONLY USED DRESSING MATERIALS

	Alginates	Biologic Dressings	Cotton Gauze Dressing	Foams	Hydrocolloidal Wafers	Hydrogel Dressing	Transparent Films
Indications	Absorption Protection	Debridement after eschar removal* Protection Test before skin grafts (pigskin and cadaver skin) Burns Dormant, nonhealing wounds that do not respond to other topical therapies	***Continuous Dry*** Absorption Protection (nonadherent contact layer) ***Continuous Wet*** Delivery of topical agent Debridement (autolysis) Protection ***Wet to Damp*** Atraumatic mechanical debridement ***Wet to Dry*** Aggressive mechanical debridement	Absorption Protection	Debridement* Absorption Protection	Debridement* Absorption Protection	Debridement* Protection (partial-thickness lesions) Secondary (cover) dressing
Advantages	Highly absorbent Biodegradable Easy application Nonadhesive Can be used as packing for deep wounds Can be used for infected wounds	Most "natural" wound covering Reduces pain Conforms to uneven wound surfaces Acts as a catalyst for healing Alternative to autograft	Readily available Good mechanical debridement *if used properly* Effective delivery of topical agents	Absorbent Insulates wound Easy application Nonadhesive (most products) Conforms to uneven wound surfaces	Absorbent Excludes bacteria Waterproof Reduces pain Easy application Easy to store	Absorbent Nonadhesive Reduces pain Conducive to use with topical agents Conforms to uneven wound surfaces Amorphous form can be used as a filler Easy to store	Wound visualization Good adhesion Waterproof Reduces pain Cost-effective Easy to store
Disadvantages	Requires secondary dressing to secure Can cause desiccation of tissue if drainage is minimal	Requires secondary dressing to secure Very expensive Skin substitutes require skill to apply	Delayed healing if used improperly Pain on removal Requires frequent dressing changes	Poor barrier function Requires secondary dressing to secure	Nontransparent Softening and loss of shape with pressure, heat, and friction Odor with dressing removal Expensive Requires use of "fillers" for deep, draining lesions	Poor barrier function Only partial wound visualization Requires secondary dressing to secure Can promote growth of *Pseudomonas* and other microorganisms	Difficult to apply properly Nonabsorbent Adhesive to normal and healing tissue Limited to superficial lesions
Dressing changes	When dressing is saturated (q3-5 days) or more frequently	Topical growth factors: Daily skin substitutes: Varies (similar to grafts)	Necrotic base: q4-6h Clean base: q12-24h	When dressing is saturated or more frequently	Necrotic base: q24h Clean base: on leakage of exudate	Necrotic base: q6-8h Clean base: q24h	Necrotic base: q24h Clean base: on leakage of exudate

*Use with caution in patients with leukopenia or vascular disease.

and delayed healing of wounds already present (see Nutritional Status, p. 1521). Severe protein deficiency inhibits all stages of the healing process and impairs local host defenses against bacterial invasion.

To promote healing, the nurse encourages the client to eat a well-balanced diet, emphasizing foods containing nutrients vital to epidermal proliferation and collagen synthesis (Table 67-7). If the client cannot eat sufficient amounts of food, nasogastric feedings and hyperalimentation via a central venous catheter may be needed to increase protein and caloric intake. Vitamin and mineral supplements also are indicated.

SURGICAL MANAGEMENT. Surgical management of a pressure ulcer includes sharp debridement of nonviable tissue and skin grafting to re-establish skin integrity in wounds that cannot heal by epithelialization and contraction.

TABLE 67-7 • FOODS THAT PROMOTE WOUND HEALING

Food	Function
PROTEIN SOURCES	
Meat	Maintenance and healing of body tissues
Fish	
Poultry	Antibody production
Milk	Energy
Cheese	
Eggs	
Soybeans	
Legumes	
Nuts	
Nutritional supplements	
CARBOHYDRATE SOURCES	
Whole grains (preferable to enriched because of higher nutritional and fiber content)	Energy
Enriched grain and cereal products	Sparing of protein (if diet does not contain sufficient nonprotein calories, protein from body tissues will be broken down to supply energy)
Fruit	
Juices	
Vegetables (especially starchy ones: corn, peas, potatoes)	Wound healing
Milk	
Desserts and sweets	
SOURCES OF VITAMIN C	
Berries	Collagen synthesis
Broccoli	Immunity
Brussels sprouts	
Cabbage	
Citrus fruits and juices	
Green peppers	
Kale	
Melons	
Spinach and dark green vegetables	
Tomatoes	
Vitamin C–enriched juices	
ZINC SOURCES	
Same as protein sources	Tissue repair (zinc-deficient diet causes poor wound healing, decreased ability to taste, and poor appetite)
Beef	
Organ meat	
Shellfish	
Salmon	
Poultry	
Cheese	Protein synthesis
Whole grains	
Dried beans	
IRON SOURCES*	
Liver	Cellular respiration
Meat	Hemoglobin synthesis
Baked beans	
Dried fruits	
Legumes	
IRON SOURCES*—cont'd	
Eggs	
Dark green leafy vegetables	
Blackstrap molasses	
Whole-grain breads and cereals	
SOURCES OF VITAMIN B_{12}	
Liver	Protein synthesis
Organ meats	
Muscle meats	
Fish	
Eggs	
Shellfish	
Milk	
Yogurt	
Cheese	
SOURCES OF VITAMIN B_6	
Meats	Amino acid metabolism
Liver	
Some vegetables (including potatoes)	
Wheat germ	
Wheat bran	
Whole-grain cereals and breads	
Fish	
Brewer's yeast	
Dried beans	
FOLATE SOURCES	
Liver	Protein synthesis
Yeast	
Leafy vegetables	
Dried beans	
Green vegetables	
Nuts	
Fresh oranges	
Whole-wheat cereals and breads	
WATER SOURCES	
Water	Maintain condition of the skin (dehydration can lead to tissue breakdown, poor appetite, and constipation)
Milk	
Juices	
Gelatin	
Tomatoes	
Citrus fruit	
Melons	
Vegetables	
Berries	
Broths	
Soups	
Tea	
Coffee	
Carbonated beverages	

From Ross, R., & Noe, J. (1983). *Chronic problem wounds.* Boston: Little, Brown & Co.
*Iron cooking utensils add iron to the diet.

PREOPERATIVE CARE. Preoperative care is focused on preparing the ulcer to accept a skin graft. The nurse monitors potential donor sites, taking care to maintain the integrity of the donor skin and to avoid minor injuries that may result in infection and graft loss.

OPERATIVE PROCEDURES. The operative procedures commonly used for surgical management of pressure ulcers include debridement and grafting. One or both of these procedures may be done.

Debridement, or sharp excision of thick, adherent wound eschar using a scalpel or scissors, is sometimes undertaken to hasten the removal of the dead tissue, a potential source of infection. Surgical debridement is indicated for severely immunosuppressed clients or those with large, full-thickness ulcers, because the extensive time required for spontaneous separation of eschar places the client at risk for systemic sepsis or prolonged hospitalization. Depending on the size and depth of the ulcer and the projected blood loss, the surgeon can perform the excision at the bedside, in the treatment room, or in an operating room.

Grafting or autografting is used for wound closure when full-thickness ulcers cannot close by second intention because of the extent of the injury or forces inhibiting contraction and when natural healing results in loss of joint function, an unacceptable cosmetic appearance, or a high potential for wound recurrence. Successful grafting of skin requires a clean and granulating or freshly excised ulcer bed. Partial-thickness (split-thickness) or full-thickness strips of skin are removed from the donor area (Figure 67-9), transferred to the ulcer, and sutured or stapled in place. Full-thickness free grafts and myocutaneous flaps are used to cover deep, massive ulcers or ulcers in which vital structures, such as bone or tendon, are exposed.

Unlike free grafts, a pedicle flap is a full-thickness flap of skin that is raised and rotated to cover the defect, with one edge of the flap still attached to the site of origin to provide a blood supply (Figure 67-10). Because all skin layers are removed, full-thickness donor sites are closed primarily or covered with additional split-thickness skin grafts. Partial-thickness donor sites heal by epithelialization if infection is avoided.

POSTOPERATIVE CARE. Postoperative graft sites are immobilized with bulky cotton pressure dressings for 3 to 5 days to allow vascularization, or "take," of the newly grafted skin. The nurse does not disturb the dressing and encourages elevation and complete rest of the grafted area. Any activity that might cause movement of the dressing against the body and separation of the graft from the wound is prohibited.

After dressings are removed, the nurse monitors the graft for indications of failure to vascularize—nonadherence to the wound or graft necrosis. If a pedicle flap has been used to cover the wound, the nurse inspects the edges of the flap frequently for changes in color. A pale flap with delayed capillary filling when blanched may have inadequate arterial perfusion. A dusky color or sharp line of color demarcation suggests inadequate venous or lymphatic drainage. Other techniques to monitor trends of blood flow in the graft, depending on the graft's location, include pulse oximetry, Doppler ultrasonography, and transcutaneous oxygen determination.

Postoperative care of donor sites aims to protect the area from injury and infection until healing can occur and to promote comfort. The client usually returns from surgery with a pressure dressing in place over the donor area to promote hemostasis. After 24 to 48 hours, this outer dressing is removed, revealing a single wound contact layer of fine-mesh gauze or synthetic mesh material.

If the donor site is treated with dry exposure, the nurse promotes air circulation to the wound by positioning the client to avoid pressure on the site and using an overbed cradle to tent the sheets. In the rare instance when heat lamps are ordered, the nurse places the 60- to 100-watt bulb at least 2 feet from the wound to prevent thermal injury to the skin. After the dressing has dried and formed a "scab," the wound is kept dry and left undisturbed until healing is evident (at 10 to 14 days). As the donor site heals, the gauze and dried blood lift away from the new epithelium beneath. Trimming the separating gauze close to the skin surface minimizes the chance of the client's catching the loose end of the dressing on an object and removing the still adherent gauze before healing is complete. Today, most surgeons prefer to dress donor sites with moisture-retentive dressings, such as synthetic transparent films, instead of the traditional dry exposure method of treatment (see Table 67-6).

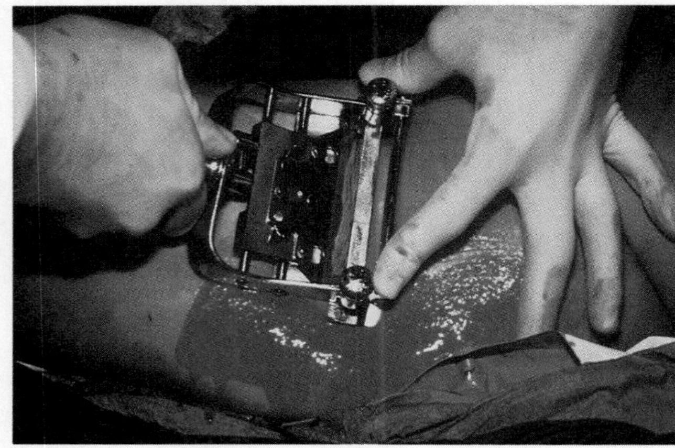

Figure 67-9 ● Removal of a partial-thickness (split-thickness) skin graft.

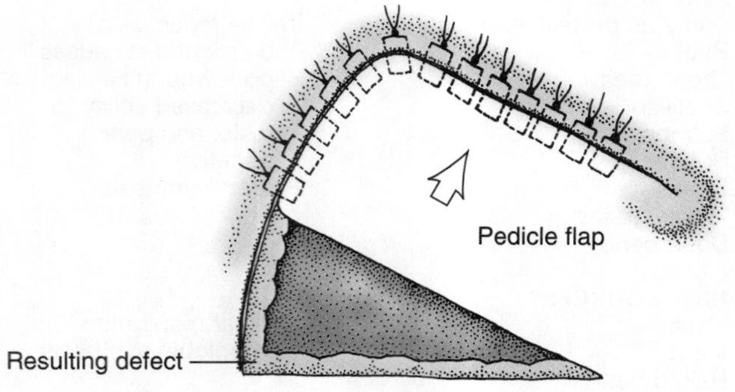

Figure 67-10 ● A full-thickness pedicle flap of skin is separated and rotated to cover the wound. Blood vessels are left intact. The resultant defect is either primarily closed or covered with skin grafts. The flap is held in place with staples or sutures.

Because exposed donor sites are initially more painful than graft sites, pain medication is administered as ordered and other comfort measures are provided as needed. The client is repositioned during the immediate postoperative period to promote comfort only if movement of the graft site can be avoided. The nurse may offer back rubs to help relieve muscle spasms that occur with bedrest and immobility. Attention must also be paid to relieving pressure over unaffected bony prominences that may lead to additional ulcers.

Graft and donor sites involving the posterior body surfaces present a particular problem. For the graft or flap to become fully vascularized or for the donor sites to dry, the client must be immobilized in a side-lying or prone position for 7 to 10 days.

An alternative to difficult positioning is the use of special low-pressure or air-fluidized beds, which not only minimize ischemia of the graft or flap while the client is supine but also help prevent breakdown of intact skin. A major limitation to the use of these beds is cost, which is usually outweighed by the potential for decreased morbidity and length of hospital stay.

RISK FOR INFECTION AND WOUND EXTENSION

PLANNING: EXPECTED OUTCOMES. The client with a pressure ulcer is expected to remain free of wound infection or systemic sepsis and to experience healing of the pressure ulcer.

INTERVENTIONS. Because of the many intrinsic factors that can affect a client's resistance to infection, the nurse closely monitors the ulcer's progress so that timely treatment with topical and systemic antibiotics can be initiated if ulcer deterioration occurs. Steps are taken to minimize introduction of pathogenic organisms to the ulcer through direct contact.

MONITORING ULCER PROGRESS. Frequent monitoring of the ulcer's appearance using objective criteria allows the nurse to evaluate response to treatment and recognize early signs of impending infection. If an ulcer shows no progress toward healing within 3 weeks, the treatment plan should be re-evaluated. Table 67-8 outlines objectives of local infection for wounds with and without tissue loss. Clients who are at highest risk for infection may have a reduced inflammatory response to infection. These clients include those who are older, have white blood cell disorders, are receiving steroid therapy, or have wounds with a compromised blood supply.

PREVENTION OF INFECTION AND WOUND EXTENSION. Complications of infection and wound extension are avoided by diligent monitoring of the ulcer's progress and by prevention of new ulcer formation. The nurse reports the following signs to the physician:

- Sudden deterioration of the ulcer, as evidenced by an increase in the size or depth of the lesion
- Changes in the color or texture of the granulation tissue
- Changes in the quantity, color, or odor of exudate

The nurse also remains alert for the classic signs of wound infection: increased erythema, edema, purulent and malodorous drainage, and tenderness of the wound margins, which may or may not be accompanied by clinical signs of bacteremia, such as fever, an elevated white blood cell count, and positive blood cultures. The nurse uses appropriate interventions to prevent the formation of new pressure ulcers and to prevent early-stage ulcers from progressing to deeper wounds (Chart 67-4; see also Chart 67-2).

MAINTAINING A SAFE ENVIRONMENT. Because of the variety of microorganisms in the hospital environment, keeping an ulcer totally free of bacteria is impossible. Optimal ulcer management is based on maintaining acceptably low levels of microorganisms through meticulous local wound care and minimizing contamination with pathogenic organisms. The nurse and assistive nursing personnel use standard precautions to prevent direct contact with ulcer secretions and cross-contamination among clients. All health care providers and assistive nursing personnel practice thorough handwashing before and after dressing changes and properly dispose of soiled dressings and linens.

Community-Based Care

Clients with pressure ulcers may be in acute care, subacute care, long-term care, or home care settings. If pressure ulcer therapy requires hospitalization, most clients with pressure ulcers are discharged before complete wound closure is obtained. Discharge may be to the home setting or to a long-term care facility, depending on the degree of debilitation and other client factors.

HEALTH TEACHING

Before the client is discharged, the client or family member or significant other who will be performing the wound care should demonstrate facility in removing the dressing, cleaning the wound, and applying the dressing. When choosing a dressing to be used at home, the nurse considers the client's or caregiver's ability to apply the dressing properly. If the client's finances are limited, the nurse also addresses the cost of the dressing material. Some dressings may be easier to apply and less expensive than other materials. At times, the more expensive dressing materials that require less frequent changing may be preferred. The nurse explains the signs and symptoms of wound infection.

The nurse encourages the client to eat a balanced diet with frequent high-protein snacks. The nurse discusses diet preferences with the client and suggests foods that promote wound healing (see Table 67-7). The physician may order vitamin and mineral supplements if there are dietary deficiencies.

If the client is incontinent, the nurse emphasizes the need to keep the skin clean and dry. If bowel and bladder training is not possible, the use of absorbent underpads, briefs, and topical moisture barrier creams and ointments is discussed as a method to reduce skin exposure to urine and feces.

HOME CARE MANAGEMENT

Care of the ulcer in the client's home is similar to care in the hospital. Most dressing supplies and pressure relief devices can be easily obtained at the local pharmacy or medical supply store. If mechanical debridement of the ulcer is still needed, a handheld shower device or forceful irrigation of the

TABLE 67-8 • MONITORING THE WOUND

Variable	Frequency of Assessment	Rationale
WOUNDS WITHOUT TISSUE LOSS		
Examples		
Surgical incisions and clean lacerations closed primarily by sutures or staples		
Observations (Using First Postoperative Dressing Change as Baseline)		
Check for the presence or absence of increased: • Localized tenderness • Swelling of the incision line • Erythema of the incision line >1 cm on each side of wound • Localized heat	At least every 24 hr until sutures or staples are removed	To detect cellulitis (bacterial infections)*
Check for the presence or absence of: • Purulent drainage from any portion of the incision site • Localized fluctuance (from fluid accumulation) and tenderness beneath a *portion* of the wound when palpated	At least every 24 hr until sutures or staples are removed	To detect abscess formation related to presence of foreign body (suture material) or deeper wound infection*
Check for the presence or absence of approximation (sealing) of wound edges with or without serosanguineous drainage.	At least every 24 hr until sutures or staples are removed	To detect potential for wound dehiscence
WOUNDS WITH TISSUE LOSS		
Examples		
Partial- or full-thickness skin loss caused by pressure necrosis, vascular disease, trauma, etc., and allowed to heal by secondary intention		
Observations		
Wound Size		
Measure wound size at greatest length and width using a metric ruler or, for asymmetric ulcers, by tracing the wound onto a piece of plastic film or sheeting (plastic template). Compare all subsequent measurements against the initial measurement.	At least every week	To detect increase in wound size and depth secondary to infectious process
Ulcer Base		
Check for the presence or absence of: • Necrotic tissue (loose or adherent) • Presence or absence of foul odor from wound when dressing is changed Note the frequency of dressing changes or dressing reinforcements owing to drainage.	At least every 24 hr	To detect the need for debridement or the response to treatment (necrotic tissue) and to detect local wound infection (frequent dressing changes and foul odor)
Wound Margins		
Check for the presence or absence of: • Erythema and swelling extending outward >1 cm from wound margins • Increased tenderness at wound margins	At least every 24 hr or at each dressing change	To detect wound infection*
Systemic Response		
Check for the presence or absence of elevated body temperature, WBCs, or positive blood culture	As needed	To detect bacteremia

WBCs, White blood cells.
*The wounds of clients who are severely immunosuppressed or those wounds with compromised blood supply may not exhibit a typical inflammatory response to local wound infection.

wound with a 35-mL syringe and 19-gauge angiocatheter can be substituted for whirlpool therapy.

Clients with chronic pressure ulcers are often depressed about their debilitated state, which may affect their compliance with wound care measures. Many clients cannot change their own dressings because of distress over an altered body image or the pain experienced with dressing removal. Others are totally dependent on family members or significant others or support personnel because of limited physical mobility or inability to reach the wound.

For some clients, drastic changes in daily activities are necessary to promote healing. Clients with pressure ulcers on the lower extremities may need frequent rest periods with leg elevation to minimize edema. Immobile clients with pressure ulcers require around-the-clock repositioning as often as every 2 to 4 hours to prevent further breakdown, which takes

CHART 67-4

BEST PRACTICE *for* Preventing Pressure Ulcers

Positioning

- Pad contact surfaces with foam, silicon gel, or air pads.
- Do not keep the head of the bed elevated above 30 degrees.
- Use a lift sheet to move client in the bed. Avoid dragging or sliding the client.
- When positioning a client on his or her side, do not position directly on the trochanter.
- Reposition an immobile client every 2 hours while in bed and every 1 hour while sitting in a chair.
- Do not place a rubber ring or doughnut under the client's sacral area.
- When moving an immobile client from a bed to another surface, use a designated slide board well lubricated with talc.
- Place pillows or foam wedges between two bony surfaces.
- Keep the client's skin directly off plastic surfaces.
- Keep the client's heels off the bed surface.

Nutrition

- Ensure a fluid intake between 2000 and 3000 mL/day.
- Help the client maintain an adequate intake of protein and calories.

Skin Care

- Use moisturizers daily on dry skin, and apply when skin is damp.
- Keep moisture from prolonged contact with skin.
  - Dry areas where two skin surfaces touch, such as the axilla and under the breasts.
  - Place absorbent pads under areas where perspiration collects.
  - Use moisture barriers on skin areas where wound drainage or incontinence occurs.
- Do not massage bony prominences.
- Humidify the room.

Skin Cleaning

- Clean the skin as soon as possible after soiling occurs and at routine intervals.
- Use a mild, heavily fatted soap.
- Use tepid rather than hot water.
- While cleaning, use the minimal scrubbing force necessary to remove soil.
- Gently pat rather than rub the skin dry.

its toll on family members or caregivers. The nurse explains the rationale for activity changes to the client and family or significant others and explores alternative ways of coping with these changes.

HEALTH CARE RESOURCES

A home care nurse may be needed to follow wound progress after the client is discharged. The hospital nurse provides details of ulcer size and appearance and any special wound care needs to the nurse in the home, who can then accurately judge changes in ulcer appearance. Chart 67-5 provides a guideline for focused assessment of the client with pressure ulcers.

To minimize waste and to help decrease the overall cost of treatment, the nurse emphasizes proper use of dressing materials. Clean tap water and nonsterile supplies are acceptable for treatment of chronic wounds in the home and are less costly than sterile products. Nonsterile dressing materials can often be purchased in bulk from a local medical supply store at reduced cost.

CHART 67-5

FOCUSED ASSESSMENT *of* Home Care Clients at Risk for Pressure Ulcer

Assess cardiovascular status:
- Presence or absence of peripheral edema
- Hand vein filling in the dependent position
- Neck vein filling in the recumbent and sitting positions
- Weight gain or loss

Assess cognition and mental status:
- Level of consciousness
- Orientation to time, place, and person
- Can the client accurately read a seven-word sentence containing no words greater than three syllables?

Assess condition of skin:
- Assess general skin cleanliness.
- Observe all skin areas, paying particular attention to bony prominences and those areas in greatest contact with the bed and other firm surfaces.
- Measure and record any areas of redness or loss of integrity.
- If possible, photograph areas of concern.
- Note presence or absence of skin tenting over the sternum or the forehead.
- Note moistness of skin and mucous membranes.
- If wounds are present, remove dressings (noting condition of dressings), cleanse the wound, and compare with previous notations of wound condition.
  - Presence, amount, and nature of exudate
  - Use a ruler to measure wound diameter and depth
  - Amount (%) and type of necrotic tissue
  - Presence of granulation/epithelium
  - Presence or absence of cellulitis
  - Presence or absence of odor

Take client's temperature.

Assess client's understanding of illness and compliance with treatment:
- Signs and symptoms to report to health care provider
- Mediation plan (correct timing and dose)
- Ambulation or positioning schedule
- Dressing changes/skin care
- Diet modifications (24-hour diet recall)

Assess client's nutritional status:
- Change in muscle mass
- Lackluster nails, sparse hair
- Recent weight loss >10% of usual weight
- Impaired oral intake
- Difficulty swallowing
- Generalized edema

The client with activity restrictions may require daily assistance from a home care aide. Consultation with a physical therapist may be appropriate to help the client and family or significant others continue rehabilitation efforts in the home.

CRITICAL THINKING CHALLENGE

In spite of preventive care, the client who had a hip replacement is being discharged to an extended care facility with a stage I pressure ulcer on her coccyx.

- What should you teach this client regarding ways to prevent extension of this ulcer?
- What information should be communicated to the new facility?
- Is there anything else you can think of to do to help this client when she leaves your unit?

For suggested answer guidelines, go to SIMON http://www.wbsaunders.com/SIMON/Iggy/.

Evaluation: Outcomes

NOC The nurse evaluates the care of the client with a pressure ulcer on the basis of the identified nursing diagnoses and collaborative problems. The expected outcomes include that the client will:

- Demonstrate skills necessary to care for the wound in the home environment
- Incorporate modifications of lifestyle related to promotion of healing in activities of daily living (ADLs)
- List the signs and symptoms of wound infection
- Make the necessary changes in dietary intake to correct any nutritional deficiencies
- Demonstrate an understanding of measures needed to prevent future episodes of skin breakdown and pressure ulcer formation
- Experience wound healing by secondary intention as evidenced by granulation, epithelialization, and resolution of wound size
- Develop skin thickness in expected range at ulcer area
- Remain tissue lesion free

COMMON INFECTIONS

OVERVIEW

Bacterial Infections

Bacterial skin lesions usually start at the hair follicle, where bacteria easily accumulate and grow in the warm, moist environment. **Folliculitis** is a superficial infection involving only the upper portion of the follicle and is usually caused by *Staphylococcus* (Figure 67-11). **Furuncles** (boils) are also caused by *Staphylococcus,* but the infection is much deeper in the follicle (Figure 67-12). **Cellulitis** is a generalized nonfollicular infection with either *Staphylococcus* or *Streptococcus* and involves the deeper connective tissue.

Minor skin trauma usually precedes the appearance of folliculitis and furuncles and may or may not be associated with the development of cellulitis. Clients may spread the infection to other parts of their bodies by scratching or rubbing the skin with fingernails that have microorganisms under them. Furuncles are more likely to occur in the presence of heat and moisture, such as in the hair-bearing skin fold areas. Cellulitis can occur as a result of secondary bacterial infection of an open wound, or it may be unrelated to skin trauma.

Viral Infections

HERPES SIMPLEX VIRUS

Herpes simplex virus (HSV) infection is the most common viral infection of adult skin. HSV infections are of two types. Type 1 (HSV 1) infections cause the classic recurring cold sore. The severity of the disease increases with age and immunosuppression. Genital herpes, caused by type 2 infection (HSV 2), is also recurrent (see Chapter 77).

After a primary infection, the virus remains in the body in a dormant state in the nerve ganglia, and the client is asymptomatic. Reactivation of the infection stimulates the virus to travel the pathway of sensory nerves to the skin, where lesions reappear. In healthy people, recurrence of HSV infection is triggered by physical or psychologic stressors, such as sunburn, trauma, fever, menses, and fatigue. The virus can also be spread by direct contact between an actively infected person and a susceptible host. *Autoinoculation,* or transfer of either viral type from one part of the body to another, is also possible.

The time span between episodes and the severity of individual attacks varies. Outbreaks of oral herpes simplex usually last 3 to 10 days, and active shedding of the virus and contagion are possible for the first 3 to 5 days. The client may experience tingling or burning of the lip before any lesion is evident.

The most common clinical presentation of HSV 1 infection is isolated or grouped vesicles on an erythematous base (Figure 67-13). The infection can occur anywhere on the skin and may be spread by respiratory droplets or by direct contact with an active lesion or virus-containing fluid (such as saliva).

Herpetic whitlow is a form of herpes simplex infection occurring on the fingertips of medical personnel who have come in contact with viral secretions. This form of herpes is a potential source of client inoculation. Immunosuppressed clients are at a particular risk for severe and persistent eruptions that can lead to life-threatening complications.

HERPES ZOSTER

Herpes zoster (shingles) is caused by reactivation of the latent varicella-zoster virus in clients who have previously had chickenpox. The dormant virus resides in the dorsal root ganglia of the sensory cranial and spinal nerves. The individual lesions of herpes zoster infections are similar to those of herpes simplex, but they have a different distribution pattern (Figure

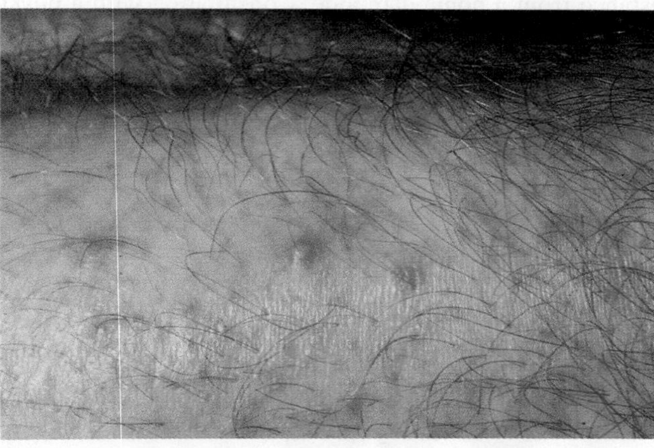

Figure 67-11 ● Folliculitis.

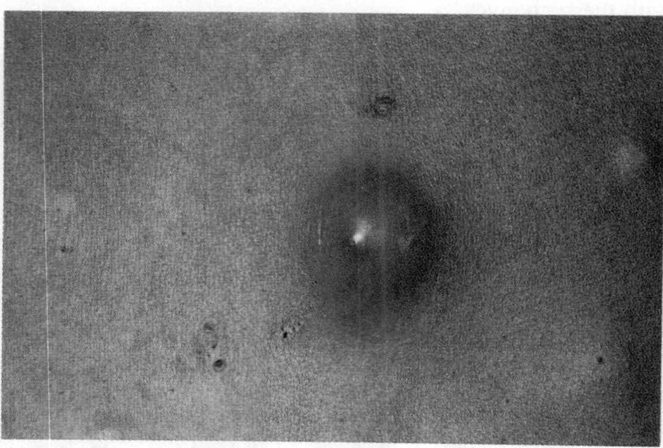

Figure 67-12 ● A furuncle.

67-14). Multiple lesions occur in a segmental distribution on the skin area innervated by the infected nerve. Herpes zoster eruptions are preceded by several days of discomfort, which may vary from minor irritation and itching to severe, deep pain. The course of eruption usually lasts several weeks. **Postherpetic neuralgia,** pain persisting after the lesions have resolved, is a common complication in older clients.

Herpes zoster is essentially a disease of immunosuppression, occurring with increased frequency and severity in older people or in anyone who is immunosuppressed for any reason. Dissemination of the virus can be accompanied by fever and malaise, often progressing to visceral involvement. Herpes zoster is contagious to people who have not been previously exposed to chickenpox.

Complications can include full-thickness skin necrosis, Bell's palsy, or ophthalmic infection and scarring if the virus is introduced into the eye.

Fungal Infections

Superficial fungal (dermatophyte) infections can differ in lesion appearance, anatomic location, and species of the infecting organism. The term *tinea* is used to describe dermatophytoses. Table 67-9 lists the corresponding anatomic locations of the various categories of infection.

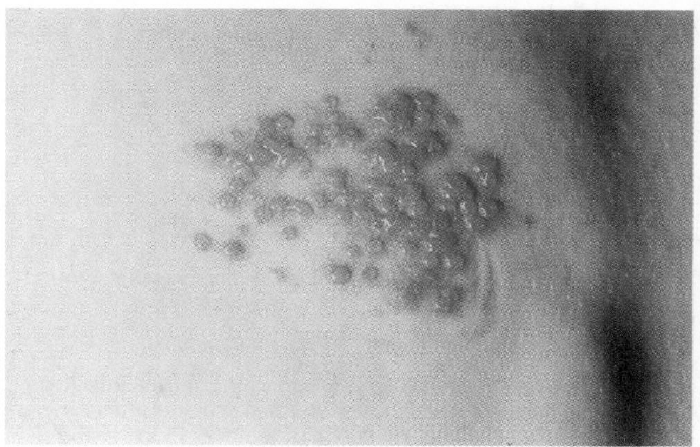

Figure 67-13 ● Herpes simplex.

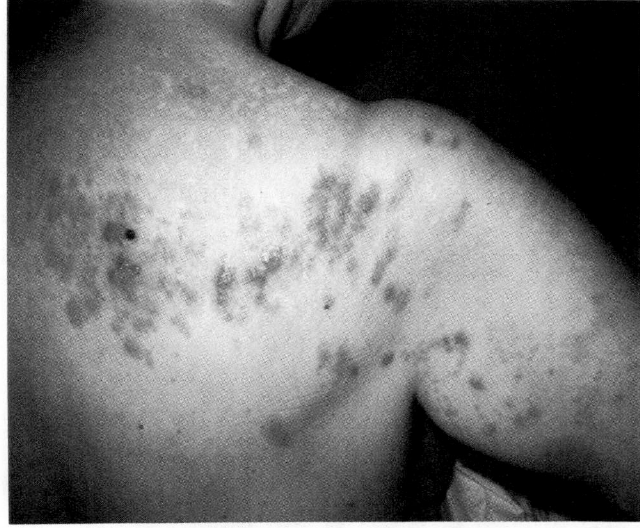

Figure 67-14 ● Herpes zoster.

Depending on the species, dermatophytes reside mainly in the soil, on animals, and on humans. Superficial infection can start only if suitable conditions exist for inoculation and maintenance of the organism in the outer layers of the skin.

Dermatophyte infections occur when the infecting organism comes in contact with an impaired skin surface in a susceptible host. Most infections are spread by direct contact with infected humans or animals. Certain types of dermatophytoses, such as tinea capitis and tinea corporis, can be transmitted by means of inanimate objects. For example, tinea capitis is associated with poor personal hygiene and the subsequent sharing of contaminated combs, brushes, hats, pillowcases, and similar objects.

COLLABORATIVE MANAGEMENT

Assessment

HISTORY

The clinical manifestations of the skin infection provide direction for collection of data to confirm a suspected diagnosis. To differentiate among the possible causes of the lesions, the nurse concentrates on risk factors associated with each type of infection. If the location and appearance of lesions suggest a bacterial infection, the nurse explores any recent history of skin trauma, as well as past or current staphylococcal or streptococcal infections. Associated symptoms of fever and malaise are also noted.

Lesions appearing on the lips, in the oral cavity, or in the genital region alert the nurse to a possible viral infection. The nurse seeks information about the following:

- A history of similar lesions in the same location
- Signs of burning, tingling, or pain
- Recent stress factors that may have precipitated the outbreak
- Recent contact with an infected person

Acknowledgment by the client of the recurrent nature of the lesions is often important in helping to differentiate viral from bacterial lesions. If herpes zoster is suspected, the nurse confirms *previous exposure to chickenpox* and asks whether the client has a history of shingles.

The type of information asked of a client with probable dermatophyte infection depends on the anatomic location of the lesions. The presence of tinea corporis and tinea capitis requires further assessment of social and environmental factors that may have contributed to inoculation, such as direct contact with an infected person, poor personal hygiene practices, or frequent contact with animals. If tinea cruris and tinea

TABLE 67-9 • TINEA INFECTIONS

Infection	Location
Tinea pedis	Feet (athlete's foot)
Tinea manus	Hands
Tinea cruris	Groin (jock itch)
Tinea corporis	Smooth skin surfaces (ringworm)
Tinea capitis	Scalp
Tinea barbae	Beard

pedis are suspected, the nurse asks the client about the type and frequency of athletic activities.

PHYSICAL ASSESSMENT/CLINICAL MANIFESTATIONS

Because most skin infections are contagious, the nurse takes necessary precautions to prevent the spread of infection when performing a physical assessment. Chart 67-6 lists the clinical manifestations of common skin infections.

LABORATORY ASSESSMENT

When pustules are present in bacterial infections, the infecting organism is confirmed by swab culture of the purulent material. Blood cultures may be helpful, especially if the client is showing clinical signs of bacteremia.

Viral infections are confirmed by *Tzanck's smear* and viral culture. **Tzanck's smear** is a cytologic examination in which cells from the base of a lesion are examined under a microscope. The presence of multinucleated giant cells confirms a viral infection.

CHART 67-6

KEY FEATURES *of* Common Skin Infections

Clinical Manifestations	Distribution
Bacterial Infections	
Folliculitis	
Isolated erythematous pustules occur singly or in groups; hairs grow from centers of many of the lesions. Occasional papules are present. There is little or no associated discomfort. There is no residual scarring.	Areas of hair-bearing skin, especially buttocks, thighs, beard area, and scalp
Furuncle	
Small, tender erythematous nodules become pus filled and more tender over time. Lesions may be single or multiple and also recurrent. Regional lymphadenopathy is sometimes present; fever is rare. Occasional scarring results.	Areas of hair-bearing skin, especially buttocks, thighs, abdomen, posterior neck regions, and axillae
Cellulitis	
Localized area of inflammation may enlarge rapidly if not treated. Redness, warmth, edema, tenderness, and pain are present. On rare occasions, blisters are present. Cellulitis is often accompanied by lymphadenopathy and fever.	Lower legs, areas of persistent lymphedema, and areas of skin trauma (leg ulcer, puncture wound, and so forth)
Viral Infections	
Herpes Simplex	
Grouped vesicles are present on an erythematous base. Vesicles evolve to pustules, which rupture, weep, and crust. Older lesions may appear as punched-out, shallow erosions with well-defined borders. Lesions are associated with itching, stinging, or pain. Secondary bacterial infection with necrosis is possible in immunocompromised clients.	Type 1 classically on the face and type 2 on the genitalia, but either may develop in any area where inoculation has occurred; recurrent infections occur repeatedly in the same skin area
Herpes Zoster	
Lesions are similar in appearance to herpes simplex and also progress with weeping and crusting. Grouped lesions present unilaterally along a segment of skin following the pathway of a spinal or cranial nerve (dermatomal distribution). Eruption is preceded by deep pain and itching. Postherpetic neuralgia is common in older adults. Secondary infection with necrosis is possible in immunocompromised clients.	Anterior or posterior trunk following involved dermatome; face, sometimes involving trigeminal nerve and eye
Fungal Infections	
Dermatophytosis	
Annular or serpiginous patches are present with elevated borders, scaling, and central clearing. Pruritus is common. Lesions may be single or multiple.	Anywhere on the body
Candidiasis	
Erythematous macular eruption occurs with isolated pustules or papules at the border (satellite lesions). Candidiasis is associated with burning and itching. Oral lesions (thrush) appear as creamy white plaques on an inflamed mucous membrane.	Skin fold areas: perineal and perianal region, axillae, beneath breasts, and between the fingers; under wet or occlusive dressings
Cracks or fissures at the corners of the mouth may be present.	Lesions possibly present on the oral or vaginal mucous membranes

Fungal infections are confirmed by a potassium hydroxide (KOH) test. Scrapings of scales from the lesions are obtained and, after preparation with KOH, examined under a microscope. The presence of fungal hyphae confirms the diagnosis. In addition to a KOH test, a fungal culture is sometimes indicated. Occasionally, a skin biopsy is performed to obtain microorganisms for identification.

Interventions

Most skin infections heal well with nonsurgical management. Surgical intervention may be required when an infectious agent is present in deep tissue layers.

NONSURGICAL MANAGEMENT. The nurse is concerned with meticulous skin care to the involved areas to facilitate resolution of lesions and adherence to general isolation precautions. In some instances, drug therapy is needed.

SKIN CARE. Clients with bacterial infections should bathe daily with an antibacterial soap. The nurse instructs the client to remove any pustules or crusts gently so that topical medications are more easily absorbed. The application of warm compresses twice a day to furuncles or areas of cellulitis often increases comfort.

The application of astringent compresses, such as Burow's solution, to viral lesions for 20 minutes three times a day promotes crust formation and healing. Compresses also relieve the irritation and pain associated with herpetic infection. The client is instructed to avoid constricting garments that might rub the lesions and increase irritation.

Most superficial skin infections resolve more quickly if the involved skin is allowed to dry between treatments. Excessive moisture, especially under occlusion, promotes growth of microorganisms. If the client is bedridden, the nurse or other assistive nursing personnel positions the client for optimal air circulation to the area and avoids occlusive dressings or garments.

ISOLATION PRECAUTIONS. The nurse takes precautions to minimize the spread of pathogenic organisms to other people. For most superficial bacterial infections, attention to proper handwashing is sufficient to prevent cross-contamination. However, when hospitalized clients are colonized with *Staphylococcus* that is resistant to antibiotic therapy, strict adherence to isolation procedures is necessary.

Of the dermatophyte infections, tinea capitis, tinea corporis, and tinea pedis show the highest rates of cross-transmission. The nurse instructs clients to avoid sharing potentially contaminated personal items, such as hairbrushes, articles of clothing, or footwear. Repeated infections transmitted by dogs or cats may mean that clients might have to get rid of a family pet to control infections.

DRUG THERAPY. Commonly used topical medications for the treatment of bacterial, viral, and fungal skin infections are listed in Chart 67-7.

Mild bacterial infections of the skin usually resolve with topical antibacterial treatment. Clients with extensive infections, including those with associated fever or lymphadenopathy, require systemic antibiotic therapy.

Acyclovir (Zovirax) is the drug of choice for the treatment of viral infections. Topical acyclovir ointment decreases the numbers of active virus on the skin surface and reduces pain in primary herpetic infections and localized lesions in immunocompromised clients. Topical treatment is of little benefit in recurrent infection. Intravenous (IV) administration is limited to severe primary infections and immunosuppressed clients with symptoms of systemic involvement.

Topical antifungal agents are indicated for clients with dermatophyte and yeast infections. An imidazole cream is applied to the infected skin at least twice a day until the lesions have cleared. To prevent recurrence, the therapy is usually continued for 1 to 2 weeks after clearing. In some instances, antifungal powders may also help to suppress fungal growth. For widespread or resistant fungal infections, systemic antifungal agents, such as ketoconazole (Nizoral), are administered.

SURGICAL MANAGEMENT. Surgery is not usually performed for a superficial skin infection, except for incision and drainage of furuncles. In severely immunocompromised clients, superficial lesions can progress to full-thickness wounds requiring surgical excision.

PARASITIC DISORDERS

Parasitic skin disorders are most often associated with poor hygiene and substandard living conditions. The nurse examines clients who show obvious signs of a self-care deficit for these contagious parasitic infections.

Pediculosis

OVERVIEW

Pediculosis refers to infestation by human lice—*pediculosis capitis* (head lice), *pediculosis corporis* (body lice), and *pediculosis pubis* (pubic, or crab, lice). Human lice are oval and measure approximately 2 to 4 mm. The female louse lays hundreds of eggs, called *nits,* which are deposited at the base of the hair shaft in hair-bearing areas.

COLLABORATIVE MANAGEMENT

The most prominent symptom of pediculosis is pruritus, which may or may not be accompanied by excoriation. In addition to causing discomfort, these parasites can also be vectors of systemic disease (e.g., typhus and recurrent fever).

Assessment

Pediculosis capitis occurs more commonly in women than in men, especially on the sides and back of the scalp. Pruritus, the result of biting of the scalp by the parasites, is intense. With severe infestation, it is possible for a secondary infection to develop from scratching.

Because the louse is difficult to see on inspection, the nurse examines the scalp for visible white flecks, the nits of the female louse. Matting and crusting of the scalp accompanied by a foul odor alert the nurse to the probability of secondary infection.

Pediculosis corporis is caused by lice that live and lay eggs in the seams of clothing. The parasites also cause itching. The only visible sign of infestation may be excoriations on the trunk, abdomen, or extremities.

Pediculosis pubis causes intense pruritus of the vulvar or perirectal region. Pubic lice, which are more compact and crablike in appearance than body lice, can be contracted from

CHART 67-7

DRUG THERAPY *for* Skin Disorders

Drug	Usual Dosage	Nursing Interventions	Rationale
ANTIBACTERIAL DRUGS			
Ointments			
Neomycin sulfate Combination antibiotics (Neosporin, Bacitracin, Polysporin, Mycitracin) Gentamicin (Garamycin) Chloramphenicol (Chloromycetin) Povidone-iodine (Betadine) Bactroban	Apply a thin layer to the affected area tid. Dressing is optional.	Gently clean affected areas with saline, half-strength peroxide, or tap water before applying ointments.	Atraumatic cleaning promotes healing by preventing further injury to skin cells. Cleaning helps to remove exudate, crusts, and residual medication and increases the effectiveness of therapy.
		Avoid rubbing ointment into skin. Apply with downward strokes in direction of hair growth.	Ointments can irritate hair follicles and lead to folliculitis.
		Assess for worsening of problem in spite of topical therapy. Discontinue use if rash appears.	Client may become allergic to active ingredients, the ointment base, or added preservatives.
Creams			
Silver sulfadiazine Silvadene, SSD, Flamazine♣)	Apply in layer approximately $^1/_{16}$-inch thick to affected areas tid and prn. Dressing is optional.	Assess for allergy to sulfa drugs.	Use should be avoided in clients with a suspected or known sulfa allergy.
		Gently clean affected areas with saline, half-strength hydrogen peroxide, or tap water before reapplying.	Cleaning removes crusts, exudate, and caked-on medication while promoting percutaneous absorption of drug.
		If affected areas are left open without dressings, reapply cream prn between cleanings to maintain a layer of cream at all times.	Cream base melts with increase in body or room temperature and is easily rubbed off with movement if left uncovered.
		Monitor white blood cell count for drop to <5000/mm³.	Use of silver sulfadiazine over large skin surface areas has been associated with a transient leukopenia (cause unknown).
ANTIFUNGAL DRUGS			
Ointments and Creams			
Clotrimazole (Lotrimin, Mycelex, Canesten♣) Nystatin (Mycolog II, Mycostatin, Nilstat) Ciclopirox olamine (Loprox) Miconazole nitrate (Monistat-Derm 2%) Econazole (Spectazole, Ecostatin♣) Tolnaftate (Tinactin, Pitrex♣) Haloprogin (Halotex♣) Undecylenic acid (Desenex) Ketoconazole (Nizoral)	Apply a thin layer to the affected area tid.	Teach the importance of thoroughly drying the skin before applying medication.	Moist environment promotes the growth of fungal organisms.
		Position bedridden clients for maximal air circulation to involved areas.	Increasing air circulation to the affected areas promotes drying.
		Emphasize wearing of nonconstricting cotton garments to absorb perspiration.	Cream base is easily removed with perspiration, decreasing the effectiveness of therapy.
Powders			
Nystatin (Mycostatin) Tolnaftate (Zeasorb-AF 1%)	Apply a thin dusting of powder to the affected area tid.	Teach the client to thoroughly dry skin before applying powder.	In addition to discouraging the growth of fungal organisms, a dry skin surface minimizes caking of powder in skin fold areas.

CHART 67-7

DRUG THERAPY *for* Skin Disorders–cont'd

Drug	Usual Dosage	Nursing Interventions	Rationale
ANTIFUNGAL DRUGS—cont'd			
Oral Preparations			
Nystatin (Mycostatin oral suspension, Nilstat oral suspension)	Rinse the mouth qid with 4-6 mL (400,000-600,000 units) and swallow.	Teach the client to coat the entire oral cavity with medication and hold the suspension in the mouth for several minutes before swallowing.	Effectiveness of medication is dependent on good contact of medication with mucous membrane surfaces.
Clotrimazole (Mycelex troche)	Take 1 troche 5 times/day.	Teach the client to let troche dissolve slowly in the mouth.	
ANTI-INFLAMMATORY DRUGS			
Potent Fluorinated Steroid Preparations			
Clobetasol propionate (Temovate 0.05%) Triamcinolone acetonide (Aristocort 0.5%, Kenalog 0.5%, Triaderm✤ 0.5%) Amcinonide (Cyclocort 0.1%) Betamethasone dipropionate (Diprosone 0.05%, Betaderm✤ 0.5%) Diflorasone diacetate (Maxiflor 0.05%, Florone 0.05%)	Apply a small amount to affected areas no more than 4 times in 24 hr.	Teach the client to use the least amount of medication possible to cover the treatment site and to use the medication *only* under the direction of a physician.	Overuse of topical steroid preparations can cause serious side effects, including skin thinning (atrophy), superficial dilated blood vessels (telangiectasia), acne-like eruptions, and adrenal suppression. The incidence of side effects increases proportionately with the potency of the steroid and is most common with prolonged widespread use of the high-potency preparations.
Halcinonide (Halog 0.025%) Fluocinonide (Lidex 0.05%, Topsyn gel✤ 0.05%, Lidemol✤ 0.05%, Topsyn✤ 0.05%) Fluocinolone acetonide (Synalar-HP 0.2%, Fluoderm✤ 0.2%) Desoximetasone (Topicort 0.25%) Betamethasone benzoate (Uticort 0.025%, Novobetamet✤ 0.025%)		Never apply highly potent steroid preparations to the face, genital area, or skin fold areas.	Absorption of topical steroids is much higher in these areas, and the associated side effects are more severe.
Medium-Potency Fluorinated Steroid Preparations			
Triamcinolone acetonide (Kenalog 0.025%, 0.1%; Aristocort 0.025%, 0.1%) Flurandrenolide (Cordran 0.5%, 0.025%) Fluocinolone acetonide (Fluonid 0.025%, Synalar 0.025%) Desoximetasone (Topicort LP 0.05%) Betamethasone valerate (Valisone 0.1%)			
Low-Potency Nonfluorinated Steroid Preparations			
Hydrocortisone 0.5%, 1.0%, 2.5% Desonide (Tridesilon) Hydrocortisone valerate (Westcort)		Teach the client to hydrate the skin before applying a topical steroid.	Skin hydration increases percutaneous absorption and maximizes the effectiveness of topical treatment.
Antiviral Drugs			
Ointments			
Acyclovir (Zovirax)	Apply to affected areas 6 times/day.	Teach the client to use topical acyclovir only under the direction of a physician for primary infections.	Topical acyclovir has no proven clinical benefit in the prevention or treatment of recurrent infections.
		Emphasize precautionary measures to prevent transmission of infection while the lesion is present.	There is no evidence that topical treatment prevents transmission of infection.

infested bed linen or during sexual intercourse. Although the louse is usually confined to the genital region, it can also infest the axillae, the eyelashes, and the chest.

Interventions

The treatment of pediculosis is chemical killing of the parasites with agents such as lindane (Bio-Well, Kwell, Kwellada) or topical malathion (Ovide, Prioderm). In the case of pediculosis capitis, areas where the client's head has rested (such as on pillows or chair backs) should also be treated. Clothing and bed linens should be washed in hot water or dry cleaned. The use of a fine-toothed comb can help remove nits from an infested scalp. In all cases of louse infestation, social contacts are treated when possible.

Scabies

OVERVIEW

Scabies is a contagious skin disease caused by mite infestations. Scabies infections are transmitted by close and prolonged contact with an infested companion or infested bedding. Infestation is common among clients of lower socioeconomic status. The scabies mite is also carried by pets and is found among schoolchildren and institutionalized older clients.

COLLABORATIVE MANAGEMENT

Scabies is characterized by epidermal curved or linear ridges and follicular papules. The pruritus experienced by clients with scabies infestation is more intense than in those with pediculosis, and clients often report that the itching becomes unbearable at night.

The visible white epidermal ridges are formed by burrowing of the mite into the outer skin layers. The nurse closely examines the skin between the fingers and on the palms and volar aspects of the wrists, where these ridges are most common. A hypersensitivity reaction to the mite results in excoriated erythematous papules, pustules, and crusted lesions found primarily on the elbows, nipples, lower abdomen, buttocks, and thighs and in the axillary folds. Male clients can also have excoriated papules on the penis.

Suspected infestation is confirmed by taking a scraping of a lesion and examining it under the microscope for mites and eggs. Close contacts are also monitored for the possibility of infestation.

Treatment consists of chemical disinfection with scabicides, such as lindane (Kwell, Kwellada) or topical sulfur preparations, with one or two daily applications. Clothes and personal items are laundered but do not need to be disinfected.

COMMON INFLAMMATIONS

OVERVIEW

The inflammatory skin conditions are characterized by a variety of nonspecific epidermal manifestations, including marked pruritus, lesions with indistinct borders, and different distribution patterns. The cause of the eruption may or may not be identifiable. Inflammatory rashes can evolve from acute to chronic conditions.

Most inflammatory rashes are related to allergic immune responses. The responses may be triggered by external skin exposure to allergens or by exposure of the internal environment to allergens and irritants. The result is tissue destruction or epidermal alteration induced by antibodies or cellular mediators of the immune system. (A more detailed description of these immune mechanisms is presented in Chapter 20.)

The specific cause of inflammatory rashes is not always known. When this is the case, the catchall diagnosis of nonspecific eczematous dermatitis, or *eczema,* is often used.

Contact dermatitis is an acute or chronic eczematous rash caused by either direct contact with an irritant substance, resulting in toxic injury to the skin, or by contact with an allergen, resulting in a cell-mediated immune reaction.

Atopic dermatitis is a chronic rash associated with a genetic predisposition to respiratory allergies and atopic skin disease. Although the exact mechanism is unknown, atopic dermatitis is exacerbated by a number of factors, including dry or irritated skin, food allergies, chemicals, or stress. (Atopic inflammatory reactions are described in Chapter 23.)

COLLABORATIVE MANAGEMENT

Assessment

Because all of the inflammatory skin eruptions have similar clinical presentations, data collected from the client are often the determining factor in identifying the cause. Although the clinical appearance of eczematous dermatitis lesions is similar, the chronicity of the disease, the distribution of lesions, and associated symptoms may vary. Chart 67-8 lists the clinical manifestations of the various types of inflammatory skin conditions. Diagnosis is based on historical and clinical data.

Interventions

If the cause of the rash is identified, avoidance therapy is used in an attempt to reverse the reaction and clear the rash. Even when the cause is unclear, certain irritants in the environment may cause the rash to worsen and increase discomfort. Additional interventions are aimed at promoting comfort through suppression of the inflammatory response.

STEROIDS. Topical, intralesional, or systemic steroids are prescribed to suppress inflammation. The vehicle used to deliver a topical steroid generally depends on the body area involved. Because a side effect of oral corticosteroid administration is adrenal suppression, clients receiving long-term therapy must taper their drug dosages rather than come to an abrupt halt.

Corticosteroids never cure. During active disease, these agents keep the disease from manifesting itself and relieve associated discomfort. The nurse can moisten dressings with warm tap water to place over topical steroid preparations for short periods to facilitate absorption.

OIL-BASED PRODUCTS. Oil-based ointments and pastes are not applied in the sweaty skin fold areas because increased maceration and blocking of pores may result in folliculitis. Instead, water-soluble creams are the vehicle of choice for these areas. Lotions and gels prevent matting of the hair and are more appropriate for hairy areas, such as the scalp. Stiff pastes are used to apply therapy to localized areas

CHART 67-8

KEY FEATURES *of* Common Inflammatory Skin Conditions

Clinical Manifestations	Distribution
Nonspecific Eczematous Dermatitis	
Evolution of lesions from vesicles to weeping papules and plaques. Lichenification occurs in chronic disease. Oozing, crusting, fissuring, excoriation, or scaling may be present. Pruritus is common.	Anywhere on the body; localized eczema commonly involves the hands or feet
Contact Dermatitis	
Localized eczematous eruption with well-defined, geometric margins that are consistent with contact by an irritant or allergen. Usually seen in the acute form, but may become chronic if exposure is repeated. Allergy to plants (e.g., poison ivy or oak) classically occurs as linear streaks of vesicles or papules.	Cosmetic/perfume allergy: head and neck Hair product allergy: scalp Shoe/rubber allergy: dorsum of feet Nickel allergy: earlobes Mouthwash/toothpaste allergy: perioral region Airborne contact allergy (e.g., paint and ragweed): generalized
Atopic Dermatitis	
Hallmark in adults is lichenification with scaling and excoriation. Extremely pruritic. Face involvement is seen as dry skin with mild to moderate erythema, perioral pallor, and skin folds beneath the eyes (Dennie-Morgan lines). Associated with linear markings on the palms.	Face, neck, upper chest, and antecubital and popliteal fossae
Drug Eruption	
Bright red erythematous macules and papules are found. Skin blisters in extreme cases.	Generalized
Lesions tend to be confluent in large areas. Moderately pruritic. Fever is rare. Dehydration and hypothermia can occur with extensive involvement. Condition clears only after offending medication has been discontinued.	Involvement begins on trunk, proceeds distally (legs are the last to be involved)

because this vehicle clings to the skin where it is applied and resists spreading to uninvolved skin.

Cream preparations are indicated in clients with acute dermatitis with oozing and weeping. Chronic dermatitis responds more favorably to oil-based ointments that seal in moisture and help combat dryness and scaling.

ANTIHISTAMINES. Antihistamines provide some relief of pruritus but may fail to keep the client totally symptom free. The sedative effects of antihistamines can be minimized if the client takes most of the daily dose near bedtime.

COMPRESSES AND BATHS. Cool, moist compresses and tepid baths with bath additives have a soothing effect, decrease inflammation, and help debride crusts and scales. Colloidal oatmeal preparations, tar extracts, cornstarch, or oils are often added to baths to relieve pruritus (see Table 67-1).

PSORIASIS

OVERVIEW

Psoriasis is a lifelong disorder characterized by exacerbations and remissions. Even though psoriasis cannot be cured, clients can usually achieve control of symptoms with proper treatment.

Pathophysiology

Psoriasis is a scaling disorder with underlying dermal inflammation. The problem involves an abnormality in the proliferation of epidermal cells in the outer skin layers. Normally, cells at the basement membrane of the epidermis take about 27 days to reach the outermost stratum corneum, where they are shed. In a person with psoriasis, the rate of cell division is speeded up so that cells are shed every 4 to 5 days.

Etiology

The cause of psoriasis is not known. A genetic predisposition has been recognized in some cases; however, often there is no family history of the disease. Many environmental factors precipitate outbreaks and influence the severity of clinical symptoms, but these vary significantly from person to person. Triggering factors may be local or systemic. A psoriatic lesion may appear after skin trauma (Koebner's phenomenon), such as surgery, sunburn, or excoriation.

Clients with psoriasis seem to improve in warmer climates, where there is more exposure to sunlight. Systemic factors that can aggravate the disease include infections (severe streptococcal throat infection, *Candida* infection, upper respiratory tract infection), hormonal changes (during puberty and menopause), psychologic stress, drugs (lithium, beta-blocking agents, indomethacin, antimalarials), obesity, and the presence of other diseases.

➤ COLLABORATIVE MANAGEMENT

Assessment

HISTORY

In addition to collecting routine epidemiologic data, the nurse asks the client about any family history of psoriasis, including the age at onset, a description of the disease progression, and the pattern of recurrences. The nurse asks the client to describe the current flare-up of psoriasis, including whether the onset was gradual or sudden, where the lesions first appeared, whether the client observed any changes in severity over time, and whether associated symptoms (e.g., fever and pruritus) are present. Possible precipitating factors are explored, including recent skin trauma, upper respiratory tract infection, recent surgeries, menopause status, past and current use of medication, and recent stress-provoking occurrences. Previous treatment modalities and the effectiveness of each in initiating and maintaining remission of the disease are investigated.

PHYSICAL ASSESSMENT/CLINICAL MANIFESTATIONS

The appearance of psoriasis and its course vary among clients. Typically, during flare-ups of the disease, lesions thicken and extend to involve new areas of the body. As psoriasis responds to treatment, individual lesions become thinner with less scaling.

PSORIASIS VULGARIS. Psoriasis vulgaris, the most common type of psoriasis, is characterized by thick erythematous papules or plaques surmounted by silvery white scales (Figure 67-15). Borders between the lesions and normal skin are sharply defined. As a result of maceration from perspiration, patches appear less red and more moist in skin fold areas. Lesions are usually distributed symmetrically; the more common sites are the scalp, elbows, trunk, knees, sacrum, and extensor surfaces of the limbs. The facial skin is rarely affected. The client may have only a few isolated lesions, or the entire skin surface may be affected.

EXFOLIATIVE PSORIASIS. Exfoliative psoriasis (erythrodermic psoriasis) is an explosively eruptive form of the disease characterized by generalized erythema and scaling without obvious lesions. The nurse examines for signs of dehydration and hypothermia or hyperthermia related to this severe inflammatory reaction. The vasodilation and increased blood flow to the skin that occur with inflammation can alter fluid volume as a result of increased evaporative water loss from the skin surface.

Interventions

The several approaches to therapy are based on the extent of disease, the client's distress, the physician's preference, and the resistance of the psoriasis to treatment. Clients must understand that no cure for psoriasis yet exists. Therapy is aimed at decreasing epidermal proliferation and underlying inflammation.

TOPICAL THERAPY. The pharmacologic and physical topical agents used to treat psoriasis are topical steroids, topical tar and anthralin preparations, and ultraviolet (UV) light.

TOPICAL STEROIDS. Corticosteroids have anti-inflammatory properties. When they are applied to psoriatic lesions, they suppress mitotic activity. The effectiveness of a topical steroid depends on its potency and ability to be absorbed into the skin. The more potent preparations are generally used to treat clients with psoriasis.

A simple procedure for enhancing the skin penetration of these agents is for the steroid to be applied directly to the skin. This step is followed by warm, moist dressings and an occlusive outer wrap of plastic film, plastic gloves, booties, or similar garments. When large surface areas are involved, occlusive therapy is limited to 12 hours per day because of the increased risk of local and systemic side effects.

TAR PREPARATIONS. When a tar preparation is applied to the skin, it suppresses mitotic activity and produces an anti-inflammatory effect. Preparations containing crude coal tar and derivations of crude coal tar are available as solutions, ointments, lotions, gels, and shampoos. The use of crude coal tar ointments is usually limited to inpatient care and special-

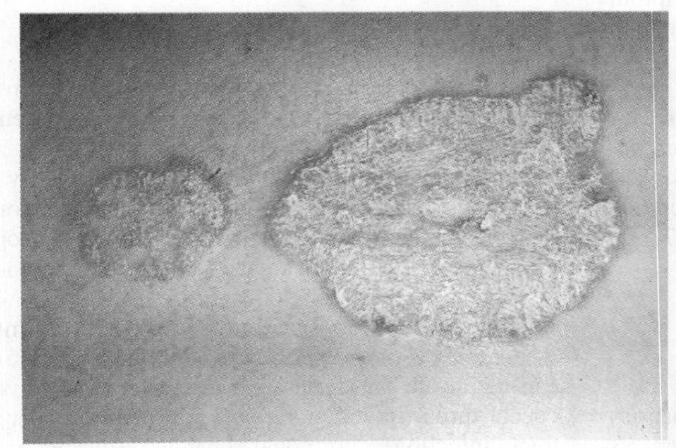

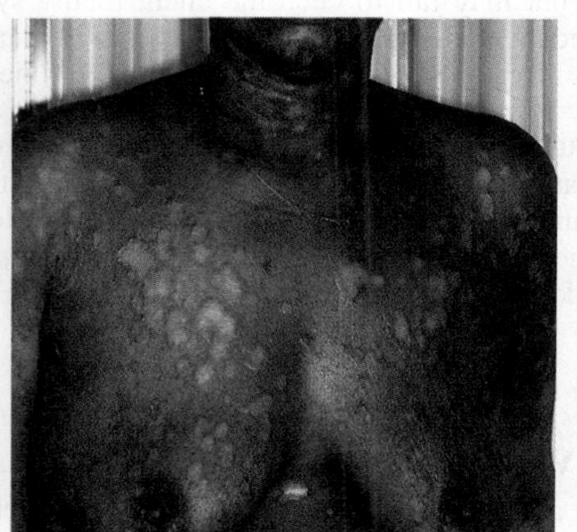

Figure 67-15 ● **A,** Psoriasis vulgaris in a Caucasian client. **B,** Psoriasis vulgaris in an African-American client.

ized outpatient treatment clinics because these ointments are messy, cause staining, and have an unpleasant odor.

Topical therapy with anthralin (Anthraforte♣, Drithocreme, Lasan), a hydrocarbon with action similar to that of tar, also relieves chronic psoriasis. Topical therapy is used in a variety of potencies alone and in combination with coal tar baths and UV light.

The nurse applies high-potency anthralin, suspended in a stiff paste, to individual lesions for short periods (not exceeding 2 hours). Because anthralin is a strong irritant and can cause chemical burns, the nurse observes for local tissue reaction and prevents inadvertent contact with uninvolved skin. Anthralin is not indicated for the treatment of acute, spreading psoriasis, because it tends to induce Koebner's phenomenon (see Skin Cancer, pp. 1546 and 1548).

Newer topical therapy with calcipotriene (Dovonex) as a cream, ointment, or lotion has proved to be effective for many clients with mild to moderate psoriasis. This drug is a synthetic form of vitamin D and is thought to regulate skin cell reproduction. Tazarotene (Tazorac), a vitamin A derivative primarily used for acne, has been helpful for treatment of psoriasis in those clients who have lesions on less than 20% of the body surface. This drug is teratogenic (can cause birth defects) even when administered topically. In addition, methotrexate delivered as a topical agent directly to lesions is undergoing study for its effectiveness in controlling psoriasis. Other immunosuppressive agents are being tested for effectiveness in a topical form.

ULTRAVIOLET LIGHT THERAPY. UV radiation is a physical agent commonly used as a topical treatment in many skin conditions, including psoriasis. Ultraviolet B (UVB) light, which produces more energy, is responsible for the obvious biologic effects of the sun, such as burning. Ultraviolet A (UVA) light emits a lower level of energy, requiring longer exposure time before cellular destruction occurs. Although the sun is the least expensive source of UV radiation, control of availability and intensity in skin treatment is best obtained with artificial light sources. These sources include high-intensity mercury vapor lamps or specially constructed cabinets containing UV tubes. *The use of commercial tanning beds is not recommended for the client with psoriasis.*

In general, UV therapy is limited by the potency and distance of the source from the skin, as well as the exposure time. Potency and distance remain constant, and the time of exposure is gradually increased to achieve a mild sunburn effect without burning or tenderness. The client's skin type, ranging from fair to darkly pigmented, affects his or her susceptibility to burning and determines the initial and subsequent exposure times. Because of the extremely high intensity of most artificial UVB light sources, daily treatments are measured in seconds of exposure; clients must wear eye protection during treatment.

The nurse teaches clients to inspect the skin carefully each day for signs of overexposure. If clients complain of tenderness on palpation and have clinical signs of severe erythema or vesicle and bullae formation, the physician must be notified promptly before therapy is resumed.

Psoralen and UVA (PUVA) treatments are more common on an outpatient basis (Figure 67-16). Clients ingest psoralen, a photosensitizing agent, 2 hours before exposure to UVA light. Because UVA light produces less energy than UVB light, the onset of erythema and skin darkening may be delayed as long as 96 hours after exposure. Treatments are limited to two to three times a week and are not given on consecutive days. Exposure is gradually increased until tanning occurs. As with UVB exposure, dosage corrections are adjusted according to the erythema reaction of normal skin, as well as the response of psoriatic lesions.

The nurse observes for generalized erythema with edema and tenderness. Treatment must be interrupted until symptoms subside. Because of the strong photosensitizing properties of psoralen, clients must wear dark glasses during treatment and for the remainder of the day.

Long-term side effects of both UVB and PUVA therapies include premature aging of the skin, actinic keratosis, and an increased incidence of skin cancer.

SYSTEMIC THERAPY. Some clients have severe psoriasis that is resistant to topical therapy. In these instances, systemic treatment with a cytotoxic agent, such as methotrexate (Folex, Mexate), is warranted. Because of the hepatotoxic side effects of methotrexate, a liver biopsy is recommended before therapy is initiated and yearly thereafter. Relatively small doses are required to obtain clearing of lesions. This treatment of last resort is contraindicated if clients have liver damage, bone marrow suppression, or impaired renal function.

Because psoriasis has an autoimmune basis, some systemic agents that induce immunosuppression are used occasionally when lesions do not respond to other therapies. Such agents include cyclosporin (Sandimmune) and azathioprine (Imuran). The many health risks associated with these therapies must be considered along with the potential benefits.

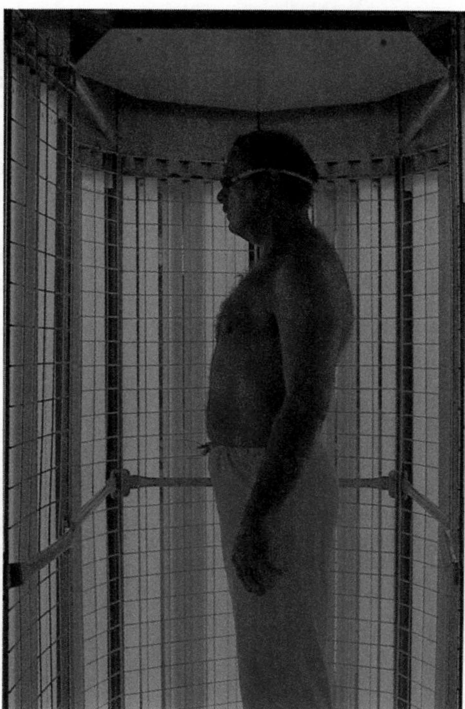

Figure 67-16 ● A client receiving psoralen and ultraviolet A treatment. (Courtesy the Department of Dermatology, Baylor College of Medicine, Houston, TX.)

EMOTIONAL SUPPORT. Often clients' self-esteem suffers not only because of the presence of skin lesions but also because of the unpleasantness associated with some of the treatment modalities. Tar not only looks dirty but also has a very unpleasant odor. Bed linen and pajamas become stained, further discouraging social interaction.

The nurse encourages contact with other clients who have similar problems. Group discussions involving family members or significant others can increase the socialization process.

The use of touch takes on an added significance for clients with psoriasis. For example, the nurse shakes the client's hand during an introduction or places a hand on the client's shoulder when explaining a procedure. The nurse does not wear gloves during these social interactions. Touch, more than any other gesture, communicates acceptance of the person and the skin problem.

BENIGN TUMORS

Cysts

OVERVIEW

Cysts are firm, flesh-colored nodules that contain liquid or semisolid material. Unlike malignant growths, which are hard and firmly attached to underlying structures, a cyst is characterized by fluctuance and mobility on palpation. Often there is a central pore through which the material can be expressed if the lesion is squeezed.

The most common cyst is an epidermal inclusion cyst. These benign growths often occur spontaneously and are asymptomatic. They can be located anywhere on the body but occur most often on the head and trunk (Figure 67-17). The most common cyst on the scalp is the sebaceous, or pilar, cyst.

COLLABORATIVE MANAGEMENT

Therapy to remove cysts is rarely indicated. If the client prefers that the cyst be removed, surgical excision with primary closure is performed with a local anesthetic agent. The surgeon removes the entire cyst wall during excision to prevent recurrence.

A pilonidal cyst is a lesion of the sacral area that is often associated with a sinus track extending into deeper tissue structures. Because the lesion's proximity to the perineum may result in secondary infection, surgical incision and drainage are necessary.

Seborrheic Keratoses

OVERVIEW

Seborrheic keratoses are a common problem of older people. These benign epidermal neoplasms are gradually acquired after middle age and are often mistaken for actinic keratoses or pigmented skin cancers. These growths may occur anywhere on the body but are more commonly found on the face, neck, upper trunk, and arms.

COLLABORATIVE MANAGEMENT

On inspection, seborrheic keratoses appear as multiple "pasted-on" papules or plaques ranging in color from flesh tones to brown or black. The surface of the lesion has a rough, greasy, wartlike texture on palpation.

Seborrheic keratoses should be removed only for cosmetic reasons or if a lesion becomes irritated from friction or excoriation. Cryosurgery or curettage with or without a local anesthetic is performed.

Keloids

OVERVIEW

A keloid is overgrowth of a scar resulting from an excessive accumulation of collagen and ground substance after skin trauma. Keloids are more common in darker-skinned people and often arise at sites of surgical incisions, burns, and ear piercing (Figure 67-18).

COLLABORATIVE MANAGEMENT

On physical examination, a keloid appears as an elevated, protruding lesion that extends well beyond the boundaries of the original injury. Treatment of these cosmetically disfiguring lesions is difficult and not always successful. Because surgical excision alone can result in a larger, more protuberant

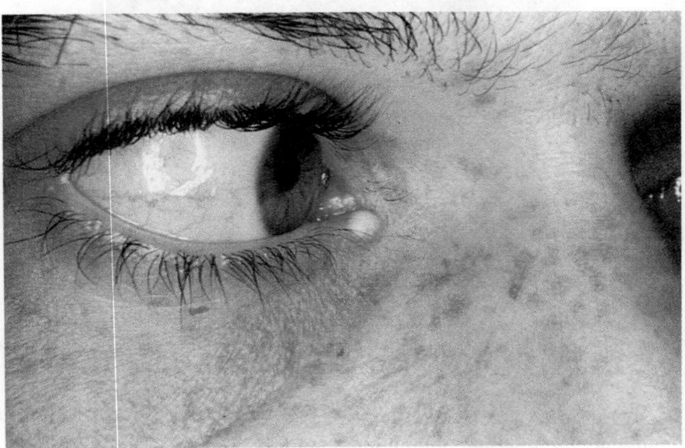

Figure 67-17 ● An epidermal inclusion cyst.

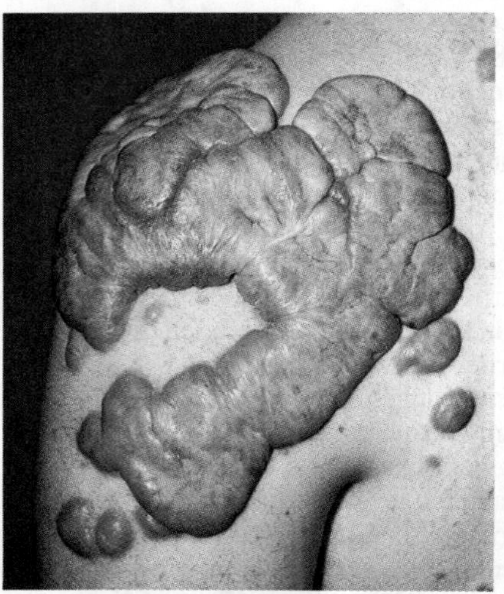

Figure 67-18 ● A keloid.

scar, surgery is usually combined with another form of therapy, such as intralesional steroid injections or low-dose radiotherapy. Pressure dressings or elastic garments worn over the skin for 1 year after excision or steroid injection may also help to keep the lesion flat.

Nevi

OVERVIEW

A **nevus,** or mole, is a benign neoplasm of the pigment-forming cells. These lesions are classified according to their location within the layers of the skin.

COLLABORATIVE MANAGEMENT

Normal nevi have regular, well-defined borders and are uniform in color, ranging from light colors to dark brown. The lesion's surface may be rough or smooth. Because about 50% of malignant melanomas arise from moles, nevi with irregular or spreading borders and those with multiple colors should be considered highly suspicious. Other abnormal findings include sudden changes in the size of the lesion and complaints of itching or bleeding.

Unsightly nevi or those subject to repeated irritation or trauma can be removed. Biopsy of any suspicious lesions is performed to rule out malignancy.

Warts

OVERVIEW

Warts, or **verrucae,** are small tumors caused by papillomavirus infection of the skin cells. They may occur singly or in groups and are classified according to their anatomic location.

Common warts are raised, flesh-colored papules with a rough surface (Figure 67-19). Although they may grow anywhere on the skin surface, they often occur on the hands and fingers.

Flat warts range in size from 2 to 4 mm. They appear as slightly elevated reddish brown or flesh-colored papules with flat tops and minimal scale. These warts often multiply and affect the hands and the face.

An often painful wart occurring on the bottom of the foot is the plantar wart. Plantar warts are covered with a thick callus that when removed reveals tiny black dots (thrombosed capillaries).

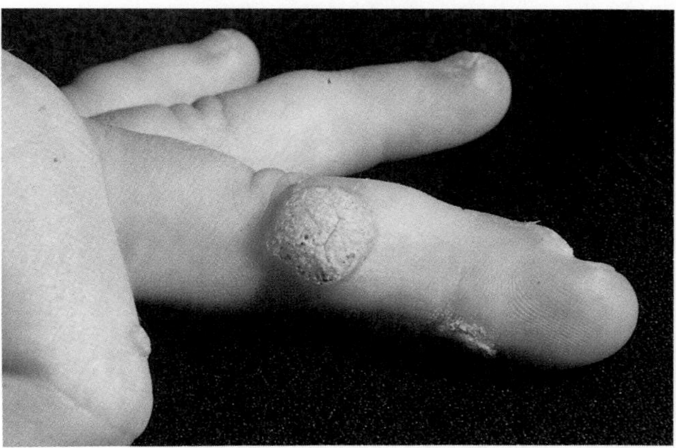

Figure 67-19 ● A common wart.

COLLABORATIVE MANAGEMENT

The treatment of warts is aimed at destroying the skin cells containing the virus, a process that can be destructive and painful. Treatment modalities include surgical excision, electrodesiccation and curettage, and cryosurgery. Cryosurgery is usually preferred because a local anesthetic is not required and scarring is less likely. Topical caustic agents, including salicylic acid and lactic acid, are also used. These agents are painted onto the surface of the lesion and result in destruction of the cells and peeling of the infected skin area.

Hemangiomas

Hemangiomas (angiomas) are blood vessel tumors and are one of the most common types of benign tumors. The clinical appearance varies from lesions that appear shortly after birth and gradually regress to those that are present at birth and gradually expand in size with growth.

Nevus flammeus is a congenital hemangioma involving the mature capillaries. These lesions are usually found on the face and the upper body. They appear as well-demarcated macular patches ranging in color from pink to bluish purple. Although nevus flammeus may gradually fade during the first years of life, a form of this neoplasm, the port-wine stain, grows with the child and remains unchanged in adult life. Port-wine stains usually occur as solitary lesions that vary in size.

The problem of nevus flammeus is cosmetic. Depending on the size of the lesion, surgical excision with or without skin grafting may be indicated. Treatment with laser therapy also is an alternative to surgery. Noninvasive treatment consists of masking the lesion by covering it with an opaque makeup.

Cherry hemangiomas are often seen in older adults. These lesions are small, dome-shaped papules ranging in color from red to purple (see Figure 66-14). Treatment is not indicated except when the client is unhappy with his or her appearance.

SKIN CANCER

OVERVIEW

Overexposure to sunlight is the major cause of skin cancer, although other factors are associated. Because sun damage is an age-related skin finding, screening for suspicious lesions is an integral part of routine physical assessment of the older adult. The most common skin cancers are actinic or solar keratosis, squamous cell carcinoma, basal cell carcinoma, and melanoma.

Pathophysiology

Actinic keratoses are premalignant lesions involving the cells of the epidermis. These lesions are common in people with chronically sun-damaged skin (see Figure 66-16). Progression to squamous cell carcinoma may occur if lesions are untreated.

Squamous cell carcinomas are cancers of the epidermis. They can invade locally and are potentially metastatic. Lesions on the ear, lip, and external genitalia are more likely to invade and metastasize than those found elsewhere on the body (Figure 67-20). Chronic skin damage from repeated injury or irritation also predisposes to this malignancy.

Basal cell carcinomas arise from the basal cell layer of the epidermis (Figure 67-21). Early malignant lesions often go unnoticed, and although metastasis is rare, underlying tissue destruction can progress to include vital structures. Genetic predisposition and chronic irritation are risk factors; however, ultraviolet (UV) radiation remains the primary carcinogen.

Melanomas are pigmented cancers originating in the melanin-producing cells of the epidermis (Figure 67-22). Risk factors include genetic predisposition, excessive exposure to UV light, and the presence of one or more precursor lesions that resemble unusual moles. *This skin cancer is highly metastatic, and a person's survival depends on early diagnosis and treatment.*

Incidence/Prevalence

The incidence of skin cancer is highest among light-skinned races and people older than 60 years of age (American Cancer Society, 2001). The incidence is higher among people who work outdoors and live at higher altitudes or lower latitudes. Occupational exposure to arsenic or other chemical carcinogens also increases risk. The incidence of malignant melanoma has rapidly increased during the past 30 years, accounting for 2% of all cancers and 1% of all cancer deaths (American Cancer Society, 2001).

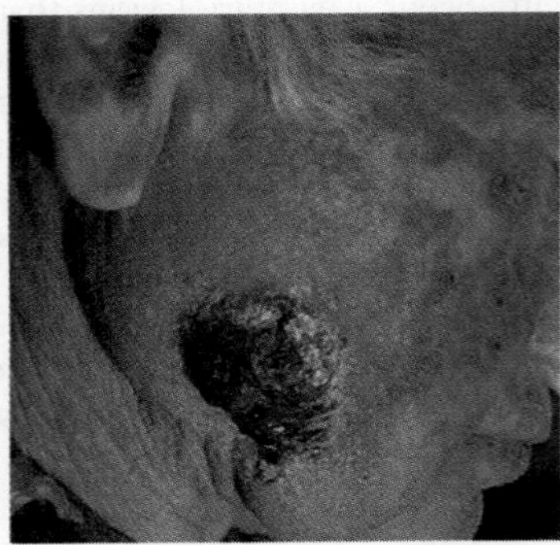

Figure 67-20 ● Squamous cell carcinoma.

The single most effective prevention strategy for skin cancer is avoiding or reducing skin exposure to sunlight. However, even when people understand the cause of skin cancer and the seriousness of the disease, preventive behaviors are not always practiced (see the Evidence-Based Practice for Nursing box on p. 1547).

COLLABORATIVE MANAGEMENT

Assessment

In addition to age and race, the nurse asks the client about any family history of skin cancer and any past surgery for removal of skin growths. Recent changes in the size, color, or sensation of any mole, birthmark, wart, or scar are also significant. The client is asked about which geographic regions he or she has lived in and where he or she currently resides. The nurse obtains information about occupational and recreational activities in relation to sun exposure, as well as any occupational history of exposure to chemical carcinogens (e.g., arsenic, coal tar, pitch, radioactive waste, and radium). The client is asked about any skin growths that are repeatedly irritated by the rubbing of clothes against them.

The skin cancers vary in their appearance and distribution. Although most skin cancers appear in sun-exposed areas of the body, the entire skin surface is inspected. The nurse systematically examines the skin for any unusual lesions, particularly moles, warts, birthmarks, and scars. Hair-bearing areas of the body, such as the scalp and genitalia, are also examined. Lesions are palpated to determine their surface texture. The location, size, color, and surface characteristics of all lesions are documented, as are any subjective reports of associated tenderness or itching.

Table 67-10 summarizes important facts about common skin cancers. Chart 67-9 lists methods of prevention that clients can use to reduce their risk for skin cancer.

Punch, shave, or excisional biopsy of suspicious lesions is necessary to confirm the diagnosis of a malignancy.

Interventions

Nonsurgical and surgical interventions are combined for the most effective management of skin cancer. Specific treatment is determined by the size and severity of the malignancy, the

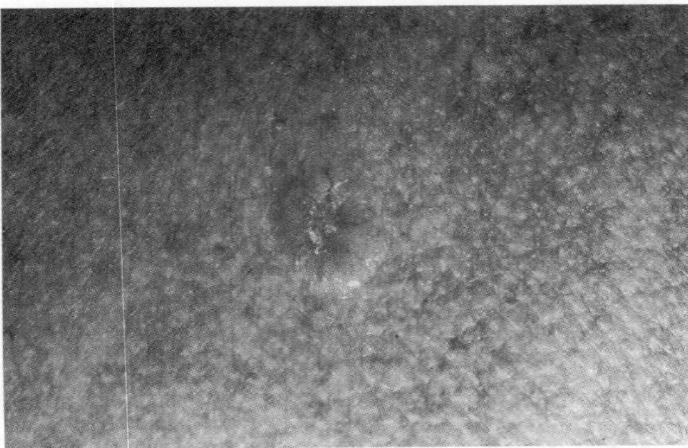

Figure 67-21 ● Basal cell carcinoma.

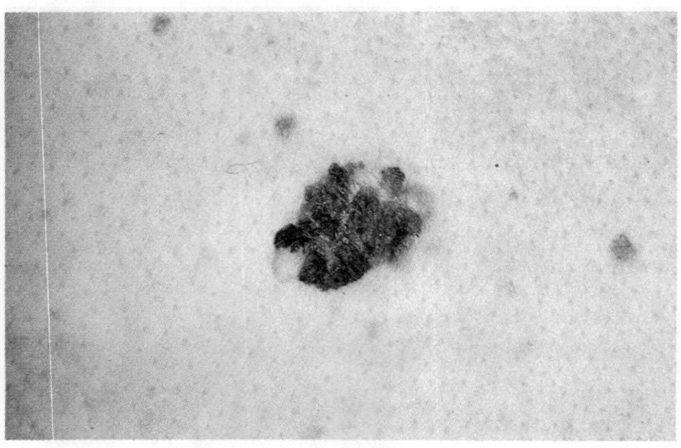

Figure 67-22 ● Melanoma.

location of the lesion, and the age and general health of the client.

NONSURGICAL MANAGEMENT

DRUG THERAPY. Topical chemotherapy with 5-fluorouracil cream is reserved for treatment of clients with multiple actinic keratoses or, in rare instances, widespread superficial basal cell carcinoma that would require several surgical procedures to eradicate. Therapy is continued for several weeks; during this time, the treated areas become increasingly tender and inflamed as the lesions crust, ooze, and erode. The nurse prepares the client for an unsightly appearance during therapy and reassures the client that the cosmetic result will be positive.

After treatment is discontinued, cool compresses and topical corticosteroid preparations help to decrease inflammation and promote comfort.

Systemic chemotherapeutic agents are rarely indicated in the treatment of cutaneous malignancy. These agents may be used, however, when the prognosis is poor, as in advanced metastatic melanoma.

Drug therapy with interferon, a biological response modifier, is now an accepted treatment after surgery for melanomas that are stage III or more advanced cancer. The client is initially started on high-dose (20,000,000 units/m^2) interferon intravenously daily for 5 days per week for 4 weeks after the surgical wound is well healed. Maintenance doses of 10,000,000 units/m^2 are continued three times per week for 1 year. The maintenance doses are administered subcutaneously, and the client must learn to self-inject the drug.

RADIATION THERAPY. Radiation therapy for malignant skin lesions is limited to older clients with large, deeply invasive basal cell tumors and to those who are poor risks for surgery. Primary malignant melanoma is resistant to radiation therapy; however, radiation therapy has proved to be of some value for clients with metastatic disease when used in combination with systemic corticosteroids.

IMMUNOTHERAPY. An experimental treatment available at some centers for clients with melanoma that has metastasized to distant sites is a melanoma vaccine. This treatment takes advantage of distinctive cell surface proteins found on some melanomas that can act like antigens. Although this form of cancer therapy is new and as yet unapproved, it shows promise for this type of cancer.

SURGICAL MANAGEMENT.

Surgical intervention ranges from local treatment of individual lesions, with minimal discomfort and positive cosmetic results, to massive excision of large areas of the skin.

CRYOSURGERY. Cryosurgery involves the local application of liquid nitrogen (−200° C) to isolated lesions, causing cell death and tissue destruction. Local anesthesia is seldom needed because clients experience only minor discomfort during the procedure. The nurse prepares clients for swelling and increased tenderness of the treated area when the skin thaws. Tissue freezing is followed in 1 or 2 days by hemorrhagic blister formation. The nurse instructs clients to clean the treatment sites with hydrogen peroxide to prevent infection. A topical antibiotic may also be ordered.

CURETTAGE AND ELECTRODESICCATION. For clients who have small lesions with well-defined borders, curettage and electrodesiccation are used to destroy the cancerous cells while minimizing damage to the surrounding uninvolved tissue. After a local anesthetic is administered, the surgeon uses a semisharp dermal curette to scrape away the cancerous tissue. After curettage is complete, the surgeon places an electric probe on the wound surface, and malignant remnants of the tumor are destroyed by thermal and mechanical energy.

Wounds treated by curettage and electrodesiccation are allowed to heal by second intention. Scarring is usually minimal. The nurse instructs clients in caring for the wound, including cleaning the wound, using prescribed antibacterial medications, and applying prescribed dressings.

EXCISION. For clients with large or poorly defined skin cancers, recurrent tumors, and deeply invasive cancers, wide excision is required to remove the malignancy. If the size and location of the lesion permit, surgical excision with primary closure is the procedure of choice. If the tumor has already been removed several times or if radiation therapy has damaged the surrounding skin, healing by second intention is indicated. This procedure allows the wound to be carefully monitored for cancer recurrence. Skin grafts and flaps are used to repair large defects with deep-tissue destruction.

EVIDENCE-BASED PRACTICE FOR NURSING

Good role modeling requires knowing your risk!

Grubbs, L., & Tabano, M. (2000). Use of sunscreen in health care professionals. *Cancer Nursing, 23*(1), 164-167.

The purpose of this descriptive study was to examine the relationship between perceived risk for skin cancer and use of sunscreen among a convenience sample of 98 health care professionals living in a high sun exposure area of the United States. The health care professionals group was made up of registered nurses, pharmacists, psychologists, nurse practitioners, and physicians. The level of education in this group was high, with 63% having postgraduate or professional degrees. Most of the participants were Caucasian women.

The study involved completion of a questionnaire that included demographic and skin cancer risk assessment questions. A total of 90 questionnaires were returned (92% response rate). The perceived risk for skin cancer among this group was 50% low perceived risk, 44% high perceived risk, and 6% neutral. The actual risk for skin cancer, based on family history, burn history, and skin type, was 7% low risk, 48% average risk, and 45% high risk. Statistical analysis confirmed that subjects at high risk and those at low risk had an accurate perception of actual risk. The subjects at average risk overwhelmingly reported their perceived risk as low. There was no relationship between perceived risk and consistent use of sunscreen.

Critique. The study was appropriately designed as a descriptive pilot study. Subject homogeneity limits the generalizability of the study results beyond this group.

Implications for Nursing. Nurses and other health care professionals are perceived by the general public as role models of healthy behaviors. With a preventable cancer, such as skin cancer, nurses can have the greatest impact by encouraging preventive practices. An inaccurate perception of personal risk and inconsistent use of protective or preventive practices reduce this positive impact.

TABLE 67-10 • COMMON SKIN CANCERS

Clinical Manifestations	Distribution	Course
ACTINIC KERATOSIS (PREMALIGNANT)		
Small (1-10 mm) macule or papule with dry, rough, adherent yellow or brown scale Base may be erythematous Associated with yellow, wrinkled, weatherbeaten skin Thick, indurated keratoses more likely to be malignant	Cheeks, temples, forehead, ears, neck, backs of hands, and forearms	May disappear spontaneously or reappear after treatment. Slow progression to squamous cell carcinoma is possible.
SQUAMOUS CELL CARCINOMA		
Firm, nodular lesion topped with a crust or with a central area of ulceration Indurated margins Fixation to underlying tissue with deep invasion	Sun-exposed areas, especially head, neck, and lower lip Sites of chronic irritation or injury (e.g., scars, irradiated skin, burns, and leg ulcers)	Rapid invasion with metastasis via the lymphatics occurs in 10% of cases. Larger tumors are more prone to metastasis.
BASAL CELL CARCINOMA		
Pearly papule with a central crater and rolled, waxy borders Telangiectasias and pigment flecks visible on close inspection	Sun-exposed areas, especially head, neck, and central portion of face	Metastasis is rare. May cause local tissue destruction. 50% recurrence rate related to inadequate treatment.
MELANOMA		
Irregularly shaped, pigmented papule or plaque Variegated colors, with red, white, and blue tones	Can occur anywhere on the body, especially where nevi (moles) or birthmarks are evident Commonly found on upper back and lower legs Soles of feet and palms in Asians and African-Americans	Horizontal growth phase followed by vertical growth phase. Rapid invasion and metastasis with high morbidity and mortality.

CHART 67-9

CLIENT EDUCATION GUIDE
Prevention of Skin Cancer

- Avoid sun exposure between 11:00 AM and 3:00 PM.
- Use sunscreens with the appropriate skin protection factor for your skin type.
- Wear a hat, opaque clothing, and sunglasses when you are out in the sun.
- Examine your body monthly for possibly cancerous or precancerous lesions.
- Seek medical advice if you note any of the following:
  - A change in the color of a lesion, especially if it darkens or shows evidence of spreading
  - A change in the size of a lesion, especially rapid growth
  - A change in the shape of a lesion, such as a sharp border becoming irregular or a flat lesion becoming raised
  - Redness or swelling of the skin around a lesion.
  - A change in sensation, especially itching or increased tenderness of a lesion
  - A change in the character of a lesion, such as oozing, crusting, bleeding, or scaling

A specialized form of excision, Mohs' surgery, is used to treat basal and squamous cell carcinomas. The cancerous tissue is sectioned horizontally in layers, and each layer is examined histologically to determine the exact location of residual tumor cells. Although the procedure is long and tedious, cure rates are higher and there is less sacrifice of healthy tissue compared with other surgical methods.

PLASTIC OR RECONSTRUCTIVE SURGERY

OVERVIEW

The aim of plastic or reconstructive surgery is to correct functional defects and alter physical appearance—processes that directly influence a person's concept of self. Unlike a medical illness that is unexpected, plastic surgery is usually an elective procedure. Surgical intervention is sought by clients who cannot perform activities of daily living (ADLs) as a result of an anatomic malformation or by those who are unsatisfied with their body image. In the United States the decision to undergo plastic surgery is often a response to established social and cultural norms. Clients become self-conscious about unsightly scars, obvious facial lesions, disproportionate anatomic features, or changes in physical features associated with aging. In some instances, severe trauma or extensive surgical excision of soft tissue leads to acquired functional defects that warrant surgical correction. For example, breast reconstruction is commonly performed after a radical mastectomy. This type of surgery not only serves an aesthetic purpose for some clients but also replaces lost anatomy and negates the need for a prosthesis.

Clients may request plastic surgery as a remedy for the normal changes in skin appearance that occur with aging. Loss of skin elasticity and redistribution of adipose tissue is progressive and especially noticeable around the eyes, near the cheeks, and on the neck. Fine facial wrinkles around the eyes and mouth are one of the first signs of aging and are followed by gradual stretching and downward displacement of the soft tissue of the lower two thirds of the face. Similar changes in skin texture contribute to wrinkling and flaccidity of the skin on the upper extremities and the chest, abdomen, buttocks, and thighs—a problem also seen after dramatic weight loss. Gradual appearance of skin lesions associated with chronic sun exposure may trouble the aging client.

COLLABORATIVE MANAGEMENT

Assessment

HISTORY

When taking a history from a client who elects to have plastic surgery, the nurse uses a nonjudgmental approach and is careful not to assume the reason for surgery on the basis of physical appearance. Often what might appear to be unsightly to the nurse is of little concern to the client, who wishes to change something else. The nurse also observes for any nonverbal communication that might establish the emotional state of the person or reveal feelings of embarrassment or guilt. The nurse encourages the client to describe the problem, including why it is bothersome and what he or she expects as a result of the change. The client is asked about both his or her health history and recent medical problems, including obesity and trauma, to predict the amount of surgery needed to correct the defect and potential complications.

PHYSICAL ASSESSMENT/CLINICAL MANIFESTATIONS

The client seeking plastic surgery may have alterations in appearance ranging from minor to significant deformity. Depending on the location of the deformity, the client may need to disrobe before the examination. The client may be embarrassed by the problem, and the nurse ensures privacy.

The nurse begins the physical assessment by closely examining the area of involvement to determine the extent of the deformity or problem. Having the client assume different normal sitting and standing postures may provide better visibility of nonfacial defects. The nurse notes any asymmetry of anatomic features, wrinkling or skin redundancy, scars or disfiguring skin marks, and obvious skin lesions.

PSYCHOSOCIAL ASSESSMENT

The nurse addresses the client's expectations of plastic surgery. Often people who seek plastic surgery have unrealistic expectations or are uncertain about what they actually want. For example, the client with minor deformities who is seeking perfection is sure to be disappointed. The client who wants an operation mainly to please the spouse or partner is also a poor candidate. His or her psychologic outlook before surgery should be positive if results are to be therapeutic.

> **CRITICAL THINKING CHALLENGE**
>
> The client is a 28-year-old woman admitted for breast augmentation surgery. After she has had her preoperative medication, she tells you that she is having this surgery because her fiance insists that she have it before their marriage. She also tells you that she is afraid to be put to sleep.
>
> - Whom should you notify about this revelation?
> - How should you document the client's concerns?
> - What is your role in this situation?

For suggested answer guidelines, go to SIMON http://www.wbsaunders.com/SIMON/Iggy/.

Interventions

SURGICAL MANAGEMENT. Depending on the planned intervention, surgery is performed either in the outpatient setting with the client under local anesthesia or in the hospital. Most clients scheduled for plastic surgery will have had several office consultations with their physician to discuss the planned intervention, possible complications, and postoperative expectations. The indications and complications of common cosmetic procedures are summarized in Table 67-11.

Many plastic surgeons use photography both as a visual aid when discussing clients' problems and as a means of documentation before and after surgical intervention. Pictures taken of clients are confidential. Showing clients pictures of other clients is done only after proper consent is obtained.

PREOPERATIVE CARE. Because of the large amount of blood loss associated with skin (particularly facial) surgery, the nurse instructs the client to avoid ingestion of salicylates for several weeks before and after the procedure. Immediate preoperative care is focused on collection of any routine laboratory test data required before general anesthesia and preparation of the operative site. In most cases, the procedure for shaving and washing the skin is dictated by the physician's preference.

Clients undergoing facial surgery, specifically **rhytidectomy** (face-lift), are often asked to wash their hair several times with antibacterial soap to decrease bacterial flora near the incision site. The nurse instructs clients to remove any makeup and avoid using face creams before surgery. If a **rhinoplasty** (reconstruction of the nose) is scheduled, the nurse prepares clients for the early postoperative period by explaining the need for nasal packing to control bleeding and by reviewing mouth-breathing techniques.

OPERATIVE PROCEDURES. Reconstructive procedures vary extensively depending on the location, purpose, and extent of reconstruction. Ironically, in performing plastic surgery, the surgeon must inflict a potentially disfiguring wound to correct existing skin deformities.

POSTOPERATIVE CARE. Postoperative care focuses on monitoring for complications associated with surgical intervention (see Chapter 19). Pressure dressings may be applied at the time of surgery and left in place for several days to control hemorrhage and edema formation. The nurse checks dressings and any nasal packing for bright red bleeding and monitors changes in vital signs and level of consciousness indicating active hemorrhage.

Repeated swallowing followed by belching after rhinoplasty is a sign of postnasal bleeding, and this sign is reported immediately to the surgeon. The client who has had breast surgery may have drains in place postoperatively, and the nurse monitors the amount and color of drainage. When the client has had any facial reconstruction, he or she is placed in a semi-Fowler's position to minimize edema and promote comfort.

Additional comfort measures, such as the application of ice packs or cold compresses, are instituted as ordered. Spe-

TABLE 67-11 • COMMON PLASTIC SURGICAL PROCEDURES

Description	Indications	Complications
BLEPHAROPLASTY		
Excision of bulging fat and redundant skin of the periorbital area with primary closure	Bags under the eyes	Hematoma Ectropion Corneal injury Visual loss (rare) Wound infection (rare)
BREAST AUGMENTATION (AUGMENTATION MAMMOPLASTY)		
Insertion of synthetic breast-shaped implants through a skin incision	Inadequate breast volume or contour	Hematoma or hemorrhage Wound infection (with gram-positive organisms) Phlebitis
BREAST REDUCTION (REDUCTION MAMMOPLASTY)		
Excision of excessive breast tissue and skin with primary closure	Hypertrophy of breast tissue caused by elevated hormone levels, endocrine abnormalities, or obesity	Hematoma or hemorrhage Nipple, areola, and skin flap necrosis Wound infection Fat necrosis Wound dehiscence
DERMABRASION		
Abrasive removal of the facial epidermis and a portion of the dermis followed by healing by second intention	Moderate to severe acne scars Deep wrinkling Multiple actinic keratoses Hyperpigmentation (postinflammatory or after the use of estrogens)	Hypertrophic scarring Altered skin pigmentation Acne flare Wound infection (rare)
RHINOPLASTY		
Removal of excessive cartilage and tissue from the nose with correction of septal defects if indicated	Disproportionate anatomy Post-traumatic nasal deformity	Hematoma or hemorrhage Ecchymosis and edema (temporary) Wound infection (with gram-positive organisms) Septal perforation Minor skin irritation
RHYTIDECTOMY (FACE-LIFT)		
Removal of excess skin and tissue from the face at the level of the hairline followed by primary closure	Excessive wrinkling or sagging of facial skin	Hematoma or hemorrhage Facial nerve damage (temporary or permanent) Wound infection Ecchymosis and edema (temporary) Skin necrosis Hair loss
LIPOSUCTION (SUCTION LIPECTOMY)		
Removal of subcutaneous fat from localized areas of accumulation such as the hips, abdomen, neck, and arms	Disproportionate distribution of adipose tissue	Hematoma Severe pain Infection Emboli Sagging of skin (if skin is not elastic enough to contract after fat removal)

cial support garments are often indicated after breast augmentation surgery to minimize edema and tension on the suture line from the weight of the breast tissue.

The nurse monitors for signs and symptoms of wound infection and progress toward healing. Of particular concern are any areas of skin necrosis or eschar formation near the operative site, a complication related to excessive tension on the suture line from edema and subsequent obstruction of microcirculation. (For a description of criteria used to monitor wound infection, see Table 67-8.)

Regardless of the planned procedure, the nurse prepares the client preoperatively for edema and discoloration of the operative site. Swelling and ecchymosis alter the facial features and may not resolve for several weeks after surgery. The client is reminded that the true results of surgery will not be visible until healing is complete, usually 6 months to a year or longer postoperatively.

OTHER SKIN DISORDERS

Acne

OVERVIEW

Acne is a red pustular eruption affecting the sebaceous glands of the skin. It is a common condition that, despite popular belief, is not confined to adolescents. Lesions result from in-

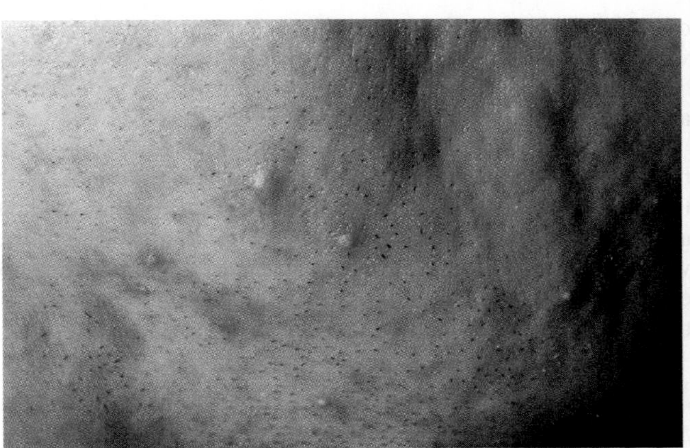

Figure 67-23 ● Acne.

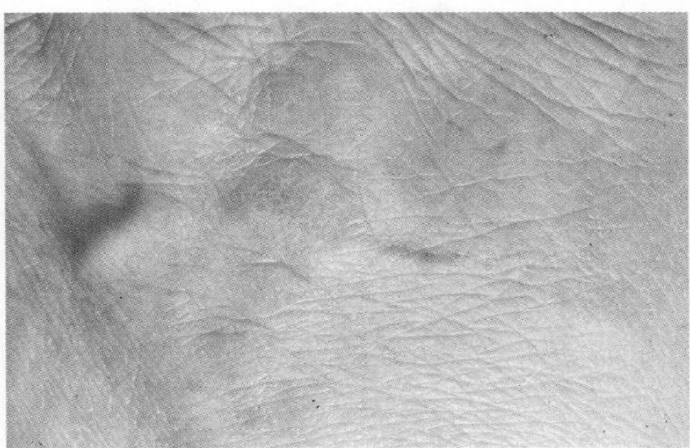

Figure 67-24 ● Lichen planus.

creased sebum production, which is stimulated by elevated androgenic hormones and obstruction of the sebaceous canal outlet. Accumulation of debris promotes bacterial growth and eventual rupture of the sebaceous gland into the surrounding dermis with inflammation.

➤ COLLABORATIVE MANAGEMENT

Acne is a progressive disorder that results in the clinical appearance of several types of lesions, including noninflammatory **comedones** (blackheads and whiteheads), inflammatory papules, pustules, and cysts. Distribution of lesions is usually limited to the face and upper trunk (Figure 67-23).

Control of the disorder is possible, with spontaneous remission occurring over time. However, severe eruptions or chronic inflammation can lead to extensive scarring.

For clients with superficial lesions and comedones, topical agents (retinoic acid, benzoyl peroxide, antibiotic solutions) are used. Systemic antibiotics, with tetracycline being the drug of choice, are indicated for those with inflammatory disease. Clients with severe acne have undergone dramatic improvement after receiving isotretinoin (Accutane, Accutane Roche✤). Side effects include elevated liver function test results; dry, chapped skin; and depression in some clients. The most important concern, however, is the teratogenic effect of systemic retinoic acid. A pregnancy test is required before therapy, and strict birth control measures must be used during therapy.

Lichen Planus

OVERVIEW

Lichen planus is a fairly common skin disorder characterized by purple, flat-topped papules that are itchy. Although viral infections and emotional stress may be possible causes, lichen planus remains an idiopathic disorder. The course of the disease can be chronic, or it can resolve spontaneously.

➤ COLLABORATIVE MANAGEMENT

Lesions of lichen planus are usually distributed over the wrists and the inner surfaces of the forearms, but they may also be present on the lower legs, genitalia, and other body areas. Oral lesions may occur alone or in combination with skin changes. Unlike the skin lesions, mucosal lesions have a characteristic white lacelike appearance; they usually occur on the buccal mucosa and are often confused with thrush (Figure 67-24).

Treatment is symptomatic. Topical steroids help to reduce inflammation, and antihistamines help to relieve itching. Occasionally, systemic steroids are prescribed when involvement is widespread, but long-term use is avoided because of the associated toxicity.

Pemphigus Vulgaris

OVERVIEW

Pemphigus vulgaris is a rare, chronic blistering disease with high morbidity and mortality. It is caused by an autoimmune disorder that occurs predominantly during middle and old age.

➤ COLLABORATIVE MANAGEMENT

The acute lesions of pemphigus vulgaris occur on nonerythematous, normal-appearing skin or mucous membrane surfaces as fragile, flaccid bullae (Figure 67-25). Disruption of the bullae leaves partial-thickness wounds that bleed, weep, and eventually form crusts.

Distribution is generalized; the initial lesions usually occur on the oral mucosa; later lesions form on the trunk. Spread of the disease is characterized by the appearance of new lesions, particularly on the face and in skin fold areas, whereas older lesions are in the process of healing. Oral lesions are common and can interfere with chewing and swallowing.

Treatment of pemphigus vulgaris is aimed at suppressing the immune response that causes the blister formation. Systemic steroids and cytotoxic agents are used to bring about remission. Topical antibiotic creams or ointments are used to minimize bacterial infection of the unhealed lesions.

Toxic Epidermal Necrolysis

OVERVIEW

Toxic epidermal necrolysis (TEN) is a rare, acute drug reaction of the skin characterized by diffuse erythema and bullae formation. Mucous membranes are often involved, and marked systemic toxicity is evident. The drugs most often im-

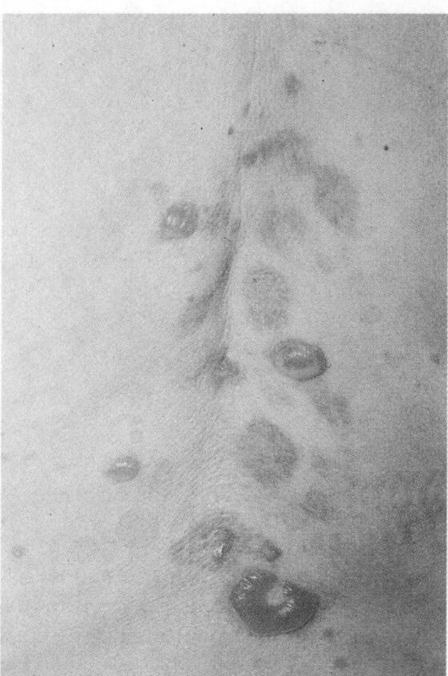

Figure 67-25 ● Pemphigus vulgaris.

plicated in triggering this disease are sulfonamides, pyrazolones, barbiturates, and antibiotics. Removal of the offending agent is usually followed by gradual healing in 2 to 3 weeks, with widespread peeling of the epidermis.

➤ COLLABORATIVE MANAGEMENT

The drug thought to be causing a toxic reaction is discontinued, and therapy is aimed at systemic support and prevention of secondary infection. Clients with TEN are often admitted to burn units, where fluid and electrolyte balance, caloric intake, and potential problems with hypothermia can be closely monitored. Topical antibacterial agents are used to suppress bacterial growth until healing occurs. Systemic steroids are not beneficial in the treatment of clients with TEN and, because of the increased risk for infection, are avoided.

Frostbite

OVERVIEW

Cold injury of the skin depends on the intensity of the external temperature, the duration of exposure to cold temperatures, and the relative hypoxia of the tissues at the time of exposure. Cell death occurs as a result of inadequate tissue oxygenation owing to cold-induced blood vessel constriction. With continued exposure to the cold, vascular necrosis and gangrene are imminent. Factors that increase the risk for cold injury are age, immobility, alcohol use, vascular disease, and psychiatric disorders.

➤ COLLABORATIVE MANAGEMENT

Acute frostbite is treated in the hospital setting, with rapid and continuous rewarming of the tissue in a water bath (90° to 107° F [32° to 42° C]) for 15 to 20 minutes or until flushing of the skin occurs. Slow thawing or interrupted periods of warmth are avoided because they can contribute to increased cellular damage. Thawing can cause considerable pain, and analgesics are administered as ordered.

After thawing, the extremity is left exposed so that local tissue changes can be monitored. Blisters are left intact. With time, the degree of actual tissue destruction becomes evident as an eschar forms. After an eschar is evident, local care of the wound is similar to that for skin trauma. Complications of cold injury include amputation, scarring, depigmentation, and thickened nail plates.

Leprosy

OVERVIEW

Leprosy (Hansen's disease) is a chronic, contagious, systemic mycobacterial infection of the peripheral nervous system with secondary skin involvement. The clinical course of the disease is either progressive or self-limiting, depending on the immunologic status of the host. Although often thought to be extinct, Hansen's disease is found in the United States; most cases are reported in Florida, Louisiana, Texas, New York, California, and Hawaii.

The exact mechanism of transmission to a susceptible host remains unknown. Clinical studies suggest transmission via the airborne route, by insects, or through direct contact with skin lesions.

➤ COLLABORATIVE MANAGEMENT

Clinical manifestations of leprosy, including any skin changes, are directly related to the degree of individual resistance to the mycobacteria:

- Localized (high-immunity) leprosy is characterized by one or two isolated, erythematous, anesthetic plaques that are hairless and sometimes scaly in texture.
- Generalized (low-immunity) leprosy involves widespread, faintly erythematous macules, papules, nodules, and plaques.
- Varying degrees of diminished skin sensation of the lesions are caused by the concomitant peripheral nerve damage.

Modern treatment is available on an outpatient basis. The aim is to control bacterial proliferation and minimize associated physical deformities. The drug of choice is dapsone (DDS; Avlosulfon), a sulfone with relatively few side effects that clients must take for life. In clients with sulfone-resistant disease, clofazimine (Lamprene) is indicated. This drug has a slow bactericidal effect on the microorganism that causes leprosy. The major side effects include severe abdominal symptoms and skin discoloration (pink to brownish black).

NAIL DISORDERS

Ingrown Toenail

OVERVIEW

Although seemingly a minor problem, an ingrown toenail **(unguis incarnatus)** can be troublesome. Pain and local infection result when the edge of the nail plate grows into the soft pulp of the toe.

➤ COLLABORATIVE MANAGEMENT

Conservative management is aimed at controlling local infection while encouraging the nail edges to grow beyond the level of the pulp, where the nail plate can be trimmed transversely. The client soaks the foot in warm water (to which an antiseptic has been added) for 20 to 30 minutes. The softened nail plate is gently lifted, and a small piece of gauze is inserted between the nail and the flesh on each side. This procedure is repeated twice daily until the nail has grown beyond the flesh so that it can be cut.

An ingrown toenail can be treated more aggressively with surgical removal of the nail plate. However, the pain of surgical removal can be severe, and recurrence is possible if the nail bed is not completely destroyed.

ONLINE RESOURCES

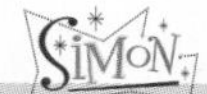

For suggested readings and Internet resources, go to http://www.wbsaunders.com/SIMON/Iggy/.

SELECTED BIBLIOGRAPHY

Asterisk indicates a classic or definitive work on this subject.

Alfonso, L., & Hogan, D. (1999). Contact dermatitis for primary care providers. *Nurse Practitioner Forum, 10*(2), 67-73.

American Cancer Society. (2001). *Cancer facts and figures—2001.* Report No. 01-300M-No. 5008.01. Atlanta: Author.

Anderson, S. (1998). Laser resurfacing: A survey of pre- and postoperative care. *Plastic Surgery Nursing, 18*(4), 229-232.

Baranoski, S. (2000). Skin tears: The enemy of frail skin. *Advances in Skin and Wound Care, 13*(3), 123-126.

Beitz, J., Fey, J., & O'Brien, D. (1998). Perceived need for education vs. actual knowledge of pressure ulcer care in a hospital nursing staff. *MEDSURG Nursing, 7*(5), 293-301.

Bergstrom, N., et al. (1998). Predicting pressure ulcer risk. *Nursing Research, 47*(5), 261-269.

Bielan, B. (2000). What's your assessment? *Dermatology Nursing, 12*(5), 350-351.

Bjorgen, S. (1998). Clinical snapshot: Herpes zoster. *American Journal of Nursing, 98*(2), 46-47.

Black, J. (1999). Malignant melanoma: An update on treatments, *Plastic Surgical Nursing, 19*(3), 143-147.

Cloote, H. (2000). Psoriasis. *Nursing Standard, 14*(45), 47-42.

Cooper, D. (1999). Wound healing: New understandings. *Nurse Practitioner Forum, 10*(2), 74-86.

Crossland, M., Shawler, L., & Boykin, J. (1998). The chronic wound. *ADVANCE for Nurse Practitioners, 6*(8), 61-65.

D'Epiro, (1999). Psoriasis: New clues to causation, new ways to treat. *Patient Care for the Nurse Practitioner, 2*(5), 42-44, 46-50.

DeBoer, S., & Zeglin, D. (2001). Necrotizing fasciitis. *American Journal of Nursing, 101*(4), 37-38.

*Fewkes, J., & Mohs, F.E. (1987). Dermatologic surgery: Microscopically controlled surgical excision (the Mohs technique). In T.B. Fitzpatrick et al. (Eds.), *Dermatology in general medicine* (3rd ed., pp. 2557-2563). New York: McGraw-Hill.

Fishman, T. (2000). Wound assessment and evaluation. *Dermatology Nursing, 12*(3), 194-195.

Goolsby, M.J. (1998). The elusive itch: Assessment, diagnosis, and management of pruritus. *ADVANCE for Nurse Practitioners, 6*(11), 61-64.

Grubbs, L., & Tabano, M. (2000). Use of sunscreen in health care professionals. *Cancer Nursing, 23*(1), 164-167.

Guyton, A., & Hall, J. (2000). *Textbook of medical physiology* (10th ed.). Philadelphia: W.B. Saunders.

Hallett, C., Caress, A., & Luker, K. (2000). Wound care in the community setting: Clinical decision-making in context. *Journal of Advanced Nursing, 31*(4), 783-793.

Harris, J. (2000). A plan to promote the prevention and early detection of melanoma. *Dermatology Nursing, 12*(5), 329-333.

Henderson, C., et al. (1997). Draft definition of stage I pressure ulcers: Inclusion of persons with darkly pigmented skin. *Advances in Wound Care, 10*(5), 16-19.

Hess, C. (2000). Skin care basics. *Advances in Skin and Wound Care, 13*(3), 127-128.

Hilton, D., Williams, L., & Nesbitt, L. (2000). Systemic glucocorticosteroid therapy in dermatology. *Dermatology Nursing, 12*(4), 258-263.

Johnson, M., Maas, M., Moorhead, S. (Eds.). (2000). *Nursing outcomes classification (NOC)* (2nd ed.). St. Louis: Mosby.

Klassen, A. (1999). Problems reported by people who request cosmetic surgery. *Plastic Surgical Nursing, 19*(4), 193-197.

Lang, P. (2000). Dermatoses in African-Americans. *Dermatology Nursing, 12*(2), 87-98.

Lapka, D. (2000). Oncology today: Skin cancer. *RN, 63*(7), 32-39.

Leber, K., Perron, V., Sinni-McKeehen, B. (1999). Common skin cancers in the United States: A practical guide for diagnosis and treatment. *Nurse Practitioner Forum, 10*(2), 106-112.

Levine, N. (2000). Exfoliative erythroderma: Skin biopsy is required to determine the cause of this pruritic eruption. *Geriatrics, 55*(8), 25.

Lookingbill, D.B., & Marks, J.G., Jr. (2000). *Principles of dermatology* (3rd ed.). Philadelphia: W.B. Saunders.

Matteson, M.A. (1997). Age-related changes in the integument. In M.A. Matteson, E.S. McConnell, & A.D. Linton (Eds.), *Gerontological nursing: Concepts and practice* (2nd ed., pp. 174-195). Philadelphia: W.B. Saunders.

McCloskey, J.C., & Bulechek, G.M. (2000). *Nursing interventions classification (NIC)* (3rd ed.). St. Louis: Mosby.

McKay, S. (2000). Why we need to worry about warts. *RN, 63*(9), 68-72.

Moss, R., Moss, C., & Broadway, D. (2000). Body contouring with ultrasound-assisted lipoplasty. *AORN Journal, 71*(2), 370-385.

Motta, G. (1997). Setting the stage for healing. *Continuing Care, 16*(3), 14-18.

Motta, G. (2000). Reimbursement relief. *Continuing Care, 19*(4), 14-16.

Nicol, N., & Boguniewicz, M. (1999). Understanding and treating atopic dermatitis. *Nurse Practitioner Forum, 10*(2), 48-55.

Palmissano, C., & Norman, R. (2000). Geriatric dermatology in chronic care and rehabilitation. *Dermatology Nursing, 12*(2), 116-123.

Peters, J. (2000). Toxic epidermal necrolysis. *Nursing Times, 96*(36), 43-44.

Pieper, B. (1998). Pressure ulcer management. *ADVANCE for Nurse Practitioners, 6*(10), 55-59.

Pirrung, M. (2001). Management of toxic epidermal necrolysis. *Journal of Intravenous Nursing, 24*(2), 107-113.

Rapaport, M. (2000). Eyelid dermatitis. *Dermatology Nursing, 12*(5), 352-354.

Rayner, V. (2000). Cosmetic rehabilitation. *Dermatology Nursing, 12*(4), 267-271.

Rivera, E., Walsh, A., & Bradley, M. (2000). Using behavior modification to promote wound healing. *Home Healthcare Nurse, 18*(9), 579-586.

Scholl, D., & Langkamp-Henken, B. (2001). Nutrient recommendations for wound healing. *Journal of Intravenous Nursing, 24*(2), 124-132.

Sheppard, C., & Brenner, P. (2000). The effects of bathing and skin care practices on skin quality and satisfaction with an innovative product. *Journal of Gerontological Nursing, 25*(10), 36-45.

Sibbald, G., et al. (2000). Preparing the wound bed: Debridement, bacterial balance, and moisture balance. *Ostomy Wound Management, 46*(11), 14-35.

*U.S. Department of Health and Human Services. (1992a). *Pressure ulcers in adults: Prediction and prevention. Clinical Practice Guideline No. 3.* Rockville, MD: Agency for Health Care Policy and Research, Public Health Service, U.S. Department of Health and Human Services.

*U.S. Department of Health and Human Services. (1992b). *Preventing pressure ulcers: A patient's guide. Clinical Practice Guideline No. 3.* Rockville, MD: Agency for Health Care Policy and Research, Public Health Service, U.S. Department of Health and Human Services.

United States Pharmacopeia Dispensing Information (USP DI): Vol. I. Drug information for the health care professional (20th ed.). (2000). Englewood, CO: Micromedix.

Whitney, J., & Heitkemper, M. (1999). Modifying perfusion, nutrition, and stress to promote wound healing in patients with acute wounds. *Heart and Lung, 28*(2), 123-133.

CHAPTER

68

Interventions for Clients with Burns

ERIC MARSH

Learning Objectives

After studying this chapter, you should be able to:

1. Identify burn clients at risk for inhalation injury.
2. Compare and contrast the clinical manifestations of superficial, partial-thickness, and full-thickness burn injuries.
3. Explain the expected clinical manifestations of neural and hormonal compensation during the emergent phase of burn injury.
4. Calculate the total body surface area involved in a burn injury.
5. Prioritize nursing care for the client during the emergent phase of burn injury.
6. Use laboratory data and clinical manifestations to determine the effectiveness of fluid resuscitation during the emergent phase of burn injury.
7. Use the Parkland formula to establish the correct rate and timing of fluid replacement.
8. Prioritize nursing care for the client during the acute phase of burn injury.
9. Explain the alteration of nutritional needs for the burn client during the acute phase of burn injury.
10. Evaluate wound healing in the client during the acute phase of burn injury.
11. Compare and contrast pain management strategies for clients in the emergent and acute phases of burn injury.
12. Describe the characteristics of infected burn wounds.
13. Explain the positioning and range-of-motion interventions for the prevention of mobility problems in the client with burns.
14. Prioritize nursing care for the client during the rehabilitation phase of burn injury.
15. Discuss the potential psychosocial problems associated with burn injury.

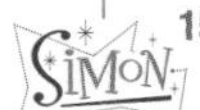

Go to http://www.wbsaunders.com/SIMON/Iggy/ for self-assessment questions related to these Learning Objectives.

Burn injuries of the skin and other tissues cause clients to experience many physiologic, metabolic, and psychologic changes. Burn injuries can range from a minor loss of small segments of the outermost layers of the skin to complex injuries involving all layers of the skin. When the skin is injured, significant fluid loss and large inflammatory responses result in altered function in most, if not all, body systems. The burn client requires complex, comprehensive care for weeks to months in order to survive the injury, reduce complications, and return to his or her best possible functional status. Collaboration with a multidisciplinary team of health care providers is essential to ensure optimal care and improve client outcomes.

INTRODUCTION TO THE BURN PROBLEM

Pathophysiology of Burn Injury

The tissue destruction caused by a burn injury can cause many local and systemic problems, including fluid and protein losses, sepsis, and disturbances of the metabolic, endocrine, respiratory, cardiac, hematologic, and immune systems. The extent of local and systemic disruption is related to many factors, including age, general health status, extent of injury, depth of injury, and area of body injured. Even after healing, the burn injury can cause late complications such as contracture formation and extensive scarring. Therefore the prevention of infection and closure of the burn wound are vitally important. A lack of or delay in healing is a key factor for all systemic disturbances and is responsible for much morbidity and mortality among clients who are burned.

INTEGUMENTARY CHANGES RESULTING FROM BURN INJURY

Anatomic Changes

The skin is the largest organ of the body (see Chapter 66). Each of its two major layers, the epidermis and dermis, has several sublayers. The epidermis, the outer layer of skin, is a superficial layer of stratified epithelial tissues approximately

0.15 mm thick (somewhat thinner in older adults and younger children). This layer can regenerate after a significant injury because the epidermal cells surrounding sweat and oil glands and hair follicles extend into dermal tissue and are responsible for the healing of partial-thickness wounds. Collectively, the sweat and oil glands and the hair follicles are referred to as **dermal appendages.** The depth of the dermal appendages varies considerably across body areas. The sweat and oil glands in the palm of the hand and the sole of the foot, for example, extend deep into the dermis. This allows for healing of fairly deep burns in these areas. The epidermis has no blood vessels and receives nutrients by diffusion from the second layer of skin, the dermis.

The basement membrane, a thin noncellular protein surface, separates the dermis from the epidermis. The dermis is sometimes called the "true skin" because it is not constantly shed and replaced; it is thicker than the epidermis and ranges in thickness from 0.60 to 1.2 mm. The dermis makes up the bulk of the skin and is composed of collagen meshes, fibrous connective tissue, and elastic fibers. Within the dermis are the functional elements of the skin: blood vessels, sensory nerves, hair follicles, lymph vessels, sebaceous glands, and sweat glands.

When burn injury occurs, the skin can regenerate as long as parts of the dermis are present. When the entire layer of dermis is burned, all epithelial cells or dermal appendages are destroyed, and the skin can no longer regenerate spontaneously. The subcutaneous tissue, or superficial fascia, varies in thickness and lies below the dermis. With deep burns, the subcutaneous tissues may be damaged, leaving bones, tendons, and muscles exposed.

Functional Changes

The skin serves multiple functions (see Table 66-1). The skin is primarily a protective barrier against injury and microbial invasion from the environment. A burn injury breaks this barrier, greatly increasing the risk for infection.

The skin also helps maintain the delicate fluid and electrolyte balance essential for life. After a burn injury, massive fluid loss occurs through evaporation. Water vapor can evaporate through burn-injured skin four times as rapidly as from intact skin. The rate of evaporation is proportional to the total body surface area burned and the depth of injury.

Skin is important in thermoregulation. Normally the body can adjust to most fluctuations in environmental temperatures because subcutaneous fat provides insulation and because blood flow to the skin changes with these fluctuations in environmental temperature. When the skin is damaged, the body cannot adjust to the loss of heat as readily, and body temperature tends to decrease.

The skin functions as an excretory organ through perspiration. Full-thickness burns destroy the sweat glands, which results in a loss of excretory ability.

The skin is the largest sensory organ of the body. Pain, pressure, temperature, and touch are sensed on the skin in normal daily activities, which allows a person to react to changes in the environment. All burn injuries are painful. With partial-thickness burns, nerve endings are exposed to the surface, which causes an increased sensitivity and a subsequent increase in pain. With full-thickness burns, nerve endings are completely destroyed. Initially these wounds are completely **anesthetic** (do not transmit sensation) when a sharp stimulus is applied. Despite this destruction, clients often complain of a dull or pressure-type of pain in these areas.

Skin exposed to sunlight produces vitamin D. The conversion of cholesterol derivatives into the active form of vitamin D is completed in the skin. Partial-thickness burns reduce the activation of vitamin D; this conversion is lost completely in full-thickness burns.

The skin is an important determinant of physical identity. The skin's cosmetic quality contributes to each person's unique appearance. With a change in appearance through a major burn, severe psychologic problems may develop.

TEMPERATURE

The temperature of the body's internal environment falls within a narrow range (approximately 84.2° to 109.4° F [29° to 43° C]) compared with the wide temperature fluctuations in the external environment. The body has several mechanisms to compensate for wide variations in external temperature. Circulating blood both provides and dissipates heat. Heat dissipation is efficient under normal conditions. When heat is applied to the skin, the temperature of the immediate subdermal layer rises rapidly. As soon as the heat source is removed, the body's compensatory mechanisms quickly return the area to a normal temperature. If the heat source is not removed, or if it is applied at a rate or level that exceeds the skin's capacity to dissipate it, cellular destruction occurs.

The skin can tolerate temperatures up to 104° F (40° C) without sustaining injury. At temperatures of 158° F (70° C) and above, cell destruction is so rapid that brief periods of exposure damage the skin down to and including the subcutaneous level. Figure 68-1 shows the relationship between temperature and exposure time for an experimental model of burn injury.

DEPTH OF BURN INJURY

The magnitude of a burn injury is based on the depth and extent of the total body surface burn. The degree of tissue destruction is determined by what agent specifically caused the burn and by the temperature and duration of exposure to the heat source.

Variations in skin thickness over different parts of the body also influence burn depth. In areas where the epidermis and dermis are thin (e.g., eyelids, ears, nose, genitalia, tops of the hands and feet, fingers, and toes), a short exposure to extreme temperatures can result in a deep burn injury. The skin is thinner in older adults, which predisposes them to increased burn severity, even at lower temperatures of shorter duration.

Burn wounds are classified as superficial-thickness wounds, partial-thickness wounds, full-thickness wounds, and deep full-thickness wounds. The partial-thickness wounds are further separated into superficial and deep subgroups. Table 68-1 characterizes the clinical differences of these burns.

The American Burn Association (ABA) describes burns as minor, moderate, or major depending on the depth, extent, and location of injury (Table 68-2). Figure 68-2 shows specific tissue layers involved with different depths of injury and describes the criteria for referral to a burn center.

SUPERFICIAL-THICKNESS WOUNDS. Of all burn types, superficial-thickness wounds have the least destruction because the epidermis is the only portion of the skin that is injured. The basal epithelial cells and basement membrane—structures necessary for the total regeneration of epithelial cells—remain present.

Superficial-thickness wounds often result from prolonged exposure to low-intensity heat (e.g., sunburn) or short (flash) exposure to high-intensity heat. Erythema with mild edema, pain, and increased sensitivity to heat occurs as a result. Peeling of dead skin **(desquamation)** occurs for 2 to 3 days after the burn, and the area rapidly heals in 3 to 5 days without a scar. No significant clinical consequences occur at this level of injury.

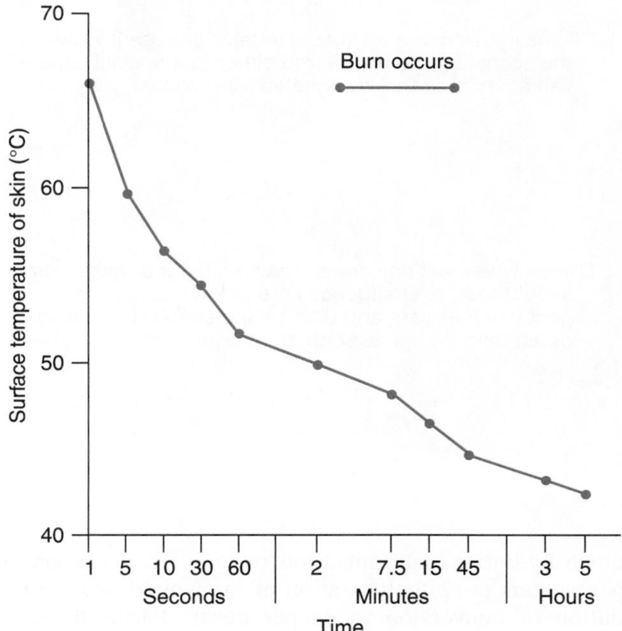

Figure 68-1 ● Relationship between intensity of heat and duration of exposure. Exposure for prolonged periods causes burns, even with milder temperatures. At more extreme temperatures, tissue damage results after only seconds. (Modified from Moritz, A.R. [1947]. Studies of thermal injuries: II. The relative importance of time and surface temperature in causation of cutaneous burns. *American Journal of Pathology, 23,* 695.)

PARTIAL-THICKNESS WOUNDS. A partial-thickness wound involves the entire epidermis and varying depths of the dermis. Depending on the amount of dermal tissue damaged, partial-thickness wounds are further subdivided into superficial partial-thickness and deep partial-thickness injuries.

SUPERFICIAL PARTIAL-THICKNESS WOUNDS. Superficial partial-thickness wounds result from either increased duration or increased intensity of exposure. These wounds are typically erythematous and moist (Figure 68-3). The classic **vesicle** (blister) forms as the stratum corneum and stratum granulosum are destroyed. When intact, the blister forms a sterile environment, which protects the wound from potential infection and excess water loss. However, large or numerous blisters are opened to promote healing and prevent immunosuppression.

Superficial partial-thickness wounds result in increased pain sensation. Nerve endings are exposed to the surface, and any stimulation (touch or temperature change) causes intense pain. With standard treatment these burns heal in 10 to 14 days with no scar, but some minor pigment changes may occur.

DEEP PARTIAL-THICKNESS WOUNDS. Deep partial-thickness wounds extend deeper into the dermal layer of the skin, and fewer healthy epidermal cells remain. The wounds usually appear red and waxy white without blisters (Figure 68-4). Edema is moderate; pain is present to a lesser degree than with superficial burns because more of the nerve endings have been destroyed. Blisters are absent because the dead tissues adhere to the underlying dermal collagen fibers.

The remaining blood supply to these areas is greatly reduced due to intense vasoconstriction. Progression to deeper injury can occur through hypoxia and ischemia. Ad-

TABLE 68-1 • CLASSIFICATION OF BURN DEPTH

Characteristic	Superficial	Partial-Thickness Superficial	Deep Partial-Thickness	Full-Thickness	Deep Full-Thickness
Color	Pink to red	Pink to red	Red to white	Black, brown, yellow, white, red	Black
Edema	Mild	Mild to moderate	Moderate	Severe	Absent
Pain	Yes	Yes	Yes	Yes and no	Absent
Blisters	No	Yes	Rare	No	No
Eschar	No	No	Yes, soft and dry	Yes, hard and inelastic	Yes, hard and inelastic
Healing time	3-5 days	~2 wk	2-6 wk	Weeks to months	Weeks to months
Grafts required	No	No	Can be used if healing is prolonged	Yes	Yes
Example	Sunburn, flash burns	Scalds, flames, brief contact with hot objects	Scalds; flames; prolonged contact with hot objects, tar, grease, chemicals	Scalds; flames; prolonged contact with hot objects, tar, grease, chemicals, electricity	Flames, electricity, grease, tar, chemicals

TABLE 68-2 • CLASSIFICATION OF BURN INJURY AND BURN CENTER REFERRAL CRITERIA

Characteristics	Comments
MINOR BURNS Deep partial-thickness burns <15% TBSA Full-thickness burns <2% TBSA No burns of eyes, ears, face, hands, feet, or perineum No electrical burns No inhalation injury No complicated concomitant injury Patient is under 60 yr and has no chronic cardiac, pulmonary, or endocrine disorder	Clients in this category should receive emergency care at the scene and be taken to a hospital emergency department. A special expertise hospital or designated burn center is not necessary.
MODERATE BURNS Deep partial-thickness burns 15%-25% TBSA Full-thickness burns 2%-10% TBSA No burns of eyes, ears, face, hands, feet, or perineum No electrical burns No inhalation injury No complicated concomitant injury Patient is under 60 yr and has no chronic cardiac, pulmonary, or endocrine disorder	Clients in this category should receive emergency care at the scene and be transferred either to a special expertise hospital or to a designated burn center.
MAJOR BURNS Partial-thickness burns >25% TBSA Full-thickness burns >10% Any burn involving the eyes, ears, face, hands, feet, perineum Electrical injury Inhalation injury Client over 60 yr of age Burn is complicated with other injuries (e.g., fractures) Client has cardiac, pulmonary, or other chronic metabolic disorders	Clients who meet *any one* of the criteria for a major burn should receive emergency care at the nearest emergency department and then be transferred to a designated burn center as soon as possible.

TBSA, Total body surface area.

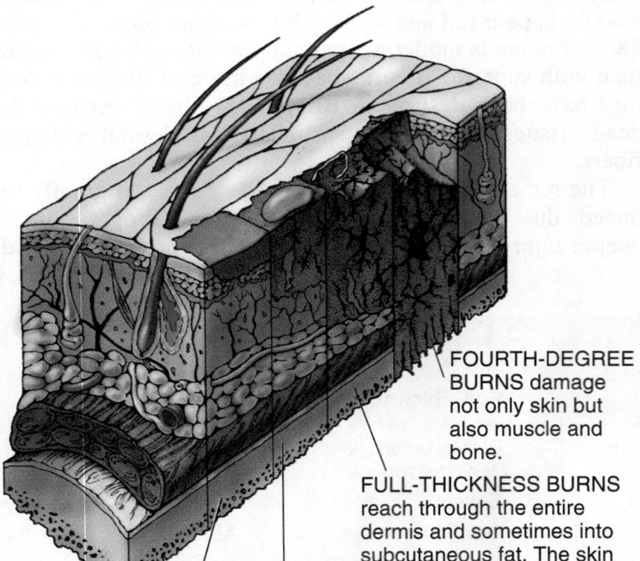

Figure 68-2 • The tissue involved in burns of various depths.

equate hydration, nutrients, and oxygen are necessary for spontaneous re-epithelialization of the wound and the prevention of conversion to deeper burns. Partial-thickness wounds can convert to full-thickness wounds when tissue damage increases with infection, hypoxia, or ischemia. Deep partial-thickness wounds generally heal in 3 to 6 weeks, but a large amount of scar formation results. Surgical intervention with skin grafting is required if healing will be prolonged.

FULL-THICKNESS WOUNDS. A full-thickness wound involves the entire epidermal and dermal layers of the skin (Figure 68-5). No living **(viable)** epidermal cells remain for re-epithelialization, and skin grafts are required in areas larger than approximately 12 to 16 cm^2. In smaller areas, secondary wound closure occurs by the growth of collagen-based scar tissue from the unburned edges inward (see Chapter 67).

The area of full-thickness injury has a hard, dry, leathery **eschar** (burn crust) that forms from coagulated particles of destroyed dermis. *The eschar is dead tissue; it must slough off or be removed from the burn wound before healing can occur.* The thick, coagulated particles often adhere to the subcutaneous layer by collagen fibers, which makes the removal of eschar difficult. Edema is a significant problem in burns and is pronounced under the eschar in a full-thickness wound. When the injury completely surrounds an extremity or the thorax **(circumferential),** circulation and ventilation may be compromised by tight eschar. **Escharotomies** (incisions through the eschar) or **fasciotomies** (incisions through eschar

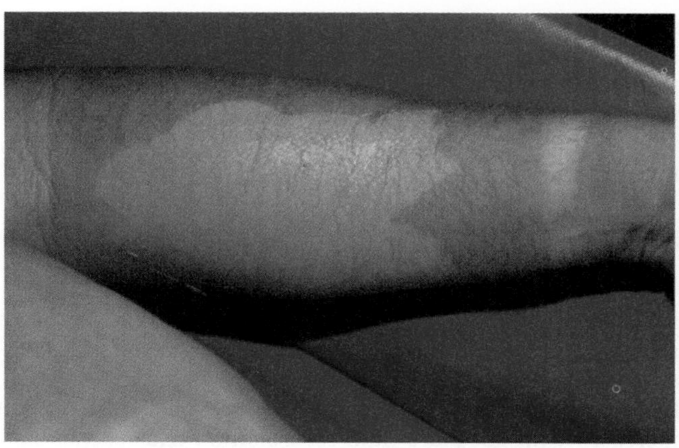

Figure 68-3 ● The typical appearance of a superficial partial-thickness burn injury.

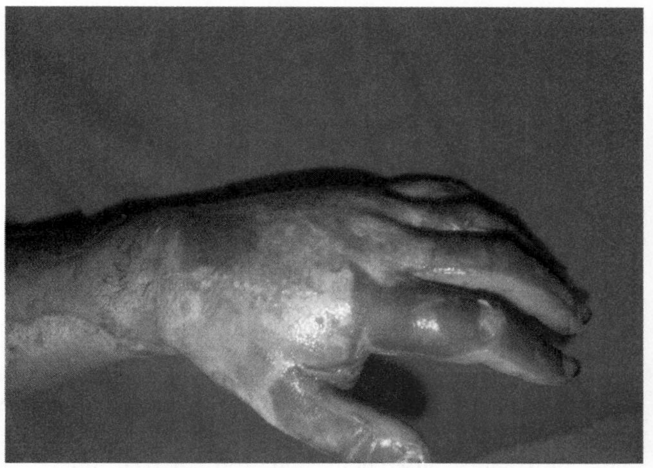

Figure 68-4 ● The typical appearance of a deep partial-thickness burn injury.

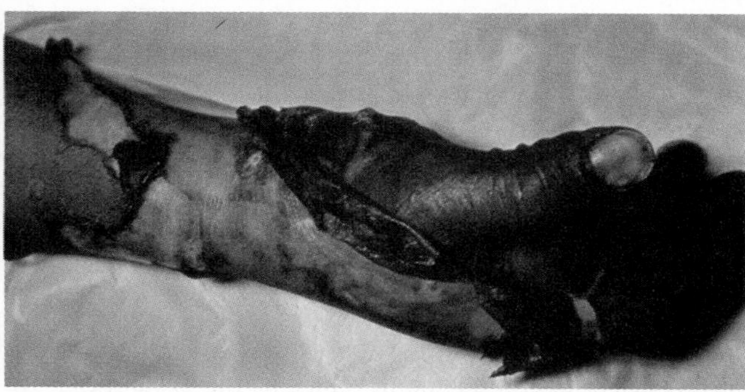

Figure 68-5 ● The typical appearance of a full-thickness burn injury.

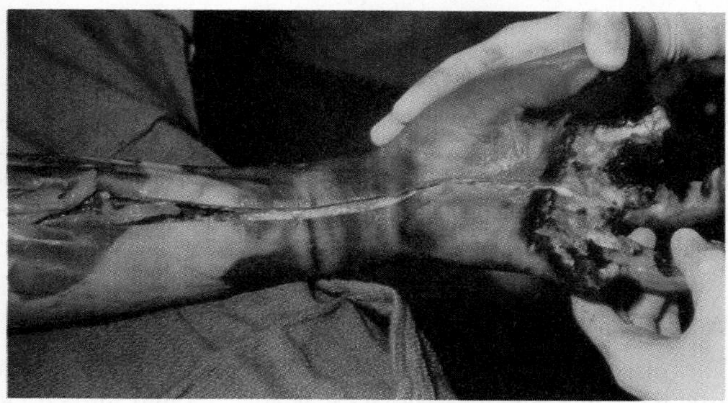

Figure 68-6 ● The typical appearance of a deep full-thickness burn injury.

and fascia) may be required to relieve pressure and allow normal perfusion and breathing (see Surgical Management [Ineffective Tissue Perfusion], p. 1572).

The color of a full-thickness burn wound may be waxy white, deep red, yellow, brown, or black. Thrombosed vessels may be present and visible beneath the surface of the burn because the dermal blood vessels are heat coagulated, causing the burned tissue to be without a blood supply **(avascular).** Sensation is minimal or absent in these areas of injury due to the destruction of nerve endings. Healing time depends on the re-establishment of an adequate blood supply within the injured areas and can range from weeks to months.

DEEP FULL-THICKNESS WOUNDS. Deep full-thickness wounds extend beyond the skin into underlying fascia and tissues. These deep injuries damage muscle, bone, and tendons and leave them exposed to the surface. These burns occur with flame, electrical, or chemical injuries. The wound is blackened and depressed, and sensation is completely absent (Figure 68-6). All full-thickness burns benefit from early excision and grafting. Grafting decreases pain and length of stay and accelerates recovery (Ramzy et al., 1999). Amputation may be required when an extremity is involved.

VASCULAR CHANGES RESULTING FROM BURN INJURIES

Major circulatory disruption occurs at the burn site immediately after a burn injury. The vessels supplying the burned skin are occluded, and blood flow through the arterial and venous channels decreases or ceases completely. Damaged macrophages within the tissues release chemicals (mediators) that initially produce vasoconstriction. Peripheral vessel thrombosis may occur; this decrease in tissue perfusion can cause necrosis, which can lead to deeper injuries in the already damaged areas.

Fluid Shift

After the initial vasoconstriction, vessels adjacent to the burn injury dilate. This leads to increased capillary hydrostatic pressure and is accompanied by increased capillary permeability (Figure 68-7). This fluid shift, also known as *third spacing* or *capillary leak syndrome,* involves a continuous leak of plasma from the intravascular space into the interstitial space. The loss of plasma fluids and proteins results in a decreased colloidal osmotic pressure in the vascular space. Leakage of fluid and electrolytes from the vascular space continues, causing significant edema formation. Fluid shift usually occurs in the first 12 hours after the burn but can continue for 24 to 36 hours.

The amount of plasma to interstitial fluid shift depends on the extent and severity of injury. Capillary leak occurs in both burned and unburned tissues when tissue damage is extensive (i.e., greater than 20% to 30% total body surface area **[TBSA]**). Peripheral edema develops as the protein-rich fluids, plasma, and electrolytes escape into the interstitial space. Tissue colloidal osmotic pressure increases as a result of the movement of proteins, increasing the third-spacing fluid shift.

Profound imbalances of fluid, electrolytes, and acid-base occur as a result of the fluid shift and other physiologic disruptions caused by injury. These imbalances usually include hypovolemia, metabolic acidosis, **hyperkalemia** (elevated blood potassium levels), and **hyponatremia** (decreased blood sodium levels). Hyperkalemia occurs as a result of direct tissue damage that releases large amounts of intracellular potassium into the vascular space; it is generally self-limiting. **Hemoconcentration** (elevated blood osmolarity, hematocrit, and hemoglobin) develops from the circulatory dehydration. Hemoconcentration increases blood viscosity, which reduces flow through small vessels and contributes to generalized tissue hypoxia.

Fluid Remobilization

The inflammatory responses gradually subside 24 to 36 hours after the injury, and the capillary leak abates. Fluid shifts back into the circulation. This fluid remobilization phase restores fluid and electrolyte levels and renal blood flow, resulting in increased urine formation and diuresis. Body weight returns to normal over several days as peripheral edema subsides.

During this phase, hyponatremia is likely to develop because of increased renal sodium excretion and the loss of sodium from wounds. Hypokalemia can occur now as potassium returns to the intracellular compartment. Anemia often develops as a result of hemodilution, but it is generally not severe enough to require blood transfusions. Transfusions are indicated if the client's hematocrit is less than 20% to 25% and is accompanied by clinical signs and symptoms of hypoxia. The exact laboratory value is not as critical as the clinical signs and symptoms. The timing of transfusions is controversial, and the trend is to limit transfusion unless absolutely necessary.

CARDIAC FUNCTION CHANGES RESULTING FROM BURN INJURY

Because of the initial fluid shifts and hypovolemia that occur after a burn injury, cardiac output decreases in spite of an increased heart rate. Cardiac output may remain depressed until 18 to 36 hours after the burn injury occurs. Cardiac output increases with adequate fluid resuscitation and reaches normal levels before plasma volume is restored completely. Appropriate fluid resuscitation and support with adequate oxygenation prevent further complications.

PULMONARY CHANGES RESULTING FROM BURN INJURY

Respiratory insufficiency (inhalation injury) rarely occurs from direct contact with flames but is caused by superheated air, steam, toxic fumes, or smoke. It is a major cause of morbidity and mortality in thermally injured clients. Pulmonary complications cause or contribute to death in 77% of clients with a combined inhalation and cutaneous burn injury (Flynn, 1999). Respiratory failure associated with burn injuries can also result from airway edema during fluid resuscitation, increased alveolar capillary permeability, circumferential chest burns that compromise breathing, and carbon monoxide toxicity.

Damage to the respiratory system from an inhalation injury can occur in the upper and major airways and the lung parenchyma. The upper airway is affected when inhaled smoke or irritants cause edema and obstructive closure of the trachea. Irritants coming in contact with the upper airway cause a reflex closure of the vocal cords. This protective mechanism results in a decrease in the amount of smoke and toxic gases entering the lungs. Although air is a poor conductor of heat, some heat does reach the upper airway, causing an inflammatory response that leads to oropharyngeal edema and potentially dangerous airway obstruction.

Major airway injury results from chemicals and toxic gases, rather than heat, that are produced from incomplete combustion. The ciliated, mucus-secreting epithelial cells lin-

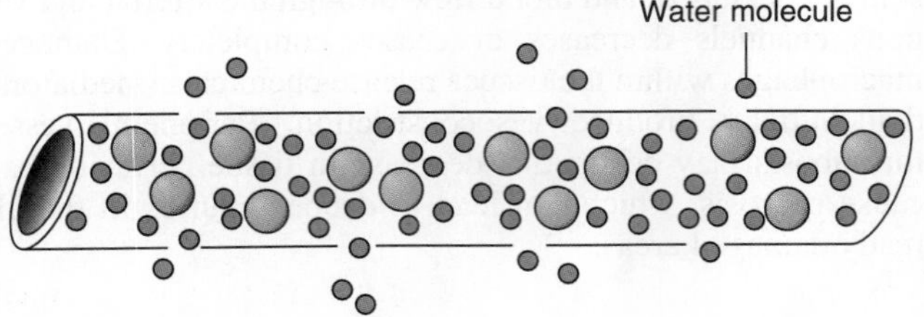

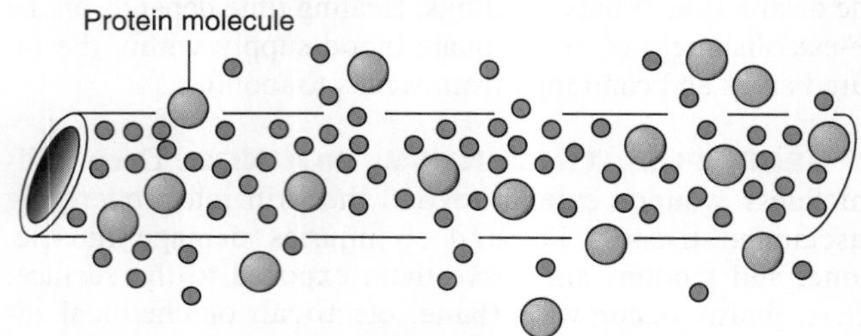

Figure 68-7 ● The vascular capillary response to burn injury (early phase).

ing the trachea normally trap bacteria and foreign materials. Smoke and products of combustion slow this activity, which allows foreign particles to enter the bronchi. The lining of the trachea and bronchi may slough 48 to 72 hours after injury, enter the airway, narrow the tracheal lumen, and obstruct the lower airways.

Parenchymal injuries result from damage to the alveolar epithelium and capillary endothelium by toxic irritants. Increased alveolar-capillary membrane permeability results in intra-alveolar edema. This edema can occur immediately or as late as 1 week after the injury. The fluid that diffuses across the membrane settles in the interstitial spaces; fibrinous membranes eventually form, which leads to respiratory distress. Progressive pulmonary failure develops with acute pulmonary insufficiency and infection.

GASTROINTESTINAL CHANGES RESULTING FROM BURN INJURY

Because of the fluid shifts and decreased cardiac output that occur after injury, blood flow is shifted to the brain, heart, and liver. Consequently other organs, including the gastrointestinal (GI) tract, have decreased perfusion. Gastric mucosal integrity and motility are impaired. The sympathetic nervous system stress response causes increased secretion of catecholamines (especially epinephrine and norepinephrine), which inhibit GI motility and reduce the flow of blood to the area. Peristalsis decreases, and a paralytic ileus may develop. Mucosal secretions and gases collect in the intestines and stomach, causing abdominal distention.

Curling's ulcer, or acute ulcerative gastroduodenal disease, may develop within 24 hours after a severe burn injury because of reduced GI perfusion and mucosal damage. The mucosal membrane normally acts as a barrier to the absorption of hydrogen ions secreted into the gastric lumen. With an alteration in gastric mucosal function, this barrier is compromised and hydrogen ion production is increased. Ulcerations may develop as a result. However, this complication has become extremely uncommon in recent years because of the use of H_2 histamine blockers such as cimetidine (Tagamet) and ranitidine (Zantac), mucoprotectants such as sucralfate (Carafate), and early enteral nutrition.

METABOLIC CHANGES RESULTING FROM BURN INJURY

A significant burn injury places the client in a hypermetabolic state. Increased secretion of catecholamines, antidiuretic hormone, aldosterone, and cortisol increase metabolism. With hypermetabolism, oxygen and calorie requirements are high.

The secreted catecholamines activate the stress response. The increased production (and loss) of heat results in protein and fat breakdown **(catabolism),** the rapid use of glucose and calories, and increased urinary nitrogen losses. The evaporated heat and water from the burn also increase metabolic and catabolic rates, which increase calorie expenditure. Depending on the extent of injury, the client's calorie requirements may be double or triple normal energy needs. These increased rates peak 4 to 12 days after the burn and can remain elevated for months until all wounds are closed.

The hypermetabolic condition also results in an increase in core body temperature. The client loses heat through the burned skin surfaces because the protective barrier is lost. Core body temperature increases as a response to the adjustment in the hypothalamus. Central thermoregulation is altered to compensate for the hypermetabolic state. There is an impaired shift in temperature; a low-grade fever can develop, which is common among clients with burn injuries. Essentially what occurs is a resetting of the body's normal temperature-regulating mechanism.

IMMUNOLOGIC CHANGES RESULTING FROM BURN INJURY

Thermal injury results in a loss of the protective barrier of the skin, which increases the risk for infection. The burn injury activates the inflammatory response but can also suppress immune function (see Chapter 20). Antibody-mediated immunity and cell-mediated immunity are both suppressed. All immune responses are therefore reduced. Topical antimicrobial agents, systemic antibiotics, general anesthesia, blood component transfusion, and the stress of surgical procedures further compromise immune function.

COMPENSATORY RESPONSES TO BURN INJURY

Any tissue injury is a threat to homeostasis and is a physiologic stressor. Two compensatory responses have immediate benefit: the inflammatory response and the sympathetic nervous system stress response. Together these responses cause the physiologic changes that result in many of the clinical manifestations seen in the first 2 to 3 days after a burn injury.

Inflammatory Compensation

The inflammatory compensatory response can be helpful by initiating healing in the injured tissues. It also is responsible for some of the serious problems that occur with the fluid shift. Inflammatory compensation causes blood vessels to leak fluid into the interstitial space and white blood cells to release chemicals that generate local tissue reactions. The inflammatory compensatory mechanisms cause the massive fluid shift, edema formation, and hypovolemia that characterize the emergent phase (first 48 hours) after a burn injury. The extent and intensity of the inflammatory response depend on the severity of the burn injury. Chapter 20 explains the inflammatory compensatory mechanisms in detail.

The inflammatory compensatory response is immediately helpful to the body when injury occurs. These actions are intended to function on a relatively local and short-term basis. When these actions are widespread and/or persistent, the tissue-damaging consequences can be severe.

Sympathetic Nervous System Compensation

The sympathetic nervous system stress response is generated by the sympathetic division of the autonomic nervous system and some components of the endocrine system when any physical or psychologic stressors are present. Changes resulting from sympathetic compensation are most evident in the cardiovascular, respiratory, and gastrointestinal systems. Fig-

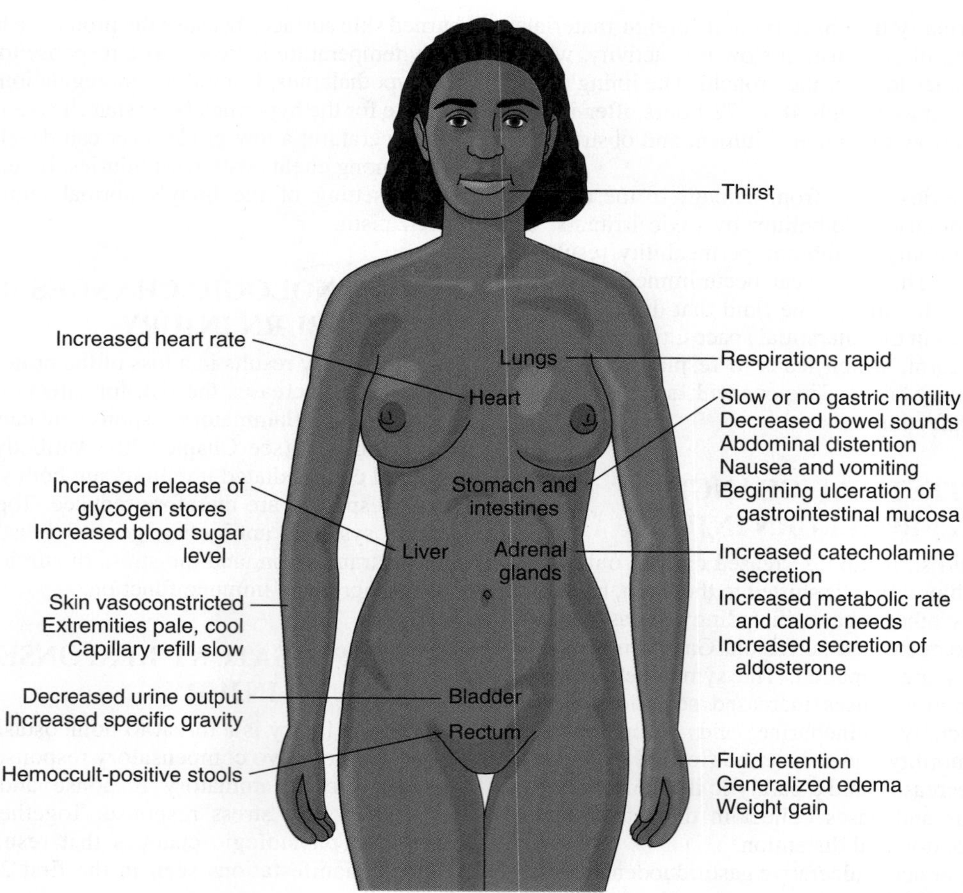

Figure 68-8 ● The physiologic actions of the sympathetic nervous system compensatory responses to burn injury (early phase).

ure 68-8 summarizes the physical consequence of sympathetic nervous system stimulation.

Etiology of Burn Injury

Burn injuries are caused by a variety of sources, including dry heat (flame), moist heat (scald), contact with hot surfaces, chemicals, electricity, and ionizing radiation. The causative agent of the injury affects both the prognosis and the treatment.

DRY HEAT

Dry heat injuries are caused by open flame. The most common causes of flame injuries are house fires and explosions. Ignited clothing from an open flame accounts for most of the injuries. Explosions usually result in flash burns because they produce a brief exposure to very high temperatures.

MOIST HEAT

Moist heat (scald) injuries are caused by contact with hot liquids. Scald injuries are most common among adults older than 65 years (Stone, Ahmed, & Evans, 2000). Hot liquid spills usually burn the upper, frontal surfaces of the body, whereas immersion scald injuries usually involve the lower portions of the body.

CONTACT BURNS

Hot metal, tar, and grease can cause full-thickness burns when they contact the skin. Hot metal injuries occur when a client places a part of the body against a hot surface, such as a space heater or iron. They also can occur in industrial settings from molten metals. Tar and asphalt temperatures usually are greater than 400° F, and significant deep injuries occur within seconds when the skin is immersed in or splashed with the agent. Hot grease injuries result from cooking agents and are usually deep because of the temperature of the grease.

CHEMICAL INJURY

A burn injury occurs when chemicals come in direct contact with the skin and epithelial tissues or are ingested. The severity of the injury depends on the duration of contact, the concentration of the chemical, the amount of tissue exposed, and the mechanisms of action of the chemical.

Chemical burns to the skin usually occur in adults in industrial settings, but they may also occur in the home from contact with products such as drain cleaner and toilet bowl cleaner.

Strong acids (e.g., hydrochloric acid, sulfuric acid) and strong alkalis (e.g., sodium hydroxide) destroy tissue by precipitation of chemical compounds in the cell, cellular dehydration, protoplasmic poisoning, and dissolution of tissue proteins. Acids cause coagulation necrosis and pain. Alkalis cause liquefaction necrosis, with deeper penetration and less pain.

ELECTRICAL INJURY

An electrical injury is considered a nonthermally induced burn; it is caused when an electrical current enters the body (Figure 68-9). Electrical injuries are serious because they damage deep structures and organs and can even result in the loss of one or more limbs. The amount of damage depends on amperage, voltage, resistance to flow, type of current, duration of contact, and the current's path through the body.

Resistance (impedance to flow) varies in different parts of the body. Nerve, muscle, and blood vessels have very low resistance and are susceptible to deep injuries. Tendons, fat, and bone have the most resistance. Skin has intermediate resistance. Wet skin has less resistance to current flow than dry, calloused areas. The higher the resistance, the greater the heat generated by the current flow and the greater the potential for soft-tissue injury.

The longer the electricity is in contact with the body, the greater the damage. The duration of contact may be increased by tetanic contractions of the strong flexor muscles in the forearm, which can prevent the person from releasing the electrical source. Severe tetanic muscle contractions have been associated with fractures of the spine and long bones, necessitating immobilization of the client with a cervical collar and backboard.

It is difficult to know the exact path a current takes in the body. The course of flow is generally defined by the locations of the "entrance" and "exit" wounds. Initially, the wounds may not be obvious. When visible, the entrance site is usually well defined and rounded. The exit site is usually explosive and surrounded by charred tissue.

Burn injuries from electricity can occur in one of three ways: *thermal burns, flash burns,* or *true electrical injury.* Thermal burns may occur when clothes ignite from heat or flames produced by electrical sparks. External burn injuries can occur when the electrical current jumps, or "arcs," between two charged surfaces. Injuries usually are severe and deep and are associated with high-tension current. True electrical injury can occur when the body makes direct contact with an electrical source. Internal damage results, and the injuries can be devastating. Damage starts on the inside and goes out; deep-tissue destruction may not be apparent initially after injury. Organs in the path of the current may become ischemic and necrotic.

RADIATION INJURY

Clients incur radiation injuries when they are exposed to large doses of radioactive material. The most common type of radiation exposure leading to tissue injury occurs in conjunction with therapeutic radiation. This injury is usually minor and rarely causes extensive skin damage.

Radiation exposure is more serious in industrial settings where radioactive energy is produced or radioactive isotopes are used. The injury depends on the amount and type of energy deposited over time. Chapter 25 discusses the penetrating ability and potential for tissue damage of alpha, beta, and gamma radiation. The severity of injury is determined by the type of radiation, distance from the source, duration of exposure, absorbed dose, and depth of penetration into the body.

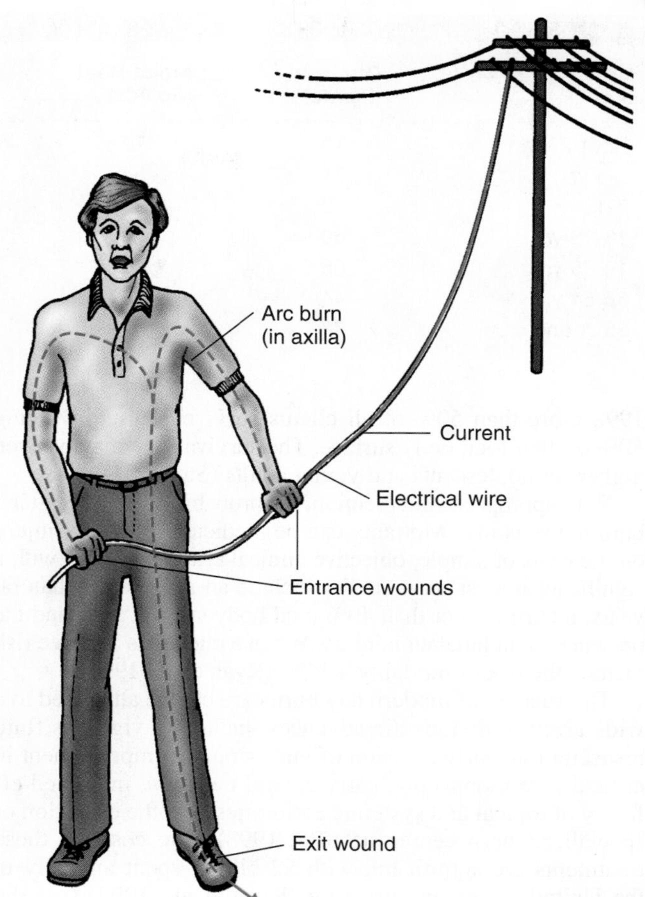

Figure 68-9 ● The mechanism of electrical injury. Currents passing through the body follow the path of least resistance to the ground.

Incidence/Prevalence of Burn Injury

Approximately 1.25 million burn injuries occur each year in the United States, leading to 600,000 emergency department visits. Of the clients who seek medical attention, approximately 45,000 require inpatient care; most are now being treated in a burn unit or center. The rest of the injuries are minor, and treatment with basic first aid at home is adequate. Approximately 3761 deaths were attributed to fires, burns, and fire-related injuries in 1996 (American Burn Association [ABA], 1999). The vast majority of these burns are attributable to house fires, and the remainder result from multiple other causes (Burn Foundation, 1999). According to the National Center for Health Statistics, there was a 40% decrease in burn deaths from 1971 to 1995.

Burns remain the sixth leading cause of accidental death in the United States. Causes vary among different age-groups (Table 68-3). The highest risk is among those 75 years and older. Males are at slightly higher risk for both fatal and nonfatal injuries resulting from fires and burns.

The probability of survival after a burn injury has improved steadily over the past 50 years. In 1945 only 50% of clients survived burns involving 40% of the total body surface. In

TABLE 68-3 • PERCENTAGE OF BURN INJURIES BY AGE IN THE UNITED STATES

Age	Dry Heat (Flame)	Moist Heat (Scalds)	Contact	Chemical	Electrical	Ionizing Radiation
Birth-23 mo	10	72	15	1	2	<1
2-4 yr	34	54	8	1	3	<1
5-12 yr	70	23	4	1	2	<1
13-18 yr	69	20	5	2	4	<1
19-35 yr	56	26	10	4	4	<1
36-54 yr	44	33	13	4	6	<1
55 yr and older	73	21	4	1	1	<1

1998 more than 50% of all clients survived burns involving 80% of their total body surface. The survival rate may be even higher for adolescents and young adults (Saffle, 1998).

With appropriate intervention, the probability of death after a burn injury is low. Mortality can be predicted soon after injury on the basis of simple, objective clinical criteria. Factors with a significant impact on mortality include an age greater than 60 years, a burn greater than 40% total body surface area, and the presence of an inhalation injury. When a client has all three risk factors, the risk of mortality is 90% (Ryan et al., 1998).

The success of modern day burn care can be attributed to a wide array of therapeutic advances, including vigorous fluid resuscitation, early excision of burn wounds, improvement in critical care monitoring, early enteral nutrition, improved efficacy of topical and systemic antibiotics, and the evolution of specialized burn centers (Saffle, 1998). The costs of these treatments are significant, with $2 billion spent annually in the United States on burn care (Ryan et al., 1998) (see the Cost of Care box at right).

WOMEN'S HEALTH CONSIDERATIONS

Burn injury during pregnancy has adverse effects on both maternal and fetal survival. The problems affecting the fetus include spontaneous labor and an increase in intrauterine fetal death due to compromised circulation. The signs of shock may not be evident until 30% to 35% of the circulating blood volume is lost. Placental-fetal perfusion depends on maternal blood pressure. Therefore if the mother has sustained a significant burn injury and develops significant hypovolemia, fetal circulation is likely to be compromised. Fetal monitoring is then necessary to determine fetal stability and/or viability.

In addition, respiratory injuries to the mother can result in trauma to the fetus due to respiratory exchange disturbances across the placental barrier, leading to hypoxia. Cesarean delivery may be indicated depending on the condition of the mother and the fetus. Each case is different, and the decision must be based on the gestational age of the fetus and the available data obtained through complete assessments of both the mother and fetus.

COST OF CARE IMPLICATIONS FOR NURSING

BURN DRESSINGS AND WOUND MANAGEMENT

Cost of Care

- Burn wound dressing materials, especially biologic materials, are expensive (range in price from $150 to more than $500 per square foot)
- Biologic materials and artificial skin are easily damaged by rough handling, nonadherence to recommended storage and use procedures, inappropriate client positioning, and contamination.
- Most burn wound dressing procedures are labor intensive and require one or more experienced burn nurses.

Implications for Nursing

Nurses need to consider the cost of materials when planning a burn wound dressing change. Only the necessary amount of materials should be prepared (thawed, etc.) for the specific individual procedure to avoid material wastage. Careful documentation at each change can assist in the communication for materials needed at the next burn wound dressing change.

Data from Burn Foundation (1999). Burn incidence and treatment in the United States, http://www.burnfoundation.org/adultfact.html; Rakel, B.A., et al. (1999). Split-thickness skin graft donor site care: A quantitative synthesis of the research. *Applied Nursing Research, 11*(4), 174-182; Ryan, C.M., et al. (1998). Estimates of the probability of death from burn injuries. *New England Journal of Medicine, 338*(6), 362-66; Winfrey, M. Cochran, M., & Hegarty, M. (1999). A new technology in burn therapy: Integra artificial skin. *Dimensions of Critical Care Nursing, 18*(1), 14-20.

EMERGENT PHASE OF BURN INJURY

OVERVIEW

Burns are often described as the most severe devastating and dehumanizing injury that a human can endure. Events within the first hour after injury can make the difference between life and death in a thermally injured client. Immediate care focuses on maintaining an open airway, ensuring adequate breathing and circulation, limiting the extent of injury, and maintaining the function of vital organs. Chart 68-1 outlines the emergency management of a burn injury.

The emergent phase is the first phase of a burn injury. It begins at the onset of injury and continues to approximately 48 hours. During this phase the injury is evaluated and immediate problems resulting from the burn, including fluid loss, edema formation, and the potential for peripheral circulatory impairment, are assessed. Interventions are initiated to resolve and/or prevent potential complications.

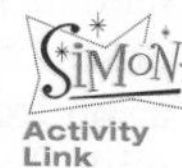

➤ COLLABORATIVE MANAGEMENT

• Assessment

HISTORY

During the emergent phase, the nurse obtains a history of the mechanism of injury and other pertinent information from the client if possible. If information cannot be obtained from the client, questions should be directed to significant others and those present at the scene of the injury. Important infor-

CHART 68-1

BEST PRACTICE *for*
Emergency Management of Burns

General Management for All Types of Burns
- Assess for airway patency.
- Administer oxygen as needed.
- Cover the client with a blanket.
- Keep the client on NPO status.
- Elevate the extremities if no fractures are obvious.
- Obtain vital signs.
- Initiate an IV line and begin fluid replacement.
- Administer tetanus toxoid for prophylaxis.
- Perform a head-to-toe assessment.

Specific Management

Flame Burns
- Smother the flames.
- Remove smoldering clothing and all metal objects.

Chemical Burns
- Brush off any dry chemicals present on the skin or clothing.
- Remove the client's clothing.
- Ascertain the type of chemical causing the burn.
- Do not attempt to neutralize the chemical unless it has been positively identified and the appropriate neutralizing agent is available.

Electrical Burns
- At the scene, separate the client from the electrical current.
- Smother any flames that are present.
- Initiate cardiopulmonary resuscitation.
- Obtain an electrocardiogram (ECG).

Radiation Burns
- Remove the client from the radiation source.
- If the client has been exposed to radiation from an unsealed source, remove the client's clothing (using tongs or lead protective gloves).
- If the client has radioactive particles on his or her skin, send the client to the nearest designated radiation decontamination center.
- Help the client to bathe or shower.

mation about the circumstances of the injury includes the time of injury, the source and cause of injury, a detailed description of how the burn occurred, and the events occurring from the time of injury until help arrived. Additional demographic data, health history (including pre-existing illness), medication use, the presence of concomitant injuries, and pain information are obtained. Potential complications associated with burn injuries must constantly be considered.

Demographic data include age, weight, and height. The rate of serious complications and death from burn injuries is greatly increased among adults over 50 years of age. Chart 68-2 summarizes the age-related differences in the older adult in response to a burn injury. The client's preburn weight is used to calculate fluid rates, energy requirements, and drug doses. The preburn weight often is referred to as "dry weight." Calculations based on a weight obtained after the initiation of fluid replacement are not accurate because of water-induced weight gain. Height is important in determining body surface area (BSA), which is used to calculate nutritional needs.

A health history, including any pre-existing illnesses, must be known for appropriate treatment to be given. The client is asked specifically about his or her history of cardiac or renal impairment and diabetes mellitus; any of these problems influence fluid resuscitation. A medication history that includes allergies,

CHART 68-2

NURSING FOCUS *on the* OLDER ADULT
Age-Related Changes That Increase Mortality and Morbidity from Burns

- The skin of an older person is thinner and more easily damaged than that of a younger person. Therefore burn injuries tend to be more extensive in older clients, even when exposure to causative agents is short.
- Healing time is slower in the older adult, which increases the risk for infection and other complications.
- Cardiac impairment in the older client with burns limits the amount and type of fluids used in resuscitation. As a result, older clients are more likely to develop complications from hypovolemic shock and inadequate renal perfusion.
- The immune responses of the older client may be reduced, which increases the risk for infection and sepsis. In addition, the older adult may not have a fever when an infection is present.
- Older adults are more likely to have a pre-existing medical condition (e.g., diabetes mellitus, cardiovascular disorders, pulmonary or renal impairment, or immunosuppression) that may further compromise vital organ function or interfere with resuscitation and treatment.

current medications, and immunization status is obtained from the client or significant other. The dose and time of the last medication taken are determined. An assessment is obtained regarding whether or not the client smokes or drinks alcohol daily; these factors can influence treatment and physical responses.

Other injuries are unusual but may occur at the time of the burn. The most common causes of associated injuries are falls and motor vehicle accidents. Such injuries often increase the morbidity and mortality of the client. A determination is made as to whether additional injuries such as fractures, chest injuries, and abdominal trauma are causing pain or discomfort.

PHYSICAL ASSESSMENT/CLINICAL MANIFESTATIONS

Physical assessment findings in the emergent phase may vary greatly from findings later in the course of the injury. A systems approach is used to ensure that no problem is missed. The systems assessed first are those that can have immediate, life-threatening alterations in function.

RESPIRATORY ASSESSMENT. Clients with major burn injuries and those with inhalation injury are at risk for respiratory complications. Respiratory manifestations commonly associated with a burn injury are presented in Chart 68-3.

DIRECT AIRWAY INJURY. The degree of inhalation damage depends on the fire source, temperature, environment, and types of toxic gases generated. Information is obtained about the source of the fire, duration of exposure, and history of being in an enclosed space. The respiratory system is assessed by visual inspection of the mouth, nose, and pharynx. Burns of the lips, face, ears, neck, eyelids, eyebrows, and eyelashes are strong indicators of exposure to flames; these burns increase the possibility of an inhalation injury. Intraoral burns and singed nasal hairs indicate potentially serious injuries. Black carbon particles in the nose and mouth along with congestion and edema of the nasal septum are indicative of smoke inhalation.

CHART 68-3

KEY FEATURES *of* Upper Airway Obstruction and Inhalation Injury

Upper Airway Obstruction
- Edema, erythema, and ulceration of airway mucosa, especially the posterior pharynx
- Increased hoarseness
- Stridor
- Any face or neck burn with edema formation
- Heat-induced intraoral injury

Inhalation Injury
- Airway injury
- Carbonaceous sputum
- Singed nasal hairs
- Bronchorrhea
- Wheezing
- Pulmonary vasoconstriction
- Reduced cardiac output
- Bronchospasm

An alteration in respiratory pattern may be indicative of pulmonary injury. The client may:
- Become progressively hoarse
- Exhibit a brassy cough
- Drool or have difficulty swallowing
- Produce expiratory sounds that include grossly audible wheezes, crowing, and stridor

Upper airway edema and inhalation injury are most notable in the trachea and mainstem bronchi. Auscultation of these areas may reveal wheezes, which are a sign of obstruction. Clients with severe inhalation injuries may sustain such progressive obstruction that within a short time they cannot force air through the narrowed airways. As a result, the wheezing sounds disappear. *This finding indicates impending airway obstruction and demands immediate intubation.* Many clients are intubated prophylactically based on suspicion of inhalation injury rather than waiting until there is significant obstruction that may make endotracheal or nasotracheal intubation difficult or impossible.

CARBON MONOXIDE POISONING. Carbon monoxide is a colorless, odorless, tasteless gas produced as a by-product of combustion. Inhalation injury presents a simultaneous risk for carbon monoxide poisoning.

When carbon monoxide is inhaled, it binds to the hemoglobin molecule 200 to 250 times more tightly than does oxygen, and carboxyhemoglobin (CoHb) is formed. This situation impairs tissue oxygen availability. CoHb reduces the oxygen-carrying capacity of hemoglobin, which results in impaired oxygen transport, decreased oxygen delivery, and an inability of the cells to use oxygen. Even though the oxygen-carrying capacity of the hemoglobin is reduced, the partial pressure of arterial oxygen (PaO_2) is normal. The vasodilating action of carbon monoxide causes the "cherry red" color in these clients. Clinical manifestations vary with the concentration of CoHb. Table 68-4 summarizes the physiologic effects of carbon monoxide poisoning.

THERMAL (HEAT) INJURY. Thermal injury to the respiratory tract results from the inhalation of superheated air or steam. The client inhales the hot air, which is rapidly cooled by the upper airway, where the most severe damage from superheated air is confined.

TABLE 68-4 • PHYSIOLOGIC EFFECTS OF CARBON MONOXIDE POISONING

Carbon Monoxide Level	Physiologic Effects
1%-10% (normal)	Increased threshold to visual stimuli Increased blood flow to vital organs
11%-20% (mild poisoning)	Headache Decreased cerebral function Decreased visual acuity Slight breathlessness
21%-40% (moderate poisoning)	Headache Tinnitus Nausea Drowsiness Vertigo Altered mental state Confusion Stupor Irritability Decreased blood pressure and increased heart rate Depressed ST segment on electrocardiogram and dysrhythmias on palpation Pale to reddish purple skin
41%-60% (severe poisoning)	Coma Convulsions Cardiopulmonary instability
61%-80% (fatal poisoning)	Death

Inhaled steam can injure the lower respiratory tract because water holds heat better than does dry air. The entire respiratory tract, up to the major bronchioles, can be damaged by steam. Ulcerations, erythema, and edema of the mouth and epiglottis are usually the first manifestations, with rapid edema formation progressing to upper airway obstruction. Stridor, hoarseness, and shortness of breath result.

SMOKE POISONING. Smoke poisoning, or chemical injury from the inhalation of combustion by-products, is the most common mechanism of inhalation injury. Toxic by-products, especially hydrogen cyanide, are produced when various structural materials (e.g., plastics) or home furnishings are burned. The most significant effects of smoke poisoning are atelectasis, pulmonary edema, and tissue anoxia.

PULMONARY FLUID OVERLOAD. Pulmonary edema can result even when the lung tissues have not sustained any direct damage. Other damaged tissues release such large quantities of vasoactive amines, leading to increased capillary permeability, that even pulmonary capillaries leak fluid into the pulmonary interstitial spaces.

Circulatory overload from fluid resuscitation may cause left-sided congestive heart failure. The circulatory overload creates such high hydrostatic pressure within pulmonary vessels that even more fluid is lost from the pulmonary vascular space into the interstitial spaces. Excess interstitial fluid makes gas exchange difficult. The client is extremely short of breath and experiences increased dyspnea in the supine position. Crackles are heard on auscultation.

EXTERNAL FACTORS. In addition to pulmonary problems, clients with burn injuries may experience respiratory difficulties as a result of external factors. The most common external factor affecting respiration is tight eschar from deep circumferential chest burns. The eschar either restricts chest movement or compresses anatomic structures in the neck and throat to such an extent that ventilation is impaired. The chest is visually inspected for ease of respiration, amount of chest movement, rate of breathing, and effort required to breathe.

CARDIOVASCULAR ASSESSMENT. Changes in the cardiovascular system begin immediately after the burn injury and include shock from various causes. Shock is a common cause of death in the immediate postburn period in clients with significant injuries. Chapter 37 discusses the pathophysiologic and compensatory mechanisms for all types of shock.

The initial cardiovascular clinical manifestations reflect hypovolemia and decreased cardiac output. The nurse notes the presence of edema and assesses cardiovascular status by measuring central and peripheral pulses, blood pressure, capillary refill, and pulse oximetry. Noninvasive blood pressure readings are inaccurate in clients with large burns involving the upper extremities (Ahrns & Harkins, 1999). This situation necessitates invasive monitoring for blood pressure measurement. Initially, tachycardia, decreased blood pressure, and diminished peripheral pulses are present. Peripheral capillary refill is slow or absent as tissue perfusion decreases. With fluid resuscitation in the initial postburn period, peripheral edema increases, as does the client's body weight.

Electrocardiographic (ECG) changes indicate electrical damage to the heart. These changes are commonly associated with electrical burn injuries or with stress that induces a myocardial infarction. Baseline ECG tracings are obtained at the time of admission to the hospital or burn center.

RENAL/URINARY ASSESSMENT. Changes in renal function with burn injury are related to decreased renal perfusion and to the presence of cellular debris. During the fluid shift of the emergent period, perfusion may not be adequate for glomerular filtration. As a result, urine output is greatly diminished compared with intravenous (IV) fluid intake. The urine is highly concentrated and has a high specific gravity.

As a result of specific tissue damage, other substances may be present in the blood that perfuses the kidney. Destroyed red blood cells release hemoglobin and potassium. When muscle damage occurs from a major burn or electrical injury, a large oxygen-carrying protein called **myoglobin** is released from damaged muscle and circulates to the kidney. Most damaged cells release protein products that form uric acid. All of these large molecules in the blood may precipitate in the kidney tubular system. This precipitation blocks filtrate flow and may contribute to severe renal dysfunction.

Renal function is assessed by accurately measuring urine output and comparing this value with fluid intake. Urine output is decreased during the first 24 hours of the emergent phase. The rate of resuscitation fluid administration should maintain adult urine output at 30 to 50 mL or 0.5 ml/kg/hr. Adequate response to fluid resuscitation is further assessed by measuring urine specific gravity and blood urea nitrogen (BUN), serum creatinine, and serum sodium levels. The urine is examined for color, odor, and the presence of particulate matter or foam.

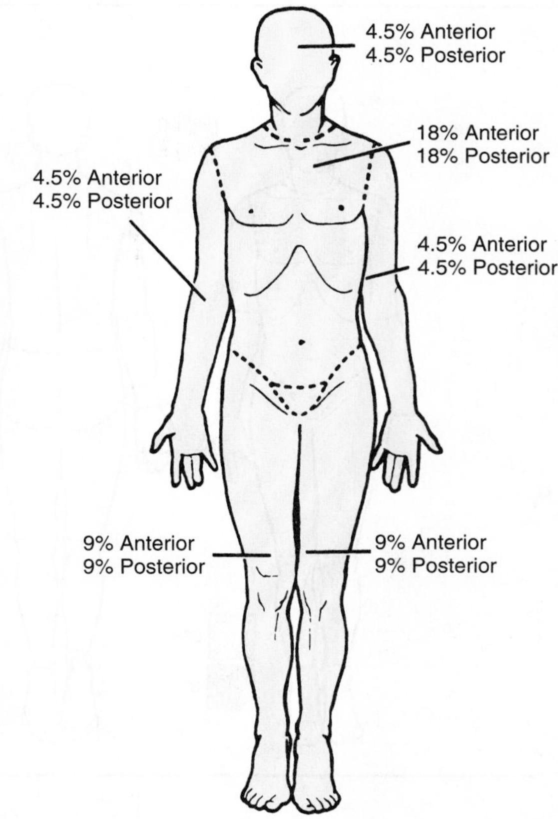

Figure 68-10 ● The rule of nines for estimating burn percentage.

INTEGUMENTARY ASSESSMENT. The skin is assessed to determine the size and depth of burn injury. The size of the injury is first estimated in comparison to the total body surface area (TBSA). For example, a burn that involves 40% of the TBSA is a 40% burn. The size of the injury is important not only for diagnosis and prognosis but also for calculating specific interventions such as drug dose, fluid replacement volumes, and caloric requirements.

The skin is inspected to identify injured areas and changes in color and appearance. Except with electrical burns, this initial size assessment usually can be made accurately with specific assessment tools and charts.

The most rapid method for calculating the size of a burn injury in adult clients whose weights are in normal proportion to their heights is the *rule of nines* (Figure 68-10). With this method, the body is divided into areas that are multiples of 9%. Although the rule of nines is useful at the site of injury and in emergency departments, overestimation of the percentage of TBSA involved can easily occur.

The Lund-Browder and Berkow methods are more accurate for evaluating the size of the injury (Figure 68-11). These methods take into account changes in body surface area from birth through adulthood.

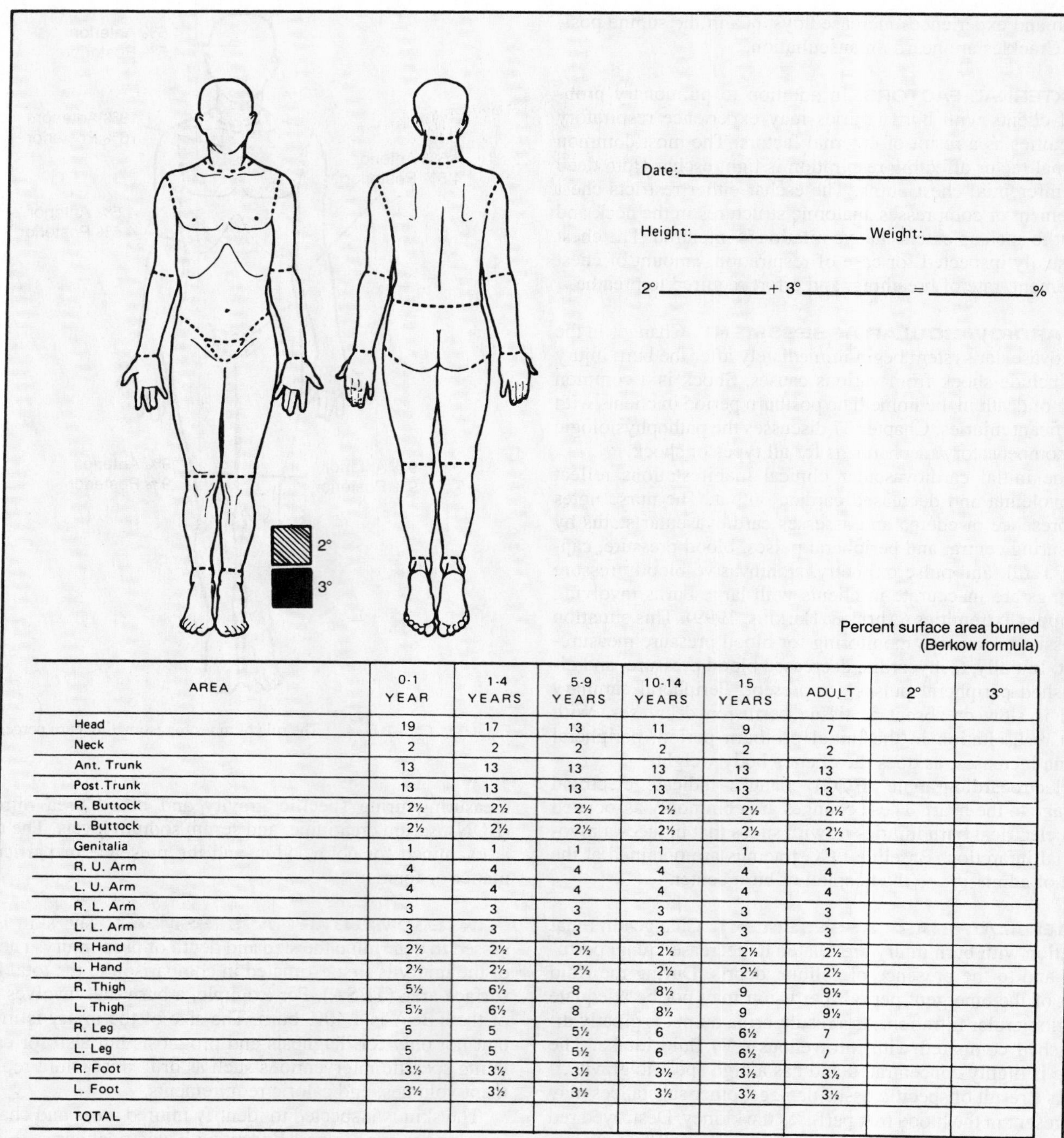

AREA	0-1 YEAR	1-4 YEARS	5-9 YEARS	10-14 YEARS	15 YEARS	ADULT	2°	3°
Head	19	17	13	11	9	7		
Neck	2	2	2	2	2	2		
Ant. Trunk	13	13	13	13	13	13		
Post.Trunk	13	13	13	13	13	13		
R. Buttock	2½	2½	2½	2½	2½	2½		
L. Buttock	2½	2½	2½	2½	2½	2½		
Genitalia	1	1	1	1	1	1		
R. U. Arm	4	4	4	4	4	4		
L. U. Arm	4	4	4	4	4	4		
R. L. Arm	3	3	3	3	3	3		
L. L. Arm	3	3	3	3	3	3		
R. Hand	2½	2½	2½	2½	2½	2½		
L. Hand	2½	2½	2½	2½	2½	2½		
R. Thigh	5½	6½	8	8½	9	9½		
L. Thigh	5½	6½	8	8½	9	9½		
R. Leg	5	5	5½	6	6½	7		
L. Leg	5	5	5½	6	6½	7		
R. Foot	3½	3½	3½	3½	3½	3½		
L. Foot	3½	3½	3½	3½	3½	3½		
TOTAL								

Figure 68-11 ● Estimation of the extent of burn injury by the Lund-Browder (Berkow) method. (*Ant.*, Anterior; *Post.*, posterior; *R.*, Right; *L.*, left; *R.U.*, right upper; *L.U.*, left upper; *R.L.*, right lower; *L.L.*, left lower.)

CHART 68-4

LABORATORY PROFILE
Burn Assessment During the Emergent Period

Test	Normal Range for Adults	Significance of Abnormal Findings
SERUM STUDIES		
Hemoglobin	11.7-15.5 g/dL (women) 13.2-17.3 g/dL (men)	Elevated as a result of fluid volume loss
Hematocrit	34%-45% (women) 39%-59% (men)	Elevated as a result of fluid volume loss
Urea nitrogen	10-20 mg/dL	Elevated as a result of fluid volume loss
Glucose	70-105 mg/dL	Elevated as a result of the stress response and increased uptake across injured tissues
ELECTROLYTES		
Sodium	136-145 mEq/L (mmol/L)	Decreased; sodium is trapped in edema fluid and lost through plasma leakage
Potassium	3.5-5.0 mEq/L (mmol/L)	Elevated as a result of disruption of the sodium-potassium pump, tissue destruction, and red blood cell hemolysis
Chloride	90-110 mEq/L (mmol/L)	Elevated as a result of fluid volume loss and reabsorption of chloride in urine
ARTERIAL BLOOD GAS STUDIES		
Pao_2	83-108 mm Hg	Slightly decreased
$Paco_2$	32-48 mm Hg	Slightly increased from respiratory injury
pH	7.35-7.45	Low as a result of metabolic acidosis
Carboxyhemoglobin	0%-10%	Elevated as a result of inhalation of smoke and carbon monoxide
OTHER		
Total protein	6-8.3 g/dL	Low; protein exudate is lost through the wound
Albumin	3.5-5.5 g/dL	Low; protein is lost through the wound and through vascular membranes because of increased permeability

Pao_2, Partial pressure of arterial oxygen; $Paco_2$, partial pressure of arterial carbon dioxide.

Because specific treatments are related to the depth of the burn injury, initial assessment of the integumentary system includes estimations of burn depth. Criteria for establishing the depth of injury are based on appearance and associated characteristics (see Depth of Burn Injury, pp. 1556-1559).

GASTROINTESTINAL ASSESSMENT. Although the gastrointestinal (GI) tract usually is not directly injured in most burn clients (except in those with chemical burns), alterations in GI function are expected. The decreased blood flow during the emergent phase may result in a loss of GI motility and paralytic ileus. The abdomen is auscultated for the presence of bowel sounds to assess GI motility. Bowel sounds are commonly diminished or absent in a client with severe burns. Associated clinical manifestations include nausea, vomiting, and abdominal distention. To prevent aspiration and remove gastric secretions, a nasogastric (NG) tube is usually placed and assessed for proper placement and patency.

Because of the potential for ulcer formation in the GI tract, the nurse examines the stool and vomitus for the presence of gross blood or other material indicative of partially digested blood. Tests for the presence of occult blood are performed.

LABORATORY ASSESSMENT

Alterations in laboratory test values are found in different phases of postburn recovery and usually indicate direct tissue damage and expected compensatory mechanisms. However, other alterations in specific laboratory findings suggest complications.

During the emergent phase and before the initiation of fluid resuscitation, venous blood analysis reflects the fluid shift and direct tissue damage. Baseline laboratory test values and early postburn variations are presented in Chart 68-4.

Changes in the total white blood cell (WBC) count and differential count reflect immune function responses to the trauma of burn injury. The burn client's total WBC count, especially the neutrophil percentage, initially rises and then drops rapidly, with a "left shift" (see Chapter 20) as the immune system becomes unable to sustain its defenses. If sepsis occurs, the total WBC count may be as low as 2000 cells/mm^3.

Additional laboratory tests that provide useful information about the burn client's status may include urine electrolyte assays, urine cultures, liver enzyme studies, and clotting studies. Drug and alcohol screens are obtained if drug or alcohol intoxication is suspected.

CULTURAL CONSIDERATIONS

For African-American clients, a sickle cell preparation may be appropriate if sickle status is unknown. Trauma often triggers a sickle cell crisis in clients who have the disease and in those who carry the trait.

RADIOGRAPHIC ASSESSMENT

Standard x-ray studies and scans do not provide direct assessment data about the burn wound. Such an assessment is not performed unless additional trauma is suspected.

OTHER DIAGNOSTIC ASSESSMENT

In addition to routine laboratory tests and examinations, specific studies of involved organs are performed. For example, when burn injuries involve the eye, an ophthalmic evaluation detects corneal damage (see Chapters 46 and 47 for specific ophthalmic evaluation procedures).

Specific diagnostic examinations can be performed when visceral organ trauma is suspected. Such examinations include intravenous pyelography (IVP), computed tomography (CT), ultrasonography, bronchoscopy, and magnetic resonance imaging (MRI) studies.

CRITICAL THINKING CHALLENGE

The client is a 22-year-old man admitted directly to the burn center after sustaining a high voltage electrical injury while attempting to remove copper at an electrical substation. He is awake and alert. He states he has a great deal of pain in his back and right arm. He has what appears to be a deep, puncture-type wound on his right thumb, and his right hand is extremely edematous. When you check his peripheral pulses, you discover an absence of the right radial and ulnar pulses. Further assessment shows a large charred exit wound in his right lower flank. The client has a 20-gauge IV line in the left hand.

- Is this client at risk for an inhalation injury? Why or Why not?
- What initial consideration must be given in moving the client from the stretcher to the bed?
- Once the client is found to have an adequate airway and level of consciousness, what is your next priority?
- The client asks, "Will I lose my arm?" What is your response?

For suggested answer guidelines, go to SIMON http://www.wbsaunders.com/SIMON/Iggy/.

Analysis

A burned client experiences dramatic changes not only in the directly damaged tissues but also in many other body systems. During the course of the illness, most burn clients experience all of the common and many of the additional nursing diagnoses listed in the following sections.

COMMON NURSING DIAGNOSES AND COLLABORATIVE PROBLEMS

The following are common nursing diagnoses for clients with burn injuries in the emergent phase who have sustained a burn injury greater than 25% of the total body surface area (TBSA):

1. Decreased Cardiac Output related to an increase in capillary permeability
2. Deficient Fluid Volume related to electrolyte imbalance, a loss of plasma volume, and inadequate fluid resuscitation
3. Ineffective Tissue Perfusion (Cerebral, Cardiopulmonary, Renal, Gastrointestinal, and Peripheral) related to decreased cardiac output, extravascular fluid shifts, hypovolemia, constriction of eschar, and edema
4. Ineffective Breathing Pattern related to respiratory distress from upper airway edema, pulmonary edema, airway obstruction, or pneumonia
5. Acute Pain and Chronic Pain related to damaged or exposed nerve endings, debridement, dressing changes, invasive procedures, and donor sites

The following are primary collaborative problems:

1. Potential for Pulmonary Edema
2. Potential for Acute Respiratory Distress Syndrome (ARDS)

ADDITIONAL NURSING DIAGNOSES AND COLLABORATIVE PROBLEMS

In addition to the common nursing diagnoses and collaborative problems, clients with burn injuries in the emergent phase may have one or more of the following:

- Excess Fluid Volume related to massive IV fluid administration
- Risk for Ineffective Thermoregulation related to hypermetabolism and a loss of the protective barrier
- Disturbed Sensory Perception related to periorbital edema or ulcerations, hospital environment, noise, infections, and dressings
- Anxiety related to initial burn trauma, threat of death, situational crisis, painful procedures, unfamiliar environment, separation from significant others, and loss of control
- Fear related to pain, knowledge deficit, therapeutic procedures, hospitalization, separation, and social re-entry

Planning and Implementation

DECREASED CARDIAC OUTPUT; DEFICIENT FLUID VOLUME; INEFFECTIVE TISSUE PERFUSION

NOC **PLANNING: EXPECTED OUTCOMES.** Following appropriate intervention, the client with a burn injury in the emergent phase is expected to (1) have cardiac output restored to normal as evidenced by blood pressure and heart rate in expected ranges and strong peripheral pulses; and (2) maintain adequate oxygenation and circulation to all vital organs as evidenced by oxygen saturation, partial pressure of arterial oxygen (Pao_2), partial pressure of arterial carbon dioxide ($Paco_2$), and arterial pH within normal limits.

INTERVENTIONS. Interventions are aimed at increasing intravascular fluid volume, supporting compensatory mechanisms, and preventing complications. Chart 68-5 lists some NIC intervention activities for the burn client with decreased cardiac output, deficient fluid volume, and ineffective tissue perfusion. Nonsurgical management is often sufficient for achieving these aims. Surgical management is required most often for full-thickness burns.

NONSURGICAL MANAGEMENT. Restoration of fluid volume and tissue perfusion can be accomplished through IV fluid therapy, plasma exchange therapy, and drug therapy.

INTRAVENOUS FLUID THERAPY. Appropriate infusion of IV fluids maintains a circulating volume sufficient for normal cardiac output, mean arterial pressure, and tissue oxygenation. Clients with burns involving 15% to 20% of the TBSA generally require IV fluid resuscitation (Shirani et al., 1996). Many formulas for calculating fluid requirements exist. Table 68-5 summarizes the formulas most commonly used for the therapy of adult clients. Although the types and amounts of electrolytes, crystalloids, and colloids vary, the ultimate purpose of all of these formulas is to prevent shock by maintaining an adequate intravascular fluid volume. The optimal formula and administration schedules remain controversial.

Resuscitation from a severe burn requires large fluid loads in a short time to maintain vital organ perfusion. The Parkland formula recommends that half of the calculated fluid volume be given in the first 8 hours after injury. The other half is administered over the next 16 hours for a total of 24 hours. In general, fluid boluses are avoided because they increase capillary hydrostatic pressure and worsen edema. In the second 24-hour period after a burn injury, the volume and content of the IV fluids are based on the client's specific volume and electrolyte imbalances and his or her response to treatment.

Most fluid replacement formulas are calculated from the time of injury and not from the time of arrival at the hospital. For example, if a burn injury occurred at 8 AM but the client was not admitted to the hospital until 10 AM, the first 8-hour period would be completed at 4 PM, or 8 hours after the injury. Thus, if resuscitation were delayed until admission to the hospital, calculated fluids would need to be administered over a 6-hour period rather than an 8-hour period. All burn resuscitation formulas are used as *guides,* with the understanding that the client's response to therapy determines ultimate fluid requirements. No single formula has been found to provide superior results over another.

The management of extensive burns may necessitate the placement of a large-bore central venous catheter so that massive fluid loads can be administered. Peripheral lines sometimes become dislodged or fluid flow is cut off because massive peripheral edema compresses the IV catheter.

CHART 68-5

NIC INTERVENTION ACTIVITIES *for* The Burn Client with Decreased Cardiac Output, Deficient Fluid Volume, and Ineffective Tissue Perfusion

Fluid Monitoring: *Collection and analysis of client data to regulate fluid balance*
- Monitor serum and urine electrolyte values, as appropriate.
- Monitor BP, heart rate, and respiratory status.
- Monitor orthostatic blood pressure and change in cardiac rhythm, as appropriate.
- Monitor weight.
- Keep an accurate record of intake and output.
- Note presence or absence of vertigo on rising.
- Monitor color, quantity, and specific gravity of urine.

Fluid Resuscitation: *Administering prescribed intravenous fluids rapidly*
- Obtain and maintain a large-bore IV.
- Administer IV fluids, as prescribed.
- Monitor hemodynamic response.
- Monitor oxygen status.
- Monitor for fluid overload.
- Monitor output of various body fluids (e.g., urine, nasogastric drainage, and chest tube).
- Monitor BUN, creatinine, total protein, and albumin levels.
- Monitor for pulmonary edema and third spacing.

Fluid Management: *Promotion of fluid balance and prevention of complications resulting from abnormal or undesired fluid levels*
- Administer IV therapy, as prescribed.
- Give fluids, as appropriate.
- Distribute the fluid intake over 24 hours, as appropriate.

NIC intervention activities selected from McCloskey, J.C., & Bulechek, G.M. (Eds.). (2000). *Nursing interventions classification (NIC)* (3rd ed.). St. Louis: Mosby.
BP, Blood pressure; *BUN,* blood urea nitrogen.

PLASMA EXCHANGE THERAPY. Shock may persist in the postburn period despite adequate fluid resuscitation. The cause of this persistent shock is unknown, but toxic serum factors have been theorized. Plasma exchange therapy is occasionally used in some burn centers for clients with massive burns who fail to respond to conventional resuscitation from burn shock.

The plasma exchange process either removes the client's plasma and replaces it with fresh frozen plasma **(plasmapheresis)** or removes the client's blood and replaces it with whole banked blood **(exchange transfusion).** Plasma exchange can decrease the amount of required fluid and increase urine output, thus helping those clients who do not respond to conventional fluid therapy.

MONITORING. Clinical criteria are monitored to determine the adequacy of fluid resuscitation. These parameters are indications of hydration and adequate tissue perfusion to the brain, heart, and kidneys. In animal studies, a 50% decrease in renal blood flow was observed while perfusion to the vital organs was preserved. These findings suggest that urine output diminishes before the compromise or loss of vital organ perfusion. During resuscitation, deviation from any of the desirable parameters suggests an inadequate or excessive amount of fluid.

Urine output is the most common and most sensitive noninvasive assessment parameter for cardiac output and tissue per-

TABLE 68-5 • COMMON FLUID RESUSCITATION FORMULAS FOR THE FIRST 24 HOURS AFTER A BURN INJURY

	Formula	Solution	Rate of Administration
Modified Brooke	0.5 mL/kg/% TBSA burn	Protenate or 5% albumin in isotonic saline	1/2 given in first 8 hr 1/2 given in next 16 hr
	1.5 mL/kg/% TBSA burn	Lactated Ringer's without dextrose	
Parkland (Baxter)	4 mL/kg/% TBSA burn for 24-hr period	Crystalloid only (lactated Ringer's)	1/2 given in first 8 hr 1/2 given in next 16 hr
Monafo		Crystalloid (hypertonic saline: sodium = 250 mEq/L)	Adjust to maintain urine output of 30 mL/hr
Modified Parkland	4 mL/kg/% TBSA burn + 15 mL/m^2 of TBSA	Crystalloid only (lactated Ringer's)	1/2 given in first 8 hr 1/2 given in next 16 hr
Winski	2 mL/kg/% burn + maintenance fluid	Crystalloid only (lactated Ringer's)	1/2 given in first 8 hr 1/2 given in next 16 hr

fusion (see Chapters 12 and 37). Regardless of the total amount of fluid calculated as appropriate to meet the fluid needs of the client, the amount of fluid administered depends on how much IV fluid per hour is required to maintain the hourly urine output at 0.5 mL/kg (30 mL/hr). Adjustment of the IV fluid rate on the basis of urine output plus serum electrolyte values is known as the **titration** of fluid to meet the perfusion needs of the client. *In clients with burns larger than 35% TBSA, the use of urine output and vital signs to guide resuscitation may be insufficient. Additional invasive monitoring of cardiopulmonary function is necessary to ensure optimal fluid resuscitation.*

Burn clients often develop severe hypovolemic shock and require invasive cardiac monitoring. With the use of modern electronic equipment (see Chapter 37), vital parameters such as central venous pressure, pulmonary artery pressures, and cardiac output can be obtained on a frequent to continuous basis. Because an adequately functioning cardiovascular system is imperative, the nurse monitors the electrocardiographic activity of clients who have sustained large burns. Rhythms that affect the mechanics of the heart (e.g., atrial fibrillation) are often present in older clients.

DRUG THERAPY. A common mistake in treatment is administering diuretics to increase urine output rather than changing the amount and rate of fluid administration. *Diuretics do not increase cardiac output; they actually decrease circulating volume and cardiac output by pulling fluid from the circulating blood volume to enhance diuresis.* This effect can cause a dangerous reduction in perfusion to other vital organs (especially the heart, lungs, and brain) and greatly increases the probability of developing a state of severe hypovolemic shock. Therefore diuretics are not generally used to improve urine output for burn clients. An exception is the client with a burn injury caused by electrical energy. Muscle and deep tissue damage can cause the release of large protein molecules (myoglobin), which precipitate in and obstruct the renal tubules. Although the diuretic mannitol (Osmitrol) is often used in this situation, it should always be given after adequate urine output has been established and is accompanied by the alkalinization of urine with sodium bicarbonate supplementation.

In some clients, particularly older adults or those with a history of cardiac disease, a complicating factor in reduced cardiac output may be congestive heart failure or myocardial infarction. Drugs that increase cardiac output, such as dopamine (Intropin), or that strengthen the force of myocardial contraction, such as digoxin (Lanoxin), may be used along with fluid therapy.

SURGICAL MANAGEMENT. The primary surgical procedure for the treatment of inadequate tissue perfusion is *escharotomy.* An incision through the burn eschar with an electrocautery device or scalpel relieves pressure caused by the restricting force of circumferential burns on the extremity or chest and improves circulation. If the pressure is not relieved, arterial compression can occur with a resultant compromise of extremity perfusion, ischemia, and possibly necrosis. Incisions are made along the medial and lateral sides of the extremity and extend into the subcutaneous tissue (Figures 68-6 and 68-12). This procedure relieves the tourniquet effect of the eschar. If tissue pressure measurements remain elevated after escharotomies, a *fasciotomy* (an incision extending through the subcutaneous tissue and fascia) may be required.

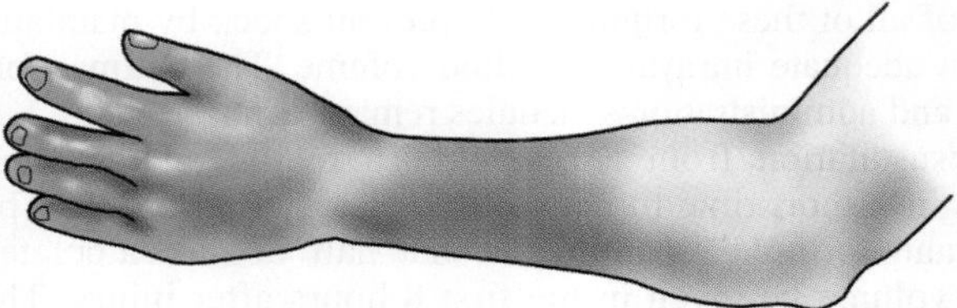

Tight, circumferential eschar restricting outward swelling as edema forms in the tissues beneath the eschar. Edema compresses blood vessels, which inhibits blood flow to the distal extremity.

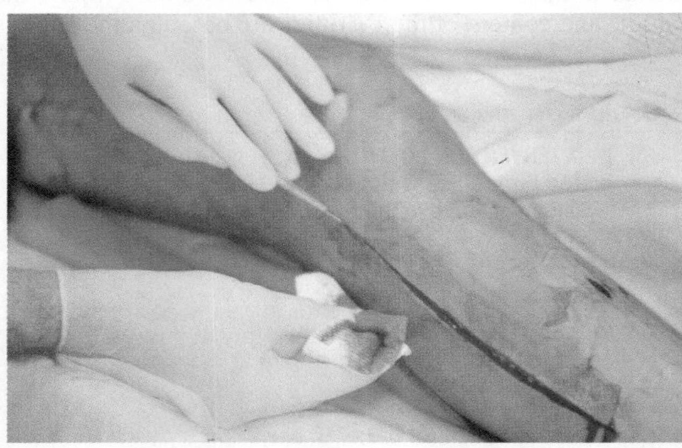

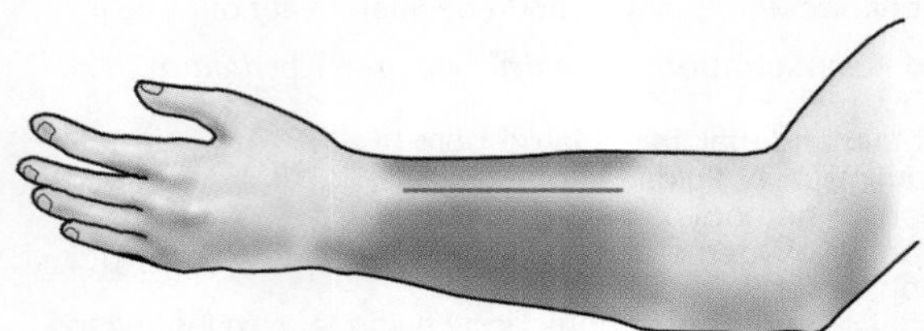

An escharotomy incision allows outward swelling of edematous tissues. Restricted blood flow through the vessels to the distal extremity is relieved.

Figure 68-12 ● Escharotomy to release circumferential burn eschar and improve circulation to a distal extremity.

Escharotomies and fasciotomies are often performed at the bedside. No anesthesia is required for escharotomy because nerve endings have been destroyed by the burn injury, but sedation and analgesia are commonly given to reduce anxiety. The nurse prepares the client by providing verbal assurance that the client will be made as comfortable as possible during the procedure. Preparation for escharotomy requires removing the dressings and thoroughly cleansing the areas to be incised. Following the procedure, topical antimicrobial agents and dressings are reapplied to the area. Escharotomy sites are carefully monitored for excessive bleeding. Fasciotomies generally require large doses of narcotics or anesthesia for pain management.

INEFFECTIVE BREATHING PATTERN

NOC **PLANNING: EXPECTED OUTCOMES.** With appropriate intervention, the client with a burn injury in the emergent phase is expected to maintain a patent airway, and have an effective breathing pattern as evidenced by maintaining oxygen saturation, PaO_2, $PaCO_2$, and arterial pH within normal limits.

INTERVENTIONS. Interventions are aimed at supporting normal pulmonary mechanisms and preventing pulmonary problems. Specific plans for pulmonary management depend on the cause of the insult and the status of the respiratory tract.

NONSURGICAL MANAGEMENT. Appropriate interventions include airway maintenance, promotion of ventilation, monitoring gas exchange, oxygen therapy, drug therapy, and positioning and deep breathing.

AIRWAY MAINTENANCE. Maintenance of the airway begins at the incident scene in an unconscious victim and may involve only a chin lift or a head tilt maneuver. Upper airway edema becomes pronounced 8 to 12 hours after the initiation of fluid resuscitation. These clients often require immediate nasal or oral intubation once signs of crowing, stridor, and dyspnea are present.

The physician performs a bronchoscopy to examine the vocal cords and airways of clients at risk for obstruction. Clients with severe smoke inhalation or poisoning may require a bronchoscopy when admitted to the hospital and routinely thereafter for examination of the respiratory tract, accurate diagnoses, deep suctioning of the lungs, and removal of sloughing necrotic tissue. The endotracheal tube is assessed frequently to ensure patency in intubated clients.

Other causes of airway obstruction are excessive secretions and sloughed tissue from damaged lungs. Suctioning is performed as indicated based on clinical assessment or clinician order. Vigorous endotracheal or nasotracheal tube suctioning is commonly performed after chest physiotherapy and aerosol treatments. Clients have reported that deep endotracheal suctioning is extremely painful. Therefore suctioning the endotracheal tube often requires increased analgesia and/or sedation.

PROMOTION OF VENTILATION. Respiration depends on skeletal muscle contractions and movement of the thoracic cavity for ventilation. Movement of the thoracic cavity can be restricted by tight dressings that cover the neck, thorax, and abdomen. The nurse observes the client for effectiveness and ease of respiratory movements and loosens tight dressings as needed to assist with ventilation.

MONITORING GAS EXCHANGE. The effectiveness of gas exchange is monitored by using laboratory tests (e.g., arterial blood gas, carboxyhemoglobin levels) and by noting physical signs such as cyanosis, disorientation, and increased pulse rate. Other data to monitor in critically ill clients include chest x-ray studies, pulmonary artery catheters, and central venous pressure measurement.

The possibility of cyanide poisoning must be considered in clients involved in house fires. An elevated plasma lactate level is a useful indicator of cyanide toxicity in clients who do not have severe burns.

OXYGEN THERAPY. Management of impaired breathing patterns includes administering humidified oxygen by face mask, cannula, or hood. Arterial oxygenation less than 60 (PaO_2 <60 mm Hg) is an indication for intubation, and mechanical ventilation is instituted. Emergency airway equipment should be located at or near the client's bedside and include oxygen, masks, cannulas, ambu bags, laryngoscope, endotracheal tubes, and equipment for tracheostomy. Chapter 32 addresses specific nursing actions for clients during mechanical ventilation.

DRUG THERAPY. When pneumonia or other pulmonary infections further impair breathing, the physician prescribes antibiotics. Antibiotic selection is based on known culture and sensitivity reports or is empirically based on a knowledge of the specific microflora of the burn unit. Impaired breathing patterns resulting from cardiac failure and increased pulmonary pressures may be treated with drugs that improve cardiac output and enhance renal excretion.

When a client's activity severely compromises respiratory mechanics, it may be necessary to use a paralytic drug, such as Atracurium (Tracrium) or Vecuronium (Norcuron). This situation is often referred to as "bucking" the ventilator. Paralytic agents remove all ventilatory control from the client and allow uninterrupted administration of artificial ventilation. *These drugs do not prevent the client from seeing and hearing or from experiencing fear, pain, and loss of control. Any client receiving neuromuscular blockade drugs must also receive agents for sedation, analgesia, and antianxiety unless clinically contraindicated. Extreme care must be taken to ensure that all alarms are operative and that clients are checked frequently, because they cannot call for help should they become extubated.*

POSITIONING AND DEEP BREATHING. To improve breathing patterns and oxygenation, the client is turned frequently and assisted out of bed to a chair as much as possible. Pulmonary hygiene techniques such as coughing and deep breathing exercises and incentive spirometry must be taught to the client and encouraged frequently. Chest physiotherapy may be helpful to facilitate the mobilization of pulmonary secretions based on the client's clinical condition and the clinician's order.

SURGICAL MANAGEMENT. A tracheostomy may be necessary in clients for whom long-term intubation is expected. A tracheostomy carries a greater risk for infection in burn clients than in nonburned clients. Emergency tracheostomies are performed when an airway becomes occluded and oral or nasal intubation cannot be achieved.

Other common surgical procedures for improving the burn client's breathing pattern include inserting chest tubes and performing an escharotomy. Chest tubes are used to reexpand the lung when a pneumothorax or hemothorax has occurred (see Chapter 30).

Tight eschar on the neck, chest, or abdomen can restrict respiratory movement. Escharotomies (described on p. 1572) can relieve this restriction and permit greater respiratory movement.

ACUTE PAIN; CHRONIC PAIN

The pain associated with burn injuries is both chronic and acute. Many factors contribute to burn pain and may be manipulated to alter the response to pain. Pain from the actual injury is compounded when painful procedures are performed. Nurses working with burn clients must often inflict pain on clients during the course of treatment. They must cope with this problem by developing strategies that allow them to rationalize the necessity for inflicting pain during procedures. One common coping mechanism is to distance oneself from the client's pain (Nagy, 1999). Accurate assessment of the client's pain before and during procedures is an essential part of pain management. In addition to more standard visual analog scales, pain assessment scales that use color or faces have been used successfully to assess pain in the client with burns (see the Evidence-Based Practice for Nursing box at right).

NOC PLANNING: EXPECTED OUTCOMES. The pain level of a client with a burn injury in the emergent phase is expected to be alleviated or reduced as evidenced by a decreased report of pain and a decreased length of pain episodes.

INTERVENTIONS. The plan for pain management is tailored to the client's tolerance for pain, coping mechanisms, and physical status.

NONSURGICAL MANAGEMENT. Interventions for the client experiencing pain include drug therapy, complementary therapy measures, and environmental manipulation.

DRUG THERAPY. Opioid and nonopioid analgesics, such as morphine sulfate, meperidine (Demerol), and nalbuphine (Nubain), are given with relative frequency throughout hospitalization. However, these drugs rarely offer more than moderate relief during acutely painful procedures, and they produce side effects of respiratory depression and diminished gastrointestinal motility.

During the emergent postburn phase, the IV route is the preferred route for administration of narcotics because of potential problems with absorption from the muscle and stomach. When these agents are administered by the intramuscular route, they remain in the spaces and do not relieve pain. In addition, when edema is present, cumulative subcutaneous or intramuscular doses are rapidly reabsorbed when the fluid shift is resolving. This delayed reabsorption can result in lethal blood levels of analgesics.

Anesthetic agents, such as ketamine (Ketalar), pentobarbital sodium (Nembutal, Novopentobarb♣), and nitrous oxide, also reduce pain. Strict protocols must be used when administering these agents to prevent serious complications.

COMPLEMENTARY AND ALTERNATIVE THERAPY. Complementary and alternative therapy measures include relaxation techniques, meditative breathing, guided imagery, music therapy, massage, and healing or therapeutic touch. Hypnosis and autohypnosis of lucid, cooperative clients can be attempted by trained therapists. Therapeutic touch, acupuncture, and acupressure are used to a limited extent for burn clients; the results are variable. Nontraditional and complementary therapy types of pain intervention are detailed in Chapter 7.

ENVIRONMENTAL MANIPULATION. The nurse can increase the client's comfort by providing a quiet environment, using nonpainful tactile stimulation, and increasing the client's control. Sleep deprivation is a significant issue for victims of burn injury. Increasing sleep or rest time in a quiet environment helps reduce the adverse effects of sleep deprivation, replenishes catecholamine stores, helps prevent critical care unit psychosis, and restores the diurnal effects of endorphins. Health care providers need to perform as many procedures as possible during the client's waking hours.

Tactile stimulation can reduce pain. The client's position is changed routinely to reduce pressure on any specific area; repositioning improves circulation to painful areas and eases pain. Massaging nonburn areas may reduce pain transmission on thick pain-sensory nerve fibers by stimulating an increased release of endorphins. Applying heat and maintaining warm room temperatures prevent shivering and stimulate the production of serotonin, which triggers the relaxation response.

To reduce anxiety and increase feelings of confidence and independence, the client is encouraged to participate in pain control measures. For example, the nurse and client make a

EVIDENCE-BASED PRACTICE FOR NURSING

What pain assessment tool is preferred by clients with burns?

Gordon, M., et al. (1998). Use of pain assessment tools: Is there a preference? *Journal of Burn Care and Rehabilitation, 19*(5), 451-454.

Pain is a major issue for clients with burns. The most commonly used method of assessing pain among burn clients is the Visual Analog Scale (VAS). This prospective, descriptive study of 40 clients with burn injuries sought to determine what pain assessment tool is perceived as most useful by clients having pain related to burn injury and burn care procedures.

Four pain assessment tools were tested: Faces Pain Rating Scale (FPRS), Adjective Pain Rating Scale (APRS), Visual Analog Scale (VAS), and Analog Chromatic Continuous Scale (ACCS). The ACCS incorporates properties of two types of scales: (1) a calibrated measure similar to the VAS ranging from "no pain" to "severe pain," and (2) a color scale ranging from light pink (no pain) through a shade of red and black (severe pain). Forty adult clients who were inpatients with burn injuries were asked to use two of the pain assessment tools for 3 consecutive days twice daily. Pain was assessed at a "quiet time" and at a time immediately following a painful activity. The 3-day assessment cycle was repeated with the remaining two pain assessment scales. Clients were asked to select the preferred type of pain assessment tool after each 3-day cycle and at the end of the test period. Most clients (35) were male; the average age was 36 years, and the average total body surface area (TBSA) injured was 20%. Overall, clients preferred the FPRS and the ACCS to the VAS and the ARPS. However, when results were compared by gender, the five women always preferred the VAS over the ACCS.

Critique. The authors initiated study in an important area of care for the client with burns. Although this study concluded that adult clients with burn injuries preferred the FPRS and ACCS to the more commonly used VAS, the results are not generalizable to all adult clients with burn injuries. The sample size was small, with a preponderance of men (35) compared to women (5). No attempt was made to correlate severity of pain with pain assessment tool preference. The study could have been strengthened by including client education or literacy level as well as by ensuring that the painful activities were similar for all clients.

Implications for Nursing. Pain management and client comfort remain important issues when caring for clients with burns. Pain assessment may not be accurate if the client experiencing the pain either does not understand the assessment tool used or finds it inadequate. Because pain is a subjective experience and pain assessment is critical to pain management, nurses could seek to individualize pain assessment by determining which pain assessment tool each client prefers and then consistently use the client-identified tool.

contract that specifies how long a painful procedure will last. This helps clients deal with the pain for that particular period. Patient-controlled analgesia (PCA) also reduces pain in burned clients. Important issues and techniques for the best use of PCA include the following: giving an initial bolus of 5 to 10 mg of morphine (or equivalent drug), increasing the PCA dose as needed to achieve pain relief, and planning for a change in dosing regimens at night (e.g., giving a bolus dose at bedtime).

SURGICAL MANAGEMENT. A technique of early surgical excision of the burn wound is used in many burn centers (see Surgical Excision, pp. 1578 and 1579). Early excision under anesthesia can reduce the pain associated with daily debridement at the bedside or during hydrotherapy.

POTENTIAL FOR PULMONARY EDEMA

PLANNING: EXPECTED OUTCOMES. With intervention, the client with a burn injury in the emergent phase is expected to be free of pulmonary edema.

INTERVENTIONS. Pulmonary edema can arise from pulmonary injury; however, pulmonary edema in the emergent phase is associated with fluid resuscitation and myocardial overload. Even a young healthy person may have some degree of ventricular insufficiency. These clients usually receive digoxin or another inotropic agent to improve left ventricular function and prevent or treat pulmonary edema. Diuretics, a mainstay of therapy for pulmonary edema from other causes, may or may not be used in the emergent phase depending on the client's vascular hydration status and renal function.

POTENTIAL FOR ACUTE RESPIRATORY DISTRESS SYNDROME

PLANNING: EXPECTED OUTCOMES. The client with a burn injury in the emergent phase is expected to have arterial blood gases (ABGs) within normal limits, maintain normal lung compliance, and be free of respiratory distress.

INTERVENTIONS. Clients who have developed acute respiratory distress syndrome (ARDS) as a result of burn injury require thorough assessments and interventions. The interventions are aimed at increasing lung compliance and improving Pa_{O_2} (partial pressure of arterial oxygen) levels.

In collaboration with the physician and respiratory therapist, the client receives positive end-expiratory pressure (PEEP) to augment the decreased lung volume by providing a continuous positive pressure in the airways and alveoli. This procedure optimizes the diffusion of oxygen across the alveolar-capillary membrane. PEEP can be combined with intermittent mandatory volume (IMV) to enhance its effectiveness.

The client's response is assessed and documented so that appropriate ventilator changes can be made. Any signs of respiratory distress and changes in respiratory patterns are documented and reported to the physician. Pulse oximetry and arterial blood gas (ABG) levels also are monitored for changes in respiratory status.

Neuromuscular blocking agents (atracurium) can be used in clients requiring mechanical ventilation to reduce or eliminate spontaneous breathing efforts and to reduce oxygen consumption (see the discussion of specific nursing care under Drug Therapy [Ineffective Breathing Pattern], p. 1573).

> **CRITICAL THINKING CHALLENGE**
>
> The client who sustained the electrical injury described earlier is started on fluid resuscitation. You notice that his urine is becoming darker and has a high specific gravity.
>
> - Do you expect that this client needs as much fluid for resuscitation as a person who has a flame burn? Why or why not?
> - What should be your first action upon viewing the change in the character of this client's urine?
> - What additional medications or adjustment(s) in resuscitation should you expect to be ordered?

For suggested answer guidelines, go to SIMON http://www.wbsaunders.com/SIMON/Iggy/.

ACUTE PHASE OF BURN INJURY

OVERVIEW

The acute phase of burn injury begins approximately 48 hours after injury and lasts until wound closure is complete. During this phase, an intense collaborative approach to care is directed toward continued assessment and maintenance of the cardiovascular and respiratory systems, as well as toward gastrointestinal and nutritional status, burn wound care, pain control, and psychosocial interventions.

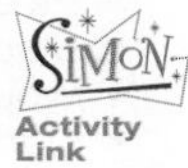
Activity Link

COLLABORATIVE MANAGEMENT

Assessment

PHYSICAL ASSESSMENT/CLINICAL MANIFESTATIONS

CARDIOPULMONARY ASSESSMENT. In the acute phase of burn injury, the physical assessment findings related to the cardiovascular and respiratory systems are directed at maintaining these systems and treating potential complications as they occur. Although airway injuries should be resolved, the client may experience pneumonia that can compromise the airway and result in respiratory failure requiring mechanical ventilation. Any cardiovascular system problems also should be resolved. However, the client is at risk for infection, which can lead to septic shock and affect cardiovascular function. The assessment and clinical interventions undertaken in the emergent phase should also be used in these isolated clinical situations.

NEUROENDOCRINE ASSESSMENT. The increased metabolic demands placed on the body after a severe burn injury can severely compromise nutritional status. The client's weight is obtained as ordered and is compared with his or her preburn weight. Body weight measurements are obtained without dressings or splints, if possible. A loss of 2% in body weight indicates a mild deficit; a weight loss of 10% or more is significant and requires the evaluation of caloric and fluid intake and appropriate modifications.

Indirect calorimetry often is used to obtain accurate calorie requirements for burn clients. This technique determines kilocalories of energy expenditure by measuring oxygen consumption (V_{O_2}) and carbon dioxide production (V_{CO_2}). Measurements are performed while the client is at rest and preferably at least 30 minutes after the most recent dressing changes or other stressful procedures. Indirect calorimetry generally is performed shortly after admission and at least once each week until the wounds are closed.

IMMUNOLOGIC ASSESSMENT. The client with a burn injury is susceptible to infection as a result of the inflammatory response and the compromise in immune function. Burn wound sepsis is a serious complication of burn injury, and infection remains the leading cause of morbidity and mortality during the acute phase of recovery. The nurse must continually assess the client for signs of local and systemic infections (Table 68-6), including changes in wound appearance, changes in neurologic and gastrointestinal function, and subtle changes in vital signs. Gram-positive, gram-negative, and fungal infections produce a variety of clinical signs and symptoms, and the nurse monitors for these differences (Table 68-7). A strict policy of meticulous handwashing for all health care providers is enforced. Aseptic technique in caring for wounds and during invasive monitoring or therapy is important in preventing hospital-acquired infections.

TABLE 68-6 • LOCAL AND SYSTEMIC SIGNS OF INFECTION

LOCAL SIGNS
- Conversion of a partial-thickness injury to a full-thickness injury
- Ulceration of healthy skin at the burn site
- Erythematous, nodular lesions in uninvolved skin and vesicular lesions in healed skin
- Edema of healthy skin surrounding the burn wound
- Excessive burn wound drainage
- Pale, boggy, dry, or crusted granulation tissue
- Sloughing of grafts
- Wound breakdown after closure
- Odor

SYSTEMIC SIGNS
- Altered level of consciousness
- Changes in vital signs (tachycardia, tachypnea, temperature instability, hypotension)
- Increased fluid requirements for maintenance of a normal urine output
- Hemodynamic instability
- Oliguria
- Gastrointestinal dysfunction (diarrhea, vomiting, abdominal distention, paralytic ileus)
- Hyperglycemia
- Thrombocytopenia
- Change in total white blood cell count (above normal or below normal)
- Metabolic acidosis
- Hypoxemia

MUSCULOSKELETAL ASSESSMENT. Clients with a burn injury are at risk for musculoskeletal problems as a result of other injuries, immobility, healing processes, and treatment. The client's musculoskeletal status is initially evaluated within the first few hours of admission to the hospital or burn center and throughout the acute phase of injury. An assessment of active and passive range of motion for all joints, including the neck, is performed. Special attention is given to joints within the burn area. Ranges and limitations are noted for future reference.

Analysis

During the acute phase of the burn injury, the client with a burn injury experiences a resolution of some earlier problems, may have initial problems that extend into the acute phase, and experiences new problems in many body systems.

COMMON NURSING DIAGNOSES AND COLLABORATIVE PROBLEMS

The following are common nursing diagnoses for clients with burn injuries in the acute phase who have sustained a burn injury greater than 25% of the total body surface area (TBSA):

1. Impaired Skin Integrity related to burn wound, graft site, or donor site
2. Risk for Infection related to impaired skin integrity, the presence of multiple invasive catheters, compromise in immune function, and nutritional compromise
3. Imbalanced Nutrition: Less than Body Requirements related to increased metabolic rate; reduced calorie intake; altered glucose, fat, and protein metabolism; and increased urinary nitrogen losses
4. Impaired Physical Mobility related to open burn wounds, pain, and scars and contractures
5. Disturbed Body Image related to changes in physical appearance and lifestyle, as well as alterations in sensory and motor function

The primary collaborative problem is Wound Care Management.

TABLE 68-7 • SIGNS AND SYMPTOMS OF SEPSIS CAUSED BY DIFFERENT ORGANISMS

Sign/Symptom	Gram-Positive	Gram-Negative	Fungal
Onset	Insidious, 2-6 days	Rapid, 12-36 hr	Delayed
Sensorium	Severe disorientation and lethargy	Mild disorientation	Mild disorientation
Ileus	Severe	Severe	Mild
Diarrhea	Rare	Severe	Occasional
Temperature	Hyperpyrexia	Hypothermia	Hyperpyrexia
Hypotension	Late	Early	Late
White blood cell count	Neutrophilia	Neutropenia	Neutrophilia
Platelets	Normal	Low	Low

ADDITIONAL NURSING DIAGNOSES AND COLLABORATIVE PROBLEMS

In addition to the common nursing diagnoses and collaborative problems, clients with burn injuries in the acute phase may have one or more of the following:

- Anticipatory Grieving related to loss of significant others, loss of possessions, physical disfigurement, and changes in body image
- Disabled Family Coping related to loss of home, family, or significant others; crises resulting from burn injury; disturbances in normal functions; role changes; and prolonged hospitalization and rehabilitation
- Ineffective Coping related to situational crises, disfigurement, separation, and sensory overload
- Self-Care Deficits (Feeding, Bathing/Hygiene, Dressing/Grooming, Toileting) related to pain; contractures; and loss of function in the hands, extremities, and other body parts
- Sexual Dysfunction related to perineal, genital, and breast burns; immobility, fatigue, and depression; and disturbance in body image
- Disturbed Sleep Pattern related to pain, treatment regimen, and environmental noise
- Social Isolation related to the protective isolation treatment regimen and alterations in physical appearance
- Deficient Knowledge related to the treatment regimen and healing process
- Potential for Pneumonia
- Potential for Septicemia

Planning and Implementation

IMPAIRED SKIN INTEGRITY; WOUND CARE MANAGEMENT

NOC **PLANNING: EXPECTED OUTCOMES.** With appropriate intervention, the client with a burn injury in the acute phase is expected to experience no further loss of skin integrity, have skin integrity restored without complications, and have skin thickness in the expected range in the burn wound area.

INTERVENTIONS. Interventions aim to preserve the integrity of nonburned skin, enhance wound healing of burned skin, and prevent complications.

NONSURGICAL MANAGEMENT. Nonsurgical burn wound management, or conservative treatment, involves removing exudates and necrotic tissue, cleaning the area, stimulating granulation and revascularization, and applying dressings. Restoration of skin, whether by natural healing or grafting, starts with the removal of eschar and other cellular debris from the burn wound. This removal is called **debridement.** Conservative treatment allows noninvasive debriding of the wound through mechanical and enzymatic actions that stimulate the separation of eschar over time. The goal is to have the wound slowly prepare itself for grafting and wound closure by a natural process.

MECHANICAL DEBRIDEMENT. Burn wounds are debrided and cleaned a minimum of once, and usually two to three times, each day during hydrotherapy (the application of water for treatment). Nurses, assistive nursing personnel, and physical therapists perform hydrotherapy daily to debride necrotic tissue and to examine the wounds. Hydrotherapy can be accomplished by immersing the client in a tub, showering the client on a specially designed table, or successively washing only small areas of the wound at the bedside if the client is too unstable to be moved. Showering enhances visualization of the wounds and allows water temperature to be kept constant.

Nurses and skilled technicians use forceps and scissors to remove loose, nonviable tissue during hydrotherapy. The care of intact blisters is controversial. At most institutions, small blisters are left alone because they serve as a protective barrier that assists with wound healing and re-epithelialization. Because the protein-filled fluid within blisters can cause some degree of immunosuppression, many institutions open larger blisters. Washcloths or gauze sponges also can facilitate the debridement of "cheesy" eschar or pseudoeschar. During hydrotherapy, the burn areas are washed thoroughly and gently with mild soap or detergent and water. The areas are then rinsed with water at room temperature.

ENZYMATIC DEBRIDEMENT. Enzymatic debridement can occur naturally by autolysis or artificially by the application of exogenous agents. **Autolysis** is the spontaneous disintegration of tissue by the action of the client's own cellular enzymes. This process is seldom used in North America for larger burns because it is slow and results in a prolonged hospital stay.

Exogenous agents, such as collagenase (Santyl), are topical enzymes used for rapid wound debridement. When these agents are applied directly to the burn wound in a once-a-day dressing change, the enzymes digest native and denatured collagen in necrotic tissues. Because collagen accounts for 75% of the dry weight of skin tissue, the ability of collagenase (Santyl) to digest collagen in the physiologic pH range makes it an important debriding agent for burn wounds. Polysporin powder is often used with this topical agent to prevent infection.

DRESSING THE BURN WOUND. After burn wounds are cleaned and debrided, topical antibiotics are reapplied to prevent infection (see Risk for Infection, p. 1579). Some type of dressing is then applied to the burn wound. Burn dressings include standard wound dressings, biologic dressings, and synthetic dressings and artificial skin. (Table 68-6 describes the characteristics of many types of dressings.)

Standard Wound Dressings. Standard wound dressings consist of multiple layers of gauze applied over the topical agent or antibiotic on the burn wound. The number of gauze layers depends on the following:

- Depth of the injury
- Amount of drainage expected
- Area injured
- Client's mobility
- Frequency of dressing changes

The gauze layers are held in place with roller-type gauze bandages applied in a distal to proximal direction or with circular net fabrics. On the client's extremities, the nurse covers gauze dressings with elastic wraps, especially if the client is ambulatory. Based on assessed needs or clinician orders, nursing personnel generally change and reapply the dressings every 8 to 24 hours after thoroughly cleaning the areas.

Biologic Dressings. Biologic dressings are materials obtained from human tissue donors (homograft or allograft) or animals (heterograft or xenograft). When applied over open wounds, a biologic dressing rapidly adheres and promotes healing or prepares the wound for permanent skin graft coverage.

Biologic materials are used in healing partial-thickness and granulating full-thickness wounds that are clean and free of eschar. Table 68-8 outlines the advantages and disadvantages of biologic dressings. The type of biologic dressing selected depends on the type of wound to be covered and the availability of the material.

Homograft. Skin for a **homograft (allograft)** is usually obtained from a cadaver and provided through a skin bank. It is fresh or frozen; frozen skin is thawed in a warm bath of sterile normal saline before application. Disadvantages to the use of homografts are the excessive costs ($750 to $1000 per square foot) and the risk of transmitting a bloodborne infection.

Heterograft. Skin for a **heterograft (xenograft)** is obtained from another species. Pigskin is the most common heterograft because of its relative compatibility with human skin. The pigskin is replaced on a continual basis until the wound heals naturally or is closed with autograft. Because pigskin does not control bacterial proliferation, it is changed frequently, usually daily.

Amniotic Membrane. Amniotic membrane is another form of biologic dressing used on burn wounds. Its large size, low cost, and availability have helped with its success. In full-thickness injuries, the amniotic membrane immediately adheres to the wound. With partial-thickness areas, the amniotic membrane is effective as a dressing until re-epithelialization occurs. The membrane may require frequent changes because it does not vascularize and has the tendency to disintegrate in 48 hours.

Cultured Skin. Cultured skin can be grown from a small biopsy specimen of epidermal cells from an unburned portion of the client's body. The cells are grown in a laboratory to produce larger epithelial sheets that can be grafted on the client to generate a permanent epidermal surface. The length of time for culturing and growing the skin is prolonged, and the epithelial sheets are not durable. Extreme care must be taken when these sheets are applied to ensure adherence and prevent sloughing. This process is also extremely costly.

Artificial Skin. Artificial skin, first developed in 1980, is an alternative approach to closure of the burn wound. This substance has two layers composed of a Silastic epidermis and a porous dermis made from bovine hide collagen and shark cartilage (Winfrey, Cochran, & Hegarty, 1999).

After the artificial skin is applied to a clean, excised wound surface, fibroblasts move into the collagen part of the artificial skin and create a fibrinous structure similar to normal dermis. The artificial dermis slowly dissolves and is replaced with normal blood vessels and connective tissue (*neodermis*). The neodermis will support a standard split-thickness autograft that is placed over it when the Silastic layer is removed.

Synthetic Dressings. Synthetic dressings consisting of solid silicone and plastic membranes (e.g., polyvinyl chloride and polyurethane) may be substituted for antimicrobial, standard, or biologic dressings. Synthetic dressings are applied directly to the surface of a clean or surgically prepared wound and remain in place until they fall off or are removed due to nonadhesion. Because many of these dressings are transparent or translucent, the nurse can inspect the wound without removing the dressing. The client experiences pain reduction at the site because these agents also prevent contact of the wound with air. These dressings may also be used to cover donor sites where skin was obtained for autografting.

A recent review of the literature found transparent film to be the best dressing for the care of donor site wounds (see the Evidence-Based Practice for Nursing box on p. 1579). Transparent film was associated with one of the fastest healing rates, a low infection rate, the least amount of associated pain, and minimal cost (Rakel et al., 1998). An additional strategy that merits consideration has been used to manage donor site pain. Topical lidocaine applied to donor harvest sites produced an analgesic effect that reduced narcotic requirements, significantly lowered pain scores, and did not produce toxic blood concentrations in clients undergoing grafting for burns involving less than 15% of the total body surface area (TBSA) (Jellish et al., 1999).

TABLE 68-8 • BIOLOGIC DRESSINGS

USES
- Debridement of untidy wounds after separation of eschar
- Promotion of re-epithelialization of deep partial-thickness wounds
- Temporary coverage after excision of the burn wound
- Protection of granulation tissue between autografts
- Test graft before autografting

ADVANTAGES
- Early adherence to the wound
- Reduction of evaporative heat loss
- Reduction of evaporate water loss
- Prevention of desiccation of granulation tissue
- Reduction of exudate protein losses
- Reduction of pain
- Assistance in wound debridement
- Enhancement of healing with partial-thickness injuries
- Protection of exposed neovascular tissue
- Inhibition of bacterial proliferation

DISADVANTAGES
- Early lysis resulting in bacterial proliferation
- Expensive
- Rejection responses
- Possible burn wound sepsis if applied over eschar
- Not readily available
- Storage (some may require refrigeration)
- Possible transmission of diseases, such as hepatitis

SURGICAL MANAGEMENT. Surgical management of burn wounds focuses on surgical excision and wound covering. Surgical excision usually occurs early in the postburn period. Grafting procedures for skin covering may be performed throughout the acute phase as burn wounds are made ready and donor sites are available. Grafting may improve function or appearance in the rehabilitative phase.

Wound covering is achieved through autografting. With autografting, viable skin from an area of the client's intact, healthy skin is transplanted to the area where a full-thickness burn wound was excised.

SURGICAL EXCISION. Surgical excision is a widely used method for managing full-thickness injuries; it is the treatment of choice for most deep partial-thickness wounds. The client is taken to the operating room as early as possible within the first 5 days after injury and as needed until complete permanent coverage has been achieved.

The burn wound is excised by either a tangential or a fascial excision technique. In the tangential technique, the surgeon excises very thin layers of the necrotic burn surface until bleeding tissue is encountered. Bleeding indicates that a viable bed of dermis or subcutaneous fat has been reached for application of the graft.

In the fascial technique, the surgeon excises the burn wound to the level of superficial fascia. Fascial excision usually is reserved for very deep and extensive burns. Blood loss is minimal, and grafting is usually successful.

WOUND COVERING. Permanent skin coverage for extensive full-thickness injuries is achieved by applying an autograft. Skin for an autograft is taken from the client's own body. The surgeon usually removes a piece of skin from a remote unburned area of the body and transplants it to cover the burn wound. Skin grafts are generally of split thickness (0.015 inch); a partial-thickness injury is formed at the site of surgical removal (the donor site). Grafts are placed either on a clean granulated bed or over a surgically excised area of burn (see also Chapter 67).

The availability of donor sites for larger burns is small. Clients with burns of a large surface area may have a mere 5% to 20% of the skin surface available to cover the 80% to 95% burned area. Coverage is accomplished in the following ways:

- Successive reharvesting of the available donor site, with time allowed between harvests for re-epithelialization and healing
- Meshing the split-thickness skin grafts (Figure 68-13) to allow a small graft to cover a larger area; although small open spaces (interstices) are present uniformly throughout the graft, healing time is slower for a meshed graft because the skin must fill in the interstices as well as attach to the granulation bed

EVIDENCE-BASED PRACTICE FOR NURSING

What is the best donor site dressing?

Rakel, B.A., et al. (1998). *Split-thickness skin graft donor site care: A quantitative synthesis of the research. Applied Nursing Research, 11*(4), 174-182.

Split-thickness skin grafting (STSG) is a commonly used reconstructive technique but is associated with a large variation in practice. The purpose of this study was to integrate and synthesize the available empirical evidence regarding STSG donor site dressings, identify which dressings are associated with the best outcomes, and provide practice recommendations. This review of 33 studies found transparent film to be the best dressing for the care of the STSG donor site wounds. Transparent film was associated with one of the fastest healing rates (9.47 days), a smooth epithelialized surface, a low infection rate (10 out of 394 patients, or 3%), the least amount of pain (1.59 on a scale of 0 to 10), and minimal cost ($.005 per square inch) when compared with other dressings.

Critique. Given that this report was a synthesis of existing data, it was impossible to match methodologies. The report limited analysis to dressings that were studied more than once. Definitions of healing varied with the dressing used and created inconsistency. Further research is needed to compare those dressings with good outcomes against each other in a randomized fashion.

Implications for Nursing. Pain associated with donor site care often becomes the primary focus of the client after the grafting procedure. A dressing for donor sites that reduces pain, has a rapid healing rate, and is inexpensive has utility in a health care environment that is focused on cost reduction without compromising quality. The dressings reviewed in this report validated the superiority of a moist healing environment. Given the vast array of available dressings, this report is helpful in identifying the best dressings based on the available data. The most interesting phenomenon is that an expensive dressing does not necessarily correlate with the best outcome.

RISK FOR INFECTION

Burn wound infection occurs through *autocontamination,* in which the client's own normal flora overgrows and penetrates the internal environment; and *cross-contamination,* in which microorganisms from another person or the environment are transferred to the client.

PLANNING: EXPECTED OUTCOMES. The client with a burn injury in the acute phase is expected to remain free from infection by cross-contamination and not experience septicemia.

INTERVENTIONS. Interventions aim to prevent infection and remove infected tissue.

NONSURGICAL MANAGEMENT. Nonsurgical management of clients at high risk for infection consists of minimizing exposure of the burn client to exogenous microorganisms, reducing the risk of autocontamination, and recognizing the signs and symptoms of infection early. Drug therapy, isolation therapy, and environmental manipulation are appropriate strategies for preventing and managing infection.

DRUG THERAPY FOR INFECTION PREVENTION. Burn wound conditions favor the growth of *Clostridium tetani.* All burn clients are at risk for this potentially fatal infectious complication. Tetanus toxoid, 0.5 mL administered intramuscularly, enhances previously acquired immunity to *C. tetani;* this is a routine prophylactic procedure when the client is admitted to the hospital. The additional administration of tetanus immune globulin (human) (Hyper-Tet) is recommended when the history of tetanus immunization is questionable.

The use of topical antimicrobial agents is one of the most important interventions for infection prevention in burn

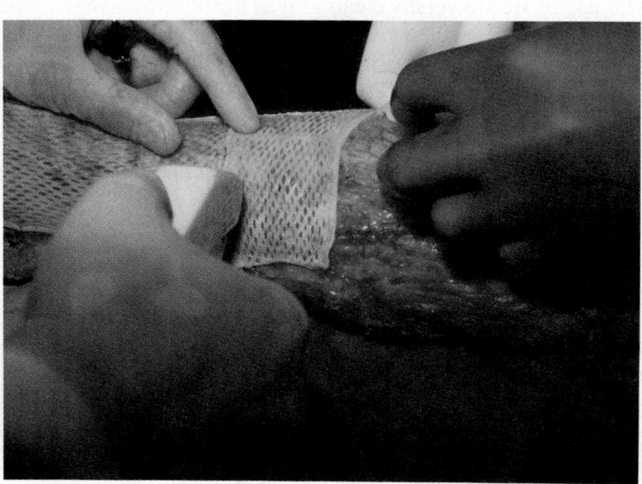

Figure 68-13 ● The typical appearance of meshed autografts.

wounds. The primary goal of topical antimicrobial therapy is to minimize bacterial proliferation into the wound and prevent systemic sepsis.

Topical antibiotics are applied by either the *open* or the *closed* technique. With the open technique, the nurse uses either aseptic or clean methods to apply the agent directly to the burn wound without further dressing the wound. The nurse cleans the wound every 8 to 24 hours and applies fresh antimicrobial agents. With the more common closed technique, the burn wound is dressed after applying the topical agents.

Topical antimicrobial drugs are not applied to freshly grafted areas because many of these agents inhibit cell growth. Chart 68-6 summarizes the characteristics of various topical antimicrobial agents; two of the more commonly used agents are silver sulfadiazine (Silvadene, Flamazine✤) and mafenide acetate (Sulfamylon).

DRUG THERAPY FOR THE TREATMENT OF INFECTION. Systemic antibiotics are ordered when burn clients experience symptoms of an actual infection, including septicemia. Broad-spectrum antibiotics are administered until the results of blood cultures and sensitivity status are available. At that time, more specific antibiotics, including the aminoglycosides such as amikacin (Amikin) or gentamicin (Garamycin, Alcomicin✤) and cephalosporins such as cephalothin (Keflin) or ceftriaxone (Rocephin), are used. Because of increased metabolism, burn clients generally require a larger than normal dose of these drugs to maintain therapeutic serum levels. If aminoglycosides are used, serial peak and trough serum levels are obtained to monitor the efficacy of treatment and evaluate potential renal toxicity.

ISOLATION THERAPY. Some clinicians believe that isolation therapy significantly reduces the incidence of cross-contamination; however, methods of isolation are varied and controversial. Some burn centers practice virtually no isolation, whereas others use near-total sterile conditions. All isolation methods for the client with burns emphasize proper and consistent handwashing as the single most effective technique for preventing the transmission of infection.

ENVIRONMENTAL MANIPULATION. All health care providers wear gloves during all contact with open wounds. The use of sterile versus clean gloves for noninvasive, routine wound care procedures varies by agency and is a matter of debate. Regardless of sterility, the nurse changes gloves when handling wounds on different areas of the body and between handling old and new dressings.

The equipment on burn units is not shared among clients. Disposable items (e.g., pillows, syringes, and dishes) are used as much as possible. The nurse assigns to each client any equipment used in daily routine care (e.g., thermometers, blood pressure cuffs, and stethoscopes). Daily cleaning of the equipment and general housekeeping are essential for environmental infection control. All equipment must be cleaned after use on one client and before use on another. Because *Pseudomonas* has been shown to sequester in plants, the presence of plants and flowers is prohibited. Some burn units do not permit clients to eat raw foods (such as salads, fruit, and pepper) to minimize exposure to exogenous microorganisms. Rugs and upholstered articles are difficult to clean and may harbor organisms; their use is also restricted.

Visitors are restricted when the client is immunosuppressed. Ill people, small children, and other clients should not come into direct contact with the burn client. Some burn units recommend that all visitors wear protective clothing (gowns, gloves, masks, and shoe and hair covers) in the room of the immunosuppressed client, but no conclusive data are available to support this approach.

SECONDARY PREVENTION/EARLY DETECTION. The burn wounds are carefully monitored on admission and at each dressing change. The wounds are examined for the following signs of infection:

- Pervasive odor
- Color changes
- Change in texture
- Purulent drainage
- Exudate
- Sloughing grafts
- Redness at the wound edges extending to nonburned skin

Laboratory cultures and biopsies are recommended. Quantitative biopsies of the eschar and granulation tissue are performed routinely and as needed to monitor the proliferation of organisms and are considered the gold standard for wound monitoring.

SURGICAL MANAGEMENT. Infected burn wounds with colony counts of or approaching 10^5 colonies per gram of tissue are life threatening, even with antibiotic therapy. Aggressive surgical excision of the burn wound may be necessary.

IMBALANCED NUTRITION: LESS THAN BODY REQUIREMENTS

NOC **PLANNING: EXPECTED OUTCOMES.** The client with a burn injury in the acute phase is expected to maintain adequate nutrient intake for meeting the body's calorie requirements as evidenced by the maintenance of normal body weight, serum albumin within expected range, and tissue healing.

INTERVENTIONS. Interventions aim to calculate the client's calorie needs and provide an adequate daily source of calories and nutrients that the client can ingest and metabolize.

Diet therapy begins with calculating the client's current daily metabolic needs and calorie requirements. Several formulas and charts are used for this calculation. Nutritional requirements for a client with a relatively large burn area can exceed 5000 kcal/day. In addition to a high-calorie intake, the burn client requires a diet high in protein for wound healing. The nurse collaborates with the dietitian and the client to plan alternatives to conventional nutritional patterns.

Oral diet therapy may be delayed for several days after the injury until the client has sufficient gastrointestinal motility. As a result, nasoduodenal tube feedings are often initiated soon after admission. The provision of early enteral feeding helps to decrease weight loss, gut atrophy, bacterial translocation, and subsequent sepsis. These feedings often are initiated within 4 hours of commencing fluid resuscitation. This type of nutritional supplement prevents nutritional deficits in critically burned clients.

CHART 68-6

TOPICAL DRUG THERAPY *for* Burns

Agent	Description	Action	Advantages	Disadvantages	Interventions
Silver sulfadiazine (Silvadene, Flamazine♣)	Nontoxic salt of silver sulfadiazine in water-based cream	Binds to bacterial cell membranes and interferes with DNA synthesis	Does not cause hypochloremia, hyponatremia, electrolyte imbalance, or kidney disease Painless Wide-spectrum antimicrobial action against gram-positive and gram-negative organisms Long shelf life Delays eschar separation to a lesser degree than do many other topical agents	Absorbed into eschar less than other agents May cause rash, pruritus, burning, and leukopenia Not consistently effective for burns covering more than 60% of the body Not effective against *Pseudomonas*	Watch for signs of infection, such as soupiness of wound area. Watch for allergic reaction causing drop in white blood cell count. Do not use if reaction to sulfonamide has occurred.
Collagenase (Santyl) with polysporin powder	Topical enzymatic debriding agent with 250 collagenase units/g of white petroleum	Digests collagen in necrotic tissue	Painless Daily dressing changes No side effects Quick debridement action Easy to apply	Expensive Use only on partial-thickness injuries	Apply only once a day.
Mafenide acetate (Sulfamylon)	Soft, white, nonstaining water-based cream	Bacteriostatic action against many gram-positive and gram-negative organisms	Effective against *Pseudomonas* Long shelf life Excellent for treating electrical burns Penetrates thick eschar	May lead to infection May cause metabolic acidosis, hyperpnea, and rash When applied, may cause pain that lasts 30-40 min	Premedicate for pain before application. Monitor blood gas and serum electrolyte levels. Do not use if sulfa drug allergy or respiratory or kidney disease is present.
Nitrofurazone (Furacin)	Cream, solution, or water-soluble powder	Wide-spectrum antibacterial	Effective against *Staphylococcus aureus* and some antibiotic-resistant organisms Causes neither pain nor maceration	May cause contact dermatitis (rare) Messy to apply in cream form May cause renal problems if used for extensive burns	Observe carefully for signs of allergic reaction and evidence of superinfections.
Povidone-iodine (Betadine)	Iodine complex available as solution, ointment, or foam	Microbicidal against gram-positive and gram-negative organisms	Effective against many infections not well controlled by silver sulfadiazine	May cause metabolic acidosis and elevated serum iodine levels May form crusts if burns are not cleaned properly Causes rash and burning in some clients Stains clothes and linen Deactivated by wound proteins	Check serum electrolyte and serum iodine levels frequently.
Gentamicin sulfate (Garamycin, Gentamar)	Available as cream or solution for topical use	Antibiotic action against organisms resistant to other agents	Effective against *Pseudomonas* Does not cause pain	May have ototoxic and nephrotoxic effects May result in resistance by certain organisms	Use with caution in clients with decreased renal function. Monitor serum and urine creatinine clearance before and during treatment.
Polymyxin B–bacitracin	Topical cream	Wide-spectrum antibacterial	Painless Effective against many gram-positive and gram-negative organisms Can be used on the face Can be placed on healed grafts to lubricate	May cause urticaria, burning, and inflammation Does not penetrate eschar	Apply q2-8h to keep areas moist.

The nurse encourages clients who can eat solid foods to ingest as many calories as possible. The client's preferences are taken into consideration for diet planning and food selection. Clients are encouraged to request food whenever they feel they can eat—not just according to the hospital's standard meal schedule. The nurse also offers frequent high-calorie, high-protein supplemental feedings. Care is taken to keep an accurate calorie count for foods and beverages that are actually ingested by the client.

Clients who cannot swallow but who have adequate gastric motility may meet calorie and nutrition needs through enteral tube feedings (see Chapter 61). Parenteral nutrition may be administered by the intravenous route when the gastrointestinal tract is not functional or when the client's nutritional requirements cannot be met by oral and enteral feeding. This method is used as a last resort because it is invasive and can lead to infectious and metabolic complications.

IMPAIRED PHYSICAL MOBILITY

NOC **PLANNING: EXPECTED OUTCOMES.** The client with a burn injury in the acute phase is expected to regain and maintain an optimal ability to move purposefully.

INTERVENTIONS. Interventions aim to maintain the client's preburn range of joint motion and prevent contracture formation.

NONSURGICAL MANAGEMENT. Nonsurgical management includes positioning, range-of-motion exercises, ambulation, and pressure dressings.

POSITIONING. Positioning is critical for clients with burn injuries because the position of comfort for the client is often one of joint flexion, which predisposes him or her to the development of contractures. Care is taken to maintain the client in a neutral body position with minimal flexion. Best practice for the prevention of contractures is presented in Chart 68-7. Splints and other conforming devices may assist in maintaining position. These devices are used most frequently on the joints of the hands, elbows, knees, neck, and axillae.

RANGE-OF-MOTION EXERCISES. Range-of-motion exercises are performed actively at least three times a day. If the client cannot move a joint actively, the nurse performs passive range-of-motion exercises. Burned hands are given special attention. The client is encouraged to perform active range-of-motion exercises for the hand, thumb, and fingers every hour while awake.

AMBULATION. Ambulation is started as soon as possible after the fluid shifts have resolved. Clients with a variety of attached equipment (IV catheters, nasogastric tubes, electrocardiographic leads, extensive dressings) can ambulate with preparation and assistance. Ambulation is performed two or three times a day and progresses in length each time. Ambulation inhibits the loss of bone density, strengthens muscles, stimulates immune function, promotes ventilation, and prevents a wide variety of complications.

PRESSURE DRESSINGS. After the graft heals, pressure dressings are implemented to assist in the prevention of contractures and tight hypertrophic scars, which can inhibit mobility. These dressings also inhibit venous engorgement and edema formation in areas with decreased lymphatic outflow. Pressure dressings may be elastic wraps or specially designed, custom-fitted, elasticized clothing that provide continuous and uniform pressure over burned surfaces. Figure 68-14 illustrates such garments. For maximal effectiveness, pressure garments should be worn at least 23 hours a day, every day, until the scar tissue is mature (12 to 24 months). Pressure garments generally cause an increase in warmth and itchiness and often are seen as very uncomfortable by the client. The nurse must reinforce to the client that wearing pressure garments is extremely beneficial in maintaining mobility and reducing hypertrophic scarring.

CHART 68-7

BEST PRACTICE *for* Positioning to Prevent Contractures

AFFECTED BODY PART	POSITION OF FUNCTION	INTERVENTIONS
Head and neck	Hyperextension	Place a towel roll under the client's neck or shoulder, or use a double mattress.
Posterior neck	Flexion	Have the client turn the head from side to side.
Upper chest and chest	Shoulder retraction	Place the client supine. Do not allow pillows. Place a folded towel under the spine, between the scapulae.
Lateral trunk	Flexion to uninvolved side	Place the client supine with the arm on the affected side up over the head.
Anterior shoulder	Abduction and external rotation	Maintain the upper arm at 90 degrees of abduction from the lateral aspect of the trunk.
Posterior shoulder	Slight flexion and interior rotation	Keep the arm slightly behind the midline.
Elbow	Extension and supination	Keep the joint in the extended position.
Wrist	30-45 degrees of extension	Use a splint.
Fingers		
MP joints	70-90 degrees of flexion	Use a splint.
PIP and DIP joints	Extended	Use a splint.
Ankle	90 degrees of dorsiflexion	Use a footboard or splint.
Legs	15-20 degrees of abduction	Place a small pillow between the legs.

MP, Metacarpal-phalangeal; *PIP,* proximal interphalangeal, *DIP,* distal interphalengeal.

SURGICAL MANAGEMENT. Surgical management is restorative rather than preventive. Surgical techniques for contracture release are most commonly performed in the neck, axilla, elbow flexion areas, and hand. Specific surgical procedures to improve movement vary for each client.

Postoperative nursing responsibilities include nonsurgical interventions to prevent contractures from reforming as well as the care of new grafts and suture lines. The nurse constantly reinforces the need for the client to comply with exercise and splinting regimens to prevent the recurrence of joint immobility.

DISTURBED BODY IMAGE

NOC **PLANNING: EXPECTED OUTCOMES.** Following intervention, the client with a burn injury in the acute phase is expected to have a positive perception of his or her own appearance and body functions as evidenced by a willingness to touch the affected body part, adjustment to changes in body function, a willingness to use strategies to enhance appearance and function, a successful progression through the grieving process, and the use of support systems.

INTERVENTIONS. Nonsurgical and surgical interventions can assist clients who experience body image disturbances as a result of burn injury.

NONSURGICAL MANAGEMENT. Understanding the stages of grief is helpful for the client, family, and nurse. The nurse assesses which stage of grief the client is currently experiencing and helps interpret his or her behaviors. The client often is unaware of or is confused by his or her feelings. The nurse reassures him or her that feelings of grief, loss, anxiety, anger, fear, and guilt are normal. The client may be grieving the loss of body parts, appearance, role identity, and social identity. The nurse seeks the help of other health care team members (e.g., psychologist, psychiatrist, social worker, or clergy or religious leader) in addressing these problems.

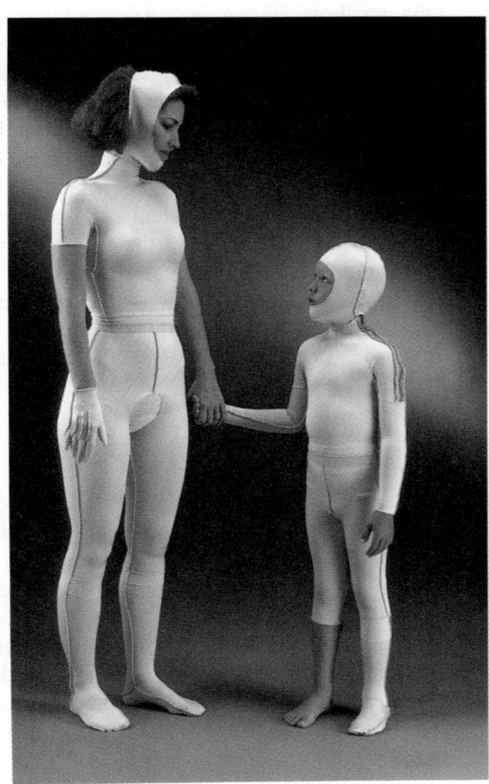

Figure 68-14 ● Models wearing pressure garments. (Courtesy Beiersdorf-Jobst, Inc., Charlotte, NC.)

The nurse accepts the physical and psychologic characteristics of the client. Clients and families are presented with realistic expected outcomes for the client's functional capacity and physical appearance. Information sessions and counseling for the family or significant others can identify previous and current patterns of support that are effective for the client and family. The nurse facilitates their use of these systems and the development of new support systems and makes referrals to specific support groups. To identify the effectiveness of such assistance and possible gaps in support, the nurse continually evaluates support resources throughout the course of illness.

Engaging in decision making and independent activities fosters feelings of self-worth, which are closely linked to body image. To this end, the nurse plans and encourages the client's participation in self-care activities. Family members are assisted in understanding that it is more beneficial for the client to perform these activities than to have them performed by someone else. Families are encouraged to include the client in family decision making to the same degree that he or she participated in this process before the injury.

SURGICAL MANAGEMENT. Reconstructive and cosmetic surgery can be performed for many years after the burn injury. Restoration of function and improvement of physical appearance through surgical techniques often increase the client's feelings of self-worth and promote a positive body image. Many clients have unrealistic expectations of reconstructive surgery and envision an appearance identical or equal in quality to the preburn state. The nurse educates the client and family about expected cosmetic outcomes.

CRITICAL THINKING CHALLENGE

The 22-year-old client who experienced an electrical injury has had his thumb and part of his right hand amputated and has had his right kidney removed. His right arm, above and below the elbow, was grafted with a split-thickness meshed graft taken from his left thigh. When you change the dressing, you note that the graft has a dusky appearance and that the edges of the graft are beginning to curl. The margins of the wound are firm and red with some purulent drainage. You also note a greenish blue color in the burned area next to the graft.

- What is your first action?
- Should range-of-motion exercises be performed for the right elbow at this time? Why or why not?
- What additional assessment data should you obtain about the graft and the surrounding burn wound?

For suggested answer guidelines, go to SIMON http://www.wbsaunders.com/SIMON/Iggy/.

REHABILITATIVE PHASE OF BURN INJURY

OVERVIEW

Although rehabilitation efforts are started from the time of admission, the technical rehabilitative phase begins with wound closure and ends when the client returns to the highest possible level of functioning. The emphasis during this phase is the psychosocial adjustment of the client, the prevention of scars and contractures, and the resumption of preburn activity, including work, family, and social roles. This phase may take years or even last a lifetime as clients adjust to permanent limitations that may not be apparent until long after the initial injury.

➤ COLLABORATIVE MANAGEMENT

Although attention initially is placed on the physical interventions for and clinical manifestations of the burn injury, psychologic care is equally important. The nurse provides psychosocial support to the client and family throughout hospitalization but more extensively throughout the rehabilitative phase.

Information from the client and family aids in the assessment and diagnosis of psychologic problems and allows treatment to be instituted. The nurse explores the client's feelings about the burn injury. It is extremely difficult for clients to concentrate on the many tasks before them when obstacles such as guilt and grief are in the forefront.

The client or family member is asked whether there is a history of psychologic or organic impairment. The type of coping mechanisms the client has used successfully during times of stress is assessed and documented to assist with a future plan of care. The nurse also assesses the client's family unit and the family members' history of interaction. The nurse determines cultural and ethnic factors and takes these into consideration when planning psychosocial interventions.

Throughout the hospitalization the client progresses through a variety of stages and exhibits a myriad of feelings, including denial, regression, and anger. The nurse accurately assesses the client's feelings during each stage so appropriate plans of care can be developed and carried out.

Community-Based Care

Discharge planning for the client with a burn injury begins at the time of admission to the hospital or burn center. In most burn centers, the multidisciplinary team meets regularly to plan for discharge. In helping the client to reach mutually established discharge goals, the team evaluates the progress of each discipline. Table 68-9 summarizes the usual discharge needs of the client with burns.

TABLE 68-9 • NEEDS TO BE ADDRESSED BEFORE DISCHARGE OF THE CLIENT WITH BURNS

- Early client assessment
- Financial assessment
- Evaluation of family resources
- Weekly discharge planning meeting
- Psychologic referral
- Client and family teaching (home care)
- Designation of principal learners (specific family members or significant others who will help with care)
- Development of teaching plan
- Training for wound care
- Rehabilitation referral
- Home assessment (on-site visit)
- Medical equipment
- Public health nursing referral
- Evaluation of community resources
- Visit to referral agency
- Re-entry programs for school or work environment
- Nursing home placement
- Environmental interventions
- Auditory testing
- Speech therapy
- Prosthetic rehabilitation

PSYCHOSOCIAL PREPARATION

During the recovery period and for some time after discharge from the hospital, clients with severe burn injuries are likely to experience psychologic problems that require psychosocial assistance. Such problems include posttraumatic stress disorder, sexual dysfunction, and severe depression. Assistance is coordinated with the client, family, and health care team. Psychosocial assistance is best provided by a professional counselor with previous experience in helping burn clients.

One specific area to be addressed with the client is the reaction of others to the sight of healing wounds and disfiguring scars. Clients with facial burns are especially subjected to stares and other forms of disquieting behavior from the general public. Visits from friends and short public appearances before discharge may help the client begin adjusting to this problem. Community reintegration programs can assist the psychosocial and physical recovery of the client with serious burns.

HOME CARE MANAGEMENT

The client with severe burns is often discharged from the acute care setting when life-threatening complications are resolved and minimal wound areas remain open. During the initial weeks at home after discharge, the client usually continues to require at least daily wound care, rehabilitative therapy, nutritional support, symptom management, and drug therapy.

Although the client usually views the prospect of going home in a positive light, the difficulties associated with physical care and the psychologic stresses associated with changes in appearance, role, function, and lifestyle are numerous and may overwhelm the client and family. Successful discharge depends on extensive planning and preparation of the client, family, and home environment through education and the involvement of appropriate support agencies and services.

Preparation for discharge includes assessment of the family and home care situation from physical and social perspectives. The nurse considers the needs of the client when evaluating the environment for cleanliness; access to bathing facilities, electricity, and running water; stairways; number of occupants; temperature control; and safety. If the burn injuries are a result of a fire at home, a new residence may need to be established.

HEALTH TEACHING

Education about burn care and living with the consequences of burn injuries begins when the client is admitted to the hospital or burn center. A weekly plan for client education is outlined; the primary goal is progression toward independence for the client and family. Critical for this goal is teaching clients, family members, or significant others to perform specific care tasks, such as dressing changes. Clients and family members first observe the nurse changing the dressings, then assist in performing the changes, and finally change the dressings independently under the supervision of the burn care nurse.

Before discharge, all people who will be involved in the client's home care participate in discharge planning and teaching sessions. In addition to details about dressing changes, the nurse explains the following:

- Signs and symptoms of infection
- Medication regimens
- Proper use of prosthetic and positioning devices
- Correct application and care of pressure garments
- Comfort measures to reduce pruritus
- Dates for follow-up appointments

HEALTH CARE RESOURCES

The nurse and health care team evaluate the family in terms of capacity and willingness to assist in providing care to the client after discharge. A visiting nurse or case manager referral can assist the family with care problems arising at home. In addition, the visiting nurse can help the family determine what special equipment, supplies, or services will be needed. The frequency of home visits depends on the client's condition and the ability of family members to function as care providers. It is imperative that the visiting nurse have extensive experience in providing burn care. The home care nurse may benefit from a brief visit to the client while in the hospital and from observing burn wound care.

The home care of a client after an extensive burn often involves daily physical therapy and rehabilitation sessions at special centers. Transportation problems are addressed and resolved before the client is discharged. In some instances, the burn center has arrangements for transportation. Some community volunteer agencies provide transportation by private car.

When rehabilitation is expected to be prolonged, the client may be discharged to a special rehabilitation facility. Before this point, the burn care nurse consults with the rehabilitation nurse or team and provides copies of the care and teaching plans used with the client.

CRITICAL THINKING CHALLENGE

The 22-year-old client who sustained an electrical injury and had his right thumb and part of his right hand amputated is being prepared for discharge. He tells you he is afraid that he will not be accepted by his friends or ever get married because of his appearance and the disability resulting from the amputation.

- Are this client's fears justified? Why or why not?
- What is your immediate response to his statements?
- What resources or referrals would be most appropriate for this client at this time?

For suggested answer guidelines, go to SIMON http://www.wbsaunders.com/SIMON/Iggy/.

Evaluation: Outcomes

NOC The nurse evaluates the care of the client with a burn injury on the basis of the identified nursing diagnoses and collaborative problems. The expected outcomes may include that the client will:

- Have cardiac output restored to normal as evidenced by blood pressure and heart rate in expected ranges and by strong peripheral pulses
- Maintain adequate oxygenation and circulation to all vital organs as evidenced by oxygen saturation, partial pressure of arterial oxygen (Pao_2), partial pressure of arterial carbon dioxide ($Paco_2$), and arterial blood pH within normal limits
- Have arterial blood gases (ABGs) within normal limits
- Have normal lung compliance
- Be free of respiratory distress
- Be free of pulmonary edema
- Be free of visceral organ damage
- Maintain stable cardiac rhythms
- Maintain a patent airway
- Have an effective breathing pattern as evidenced by maintaining oxygen saturation, Pao_2, $Paco_2$, and an arterial blood pH within normal limits
- Have pain alleviated or reduced as evidenced by a decreased report of pain and a decreased length of pain episodes
- Experience no further loss of skin integrity
- Have skin integrity restored without complications
- Have skin thickness in the expected range in the burn wound area
- Remain free from infection by cross-contamination
- Not experience septicemia
- Maintain an adequate nutrient intake for meeting the body's calorie requirements as evidenced by maintenance (achievement) of normal weight, serum albumin within expected range, and tissue healing
- Regain and maintain an optimal ability to move purposefully
- Have a positive perception of his or her own appearance and body functions
- Willingly touch affected body parts
- Accept altered appearance as a result of the burn injury
- Successfully progress through the grieving process
- Use support systems

ONLINE RESOURCES

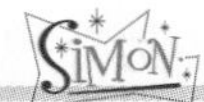

For suggested readings and Internet resources, go to http://www.wbsaunders.com/SIMON/Iggy/.

SELECTED BIBLIOGRAPHY

Asterisk indicates a classic or definitive work on this subject.

Ahrns, K.A., & Harkins, D.R. (1999). Initial resuscitation after burn injury: Therapies, strategies and controversies. *AACN Clinical Issues: Advanced Practice in Acute and Critical Care, 10*(1), 46-60.

American Burn Association. (1999). U.S. trauma and burn statistics; http://www.ameriburn.org.

Atkins, S. (1999). Burns assessment and initial management. *Nursing Times, 95*(35), 46-48.

*Baud, F.J., et al. (1991). Elevated blood cyanide concentrations in victims of smoke inhalation. *New England Journal of Medicine, 325*(25), 1761-1766.

Burn Foundation. (1999). Burn incidence and treatment in the United States; http://www.burnfoundation.org/adultfact.html.

*Cadier, M., & Shakespear, P. (1995). Burns in octogenarians. *Burns, 21*(3), 200-204.

*Covington, D., Wainwright, D., & Parks, D. (1996). Prognostic indicators in the elderly patient with burns. *Journal of Burn Care and Rehabilitation, 17*(3), 222-230.

*Dries, D.J., & Waxman, K. (1991). Adequate resuscitation of burn patients may not be measured by urine output and vital signs. *Critical Care Medicine, 19*(3), 327-329.

Flynn, M. (1999). Identifying and treating inhalation injuries in fire victims. *DCCN: Dimensions of Critical Care Nursing, 18*(4), 18-23.

Fowler, A. (1998). Nursing management of minor burn injuries. *Nursing Standard, 12*(49), 47-52, 55-56.

Gordon, M., et al. (1998). Use of pain assessment tools: Is there a preference? *Journal of Burn Care & Rehabilitation, 19*(5), 451-454.

Greenfield, E., & McManus, A. (1997). Infectious complications: Prevention and strategies for their control. *Nursing Clinics of North America, 32*(2), 297-309.

*Hansbrough, J., et al. (1995). Wound healing in partial-thickness burn wounds treated with collagenase ointment versus silver sulfadiazine cream. *Journal of Burn Care and Rehabilitation, 16*(3), 241-247.

Hunt, J., et al. (2000). Occupation-related burn injuries. *Journal of Burn Care: Rehabilitator 21*(4), 327-332.

Iraniha, S., et al. (2000). Determination of burn depth with noncontact ultrasonography. *Journal of Burn Care and Rehabilitation, 21*(4), 333-338.

Jellish, W.S., et al. (1999). Effect of topical local anesthetic application to skin harvest sites for pain management in burn patients undergoing skin-grafting procedures, *Annals of Surgery, 229*(1), 115-120.

Jordan, B., & Harrington, D. (1997). Management of the burn wound. *Nursing Clinics of North America, 32*(2), 251-273.

Kagan, R., & Smith, S. (2000). Evaluation and treatment of thermal injuries. *Dermatology Nursing, 12*(5), 334-335, 338-344, 347-350.

*Kealey, G. (1995). Pharmacologic management of background pain in burn victims. *Journal of Burn Care and Rehabilitation, 16*(3), 358-362.

Kraft, P. (2000). The osmotic shift. *Journal of Intravenous Nursing, 23*(4), 220-224.

*Kravitz, M., et al. (1989). A randomized trial of plasma exchange in the treatment of burn shock. *Journal of Burn Care and Rehabilitation, 10*(1), 17-26.

*Latarjet, J., & Choinere, M. (1995). Pain in burn patients. *Burns, 21*(5), 344-348.

Lawrence, J.W., et al. (1998). Sleep disturbance after burn injury: A frequent yet understudied complication. *Journal of Burn Care & Rehabilitation, 19*(6), 480-486.

*Marvin, J.A., et al. (1996). Pain response and control. In D.L. Herndon (Ed.), *Total Burn Care,* Philadelphia: W.B. Saunders.

Mayes, T., Gottschlich, M., & Warden, G. (1997). Clinical nutrition protocols for continuous quality improvements in the outcomes of patients with burns. *Journal of Burn Care and Rehabilitation, 18*(4), 365-368.

McCain, D., & Sutherland, S. (1998). Skin grafts for patients with burns. *American Journal of Nursing, 98*(7), 34-38.

Mertens, D., Jenkins, M., & Warden, G. (1997). Outpatient burn management. *Nursing Clinics of North America, 32*(2), 343-364.

*Moritz, A.R. (1947). Studies of thermal injuries: II. The relative importance of time and surface temperature in the causation of cutaneous burns. *American Journal of Pathology, 23,* 695.

Nagy, S. (1999). Strategies used by burn nurses to cope with the infliction of pain on patients. *Journal of Advanced Nursing, 29*(6), 1427-1433.

*Nguyen, T.T., et al. (1996). Current treatment of severely burned patients. *Annals of Surgery, 223*(1), 14-25.

The physiology of burns. (1999). *Nursing Times, 95*(34), 30.

Rakel, B.A., et al. (1998). Split-thickness skin graft donor site care: A quantitative synthesis of the research, *Applied Nursing Research, 11*(4), 174-182.

Ramzy, P.I., Barret, J.P., & Herndon, D.N. (1999). Thermal injury. *Critical Care Clinics, 15*(2), 333-352.

*Rodriguez, D. (1996). Nutrition in patients with severe burns: State of the art. *Journal of Burn Care and Rehabilitation, 17*(1), 62-70.

Ryan, C.M., et al. (1998). Estimates of the probability of death from burn injuries. *New England Journal of Medicine, 338*(6), 362-66.

Saffle, J.R. (1998). Predicting outcome of burns. *New England Journal of Medicine, 338*(6), 387-388.

Scholl, D., & Langkamp-Henken, B. (2001). Nutrient recommendations for wound healing. *Journal of Intravenous Nursing, 24*(2), 124-132.

Sheridan, R. (2000). Evaluating and managing burn wounds. *Dermatology Nursing, 12*(1), 17-28.

*Shirani, K.Z., et al. (1996). Update on current therapeutic approaches in burns. *Shock, 5*(1), 4-16.

Sibbald, G., et al. (2000). Preparing the woundbed: Debridement, bacterial balance, and moisture balance. *Ostomy Wound Management, 46*(4), 14-35.

Stone, M., Ahmed, J., & Evans, J. (2000). The continuing risk of domestic hot water scalds to the elderly. *Burns, 26*(4), 347-350.

Wiebelhaus, P., & Hansen, S. (2001). What you should know about managing burn emergencies. *Nursing2001, 31*(1), 36-41.

Winfree, J., & Barillo, D. (1997). Nonthermal injuries. *Nursing Clinics of North America, 32*(2), 275-296.

Winfrey, M. Cochran, M., & Hegarty, M. (1999). A new technology in burn therapy: Integra artificial skin. *Dimensions of Critical Care Nursing, 18*(1), 14-20.

UNIT 15

PROBLEMS OF EXCRETION

Management of Clients with Problems of the Renal/Urinary System

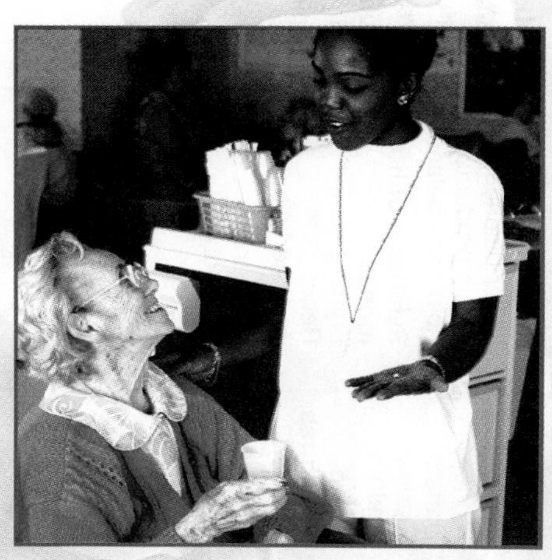

PROBLEMS OF EXCRETION: RENAL/URINARY ■ Core Concepts Grid

Anatomy	Physiology	Pathophysiology	History	Physical Exam	Diagnostic Tests	Interventions	Pharmacology
• **Macro-structures** Kidneys Ureters Bladder Urethra • **Micro-structures** Cortex Medulla Pelvis Glomerulus Nephron	• **Regulation** Water balance Waste products Acid-base balance • **Synthesis of hormones** Erythropoietin Renin Activated vitamin D • **Glomerular filtration**	• **Obstruction** • **Inflammation** • **Infection** • **Trauma** • **Tumors** • **Metabolic acidosis**	• **Client history** Past renal problems Difficulty with urination Change in urinary elimination pattern Pain Hypertension • **Family history** Diabetes mellitus Hypertension • **Social history** Alcohol/drug use Occupation Age	• **Skin** Color/turgor Moisture • **Eyes** Conjunctiva • **Mouth** Moisture/color Ulceration • **Chest** Shape Pulsation • **Periphery** Color Hair distribution Striae/edema Pulses/rashes • **Abdomen** Striae/tenderness over kidney Bruits over renal artery	• **Urinalysis** • **Specific gravity** • **Sediment** • **Serum creatinine** • **Blood urea nitrogen (BUN)** • **Uric acid** • **Scans** • **Renal arteriogram** • **Kidney, ureter, and bladder (KUB)** • **Sonograms** • **Intravenous pyelography (IVP)** • **Biopsy** • **Creatinine clearance** • **Serum pH** • **Cystoscopy**	• **Fluid regulation** • **Dialysis** Hemodialysis Peritoneal dialysis Continuous ambulatory peritoneal dialysis (CAPD) • **Renal transplantation** • **Extracorporeal shock wave lithotripsy (ESWL)** • **AV fistula** • **AV shunt** • **Therapeutic diet** • **Fluids, as appropriate** • **Lithotripsy** • **Health teaching** • **Bladder training** • **Skin care** • **Urinary catheter care**	• **Diuretics** • **Anti-inflammatories** • **Antibiotics** • **Immunosuppressive agents** • **Calcium replacement agents** • **Hormone replacement agents** • **Chelating agents** • **Phosphorus-binding agents** • **Anticholinergics** • **Skin barrier topical agents**

CHAPTER 69

Assessment of the Renal/Urinary System

CHRIS WINKELMAN

Learning Objectives

After studying this chapter, you should be able to:

1. Compare and contrast kidney function with functions of the ureters, bladder, and urethra.
2. Describe the roles of the afferent and efferent arterioles in glomerular filtration.
3. Explain the influence of antidiuretic hormone and aldosterone on urine formation and composition.
4. Describe age-related changes in the renal/urinary system.
5. Use laboratory data to distinguish between dehydration and renal impairment.
6. Describe how to obtain a sterile urine specimen from a client with a Foley catheter.
7. Identify teaching priorities for a client who needs to obtain a 24-hour urine specimen.
8. Identify teaching priorities for a client who needs to obtain a "clean catch" urine specimen.
9. Describe the correct techniques to use in physically assessing the renal system.
10. Prioritize nursing care for the client during the first 24 hours following a renal arteriogram.

SIMON

Go to http://www.wbsaunders.com/SIMON/Iggy/ for self-assessment questions related to these Learning Objectives.

Kidneys contribute to health in several ways. Their primary role is to maintain body fluid volume and composition and to filter waste products for elimination. The kidneys also help regulate blood pressure, participate in acid-base balance, produce erythropoietin for red blood cell synthesis, and metabolize vitamin D to an active form.

The renal system includes the kidneys and the entire urinary tract. The ureters, bladder, and urethra provide a drainage route for the excretion of urine. Structural or functional problems in the kidney or urinary tract usually alter fluid, electrolyte, and acid-base balance.

Assessment of the client at risk for or with actual problems of the renal system begins with a history and physical assessment. A clear understanding of the anatomy, physiology, and diagnostic tests of the renal system will help the nurse in problem solving about renal function in the clinical setting. It will also assist the nurse in teaching the client about the purpose of tests or procedures and in physically and emotionally preparing the client for assessment.

ANATOMY AND PHYSIOLOGY REVIEW

Kidneys

Structure

GROSS ANATOMY

Normally, two kidneys are located in the **retroperitoneal space** (behind the peritoneum, not really in the abdominal cavity), one on either side of the vertebral column (Figure 69-1). The adult kidney is 4 to 5 inches (11 to 13 cm) long, 2 to 3 inches (5 to 7 cm) wide, and about 1 inch (2.5 to 3 cm) thick. It weighs about 8 ounces (250 g). The left kidney is slightly longer and narrower than the right kidney. Kidney size is usually determined via ultrasound. Larger-than-usual kidneys may indicate renal obstruction or polycystic disease, whereas smaller-than-usual kidneys may indicate chronic renal disease.

Several layers of protective, supportive tissue surround the kidney. On the outer surface of the kidney is a layer of fibrous tissue called the **renal capsule** (Figure 69-2). This capsule covers most of the kidney except the **hilum,** the area in which the renal artery enters and the renal vein and ureter exit. The renal capsule is surrounded by layers of fat and connective tissue (Gerota's fascia).

Lying beneath the renal capsule is functional renal tissue composed of two distinct sections: the cortex and the medulla. The **renal cortex,** or outer tissue layer, is in direct contact with the renal capsule. The **medulla,** or medullary tissue, lies below the cortex in the shape of many fans. Each "fan" is called a **pyramid,** and there are 12 to 18 pyramids per kidney. The **renal columns** (columns of Bertin) are cortical tissue that dip down into the interior of the kidney and separate the pyramids.

The tip, or end, of each pyramid is called the **papilla.** The papillae drain urine into the collecting system. A cuplike structure called a **calyx** collects the urine at the end of each papilla. The calices merge together to form the **renal pelvis,** which narrows to become the ureter.

The kidneys receive 20% to 25% of the total cardiac output. Renal blood flow per minute varies from about 600 to 1300 mL/min. The blood supply to each kidney is usually delivered by a single **renal artery,** which branches from the abdominal aorta (Table 69-1). The renal artery separates into progressively smaller arteries, supplying all areas of the renal tissue (**parenchyma**) and the nephrons. The smallest arteries, the afferent arterioles, feed the nephrons directly to form urine.

Venous blood from the kidneys starts with the capillaries surrounding each nephron. These capillaries drain into progressively larger veins, with blood eventually returned to the inferior vena cava through the renal vein.

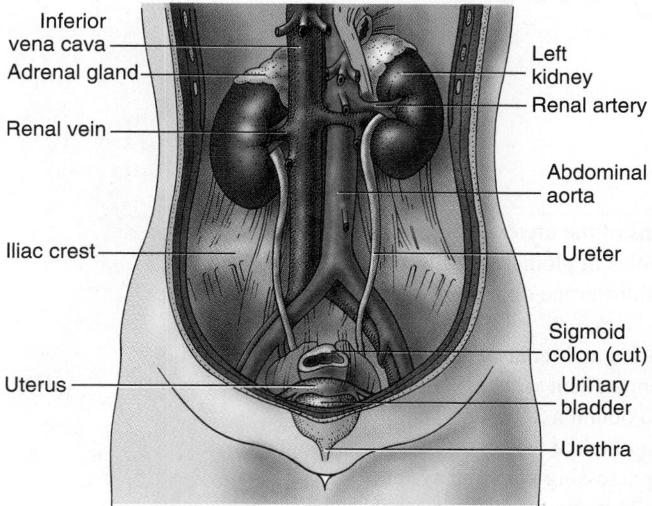

Figure 69-1 ● Anatomic location of organs of the renal/urinary system.

MICROSCOPIC ANATOMY

The **nephron** is the functional unit of the kidney, and it is here that urine is actually formed from blood. There are about 1 million nephrons per kidney, and each nephron separately makes urine from blood.

There are two types of nephrons: cortical nephrons and juxtamedullary nephrons. The cortical nephrons are short, with all parts located in the renal cortex. The juxtamedullary nephrons (about 20% of all nephrons) are longer, and their tubes and associated blood vessels dip deeply into the

TABLE 69-1 • THE SEQUENCE OF RENAL BLOOD FLOW FROM THE RENAL ARTERY TO THE RENAL VEIN
1. Renal artery
2. Interlobar artery
3. Arcuate artery
4. Interlobular artery
5. Afferent arteriole
6. Glomerulus
7. Efferent arteriole
8. Peritubular capillaries or vasa recta
9. Stellate vein
10. Interlobular vein
11. Arcuate vein
12. Interlobar vein
13. Renal vein

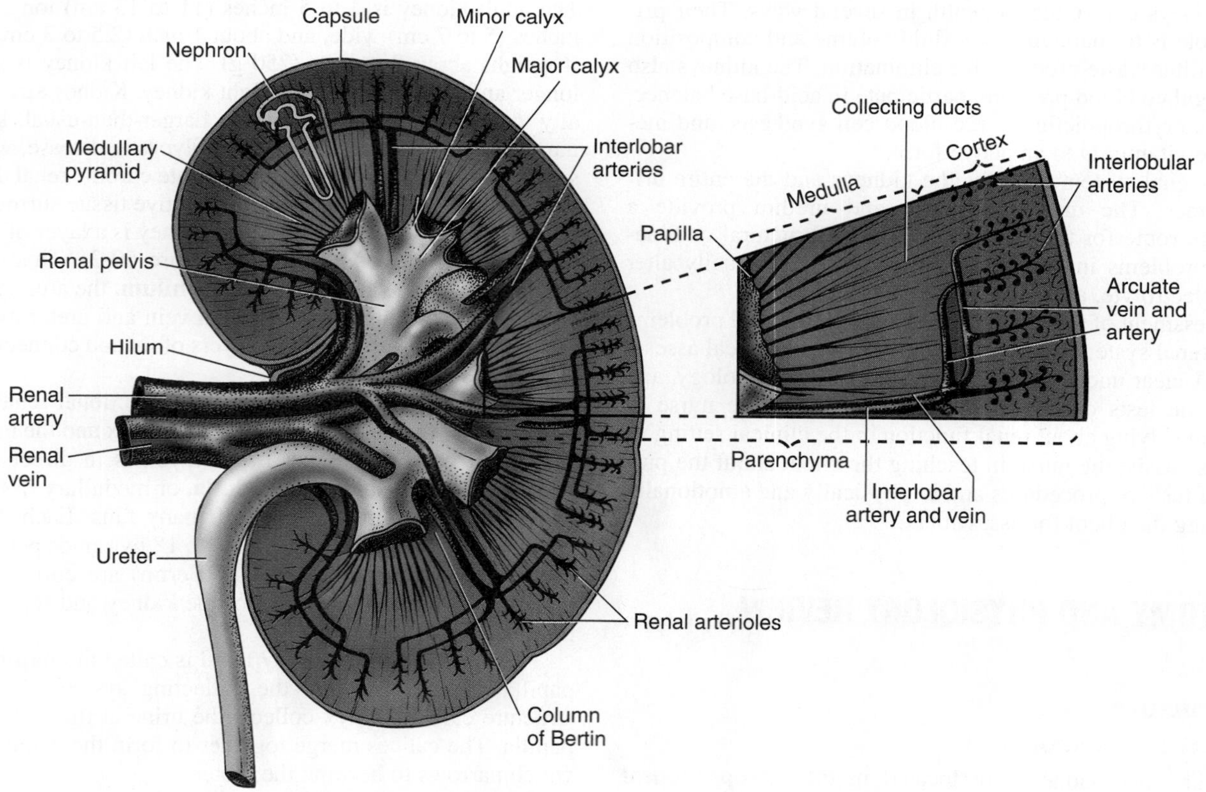

Figure 69-2 ● Bisection of the kidney showing the major structures of the kidney.

medulla. The purpose of the juxtamedullary nephrons is to concentrate urine during times of low fluid intake. The ability to concentrate urine allows for the maximum excretion of waste products with less fluid loss.

Blood supply to the nephron is delivered via the **afferent arteriole,** the smallest, most distal portion of the renal arterial system. From the afferent arteriole, blood flows into the **glomerulus,** a series of specialized capillary loops. It is through these capillaries that water and small particles are filtered from the blood to make urine. The remaining blood exits the glomerulus via the **efferent arteriole.** From the efferent arteriole, blood exits into one of two additional capillary systems:

- The **peritubular capillaries** around the tubular component of cortical nephrons
- The **vasa recta** around the tubular component of juxtamedullary nephrons

Each nephron is a tubular structure with distinct parts (Figure 69-3). The tubular component of the nephron begins with **Bowman's capsule,** a saclike structure that surrounds the glomerulus. The tubular tissue of Bowman's capsule narrows into the **proximal convoluted tubule (PCT).** The PCT twists and turns, finally straightening into the descending limb of the **loop of Henle.** The descending loop of Henle dips in the direction of the medulla but forms a hairpin loop and comes back up into the cortex.

As the loop of Henle changes direction, two segments are identified in the ascending limb of the loop of Henle: the thin and thick segments. The **distal convoluted tubule (DCT)** is formed from the thick segment of the ascending limb of the loop of Henle. The DCT ends in one of many **collecting ducts** located in the kidney tissue. The urine in the collecting ducts passes through the papillae and empties into the renal pelvis.

A series of specialized cells located in the afferent arteriole, efferent arteriole, and DCT are collectively known as the **juxtaglomerular complex** (Figure 69-4). The specialized cells in this area are the **renin-producing cells,** which produce and store renin. **Renin** is a hormone that helps to regulate blood flow, glomerular filtration rate (GFR), and systemic blood pressure. Renin is secreted when special cells in the DCT called the **macula densa** sense changes in blood volume and pressure. The macula densa lies next to the renin-producing granular cells of both afferent and efferent arterioles. Renin is secreted when the macula densa cells sense that blood volume, blood pressure, or blood sodium levels are low. Renin then converts angiotensinogen into angiotensin I. This leads to a series of reactions that cause secretion of the hormone **aldosterone** (Figure 69-5). Aldosterone increases kidney reabsorption of sodium and water, restoring blood pressure, blood volume, and blood sodium levels. (See Chapter 11 for a more complete description of the renin-angiotensin-aldosterone pathway).

Microscopically, the glomerular capillary wall has three layers (Figure 69-6): the endothelium, the basement membrane, and the epithelium. The endothelial and epithelial cells lining the glomerular capillary are separated by pores that filter water and small particles from the blood into Bowman's capsule. This fluid is called the **filtrate,** or early urine.

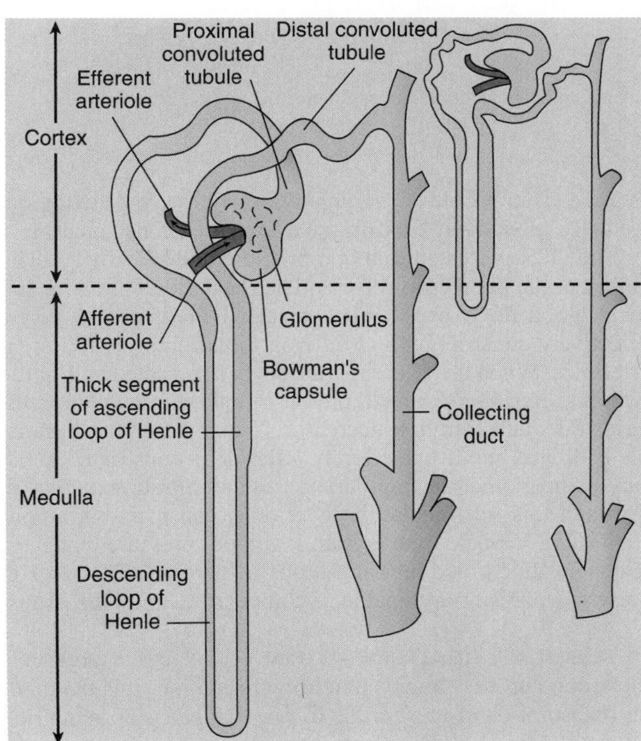

Figure 69-3 ● Anatomy of the nephron, the functional unit of the kidney. Note that the particular nephron labeled here is a juxtamedullary nephron.

Function

The kidneys have both regulatory and hormonal functions. The regulatory functions control fluid, electrolyte, and acid-base balance. The hormonal functions control red blood cell formation, blood pressure, and vitamin D activation.

REGULATORY FUNCTIONS

The physiologic processes responsible for maintaining fluid, electrolyte, and acid-base balance are glomerular filtration,

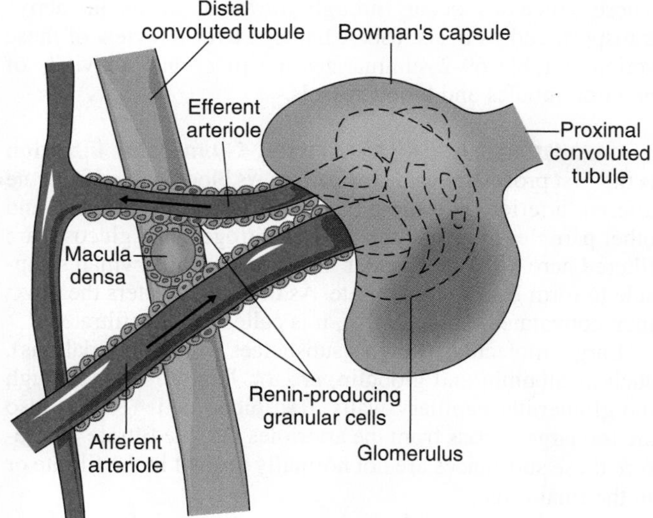

Figure 69-4 ● The juxtaglomerular complex showing juxtaglomerular cells and the macula densa.

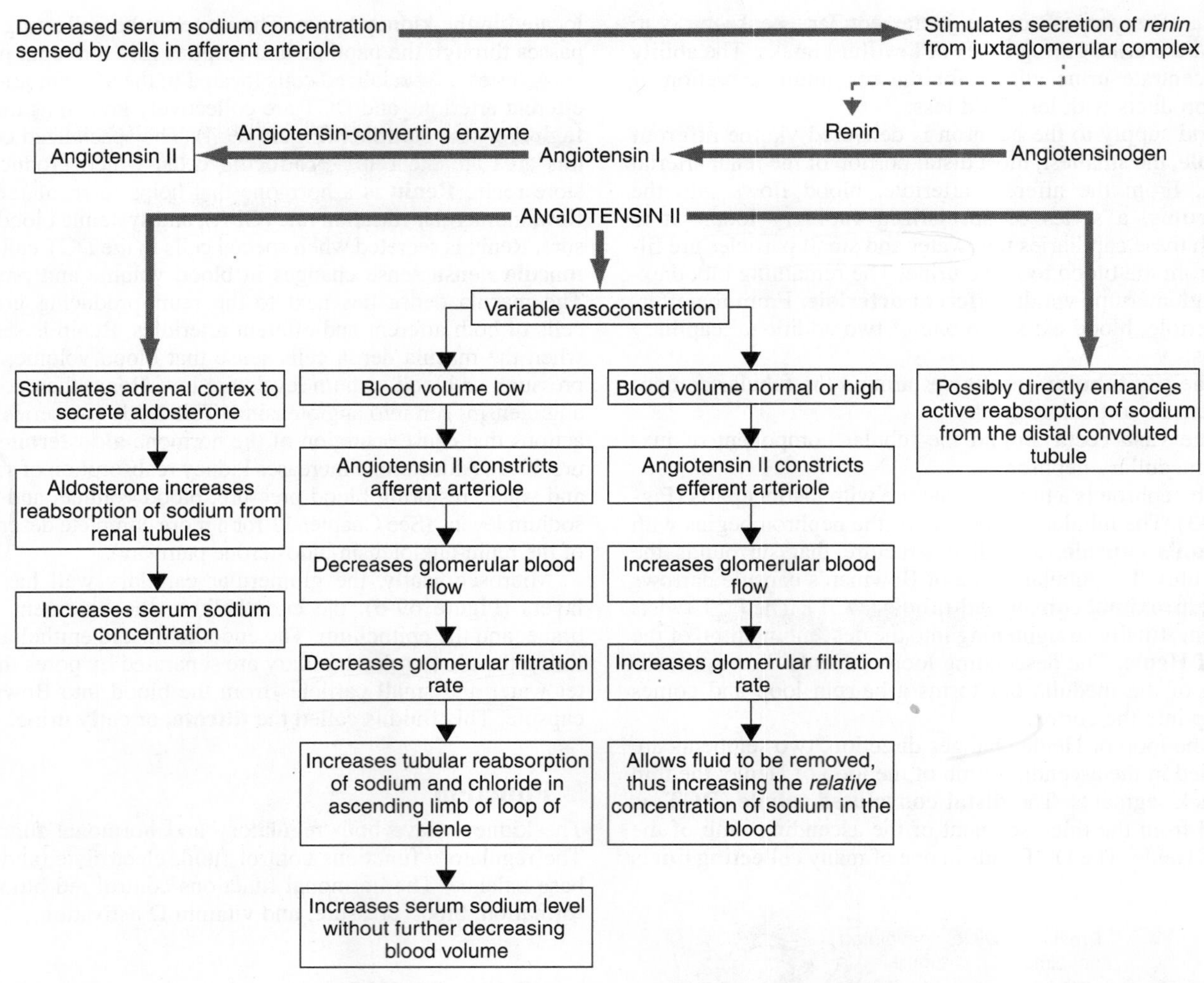

Figure 69-5 ● The role of aldosterone, angiotensinogen, angiotensin I, and angiotensin II in the renal regulation of water and sodium.

tubular reabsorption, and tubular secretion (Figure 69-7). These processes occur through filtration, diffusion, active transport, and osmosis. (See Chapter 11 for a review of these actions.) Table 69-2 summarizes the functional activities of nephron tubules and blood vessels.

GLOMERULAR FILTRATION. Glomerular filtration is the first process in urine formation. As blood passes from the afferent arteriole into the glomerulus, water, electrolytes, and other particles (e.g., creatinine, urea nitrogen, and glucose) are filtered across the glomerular membrane into Bowman's capsule to form *glomerular* filtrate. As the filtrate enters the proximal convoluted tubule (PCT), it is called *tubular* filtrate.

Large–molecular weight substances (>69,000 daltons), such as albumin and globulin, are too large to filter through the glomerular capillary walls. Red blood cells (RBCs) also are too large to pass from the arterioles into the filtrate. Therefore these substances are not normally present in the filtrate or in the final urine.

Approximately 180 L of glomerular filtrate is formed from the blood each day. The rate of filtration is often expressed in milliliters per minute. A normal glomerular filtration rate (GFR) averages 125 mL/min. If all filtrate were to be excreted as urine, death would occur quickly from massive dehydration. Actually, only about 1 to 3 L are excreted each day as urine.

The GFR is related to blood pressure and blood flow. The ability of the kidneys to self-regulate renal blood pressure and renal blood flow keeps GFR constant. GFR is controlled by selectively constricting and dilating the afferent and efferent arterioles. When the afferent arteriole is constricted and/or the efferent arteriole is dilated, pressure in the glomerular capillaries falls and filtration decreases. When the afferent arteriole is dilated and/or the efferent arteriole is constricted, pressure in the glomerular capillaries rises and filtration increases. Through this self-regulation the kidney can maintain a constant GFR, even when systemic blood pressure changes. When systolic blood pressure drops below about 70 mm Hg, these mechanisms are unable to compensate, and GFR stops.

TUBULAR REABSORPTION. Tubular reabsorption is the second process involved in urine formation. It is the tubular reabsorption of most of the filtrate that keeps normal urine output at 1 to 3 L/day and prevents dehydration. As the filtrate passes through the tubular component of the nephron, the kidney reabsorbs variable amounts of water and electrolytes. Reabsorption returns particles **(solutes)** and water to the blood.

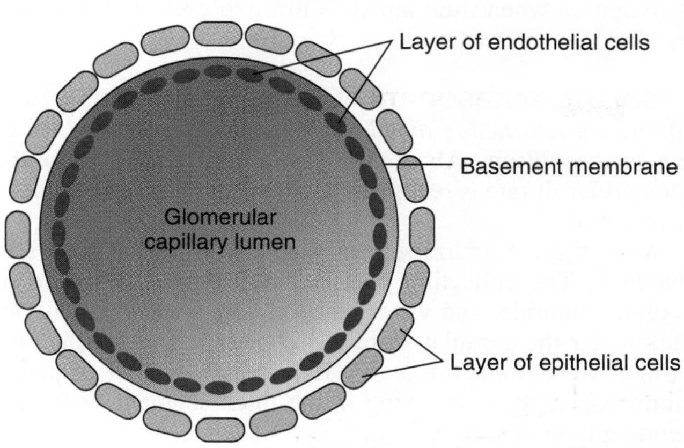

Figure 69-6 ● Glomerular capillary wall.

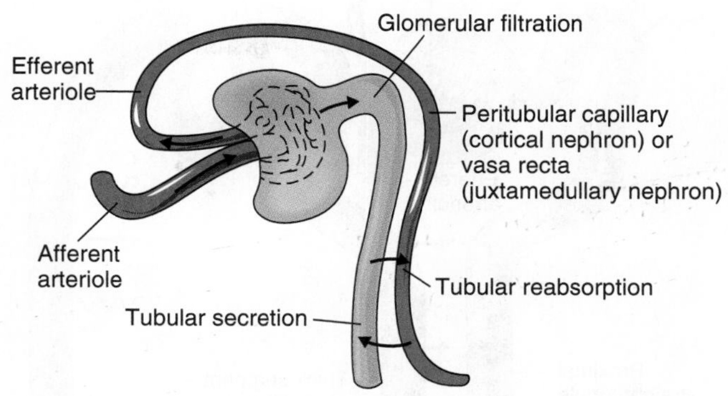

Figure 69-7 ● Glomerular filtration, tubular reabsorption, and tubular secretion.

TABLE 69-2 ● VASCULAR AND TUBULAR COMPONENTS OF THE NEPHRON

Structure	Anatomic Features	Physiologic Aspects
VASCULAR COMPONENTS		
Afferent arteriole	Delivers arterial blood from the branches of the renal artery into the glomerulus	Autoregulation of renal blood flow via vasoconstriction or vasodilation Renin-producing granular cells
Glomerulus	Capillary loops with thin semipermeable membrane	Site of glomerular filtration Glomerular filtration occurs when hydrostatic pressure (blood pressure) is greater than opposing forces (tubular filtrate and oncotic pressure)
Efferent arteriole	Delivers arterial blood from the glomerulus into the peritubular capillaries or the vasa recta	Autoregulation of renal blood flow via vasoconstriction or vasodilation Renin-producing granular cells
Peritubular capillaries (PTCs) and vasa recta (VR)	PTCs: surround tubular components of cortical nephrons VR: surround tubular components of juxtamedullary nephrons	Tubular reabsorption and tubular secretion allow movement of water and solutes to or from the tubules, interstitium, and blood
TUBULAR COMPONENTS		
Bowman's capsule (BC)	Thin membranous sac surrounding $^7/_8$ of the glomerulus	Collects glomerular filtrate (GF) and funnels GF into the tubule
Proximal convoluted tubule (PCT)	Evolves from and is continuous with Bowman's capsule Specialized cellular lining facilitates tubular reabsorption	Site for reabsorption of sodium, chloride, water, glucose, amino acids, potassium, calcium, bicarbonate, phosphate, and urea
Loop of Henle		
Descending limb (DL)	Continues from PCT Juxtamedullary nephrons dip deep into the medulla Permeable to water, urea, and sodium chloride	Regulation of water balance
Ascending limb (AL)	Emerges from DL as it turns and is redirected up toward the renal cortex	Potassium and magnesium reabsorption in the thick segment Thin segment is impermeable to water
Distal convoluted tubule (DCT)	Evolves from AL and twists so the macula densa cells lie adjacent to the juxtaglomerular cells of afferent arteriole	Site of additional water and electrolyte reabsorption, including bicarbonate Potassium and hydrogen secretion
Collecting ducts	Collects formed urine from several tubules and delivers it into the renal pelvis	Receptor sites for antidiuretic hormone regulation of water balance

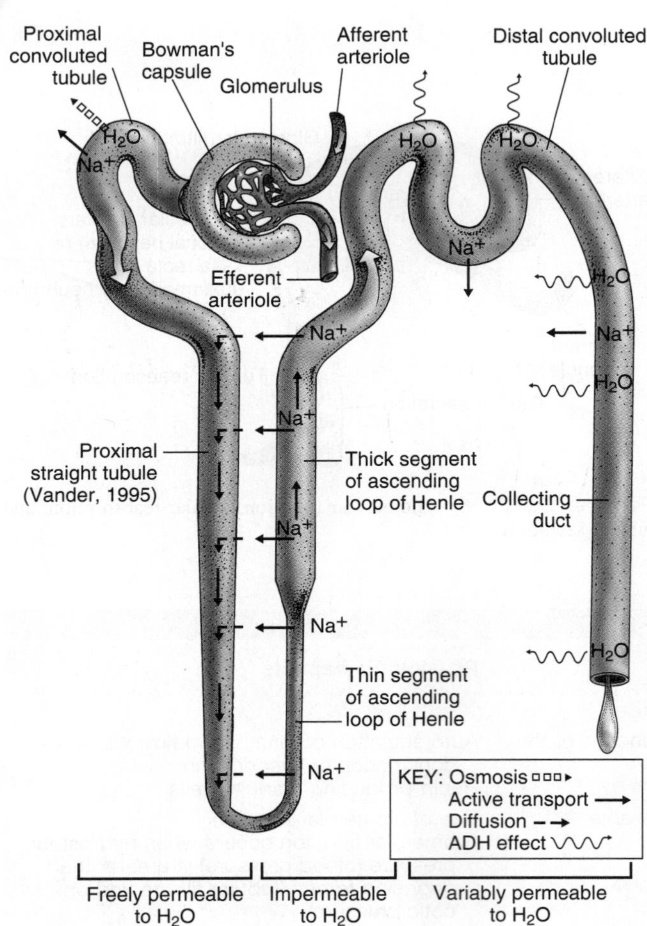

Figure 69-8 ● Sodium and water reabsorption by the tubules of a cortical nephron.

Reabsorption occurs *from the filtrate* across the tubular lumen of the nephron and into the blood of the peritubular capillaries. The PCT reabsorbs approximately 65% of the total glomerular filtrate.

WATER REABSORPTION. The tubules reabsorb more than 99% of all filtered water back into the body (Figure 69-8). Most water reabsorption from the filtrate into the plasma occurs as the filtrate passes through the PCT. Water reabsorption continues as the filtrate flows down the descending loop of Henle. The thin segment of the ascending loop of Henle is *not* permeable to water.

The distal convoluted tubule (DCT) is potentially permeable to water, and therefore water reabsorption can occur as the filtrate continues to flow through the tubule. The membrane of the DCT may be made more permeable to water through the influence of the hormones **antidiuretic hormone (ADH)** and aldosterone. ADH increases the permeability of the membrane to water and enhances water reabsorption. Aldosterone promotes the reabsorption of sodium in the DCT; water reabsorption occurs as a result of the movement of sodium (where sodium goes, water follows).

The ability of the kidneys to vary the volume or concentration of urine helps regulate total water balance regardless of water intake. In this way, the healthy kidney can prevent dehydration when fluid intake is low and prevent circulatory overload when fluid intake is excessive.

SOLUTE REABSORPTION. Some particles in the tubular filtrate are *returned to the blood.* This process is called **tubular reabsorption.** About 50% of all urea present in the glomerular filtrate is reabsorbed, but virtually no creatinine is reabsorbed.

Most sodium, chloride, and water reabsorption occurs in the PCT. The collecting ducts are the other major site of sodium, chloride, and water reabsorption, which usually occurs under the stimulation of aldosterone. Potassium is also primarily reabsorbed in the PCT, with 20% to 40% of potassium reabsorption occurring in the thick segment of the ascending loop of Henle.

Bicarbonate, calcium, and phosphate are reabsorbed in the PCT, with a little additional reabsorption occurring in the ascending loop of Henle and the DCT. The reabsorption of bicarbonate helps neutralize acids and maintain a normal blood pH. Calcium reabsorption and excretion is controlled by circulating calcitonin and parathyroid hormone (PTH) levels (see Chapter 13).

The kidney reabsorbs some of the glucose filtered from the blood. However, there is a limit to how much glucose the kidney can reabsorb. This limit is called the **renal threshold** for glucose reabsorption or the **transport maximum** for glucose reabsorption. The usual renal threshold for glucose is about 220 mg/dL. This means that at a blood glucose level of 220 mg/dL, all glucose is reabsorbed from the filtrate and returned to the blood. When blood glucose levels are greater than 220 mg/dL, some glucose stays in the filtrate and is present in the urine. Normally, almost all glucose and any filtered amino acids or proteins are reabsorbed.

TUBULAR SECRETION. Tubular secretion is a third process involved in urine formation. Like glomerular filtration, it is a process by which substances may move *from the blood* into the tubular filtrate. During tubular secretion, molecules pass from the peritubular capillaries, across capillary membranes, and into the cells that line the tubules. From the cells these substances are moved into the urine to be excreted from the body. Potassium (K^+) and hydrogen ions (H^+) are some of the substances moved in this way to maintain homeostasis of electrolytes and pH.

HORMONAL FUNCTIONS

The kidneys produce renin, prostaglandins, bradykinin, erythropoietin, and activated vitamin D (Table 69-3). Other secretions, such as the kinins, influence renal blood flow and capillary permeability. The kidneys also have a role in the breakdown and excretion of insulin.

RENIN PRODUCTION. As discussed earlier under Microscopic Anatomy (pp. 1590 and 1591), renin assists in the regulation of blood pressure. Renin is formed and released when there is a decrease in blood flow, volume, or pressure through the renal arterioles or when a decrease in the sodium ion concentration of the tubular filtrate is detected through the receptors of the juxtaglomerular complex.

TABLE 69-3 • RENAL HORMONE PRODUCTION AND HORMONES INFLUENCING RENAL FUNCTION

	Site	Action
RENAL HORMONE PRODUCTION		
Renin	Renin-producing granular cells	Raise blood pressure as result of angiotensin (local vasoconstriction) and aldosterone (volume expansion) secretion
Prostaglandins	Renal tissues	Regulate intrarenal blood flow by vasodilation or vasoconstriction
Bradykinins	Juxtaglomerular cells of the arterioles	Increases blood flow (vasodilation) and vascular permeability
Erythropoietin	Renal parenchyma	Stimulates bone marrow to make red blood cells
Activated vitamin D	Renal parenchyma	Promotes absorption of calcium in the gastrointestinal tract
HORMONES INFLUENCING RENAL FUNCTION		
Antidiuretic hormone (ADH, vasopressin)	Released from posterior pituitary	Makes DCT and CD permeable to water to maximize reabsorption and produce a concentrated urine
Aldosterone	Released from adrenal cortex	Promotes sodium reabsorption and potassium secretion in DCT and CD; water and chloride follow sodium movement
Natriuretic hormones	Cardiac atria, brain	Cause tubular secretion of sodium

DCT, Distal convoluted tubule; *CD,* collecting ducts.

The release of renin stimulates the production of *angiotensin II* through a series of metabolic steps (see Figure 69-5). Angiotensin II increases systemic blood pressure through powerful vasoconstrictive effects and stimulates the release of aldosterone from the adrenal cortex. Aldosterone increases the reabsorption of sodium in the distal tubule of the nephron. Therefore more water is reabsorbed and blood pressure is increased because of increases in blood volume expansion. When renal blood flow is diminished, this renin-angiotensin-aldosterone system of blood pressure regulation influences the autoregulatory blood pressure processes within the nephron as well as systemic blood pressure (see also Chapter 11).

PROSTAGLANDIN PRODUCTION. Prostaglandins are produced in a variety of tissues, including the kidney. Specific prostaglandins produced in the kidney are prostaglandin E_2 (PGE_2) and prostacyclin (PGI_2). These prostaglandins help regulate glomerular filtration, kidney vascular resistance, and renin production. PGE_2 acts on the distal tubule and collecting duct to inhibit ADH secretion, decrease membrane permeability, and promote sodium and water excretion.

BRADYKININ PRODUCTION. The presence of angiotensin II, prostaglandins, and ADH stimulates the release of bradykinin in the renal system. **Bradykinin** dilates the afferent arteriole and increases capillary membrane permeability to some solutes. These actions maintain kidney blood flow and tubular function even when other conditions cause systemic vasoconstriction.

ERYTHROPOIETIN PRODUCTION. Erythropoietin is produced and released in response to decreased oxygen tension in the renal blood supply. Erythropoietin stimulates red blood cell (RBC) production in the bone marrow. When kidney tissue is destroyed or nonfunctional, erythropoietin production decreases and the person becomes anemic.

VITAMIN D ACTIVATION. A series of metabolic changes are necessary for vitamin D, a hormone, to become active. Metabolic conversions take place in the skin through exposure to ultraviolet light and then in the liver. From there, vitamin D is converted to its active form (1,25-dihydroxycholecalciferol) in the kidney. Activated vitamin D is necessary to absorb calcium in the gastrointestinal tract and is critical in the regulation of calcium balance.

Ureters

Structure

Each kidney has a single ureter, a hollow tubelike structure that connects the renal pelvis with the urinary bladder. The ureter is about ½ inch (1.25 cm) in diameter and about 12 to 18 inches (30 to 45 cm) in length.

The diameter of the ureter narrows in three areas:

- In the upper third of the ureter, at the point at which the renal pelvis becomes the ureter, is a narrowing known as the **ureteropelvic junction (UPJ).**
- The ureter also narrows as it arches toward the abdominal wall (aortoiliac bend).
- Each ureter then narrows upon entering the posterior wall of the urinary bladder at an oblique angle; this point is referred to as the **ureterovesical junction (UVJ).**

The ureter tunnels through bladder tissue for a few centimeters before opening into the bladder in an area referred to as the **trigone** (Figure 69-9).

The ureter is composed of three layers: an inner lining of mucous membrane **(urothelium),** a middle layer of smooth muscle fibers, and an outer layer of fibrous tissue. The outer layer of the ureter contains the blood supply. The middle layer of ureteral tissue contains longitudinal and circular muscle fibers. These muscle fibers are under the control of a variety of nerve pathways from the lower spinal cord.

Function

Rapid peristaltic contractions of the smooth muscle in the ureter move urine from the renal pelvis of the kidney to the bladder. Stretch receptors in the renal pelvis regulate ureteral peristalsis. For example, a large volume of urine in the renal pelvis stimulates the stretch receptors, which respond by causing an increase in ureteral peristalsis.

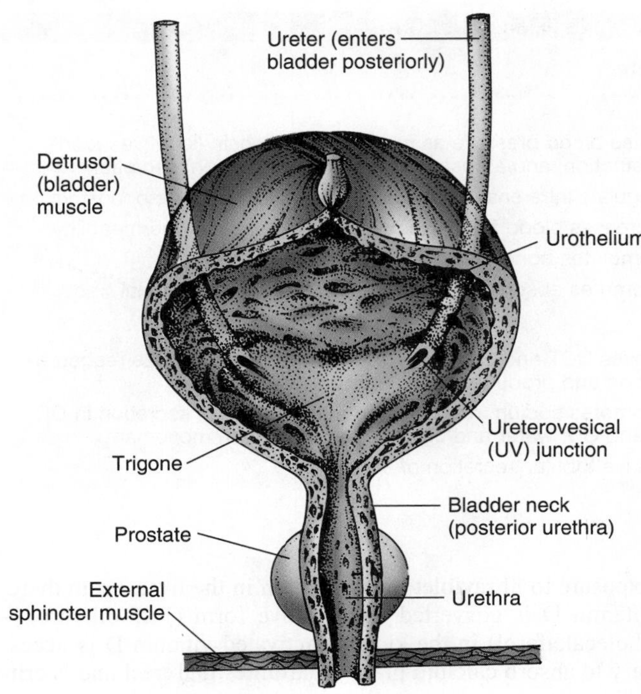

Figure 69-9 ● Gross anatomy of the urinary bladder.

Urinary Bladder

Structure

The urinary bladder is a muscular sac. The upper surface lies next to the peritoneal cavity. In men, the bladder is in front of the rectum. In women, the bladder is in front of the vagina. The bladder lies directly behind the pubic symphysis, the connecting point for pelvic bone structures.

The bladder is composed of the **body** (the rounded sac portion) and the **bladder neck** (posterior urethra), which connects to the bladder body. The bladder has three linings, an inner lining of epithelial cells **(urothelium),** middle layers of smooth muscle **(detrusor muscle),** and an outer lining. The **trigone** is an area on the inner aspect of the posterior bladder wall between the points of ureteral entry (ureterovesical junctions [UVJs]) and the urethra.

The **internal urethral sphincter** is composed of the smooth detrusor muscle of the bladder neck and elastic tissue. The **external urethral sphincter** is composed of skeletal muscle that surrounds the urethra. In men, the external sphincter surrounds the urethra at the base of the prostate gland. In women, the external sphincter is at the base of the bladder. The pudendal nerve from the spinal cord controls the external sphincter.

Function

The urinary bladder is a site for the temporary storage of urine. The bladder also provides continence and enables micturition (voiding). The secretions of the bladder lining resist bacteria.

Bladder continence is achieved during filling through the combination of detrusor muscle relaxation, internal sphincter muscle tone, and external sphincter contraction. As the bladder fills with urine, stretch sensations are transmitted to segments of spinal sacral nerves S2 and S3.

MAINTAINING CONTINENCE

Continence is maintained by the interaction of the nerves that control the muscles of the bladder, bladder neck, urethra, the pelvic floor, as well as by factors that close the urethra. During bladder filling, the sympathetic nervous system fibers prevent detrusor muscle contraction. These control centers are located in the cerebral cortex, the brainstem, and the sacral part of the spinal cord. For urethral closure to be adequate for continence, the mucosal surfaces must be in contact and must be adhesive. Contact depends on the structural and functional integrity of the involved nerves and muscles. Adhesion depends on the adequate secretion of mucus-like substances.

MICTURITION

Micturition (voiding) is a reflex of parasympathetic control that stimulates contraction of the detrusor muscle at the same time as relaxation of the external sphincter and the muscles of the pelvic floor. With detrusor muscle contraction, the UVJ of the ureter closes, and the normally round bladder assumes the shape of a funnel. Voiding is a voluntary act as the result of a learned response and is controlled by the cerebral cortex and the brainstem. Contraction of the external sphincter inhibits the micturition reflex and prevents voiding.

Urethra

Structure

The urethra is a narrow, tubelike structure lined with mucous membranes and epithelial cells. The **urethral meatus,** or opening, is the terminal point of the urethra. In men, the urethra is about 6 to 8 inches (15 to 20 cm) long, with the urethral meatus is located at the tip of the penis. Three sections make up the male urethra:

- The prostatic urethra, which traverses the prostate gland from the urinary bladder
- The membranous urethra, which traverses the wall of the pelvic floor
- The cavernous urethra, which is external and extends through the length of the penis

In women, the urethra is about 1 to 1.5 inches (2.5 to 3.75 cm) long and exits the urinary bladder through the pelvic floor. The urethral meatus lies slightly below the clitoris and directly in front of the vagina and rectum.

Function

The urethra is a tube for eliminating urine from the body. The passing of urine normally removes bacteria from the urethra.

Renal/Urinary System Changes Associated with Aging

Renal Changes

Structural and functional changes occur in the kidney as a result of the aging process. These changes often have clinical significance. The kidney loses cortical mass and gets smaller by 80 years of age. This cortical loss is caused by reduced re-

CHART 69-1

NURSING FOCUS *on the* OLDER ADULT

Changes in the Renal/Urinary System Related to Aging

Physiologic Change	Nursing Implications	Rationale
Decreased glomerular filtration rate (GFR)	Monitor hydration status.	With aging, the ability of the kidneys to regulate water balance is decreased.
	Ensure adequate fluid intake.	The kidneys are less able to conserve water when necessary.
	Administer potentially nephrotoxic agents or medications carefully.	Dehydration results in decreased renal blood flow and increases the nephrotoxic potential of many agents. Acute or chronic renal failure may result.
Nocturia	Ensure adequate nighttime lighting and a hazard-free environment.	Nocturia may occur from decreased renal concentrating ability associated with aging.
	Ensure the availability of a toilet, bedpan, or urinal.	The desire to maintain continence prompts individuals to seek the bathroom. Falls and injuries are common among older clients seeking bathroom facilities.
	Discourage excessive fluid intake for 2-4 hr before the client retires for the evening.	Excessive fluid intake at nighttime may increase nocturia.
Decreased bladder capacity	Encourage the client to use the toilet, bedpan, or urinal at least q2h. Respond as soon as possible to the client's indication of the need to void.	By emptying the bladder on a regular basis, urinary incontinence from overflow may be avoided.
Weakened urinary sphincter muscles and shortened urethra in women	Respond as soon as possible to the client's indication of the need to void.	A quick response may alleviate episodes of urinary stress incontinence.
	Provide thorough perineal care after each voiding.	The shortened urethra increases the potential for bladder infections. Good perineal hygiene may prevent skin irritations and urinary tract infection (UTI).
Tendency to retain urine	Observe the client for urinary retention (e.g., bladder distention) or urinary tract infection (e.g., dysuria, foul odor, confusion).	Urinary stasis may result in a UTI. UTIs may become bloodstream infections, resulting in septicemia or septic shock.
	Provide privacy, assistance, and voiding stimulants such as warm water over the perineum as needed.	Nursing interventions can help to initiate voiding.

nal blood flow. The medulla appears not to be affected by aging, and the juxtamedullary nephrons are generally preserved. However, the glomerular and tubular basement membranes thicken, reducing filtrating ability. Both the number of glomeruli and their surface area decrease with aging. The length of the tubules also decreases.

Kidney function also changes with aging (Chart 69-1). Blood flow to the kidney decreases by about 10% per decade as blood vessels thicken and become more rigid. Glomerular filtration rate (GFR) decreases with advancing age and more rapidly after 45 years of age. By age 65 years, the GFR decreases to approximately 65 mL/min (roughly half the rate in a young adult). This decline is more rapid in clients with diabetes or hypertension.

Tubular changes with aging are shown by a decreased ability to concentrate urine, resulting in **nocturia** (increased need to urinate at night). The excretion and regulation of sodium, acids, and bicarbonate remain effective but are less efficient because homeostasis is slower. Along with an age-related impairment in the thirst mechanism, these changes may be associated with an increased incidence of dehydration and hypernatremia (increased blood sodium levels) in the older adult (Brenner, 2000). Hormonal changes include a decrease in renin secretion, aldosterone levels, and activation of vitamin D.

CULTURAL CONSIDERATIONS

African Americans experience more rapid age-related decreases in GFR than do Caucasians (Brenner, 2000). The renal excretion of sodium is less effective in hypertensive African Americans who have high sodium intake, and the kidneys have approximately 20% less blood flow as a result of anatomic changes in small renal vessels (Shulman & Hall, 1991).

Urinary Changes

Changes in the elasticity of the detrusor muscle may cause decreased bladder capacity and a decreased ability to retain urine. The sensation of the urge to void may cause immediate bladder emptying because the urinary sphincters lose muscle tone and often become weaker with age. In women, weakening muscles shorten the urethra, which contributes to incontinence. In men, an enlarged prostate gland causes difficulty in starting the urine stream and may cause urinary retention.

ASSESSMENT TECHNIQUES

History

One way to assess renal and urologic function is to use Gordon's Functional Health Patterns (Gordon, 2000). The patterns most pertinent to the renal system are Nutritional/Metabolic and Elimination (Chart 69-2).

DEMOGRAPHIC DATA

Age, gender, race, and ethnicity are important in the overall history of the client with suspected renal or urinary dysfunction. A sudden onset of hypertension in clients older than 50 years of age suggests possible kidney disease. Clinical evidence of adult polycystic kidney disease typically occurs in clients in their 40s or 50s. In men older than 50 years, altered urine patterns suggest prostatic disease.

Anatomic gender differences make some disorders worse or more common. For example, men rarely have urinary tract infections unless there are abnormalities, such as ureteral reflux or prostatic enlargement. Women have a shorter urethra and therefore more commonly experience **cystitis** (bladder infection) because bacteria pass more readily into the bladder.

CULTURAL CONSIDERATIONS

End-stage renal disease (ESRD) is three to four times more common in African Americans, Native Americans, and Mexican Americans than in Caucasians. A history of hypertension or diabetes mellitus (both associated with renal disease) is also common in these groups.

PERSONAL AND FAMILY HISTORY

The family history of the client with a suspected kidney or urologic problem is significant because some disorders have a familial inheritance pattern. The client is asked whether his or her siblings, parents, parents' siblings, or grandparents have had renal problems. Past terms used for kidney disease include Bright's disease, nephritis, and nephrosis. Clients may use these terms to describe kidney disease as it was known by their parents or grandparents in the earlier part of the twentieth century. Adult polycystic kidney disease can occur in clients of either gender.

The client is asked about any previous renal or urologic disorders, including tumors, infections, stones, or urologic surgery. A history of any chronic health problems, such as diabetes mellitus or hypertension, may contribute to the development of renal disease.

The nurse identifies all of the client's prescription medications. The client is asked about their duration of use and whether any recent changes in medications have been prescribed. Drugs prescribed for diabetes mellitus, hypertension, cardiac disorders, hormonal disorders, cancer, arthritis, and psychiatric disorders are potential causes of renal dysfunction. Antibiotics taken for infections, such as gentamicin (Garamycin, Cidomycin✦), may also produce sudden renal dysfunction.

The use of over-the-counter (OTC) drugs or agents, including vitamin and mineral supplements and replacements, laxatives, analgesics, and nonsteroidal anti-inflammatory drugs (NSAIDs) is explored. Many of these drugs affect renal function. The long-term use of NSAIDs, especially combination agents, can seriously reduce renal function.

CHART 69-2

RENAL/URINARY ASSESSMENT
Using Gordon's Functional Health Patterns

Nutritional/Metabolic Pattern

What is your typical daily food intake? Describe a day's meals, snacks, and vitamins.
How much salt do you typically add to your food? Do you use salt substitutes?
How is your appetite?
Have you experienced any nausea or vomiting?
What is your typical daily fluid intake?
What types of fluids do you drink (water, juices, soft drinks, coffee, tea)?
How much fluid do you drink each day?
Have you had any recent change in your weight? Weight gain? Weight loss? How much?
Have you noticed a change in the tightness of your rings or shoes? Tighter? Looser?
Have you noticed any skin changes lately? More dry? Less Dry? Itchy?

Elimination Pattern

What is your usual bowel elimination pattern? Frequency? Character? Discomfort? Laxatives?
What is your usual urinary elimination pattern? Frequency? Amount? Color? Odor? Control?
Have you noticed a change in the amount of urine?
Do you have any problem with excessive perspiration?
Do you have any other type of drainage?

Based on Gordon, M. (2000). *Manual of nursing diagnosis* (9th ed.). St. Louis: Mosby.

The client is specifically asked whether he or she has ever been told about the presence of protein or albumin in the urine. The question "Have you ever been told that your blood pressure is high?" may prompt a vastly different response than "Do you have high blood pressure?" The nurse also asks female clients about health problems associated with pregnancy (e.g., proteinuria, high blood pressure, gestational diabetes, and urinary tract infections). Additional information is obtained about the following:

- Chemical or environmental toxin exposure in occupational or other settings
- Recent travel to geographic regions that pose infectious disease risks
- Recent physical injuries
- Trauma
- Sexual contacts
- A history of altered patterns of urinary elimination

DIET HISTORY

The client with known or suspected renal or urologic disorders is asked about his or her usual diet and any recent changes in the diet. The excessive intake or omission of certain categories of foods is noted. Information about food and fluid intake is obtained. If the client has followed a diet for weight reduction, the details of the diet plan are pertinent. A high-protein intake can result in temporary renal problems. Clients susceptible to **calculi** (stone) formation who ingest large amounts of calcium-containing products or have an insufficient fluid intake may form new stones.

Changes in appetite, alterations in taste acuity, and an inability to discriminate tastes are important. These symptoms are associated with the accumulation of nitrogenous waste products from renal failure. Changes in thirst or fluid intake may also produce changes in urine output or other evidence of urologic disorders. Endocrine disorders may also produce changes in thirst, fluid intake, and urine output (see Chapter 63).

SOCIOECONOMIC STATUS

The socioeconomic status of the client may influence health care practices. People with limited income or no health insurance often ignore physical ailments or delay seeking health care because they lack the funds to pay for diagnostic tests or treatment. They may also have difficulty following medical advice, having prescriptions filled, and keeping follow-up appointments.

The information that a client has about the disease and its symptoms may relate to educational level. Educational level may also affect health-seeking practices. Recurring urinary tract infections often result from inadequate or incomplete treatment, including lack of follow-up to ensure eradication. The lack of money to pay for antibiotics or nutritious foods or the lack of knowledge or motivation to select healthful foods may inhibit full recovery.

The client's health beliefs affect the approach to health and illness. Cultural background or religious affiliation may influence the belief system.

The language used by clients may be different from that used by the health care professional. Anatomic or medical terms may have no meaning for the client (Table 69-4). When obtaining a history, the nurse listens to and explores the terms used by the client. By using the client's own terms, the nurse may help him or her to provide a more complete and thorough description of the problem. This technique may increase the amount of information communicated and decrease the client's discomfort when discussing bodily functions.

CURRENT HEALTH PROBLEMS

The effects of renal failure result in changes in all body systems. Therefore all of the client's current health problems are documented. The client is encouraged to describe all health concerns, because some renal and urologic disorders are associated with symptoms that are related to other body systems or that occur as generalized problems. Recent upper respiratory problems, generalized musculoskeletal discomfort, or gastrointestinal (GI) problems may be related to problems of kidney function.

The kidney and urologic system are assessed specifically. The client is asked about any changes in the appearance (color, odor, clarity) of the urine, pattern of urination, ability to initiate or control voiding, and other unusual symptoms. Urine that is reddish, dark brown or black, greenish, or otherwise different from the usual yellowish, straw color usually prompts the client to seek health care assistance. Urine typically has a mild but distinct odor of ammonia. An increase in the intensity of color, a change in odor quality, or a decrease in urine clarity may suggest infection.

The client is asked about changes in urination patterns, such as nocturia, frequency, or an increase or decrease in the amount of urine. The normal urine output for adults is 1 mL/kg/hr, or approximately 1500 to 2000 mL/day. The client usually does not know the exact amount of urine produced; a bladder diary may provide useful data (see the Evidence-Based Practice for Nursing box above). The nurse also asks the following:

- If the client has difficulty initiating urine flow
- If a burning sensation or other discomfort is present on urination
- If the force of the urine stream is decreased (in men)

The nurse asks about any loss of urinary continence. Situations that increase intra-abdominal pressure (e.g., coughing and sneezing) may result in the involuntary passage of urine. Clients may also report a persistent dribbling of urine.

TABLE 69-4 • COMMONLY USED RENAL AND URINARY TERMS

anuria Total urine output of less than 100 mL in 24 hours
azotemia Increased blood urea nitrogen and serum creatinine levels suggestive of renal impairment but without outward symptoms of renal failure
dysuria Discomfort or pain associated with micturition
frequency Feeling the need to void often, usually voiding small amounts of urine each time; may void every hour or even more frequently than hourly
hesitancy Difficulty in initiating the flow of urine, even when the bladder has sufficient urine to initiate a void and the sensation of the need to void is present
micturition The act of voiding
nocturia Awakening prematurely from sleep because of the need to empty the bladder
oliguria Decreased urine output; total urine output between 100 and 400 mL in 24 hours
polyuria Increased urine output; total urine output usually greater than 2000 mL in 24 hours
uremia Full-blown signs and symptoms of renal failure; sometimes referred to as the uremic syndrome, especially if the cause of the renal failure is unknown
urgency A sudden onset of the feeling of the need to void immediately; may result in incontinence if the client is unable to locate or get to toileting facilities quickly

EVIDENCE-BASED PRACTICE FOR NURSING

How does one assess a urinary elimination problem?

Pfister, S.M. (1999). Bladder diaries and voiding patterns in older adults. *Journal of Gerontological Nursing, 25*(3), 36-41.

The purpose of this article is to describe how a bladder diary was used in research with residents of retirement settings. Bladder diaries are similar to intake and output records but are self-recorded by clients. It reviews different methods of collecting information about fluid consumed and urine eliminated. The narrative details the written record used by 51 subjects in a self-care community of retired individuals and the instructions given to participants so as to yield specific and accurate information.

The author concludes that bladder diaries were used successfully and allow both the client and health care provider to visualize daily voiding patterns. Based on bladder diary data, nurses can diagnose, plan, and intervene to manage voiding problems such as incontinence.

Critique. The clients in this study were physically mobile, able to write, and cognitively intact. Although self-reported bladder diaries may not apply to all clients with elimination problems, the forms and techniques described in this report specify a useful assessment tool that can be used in a variety of community settings.

Implications for Nursing. Bladder diaries can assist the nurse and client in determining the patterns of intake and voiding. Diaries can also be used to evaluate responses to interventions.

The onset of pain in the flank, in the lower abdomen or pelvic region, or in the perineal area is often of great concern and usually prompts the client to seek assistance. The nurse inquires about the onset, intensity, and duration of the pain, its location, and its association with any activity or event.

Pain associated with renal or ureteral irritation is often severe and spasmodic. Pain that radiates into the perineal area, groin, scrotum, or labia is described as **renal colic.** Renal colic pain is usually associated with distention or spasm of the ureter, such as in an obstruction or the passing of a stone. Renal colic pain may be intermittent or continuous and may even be systemic with pallor, diaphoresis, and hypotension. These general symptoms occur because of the location of the nerve tracts associated with the kidneys and ureters.

Because the kidneys are close to the GI organs and the nerve pathways are similar, GI symptoms may be part of the client's presenting history. These **renointestinal reflexes** often complicate the detailed description of the renal problem.

Uremia results from the accumulation of nitrogenous waste products in the blood, a result of renal failure. Symptoms include anorexia, nausea and vomiting, muscle cramps, **pruritus** (itching), fatigue, and lethargy.

Physical Assessment

The physical assessment of the client with a known or suspected renal or urologic disorder includes an assessment of general appearance, a general review of body systems, and specific structure and functions of the renal/urinary systems.

The nurse assesses the general appearance of the client and checks for a yellowish skin color and the presence of any rashes, bruising, or other discoloration. The skin and tissues may show edema, which with renal disorders may be detected in the **pedal** (foot), **pretibial** (shin), sacral tissues, and around the eyes. The lungs are auscultated to determine whether fluid is present. Weight and blood pressure measurements are obtained for comparison purposes.

The nurse assesses the client's general level of consciousness and level of alertness, noting deficits in concentration, thought processes, or memory. Family members may report subtle changes. Such cognitive changes may be the result of an insufficient clearance of waste products when renal disease is present.

ASSESSMENT OF THE KIDNEYS, URETERS, AND BLADDER

Assessment of the kidneys, ureters, and bladder is performed in conjunction with an abdominal assessment. Auscultation is performed before percussion and palpation because these activities can enhance bowel sounds and obscure abdominal vascular sounds.

Inspection

The nurse inspects the abdomen and the flank regions with the client in both the supine and the sitting position. The client is observed for asymmetry (e.g., swelling) or discoloration (e.g., bruising or redness) in the flank region, especially in the area of the **costovertebral angle (CVA).** The CVA is located between the lower portion of the twelfth rib and the vertebral column.

Auscultation

The nurse listens for a bruit over each renal artery on the midclavicular line. A **bruit** is an audible swishing sound produced when the volume of blood or the diameter of the blood vessel changes. A bruit is usually associated with blood flow through a narrowed vessel, as in renal artery stenosis.

Palpation

Renal palpation identifies masses and areas of tenderness in or around the kidney. The abdomen is lightly palpated in all quadrants. The nurse asks about areas of tenderness or discomfort and examines nontender areas first. The outline of the bladder may be seen as high as the umbilicus in clients with severe bladder distention. Special training and practice under the guidance of a qualified practitioner are necessary; therefore appropriate education is essential before attempting the procedure. If tumor or aneurysm is suspected, palpation may harm the client.

Because the kidneys are deep, posterior structures, palpation is easier in thin clients who have little abdominal musculature. For palpation of the right kidney, the client assumes a supine position while the nurse places one hand under the right flank and the other hand over the abdomen below the lower right part of the rib cage. The lower hand raises the flank, and the upper hand depresses the anterior abdomen as the client takes a deep breath (Figure 69-10). The left kidney is deeper and rarely palpable. A transplanted kidney is readily palpable in either the lower right or left abdominal quadrant. The kidney should feel smooth, firm, and nontender.

Percussion

A distended bladder sounds dull when percussed. After gently palpating to determine the general outline of the distended bladder, the nurse begins percussion on the skin of the lower abdomen and continues in the direction of the umbilicus until dull sounds are no longer produced.

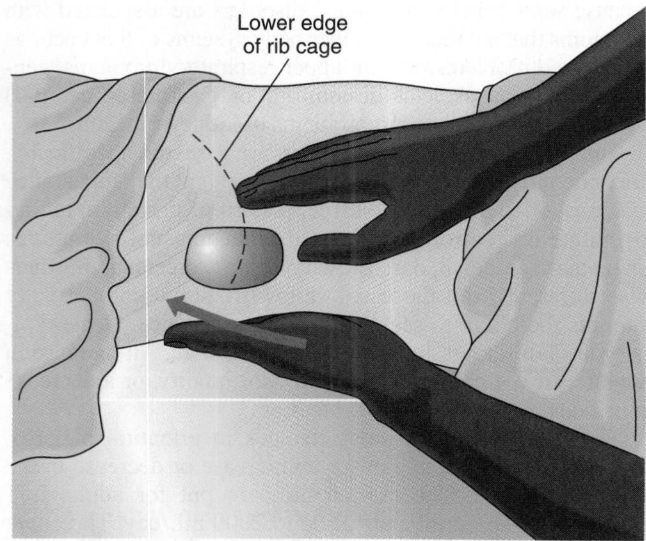

Figure 69-10 ● Advanced technique for palpation of the kidney.

If the client identifies flank pain or tenderness, the nontender flank is percussed first. The client assumes a sitting, side-lying, or supine position, and the nurse forms one hand into a clenched fist. The heel of the other hand and the little finger form a flat area with which a firm thump to the CVA area can be quickly administered. Costovertebral tenderness is highly suggestive of kidney infection or inflammation. Clients with inflammation or infection in the kidney or adjacent structures may describe their pain as severe or as a constant, dull ache.

ASSESSMENT OF THE URETHRA

Using a good light source and wearing gloves, the nurse inspects the urethra by examining the meatus and surrounding tissues. Any unusual discharge such as blood, mucus, and purulent drainage is noted. The skin and mucous membranes of surrounding tissues are inspected, and the presence of lesions, rashes, or other abnormalities of the penis or scrotum or of the labia or vaginal orifice is documented. Urethral irritation is suspected when the client reports discomfort with urination.

Psychosocial Assessment

Concerns about the urologic system may evoke fear, anger, embarrassment, anxiety, guilt, or sadness in the client. Childhood learning often includes privacy with regard to urination habits. Urologic disorders may stimulate previously forgotten memories of difficult toilet training and bedwetting or of childhood experiences of exploring one's body. The client may ignore symptoms or delay seeking health care because of emotional responses or cultural taboos about the urogenital area.

CRITICAL THINKING CHALLENGE

The client is a 62-year-old woman who has had a backache in the lower left flank area for a month. She has been seen by an orthopedic specialist, who has determined the pain is not from a strained muscle or spinal problem. This women is about 5 feet tall and weighs 95 pounds.

- What personal or demographic data should you obtain?
- What additional questions should you ask this client regarding her pain?
- How would you proceed in gathering physical assessment data?

For suggested answer guidelines, go to SIMON http://www.wbsaunders.com/SIMON/Iggy/.

Diagnostic Assessment

LABORATORY TESTS

Blood Tests

SERUM CREATININE

Serum creatinine is a measurement of the end product of muscle and protein metabolism. Creatinine is filtered by the kidneys and excreted in the urine. Because muscle mass and metabolism are usually constant, the serum creatinine level is an excellent indicator of kidney function. Normal serum creatinine levels vary with age, gender, and body muscle mass. The normal serum creatinine value is slightly higher in adult men than in adult women (Chart 69-3). In general, men have a larger muscle mass than do women, but there are exceptions. Muscle mass and the amount of creatinine produced diminish with age. Because of decreased rates of creatinine clearance, however, the serum creatinine level remains relatively constant in older adults unless renal disease is present.

No common pathologic condition other than renal disease results in an increase in serum creatinine level. The serum creatinine level does not increase until at least 50% of the renal function is lost, and therefore *any* elevation of serum creatinine values is important.

BLOOD UREA NITROGEN

Blood urea nitrogen (BUN) measures the renal excretion of urea nitrogen, a by-product of protein metabolism in the liver. Urea nitrogen is produced primarily from food sources of pro-

CHART 69-3

LABORATORY PROFILE
Renal Function Blood Studies

Test	Normal Range for Adults	Significance of Abnormal Findings
Serum creatinine	*Males:* 0.6-1.2 mg/dL (80-115 mmol/L) *Females:* 0.5-1.1 mg/dL (44-97 mmol/L) *Older Adults:* may be decreased	An *increased level* indicates renal impairment. A *decreased level* may be caused by a decreased muscle mass.
Blood urea nitrogen (BUN)	10-20 mg/dL (2.1-7.1 mmol/L) *Older Adult:* 60-90 yr: 8-23 mg/dL (2.9-8.2 mmol/L); over 90 yr: 10-31 mg/dL (3.6-11.1 mmol/L)	An *increased level* may indicate hepatic or renal disease, dehydration or decreased renal perfusion, a high-protein diet, infection, stress, steroid use, GI bleeding, or other situations in which there is blood in body tissues. A *decreased level* may indicate malnutrition, fluid volume excess, or severe hepatic damage.
BUN/creatinine ratio	Mass ratio: 12:1 to 20:1; mole ratio: 48.5:1 to 80.8:1	An *increased ratio* may indicate fluid volume deficit, obstructive uropathy, catabolic state, or a high-protein diet. A *decreased ratio* may indicate fluid volume excess or acute renal tubular acidosis. *No change* in the ratio with increases in both the BUN and creatinine levels indicates renal impairment.

Data from Pagana, K.D., & Pagana, T.J. (1999). *Diagnostic testing and nursing implications: A case study approach* (5th ed.). St. Louis: Mosby.
GI, Gastrointestinal.

tein, which undergo metabolism by the liver. The kidneys filter urea nitrogen from the blood and excrete the nitrogenous waste in urine. BUN levels indicate the extent of renal clearance of this nitrogenous waste product.

Other factors may influence the BUN level, and therefore an elevation does not always represent renal disease (see Chart 69-3). For example, rapid cell destruction from infection or steroid therapy may elevate BUN level. In addition, blood is a protein. If blood is present in body tissues, the reabsorption of the blood protein is processed by the liver, resulting in an increased BUN level.

The liver must function properly to produce urea nitrogen. When liver and kidney dysfunction are both present, urea nitrogen levels are actually decreased; this decrease reflects the liver failure but not the kidney failure. The BUN level is not always elevated with kidney disease and is not the most reliable indicator of kidney function. However, an elevated BUN level is highly *suggestive* of kidney dysfunction.

RATIO OF BLOOD UREA NITROGEN TO SERUM CREATININE

The BUN/creatinine ratio determines whether factors such as dehydration or lack of renal perfusion are causing the elevated BUN level. When a blood volume deficit (dehydration) or hypoperfusion exists, the BUN level rises more rapidly than the serum creatinine level. As a result, the ratio of BUN to creatinine is *increased.*

When both the BUN and serum creatinine levels increase at the same rate, the BUN/creatinine ratio remains normal. However, the elevated serum creatinine and BUN levels suggest renal dysfunction that is not related to acute volume depletion or hypoperfusion.

Urine Tests

URINALYSIS

Urinalysis is a usual part of any complete physical examination but is particularly useful for clients with suspected kidney or urologic disorders (Chart 69-4). Ideally, the urine specimen is collected at the first morning's voiding; specimens obtained at other times may not be adequately concentrated. The specimen may be collected by several techniques (Table 69-5).

COLOR, ODOR, AND TURBIDITY. The color of urine is derived from urochrome pigment. Variations in color may result from increased levels of urochrome or other pigments, changes in the concentration or dilution of the urine, and the presence of drug metabolites in the urine. Urine smells faintly like ammonia and is normally clear without **turbidity** (cloudiness) or haziness.

SPECIFIC GRAVITY. The specific gravity of urine measures the concentration or density of urine compared to water. The specific gravity of urine ranges from 1.000 (the specific gravity of water) to greater than 1.035. In kidney disease, increases and decreases in specific gravity may not reflect systemic fluid volume. For example, dilute urine with a decreased specific gravity may occur in a dehydrated client who has a lack of nephron receptors for antidiuretic hormone.

An *increase* in specific gravity occurs with dehydration, decreased kidney perfusion, or the presence of antidiuretic hormone (ADH). (ADH production is normally increased with stress, surgery, anesthetic agents, and certain drugs such as morphine and oral antidiabetic agents.) In each of these situations the expected kidney response is to reabsorb water and decrease urine output. As a result, the urine produced is more concentrated.

A *decrease* in specific gravity occurs with increased fluid intake, diuretic administration, and diabetes insipidus. In each of these situations, the normal kidney response is to excrete more water; thus urine output is increased. In kidney disease, the specific gravity decreases because there is less solute, and it does not vary with changes in plasma osmolality (e.g., it becomes fixed).

pH. A pH value less than 7 is considered acidic, and a value greater than 7 is considered alkaline. Various factors influence the acidity or alkalinity of urine. A diet high in certain fruits and vegetables results in a more alkaline urine, whereas a high-protein diet produces a more acidic urine. The presence of *Escherichia coli* in the urine also results in an acidic urine.

Urine specimens become more alkaline when left standing unrefrigerated for more than 1 hour, if urea-splitting bacteria are present, or if a specimen is left uncovered. Alkaline urine increases cell breakdown; thus the presence of red blood cells may be missed on analysis. The nurse ensures that urine specimens are covered and delivered to the laboratory promptly or refrigerated. During metabolic or respiratory acidosis or alkalosis, the kidneys, along with blood buffers and the lungs, should respond appropriately to maintain a normal serum pH. Chapters 15 and 16 discuss acid-base balance and imbalance.

GLUCOSE. Glucose is filtered at the glomerulus and is reabsorbed in the proximal tubule of the nephron. When the blood glucose level rises above 220 mg/dL, the renal threshold for reabsorption is usually exceeded, and glucose is excreted in the urine. Variations in the renal threshold for glucose occur in many clients, such as those who experience any infection or those who have had diabetes mellitus for a number of years. It is possible that their serum glucose level may be high (e.g., greater than 400 mg/dL), and glucose may still not be present in the urine.

KETONE BODIES. Three types of ketone bodies are acetone, acetoacetic acid, and beta-hydroxybutyric acid. **Ketone bodies** are by-products of the incomplete metabolism of fatty acids. Normally there are no ketones in urine. Ketone bodies are produced when fat sources are used instead of glucose to provide cellular energy. When ketones are present in the blood, they are partially excreted in the urine.

PROTEIN. Protein, such as albumin, is not normally present in the urine. Levels greater than 300 mg/24 hr, or 200 μg/min, are abnormal. The glomerular membrane is semipermeable to small molecules; protein molecules are too large to pass through this semipermeable membrane. When permeability of the glomerular membrane is increased, protein molecules pass through and are excreted in the urine. Increased glomerular membrane permeability may be caused by infection, inflammation, or immunologic problems. Certain systemic processes result in the production of abnormal proteins, such as globulin. These proteins are not detected with routine

CHART 69-4

LABORATORY PROFILE
Urinalysis

Test	Normal Range for Adults	Significance of Abnormal Findings
Color	Pale yellow	*Dark amber* indicates concentrated urine. *Very pale yellow* indicates dilute urine. *Dark red or brown* indicates blood in the urine; brown also may indicate increased urinary bilirubin level; red may also indicate the presence of myoglobin. *Other color changes* may result from diet or medications.
Odor	Specific aromatic odor, similar to ammonia	*Foul smell* indicates possible infection, dehydration, or ingestion of certain foods or drugs.
Turbidity	Clear	*Cloudy urine* indicates infection or sediment or high levels of urinary protein.
Specific gravity	Usually 1.010-1.025; possible range 1.000-1.030; after 12-hr fluid restriction >1.025 *Older adult:* Decreased because of decreased concentrating ability	*Increased* in decreased renal perfusion, inappropriate antidiuretic hormone secretion, or congestive heart failure. *Decreased* in chronic renal insufficiency, diabetes insipidus, malignant hypertension, diuretic administration, and lithium toxicity.
pH	Average: 6; possible range: 4.6-8	*Changes* are caused by diet, the administration of medications, infection, freshness of the specimen, acid-base imbalance, and altered renal function.
Glucose	<0.5 g/day (<2.78 mmol/L)	*Presence* reflects hyperglycemia or a decrease in the renal threshold for glucose.
Ketones	None	*Presence* reflects incomplete metabolism of fatty acids, as in diabetic ketoacidosis, prolonged fasting, anorexia nervosa.
Protein	8-18 mg/dL (10-140 mg/L)	*Increased amounts* may indicate stress, infection, recent strenuous exercise, or glomerular disorders.
Bilirubin (urobilinogen)	None	*Presence* suggests hepatic or biliary disease or obstruction.
Red blood cells (RBCs)	0-2 per high-power field	*Increased* amounts are normal with indwelling or intermittent catheterization or menses but may reflect tumor, stones, trauma, glomerular disorders, cystitis, or bleeding disorders.
White blood cells (WBCs)	Males: 0-3 per high-power field Females: 0-5 per high-power field	*Increased* amounts may indicate an infectious or inflammatory process anywhere in the renal/urinary tract, renal transplant rejection, fever, or exercise.
Casts	A few or none, composed of RBC or WBC, protein, or tubular cell casts	*Increased amounts* indicate the presence of bacteria or protein, which is seen in severe renal disease and could also indicate urinary calculi.
Crystals	None	*Presence* of normal or abnormal crystals may indicate that the specimen has been allowed to stand.
Bacteria	<1000 colonies/mL	*Increased amounts* indicate the need for urine culture to determine the presence of urinary tract infection.
Parasites	None	*Presence* of *Trichomonas vaginalis* indicates infection, usually of the urethra, prostate, or vagina.
Nitrates	None	*Presence* suggests bacteria, usually *Escherichia coli.*

urinalysis procedures; urine protein electrophoresis or other tests are necessary to detect these unusual proteins.

A random finding of proteinuria followed by a series of negative (normal) findings does not imply renal disease. If infection is suspected to be the cause of the proteinuria, urinalyses after elimination of the infection should be negative for protein. Persistent proteinuria needs further investigation.

Microalbuminuria is the presence of albumin in the urine that is not measurable by a urine dipstick or conventional urinalysis procedures. Specialized immunoassay tests can quickly analyze a freshly voided urine specimen for microscopic levels of albumin. The normal microalbumin levels in a freshly voided random specimen should range between 2.0 to 20 mg/mmol for men and 2.8 to 28 mg/mmol for women. Higher levels indicate microalbuminuria and could mean the presence of very early kidney disease, especially in clients with diabetes mellitus. For 24-hour urine specimens, levels of 30 to 300 mg/24 hr, or 20 to 200 μg/min, indicate microalbuminuria.

SEDIMENT. Urine sediment refers to particles in the urine. These particles include cells, casts, crystals, and bacteria.

CELLS. Types of cells abnormally present in the urine may include tubular cells (from the tubule of the nephron), epithelial cells (from the lining of the urinary tract), red blood cells (RBCs), and white blood cells (WBCs).

CASTS. Casts are structures formed around other particles. There may be casts of cells, bacteria, or protein. When casts are formed, there is a clumping or agglutination of the element, and gelatinous substances form the surrounding

TABLE 69-5 • COLLECTION OF URINE SPECIMENS

Nursing Interventions	Rationale
VOIDED URINE	
Collect the first specimen voided in the morning.	Urine is more concentrated in the early morning.
Send the specimen to the laboratory as soon as possible.	After urine is collected, cellular breakdown results in more alkaline urine.
Refrigerate the specimen if a delay is unavoidable.	Refrigeration delays the alkalinization of urine. Bacteria are more likely to multiply in an alkaline environment.
CLEAN-CATCH SPECIMEN	
Explain the purpose of the procedure to the client.	Correct technique is needed to obtain a valid specimen.
Instruct the client to self-clean before voiding.	
Instruct the female client to separate the labia and use the sponges and solution provided to wipe with three strokes over the urethra. The first two wiping strokes are over each side of the urethra; the third wiping stroke is centered over the urethra (from front to back).	Surface cleaning is necessary to remove secretions or bacteria from the urethral meatus.
Instruct the male client to retract the foreskin of the penis and to similarly clean the urethra, using three wiping strokes with the sponge and solution provided (from the head of the penis downward).	
Instruct the client to initiate voiding after cleaning. The client then stops and resumes voiding into the container. Only 1 ounce (30 mL) is needed; the remainder of the urine may be discarded into the commode.	A midstream collection further removes secretions and bacteria because urine flushes the distal portion of the internal urethra. An improperly collected specimen may result in inappropriate or incomplete treatment.
Ensure that the client understands the procedure.	The client's understanding and the nurse's assistance ensure proper collection.
Assist the client as needed.	
CATHETERIZED SPECIMEN	
For nonindwelling (straight) catheters:	The one-time passage of a urinary catheter may be necessary to obtain an uncontaminated specimen for analysis or to measure the volume of residual urine.
Avoid routine use.	These procedures minimize bacterial entry.
Follow the facility's procedures for catheterization technique.	
For indwelling catheters:	Collection of urine from an indwelling catheter or tubing is performed when clients have catheters for continence or long-term urinary drainage.
Apply a clamp to the drainage tubing, distal to the injection port.	Clamping allows urine to collect in the tubing at the location where the specimen is obtained.
Clean the injection port cap of the catheter drainage tubing with an appropriate antiseptic. Povidone-iodine solution or alcohol is acceptable.	Surface contamination is prevented by following the cleaning procedures.
Insert a sterile 5-mL syringe into the port and aspirate the quantity of urine required.	A minimum of 5 mL is needed for culture and sensitivity (C&S) testing.
Inject the urine sample into a sterile specimen container.	A sterile container is used for C&S specimens.
Remove the clamp to resume drainage.	
Properly dispose of the syringe.	
24-HOUR URINE COLLECTION	
Instruct the client thoroughly.	A 24-hr collection of urine is necessary to quantify or calculate the rate of clearance of a particular substance.
Provide written materials to assist in instruction.	Instructional materials for clients, signs, and so on remind clients and staff to ensure that the total collection is completed.
Place signs appropriately.	
Inform all personnel or family caregivers of test in progress.	
Check laboratory or procedure manual on proper technique for maintaining the collection (e.g., on ice, in a refrigerator, or with a preservative).	Proper technique prevents breakdown of elements to be measured.
On initiation of the collection, ask the client to void, discard the urine, and note the time. If a Foley catheter is in use, empty the tubing and drainage bag at the start time and discard the urine.	Proper techniques ensure that *all* urine formed within the 24-hr period is collected.
Collect all urine for the next 24 hr.	
24 hr after initiation, ask the client to empty the bladder and add that urine to the container.	
Do not remove urine from the collection container for other specimens.	Urine in the container is not considered a "fresh" specimen and may be mixed with preservative.

CHART 69-5

LABORATORY PROFILE
24-Hour Urine Collections

Component	Normal Range for Adults	Significance of Abnormal Findings
Creatinine	0.8-2 g/24 hr *Males:* 1-2 g/24 hr or 14-26 mg/kg/24 hr (124-230 μmol/kg/24 hr or 7.1-17.7 mmol/24 hr) *Females:* 0.6-1.8 g/24 hr or 11-20 mg/kg/24 hr (97-177 μmol/kg/24 hr or 5.3-15.9 mmol/24 hr) *Older adults:* 10 mg/kg/24 hr (88.4 μmol/kg/24 hr) at 90 yr	*Decreased amounts* indicate a deterioration in renal function caused by renal disease, shock, hypovolemia, or any condition affecting muscle. *Increased amounts* occur with infections, exercise, diabetes mellitus, and meat meals.
Urea nitrogen	12-20 g/24 hr (0.43-0.71 mmol/24 hr)	*Decreased amounts* occur when renal damage or liver disease is present. *Increased amounts* commonly result from a high-protein diet, dehydration, trauma, or sepsis.
Sodium	40-220 mEq/24 hr (40-220 mmol/24 hr)	*Decreased amounts* are seen in hemorrhage, shock, hyperaldosteronism, and prerenal acute renal failure. *Increased amounts* are common with diuretic therapy, excessive salt intake, hypokalemia, and acute tubular necrosis.
Chloride	110-250 mEq/24 hr (110-250 mmol/24 hr) *Older adults:* 95-195 mEq/24 hr (95-195 mmol/24 hr)	*Decreased amounts* are seen in certain renal diseases, malabsorption syndrome, pyloric obstruction, prolonged nasogastric tube drainage, diarrhea, diaphoresis, congestive heart failure, and emphysema. *Increased amounts* are seen with hypokalemia, adrenal insufficiency, and massive diuresis.
Calcium	100-400 mg/24 hr (2.50-7.50 mmol/kg/24 hr)	*Decreased amounts* are often associated with hypocalcemia, hypoparathyrodism, nephrosis, and nephritis. *Increased amounts* are commonly seen with calcium renal stones, hyperparathyroidism, sarcoidosis, certain cancers, immobilization, and hypercalcemia.
Total catecholamines*	<100 μg/24 hr (<591 mmol/24 hr)	*Increased amounts* occur with pheochromocytoma, neuroblastomas, stress, or strenuous exercise.
Protein	1-14 mg/dL (10-140 mg/L) or 50-80 mg/24 hr at rest	*Increased amounts* indicate glomerular disease, nephrotic syndrome, diabetic nephropathy, urinary tract malignancies, and irritations.

*Epinephrine and norepinephrine only; dopamine is not measured.

structure, a cast. Casts are described by the type of element in the structure (e.g., RBC cast, WBC cast, tubular epithelial cast) or the stage of degeneration. The degeneration of casts refers to the stage of breakdown of the internal element. Casts are described as "granular" (coarse or fine) and "waxy."

CRYSTALS. Crystals in the urine come from various salts. These particles may be a result of diet, drugs, or disease. The salts may be composed of calcium, oxalate, urea, phosphate, magnesium, or other substances. Certain drugs, such as the sulfates, can also produce crystals.

BACTERIA. Bacteria in a urine sample multiply quickly, so the specimen must be analyzed promptly. Normally urine is sterile, but it can be contaminated easily by perineal bacteria or airborne pathogens during collection.

URINE FOR CULTURE AND SENSITIVITY

The nurse may collect a sample of urine for laboratory determination of the number and types of pathogens present. The presence of clinical symptoms and unexplained bacteria in a urinalysis specimen are indications for urine culture and sensitivity testing. When bacterial colonies are present, they are placed in a medium containing different antibiotic drugs to determine which drugs are effective in killing or stopping the growth of the bacteria (sensitivity). Those drugs to which the microorganisms are sensitive or resistant are reported to guide decisions about needed therapy. A clean-catch or catheter-derived specimen is always preferred for culture and sensitivity testing.

COMPOSITE URINE COLLECTIONS

When ordered, urine collections are made for a number of hours (e.g., 24 hours) for laboratory quantitative and qualitative analysis of one or more substances. Collections are often ordered to measure levels of urinary creatinine or urea nitrogen, sodium, chloride, calcium, catecholamines, or other components (Chart 69-5). For a composite urine specimen, *all* urine within the designated time frame must be collected (see Table 69-5). If other voided or catheterized specimens must be obtained while the collection is in progress, the nurse measures and appropriately documents the amount collected but not added to the timed collection.

The urine collection may need to be refrigerated or stored on ice to prevent changes in the urine during the collection time. The nurse follows the procedure from the laboratory for urine storage. The urine collection must be free from fecal contamination. Menstrual blood and toilet tissue also contaminate the specimen and can invalidate the results.

The collection of urine for a 24-hour period is often more difficult than it seems. With hospitalized clients, the cooperation of staff personnel, the client, family members, and visitors is essential. Placing signs in the bathroom, instructing the client and family, and emphasizing the need to save the urine are helpful.

CREATININE CLEARANCE TEST

Creatinine clearance is a calculation of glomerular filtration rate. It is the best indication of overall kidney function. The amount of creatinine cleared from the blood (e.g., filtered into the urine) is measured in the total volume of urine excreted in a defined period. A urine specimen for a creatinine clearance test is usually collected for 24 hours, but it can be collected for shorter periods (e.g., 8 or 12 hours). The calculation requires a comparison with the blood creatinine level, and therefore a blood specimen for creatinine must also be collected.

The laboratory or the physician calculates the creatinine clearance. Because the client's age, gender, height, weight, diet, and activity level influence the expected amount of creatinine to be excreted, these variables are considered in the interpretation of creatinine clearance test results.

The following formula is used to calculate creatinine clearance:

$$\text{Creatinine clearance} = U \times V/P \times T$$

where U is creatinine in urine (mg/dL), V is volume of urine (mL/24 hr), P is creatinine in plasma or blood (mg/dL), and T is time (minutes).

The rate of creatinine clearance is expressed as milliliters per minute per 1.73 m^2 of body surface area. The range for normal creatinine clearance is 90 to 139 mL/min for adult males and 80 to 125 mL/min for females.

Creatinine clearance measurements are necessary to determine the client's current kidney function. Decreases in the creatinine clearance rate may require modification of drug dosing and often signifies the need for further investigation of the cause of kidney deterioration.

URINE ELECTROLYTES

Urine samples may be collected for the analysis of urine electrolyte levels (e.g., sodium and chloride). Normally the amount of sodium excreted in the urine is nearly equal to that consumed. Urine sodium levels of less than 10 mEq/L indicate that the tubules are functioning to conserve (reabsorb) sodium.

OSMOLALITY

Osmolality is a measure of the concentration of particles in solution, in this case the concentration of solutes in urine. These solutes include electrolytes and solutes such as glucose, urea, and creatinine.

BLOOD/PLASMA OSMOLALITY. The kidneys excrete or reabsorb water to maintain a blood osmolality in the range of 285 to 295 mOsm/kg. Osmolality is slightly higher in older adult clients (285 to 301 mOsm/kg). When blood osmolality is decreased, the release of antidiuretic hormone (ADH) is inhibited. Without ADH, the distal tubule and collecting ducts are *not* permeable to water. As a result, water is *excreted,* not reabsorbed, and blood osmolality increases. When blood osmolality increases, ADH is produced. With ADH production, the distal tubule is made permeable to water. Consequently, water is reabsorbed, and blood osmolality decreases.

URINE OSMOLALITY. Urine osmolality can vary from 50 to 1400 mOsm/kg water, depending on the clinical and hydration status of the client and the functional status of the kidneys. With average fluid intake, the range for urine osmolality is 300 to 900 mOsm/kg water. The fixed acids and other wastes that are continually produced constitute a solute load that must be excreted in the urine on a regular basis. This is referred to as *obligatory solute excretion.* If the client has lost excessive fluids, the renal response is to conserve water, preserve blood osmolality, and excrete small amounts of highly concentrated urine. Many factors such as diet, medications, and activity can influence urine osmolality. Thus increased urine osmolality reflects a concentrated urine with less water than solutes. A decreased urine osmolality reflects a dilute urine with more water than solutes.

RADIOGRAPHIC EXAMINATIONS

Radiographic and other special procedures are used to diagnose abnormalities within the genitourinary system (Table 69-6). The nurse explains the procedures thoroughly to the client, prepares the client, and provides postprocedural care.

Kidney, Ureter, and Bladder X-Ray Examination

Radiographic examination of the kidneys, ureters, and bladder (KUB) is a plain film of the abdomen taken without any specific client preparation. The KUB study shows gross anatomic features and may show obvious stones, strictures, calcifications, or obstructions in the urinary tract. This test identifies the organs' shape, size, and relationship to other parts of the urinary tract. Other tests are necessary for diagnosis of functional or structural abnormalities.

There is no discomfort or risk from this procedure. The nurse tells the client that the films will be taken while the client is in a supine position. No specific postprocedure care is necessary.

Intravenous Urography

Other names for intravenous urography include excretory urography and (the older term) intravenous pyelography (IVP).

CLIENT PREPARATION. Before urography, the nurse assesses the client (Chart 69-6), institutes bowel preparation, and teaches the client. Allergy information is reported to the physician. Contrast reactions can be minor (nausea and vomiting, urticaria, itching, sneezing), moderate (nephrotoxic effects, congestive heart failure, pulmonary edema), or severe

TABLE 69-6 • COMMON RADIOLOGIC AND SPECIAL DIAGNOSTIC TESTS FOR CLIENTS WITH DISORDERS OF THE RENAL/URINARY SYSTEM

Test	Purpose	Comments
Radiography of kidneys, ureters, and bladder (KUB) (plain film of abdomen)	To screen for the presence of two kidneys To measure the kidneys' size To detect gross obstruction	
Excretory urography	To measure the kidneys' size To detect obstruction To assess parenchymal mass	Radiopaque contrast media may cause an allergic (hypersensitivity) reaction in iodine-sensitive clients. Contrast agent is also hypertonic and increases the risk of acute renal failure in adults with serum creatinine levels greater than 1.5 mg/dL, diabetes mellitus, multiple myeloma, or dehydration. Nephrotoxic complications can be prevented by parenteral fluid administration, the use of mannitol, and daily monitoring of serum creatinine levels.
Nephrotomography	To assess various planes of kidney tissue for cysts, tumors, or calculi	Same as for excretory urogram.
Computed tomography (CT)	To measure the size of the kidneys To evaluate contour to assess for masses or obstruction	Contrast medium may provoke acute renal failure. See comments with excretory urography for high-risk clients and preventive measures related to contrast. May be performed without contrast medium and still obtain adequate visualization.
Cystography and cystoscopy	To identify abnormalities of the bladder wall and urethral and ureteral occlusions To treat small obstructions or lesions via fulguration, lithotripsy, or removal with a stone basket	Instrumentation of the urinary tract increases the risk of infection. Monitor for infection for 48-72 hr after the procedure.
Voiding cystourethrography (VCUG)	To outline the bladder's contour and to detect urinary reflux from vesicourethral junctions	The risk of infection is similar to that in cystography because urinary catheterization is necessary. Monitor for postprocedure infection.
Renal arteriography	To identify vascular abnormalities within each kidney and adjacent aorta	Contrast medium may provoke acute renal failure. See comments with excretory urography for high-risk clients and preventive measures related to contrast. Essential for diagnosis and treatment of some vascular abnormalities, such as renal artery stenosis. Monitor for bleeding after the procedure.
Ultrasonography (US)	To identify the size of the kidneys or obstruction in the kidneys or the lower urinary tract May detect tumors or cysts	Ultrasonography entails minimal risk to the client. Ultrasonography is a good alternative to excretory urography.
Renography (Renal scan)	To assess renal blood flow	Radioactive material is used for this test. Captopril or another angiotensin-converting enzyme (ACE) inhibitor may be used, placing the client at risk for severe hypotensive reactions during and following this procedure.

(bronchospasm, anaphylaxis). If the diagnostic test is to be performed in the presence of minor allergy, the physician orders preprocedural medications such as a steroid (methylprednisolone or prednisone), and an antihistamine (diphenhydramine hydrochloride [Benadryl, Allerdryl✱]) to suppress the allergic response (Cohan & Ellis, 1997). The nurse explains the rationale for the procedure to the client.

Procedures to ensure that films provide adequate visualization vary according to the radiologist's preferences. Some radiologists recommend a light evening meal or clear liquids, then fasting (NPO status) from midnight on the night before the procedure. Others recommend increased fluid intake to prevent dehydration up until the time of the procedure. Because of the possibility of a vomiting reaction to the intravenous (IV) contrast, however, the physician may prefer the client to remain on NPO status at least a few hours before the procedure. The physician orders hydration with IV fluids as indicated.

The physician orders a bowel preparation to remove fecal contents, fluid, and air from the gut, which permits an adequate outline of the lower poles of the kidneys, ureters, and bladder. Bowel preparation procedures vary but usually include the use

CHART 69-6

BEST PRACTICE *for*
Assessing the Client About to Undergo a Diagnostic Test or Interventional Procedure Using Contrast Media

Before the procedure:

- Ask the client if he or she has ever had a reaction to contrast media. (Such a client has the highest risk for having another reaction.)
- Ask the client about a history of asthma. (Clients with asthma have been shown to be at greater risk for contrast reactions than the general public; when reactions do occur, they are more likely to be severe.)
- Ask the client about known hay fever or food or medication allergies, especially to seafood, eggs, milk, or chocolate. (Contrast reactions have been reported to be as high as 15% in these clients.)
- Ask the client to describe any specific allergic reactions (e.g., hives, facial edema, difficulty breathing, bronchospasm).
- Assess for a history of renal insufficiency and for conditions that have been implicated in increasing the chance of developing renal failure after contrast media (e.g., diabetic nephropathy, class IV heart failure, dehydration, concomitant use of potentially nephrotoxic medications such as the aminoglycosides or NSAIDs, and cirrhosis).
- Ask the client if he or she is taking metformin (Glucophage). (Metformin must be discontinued at least 48 hours before any study using contrast media because the life-threatening complication of lactic acidosis, although rare, could occur.)
- Assess hydration status by checking blood pressure, heart and respiratory rates, mucous membranes, skin turgor, and urine concentration.
- Ask the client when he or she last ate or drank anything.

From Cohan, R.H., & Ellis, J.H. (1997). Iodinated contrast material in uroradiology. Choice of agent and management of complications. *Urologic Clinics of North America, 24*(3), 471-491.
NSAIDS, Nonsteroidal anti-inflammatory drugs.

of laxatives the day before the procedure. Enemas also may be prescribed but are controversial because air and fluid can be introduced with inadequate expulsion of fecal contents.

CONSIDERATIONS FOR OLDER ADULTS

Bowel preparation procedures increase the risk for dehydration, especially in older clients. To help prevent dehydration, the nurse contacts the testing department and requests that urograms be scheduled early in the day for older clients.

The contrast medium (dye) is potentially nephrotoxic. The risk for *contrast-induced renal failure* is greatest in clients who are older or dehydrated, who have some renal insufficiency (e.g., serum creatinine levels greater than 1.5 mg/dL), or who are also taking other nephrotoxic drugs. These clients usually require additional IV fluids before the procedure to maintain hydration and to decrease the nephrotoxic risk. Diuretics may be administered immediately after the dye is injected to enhance its excretion.

The nurse instructs the client in the preparation procedures for the urogram and explains the procedure so he or she knows what to expect in the examination room (Chart 69-7). The nurse intervenes on behalf of the client to ensure that questions are answered *before* the procedure.

CHART 69-7

CLIENT EDUCATION GUIDE
Excretory Urogram

- The urogram outlines your urinary tract and helps determine any problems there.
- Notify your nurse or physician if you have had any reactions (allergic or otherwise) to any food or drugs, especially shellfish (shrimp, scallops, crab, lobster, and so on) or iodine, or to x-ray "dyes" such as contrast media; if you have a history of asthma; or if you are taking metformin (Glucophage) or Glucovance.
- The day before the test, follow the instructions about changes in your diet and fluid intake to be sure that as much information as possible is gained from the test.
- After you start the bowel preparation, you may need to be close to toileting facilities. The preparation medications usually work quickly.
- You will be lying on an x-ray table with the x-ray machine above you for most of the procedure.
- A pressure band, similar to a large blood pressure cuff, may be placed around your stomach or abdomen to help obtain better x-ray pictures.
- If you do not already have an IV access site, one will be started to give you the contrast agent.
- After the contrast is injected, you may feel a sense of warmth or heat as it travels throughout your body. You also may have a taste in your mouth that is sometimes described as metallic. These sensations last only a few seconds or minutes.
- When the pressure band is inflated, you may feel some tightness around your abdomen. The sensation is similar to the feeling on your arm when you have your blood pressure taken.
- A series of x-ray pictures will be taken. You may be asked to empty your bladder and return to the table for more films. You also may be asked to have a standing film taken.
- After the test is completed, you are usually able to resume your normal activities and diet.
- The contrast will be excreted normally in your urine. You will not notice any change in the color or characteristics of your urine.
- Please do not hesitate to ask your nurse, physician, or x-ray technologist any question, no matter how slight the question may seem to you. It is important that you have as much understanding as possible.

PROCEDURE. A radiopaque contrast medium (dye) is injected intravenously with the client in a supine position. As blood (with the dye) rapidly circulates into the kidney blood vessels and is filtered by the glomeruli, the dye is excreted in the urine. A series of x-ray films are taken at various times after injection. When ordered, nephrotomograms are taken at the same time as the urogram. Tomograms provide images of different planes of tissue and show any abnormalities present at varying depths. The technologist then asks the client to empty the bladder and return for a few more films. An outline of the kidneys, ureters, and bladder results as urine containing the dye is excreted.

The urogram provides information about the following:

- The number, size, shape, and location of the kidneys
- The adequacy of uptake (filling) and the rate of excretion of contrast medium
- The number, size, location, appearance, and patency of the calices, pelves, and ureters
- The size, location, and nature of the urinary bladder

FOLLOW-UP CARE. After the urogram, the nurse monitors the client for altered renal function and other effects from the dye. Adequate hydration is ensured by encouraging the client to take fluid orally or by administering IV fluids. Hydration decreases the risk for renal deterioration. Blood creatinine levels are monitored to determine ongoing renal function.

Computed Tomography

CLIENT PREPARATION. The nurse informs the client that a computed tomography (CT) scan is performed to provide three-dimensional information about the kidneys, ureters, bladder, and surrounding tissues. A CT scan is usually performed after other diagnostic procedures and can provide information about tumors, cysts, abscesses, other masses, obstruction, and certain blood vessel abnormalities.

A bowel preparation with laxatives or an enema and a light meal the evening before the procedure is needed. The client is given nothing by mouth (NPO status) after midnight on the night before the examination. For clients having the CT scan with dye, the physician orders preprocedural IV hydration. The nurse assesses for any allergy to dye and intervenes as with IV urography.

PROCEDURE. The CT scan is performed in a special room, usually in the radiology department. An IV injection of radiopaque dye may be administered before starting the imaging procedures. The use of dye may be eliminated in clients at risk for contrast media–induced acute renal failure, but the images produced are less distinct. Tomograms are obtained at various levels.

FOLLOW-UP CARE. No special follow-up care is necessary unless a dye was used. In that case, the follow-up care is the same as for IV urography.

Cystography and Cystourethrography

CLIENT PREPARATION. The nurse explains the procedure to the client undergoing a cystography or cystourethrography. A urinary catheter is temporarily needed to instill a contrast medium (dye). The dye is necessary for visualization of the lower urinary tract.

PROCEDURE. In both cystography and cystourethrography, dye is instilled into the bladder via a urethral catheter. After bladder filling, a variety of films are obtained from the front, back, and side positions. For the voiding cystourethrogram (VCUG), the client is requested to void, and films are taken during the voiding. A VCUG is obtained to determine whether a vesicoureteral reflux is present. The cystogram is often indicated in cases of trauma when urethral or bladder injury is suspected.

FOLLOW-UP CARE. The nurse monitors for the development of infection as a result of catheterization. In this test, the dye is not nephrotoxic because it is not injected into the bloodstream. Fluid intake is encouraged to dilute the urine and reduce the burning sensation from catheter irritation after removal. Because pelvic or urethral trauma may be present, the nurse also monitors for changes in urine output.

OTHER RENAL DIAGNOSTIC TESTS

Renal Arteriography (Angiography)

CLIENT PREPARATION. The nurse informs the client that an arteriography is used to assess the arterial blood supply of the kidneys. A bowel preparation is given to remove fecal contents, gas, and fluid. A light evening meal is given, and the client is on NPO status until after the procedure. An IV may be placed before the procedure. IV fluids are often given to ensure adequate hydration because a contrast medium (dye) is used as part of the procedure.

The nurse reviews the procedure with the client, answers questions, and reviews the medication regimen and blood study results as indicated. For example, the nurse reviews the prothrombin time if the client has been taking warfarin sodium (Coumadin, Warfilone♣). The client also signs an informed consent statement. Renal arteriography is performed to explore suspected causes of decreased renal function such as renovascular hypertension, other vessel abnormalities, and bleeding from trauma.

PROCEDURE. The injection of a radiopaque dye into the renal arteries requires entry into an artery, usually the femoral artery in the groin. After the client is sedated and the skin is prepared and draped, the radiologist injects a local anesthetic. An arterial puncture is then performed through which the angiographic catheter is inserted.

Using fluoroscopy, the radiologist guides the catheter into the abdominal aorta and the renal artery. When the tip of the catheter is positioned at each renal artery, the radiologist injects dye and films are taken. The speed of distribution of the dye and any areas of blood vessel narrowing are noted. Arterial blockage is noted when the dye fails to circulate within the kidney. **Extravasation** (infiltration) of dye into surrounding tissue indicates vessel rupture, which could be present after trauma.

Visualization of the renal vessels can be improved by using a digital subtraction technique. In the digital subtraction arteriogram (DSA), a computer is used to "subtract out" loops of bowel, ribs, and other structures normally seen on the x-ray film. As a result, even the small-vessel images are improved. In addition, the use of a smaller amount of dye means less risk for nephrotoxicity. DSA procedures may not provide sufficient detail for surgical intervention when used without full arteriography.

FOLLOW-UP CARE. Bleeding from the catheter insertion site and dye-induced reactions are the two most common complications of renal arteriography. The nurse monitors the catheter insertion site for signs of bleeding or swelling. A pressure dressing may have been placed as a preventive measure before the client returned to the nursing area. The nurse ensures that a 5-pound sandbag and ice are available in case of emergency.

The vital signs are monitored as per the physician's order or according to the agency's policy, usually every 15 minutes for 1 hour, then every 30 minutes for 2 hours, then every hour for 4 hours, and then every 4 hours. The nurse checks the temperature and color of the extremities and distal pulses. A sudden absence of pulses in the catheterized vessel may reflect hematoma formation or embolization. Hemoglobin and hematocrit levels are monitored closely for 24 hours after the procedure, usually every 6 hours.

The period of absolute bedrest (to prevent bleeding) after arteriography varies. In general, bedrest is maintained for 4 to 6 hours. The nurse instructs the client about the importance of keeping the leg in a straight position for those 4 to 6 hours. A restraint may be used on the leg with the client's consent. Ankle flexing and weight shifting are encouraged to prevent deep vein thrombosis. If there is no evidence of bleeding after 4 to 6 hours, the client may be permitted to stand to void or may use a bedside commode.

Serum creatinine tests are ordered for several days after the arteriogram to determine whether the procedure has affected kidney function. For some clients with renal insufficiency, the administration of dye may cause an episode of acute renal failure sufficient to require short-term dialysis. Because the test is used to provide information for interventions to restore blood flow and thus preserve kidney function, many clients are willing to accept the risk of short-term dialysis to prevent the need for permanent dialysis. The client is urged to drink fluids after the procedure to ensure adequate excretion of the dye.

Renal Biopsy

CLIENT PREPARATION. The nurse explains that a biopsy of the kidney is performed to determine a pathologic reason for unexplained renal dysfunction and to direct or change a course of therapy. The client signs an informed consent or operative permit.

In a closed biopsy, the physician obtains kidney tissue samples **percutaneously** (through the skin and other tissues). In an open biopsy, the tissues are obtained surgically. Factors to consider include the number of kidneys, the ability of the client to cooperate, and the need for abdominal surgical exploration. If a percutaneous biopsy is selected, the client must have two kidneys, be able to breathe comfortably in a prone position for 30 to 45 minutes, and be able to hold his or her breath on request for several seconds. The client is on NPO status for 4 to 6 hours before the procedure in case a major complication requires immediate surgery.

An open renal biopsy is performed when cancer is suspected or when the client has only one kidney, cannot hold his or her breath, or is unable to tolerate a prone position. If abdominal surgery is necessary for other reasons and a renal biopsy is also needed, the nephrologist may request the surgeon to perform the biopsy, thereby eliminating the need for a second procedure. If an open biopsy is performed, client preparation is the same as for general surgery and anesthesia (see Chapter 17).

Because of the risk for postprocedure bleeding, coagulation studies such as platelet count, activated partial thromboplastin time (aPTT), prothrombin time (PT), and bleeding time are performed before surgery. A blood transfusion may be needed to correct a low hemoglobin level before biopsy. Hypertension and uremia increase the risk for bleeding and the physician may order antihypertensive medications or dialysis before a biopsy.

PROCEDURE. Immediately before a percutaneous biopsy, the nurse asks the client to void to decrease the possibility of puncturing the bladder. The left kidney is biopsied because it is closer to the skin and is not near the liver. The exact position of the kidney is determined via fluoroscopic or ultrasonographic examination or by radionuclide scan. In some clients the nephrologist may locate the kidney by using landmarks from previous images. In other clients the closed biopsy is performed directly during fluoroscopy or ultrasonographic examination.

For a closed biopsy, the client is placed in a prone position. A roll of padding is placed under the client's abdomen to angle the kidney closer to the skin. The skin is prepared and draped, and a local anesthetic is injected. The depth of the kidney is identified by inserting a thin-gauge spinal needle. Movement of the spinal needle with breathing helps to determine that the capsule of the kidney has been located. A specially designed trocar is inserted in the path established by the spinal needle. While the client holds his or her breath, tissue is obtained by inserting the biopsy needle through the trocar and capsule into the kidney cortex. Automated spring-loaded and smaller biopsy needles have improved the tissue samples obtained. Ideally, three tissue specimens are obtained.

FOLLOW-UP CARE. After a closed percutaneous biopsy, the major risk is bleeding from the biopsy site. For 24 hours after the biopsy, the nurse monitors the dressing site, vital signs, urinary output, hemoglobin level, and hematocrit (as for postarteriography protocols). Even if the dressing is dry and there is no hematoma, the client could be bleeding from the site. An internal bleed is not readily visible but is suspected with flank pain, decreasing blood pressure, decreasing urine output, or other signs of hypovolemia or shock.

The client follows a plan of strict bedrest, lying in a supine position with a back roll for additional support for at least 6 hours after the biopsy. The head of the bed may be elevated, and the client may resume oral intake of food and fluids. After 6 hours, the client may have limited bathroom privileges if there is no evidence of bleeding.

The nurse monitors for hematuria, the most common complication of a percutaneous renal biopsy. Hematuria occurs microscopically in almost all clients, whereas 5% to 9% have gross hematuria. This problem usually resolves spontaneously 48 to 72 hours after the biopsy but can persist for 2 to 3 weeks. In rare cases, transfusions and surgery are required. There should be no obvious blood clots in the urine.

The client may have some local discomfort after the percutaneous renal biopsy. If aching originates at the biopsy site and begins to radiate to the flank and around the front of the abdomen, the nurse suspects an onset of bleeding or the development of a perinephric hematoma. This pattern of discomfort with bleeding occurs because blood in the perirenal tissues and musculature increases pressure on local nerve tracts.

If bleeding occurs, IV fluid, packed red blood cells, or both may need to be administered to restore blood pressure. In general, a small amount of bleeding creates enough pressure to compress bleeding sites; this is called a **tamponade effect.** If tamponade does not occur and bleeding becomes extensive, surgical intervention for hemostasis or even nephrectomy may be necessary. A perinephric hematoma may become infected, requiring treatment with antibiotics and surgical drainage.

If no bleeding occurs, the client can resume general activities after 24 hours. The nurse instructs him or her to avoid lifting heavy objects, exercising, or performing other strenuous activities for 1 to 2 weeks after the biopsy procedure. Driving may also be restricted.

Refer to Chapter 19 for general postoperative care for the client undergoing an open renal biopsy.

Renography (Kidney Scan)

CLIENT PREPARATION. The nurse explains to the client that a kidney scan is performed to provide general information about renal blood flow. A small amount of radioactive material, a radionuclide, is used. The nurse reassures the client that there is generally no danger from the small amount of radioactive material present in the agent.

PROCEDURE. For a kidney scan, the radionuclide is injected intravenously. After injection, the radionuclide is absorbed into kidney tissue and gives off low-level radioactive emissions **(scintillations).** The amount of emission is measured by a scintillator or a scintillation counter. A specially designed camera records the emissions and produces an image. At the same time, the rate and location of the emissions are recorded by computer, and information about renal blood flow, or glomerular filtration, is provided.

In some cases captopril (Capoten), an antihypertensive agent, is administered at the start of the procedure to change blood flow in the kidney. This procedure is known as a Captopril Renal Scan. The drug can cause severe hypotension during and after the procedure.

FOLLOW-UP CARE. If the client is able, urination into a commode is acceptable without risk from the small amount of radioactive material to be excreted. If the client is incontinent, the nurse changes the bed linens promptly and wears gloves to maintain standard precautions. If captopril was used during the procedure, the client's blood pressure is assessed frequently. The client is cautioned about rapid position changes and the risk for falling associated with orthostatic (positional) hypotension.

Ultrasonography

CLIENT PREPARATION. The nurse informs the client that ultrasonography does not cause discomfort and is without risk. This test involves applying sound waves to structures of different densities to produce images of the kidneys, ureters, and bladder and surrounding tissues. Ultrasonography allows assessment of kidney size, cortical thickness, and status of the calices. The test can be used to identify obstruction in the urinary tract, tumors, cysts, and other masses without the use of nephrotoxic contrast material (dye).

PROCEDURE. The client undergoing renal ultrasound is usually placed on a table in a prone position. A sonographic gel is applied to the skin over the back and flank areas to promote the conduction of sound waves. A transducer in contact with and moving across the skin delivers sound waves and measures the echoes. Images of the internal structures are produced.

FOLLOW-UP CARE. Skin care to remove the gel is all that is necessary after ultrasonography.

OTHER URINARY TRACT DIAGNOSTIC TESTS

Cystoscopy and Cystourethroscopy

CLIENT PREPARATION. Cystoscopy and cystourethroscopy are considered operative procedures and thus require completion of a preoperative checklist and an informed consent statement. The nurse provides a complete description of and reasons for the procedure. Cystoscopy may be performed for diagnosis or treatment. Diagnostic indications include examination for bladder trauma (cystoscopy) or urethral trauma (cystourethroscopy) and identification of the causes of urinary tract obstruction from stones or tumors. Cystoscopy may be indicated to remove bladder tumors or an enlarged prostate gland.

Cystoscopy may be performed under general or local anesthesia with sedation. The client's age, general health, and expected duration of the procedure are some of the considerations in the decision about anesthesia. A light evening meal may be eaten. Usually the client is on NPO status after midnight on the night before the cystoscopy. A bowel preparation with laxatives or enemas is performed the evening before the procedure.

PROCEDURE. The cystoscopic examination is performed in a specially designed cystoscopic examination room. If the procedure is performed in a surgical suite under general anesthesia, traditional surgical support personnel are present. This procedure is more often performed in outpatient settings, such as a clinic, an ambulatory surgery or short-procedure unit, or a urologist's office.

The client is assisted onto a table and, after sedation, is placed in the lithotomy position. After the administration of anesthesia, skin cleaning, and draping, a cystoscope is inserted via the urethra into the urinary bladder. If visualization of the urethra is also indicated, a urethroscope is used. Examinations commonly include the use of both the cystoscope and the urethroscope.

FOLLOW-UP CARE. After cystoscopic examination with general anesthesia, the client is returned to a postanesthesia care unit (PACU) or area. If local anesthesia and sedation were used, the client may be returned directly to the hospital room. Clients undergoing cystoscopic examinations as outpatients are transferred to an area for monitoring before discharge to home. The nurse monitors the client for airway patency and breathing, alterations in vital signs (including temperature), and changes in urine output. The nurse also observes for the complications of bleeding and infection.

A catheter may or may not be present after cystoscopy. The client without a catheter has urinary frequency due to irritation from the catheter. The urine may be pink tinged, but gross bleeding is not expected. Bleeding or the presence of clots may obstruct the catheter and decrease urine output. The nurse monitors urine output and notifies the physician of obvious blood clots or a decreased or ceased urine output. The Foley catheter is irrigated with sterile saline, as ordered. The physician is notified if the client has a fever (with or without chills) or an elevated white blood cell (WBC) count, which suggests infection. The client is encouraged to take oral fluids to promote adequate urine output (which helps prevent clotting) and to reduce the burning sensation on urination.

Retrograde Procedures

CLIENT PREPARATION. The client is prepared for retrograde procedures (retrograde pyelography, retrograde cystography, and retrograde urethrography) in a manner similar to that for the cystoscopic examination. **Retrograde** means going against the normal flow of urine. The nurse explains that a retrograde examination of the ureters and pelves **(pyelogram),** the bladder **(cystogram),** and the urethra **(urethrogram)** involves the direct injection of radiopaque contrast medium (dye) into the lower urinary tract. Because the dye is instilled directly to obtain an outline of the structures desired, the dye does not enter the bloodstream. Therefore the client is not at risk for dye-induced acute renal failure or a systemic allergic response.

PROCEDURE. Retrograde films are obtained during the cystoscopic examination. After placement of the cystoscope by the urologist, catheters are placed into each ureter, and contrast medium is instilled into each ureter and renal pelvis. The catheters are removed by the urologist, and films are taken by the radiology technician to outline these structures as the dye is excreted. The procedure identifies any obstruction or structural abnormality.

For clients undergoing retrograde cystoscopy or urethrography, contrast medium is instilled similarly into the bladder or urethra. Cystography and urethrography also identify structural abnormalities, such as fistulas, diverticula, and tumors.

FOLLOW-UP CARE. After retrograde procedures, the nurse monitors the client for the development of infection as a result of instrumentation of the urinary tract. Because these procedures are performed during cystoscopic examination, follow-up care is the same as that for cystoscopy.

Urodynamic Studies

Urodynamic studies describe the processes of voiding and include the following:

- Tests of bladder capacity, pressure, and tone
- Studies of urethral pressure and urine flow
- Examination of the function of perineal voluntary muscles

These tests are often used along with excretory urographic or cystoscopic procedures to evaluate problems with urine flow.

CYSTOMETROGRAPHY

CLIENT PREPARATION. The nurse explains that the purpose of a cystometrogram (CMG) is to determine the effectiveness and sensitivity of the bladder wall (detrusor) muscle. Determinations about bladder capacity, bladder pressure, and voiding reflexes may be made with these measurements of detrusor muscle quality. A urinary catheter may be needed temporarily during the procedure.

PROCEDURE. The nurse asks the client to void normally. The nurse records measurements of the amount, rate of flow, and time of voiding. A urinary catheter is inserted to measure the residual bladder urine volume. The cystometer is attached to the catheter, and fluid is instilled via the catheter into the bladder. The point at which the client first notes a feeling of the urge to void and the point at which the client notes a strong urge to void are recorded. Bladder capacity and bladder pressure readings are recorded graphically. The client is asked to void when the bladder instillation is complete (about 500 mL). The urinary residual after voiding is noted, and the catheter is removed. Electromyography of the perineal muscles may also be performed during the cystometric examination.

FOLLOW-UP CARE. As with any instrumentation of the urinary tract, the nurse monitors for infection. The client's temperature, the characteristics of the urine, and the amount of urine output are recorded.

URETHRAL PRESSURE PROFILE

CLIENT PREPARATION. The nurse explains that a urethral pressure profile (also called a urethral pressure profilometry [UPP]) can provide information about the nature of urinary incontinence or urinary retention. A urinary catheter may be temporarily placed during the procedure.

PROCEDURE. A special catheter with pressure-sensing capabilities is inserted into the bladder. Variations in the pressure of the smooth muscle of the urethra are recorded as the catheter is slowly withdrawn.

FOLLOW-UP CARE. As with other studies involving instrumentation of the urinary tract, the client is monitored for the development of infection.

ELECTROMYOGRAPHY

CLIENT PREPARATION. The nurse explains that electromyography (EMG) of the perineal muscles may be useful in evaluating the strength of the muscles used in voiding. This information may assist in identifying methods of improving continence. The nurse informs the client that some temporary discomfort may accompany placement of the electrodes.

PROCEDURE. In EMG of the perineal muscles, electrodes are placed in either the rectum or the urethra to measure muscle contraction and relaxation.

FOLLOW-UP CARE. After the completion of EMG, the nurse administers analgesics to promote the client's comfort. Any discomfort is usually mild and of short duration.

URINE STREAM TEST

CLIENT PREPARATION. The nurse explains that a urine stream test evaluates pelvic muscle strength and the effectiveness of pelvic muscles in interrupting the flow of urine. It is useful in evaluating urinary incontinence.

PROCEDURE. Three to five seconds after urination begins, the examiner gives the client a signal to stop urine flow. The length of time required to interrupt the flow of urine is recorded.

FOLLOW-UP CARE. Cleansing of the perineal area, as after any voiding, is all that is necessary after the urine stream test.

CRITICAL THINKING CHALLENGE

The client, a 62-year-old woman with type 2 diabetes, is scheduled to have a percutaneous biopsy of the left kidney. She asks you whether she should take her oral antidiabetic medicine in the morning before the procedure. She also asks if the procedure will be painful and if she can attend her card party the evening after the procedure.

- Should this client take her usual antidiabetic medication before the procedure? Why or why not?
- What will you tell this client about activity restrictions?
- How will you reassure this client about pain management during and after the procedure?

For suggested answer guidelines, go to 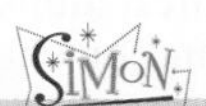 http://www.wbsaunders.com/SIMON/Iggy/.

ONLINE RESOURCES

For suggested readings and Internet resources, go to http://www.wbsaunders.com/SIMON/Iggy/.

SELECTED BIBLIOGRAPHY

Asterisk indicates a classic or definitive work on this subject.

Beck, L.H. (1998). Changes in renal function with aging. *Clinics in Geriatric Medicine, 14*(2), 199-209.

Brenner, B.M. (Eds.). (2000). *Brenner & Rector's The kidney* (6th ed.). Philadelphia: W.B. Saunders.

Cohan, R.H., & Ellis, J.H. (1997). Iodinated contrast material in uroradiology: Choice of agent and management of complications. *Urologic Clinics of North America, 24*(3), 471-491.

*Driver, D.S. (1996). Renal assessment: Back to basics. *American Nephrology Nurses' Association Journal, 23*(4), 361-368.

Duthrie, E.H., & Katz, P.R. (1998). *Practice of geriatrics* (3rd ed.). Philadelphia: W.B. Saunders.

Gordon, M. (2000). *Manual of nursing diagnosis* (9th ed.). St. Louis: Mosby.

Guyton, A.C., & Hall, J.E. (2000). *Textbook of medical physiology* (10th ed.). Philadelphia: W.B. Saunders.

*Holechek, M.J. (1992). Glomerular filtration and renal hemodynamics. *American Nephrology Nurses' Association Journal, 19*(3), 237-245.

Jarvis, C. (2000). *Physical examination and health assessment* (3rd ed.) Philadelphia: W.B. Saunders.

Krop, J.S., et al. (1999). A community-based study of the explanatory factors for the excess risk for early renal function decline in blacks vs whites with diabetes: The atherosclerosis risk in communities study. *Archives of Internal Medicine, 159*(15), 1777-1783.

*Lancaster, L.E. (Ed.). (1995). *Core curriculum for nephrology nursing* (3rd ed.). Pitman, NJ: A.J. Janetti.

Little, C. (2000). Renovascular hypertension. *American Journal of Nursing, 100*(2), 46-51.

Pagana, K., & Pagana, T. (1999). *Diagnostic testing and nursing implications: A case study approach.* St. Louis: Mosby.

Pfister, S.M. (1999). Bladder diaries and voiding patterns in older adults. *Journal of Gerontological Nursing, 25*(3), 36-41.

*Preisig, P. (1994). Renal acidification. *American Nephrology Nurses' Association Journal, 21*(4), 251-257.

*Radke, K.J. (1994). The aging kidney: Structure, function, and nursing practice implications. *American Nephrology Nurses' Association Journal, 21*(4), 181-193.

Shinopulos, N. (2000). Bedside urodynamic studies: Simple testing for urinary incontinence. *The Nurse Practitioner, 25*(6), 19-20, 22, 25-26, 28, 33-34, 37.

*Shulman, N.B., & Hall, W.D. (1991). Renal vascular disease in African-Americans and other racial minorities. *Circulation, 83*(4), 1477-1479.

Stanton, B.A., & Koeppen, B.M. (1998). The kidney. In R.M. Berne et al. (Eds.), *Physiology* (4th ed.). St. Louis: Mosby.

Stark, J. (1998). Interpretation of BUN and creatinine. *Critical Care Nursing Clinics of North America, 10*(4), 491-496.

U.S. Renal Data Systems. (1999). *USRDS 1999 annual data report.* Bethesda, MD: The National Institutes of Health, National Institute of Diabetes and Digestive and Kidney Diseases.

*Valtin, H., & Schafer, J.A. (1995). *Renal function* (3rd ed.). Boston: Little, Brown.

Walsh, P.C., et al. (1998). *Campbell's urology* (7th ed.). Philadelphia: W.B. Saunders.

*Yucha, C., & Keen, M. (1996). Renal regulation of extracellular fluid volume and osmolality. *American Nephrology Nurses' Association Journal, 23*(5), 487-497.

CHAPTER 70

Interventions for Clients with Urinary Problems

CHRIS WINKELMAN

Learning Objectives

After studying this chapter, you should be able to:

1. Describe the clinical manifestations of cystitis.
2. Prioritize educational needs for a person at risk for cystitis.
3. Compare and contrast the pathophysiology and manifestations of stress incontinence, urge incontinence, overflow incontinence, mixed incontinence, and functional incontinence.
4. Prioritize educational needs for the client taking sulfonamide antibiotics for a urinary tract infection.
5. Describe the techniques used to assess pelvic floor strength in the client who is experiencing some incontinence.
6. Explain the proper application of exercises to strengthen pelvic floor muscles.
7. Explain the drug therapy for different types of incontinence.
8. Prioritize nursing care for the client with renal colic.
9. Describe the common clinical manifestations of bladder cancer.
10. Develop a teaching plan for a client who has had a urinary diversion for bladder cancer.

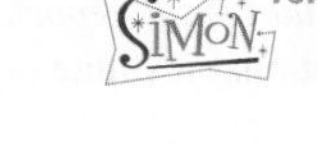

Go to http://www.wbsaunders.com/SIMON/Iggy/ for self-assessment questions related to these Learning Objectives.

Urinary disorders affect the storage or elimination of urine. Both acute and chronic urinary problems are common and costly. More than 20 million people in the United States annually experience urinary tract infections, cystitis, kidney and ureter stones, or urinary incontinence (U.S. Renal Data Systems, 1999). Although life-threatening complications are rare with urinary disorders, clients experience significant functional, physical, and psychosocial changes that adversely affect quality of life. Nursing interventions are directed toward prevention, detection, and management of urologic disorders.

INFECTIOUS DISORDERS

Infections of the urinary tract and kidneys occur often. Symptoms of urinary tract infection (UTI) account for more than 6.5 million health care visits annually in the United States, and 1.5 million hospital discharges involve a diagnosis of UTI (Centers for Disease Control and Prevention [CDC], 2001). In the hospital, UTIs are the most prevalent nosocomial infection (Warren, 1997). Total direct and indirect costs for urologic disorders are estimated at nearly $200 million dollars each year.

The primary site of the infectious process describes infections in the urinary tract. Acute infections in the lower urinary tract include urethritis (urethra), cystitis (bladder), and **prostatitis** (prostate gland). **Acute pyelonephritis** is an upper urinary tract (kidney) infection. It is important to determine the site of infection, since both the site of infection and the specific type of bacteria present determine treatment. A number of structural or functional abnormalities of the urinary tract and characteristics of the urine are thought to predispose clients to UTIs (Table 70-1).

Cystitis

OVERVIEW

Cystitis is an inflammation of the urinary bladder. It can be caused by infection from bacteria, viruses, fungi, or parasites. Infectious cystitis is the most common of the UTIs. Noninfectious cystitis is caused by chemicals or radiation. Interstitial cystitis is an inflammatory process of unknown etiology.

Pathophysiology

Infectious agents, most commonly bacteria, typically move up the urinary tract from the external urethra to the bladder. Less typically, spread of infection through the blood and lymph fluid can occur. Once bacteria enter the urinary tract, several factors influence the outcome (Table 70-2).

Asymptomatic bacteriuria is more common in older adults and is generally considered a benign condition. No studies have demonstrated a relationship between asymptomatic bacteriuria and progression to acute infection or renal insuffi-

TABLE 70-1 • FACTORS CONTRIBUTING TO URINARY TRACT INFECTIONS

Factor	Mechanism	Interventions
Obstruction	Incomplete bladder emptying creates a continuous pool of urine where bacteria can grow, prevents flushing out of bacteria, and allows bacteria to ascend more easily to higher structures.	Relieve or bypass the obstruction to promote complete bladder emptying.
	Bacteria have a greater chance of multiplying the longer they remain in residual urine.	Increase liquids to dilute urine and encourage more frequent voiding.
	Overdistention of the bladder damages the mucosa and allows bacteria to invade the bladder wall.	Use intermittent catheterization to keep the bladder from becoming distended.
Calculi	Large calculi can cause obstruction to urine flow.	Remove calculi and/or treat the underlying condition that causes the calculi to form.
	The rough surface of a calculus irritates mucosal surfaces and creates a spot where bacteria can establish and grow.	
	Bacteria can live within calculi and cause reinfection.	
Vesicoureteral reflux	Bacteria-laden urine is forced backward from the bladder up into the ureters and kidneys, where pyelonephritis can develop.	The affected ureters may be able to be surgically reimplanted in the bladder to eliminate the reflux.
	Reflux of sterile urine can cause renal scarring, which may promote renal dysfunction.	
Diabetes mellitus	Excess glucose in urine provides a rich medium for bacterial growth.	Maintain good glucose control in clients with diabetes.
	Peripheral neuropathy affects bladder innervation and leads to a flaccid bladder and incomplete bladder emptying.	
Characteristics of urine	Alkalotic urine promotes bacterial growth.	Acidify urine by taking vitamin C tablets, not citrus fruits. Such fruits make the urine alkaline.
	Concentrated urine promotes bacterial growth.	Increase urine dilution by increasing fluid intake.
Gender	Female clients are susceptible to periurethral colonization with coliform bacteria.	Explain the importance of perineal hygiene (wiping front to back) to prevent large amounts of coliform bacteria from remaining in the perineal area.
	Bladder displacement during pregnancy predisposes women to cystitis and the development of pyelonephritis.	Routine monitoring of pregnant women for UTIs prevents complications.
	A diaphragm or pessary that is too large can cause an obstruction to urine flow or trauma to the urethra.	Be sure diaphragms and pessaries are properly fitted.
Age	Obstruction may be caused by incomplete bladder emptying as a result of an enlarged prostate in men and cystocele and prolapse in women.	Do not rush older clients during toileting; provide regular and private toileting times to promote complete bladder emptying.
	Neuromuscular conditions that cause incomplete bladder emptying, such as Parkinson's disease and strokes, affect older adults more frequently.	Straight catheter for residual and Credé maneuver to promote more complete emptying.
	The use of anticholinergic medications in older adults contributes to delayed bladder emptying.	Monitor and report this medication side effect.
	Fecal incontinence contributes to poor perineal hygiene.	Promptly clean clients after episodes of incontinence.
	Hypoestrogenism in older women adversely affects the cells of the vagina and urethra, making them more susceptible to infections.	Give vaginal estrogen cream as directed to improve the health of the client's vaginal and urethral cells.
Sexual activity	Irritation of the perineum and urethra during intercourse can promote migration of bacteria from the perineal area to the urinary tract in some women.	Empty the bladder before and after intercourse. Drink 8 oz of fluid (especially water) after intercourse.
	Spermicides can alter vaginal pH, increasing potential numbers of pathogens.	Consider alternate method of birth control if experiencing repeated UTIs.
	Inadequate vaginal lubrication may exacerbate potential urethral irritation.	Use an artificial vaginal lubricant.
	Bacteria may be introduced into the man's urethra during anal intercourse or during vaginal intercourse with a woman who has a bacterial vaginitis.	Use a condom.

TABLE 70-2 • IMPORTANT FACTORS INFLUENCING THE OUTCOME OF URINARY TRACT INFECTIONS

Facilitating Aspects	Protective Aspects
ANATOMY	
Females: Short length of the urethra and its proximity to the vagina and rectum facilitate colonization of coliform bacteria. *Males:* With age, the prostate enlarges and may obstruct the normal flow of urine, producing stasis.	*Males:* Long length of the urethra and its distance from the rectum provide protection from colonization with coliform bacteria.
PHYSIOLOGY	
Females: Pregnancy predisposes a woman to ureteral reflux and subsequent pyelonephritis; with age the decline in estrogen facilitates colonization of *E. coli.* *Males:* With age, prostatic secretions lose their antibacterial characteristics and predispose to bacterial proliferation in the urine.	*Females:* Well-estrogenized mucosa in the urethra and trigone may inhibit bacterial colonization. *Males:* Normal prostatic secretions inhibit bacterial growth. *Both males and females:* Mucin is produced by urothelial cells lining the bladder—this helps to maintain mucosal integrity and prevent cellular damage; mucin may also prevent bacteria from adhering to urothelial cells.
TRAUMA	
Females: Vaginal penetration with sexual intercourse may traumatize the urethra and bladder base, leading to postcoital (or honeymoon) cystitis; a vaginal diaphragm that is too large can place pressure on the urethra, causing trauma; vaginal childbirth can cause permanent damage to the urethra. *Males:* Sexually transmitted diseases may cause urethral strictures that obstruct the flow of urine and predispose to urinary stasis. *Both males and females:* Urethral instrumentation (such as catheterization) may disturb the urothelial surface and predispose to adherence of bacteria that would ordinarily not be pathogenic.	*Females:* Adequate lubrication, either natural or artificial, with intercourse may prevent any trauma.
INFECTIOUS AGENT	
Some organisms are better able to adhere to host cells and secrete substances that induce inflammation.	A small inoculum (number of microorganisms introduced into the body) is more easily flushed away by the flow of urine.

ciency in clients without obstructive conditions, reflux, stones, or diabetes mellitus.

Etiology

The most common pathogens in infectious cystitis are organisms from the gastrointestinal (GI) tract. It is estimated that 90% of UTIs are caused by *Escherichia coli.* Other, less common infective organisms include *Staphylococcus saprophyticus, Klebsiella pneumoniae,* and organisms from the *Proteus* and *Enterobacter* species.

In most cases, GI organisms first grow in the perineal area; then move into the urethra as a result of irritation, trauma, or instrumentation of the urinary tract (i.e., catheterization); and ascend to the bladder. Catheters are the most common predisposing factor for UTIs in the hospital setting. Within 48 hours of catheter insertion, bacterial colonization begins. About 50% of clients with indwelling catheters become infected within 1 week of catheterization. The etiology of catheter-related infections varies between genders. Bacteria from a female client's perineal area are more likely to adhere to the outer surface of the catheter and then ascend to the bladder. In male clients, bacteria tend to gain access to the bladder from inside the lumen of the catheter (Warren, 1997). Any break in the closed urinary drainage system provides an opportunity for bacteria to adhere to and migrate through the urinary tract. Best practices to minimize the risk of catheter contamination are listed in Chart 70-1.

Organisms other than bacteria can cause cystitis. Fungal infections, such as those caused by *Candida,* may develop during long-term antibiotic therapy, since antibiotics alter normal flora. Clients who are severely immunocompromised and have decreased resistance to infection, are receiving glucocorticosteroids or other immunosuppressive agents, or have diabetes mellitus or acquired immunodeficiency syndrome (AIDS) are also at risk for fungal UTIs.

Viral and parasitic infections are rare and usually accompany an infection in another site. For example, *Trichomonas,* a parasite found in the vagina, can also be found in the urine. Treatment of the vaginal infection (see Chapter 75) is usually sufficient to treat the UTI.

Noninfectious cystitis may result from chemical exposure, such as to drugs (e.g., cyclophosphamide [Cytoxan, Procytox♣]), from radiation therapy, and from immunologic responses, as with systemic lupus erythematosus (SLE).

Interstitial cystitis is a relatively rare, chronic inflammation of the bladder. The condition affects women more often than men (in a 12:1 ratio), and the diagnosis is difficult to make. The symptoms are identical to those of simple cystitis, but the urgency and bladder pain are more intense (Thompson & Christmas, 1996).

Although cystitis is not life threatening, infectious cystitis can lead to life-threatening complications, including pyelonephritis and sepsis. There is considerable debate about the risk for kidney tissue damage and subsequent kidney failure as a result of bacteria ascending from the bladder to the kidney. Most experts believe that severe deterioration of renal function is a rare complication without one or more predisposing factors, such as anatomic abnormalities, pregnancy, obstruction, reflux, calculi, or diabetes mellitus.

The spread of the infecting agent from the urinary tract to systemic circulation is termed **urosepsis. Sepsis** from any

CHART 70-1

BEST PRACTICE *for* Minimizing Catheter-Related Infection

- Avoid long-term use (>3 days) during active illness or perioperatively.
- Use aseptic routine when handling catheter devices; manipulation can promote an environment favorable to pathogens.
- Use strict sterile technique to insert the catheter (in the hospital setting); a break in technique can introduce pathogens into the urinary tract.
- Ensure that catheter tubing connections are sealed securely; disconnections can introduce pathogens into the urinary tract.
- Keep urine collection bags below the level of the bladder at all times; elevating the collection bag above the bladder causes reflux of pathogens from the bag into the urinary tract.
- Secure the catheter to the client's thigh (female) or lower abdomen (male); catheter movement can cause urethral friction and irritation.
- Perform daily catheter care by washing the perineum and proximal portion of the catheter with soap and water, drying gently (removes pathogens and reduces pathogenic population).
- *Application of antiseptic solutions or antibiotic ointments to the perineal area of catheterized clients has not been demonstrated to have any beneficial effect.*

source is a systemic infection that can lead to overwhelming organ failure, shock, and death. The most common cause of sepsis in the hospitalized client is a UTI (Warren, 1997). Sepsis is associated with high mortality and prolonged hospitalization (see Chapter 37).

Incidence/Prevalence

The incidence of UTI is second only to that of upper respiratory infections in primary care. Clients who have the symptoms of **frequency** (an urge to urinate frequently in small amounts), **dysuria** (pain and/or burning with urination), and **urgency** (the feeling that urination will occur immediately) account for more than 5 million health care visits annually. Approximately 50% of these clients will have a confirmed UTI. Recurrent infections account for an unknown number of these visits (CDC, 2001).

WOMEN'S HEALTH CONSIDERATIONS

The prevalence of UTIs varies with age and gender. Generally, women are more commonly affected with UTIs than men. In men 65 to 70 years old, the incidence of UTI is 3%; after age 70, however, the incidence is 20%. In women over the age of 80, the prevalence rises from 20% to 50% (Duffield, 1997). It is believed that skin and mucous membrane changes from a lack of estrogen account for much of the increased risk.

COLLABORATIVE MANAGEMENT

Assessment

PHYSICAL ASSESSMENT/CLINICAL MANIFESTATIONS

Frequency, urgency, and dysuria are the primary clinical manifestations of a urinary tract infection (UTI), but other signs and symptoms may be present (Chart 70-2). Urine may be cloudy, foul smelling, or blood tinged. Identifying risk factors contributing to UTI are included in the assessment (see Table 70-1).

CHART 70-2

KEY FEATURES *of* Urinary Tract Infection

Common Clinical Manifestations

- Frequency
- Urgency
- Dysuria
- Hesitancy or difficulty in initiating urine stream
- Low back pain
- Nocturia
- Incontinence
- Retention
- Suprapubic tenderness or fullness
- Feeling of incomplete bladder emptying

Rare Clinical Manifestations

- Fever
- Chills
- Nausea
- Vomiting
- Malaise
- Flank pain

Atypical Clinical Manifestations That May Occur in the Older Adult

- The only symptom may be something as vague as increasing mental confusion or frequent, unexplained falls.
- A sudden onset of incontinence or a worsening of incontinence may be the only symptom of an early UTI.
- Fever, tachycardia, tachypnea, and hypotension, even without any urinary symptoms, may be signs of urosepsis.
- Loss of appetite, nocturia, and dysuria are common symptoms.

UTI, Urinary tract infection.

Before performing the physical assessment, the nurse asks the client to void so that the urine can be examined and the bladder emptied before palpation. The nurse assesses vital signs to help rule out sepsis, inspects the lower abdomen, and palpates the urinary bladder. Distention after voiding indicates incomplete bladder emptying.

Using standard precautions (see Chapter 26), the nurse notes inflammation and any skin lesions around the urethral meatus and vaginal introitus (opening). Female clients often report "burning with urination" when normal, acidic urine touches labial tissues that are inflamed and ulcerated by vaginal infections or sexually transmitted diseases (STDs). Privacy is maintained with drapes during the examination.

The prostate is palpated by rectal examination for size, alteration in contour, and any evidence of tenderness. The physician or advanced-practice nurse performs the rectal prostate assessment.

LABORATORY ASSESSMENT

Laboratory evaluation for a UTI is usually a urinalysis with a microscopic count of bacteria, white blood cells (WBCs), and red blood cells (RBCs). The presence of 100,000 colonies/mL and/or the presence of WBCs **(pyuria)** indicate an infection. A urinalysis is performed on a clean-catch midstream specimen. If the client cannot produce a clean-catch specimen, the nurse may need to obtain the specimen with a small-caliber (6 Fr) urethral catheter. For a routine urinalysis, 10 mL of urine is required; smaller quantities are sufficient for culture.

A urine culture confirms the type of microorganism and the number of colonies. Urine culture is expensive and takes 48 hours to obtain results. It is indicated when the UTI is complicated or not responsive to usual therapy or if the diagnosis is uncertain. The presence of a UTI is confirmed when there are more than 10^5 colony-forming units in the urine from any client, although in a symptomatic client as few as 10^3 colony-forming units may be diagnostic. Multiple organisms in low colony counts generally indicate a contaminated specimen.

Sensitivity testing follows culture results, especially when complicating factors are present, such as stones or recurrent infection, or when the client is older.

Occasionally the serum WBC count may be elevated, with the differential WBC count showing "left shift." This shift indicates that the number of immature WBCs is increasing in response to the infectious organisms. Consequently, the number of bands, or immature WBCs, is elevated. Left shift most commonly occurs with urosepsis and rarely occurs with uncomplicated cystitis.

OTHER DIAGNOSTIC ASSESSMENT

The clinician usually bases the diagnosis of cystitis on the history, physical examination, and laboratory data. If urinary retention and obstruction to urinary outflow are suspected, urography, abdominal sonography, or computed tomography (CT) may be needed to determine the site of obstruction or the presence of calculi. Voiding cystourethrography (see Chapter 69) is used for the diagnosis of suspected cases of vesicoureteral reflux.

Cystoscopy (see Chapter 69) is often performed when there is a history of recurrent UTIs (more than three or four a year). The urine is sterilized with antibiotic therapy before the procedure so that the risk of sepsis is not increased. Cystoscopy can identify abnormalities that may have contributed to the development of cystitis. These abnormalities include bladder calculi, bladder diverticula, urethral strictures, foreign bodies (such as sutures from previous surgery), and **trabeculation** (an abnormal thickening of the bladder wall caused by urinary retention and obstruction). Retrograde pyelography, along with the cystoscopic examination, produces outlines and images of the drainage tract. Areas of obstruction or malformation and the presence of reflux are then identified early.

Cystoscopy is the only means of accurately diagnosing interstitial cystitis. A urinalysis may show WBCs and RBCs but no bacteria. Classic findings in interstitial cystitis include a small-capacity bladder, the presence of **Hunner's ulcers** (a type of bladder lesion), and small hemorrhages after bladder distention.

Interventions

NONSURGICAL MANAGEMENT

DRUG THERAPY. Medications prescribed to treat bacteriuria and promote comfort in the client with cystitis include urinary antiseptics or antibiotics, analgesics, and antispasmodics. The clinician prescribes antibiotics to treat any infection (Chart 70-3). Antifungal agents are administered when the infecting organism is a fungus. Amphotericin B is most often given in daily bladder instillations, and ketoconazole (Nizoral) is given in oral or parenteral form. The antispasmodic agents decrease bladder spasm and promote complete bladder emptying.

Antibiotic therapy is the usual prescription for a UTI (see Chart 70-3). Guidelines for UTIs in women indicate that a 3-day course of trimethoprim/sulfamethoxazole or fosfomycin is effective in eradicating an uncomplicated, community-acquired UTI (Houston, 1999). These shorter courses increase compliance and reduce cost. A longer treatment course of 7 to 21 days with oral or parenteral antibiotics is required for hospitalized clients; those with complicating factors, such as indwelling catheters or calculi; and those with a history of diabetes or immunosuppression.

> **WOMEN'S HEALTH CONSIDERATIONS**
> Pregnant women require vigorous intervention when bacteriuria is identified because of the tendency of simple cystitis to lead to acute pyelonephritis. Pyelonephritis in pregnancy can cause preterm labor and deleterious effects on the fetus.

Long-term antibiotic therapy is recommended for the treatment of chronic, recurring infections caused by structural abnormalities or calculi. Trimethoprim 100 mg daily may be prescribed for long-term management of the older client with frequent UTIs (Duffield, 1997). For women who experience recurrent UTIs after sexual intercourse, 1 low-dose tablet of nitrofurantoin (Macrodantin, Nephronex♣, Novofuran♣) after intercourse is often recommended.

NIC ***URINARY ELIMINATION.*** The goal is to maintain an optimal urinary elimination pattern. Interventions for the management of cystitis are highlighted in Chart 70-4.

DIET THERAPY. The diet should include all food groups and include a number of calories for the increased metabolic processes associated with infection. Unless medically contraindicated, fluid intake needs to be at least 2 to 3 L/day for adequate flushing of urine through the system. Evidence suggests that 300 mL of cranberry juice consumed daily decreases bacterial adherence to the urinary tract, decreasing the incidence of UTIs in some clients. Cranberry juice must be consumed for 3 to 4 weeks to be effective (Walsh et al., 1998).

OTHER PAIN RELIEF MEASURES. A warm sitz bath taken two or three times a day for 20 minutes may provide comfort and some relief of local symptoms. If burning with urination is severe or urinary retention occurs, the nurse instructs the client to sit in the sitz bath and urinate into the warm water.

SURGICAL MANAGEMENT. Surgical interventions for clients with cystitis treat the conditions that predispose to recurrent UTIs (e.g., removal of obstructions, treatment of calculi, and repair of vesicoureteral reflux). Procedures may include cystoscopy (see Chapter 69) to identify and remove calculi or obstructions.

Community-Based Care

The nurse assesses the client's level of understanding from his or her description of the problem. The client's knowledge about factors contributing to the development of cystitis is the basis on which further teaching interventions are planned.

CHART 70-3

DRUG THERAPY *for* Urinary Tract Infection

Drug	Usual Dosage	Nursing Interventions	Rationale
ANTIMICROBIALS			
Quinolones		Avoid use in pregnancy and those <18 yr.	Can interfere with cartilage formation in weight-bearing joints.
Ciprofloxacin (Cipro)	250 mg bid PO for 3 days with uncomplicated cystitis, for 7 days with complicated cystitis, and for 10-14 days with uncomplicated pyelonephritis	Avoid taking with aluminum- or magnesium-containing antacids. Give 1 hr before or 2 hr after food or drink. Avoid caffeinated beverages, and use with caution in clients receiving theophylline.	Food, calcium, and antacids interfere with drug adsorption. Quinolones prolong the half-life of caffeine and theophylline.
Lomefloxacin (Maxaquin)	400 mg qd PO for 3 days for uncomplicated cystitis, for 7 days for complicated cystitis, and for 10-14 days for uncomplicated pyelonephritis	As above. Avoid the sun.	As above. Drug causes photosensitivity.
Levofloxacin (Levaquin)	250 mg qd PO for 3 days for uncomplicated cystitis, for 7 days for complicated cystitis, and for 10-14 days for uncomplicated pyelonephritis	As above. Avoid the sun.	As above. Drug causes photosensitivity.
Norfloxacin (Noroxin)	400 mg bid PO for 3 days for uncomplicated cystitis, for 7 days for complicated cystitis, and for 10-14 days for uncomplicated pyelonephritis	As above.	As above.
Ofloxacin (Floxin)	200 mg bid PO for 3 days for uncomplicated cystitis, for 7 days for complicated cystitis, and for 10-14 days for uncomplicated pyelonephritis	As above.	As above.
Sparfloxacin (Zagam)	400 mg PO for 1 day, then 200 mg/day for 2 days for uncomplicated cystitis, for 7 days for complicated cystitis, and for 10-14 days for uncomplicated pyelonephritis	As above.	As above.
Penicillins		Inquire about penicillin allergy.	
Amoxicillin (Amoxil)	500 mg bid PO for 3 days	Give with food.	Food reduces GI upset.
Amoxicillin/clavulanate (Augmentin, Clavulin♣)	500 mg bid PO for 3 days	Give with food.	Food reduces GI upset.
Cephalosporins		Inquire about allergy to cephalosporin or penicillin.	There is a 1% to 20% cross-reactivity between penicillin and cephalosporins.
Cefadroxil (Duricef)	1000 mg qd PO for 3 days for uncomplicated cystitis, or 1000 mg bid for 10 days for complicated cystitis		
Cefixime (Suprax)	400 mg PO qd for 3 days for uncomplicated cystitis, for 7 days for complicated cystitis, and for 10-14 days for uncomplicated pyelonephritis		
Fosfomycin (Monurol)	3 g PO (1 packet) as a single dose	Avoid use of GI drugs during dosing.	Less effective if given with drugs that increase GI motility.

GI, Gastrointestinal; *G6PD*, glucose-6-phosphate dehydrogenase deficiency.

Continued

CHART 70-3

DRUG THERAPY *for* Urinary Tract Infection—cont'd

Drug	Usual Dosage	Nursing Interventions	Rationale
SULFONAMIDE			
Trimethoprim/ sulfamethoxazole (Bactrim, Septra, Sulfatrim Roubac✤)	1 double-strength tablet (DS or 160/800 mg), for 3 or 10 days for uncomplicated cystitis, or single-strength PO (80/400 mg) after coitus for prophylaxis	Provide adequate fluid intake. Avoid ascorbic acid and ammonium chloride that acidify the urine.	Sulfa can crystallize in acidic or concentrated urine.
		Use with caution in clients with asthma, G6PD deficiency, or multiple allergies.	Sulfa allergies are relatively common; monitor client for potential reaction.
URINARY ANTISEPTIC			
Nitrofurantoin (Macrobid Macrodantin, Nephronex✤, Novofuran✤)	*Macrobid:* 100 mg bid PO for 7 days *Macrodantin:* 100 mg qid PO for 7 days	Give with food or milk. Monitor for flu-like symptoms in older clients and in those with pulmonary disease.	Food or milk decreases GI upset. Rare case of interstitial pneumonitis can occur in susceptible clients.
ANALGESIC			
Phenazopyridine (Pyridium, Phenazo✤)	100-200 mg PO tid for 2-3 days	Give with food. Advise client that urine will become red or orange.	Food helps reduce GI upset. Urine discoloration is normal.
		Help the client to understand the difference between a urinary analgesic and antibiotic.	A complete dosing schedule is not necessary.
ANTISPASMODIC			
Hyoscyamine (Anaspaz, Cystospaz-M, others)	0.125-0.5 PO tid and hs	Assess for safety, constipation, and urinary retention.	Anticholinergics cause drowsiness, blurred vision, dry mouth, constipation, and urinary retention.

GI, Gastrointestinal; *G6PD,* glucose-6-phosphate dehydrogenase deficiency.

CHART 70-4

NIC INTERVENTION ACTIVITIES *for* The Client with a Urinary Tract Infection

Urinary Elimination Management: *Maintenance of an optimum urinary elimination pattern*
- Monitor urinary elimination, including frequency, consistency, odor, volume, and color, as appropriate.
- Teach client signs and symptoms of urinary tract infection.
- Obtain midstream voided specimen for analysis, as appropriate.
- Refer to physician if signs and symptoms of urinary tract infection occur.
- Instruct to respond immediately to urge to void, as appropriate.
- Teach client to drink 8 ounces of liquid with meals, between meals, and in early evening.
- Assist client with development of toileting routine, as appropriate.

NIC intervention activities selected from McCloskey, J.C., & Bulechek, G.M. (Eds.). (2000). *Nursing interventions classification (NIC)* (3rd ed.). St. Louis: Mosby.

The client is instructed in self-administration of medications. Appropriate spacing of doses throughout the day and the need to complete all of the prescribed medication are stressed. If the drug will change the color of the urine, as it does with phenazopyridine (Pyridium, Pyronium), the nurse informs the client to expect this occurrence. The nurse offers techniques for remembering the medication schedule, such as the use of a daily calendar or the association of medications with usual activities (e.g., mealtimes).

Clients may associate symptoms of discomfort with sexual activities and experience feelings of guilt and embarrassment. Frank and sensitive discussions with a woman who experiences frequent recurrences of UTI after sexual intercourse can help her find appropriate techniques to handle the problem (see Table 70-1). The nurse explores with the woman the factors that contribute to her postcoital infections, such as diaphragm use and her general resistance to infection. The client is reminded that vigorous cleaning of the perineum with harsh soaps and vaginal douching may irritate the perineal tissues and actually increase the risk of UTI. At the client's request, the nurse discusses the problem with the client and her partner to help them find ways of maintaining their intimate relationship. Chart 70-5 gives other specific instructions for preventing UTIs.

Urethritis

OVERVIEW

Urethritis is an inflammation of the urethra that causes symptoms similar to urinary tract infection (UTI). In male clients, signs and symptoms of urethritis are burning or difficulty with urination and usually a discharge from the urethral meatus. The most common cause of urethritis in men is sexually transmitted diseases (STDs): gonorrhea or nonspecific urethritis caused by *Ureaplasma* (a gram-negative bacterium),

CHART 70-5

CLIENT EDUCATION GUIDE
Preventing a Urinary Tract Infection

- Drink 2 to 3 L of fluid every day.
- Drink 300 mL of cranberry juice daily.
- Be sure to get enough sleep, rest, and nutrition daily.
- [For women] Clean your perineum (the area between your legs) from front to back.
- [For women] Avoid irritating substances, such as bubble bath, nylon underwear, and scented toilet tissue. Wear loose-fitting cotton underwear.
- [For women] Empty your bladder before and after intercourse.
- If you experience burning when you urinate, if you have to urinate frequently, or if you find it difficult to begin urinating, notify your physician or other health care provider right away, especially if you have a chronic medical condition (such as diabetes).
- Empty your bladder as soon as you feel the urge to urinate.
- Empty your bladder regularly (e.g., every 4 hours), even if you do not feel the urge to urinate.
- You may try the following home therapies:
  - Apple cider vinegar, 2 tablespoons three times per day in juice.
  - Echinacea (herb), one dropperful three times per day in juice or herbal tea (Duffield, 1997).
  - Vitamin C 500 mg/day to acidify the urine.
- To prevent recurrent infection:
  - Take your medication as directed even after the symptoms go away.
  - Schedule a follow-up appointment for 10 to 14 days after you finish taking your medication. At your follow-up visit, another urine sample may be taken for analysis or culture.

Chlamydia (a prevalent sexually transmitted gram-negative bacterium), or *Trichomonas vaginalis* (a protozoan found in both the male and female genital tract).

In female clients, urethritis causes symptoms similar to those of bacterial cystitis. Urethritis is known by several synonyms: *pyuria-dysuria syndrome, frequency-dysuria syndrome, trigonitis syndrome,* and *urethral syndrome.* Urethritis is most common in postmenopausal women and is probably caused by tissue changes related to low estrogen levels.

COLLABORATIVE MANAGEMENT

Assessment

The nurse asks the client about a history of STD, painful or difficult urination, discharge from the penis or vagina, and internal discomfort in the lower abdomen. Urinalysis may show **pyuria** (white blood cells [WBCs]) without a significant number of bacteria; however, results of urethral culture may indicate an STD. In female clients, the diagnosis may be made by exclusion when urinalysis and urethral culture are negative for bacteria and symptoms persist. In such cases, pelvic examination may show symptoms of **hypoestrogenism** (tissue changes from low estrogen levels) in the vagina; cystourethroscopy may show hypoestrogenism with inflammation of urethral tissues.

Interventions

STDs and infectious processes are treated with appropriate antibiotic therapy. Further information on STDs can be found in Chapter 74.

Postmenopausal women with urethral syndrome often have improvement in their urethral symptoms with the use of estrogen vaginal cream. Estrogen cream applied locally to the vagina increases the amount of estrogen in the urethra as well, and irritating symptoms are reduced.

NONINFECTIOUS DISORDERS

Urethral Strictures

OVERVIEW

Urethral strictures are narrowed areas of the urethra. These problems may be caused by complications of an STD (usually gonorrhea) and from trauma during catheterization, urologic instrumentation, or childbirth. Strictures occur more often in men than in women and may be an important factor in other urologic conditions, such as recurrent UTIs, urinary incontinence, and urinary retention.

COLLABORATIVE MANAGEMENT

The most common symptom of urethral stricture is obstruction to the flow of urine; strictures rarely cause pain. Because stasis of urine can result when flow is obstructed, the client with a stricture is more likely to develop a UTI and have overflow incontinence. **Overflow incontinence** is the involuntary loss of urine when the bladder is overdistended. The nurse assesses the client for these two problems.

A urethral stricture is usually treated surgically. Dilation of the urethra (using a local anesthetic) is a temporary measure, not a curative one. The best chance of long-term cure is with **urethroplasty,** a surgical procedure in which the affected area is removed or grafted to create a larger opening for the passage of urine. The recurrence rate with surgical interventions is still high, and most clients need repeated procedures.

Urinary Incontinence

OVERVIEW

Continence (control over the time and place of urination) is a unique accomplishment of humans and certain domestic animals. Continence is a learned behavior whereby a person can suppress the urge to urinate until a socially appropriate (culturally prescribed) location is available (e.g., a toilet). Efficient bladder emptying (i.e., coordination between bladder contraction and urethral relaxation) is required for continence. Continence is learned in early childhood through toilet training and is generally accomplished by age 5 years.

Incontinence is an involuntary loss of urine severe enough to cause social or hygienic problems. Incontinence is *not* a normal consequence of aging or childbirth. Because of the stigma associated with incontinence and the belief that it is normal in the older adult, incontinence is one of the most underreported health problems. Many people suffer in silence, socially isolated and unaware that treatment is available.

The Agency for Healthcare Research and Quality (AHRQ) (formerly the Agency for Health Care Policy and Research [AHCPR]) chose urinary incontinence as one of its first topics for Clinical Practice Guidelines. The agency's goal is to educate the public and health care professionals about assessment and management of this condition (AHCPR, 1992, 1996).

TABLE 70-3 • TYPES OF URINARY INCONTINENCE

Type	Definition/Description	Cause	Clinical Manifestations
Stress incontinence	The involuntary loss of urine during activities that increase abdominal and detrusor pressure Clients cannot tighten the urethra sufficiently to overcome the increased detrusor pressure; leakage of urine results	Weakening of bladder neck supports; associated with childbirth Intrinsic sphincter deficiency caused by such congenital conditions as epispadias (abnormal location of the urethra on the dorsum of the penis) or myelomenigocele Acquired anatomic damage to the urethral sphincter (from repeated incontinence surgeries, prostatectomy, radiation therapy, and trauma)	Urine loss with physical exertion, cough, sneeze, or exercise Usually only small amounts of urine are lost with each exertion Normal voiding habits (≤8 times per day, 2 or fewer times per night) Postvoid residual usually ≤50 mL Pelvic examination shows hypermobility of the urethra or bladder neck with Valsalva maneuvers
Urge incontinence	The involuntary loss of urine associated with a strong desire to urinate Clients cannot suppress the signal from the bladder muscle to the brain that it is time to urinate	Unknown	An abrupt and strong urge to void May have loss of large amounts of urine with each occurrence
Detrusor hyperreflexia (reflex incontinence)	The abnormal detrusor contractions result from neurologic abnormalities	Central nervous system (CNS) lesions from stroke, multiple sclerosis, and parasacral spinal cord lesions Local irritating factors such as caffeine, medications, or bladder tumor	Postvoid residual >50 mL
Detrusor	No associated neurologic abnormality	Unknown	Postvoid residual ≤50 mL
Overflow incontinence	The involuntary loss of urine associated with overdistention of the bladder when the bladder's capacity has reached its maximum	Diabetic neuropathy; side effects of medication; after radical pelvic surgery or spinal cord damage; outlet obstruction	Bladder distention, often up to the level of the umbilicus Constant dribbling of urine
	The urethra is obstructed, so it fails to relax sufficiently to allow urine to flow, resulting in incomplete bladder emptying or complete urinary retention, causing overflow incontinence	Causes external to the mechanism of the urethra include an enlarged prostate (male clients) and large genital prolapse (female clients) When the cause is intrinsic to the urethra, abnormal contraction of the skeletal muscle occurs, causing obstruction; this condition, called *detrusor dyssynergia,* is seen in clients with spinal cord injuries and multiple sclerosis	

Pathophysiology

Continence occurs when pressure in the urethra is greater than pressure in the bladder. For normal voiding to occur, the urethra must relax and the bladder must contract with sufficient pressure and duration to empty completely. Voiding should occur in a smooth and coordinated manner under a person's conscious control. The symptom of urinary incontinence has several possible causes and can be either temporary or chronic (Table 70-3). Temporary causes of incontinence are usually external to the urinary tract and involve no disorder of the urinary tract itself. The most common forms of urinary incontinence in adults are stress incontinence, urge incontinence, overflow incontinence, functional incontinence, and a mixed form.

STRESS INCONTINENCE

The urethra can be relaxed and tightened under conscious control because skeletal muscles of the pelvic floor surround it. When a person feels the urge to urinate, the conscious contraction of the urethra can override a bladder contraction if the urethral contraction is strong enough.

Clients who suffer from *stress incontinence* cannot tighten the urethra sufficiently to overcome the increased detrusor pressure. Stress incontinence is common after childbirth, when the pelvic muscles are stretched and weakened from pregnancy and delivery. The weakened pelvic floor contributes to mobility and displacement of the urethra during exertion. If the pelvic muscles are not properly strengthened, this condition continues. Decreasing amounts of estrogen after menopause also contribute to stress incontinence. Vaginal, urethral, and pelvic floor muscles become thin and weak without estrogen. Stress incontinence is the most common form of incontinence in women.

URGE INCONTINENCE

Bladder contractions are perceived as an urge to urinate. When the bladder is full, contraction of the smooth muscle fibers of the

TABLE 70-3 • TYPES OF URINARY INCONTINENCE—cont'd

Type	Definition/Description	Cause	Clinical Manifestations
Mixed incontinence	A combination of stress, urge, and overflow incontinence	As with each separate disorder	As with each separate disorder
Functional incontinence	Leakage of urine caused by factors other than disease of the lower urinary tract		Quantity and timing of urine leakage vary; patterns are difficult to discern
Transient causes	Transient causes will improve with treatment of the underlying condition	Loss of cognitive functioning Loss of awareness that urination is to occur in a socially acceptable place	Altered mental state, as in delirium, confusion, depression, dementia, sepsis, mental illness, or severe psychologic stress
		Abnormal openings in the urinary tract, such as a fistula or diverticulum	Urinary drainage noted from areas other than the urinary meatus
		Medications, such as sedatives, hypnotics, diuretics, anticholinergics, decongestants, antihypertensives, and calcium channel blockers	Some medications cause altered mental state; others cause increased urine production
		Diabetes insipidus or psychogenic polydipsia	Increased urine output
		Inability to get to toileting facilities	Restraints, restricted mobility
		Direct bladder pressure or urethral obstruction	Constipation or fecal impaction
Permanent causes	Permanent causes are organic but may be improved with treatment	Cognitive impairment Traumatic or surgical effects Those factors contributing to stress incontinence, urge incontinence, and overflow incontinence Structural or functional defects of the bladder or the sphincters Injuries or diseases of the spinal cord, brainstem, or cerebral cortex (neurogenic bladder) Congenital defects, including exstrophy of the bladder (bladder turned "inside out") and spina bifida	Clinical manifestations depend on the cause

bladder detrusor muscle normally signals the brain that it is time to urinate. Continent persons override that signal and relax the detrusor muscle for the time it takes to locate a toilet. Those who suffer from urge incontinence cannot suppress the signal. Abnormal detrusor contractions may be a result of neurologic abnormalities or may occur with no known abnormality.

OVERFLOW INCONTINENCE

When the detrusor muscle fails to respond by contracting, the bladder becomes overdistended. Overflow incontinence (also known as reflex incontinence) occurs when the bladder has reached its absolute maximal capacity and some urine must leak out to prevent bladder rupture. Causes for the underactive **(acontractile)** bladder may or may not be determined.

The urethra can also be obstructed so that it fails to relax enough to allow urine flow. Incomplete bladder emptying or complete urinary retention due to urethral obstruction results in overflow incontinence.

MIXED INCONTINENCE

Many clients with urinary incontinence fall into the mixed category. Their signs and symptoms have aspects of more than one of the major subtypes. This category is more common in older women.

FUNCTIONAL INCONTINENCE

Factors other than the abnormal function of the bladder and urethra also result in functional incontinence. The most common factor is a loss of cognitive function in clients affected by dementia. To maintain continence, a person must be aware that urination needs to occur in a socially acceptable place; clients with dementia may not have that awareness.

Etiology

Incontinence may have temporary or permanent causes. Evaluation of the incontinent client means considering all possible causes, beginning with those that are temporary and correctable. Surgical and traumatic causes of urinary incontinence are usually related to procedures or surgery in the lower pelvic structures, areas that are richly supplied by complex nerve pathways. Radical urologic, prostatic, and gynecologic procedures associated with pelvic cancers may result in postsurgical urinary incontinence. Trauma that injures segments S2 to S4 of the spinal cord may cause incontinence from interruption of normal nerve pathways.

Inappropriate bladder contraction may result from disorders of the brain and nervous system or from bladder irritation due to chronic infection, stones, chemotherapy, or radiation therapy. Failure of bladder contraction accompanies the autonomic neuropathy associated with diabetes mellitus and syphilis.

Costs associated with incontinence are enormous. The Cost of Care box below gives information about the individual and institutional considerations in providing continence care.

CONSIDERATIONS FOR OLDER ADULTS
Numerous factors contribute to the increased incidence of urinary incontinence in older adults (Chart 70-6). An older person may have decreased mobility from disease, neurologic dysfunction, or musculoskeletal degeneration. In the hospital or extended care setting, mobility is further limited when the older client is restrained or placed on bedrest. Vision and hearing impairments may also prevent the client from locating a call bell to notify the nurse or assistive nursing personnel of the need to void. The nurse assesses for these factors and, if possible, minimizes them to prevent urinary incontinence.

Incidence/Prevalence

Urinary incontinence is a significant health problem that affects more than 13 million people of all ages in the United States (AHCPR, 1996); about 85% are women. The disorder is particularly common in older adults, including 15% to 30% of community-dwelling older people and at least one half of all nursing home residents (AHCPR, 1996).

In adult clients under 65 years of age, urinary incontinence occurs twice as often in women as in men. Incontinence in women of this age may occur after one or more pregnancies. Men in this age-group rarely experience urinary incontinence unless they have prostate disease or a spinal cord injury.

COST OF CARE
IMPLICATIONS FOR NURSING

INCONTINENCE

Cost of Care

- $16.4 billion is spent every year in the United States on incontinence-related care
  - $11.2 billion is spent for community-based programs and at-home care.
  - $5.2 billion is spent in long-term care facilities.
- $1.1 billion is spent every year on disposable continence care products for adults.
- The urologic diagnostic evaluation for incontinence ranges between $400 and $2000.
- Implementation of the Agency for Healthcare Research and Quality (AHRQ) Clinical Practice Guidelines for Urinary Incontinence has yielded significant cost savings.
  - Over a 14-month period, use of the guidelines helped one nursing home reduce the number of incontinent residents by 65%.
  - Diagnostic tests recommended by the guidelines average $100.
  - One nurse practitioner reported a cure of or improvement in incontinence problems in 98% of her clients through use of the behavioral methods recommended in the guidelines.

Implications for Nursing

Because of the high cost and prevalence of incontinence in the United States, nurses need to become familiar with the evidence-based Clinical Practice Guidelines for Urinary Incontinence. Competence in implementing the guidelines can reduce the financial, functional, and psychosocial burden of this common disorder.

Data from Jirovec, M.M., Wyman, J.F., & Wells, T.J. (1998). Addressing urinary incontinence with educational continence-care competencies. *Image: The Journal of Nursing Scholarship, 30*(4), 375-378; and Agency for Health Care Policy and Research. (1996). *Urinary incontinence in adults: Acute and chronic Management. Clinical practice guideline.* AHCPR Pub. No. 96-0682. Rockville, MD: Agency for Health Care Policy and Research, Public Health Service, U.S. Department of Health and Human Services; http://www.ahcpr.gov/clinic/uhistory.html (Clinical Practice Guidelines Online Urinary Incontinence Guideline: Real World Examples of Use).

COLLABORATIVE MANAGEMENT

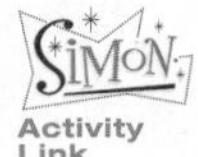

Assessment

HISTORY

The nurse asks, "Do you ever leak urine?" If the answer is yes, the nurse proceeds with a focused assessment (Chart 70-7). Incontinence may be underreported because health care professionals do not question clients about urine loss. It is not safe to assume that clients will volunteer the information without specifically being asked.

PHYSICAL ASSESSMENT/CLINICAL MANIFESTATIONS

The nurse assesses the abdomen to estimate suprapubic fullness, to rule out palpable hard stool, and to evaluate bowel sounds. With a physician's order, the nurse determines the amount of postvoid residual urine by catheterizing the client immediately after voiding. In some facilities, the nurse estimates the postvoid residual amount with a pelvic ultrasonographic scanner (AHCPR, 1996). Urinary incontinence is confirmed by evaluating the force and character of the urine stream during voiding by the client. Asking the client to cough while wearing a perineal pad may be useful in evaluating stress incontinence; a wet pad with forceful coughing may indicate stress incontinence (see the Evidence-Based Practice for Nursing box on p. 1625). A cystometrogram (see Chapter 69) is used as the basic diagnostic study in most cases (Walsh et al., 1998).

CHART 70-6

NURSING FOCUS *on the* OLDER ADULT
Factors Contributing to Urinary Incontinence*

MEDICATIONS
- Central nervous system depressants, such as opioid analgesics, decrease the client's level of consciousness and the urge to void, and they contribute to constipation.
- Diuretics cause frequent voiding, often of large amounts of urine.
- Multiple medications can contribute to changes in mental status or mobility, and they can irritate the bladder.

DISEASE
- Cerebrovascular accidents and other neurologic disorders decrease mobility, sensation, or cognition.
- Arthritis decreases mobility and causes pain.
- Parkinson's disease causes muscle rigidity and an inability to initiate movement.

DEPRESSION
- Depression decreases the energy necessary to maintain continence.
- Decreased self-esteem and feelings of self-worth decrease the importance to the client of maintaining continence.

INADEQUATE RESOURCES
- Clients who have glasses or use a cane, walker, or slippers may be afraid to ambulate.
- Products that help clients manage incontinence are often costly.
- No one may be available to assist the client to the bathroom or help with incontinence products.

*These factors are in addition to the physiologic changes of aging given in Chapter 5.

For women, the nurse inspects the external genitalia to determine whether there is apparent urethral or uterine prolapse, **cystocele** (herniation of the bladder into the vagina), or **rectocele.** These conditions occur because of pelvic floor muscle weakness. An advanced-practice nurse puts on an examination glove and inserts two fingers into the vagina to assess the strength of these muscles. Strength is described as weak, adequate, or strong on the basis of the amount of pressure felt by the nurse as the client tightens her vaginal muscles. The color, consistency, and odor of any secretions from the genitourinary orifices are described and documented. The urine stream interruption test (see Chapter 69) is another method of determining pelvic muscle strength. For men, the nurse inspects the urethral meatus for any discharge.

A digital rectal examination is performed on both male and female clients. The digital rectal examination may provide information about the integrity of the nerve supply to the bladder. The examiner determines whether there is tactile sensation in the anorectal area by noting whether the rectal sphincter is relaxed or contracted on digital insertion. Because nerve supply to the bladder is similar to nerve supply to the rectum, the presence of tactile sensation and a rectal sphincter that contracts suggest that the nerve supply to the bladder is intact. During rectal examination, the nurse also notes any fecal impaction. Enlargement of the prostate is assessed in men by the physician or advanced-practice nurse.

CHART 70-7

FOCUSED ASSESSMENT *of* The Client with Urinary Incontinence

Note the presence of risk factors for urinary incontinence:
- Age
- If female, menopausal status
- Neurologic disease
  - Parkinson's disease
  - Dementia
  - Multiple sclerosis
  - Stroke
  - Spinal injury
- Diabetes mellitus
- Childbirth
- Urologic procedures
- Medications
- Bowel patterns
- Stress/anxiety level

Detail the symptoms of urinary incontinence:
- Leakage
- Frequency
- Urgency
- Nocturia
- Sensation of full bladder before leakage

Obtain a 24-hour intake and output record:
- Time and amount of oral intake and continent voidings
- Time and estimated amount of incontinent leakages
- Activity around the time of leakage

Assess client's:
- Mobility
- Self-care ability
- Cognitive ability
- Communication patterns

Assess the environment for barriers to toileting:
- Privacy
- Restrictive clothing
- Access to toilet

Data from Jirovec, M.M., Wyman, J.F., & Wells, T.J. (1998). Addressing urinary incontinence with educational continence-care competencies. *IMage: The Journal of Nursing Scholarship, 30*(4), 375-378; and Agency for Health Care Policy and Research. (1996). *Urinary incontinence in adults: Acute and chronic management. Clinical practice guideline.* AHCPR Pub. No. 96-0682. Rockville, MD: Agency for Health Care Policy and Research, Public Health Service, U.S. Department of Health and Human Services; http://www.ahcpr.gov/clinic/uhistory.html (Clinical Practice Guidelines Online: Urinary Incontinence Guideline: Real World Examples of Use).

LABORATORY ASSESSMENT

A urinalysis is inexpensive and useful to rule out infection. This test is the first step in the assessment of incontinent clients of any age. The presence of red blood cells (RBCs), white blood cells (WBCs), leukocyte esterase, or nitrites is an indication for culturing the urine. Any infection is treated before further assessment of incontinence.

RADIOGRAPHIC ASSESSMENT

Radiographic assessment is rarely indicated unless surgery is being considered. Excretory urography is the most useful for locating the kidneys and ureters. A voiding cystourethrogram (VCUG) may be performed to assess the size, shape, support, and function of the bladder; look for obstruction (especially prostate obstruction in men); and assess for postvoid residual (PVR) with a postvoid film. An assessment of PVR also can be made with a portable ultrasonographic bladder scanner.

OTHER DIAGNOSTIC ASSESSMENT

Clients who have unusual symptoms, medical complications, or a history of failed incontinence surgery often undergo urodynamic studies to determine the cause of their incontinence. A urodynamic evaluation is not a standardized procedure and may consist of any combination of the following tests:

- Cystourethroscopy to examine the inside of the bladder and urethra directly
- Cystometrogram (CMG) to measure the pressure inside the bladder as it fills
- Urethral pressure profilometry (UPP) to measure the pressure in the urethra in relation to the bladder pressure during various activities

EVIDENCE-BASED PRACTICE FOR NURSING

"Low-tech" tests can be reliable

Swift, S.E., & Yoon, E.A. (1999). Test-retest reliability of the cough stress test in the evaluation of urinary incontinence. *Obstetrics and Gynecology, 94*(1), 99-102.

The goal of this descriptive study was to determine whether a forceful cough initiated in a standing woman with a full bladder would reliably demonstrate results of urine leakage at two different times. Of the 50 women studied, 35 had a positive cough stress test initially and 33 (91%) had a positive cough stress test 1 to 4 weeks later (no treatment occurred between tests). The reliability was highest in those subjects with pure stress incontinence, but the test was also fairly reliable (80%) in those subjects with mixed incontinence.

Critique. The sample size was adequate for the design of the study. No attempt was made to ensure that the bladder volumes were the same at the time of the two testing periods for each subject.

Implications for Nursing. A cough stress test is inexpensive and does not rely on technology or site. It can aid the clinician in differentiating between stress and urge incontinence. Knowing that the test is reliable in assessing the presence of stress and mixed incontinence, it may also be useful in determining client response to treatment. That is, after intervention, if a cough test is negative, one may be more likely to consider the intervention successful and continue that plan of care.

- Uroflowmetry to measure speed and completeness of bladder emptying

Testing may take several hours and more than one visit (see Chapter 69).

Electromyography (EMG) of the pelvic muscles may be a part of the urodynamic studies. A perineometer is a tampon-shaped instrument inserted into the vagina to measure the strength of pelvic muscle contractions. The graph can be used to demonstrate the amplitude of muscle contraction to the client as a method of biofeedback.

CRITICAL THINKING CHALLENGE

You are assigned to care for an older client in the community who is recovering from right total hip replacement surgery. She has a history of diabetes mellitus. She is able to care for herself but is using a walker for ambulation as she recovers. When you ask how things are going, she confides that she has a terrible rash on her "bottom" because "I leak urine so terribly since the surgery."

- What is your next step?
- How might this client's other medical diagnosis and her current health status affect the physical assessment?

For suggested answer guidelines, go to SIMON http://www.wbsaunders.com/SIMON/Iggy/.

Analysis

COMMON NURSING DIAGNOSES AND COLLABORATIVE PROBLEMS

The following are priority nursing diagnoses for clients with urinary incontinence (AHCPR, 1996):

1. Stress Urinary Incontinence related to weak pelvic muscles and structural supports
2. Urge Urinary Incontinence related to decreased bladder capacity, bladder spasms, and neurologic impairment
3. Reflex Urinary Incontinence related to incomplete bladder emptying
4. Mixed or Total Urinary Incontinence related to multiple causes
5. Functional Urinary Incontinence related to cognitive, motor, or sensory deficits

ADDITIONAL NURSING DIAGNOSES AND COLLABORATIVE PROBLEMS

In addition to the common nursing diagnoses, clients with urinary incontinence may have one or more of the following:

- Social Isolation related to altered state of wellness or fear of embarrassment
- Risk for Impaired Skin Integrity related to external risk factors, such as urinary excretions
- Disturbed Body Image related to odor, need to alter clothing selections, or need to wear protective briefs or supplies
- Risk for Infection related to retained or refluxing urine

Planning and Implementation

Several interventions are useful for each type of incontinence and for mixed incontinence. Collaborative management uses these interventions, as well as medication, surgical repair, and diet therapy.

STRESS URINARY INCONTINENCE

PLANNING: EXPECTED OUTCOMES. The client with urinary incontinence is expected to have fewer episodes of stress incontinence or a decreased amount of urine lost with each episode.

INTERVENTIONS. Initial interventions for clients with stress incontinence include diary keeping, behavioral interventions, and medications. Surgery is reserved as an option. The nurse explains the purpose of a detailed diary in which the client records times of urine leakage, activities, and foods eaten. The diary is then used by the health care practitioner to plan and evaluate interventions. Collection devices, absorbent pads, and undergarments may be used during the sometimes lengthy process of assessment and treatment and by those clients who elect not to pursue further interventions.

NONSURGICAL MANAGEMENT. Drug therapy and behavioral interventions (primarily diet and exercise) for stress incontinence require active participation on the part of the client for success. The ongoing availability of a nurse to provide encouragement, clarification, and support is extremely valuable for maximizing the effects of all interventions.

EXERCISE THERAPY. Pelvic floor **(Kegel)** exercises for female clients with stress incontinence are designed to strengthen the muscles of the pelvic floor (circumvaginal muscles). These muscles become strengthened, as any other skeletal muscle does, by frequent, systematic, and repeated contractions.

The most important step in teaching pelvic muscle exercises is to help the client become aware of which muscle to exercise. During the pelvic examination in women and the rectal examination in men or women, the nurse instructs the client to tighten the pelvic muscles around the examiner's fingers. The nurse then provides feedback about the strength of the contraction. Biofeedback devices, such as electromyography (EMG) or perineometers (see earlier discussion), measure the strength of contraction. Retention of a vaginal weight is also evidence that the client has identified the proper muscle. The ability to start and stop the urine stream or stop the passage of flatus is further evidence that the client has correctly identified the pelvic muscles.

Instructions for pelvic muscle exercises are given in Chart 70-8. Although improvement may take several months, most clients notice a significant change after 6 weeks. Clients may need to continue the exercises to maintain the improvement (AHCPR, 1996).

DIET THERAPY. A diet plan to encourage weight reduction is helpful for obese clients because stress incontinence is made worse by increased abdominal pressure from obesity. The nurse instructs the client to avoid alcohol and caffeine (bladder irritants) and refers him or her to the dietitian as needed.

DRUG THERAPY. Because bladder pressure is greater than urethral resistance in clients with stress incontinence, medications may be prescribed to increase the resistance of the urethra (Chart 70-9). Beta-adrenergic blocking agents, such as propranolol (Inderal, Detensol✤), have not been ade-

CHART 70-8

CLIENT EDUCATION GUIDE
Pelvic Muscle Exercises

- The pelvic muscles are composed of a sling of muscles that support your bladder, urethra, and vagina. Like any other muscles in your body, you can make your pelvic muscles stronger by alternately contracting (tightening) and relaxing them in regular exercise periods. By strengthening these muscles, you will be able to stop your urine flow more effectively.
- *To identify your pelvic muscles,* sit on the toilet with your feet flat on the floor about 12 inches apart. Begin to urinate, then try to stop the urine flow. Do not strain down, lift your bottom off the seat, or squeeze your legs together. When you start and stop your urine stream, you are using your pelvic muscles.
- *To perform pelvic muscle exercises,* tighten your pelvic muscles for a slow count of 10, then relax for a slow count of 10. Do this exercise 15 times while you are lying down, sitting up, and standing (a total of 45 exercises). Repeat, this time rapidly contracting and relaxing the pelvic muscles 10 times. This should take no more than 10 to 12 minutes for all three positions, or 3.5 to 4 minutes for each set of 15 exercises.
- Begin with 45 exercises a day in three sets of 15 exercises each. You will notice faster improvement if you can do this twice a day, or a total of 20 minutes each day. Remember to exercise in all three positions so your muscles learn to squeeze effectively despite your position. At first, it is helpful to have a designated time and place to do these exercises because you will have to concentrate to do them correctly. After you have been doing them for several weeks, you will notice improvement in your control of urine; however, many people report that improvement may take as long as 3 months.

quately tested in controlled trials and thus are not recommended for the treatment of incontinence (AHCPR, 1996).

Estrogen is used to treat postmenopausal women with stress incontinence, although its exact mechanism of action is unknown. Estrogen may increase the blood flow and tone of the circumvaginal and periurethral muscles, thus improving the client's ability to contract those muscles during times of increased intra-abdominal stress.

VAGINAL CONE THERAPY. Vaginal cones are a set of five small, cone-shaped weights. They are of equal size but of varying weights and are used with pelvic muscle exercise. The woman inserts the lightest cone, labeled 1, into her vagina (Figure 70-1), with the string to the outside, for a 1-minute test period. If she can hold the first cone in place without its slipping out while she walks around, she proceeds to the second cone, labeled 2, and repeats the procedure. The client begins her treatment with the heaviest cone she can comfortably hold in her vagina for the 1-minute test period. Treatment periods are 15 minutes twice a day. When she can comfortably hold the cone in her vagina for the 15-minute period, the client progresses to the next heaviest weight. Treatment is completed with the cone labeled 5.

Several studies have shown weighted vaginal cones to be helpful in strengthening the pelvic muscles and decreasing stress incontinence (AHCPR, 1996). Further research is needed, however, before recommending the weights to clients with pelvic prolapse. Vaginal cones are available without prescription, and the cost may be reimbursable by some health insurance companies.

OTHER THERAPY. Other types of interventions for stress incontinence include behavior modification, psychotherapy,

CHART 70-9

DRUG THERAPY *for* Urinary Incontinence

Drug	Usual Dosage	Nursing Interventions	Rationale
Estrogen (Premarin, C.E.S.✤)	0.3-1.25 mg daily PO 1-2 g qod per vagina	Report any unusual vaginal bleeding or calf pain.	Estrogen use can increase the risk of endometrial cancer and thrombophlebitis.
Anticholinergics/ antispasmodics		Check the client's intraocular pressure before starting the regimen.	Anticholinergics can increase intraocular pressure and are contraindicated in the presence of narrow-angle glaucoma.
Propantheline (Pro-Banthine, Propanthel✤)	7.5-30 mg tid/qid PO		
Oxybutynin (Ditropan)	2.5-5 mg tid/qid PO	Offer fluids and hard candy to moisten the mouth.	Anticholinergics cause extreme dryness of the mouth.
Dicyclomine hydrochloride (Bentyl, Di-Spaz, Bentylol✤, Formulex✤, Lomine✤)	10-20 mg tid PO	Give the drug between meals.	Food interferes with absorption of the drug.
		Increase fluids and fiber in the client's diet.	Anticholinergics decrease GI motility and can cause constipation.
Tricyclic antidepressants		Administer the full dose at bedtime if possible and warn clients that dizziness may occur on arising in the morning.	Tricyclics have a high potential to cause postural hypotension.
Imipramine (Tofranil, Novo-Pramine✤)	25-100 mg daily PO		
Desipramine (Norpramin)	10-25 mg tid PO	Warn clients about other anticholinergic and alpha-adrenergic side effects.	Tricyclics have a combination of anticholinergic and alpha-adrenergic effects.
Nortriptyline (Pamelor)	10-25 mg tid PO		

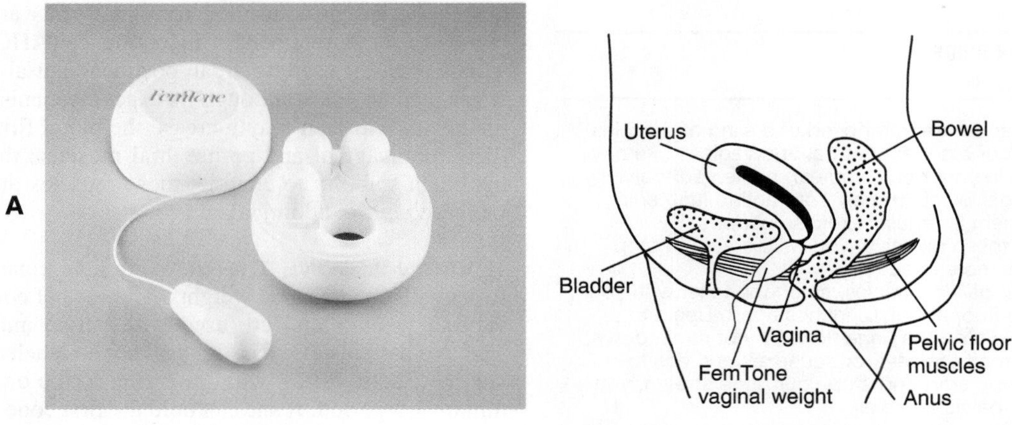

Figure 70-1 ● **A,** FemTone vaginal weights, or cones. The number on the top of each cone represents increasing weight up to the heaviest cone, a *5*. **B,** Diagram showing the correct positioning of a vaginal weight, or cone, in place. (**A** courtesy Convatec, a Bristol-Myers Squibb Company, a division of E.R. Squibb & Sons, Inc., Princeton, NJ; **B** from Convatec [1996]. *FemTone vaginal weights: A training aid for pelvic floor exercises* [brochure]. Princeton, NJ: Author.)

and electrical stimulation devices to strengthen urethral contractions. A variety of intravaginal and intrarectal electrical stimulation devices have been used to treat neurologically and nonneurologically impaired clients with varying degrees of success. More research is needed to determine the ideal level of stimulation and methods of reducing the associated discomfort before electrical stimulation becomes a standard treatment for incontinence.

The Reliance insert is like a tiny tampon that the client inserts into the urethra. After insertion, the client inflates a tiny balloon, which rests at the bladder neck and prevents the flow of urine. To void, the client pulls a string to deflate the balloon and removes the device. The applicator is reusable, although the tampon part is disposed of after each void (Gallo, 1997).

SURGICAL MANAGEMENT. Stress incontinence may be surgically corrected by vaginal, abdominal, or retropubic procedures. Success rates vary between 50% and 90% for most procedures, but these rates are difficult to evaluate because of the varying definitions of "cure" in the studies. Furthermore, cure may vary between short-term and long-term (over 5 years) results. In addition, published complication rates are significant, ranging from less than 2% for collagen or siloxane injection to 50% for bladder neck suspension.

PREOPERATIVE CARE. The nurse instructs the client about the surgical procedure and clarifies events surrounding the surgery. Extensive urodynamic testing (see Chapter 69) is often performed before surgery, and the need for such thorough assessment should be explained to the client.

OPERATIVE PROCEDURES. The surgical procedures used for women are designed to reposition the urethra and bladder, change the structure of the involved tissues, or insert artificial devices to improve function (Table 70-4).

POSTOPERATIVE CARE. After surgery, the nurse assesses for and intervenes to prevent or detect complications. For prevention of unnecessary movement or traction on the bladder neck, the urethral catheter is secured with tape or a tube holder. If a suprapubic catheter is present instead of a urethral catheter, the dressing is monitored for leakage of urine, as well as serosanguineous drainage. Catheters are usually in place until the client can urinate easily and has postvoid residual urine of less than 50 mL. (See Chapters 17 and 19 for a thorough discussion of general preoperative and postoperative care.)

URGE URINARY INCONTINENCE

PLANNING: EXPECTED OUTCOMES. The client with urinary incontinence is expected to use techniques to prevent or manage urge incontinence.

INTERVENTIONS. Interventions for clients with urge incontinence, sometimes called "overactive bladder" by the lay public, include behavioral interventions and medications. Surgery is not recommended for treatment of this condition. Collection devices and absorbent pads and undergarments may be used.

DRUG THERAPY. Because the hypertonic bladder contracts involuntarily in clients with urge incontinence, medications that relax the smooth muscle and increase the bladder's capacity are prescribed (see Chart 70-9).

The most effective medications are anticholinergics, such as propantheline (Pro-Banthine, Propanthel♣), and anticholinergics with smooth muscle relaxant properties, such as oxybutynin (Ditropan) and dicyclomine hydrochloride (Bentyl, Formulex♣, Spasmoban♣, Viscerol♣). Anticholinergics have serious side effects and are therefore used in conjunction with behavioral interventions. These agents inhibit the cholinergic fibers that stimulate bladder contraction. Tricyclic antidepressants with anticholinergic and alpha-adrenergic agonist activity, such as imipramine (Tofranil, Novopramine♣), have been used successfully. Other drugs, such as flavoxate (Urispas) and the antihistamines, nonsteroidal anti-inflammatory agents, beta-adrenergic agonists, and calcium channel blockers, have not been studied well enough for their use to be recommended (AHCPR, 1996).

TABLE 70-4 • SURGICAL PROCEDURES FOR STRESS INCONTINENCE

Procedure	Purpose	Nursing Considerations
Anterior vaginal repair (colporrhaphy)	Elevates the urethral position and repairs any cystocele	Because the operation is performed by vaginal incision, it is often done in conjunction with a vaginal hysterectomy. Recovery is usually rapid, and a urethral catheter is in place for 24-48 hr.
Retropubic suspension (Marshall-Marchetti-Krantz or Burch colposuspension)	Elevates the urethral position and provides longer-lasting results	The operation requires a low abdominal incision and a urethral or suprapubic catheter for several days postoperatively. Recovery takes longer, and urinary retention and detrusor instability are the most frequent complications.
Needle bladder neck suspension (Pereyra or Stamey procedure)	Elevates the urethral position and provides longer-lasting results without a long operative time	The combined vaginal approach with a needle and a small suprapubic skin incision does not allow direct vision of the operative site; however, the high complication rates may be due to the selection of clients who, because of their medical condition, are not good candidates for longer retropubic procedures.
Pubovaginal sling procedures	A sling made of synthetic or fascial material is placed under the urethrovesical junction to elevate the bladder neck	The operation uses an abdominal, vaginal, or combined approach to treat intrinsic sphincter deficiencies. Temporary or permanent urinary retention is common postoperatively.
Artificial sphincters	A mechanical device to open and close the urethra is placed around the anatomic urethra	The operation is done more frequently in men. The most common complications include mechanical failure of the device, erosion of tissue, and infection.
Periurethral injection of collagen or siloxane	Implantation of small amounts of an inert substance through several small injections provides support around the bladder neck	The procedure can be done in an ambulatory care setting and can be repeated as often as necessary. Certain compounds may migrate after injection; an allergy test to bovine collagen must be performed before implantation.

Data from Schultz, J.A., & Drutz, H.P. (1999). The surgical management of recurrent urinary stress incontinence. *Current Opinions in Obstetrics and Gynecology, 11*(5), 489-494; and Lightner, D.J., & Itano, N.M. (1999). Treatment options for women with stress urinary incontinence. *Mayo Clinic Proceedings, 74*(11), 1149-1156.

DIET THERAPY. The nurse instructs the client to avoid foods that have a direct bladder-stimulating or diuretic effect, such as caffeine and alcohol. Spacing fluids at regular intervals throughout the day (e.g., 120 mL every hour or 240 mL every 2 hours) and limiting fluids after the dinner hour (e.g., only 120 mL at bedtime) help avoid placing a fluid overload on the bladder and allow urine to accumulate at a steady pace.

BEHAVIORAL INTERVENTIONS. Behavioral interventions for urge incontinence include bladder training, habit training, exercise therapy, and electrical stimulation.

NIC interventions for urinary bladder training and urinary habit training are presented in Chart 70-10. It can be difficult for clients to understand these interventions because they involve a significant amount of participation on their part. The ongoing availability of a nurse to provide encouragement, clarification, and support is extremely valuable for maximizing the effects of all interventions. Behavioral interventions are often combined with drug therapy for maximal effect.

NIC ***BLADDER TRAINING.*** Bladder training is primarily an education program for the client that begins with a thorough explanation of the problem of urge incontinence. Instead of the bladder being in control of the client, the client learns to control the bladder. For the program to succeed, he or she must be alert, aware, and able to resist the urge to urinate.

A regular schedule for voiding is established, beginning with the longest interval that is comfortable for the client, even if the interval is only 30 minutes. The nurse instructs the client to void every 30 minutes and ignore any urge to urinate between the mandated intervals. Once the client is comfortable with the initial schedule, the interval is increased by 15 to 30 minutes; the new schedule is followed until the client again achieves success. As he or she progressively increases the voiding interval, the bladder gradually tolerates more volume. The client is taught relaxation and distraction techniques to maximize success in the retraining. The nurse provides positive reinforcement for maintaining the prescribed schedule.

NIC ***HABIT TRAINING.*** Habit training (scheduled toileting) is a variation of bladder training that has been successful in reducing incontinence in cognitively impaired clients. To use habit training, caregivers assist the client in voiding at specific times (e.g., every 2 hours on the even hours) in an effort to get him or her to the toilet before incontinence can occur. There is no effort to increase bladder capacity by gradually lengthening the voiding intervals.

Prompted voiding, a supplement to habit training, attempts to increase the client's awareness of the need to void and to prompt him or her to ask for toileting assistance. Habit training otherwise relies completely on a time schedule.

EXERCISE THERAPY. Pelvic muscle exercises for urge incontinence have been helpful and are taught in the same way as for stress incontinence (see Chart 70-8). Improved urethral resistance enhances the client's ability to overcome abnormal detrusor contractions long enough to get to the toilet.

ELECTRICAL STIMULATION. A variety of intravaginal and intrarectal electrical stimulation devices have been used to treat both urge and stress incontinence.

CHART 70-10

NIC INTERVENTION ACTIVITIES *for* The Client with Urinary Incontinence

Urinary Bladder Training: *Improving bladder function for those with urge incontinence by increasing the bladder's ability to hold urine and the client's ability to suppress urination*

- Determine ability to recognize urge to void.
- Keep a continence specification record for 3 days to establish voiding pattern.
- Establish interval of initial toileting schedule, based on voiding pattern.
- Establish beginning and ending time for toileting schedule if not for 24 hours.
- Establish interval for toileting of not less than 1 hour and preferably not less than 2 hours.
- Toilet client or remind client to void at prescribed intervals.
- Provide privacy for toileting.
- Use power of suggestion (e.g., running water or flushing toilet) to assist client to void.
- Avoid leaving client on toilet for more than 5 minutes.
- Reduce toileting interval by 1/2 hour if client is unable to void at two or more scheduled toileting times.
- Increase toileting interval by 1 hour if client has no incontinence episodes for 3 days until optimal 4-hour interval is achieved.
- Teach the client to consciously hold urine until the scheduled toileting time.
- Discuss daily record of continence with client to provide reinforcement.

Urinary Habit Training: *Establishing a predictable pattern of bladder emptying to prevent incontinence for persons with limited cognitive ability who have urge, stress, or functional incontinence*

- Keep a continence specification record for 3 days to establish voiding pattern.
- Establish interval of initial toileting schedule based on voiding pattern and usual routine (e.g., eating, rising, and retiring).
- Establish beginning and ending time for toileting schedule if not for 24 hours.
- Establish interval for toileting of preferably not less than 2 hours.
- Assist client to toilet and prompt to void at prescribed intervals.
- Provide privacy for toileting.
- Use power of suggestion (e.g., running water or flushing toilet) to assist client to void.
- Avoid leaving the client on the toilet for more than 5 minutes.
- Reduce toileting interval by 1/2 hour if there are more than two incontinence episodes in 24 hours.
- Maintain toileting interval if there are two or fewer incontinence episodes in 24 hours.
- Increase toileting interval by 1/2 hour if client has no incontinence episodes for 48 hours until optimal 4-hour interval is achieved.
- Discuss daily record of continence with staff to provide reinforcement and encourage compliance with toileting schedule.
- Maintain scheduled toileting to assist in establishing and maintaining voiding habit.
- Give positive feedback or positive reinforcement (e.g., 5 minutes of social conversation) to client when voids at scheduled toileting times, and make no comment when client is incontinent.

Urinary Catheterization: Intermittent: *Regular periodic use of a catheter to empty the bladder*

- Teach client/family the purpose, supplies, method, and rationale of intermittent catheterization.
- Teach client/family clean intermittent catheterization technique.
- Provide quiet private room for the procedure.
- Demonstrate procedure and have a return demonstration, as appropriate.
- Determine catheterization schedule based on comprehensive urinary assessment.
- Adjust frequency of catheterization to maintain output of 300 mL or less.
- Maintain client on prophylactic antibacterial therapy for 2 to 3 weeks at initiation of intermittent catheterization, as appropriate.
- Complete a urinalysis about every 2 weeks to 1 month.
- Establish a catheterization schedule based on individual needs.
- Maintain a detailed record of catheterization schedule, fluid intake, and output.
- Teach client/family signs and symptoms of urinary tract infection.
- Monitor color, odor, and clarity of urine.

NIC intervention activities selected from McCloskey, J.C., & Bulechek, G.M. (Eds.). (2000). *Nursing interventions classification (NIC)* (3rd ed.). St. Louis: Mosby.

REFLEX URINARY INCONTINENCE

PLANNING: EXPECTED OUTCOMES. The client with urinary incontinence is expected to achieve continence by keeping urine volume in the bladder within normal limits, preventing bladder overdistention.

INTERVENTIONS. Interventions for the client with reflex (overflow) incontinence caused by obstruction of the bladder outlet may include surgery to relieve the obstruction. The most common surgical procedures are removal of the prostate (see Chapter 76) and repair of genital prolapse (see Chapter 75). For overflow incontinence related to detrusor muscle inadequacy, the most effective method of treatment is intermittent catheterization. Behavioral interventions such as bladder compression and intermittent self-catheterization are the primary management techniques for urinary retention leading to overflow incontinence.

DRUG THERAPY. Medications are prescribed for short-term management of urinary retention, often postoperatively. They are not indicated in long-term management of the hypotonic bladder resulting in overflow incontinence. The most commonly used medication is bethanechol chloride (Urecholine), a cholinergic agent that increases bladder pressure.

BEHAVIORAL INTERVENTIONS. The mainstays of behavioral interventions include methods for bladder compression and intermittent self-catheterization.

BLADDER COMPRESSION. Techniques that promote bladder emptying include the Credé method, the Valsalva maneuver, double-voiding, and splinting.

In the Credé method, the nurse instructs the client in external compression of the urinary bladder or parasympathetic stimulation via tugging at pubic hair or massaging the genital area. These techniques manually assist the bladder in emptying. In the Valsalva maneuver, breathing techniques increase intrathoracic and intra-abdominal pressure. This increased pressure is then directed toward the bladder during exhalation. With the technique of double-voiding, the client empties the bladder and then, within a few minutes, consciously attempts a second bladder emptying.

For women who have a severe cystocele (prolapse of the bladder into the vagina), a technique called *splinting* both compresses the bladder and moves the obstruction out of the way. The woman inserts her own fingers into her vagina, gently pushes the cystocele back into the vagina, and begins to urinate.

NIC ***INTERMITTENT SELF-CATHETERIZATION.*** NIC interventions for intermittent urinary catheterization are presented in Chart 70-10. The nurse teaches intermittent self-catheterization to clients with long-term problems of incomplete bladder emptying. Techniques of self-catheterization are well established and can be learned fairly easily. The nurse remembers the following important points in teaching this technique:

- Proper handwashing and cleaning of the catheter reduce the frequency of infection.
- A small lumen and adequate lubrication of the catheter prevent urethral trauma.
- A regular schedule for bladder emptying prevents overdistention of the bladder with subsequent mucosal trauma.

Clients must be able to understand instructions and have the manual dexterity to manipulate the catheter. Caregivers or family members in the home can also be taught to perform straight catheterization using a clean (rather than sterile) technique with good outcomes.

FUNCTIONAL URINARY INCONTINENCE

PLANNING: EXPECTED OUTCOMES. The client with urinary incontinence is expected to use methods of urine containment or collection that ensure dryness until the underlying cause of the incontinence is treated.

INTERVENTIONS. Causes of functional (or chronic intractable) incontinence vary greatly; some are reversible, and others are not. The primary focus of intervention is treatment of reversible causes. When incontinence is not reversible, urinary habit training (see Habit Training, p. 1629) is done to establish a predictable pattern of bladder emptying to prevent incontinence regardless of the cause(s). A final strategy focuses on containment of the urine and protection of the client's skin. Nonsurgical interventions include applied devices, containment, and urinary catheterization.

APPLIED DEVICES. Applied devices include intravaginal pessaries for women and penile clamps for men. The intravaginal pessary supports the uterus and vagina and helps maintain the correct position of the bladder. (See Chapter 75 for further discussion of pessaries.) The penile clamp is applied externally to compress the urethra and prevent leakage of urine.

The dangers of pessaries and penile clamps include damage to the tissues and infection from constant pressure in sensitive areas. Both devices require that the client have manual dexterity or a caregiver who applies and removes the device. The clinician prescribes the device, and the nurse instructs the client or caregivers in its use. Male clients may use an external collecting device, such as a condom catheter. Design of a suitable external collecting device for women has not been as successful.

CONTAINMENT. Absorbent pads and briefs are designed to collect urine and keep the client's skin and clothing dry. A variety of types and sizes of pads are available:

- Shields or liners inserted inside a panty
- Undergarments consisting of full-sized pads with waist straps
- Plastic-lined protective underpants with or without elastic legs
- Combination pad and pant systems
- Absorbent bed pads

A major concern with the use of protective pads is the risk that skin breakdown will occur. Materials and costs vary; some are reusable, and others are disposable. The disposal of these products raises ecologic concerns. Newer, more absorbent products are coming on the market as manufacturers take advantage of the growth of the "adult diaper" market. The nurse avoids use of the word "diaper," however, because of the usual association of diapers with a baby.

URINARY CATHETERIZATION. Catheterization for the control of incontinence may be intermittent or involve placement of an indwelling catheter. Intermittent self-catheterization is preferred to placement of an indwelling catheter because of the decreased likelihood of infection. Indwelling urinary catheters should be used temporarily and only when all other alternatives have been tried and have been unsuccessful. A long-term indwelling urinary catheter is appropriate for clients with skin breakdown who need a dry environment for healing, clients who are terminally ill and need comfort, and clients who are acutely or critically ill and require careful measurement of urine output.

CRITICAL THINKING CHALLENGE

Your client is diagnosed with mixed stress and urge incontinence. Her environment has no barriers to toileting, and she is able to ambulate in her home with the walker. Your client reports drinking about four cups of coffee daily.

- What effect does coffee have on continence?
- What exercises can you teach and reinforce in relation to continence care?
- How can you help evaluate your client's response to exercise and/or prescribed medication to improve continence?

For suggested answer guidelines, go to SIMON http://www.wbsaunders.com/SIMON/Iggy/.

Community-Based Care

Community-based care for the client with urinary incontinence considers his or her personal, physical, emotional, and social resources. Important personal resources for self-care include mobility, vision, and manual dexterity. The nurse considers who will be the primary caregiver and what environmental circumstances or factors will influence the effectiveness of the plan.

HEALTH TEACHING

The nurse teaches the client and family or significant others about the cause of the identified type of urinary incontinence and discusses treatment options available for its management. The teaching plan addresses the prescribed medications (purpose, dosage, method and route of administration, and expected and potential side effects). The client and family are also instructed about the importance of weight reduction and dietary modification to assist with control of urinary incontinence.

When external devices or protective pads are needed, the nurse describes the possible options, discusses the advantages and disadvantages of each, and helps the client make a selection that considers lifestyle and resources. For clients who will use intermittent catheterization or those with artificial urinary sphincters, the nurse demonstrates the appropriate technique to the client or caregiver. Return demonstrations are evaluated for correct technique. Chart 70-11 also addresses teaching.

The embarrassment experienced by incontinent clients can be devastating to their self-esteem, body image, and interpersonal relationships. The unpredictability of incontinence creates anxiety. Clients are often embarrassed to seek help, and even when resources are identified, they may need assistance to feel comfortable in using the resources. Even buying supplies in the local drugstore or grocery store can be perceived as a threat to their privacy.

The nurse assists in psychosocial preparation by accepting and acknowledging the personal concerns of the client and caregiver. These concerns must never be minimized or made to seem trivial. The nurse helps the client learn methods of controlling or managing the fear or anxiety. As the client learns the specifics of the plan that will allow control of urinary incontinence, the confidence to resume psychosocial interactions should return.

CHART 70-11

CLIENT EDUCATION GUIDE
Urinary Incontinence

- Maintain a normal body weight to reduce the pressure on your bladder.
- Do not try to control your incontinence by limiting your fluid intake. Adequate fluid intake is necessary for kidney function and health maintenance.
- If you have a catheter in your bladder, follow the instructions given to you about maintaining the sterile drainage system.
- If you are discharged with a suprapubic catheter in your bladder, inspect the entry site for the tube daily, clean the skin around the opening gently with warm soap and water, and place a sterile gauze dressing on the skin around the tube. Report any redness, swelling, drainage, or fever to your physician.
- Do not put anything into your vagina, such as tampons, medications, hygiene products, or exercise weights, until you check with your physician at your 6-week checkup after surgery.
- Do not have sexual intercourse until after your 6-week postoperative checkup.
- Do not lift or carry anything heavier than 5 pounds or participate in any strenuous exercise until your physician gives you postoperative clearance. In some cases, this could be as long as 3 months.
- Avoid exercises, such as running, jogging, step or dance aerobic classes, rowing, cross-country ski or stairclimber machines, and mountain biking. Brisk walking without any additional hand, leg, or body weights is allowed. Swimming is allowed after all drains and catheters have been removed and your incision is completely healed.
- If Kegel exercises are recommended, ask your nurse for specific instructions.

HOME CARE MANAGEMENT

The home environment is assessed for barriers that impede access to the toileting facilities. Environmental hazards that might slow walking or contribute to injury are eliminated. These hazards might include small area rugs (throw rugs), tables or chairs with legs that extend into the walking area, slippery waxed or polished floors, and inadequate lighting.

If the client must climb stairs to reach a bathroom, handrails should be installed and stairs should be kept free of obstacles. Toilet seat extenders may help provide the appropriate level of seating so that maximal abdominal pressure may be applied to encourage voiding. Portable commodes may be obtained for homes in which ambulatory access to toilets is impractical or impossible. Physical and occupational therapists are valuable resources for assisting with home care management.

HEALTH CARE RESOURCES

Referral to home care agencies for assistance with personal care and to continence clinics that specialize in evaluation and treatment may be helpful. In many continence clinics, nurses collaborate with physicians and other health care professionals to evaluate and manage clients. The treatment plan is specific for each client; supplies and products are custom selected.

Clients benefit emotionally from education and from the support of others who experience similar concerns. The National Association for Continence (NAFC) and the Simon Foundation for Continence publish newsletters with informative articles and educational materials written with simple, easy-to-understand explanations. The Agency for Healthcare Research and Quality (AHRQ) has also published a caregiver guide (AHCPR Pub. No. 96-0683) for the public that is available on the Internet or by calling (800) 358-9295. Local hospitals, in collaboration with the NAFC, may conduct local support groups.

Evaluation: Outcomes

The nurse evaluates the care of the client with urinary incontinence on the basis of the identified nursing diagnoses and collaborative problems. The expected outcomes are that the client will:

- Describe the type of urinary incontinence experienced
- Demonstrate knowledge of proper use of medications and correct procedures for self-catheterization, use of the artificial sphincter, or care of an indwelling urinary catheter
- Demonstrate effective use of the selected exercise or bladder training program
- Select and use incontinence devices and products
- Have a reduction in the number of incontinence episodes

Urolithiasis

OVERVIEW

Urolithiasis is the presence of **calculi** (stones) in the urinary tract. Stones are generally asymptomatic until they pass into the lower urinary tract, where they can cause excruciating pain. The term **nephrolithiasis** describes a condition in which stones form in the kidney. Formation of stones in the ureter is **ureterolithiasis.**

Pathophysiology

Urologic stones result from a variety of metabolic disorders. However, the exact mechanism of stone formation, commonly referred to as stone disease, is not entirely understood. Everyone excretes crystals in the urine at some time, but fewer than 10% of people form calculi. About 75% of calculi contain calcium as one component of the stone complex, which may be calcium oxalate or calcium phosphate (Hruska, 1996). Struvite (15%), uric acid (8%), and cystine (3%) make up the less common stones (Balaji & Menon, 1997).

Formation of stones seems to involve three conditions:

- Slow urine flow, resulting in supersaturation of the urine with the particular element (such as calcium) that first becomes crystallized and later becomes the stone
- Damage to the lining of the urinary tract (i.e., from crystals)
- Decreased inhibitor substances in the urine that would otherwise prevent supersaturation and crystal aggregation

High urine acidity (as with uric acid and cystine stones) or alkalinity (as with calcium phosphate and struvite stones) also contributes to stone formation.

One example of a metabolic problem causing stone formation begins when excessive amounts of calcium are absorbed through the intestinal tract (the most common cause of hypercalciuria). As blood circulates through the kidneys, the excess calcium is filtered into the urine, causing supersaturation of calcium in the urine. If fluid intake is inadequate, such as when a client is dehydrated, supersaturation is more likely to occur, and there is an increased risk of calcium combining with another compound to form a larger molecule. The calcium complex often serves as a center for additional deposition, and eventually a stone forms.

Stones that form in the kidney and then pass into the ureter often lodge in the ureteropelvic angle, the aortoiliac bend, or the ureterovesical angle. When the calculus occludes the ureter and blocks the flow of urine, the ureter dilates. An enlargement of the ureter is called **hydroureter.**

The pain associated with ureteral spasm is excruciating and may cause the client to go into shock from stimulation of nearby sympathetic nerves. In addition, **hematuria** (bloody urine) may result from damage to the urothelial lining. If the obstruction is not removed, urinary stasis may result in infection and impair kidney function on the side of the blockage. As the blockage persists, **hydronephrosis** (enlargement of the kidney caused by blockage of urine lower in the tract and filling of the kidney with urine) and irreversible kidney damage, although rare, may develop.

Etiology

The cause of urolithiasis is unknown, although several hypotheses have been suggested. At least 90% of clients with calculi have a contributing metabolic risk factor. Table 70-5 summarizes the known metabolic defects that commonly cause stone formation.

A diet high in calcium is not believed to cause stones unless a metabolic defect or renal tubular defect already exists. Even in clients with a history of nephrolithiasis, taking calcium citrate supplements does not cause new stone formation (Parivar, Low, & Stoller, 1996). Urinary stasis, urinary retention, immobilization, and dehydration all contribute to a calculus-forming environment. Except for the use of the thiazides for calcium oxalate stones, diuretics can cause volume depletion and thus may promote the formation of calculi.

Incidence/Prevalence

The incidence of stone disease in the adult population is relatively high and varies with geographic location, race, and family history. About 12% of adults will have at least one episode of renal stone disease. Overall, the incidence is higher in men; however, struvite calculi are twice as common in women. Recurrence rates vary, depending on the type of treatment. The recurrence rate of untreated calcium oxylate stones is 35% to 50% in 5 to 10 years. A higher recurrence of stones is found in those clients with a family history of stone disease and those who had their first occurrence by age 25 years.

CULTURAL CONSIDERATIONS

There is an increased incidence of stone disease in the southeastern United States and a rising incidence in Japan and Western Europe. Calcium stone disease is more common in men than in women and tends to occur in young adults or during early middle adulthood. Stone disease in African Americans is uncommon (Hruska, 1996). Cystinuria is more common among Jews of Libyan extraction (Rutchik & Resnick, 1997).

TABLE 70-5 • METABOLIC DEFECTS THAT COMMONLY CAUSE CALCULI

Metabolic Deficit	Etiology
Hypercalcemia	
Primary	Absorptive: increased intestinal calcium absorption Renal: impaired renal tubular resorption of calcium
Secondary	Resorptive: hyperparathyroidism, vitamin D intoxication, renal tubular acidosis, prolonged immobilization
Hyperoxaluria	
Primary	Genetic: autosomal recessive trait resulting in high oxalate production
Secondary	Dietary: excess oxalate from foods such as spinach, rhubarb, Swiss chard, cocoa, beets, wheat germ, pecans, peanuts, okra, chocolate, and lime peel
Hyperuricemia	
Primary	Gout is an inherited disorder of purine metabolism (20% of clients with gout have uric acid calculi)
Secondary	Increased production or decreased clearance of purine from myeloproliferative disorders, thiazide diuretics, carcinoma
Struvite	Made of magnesium ammonium phosphate and carbonate apatite; formed by urea splitting by bacteria, most commonly, *Proteus mirabilis;* needs an alkaline urine to form
Cystinuria	Autosomal recessive defect of amino acid metabolism that precipitates insoluble cystine crystals in the urine

➤ COLLABORATIVE MANAGEMENT

Assessment

HISTORY

The client is asked about a personal or family history of urologic stones. A diet history, including fluid intake patterns, is also obtained. If the client has a history of calculus formation, the nurse asks about past treatment, whether chemical analysis of the stone was performed, and what preventive measures the client follows.

PHYSICAL ASSESSMENT/CLINICAL MANIFESTATIONS

The major clinical manifestation of calculi is severe pain, commonly called **renal colic.** Flank pain suggests that the stone is in the kidney or upper ureter. Flank pain that radiates abdominally or into the scrotum and testes or the vulva suggests that stones are in the ureters or bladder. Pain is most intense when the stone is moving or when the ureter is obstructed (Walsh et al., 1998).

Renal colic begins suddenly and is usually described as "unbearable." Nausea, vomiting, pallor, and diaphoresis often accompany the pain. A large stationary stone in the kidney (staghorn calculus), however, rarely causes much pain. Frequency and dysuria occur when a stone reaches the bladder.

Hematuria is a common finding; blood may make the urine appear smoky or rusty. Increased turbidity and odor are associated with infectious processes that may accompany urolithiasis. **Oliguria** (scant urine output) or **anuria** (absence of urine output) suggests obstruction, possibly at the bladder neck or urethra. Obstruction of the urinary tract is an emergency and must be treated immediately to preserve kidney function.

The nurse examines the client to detect bladder distention. The physical examination may reveal pale, ashen, diaphoretic skin; the client may suffer from excruciating pain. Vital signs may be moderately elevated with pain; body temperature and pulse are elevated with infection. Blood pressure may decrease markedly if the severe pain causes shock.

LABORATORY ASSESSMENT

Urinalysis may show red blood cells (RBCs), white blood cells (WBCs), and bacteria. RBCs are most likely the result of direct trauma, caused by the stone, on the endothelial lining of the ureter, bladder, or urethra. WBCs and bacteria may be present as a result of urinary stasis. Urine culture reveals infection (associated with struvite stones); sensitivity studies of the culture identify antibiotic effectiveness. Microscopic examination of the urine may identify crystals from which stones could form. Urinary pH is measured to determine acidity or alkalinity.

The serum WBC count is elevated with infection. Increases in the serum calcium, serum phosphate, or serum uric acid levels suggest that excess minerals are present and may contribute to stone formation.

RADIOGRAPHIC ASSESSMENT

Stones are easily seen on x-ray films of the kidneys, ureters, and bladder (KUB); IV urograms; or computed tomography (CT) scans. The primary purpose of these radiographic procedures is to confirm the presence and location of the calculi.

The urogram is useful for identifying whether urinary tract obstruction is present; however, because of the risk of acute renal failure induced by contrast media, other diagnostic tests may be chosen for high-risk clients (older adults and clients who have diabetes mellitus, multiple myeloma, or elevated serum creatinine levels). CT is generally needed to identify cystine or uric acid stones, neither of which are visible on x-ray examination.

OTHER DIAGNOSTIC ASSESSMENT

Renal ultrasonography produces images from sound waves. Structures of varying density are reproduced. Solid structures, such as stones, are extremely dense; therefore the images of stones are clear. The identification of small stones and their exact location, however, may not be as precise as desired.

Interventions

Nursing interventions are focused on pain management and prevention of infection and urinary obstruction. The majority of clients will be able to expel the stone without invasive procedures. The most important factors regarding whether a stone will pass on its own are its composition, size, and location. The larger the stone and the higher up in the urinary tract it is, the less likely it is to be passed. Other interventions may be necessary when the client does not pass the stone spontaneously (Figure 70-2).

PAIN RELIEF MEASURES. Nonsurgical and surgical approaches are used to assist the client with a kidney stone in achieving an acceptable degree of pain relief.

NONSURGICAL MANAGEMENT

DRUG THERAPY. Pain is usually most severe in the first 24 to 36 hours. Opioid analgesics are often required to control the moderately severe to severe pain caused by stones in the urinary tract. Opioid agents, such as morphine sulfate (Statex✥), are often administered intravenously so that prompt and adequate absorption is ensured. Nonsteroidal anti-inflammatory drugs such as ketorolac (Toradol) in the acute phase may be quite effective.

Control of pain is more effective when medications are given at regularly scheduled intervals or via a constant delivery system (e.g., skin patch) instead of as needed (prn). Spasmolytic agents, such as oxybutynin chloride (Ditropan) and propantheline bromide (Pro-Banthine, Propanthel✥), are extremely important for the relief and control of pain (see Chart 70-9). The nurse administers the medication and assesses the response by asking the client to rate the discomfort on a rating scale.

COMPLEMENTARY AND ALTERNATIVE THERAPY. Relaxation techniques, such as hypnosis and imagery, therapeutic or healing touch, and acupuncture, can relieve pain. Clients often have great difficulty finding a comfortable position in which to relax; assisting the client with positioning can often aid in relaxation. Breathing techniques, such as those used in childbirth, can also help clients to relax.

OTHER MANAGEMENT TECHNIQUES. Avoiding overhydration in the acute phase helps to make the spontaneous passage of a stone less painful (Singal & Denstedt, 1997). The nurse strains the urine to monitor for excretion of the calcu-

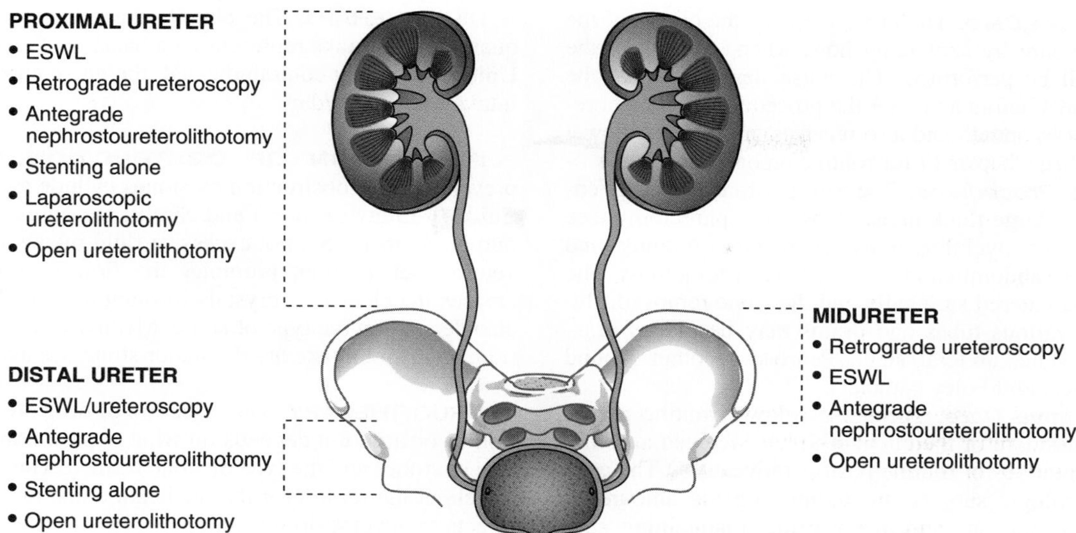

Figure 70-2 ● Treatment options for ureteral stones. (ESWL, Extracorporeal shock wave lithotripsy.) (From Singal, R.K., & Denstedt, J.D. [1997]. Contemporary management of ureteral stones. *Urologic Clinics of North America, 24*[1], 59-70.)

lus. Any stones obtained are sent to the laboratory for analysis; preventive therapy is based on stone composition.

EXTRACORPOREAL SHOCK WAVE LITHOTRIPSY. **Lithotripsy,** also known as extracorporeal shock wave lithotripsy (ESWL), is the application of sound, laser, or dry shock wave energies (electrohydraulic, electromagnetic, or piezoelectric) to break the stone into small fragments. The client receives conscious sedation and lies on a flat x-ray–type table with the lithotriptor aimed at the stone, which is visualized by fluoroscopy. A local anesthetic cream is applied to the skin focal site 45 minutes before the procedure.

During the procedure, cardiac rhythm is monitored by electrocardiography (ECG), and the shock waves are administered in synchrony with the R wave; 500 to 1500 shock waves are administered in 30 to 45 minutes. Continuous ECG monitoring for dysrhythmia and fluoroscopic observation for destruction of the stone are maintained.

After lithotripsy, the nurse may strain the urine to monitor the elimination of stone fragments. Some bruising may occur on the flank of the affected side after extracorporeal shock wave lithotripsy (ESWL).

Occasionally a stent is placed in the ureter before ESWL to facilitate passage of the stone fragments. Cystine stones are generally resistant to ESWL.

SURGICAL MANAGEMENT. Various minimally invasive surgical and open surgical procedures are indicated if urinary obstruction occurs or if the stone is too large to be passed spontaneously.

MINIMALLY INVASIVE SURGICAL PROCEDURES. Minimally invasive surgical (MIS) procedures include stenting, retrograde ureteroscopy, percutaneous antegrade nephrostoureterolithotomy, and laparoscopic ureterolithotomy.

Stenting. A stent is a small tube that is placed in the ureter through the endoscopic procedure of ureteroscopy. The stent dilates the ureter and creates a passageway for the stone or stone fragments. This procedure prevents the passing stone from coming in contact with the ureteral mucosa, thereby reducing pain. A Foley catheter also may be placed to facilitate passage of the stone through the urethra.

Retrograde Ureteroscopy. Retrograde ureteroscopy is an endoscopic procedure. The ureteroscope is passed through the urethra and bladder into the ureter. Once the stone is seen, it can be removed using grasping baskets, forceps, or loops. Through the ureteroscope, lithotripsy also can be performed. A Foley catheter also may be placed to facilitate passage of the stone fragments through the urethra.

Percutaneous Antegrade Nephrostoureterolithotomy. In percutaneous antegrade nephrostoureterolithotomy, the client lies prone or laterally and receives general anesthesia. The physician identifies the ideal kidney entry point with fluoroscopy and then passes a needle into the collecting system of the kidney. Once a tract has been made in the kidney, other equipment, such as an **intracorporeal** (inside the body) ultrasonic or laser lithotriptor, can be used to break up and remove the stone. An endoscope with a special attachment to grasp and extract the stone also could be used. Often a nephrostomy tube is left in place initially to prevent the stone fragments from passing through the normal urinary tract.

The nurse provides routine nephrostomy tube care and monitors the client for complications after the procedure. Possible complications include bleeding at the site or through the tube, pneumothorax, and infection.

Laparoscopic Ureterolithotomy. Laparoscopic ureterolithotomy uses a laparoscope to access the ureters. The surgeon enters the ureter and removes, fragments, and vaporizes the stone with the laser. Preoperative and postoperative care is the same as for any laparoscopic procedure.

OPEN SURGICAL PROCEDURES. After failed attempts to remove the stone through other methods, or when risk of a lasting injury to the ureter or kidney is possible, an **open ureterolithotomy** (into the ureter), **pyelolithotomy** (into the kidney pelvis), or **nephrolithotomy** (into the kidney) procedure may be indicated. These procedures are used for a large or impacted stone.

Preoperative Care. The nurse prepares the client for the selected procedure by explaining how, when, and where the procedure will be performed. The nurse describes what the client can expect before and after the procedure. The client receives nothing by mouth and also receives preoperative bowel preparation. (See Chapter 17 for routine preoperative care.)

Operative Procedures. The retroperitoneal area is entered through a large flank incision, as for nephrectomy (see Chapter 71), for pyelolithotomy or nephrolithotomy and through a lower abdominal incision for ureterolithotomy. The urinary tract is entered surgically and the stone removed. Before closure, various tubes and drains may be placed (e.g., nephrostomy tube, ureteral stent, Penrose or other wound drainage device, and Foley catheter).

Postoperative Care. The nurse follows routine procedures for assessment of the client who has received anesthesia. (See Chapter 19 for routine postoperative care.) The concerns after urologic surgery are monitoring the amount of bleeding from incisions and in the urine, maintaining adequate urine output, straining the urine to monitor the elimination of stone fragments, and assisting the client in preventing future stones through dietary modification.

INFECTION PREVENTION. Control of infections before invasive and noninvasive procedures is critical for the prevention of urosepsis. Interventions include the administration of appropriate antibiotics, either to eliminate an existing infection or to prevent new infections, and the maintenance of adequate nutrition and fluid intake. Because infection is always a component of struvite stone formation, the health care team plans for long-term prevention.

DRUG THERAPY. The clinician initially prescribes broad-spectrum antibiotics, such as the aminoglycosides (e.g., gentamicin [Garamycin]) and cephalosporins (e.g., cephalexin [Keflex, Novo-Lexin✦]), for treatment of infections occurring with urologic stone disease. The broad coverage is effective against gram-negative bacilli. After the results of the culture and sensitivity (C&S) studies are obtained, the clinician can select more specific antibiotics. C&S studies may be done 48 hours after the initiation of antibiotic therapy and again 48 hours after the conclusion of the prescribed course of therapy.

Blood levels of certain antibiotics, such as the aminoglycosides, are measured to ensure that appropriate levels of the antibiotic have been reached. If the desired blood level of these antibiotics is exceeded, toxic effects and kidney damage may result. If the blood level of the antibiotic is inadequate, microorganisms may not be completely eliminated. New clinical evidence of an infection (such as chills, fever, or altered mental status) warrants the collection of a urine sample for repeated C&S tests.

For the client with struvite stones, the primary care provider prescribes periodic and long-term monitoring of the urine for infection. Commonly, urine cultures are ordered monthly for 3 months, then quarterly for 1 year. Drugs that prevent bacteria from splitting urea, such as acetohydroxamic acid (Lithostat) and hydroxyurea (Hydrea), are often prescribed on a long-term basis for clients with struvite stones. The primary care provider monitors the serum creatinine with acetohydroxamic acid; its administration is contraindicated for levels above 2 mg/dL. The nurse reviews interventions aimed at preventing urinary tract infection (UTI) (see Interventions [Cystitis], p. 1618).

DIET THERAPY. The client's diet ideally includes adequate calorie intake representing a balance of all food groups. Unless medically contraindicated, the nurse encourages fluid intake of 2 to 3 L/day.

PREVENTION OF OBSTRUCTION. Measures to prevent urinary obstruction by stones include a high intake of fluids (3 L/day or more) and careful measures of intake and output. A liberal but not excessive fluid intake assists in preventing dehydration, promotes the flow of urine, and decreases the chance of crystals forming a stone. Interventions also depend on the type of stone. Medications, diet modification, and fluid intake are the major strategies available.

DRUG THERAPY. The selection of drugs for the prevention of obstruction depends on what is promoting the formation of stones and the type of stone formed. The nurse teaches the client the reason for the medication and assesses for side effects or adverse drug reactions.

CALCIUM-CONTAINING STONES. Drugs to treat **hypercalciuria** (high levels of calcium in the urine) may include thiazide diuretics (e.g., chlorothiazide [Diuril] or hydrochloro-thiazide [HydroDiuril, Natrimax✦, Urozide✦]), orthophosphate, and sodium cellulose phosphate. The thiazide diuretics promote calcium resorption from the renal tubules back into the body, thereby preventing excess calcium loads in the urine. Orthophosphate affects normal calcium-phosphorus metabolism, resulting in decreased urinary saturation of calcium oxalate. Sodium cellulose phosphate reduces intestinal absorption of calcium.

OXALATE-CONTAINING STONES. For clients with **hyperoxaluria** (high levels of oxalic acid in the urine), allopurinol (Zyloprim) and vitamin B_6 (pyridoxine) are used.

URIC ACID–CONTAINING STONES. For clients with chronic gout, allopurinol helps prevent the formation of **urate** (uric acid) stones. To alkalinize the urine, medications such as potassium citrate, 50% sodium citrate, and sodium bicarbonate may be used. The desired urinary pH is 6 to 6.5. Because the normal urinary pH averages 5 to 6, these desired values are termed "alkaline."

CYSTINE-CONTAINING STONES. For clients with **cystinuria** (high levels of cystine in the urine), alpha-mercaptopropionylglycine (AMPG) and captopril (Capoten) have both been found to lower urinary cystine levels. Their use is reserved for when hydration and alkalinization of the urine have not been successful.

DIET THERAPY. Diet modification depends on the type of stone formed (Table 70-6). The nurse consults the dietitian to plan the appropriate diet for the client.

OTHER MEASURES. The nurse encourages the client to ambulate frequently. Ambulation promotes passage of stones and reduces the possibility of calcium resorption from the bones. The nurse checks the pH of the urine daily and strains the urine with filter paper to collect passed fragments of stones.

HEALTH TEACHING. Key points of health teaching are described in Chart 70-12. The client often experiences tremendous anxiety and fear that a stone and its related pain may re-

TABLE 70-6 • DIETARY TREATMENT FOR RENAL STONES

Stone Type	Dietary Interventions	Rationale
Calcium oxalate	Avoid oxalate sources, such as spinach (see also Table 70-5).	Reduction of urinary oxalate content may help prevent these stones from forming. Urinary pH is not a factor.
Calcium phosphate	Decrease intake of foods high in protein.	Reduction of protein intake reduces acidic urine and prevents calcium precipitation.
	Some clients may benefit from a reduced calcium intake (milk, other dairy products).	Reduction of urine calcium concentration may prevent calcium precipitation and crystallization.
Struvite (magnesium ammonium phosphate)	Limit high-phosphate foods, such as dairy products, red and organ meats, and whole grains.	Reduction of urinary phosphate content may help prevent these stones from forming.
Uric acid (urate)	Decrease intake of purine sources, such as organ meats, poultry, fish, gravies, red wines, and sardines.	Reduction of urinary purine content may help prevent these stones from forming.
Cystine	Encourage PO fluids, up to 3 L/day.	Increased fluid helps dilute the urine and prevent the cystine crystals from forming.

CHART 70-12

CLIENT EDUCATION GUIDE
Urinary Calculi

- Finish your entire prescription of antibiotics to ensure that you will not get a urinary tract infection.
- You may resume your usual daily activities.
- Remember to balance regular exercise with sleep and rest.
- You may return to work 2 days to 6 weeks after surgery, depending on the type of intervention, your personal tolerance, and your physician's directives.
- Depending on the type of stone you had, your diet may be restricted to prevent further stone formation.
- Remember to drink at least 3 L of fluid a day to dilute potential stone-forming crystals, prevent dehydration, and promote urine flow.
- Monitor urine pH as directed (may be up to three times per day).
- You can expect bruising after lithotripsy. The bruising may be quite extensive and may take several weeks to resolve.
- Your urine may be bloody for several days after surgery.
- Pain in the region of the kidneys or bladder may signal the beginning of an infection or the formation of another stone. Report any pain, fever, chills, or difficulty with urination immediately to your physician or nurse.
- Keep follow-up appointments to check on infection, have repeat cultures done, and so forth.

TABLE 70-7 • STAGING OF BLADDER CANCER

PRIMARY TUMOR (T)	
T_X	Primary tumor cannot be assessed
T_0	No evidence of primary tumor
T_{IS}	Carcinoma in situ: "flat tumor"
T_1	Tumor invades submucosa (subepithelial connective tissue)
T_2	Tumor invades superficial muscle (inner half)
T_3	Tumor invades deep muscle or perivesical fat
T_{3a}	Tumor invades deep muscle (outer half)
T_{3b}	Tumor invades perivesical fat
T_4	Tumor invades any of the following: prostate, uterus, vagina, pelvic wall, abdominal wall
T_{4a}	Tumor invades prostate, uterus, vagina
T_{4b}	Tumor invades pelvic or abdominal wall
LYMPH NODE (N)	
N_X	Regional lymph nodes cannot be assessed
N_0	No regional lymph node metastasis
N_1	Metastasis in a single lymph node, 2 cm or less in greatest dimension
N_2	Metastasis in a single lymph node, more than 2 cm but not more than 5 cm in greatest dimension, or multiple lymph nodes, none more than 5 cm in greatest dimension; pelvic only
DISTANT METASTASIS (M)	
M_X	Presence of distant metastasis cannot be assessed
M_0	No distant metastasis
M_1	Distant metastasis or nodes positive above aortic bifurcation

Modified from American Joint Committee on Cancer. (1992). In O.H. Beahrs (Ed.), *Manual for staging of cancer* (4th ed.). Philadelphia: Lippincott-Raven; and Bennett, J.C., & Plum, F. (Eds.). (1996). *Cecil textbook of medicine* (20th ed.). Philadelphia: W.B. Saunders.

cur. In addition to anxiety about the pain, the possibility of repeated surgical interventions or permanent and serious kidney damage is of tremendous concern. Psychosocial preparation is generally enhanced when clients know what to expect and what actions to take should the unexpected develop. The nurse reassures the client that preventive and health promotion activities are designed to prevent recurrence.

Urothelial Cancer

OVERVIEW

Urothelial cancers are malignant tumors of the urothelium, which is the lining of transitional cells in the kidney, renal pelvis, ureters, urinary bladder, and urethra. Most urothelial tumors occur in the urinary bladder. Consequently, the general term *bladder cancer* is sometimes used to describe this pathologic condition.

In the United States, approximately 72% of urinary tract cancers occur as transitional cell carcinomas in the bladder (American Cancer Society [ACS], 2001). The second most common site of urinary tract cancer is the kidney and renal pelvis (27%). Squamous cell carcinoma accounts for approximately 5% of all bladder cancers.

Urothelial tumors are generally low grade, have multiple points of origin **(multifocal),** and are recurrent. Once the tumors spread beyond the transitional cell layer, they tend to be highly invasive and metastatic. Because of the multifocal, recurrent nature of the disease, clients with superficial tumors may experience recurrence up to 10 years after being tumor free.

Table 70-7 shows the staging of bladder cancer. Tumors confined to the mucosa are treated by simple excision, whereas carcinoma in situ (CIS), or stage T_{IS}, is generally treated with excision plus **intravesical** (inside the bladder) chemotherapy. Disease that has spread beyond CIS is treated with more extensive resection, often a **radical cystectomy** (removal of the bladder and surrounding tissue) with urinary diversion. Chemotherapy and radiotherapy are used in addition to surgery. When the tumor remains unchecked, it can invade surrounding structures, metastasize to distant sites (liver, lung, and bone), and ultimately lead to death.

Exposure to environmental toxins, particularly the chemicals used in the rubber, paint, electric cable, and textile industries, is highly associated with bladder cancer. The greatest risk factor for bladder cancer is tobacco use. Other risks include *Schistosoma haematobium* (a parasite) infection, excessive use of phenacetin compounds, and long-term administration of cyclophosphamide (Cytoxan, Procytox✤).

There are approximately 54,300 new cases of bladder cancer diagnosed each year in the United States and approximately 12,400 deaths per year from the disease (ACS, 2001). The condition is rare in adults younger than age 40, and there is a substantial increase in incidence after age 60.

COLLABORATIVE MANAGEMENT

Assessment

PHYSICAL ASSESSMENT/CLINICAL MANIFESTATIONS

The nurse inquires about the client's perception of general health. The gender and age of the client are documented. The nurse inquires about active and passive exposure to cigarette smoke. To detect potentially harmful environmental agents, the nurse asks the client to describe his or her occupation in detail. He or she is also asked to describe any change in the color, frequency, or amount of urine and any abdominal discomfort.

The overall appearance of the client is observed, especially skin color and general nutritional status. The nurse inspects, percusses, and palpates the abdomen for asymmetry, tenderness, and bladder distention.

The urine is examined for color and clarity. Hematuria is the predominant sign associated with bladder cancer; it may be gross or microscopic and is usually painless and intermittent. Dysuria, frequency, and urgency are usual symptoms when infection or obstruction is also present.

PSYCHOSOCIAL ASSESSMENT

The nurse assesses the client's emotions, including his or her response to known or suspected bladder cancer, and notes anxiety, fear, sadness, anger, or guilt. Early symptoms are painless, and many clients ignore hematuria because it is intermittent. Clients also may be reluctant to seek treatment because they suspect a sexually transmitted disease (STD). Consequently, they may experience guilt or anger about their own delays in seeking medical attention.

The nurse assesses the client's personal methods of coping and the degree of evident support from family or significant others. Social interaction and active role relationships with others may provide support and motivation for coping with convalescence.

DIAGNOSTIC ASSESSMENT

The only significant finding on a routine urinalysis is generally gross or microscopic hematuria. Cytologic testing on voided urine specimens is not usually helpful. Bladder-wash specimens and bladder biopsies are the most sensitive and specific tests for cancer.

Cystoscopy with retrograde pyelography is the primary method for evaluation of painless hematuria. A closed biopsy of a visible bladder tumor can be performed during cystoscopy. This is essential for staging and is usually performed in a day-surgery unit before admission to the hospital for treatment. Excretory urography is useful in identifying obstructions, especially at the ureterovesical junction. The computed tomography (CT) scan shows tumor invasion of surrounding tissues.

Ultrasonography shows masses but is less valuable for tumor staging. Magnetic resonance imaging (MRI) may help in the assessment of deep, invasive tumors.

Interventions

Therapy for the client with bladder cancer usually begins with surgical removal of the tumors for diagnosis and staging of disease. For tumors extending beyond the mucosa, surgery is followed by intravesical chemotherapy or immunotherapy. High-grade or recurrent tumors are treated with more radical surgery plus intravesical chemotherapy and/or radiotherapy. Systemic chemotherapy is reserved for clients with distant metastases. (See Chapter 25 for general care of the client receiving chemotherapy or radiation therapy.)

NONSURGICAL MANAGEMENT. Prophylactic immunotherapy with intravesical instillation of bacille Calmette-Guérin (BCG), a compound used to vaccinate against tuberculosis in some countries, is used to prevent tumor recurrence of superficial cancers (stage T_1 or lower). This procedure has been more effective than single-agent chemotherapy; side effects, however, are comparable.

Multiagent systemic chemotherapy is successful in prolonging life after distant metastasis has occurred but is rarely curative. Radiation therapy has also been successful in prolonging life.

SURGICAL MANAGEMENT. The type of surgery for bladder cancer depends on the type and stage of the cancer and the client's general health status. Complete cystectomy with extensive surgical removal of surrounding muscle and tissue offers the best chance of a cure for large, invasive bladder cancers.

PREOPERATIVE CARE. Specific client education depends on the type and extent of the planned surgical procedure. The nurse coordinates preoperative education with the physician and enterostomal (ET) therapist. The nurse discusses the type of urinary diversion and the selection of a site for the stoma. The goal is for the client to have a positive attitude about body image and a positive self-image. The nurse intervenes with educational counseling to ensure accurate understanding about self-care practices, methods of pouching, control of urine drainage, and minimization of odor.

The site selected for the stoma should be visible and avoid folds of skin, bones, and scar tissue. When possible, the client's waistline or belt area is avoided. The nurse prepares the client for the number and type of drains that will be present postoperatively. General preoperative care is discussed in Chapter 17.

OPERATIVE PROCEDURES. Transurethral resection of the bladder tumor (TURBT) or partial cystectomy is performed for small, early, superficial tumors. In a partial (segmental) cystectomy, a portion of the urinary bladder is removed. This procedure is generally used when there is only a single isolated bladder tumor.

When the entire bladder must be removed (complete cystectomy), the ureters are diverted into a collecting reservoir. Techniques for urinary diversion are illustrated in Figure 70-3. With an ileal conduit, the ureters are surgically implanted in a portion of the ileum, and urine is collected in a pouch on the skin around the stoma. Increasingly, continent reservoirs are being used. With cutaneous ureterostomy or ureteroureterostomy, the ureter opening is brought out onto the skin. The cutaneous ureterostomies may be located on either side of the abdomen or side by side.

POSTOPERATIVE CARE. After cutaneous ureterostomy, as with the ileal conduit, an external pouch covers the ostomy to collect urine. The nurse collaborates with the enterostomal therapist and focuses care on the wound, the skin, and urinary drainage. (See Chapters 56 and 57 for ostomy care.)

The client with a Kock's pouch, a continent reservoir, may have a Penrose drain and a plastic Medena catheter in the stoma. The drain removes lymphatic fluid or other secretions; the catheter ensures urine drainage so that suture lines may heal. The physician orders irrigation of the catheter to ensure patency. General postoperative care is discussed in Chapter 19.

Community-Based Care

HEALTH TEACHING

The nurse educates the client and family or significant others about medications, diet and fluid therapy, the use of external pouching systems, and the technique for catheterization of a continent reservoir.

With some procedures, the client may require electrolyte replacements to prevent long-term deficits. The nurse instructs the client to avoid foods that are known to produce gas if the urinary diversion uses the gastrointestinal (GI) tract. When the intestinal production of gas is minimized, flatus will not result in incontinence.

The nurse also instructs the client and family or significant others about any changes in self-care activities related to the urinary diversion. In conjunction and collaboration with the enterostomal therapist, the nurse demonstrates external pouch application, local skin care, pouch care, methods of adhesion, and drainage mechanisms. If a Kock's pouch has been created, the client is instructed about the technique of catheterization. For all instruction, the nurse observes at least one return demonstration by the client or the family caregiver. The client ideally assumes responsibility for self-care before discharge.

The nurse assists the client in preparing psychologically for the impact of urinary diversion on self-image, body image, sexual functioning, and self-esteem. Counseling provides information and support so that the feelings of powerlessness may be minimized.

Through discussions with the client about usual social situations, the nurse helps the client gain control over new toileting practices. Men with a urinary diversion into the sigmoid colon need to learn a new habit of sitting to urinate. For clients of either gender, the nurse promotes confidence in social situations by encouraging frequent emptying of urinary collection devices before traveling or attending social functions or events. Resumption of sexual activity is a major concern for many adult clients, regardless of age; this topic needs to be addressed openly and with sensitivity. Cystectomy causes physiologic impotence in men, but treatment is available (see Chapter 76).

HEALTH CARE RESOURCES

The United Ostomy Association and the American Cancer Society units and chapters have educational materials that may be useful to clients. In some areas, local support groups have meetings to assist others and to send visitors to provide peer counseling and support. Home care personnel may assist with follow-up, easing the transition from hospital to home. The Wound, Ostomy, and Continence Nurses Society provides educational programs and a journal devoted to the care of clients with ostomies.

Bladder Trauma

OVERVIEW

Bladder trauma can be caused by penetrating or blunt injury to the lower abdomen. Penetrating lower abdominal injury may occur by stabbing, gunshot wound, or other trauma in which objects pierce the abdominal wall. A fractured pelvis with puncture of the bladder by bone fragments is the most common cause of bladder trauma. Bladder trauma may also be a result of sexual assault.

Blunt trauma compresses the abdominal wall and the bladder. A seat belt may compress the bladder hard enough to cause injury, especially if the bladder is full or distended.

COLLABORATIVE MANAGEMENT

Assessment

Clients with a penetrating bladder wound often have anuria or hematuria. In the emergency department, initial assessment includes inspection of the urinary meatus for blood.

Diagnostic tests include cystography and voiding cystourethrography (VCUG). If renal or ureteral trauma is suspected, IV urography is scheduled before cystography so that any leakage of bladder contrast medium does not mask the outlines of the kidneys or ureters. The cystogram shows whether there is a defect in bladder filling; the voiding cystourethrogram defines bladder emptying.

Interventions

Bladder trauma, other than a simple contusion, requires surgical intervention. Stabilization of any fractures usually precedes bladder repair. Surgical interventions include procedures to repair the anterior or posterior bladder wall and peritoneal membrane. In general, repairs of the bladder are accomplished by closure procedures.

The client with an anterior bladder wall injury commonly has a Penrose drain and a Foley catheter in place postoperatively; the client with a posterior bladder wall injury has a

Ureterostomies divert urine directly to the skin surface through a ureteral skin opening (stoma). After ureterostomy, the client must wear a pouch.

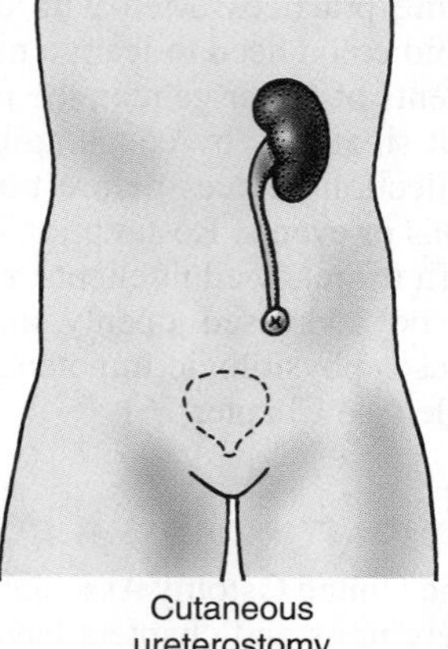

Cutaneous ureterostomy

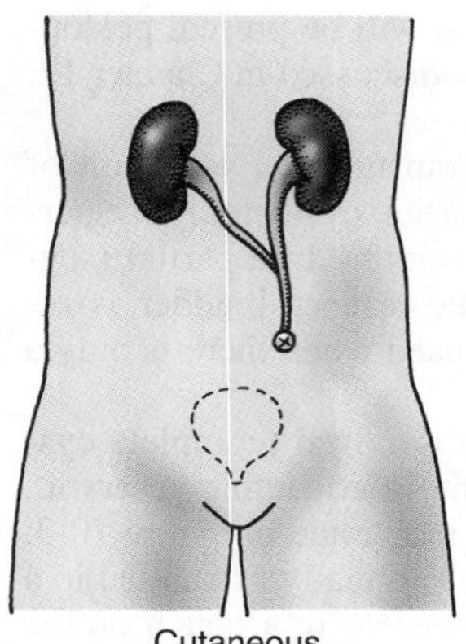

Cutaneous ureteroureterostomy

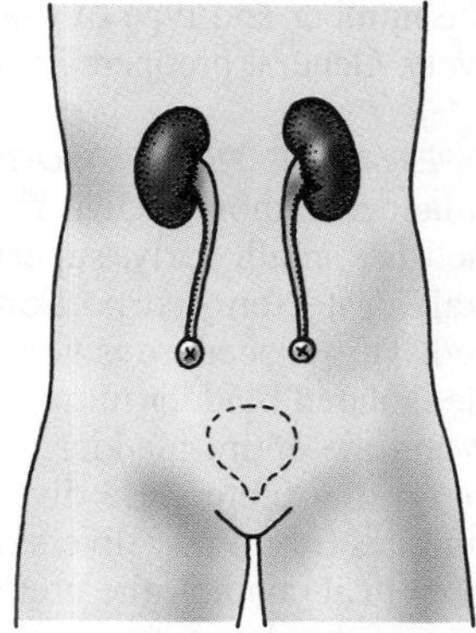

Bilateral cutaneous ureterostomy

Conduits collect urine in a portion of the intestine, which is then opened onto the skin surface as a stoma. After the creation of a conduit, the client must wear a pouch.

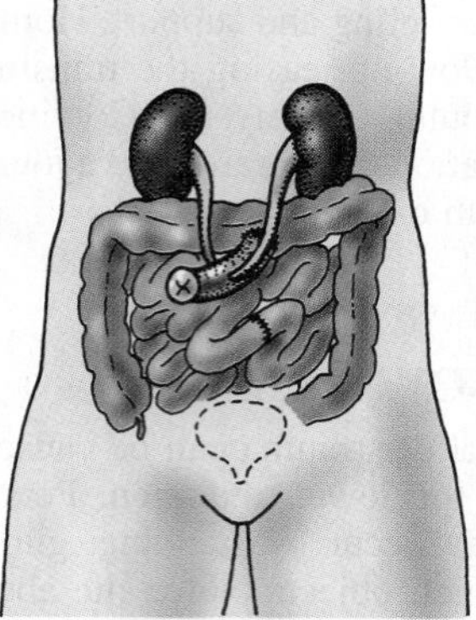

Ileal (Bricker's) conduit

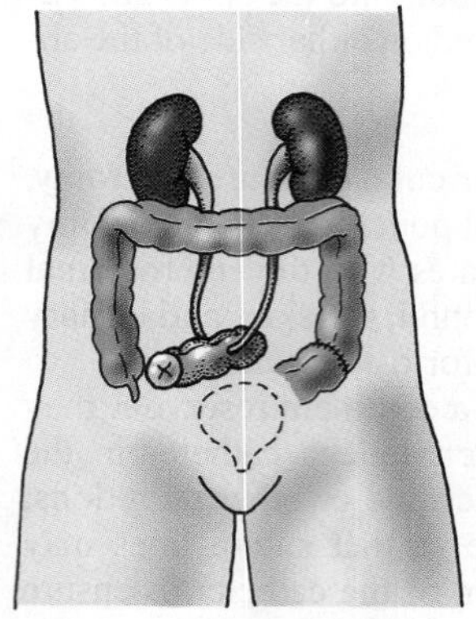

Colon conduit

Ileal reservoirs divert urine into a surgically created pouch, or pocket, that functions as a bladder. The stoma is continent, and the client removes urine by regular self-catheterization.

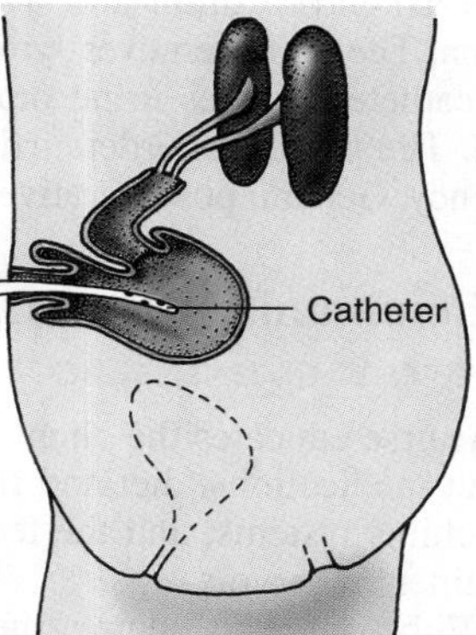

Continent internal ileal reservoir (Kock's pouch)

Sigmoidostomies divert urine to the large intestine, so no stoma is required. The client excretes urine with bowel movements, and bowel incontinence may result.

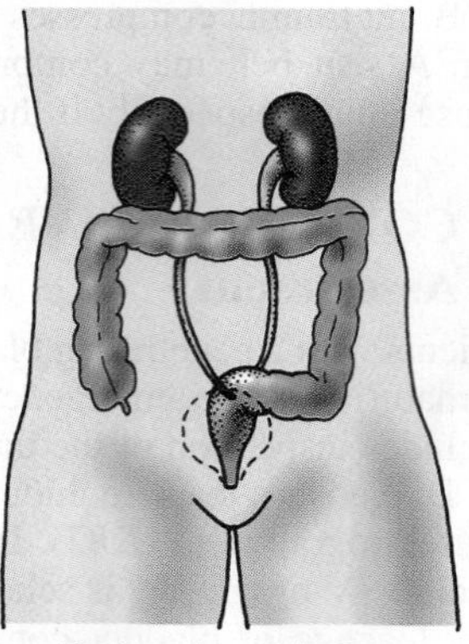

Ureterosigmoidostomy

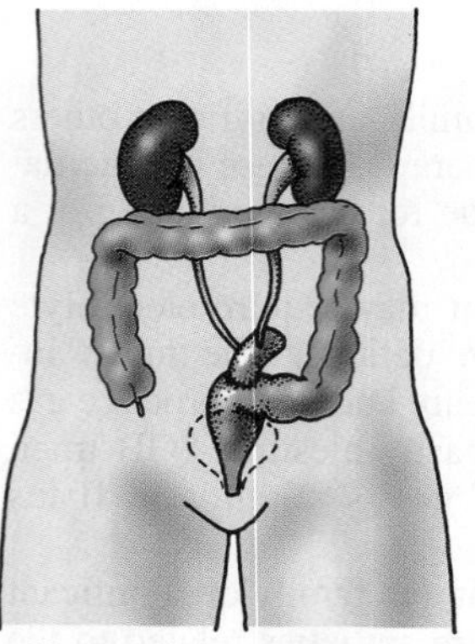

Ureteroiliosigmoidostomy

Figure 70-3 ● Urinary diversion procedures used in the treatment of bladder cancer.

Penrose drain and Foley or suprapubic catheter. In some instances, vaginal or rectal fistulas may also require repair.

Psychosocial support is critical for clients who have sustained traumatic injuries. The nurse refers the client to appropriate resources to assist in dealing with potential psychosocial issues.

ONLINE RESOURCES

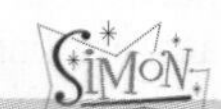

For suggested readings and Internet resources, go to http://www.wbsaunders.com/SIMON/Iggy/.

SELECTED BIBLIOGRAPHY

Asterisk indicates a classic or definitive work on this subject.

*Adams, D.H., & Abernathy, B.B. (1996). Laser ureterolithotripsy for cystine calculi. *AORN Journal, 64*(6), 924, 926-927, 929-930.

*Agency for Health Care Policy and Research. (1992). *Urinary incontinence in adults. Clinical practice guideline.* AHCPR Pub. No. 92-0038. Rockville, MD: Agency for Health Care Policy and Research, Public Health Service, U.S. Department of Health and Human Services.

*Agency for Health Care Policy and Research. (1996). *Urinary incontinence in adults: Acute and chronic management. Clinical practice guideline.* AHCPR Pub. No. 96-0682. Rockville, MD: Agency for

Health Care Policy and Research, Public Health Service, U.S. Department of Health and Human Services.

American Cancer Society. (2001). *Cancer facts and figures—2001.* Report No. 01-300M-No. 5008.01. Atlanta: Author.

Balaji, K.C., & Menon, M. (1997). Mechanism of stone formation. *Urologic Clinics of North America, 24*(1), 1-11.

Centers for Disease Control and Prevention. (May 2001); www.cdc.gov/nchs.

Cohen, M., & Rothmann, M. (2001). Gemcitabine and cisplatin for advanced metastatic bladder cancer. *Journal of Clinical Oncology, 19*(4), 1229-1231.

Diering, C., & Palmer, M. (2001). Professional information about urinary incontinence on the World Wide Web: Is it timely? Is it accurate? *Journal of Wound, Ostomy, and Continence Nursing, 28*(1), 55-62.

Duffield, P. (1997). Urinary tract infections in the elderly. *ADVANCE for Nurse Practitioners, 5*(4), 30-32.

Gallo, M. (1997). Quality of life improvement and the reliance urinary control insert. *Urologic Nursing, 17,* 146-153.

Houston, M. (1999). Uncomplicated urinary tract infection in women: Diagnostic and therapeutic recommendations by the Institute for Clinical Systems Integration. *Postgraduate Medicine, 105*(5), 181-183, 187-188.

*Hruska, K. (1996). Renal calculi. In J.C. Bennett & F. Plum (Eds.), *Cecil textbook of medicine* (20th ed.). Philadelphia: W.B. Saunders.

Jay, J., & Staskin, D. (1998). Urinary incontinence: Strategies for effective diagnosis and management. *ADVANCE for Nurse Practitioners, 6*(10), 32-37.

Jirovec, M.M., Wyman, J.F., & Wells, T.J. (1998). Addressing urinary incontinence with educational continence-care competencies. *Image: The Journal of Nursing Scholarship, 30*(4), 375-378.

Johnson, S. (2000). From incontinence to confidence. *American Journal of Nursing, 100*(2), 69-76.

Johnson, V. (2001). Effects of a submaximal exercise protocol to recondition the pelvic floor musculature. *Nursing Research, 50*(1), 33-41.

Kee, J.L. (1998). *Handbook of laboratory and diagnostic tests with nursing implications* (3rd ed.). Stamford, CN: Appleton & Lange.

Kincade, J., Peckous, B., & Busby-Whitehead, J. (2001). A pilot study to determine predictors of behavioral treatment completion for urinary incontinence. *Urologic Nursing, 21*(1), 39-44.

Kirton, C.A. (1997). Assessing for bladder distension. *Nursing97, 27*(4), 64.

Krautschick, A.W. (1999). Metabolic evaluation and medical therapy for stone formation. *Current Opinions in Urology, 9*(4), 335-338.

Lightner, D.J., & Itano, N.M. (1999). Treatment options for women with stress urinary incontinence. *Mayo Clinic Proceedings, 75*(11), 1149-1156.

Lingappa, V. (2000). Renal disease. In S. McPhee, V. Lingappa, & W. Ganong (Eds.), *Pathophysiology of disease* (3rd ed.). New York: Lange Medical Books/McGraw-Hill.

*Lowe, A., & Gabriel, L.S. (1993). Laser lithotripsy: Patient care, staff education. *AORN Journal, 58*(5), 961-964, 966, 968-969.

Lyons, S., & Specht, J. (2000). Prompted voiding protocol for individuals with urinary incontinence. *Journal of Gerontological Nursing, 20*(6), 5-13.

Marchiondo, K. (1998). A new look at urinary tract infection. *American Journal of Nursing, 98*(3), 34-39.

McCloskey, J.C., & Bulechek, G.M. (2000). *Nursing interventions classification (NIC)* (3rd ed.). St. Louis: Mosby.

*Parivar, F., Low, R.K., & Stoller, M.L. (1996). The influence of diet on urinary stone disease. *Journal of Urology, 155,* 432-440.

Parker, S.L., et al. (1997). Cancer statistics, 1997. *CA: A Cancer Journal for Clinicians, 47*(1), 5-27.

Renner, C., & Rassweiler, J. (1999). Treatment of renal stones by extracorporeal shock wave lithotripsy. *Nephron, 81*(Suppl. 1), 71-81.

Resnick, M.I. (Ed.). (1997). Urolithiasis. *Urologic Clinics of North America, 24*(1), entire issue.

Ruml, L.A., Pearle, M.S., & Pak, C.Y.C. (1997). Medical therapy: Calcium oxalate urolithiasis. *Urologic Clinics of North America, 24*(1), 117-133.

Rutchik, S.D., & Resnick, M.I. (1997). Cystine calculi. *Urologic Clinics of North America, 24*(1), 163-171.

Scheinman, S.J. (1999). Nephrolithiasis. *Seminars in Nephrology, 19*(4), 381-388.

Schulz, J.A., & Drutz, H.P. (1999). The surgical management of recurrent stress urinary incontinence. *Current Opinions in Obstetrics and Gynecology, 11*(5), 489-494.

Schwartz, B.F., & Stoller, M.L. (1999). Nonsurgical management of infection-related renal calculi. *Urologic Clinics of North America, 26*(4), 765-778.

Singal, R.K., & Denstedt, J.D. (1997). Contemporary management of ureteral stones. *Urologic Clinics of North America, 24*(1), 59-70.

Sirls, L.T., & Rashid, T. (1999). Geriatric urinary incontinence. *Geriatric Nephrology and Urology, 9*(2), 87-99.

Smith, D. (1998). A continence care approach for long-term care facilities. *Geriatric Nursing, 19*(2), 81-86.

Stockert, P.A. (1999). Getting UTI patients back on track. *RN, 62*(3), 49-54.

Strangio, L. (1997). Interventional uroradiologic procedures. *AORN Journal, 66*(2), 286-290, 292-294.

Suchinski, G.A., et al. (1999). Treating urinary tract infections in the elderly. *Dimensions in Critical Care Nursing, 18*(91), 21-27.

Swift, S.E., & Yoon, E.A. (1999). Test-retest reliability of the cough stress test in the evaluation of urinary incontinence. *Obstetrics and Gynecology, 94*(1), 99-102.

*Thompson, A.C., & Christmas, T.J. (1996). Interstitial cystitis: An update. *British Journal of Urology, 78*(6), 813-820.

United States Pharmacopeia Dispensing Information (USP DI): Vol. I. Drug information for the health care professional (20th ed.). (2000). Englewood, CO: Micromedix.

U.S. Renal Data Systems. (1999). *USRDS 1999 annual data report.* Bethesda, MD: The National Institutes of Health, National Institute of Diabetes and Digestive and Kidney Diseases.

Vaughn, D., & Malkowicz, S. (2001). Recent advances in bladder cancer chemotherapy. *Cancer Investigation, 19*(1), 77-85.

Walsh, P.C., et al. (1998). *Campbell's urology* (7th ed.). Philadelphia: W.B. Saunders.

Warren, J.W. (1997). Catheter-associated urinary tract infections. *Infectious Disease Clinics of North America, 11*(93), 609-622.

Warren, J.W., et al. (1999). Guidelines for antimicrobial treatment of uncomplicated acute bacterial cystitis and acute pyelonephritis in women. *Clinics in Infectious Disease, 29*(4), 745-758.

Young-McCaughan, S. (1999a). Invasive bladder cancer. In C. Miaskowski & P. Buchsel (Eds.), *Oncology nursing: Assessment and clinical care* (pp. 1055-1087), St. Louis: Mosby.

Young-McCaughan, S. (1999b). Superficial bladder cancer. In C. Miaskowski & P. Buchsel (Eds.), *Oncology nursing: Assessment and clinical care* (pp. 1031-1055), St. Louis: Mosby.

Zagoria, R.J. (Ed.). (1997). Uroradiology. *Urologic Clinics of North America, 24*(3), entire issue.

CHAPTER

71

Interventions for Clients with Renal Disorders

CHRIS WINKELMAN

Learning Objectives

After studying this chapter, you should be able to:

1. Prioritize nursing care for the client with polycystic kidney disease.
2. Describe the clinical manifestations of hydronephrosis.
3. Identify clients at risk for pyelonephritis.
4. Use laboratory data and clinical manifestations to determine the effectiveness of therapy for pyelonephritis.
5. Compare and contrast the pathophysiology and clinical manifestations of acute glomerular nephritis and nephrotic syndrome.
6. Prioritize nursing care for the client during the first 24 hours after a nephrectomy.
7. Explain how diabetic nephropathy can affect glucose metabolism and control in the client with diabetes mellitus.
8. Develop a teaching plan for the client who has had a nephrectomy for renal cell carcinoma.

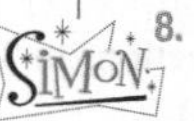

Go to http://www.wbsaunders.com/SIMON/Iggy/ for self-assessment questions related to these Learning Objectives.

Renal disorders interfere with the ability of the kidney to filter wastes and to balance fluid and solutes. The kidneys work in an integrated way with so many other organ systems; therefore a renal disorder can significantly affect systemic health and lead to life-threatening outcomes. Renal disorders can be categorized as congenital, obstructive, infectious, glomerular, and degenerative. Renal tumors and renal trauma are also described in this chapter.

CONGENITAL DISORDERS

Polycystic Kidney Disease

OVERVIEW

Polycystic kidney disease (PKD) is one of the most common inherited disorders and affects 250,000 to 500,000 people in the United States. It can be inherited as either an autosomal dominant trait or, less commonly, as an autosomal recessive trait. People who inherit the recessive form of PKD usually die in early childhood. The 5% to 10% incidence of PKD in clients with no family history occurs as a result of a spontaneous genetic mutation. PKD is more common in Caucasians than in people of other races.

Pathophysiology

Fluid-filled cysts in the epithelial cells of the nephron characterize PKD. In the dominant form only 5% to 10% of nephrons may be involved until the fourth decade of life, whereas in the autosomal recessive form nearly 100% of nephrons are involved at birth. Cysts develop as a result of kidney cell proliferation, altered secretion, and abnormal cell matrix biology (Avner, et al., 1999; Calvet & Grantham, 2001).

Cysts can develop anywhere in the nephron. Over time, small cysts become progressively larger (up to a few centimeters in diameter) and more widely distributed; the glomerular and tubular membranes are damaged. As the cysts become filled with fluid, the nephron functions of filtration, reabsorption, and secretion become less effective.

The kidney tissue is eventually replaced by nonfunctioning cysts, which look like a cluster of grapes (Figure 71-1). The kidneys are grossly enlarged; each cystic kidney may enlarge to two or three times its normal size, becoming as large as a football. Other abdominal organs are displaced, and the client has considerable discomfort. The fluid-filled cysts are also prone to infection, rupture, and bleeding.

More than 60% of clients with PKD have high blood pressure. The cause of hypertension in this disorder is thought to be related to renal ischemia from the enlarging cysts. As the vessels are compressed and renal blood flow decreases, the renin-angiotensin system is activated, raising blood pressure. Control of hypertension is a top priority because proper treatment can interrupt the vasoconstriction that leads to renal ischemia.

Cysts may also occur in other tissues, such as the liver, blood vessels of the brain, and cardiac blood vessels. Cysts may alter liver function or result in spontaneous rupture of

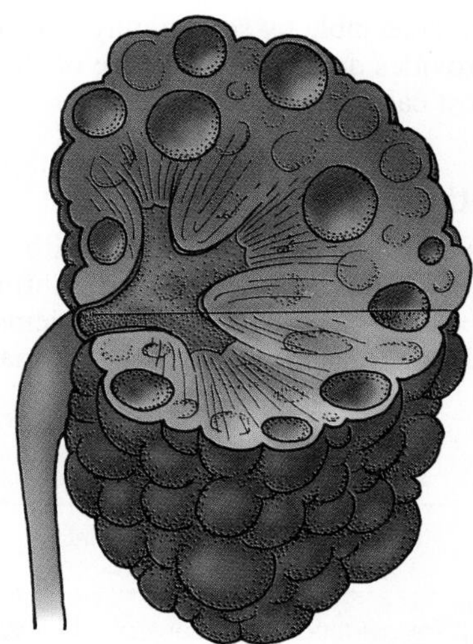

Figure 71-1 ● Polycystic kidney.

vascular cysts (*berry aneurysms*) in the brain, causing sudden death. For reasons as yet unknown, kidney stones occur in 8% to 36% of the clients with PKD. Heart valve abnormalities (e.g., mitral valve prolapse), left ventricular hypertrophy, and colonic diverticuli also are more prevalent in clients with PKD.

Etiology

PKD has at least two inherited forms. Men and women have an equal chance of inheriting the disease because the gene responsible for PKD is not located on the sex chromosomes. The offspring of parents who have PKD have a 50% probability of inheriting the gene that causes the autosomal dominant form of the disease.

Manifestations of autosomal dominant polycystic kidney disease (ADPKD) usually do not appear until the fourth decade of life. Half of the affected people develop renal failure by age 50 years. ADPKD-1 is the most severe form both in disease progression and in mortality. ADPKD-2 involves a slower rate of cystic formation and growth, resulting in a delayed progression to renal failure and other complications.

At present, there is no way to prevent PKD, although early detection and management of hypertension may slow the progression of renal impairment. Genetic counseling and evaluation may be useful for adults who have one parent or both parents with PKD. For those whose clinical symptoms do not appear until after the childbearing years, offspring can be included in genetic counseling sessions.

COLLABORATIVE MANAGEMENT

Assessment

HISTORY

The nurse explores the family history of a client with suspected or actual PKD and asks whether either parent was known to have PKD or whether there is any family history of kidney disease. The age at which signs and symptoms developed in the parent and any related complications may have prognostic significance. The client is asked about constipation, abdominal discomfort, a change in urine color or frequency, high blood pressure, headaches, and a family history of sudden death from a stroke.

CHART 71-1

KEY FEATURES *of* Polycystic Kidney Disease

- Abdominal or flank pain
- Hypertension
- Nocturia
- Increased abdominal girth
- Constipation
- Bloody or cloudy urine
- Kidney stones

PHYSICAL ASSESSMENT/CLINICAL MANIFESTATIONS

Chart 71-1 lists key features of PKD. Pain is the presenting symptom in 20% to 30% of clients and is noted in at least 60%. The nurse inspects the abdomen. A protruding and distended abdomen is common as the cystic kidneys swell and push the abdominal contents forward. Polycystic kidneys are easily palpated because of their increased size. The nurse proceeds with *gentle* abdominal palpation because the cystic kidneys and nearby tissues may be tender, and palpation is uncomfortable.

The client also may have flank pain as a dull ache or as sharp and intermittent discomfort. Dull and aching pain is caused by increased kidney size with distention or from infection within the cyst. Sharp, intermittent pain occurs in response to a ruptured cyst or the presence of a stone. When a cyst ruptures, the client may notice bright red or cola-colored urine. The nurse suspects infection if the urine is cloudy or foul smelling or if there is **dysuria** (pain on urination).

Nocturia (the need to urinate excessively at night) may be an early disease sign and occurs because of decreased renal concentrating ability. As renal function further declines, the client experiences increasing hypertension, edema, and uremic symptoms such as anorexia, nausea, vomiting, pruritus, and fatigue (see Chapter 72). Because berry aneurysms often occur in clients with PKD, a severe headache with or without neurologic or vision alterations deserves particular attention.

PSYCHOSOCIAL ASSESSMENT

As an inherited disorder, PKD may cause complex psychosocial responses. The client often has had direct experience with the effects and consequences of the disease in other close family members. He or she may have had a parent who died or other close relatives who required dialysis or transplantation. While obtaining the family history, the nurse listens carefully for spoken and unspoken feelings of anger, resentment, hostility, futility, sadness, or anxiety; such feelings may need further exploration. The focus may be one or both parents or the process of diagnosis and treatment. Feelings of guilt and concern for the client's own children may further complicate the adjustment.

DIAGNOSTIC ASSESSMENT

Urinalysis usually reveals **proteinuria** (protein in the urine) once the glomeruli are involved. Hematuria may be gross or microscopic. Bacteria in the urine suggest an infection, usually in the cysts. A urine sample for culture and sensitivity testing is obtained when there is clinical or laboratory evidence of infection. As kidney function deteriorates, serum creatinine and blood urea nitrogen (BUN) levels rise. With worsening kidney function, the 24-hour creatinine clearance decreases. Renal handling of sodium may cause either sodium losses or sodium retention.

Diagnostic studies include renal sonography, computed tomography (CT), and magnetic resonance imaging (MRI). Small cysts are detectable by sonography, CT, or MRI. Renal sonography provides diagnostic evidence of PKD, with minimal risk in most cases.

Interventions

Common nursing diagnoses for the client with polycystic kidney disease (PKD) include Acute Pain, Chronic Pain, and Constipation. Common collaborative problems include Potential for Infection, Hypertension, Stone Formation, or Renal

CHART 71-2

NIC INTERVENTION ACTIVITIES *for* The Client with Renal Problems

Pain Management: *Alleviation of pain or a reduction in pain to a level of comfort that is acceptable to the client.*
- Observe for nonverbal cues of discomfort, especially in those unable to communicate effectively.
- Assure client attentive analgesic care.
- Consider cultural influences on pain response.
- Utilize a developmentally appropriate assessment method that allows for monitoring of change in pain (e.g., flow sheet, daily diary).
- Control environmental factors that may influence the client's response to discomfort.
- Consider type and source of pain when selecting pain relief strategy.
- Provide the person optimal pain relief with prescribed analgesics.
- Implement the use of patient-controlled analgesia (PCA), if appropriate.
- Use pain control measures before pain becomes severe.
- Evaluate the effectiveness of the pain control measures used through ongoing assessment of the pain experience.
- Institute and modify pain control measures on the basis of the client's response.

Bowel Management: *Establishment and maintenance of a regular pattern of bowel elimination.*
- Note pre-existent bowel problems, bowel routine, and use of laxatives.
- Teach client about specific foods that are assistive in promoting bowel regularity.
- Initiate a bowel training program, as appropriate.
- Instruct client in foods high in fiber, as appropriate.
- Evaluate medication profile for gastrointestinal side effects.

Medication Management: *Facilitation of safe and effective use of prescription and over-the-counter drugs.*
- Monitor client for the therapeutic effect of the medication.
- Monitor for signs and symptoms of drug toxicity.
- Monitor for adverse effects of the drug.
- Develop strategies with the client to enhance compliance with prescribed medication regimen.
- Teach the client and/or family members the expected action and side effects of the medication.
- Instruct client when to seek medical attention.

Energy Management: *Regulating energy use to treat or prevent fatigue and optimize function.*
- Determine client's physical limitations.
- Determine client's/significant other's perceptions of causes of fatigue.
- Encourage verbalization of feelings about limitations.
- Determine what and how much activity is required to build endurance.
- Monitor nutritional intake to ensure adequate energy resources.
- Monitor client for evidence of excess physical and emotional fatigue.
- Monitor cardiorespiratory response to activity (e.g., tachycardia, other dysrhythmias, dyspnea, diaphoresis, pallor, hemodynamic pressures, and respiratory rate).
- Monitor location and nature of discomfort or pain during movement/activity.
- Promote bedrest/activity limitation (e.g., increase number of rest periods).
- Encourage alternate rest and activity periods.
- Provide calming diversional activities to promote relaxation.
- Plan activities for periods when the client has the most energy.
- Assist with regular physical activities (e.g., ambulation, transfers, turning, and personal care), as needed.
- Encourage physical activity (e.g., ambulation or performance of activities of daily living, consistent with client's energy resources).

Fluid Monitoring: *Collection and analysis of client data to regulate fluid balance.*
- Monitor weight.
- Monitor intake and output.
- Monitor serum and urine electrolyte values, as appropriate.
- Monitor serum albumin and total protein levels.
- Monitor serum and urine osmolality levels.
- Keep an accurate record of intake and output.
- Monitor for distended neck veins, crackles in the lungs, peripheral edema, and weight gain.
- Restrict and allocate fluid intake, as appropriate.
- Administer pharmacologic agents to increase urine output, as appropriate.
- Administer dialysis, as appropriate, noting client response.

Urinary Retention Care: *Assistance in relieving bladder distension.*
- Provide privacy for elimination.
- Provide Credé maneuver, as necessary.
- Use double voiding technique.
- Insert urinary catheter, as appropriate.
- Monitor degree of bladder distension by palpation and percussion.
- Catheterize for residual, as appropriate.
- Implement intermittent catheterization, as appropriate.

Infection Protection: *Prevention and early detection of infection in a client at risk.*
- Monitor for systemic and localized signs and symptoms of infection.
- Maintain asepsis for client at risk.
- Inspect condition of any surgical incision/wound.
- Instruct client to take antibiotics as prescribed.
- Obtain cultures, as needed.

NIC intervention activities selected from McCloskey, J.C., & Bulechek, G.M. (Eds). (2000). *Nursing interventions classification (NIC)* (3rd ed.). St. Louis: Mosby.

Failure. Chart 71-2 lists some NIC interventions for clients with renal disorders. (See Chapter 70 for information on renal infections and stone formation. See Chapter 72 for care of the client with renal failure.)

PAIN

NIC *PAIN MANAGEMENT; ANALGESIC ADMINISTRATION.* Comfort strategies include pharmacologic, physical, and integrative approaches. A combination may be most effective. Nonsteroidal anti-inflammatory agents (NSAIDs) are used cautiously because of their tendency to adversely affect renal function. Aspirin-containing compounds are avoided to prevent an increased potential for bleeding.

If cyst infection is the cause of discomfort, the physician orders a lipid-soluble antibiotic such as trimethoprim/sulfamethoxazole (Bactrim, Septra, Trimpex) or ciprofloxacin (Cipro), which penetrate the cyst wall. Monitoring serum creatinine levels is necessary because antibiotic therapy can be nephrotoxic. Applying dry heat to the abdomen or flank may promote comfort when renal cysts are infected. When pain is severe or debilitating, cysts can be decompressed with percutaneous needle aspiration and drainage.

The nurse teaches the client methods of enhancing relaxation and promoting comfort via deep breathing, guided imagery, or other relaxation strategies. The overall goal is client self-management. (See Chapter 7 for pain management.)

CONSTIPATION

NIC *BOWEL MANAGEMENT.* The nurse also teaches the client how to prevent constipation. The teaching plan covers adequate fluid intake, the role of increased dietary fiber when fluid intake is more than 2500 mL/24 hr, and the need for regular exercise to achieve regular bowel elimination. The nurse explains that pressure on the large intestine may further impede peristalsis as the polycystic kidneys increase in size. Consequently, the client should know that these recommendations for bowel management might change, particularly if renal failure also develops. The nurse also advises about the appropriate use of stool softeners and bulk agents, including the careful use of laxatives, to prevent complications related to chronic constipation.

HYPERTENSION AND RENAL FAILURE

NIC *TEACHING: DISEASE PROCESS; TEACHING: PRESCRIBED MEDICATION.* Blood pressure control is necessary to minimize cardiovascular complications and slow the progression of renal dysfunction. Nursing interventions include education to promote self-management and understanding (see Chapter 36 for more information on hypertension). When renal impairment is evident through a decreased concentrating ability (e.g., nocturia, low urine specific gravity), the nurse encourages the client to drink at least 2 L of fluid per day to prevent fluid volume deficit, which could further affect renal function. Restricting excess dietary sodium intake may control blood pressure. Because fluid volume intake is not restricted, intravascular volume depletion and decreased renal perfusion does not occur.

Medications for blood pressure control include antihypertensive agents and diuretics. Antihypertensive agents include angiotensin-converting enzyme (ACE) inhibitors, calcium channel blockers, beta blockers, and vasodilators (see Chart 36-2). ACE inhibitors show promise in controlling the epithelial-proliferative aspects of PKD and in reducing microalbuminuria (Torra, 1999). If PKD progresses to chronic renal failure or end-stage renal disease, treatment approaches are similar to those in Chapter 72.

The nurse teaches the client, family, or significant other how to measure and record blood pressure. The nurse also helps the client establish a schedule for self-administering medications, monitoring daily weights, and keeping blood pressure records (Chart 71-3). The potential side effects of the medications are explained. The nurse makes written materials, such as medication teaching cards and booklets, available.

A low-sodium diet is often prescribed to control the hypertension that usually accompanies PKD. However, some clients may experience salt wasting and do not require a sodium-restricted diet. As the disease progresses, the physician may limit the client's protein intake to slow the development of renal failure. The nurse assists the client, family, or significant other in understanding the recommended diet plan and clarifies its rationale. The nurse works closely with the dietitian to foster the client's understanding. The nurse may also initiate a referral for nutritional counseling.

Health Care Resources

The Polycystic Kidney Research Foundation conducts research and provides education about PKD. Many publications are available on request; there is a fee for some materials. Chapters of the National Kidney Foundation (NKF) and the American Association of Kidney Patients (AAKP) may also provide resources for client information and support.

OBSTRUCTIVE DISORDERS

Hydronephrosis, Hydroureter, and Urethral Stricture

OVERVIEW

Hydronephrosis and hydroureter are disorders usually associated with the obstruction of urine outflow. Urethral strictures also obstruct outflow. Prompt recognition and treatment are crucial to prevent permanent renal damage.

In **hydronephrosis,** the kidney becomes enlarged as urine accumulates in the pelvis and kidney tissue. Because the ca-

CHART 71-3

CLIENT EDUCATION GUIDE
Polycystic Kidney Disease

- Measure and record your blood pressure daily.
- Take your temperature if you suspect you have a fever.
- Weigh yourself every day at the same time of day and with the same amount of clothing, notify your physician or nurse if you have a sudden weight gain.
- Limit your intake of salt to help control your blood pressure.
- Notify your physician or nurse if your urine is foul smelling or if there is blood in your urine.
- Notify your physician or nurse if you have a headache that does not go away or if you have visual disturbances.
- Monitor bowel movements to prevent constipation.

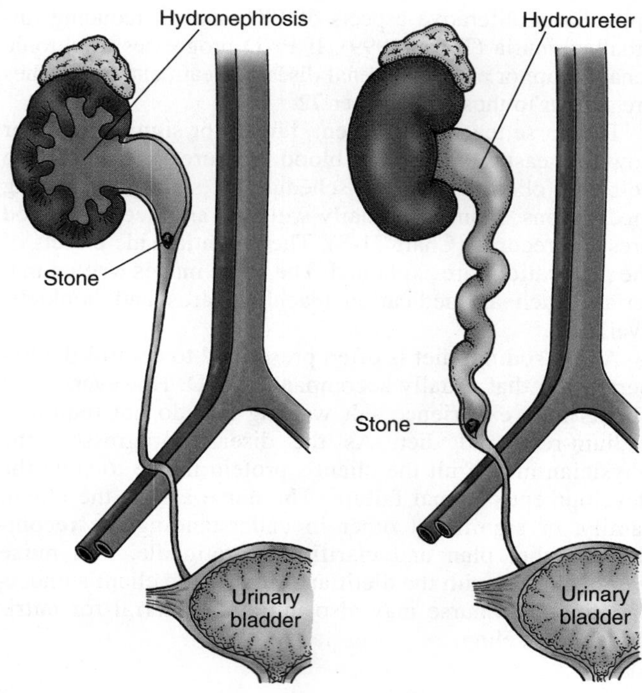

Figure 71-2 ● Hydronephrosis is caused by obstruction in the upper part of the ureter; hydroureter is caused by obstruction in the lower part of the ureter.

pacity of the renal pelvis is normally 5 to 8 mL, obstructions within it or at the ureteropelvic junction (UPJ) quickly result in renal pelvic distention. Kidney medullary pressure increases as the volume of urine increases. Over time, sometimes in only a matter of hours, the blood vessels and renal tubules can be damaged extensively (Figure 71-2).

In clients with **hydroureter,** the pathophysiologic effects are similar but the obstruction is lower in the urinary tract. The ureter is most likely to become obstructed where the iliac vessels cross or at the ureterovesical entry. Dilation of the ureter above the point of obstruction results in enlargement as urine continues to accumulate (see Figure 71-2).

In a client with a **urethral stricture,** the obstruction is very low in the urinary tract; this causes bladder distention to occur before hydroureter and hydronephrosis. The problems and kidney damage are similar without prompt treatment.

A urinary obstruction can cause structural damage when pressure builds up directly on tissue. Tubular filtrate pressure also increases within the nephron as drainage through the collecting system is impaired. With this added pressure, glomerular filtration decreases or ceases, and renal failure results. Nitrogenous waste products (urea, creatinine, and uric acid) and electrolytes (sodium, potassium, chloride, and phosphorus) are retained in the serum, and renal regulation of acid-base balance is impaired.

Disorders that can cause hydronephrosis or hydroureter include tumors, stones, trauma, congenital structural defects, and retroperitoneal fibrosis. Early treatment of the causes can prevent hydronephrosis and hydroureter and thus prevent permanent renal damage. The specific time needed to prevent permanent damage varies and depends on the client's underlying renal status. Permanent damage may occur in less than 48 hours in some clients and after several weeks in other clients.

COLLABORATIVE MANAGEMENT

Assessment

The nurse obtains a history from the client, focusing on known renal or urologic disorders. A history of childhood urinary tract problems may signal the presence of previously unidentified structural defects. The nurse inquires about the client's pattern of urination, especially its amount, frequency, color, clarity, and odor. The client is asked about recent flank or abdominal pain. Chills, fever, and malaise may be present with a urinary tract infection (UTI).

The nurse inspects each flank to identify asymmetry, which may occur with a renal mass, and *gently* palpates the client's abdomen to identify any areas of tenderness. The urinary bladder is also palpated and percussed to detect distention. Gentle pressure on the abdomen may cause urine leakage, which reflects a full urinary bladder and possible obstruction of the bladder/urethral junction.

Urinalysis may show bacteria or white blood cells if infection is present. When urinary tract obstruction is prolonged, microscopic examination may reveal tubular epithelial cells. The chemical analysis of serum is normal unless decreased glomerular filtration has occurred; serum creatinine and blood urea nitrogen (BUN) levels increase with a decreased glomerular filtration rate (GFR). Serum electrolyte levels may also be altered and indicate hyperkalemia, hyperphosphatemia, hypocalcemia, and metabolic acidosis (bicarbonate deficit).

Intravenous urography reveals ureteral or renal pelvis dilation. Urinary outflow obstruction may be revealed by sonography (renal echography) or computed tomography (CT).

Interventions

NIC **FLUID MONITORING; URINARY RETENTION CARE; INFECTION PROTECTION.** Urinary retention and potential for infection are the primary problems. Failure to treat the cause of urinary obstruction may lead to infection and renal failure. Surgery is usually required to remove or reduce the cause of the obstruction.

INFECTIOUS DISORDERS

The urinary system is normally one in which a sterile body fluid (urine) is excreted. The unobstructed and complete passage of urine from the renal and urinary systems is critical to the sterility of the urinary tract. When a structural abnormality (either congenital or acquired) is present, the potential for degenerative changes from infection is dramatically increased. **Urinary tract infection (UTI)** usually refers to infections in this sterile system. **Pyelonephritis** is a bacterial infection within the kidney and renal pelvis—the *upper* urinary tract. Infections within the *lower* urinary tract are described in Chapter 70.

Pyelonephritis

OVERVIEW

With improved diagnostic techniques and a better understanding of the inflammatory response, pyelonephritis has come to refer to active microorganisms or the effects of kidney infections. **Acute pyelonephritis** is the condition resulting from an active bacterial infection, whereas **chronic pyelonephritis** results from repeated or continued upper urinary tract infections or infectious sequelae. Chronic pyelonephritis is usually associated with an anatomic urinary tract anomaly, urinary obstruction or, most commonly, vesicoureteral reflux. The vesicoureteral junction is the point at which the ureter joins the bladder. Reflux refers to the reverse (e.g., backward, upward, ascending) flow of urine toward the renal pelvis and kidney.

Pathophysiology

In pyelonephritis, microorganisms usually ascend from the lower urinary tract into the renal pelvis. Infection from organisms carried in the blood **(hematogenous)** may occur, but they occur with much less frequency. Bacteria activate the inflammatory response, and local edema results.

Acute pyelonephritis involves acute interstitial inflammation, tubular cell necrosis, and a tendency for abscess formation. Abscesses, pockets of localized infection, can appear in the capsule, cortex, or medulla. The pattern of infection within the kidney is not uniform; normal tissue and tubules can lie next to infected areas. Fibrosis or scar tissue develops as the inflammatory process subsides. The calices become blunted, and scars develop in the interstitial tissue.

Vesicoureteral and intrarenal reflux of infected urine are the major mechanisms responsible for chronic pyelonephritis. Some papillae in the kidney do not close with increased intracaliceal pressure, causing intrarenal reflux. Refluxing papillae are most often located in the upper and lower poles of the kidney and therefore are more susceptible to chronic pyelonephritis. Inflammation, fibrosis, and deformity of the renal pelvis and calices are evident. Repeated or continuous infectious produce additional scar tissue. Vascular, glomerular, and tubular changes within the scars can occur. Filtration, reabsorption, and secretion are eventually impaired, and renal function is diminished (Figure 71-3).

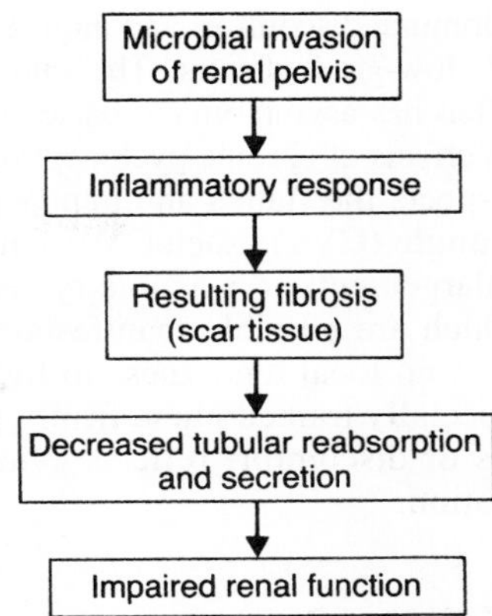

Figure 71-3 ● Pathophysiology of pyelonephritis.

Etiology

Single episodes of *acute* pyelonephritis may result from the entry of bacteria associated with pregnancy, obstruction, or reflux. *Chronic* pyelonephritis is usually associated with structural abnormalities and/or obstruction with reflux. Vesicoureteral reflux or obstruction leading to chronic pyelonephritis is often due to stones, obstruction, or neurogenic impairment involving the voiding mechanism. Reflux is more common in children, who as adults often have scarring associated with chronic pyelonephritis. Clients who develop chronic pyelonephritis without having reflux as a child are usually adults with a history of spinal cord injury, bladder tumor, prostatic hypertrophy, or urinary tract stones.

Acute or chronic pyelonephritis is more likely to occur in clients who have undergone manipulation of the urinary tract (e.g., placement of a urinary catheter), those who have diabetes mellitus or chronic renal calculi, or those who overuse analgesics. In clients with diabetes mellitus, the development and progression of bladder atony increase the tendency to develop pyelonephritis. In clients with chronic stone disease, calculi provide a site for ongoing infection and resultant renal scarring. Nonsteroidal anti-inflammatory drug (NSAID) use has been associated with papillary necrosis, which then permits reflux.

The most common pyelonephritis-causing organism is *Escherichia coli. Enterococcus faecalis* is typical in hospitalized clients. Both are organisms of the gastrointestinal tract. Non–*E. coli* organisms such as *Proteus mirabilis, Klebsiella,* and *Pseudomonas aeruginosa* and the more antibiotic-resistant organisms are also causes of pyelonephritis in hospitalized clients. When the infection is bloodborne, common infecting organisms include *Staphylococcus aureus* and the *Candida* and *Salmonella* species.

Theories of noninfectious or idiopathic causes of intrarenal scarring and the eventual outcome of pyelonephritis include an antibody reaction, cell-mediated immunity against the bacterial antigens, or an autoimmune reaction.

Incidence/Prevalence

The exact incidence and prevalence of pyelonephritis are not known; this diagnosis is not separately reported from all urinary tract infections. Acute urinary conditions of the kidneys or urinary tract, nephritic syndrome, urethral stricture, and cystitis account for more than 7 million new cases annually in noninstutionalized Americans (NIDDK National Kidney and Urologic Diseases Information Clearinghouse, 1999). Women overall have more cases of pyelonephritis. After age 65, rates for men increase greatly because of the increased incidence of prostatitis.

COLLABORATIVE MANAGEMENT

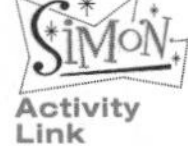

Assessment

HISTORY

The nurse asks about a history of urinary tract infections (UTIs), diabetes mellitus, stone disease, and other structural or functional abnormalities of the genitourinary tract. The nurse attempts to determine whether the UTIs were associated with pregnancy and asks the client about any previous experiences with pyelonephritis or similar symptoms. Recurrences are common and may lead to a deterioration of renal function.

PHYSICAL ASSESSMENT/CLINICAL MANIFESTATIONS

The nurse asks the client about specific symptoms associated with acute pyelonephritis (Chart 71-4). Chronic pyelonephritis has a less dramatic clinical presentation; signs and symptoms are usually related to the infection or renal function. The nurse asks the client to describe any vague or nonspecific urinary symptoms or abdominal discomfort and inquires about any history of repeated, low-grade fevers. The client with chronic pyelonephritis often has asymptomatic bacteremia. Chart 71-5 outlines the renal effects of chronic pyelonephritis.

The nurse inspects the flanks and gently palpates in the **costovertebral angle (CVA).** Each CVA is inspected to determine any enlargement or asymmetry, edema, or erythema, all of which are possible manifestations of inflammation. If there is no local tenderness to light palpation in either CVA, a specially trained nurse firmly percusses each area. Tenderness or discomfort reflects evidence of infection or inflammation.

PSYCHOSOCIAL ASSESSMENT

As with any disorder associated with the genitourinary tract, the client may have feelings of anxiety, embarrassment, or guilt. The nurse listens carefully to the client's description for evidence of generalized anxiety or specific fears and prevents embarrassment during assessment. Feelings of guilt, often associated with sexual habits or practices, may be masked through denial (e.g., delay in seeking treatment) or through vague, nonspecific responses to specific or direct questions. The nurse encourages clients to tell their own story in familiar, comfortable language.

LABORATORY ASSESSMENT

A urinalysis shows white blood cells and bacteria. The urine is analyzed to determine whether gram-positive or gram-negative organisms are responsible for the infection. The urine sample for culture and sensitivity testing, obtained by the clean-catch method, reveals the bacterial species and susceptibility or resistance of the specific organism to various antibiotics. In clients with recurrent episodes of pyelonephritis or upper UTIs, more specific testing of bacterial antigens and antibodies may help determine whether the same organism is responsible for the recurrent infections.

Blood cultures are examined for specific pathogenic microorganisms. Nonspecific serologic tests include the C-reactive protein and erythrocyte sedimentation.

RADIOGRAPHIC ASSESSMENT

An x-ray examination of the kidneys, ureters, and bladder (KUB) and intravenous (IV) urography are performed initially to determine the presence of stones or obstructions. A cystourethrogram is also indicated for some clients. These radiographic procedures define urinary tract structures and identify any structural defects. Specific defects to be identified include foreign bodies, such as stones; obstruction to the outflow of urine, such as tumors, structural defects, or prostate enlargement; and urine reflux associated with incompetent ureterovesical valve closure. (See Chapter 69 for more information on radiographic diagnostic assessment.)

OTHER DIAGNOSTIC ASSESSMENT

Several other diagnostic tests are currently being researched, including examining antibody-coated bacteria in urine, certain enzymes (e.g., lactate dehydrogenase isoenzyme 5), and radionuclide scintillation (e.g., gallium scan). Examining urine for antibody-coated bacteria is useful in identifying clients who may need long-term antibiotic therapy. High-molecular-weight enzymes in urine, such as lactate dehydrogenase isoenzyme 5, are present with any process associated with renal tissue deterioration and give trend data. The gallium scan can identify active pyelonephritis or abscesses in the perinephric region.

CRITICAL THINKING CHALLENGE

You are assigned to admit a 28-year-old woman who is 26 weeks pregnant. She complains of flank and CVA pain, dysuria, urgency, nocturia, and frequency: "I have to pee all the time, all night long, too, and it hurts!" She complains of nausea: "I thought morning sickness would be gone by now." She also reports fatigue: "Usually I can work a 10-hour day without even a bathroom break. I stayed in bed the past two days. My husband insisted I go to the emergency department this morning." She states, "I hope you can help me; I've never had anything like this before." Her vital signs are: heart rate, 110; blood pressure, 110/50; respirations, 20; and temperature 38° C. Her urinalysis is cloudy, amber, and foul smelling, with white blood cells and gram-negative bacteria.

- What signs and symptoms support a diagnosis of a lower UTI (e.g., cystitis)? Pyelonephritis? Both?
- What risk factors for pyelonephritis are present for this client?

For suggested answer guidelines, go to SIMON http://www.wbsaunders.com/SIMON/Iggy/.

Analysis

COMMON NURSING DIAGNOSES AND COLLABORATIVE PROBLEMS

The primary common nursing diagnosis for the client with pyelonephritis is Acute Pain (Flank and Abdominal) related to inflammation and infection. A common collaborative problem is Potential for Renal Failure.

CHART 71-4

KEY FEATURES *of* Acute Pyelonephritis

- Fever
- Chills
- Tachycardia and tachypnea
- Flank, back, or loin pain
- Tender costal vertebral angle (CVA)
- Abdominal, often colicky, discomfort
- Nausea and vomiting
- General malaise or fatigue
- Burning, urgency, or frequency of urination
- Nocturia

CHART 71-5

KEY FEATURES *of* Chronic Pyelonephritis

- Hypertension
- Inability to conserve sodium
- Decreased concentrating ability (nocturia)
- Tendency to develop hyperkalemia and acidosis

ADDITIONAL NURSING DIAGNOSES AND COLLABORATIVE PROBLEMS

In addition to the common nursing diagnoses and collaborative problems, clients with pyelonephritis may have one or more of the following:

- Infection or Risk for Infection related to inadequate primary defenses (urinary stasis) or instrumentation
- Deficient Knowledge regarding the medical diagnosis and therapy related to lack of information resources
- Activity Intolerance related to fatigue, debilitation, and generalized weakness associated with the infection
- Fear of development of chronic renal failure related to an inability to control recurrent infections
- Hyperthermia related to increased metabolic rate from infection

An additional collaborative problem is Potential for Sepsis and Septic Shock.

Planning and Implementation

ACUTE PAIN

NOC **PLANNING: EXPECTED OUTCOMES.** The client with pyelonephritis is expected to report that he or she has achieved a state of comfort that allows for adequate rest, nutrition, and activity.

INTERVENTIONS

NIC **PAIN MANAGEMENT.** Interventions may be nonsurgical or surgical. The availability and success of several noninvasive techniques that result in stone crushing, such as extracorporeal shock wave lithotripsy and percutaneous ultrasonic pyelolithotomy (see Chapter 70), have decreased the need for surgery.

NONSURGICAL MANAGEMENT. Nonsurgical interventions include the use of medications, diet and fluid therapy, and educational counseling to ensure the client's understanding about the treatment.

DRUG THERAPY

NIC ***Medication Management.*** Antibiotics are ordered to treat the infection. Initially, the antibiotics are broad spectrum. With urine and blood culture and sensitivity results, the physician may order a more specific antibiotic. Urinary antiseptic medications (e.g., nitrofurantoin [Macrodantin]) may also be prescribed to provide comfort.

DIET THERAPY

Fluid Monitoring; Teaching: Prescribed Diet. For healing to occur, the client's nutritional intake must include adequate numbers of calories and all food groups. Fluid intake is recommended at 2 to 3 L/day unless medically contraindicated.

SURGICAL MANAGEMENT. Surgical interventions may be needed to correct structural abnormalities causing urine reflux or obstruction of urine outflow or to eradicate the source of intractable infection.

PREOPERATIVE CARE. Antibiotics are given, usually intravenously, to achieve adequate blood levels or sterile blood culture results. The nurse also teaches the client the nature and purpose of the proposed surgery, the expected outcome, and expectations of how the client can participate.

OPERATIVE PROCEDURES. The surgical procedures may be one of the following: **pyelolithotomy** (stone removal from the renal pelvis), **nephrectomy** (removal of the kidney), ureteral diversion, or reimplantation of ureter to restore proper bladder drainage.

A pyelolithotomy is indicated for removal of a large stone in the renal pelvis that blocks urine flow and causes infection. Nephrectomy is considered a last resort when all other measures to eradicate infection have failed. For clients with incompetent ureterovesical valve closure or dilated ureters, **ureteroplasty** (repair or revision) or ureteral reimplantation (through another site in the posterior bladder wall) preserves renal function and eliminates infections.

POSTOPERATIVE CARE. See Chapter 70 for postoperative nursing care for the client undergoing urologic surgery.

POTENTIAL FOR RENAL FAILURE

PLANNING: EXPECTED OUTCOMES. It is expected that the client under treatment for pyelonephritis will conserve existing renal function for as long as possible and then experience a slow progression of renal failure once the process of renal failure begins.

INTERVENTIONS. The physician or nurse practitioner orders specific antibiotics to treat the infection. The nurse stresses the importance of taking all the medication as directed. The nurse also discusses with the client and family the importance of regular follow-up examinations and completing diagnostic tests as recommended.

Control of blood pressure is necessary to minimize the progression of renal dysfunction. When renal impairment is evident through a decreased concentrating ability (e.g., nocturia, low urine specific gravity), the nurse encourages the client to drink at least 2 L of fluid per day to prevent fluid volume deficit, which could further affect renal function. When dietary protein is restricted to delay the onset of renal failure, the nurse refers the client to the dietitian as needed. Other interventions related to the progression of chronic renal failure are covered in Chapter 72.

Community-Based Care

Acute or chronic pyelonephritis causes fear and anxiety in the client and family. The severity of the acute process and its potential to develop into a chronic process are quite frightening. Both the client and the family require reassurance that treatment and preventive measures can be accomplished.

HEALTH TEACHING

After assessing the client's and family's understanding of pyelonephritis and the suggested treatment, the nurse explains the following:

- Medication administration (purpose, timing, frequency, duration, and possible side effects)
- The role of nutrition and adequate fluid intake
- The need for a balance between rest and activity, including any limitations after surgery
- The signs and symptoms of disease recurrence
- The use of previously successful coping mechanisms

The nurse advises the client to complete all prescribed antibiotic regimens and instructs the client to report any side effects or unusual symptoms to the prescribing health team member rather than suspend the regimen. The client and family are referred for nutritional counseling as needed, because many clients have special nutritional requirements, such as those caused by diabetes mellitus or pregnancy.

HOME CARE MANAGEMENT

If no surgery is performed, the client may need assistance with self-care, nutrition, and medication administration at home. If surgical intervention is necessary, the client may require help with incision care, self-care, and transportation for follow-up medical appointments.

HEALTH CARE RESOURCES

The client may also briefly need a community health nurse to help administer medications or nutrition at home. Housekeeping services may also be helpful while the client is regaining strength.

Evaluation: Outcomes

NOC The nurse evaluates the care of the client with pyelonephritis on the basis of the identified nursing diagnoses and collaborative problems. Expected outcomes may include that the client will:

- Demonstrate methods of enhancing comfort
- Report that pain is controlled
- Express satisfaction with pain control
- Describe the role of antibiotics and self-administration of medications
- Explain and offer techniques to ensure adequate nutrition and hydration
- Describe the plan for posttreatment follow-up, including knowledge of recurrent symptoms
- Modify the prescribed regimen as directed by a health care professional

CRITICAL THINKING CHALLENGE

Your client is prescribed IV ciprofloxacin (Cipro) for pyelonephritis. She is also prescribed 25 mg meperidine every 3 hours prn for her pain. Radiographic studies are deferred at this time because of her pregnancy. A urine culture indicates that the infecting organism is *E. coli,* and the sensitivity of the bacteria to ciprofloxacin is confirmed. After 3 days her pain is absent, her fever is resolved, and her urinary symptoms are clearing. She is to be discharged today and is to continue taking her antibiotic orally at home. A follow-up medical visit is scheduled in 7 days.

- What discharge planning and health care teaching are indicated at this time?

For suggested answer guidelines, go to SIMON http://www.wbsaunders.com/SIMON/Iggy/.

Renal Abscess

OVERVIEW

An **abscess** is a collection of fluid and cells caused by an inflammatory response to bacteria. An abscess may occur within the renal parenchyma (renal abscess), in the renal and Gerota's fascia (perinephric abscess), or in the flank. An abscess is suspected when fever and symptoms are not relieved promptly by antibiotic therapy.

COLLABORATIVE MANAGEMENT

A renal or perirenal abscess is readily diagnosed via sonography or a computed tomography (CT) scan. Arteriography and radionuclide scintillation methods (e.g., gallium scan) also may be useful for diagnosis. Symptoms of renal abscess include fever, flank pain, and general malaise. Local flank edema and erythema may be observed.

Drainage by surgical incision or needle aspiration is often necessary. Appropriate broad-spectrum antibiotics are also prescribed.

Renal Tuberculosis

OVERVIEW

The genitourinary tract is the most common extrapulmonary site of tuberculosis. Approximately 10% of new cases of tuberculosis are extrapulmonary (Tolkoff-Rubin, Cotran, & Rubin, 2000). Tuberculosis of the kidney is sometimes called *granulomatous nephritis.* After *Mycobacterium tuberculosis* invades the kidneys, usually by a bloodborne route, an inflammatory response is activated and forms scar tissue **(granuloma)** that replaces normal kidney tissue.

COLLABORATIVE MANAGEMENT

Clients may experience urinary frequency, dysuria, hematuria and/or proteinuria, flank pain or renal colic secondary to the passage of clots or stones, pyuria, and hypertension. Skin test (e.g., purified protein derivative [PPD]) or chest x-ray film evidence of tuberculosis may or may not be present.

Clients with current or previous pulmonary tuberculosis who show signs of unexplained fever, hematuria, and sterile pyuria are at high risk for renal tuberculosis. The diagnosis is made through a urine culture of three clean-catch, first-morning specimens. Other genitourinary sites for tuberculosis include the prostate, epididymis, ureters, testes, bladder, and seminal vesicles.

Antitubercular therapy is the primary treatment. Recommendations include a 2-month course of rifampin, isoniazid, and pyrazinamide followed by 4 months of rifampin and isoniazid. Three to six more months of rifampin and isoniazid may be recommended for men who may be harboring the organism in the prostate (Tolkoff-Rubin, Cotran, & Rubin, 2000).

Complications include the loss of renal function, nephrolithiasis, obstructive uropathy, and bacterial superinfection of the urinary tract. Surgical excision of diseased tissue may be indicated to preserve renal function.

IMMUNOLOGIC RENAL DISORDERS

Glomerulonephritis is the third leading cause of end-stage renal disease (ESRD). Approximately 1% of all ESRD cases are attributed to one of the primary or secondary causes of glomerulonephritis (NIDDK, 1999).

Both primary and secondary diseases or syndromes result in glomerular injury. Glomeruli are usually involved in primary disease (Table 71-1); the extrarenal effects of primary disease stem from the glomerular injury. Most primary diseases and syndromes have an immunologic component, and many have an underlying genetic basis. Secondary glomerular disease refers to the situation in which glomerular involvement is part of another disease. For example, certain systemic diseases and infections can have renal effects and cause glomerular injury (Table 71-2). Some of the conditions causing secondary glomerular disease include systemic lupus erythematosus and diabetic nephropathy.

Each primary or secondary disease or syndrome has a specific pathophysiology and associated clinical manifestations. Their *glomerular* effects are caused by injury to the glomeruli and result in proteinuria, hematuria, decreased glomerular filtration rate (GFR), edema, and hypertension due to sodium retention. The extent and duration of renal injury, prognosis, and specific known cause vary considerably among these syndromes.

Immunologic changes may result in injury to the glomeruli, interstitium, and/or tubules, and the effects may be acute or chronic. Both antibody and cellular immune responses are involved. The resultant renal disorder may be a systemic disease or localized in the kidneys.

Most forms of glomerulonephritis are associated with an accumulation of immune complexes in the glomeruli (Figure 71-4). An immune complex is made up of antigen and antibody. The antigen can be normal kidney tissue such as the glomerular basement membrane, tubular basement membrane, or mesangium, or it can be dissolved in a body fluid (e.g., blood). Bacteria and viruses are also examples of antigens. Increasingly, exposure to bacteria, viruses, drugs, or other toxins is believed to be the trigger for glomerular injury.

Antibody reaction with antigen can lead to immune complex formation either directly in or deposited in glomerular tissue. The immune complexes activate many mediators—including complement, leukocytes, and coagulation proteins—that are responsible for the resultant renal tissue injury. Some of the major responses causing tissue injury include damage to cell membranes, local edema, movement of white blood cells to the site of inflammation, and activation of platelets.

TABLE 71-1 • PRIMARY GLOMERULAR DISEASES AND SYNDROMES

- Acute glomerulonephritis
- Rapidly progressive glomerulonephritis (RPGN)
- Chronic glomerulonephritis
- Nephrotic syndrome
- Persisting urinary abnormalities with few or no symptoms

TABLE 71-2 • SECONDARY GLOMERULAR DISEASES AND SYNDROMES

- Systemic lupus erythematosus (SLE)
- Schönlein-Henoch purpura
- Goodpasture's syndrome
- Systemic necrotizing vasculitis
- Wegener granulomatosis
- Periarteritis nodosa (also called polyarteritis nodosa)
- Amyloidosis
- Diabetic glomerulopathy
- HIV-associated nephropathy
- Alport syndrome
- Multiple myeloma
- Viral hepatitis B
- Viral hepatitis C
- Cirrhosis
- Sickle-cell disease
- Nonstreptococcal postinfectious acute glomerulonephritis (GN)
- Infective endocarditis
- Hemolytic-uremic syndrome
- Thrombotic thrombocytopenic purpura (TTP)

Acute Glomerulonephritis

OVERVIEW

An infection often occurs before the renal manifestations of acute glomerulonephritis (GN). The onset of symptoms averages 10 days from the time of infection; there is a broad range of illness severity but recovery is usually complete and quick. The term *acute nephritic syndrome* also describes this disorder.

Most causes of acute GN are postinfectious (Table 71-3) or are related to other systemic diseases (see Table 71-2). The incidence of acute GN is unknown, but poststreptococcal GN is more common in males.

COLLABORATIVE MANAGEMENT

Assessment

HISTORY

The nurse asks about recent infections, particularly of the skin or upper respiratory tract, and about recent travel or other activities with possible exposure to viruses, bacteria, fungi, or parasites. Recent illnesses, surgery, or other invasive procedures may suggest infections. The nurse also asks about any known systemic diseases, such as systemic lupus erythematosus (SLE), which could cause acute GN.

PHYSICAL ASSESSMENT/CLINICAL MANIFESTATIONS

The nurse inspects the client's skin for lesions or recent incisions and the face, eyelids, hands, and other areas for edema (present in approximately 75% of the clients with acute GN).

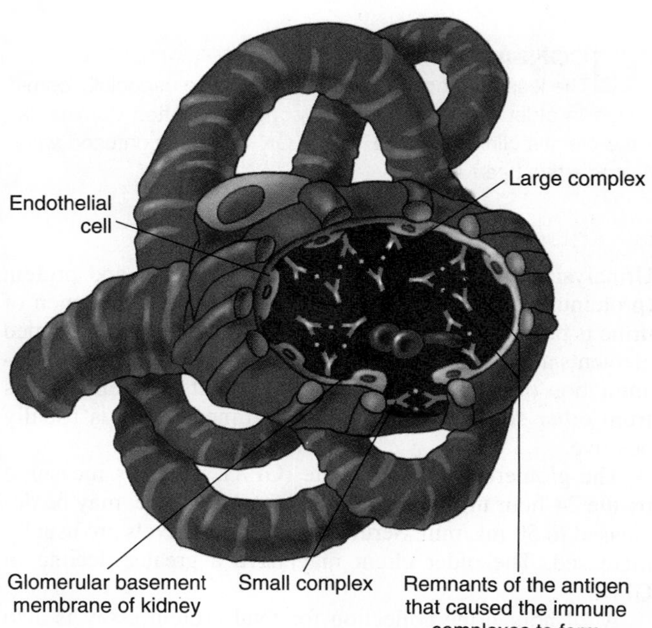

Figure 71-4 • An immune complex precipitating in the glomerulus of a client with glomerulonephritis.

TABLE 71-3 • INFECTIOUS CAUSES OF ACUTE GLOMERULONEPHRITIS

- Group A beta-hemolytic *Streptococcus*
- Staphylococcal or gram-negative bacteremia or sepsis
- Pneumococcal, *Mycoplasma,* or *Klebsiella* pneumonia
- Syphilis
- Visceral abscesses
- Infective endocarditis
- Hepatitis B
- Infectious mononucleosis
- Measles
- Mumps
- Rocky Mountain spotted fever
- Cytomegaloviral (CMV) infection
- Histoplasmosis
- Toxoplasmosis
- Varicella
- *Chlamydia psittaci* infection
- Coxsackievirus infection
- Any bacterial, parasitic, fungal, or viral infection (potentially)

In assessing for circulatory congestion and fluid overload (which often accompanies the sodium and fluid retention associated with acute GN), the client is asked about any difficulty in breathing, nocturnal or exertional dyspnea, or orthopnea. The nurse also assesses for crackles in the lung fields, an S_3 heart sound (gallop rhythm), and neck vein distention.

The nurse asks about changes in urination pattern and any change in urine color. Microscopic hematuria occurs up to 66% of the time, and clients often describe their urine as smoky, reddish-brown, rusty, or cola colored. The client is asked about dysuria or oliguria. He or she is weighed because changes in urine output may result in fluid retention.

The blood pressure is measured and compared with the client's baseline blood pressure. Mild to moderate hypertension often accompanies acute GN due to sodium and fluid retention. The client may have symptoms of fatigue, a lack of energy, anorexia, nausea, and/or vomiting if uremia from renal failure is present.

CONSIDERATIONS FOR OLDER ADULTS

The less common signs of acute GN are especially common in older adults. Circulatory congestion often dominates the client's clinical picture. Acute GN is easily confused with congestive heart failure.

LABORATORY ASSESSMENT

Urinalysis reveals red blood cells **(hematuria)** and protein (proteinuria). Examination of an early morning specimen of urine is preferred because the urine is most acidic and formed elements are more intact at that time. Further microscopic examination often reveals red blood cell casts as well as casts from other substances. The urine sediment assay is usually positive.

The glomerular filtration rate (GFR), which is measured by the 24-hour urine test for creatinine clearance, may be decreased to 50 mL/min. Serum urea nitrogen levels are usually increased. The older client may have a greater decline in GFR.

A 24-hour urine collection for total protein assay is also obtained. The protein excretion value for clients with acute GN may be increased to values of 500 mg to 3 g/24 hr in more than 75% of clients. Serum albumin levels may be decreased because of the large amount of protein lost in the urine and because of fluid retention (dilutional value).

Specimens from the blood, skin, or throat are obtained for culture, if indicated. Other serologic tests include antistreptolysin-O titers, C3 complement levels, cryoglobulins (immunoglobulin G [IgG]), antinuclear antibodies (ANAs), and circulating immune complexes.

Antistreptolysin-O titers are increased after group A beta-hemolytic *Streptococcus* infections. Complement levels are decreased when the complement system is activated. Type III cryoglobulins may be found during acute illness. ANAs suggest an autoimmune response, and SLE is only one possibility. Circulating immune complexes containing IgG and C3 are often detected.

OTHER DIAGNOSTIC ASSESSMENT

A percutaneous renal biopsy may provide a precise diagnosis of the pathologic condition, assist in determining the prognosis, and help outline treatment (see Chapter 69). The specific tissue morphology is determined by light microscopy, immunofluorescent stains, and electron microscopy to identify the type of cellular proliferation (light microscopy), the presence of immunoglobulins (immunofluorescence), or the specific type of tissue deposits (electron microscopy).

Interventions

Interventions focus on treating the underlying infectious process, preventing complications, and providing appropriate client education.

MANAGEMENT OF INFECTION

NIC ***MEDICATION MANAGEMENT.*** Treatment for cases of acute GN with an infectious cause would be the appropriate anti-infective. Penicillin, erythromycin, or azithromycin are usually prescribed for poststreptococcal GN. The nurse checks the client's known allergies before administering any medication. To prevent infection spread, the physician may order anti-infective drugs for persons in immediate close contact with the client. The nurse stresses personal hygiene and basic infection control principles (e.g., handwashing) to prevent spread of the organism.

PREVENTION OF COMPLICATIONS. For clients with circulatory congestion, hypertension, and edema, the physician orders diuretics and a sodium and water restriction. Antihypertensive medications may be needed to control hypertension (see Chart 36-3). The usual fluid allowance is equal to the 24-hour urine output plus 500 to 600 mL for insensible fluid losses. Clients with oliguria also usually have increased serum levels of potassium and blood urea nitrogen (BUN). Potassium and protein intake may be restricted to prevent hyperkalemia and additional uremic manifestations of the elevated BUN.

Nausea, vomiting, or anorexia indicates that uremia is interfering with nutrition. Dialysis is necessary if uremic symptoms or fluid volume excess cannot be controlled (see Chapter 72). **Plasmapheresis** (removal and filtering of the plasma to eliminate antibodies) also may be attempted (see Chapter 40); steroids are not usually helpful.

NIC **ENERGY MANAGEMENT.** To conserve and maintain the client's energy, the nurse assists him or her in maintaining a restful environment, balancing activity and rest, and coordinating necessary assessments and treatments. The client also needs to minimize emotional stress, and the nurse encourages him or her to practice relaxation techniques and to participate in diversional activities.

CLIENT EDUCATION. The nurse instructs the client, family, or significant other about the purpose and desired effects of prescribed medications, the dosage and route of administration, and potential adverse side effects. The nurse ensures that the client and family understand dietary or fluid modifications, including methods of detecting fluid retention. The client is advised to measure his or her weight and blood pressure daily at the same time each day and to notify the primary care provider of sudden increases in weight or of any increase in blood pressure.

If short-term dialysis is required to control fluid volume excess or uremic symptoms, the nurse explains peritoneal or vascular access care and dialysis schedules and routines (also see Chapter 72).

Rapidly Progressive Glomerulonephritis

Rapidly progressive glomerulonephritis (RPGN), a variant of acute nephritis, is also called *crescentic glomerulonephritis* because of the usual accumulation of crescent-shaped cells in Bowman's capsule. RPGN develops over several weeks or months and is associated with a significant loss of renal function. Clients can become quite ill quickly and have signs and symptoms of renal failure: fluid volume excess with hypertension and oliguria, electrolyte imbalances, and uremic symptoms.

A previous infection or multisystem disease, such as systemic lupus erythematosus (SLE), is sometimes identified in the client's recent history. The renal deterioration often progresses to nonreversible end-stage renal disease (ESRD).

Chronic Glomerulonephritis

OVERVIEW

Chronic glomerulonephritis, or *chronic nephritic syndrome,* refers to renal deterioration or failure that develops over 20 to 30 years or even longer. The exact onset of the disorder is rarely identified. In many instances the cause of the disease is not known because the kidneys are atrophied and tissue is not available for biopsy or diagnosis. Mild proteinuria and hematuria, hypertension, and occasional edema are often the only manifestations.

Although the exact pathogenesis is not known, changes in the renal parenchyma may result from hypertension, intermittent or recurrent parenchymal infections and inflammation, and altered metabolism and hemodynamics. Kidney tissue atrophies, and the functional mass of nephrons decreases significantly. The cortex of the parenchyma is thinned, but the calices and pelves are normal. Tissue obtained by renal biopsy in the late stages of atrophy may reveal hyalinization of the glomeruli, loss of tubules, and fibrosis of the kidney tissue. Immunofluorescent examination and electron microscopy may reveal residual effects of immune complex deposition.

The loss of nephrons results in decreased glomerular filtration. Hypertension with sclerosis of the renal arterioles is often present. The glomerular injury also causes proteinuria because of increased permeability of the glomerular capillaries. Chronic glomerulonephritis eventually results in chronic renal failure (see Chapter 72).

COLLABORATIVE MANAGEMENT

Assessment

HISTORY

The nurse asks the client about previously identified health problems, including systemic diseases, renal or urologic disorders, childhood infectious diseases (e.g., streptococcal infections), and recent exposures to infections. The client is asked about his or her overall health status and whether increasing fatigue and lethargy have been experienced.

The client's pattern of voiding is noted; the nurse asks whether the frequency of voiding has increased or the quantity of urine has decreased. The client is asked about changes in urine color, odor, or clarity and is asked about dysuria and continence.

Because edema can result from oliguria and fluid volume excess, the nurse also asks about the client's general comfort and any dyspnea at rest or with exertion.

The nurse asks about and observes changes in mental functioning, such as irritability or an inability to read or to perform job-related functions or other processes requiring mental concentration. Changes in memory and the ability to concentrate occur with the waste product accumulation that accompanies renal failure.

PHYSICAL ASSESSMENT/CLINICAL MANIFESTATIONS

The nurse assesses for signs of systemic circulatory overload by auscultating lung fields to detect crackles, observing the quality of respirations, measuring blood pressure and weight, and auscultating the heart to describe rate, rhythm, and the presence of an S_3 heart sound. The nurse inspects the neck veins to identify venous engorgement and checks for edema in the pedal, pretibial, and presacral tissues.

The nurse notes changes due to uremia, such as slurred speech, ataxia, tremors, or **asterixis** (flapping tremor of the fingers or the inability to maintain a fixed posture with the arms extended and wrists hyperextended). The nurse inspects the client's skin for a yellowish color, texture, ecchymoses, rashes, or eruptions. Areas of dryness and breaks that may have resulted from scratching are noted.

DIAGNOSTIC ASSESSMENT

Urine output may decrease, but gross visual changes in urine are unusual unless there is an associated urinary tract infection (UTI). Urinalysis commonly shows proteinuria, usually less than 2 g in a 24-hour collection; the specific gravity is usually fixed at a constant level of dilution (around 1.010). There may be red blood cells and casts in the urine, which suggests chronic renal disease processes.

The glomerular filtration rate (GFR) is measured by creatinine clearance and is reduced from the normal range of 105 to 120 mL/min. The serum creatinine level is elevated and varies depending on the client's muscle mass. Serum creatinine levels are usually greater than 6 mg/dL but may be as high as 30 mg/dL or more. Blood urea nitrogen (BUN) is increased and varies in relation to the dietary protein intake; BUN levels are often between 100 and 200 mg/dL.

Serum electrolyte levels may be abnormal as a result of decreased renal function. Sodium retention is common, but dilution of the plasma from excess fluid results in an apparently normal serum sodium level (135 to 145 mEq/L) or a dilutional hyponatremia (<135 mEq/L). When oliguria develops, potassium retention occurs; hyperkalemia is present when levels exceed 5.4 mEq/L. Hyperphosphatemia develops with serum levels greater than 4.7 mg/dL. Serum calcium levels are usually at the lower end of the normal range or are slightly below normal.

A base deficit with a decrease in serum carbon dioxide (CO_2) occurs with respiratory compensation by hyperventilation in response to metabolic acidosis. If respiratory compensation is present, the pH of arterial blood is between 7.35 and 7.45. A pH of less than 7.35 signifies inadequate respiratory compensation for metabolic acidosis (see Chapter 16).

In clients with chronic glomerulonephritis, the kidneys appear to be small when observed by x-ray or IV urography and when measured by sonography or computed tomography (CT).

A renal biopsy is important in the early stages of glomerulonephritis, when proteinuria or hematuria is initially present. Changes include an increase in the number and types of cells infiltrating the glomerular tissue, deposition of immune complexes, and vessel sclerosis. A renal biopsy (percutaneous or open) is rarely performed for clients once glomerulonephritis progresses to ESRD because the kidneys are too small to obtain tissue.

Interventions

Interventions focus on slowing the progression of the disease and preventing complications. Treatment consists of dietary modification, fluid intake sufficient to prevent reduced blood flow volume to the kidneys, and medication therapy to temporarily control the symptoms of uremia. Eventually, the client requires dialysis or transplantation to prevent death from the numerous potential systemic effects of uremia. (Nursing care for the client with ESRD requiring dialysis or transplantation is discussed in Chapter 72.)

Nephrotic Syndrome

OVERVIEW

Nephrotic syndrome (NS) is a condition of increased glomerular permeability that causes massive proteinuria, edema, and hypoalbuminemia. Many agents, diseases, and physiologic processes are implicated as possible causes of NS.

Glomerular membrane changes from immune processes permit protein loss into urine. With this loss, plasma albumin levels decrease and edema develops. Altered liver activity results in elevated lipid production.

COLLABORATIVE MANAGEMENT

The primary feature of nephrotic syndrome is severe proteinuria (>3.5 g of protein in 24 hours). Clients diagnosed with NS also often have hypoalbuminemia (serum albumin <3 g/dL), hyperlipidemia, lipiduria, edema, and hypertension (Chart 71-6). Renal vein thrombosis often occurs at the same time as

CHART 71-6

KEY FEATURES *of* Nephrotic Syndrome

- Massive proteinuria
- Hypoalbuminemia
- Edema
- Hyperlipidemia
- Increased coagulation
- Infection

NS—either as a cause or as an effect. Clot development is not clearly understood. NS may progress to ESRD, but progression is not inevitable.

Treatment varies depending on the specifics of the glomerulopathy identified by renal biopsy. Some immunologic processes may respond to steroids or cytotoxic agents. Dietary modification is often prescribed. If the glomerular filtration rate (GFR) is normal, proteins should contain all essential amino acids; if the GFR is decreased, dietary protein intake is decreased. Mild diuretics (Chart 71-7) and dietary sodium restriction may be needed to control edema and hypertension. The nurse assesses the client to ensure that plasma volume depletion does not occur; hemodynamic changes and acute renal failure may be avoided if renal perfusion can be maintained.

IMMUNOLOGIC INTERSTITIAL AND TUBULOINTERSTITIAL DISORDERS

Interstitial and tubulointerstitial disorders in the kidney may be immunologically mediated; renal changes may be acute or chronic. The acute effects are often associated with medications such as penicillin-like antibiotics, sulfonamides, or nonsteroidal anti-inflammatory drugs (NSAIDs). Chronic interstitial nephritis has many causes, including analgesic nephropathy, complement activation, the medication cyclosporin, polycystic kidney disease, systemic lupus erythematosus, sarcoidosis, multiple myeloma, sickle cell disease, obstructive disorders, and radiation nephritis. Drug-induced problems are often associated with rash or eosinophilia. Fever is common in idiopathic forms of interstitial nephritis. Progression to ESRD is likely unless the offending agent can be identified and removed.

DEGENERATIVE DISORDERS

Degenerative disorders that cause changes in renal function are usually associated with the damage or effects caused by a multisystem disorder. Many of these degenerative disorders result from changes in kidney blood vessels.

Nephrosclerosis

OVERVIEW

Nephrosclerosis is a problem of changes in the nephron blood vessels. Vessel walls thicken, and the vessel lumen narrows. As a result, renal blood flow is decreased and kidney tissue is chronically hypoxic. Ischemia and fibrosis develop over time.

Nephrosclerosis is associated with all types of hypertension, atherosclerosis, and a history of diabetes mellitus. The more severe the hypertension, the greater the risk for extensive kidney damage. Nephrosclerosis is rarely seen when blood pressure is consistently below 160/110 mm Hg. The changes associated with hypertension may be reversible or

CHART 71-7

DRUG THERAPY *for* Diuretics Used to Increase Urine Output

Drug	Usual Dosage	Indication	Nursing Interventions	Rationale
OSMOTIC DIURETICS (act on glomerulus and renal tubular system)				
Mannitol (Osmitrol✱), urea	50-100 g IV as a 5%-25% solution	Causes rapid diuresis (e.g., after contrast media infusion)	Measure fluid intake and output.	Severe dehydration is possible. Mannitol may crystallize while on the shelf.
			Check vial for crystals. If crystals are present, warm vial between the hands.	Crystals will dissolve with body warmth.
			Administer through a filter.	This will prevent remaining crystals from entering the body.
THIAZIDE AND THIAZIDE-LIKE DIURETICS (act on cortical diluting site of ascending limb of loop of Henle)				
Chlorothiazide (Diuril)	250 mg PO, IV once to four times/day	Hypertension	Observe for signs and symptoms of electrolyte imbalance	Common complications include hypokalemia and hypercalcemia.
Hydrochlorothiazide (HydroDIURIL, Apo-Hydro✱, Urozide✱)	25-100 mg PO once or twice daily	Congestive heart failure (CHF) with edema	Monitor heart sounds for S_3, lung sounds for crackles and other signs of CHF.	Ongoing monitoring detects complications and helps ensure prompt treatment.
Chlorthalidone (Hygroton, Uridon✱)	25-100 mg PO daily	Edema, hypertension	Do not give with NSAIDs.	An increased diuretic effect is seen with concomitant use of NSAIDs.
Metolazone (Zaroxolyn)	5-20 mg PO daily	Edema, hypertension	Do not give with NSAIDs.	
LOOP DIURETICS (act on ascending limb of loop of Henle)				
Furosemide (Lasix, Furoside✱)	20-80 mg PO, IV once or twice daily; maximum dose 600 mg/day	Hypertension	Observe for orthostatic hypotension.	An early sign of rapid fluid volume depletion may be orthostatic hypotension.
Bumetanide (Bumex)	0.5-2 mg PO daily	CHF	Monitor for possible hyponatremia and hypokalemia.	These agents increase excretion of both sodium and potassium.
Ethacrynic acid (Edecrin)	50-200 mg PO daily	Edema (when creatinine clearance is <25-50 mL/min)	Monitor older clients closely for excessive diuresis.	Older adults are susceptible to the effects of rapid fluid changes.
POTASSIUM-SPARING DIURETICS (act on distal convoluted tubule)				
Spironolactone (Aldactone, Novospiroton✱)	25-200 mg PO once or twice daily	Primary aldosteronism	Observe for signs and symptoms of electrolyte imbalance.	Hyperkalemia with cardiac manifestations is a common complication.
Triamterene (Dyrenium)	25-100 mg once or twice daily; maximum dose 300 mg/day	Hypertension (with other drugs to decrease potassium loss)	Teach client to avoid unprotected sun exposure.	Photosensitivity reactions are possible.
Amiloride (Midamor✱)	5-10 mg daily	Edema, hypertension	Give with food or milk.	Stomach upset is possible.

NSAID, Nonsteroidal anti-inflammatory drug.

may progress to end-stage renal disease (ESRD) within months or years.

Hypertension is the second leading cause of ESRD. Approximately 30% of clients requiring lifesaving renal replacement therapy (e.g., dialysis or transplantation) have hypertension as the cause of their renal failure (NIDDK, 1999).

CULTURAL CONSIDERATIONS

Hypertension is more common in African Americans, and the risks of ESRD from hypertension are also greater for African Americans (Bakris et al., 2000). Between the ages of 25 and 45 years, the ratio of African Americans to Caucasians at risk for ESRD from hypertension is nearly 20:1 (Richardson & Piepho, 2000). These findings do not suggest that ESRD from nephrosclerosis does not occur in Caucasians but rather that affected Caucasians are likely to be older.

COLLABORATIVE MANAGEMENT

Treatment aims to control high blood pressure and preserve renal function. Although many antihypertensive drugs may lower blood pressure, the client's response is important in ensuring long-term adherence to the prescribed therapy. Factors promoting adherence include regimen simplicity (e.g., once-a-day dosing), low cost, and minimal side effects.

Lack of basic knowledge or misinformation about hypertension poses additional challenges to nurses and all health care providers working with hypertensive clients. When evidence of renal disease occurs, adherence to therapy is even more important for preserving health.

Many medications can control high blood pressure (see Chart 36-2); more than one agent may be necessary. Angiotensin-converting enzyme (ACE) inhibitors are particularly useful in reducing hypertension and preserving renal function. Diuretics can maintain fluid and electrolyte balance in the presence of renal insufficiency. Caution is required to prevent hyperkalemia when potassium-sparing diuretics (e.g., triamterene or spironolactone) or combination agents containing a potassium-sparing diuretic are used for clients with known renal disease.

Renovascular Disease

OVERVIEW

Pathologic processes affecting the renal arteries may result in severe lumen narrowing and drastically reduced blood flow to the renal parenchyma. Uncorrected renovascular disease, such as renal artery stenosis or thrombosis, causes ischemia and atrophy of renal tissue.

Renovascular disease is suspected with a sudden onset of hypertension, particularly in clients older than 50 years. Clients with high blood pressure but with a negative family history for hypertension may also be considered potential candidates for renal artery stenosis (RAS).

RAS from atherosclerosis or fibromuscular hyperplasia (increased amount of tissue) is the primary cause of renovascular disease. Other causes include thrombosis and renal aneurysms.

Atherosclerotic changes in the renal artery are often associated with sclerosis in the aorta and other major vessels. Changes in the renal artery are close to where the renal artery and aorta meet. Fibrotic changes of the vessel wall occur throughout the length of the renal artery.

COLLABORATIVE MANAGEMENT

Assessment

Key features of renovascular disease are listed in Chart 71-8. The onset of hypertension is usually after age 40 to 50 years, and the family history is often negative for hypertension. Diagnosis is made by renal arteriography; measurement of renal vein renin levels provides additional evidence but may not be confirmatory. A renal arteriogram visualizes the renal vasculature and offers critical information for invasive treatment. The comparison of renal vein renin levels *may* reveal which kidney is producing more renin.

Interventions

Visualization of the type of defect, extent of narrowing, and surrounding vasculature is critical to decide treatment intervention. The client's overall condition and the size of the atrophied kidney further influence decisions about intervention.

RAS may be treated by drugs to control high blood pressure and by percutaneous transluminal balloon angioplasty or by surgical bypass procedures to restore the renal blood supply. Drugs may control high blood pressure but may not lead to long-term preservation of kidney function. In young and middle-aged adults, a lifetime of treatment with multiple agents for high blood pressure may make treatment difficult and the outcomes uncertain.

CHART 71-8

KEY FEATURES *of* Renovascular Disease

- Significant, difficult to control blood pressure
- Elevated serum creatinine
- Decreased creatinine clearance

Balloon angioplasty is considered less risky and requires much less time for recovery than does renal artery bypass surgery (see Chapter 36). Renal artery bypass surgery is a major procedure and involves at least 2 months for convalescence. A bypass may be performed for either one or both renal arteries. The surgeon inserts a synthetic graft that redirects blood flow from the abdominal aorta into the renal artery, beyond the area of stenosis. Increasingly, splenorenal bypass procedures can also restore renal blood flow. Technically, the process is similar to other arterial bypass procedures (see Chapter 36).

For clients with RAS, the diagnostic and treatment alternatives present tremendous decisional conflict. Clients often experience a deterioration of renal function, as noted by elevated serum creatinine levels and decreased creatinine clearance. These clients are at increased risk for acute renal failure from the administration of nephrotoxic agents such as radiopaque contrast media and from possible intraoperative hypotensive episodes. However, no treatment probably means that dialysis is inevitable.

Diabetic Nephropathy

OVERVIEW

Diabetes mellitus is the leading cause of end-stage renal disease (ESRD) among Caucasians in the United States. Approximately 36% of clients requiring dialysis or renal transplantation have diabetes mellitus as the primary contributing factor (NIDDK, 1999). The cost of preventing or reducing renal problems among clients with diabetes is offset by the high cost of treating severe renal disease (see the Cost of Care box on p. 1657). Diabetic nephropathy may result from type 1 or type 2 diabetes mellitus. Diabetic renal disease is influenced by the extent, duration, and effects of atherosclerosis, hypertension, and autonomic neuropathy, which promotes bladder atony, urinary stasis, and urinary tract infection.

Immunologic response mechanisms have also been implicated in glomerular basement membrane thickening and other changes in clients with diabetic renal disease. Investigations continue to explore if defects are the result of genetic or metabolic disturbances.

COLLABORATIVE MANAGEMENT

Diabetic nephropathy is a *microvascular* complication of diabetes defined by persistent albuminuria (as shown by dipstick or a urinary albumin excretion rate above 0.3 g/dL), without evidence of other renal disease. A diagnosis of renal disease in clients with diabetes mellitus is made on the basis of the history and clinical examination. Diabetic renal disease is progressive (Table 71-4).

COST OF CARE IMPLICATIONS FOR NURSING

DIABETES AND RENAL DISEASE

Cost of Care

- A common complication of both type I and type 2 diabetes mellitus (DM) is nephropathy leading to end-stage renal disease.
- Diabetic clients are five times more likely to develop end-stage renal disease than others in their cohort.
- Abnormal renal function increases diabetes treatment costs by $1337 and advanced renal disease by $3979 per individual treated.
- Intensive therapy was shown by the Diabetes Control and Complications Trial to avert complications in type 1 DM; a similar trial is examining the effects of tight control on type 2 DM clients.

Implications for Nursing

Although the cost of maintaining tight control is two to three times the costs of conventional therapy, economic modeling predicts that tight control could reduce end-stage renal disease from 24% to 7%. Thus the costs of maintaining tight control are offset by the savings related to a reduced need for the diagnosis and treatment of DM-related renal disease.

Renal disease is an expensive diagnosis, not only in dollar costs but also in social, psychologic, and functional costs as patients undergo extensive diagnostic workups and work-limiting treatments. Preventing the renal complications of DM saves money; it also saves individuals from a heavy biopsychosocial burden.

Data from Brown, J.B., Pedula, K.L., & Baskt, A.W. (1999). The progressive cost of complications in type 2 diabetes mellitus. *Archives of Internal Medicine, 159*(16), 1873-1880; Herman, W.H. & Eastman, R.C. (1998). The effects of treatment on the direct costs of diabetes. *Diabetes Care, 21*(Suppl. 3), C19-C24; Nathan, D.M. (1993). Diabetes Control and Complications Trial Research Group: The effect of long-term intensified insulin treatment on development of microvascular complications of diabetes. *New England Journal of Medicine, 329*,(14) 977-986; and Ramsy, S.D., et al. (1999). Patient-level estimates of the cost of complications in diabetes in a managed-care population. *Pharmacoeconomics, 16*(3), 285-295.

TABLE 71-4 • THE STAGES OF PROGRESSION OF TYPE 1 DIABETIC RENAL DISEASE

- **Stage I, at the time diabetes is diagnosed.** Kidney size and glomerular filtration rate are increased. Blood sugar control can reverse the changes.
- **Stage II, 2 to 3 years after diagnosis.** Glomerular and tubular capillary basement membrane changes result in microscopic changes, with loss of filtration surface area and scar formation. Glomerular changes are referred to as glomerulosclerosis.
- **Stage III, 7 to 15 years after diagnosis.** Microalbuminuria is present. The glomerular filtration rate (GFR) may still be normal or may be increased.
- **Stage IV.** Albuminuria is detectable by dipstick. GFR is decreased. Blood pressure is increased, and retinopathy is present.
- **Stage V.** GFR decreases at an average rate of 10 mL/min/yr.

Structural and functional changes occur in the kidneys of diabetic clients. Initially, kidney size is slightly increased and glomerular filtration rates (GFR) are higher than normal. A radioimmunoassay of urine detects the microlevels of albumin associated with albuminuria. Progressive renal damage occurs before dipstick procedures can detect protein in the urine. For most clients, proteinuria (albuminuria) indicates the need for a renal biopsy for further diagnosis. For the client with diabetes, observed microvascular changes in the retina correlate well with the renal microvascular changes. Examination of the retina showing capillary leakage, fibrosis, and the typical changes of diabetic retinopathy eliminates the need for a risky renal biopsy.

EVIDENCE-BASED PRACTICE FOR NURSING

Does a multidisciplinary case management approach affect patient outcomes?

Harris, L.E., et al. (1998). Effects of multidisciplinary case management in patients with chronic renal insufficiency. *American Journal of Medicine, 195*(6), 464-471.

Case management has been recommended to improve clients' outcomes. In one setting, 437 clients with chronic renal insufficiency were enrolled in an intensive, multidisciplinary case management program for 2 years. A similar number received usual care in an urban, academic, general medicine practice. There were no differences in renal function, health services use, and mortality in the first, second, third, or fifth year of enrollment. The authors conclude that the intensive, multidisciplinary case-management intervention had no effect on the outcomes of care among primary care clients with established chronic renal insufficiency.

Critique. Both clients and practitioners knew which clients were receiving intensive case management; those in the control group may have modified their interventions (either client initiated or practitioner initiated) to demonstrate "equal" competence in care and practice. Most clients in the United States do not receive care in an urban, academic setting; these findings may not be reproducible in a community or rural setting.

Implications for Nursing. The potential benefits of assembling a multidisciplinary team to evaluate and manage the care of clients with chronic renal insufficiency were not supported. Individual practices may be a key factor in influencing the early diagnosis and accurate treatment of renal insufficiency. Further examination is essential to identify provider differences that positively influence client outcomes.

As with nephrotic syndrome, proteinuria may be mild, moderate, or severe. Clients with diabetes mellitus are always considered to be at risk for renal failure. If possible, nephrotoxic agents (e.g., radiopaque contrast media or aminoglycosides) and fluid volume deficit are avoided. Clients with worsening renal function may begin to have frequent hypoglycemic episodes and a decreased need for insulin or oral antihyperglycemic agents. The nurse explains to the client that the kidneys metabolize and excrete insulin. When renal function deteriorates, the insulin is available for a longer time and thus less of it is needed. Unfortunately, many clients believe this means their diabetes mellitus is improving. The result is accelerated progression to ESRD. (See Chapter 65 for more information on diabetic nephropathy.)

Care of the client with chronic renal insufficiency is thought to be more effective when a multidisciplinary case management approach is used. Research has not demonstrated a clear advantage to such an approach (see the Evidence-Based Practice for Nursing box above).

TUMORS

Cysts and Benign Tumors

OVERVIEW

Benign urinary tract growths include cysts and tumors of the renal parenchyma or urinary bladder. Because malignant growths may occur within cystic structures, a thorough evaluation is essential.

A simple renal cyst grows out of renal parenchymal tissue, usually the *cortical* tissue. The cyst is filled with fluid and can cause local tissue destruction as it enlarges. Many cysts cause no symptoms and are discovered accidentally during fluoroscopic examination or autopsy.

Although the exact cause is unknown, cysts are usually considered a structural defect that occurs prenatally. The etiology and incidence of benign tumors is also unknown. Thus far there are no recognized methods of prevention.

COLLABORATIVE MANAGEMENT

Diagnosis of a simple renal cyst involves IV urography, sonography, and computed tomography (CT). If the cyst appears to be filled with fluid at urographic examination, a sonography is generally recommended; if the cyst appears denser, a CT scan is needed.

Treatment may consist of percutaneous aspiration of a fluid-filled cyst or surgical exploration with the potential for total or subtotal nephrectomy.

Renal Cell Carcinoma

OVERVIEW

Renal cell carcinoma is also referred to as *adenocarcinoma of the kidney.* As with other malignancies, the healthy tissue of the kidney is replaced and displaced by cancer cells. Although the exact mechanism is not known, the tumor cells are thought to originate in the proximal convoluted tubules of the nephron.

Systemic effects occurring with the cancer are called **paraneoplastic syndromes** and include anemia, erythrocytosis, hypercalcemia, liver dysfunction with elevated liver enzymes, hormonal effects, increased sedimentation rate, and hypertension.

Anemia and erythrocytosis may appear contradictory: There is some blood loss from hematuria, but the amount lost is not sufficient to cause anemia. Erythrocytosis may be caused by erythropoietin production in the tumor cells. Hypertension may result from increased renin.

Parathyroid hormone produced by tumor cells may be the cause of hypercalcemia; other hormone alterations include increased renin levels (causing hypertension) and increased human chorionic gonadotropin (hCG) levels, which are accompanied by decreased libido and changes in secondary sex characteristics. The cause of the increased sedimentation rate and changes in liver function studies is not known.

Renal tumors are categorized into four stages (Table 71-5). Complications include metastasis and urinary tract obstruction. Metastasis usually occurs via the blood or lymph to the adrenal gland, liver, lungs, long bones, or the other kidney. When the tumor surrounds a ureter, hydroureter and urinary tract obstruction may result.

The exact cause of renal cell carcinoma is unknown, but links to tobacco use and exposure to chemicals such as lead, phosphate, and cadmium have been observed. Other studies suggest the possibility of hereditary influences.

Renal malignancies account for approximately 2% of reported cancers, with about 28,800 new cases and 11,300 deaths annually in the United States. The 5-year survival rate is 60% in the United States (Bonsib, 1999). Renal cell carcinoma usually affects clients between 55 and 60 years of age.

TABLE 71-5 • STAGING RENAL TUMORS

- **Stage I.** Tumors of up to 2.5 cm within the capsule of the kidney; the renal vein, perinephric fat, and adjacent lymph nodes have no tumor.
- **Stage II.** Tumors are larger than 2.5 cm and extend beyond the capsule but are within Gerota's fascia; the renal vein and lymph nodes are not involved.
- **Stage III.** Tumors extend into the renal vein and/or lymph nodes.
- **Stage IV.** Tumors include invasion of adjacent organs beyond Gerota's fascia or metastasis to distant tissues.

COLLABORATIVE MANAGEMENT

Assessment

HISTORY

The nurse asks the client for specific information, including age, known risk factors (e.g., smoking or environmental exposures), history of weight loss, changes in urine color, abdominal or flank discomfort, and fever. The cause of fever is unknown, but pyrogens produced by the tumor cells have been implicated.

PHYSICAL ASSESSMENT/CLINICAL MANIFESTATIONS

Presentations of renal carcinoma are seen only in 5% to 10% of clients and include flank pain, gross hematuria, and a palpable renal mass. The nurse asks about the nature of the flank or abdominal discomfort; clients typically describe the pain as dull and aching. The pain may be more intense if bleeding into the tumor occurs. The nurse inspects the flank, noting asymmetry or obvious protrusions. An abdominal mass may be detected through *gentle* palpation. A renal bruit may be heard on auscultation.

Hematuria is a *late* common sign. Blood in the urine may be grossly observable as bright red flecks or clots, or the urine may appear smoky or cola colored. Without gross hematuria, microscopic examination may or may not reveal red cells.

The skin is inspected for pallor, darkening of the nipples and breast enlargement (in men). Other findings may include muscle wasting, weakness, generally poor nutritional status, and weight loss. All tend to occur late in the disease.

DIAGNOSTIC ASSESSMENT

Urinalysis may reveal red blood cells. Hematologic studies reveal decreased hemoglobin and hematocrit values, hypercalcemia, increased erythrocyte sedimentation rate, and increased levels of adrenocorticotropic hormone, human chorionic gonadotropin (hCG), cortisol, renin, and parathyroid hormone.

Renal masses may be detected by surgical exploration, IV urogram with nephrograms, or sonography. The mass and surrounding structures may be further delineated by CT with contrast or magnetic resonance imaging (MRI). Staging or determining the extent of tumor spread is best accomplished with renal arteriography and renal venography.

Interventions

Interventions focus on controlling the cancer and preventing metastasis.

NONSURGICAL MANAGEMENT. Chemotherapy with a variety of agents has had limited effectiveness. The Food and Drug Administration (FDA) has approved expanded clinical trials for the study of interleukin-2 (IL-2), a biologic response modifier (see Chapters 20 and 25). Interferon (INF) and tumor necrosis factor (TNF) are also being used investigationally. Studies with lymphokine-activated killer (LAK) cells and tumor-infiltrating lymphocytes (TIL) are in the clinical trial stage.

SURGICAL MANAGEMENT. Renal cell carcinoma is usually treated surgically by **nephrectomy** (kidney removal) when pain, bleeding, or tumor spread cannot be controlled otherwise.

PREOPERATIVE CARE. The client is instructed about surgical routines (see Chapters 17, 18, and 19). The nurse explains the probable site of incision and the postoperative dressings, drains, or other equipment needed and reassures the client about pain relief. Preoperative care includes administering blood and fluids to achieve hemodynamic stabilization.

OPERATIVE PROCEDURE. The client is placed in the lateral position with the operative kidney uppermost; after positioning the arms and legs, the client's trunk area is flexed to increase exposure of the kidney area. Removal of the eleventh or twelfth rib is needed to provide better access to the kidney. The surgeon removes the entire kidney, renal artery and vein, and surrounding Gerota's fascia after ligation of the ureter. The adrenal gland is left intact. A drain may be placed in the wound before closure.

When a *radical* nephrectomy is performed, the periaortic lymph nodes are also removed. the surgical approach may be transthoracic (as discussed in the previous paragraph), lumbar, or transabdominal depending on the size and location of the lesion. Radiation therapy may follow a radical nephrectomy. Studies are ongoing to identify the effectiveness of adjuvant therapy (e.g., chemotherapy).

POSTOPERATIVE CARE. Refer to Chapter 19 for postoperative care. Assessment of urologic and renal function is essential to determine function in the remaining kidney.

Monitoring. The nurse observes the client's abdomen for distention from bleeding and symptoms of adrenal insufficiency. The nurse observes the bed linens under the supine client, because bleeding may be present. Hemorrhage or adrenal insufficiency may be accompanied by hypotension, a decrease in urine output, and an altered level of consciousness.

A decrease in blood pressure is one of the earliest signs of both hemorrhage and adrenal insufficiency; in clients with hypotension, urine output also decreases immediately. Large water and sodium losses in the urine occur in clients with adrenal insufficiency; consequently, a large urine output is followed by hypotension and subsequent oliguria (<400 mL/24 hr or less than 25 mL/hr). The physician may prescribe IV replacement of fluids and the administration of packed red blood cells.

The second kidney is expected to provide adequate renal function. The nurse assesses urine output hourly for the first 24 hours postoperatively; a urine flow of 30 to 50 mL/hr is acceptable. Flow rates of less than 25 to 30 mL/hr suggest a decrease in renal perfusion. Initially, the postoperative hemoglobin level, hematocrit values, and white blood cell count may be measured every 6 to 12 hours.

The nurse monitors the client's temperature, pulse rate, and respiratory rate at least every 4 hours; careful measurement and recording of fluid intake and output are critical. The client is weighed daily.

The client may be in a special care unit for 24 to 48 hours postoperatively for monitoring of bleeding and/or adrenal insufficiency. A drain placed near the site of incision removes residual fluid. Because of the discomfort associated with lung expansion, the client is susceptible to atelectasis. Fever, chills, thick sputum, or decreased breath sounds suggest pneumonia.

Pain Management. After surgery, opioid analgesics (e.g., meperidine [Demerol], hydromorphone [Dilaudid], and morphine sulfate [Statex🍁]) are given parenterally. The incision site, in which the major muscle groups associated with breathing and movement are involved, necessitates the liberal use of analgesic agents. These medications may be required for 3 to 5 days for pain management. Oral analgesic agents may be considered when the client is permitted to eat and drink.

Prevention of Complications. One or more antibiotics may be prescribed for intraoperative and postoperative prophylaxis. These agents are usually given as single-dose prescriptions. The need for additional antibiotics is based on clinical and laboratory evidence of infection. Steroid replacements may be necessary in adrenal insufficiency.

RENAL TRAUMA

OVERVIEW

Trauma to one or both kidneys is always a concern in penetrating wounds or blunt injuries to the back, flank, or abdomen. Injury to the kidney can be minor, major, or pedicle (Figure 71-5). Strategies to prevent trauma are reviewed in Chart 71-9.

Minor injuries include contusions, small lacerations, and disruption of the integrity of the parenchyma and the calyx (forniceal disruption). In a person with a contusion, one or both kidneys sustained a bruise because of the major impact. Small blood vessels may be damaged, causing some hematuria. One or more small lacerations may result in small, localized hematomas. There may also be a small hematoma at the site of forniceal disruption. Common causes include falls, contact sports, and blows to the back and torso.

Major injuries involve lacerations to the cortex, medulla, or one of the segmental branches of the renal artery or vein. Deep parenchymal injuries may extend throughout the kidney and result in hematomas contained within or disrupting the capsule. Other parenchymal injuries involve the cortex and cause shattering of tissue, resulting in either an intact or a disrupted capsule.

A major injury is most likely to follow a penetrating abdominal, flank, or back wound (such as seen with gunshot wounds, knife wounds, or motor vehicle accidents). Bleeding is extensive, and surgical exploration is often required. Because of the hemorrhage, hypoperfusion of renal parenchyma can produce short-term or long-term renin-induced hypertension.

Pedicle injuries involve a laceration or disruption of the renal artery and/or renal vein. Hemorrhage is extensive and rapid, and death may ensue quickly unless diagnosis and intervention are prompt.

MINOR TRAUMA

Contusion

Cortical laceration

Fornical disruption

PEDICLE INJURY

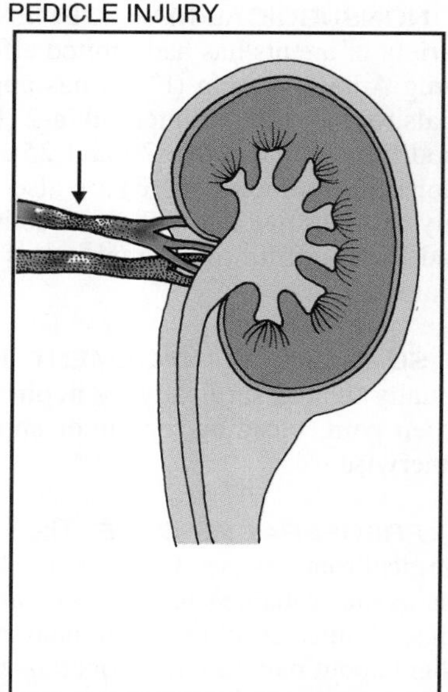

MAJOR TRAUMA

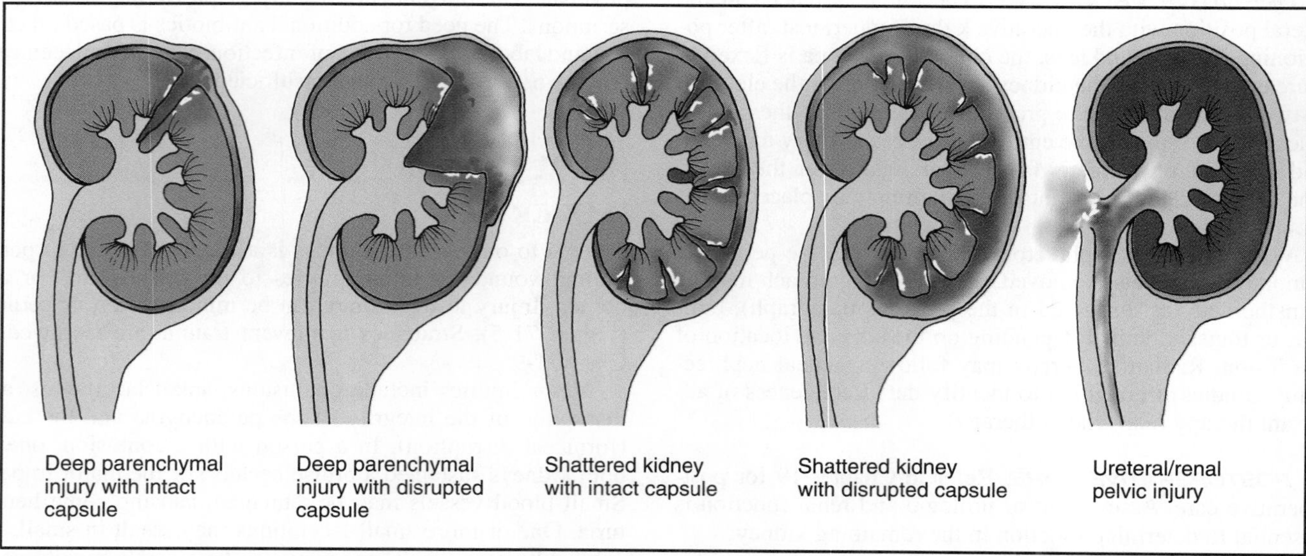

Figure 71-5 ● Common types and locations of renal trauma.

CHART 71-9

CLIENT EDUCATION GUIDE
Preventing Renal and Genitourinary Trauma

- Wear a seat belt.
- Practice safe walking habits.
- Use caution when riding bicycles and motorcycles.
- Wear appropriate protective clothing when participating in contact sports.
- Avoid all contact sports and high-risk activities if you have only one kidney.

➤ COLLABORATIVE MANAGEMENT

● Assessment

The nurse obtains a history of the client's usual health status and the events surrounding the trauma from the client, a witness, or emergency personnel. Critical assessment information includes a history of renal or urologic disease, surgical intervention, or systemic health problems (e.g., diabetes mellitus or hypertension).

Ureteral and/or renal pelvic injury may cause diffuse abdominal pain, local collections of urine, and infection. The nurse asks the client about pain, specifically flank or abdominal pain, and solicits a description: Is the pain dull? Sharp? Constant? Intermittent? Aggravated by coughing?

The nurse measures the client's blood pressure and apical and peripheral pulse rates, respiratory rate, and temperature. The right and left flanks are inspected to determine asymmetry or penetrating injuries of the lower thorax or back. Similarly, the nurse inspects the abdomen for ecchymoses, percusses the abdomen for distention, and observes for penetrating wounds. The urethra is inspected for gross bleeding.

Urinalysis commonly reveals hemoglobin or red blood cells from the rupture of small or large renal blood vessels.

Microscopic examination of the urine may also show red blood cell casts, which suggest tubular damage. Hemoglobin and hematocrit values decrease with blood loss; the white blood cell count is elevated with inflammation or infection.

Fluoroscopic procedures include IV urography, renal arteriography, and computed tomography (CT). A urogram reveals the number of kidneys and the integrity and patency of the collecting system. Renal sonography is an alternative diagnostic procedure to a urogram that avoids radiopaque contrast media exposure to clients with elevated serum creatinine levels.

Renal arteriography reveals the number of kidneys and, more specifically, the blood supply to each. In clients with pedicle injuries, the contrast media used in arteriography extravasates from the ruptured vessels, and the renal parenchyma is not visualized. The CT scan shows the location of the injury and vascular and tissue integrity. Intracapsular and extracapsular hematomas are readily observable on the CT scan.

Interventions

Nursing diagnoses for the client with renal trauma include Ineffective (Renal) Tissue Perfusion, Anxiety, Pain, Impaired Urinary Elimination, Post-Trauma Syndrome, and Risk for Infection. Interventions include medications for vascular support, fluids to restore fluid volume, and surgery when indicated.

NONSURGICAL MANAGEMENT

DRUG THERAPY. Prescribed IV dopamine (Revimine✤, others) supports renal perfusion. Coagulation factors such as vitamin K and platelets are assessed and administered as needed.

FLUID THERAPY. Fluid administration to restore circulating blood volume is critical for renal tissue perfusion. *Crystalloid* solutions replace water and some electrolytes and include 0.9% sodium chloride (NSS), 5% dextrose in 0.45% sodium chloride, and Ringer's solution. When significant bleeding has occurred, whole blood or packed red cell replacement restores the oxygen-carrying capacity of hemoglobin. *Plasma volume expanders,* such as dextran or albumin, help re-establish plasma oncotic pressure and minimize fluid shift from the intravascular to the interstitial fluid space.

During fluid resuscitation or restoration, the nurse administers fluid at the prescribed rate and monitors the client for hemodynamic instability. The nurse also monitors vital signs as often as every 5 to 15 minutes and measures and records urine output hourly. Urine output should be greater than 25 to 30 mL/hr.

SURGICAL MANAGEMENT. Surgical interventions may include nephrectomy and partial nephrectomy. For clients with major vascular tearing, the kidney may be surgically removed, repaired through revascularization techniques, and then reimplanted. The repair of kidney tissue outside the client is called *bench surgery.* Autotransplantation is transplantation of one's own kidney.

Community-Based Care

The nurse instructs the client, family, or significant other about the effects of the injury and how to assess for infection or other complications, such as the onset of bleeding or urinary retention. The client is instructed to observe the pattern and frequency of urination and to note whether the color, clarity, and amount appear normal. The nurse also instructs the client to seek medical attention if these characteristics change significantly and if a feeling of bladder distention or inadequate bladder emptying occurs, which suggests an obstruction. Chills, fever, lethargy, and/or cloudy, foul-smelling urine may suggest a urinary tract infection. The nurse warns the client not to ignore these symptoms and to seek medical care promptly if they occur.

ONLINE RESOURCES

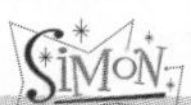

For suggested readings and Internet resources, go to http://www.wbsaunders.com/SIMON/Iggy/.

SELECTED BIBLIOGRAPHY

Asterisk indicates a classic or definitive work on this subject.

*Adler, S.G., Cohen, A.H., & Glassock, R.J. (1996). Secondary glomerular diseases. In B.M. Brenner & F.C. Rector (Eds.), *Brenner & Rector's the kidney* (5th ed., pp. 1498-1596). Philadelphia: W.B. Saunders.

Agodoa, L. (1998). African-American study of kidney disease and hypertension (AASK): Clinical trial update. *Ethnic Disease, 8*(2), 249-253.

American Cancer Society. (2001). *Cancer facts and figures 2001.* 01-300M-NO.5008.01. Atlanta: Author.

Avner, E.D., et al. (1999). Cellular pathophysiology of cystic kidney disease: Insight into future therapies. *International Journal of Developmental Biology, 43*(5 Spec. No.), 457-461.

Bakris, G. et al. (2000). Preserving renal function in adults with hypertension and diabetes: A consensus approach. National Kidney Foundation Hypertension and Diabetes Executive Committees Working Group. *American Journal of Kidney Disease, 36*(3), 646-661.

Bernini, G., et al. (1998). Treatment of renovascular disease and of renovascular hypertension. *Journal of Nephrology, 11*(6), 311-317.

Bleyer, A.J., & Appel, R.G. (1999). Risk factors associated with hypertensive nephrosclerosis. *Nephron, 82*(30), 193-198.

Bonsib, S.M. (1999). Risk and prognosis in renal neoplasms. A pathologists prospective. *Urologic Clinics of North America, 26*(3), 643-660, viii.

Brater, D.C. (1999). The use of diuretics in cirrhosis and nephrotic syndrome. *Seminars in Nephrology, 19*(6), 575-580.

Brown, J.B., Pedula, K.L., Baskt, A.W. (1999). The progressive cost of complications in type 2 diabetes mellitus. *Archives of Internal Medicine, 159*(16), 1873-1880.

Calvet, J., & Grantham, J. (2001). The genetics and physiology of polycystic kidney disease. *Seminars in Nephrology, 21*(2), 107-123.

Connolly, A., & Thorp, J.M. (1999). Urinary tract infections in pregnancy. *Urology Clinics of North America, 26*(4), 779-787.

Coresh, J., & Jaar, B. (1997). Further trends in the etiology of end-stage renal disease in African-Americans. *Current Opinions in Nephrology & Hypertension, 6*(3), 243-249.

Crook, E.D. (1999). The role of hypertension, obesity, and diabetes in causing renal vascular disease. *American Journal of Medical Science, 17*(3), 183-188.

*Duley, I., & Gabow, P. (1990). *PKD patient's manual: Understanding and living with autosomal dominant polycystic kidney disease.* Kansas City, MO: PKD Foundation.

Falk, J., Jennett, J., & Nachman, S. (2000). Primary glomerular disease. In B.M. Brenner & S.A. Levine (Eds.), *Brenner & Rector's the kidney* (6th ed., pp. 1263-1349). Philadelphia: W.B. Saunders.

Fliser, D., & Ritz, E. (1998). Does essential hypertension cause progressive renal disease? *Journal of Hypertension Supplement, 16*(4), S13-S15.

Fogo, A.B. (1999). Current concepts in glomerulosclerosis. *American Journal of Kidney Disease, 34*(5), liv-lvi.

Germino, G.G. (1997). Autosomal dominant polycystic kidney disease: A two-hit model. *Hospital Practice, 32*(3), 81-82, 85-88, 91-92, 95-97, 102.

Golan, L., Birkmeyer, J.D., Welch, H.G. (1999). The cost-effectiveness of treating all patients with type 2 diabetes with angiotensin-converting enzyme inhibitors. *Annals of Internal Medicine, 131*(9), 660-667, editorial 707-708.

Gonzalez, R.P., et al. (1999). Surgical management of renal trauma: Is vascular control necessary? *Journal of Trauma, 47*(6), 1039-1042, discussion 1042-1044.

Grist, T.M. (1999). Magnetic resonance angiography of renal artery stenosis. *Coronary Artery Disease, 10*(3), 151-156.

Harris, L.E., et al. (1998). Effects of multidisciplinary case management in patients with chronic renal insufficiency. *American Journal of Medicine, 195*(6), 464-471.

Hartman, D.S., & Stagg, P.L. (1998). Diagnosis please. Case 3: Renal tuberculosis. *Radiology, 209*(1), 69-72.

Hartmann, J.S. & Bokemeyer, C. (1999). Chemotherapy for renal cancer. *Anticancer Research, 19*(2C), 1541-1543.

Herman, W.H. & Eastman, R.C. (1998). The effects of treatment on the direct costs of diabetes. *Diabetes Care, 21*(Suppl. 3), C19-C24.

Ichigi, Y., et al. (1999). Significance of hematoma size for evaluating the grade of blunt renal trauma. *International Journal of Urology, 6*(10), 502-508.

Kelly, C.J., & Neilson, E.G. (2000). Tubulointerstitial diseases. In B.M. Brenner & S.A. Levine (Eds.), *Brenner & Rector's the kidney* (6th ed., pp. 1506-1536). Philadelphia: W.B. Saunders.

Knudson, M.M., & Maull, K.I. (1999). Nonoperative management of solid organ injuries: Past, present, and future. *Surgery Clinics of North America, 79*(6), 1357-1371.

Krautschick, A.W. (1999). Metabolic evaluation and medical therapy for stone formation. *Current Opinion in Urology, 9*(4), 335-338.

*Lancaster, L.E. (Ed.). (1995). *Core curriculum for nephrology nursing* (3rd ed.). Pitman, NJ: A.J. Jannetti.

Laragh, J.H., & Blumenfeld, J.D. (2000). Essential hypertension. In B.M. Brenner & S.A Levine (Eds.), *Brenner & Rector's the kidney* (6th ed., pp. 1967-2006). Philadelphia: W.B. Saunders.

*Letizia, M., & Conway, A.M. (1996). Interleukin-2 therapy for renal cell cancer. *Critical Care Nurse, 16*(5), 20-26, 30-32, 34-35.

Levy, A.S., et al. (1999). Dietary protein restriction and the progression of chronic renal disease: What have all the results of the MDRD study shown? Modification of Diet in Renal Disease Study Group. *Journal of the American Society of Nephrology, 10*(11), 2426-2439.

Lewis, J.B., et al. (1999). Effect of intensive blood pressure control on the course of type 1 diabetic nephropathy: Collaborative Study Group. *American Journal of Kidney Disease, 34*(5), 809-817.

Little, C. (2000). Renovascular hypertension. *American Journal of Nursing, 100*(2), 46-51.

Losito, A., et al. (1999). Survival of patients with renovascular disease and ACE inhibition. *Clinics in Nephrology, 52*(6), 339-343.

McCarthy, S., & McMullen, M. (1997). Autosomal dominant polycystic kidney disease: Pathophysiology and treatment. *American Nephrology Nurses' Association Journal, 24*(1), 45-53.

McCloskey, J., & Bulechek, G. (2000). *Nursing interventions classification (NIC)* (3rd ed.). St. Louis: Mosby.

*McKinney, B. (1996). When this rare cancer strikes: Renal cell carcinoma. *RN, 59*(12), 36-41, 51.

Mihara, S., et al. (1999). Early detection of renal cell carcinoma by ultrasonographic screening based on the results of 13 years of screening in Japan. *Ultrasound in Medicine and Biology, 25*(7), 1033-1039.

Morganti, A., et al. (1999). Renovascular hypertension: Clinical and diagnostic clues. *Annals of Urologie, 33*(3), 137-143.

Nangaku, M., Pippin, J., & Couser, W.G. (1999). Complement membrane attack complex (C5b-9) mediates interstitial disease in experimental nephrotic syndrome. *Journal of the American Society of Nephrology, 10*(11), 2323-2331.

*Nathan, D.M. (1993). Diabetes Control and Complications Trial Research Group: The effect of long-term intensified insulin treatment on development of microvascular complications of diabetes. *New England Journal of Medicine, 329*(14), 977-986.

Nickeleit, V., et al. (1999). Nephrotic syndrome in an adult: The ongoing saga of fibrils versus microtubules. *American Journal of Kidney Disease, 34*(6), 1146-1151.

Nicolau, C., et al. (1999). Autosomal dominant polycystic kidney disease types 1 and 2: Assessment of US sensitivity for diagnosis. *Radiology, 213*(1), 273-276.

NIDDK National Kidney and Urologic Diseases Information Clearinghouse. (1999). *Kidney and Urologic Diseases Statistics for the United States.* Bethesda, MD: U.S. Government NIH Pub. No. 99-3895.

Parker, S.L., et al. (1997). Cancer statistics, 1997. *CA: A Cancer Journal for Clinicians, 47*(1), 5-27.

*Pasternack, M.S., & Rubin, R.H. (1993). Urinary tract tuberculosis. In R.W. Schrier & C.W. Gottschalk (Eds.), *Diseases of the kidney* (5th ed., pp. 909-928). Boston: Little, Brown.

Ramsy, S.D., et al. (1999). Patient-level estimates of the cost of complications in diabetes in a managed-care population. *Pharmacoeconomics, 16*(3), 285-295.

Rees, C.R. (1999). Stents for atherosclerotic renovascular disease. *Journal of Vascular Interventional Radiology, 10*(6), 689-705.

Richardson, A., & Piepho, R. (2000). Effect of race on hypertension and antihypertensive therapy. *International Journal of Clinical Pharmacology, 38*(2), 75-79.

Ritz, E., et al. (1999). End-stage renal failure in type 2 diabetes: A medical catastrophe of worldwide dimensions. *American Journal of Kidney Disease, 34*(5), 795-808.

Roberts, J.A. (1999). Management of pyelonephritis and upper urinary tract infections. (1999). *Urology Clinics of North America, 26*(4), 753-763.

Rodriguez-Itrube, B. (2000). Post-infectious glomerulonephritis. *American Journal of Kidney Disease, 35*(1), xlvi-xlviii.

Rosenberg, M. (1999). Pharmacoeconomics of treating uncomplicated urinary tract infections. *International Journal of Antimicrobial Agents, 11*(3-4), 247-251, discussion 261-264.

*See, W.A., & Williams, R.D. (1992). Tumors of the kidney, ureter, and bladder. *Western Journal of Medicine, 156*(5), 523-534.

Seedat, Y.K. (1999). Improvement in treatment of hypertension has not reduced the incidence of end-stage renal disease. *Journal of Human Hypertension, 13*(11), 747-751.

Sessa, A., et al. (1999). Renal-retinal diabetic syndrome. *Nephron, 83*(3), 285-286.

*Smith, M.F. (1990). Renal trauma: Adult and pediatric considerations. *Critical Care Nursing Clinics of North America, 2*(10), 67-77.

*Sommers, M. S. (1990). Blunt renal trauma. *Critical Care Nurse, 10*(3), 38-49.

Sorcini, A., & Libertino, J.A. (1999). Vascular reconstruction in urology. *Urologic Clinics of North America, 26*(1), 219-234, x-xi.

Stuart, R. & Nigam, S. (2000). Developmental biology of the kidney. In B.M. Brenner and S.A. Levine (Eds.), *Brenner & Rector's the kidney* (6th ed., pp. 68-92). Philadelphia: W.B. Saunders.

Tolkoff-Rubin, N., Cotran, R., & Rubin, R. (2000). Urinary tract infection, pyelonephritis, and reflux nephropathy. In B.M. Brenner & S.A. Levine (Eds.), *Brenner & Rector's the kidney* (6th ed., pp. 1449-1508). Philadelphia: W.B. Saunders.

Torra, R. (1999). Autosomal dominant polycystic kidney disease, type 2 (PKD2 disease). *Advances in Nephrology Necker Hospital, 29*(11), 277-287.

*Torres, V.E. (1996). Polycystic kidney disease: Guidelines for family physicians. *American Family Physician, 53*(3), 847-850.

Torres, V.E. (1999). Extrarenal manifestations of autosomal dominant polycystic kidney disease. *American Journal of Kidney Disease, 34*(6), xlv-xlvii.

U.S. Renal Data Systems. (1999). *USRDS 1999 annual data report.* Bethesda, MD: The National Institutes of Health, National Institute of Diabetes and Digestive and Kidney Diseases.

*Watson, M., & Torres, V. (Eds.). (1996). *Polycystic kidney disease.* New York: Oxford University Press.

Weir, M.R., & Dzau, V.J. (1999). The renin-angiotensin-aldosterone system: A specific target for hypertension management. *American Journal of Hypertension, 12*(12 Pt. 3), 105S-213S.

*Wong, J.M., et al. (1991). Surgery after failed percutaneous renal artery angioplasty. *Journal of Vascular Surgery, 30*(3), 468-482.

Zuccala, A., & Zucchelli, P. (1998). Ischemic nephropathy: Diagnosis and treatment. *Journal of Nephrology, 11*(6), 318-324.

CHAPTER 72

Interventions for Clients with Acute and Chronic Renal Failure

CONSTANCE VISOVSKY

Learning Objectives

After studying this chapter, you should be able to:

1. Compare and contrast the pathophysiology and causes of chronic renal failure (CRF) and acute renal failure (ARF).
2. Identify clients at risk for development of ARF.
3. Identify clients at risk for development of CRF.
4. Use laboratory data and clinical assessment to determine the effectiveness of therapy for renal failure.
5. Discuss interventions to prevent ARF.
6. Prioritize nursing care for the client with ARF.
7. Compare the clinical manifestations of stage I, stage II, and stage III CRF.
8. Discuss the mechanisms of peritoneal dialysis (PD) and hemodialysis (HD) as renal replacement therapies.
9. Prioritize nursing care for the client with end-stage renal disease.
10. Prioritize teaching needs for the client using continuous ambulatory PD.
11. Prioritize teaching needs for the client with a permanent vascular access for long-term HD.
12. Compare and contrast the dietary modifications needed for the client undergoing HD with those for the client undergoing PD.
13. Plan prevention strategies for the complications of PD.
14. Discuss the criteria for kidney donation.
15. Prioritize nursing care for the client during the first 24 hours after kidney transplantation.

SIMON

Go to http://www.wbsaunders.com/SIMON/Iggy/ for self-assessment questions related to these Learning Objectives.

Acute and chronic renal failure have become increasingly more common in the United States, resulting in considerable morbidity and mortality. Acute renal failure is responsible for 7% of all hospital admissions, and the prevalence of end-stage renal disease has virtually doubled in the last decade (Stark, 1998; U.S. Renal Data Systems, 1999). There are many causes of renal failure, but complications related to poorly controlled diabetes remain the most common cause.

The functions of the kidney are excretion of waste, water and salt regulation, maintenance of acid balance, and hormone secretion. When renal function deteriorates gradually, as occurs with most causes of chronic renal failure, 90% to 95% of the nephrons must be destroyed before significant renal failure is evident. The client may have many years of decreased renal reserve and chronic renal insufficiency before the uremia of end-stage renal failure develops. During this time of decreased renal reserve and chronic renal insufficiency, the client is at increased risk for acute renal failure because of the diminished availability of functioning nephrons.

When renal deterioration is sudden, the capacity of the functioning nephrons is exceeded more quickly, and renal failure may develop with the loss of only 50% of functioning nephrons. Acute renal failure and chronic renal failure are compared in Table 72-1. Acute renal failure affects *many* body systems; chronic renal failure affects *every* body system. The abnormalities are primarily related to the effects of the following:

- Fluid volume excess
- Electrolyte and acid-base abnormalities
- Accumulated nitrogenous wastes
- Hormonal inadequacies

When renal function decreases to the point where the kidneys can no longer meet the body's homeostatic demands, re-

TABLE 72-1 • CHARACTERISTICS OF ACUTE AND CHRONIC RENAL FAILURE

Characteristic	Acute Renal Failure	Chronic Renal Failure
Onset	Sudden (hours to days)	Gradual (months to years)
Percentage of nephron involvement	~50%	90%-95%
Duration	2-4 wk; less than 3 mo	Permanent
Prognosis	Good for return of renal function with supportive care; high mortality in some situations	Fatal without a renal replacement therapy, such as dialysis or transplantation

nal replacement therapy is required to prevent death from potentially life-threatening consequences.

ACUTE RENAL FAILURE

OVERVIEW

Acute renal failure (ARF) is a rapid decrease in renal function, leading to the accumulation of metabolic waste in the body. ARF can result from conditions that cause inadequate kidney perfusion **(prerenal failure);** damage to the glomeruli, interstitium, or tubules **(intrarenal failure);** or obstruction **(postrenal failure)** (Kelly, 1997). ARF in clients with chronic renal insufficiency (CRI) may result in **end-stage renal disease (ESRD)** or may resolve to nearly the pre-ARF level of renal function. Many factors contribute to renal insults resulting in ARF, but the acute syndrome may be reversible.

Pathophysiology

The pathophysiologic process of ARF is related to the cause of the sudden decrease in kidney function and the involved site or sites of the kidney. Hypoperfusion, toxins, tubular ischemia, infections, and obstruction have different effects on the renal system. Any of these processes can result in a decreased glomerular filtration rate (GFR), alterations in renal tubular cell membrane integrity, and tubular lumen obstruction.

With acute hypoperfusion, autoregulatory responses (i.e., renal vasoconstriction, activation of renin-angiotensin-aldosterone, and release of antidiuretic hormone [ADH]) increase blood volume and improve renal perfusion. However, these compensatory mechanisms cause urine volume to fall, resulting in **oliguria** (urine output less than 400 mL/day). Tubular cell injury is more likely to occur from the increasing ischemia related to hypoperfusion. Toxins can cause vasoconstrictive responses in the kidney, leading to reduced renal blood flow and renal ischemia.

Interstitial inflammatory changes resulting from infection, drugs, or infiltrating tumors result in immune-mediated changes in renal tissue. With extensive tubular damage, sloughing of tubular cells and other formed elements (e.g., red blood cell [RBC] casts) may obstruct the tubular lumen and prevent the formation or outflow of urine. Obstruction anywhere within the genitourinary tract eventually results in full or partial obstruction to the formation and outflow of urine.

When intratubular pressure exceeds glomerular hydrostatic pressure, glomerular filtration ceases. This process causes a progressive elevation of the serum blood urea nitrogen (BUN) and creatinine levels. When the BUN rises faster than the serum creatinine level, the cause is usually related to protein catabolism or volume depletion. When both the BUN and creatinine levels rise and the ratio between the two remains constant, renal failure is present.

TYPES OF ACUTE RENAL FAILURE

Several syndromes describe the types of ARF. These include prerenal azotemia, intrarenal (intrinsic) ARF, and postrenal azotemia. Table 72-2 summarizes the pathologic changes and causes of ARF.

Prerenal azotemia can be reversed by establishing normal intravascular volume, increasing blood pressure and cardiac output. Prolonged, untreated hypoperfusion can lead to severe ischemic injury and intrarenal failure.

The term *intrarenal ARF* is often shortened to just *ARF* in the clinical setting. Other terms include **acute tubular necrosis (ATN)** and **lower nephron nephrosis.** Infections (bacteria, viral, fungal, or endotoxin), drugs (especially aminoglycoside antibiotics and nonsteroidal anti-inflammatory drugs [NSAIDs]), and infiltrating tumors (e.g., lymphomas or leukemias) can cause acute interstitial nephritis. Inflammation of the glomeruli (glomerulonephritis) or of the small vessels of the kidneys (vasculitis) or a major obstruction to blood flow can also cause intrarenal ARF.

Postrenal azotemia develops from obstruction to the outflow of formed urine anywhere within the genitourinary tract.

PHASES OF ACUTE RENAL FAILURE

When a client's renal function has been compromised, the phases of ARF begin (Table 72-3). Increasing numbers of clients have a *nonoliguric* form of ARF. The description of the phases of this form of ARF are similar to those described in Table 72-3 except for the references to urine output. In addition, the treatment of these clients is less complicated because renal replacement therapy is rarely needed. Interventions to restore circulating volume, improve cardiac output, or reestablish blood pressure may prevent progression of the phases when renal hypoperfusion is present.

Etiology

Many types of renal insults can lead to reduced renal function. Severe hypotension from excessive blood loss or dehydration results in hypoperfusion of blood to the kidneys and can lead to prerenal ARF. Cardiac disease or heart failure also results in decreased renal perfusion. The client may be oliguric, or even anuric (less than 100 mL/24 hr), if the dehydration or renal blood flow obstruction is severe. The following are other conditions that precipitate ARF:

- Nephrotoxic agents (antibiotics, NSAIDs) (Table 72-4)
- Disseminated intravascular coagulation (DIC)

TABLE 72-2 • CAUSES OF THE THREE TYPES OF ACUTE RENAL FAILURE

Pathologic Change	Causes
PRERENAL	
Decreased blood flow to the kidneys leading to ischemia in the nephrons; prolonged hypoperfusion can lead to tubular necrosis and ARF	Conditions that cause decreased cardiac output Shock CHF Pulmonary embolism Anaphylaxis Pericardial tamponade Sepsis
INTRARENAL (INTRINSIC)	
Actual tissue damage to the kidney caused by inflammatory or immunologic processes or from prolonged hypoperfusion	Acute interstitial nephritis Exposure to nephrotoxins Acute glomerulonephritis Vasculitis Hepatorenal syndrome ATN Renal artery or vein stenosis/thrombosis
POSTRENAL	
Obstruction of the urine collecting system anywhere from the calyces to the urethral meatus Obstruction of the bladder must be bilateral to cause postrenal failure unless only one kidney is functional	Urethral or bladder cancer Renal calculi Atony of bladder Prostatic hyperplasia or cancer Cervical cancer Urethral stricture

ARF, Acute renal failure; *CHF,* congestive heart failure; *ATN,* acute tubular necrosis.

TABLE 72-3 • THE PHASES OF OLIGURIC ACUTE RENAL FAILURE

Phase	Description	Characteristics	Duration
Onset phase	Begins with the precipitating event and continues until oliguria develops.	The gradual accumulation of nitrogenous wastes, such as serum creatinine and BUN, may be noted.	Can last hours to several days.
Oliguric phase	Characterized by a urine output of 100-400 mL/24 hr that does not respond to fluid challenges or diuretics.	Laboratory data include increasing serum creatinine and BUN levels, hyperkalemia, bicarbonate deficit (metabolic acidosis), hyperphosphatemia, hypocalcemia, and hypermagnesemia. Sodium retention occurs, but this is masked by the dilutional effects of water retention. Urinary indices are typically low and fixed; regulation of water balance by the kidneys is impaired, so urine specific gravity and urine osmolality will not vary as plasma osmolality changes.	Typically lasts 8-15 days but can last for several weeks, especially in older clients or those having pre-existing renal insufficiency.
Diuretic phase (high-output phase)	Often has a prompt onset, with urine flow increasing rapidly over a period of several days. The diuresis can result in an output of up to 10 L/day of dilute urine.	Electrolyte losses typically precede clearance of nitrogenous wastes. Later in the diuretic phase, the BUN level starts to fall and continues to fall until the level reaches normal limits or reaches a plateau. Normal renal tubular function is reestablished during this phase.	Usually occurs 2-6 wk after the onset of oliguric acute renal failure and continues until the BUN level ceases to rise.
Recovery phase (convalescent phase)	In this phase, the client begins to return to normal levels of activity.	The client functions at a lower energy level and has less stamina than before the illness. Residual renal insufficiency may be noted through regular monitoring of renal function. Renal function may never return to preillness levels, but renal function sufficient for a long and healthy life is likely.	Renal function may continue to improve for up to 12 mo after oliguric acute renal failure began. The client is particularly vulnerable to additional renal injury during this time.

BUN, Blood urea nitrogen.

- Obstruction by thrombosis or stenosis
- Uric acid crystals or other obstructing precipitates
- Acute hemolytic transfusion reactions
- Complications of infection (e.g., endotoxins or sepsis)
- Acute glomerulonephritis
- Vasculitis
- Severe hypertension
- Hepatorenal syndrome of cirrhosis

Incidence/Prevalence

ARF affects 20% of all critically ill clients and carries a 50% to 80% mortality rate (Stark, 1998). Eighty percent of ARF episodes are due to ATN and exacerbations of CRI. Volume depletion leading to prerenal azotemia is the most common cause of acute renal deterioration and is reversible in most cases with prompt intervention.

For clients surviving the precipitating event, the opportunity for return of renal function is good. Complications during the course of ARF can vastly increase mortality. Bloodstream infections associated with central and peripheral lines and the pulmonary system are most often involved in complications. However, the highest mortality occurs with trauma (70%) and surgery. ARF caused by nephrotoxic substances is associated with the lowest rates (10% to 26%) of recovery. The prognosis for ARF caused by obstruction or glomerulonephritis is much better.

COLLABORATIVE MANAGEMENT

Prevention

Nurses have an essential role in the prevention of acute renal failure (ARF). The nurse notes the signs of impending renal dysfunction through careful physical assessment and close monitoring of laboratory values. Prompt recognition and correction of extrarenal problems usually restore renal function before tissue damage can occur. Careful physical assessment is required to evaluate the client's fluid status. Intake and output records and body weights can assist in identifying trends in fluid balance. If vascular volume is depleted, decreased urine output, postural hypotension, and tachycardia will be present. Prompt fluid resuscitation for clients in the prerenal stage can prevent intrarenal problems that can lead to renal tissue damage and renal failure.

The nurse also monitors laboratory values for any changes that reflect compromised renal function. Decreased urine specific gravity indicates a loss of urine-concentrating ability and is the earliest sign of renal tubular damage. Other laboratory values that are helpful in monitoring renal function include serum creatinine, urine and serum electrolytes, and blood urea nitrogen (BUN).

The nurse is aware of nephrotoxic substances that the client may ingest or be exposed to (see Table 72-4). The nurse questions orders for potentially nephrotoxic drugs, and the ordered dose is validated before the client receives the drug. Antibiotics are the most likely drug group to have nephrotoxic side effects. NSAIDs may cause or potentiate the risk for ARF. Combinations of drugs can cause synergistic reactions, further increasing the risk for ARF. If a client must receive a potentially nephrotoxic drug, the nurse monitors laboratory values, including BUN, creatinine, and drug peak and trough levels, closely for indications of actual or potential renal dysfunction.

TABLE 72-4 • SOME POTENTIALLY NEPHROTOXIC SUBSTANCES

DRUGS

Antibiotics/Anti-infectives
- Amphotericin B
- Colistimethate
- Methicillin
- Polymyxin B
- Rifampin
- Sulfonamides
- Tetracycline hydrochloride
- Vancomycin

Aminoglycoside Antibiotics
- Gentamicin
- Kanamycin
- Neomycin
- Netilmicin sulfate
- Tobramycin

Antineoplastics
- Cisplatin
- Cyclophosphamide
- Methotrexate

Other Drugs
- Acetaminophen
- Captopril
- Cyclosporine
- Fluorinate anesthetics
- Indomethacin
- D-Penicillamine
- Phenazopyridine hydrochloride
- Quinine

OTHER SUBSTANCES

Organic Solvents
- Carbon tetrachloride
- Ethylene glycol

Nondrug Chemical Agents
- Radiographic contrast dye
- Pesticides
- Fungicides
- Myoglobin (from breakdown of skeletal muscle)

Heavy Metals and Ions
- Arsenic
- Bismuth
- Copper sulfate
- Gold salts
- Lead
- Mercuric chloride

Assessment

HISTORY

The accurate diagnosis of ARF, including its type and its cause, largely depends on a detailed history. The history must include questions relating to the potential causes of ARF. The client is asked about exposure to nephrotoxins, recent surgery or trauma, transfusion, or other factors that might lead to renal ischemia. A medication history is also important, since treatment with certain anti-infectives, aminoglycoside antibiotics, angiotensin-converting enzyme (ACE) inhibitors, and NSAIDs can cause prerenal failure. Exposure to radiographic contrast medium can precipitate ARF, especially in older clients with reduced renal reserve. In some situations, ARF must be differentiated from chronic renal insufficiency (CRI). In these cases, the nurse asks about known renal diseases; systemic diseases, such as diabetes mellitus and systemic lupus erythematosus and other connective tissue diseases; and chronic hypertension.

To identify possible acute glomerulonephritis, questions about acute illnesses such as influenza, colds, gastroenteritis, and sore throats or pharyngitis, as well as the presence of cocoa-colored urine (hematuria), are included.

Reversible prerenal azotemia may be suspected after hypotension, hemorrhage or shock, burns, congestive heart failure (CHF), or any situation in which the client experiences intravascular volume depletion. Phosphorus-containing bowel preparations and being allowed nothing by mouth (NPO) preoperatively, in conjunction with the fluid losses of most surgical procedures, are sufficient to cause prerenal azotemia in many clients (Orias, Mahnensmith, & Perazella, 1999).

Postrenal azotemia can be identified by focusing on any history of obstructive disease processes that would be manifested as difficulty in starting the urine stream, changes in the amount or appearance of the urine, narrowing of the urine stream, nocturia, urgency, or symptoms of renal calculi. The nurse also notes any history of malignant carcinoma that may cause bilateral obstruction.

Because of the widely varied causes and the potentially reversible nature of the illness, the nurse obtains or validates a detailed history when ARF is suspected.

PHYSICAL ASSESSMENT/CLINICAL MANIFESTATIONS

The clinical manifestations of ARF are related to azotemia, as well to as the underlying cause (Chart 72-1). Signs and symptoms of *prerenal* azotemia are hypotension, tachycardia, decreased urine output, decreased cardiac output, decreased central venous pressure (CVP), and lethargy. The general clinical appearance of a client with prerenal azotemia is similar to that of a client with heart failure or dehydration, depending on the cause of the renal compromise.

Intrarenal (intrinsic) ARF usually involves damage to the glomeruli, interstitium, or tubules. Classic manifestations include oliguria or **anuria** (absence of urine), edema, hypertension, tachycardia, shortness of breath, jugular venous distention, elevated CVP, weight gain, rales or crackles, anorexia, nausea, vomiting, and lethargy or varying levels of consciousness. Clinical manifestations of electrolyte abnormalities, such as electrocardiographic (ECG) changes, may also be present.

CHART 72-1

KEY FEATURES *of* Acute Renal Failure

Prerenal Azotemia
- Hypotension
- Tachycardia
- Decreased cardiac output
- Decreased central venous pressure
- Decreased urine output
- Lethargy

Intrarenal (Intrinsic) ARF and Postrenal Azotemia
- Renal manifestations
  - Oliguria or anuria
  - Increased urine specific gravity
- Cardiac manifestations
  - Hypertension
  - Tachycardia
  - Jugular venous distention
  - Increased central venous pressure
  - ECG changes: tall T waves
- Respiratory manifestations
  - Shortness of breath
  - Orthopnea
  - Rales or crackles
  - Pulmonary edema
  - Friction rub
- Gastrointestinal manifestations
  - Anorexia
  - Nausea
  - Vomiting
  - Flank pain
- Neurologic manifestations
  - Lethargy
  - Headache
  - Tremors
  - Confusion
- General manifestations
  - Generalized edema
  - Weight gain

ARF, Acute renal failure; *ECG,* electrocardiogram.

In clients with *postrenal* azotemia, the nurse monitors for oliguria or intermittent anuria, symptoms of uremia, and lethargy. The nurse reports changes in the character of the urine stream or difficulty starting urination.

LABORATORY ASSESSMENT

The numerous alterations in laboratory values in the client with ARF are similar to those occurring in chronic renal failure (CRF) (Chart 72-2; see also Laboratory Assessment [Chronic Renal Failure], p. 1681). The nurse can expect to find rising BUN and creatinine levels, and abnormalities in serum electrolytes. Table 72-5 shows the effects of renal failure on electrolyte values. Clients with ARF, however, typically do *not* experience the anemia associated with CRF unless there is hemorrhagic blood loss. However, uremic hemolysis secondary to severe azotemia can develop and may be the cause of anemia in the early phase of ARF.

In the early phases of ARF, urinalysis and microscopic examination of urine may provide diagnostic information. Urine sodium levels are often less than 10 to 20 mEq/L in clients with prerenal azotemia. In prerenal azotemia, the urine is often concentrated, with a specific gravity greater than 1.020. The presence of urine sediment (red blood cells [RBCs], RBC casts, tubular cells), myoglobin, or hemoglobin; a urinary sodium level lower than 40 mEq/L; and a specific gravity of 1.010 are indicative of intrarenal failure. In postrenal failure, urinary sodium levels may be normal to 40 mEq/L, with a specific gravity of 1.000 to 1.010.

RADIOGRAPHIC ASSESSMENT

X-ray studies help to determine the cause of ARF. A flat-plate x-ray film of the abdomen is obtained to determine the size of the kidneys. In the absence of underlying renal disease, normal-size kidneys are expected. Enlarged kidneys, possibly due to obstruction, may result from hydronephrosis. This x-ray finding may also illustrate obstructing calculi in the renal pelvis, ureters, or bladder.

Renal ultrasonography is a noninvasive procedure using high-energy sound waves. It is useful in the diagnosis of urinary tract obstruction. Dilation of the renal calyces and collecting ducts, as well as calculi, can be detected.

Computed tomography (CT) scans without contrast dye can be obtained to identify obstruction or tumors. Contrast media are usually avoided to prevent further renal damage. A sonogram is generally preferred to the intravenous pyelogram (IVP) to determine kidney size and the patency of the ureters.

Aortorenal angiography may be used to examine renal blood vessels and blood flow. The procedure involves the necessary risk of using contrast media but can reveal any occlusion of major renal vessels by thrombus, embolus, or stenosis. Cystoscopy or retrograde pyelography may be indicated to identify possible obstructive lesions in the urinary tract.

OTHER DIAGNOSTIC ASSESSMENT

Renal biopsy may be performed if the primary cause is uncertain, an immunologic disease is suspected, or the reversibility of the renal failure needs to be determined after ARF has persisted for an extended period. The nurse assists with many of the diagnostic studies, prepares the client before

CHART 72-2

LABORATORY PROFILE
Renal Failure

Test	Normal Range for Adults	Values in Renal Failure	Comments
TESTS TO EVALUATE REMOVAL OF NITROGENOUS WASTES			
Serum creatinine	0.6-1.1 mg/dL (women) 0.9-1.3 mg/dL (men) *Older adults:* Decreased	***In Chronic Renal Failure*** May increase by 0.5-1.0 mg/dL every 1-2 yr May be as high as 15-30 mg/dL *before* symptoms of CRF are present ***In Acute Renal Failure*** Gradual increase of 1-2 mg/dL every 24-48 hr May increase 1-6 mg/dL in 1 wk or less	Consistently elevated levels indicate decreased renal function. Serum creatinine levels are used to evaluate the effectiveness of dialysis treatments.
Blood urea nitrogen	6-20 mg/dL *Older adults:* May be slightly increased	***In Chronic Renal Failure*** May reach 180-200 mg/dL *before* symptoms develop ***In Acute Renal Failure*** Often increases by 10-20 mg/dL at same pace as serum creatinine level May reach 80-100 mg/dL within 1 wk	Increases depend on protein intake and other factors (see text). Rate of increase is controlled by limiting protein intake. This intervention is believed to decrease the rate of onset of systemic symptoms, such as anorexia, nausea, and vomiting. Elevations have multiple causes, including diminished renal function, excessive protein intake, sepsis, GI bleeding, dehydration, and tissue catabolism.
ELECTROLYTE STUDIES			
Serum sodium	136-145 mEq/L; 136-145 mmol/L (SI units)	Normal or decreased	Clients with renal failure retain sodium. With associated water retention, serum sodium levels seem normal. With excessive water retention, serum sodium levels seem decreased owing to hemodilution. Assess the client for evidence of fluid volume excess: edema, weight increase, or elevation of diastolic blood pressure. Limit fluid intake as directed. Avoid excessive sodium intake. Monitor for signs of hypernatremia: dry skin, excessive thirst, dry mucous membranes, elevated body temperature, and flushed skin. Client may need diuretics or dialysis.
Serum potassium	*Male:* 3.5-5.0 mmol/L (SI units) *Female:* 3.4-4.4 mmol/L (SI units)	Increased	Advise the client to avoid salt substitutes and to limit potassium-containing foods. Monitor for rapidly increasing serum potassium levels in ARF. ECG changes occur with serum potassium levels ≥6.5. Monitor for signs of hyperkalemia: dizziness, weakness, cardiac irregularities, muscle cramps, diarrhea, and nausea. May require administration of sodium polystyrene sulfonate (Kayexalate) or other treatment.

GI, Gastrointestinal; *ARF,* acute renal failure; *ECG,* electrocardiogram; *CRF,* chronic renal failure; *RBCs,* red blood cells; *WBCs,* white blood cells; *GFR,* glomerular filtration rate.

Continued

CHART 72-2

LABORATORY PROFILE
Renal Failure—cont'd

Test	Normal Range for Adults	Values in Renal Failure	Comments
Serum phosphorus (phosphate)	3.0-4.5 mg/dL; 0.97-1.45 mmol/L (SI units) *Older adults:* May be slightly decreased	Increased	Short-term increases have potential to cause rapid decrease in serum calcium level and cardiac rhythm disturbances. Long-term increases demineralize bones of calcium and enhance fracture potential. Phosphate-binding medications help control hyperphosphatemia and prevent calcium depletion from the bones.
Serum calcium	Total calcium: 9.0-10.5 mg/dL; 2.25-2.75 mmol/L (SI units) Ionized calcium: 4.60-5.08 mg/dL; 1.15-1.27 mmol/L (SI units) *Older adults:* Slightly decreased	Decreased	Decreases in ARF may necessitate replacement. Decreases in CRF may only be slight and may or may not necessitate replacement. As the serum phosphate level increases, the serum calcium level decreases. Chronic calcium deficiency leads to renal osteodystrophy. Control of phosphate excess is usually essential before calcium replacement is initiated. Monitor for signs and symptoms of hypocalcemia: abdominal cramps, hyperactive reflexes, tingling in fingertips, and spasms in feet and wrists (see also Chapter 13).
Serum magnesium	1.2-2.0 mEq/L; 0.66-1.07 mmol/L (SI units)	Increased	Advise the client to avoid compounds containing magnesium (e.g., laxatives).
Serum carbon dioxide combining power (bicarbonate)	23-29 mEq/L (venous); 23-29 mmol/L (SI units)	Decreased	Replace bicarbonate. Monitor respiratory rate and depth. Monitor for decreased orientation.
Arterial blood pH	7.31-7.42	Decreased (in metabolic acidosis) or normal	The respiratory system attempts to compensate by hyperventilation (increased rate and depth of respiration). Values are within the normal range if blood buffers and lungs can compensate. Monitor breathing rate and depth. Monitor level of consciousness.
Arterial blood bicarbonate (HCO_3^-)	21-28 mEq/L	Decreased	Provide replacement PO, IV, or by hemodialysis or peritoneal dialysis.
Arterial blood $PaCO_2$	*Male:* 35-48 mm Hg *Female:* 32-45 mm Hg	Decreased	Monitor for respiratory fatigue (the client breathes more rapidly and deeply to "blow off" carbon dioxide).
OTHER BLOOD STUDIES			
Hemoglobin	11.7-15.5 g/dL (women); 7.4-9.9 mmol/L (SI units) 13.2-17.3 g/dL (men); 8.7-11.2 mmol/L (SI units) *Older adults:* Slightly decreased	Decreased	Decreased levels indicate anemia. Monitor for pallor, weakness, lethargy, dizziness, possible shortness of breath, and activity intolerance.
Hematocrit	*Female:* 35%-45% *Male:* 39%-49% *Older adults:* May be slightly decreased	Decreased to 20%	Same as for hemoglobin. With erythropoietin therapy, may be able to obtain levels as high as 36%.

GI, Gastrointestinal; *ARF,* acute renal failure; *ECG,* electrocardiogram; *CRF,* chronic renal failure; *RBCs,* red blood cells; *WBCs,* white blood cells; *GFR,* glomerular filtration rate.

CHART 72-2

LABORATORY PROFILE
Renal Failure—cont'd

Test	Normal Range for Adults	Values in Renal Failure	Comments
URINALYSIS*			
Specific gravity	Usually 1.016-1.022; possible range: 1.001-1.035	Usually decreased and fixed	Reflects inability of the tubules to produce a concentrated or diluted urine in response to changes in plasma osmolality. Monitor for fluid volume deficit or excess.
pH	Average: 5.5-6; possible range: 4.5-8	May be fixed; pH does not change with dietary changes	Collect a freshly voided specimen for testing
Glucose	None or <15 mg/dL Usually detectable in urine of nondiabetic clients when blood level is 160-180 mg/dL	Increased	The renal threshold is often increased; therefore the blood glucose level may be >160-180 mg/dL before glucose is detectable in the urine. Monitor *blood* glucose levels.
Protein	2-8 mg/dL	Increased when there is glomerular damage or disease	Increases may be an incidental and benign finding. Transient increases occur with extreme exercise, fever, stress, or infection. Persistent proteinuria requires 24-hr collection for determination of total quantity excreted. Persistent proteinuria may indicate a serious renal problem. Instruct the client about the need for follow-up. Instruct the client in the correct procedure for collection of 24-hr specimen (see Chapter 69).
Occult blood	No RBCs or occasionally 2 or 3 RBCs per high-power field No hemoglobin	More than 2 or 3 RBCs per high-power field Detectable hemoglobin	Hemoglobin is detectable when hemolysis of RBCs has occurred. Intact RBCs are only detectable with microscopic examination. Collect a freshly voided specimen for testing.
WBCs	0-5 per high-power field	Increased in urinary tract infection	Often indicates need for urine culture.
Bacteria	Less than 1000 colonies/mL	Increased in the presence of infection, with or without an increase in WBCs	Obtain urine culture.
Casts	None or a few; composed of RBCs, WBCs, protein, or tubular cell casts such as hyaline	Casts present	Casts may be a benign occurrence or may signify that some renal injury or disease is present. Collect a freshly voided specimen for direct microscopic examination.
Creatinine clearance	97-137 mL/min (men) 88-128 mL/min (women) *Older adults:* Progressively decreased with advancing age	Decreased	Change reflects decreases in GFR. Creatinine clearance is determined from a 24-hr urine collection and a serum creatinine value.

GI, Gastrointestinal; *ARF,* acute renal failure; *ECG,* electrocardiogram; *CRF,* chronic renal failure; *RBCs,* red blood cells; *WBCs,* white blood cells; *GFR,* glomerular filtration rate.
*Urine may become cloudy with heavy sediment. Urine output and appearance vary, depending on remaining renal function.

TABLE 72-5 • EFFECTS OF RENAL FAILURE ON ELECTROLYTE BALANCE

Electrolyte	Effects of Renal Failure	Problems	Treatments
Potassium	Retained with oliguria	Hyperkalemia Cardiac dysrhythmias Asystole	Kayexalate, PO or rectal Regular IV insulin with 5% to 50% dextrose IV calcium gluconate Dialysis
Sodium	Retained	Dilutional hyponatremia Fluid volume excess Hypertension Congestive heart failure Pulmonary edema	Diuretics until no longer responsive Dialysis Fluid restriction Sodium restriction
Phosphate	Retained	Hyperphosphatemia Metastatic calcium phosphate deposits Renal bone disease	Phosphate-binding agents Limit phosphorus intake Vitamin D analogs
Calcium	Decreased gastrointestinal absorption Binds to phosphate	Bone demineralization Pathologic fractures	Replace vitamin D Calcium supplements
Hydrogen	Retained	Binds with bicarbonate for excretion through respiratory compensation	Dialysis Bicarbonate supplements
Bicarbonate	Depleted	Used for blood buffering to prevent metabolic acidemia	Dialysis Bicarbonate supplements
Magnesium	Retained	Potential for hypermagnesemia	Avoid magnesium-containing antacids and laxatives

the test, and provides follow-up care. The nurse must be aware of all test results and understand how they may affect the treatment regimen. (See Chapter 69 for a detailed discussion of renal diagnostic tests.)

Interventions

The primary nursing diagnosis and collaborative problems for the client with acute renal failure (ARF) are Excess Fluid Volume, Potential for Pulmonary Edema, and Potential for Electrolyte Imbalances. The client with ARF may pass from the oliguric phase (in which fluid and electrolytes are retained) to the diuretic phase. If the client moves to the diuretic phase, hypovolemia and electrolyte *loss* are the primary problems. As a result, the client in the diuretic phase of ARF needs a plan of care that focuses on fluid and electrolyte *replacement* and monitoring.

These examples of output variation reflect the continually changing nature of ARF and the need for the plan of care to be constantly updated to reflect the client's movement through the stages of the disease process. Drug therapy, diet therapy, and renal replacement therapy (peritoneal dialysis [PD], hemodialysis [HD], or hemofiltration) are commonly employed in the management of ARF.

DRUG THERAPY. Clients with ARF receive numerous medications. As kidney function changes, the physician often modifies drug doses. The nurse is knowledgeable about the site of drug metabolism and is especially careful when administering medications. The nurse constantly monitors for possible side effects and interactions of the drugs the client with ARF is receiving (Chart 72-3; see also Drug Therapy under Chronic Renal Failure, p. 1685). Diuretics may be used to increase urine output.

In clients with prerenal azotemia, fluid challenges and diuretics are often used to promote renal perfusion. In clients without signs and symptoms of fluid volume excess, 500 to 1000 mL of normal saline may be infused over a 1-hour period. In prerenal azotemia, the client should respond to the fluid challenge by producing urine soon after the initial bolus. Diuretics such as furosemide (Lasix) may also be ordered in conjunction with a fluid bolus. If oliguric renal failure is diagnosed, the fluid challenges and diuretics are discontinued. The physician may prescribe low-dose (1 to 3 μg/kg) dopamine in a continuous infusion to enhance renal perfusion and/or increase blood pressure (Zellner, 1999) (Chart 72-4). These clients often require central venous pressure (CVP) monitoring or measurement of pulmonary arterial pressure by means of a Swan-Ganz catheter for a more exact evaluation of their hemodynamic status. They also require constant nursing supervision for assessment of the response to fluid and drug administration. The nurse carefully monitors for signs of possible fluid overload.

Calcium channel blockers may be used to treat ARF resulting from nephrotoxic acute tubular necrosis (ATN) by preventing the influx of calcium into the kidney cells, thereby maintaining cell integrity and improving the glomerular filtration rate (GFR).

DIET THERAPY. Clients who have ARF often have a high rate of catabolism. The exact mechanism for this state is not well understood. Increases in catabolism may be related to the stress of a critical illness, causing an increase in levels of circulating catecholamines, cortisol, and glucagon, all of which stimulate catabolism. The rate of catabolism is correlated with the severity of uremia and azotemia. This hypercatabolic state causes the breakdown of muscle for protein, which leads to an increase in azotemia and an even more elevated serum blood urea nitrogen (BUN) level.

If the client with ARF has an adequate dietary intake (see Imbalanced Nutrition: Less Than Body Requirements [Chronic Renal Failure] , p. 1682), nutritional support may

CHART 72-3

DRUG THERAPY *for* Renal Failure

Drug	Usual Dosage	Indications	Nursing Interventions	Rationale
CARDIOTONICS				
Digoxin (Lanoxin, Novodigoxin♣)	0.125-0.25 mg PO or IV daily or every other day *Older adults:* 0.0625-0.125 PO or IV daily or every other day	Decreased stroke volume Decreased strength of cardiac contractions	Monitor for signs of digoxin toxicity and hypokalemia.	Digoxin remains in the body longer when renal function is impaired.
			Monitor for bradycardia (pulse <50-60 beats/min).	Bradycardia is a sign of digoxin toxicity.
			Monitor serum drug levels.	A toxic digoxin level is >2.5 ng/mL.
VITAMINS AND MINERALS				
Folic acid (vitamin B_9, Folvite, Novofolacid♣)	0.1 mg PO, SC, or IM daily	Dietary supplement	Usually given after dialysis.	Water-soluble vitamins are removed during dialysis.
Ferrous sulfate (Feosol, Novoferrosulfa♣)	325 mg tid or qid PO	Anemia	Monitor for constipation.	Constipation is a frequent and uncomfortable side effect associated with oral iron supplements.
			Note any change in the stools, which normally become blackish green.	The color is caused by the presence of unabsorbed iron and is harmless.
BIOLOGIC RESPONSE MODIFIERS				
Erythropoietin alpha (Epogen, Procrit)	50-100 units/kg IV or SC 3 times/wk	Anemia associated with CRF	Monitor hematocrit twice weekly until maintenance dose is achieved.	The dose is based on response as measured by hematocrit changes.
			Monitor blood pressure.	Rapid rise in hematocrit can cause hypertension.
PHOSPHATE BINDERS				
Aluminum hydroxide gel (Amphojel, AlternaGEL, Alu-Cap, Nephrox) Aluminum carbonate gel (Basaljel)	500 mg-2 g bid-qid PO as tablets, capsules, or oral suspension	Phosphate binder Prevention of renal osteodystrophy	Monitor for constipation, which occurs frequently.	Constipation is a frequent side effect of many drugs that bind phosphorus.
			Monitor for signs of hypophosphatemia.	These drugs can prevent intestinal absorption of phosphorus to the extent that the client develops hypophosphatemia.
			Monitor serum aluminum levels.	Aluminum toxicity may cause bone disease and dementia.
Sevelamer hydrochloride (Renagel)	Serum phosphorus 6.0-7.5 mg/dL; 2 capsules tid Serum phosphorus 7.6-8.9 mg/dL; 3 capsules tid Serum phosphorus >9.0 mg/dL; 4 capsules tid	Hyperphosphatemia	Give with meals	Drug binds with phosphorus in food, preventing absorption.
			Tell client to swallow capsule whole; do not chew.	Drug expands when capsule is broken.
			Monitor serum phosphorus levels.	Drug can cause hypophosphatemia.
Calcium carbonate (Tums, OsCal, CalciChew)	1-3 PO daily in divided doses tid or qid	Dietary supplement Phosphate binder	Give only when serum phosphate levels are normal. Monitor for hypercalcemia, constipation, and soft-tissue calcifications	Calcium supplements may cause a *decrease* in serum phosphate levels because these two minerals exist in blood in a balanced, *reciprocal* relationship.
			Give after meals.	Giving binders after meals enhances binding capacity.
STOOL SOFTENERS AND LAXATIVES				
Docusate sodium (Colace) Bisacodyl (Dulcolax, Bisco-Lax, Laxit♣)	100-300 mg daily 5-10 mg PO or PR daily or every other day	Prevention of constipation caused by limited fluid intake, iron supplements, and phosphate binders	Observe for abdominal cramps and diarrhea.	These gastrointestinal effects indicate drug overdose.
			Monitor bowel movements.	Monitoring bowel movements is a way of determining medication effectiveness.

CHART 72-4

BEST PRACTICE *for* Administering Renal-Dose Dopamine

- Take an accurate weight because the dose is ordered according to the client's weight.
- Know the hospital's policy regarding who is responsible for calculating the rate of infusion (i.e., physician, pharmacist, or nurse). Renal-dose dopamine is 1 to 5 μg/kg body wt/min but is converted to mL/min for an IV infusion.
- Before hanging the dopamine infusion, double-check the amount of dopamine added to the solution, the total volume of solution (usually 250 mL), and the calculation milliliters per minute.
- Do not hang the dopamine infusion until all questions about the calculation are clarified.
- If dopamine is to be infused into a peripheral vein, be sure that the line is intact and secured.
- Once the infusion is started, check the client's blood pressure and pulse per hospital policy or the physician's orders, usually at least every 2 hours.
- Notify the physician of changes in vital signs per policy or the physician's orders.
- Monitor the IV site frequently for clinical manifestations of infiltration.
- If infiltration occurs, stop the infusion but do not discontinue the IV catheter. Prepare for phentolamine (Regitine, Rogitine♣) administration through the IV catheter and subcutaneously into the infiltrated tissue.

not be necessary. The health care provider may order a consultation with a dietitian, who will calculate the client's caloric requirements. In conjunction with the dietitian, the health care provider will order a diet with specific levels of protein and sodium and the amount of fluids required. If the client does not require dialysis, 0.6 g/kg of body weight or 40 g/day of protein is ordered. For clients needing dialysis, the protein level needed will range from 1 to 1.5 g/kg. The amount of dietary sodium ranges from 60 to 90 mEq. In the presence of hyperkalemia, dietary potassium is restricted to 60 to 70 mEq. The amount of fluid permitted is generally calculated to equal the urine volume plus 500 mL. The nurse continually assesses oral intake to make certain that sufficient calories are consumed.

Many clients with ARF are too ill or too anorexic to eat sufficient food. For these clients, some form of nutritional support (e.g., total parenteral nutrition [TPN] or hyperalimentation) must be initiated to avoid catabolism. The goals of nutritional support in ARF are to provide sufficient nutrients to maintain or improve nutritional status, to preserve lean body mass, to restore or maintain fluid balance, and to preserve renal function.

If TPN is administered, the solutions may be formulated to meet the client's specific needs. Because kidney function is unstable in ARF, the nurse constantly monitors the serum electrolyte concentrations and facilitates revisions in the hyperalimentation solution as needed. In addition to TPN, intravenous (IV) fat emulsion (Intralipid) infusions provide a nonprotein source of calories. In uremic clients, fat emulsions can be used in place of glucose to avoid the problems associated with excessive sugars.

DIALYSIS THERAPIES. Hemodialysis (HD) and peritoneal dialysis (PD) may be implemented for clients with ARF if necessary. Until recently, intermittent hemodialysis (IHD) has been the most common treatment of ARF. The following are indications for dialysis in ARF:

- Uremia
- Persistent hyperkalemia
- Uncompensated metabolic acidosis
- Fluid volume excess unresponsive to diuretics
- Uremic pericarditis
- Uremic encephalopathy

Immediate vascular access for HD in clients with ARF is established by placement of a dual- or triple-lumen catheter specifically designed for HD. For HD that is expected to be necessary for several weeks, the catheter is usually placed into the subclavian or internal jugular vein. If only one or two treatments are expected to be necessary, as for removal of drugs or toxins by hemoperfusion, a femoral site may be selected. Longer use of the femoral site is generally discouraged because of positioning limitations (i.e., required immobility) and other potential complications, such as hematomas and infection. Repeated cannulation of the femoral site also increases the risk for hematoma formation and makes repeated use of the vein impossible.

The subclavian vein is often preferred over femoral vein cannulation because the catheter can be left in place between dialysis treatments. This placement is also a disadvantage, however, because the longer the catheter is left in place, the greater is the chance for infection. The subclavian dialysis catheter (Figure 72-1) is inserted at the bedside. A physician performs the sterile procedure, and then the catheter is covered with a sterile dressing. Catheter placement is checked by chest x-ray examination before its use.

HD catheters have two lumens separating the outflow and inflow extensions of the catheter. Consequently, the continuous outflow of blood to be dialyzed is separated from the dialyzed blood returned through the inflow port and lumen. A triple-lumen catheter for HD is now available. The third lumen provides a port for drawing venous blood or administering medication and fluid without interruption of the dialysis lumens.

PD may also be used in the treatment of ARF, but its use may be limited in the critically ill, since mechanically ventilated clients may not be able to tolerate the accompanying abdominal distention, and since its use requires an intact, uninfected abdominal cavity (Giuliano & Pysznik, 1998). PD uses the peritoneum as a semipermeable membrane for which dialysate is infused through a catheter implanted in the peritoneum. A more complete discussion of PD is provided later in this chapter under Chronic Renal Failure, pp. 1694-1697).

CONTINUOUS RENAL REPLACEMENT THERAPIES. Currently, continuous renal replacement therapies (CRRTs) have become the standard treatment for ARF. Renal replacement therapies in the form of hemofiltration may be better tolerated than HD for clients who are critically ill, since rapid shifts of fluids and electrolytes associated with HD are avoided (Giuliano & Pysznik, 1998).

Continuous arteriovenous hemofiltration (CAVH) and continuous arteriovenous hemodialysis and filtration (CAVHD) provide additional renal replacement therapies for clients with ARF. These procedures share some similarities with HD, but their use and indications are specific and limited.

CAVH is indicated for clients who are fluid volume overloaded, resistant to diuretics, and hemodynamically unstable. The implementation of CAVH requires the placement of both arterial and venous catheters to provide adequate filtration

A

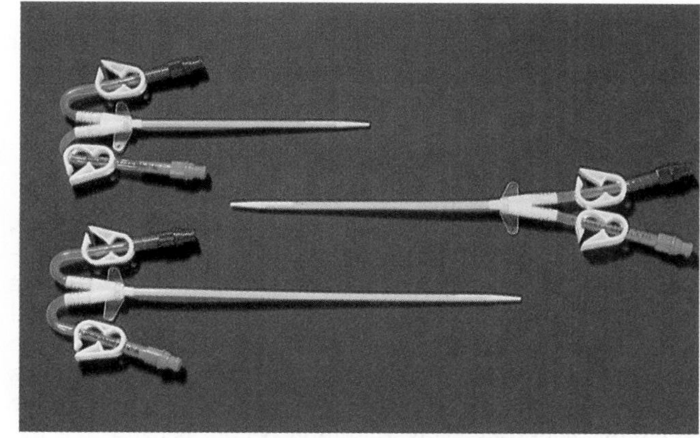

B

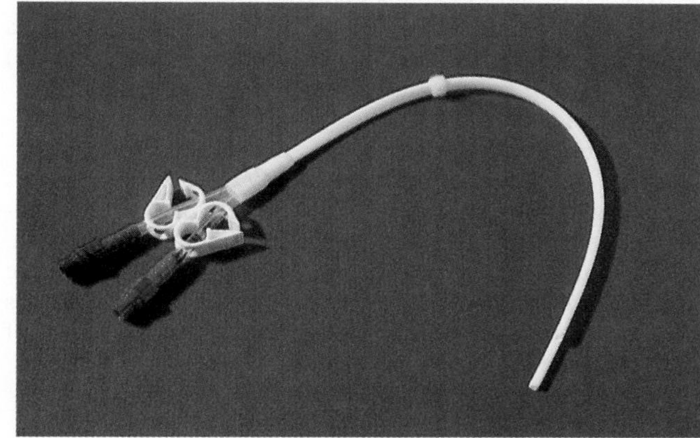

Figure 72-1 ● Subclavian dialysis catheters. These catheters are radiopaque tubes that can be used for hemodialysis access. The Y-shaped tubing allows arterial outflow and venous return through a single catheter. **A,** Mahurkar catheters, made of polyurethane and used for short-term access. **B,** A PermCath catheter, made of silicone and used for long-term access. (Courtesy Kendall Company, Bothell, WA.)

and a mean arterial pressure of at least 60 mm Hg. CAVH removes large amounts of plasma water and solutes on a continuous basis. When large volumes of plasma water are removed, electrolytes are also removed. Electrolytes are replaced through prescribed amounts of IV electrolyte solution. The most significant disadvantage of arteriovenous (AV) filtration is the risk of bleeding associated with anticoagulants used to prevent membrane clotting (Craig, 1998).

A double-lumen dialysis catheter inserted into a large vein (subclavian, jugular) provides access for CAVHD. CAVHD uses a **dialysate** (a solution composed of water, glucose, sodium chloride, potassium, magnesium, calcium, and bicarbonate) delivery system to remove nitrogenous or other waste products in addition to fluid in clients with limited cardiac output, those with significant hypotension, or those who have been unresponsive to diuretic therapy. The conventional form of HD would not be tolerated, and PD would probably be inadequate for the fluid removal required.

Continuous venovenous hemofiltration (CVVH) is often considered to be the treatment of choice for critically ill clients. CVVH requires only a double-lumen venous catheter for access and is powered by a pump, making the rate of filtration more reliable than that of the mean arterial pressure (Giuliano & Pysznik, 1998). There is a risk of air embolus associated with the pump, but most pumps are equipped with alarms that detect air. These systems also require the use of anticoagulants, but at lower doses than needed for AV systems. These procedures are performed in a critical care unit, and clients require continuous nursing care.

POSTHOSPITAL CARE. The posthospital care for a client with ARF varies widely, depending on the status of the disease when the client is discharged. The course of ARF varies, with recovery lasting up to several months. If the renal failure is resolving, follow-up care is often provided by a nephrologist or by the family physician in consultation with the nephrologist. On occasion, however, ARF results in permanent renal damage and the need for chronic dialysis or even transplantation. In these cases, the posthospital care may be as extensive and multifaceted as it is for any other client with chronic renal failure (CRF) (see Community-Based Care [Chronic Renal Failure], p. 1700).

If the ARF is in the process of resolving, the follow-up care may involve a variety of services. Frequent medical visits are necessary, as are routine laboratory blood and urine tests to monitor renal function. Consultation with a dietitian may be needed to modify the client's diet according to the degree of renal function and ongoing nutritional requirements. Clients continuing dialysis after discharge must be taught to limit foods high in potassium and sodium and to observe protein restrictions. In addition, education concerning the need for limited fluid intake may be necessary.

Some clients may need some form of temporary dialysis until their kidneys can metabolize fluid and waste products independently. The dialysis begun while the client was hospitalized may be continued at an outpatient dialysis center for as long as necessary. Teaching concerning the type of dialysis, care of vascular access sites, dietary restrictions, fluid restrictions, and prevention of complications is ongoing throughout the recovery phase. Depending on their level of independence and family support, some clients may also need home care nursing or social work assistance.

CHRONIC RENAL FAILURE

OVERVIEW

In contrast to the ability of the kidneys to regain function following acute renal failure (ARF), chronic renal failure (CRF) represents a clinical syndrome of progressive, irreversible kidney injury. When kidney function is inadequate for sustaining life, CRF is referred to as end-stage renal disease (ESRD). Terms associated with renal failure include **azotemia** (accumulation of nitrogenous waste products in the bloodstream), **uremia** (azotemia with clinical symptoms [Chart 72-5]), **uremic syndrome** (the diverse systemic clinical and laboratory manifestations associated with ESRD), and *renal replacement therapy* (hemodialysis [HD], peritoneal dialysis [PD], renal transplantation; necessary to sustain life in clients with renal failure). ARF and CRF are compared in Table 72-1.

Pathophysiology

STAGES OF RENAL FAILURE

The kidneys tend to fail in an organized fashion. The client's progression toward ESRD usually begins with a gradual decrease in renal function of 30% to 50% (Table 72-6). Initially,

CHART 72-5

KEY FEATURES *of* Uremia

- Metallic taste in the mouth
- Anorexia
- Nausea
- Vomiting
- Muscle cramps
- Itching
- Fatigue and lethargy
- Hiccups
- Edema
- Dyspnea
- Muscle cramps
- Paresthesias

TABLE 72-6 • PROGRESSION TOWARD CHRONIC RENAL FAILURE

STAGE I: DIMINISHED RENAL RESERVE
- Renal function is reduced, but no accumulation of metabolic wastes occurs.
- The healthier kidney compensates for the diseased kidney.
- Ability to concentrate urine is decreased, resulting in nocturia and polyuria.
- A 24-hour urine collection for creatinine clearance is necessary to detect that renal reserve is less than normal.

STAGE II: RENAL INSUFFICIENCY
- Metabolic wastes begin to accumulate in the blood because the unaffected nephrons can no longer compensate.
- Responsiveness to diuretics is decreased, resulting in oliguria and edema.
- The degree of insufficiency is determined by decreasing the GFR and is classified as mild, moderate, or severe.
- Treatment is medical.

STAGE III: END-STAGE RENAL DISEASE
- Excessive amounts of metabolic wastes such as urea and creatinine accumulate in the blood.
- The kidneys are unable to maintain homeostasis.
- Treatment is by dialysis or other renal replacement therapy.

GFR, Glomerular filtration rate.

there is a *diminished renal reserve.* A 24-hour urine specimen for monitoring creatinine clearance is necessary to detect that renal reserve is less than normal. In this stage, reduced renal function occurs without any measurable accumulation of metabolic wastes in the serum because of the ability of the unaffected nephrons to compensate for the decreased functioning of the diseased nephrons. Renal damage is accompanied by an elevation in the systemic blood pressure, resulting in an increase in the pressure within the glomerular apparatus and the remaining unaffected nephrons. Eventually, the unaffected nephrons may be damaged by long-term exposure to this increased pressure, leading to the progressive renal damage characteristic of CRF. However, under stressful conditions, such as infection, fluid overload, or dehydration, renal function at this stage can appear compromised.

In the next stage, *renal insufficiency,* metabolic wastes begin to accumulate in the blood because the healthier kidney tissue can no longer compensate for the loss of nonfunctioning nephrons. Levels of blood urea nitrogen (BUN), serum creatinine, uric acid, and phosphorus are increasingly elevated in relation to the degree of renal function loss. Careful nursing and medical management of fluid volume, blood pressure, electrolytes, dietary intake, and medication administration may slow the progression of renal failure.

Many clients ultimately progress to *end-stage renal disease (ESRD).* Excessive amounts of nitrogenous wastes, such as urea and creatinine, accumulate in the blood, and the kidneys cannot maintain homeostasis. Initially, severe fluid overload and electrolyte and acid-base imbalances occur. Without renal replacement therapy, fatal complications are likely.

PATHOLOGIC ALTERATIONS

Renal dysfunction causes multiple pathologic situations, including disruptions in the glomerular filtration rate (GFR), abnormalities of urine production and water excretion, electrolyte imbalances, and metabolic abnormalities. The kidneys can maintain an effective GFR until 70% to 80% of renal function is lost. Homeostasis is maintained until late in the course of renal failure. When less than 20% of the nephrons are functional, the GFR is altered despite hypertrophy of the remaining nephrons. This alteration occurs because the hypertrophied nephrons can maintain the excretion of solutes or waste products only by decreasing water reabsorption. As a result, **hyposthenuria** (the loss of urine concentrating ability) and *polyuria* (increased urine output) occur. Both hyposthenuria and polyuria are early signs of CRF and, if the problem is untreated at this stage, can cause severe dehydration.

As the disease progresses, the ability to dilute the urine is increasingly diminished, resulting in urine with a fixed osmolality **(isosthenuria).** As renal function continues to diminish, the concentration of urea is increased in the blood, and urine output decreases. When renal function deteriorates to this level, the client is at risk for fluid overload because of loss of adequate urine output.

METABOLIC ALTERATIONS

UREA AND CREATININE. Renal failure also causes disturbances in urea and creatinine excretion. Creatinine is derived from creatine and phosphocreatine, which are present in skeletal muscle. The normal rate of creatinine excretion depends on muscle mass, physical activity, and diet. Without major alterations in the diet or physical activity, the serum creatinine level remains relatively constant. Creatinine is partially excreted by the renal tubules, and a decrease in renal function leads to a buildup of serum creatinine. Urea is the primary product of protein metabolism and is excreted by the kidneys. The BUN level normally varies directly with protein intake.

An important method for accurately estimating the GFR is to monitor the creatinine clearance of the kidneys. As renal function and glomerular filtration diminish, creatinine clearance decreases and the serum creatinine level rises (see Chapter 69).

SODIUM. In addition to decreased BUN and creatinine excretion, alterations in sodium excretion are common. Early in chronic renal failure (CRF), the client is particularly susceptible to hyponatremia (sodium depletion) because, although a diminishing number of nephrons are reabsorbing sodium at their maximal ability, there is an obligatory loss of sodium in urine production. Thus the polyuria often seen in early renal failure also causes sodium depletion.

In the later stages of renal failure, the capacity of the kidneys to excrete sodium diminishes as urine production decreases. As a result, sodium retention can occur with only modest increases in dietary sodium intake and can lead to severe fluid and electrolyte imbalances (see Chapters 12 and 13). Sodium retention manifests as hypertension and edema.

Despite the sodium retention, the concurrent retention of water results in an *apparently* normal serum sodium level; dilutional hyponatremia is likely, since fluid volume excess develops (see Table 72-5).

POTASSIUM. The kidney is the primary organ responsible for potassium excretion. Any increase in potassium load during the later stages of renal disease can lead to hyperkalemia (excessive potassium retention). Normal serum potassium levels of 3.5 to 5 mEq/L are maintained until the 24-hour urine output falls below 500 mL with a decreased GFR. When hyperkalemia develops, serum levels are quickly elevated and may be 7 to 8 mEq/L or higher. Severe electrocardiographic (ECG) changes result from this elevation, increasing the risk of fatal dysrhythmias. Other factors contributing to hyperkalemia in renal failure include ingestion of potassium in medications, failure to restrict potassium in the diet, excessive tissue breakdown secondary to the hypercatabolic state, blood transfusions, and excessive bleeding or hemorrhage. (See Chapter 13 for further discussion of hyperkalemia.)

ACID-BASE BALANCE. In the early stages of renal disease, loss of functioning nephrons causes little change in blood pH because the remaining nephrons increase their rate of acid excretion. As the loss of nephrons continues, the kidneys cannot compensate and acid excretion is restricted; a *bicarbonate deficit* or *metabolic acidosis* results (see Chapter 16).

Many factors contribute to metabolic acidosis in renal failure. First, the kidney becomes unable to excrete excessive hydrogen ions. Normally, renal tubular cells secrete hydrogen ions into the tubular lumen for excretion, but ammonia and bicarbonate are required in order for excretion to take place. In clients with renal failure, the kidney's ability to produce ammonia is decreased, and the normal reabsorption of filtered bicarbonate does not occur. This process leads to a buildup of hydrogen ions for which the supply of bicarbonate and other buffering bases is inadequate. As a result, there is a base (bicarbonate) deficit in an environment with excess acid. In the presence of hyperkalemia, renal ammonium production and excretion are inhibited further.

As renal failure advances and acid retention increases, respiratory compensation is essential for maintenance of a blood pH compatible with life. The respiratory system compensates for the decreased pH by increasing the rate and depth of breathing to excrete carbon dioxide through the lungs. This pattern of breathing, called **Kussmaul respiration,** is increasingly apparent when worsening renal failure results in respiratory alkalosis. Serum bicarbonate measures the extent of metabolic acidosis (bicarbonate deficit). Individuals with CRF usually require treatment with alkali replacement to counteract acidosis.

CALCIUM AND PHOSPHATE. A complex, balanced reciprocal relationship between calcium and phosphate is influenced by vitamin D (see Chapter 13). Vitamin D facilitates calcium absorption in the intestines, and the kidney produces 1,25-dihydroxycholecalciferol, a hormone needed to create active vitamin D.

In renal failure, phosphate retention and a deficiency of active vitamin D contribute to the disruption in calcium and phosphate balance and metabolism. Normally, excessive dietary phosphate is excreted by the kidneys in the urine.

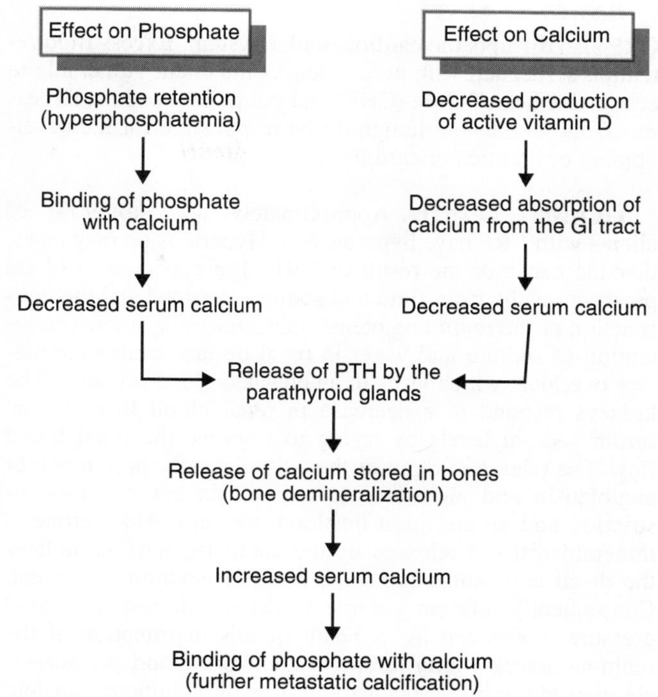

Figure 72-2 ● The effects of renal failure on phosphate and calcium balance. (*GI,* Gastrointestinal; *PTH,* parathyroid hormone.)

Parathyroid hormone (PTH) regulates the amount of phosphate in the blood by causing tubular excretion of phosphate when there is a serum phosphate excess. One of the initial effects of decreased renal function is decreased phosphate excretion due to a diminished GFR (Figure 72-2). As plasma phosphate levels increase (causing hyperphosphatemia), calcium levels decrease (causing hypocalcemia). Chronic hypocalcemia results in chronic stimulation, hyperplasia, and hypertrophy of the parathyroid glands. Under the influence of additional PTH, calcium is released from storage areas in bones **(bone resorption),** which results in demineralization. The additional calcium is needed to compensate, or balance, excess plasma phosphate concentration. The problem of hypocalcemia is compounded because decreased renal function also causes decreased production of active vitamin D. Thus less calcium is absorbed through the intestinal mucosa in the absence of sufficient vitamin D.

The pathologic process in bone metabolism and structure caused by hypocalcemia and hyperphosphatemia is called **renal osteodystrophy.** Skeletal demineralization resulting from hyperparathyroidism may be manifested as bone pain, sclerosis of the spine, pseudofractures, demineralization of parts of the skull, osteomalacia, resorption of bone, or loss of the lamina dura in the teeth.

Metastatic calcifications, crystals formed from excessive calcium phosphate, may precipitate in various parts of the body. When the plasma concentration of the calcium-phosphate product (serum calcium concentration times serum phosphate concentration) exceeds 70 mg/dL, the crystals may lodge in the kidneys, heart, lungs, major blood vessels, joints, eyes (causing conjunctivitis), and brain. Uremic pruritus is also believed to be the result of calcium-phosphate imbalances and excess PTH production.

CARDIAC ALTERATIONS

CRF also disrupts the cardiovascular system. Excess fluid retention associated with uremia leaves the client vulnerable to congestive heart failure (CHF) and pulmonary edema. Excess metabolic toxins are thought to be responsible for the development of uremic pericarditis.

HYPERTENSION. Approximately 80% to 90% of clients with CRF have hypertension. Hypertension may be either the cause or the result of CRF. The elevation in blood pressure results from fluid and sodium overload and the malfunction of the renin-angiotensin-aldosterone system. The retention of sodium and water in renal disease causes circulatory overload, which leads to an elevated blood pressure. The kidneys respond to a decrease in renal blood flow or low serum sodium levels by trying to improve the renal blood flow. The release of renin further stimulates the production of angiotensin and aldosterone. Angiotensin causes vasoconstriction and an elevation in blood pressure. Aldosterone, a mineralocorticoid released by the adrenal glands, stimulates the distal convoluted tubule to reabsorb sodium and water. Consequently, plasma volume is expanded, and the blood pressure is elevated. As a result of this malfunction of the renin-angiotensin-aldosterone system, the blood pressure is elevated either by vasoconstriction or by volume expansion. The kidneys do not recognize the increase in blood pressure and continue to produce renin. The result is severe hypertension that is difficult to treat and that ultimately worsens renal function. Many clients with CRF also have cardiomyopathy and left ventricular hypertrophy as a consequence of prolonged hypertension.

HYPERLIPIDEMIA. CRF is associated with alterations in the metabolism of lipoproteins. Increased triglyceride, total cholesterol, and low-density lipoprotein levels are seen with a corresponding reduction in high-density lipoprotein levels. CRF renders individuals at increased risk for coronary artery disease and acute cardiac events.

CONGESTIVE HEART FAILURE. Many clients with renal failure have some form of myocardial dysfunction. CRF causes an increased workload on the heart because of anemia, hypertension, and fluid overload. Left ventricular hypertrophy and CHF are common manifestations of late end-stage renal disease (ESRD). Uremia itself may cause uremic cardiomyopathy, the uremic toxin effect on the myocardium. CHF is also common in these clients because of the presence of hypertension and coronary artery disease. Cardiac disease is the leading cause of death in clients with ESRD (U.S. Renal Data Systems, 1999).

UREMIC PERICARDITIS. Pericarditis also occurs in clients with CRF. If it is not treated effectively, this inflammation of the pericardium can lead to pericardial effusion, cardiac tamponade, and death. The pericardial sac becomes inflamed and irritated by uremic toxins or infection. Signs and symptoms include localized, severe chest pain, an increased pulse rate, a low-grade fever, and an intermittent and transient pericardial friction rub that can be heard on auscultation.

As the pericarditis continues and the pericardial effusion worsens, dysrhythmias may develop; heart tones become softer and less audible, the blood pressure decreases, and the client may experience shortness of breath. Progressive pericardial effusion results in cardiac tamponade, a medical and surgical emergency in which pulse pressure diminishes and bradycardia or asystole results. Treatment of pericardial tamponade involves removal of pericardial fluid by placement of a needle, catheter, or drainage tube into the pericardium or pericardiectomy with pericardial drainage. The incidence of uremic pericarditis has diminished with the initiation of early, aggressive dialysis.

HEMATOLOGIC ALTERATIONS

Anemia is the primary hematologic abnormality in clients with CRF. Normochromic, normocytic anemia is a common manifestation of CRF and contributes to the client's symptoms. The causes include a decreased erythropoietin level with resulting decreased red blood cell (RBC) production, decreased RBC survival time resulting from uremia, iron and folic acid deficiencies, and impaired platelet function as a result of uremic toxins.

GASTROINTESTINAL ALTERATIONS

Uremia can affect all levels of the gastrointestinal (GI) system. The normal flora of the oral cavity is altered in uremia. The mouth normally contains the enzyme urease, which hydrolyzes urea. The ammonia generated from this reaction contributes to uremic halitosis and may also cause uremic **stomatitis** (mouth inflammation).

Anorexia, nausea, vomiting, and hiccups are relatively common in clients with uremia. The specific cause of these symptoms is uncertain but may be related to increased nitrogenous waste levels (i.e., blood urea nitrogen [BUN] and creatinine levels) and metabolic acidosis.

Peptic ulcer disease is also common in clients with uremia; however, the exact cause is unclear. Uremic colitis with profound watery diarrhea or constipation may also be present in clients with uremia. Ulcerations may occur in the stomach or small or large intestine, causing erosion of blood vessels. The blood loss caused by these erosions may result in melena or, in more serious cases, may progress to hemorrhagic shock from severe GI bleeding.

Etiology

The etiology of CRF is complex (Table 72-7). There are more than 100 different disease processes that can result in progressive loss of renal function (see also Chapter 71). However, diabetes and hypertension are the most common causes of CRF.

Incidence/Prevalence

The number of clients with CRF is continually increasing. The 1999 U.S. Renal Data Systems annual report suggests that more than 307,000 people in the United States are receiving treatment for ESRD. In 1999 the reported incidence of renal disease (i.e., new clients requiring renal replacement therapy) was 79,102. There were more than 57,000 deaths in 1999 related to ESRD. Three primary causes of ESRD include diabetes mellitus (40%), hypertension (27%), and

TABLE 72-7 • SELECTED CAUSES OF CHRONIC RENAL FAILURE

MORPHOLOGIC	ETIOLOGIC
Glomerular Disease	*Infection*
• Glomerulonephritis	• Pyelonephritis
• Basement membrane disease	• Tuberculosis
• Goodpasture's syndrome	*Systemic Vascular Disease*
• Intercapillary glomerulosclerosis	• Intrarenal renovascular hypertension
Tubular Disease	• Extrarenal renovascular hypertension
• Chronic hypercalcemia	*Metabolic Renal Disease*
• Chronic potassium depletion	• Amyloidosis
• Franconi's syndrome	• Gout (hyperuricemic nephropathy)
• Heavy metal (lead) poisoning	• Diabetic nephropathy
Vascular Disease of the Kidney	• Milk-alkali syndrome
• Ischemic disease of the kidney	• Sarcoidosis
• Bilateral renal artery stenosis	*Connective Tissue Disease*
• Nephrosclerosis	• Progressive systemic sclerosis
• Hyperparathyroidism	• Systemic lupus erythematosus
Urinary Tract Disease	• Polyarteritis
• Obstructive uropathy	
Congenital Anomalies	
• Hypoplastic kidneys	
• Medullary cystic disease	
• Polycystic kidney disease	

NOTE: List is not all-inclusive.

glomerulonephritis (11%). There is a higher incidence of ESRD in men than in women (U.S. Renal Data Systems, 1999). The greatest increase in ESRD is in those 65 years of age and older. More than 221,000 people were estimated to be receiving renal replacement therapy in the United States in 1999 (U.S. Renal Data Systems, 1999). Chart 72-6 addresses prevention of renal and urinary problems.

CULTURAL CONSIDERATIONS

Significant racial differences can be observed in the incidence of ESRD. The highest incidence of ESRD is in African Americans, followed by Native Americans and Asians. Caucasians have the lowest incidence of the disease (U.S. Renal Data Systems, 1999).

➤ COLLABORATIVE MANAGEMENT

Assessment

HISTORY

When taking a history from a client with suspected chronic renal failure (CRF), the nurse focuses on the signs and symptoms of CRF. The client's age and gender are noted. The nurse obtains accurate weight and height measurements and inquires about usual weight and recent weight gain or loss. Weight gain may indicate cardiovascular overload and fluid retention caused by poorly functioning kidneys. Weight loss may be the result of anorexia associated with the uremic syndrome.

CHART 72-6

CLIENT EDUCATION GUIDE
Prevention of Renal and Urinary Problems

- Be alert to the general appearance of your urine. Note any changes in its color, clarity, or odor.
- Changes in the frequency or volume of urine passage occur with changes in fluid intake. More frequent, or infrequent, voiding not associated with changes in fluid intake may signal potential problems.
- Any discomfort or distress with the passage of urine is not normal. Pain, burning, urgency, aching, or difficulty with initiating urine flow or complete bladder emptying is of some concern.
- The kidneys need $1\frac{1}{2}$ to 2 quarts of fluid a day to flush out your body wastes. Water is the ideal flushing agent.
- Changes in kidney function are often silent for many years. Periodically ask your health care provider to measure your kidney function with a blood test (serum creatinine) and a urinalysis.
- If you have a history of renal disease, diabetes mellitus, or hypertension (high blood pressure), or a family history of kidney disease, you should know your serum creatinine level and your 24-hour creatinine clearance. At least one checkup per year that includes laboratory blood and urine testing of kidney function is recommended.
- If you are identified as having decreased kidney function, ask about whether any prescribed medication, diet, diagnostic test, or therapeutic procedure will present a risk to your current kidney function. Check out all nonprescription medications with your physician or pharmacist before using them.

The nurse also obtains a complete history of known renal or urologic disorders, long-term health problems, medication use, and current health conditions. The client is asked about knowledge of any existing renal disease or family history of renal disease, which might indicate a hereditary disorder. A history of kidney infection or renal calculi could imply past kidney damage. It is important to explore long-term health problems because illnesses such as hypertension, diabetes, systemic lupus erythematosus, arthritis, cancer, and tuberculosis can contribute to decreased renal function.

The nurse documents use of both prescription and over-the-counter medications because many medications are potentially nephrotoxic and can cause renal damage.

The nurse examines the client's dietary or nutritional habits and discusses any present GI problems. A change in the taste of foods often accompanies renal failure. Clients may note that sweet foods are not as appealing or that certain foods, especially meats, leave a metallic taste in the mouth. The client is asked specifically about a history of GI problems, such as nausea, vomiting, anorexia, hiccups, diarrhea, or constipation. Any of these manifestations can be the result of the buildup of nitrogenous or other metabolic wastes that the body cannot excrete because of renal malfunction.

The nurse questions the client about his or her current energy level and any recent injuries or bleeding. Changes in the client's daily routine are explored as a possible *result* of physical fatigue. Weakness, drowsiness, and shortness of breath are typical and suggest impending pulmonary edema or neurologic degeneration. The nurse asks specifically about abnormal bruising or bleeding, which may be the result of hematologic changes associated with uremia.

The nurse discusses the client's urinary elimination in detail, including frequency of urination, appearance of the urine, and any difficulty starting or controlling urination. This information can help identify existing urologic disorders that may influence the preservation of existing renal function.

PHYSICAL ASSESSMENT/CLINICAL MANIFESTATIONS

Chronic renal failure (CRF) results in many multisystem manifestations (Chart 72-7). Clinical manifestations of CRF or uremia are associated with changes in fluid volume and chemical composition. The specific causes of many of these manifestations are not known.

NEUROLOGIC MANIFESTATIONS. Neurologic manifestations of the uremic syndrome of CRF are numerous (see Chart 72-7) and vary widely, depending on nitrogenous waste products, acid-base imbalances, and electrolyte imbalances. The nurse observes for neurologic signs, ranging from lethargy to seizures or coma, indicating uremic encephalopathy. In addition, the nurse assesses for sensory changes that generally appear in a glove and stocking distribution over the lower extremities and examines for weakness in the upper or lower extremities (i.e., uremic neuropathy).

If untreated, uremic encephalopathy progresses to seizures and coma. Dialysis is the treatment of choice for neurologic disturbances associated with CRF. The manifestations of uremic encephalopathy resolve with the initiation of dialysis. However, improvement in uremic neuropathy is limited if the neuropathy is severe and motor function is already impaired.

CARDIOVASCULAR MANIFESTATIONS. The clinical manifestations of CRF and uremia lead to specific cardiovascular abnormalities of fluid volume excess, hypertension, congestive heart failure (CHF), uremic pericarditis, and cardiac dysrhythmias associated with hyperkalemia. The nurse assesses for signs of a diminished ability to excrete salt and water. The resulting circulatory fluid overload, if untreated, can lead to CHF, pulmonary edema, peripheral edema, and hypertension.

The nurse assesses heart rate and rhythm, listening for extra beats (particularly an S_3), irregular patterns, or a pericardial friction rub. Unless a hemodialysis (HD) vascular access has been previously created, blood pressure is measured in each arm. The nurse assesses the jugular veins for distention and assesses for the presence of pedal, pretibial, presacral, and periorbital edema. Shortness of breath with exertion and paroxysmal nocturnal dyspnea (PND) suggest fluid volume excess.

RESPIRATORY MANIFESTATIONS. Respiratory manifestations of CRF vary widely among clients (e.g., breath that smells like urine [*uremic fetor* or uremic halitosis], deep sighing, yawning, shortness of breath). The nurse notes the rhythm, rate, and depth of breathing. Tachypnea (increased rate of breathing) and hyperpnea (increased depth of breathing) are respiratory compensation mechanisms for worsening metabolic acidosis.

With severe metabolic acidosis, the nurse may observe extreme hyperventilation or Kussmaul respiration. A few clients have hilar pneumonitis, or *uremic lung*. In these clients, the nurse assesses for thick sputum, minimal coughing, an increased respiratory rate, and an elevated temperature. A pleural friction rub may be heard with a stethoscope. Clients often have pleuritic pain with breathing. The nurse auscultates the lungs for crackles, which indicate fluid volume overload.

HEMATOLOGIC MANIFESTATIONS. Hematologic abnormalities include anemia and abnormal bleeding. The nurse notes indicators of anemia, including fatigue, pallor, lethargy, weakness, shortness of breath, and dizziness. The

CHART 72-7

KEY FEATURES *of* Chronic Renal Failure

Neurologic Manifestations
- Lethargy and daytime drowsiness
- Inability to concentrate or decreased attention span
- Seizures
- Coma
- Slurred speech
- Asterixis
- Tremors, twitching, or jerky movements
- Myoclonus
- Ataxia (alteration in gait)
- Paresthesias

Cardiovascular Manifestations
- Cardiomyopathy
- Hypertension
- Peripheral edema
- Congestive heart failure
- Uremic pericarditis
- Pericardial effusion
- Pericardial friction rub
- Cardiac tamponade

Respiratory Manifestations
- Uremic halitosis
- Tachypnea
- Deep sighing, yawning
- Kussmaul respirations
- Uremic pneumonitis
- Shortness of breath
- Pulmonary edema
- Pleural effusion
- Depressed cough reflex
- Crackles

Hematologic Manifestations
- Anemia
- Abnormal bleeding and bruising

Gastrointestinal Manifestations
- Anorexia
- Nausea
- Vomiting
- Metallic taste in the mouth
- Changes in taste acuity and sensation
- Uremic colitis (diarrhea)
- Constipation
- Uremic gastritis (possible GI bleeding)
- Uremic fetor
- Stomatitis
- Diarrhea

Urinary Manifestations
- Polyuria, nocturia (early)
- Oliguria, anuria (later)
- Proteinuria
- Hematuria
- Diluted, strawlike appearance

Integumentary Manifestations
- Decreased skin turgor
- Yellow-gray pallor
- Dry skin
- Pruritus
- Ecchymosis
- Purpura
- Soft-tissue calcifications
- Uremic frost (late, premorbid)

Musculoskeletal Manifestations
- Muscle weakness and cramping
- Bone pain
- Pathologic fractures
- Renal osteodystrophy

Reproductive Manifestations
- Decreased fertility
- Infrequent or absent menses
- Decreased libido
- Impotence

GI, Gastrointestinal.

presence of abnormal bleeding is assessed by observing for bruising, petechiae, purpura, ecchymoses (confluent bruises), mucous membrane bleeding in the nose or gums, abnormal vaginal bleeding, or gastrointestinal (GI) bleeding (often demonstrated by black tarry stools [melena]).

GASTROINTESTINAL MANIFESTATIONS. The nurse assesses for a foul odor to the breath, mouth ulceration, or mouth inflammation and notes any vomiting. Abdominal pain or cramping may be associated with uremic colitis. Stools may test positive for blood.

URINARY MANIFESTATIONS. The urinary findings in renal failure reflect the kidneys' decreasing functioning. At first, changes occur in the amount, frequency, and appearance of the urine. Many etiologic features of chronic renal disease result in proteinuria; some cause hematuria.

The quantity and composition of the urine change as renal function deteriorates. With the onset of end-stage renal disease (ESRD), the urine may become more dilute and clearer, reflecting a diminished glomerular filtration rate (GFR). The nurse must be aware that the actual urine output in a client with CRF varies with the amount of remaining renal function. The client with ESRD usually has oliguria, but some clients will remain relatively nonoliguric, producing 1 L or more per 24 hours. Urine volume produced per day will probably change again after dialysis is initiated.

INTEGUMENTARY MANIFESTATIONS. There are several dermatologic manifestations of CRF. In clients with uremia, deposition of urochrome pigment in the skin results in a yellowish coloration. Some African Americans report a darkening of the skin. The anemia of CRF causes a sallowness to the quality of the color, which some people describe as a faded suntan. This is most noticeable in lighter-skinned clients.

Skin oils and turgor are decreased in clients with uremia. One of the most uncomfortable problems of uremia is severe **pruritus** (itching). The nurse also assesses for bruises **(ecchymoses),** purple patches **(purpura),** and occasionally, drug-induced rashes.

Uremic frost, a layer of urea crystals from evaporated perspiration, may appear on the face, eyebrows, axilla, and groin in clients with advanced uremic syndrome.

PSYCHOSOCIAL ASSESSMENT

CRF and its treatment disrupt more aspects of a client's life than almost any other illness. Nurses are in a unique position to evaluate the client with newly diagnosed renal failure and to assist with these adjustments.

Psychosocial assessment and support are part of the nurse's role from the time that CRF is first diagnosed. Initially, the nurse asks about the client's understanding of the diagnosis and its implications for treatment regimens (e.g., diet, medication, and dialysis). The nurse assesses for any signs of anxiety and for the coping mechanisms used by the client or family members. Some of the psychosocial aspects altered by CRF include family relations, social activity, work patterns, body image, and sexual activity. The chronicity of ESRD, the variety of treatment options, and the uncertainties surrounding the course of the disease and its treatment necessitate an ongoing psychosocial assessment.

LABORATORY ASSESSMENT

CRF results in serious abnormalities in many laboratory values (see Chart 72-2). The following blood values are routinely monitored in clients with CRF: creatinine, blood urea nitrogen (BUN), sodium, potassium, calcium, phosphate, bicarbonate, hemoglobin, and hematocrit.

Initially, a urinalysis is performed, and a 24-hour urine specimen for creatinine and urea clearance is obtained. In the early stages of renal insufficiency, urinalysis can reveal key indicators of kidney function. Urinalysis may show excessive protein, glucose, red blood cells (RBCs), white blood cells (WBCs), and decreased or fixed specific gravity. Urine osmolality is usually decreased. A 24-hour creatinine clearance is calculated after serum and urinary creatinine levels are collected and quantified. These data, along with information on body weight and height, are used to calculate renal creatinine clearance. As renal failure progresses, the urine output may decrease dramatically.

Trends in renal function and progressive deterioration are typically monitored by measurements of the serum creatinine and BUN levels. Serum creatinine levels may increase gradually over a period of years, reaching levels of 15 to 30 mg/dL or more, depending on the client's muscle mass. Urea nitrogen levels are directly related to dietary protein intake. Without dietary protein restriction, BUN levels are typically 10 to 20 times the value of the serum creatinine level. As dietary protein is increasingly restricted in an attempt to slow the rate of progression of renal failure, BUN levels remain elevated but less than the 10:1 to 20:1 ratio of nonprotein-restricted clients. Other factors affect the level of BUN, and the nurse must consider these for a complete assessment. Chapter 69 describes the factors influencing BUN levels, as well as the interpretation of serum creatinine and creatinine clearance.

RADIOGRAPHIC ASSESSMENT

X-ray findings in clients with CRF are few. Bone radiographs of the metacarpals and phalanges of the hand can reveal the presence of renal osteodystrophy. With established ESRD, the kidneys are atrophic and may be 8 to 9 cm or less. This diminished size is usually the result of renal tubular atrophy and fibrosis. If obstructive uropathy is a possible factor contributing to deterioration of renal function that is more rapid than expected, a renal ultrasound or computed tomography (CT) scan without contrast media may be obtained. (See Chapter 69 for a complete description of renal diagnostic tests.)

CRITICAL THINKING CHALLENGE

You are gathering the initial history for a 67-year-old African-American client admitted to your unit with suspected CRF. The client tells you that he has a history of diabetes, gout, and peptic ulcer disease. He also states that he has noted a 7-pound weight gain over the last 4 weeks.

- What other questions should you ask this client regarding his symptoms?
- What risk factors for the development of CRF are noted in his past medical history?
- What cardiac and respiratory manifestations may you find on physical examination of this client?

For suggested answer guidelines, go to SIMON http://www.wbsaunders.com/SIMON/Iggy/.

Analysis

The client with chronic renal failure (CRF) has usually experienced a progressive degeneration of renal function and is often hospitalized for evaluation and modification of the treatment plan. The focus of care is to control or manage symptoms and prevent complications.

COMMON NURSING DIAGNOSES AND COLLABORATIVE PROBLEMS

The following are priority nursing diagnoses for clients with CRF:

1. Imbalanced Nutrition: Less Than Body Requirements related to nausea and vomiting, decreased appetite, effects of a catabolic state, decreased level of consciousness, altered taste sensations, or dietary restrictions
2. Excess Fluid Volume related to compromised regulatory mechanisms (inability of the kidneys to maintain body fluid balance)
3. Decreased Cardiac Output related to reduction in stroke volume as a result of electrical malfunction (dysrhythmias) and mechanical malfunction (increased preload [volume excess] and increased afterload [increased peripheral vascular resistance])
4. Risk for Infection related to inadequate primary defenses (broken skin), chronic disease, or malnutrition
5. Risk for Injury related to internal biochemical risk factors associated with renal failure (increased susceptibility to bleeding, falls, and pathologic fractures) and external risk factors, such as drugs
6. Fatigue related to altered metabolic energy production, imbalance between oxygen supply and demand, and anemia
7. Anxiety related to threat to or change in health status, socioeconomic status, relationships, role functioning, support systems, or self-concept; situational crisis; threat of death; lack of knowledge (procedures, diagnostic tests, disease process, renal replacement therapy); loss of control; feelings of failure; or disrupted family life

The primary collaborative problem is Potential for Pulmonary Edema.

ADDITIONAL NURSING DIAGNOSES AND COLLABORATIVE PROBLEMS

In addition to the common nursing diagnoses and collaborative problems, clients with CRF may have one or more of the following:

- Diarrhea related to chemical or electrolyte imbalances, fear, anxiety, or side effects of medications
- Impaired Oral Mucous Membrane related to parotid gland changes, limited fluid intake, malnutrition, and elevated levels of uremic toxins
- Impaired Skin Integrity related to altered chemical balance and uremic toxins
- Social Isolation related to illness or alterations in physical appearance
- Interrupted Family Processes related to situational crisis, reduced income, unemployment, or effects of chronic illness
- Sexual Dysfunction related to altered body function (decreased libido and/or impotence) from disease and/or effects of medications, depression, or disturbance in self-esteem or body image
- Disturbed Thought Processes related to irritation, central nervous system (CNS) depression, side effects of medications, sleep deprivation, or clinical depression
- Deficient Knowledge (disease process, care regimen, and follow-up care) related to lack of informational resources and magnitude of the care issues
- Potential for Sepsis
- Potential for Malnutrition
- Potential for Electrolyte Imbalances
- Potential for Metabolic Acidosis
- Potential for Gastrointestinal (GI) Bleeding

Planning and Implementation

The Concept Map on p. 1683 addresses assessment and nursing care issues related to clients who have renal failure that has progressed to end-stage renal disease (ESRD).

IMBALANCED NUTRITION: LESS THAN BODY REQUIREMENTS

PLANNING: EXPECTED OUTCOMES. The client with CRF is expected to attain and maintain the following:

- Adequate nutritional status
- Ideal body weight for age, height, and body build
- Laboratory values within safe levels

INTERVENTIONS. The nutritional requirements and dietary restrictions for the client with renal failure vary according to the degree of decrease in renal function and the type of dialysis performed, if any (Table 72-8).

NIC **NUTRITION THERAPY.** The purpose of nutrition therapy is the administration of food and fluids to support the metabolic processes of a client who is malnourished or at high risk of becoming malnourished. Clients begun on hemodialysis (HD) have an increase in catabolism and subsequent decrease in intake that often results in a loss of lean body mass. NIC interventions for nutrition therapy are summarized in Chart 72-8.

The client is referred to a registered dietitian for dietary teaching and planning. The nurse in collaboration with the dietitian instructs the client about alterations in the diet that are necessary as a result of CRF. Dietary alterations include control of protein intake; limitation of fluid intake; restriction of potassium, sodium, and phosphorus intake; administration of appropriate vitamin and mineral supplements; and provision of adequate calories to meet metabolic demand.

If adequate calories are not supplied, the body will use tissue protein for energy, which leads to a negative nitrogen balance and malnutrition. The dietitian assists in determining the number of calories and types of nutrients needed to meet nutritional requirements.

PROTEIN RESTRICTION. There is some evidence to suggest that early implementation of a protein-restricted diet prevents some of the symptoms associated with CRF and may preserve kidney function. Dietary protein is restricted on the basis of the degree of renal insufficiency and the severity of the symptoms in accordance with the belief that the accumulation of waste products from protein metabolism is the pri-

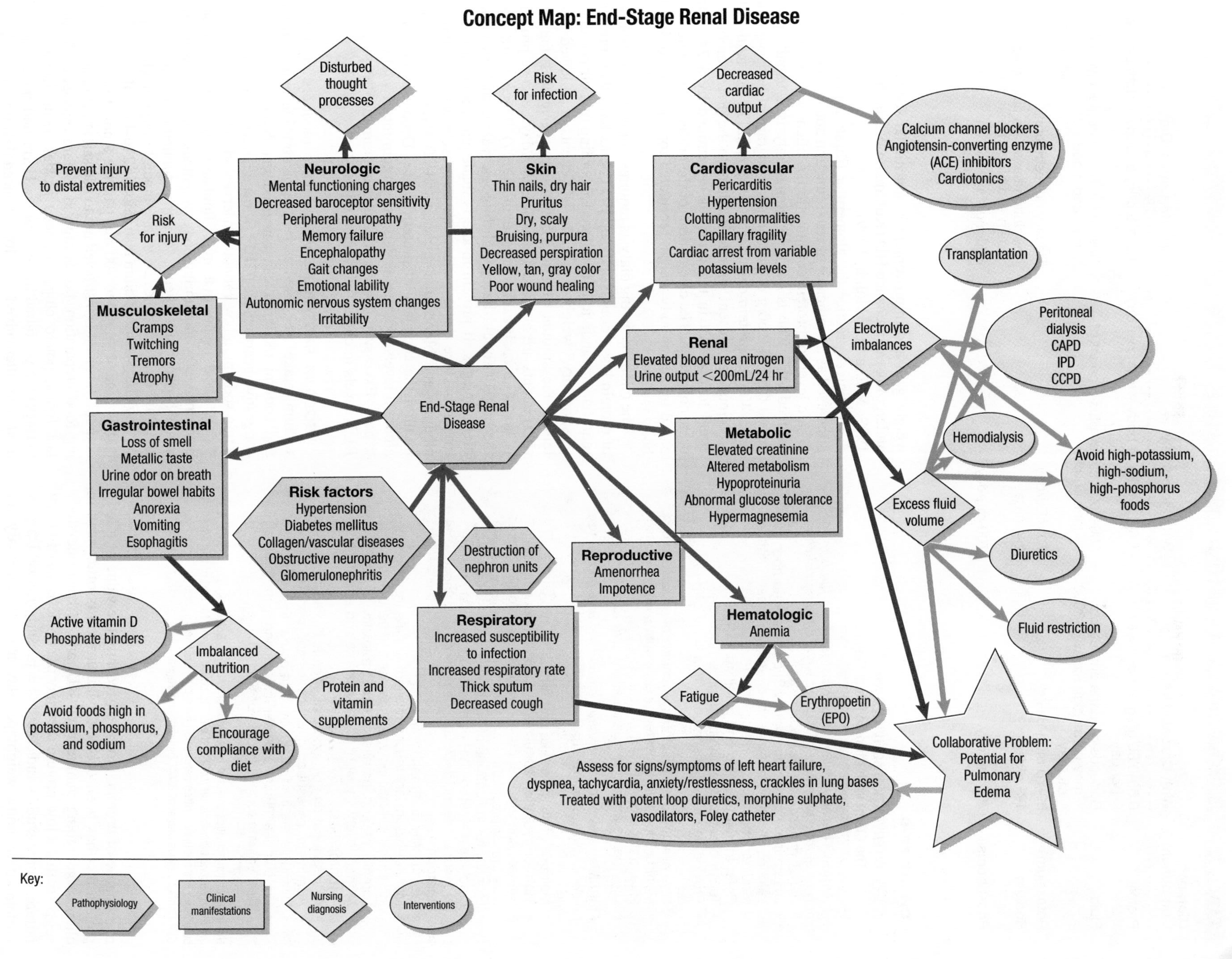
Concept Map: End-Stage Renal Disease
Disturbed thought processes
Risk for infection
Decreased cardiac output
Calcium channel blockers
Angiotensin-converting enzyme (ACE) inhibitors
Cardiotonics
Prevent injury to distal extremities
Risk for injury
Neurologic
Mental functioning charges
Decreased baroceptor sensitivity
Peripheral neuropathy
Memory failure
Encephalopathy
Gait changes
Emotional lability
Autonomic nervous system changes
Irritability
Skin
Thin nails, dry hair
Pruritus
Dry, scaly
Bruising, purpura
Decreased perspiration
Yellow, tan, gray color
Poor wound healing
Cardiovascular
Pericarditis
Hypertension
Clotting abnormalities
Capillary fragility
Cardiac arrest from variable potassium levels
Transplantation
Musculoskeletal
Cramps
Twitching
Tremors
Atrophy
Renal
Elevated blood urea nitrogen
Urine output <200mL/24 hr
Electrolyte imbalances
Peritoneal dialysis
CAPD
IPD
CCPD
End-Stage Renal Disease
Gastrointestinal
Loss of smell
Metallic taste
Urine odor on breath
Irregular bowel habits
Anorexia
Vomiting
Esophagitis
Metabolic
Elevated creatinine
Altered metabolism
Hypoproteinuria
Abnormal glucose tolerance
Hypermagnesemia
Hemodialysis
Avoid high-potassium, high-sodium, high-phosphorus foods
Excess fluid volume
Risk factors
Hypertension
Diabetes mellitus
Collagen/vascular diseases
Obstructive neuropathy
Glomerulonephritis
Destruction of nephron units
Reproductive
Amenorrhea
Impotence
Diuretics
Active vitamin D
Phosphate binders
Imbalanced nutrition
Respiratory
Increased susceptibility to infection
Increased respiratory rate
Thick sputum
Decreased cough
Hematologic
Anemia
Fluid restriction
Fatigue
Erythropoetin (EPO)
Avoid foods high in potassium, phosphorus, and sodium
Encourage compliance with diet
Protein and vitamin supplements
Collaborative Problem: Potential for Pulmonary Edema
Assess for signs/symptoms of left heart failure, dyspnea, tachycardia, anxiety/restlessness, crackles in lung bases
Treated with potent loop diuretics, morphine sulphate, vasodilators, Foley catheter
Key:
Pathophysiology
Clinical manifestations
Nursing diagnosis
Interventions

TABLE 72-8 • DIETARY RESTRICTIONS FOR THE CLIENT WITH RENAL FAILURE

Dietary Component	With Chronic Uremia	With Hemodialysis	With Peritoneal Dialysis
Protein	0.55-0.60 g/kg of body weight per day	1.0-1.5 g/kg of body weight per day	1.2-1.5 g/kg of body weight per day
Fluid	Depends on urine output, but may be as high as 1500-3000 mL/day	500-700 mL/day plus amount of urine output	Restriction based on fluid weight gain and blood
Potassium	60-70 mEq/day	70 mEq/day	Usually no restriction
Sodium	1-3 g/day	2-4 g/day	Restriction based on fluid weight gain and blood pressure
Phosphorus	700 mg/day	700 mg/day	800 mg/day

CHART 72-8

NIC INTERVENTION ACTIVITIES *for* The Client with Chronic Renal Failure

Nutrition Therapy: *Administration of food and fluids to support metabolic processes of a client who is malnourished or at high risk of becoming malnourished*
- Determine—in collaboration with dietitian—number of calories and type of nutrients needed to meet nutritional requirements.
- Refer to diet teaching and planning, as needed.
- Teach client and family about prescribed diet.
- Provide needed nourishment within limits of prescribed diet.
- Give client and family written examples of prescribed diet.
- Monitor food/fluid ingested and calculate daily caloric intake, as appropriate.
- Offer herbs and spices as an alternative to salt.

Fluid Management: *Promotion of fluid balance and prevention of complications resulting from abnormal or undesired fluid levels.*
- Maintain accurate intake and output record.
- Monitor hydration status (e.g., moist mucous membranes, adequacy of pulses, and orthostatic blood pressure), as appropriate.
- Monitor for indications of fluid overload/retention (e.g., crackles, elevated CVP or pulmonary capillary wedge pressure, edema, neck vein distention, and ascites), as appropriate.
- Weigh daily and monitor trends.
- Monitor laboratory results relevant to fluid retention (e.g., increased specific gravity, increased BUN, decreased hematocrit, and increased urine osmolality levels).
- Monitor client's weight change before and after dialysis, if appropriate.
- Assess location and extent of edema, if present.
- Administer prescribed diuretics, as appropriate.
- Distribute the fluid intake over 24 hours, as appropriate.
- Consult health care provider if signs and symptoms of fluid volume excess persist or worsen.

NIC intervention activities selected from McCloskey J.C., & Bulechek, G.M. (2000). *Nursing interventions classification (NIC)* (3rd ed.). St. Louis: Mosby. No part of this work is to be altered without prior written permission from the Publisher.
CVP, Central venous pressure; *BUN,* blood urea nitrogen.

mary cause of uremia. However, recently the value of a low-protein diet has been debated. Malnutrition is often seen in clients undergoing maintenance HD, and at least one study suggests that a low-protein diet may not be necessary in renal failure. Some studies indicate that a prescription of 1.5 g of protein/kg of body weight per day may be necessary for weight gain and improvement in nutritional status in clients undergoing maintenance HD (Kuhlmann, Schmidt, & Kohler, 1999; Mehrotra & Nolph, 1999).

In clinical practice the glomerular filtration rate (GFR) is often used as an indicator of renal function and can be a guide to safe levels of protein consumption. A client with a severely reduced GFR who is *not* undergoing dialysis is usually permitted 0.55 to 0.60 g of protein per kilogram of body weight (e.g., 40 g of protein daily for a 150-pound [70-kg] adult). If proteinuria is present, protein is added to the diet in amounts equal to that lost in the urine, as determined by a 24-hour urine collection. The calculation for the protein requirement is based on actual body weight (corrected for edema), not ideal body weight.

The client receiving dialysis requires more protein because of protein loss through dialysis. HD clients have their protein requirements individually tailored according to their postdialysis, or "dry," weight. Typically, HD clients are allowed protein in the amount of 1 to 1.5 g/kg/day; peritoneal dialysis (PD) clients are allowed 1.2 to 1.5 g/kg/day because protein is lost with each exchange (Levine, 1997). Three fourths of the protein should be of high biologic value, such as milk, meat, or eggs. If protein intake is inadequate, a negative nitrogen balance develops and causes muscle wasting. Serum albumin and blood urea nitrogen (BUN) levels are used to monitor the adequacy of protein intake. Decreases in serum albumin levels indicate inadequate protein intake and malnutrition. Excessive protein intake can dramatically increase BUN levels in clients with renal failure.

SODIUM RESTRICTION. The nurse monitors fluid and sodium intake. In clients with little or no urine output, fluid and sodium retention can cause edema, hypertension, and congestive heart failure (CHF). Most clients with renal failure retain sodium; a few cannot conserve sodium.

The client's status in terms of fluid and sodium retention can be estimated by monitoring body weight and blood pressure. In nondialyzed uremic clients, sodium is limited to 1 to 3 g daily, and fluid intake depends on urine output. In oliguric clients receiving dialysis, the sodium restriction is 2 to 4 g daily; fluid intake is limited to 500 to 700 mL plus the amount of any urine output. The client is instructed not to add salt at the table or during food preparation. Foods high in sodium (processed foods, fast foods, potato chips, pretzels, pickles, ham, bacon, and sausage) are permitted in moderation. Herbs and spices can be used as an alternative to salt for enhanced flavoring of food.

POTASSIUM RESTRICTION. The nurse monitors potassium intake because hyperkalemia can cause dangerous cardiac dysrhythmias. Cardiac rhythm is monitored for the tall, peaked T waves characteristic of hyperkalemia; the serum potassium level is also documented. The client with advanced CRF is instructed to limit potassium intake to 60 to 70 mEq/day. The labels of seasoning agents are carefully inspected for sodium and potassium content. Clients are instructed to avoid salt substitute agents, many of which are composed of potassium chloride, if oliguria is present. Clients receiving PD or who are producing urine may not need dietary potassium restrictions.

PHOSPHORUS RESTRICTION. Control of phosphate levels is begun early in renal failure to avoid osteodystrophy. The nurse monitors serum phosphate levels, and the physician may order dietary phosphorus restrictions and medications to assist with phosphate control. Phosphate binders must be taken at mealtime. Most clients with kidney disease already restrict their protein intake, and because high-protein foods are high in phosphorus, their phosphorus consumption is also reduced. Chapter 11 lists foods high in potassium, sodium, and phosphorus.

VITAMIN SUPPLEMENTATION. Most clients with renal failure require daily vitamin and mineral supplementation. Low-protein diets are usually deficient in vitamins, and water-soluble vitamins are removed from the blood during dialysis. In addition, anemia is a chronic problem in clients with renal failure because of the limited iron content of low-protein diets and decreased erythropoietin production by the kidneys. Thus supplemental iron is needed. Calcium and vitamin D supplements may also be required, depending on the client's serum levels and bone status.

INDIVIDUALIZATION OF THE DIET. Clients undergoing PD require a slightly different diet from those undergoing HD. Because protein is lost with the dialysate in PD, a major nutritional problem for these clients is replacing lost protein. In many cases, 1.2 to 1.5 g of protein per kilogram of body weight per day is recommended. The anorexia that often accompanies advanced renal disease requires clients to consume a diet with sufficient protein that includes high-calorie enteral supplements. The amount of sodium restriction varies with fluid weight gain and blood pressure. There is usually no need to restrict dietary potassium because the dialysate is potassium free. The potassium restriction, if any, is determined by the serum potassium level.

The nurse plays a vital role in managing the client's diet. In collaboration with the dietitian, the nurse provides teaching and performs ongoing assessments of the client's comprehension of and compliance with dietary regimens. Written examples of the prescribed diet can be given to the client and family. The nurse and dietitian can help clients adapt the diet to their budget, ethnic background, and food preferences to maximize caloric intake within the diet's restrictions.

EXCESS FLUID VOLUME

PLANNING: EXPECTED OUTCOMES. The client with chronic renal failure (CRF) is expected to:

- Achieve and maintain an acceptable fluid balance
- Minimize the risk of complications from fluid imbalances

INTERVENTIONS. Management of the client with CRF includes drug therapy, diet therapy, fluid restriction, and dialysis. Diet therapy is discussed under Imbalanced Nutrition: Less Than Body Requirements, p. 1682, and dialysis is discussed under Renal Replacement Therapies, p. 1688).

NIC **FLUID MANAGEMENT.** The purpose of fluid management is the promotion of fluid balance and the prevention of complications resulting from abnormal or undesired fluid levels (see Chart 72-8). The nurse monitors the client's intake and output and hydration status. In addition, the nurse assesses for signs and symptoms indicative of fluid volume excess, such as crackles in the bases of the lungs, edema, and distended neck veins.

DRUG THERAPY. Diuretics are prescribed for clients with renal insufficiency when needed for treatment of fluid retention or to help control blood pressure. The diuresis produced from these drugs is useful in treating fluid overload in clients who still have some urine output. Diuretics are seldom used in clients with end-stage renal disease (ESRD) after dialysis has been initiated because, as kidney function diminishes, these drugs can have harmful side effects, including nephrotoxic and ototoxic effects.

The nurse uses daily weight measurements and intake and output records as important sources of assessment data. Daily weight gain generally indicates fluid retention rather than true body weight gain. The nurse estimates the amount of fluid retained: 1 kg of weight equals approximately 1 L of fluid retained. Daily weights are taken at the same time each day, on the same scale, with the client wearing the same amount of clothing, and after the bladder has been emptied if the client is not anuric. The weight is monitored for changes before and after dialysis.

FLUID RESTRICTION. The amount of fluid restriction ordered is discussed under Sodium Restriction, p. 1684. The nurse considers all forms of intake, including oral, intravenous, and fluid or medication administration through gastrointestinal (GI) tubes, when calculating fluid intake. The nurse assists the client in distributing fluid intake by mouth over a 24-hour period. The client's response to fluid restriction is monitored, and the health care provider is notified if signs and symptoms of fluid volume excess persist or worsen.

DECREASED CARDIAC OUTPUT

NOC **PLANNING: EXPECTED OUTCOMES.** The client with CRF is expected to attain and maintain normal sinus rhythm, adequate cardiac output, and blood pressure in expected ranges.

INTERVENTIONS. Many clients with long-standing hypertension have renal insufficiency, and some progress to CRF and ESRD. Therefore the control of hypertension is an essential factor in preserving renal function. To control hypertension, the physician may order calcium channel blockers, angiotensin-converting enzyme (ACE) inhibitors, alpha-adrenergic and beta-adrenergic blockers, and vasodilators. Recent studies have documented the effectiveness of ACE inhibitors, as compared with other antihypertensives, in slowing the progression of renal failure (Levine, 1997). More information on the specific medications can be found in Chapter 36. Indications vary, depending on the client, and these drugs are used carefully to avoid hyperkalemia and hypotension. Various combinations and doses may be tried until blood pressure control is adequate and side effects are minimized. Calcium channel blockers seem to improve the GFR and renal blood flow.

The client and family or significant others are instructed to measure blood pressure. The nurse evaluates the client's ability to measure and record blood pressure accurately using the client's own equipment. The nurse periodically rechecks measurement accuracy. In addition to accurate measurement of blood pressure, the client and family must understand the relationship of blood pressure control and regulation to diet and medication therapy. The nurse further instructs the client to measure weight daily and to bring records of blood pressure measurements and weights for discussion with the physician, nurse, or dietitian.

The nurse assesses and monitors, on an ongoing basis, for signs and symptoms of decreased cardiac output, heart failure, congestive heart failure (CHF), and dysrhythmias. These topics are discussed in Chapters 33 through 35.

RISK FOR INFECTION

PLANNING: EXPECTED OUTCOMES. The client with CRF is expected to remain free of infection.

INTERVENTIONS. The nurse or assistive nursing personnel provides meticulous care to any areas where skin integrity has been broken (incisions, site of drains, puncture sites, cracked or excoriated skin, pressure sores) and provides good basic preventive skin care. For clients undergoing dialysis, the nurse also inspects the vascular access site or PD catheter insertion site. These areas are assessed on an ongoing basis for redness, swelling, pain, and drainage. Vital signs are monitored for any signs or symptoms of infection.

RISK FOR INJURY

PLANNING: EXPECTED OUTCOMES. The client with chronic renal failure (CRF) is expected to remain free of injury (will not fall or experience injury from a fall and will not experience pathologic fractures, bleeding, or toxic effects of medications administered in the presence of CRF).

INTERVENTIONS. Managing drug therapy in clients with CRF is a complex and ongoing clinical problem. Many over-the-counter drugs contain ingredients that may affect renal function. Therefore it is important to obtain a detailed drug history. The nurse must be aware of the use of each drug, its side effects, and the site of metabolism. The nurse, in conjunction with the physician and pharmacist, monitors the client closely for drug-related complications and adjusts dosages accordingly.

Certain medications must be avoided, and the dosages of others must be adjusted according to the degree of remaining renal function. As the client's renal function decreases, repeated dosage adjustments are necessary. The nurse assesses for side effects and signs of drug toxicity and notifies the physician as appropriate.

A number of medications are routinely administered to clients with renal failure (see Chart 72-3). The nurse giving these medications understands the rationale for administration and the nursing interventions for each drug. Many clients have some degree of cardiac disease and may require cardiotonic drugs, such as digoxin. Clients with decreased renal function are particularly susceptible to digoxin toxicity because the drug is excreted by the kidneys. The nurse caring for clients with CRF who are receiving any digitalis derivative, including digoxin, monitors for signs of toxicity, such as nausea, vomiting, anorexia, visual disturbances, restlessness, headache, fatigue, confusion, cardiac irregularities (particularly bradycardia [pulse rate, 50 to 60 beats/min] and tachycardia [pulse rate, 100 beats/min]), and serum drug levels above therapeutic range. In addition, serum levels of potassium are monitored closely in any client receiving cardiotonic medications.

Drugs to control an excessively high phosphate level include phosphate-binding compounds. Calcium acetate, calcium carbonate, and aluminum hydroxide are used as phosphate-binding agents in clients with renal failure. These drugs treat the metabolic complications that if untreated may lead to renal osteodystrophy and related injuries. To prevent further complications, the nurse stresses the importance of these and all medications.

Hypercalcemia (excessively high serum calcium levels) is a possible complication for clients taking calcium-containing compounds to control phosphate excess. **Hypophosphatemia** (low serum phosphorus levels) is also a possible outcome of phosphate binding but is typically also associated with phosphate depletion in clients who are not eating adequately but are continuing to take phosphate-binding medications. In clients taking aluminum-based phosphate binders for prolonged periods, retention and deposition of aluminum may cause bone disease or neurologic manifestations that may not be reversible. The nurse monitors the client for evidence of muscle weakness, anorexia, malaise, tremors, or bone pain.

Clients with renal disease should avoid antacid compounds containing magnesium. Clients with renal failure cannot excrete magnesium and thus should avoid additional intake.

In addition to the drugs used to treat renal failure, the use of other medications requires special consideration. These medications include antibiotics, opioids, antihypertensives, diuretics, insulin, and heparin.

Many antibiotics are safe for clients with renal failure, but those excreted primarily by the kidneys require dose modification. To prevent complications of bloodstream infections from oral cavity bacteria, prophylactic antibiotic treatment is routinely given to clients with CRF before any dental procedures. The antibiotic and protocol used vary with the client's needs and the physician's preference.

The nurse administers opioid analgesics cautiously in clients with renal failure because the effects often last much longer than in people with healthy kidneys. Clients with uremia are particularly sensitive to the respiratory depressant effects of these drugs. Because opioids are metabolized by the liver and not the kidneys, the dose recommendations are often the same regardless of the level of renal function. The nurse monitors these clients closely after opioid administration and evaluates the need for additional administration on the basis of the client's reaction to the drug.

As renal disease progresses, the client with diabetes mellitus often requires modification of an insulin or oral antidiabetic drug dose because of decreased insulin metabolism by failing kidneys. Frequent blood glucose determinations are obtained to evaluate the client's insulin or oral agent needs. Urine glucose measurements are less accurate when renal disease is present.

Because of poor platelet function and capillary fragility in renal failure, heparin and other anticoagulants are used cautiously.

FATIGUE

NOC **PLANNING: EXPECTED OUTCOMES.** The client with chronic renal failure (CRF) is expected to conserve energy by balancing activity and rest in order to be able to perform self-care and activities of daily living.

INTERVENTIONS. All clients with renal dysfunction are given some type of vitamin and mineral supplement. Because of diet restrictions and vitamin losses associated with both peritoneal dialysis (PD) and hemodialysis (HD), water-soluble vitamins must be replaced. The nurse avoids giving the client these vitamin supplements before HD treatment because they will be dialyzed out of the body and the client will receive no benefit.

The anemic client with CRF is treated with recombinant erythropoietin (erythropoietin alfa [Epogen, Procrit]). The goal of erythropoietin therapy is to achieve a hematocrit of 30% to 35%. For erythropoietin to stimulate bone marrow to produce red blood cells (RBCs), clients must have adequate iron stores. In addition, chronic administration of erythropoietin can deplete iron stores, necessitating iron supplementation. Many who receive epoetin alfa report improved appetite and sexual function along with decreased fatigue; in some clients, hypertension associated with a rise in hematocrit has been reported. The improved appetite may challenge clients in their attempts to maintain dietary protein, potassium, and fluid restrictions and necessitates additional education.

ANXIETY

NOC **PLANNING: EXPECTED OUTCOMES.** The client with CRF is expected to eliminate or reduce feelings of apprehension and tension from an unidentified source as evidenced by:

- Seeking information to reduce anxiety
- Using effective coping strategies
- Reporting an absence of physical manifestations of anxiety

INTERVENTIONS. The nurse has the most frequent contact with the client with CRF when the client is hospitalized or undergoing in-center dialysis treatments. Thus nurses perform an ongoing assessment of the client's anxiety level to determine the level of nursing intervention required. The nurse observes the client's behavior for physical cues indicating anxiety (e.g., an anxious facial expression or gestures and an increased pulse rate). In addition, the nurse evaluates the support systems, as evidenced by the involvement of family and friends with the client's care.

Unfamiliar settings and situations, and lack of knowledge about treatments and tests can increase the client's anxiety level. The nurse explains all procedures, tests, and treatments. The client's knowledge deficits concerning normal renal function and renal failure are identified. Evaluating the client's current knowledge avoids needless repetition during teaching sessions. The nurse provides instruction appropriate to the client's needs and ability to understand. By explaining the disease process, the nurse enhances the client's acceptance and decreases anxiety.

The nurse provides continuity of care, whenever possible, to establish a consistent nurse-client relationship to decrease anxiety and promote discussions of client and family concerns. As the nurse-client relationship develops, the client is encouraged to discuss current problems or concerns. A multidisciplinary team of professionals participates to provide support and counseling for the client and family, often over many years of treatment.

The nurse encourages the client to ask questions and discuss fears about the diagnosis of renal failure. An open atmosphere that allows for discussion can decrease anxiety level. Nurses also facilitate discussions with family members or significant others concerning the prognosis and the potential impact on the client's lifestyle.

POTENTIAL FOR PULMONARY EDEMA

PLANNING: EXPECTED OUTCOMES. The client with CRF is expected to remain free of pulmonary edema. A secondary outcome is to maintain optimal fluid volume balance through dialysis and pharmacologic measures, thus preventing the onset of pulmonary edema.

INTERVENTIONS. In the client with CRF, pulmonary edema can result from either of two distinct mechanisms: left-sided heart failure or microvascular injury. In left-sided heart failure, the heart is unable to adequately eject blood from the left ventricle, leading to an increase in hydrostatic pressure. The increased pressure allows fluid to cross the capillaries into the pulmonary interstitium. Pulmonary edema can also occur from injury to the vascular endothelium or alveolar epithelial cells secondary to uremia. Fluids then leak into the interstitial space and ultimately into the alveoli.

The nurse assesses the client for early signs of pulmonary edema, such as restlessness, heightened anxiety, tachycardia, dyspnea, and crackles that begin at the base of the lungs. As pulmonary congestion worsens, the level of fluid in the lungs rises. Auscultation will reveal increased rales, decreased air exchange, and dullness to percussion at the upper limits of fluid collection. The client may expectorate frothy, blood-tinged sputum. With further cardiac and respiratory compromise, the client can become diaphoretic and cyanotic.

The client who develops pulmonary edema is often admitted to the intensive care unit for aggressive treatment, which includes continuous cardiac monitoring. The client is placed in a high Fowler's position and given oxygen to maximize lung expansion and improve gas exchange. Drug therapy with renal failure and pulmonary edema is difficult at best because of the potential adverse effects of drugs on the kidneys. Treatment of pulmonary edema involves the administration of potent loop diuretics, such as furosemide (Lasix). Furosemide dosing usually begins at 40 mg, administered intravenously over a 1- to 2-minute period. This dose may be repeated in 30 minutes if no response is elicited. For clients already receiving maintenance doses of furosemide, an IV dose equivalent to the oral maintenance dose is given; it is doubled in 30 minutes if no response is seen (Johnson & Lalonde, 1997). Renal impairment multiplies the risk of ototoxicity with the use of furosemide; thus IV doses are given cautiously.

Morphine sulfate 1 to 2 mg administered intravenously is usually prescribed to reduce myocardial oxygen demand by reducing ventricular preload and to provide vasodilation and sedation. The dose is adjusted to achieve the desired response, but the potential for respiratory depression exists. Therefore the nurse monitors the client's respiratory rate and blood pressure closely. To further decrease hydrostatic pressure, a continuous infusion pump may administer a vasodilator, such as nitroglycerin. Vital signs are monitored vigilantly, since these drugs in combination may result in severe hypotension.

Nursing interventions include Foley catheter placement and frequent assessment of urine output to gauge the effectiveness of diuretic therapy. Diuresis usually begins within 5 minutes of administration of IV furosemide. Urine output is measured every 15 to 30 minutes during the acute episode and every hour thereafter until the client is stabilized. In addition, the nurse assesses breath and heart sounds for improvement in crackles and for the presence of an S_3, indicating fluid overload.

The nurse monitors serum chemistry results for electrolyte imbalances and reports abnormalities to the appropriate health care provider so that correction of imbalances can be initiated. Continuous cardiac monitoring is initiated to identify potential dysrhythmias. Oxygen saturation levels are monitored by pulse oximetry and arterial blood gas values. The oxygen delivery system is adjusted to maintain adequate oxygen saturation levels. The nurse monitors the client for deterioration, manifested as increasing pulmonary congestion and hypoxemia. It may be necessary to intubate the client and mechanically ventilate the lungs at this point to prevent death.

Clients with CRF are at increased risk for developing pulmonary edema, since they may present with precipitating fluid volume overload and existing cardiac compromise secondary to hypertension and volume overload. Such clients are less likely to respond quickly to treatment and are more likely to develop adverse effects from pharmacologic agents as a result of renal impairment. Occasionally, ultrafiltration may be used to further reduce fluid volume.

TABLE 72-9 • A COMPARISON OF HEMODIALYSIS AND PERITONEAL DIALYSIS AS RENAL REPLACEMENT TREATMENT OPTIONS

Hemodialysis	Peritoneal Dialysis
ADVANTAGES	
More efficient clearance	Easy access
Short time needed for treatment	Few hemodynamic complications
COMPLICATIONS	
Disequilibrium syndrome	Protein loss
Muscle cramps	Peritonitis
Hemorrhage	Hyperglycemia
Air embolus	Respiratory distress
Hemodynamic changes (hypotension, cardiac dysrhythmias, and anemia)	Bowel perforation
CONTRAINDICATIONS	
Hemodynamic instability	Extensive peritoneal adhesions
	Peritoneal fibrosis
	Recent abdominal surgery
ACCESS	
Vascular access route	Intra-abdominal catheter
PROCEDURE	
Complex	Simple
Specially trained registered nurses required	Training less complex than for hemodialysis
NURSING IMPLICATIONS	
Vascular access care	Abdominal catheter care
Restrict diet	More flexible diet

Renal Replacement Therapies

Renal replacement therapy is required only when the clinical and laboratory manifestations of renal failure present complications that are potentially life threatening or that pose continuing discomfort to the client. When the client can no longer be managed with conservative therapies, such as diet, medication, and fluid restriction, dialysis is indicated. Transplantation may be discussed at any time.

HEMODIALYSIS

Hemodialysis (HD) is one of several renal replacement therapies used for the treatment of renal failure (Table 72-9). Dialysis removes excess fluids and waste products and restores chemical and electrolyte balance. HD involves the extracorporeal (outside of the body) passage of the client's blood through a semipermeable membrane that serves as an artificial kidney.

CLIENT SELECTION. Any client may be considered for HD therapy. Initiation of renal replacement therapy depends on the symptoms of the client, not on the creatinine clearance. Dialysis is initiated immediately for clients who exhibit the following: fluid overload refractory to diuretics, presence of pericarditis, uncontrolled hypertension, neurologic manifestations, and development of bleeding diathesis. More commonly, dialysis is started when clients have signs of symptom progression, such as nausea and vomiting, decreased attention span, decreased cognition, worsening anemia, and pruritus (Levine, 1997).

The duration of survival after HD depends on the client's age, the cause of renal failure, and the presence of other diseases, such as coronary artery disease, hypertension, or diabetes. The following are general guideline requirements for appropriate client selection:

- Presence of fatal, irreversible renal failure when other therapies are unacceptable or ineffective
- Absence of illnesses that would prevent or seriously complicate HD
- Expectation of rehabilitation
- The client's acceptance of the regimen

DIALYSIS SETTINGS. Clients may receive HD treatments in any of several settings, depending on specific needs. They may be dialyzed in an acute care (hospital-based) center if they have recently begun treatment or have complicating conditions that require close nursing or medical supervision. Stable clients with chronic renal failure (CRF) may be hemodialyzed in a freestanding HD center in the community when they no longer require intensive supervision. Stable clients may participate in complete or partial self-care in an outpatient center or with in-home HD.

In-home HD offers the least disruptive form of therapy and allows for the most adaptation of the regimen to the client's lifestyle. Unfortunately, many clients cannot participate in in-home dialysis because they lack a reliable and consistent partner to administer the therapy and manage the dialysis machine. For some clients and partners, the responsibilities of in-home dialysis are extremely stressful, so that this option is less desirable. In addition, a water treatment system must be installed in the home to provide a safe, clean water supply for the dialysis process.

Regardless of the setting for therapy, the client needs ongoing nursing support and intervention to maintain this complex and lifesaving treatment.

PROCEDURE. The principles of HD are based on the passive transfer of toxins, which is accomplished by diffusion. **Diffusion** is the movement of molecules from an area of higher concentration to an area of lower concentration. The rate of diffusion is affected by numerous factors. Diffusion during dialysis occurs more rapidly when the membrane pores are large, there is a large surface area of membrane, the temperature of the solutions is higher, and there is a greater difference in the solute concentrations. Molecules that are too large, such as RBCs and plasma proteins, cannot pass through the membrane.

When HD is initiated, blood and dialysate flow in opposite directions from their respective sides of an enclosed semipermeable membrane. The dialysate is a balanced mix of electrolytes and water that closely resembles human plasma. On the other side of the membrane is the client's blood, which contains metabolic waste products, excess water, and excess electrolytes. During HD, the waste products move from the blood into the dialysate because of the difference in their concentrations (diffusion). Excess water is also removed from the blood into the dialysate **(osmosis).** Electrolytes can move in either direction, as needed, and take some fluid with them. Potassium and sodium typically move out of the plasma into the dialysate, whereas bicarbonate and calcium move from the dialysate into the plasma. This process continues as the blood and the dialysate are circulated past the membrane for a preset length of time. Water volume may be removed from the plasma by applying positive or negative pressure to the system.

The components of an HD system include a dialyzer, dialysate, vascular access routes, and an HD machine. The artificial kidney, or **dialyzer** (Figure 72-3), has four components: a blood compartment, a dialysate compartment, a semipermeable membrane, and an enclosed structure to support the membrane.

Dialysate is made from clear water and chemicals and is free of any metabolic waste products or drugs. Because bacteria and other microorganisms are too large to pass through the membrane, dialysate does not need to be sterile. The water used in dialysate must meet specific standards, and water treatment systems are used to ensure a safe water supply. The dialysate composition may be altered according to the client's needs for treatment of electrolyte imbalances. During HD, the dialysate is warmed to approximately 100° F (37. 8° C) to increase the efficiency of diffusion and to prevent a decrease in blood temperature.

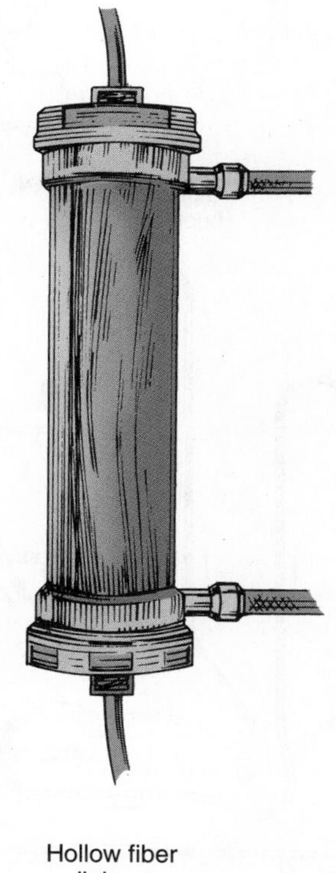

Figure 72-3 ● Artificial kidney (dialyzer) used in hemodialysis.

An essential function of an HD machine is the monitoring for potential problems, including the following:

- Changes in dialysate temperature
- Presence of air in the blood tubing
- A blood leak in the dialysate compartment
- Changes in the pressure or composition within the blood and the dialysate compartments

If any of these problems are detected, an alarm alerts the nurse. The monitoring systems protect the client from life-threatening complications that can result if these technical problems are not corrected.

All models of HD machines function, in principle, as illustrated in Figure 72-4. Figure 72-5 shows one type of machine. The duration and frequency of HD treatments depend on the amount of metabolic waste to be cleared, the clearance capacity of the dialyzer, and the amount of fluid to be removed. Most dialyzers provide sufficient clearance to limit the total number of hours of dialysis to about 12 hours a week. This time is usually divided into three 4-hour treatments a week. For clients with less muscle or more ongoing urine production, two 5- to 6-hour treatments a week may be adequate. If the client gains large amounts of fluid weight, a longer treatment time may be needed to remove the fluid without hypotension or severe side effects.

ANTICOAGULATION. To prevent blood clots from forming within the dialyzer membrane and the blood tubing, anticoagulation with heparin is necessary during HD treatments. Heparin, a short-acting anticoagulant, inhibits the tendency of blood to clot when it comes in contact with foreign surfaces. There is considerable variability among clients in

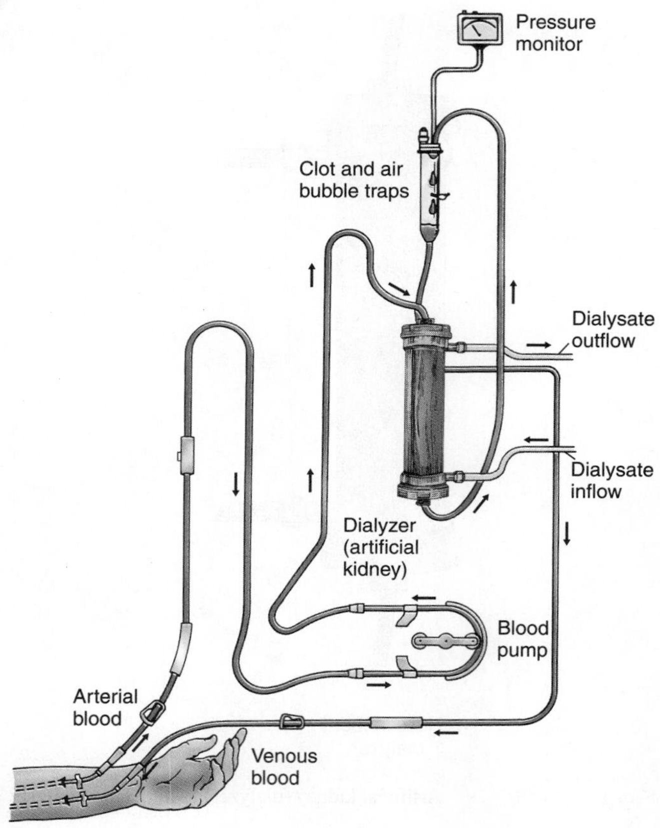

Figure 72-4 ● A hemodialysis circuit.

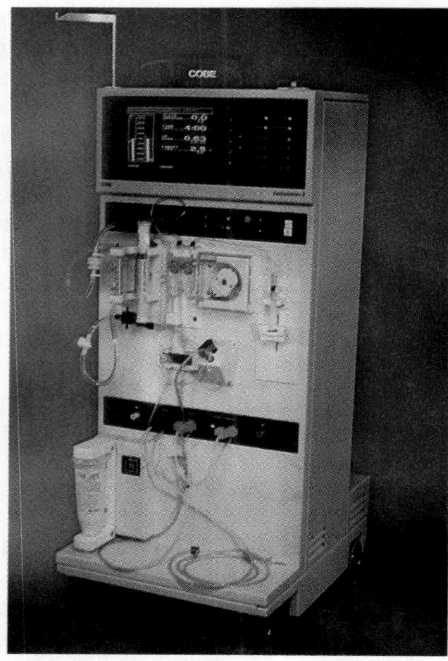

Figure 72-5 ● A hemodialysis machine. (Courtesy Gambro Healthcare.)

their anticoagulation response and elimination of heparin. The heparin dose must be adjusted on the basis of each client's need. Clients receiving erythropoietin may need more heparin.

Heparin remains active in the body for 4 to 6 hours after administration, making the client at risk for hemorrhage during and immediately after HD treatments. The client must avoid any invasive procedures during that time. Thus the nurse monitors closely for any signs of bleeding or hemorrhage. Clotting tendencies can be monitored during HD with a bedside machine (such as the Hemochron), by whole-blood clotting times (Lee-White clotting test), or by activated partial thromboplastin times (aPTT) during and after HD. Protamine sulfate is given as an antidote to neutralize heparin's anticoagulant activity when necessary.

VASCULAR ACCESS. For hemodialysis (HD) to be performed, a vascular access route is required (Table 72-10). Dialysis treatments necessitate the easy availability of a large amount of blood flow—at least 250 to 300 mL/min, usually for a period of 3 to 4 hours. Normally, the body cannot provide this type of circulatory access without surgical revision of blood vessels.

LONG-TERM VASCULAR ACCESS. An internal access is preferred for most clients undergoing long-term HD (see Table 72-10). There are two common choices: an internal arteriovenous (AV) fistula or an AV graft (Figure 72-6). *AV fistulas* are formed by connecting **(anastomosis)** an artery to a vein. The most commonly used vessels are the radial or brachial artery and the cephalic vein of the nondominant arm. This process increases the blood flow through the vein to 250 to 400 mL/min, the amount required for dialysis to be effective.

Some time is necessary for an AV fistula to develop, and the amount of time required for the fistula to "mature" varies. Primary AV fistulas may not be suitable for use for as long as 4 months. Therefore vascular access must be planned accordingly. As the fistula matures, the increased pressure of the arterial blood flow into the vein causes the vessel walls to thicken. This thickening increases their strength and suitability for repeated cannulation.

To obtain access to a fistula, the nurse cannulates it or inserts two needles, one toward the venous blood flow and one toward the arterial blood flow. This procedure allows the HD machine to draw the blood out through the arterial needle and return it through the venous needle. The client may require a temporary vascular access (AV shunt or HD catheter) for HD treatments until the fistula is ready for use.

AV grafts are used when the AV fistula does not develop or when complications of the AV fistula limit continued use. The polytetrafluoroethylene (PTFE) graft is a synthetic material (Gore-Tex). This type of graft is commonly used in older clients undergoing HD.

PRECAUTIONS. Several precautions must be observed to ensure the functioning of an internal AV fistula or AV graft. First, the nurse assesses for adequate circulation in the fistula or graft, as well as in the distal portion of the extremity. The nurse then checks for a bruit or a thrill by auscultation or palpation over the access site. Repeated compression can result in the loss of the vascular access; therefore the nurse avoids taking the blood pressure in the arm with the vascular access unless absolutely necessary. The AV fistula or graft is *not* used for administration of IV fluids; venipuncture is avoided anywhere in the arm used for HD access. Chart 72-9 lists best practices for care of the client with an HD access.

TABLE 72-10 • TYPES OF VASCULAR ACCESS FOR HEMODIALYSIS

Access Type	Description	Location	Initial Use
PERMANENT			
AV fistula	An internal anastomosis of an artery to a vein	Forearm	2-4 mo or longer
AV graft	Synthetic vessel tubing tunneled beneath the skin, connecting an artery and a vein	Forearm Upper arm Inner thigh	1-2 wk
Dual-lumen hemodialysis catheter	An extended-use catheter, surgically tunneled under the skin with a barrier cuff	Subclavian vein	Immediately postoperatively and after x-ray confirmation of placement
TEMPORARY			
Hemodialysis catheter (dual- or triple-lumen)	A specially designed catheter with two or three lumens Two lumens are for blood outflow and inflow for hemodialysis; a third lumen allows venous access without accessing dialysis lumens	Subclavian, internal jugular, or femoral vein	Immediately after insertion and x-ray confirmation of placement
AV shunt (relatively uncommon)	An external loop of Silastic tubing connecting an artery and a vein Each section of tubing is sutured into a vessel and brought through a skin stab wound	Forearm	Immediately after insertion

AV, Arteriovenous.

COMPLICATIONS. Complications can occur regardless of the type of access. The most common problems include thrombosis or stenosis, infection, aneurysm formation, ischemia, and high-output heart failure.

Thrombosis, or clotting, is the most frequent complication. Some clients are more susceptible to clotting than are others and may be given anticoagulants. Surgical declotting or revision of stenotic areas is typically performed in the surgical suite with the use of local anesthesia.

Most infections that occur in clients undergoing long-term HD involve the vascular access. The most common organism causing infection is *Staphylococcus aureus,* which can be introduced by punctures for dialysis access. The nurse limits the incidence of infections by using careful sterile technique before needle cannulation (Table 72-11).

Aneurysms can form in any internal fistula and are caused by repeated needle punctures at the same site. Aneurysms that appear to be increasing in size may cause loss of the fistula's function and require surgical repair.

Ischemia occurs in a few clients with vascular access when the formation of the fistula causes a decrease in arterial blood flow to areas distal to the fistula. Ischemic symptoms *(steal syndrome)* vary from cold or numb fingers to gangrene. If the collateral circulation is inadequate, the existing fistula may need to be ligated and a new fistula created in another area for circulation to be preserved in the extremity.

The shunting of blood directly from the arterial system to the venous system, through the fistula, can cause high-output heart failure in clients with a limited cardiac reserve (see Chapter 35). This complication occurs rarely, but if it does, the fistula may need to be revised to decrease the blood flow from the arterial supply.

TEMPORARY VASCULAR ACCESS. The first type of vascular access developed was the external *arteriovenous (AV) shunt* (Figure 72-7; see also Table 72-10), but it is rarely used today. To create a shunt, the surgeon places a piece of silicone rubber (Silastic) tubing into an artery and a second piece into an adjacent vein. The tubings are connected externally to provide a readily available vascular access. The arterial limb is used to obtain the blood for passage through the artificial kidney (dialyzer membrane), and the venous limb is used to return the blood to the client's body after each pass through the dialyzer.

Temporary vascular access with special catheters has replaced the use of the AV shunt for most clients requiring immediate HD. A catheter designed for HD may be inserted into the subclavian, internal jugular, or femoral vein if no permanent vascular access is available for use (see Dialysis Therapies, pp. 1674 and 1675). The lumens of these devices are considerably smaller than the permanent accesses, and the duration of each dialysis session is increased (usually requires 4 to 8 hours).

POSTDIALYSIS NURSING CARE. The nurse closely monitors the client immediately after dialysis and for several hours afterward for any side effects from the treatment. The more common clinical manifestations of complications include hypotension, headache, nausea, malaise, vomiting, dizziness, and muscle cramps.

The nurse obtains vital signs and weight for comparison with predialysis measurements. Blood pressure and weight are expected to be reduced as a result of fluid removal. Excessive hypotension may require rehydration with IV fluids, such as normal saline. The client's temperature may also be elevated, because the dialysis machine warms the blood slightly. If the temperature is elevated excessively, sepsis is suspected and a blood sample is obtained, as ordered, for culture and sensitivity determinations.

The heparinization required for hemodialysis (HD) increases the clotting time and thus the risk for excessive bleeding. *All invasive procedures must therefore be avoided for 4 to 6 hours after dialysis, and the nurse continually monitors the*

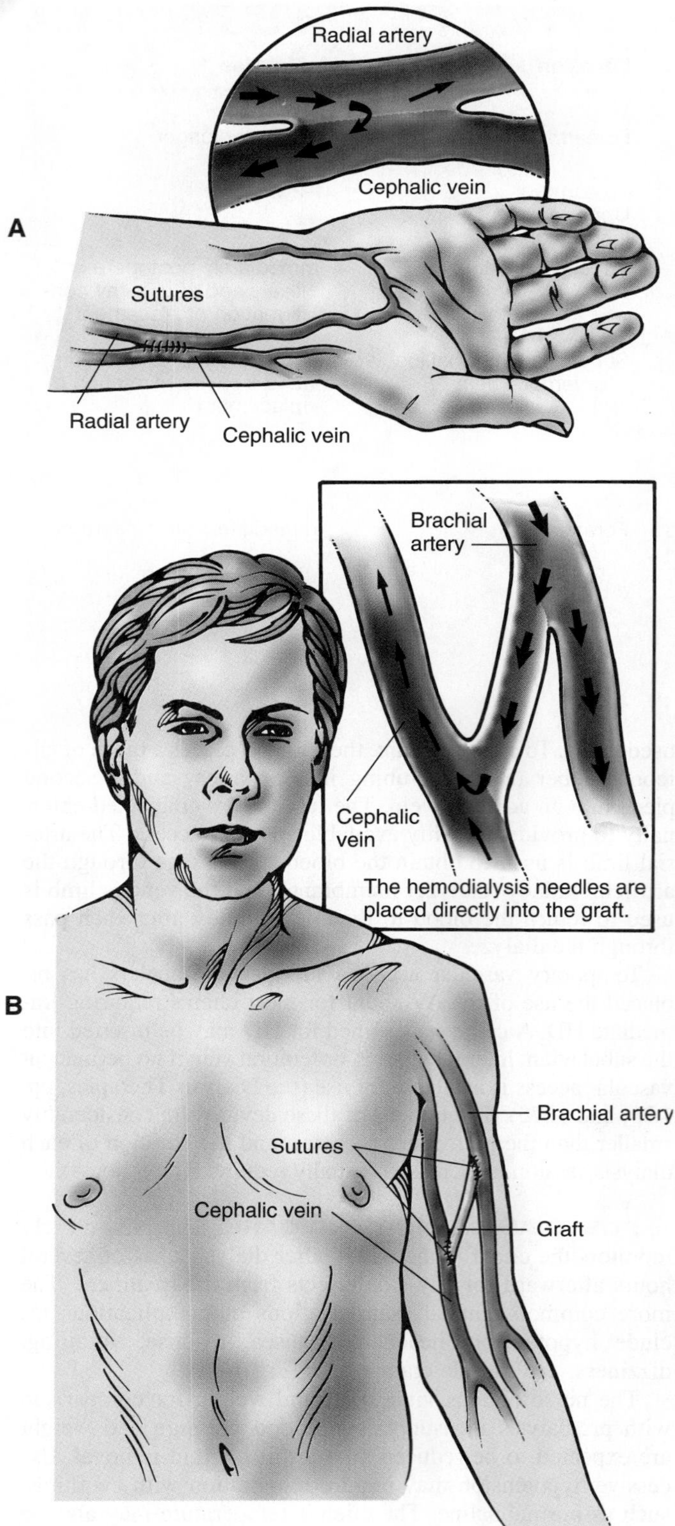

Figure 72-6 ● Options for long-term vascular access for hemodialysis. **A,** A surgically created venous fistula. The increased pressure from the artery forces blood into the vein. This process causes the vein to dilate enough for fistula needles to be placed for hemodialysis. When the vein dilates in this matter, the fistula is said to be "developed." **B,** A surgically placed straight vascular graft in the upper arm. The graft creates a shunt between arterial and venous blood.

client for signs of hemorrhage during dialysis and for 1 hour after dialysis (Chart 72-10).

COMPLICATIONS. A variety of fluid-related and infectious complications can occur from HD. The most common complications include disequilibrium syndrome and acquisition of viral infections.

Dialysis disequilibrium syndrome may develop during HD or after HD has been completed. The cause is unknown but may be due to the rapid decrease in blood urea nitrogen (BUN) levels during HD. These changes in urea levels can cause cerebral edema, which leads to increased intracranial pressure. Neurologic complications can result (headache, nausea, vomiting, restlessness, decreased level of consciousness, seizures, coma, or death).

Early recognition by the nurse of the signs of the syndrome and appropriate treatment with anticonvulsant medications and barbiturates may prevent a life-threatening situation. Dialysis disequilibrium syndrome may be avoided, or minimized, by introducing HD for short periods initially with low blood flows so that rapid changes in plasma composition are avoided.

Infectious diseases transmitted by blood transfusion are another serious complication associated with long-term HD. Two of the most serious blood-transmitted infections are hepatitis and human immunodeficiency virus (HIV).

Hepatitis infection in clients with chronic renal failure (CRF) has decreased in recent years, paralleling the decrease in blood transfusion requirement for these clients because of the availability of erythropoietin therapy. Yet, because of the blood access and the risk of microscopic exposure, hepatitis continues to be a problem for clients undergoing HD. The hepatitis B virus can be transmitted through the use of contaminated needles or instruments, by entry of contaminated blood through open wounds in the skin or mucous membranes, or through transfusion of blood contaminated with the virus.

CHART 72-9

BEST PRACTICE *for*
Caring for the Client with an Arteriovenous Fistula, Arteriovenous Graft, or Arteriovenous Shunt

- Do not take blood pressure readings using the extremity in which the vascular access is placed.
- Do not perform venipunctures or start an IV line in the extremity in which the vascular access is placed.
- Palpate for thrills and auscultate for bruits every 4 hours while the client is awake.
- Assess the client's distal pulses and circulation.
- Elevate the affected extremity postoperatively.
- Encourage routine range-of-motion exercises.
- Check for bleeding at needle insertion sites or shunt tubing insertion sites. (Keep small clamps handy on the dressing of the AV shunt.)
- Assess for signs and symptoms of infection at needle sites and shunt tubing insertion sites.
- Instruct the client not to carry heavy objects or anything that compresses the extremity in which the vascular access if placed.
- Instruct the client against sleeping with his or her body weight on top of the extremity in which the vascular access is placed.

AV, Arteriovenous.

The incubation period for acute hepatitis is 6 weeks to 6 months. Thus the nurse continually monitors the client undergoing HD who is receiving frequent transfusions for signs of hepatitis virus infection (see Chapter 59).

HIV is a bloodborne and body fluid–borne virus with some potential threat to clients undergoing HD. Fortunately, the risks of HIV transmission are minimized by the consistent practice of standard precautions (blood and body fluids), routine screening of donated blood for HIV, and decreased numbers of blood transfusions for clients with end-stage renal disease (ESRD). Despite this progress, however, an unknown number of clients may have already been infected with the HIV virus. Clients who have been undergoing HD and who received frequent transfusions during the early to mid-1980s are at risk for acquired immunodeficiency syndrome (AIDS) (see also Chapter 22).

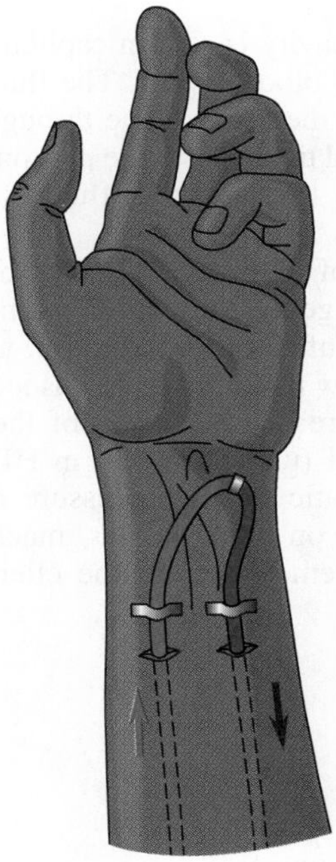

Figure 72-7 • An arteriovenous shunt in the forearm. One part of the shunt cannula is placed in an artery; the other part in a vein. The ends of the shunt cannula are joined when dialysis is not in progress.

CRITICAL THINKING CHALLENGE

Your client has been diagnosed as having ESRD. The health care provider has ordered dietary teaching. In addition, your client will begin outpatient HD three times per week.

- What instructions should you provide regarding the dietary and fluid needs for this client?
- What complications should you monitor the client for during and immediately following dialysis?

For suggested answer guidelines, go to SIMON http://www.wbsaunders.com/SIMON/Iggy/.

CONSIDERATIONS FOR OLDER ADULTS

There is a greater occurrence of ESRD in individuals 65 to 69 years of age. In the past decade there has been an 8% increase in the incidence of ESRD in individuals ages 45 to 65, and a 14% increase in those 75 years of age and older (USRSD, 1999). In addition, clients over age 65 who are receiving dialysis treatments are more at risk for dialysis-induced hypotension.

CHART 72-10

BEST PRACTICE *for*
Caring for the Client Undergoing Hemodialysis

- Weigh the client before and after dialysis.
- Know the client's dry weight.
- Discuss with the physician whether any of the client's medications should be withheld until after dialysis.
- Be aware of events that occurred during the dialysis treatment.
- Measure blood pressure, pulse rate, respirations, and temperature.
- Assess for symptoms of orthostatic hypotension.
- Assess the vascular access site.
- Observe for bleeding.
- Assess the client's level of consciousness and assess for headache, nausea, and vomiting.

TABLE 72-11 • NURSING MEASURES FOR PREVENTION OF COMPLICATIONS IN HEMODIALYSIS VASCULAR ACCESS

Access Type	Bleeding	Infection	Clotting
AV fistula or AV graft	Apply pressure to the needle puncture sites.	Ensure adequate site cleaning before cannulation.	Avoid constrictive devices. Rotate needle insertion sites with each hemodialysis treatment. Assess for thrill and bruit.
AV shunt	Keep clamps available.	Perform exit site care 3 times/wk.	Avoid constrictive devices. Assess for thrill and bruit.
Hemodialysis catheters (temporary and permanent)	Monitor the access site.	Use aseptic technique. Change the dressing 3 times/wk.	Place a heparin or heparin/saline dwell solution after hemodialysis treatment. Not used between treatments.

AV, Arteriovenous.

PERITONEAL DIALYSIS

Peritoneal dialysis (PD) takes place within the peritoneal cavity. PD is slower than hemodialysis (HD), however, and more time is needed for the same effect to be obtained.

CLIENT SELECTION. Most clients with chronic renal failure (CRF) can select either HD or PD. For clients who are hemodynamically unstable and for those who cannot tolerate systemic anticoagulation, PD is less hazardous than HD. The lack of vascular access due to inadequate vessels may eliminate HD as an option. In addition, some clients with a new arteriovenous (AV) fistula receive PD while waiting for the access to mature for HD. PD is also often the treatment of choice in the older adult and pediatric populations because it offers more flexibility if the client's status changes frequently.

In some relatively rare situations, PD cannot be performed, usually because of peritoneal adhesions or intra-abdominal surgery in the peritoneal cavity. In these cases, the peritoneal membrane's surface area has been reduced too much to allow for adequate dialysis exchange. In other cases, peritoneal membrane fibrosis may occur after repeated infections, which decreases membrane permeability despite adequate surface area.

PROCEDURE. The surgical insertion of a siliconized rubber (Silastic) catheter into the abdominal cavity is required to allow the infusion of dialyzing fluid (dialysate) (Figure 72-8). According to the physician's order, 1 to 2 L of dialysate is infused by gravity *(fill)* into the peritoneal space over a 10- to 20-minute period, according to the client's tolerance. The fluid *dwells* in the cavity for a specified time ordered by the physician. The fluid then flows out of the body *(drain)* by gravity into a drainage bag. The peritoneal outflow contains the dialysate in addition to the excess water, electrolytes, and nitrogenous waste products that have accumulated in the body. The dialyzing fluid is called peritoneal *effluent* on outflow. The three phases of the process (infusion, or "fill"; dwell; and outflow, or drain) are considered one PD exchange. The number and frequency of PD exchanges are prescribed by the physician, depending on the clinical manifestations and laboratory data.

PROCESS. PD occurs through diffusion and osmosis across the semipermeable peritoneal membrane and adjacent capillaries. The peritoneal membrane is large and porous. It allows solutes, which carry fluid with them, to move by an osmotic gradient from an area of higher concentration in the body (blood) to an area of lower concentration in the dialyzing fluid.

The peritoneal cavity is rich in capillaries and provides a ready access to the blood supply. The fluid and waste products dialyzed from the client move through the blood vessel walls, the interstitial tissues, and the peritoneal membrane and are removed when the dialyzing fluid is drained from the body.

The efficiency of PD can be affected by numerous situations, such as changes in the peritoneal membrane's permeability caused by infection or irritation, and changes in the capillary blood flow resulting from vasoconstriction, vascular disease, or decreased perfusion of the peritoneum. Excess water removal (ultrafiltration) in HD is accomplished by use of hydrostatic positive pressure or transmembrane negative pressure on the dialysis machine. In PD, the amount of water removed from the client depends on the

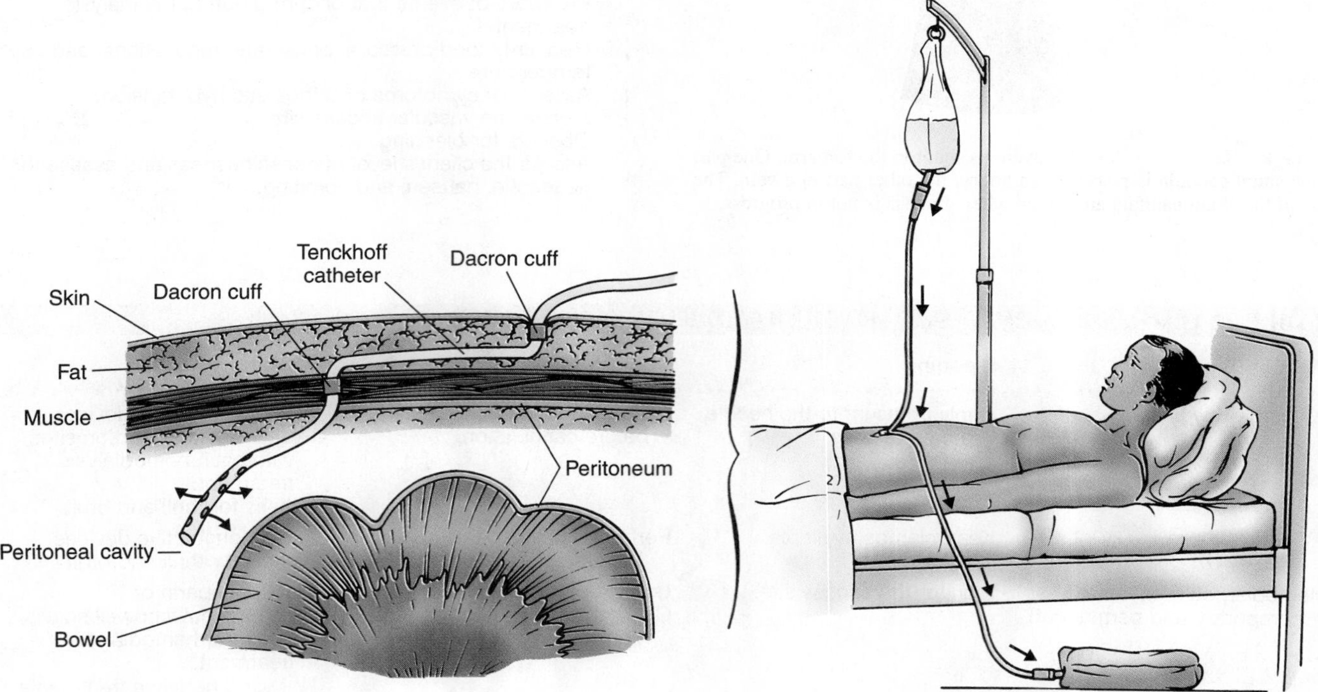

Figure 72-8 ● Manual peritoneal dialysis via an implanted abdominal catheter (Tenckhoff catheter).

concentration of the dialysate. Increasing the glucose concentration of the dialysate makes the solution increasingly more hypertonic. The more hypertonic the solution, the greater the osmotic pressure for ultrafiltration and thus the greater the amount of fluid removed from the client during an exchange. The physician orders the dialysate concentration on the basis of the client's fluid status.

MEDICATION ADDITIVES. Heparin may be added to the dialysate to prevent fibrin clot formation in the catheter or tubing; this intraperitoneal (IP) heparin administration is necessary only after new catheter placement or with the occurrence of peritonitis. There is no systemic absorption of heparin with IP administration, so clotting studies are not needed.

Other agents that may be administered by the IP route include potassium chloride and antibiotics. Commercially prepared dialysate does not contain potassium chloride. Some clients will need potassium chloride added to the dialysate so that the dialysate does not excessively deplete potassium from the plasma. Oral potassium supplements may be prescribed in selected clients. The physician may order IP administration of antibiotics (e.g., gentamicin, vancomycin, cephalosporins) when peritonitis is present or suspected. The combination of potassium chloride and antibiotics in the same bag of dialysate is not recommended, because chemical interactions may limit effectiveness.

TYPES OF PERITONEAL DIALYSIS. Many types of PD are available, including continuous ambulatory PD, multiple-bag continuous ambulatory PD, automated PD, intermittent PD, and continuous-cycle PD. The selection of the type depends on the client's ability and lifestyle.

CONTINUOUS AMBULATORY PERITONEAL DIALYSIS. In continuous ambulatory peritoneal dialysis (CAPD), the client performs self-dialysis by infusing four 2-L exchanges of dialysate into the peritoneal cavity, where the dialysate remains for 4 to 8 hours, 7 days a week. During the dwell period, the client can choose a continuous connect system or a disconnect system.

With the continuous *connect* system (straight transfer set), the dialysate bag is usually attached to the catheter by 48-inch (122-cm) tubing; the empty bag and tubing are folded and worn beneath the clothing until they are used for outflow. After draining, the client removes the bag and connects a new bag to repeat the process.

With the *disconnect system* (Y-transfer set), the client removes the connecting tubing and empty dialysate bag after inflow and attaches a protective cap to the PD catheter junction. The disconnect system eliminates the need to wear the tubing and bag but requires opening the system two extra times with each exchange. This opening of the system increases the potential for contamination and infection.

With CAPD treatment, no machine is necessary, and client independence is encouraged. Theoretically, no partner is required. However, many home training programs suggest that a partner be trained in CAPD as a support for the client should illness or temporary disability occur. Devices to assist in the safe, uncontaminated connection of the tubing spike with the dialysate bag are increasingly in use. These devices can be considered for clients with impaired vision, limited manual dexterity, or decreased upper extremity strength. CAPD offers the advantage of constant removal of fluid and wastes and more nearly resembles renal function than does HD. Some clients continue to perform their own exchanges while hospitalized.

MULTIPLE-BAG CONTINUOUS AMBULATORY PERITONEAL DIALYSIS. For those who are unable to perform self-CAPD in the acute care setting, a multiple-bag CAPD (MB-CAPD) system allows continuation of CAPD. With MB-CAPD, a manifold of tubing connected to the dialysate and hanging on a portable pole is attached to the PD catheter by connecting tubing (see Figure 72-8). The nurse inflows the dialysate at the prescribed time, allows the dwell, and initiates the outflow for each exchange. The MB-CAPD system permits mobility for the ambulatory client and provides for continuous PD.

AUTOMATED PERITONEAL DIALYSIS. An automated cycling machine that provides for dialysate inflow, dwell, and outflow according to preset times and volumes may be used. A warming chamber for dialysate is part of the machine. Automated peritoneal dialysis (APD) may be used in the acute care setting, the outpatient dialysis center, or the client's home. The functions are performed in response to machine programming that can be individualized for the client's specific needs. A typical prescription calls for 30-minute exchanges (10/10/10 for inflow, dwell, and outflow) for a period of 8 to 10 hours. The machines have numerous safety monitors and alarms and are relatively simple to learn to use.

APD has several distinct advantages. It permits the performance of in-home dialysis while the client sleeps, allowing him or her to be dialysis free during waking hours. Also, because the number of connections and disconnections are fewer with APD, the incidence of peritonitis has been reduced. Finally, APD provides a means by which increased volumes of dialysis solution can be administered to clients who require higher clearances (Levine, 1997).

INTERMITTENT PERITONEAL DIALYSIS. Intermittent peritoneal dialysis (IPD) combines the principles of an osmotic pressure gradient and true dialysis. The client usually requires exchanges of 2 L of dialysate at 30- to 60-minute intervals, allowing 15 to 20 minutes of drain time. For most anuric clients, 30 to 40 exchanges of 2 L three times weekly are sufficient. IPD treatments can be automated or manual.

CONTINUOUS-CYCLE PERITONEAL DIALYSIS. Continuous-cycle peritoneal dialysis (CCPD) also uses an automated cycling machine. Exchanges occur at night while the client sleeps. The final exchange of the night is left to dwell through the day and is drained the next evening as the process is repeated. CCPD offers the advantage of 24-hour dialysis, as in CAPD, but the sterile catheter system is less often violated.

COMPLICATIONS. Complications are possible with PD, but many can be treated or prevented with careful nursing care.

PERITONITIS. The major complication of PD is peritonitis. The most common cause of peritonitis is contamination of the connection site during an exchange. This infection of the peritoneum is manifested by cloudy dialysate outflow (effluent), fever, rebound abdominal tenderness, abdominal pain, general malaise, nausea, and vomiting.

When peritonitis is suspected, the nurse sends a specimen of the dialysate outflow for culture and sensitivity study, Gram stain, and cell count to identify the infecting organism so that an appropriate antibiotic can be ordered. Procedures for routine or periodic culturing of PD effluent vary with institutional practice. In today's era of cost containment, routine practices are less likely to be the norm. Cloudy or opaque effluent is the earliest sign of peritonitis. Thus nursing observations are key to the detection and identification of peritonitis. The best treatment of peritonitis is prevention. The nurse must maintain meticulous sterile technique when caring for the PD catheter and when hooking up or clamping off dialysate bags (Chart 72-11).

PAIN. Pain during the inflow of dialysate is common during the first few exchanges because of peritoneal irritation; however, it disappears after a week or two. Cold dialysate aggravates discomfort. Thus the dialysate bags should be warmed before instillation by use of a heating pad to wrap the bag or by use of the warming chamber of the automated cycling machine. *Microwave ovens are not recommended for the warming of dialysate because of their unpredictable warming patterns and temperatures.*

EXIT SITE AND TUNNEL INFECTIONS. The normal exit site from a PD catheter should be clean, dry, and without pain or evidence of inflammation. Exit site infections (ESIs) are associated with all types of PD catheters. Such infections can be difficult to treat and can become chronic. Exit site and tunnel infections cause increased morbidity, since they can lead to peritonitis, catheter failure, and hospitalization. Dialysate leakage and pulling or twisting of the catheter can predispose the client to ESIs. A Gram stain and culture should be performed when exit sites have purulent drainage.

Tunnel infections occur in the path of the catheter from the skin to the cuff. Signs of infection include redness, tenderness, and pain. ESIs are treated with antimicrobials; however, deep cuff infections usually require catheter removal.

CHART 72-11

BEST PRACTICE *for*
Caring for the Client with a Peritoneal Dialysis Catheter

- Mask yourself and your client. Wash your hands.
- Put on sterile gloves. Remove the old dressing. Remove the contaminated gloves.
- Assess the area for signs of infection, such as swelling, redness, or discharge around the catheter site.
- Use aseptic technique:
  Open the sterile field on a flat surface and place two precut 4 × 4 inch gauze pads on the field.
  Place three cotton swabs soaked in povidone-iodine on the field. Put on sterile gloves.
- Use cotton swabs to clean around the catheter site. Use a circular motion starting from the insertion site and moving away toward the abdomen. Repeat with all three swabs.
- Apply precut gauze pads over the catheter site. Tape only the edges of the gauze pads.

INSUFFICIENT FLOW OF THE DIALYSATE. Constipation is the primary cause of inflow or outflow problems. To prevent constipation, the physician orders a bowel preparation before placing the PD catheter. Colon evacuation before the initiation of PD may also prevent constipation. A high-fiber diet and stool softeners are often needed for ongoing prevention. Other causes of inflow or outflow difficulty include kinking or clamped connection tubing, the client's positioning, fibrin clot formation, and PD catheter migration.

Because outflow drainage is by gravity, the nurse ensures that the drainage bag is lower than the client's abdomen. The nurse inspects the connection tubing and PD system for kinking or twisting and rechecks to make sure that clamps are open. If inflow or outflow drainage is still inadequate, the nurse attempts to stimulate inflow or outflow by repositioning the client. Turning the client to the other side or making sure that he or she is in good body alignment may help. Having the client in a supine low-Fowler's position seems to minimize the buildup of intra-abdominal pressure. Increased intra-abdominal pressure that occurs in the sitting or standing position, or with coughing, contributes to leakage at the PD catheter site.

Fibrin clot formation may occur after PD catheter placement or with the onset of peritonitis. Careful milking of the tubing may dislodge the fibrin clot and facilitate inflow and outflow. Radiographic examination is needed to identify PD catheter migration out of the pelvic area. If migration has occurred, the physician repositions the PD catheter.

DIALYSATE LEAKAGE. When dialysis is initiated, small volumes of dialysate are used. It may take clients 1 to 2 weeks to tolerate a full 2-L exchange without leakage around the catheter site. Leakage tends to occur most often in obese or diabetic clients, older adults, and those on long-term steroid therapy (Levine, 1997). Dialysate leakage presents as clear fluid emitting from the catheter exit site. During this time, clients may require hemodialysis (HD) support.

OTHER COMPLICATIONS. The PD effluent (outflow drainage) is expected to be relatively clear and light yellow. The nurse notes any change in the color of the outflow. With the initial exchanges, the outflow may be bloody. The physician may order several in-and-out exchanges of unwarmed dialysis solution in an effort to clear the dialysate of blood. In these cases, the client's hematocrit, pulse, and blood pressure are closely monitored. If the drainage return is brown, a bowel perforation must be suspected. Similarly, if the outflow is the same color as urine and has the same glucose concentration, a possible bladder perforation should be investigated. If the drainage is cloudy or opaque, an infection is suspected.

NURSING CARE DURING PERITONEAL DIALYSIS. In the hospital setting, peritoneal dialysis (PD) is routinely initiated and monitored by the nursing staff. Before the treatment, the nurse evaluates baseline vital signs, including blood pressure, apical and radial pulse rates, temperature, quality of respirations, and breath sounds. The client is weighed, always on the same scale, before beginning the procedure and at least every 24 hours while receiving treatment. Baseline laboratory value determinations, such as electrolyte and glucose levels, are also essential and are repeated at least daily during the PD treatment.

During PD, the nurse continually monitors the client. Vital signs are taken regularly and recorded on a flow sheet. For the first few exchanges, the nurse records the vital signs every 15 minutes. The nurse also performs an ongoing assessment of the client for signs of respiratory distress, pain, or discomfort. The abdominal dressing around the catheter exit site is checked frequently for wetness. The nurse monitors dwell time and initiates outflow. The physician orders dwell time according to the client's needs for fluid removal and electrolyte balance.

For hourly exchanges, dwell time usually ranges from 20 to 40 minutes. Glucose absorption may occur in some clients, and blood glucose assessment is necessary. The outflow should be a continuous stream after the clamp is completely open. The total amount of outflow is recorded accurately after each exchange. Accurate inflow and outflow records are maintained when hourly PD exchanges are done. When outflow is less than inflow, the difference is equal to the amount absorbed or retained by the client during dialysis and should be counted as intake. For clients performing self-CAPD, or when the MB-CAPD system is used, a daily weight is used to monitor fluid status. A visual inspection of the outflow bag and daily weights may be sufficient to note the adequacy of the return.

RENAL TRANSPLANTATION

Dialysis and transplantation are life-sustaining treatments for end-stage renal disease (ESRD); transplantation is not considered a "cure." It is up to each client, in consultation with nephrology personnel, to determine which type of therapy is best suited to that client's physical condition and lifestyle. In 2001, 13,290 kidney transplants were performed. Currently, more than 48,000 people are awaiting renal transplantation in the United States alone (United Network for Organ Sharing [UNOS], 2001).

CANDIDATES. Candidates for transplantation must be free of medical problems that might increase the risks associated with the procedure. The usual age range for clients undergoing transplantation is 2 to 70 years of age. In clients older than 70 years of age, the risk of complications increases, but clients older than 70 years of age are considered on an individual basis. A thorough body systems assessment of the client is performed before the client is considered for transplantation (see the Legal/Ethical Issues in Health Care box at right). The process of transplantation can place a life-threatening stress on the cardiac system in clients with advanced, uncorrectable cardiac disease. Thus these clients are usually excluded from consideration for transplantation. Contraindications for transplantation include metastatic malignant neoplasms, chronic infection, severe cardiovascular disease unresponsive to treatment, and severe psychosocial problems such as chemical dependency (Bartucci, 1999). In addition, longstanding disease of the pulmonary system increases the risk of morbidity and mortality owing to respiratory tract infections after transplantation. Clients with diseases of the gastrointestinal (GI) system may require treatment before consideration for transplantation. Such problems as peptic ulcer and diverticulosis can be severely aggravated by the large doses of steroids used after transplantation.

The urinary system must be completely evaluated to ensure its ability to manage normal urine flow. Many clients with ESRD have not used their lower urinary tract for extended periods, and ureteral or bladder abnormalities may require surgical correction before renal transplantation.

Metabolic diseases, such as diabetes mellitus, gout, and hyperparathyroidism, cause even greater risks. These clients can still accept a renal transplant, but careful observation and management are necessary to limit complications. Other conditions that may complicate transplantation include malignant neoplasm and inflammatory disease. Clients with a recent history of a malignant tumor are usually treated with dialysis because of the shortage of donor organs, the possibility that the cancer could attack the transplanted kidney, and the limited life expectancy of these clients. In addition, the immunosuppressive agents used after transplantation increase the risk for cancer recurrence. If more than 2 to 5 years have passed since eradication of the cancer, the client can be considered for a transplant.

Other complicating conditions are considered on an individual basis, depending on the client's current health status. Renal transplantation can be considered for most of those with ESRD and may prove to be the optimal therapy for many people (see the Evidence-Based Practice for Nursing box on p. 1698).

DONORS. The sources of donor kidneys are living donors, non–heart-beating donors (NHBDs), and cadaveric donors. The available kidneys are matched on the basis of immunologic similarity between the donor and the recipient. Living donors are most often blood relatives, but in recent years, unrelated donors have been used. NHBDs are persons declared dead by cardiopulmonary criteria. Kidneys from NHBDs are harvested immediately after death in cases where clients have previously given consent for organ donation and

LEGAL/ETHICAL ISSUES IN HEALTH CARE

UNEQUAL ACCESS TO KIDNEY TRANSPLANTATION

There is evidence to suggest that individuals who are insured by Medicaid alone may not be placed on the kidney transplant waiting list. Medicare covers most, but not all, Americans with end-stage renal disease (ESRD). In a retrospective study of all California ESRD clients under 65 years of age who were eligible for Medicare or Medicaid, an analysis was done to determine the importance of health insurance status in relation to kidney transplantation.

The findings of this study suggest that placement on the kidney transplant waiting list is associated with insurance status. In California, clients undergoing dialysis who are ineligible for Medicare coverage are more likely to be poor, female, and members of a minority group. These individuals are also much less likely to be placed on a kidney transplant waiting list. However, once placed on the waiting list, insurance status does not affect access to cadaveric transplantation. It is possible that potential loss of insurance following transplantation, cultural barriers, and educational factors are explanatory factors.

Data from Thamer, M. et al. (1999). Unequal access to cadaveric kidney transplantation in California based on insurance status. *Health Services Research, 34*(4), 879-898.

EVIDENCE-BASED PRACTICE FOR NURSING

Does race or gender affect quality of life in nondiabetic kidney transplant recipients?

Johnson, C., et al. (1998). Racial and gender differences in quality of life following kidney transplantation. *Image: The Journal of Nursing Scholarship, 30*(2), 125-130.

The purpose of this descriptive, prospective clinical study was to determine if race or gender affected changes in quality of life (QOL) reported by nondiabetic kidney transplant recipients before transplantation and 6 and 12 months after transplantation. The convenience sample obtained for this study consisted of 90 subjects (63 men, 27 women), of whom 36 were African Americans and 55 were Caucasians ages 19 to 67 years. None of the subjects had a history of diabetes.

The Sickness Impact Profile (SIP), Ferrans and Powers Quality of Life Index (QLI), and Adult Self-Image Scales (ASIS) were administered to clients before transplantation and 6 months and 12 months after transplantation. The SIP was used to capture dimensions of QOL related to functional disability, the QLI was used to assess health-focused QOL, and the ASIS was used to determine the psychoemotional aspects of QOL.

QOL scores improved overall for both racial and gender groups after kidney transplantation. African Americans appeared to improve less than Caucasians in such areas as self-image and emotional behavior; however, they had higher baseline scores in these areas as compared with Caucasians. African Americans appeared to suffer more functional impairment before transplantation and demonstrated less improvement following transplantation as compared with Caucasians. Overall, women's scores on QOL measures tended to be lower than those of men.

Possible explanations for the racial differences observed in baseline functional status may relate to poorer socioeconomic status and less access to health care. The higher affective scores of African Americans may be related to spiritual factors. Whereas men seemed to regain independence and improved self-image after transplantation, women may have had more difficulty in adjusting to physical changes and the immunosuppressant regimen. The authors suggest that nurses should consider sociocultural influences and functional concerns of African Americans and women.

Critique. Quality of life has become an important consideration for many individuals in making health care decisions. It is also an important outcome in the evaluation of new therapies. The convenience sample makes it difficult to generalize the results to other kidney transplant recipients, particularly since the majority of transplants are performed on people with diabetes. In addition, the relatively higher baseline scores of the African Americans on the ASIS and QLI may have made comparing QOL scores between races unreliable. Additional studies are needed to lend support to these findings.

Implications for Nursing. Sociocultural and economic factors and gender need to be considered in preparing clients for transplant surgery. Nurses may need to design education interventions that prepare clients for what to expect and how to manage their differing recovery trajectories.

no longer seek active treatment or by in situ preservation in which a cool preservation solution is infused via a catheter inserted into the abdominal aorta after death is declared. Cadaveric donors are usually individuals who suffered irreversible brain injury, typically as a result of trauma. This type of donor must be maintained on a ventilator and have sufficient cardiovascular functioning in order for the kidneys to remain transplantable (Bartucci, 1999).

The size of the kidney is seldom a problem in adults. Pediatric cadaveric kidneys hypertrophy to accommodate adult needs within a few months.

Organs from living *related* donors (LRDs) provide the highest rates of renal graft survival (90%). Donors are usually at least 18 years old because of legal requirements and are seldom older than 65 years of age. General physical criteria for donors include the following:

- Absence of systemic disease and infection
- No history of cancer
- Absence of hypertension and renal disease
- Adequate renal function as evidenced by diagnostic studies

In addition, LRDs must express a clear understanding of the associated surgery and a willingness to give up a kidney. Some transplant centers also require a psychiatric evaluation to determine the motivation of the donor.

Because of advances in immunosuppressant therapy and medical management, the United Network of Organ Sharing (UNOS) reported 1-year renal transplant graft survival to be 90% for all centers in the United States (UNOS, 2001).

PREOPERATIVE CARE. Many issues must be decided before transplantation. Some issues are related to client health and others to the actual transplant procedure. The Clinical Pathway on pp. 1848-1851 highlights care needs for the client undergoing renal transplantation.

IMMUNOLOGIC STUDIES. The major barrier to successful renal transplantation after a suitable donor kidney is available is the body's ability to identify and reject tissue that is not its own. This immunologic process attacks the transplanted kidney and renders it nonfunctional. For immunologic contraindications to be overcome, in-depth tissue typing is done on all candidates for transplantation. These studies include simple ABO blood group typing for compatible blood transfusions and human leukocyte antigen (HLA) studies, as well as other tests. The HLAs have become the principal histocompatibility system used to match transplant recipients with compatible donors. The more similar the antigens of the donor are to those of the recipient, the more likely it is that the transplant will be successful and immunologic rejection will be avoided. Research is ongoing in immunology, and new information in this area could increase the success rate of organ transplantations in the future (see Chapter 20).

SURGICAL TEAM. The surgical team is a group of specialists trained in transplantation procedures. The team includes operating room nurses (circulating and scrub nurses), clinical nurse specialists, and preoperative nurses, as well as transplant surgeons, anesthesiologists, and nephrologists. The role of the preoperative nurse includes the following:

- Teaching about the procedure and postoperative care
- In-depth client assessment
- Coordination of diagnostic tests
- Development and implementation of treatment plans

The transplant recipient usually requires dialysis within 24 hours of the surgery. In addition, the recipient often receives a blood transfusion before surgery. Current research favors donor-specific transfusions, in which blood from the kidney donor is transfused into the recipient. This procedure has resulted in increased graft survival, especially of organs from LRDs.

OPERATIVE PROCEDURES. The donor nephrectomy procedure varies depending on whether the donor is an

NHBD, cadaveric donor, or living donor. The NHBD or cadaveric donor nephrectomy is conducted as a sterile autopsy in the operating room. All arterial and venous vessels and as long a piece of ureter as possible are carefully preserved. After removal, the kidneys are preserved until time for implantation into the recipient. The technique for kidney removal from living donors requires greater surgical care and is a delicate procedure lasting 3 to 4 hours. A flank incision is used, and care is taken to avoid scarring. Donors usually experience more pain than do recipients. They also need special nursing care and support for the psychologic adjustment to loss of a body part.

The transplantation surgery usually takes 4 to 5 hours. The transplanted kidney is usually placed in the right anterior iliac fossa (Figure 72-9) instead of the usual anatomic position. This placement allows easier anastomosis of the ureter and the renal artery and vein, and it also allows for assessment by palpation. The recipient's own nonfunctioning kidneys are not usually removed unless chronic infection in one or both kidneys would compromise overall recovery. The client is then taken to the postanesthesia unit and then, when stable, to a designated surgical unit in the transplant center or to a critical care unit.

POSTOPERATIVE CARE. Postoperative care of the kidney transplant recipient requires that nurses be knowledgeable about the expected clinical findings and potential complications unique to this population. Nursing care includes ongoing physical assessment with an emphasis on evaluation of renal function. The transplant recipient requires particularly close attention because the immunosuppressive drug therapy to prevent tissue rejection causes impaired healing and an increased susceptibility to infection. Careful urologic management is essential to graft success. These clients always have a large indwelling (Foley) catheter for accurate measurements of urine output and decompression of the bladder and to prevent stretch on suture and anastomosis sites on the bladder. An abrupt decrease in urine output is significant, since it can herald the onset of complications such as rejection, acute tubular necrosis (ATN), thrombosis, or obstruction. The urine color is carefully monitored (usually hourly). The urine is initially pink and bloody, but it gradually returns to normal over a period of several days to several weeks, depending on renal function. A continuous bladder irrigation is occasionally prescribed to decrease the formation of blood clots, which could increase pressure in the bladder and jeopardize the graft. Routine catheter care is performed to minimize contamination of the catheter; the nurse adheres to the agency's policy. The catheter is removed as soon as possible to avoid infection, usually 3 to 7 days postoperatively. The nurse is also responsible for obtaining daily urine tests, including urinalysis, glucose determinations, tests for the presence of acetone, culture, and specific gravity measurement.

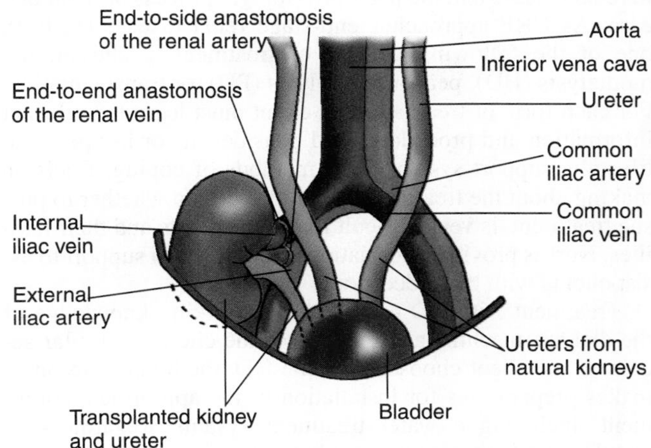

Figure 72-9 ● Placement of a transplanted kidney in the right iliac fossa.

During the postoperative period, the function of the transplanted kidney (renal graft) can result in either oliguria or diuresis. Oliguria may occur as a result of ischemia and ATN, rejection, or other complications. To increase urine output, the physician may order diuretics and osmotic agents, such as mannitol. The nurse and the physician carefully monitor the client's fluid status because fluid overload can cause hypertension, congestive heart failure (CHF), and pulmonary edema. Daily weight measurement, frequent blood pressure readings, and careful intake and output measurements are required to evaluate fluid status.

Instead of oliguria, the client may have diuresis, especially with a transplanted kidney from a living related donor (LRD). The nurse carefully monitors fluid intake and output and observes for electrolyte imbalances, such as hypokalemia and hyponatremia. Hypovolemia from excessive diuresis may cause hypotensive episodes. The nurse strives to prevent this situation because decreased blood pressure also decreases the oxygen and blood supply to the new kidney, which can threaten graft survival.

COMPLICATIONS. Unfortunately, numerous potential complications are associated with transplantation surgery.

REJECTION. The most common and the most threatening complication of renal transplantation is rejection. Rejection is the leading cause of graft loss. A reaction occurs between the antigens in the transplanted kidney and the antibodies and cytotoxic T-cells in the recipient's blood. These immunologic substances treat the new kidney as a foreign invader and cause tissue destruction, thrombosis, and eventual necrosis of the kidney. The three types of rejection are hyperacute, acute, and chronic. Acute rejection is the most common type in the transplant client. It is treated with increased immunosuppressive therapy and can be reversible. Rejection can be diagnosed by clinical manifestations, a renal scan, and renal biopsy. Table 72-12 summarizes the characteristics of the three types of rejection; Chapter 20 discusses their pathophysiology and treatment.

ACUTE TUBULAR NECROSIS. Prolonged preservation of cadaveric kidneys before transplantation can result in ischemic damage that is manifested as acute tubular necrosis (ATN). These clients usually need to be dialyzed until urine output becomes sufficient and the blood urea nitrogen (BUN) and creatinine normalize. Because ATN is often difficult to distinguish from acute rejection, clients need to undergo weekly biopsies to assess the need for further immunosuppression if rejection is occurring.

THROMBOSIS. Thrombosis may occur during the first 2 to 3 days following transplantation. A sudden decrease in

TABLE 72-12 • A COMPARISON OF HYPERACUTE, ACUTE, AND CHRONIC POST-TRANSPLANT REJECTION

Hyperacute Rejection	Acute Rejection	Chronic Rejection
ONSET		
Within 48 hr after surgery	1 wk to 2 yr postoperatively (most common in first 2 wk)	Occurs gradually during a period of months to years
CLINICAL MANIFESTATIONS		
Increased temperature Increased blood pressure Pain at transplant site	Oliguria or anuria Temperature over 100° F (37.8° C) Increased blood pressure Enlarged, tender kidney Lethargy Elevated serum creatinine, BUN, potassium levels Fluid retention	Gradual increase in BUN and serum creatinine levels Fluid retention Changes in serum electrolyte levels Fatigue
TREATMENT		
Immediate removal of the transplanted kidney	Increased doses of immunosuppressive drugs	Conservative management until dialysis is required

BUN, Blood urea nitrogen.

urine production or output may signal impaired perfusion resulting from thrombosis. Ultrasound examination of the kidney will reveal decreased or absent blood supply, and emergency surgery is required to prevent further ischemic damage or loss of the graft (Bartucci, 1999).

RENAL ARTERY STENOSIS. Stenosis of the renal artery is detected by identification of hypertension, a bruit over the artery anastomosis site, and decreased renal function. The involved artery must be surgically resected and the kidney anastomosed to another artery. Clients with vascular complications nearly always require surgical intervention. Other vascular problems include vascular leakage or thrombosis, both of which require an emergency transplant nephrectomy.

OTHER COMPLICATIONS. Other complications may involve the wound or genitourinary tract. Wound complications, such as hematomas, abscesses, and lymphoceles, can become a medium for infection and can place external pressure on the new kidney. Infection is a significant cause of morbidity and mortality in the transplant recipient. Prevention of infection is paramount. Strict aseptic technique and handwashing must be rigorously enforced. Because of immunosuppression, transplant recipients may not present with typical signs of infection. Low-grade fevers, mental status changes, and vague complaints of discomfort may be present before sepsis. Nurses play a pivotal role in the early detection of infection.

Genitourinary tract complications include ureteral leakage, fistula, or obstruction; calculus formation; bladder neck contracture; scrotal swelling; and graft rupture. Surgical intervention may be required.

IMMUNOSUPPRESSIVE DRUG THERAPY. The success of renal transplantation depends on changing the client's immunologic response so that the new kidney is not rejected as a foreign organ. The nurse administers and is aware of the immunosuppressive drugs that protect the transplanted organ. These drugs include corticosteroids, antilymphocyte preparations, monoclonal antibodies, and cyclosporine (Cyclosporin A). Chapter 20 discusses the mechanisms of action for these agents and the associated client responses. Clients who must take immunosuppressant medications are vulnerable to infection secondary to myelosuppression. Clients are at risk for developing a number of fatal viral, fungal, bacterial, or protozoal infections (Giuliano & Sims, 1999).

Community-Based Care

HOME CARE MANAGEMENT

Because of the complex nature of chronic renal failure (CRF), its progressive course, and multiple treatment modalities, a case manager may be useful in the planning, coordination, and evaluation of care. As the renal disease progresses, the client is seen by a physician or nurse practitioner regularly and may have frequent hospitalizations. The nurse, in conjunction with the dietitian and social worker, evaluates the home environment and determines special equipment needs before discharge. Once the client is discharged, home care nurses may direct care and monitor progress Chart 72-12 provides a focused assessment guideline for the client after renal transplantation.

The nurse provides ongoing health teaching about the diet in renal disease and the pathophysiologic process of renal disease. As CRF approaches end-stage renal disease (ESRD), one of the following courses of treatment is chosen: hemodialysis (HD), peritoneal dialysis (PD), or transplantation. For each form of treatment, the client must learn the relevant information and procedures and consider his or her personal lifestyle, support systems, and methods of coping. Decision making about the treatment modality, or even whether to pursue treatment, is very difficult for many clients and their families. Nurses provide information and emotional support to assist clients with these decisions.

Treatment with HD necessitates a working knowledge of the dialysis machine and the care of the client's vascular access. If the client chooses in-home HD, the home care nurse makes preparations for installation of the appropriate equipment, including a water treatment system. Regardless of whether the treatment is provided at home or in a center, the nurse provides ongoing physical assessment and health teaching to promote maximal independence at home.

CHART 72-12

FOCUSED ASSESSMENT *of* Home Care Clients with Chronic Renal Failure

Assess cardiovascular and respiratory status, including:
- Vital signs, with special attention to blood pressure
- Presence of S_3 and/or pericardial friction rub
- Presence of chest pain
- Presence of edema (periorbital, pretibial, sacral)
- Jugular vein distention
- Presence of dyspnea
- Presence of crackles, beginning at the bases and extending upward

Assess nutritional status, including:
- Weight gain or loss
- Presence of anorexia, nausea, or vomiting

Assess renal status, including:
- Amount, frequency, and appearance of urine (in nonanuric clients)
- Presence of bone pain
- Presence of hyperglycemia secondary to diabetes

Assess hematologic status, including
- Presence of petechiae, purpura, ecchymoses
- Presence of fatigue or shortness of breath

Assess gastrointestinal status, including:
- Presence of stomatitis
- Presence of melena

Assess integumentary status, including:
- Skin integrity
- Presence of pruritus
- Presence of skin discoloration

Assess neurologic status, including
- Changes in mental status
- Presence of seizure activity
- Presence of sensory changes
- Presence of lower extremity weakness

Assess laboratory data, including:
- BUN
- Serum creatinine
- Creatinine clearance
- CBC
- Electrolytes

Assess psychosocial status, including:
- Presence of anxiety
- Presence of maladaptive behavior

BUN, Blood urea nitrogen; *CBC,* complete blood count.

The client receiving PD needs extensive training in the procedure. The client also needs assistance in obtaining equipment and the numerous supplies involved. Home care nurses perform physical assessments, monitor vital signs, assess compliance with drug and diet regimens, and carefully monitor for signs and symptoms of peritonitis.

The nurse plays a vital role in the long-term care of the client with a renal transplant. This client is usually discharged 3 to 4 weeks after surgery. Meticulous maintenance of prescribed immunosuppressive drug therapy is essential for the survival of the renal graft. Thus the nurse facilitates acceptance and understanding of this regimen as a part of daily life. The nurse also carefully monitors for signs of graft rejection and for complications, such as infection.

HEALTH TEACHING

Health teaching is a primary function of nurses caring for clients with any form of renal disease. The home care nurse collaborates with other members of the health care team, especially the dietitian, pharmacist, and physician, to instruct clients and family members or significant others in all aspects of diet therapy, necessary drug therapy, and associated renal pathologic changes. Clients and family members are taught to report signs and symptoms of complications, such as fluid overload and infection. When a client requires a more advanced form of therapy, such as dialysis or transplantation, the teaching focuses on the chosen therapeutic intervention.

HD is the most complex form of therapy for the client and family to understand. Even if clients receive HD in a dialysis center instead of at home, they are usually expected to have some knowledge of the HD machine. The client or a family member or other caregiver must be taught to care for the vascular access and to report signs of infection and stenosis. The client who plans to have in-home HD will need a partner. Both the client and the partner must be completely educated in the entire process of HD and must be able to perform it independently before the client is discharged from the HD center or hospital HD unit.

PD involves extensive health teaching. This instruction can be given to the client alone or to the client and a family member or other caregiver if the client cannot perform the procedure. The nurse emphasizes sterile technique because peritonitis is the most common complication of PD performed at home. The nurse instructs clients to report the signs and symptoms associated with peritonitis. They should report the presence of cloudy effluent and abdominal pain, especially when accompanied by rebound tenderness. Clients are taught that cloudy effluent needs to be analyzed promptly. A specimen is sent by the home care nurse for culture and sensitivity, cell count, and Gram stain to identify the causative organism. Clients are taught that peritonitis is treated with antimicrobial therapy, usually given by the intraperitoneal (IP) route. To prevent peritonitis, they are taught how breaks in aseptic technique can occur, resulting in peritonitis. In addition, to eradicate the infection, nurses must educate clients about the importance of completing the antibiotic regimen. Nurses need to teach that repeated episodes of peritonitis can result in diminished ultrafiltration capability, which may necessitate transfer to HD.

The client receiving a renal transplant also needs extensive health teaching. The nurse provides instruction about drug regimens, home monitoring, immunosuppression, signs and symptoms of rejection, infection, and prescribed changes in the diet and activity level.

PSYCHOSOCIAL PREPARATION

The nurse provides psychologic support for the client and family or significant others. The nurse facilitates the client's adjustment to the diagnosis of renal failure and eventual acceptance of the treatment regimens.

For many clients, the reduction of uremic symptoms in the initial weeks and months of dialysis treatment creates a sense of euphoria and well-being (the "honeymoon" period). They feel better physically, their mood may be happy and hopeful, and they tend to overlook the inconvenience and discomfort of frequent dialysis treatments. The nurse realizes that this mood is temporary and uses the time to initiate health care teaching. The nurse stresses that although the client's uremic symptoms have diminished, the client will not return completely to the previous state of well-being. The client and the family may have looked on dialysis as a cure instead of a required lifelong treatment.

Many clients enter a phase of discouragement and disillusionment sometime during the first year of treatment; this may last a few months to a year or longer. The difficulties of incorporating dialysis into daily life are staggering, and clients often become disappointed and depressed as the problems become apparent. During this time, they may struggle against the idea of having to be permanently dependent on a disruptive therapy. The fear of rejection by health staff and family members or significant others reinforces feelings of helplessness and dependence. Some people retreat into complete or partial denial of the disease and the need for treatment. They may deny the need for dialysis or may not comply with medication administration and dietary restrictions. Nurses who work with these clients need to monitor any maladaptive behaviors that may contribute to noncompliance and suggest psychiatric referrals. Nurses and family members should focus on the positive aspects of the treatments. The nurse continues health care education with clients as active participants and decision makers.

Most clients with chronic renal failure (CRF) eventually enter a phase of acceptance or, at least, resolution. The prospect of a chronic illness may be devastating for some people, and each person reacts differently. To make this long-term adaptation, the client must adjust to continuous change, but specific concerns depend on the current physical status and particular treatment method.

After clients have accepted or become resigned to the chronicity of their disease, they usually attempt to return to their previous activities. Resuming the previous level of activity, however, may not be possible. The nurse and other health care professionals can help clients to establish realistic goals that allow them to lead active, productive lives.

HEALTH CARE RESOURCES

Professionals from various disciplines are valuable resources for the client with renal failure. Home care nurses are often required to monitor the client's status and evaluate maintenance of the prescribed treatment regimen (HD or PD). A client with advanced renal failure may need the assistance of a home care aide in performing the activities of daily living. Social services personnel are usually involved because of the complex process of applying for financial aid to pay for the required medical care (see the Cost of Care box above). To increase the functional capacity of the client, a physical therapist may be beneficial. Consultation with a dietitian will assist the client and family members in understanding the special dietary needs. A psychiatric evaluation may be needed to assist with depressive symptoms and maladjustment. Clergy and pastoral care specialists offer spiritual support.

Clients with CRF are routinely observed by a physician, usually a nephrologist. Such organizations as the National Kidney Foundation (NKF), the American Kidney Fund, and the National Association of Patients on Hemodialysis and Transplantation (NAPHT) may be helpful to clients and families.

Evaluation: Outcomes

NOC The nurse evaluates the care of the client with chronic renal failure (CRF) on the basis of the identified nursing diagnoses and collaborative problems. The expected outcomes are that the client will:

- Achieve and maintain appropriate fluid volume
- Maintain serum electrolyte levels in expected ranges

COST OF CARE / IMPLICATIONS FOR NURSING

ECONOMIC COST OF END-STAGE RENAL DISEASE

Cost of Care

- Public and private funds totaling $15.6 billion were spent in the treatment of ESRD in 1997.
- Payments to skilled nursing facilities, home care, and hospice for the care of individuals with ESRD account for 6.3% of total costs.
- Medicare spending for the care of individuals with ESRD from 1993 to 1997 totaled $44.93 billion.
- Medicare payments for kidney donor acquisitions are estimated to be $25,000 per acquisition.
- Health maintenance organizations (HMO) payments for the treatment of clients with ESRD average approximately $1438 to $2040 per month.

Implications for Nursing

ESRD has increased steadily since 1993. The chronic nature of the disease, with its relatively high morbidity and mortality rates, suggests a role for nurses in the prevention of renal impairment through rigorous teaching and follow-up of clients with diabetes and hypertension. Teaching efforts by nurses should also target those already diagnosed with the disease to prevent further decline to kidney function.

Data from U.S. Renal Data Systems. (1999). *USRDS 1999 annual data report.* Bethesda, MD: National Institutes of Health, National Institute of Diabetes and Digestive and Kidney Diseases.
ESRD, End-stage renal disease.

- Maintain heart rate and blood pressure in expected ranges
- Comply with the prescribed dietary regimen
- Maintain an adequate nutritional status
- Seek information to reduce anxiety
- Use effective coping strategies
- Report an absence of physical manifestations of anxiety

ONLINE RESOURCES

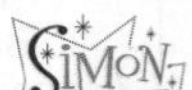

For suggested readings and Internet resources, go to http://www.wbsaunders.com/SIMON/Iggy/.

SELECTED BIBLIOGRAPHY

Asterisk indicates a classic or definitive work on this subject.

Baer, C. (1998). Care of the critically ill chronic renal failure patient: Crisis, challenges and choices. *Critical Care Nursing Clinics of North America, 10*(4), 433-448.

Baker, J., & Thomas, A. (2001). Progressive renal insufficiency program planning: A technique for evaluation and improvement. *Nephrology Nursing Journal, 28*(1), 13-18.

Bartucci, M.R. (1999). Kidney transplantation: State of the art. *AACN Clinical Issues: Advanced Practice in Acute and Critical Care, 10*(2), 153-163.

Behrens, J. (2001). Assessing anemia secondary to hemolysis in hemodialysis patients. *Nephrology Nursing Journal, 28*(2), 253-258.

Bonventre, J. (1998). Ischemic acute renal failure. In J.L. Jameson (Ed.), *Principles of molecular medicine* (pp. 651-657). Totowa, N.J.: Humana Press.

Brundage, D., & Linton, A.D. (1997). Age-related changes in the genitourinary system. In M.A. Matteson, E.S. McConnell, & A.D. Linton (Eds.), *Gerontological nursing: Concepts and practice* (2nd ed., pp. 342-343). Philadelphia: W.B. Saunders.

Craig, M. (1998). Continuous venous to venous hemofiltration. Implementing and maintaining a program: Examples and alternatives. *Critical Care Clinics of North America, 10*(2), 219-233.

Curtin, R.B., Svarstad, B., & Keller, T. (1999). Hemodialysis patients' noncompliance with oral medications. *ANNA Journal, 26*(3), 307-316.

Giuliano, K., & Pysznik, E. (1998). Renal replacement therapy in critical care: Implementation of a unit-based continuous venovenous hemodialysis program. *Critical Care Nurse, 18*(1), 40-51.

Giuliano, K., & Sims, T.W. (1999). Transplant issues: Infections and immunosuppressant drugs. *Dimensions of Critical Care Nursing, 18*(2), 16-19.

Hayes, D. (2000). Caring for your patient with a permanent renal dialysis access. *Nursing2000, 30*(3), 41-46.

Johnson, C., et al. (1998). Racial and gender differences in quality of life following kidney transplantation. *Image: The Journal of Nursing Scholarship, 30*(2), 125-130.

Johnson, J., & Lalonde, R. (1997). Congestive heart failure. In J.T. Dipiro et al. (Eds.), *Pharmacotherapy: A pathophysiologic approach* (3rd ed., pp. 219-256). New York: McGraw-Hill.

Kearney, K. (2000). Dialysis disequilibrium syndrome. *American Journal of Nursing, 100*(2), 53-54.

Kellum, J. (2000). An evaluation of pharmacological strategies for the prevention and treatment of acute renal failure. *Drugs, 59*(1), 79-91.

Kelly, M. (1997). Acute renal failure. *American Journal of Nursing, 97*(3), 32-34.

King, B. (2000). Meds and the dialysis patient. *RN, 63*(7), 54-59.

Kuhlmann, M.K., Schmidt, F., & Kohler, H. (1999). High protein/energy vs. standard protein: Energy nutritional regimen in the treatment of malnourished hemodialysis patients. *Mineral and Electrolyte Metabolism, 25*(4-6), 306-310.

Levine, D.Z. (1997). *Caring for the renal patient* (3rd ed.). Philadelphia: W.B. Saunders.

McAlpine, L. (1998a). CAVH: Principles and practical applications. *Critical Care Nursing Clinics of North America, 10*(2), 179-189.

McAlpine, L. (1998b). CAVHD: Transitioning from CAVH. *Critical Care Nursing Clinics of North America, 10*(2), 191-195.

Mehrotra, R., & Nolph, K.D. (1999). Low protein diets are not needed in chronic renal failure. *Mineral and Electrolyte Metabolism, 25*(4-6), 311-316.

Mehta, R., & Letteri, J. (1997). Current status of renal replacement therapy for acute renal failure: A survey of US nephrologists. The National Kidney Foundation Council on Dialysis. *American Journal of Nephrology, 19*(3), 377-382.

Orias, M., Mahnensmith, R., & Perazella, M. (1999). Extreme hyperphosphatemia and acute renal failure after a phosphorus-containing bowel regimen. *American Journal of Nephrology, 19*(1), 60-63.

Politoski, G., et al. (1998). Continuous renal replacement therapy, *Critical Care Nursing Clinics of North America, 10*(2), 171-177.

Ray, T. (2000). Chronic and acute renal failure: Primary care issues. *ADVANCE for Nurse Practitioners, 8*(8), 69-72.

Sehgal, A.R. (2000). Outcomes of renal replacement therapy among blacks and women. *American Journal of Kidney Diseases, 35*(4 Suppl. 1), S148-S152.

Sosa-Guerrero, S., & Gomez, N. (1997). Dealing with end-stage renal disease. *American Journal of Nursing, 97*(10), 44-50.

Stark, J. (1998a). Acute renal failure: Focus on advances in acute tubular necrosis. *Critical Care Nursing Clinics of North America, 10*(2), 159-170.

Stark, J. (1998b). The interrelationship between renal and cardiac function. *Critical Care Clinics of North America, 10*(4), 411-419.

Thamer, M., et al. (1999). Unequal access to cadaveric kidney transplantation in California based on insurance status. *Health Services Research, 34*(4), 879-900.

Tran, M., & Rutecki, G. (2000). Renal disease: Tips on prevention and early recognition. *Consultant, 40*(2), 222-229.

United Network for Organ Sharing online. (2001). http://www.unos.org.

U.S. Renal Data Systems. (1999). *USRDS 1999 annual data report.* Bethesda, MD: National Institutes of Health, National Institute of Diabetes and Digestive and Kidney Diseases.

Wade-Elliott, R. (1999). Caring for the elderly with renal failure: Gastrointestinal changes. *ANNA Journal, 26*(6), 563-569.

White, V. (1997). Hyperkalemia. *American Journal of Nursing, 97*(6), 35.

Zellner, K. (1999). Acute tubular necrosis. *RN, 62*(2), 42-45.

UNIT

16

PROBLEMS OF REPRODUCTION

Management of Clients with Problems of the Reproductive System

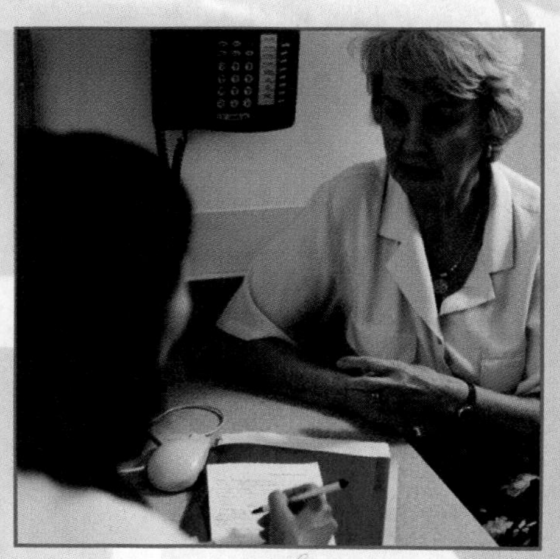

PROBLEMS OF REPRODUCTION ■ Core Concepts Grid

Anatomy	Physiology	Pathophysiology	History	Physical Exam	Diagnostic Tests	Interventions	Pharmacology
• **Female** Ovaries Fallopian tubes Uterus Vagina • **Male** Penis Scrotum Testes Ducts • **Breasts**	• **Procreation** • **Nurturing** • **Sexual pleasure** • **Urinary elimination**	• **Infection** • **Obstruction** • **Inflammation** • **Tumors**	• **Client history** Past problems Contraceptives Obstetric history Self-examination Breast Testes Difficult/painful urination Menstrual history Erectile dysfunction Renal/endocrine dysfunction Hypertension • **Family history** Cancer Thyroid Diabetes • **Social history** Sexual history Alcohol use Smoking Exposure to sexually transmitted disease (STDs) Age Race	• **Skin/hair distribution** • **Skin ulceration/ rashes/color** • **Discharge** Vagina Penis Nipple • **Hernia** • **Breasts** Size Shape Masses	• **Mammography** • **Ultrasonography** • **Pap smear** • **Estrogen levels** • **Androgen levels** • **Venereal Disease Research Laboratory (VDRL) test** • **Fluorescent Treponemal Antibody Absorption (FTA-ABS) test** • **Gram stain** • **Acid phosphate** • **Prostate-specific antigen (PSA)** • **Carcinoembryonic antigen (CEA)**	• **Radiation therapy** • **Client education** Self-examination Breast Testes Safer sex Hormone replacement therapy (HRT) Kegel exercises • **Bladder irrigations** • **Urinary catheter care** Foley (3-way) Suprapubic • **Penile implants** • **Postoperative care and monitoring for complications (e.g., hemmorrhage)** • **Sperm banking** • **Emotional support** • **Health teaching**	• **Antibiotics** • **Antivirals** • **Antiprotozoals** • **Antifungals** • **Hormone replacement therapy** • **Anti-impotence agents** • **Chemotherapeutic agents**

CHAPTER 73

Assessment of the Reproductive System

DEITRA L. LOWDERMILK

Learning Objectives

After studying this chapter, you should be able to:

1. Review the anatomy and physiology of the reproductive system.
2. Discuss the components of a health history for reproductive health problems using Gordon's Functional Health Patterns.
3. Interpret common reproductive diagnostic tests.
4. Describe the client preparation for common reproductive diagnostic tests.
5. Develop a teaching plan for clients undergoing endoscopic studies for reproductive health problems.
6. Explain the importance of selected reproductive tests in promoting and maintaining health (e.g., mammogram).

SIMON

Go to http://www.wbsaunders.com/SIMON/Iggy/ for self-assessment questions related to these Learning Objectives.

The nurse is often the first health care professional to assess the client with a reproductive system disorder. Basic assessment of the male and female reproductive systems should be part of every complete physical examination. The nurse should be comfortable with his or her sexuality and be nonjudgmental about variations in sexual practices.

This chapter describes basic reproductive system assessment. Chapters 74 and 76 provide additional assessment data. The student is also referred to a fundamentals or basic nursing text for information on human sexuality.

ANATOMY AND PHYSIOLOGY REVIEW

Structure and Function of the Female Reproductive System

Females begin to develop secondary sex characteristics at a wide range of ages. The average age for a girl to begin pubertal development is 11 years. Delayed puberty may be caused by the following:

- A familial history of late growth
- A low percentage of body fat
- Abnormalities of the pituitary gland, ovaries, or hypothalamus
- Congenital structural abnormalities

EXTERNAL GENITALIA

The external female genitalia, or **vulva,** extends from the mons pubis to the anal opening. The mons pubis is a fat pad that covers the symphysis pubis and protects it during coitus (sexual intercourse). The mons becomes prominent and covered with hair during puberty.

The **labia majora** are two vertical folds of adipose tissue that extend posteriorly from the mons pubis to the perineum. Because fatty tissue deposits vary among individuals, the size of the labia majora varies. The skin over the labia majora is usually darker than the surrounding skin and is highly vascular. The labia become prominent during puberty and develop hair on the outer surfaces. The labia majora protect inner vulval structures and enhance sexual arousal.

The labia majora surround two thinner, vertical folds of reddish epithelium called the **labia minora.** The labia minora are highly vascular and have a rich nerve supply. Emotional or physical stimulation produces marked swelling and sensitivity. Numerous sebaceous glands in the labia minora lubricate the entrance to the vagina.

Anteriorly, the labia minora form the prepuce (the hood of the clitoris) and the frenulum (a fold connecting the undersurface of the clitoris with the labia minora). Posteriorly, the labia minora join to form a thin, flat tissue called the fourchette. The clitoris is a small, cylindric organ located beneath the prepuce that is composed of erectile tissue with a high concentration of sensory nerve endings. During sexual arousal, the clitoris becomes larger and increases sexual sensation.

The vestibule is a longitudinal area between the labia minora, the clitoris, and the fourchette. This area contains Bartholin's glands and the openings of the urethra, Skene's glands (paraurethral glands), and vagina. The two Bartholin's glands, located deeply posterior on both sides of the vaginal opening, secrete lubrication fluid during sexual excitement. Their ductal openings are usually not visible.

The connective tissue that partly or wholly occludes the vaginal opening in the vestibule is called the hymen. The hymen can tear during strenuous exercise, masturbation, coitus, or tampon insertion.

The area between the fourchette and the anus is the perineum. The skin of the perineum covers the muscles, fascia, and ligaments that support the pelvic structures and provide voluntary control of the vagina and of the urinary and anal sphincters.

INTERNAL GENITALIA

The internal female genitalia are shown in Figure 73-1.

Vagina

The **vagina** is a collapsible hollow tube that extends from the vestibule to the uterus. In addition to being the channel for the passage of the menstrual flow, the vagina allows reception of the penis during intercourse and passage of the fetus during a vaginal birth. Squamous epithelium and abundant blood vessels line the thin, muscular vaginal walls of the vagina that lie in transverse folds (rugae) during the reproductive years and are highly distensible (stretchable). Estrogen deprivation occurring during postpartum periods, lactation, and menopause causes the vaginal wall to become dry and thinner and the rugae to become smoother. There are few sensory nerve endings in the lower vaginal segment.

The amounts of glycogen and lubricating fluid secreted by the vaginal epithelium are influenced by ovarian hormones. Döderlein's bacilli, the normal vaginal flora, interact with the secreted glycogen to produce lactic acid and maintain an acidic pH (4 to 5) in the vagina. This acidity reduces the vagina's susceptibility to infection.

At the upper end of the vagina, the uterine cervix projects into a cup-shaped vault of thin vaginal tissue. The recessed pockets around the cervix (the fornices) permit palpation of the internal pelvic organs. The posterior area is clinically significant because it provides access into the peritoneal cavity (through Douglas' cul-de-sac) for diagnostic or surgical purposes.

Uterus

The **uterus** is a thick-walled, muscular organ attached to the upper end of the vagina. This inverted pear–shaped organ is located within the true pelvis, between the bladder and the rectum. The uterus is composed of the corpus (body) and the cervix; these areas are separated by a constricted region called the isthmus. Functionally, the uterus responds to hormonal stimulation and prepares to receive, nurture and, finally, expel the products of conception.

The size of the uterus depends on the woman's developmental stage and obstetric history. In women who have never been pregnant, the average uterine dimensions are 3½ inches × 2 inches × 1 inch (7.5 cm × 5 cm × 2.5 cm).

CORPUS

The upper segment of the uterine body, between the insertion sites of the fallopian tubes, is referred to as the fundus. Although the uterus is a hollow organ, its walls are in such close proximity in the nonpregnant state that its cavity is merely a

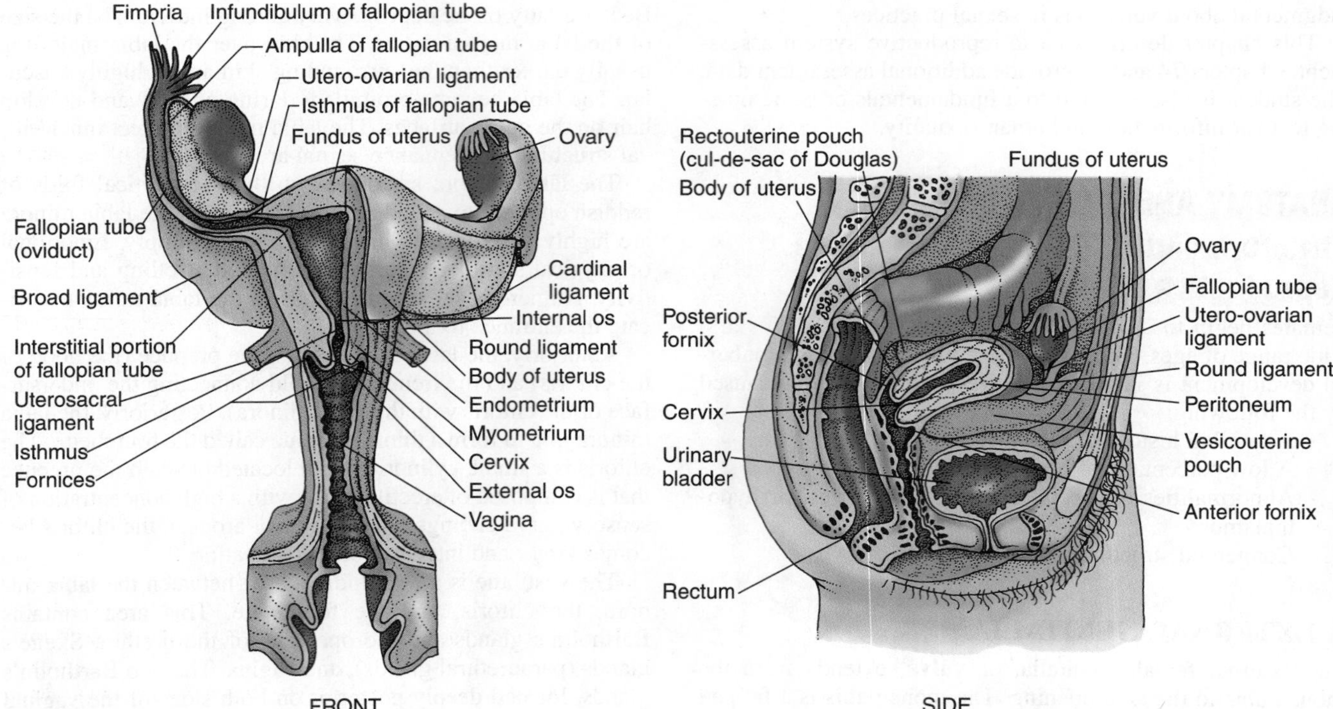

Figure 73-1 ● Internal female genitalia.

slit. The uterine walls are composed of three layers: the peritoneum, the myometrium, and the endometrium.

The peritoneum is the outer layer that separates the uterus from the abdominal cavity. The pouch formed by the peritoneum, where it lines the anterior uterus and extends to the top of the bladder, is called the vesicouterine pouch. The rectouterine pouch (also referred to as Douglas' cul-de-sac or the posterior cul-de-sac) is the posterior peritoneal pocket, between the rectum and the posterior uterine and vaginal walls.

The myometrium is the thick middle layer of the body of the uterus and is made up of three layers of smooth muscle fibers. These muscle fibers are arranged in opposing directions and are interlaced with blood vessels. Contraction of these muscle fibers can expel the products of conception and can constrict the blood vessels to control bleeding after childbirth.

The inner mucosal layer of the uterine body is the endometrium. The cyclic activity of estrogen and progesterone produces great variation in the thickness of this tissue (from 0.5 to 5 mm). The endometrium consists of a single layer of epithelial cells that cover tubular uterine glands, a spongy stroma (connective tissue framework), and a vascular network. The uterine glands secrete an alkaline fluid that keeps the cavity moist. All but the deepest layer of endometrium is shed during menses and after the delivery of a fetus.

CERVIX

The **cervix** lies below the isthmus of the uterus and extends into the vagina. The cervix provides a canal for the entry of sperm into the uterus and for the passage of menstrual flow, secretes mucus; it also provides a barrier to ascending vaginal bacteria. In addition, sphincter-like fibers that comprise the cervix hold the products of conception in the uterine cavity or stretch to permit vaginal birth.

The cervical portion of the uterus is approximately 1 inch (2.5 cm) long. The upper boundary is the internal os. The lower boundary, the external os, projects into the vaginal fornix. In the nonpregnant woman, the cervix around the external os is usually smooth, firm, and pink. A woman who has borne a child has a small, transverse, slitlike external os. A woman who has not had a child has a circular os. The endocervical canal connects the internal os with the external os and provides access from the vagina to the uterine cavity.

The outer cervix is covered with squamous epithelium, whereas the inner cervix is covered with columnar epithelium. These two types of cells meet at the squamocolumnar junction, which is usually located inside the cervical os. This is the site for Papanicolaou testing (see the later discussion on p. 1721).

CONNECTIVE TISSUE SUPPORT

The uterus is supported by the broad, round, uterosacral, and cardinal ligaments and by the muscles of the pelvic floor (see Figure 73-1).

Fallopian Tubes

The **fallopian tubes** (uterine tubes) insert into the fundus of the uterus and extend laterally to a site near the ovaries. Functionally, the uterine tubes provide a duct between the ovaries and the uterus for the passage of ova and sperm. In most cases, the ovum is fertilized in these tubes.

Each tube is about 3⅛ to 5½ inches (8 to 14 cm) long and is covered by one of the peritoneal folds of the broad ligament. The tubes are lined with longitudinal folds of ciliated and secretory columnar epithelial cells. Rhythmic contractions of the musculature of the tubes vary in response to the ovarian cycle. The tubal contractions and the current produced by the movement of cilia transport the ovum to the uterus.

The uterine tubes are divided into four anatomic sections (see Figure 73-1). The interstitial portion is the most proximal to the uterus, the isthmus and the ampulla are the middle segments, and the infundibulum is the most distal portion.

The fimbriated ends of the infundibulum extend almost to each ovary and facilitate the capture of a released ovum during ovulation.

Ovaries

The **ovaries** are a pair of almond-shaped organs situated near the lateral walls of the upper pelvic cavity. They are approximately ⅛ inch x ⅞ inch x ⅜ inch (0.3 cm x 2 cm x 1 cm) but are significantly smaller after menopause. Functionally, these small organs develop and release ova. The cyclic maturation of a dominant follicle (the graafian follicle) and the subsequent release of the ovum is referred to as ovulation. The ovaries also produce the sex steroid hormones (estrogen, progesterone, androgen, and relaxin). Adequate amounts of these steroidal sex hormones are necessary for normal female growth and development and for the maintenance of a pregnancy.

Breasts

The female breasts are a pair of mammary glands that develop in response to secretions from the hypothalamus, pituitary gland, and ovaries. Functionally, the breasts are an accessory of the reproductive system meant to nourish the infant after birth. They also function as an organ for sexual arousal in the mature adult.

The breasts are located between the second and sixth ribs, between the edge of the sternum and the midaxillary line. About two thirds of the breast diameter is over the greater pectoral muscle, and one third is superficial to the anterior serratus muscle.

STRUCTURE

The structure of a mature female breast is shown in Figure 73-2. The nipple rises from the center of the pigmented areola, which is usually located slightly lateral to the midline of each breast. Montgomery's glands are small, round sebaceous glands that appear as elevations on the areola. These glands are thought to secrete a fatty substance that protects the nipple during breastfeeding.

Breast tissue is composed of a network of glandular and ductal tissue, fibrous tissue, and fat. The proportion of each component of breast tissue depends on genetic factors, nutrition, age, and obstetric history. The breast is supported by Cooper's suspensory ligaments that are attached to underlying muscles.

The breasts may not develop symmetrically during puberty but are usually symmetric in size and contour by adulthood. It is not unusual for the breast on the woman's dominant side (on

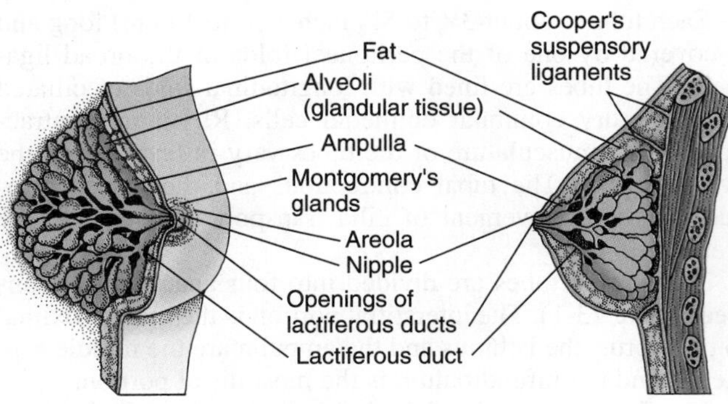

Figure 73-2 ● Structure of the mature female breast.

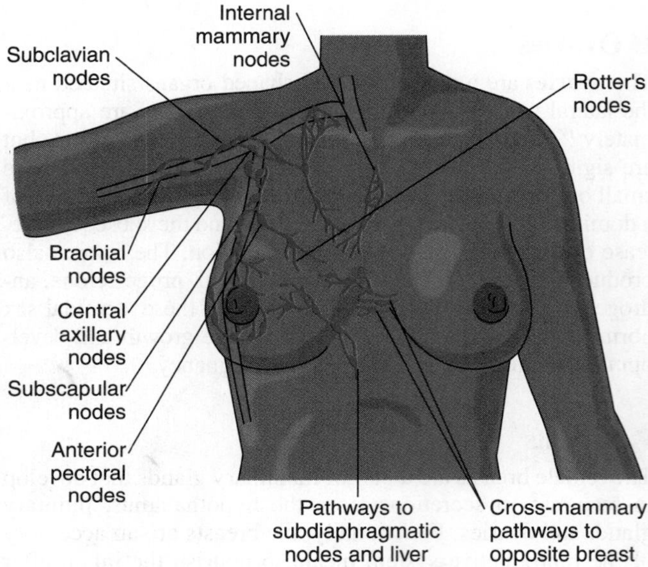

Figure 73-3 ● Lymphatic drainage of the female breast.

the basis of right-handedness or left-handedness) to appear larger because of the more developed pectoral muscle base.

In many women the breasts become slightly larger and tender during the premenstrual period. The tissue may also feel nodular at this time. Increasing levels of estrogen and progesterone 3 to 4 days before menses affect the breasts by increasing vascularity, inducing the growth of the ducts and alveoli, and promoting water retention.

BLOOD SUPPLY

The abundant blood supply to the breasts comes from branches of the internal mammary and lateral thoracic arteries. The veins of the breast connect with the superior vena cava. Much of the lymph drains through an extensive network that is radial to the axilla (Figure 73-3).

Menstruation and Menopause

NORMAL MENSTRUAL CYCLE

Menstruation is the cyclic shedding of the endometrial lining of the uterus. The term *menarche* refers specifically to the female's first menstruation and is one sign of puberty. Most girls begin to menstruate between 10 and 16 years of age.

The occurrence of cyclic menstruation and reproduction depends on maturation of the hypothalamic-pituitary-ovarian-uterine axis. Normally this cycle is not achieved for the first 1 to 2 years after menarche. The first menstrual cycles are typically anovulatory and irregular.

The menstrual cycle is under a feedback control system of three interrelated cycles:

- The hypothalamic-pituitary cycle
- The ovarian cycle
- The uterine (or endometrial) cycle

The relationship of these cycles is illustrated in Figure 73-4.

The idealized menstrual cycle is 28 days, but variations are normal. The first day of the menstrual cycle is calculated as the first day of monthly menstrual bleeding. The menstrual flow is referred to as the menses. Ovulation occurs approximately 14 days before the beginning of the next menstrual cycle. Regular menstrual cycles indicate normal sex hormone production and the occurrence of ovulation. Variations in the length of the menstrual cycle occur in response to variations in the length of the preovulatory stage compared with the postovulatory stage.

MENOPAUSE AND THE CLIMACTERIC

Natural Menopause

Menopause is the biologic end of reproductive ability, but the term applies to only the last menstrual period. The actual date of menopause cannot be determined until at least 1 year has passed without menses. The phase of a woman's life from the initial decline in the amount of estrogen produced by the ovaries to the cessation of symptoms produced by this phenomenon is called the *climacteric.* Lay terminology for this phase is "the change of life." Menopause is only one sign of the climacteric.

The follicles in the ovary atrophy continuously during a woman's life span. The progressive decline in the number of follicles that can produce estrogen in response to pituitary hormones causes the woman (usually between 40 and 50 years of age) to begin to notice physical changes in her body. Levels of estrogen and progesterone diminish gradually until the effect of these hormones on the endometrial lining of the uterus ceases. At the same time, the low levels of the ovarian hormones continue to stimulate the hypothalamic-pituitary axis. The anterior pituitary secretes high levels of follicle-stimulating hormone (FSH) and luteinizing hormone (LH) after menopause.

For a time, the inner core of the ovary produces androstenedione (a weak male hormone) and testosterone. Eighty percent of the androstenedione is produced by the adrenal glands. When the ovarian core ceases to function, the adrenal cortices are the only source of steroids. The production of androstenedione is significant, especially after menopause, because it is converted to a form of estrogen (estrone) in body fat. Consequently, women with a greater percentage of body fat have higher estrone levels after menopause.

During the climacteric, a woman experiences irregular menstrual and ovarian cycles. Ovulation often fails to occur. The menstrual flow may be lighter or heavier during these irregular cycles.

Decreased amounts of estrogen affect sites in the body other than the reproductive system, such as bone density and cardiovascular function. The uterus, cervix, ovaries, labia, and

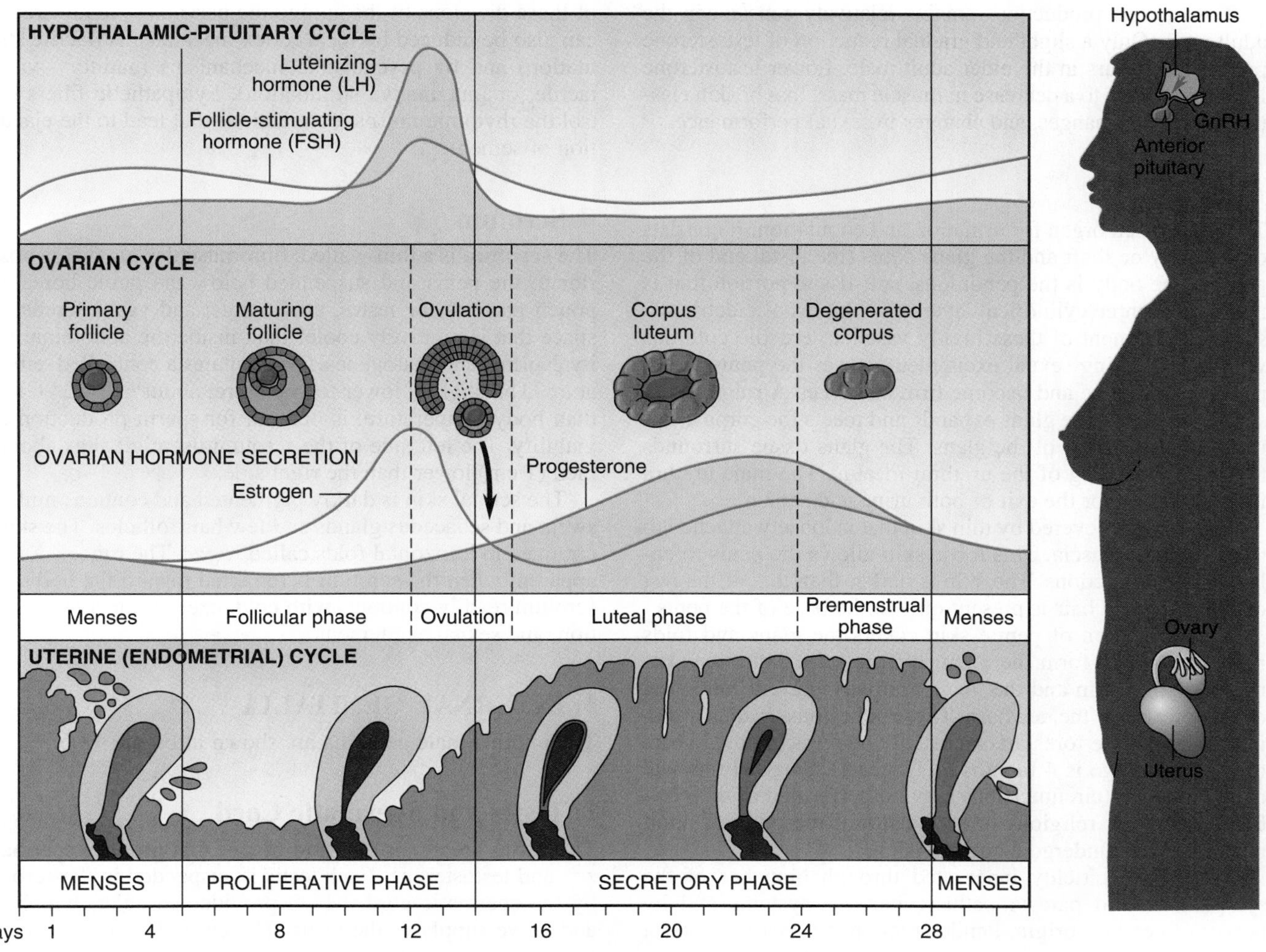

Figure 73-4 ● Interrelationships of the events of the menstrual cycle. (*GnRH,* Gonadotropin-releasing hormone.)

clitoris shrink in size. The low estrogen levels cause the vagina to narrow and shorten. The vaginal mucosa becomes thin and dry, which makes intercourse uncomfortable. The muscular support to the pelvis becomes more relaxed. The loss of tone also affects bladder support.

Bone density is a concern after estrogen production decreases. Estrogen is needed by bone tissue for calcium uptake. It also increases the metabolism of vitamin D, which is needed for the absorption of calcium from the intestines. Bone density decreases in clients with decreased calcium uptake. The reduction in the amount of bone mass is called **osteoporosis** (see Chapter 51).

One of the most common symptoms that occur during the climacteric are hot flashes, which are caused by vasomotor instability. Their cause is not clear, but it is thought that surges of FSH and LH on the hypothalamus cause vasodilation and increased heat production (Fogel, 2000). In addition to physical changes during the climacteric, the woman may also experience emotional changes (including mood changes) and fatigue.

Artificial Menopause

Menopause may occur for reasons other than the natural physiologic changes of the climacteric. Artificial menopause is the cessation of menstruation by some artificial means, such as an oophorectomy (surgical removal of the ovaries) or radiation to the ovaries. A premenopausal woman who experiences artificial menopause from removal of her ovaries may need estrogen and progesterone therapy.

Structure and Function of the Male Reproductive System

EXTERNAL GENITALIA

The external male genitalia undergo multiple changes during puberty. The first visible sign of pubescence is enlargement of the scrotum and testes, which typically occurs between 11 and 13½ years of age.

These changes occur in response to an increase in testosterone production at puberty. The release of gonadotropin-releasing hormone (GnRH) from the male's hypothalamus stimulates the anterior pituitary to secrete LH and FSH. As the levels of the gonadotropins increase, the amount of testosterone significantly increases. Other signs of puberty that relate to testosterone production are the growth of axillary hair, lengthening and thickening of the vocal cords, increased sebaceous gland activity, and a general increase in muscle mass and body size.

Testosterone production remains relatively constant in the adult male. Only a slight and gradual reduction of testosterone production occurs in the older adult male. Lower testosterone levels contribute to a decrease in muscle mass, loss of skin elasticity, postural changes, and changes in sexual performance.

Penis

The **penis** is an organ for urination and copulation. It consists of the body or shaft and the glans penis (the distal end of the penis). The body is the pendulous, soft-tissue portion that is made up of three cylindrical layers or columns of erectile tissue. Engorgement of these highly vascular, erectile columns with blood during sexual excitement causes the penis to expand and elongate and become firm and erect. A ridge of tissue forms where the glans expands and meets the corpus; this is called the corona of the glans. The glans tissue surrounds the slitlike opening of the urethral meatus. The male urethra is the pathway for the exit of both urine and semen.

The penis is covered by thin skin that is loosely attached to the underlying fascia. This loose skin allows the penis to enlarge during erections. The skin is darker than that of the rest of the body, and hair is present only at the base of the penis.

A continuation of penile skin covers the glans and folds back on itself to form the prepuce (foreskin). Adhesions between the foreskin and the glans normally prevent retraction of the foreskin in the newborn. These adhesions gradually disintegrate, and the foreskin can usually be retracted by 3 years of age (the range is 4 months to 13 years). Surgical removal of the prepuce (circumcision) may be performed in the newborn period for religious or sociocultural reasons. An adult male may also undergo a circumcision.

The penis is richly innervated through branches of the sympathetic and parasympathetic nervous systems and by nerves of cerebral origin. Penile erection is under the control of these divisions of the autonomic nervous system. Erection can also be induced by local reflex mechanisms (tactile stimulation) and by psychogenic mechanisms (auditory, visual, tactile, or imaginative stimulation). Sympathetic fibers control the rhythmic muscle contractions that lead to the ejaculation of semen.

Scrotum

The **scrotum** is a thin-walled, fibromuscular sac that is posterior to the penis and suspended below the pubic bone. The pouch protects the testes, epididymis, and vas deferens in a space that is relatively cooler than inside the abdominal cavity. Normal spermatogenesis necessitates a controlled temperature. The slightly lower temperature, about 6° F (2° C) less than body temperature, is optimal for sperm production and viability. The left side of the scrotum usually hangs about 3/8 inch (1 cm) lower than the right side.

The scrotal skin is darkly pigmented and contains multiple sweat and sebaceous glands and few hair follicles. The skin is arranged in horizontal folds called *rugae.* The rugae are more apparent when the scrotum is retracted toward the body. The scrotum readily contracts with cold, exercise, tactile stimulation, and sexual excitement.

INTERNAL GENITALIA

The internal male genitalia are shown in Figure 73-5.

Testes and Spermatic Cord

The **testes** are a pair of ovoid organs that produce spermatozoa and testosterone. Each testis is suspended in the scrotum by the spermatic cord, which provides vascular, lymphatic, and nerve supply to the testis. The cord also covers the epi-

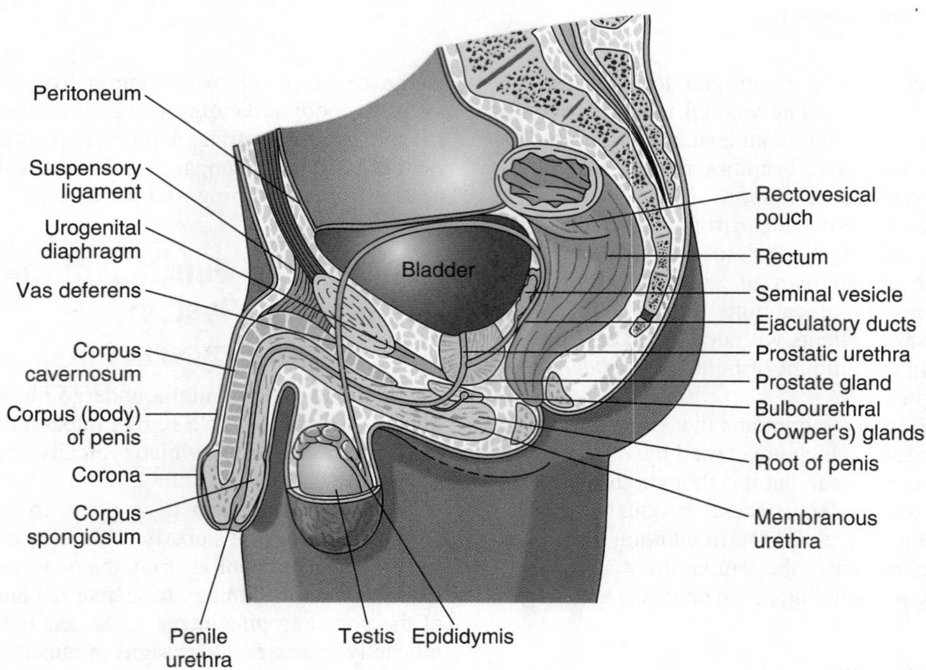

Figure 73-5 ● Internal male genitalia.

didymis and a portion of the vas deferens. The cord and testes are encircled by layers of spermatic fascia and cremaster muscle. Sympathetic nerve fibers are located on the arteries in the cord, and sympathetic and parasympathetic fibers are on the vas deferens. When the testes sustain a trauma, these autonomic nerve fibers transmit excruciating pain and a nauseating sensation.

EPIDIDYMIS

The epididymis is the first portion of a ductal system that transports sperm from the ductules of the testes to the urethra; it also aids in maturation of the sperm. The epididymis is comma shaped, lies posterolateral to one side of each testis, and is divided into a head, body, and tail.

The head of the epididymis attaches to the posterior aspect of the testis. The body descends against the lateral wall of the testis. At the lower border of the testis, the tail folds back over on itself and ascends toward the spermatic cord. The tail merges gradually into the vas deferens and provides storage for maturing sperm.

VAS DEFERENS

The vas deferens, or ductus deferens, is a firm, muscular tube about 17¾ inches (45 cm) long that continues from the tail of each epididymis. The terminal end of each vas deferens is a major reservoir for sperm and tubular fluids. They merge with ducts from the seminal vesicle to form the ejaculatory ducts at the base of the prostate gland. Sperm from the vas deferens and nutritive secretions from the seminal vesicles are transported through the ejaculatory duct to mix with prostatic fluids in the prostatic urethra.

Although the vas deferens secretes a small amount of fluid to support the sperm, its main function is to transport sperm from the epididymis to the ejaculatory ducts. In contrast to the movement of sperm through the epididymis by ciliary action, transport of sperm through the vas deferens occurs by means of peristaltic contractions of the ducts. A vasectomy, the surgical procedure for male sterilization, prevents only the passage of sperm to the ejaculatory ducts. It does not prevent the production of sperm, does not limit the erection of the penis, and does not greatly decrease the total amount of semen. Unexpelled sperm degenerate and are reabsorbed within the epididymis and the distal portion of the vas deferens.

Seminal Vesicles and Ejaculatory Ducts

The seminal vesicles are paired glands that secrete a major portion of the volume of the ejaculate. They are located behind the bladder near the prostate gland and are separated from the rectum by the rectovesical pouch. Each vesicle ends in a small duct that joins that of the ampulla of the vas deferens to form an ejaculatory duct. The two ejaculatory ducts are slender tubes that descend through the prostate gland; they end in slitlike openings in the prostatic urethra.

Prostate Gland

The **prostate gland** is the largest accessory gland of the male reproductive system. It is a chestnut-shaped, glandular, and fibromuscular organ. Functionally, it secretes a milky alkaline fluid that adds bulk to the semen, enhances sperm motility, and neutralizes acidic vaginal secretions.

During emission, the first stage of the male orgasm, the smooth muscle of the prostate gland contracts and secretes its fluid at the same time as the vas deferens. Fluid from the prostate gland contributes 20% to 30% of the total ejaculate. The average pH of the combined secretions of semen is approximately 7.5, whereas secretions from the vagina normally have a pH of 3.5 to 4. Sperm need a surrounding fluid pH of 6 to 6.5 before they become optimally motile.

The prostate gland is approximately the size of an adult testis. It is situated between the neck of the bladder and the urogenital diaphragm. The prostate gland is separated from the anterior wall of the rectum by a thin fascial sheath that is part of the rectovesical septum. The prostate gland can be palpated through the rectum and should not project more than ⅜ inch (1 cm) into the rectal lumen.

As men age, the prostate gland becomes clinically significant. The gland is small at birth, but during puberty it rapidly enlarges to its normal adult size. By age 50 or 60 years, about 80% of men have an enlarged prostate (benign prostatic hyperplasia), which can cause urinary problems (Barkauskas et al., 1998).

Prostatic function depends on adequate levels of testosterone. As men age, testicular production of testosterone decreases.

Bulbourethral (Cowper's) Glands

Semen is ejaculated through the prostatic urethra, membranous urethra, and penile urethra. The bulbourethral glands are two yellow, pea-sized glands located posterior to the membranous urethra and connected to the penile portion of the urethra by ducts. The bulbourethral glands secrete an alkaline mucus into the penile urethra during emission. The mucus mixes with the sperm and other glandular secretions to form the semen. The bulbourethral glands contribute about 5% to 6% of the total ejaculate. The alkalinity of the mucus further protects the sperm against the relative acidity within the urethra.

Reproductive Changes Associated with Aging

Age affects the function of both the male and the female reproductive systems. After puberty, hormones produced by the gonads affect the normal functioning of many body systems. Many changes in the reproductive system are evident in older adults (Chart 73-1).

ASSESSMENT TECHNIQUES

History

DEMOGRAPHIC DATA

The nurse uses data about the client's age, sex, and culture to assess the risk for certain diseases. The nurse considers the client's age in evaluating the reproductive system. The age at which secondary sex characteristics developed in the client are compared with the established normal ranges for males or females.

CHART 73-1

NURSING FOCUS *on the* OLDER ADULT
Changes in the Reproductive System Related to Aging

Physiologic Change	Nursing Implications	Rationale
WOMEN		
Graying and thinning of the pubic hair Decreased size of the labia majora and clitoris	Discuss changes with the client (applies to all structures for both women and men).	Education helps prevent problems with body image (applies to all structures for both women and men).
Drying, smoothing, and thinning of the vaginal walls	Provide information about estrogen replacement therapy and water-soluble lubricants.	Education enables the client to make informed decisions about the treatment of vaginal dryness, which can cause painful intercourse.
Decreased size of the uterus Atrophy of the endometrium Decreased size and marked convolution of the ovaries Loss of tone and elasticity of the pelvic ligaments and connective tissue	Provide information about Kegel exercises to strengthen pelvic muscles. Urinary incontinence can be a major problem.	Strengthening exercises may prevent or reduce pelvic relaxation and urinary incontinence.
Increased flabbiness and fibrosity of the breasts, which hang lower on the chest wall; decreased erection of the nipples	Teach or reinforce the importance of breast self-examination (BSE).	BSE may detect lumps or other changes that may indicate the presence of cancer.
MEN		
Graying and thinning of the pubic hair Increased pedulousness of the scrotum and loss of rugae	Teach or reinforce the importance of testicular self-examination (TSE).	TSE may detect changes that may indicate cancer.
Prostate enlargement, with an increased likelihood of urethral obstruction	Teach the client the signs of urethral obstruction and the importance of prostate cancer screening.	Education helps the client detect enlargement or obstruction, which may indicate the presence of cancer.

CULTURAL CONSIDERATIONS

Cultural influences and expectations account for variations in acceptable gender-related and sexual identity. A child's attitude and behavior about the meaning and use of the genitals begin in infancy and are modeled on the behavior of significant adults. Religious dictates often parallel those of a specific culture and strongly affect sexual activity. A person's religious beliefs often influence specific sexual practices, the acceptable number of partners, contraceptive use, and specific treatments to terminate a pregnancy, end fertility, or remove barriers to infertility (Geissler, 1999).

Ethnicity often has an epidemiologic influence on particular diseases. For instance, the incidence of cancer of the reproductive system (excluding breast cancer) and associated death rates are higher for African Americans than for Caucasians (American Cancer Society [ACS], 1999).

PERSONAL AND FAMILY HISTORY

Personal History

The nurse assesses the client's health habits, such as diet, sleep, and exercise patterns. Low levels of body fat may be related to ovarian dysfunction. The nurse also determines the client's alcohol, tobacco, and drug use because libido, spermatogenesis, and potency can be affected by such substances (Nichols & Lowdermilk, 2000).

The client's personal medical history provides data about his or her general health. Certain childhood illnesses can have an effect on the reproductive system. Females need to be screened for sufficient rubella titers and should be treated, if necessary, to prevent possible teratogenic effects on their unborn children if they get rubella during the first trimester of pregnancy. Mumps or smallpox in the postpubertal male may cause orchitis (painful inflammation and swelling of the testes) and occasionally leads to testicular atrophy and sterility.

The nurse also assesses for a history of major adult illnesses or chronic illnesses that may severely affect reproductive function. Endocrine disorders may affect the hypothalamic-pituitary-gonadal axis of the male or female. Almost any disease that disturbs a woman's metabolism or nutrition can depress ovarian function and cause amenorrhea. A history of infertility and failure of ovulation is associated with a greater risk for endometrial cancer. Clients with diabetes mellitus may experience physiologic changes such as vaginal dryness or impotence.

Some pre-existing cancers increase a woman's risk for developing other reproductive system cancers. Chronic disorders of the nervous system, respiratory system, or cardiovascular system can alter the sexual response. Some drugs (antihypertensives, opioids, monoamine oxidase inhibitors, histamine antagonists) may impair fertility (Nichols & Lowdermilk, 2000).

Reproductive system dysfunction can also result from irradiation, prolonged use of corticosteroids, exogenous estrogen or testosterone use, and chemotherapeutic agents.

In addition, past severe infections can alter a person's reproductive ability. For example, pelvic inflammatory disease or a ruptured appendix followed by peritonitis can cause strictures or adhesions in the fallopian tubes and pelvic scarring. Salpingitis (tubal infection) is most often caused by *Neisseria gonorrhoeae* infection and often results in female infertility. Infections or prolonged fever in males may damage sperm production or cause obstruction of the seminal tract, which leads to infertility. The nurse explores the client's history of surgeries, serious injuries, current medications, and allergies; each of these can affect reproductive structure or function.

Genitoreproductive History

The nurse completes a genitoreproductive history for both male and female clients. Chart 73-2 describes assessment data using Gordon's Functional Health Patterns.

FEMALE CLIENT

The nurse asks the female client about her menses, including age of menarche, cycle frequency and duration, amount of flow, spotting between periods, dysmenorrhea (painful menstrual periods), and premenstrual symptoms.

If the client is of menopausal age, the nurse determines the date of her last menstrual period, the presence of climacteric symptoms, and any medications or alternative therapies used for these symptoms. The nurse asks all women about the presence of vaginal discharge, a history and treatment of sexually transmitted diseases, the date and the result of her last Papanicolaou (Pap) test, breast self-examination practices, and vulvar self-examination practices.

The nurse also obtains an obstetric history. Women who have never had children have higher rates of ovarian, endometrial, and breast cancer than do multiparous women. If the woman has ever been pregnant, the nurse asks about the outcome of the pregnancies. In addition, the nurse collects information about the date and mode of deliveries or termination of the pregnancy; complications during pregnancy, labor, and delivery; birth weight and gestational age of the infants; and the condition of the infants at birth and at present.

The nurse also collects data about sexual activity. Heterosexual activity should not be assumed. Gay issues are often not assessed by the nurse or discussed by the client. The nurse explores information about sexual practices in a nonjudgmental manner.

An early age at first intercourse and multiple sex partners are associated with an increased risk of cervical cancer. The client is asked about satisfaction with sexual response, any pain or bleeding with sexual intercourse, and contraceptive use. Religious beliefs or type of sex (oral, anal, or vaginal) may dictate the contraceptive practices for a couple. Assessment for abuse may also be included at this point of the interview.

MALE CLIENT

The nurse asks the male client about testicular changes and self-examination practices, problems with urination, discharge from the penis, rectal problems, history and treatment of sexually transmitted diseases, and symptoms related to hernias.

The nurse also inquires about sexual functioning. Reproductive history and contraceptive use; current problems or changes in sexual response; any difficulty with erection, ejaculation, or infertility; and the use of medications or treatments also direct the physical assessment. The type of sex practiced also allows the nurse to focus on the body area involved.

Family History

The family history, including that of the parents, grandparents, siblings, and spouse, helps to determine the client's risk for conditions that affect reproductive system functioning. A delayed or early development of secondary sex characteristics may be a familial pattern.

The current age and state of health of the living members of the extended family are of interest. The cause of and age at death of specific family members may also be important. Evidence of serious diseases in family members (e.g., diabetes, cardiovascular disease, hypertension, renal disease, cancer, and complications of pregnancy) allows the nurse to better interpret the client's presenting symptoms. For example, daughters of women who were given diethylstilbestrol (DES) to control bleeding during pregnancy have an increased risk for infertility and reproductive tract carcinomas.

CHART 73-2

REPRODUCTIVE ASSESSMENT
Using Gordon's Functional Health Patterns

Health Perception/Health Management Pattern

Has anyone in your family had cancer of the breast or reproductive organs? Who and what type of cancer?

If you engage in sexual activities, do you practice "safer" sex?

What do you do to keep healthy—regular health checkups, self-examination (breast, genital [vulvar, testicular]), healthy diet, exercise, use of medications or alternative therapies, use of alcohol, tobacco, or street drugs?

Sexuality-Reproductive Pattern

Male and Female: Are you sexually active? Do you find your sexual relationship satisfying? Have there been any changes in your relationship? Are you having any problems in your sexual relationship?

Do you use contraceptives? If so, do you have any problems with the method of contraception?

Have you had any sexually transmitted diseases? If yes, when, and what type did you have?

Female: When did you first start menstruating? When was your last menstrual period? Do you have any menstrual problems?

Have you ever been pregnant? If so, how many times, and what were the outcomes?

Have you had any symptoms of menopause?

Male: Do you have any problems with getting and maintaining an erection, or do you have difficulty with ejaculation?

Have you ever had a hernia or pain in the groin?

Self-Perception/Self-Concept Pattern

How would you describe yourself? Do you feel good or not so good about yourself?

Have you experienced changes in your body appearance or function? If so, are these problematic for you? Have you felt anxious, fearful, or depressed about these changes?

Based on Gordon, M. (2000). *Manual of nursing diagnosis* (9th ed.). St Louis: Mosby.

DIET HISTORY

A diet history is often critical for the correct interpretation of presenting symptoms of the reproductive system. For instance, fatigue and a lack of sexual interest may be associated with poor diet and anemia. Obesity raises the risk for uterine cancer. High-fat diets may increase the risk for cancer of the breast, ovary, and prostate gland (ACS, 1999). The nurse asks the client to recall his or her dietary intake for a recent 24-hour period to estimate the quality of the diet.

The nurse compares the client's height, weight, and body mass index with the dietary recall. The client may be hesitant to divulge practices such as bingeing, purging, anorexic behaviors, or excessive exercise; however, these practices may affect the reproductive system. A certain level of body fat and weight is necessary for the onset of menses and the maintenance of regular menstrual cycles. A decreased amount of body fat is associated with insufficient estrogen levels for the maintenance of normal ovulatory cycles.

Women have special dietary needs. The diet of women who use oral contraceptives should reflect increased sources of folic acid and vitamins B_6, B_{12}, and C. Heavy menstrual bleeding, particularly in women who have intrauterine devices, may necessitate oral iron supplements. All women need to be aware of their body's need for calcium. Although adequate calcium intake throughout life is optimal, it is especially important during the premenopausal and postmenopausal periods. A woman's bone density decreases because of the decreased production of estrogen during the climacteric, and this predisposes her to osteoporosis and fractures (see Chapter 51).

SOCIOECONOMIC STATUS

The social history of the client provides insight into the whole person, including stressors, job history, education, and support systems. The nurse asks about smoking and the use of substances such as alcohol and drugs. All of these factors can influence the health of the reproductive system.

Stressors

Stress has long been associated with menstrual and ovulatory irregularities. The nurse asks about leisure time activities that pose a high risk of injury to the reproductive system. For example, men who lounge for long periods in hot tubs or saunas may experience decreased sperm production. Women who exercise or train vigorously have reduced percentages of body fat and a higher degree of menstrual irregularities (West, 1998).

Occupation

The client's work may directly affect the reproductive system. Routine occupational exposure to potential teratogenic substances (agents capable of producing birth defects in offspring) results in a higher incidence of abnormal sperm cellular features and low sperm counts in men or miscarriages in women. People who work around certain chemicals, radiation, and heavy metals are at risk. Trauma and exposure to extremely high temperatures in the workplace are potential causes of male infertility. Exposure to some industrial agents, such as cadmium, may be related to the development of carcinomas of the reproductive system.

Education

The nurse assesses the educational level of the client to individualize health teaching. Lay language for body parts and functions is commonly used when discussing the reproductive system. The nurse must be familiar with such terms and be comfortable in their use. Clients may try to evoke a particular response in the nurse by using certain words, or they may have no other terminology to express the problem. The nurse who responds with shock or disdain displays a judgmental attitude that hinders successful data gathering. Health care professionals can use teaching opportunities to provide more appropriate terminology.

Support Systems

The client's general satisfaction with life and the support systems available can directly relate to the current health problem. Questions designed to elicit information about daily routines often give insight into the client's perception of the quality of life and outlook for the future.

CURRENT HEALTH PROBLEM

If a client seeks medical attention for a problem related to the reproductive system, the nurse asks additional questions to explore the chief complaint. Most complaints concern pain, bleeding, discharge, masses, and reproductive functioning (Chart 73-3).

Pain

Pain related to reproductive system disorders may be confused with that associated with gastrointestinal or urinary tract problems. The client needs to describe the nature of the pain, including its type, intensity, timing and location, duration, and relationship to menstrual, sexual, urinary, or gastrointestinal function. Factors that exacerbate or give relief are also assessed.

Reproductive system disorders can be multifaceted; the nurse should not assume that the initial medical diagnosis is conclusive.

Bleeding

Heavy bleeding or a lack of bleeding may concern the client. The possibility of pregnancy is considered in any sexually ac-

CHART 73-3

BEST PRACTICE *for* Client Complaints Related to the Reproductive System

COMPLAINT	NURSING ASSESSMENT
Pain	Type and intensity of pain Location and duration of pain Factors that relieve or worsen pain Relationship to menstrual, sexual, urinary, or gastrointestinal function Medications
Bleeding	Presence or absence of bleeding Character and amount of bleeding Relationship of bleeding to events or other factors (e.g., menstrual cycle) Onset and duration of bleeding Presence of associated symptoms, such as pain
Discharge	Amount and character of discharge Presence of genital lesions, bleeding, itching, or pain Presence of symptoms or discharge in sexual partner
Masses	Location and characteristics of mass Presence of associated symptoms, such as pain Relationship to menstrual cycle

tive woman with amenorrhea. Any postmenopausal bleeding needs to be evaluated. The nurse asks the client to describe the amount and character of abnormal bleeding from the vagina or penis. The nurse asks when the bleeding occurs in relation to certain events, such as the menstrual cycle or menopause, intercourse, trauma, and strenuous exercise. In addition, the nurse notes the presence of associated symptoms, such as pain, cramping or abdominal fullness, a change in bowel habits, urinary difficulties, and weight changes. Many factors can cause bleeding, and therefore the nurse considers sources other than the genital tract.

Discharge

Discharge from either the male or female reproductive tract can cause severe irritation of the surrounding tissues, itching, pain, embarrassment, and anxiety.

The nurse asks about the amount, color, consistency, odor, and chronicity of the discharge. Medications (e.g., antibiotics) and clothing (e.g., tight jeans and noncotton underwear) may also initiate or exacerbate genital discharge. Many types of discharge are caused by sexually transmitted diseases. The localization of these infections in the body depends on the client's sexual practices. The nurse questions the client about lesions, bleeding, itching, pain related to the genitals and orifices used during sexual activity, and the presence of symptoms in the sexual partner.

Masses

Any reported masses in the breasts, testes, or inguinal area need to be evaluated. Some masses change in character or size, and the client can often relate these changes to menstrual cycles, heavy lifting, straining, or trauma. The nurse inquires about associated symptoms such as tenderness, heaviness, pain, dimpling, and tender lymph nodes.

CRITICAL THINKING CHALLENGE

An 18-year-old woman has come to the clinic with a complaint of menstrual problems. A 47-year-old woman has also visited the clinic because she thinks she is going through menopause.

- What assessment questions would be the same for these clients?
- What assessment questions would be different for these clients?

For suggested answer guidelines, go to SIMON http://www.wbsaunders.com/SIMON/Iggy/.

Physical Assessment

ASSESSMENT OF THE FEMALE REPRODUCTIVE SYSTEM

Examination of the breasts, axillae, and lymph nodes often precedes that of the anterior thorax in a complete physical examination. Inspection of the female genitalia and the pelvic examination are usually performed at the end of the physical examination. The client is often more apprehensive about these portions of the examination than about any other segment. Pain or lack of privacy during previous pelvic or breast examinations may prevent the client from relaxing.

The nurse can show the equipment to be used, along with three-dimensional models to demonstrate the assessment procedures. Relaxation and breathing techniques can be taught to enhance the client's sense of control. The nurse informs the client about what is going to be done and what she may feel as the examination proceeds. This information allows the client to incorporate learned coping mechanisms more successfully than if she were not expecting any discomfort. If the client displays signs of pain or exceptional concern during the procedures, the nurse should stop and make adjustments in the assessment plan or techniques. For example, clients who have been sexually abused may become upset during pelvic examinations (Heritage, 1998). The presence of a support person may also be of benefit to the client during the examination.

A pelvic examination is recommended every 1 to 3 years for women older than 18 years and for younger, sexually active adolescents (U.S. Department of Health and Human Services, 1997). A pelvic examination is indicated to assess the following:

- Menstrual irregularities
- Unexplained abdominal pain
- Vaginal discharge or infection
- Appropriateness of a desired contraceptive
- Rape trauma
- Physical changes in the vagina, cervix, uterus, and adnexa
- Infertility

The woman should not douche for at least 24 hours before the pelvic examination, because doing so may prevent an accurate evaluation of smears, cultures, and cytologic data.

Before the pelvic and breast examinations, the nurse asks the client to empty her bladder and to undress completely. The woman is adequately draped to protect modesty throughout the examination. If she is not wearing a gown, a small towel can be placed over the breasts under the larger drape. Drapes are removed only over the region being examined and are replaced when that area has been examined. Drapes that prevent eye contact between the examiner and the client dehumanize the client and prevent successful assessment of comfort during the examination. Mirrors can be used to facilitate teaching if the client so desires. The examination is performed in a room with adequate lighting for body inspection, a comfortable temperature, and the assurance of privacy.

Breast Examination

The physical examination of the reproductive system often includes the breasts (see Chapter 74).

Abdominal Examination

After the breast examination, the examiner generally completes the thoracic and cardiovascular examinations and then inspects, auscultates, and palpates the abdomen. The client's arms should be at her sides or over her chest to allow better relaxation of the abdominal muscles. During the gynecologic examination, the health care provider palpates for symptomatic and asymptomatic abdominopelvic masses. A mass can be of reproductive, gastrointestinal, or urinary tract origin. Careful history taking combined with the physical examination can usually determine the origin of a mass. Gynecologic masses, such as ovarian and adnexal masses, can be further differentiated from lesions on the body of the uterus during the bimanual portion of the pelvic examination.

Examination of the External Genitalia

After the abdominal examination, the nurse prepares the client for the inspection of the external genitalia and the pelvic examination. The nurse assists the woman into the lithotomy position and asks her to place her arms at her sides or over her chest. The client's buttocks extend slightly beyond the edge of the table, and her thighs are abducted. The nurse prepares all equipment for the vaginal and speculum examination and cytologic studies. The examiner wears gloves to protect against possible disease and potential cross-contamination from other clients. The client is informed that the genitalia will be touched and separated.

The initial inspection and palpation of the external genitalia provide an assessment of age-appropriate development. Hair color and distribution over the symphysis pubis and vulva suggest the woman's age and hormonal functioning. The pubic hair is inspected for the presence of lice or scabies. The skin and mucosa of the vulva are inspected in a systematic pattern from anterior to posterior for signs of inflammation, infestation, swelling, lesions, and discharge.

The paraurethral glands (Skene's glands) are barely visible on either side of the urethral meatus. If infection is suspected, the urethra should be gently "milked" by inserting the index finger into the vagina and gently pressing its pad against the anterior vaginal wall as the finger is being withdrawn. This procedure usually produces no pain or discharge unless there is inflammation or infection. The openings of the ducts from the Bartholin's glands cannot be visualized. The examiner carefully palpates the area just outside the lower vaginal orifice to assess for inflammation, tenderness, or swelling. Any discharge elicited from these ducts is cultured, because these structures are often involved in gonorrheal infections.

The examination of the external female genitalia is an excellent time for teaching about **vulvar self-examination (VSE).** The incidence of precancerous conditions and infectious diseases of the vulva is increasing, especially in young women (Lowdermilk, 2000). VSE can easily be taught and can lead to early diagnosis of vulvar conditions (Chart 73-4).

Perineal support and the strength of the vaginal walls are assessed by asking the woman to squeeze the vaginal opening closed after the examiner has inserted two fingers. The client is then asked to strain downward while the examiner assesses for urinary incontinence or any bulging of the anterior or posterior vaginal walls that would indicate a cystocele or rectocele, respectively.

Pelvic Examination

EXAMINATION WITH A SPECULUM

After the correct speculum size is selected, the speculum may be warmed and lubricated with warm water. Lubricant should not be used if cytologic studies are to be collected because it interferes with specimen analysis. The woman should be told when the speculum is going to be inserted. The examiner's fingers can ease insertion of the speculum by pressing down on the perineal body just inside of the vaginal orifice (Figure 73-6, step 1). The woman can also be asked to breathe slowly and to bear down. The examiner inserts the closed speculum in an oblique position, with the pressure exerted toward the posterior vaginal wall. The examiner removes his or her fingers. The examiner then rotates the closed blades of the speculum to a horizontal position while inserting the speculum to its full length (see Figure 73-6, step 2). The blades are opened, and the speculum is maneuvered to enable visualization of the cervix. The examiner locks the blades in place by tightening the thumbscrew of the speculum (see Figure 73-6, step 3).

CHART 73-4

CLIENT EDUCATION GUIDE
Vulvar Self-Examination

- Perform a vulvar self-examination monthly between menstrual periods if you are older than 18 years or if you are sexually active.
- Sit in a well-lighted area on a soft surface (bed or carpeted floor).
- Use a handheld mirror to visualize your external genitalia.
- Examine the area around the vaginal opening from the mons pubis to the perianal area.
- Feel and visually inspect the area.
- Report to your health care provider new nodes, warts, growths of any type, ulcers, sores, blisters, change in skin color, painful areas, areas of itching or inflammation, or any change in vaginal discharge.

The examiner inspects the cervix for color, shape, and dilation of the os; erosions; nodules; masses; discharge; and bleeding.

Herpes simplex, syphilis, and carcinomas can produce characteristic lesions on the cervix. Specimens are obtained from the cervix, endocervix, and vaginal pool for cytologic studies (see Microscopic Studies, p. 1722). After completion of the cervical examination, the examiner loosens the thumbscrew of the speculum to close the blades and slowly rotates the speculum to a vertical position as it is withdrawn. The examiner inspects the vaginal tissue for lesions or inflammation during withdrawal.

BIMANUAL EXAMINATION

After withdrawing the speculum, the examiner proceeds with the bimanual examination. Using a new glove and lubricant, the examiner stands and inserts one or two fingers of one hand into the client's vagina (Figure 73-7). The examiner palpates the posterior vaginal wall and checks for masses or tenderness. The cervix and fornix around the cervix are identified. The examiner places the opposite hand on the client's abdomen—between her umbilicus and symphysis pubis—and presses downward. The examiner lifts the cervix and uterus with the pelvic hand toward the abdominal hand to trap the uterus and adnexa for assessment by palpation. The examiner assesses the size, shape, consistency, location, and mobility of the uterus and for any tenderness or masses. To palpate each ovary and tube, the examiner presses the abdominal hand into the right or left lower quadrant. The fingers in the fornix are used to palpate the ovaries and adnexa against the opposite hand.

Obesity or tense abdominal muscles may prevent the examiner from locating the ovaries. If palpable, the ovaries are 3 cm long, 2 cm wide, and 1 cm thick; they are ovoid, feel firm and smooth, and may feel somewhat tender. The uterine tubes are not usually palpable. Ovarian cysts may be painful

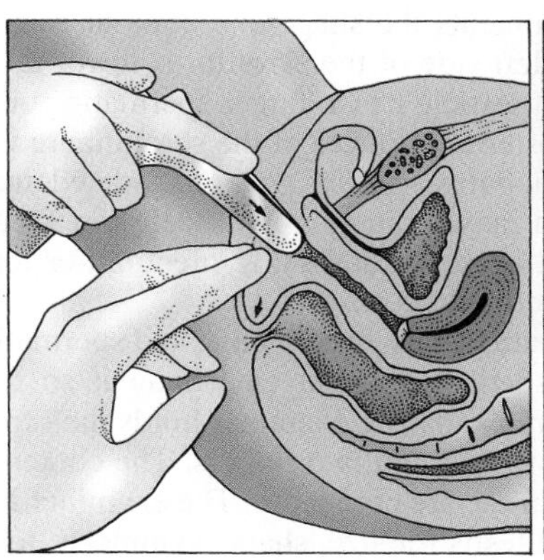

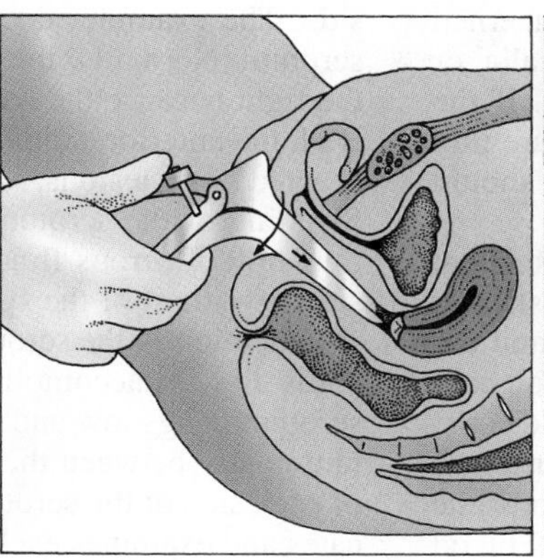

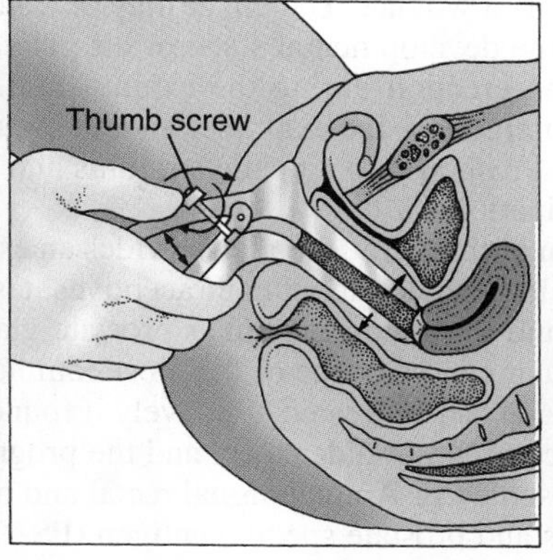

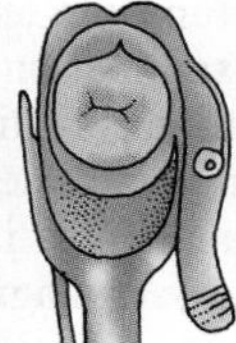

1. With the speculum blades positioned vertically, the nurse presses down on the perineal body just inside the vagina as the speculum is inserted.

2. The nurse removes the fingers from the vagina while continuing to insert the closed blades of the speculum to their full length and rotating them into a horizontal position.

3. The nurse opens the blades and maneuvers the speculum for optimal visualization of the cervix, then tightens the thumb screw to lock the blades in place.

View of the cervix through the speculum

Figure 73-6 ● Internal examination of the cervix.

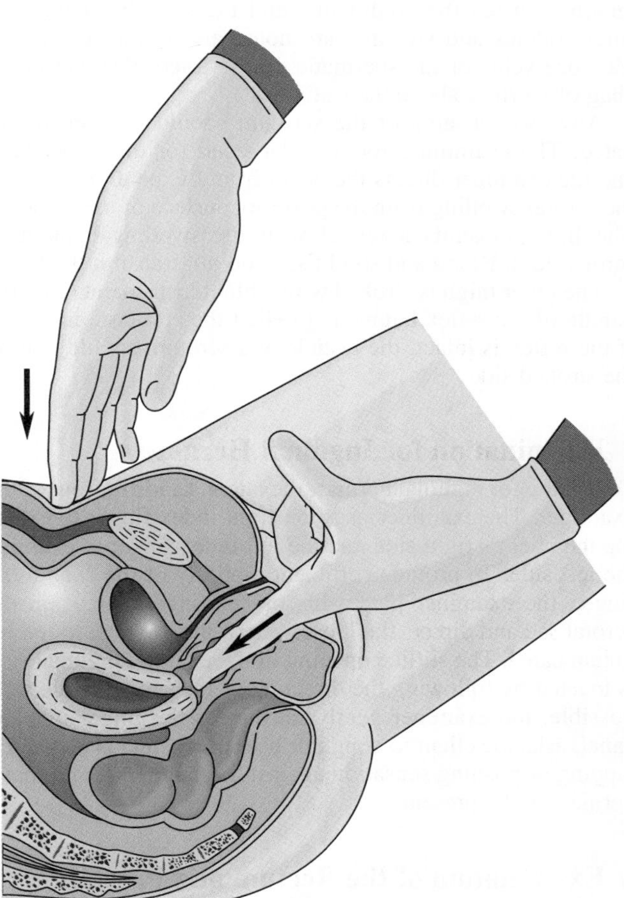

Figure 73-7 ● Technique of bimanual pelvic examination.

and recurrent in premenopausal women. An ovarian cyst smaller than 2 inches (5 cm) in diameter is usually functional and responds to hormonal influence. Cysts larger than 2⅜ inches (6 cm) in diameter are possible neoplasms. The ovaries are normally atrophied and not palpable 3 to 5 years after menopause; therefore any palpable structure in the adnexa of postmenopausal women suggest cancer.

RECTOVAGINAL EXAMINATION

The rectovaginal and rectal examination is the last segment of the pelvic examination. The examiner changes and lubricates the glove and places the middle finger in the rectum and the index finger in the vagina. Insertion of the rectal finger is facilitated if the client strains and relaxes the anal sphincter. The procedure for the bimanual examination is repeated. The posterior vaginal and uterine walls are palpated through the rectal mucosa. This examination is especially helpful in assessing a retroflexed or retroverted uterus. The examiner can assess the tissue structure between the vagina and the rectum by palpating between the two fingers. The vaginal finger is removed and folded into the palm. The rectal finger is rotated as it is withdrawn; any fecal material that remains on the glove may be tested for occult blood.

After the examination, the foot of the examining table is raised. The client's feet are lowered from the stirrups at the same time to reduce strain on the perineal muscles and lumbosacral ligaments. Nurses should be aware that some clients experience orthostatic (postural) hypotension if they sit up too quickly. The nurse evaluates the client for signs of dizziness before letting her get off the examining table. The nurse provides appropriate supplies, such as perineal wipes and perineal napkins or minipads. The nurse allows the client privacy for dressing and is available to answer questions and provide support.

ASSESSMENT OF THE MALE REPRODUCTIVE SYSTEM

Unless a male client seeks health care for a genital tract problem, inspection and palpation of the male genitalia and rectum may not be performed during physical examinations, depending on the health care setting and the age of the client. Male clients are often embarrassed and anxious when the reproductive system is assessed. This concern may be compounded when the examiner is a woman. The client may be concerned about discomfort, the developmental stage of his genitalia, or the likelihood of an erection during the examination. If the client does have an erection, the examiner should assure him that this is a normal response to a tactile stimulus and should continue the examination.

The examination of the male genitalia provides an excellent opportunity to teach the client about contraceptives, testicular self-examination, and the need for regular prostate gland examinations. Testicular cancer is one of the most common cancers in young men and can be treated effectively if found early. Prostate cancer is common in older men, and the prognosis is favorable if diagnosed early. Annual digital rectal and prostate gland examinations and prostate specific antigen (PSA) blood tests are recommended for men older than 50 years with a life expectancy of at least 10 years (ACS, 1999).

The examiner wears gloves to protect against possible infection. The examination room should offer the client privacy and a comfortable temperature. Proper light sources are mandatory for the inspection. The client undresses completely but should be given a gown to wear because the genitalia and buttocks need to be exposed. As with examinations of other body systems, the examiner explains each step of the assessment procedure before performing it. The client needs to be reassured that the examiner will stop and change the assessment plan or technique if the client perceives pain during the examination. Relaxation techniques and support during the examination can increase the tolerance of minimal discomfort.

Examination of the External Genitalia

The client may be in a lying or a standing position for inspection and palpation of the external genitalia. The examiner is seated on a chair in front of the client. A general observation is made of the secondary sex characteristics. The examiner notes the age appropriateness of the developmental stage, including the distribution pattern of the pubic hair, the descent and size of the testes, and the size of the scrotum and penis. Pubic hair is inspected for the presence of lice or scabies.

The examiner inspects the skin of the penis for intactness; the dorsal vein should be apparent. Any lesions or ulcers on the penis are noted, and a specimen may be scraped for cytologic study. If the client has not been circumcised, he is asked to retract the foreskin. This should be accomplished easily unless the client has phimosis (a tight prepuce that cannot be retracted). The examiner inspects the glans penis for possible inflammation, fungal infection, syphilitic chancres, and carcinomas. Smegma, a white, cheesy secretion from the sebaceous glands in the glans, may accumulate under the prepuce. This secretion is not present in the circumcised male.

The glans is also inspected for placement of the urinary meatus. Positions other than at the distal end of the glans are abnormal. By compressing the glans between the thumb and index finger, the examiner separates the meatus and can determine whether any discharge is present. Urethral discharge is not normal, and a specimen should be obtained for culture. The foreskin is replaced if it has been retracted. The body of the penis is palpated between the examiner's thumb and first two fingers; the examiner notes tenderness, hard areas under the skin, and signs of inflammation.

Inspection of the scrotum and inguinal areas is best accomplished by having the client hold the penis up and to the side. The examiner documents the shape and contour of the scrotum. Normally, the left side of the scrotum is lower than the right because the left testicle has a longer spermatic cord. Both the anterior and posterior surfaces of the scrotum are inspected for lesions, nodules, rashes, pain, and edema. Swelling of the scrotum may indicate a hydrocele (an accumulation of serous fluid in the scrotal sac), infection, or torsion (twisting) of the spermatic cord.

Palpation of the scrotum, testes, epididymis, and spermatic cords is best accomplished in a warm environment so the scrotum hangs low and relaxed. The examiner holds the scrotum gently between the thumb and two fingers. The contents of each side of the scrotal sac are compared. The examiner locates and examines each testis for size, shape, symmetry, tenderness, nodules, and consistency.

The normal testis has smooth borders, is somewhat sensitive to light palpation, and feels rubbery. The epididymis can be palpated on the posterior surface of the testis. It is examined for size, shape, and tenderness. In clients with infection of the epididymis, its outline is indistinguishable from that of the testis. The examiner palpates the spermatic cord along its length between the epididymis and the superficial inguinal ring; nodules and swelling are noted and further evaluated. Varicose veins of the spermatic cord (varicocele) feel like a "bag of worms" above the testis.

Any swollen area of the scrotum should be transilluminated. The examining room is darkened for this procedure, and the examiner directs the beam from the penlight through the scrotal swelling from the posterior surface of the scrotum. The light transmits a red glow if the swelling contains a serous fluid. Blood and solid tissue do not transmit the light.

The inner thigh is stroked with a blunt instrument (e.g., the handle of the reflex hammer) to elicit the cremasteric reflex. If the reflex is intact, the testicle and scrotum should rise on the stroked side.

Examination for Inguinal Hernia

To palpate for inguinal hernias, the client stands in front of the examiner. The examiner uses the right index finger to examine the client's right side and the left index finger to examine the left side. To provide sufficient mobility of the examining finger, the examiner places his or her fingertip low on the scrotal sac and directs the loose skin of the sac toward the inguinal canal. The slitlike opening of the external inguinal ring is located by following the direction of the spermatic cord. If possible, the examiner gently introduces the finger into the canal, asks the client to cough or bear down, and is alert for a tapping or pushing sensation against the finger—a sign that a hernia may be present.

Examination of the Rectum and Prostate

The final assessment of the male reproductive system includes an examination of the rectum and the prostate gland. This examination can be performed with the client in a knee-chest position, in a lithotomy position, in a left lateral with knees flexed position, or standing and leaning over the examining table with the feet turned inward to relax the buttocks.

Proper lighting is necessary for visualization of the anus and surrounding tissue. The examiner notes any lesions, ulcerations, masses, or fissures.

To assess the prostate gland, the examiner presses the pad of a well-lubricated, gloved index finger against the anus. As the sphincter relaxes, the finger is slowly inserted in the direction of the umbilicus and is rotated to palpate the anterior rectal wall. The posterior surface of the prostate gland is felt extending less than 3/8 inch (1 cm) into the rectum. The client is informed that he may feel an urge to urinate as the prostate is being examined but that he will not do so. The examiner notes the size of the lateral prostate lobes and their contour and consistency. The prostate should feel firm (the consistency has been equated to that of a pencil eraser), smooth, and slightly mobile. It should be nontender across its diameter.

The examiner extends the finger further to attempt to palpate the seminal vesicles, which are palpable only if they are inflamed. If any discharge is secreted from the penis during palpation of the prostate gland and seminal vesicles, specimens are obtained for culture and microscopic examination. The examining finger is withdrawn, and any fecal material may be tested for occult blood.

Psychosocial Assessment

The psychosocial assessment may suggest some contributory factors to the client's illness. During the social history, the nurse asks about the client's sources of support, strengths, and likely reactions to illness or dysfunction.

A client's personal history or beliefs may negatively influence his or her ability to enjoy a satisfactory sexual life. These factors may include the following:

- Sexual trauma or abuse inflicted during childhood or adulthood
- Punishment or reproach for masturbation
- Psychologic trauma
- Cultural influences, such as the idea of female passivity during intercourse
- Concerns about sexual partners or sexual lifestyle
- Use of alcohol or street drugs

Fears may affect the client's satisfaction with sexuality or body image. He or she may also be concerned about the potential or actual reaction of family members to reproductive health problems (see Chart 73-2).

Diagnostic Assessment

LABORATORY TESTS

Papanicolaou Test

The **Papanicolaou test,** or **Pap smear,** is a cytologic study that is effective in detecting precancerous and cancerous cells from the cervix. Health care providers vary in their recommendations for the frequency of routine Pap tests. The American Cancer Society (ACS) advises all asymptomatic women who have been or are sexually active to have an annual Pap test. After three or more consecutive negative test results, Pap tests may be performed less frequently (ACS, 1999). However, many clinicians continue to suggest that the test be performed annually during routine physical examinations.

Cytologic examinations can also detect viral, fungal, and parasitic disorders. Examination of cells from the vaginal walls can evaluate the function of steroid hormones.

CLIENT PREPARATION. The Pap test should be scheduled between the client's menstrual periods so that the menstrual flow does not interfere with the test interpretation. The woman should not douche, use vaginal medications or deodorants, or have sexual intercourse for at least 24 hours before the test.

The nurse assists the woman into the lithotomy position. Relaxation techniques, including concentrating on breathing patterns or a visual focal point, may be valuable for the apprehensive client. All steps of the examination are explained to the client before they are performed.

PROCEDURE. The examiner first inserts a speculum into the vagina. For the conventional Pap smear, the cervix is visualized and then scraped with one of the various sampling tools available, such as a cytology brush, cotton-tipped applicator, endocervical aspirator, or wooden or plastic spatula. The use of brushes improves the quality of cells obtained for analysis (Seidel, 1999).

The examiner takes one sample from the endocervical canal and a second from the ectocervical and squamocolumnar junction (Figure 73-8). Both specimens are immediately transferred to glass slides and are either sprayed with or immersed in a fixative solution. If the smear is allowed to dry on the slide before the fixative is applied, the diagnosis will be inaccurate. The slides are sent to a laboratory for interpretation.

The ThinPrep Pap Test is an improved method of preserving the sample. After the sample has been obtained, the health care provider rinses the cells into a vial filled with a preserving solution. The vial is sent to the laboratory, where an automated instrument gently separates the cells from blood and mucus. The thinner layer of cells can then be better visualized under a microscope, which improves the accuracy of the test.

FOLLOW-UP CARE. The nurse can provide the client with a perineal pad after the procedure to protect her clothes from any bleeding from the cervix. The test results are shared with the client in person, by telephone, or by letter. If a woman's smear has demonstrated atypical cells, she is encouraged to have follow-up testing.

Blood Studies

PITUITARY GONADOTROPIN

Determinations of the quantitative levels of follicle-stimulating hormone (FSH), luteinizing hormone (LH), and prolactin are helpful in the diagnosis of male and female reproductive tract disorders. The serum levels are measured by the radioimmunoassay method. No dietary restrictions are necessary before the test. Chart 73-5 gives the normal values and the significance of abnormal findings.

STEROID HORMONES

The radioimmunoassay technique can detect estrogen, progesterone, and testosterone levels in adult men and women.

SEROLOGIC TESTS

Serologic blood studies detect antigen-antibody reactions that occur in response to foreign organisms. This form of diagnostic testing is beneficial only after an infection has be-

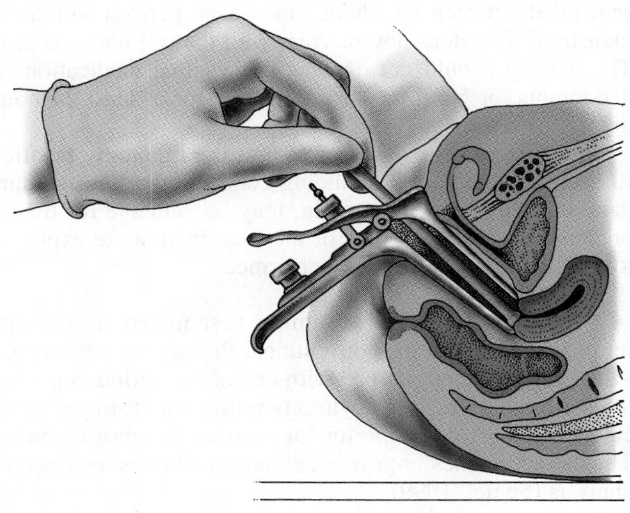

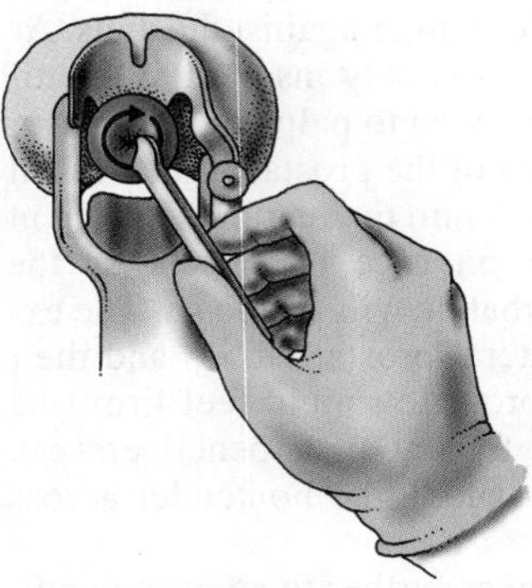

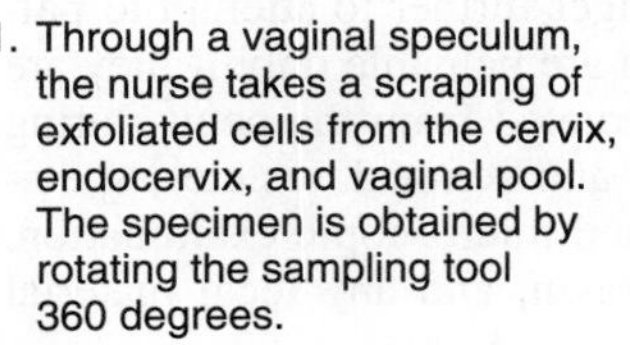

1. Through a vaginal speculum, the nurse takes a scraping of exfoliated cells from the cervix, endocervix, and vaginal pool. The specimen is obtained by rotating the sampling tool 360 degrees.

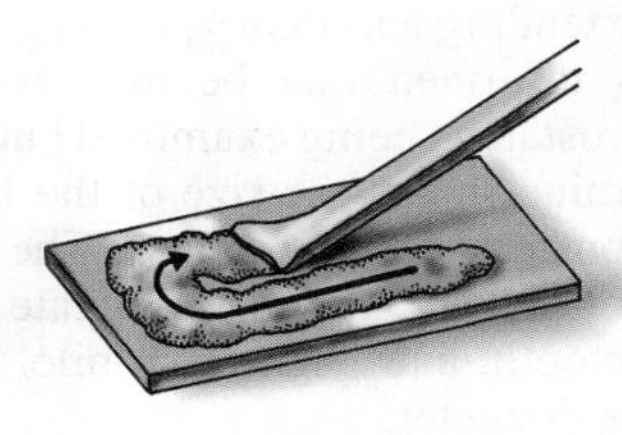

2. The nurse immediately transfers the specimens to a glass slide and applies a fixative solution.

Figure 73-8 ● Procedure for obtaining a cervical smear (Pap test).

come well established. Serologic testing can be used in the evaluation of exposure to organisms causing syphilis and rubella and to herpes simplex virus type 2 (HSV2). Results may be read as nonreactive, weakly reactive, or reactive. A single titer is not as revealing as serial titers, which can detect the rise in antibody reactions as the body continues to fight the intruder.

SYPHILIS DETECTION

The VDRL (Venereal Disease Research Laboratory) test, Serologic Test for Syphilis (STS), and the Rapid Plasma Reagin Test (RPR) are serologic tests used to detect, confirm, and monitor cases of syphilis. These tests are recommended for all pregnant women and persons at high risk for syphilis (Centers for Disease Control and Prevention [CDC], 1998). These nontreponemal antigen tests are used to screen for the presence of nonspecific reagin antibodies that appear and increase in titer after infection. They are not absolutely specific or sensitive for syphilis, but they are economical and highly diagnostic. Some acute and chronic conditions that cause false-positive results are the following:

- Tuberculosis
- Infectious mononucleosis
- Recent smallpox vaccination
- Rheumatoid arthritis
- Systemic lupus erythematosus
- Subacute bacterial endocarditis
- Hepatitis
- Recent ingestion of alcohol

Test results vary with the stage of syphilis. The serologic test result is usually positive about 2 weeks after the client has become infected. If the primary syphilis is treated, the serologic titers almost always return to nonreactive levels within 4 months.

If the VDRL or RPR test is positive, the diagnosis must be confirmed by a more specific test for *Treponema pallidum,* such as the fluorescent treponemal antibody absorption test (FTA-ABS). This expensive and time-consuming test becomes positive 4 to 6 weeks after infection. Most positive test results for *Treponema pallidum* remain positive for the rest of the infected person's life.

PROSTATE-SPECIFIC ANTIGEN

The prostate-specific antigen (PSA) test is used to screen for prostate cancer and to monitor the disease after treatment. PSA levels of <4 ng/mL are normal; elevated PSA levels are associated with prostate cancer. If combined with a digital rectal examination, almost 90% of all prostate cancers can be detected (Pagana & Pagana, 1998).

Urinalysis for Steroid Hormones

The health care provider may order 24-hour urine samples for levels of total estrogens and pregnanediol (a urinary byproduct of progesterone) to detect ovulation.

Microscopic Studies

WET PREPARATION (WET SMEARS)

The examiner can obtain secretions from the vaginal pool at the beginning of a speculum examination. Specimens can also be obtained from the vaginal walls, labia, or vulva during the examination. The specimens are placed on glass slides and are treated with a wet preparation such as saline and potassium hydroxide (KOH). The slides are examined under a microscope to confirm or rule out the presence of a pathogen. Table 73-1 presents the common types of wet preparations used to diagnose selected vaginal problems.

CULTURES

Cultures identify pathogenic organisms and are used to determine the appropriate antibiotic therapy. The examiner obtains specimens for culture analysis from any discharge or orifice of the male or female reproductive system. The health care provider orders routine bacteriologic cultures and antibiotic

CHART 73-5

LABORATORY PROFILE
Reproductive Assessment

Test	Normal Range for Adults	Significance of Abnormal Findings
SERUM STUDIES		
Follicle-stimulating hormone (FSH) (Follitropin)	*Men:* 1.42-15.4 mIU/mL *Women:* follicular phase, 1.37-9.9 mIU/mL; midcycle, 6.17-17.2 mIU/mL; luteal phase, 1.09-9.2 mIU/mL; post-menopause, 19.3-100.6 mIU/mL	Decreased levels indicate possible infertility, anorexia nervosa, neoplasm Elevations indicate possible Turner's syndrome
Luteinizing hormone (LH) (Lutropin)	*Men:* 1.24-7.8 mIU/mL *Women:* follicular phase, 1.68-15 mIU/mL; midcycle, 21.9-56.6 mIU/mL; luteal phase, 0.61-16.3 mIU/mL; post-menopause, 14.2-52.3 mIU/mL	Decreased levels indicate possible infertility, anovulation Elevations indicate possible ovarian failure, Turner's syndrome
Prolactin	*Men:* 0-20 ng/mL *Women:* 0-20 ng/mL *Pregnant women:* 20-400 ng/mL	Elevations indicate possible galactorrhea (breast discharge), pituitary tumor, disease of hypothalamus or pituitary gland, hypothyroidism
Estradiol	*Men:* 10-50 pg/mL *Women:* follicular phase, 20-350 pg/mL; midcycle, 150-750 pg/mL; luteal phase, 30-450 pg/mL; postmenopause, ≤20 pg/mL	Elevations of estradiol, total estrogens, and estriol in men indicate possible gynecomastia, decreased body hair, increased fat deposits, feminization
Total estrogens	*Men:* 20-80 pg/mL *Women:* follicular phase, 60-200 pg/mL; luteal phase, 160-400 pg/mL; post-menopause, <130 pg/mL	Elevations of estradiol, total estrogens, and estriol in women indicate possible uterine cancer, precocious puberty, cystic breast disease, corpus luteum cysts
Estriol	*Men and nonpregnant women:* <2.0 ng/dL	Decreased levels of estradiol, total estrogens, and estriol in women indicate possible amenorrhea, climacteric, impending abortion, hypothalamic disorders
Progesterone	*Men:* 10-50 ng/dL *Women:* follicular phase, <50 ng/dL; luteal phase, 300-2500 ng/dL	Decreased levels in women indicate possible inadequate luteal phase, amenorrhea Elevations in women indicate possible ovarian luteal cysts
Testosterone	*Men:* 280-1100 ng/dL *Women:* 15-70 ng/dL	Decreased levels in men indicate possible hypogonadism, Klinefelter's syndrome, hypopituitarism, orchidectomy Elevations in women indicate possible adrenal neoplasm, polycystic ovaries, ovarian tumors
URINE STUDIES		
Total estrogens	Men: 4-23 μg/24 hr *Women:* follicular phase, 7-65 μg/24 hr; luteal phase, 8-135 μg/24 hr; post-menopause, 0-10 μg/24 hr	Elevations indicate possible testicular tumors, adrenal tumors, ovarian tumors, pregnancy Decreased levels indicate possible ovarian dysfunction, intrauterine death, menopause
Pregnanediol	*Men:* 0-1.9 mg/24 hr *Women:* follicular phase, <2.6 mg/24 hr; luteal phase, 2.6-10.6 mg/24 hr	Elevations indicate possible luteal ovarian cysts, ovarian neoplasms, adrenal disorders Decreased levels indicate possible amenorrhea
17-Ketosteroids	*Men (20-50 yr):* 7-25 mg/24 hr *Women (20-50 yr):* 4-15 mg/24 hr Values decrease with age	Elevations indicate possible Cushing's syndrome, increased androgen or cortisol production, severe stress Decreased levels indicate possible Addison's disease, hypopituitarism

Data from Pagana, K.D., & Pagana, T.J. (1998). *Mosby's manual of diagnostic and laboratory tests.* St. Louis: Mosby.
mIU/mL, IU/L; *1 ng,* 1 nanogram or 1 billionth of a gram; *1 pg,* 1 picogram or 1 trillionth of a gram; *μg,* 1 microgram or 1 millionth of a gram.

sensitivity studies when a nonspecific bacterial infection is suspected.

The culture to detect *Neisseria gonorrhoeae* is one of the most important in evaluating the reproductive system. This culture is the only means of confirming a diagnosis of gonorrhea in asymptomatic women. Specimens from male clients can be taken directly from any penile discharge. In women, cervical cultures can be taken after the Pap test is obtained. Additional specimens from males or females can also be obtained from the urethra, rectum, and oropharynx. The swab is then placed in a culture tube and sent to the laboratory for incubation and analysis.

Cultures to detect *Chlamydia trachomatis* use antigen detection methods. Tissue cultures are the most accurate but take several days for results. Less expensive and more widely available are a direct immunofluorescent test and an enzyme-linked immunosorbent assay (ELISA) (Pagana & Pagana, 1998). Nucleic acid amplification tests can be used to detect

TABLE 73-1 • WET PREPARATIONS USED FOR THE DIAGNOSIS OF COMMON VAGINAL PROBLEMS

Wet Preparation	Problems
Normal saline	Cervicitis Trichomoniasis Bacterial vaginosis Atrophic vaginitis
Potassium hydroxide (KOH)	Candidiasis *(Candida albicans, Monilia)* Bacterial vaginosis
Gram stain	Mucopurulent cervicitis

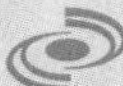
CRITICAL THINKING CHALLENGE

- What laboratory or diagnostic tests would be useful in evaluating a young adult's complaint of menstrual irregularity?
- What laboratory or diagnostic tests would be useful in evaluating a client experiencing menopausal symptoms?

For suggested answer guidelines, go to SIMON http://www.wbsaunders.com/SIMON/Iggy/.

N. gonorrhoeae and C. trachomatis in first-voided urine specimens or in specimens collected from the cervix (CDC, 1998).

RADIOGRAPHIC EXAMINATIONS

General X-ray Studies

A kidney, ureter, and bladder (KUB) study is an x-ray study of the abdomen that shows these structures and is used in the assessment of disorders of either the male or female reproductive system. Pelvic masses, calcified tumors or fibroids, dermoid cysts, and metastatic bone changes may be evident. Urologic studies may enhance the film by the use of contrast media. No specific client preparation is needed.

Bone scans, intravenous (IV) pyelograms, barium enema studies, and chest films are also included in the workup of the client with suspected metastatic cancer. They help to determine the extent of the metastasis and obstruction or displacement of the organs. These tests are discussed elsewhere in this text.

Computed Tomography

Computed tomography (CT) scans for reproductive system disorders primarily involve the abdomen and the pelvis. They can detect and evaluate masses and lymphatic enlargement from metastasis. This scan can differentiate solid tissue masses from cystic or hemorrhagic structures.

Hysterosalpingography

A **hysterosalpingogram** is an x-ray study of the cervix, uterus, and fallopian tubes and is performed after the injection of a contrast medium. This test is used in infertility workups to evaluate tubal anatomy and patency and uterine abnormalities such as fibroids, tumors, and fistulas. The study should not be attempted for at least 6 weeks after abortion, delivery, or dilation and curettage. Other contraindications include reproductive tract infection or uterine bleeding.

CLIENT PREPARATION. The examination should be scheduled in a radiology department 2 to 5 days after the end of the client's normal menses. The scheduling is important to prevent the accidental flushing of a fertilized ovum from the fallopian tube or the exposure of a fetus to radiation.

The client is usually instructed to take a laxative the evening before the test, followed by an enema or rectal suppository on the morning of the examination. These procedures reduce the distortion of the x-rays by gas shadows.

On the day of the examination, the date of the client's last menstrual period is confirmed and recorded in the medical record. The woman is assessed for an allergy to iodine dye or shellfish. She signs a consent form for the procedure. Because discomfort is anticipated during the examination, she may be premedicated with analgesics or nonsteroidal anti-inflammatory drugs. She should be informed that she may experience some nausea and vomiting, abdominal cramping, or faintness. The nurse provides support and assistance with relaxation techniques.

PROCEDURE. The client is placed in the lithotomy position. A speculum is inserted, and the cervix is visualized. Radiopaque oil or water-soluble dye is injected through the cervix to fill and highlight the interior of the cervix, uterus, and fallopian tubes. If the fallopian tubes are patent, the contrast material spills into the peritoneal cavity. Usually, only two or three films are taken to show the path and distribution of the contrast medium.

FOLLOW-UP CARE. The client may experience pelvic pain after the study and should receive medications accordingly. She may also experience referred shoulder pain because of irritation of the phrenic nerve caused by the dye. The nurse provides a perineal pad after the test to prevent the soiling of clothes as the dye drains from the cervix. The woman is instructed to contact her health care provider if bloody discharge continues for 4 days or longer and to report any signs of infection, such as lower quadrant pain, fever, malodorous discharge, and tachycardia.

Mammography

Mammography is an x-ray study of the soft tissue of the breast. Mammograms assess differences in the density of breast tissue. They are especially helpful in evaluating poorly defined masses, multiple masses or nodules, nipple changes or discharge, skin changes, and pain.

Mammography can detect many cancers that are not palpable by physical examination; however, some actual cancers are shown as benign by mammography.

In young women's breasts there is little difference in the density between normal glandular tissue and malignant tumors, which makes the mammogram less useful for the discovery and diagnosis of breast masses in these women. For that reason, annual screening mammograms are not recommended for women under 40 years of age (ACS, 1999). In older women, the percentage of fatty tissue is higher and the fatty tissue appears lighter than neoplasms. Cancer and cysts may have the same density. However, cysts usually have smooth borders, and neoplasms often have starburst-shaped margins.

CLIENT PREPARATION. No dietary restrictions are necessary before the mammogram. The woman is asked not to use creams, powders, or deodorant on the breasts or underarm areas before the study, because aluminum chlorhydrate can mimic calcium clusters. If there is any possibility that the client is pregnant, the test should be rescheduled. The purpose of the examination and its anticipated discomforts should be explained. A cover gown and adequate privacy for the client to undress above the waist are provided. The client also needs appropriate support and may need time to express her concerns about the mammogram and the presence of any lumps. Because this is a time when the client is anxious about the health of her breasts, it is an excellent opportunity to teach or reinforce the importance of breast self-examination.

PROCEDURE. The technician positions the client next to the x-ray machine with one breast exposed. A film plate and the platform of the machine are placed on opposite sides of the breast to be examined. The technician includes as much breast tissue as possible between the plates. The woman may experience some temporary discomfort when the breast is compressed during the positioning and the test. The test takes approximately 15 minutes, but the client is usually asked to wait until the films are developed in case a view needs to be repeated. Mammography usually necessitates two low-dose x-ray views of each breast: a view from the side and a view from above.

FOLLOW-UP CARE. If the results are not communicated at the time of the mammogram, the woman should know when to expect the report. She should be assessed for her knowledge of breast self-examination and given instructions if needed.

OTHER DIAGNOSTIC TESTS

Ultrasonography

Ultrasonography is a nonradiographic diagnostic technique that is routinely used to assess reproductive problems such as uterine fibroids, ovarian cysts, and pelvic masses. It can be used to locate intrauterine devices and to monitor the progress of tumor regression after medical treatment. Ultrasonography is also useful in differentiating solid tumors from cysts in breast examinations (Pagana & Pagana, 1998).

No specific preparations are necessary for this study. The client should have a full bladder to enable visualization of the uterus and to make the location of other structures more distinct with abdominal ultrasonography; a full bladder is not necessary for transvaginal scans.

For an abdominal or breast scan, the technician exposes the area and applies oil or gel to the area to be scanned. These substances provide better transmission of sound waves from the transducer through the client's skin. The transducer is moved in a linear pattern across the abdomen to outline and define soft-tissue masses and to differentiate tumor types, ascites, and encapsulated fluid.

For a transvaginal scan, the transducer is covered with a condom or vinyl glove into which transmission gel has been placed. The transducer is then inserted in the vagina. The client is often interested in the oscilloscope screen and appreciates a brief explanation of the landmarks and structures visualized. There is no special follow-up care for the client after this procedure except to provide wipes to remove the gel.

EVIDENCE-BASED PRACTICE FOR NURSING

Mailing informational handouts before colposcopy can increase knowledge

Tomaino-Brunner, C., et al. (1998). Can precolposcopy education increase knowledge and decrease anxiety? *Journal of Obstetric, Gynecologic, and Neonatal Nursing, 27*(6), 636-645.

Referral for colposcopy is the usual follow-up for women with abnormal Papanicolaou (Pap) tests. Previous studies have found that women expressed little understanding of the procedure before the appointment.

This randomized, controlled study investigated the impact of an informational handout about colposcopy on knowledge and anxiety levels. This handout was mailed to inner-city women scheduled for the procedure. The sample included 58 women in the intervention group and 55 women in the control group who did not receive the mailing. Knowledge was measured by content analysis of interviews held at the clinic at the time of the colposcopy; anxiety was measured using the Spielberger State/Trait Anxiety Inventory. Results indicated that 72% of the intervention group understood what a colposcopy was compared to 42% of the control group. No significant differences were found in mean anxiety scores between the groups.

Critique. This experimental, randomized controlled study of a small sample of inner city women did not include a pretest-posttest design, and therefore the knowledge and anxiety levels of the women before the intervention are not known. Further study is needed to understand what interventions can decrease anxiety about colposcopy.

Implications for Nursing. This study has implications for client education. Mailing a handout on colposcopy or other procedures shortly before the appointment is a simple yet effective method of providing information to clients. Because client education is an important nursing function, nurses need to be able to use a variety of methods to meet individual client needs.

Magnetic Resonance Imaging

Magnetic resonance imaging (MRI) uses a magnetic field and radiofrequency energy to scan for pelvic tumors. This scan effectively distinguishes between normal and malignant tissues. MRIs are also being investigated for use in the diagnosis of breast cancer (Mishell et al., 1997).

Endoscopic Studies

COLPOSCOPY

The colposcope allows three-dimensional magnification and intense illumination of epithelium with suspected disease. **Colposcopy** is suited for inspection of the cervical epithelium, vagina, and vulvar epithelium. This procedure can locate the exact site of precancerous and malignant lesions for biopsy.

CLIENT PREPARATION. The woman is placed in the lithotomy position and provided the same support as for a pelvic examination. The client should not douche or use vaginal preparations for 24 to 48 hours before the examination. This relatively painless procedure is usually better tolerated if it is explained in advance and if the instrument is shown to the client (see the Evidence-Based Practice for Nursing box above).

A colposcopy provides accurate site selection for tissue biopsy, and therefore the client should also be prepared for a biopsy. Materials necessary for cytologic studies and biopsy should be readily available.

PROCEDURE. The physician locates the cervix, or vaginal site, through a speculum examination. Lubricants other than water should not be used. Cells in the area may be stained or left unstained to enhance visualization. The physician cleans the cervix of secretions and moistens the cervix with normal saline. This allows for better visualization of vascular patterns and the junction between the columnar epithelium and the squamous epithelium. Acetic acid, 3%, applied to the cervix acts as a mucolytic agent to draw moisture from the tissue and to accentuate important morphologic features. The physician then uses a colposcope or colpomicroscope to inspect the area in question. A biopsy may also be taken if abnormal cells are seen (see discussion on cervical biopsy on p. 1727).

FOLLOW-UP CARE. After the procedure, the nurse assists the woman as for a pelvic examination and provides supplies to clean the perineum. The nurse also gives her a perineal pad to absorb any dye or discharge. If procedures other than direct visualization were performed, follow-up care needs to be revised appropriately.

LAPAROSCOPY

Laparoscopy is a highly accurate diagnostic tool for exploring the pelvic cavity. This procedure can rule out an ectopic pregnancy, evaluate ovarian disorders and pelvic masses, and aid in the diagnosis of infertility and unexplained pelvic pain. Laparoscopy is also used during surgical procedures such as the following:

- Tubal sterilization
- Ovarian biopsy
- Cyst or graafian follicle aspiration (to retrieve ova for in vitro fertilization)
- Lysis of adhesions around the fallopian tubes
- Retrieval of "lost" intrauterine devices

A **laparoscopy** is preferable to a laparotomy for minor surgical procedures because it necessitates only a small infraumbilical incision, involves less discomfort, and does not require hospitalization.

CLIENT PREPARATION. The physician explains the procedure, risks (complications associated with the use of general anesthesia, postoperative shoulder pain, and the rare occurrence of infection or electric burns), and anticipated discomforts and obtains the client's consent. The procedure can be performed with either a regional or general anesthetic. Clients should expect mild discomfort from the incision site and may experience referred shoulder pain from phrenic nerve irritation (Nichols & Lowdermilk, 2000).

PROCEDURE. The client is anesthetized and placed in the lithotomy position. A urinary catheter is inserted to drain the bladder. The operating table is placed in a slight Trendelenburg position to cause the intestines to fall away from the pelvis. The cervix is held with a cannula to allow movement of the uterus during laparoscopy (Figure 73-9). The surgeon inserts a needle below the umbilicus to infuse carbon dioxide into the pelvic cavity; this distends the abdomen and permits better visualization of the organs. The surgeon inserts a trocar and a cannula into an infraumbilical incision. After the trocar and cannula are in place in the abdominal cavity, the surgeon removes the trocar and inserts the laparoscope. The surgeon can thus visualize the pelvic cavity and reproductive organs. Further instrumentation is possible through a second small incision. The laparoscope is removed at the end of the procedure, and the abdomen is deflated. The physician usually closes the incision with absorbable sutures and dresses the area with an adhesive bandage.

FOLLOW-UP CARE. The client requires postoperative care similar to that for other clients after general anesthesia but is usually discharged on the day of the surgery. Discomfort from the incision is usually alleviated by the administration of oral analgesics. The greatest discomfort is due to referred shoulder pain caused by residual gas in the peritoneal cavity. Most of these sensations disappear within 48 hours. Clients are instructed to change the small adhesive bandage as needed and to observe the incision for signs of infection or hematoma. The client should avoid strenuous activity for the first week after the procedure.

HYSTEROSCOPY

Hysteroscopy is an endoscopic examination that permits visualization of the interior of the uterus and the cervical canal. The hysteroscope includes a lens with fiberoptic lighting; an aqueous solution of carbon dioxide is the medium used to distend the uterus. Hysteroscopy can be used for the removal of intrauterine devices and as a complement to other diagnostic tests for infertility and unexplained bleeding.

CLIENT PREPARATION. The surgeon informs the client of all aspects of the procedure and obtains consent. The client receives the same preparation as for a pelvic examination. The procedure is best performed 5 days after menses have ceased to eliminate the possibility of pregnancy. The

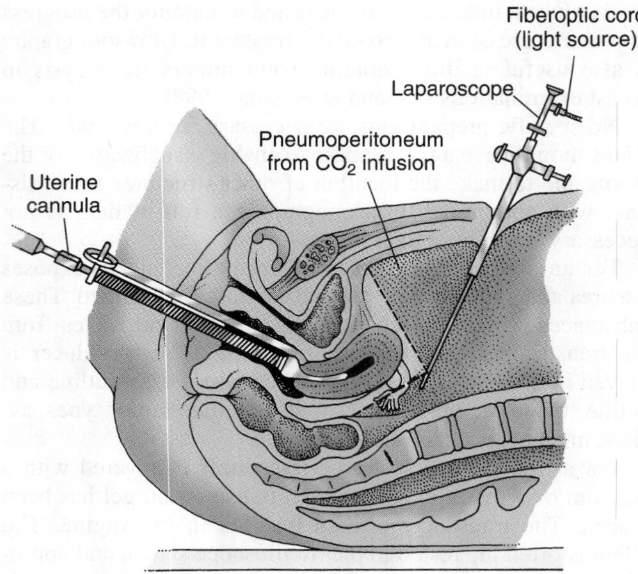

Figure 73-9 • Laparoscopy.

client is placed in the lithotomy position and is usually anesthetized with a pericervical or other regional block.

PROCEDURE. After the client is anesthetized, the cervix is dilated. The physician inserts the hysteroscope through the cervix. Because a medium distends the uterus, cells can be pushed through the fallopian tubes and into the pelvic cavity. Therefore hysteroscopy is contraindicated in clients with suspected cervical or endometrial cancer, in clients with infection of the upper reproductive tract, and in pregnant clients.

FOLLOW-UP CARE. Care is the same as that after a pelvic examination. Analgesics may be ordered if the client experiences cervical and uterine cramping. Shoulder pain may be present for up to 24 hours if carbon dioxide was used to distend the uterus during the procedure.

Biopsy Studies

CERVICAL BIOPSY

In a cervical biopsy, cervical tissue is removed for additional cytologic study. A biopsy is definitely indicated in a client with an identifiable cervical lesion, regardless of the cytologic findings. The physician usually performs a biopsy in conjunction with colposcopy as a follow-up to a suspicious Pap test finding. This procedure may be performed in the health care provider's office.

Several techniques can be used for a cervical biopsy. If a lesion is clearly visible, an endocervical curettage can be performed as an outpatient procedure and with little or no anesthetic. Conization (removal of a cone-shaped sample of tissue) and loop electrosurgical excision procedures (LEEP) are usually not done unless the cervical biopsy is positive or the results of the colposcopy are unsatisfactory (Lowdermilk, 2000). Conization, if performed, can be done as a cold-knife procedure, a laser excision, or an electrosurgical incision.

CLIENT PREPARATION. The client should be scheduled for the biopsy in the early proliferative phase of the menstrual cycle, when the cervix is least vascular. The selected procedure should be explained to the client. Because a biopsy evaluates potentially malignant cells, most women become anxious and need time to discuss their feelings and fears. The use of relaxation techniques may facilitate comfort. The nurse assists the client into the lithotomy position and prepares her in the same way as for a pelvic examination. Further preparation depends on the type of procedure to be performed.

PROCEDURE. The physician may anesthetize the client according to the needs of the chosen procedure. The physician visualizes the cervix and obtains the tissue sample. All specimens are immediately placed into a formalin solution.

FOLLOW-UP CARE. The type of anesthetic used for the procedure determines the type of immediate postoperative care provided by the nurse. Discharge instructions are listed in Chart 73-6.

ENDOMETRIAL BIOPSY AND ASPIRATION

Both endometrial biopsy and aspiration are used to obtain cells directly from the lining of the uterus in women at risk for cancer of the endometrium. Endometrial biopsy is also valuable for assessing functional menstrual disturbances (especially anovulatory bleeding) and infertility (corpus luteum dysfunction).

When menstrual disturbances are being evaluated, the biopsy is generally done in the immediate premenstrual period to serve as an index of progesterone influence and ovulation. A biopsy performed in the second half of the menstrual cycle (approximately days 21 and 22) evaluates corpus luteum function and the presence or absence of a persistent secretory endometrium. Postmenopausal women may undergo biopsies at any time.

CLIENT PREPARATION. Menstrual data are obtained from the client and included on the specimen slip for the pathologist. The client is given the same preparation as for a pelvic examination. The nurse advises her that she may experience some cramping when the cervix is dilated. Analgesia before the procedure and relaxation and breathing techniques during the procedure are often of value.

PROCEDURE. An endometrial biopsy is often performed as an office procedure with or without anesthesia. After the uterus is sounded (measured) and the cervix sufficiently dilated, the physician inserts the curette or intrauterine cannula into the uterus. The physician withdraws a portion of the endometrium either with the cuplike end of the curette or with suction aspiration equipment. The client experiences moderate cramping. The specimens are placed in a formalin solution and sent for histologic examination.

FOLLOW-UP CARE. The client is allowed to rest on the examining table until the cramping has subsided. A perineal pad and a wipe to clean the perineum are provided. Spotting may be present for 1 to 2 days, but any signs of infection or excessive bleeding should be reported to the physician. The client is informed to refrain from intercourse or douching until all discharge has ceased. Results of the biopsy are usually available within 72 hours.

BREAST BIOPSY AND ASPIRATION

An incisional biopsy is the surgical removal of tissue from a breast mass. An excisional biopsy removes the mass itself for histologic (cellular) evaluation. Aspiration biopsy is the removal of fluid or tissue from the breast mass through a large-

CHART 73-6

CLIENT EDUCATION GUIDE
The Client Recovering from Cervical Biopsy

- Do not lift any heavy objects until the site is healed (about 2 weeks).
- Rest for 24 hours after the procedure.
- Report any excessive bleeding (more than that of a normal menstrual period) to your health care provider.
- Report signs of infection to your health care provider.
- Do not douche, use tampons, or have vaginal intercourse until the site is healed (about 2 weeks).
- Keep the perineum clean and dry by using antiseptic solution rinses (as directed by your health care provider) and changing pads frequently.

bore needle. Figure 73-10 shows these three types of breast biopsy.

Any breast mass needs to be evaluated further for the possibility of cancer. Fibrocystic lesions, fibroadenomas, and intraductal papillomas can be differentiated by biopsy. Any discharge from the breasts is examined histologically.

CLIENT PREPARATION. The instructions to the client depend on the type of biopsy and the type of anesthesia. The woman is told to expect pulling or probing sensations during the procedure.

PROCEDURE. Aspiration biopsy is often performed in an outpatient setting without an anesthetic. The mass is located by palpation of the breast. The surgeon then directs the needle into the lump and aspirates the contents into the syringe. The contents are placed on a slide for Pap evaluation. Fluid from benign cysts may appear clear to dark green-brown; bloody fluid suggests cancer. If no fluid is aspirated, the tumor should be examined by incisional biopsy.

Incisional or excisional biopsies are typically performed as same-day procedures with local or general anesthesia. The tumor specimen is evaluated by the frozen section technique. If cancer is found, the physician sends the tissue to the laboratory for estrogen receptor analysis.

FOLLOW-UP CARE. Postoperative discomfort is usually mild and is controlled with analgesic administration or the use of a heating pad. The client is taught how to assess the incisional site for bleeding and edema. A properly supportive bra should be worn continuously by the woman for 1 week postoperatively. The woman should avoid cold temperatures to prevent nipple contractions that can cause stress on the incision. Numbness around the biopsy site may last 2 to 3 months. The woman should also be assessed about her knowledge of breast self-examination and given instructions if needed. If a malignancy is identified, the woman will need emotional support as well as information about follow-up treatment alternatives.

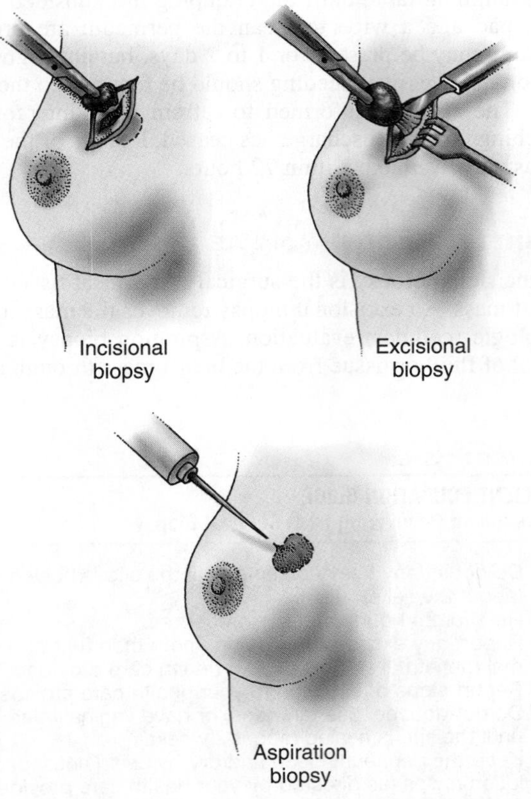

Figure 73-10 ● Breast biopsy techniques.

NEEDLE BIOPSY OF THE PROSTATE

When prostate cancer is suspected, the physician performs a needle aspiration biopsy of the prostate gland to retrieve cells for histologic study. This procedure is often performed at the same time as cystoscopy, with the client under anesthesia. The physician can perform needle biopsies without anesthesia or with the client under local anesthesia.

CLIENT PREPARATION. Preparation for the procedure depends on the technique used to puncture the gland. The nurse provides data on the expected discomforts. The nurse can also teach breathing and relaxation techniques for use during the examination. Because the purpose of this procedure is to evaluate prostate cells for potential malignancy, the man needs support and time to discuss his fears. Preparation for a transrectal biopsy involves the use of cleansing enemas and the administration of prophylactic antibiotics to reduce the risk of bacterial contamination of the bloodstream or prostate tissue. Local anesthesia is used at the site of transperineal biopsy.

PROCEDURE. The nurse places the client in the same position as for a rectal examination. After injecting a local anesthetic for the transperineal biopsy, the physician places a finger in the rectum to help guide the needle to the prostate. For the transrectal biopsy, the physician places the needle against the examining finger and then inserts it into the rectum to the prostate. From this site, the needle is advanced through the rectal mucosa and into the prostate gland. The aspiration may be repeated several times to obtain a satisfactory specimen.

FOLLOW-UP CARE. Sepsis is a potentially life-threatening complication of transrectal biopsy. Any signs of infection or septic shock must be reported immediately. Prophylactic antibiotics are usually prescribed.

ONLINE RESOURCES

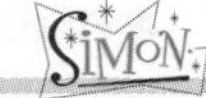

For suggested readings and Internet resources, go to http://www.wbsaunders.com/SIMON/Iggy/.

SELECTED BIBLIOGRAPHY

Asterisk indicates a classic or definitive work on this subject.

American Cancer Society. (1999). *Cancer facts and figures, 1999.* New York: Author.

American College of Obstetricians and Gynecologists. (1997). *Committee opinion: Routine cancer screening.* Washington, D.C.: Author.

Angard, N. (1999). Diagnosis infertility. *AWHONN's Lifelines, 3*(3), 22-29.

Apgar, B. (1997). Dysmenorrhea and dysfunctional bleeding. *Primary Care, 24*(1), 161-168.

Barkauskas, V., et al. (1998). *Health and physical assessment* (2nd ed.). St. Louis: Mosby.

Centers for Disease Control and Prevention. (1998). Guidelines for the treatment of sexually transmitted diseases. *Morbidity & Mortality Weekly Report, 47*(RR-1), 1-116.

*Cook, M. (1994). Nursing assessment for the older woman. *RN, 57*(9), 40-43.

DiSaia, P., & Creasman, W. (1997). *Clinical gynecologic oncology* (5th ed.). St. Louis: Mosby.

Fernandez, M., Tortolero-Luna, G., & Gold, R. (1998). Mammography and Pap test screening among low-income foreign-born Hispanic women in the USA. *Cadernas de Saude Publica, 14*(Suppl. 3), 133-147.

Fishwick, N. (1998). Assessment of women for partner abuse. *Journal of Obstetric, Gynecologic, and Neonatal Nursing, 27*(6), 661-670.

Fogel, C. (2000). Common reproductive concerns. In D. Lowdermilk, S. Perry, & I. Bobak (Eds.), *Maternity and women's health care* (7th ed., pp. 115-143). St. Louis: Mosby.

Fogel, C., & Woods, N. (in press). *Women's health care: A comprehensive handbook* (2nd ed.). Thousand Oaks, CA: Sage.

*Geissler, E. (1999). *Pocket guide to cultural assessment* 2nd ed. St. Louis: Mosby.

Gordon, M. (2000). *Manual of nursing diagnosis* (9th ed.). St. Louis: Mosby.

Heritage, C. (1998). Working with childhood sexual abuse survivors during pregnancy, labor, and birth. *Journal of Obstetric, Gynecologic, and Neonatal Nursing, 27*(6), 671-677.

Higgins, P., & Smith, P. (1997). Assessing cervical cancer risks. *AWHONN's Lifelines, 1*(6), 43-47.

Lawson, E. (1998). A narrative analysis: A black woman's perception of breast cancer risks and early breast cancer detection. *Cancer Nursing, 21*(6), 421-429.

Lowdermilk, D. (1997). Caring for women with sexual and reproductive system disorders. In J. Luckmann (Ed.). *Saunders manual of nursing care.* (pp. 1441-1495). Philadelphia: W.B. Saunders.

Lowdermilk, D. (2000). Structural disorders and neoplasms of the reproductive system. In D. Lowdermilk, S. Perry, & I. Bobak (Eds.), *Maternity and women's health care* (7th ed., pp. 268-302). St. Louis: Mosby.

Lowdermilk, D. (in press). Reproductive surgery. In C. Fogel, & N. Woods (Eds.), *Women's health care: A comprehensive handbook* (2nd ed.). Thousand Oaks, CA: Sage.

Mishell, D., et al. (1997). *Comprehensive gynecology.* (3rd ed.). St. Louis: Mosby.

Morrell, V. (1997). Basic infertility assessment. *Primary Care, 21*(1), 195-204.

National Women's Health Resource Center. (1999). Breast health. *National Women's Health Report, 17*(5), 1-11.

Nichols, A., & Lowdermilk, D. (2000). Infertility. In D. Lowdermilk, S. Perry, & I. Bobak (Eds.), *Maternity and women's health care* (7th ed., pp. 206-224). St. Louis: Mosby.

Pagana, K.D., & Pagana, T.J. (1998). *Mosby's manual of diagnostic and laboratory tests.* St. Louis: Mosby.

Plourd, D. (1997). Practical guide to diagnosing and treating vaginitis. *Medscape Women's Health, 2*(2), 2.

Sampselle, C., et al. (1999). Continence for women: Evidence-based practice. *Journal of Obstetric, Gynecologic, and Neonatal Nurses, 28*(6 Suppl. 1), 25-33.

Schweitzer, M., et al. (1998). Cost-effectiveness of detecting breast cancer in lower socioeconomic status African-American and Hispanic women through mobile mammogram services. *Medical Care Research and Review, 55*(1), 99-115.

Seidel, H.M., et al. (1999). *Mosby's guide to physical examination* (4th ed.). St. Louis: Mosby.

Sinclair, B. (2000). Health promotion and prevention. In D. Lowdermilk, S. Perry, & I. Bobak (Eds.), *Maternity and women's health care* (7th ed., pp. 68-87). St. Louis: Mosby.

Snell, L. (2000). Problems of the breast. In D. Lowdermilk, S. Perry, & I. Bobak (Eds.), *Maternity and women's health care* (7th ed., pp. 247-266). St. Louis: Mosby.

Tomaino-Brunner, C., et al. (1998). Can precopolscopy education increase knowledge and decrease anxiety? *Journal of Obstetric, Gynecologic, and Neonatal Nursing, 27*(6), 636-645.

U.S. Department of Health and Human Services, Public Health Service. (1997). *Clinician's handbook of preventive medicine.* Washington, D.C.: U.S. Government Printing Office.

West, R. (1998). The female athlete: Disordered eating, amenorrhea, and osteoporosis. *Sports Medicine, 26*(2), 63-71.

Youngkin, E., & Davis, M. (1998). *Women's health: A primary care clinical guide* (2nd ed.). Stamford, CT: Appleton & Lange.

Zdanuk, J. (2000). Assessment of women. In D. Lowdermilk, S. Perry, & I. Bobak (Eds.), *Maternity and women's health care* (7th ed., pp. 88-114). St. Louis: Mosby.

CHAPTER 74

Interventions for Clients with Breast Disorders

AMY NICHOLS • DONNA D. IGNATAVICIUS

Learning Objectives

After studying this chapter, you should be able to:

1. Describe the three-pronged approach to early detection of breast masses: mammography, clinical breast examination, and breast self-examination (BSE).
2. Teach a client how to do BSE.
3. Explain the options available to a woman at high genetic risk for breast cancer.
4. Compare and contrast assessment findings associated with benign and malignant breast lesions.
5. Analyze assessment data to determine priority nursing diagnoses and collaborative problems for a woman with breast cancer.
6. Develop a plan of care for a client with breast cancer.
7. Discuss the psychosocial aspects related to having breast cancer and undergoing surgery for breast cancer.
8. Formulate a community-based teaching plan for clients undergoing surgery for breast cancer.

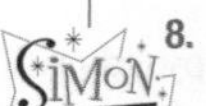

Go to http://www.wbsaunders.com/SIMON/Iggy/ for self-assessment questions related to these Learning Objectives.

Breast cancer is the most commonly diagnosed cancer in women in the Western world, with more than 180,000 new cases identified annually and more than 40,000 deaths in the United States alone (Nass & Davidson, 1999). Although breast disorders affect both men and women, women are most often affected. The most common sign or symptom associated with a breast disorder is a palpable mass. The discovery of a mass in a woman's breast, whether the discovery is by the woman herself, her partner, or a health care provider, is a frightening experience. Even if the woman is aware that 90% of all breast lumps are benign, she may fear that the lump is cancerous. This fearful reaction accompanies the woman through the period of diagnosis, decision making, and treatment. Regardless of the severity of the diagnosis, the nurse must incorporate the physiologic and emotional factors involved to provide effective nursing care.

PREVENTION AND EARLY DETECTION OF BREAST MASSES

Early detection by screening for breast masses involves a three-pronged approach: mammography, breast self-examination, and clinical breast examination.

Mammography

The American Cancer Society (ACS), the National Cancer Institute (NCI), the National Comprehensive Cancer Network (NCCN), the American College of Radiology (ACR), and the American College of Physicians (ACP) have established guidelines for breast cancer screening. Most recommend a baseline screening **mammogram** (x-ray examination of the breast) at the age of 40 years and yearly screening for women beginning between the ages of 40 and 50 (Table 74-1).

Evidence-based data support a significant reduction in breast cancer mortality as a result of annual or biennial mammography and clinical breast examination (CBE) for asymptomatic women between the ages of 50 and 69 years. Champion (1995) conducted a study to determine what influences mammogram compliance and how compliance rates can be improved. Barriers to mammography may include fear of radiation, fear of results, concern about pain, and knowledge deficit. Compliance with mammogram guidelines has been significantly associated with health care provider recommendations for mammography (Champion, 1995).

Other factors influencing whether women have screening mammograms include accessibility and client cost. Not all health insurers pay for mammography. The Breast and Cervical Cancer Mortality Prevention Act of 1990 was established to provide screening services to medically underserved women after a 1992 National Health Interview Survey indicated that only 35% of women older than age 50 years had received a screening mammogram during the previous year. Currently, a number of state and federal programs that target low-income women are available in many areas of the United States.

Breast Self-Examination

Breast self-examination (BSE) is an inexpensive means for detecting breast cancer that has been encouraged by health

TABLE 74-1 • BREAST CANCER SCREENING GUIDELINES FOR ASYMPTOMATIC WOMEN AGE 40 YEARS OR OLDER

Screening Modality	ACS, ACR	NCI	NCCN	ACP
Two-view mammography	Annual Begin at age 40 yr No upper age	Biennial Begin at age 40 yr Upper age, 69 yr	Biennial Begin at age 40 yr No upper age	Annual Begin at age 50 yr Upper age, 74 yr
Clinical breast examination	Annual	Encourage	Annual	Encourage
Breast self-examination	Monthly	Encourage	Encourage	Encourage

From Overmoyer, B. (1999). Breast cancer screening. *Medical Clinics of North America, 83*(6), 1143-1460.
ACS, American Cancer Society; *ACR,* American College of Radiology; *NCI,* National Cancer Institute; *NCCN,* National Comprehensive Cancer Network; and *ACP,* American College of Physicians.

EVIDENCE-BASED PRACTICE FOR NURSING

Does special training improve the proficiency of breast self-examination?

Bragg Leight, S., et al. (2000). The effect of structured training on breast self-examination search behaviors as measured using biomedical instrumentation. *Nursing Research, 49*(5), 283-289.

Although breast self-examination (BSE) has been recommended for many years as a complement to the professional examination and mammography, only a small percentage of women in the United States report doing monthly BSE. The authors describe a study in which they asked 41 young women to participate in a structured training protocol for BSE instruction. Using biomedical instrumentation, the researchers evaluated the depth of breast palpation and the duration of the examination. The results showed that with individualized instruction, the examination was much more thorough for both palpation and duration.

Critique. This study was a small descriptive study that cannot be generalized to the female population. However, it demonstrates that individualized education may make a difference in compliance and thoroughness of the examination. Since the study subjects were young, the study should be replicated to represent a better cross-section of ages and cultures.

Implications for Nursing. Nurses are in a unique position to provide individualized instruction to their clients of any age in any setting. One-on-one training with follow-up may be the most successful way to increase participation in this very important health promotion practice.

care providers for decades. The goal of screening for breast cancer is *early detection.* Detection of breast cancer before axillary node invasion increases the chance of survival. BSE, used in conjunction with mammography and CBE, is extremely effective in detecting early breast cancer and reducing mortality rates. BSE *alone* as a screening technique has not been of equal value. The American Cancer Society recommends that all women older than age 20 years practice BSE monthly. Most women have heard of BSE, but many do not practice it regularly or proficiently (see the Evidence-Based Practice for Nursing box above). The reasons for nonpractice of BSE and the best methods for teaching BSE continue to be researched.

Whether the client seeks health care because she has found a breast lump, because she needs a routine physical examination, or because she has an unrelated health problem, the nurse's encounter with her provides an excellent opportunity to teach BSE. Health care providers must not assume that women who practice BSE do so competently and regularly. Also, most women prefer individualized instruction to learning from pamphlets and magazines. Women who are taught

CONSIDERATIONS FOR OLDER ADULTS

With the projected increase in the older adult population, especially women, during the next half-century, breast cancer will be an even greater health concern. The current recommendation is BSE monthly, CBE yearly, and mammography every 1 to 2 years for women age 65 years and older. Older women may be more resistant to practicing BSE if they have yearly CBE performed by their health care provider. Health teaching to promote compliance and competence in BSE is extremely important in this soon-to-be high-risk group.

CULTURAL CONSIDERATIONS

One of the national health objectives for the year 2010 is the prevention of cancer in minority ethnic populations. Some progress has been made in the area of research to examine the variables associated with BSE in minority women. Research results from one study population of Chinese-American women indicated that only 15% of the women studied practiced BSE monthly, and 48% reported never having done BSE. Although the majority of these women recognized the efficacy of BSE, perceived competency in the technique was the variable that most influenced whether they regularly performed BSE (Lu, 1995). A more recent study by Facione et al. (2000) found that Chinese-American women believe that they are not likely to get breast cancer and that cancer is linked to tragic luck. If they have symptoms suggestive of breast cancer, they are likely to delay Western treatment in favor of Chinese medicine to conserve money and modesty.

In similar studies of African-American women, 63% were found to practice BSE monthly and 76% had yearly CBE; however, only 20% had a mammogram according to age-related guidelines (Phillips & Wilbur, 1995). Like Chinese-American women, African-American women believe in chance and doubt the value of early diagnosis and treatment (Barroso et al., 2000). Culturally sensitive strategies need to be used to increase breast cancer awareness and screening practices among these culturally diverse groups (see Chapter 6).

by a health care provider on an individual or group basis practice BSE more often, more proficiently, and more confidently.

PREPARATION FOR TEACHING BREAST SELF-EXAMINATION

Before teaching BSE, the nurse assesses the psychologic factors influencing the client's motivation to practice BSE. Lack of knowledge about the technique and the benefits of early detection, uneasiness about self-assessment, and lack of confidence in self-assessment may be reasons why women fail to perform BSE regularly. The nurse stresses that treatment for breast cancer is more successful the earlier the disease is detected. It is also important for the client to develop confidence in her ability to detect breast changes. It should be emphasized to the client that a yearly breast examination by a health care provider cannot substitute for BSE.

BSE is used as an assessment tool for detecting cancer but does nothing to prevent breast cancer. Therefore the asymptomatic woman, when choosing whether to practice BSE, may think, "What's the use? It won't keep me from getting breast cancer." Again, the nurse can emphasize the advantages of early detection in terms of outcome and help the client to review risk factors to determine her risk of developing breast cancer. Women must believe that there are benefits to practicing BSE and that the barriers to practicing it are minimal. Addressing these issues will increase the client's knowledge and practice of BSE.

Discussing the client's fears, beliefs, and concerns about breast disease and BSE with her is an important step. Assessment for the presence of risk factors for breast cancer and a history of previous breast problems is essential. Proper timing for BSE should also be discussed. Premenopausal women should examine their breasts 1 week after the menstrual period. At this time, hormonal influence on breast tissue is minimal, so that fluid retention and tenderness are reduced. For these same reasons, if possible, the best time of the month to schedule a mammogram is also 1 week after the menstrual period. Women whose breast tissue is no longer influenced by hormonal fluctuations, such as after a hysterectomy or menopause, should pick a day each month when they will do BSE, such as the first day of the month. Clients who verbalize the need for monthly BSE, the need for yearly CBE, and the mammogram recommendations appropriate for their age demonstrate that client education has been successful.

TEACHING BREAST SELF-EXAMINATION

The setting in which BSE is demonstrated should be private and comfortable. The woman is asked to undress from the waist up and provided with a gown and sheet. Before teaching the technique of breast palpation, the nurse assesses the client's technique by asking her to demonstrate her own method. If the woman is unsure or has not performed BSE before, the nurse can slowly lead her through the examination while explaining the rationale for the technique and answering questions. It is also helpful for the nurse to point out different findings at this time, especially those that the client might perceive as abnormal. For example, nodular breast tissue may normally feel lumpy, which conjures up visions of widespread cancer in the unknowledgeable woman. Placing the client's hand directly on the involved area and showing her precisely what is normal for her can build self-confidence.

The nurse points out the inframammary ridge, the area of the breast where the skin folds under the breast. This thickened area may be perceived as a lump instead of a normal finding. In thin or small-breasted women, the ribs may be mistaken for masses. The nurse shows the client how to follow the rib to the sternum to be sure that what she is feeling is bone and not breast tissue. The client is taught to stand in front of a mirror to inspect the breast for abnormalities. She should raise her arms above her head and press her hands on her hips to emphasize any changes in the shape of the breasts. The breasts are examined in a lying position and while bathing or showering.

The nurse also demonstrates two other aspects of the examination: the amount of pressure needed and the correct position of the hands. The finger pads, which are more sensitive than the fingertips, are used when palpating the breasts. The finger pads should press firmly enough to detect the underlying tissue. However, the client should be instructed not to compress the tissue on the ribs, since this may falsely feel like a mass.

Use of teaching models of normal and abnormal breasts is helpful when teaching BSE. The nurse demonstrates the correct technique of examining the breasts with the arm overhead while lying down instead of having the arm by the side. Showing the difference in the two techniques, especially in large-breasted women, reveals the advantage of using the correct method, which spreads the tissue over the chest wall for more effective palpation.

Clinical Breast Examination

Clinical breast examination (CBE) is typically performed by advanced-practice nurses and physicians. However, nurses in general practice who are skilled in the technique can perform this examination. The examination can be done before, after, or during the teaching session. The same guidelines of providing a private and comfortable setting, maintaining dignity, and allowing time for discussion apply.

Taking a breast history is vital. Results may be recorded on a breast evaluation form, which is a part of the client's record (Figure 74-1). This record helps the nurse establish the relative risk for breast disease and the need for follow-up diagnostic tests, such as mammograms, and teaching.

The physical assessment begins with inspection. The woman undresses from the waist up and first sits or stands with her hands by her sides. The examiner inspects the breasts for symmetry and size, contour, skin changes (color, texture, and venous patterns), nipple changes, and lesions.

One breast may be larger than the other, and inverted nipples are not uncommon. The nurse asks the client whether these findings are normal for her. Any change in symmetry may indicate a problem. The contour should be even, and the skin should have a smooth texture. Venous patterns may be visible but should be similar bilaterally. The nipples and areola should be equal or nearly equal in size and should be a similar color. The nipples may be wrinkled or smooth, and Montgomery's tubercles on the areola are normal. Supernumerary nipples (extra nipples), although rare, are also normal. If a mass is palpated, the examiner notes its position by visualizing the breast as a clock face and noting the "area of the clock" where the mass is located. If it is necessary to move the arms away from the body, the woman should rest her arm on the examiner's to prevent flexion of the underlying muscles. While the arms are by the side and relaxed, the axillae can be palpated. The examiner palpates the axilla and the area above and below the clavicle for enlarged lymph nodes. The woman is then asked to raise her arms over her head, which exposes the sides and underneath portions of the breast for inspection. Finally, she is asked to place her hands on her hips and press, thus flexing the pectoral muscles. This action accentuates skin dimpling, retractions, or masses.

CLIENT'S NAME ______ Sex ______ Race ______ Age ______
Weight ______ Ideal Weight ______ Marital Status ______

HISTORY	Yes	No	Comments
Family history of breast cancer			
Personal history of breast cancer			
Previous mammograms			
Previous biopsy (findings)			
Nipple discharge			
Hormone use (specify)			
BSE Practice			
High-fat diet			
ETOH/smoking			
Current medications (list)			

Age at menses ______ Age at menopause ______

COMMENTS ______

PHYSICAL FINDINGS

Mammogram Report ______
Biopsy/Cytology Results ______
BSE Return Demonstration ______
Plan ______

CLIENT EDUCATION ______

Figure 74-1 ● A breast evaluation form.

The remainder of the examination is done with the client lying supine. The examiner places a pillow or rolled sheet under the client's shoulder, and the arm on that side is raised above the head. Each breast is palpated separately while the other breast remains covered. If the woman has identified a problem in one breast, the other, "normal" breast is examined first to establish a baseline for comparison.

The examiner palpates in a vertical pattern, in a horizontal pattern, or in concentric circles, covering every inch of the breast tissue, including the tail of Spence, which extends from the upper outer quadrant of the breast into the axilla. Supraclavicular lymph nodes are palpated for the presence of enlarged nodes by hooking the fingers over the clavicle.

Finally, the nipple is gently compressed to detect the presence of a discharge. If a discharge is produced, the examiner notes the "area of the clock" where the breast was compressed when the discharge was released. If there is a history of discharge, the client may be able to express the discharge more successfully than the examiner can and may be asked to do so.

Discovery of a suspicious lesion or discharge during the examination requires consultation or referral to a health care provider who specializes in caring for breast disorders. Follow-up usually involves mammography and possibly ultrasound. If there is a dominant mass or a suspicious clinical picture, the woman should be referred for biopsy even if the mammogram is negative.

CONSIDERATIONS FOR OLDER ADULTS

As women age, the breast tissue becomes flattened and elongated and is suspended loosely from the chest wall. On palpation the breast tissue of the older woman will have a finer, more granular feel than the lobular feel in a younger woman. The inframammary ridge may be more prominent as a result of atrophy of the breast tissue. Breast examination in older clients may be easier because of tissue atrophy and relaxation of the suspensory ligaments (Cooper's ligaments).

WOMEN AT HIGH GENETIC RISK FOR BREAST CANCER

A woman is considered to be at high genetic risk for breast cancer if her family history suggests a predisposition to the disease. Family history includes multiple relatives with breast cancer, early age at diagnosis, and in some families, ovarian cancer. Currently, inherited mutations in several genes are known to be manifested in hereditary patterns of breast cancer. The most common genes tested for breast cancer are BRCA1 and BRCA2. Mutations in these genes could account for 40% to 50% of hereditary breast cancers in the United States (Couch, DeShano, & Blackwood, 1997; Couch & Hartmann, 1998; Frank, Manley, & Olopade, 1998).

Cancer Surveillance

Cancer surveillance is currently the prevention option preferred by most high-risk women. Cancer surveillance is also referred to as "secondary prevention" and is used to detect cancer early in the initial stages. For breast cancer surveillance in high-risk women, the same combination of breast self-examination (BSE), clinical breast examination (CBE), and mammography are recommended as in the asymptomatic population. The difference for high-risk women is in the timing of examinations and starting age of mammography. The Cancer Genetics Studies Consortium, organized by the National Human Genome Research Institute, convened a task force to make recommendations for the management of women with BRCA1 and BRCA2 mutations (Burke, Daly, & Garber, 1997). The recommendations include monthly BSE beginning at age 18 to 21 years, CBE every 6 to 12 months beginning at age 25 to 35, and annual mammography beginning at age 25 to 35.

Prophylactic Mastectomy

Prophylactic **mastectomy** (surgical breast removal) is another option for reducing the risk of breast cancer. Although prophylactic mastectomy has been an option for decades, little information has been available until now regarding the long-term outcome of women who have elected to undergo this procedure (American Society of Clinical Oncology, 1998; Burke et al., 1997). Even though a woman may elect to undergo a prophylactic mastectomy, there is a small risk that breast cancer will develop in residual breast glandular tissue, because no mastectomy reliably removes all mammary tissue (Hartmann et al., 1999).

Chemoprevention

The third management option for women at high risk for breast cancer is **chemoprevention** with the prophylactic use of the drug known as tamoxifen citrate (Nolvadex, Tamofen✤, Tamone✤). In three clinical trials in which tamoxifen was introduced as a breast cancer chemopreventive, tamoxifen citrate was indicated to reduce the incidence of breast cancer in women at high risk for breast cancer (Fisher, Costantino, & Wickerman, 1998; Veronesi et al., 1998). Although the drug treatment was successful, there were drawbacks. Women who were treated with tamoxifen complained of many serious side effects, and the medication treatment is very expensive (Fisher, Costantino, & Wickerman, 1998).

BENIGN BREAST DISORDERS

Most breast lumps are benign. Because the incidence of breast disease is related to age, breast disorders are described in an age-related order (Table 74-2).

Fibroadenoma

Fibroadenomas are the most common cause of breast masses during adolescence, although they may occur into the 30s. A fibroadenoma is a solid, slowly enlarging, benign mass of connective tissue that is unattached to the surrounding breast tissue and is typically discovered by the client herself. Although the immediate fear is that of breast cancer, only 0.9% of these masses are malignant. The mass is usually round, firm, easily movable, nontender, and clearly delineated from the surrounding tissue.

Fibroadenomas are usually located in the upper outer quadrant of the breast; multiple masses may be present in 10% to 15% of cases (Dent & Cant, 1999). Enlargement is more likely in pregnancy. The health care provider may order a breast ultrasound examination or may perform a needle aspiration to establish whether the lump is cystic or solid. If the lesion is solid, outpatient excision using local anesthesia is the treatment of choice.

CULTURAL CONSIDERATIONS

Fibroadenomas are most common in African-American women and tend to occur at an earlier age in African-American women than in women of other ethnic backgrounds (Tierney et al., 1995).

Fibrocystic Breast Disease

OVERVIEW

Fibrocystic changes, or physiologic nodularity of the breast, often referred to as **fibrocystic breast disease (FBD),** are the most common breast problem of women between the ages of 20 and 30 years. Over the life span, approximately 90% of women will have fibrocystic changes. Fibrocystic changes may proceed through several clinical stages or may present in only one form.

TABLE 74-2 • TYPICAL PRESENTATION OF BENIGN BREAST DISORDERS

Breast Disorder	Description	Incidence
Fibroadenoma	Most common benign lesion; solid mass of connective tissue that is unattached to the surrounding tissue	During teenage years into the 30s
Fibrocystic breast disease (FBD)	*First stage:* Characterized by premenstrual bilateral fullness and tenderness *Second stage:* Presence of bilateral, multicentric nodules *Third stage:* Presence of microscopic and macroscopic cysts	Late teens and 20s
Ductal ectasia	Hard, irregular mass or masses with nipple discharge, enlarged axillary nodes, redness, and edema; difficult to distinguish from cancer	Women approaching menopause
Intraductal ectasia	Mass in duct that results in nipple discharge; mass is usually not palpable	Women ages 40 to 55 yr

Data from National Cancer Institute.

The first stage commonly occurs between the late teens and early 20s. Premenstrual bilateral fullness and tenderness are present, especially in the outer upper quadrant. Symptoms usually resolve after menstruation and then recur before the next menstrual period in a cyclic fashion.

The second stage usually occurs in the late 20s and throughout the 30s. Bilateral multicentric nodular areas that feel like small marbles can be felt and accompany the fullness and soreness.

The third stage generally occurs between the ages of 35 and 55 years. Microscopic or macroscopic cysts generally appear suddenly and are associated with pain, tenderness, or burning. They are usually three-dimensional, smooth, mobile, and well delineated. Although the cysts may recede somewhat before menstruation, they do not disappear completely. Mammography is generally indicated, and fine-needle aspiration may be performed. Older clients receiving hormone replacement therapy may develop painful, fluid-filled cysts. Biopsy is indicated in the following situations:

- The aspirated fluid is bloody.
- No fluid is aspirated.
- The mammogram shows suspicious findings.
- A mass remains palpable after aspiration.
- The cytologic study of the aspirated fluid reveals malignant cells.

Although the cause of fibrocystic breast changes is unknown, the condition seems to be related to normal fluctuations in estrogen levels during the menstrual cycle. Symptoms usually resolve after menopause in the absence of estrogen supplementation.

➤ COLLABORATIVE MANAGEMENT

Medical management of FBD is generally symptomatic. Hormonal manipulation has been the primary means of pharmacologic intervention. Oral contraceptives can suppress oversecretion of estrogen, and progestins may be used to correct luteal insufficiency. Danazol (Danocrine, Cyclomen🍁) suppresses ovarian function and estrogen stimulation of breast tissue. However, because hormonal therapy with danazol will not cure FBD, and because its side effects are undesirable, it is generally used only in clients with recurrent and unusually severe fibrocystic disease.

Medical management may also include the use of vitamins C, E, and B complex. The health care provider may prescribe diuretics to decrease premenstrual breast engorgement. Clients are counseled to avoid the use of caffeine; however, the role of caffeine in FBD is controversial.

The client is encouraged to continue prescribed medical interventions and monitors the effectiveness of these interventions. The nurse suggests supportive measures, such as the use of mild analgesics or limiting salt intake before menses, to help decrease swelling. The client may want to wear (both day and night) a well-padded, supportive brassiere to decrease tension on ligaments. Local application of ice or heat may provide temporary relief of pain. The nurse promotes the practice of BSE and teaches the procedure when necessary.

Ductal Ectasia

Ductal ectasia is a benign breast problem that is usually seen in women approaching menopause. The disease is caused by dilation and thickening of the collecting ducts in the subareolar area. These ducts become distended and filled with cellular debris, which activates an inflammatory response. Two clinical signs result from these changes:

- A mass develops that feels hard, has irregular borders, and may be tender.
- A greenish brown nipple discharge, enlarged axillary nodes, and redness and edema over the site of the mass are noted.

These masses are often difficult to distinguish from breast cancer. Because the risk for breast cancer is increased in the menopause age-group, accurate diagnosis is vital. A microscopic examination of the nipple discharge is performed to detect any atypical or malignant cells, and the affected area is excised. Nursing care is directed at alleviating the anxiety associated with the threat of breast cancer and at supporting the woman through the diagnostic and treatment procedures.

Intraductal Papilloma

Intraductal papilloma, like ductal ectasia and breast cancer, occurs primarily in women ages 40 to 55 years. A benign process in the epithelial lining of the duct forms a papilloma, or pedunculated outgrowth of tissue. As the papilloma grows, trauma and erosion within the duct result in a serosanguineous or serous nipple discharge. A mass is rarely palpable.

Diagnosis is aimed first at ruling out breast cancer. Microscopic examination of the nipple discharge and surgical excision of the mass and ductal area are usually indicated.

Issues of Large-Breasted Women

Although Western society emphasizes large breasts as positive attributes, women with excessive breast tissue experience difficulties and discomfort. For instance, because fashion is directed at the small-breasted figure, a woman with large breasts may have difficulty finding clothes that fit well and in which she feels attractive. The breast size may be disproportionate to the rest of the body, which adds to the problem of finding clothes that fit. Brassieres are expensive and may have to be specially ordered, and the straps create large dents in the shoulders. In addition, many large-breasted women experience fungal infections under the breasts because it is difficult to keep this area dry and exposed to air.

Backaches from the added weight are also common. The only alternative for this condition, if well-fitting brassieres do not help and obesity is not part of the problem, may be breast reduction surgery. The surgeon removes excess breast tissue, repositions the nipple, and repositions the resultant skin flaps to produce the optimal cosmetic effect. This operation is a major surgical procedure and is termed a **reduction mammoplasty.**

The decision to undergo the procedure is usually made after years of living with the discomfort of excessive breast size. The nurse may be involved in the decision-making stage by listening to the client verbalize her feelings and providing information as appropriate. The postoperative diagnoses and goals are consistent with those for the woman undergoing reconstructive surgery (see Breast Reconstruction, p. 1744).

Gynecomastia

Gynecomastia literally means "female breasts" and is a symptom rather than a disease. It is usually a benign condition of breast enlargement in *men* (Figure 74-2). However, gynecomastia can be a result of a primary cancer such as lung cancer. The enlargement is usually bilateral, but enlargement is asymmetric in about 10% of cases. The condition is caused by proliferation of the glandular tissue, including the mammary ducts and ductal stroma. In many instances, it is difficult to distinguish gynecomastia from breast enlargement related to excess adipose tissue. Etiologic factors of gynecomastia include drugs; aging; obesity; underlying diseases causing estrogen excess, such as malnutrition, liver disease, or hyperthyroidism; and androgen deficiency states, such as age or chronic renal failure.

Although gynecomastia is not common, men with abnormal breast findings, especially a breast mass, are carefully evaluated for breast cancer.

BREAST CANCER

OVERVIEW

Breast cancer is the most commonly diagnosed cancer in women and is currently a leading cause of cancer mortality in women, second only to lung cancer. The ultimate goal of early diagnosis is to reduce mortality by identifying women at risk for breast cancer and predicting the prognosis and response to different therapies. Many of the current therapies for breast cancer are standard cytotoxic agents that treat all types of cancer; however, the increased use of the antiestrogen medication tamoxifen has been shown to be effective in the battle against breast cancer. Because of the high incidence of the disease, almost every woman has had a close personal association with another woman with the disease. Thus most women have strong reactions to the threat of breast cancer. These reactions greatly influence a woman's health habits, including breast self-examination (BSE) and her readiness to seek care when a suspicious area is discovered.

Until prevention becomes a viable option, early detection is the key to better treatment and survival. Statistics support the advantages of early detection and treatment. The most reliable indicator of prognosis is related to the stage of the breast cancer at the time of diagnosis. Localized breast cancer with no regional spread is associated with a clinical cure rate of 75% to 90%. If the woman has a small tumor with no evidence of axillary node involvement, the 5-year survival rate is 90%. The 5-year survival rate drops to 40% to 50%, with a 10-year survival rate of 25%, when the axillary lymph nodes are involved (Tierney et al., 1995). Breast cancer is the second leading cause of cancer deaths in women in the United States and is the leading cause of cancer deaths in the 35- to 54-year-old age-group.

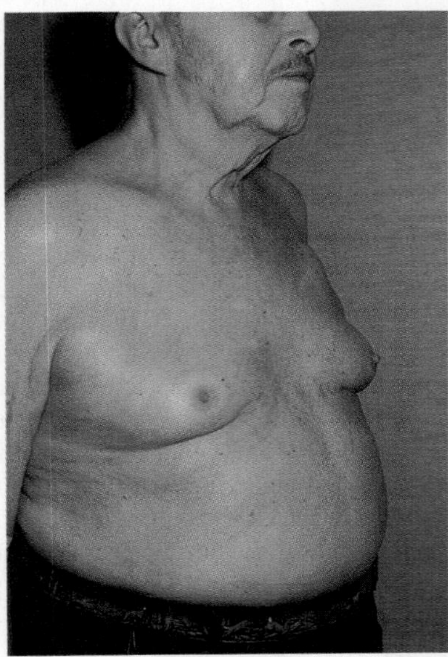

Figure 74-2 ● Gynecomastia. (From Swartz, M.H. [1998]. *Textbook of physical diagnosis: History and examination* [3rd ed.]. Philadelphia: W.B. Saunders.)

Pathophysiology

TYPES OF BREAST CANCER

There are many pathologic types of breast cancer, but the most common, accounting for more than 80% of cases, is *infiltrating ductal carcinoma.* As the name implies, the disease originates in the mammary ducts and specifically grows in the epithelial cells lining these ducts. The rate of cancer growth varies and partially depends on hormonal influences. It takes an estimated 5 to 9 years for a cancer cell to divide and result in a lesion large enough to be clinically palpable.

As long as the cancer remains within the duct, it is considered **noninvasive.** The cancer is classified as **invasive** when it penetrates the tissue surrounding the duct. Most breast cancers arise from the intermediate ducts and are invasive. Once invasive, the cancer grows into the tissue around it in an irregular pattern; for this reason, once the lesion is palpable, it is felt as an irregular, poorly defined mass.

As the tumor continues to grow, fibrosis develops around the cancer. This fibrosis may cause shortening of Cooper's ligaments and the resulting characteristic skin dimpling that is seen with more advanced disease.

COMPLICATIONS OF BREAST CANCER

The tumor also invades the lymphatic channels, blocking skin drainage and causing skin edema and an orange peel appearance of the skin **(peau d'orange).** Invasion of the lymphatic channels carries tumor cells to the lymphatic nodes, including those in the axillary region. For this reason, pathologic examination of the axillary nodes is imperative for staging the disease. The tumor eventually replaces the skin itself, and ulceration of the overlying skin occurs. Metastases result from seeding of the cancer cells into the blood and lymph systems, which permits spread of these cells to distant sites. The most common sites of metastatic disease from breast cancer are bone, lungs, brain, and liver.

The course of metastatic breast cancer is related to the site affected and to the function impaired. The pathophysiologic process of cancer is further described in Chapter 25.

BREAST CANCER IN MEN

About 1% of all cases of breast cancer occur in men. The average age of onset is 60 years. Men usually present with a hard, nonpainful, subareolar mass, and gynecomastia may be present. Occasionally the man may present with a nipple discharge, retraction, erosion, or ulceration. Although nipple discharge is not a common presenting symptom, about 75% of the men who present with nipple discharge are diagnosed with breast carcinoma. Breast cancer in men is staged the same as in women. However, the prognosis even for stage I breast cancer is worse for men. Five-year survival rates for stage I breast cancer in men are 58%; 5-year survival rates decrease to 38% for stage II disease (Tierney et al., 1995). Breast cancer in men is often a disseminated disease, which accounts for lower survival rates. Treatment of men with breast cancer parallels that of women at a similar stage of disease.

Etiology

There is no single known etiologic agent for breast cancer. Breast cancer can be attributed to multiple factors (Table 74-3).

Women with a familial history of breast cancer, particularly a history of a first-degree relative (mother, sister, or daughter) with premenopausal breast cancer, have a threefold risk increase. This risk is further increased if the relative had breast cancer bilaterally or before age 50 years. Ninety percent of clients with breast cancer have no familial history. Seventy percent of women over the age of 50 who are diagnosed with breast cancer have no identifiable risk factor for the development of the disease other than age and gender (Shapiro & Clark, 1995). Family history includes multiple relatives with breast cancer, early age at diagnosis, and in some families, ovarian cancer.

As discussed earlier, inherited mutations in several genes are known to be manifested in hereditary patterns of breast cancer. Breast cancer, however, is not an exclusively inherited, genetic disease. Exposure to high-dose ionizing radiation (especially before the age of 20 years), early menarche (before age 12), and late menopause (after age 50) are associated with an increased risk of breast cancer. A history of previous breast cancer, nulliparity (no pregnancies), and first birth after age 30 years are also considered to heighten risk.

Questionable risk factors include a diet high in animal fats, a diet low in fiber, alcohol consumption, and long-term estrogen replacement therapy (Leslie, 1995). Studies have shown a small increase in the risk of breast cancer in perimenopausal women receiving hormone replacement therapy (HRT) after 5 or more years of use. The risks of HRT must be weighed against the benefits. The benefits of HRT are a decreased risk of heart disease and osteoporosis and the control of menopausal symptoms. Decisions related to the use of HRT must be individualized on the basis of the client's risk profile.

TABLE 74-3 • RISK FACTORS FOR BREAST CANCER

Factor	Degree of Risk	Comments
Female gender	Increased	99% of all breast cancers occur in women.
History of a previous breast cancer	Increased	The risk of developing a cancer in the opposite breast is 5 times greater than for the average population at risk.
Age >40 yr	Increased	Incidence increases with age and peaks in the fifth decade.
Menstrual history Early menarche or late menopause or both	Increased	The risk of breast cancer rises as the interval between menarche and menopause increases; shortening the interval by mastectomy reduces the risk, especially if performed in women younger than age 35 yr.
Reproductive history Nulliparity First child born after age 30 yr	Increased	Childless women have an increased risk, as do women who bear their first child near or after age 30 yr.
Family history Mother or sister or both	Increased	Risk increases 2 to 3 times if the mother or a sister has had breast cancer and is further increased if the relative was diagnosed during the premenopausal state and if the cancer was bilateral.
Diet	Controversial	Animal data and descriptive epidemiology of breast cancer incidence strongly suggest an association of dietary factors, specifically a high-fat diet, with an increased risk of breast cancer. The National Academy of Science recommends decreasing total fat intake to 30% of available calories.
Alcohol	Unknown	A suggested small increase in risk with moderate alcohol consumption has been reported, although limitations in methodology have been cited and results require confirmation.
Obesity	Controversial	Weight, height, obesity, and increased body mass have been reported to be associated with an increased risk of breast cancer.
Ionizing radiation	Increased	Three groups of women who received low-level radiation exposure demonstrated an increased breast cancer risk, which was particularly notable if the exposure occurred in the early years (before age 30 yr).
Benign breast disease	None	Fibrocystic breast disease is not associated with breast cancer. However, biopsy-proven atypical hyperplasia is associated with an increased risk.
Oral contraceptives	None	There is no evidence yet to suggest a causal relationship between oral contraceptives and the incidence of and survival from breast cancer.
Exogenous hormones	Controversial	Several studies report no link with replacement hormones and breast cancer, and those that do appear to identify only subsets of clients at risk: those who have taken replacement estrogens for more than 5 yr and those who have taken large cumulative doses.

Modified from McCorkle, R., et al. (1996). *Cancer nursing: A comprehensive textbook* (2nd ed.). Philadelphia: W.B. Saunders.

TABLE 74-4 • AGE-RELATED RISK FOR BREAST CANCER

Age (yr)	Breast Cancer Risk
25	1 in 19,608
30	1 in 2525
35	1 in 622
40	1 in 217
45	1 in 93
50	1 in 50
55	1 in 33
60	1 in 24
65	1 in 17
70	1 in 14
75	1 in 11
80	1 in 10
85	1 in 11
In a lifetime	1 in 8

Data from National Cancer Institute.

Being an older woman is the primary risk factor, although some women are at higher risk than others. As age increases, so does risk. More than 85% of clients are diagnosed after age 45 years. Obesity may be a factor associated with the development of breast cancer in postmenopausal women. Other genetic and environmental risk factors are listed in Table 74-3.

Incidence/Prevalence

Each year an estimated 184,000 women and 1400 men are diagnosed with breast cancer in the United States. Of these, approximately 46,000 women and 400 men die of the disease (Wingo et al., 1995). Although these numbers are staggering, there is a trend toward earlier diagnosis. In 1993, 75% of newly diagnosed breast cancers were stage I or II; in addition, negative nodes were found in one third of all breast cancers (Moore & Kinne, 1995). Breast cancer accounts for 1 in 4 cancers in women. It occurs most commonly in older adults, and its prevalence increases with age. With the aging female population, health care researchers are predicting a rise in the incidence of breast cancer in women over 67 years of age. By age 85 years, each American woman faces a 1-in-9 risk of being diagnosed with breast cancer. One of every eight American women will develop breast cancer in her lifetime (Table 74-4).

CULTURAL CONSIDERATIONS

The mortality rate of breast cancer is higher in African-American women. Overall, cancer remains a major public health problem for African Americans despite decreases in mortality for specific cancers. Although the incidence of breast cancer is lower in African Americans than in Caucasians, death rates are higher for African-American women at every stage of the disease. The 5-year survival rate for African Americans is 62% as compared with 79% for Caucasians (Allen & Phillips, 1997). Research suggests that poverty, less education, and inadequate access to screening are related to higher cancer morbidity and mortality rates in African Americans (Wingo et al., 1996).

Like the African-American female population, Latino and Hispanic women have a lower incidence of breast cancer than Caucasians but a higher death rate. The differences in survival rates reflect the stage at which the cancer is diagnosed. Breast cancer is the most common cancer in Asian and Pacific Island women; the death rates are higher for Hawaiian women than for all other ethnic groups (Allen & Phillips, 1997).

➤ COLLABORATIVE MANAGEMENT

Assessment

HISTORY

The initial history may be taken after a mass has been discovered but before definitive diagnosis has been made, or the history may be obtained at the time the woman is seen for treatment of an identified cancer. The history should focus on three major areas: risk factors, the breast mass, and health maintenance practices.

RISK FACTORS. In the first area of assessment, the nurse records age, gender, marital status, weight, and height. Marital status and identification of the client's primary support person provide information about those to be included in the woman's care, teaching, and support. The nurse obtains specific information on personal and family histories of breast cancer. In addition to increasing the woman's own risk, these factors also affect any sister's or daughter's risk and should be incorporated into later counseling.

The gynecologic/obstetric history includes the following:
- Age at menarche
- Age at menopause
- Symptoms of menopause
- Age at first child's birth
- Number of children

Prolonged hormonal stimulation (e.g., early menses and/or late menopause) increases a woman's risk, as does birth of the first child after age 30 years and nulliparity.

HISTORY OF THE BREAST MASS. The second area of assessment focuses on the history of the breast mass. The history reveals not only the course of the disease but also data related to health care–seeking practices and health-promoting behaviors.

Knowledge of how, when, and by whom the mass was discovered and the interval between discovery and seeking care is crucial. If the woman found the mass, was it discovered through breast self-examination (BSE) or by accident? The answer to this question might alert the nurse to the need for discussion and teaching about BSE regardless of whether the mass proves to be malignant. What was the time interval between discovery and seeing the health care provider? If there was a delay, what caused it? These questions are linked to the psychosocial assessment but also reveal the length of time that the tumor has been present. The nurse notes procedures directed at diagnosing this problem and others in the past. Finally, a review of systems focusing on the most common areas for metastases is made.

HEALTH MAINTENANCE PRACTICES. The third area of assessment includes health maintenance practices. In addition to questioning the client about the knowledge, practice, and regularity of BSE, the nurse takes a mammographic history. The existence of previous mammograms allows the health care provider to compare current mammograms with past ones to facilitate diagnosis.

A brief diet history, in which the client is asked to recall a typical day's menu and alcoholic intake per week, reveals the usual intake of fat and alcohol. A high alcohol and fat intake *may* increase the risk of breast cancer.

The nurse asks the client what types of medications she uses, specifically, hormonal supplements, such as estrogen. Estrogen can be administered orally, intravaginally, or via a transdermal patch. The nurse documents the type and form of hormones (birth control pills, supplements) and length of use. Postmenopausal use of estrogen creams intravaginally is not uncommon and should be considered a major source of estrogen.

PHYSICAL ASSESSMENT/CLINICAL MANIFESTATIONS

The approach to physical assessment is discussed earlier under Breast Self-Examination (p. 1730) and under Clinical Breast Examination (p. 1732). The nurse notes specific information about the breast mass (Chart 74-1). The mass is described in the chart in terms of location (using the "face of the clock" method), shape, size, consistency, and fixation to the surrounding tissues.

Any skin change, such as **peau d'orange** (dimpling, orange peel appearance), increased vascularity, nipple retraction, or ulceration, can indicate advanced disease and needs to be documented. The nurse examines the axillary and supraclavicular areas thoroughly by palpating deeply for enlarged lymph nodes and noting their presence and location in the client's record. The presence of pain or soreness in the affected breast is evaluated. After gathering this information, the nurse draws a diagram on the chart (see Figure 74-1) that will be helpful for others involved in the client's care.

PSYCHOSOCIAL ASSESSMENT

The client with potential or diagnosed breast cancer faces three major issues: the fear of cancer; threats to body image, sexuality, intimate relationships, and survival; and decisional conflict related to treatment options.

The woman will need information about how advanced the disease is, the likelihood of cure, treatment options and side effects, how treatment will affect her life and self-image, how her family or significant others will be affected, and home self-care. A woman's previous experience with cancer, and especially with other women with breast cancer, influences her reactions to the disease. The client is asked whether she has known anyone with breast cancer and what types of experiences she has had with breast disease and cancer in general. The nurse explores the woman's feelings about the disease because her choices of treatment, her recovery, and her ability to learn are greatly influenced by these emotions. The client's and family's knowledge of breast cancer, the stage of the disease, and treatment options are assessed. The client's level of education is a significant influencing factor in her treatment choices for stage I breast cancer. Her perception of her situation is often influenced by outdated information. Perhaps she knew someone who had a Halsted radical mastectomy 30 years ago and associates breast surgery with the chest deformity and lymphedema experienced by that woman. Dispelling misconceptions by providing current information can affect her attitude in a positive way.

The nurse may also assess the client with breast cancer for problems related to sexuality. Three critical areas of distress—psychologic, physiologic, and relational—contribute to the psychosexual morbidity of these clients. The nurse should inquire about the frequency of, and the client's satisfaction with, sexual relations with her partner. The client should reflect on the relationship with the partner and be asked if and how the breast cancer has changed the intimate relations with, sexual function of, or types of touch by the partner.

The need for additional resources is also evaluated at this time. Will extra psychologic counseling be needed? Are there financial concerns that need to be discussed with social services? Will the client's spouse, family, or friends support her throughout this period? How much support and teaching do they need? When does the client expect to hear about her pathology results, and whom would she like to have with her when she hears the results? Answers to these types of questions provide guidelines in establishing expected outcomes and in planning nursing care.

CHART 74-1

BEST PRACTICE *for* Assessing a Breast Mass

- Identify the location of the mass by using the "face of the clock" method.
- Describe the shape, size, and consistency of the mass.
- Assess whether the mass is fixed or movable.
- Note any skin changes around the mass, such as dimpling *(peau d'orange)*, increased vascularity, nipple retraction, and ulceration.
- Assess the adjacent lymph nodes, both axillary and supraclavicular nodes.
- Ask the client if she experiences pain or soreness in the area around the mass.

LABORATORY ASSESSMENT

The diagnosis of breast cancer relies primarily on pathologic examination of tissue from the breast mass. Serum-based laboratory tests are not used routinely to aid in this diagnosis; however, radioimmunoassay (RIA) is being used in research to detect and monitor breast cancer. Studies to identify breast cancer tumor markers are currently being conducted. One breast cancer tumor marker is 5-hydroxymethyl-2-deoxyuridine (Djuric et al., 1996).

After the presence of cancer is established, laboratory tests, including pathologic examination of the lymph nodes, help detect possible metastases. Elevated liver enzyme levels indicate possible liver metastases, and increased serum calcium and alkaline phosphatase levels suggest bone metastases.

RADIOGRAPHIC ASSESSMENT

Mammography is the most sensitive screening tool for breast cancer. However, it must be combined with BSE for optimal early detection and with clinical breast examination (CBE) for full interpretation of the findings. These three methods together are effective in detecting breast cancer as early as possible. The uniqueness of mammography results from its ability to reveal preclinical lesions (masses too small to be palpated manually). Client preparation and the procedure for mammography are discussed in Chapter 73.

Other radiographic procedures may be used preoperatively to rule out metastases. A chest x-ray examination to screen for lung metastases is routine. Bone, liver, and brain scans and computed tomography (CT) scans of the chest and abdomen can reveal distant metastases.

OTHER DIAGNOSTIC ASSESSMENT

Ultrasonography of the breast is an additional diagnostic tool used to clarify findings on mammography. If the mammogram reveals a lesion, ultrasonography is helpful in differentiating a fluid-filled cyst from a solid mass.

Postoperative pathologic examination of the breast tissue, or **breast biopsy,** is the key to diagnosis of breast cancer. It is estimated that as many as 1.8 million breast biopsies are performed each year (Shapiro & Clark, 1995). Breast tissue is obtained by one of several types of biopsies (see Chapter 73).

Several other tests are useful for establishing the stage of disease and prognosis after the diagnosis is made. These tests include a pathologic examination of the lymph nodes on the affected side. Other prognostic factors include the following (Donegan & Spratt, 1995):

- Estrogen and progesterone receptors
- S-phase index, or growth rate (done by flow-cytometric determinations of the S-phase fraction)
- DNA ploidy (the amount of DNA in a tumor cell as compared with a normal cell)
- Histologic or nuclear grade

Estrogen and progesterone receptors are cytoplasmic proteins present in and on the surface of breast cancer cells that bind to estrogen and progesterone. When estrogen and progesterone bind to the cell, the cell's activity is thought to change. A tumor that contains receptors capable of binding with circulating hormones, specifically estrogen and progesterone, is estrogen receptor (ER) positive. More postmenopausal women than premenopausal women are ER positive. Women with ER-positive tumors respond better to adjuvant therapy and usually survive longer.

The receptor status also predicts which women will respond to hormonal manipulation as a treatment. Thymidine labeling index, ploidy factor (deoxyribonucleic acid [DNA] content), and calculation of the number of cells in S phase by flow cytometry can reveal the growth rate of cells. Tumors with a high growth rate index and altered DNA content are associated with a worse prognosis (Donegan & Spratt, 1995).

Tumor cells are also examined for specialization or differentiation. Because well-differentiated tumors tend to be less aggressive than poorly differentiated ones, a woman with a well-differentiated breast cancer has a better prognosis than the woman with a poorly differentiated tumor.

As mentioned earlier, several procedures related to specific sites of possible metastases also help establish the stage or progression of the breast cancer. Figure 74-3 illustrates the four stages of breast cancer.

Analysis

COMMON NURSING DIAGNOSES AND COLLABORATIVE PROBLEMS

A common nursing diagnosis for clients with breast cancer is Anxiety related to the diagnosis of cancer.

A common collaborative problem is Potential for Metastasis.

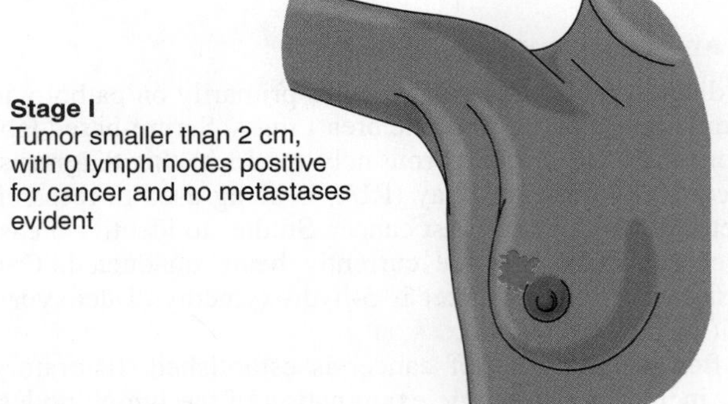

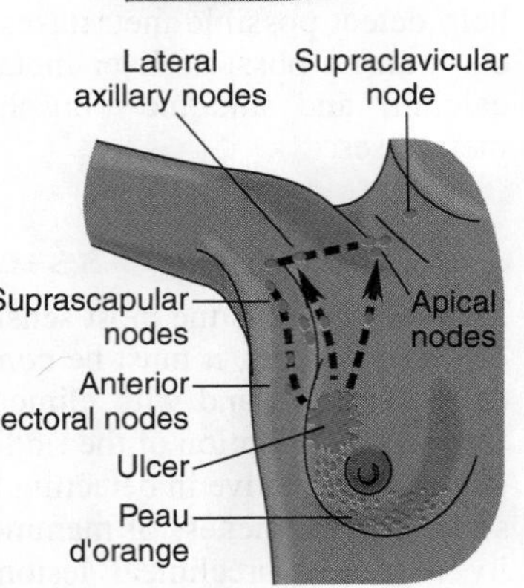

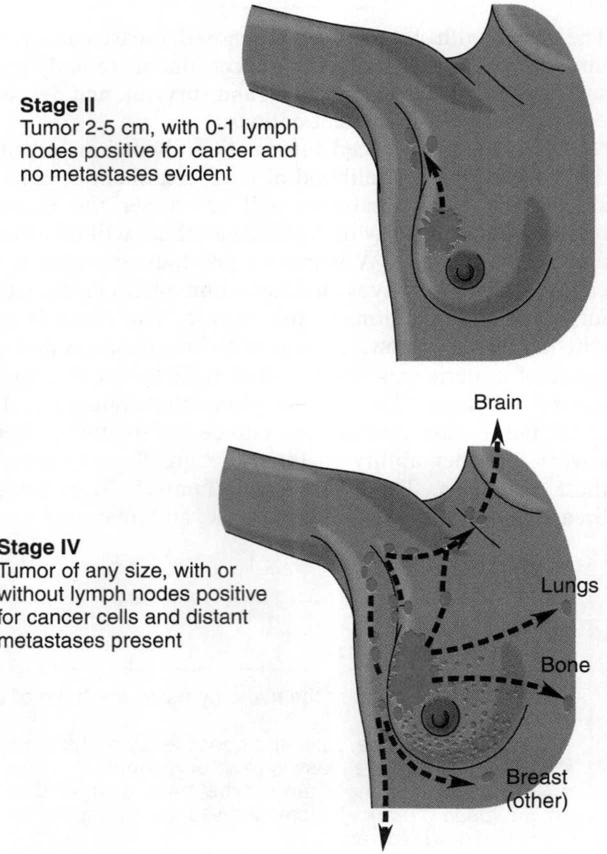

Figure 74-3 ● Staging of breast cancer.

ADDITIONAL NURSING DIAGNOSES AND COLLABORATIVE PROBLEMS

In addition to the common nursing diagnoses and collaborative problems, clients with breast cancer (particularly advanced breast cancer) may have one or more of the following:

- Anticipatory Grieving related to loss and possible or impending death
- Acute Pain related to tumor compression on nerve endings
- Disturbed Sleep Pattern related to pain and anxiety
- Disturbed Body Image related to loss of a body part
- Sexual Dysfunction related to body image or self-esteem disturbance

Planning and Implementation

ANXIETY

NOC **PLANNING: EXPECTED OUTCOMES.** The client with breast cancer is expected to seek information to reduce anxiety, control anxiety responses, and use effective coping strategies throughout the treatment period by participating in decision making, discussing concerns, and learning self-care measures.

INTERVENTIONS. The woman with breast cancer is usually admitted to the health care facility with a definitive diagnosis established through an outpatient biopsy of the mass. The practice of admitting a woman with a suspicious lesion and using general anesthesia for a biopsy, frozen section, and possible mastectomy has largely been abandoned. Women who have an interval between the biopsy and treatment, during which they actively participate in the choice of treatment, cope more effectively after surgery, no matter which treatment is chosen.

NIC **ANXIETY REDUCTION.** The anxiety for the woman with breast cancer begins the moment the lump is discovered. The level of anxiety may be related to past experiences and personal associations with the disease. Many women also have an intuitive feeling about the diagnosis even before it has been established. The clinical likelihood that the lesion is or is not cancer is irrelevant to the level of fear. The client's perceptions of her own situation and personal level of anxiety are assessed. The nurse allows the client to ventilate these feelings even if a diagnosis has not been established (Chart 74-2).

CHART 74-2

NIC INTERVENTION ACTIVITIES *for* The Client with Breast Cancer

Anxiety Reduction: *Minimizing apprehension, dread, foreboding, or uneasiness related to an unidentified source of anticipated danger*

- Listen attentively.
- Use calm, reassuring approach.
- Provide factual information concerning diagnosis, treatment, and prognosis.
- Encourage verbalization of feelings, perceptions, and fears.
- Identify when level of anxiety changes.
- Support the use of appropriate defense mechanisms.
- Determine client's decision-making ability.

NIC intervention activities selected from McCloskey, J.C., & Bulechek, G.M. (2000). *Nursing interventions classification (NIC)* (3rd ed.). St. Louis: Mosby. No part of this work is to be altered without prior written permission from the Publisher.

If the mass has been diagnosed as cancer, many women feel a partial sense of relief to be dealing with a known entity. A feeling of shock or disbelief may predominate. It is difficult to accept a diagnosis of cancer when one feels basically well. Clients and their families or significant others deal in individual ways with the mix of feelings, which include shock, disbelief, and grief. Some may want to read and discuss any available information. Others may want to know as little as possible and resent attempts at teaching. Although one woman may want to talk at length about her concerns, another may want to be alone. Flexibility is the key to nursing care; the nurse adjusts the approach to care as the client's emotional state changes. An integral part of the plan to meet these emotional needs is the use of outside resources. Most health care providers view such groups as the American Cancer Society's Reach to Recovery as a source of support in the postoperative period, but the nurse can suggest these groups in the preoperative phase.

Health care providers working with breast cancer clients may know other clients willing to make a preoperative visit. These resource people may be chosen on the basis of the client's concerns. The woman who is worried in particular about the side effects of radiation therapy may benefit more from talking to someone who has undergone radiation than from talking to the nurse about secondhand experiences.

In addition to Reach to Recovery, formal and informal community support groups, such as ENCORE (Encouragement, Normalcy, Counseling, Opportunity, Reaching Out, and Energies Revived), may be available. These groups can be reached through the health care provider or by word of mouth.

POTENTIAL FOR METASTASIS

PLANNING: EXPECTED OUTCOMES. The client with breast cancer is expected to remain free of metastases or recurrence of disease.

INTERVENTIONS. There has been significant controversy in the past about the treatment of breast cancer. Until about 1950 the Halsted radical mastectomy was considered the treatment of choice. Gradually the modified radical mastectomy became popular. More recently, evidence has been presented that supports less traumatic procedures as having comparable survival rates. Because of the various options, the woman with breast cancer often faces difficult decisions.

Although most women with metastatic breast cancer eventually succumb to the disease, chemotherapy, hormonal therapy, radiotherapy, and limited surgery are all effective treatment modalities for palliative care, improvement in quality of life, and prolongation of life (Hortobagyi, 1998). Once cancer is found, the extent and location of metastases determine the overall therapeutic strategy. Treatment should be tailored specifically to each client, taking into account other comorbidities and the client's ability to tolerate a particular therapy. Most important, the nurse should thoroughly understand an individual's specific goals and the particular outcome she seeks from therapy.

NONSURGICAL MANAGEMENT. For clients with late-stage breast cancer, nonsurgical treatment may be the only alternative. If the disease is in a late stage, such as stage IV, with the presence of confirmed metastasis, or if the client cannot withstand a major surgical procedure, the tumor may be removed with a local anesthetic. Follow-up treatment may include hormonal therapy, chemotherapy, and sometimes radiation. If the tumor is attached to the skin or the underlying muscle, resection may be impossible. Follow-up therapy involves radiation, usually in conjunction with chemotherapy. Chapter 25 describes the nursing care associated with chemotherapy and radiation.

SURGICAL MANAGEMENT. The most common types of breast surgery are illustrated in Figure 74-4. Although controversy exists concerning the best treatment for a malignant mass, many experts agree that the mass itself should be removed to reduce the risk of local recurrence. Removal of the axillary lymph nodes for staging purposes may also be recommended. Axillary lymph node dissection (ALND) is usually performed for clients with palpable axillary lymph nodes;

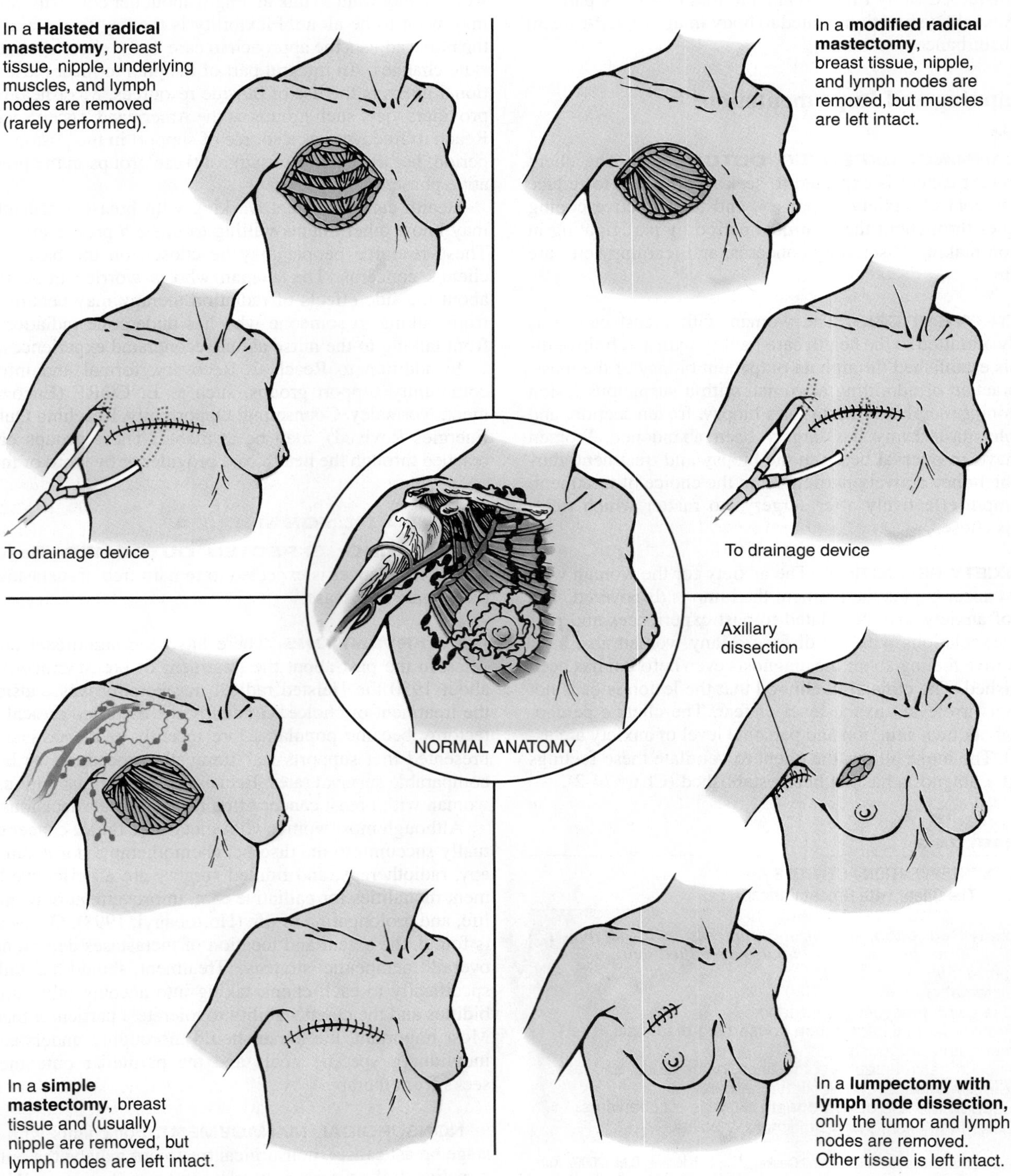

Figure 74-4 ● Surgical management of breast cancer.

it is unclear if clients with nonpalpable nodes should also have ALND.

PREOPERATIVE CARE. Care of the woman facing surgery for breast cancer focuses on psychologic preparation and preoperative teaching. The issues related to anxiety and lack of knowledge are primary. Efforts are directed toward educating the client, including the husband or significant other, who may be experiencing similar stress and confusion.

The type of procedure is reviewed. Open-ended questions (e.g., "What type of surgery are you having? Can you explain what will happen?") are used. This questioning helps the nurse assess the client's level of knowledge and allows for additional explanations as needed. The client should be knowledgeable about the type of procedure. Specific postoperative information, such as the following, is also provided:

- The need for a drainage tube
- The location of the incision
- Mobility restrictions
- The length of the hospital stay (if any)
- The possibility of additional medical therapy
- Basic preoperative and postoperative information needed by any surgical client (see Chapters 17 and 19)

Because of short hospital stays or same-day surgery procedures, preoperative teaching should be supplemented with written materials for the client and family to take home as references and should include who to call should there be any complications. The nurse helps the client address body image issues before surgery to correct misconceptions about postoperative appearance and to begin adjusting to changes after surgery. If available, clients and their caregivers may attend preoperative classes in an ambulatory care setting, such as a surgical clinic, to promote successful early discharge from the hospital. Preoperative programs that provide emotional support, information, and opportunities for discussion related to sexuality, body image, preoperative instructions, and postoperative care enhance the care of the short-stay mastectomy client.

OPERATIVE PROCEDURES. During **breast-conserving surgery,** the surgeon removes the bulk of the tumor; typically, radiation therapy follows to eradicate residual tumor cells. Radiation therapy plays a critical role in the therapeutic regimen and is effective treatment for nearly all sites where breast cancer can metastasize. The most common site for metastasis is to bone tissue.

The following types of breast-conserving surgery are used as primary treatment for stage I and stage II breast cancer:

- **Lumpectomy,** also known as tylectomy or local excision, is gross resection of the tumor.
- **Partial mastectomy,** which includes wide excision, quadrantectomy, or segmental mastectomy, is removal of the portion of the breast that contains the tumor.

Breast-conserving procedures are usually performed in same-day surgical settings. The breast-conserving approach offers 5- and 10-year survival and local recurrence rates at least equivalent to those of the modified radical mastectomy. The cosmetic results have been good to excellent, and other long-term problems are comparable to those of more radical procedures. For many women, the psychologic benefits of avoiding breast removal are significant and lead them to choose this option.

The **modified radical mastectomy** does *not* conserve the breast; the affected breast is completely removed. This procedure differs from the older Halsted radical mastectomy in that the surgeon leaves the pectoral muscles and nerves intact. Thus the breast tissue and skin and the axillary nodes are removed, and the underlying muscles are left in place. The typical incision is a 5- to 6-inch-long elliptic incision from the midchest to the axilla (see Figure 74-4). If reconstruction is to follow the procedure, the plastic surgeon may recommend a different location for the incision. When reconstruction is to be performed at the same time as the mastectomy, less invasive techniques, such as incising a 1.5-inch flap of skin around the nipple (excising the same amount of breast tissue as with conventional mastectomy), may be performed. Skin flaps or implants may be used to create a breast mound at the time of the original procedure.

The use of carbon dioxide laser procedures in place of cutting and cauterizing for mastectomies is an option that is becoming more available. Advantages of laser procedures include less blood loss and faster recovery.

POSTOPERATIVE CARE. Postoperative and home care of the woman undergoing a modified radical mastectomy or breast-conserving surgery is provided in the Client Care Plan on pp. 1744 and 1745. Before the woman returns from surgery, the nurse places a sign over the client's bed to warn nurses and other personnel to avoid using the affected arm for taking blood pressure measurements, giving injections, or drawing blood. The woman returns from the postanesthesia care unit (PACU) as soon as vital signs return to baseline levels and if no complications have occurred. On the client's return, the nurse focuses on maintaining physiologic stability and comfort. Vital signs are usually assessed on a schedule of decreasing frequency, such as every 30 minutes for two times, every hour for two times, and then every 4 hours. During these checks, the nurse or assistive nursing personnel assesses the dressing for bleeding.

Care of Drainage Tubes. During a modified radical mastectomy, the surgeon places one or two drainage tubes, usually Jackson-Pratt drains, under the skin flaps and attached to a small collection chamber. Gentle suction is exerted, and fluid that would accumulate under the flaps and delay healing is collected. Various drains are available, but all allow the drainage to be seen and measured. When taking vital signs, the nurse or assistive nursing personnel monitors the drain for the amount and color of drainage and adds this information to the intake and output record. Clients undergoing a lumpectomy may also have drainage tubes (usually Jackson-Pratt drains) placed if the lump is large or if axillary node dissection is performed.

The nurse or assistive nursing personnel continues to measure the amount of wound drainage, although measurements of general fluid intake and output are usually discontinued by the first postoperative day. The nurse observes the wound for signs of swelling and infection throughout the client's recovery. Drainage tubes are removed by the surgeon when drainage is less than 50 mL in 24 hours. With short hospital stays, drainage tubes are usually removed about 1 week after hospital discharge, when the client returns for her first postoperative office visit. The nurse informs the client that although these tubes lie just under the skin, removal may be painful.

CLIENT CARE PLAN • CARE OF THE CLIENT AFTER MASTECTOMY OR BREAST-CONSERVING SURGERY

NURSING DIAGNOSIS NO. 1 • Acute Pain related to tissue trauma from surgery

Expected Outcomes	Nursing Interventions	Rationale
The client will experience no pain or unnecessary discomfort.	Assess for pain and identify possible causes. Assess for sensation changes in the arm and the incision.	Thorough assessment allows identification of and appropriate intervention for the specific cause of pain.
	Reduce anxiety by reorienting the client to surroundings and explaining procedures, dressings, drains, and other equipment. D	Anxiety and fear of the unknown decrease the pain threshold.
	Medicate as appropriate with analgesics, as ordered.	Pain medications decrease the perception of pain.
	Position the client on the back or the unaffected side, with the arm on the affected side elevated on a pillow. D	Elevation of the arm decreases swelling, which might cause discomfort.
	Check drains and dressings for constriction, position, and functioning.	Impeded circulation or swelling under the skin flap caused by obstruction of the drain causes pain.
	Explain the potential for phantom sensations of the missing breast. Explain the potential for numbness in the arm and in the incision.	Previous knowledge of the event decreases anxiety when the event occurs.

NURSING DIAGNOSIS NO. 2 • Risk for Ineffective Tissue Perfusion related to edema or bleeding

Expected Outcomes	Nursing Interventions	Rationale
The client will maintain adequate tissue perfusion.	Assess the client for signs of shock (decreased blood pressure, increased pulse, decreased urine output, confusion).	These signs indicate shock.
	Check the dressing and the sheet under the client for bleeding.	Bleeding may stain the dressing or seep under the dressing and be unnoticed unless the bed is checked.
	Empty and record the drainage in the drainage container. Report excessive amounts of and changes in drainage.	Excessive drainage indicates hemorrhage.
	Assess the operative site for swelling or the presence of fluid collection under the skin flaps.	Collection of fluid under the skin flaps disrupts healing and may indicate a malfunctioning drainage device or bleeding.

D indicates tasks that can be delegated to assistive nursing personnel.

Comfort Measures. The nurse or assistive nursing personnel assesses the client's position to ensure that the drainage tubes or collection device will not be pulled or kinked. The client should sit with the head of the bed up at least 30 degrees, with the affected arm (the arm on the same side as the axillary dissection) elevated on a pillow, while awake. Keeping the affected arm elevated promotes lymphatic fluid return after removal of axillary lymph nodes and channels. Other basic comfort measures, such as repositioning and pain medications, as prescribed, are provided on a regular basis until pain ceases.

Mobility and Diet. The hospital stay after a modified radical mastectomy is short—typically same-day or overnight—and recovery is usually not complicated. Because some managed care companies will not authorize an overnight stay in the hospital following a mastectomy, several states have enacted legislation mandating inpatient benefits. The client who chooses an early discharge should have a home care visit within 24 hours of the discharge.

Ambulation and a regular diet are resumed by the day after surgery. While the client is in an upright position, the arm on the affected side may need to be supported at first. Gradually the arm should be allowed to hang straight by the side while the client is walking. The nurse teaches the client to avoid the hunched-back position with the arm flexed because of the risk of elbow contractures. Beginning exercises that do not stress the incision can usually be started on the first postoperative day. These exercises include squeezing the affected hand around a soft, round object (a ball or rolled washcloth) and flexion/extension of the elbow. The progression to more strenuous exercises depends on the subsequent procedures planned (such as reconstruction) and the surgeon's orders.

As soon as the woman is fully ambulatory and eating well and her postoperative pain is under control, she is discharged to continue recuperation at home. Typical instructions for postmastectomy exercises are provided in Chart 74-3.

BREAST RECONSTRUCTION. Breast reconstruction has undergone a dramatic evolution in the last 20 years with substantial improvement in the quality, predictability, and complication rate of the procedures used to reconstruct the breast. Clients now present to the reconstructive surgeon with definite ideas regarding the type of reconstruction, timing of the procedure, and technique desired. With this trend, more women want immediate breast reconstruction using their own tissue (autogenous reconstruction). In addition, instantaneous

CLIENT CARE PLAN • CARE OF THE CLIENT AFTER MASTECTOMY OR BREAST-CONSERVING SURGERY—cont'd

NURSING DIAGNOSIS NO. 3 • Impaired Physical Mobility related to pain and tissue trauma

Expected Outcomes	Nursing Interventions	Rationale
The client will experience a return of mobility to her preoperative level.	Tell the client that flexion and extension of the fingers and wrist can begin immediately postoperatively. Encourage gentle use of the arm for activities of daily living. Limited exercises include: Range of motion for the hand, wrist, and elbow Squeezing a ball Flexing the fingers Touching the hand to the shoulder and circular wrist motion	Early use of the hand and arm muscles and joints prevents muscle atrophy and contractures and enhances fluid return.
	Teach appropriate exercises, and ask the client to begin performing exercises 1 week after surgery or when sutures and drains are removed.	Active range-of-motion exercises preserve the range of motion in the client's arm in which axillary dissection was done.
	Inform the client about Reach to Recovery or a similar organization, and contact the organization with the client's permission to arrange a home visit.	Reach to Recovery provides volunteers and written materials on exercises that are safe to perform at home.
	Encourage the client to use an upright posture with the shoulders held back and the arm by the side while walking and standing. D	The tendency is to hold the arm bent across the waist and to stoop over, which results in elbow and shoulder contractures.

NURSING DIAGNOSIS NO. 4 • Risk for Infection related to disruption in skin integrity

Expected Outcomes	Nursing Interventions	Rationale
The client will have an incision that remains free of infection.	Assess for signs of infection and swelling.	Infection and collection of serosanguineous fluid delay wound healing and disrupt adhesion of the skin flaps.
	Teach the client measures to reduce the risk of infection: Avoid taking blood pressure, drawing blood, and giving injections in the operative arm. Avoid injury to the arm, such as burns, scratches, insect bites, and scrapes. Treat injuries immediately to avoid infection.	Injury and infection in the operative arm increase the risk of lymphedema related to removal of lymph nodes.
	Encourage the client to look at the incision before discharge from the hospital, and explain signs of infection, including redness, heat, swelling, and wound discharge.	Discharge usually occurs before complete healing. The client or some other responsible person must monitor wound healing.
	Instruct the client to notify the physician if swelling, redness, or pain occurs.	Early intervention may prevent disruption of the skin flaps.

D indicates tasks that can be delegated to assistive nursing personnel.

breast reconstruction, both autogenous and prosthetic, has been shown to lessen the psychologic strain associated with undergoing a mastectomy.

The surgeon should offer the option of breast reconstruction before surgery is performed. If the client does not choose immediate reconstructive surgery, a temporary prosthesis is given to the client. Some surgeons allow women to use a temporary prosthesis in the immediate postoperative period as a component of the postoperative dressing. If this is the case, the client returns from surgery with a surgical brassiere and temporary sterile prosthesis in place. The nurse or social worker can refer the client to the American Cancer Society's Reach to Recovery program. In this program, a volunteer who has had breast cancer surgery visits the client at home, offering information on breast forms, clothing, coping with breast cancer, and possible reconstructive options. For this intervention to be as therapeutic as possible, the volunteer should be about the same age as the client and have experienced the same surgical procedure.

The client's level of satisfaction with her prosthesis is evaluated several weeks postoperatively. The nurse assesses the client's attitude by asking about plans for restoring appearance postoperatively. Although reconstruction is not appropriate for some clients and others may not be interested in it, the surgeon should discuss the indications and contraindications, advantages and disadvantages, and typical postoperative recovery. If immediate reconstruction is chosen, the surgeon should be aware of this preoperatively so that the surgeon's plans can be coordinated with those of the plastic surgeon.

Several procedures are available for restoring the appearance of the breast (Table 74-5). Reconstruction may begin during the original operative procedure or later in one to several stages. The following are some of the more common techniques:

- Use of a flap of skin and muscle from the abdomen, back, or hip to create a breast mound
- Placement of a saline- or gel-filled prosthesis
- Use of progressive tissue expanders to slowly create a pocket under the mastectomy site for placement of a permanent implant

Reconstruction of the nipple-areola complex is the last stage in the reconstruction of the breast. If necessary, a new

CHART 74-3

CLIENT EDUCATION GUIDE
Postmastectomy Exercises

Hand Wall Climbing
- Face the wall, and put the palms of your hands flat against the wall at shoulder level.
- Flex your fingers so that your hands slowly "walk" up the wall.
- Stop when your arms are fully extended.
- Slowly "walk" your hands back down the wall until they return to shoulder level.

Pulley Exercise
- Drape a 6-foot-long rope over a shower curtain rod or over the top of a door. If you use a door for this exercise, have someone put a nail or hook at the top of the door so that the rope does not slip off.
- Grab the ends of the rope, one in each hand, and extend your arms out to your sides until they are straight.
- Keeping your arms straight, pull down with your left arm to raise your right arm as high as you can.
- Pull down with your right arm to raise your left arm as high as you can.

Rope Turning
- Tie a rope to the knob of a closed door.
- Hold the other end of the rope and step back from the door until your arm is almost straight out in front of you.
- Swing the rope in a circle. Start with small circles and gradually increase to larger circles as you become more flexible.

nipple may be created with tissue from the other nipple or from other body tissue, such as the labia or inner thigh. In some cases, the client's natural nipple can be reattached to another part of the body if the reconstruction is planned for a later date.

In June 1992, the Food and Drug Administration (FDA) restricted the use of silicone gel implants to women in FDA-approved safety studies. The studies were open to women seeking implants after breast cancer surgery or traumatic injury (MacMahon, 1992). The restriction of silicone implants resulted from complaints that silicone leakage caused clients to experience connective tissue diseases, such as systemic lupus erythematosus, or other vague physical symptoms. In mid-1994, silicone gel implants were once again permitted for use in breast reconstruction, but not in breast augmentation (enlargement) (Corral & Mustoe, 1996).

The transverse rectus abdominis myocutaneous (TRAM) flap, a commonly used method of reconstruction, provides women with naturally appearing breasts without the risks associated with the silicone gel implant. This procedure has largely replaced the prosthetic implant as the first choice for breast reconstruction and can be combined with tissue expanders and implants to obtain symmetry (Moran et al., 2000). Postoperative nursing care of the woman who has undergone breast reconstruction is outlined in Chart 74-4.

ADJUVANT THERAPY. The decision to follow the original surgical procedure with chemotherapy, radiation, or hormonal therapy is based on the following:

- The stage of the disease
- The client's age and menopausal status
- Client preferences
- Pathologic examination
- Hormone receptor status

The purpose of adjuvant therapy is to decrease the risk of recurrence for the client who has no evidence of but is at risk for metastasis or to prolong survival after metastasis occurs. Adjuvant therapy for stage I and stage II (early-stage) breast cancer consists of breast-conserving surgery and postoperative radiotherapy or modified radical mastectomy. Women who have estrogen receptor (ER)–positive tumors are given tamoxifen (Nolvadex, Tamofen♣). This estrogen antagonist blocks the estrogen receptor sites in the tumor cells, thereby inhibiting growth. When this therapy is appropriate, the response rate is 50% to 60%.

Therapy for stage III, or locally advanced, breast cancer is still controversial. Treatment usually includes surgery (if the tumor is operable) and chemotherapy with or without radiotherapy. Although chemotherapeutic regimens differ among treatment centers, multiple-agent combinations are used. A common example of such a combination is cyclophosphamide (Cytoxan, Neosar, Procytox♣), methotrexate (Folex, Mexate), and fluorouracil (5-FU, Adrucil). The length of treatment may also vary. Autologous and allogeneic bone marrow transplantation (stem cell transplantation) and preoperative chemotherapy are being investigated as early treatment for women who have a high risk for recurrence or advanced disease (Smith, 1996). Autologous bone marrow transplantation (taken from the client's bone marrow), peripheral blood stem cell transplantation (taken from the client's circulating blood), or allogeneic bone marrow transplantation (taken from a healthy donor's bone marrow or peripheral blood) may be performed as a means of rescue following very high doses of chemotherapy or radiation. These procedures decrease the expected morbidity and mortality related to adjuvant therapy.

Before planning care and teaching for the breast cancer client undergoing chemotherapy, the nurse knows the specific agents to be used and their properties. A discussion of the care of the client undergoing chemotherapy and a discussion of the care of the client undergoing bone marrow transplantation are given in Chapter 25.

Community-Based Care

HOME CARE MANAGEMENT

Home care preparation should be initiated when the decision to have surgical therapy is made. Referral to a case manager can ensure that the educational needs of the client are met early in the perioperative period. The preadmission testing center or the surgeon could make referrals. Preoperative teaching and arrangements for home care management and referrals (Reach to Recovery, social services, home care) can be initiated before hospitalization. Planning ahead for the client's discharge needs facilitates discharge.

The client who has undergone breast surgery can be discharged to the home setting unless other physical disabilities exist. Some are discharged 1 to 2 days after surgery, with Jackson-Pratt or other types of drains in place. The current trend, however, is to be discharged to home on the same day that surgery is performed. These clients need assistance at home with drain care, dressings, and activities of daily living because of pain and impaired range of motion of the affected arm. Summaries of discharge instructions are given in Charts 74-5 and 74-6.

It is not necessary to modify the home for the client after breast surgery. Activities involving stretching or reaching for

TABLE 74-5 • EXAMPLES OF BREAST RECONSTRUCTION PROCEDURES

Procedure	Description	Procedure	Description
Implantation	An implant matching the size of the other breast is placed under the muscle on the operative side to create a breast mound. 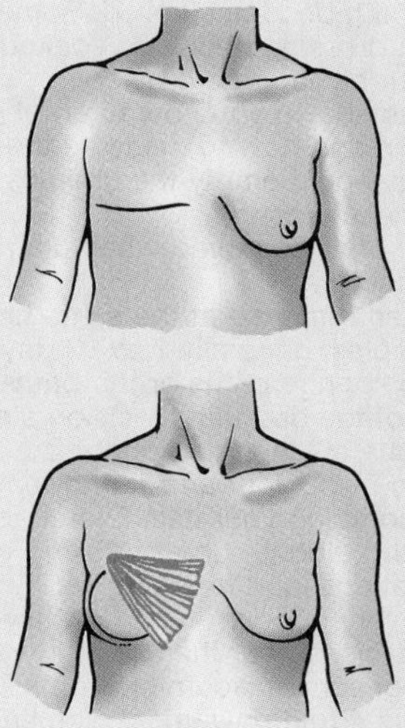	Myocutaneous flaps	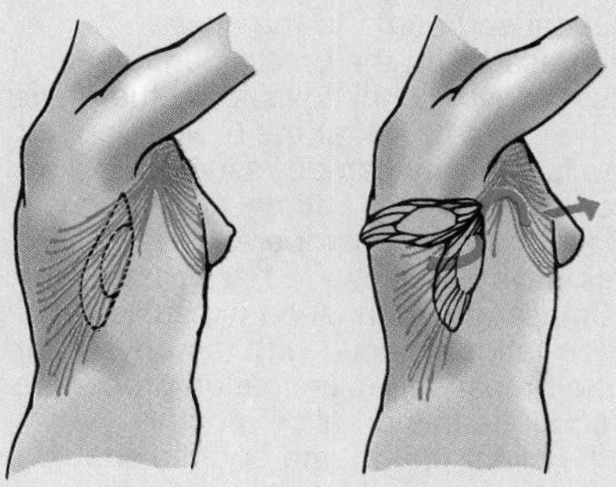 A flap of skin, fat, and muscle is transferred from the donor site to the operative area. The flap contains an appropriate amount of fat to match the other breast and is similar in appearance to breast tissue. A blood supply is established by reanastomosis of vessels from the operative area to those with the flap when possible. A new nipple may be created with tissue from the other nipple, labia, or thigh. Nipples can also be created by tattooing. 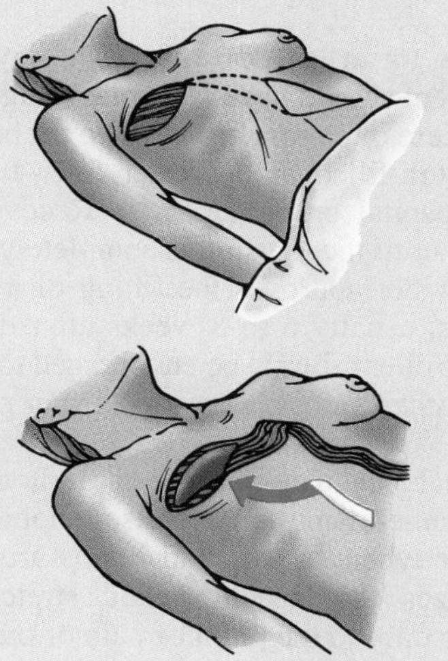
Tissue expansion	A tissue expander is placed under the muscle and gradually expanded with saline to stretch the overlying skin and create a pocket. After several weeks, the tissue expander is exchanged for an implant. 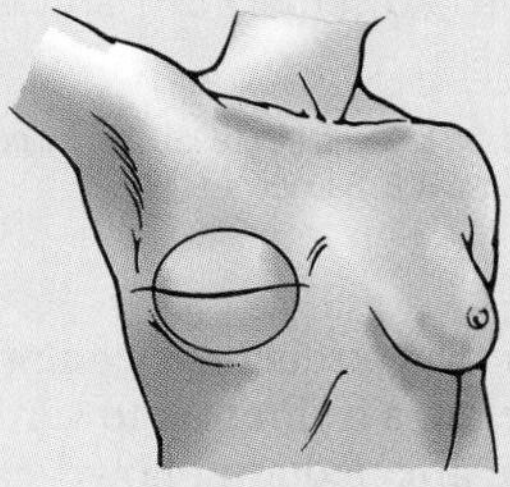		

Latissimus dorsi musculocutaneous flap

Abdominal myocutaneous flap

heavy objects should be avoided. This restriction can be discussed with a family member or significant other who can perform these tasks or place the objects within easy reach of the client.

HEALTH TEACHING

The teaching plan for the client after surgery includes the following:

- Measures to optimize a positive body image
- Information to enhance interpersonal relationships and roles
- Exercises to regain full range of motion
- Measures to prevent infection of the incision
- Measures to avoid injury, infection, and subsequent swelling of the affected arm
- Care of the incision and drainage device

PHYSICAL CARE. The nurse has the opportunity to explain incisional care. The client may wear a light dressing to prevent irritation. The nurse explains that no lotions or ointments should be used on the area and that the use of deodorant under the affected arm should be delayed until healing is complete. Although swelling and redness of the scar itself are normal for the first few weeks, swelling, redness, increased heat, and tenderness of the surrounding area indicate infection and should be reported to the surgeon. If a lymph node dissection was performed, the client should elevate the affected

CHART 74-4

BEST PRACTICE *for*
Postoperative Care of the Client After Breast Reconstruction

- Assess the incision and flap for signs of infection (excessive redness, drainage, odor) during dressing changes.
- Assess the incision and flap for signs of poor tissue perfusion (duskiness, decreased capillary refill) during dressing changes.
- Avoid pressure on the flap and suture lines by positioning the client on her nonoperative side and avoiding tight clothing.
- Monitor and measure drainage in collection devices, such as Jackson-Pratt drains.
- Teach the client to return to her usual activity level gradually and to avoid heavy lifting.
- Avoid sleeping in the prone position.
- Avoid participation in contact sports or other activities that could cause trauma to the chest.
- Minimize pressure on the breast during sexual activity.
- Refrain from driving until advised by the physician.
- Remind the client to ask at the 6-week postoperative visit when full activity can be resumed.
- Reassure the client that optimal appearance may not occur for 3 to 6 months postoperatively.
- If implants have been inserted, teach the proper method of breast massage to enhance expansion and prevent capsule formation (consult with the physician).
- Review the breast self-examination procedure and the need to continue this practice monthly.
- Remind the client that mammograms should be scheduled at least yearly for the rest of her life.

arm on a pillow for at least 30 minutes a day for the first 6 months. The client should have someone bring a loose-fitting, nonwired brassiere or camisole for her to try before discharge with a soft cotton-filled or polyester fiber–filled form supplied by the hospital or by Reach to Recovery. The client wears this form until the incision is completely healed and the health care provider approves the fitting of a more sophisticated prosthesis, usually 6 to 8 weeks after discharge. After going home, the client should be encouraged to dress in loose-fitting street clothes, not pajamas, to further enhance a positive self-image.

Exercises that began in the hospital should continue at home. Active range-of-motion exercises should begin 1 week after surgery or when sutures and drains are removed. The nurse emphasizes that reaching and stretching exercises should continue only to the point of pain or pulling, never beyond that. ENCORE, a YWCA program, is appropriate for women as early as 3 weeks postoperatively and includes exercise to music, exercise in water, and psychologic support. Before discharge, the surgeon may prescribe precautions or limitations specific to plans for future procedures, such as reconstruction.

The nurse provides information needed to help the client avoid infection and subsequent lymphedema of the affected arm after the mastectomy. The client should avoid having blood pressure measurements taken on, having injections in, and having blood drawn from the arm on the side of the mastectomy. The client should wear a mitt when using the oven, wear gloves when gardening, and treat cuts and scrapes appropriately. If lymphedema occurs, the arm should be elevated when possible and special attention paid to the above-mentioned warnings. In addition, if lymphedema occurs, it can be managed with the use of an arm sleeve (similar to a Ted or Jobst stocking) or a sequential compression device. Management of lymphedema is directed toward measures that promote drainage of the affected arm; however, prevention is the best cure.

CHART 74-5

CLIENT EDUCATION GUIDE
Recovery from Breast Cancer Surgery

- There may be a dry gauze dressing over the incision when you leave the hospital. You may change this dressing if it becomes soiled.
- A small, dry dressing will be around the site where a drain is placed. Often there is some leakage of fluid around the drain. Check the gauze dressing for drainage, and change it if it becomes soiled. Some leakage is normal, but if the dressing becomes soaked more than once a day, call your health care provider.
- Your nurse has shown you how to empty the reservoir from your drain and how to measure the volume of drainage. You should empty the drain twice a day and record the measurements.
- Drains are generally removed when drainage is less than 50 mL in 24 hours.
- Drains are often removed at the same time as the stitches or staples, generally 7 to 10 days after surgery.
- You may take sponge baths or tub baths, making certain that the area of the drain and incision stays dry. You may shower after the stitches and drains are removed.
- You can begin using your arm for normal activities, such as eating or combing your hair. Exercises involving the wrist, hand, and elbow, such as flexing your fingers, circular wrist motions, and touching your hand to your shoulder, are very good. You can usually resume more strenuous exercises after the drains have been removed.
- You can expect some discomfort or mild pain after surgery, but within 4 to 5 days most women have no need for pain medication or require medication only at bedtime.
- Numbness in the area of the surgery and along the inner side of the arm from the armpit to the elbow occurs in virtually all women. It is the injury to the nerves that causes sensation to the skin in those areas. Women have described sensations of heaviness, pain, tingling, burning, and "pins and needles." These sensations change over the months and usually resolve by 1 year.
- Pamphlets on exercises, hand and arm care, and general facts about breast cancer are available from your nurse or volunteer visitor. The American Cancer Society has volunteers who have had surgery similar to yours and are available to visit you.

Modified from McCorkle, R., Baird, S., & Grant, M. (1996). *Cancer nursing: A comprehensive approach* (2nd ed.). Philadelphia: W.B. Saunders.

PSYCHOSOCIAL MANAGEMENT. Concerns about appearance after surgery are common and are often a threat to the client's self-concept as a woman. Before breast surgery, the woman and her partner can benefit from an explanation of the expected postoperative appearance. After a modified radical mastectomy, the chest wall is fairly smooth and has a horizontal incision from the axilla to the midchest area. After breast-conserving surgery, scars vary according to the amount of breast tissue removed. Scars may be red and raised at first, but these characteristics diminish in the first few months. After surgery, the nurse encourages the woman to look at her incision before she goes home and offers to be present when she does so.

Much of one's body image is a reflection of how others respond. Therefore the response of the client's family or partner to

CHART 74-6

FOCUSED ASSESSMENT *of* Home Care Clients Recovering from Breast Cancer Surgery

Assess cardiovascular, respiratory, and urinary status, including:
- Vital signs
- Lung sounds
- Urine output patterns

Assess for pain and effectiveness of analgesics.

Assess dressing and incision site for:
- Excess drainage
- Signs and symptoms of infection
- Wound healing
- Intact staples

Assess drain and site for:
- Drainage around drain site and in drain
- Color and amount of drainage
- Signs and symptoms of infection

Review client's recordings of drainage.

Evaluate ability to care for and empty drain.

Assess status of affected extremity, including:
- Range of motion
- Ability to perform exercise regimen
- Lymphedema

Assess nutritional status, including:
- Food and fluid intake
- Presence of nausea and vomiting
- Bowel sounds

Assess functional ability, including:
- Activities of daily living
- Mobility and ambulation

Assess home environment, including:
- Safety
- Structural barriers

Assess client's compliance and knowledge of illness and treatment plan, including:
- Follow-up appointment with surgeon
- Signs and symptoms to report to health care provider
- Hand and arm care guidelines
- Referral to Reach to Recovery

Assess client and caregiver coping skills:
- Determine if client has looked at incision site
- Assess client's reaction to incision site

the surgery is crucial in determining the effect on self-concept. These people may also need the support of the nurse. They may have concerns about their ability to accept the changes and need to discuss these feelings with an objective listener. They may also need help with communicating their feelings, both negative and positive, with their loved one. Involving them in teaching may also help reinforce learning and increase retention.

Sexual concerns should be discussed before discharge. Sexual intercourse can be resumed whenever the client is comfortable. Clients may prefer to lay a pillow over the surgical site or wear a bra or camisole to prevent contact with the surgical site during intercourse. The client may be embarrassed to broach the topic, and the nurse should be sensitive to possible concerns and approach the subject first.

For women of childbearing age (approximately 25% of breast cancer clients), issues related to childbearing may be a concern. Some providers believe that the woman who has had breast cancer should wait 2 to 3 years after completing treatment to attempt pregnancy. Others, however, suggest no waiting period, since recurrences could happen at any time (Shapiro & Clark, 1995). Chemotherapy and radiation are considered serious **teratogenic** (birth defect–causing) agents, and sexually active clients receiving chemotherapy or radiotherapy must use birth control during therapy. The method and length of birth control is discussed with the health care provider.

HEALTH CARE RESOURCES

Resources available to the client after discharge include personal support and community programs. After discharge, the spouse or significant other may need help in planning support for home responsibilities. For example, a partner who may be assuming additional duties at home and work may feel stressed. Exploring temporary relief resources for child care, cleaning, or cooking may be helpful until the woman regains her previous energy level. Discussing the need for ongoing emotional support is also beneficial to both the client and her partner. Leaving the hospital and appearing normal do not end the anxiety and fear. Identifying a support person with whom the client or couple can explore these feelings and discussing the need to ventilate feelings enhance personal and family recovery.

As mentioned, Reach to Recovery and ENCORE are two community resources for women with breast cancer. Reach to Recovery provides a volunteer who visits the client in the hospital or at home. She brings a personal message of hope, informational materials on breast cancer recovery, and a soft, temporary breast form. Some communities offer additional resources such as support groups and exercise classes.

Evaluation: Outcomes

NOC The nurse evaluates the care of the client with breast cancer on the basis of the identified nursing diagnoses and collaborative problems. The expected outcomes include that the client will:
- Demonstrate the correct method of breast self-examination (BSE) and practice BSE on a monthly basis
- Comply with guidelines for mammography and professional examination
- Be able to cope with the diagnosis, as shown by her use of social support, use of information to deal with uncertainty, absence of physical signs of anxiety, and verbal confirmation of feeling calm
- State that she feels positive about her self-image
- Regain full range of motion of the affected arm
- Remain free from lymphedema or infection

ONLINE RESOURCES

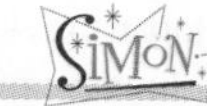

For suggested readings and Internet resources, go to http://www.wbsaunders.com/SIMON/Iggy/.

SELECTED BIBLIOGRAPHY

Asterisk indicates a classic or definitive work on this subject.

Allen, K.M., & Phillips, J.M. (1997). *Women's health across the lifespan.* Philadelphia: J.B. Lippincott.

American Society of Clinical Oncology. (1998). *American Society of Clinical Oncology curriculum: Cancer genetics and cancer predisposition testing.* Alexandria, VA: Author.

*Baron, R.H., & Walsh, A. (1995). Nine facts everyone should know about breast cancer. *American Journal of Nursing, 95*(7), 29-33.

Barroso, J., et al. (2000). Comparison between African-American and white women in their beliefs about breast cancer and their health locus of control. *Cancer Nursing, 23*(4), 268-276.

*Bostwick, J. (1995). Breast reconstruction following mastectomy. *CA: A Cancer Journal for Clinicians, 45*(5), 289-303.

Bragg Leight, S., et al. (2000). The effect of structured training on breast self-examination search behaviors as measured using biomedical instrumentation. *Nursing Research, 49*(5), 283-289.

Burke, W., et al. (1997). Recommendations for follow-up care of individuals with an inherited predisposition to cancer: BRCA1 and BRCA2. *JAMA, 227*(12), 997-1003.

Cha, C., Kennedy, G., & Niederhuber, J. (1999). Metastatic breast cancer. *Surgical Clinics of North America, 79*(5), 1117-1136.

*Champion, V. (1995). Development of a benefits and barriers scale for mammography utilization. *Cancer Nursing, 18*(1), 53-59.

*Corral, C., & Mustoe, T. (1996). Controversy in breast reconstruction. *Surgical Clinics of North America, 76*(2), 310-312.

Couch, F.J., & Hartmann, L.C. (1998). BRCA1 testing advances and retreats. *Journal of the American Medical Association, 279*(12), 955-956.

Couch, F.J., et al. (1997). BRCA1 mutations in women attending clinics that evaluate the risk of breast cancer. *New England Journal of Medicine, 336*(20), 1409-1415.

Dent, D.M., & Cant, P.F. (1999). Fibroadenoma. *World Journal of Surgery, 13*(6), 706-710.

*Djuric, Z., et al. (1996). Levels of 5-hydroxymethyl-2-deoxyuridine in DNA from blood as a marker of breast cancer. *Cancer, 77*(4), 691-696.

*Donegan, W.L, & Spratt, J.S. (1995). *Cancer of the breast* (4th ed.). Philadelphia: W.B. Saunders.

Facione, N.C., et al. (2000). Perceived risk and help-seeking behavior for breast cancer: A Chinese-American perspective. *Cancer Nursing, 23*(4), 258-267.

Fisher, B., et al. (1998). Tamoxifen for prevention of breast cancer: Report of the National Surgical Adjuvant Breast and Bowel Project P-1 Study. *Journal of the National Cancer Institute, 90*(18), 1371-1388.

Frank, T.S., et al. (1998). Sequence analysis of BRCA1 and BRCA2: Correlation of mutations with family history and ovarian cancer risk. *Journal of Clinical Oncology 16*(7), 2417-2425.

Gaston-Johansson, F., et al. (2000). The effectiveness of the comprehensive coping strategy on clinical outcomes in breast cancer autologous bone marrow transplantation. *Cancer Nursing, 23*(4), 277-285.

*Giomuso, C.B., & Suster, V. (1994). Free flap breast reconstruction. *MEDSURG Nursing, 3*(1), 9-22.

*Gould, K., Gates, M.L., & Miaskowski, C. (1995). Breast cancer prevention: A summary of the chemoprevention trial with tamoxifen. *Oncology Nursing Forum, 21*(5), 835-840.

Hansen, N., & Morrow, M. (1998). Breast disease. *Medical Clinics of North America, 82*(2), 203-222.

Hartmann, L., et al. (1999a). Clinical options for women at high risk for breast cancer. *Surgical Clinics of North America, 79*(5), 1189-1204.

Hartmann, L., et al. (1999b). Efficacy of bilateral prophylactic mastectomy in women with a family history of breast cancer. *New England Journal of Medicine, 340*(2), 77-84.

Hilton, B.A., et al. (2000). Men's perspectives on individual and family coping with their wives' breast cancer and chemotherapy. *Western Journal of Nursing Research, 22*(4), 438-459.

Horden, A. (2000). Intimacy and sexuality for the woman with breast cancer. *Cancer Nursing, 23*(3), 230-236.

Hortobagyi, G. (1998). Treatment of breast cancer, *New England Journal of Medicine, 339*(4), 974-984.

*Hoskins, K.F., et al. (1996). Assessment and counseling for women with a family history of breast cancer: A guide for clinicians. *Journal of the American Medical Association, 273*(7), 577-585.

Jeffries, E. (1997). Home healthcare for patients receiving one-day mastectomy. *Home Healthcare Nurse, 115*(1), 31-37.

Kimmick, G., & Balducci, L. (2000). Breast cancer and aging. *Hematology/Oncology Clinics of North America, 14*(1) 213-234.

Kraus, P.L. (1999). Body image, decision making, and breast cancer treatment. *Cancer Nursing, 22*(6), 421-427.

Landis, S.H., et al. (1999). Cancer statistics. *CA: A Cancer Journal for Clinicians, 49*(1), 8-31.

Leitch, A.M., et al. (1997). American Cancer Society guidelines for the early detection of breast cancer: Update 1997, *CA: A Cancer Journal for Clinicians, 47*(3), 150-153.

*Leslie, N.S. (1995). Role of the nurse practitioner in breast and cervical cancer prevention. *Cancer Nursing, 18*(4), 251-257.

Lessick, M., Wickham, R., & Rehwaldt, M. (1997). Breast and ovarian cancer: Genetic update and implications for nursing. *MEDSURG Nursing 6*(6), 341-349.

*Lu, Z.J. (1995). Variables associated with breast self-examination among Chinese women. *Cancer Nursing, 18*(1), 29-34.

*Luker, K.A., et al. (1996). Information needs and sources of information for women with breast cancer: A follow up study. *Journal of Advanced Nursing, 23*(3), 487-495.

*MacMahon, A.T. (1992). FDA limits access to breast implants. *NAACOG Newsletter, 19*(6), 3.

Malone, K., et al. (1998). BRCA1 mutations and breast cancer in the general population: Analyses in women before age 35 years and in women before age 45 years with first-degree family history. *Journal of the American Medical Association, 279*(12), 922-929.

*Moore, M.P., & Kinne, D. (1995). The surgical management of primary invasive breast cancer. *CA: A Cancer Journal for Clinicians, 45*(5), 278-288.

Moran, S.L., et al. (2000). TRAM flap breast reconstruction with expanders and implants. *AORN Journal, 71*(2), 354-362.

Mushin, A.I., & Fintor, L. (1997). Is screening for breast cancer cost-effective? *Cancer, 69*(12), 1957-1962.

Nass, S., & Davidson, N. (1999). The biology of breast cancer. *Hematology/Oncology Clinics of North America, 17*(2), 311-327.

NCCN practice guidelines: Screening for and evaluation of suspicious breast lesions. (1998). *Oncology, 12*(2), 89-138.

Nogueira, S.M., & Appling, S.E. (2000). Breast cancer: Genetics, risks, and strategies. *Nursing Clinics of North America, 35*(3), 663-669.

Overmoyer, B. (1999). Breast cancer screening. *Medical Clinics of North America, 83*(6), 1143-1460.

*Phillips, J.M., & Wilbur, J. (1995). Adherence to breast cancer screening guidelines among African-American women of differing employment status. *Cancer Nursing, 18*(4), 258-269.

*Shapiro, T., & Clark, P. (1995). Breast cancer: What the primary care provider needs to know. *Nurse Practitioner, 20*(3), 39-40, 42.

*Smith, R.J. (1996). Buying more time in less time: Case management and bone marrow transplantation. *Case Manager, 7*(1), 77-83.

Templeman, C., & Hertweck, S. (2000). Breast disorders in the pediatric and adolescent patient. *Obstetric and Gynecology Clinics, 27*(1), 19-31.

*Tierney, L., et al. (1995). *Current medical diagnosis and treatment.* Norwalk, CT: Appleton & Lange.

Veronesi, U., et al. (1998). Prevention of breast cancer with tamoxifen. *Lancet 352*(9122), 93-97.

*Walkenstein, M. (1995). Surgical clinical nurse specialist facilitates discharge of patients undergoing breast surgery. *Oncology Nursing Forum, 22*(1), 147-148.

Weber, E.S. (1997). Questions and answers about breast cancer diagnosis. *American Journal of Nursing, 97*(10), 34-38.

*Wingo, P.A., et al. (1995). Cancer statistics, 1995. *CA: A Cancer Journal for Clinicians, 45*(1), 8-30.

*Wingo, P.A., et al. (1996). Cancer statistics for African Americans, 1996. *CA: A Cancer Journal for Clinicians, 46*(2), 113-125.

CHAPTER

75

Interventions for Clients with Gynecologic Problems

AMY NICHOLS • DONNA D. IGNATAVICIUS

Learning Objectives

After studying this chapter, you should be able to:

1. Compare and contrast common menstrual cycle disorders.
2. Discuss common assessment findings associated with menopause.
3. Develop a teaching plan for a client with a vaginal inflammation or infection.
4. Prioritize postoperative care for the client undergoing an anterior and/or posterior repair.
5. Analyze assessment data for clients with leiomyomas to determine nursing diagnoses and collaborative problems.
6. Formulate a plan of care for a client undergoing a hysterectomy.
7. Identify the risk factors for gynecologic cancers.
8. Discuss the psychosocial issues associated with gynecologic cancers.
9. Explain the purpose of radiation and chemotherapy for clients with gynecologic cancers.
10. Develop a community-based plan of care for clients with gynecologic cancers.

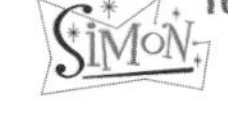

Go to http://www.wbsaunders.com/SIMON/Iggy/ for self-assessment questions related to these Learning Objectives.

The most common reasons for seeking gynecologic care are pain, vaginal discharge, and bleeding. Nurses can play an important role in assessing gynecologic disorders by being knowledgeable about disease presentation, being sensitive to the client's complaints, and encouraging discussion about menstrual or other reproductive problems. Educating women about their bodies, helping them to recognize when professional help should be sought, and teaching them how to make informed decisions about treatments are major goals for nurses working with female clients in any setting. Nurses also need to assess the effects of gynecologic problems on sexual health.

MENSTRUAL CYCLE DISORDERS

Primary Dysmenorrhea

OVERVIEW

Dysmenorrhea, or painful menstrual flow, is one of the most common gynecologic problems, occurring most often in women in their teens and early 20s. More than 50% of all women report some degree of dysmenorrhea, but only a small percentage are not able to function. Primary dysmenorrhea is not associated with pelvic pathologic changes, whereas secondary dysmenorrhea usually begins with an underlying disease condition.

Primary dysmenorrhea usually occurs after ovulation is established. Dysmenorrhea is painful uterine cramping characterized by spasmodic lower abdominal pain that begins with the onset of menstrual flow, and lasts 12 to 48 hours. The pain often radiates to the lower back and thighs; nausea and vomiting, fatigue, and nervousness may accompany the pain. Less common clinical manifestations include headache, syncope, diarrhea, bloating, and breast tenderness.

Most researchers believe that the cause of primary dysmenorrhea is increased production and release of uterine prostaglandins. Prostaglandins are produced by the endometrium during the luteal phase of the menstrual cycle, and the levels peak at the onset of menses. Excessive prostaglandin levels stimulate the myometrium and cause severe spasms, which constrict uterine blood flow, resulting in ischemia and pain.

➤ COLLABORATIVE MANAGEMENT

● Assessment

A thorough history of the client includes the following:

- The age at menarche (onset of menstruation)
- Characteristics of menstruation
- Obstetric history
- Contraceptive history
- The type of pain
- Previous therapy
- The need for contraception

The client is asked whether she has any conditions suggestive of pelvic problems. To plan care, the nurse assesses emotional factors, such as the individual woman's response to dysmenorrhea, her attitudes about menstruation, and the extent to which dysmenorrhea is perceived to disrupt her life.

Interventions

Interventions for primary dysmenorrhea include prevention, education, support, and therapeutic measures that are tailored to each woman's needs. Prostaglandin synthetase inhibitors (nonsteroidal anti-inflammatory drugs [NSAIDs]), such as ibuprofen (Motrin, Apo-Ibuprofen🍁) and naproxen sodium (Anaprox, Naprosyn), are currently recommended for pain relief. In addition, numerous over-the-counter ibuprofen products, such as Advil and Nuprin, provide pain relief for many clients with primary dysmenorrhea. Aspirin is a mild prostaglandin synthetase inhibitor and may relieve mild dysmenorrhea. All of these drugs can cause gastrointestinal (GI) distress and should therefore be taken with meals or milk.

Before treatment, the health care provider must assess the client's contraception needs. When contraception is not needed, prostaglandin synthetase inhibitors are the treatment of choice because they are required only for the duration of symptoms. If contraception is a consideration, ovulation suppression with oral contraceptives is the treatment of choice.

COMPLEMENTARY AND ALTERNATIVE THERAPIES. Complementary therapies that may alleviate or prevent pain include acupressure, aerobic exercise, swimming, yoga or other meditation, application of heat or cold, massage, biofeedback, and relaxation techniques. Dietary measures for the prevention of pain may include increasing the intake of vitamin B_6, calcium, magnesium, and protein and reducing the intake of sodium to reduce fluid retention.

Premenstrual Syndrome

OVERVIEW

The syndrome experienced by menstruating women in which adverse symptoms recur regularly in the luteal phase of each menstrual cycle has been recognized as **premenstrual syndrome (PMS).** Approximately 5% of menstruating women experience severe premenstrual symptoms; many more have moderate symptoms. Fortunately, because considerable progress has been made in understanding PMS, most affected women can be helped.

PMS is a collection of symptoms that are cyclic in nature. These symptoms are followed by relief with menses and a symptom-free phase. PMS affects women of all races, socioeconomic levels, and educational levels. It seems to be more prevalent in women 30 to 40 years old. The severity increases with aging until menopause. Women are at greater risk for PMS after pregnancy, childbirth, and tubal ligation; during the perimenopausal years; and during major life stresses.

Currently, there is no agreement on a single set of diagnostic criteria for PMS. Three elements are found in defining PMS: symptoms, severity level, and timing. Many women report experiencing six or more symptoms across emotional, physical, and cognitive categories.

Emotional symptoms include irritability, easily precipitated crying spells, low self-esteem, anxiety, and depression. Somatic or physical symptoms include breast tenderness, bloating, fluid retention, increased appetite and food cravings, insomnia, fatigue, hot flashes, headaches, and musculoskeletal discomfort. Cognitive problems include short-term memory problems, difficulty concentrating, and unclear thinking.

➤ COLLABORATIVE MANAGEMENT

Assessment

There is no reported objective means of diagnosing PMS. Some researchers have attempted to differentiate premenstrual patterns. Determining the timing of the symptoms is as critical as noting the type of symptoms. The most effective and readily available assessment tool is a menstrual chart. The nurse instructs the client to keep a chart for at least three consecutive cycles, showing the length of the menstrual cycle, the duration of bleeding, and the occurrence of symptoms. If the woman has PMS, the symptoms recur during the luteal phase (from ovulation to menstruation), which is followed by a symptom-free period (at least 7 days). When taking a menstrual history, the nurse also assesses to what extent the woman believes that her activities of daily living (ADLs) are disrupted by the symptoms. Often reassurance that the symptoms are legitimate and that other women share these problems can help the client learn more about PMS. Clinical manifestations vary greatly among women and affect many body systems (Chart 75-1).

Interventions

Management of PMS focuses on eliminating the uncomfortable symptoms. The syndrome is highly individualized; however, one of the most important interventions is education.

CHART 75-1

KEY FEATURES *of* Premenstrual Syndrome

Dermatologic Manifestations
- Acne
- Urticaria
- Herpes

Respiratory Manifestations
- Sinusitis
- Asthma
- Rhinitis
- Colds

Urologic Manifestations
- Oliguria
- Cystitis
- Enuresis
- Urethritis

Ophthalmologic Manifestations
- Conjunctivitis
- Styes
- Glaucoma

Neurologic Manifestations
- Headaches
- Migraine
- Syncope
- Vertigo
- Numbness of hands and feet
- Epilepsy (if susceptible)

Metabolic Manifestations
- Edema
- Breast tenderness

Emotional or Psychologic Manifestations
- Depression
- Irritability
- Tension
- Panic attacks
- Change in libido
- Mood swings
- Anxiety

Behavioral Manifestations
- Lowered work performance
- Food cravings
- Alcohol and drug overindulgence
- Confusion
- Sleeplessness
- Lack of coordination
- Suicide
- Lethargy
- Child abuse
- Assaultive behavior

Other Manifestations
- Allergies
- Hypoglycemia
- Joint pain
- Backache
- Palpitations
- Water retention

Each woman needs information about her body, especially the menstrual cycle, so that she can begin to understand the physiologic basis of PMS.

Women may need to express their feelings and discuss their experiences with PMS. Self-help groups and support groups are helpful resources. These groups also encourage significant others to participate, because PMS usually affects not only the woman but also her family and friends. For example, increased family conflict, communication problems with family and friends, and decreased family cohesion occur. Other coping strategies for the woman with PMS may include spiritual support, especially participating in religious services and seeking advice from spiritual leaders.

DIET THERAPY. Diet and nutrition are also important in managing PMS. If hypoglycemia (low blood glucose) occurs, the nurse instructs the woman to eat six small meals a day and to limit her intake of sugar, red meat, alcohol, coffee, tea, and chocolate.

Eliminating caffeine may help reduce irritability. Salt and sodium intake should be limited if edema occurs. Calcium, magnesium, and vitamins A, B_6, and C have also been used for relief of PMS.

DRUG THERAPY. Drug therapy remains controversial, but some treatments have been effective. Mild potassium-sparing diuretics taken for 10 days before menstruation can provide relief for some women. Women may need to increase their intake of potassium-containing foods if they are receiving this therapy.

Progesterone may relieve physical and psychologic symptoms. Natural progesterone is preferable to synthetic progesterone, even though the drug must be specially made by a pharmacist at the time prescribed. The daily dosage is 50 to 100 mg IM from ovulation to menstruation. Long-term side effects are unknown.

Bromocriptine mesylate (Parlodel) 2.5 mg two or three times a day with meals during the luteal phase can relieve breast symptoms. The side effects (lightheadedness and hypotension) may not be well tolerated. Other drugs for PMS that have been used include birth control pills, gonadotropin-releasing hormone (GnRH) agonists, antidepressants, and prostaglandin inhibitors, such as nonsteroidal anti-inflammatory drugs (NSAIDs).

Amenorrhea

OVERVIEW

Amenorrhea (the absence of menstrual periods) can be either primary (menstruation that has failed to occur by age 16 years) or secondary (menstruation that has started but has since stopped and has not recurred for at least 3 months). Primary amenorrhea is often associated with anomalies of the reproductive tract, and the prognosis for fertility is usually poor. Secondary amenorrhea is probably due to a functional disorder, and the prognosis for fertility is better. Amenorrhea can cause a woman much distress and concern.

Menstruation is a complex series of events that rely on the interplay of the hypothalamic, pituitary, ovarian, and endometrial functions. Dysfunction related to any of these four factors may cause amenorrhea (Table 75-1). Primary amenorrhea is relatively uncommon. Congenital factors are responsible for about two thirds of cases, and the remaining one third of cases are caused by ovarian, pituitary, or hypothalamic disease. Pregnancy, lactation (breastfeeding), and menopause are the most common physiologic causes of secondary amenorrhea.

COLLABORATIVE MANAGEMENT

Assessment

The nurse assesses both the menstrual history and the obstetric history and asks about possible sexual activity and symptoms of pregnancy. A medical history may identify a systemic disease as a cause of amenorrhea. The nurse asks about current eating habits and any history of dieting because both obesity and starvation (e.g., anorexia nervosa) can contribute to amenorrhea. Strenuous exercise associated with competitive athletics, such as long-distance running, can cause stress or a reduction in body fat, resulting in amenorrhea. The nurse assesses hormone deficiencies, such as those associated with menopause that can cause hot flashes and vaginal dryness. Women should be questioned about their ingestion of drugs (e.g., oral contraceptives, phenothiazines, and antihypertensives) and recent stressors. The nurse is also alert for signs of **galactorrhea** (watery or milky breast secretions in nonbreastfeeding or women who have not been pregnant and **hirsutism** (unusual hair growth in women), both of which are related to polycystic ovary disease and subsequent amenorrhea.

Interventions

The nurse's primary roles in implementing care are to explain amenorrhea in easily understandable terms and to answer questions about tests and treatments. Counseling and emo-

TABLE 75-1 • COMMON CAUSES OF AMENORRHEA

PRIMARY
- Congenital anomalies
- Hypothalamic and pituitary disorders, such as delayed puberty
- Systemic disease
  - Thyroid and adrenal dysfunction
  - Diabetes mellitus
  - Extreme malnutrition
- Ovarian disease
- Malformations of the reproductive tract

SECONDARY
- Pregnancy
- Menopause
- Lactation
- Cervical stenosis
- Polycystic ovary disease
- Pituitary tumor or insufficiency
- Psychogenic stress
- Excessive physical activities
- Medications
  - Antihypertensive agents
  - Birth control pills
  - Phenothiazines
- Nutritional disorders
  - Obesity
  - Anorexia nervosa
  - Sudden weight loss
- Ovarian disease, failure, or destruction

tional support must be provided. Amenorrhea may be a threat to a woman's self-concept; she usually needs to ventilate her feelings about sexuality or fertility.

Interventions for specific causes of amenorrhea are based on each woman's needs. Medical and surgical management of amenorrhea is directed at the underlying causes. Treatment includes hormone replacement, ovulation stimulation, and periodic progesterone withdrawal.

Postmenopausal Bleeding

OVERVIEW

Postmenopausal bleeding (vaginal bleeding occurring after a 12-month cessation of menses after the onset of menopause) is a symptom rather than a medical diagnosis. Bleeding is considered serious and should be evaluated. Gynecologic cancer occurs in 20% to 40% of women who experience postmenopausal bleeding.

Postmenopausal bleeding can be caused by numerous benign and malignant conditions (Table 75-2). The three most common causes are atrophic vaginitis, cervical polyps, and endometrial hyperplasia.

In a client with **atrophic vaginitis,** the vaginal mucosa is thin and dry and is easily traumatized by sexual intercourse and infection, causing spotting. Cervical polyps are usually soft, red, oval tissue masses that appear within the cervical canal, and they may bleed spontaneously or after intercourse.

The most serious cause of postmenopausal bleeding is **endometrial hyperplasia** (tissue overgrowth), a precursor of endometrial cancer. Bleeding is caused by declining ovarian function that leads to prolonged estrogen stimulation, producing the hyperplasia that eventually breaks down and bleeds. Estrogen stimulation can also be caused by estrogen replacement therapy (ERT).

Because many women who report postmenopausal bleeding need medical or surgical interventions, assessment is the major focus. The nurse assesses the menstrual history and family history initially, including the following:

- The client's age at menopause
- The frequency and amount of bleeding
- Previous bleeding episodes
- Use of medications (especially estrogen-only [unopposed estrogen] replacement therapy [ERT])
- Gastrointestinal (GI) or genitourinary symptoms

The nurse also identifies women who are at high risk for endometrial cancer (e.g., women who are obese, hypertensive, or diabetic or who have never had children).

Urine and stool specimens can be collected and tested for blood to differentiate other sources of bleeding. Blood specimens may be drawn for hemoglobin or hematocrit determinations, because clients are often anemic as a result of excessive bleeding. The nurse can prepare the woman for physical and pelvic examinations, including obtaining a specimen for a Papanicolaou (Pap) test, or smear, to evaluate the cause of bleeding.

TABLE 75-2 • COMMON CAUSES OF POSTMENOPAUSAL BLEEDING

BENIGN	MALIGNANT
• Atrophic vaginitis	• Endometrial cancer
• Cervical polyps	• Cervical cancer
• Endometrial hyperplasia	• Ovarian cancer
• Uterine fibroids	• Vaginal cancer
• Cervical erosion	• Tubal cancer
• Estrogen therapy	

COLLABORATIVE MANAGEMENT

Nursing interventions focus on providing information and support for diagnostic and treatment procedures directed at the specific causes of bleeding. An endometrial biopsy can evaluate the presence of malignancy. A diagnostic dilation and curettage (D&C) procedure can be used to determine malignancy (see Dysfunctional Uterine Bleeding, p. 1756). Atypical hyperplasia is often treated with a hysterectomy (see Uterine Leiomyomas, p. 1764). Malignancy is usually treated with a combination of surgery, radiation therapy, and chemotherapy (see Endometrial Cancer, p. 1769).

The medical treatment of a woman receiving unopposed estrogen therapy may include the monthly administration of progesterone daily for the last 10 days of the estrogen therapy (days 16 to 25) or a once-per-month intramuscular (IM) progesterone injection. This treatment can reduce the abnormal endometrial proliferation and is suggested for the prevention of endometrial and breast cancer.

Atrophic vaginitis is managed by the administration of estrogen via the vaginal, oral, transdermal, or subdermal route. The nurse teaches the client about ERT (Chart 75-2). Women who use vaginal estrogen cream need to be aware that it can cause systemic effects. Women who take estrogen may be at risk for gallbladder disease, hypertension, breast cancer, endometrial cancer, and coronary artery disease.

CHART 75-2

CLIENT EDUCATION GUIDE
Estrogen Replacement Therapy

For All Types of Estrogen Replacement Therapy
- Call your health care provider if you have pain in your calves or groin, if you suddenly become short of breath, if you have abnormal vaginal bleeding, if you feel a lump in your breast, if you have a severe headache, or if you feel weak or numb in your arms or legs.
- Use sunscreen if you are in the sun for a prolonged period.
- Keep appointments for checkups.
- If your health care provider has prescribed progesterone to decrease your risk of endometrial cancer, take it as prescribed.

For Oral Therapy
- Take 1 pill a day for the first 25 days each month.
- If you feel nauseated or have intestinal upset, take your medication with food.

For Transdermal or Subdermal Administration
- Rotate the sites for the patches or injections to avoid skin irritation.
- Change the patches twice a week or according to your prescribed schedule.

For Vaginal Therapy
- Use an applicator to insert the suppository or cream daily as prescribed.
- You may need to wear a minipad to protect your clothing from soiling or staining by the drug.

Endometriosis

OVERVIEW

Endometriosis is usually a benign disease characterized by implantation of endometrial tissue outside the uterine cavity. The tissue typically appears on the ovaries and the cul-de-sac and less commonly on other pelvic organs and structures (Figure 75-1). A "chocolate" cyst is an area of endometriosis inside an ovary.

Endometrial tissue located outside the endometrium responds similarly to the endometrium to hormonal stimulation and goes through the same cyclic changes. Bleeding occurs at the site of implantation, and the blood is trapped in the tissues; scarring and adhesions result as the blood is reabsorbed. Endometriosis progresses slowly. It regresses during pregnancy and at menopause. Rarely does endometriosis become a malignant disease.

The cause of endometriosis is unknown. The most accepted theories of causation are transportation and formation. There are two transportation theories: (1) implantation and (2) vascular and lymphatic dissemination. The implantation theory holds that endometrial tissue flows back through the fallopian tubes during menstruation and then implants on pelvic structures. Proponents of the vascular and lymphatic dissemination theory advocate that endometrial glands are transported through the vascular and lymphatic system to foreign locations. This latter theory may explain implantation in areas outside the pelvis, such as the lungs and the kidneys. Formation theories propose that endometrial tissue develops spontaneously outside the uterus.

Endometriosis occurs most often in women in their 30s and 40s; rarely does it appear before age 20. It is most common in women who have not been pregnant and in those whose mothers had endometriosis.

COLLABORATIVE MANAGEMENT

Assessment

The nursing assessment should be as detailed as possible and include the client's menstrual history, her sexual history, and the characteristics of bleeding. Pain is the most common symptom of endometriosis. The pain usually peaks just before the menstrual flow. Pain is usually located in the lower abdomen, causing many women to feel a sense of rectal pressure. The degree of pain is not related to the extent of the endometriosis but is related to the site. Often women with minimal disease have more severe pain than do women with extensive disease. Other clinical manifestations include dyspareunia (painful sexual intercourse), painful defecation, sacral backache, hypermenorrhea (excessive, prolonged, or frequent bleeding), and infertility.

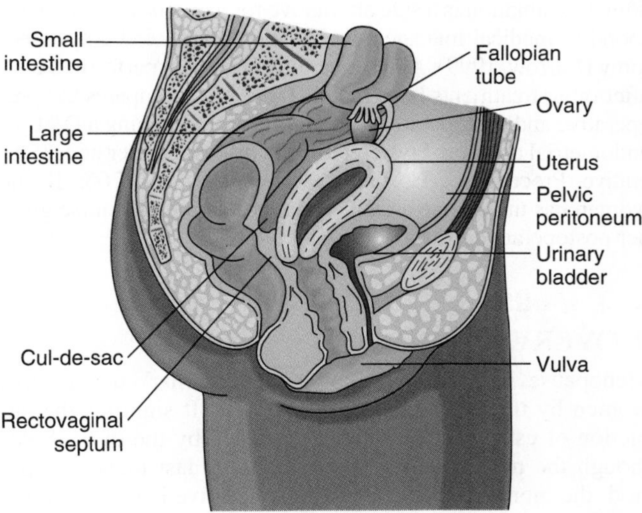

Figure 75-1 ● Common sites of endometriosis.

A pelvic examination may reveal pelvic tenderness, nodular uterosacral ligaments, and fixed or limited movement of the uterus. Psychosocial assessment may reveal anxiety because of uncertainty about the diagnosis. The woman may also have concerns about her self-concept if she is infertile and wants to become pregnant.

Diagnostic studies include blood tests (erythrocyte sedimentation rate [ESR] and white blood cell [WBC] count) to rule out pelvic inflammatory disease (PID). Ultrasonography is used to confirm or delineate pelvic masses that might be mistaken for endometriosis. Laparoscopy is the key diagnostic procedure for pelvic endometriosis. Examination of tissue specimens obtained during laparoscopy can confirm the diagnosis.

Interventions

Medical (hormonal) and surgical management may be used, depending on the symptoms, the extent of disease, and the client's desire for childbearing. Nursing management is aimed at the following:

- Reducing pain
- Restoring sexual function that was impaired by **dyspareunia** (painful sexual intercourse)
- Alleviating anxiety related to the clinical manifestations of the disease and the uncertainty of the diagnosis
- Eliminating the client's knowledge deficit about the disease or its treatment
- Alleviating fear related to the possibility of laparoscopy or surgery
- Preventing self-esteem disturbance related to infertility

Several organizations, including the Endometriosis Society and RESOLVE (an organization for infertile couples), offer additional information on endometriosis that may be helpful in planning care.

NONSURGICAL MANAGEMENT. Nonsurgical management involves the use of mild analgesics or nonsteroidal anti-inflammatory drugs (NSAIDs) for pain relief. The health care provider also uses hormonal therapies to relieve pain by suppressing ovulation. The hormonal therapies produce pseudopregnancy, pseudomenopause, or medical oophorectomy.

Pseudopregnancy is induced with oral contraceptives or progesterone. The health care provider usually prescribes a 6-month course of a low-dose estrogen oral contraceptive, followed by cyclic oral contraceptive use or therapy with progesterone alone.

The second hormonal treatment causes ovarian suppression, or pseudomenopause, by the use of danazol (Danocrine, Cyclomen🍁), an antigonadotropin testosterone derivative. This therapeutic approach is the current choice of many health care providers, but it is expensive ($120 to $180 per month) and may cause undesirable side effects, including acne, hirsutism (abnormal hair growth in unwanted areas), weight gain, decreased breast size, and hot flashes.

The third hormonal treatment is the use of gonadotropin-releasing hormone (GnRH) agonists to produce a reversible medical oophorectomy. The drug can be administered by IM or subcutaneous injection or by nasal spray. Side effects include hot flashes, vaginal dryness, and insomnia.

COMPLEMENTARY AND ALTERNATIVE THERAPIES. Therapies that can relieve pain include the application of a heating pad to the abdomen or sacrum, relaxation techniques, yoga, and biofeedback. These approaches may decrease muscle tissue hypoxia and hypertonicity and relieve ischemia by increasing blood flow to the affected areas.

SURGICAL MANAGEMENT. Surgical management of endometriosis for a woman who wants to remain fertile is conservative and involves removal of endometrial implants and adhesions. The surgeon may use a carbon dioxide laser to treat endometriosis by vaporizing adhesions and endometrial implants. If the client does not wish to have children, the uterus and ovaries may be removed.

Dysfunctional Uterine Bleeding

OVERVIEW

Dysfunctional uterine bleeding (DUB), a nonspecific diagnostic term, is bleeding that is excessive or abnormal in amount or frequency without predisposing anatomic or systemic conditions. DUB occurs most often at either end of the span of a woman's reproductive years—when ovulation is becoming established or when it is becoming irregular at menopause.

Normally, the menstrual cycle represents a series of complex hormonal events related to balanced hypothalamic, pituitary, ovarian, and uterine functions. Menses, the sloughing of the endometrial lining, is an expected result. DUB occurs when there is a breakdown of these functions, causing hormonal imbalance.

The mechanism of DUB is unknown, but several theories have linked it with endometrial or myometrial dysfunction. Excessive fibrinolytic activity in the endometrium and changes in prostaglandin production in the uterus may also cause DUB.

Generally, DUB occurs in the absence of ovulation when the absence is associated with ovarian dysfunction. Estrogen stimulation of the endometrium is prolonged, and the endometrium grows past its hormonal support, causing bleeding and desquamation (shedding of uterine lining).

Anovulatory DUB during the reproductive years is associated with the following:

- Polycystic ovary disease
- Stress
- Extreme weight changes
- Long-term drug use (e.g., anticholinergics, morphine, or oral contraceptives)

Ovulatory causes of DUB are uncommon and are related to a dysfunctional corpus luteum, irregular maturation, and shedding of the endometrium.

COLLABORATIVE MANAGEMENT

Assessment

When interviewing a woman with DUB, the nurse takes a complete menstrual history. The client is also asked about illnesses, variations in weight or diet, exercise, drug ingestion, and whether she has pain.

During the physical assessment, the nurse observes for symptoms of anemia or systemic disease, such as the following:

- Renal or hepatic disease
- Obesity
- Undernutrition
- Abnormal hair growth related to hormonal dysfunction
- Evidence of abdominal pain or masses

An examination that includes inspection of the external genitalia and a bimanual pelvic and rectal examination is essential to identify lesions or tenderness. A physician, a nurse practitioner, or a nurse midwife performs the internal pelvic examination.

Pelvic ultrasonography and hysteroscopy may be performed. In addition, the surgeon usually does an endometrial biopsy by suction aspiration or dilation and curettage (D&C). These are important procedures for women older than 40 years of age, who are at greater risk for endometrial cancer.

Interventions

NONSURGICAL MANAGEMENT. Nonsurgical management is usually the treatment of choice, although surgery may be needed to treat DUB. Most women can be treated successfully with hormonal manipulation. For those with anovulatory DUB, the health care provider typically prescribes medroxyprogesterone acetate (Depo-Provera) or combination oral contraceptives. If the client takes oral contraceptives, she should take 1 pill a day for 21 or 28 days, beginning on the first day of the menstrual cycle. Medroxyprogesterone is taken on days 16 to 25 of each month. Monthly withdrawal bleeding is expected with both therapies.

Women with ovulatory DUB may be treated with progestins during the luteal phase, oral contraceptives, prostaglandin inhibitors, or danazol. The nurse explains the desired and side effects of these drugs and evaluates the woman's knowledge of the effects, dosage, and administration schedule.

SURGICAL MANAGEMENT. Surgical management includes D&C, laser or balloon endometrial ablation, and hysterectomy. A D&C is usually used to treat an acute episode of bleeding, but the problem often returns. Laser or balloon endometrial ablation is a safe alternative for women who do not respond to medical management or who do not need a hysterectomy (Barrow, 1999). A hysterectomy is usually performed only after other treatments have failed. Table 75-3 compares the preoperative and postoperative care of clients undergoing a D&C or endometrial ablation. Hysterectomy is discussed later under Operative Procedures (Uterine Leiomyomas), p. 1766. If the woman has undergone a D&C or laser ablation, the nurse gives her postoperative instructions (Chart 75-3).

Menopause

OVERVIEW

Menopause is a normal biologic event marked for most women by the end of menstrual periods. It signifies the depletion of estradiol, a hormone produced by the ovaries. Although the meaning of menopause is the last menstrual period, the more clinically relevant perspective is to look at the months or years surrounding this event.

During the past decade there has been an explosion of interest among health care providers about all aspects of

TABLE 75-3 • NURSING CARE OF CLIENTS UNDERGOING SURGERY FOR DYSFUNCTIONAL UTERINE BLEEDING

	Dilation and Curettage (D&C)	Endometrial Ablation
Usual site	Outpatient	Outpatient
Anesthesia	Local, regional, general	Regional, general
Procedure	The cervical os is dilated; the endometrium is scraped.	The laser fiber is passed into the uterus through a hysteroscope; the endometrium is destroyed by laser energy, and tissues are removed by irrigating the uterine cavity with saline.
Preoperative care	Assess the client's knowledge of the procedure. The client is NPO after midnight. Teach postoperative expectations.	Same as for D&C The client may be given danazol or GnRH agonist for 1 month before surgery to decrease endometrial thickness. Counsel the client about the likelihood of sterility as a result of uterine scarring.
Postoperative care	Monitor vital signs every 15 min until they are stable. Assess the need for pain relief. Assess for vaginal bleeding. Expect discharge when the client is stable.	Same as for D&C Same as for D&C Assess for spotting and vaginal drainage. Same as for D&C

GnRH, Gonadotropin-releasing hormone.

CHART 75-3

CLIENT EDUCATION GUIDE
Endometrial Ablation and Dilation and Curettage

Endometrial Ablation
- Spotting and vaginal drainage are normal for several days after the procedure.
- If you have abdominal cramping, take mild analgesics, such acetaminophen (Tylenol, Atasol♣), or prostaglandin inhibitors, such as ibuprofen (Motrin).
- You can return to your normal activities within 2 or 3 days.
- You will probably be sterile because of uterine scarring.

Dilation and Curettage
- Take your temperature once a day for the next 2 days. If your oral temperature is more than 100° F (38° C), call the clinic or your doctor.
- Avoid sexual intercourse, tub bathing, and the use of tampons for 2 weeks to allow healing and prevent infection.
- Slight bleeding is normal. However, if bleeding is as heavy as during your normal menstrual period or if bleeding lasts longer than 2 weeks, call the clinic or health care provider.
- You can use a heating pad or hot water bottle to relieve abdominal cramping if it occurs.
- You can take mild analgesics, such as acetaminophen, for pain.

menopause—endocrinologic, metabolic, pathologic, sociocultural, and psychologic. Of particular interest for clinicians is the role of hormone replacement therapy (HRT) in the management of symptoms.

Much present-day interest in menopause is directed at the postmenopausal period and the medical illnesses common to postmenopausal women that may be affected by hormonal change. The most commonly discussed conditions are osteoporosis, coronary heart disease, and breast and endometrial cancer; interest in the effects of hormones on Alzheimer's disease has also emerged.

Women experience menopause as individuals, and care should be taken not to make generalizations. Women become menopausal in a variety of ways, including through surgery when the uterus and ovaries are removed and through medical treatment for cancer. Natural menopause is experienced across a wide age range, occasionally as early as the 30s or 40s or as late as the 60s. The average age at which women experience their last menstrual period is between 50 and 52 years. All women under 40 who experience an early menopause, regardless of cause, are at higher than average risk for osteoporosis and osteoporosis-related fractures and may be at higher risk for cardiovascular disease. HRT is therefore particularly important in this group.

Several factors have been identified that may affect the timing of menopause. These include the following:

- Genetic influence
- Early **menarche** (beginning of menses)
- Hysterectomy
- Smoking
- Cancer treatment (chemotherapy or radiation)

COLLABORATIVE MANAGEMENT

Assessment

Menopause transition, or **perimenopause,** refers to the changes in spontaneous ovarian function that precede the last menstrual period and occur gradually. Common clinical characteristics of the transition are a change in the woman's usual menstrual periods and the beginning of vasomotor symptoms, such as hot flashes and night sweats. These symptoms may disturb the woman's usual sleep pattern. Vaginal dryness and mood changes may also occur. The nurse asks the client about these changes and reassures her that they are normal during perimenopause.

The most common early change in the bleeding pattern is a shortening of the time between menstrual periods, which is sometimes accompanied by an increase in menstrual flow. As the transition evolves, approximately 70% of women find that their periods become lighter and farther apart until they finally stop.

Some women simply stop menstruating without further change. The remaining women experience heavier bleeding, which can be either regularly timed or unpredictable. In addition, abnormal bleeding in this age-group can be caused by endometrial cancer, endometrial polyps, or uterine leiomyomas (tumors).

Most women pass through the menopause transition and into the postmenopause phase with minimal symptoms and never seek treatment for menopause-related problems. Approximately 20% of women, however, seek care for one or more of the symptoms discussed in this section, which are directly related to menopause.

Interventions

Hormone replacement therapy (HRT), a combination of estrogen and progestin (progesterone), is the primary medical intervention for menopause. Estrogen given alone can cause gynecologic cancers and thromboembolitic conditions, such as deep vein thrombosis.

Estrogen is available as oral, transdermal, intravaginal, and intramuscular preparations. The oral estrogens have generally equivalent effects on symptoms and equivalent medical risk factors, so the choice of preparation for most women can be based on cost and individual side effect experience (Johnson, 1998). Transdermal estrogen offers a useful alternative route of administration for women who prefer not to take pills, who cannot tolerate oral therapy because of gastrointestinal (GI) side effects, or who have liver function test abnormalities, elevated triglycerides, or other conditions in which a first-pass hepatic effect is best avoided (Johnson, 1998). Side effects of estrogen occur and persist in approximately 10% of women.

The most common complaints are bloating, nausea, and breast tenderness. These symptoms often resolve after a few months of estrogen use.

> **CRITICAL THINKING CHALLENGE**
>
> As you are admitting a middle-aged woman to your hospital unit for cellulitis, she mentions that she thinks she is going through menopause. She complains that she gets hot flashes, is very moody, and cries a lot. She has been hesitant to tell her physician because she kept hoping that the symptoms would cease.
>
> - How should you respond to the woman at this time?
> - What other data should you obtain during the nursing history?
> - What options will the health care provider have in treating the client's symptoms?

For suggested answer guidelines, go to SIMON http://www.wbsaunders.com/SIMON/Iggy/.

INFLAMMATIONS AND INFECTIONS

Vaginal discharge and itching are two of the most common complaints of female clients. Women may need information from their health care provider about the normal vaginal physiology, causes of symptoms, and methods of treatment. The nurse must be well informed about these topics to provide comprehensive care to clients with vaginal infections.

Vaginal infections are sometimes considered sexually transmitted diseases (STDs) because their causative organisms may be transmitted to sexual partners. However, infections can develop without sexual contact, and sexual partners do not always become infected. True STDs, such as gonorrhea, syphilis, chlamydial infection, and herpes simplex virus infection, are discussed in Chapter 77. Acquired immunodeficiency syndrome (AIDS) is covered in Chapter 23.

Simple Vaginitis

OVERVIEW

Vaginitis can develop whenever there is a disturbance of the balance of hormones and bacterial interaction in the vagina as a result of one or more of the following:

- Changes in the normal flora
- Alkaline pH
- Insertion of foreign bodies, such as tampons and condoms
- Chemical irritations, such as from douches or sprays
- Medications, especially antibiotics

Vaginitis is an inflammation of the lower genital tract. The nurse completes the assessment of vaginitis by asking questions about the symptoms, assisting with a pelvic examination, and obtaining vaginal smears for laboratory testing (Chart 75-4). The nurse is nonjudgmental and reassuring during the assessment because the client may be embarrassed or afraid to discuss her symptoms.

COLLABORATIVE MANAGEMENT

Interventions for vaginitis depend on the causes and the specific vaginal infection (Table 75-4). A woman's proper health habits can be beneficial to treatment. Therefore she should get enough rest and sleep, observe good dietary habits, get regular exercise, and use good personal hygiene. Popular, but not scientifically tested, hygiene practices to prevent vaginitis include the following:

- Perineal cleaning (wiping front to back) after urinating or defecating
- Wearing cotton underwear
- Avoiding strong douches and feminine hygiene sprays
- Avoiding tight-fitting pants

If antibiotics are prescribed, eating yogurt or taking *Lactobacillus* culture (Lactinex) tablets may help restore the natu-

> **CHART 75-4**
>
> **BEST PRACTICE *for***
> **Care of the Client with Simple Vaginitis**
>
> In taking a client history, ask about:
> - Onset of symptoms
> - Characteristics of the discharge, especially the color and odor
> - Associated symptoms such as itching and dysuria
> - Types of contraceptives used
> - Recent use of antibiotics
> - Client's sexual activity
> - Any history of vaginal infection
> - Client's hygiene practices: douching and using tampons
>
> In performing a physical examination:
> - Palpate the abdomen for tenderness or pain.
> - Inspect the external genitalia for erythema, edema, excoriation, odor, and discharge.
> - If you are qualified, perform a speculum examination to visualize the vagina and cervix, and note the source of any discharge or inflammation.
>
> If you are qualified, perform the following laboratory tests, as ordered: a saline or potassium hydroxide wet smear and a nitrazine paper test of vaginal pH.

TABLE 75-4 • COMMON VAGINAL INFECTIONS

	Assessment		
Sexual Transmission	**Physical Findings**	**Laboratory Findings**	**Drug Therapy**
***CANDIDA ALBICANS* INFECTION**			
Unlikely	Odorless, white, curdlike discharge Patches on vaginal walls and cervix Inflamed vaginal walls and cervix Itching	Hyphae and spores visible on potassium hydroxide wet slide Vaginal pH 4.5 or less	Miconazole nitrate (Monistat), clotrimazone (Gyne-Lotrimin), or nystatin (Mycostatin) vaginal creams or suppositories for 7 days Terconazole (Terazol) cream or suppositories for 7 days or double strength for 3 days Tioconazole (Vagistat) single-dose vaginal application
***TRICHOMONAS VAGINADIS* INFECTION**			
Yes	None or fishy Itching Strawberry spot on vaginal surface and cervix	Flagellated, pear-shaped protozoa on saline wet slide Vaginal pH 6-7	Oral metronidazole (Flagyl), single 2-g dose for client and sexual partners
BACTERIAL VAGINOSIS/*GARDNERELLA VAGINALIS* INFECTION			
Yes	Gray-white or green discharge Fishy odor Itching Normal vaginal mucosa 10%-40% asymptomatic	"Clue" cells on examination of saline wet slide Positive "whiff" test finding Vaginal pH 5-6	Oral metronidazole 500 mg qid for 7 days, or ampicillin or tetracycline Clindamycin 450 mg qid for 7 days
CERVICITIS			
Yes	Mucopurulent discharge from endocervix Pelvic pain, postcoital and intermenstrual bleeding The cervix may be inflamed and bleed when touched	Need to rule out herpes, gonorrhea, and chlamydial infection Vaginal pH 4.5 or less	Depends on diagnosis
ATROPHIC VAGINITIS			
No	Pale, thin, dry mucosa Itching No odor Scant white, yellow, gray, or green discharge Dyspareunia, postcoital bleeding	Parabasal cells Leukocyte predominance Vaginal pH 6	Topical conjugated estrogen cream 1/2 to 1 application at night for 7 nights, then twice weekly

ral flora (Döderlein's bacilli) of the vagina. Education of the client focuses on preventive measures and on information about infection transmission (Chart 75-5).

Vulvitis

OVERVIEW

Vulvitis is an inflammatory condition of the vulva that is associated with symptoms of pruritus (itching) and a burning sensation. The vulvar skin is sensitive to hormonal, metabolic, and allergic influences. Symptoms can be caused by systemic conditions, direct contact with irritants, and extension of infection from the vagina.

The most common skin disease affecting the vulva is contact dermatitis, which can be caused by an irritant, such as feminine hygiene sprays, fabric dyes, soaps and detergents, or allergens. Primary infections that affect the vulva include herpes genitalis and condylomata acuminata (venereal warts) (see Chapter 77). Secondary infections of the vulva are caused by organisms responsible for the numerous types of vaginitis, including candidiasis in diabetic women. Pediculosis pubis (crab lice infestation) and scabies (itch mite infestation) are common parasitic infestations of the skin of the vulva. Other causes of vulvitis include the following:

- Atrophic vaginitis
- Vulvar kraurosis (postmenopausal disorder causing dryness and atrophy)
- Vulvar leukoplakia (postmenopausal atrophy and thickening of vulvar tissues)
- Cancer
- Urinary incontinence

COLLABORATIVE MANAGEMENT

Assessment of the woman usually identifies symptoms of itching and burning sensation. Erythema (redness), edema, and superficial skin ulcers also may be present. Some women may have an itch-scratch-itch cycle, in which the itching

CHART 75-5

CLIENT EDUCATION GUIDE
Vaginal Infections

- Your risk of getting vaginal infections increases if you have sex with more than one person.
- When you have a vaginal infection, do not have sexual intercourse, or at least make sure that your partner wears a condom.
- Sexual partners may need to be treated for infection.
- The only way to identify what infection you have is to be examined by a health care provider and to get the results of laboratory tests.
- Take your medicine as prescribed, not just until your symptoms go away.

CHART 75-6

BEST PRACTICE *for*
Prevention of Vulvitis

- Wear cotton underwear.
- Avoid wearing tight clothing, such as pantyhose or tight jeans, because they can cause chafing. You can also get hot and sweaty, which can cause an infection.
- Always wipe front to back after having a bowel movement or urinating.
- Do not douche or use feminine hygiene sprays.
- If your sexual partner has an infection of his sex organs, do not have intercourse with him until he has been treated.
- You are more likely to get an infection if you are pregnant, have diabetes, take oral contraceptive drugs, or are menopausal.
- Practice vulvar self-examination monthly (see Chapter 73).

leads to scratching, which causes excoriation that then must heal. As healing takes place, itching occurs again, which leads to further scratching. If the cycle is not interrupted, the condition may become chronic, causing the vulvar skin to become white and thickened (leathery). This skin is dry and scaly and cracks easily, increasing the woman's chances of infection.

Medical treatment of clients with vulvitis depends on the cause. Nursing interventions to relieve itching include applying wet compresses, sitz baths for 30 minutes several times a day, and the application of prescribed topical medications, such as hydrocortisone and fluorinated corticosteroids (betamethasone valerate [Valisone, Betaderm♣] or fluocinolone acetonide [Synalar, Fluoderm]).

The health care provider prescribes oral antibiotics if infection is the underlying cause. Removal of any irritant or allergen, such as by changing detergents, should be encouraged. Treatment of pediculosis and scabies is instituted if needed and includes applying lindane (1% gamma benzene hexachloride [Kwell, Kwellada♣]) lotion, shampoo, or cream to the affected area as directed; cleaning affected clothes, bedding, and towels; and disinfecting the home environment (lice cannot live for more than 24 hours away from the body).

If the vulvitis is chronic or severe, laser therapy (see p. 1774) or a "skinning" vulvectomy (see p. 1779) may be performed. Preventive measures that may be helpful for vulvitis are listed in Chart 75-6.

Toxic Shock Syndrome

OVERVIEW

Toxic shock syndrome (TSS) was not commonly recognized by health care providers until 1980, when it was found to be related to menstruation and tampon use. Other conditions that have been associated with TSS include surgical wound infection, nonsurgical focal infections, postpartum conditions, and nonmenstrual vaginal conditions. Use of the diaphragm, cervical cap, and vaginal contraceptive sponge has also been linked to TSS.

The pathophysiology of TSS is not clearly understood. Certain strains of *Staphylococcus aureus* produce a toxin that has been associated with the symptoms of TSS. Numerous theories have been reported to explain the mechanism of *S. aureus* absorption in TSS. The vagina may be highly susceptible to the toxin released by *S. aureus.*

In menstrually related TSS, the theories about the mechanisms of absorption focus on tampon use. Risk for TSS is related to the degree of absorbency of the tampon. The following are possible explanations:

- Toxins readily cross the vaginal mucosa.
- Highly absorbent tampons rub the vaginal walls and cause ulceration, which allows transport of the toxins.
- Prolonged or continued tampon use can cause chronic vaginal ulcerations through which *S. aureus* is absorbed.
- Plastic tampon inserters can cause ulceration through which toxins are transported.
- Toxin producing *S. aureus* has a growth requirement for magnesium (some tampons contain magnesium).

COLLABORATIVE MANAGEMENT

Influenza-like symptoms for the first 24 hours are common. The abrupt onset of a high temperature associated with a headache, sore throat, vomiting, diarrhea, generalized rash, and hypotension are often present. The most common clinical manifestations are skin changes (initially a rash resembling a severe sunburn that changes to a macular erythema similar to a drug-related rash). Because not all women experience all of these clinical manifestations, the criteria established by the U.S. Centers for Disease Control and Prevention (CDC) are used in epidemiologic studies to verify cases of TSS (Chart 75-7).

Management in the primary care setting focuses on client education and prevention. The nurse instructs the client on the prevention of TSS related to the use of tampons, vaginal sponges, and diaphragms (Chart 75-8).

Primary treatment in the acute care setting includes fluid replacement because dehydration and electrolyte imbalance result from vomiting and diarrhea. The health care provider also prescribes antibiotics if the penicillin-resistant strain of *S. aureus* is the cause of TSS. Other measures may include administering transfusions to reverse low platelet counts, corticosteroids to treat skin changes, and drugs to treat hypotension.

PELVIC STRUCTURE SUPPORT PROBLEMS

Uterine Prolapse

OVERVIEW

Three stages of **uterine prolapse** have been described according to the degree of descent of the uterus (Figure 75-2). Prolapse of the uterus can be caused by congenital defects, persistent high levels of intra-abdominal pressure related to

CHART 75-7

KEY FEATURES *of* Toxic Shock Syndrome

- Fever (temperature > 102° F [38.9° C]
- Diffuse rash resembling sunburn
- Peeling of skin—primarily the soles of the feet and the palms of the hands—1 to 2 weeks after the onset of the illness
- Hypotension (systolic blood pressure <90 mm Hg or orthostatic syncope)
- Involvement of three or more of the following:
  - Gastrointestinal system: vomiting, diarrhea at the onset of the syndrome
  - Musculoskeletal system: severe aching or a serum creatinine phosphatase level twice the normal level
  - Respiratory system: acute respiratory distress syndrome (ARDS)
  - Renal/urinary system: decreased urine output, pyuria
  - Cardiovascular system: decreased left ventrical contractility; ischemic changes shown on the electrocardiogram
  - Liver: total bilirubin, aspartate aminotransferase (serum glutamic-oxaloacetic transaminase), and alanine aminotransferase (serum glutamic-pyruvic transaminase) levels elevated; jaundice; disseminated intravascular coagulation (DIC)
  - Hematologic system: platelet levels below normal
  - Central nervous system: disorientation, altered consciousness in the absence of fever or hypertension
  - Mucous membranes: hyperemia of the vaginal walls, the throat, or the conjunctiva of the eye
- Negative results for the following: Rocky Mountain spotted fever, measles, scarlet fever, and throat, blood, and cerebrospinal fluid cultures
- Positive culture for *Staphylococcus aureus* from blood, urine, or stool

CHART 75-8

CLIENT EDUCATION GUIDE
Prevention of Toxic Shock Syndrome

Tampon Use
- Wash your hands before inserting a tampon.
- Do not use a tampon if it is dirty.
- Insert the tampon carefully to avoid injuring the delicate tissue in your vagina.
- Change your tampon every 3 to 6 hours.
- Do not use superabsorbent tampons.
- Use sanitary napkins at night.
- Call your health care provider if you suddenly experience a high temperature, vomiting, or diarrhea.
- Do not use tampons at all if you have had toxic shock syndrome.
- Not using tampons almost guarantees that you will not get toxic shock syndrome.

Vaginal Sponge Use
- Wash your hands before inserting a vaginal sponge.
- Use only clean water to wet the sponge.
- Do not use the sponge if it is dirty.
- Do not use the sponge for more than 30 hours at a time
- Call your health care provider if you have two or more symptoms of toxic shock syndrome.

Diaphragm Use
- Wash your hands and the diaphragm before insertion.
- Remove the diaphragm within 24 hours after intercourse.
- Do not use the diaphragm during your menstrual period.
- After you take out the diaphragm, wash it with mild soap, rinse it, and dry it. Coating the diaphragm with a small amount of cornstarch will absorb any excess water and prevent damage to the latex rubber. Store it in a clean, dry place.

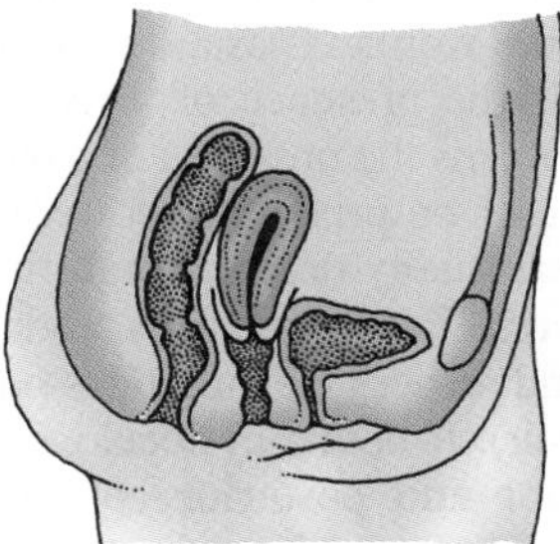

In **grade I uterine prolapse**, the uterus bulges into the vagina, but the cervix does not protrude through the entrance to the vagina.

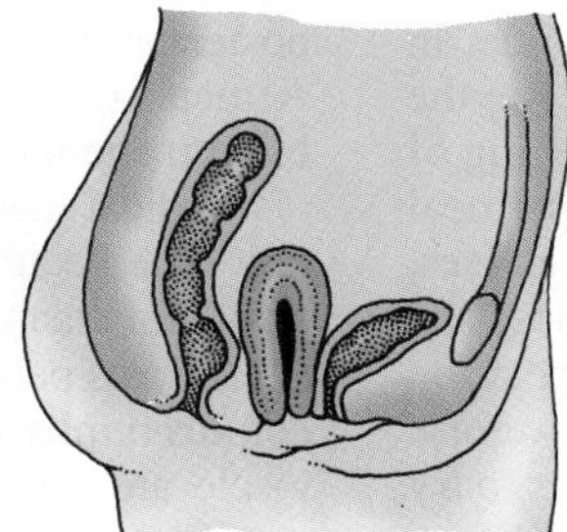

In **grade II uterine prolapse**, the uterus bulges farther into the vagina, and the cervix protrudes through the entrance to the vagina.

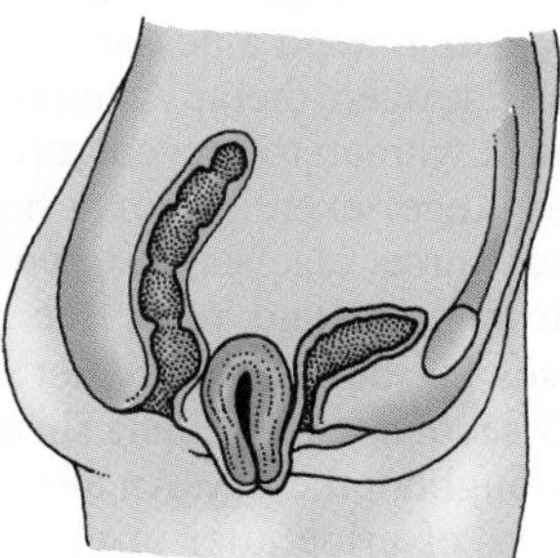

In **grade III uterine prolapse**, the body of the uterus and the cervix protrude through the entrance to the vagina. The vagina is turned inside out.

Figure 75-2 ● Types of uterine prolapse.

heavy physical labor or exertion, or any other event that weakens the pelvic supports.

CONSIDERATIONS FOR OLDER ADULTS

Prolapse is often a complication of childbirth injuries and repetitive stresses occurring many years later, but it also occurs in older adults who have never had children. The pelvic floor that supports the uterus is weakened by aging.

COLLABORATIVE MANAGEMENT

Assessment findings include the client's verbalization of feeling as if "something is in my vagina," dyspareunia (painful sexual intercourse), backache, a feeling of heaviness or pressure in the pelvis, and bowel or bladder problems (if cystocele or rectocele is also present). A pelvic examination may reveal a protrusion of the cervix when the woman is asked to bear down.

Interventions are based on the degree of prolapse. Conservative treatment, such as the use of pessaries, is preferred over surgical treatment when possible. Vaginal hysterectomy with repair is the usual surgical procedure (see Operative Procedures [Uterine Leiomyomas], p. 1766). Before surgical intervention, the nurse questions the woman about her desire for future childbearing (surgery may be delayed) and her desire for sexual intercourse. Surgery usually shortens and narrows the vagina, possibly causing painful intercourse.

Whenever the uterus is displaced, other structures, such as the bladder, rectum, and small intestine, are affected and can protrude through the vaginal walls.

Cystocele

OVERVIEW

A **cystocele** is a protrusion of the bladder through the vaginal wall (Figure 75-3). It is due to weakened pelvic structures. This protrusion can be caused by obesity, advanced age, childbearing, or genetic predisposition. The development of a cystocele is more noticeable in the postmenopausal years, when estrogen loss also weakens tissue supports and can cause relaxation of the supports.

COLLABORATIVE MANAGEMENT

Assessment findings may include the following:

- Difficulty in emptying the bladder
- Urinary frequency and urgency
- Urinary tract infection
- Stress urinary incontinence (loss of urine during stressful activities such as laughing, coughing, sneezing, or lifting heavy objects)

A pelvic examination reveals a significant bulge of the anterior vaginal wall when the woman is asked to bear down. Diagnostic tests that may be ordered include cystography (to show the presence of bladder herniation), measurement of residual urine by catheterization, and urine culture and sensitivity testing (which may reveal infection caused by urinary retention).

If the client is asymptomatic or has mild symptoms, medical management is usually conservative. The health care provider may recommend a pessary to support the bladder in some clients. Estrogen therapy might be prescribed for the postmenopausal woman to prevent atrophy and weakening of vaginal walls. Kegel exercises may help strengthen perineal muscles. The nurse teaches the woman Kegel exercises, telling her to tighten and relax the perineal muscles; the woman presses the buttocks together and holds the position for at least 5 seconds. The client should repeat the exercise frequently throughout the day. An alternative exercise is to try to stop the flow of urine after urination has started and then hold the position for a few seconds before letting the urine flow again.

The health care provider may recommend surgery for severe symptoms. An **anterior colporrhaphy** (anterior repair) tightens the pelvic muscles for better bladder support. A vaginal surgical approach is used. Nursing care of a woman undergoing an anterior repair is similar to that for a woman undergoing a vaginal hysterectomy (see Operative Procedures [Uterine Leiomyomas], p. 1766).

Postoperatively, the nurse instructs the client to limit her activities, not lift anything heavier than 5 pounds, avoid strenuous exercises, and avoid sexual intercourse for 6 weeks. The woman should notify her health care provider if she has signs of infection, such as fever, persistent pain, or purulent, foul-smelling discharge. The client should keep her follow-up appointment after surgery.

Rectocele

OVERVIEW

A **rectocele** is a protrusion of the rectum through a weakened vaginal wall (see Figure 75-3). This usually results from the pressure of a baby's head during a difficult delivery, a traumatic forceps delivery, or a congenital defect of the supporting tissues. Symptoms do not typically appear until the woman is older than 35 years of age.

COLLABORATIVE MANAGEMENT

The woman's history may reveal symptoms of constipation, hemorrhoids, fecal impaction, and feelings of rectal or vaginal fullness. A pelvic examination may show a bulge of the posterior vaginal wall when the woman is asked to bear down. A rectal examination reveals the presence of a rectocele. A barium enema study also confirms the presence of a rectocele.

Medical management focuses on promoting bowel elimination. The health care provider usually orders a high-fiber diet, stool softeners, and laxatives. The surgical procedure that strengthens pelvic supports and reduces the bulging is **posterior colporrhaphy** (posterior repair). If both a cystocele and a rectocele are present, an **anterior and posterior colporrhaphy (anterior and posterior [A&P] repair)** is performed.

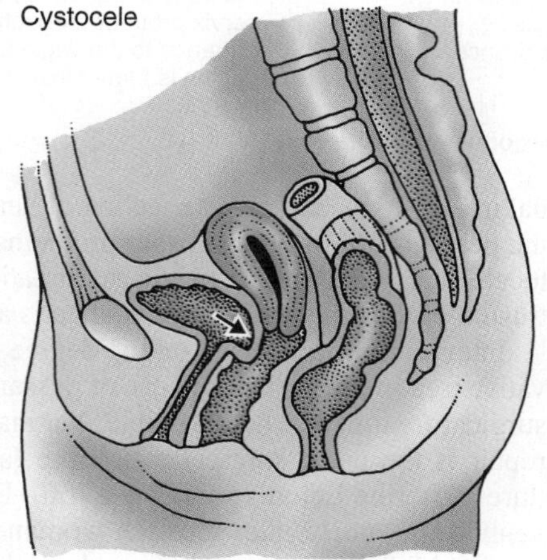

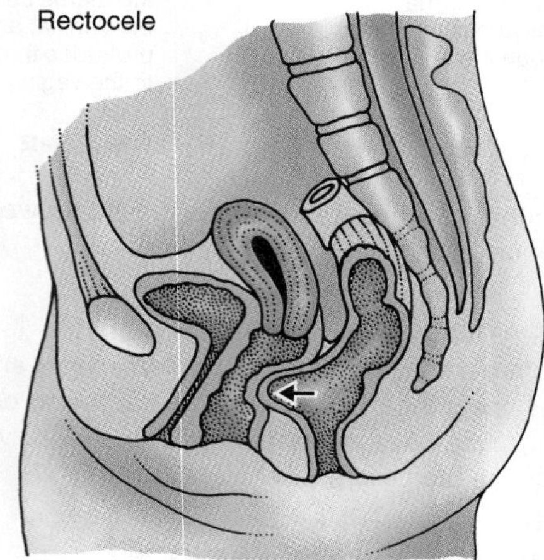

Figure 75-3 ● In cystocele, the urinary bladder is displaced downward, causing bulging of the anterior vaginal wall. In rectocele, the rectum is displaced, causing bulging of the posterior vaginal wall.

The nursing care after a posterior repair is similar to that after any rectal surgery. Postoperatively, the woman is usually given a low-residue diet to prevent bowel movements and allow time for the incision to heal. The woman is told not to strain when she does have a bowel movement so that she does not put pressure on the suture line. Bowel movements are often painful, and the client may need pain medication before having a bowel movement. Sitz baths may relieve discomfort. Postoperative instructions for the client undergoing a posterior repair are similar to those for an anterior repair.

Fistulas

OVERVIEW

Fistulas are abnormal openings between two adjacent organs or structures. Vaginal fistulas can occur between the vagina and the urethra (urethrovaginal), the vagina and the bladder (vesicovaginal), or the vagina and the rectum (rectovaginal). Trauma is the primary cause of fistulas, although they can result from complications of surgery, vaginal delivery complications, malignancy, or radiation therapy for cancer.

COLLABORATIVE MANAGEMENT

Symptoms depend on the location of the fistula. A fistula should be considered as a possible cause if a woman's history includes the following complaints:

- Leakage of urine, flatus, or feces into the vagina
- Irritation or excoriation of the vulva and vaginal tissues
- An unpleasant odor (fecal or urine) in the vagina
- A feeling of wetness or dribbling in the vagina

Women who have fistulas may be embarrassed to seek help until symptoms are severe. The client may withdraw from social activities or from relationships with significant others as the symptoms become more difficult to manage.

Management depends on the fistula's location. Surgery is not recommended if infection or inflammation is present. Surgery may not be successful. Nursing care focuses on assisting the woman with the frequent and time-consuming perineal hygiene, including sitz baths; perineal cleaning with mild, unscented soap and water; and low-pressure douching with commercial deodorizing solutions or homemade solutions (1 teaspoon [5 mL] of nonchlorine household bleach to 1 quart [approximately 1 L] of water). The woman may need to wear sanitary napkins or disposable undergarments (such as Depends) if there is leakage of urine or feces. Other beneficial treatments may include the application of A and D ointment to excoriated tissues.

If the fistula is repaired surgically, nursing care focuses on preventing infection and avoiding stress on the repaired area (low-residue diet and administration of stool softeners for 2 weeks after rectovaginal fistula repair). Nursing care and postoperative teaching are similar to the care and teaching of the client who has a cystocele or rectocele repair (see p. 1762).

BENIGN NEOPLASMS

Functional Ovarian Cysts

Functional **ovarian cysts** can occur in a woman of any age but are rare after menopause.

FOLLICULAR CYSTS

Follicular cysts usually occur in young, menstruating females. These cysts are nonneoplastic and do not grow without hormonal influences. A cyst can develop when a mature follicle fails to rupture or an immature follicle fails to reabsorb follicular fluid during the second half of the menstrual cycle. The cyst is usually small (2.4 to 3.2 inches [6 to 8 cm]) and may be asymptomatic unless it ruptures. Rupture of a follicular cyst or torsion (twisting) may cause acute, severe pelvic pain. The pain usually resolves after several days of bedrest and the administration of mild analgesics. If the cyst does not rupture, it usually disappears within two or three menstrual cycles without medical intervention. If the cyst does not shrink, the health care provider may prescribe oral contraceptive pills for one or two menstrual cycles to depress ovulation. When the cyst is managed conservatively, follow-up care is necessary to confirm that it has disappeared.

If the cyst is larger than 6 to 8 cm, a neoplasm may be suspected, and further evaluation by ultrasonography or laparoscopy is necessary. Larger cysts are often associated with menstrual irregularities.

Surgery is recommended only before puberty, after menopause, or when cysts are larger than 3.2 inches (8 cm). A cystectomy (removal of the cyst) is recommended instead of an oophorectomy (removal of the ovary).

CORPUS LUTEUM CYSTS

Corpus luteum cysts occur after ovulation and are often associated with increased secretion of progesterone. The cysts are usually small, averaging 1.5 inches (4 cm). They are purplish red as a result of hemorrhage within the corpus luteum. Corpus luteum cysts are associated with a delay in the onset of menses and irregular or prolonged flow. They may be accompanied by unilateral low abdominal or pelvic pain that is usually described as dull or aching. If the cyst ruptures, intraperitoneal hemorrhage can occur.

Corpus luteum cysts may disappear in one or two menstrual cycles or with suppression of ovulation. The treatment is the same as that for follicular cysts.

THECA-LUTEIN CYSTS

Theca-lutein cysts are the least common of the functional cysts. They are associated with hydatidiform mole (molar pregnancy), occurring in 50% of these complicated pregnancies. Theca-lutein cysts develop as a result of prolonged stimulation of the ovaries by excessive amounts of human chorionic gonadotropin (hCG).

Theca-lutein cysts regress spontaneously within 3 months with the removal of the molar pregnancy or the source of excessive hCG. No other treatment is usually necessary.

POLYCYSTIC OVARY

Polycystic ovary, or Stein-Leventhal syndrome, results when elevated levels of luteinizing hormone (LH) cause hyperstimulation of the ovaries, which produces multiple cysts on one or both ovaries. High levels of estrogen are produced by these cysts and are unopposed by postovulatory progesterone. Endometrial hyperplasia (tissue overgrowth) or even carcinoma may result.

A typical client is obese, is hirsute (hairy), has irregular menses, and may be infertile because of lack of ovulation. Treatment depends on which disorder is of greatest concern to the woman. The best treatment is the administration of oral contraceptives because they inhibit LH production. The health care provider may advise a woman who is older than 35 years of age and no longer desires childbearing to undergo a **bilateral salpingo-oophorectomy (BSO)** (removal of both tubes and ovaries) and **hysterectomy** (removal of the uterus and cervix). Women who desire fertility can be treated with drugs such as clomiphene citrate (Clomid) to stimulate ovulation.

Other Benign Ovarian Cysts and Tumors

DERMOID CYSTS

Dermoid cysts are the most common germ cell tumors and are benign in more than 99% of cases. These cysts are the most common ovarian tumors of childhood, although they can develop in a female of any age.

Dermoid cysts may contain hair, sebaceous material, teeth, and other calcifications. They are usually asymptomatic unless they grow large and put pressure on other organs, such as the bladder and the bowel. The cysts develop bilaterally in some cases. They are often attached to the ovary by a pedicle (stalk).

Management of dermoid cysts is by surgical removal (cystectomy). If the cysts are not removed, they usually continue to grow and rupture, causing hemorrhage and infection.

OVARIAN FIBROMAS

Fibromas are the most common benign, solid ovarian neoplasms. These pearly white tumors of connective tissue origin have a low potential for becoming malignant. Fibromas can range in size from a small nodule to a mass weighing more than 50 pounds (22.7 kg). The average size is 2.4 inches (6 cm) in diameter, slightly smaller than a tennis ball. Ninety percent of fibromas are unilateral. On examination, they feel firm, have a slightly irregular contour, and are mobile. Fibromas greater than 6 cm in diameter may be associated with ascites and may cause feelings of pelvic pressure or abdominal enlargement. Unless rupture or torsion occurs, the neoplasm is usually asymptomatic. Fibromas often occur postmenopausally.

Solid ovarian neoplasms are surgically removed. The surgeon may perform an oophorectomy for borderline tumors (when there is a question of possible malignancy). Nursing care of a woman undergoing an oophorectomy is similar to that for a woman undergoing a tubal ligation. When both ovaries are removed, surgery-induced menopause occurs in a premenopausal women. As a result, a woman often experiences decreased vaginal lubrication, hot flashes, and atrophy of the vaginal epithelium. These symptoms may be treated with estrogen replacement therapy (ERT) (see Chart 75-2).

EPITHELIAL OVARIAN TUMORS

Epithelial ovarian tumors, serous and mucinous cystadenomas, occur in women between the ages of 30 and 50 years. Serous cystadenomas usually occur bilaterally and are more likely to become malignant than mucinous cystadenomas. Both tumors can be irregular and smooth, but mucinous cystadenomas tend to grow large, some to more than 100 pounds (45 kg).

Management of cystadenomas is usually by unilateral salpingo-oophorectomy (surgical removal of a fallopian tube and ovary), because it is often impossible to tell whether the tumor is benign or malignant. Small cystadenomas may be removed by cystectomy, but the larger ones are difficult to resect from the ovary.

Uterine Leiomyomas

OVERVIEW

Leiomyomas, also called **myomas** and **fibroids,** are the most commonly occurring pelvic tumors. They are benign, slow-growing solid tumors of the uterus.

Pathophysiology

Leiomyomas initially develop from the uterine myometrium. As they grow, fibroids stay attached to the myometrium by means of a pedicle. Leiomyomas are classified according to their position in the layers of the uterus and their anatomic position. The most common types of leiomyomas are intramural, submucosal, and subserosal (Figure 75-4).

Intramural leiomyomas are contained in the uterine wall within the myometrium. Submucosal leiomyomas protrude into the cavity of the uterus. Subserosal leiomyomas protrude through the outer surface of the uterine wall. Subserosal leiomyomas may grow laterally and extend to the broad ligament.

Although most fibroids develop within the uterine wall, about 5% may appear in the cervix. Rarely, a fibroid breaks off the pedicle and attaches to other tissues (parasitic fibroid).

Etiology

The cause of leiomyomas is not precisely known. Leiomyomas usually result from a localized proliferation of smooth muscle cells in their initial stages. The stimulus for proliferation may be physical or mechanical and may operate at points of maximal stress within the myometrial layer of the uterine wall. Because there are multiple points of stress caused by the contractions of the uterine muscle, multiple fibroids develop. The growth of leiomyomas may be related to estrogen stimulation; fibroids often enlarge during pregnancy and diminish in size after menopause.

Incidence/Prevalence

Leiomyomas occur in approximately 20% to 30% of women older than age 30. The rationale for why leiomyomas develop in some women and not in others is not known.

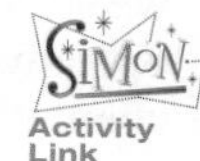

COLLABORATIVE MANAGEMENT

Assessment

HISTORY

Although most women with uterine leiomyomas are asymptomatic, abnormal bleeding is the most common complaint. Because African-American women and premenopausal women are at greatest risk for leiomyomas, any presence of

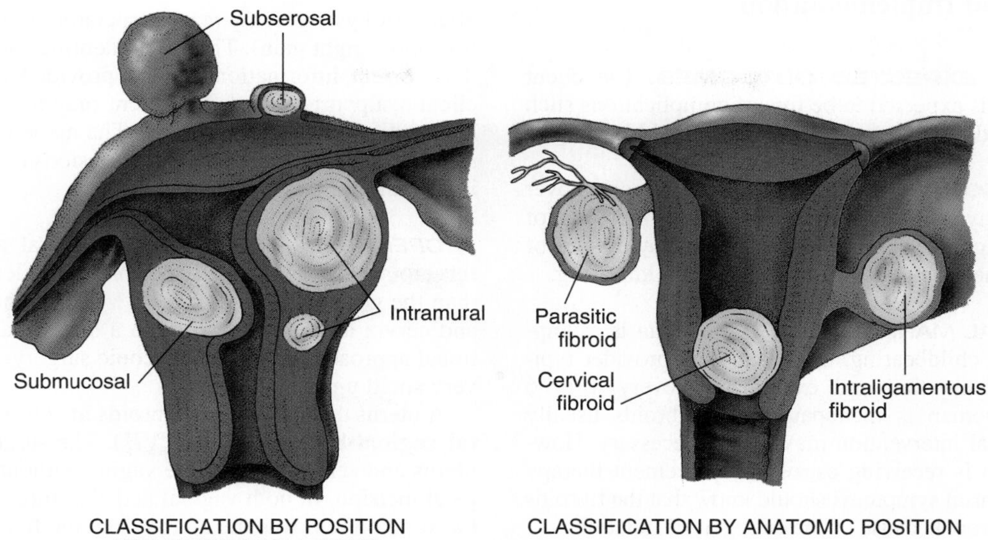

Figure 75-4 ● Classification of uterine leiomyomas.

abnormal bleeding should be discussed. There may be an increase in menstrual bleeding **(menorrhagia),** the bleeding may occur between menstrual periods **(metrorrhagia),** or it may be continuous.

PHYSICAL ASSESSMENT/CLINICAL MANIFESTATIONS

Women with fibroids do not usually complain of pain, although acute pain may occur with torsion (twisting) of the fibroid on the pedicle. A woman may report a feeling of pelvic pressure, constipation, or urinary frequency or retention. These symptoms result when an enlarged fibroid presses on other organs. The client may also notice that her abdomen has increased in size with or without noticeable weight gain. Dyspareunia (painful sexual intercourse) and infertility have also been associated with leiomyomas.

Abdominal, vaginal, and rectal examinations usually establish the presence of a uterine enlargement that may indicate a leiomyoma. However, other diagnostic procedures may be ordered to differentiate benign lesions from malignant ones.

PSYCHOSOCIAL ASSESSMENT

A woman who is symptomatic may fear that she has a malignancy. She may be anxious about abnormal bleeding or her failure to conceive. She may also be concerned if surgical procedures are recommended. The nurse assesses the woman's feelings and concerns about her symptoms and fears of the unknown. If surgery is recommended, the significance of the loss of the uterus for the woman is explored.

LABORATORY ASSESSMENT

A complete blood count identifies iron deficiency anemia (related to bleeding). A pregnancy test may be done to determine whether pregnancy is the cause of the uterine enlargement. An endometrial biopsy may be performed to determine whether the lesion is malignant.

RADIOGRAPHIC ASSESSMENT

Computed tomography (CT) may be of some value. However, CT scans do not differentiate between benign and malignant myomas.

OTHER DIAGNOSTIC ASSESSMENT

Ultrasonography may be useful in differentiating other causes of pelvic masses, including ovarian masses and pregnancy. Culdoscopy or laparoscopy may also be of value in differentiating a uterine fibroid from an ovarian mass. These tests are described in Chapter 73.

Analysis

COMMON NURSING DIAGNOSES AND COLLABORATIVE PROBLEMS

The most common collaborative problem for clients with leiomyomas is Potential for Hemorrhage.

ADDITIONAL NURSING DIAGNOSES AND COLLABORATIVE PROBLEMS

In addition to the common collaborative problems, clients with leiomyomas may have one or more of the following:

- Fear and Anxiety related to an uncertain diagnosis and potential surgical treatment
- Acute Pain related to pressure from tumors
- Anticipatory Grieving or Dysfunctional Grieving related to perceived or actual loss of the uterus or reproductive function
- Sexual Dysfunction related to dyspareunia
- Ineffective Coping related to depression as a response to treatment

Planning and Implementation

POTENTIAL FOR HEMORRHAGE

PLANNING: EXPECTED OUTCOMES. The client with leiomyomas is expected to be free of complications such as hemorrhage and severe anemia from abnormal bleeding.

INTERVENTIONS. Observation of the leiomyomas over time, myomectomy, and hysterectomy are the methods of management. The choice depends on the size and symptoms of the fibroids and the woman's desire for future childbearing.

NONSURGICAL MANAGEMENT. If the client is asymptomatic or desires childbearing, the health care provider typically suggests observation and examination every 4 to 6 months. If the woman is menopausal, the fibroids usually shrink, and surgical intervention may not be necessary. However, a client who is receiving estrogen replacement therapy (ERT) for menopausal symptoms should know that the fibroids may continue to grow because of the estrogen stimulation.

SURGICAL MANAGEMENT. The treatment of leiomyomas depends on whether future childbearing is desired, the age of the woman, the size of the fibroids, and the clinical manifestations. If the woman desires childbearing, the surgeon may perform a **myomectomy** (the removal of leiomyomas with preservation of the uterus) regardless of the size, number, or location of the fibroids. The surgeon may use a laser to remove the tumors. Myomectomy is usually performed in the proliferative phase of the menstrual cycle to minimize blood loss and to avoid the possibility of interrupting an unsuspected pregnancy. A small percentage of leiomyomas that are removed recur. Nursing care is similar to that of a woman undergoing a hysterectomy, as described later in this section under Operative Procedures.

> **CONSIDERATIONS FOR OLDER ADULTS**
> Hysterectomy is the usual surgical management in the older woman who has multiple symptomatic leiomyomas. (The care of a woman undergoing a traditional total abdominal hysterectomy is described in the Clinical Pathway on pp. 1853-1854.)

PREOPERATIVE CARE. Preoperative teaching by the physician begins in his or her office. The physician's office nurse makes sure that the client can describe all of the options for surgery, the advantages and risks of surgery, preoperative and postoperative procedures, and recovery needs. With this information, the woman can make an informed consent to surgery.

Preoperative teaching is usually done on an individual basis. The nurse should explain routine preoperative procedures, including laboratory tests for baseline data and the administration of medications such as prophylactic antibiotics.

The client will need preparation for postoperative measures, including turning, coughing, deep breathing exercises (TCDB), and incentive spirometry; early ambulation; and the need for pain relief. Psychologic assessment is essential. The nurse first explores the significance of the loss of the uterus for the client. She may feel a great loss if she wishes to retain her childbearing ability, relates her uterus to her self-image and femininity, or believes that her sexual function is related to her uterus. Often a woman has misconceptions about the effects of hysterectomy (e.g., associating it with masculinization and weight gain). The nurse identifies misconceptions so that correct information can be provided and assesses the client's support system. The client may fear rejection by her husband or other sexual partner. The nurse encourages inclusion of the partner in all teaching sessions unless this practice is not culturally acceptable.

OPERATIVE PROCEDURES. A **total abdominal hysterectomy (TAH)** is usually performed for leiomyomas larger than the gestational size of a 12-week pregnancy. The uterus and cervix are removed through a horizontal incision (traditional approach) or via laparoscopic surgery, which requires a very small umbilical incision.

A uterus that has smaller fibroids may be removed via a **total vaginal hysterectomy (TVH).** The surgeon removes the uterus and cervix through the vagina without an external surgical incision. In both vaginal and abdominal hysterectomies, the surgeon removes the uterus from the five supporting ligaments, which are then attached to the vaginal cuff so that normal depth of the vagina is maintained (Table 75-5).

In some cases (e.g., treatment of submucous fibroids and menorrhagia), hysterectomy has been replaced by minimally invasive uterine surgery such as a **transcervical endometrial resection (TCER).** A hysteroscope is inserted into the uterus, and the endometrium is destroyed, usually with a diathermy resectoscope (similar to the scope used with prostate surgery). Complications specific to hysteroscopic surgery include the following:

- Fluid overload (fluid used to distend the uterine cavity can be absorbed)
- Embolism
- Hemorrhage
- Perforation of the uterus, bowel, or bladder and ureter injury
- Persistent increased menstrual bleeding
- Incomplete suppression of menstruation

These complications occur less commonly when the procedure is performed by an experienced surgeon. In addition, there is a small risk of subsequent pregnancy and the possibility of cancer developing in the scar. Hysterectomy is still

TABLE 75-5 • COMMON GYNECOLOGIC SURGERIES

TOTAL HYSTERECTOMY
All of the uterus, including the cervix, is removed. The procedure may be vaginal abdominal or laparoscopic.

SUBTOTAL HYSTERECTOMY
All of the uterus, except the cervix, is removed. This procedure is rarely performed.

BILATERAL SALPINGO-OOPHORECTOMY
Fallopian tubes and ovaries are removed.

PANHYSTERECTOMY
Total abdominal hysterectomy and bilateral salpingo-oophorectomy. The uterus, ovaries, and fallopian tubes are removed adominally.

RADICAL HYSTERECTOMY
All of the uterus is removed abdominally. The lymph nodes, the upper third of the vagina, and the surrounding tissues (parametrium) are also removed.

the procedure of choice for women who have coexisting problems, especially those with malignancy or symptomatic uterovaginal prolapse.

POSTOPERATIVE CARE. Postoperative care of the woman who has undergone a TAH is similar to that of any client who has undergone abdominal surgery (see Chapter 19). For clients who have undergone an abdominal hysterectomy, the nurse (Chart 75-9):

- Assesses vaginal bleeding (there should be less than one saturated perineal pad in 4 hours)
- Assesses abdominal bleeding at the incision site (a small amount is normal)
- Checks the incision for intactness
- Maintains the urethral catheter (Foley catheter), if placed, usually for 24 hours or less for a traditional surgical approach
- Offers pain medications as ordered for the abdominal pain

Specific interventions for a vaginal hysterectomy include the following:

- Assessment of vaginal bleeding (there should be less than one saturated pad in 4 hours)
- Foley catheter care
- Perineal care (sitz baths or ice packs)

The surgeon usually removes the abdominal sutures or clips at the time of the first postoperative visit, whereas vaginal sutures are usually absorbed. The nurse recognizes and monitors for complications associated with hysterectomies (Table 75-6).

CHART 75-9

FOCUSED ASSESSMENT *of* The Client After Total Abdominal Hysterectomy

Assess cardiovascular, respiratory, renal, and gastrointestinal status, including:
- Vital signs
- Heart, lung, and bowel sounds
- Urine output
- Temperature and color of the skin
- Red blood cell, hemoglobin, and hematocrit levels
- Activity tolerance
- Dressing and drains for color and amount of drainage
- Peripads for vaginal bleeding and clots
- Fluid intake (IVs until bowel sounds return and client is tolerating oral intake)
- Signs of thrombophlebitis

Use the following interventions to prevent postoperative complications:
- Cough and deep breathing exercises
- Incentive spirometry
- Sequential compression devices
- Ambulation
- Avoidance of heavy lifting or strenuous activity

Assess the home care teaching needs of the client related to the illness and surgery, including:
- Physiologic effects of the surgery
- Signs of symptoms to report
- Side or toxic effects of medications
- Activity limitations related to driving and use of stairs
- Follow-up care
- Postoperative restrictions related to sexual activity, use of tampons, and bathing
- Care of wound and/or drains

Assess the client's coping skills and reaction to the diagnosis and surgical procedure.

CRITICAL THINKING CHALLENGE

You are a nurse in the postanesthesia care unit (PACU) assigned to the care of an older adult who has undergone a total abdominal hysterectomy and bilateral salpingo-oophorectomy via a horizontal abdominal incision. On initial assessment, you note that her vital signs are within baseline, the dressing is dry and intact, and she has a scant amount of blood on her perineal pad. Immediately before she is to be transferred to the surgical unit, you find that her blood pressure has dropped from 124/78 to 108/60. Her pulse has increased from 80 to 96 within the past hour.

- Should you continue with plans to transfer the client to the surgical unit, since her vital signs are still within normal limits? Why or why not?
- What other assessments should you perform at this time?
- What might explain the change in her vital signs?

For suggested answer guidelines, go to SIMON http://www.wbsaunders.com/SIMON/Iggy/.

CONSIDERATIONS FOR OLDER ADULTS

Older women are more at risk for all complications, particularly pulmonary embolism. Obese women are more at risk for thromboembolism. Psychologic complications can occur with both abdominal and vaginal procedures. Depression is the most frequent reaction reported. Other reactions are perceived loss of femininity and decreased libido. Loss of femininity may be the problem if a woman was interested in her appearance before surgery but afterward has no interest, even when she is feeling better. Decreased sexual desire is often temporary, if it occurs, and is usually related to discomfort.

Community-Based Care

The client with uterine leiomyomas is managed on an ambulatory care basis unless surgical intervention is required. After hospital discharge, the client typically returns to her home.

HOME CARE MANAGEMENT

Planning for home care management begins at the time of admission. The woman is usually discharged to the home setting 1 to 2 days after a traditional TAH, depending on the age and

TABLE 75-6 • COMMON POSTOPERATIVE COMPLICATIONS OF TRADITIONAL ABDOMINAL AND VAGINAL HYSTERECTOMIES

TRADITIONAL ABDOMINAL HYSTERECTOMY
- Intestinal obstruction (paralytic ileus)
- Thromboembolism
- Atelectasis
- Pneumonia
- Wound dehiscence (especially in obese clients)
- Urinary retention

VAGINAL HYSTERECTOMY
- Hemorrhage
- Urinary tract complications, especially infection or retention
- Wound infection
- Urinary retention

general health of the client. TVH, laparoscopic surgery, or TCER may be performed as same-day surgery in an ambulatory setting. The client undergoing a hysterectomy should be told to avoid or limit stair climbing for 1 month. She is advised to avoid tub baths (which may promote infection) and sitting for long periods (which causes pooling of blood in the pelvic vessels). The nurse also teaches the client to avoid engaging in strenuous activity or lifting anything weighing more than 5 pounds (2.3 kg). Some health care providers also restrict driving for 4 to 6 weeks.

HEALTH TEACHING

The nurse teaches the woman who has undergone a hysterectomy about the following (see Chart 75-9):

- The physical changes to be expected
- Exercise and activities
- Diet
- Sexual activity
- Wound care (if any)
- Complications
- Follow-up care

The physical changes include cessation of menses, inability to become pregnant, weakness and fatigue during convalescence (may last 2 to 3 months), and absence of menopausal symptoms unless the ovaries are also removed. Moderate exercise, such as walking, is encouraged, but active sports, such as jogging and aerobic exercise, should be avoided for at least 1 month.

The nurse teaches the client to consume foods that aid in healing tissues, such as foods high in protein, iron, and vitamin C. The nurse also reminds her to avoid sexual intercourse for 4 to 6 weeks. The first coital activity may cause some tenderness or pain because the vaginal walls are tight and need to be stretched. Water-soluble lubricants can decrease discomfort. The client should be taught the signs of complications, particularly infection. An appointment for follow-up medical care is scheduled for 1 week postoperatively.

Women who have undergone a hysterectomy need information about possible emotional reactions. Generally, women adjust well to surgery if they:

- Have completed childbearing
- Work
- Have interests outside the home
- Have no misconceptions about the effects of hysterectomy
- Have support from the family, especially the husband or their sexual partner

Reactions may be different after vaginal and abdominal procedures, because women who have undergone a vaginal hysterectomy have no external focus (no obvious change in body image) for their feelings. Psychologic reactions can occur 3 months to 3 years after surgery. Women identified as being at high risk for psychologic problems may need long-term follow-up care or referral. Women may need to be counseled about signs of depression. Intermittent sadness is normal, but continued feelings of low self-esteem or loss of interest or pleasure in usual activities and pastimes is not normal and should be evaluated. The incidence of psychologic reactions often decreases after the nurse provides written materials and discusses the positive forces in the client's life with her and her family or significant others.

HEALTH CARE RESOURCES

Usually no special home equipment is needed for a woman who has undergone a hysterectomy. A home care nurse may be needed to assess and monitor the older client's postoperative progress if other conditions (e.g., uncontrolled diabetes) are present. Financial assistance may be needed, and referral to the hospital's department of social services or case management department may be indicated if the woman has no insurance coverage. The nurse can provide a referral for psychologic or sexual counseling if potential problems are identified before discharge.

Evaluation: Outcomes

NOC The nurse evaluates the care of the client who has undergone surgery for leiomyomas on the basis of the identified nursing diagnoses and collaborative problems. The expected outcomes include that the client will:

- Be free of hemorrhage
- State the role of the reproductive system and the changes that occur after a hysterectomy (without misconceptions)
- Recover from surgery without complications
- Demonstrate a positive psychologic adjustment to surgery as evidenced by the absence of depression and the presence of a positive self-concept
- Resume sexual activities at her previous level of satisfaction

Bartholin's Cysts

OVERVIEW

Bartholin's cysts are one of the most common disorders of the vulva. The cysts result from obstruction of a duct. The secretory function of the gland continues, and the fluid fills up the obstructed duct. The cause of the obstruction may be infection, congenital stenosis or atresia, thickened mucus near the ductal opening, or mechanical trauma, such as lacerations or episiotomy.

COLLABORATIVE MANAGEMENT

Assessment

The client may be asymptomatic if the cyst is small, but a history may reveal complaints of dyspareunia, inadequate genital lubrication, or a mass in the perineal area. A large cyst usually causes constant localized pain and may cause difficulty walking or sitting. Physical examination of the vulva reveals a swelling immediately beneath the skin in the posterior portion of the vulva. The cyst may appear brown or sanguineous, depending on its contents. Usually the cyst is unilateral and ranges from ⅜ to 4 inches (1 to 10 cm) in size.

If the cyst is draining, the health care provider usually requests that the fluid be sent to the laboratory for culture (for gonorrhea and aerobic and anaerobic organisms) and sensitivity testing. If the woman is older than 40 years of age, a specimen of the cyst should be sent for pathologic examination to determine whether the lesion is benign or malignant.

Interventions

If the woman is asymptomatic, no interventions are necessary. If the cysts are symptomatic, simple incision and drainage

(I&D) may provide temporary relief; however, cysts tend to recur as the opening of the duct becomes obstructed again. Usually the health care provider establishes a permanent opening for drainage. Marsupialization (formation of a pouch that is a new duct opening) is accomplished using local, regional, or general anesthesia. Any postoperative discomfort may be relieved by the administration of analgesics and sitz baths. The health care provider may prescribe prophylactic antibiotics.

Bartholin's cysts may become infected. Abscesses are formed when bacteria, such as *Escherichia coli* or *Staphylococcus aureus,* enter the duct, resulting in infection that closes the duct. An abscess usually ruptures spontaneously within 72 hours of formation. Interventions for the woman with an abscess include the administration of analgesics and application of moist heat (sitz baths or hot wet packs) to the vulva. The health care provider usually orders broad-spectrum antibiotics to treat the infection. I&D of the abscess may provide temporary relief.

The health care provider may totally excise the Bartholin's glands in women older than 40 years of age when cancer is suspected or if repeated infections with abscess formation occur. Postoperative interventions include the following:

- Application of ice packs or sitz baths several times a day for comfort and promotion of healing
- Administration of analgesics for pain, if needed
- Prophylactic administration of antibiotics
- Assessment of the incision for signs of healing or infection

Cervical Polyps

Cervical polyps are pedunculated (on stalks) tumors arising from the mucosa and extending to the opening of the cervical os. The cause is unknown, although polyps result from a hyperplastic condition of the endocervical epithelium. They may also be due to inflammation. Polyps are the most common benign neoplastic growth of the cervix. Cervical polyps are most common in multiparous women older than 40 years of age.

A woman may be asymptomatic, or a history may reveal complaints of premenstrual or postmenstrual bleeding or bleeding after coitus. A speculum examination may reveal small (3/8 to 1½-inch [1- to 4-cm]) single or multiple polyps. They are bright red; have a soft, fragile consistency; and may bleed when touched.

Polyp removal is easily accomplished as an office procedure. The base of the polyp can be grasped with a clamp, and the polyp can be twisted off and sent to the pathology laboratory for evaluation. Electrocautery or chemical cautery usually stops any bleeding at the site of removal. After the procedure, the nurse may instruct the client to avoid tampon use, douches, and sexual intercourse for a week or until healing has taken place.

MALIGNANT NEOPLASMS

Endometrial Cancer

OVERVIEW

Endometrial cancer (cancer of the uterus) is one of the most commonly occurring reproductive cancers (American Cancer Society, 2000). This type of cancer is asymptomatic in its early development and has a good prognosis in 80% to 90% of cases.

CONSIDERATIONS FOR OLDER ADULTS

Endometrial cancer is a slow-growing tumor primarily occurring in postmenopausal women. The average age at onset is 61 years. The incidence declines after the age of 70 years (DeStefano & Bertin-Matson, 1996).

Pathophysiology

Adenocarcinoma of the endometrium accounts for 75% to 80% of all endometrial cancers. It arises from the glandular component of the endometrial mucosa and may be preceded by endometrial hyperplasia (tissue overgrowth). The initial growth of the cancer is within the uterine cavity, followed by extension into the myometrium and the cervix. Spread outside the uterus occurs as follows:

- Through lymphatic spread to the ovaries and parametrial, pelvic, inguinal, and para-aortic lymph nodes
- By hematogenous metastasis (spread by blood) to the lungs, liver, or bone
- By transtubal or intra-abdominal spread to the peritoneal cavity

Etiology

Risk factors associated with endometrial cancer include obesity, diabetes mellitus, hypertension, a history of uterine polyps, a history of infertility, nulliparity and polycystic ovary disease. Estrogen stimulation, including unopposed menopausal estrogen replacement therapy (ERT), late menopause (after age 52 years), postmenopausal bleeding, and a family history of uterine cancer also predispose a woman to endometrial cancer. Table 75-7 compares the risk factors for endometrial cancer with those for other female reproductive cancers.

Incidence/Prevalence

The National Cancer Institute (NCI) estimates that more than 35,000 new cases of endometrial cancer occur annually in the United States (American Cancer Society, 2000). Thus about 1 of every 100 women in the United States has endometrial cancer.

CULTURAL CONSIDERATIONS

Endometrial cancer occurs more often in Caucasian women than in African-American women and typically in postmenopausal women ages 50 to 65 years. Survival rates differ between Caucasian and African-American women with endometrial cancer; Caucasian women have higher survival rates (American Cancer Society, 2000). The difference in survival rates appears to be related to the occurrence of higher-grade lesions and more aggressive cell types in African-American women.

COLLABORATIVE MANAGEMENT

Assessment

The primary symptom of endometrial cancer is postmenopausal bleeding. In addition, the woman may complain of a watery, serosanguineous vaginal discharge, low back or

TABLE 75-7 • RISK FACTORS FOR CANCERS OF THE REPRODUCTIVE SYSTEM

Risk Factor	Endometrial Cancer	Cervical Cancer	Ovarian Cancer	Vulvar Cancer	Vaginal Cancer	Fallopian Tube Cancer	Gestational Trophoblastic Disease
Age	50-65 yr of age	CIS: 30-40 yr of age Invasive: 40-60 yr of age	Infrequent before 35 yr of age; range usually is 40-65 yr of age	After 40 yr of age; peak is 60-70 yr of age	Most after 50 yr of age; adenocarcinoma: 14-30 yr of age	After 50 yr of age; range is 18-80 yr of age	After 40 yr of age; before 20 yr of age
Family history	Increased risk	—	Increased risk	—	DES exposure in utero	—	—
Personal history	Diabetes, hypertension	—	Breast, bowel, or endometrial cancer	Cervical cancer, diabetes, vulvar disease	Vulvar or cervical cancer	Ovarian or uterine cancer, infertility	Previous molar pregnancy (3%-5%)
Race	Caucasians	African Americans, Native Americans	Caucasians	—	—	—	Asian-Americans; Mexican-Americans
Mother's age at birth	—	<18 yr	>30 yr	—	—	—	—
Body size	Obesity	—	—	Possibly obesity	—	—	—
Parity	Nulliparity	Multiparity	Nulliparity	—	Multiparity	Nulliparity	—
Estrogen use	Prolonged use; >3 yr menopausally	Possibly long-term birth control pill use	—	—	—	—	—
Smoking	Possibly increased risk	Possibly double the risk	—	—	—	—	—
Infection (STD)	—	Possibly STD (herpes simplex virus type 2 or papillomavirus infection)	—	Possibly STD (papillomavirus infection)	STD (herpes simplex virus type 2 or papillomavirus infection)	PID, chronic salpingitis	Exposure to infectious agents

CIS, Carcinoma in situ; *DES*, diethylstilbestrol; *PID*, pelvic inflammatory disease; *STD*, sexually transmitted disease.

abdominal pain, and low pelvic pain (caused by pressure of the enlarged uterus). A pelvic examination may reveal the presence of a palpable uterine mass or uterine polyp. The uterus is enlarged if the cancer is in an advanced stage.

Before a diagnosis is made, the client may deny that the symptoms are related to cancer. During the diagnostic phase, the woman may express fears and concerns about having a malignancy. After the diagnosis is confirmed, she may express disbelief, anger, depression, anxiety, or withdrawal behaviors.

The health care provider orders basic diagnostic tests to determine the client's overall status. The results of the tests may also indicate the presence of metastasis. These tests include the following:

- Chest x-ray examination to detect metastasis
- Intravenous pyelography (IVP), or excretory urography, to assess renal function and to assess for renal metastasis
- Barium enema study to assess for intestinal metastasis
- Computed tomography (CT) of the pelvis to identify the origin and spread of the tumor
- Lymphangiography to assess for lymph node metastasis
- Liver and bone scans to assess for distant metastasis

Fractional dilation and curettage (D&C [scraping individual sections of the uterus]) and endometrial biopsy are the definitive diagnostic procedures for endometrial cancer. Other tests that may be useful for some clients include proctosigmoidoscopy, ultrasonography, and hysteroscopy (examination of the uterus via an endoscope).

Interventions

Nonsurgical interventions (radiation therapy and chemotherapy) and surgery may be used alone or in combination, depending on the stage of the cancer.

NONSURGICAL MANAGEMENT. Radiation therapy and chemotherapy are the two major nonsurgical methods used to treat endometrial cancer.

RADIATION THERAPY. The health care provider orders radiation therapy (external and internal) if the stage of cancer is hard to determine and if surgery is planned for stage II and III cancers. Clients usually receive radiation therapy for 6 weeks preoperatively to destroy cancer cells in the pericervical lymphatics and to inhibit recurrence.

Intracavitary Radiation. If intracavitary radiation therapy (IRT [brachytherapy]) is selected, the radiologist places an applicator within the woman's uterus through the vagina while she is anesthetized. After the correct position of the applicator is confirmed by x-ray examination, the client is taken to the hospital room and a radiologist places a radioactive isotope in the applicator, which remains for 1 to 3 days. Before the procedure, the nurse instructs the client on postprocedure activities, such as deep breathing and leg exercises. While the radioactive implant is in place, the woman is strictly isolated, usually in a private room. The nurse informs the client that she is restricted to bedrest on her back with the head of the bed flat or slightly elevated (20 degrees or less). Movement in bed is restricted to prevent dislodgment of the radioactive source.

A Foley catheter is inserted into the bladder to prevent dislodgment of the implant, which can be caused by a full bladder or attempts to void. The nurse carefully assesses the skin for breakdown over bony pressure points during the activity restriction period. The client is usually placed on a low-residue diet (to prevent bowel movements that might dislodge the implant), and fluid intake is encouraged (to prevent stasis of urine and possible infection). The health care provider usually prescribes the following:

- Antiemetics
- Broad-spectrum antibiotics (to prevent bladder infections)
- Tranquilizers (to help the client relax)
- Analgesics
- Heparin or Lovenox (to prevent thromboembolism)
- Antidiarrheal medications (to prevent bowel movements)

Radiation precautions are practiced while the implant is in place. The nurse organizes care so that minimal time is spent at the bedside. Care is given as far away from the radioactive source as possible and behind lead shields when possible. Nurses who are pregnant or attempting to become pregnant should not be assigned to these clients. Visitors are restricted to brief visits, and pregnant women and children younger than 18 years should not be allowed to visit.

External Radiation. External radiation therapy may be used to treat all stages of endometrial cancer. It is usually used in combination with surgery, preoperatively or postoperatively. Depending on the extent of the tumor, external radiation is given on an ambulatory care basis for 4 to 6 weeks. The lateral extensions of the tumor in the parametrium and pelvic wall nodes are irradiated (see also Chapter 25). Specific instructions for the woman undergoing external radiation for endometrial cancer include monitoring for signs of skin breakdown, especially in the perineal area, no sunbathing, and no bathing over the markings outlining the treatment site. The nurse informs the client that cystitis and diarrhea are common complications, as are nutritional problems that result from anorexia.

CHEMOTHERAPY. Chemotherapy is used as a palliative treatment in advanced and recurrent disease. Chemotherapeutic agents used for palliative treatment of endometrial cancer include doxorubicin (Adriamycin), cisplatin, and cyclophosphamide (Cytoxan, Procytox✤). These agents are used as single agents or in combination, and the length of treatment and dosage are determined by the woman's response to treatment. Chapter 25 discusses nursing interventions for clients receiving chemotherapy.

OTHER DRUG THERAPY. The health care provider may choose progestational therapy for stage I and II cancers that are estrogen dependent and for palliative treatment of stage IV cancer. The hormones commonly prescribed are medroxyprogesterone acetate (Depo-Provera) and megestrol acetate (Megace). Tamoxifen citrate (Nolvadex✤, Tamofen✤), an antiestrogen, is also used. The progestational agents do not cause acute side effects, but nausea and vomiting and hot flashes are associated with tamoxifen.

SURGICAL MANAGEMENT. The surgeon typically performs a total abdominal hysterectomy (removal of the uterus and cervix) and bilateral salpingo-oophorectomy (removal of both tubes and ovaries) for stage I tumors without cervical involvement. A radical hysterectomy (see Table 75-5) with bilateral pelvic lymph node dissection is performed for stage II cancer. Nursing care for a radical hysterectomy is essentially the same as that for a total abdominal hysterectomy except that the woman's hospitalization is usually longer and her convalescence may be extended.

PSYCHOSOCIAL SUPPORT. Women need to discuss their concerns about the presence of cancer and the potential for recurrence. The nurse provides emotional support and tries to create an atmosphere that encourages the woman to ask questions or express her fears and concerns. Family members or significant others are included in discussions when possible.

Reactions to radiation therapy vary. Some women may feel radioactive or "unclean" after treatments and may exhibit withdrawal behaviors. The nurse needs to correct such misconceptions.

Women who have chemotherapy may be upset if alopecia (hair loss) occurs. The nurse warns the client of this possibility before treatment starts. Wigs, scarves, or turbans can be worn until regrowth occurs.

Community-Based Care

The client with endometrial cancer is managed at home unless surgery is indicated. After surgery, the client is usually discharged to her home.

HOME CARE MANAGEMENT

Home care after surgery for endometrial cancer is the same as that after a hysterectomy (see Operative Procedures [Uterine Leiomyomas], p. 1766). Women who are receiving chemotherapy or external radiation therapy are usually treated on an ambulatory care basis, which may mean that the woman and her family have to plan daily activities around trips to the clinic or the health care provider's office. If the tumor recurs and cure is not likely, the client and her family need to think about hospice care and whether the woman can be cared for in the home.

HEALTH TEACHING

For the woman who has undergone a hysterectomy for endometrial cancer, the teaching plan is the same as that for the woman who has undergone a hysterectomy for uterine leiomyomas (see Postoperative Care, p. 1767). Side effects to report to the health care provider include vaginal or rectal bleeding, foul-smelling discharge, abdominal pain or distention, and hematuria.

The high dose of radiation causes sterility, and vaginal shrinkage can occur. Vaginal dilators can be used with water-soluble lubricants for 10 min/day until sexual activity resumes (in 10 days to 6 weeks). The woman is not radioactive, and her partner will not "catch" cancer from engaging in sexual intercourse. A normal diet may be resumed.

All prescribed medications are reviewed, including the dosage and schedule of administration, therapeutic effects, and side effects. The nurse also emphasizes the importance of keeping appointments for follow-up care.

Often women experience emotional crises because of the physical effects of cancer treatments. Radical hysterectomy may be seen as mutilating, and chemotherapy may affect the woman's body image if hair loss occurs. A woman may exhibit a grief reaction to this perceived change in body image. The feelings of loss depend on the visibility of the loss, the function of the loss, and the amount of emotional investment. The nurse may need to help the woman adapt to the body changes. One way to do this is to encourage self-care as soon as the woman's condition is stable. A calm, accepting attitude may also be helpful.

Death can occur with or without treatment. Women and their families or significant others have concerns about recurrence. All want to pass the 5-year survival mark without a recurrence. If there is a recurrence, the woman may be hostile and may exhibit characteristics of a grief reaction. The nurse encourages clients to ventilate their feelings. Response to loss and grieving are discussed in Chapter 9.

HEALTH CARE RESOURCES

In the United States, local American Cancer Society chapters provide written materials about endometrial cancer, as well as information about local support groups. If the client is in the terminal stages of cancer, hospice care may be appropriate (see Chapter 9). If nursing care is needed at home, the hospital nurse or case manager refers the client and her family to a community health or home care agency. A referral to a social services agency may be needed if the woman is unable to meet the financial demands of treatment and long-term follow-up.

Cervical Cancer

OVERVIEW

Cervical cancer is one of the most common reproductive cancers among women in the United States. Cervical cancer is also the third most common cause of death related to reproductive cancers (American Cancer Society, 2000). Death rates for cervical cancer have dropped 50% in the past two decades, primarily because of the availability of Pap tests for screening of premalignant cervical changes. However, among some ethnic/racial groups, Pap smears are not common as a screening test for cervical cancer. For example, in a study by Kim et al. (1999), only 34% of Korean-American women in the sample reported having a Pap smear (see the Evidence-Based Practice for Nursing box on p. 1773).

Pathophysiology

Cervical cancer may be described as preinvasive or invasive. Preinvasive cancer is limited to the cervix; invasive cancer is in the cervix and other pelvic structures. Preinvasive lesions usually originate in the area called the *transformation zone* (Figure 75-5). This area includes the squamocolumnar junction, which is located near the external cervical os, where changes in the squamous and columnar (glandular) epithelium normally occur. Abnormal squamous epithelium can also be found in this zone. These cells can develop into invasive carcinoma.

These premalignant changes can be described on a continuum from dysplasia—the earliest premalignant change—to carcinoma in situ (CIS), the most advanced premalignant change. Preinvasive cancers can also be designated by the term *cervical intraepithelial neoplasia (CIN)* and classified according to severity:

- CIN I: mild
- CIN II: moderate
- CIN III: severe to carcinoma in situ

Squamous cell cancers spread by direct extension to the vaginal mucosa, lower uterine segment, parametrium, pelvic wall, bladder, and bowel. Metastasis is usually confined to the pelvis, but distant metastases can occur through lymphatic spread and, rarely, via the circulatory system to the liver, lungs, or bones. Table 75-8 shows the clinical stages of cancer of the cervix.

Etiology

The exact cause of squamous cell cervical cancer is unknown, but numerous factors may be involved. An association has been identified with early and frequent sexual contact and with viral infections of the cervix, such as herpes simplex virus type 2, cytomegalovirus, and papillomavirus.

Risk factors associated with cervical cancer include low socioeconomic status, early age at first sexual contact or first pregnancy, multiple sexual partners, and intrauterine exposure to diethylstilbestrol (DES). Other possible risk factors include sexual intercourse with men whose previous sexual partners had cervical cancer, use of oral contraceptives, cigarette smoking, and vitamin A and C deficiencies. Nulliparity and diabetes mellitus are also associated with adenocarcinoma of the cervix.

EVIDENCE-BASED PRACTICE FOR NURSING

Do Korean-American women have Pap smears for screening of cervical cancer?

Kim, K., et al. (1999). Cervical cancer screening knowledge and practices among Korean-American women. *Cancer Nursing, 22*(4), 297-302.

The nursing researchers in this study surveyed 159 Korean-American women between 40 and 69 years of age to determine if they knew what a Pap smear was and if they had ever had one. The 1987 Cancer Control Supplement questionnaire was translated into Korean and used to collect the data. Twenty-six respondents had never heard of the Pap smear, and only 34% reported ever having one. The most commonly cited reason for not having a Pap test was the absence of disease symptoms.

Critique. The researchers undertook a study to examine possible differences among a group of non-Caucasian women. Although this was a descriptive study, it paves the way for further study of other non-Caucasian health practices.

Implications for Nursing. The findings of this study have implications for nurses who work with this population and other culturally diverse groups. Health education about Pap smears is crucial if cervical cancer is to be found in its earliest stage to ensure a positive outcome. Some subjects thought that the Pap smear was appropriate as a treatment rather than a health promotion/illness prevention intervention.

CULTURAL CONSIDERATIONS

The rate of cervical cancer is twice as high for African-American women as for Caucasian women. The mortality rate is more than twice as high for African-American women as for Caucasian women (American Cancer Society, 2000).

Incidence/Prevalence

The National Cancer Institute (NCI) estimates that there are more than 14,000 new cases of cervical cancer (excluding CIS) and more than 4400 deaths in the United States annually. Although the rate of invasive cervical cancer has decreased over the last several decades, it has increased in recent years in women younger than 50 years of age (American Cancer Society, 2000).

CIN occurs mainly in young women; the peak incidence of dysplasia occurs in clients in their mid-20s. CIS occurs in

TABLE 75-8 • CLINICAL STAGES OF CANCER OF THE CERVIX

Stage	Characteristics
I	Carcinoma is strictly confined to cervix (extension to corpus should be disregarded)
Ia	Preclinical carcinoma
Ia1	Minimal microscopically evident stromal invasion
Ia2	Microscopic lesions no more than 5-mm depth measured from base of epithelium surface or glandular surface from which it originates, and horizontal spread not to exceed 7 mm
Ib	All other cases of stage I; occult cancer should be marked "occ"
II	Carcinoma extends beyond cervix but has not extended to pelvic wall; it involves vagina, but not as far as lower third
IIa	No obvious parametrial involvement
IIb	Obvious parametrial involvement
III	Carcinoma has extended to pelvic wall; on rectal examination, there is no cancer-free space between tumor and pelvic wall; tumor involves lower third of vagina; all cases with hydronephrosis or nonfunctioning kidney should be included unless they are known to be due to another cause
IIIa	No extension to pelvic wall, but involvement of lower third of vagina
IIIb	Extension to pelvic wall, or hydronephrosis or nonfunctioning kidney due to tumor
IV	Carcinoma has extended beyond true pelvis or has clinically involved mucosa of bladder or rectum
IVa	Spread of growth to adjacent pelvic organs
IVb	Spread to distant organs

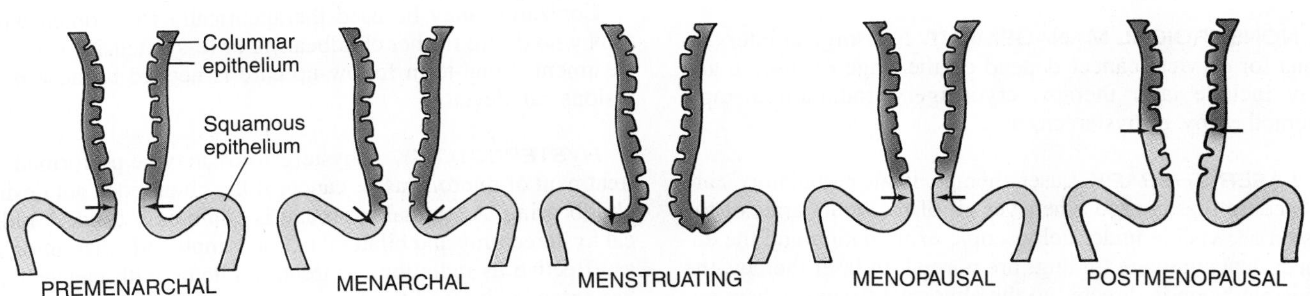

Figure 75-5 • The location of the transformation zone at various stages of adult development.

women about 30 years old, and invasive cancer occurs most commonly in the late 40s.

➤ COLLABORATIVE MANAGEMENT

Assessment

The woman who has preinvasive cancer is often asymptomatic. The classic symptom of invasive cancer is painless vaginal bleeding. The bleeding may start as spotting between menstrual periods or after coitus or douching. As the malignancy grows, the bleeding increases in frequency, duration, and amount. It may become continuous.

The woman may also complain of a watery, blood-tinged vaginal discharge that may become dark and foul smelling as the disease progresses. Leg pain (along the sciatic nerve) or unilateral swelling of a leg may be a late symptom or may indicate recurrent disease. Other signs of recurrence or metastasis (spread) may include unexplained weight loss, pelvic pain (caused by pressure of the tumor on the bladder or the bowel), dysuria (painful urination), hematuria (bloody urine), rectal bleeding, chest pain, and coughing. A physical examination may not reveal any abnormalities in early preinvasive cervical cancer; the internal pelvic examination may identify late-stage disease.

Laboratory assessment of the woman begins with a Pap smear. If the results are abnormal, the smear is repeated before further studies are done. If abnormal tissue is detected on a subsequent Pap test, further testing is done. If invasive cervical cancer is diagnosed, laboratory tests such as those described earlier for the investigation of endometrial cancer are performed (see Assessment, p. 1769).

The health care provider may perform a colposcopic examination to view the transformation zone, where dysplasia, cervical intraepithelial neoplasia (CIN), and carcinoma in situ (CIS) usually originate. If abnormal tissue is recognized, multiple biopsies of the cervical tissue are performed (see Chapter 73).

The health care provider usually performs an endocervical curettage (scraping of the endocervix from the internal to the external os) as well. Because this procedure is uncomfortable, the nurse may need to encourage the woman to use relaxation or breathing exercises to cope with the cramping and pain. A small amount of bleeding is expected and may occur for up to 2 weeks after the biopsies.

Interventions

Nursing care of the client with cervical cancer is similar to that for endometrial cancer. The only interventions discussed here are those that differ from those for the client with endometrial cancer.

NONSURGICAL MANAGEMENT. Nonsurgical interventions for cervical cancer depend on the stage of disease and may include laser therapy, cryosurgery, radiation therapy, chemotherapy, or hysterectomy.

LASER THERAPY. Laser therapy is an ambulatory care procedure that is used whenever all of the boundaries of the lesion are visible under colposcopic examination and the endocervical curettage findings are normal. In laser therapy, the invisible beam is directed to the abnormal tissues, where energy from the beam is absorbed by the fluid in the tissues, causing them to vaporize. There is usually a small amount of bleeding associated with the procedure. The woman may have a slight vaginal discharge, and healing occurs in 6 to 12 weeks.

CRYOSURGERY. Cryosurgery is another common treatment for CIN. A probe is placed against the cervix to cause freezing of the tissues and subsequent necrosis. Although this treatment can also be considered a type of surgery, no anesthesia is required. After the procedure, the client may experience slight cramping. The woman has a heavy watery discharge for several weeks after the procedure; she should avoid sexual intercourse and the use of tampons while discharge is present because the cervix is friable and these precautions will decrease the risk of infection.

RADIATION THERAPY. Most women with invasive cervical cancer are treated with radiation. For cancer that has extended beyond the cervix but not to the pelvic wall, radiation therapy is as effective as a radical hysterectomy. Intracavitary and external radiation therapies are used in combination, depending on the extent and location of the lesion. Intracavitary implants (brachytherapy) are usually used for lesions that have extended beyond the pelvic wall. External therapy is often given first to shrink the tumor and increase the effectiveness of the implant. Nursing care related to radiation therapy is presented in the earlier discussion of endometrial cancer (see p. 1771) and in Chapter 25.

CHEMOTHERAPY. Chemotherapeutic agents have generally performed poorly in the treatment of cervical cancer. These agents are usually reserved for unresectable recurrent tumors or disseminated metastatic disease (DeStefano & Bertin-Matson, 1996). Two drugs that have shown some response are cisplatin and 5-fluorouracil (5-FU).

SURGICAL MANAGEMENT. The surgical procedure for cervical cancer depends on the extent of the disease and whether the client wants to have children.

CONIZATION. Conization is the definitive treatment for clients with microinvasive cervical cancer. This procedure is done when the lesion cannot be visualized by colposcopic examination. A cone-shaped area of cervix is removed surgically and sent to the laboratory to determine the extent of the malignancy. Potential complications associated with conization include hemorrhage, uterine perforation, incompetent cervix, cervical stenosis (hardening), and preterm labor for future pregnancies.

Conization may be used therapeutically for women with CIN who desire further childbearing or less extensive surgical treatment. Long-term follow-up care is needed because new lesions can develop.

HYSTERECTOMY. A hysterectomy may be performed as treatment of microinvasive cancer if the client does not desire childbearing. A vaginal approach is commonly used. A radical hysterectomy and bilateral pelvic lymph node dissection is as effective as radiation for treating clients with cancer that has extended beyond the cervix but not to the pelvic wall. Information about hysterectomy is found under Operative Procedures (Uterine Leiomyomas), p. 1766.

PELVIC EXENTERATION. One of the most radical surgical procedures is **pelvic exenteration.** It is performed for recurrent cancers if there is no evidence of tumor outside the pelvis and no lymph node involvement.

Preoperative Care. Nursing care of the woman scheduled for exenteration includes assessment of preoperative anxiety, concerns about the impact on sexual function, and the ability to adjust to her altered body image. The nurse involves family members or significant others in discussions about postoperative expectations. Physical preparation includes selection of stoma sites, extensive bowel preparation, and extensive radiographic and laboratory tests to assess for spread of cancer outside the pelvis. The nurse teaches the client about the following:

- Postoperative recovery in a critical care unit
- Pain management
- Presence of numerous intravenous (IV) and arterial catheters
- Nasogastric suction
- Colostomy and/or urinary diversion (e.g., ileal conduit, Kock ileal urinary pouch)

Operative Procedures. There are three types of exenteration: anterior, posterior, and total (Figure 75-6). Anterior exenteration is the removal of the uterus, cervix, ovaries, fallopian tubes, vagina, bladder, urethra, and pelvic lymph nodes. Posterior exenteration is the removal of the uterus, cervix, ovaries, fallopian tubes, descending colon, rectum, and anal canal. Total exenteration is a combination of anterior and posterior procedures. When the bladder is removed, urine is diverted through a urinary diversion (e.g., ileal conduit or Kock ileal urinary pouch). When the colon, rectum, and anal canal are removed, a colostomy is created for passage of feces. The stomas are located on the abdomen—the colostomy on the left and the ileal conduit on the right.

Postoperative Care. After surgery, the client often is admitted to a critical care unit for the first 1 to 2 days because of the high risk for complications resulting from the massive tissue resection. The nurse assesses for the following:

- Cardiovascular complications such as hemorrhage and shock
- Pulmonary complications such as atelectasis and pneumonia
- Fluid and electrolyte imbalances such as metabolic acidosis or alkalosis and dehydration
- Renal or urinary complications
- Pain

The nurse or assistive nursing personnel also assists with deep breathing and coughing hourly, monitors urine output and specific gravity, monitors parenteral nutrition, and provides colostomy and urinary diversion care.

Once the client's condition is stable, she returns to the regular postoperative unit. The nurse continues postoperative interventions. During the recovery period, the nurse assesses for the following:

- Late cardiovascular complications such as deep vein thrombosis and pulmonary emboli
- Gastrointestinal (GI) complications such as paralytic ileus
- Wound infections
- Wound dehiscence or evisceration
- Pain

The nurse administers prophylactic heparin or low-molecular weight heparin (enoxaparin [Lovenox]) and maintains the use of antiembolism stockings or sequential compression devices (SCDs) for the prevention of thrombosis, as ordered. The nurse also auscultates the lungs frequently, assesses for the presence of bowel sounds and wound infection, administers antibiotics as prescribed, and manages pain with a gradual withdrawal of opioid analgesics.

After the surgeon removes the operative dressings, perineal irrigations may be implemented. Irrigation is usually done with normal saline solution applied with an Asepto syringe. This is followed by drying of the perineum with a heat lamp (25 W at a distance of 18 inches [45 cm]) or a hair dryer (using warm air). Care must be taken to avoid burning the

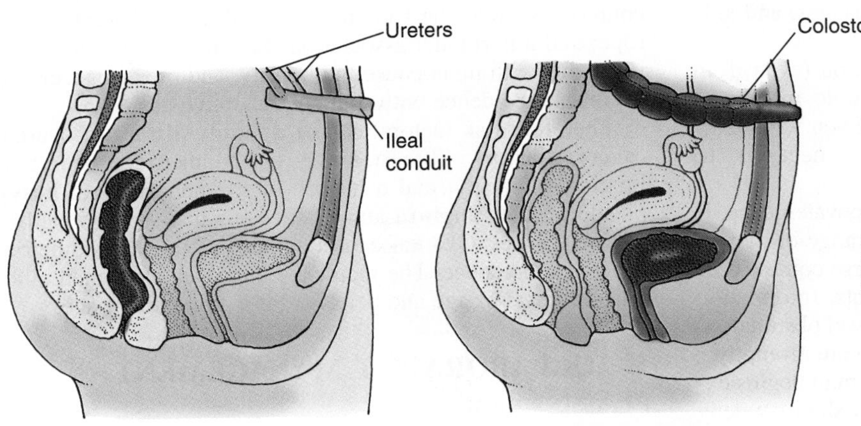

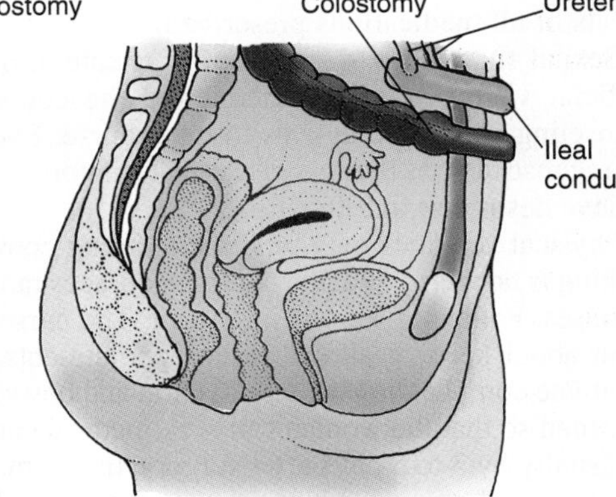

Anterior exenteration is removal of all pelvic organs except the descending colon, rectum, and anal canal. Urine can be diverted into an ileal conduit or urinary Kock pouch.

Posterior exenteration is removal of all pelvic organs except the bladder. A colostomy is created for the passage of feces.

Total exenteration is removal of all pelvic organs with creation of an ileal conduit or urinary Kock pouch and a colostomy.

Figure 75-6 ● Pelvic exenteration.

client. Sitz baths may be ordered as tolerated. (Postoperative care of clients with colostomies and urinary diversions is discussed elsewhere in this text).

Community-Based Care

If the client has undergone a hysterectomy, the discharge planning is similar to that described for endometrial cancer. For the client who has undergone a pelvic exenteration, the discharge planning is more involved.

HOME CARE MANAGEMENT

The client who has undergone a pelvic exenteration is usually in the hospital for at least 1 week postoperatively. She may be discharged to a skilled nursing facility or subacute unit for continued recovery and care or may be discharged directly to home. When the client returns home, she needs assistance. She is not able to engage in strenuous activities associated with most household work for up to 6 months. The family may need to consider outside help if there is no one in the family who can assume household responsibilities.

No special equipment is needed in the home, although a convoluted foam mattress or other special pressure-relieving device may be placed on the bed to prevent skin breakdown and to increase comfort. Colostomy and ureterostomy pouches and equipment for changing the pouches can be purchased in local pharmacies.

HEALTH TEACHING

The nurse teaches the woman who has undergone a pelvic exenteration how to manage new functions with equipment (colostomy and urinary diversion) and to perform activities of daily living (ADLs) and self-care. The perineal opening may drain mucus for several months to a year. The client can wear sanitary napkins (minipads or maxipads) if they are beltless (so as not to interfere with the stomas). The woman may need help in adjusting her diet to maintain high nutritional requirements for healing while selecting foods that are tolerated. The woman should be able to state the effects, dosages, and side effects of all medications prescribed.

Sexual function is different after exenteration (even if an artificial vagina is constructed), and the couple may need counseling about alternatives to intercourse. Even with vaginal reconstruction, the use of vaginal dilators is necessary to achieve desired sexual function.

Physical activities may be limited during convalescence. If walking is not permitted, the nurse encourages range-of-motion exercises. Follow-up care is important. The nurse counsels the client about keeping all follow-up appointments. Information about late complications (e.g., infection and bowel obstruction) is needed so that the woman can seek medical care promptly.

Usually by 3 to 5 days after surgery, the woman begins expressing grief about her body changes. At first she may deny changes by refusing to look at the wound or stoma sites. Later she may become depressed or withdrawn or even angry or hostile. She may then move to reality testing by asking questions about her care, watching the nurses do wound care, and becoming actively involved in self-care.

The woman may have mood swings, and the nurse is alert when the woman becomes depressed so that interventions can be implemented. The woman needs intense emotional support if she is to adapt to her altered body image and functions.

Unless the woman has vaginal reconstruction after anterior or total pelvic exenteration, she is not able to have vaginal intercourse. The nurse must assess the need for sexual counseling by listening for cues about altered perceptions of body image and anxiety about her sexual partner's response. Further sexual counseling may be needed to provide information on alternative methods of sexual gratification.

HEALTH CARE RESOURCES

Resources for the woman who has cervical cancer are similar to those for the woman with endometrial cancer.

Ovarian Cancer

OVERVIEW

Ovarian cancer is the leading cause of death from female reproductive malignancies. Death rates have risen during the past four decades, and it is projected that 1 of every 70 women will develop ovarian cancer sometime in her life (American Cancer Society, 2000). Survival rates continue to be low because ovarian cancer is poorly detected in its early stages.

Of all ovarian cancers, 85% are epithelial tumors; the most common type is serous adenocarcinoma. These tumors grow rapidly, spread quickly, and are often bilateral. Of all epithelial tumors, ovarian tumors are associated with the worst prognosis.

The cancer spreads by several mechanisms:

- Direct spread to other organs in the pelvis that are in close proximity to the ovary (e.g., uterus, bladder, and colon)
- Distal spread through lymphatic drainage (via para-aortic and iliac lymph nodes to the rest of the pelvis, abdomen or liver, lung, or bones)
- Peritoneal seeding (malignant spread of free-floating cells, usually after the development of ascites)

The cause of ovarian cancer is not precisely known. Suggested etiologic theories include a familial association; an environmental association related to products of industry in countries such as the United States and those of western Europe; and a hormonal association, as evidenced by increased incidence with menopause, nulliparity, and breast cancer and decreased incidence with oral contraceptive use.

Therefore risk factors include a family history of ovarian cancer; a history of breast, bowel, or endometrial cancer; nulliparity; infertility; and a history of dysmenorrhea or heavy bleeding. Diets high in animal fat have also been linked to ovarian cancer. Ovarian cancer ranks second to endometrial cancer in incidence. The incidence increases in women older than 40 years of age and peaks at 50 to 55 years of age.

COLLABORATIVE MANAGEMENT

Assessment

Women with ovarian cancer may complain of abdominal pain or swelling or have vague symptoms of abdominal discomfort, such as dyspepsia, indigestion, gas and distention, and other mild gastrointestinal (GI) disturbances. The woman may have a history of ovarian imbalance, such as evidenced by premenstrual tension, heavy menstrual flow, or dysfunctional bleeding.

The only sign may be an abdominal mass, which may be noticed only after it reaches a size of 6 inches (15 cm). Most pelvic examinations do not identify abnormalities. However, an enlarged ovary found postmenopausally should be evaluated as though it were malignant.

The woman with ovarian cancer has concerns similar to those described for the woman with endometrial cancer. Because the malignancy is usually diagnosed in an advanced stage, fears of death and dying are common and may be more of a concern than the proposed treatments.

Cytologic examination has limited application because a Pap smear is abnormal in only 20% to 30% of women with ovarian cancer, even in advanced cases. Diagnosis depends on surgical exploration. Usually a complete laboratory workup is done before exploratory surgery, including a complete blood count, urinalysis, and liver studies if ascites occurs.

The level of ovarian antibody designated as CA-125 may be elevated if ovarian cancer is present. This test may be useful to monitor a woman's progress after treatment but may not be as useful for diagnostic purposes.

Ultrasonography, intravenous pyelography (IVP), computed tomography (CT), and radiography are used in detecting ovarian tumors. In addition, a barium enema study and an upper GI radiographic series can be performed to rule out tumor in the adjacent structures.

Exploratory laparotomy is performed to diagnose and stage ovarian tumors. Ovarian cancer is the only neoplasm that is staged when it is removed (Table 75-9).

TABLE 75-9 • STAGING CLASSIFICATION OF OVARIAN CANCER

Stage	Characteristics
I	Growth limited to ovaries
Ia	Growth limited to one ovary; no ascites; no tumor on external surface; capsule intact
Ib	Growth limited to both ovaries; no ascites; no tumor on external surfaces; capsules intact
Ic	Tumor either stage Ia or Ib, but with tumor on surface of one or both ovaries, or with capsule ruptured, or with ascites present containing malignant cells, or with positive peritoneal washings
II	Growth involving one or both ovaries with pelvic extension
IIa	Extension and/or metastases to uterus and/or tubes
IIb	Extension to other pelvic tissues
IIc	Tumor either stage IIa or IIb, but with tumor on surface of one or both ovaries, or with capsule(s) ruptured, or with ascites present containing malignant cells or with positive peritoneal washings
III	Tumor involving one or both ovaries with peritoneal implants outside pelvis and/or positive retroperitoneal or inguinal nodes; superficial liver metastasis but with histologically proven malignant extension to small bowel or omentum
IIIa	Tumor grossly limited to true pelvis with negative nodes but with histologically confirmed microscopic seeding of abdominal peritoneal surfaces
IIIb	Tumor of one or both ovaries with histologically confirmed implants of abdominal peritoneal surfaces, none exceeding 2 cm in diameter; nodes are negative
IIIc	Abdominal implants greater than 2 cm in diameter and/or positive retroperitoneal inguinal nodes
IV	Growth involving one or both ovaries with distant metastases; if pleural effusion is present, there must be positive cytologic findings to allot a case to stage IV; Parenchymal liver metastasis equals stage IV

Interventions

Nursing care of the woman with ovarian cancer is similar to that of the woman with endometrial or cervical cancer. The options for treatment depend on the extent of the cancer and include chemotherapy (systemic or intraperitoneal), immunotherapy, radiation therapy (external or intraperitoneal), and surgery.

NONSURGICAL MANAGEMENT. Chemotherapy and radiation therapy are the two most common nonsurgical options for ovarian cancer.

CHEMOTHERAPY. The health care provider usually prescribes chemotherapeutic agents postoperatively for all stages of ovarian cancer, although their purpose is usually palliative for stage IV tumors. Cisplatin, carboplatin, paclitaxel (Taxol), isofamide, doxorubicin (Adriamycin), hexamethylmelamine, methotrexate, and 5-fluorouracil (5-FU) have been used as single agents for treating ovarian cancer (DeStefano & Bertin-Matson, 1996). Combinations of agents seem to obtain higher response rates, especially if cisplatin is one of the drugs used.

Chemotherapy is usually administered every 3 to 4 weeks for 1 week and can be administered on an inpatient or an ambulatory basis. Intraperitoneal chemotherapy is the instillation of chemotherapeutic agents into the abdominal cavity. With the use of this method, it is believed that the cytotoxic effects of the drugs on the tumor are increased. Immunotherapy is also used to treat ovarian cancer. It alters the immunologic response of the ovary and promotes tumor resistance.

RADIATION THERAPY. External radiation therapy is used postoperatively if tumors have invaded other organs. It may be given with chemotherapy or alone (see Chapter 25). Radioactive colloids have also been injected into the abdomen to increase survival rates. A primary beta-emitter, ^{32}P, is injected through a catheter placed during surgery. After instillation, the woman is asked to turn frequently for 1½ to 2 hours to facilitate the distribution of the radioactive colloids throughout the peritoneal cavity (e.g., turning to the right, to the left, head down, feet down, prone, and supine).

SURGICAL MANAGEMENT. Total abdominal hysterectomy and bilateral salpingo-oophorectomy is the surgical procedure for all stages of ovarian cancer. In clients with stage III or IV cancer, the goal is to remove as much of the cancer as possible because it has spread to adjacent organs. Nursing care of the woman is similar to that of the woman undergoing a hysterectomy for uterine leiomyomas.

A second-look procedure (laparoscopy or laparotomy) is performed, usually after 1 year of chemotherapy, to confirm the absence or presence of tumor and to remove any new or residual tumor if it was too large to be removed at the first operation. Nursing care is similar to that of the client after any major abdominal surgery.

The woman who is faced with the diagnosis of advanced ovarian cancer may be concerned about dying. She needs to be encouraged to ventilate her feelings about her diagnosis. Realistic assurance, as well as accurate information about treatments, can be provided. Often providing the woman with information about ovarian cancer and its treatment decreases her fears. Providing continuity of care, with at least one regular caregiver, may be helpful. The nurse encourages the client to use her support system, including family members, friends, and a spiritual leader, such as a rabbi or other clergy member. A visit from another woman who has survived a similar disease may decrease fears.

If there is recurrence, the woman may deny symptoms at first or express feelings of anger and grief. The family is often fearful of the outcome. The nurse needs to provide encouragement and support during this difficult time and help the woman and her family or significant others work through their grief and prepare for death.

Vulvar Cancer

OVERVIEW

Vulvar cancer represents only 4% of all gynecologic malignancies, even though it ranks fourth in occurrence. Vulvar cancer is slow growing, stays localized for a long time, and metastasizes late. Vulvar cancer occurs most commonly in women 50 to 70 years of age. More than 50% of the cases of vulvar cancer occur in women older than 60 years of age. Of all vulvar cancers, 90% are squamous cell carcinomas. The other 10% consist of adenocarcinomas, sarcomas, and Paget's disease. Most vulvar cancers develop in the absence of premalignant changes in the epithelium, but occasionally they develop and spread similarly to cancer of the cervix.

The first change is usually vulvar atypia or mild dysplasia (vulvar intraepithelial neoplasia [VIN] I), followed by moderate dysplasia (VIN II) and then severe dysplasia or carcinoma in situ (VIN III) until the lesion becomes invasive. Vulvar cancer can spread directly to the urethra, the vagina, or the anus and through the lymphatic system to the inguinal, femoral, and deep iliac pelvic nodes.

The cause of vulvar cancer is unknown. There is no proven relationship with sexually transmitted diseases (STDs), although a history of condylomata acuminata (venereal warts) may be present. A strong relationship exists between vulvar cancer and herpes simplex type II, human papillomavirus, and capsid antigen. Obesity, hypertension, diabetes, smoking, and granulomatous disease of the vulva have been suggested as possible causes, but no scientific data support these suggestions.

Vulvar cancer seldom occurs before age 40 years, although studies have found premalignant changes in women in their 20s and 30s. This increase may be linked to the increase in sexually transmitted infections.

The prognosis for vulvar cancer is related to the stage of the cancer and whether cancer is present in the lymph nodes. Guidelines for the early detection and prevention of vulvar cancer include performing monthly vulvar self-examination, having an annual pelvic examination, and practicing "safe sex."

➤ COLLABORATIVE MANAGEMENT

Assessment

Women with vulvar lesions are likely to report irritation or itching in their perineal area. Sometimes they describe a "sore that will not heal." Bleeding is a late symptom. Women usually try to treat themselves before seeking medical help. Often a lesion has been present for months. Embarrassment has been suggested as the reason why older women delay seeking medical attention.

Pelvic examinations usually reveal multifocal lesions, the majority of which develop on the labia. The lesions may be whitish or reddish, and the vulvar skin may be excoriated as a result of irritation.

The woman may be anxious or fearful about the diagnosis of cancer. She may have fears that her partner will reject her because of the diagnosis, or she may worry about disfigurement related to surgery. The nurse needs to assess the woman's past experiences in coping with stressful situations and whether she has the psychologic resources to cope with the present crisis.

A Pap smear and colposcopic examination of the vulva (see Assessment [Cervical Cancer], p. 1774) may aid in diagnosis. A toluidine blue test may be used to identify abnormal cells for biopsy. A 1% aqueous solution of toluidine blue is applied to the vulva and allowed to dry. Then a 1% acetic acid solution is applied. Biopsy of the areas that remain blue is performed. The test chemical stains nuclei in the superficial epithelium, where cells do not normally contain nuclei. An abnormal finding does not necessarily indicate malignancy, because ulcerations also stain.

A biopsy of the lesion is necessary for diagnosis. This is easily accomplished with a Keyes dermal punch (a device that removes a disk of tissue). Depending on the site of the lesion, one or more biopsy specimens may be taken.

Interventions

Nursing care of the client with vulvar cancer is similar to that for endometrial cancer; only the interventions that differ are discussed.

NONSURGICAL MANAGEMENT. Nonsurgical management of vulvar cancer depends on the extent of the spread and may include laser therapy, chemotherapy, and radiation therapy.

LASER THERAPY. If a woman has premalignant vulvar lesions, laser therapy may be used (see p. 1774). The treatment is usually done on an outpatient basis; local, regional, or general anesthesia is used. Healing occurs over a period of several weeks, and usually the lesions are removed without scarring.

CHEMOTHERAPY. Chemotherapy in the form of a topical application of 5-FU has been used to treat carcinoma in situ successfully. However, the treatment causes severe vulvar edema and pain and is not often used.

RADIATION THERAPY. External radiation therapy to the deep pelvic nodes may be used postoperatively (see earlier discussion of endometrial cancer [p. 1771] and Chapter 25). Radiation treatments cause ulceration and dermatitis, which can be uncomfortable for the woman.

SURGICAL MANAGEMENT. The surgeon performs a vulvectomy to remove the cancerous vulvar lesions.

PREOPERATIVE CARE. The woman needs a complete explanation of the extent of the surgical procedure to be performed and information about preoperative and postoperative procedures (see Chapters 17 and 19). Specific preoperative care for a vulvectomy may include an abdominal or perineal shave, an enema, douching, and insertion of an indwelling catheter into the bladder.

OPERATIVE PROCEDURES. Several surgical procedures are effective for the treatment of vulvar cancer. A local wide excision may be used to remove the abnormal area (for carcinoma in situ [CIS]). A simple vulvectomy (removal of the vulva, the labia majora, the labia minora, and possibly the clitoris) may also be performed for CIS, but this disfiguring surgery is used less often today. Instead, a **skinning vulvectomy**—the removal of superficial vulvar skin (without removal of the clitoris) and replacement of removed skin with split-thickness grafts—is performed (Figure 75-7). Sexual function is less affected, and the appearance of the vulva is less changed.

For invasive cancer, the surgery most often recommended is the modified radical or **radical vulvectomy** (removal of the entire vulva—skin, labia, clitoris, subcutaneous tissues, and possibly inguinal and femoral node dissection), depending on node involvement (see Figure 75-7).

POSTOPERATIVE CARE. Postoperatively, the woman can expect to have multiple suction drains (Hemovac or Jackson-Pratt drains) in the inguinal or vulvar areas for wound drainage for 7 to 10 days. A pressure-reducing mattress may be placed on the bed to prevent pressure ulcers and increase comfort. A bed cradle may be used to keep linens off the incision site. The client usually wears antiembolism stockings or sequential compression devices to prevent thromboembolism and leg edema.

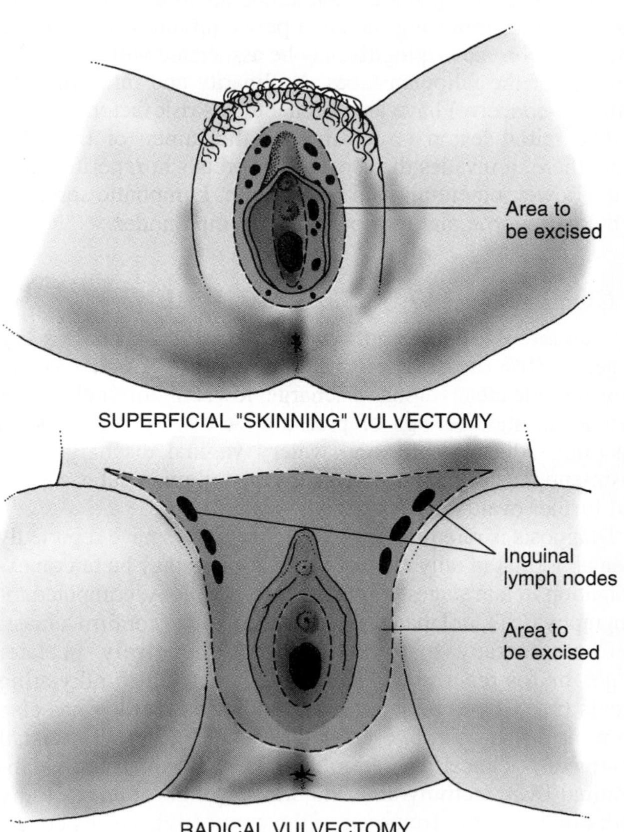

Figure 75-7 ● Vulvectomy.

Providing Wound Care. The major focus of nursing care is wound healing. The nurse changes the dressings over the incision frequently because of the amount of wound drainage and the risk of infection. Wound complications, such as infection and dehiscence, often occur after vulvectomies; subsequently, the healing process may take up to 6 months. Meticulous wound care is necessary and usually involves debridement. The nurse typically uses normal saline solution, which may be applied with an Asepto bulb syringe or a water pick (on low speed). The wound is then dried with a heat lamp or air dried with a hair dryer (using warm air). Wound care is usually done three or four times a day.

Diet in the postoperative period should include foods rich in vitamin C, iron, and protein to promote wound healing.

Promoting Urinary and Bowel Elimination. The Foley catheter remains in the bladder for 7 to 10 days to prevent ureteral stenosis and incontinence. After the catheter is removed, the urine stream may be deflected down the leg as a result of edema or even may be uncontrolled. Having the woman stand while voiding may decrease the incidence of these annoying problems. Antiperistaltic medications are usually given for 7 to 10 days to prevent defecation and decrease the risk of wound infection. Then stool softeners may be given to prevent straining and decrease discomfort related to bowel movements. Perineal care or sitz baths after voidings or bowel movements may prevent contamination of the incision site.

Managing Pain. Postoperative discomfort is usually controlled with analgesics during the first couple of days after surgery. Medicating for pain before wound care may help the woman relax and tolerate the procedure with less distress.

Addressing Sexuality. The woman needs complete explanations of the changes that occur as a result of surgery. If a radical vulvectomy is done, the clitoris is removed and loss of orgasm usually occurs. Dyspareunia may result from any of the surgical procedures. Vaginal dilators may be useful to stretch the remaining vaginal tissues. Discomfort can also be reduced during sexual intercourse by having the couple use water-soluble lubricants or a side-lying position. The couple may need counseling about alternatives to vaginal intercourse. The woman may need to be encouraged to express feelings of grief related to her loss of normal sexual function.

A vulvectomy can be devastating to a woman's self-concept. She often has a grief reaction related to the loss of the vulva and subsequent disfigurement. She may fear rejection from her sexual partner or significant others and may be reluctant to make herself vulnerable by getting involved in any relationship. Fears of recurrence or metastasis may be present. The nurse's role is one of support. The woman needs encouragement to vent her feelings and concerns about her perceived or actual losses and body changes. Family members or significant others should be encouraged to share their feelings and concerns with the woman. A visit by a woman who has successfully recovered from similar surgery could be beneficial.

Vaginal Cancer

OVERVIEW

Primary invasive vaginal cancer is rare, accounting for less than 2% of all gynecologic cancers. Usually vaginal cancer is an extension of cervical, endometrial, or vulvar cancers. Most vaginal cancers are squamous cell carcinomas that develop in the upper one third of the vagina. They occur most often in women older than 50 years of age; 90% of cases are found postmenopausally. Adenocarcinoma of the vagina is found in females between the ages of 14 and 30 years and is associated with intrauterine exposure to diethylstilbestrol (DES) as a result of maternal ingestion during pregnancy.

The cause of vaginal cancer is unknown. Predisposing factors include repeated pregnancies; vaginal trauma; sexually transmitted diseases (STDs), especially syphilis and herpes simplex virus type 2 and papillomavirus infections; and prior radiation.

The spread of vaginal cancer depends on the location of the tumor. Upper vaginal lesions spread in the same manner as cervical cancer, whereas lower lesions spread similarly to vulvar cancer. Because of the rich lymphatic drainage in the vaginal area, metastasis can occur early.

COLLABORATIVE MANAGEMENT

Assessment

Premalignant lesions (vaginal intraepithelial neoplasia) are usually asymptomatic. An abnormal Pap smear is the most common presenting problem. Uncommon or late symptoms include pain, foul-smelling vaginal discharge, painless vaginal bleeding, pruritus, and urinary symptoms attributable to the pressure of the lesion on the bladder.

A pelvic examination may reveal a lesion. Premalignant changes are diagnosed through colposcopic examination and biopsy.

Interventions

Both nonsurgical and surgical interventions may be used to treat women with vaginal cancer.

NONSURGICAL MANAGEMENT. Noninvasive malignancy and early-stage vaginal cancers may be treated nonsurgically with a variety of techniques. Laser therapy (see p. 1774) may be used. The health care provider stains the abnormal tissues with an iodine solution to identify the area for treatment. A vaginal discharge may be present for several days after treatment, and healing normally takes a few weeks. Close follow-up is necessary and includes a Pap smear and colposcopic examination every 4 months for 1 year and then every 6 to 12 months.

Local application of 5-fluorouracil (5-FU) cream to the vagina daily for 1 week is another treatment option. This chemotherapeutic agent is irritating to the skin, and often zinc oxide ointment is recommended for application to the vulvar area. The treatment is repeated in 3 to 4 weeks, and follow-up is the same as that for laser therapy.

Radiation therapy can be used for all stages of vaginal cancer. Intracavitary radiation therapy (IRT, brachytherapy) is usually used alone for the treatment of cancer limited to the vaginal wall, and external radiation therapy is combined with IRT for the treatment of cancer that extends beyond the vaginal wall. Complications of radiation therapy include vaginal stenosis, adhesions, and discharge. Women need to use vaginal dilators after treatment, and assessment for sexual dysfunction is suggested.

Chemotherapy may be used for recurrent disease, although there is no effective therapy.

SURGICAL MANAGEMENT. A local wide excision may be performed for localized lesions. A partial or total **vaginectomy** (removal of part or all of the vagina) may be done for invasive disease. Vaginectomy affects sexual function. Without surgical reconstruction, vaginal intercourse is impossible. The woman and her sexual partner need counseling about alternative activities for achieving sexual satisfaction. A radical hysterectomy or pelvic exenteration may also be performed, depending on the extent of the cancer.

Preventive and early detection measures for vaginal cancer are to avoid taking DES during pregnancy (to prevent one's daughter from developing cancer) and to continue to have Pap screening and pelvic examinations after menopause on a regular basis.

Fallopian Tube Cancer

OVERVIEW

Fallopian tube cancer is the rarest of gynecologic cancers; it is associated with an incidence of less than 1%. It occurs in women older than 50 years of age; 80% to 90% of cases result from metastasis from ovarian and endometrial cancers.

The cause of squamous cell fallopian tube cancer is unknown. It has been suggested that pelvic inflammatory disease (PID) and chronic salpingitis may be associated with adenocarcinomas of the fallopian tubes. Nulliparity and infertility (inability to conceive) have also been cited as risk factors.

The initial lesion is confined to the lumen of the tube. From there, it invades the serosa and spreads intraperitoneally to the bowel, omentum, and peritoneum. Lymphatic spread is to the para-aortic and retroperitoneal lymph nodes.

COLLABORATIVE MANAGEMENT

Women are usually asymptomatic until the tumor is in a late stage. In 50% of the cases, bleeding is present. Other symptoms include clear vaginal discharge, lower abdominal pain or distention, and feelings of pressure. A history of abnormal bleeding, adnexal pain, and watery vaginal discharge in a postmenopausal woman may suggest fallopian tube cancer, and further evaluation is needed.

Diagnosis is rare preoperatively. Pap smears have reportedly been abnormal in only 10% of cases. A mass may be felt on examination in late stages. Vaginal ultrasonography, computed tomography (CT), or laparoscopy may be used to confirm a mass.

Chemotherapy may be used postoperatively in later stages or for recurrence. The lesions respond to alkylating agents (see Chapter 25). External radiation therapy has also been used postoperatively for late-stage tumors. The usual treatment of cancer limited to the fallopian tube is a total abdominal hysterectomy and bilateral salpingo-oophorectomy with omentectomy (removal of the connective tissues covering these organs). Care of the woman with fallopian tube cancer is similar to that described earlier for cancer of the ovary (see Interventions [Ovarian Cancer], p. 1777).

ONLINE RESOURCES

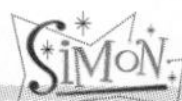

For suggested readings and Internet resources, go to http://www.wbsaunders.com/SIMON/Iggy/.

SELECTED BIBLIOGRAPHY

Asterisk indicates a classic or definitive work on this subject.

American Cancer Society. (2000). *Cancer facts and figures—2000.* Report No. 00-300M-No. 5008.00. Atlanta: Author.

*Baird, G. (1996). Advances in gynaecology. *The Practitioner, 240,* 90-95.

*Barrett, R.J., et al. (1995). Endometrial cancer: Stage at diagnosis and associated factors in black and white patients. *American Journal of Obstetrics and Gynecology, 173*(2), 414-422.

Barrow, C. (1999). Balloon endometrial ablation as a safe alternative to hysterectomy. *AORN Journal, 70*(1), 80, 83-86, 89-90.

*Chuong, C.J., Pearsall-Otey, L.R., & Rosenfeld, B.L. (1995). A practical guide to relieving PMS. *Contemporary Nurse Practitioner, 1*(3), 31-37.

*DeStefano, M.S., & Bertin-Matson, K. (1996). Gynecologic cancers. In R. McCorkle et al. (Eds.), *Cancer nursing: A comprehensive textbook* (2nd ed., pp. 698-727). Philadelphia: W.B. Saunders.

*Jarrett, M., et al. (1996). Relationship between gastrointestinal and dysmenorrheic symptoms at menses. *Research in Nursing and Health, 19*(1), 45-51.

Jennings-Dozier, K. (1999). Predicting intentions to obtain a Pap smear among African American and Latina women: Testing the theory of planned behavior. *Nursing Research, 48*(4), 198-205.

Johnson, S. (1998). Menopause and hormone replacement therapy. *Medical Clinics of North America, 82*(2), 297-320.

Kim, K., et al. (1999). Cervical cancer screening knowledge and practices among Korean-American women. *Cancer Nursing, 22*(4), 297-302.

Lessick, M., Wickham, R., & Rehwaldt, M. (1997). Breast and ovarian cancer: Genetic update and implications for nursing. *MEDSURG Nursing, 6*(6), 341-349.

*Lowdermilk, D.L. (1995). Reproductive surgery. In C.I. Fogel & N.F. Woods (Eds.), *Women's health care* (pp. 629-650). Springhouse, PA: Springhouse.

Mazmanian, C.M. (1999). Hysterectomy: Holistic care is key. *RN, 62*(6), 32-35.

McCance, K.L., & Huether, S.E. (1998). *Pathophysiology: The biological basis for disease in adults and children* (3rd ed.). St. Louis: Mosby.

Pearl, M.L., et al. (1999). Transcutaneous electrical nerve stimulation as an adjunct for controlling chemotherapy-induced nausea and vomiting in gynecologic oncology. *Cancer Nursing, 22*(4), 307-311.

*Rose, P.G. (1996). Endometrial carcinoma. *New England Journal of Medicine, 335*(9), 640-649.

Scura, K.W., & Whipple, B. (1997). How to provide better care for the postmenopausal woman. *American Journal of Nursing, 97*(4), 36-44.

Shurpin, K. (1997). Clinical snapshot: Ovarian cancer. *American Journal of Nursing, 97*(4), 34-35.

Taylor, L.K., et al. (1998). The effect of music in the postanesthesia care unit on pain levels in women who have had abdominal hysterectomies. *Journal of Perianesthesia Nursing, 13*(2), 88-94.

Wade, J., et al. (2000). Hysterectomy: What do women need and want to know? *Journal of Obstetric, Gynecologic, and Neonatal Nursing, 29*(1), 33-42.

CHAPTER 76

Interventions for Male Clients with Reproductive Problems

LORI KLINGMAN

Learning Objectives

After studying this chapter, you should be able to:

1. Describe common physical assessment findings for the client with benign prostatic hyperplasia (BPH).
2. Discuss options for nonsurgical and surgical management of the client with BPH.
3. Develop a postoperative plan of care for a client undergoing a transurethral resection of the prostate (TURP).
4. Identify the procedures for prostate cancer screening.
5. Explain the role of hormonal therapy in treating prostate cancer.
6. Describe the options for treating erectile dysfunction.
7. Discuss the cultural considerations related to male reproductive problems.
8. Analyze assessment data to determine priority nursing diagnoses and collaborative problems for a man with testicular cancer.
9. Develop a plan of care for a client with testicular cancer.
10. Formulate a community-based teaching plan for continuing care of clients with testicular cancer.
11. Compare and contrast hydrocele, spermatocele, and varicocele.
12. Discuss issues related to sexuality and body image for a man experiencing male reproductive health problems.

SIMON

Go to http://www.wbsaunders.com/SIMON/Iggy/ for self-assessment questions related to these Learning Objectives.

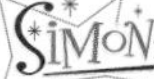

Nurses need to know about the anatomy and physiology of male reproductive functions so that they can instruct clients about the impact of a disease process or treatment on their reproductive ability. The nurse includes the client and his spouse, sexual partner, or significant other in the decision-making process and works with members of the interdisciplinary team in providing collaborative care.

BENIGN PROSTATIC HYPERPLASIA

OVERVIEW

The prostate gland is the major accessory sex gland of the male. It is often a site of infection and benign and malignant neoplasms, all of which can affect urinary elimination.

Pathophysiology

In a young adult male, the prostatic capsule is thin and is attached to the underlying tissue. As the man ages, the glandular units in the prostate begin to undergo tissue **hyperplasia** (an abnormal increase in the number of cells), resulting in prostatic **hypertrophy** (enlargement). Although benign prostatic hypertrophy is the more common term used to describe this phenomenon, **benign prostatic hyperplasia (BPH)** is the correct term for the pathologic process.

When the prostate gland enlarges, it extends upward, into the bladder, and inward, narrowing the prostatic urethral channel, and obstructs the outflow of urine by encroaching on the bladder opening (Figure 76-1). In response to this outlet resistance, the bladder is affected in several ways (Figure 76-2). First, it may become hyperirritable, which produces urgency and frequency. As the bladder tries to compensate for its increased workload, muscles in the bladder wall hypertrophy and may develop cellules and diverticula. If allowed to continue, this obstruction of urine flow can cause a gradual dilation of the ureters **(hydroureter)** and kidneys **(hydronephrosis).** The enlarged prostate may also obstruct the bladder neck or the prostatic urethra, leading to urinary retention or incomplete bladder emptying. Overflow urinary incontinence is common; the urine "leaks" around the enlarged prostate, causing dribbling. Urinary stasis can result in urinary tract infections.

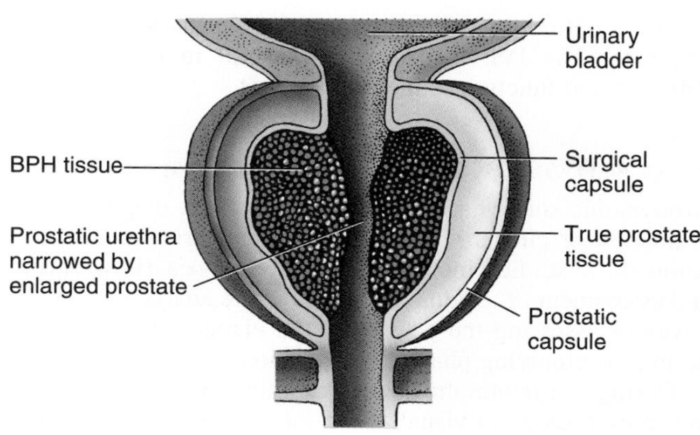

Figure 76-1 ● Benign prostatic hyperplasia (BPH) grows inward, causing narrowing of the urethra.

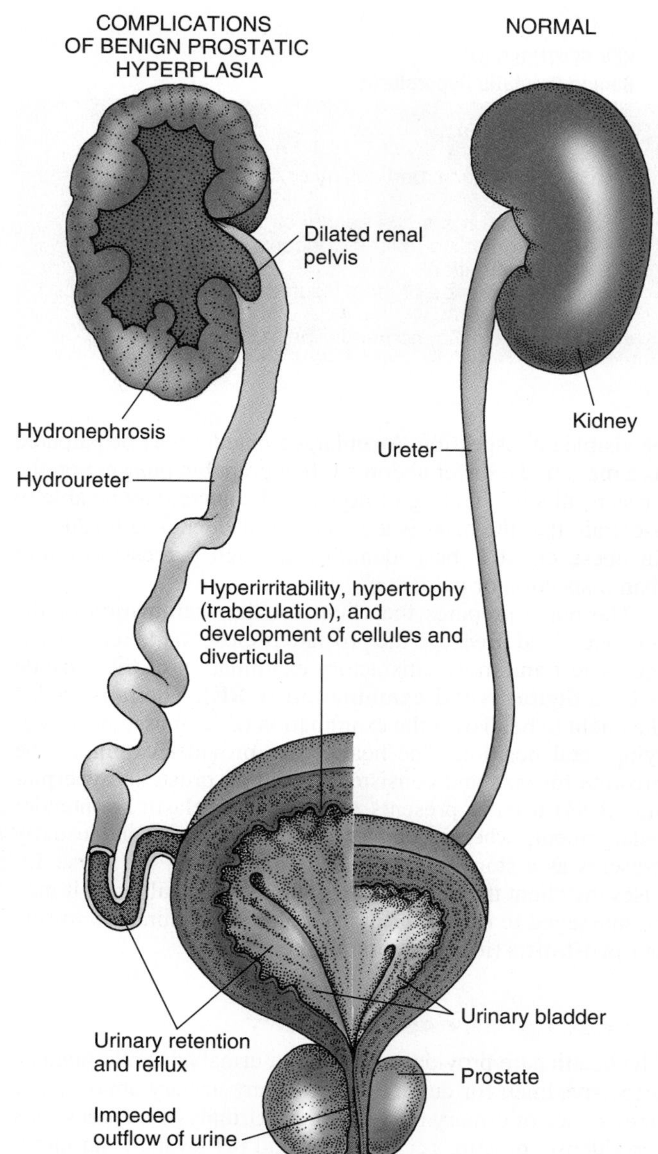

Figure 76-2 ● Potential complications of benign prostatic hyperplasia. The right side of the illustration shows a normal male urologic system. The left side shows potential complications.

Etiology

The exact cause of BPH remains unknown. Because the development of BPH is almost universal in older men, several theories have been examined:

- The effect of chronic inflammation of the prostate gland
- The role of general metabolic and nutritional factors (diet)
- The possible contribution of atherosclerosis

Demographic data (such as race) and social factors (such as socioeconomic status and heredity) have been examined as predictors for the development of BPH. Although these theories continue to be investigated, it is thought that BPH results from a systemic hormonal alteration. Support for this theory is based on the observations that aging is the major contributing factor and that another factor is the presence of testicular androgen. BPH does not occur in men who have been castrated before puberty (testicular androgen is absent). Men with BPH experience a regression of BPH after a bilateral orchiectomy (testicular androgen is removed).

Incidence/Prevalence

CONSIDERATIONS FOR OLDER ADULTS

The incidence of BPH consistently increases with age. Characteristically, BPH is a disease of men older than 40 years of age, with an increase in incidence occurring with each decade of life. By age 50, at least 50% of all men have some degree of BPH, although not all are symptomatic (Matteson, McConnell, & Linton, 1997).

COLLABORATIVE MANAGEMENT

Assessment

HISTORY

The nurse pays particular attention to the client's report of his urinary pattern. Commonly, the client complains of frequency, **nocturia** (voiding at night), and other symptoms of bladder neck obstruction known as **lower urinary tract symptoms (LUTS)** (Holtgrave, 1998). The symptoms of LUTS include hesitancy, intermittency, diminished force and caliber of the urinary stream, a sensation of incomplete bladder emptying, and postvoid dribbling. If frequency and nocturia are not accompanied by symptoms of restricted flow, the possibility of a nonobstructive etiology, such as infection, is considered.

The nurse questions whether the client has experienced any **hematuria** (blood in the urine) when initiating or at the end of urination. BPH is a common cause of hematuria in men older than 60 years of age.

PHYSICAL ASSESSMENT/CLINICAL MANIFESTATIONS

The client is instructed to void before the physical assessment. The nurse inspects, palpates, and percusses the abdomen for any evidence of a distended bladder. Normally, the bladder must contain 150 mL of urine to allow its palpation and percussion. A bladder with a larger amount of urine may

CHART 76-1

KEY FEATURES *of* Benign Prostatic Hyperplasia

- Urinary frequency
- Nocturia
- Urinary hesitancy, particularly on initiation of voiding
- Hematuria
- Diminished force of the urinary stream
- Postvoid dribbling (overflow incontinence)
- Bladder distention
- Possible evidence of renal insufficiency, including edema, pallor, and pruritus
- A uniform, elastic, nontender palpable prostate

be visible on inspection. An enlarged bladder may be palpated as a mass in the lower abdomen. If suprapubic pressure on the mass results in a feeling of urgency, the nurse may be able to ascertain that the mass is a distended bladder. The bladder of an obese client is best identified through percussion rather than inspection or palpation.

The nurse prepares the client for the examination of the prostate gland. Because the prostate is close to the rectal wall, the easiest and most satisfactory examination of the prostate is by a **digital rectal examination (DRE).** The nurse helps the client to bend over the examination table or assume a side-lying fetal position. The health care provider examines the prostate for size and consistency. Benign prostatic hyperplasia (BPH) usually presents as a uniform, elastic, nontender enlargement, whereas cancer of the prostate gland usually presents as a stony-hard nodule (Chart 76-1). The nurse advises the client that after the prostate gland is palpated, it may be massaged to obtain a fluid sample for examination to rule out **prostatitis** (inflammation of the prostate).

LABORATORY ASSESSMENT

The health care provider may order a urinalysis and obtains a urine specimen for culture to detect any urinary abnormality or evidence of urinary tract infection. Urinalysis includes tests for glucose, protein, occult blood, and pH levels. If an infection is present, the specimen may contain white blood cells (WBCs) (pus) or red blood cells (RBCs).

Blood studies that may be performed at the initial evaluation, depending on the client's condition and third-party payer, include the following:

- A complete blood count (CBC) to evaluate any evidence of infection or anemia
- Blood urea nitrogen (BUN) and serum creatinine determinations to evaluate renal function
- A prostate-specific antigen (PSA) and a serum acid phosphatase measurement if a prostatic malignancy is suspected (see Prostate Cancer Screening, p. 1790).

If the health care provider expresses prostatic fluid during the examination, the fluid is sent to the laboratory for microscopic examination and cultures.

RADIOGRAPHIC ASSESSMENT

...gic studies that may be conducted in the workup of the ...th suspected BPH include x-ray studies of the kidneys, ...d bladder (KUB) and intravenous pyelography (IVP).

The KUB outlines the structure of the urinary tract in the abdomen. The IVP is particularly useful in revealing the structure and function of the urinary tract.

OTHER DIAGNOSTIC ASSESSMENT

Urodynamic studies are very important in the diagnosis and evaluation of clients with bladder neck obstruction. Urodynamic flow studies include flow rate analysis **(flowmetry)** and assessment of residual urine. Flow rate analysis is simply a way of assessing the activity of the bladder and the outlet during the emptying phase of micturition.

During a cystourethroscopic examination, the physician uses a cystoscope to visualize the interior of the bladder, the bladder neck, and the urethra. This examination is necessary to study the presence and effect of bladder neck obstruction. The procedure is usually done in an ambulatory care setting.

Residual urine may be determined by catheterizing the client immediately after he voids. As an alternative, because the client always voids before cystourethroscopy, residual urine may be measured at that time.

Interventions

Traditionally, the only effective treatment for the relief of the symptoms caused by BPH has been surgical, although some clients can be managed without surgery.

NONSURGICAL MANAGEMENT. Medical management of BPH includes drug therapy and other measures to minimize obstruction.

DRUG THERAPY. The health care provider may prescribe finasteride (Proscar) to shrink the prostate gland and improve urine flow. Finasteride lowers the level of **dihydrotestosterone (DHT),** a major cause of prostate growth. In some men, decreasing the DHT levels can shrink the enlarged prostate. The client may need to take the drug for as long as 6 months before any improvement occurs. The major side effects of the drug are erectile dysfunction (ED) and decreased libido, although these effects are not common.

The presence of alpha-adrenergic receptors in the prostatic smooth muscle makes it treatable by alpha-blocking agents, such as terazosin (Hytrin), doxazosin (Cardura), and tamsulosin (Flomax). When alpha-blocking agents are given, the prostate gland constricts, thereby reducing urethral pressure, improving urine flow, and decreasing residual mass. A variety of hormonal agents, including estrogens and androgens, alone or in combination, also have been used in attempts to alter BPH and its effects on voiding. This type of hormonal manipulation has usually not been successful.

COMPLEMENTARY AND ALTERNATIVE THERAPIES. Health care providers in Europe have successfully treated benign BPH with saw palmetto extract, a natural herb, for many years. In the United States most health care providers have been reluctant to recommend the herb because of lack of adequate clinical research on its effectiveness. Despite this trend, many men with early to moderate BPH believe that saw palmetto has relieved their symptoms and prefer this treatment over prescription drugs or surgery. A study in the United States by Marks at al. (2000) found that a saw palmetto herbal blend was a safe, highly desirable option for men with BPH. The herb caused epithelial tissue contraction in the prostate gland.

OTHER MEASURES. Some nonsurgical measures seem to minimize obstructive symptoms, including those that cause the release of prostatic fluid, such as prostatic massage, frequent sexual intercourse, and masturbation. These measures are very helpful for the client whose urinary obstructive symptoms have resulted from an enlarged prostate with a large amount of retained prostatic fluid. The nurse instructs the client to avoid drinking large amounts of fluid in a short time; to avoid alcohol, diuretics, and caffeine; and to void as soon as the urge is felt. These measures are aimed at preventing overdistention of the bladder, which may result in loss of detrusor muscle tone. Clients should also avoid any medications that can cause urinary retention, especially anticholinergics, antihistamines, and decongestants. The nurse emphasizes the importance of telling the health care provider about the diagnosis of BPH so that these drugs will not be prescribed.

SURGICAL MANAGEMENT. Because most older men have some evidence of BPH, the mere presence of the condition does not mean that the client requires surgical intervention. Some or all of the following criteria are typically present when surgical intervention is considered necessary:

- Acute urinary retention
- Chronic urinary tract infections secondary to residual urine in the bladder
- Hematuria
- Hydronephrosis
- Bladder neck obstruction symptoms that are worrisome to the client, such as urinary frequency and nocturia

The goals of surgical intervention are to relieve the symptoms associated with bladder neck obstruction and to improve the quality of the client's life by allowing him to void at normal intervals while retaining adequate urinary control and normal sexual functioning.

PREOPERATIVE CARE. When planning surgical interventions, the physician considers the client's general physical condition, the size of the prostate gland, and the client's preference.

CONSIDERATIONS FOR OLDER ADULTS

The client is thoroughly evaluated for any other diseases that are common in older persons, such as cardiovascular disease, chronic pulmonary disease, diabetes mellitus, or renal disease. If the client has renal disease, the nurse or physician may insert a Foley catheter. The client's intake, output, and serum electrolyte and creatinine levels are closely monitored until renal status has improved. In some cases, a thorough workup and evaluation of the client's medical condition may indicate that surgery would be too risky. In such cases, bladder neck obstruction may be relieved by permanent Foley drainage. The physician also assesses for the presence of urinary tract infection and treats any infection before performing surgery.

Preoperatively, the client may have many fears and misconceptions about prostatic surgery, such as automatic loss of sexual functioning or permanent incontinence. The nurse assesses the client's anxiety, corrects any misconceptions about the surgery, and provides accurate information to him and his family or significant others. Regardless of the type of surgery to be performed, the nurse provides information about anesthesia (see Chapter 19). The client may have concurrent medical problems that put him at risk for complications of general anesthesia and may be advised to have epidural anesthesia. Epidural anesthesia may be used for any of the procedures and is the most commonly used type of anesthesia for a transurethral resection of the prostate. Because the client is awake, it is easier to assess for hyponatremia, fluid overload, and water intoxication.

The nurse also includes the topic of urinary catheters in the preoperative teaching plan. After prostatic surgery, all clients have an indwelling urethral (Foley) catheter for at least a day. The nurse instructs the client that he may also have continuous bladder irrigation (CBI) and traction on the catheter, but this may not be known until the client returns from the postanesthesia care unit (PACU). The nurse also explains before surgery that it is normal postoperatively for the urine to be blood tinged. Small blood clots and tissue debris may pass while the catheter is in place and immediately after it is removed.

OPERATIVE PROCEDURES. Several surgical procedures are possible for removing the hypertrophied portion of the prostate gland (Figure 76-3). In all approaches, the surgeon removes the hyperplastic tissue and leaves the prostatic capsule.

In the last few years, a variety of less invasive surgical procedures for BPH have emerged. These procedures include transurethral thermotherapy, transurethral needle ablation, visual laser ablation, and electrovaporization (using electrocautery) of the prostate. The advantages of these minimally invasive procedures are that the client can be discharged from the hospital within 24 hours with a Foley catheter because there is minimal postoperative bleeding. Postoperatively, the nurse teaches the client to monitor for catheter patency, hematuria, and infection. Clients and their caregivers should also be told that delayed hematuria and urinary retention may occur days to weeks after the electrovaporization procedure (Gray & Allensworth, 1999).

Transurethral Resection of the Prostate. The traditional **transurethral resection of the prostate (TURP)** is a "closed" surgical procedure and is still commonly performed. The prostate may also be removed using an "open" procedure because of the need for a surgical incision. The choice of procedure depends on the following:

- The size of the prostate gland
- The location of the enlargement
- Whether surgery on the bladder is also needed
- The client's age and physical condition

To perform the TURP procedure, the most common type of prostatic surgery, the surgeon inserts a resectoscope (an instrument similar to a cystoscope, but with a cutting and cauterizing loop) through the urethra. The enlarged portion of the prostate gland is then resected in small pieces (prostate chips).

The surgeon chooses this procedure when the major enlargement exists in the medial lobe of the prostate that directly surrounds the urethra and when the amount of tissue to be removed is relatively small. A TURP is safer for the client who is at high risk for open surgery because a surgical incision is not necessary. Hospitalization and convalescence are shorter than with any other type of **prostatectomy** (prostate removal).

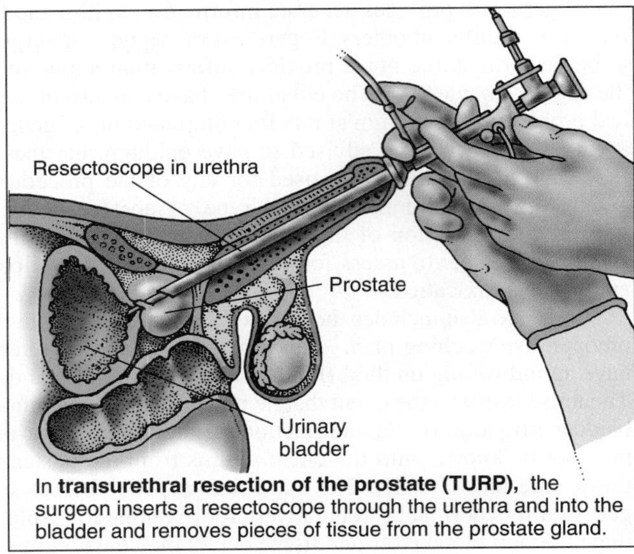

In **transurethral resection of the prostate (TURP),** the surgeon inserts a resectoscope through the urethra and into the bladder and removes pieces of tissue from the prostate gland.

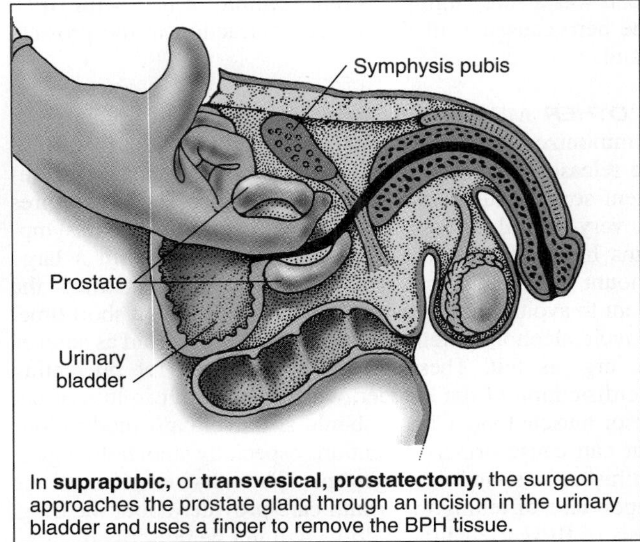

In **suprapubic,** or **transvesical, prostatectomy,** the surgeon approaches the prostate gland through an incision in the urinary bladder and uses a finger to remove the BPH tissue.

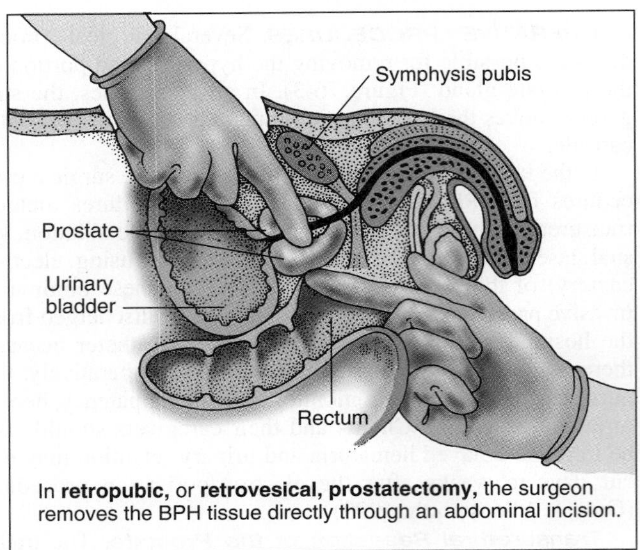

In **retropubic,** or **retrovesical, prostatectomy,** the surgeon removes the BPH tissue directly through an abdominal incision.

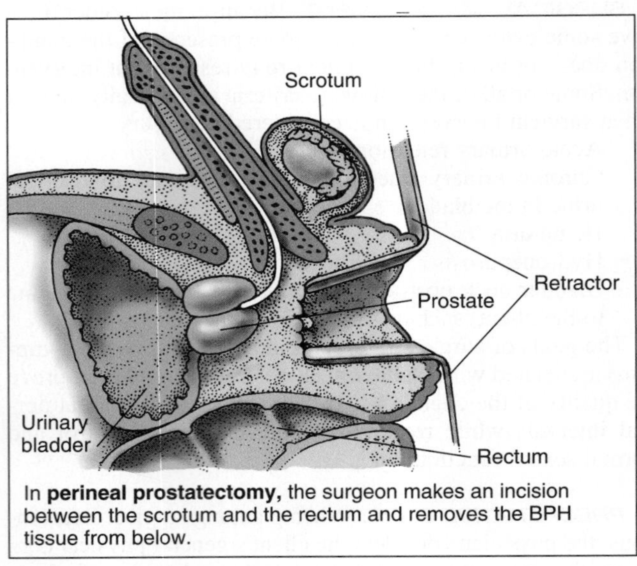

In **perineal prostatectomy,** the surgeon makes an incision between the scrotum and the rectum and removes the BPH tissue from below.

Figure 76-3 ● Prostatectomy procedures. (*BPH,* Benign prostatic hyperplasia.)

The disadvantage of a TURP is that because only small pieces of the gland are removed, prostatic tissue may grow back, resulting in recurrent urinary obstruction and necessitating additional TURPs. There is also the possibility of urethral trauma from the resectoscope, with resultant urethral strictures.

Suprapubic Prostatectomy. **Suprapubic,** or transvesical, **prostatectomy** is performed when the prostate is larger than the surgeon believes can be removed transurethrally and if the client has any coexisting bladder abnormalities that can be treated concurrently.

The surgeon makes a low, horizontal abdominal incision just above the symphysis pubis and exposes the bladder. The bladder is then distended with fluid, and a small incision is made in the bladder wall. The prostate gland is removed through the bladder cavity, and any bladder disease is treated at this time.

The ability to treat bladder problems is the major advantage of suprapubic prostatectomy because an incision is made into the bladder to reach the prostate. The following are disadvantages:

- An abdominal incision and an incision into the bladder are necessary.
- The client has a suprapubic tube in place postoperatively.
- There is an increased risk of urinary tract infection, incontinence, bladder spasms, and hemorrhage.
- The surgery is more painful.
- Convalescence is longer than with a TURP.

Retropubic Prostatectomy. **Retropubic,** or extravesical, **prostatectomy** may be selected when the prostate is too large to be resected via the transurethral approach but no coexisting bladder abnormalities have been identified. The surgeon makes an abdominal incision above the symphysis pubis to expose the prostate gland. A small incision is made in the prostate gland, and the gland is removed. The difference between the suprapubic and the retropubic approaches is the bladder incision.

Perineal Prostatectomy. Perineal prostatectomy is performed primarily to:

- Remove an enlarged prostate gland that is filled with calculi (stones)
- Treat prostatic abscesses that have not responded to conservative treatment
- Repair complications, such as lacerations in the prostatic capsule, that may have occurred during a different type of prostatectomy
- Treat clients who are poor surgical risks

The client is placed in an exaggerated lithotomy position, and the knees are positioned on the chest. The surgeon makes a U-shaped incision between the ischial tuberosities, the scrotum, and the rectum. The prostatic capsule is then opened and enucleated. This type of prostatectomy provides a direct anatomic approach to the prostate gland.

The major disadvantage of this procedure is the loss of sexual potency resulting from damage to the pudendal nerve. Clients with peripheral vascular disease or chronic pulmonary problems cannot tolerate the exaggerated lithotomy position and are not candidates for a perineal prostatectomy. Other disadvantages of this procedure include a greater risk for infection, the possibility of damage to the rectum and anal sphincter, and the possibility of urinary incontinence. For these reasons, this surgical approach is not commonly used.

POSTOPERATIVE CARE. The general postoperative care for the client who has undergone prostatic surgery is similar regardless of the type of procedure done and the type of anesthesia used (see Chapter 19). However, the nurse is aware of several differences as they affect nursing care.

Nursing Care After a Transurethral Resection of the Prostate. After a TURP, the surgeon inserts a three-way Foley catheter with a 30- to 45-mL retention balloon through the urethra into the bladder (Figure 76-4). The catheter is pulled down into the prostatic fossa to help prevent bleeding. The surgeon often applies traction on the catheter by pulling it taut and taping it to the client's abdomen or thigh.

Catheter Care and Continuous Bladder Irrigation. If the catheter is taped to the client's thigh, the nurse instructs him to keep his leg straight. The surgeon determines when the traction should be removed; usually it is removed on the first postoperative day.

The nurse explains that because of the Foley catheter's large diameter and the pressure of the retention balloon on the internal sphincter of the bladder, the client will continually feel the urge to void. This is a normal sensation and not a surgical complication. The nurse advises the client not to try to void around the catheter, which causes the bladder muscles to contract and may result in painful bladder spasms. He is reassured that an antispasmodic medication can be given to keep him comfortable.

> **CONSIDERATIONS FOR OLDER ADULTS**
> When caring for older men who may become confused after surgery, the nurse reorients them frequently and reminds them not to pull on the catheter (Chart 76-2). If the client is restless or "picks" at tubes, the nurse may provide a familiar object, such as a family picture, for him to hold on to for distraction and a feeling of security. If possible, the client should not be restrained; other alternatives should be tried first.

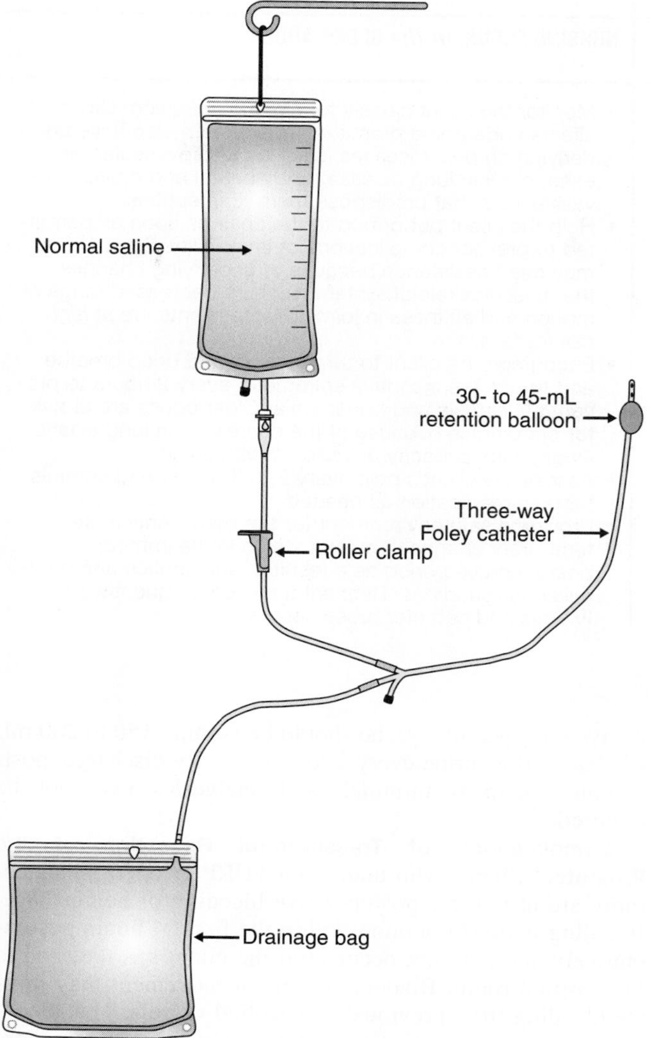

Figure 76-4 ● Continuous bladder irrigation.

Continuous bladder irrigation (CBI) with normal saline or other solution, as ordered by the physician, may keep the catheter free of obstruction and facilitates detection of obstruction or other complications. The nurse adjusts the irrigation fluid rate to maintain a colorless or light pink drainage return. (For the nursing care of the client undergoing CBI, see Chart 76-3.) The continuous irrigation is usually discontinued 24 hours after a TURP. The Foley catheter is usually removed when CBI is discontinued.

Postcatheterization Care. When the Foley catheter is removed, the client may experience some burning on urination, as well as some urinary frequency, dribbling, and leakage. The nurse reassures the client that these symptoms are normal and will subside. The client may also pass small clots and tissue debris for several days after the TURP. The nurse instructs him to increase fluid intake to a minimum of 2000 to 2500 mL/day, which helps to decrease the dysuria and to keep the urine clear. An older client who has renal disease or who is susceptible to congestive heart failure may not be able to tolerate this much fluid. By the time of discharge (usually

CHART 76-2

NURSING FOCUS *on the* OLDER ADULT
Prostate Surgery

- Monitor the client closely for signs of infection. Older clients undergoing prostate surgery often also have underlying chronic diseases (such as cardiovascular disease, chronic lung disease, or diabetes) and multiple invasive lines that predispose them to infections.
- Help the client out of bed to the chair as soon as permitted to prevent complications of immobility. Older clients may need assistance because of underlying changes in the musculoskeletal system, such as decreased range of motion and stiffness in joints. These clients are at *high risk* for falls.
- Encourage the client to turn, cough, and deep breathe and to use the incentive spirometer every 2 hours to prevent atelectasis and pneumonia. Older adults are at risk for pneumonia because of the decreases in lung elasticity and vital capacity associated with aging.
- Assess the client's pain every 2 to 3 hours, and administer pain medication as needed.
- Provide a safe environment for the client. Anticipate a temporary change in mental status in the immediate postoperative period as a result of anesthetics and unfamiliar surroundings. Reorient the client frequently. Keep IV lines and catheter tubes secure.

2 days postoperatively), he should be voiding 150 to 200 mL of clear yellow urine every 3 to 4 hours. By discharge, postoperative pain is minimal, and analgesics may not be required.

Complications of Transurethral Resection of the Prostate. Clients who undergo a TURP or open prostatectomy are at risk for postoperative bleeding or hemorrhage. Bleeding is most common within the first 24 hours postoperatively and may not occur until the client has returned to his hospital room. Bladder spasms or movement may initiate bleeding from previously controlled vessels. This bleeding may be arterial or venous, but venous bleeding is more common.

The nurse or assistive nursing personnel monitors the client's urine output every 2 hours and vital signs every 4 hours. If the bleeding is arterial, the nurse will notice that the urinary drainage is bright red or ketchup-like with numerous clots. If arterial bleeding occurs, the nurse notifies the surgeon immediately and increases the CBI rate or intermittently irrigates the catheter with normal saline solution. The surgeon may order aminocaproic acid (Amicar) to control bleeding. The nurse keeps in mind that if the medication does not work, surgical intervention may be necessary to clear the bladder of clots and to stop the arterial bleeding.

If the bleeding is venous, the urine output will be burgundy, with or without any change in vital signs. The nurse informs the client's surgeon of any of the signs and symptoms of bleeding. The surgeon may apply traction on the catheter for a few hours, which may control venous bleeding. The nurse assesses the success of this procedure in stopping the bleeding and is aware that the traction on the catheter is quite uncomfortable and increases the risk of bladder spasms. The physician usually orders analgesics or antispasmodics, such as dicyclomine hydrochloride (Bentyl, Antispas, Formulex♣, Lomine♣), oxybutynin (Ditropan), or belladonna and opium (B&O) suppositories, to decrease painful bladder spasms.

CHART 76-3

BEST PRACTICE *for*
Care of the Client with Continuous Bladder Irrigation

- Use normal saline solution for the bladder irrigant unless otherwise ordered by the physician. Normal saline solution is isotonic.
- Adjust the rate of the irrigation solution to the physician's specifications. The physician may order a solution rate that keeps the output clear and free of clots.
- Monitor the color, consistency, and amount of urine output.
- Check the drainage tubing frequently for external obstructions (such as kinks) and internal obstructions (such as blood clots and decreased output).
- Assess the client for complaints of bladder spasms, which may indicate obstruction.
- If the urinary catheter is obstructed, turn off the continuous bladder irrigation (CBI) and irrigate the catheter with 30 to 50 mL of normal saline solution using a large piston syringe.
- Notify the physician immediately if the obstruction does not resolve by hand irrigation or if the urinary return becomes "ketchupy."

The nurse closely monitors the client's hemoglobin (Hgb) and hematocrit (Hct) levels for anemia as a result of blood loss. Some clients may require blood transfusions to return the Hgb and Hct values to baseline levels.

Nursing Care After Suprapubic Prostatectomy. If the client has undergone a suprapubic prostatectomy, a **suprapubic catheter,** in addition to a Foley catheter, will be in place. Each catheter is connected to a separate closed drainage system and drains the bladder via gravity. The nurse is aware that catheter traction is not effective for the client who experiences postoperative bleeding after a suprapubic prostatectomy. Such a client needs brisk CBI via the catheter. If the CBI does not control the postoperative bleeding, the client needs surgical intervention.

If the client has an suprapubic catheter in place, the Foley catheter is generally removed on the second postoperative day. After the Foley catheter is removed, the nurse clamps the suprapubic catheter and the client attempts to void. After the client has urinated, the nurse checks the residual urine in the bladder by unclamping the suprapubic tube. The client may be discharged from the hospital with a suprapubic catheter in place. When the client consistently empties his bladder and the residual urine in the bladder is 75 mL or less, the suprapubic catheter is then removed. An antimicrobial ointment may be applied daily to the site, depending on hospital policy or the physician's order.

The client with a suprapubic catheter in place is at increased risk for bladder spasms. The incision dressing for these clients should be observed and changed more frequently than for clients who do not have an incision drain, because the dressing becomes saturated with urine until the incision heals. If the suprapubic drain is not connected to gravity drainage, the nurse may enclose the drain with an ostomy bag to measure the output accurately and to prevent any skin problems or breakdown.

Nursing Care After Retropubic Prostatectomy. After a retropubic prostatectomy, the urinary sphincter muscles are seldom damaged, the bladder is not entered, and no urinary drainage should be seen on the abdominal dressing. The nurse notifies the client's surgeon of any urinary or purulent drainage, fever, or increased pain because these symptoms indicate a serious complication such as a deep wound infection or pelvic abscess.

Nursing Care After Perineal Prostatectomy. After the perineal approach to prostatectomy, the client has an incision dressing and may or may not have an incision drain. The use of rectal thermometers and rectal tubes and enemas are contraindicated because they may cause trauma or bleeding.

CRITICAL THINKING CHALLENGE

You are caring for a man who has just been admitted to your surgical unit after a TURP. The nurse from the postanesthesia care unit (PACU) reported that the urine that was draining was pinkish and that he was undergoing CBI. When you check his urine output, you notice that his Foley catheter is not draining and that there are several large, bright red blood clots in his drainage bag.

- What other assessments should you make at this time?
- What action should you take as soon as possible?

For suggested answer guidelines, go to SIMON http://www.wbsaunders.com/SIMON/Iggy/.

Community-Based Care

The client with benign prostatic hyperplasia (BPH) is typically managed at home. Clients who have surgery are also discharged to their home.

HEALTH TEACHING

After any type of prostatectomy, some clients, and especially those who have undergone a transurethral resection of the prostate (TURP), may experience some temporary loss of control of urination or a dribbling of the urine. The client is reassured that these symptoms are almost always temporary and will resolve. The nurse assists the client and his family or significant others in devising ways to keep his clothing dry until sphincter control returns. He is instructed to contract and relax his sphincter frequently to re-establish urinary control (Kegel exercises). External urinary (condom or Texas) catheters are not used except in extreme cases, because they may give the client a false sense of security and delay his urinary control.

The nurse provides specific instructions for each client on the basis of the type of surgical procedure performed and any further interventions he may need in the future. Discharge instructions for a client undergoing surgery of the prostate gland are listed in Chart 76-4.

The client who undergoes prostatic surgery usually needs emotional support. The client who undergoes a perineal prostatectomy is at risk for permanent sexual dysfunction. The nurse informs the client of the options, such as a penile prosthesis, that are available to treat erectile dysfunction (ED) (see Interventions [Erectile Dysfunction], p. 1794).

Other surgical procedures for prostate removal should not cause physiologic ED. However, some clients may have functional ED for a short time after surgery during the recovery phase.

CHART 76-4

CLIENT EDUCATION GUIDE
Care After a Transurethral Resection of the Prostate

- Drink 12 to 14 glasses of water each day, preferably before 8 PM, *unless otherwise contraindicated.*
- Use alcohol, caffeinated beverages, and spicy foods in moderation to avoid overstimulation of your bladder.
- If your urine becomes bloody, rest quietly and increase your fluid intake. If the bleeding does not subside shortly, contact your doctor.
- Avoid strenuous activities, such as driving and working, during the first 2 to 3 weeks after surgery.
- Schedule a follow-up appointment with your doctor after you leave the hospital.

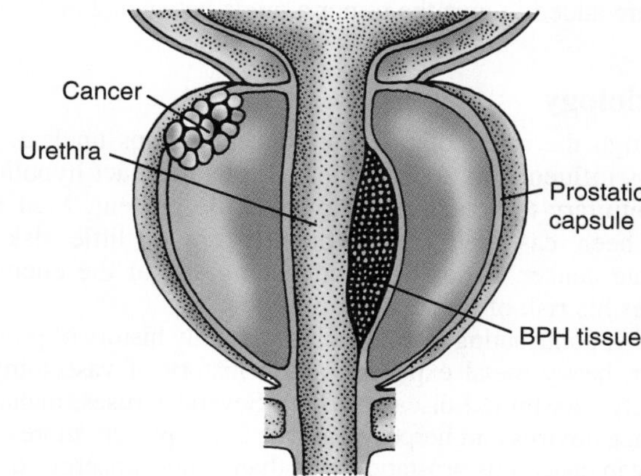

Figure 76-5 ● The prostate gland with cancer and benign prostatic hyperplasia (BPH). Note that cancer normally arises in the periphery of the gland, whereas BPH occurs in the center of the gland.

HOME CARE MANAGEMENT

Unless there is a complication of surgery, such as a wound infection or an unusual problem with voiding, the client does not have a dressing or indwelling catheter at the time of discharge. In some cases, the suprapubic tube may remain in place for several weeks after discharge.

PROSTATE CANCER

OVERVIEW

Prostate cancer is the most common cancer among American men, other than skin cancer, and follows lung cancer as the second leading cause of cancer deaths in this group (American Cancer Society, 2000).

Pathophysiology

Of all cancers of the prostate, 95% are adenocarcinomas. These adenocarcinomas arise from the epithelial cells of the prostate and are usually located in the posterior lobe or outer portion of the gland (Figure 76-5). The remaining types of prostatic neoplasms are classified as *nonepithelial* carcinomas and include ductal carcinomas, transitional cell carcinomas, squamous cell carcinomas, and sarcomas.

Of all malignancies, prostate cancer is one of the slowest growing and metastasizes in a fairly predictable pattern. The most common sites of metastatic spread are the prostatic and perivesicular lymph nodes, the pelvic lymph nodes, bone marrow, and the bones of the pelvis, sacrum, and lumbar spine.

Metastatic involvement of the visceral organs tends to occur late in the natural history of the disease. The most common sites for metastatic prostate cancer are the lungs, liver, adrenals, and kidneys.

Tumor grade is an important variable in the management of prostate cancer. Grading is the pathologist's interpretation of the aggressiveness of the cancer. Usually the Gleason grading system is used. Normal prostate tissue cells are given a score of 1 (best), and abnormal cells are given a score of 5 (worst). The scores of the two most common cell types found in the specimen are added to give the tumor a grade between 2 and 10.

Etiology

Although the cause of prostate cancer remains unclear, two factors influence its development. First, an intact hypothalamic-pituitary-testicular pathway must be present. Men who have been castrated before puberty are at little risk for prostate cancer. Second, the advancing age of the client increases his risk of prostate cancer.

Other contributing factors include a family history of prostate cancer, heavy metal exposure, and a history of vasectomy or sexually transmitted disease (STD). Several viruses, including cytomegalovirus and herpesvirus type 2, are present more commonly in cancerous prostatic tissue than in noncancerous tissue.

The relationship between benign prostatic hyperplasia (BPH) and cancer of the prostate is controversial. Although some researchers say that BPH and cancer of the prostate are unrelated diseases, others suggest that cancer is more likely to occur within or adjacent to any proliferative cell population (Haas & Sakr, 1997).

Incidence/Prevalence

Prostate cancer is the sixth most common cancer in the world and the fourth most common in men. Incidence rates have been influenced by the diagnosis of latent cancers found during screening of asymptomatic men. Developing countries in Africa, South America, and the Caribbean have a very high incidence of the disease. In contrast, the rate is low in Asian countries.

In the United States the introduction of screening with prostate-specific antigen (PSA) has resulted in the doubling of cases diagnosed between 1984 and 1992. If the rate continues to increase, almost 1 million new cases per year could be expected by 2010 (Parkin et al., 1999).

CONSIDERATIONS FOR OLDER ADULTS

The incidence of prostate cancer increases with age. More than 75% of all prostate cancers are diagnosed in men over 65 years of age (American Cancer Society, 2000).

CULTURAL CONSIDERATIONS

African-American men have the highest prostate cancer incidence rates in the world. Associated mortality rates are twice those of Caucasian men (von Eschenbach et al., 1997). African-American men tend to be affected at an earlier age and have more advanced disease at the time of diagnosis. Lack of cancer awareness has been identified as a cause of increased mortality rates (Collins, 1997). Prostate cancer also occurs more often in Scandinavians than in Caucasians.

Hispanic and Asian-American men have lower rates of prostate cancer than Caucasian men and lower mortality rates, implying cultural, genetic, or lifestyle variables (Huff & Kline, 1999).

COLLABORATIVE MANAGEMENT

Assessment

As with any cancer, accurate staging is necessary for treatment planning and for monitoring the clinical course of the disease. As in BPH, the first symptoms that the client may experience are related to bladder neck obstruction, such as difficulty in initiating urination, recurrent bladder infections, and urinary retention. Gross, painless hematuria is the most common presenting clinical manifestation.

At times, a client may be undergoing intervention for BPH and is discovered to have cancer of the prostate. Bone pain is a symptom of a more advanced stage of prostate cancer. The client who has symptoms of urinary obstruction (urinary hesitancy, back pain) and bone pain is most likely to have metastatic disease at diagnosis.

PROSTATE CANCER SCREENING

The most effective procedures for screening for cancer of the prostate are the **digital rectal examination (DRE)** and the PSA test. In 1997 the American Cancer Society updated its guidelines for cancer screening (Chart 76-5). Beginning at age 50 years, all men should have an annual DRE and PSA test (Mettlin, 1997). Men at high risk for prostate cancer, including African Americans or men with a history of prostate cancer in first-degree relatives, should consider screening at an earlier age. On rectal examination, a prostate that is found to be stony hard and with palpable irregularities or indurations is suspected to be malignant.

Prostate-specific antigen (PSA) is a highly immunogenic glycoprotein produced solely by the prostate. The normal

CHART 76-5

CLIENT EDUCATION GUIDE
1997 American Cancer Society Prostate Screening and Detection Guidelines

- An annual digital rectal examination (DRE) and prostate-specific antigen (PSA) test should be offered to:
  - Men beginning at age 50 years
  - Men who have a life expectancy of at least 10 years
  - Younger men who are at high risk (at least by age 45 years)
- Men at high risk include those with a strong familial predisposition (e.g., two or more first-degree relatives with prostate cancer) and African-American men.
- DRE should be performed by health care professionals skilled in recognizing subtle prostate abnormalities.
- DRE is less effective than PSA in detecting prostate cancer. An abnormal PSA test result is a value above 4.0 ng/mL.

level of PSA established by the American Cancer Society is a value of less than 4 ng/mL. PSA levels are elevated in clients with increased prostatic tissue as a result of various conditions, including carcinoma of the prostate, benign prostatic hyperplasia (BPH), prostatic infarction, and prostatitis.

PSA blood levels should never be used as a screening test without a physical examination of the prostate. The PSA serum level was never meant to replace the DRE, but to be used in conjunction with it. Twenty-five percent of clients with prostate cancer have PSA levels less than 4 ng/mL (Mettlin, 1997).

PSA is not elevated in healthy men or in men with carcinomas other than prostate carcinoma. However, the normal PSA level is slightly higher in older adults and in African Americans. An elevated PSA level should decrease a few days after a prostatectomy. An increase in the PSA level at postoperative visits usually indicates that the disease has recurred.

CULTURAL CONSIDERATIONS

The participation rate of African-American men in prostate cancer screening programs remains very low. A nursing study by Collins (1997) showed that educational intervention had a positive effect on short-term knowledge and awareness of prostate cancer by African-American men (see the Evidence-Based Practice for Nursing box below).

After screening by DRE and PSA, some clients undergo a **transrectal ultrasound** study of the prostate, although its effectiveness is controversial. The urologist inserts a small probe into the rectum and obtains an ultrasonogram of the prostate. A specimen for biopsy may also be obtained with the rectal probe.

When the diagnosis of prostatic cancer is suspected, a biopsy is necessary for confirmation. Prostatic ultrasonography may be performed to isolate the area of the prostate for biopsy. One of several procedures may be used to obtain the biopsy specimen. The most common procedure is the needle-core or aspiration biopsy.

EVIDENCE-BASED PRACTICE FOR NURSING

Educating African-American men about early detection of cancer

Collins, M. (1997). Increasing prostate cancer awareness in African American men. *Oncology Nursing Forum, 24*(1), 91-95.

The intent of this study was to assess the effect of an educational program about prostate cancer on the knowledge level of African-American men. A convenience sample of 75 men between the ages of 23 and 83 years completed a preintervention and postintervention questionnaire. The findings were positive in that test scores improved after the educational session.

Critique. Although a convenience sample was used, the researcher addressed a major health concern (i.e., the lack of knowledge and participation of African-American men in prostate screening programs). Unfortunately, only short-term retention was evaluated. A follow-up test weeks or months later could determine the lasting effects of education. The sample could also be followed to see if they participated in prostate screening as a result of learning more about prostate cancer.

Implications for Nursing. Nurses have to continue their efforts to educate the public, especially high-risk groups, about the need for prevention and early detection of all types of cancers. African-American men are at the highest risk for prostate cancer.

After the diagnosis of prostate cancer is made, the client undergoes radiographic and blood studies to ascertain the extent of the disease. Common tests include computed tomography (CT) of the pelvis and abdomen and magnetic resonance imaging (MRI) to assess the status of the pelvic and para-aortic lymph nodes. A bone scan is performed to find any evidence of metastatic disease. Hepatomegaly or abnormal results of liver function studies indicate a need for further evaluation for the presence of liver metastases.

Most clients with advanced prostate cancer also have elevated levels of **serum acid phosphatase.** Approximately 90% of clients with prostate cancer metastatic to the bone have elevated **serum alkaline phosphatase** levels.

Interventions

Management of the client with prostate cancer includes surgery, radiation therapy, and drug therapy. Management is based on the extent of the disease and the client's physical condition. The client may undergo surgery for a tumor biopsy, staging and removal of the tumor, or palliation to control the spread of disease or relieve distressing symptoms. The health care provider and client must weigh the benefits of treatment against potential adverse effects such as incontinence and erectile dysfunction (ED).

SURGICAL MANAGEMENT. Because as many as 30% of localized prostate cancers are resistant to radiation, surgery is the standard treatment and is therefore presented first. The surgical approaches for prostatectomy in the client with prostate cancer are similar to those for BPH (see Surgical Management [Benign Prostatic Hyperplasia], p. 1785). In most cases, however, the surgical procedure is much more extensive and includes a **pelvic lymphadenectomy** (removal of pelvic lymph nodes).

Clients who have stage 0 cancer of the prostate require only close follow-up by their health care provider. If obstruction recurs, repeated needle biopsies or transurethral resections of the prostate (TURPs) should be part of the screening.

RADICAL PROSTATECTOMY. Clients with more severe disease typically undergo a radical prostatectomy via a retropubic, perineal, or suprapubic approach. In the radical prostatectomy, instead of removing only the prostate gland, as in the procedure for BPH, the surgeon removes the entire gland along with the prostatic capsule, the cuff at the bladder neck, the seminal vesicles, and the regional lymph nodes. The remaining urethra is anastomosed to the bladder neck. The removal of tissue at the bladder neck allows the seminal fluid to travel upward into the bladder rather than down the urethral tract, resulting in retrograde ejaculations. The client is sterile, but his ability to have an erection and an orgasm should not be permanently impaired.

Sexual Dysfunction. The surgeon advises clients who are undergoing radical perineal prostatectomy that they may have ED after the surgery. This consequence is directly related to any damage done to the pudendal nerve (which is necessary for erection and orgasm) during the surgery.

The surgeon may perform a nerve-sparing prostatectomy in the following cases:

- There is no evidence of disease in adjacent lymph nodes.
- Serum acid phosphatase levels are not elevated.
- There is no clinical evidence of cancer extension beyond the prostate gland.

As the name of the procedure implies, the surgeon keeps the nerves responsible for penile erection intact. After surgery, the client may experience temporary ED, but normal function usually returns in 3 to 12 months.

Urinary Incontinence. Because the internal and external sphincters of the bladder lie close to the prostate gland, urinary incontinence can be another complication of a radical prostatectomy. The nurse teaches the client perineal exercises to help facilitate the return of urinary continence after surgery or after removal of the Foley catheter. To perform the exercises, the client contracts and relaxes the perineal and gluteal muscles in several ways. For one of the exercises, the nurse teaches the client to:

1. Tighten the perineal muscles for 3 to 5 seconds as if to prevent voiding, then relax
2. Bear down as if having a bowel movement
3. Relax and repeat the exercise

The nurse shows the client how to inhale through pursed lips while tightening the perineal muscles and how to exhale when he relaxes. To regain urinary control, the client can also practice holding an object, such as a pencil, in the fold between the buttock and the thigh. He may also sit on the toilet with his knees apart while voiding and start and stop his stream several times. Chart 76-6 summarizes the most important aspects of postoperative nursing care for the client who has undergone a radical prostatectomy.

Complementary and Alternative Therapies for Incontinence. Biofeedback has been successfully used as a noninvasive treatment for incontinence after radical prostatectomy. In a nursing study by Jackson et al. (1996), 27 postoperative radical prostatectomy clients were treated by biofeedback for urinary incontinence. Forty-eight percent of the sample had complete success, 26% had significant improvement but were not completely dry, and 26% experienced failure. The authors concluded that biofeedback training can work as a first-line option for most clients if they are motivated to decrease their incontinence.

Other Measures for Incontinence. If the client cannot recover urinary continence, an artificial urinary sphincter may be surgically implanted (Figure 76-6). Artificial sphincters have been more successful in males than in females, possibly because of the difference in urethral length.

After the sphincter has been implanted, the nurse instructs the client to report any complications, such as fever, pain on inflation of the device, edema or cellulitis in the genitalia, or recurrence of incontinence, indicating a possible mechanical malfunction in the system.

CRYOSURGICAL ABLATION. A newer, minimally invasive procedure that is becoming more popular as an alternative to radical prostatectomy is cryosurgical ablation of the prostate. During surgery, the client is placed in the lithotomy position to facilitate placement of the transrectal ultrasound probe. The probe helps determine the size of the prostate and the subsequent number of small cryoprobes that are positioned around the prostate gland. Liquid nitrogen freezes the gland, whose dead cells are then absorbed by the body.

The primary advantages of this procedure are minimal blood loss, minimal postoperative pain, decreased risk for postoperative urinary incontinence, and a short hospital stay. Most clients are permitted to return to their usual activity level in about 1 week after surgery. The procedure can be repeated if necessary (Schmidt et al., 1998).

BILATERAL ORCHIECTOMY. Unlike radical prostatectomy, **bilateral orchiectomy** (removal of both testes) is palliative

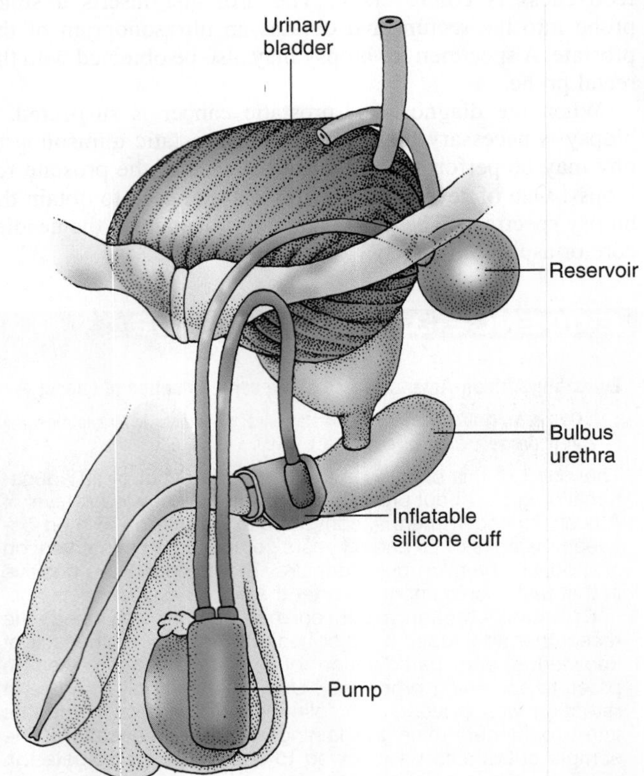

Figure 76-6 ● An artificial urinary sphincter is a fluid-filled system with a silicone cuff that surrounds the urethra and functions as a urinary sphincter. A pump is placed in the scrotum, and a fluid reservoir is placed in the abdomen. When the pump is squeezed, fluid leaves the urethral cuff and flows into the reservoir, allowing the client to empty his bladder.

CHART 76-6

BEST PRACTICE *for*
Care of the Client After a Radical 794

- Encourage the client to use patient-controlled analgesia (PCA) as needed. The PCA device may be used through the second postoperative day.
- Keep the client on bedrest on the day of surgery. Help the client to get out of bed and ambulate for a short distance by the first postoperative day.
- Maintain the sequential compression device until the client begins to ambulate. Apply antiembolic stockings until discharge.
- Monitor the client for deep vein thrombosis and pulmonary embolus.
- Keep an accurate record of intake and output, including Jackson-Pratt or other drainage device drainage.
- Keep the urinary meatus clean using soap and water.
- Avoid rectal procedures or treatments.
- Teach the client how to care for the urinary catheter because he will be discharged with the catheter in place.
- Teach the client how to use a leg bag.
- Emphasize the importance of not straining during bowel movement. Advise the client to avoid suppositories or enemas.
- Remind the client about the importance of follow-up appointments with the physician to monitor progress.

surgery. The intent of the surgery is not to cure the disease but to arrest its spread by removing testosterone. This procedure is described later in this chapter under Testicular Cancer, p. 1798.

NONSURGICAL MANAGEMENT. Nonsurgical management is usually done as an adjunct to surgery but may be done as an alternative intervention. Modalities include radiation therapy and drug therapy.

RADIATION THERAPY. External beam radiation therapy is important in the treatment of prostate cancer. It is performed for the following purposes:

- As an alternative curative treatment to surgery for locally contained tumors
- As an adjunct to radical prostatectomy when surgical margins or regional lymph nodes show malignancy postoperatively
- For palliation of the client's symptoms

Palliative radiation therapy alleviates pain caused by skeletal metastases and relieves ureteral or bladder neck obstruction.

Another popular treatment is ultrasonically guided iodine-125 or pallidium-103 **interstitial brachytherapy** (radiation therapy) or radioactive **seed implantation.** These procedures are done on an ambulatory care basis and are the most cost-effective treatment for early-stage prostate cancer. The client is reassured that these treatments are safe and well tolerated with minimal complications.

DRUG THERAPY. Drug therapy may consist of either hormonal therapy or chemotherapy. A vaccine to prevent prostate cancer is also being investigated (Tjoa et al., 1999).

Hormonal Therapy. Because prostate cancer is hormone dependent, clients with extensive tumors or those with metastatic disease are usually managed by androgen deprivation. Manipulating the hormonal environment in the client may be accomplished in two ways:

- The testosterone influence can be removed by a bilateral orchiectomy.
- Estrogens or gonadotropin-releasing hormone (GnRH) agonist analogs can be administered (Chart 76-7).

Estrogens such as diethylstilbestrol (DES) inhibit the release of luteinizing hormone (LH) from the pituitary gland. Clients with significant cardiovascular disease may not be candidates for estrogen therapy because of the side effects of estrogens, such as sodium and water retention and thromboembolic episodes. Other hormonal drugs, such as megestrol (Megace) and medroxyprogesterone (Depo-Provera), are sometimes used if first-line hormonal treatments lose their effectiveness.

Leuprolide acetate (Lupron), a GnRH agonist analog (which suppresses LH release by the pituitary), also reduces serum testosterone levels without any of the estrogenic side effects of DES. Flutamide (Eulexin, Euflex✤), an oral androgen-blocking agent, inhibits tumor progression by blocking the uptake of testicular and adrenal androgens at the prostate tumor site.

The health care provider may prescribe goserelin acetate (Zoladex), a potent GnRH agonist analog, for palliation of advanced prostatic carcinoma. This drug is an alternative treatment when orchiectomy or estrogen administration is neither acceptable nor indicated for the client.

Chemotherapy. Systemic cytotoxic chemotherapy has not proved effective in the treatment of prostate cancer. It is used for the client who fails to respond to hormonal manipulation. Unfortunately, only a small percentage of clients respond to cytotoxic chemotherapy with a partial shrinkage of their tumors, and the response usually lasts only a few months. (See Chapter 25 for a discussion of chemotherapy.)

Community-Based Care

Nursing management of the client with prostate cancer always includes his spouse or sexual partner. Clients with prostate cancer may require nursing interventions in a wide variety of settings—at the hospital, the radiation therapy department, the oncologist's office, or home—and at any stage of the disease process. Ongoing care of the client undergoing surgery is similar to that described under Community-Based Care for benign prostatic hyperplasia, p. 1789. Major quality-of-life issues facing the client with prostate cancer include body image, sexuality, and the impact of the cancer diagnosis on his life.

ERECTILE DYSFUNCTION

OVERVIEW

Erectile dysfunction (ED), previously known as **impotence,** is the inability to achieve or maintain an erection for sexual intercourse. It affects approximately 10 to 20 million

CHART 76-7

DRUG THERAPY *for* Prostate Cancer: Commonly Used Drugs

Drug	Usual Dosage	Nursing Interventions
Leuprolide acetate (Lupron)	7.5 mg q mo IM	Use at least a 22-gauge needle. Mix the solution well; it is a milky suspension. Observe for side effects, including "hot flashes" and sweating. Be aware that the client's symptoms may temporarily worsen, caused by a temporary testosterone increase.
Flutamide (Eulexin, Euflex✤)	750 mg in 3 daily divided doses PO	Teach the client that side effects include "hot flashes," loss of libido, and impotence. Diarrhea and nausea with vomiting are less common.
Goserelin acetate (Zoladex)	3.6 mg every 28 days SC	The prefilled syringe cannot be aspirated. If a blood vessel is damaged, blood will enter the syringe. Teach the client that side effects include "hot flashes," sexual dysfunction, and decreased erections.

men in the United States (Colpo, 1998). During the last decade, there has been a major change in the management of men with ED as a result of increased understanding of the physiology of erectile function and the development of new, effective therapies. There are two classes of ED: organic and functional.

Organic Erectile Dysfunction

Organic ED is characterized by a gradual deterioration of function. The man first notices diminishing firmness and a decrease in frequency of erections. Causes include the following:

- Inflammation of the prostate, urethra, or seminole vesicles
- Surgical procedures such as prostatectomy
- Pelvic fractures
- Lumbosacral injuries
- Vascular disease, including hypertension
- Chronic neurologic conditions, such as Parkinson's disease or multiple sclerosis
- Endocrine disorders, such as diabetes mellitus or thyroid disorders
- Smoking and alcohol consumption
- Medications
- Poor overall health that prevents sexual intercourse

Functional Erectile Dysfunction

If the client has episodes of ED, it usually has a functional (psychologic) cause. Men with **functional ED** have normal nocturnal (nighttime) and morning erections. Presentation of symptoms is usually sudden and preceded by a period of high stress.

COLLABORATIVE MANAGEMENT

Assessment

For a man to have an erection, he must have normal innervation and a normal **libido** (sex drive). Therefore a medical, social, and sexual history along with a complete physical examination is necessary. The first step is to determine if there is an organic cause. Diagnostic testing is done to rule out possible organic causes, as described in the preceding section.

If test results are negative, then the diagnostic evaluation focuses on the specific causes that may have been indicated in the health care provider's medical history. For example, hormone testing is used for clients who have a poor libido, small testicles, or a diminished beard growth. Serum levels of testosterone and gonadotropins are also measured.

Duplex Doppler ultrasonography is another test to evaluate ED. It provides information about arterial and venous blood flow to the penis. It can also be used to determine the best treatment for ED. A **nocturnal penile tumescence test** that measures nighttime erections is done in a sleep laboratory. Usually an erection is expected with each rapid eye movement (REM) episode. This study can determine if ED is caused by an organic or functional problem. If the man has nocturnal erections, the ED is functional. Sexual counseling is needed in this case, and the client is referred to a certified sexual therapist.

Interventions

Current methods of treatment include vacuum devices, intracorporal injections, intraurethral applications, prostheses, and oral medications.

VACUUM DEVICES. **Vacuum devices** have been used for many years. The basic design of any model is a cylinder that fits over the penis and sits firmly against the body. Using a pump, a vacuum is created to draw blood into the penis to maintain an erection. The cylinder is then removed. The advantage of this procedure is that the device is easy and safe to use. The disadvantage is its clumsiness and lack of spontaneity. In addition, the man may experience pain from the rubber ring or from pumping the device too quickly. The ring should be removed after an hour, or tissue damage may occur. Most insurance companies pay for this device, which typically costs between $350 and $500.

INTRACORPORAL INJECTIONS. In the 1980s it was discovered that injecting the penis with vasoconstrictive drugs would make the penis erect. The most common agents used for this purpose today are papaverine and phentolamine (Regitine). These drugs may be used alone but are most often given in combination. Adverse effects include priapism (prolonged erection), penile scarring, bleeding, bruising at the injection site, pain, and infection.

INTRAURETHRAL APPLICATIONS. In a single-use urethral suppository, alprostadil (Muse) is self-administered with an applicator. The drug is absorbed into the corpora, which causes an erection in about 10 minutes. Advantages include the simplicity of the procedure and noninvasiveness. Disadvantages are a decrease in spontaneity, burning of the urethra, syncope ("blackout") after the application, and cost.

PROSTHESES. **Penile implants** have been used for more than 20 years and are still used when other modalities fail. The three-piece inflatable device is the most commonly implanted prosthesis. This surgical procedure is performed on an ambulatory basis. To inflate the prosthesis, the man squeezes the pump located in the scrotum. To deflate the prosthesis, a release button is activated. Advantages include the man's ability to control his erections. The major disadvantage is that the device is permanent.

Postoperatively, the nurse gives the client instructions for home care. These instructions are similar to postoperative instructions for any client, including observation for bleeding and infection.

ORAL THERAPIES. The most promising oral medication to treat ED is sildenafil (Viagra), used to treat both types of the problem. Clients are instructed to take the pill 1 hour before sexual intercourse. Sexual stimulation is needed within a half hour to 1 hour to promote the erection. Because the erection occurs more naturally when compared with other treatment options, most men and their partners prefer this option.

Clients should abstain from alcohol before sexual intercourse because it may impair the ability to have an erection. Common side effects of the drug include headaches, facial flushing, and diarrhea. If more than 1 pill a day is being taken, leg and back cramps, nausea, and vomiting may be added to the more common side effects. Men who take nitrates should not take Viagra because of vasodilation effects.

TESTICULAR CANCER

OVERVIEW

Although malignant tumors of the testis are rare and represent less than 2% of all cancers in men, testicular cancer is the most common malignancy in males ages 15 to 35 years (American Cancer Society, 2000). Testicular cancer strikes young men at a productive time of life and thus has significant economic, social, and psychologic impact on the client and his family or significant others. However, with the advent of combination chemotherapy and earlier detection by testicular self-examination (TSE) (Chart 76-8), this form of cancer can be one of the most curable solid neoplasms.

Pathophysiology

Primary testicular cancers fall into two major groups:

- Germinal tumors arising from the sperm-producing germ cells
- Nongerminal tumors arising from the other structures in the testes

Germinal tumors are the most common type of testicular tumors, accounting for more than 95% of cases.

GERMINAL TUMORS

Germinal tumors of the testis are classified into two broad categories: seminomas and nonseminomas (Table 76-1).

SEMINOMAS. The most common type of testicular tumor is **seminoma.** Clients with pure seminomatous tumors have the most favorable prognoses because the tumors generally remain localized and metastasize late. In most clients with seminomatous testicular tumors, seminomas are diagnosed when they are confined to the testicles and retroperitoneal lymph nodes. These tumors also respond extremely well to radiation therapy. Clients with early-stage seminomas have about a 95% 5-year survival rate with surgery (orchiectomy) and radiation therapy (American Cancer Society, 2000).

NONSEMINOMAS. Nonseminomatous germ cell tumors include three types: embryonal carcinoma, teratoma, and choriocarcinoma.

These tumors are made up of cells that are not as sensitive to treatment with radiation therapy. They are treated with surgery or chemotherapy, depending on the extent of the disease at presentation.

Pure embryonal carcinomas are common in young men between the ages of 19 and 26 years. Embryonal carcinomas tend to spread earlier than seminomas and usually first affect the retroperitoneal lymph nodes. This type of tumor may also spread via the bloodstream to other sites in the body, such as the lung or the liver. Pure teratomas rarely occur. They are usually found mixed with other types of testicular tumors. Choriocarcinoma is a lethal type of nonseminomatous cancer, which spreads rapidly throughout the body. Clients with choriocarcinomas almost always have metastatic disease at the initial diagnosis because choriocarcinoma spreads via the hematogenous route rather than via the lymphatic system.

MIXED CELL TYPES. Testicular cancers with a mixture of cell types are also common. Almost any combination of germ cell tumors is possible, but the most common combination is embryonal carcinoma and teratoma *(teratocarcinoma).* About 25% of all testicular cancers are teratocarcinomas.

NONGERMINAL TUMORS

The remaining 5% of testicular tumors arise from the nongerminal elements in the testes, such as the interstitial cells or cells that make up fibrous or vascular networks. Nongerminal testicular neoplasms are classified as either *interstitial cell tumors* or *androblastomas* (testicular adenomas).

Interstitial cell tumors arise from the Leydig cells, which secrete testosterone into the bloodstream. These tumors are rare and usually benign. They may secrete an excessive amount of androgenic hormones, which cause young boys with such tumors to undergo early puberty.

Androblastomas are also rare and usually benign. They sometimes secrete estrogen, which accounts for the feminization and gynecomastia (breast enlargement) occasionally seen in these clients.

Etiology

The cause of testicular cancer is unknown. The risk for testicular tumors is reported to be higher in males who have an undescended testis **(cryptorchidism).** In males with cryptorchidism, the testicular cancer usually develops in the undescended testis (80%), and there is a 25% chance of cancer developing in the normally descended testis. Seminoma is the most common type of testicular cancer associated with cryptorchidism. The undescended testis undergoes gradual involution and degeneration over time, which may contribute to

CHART 76-8

CLIENT EDUCATION GUIDE
Testicular Self-Examination

- Examine your testicles monthly immediately after a bath or a shower, when your scrotal skin is relaxed.
- Examine each testicle by gently rolling it between your thumbs and fingers. Testicular tumors tend to appear deep in the center of the testicle.
- Report any lump or swelling to your doctor as soon as possible.

TABLE 76-1 • CLASSIFICATION OF TESTICULAR TUMORS

GERMINAL (GERM CELL) TUMORS
- Seminoma
- Nonseminoma
    - Embryonal carcinoma
    - Teratoma
    - Choriocarcinoma

NONGERMINAL (NON–GERM CELL) TUMORS
- Intestinal cell tumor
- Androblastoma

tumor development. It is not known why the normally descended testis is at risk for cancer. Brothers and close male relatives of clients with testicular cancer have a slightly greater risk of testicular cancer than the general population.

Although a history of trauma or infection is common in clients with testicular cancer, neither has been established as a cause of testicular cancer and may be coincidental findings at the time of the testicular examination. The client with a history of trauma or infection should be examined by a health care provider after the acute episode subsides to rule out the existence of a tumor.

Testicular cancer is rarely bilateral. There is only a minute chance that a client with a tumor in one testis will have another primary testicular tumor in the other testis. In rare instances, leukemias, lymphomas, plasmacytomas, and metastatic carcinomas may involve the testes. A client with bilateral testicular tumors is more likely to have metastatic disease to the testes than bilateral primary testicular tumors.

Incidence/Prevalence

In the United States it is estimated that 7400 new cases of testicular cancer will be diagnosed each year, and an estimated 300 men will die of the disease. This cancer is the most common solid tumor diagnosed in men between the ages of 15 and 40 years. Testicular cancer can occur during infancy and middle age (after age 50); however, the peak incidence is between the ages of 18 and 40 years (American Cancer Society, 2000).

CULTURAL CONSIDERATIONS

Testicular cancer occurs most often in Caucasians and is rare in African Americans (American Cancer Society, 2000).

COLLABORATIVE MANAGEMENT

Assessment

HISTORY

When taking a history from a client with a suspected testicular tumor, the nurse keeps the risk factors in mind. Basic but important data to collect are age and race, because the disease occurs most often in young Caucasian males. The nurse is also alert to other risk factors, including a history or presence of an undescended testis and a family history of testicular cancer.

The nurse then assesses the client's family situation. Is the client married? Does he have children? Does he want children in the future? Depending on the treatment plan chosen, would he be interested in sperm storage in a sperm bank?

If the client has one healthy testis, he can function sexually and may not have any reproductive dysfunction. If the client undergoes a retroperitoneal lymph node dissection or chemotherapy, he may become sterile because of treatment effects on the sperm-producing cells or surgical trauma to the sympathetic nervous system, resulting in retrograde ejaculations.

PHYSICAL ASSESSMENT/CLINICAL MANIFESTATIONS

The testes, lymph nodes, and abdomen are thoroughly examined. The health care provider or generalist nurse palpates the testes for lumps or swelling (Chart 76-9). The presence of any palpable lymphadenopathy, abdominal masses, or gynecomastia (enlarged breasts) usually indicates metastatic disease.

CHART 76-9

FOCUSED ASSESSMENT *of* A Male Client with a Testicular Lump

Obtain a medical history from the client:
- When was the lump discovered?
- Are there any other symptoms (sensation of heaviness, dragging in testicle, pain, discharge from penis)?
- Is there a history of cryptorchidism?

Assess the genital system. Always wear gloves during the examination of the male genitalia.
- Inspect and palpate the scrotal contents. Have the client perform a Valsalva maneuver, and palpate for a varicocele.
- Any lump or enlargement that does not transilluminate should be suspected as malignant.

Palpate for any enlarged lymph nodes. Most common lymphadenopathy is in the inguinal or supraclavicular regions.

Assess the abdomen for a possible mass or hepatomegaly.

PSYCHOSOCIAL ASSESSMENT

Because the diagnosis of testicular cancer usually occurs in the young adult, the nurse pays close attention to the psychosocial ramifications of the disease. Even if the cancer is detected at an early stage and the client is cured after orchiectomy, he may be afraid that he will be sexually handicapped. Even if the client's disease is arrested with surgery, radiation, or chemotherapy, he may think of himself as less than a whole man. These fears can disrupt the psychosocial and sexual development of the young male and can threaten the identity of adult males. The client may be afraid that he will not be able to perform sexually, will no longer be sexually attractive or desirable, and will face rejection. Feelings of sexual inadequacy may be denied, repressed, or displaced, causing increased stress on the man's personal and work relationships.

The nurse performs a psychosocial assessment of these clients on a routine basis because problems may arise at any time. The nurse also makes referrals to other resources as appropriate.

LABORATORY ASSESSMENT

An important diagnostic indicator for the client with a testicular mass is the presence of any serum or urinary marker proteins (tumor markers) that are often produced by testicular cancers. Benign testicular tumors *never* cause an elevation in the levels of any of these marker proteins.

The primary tumor markers for testicular cancer are **alpha-fetoprotein (AFP)** and the beta subunit of human chorionic gonadotropin (hCG). Approximately 90% of clients with nonseminomatous testicular tumors (embryonal carcinoma, teratoma, or choriocarcinoma) initially have elevated serum levels of AFP, hCG, or both. Clients with a pure seminoma do not have an elevated AFP level, and only 10% have a slightly elevated hCG level. This level resolves after orchiectomy.

If a client has a diagnosis of seminoma and also has an elevated AFP level, the tumor specimen must be re-examined for evidence of a component of nonseminomatous cancer. This step is necessary because the treatments differ for seminomatous and nonseminomatous tumors.

AFP and hCG determinations are also used to evaluate responses to therapy for testicular cancer and to document the presence of residual or recurrent disease. With effective treatment, the levels of abnormal markers fall. The persistence of elevated levels of markers after orchiectomy is substantive evidence that the client has metastatic disease, even if results of clinical staging procedures (x-ray studies and scans) are normal. The reappearance of the tumor markers heralds a recurrence of the cancer. Therefore marker levels must be monitored regularly during the follow-up of clients treated for testicular cancer.

OTHER DIAGNOSTIC ASSESSMENT

After the diagnosis of testicular cancer, the client should have a computed tomography (CT) scan of the abdomen and the chest, or chest tomograms, to identify any small lesions not apparent on conventional x-ray films or physical assessment.

Magnetic resonance imaging (MRI) is used to detect enlarged lymph nodes and abnormal nodules in certain organs that may indicate metastasis from the testicles. Chest x-ray studies and bone scans may also be performed if metastasis is suspected.

Clients with a pure seminoma may undergo bipedal lymphangiography as part of the staging workup to assess for any evidence of retroperitoneal lymph node involvement. Lymphangiograms are also valuable in determining the extent of radiation therapy fields.

Analysis

COMMON NURSING DIAGNOSES AND COLLABORATIVE PROBLEMS

A common nursing diagnosis in clients with testicular cancer is Risk for Sexual Dysfunction related to disease or treatment. A common collaborative problem is Potential for Metastasis.

ADDITIONAL NURSING DIAGNOSES AND COLLABORATIVE PROBLEMS

In addition to the common nursing diagnoses and collaborative problems, clients with testicular cancer may have one or more of the following:

- Dysfunctional Grieving or Anticipatory Grieving related to loss of a body part or changes in body function
- Disturbed Body Image related to the diagnosis of cancer and its treatment
- Acute or Chronic Pain related to tumor compression or effects of metastasis
- Anxiety related to the diagnosis of cancer

Planning and Implementation

RISK FOR SEXUAL DYSFUNCTION

NOC **PLANNING: EXPECTED OUTCOMES.** The client with testicular cancer is expected to identify potential or actual alterations in reproductive function and identify alternative methods of meeting reproductive needs if necessary.

INTERVENTIONS. At the time of diagnosis, the incidence of **oligospermia** (low sperm count) and **azoospermia** (minimal sperm) is increased in clients with testicular cancer. This finding may be due to the disease process itself and to stress, but the exact reasons are unknown. The client may not discover that he is oligospermic or azoospermic until he has a presurgery sperm count.

> **CHART 76-10**
>
> **CLIENT EDUCATION GUIDE**
> **Sperm Banking**
>
> - You may want to investigate sperm storage in a sperm bank as a way to preserve your sperm for future use.
> - No one knows how long sperm can be stored successfully, but pregnancies have resulted from sperm stored for longer than 10 years.
> - Check with the sperm bank to see how much it charges to process and store your sperm and to see whether you must pay when the service is provided.
> - Investigate whether your health insurance company will reimburse you for sperm collection and storage.

Male cancer clients who are not candidates for sperm storage in a sperm bank may select from other options such as donor insemination, adoption, or not fathering children. The nurse initiates health teaching about reproduction, fertility, and sexuality in the pretreatment phase. Normal reproductive function is reviewed, as well as the possible effects of cancer and its treatment on reproductive function. The nurse explains various reproductive options (e.g., sperm banks and artificial insemination) (Chart 76-10). The sperm bank facility provides comprehensive information on semen collection, storage of semen, the storage contract, costs, and the insemination process.

When preparing the client for the collection and storage of sperm, the nurse assumes the role of client advocate and keeps in mind the effect of the cancer diagnosis on the client. The psychologic benefit of having stored sperm may be important for the client and may influence his response to treatment. Knowing that the potential for being a father still exists may help the client cope with other assaults to his masculinity, such as alopecia or erectile dysfunction (ED).

The client should arrange for semen storage as soon as possible after diagnosis. Sperm collection should be completed *before* he begins radiation therapy or chemotherapy or undergoes a radical retroperitoneal lymph node dissection. After radiation therapy or chemotherapy has been implemented, the client may be at increased risk for producing mutagenic sperm, which may not be viable or may result in fetal abnormalities.

The recommended number of samples to optimize the chances of later fertilization is three to six ejaculates, collected 2 to 4 days apart. The process of sperm collection can delay treatment for as long as 1 month, especially if the client is still recovering from surgery and multiple procedures or tests. The client's diagnosis (e.g., acute leukemia, sarcoma, advanced lymphoma, or testicular cancer) and his physical condition may not allow treatment to be postponed, thus making sperm storage an unfeasible reproductive option.

POTENTIAL FOR METASTASIS

PLANNING: EXPECTED OUTCOMES. The client with testicular cancer is expected not to experience complications of the tumor, including metastasis or recurrence of disease.

INTERVENTIONS. A combination of nonsurgical and surgical management is often necessary to prevent metastatic disease (or to alleviate symptoms associated with it) and to bring about tumor regression. The nurse explains the interventions for treating testicular cancer.

NONSURGICAL MANAGEMENT. Chemotherapy and radiation therapy are indicated for nonsurgical management of clients at high risk for metastatic disease or those with metastatic disease.

CHEMOTHERAPY. Combination chemotherapy may be used as adjuvant therapy for *nonseminomatous* testicular tumors or as primary treatment when there is evidence of metastatic disease. Combination chemotherapy is dramatically effective in treating nonseminomatous testicular cancer, particularly if cisplatin (Platinol) is used. This agent is necessary in any successful combination chemotherapy regimen for treating testicular cancer.

The following are other drugs commonly used in combination with cisplatin:

- Bleomycin sulfate (Blenoxane)
- Vinblastine sulfate (Velban, Velbe✤)
- Etoposide (VP-16, VePesid)
- Dactinomycin (Cosmegen)
- Cyclophosphamide (Cytoxan, Procytox✤)
- Doxorubicin (Adriamycin)

The specific combination of drugs, the route of administration, and the frequency, cycling, and duration of treatment can vary considerably from client to client, depending on the extent of the disease and the protocol being followed by the health care provider. Chapter 25 discusses the nursing care of the client receiving chemotherapy.

RADIATION THERAPY. After orchiectomy (removal of one or both testes), external beam radiation therapy is the treatment of choice for clients with pure seminomatous testicular cancer because of the marked radiosensitivity of this type of testicular cancer. If radiation therapy is administered, a staging lymphangiogram is used to determine the treatment portals. An advantage of using radiation therapy instead of radical lymph node dissection is that reproductive function is preserved because surgical dissection of the sympathetic ganglia is avoided.

For the client undergoing radiation therapy to the retroperitoneal lymph nodes, the remaining testis is shielded with a lead cup to preserve reproductive function. Yet, even with these precautions, the client may have transient oligospermia (a decreased sperm count) as a result of radiation scatter. Normally, the sperm count returns to the pretreatment level within 24 to 30 months after the radiation treatment is completed. If metastases develop outside the lymphatic system, the client may still be cured with radiation therapy if the area of involvement is limited. If lymphatic involvement is extensive, or if the visceral organs are involved, the health care provider uses combination chemotherapy similar to that for nonseminomatous testicular cancer.

STEM CELL TRANSPLANTATION. Studies are being conducted to explore whether high-dose chemotherapy with stem cell transplantation may be valuable in treating men with advanced germ cell cancer. In this procedure, the client's blood-forming stem cells are removed from the bone marrow and preserved by freezing while the client receives high-dose chemotherapy. Once the chemotherapy is completed, the stem cells are returned to the client. This procedure helps to prevent the infection and anemia that accompany chemotherapeutic drug use.

SURGICAL MANAGEMENT. The physician performs a unilateral orchiectomy for diagnosis and uses primary surgical management. Clients with testicular cancer may also undergo a radical retroperitoneal lymph node dissection. Using this procedure, the physician can accurately stage the disease and debulk (reduce) the tumor volume so that chemotherapy or radiation therapy is more effective.

PREOPERATIVE CARE. Like most clients with cancer, the client with testicular cancer is usually apprehensive. The nurse offers support and reinforces the teaching provided by the surgeon.

The client's postoperative needs should be anticipated and planned for before surgery. The physician's office nurse or case manager informs the client and his family or significant others about what to expect after surgery. The surgical incision for a retroperitoneal lymph node dissection is extensive. Depending on the extent of the dissection and the need for surgical exploration, the surgeon might make not only a midline incision but also a transthoracic incision or a combination of the two incisions (thoracoabdominal).

The nurse informs the client that radical retroperitoneal lymph node dissections are relatively long operations, lasting 6 to 12 hours. These clients need close and frequent observation, which may be done by nurses in a critical care unit.

OPERATIVE PROCEDURES. To perform a radical retroperitoneal lymph node dissection, the surgeon removes the retroperitoneal nodes in the iliac and lumbar regions. Because the blood supply and the lymphatic vessels of the testes and kidneys are directly related, an extensive midline incision from the xiphoid process to the pubis is necessary. After mobilization of the colon, the surgeon removes the perinephric nodes along with the nodes near the aorta and both renal hila. The node dissection also includes the inguinal area on the affected side. During the lymphadenectomy, the sympathetic ganglia around the lower lumbar lymphatics are dissected. The removal of the sympathetic ganglia abolishes peristalsis in the ductus deferens and contractions of the seminal vesicles. This disruption results in sterility because the client's ejaculate no longer contains sperm. The surgery, however, usually does not interfere with the client's ability to have a normal erection and does not affect his ability to experience orgasm.

A gel-filled silicone prosthesis can usually be surgically implanted into the scrotum at the time of the orchiectomy or later, if the client desires. The nurse reassures the client that this procedure does not impair fertility or sexual function; the client cosmetically appears to have two testes.

POSTOPERATIVE CARE. Because of the length of the surgery, the manipulation of the abdominal and retroperitoneal viscera, and the loss of a major part of the lymphatic fluid, nodes, and channels, the nurse observes and assesses the client for any of the complications of major abdominal surgery. The nurse intervenes for any of the following expected problems:

- Pain from surgical incisions
- Immobility related to prolonged maintenance of surgical positioning and postoperative pain
- Injuries related to any invasive catheters or tubes

The client is usually hospitalized for 3 to 4 days after a radical retroperitoneal lymph node dissection. During this time, the nurse explains care after discharge.

CRITICAL THINKING CHALLENGE

While visiting your sister, she confides that her husband has just been diagnosed with early-stage testicular cancer. She wants to have children and is very concerned about her husband's future and the possibility of starting a family. She was told by the physician that there are several options for treatment and having a family, but she is confused and scared.

- What reassurance can you give your sister at this time?
- How will they be able to have children if he is treated for cancer?
- What options will your brother-in-law have to treat his cancer?

For suggested answer guidelines, go to SIMON http://www.wbsaunders.com/SIMON/Iggy/.

Community-Based Care

After an orchiectomy, the client is typically hospitalized for 1 to 2 days. This period may need to be extended if he must undergo additional surgery or chemotherapy. Because it may not be known until after the orchiectomy whether the client has cancer, what type of testicular cancer he has, or if he needs additional surgery or treatment with radiation therapy or chemotherapy, specific discharge planning may need to be deferred until the postoperative period.

HEALTH TEACHING

For the client who has undergone testicular surgery, the nurse emphasizes the importance of scheduling a follow-up visit with the physician, who will examine the incision for healing and complications. The nurse instructs the client to notify the physician if any of the following symptoms occurs before the scheduled appointment: chills, fever, increasing tenderness or pain around the incision, drainage, or dehiscence of the incision.

These symptoms may indicate the presence of an infection for which medical attention is needed. The nurse instructs the client that he will be able to resume most of his usual activities within 1 week after discharge, except for lifting heavy objects (objects weighing 20 pounds [9.1 kg]) or stair climbing. The nurse also reminds him to ask his physician when strenuous activities may be resumed.

The client who has undergone an orchiectomy is informed that he may make arrangements with his physician to have a silicone prosthesis inserted into the scrotum if a prosthesis was not inserted during the orchiectomy.

The nurse also explains the importance of performing monthly testicular self-examination (TSE) on the remaining testis and scheduling follow-up examinations with the physician. The client who has had testicular cancer should schedule determinations of urinary and serum levels of tumor markers and computed tomography (CT) or magnetic resonance imaging (MRI) studies as part of his routine follow-up for a minimum of 3 years.

Depending on the pathologic findings and the stage of the cancer, the client may need further treatment. This information may not be available at the time of discharge. If it is known that the client needs further surgery, he and his family need information about the future surgery. If it is known that he must undergo radiation therapy or chemotherapy, he needs education about a radiation therapy and chemotherapy regimen.

The client who undergoes treatment for testicular cancer may need emotional support. If permanent sterility occurs and sperm storage has not been feasible, the man may need counseling about other reproductive options.

HOME CARE MANAGEMENT

After a unilateral orchiectomy, unless the client has a wound complication, he is discharged without a dressing on the inguinal incision. The client may want to wear a dressing to prevent his clothing from rubbing on the sutures and producing irritation. Because his sutures are intact at the time of discharge, he is told that they will be removed in the physician's office 7 to 10 days postoperatively.

HEALTH CARE RESOURCES

The client may be referred to agencies or support groups such as the American Fertility Society or RESOLVE (an organization for infertile couples).

Evaluation: Outcomes

NOC The nurse evaluates the care of the client who has been treated for testicular cancer on the basis of the identified nursing diagnoses and collaborative problems. The expected outcomes include that the client will:

- Not experience a recurrence of cancer or metastases
- Accept body image changes and show adaptation to his altered self-concept
- Verbalize feelings of grief
- Recover from surgery, chemotherapy, or radiation therapy without complications
- Verbalize an understanding of the effects of surgery or radiation therapy on sexual function and identify alternative methods of meeting reproductive needs

OTHER COMMON PROBLEMS AFFECTING THE TESTES AND ADJACENT STRUCTURES

Problems that develop inside the scrotum usually occur as a mass or as scrotal edema. Some problems produce pain, but others do not. Figure 76-7 shows some of the most common conditions found in the male, including hydrocele, spermatocele, varicocele, and scrotal trauma.

Hydrocele

OVERVIEW

A **hydrocele** is a cystic mass, usually filled with straw-colored fluid, that forms around the testis (see Figure 76-7). It results from a disorder in the lymphatic drainage of the scrotum, causing a swelling of the tunica vaginalis, which surrounds the testes. Unless the swelling becomes large and uncomfortable or begins to compromise the circulation to the testis, no treatment is necessary.

COLLABORATIVE MANAGEMENT

A hydrocele may be aspirated via a needle and syringe, or it may be removed surgically. To correct a hydrocele surgically,

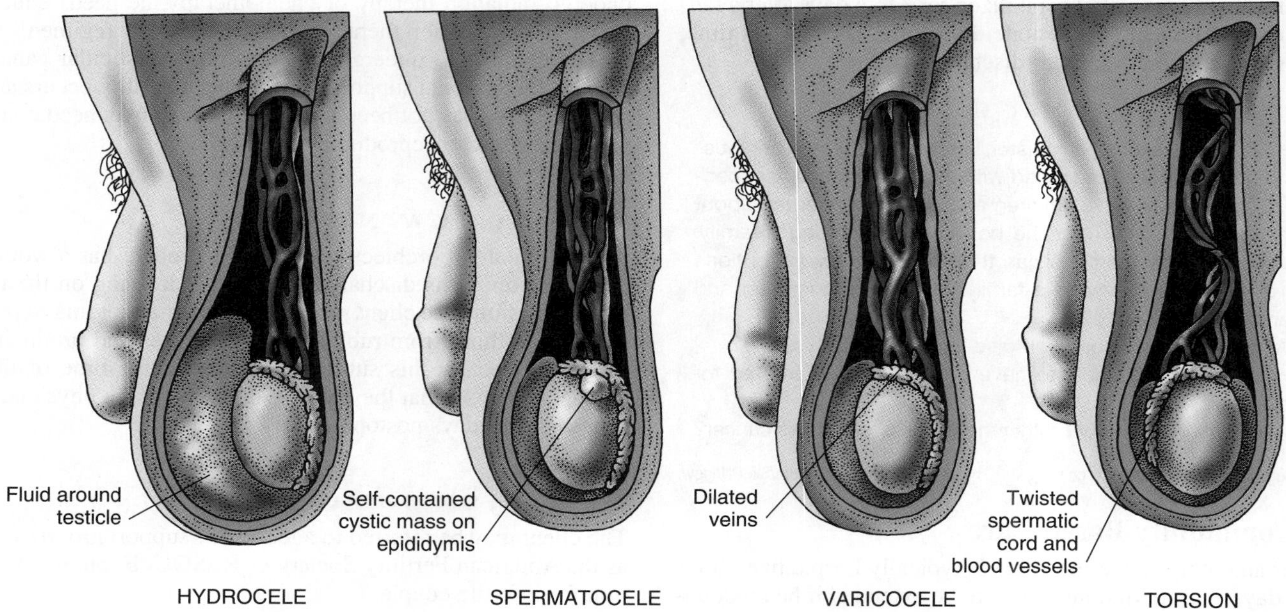

Figure 76-7 ● Common problems affecting the testes and adjacent structures.

the physician makes an incision in the scrotum and removes the hydrocele. The client may or may not return from the operating suite with a drain at the incision site. Typically, hydrocelectomies are performed on an outpatient basis; if the client requires hospitalization, it is for only 1 or 2 days. The nurse instructs the client that if an incision drain is present, there may be some serosanguineous drainage for the first 24 to 48 hours after surgery. The nurse also explains the importance of wearing a scrotal support. The scrotal support keeps the scrotal dressing in place and keeps the scrotum elevated, which helps to prevent edema.

Clients vary considerably in the degree of pain that they experience with this surgery. The nurse assesses and observes the client for pain every 2 to 3 hours in the immediate postoperative period. Moderate incision pain is expected for approximately 24 hours after surgery and should markedly decrease within 1 or 2 days. If the client's pain does not resolve within this time, the nurse is alert to the possible development of wound complications.

The client is instructed to schedule a follow-up visit with the surgeon to have the wound evaluated for healing. The nurse stresses the importance of continuing to wear a scrotal support to promote drainage and comfort. The scrotum can remain swollen from residual inflammation and edema for as long as several weeks. The client is reassured that this swelling is normal and eventually subsides.

Spermatocele

A **spermatocele** is a sperm-containing cystic mass that develops on the epididymis alongside the testicle (see Figure 76-7). Normally, spermatoceles remain small and asymptomatic, and no interventions are necessary. If the spermatocele becomes large enough to cause discomfort to the client, a spermatocelectomy is performed. In this simple procedure, the spermatocele is excised through a small scrotal incision. Routinely, no incision drain is used because drainage and swelling are minimal.

Varicocele

OVERVIEW

A **varicocele** is a cluster of dilated veins posterior to and above the testis (see Figure 76-7). The diagnosis is made by scrotal palpation, particularly when the client performs a Valsalva maneuver. The scrotum feels "wormlike" when palpated. Varicoceles can be either unilateral or bilateral, but most are unilateral and on the left side of the scrotum. In many cases, varicoceles are asymptomatic, with no treatment required. In a few men, varicoceles are painful and must be removed surgically.

Varicoceles can also cause infertility. It is thought that the increase in scrotal temperature resulting from the venous stasis near the testis is the cause of the altered spermatogenesis.

COLLABORATIVE MANAGEMENT

A **varicocelectomy** (surgical removal of the varicocele) is usually performed through an inguinal incision, in which the spermatic veins are ligated in the cord, or through an incision adjacent to the superior iliac spine, in which the spermatic veins are ligated in the retroperitoneal space. A varicocelectomy may be done on an ambulatory care basis, or the client may be hospitalized overnight.

Before surgery, the nurse explains to the client that persistent venous congestion of the scrotum is common after this type of surgery because of the changed circulation in the area. To promote drainage of the scrotum, a rolled towel is placed under the scrotum while the client is in bed. The nurse may also apply ice to the scrotum if necessary. Any intervention that facilitates drainage and decreases swelling from the area promotes relief. The nurse instructs the client about the importance of wearing a scrotal support while ambulating.

At the time of discharge, the nurse instructs the client to make a follow-up appointment with the surgeon to have the sutures removed. The nurse also reminds him to notify the physician of any increasing discomfort at the incision site or in the scrotum, which might indicate an infection. Increasing scrotal discomfort can mean that the circulation to the testis has been impaired. Testicular atrophy, a rare complication of a varicocelectomy, may occur if the blood supply to the testis becomes insufficient.

Scrotal Trauma

Because of the mobility of the scrotum, scrotal injuries are relatively rare. Torsion of the testes involves the twisting of the spermatic cord and occurs most often during puberty (see Figure 76-7). Torsion may occur after strenuous exercise or trauma, or it may develop spontaneously. Because the testes are sensitive to any decrease in blood flow, torsion of the testis is considered a surgical emergency. The client experiences pain, which does not subside with scrotal elevation. In addition to pain, he usually complains of nausea and vomiting.

In addition to caring for the client's physical needs, the nurse is also attuned to his psychosexual needs. Of primary concern to the male client with an injury to his external genitalia are his masculinity and sexuality. The nurse is prepared to use crisis intervention techniques and is knowledgeable about sexuality in order to help the client adjust to an injury in the genital area.

At discharge, the nurse instructs the client to maintain ice to the scrotum for at least 72 hours and elevate the scrotum to minimize edema. The client should avoid lifting heavy objects for 4 to 6 weeks, limit stair climbing, and suspend strenuous physical activity for 1 month. The client is also reminded to wear a scrotal support for at least 3 weeks (Miller, 1999).

Cryptorchidism

An undescended testis, or **cryptorchidism,** is mainly a pediatric problem. Three percent of full-term male infants and 20% of premature infants have an undescended testis. In 80% of cases, the undescended testis descends spontaneously during the infant's first year. If an adult has cryptorchidism, an **orchidopexy** (surgical placement of the testicle into the scrotum) may be performed for cosmetic and psychosexual reasons. The surgery may also prevent the adverse effect of body temperature on spermatogenesis and reduce the risk of testicular cancer. As an alternative, an orchiectomy of the cryptorchid testicle may be recommended.

During an orchidopexy, the client is placed in a supine position. The surgeon makes an inguinal incision, and the spermatic cord is released from the surrounding fascia to obtain maximal length. The surgeon then creates a dartos pouch and places the testis between the skin and the dartos muscle of the scrotum. The tunica albuginea of the testis is sutured to the dartos muscle of the scrotum. The inguinal incision and the scrotal incision (if there is one) are then closed, and a dressing is applied. If there is an incision in the scrotum, it is also covered with a dressing and the client is instructed to wear a scrotal support.

Cancer of the Penis

OVERVIEW

Cancer of the penis represents less than 1% of all malignancies in men in the United States.

> **CULTURAL CONSIDERATIONS**
> Epidermoid carcinoma is the most common cancer of the penis. In countries where circumcision is not practiced, such as India, China, and Africa, this type of cancer represents 12% of all cancers (American Cancer Society, 2000).

COLLABORATIVE MANAGEMENT

Assessment

Carcinoma of the penis usually occurs as a painless, wartlike growth or ulcer on the glans under the prepuce (foreskin) and may initially be mistaken for a venereal wart. A penile carcinoma may also appear as a reddened lesion with plaque.

Interventions

Small lesions involving only the skin may be controlled by excisional biopsy. When the lesion is not curable by excisional biopsy or radiation therapy, a **penectomy** (partial or total removal of the penis) may be required.

PARTIAL PENECTOMY. When the lesion is limited to the glans, a partial penectomy is performed. The client is placed in the lithotomy position, and a tourniquet is applied around the penis. The surgeon makes an incision to amputate a portion of the corpus cavernosum and the corpus spongiosum. The urethra is anastomosed to the skin, and a dressing is applied. A Foley catheter is in place for 3 to 5 days after surgery until the edema surrounding the urethra subsides. The nurse assesses the dressing for drainage, which should be minimal. The catheter is checked for patency every 4 hours for the first postoperative day.

TOTAL PENECTOMY. A total penectomy is required when the lesion has penetrated the shaft of the penis or when the tumor has recurred after a partial penectomy or radiation therapy. The client is placed in the lithotomy position. The surgeon makes an incision from the pubic bone, which encircles the penis and extends into the perineum. The bases of both corpora cavernosa are exposed and excised, and the penis is amputated. The surgeon places an incision drain in the wound before it is sutured. Clients who undergo a total penectomy also have a perineal urethrotomy (anastomosis of the urethra to the skin in the perineum) for urinary drainage.

After a total penectomy, the nurse observes the incision dressing every 2 to 4 hours during the first 24 to 48 hours. There may be a moderate amount of serosanguineous drainage from the incision drains.

The nurse is aware that regardless of how accepting the client may appear preoperatively, he may experience severe emotional problems postoperatively. After a partial penectomy, the client must adjust to considerable changes in body image and sexuality. The nurse encourages him to verbalize his feelings about the loss of his penis. After a total penectomy, the client can no longer have penile-vaginal or penile-anal intercourse and cannot urinate in a standing position. It is difficult for most clients to accept the possibility that they might die because of a lesion on the penis, especially because they are rarely experiencing any systemic cancer symptoms and are otherwise healthy. The nurse helps the client realize that the removal of his penis may save his life. The nurse is aware of the possibility of suicide attempts, since the client's penis may be more important to him than his life. The nurse may be the one to detect the need for professional psychologic assistance for the client or his partner. Early interventions by the nurse can make a tremendous difference in the client's or partner's well-being.

Circumcision (the surgical removal of the prepuce from the penis) in infancy almost eliminates the possibility of penile cancer in that chronic irritation and inflammation of the glans penis predispose uncircumcised men to penile cancer. Because of the ongoing controversy about neonatal circumcision, the nurse teaches both men and new mothers of boys that strict personal hygiene is an important preventive measure against penile cancer.

Phimosis

In a man with **phimosis,** the prepuce is constricted so that it cannot be retracted over the glans. Because of the recent trend away from routine circumcision of newborns, the nurse instructs new mothers, male children, and adult men about the importance of cleaning the prepuce. Phimosis is corrected by circumcision.

Circumcision

OVERVIEW

Circumcision (the surgical removal of the prepuce or foreskin) in the adult male is usually done for medical reasons, such as to correct phimosis and to eliminate the infections that often result from this condition.

COLLABORATIVE MANAGEMENT

Circumcision in the adult male is usually performed in a same-day surgical setting. If the client has a dressing, the nurse instructs him to soak in a warm bath that evening to allow the dressing to loosen. If the dressing falls off before the next day, the client is cautioned not to replace it. The nurse explains that the sutures will be absorbed and need not be removed. No residual or side effects result from this surgery, and the client should be able to resume his normal activities within 1 week; sexual intercourse may be resumed after 1 to 2 weeks.

The client may be discharged with a prescription for a barbiturate sleeping medication to be taken for several nights postoperatively. The nurse emphasizes that barbiturate sleeping medications suppress the rapid-eye-movement (REM) phase of sleep so that normal nocturnal erections do not occur. This prevents any tension on the sutures by an erection.

Nonbarbiturate sleeping medications do not inhibit the nocturnal erection pattern. The nurse explains the relationship between barbiturate sleeping medications and nocturnal erections because the client may not comply with the instructions to take the medication, especially if he is not having any difficulty sleeping.

The nurse advises the client to notify his physician if he has any wound complications, such as swelling at the incision area of drainage, and to schedule a postoperative office visit.

Priapism

OVERVIEW

Priapism is an uncontrolled and long-maintained erection without sexual desire, which causes the penis to become large, hard, and painful. Priapism affects the two corpora cavernosa; the corpus spongiosum and glans penis are not affected.

Priapism can occur from neural, vascular, or pharmacologic causes, including the following:

- Thrombosis of the veins of the corpora cavernosa (usually resulting from trauma)
- Leukemia
- Sickle cell anemia
- Diabetes
- Malignancies

Sickle cell disease causes priapism through the accumulation of erythrocytes within the corporal bodies. Leukemia may cause priapism because the increased number of white blood cells (WBCs) permits persistent engorgement of the corporal bodies. Malignancies may also infiltrate the corporal bodies, causing persistent engorgement. Priapism can also result from an abnormal neurogenic reflex, psychotropic medications, antidepressants, and antihypertensive medications.

COLLABORATIVE MANAGEMENT

Priapism is considered a urologic emergency because the circulation to the penis may be compromised and the client may not be able to void with an erect penis. The goal of medical intervention is to improve the venous drainage of the corpora cavernosa. Conservative measures involve prostatic massage, sedation, and bedrest.

Meperidine (Demerol) is usually administered immediately because of its hypotensive effect. Warm enemas may be given to bring about venous dilation and thus increase the outflow of the trapped blood. Urinary catheterization is required if the client cannot void.

If conservative therapy is unsuccessful, treatment may proceed to aspiration of the corpora cavernosa with a large-bore needle or surgical intervention. The priapism should be resolved within the first 24 to 30 hours to prevent penile ischemia, gangrene, fibrosis, and impotence. If a cause of priapism is identified, treatment is directed toward that underlying cause.

The nurse who is caring for the client with priapism is sensitive to his emotional needs. The client may be uncomfortable and in crisis but at the same time embarrassed by his erection and loss of control. The nurse reassures the client that he or she understands that the client is not in control of his erection and provides him with privacy.

Prostatitis

OVERVIEW

A number of inflammatory conditions can affect the prostate gland, causing **prostatitis.** The most common is abacterial prostatitis.

Abacterial Prostatitis

Abacterial prostatitis can occur after a viral illness or may be associated with sexually transmitted diseases (STDs), especially in young males. In many instances, an exact cause of the perineal discomfort cannot be found. The prostatitis can be related to psychosexual problems. The term *prostatodynia* is sometimes used to described this condition.

Bacterial Prostatitis

Bacterial prostatitis is usually associated with urethritis or an infection of the lower urinary tract. Organisms may reach the prostate via the bloodstream or the urethra. The most common organisms are *Escherichia coli, Enterobacter, Proteus,* and group D streptococci. Acute bacterial prostatitis may be manifested by fever, chills, **dysuria** (painful urination), urethral discharge, and a boggy, tender prostate.

Gentle palpation of the prostate usually results in a urethral discharge, which is evidenced by white blood cells (WBCs) in the prostatic secretions.

COLLABORATIVE MANAGEMENT

The client with chronic prostatitis usually complains of backache, perineal pain, mild dysuria, and urinary frequency; hematuria may be present. The prostate may feel irregularly enlarged, firm, and slightly tender when palpated. Complications of prostatitis are epididymitis (inflammation of the epididymis) and cystitis (inflammation of the bladder). A rare complication is a prostatic abscess. The client with either acute or chronic bacterial prostatitis is likely to experience urinary tract infections. Sexual functioning may be diminished because of discomfort.

Early diagnosis and treatment of prostatitis with antimicrobials, such as carbenicillin indanyl sodium (Geocillin, Geopen Oral), or fluoroquinolones (ciprofloxacin [Cipro]), can help prevent an abscess. The nurse emphasizes the importance of comfort measures, such as sitz baths, and taking prescribed antibiotics on schedule. The physician orders stool softeners to prevent straining and rectal irritation of the prostate during a bowel movement. Analgesics may be used for symptomatic relief.

The nurse instructs the client with chronic prostatitis about the long-term nature of the problem. Because prostatitis can cause other urinary tract infections, the nurse explains the importance of increasing fluid intake and long-term antibiotic therapy (therapy lasting 30 days). Because trimethoprim (Bactrim✤, Septra) diffuses into the prostatic fluid, it is the antibiotic of choice. The nurse instructs the client about activities that drain the prostate (sexual intercourse, masturbation, and prostatic massage), which may help in the management of chronic prostatitis.

Epididymitis

OVERVIEW

Epididymitis, an infection of the epididymis, may result from an infection of the prostate. It used to be a frequent complication of gonorrhea. Although not common, epididymitis can also be a complication of long-term use of an indwelling Foley catheter, prostatic surgery, or a cystoscopic examination.

In men younger than 35 years of age, the major causative organism in epididymitis is *Chlamydia trachomatis,* which is transmitted sexually (see Chapter 77). The infective organism passes upward through the urethra and the ejaculatory duct, then along the vas deferens to the epididymis.

The client with epididymitis usually complains of pain along the inguinal canal and along the vas deferens, followed by pain and swelling in the scrotum and the groin. If epididymitis is untreated, the epididymis becomes swollen and painful, and the client's temperature may become elevated. Pyuria and bacteriuria may develop, with resultant chills and fever. An abscess may form, necessitating an orchiectomy (removal of one or both testes).

COLLABORATIVE MANAGEMENT

The nurse instructs the client with epididymitis to remain in bed with his scrotum elevated on a towel to prevent traction on the spermatic cord, to facilitate venous drainage, and to relieve pain. The client may be given antibiotics until all acute symptoms of inflammation are gone. If the epididymitis is chlamydial or gonorrheal in origin, the client's sexual partners are also treated with antibiotics.

The client may find other comfort measures effective, such as applying cold compresses or ice to the scrotum intermittently and taking sitz baths. The nurse advises him to avoid lifting, straining, or sexual activity until the infection is under control (which may take as long as 4 weeks).

In clients with epididymitis, there must always be the suspicion of a testicular tumor, especially if the condition does not resolve in a week or two. Ultrasound study is often done to rule out an abscess or tumor. Clients with recurrent or chronic painful conditions may require an epididymectomy (excision of the epididymis from the testicle).

Orchitis

Orchitis, or acute testicular inflammation, may result from trauma or infection. The infection may be caused by the direct spread of bacteria through the urethra or by an infection elsewhere in the body, such as pneumonia, tuberculosis, gonorrhea, syphilis, or mumps. It is rare that the testes alone are involved; usually both the testes and the epididymis are involved (epididymo-orchitis).

Orchitis may be unilateral or bilateral. If the orchitis is bilateral, the client is at increased risk for sterility because of the testicular atrophy and fibrosis that occur during healing.

The signs and symptoms of orchitis are the same as those of epididymitis (scrotal pain and edema). In addition, the client may experience nausea and vomiting and pain radiating to the inguinal canal.

The treatment of orchitis is the same as for epididymitis and includes the following:

- Bedrest with scrotal elevation
- Application of ice
- Administration of analgesics and antibiotics

Mumps orchitis, which occurs in approximately 20% of males who have mumps after puberty, is usually bilateral, and orchitis symptoms develop 4 to 6 days after the parotitis. Any postpubertal male who has not had mumps and is exposed to or contracts mumps is usually given gamma globulin. Although gamma globulin does not prevent mumps, the clinical course of the disease is likely to be less severe, with fewer complications. Childhood vaccination against mumps is an important preventive measure.

ONLINE RESOURCES

For suggested readings and Internet resources, go to http://www.wbsaunders.com/SIMON/Iggy/.

SELECTED BIBLIOGRAPHY

Asterisk indicates a classic or definitive work on this subject.

American Cancer Society. (2000). *Cancer facts and figures—2000.* Report No. 00-300M-No. 5008.00. Atlanta: Author.

Collins, M. (1997). Increasing prostate cancer awareness in African American men. *Oncology Nursing Forum, 24*(1), 91-95.

Colpo, L. (1998). Evaluation, treatment, and management of erectile dysfunction: An overview. *Urologic Nursing, 18*(2), 100-106.

Gray, M., & Allensworth, D. (1999). Electrovaporization of the prostate: Initial experiences and nursing management. *Urology Nursing, 19*(1), 25-31.

Haas, G.P., & Sakr, W. (1997). Epidemiology of prostate cancer. *CA: A Cancer Journal for Clinicians, 47*(5), 273-285.

Holtgrave, H. (1998). Current trends in management of men with lower urinary tract symptoms and benign prostatic hyperplasia. *Urology, 51* (Suppl. 4A), 1-7.

Huff, R., & Kline, M. (1999). *Promoting health in multicultural populations.* London: Sage.

*Jackson, J., et al. (1996). Biofeedback: A noninvasive treatment for incontinence after radical prostatectomy. *Urology Nursing, 16*(2), 50-54.

Klingman, L. (1999). Assessing the male genitalia. *American Journal of Nursing, 99*(7), 47-50.

Marks, L.S., et al. (2000). Effects of a saw palmetto herbal blend in men with symptomatic benign prostatic hyperplasia. *Journal of Urology, 163*(5), 1451-1456.

Matteson, M.A., McConnell, E.S., & Linton, A.D. (1997). *Gerontological nursing: Concepts and practices* (2nd ed.). Philadelphia: W.B. Saunders.

Mettlin, C. (1997). The American Cancer Society National Prostate Cancer Detection Project and national patterns of prostate cancer detection and treatment. *CA: A Cancer Journal for Clinicians, 47*(5), 265-272.

Miller, K. (1999). Emergency! Testicular torsion: A surgical emergency primarily affecting young men. *American Journal of Nursing, 99*(6), 33.

Parkin, D., et al. (1999). Global cancer statistics. *CA: A Cancer Journal for Clinicians, 49*(1), 33-64.

Pickett, M., et al. (2000). Prostate cancer elder alert: Living with treatment choices and outcomes. *Journal of Gerontological Nursing, 26*(2), 22-34.

Redmond, M.C. (1998). Ultrasonically guided interstitial brachytherapy for prostate cancer: Care of the patient in ambulatory surgery. *Journal of Perianesthesia Nursing, 13*(3), 156-164.

Schmidt, J., Doyle, J., & Larison, S. (1998). Prostate cryoablation: Update 1998. *CA: A Cancer Journal for Clinicians, 48*(4), 239-253.

Tingen, M., et al. (1998). Perceived benefits: A predictor of participation in prostate cancer screening. *Cancer Nursing, 21*(5), 349-357.

Tjoa, B., et al. (1999). Dendritic cell-based immunotherapy for prostate cancer. *CA: A Cancer Journal for Clinicians, 49*(2), 117-128.

von Eschenbach, A., et al. (1997). American Cancer Society guideline for the early detection of prostate cancer: Update 1997. *CA: A Cancer Journal for Clinicians, 47,* 261-264.

Weinrish, S.P., et al. (2000). Barriers to prostate screening. *Cancer Nursing, 23,* 117-121.

CHAPTER 77

Interventions for Clients with Sexually Transmitted Diseases

SHIRLEY E. VAN ZANDT

Learning Objectives

After studying this chapter, you should be able to:

1. Explain how sexually transmitted diseases (STDs) can be prevented.
2. Compare and contrast the stages of syphilis.
3. Prioritize nursing care for the client with syphilis at each stage.
4. Identify the role of drug therapy in managing clients with genital herpes.
5. Discuss the psychosocial effects of having an STD.
6. Develop a teaching plan for clients diagnosed with gonorrhea.
7. Describe the assessment findings that are typical in clients with *Chlamydia trachomatis* infection.
8. Analyze assessment data to determine common nursing diagnoses for women with pelvic inflammatory disease (PID).
9. Formulate a collaborative plan of care for a client with PID.
10. Develop a community-based teaching plan for clients with PID.
11. Evaluate care for a client with PID.
12. Identify common causes of vaginal infections.

SIMON

Go to http://www.wbsaunders.com/SIMON/Iggy/ for self-assessment questions related to these Learning Objectives.

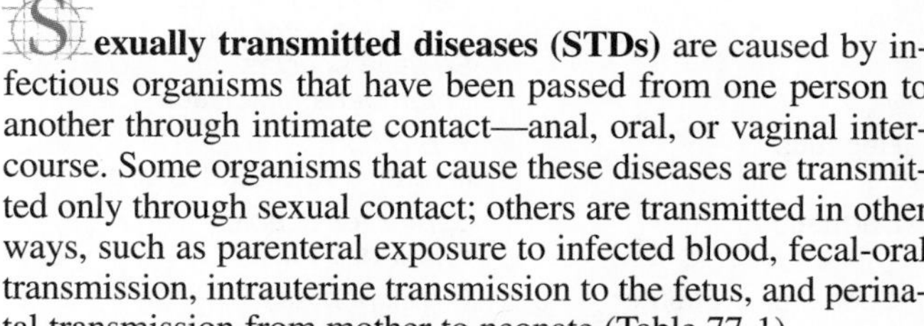

Sexually transmitted diseases (STDs) are caused by infectious organisms that have been passed from one person to another through intimate contact—anal, oral, or vaginal intercourse. Some organisms that cause these diseases are transmitted only through sexual contact; others are transmitted in other ways, such as parenteral exposure to infected blood, fecal-oral transmission, intrauterine transmission to the fetus, and perinatal transmission from mother to neonate (Table 77-1).

The list of STDs continues to grow because of improved diagnostic techniques, an increased number of organisms and systemic diseases that can be sexually transmitted, and sexual attitudes and practices. In the United States, sexual issues are often controversial. The nurse must respect the choices that clients make, and provide confidentiality (see the Legal/Ethical Issues in Health Care box on p. 1806).

The prevalence of STDs is a major health concern worldwide. Increasing population, cultural factors (e.g., later marriages), political and economic policies, and human physiology patterns such as earlier menarche affect the prevalence of STDs in any given geographic area. Sexual attitudes and behaviors and access to care play a major role in the risk of acquiring an STD (Amaral, 1998). STDs also cause complications that can contribute to severe physical and emotional suffering, including infertility, ectopic pregnancy, cancer, and death. Some of the most common complications caused by sexually transmitted organisms are listed in Table 77-2.

STDs and acquired immunodeficiency syndrome (AIDS) are reportable to local health authorities in every state. Some STDs, such as genital herpes, may or may not be reported, depending on local legal requirements. Chlamydial infection is now reportable in most states (Centers for Disease Control and Prevention [CDC], 1998). Rigorous reporting and follow-up efforts by federal and local public health departments and health care providers is one intervention for decreasing the incidence of STDs.

Nurses in a variety of community settings are responsible for identifying clients at risk for STDs, caring for clients with diagnosed STDs, and preventing further cases through education and case finding. Nurses in secondary and tertiary care settings, such as hospitals, also have a responsibility to recognize clients who are at risk for or who have symptoms of STDs. Nurses also need to be aware of the individual and societal costs of the care of clients with STDs (see the Cost of Care box on p. 1807).

The Centers for Disease Control and Prevention (CDC) regularly updates its guidelines for treatment of STDs. The 1998

TABLE 77-1 • SEXUALLY TRANSMITTED DISEASES

- Human immunodeficiency virus infection
- Chancroid
- Syphilis
- Lymphogranuloma venereum
- Genital herpes simplex virus infection
- Genital warts
- Gonococcal infection
- Chlamydial infection
- Nongonococcal urethritis
- Mucopurulent cervicitis
- Epididymitis
- Pelvic inflammatory disease
- Sexually transmitted enteritis
- Sexually transmitted proctitis
- Trichomoniasis
- Candidal infection
- Bacterial vaginosis
- Viral hepatitis
- Cytomegalovirus infection
- Ectoparasitic infection
  - Pediculosis pubis
  - Scabies

From Centers for Disease Control and Prevention. (1998). 1998 guidelines for treatment of sexually transmitted diseases. *Morbidity and Mortality Weekly Report, 47*(No. RR-1), 1-103.

LEGAL/ETHICAL ISSUES IN HEALTH CARE

SEXUAL DECISION MAKING AND CONFIDENTIALITY FOR CLIENTS WITH SEXUALLY TRANSMITTED DISEASES

Sexual issues are surrounded with much controversy in the United States. Personal values, cultural mores, and public health standards often collide as clients make decisions about their sexual health. Americans hold strongly to the principle of autonomy. Autonomy in sexual decision making (e.g., about whether to be sexually active, how to choose sexual partners, and the type of sexual behavior that is appropriate) is held as a high value. The parental right to know about a minor's sexual activity is debated as one challenge to this principle of autonomy. The standard of confidentiality protects this principle of autonomy in some clinical situations and under some state laws.

As nurses aim to respect this principle of autonomy about sexual decision making and confidentiality, they can be challenged by the public health concerns of protecting the health of the entire community versus the autonomy of the individual to make his or her own decisions. Increasing rates of chlamydial infection, especially in the teenage population, with the costly risk of infertility complications, make this notion of autonomy in sexual decision making more problematic. Clients who refuse to discuss their sexually transmitted disease with their partners, or partners who choose not to get tested or treated pose additional challenges to our respect for autonomy in light of the overwhelming public health concerns. Nurses are conflicted in their commitment to both confidentiality (autonomy) and promotion of the public's health (beneficence).

TABLE 77-2 • COMPLICATIONS CAUSED BY SEXUALLY TRANSMITTED ORGANISMS

Complication	Causative Organisms
Salpingitis, infertility, and ectopic pregnancy	*Neisseria gonorrhoeae* *Chlamydia trachomatis* *Mycoplasma hominis* *Ureaplasma urealyticum*
Reproductive loss (abortion/miscarriage)	*N. gonorrhoeae* *C. trachomatis* Herpes simplex virus *M. hominis* *U. urealyticum* *Treponema pallidum*
Puerperal infection	*N. gonorrhoeae* *C. trachomatis*
Perinatal infection	Hepatitis B virus Human immunodeficiency virus Human papillomavirus *N. gonorrhoeae* *C. trachomatis* Herpes simplex virus *T. pallidum* Cytomegalovirus Group B streptococcus
Cancer of genital area	*C. trachomatis* Herpes simplex virus Human papillomavirus
Male urethritis	*M. hominis* Herpes simplex virus *N. gonorrhoeae* *C. trachomatis* *U. urealyticum*
Vulvovaginitis	Herpes simplex virus *Trichomonas vaginalis* Bacteria causing vaginosis *Candida albicans*
Cervicitis	*N. gonorrhoeae* *C. trachomatis* Herpes simplex virus
Proctitis	*N. gonorrhoeae* *C. trachomatis* Herpes simplex virus *Campylobacter jejuni* *Shigella* species *Entamoeba histolytica*
Hepatitis	*T. pallidum* Hepatitis A, B, and C virus
Dermatitis	*Sarcoptes scabiei* *Phthirus pubis*
Genital ulceration or warts	*C. trachomatis* Herpes simplex virus Human papillomavirus *T. pallidum* *Haemophilus ducreyi* *Calymmatobacterium granulomatis*

COST OF CARE IMPLICATIONS FOR NURSING

SEXUALLY TRANSMITTED DISEASES

Cost of Care

- Estimates of annual direct and indirect costs for sexually transmitted diseases (STDs) and their complications in 1994 were $9.9 billion as compared with the national public investment of $231 million in STD prevention (Hein, 1998).
- The Institute of Medicine has estimated that the sequelae of *Chlamydia trachomatis* infections in women (i.e., PID, infertility, and ectopic pregnancy) result in an estimated $4 billion in health care costs per year (Stamm, 1999).
- Approximately $5.5 billion is spent on PID and its sequelae a year (Paavonen, 1998).
- Managed care poses some new obstacles to prevention of STDs. An emphasis on short-term cost savings, differences in technical capabilities for diagnosis and treatment, and challenges to reliable follow-up because partners of those infected may not be members of the same health plan may undermine public health strategies of the past.
- Costs of individual antibiotics used to treat STDs may be a hindrance to proper treatment, especially for the rapidly increasing uninsured segment of the U.S. population.

Costs (Wholesale) of Oral Medications*

ORAL DRUGS	APPROXIMATE COST OF DRUG PER DOSE	APPROXIMATE COST FOR COURSE OF TREATMENT
Acyclovir 200 mg 5 times/day for 10 days	$1.14	$57.00
Azithromycin 1 g once (4 tablets, 250 mg each)	$24.80	$24.80
Cefixime 400 mg once	$6.90	$6.90
Ciprofloxacin 500 mg once	$3.74	$3.74
Clindamycin 450 mg qid for 14 days	$1.56	$87.36
Doxycycline 100 mg bid for 7 days	$0.11	$1.54
Famciclovir 125 mg bid for 5 days	$1.59	$15.90
Metronidazole 500 mg bid for 14 days	$0.06	$1.68
Ofloxacin 400 mg once	$4.34	$4.34
Valacyclovir 500 mg bid for 5 days	$2.82	$28.20

Implications for Nursing

Nurses have a unique role in the prevention and early detection of STDs. Their role has high potential for decreasing the cost of disease to the nation and individuals. Ongoing education with clients about their risk of contracting or transmitting a disease and methods of prevention is essential. Discussing the cost, both financial and emotional, of STDs, including the cost of unintended infertility, is part of the nurse's teaching to clients. Nurses include thorough health histories in their assessment of clients. This information may be more revealing in terms of the client's ability to prevent or treat disease than what other members of the health care team have been able to elicit.

Since most clients are treated for STDs as outpatients, assessing the client's ability to pay for medication and access and pay for follow-up care is a significant part of the nurse's assessment and intervention.

*Modified from Bartlett, J.G. (1998). *Pocket book of infectious disease therapy.* Baltimore: Williams & Wilkins

WOMEN'S HEALTH CONSIDERATIONS

Women are at the greatest risk for health problems caused by STDs. Pregnancy and adolescence substantially increase the risk of transmission and complications. Because of differences in the physiology of reproductive structures, women have greater rates of transmission of STDs if exposed. Adolescence tends to be a time of risk taking. Young women who are sexually active have more frequent unprotected sexual intercourse than their older counterparts because of the following:

- Lack of knowledge about the risk of disease
- Their belief that they are not vulnerable to disease
- Alcohol consumption, which promotes risky sexual behavior

The rates of many STDs are highest among adolescents, more frequently in adolescent females (CDC, 1998). Postmenopausal women also may be at high risk for STDs, since many do not use barrier protection because of age-related infertility. Mucosal tears from vaginal atrophy in postmenopausal women may also place them at greater risk (Rosen & Brown, 1998b).

Women have more asymptomatic infections that may delay diagnosis and treatment. This delay increases the likelihood of more serious problems, including irreversible damage to reproductive organs and systemic illness. Embarrassment, denial, or fear about STDs may further delay treatment, increasing the potential for serious complications.

guidelines provide information, treatment standards, and counseling advice to help decrease the spread of STDs (CDC, 1998).

ACQUIRED IMMUNODEFICIENCY SYNDROME

Acquired immunodeficiency syndrome (AIDS), a disease caused by infection with the human immunodeficiency virus (HIV), is a disorder of immunosuppression affecting the body's ability to fight disease. HIV is transmitted through infected body fluids (e.g., semen, vaginal secretions, blood and blood products, breast milk) infected with HIV. People at high risk include the following (Youngkin & Davis, 1998):

- People who engage in anal sexual activity
- People who share needles
- People who have unprotected sexual intercourse with multiple partners
- People who have unprotected sexual intercourse with partners infected with HIV
- Infants born to women who are infected with HIV
- People who have hemophilia or other clotting disorders
- People who used untested blood and blood products before 1985
- Health care workers
- Sexual partners of anyone at risk for HIV (of both sexes)

Because HIV affects the immune system and can be transmitted in ways other than by sexual contact, it is discussed in detail in Chapter 22.

INFECTIONS ASSOCIATED WITH ULCERS

Syphilis

OVERVIEW

Syphilis is a complex sexually transmitted disease (STD) that can become systemic and cause serious complications and even death. Before penicillin was available in the 1940s, syphilis af-

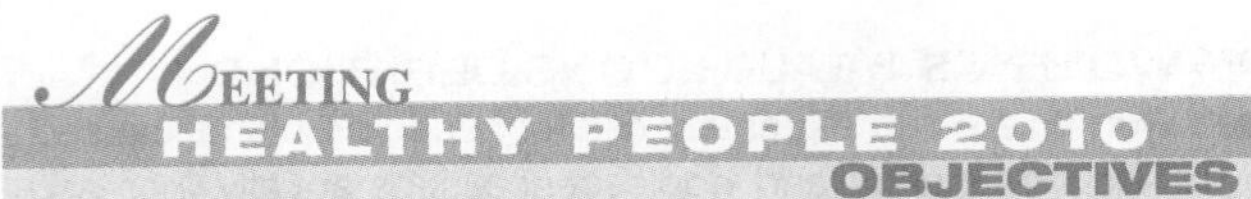

SEXUALLY TRANSMITTED DISEASES

Objective 25.3: Eliminate sustained domestic transmission of primary and secondary syphilis.

Objective 25.6: Reduce the proportion of females who have ever required treatment for pelvic inflammatory disease.

- Teach sexually active clients of all ages to use protection during sexual intercourse.
- Teach clients how and when to use condoms.
- Educate clients and partners about the medical complications of STDs and pelvic inflammatory disease (PID).
- Target non-Caucasian groups for education and screening because these groups have the highest incidence of STDs and PID.
- Target clients who are substance abusers for education and screening because they have a high incidence of STDs and PID.
- Participate in health fairs and surveillance programs to screen at-risk groups.

fected nearly 25% of the U.S. population. Between 1958 and 1990 there was no appreciable change or improvement in the rates of syphilis despite successful treatment. However, in 1990 the number of cases increased to a post–World War II peak of over 50,000. Since 1990 there has been a steady *decrease* in cases, with only 6993 primary and secondary cases reported in 1998 (CDC, 1999). One of the Healthy People 2010 objectives is to eliminate syphilis in the United States (see the Meeting Healthy People 2010 Objectives box above).

The causative organism of syphilis is *Treponema pallidum,* a spirochete with a slender, spiral shape that resembles a corkscrew. Nonpathogenic *Treponema* species are found in the mouth, intestinal tract, and genital areas of people and animals. Although the organism can be seen only with a dark-field microscope, several serologic tests may be used to screen for the presence of syphilis antigen/antibody. *T. pallidum* is susceptible to dry air or any known disinfectant. The organisms die within hours at temperatures of 105.8° to 107.6° F (41° to 42° C) and are not airborne. The infection is usually transmitted by sexual contact, but transmission can occur through close body contact and kissing.

Syphilis progresses through stages: primary, secondary, latency, and tertiary.

Primary Syphilis

The appearance of an ulcer, called a **chancre,** is the first sign of syphilis. The chancre develops at the site of inoculation, or entry, of the organism from 10 to 90 days after exposure (3 weeks is average). Chancres may be found on any area of the skin or mucous membranes but most frequently occur on the genitalia, lips, nipples, and hands and in the oral cavity, anus, and rectum.

During this highly infectious stage, the chancre begins as a small papule. Within 3 to 7 days, it breaks down into its characteristic appearance: a painless, indurated, smooth weeping lesion. Regional lymph nodes enlarge, feel firm, and are not painful. Without treatment, the chancre usually disappears within 6 weeks. However, the organism spreads throughout the body, and the client is still considered infectious.

Secondary Syphilis

Secondary syphilis develops 6 weeks to 6 months after the onset of primary syphilis. Secondary syphilis is a systemic disease, since the spirochetes circulate throughout the bloodstream. Clinical manifestations include malaise, low-grade fever, headache, muscular aches and pains, and sometimes a sore throat.

These symptoms are frequently mistaken for those of influenza. A generalized rash develops, which involves the palms and soles of the feet. Although there is no typical appearance of the rash, it tends to evolve sequentially from papules to squamous papules to pustules. Other skin lesions can include psoriasis-like rashes, wartlike lesions (condyloma lata), and mucous patches. The lesions are highly contagious and should not be touched without gloves. The rash subsides spontaneously in 4 to 12 weeks.

Early and Late Latent Syphilis

After the second stage of syphilis, there is a period of latency. *Early* latent syphilis occurs during the first year after infection, and infectious lesions can recur. *Late* latent syphilis is a disease of more than 1 year's duration after infection. This stage is noninfectious except to the fetus of a pregnant woman. Clients with latent syphilis may or may not have reactive serologic test findings.

Tertiary Syphilis

Tertiary, or late, syphilis occurs after a highly variable period, from 4 to 20 years. This stage develops in untreated cases and can mimic almost any pathologic condition, since virtually any organ system can be affected. The following are manifestations of late syphilis:

- Benign lesions (gummas) of the skin, mucous membranes, and bones
- Cardiovascular syphilis, usually in the form of aortic valvular disease and aortic aneurysms
- Neurosyphilis, which includes central nervous system involvement (e.g., meningitis, sensorineural hearing loss, generalized paresis)

CULTURAL CONSIDERATIONS

Specific ethnic groups in the United States seem to be more affected by syphilis than Caucasians. Primary and secondary syphilis rates of African Americans are nearly 60 times those of Caucasians, and the rates of Hispanics are 4 times those of Caucasians (Rosen & Brown, 1998a).

COLLABORATIVE MANAGEMENT

Assessment

Assessment of the client presenting with symptoms of syphilis begins with a history to gather information about the lesions or rash noticed. The history should include a risk assessment and sexual history and whether previous testing or treatment for syphilis or other STDs has ever been done (Chart 77-1). The nurse asks about allergic reactions to drugs, especially penicillin. A woman may present with complaints of inguinal lymph node enlargement, the location that drains the area of the vagina and cervix. She may state a history of sexual contact with a male partner who had an ulcer that she

CHART 77-1

FOCUSED ASSESSMENT *of* The Client with a Sexually Transmitted Disease

Assess history of present illness:
- Chief complaint
- Symptoms by quality and quantity, precipitating and palliative factors
- Any treatments taken (self-prescribed or over-the-counter products)

Assess past medical history:
- Major health problems—including any history of STDs/PID
- Surgeries—obstetric and gynecologic

Assess current health status:
- Menstrual history for irregularities
- Sexual history
  - Type and frequency of sexual activity
  - Number of sexual contacts
  - Sexual orientation
- Contraceptive history
- Medications
- Allergies
- Lifestyle risks—drugs, alcohol, tobacco

Assess preventive health care practices:
- Having Pap smears
- Regular STD screening
- Use of barrier contraceptives to prevent STDs and pregnancy

Assess physical examination findings:
- Vital signs
- Oropharyngeal findings
- Abdominal findings
- Genital or pelvic findings
- Anorectal findings

Assess laboratory data:
- Urinalysis
- Hematology
- Cervical and/or urethral, oral, rectal specimens
- Lesion samples for microbiology/virology
- Pregnancy testing

STDs, Sexually transmitted diseases; *PID,* pelvic inflammatory disease.

noticed during the encounter. Men usually discover the chancre on the penis or scrotum.

A physical examination, including inspection and palpation, is then conducted to identify manifestations of syphilis. Gloves should be worn while palpating any lesions because of the highly contagious treponemes that are present. Women frequently have the chancre on areas that are not easily visible to them, such as the vagina or cervix. Rashes of any type should be noted because of the variable presentation of secondary syphilis

After the physical examination, the physician, nurse practitioner, or nurse-midwife obtains a specimen of the chancre for examination under a darkfield microscope. Diagnosis of primary or secondary syphilis is confirmed if *T. pallidum,* the characteristic spirochete, is present. If the first slide is negative for *T. pallidum,* the procedure should be repeated in 3 days because many conditions can cause a false-negative result.

Blood tests are also used to diagnose syphilis. The usual screening test is the Venereal Disease Research Laboratory (VDRL) serum test. This test is based on an antibody-antigen reaction that determines both the presence and the amount of antibodies produced by the body in response to an infection by *T. pallidum.* The VDRL test becomes reactive 2 to 6 weeks after infection. VDRL titers are also used to monitor the effectiveness of treatment. The antibodies are not specific to *T. pallidum,* and false-positive reactions can occur frequently from such conditions as drug addiction, cancer, hepatitis, some viral diseases, and systemic lupus erythematosus (SLE).

If a positive VDRL result is obtained, the health care provider orders a more specific test, such as the *fluorescent treponemal antibody absorption (FTA-ABS)* test or the *microhemagglutination assay for T. palladium* (MHA-TP), to confirm the infection. These tests are more sensitive for all stages of syphilis, although false-positive results may still occur.

Interventions

The health care provider prescribes antibiotic therapy for the client with syphilis. The drug therapy of choice is benzathine penicillin G. Allergic reactions to the antibiotic occur frequently, and the nurse monitors for these signs and symptoms. Penicillin desensitization is recommended for penicillin-allergic clients. The client who has never had penicillin previously should have a skin test before receiving a penicillin injection. All clients who have received injections of antibiotics should remain at the health care agency for at least 30 minutes so that signs of a severe and immediate allergic reaction can be detected. If an allergic reaction does occur, treatment can begin immediately. The most severe reaction is anaphylaxis. All nurses working in clinics or physicians' offices where injections of penicillin are given should be familiar with the symptoms and treatment of anaphylaxis.

The **Jarisch-Herxheimer reaction** may also follow antibiotic therapy for syphilis. This reaction is due to the rapid release of products from the disruption of the cells of the organism. Onset occurs within 2 hours after therapy, with a peak at 4 to 8 hours. Symptoms include generalized aches and pain at the injection site, vasodilation and hypotension, and a rise in temperature. These symptoms do not always occur and generally are benign. This reaction may be treated symptomatically with analgesics and antipyretics.

Nursing interventions are based on information gained during the history and physical assessment. Common nursing diagnoses for clients with syphilis, as well as STDs in general, are listed in Table 77-3.

The nurse reinforces the information provided to the client about the cause of infection (sexual transmission); treatment, including side effects, possible complications of untreated or incompletely treated disease; and the need for follow-up care. All sexual partners must be adequately treated as soon as possible. Sensitive discussion with the client about the importance of partner notification and treatment should include the risk of reinfection if the partner goes untreated. The nurse informs the client that the disease must be reported to the local health authority and that all information will be held in strict confidence. The client must be encouraged to provide accurate information for this follow-up to ensure that all at-risk partners are treated appropriately. The nurse provides a setting that offers privacy and encourages open discussion.

The client is urged to comply with the treatment regimen, which includes follow-up visits. Sexual abstinence until the treatment is completed is urged. Prevention of infection with other STDs must be frankly discussed.

The emotional responses to syphilis vary and may include feelings of fear, depression, guilt, and anxiety. Clients may experience guilt if they have infected others or anger if they

TABLE 77-3 • SELECTED NURSING DIAGNOSES FOR CLIENTS WITH SEXUALLY TRANSMITTED DISEASES

- Risk for Injury related to the disease process
- Ineffective Coping related to fear, guilt, or anger
- Noncompliance related to treatment and/or partner follow-up
- Sexual Dysfunction related to fear of transmission
- Impaired Skin Integrity related to the presence of genital ulcers, warts, or rash
- Ineffective Health Maintenance related to Deficient Knowledge about the mode of transmission, disease process, or need for treatment
- Impaired Social Interaction related to social stigma
- Acute Pain related to the infection process
- Anxiety related to possible infertility as a result of having an STD
- Chronic Low Self-Esteem/Situational Low Self-Esteem related to the effects of having an STD

have been infected by a partner. If further psychosocial interventions are necessary, the nurse encourages the client to discuss these feelings or refers him or her to other resources such as psychotherapy groups, self-help support groups, or STD clinics.

CHART 77-2

BEST PRACTICE *for* Care of the Client with Genital Herpes

- Administer oral analgesics as prescribed.
- Apply local anesthetic sprays or ointments as prescribed.
- Apply ice packs or warm compresses to the client's lesions.
- Administer sitz baths three or four times a day.
- Encourage an increase in fluid intake.
- Encourage frequent urination.
- Pour water over the client's genitalia while the client is voiding, or encourage voiding while the client is sitting in a tub of water or standing in a shower.
- Catheterize the client as necessary.
- Encourage genital hygiene, and encourage keeping the skin clean and dry.
- Wash hands thoroughly after contact with lesions, and launder towels that have had direct contact with lesions.
- Wear gloves when applying ointments.
- Advise the client to avoid sexual activity when lesions are present.
- Advise the client to use latex or polyurethane condoms during all sexual exposures.
- Instruct the client in the use, side effects, and risks versus benefits of antiviral agents.

Genital Herpes

OVERVIEW

Genital herpes (GH) is an acute, recurring, incurable viral disease. Two serotypes of herpes simplex virus (HSV) affect the genitalia: type 1 (HSV-1) and type 2 (HSV-2). Most nongenital lesions, such as cold sores, are caused by HSV-1; HSV-2 causes most of the genital lesions. However, this differentiation is academic, since the transmission, symptoms, diagnosis, and treatment are identical for the two types. Either type can produce oral or genital lesions through oral-genital contact with an infected person.

On the basis of serologic studies, not symptoms, 45 million persons in the United States may have HSV-2 (CDC, 1998). HSV-2 is believed to cause 70% to 95% of the primary episodes of GH and recurs more frequently than HSV-1. Approximately 32% of the U.S. population was reported to have acquired HSV-2 by the early 1990s (Schaffer, 1998). Most people infected with HSV have not received a diagnosis because they have mild symptoms and shed virus intermittently.

The incubation period is 2 to 20 days, with the average period being 1 week. Many people are asymptomatic during the primary infection, but symptoms, if they occur, are usually most severe during this first infection and infrequently require hospitalization.

Itching or a tingling sensation may be felt in the skin 1 to 2 days before an outbreak. These sensations are followed by the appearance of vesicles (blisters) in a characteristic cluster on the penis, scrotum, vulva, perineum, vagina, cervix, or perianal region. The vesicles rupture spontaneously in a couple of days and leave painful erosions. These lesions can become extensive, and other symptoms, such as headaches, fever, general malaise, and inguinal lymphadenopathy, may be present. Urination may be painful, and clients with urinary retention may require catheterization. Lesions resolve within 2 to 6 weeks.

After the lesions heal, the virus remains in a dormant state in the nerve ganglia (specifically, in the sacral ganglia). Periodically, the virus may activate, and symptoms recur. These recurrences may be stimulated by many factors, including stress, fever, sunburn, poor nutrition, menses, and sexual activity.

Recurrences are not caused by reinfection. Recurrent episodes are usually less severe and of shorter duration than the primary infection; there may not even be symptoms at all. Occasionally, HSV infection may become active without producing apparent clinical manifestations. However, there is viral shedding, and the client is infectious. Long-term complications of GH include the risk of neonatal transmission and an increased risk of acquiring HIV infections. The risk of transmission to the neonate is greater in a pregnant woman who has a primary infection than in one who has a recurrence.

COLLABORATIVE MANAGEMENT

Assessment

The diagnosis of GH is usually based on the client's history and physical examination and is confirmed through a viral culture (see Chart 77-1). Cultures are most accurate if specimens are obtained within 48 hours of the first outbreak of the blisters. Fluid from inside the vesicle should be obtained to ensure a correct diagnosis. GH is frequently diagnosed presumptively by the health care provider if the presenting signs and symptoms are classic.

Interventions

Treatment of HSV-infected clients is usually symptomatic. The goals of collaborative management are to decrease the discomfort from painful ulcerations, to promote healing without secondary infection, to decrease viral shedding, and to prevent transmission of the infection (Chart 77-2).

DRUG THERAPY. Antiviral drugs are used to treat GH. The drugs do not cure the infection but do decrease the severity, accelerate the healing, and decrease the frequency of re-

CHART 77-3

DRUG THERAPY *for* Genital Herpes: First Clinical Episode of Genital Herpes

Drug	Dosage	Nursing Interventions	Rationale
Acyclovir (Zovirax, Avirax✤)	400 mg tid PO for 7-10 days	Instruct client that nausea and vomiting may occur when taking the drug.	The client is prepared for possible side effect.
	Or 200 mg 5 times/day PO for 7-10 days	Same as above.	Same as above.
Famciclovir (Famvir)	250 mg tid PO for 7-10 days	Instruct client that the drug is most effective if started within the first 48 hours of symptoms.	Efficacy has not been established for the first dose started more than 72 hours after the onset of symptoms.
Valacyclovir (Valtrex)	1 g bid PO for 7-10 days	Observe for side effects, including gastrointestinal disturbances, headaches, and dizziness.	The client is prepared for possible side effects.

current outbreaks. Topical therapy is not as effective as oral therapy. Acyclovir (Zovirax, Avirax✤), famciclovir (Famvir), or valacyclovir (Valtrex) may be used. The differences in these drugs are primarily in cost and frequency of use. Dosage and length of treatment differ for primary outbreaks (lasting 7 to 10 days) and recurrent outbreaks (lasting 5 days) (Chart 77-3). Mild recurrent episodes do not benefit appreciably from antiviral treatment, and their cost seems to outweigh their benefit. Therapy for severe recurrent outbreaks may be beneficial if it is started within 2 days of the appearance of lesions.

Clients who have frequent recurrences (more than six in a year) may benefit from daily suppressive treatment with any of the antivirals mentioned. Long-term safety and efficacy has been established for up to 6 years with acyclovir and for 1 year with valacyclovir and famciclovir. Clients receiving continuous therapy should stop after 1 year for reassessment of recurrences.

The cost of care for clients with GH is enormous, making it a major public health problem with a large economic burden. In 1999 the direct medical costs in the United States were estimated at $207 million. Of that amount, health care provider visits accounted for 36%, and drug therapy accounted for 64% (Tao et al., 2000).

NURSING MANAGEMENT. Nursing management includes client counseling and education about the infection, the potential for recurrent episodes, viral shedding even when clients are asymptomatic, and sexual transmission. Discussion about sexual activity is extremely important. The nurse reminds clients to abstain from sexual activity while lesions are present. Condom use during all sexual exposures is urged because of the increased risk of HSV transmission, since viral shedding can occur even when lesions are not present. The nurse teaches the client about how and when to use condoms (Chart 77-4).

The nurse also emphasizes the risk of fetal infection to all clients, both male and female. Women and men who have genital herpes need to inform the maternity care provider of their history during future pregnancies.

The nurse also assesses the client's psychologic responses to the diagnosis of genital herpes. Many clients are initially shocked and need reassurance that they can manage the disease. Infected clients have reported feelings of disbelief, uncleanness, isolation, and loneliness. They have also reported anger at their partners for transmitting the infection or fear of rejection by partners because they have the infection. The nurse helps clients cope with the diagnosis by being sensitive and supportive during assessments and interventions. Social supports should be encouraged, and referrals to support groups such as HELP (local support groups of the National Herpes Resource Center) may be beneficial. Symptomatic care may include oral analgesics, topical anesthetics, sitz baths, and increased oral fluid intake.

CHART 77-4

CLIENT EDUCATION GUIDE
Use of Condoms

- Use latex or polyurethane condoms rather than natural membrane condoms.
- Use a condom with every sexual encounter.
- Female condoms—polyurethane sheaths in the vagina—are effective in preventing transmission of viruses, including HIV.
- Condoms infrequently (2 per 100) break during sexual intercourse, unless used incorrectly.
- Keep condoms (especially latex) in a cool, dry place, out of direct sunlight.
- Do not use condoms that are in damaged packages or that are brittle or discolored.
- Always handle a condom with care to avoid damaging it with fingernails, teeth, or other sharp objects.
- Put condoms on before any genital contact. Hold the condom by the tip and unroll it on the penis. Leave a space at the tip to collect semen.
- If you use a lubricant with condoms, make sure that the lubricant is water based and washes away with water. Oil-based products may damage latex condoms.
- Use of spermicide with condoms, either lubricated condoms or vaginal application, has not been proved to be more or less effective against STDs than use without spermicide. Spermicide does provide added protection against pregnancy. Spermicide-coated condoms have been associated with *Escherichia coli* urinary tract infections in women.
- If a condom breaks, replace it immediately.
- After ejaculation, withdraw the erect penis carefully, holding the condom at the base of the penis to prevent the condom from slipping off.
- Never use a condom more than once.

Modified from Centers for Disease Control and Prevention. (1998). 1998 guidelines for treatment of sexually transmitted diseases. *Morbidity and Mortality Weekly Report, 47*(No. RR-1), 1-103.

Lymphogranuloma Venereum

OVERVIEW

Lymphogranuloma venereum (LGV) is the result of genital inoculation with one of three serotypes of *Chlamydia trachomatis,* which is spread systemically until it localizes in the genital or rectal lymph nodes. The incubation period is 3 to 30 days. The primary lesion, at the point of inoculation, is transient and painless and is not usually noticed by the client. The lesion usually appears on the penis in men and on the vaginal wall in women; however, sores may also be located in the mouth and rectum. Five times as many men are diagnosed with this disease as women.

Lesions vary in form from herpes-like blisters (vesicles), to ulcers, papules, or pustules. Within 1 to 2 weeks after the appearance of the primary lesion, secondary signs of infection appear. Lymphadenopathy (primarily inguinal) is present, and symptoms of headache, malaise, arthralgia, and anorexia may occur. Most clients seek care at this point. Lymphadenopathy can recede or develop into abscesses. When the abscesses rupture, healing occurs slowly. Sinus tracts, formed as a result of the infection, drain thick, viscous pus for several weeks, leaving behind deep scars.

Complications of the infection can be chronic lymphadenopathy, fistulas, rectal strictures, and proctitis. Systemic involvement can also cause carditis, arthritis, and pneumonia.

> **CULTURAL CONSIDERATIONS**
> LVG has a worldwide distribution, but it occurs primarily in South America, Southeast Asia, India, and East and West Africa and rarely in the United States. Cases in the United States usually occur in clients who have visited these countries or had sexual contact with someone who is from or has traveled to or from these areas (Kellock et al., 1997).

COLLABORATIVE MANAGEMENT

The diagnosis of LGV is usually made on physical examination and serologic testing. The serologic test, an antibody complement fixation test (LGV-CF), is considered diagnostic if the titer is higher than 1:64. Cultures from the enlarged lymph nodes, although technically difficult and expensive, are considered the "gold standard" if the organism can be isolated, which occurs only 50% of the time (Rosen & Brown, 1998).

The health care provider prescribes doxycycline (Monodox, Doxy-Caps, Doxycin✤) 100 mg twice a day orally or tetracycline (Tetracyn, Tetram, Nu-Tetra✤, Apo-Tetra✤) 500 mg four times a day orally for 21 days. Antibiotic treatment cures the infection and prevents further tissue damage. Infected lymph nodes may be aspirated by needle or incised and drained to prevent ulcer formation. Surgical intervention may be required for late complications, such as perianal or perirectal strictures and fistulas. Nursing management and client education is similar to that for syphilis. Sexual partners should be tested for cervical or urethral chlamydial infection and treated if they had sexual contact with the client during the 30 days before the client's onset of symptoms.

Chancroid

OVERVIEW

Painful genital ulcerations characterize **chancroid.** Genital lesions and inguinal lymphadenopathy without systemic illness are the usual presentation. Although chancroid has a worldwide distribution, it is most common in developing tropical and subtropical countries, such as Africa, the West Indies, and Asia, but is endemic in parts of the United States. Chancroid is a cofactor for HIV transmission, leading to high rates of HIV infection of those with chancroid. Estimates of 10% of clients with chancroid being co-infected with syphilis and herpes simplex virus have been made. This co-infection appears to be the result of the open genital lesions. Uncircumcised men may be at greater risk for infection than circumcised men.

The incubation period for chancroid varies from 3 to 10 days. A tender papule appears at the site of inoculation. This lesion rapidly breaks down to form an irregularly shaped, deep ulcer that has a purulent discharge and bleeds easily.

Complications include inguinal adenitis, balanitis, phimosis, and urethral fistulas. Chancroids differ from chancres caused by syphilis in that chancroids are soft and painful. Transmission of the disease is through contact with the ulcer or with the discharge from the infected local lymph glands during sexual activity.

COLLABORATIVE MANAGEMENT

Cultures from the ulcers can isolate the *Haemophilus ducreyi* organism. Gram staining of the exudate from the ulcer can be difficult because of polymicrobial contamination, but the gram-negative rods may be seen. Usually the diagnosis is based on clinical signs, the exclusion of syphilis and herpes by appropriate testing, and a positive culture.

Management for chancroid consists of azithromycin (Zithromax) 1 g in a single dose orally, ceftriaxone (Rocephin) 250 mg in a single dose intramuscularly, ciprofloxacin (Cipro) 500 mg twice a day orally for 3 days, or erythromycin (E-Mycin, Apo-Erythro✤) 500 mg four times a day orally for 7 days. These antibiotics cure the infection, resolve the symptoms, and prevent further transmission. Clients should be observed periodically by a physician or nurse practitioner until ulcers heal, usually in 7 days. Client education is similar to that for syphilis. Sexual contacts must be located and treated whether or not they are symptomatic. The nurse's responsibility in management of the client with chancroid is similar to that for other sexually transmitted diseases (STDs).

Granuloma Inguinale

OVERVIEW

The causative organism of granuloma inguinale, or donovanosis, is *Calymmatobacterium granulomatis.* A nodule appears at the site of inoculation after 1 to 12 weeks. This lesion ulcerates, and others are formed; they grow together, becoming a spreading ulcer on the genitalia. Left untreated, these lesions can be mutilating. Regional lymphadenopathy does not occur. The ulcerated lesions bleed easily on contact.

> **CULTURAL CONSIDERATIONS**
> Granuloma inguinale is endemic in parts of Australia (among the central aborigines) and common in Africa, Southeast Asia, southern India, and New Guinea. Occurrence in the United States, Japan, and Europe is rare.

COLLABORATIVE MANAGEMENT

Biopsy and cytologic smears from the ulcers are the only conclusive methods for diagnosis. Definitive diagnosis depends on finding characteristic Donovan bodies in these samples. This can be difficult, and frequently treatment will be given empirically before results of these tests are available.

Granuloma inguinale is treated with 1 tablet of trimethoprim/sulfamethoxazole (Bactrim✱, Septra) double strength twice a day orally or doxycycline 100 mg twice a day orally for a minimum of 3 weeks. Treatment needs to continue until all the lesions are completely healed. Relapse can occur within 6 to 18 months, even after successful initial treatment.

Sexual contacts within 60 days of the onset of symptoms or those displaying any signs or symptoms should be treated.

The nurse's responsibility in management of the client with granuloma inguinale is similar to that for other STDs. A thorough history that includes sexual contacts, travel abroad, and contact with partners who may have traveled to or are from endemic areas is taken (see Chart 77-1). Collecting the history about genital lesions that may have disappeared or changed is essential diagnostic information that can be used in collaboration with the health care provider.

The nurse explains cultures, biopsies, or other diagnostic tests that will be done to make a correct diagnosis. Comfort measures and emotional support need to be provided, since some procedures may be invasive or painful. The nurse teaches the client about the diagnosis, the risk for complications if granuloma inguinale is left untreated or incompletely treated, and the antibiotics prescribed.

The client should be encouraged to provide the names of sexual contacts for follow-up and treatment. Concerns about coping with the disease may arise; the nurse encourages the client to verbalize concerns and/or refers him or her for further counseling. Because these infections are relatively rare, the client may experience the added discomfort and inconvenience of being evaluated by specialists to get a correct diagnosis, which may contribute to his or her anxiety.

INFECTIONS OF THE EPITHELIAL STRUCTURES

Condylomata Acuminata

OVERVIEW

Condylomata acuminata (also known as genital *warts*) are caused by certain types of human papillomavirus (HPV). At least 6 of the approximately 70 HPV genotypes are found on the skin of the genitalia. Some of these are considered high risk in their association with genital cancers. Genital warts are the most common sexually transmitted viral disease and are often seen with other infections. Approximately 20% to 40% of the sexually active population in the United States is thought to be infected with HPV (Beutner et al., 1999). Sites commonly affected include the urinary meatus, labia, vagina, cervix, penis, scrotum, anus, and perineal area. Pregnancy seems to lead to increased growth of the lesions. The incubation period is usually 2 to 3 months.

The genital warts are initially single, small papillary growths that may grow into large cauliflower-like masses. Bleeding may occur if the wart is disrupted. Warts may regress spontaneously without treatment.

HPV infection is strongly associated with genital dysplasia and cervical carcinoma. A Pap smear is useful in the isolation and diagnosis of HPV from the cervix. HPV can also be detected in genital swab specimens using a more sensitive polymerase chain reaction (PCR) assay. A specimen for biopsy is obtained from any atypical, pigmented, or persistent warts.

➤ COLLABORATIVE MANAGEMENT

Assessment

The diagnosis of condylomata acuminata is made by examination of the lesions, which appear wartlike. To rule out the presence of other infections, a VDRL test and cultures for chlamydial infection and gonorrhea are obtained. A Pap smear is obtained to assess for cervical dysplasia (abnormal tissue growth). If lesions bleed easily or appear to be infected, a biopsy may be done to rule out other pathologic conditions. Colposcopy with biopsies is recommended for assessment of lesions that appear atypical, lesions that do not respond to treatment, and any lesions on the cervix.

Interventions

The goals of management are to remove the warts, treat the symptoms, and prevent progression of neoplasias. No therapy has been shown to eradicate HPV; therefore recurrences after treatment are likely.

The treatment options for external warts are client applied or provider applied. Clients may apply podofilox 0.5% solution or gel twice a day for 3 days with no treatment for the next 4 days. This regimen should be repeated for four cycles. Another option is imiquimod 5% cream applied topically at bedtime three times a week for up to 16 weeks.

Cryotherapy, podophyllin, and trichloroacetic acid (TCA) are relatively inexpensive provider-applied treatments. Cryotherapy (freezing), usually with liquid nitrogen, can be used every 1 to 2 weeks until lesions are resolved. Podophyllin resin 10% to 25% in a compound of tincture of benzoin can be applied weekly but needs to be washed off 1 to 4 hours after application. Trichloroacetic acid (80% to 90%) can be applied weekly. Extensive warts have been treated with the carbon dioxide laser or by surgical removal.

For effective management of condylomata acuminata, sexual partners must also be treated. Clients should avoid intimate sexual contact until external lesions are healed.

Nursing management focuses on client education about the mode of transmission, incubation period, treatment, and complications. Reinforcing instructions about local care of the lesions or patient-applied treatment is essential. After treatment with cryotherapy, podophyllin, or TCA, clients may experience discomfort, bleeding or discharge from the site, or sloughing of parts of warts. The nurse instructs the client to keep the area clean (shower or bath) and dry, and to be alert for any signs or symptoms of infection or side effects of the treatment.

Condoms are recommended to help reduce transmission (see Chart 77-4). Clients need to know that recurrence is likely and that repeated treatments may be necessary. The nurse encourages women who have had condylomata acuminata to have an annual Pap smear. As with other STDs, emotional support is needed, and a referral for counseling may help.

Gonorrhea

OVERVIEW

Gonorrhea continues to be the most reported communicable disease in the United States and may be on the rise. An estimated 600,000 new infections occur each year. The incidence is highest in sexually active people between the ages of 15 and 19 years. This bacterial infection occurs in men and women, and infants can be infected during childbirth. The causative organism is *Neisseria gonorrhoeae,* a gram-negative intracellular diplococcus. *N. gonorrhoeae* is transmitted by direct sexual contact with mucosal surfaces (vaginal intercourse, orogenital or anogenital contact) or, in the neonate, through an infected birth canal). Although the organism has been found on inanimate surfaces where it has been artificially inoculated, there is no evidence that transmission occurs naturally in this manner.

The initial symptoms of gonorrhea may appear 3 to 10 days after sexual contact with an infected person. The infection can be asymptomatic in both men and women, but women have asymptomatic, or silent, infections more often than men do. If symptoms are present, men most likely notice dysuria and a penile discharge that can be either profuse yellowish green fluid or scant clear fluid. The urethra is the site most commonly affected, but infection can extend to the prostate, the seminal vesicles, and the epididymis. Men seek curative treatment sooner, usually because they are symptomatic, and thereby avoid some of the serious complications. Women may report a change in vaginal discharge (yellow, green, profuse, odorous), urinary frequency, or dysuria. The cervix and urethra are the most common sites of infection. Gonorrhea can sit asymptomatically in the cervix and be transmitted or progress without warning. Ascending spread of the gonococci can cause pelvic infection (pelvic inflammatory disease [PID]), endometritis (endometrial infection), salpingitis (fallopian tube infection), and/or pelvic peritonitis. Both symptomatic and asymptomatic infections can lead to PID and tubal scarring. Rare sequelae of gonorrhea include arthritis, meningitis, perihepatitis, and disseminated infection. Neonates contacting the infection at birth can develop conjunctivitis and blindness.

Anal manifestations may include anal itching and irritation, rectal bleeding or diarrhea, and painful defecation. Oral manifestations are related to pharyngeal infection. Symptoms are seldom noted but may include a sore throat, ulcerated lips, tender gingivae, and vesicles in the oropharynx. Figure 77-1 shows common sites of gonococcal infections.

Asymptomatic clients may be found to have positive cultures for gonorrhea when they present to a health care facility for routine physical examination, for hospital admission, or for preoperative assessments. Others may present to the

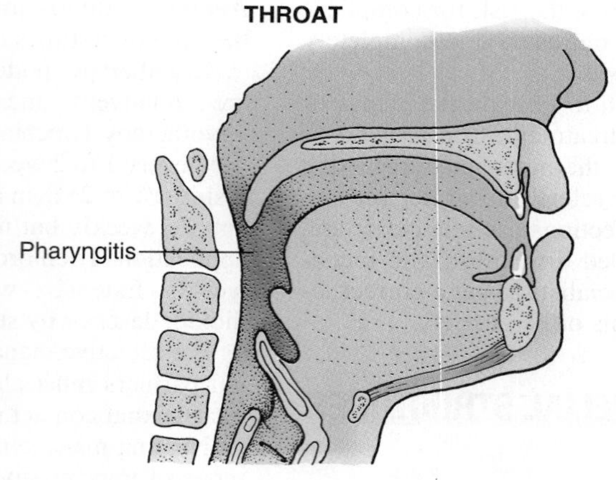

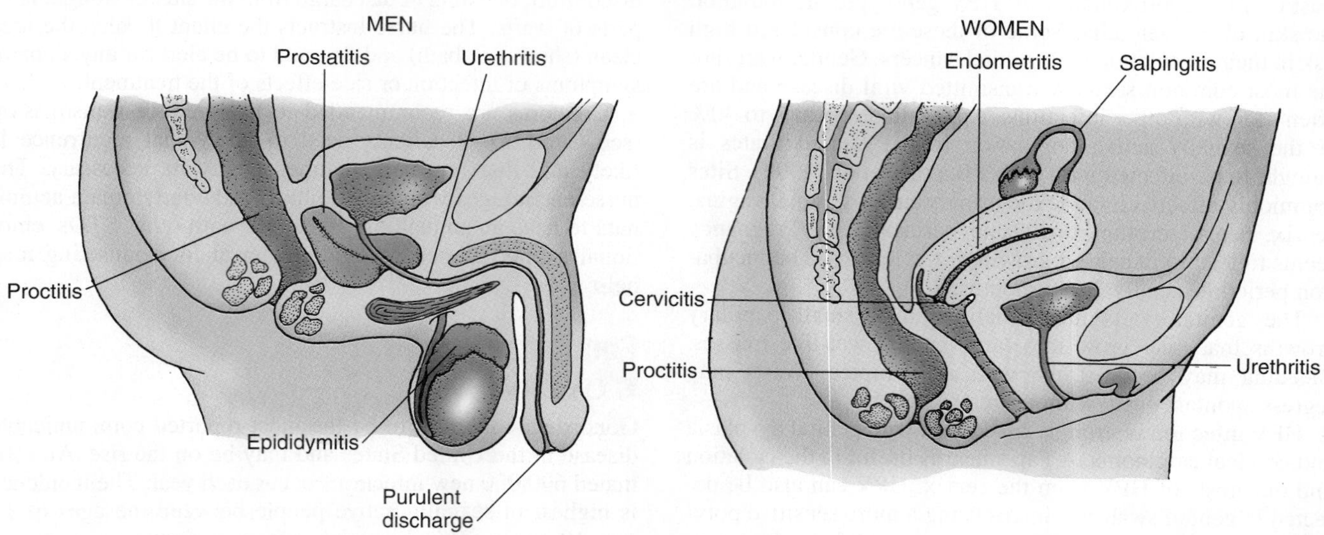

Figure 77-1 ● Some areas of involvement with gonorrhea in men and women.

health care agency because the sexual partner has been diagnosed with the infection. Screening all sexually active men and women for gonorrhea is a useful public health tool to avoid spread of asymptomatic infection.

CULTURAL CONSIDERATIONS

In 1998 in the United States, African Americans had 61% of the reported cases of gonorrhea, Caucasians had 11%, and Hispanics had 5%, with rates in women nearly equal to those of men (CDC, 1999).

COLLABORATIVE MANAGEMENT

Assessment

A complete history includes reviewing possible symptoms of gonorrhea, taking a sexual history that includes sexual orientation and sites of intercourse, and assessing for allergies to antibiotics (see Chart 77-1). The nurse's nonjudgmental approach helps elicit appropriate and complete information. These techniques may decrease the client's anxiety and fear about having a sexually transmitted disease (STD).

Physical assessment includes inspection for discharge from the urethra, cervix, and rectum. Palpation of the lower abdomen may reveal tenderness. Fever may be present, especially in complicated infections.

Definitive diagnosis involves laboratory testing. Identification of gonorrhea in men can be made with smears of the discharge that has been swabbed onto a glass slide, dried, and Gram stained. The presence of gram-negative diplococci is diagnostic for gonococcal urethritis. Gram stains are 50% to 70% sensitive and 97% specific for gonorrhea. Gram staining allows for immediate diagnosis and earlier treatment.

Smears do not confirm the diagnosis in women, because the female genital tract normally harbors organisms that resemble *N. gonorrhoeae.* Cultures provide a more definitive diagnosis and are the most reliable method of confirming a diagnosis for men and women. The sensitivity of cultures is 80% to 90%.

A specimen is obtained from the male urethra or the female cervix and inoculated onto Thayer-Martin (chocolate agar) culture medium. The medium must be placed in a carbon dioxide–rich environment for the organism to grow. Depending on the history given by the client, culture specimens may also be obtained from the throat and rectum. After 24 to 48 hours, the culture is examined for the presence of gram-negative diplococci.

Direct fluorescent antibody tests, collected on a swab as with cultures, are available and are very sensitive and specific. First-voided urine specimens tested by the multiplex PCR methodology are an additional highly sensitive and specific method for screening and diagnosing *N. gonorrhoeae* (and *Ureaplasma urealyticum, Chlamydia trachomatis, and Mycoplasma genitalium* all in one specimen) (Mahoney et al., 1997).

All clients with gonorrhea should be tested for syphilis, chlamydial infection, hepatitis B and C, and HIV infection because they may have been exposed to these STDs as well. Sexual partners who have been exposed in the last 30 days should be examined, and specimens for culture should be obtained.

Interventions

The health care provider treats uncomplicated gonorrhea with antibiotics. Treatment has changed because of penicillin-resistant strains and now quinolone-resistant strains of *N. gonorrhoeae.* Chlamydial infections are frequently found in clients with gonorrhea. Management for gonorrhea includes medications that also eradicate *Chlamydia.*

DRUG THERAPY. Drug therapy recommended by the Centers for Disease Control and Prevention (CDC) is cefixime (Suprax) 400 mg orally, ceftriaxone (Rocephin) 125 mg intramuscularly, ciprofloxacin (Cipro) 500 mg orally, *or* ofloxacin (Floxin) 400 mg orally, *each* in a single dose *plus* azithromycin (Zithromax) 1 g in a single dose orally *or* doxycycline (Monodox, Doxy-Caps, Doxycin✱) 100 mg twice a day orally for 1 week. The quinolones (ciprofloxacin, ofloxacin) are contraindicated in clients younger than 18 years of age. These combinations seem to be effective for all mucosal gonorrheal infections; treatment failure is rare. Sexual partners must be treated as well. A test of cure is not required, but the client is advised to return for a follow-up examination if symptoms persist after treatment. Reinfection is frequently the cause of these symptoms and indicates a need for more education of the client and sexual partner.

Gonorrheal infections that have become systemic may develop abruptly. Symptoms of disseminated gonococcal infection (DGI) may include fever, chills, skin lesions on distal parts of extremities, and asymmetric arthralgias with or without joint swelling, heat, or erythema. Treatment includes intravenous (IV) or intramuscular antibiotic therapy (ceftriaxone 1 g every 24 hours). If symptoms resolve within 24 to 48 hours, the client may be discharged to home to continue oral antibiotic therapy for at least 1 week.

Meningitis and endocarditis occur rarely. Hospitalization for these clients is recommended for the initial treatment, especially if endocarditis or meningitis is suspected. Treatment is with IV antibiotic therapy, usually ceftriaxone 1 to 2 g every 12 hours. If meningitis or endocarditis is present, therapy should be continued for 10 to 14 days for meningitis and at least 4 weeks for endocarditis. Infectious disease specialists are consulted for management of these infections.

HEALTH TEACHING. Nursing interventions focus on health teaching about transmission and treatment of gonorrhea. Clients must understand why medications should be taken for the prescribed time for maximal effectiveness. The nurse discusses the possibility of reinfection. Clients should avoid sexual activity until the antibiotic therapy is completed and they no longer have symptoms. Men and women are urged to use condoms, especially if abstinence is not possible. The nurse explains that gonorrhea is a reportable disease. All sexual contacts need to be examined and treated for both gonorrhea and chlamydial infection.

When a diagnosis of gonorrhea is made, clients may have feelings of fear or guilt. They may be concerned that they have contracted other STDs or see the disease as a punishment for promiscuity or "unnatural" sex acts. They may believe that acquiring gonorrhea (or any STD) is a risk that they must take to pursue their desired lifestyle. Such feelings can impair relationships with sexual partners. The nurse encourages expression of feelings during assessments and teaching sessions. Privacy for client teaching and maintenance of confidentiality of medical records are important nursing interventions in meeting the client's psychosocial needs.

CRITICAL THINKING CHALLENGE

A middle-aged woman visits her gynecologist with complaints of a greenish yellow, odorous vaginal discharge that is very irritating and itchy. On examination, the physician suspects gonorrhea and asks her about sexual activity. She states that she has been married for 32 years and has never had sexual intercourse with any man other than her husband. Laboratory tests confirm the STD diagnosis.

- What questions will you need to ask the client at this time?
- How do you think she became infected with the disease?
- What emotional support will she need as she begins treatment for gonorrhea?

For suggested answer guidelines, go to SIMON http://www.wbsaunders.com/SIMON/Iggy/.

Chlamydial Infection

OVERVIEW

Chlamydia trachomatis is the most common sexually transmitted infection in the United States. The disease is now reportable to local health departments in almost all states. More than 500,000 acute infections are reported annually, but estimates of 3 million genital infections per year have been made (Groseclose et al., 1999). Asymptomatic infections, perhaps in up to 80% of women infected with *C. trachomatis,* account for most of this difference. In men, about 10% to 20% of the cases of nongonococcal urethritis are caused by *C. trachomatis.* In women, 20% to 40% of those infected with *C. trachomatis* develop pelvic inflammatory disease (PID), discussed on pp. 1817-1823. Transmission to the newborn can occur during vaginal delivery, with resultant neonatal eye infections and pneumonia.

C. trachomatis invades the columnar epithelial tissues in the reproductive tract and causes clinical manifestations similar to those of gonorrheal infections. The incubation period ranges from 1 to 3 weeks, but the pathogen may be present in the genital tract for months without producing symptoms. The average duration of infection before diagnosis has been estimated to be about 1 year in women and 5 months in men because of its frequent asymptomatic status (Groseclose et al., 1999).

In men, the primary symptom is nongonococcal urethritis, accompanied by dysuria, frequent urination, and a mucoid discharge that is more watery and less copious than a gonorrheal discharge. Some men have the discharge only in the morning on arising. Complications include epididymitis, prostatitis, infertility, and Reiter's syndrome, a type of connective tissue disease (see Chapter 21).

In contrast, up to 80% of women may have no symptoms. Women with symptoms have a mucopurulent cervicitis that presents with a change in vaginal discharge, easily induced cervical bleeding, urinary frequency, and abdominal discomfort or pain. The vaginal discharge typically becomes yellow and more opaque (Sellors et al., 2000). Complications of infection with *C. trachomatis* include salpingitis, PID, ectopic pregnancy, and infertility.

COLLABORATIVE MANAGEMENT

Assessment

A complete history, including medical, menstrual, and sexual history is obtained from the client (see Chart 77-1). The nurse asks about the following:

- Presence of symptoms
- Any history of sexually transmitted diseases (STDs)
- Whether sexual partners have had symptoms or have a history of STDs

The nurse understands that many women with chlamydial infections are asymptomatic and that a history may reveal only risk factors associated with *C. trachomatis.* These factors include pregnancy, age younger than 20 years, being unmarried, nulliparity, having a higher number of sexual partners or a new sexual partner, use of a nonbarrier method of birth control (hormonal, intrauterine device [IUD]), and concurrent gonorrhea. As with all interviews concerning sexual behavior, the nurse uses a nonjudgmental approach and provides privacy and confidentiality.

Diagnosis of chlamydial infections is made by sampling cells from the endocervix and/or urethra. Since chlamydiae are obligate intracellular pathogens, host cells that harbor the organism (or parts of it) are required in the sample. Gram staining of urethral or cervical samples can help exclude gonorrhea. The presence of polymorphonuclear leukocytes and the absence of gram-negative intracellular diplococci (suggestive of gonorrhea) points to a chlamydial infection. Absolute diagnosis of chlamydial infection is made with a tissue culture. Culture for *Chlamydia,* which detects 70% to 80% of cervical infections with *C. trachomatis,* has been the "gold standard." Special transport medium is required.

Two enzyme immunoassay tests can be performed easily, less expensively, and more quickly than cultures: the Chlamydiazyme, an enzyme-linked immunoassay (ELISA), and the MicroTrak, a direct fluorescent antibody test (DFA); these tests detect about 60% to 90% of infections.

DNA probe (GenProbe) testing also detects 60% to 90% of infections. Newer genetic amplification tests or DNA amplification tests (ligase chain reaction [LCR] and polymerized chain reaction [PCR]) appear able to detect more than 90% to 95% of infections and can be done additionally on urine but are more expensive (Mahoney et al., 1997). If affordable, these tests are the best choice. Specimens with cervical or urethral secretions, obtained with swabs, are used.

Screening asymptomatic women who may have risk factors for having chlamydial infections is strongly encouraged. Screening adolescents every 6 months regardless of other risk factors is now being recommended by some experts (see Evidence-Based Practice for Nursing box on p. 1817).

Interventions

The treatment of choice for chlamydial infections is azithromycin (Zithromax) 1 g in a single dose or doxycycline (Monodox, Doxy-Caps, Doxycin♣) 100 mg twice a day for 7 days. The one-dose course, although more expensive, is preferred because of the ease in completing the treatment. Administering the drug while in the health care facility helps ensure compliance. Sexual partners should be tested and treated if at all possible.

Client education is an important nursing intervention. The nurse explains the following:

- The mode of disease transmission
- The incubation period
- Signs and symptoms, including the possibility of asymptomatic infections
- Medical treatment

EVIDENCE-BASED PRACTICE FOR NURSING

Sexually active adolescent females are recommended to have screening for *Chlamydia* every 6 months regardless of other risk factors

Burnstein, G.R., et al. (1998). Incident *Chlamydia trachomatis* infections among inner-city adolescent females. *Journal of the American Medical Association, 280*(6), 521-526.

Adolescents are at highest risk for *Chlamydia trachomatis* infection for multiple reasons. Chlamydial infection is an important preventable cause of pelvic inflammatory disease (PID) and subsequent infertility. Since sexually transmitted disease (STD) prevention and screening are the responsibility of those providing care in many settings, identifying adolescent females at risk for infection is an important practice issue.

A consecutive convenience sample of 3202 sexually active females, 12 to 19 years old, who were seen at an urban health department family planning or STD clinic or school-based clinic, were screened. Specimens (cervical or urine) for *Chlamydia* testing were obtained as part of the standard care after informed consent was received. Demographic and behavioral data were collected that included age, race or ethnicity, reason for testing or examination (e.g., STD contact, STD symptoms, asymptomatic screening), and prior STD history. The adolescents were asked about sexually risky behaviors in the previous 90 days (i.e., new or multiple partners, inconsistent condom use). They were tested again on repeat visits, which ranged from 1 to 9 visits per woman. The median time between visits was 4 months.

Twenty-nine percent of all adolescent females tested were positive for *Chlamydia,* which is a higher percentage than in other populations of adolescent women that have been studied. Fourteen-year-olds had the highest proportion of positive test results; 24% tested positive on their first visit, and 14% tested positive on a repeat visit. This study confirmed that risk factors failed to identify a high-risk subgroup needing targeted screening. For adolescents who had initially had a negative test, the mean time until they had a positive result was 7.2 months. For those with a previous positive test result, the median time until a repeat positive test was 4.1 months. The researchers therefore recommend screening all sexually active adolescent females every 6 months regardless of their risk.

Critique. This well-designed study demonstrates that previous recommendations for *Chlamydia* screening based on risk factors may not be appropriate for the adolescent female population. A limitation of the study is that the study sample was racially and socioeconomically homogeneous. More study needs to be done with ethnically diverse populations using the newer, more sensitive nucleic acid amplification tests used in this study.

Implications for Nursing. Nurses educating clients about STD risk and need for screening have new data on which to base their recommendations. Adolescent females are at greatest risk for acquiring chlamydial infections. Nurses in every setting should view this age-group as a high-risk subset that needs additional education on STD prevention, as well as screening every 6 months.

- The need for abstinence from sexual intercourse until the client and partner(s) have completed treatment (7 days from the start of treatment, including a single-dose regimen)
- The fact that no test of cure is required
- The need to return for evaluation if symptoms recur or new symptoms develop
- Possible complications of untreated or inadequately treated infection

Psychosocial support is similar to that discussed in the previous section on gonorrhea.

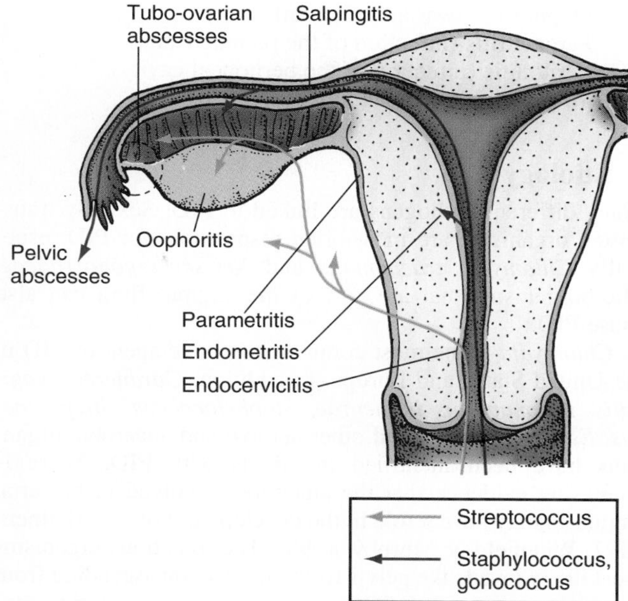

Figure 77-2 ● The spread of pelvic inflammatory disease.

OTHER GYNECOLOGIC CONDITIONS

Pelvic Inflammatory Disease

OVERVIEW

Pelvic inflammatory disease (PID) is considered a costly gynecologic health problem in the United States, affecting over 1 million women annually (see the Cost of Care box on p. 1807). It is an infectious process that may involve one or more pelvic structures, including the uterus, fallopian tubes, and adjacent pelvic structures. The most common site is the fallopian tube.

Many practitioners use the terms *PID* and *salpingitis* synonymously for acute infections. PID is one of the leading causes of infertility and is related to the rise in the number of ectopic pregnancies reported in the United States. PID is generally viewed as an acute syndrome resulting in tenderness in the tubes and ovaries (adnexa) and low, dull abdominal pain. However, many women experience only mild discomfort or menstrual irregularity; others experience no symptoms at all—so-called silent or subclinical PID. Diagnosis and treatment of PID in these women is a challenge to health care providers. Irreversible scarring or stricture, causing sterility, may occur before PID is diagnosed.

Pathophysiology

PID is a complex process in which organisms from the lower genital tract migrate from the endocervix upward through the endometrial cavity to the fallopian tubes. The spread of infection to other organs of the upper genital tract occurs by way of direct contact with mucosal surfaces or through the fimbriated ends of the tubes to the ovaries, parametrium, and peritoneal cavity (Figure 77-2). Resultant infections include the following:

- Endometritis (infection of the endometrial cavity)
- Salpingitis (inflammation of the fallopian tubes)

- Oophoritis (ovarian infection)
- Parametritis (infection of the parametrium)
- Peritonitis (infection of the peritoneal cavity)
- Tubal or tubo-ovarian abscess

Etiology

Many different pathogens are linked to PID. Sexually transmitted organisms are most often responsible for PID, especially *Chlamydia trachomatis* and *Neisseria gonorrhoeae.* Microorganisms that are part of the vaginal flora can also cause PID.

Chlamydia is the most common causative agent of PID in the United States and Europe. In addition, *Gardnerella vaginalis, Haemophilus influenzae, Staphylococcus, Streptococcus, Escherichia coli,* and other aerobic and anaerobic organisms have been identified in clients with PID. There is increasing evidence that the anaerobes involved in bacterial vaginosis may have a role in the development of PID (Peipert, 1997; Winefield & Murphy, 1998). The infectious organisms most likely invade the pelvis from an infection ascending from the vagina or cervix. Infections have been spread during sexual intercourse, during childbirth (including the postpartum period), and after abortion. Rarely do infections result from transperitoneal spread from a ruptured appendix or intra-abdominal abscess.

Incidence/Prevalence

The incidence of PID is on the rise. Accurate rates are unavailable because PID is not a reportable disease. Many of the same factors that place women at risk for STDs also place them at risk for PID.

Risk factors for sexually active women include the following:

- Age less than 20 years
- Multiple sexual partners
- Intrauterine device (IUD) in place
- Use of vaginal douches
- Smoking
- Chlamydial or gonococcal infection; bacterial vaginosis
- A history of sexually transmitted diseases (STDs)
- A history of PID

COLLABORATIVE MANAGEMENT

Activity Link

Assessment

HISTORY

The nurse obtains a complete medical, family, menstrual, obstetric, and sexual history, including a history of previous episodes of pelvic inflammatory disease (PID) or other sexually transmitted infections (see Chart 77-1). The nurse also assesses for contraceptive use (especially the intrauterine device), a history of reproductive surgery, and other risk factors previously identified. The possibility of sexual abuse should be raised.

One of the most frequent symptoms of PID is lower abdominal pain. Other symptoms include menstrual irregularities or abnormal vaginal bleeding, dysuria, an increase or change in vaginal discharge, dyspareunia, malaise, fever, and chills.

> **CRITICAL THINKING CHALLENGE**
>
> A 28-year-old married woman comes to the women's health clinic with low abdominal discomfort, dysuria, and intermenstrual (breakthrough bleeding), which she has had for 1 month. She also reports new vaginal discharge for the last week but seems reluctant to discuss her symptoms further.
>
> - What critical client history questions should you ask this client about her symptoms?
> - What questions should you ask as part of her sexual history?
> - If the client refuses to answer, what should you do?

For suggested answer guidelines, go to SIMON http://www.wbsaunders.com/SIMON/Iggy/.

PHYSICAL ASSESSMENT/CLINICAL MANIFESTATIONS

On physical assessment, the nurse may observe the client's discomfort with movement. Often the client will have a hunched-over gait that she uses to intuitively protect her abdomen. She may find it difficult to independently get on the examination table or stretcher. She may be fatigued, diaphoretic, and hyperthermic.

On abdominal assessment, the nurse notes lower abdominal tenderness, possibly with rigidity or rebound tenderness. A pelvic examination by the health care provider may reveal yellow or green cervical discharge and a reddened or friable cervix (a cervix that bleeds easily). On bimanual examination, uterine or cervical tenderness with motion and tender adnexa (tubes and ovaries) are typically present. If the client is using an IUD for contraception, the device should be removed at the time of the examination if possible. Ectopic pregnancy and appendicitis must be ruled out as potential causes of the pain.

PSYCHOSOCIAL ASSESSMENT

The woman who presents with symptoms of PID is usually anxious and fearful of the examination and unknown diagnosis. She may need much reassurance and support during the physical examination because the abdomen is likely to be quite tender and she may wish to avoid further pain. An explanation of what is taking place often helps promote cooperation during the examination.

Because PID is most frequently associated with an STD, the woman may feel embarrassed or uncomfortable discussing her symptoms or history. The nurse uses a nonjudgmental approach and encourages the client to express her feelings and concerns. The client's ability to follow through with the treatment plan (taking antibiotics, resting, returning for follow-up evaluation in 48 hours) is essential in deciding if ambulatory care treatment is appropriate.

LABORATORY ASSESSMENT

The health care provider typically obtains cultures of the cervix, urethra, and rectum to determine the presence of *N. gonorrhoeae* or *C. trachomatis.* The white blood cell (WBC) count and erythrocyte sedimentation rate (ESR) may be elevated but are not sensitive enough by themselves for diagnosis of PID. Gram stains of endocervical secretions may show the presence of *N. gonorrhoeae.* A sensitive test that detects human chorionic gonadotropin in urine or blood should be performed to determine if the client is pregnant. Microscopic examination of vaginal discharge should be done to evaluate for signs of infection. The presence of more than 10 WBCs/HPF (high-power field) in vaginal discharge correlates with infection. Bacterial vaginosis can be found by observing the diagnostic clue cells.

OTHER DIAGNOSTIC ASSESSMENT

Abdominal ultrasonography is not helpful in establishing the diagnosis of PID, since it is usually normal. Sonography has been found to be useful in the diagnosis of appendicitis and tubo-ovarian abscesses that need to be ruled out when the diagnosis of PID is made. Transvaginal ultrasound has been used in some cases to detect tubal enlargement and tubal wall thickening associated with PID.

Laparoscopy, although expensive, invasive, and requiring anesthesia, is most definitive, giving an immediate, accurate diagnosis through direct inspection of the tubes and ovaries. Magnetic resonance imaging (MRI) and endometrial biopsy have been used to increase the accuracy of the diagnosis.

Because of great variations in client signs and symptoms, the diagnosis of acute PID is difficult. Because women may display subtle symptoms not typical of PID, delay in diagnosis and treatment may add to the sequelae of PID in the upper genital tract. Laparoscopy is considered the definitive diagnostic tool for PID but is not usually feasible. Therefore PID is diagnosed on the basis of clinical signs and symptoms. The Centers for Disease Control and Prevention (CDC) has set minimum criteria for the diagnosis of PID, but there are no laboratory or physical examination techniques that alone are both sensitive and specific for the diagnosis of acute PID. The CDC recommends empiric treatment of PID with antibiotics if all of the minimum criteria have been met and no other causes of illness can be found (Table 77-4).

TABLE 77-4 • DIAGNOSTIC CRITERIA FOR PELVIC INFLAMMATORY DISEASE

MINIMUM CRITERIA FOR INITIATING EMPIRIC TREATMENT FOR PELVIC INFLAMMATORY DISEASE
- Lower abdominal tenderness *and*
- Adnexal tenderness *and*
- Cervical motion tenderness (chandelier sign)

ADDITIONAL CRITERIA TO INCREASE THE SPECIFICITY OF THE DIAGNOSIS OF PID
- Oral temperature >101° F (>38.3° C)
- Abnormal cervical or vaginal discharge
- Elevated erythrocyte sedimentation rate
- Elevated C-reactive protein
- Laboratory documentation of cervical infection with *Neisseria gonorrhoeae* or *Chlamydia trachomatis*

DEFINITIVE CRITERIA FOR DIAGNOSING PID, WARRANTED IN SELECTED CASES
- Histopathologic evidence of endometritis on endometrial biopsy
- Transvaginal sonography or other imaging techniques showing thickened fluid-filled tubes with or without free pelvic fluid or tubo-ovarian complex
- Laparoscopic abnormalities consistent with PID

Modified from Centers for Disease Control and Prevention. (1998). 1998 guidelines for treatment of sexually transmitted diseases. *Morbidity and Mortality Weekly Report, 47*(No. RR-1), 1-103.
PID, Pelvic inflammatory disease.

CRITICAL THINKING CHALLENGE

On your initial physical assessment, you find that the 28-year-old married client has an oral temperature of 100.2° F (37.9° C). The abdominal assessment is significant for grimacing and holding the abdomen as the woman moves onto the examination table. Her abdomen is tender in the suprapubic and right lower quadrant areas. The nurse practitioner plans to perform the pelvic examination.

- What further physical assessment and laboratory data should be obtained?
- When she learns that she has PID, the woman begins to cry and then yells, "I can't have that. Only loose women have that!" How would you respond to this statement?

For suggested answer guidelines, go to SIMON http://www.wbsaunders.com/SIMON/Iggy/.

Analysis

COMMON NURSING DIAGNOSES AND COLLABORATIVE PROBLEMS

The primary collaborative problem for clients with pelvic inflammatory disease (PID) is Infection related to invasion of pelvic organs by pathogens.

The following are common nursing diagnoses for clients with PID:

1. Acute Pain related to the effects of the infectious process
2. Anxiety related to possible infertility as a result of infection

ADDITIONAL NURSING DIAGNOSES AND COLLABORATIVE PROBLEMS

In addition to the common nursing diagnoses and collaborative problems, clients with PID may have one or more of the following:

- Altered Health Maintenance related to knowledge deficit about risks, prevention, symptoms, treatment, and effects of PID
- Chronic Pain related to recurrent PID episodes
- Sexual Dysfunction related to the effects of the infectious process
- Situational Low Self-Esteem/Chronic Low Self-Esteem related to feeling guilty for having PID (associated with sexual transmission)

Planning and Implementation

INFECTION

PLANNING: EXPECTED OUTCOMES. The client with PID is expected to have her infection resolve as evidenced by (1) a decrease in pain and tenderness of the pelvis, (2)being afebrile, and (3) resolution of other associated symptoms (vaginal discharge, positive cultures).

INTERVENTIONS. Infection control is accomplished by the administration of antibiotics, self-care measures, and surgical intervention if needed (Chart 77-5).

NIC **INFECTION CONTROL.** Uncomplicated PID is usually treated on an ambulatory care basis. The CDC recommends hospitalization for PID if the client:

- Has appendicitis, ectopic pregnancy, or other surgical emergency that has not been excluded

CHART 77-5

NIC INTERVENTION ACTIVITIES *for* The Client with Pelvic Inflammatory Disease

Infection Control: *Minimizing the acquisition and transmission of infectious agents*
- Encourage rest.
- Encourage fluid intake, as appropriate.
- Administer antibiotic therapy, as appropriate. *Or*
- Instruct client to take antibiotics, as prescribed.
- Promote appropriate nutritional intake.
- Teach client and family about signs and symptoms of infection and when to report them to the health care provider.
- Teach client and family members how to avoid infections.

Anxiety Reduction: *Minimizing apprehension, dread, foreboding, or uneasiness related to an unidentified source of anticipated danger*
- Create an atmosphere to facilitate trust.
- Listen attentively.
- Encourage verbalization of feelings, perceptions, and fears.
- Provide factual information concerning diagnosis, treatment, and prognosis.
- Instruct client on the use of relaxation techniques.

- Is pregnant
- Does not respond clinically to oral antibiotic therapy
- Is unable to follow or tolerate an outpatient regimen
- Has severe illness, nausea and vomiting, or high fever
- Has a tubo-ovarian abscess
- Is immunodeficient (e.g., has HIV infection with low CD4 counts, is taking immunosuppressive therapy, or has another disease)

Drug therapy consists of oral and possibly intramuscular or IV antibiotics (Chart 77-6). Oral treatment lasts for 14 days. All clients should be re-evaluated 48 to 72 hours after antibiotic therapy is started. If the infection has not responded to treatment, the client may need to be hospitalized for IV antibiotic therapy and further evaluation.

Inpatient therapy initially involves a combination of several IV antibiotics until the client has shown signs of clinical improvement, such as decreased abdominal tenderness, for at least 24 hours. Then oral antibiotics can be continued until the course of treatment has lasted 14 days.

When a client is treated as an outpatient, she should be encouraged to rest, abstain from sexual intercourse, and check her temperature twice a day. She will need to be seen by the health care provider 48 to 72 hours from starting the antibiotics and then 1 and 2 weeks from the time of the initial diagnosis.

In a small number of clients, the pain and tenderness may not be relieved by antibiotic therapy. The surgeon may perform a laparotomy to remove an abscess or a pelvic mass through a subumbilical incision that is several inches long to provide better access to the fallopian tubes. Preoperatively, the nurse provides information about hospital routines and procedures. General preoperative care is described in Chapter 17.

The postoperative care of the woman with PID is similar to that of any client after abdominal surgery. One difference is that the client with PID may have a wound drain in place for drainage of abscess fluid that may not have been completely removed during surgery. The nurse observes, measures, and records wound drainage every 4 to 8 hours as ordered.

ACUTE PAIN

NOC PLANNING: EXPECTED OUTCOMES. The client with PID is expected to report or demonstrate reduced pain and increased comfort as indicated by decreased restlessness; decreased blood pressure, heart rate, and respiratory rate; and decreased facial expressions of pain.

INTERVENTIONS. Pain management of PID begins with treatment of the infection. Antibiotic treatment relieves pain. If the client is ill enough to be hospitalized, parenteral antibiotic administration is usually chosen. Oral therapy can begin once the client's clinical status has shown improvement for at least 24 hours. Doxycycline (Monodox, Doxy-Caps, Doxycin✤) is usually given orally because of the pain associated with parenteral administration but is given as part of a parenteral inpatient regimen.

Other pain relief measures include taking analgesics or sitz baths and applying heat to the lower abdomen or back. Bedrest in a semi-Fowler's position promotes gravity drainage and consolidation of the infection that may relieve pain as well.

ANXIETY

NOC PLANNING: EXPECTED OUTCOMES. The client with PID is expected to take actions to reduce anxiety about infertility as indicated by identifying effective coping patterns, verbalizing a sense of control, using available social support, using effective coping strategies, and seeking professional help as appropriate.

INTERVENTIONS. Infertility is the most common complication of PID and affects at least 15% to 25% of women who have had at least one episode of PID. Nursing interventions are aimed at seeking to understand the client's perspective on the diagnosis and future complications.

NIC ANXIETY REDUCTION. If the client has anxiety, the nurse tries to provide an atmosphere in which she feels comfortable expressing her feelings and asking questions. The nurse provides information about the diagnosis, treatment, and prognosis. Providing information about the advantages of early diagnosis and treatment (possibly limiting damage to one area of the pelvis) and the advances in treatments for infertility may reassure the client. The nurse helps the client assess the emotional support available from family members or significant others. Relaxation techniques may be useful to decrease the anxiety (see Chart 77-5).

Community-Based Care

The client with pelvic inflammatory disease (PID) needs to have regular follow-up with her health care provider to assess for complications and ensure that the infection has resolved. The ongoing role of the nurse is to vigilantly assess for any continued risk of contracting PID again, signs of persistent or recurrent infection, and ongoing education to prevent expo-

CHART 77-6

DRUG THERAPY *for* Acute Pelvic Inflammatory Disease

Drug	Dosage	Nursing Interventions	Rationale
PARENTERAL TREATMENT			
Regimen A			
Cefotetan (Cefotan)	2 g every 12 hr IV, which can be changed to oral therapy after 24 hr of clinical improvement	Assess the client for rash, itching, and hypotension.	Assessment detects adverse reactions.
Or			
Cefoxitin (Mefoxin)	2 g IV every 6 hr, which can be changed to oral therapy after 24 hr of clinical improvement	Assess the client for rash, itching, and hypotension. Observe the IV site for signs of redness, heat, and tenderness.	Assessment detects adverse reactions. Phlebitis can be detected.
Plus			
Doxycycline (Monodox, Doxy-Caps, Doxycin♣)	100 mg every 12 hr IV or PO for 14 days. (Orally is preferred because of the pain associated with infusion.)	Assess the client for rash, nausea, and diarrhea. Encourage fluid intake. Instruct the client about possible photosensitivity. Instruct the client that it is beneficial to take the drug with food.	Assessment detects drug side effects. Fluid intake decreases esophageal irritation. This precaution prevents sunburning by limiting the client's exposure to the sun. Food decreases gastrointestinal upset.
Regimen B			
Clindamycin (Cleocin)	900 mg every 8 hr IV	Observe the client for rash and urticaria. Observe the client for hypotension, dyspnea, and restlessness. Observe the client for diarrhea. Observe the IV site for redness, heat, and tenderness.	Adverse reactions are detected. Anaphylactic reaction is detected. This precaution avoids pseudomembranous colitis. Phlebitis can be detected.
Plus			
Gentamicin (Garamycin IV)	2 mg/kg once IV or IM followed by 1.5 mg/kg every 8 hr IV or IM until there have been signs of clinical improvement for 24 hr	Encourage oral intake of fluids. Observe the IV site for redness, heat, and tenderness. Measure fluid intake and output. Observe the client for hearing loss, fever, or decreased renal function. Draw serum for peak and trough levels.	Fluid intake prevents irritation to renal tubules. Phlebitis can be detected. Oliguria or anuria can be detected. Ototoxicity, nephrotoxicity, and fever are known side effects. Serum levels can vary, and drug has low threshold for toxic level.
Then			
Doxycycline (Monodox, Doxy-Caps, Doxycin♣)	100 mg bid PO to complete a total of 14 days of treatment	See above for doxycycline.	See above for doxycycline.
Or			
Clindamycin (Cleocin)	450 mg qid PO to complete a total of 14 days of treatment	Give with 8 oz of water. See above for clindamycin.	Water decreases esophageal irritation. See above for clindamycin.

Modified from Centers for Disease Control and Prevention (1998). 1998 guidelines for treatment of sexually transmitted diseases. *Morbidity and Mortality Weekly Report, 47*(No. RR-1), 1-103.

Continued

CHART 77-6

DRUG THERAPY *for* Acute Pelvic Inflammatory Disease—cont'd

Drug	Dosage	Nursing Interventions	Rationale
ORAL TREATMENT			
Regimen A			
Ofloxacin (Floxin)	400 mg bid PO for 14 days	Monitor the serum level if the client is taking theophylline.	This drug raises the serum level of theophylline.
		Do not administer this drug to clients <18 yr of age.	The safety of this drug has not been established in clients <18 yr of age.
		Administer or instruct the client to take this drug on an empty stomach.	Food decreases this drug's absorption.
Plus			
Metronidazole (Flagyl, Novonidazol✤)	500 mg bid PO for 14 days	Monitor the serum level if the client is taking lithium.	This drug raises the serum level of lithium.
		Avoid alcohol within 24 hr of use.	Avoids disulfiram (Antabuse)–like effect.
Regimen B			
Ceftriaxone (Rocephin)	250 mg once IM	Give deep IM injection in the outer upper quadrant of the gluteus maximus.	Local irritation is avoided, and drug absorption is increased.
		Watch for fever, chills, and nausea.	Allergic reactions can be detected.
		Tell the client that the injection may be painful.	The client is prepared for discomfort related to the inflammatory reaction.
Or			
Cefoxitin (Mefoxin)	2 g once IM	Give deep IM injection in the outer upper quadrant of the gluteus maximus.	Local irritation is avoided, and drug absorption is increased.
		Watch for fever, chills, and nausea.	Allergic reactions can be detected.
		Tell the client that the injection may be painful.	The client is prepared for discomfort related to the inflammatory reaction.
Plus			
Probenecid (Benemid, Benuryl✤)	1 g once PO concurrently	Give with food.	Taking the medication with food avoids gastrointestinal upset.
		Encourage fluid intake (10 glasses a day).	Fluid intake prevents formation of kidney stones.
Or			
Other parenteral third-generation cephalosporin (e.g., ceftizoxime or cefotaxime)			
Plus			
Doxycycline (for all of the above regimens)	100 mg bid PO for 14 days	See above for doxycycline.	See above for doxycycline.

Modified from Centers for Disease Control and Prevention (1998). 1998 guidelines for treatment of sexually transmitted diseases. *Morbidity and Mortality Weekly Report, 47*(No. RR-1), 1-103.

sure to and infection with all STDs (e.g., a decrease in the number of partners, consistent condom use). The nurse establishes an atmosphere of trust that encourages the client to return frequently, if needed, for education or reassurance.

HEALTH TEACHING

Client teaching focuses on providing information about PID, identifying recurrences (persistent pain, dysmenorrhea, low backache, fever), and urging early treatment to prevent complications. The nurse also reviews teaching for oral antibiotic therapy (Chart 77-7).

The client needs to be counseled to contact her sexual partner(s) for examination and treatment. The partner is usually given treatment for gonorrhea and chlamydial infection. The nurse reminds her client about follow-up care and counsels her about the complications that can occur after an episode of PID, including increased risk for recurrence of PID, increased risk for ectopic pregnancy, increased risk for infertility, and chronic pelvic pain.

CHART 77-7

CLIENT EDUCATION GUIDE
Oral Antibiotic Therapy for Sexually Transmitted Diseases

- Take your medicine for the number of times a day it is prescribed and until it is completed.
- Your sexual partner must be tested and may need to be treated.
- Be sure to return for your follow-up appointment after completing your antibiotic treatment.
- Call if you have any questions or concerns.
- Do not have sex until after you complete your antibiotic therapy. If your partner is being treated, you can go back to having sex together 48 hours after he or she starts taking antibiotics if you use a condom.
- Drink at least 8 to 10 glasses of fluid a day while taking your antibiotics.
- Do not take antacids containing calcium, magnesium, or aluminum, such as Tums, Maalox, or Mylanta, with your antibiotics. They may decrease the effectiveness of the antibiotic.
- Take your antibiotics on an empty stomach unless your health care provider instructs you to take them with food.

If the client desires contraception, the nurse discusses methods that may decrease the risk of future episodes of PID, such as oral contraceptive pills, barrier methods in combination with spermicides containing nonoxynol 9, and tubal ligation.

Counseling is also given to help the client understand lifestyle factors that heighten the risk for recurrent episodes of PID, including sexual intercourse with multiple partners and vaginal douching.

Psychosocial concerns may require teaching and counseling as well. A client who has PID may exhibit a variety of feelings (guilt, disgust, anger) about having a condition that may have been transmitted to her sexually. These feelings may affect her relationship with significant others and future sexual relationships. She may also have concerns about future fertility if PID has caused damage or scarring of the fallopian tubes and other reproductive organs. The nurse provides emotional support and allows time for the client to express her feelings.

HOME CARE MANAGEMENT

Parenteral antibiotic therapy may be administered at home, but usually the health care provider changes the treatment regimen to oral antibiotics before hospital discharge (see Planning and Implementation, p. 1819).

HEALTH CARE RESOURCES

If infertility is a result of PID, the client may need referral to a clinic specializing in infertility treatment and counseling. The client can also contact support groups for infertile couples; such groups exist in many local communities.

The costs of antibiotics for care of clients with PID and other STDs may be a concern for those who are uninsured or underinsured. The case manager, social worker, or ambulatory care nurse seeks community resources for free or discounted medications for clients with financial limitations.

Evaluation: Outcomes

NOC The nurse evaluates the care of the client with PID on the basis of the identified nursing diagnoses and collaborative problems. The expected outcomes include that the client will:

- Show evidence that the infection has resolved by (1) a decrease in pain and tenderness of the pelvis, (2) being afebrile, and (3) resolution of other associated symptoms (vaginal discharge, positive cultures)
- Report or demonstrate that pain is relieved or reduced and that she feels more comfortable
- Take action to manage anxiety about future infertility
- Describe the risk factors, signs and symptoms, management, and effects of PID
- Resume usual sexual activities without discomfort
- Express her feelings about having an infection that was probably caused by a sexually transmitted organism

SEXUALLY TRANSMITTED VAGINAL INFECTIONS

Vaginal infections, which are associated with discharge and vaginal irritation, are frequent and recurring problems for sexually active women. The following are common causes of vaginal infection:

- *Trichomonas vaginalis*
- *Candida,* primarily *C. albicans*
- Bacteria that produce bacterial vaginosis, including *Gardnerella vaginalis* and anaerobes

These infections can be spread by sexual contact. Men can also acquire these infections but are not always symptomatic. Several studies have shown that *T. vaginalis* is common in men, especially those who have other STDs, such as *Chlamydia trachomatis* (Bachmann et al., 2000; Joyner et al., 2000). However, because most of these infections are usually seen more commonly in women, assessments and interventions are discussed with other causes of vaginitis in Chapter 75.

Trichomoniasis and candidal infections are limited to the vagina. They can be very irritating and bothersome but will not cause any long-term sequela. The partner must also be treated for trichomoniasis if the infection is to be resolved. Candidiasis does not usually require partner treatment, but if the male partner is symptomatic (irritation of the genital skin), then treatment is indicated.

Bacterial vaginosis (BV) has been implicated in upper genital tract infections. Women undergoing surgery of the upper genital tract should be evaluated and treated if BV is found (Peipert et al., 1997). There has also been evidence that BV in pregnancy can lead to preterm labor and premature delivery. This has been controversial, but evaluation for BV during pregnancy has been suggested.

HEPATITIS B AND C

In the United States, 30% to 60% of the new cases of hepatitis B and in 15% to 20% of the new cases of hepatitis C are transmitted sexually. Each year an estimated 240,000 new cases of hepatitis B virus (HBV) and 36,000 new cases of hepatitis C (HCV) occur. Of those infected as adults, 1% to 6% of those with HBV and 75% to 85% of those with HCV develop chronic hepatitis, which can lead to cirrhosis and primary hepatocellular carcinoma. Each year approximately

6000 people die from HBV and 8000 to 10,000 die from HCV (CDC, 1998a; CDC, 1998b). Hepatitis is discussed further in Chapter 59.

Prevention of sexually transmitted diseases (STDs) should include educating clients about the risks of contracting hepatitis B and C. Screening for STDs should include serum evaluation for hepatitis B and C. Hepatitis B vaccine, a series of three injections over a period of 6 months, is now recommended for all newborns, children 11 to 12 years of age if they have not already received the vaccine, and adolescents and adults at high risk for STDs.

ONLINE RESOURCES

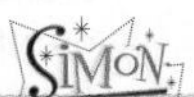

For suggested readings and Internet resources, go to http://www.wbsaunders.com/SIMON/Iggy/.

SELECTED BIBLIOGRAPHY

Asterisk indicates a classic or definitive work on this subject.

Amaral, E. (1998). Current approaches to STD management in women. *International Journal of Gynecology and Obstetrics, 63*(Suppl. 1), S183-S189.

Bachmann, L.H., et al. (2000). Risk and prevalence of treatable sexually transmitted diseases at a Birmingham substance abuse treatment facility. *American Journal of Public Health, 90*(10), 1615-1618.

Bartlett, J.G. (1998). *Pocket book of infectious disease therapy.* Baltimore: Williams & Wilkins.

Barton, S.E. (1998). Herpes management and prophylaxis. *Dermatologic Clinics, 16*(4), 799-803.

Beutner, K.R., et al. (1999). Genital warts and their treatment. *Clinical Infectious Diseases, 28*(Suppl. 1), S37-S56.

Black, C.M. (1997). Current methods of laboratory diagnosis of *Chlamydia trachomatis* infections. *Clinical Microbiology Review, 10*(1), 160-184.

Bob, P.S.S., & Famolare, N.E. (1998). Teaching and communication strategies: Working with the hospitalized adolescent with pelvic inflammatory disease. *Pediatric Nursing, 24*(1), 17-20, 29-30.

Burnstein, G.R., et al. (1998). Incident *Chlamydia trachomatis* infections among inner-city adolescent females. *Journal of the American Medical Association,, 280*(6), 521-526.

Carrico, C.W. (1999). Impact of sonography on the diagnosis and treatment of acute lower abdominal pain in children and young adults. *American Journal of Roentgenology, 172*(2), 513-516.

Centers for Disease Control and Prevention. (1997). *Chlamydia trachomatis* genital infections—United States, 1995. *Journal of the American Medical Association, 277*(12):952-953.

Centers for Disease Control and Prevention. (1998a). 1998 guidelines for treatment of sexually transmitted diseases. *Morbidity and Mortality Weekly Report, 47*(RR-1), 1-103.

Centers for Disease Control and Prevention. (1998b). Recommendations for prevention and control of hepatitis C virus (HCV) infection and HCV-related chronic disease. *Morbidity and Mortality Weekly Report, 47*(RR-19), 1, 7-8.

Centers for Disease Control and Prevention. (1999). Primary and secondary syphilis—United States, 1998. *Morbidity and Mortality Weekly Report, 48*(39), 873-878.

Centers for Disease Control and Prevention. (2001). Tracking the hidden epidemics: Trends in STDs in the United States 2000; www.cdc.gov/nchstp/dstd/Stats_Trends/Trends2000.pdf.

Cohen, C.R., & Brunham, R.C. (1999). Pathogenesis of chlamydia induced pelvic inflammatory disease. *Sexually Transmitted Infections, 75*(1), 21-24.

Daley, E.M. (1998). Clinical update on the role of HPV and cervical cancer. *Cancer Nursing, 21*(1), 31-35.

Faro, S. (1998). Sepsis in obstetric and gynecologic patients. *Current Clinical Topics in Infectious Disease, 19,* 60-82.

Groseclose, S.L., et al. (1999). Estimated incidence and prevalence of genital *Chlamydia trachomatis* infections in the United States, 1996. *Sexually Transmitted Diseases, 26*(6), 339-344.

Hein, K. (1998). Health policy implications of emerging infections. *Emerging Infectious Diseases, 4*(3), 1-5.

Joyner, J.L., et al. (2000). Comparative prevalence of infection with *Trichomonas vaginalis* among men attending a sexually transmitted disease clinic. *Sexually Transmitted Diseases, 27*(4), 236-240.

Kellock, D.J., et al. (1997). Biopsy, serology, and molecular biology, *Genitourinary Medicine, 73*(5): 399-401.

Mahoney, J.B., et al. (1997). Detection of Chlamydia trachomatis, Neisseria gonorrhoeae, Ureaplasma urealyticum, and Mycoplasma genitalium in first-void urine specimens by multiplex polymerase chain reaction. *Molecular Diagnosis, 2*(3), 161-168.

Marr, L. (1998). *Sexually transmitted diseases: A physician tells you what you need to know.* Baltimore: Johns Hopkins University Press.

McOwan, A.G., Broughton, C., & Robinson, A.J. (1999). Advising patients with genital warts: A consensus approach. *International Journal of STD and AIDS, 10*(9), 619-622.

*Morse, S.A., Moreland, A.A., & Holmes, K.K. (1996). *Atlas of sexually transmitted diseases and AIDS* (2nd ed.). London: Mosby-Wolfe.

Norton, N.J. (1998). Coping with HPV: How to help a patient diagnosed with this sexually transmitted disease. *Nursing98, 28*(9), 73-74.

Paavonen, J. (1998). Pelvic inflammatory disease: from diagnosis to prevention. *Dermatologic Clinics, 16*(4), 747-756.

Peipert, J.F., et al. (1997). Bacterial vaginosis as a risk factor for upper genital tract infection. *American Journal of Obstetrics and Gynecology, 177*(5), 1184-1187.

Rosen, T., & Brown, T.J. (1998a). Cutaneous manifestations of sexually transmitted diseases, *Medical Clinics of North America, 82*(5), 1081-1104.

Rosen, T., & Brown, T.J. (1998b). Genital ulcers—Evaluation and treatment. *Dermatologic Clinics, 16*(4), 673-685.

Schaffer, S.D. (1998). Vaginitis and sexually transmitted diseases. In E.Q. Youngkin & M.S. Davis (Eds.), *Women's health care: A primary care clinical guide* (2nd ed., pp. 265-299). Stamford, CT: Appleton & Lange.

Schmid, G.P. (1999). Treatment of chancroid. *Clinical Infectious Diseases, 28*(Suppl. 1), S14-S20.

Sedlacek, T.V. (1999). Advances in the diagnosis and treatment of human papillomavirus infections. *Clinical Obstetrics and Gynecology, 42*(2), 206-220.

Sellors, J.W., et al. (2000). A new visual indicator of chlamydial cervicitis? *Sexually Transmitted Infections, 76*(1), 46-48.

Stamm, W.E. (1999). Chlamydia trachomatis infections: Progress and problems. *Journal of Infectious Diseases, 179*(Suppl. 2), S380-383.

Stanberry, L.R. (1998). Control of STDs: The role of prophylactic vaccines against herpes simplex virus. *Sexually Transmitted Infections, 74*(6), 391-394.

Tao, G., et al. (2000). Medical care expenditures for genital herpes in the United States. *Sexually Transmitted Diseases, 27*(1), 32-38.

Winefield, A.D., & Murphy, S.A. (1998). Bacterial vaginosis: A review. *Clinical Excellence for Nurse Practitioners, 2*(4), 212-217.

Youngkin, E.Q., & Davis, M.S. (1998). *Women's health care: A primary care clinical guide* (2nd ed.), 1998, Stamford, CT: Appleton & Lange.

APPENDIXES

Abbreviations

AAA	abdominal aortic aneurysm
AACN	American Association of Critical Care Nurses
AAKP	American Association of Kidney Patients
ABC	airway, breathing, and circulation
ABG	arterial blood gas
ABI	ankle-brachial index
ABPM	ambulatory blood pressure monitoring
ABVD	Adriamycin, bleomycin, vinblastine, dacarbazine
AC	assist-control; alternating current
ACE	angiotensin-converting enzyme
ACh	acetylcholine
AChRAb	acetylcholine receptor antibody
ACL	anterior cruciate ligament
ACLS	advanced cardiac life support
ACS	acute compartment syndrome; American Cancer Society
ACTH	adrenocorticotropic hormone
ADC	AIDS dementia complex
ADH	antidiuretic hormone
ADL	activities of daily living
ADP	adenosine diphosphate
ADPKD	autosomal-dominant polycystic kidney disease
AED	automatic external defibrillation
aFP	alpha-fetoprotein
AGC	absolute granulocyte count
AGN	acute glomerulonephritis
AGR	abdominal/gluteal ratio
AHA	American Heart Association
AHRQ	Agency for Healthcare Research and Quality
AIDS	acquired immunodeficiency syndrome
AIVR	accelerated idioventricular rhythm
AJCC	American Joint Committee on Cancer
AKA	above-knee amputation
AL	ascending limb
ALA	American Lung Association
ALG	antilymphocyte globulin
ALL	acute lymphocytic leukemia
ALP	alkaline phosphatase
ALS	amyotrophic lateral sclerosis
AMI	antibody-mediated immunity
AML	acute myelocytic leukemia
AMSN	Academy of Medical-Surgical Nurses
ANA	American Nurses' Association; anti-nuclear antibody
ANC	absolute neutrophil count
ANOVA	analysis of variance
ANP	atrial natriuretic peptide
ANS	autonomic nervous system
AORN	Association of periOperative Room Nurses
AP	anteroposterior
APSAC	anisoylated plasminogen streptokinase activator complex
APSGN	acute poststreptococcal glomerulonephritis
aPTT	activated partial thromboplastin time
ara-A	adenine arabinoside
ARDS	acute respiratory distress syndrome
ARF	acute renal failure
ASA	acetylsalicylic acid
ASPEN	American Society of Parenteral and Enteral Nutrition
AST	aspartate aminotransferase
ATG	antithymocyte globulin
ATN	acute tubular necrosis
ATP	adenosine triphosphate
ATPase	adenosine triphosphatase
AV	atrioventricular, arteriovenous
AVM	arteriovenous malformation
AVN	avascular necrosis
AZA	azathioprine
AZT	azidothymidine (zidovudine)
BBIAT	Baird Body Image Assessment Tool
BC	Bowman's capsule
BCG	bacille Calmette-Guérin
BCNU	carmustine
BCS	Body Cathexis Scale
BE	barium enema
BGMS	blood glucose monitoring strip
bid	*bis in die* (twice a day)
BKA	below-knee amputation
BMI	body mass index
BMT	bone marrow transplantation
BP	blood pressure
BPEG	British Pacing and Electrophysiology Group
BPH	benign prostatic hyperplasia (hypertrophy)
BPM	breaths per minute; beats per minute
BRM	biologic response modifier
BSE	breast self-examination
BSI	body substance isolation
BSO	bilateral salpingo-oophorectomy
BUN	blood urea nitrogen
c	cup(s)
C&S	culture and sensitivity
CABG	coronary artery bypass graft
CAD	computer-assisted design; coronary artery disease
CAH	chronic active hepatitis
CAL	chronic airflow limitation
CALLA	common acute lymphoblastic leukemia antigen
CAM	complementary and alternative medicine
cAMP	cyclic adenosine monophosphate
CAPD	continuous ambulatory peritoneal dialysis
CAVH	continuous arteriovenous hemofiltration
CAVHD	continuous arteriovenous hemofiltration and dialysis
CBC	complete blood count
CBD	common bile duct
CBE	charting by exception
CBI	continuous bladder irrigation
CBS	chronic brain syndrome
CCA	circumflex coronary artery
CCP	critical closing pressure
CCPD	continuous-cycle peritoneal dialysis
CD	Cotrel-Dubousset; collecting duct

CD4 cluster of differentiation 4
CDC Centers for Disease Control and Prevention; chenodeoxycholic acid
CEA carcinoembryonic antigen
CFU colony-forming unit
CGN chronic glomerulonephritis
CHF congestive heart failure
CIC Certified in Infection Control
CIN cervical intraepithelial neoplasia
CIS carcinoma in situ
CK creatine kinase
CLE centrilobular emphysema
CLL chronic lymphocytic leukemia
cm centimeter(s)
CMG cystometrogram
CMI cell-mediated immunity
CML chronic myelocytic leukemia
CMS circulation, movement, sensation
CMV cisplatin, methotrexate, vinblastine; cytomegalovirus
CNS central nervous system
CO cardiac output
COHb carboxyhemoglobin
COLD chronic obstructive lung disease
COPD chronic obstructive pulmonary disease
COPES Family Crisis-Oriented Personal Evaluation Scale
CPAP continuous positive airway pressure
CPB cardiopulmonary bypass
CPK creatine phosphokinase
CPM continuous passive motion
CPN chronic pyelonephritis
CPO certified prosthetist-orthotist
CPP cerebral perfusion pressure
CPR cardiopulmonary resuscitation
cps cycles per second
CQI continuous quality improvement
CREST calcinosis, Raynaud's phenomenon, esophageal dysfunction sclerodactyly, telangiectasia
CRF chronic renal failure
CRH corticotropin-releasing hormone
CRI chronic renal insufficiency
CRNA Certified Registered Nurse Anesthetist
CS crush syndrome
CSA cyclosporine A
CSF cerebrospinal fluid
CST Certified Surgical Technologist
CT computed tomography
CTD connective tissue disease
CTS carpal tunnel syndrome
CVA cerebrovascular accident (stroke); costovertebral angle
CVC central venous catheter
CVP central venous pressure
D&C dilation and curettage
DARE Drug Awareness Resistance Education
dB decibel(s)
DCCT Diabetes Control and Complications Trial
DCM dilated cardiomyopathy
DCT distal convoluted tubule
DDAVP desmopressin acetate
ddI dideoxyinosine (didanosine)
DDS dapsone
DES diethylstilbestrol
DHE dihydroergotamine
DHHS (US) Department of Health and Human Services
DHT dihydrotestosterone
DI diabetes insipidus
DIC disseminated intravascular coagulation
DIP distal interphalangeal joint
DJD degenerative joint disease
dL deciliter(s)
DL descending limb
DLCO diffusion capacity for carbon monoxide
DLE discoid lupus erythematosus
DNA deoxyribonucleic acid
DNP dinitrophenol
DNR do not resuscitate
DOE dyspnea on exertion
DP dopamine
DPOA durable power of attorney
DRE digital rectal examination
DRG diagnosis-related group
DS double-strength
DSA digital subtraction angiography
DTIC dacarbazine
DTR deep tendon reflex
DUB dysfunctional uterine bleeding
DVT deep vein thrombosis
EAT Eating Attitudes Test
EBL estimated blood loss
EBV Epstein-Barr virus
ECCC Emergency Cardiac Care Committee
ECCE extracapsular cataract extraction
ECF extracellular fluid
ECG electrocardiogram
EDI Eating Disorder Inventory
EGD esophagogastroduodenoscopy
EHDP etidronate disodium
EIA enzyme immunoassay
ELISA enzyme-linked immunosorbent assay
EMD electromechanical dissociation
EMG electromyography
EMS emergency medical services
EMT Emergency Medical Technician
ENCORE encouragement, normalcy, counseling, opportunity, reaching out, revived energies
ENG electronystagmography
ENT ear, nose, and throat
EOM extraocular movement
EPO erythropoietin
EPS electrophysiologic study
ER estrogen receptor
ERCP endoscopic retrograde cholangiopancreatography
ERS endoscopic retrograde sphincterotomy
ERT estrogen replacement therapy
ESR erythrocyte sedimentation rate
ESRD end-stage renal disease
ET Enterostomal Therapist; endotracheal tube
ETDR early treatment diabetic retinopathy
ETT exercise tolerance test
EVS early vitrectomy study
FACT fruits, animals, colors, and towns
FAM fluorouracil, Adriamycin, and mitomycin C
FANA fluorescent antinuclear antibody
FAST fluoroallergosorbent test
FBD fibrocystic breast disease
FBSS failed back surgery syndrome
FDA (US) Food and Drug Administration
FEF forced expiratory flow
FES fat embolism syndrome
FEV forced expiratory volume
FEV_1 forced expiratory volume in one second
FEV_1/FVC ratio of expiratory volume in one second to forced vital capacity

FFP	fresh frozen plasma
FIM	Functional Independence Measure
FIO_2	fraction of inspired oxygen
FNB	Food and Nutrition Board
FNCR	Family Nursing Chart Review
FOBT	fecal occult blood test
FR	flutter rate
Fr	French
FRC	functional residual capacity
FS	full-strength
FSBS	fingerstick blood sugar
FSH	follicle-stimulating hormone
ft	foot (feet)
FTA-ABS	fluorescent treponemal antibody absorption test
5-FU	5-fluorouracil
FUDR	floxuridine
FVC	forced vital capacity
FWB	full weight-bearing
g/day	gram(s) per day
g	gram(s)
G6PD	glucose-6-phosphate dehydrogenase
GABA	gamma-aminobutyric acid
GAS	general adaptation syndrome
GB	gallbladder
GBS	Guillain-Barré syndrome
GCS	Glasgow Coma Scale
GCSF	granulocyte colony-stimulating factor
GDM	gestational diabetes mellitus
GE	gastroenteritis
GF	glomerular filtrate
GFR	glomerular filtration rate
GH	growth hormone
GH-IH	growth hormone–inhibiting hormone
GH-RH	growth hormone–releasing hormone
GI	gastrointestinal
GM-CSF	granulocyte-macrophage colony-stimulating factor
Gn-RH	gonadotropin-releasing hormone
GSW	gunshot wound
GVHD	graft-versus-host disease
Gy	Gray(s)
h	hour(s)
HAT	hearing assessment test
Hb	hemoglobin
HBIG	hepatitis B immunoglobulin
HBO	hyperbaric oxygen
HBV	hepatitis B virus
hCG	human chorionic gonadotropin
HCM	hypertrophic cardiomyopathy
Hct	hematocrit
HCV	hepatitis C virus
HD	hemodialysis
HDL	high-density lipoprotein
HDV	hepatitis delta virus
HEPA	high-efficiency particulate air
HEV	hepatitis E virus
Hgb	hemoglobin
HIDA	hepatobiliary iminodiacetic acid analog (radionuclide labeled with technetium-99m)
HIP	Help for Incontinent Persons
HITT	heparin-induced thrombocytopenia/thrombosis
HLA	human leukocyte antigen
HMO	health maintenance organization
HPA	hypothalamic-pituitary-adrenal
HPV	human papillomavirus
HR	heart rate
HSV	herpes simplex virus
5-HT	5-hydroxytryptamine (serotonin)
HTLV	human T-cell lymphotropic virus
Hz	Hertz
I&D	incision and drainage
IABP	intra-aortic balloon pumping
IBS	irritable bowel syndrome
IBW	ideal body weight
ICD	implantable cardioverter-defibrillator
ICE	Institutional Ethics Committee
ICF	intracellular fluid
ICHD	Intersociety Commission for Heart Disease
ICP	intracranial pressure
ICS	intercostal space
ICU	intensive care unit
IF	interstitial fluid
Ig	immunoglobulin
IHSS	idiopathic hypertrophic subaortic stenosis
IL	interleukin
IL-2	interleukin-2
IL-3	interleukin-3
IL-4	interleukin-4
IL-5	interleukin-5
IL-8	interleukin-8
IM	intramedullary rod; intramuscular
IMF	intermaxillary fixation
IMV	intermittent mandatory ventilation
INF	interferon
INR	International Normalized Ratio
IOL	intraocular lens
IOP	intraocular pressure
IP	intraperitoneal
IPD	intermittent peritoneal dialysis
IPG	impedance plethysmography
IRT	intracavitary radiation therapy
IS	incentive spirometer
ITH	idiosyncratic toxic hepatitis
ITP	idiopathic thrombocytopenic purpura
IU	International Unit(s)
IUD	intrauterine device
IU/L	International Unit(s) per liter
IV	intravenous
IVC	inferior vena cava
IVP	intravenous pyelography
JCAHO	Joint Commission on the Accreditation of Healthcare Organizations
JGC	juxtaglomerular cell
JVD	jugular-venous distention
JVP	jugular venous pressure
KCS	keratoconjunctivitis sicca
kg	kilogram(s)
kJ	kilojoule(s)
KS	Kaposi's sarcoma
KUB	kidneys, ureters, and bladder
KW	Keith-Wagner classification
LAC	long arm cast
LAD	left anterior descending
LAK	lymphokine-activated killer (cell)
LAP	leukocyte alkaline phosphatase
LAS	localized adaptation syndrome
LATS	long-acting thyroid stimulator
LBP	low back pain
LCA	left coronary artery
LDH	lactate dehydrogenase
LDL	low-density lipoprotein
LE	lupus erythematosus; lower extremity
LES	lower esophageal sphincter
LGV	lymphogranuloma venereum
LH	luteinizing hormone
LL	left lateral

LLC long leg cast
LLQ left lower quadrant
LMN lower motor neuron
LOA leave of absence
LOC level of consciousness
LORS Level of Rehabilitation Scale
LP lumbar puncture, light perception
LPS lipopolysaccharide
LR lactated Ringer's (solution)
LRD living related donor
LTC long-term care
LUQ left upper quadrant
LVD left ventricular dysfunction
LVEDP left ventricular end-diastolic pressure
mA milliampere(s)
MAC *Mycobacterium avium* complex
MAO monoamine oxidase
MAP mean arterial pressure
MAST military antishock trousers
MAT multifocal atrial tachycardia
MB-CAPD multiple-bag continuous ambulatory peritoneal dialysis
MCA middle cerebral artery
MCH mean corpuscular hemoglobin
MCHC mean corpuscular hemoglobin concentration
MCL modified chest lead
MCP metacarpophalangeal
M-CSF monocyte-macrophage colony-stimulating factor
MCV mean corpuscular volume
MD muscular dystrophy
MDF myocardial depressant factor
MDI metered-dose inhaler
MEN multiple endocrine neoplasia
mEq milliequivalent(s)
mEq/L milliequivalent(s) per liter
MFH malignant firous histiocytoma
μg microgram(s)
mg milligram(s)
MG myasthenia gravis
mg/dL milligram(s) per deciliter
MH malignant hyperthermia
MHAUS Malignant Hyperthermia Association of the United States
MHC major histocompatibility complex
MI myocardial infarction
MICU medical intensive care unit
MIH melanocyte-inhibiting hormone
min minute(s)
mL milliliter(s)
mL/kg milliliter(s) per kilogram
mm millimeter(s)
mm Hg millimeter(s) of mercury
mmol millimole(s)
mmol/L millimoles per liter
MMPI Minnesota Multiphasic Personality Inventory
MMSE Mini-Mental State Examination
MMV maximum mandatory ventilation
MODY maturity-onset diabetes of the young
MOPP mechlorethamine, Oncovin, procarbazine, prednisone
mOsm milliosmole(s)
mOsm/L milliosmole(s) per liter
MRB manual resuscitation bag
MRC Medical Research Council
MRI magnetic resonance imaging
MS multiple sclerosis; morphine sulfate
msec millisecond(s)
MSH melanocyte-stimulating hormone
MTP metatarsophalangeal
MTX methotrexate
mU milliunit(s)
mU/mL milliunit(s) per milliliter
MUGA multigated angiography
mV millivolt(s)
MVA motor vehicle accident
MVAC methotrexate, vinblastine, Adriamycin, cisplatin
NANDA North American Nursing Diagnosis Association
NAON National Association of Orthopaedic Nurses
NAPHT National Association of Patients on Hemodialysis and Transplantation
NASPE North American Society for Pacing and Electrophysiology
NCI National Cancer Institute
NE norepinephrine
ng nanogram(s)
NG nasogastric
NHANES National Health and Nutrition Examination Survey
NHIF National Head Injury Foundation
NIC Nursing Interventions Classification
NK natural killer (cell)
NKF National Kidney Foundation
NLN National League for Nursing
NRC/NAS National Research Council/National Academy of Sciences
NS nephrotic syndrome; normal saline
NSAID nonsteroidal anti-inflammatory drug
NSNA National Student Nurse Association
NSR normal sinus rhythm
NTP noninvasive temporary pacing
NWB non-weight-bearing
NYHA New York Heart Association
OA osteoarthritis
OBS organic brain syndrome
OCG oral cholecystogram
OD oculus dexter (right eye)
OFP Optimal Functioning Plan
OI osteogenesis imperfecta
OR operating room
ORIF open reduction, internal fixation
ORT oral rehydration therapy; operating room technician
OS oculus sinister (left eye)
OSHA (US) Occupational Safety and Health Administration
OT occupational therapist
OTC over-the-counter
oz ounce(s)
PA posteroanterior; physician's assistant
PAB prealbumin
PAC premature atrial complex
$Paco_2$ partial pressure of arterial carbon dioxide
PACU postanesthesia care unit
Pao_2 partial pressure of arterial oxygen
Pap Papanicolaou (test, smear)
PAP pulmonary artery pressure
PASG pneumatic antishock garment
PAT paroxysmal atrial tachycardia
PAWP pulmonary artery wedge pressure
PCA patient-controlled analgesia; patient care assistant
PCAC Patient Care Advisory Committee
PCM protein-calorie malnutrition
PCN penicillin
PCP *Pneumocystis carinii* pneumonia
PCR polymerase chain reaction
PCT proximal convoluted tubule

PD	peritoneal dialysis
PE	pulmonary embolism; pharyngoesophageal
PEA	pulseless electrical activity
PEEP	positive end-expiratory pressure
PERRLA	pupils equal, round, and reactive to light and accommodation
PES	problem, etiology, symptoms
PES-EO-IO	problem, etiology, signs and symptoms; expected outcome, interventions, outcome
PET	positron emission tomography
PFT	pulmonary function test
PGE_2	prostaglandin E_2
PGI_2	prostaglandin I_2 (prostacyclin)
pH	the negative logarithm of the hydrogen ion concentration
PHP	plasma hydrostatic pressure
PHS	Public Health Service
PICC	peripherally inserted central catheter
PID	pelvic inflammatory disease
PIE	plan, interventions, evaluation
PIH	prolactin-inhibiting hormone
PIP	proximal interphalangeal; peak inspiratory pressure
PJC	premature junctional complex
PJT	premature junctional tachycardia
PKD	polycystic kidney disease
PLE	panlobular emphysema
PLP	phantom limb pain
PMI	point of maximal impact
PMN	polymorphonuclear cell
PMR	progressive muscle relaxation; polymyalgia rheumatica
PMS	premenstrual syndrome
PMT	premenstrual tension
PND	paroxysmal nocturnal dyspnea
PNS	parasympathetic nervous system; peripheral nervous system
PO	*per os* (by mouth)
POAG	primary open-angle glaucoma
POC	point-of-care
POR	problem-oriented record
PPD	purified protein derivative
ppm	parts per million
PPM	pulses per minute
PPN	partial parenteral nutrition
PPS	post-polio sequelae (syndrome)
PRL	prolactin
PRN	*pro re nata* (as needed)
PSA	prostate-specific antigen
PSE	portal-systemic encephalopathy
PSS	progressive systemic sclerosis
PSV	pressure support ventilation
PSVT	paroxysmal supraventricular tachycardia
PT	physical therapy; physical therapist; prothrombin time
PTA	percutaneous transluminal angioplasty; peritonsillar abscess
PTC	peritubular capillary
PTCA	percutaneous transluminal coronary angioplasty
PTFE	polytetrafluoroethylene
PTH	parathyroid hormone (parathormone)
PTT	partial thromboplastin time
PTU	propylthiouracil
PUD	peptic ulcer disease
PULSES	physical condition, upper limb function, lower limb function, sensory components, excretory function, support factors
PUVA	psoralen and ultraviolet A
PV	polycythemia vera
PVC	premature ventricular contraction
PVD	peripheral vascular disease
PVR	postvoiding residual
PVS	persistent vegetative state
PWB	partial weight-bearing
q	*quaque* (every)
qd	*quaque die* (every day)
qid	*quater in die* (four times a day)
qod	every other day
QOL	quality of life
QOLY	Quality of Life Year(s)
RA	rheumatoid arthritis
rad	radiation absorbed dose
RAI	radioactive iodine
RAIU	radioactive iodine uptake
RAS	reticular activating system
RBC	red blood cell
RCA	right coronary artery
RDA	recommended daily allowance; recommended dietary allowance
REM	rapid eye movement
RFUT	radiofibrinogen uptake test
RIA	radioimmunoassay
RIND	reversible ischemic neurologic deficit
RL	right lateral
RLQ	right lower quadrant
RNA	ribonucleic acid
RNI	Recommended Nutrient Intake
ROM	range of motion
RPGN	rapidly progressive glomerulonephritis
RSD	reflex sympathetic dystrophy
RTA	renal tubular acidosis
RUQ	right upper quadrant
RV	residual volume
SA	sinoatrial
SAC	short arm cast
SAECG	signal-averaged electrocardiography
SAM	smoking-attributable mortality
Sao_2	saturation of arterial oxygen
SBE	subacute bacterial endocarditis
SBFT	small bowel follow-through
SC	subcutaneous
SCD	sequential compression device
SCI	spinal cord injury
SCID	severe combined immunodeficiency
SCS	Self-Cathexis Scale
SDA	same-day admission
SDAT	senile dementia Alzheimer's type
SDS	same-day surgery
SEAPort	side-entry access port
sec	second(s)
SEP	somatosensory evoked potential
SF6	sulfahexafluoride
SFA	superficial femoral artery
SGOT	serum glutamic-oxaloacetic transaminase
SI	Système International d'Unites
SIADH	syndrome of inappropriate antidiuretic hormone
SIMV	synchronized intermittent mandatory ventilation
SLC	short leg cast
SLE	systemic lupus erythematosus
SLP	speech/language pathologist
SLR	straight-leg raise
SMI	sustained minimal inspiration; self-management inventory
SMR	submucous resection
SMX	sulfamethoxazole
SNF	skilled nursing facility

SNS	sympathetic nervous system
SOAP	subjective data, objective data, analysis, plan
SOAPIER	subjective data, objective data, analysis, plan, interventions, evaluation, revision of plan
SP	suprapubic
SPD	supply processing and distribution
SPECT	single photon emission computed tomography
SPEP	serum protein electrophoresis
SPF	suntan photoprotection factor
SSKI	saturated solution of potassium iodide
STA	superficial temporal artery
STD	sexually transmitted disease
STS	serologic test for syphilis
STSG	split-thickness skin graft
SV	stroke volume
SVC	superior vena cava
T&A	tonsillectomy and adenoidectomy
T_3	triiodothyronine
T_3RU	triiodothyronine resin uptake
T_4	thyroxine
TAF	tumor angiogenesis factor
TAH	total abdominal hysterectomy
TB	tuberculosis
TBI	total body irradiation
TBSA	total body surface area
tbsp	tablespoon(s)
TCDB	turn, cough, and deep breathe
TCT	thyrocalcitonin
TDT	terminal deoxynucleotidyl transferase
TED	thromboembolic device
TEE	transesophageal echocardiography
TEF	tracheosophageal fistula
TEN	toxic epidermal necrolysis
TENS	transcutaneous electrical nerve stimulation
THA	tetrahydroaminoacridine
THP	tissue hydrostatic pressure
THR	total hip replacement
TIA	transient ischemic attack
TIBC	total iron-binding capacity
tid	*ter in die* (three times a day)
TJR	total joint replacement
TKR	total knee replacement
TLC	total lung capacity; total lymphocyte count
TLS	tumor lysis syndrome
TLSO	thoracic lumbar sacral orthosis (thoracolumbosacral orthosis)
TMJ	temporomandibular joint
TMP	trimethroprim
TNF	tumor necrosis factor
TNM	tumor, node, metastasis
TOP	tissue osmotic pressure
TOPS	Take Off Pounds Sensibly
t-PA	tissue plasminogen activator
TPI	treponemal immobilization (test)
TPN	total parenteral nutrition
TQM	total quality management
TRH	thyrotropin-releasing hormone
TSE	testicular self-examination
TSH	thyroid-stimulating hormone
TSI	thyroid-stimulating immunoglobulin
TSM	transparent semipermeable membrane
tsp	teaspoon(s)
TSS	toxic shock syndrome
TTD	transtelephonic defibrillation/monitoring
TTO	transtracheal oxygen
TTP	thrombotic thrombocytopenic purpura
TURBT	transurethral resection of bladder tumor
TURP	transurethral resection of the prostate
TVH	total vaginal hysterectomy
UGI	upper gastrointestinal
UMN	upper motor neuron
UPJ	ureteropelvic junction
UPP	urethral pressure profilometry
US	ultrasonography
USDA	United States Department of Agriculture
UTI	urinary tract infection
UV	ultraviolet
UVA	ultraviolet A
UVB	ultraviolet B
UVJ	ureterovesical junction
VAD	venous access device
VADS	Visual Analog Dyspnea Scale
VAS	visual analog scale
VC	vital capacity
VCUG	voiding cystourethrogram
VDRL	Venereal Disease Research Laboratory (test)
VEP	visual evoked potential
VF	ventricular fibrillation
VLS	vascular leak syndrome
VMA	vanillylmandelic acid
$\dot{V}O_2$	oxygen consumption
VOD	veno-occlusive disease
VPB	ventricular premature beat
$\dot{V}/\dot{Q}$	ventilation-perfusion
VR	vasa recta
VSE	vulvar self-examination
VT	ventricular tachycardia
V_T	tidal volume
VZV	varicella-zoster virus
WAIS	Wechsler Adult Intelligence Scale
WBC	white blood cell
WHO	World Health Organization
WHR	waist-to-hip ratio

APPENDIX 2

Screening Guidelines for Secondary Prevention of Selected Cancers in Asymptomatic People

Cancer	Screening Test*
Breast cancer	Breast self-examination (monthly) Clinical examination (yearly) Mammography (baseline at age 35, every 2 years for ages 40-49, yearly after age 50)
Cervical cancer	Papanicolaou test and pelvic examination (yearly for sexually active women)
Ovarian cancer	Pelvic examination (yearly for women over age 40) Pelvic ultrasonography and blood test for CA-125 (yearly for women at high-risk)
Prostate cancer	Digital rectal examination and blood test for prostate-specific antigen (yearly starting at age 40)
Testicular cancer	Testicular self-examination (monthly after puberty) Clinical examination (yearly)
Colorectal cancer	Digital rectal examination and stool blood test (yearly starting at age 40) Colonoscopy (yearly starting at age 50)
Skin cancer	Visual self-examination of skin lesions (monthly for all ages) Clinical examination (yearly)

*Recommended frequency of screening tests varies by agency, preference of the health care provider, and individual client risk.

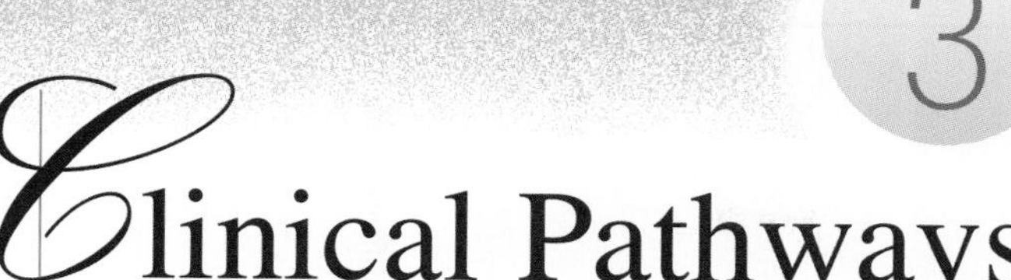

Clinical Pathways

Clinical Pathway ■ ANKLE SPRAIN CONTINUUM OF CARE

This pathway is designed to help you understand how to care for your ankle sprain during the initial healing phase and the rehabilitation phase. It is important for you to understand what to expect and to be able to participate actively in your recovery.

	Initial Healing Phase	Rehabilitation Phase
PAIN MANAGEMENT	Swelling increases the amount of pain in the ankle. Keep swelling down to reduce your pain. Use pain medicine prescribed by your doctor.	Ask your doctor about medicine you may buy without a prescription for pain management.
SWELLING	**RICE** **Rest** the ankle; use crutches if directed by your doctor. Limit walking to activity that is absolutely necessary. **Ice** the ankle for the first 24 hr after injury. Then use ice on the ankle 3-4 times a day for 20 min until swelling is no longer a problem. *Caution: Do not place ice directly on skin; always place towel between ice and skin.* **Compression** on the ankle with an elastic wrap or a brace if ordered by your doctor. *Caution: If the foot or toes become numb, call your doctor.* **Elevate** your ankle above your heart whenever possible (ankle above knee, knee above heart).	Swelling may occur after exercise or after standing or walking long distances. Continue to use ice and elevation after long periods of standing or walking to reduce swelling.
WALKING	Walk only when absolutely necessary. Use crutches or a cane if prescribed by your doctor. Use crutches properly, with weight on the ankle only as prescribed by your doctor. Use a brace only if prescribed by your doctor.	Walking on flat, level surfaces decreases the chance of reinjuring the ankle. Use a brace only if prescribed by your doctor.
DAILY ACTIVITIES	You may be limited in the distance you can walk because of pain or difficulty in walking with crutches. Plan your activities with frequent rest periods. Plan times for elevation of your ankle throughout the day.	Perform strengthening exercises as directed by your doctor or therapist. Return to normal walking pattern (avoid limping) as pain and swelling disappear.
PREVENTION		Prevent injury by avoiding potholes and uneven walking surfaces.

From Maher, A.B., Salmond, S.W., & Pellino, T. (1998). *Orthopaedic nursing* (2nd ed.). Philadelphia, W.B. Saunders.

CATHOLIC MEDICAL CENTER—MANCHESTER, NH.

Clinical Pathway ■ **CORONARY ARTERY BYPASS**

Name: ____________ Allergies: ____________

Admission date: ____________ Admitting diagnosis: ____________

Significant other: ____________ Can be reached at: home # ________ other # ________

DISCHARGE GOAL ☐ HOME ☐ SNF/REHAB

Addressograph

Day Prior to Surgery

Outcome	Standard	Completed date/time/initial	Misc. Information.
Appropriate lab/diagnostic testing is completed with results available on chart	If not done in the preceeding 15 days: CBC, chemistry group (CGR), U/A, PT, PTT, ECG, chest PA and lateral		BUN: ______ Creatinine: ______
Blood products are available as ordered for surgery	Day prior to surgery: type and crossmatch ____ units of PRBCs or type and screen ____ units of PRBCs		Hgb: ____ Hct: ____ Potassium: ______
Risk of stroke is reduced	Carotid ultrasound studies to be done on all clients 60 years or older ☐ done ☐ N/A ☐ report on chart for OR		Ejection fraction ______
Client is educated to enhance understanding of surgery and the immediate postoperative period prior to discharge IS goal: ____ mL IS achieved: ____ mL	Consult Cardiac Health and Wellness for preop teaching Preop teaching is completed prior to surgery, including significant others whenever possible Consult respiratory therapy for IS teaching Respiratory therapist completes instruction with client able to return demonstration	______ ______ ______ ______	Past medical history:
Discharge planning starts on admission to the hospital; clients' needs are identified at the earliest possible date Spiritual needs are assessed on admission	Diabetics will be referred to the Diabetic Institute ☐ done ☐ N/A Social Service is consulted for all clients who will require SNF or VNA service or those with financial concerns ☐ done ☐ N/A Pastoral Care is consulted to meet spiritual needs ☐ done ☐ N/A		Current problem list:
Nursing history and physical exam is completed within 4 hours	Nursing assessment and history is completed; abnormal findings are communicated to the physician; appropriate interventions occur Current medications needing to be resumed after surgery include: ______		
pHisoHex scrub and shower to entire body is completed evening before surgery and after prep AM of surgery	pHisoHex scrub and ☐ shower or ☐ bed bath is done evening prior to surgery pHisoHex scrub and ☐ shower or ☐ bed bath is done AM of surgery after prep	______ ______	Medication list from home:
Prep of lower neck, chest, pubic area, groin, both wrists, and both legs to below ankle	Each client will be prepped for surgery as close to surgery as possible; standard prep will be done as a wet prep with a razor Physician is notified of any skin/skin integrity issues Area prepped/abnormal skin findings are documented in this space ______ ______		

Courtesy of Catholic Medical Center, Manchester NH.

Yes	No	N/A	Preoperative Check List
			Permits signed ☐ Operative ☐ Anesthesia ☐ Blood
			☐ ID bracelet on ☐ Blood band on Blood available ☐ yes ☐ no _____ units _____ T&S
			Allergies (including dyes, latex, tape, prep solutions)
			Medex, Addressograph card, operating note, and anesthesia record on chart
			Significant medical history (diabetic, cardiac, seizures, pulmonary, ETOH, renal)
			Sensory/motor impairment noted; include inability to stand, speak, hear, see, decreased level of awareness
			Permanent pacemaker/AICD
			Client NPO after midnight
			Rings, hairpins, accessories, makeup, and nail polish removed
			Eyeglasses/contact lenses/dentures removed
			Current blood work U/A, ECG, chest x-ray reports, history and physical, and consults on chart Glucose-AccuChek if diabetic __________
			Height _____ Weight _____
			Pre-op medications given, vital signs taken and recorded T _____ P _____ R _____ BP _____
			Old records with chart
			Skin breakdown present? If yes, location: __________
			Shave prep completed and checked
			Foley drainage bag emptied
			Client had pHisoHex scrub and shower or bed bath evening before and AM of surgery
			Chest x-rays brought by client sent to OR with client chart
			Cath report on chart
			Carotid ultrasounds report on chart

Nurses signature: __________ Date __________

DATE: _____ ROOM FROM: _____ TO: _____
MEDS: CASSETTE: _____ REFRIG: _____ OWN: _____
DENTURES: __________
PROSTHESIS: __________
GLASSES: _____ WATCH: _____
HEARING AID: _____ RINGS: _____
JEWELRY: __________

OTHER: __________

Transferring Unit Sig: __________
Receiving Unit Sig: __________
Messenger Sig: __________

DATE: _____ ROOM FROM: _____ TO: _____
MEDS: CASSETTE: _____ REFRIG: _____ OWN: _____
DENTURES: __________
PROSTHESIS: __________
GLASSES: _____ WATCH: _____
HEARING AID: _____ RINGS: _____
JEWELRY: __________
OTHER: __________

Transferring Unit Sig: __________
Receiving Unit Sig: __________
Messenger Sig: __________

The following items have been sent home with:
Print name: __________ Telephone # __________

Signature: __________ Date __________
Witness: __________

CVSPCU Clinical Pathway for the CABG

Outcomes	Interventions	Surgical Day	POD 1	POD 2	POD 3	Day
Client is hemodynamically stable as evidenced by SBP 90-150; DBP 50-90, HR 60-100 beats/min and stable rhythm, temp 99° F	1. Cardiac monitor/assess pattern q4h × 48 hr 2. Assessment q4h × 48 hr then q shift until discharge 3. Obtain CSP on POD 2 4. D/C pacing wires on POD 3					
Respirations are 12-22/min at rest with regular rhythm and clean lung sounds	1. Cont. resp. care postextubation cardiac surgery protocol orders 2. O_2 as ordered 3. Assess lung sounds and obtain O_2 sats q4h × 48 hr then q shift 4. IS/CDB qh WA 5. If wheezes or rales present, refer to respiratory protocol 6. Obtain CXR on POD 2					
Client returns to baseline neuro status	1. Assess q4h × 48 hr then q shift till discharge					
Client will indicate adequate pain relief	1. Assess for pain q2-4h 2. MSO_4 SC for pain × 24 hr then PO analgesia through discharge and document effect					
Chest tube drainage will be <50 mL/hr Maintain Hct >24	1. CT to 20 cm H_2O seal suction 2. Check patency q1-2h 3. Measure and document drainage q1-2h 4. Consider removal when drainage ___ mL/hr or less					
Wound drainage within normal limits	1. Assess drainage q4h and change dressings prn 2. Remove dressings on POD 2 3. Apply TEDS on POD 2					
Client tolerates diet as ordered Client is free of nausea/vomiting after appropriate medication Client will have BM prior to discharge	1. Assess bowel sounds q4h × 48 hr then q shift 2. Clear liquid/diet as tolerated 3. Stool softeners/consider laxatives					
Client tolerates progressive activity Client remains free from injury	1. Phase I activity 2. Ambulate 50-500 feet tid 3. Stairs if able					
Client will maintain adequate urine output as evidenced by I&O balance Fluid restriction maintained as ordered	1. I&O q4h 2. Daily weights 3. D/C Foley POD # 4. 2000 mL/24 hr fluid restriction					
Client/SO demonstrates understanding of procedures, CV surgical routine, and plan of care	1. Review plan of care with client/SO 2. Review meds with client/SO 3. Client/SO attends discharge/dietary classes 4. Client receives diabetic teaching if indicated					
Client/SO demonstrates effective coping mechanism and verbalizes a discharge plan	1. Psychologic assessment 2. Review discharge plan 3. Review referral needs daily: Social Service Case Manager Diabetic Dietary Pastoral PT OT					

Courtesy of Catholic Medical Center, Manchester NH.

Coronary Artery Bypass Pathway Day of Surgery

Date: ______________

Admit time: ______________ Extubation time: ______________ Discharge time: ______________

☐ Hour 1 ☐ Hour 0 through 4	Hour 2 through 4 Hour 5 through 12	Hour 4 through 8 Hour 13 through 18	Hour 8 through 12 Hour 19 through 24
HEMODYNAMICS Management of hemodynamic parameters ☐ • Protocol(s) initiated to achieve hemodynamic stability	**HEMODYNAMICS** Wean vasoactive meds ☐ • Follow inotrope, vasoactive, pacing, and volume protocols	**HEMODYNAMICS** Hemodynamics stable rhythm with HR producing SBP ≥90, DBP 45-90 ☐ • Wean vasoactive meds Pacer thresholds determined ☐ • Follow standards of care	**HEMODYNAMICS** Hemodynamics stable rhythm with HR producing SBP ≥ 90, DBP 45-90 ☐ • Off vasoactive medications • A line D/C according to protocol • PA line D/C according to protocol
RESPIRATORY Extubation protocol initiated ☐	**RESPIRATORY** Weaning from ventilator ☐ • Follow extubation protocol	**RESPIRATORY** Extubated: Spo2 ≥92% on FIO_2 ≤60% and RR < 25 beats/min and unlabored ☐ • Follow extubation protocol • Initiate postextubation cardiac surgery treatment protocol ☐	
LABS AND DIAGNOSTICS Appropriate labs/diagnostics obtained ☐ • Follow labs and diagnostic protocol	**LABS AND DIAGNOSTICS** Appropriate labs/diagnostics obtained ☐ • Follow labs and diagnostic protocol		
METABOLIC K repletion ☐ • K^+ replacement protocol initiated Rewarming ☐ • Protocol for management of hypothermia initiated	**METABOLIC** Return to baseline neuro status ☐ Temp ≥36° C ☐ • Continue with hypothermia protocol	**METABOLIC** $K^+ \geq 4.0$ ☐ • Follow K^+ replacement protocol	
PAIN MANAGEMENT Pain protocol initiated ☐	**PAIN MANAGEMENT** Pain controlled by meds ☐ • Continue pain protocol	**PAIN MANAGEMENT** Pain controlled by meds ☐ • Continue pain protocol	**PAIN MANAGEMENT** Pain controlled by meds ☐
		MOBILITY Dangled ☐	**MOBILITY** Up to chair ☐
MISC Significant other contact/visit ☐ Safety protocol initiated ☐ Follow standards of care ☐		**MISC** Clear liquids tolerated ☐	**MISC** Ready for transfer ☐ • Documentation completed • Referrals initiated • Family/significant others notified • Report called to receiving RN

Clinical Pathway ■ ENDOVASCULAR STENT GRAFT

TIME FRAME LOCATION	Hospital Day *Day of Procedure*	Hospital Day *POD 1*	Hospital Day *POD 2*	Hospital Day *POD 3*
Client Satisfaction	**"What can we do to enhance your stay with us?"**	**"What can we do to enhance your stay with us?"**	**"What can we do to enhance your stay with us?"**	**"What can we do to enhance your stay with us?"**
Discharge Planning	Assess discharge needs Assess need for social worker or case manager Identify caregiver	Determine discharge plans and confirm with client and caregiver		
Client Education	Assess client and caregiver learning needs	Provide discharge instructions Instruct no lifting or straining at stools Review risk factors; offer smoking cessation information if smoker	Reinforce discharge instructions	
Tests/Procedures/ Consults	CBC, BMP, ECG, KUB in PACU	CBC, BMP, ABI, ultrasound of abdomen, spiral CT Test all stools for blood	CBC, BMP Test all stools for blood	
Allied Health Interventions		PT/OT consult for mobility Consult nutritional therapy if needed Consult respiratory therapy if needed		
Nursing/Medical Interventions	PACU 4 to 6 hr Bedrest with head of bed elevated Vital signs every $1/2$ hr times 4 and then every hr until discharge to regular nursing unit Check bilateral groin/angioplasty site every $1/2$ hr times 4 and then every hr until discharge to regular nursing unit Check peripheral pulses every 4 hr NPO, IV/Fluid for hydration, I&O Foley catheter Assess skin integrity Neurologic checks every 2 hr Pressure dressings to bleeding sites Assess pain every 4 hr and maintain pain level <5 on pain scale (1 to 10) with analgesics Encourage coughing and deep breathing every 1 hr while awake DVT prophylaxis, pneumatic antiembolism sleeves to the legs, SC heparin	Vital signs every shift Check bilateral groin/angioplasty site every shift Check peripheral pulses every shift Discontinue IV fluids and foley catheter Remain NPO until spiral CT and ultrasound of abdomen complete, then advance diet as tolerated Assess skin integrity Assess pain every 4 hr and maintain pain level <5 on pain scale (1 to 10) with analgesics Encourage coughing and deep breathing every 1 hr while awake Ambulate tid	Vital signs every shift Assess peripheral pulses and angioplasty site every shift Return to pre-op diet Activity up ad lib DVT prophylaxis Discontinue saline lock when client is discharged to home	
Outcome Criteria	Client/family satisfaction addressed PACU discharge criteria met Hemodynamically stable Bleeding controlled, pain controlled Maintain urine output >240 mL for 8 hr	Client/family satisfaction addressed Vital signs stable Pain controlled Tolerates diet Tolerates activity Fluid/electrolyte balanced	Client/family satisfaction addressed Discharge criteria for home met	Client/family satisfaction addressed

University of Maryland Medical System

CLINICAL PATHWAY :
Ischemic Cerebral Infarction (Mild, moderate)
[Page 2; 1/00 Revision]

Addressograph

Day #1 Neuro IMC/Gudelsky 5 **Targeted LOS ≤ 5 days VARIANCE AND ACTIONS DATE:____**

TESTS CD, and transthoracic echo within 24 hours of admission
TCD if indicated

ASSESSMENT Weight on admission
EKG monitoring for arrhythmias
I & O
Fingersticks q6h if diabetic
Assess chronic med regimen (MD/Pharmacist)
VS & neuro checks q1-2h
Pulse oximetry
Assess voiding
Heme test all stools for patients on thrombolytics
Preliminary swallow assessment by nursing; **if swallowing problems identified, request swallow eval**

TREATMENTS ○Aspiration precautions until swallowing cleared
NGT if fail swallowing eval or if otherwise warranted
Saline lock or IV
Venodynes
Fall precautions
Soft care mattress if indicated

MEDS ○Resume chronic meds, except for BP & DM: list to right
○**Thrombolytic or Neuroprotective agents as per standing order sets *(list drugs given to right)***
○Aspirin, ticlopidine, IV heparin, & warfarin on hold for 24 hrs after thrombolytic therapy or study drug infusion
○Heparin at ______units/hr (15 units/kg, starting dose; see dosing card)
○Warfarin_____mg po qhs *or*
○Aspirin____mg po___ *or*
○IV labetalol/hydralazine prn
○Other HTN agents as prescribed (list to right)
○Ticlopidine 250 mg po bid *or* ○Lipid lowering agent as prescribed
○Clopidogrel 75 mg qd
○IV fluids if indicated
○Saline lock flush
○Insulin sliding scale, if applicable
○Sucralfate 1 gm po ac & hs *or* ○Antacid:_________(list)
○Nizatidine 150 mg po bid
○Colace 100 mg po bid
○MOM 10 ml q pm prn
○Tylenol po/pr/NG q4h prn
○Heparin 5000U subq bid for DVT prophylaxis if not on heparin IV
○Diphenhydramine 12.5-25 mg po/NG in pm for sleep

DIET NPO until preliminary swallowing assessment

ACTIVITY Bedrest except for PT eval

TEACHING ○Orientation to unit
○Advance directives
○Diagnostic tests: TCD & CD, TTE
○Request family to bring in list of meds
○Passive ROM exercises with patient/family
○Anticipated LOS & DC plng process (review pathway as appropriate)
○Review content of handouts: ○Krames booklet pp. 1-4 on coping, recovery, and stroke affects, ○Stroke a Med Emergency, ○Warning Signs
○Include note "see pathway" on Multidiscip Educ Summary Form

DISCHARGE PLANNING RN completion of intake/triage form
○Case manager initiation of discharge planning within 48° of admission

EXPECTED OUTCOMES □Neuro status stable
□Vital signs stable
□Free from aspiration
□Voiding spontaneously
□Controlled fingersticks, if applicable
□No evidence of DVT or PE
□Free from falls
□No evidence of bleeding
□PTT approaching therapeutic goal if on IV heparin
□Completes TCD, CD, and TTE within 24 hours of admission
□Verbalizes understanding of diagnostic tests; □explains stroke effects and warning signs
□Returns demonstration of ROM exercises

***DAILY EVALUATION*: Did patient meet expected outcomes?**
YES__ NO__ (If NO, document under `variance and action')
YES__ NO__

Admitted from: ___________
Date and time of symptom onset: __________

Rxs/drug study prior to inpatient admission:
__ **IV rt-PA (0-3 hr)**__ **Citicoline**
__ **BMS 204352** __ **Other:** _____

Neuro deficits present on admission:

If foley catheter inserted, document need for insertion:

SIGNATURES: (RNs/PT/OT/Speech/Nutrition/SW/Case Manager)
7A-7P________________________/Date:______
7P-7A________________________/Date:______
Team_________________________/Date:______

This clinical pathway is intended as a general guideline. Patient care continues to require individualization based on patient needs and responses. 4/95, rev. 12/98

UNIVERSITY OF MARYLAND MEDICAL SYSTEM

CLINICAL PATHWAY:
Ischemic Cerebral Infarction (Mild, moderate)
[Page 3, 1/00 Revision]

Addressograph

Day #2 Neuro Stepdown/Gudelsky 5 **VARIANCE AND ACTIONS DATE:__**

TESTS Fasting lipid panel
PTT q6h after any heparin dose change INR qd in am if on warfarin
If no etiology established, proceed to MRI/A, TEE, and/or further lab testing as indicated (list tests ordered/requested to right)

ASSESSMENT Social Work assessment completed
OT, PT, Speech and language assessments initiated if patient stable or improving
Nutrition screening
Neuropsych consult if indicated
VS & neuro checks q2h
I&O; assess voiding
EKG monitoring
Pulse oximetry
Heme test stools if on heparin
Fingersticks q6h if diabetic, ac & hs if eating
Assess for orthostatic changes if OOB
Continued need for monitored bed documented (MD)

Neuro deficits:

TREATMENTS Venodynes
Fall precautions: Level I/II
Soft care mattress if indicated
Saline lock
Passive ROM exercises by patient/family

MEDS ○Resume chronic meds: list to right
○Resume po BP meds if tolerates po well: list to right
○Heparin at ______units/hr as per protocol; see dosing card
○Warfarin____mg po qhs *or*
○IV Labetalol/hydralazine prn
○Aspirin____mg po___ *or*
○Other HTN agents (list to right)
○Ticlopidine 250 mg po bid c food *or*
○Lipid lowering agent as prescribed
○Clopidogrel 75 mg po qd
○IV fluids if indicated or ○Saline lock flush
○Sucralfate 1 gm po ac & hs *or* ○Antacid:__________(list)
○Nizatidine 150 mg po bid
○Colace 100 mg po bid
○MOM 10 ml q pm prn
○Tylenol po/pr/NG q4h prn
○Heparin 5000U subq bid or DVT prophylaxis if not on heparin IV
○Insulin sliding scale, if applicable
○Diphenhydramine 12.5-25 mg po/NG in pm for sleep

DIET Cardiac diet unless otherwise ordered/recommended by Nutrition &/or Speech

ACTIVITY Progress with activity as ordered (with supervision) *or OOB in chair unless medically contraindicated*

TEACHING ○Diagnostics--MRI/A if test ordered
○Review content of handouts: ○Krames' Brain Attack brochure pp 5-9,
○Antiplatelet/anticoagulation therapy (AHA ho), ○Nutrition tips, ○MRI

DISCHARGE PLANNING
On-going discharge planning with case manager
Transfer to floor if medically stable

EXPECTED OUTCOMES ☐Neuro status stable
☐Vital signs stable
☐Free from aspiration
☐Voiding spontaneously
☐No evidence of DVT or PE
☐Controlled fingersticks, if applicable
☐Tolerates being OOB
☐Free from falls
☐No evidence of bleeding
☐PTT within desired therapeutic range if on IV heparin
☐Successfully completes MRI/A if ordered
☐PT, OT, Speech evaluations initiated for stable/improving cases
☐Patient/family describe ☐purpose of antiplatelet/anticoagulation therapy and ☐stroke affects on speech/language, swallow, and motor function

DAILY EVALUATION: **Did patient meet expected outcomes?**
YES__ NO__ (If NO, document under `variance and action')
YES__ NO__

SIGNATURES: (RNs/PT/OT/Speech/Nutrition/SW/Case Manager)
7A-7P________________ /Date:______
7P-7A________________ /Date:______
Team________________ /Date:______

This clinical pathway is intended as a general guideline. Patient care continues to require individualization based on patient needs and responses. 4/95, rev. 12/98

UNIVERSITY OF MARYLAND MEDICAL SYSTEM

Addressograph

CLINICAL PATHWAY:
Ischemic Cerebral Infarction (Mild, moderate)
[Page 4, 1/00 Revision]

Day #3 Gudelsky 5

VARIANCE AND ACTIONS

TESTS

○**During resident rounds, review diagnostic test results & probable etiology; develop plans for further stroke workup (TEE, angio etc) and therapy (medications, diet, surgery)**
PTT q6h after any heparin dose change
INR qd if on warfarin

ASSESSMENT ○OT/○PT/○Speech evaluations completed

Neuro deficits:

VS & neuro checks q2-8h
I&O if still indicated
Fingersticks ac & hs if diabetic and eating
Heme test stools if on heparin
Assess for orthostatic changes when OOB
Nutrition screening completed
Consultation for carotid endarterectomy if indicated

TREATMENTS Venodynes
Fall precautions
Soft care mattress
○OT/○PT/○Speech/lang Rx initiated if applicable

MEDS ○Chronic meds: list to right (if different than previous page)
○Resume po BP meds if tolerates po well: list to right
○Heparin at ______units/hr as per protocol; see dosing card
○Warfarin_____mg po qhs *or*
○IV Labetalol/hydralazine prn
○Aspirin___mg po___ *or*
○Other HTN agents (list to right)
○Ticlopidine 250 mg po bid c food
○Lipid lowering agent as prescribed
○Clopidogrel 75 mg po qd
○IV fluids if indicated/○Saline lock flush
○Sucralfate 1 gm po ac & hs* *or*
○Antacid:_________(list)*
○Nizatidine 150 mg po bid*
○Colace 100 mg po bid
○MOM 10 ml q pm prn
○Tylenol po/pr/NG q4h prn
○Heparin 5000U subq bid or DVT prophylaxis if not on heparin IV
○Insulin sliding scale, if applicable
○Diphenhydramine 12.5-25 mg po/NG in pm for sleep

***DC if tolerates po well**

DIET Cardiac diet unless otherwise ordered

ACTIVITY OOB with supervision

TEACHING ○Review content in the following handouts: ○Krames' Brain Attack brochure pp. 10-13, ○cholesterol, ○cholesterol lowering, ○BP
○Any further diagnostic tests (TEE etc)
○Nutrition education, if appropriate (consult)

DISCHARGE PLANNING
On-going discharge planning with case manager; identify discharge disposition
Discuss anticipated discharge date/location with resident/attending and family members

EXPECTED OUTCOMES
□Probable stroke etiology established and stroke prophylaxis initiated
□Neuro status stable or improving
□Vital signs stable
□Voiding spontaneously
□No evidence of DVT or PE
□Free from aspiration
□Tolerates increased activity
□Controlled fingersticks, if applicable
□Free from falls
□PTT within therapeutic range if on heparin
□BM every 3rd day
□OT/PT/Speech evaluations completed
□Patient/family describe purpose of lipid lowering agents and importance of HTN control

***DAILY EVALUATION*: Did patient meet expected outcomes?**
YES__ NO__ (If NO, document under `variance and action')
YES__ NO__

SIGNATURES: (RNs/PT/OT/Speech/Nutrition/SW/Case Manager)
7A-7P________________________/Date:________
7P-7A________________________/Date:________
Team________________________/Date:________

This clinical pathway is intended as a general guideline. Patient care continues to require individualization based on patient needs and responses. 4/95, rev. 12/98

UNIVERSITY OF MARYLAND MEDICAL SYSTEM

Addressograph

CLINICAL PATHWAY:

Ischemic Cerebral Infarction (Mild, moderate)

[Page 5, 1/00 Revision]

Day #4 Gudelsky 5

VARIANCE AND ACTIONS DATE:______

TESTS PTT q6h after any heparin dose change
INR qd in am in on warfarin

ASSESSMENT VS & neuro checks q4-8h
Fingersticks ac & hs if diabetic & eating
Heme test stools if on IV heparin therapy
Check for orthostatic changes when OOB

Neuro deficits:

TREATMENTS IV > saline lock if po intake adequate
Venodynes if still indicated
Soft care mattress if indicated
OOT Rx
Fall precautions
OPT Rx
OST Rx

MEDS OChronic meds: list to right if different than previous page
OAntihypertensive po as ordered: list to right
OHeparin at ______units/hr as per protocol; see dosing card
OWarfarin_____mg po qhs *or* OAspirin____mg po___ *or* OTiclopidine 250 mg po bid c food *or* Clopidogrel 75 mg po qd
OIV fluids if indicated
OSucralfate 1 gm po ac & hs* *or*
ONizatidine 150 mg po bid*
OMOM 10 ml q pm prn
OSaline lock flush
OAntacid:_________(list)*
OColace 100 mg po bid
OTylenol po/pr/NG q4h prn
OLipid lowering agent as prescribed
OHeparin 5000U subq bid or DVT prophylaxis if not on heparin IV
OInsulin sliding scale, if applicable
ODiphenhydramine 12.5-25 mg po/NG in pm for sleep

***DC if tolerates po well**

DIET Cardiac diet unless otherwise ordered

ACTIVITY OOB as tolerated

TEACHING OComplete teaching from Krames' brochure, pp. 14-16
OCheck with MD regarding meds patient to continue on after discharge
ODiscuss content of specific med handouts for stroke prophylaxis and lipid lowering agents to be discharged on; assess patient/family ability to read handouts
OSmoking cessation handout if applicable
OLevel of supervision needed in the home

DISCHARGE PLANNING
On-going discharge planning with case manager
Home Health assessment for patients being discharged home
Discuss anticipated discharge date and time with pt/family

EXPECTED OUTCOMES
☐Stroke etiology established (MD)
☐Vital signs stable
☐No evidence of DVT or PE
☐No evidence of bleeding
☐Controlled fingersticks, if applicable
☐Neuro status stable or improving
☐Voiding spontaneously
☐Free from aspiration
☐Free from infection
☐Free from falls
☐PTT within desired range, INR 2-3 if on warfarin
☐Patient/family state name, dosage, frequency, purpose, possible side effects, and lab monitoring needs of/for prescribed medications incl those for stroke prophylaxis and lipid lowering

DAILY EVALUATION: **Did patient meet expected outcomes?**
YES__ NO__ (If NO, document under `variance and action')
YES__ NO__

SIGNATURES: (RNs/PT/OT/Speech/Nutrition/SW/Case Manager)
7A-7P______________________________ /Date:______
7P-7A______________________________ /Date:______
Team______________________________ /Date:______

This clinical pathway is intended as a general guideline. Patient care continues to require individualization based on patient needs and responses. 4/95, rev. 12/98

UNIVERSITY OF MARYLAND MEDICAL SYSTEM

Addressograph

CLINICAL PATHWAY:
Ischemic Cerebral Infarction (Mild, Moderate)
[Page 6, 1/00 Revision]

Day #5 Gudelsky 5

VARIANCE AND ACTIONS DATE:___

TESTS CBC if on ticlopidine INR qd in am if on warfarin
Determine if any other labs needed prior to discharge

ASSESSMENT VS & neuro checks q8h
Assessment and documentation of patient ability to sit in chair at least 1 hr (if patient going to inpatient rehab)

Neuro deficits:

TREATMENTS Safety evaluations by therapies as indicated
Venodynes Fall precautions Soft care mattress
PT Rx OT Rx ST Rx

MEDS O Chronic meds: list to right if different than previous pages
O Antihypertensive po as ordered: list to right
O Heparin at ______units/hr as per protocol; see dosing card
O Warfarin_____mg po qhs *or* O Aspirin___mg po___ *or* O Ticlopidine 250 mg po bid with food *or* O Clopidogrel 75 mg po qd
O IV fluids if indicated O Saline lock flush
O Colace 100 mg po bid O MOM 10 ml q pm prn
O Tylenol po/pr/NG q4h prn O Insulin sliding scale, if applicable
O Lipid lowering agent as prescribed
O Heparin 5000U subq bid or DVT prophylaxis if not on heparin IV
O Diphenhydramine 12.5-25 mg po/NG in pm for sleep

DIET Cardiac diet unless otherwise ordered

ACTIVITY OOB as tolerated

TEACHING O Evaluate patient/family understanding of content in Krames brochure on Brain Attack and prescribed medications; reinforce as necessary
O Discuss plans for medical follow-up
Include note "see pathway" on Multidiscip Educ Summary Form

DISCHARGE PLANNING On-going discharge planning with case manager
O Final arrangements with Home Health/Rehab facility if indicated
O Insurance coverage for rehab/home health services reviewed with pt/family if indicated
O Arrange outpatient therapy if needed
O Discuss planned time of discharge with family; O give prescriptions to family member
O Schedule follow up appointments, including Neuro Ambul Center
If dc'd on ticlopidine, arrange follow-up CBCs and make application to Roche-Centex for financial support if indicated
If dc'd home on warfarin, referral form completed and faxed to AC clinic and follow-up appointment made for labs unless being done by home health
MD & RN discharge summaries

EXPECTED OUTCOMES
☐ Neuro status stable or improving ☐ Vital signs stable
☐ Voiding spontaneously ☐ BM every 3rd day
☐ No evidence of DVT or PE ☐ Free from aspiration
☐ Controlled fingersticks, if applicable ☐ Free from falls
☐ PTT within desired range, INR 2-3 if on warfarin
☐ Increased participation in ADLs
☐ Patient/family verbalize understanding of discharge instructions & medication counselling, & plans for further testing & follow-up
☐ Pt aware of insurance benefits for ongoing care needs
☐ Referrals made to hospital/community resources

DAILY EVALUATION: **Did patient meet expected outcomes?**
YES__ NO__ (If NO, document under `variance and action')
YES__ NO__

SIGNATURES: (RNs/PT/OT/Speech/Nutrition/SW/Case Manager)
7A-7P________________________/Date:__________ 7P-
7A________________________/Date:__________
Team________________________/Date:__________

This clinical pathway is intended as a general guideline. Patient care continues to require individualization based on patient needs and responses. 4/95, rev. 12/98

UNIVERSITY OF MARYLAND MEDICAL SYSTEM

CLINICAL PATHWAY:
Ischemic Cerebral Infarction (Mild, moderate)

[Page 7, 1/00 Revision]

Addressograph

Discharge

VARIANCE AND ACTIONS DATE:____

TESTS

If on Ticlopidine, CBC with diff arranged for every 2 weeks until the end of 3 months of therapy
If on warfarin and INR not stable at discharge, INR scheduled twice weekly x 2; then every week x 3; then every 3-4 weeks
If on warfarin and INR is stable at discharge, INR scheduled every 5-6 weeks

ASSESSMENT

VS and neuro checks prior to discharge
Assessment of home health needs by liaison RN

Neuro deficits remaining at discharge:

TREATMENTS

Fall precautions
Seizure precautions, if indicated
Continuing PT/OT/Speech after discharge if indicated

MEDS O Chronic meds

O Antihypertensive po as ordered: list to right
O Saline lock flush
O Warfarin ___mg po qhs *or* O Aspirin____ mg po___ *or* O Ticlopidine 250 mg po bid c meals *or* O Clopidogrel 75 mg po qd
O Lipid lowering agent as prescribed
O Colace 100 mg po bid
O MOM 10 ml q pm prn
O Dulcolax supp prn
O Tylenol prn
O Insulin sliding scale, if applicable

Medications at discharge (list):

DIET As recommended by Nutrition &/or Speech

ACTIVITY OOB as tolerated

TEACHING Reinforce discharge instructions as needed
Level of supervision needed in home

DISCHARGE PLANNING

Home Health referral if not being discharged to transitional or acute rehab, or skilled facility
Discharge summary completed and chart dictated
O Clerk to set follow-up appointment at Neuro Ambul Center (fax request after hours)

Appointments scheduled for: Neuro Ambulatory Center __, AC Clinic __, Internal Med/Fam Practice __, Hypertension Clinic __, Diabetes Clinic __, PT __, OT __, Speech __, Other (please list):

Discharge date and time: ***(goal < 12 N)*****________**
Discharge location and level of care (acute rehab, transitional/subacute rehab): ________

EXPECTED OUTCOMES

☐ Neuro status stable
☐ BP controlled
☐ Maximum participation in ADLs
☐ Free from falls
☐ Free from aspiration
☐ Controlled fingersticks, if applicable
☐ Patient/family understands discharge instructions, including plans for follow-up and further testing if indicated
☐ WBC $> 4.2 \times 10^3/mm^3$ with neutrophils $> 1200/mm^3$ if on Ticlopidine
☐ INR 2-3 if on warfarin

DAILY EVALUATION**: Did patient meet expected outcomes?**
YES__ NO__ (If NO, document under `variance and action')
YES__ NO__

SIGNATURES:
7A-7P________________
7P-7A________________

This clinical pathway is intended as a general guideline. Patient care continues to require individualization based on patient needs and responses. 4/95, rev. 12/98

NOTE: **FAX this page at time of patient discharge to Neuro Ambul Center, 8-1149, ATTN: J. Valino, RN**

NOTE: **Send/keep copy of pathway on C5 upon patient's discharge**

UNIVERSITY OF MARYLAND MEDICAL SYSTEM

CLINICAL PATHWAY:
Ischemic Cerebral Infarction (Mild, moderate)

[Page 8, 1/00 Revision]

Addressograph

Home Home Health/Rehab

	VARIANCE AND ACTIONS DATE:______
TESTS If on ticlopidine, CBC with diff arranged for every 2 weeks until the end of 3 months of therapy If on warfarin and INR not stable at discharge, INR twice weekly x 2; then every week x 3; then every 3-4 weeks If on warfarin and INR is stable at discharge, INR every 5-6 weeks INR results to be sent STAT to neuro attending/primary care MD as arranged prior to discharge	
ASSESSMENT ○Home Health RN assessment for neuro worsening, blood pressure and blood sugar stability, home environment (incl. function and safety in home and supports available), any needs for durable medical equipment, safety or adaptive devices, compliance with diet and medication regimen, sufficiency of intake & output, therapeutic blood levels if applicable Primary Care and Neuro Ambul Center follow-up visits Nutrition, DM, and HTN follow-up visits as indicated Screen for depression Driving evaluation, if indicated Social Work referrral if indicated Transportation needs for health care follow-up assessed	
TREATMENTS PT, OT, Speech therapies as indicated Institute treatment of depression if indicated	
MEDS ○ All meds, list to right:	
DIET Cardiac diet	
ACTIVITY Increasing activity as tolerated	
TEACHING Needs for medical follow-up Results of lab tests and any necessary medication adjustments Activity prescription Safety and ADL adaptation in home Driving and return to work status	
DISCHARGE PLANNING Home Health follow-up after discharge if not being transferred to transitional or acute rehab, or skilled facility Summary note from home health/rehab to Neuro Ambul Center/attending MD Vocational rehab referral, if indicated	
EXPECTED OUTCOMES ☐Neuro status stable ☐Maximum participation in ADLs ☐Free from falls ☐Tolerating medication therapy ☐WBC > 4.2 X 10^3/mm^3 with neutrophils > 1200/mm^3, if on Ticlopidine ☐INR 2-3 if on warfarin ☐Treatment for depression begun (if indicated) and patient free from adverse side effects ☐Patient medical follow-up appointment date and transportation arranged	
EVALUATION: **Did patient meet expected outcomes?** YES__ NO__ (If NO, document under `variance and action')	**SIGNATURES:**

This clinical pathway is intended as a general guideline. Patient care continues to require individualization based on patient needs and responses. 4/95, rev. 3/97

NOTE: **At completion of home health visits/rehab stay, FAX copy of summary note of outcomes achieved and plans for follow-up to Neuro Ambulatory Center, ATTN: J. Valino, RN at 328-1149.**

UNIVERSITY OF MARYLAND MEDICAL SYSTEM

CLINICAL PATHWAY:
Ischemic Cerebral Infarction (Mild, Moderate)
[Page __, 1/00 Revision]

Extended Stay

Addressograph

Day #___ Gudelsky 5

VARIANCE AND ACTIONS DATE:___

*****Note reason(s) for extended stay and actions being taken to address variances*** (use back of form if necessary)

TESTS CBC if on ticlopidine INR qd in am if on warfarin
Determine if any other labs needed prior to discharge

ASSESSMENT VS & neuro checks q8h
Heme test stools if on IV heparin

TREATMENTS Safety evaluations by therapies as indicated
Venodynes Fall precautions Soft care mattress
PT Rx OT Rx ST Rx

MEDS OChronic meds: list to right if different than previous pages

OHeparin at ______units/hr as per protocol
OWarfarin_____mg po qhs *or*
OASA____mg po___ *or*
OTiclopidine 250 mg po bid c food *or*
OClopidogrel 75 mg po qd
OHeparin 5000U subq bid if not on Heparin IV
OIV Labetalol/hydralazine prn
OOther HTN agents (list to right)
OLipid lowering agent as prescribed
OIV fluids if indicated/OSaline lock flush
OInsulin sliding scale, if applicable
OSucralfate 1 gm po ac & hs or OAntacid:__________(list)
ONizatidine 150 mg po bid
OColace 100 mg po bid
OMOM 10 ml q pm prn
OTylenol po/pr/NG prn
ODiphenhydramine 12.5-25 mg po/NG in pm for sleep

DIET As recommended by Nutrition &/or Speech

ACTIVITY OOB as tolerated

TEACHING OComplete review of Krames' Brain Attack brochure with patient and family
Other (list):

DISCHARGE PLANNING

OFamily/team meeting as needed to discuss discharge plans
OFinal arrangements with rehab facility if indicated
OInsurance coverage for rehab/home health services reviewed with pt/family if indicated
OArrange outpatient therapy if needed
OPrescriptions to family member
Schedule follow up appointments, including Neuro Ambulatory Center
If on Ticlopidine or Warfarin, arrange appointment for blood work
MD & RN discharge summaries

EXPECTED OUTCOMES

☐Neuro status stable or improving
☐Voiding spontaneously
☐No evidence of DVT or PE
☐Controlled fingersticks, if applicable
☐Vital signs stable
☐BM every 3rd day
☐Free from aspiration
☐Free from falls
☐PTT within desired range, INR 2-3 if on warfarin
☐Increased participation in ADLs
☐Demonstrates understanding of discharge instructions & medication counselling, & plans for further testing & follow-up
☐Pt aware of insurance benefits for ongoing care needs
☐Referrals made to hospital/community resources

***DAILY EVALUATION*: Did patient meet expected outcomes?**
YES__ NO__ (If NO, document under `variance and action')
YES__ NO__

SIGNATURES: (RNs/PT/OT/Speech/Nutrition/SW/Case Manager)

This clinical pathway is intended as a general guideline. Patient care continues to require individualization based on patient needs and responses. 4/95, rev. 12/98

Addressograph

CLINICAL PATHWAY: Mild/moderate ischemic cerebral infarction

Date/Time	VARIANCE NOTES
	Signature:____________________
	Signature:____________________

University Hospitals
of Cleveland

CARE PATH NAME: KIDNEY TRANSPLANT
DRG: ELOS: 7 Days
Expected Disposition: Home
Surgery Date: ___/___/___
Pre-Op Dry Weight: ____ Kg

Collaborative Problem List
1. Impaired Home Maintenance Management
2. Potential for Infection
3. Knowledge Deficit
4. Fluid and Electrolyte Imbalance
5. Plan Management
6.
7.

Focus	Pre-Op Date: __/__/__	Day of Surgery Date: __/__/__	Post-Op to Day 1 Date: __/__/__	Post-Op to Day 2 Date: __/__/__	Post-Op to Day 3 Date: __/__/__	Post-Op to Day 4 Date: __/__/__
Laboratory Tests/ Procedures	• Chem 23 • CBC + Diff • PT/PTT • Urine C&S • T&C 2u PRBC • Check CMV status • Chemstick of diabetic • CMV IgG quantitative	• Immediately post-op: Chem 7, CBC • 8 hours post-op: Chem 7, CBC • CXR on arrival to PACU	• CBC + Diff • Chem 23 • CD3 level if on OKT3 • CXR • Ultrasound as indicated per protocol	• Chem 7 → • Urine for bacteria/fungus • CBC (Diff if on OKT3) → • CD3 level if on OKT3 → • CYA level starting day 2 of therapy →		• Chem 23
Consults/ Referrals			• Consider PT Consult • Dietary screen and evaluation			
Physical Assessment	• VS q 4 h • Weight • Baseline skin assessment • Renal assessment regarding need for dialysis	• BP, AP, Rq 1/2 h until stable then q 2 h-q 4 h then q 4 h prn • Temp. immediately and q 2 h x 16 h then q 4 h • CVP q 2-4 x 16 h then q 4 h • Pulse ox baseline and prn → • Urine output q 1 h x 24 h then q 4 h x 24 then qs	• VS q 4 h with CVP • Urine output q 4 h weight • Bowel sounds	• VS q 4 h • I&O q shift → • Weight → • Pulse ox x 2	• VS q shift →	
Activity	• Up ad lib	• Bed rest	• Out of bed → chair			
Treatments	• Fleets enemas x 2 • Hibiclens shower • SCDs with patient to OR • Apply Teds pre-op	• O2 per order, wean as tolerated • CVP dressing • JP dressing → • Incision dressing • Incentive spirometry q 1 h W/A → • Foley care → • Guaiac stools → • SCDs and Teds →	• D/C O2 if RA pulse ox > 92% • Incision care	• Up with assistance • CVP dressing • D/C JP if output < 30 cc → • Remove incision dressing	• Out of bed ad lib → • Incentive spirometry q 2 h W/A →	• CVP dressing • D/C Foley
Diet	• NPO	• NPO, ice chips • Advance as tolerated	• Diabetic/or any other diet restrictions as indicated →			
Medications	• On call to OR: Antibiotic Solumedrol 250 mg IV Imuran 5 mg/kg IV maximum dose — 500 mg • Induction options: OKT3, ATG, Cyclosporine, MMF, Neoral	• Solumedrol 60 mg q 6 h IV → • Antibiotic • Fluid replacements	• Imuran or Mycophenolate → • OKT3, ATG, Cyclosporine, Neoral • Gancyclovir 2.5 mg/kg qd if CMV (+) or CMV (−) receiving (+) organ • MSO4 PRN	• Solumedrol 60 mg IV q 8 h • OKT3, ATG, Cyclosporine, Neoral → • Gancyclovir → • Bactrim ss or Trimethoprim qd → • Colace → • Clotrimazole → • Acyclovir → • Zantac →	• Solumedrol 60 mg IV q 12 h • Tylenol #3 • CytoGam if donor CMV (+) and recipient (−)	• Prednisone 1 mg/kg/day • OKT3, CYA, or ATG • Tylenol or Darvon

University Hospital's carepaths have been developed to assist clinicians in patient management and clinical decision-making. The carepaths are intended to meet the needs of patients in most circumstances. They are not intended to replace a clinician's judgment or establish a protocol for all patients with this diagnosis.
SP-9601 (01/05/96)

Courtesy University Hospitals of Cleveland.

Focus	Pre-Op Date: __/__/__	Day of Surgery Date: __/__/__	Post-Op to Day 1 Date: __/__/__	Post-Op to Day 2 Date: __/__/__	Post-Op to Day 3 Date: __/__/__	Post-Op to Day 4 Date: __/__/__
Patient/ Family Teaching	• View pre-op transplant video • Orient to Tower 9		• Give teaching materials to patient • Renal transplant booklet • Preprinted cards • I&O sheet • Outcome criteria form	• Review of meds and teaching material with patient/family →	→	• Continued review and if ready, take test
Discharge Planning		• Social Worker review notes from information appointments	• Review chart, interview RN and patient → • Collect psychosocial data (insurance, financial issues discharge needs) →	→	• Initial note in chart • Discuss prescription plan	• Arrange financial applications • Begin arranging prescription plans • Meet/talk with family prn • Consult/refer to other disciplines prn • For patients using mail order program, arrange forms with physicians
				• Psychosocial assessment, support and education/ information →	→	→
Intermediate Outcomes	1. Viewed video 2. Negative crossmatch	1. Hemodynamically stable 2. CVP 10-12 3. Euvolemic with fluid replacements 4. Vital signs returned to baseline 5. K + < 6.0 6. Equal and clear breath sounds 7. Pain controlled	1. Hemodynamically stable 2. CVP 10-12 3. Euvolemic with or without fluid replacements 4. Vital signs at baseline 5. Decrease in BUN and Cr from pre-op 6. Equal and clear breath sounds 7. Pain controlled 8. Teaching material given to patient/family 9. Immunosuppression dosages adjusted	1. Hemodynamically stable 2. Euvolemic without fluid replacements 3. Decrease in BUN and Cr 4. Electrolytes WNL 5. Equal and clear breath sounds 6. Pain controlled 7. Ambulating 8. Tolerating oral meds and diet 9. Teaching begun 10. JP removed if drainage is < 30 cc for 24 h 11. Immunosuppression dosages adjusted 12. Wound dry and approximated	1. Hemodynamically stable 2. Euvolemic 3. Decrease in BUN and Cr 4. Electrolytes WNL 5. Equal and clear breath sounds 6. Pain controlled 7. Actively participates in ADLs 8. Ambulates at baseline 9. Has bowel movement 10. Initial Social Worker note in chart 11. Teaching continues 12. JP removed if drainage is < 30 cc for 24 h 13. Immunosuppression dosages adjusted 14. Wound dry and approximated	1. Hemodynamically stable 2. Euvolemic 3. Decrease in BUN and Cr 4. Electrolytes WNL 5. Equal and clear breath sounds 6. Actively participates in ADLs 7. Pain controlled 8. Ambulates at baseline 9. Has bowel movement 10. Teaching continues 11. Foley discontinued 12. JP removed if drainage is < 30 cc for 24 h 13. Immunosuppression dosages adjusted 14. Wound dry and approximated 15. Financial and prescription arrangements made
Intermediate Outcomes RN Signature Days	☐ Met ☐ Not Met (see notes) #s not met ____ Signature ____	☐ Met ☐ Not Met (see notes) #s not met ____ Signature ____	☐ Met ☐ Not Met (see notes) #s not met ____ Signature ____	☐ Met ☐ Not Met (see notes) #s not met ____ Signature ____	☐ Met ☐ Not Met (see notes) #s not met ____ Signature ____	☐ Met ☐ Not Met (see notes) #s not met ____ Signature ____
Intermediate Outcomes RN Signature Evenings	☐ Met ☐ Not Met (see notes) #s not met ____ Signature ____	☐ Met ☐ Not Met (see notes) #s not met ____ Signature ____	☐ Met ☐ Not Met (see notes) #s not met ____ Signature ____	☐ Met ☐ Not Met (see notes) #s not met ____ Signature ____	☐ Met ☐ Not Met (see notes) #s not met ____ Signature ____	☐ Met ☐ Not Met (see notes) #s not met ____ Signature ____
Intermediate Outcomes RN Signature Nights	☐ Met ☐ Not Met (see notes) #s not met ____ Signature ____	☐ Met ☐ Not Met (see notes) #s not met ____ Signature ____	☐ Met ☐ Not Met (see notes) #s not met ____ Signature ____	☐ Met ☐ Not Met (see notes) #s not met ____ Signature ____	☐ Met ☐ Not Met (see notes) #s not met ____ Signature ____	☐ Met ☐ Not Met (see notes) #s not met ____ Signature ____

University Hospital's carepaths have been developed to assist clinicians in patient management and clinical decision-making. The carepaths are intended to meet the needs of patients in most circumstances. They are not intended to replace a clinician's judgment or establish a protocol for all patients with this diagnosis.

SP-9601 (01/05/96)

Focus	Post-Op Day 5 Date: ___/___/___	Post-Op Day 6 Date: ___/___/___	Post-Op Day 7 Date: ___/___/___
Laboratory/ Tests/ Procedures	• CBC (Diff on OKT3) → • Chem 7 → • CD3 level if on OKT3 → • CYA level →	→	→
Consults/ Referrals	• Consider Home Team referral		
Physical Assessment	• VS qs → • I&O qs → • Weight →	→	→
Activity	• OOB ad lib →	→	→
Treatments	• Guaiac stools → • Incentive spirometry q 2 h W/A	• CVP dressing	• D/C central line
Diet	• Diabetic or any other diet restriction as indicated →	→	→
Medications	• Prednisone — taper as indicated → • Imuran or Mycophenolate → • OKT3, ATG, Neoral, or Cyclosporine → • Gancyclovir → • Bactrim → • Colace → • Clotrimazole → • Acyclovir → • T3 or Darvon → • Zantac →	→	• D/C Ganciclovir • Acyclovir **SrCr** / **Dosage** < 1.4 / 800 mg po q 6 h 1.5-2.5 / 800 mg po q 8 h 2.6-4.5 / 800 mg po q 12 h > 4.5 / 800 mg po q 24 h HD / 800 mg po q 48 h

University Hospital's carepaths have been developed to assist clinicians in patient management and clinical decision-making. The carepaths are intended to meet the needs of patients in most circumstances. They are not intended to replace a clinician's judgment or establish a protocol for all patients with this diagnosis.

SP-9601 (01/05/96)

Courtesy University Hospitals of Cleveland.

Focus	Post-Op Day 5 Date: ___/___/___	Post-Op Day 6 Date: ___/___/___	Post-Op Day 7 Date: ___/___/___
Patient/ Family Teaching	• Take test • Diet teaching prn	• Review material as needed and retake test if needed	• Review homegoing med dosages, clinic and lab test follow-up appointments
Discharge Planning	• Arrange financial applications • Arrange prescription plans • Meet/talk with family prn • Consult/refer to other disciplines prn • Other D/C plans • Psychosocial assessment, support, and education/information	• Transportation arrangements prn → • Other D/C plans carried out prn → • Final note in chart with D/C plan Psychosocial assessment, support, and education/information →	→
Homegoing Medications	• Mail order prescription forms completed and faxed by 2:00 PM. (If weekend/ holiday D/C anticipated must do this by 2:00 PM, Friday)	• Delivery of medications prn →	→
Intermediate Outcomes	1. Hemodynamically stable → 2. Euvolemic → 3. Electrolytes WNL → 4. Independent in ADLs and ambulation → 5. Has bowel movement → 6. Test taken and passed with 90% or continue med review 7. Scale and thermometer arranged for home 8. JP removed if drainage is < 30 cc for 24 h 9. Immunosuppression dosage assessed → 10. Financial and prescription plans arranged 11. Cyclosporine levels assessed and adjusted	1. Therapeutic cyclosporine level 2. Homegoing meds obtained 3. Test taken and passed with 90%	1. D/C to home with written instructions 2. Medications available to take at home 3. Refer to discharge order form
Intermediate Outcomes RN Signature Days	☐ Met ☐ Not Met (see notes) #s not met ______ Signature ______	☐ Met ☐ Not Met (see notes) #s not met ______ Signature ______	☐ Met ☐ Not Met (see notes) #s not met ______ Signature ______
Intermediate Outcomes RN Signature Evenings	☐ Met ☐ Not Met (see notes) #s not met ______ Signature ______	☐ Met ☐ Not Met (see notes) #s not met ______ Signature ______	☐ Met ☐ Not Met (see notes) #s not met ______ Signature ______
Intermediate Outcomes RN Signature Nights	☐ Met ☐ Not Met (see notes) #s not met ______ Signature ______	☐ Met ☐ Not Met (see notes) #s not met ______ Signature ______	☐ Met ☐ Not Met (see notes) #s not met ______ Signature ______

University Hospital's carepaths have been developed to assist clinicians in patient management and clinical decision-making. The carepaths are intended to meet the needs of patients in most circumstances. They are not intended to replace a clinician's judgment or establish a protocol for all patients with this diagnosis.

SP-9601 (01/05/96)

Clinical Pathway ■ LAPAROSCOPIC CHOLECYSTECTOMY

Aspect of Care	Preadmission/Preoperative	Preoperative/DOS	Postoperative
ASSESSMENT	Physician assessment	Preoperative check, nursing assessment, psychosocial assessment	Vital signs, intake and output; assess abdomen, bowel sounds, pain, breath sounds, incisions
TEACHING	Education by physician; review clinical pathway with client and family	Teach/demonstrate turning, coughing, and deep breathing	Review discharge information: pain control, activity, wound care, complications
CONSULTS	Anesthesia if indicated; social worker, dietitian, spiritual guide		
LABORATORY TESTS AND DIAGNOSTIC TESTS	CBC, ECG if age >40 yr; liver/pancreas screen		If indicated: CBC, H&H
MEDICATIONS	Assess allergies; identify home medications	Preoperative medications taken at home; IVF antibiotic per hospital protocol	Analgesic, antiemetic
TREATMENT/ INTERVENTIONS	NPO after midnight		Elevate head of bed; Band-Aids, turning, coughing, and deep breathing; emotional support Encourage fluids, solid food per client choice
ACTIVITY	Activity ad lib		Progressive ambulation
DISCHARGE PLANNING	Determine needs: transportation, financial, home care		Arrangements made on basis of preoperative assessment needs; follow-up appointment with physician

Modified from *Clinical path: Outpatient laparoscopic cholecystectomy.* (1995). Asheville, NC: Saint Joseph's Hospital; and Ignatavicius, D.D., & Hausman, K.A. (1995). *Clinical pathways for collaborative practice.* Philadelphia: W.B. Saunders.

Clinical Pathway ■ **CARE PATH NAME: TOTAL ABDOMINAL HYSTERECTOMY**

☐ With Burch ☐ Without Burch

DRG: 353-358 ELOS: 2 Days
Expected Disposition: Home

Collaborative Problem List
1. Discharge Planning
2. Pain/Comfort Management
3. Coping Response to Surgery/Diagnosis
4. ______________________

Focus	Preadmission	Day of Surgery	Post-Op Day 1	Post-Op Day 2
LABORATORY/ TESTS/ PROCEDURES	☐ Blood work ☐ <40 years Hct ☐ >40 years SMA 6, CBC ☐ EKG if >40 years ☐ CXR if >60 years ☐ Type and screen		☐ CBC	
CONSULTS/ REFERRALS/	☐ Anesthesia Consult ☐ Nursing Consult		☐ Primary RN	
PHYSICAL ASSESSMENT	☐ H & P obtained	☐ VS per post-op routine ☐ Routine post-op assessment ☐ I/O	☐ VS Q shift ☐ Q shift assessment ☐ I/O ☐ Weight	☐ VS Q shift ☐ Q shift assessment ☐ I/O ☐ Weight
DIAGNOSIS:			☐ Fever assessment (if temp >39° C) ☐ Exam ☐ Cultures of surgical area ☐ CBC with diff ☐ Blood cultures	☐ Fever assessment (if temp >38.5° C) ☐ Exam ☐ Cultures of surgical area ☐ CBC with diff ☐ Blood cultures
ACTIVITY	☐ Ad lib	☐ Dangle at bedside or OOB to chair	☐ OOB to chair	☐ Ambulate QID
TREATMENTS	☐ Instruction on IS ☐ Review of procedure	☐ IS/C&DB Q 1 h WA ☐ Foley ☐ SCD's ☐ Drains: **BURCH ONLY:** ☐ Suprapubic Catheter	☐ IS/C&DB Q 1 h WA ☐ D/C Foley ☐ SCD's ☐ Drains: **BURCH ONLY:** ☐ Suprapubic Catheter	☐ IS/C&DB Q 1 h ☐ D/C Drains: **BURCH ONLY:** ☐ Suprapubic Catheter ☐ Monitor postvoid residuals ☐ Begin clamp routine 24 h after surgery if no hematuria
DIET	☐ NPO pre-op	☐ Ice chips ☐ Clear liquids	☐ Advanced as tolerated	☐ House diet
MEDICATIONS		☐ PCA protocol ☐ Epidural protocol ☐ IV pain meds ☐ IV antibiotics: ☐ IVF:	☐ D/C PCA at 08:00 ☐ D/C Epidural ☐ IV pain meds to PO ☐ IVF: ☐ Heplock when taking PO	☐ PO meds ☐ D/C HL

Courtesy University Hospitals of Cleveland.
University Hospitals' carepaths have been developed to assist clinicians in patient management and clinical decision-making. The carepaths are intended to meet the needs of patients in most circumstances. They are not intended to replace a clinician's judgment or establish a protocol for all patients with that diagnosis.

Clinical Pathway ■ **CARE PATH NAME: TOTAL ABDOMINAL HYSTERECTOMY (CONTINUED)**

☐ With Burch ☐ Without Burch

DRG: 353-358 ELOS: 2 Days
Expected Disposition: Home

Collaborative Problem List
1. Discharge Planning
2. Pain/Comfort Management
3. Coping Response to Surgery/Diagnosis
4. ____________

Focus	Preadmission	Day of Surgery	Post-Op Day 1	Post-Op Day 2
DISCHARGE PLANNING/ TEACHING	☐ Discharge Planning Review: ☐ Pre-op checklist ☐ Advanced directives ☐ Client care path pamphlet ☐ Determine services needed ☐ Client lives alone ☐ Client lives with others Support person: Phone number:	☐ Client lives alone ☐ Client lives with others Support person: Phone Number:	Provide Homegoing Instructions: ☐ Hysterectomy PI-128 ☐ "Women and AIDS" pamphlet ☐ Breast self exam pamphlet ☐ Hormone replacement therapy ☐ Instruct on pericare **BURCH ONLY:** ☐ Clamp Routine PI Sheets	☐ Review home-going instructions.
INDIVIDUALIZED CARE FOCUS				
INTERMEDIATE OUTCOMES	☐ Client able to explain home-going plan ☐ Client able to describe procedure(s) to be performed ☐ Client states she has participated in decision making and plan	☐ Afebrile ☐ Client states pain is adequately controlled ☐ Client shows no evidence of post-op complications	☐ Able to void without difficulty ☐ Afebrile or temp <38° with normal WBC ☐ Tolerating PO fluids ☐ Ambulates with assistance ☐ Client states pain is adequately controlled with PO pain medication	☐ Ambulates independently ☐ Has had a bowel movement and/or passed flatus ☐ Tolerates house diet ☐ Client able to describe procedure(s) performed ☐ Client able to describe pericare ☐ Client able to explain all discharge instructions **BURCH ONLY:** ☐ Able to measure and record postvoid residuals

Discharge Outcomes:	Met	Not Met	Comments	Dat/Initials
1. Abdominal incision approximated and healing				
2. Has minimal, odorless vaginal discharge				
3. Able to describe/perform pericare				
4. Has functional pattern for bladder and bowel				
5. Maintains adequate nutritional intake				
6. Pain controlled by oral medication				
7. States use of homegoing medications				
8. Describes plan for follow-up care				
9. Describes feeling about effects of surgery on health and sexuality				
10. Identifies support systems and resources available to her after discharge				
11. Afebrile or Temp <38° C with normal WBC				
12. **BURCH ONLY:** Able to demonstrate clamp routine				

Courtesy University Hospital of Cleveland.
University Hospitals' carepaths have been developed to assist clinicians in patient management and clinical decision-making. The carepaths are intended to meet the needs of patients in most circumstances. They are not intended to replace a clinician's judgment or establish a protocol for all patients with that diagnosis.

Clinical Pathway ■ **Ventilator-Dependent Clients with a Tracheostomy or Endotracheal Tube**

Phase I Acute Ventilatory Support	Phase II Ventilatory Support	Phase III Weaning	Phase IV Resolution
DIAGNOSTIC TESTS, LABORATORY VALUES, AND PROCEDURES			
ABG analysis CXR SMA-7 Pulse oximetry CBC SMA-12 ECG Sputum culture and sensitivity after 72 hr ETT Blood cultures as needed Phosphorus 4 times daily if on TF or TPN for first week Prealbumin prn	Pulmonary mechanics ECG prn SMA-7 ABG prn CBC SMA-12 weekly Pulse oximetry CXR 24-hr urine urea nitrogen prn (if no renal failure) Prealbumin prn	Pulmonary mechanics ECG prn SMA-7 ABG prn CBC SMA-12 weekly Pulse oximetry CXR 24-hr urine urea nitrogen prn (if no renal failure) Prealbumin prn	Pulmonary mechanics Pulse oximetry prn
CONSULTS			
Pulmonologist consultation if intubated after 72 hr or if reintubation is required Assess need for swallow/speech consultation Nutritional support dietitian Respiratory care clinician Social worker: Supportive counseling/crisis intervention	Physical medicine and rehabilitation Physical therapy Occupational therapy Swallow/speech consultation Social worker: Supportive counseling/ crisis intervention Social worker assesses client's and family's resource needs	Physical medicine and rehabilitation Social worker: Supportive counseling Social worker to evaluate client for placement options	
TREATMENTS			
Svo_2 prn Mechanical ventilation Respiratory treatments Secretion management Tracheostomy after ETT in place × 7 days GI protection (histamine blockers/carafate) Sedation prn Diuretics prn Vasopressors Vasoactive infusions Daily weight Special bed prn Foley Swallowed/dysphagia assessment IV medications Packed cells prn Antibiotics prn Paralytics prn I&O hourly Suction prn	Respiratory treatments Packed cells prn Secretion management Antibiotic prn Sedation prn Diuretics prn Tracheostomy care Daily weight Suction prn I&O Foley Evaluate need for permanent IV access	Respiratory treatments Packed cells prn Secretion management Antibiotic prn Diuretics prn Tracheostomy care Daily weight Suction prn I&O D/C Foley prn If prolonged TFs, evaluate need for PEG Evaluate continued need for IV access	Tracheostomy collar Decannulator Extubator Continue vent and slow wean Daily weight I & O every 8 hr Suction prn

Clinical Pathway ■ VENTILATOR-DEPENDENT CLIENTS WITH A TRACHEOSTOMY OR ENDOTRACHEAL TUBE (CONTINUED)

Phase I Acute Ventilatory Support	Phase II Ventilatory Support	Phase III Weaning	Phase IV Resolution
DIET			
Nutritional assessment TPN/TF TF preferred	If on TPN, transition to TF Reassess nutritional status every 10 days	Transition to PO diet if no dysphagia Reassess nutritional status every 10 days	Continue PO diet or TF
ACTIVITY			
Bedrest Passive range of motion every 4 hr Increase activity as tolerated	Up on side of bed with assistance Foot support Up in chair if tolerated Active range of motion	Up in chair 3 times daily Increase ambulation	Up in chair 3 times daily for increased time Increased ambulation Increased client involvement in self-care activities
TREATMENT			
Establish a communication mode with the client Orient client to environment Orient family to environment, procedures, client's current condition and prognosis, care needs, and hospital policy	Keep client and family updated about client's condition, new and continuing procedures, treatment plans, and changes in care needs	Teach client and family about weaning procedures and expected responses	Keep client and family informed regarding progress, changes in treatment plan, expected responses, new equipment or personnel
DISCHARGE PLANNING			
Family members and social worker Assessment of resources and a discharge plan appropriate and individualized to the expected outcomes for the ventilator-dependent client	Inform social worker of client's progress Social worker to assess client's and family's resource needs; explore rehabilitation and long-term insurance coverage	Keep social worker updated about client's progress Social worker to evaluate client for placement options Social worker to initiate referrals	Social worker to finalize client's transportation and disposition Social worker to finalize arrangements for needed equipment, home health services, and follow-up care

INDEX

A

b indicates boxed material, *c* indicates charts, *f* indicates illustrations, and *t* indicates tables.

C

D

G

H

M

N

O

P

Q

R

S

V

Communication Quick Reference for Spanish-Speaking Clients—cont'd

OBTAINING BLOOD FROM A FINGER STICK

I need to take a few drops of blood from your finger.	Necesito sacarle unas gotas de sangre de uno de sus dedos.	*Neh-seh-SEE-toh sah-KAHR-leh OO-nahs GOH-tahs deh SAHN-greh deh OO-noh deh soos DEH-dohs.*

OBTAINING A URINE SAMPLE

We also need a urine sample.	También necesitamos una muestra de la orina.	*Tahm-BYEHN neh-seh-see-TAH-mohs OO-nah MWEHS-trah deh lah oh-REE-nah.*
It has to be from the middle of the stream.	Tiene que ser de la mitad del chorro.	*TYEH-neh keh sehr deh lah mee-TAHD dehl CHOH-rroh.*
Put the urine in this cup.	Ponga la orina en este vaso.	*POHN-gah lah oh-REE-nah ehn EHS-teh VAH-soh.*

OBTAINING A STOOL SPECIMEN

I need a sample of your stool.	Necesito una muestra de su excremento.	*Neh-seh-SEE-toh OO-nah MWEHS-trah deh soo ehks-kreh-MEN-toh.*
Please put a small amount in this cup.	Por favor ponga un poco en este vaso.	*Pohr fa-VOHR POHN-gah oon POH-koh ehn EHS-teh VAH-soh.*

OBTAINING A SPUTUM SPECIMEN

I need a sample of your sputum.	Necesito una muestra de su esputo.	*Neh-seh-SEE-toh OO-nah MWEHS-trah deh soo ehs-POO-toh.*
Please spit in this cup.	Por favor, escupa en este vaso.	*Pohr fah-VOHR, ehs-KOO-pah ehn EHS-teh VAH-soh.*

ORDERS

You need . . .	Necesita . . .	*Neh-seh-see-TAH . . .*
a bandage.	un vendaje.	*oon behn-DAH-heh.*
a blood transfusion.	una transfusión de sangre.	*OO-nah trahns-foo-SEE-ohn deh SAHN-greh.*
a cast.	una armadura de yeso.	*OO-nah ahr-mah-DOO-rah deh YEH-soh.*
gauze.	la gasa.	*lah GAH-sah.*
intensive care.	el cuidado intensivo.	*ehl kwee-DAH-doh een-tehn-SEE-boh.*
intravenous fluids.	los líquidos intravenosos.	*lohs LEE-kee-dohs een-trah-beh-NOH-sohs.*
an operation.	una operación.	*OO-nah oh-peh-rah-see-OHN.*
physical therapy.	la terapia física.	*lah teh-RAH-pee-ah FEE-see-kah.*
a shot.	una inyección.	*OO-nah een-yehk-see-OHN.*
x-rays.	los rayos equis.	*lohs RAH-yohs EH-kees.*
We're going to . . .	Vamos a . . .	*VAH-mohs ah . . .*
change the bandage.	cambiarle el vendaje.	*kahm-bee-AHR-leh ehl behn-DAH-heh.*
give you a bath.	darle un baño.	*DAHR-leh oon BAH-nyoh.*
take out the I.V.	sacarle el tubo intravenoso.	*sah-KAHR-leh ehl TOO-boh een-trah-beh-NOH-soh.*

DESCRIPTION OF TUBES

The tube in your . . .	El tubo en su . . .	*Ehl TOO-boh ehn soo . . .*
arm is for I.V. fluids.	brazo está para los líquidos intravenosos.	*BRAH-soh ehs-TAH PAH-rah LEE-kee-dohs een-trah-beh-NOH-sohs.*
bladder is for urinating.	vejiga es para orinar.	*beh-HEE-gah ehs PAH-rah oh-ree-NAHR.*
stomach is for the food.	estómago es para la comida.	*ehs-TOH-mah-goh ehs PAH-rah lah koh-MEE-dah.*
throat is for breathing.	garganta es para respirar.	*gahr-GAHN-tah ehs PAH-rah rehs-pee-RAHR.*

Communication Quick Reference for Spanish-Speaking Clients

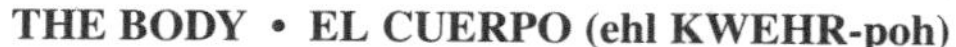

THE BODY • EL CUERPO (ehl KWEHR-poh)

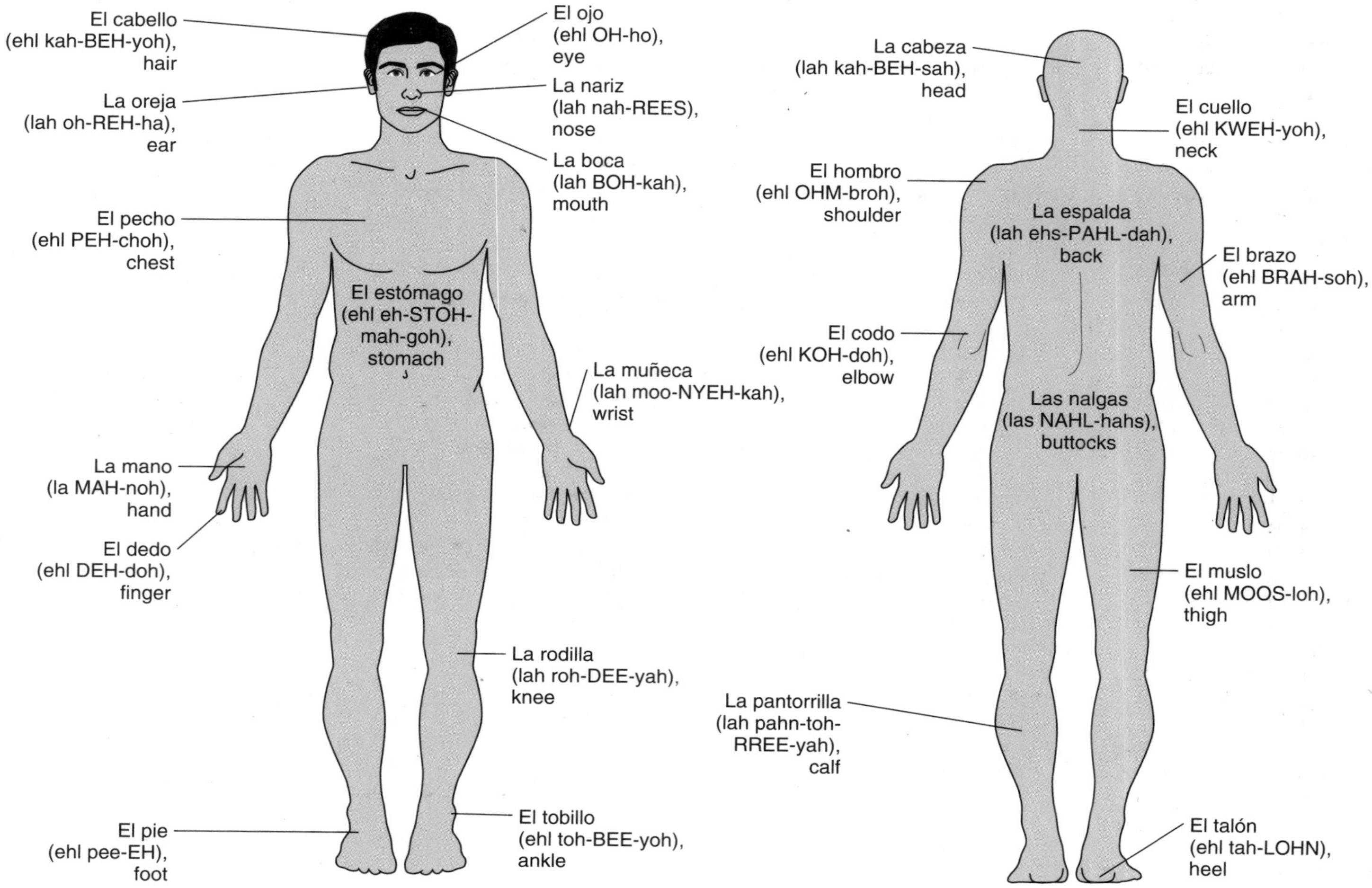

El cabello (ehl kah-BEH-yoh), hair
El ojo (ehl OH-ho), eye
La oreja (lah oh-REH-ha), ear
La nariz (lah nah-REES), nose
La boca (lah BOH-kah), mouth
El pecho (ehl PEH-choh), chest
El estómago (ehl eh-STOH-mah-goh), stomach
La muñeca (lah moo-NYEH-kah), wrist
La mano (la MAH-noh), hand
El dedo (ehl DEH-doh), finger
La rodilla (lah roh-DEE-yah), knee
El pie (ehl pee-EH), foot
El tobillo (ehl toh-BEE-yoh), ankle
La cabeza (lah kah-BEH-sah), head
El cuello (ehl KWEH-yoh), neck
El hombro (ehl OHM-broh), shoulder
La espalda (lah ehs-PAHL-dah), back
El brazo (ehl BRAH-soh), arm
El codo (ehl KOH-doh), elbow
Las nalgas (las NAHL-hahs), buttocks
El muslo (ehl MOOS-loh), thigh
La pantorrilla (lah pahn-toh-RREE-yah), calf
El talón (ehl tah-LOHN), heel

COMMON INSTRUCTIONS TO BE USED WITH THE BODY PARTS

Move the, Mueva *(mooh-EH-bah)*
Touch the, Toque *(TOH-keh)*
Point to the, Señale *(seh-NYAH-leh)*

MORE PARTS OF THE BODY

Armpit, la axila *(lah ahk-SEE-lah)*
Breasts, los senos *(lohs SEH-nohs)*
Collarbone, la clavícula *(lah klah-BEE-koo-lah)*
Diaphragm, el diafragma *(ehl dee-ah-FRAH-mah)*
Forearm, el antebrazo *(ehl ahn-teh-BRAH-soh)*
Groin, la ingle *(lah EEN-gleh)*
Hip, la cadera *(lah kah-DEH-rah)*
Kneecap, la rótula *(lah ROH-too-lah)*
Nail, la uña *(lah OON-yah)*
Pelvis, la pelvis *(lah PEHL-beece)*
Rectum, el recto *(ehl REHK-toh)*
Rib, la costilla *(lah koh-STEE-yah)*
Spine, el espinazo *(ehl ehs-pee-NAH-soh)*
Throat, la garganta *(lah gahr-GAHN-tah)*
Tongue, le lengua *(lah LEHN-gwah)*

ORGANS

Appendix, el apéndice *(ehl ah-PEHN-dee-seh)*
Bladder, la vejiga *(lah beh-HEE-gah)*
Brain, el cerebro *(ehl seh-REH-broh)*
Colon, el colon *(ehl KOH-lohn)*
Esophagus, el esófago *(ehl eh-SOH-fah-goh)*
Gallbladder, la vesícula biliar *(lah beh-SEE-koo-lah bee-lee-AHR)*
Genitals, los genitales *(lohs heh-nee-TAH-lehs)*
Heart, el corazón *(ehl koh-rah-SOHN)*
Kidney, el riñón *(ehl ree-NYOHN)*
Large intestine, el intestino grueso *(ehl een-tehs-TEE-noh groo-EH-so)*
Liver, el hígado *(ehl EE-gah-doh)*
Lungs, los pulmones *(lohs pool-MOH-nehs)*
Pancreas, el páncreas *(ehl PAHN-kreh-ahs)*
Small intestine, el intestino delgado *(ehl een-tehs-TEE-noh dehl-GAH-doh)*
Spleen, el bazo *(ehl BAH-soh)*
Thyroid gland, la tiroides *(lah tee-ROH-ee-dehs)*
Tonsils, las amígdalas *(lahs ah-MEEG-dah-lahs)*
Uterus, el útero *(ehl OO-teh-roh)*

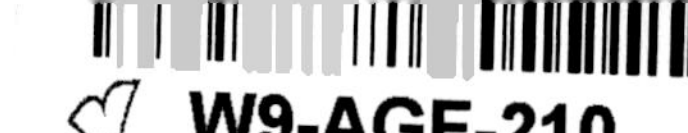

GASTROENTEROLOGY

GYNECOLOGY AND OBSTETRICS

HEMATOLOGY/ONCOLOGY

INFECTIOUS DISEASES

MISCELLANEOUS

NEPHROLOGY

NEUROLOGY

Don't Forget Your Online Access to

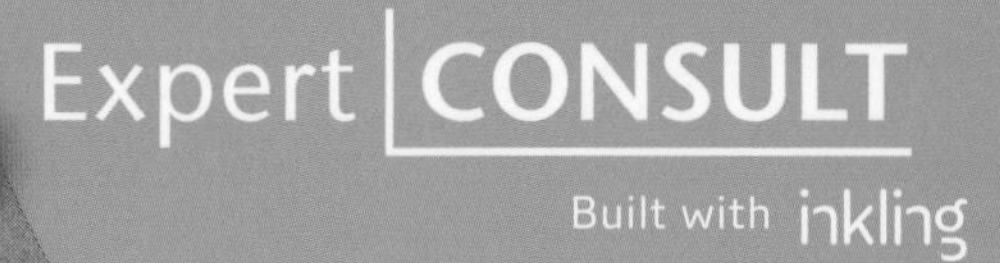

Elsevier | ExpertConsult.com

Enhanced eBooks for medical professionals

Compatible with PC, Mac®, most mobile devices, and eReaders, Expert Consult allows you to browse, search, and interact with this title – online *and* offline. Redeem your PIN at expertconsult.com today!

Start using these innovative features today:

- Seamless, real-time integration between devices
- Straightforward navigation and search
- Notes and highlights sharing with other users through social media
- Enhanced images with annotations, labels, and hot spots for zooming on specific details *
- Live streaming video and animations *
- Self-assessment tools such as questions embedded within the text and multiple-format quizzes *

** some features vary by title*

PIN REDEMPTION INSTRUCTIONS

1. Login or Sign Up at ExpertConsult.com
2. Scratch off your PIN code below
3. Enter PIN into the "Redeem a Book Code" box
4. Click "Redeem"
5. Go to "My Library"

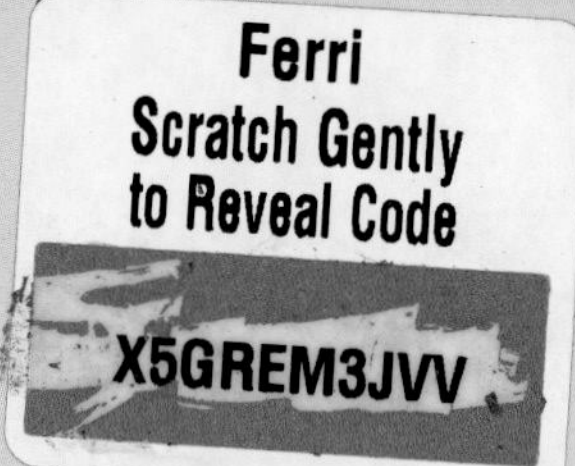

For technical assistance: Email: online.help@elsevier.com;
Call: within the US and Canada: 800-401-9962;
outside the US and Canada: +1-314-447-8200

2015

Ferri's CLINICAL ADVISOR

5 Books in 1

FRED F. FERRI, M.D., F.A.C.P.
Clinical Professor
Alpert Medical School
Brown University
Providence, Rhode Island

ELSEVIER
MOSBY

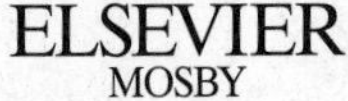

1600 John F. Kennedy Blvd.
Ste 1800
Philadelphia, PA 19103-2899

FERRI'S CLINICAL ADVISOR 2015: 5 BOOKS IN 1
ISBN: 978-0-323-08375-1
ISSN: 1541-4515

Notices

Knowledge and best practice in this field are constantly changing. As new research and experience broaden our understanding, changes in research methods, professional practices, or medical treatment may become necessary.

Practitioners and researchers must always rely on their own experience and knowledge in evaluating and using any information, methods, compounds, or experiments described herein. In using such information or methods they should be mindful of their own safety and the safety of others, including parties for whom they have a professional responsibility.

With respect to any drug or pharmaceutical products identified, readers are advised to check the most current information provided (i) on procedures featured or (ii) by the manufacturer of each product to be administered, to verify the recommended dose or formula, the method and duration of administration, and contraindications. It is the responsibility of practitioners, relying on their own experience and knowledge of their patients, to make diagnoses, to determine dosages and the best treatment for each individual patient, and to take all appropriate safety precautions.

To the fullest extent of the law, neither the Publisher nor the authors, contributors, or editors, assume any liability for any injury and/or damage to persons or property as a matter of products liability, negligence or otherwise, or from any use or operation of any methods, products, instructions, or ideas contained in the material herein.

ISBN: 978-0-323-08375-1
ISSN: 1541-4515

Senior Content Strategist: Suzanne Toppy
Content Development Specialist: Lauren Boyle
Publishing Services Manager: Patricia Tannian
Project Manager: Kate Mannix
Design Direction: Steven Stave

Printed in the United States of America

Last digit is the print number: 9 8 7 6 5 4 3 2 1

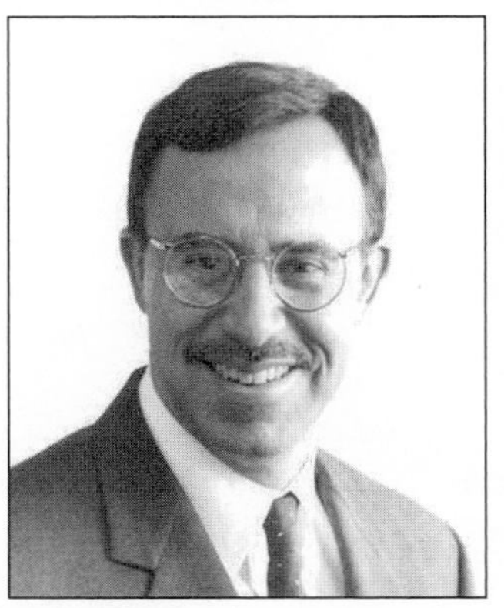

RUBEN ALVERO, M.D.
Director
Assisted Reproductive Technologies
Division Director REI
Vice Chairman for Education
Department of Obstetrics and Gynecology
University of Colorado Denver
Aurora, Colorado
SECTION I

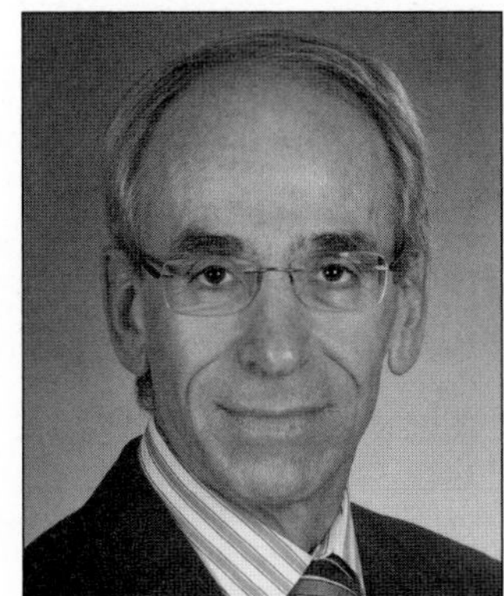

RICHARD J. GOLDBERG, M.D., M.S.
Psychiatrist-in-Chief
Rhode Island Hospital and the Miriam Hospital
Professor
Department of Psychiatry and Human Behavior
Alpert Medical School
Brown University
Providence, Rhode Island
SECTION I

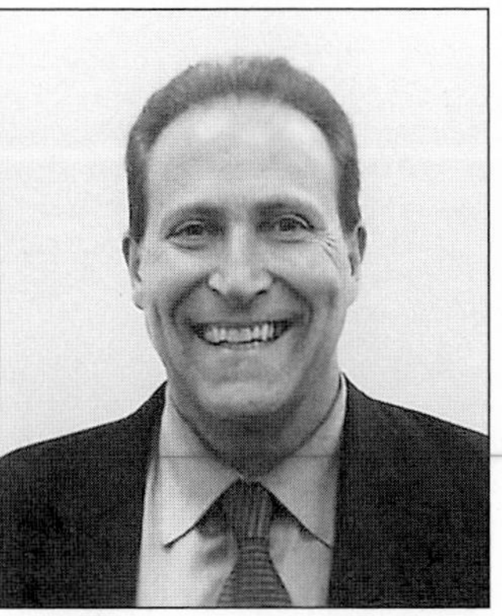

FRED F. FERRI, M.D., F.A.C.P.
Clinical Professor
Alpert Medical School
Brown University
Providence, Rhode Island
SECTION I

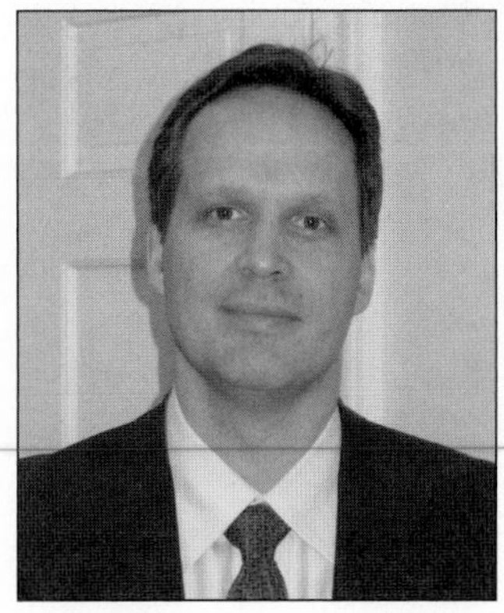

HARALD ALEXANDER HALL, M.D.
Director
Rheumatology Fellowship Program
Roger Williams Medical Center
Providence, Rhode Island
Assistant Professor of Medicine
Boston University School of Medicine
Boston, Massachusetts
SECTION I

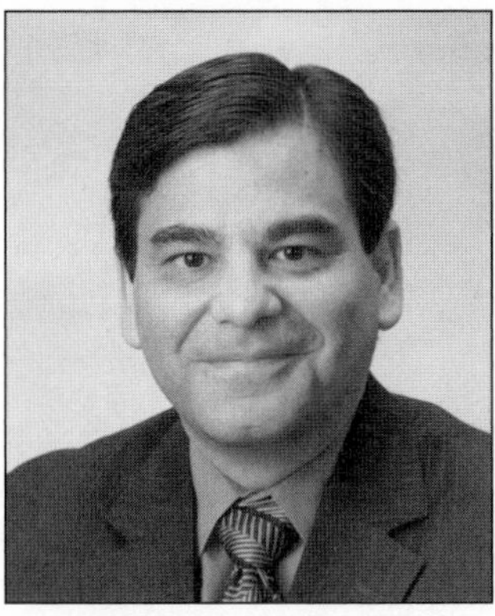

GLENN G. FORT, M.D., M.P.H., F.A.C.P., F.I.D.S.A.
Clinical Associate Professor of Medicine
Alpert Medical School
Brown University
Providence, Rhode Island Chief
Infectious Diseases
Our Lady of Fatima Hospital
North Providence, Rhode Island
SECTION I

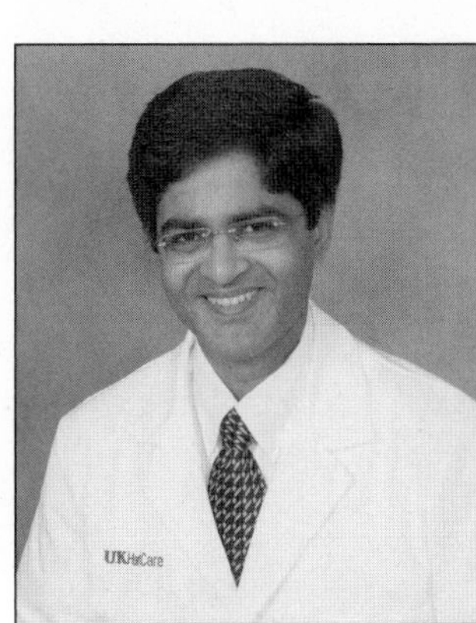

SACHIN KEDAR, M.B.B.S., M.D.
Assistant Professor of Neurology and Ophthalmology
Director, Neurology Residency Program
Director, Neuro-ophthalmology Service
University of Kentucky College of Medicine
Lexington, Kentucky
SECTION I

Section Editors

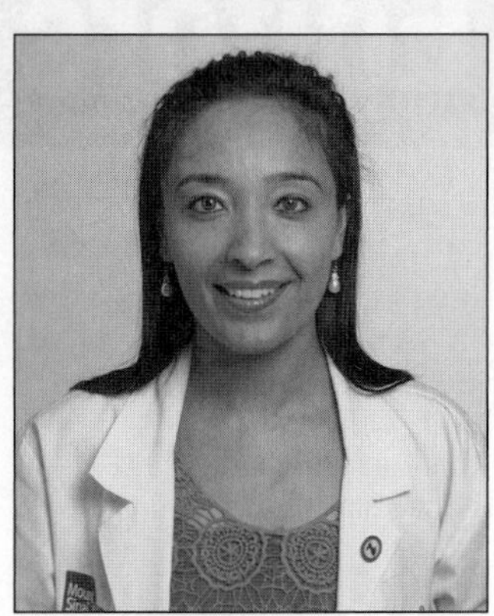

GAGAN D. SAHNI, M.D., F.A.C.C., F.A.C.P.
Associate Professor
Cardiovascular Institute
Mount Sinai Hospital Center
New York, New York
SECTION I

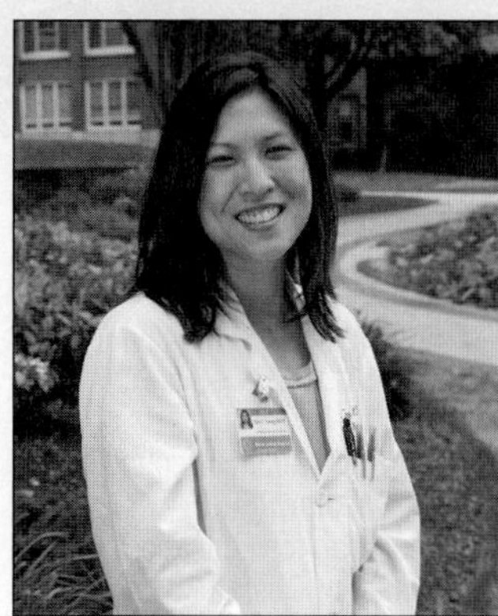

IRIS L. TONG, M.D.
Director, Women's Primary Care
Women's Medicine Collaborative
Assistant Professor
Department of Medicine
Alpert Medical School
Brown University
Providence, Rhode Island
SECTION I

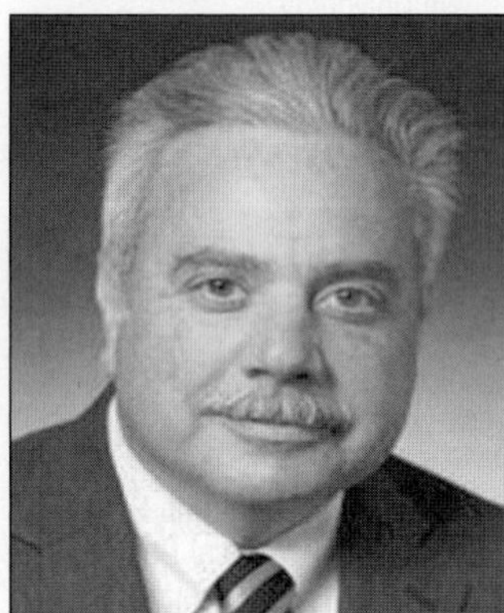

STEVEN M. SEPE, M.D., PH.D.
Chairman
Department of Medicine
Roger Williams Medical Center
Clinical Professor of Medicine
Assistant Dean
Boston University School of Medicine
Providence, Rhode Island

SONYA S. ABDEL-RAZEQ, M.D.
Clinical Assistant Instructor
Department of Obstetrics and Gynecology/Resident Education
State University of New York at Buffalo
Women's and Children's Hospital
Buffalo, New York

TONY ABDO, M.D.
Internal Medicine Resident
Roger Williams Medical Center
Boston University School of Medicine
Providence, Rhode Island

ABDULRAHMAN ABDULBAKI, M.D.
Fellow, Cardiology
Louisiana State University and Health Science Center
Shreveport, Louisiana

SADDAM SALEH ABISSE, M.D.
Cardiovascular Fellow
Warren Alpert Medical School
Brown University
Rhode Island Hospital
Providence, Rhode Island

CATHLEEN ADAMS, M.D.
Department of Psychiatry
Rhode Island Hospital
Providence, Rhode Island

WAFFIYAH AFRIDI, M.D.
Fellow, Rheumatology
Rhode Island Hospital
Alpert Medical School
Brown University
Providence, Rhode Island

MEGHA AGARWAL, M.D.
Cardiology Fellow
Department of Medicine
University of California, Irvine
Orange, California

TANYA ALI, M.D.
Clinical Assistant Professor of Medicine
Department of Medicine
Alpert Medical School
Brown University
Providence, Rhode Island

PHILIP J. ALIOTTA, M.D., M.S.H.A., F.A.C.S.
Clinical Instructor
Department of Urology
School of Medicine and Biomedical Sciences
State University of New York at Buffalo
Buffalo, New York
Medical Director
Center for Urologic Research of Western New York
Williamsville, New York

RUBEN ALVERO, M.D.
Professor, Obstetrics and Gynecology
Director, Assisted Reproductive Technologies
Section Head, Reproductive Endocrinology and Infertility
Vice Chair for Education
University of Colorado Denver
Aurora, Colorado

SRIVIDYA ANANDAN, M.D.
Attending Physician
Internal Medicine
Harvard Vanguard Medical Associates
Quincy, Massachusetts

MEL L. ANDERSON, M.D., F.A.C.P.
Assistant Professor of Medicine
University of Colorado School of Medicine
Denver Veterans Affairs Medical Center
Denver, Colorado

THOMAS J.T. ANDERSON, M.D.
Intern, Internal Medicine
Boston University School of Medicine
Boston, Massachusetts
Roger Williams Medical Center
Providence, Rhode Island
Resident, Diagnostic Radiology
Beth Israel Deaconess Medical Center
Harvard Medical School
Boston, Massachusetts

LAURA M. ANDOLINA, M.S., C.G.C.
Clinical Instructor of Pediatrics
State University of New York at Buffalo
School of Medicine and Biomedical Sciences
Buffalo, New York

KATHRYN TAYLOR ANILOWSKI, M.S., P.T., C.L.T.-L.A.N.A., A.B.D. CANDIDATE
Physical Therapist
Kinder Touch Lymphedema Center
Saratoga Springs, New York

ANNGENE G. ANTHONY, M.D., M.P.H., F.A.A.F.P.
Attending Physician
Family Medicine
Morrison Memorial Hospital
Morristown, New Jersey

MICHELLE S. ANVAR, M.D.
Assistant Professor of Medicine
General Internal Medicine
The Warren Alpert Medical School of Brown University
Rhode Island Hospital
Providence, Rhode Island

ETSUKO AOKI, M.D., PH.D.
Assistant Professor
Department of Leukemia/General Internal Medicine
The University of Texas M.D. Anderson Cancer Center
Houston, Texas

Contributors

GRAYSON ARMSTRONG, B.A.
Medical Student
The Warren Alpert Medical School of Brown University
Providence, Rhode Island
MPH Candidate
Health Care Management and Policy
Harvard School of Public Health
Boston, Massachusetts

RABIA ARSHAD, M.D.
Attending Cardiologist
Cardiology
Mercy Medical Center
Canton, Ohio

WISSAM S.Z. ASFAHANI, M.D.
Department of Neurosurgery
University of Kentucky
Lexington, Kentucky

MOHAMMAD ASHKIANI, M.D.
PGY-2 Internal Medicine Resident
The Warren Alpert Medical School of Brown University
Providence, Rhode Island
Memorial Hospital of Rhode Island
Pawtucket, Rhode Island

DANIEL K. ASIEDU, M.D., PH.D., F.A.C.P.
Clinical Instructor of Medicine
Alpert Medical School
Brown University
Staff Physician
Coastal Medical, Inc.
Providence, Rhode Island

SUDEEP KAUR AULAKH, M.D., C.M., F.R.C.P.C.
Director of Ambulatory Education, Baystate Internal Medicine Residency
Co-Director, Baystate Primary Care Residency
Baystate Medical Center
Springfield, Massachusetts
Medical Director, Physician Assistant Program
Bay Path College
Longmeadow, Massachusetts
Assistant Professor of Medicine
Tufts University School of Medicine
Boston, Massachusetts

CRISOSTOMO R. BALIOG Jr., M.D.
Assistant Professor
Department of Internal Medicine
University of South Alabama College of Medicine
Mobile, Alabama

PRIYA BANSAL, M.D., M.P.H.
Physician
Internal Medicine
Miriam Hospital/Rhode Island Hospital
Providence, Rhode Island

LUKE BARRÉ, M.D.
Instructor, Department of Medicine
Boston University School of Medicine
Medical Resident
Department of Medicine
Roger Williams Medical Center
Providence, Rhode Island

ROWLAND P. BARRETT, PH.D.
Associate Professor of Psychiatry & Human Behavior
Alpert Medical School
Brown University
Providence, Rhode Island

KERRI BATRA, M.D.
Assistant Professor of Medicine
The Warren Alpert Medical School of Brown University
Rheumatologist
Women's Medicine Collaborative
Miriam Hospital
Providence, Rhode Island
Rheumatologist
Milford Regional Medical Center
Milford, Massachusetts

OMRI BERGER, M.D.
Fellow, Psychiatry and the Law Program
Department of Psychiatry
University of California, San Francisco
San Francisco, California

ARNALDO A. BERGES, M.D.
Rhode Island Hospital
Assistant Clinical Professor
Department of Psychiatry and Human Behavior
Alpert Medical School
Brown University
Providence, Rhode Island

VICKY BHAGAT
PGY-1
Internal Medicine
Boston University
Boston, Massachusetts
Roger Williams Medical Center
Providence, Rhode Island

RAHUL BHARDWAJ, M.D.
Cardiology Fellow
Department of Medicine
University of California, Irvine
Orange, California

RACHAEL M. BIANCUZZO, M.S.I.V.
Medical Student, M.S.I.V.
Department of Medicine
University of New England College of Osteopathic Medicine
Biddeford, Maine
Medical Student, M.S.I.V.
Department of Internal Medicine
Roger Williams Medical Center
Providence, Rhode Island

COURTNEY CLARK BILODEAU, M.D.
Assistant Clinical Professor
Department of Medicine
The Warren Alpert Medical School of Brown University
Attending Physician
Department of Medicine
Miriam Hospital
Providence, Rhode Island

KENNETH D. BISHOP, M.D., PH.D.
Fellow
Division of Hematology/Oncology
Brown University
Providence, Rhode Island

MICHAEL BLUNDIN, M.D.
Pulmonary and Critical Care
Rhode Island Hospital
Providence, Rhode Island

SHEENAGH M. BODKIN, M.D.
Women's Primary Care
Women's Medicine Collaborative
Providence, Rhode Island

NIRALI BORA, M.D.
Assistant Clinical Instructor of Family Medicine
Alpert Medical School
Brown University
Providence, Rhode Island
Memorial Hospital of Rhode Island
Pawtucket, Rhode Island

JEFFREY M. BORKAN, M.D., PH.D.
Professor and Chair
Department of Family Medicine
Memorial Hospital of Rhode Island
Pawtucket, Rhode Island
Alpert Medical School
Brown University
Providence, Rhode Island

ALEXANDRA BOSKE, M.D.
Director of Inpatient Neurology
Stroke Program Director
Saint David's Round Rock Medical Center
Round Rock, Texas

LYNN BOWLBY, M.D., F.A.C.P.
Medical Director
Duke Outpatient Clinic (DOC)
Duke Internal Medicine Residency Program
Durham, North Carolina

MARK F. BRADY, M.D., M.P.H., M.M.S., D.T.M.&H.
Attending Physician
Emergency Medicine
Baptist Memorial Hospital
Memphis, Tennessee

MANDEEP K. BRAR, M.D.
Clinical Assistant Professor
Department of Obstetrics and Gynecology
State University of New York at Buffalo
Buffalo, New York

KEITH BRENNAN, M.D.
Doctor, Internal Medicine
Boston University
Boston, Massachusetts
Roger Williams Medical Center
Providence, Rhode Island

ELIZABETH J. BROWN, M.D.
Assistant Clinical Instructor of Family Medicine
Memorial Hospital of Rhode Island
Pawtucket, Rhode Island
Alpert Medical School
Brown University
Providence, Rhode Island

GAVIN BROWN, M.D.
General Neurologist
Laureate Medical Group at Northside Hospital
Atlanta, Georgia

JENNIFER BUCKLEY, M.D.
Clinical Assistant Professor of Family Medicine
Memorial Hospital of Rhode Island
Pawtucket, Rhode Island
Brown University
Providence, Rhode Island

JONATHAN BURNS, M.A., M.D.
Clinical Instructor in Ambulatory Care and Prevention
Harvard Medical School
Boston, Massachusetts
Staff Physician
Family Medicine
Cambridge Health Alliance
Cambridge, Massachusetts

D. BRANDON BURTIS, D.O.
Assistant Professor
Department of Neurology
College of Medicine
University of Florida
Gainesville, Florida

DOUGLAS BURTT, M.D.
Clinical Assistant Professor of Medicine
Division of Cardiology
Alpert Medical School
Brown University
Providence, Rhode Island

STEVEN BUSSELEN, M.D.
Medical Director
Tri-Town Health Center
Johnston, Rhode Island

ROBERT BUTLER, M.D.
Resident
The Warren Alpert School of Medicine of Brown University
Providence, Rhode Island

CLAUDIA RODRIGUEZ CABRERA, M.D.
Internal Medicine Residency Program Director
Hospital Regional Universitario de Jose Maria Cabral y Baez
Clinical Parasitology, Department of Medicine
Universidad Tecnológica de Santiago
Santiago, Dominican Republic

ANDREW CARAGANIS, M.D.
PGY-2 Internal Medicine
Roger Williams Medical Center
Providence, Rhode Island

CAROLINA S. CEREZO, M.D., F.A.A.P.
Department of Pediatrics
Rhode Island Hospital
Assistant Professor of Pediatrics
The Warren Alpert Medical School of Brown University
Providence, Rhode Island

JOSHUA CHALKLEY, M.S., D.O.
Department of Neurology
University of Kentucky Medical Center
Lexington, Kentucky

Contributors

PHILIP A. CHAN, M.D., M.S.
Infectious Disease Medicine
Miriam Immunology Clinic
The Miriam Hospital
Providence, Rhode Island

SAURAV CHATTERJEE, M.D.
Fellow, Preventive Cardiology
Providence VA Medical Center
Alpert Medical School
Brown University
Providence, Rhode Island

SUNIT-PREET CHAUDHRY, M.D.
Department of Cardiology
Rhode Island Hospital
Brown University
Providence, Rhode Island

VICKY CHENG, M.D.
Assistant Professor of Medicine (Clinical)
The Warren Alpert Medical School of Brown University
Providence, Rhode Island

SARAH L. CHISHOLM, M.D.
Resident Physician
Department of Obstetrics and Gynecology
University of Colorado Hospital
Denver, Colorado

NEELESH LALJI CHUDASAMA, M.D.
Postdoctoral Clinical Fellow
Division of Cardiology, Department of
Internal Medicine
New York Presbyterian Hospital
Columbia University Medical Center
New York, New York

JONATHAN P. CLARKE, M.D.
Department of Internal Medicine
Roger Williams Medical Center
Providence, Rhode Island

LISA COHEN, PHARM.D.
Associate Professor of Pharmacy
Department of Pharmacy Practice
University of Rhode Island
Kingston, Rhode Island
Research Pharmacist
Veterans Affairs Medical Center
Providence, Rhode Island

KAILA COMPTON, M.D., PH.D.
Attending Psychiatrist
Alta Bates/Herrick Hospital,
Berkeley, California

JESSICA CORWIN, M.D., M.P.H.
The Permanente Medical Group
Northern California

BRIAN J. COWLES, PHARM.D.
Assistant Professor of Pharmacy
Department of Pharmacy Practice,
Albany College of Pharmacy and Health Sciences
Colchester, Vermont

DAN A. CRISTESCU, M.D.
Arthritis Associates and Osteoporosis Center of Colorado Springs
Colorado Springs, Colorado

PATRICIA CRISTOFARO, M.D.
Assistant Professor of Medicine
Alpert Medical School
Brown University
Physician
Providence VA Medical Center
Providence, Rhode Island

JOANNE SZCYGIEL CUNHA, M.D.
Fellow, Department of Rheumatology
The Warren Alpert School of Medicine of Brown University
Providence, Rhode Island

STEPHANIE A. CURRY, M.D.
Department of Internal Medicine
Roger Williams Medical Center,
Boston University School of Medicine
Boston, Massachusetts

ALICIA J. CURTIN, PH.D., G.N.P.
Assistant Professor
Division of Geriatrics
Alpert Medical School
Brown University
Providence, Rhode Island

CATHERINE D'AVANZATO, M.S.
Psychology Fellow
Rhode Island Hospital
Department of Psychiatry and Human Behavior
The Warren Alpert School of Medicine of Brown University
Providence, Rhode Island

ALI DAHHAN, M.D.
Staff Physician
Department of Internal Medicine
Carver College of Medicine
University of Iowa
Iowa City, Iowa

KRISTY L. DALRYMPLE, PH.D.
Assistant Professor (Research)
Alpert Medical School
Brown University
Staff Psychologist
Rhode Island Hospital
Providence, Rhode Island

GEORGE T. DANAKAS, M.D., F.A.C.O.G.
Clinical Assistant Professor
Department of Obstetrics and Gynecology
State University of New York at Buffalo
Buffalo, New York

ALEXANDRA DEGENHARDT, M.D., M.M.S.
Director
Multiple Sclerosis Center
Pen Bay Medical Center
Rockport, Maine

JOSEPH A. DIAZ, M.D., M.P.H.
Associate Professor of Medicine
Department of Medicine
Alpert Medical School
Brown University
Providence, Rhode Island
Department of Medicine
Memorial Hospital of Rhode Island
Pawtucket, Rhode Island

MICHAEL R. DOBBS, M.D.
Associate Professor of Neurology
Vice-Chair for Clinical Operations
Medical Director
Stroke Care
Chandler Medical Center
University of Kentucky
Lexington, Kentucky

NATHALIA DOOBAY, D.P.M.
Department of Podiatric Surgery
Roger Williams Medical Center
Providence, Rhode Island

AMANDA C. DORAN, M.D., PH.D.
Cardiology Fellow
Department of Medicine, Division of Cardiology
Columbia University
New York Presbyterian Hospital
New York, New York

WILLIAM F. DOTSON II, M.D.
Neurophysiology Fellow
Department of Neurology
Medical University of South Carolina
Charleston, South Carolina

ANDREW DUKER, M.D.
Assistant Professor of Neurology and Rehabilitation Medicine
University of Cincinnati
Cincinnati, Ohio

STUART J. EISENDRATH, M.D.
Professor of Clinical Psychiatry
Director of the UCSF Depression Center
University of California, San Francisco
San Francisco, California

CHRISTINE EISENHOWER, PHARM.D.
Clinical Assistant Professor
Pharmacy Practice
University of Rhode Island College of Pharmacy
Kingston, Rhode Island
Clinical Pharmacist
PACE Organization of Rhode Island
Providence, Rhode Island

PAMELA ELLSWORTH, M.D.
Professor of Urology
Chief of Pediatric Urology
Department of Urology
UMass Memorial Medical Center
Worchester, Massachusetts

MICHAEL ENGELS, M.D.
Internal Medicine Resident
Warren Alpert Medical School
Brown University
Rhode Island Hospital
Providence, Rhode Island

PATRICIO SEBASTIAN ESPINOSA, M.D., M.P.H.
Visiting Associate Professor of Neurology
Department of Neurology
Universidad San Francisco de Quito
Quito, Ecuador
Division Director
Neurology
North Oaks Neuroscience Institute
Hammond, Louisiana

VALERIA FABRE, M.D.
Infectious Disease Fellow
Department of Infectious Diseases
Johns Hopkins University
Baltimore, Maryland

MARK J. FAGAN, M.D.
Director
Medical Primary Care Unit
Rhode Island Hospital
Professor of Medicine
Alpert Medical School
Brown University
Providence, Rhode Island

LIORA FARBER, M.D.
Department of Internal Medicine
Roger Williams Medical Center
Providence, Rhode Island

TIMOTHY W. FARRELL, M.D.
Assistant Professor of Medicine (Clinical)
Division of Geriatrics
Adjunct Assistant Professor of Family Medicine
Department of Family & Preventive Medicine
University of Utah School of Medicine
Salt Lake City, Utah

FRED F. FERRI, M.D., F.A.C.P.
Clinical Professor
Alpert Medical School
Brown University
Providence, Rhode Island

HEATHER FERRI, D.O.
Medical Resident
Department of Medicine
The Warren Alpert Medical School of Brown University
Rhode Island Hospital
Providence, Rhode Island

ANTONELLA FINE, M.D.
Resident, Internal Medicine
The Warren Alpert Medical School of Brown University
Rhode Island Hospital
Providence, Rhode Island

BARRY FINE, M.D., PH.D.
Fellow in Cardiovascular Medicine
Department of Cardiology
Columbia University
Clinical Fellow
Department of Medicine
New York Presbyterian Hospital
New York, New York

Contributors

GLEN FINNEY, M.D.
Assistant Professor
Department of Neurology
College of Medicine
University of Florida
Gainesville, Florida

STACI A. FISCHER, M.D., F.A.C.P., F.I.D.S.A.
Associate Professor of Medicine
Division of Infectious Diseases
Alpert Medical School
Brown University
Director, Transplant Infectious Diseases
Transplant Services and Medicine
Rhode Island Hospital
Providence, Rhode Island

TAMARA G. FONG, M.D., PH.D.
Assistant Professor of Neurology
Harvard Medical School,
Staff Neurologist
Beth Israel Deaconess Medical Center
Assistant Scientist, Aging Brain Center
Institute for Aging Research, Hebrew SeniorLife
Boston, Massachusetts

AMBER N. FONTENOT FERRISS, M.D.
Anschutz Medical Campus
University of Colorado Denver
Denver, Colorado

MICHELLE FORCIER, M.D., M.P.H.
Associate Professor of Pediatrics
Division of Adolescent Medicine
Alpert Medical School
Brown University
Providence, Rhode Island

FRANK G. FORT, M.D., F.A.C.S., R.PH.S.
Medical Director
Capital Region Vein Centre
Schenectady, New York

GLENN G. FORT, M.D., M.P.H., F.A.C.P., F.I.D.S.A.
Clinical Associate Professor of Medicine
Alpert Medical School
Brown University
Providence, Rhode Island
Chief
Infectious Diseases
Our Lady of Fatima Hospital
North Providence, Rhode Island

DAVID J. FORTUNATO, M.D., F.A.C.C.
Clinical Associate Professor of Medicine
Alpert Medical School
Brown University
Cardiology Section
Providence VA Medical Center
Providence, Rhode Island

KYLE FRANCO, PHARM.D. CANDIDATE
Student Pharmacist
College of Pharmacy
University of Rhode Island
Kingston, Rhode Island

JUSTIN F. FRASER, M.D.
Assistant Professor of Cerebrovascular, Endovascular, and Skull Base Surgery
Department of Neurological Surgery
University of Kentucky
Lexington, Kentucky

SAINATH GADDAM, M.D.
Fellow, Preventive Cardiology
Providence VA Medical Center,
Alpert Medical School
Brown University,
Providence, Rhode Island

ANTHONY GALLO, M.D.
Assistant Clinical Professor of Psychiatry
Alpert Medical School
Brown University
Providence, Rhode Island

MARINA GARAS, B.S., OMS-III
College of Osteopathic Medicine
University of New England
Biddeford, Maine
Department of Internal Medicine
Roger Williams Medical Center
Boston University School of Medicine
Providence, Rhode Island

LEANNA R. GARBUS, OMS-II
University of New England College of Osteopathic Medicine
Biddeford, Maine

PAUL F. GEORGE, M.D.
Assistant Professor of Family Medicine
Alpert Medical School
Brown University
Providence, Rhode Island

JOYDEEP GHOSH, M.D., F.A.C.C.
Assistant Professor of Medicine
Columbia Presbyterian Medical Center
New York, New York

CINDY GLEIT, M.D.
Assistant Clinical Instructor
Department of Family Medicine
Alpert Medical School
Brown University
Providence, Rhode Island

RICHARD J. GOLDBERG, M.D., M.S.
Psychiatrist-in-Chief
Rhode Island Hospital and The Miriam Hospital
Professor
Department of Psychiatry and Human Behavior
Alpert Medical School
Brown University
Providence, Rhode Island

ALLA GOLDBURT, M.D.
Resident, Family Medicine
Memorial Hospital of Rhode Island
Pawtucket, Rhode Island

GEETHA GOPALAKRISHNAN, M.D.
Associate Professor of Medicine
Alpert Medical School
Brown University
Providence, Rhode Island

PAUL GORDON, M.D.
Clinical Assistant Professor of Medicine
Division of Cardiology
Alpert Medical School
Brown University
Providence, Rhode Island

NANCY R. GRAFF, M.D.
Professor of Pediatrics
University of California, San Diego
San Diego, California

JOHN A. GRAY, M.D., Ph.D.
Assistant Professor
Department of Neurology
Center for Neuroscience
University of California, Davis
Davis, California

ELLIOTT M. GROVES, M.D., M.Eng.
Cardiology Fellow
Department of Medicine
University of California, Irvine
Orange, California

STEPHEN L. GRUPKE, M.D., M.S.
Resident
Department of Neurological Surgery
University of Kentucky
Lexington, Kentucky

PATAN GULTAWATVICHAI, M.D.
Department of Internal Medicine
Roger Williams Medical Center
Providence, Rhode Island

PRIYA SARIN GUPTA, M.D., M.P.H.
Fellow, Adolescent Medicine
Division of General Pediatrics and
Adolescent Medicine
Johns Hopkins Hospital
Baltimore, Maryland

NAWAZ HACK, M.D.
Doctor of Neurology
Adjunct Postclinical Doctoral Fellow in
Movement Disorders
University of Florida
Gainesville, Florida

HARALD A. HALL, M.D.
Assistant Professor of Medicine
Boston University School of Medicine
Director, Rheumatology Fellowship Program
Roger Williams Medical Center
Rheumatology Section Chief
Providence VA Medical Center
Providence, Rhode Island

LEO HAN, M.D.
Resident, Obstetrics and Gynecology
University of Colorado
Aurora, Colorado

SAJEEV HANDA, M.D., S.F.H.M.
Director
Division of Hospital Medicine
Rhode Island Hospital
Clinical Assistant Professor of Medicine
Alpert Medical School
Brown University
Providence, Rhode Island

ERICA J. HARDY, M.D., M.M.S.
Assistant Professor of Medicine (Clinical)
The Warren Alpert School of Medicine of Brown University
Attending Physician
Department of Infectious Diseases and Obstetric Medicine
Women & Infant's Hospital
Providence, Rhode Island

TAYLOR HARRISON, M.D.
Assistant Professor of Neurology
Department of Neurology
Emory University
Atlanta, Georgia

DON HAYES, Jr., M.D., M.S.
Associate Professor
Departments of Pediatrics and Internal Medicine
The Ohio State University
Section of Pulmonary Medicine
Nationwide Children's Hospital
Division of Pulmonary, Allergy, Critical Care, and Sleep Medicine
The Ohio State University Wexner Medical Center
Columbus, Ohio

R. SCOTT HOFFMAN, M.D.
Assistant Clinical Professor
Ophthalmology and Visual Sciences
University of Louisville
Physician, Ophthalmologist
Doctors Eye Institute
Louisville, Kentucky

DAWN HOGAN, M.D.
Clinical Assistant Professor of Family Medicine
Alpert Medical School,
Brown University
Providence, Rhode Island

N. WILSON HOLLAND, M.D., F.A.C.P., A.G.S.F.
Associate Professor of Medicine
Division of Geriatrics and Gerontology
Emory University School of Medicine
Acting Designated Learning Officer
Atlanta Veterans Administration Medical Center
Atlanta, Georgia

SUSIE L. HU, M.D.
Assistant Professor of Medicine
Division of Renal Diseases
Department of Internal Medicine
Alpert Medical School
Brown University
Rhode Island Hospital
Providence, Rhode Island

ANNE L. HUME, PHARM.D.
Professor of Pharmacy
Department of Pharmacy Practice,
University of Rhode Island
College of Pharmacy
Kingston, Rhode Island,
Adjunct Professor of Family Medicine
Memorial Hospital of Rhode Island
Pawtucket, Rhode Island

SHARLISA WALLER HUTSON, M.D.
T.C. Thompson Children's Hospital
Elranger Hospital
Chattanooga, Tennessee

RICHARD S. ISAACSON, M.D.
Associate Professor of Clinical Neurology
Vice-Chair of Education
Miller School of Medicine
University of Miami
Miami, Florida

AHMAD M. ISMAIL, M.D.
Academic Hospitalist
Memorial Hospital of Rhode Island
Pawtucket, Rhode Island
Assistant Program Director
Internal Medicine Residency Program
Alpert Medical School
Brown University
Providence, Rhode Island

JENNIFER JANTZ, M.D.
Brown Cardiology Fellow
Rhode Island Hospital
Brown University
Providence, Rhode Island

NOEL S.C. JAVIER, M.D.
Clinical Assistant Professor of Medicine and Pediatrics
Alpert Medical School
Brown University
Providence, Rhode Island

JENNIFER JEREMIAH, M.D.
Clinical Associate Professor of Medicine
Alpert Medical School
Brown University
Providence, Rhode Island

MICHAEL P. JOHNSON, M.D.
Staff Physician
Division of General Internal Medicine
Rhode Island Hospital
Assistant Professor of Medicine
Brown University
Providence, Rhode Island

KIMBERLY JONES, M.D.
Associate Professor of Child Neurology
Department of Neurology
University of Kentucky
Lexington, Kentucky

LUCY KALANITHI, M.D.
Postdoctoral Fellow
Stanford Clinical Excellence Research Center
Stanford University School of Medicine
Stanford, California

SIDDHARTH KAPOOR, M.D.
Assistant Professor of Neurology
Director, Headache Medicine
Program Director, Fellowship in Headache Medicine
Department of Neurology
University of Kentucky College of Medicine
Lexington, Kentucky

CLAIRE KASSAKIAN, M.D.
Fellow
Department of Nephrology and Hypertension
Alpert Medical School of Brown University
Providence, Rhode Island

EMILY R. KATZ, M.D.
Director
Child & Adolescent Psychiatry Consultation-Liaison Service
Hasbro Children's Hospital
Rhode Island Hospital
Assistant Professor (Clinical) of Psychiatry and Human Behavior
Alpert Medical School
Brown University
Providence, Rhode Island

ALI KAZIM, M.D.
Clinical Associate Professor
Department of Psychiatry
David Geffen School of Medicine at UCLA
Los Angeles, California
Associate Chief of Mental Health
Sepulveda Veterans Administration Ambulatory Health Care
Sepulveda, California

SACHIN KEDAR, M.B.B.S., M.D.
Assistant Professor of Neurology and Ophthalmology
Director, Neurology Residency Program
Director, Neuro-ophthalmology Service
University of Kentucky College of Medicine
Lexington, Kentucky

BROOKE E. KEELEY, D.P.M.
Podiatric Surgeon
Department of Surgery
Newport Hospital
Newport, Rhode Island
South County Hospital
Wakefield, Rhode Island
The Miriam Hospital
PMS-3 Surgical Resident Training
Roger Williams Medical Center
Providence, Rhode Island

BEVIN KENNEY, M.D.
Instructor in Medicine
Harvard Medical School
Internist
Department of Medicine
Brigham and Women's Hospital
Boston, Massachusetts

BYUNG KIM, M.D.
Internal Medicine Chief Resident
Roger Williams Medical Center
Boston University School of Medicine
Boston, Massachusetts

JIN KYUNG KIM, M.D., PH.D., F.A.C.C.
Assistant Professor of Medicine
Department of Medicine
University of California, Irvine
Orange, California

WAN J. KIM, M.D.
Department of Obstetrics and Gynecology
Kaiser Permanente
Hayward Medical Center
Hayward, California

ROBERT M. KIRCHNER, M.D.
Fellow, Cardiology
Division of Cardiology
Alpert Medical School
Brown University
Providence, Rhode Island

MELVYN KOBY, M.D.
Associate Clinical Professor of Medicine
Department of Ophthalmology
University of Louisville School of Medicine
Louisville, Kentucky

ROBERT KOHN, M.D.
Professor
Department of Psychiatry and Human Behavior
The Warren Alpert School of Medicine
Brown University
Providence, Rhode Island

ARAVIND RAO KOKKIRALA, M.D.
Cardiology Staff
Providence VA Medical Center
Providence, Rhode Island

KRISTINA KRAMER, M.D.
Medical Director
Intensive Care Unit
John Muir Medical Center
Walnut Creek, California

PRASHANTH KRISHNAMOHAN, M.B.B.S., M.D.
Resident Physician
Department of Neurology
University of Kentucky
Lexington, Kentucky

DEEPA KUMARAIAH, M.D., M.B.A.
Clinical Cardiology Fellow
Department of Cardiology
Columbia University Medical Center
New York, New York

DAVID I. KURSS, M.D., F.A.C.O.G.
Clinical Assistant Professor
Department of Obstetrics and Gynecology,
State University of New York at Buffalo
Buffalo, New York
Medical Director
Women's Wellness Center of Western New York
Williamsville, New York

CINDY LAI, M.D.
Associate Professor of Clinical Medicine
Intersessions Course Director
Site Director
Medicine Clerkships
University of California, San Francisco
San Francisco, California

EDWARD V. LALLY, M.D.
Director
Division of Rheumatology
Rhode Island Hospital
Professor of Medicine
Department of Rheumatology
Brown University
Providence, Rhode Island

SYDE RIZWAN LATIF, M.D.
Clinical Fellow
Department of Medicine
Division of Cardiovascular Medicine
University of California, Davis, Medical Center
Sacramento, California

QUANG P. LE, M.D., M.P.H.
Department of Same Day Services
Tufts University School of Medicine
St. Vincent Hospital
Medical Director
Le & Chang Family Urgent Care
Worcester, Massachusetts

KACHIU LEE, B.A.
Clinical Fellow in Dermatology and Laser Medicine
Department of Dermatology
Massachusetts General Hospital
Harvard Medical School
Boston, Massachusetts

ANDRE LEVCHENKO, PH.D.
Professor of Biomedical Engineering
Johns Hopkins University
Baltimore, Maryland

DONITA DILLON LIGHTNER, M.D.
Assistant Professor of Pediatric Neurology
Department of Neurology,
University of Kentucky
Lexington, Kentucky

RICHARD LONG, M.D.
Associate Professor of Family Medicine
Director of Maternal and Child Health
Department of Family Medicine
Boston University School of Medicine
Department of Family Medicine
Boston Medical Center
Boston, Massachusetts

ELIZABETH A. LOWENHAUPT, M.D., F.A.A.P.
Associate Training Director
Child Psychiatry Fellowship & Triple Board Residency
Director, Medical Student Education in Child & Adolescent Psychiatry
Director of Psychiatric Services, Rhode Island Training School
Clinical Assistant Professor, Department of Psychiatry and Human Behavior
Rhode Island Hospital
Brown University,
Providence, Rhode Island

AMY L. LUNDHOLM, M.D.
Fellow
Department of Rheumatology
Roger Williams Medical Center
Providence, Rhode Island

SUSANNA R. MAGEE, M.D., M.P.H.
Assistant Professor
Department of Family Medicine
Alpert Medical School
Brown University
Providence, Rhode Island
Director of Maternal and Child Health
Memorial Hospital of Rhode Island
Pawtucket, Rhode Island

MICHAEL MAHER, M.D.
Assistant Professor of Internal Medicine
Brown University School of Medicine
Rhode Island Hospital
Providence, Rhode Island

MARTA MAJCZAK, M.D.
Child and Adolescent Psychiatrist
Bradley Hospital
Clinical Assistant Professor of Psychiatry and Human Behavior
Brown University
Providence, Rhode Island

MONZR M. AL MALKI, M.D.
Instructor
Department of Hematology and Hematopoietic Cell Transplantation
City of Hope National Medical Center
Duarte, California

ATIZAZUL H. MANSOOR, M.D., F.A.C.C.
Department of Cardiovascular Diseases
Pinnacle Health Cardiovascular Institute
Pinnacle Hospitals
Harrisburg, Pennsylvania

MICHAEL A. MARSH, M.D.
Chief Medical Resident
Internal Medicine
Roger Williams Medical Center
Providence, Rhode Island

ELISABETH B. MATSON, D.O.
Rheumatologist
Exeter, New Hampshire

KATE MAVRICH, M.D.
Assistant Professor (Clinical)
Department of Medicine
Alpert Medical School
Brown University
Providence, Rhode Island

LAUREN MAY, M.D.
Resident in Obstetrics and Gynecology,
Department of Obstetrics and Gynecology
University of Colorado
Aurora, Colorado

ALISON C. MAY, M.D.
Department of Psychiatry
VA Medical Center,
Clinical Instructor
University of California, San Francisco,
San Francisco, California

MAITREYI MAZUMDAR, M.D., M.P.H., M.Sc.
Assistant Professor of Neurology
Harvard Medical School
Staff Physician
Department of Neurology
Boston's Children's Hospital
Assistant Professor
Department of Environmental Health
Harvard School of Public Health
Boston, Massachusetts

NADINE MBUYI, M.D.
Resident Physician
Department of Internal Medicine
Boston University School of Medicine
Boston, Massachusetts
Roger Williams Medical Center
Providence, Rhode Island

RUSSELL J. MCCULLOH, M.D.
Assistant Professor
Department of Pediatric Infectious Diseases
Children's Mercy Hospitals and Clinics
University of Missouri-Kansas City
Kansas City, Missouri
University of Kansas School of Medicine
Kansas City, Kansas

KELLY A. MCGARRY, M.D.
Program Director
General Internal Medicine Residency Program
Rhode Island Hospital
Associate Professor of Medicine
Alpert Medical School
Brown University
Providence, Rhode Island

LYNN MCNICOLL, M.D., F.R.C.P.C.
Assistant Professor of Medicine (Clinical)
Alpert Medical School
Brown University
Geriatrician
Division of Geriatrics
Rhode Island Hospital
Providence, Rhode Island

ERIN MEDLIN, M.D.
Clinical Instructor, Gynecologic Oncology
Department of Obstetrics and Gynecology
University of Wisconsin School of Medicine and Public Health
Madison, Wisconsin

AKANKSHA MEHTA, M.D.
Senior Associate in Urology
Emory University School of Medicine
Atlanta, Georgia

DANIEL E. MENDEZ-ALLWOOD, M.D.
Rheumatologist
Salem, Oregon

ALVARO MENENDEZ, M.D.
Internal Medicine Resident Physician
Department of Internal Medicine
Roger Williams Medical Center
Providence, Rhode Island

LONNIE R. MERCIER, M.D.
Clinical Instructor
Department of Orthopedic Surgery,
Creighton University School of Medicine
Omaha, Nebraska

VEERANNA MERLA, M.D.
Assistant Professor
Department of Cardiology
Columbia University
Attending
Medicine and Cardiology
New York Presbyterian Hospital
New York, New York

HASSAN MNHAS, M.D.
Child and Adolescent Psychiatry Fellow
Rhode Island Hospital
Brown University
Providence, Rhode Island

NADEEM MOHAMMED, M.D.
PGY-1 Internal Medicine
Roger Williams Medical Center
Boston University
Providence, Rhode Island

THERESA A. MORGAN, PH.D., M.PHIL.
Resident in Clinical Psychology
Alpert Medical School,
Brown University
Department of Psychiatry
Rhode Island Hospital
Providence, Rhode Island

NADIA MUJAHID, M.D.
Co-Director, Geriatric Fracture Program,
Assistant Professor of Medicine (Clinical)
The Warren Alpert Medical School of Brown University
Geriatrician
Division of Geriatric and Palliative Care Medicine
Rhode Island Hospital
Providence, Rhode Island

CATHERINE ELIAS NAJEM, M.D.
Resident, Internal Medicine
Roger Williams Medical Center
Clinical Research Assistant
Rheumatology Department
Boston University School of Medicine
Providence, Rhode Island

BILAL H. NAQVI, M.D.
Hematologist/Oncologist
Marshfield Clinic Regional Cancer Center
Eau Claire, Wisconsin

UZMA NASIR, M.D.
Assistant Professor
Department of Pain Management and Anesthesiology
Stony Brook University
Stony Brook, New York

JUDY NEE, M.D.
Fellow, Gastroenterology
Alpert Medical School
Brown University
Providence, Rhode Island

TAKUMA NEMOTO, M.D.
Research Associate Professor of Surgery
State University of New York at Buffalo
Buffalo, New York

MELISSA NOTHNAGLE, M.D., M.SC.
Director, Family Medicine Residency
Associate Professor of Family Medicine
The Warren Alpert Medical School of Brown University
Providence, Rhode Island
Residency Director
Family Medicine
Memorial Hospital of Rhode Island
Pawtucket, Rhode Island

PATRICK NSEREKO, M.D.
Resident
Boston University School of Medicine
Boston, Massachusetts
Resident, Internal Medicine
Roger Williams Medical Center
Providence, Rhode Island

GAIL M. O'BRIEN, M.D.
Alliance Internal Medicine
Edgartown, Massachusetts

ALEXANDER B. OLAWAIYE, M.D.
Fellow
Division of Gynecologic Oncology
Vincent Department of Obstetrics, Gynecology and Reproductive Biology
Massachusetts General Hospital
Harvard Medical School
Boston, Massachusetts

MICHAEL K. ONG, M.D., PH.D.
Associate Professor in Residence
UCLA Division of General Internal Medicine/Health Services Research
David Geffen School of Medicine
University of California, Los Angeles
Greater Los Angeles VA Health Care System
Los Angeles, California

STEVEN M. OPAL, M.D.
Professor of Medicine
Infectious Disease Division
Alpert Medical School
Brown University,
Providence, Rhode Island

LINDSAY M. ORCHOWSKI, PH.D.
Staff Psychologist
Rhode Island Hospital
Assistant Professor (Research)
The Warren Alpert Medical School of Brown University
Providence, Rhode Island

JOSEPH R. OWENS, M.D.
Georgetown Neurology
Georgetown, Kentucky

AMAR OZA, M.D.
Resident, Internal Medicine
Brown University
Rhode Island Hospital
Providence, Rhode Island

PAOLO G. PACE, M.A.Sc., M.D
Resident Physician
Department of Internal Medicine
Roger Williams Medical Center
Providence, Rhode Island

CRISTINA ANTONIO PACHECO, M.D.
Clinical Assistant Professor
Department of Family Medicine
Alpert Medical School
Brown University,
Providence, Rhode Island

LISA PAPPAS-TAFFER, M.D.
Assistant Professor of Dermatology
The University of Pennsylvania
Perelman Center for Advanced Medicine & The Hospital of the University of Pennsylvania
Veterans Affairs Hospital
Philadelphia, Pennsylvania

ALEEMA PATEL, M.D.
Medicine Preliminary Intern
Boston University
Boston, Massachusetts
Roger Williams Medical Center
Providence, Rhode Island
Resident Physician
Department of Radiology
The University of Texas Health Science Center at San Antonio
San Antonio, Texas

BIRJU B. PATEL, M.D., F.A.C.P.
Assistant Professor of Medicine
Department of Medicine
Division of Geriatrics and Gerontology
Emory University School of Medicine
Atlanta Veterans Affairs Medical Center
Director, Bronze Geriatric Outpatient Clinic
Co-Consultant Network Geriatrics and Extended Care
Atlanta, Georgia

HEMALI PATEL, M.D.
Assistant Clinical Professor
Department of Medicine
University of Colorado
Boulder, Colorado

PRANAV M. PATEL, M.D., F.A.C.C., F.S.C.A.I.
Interim Chief of Cardiology
Associate Professor of Medicine
University of California, Irvine
Irvine, California

ELENI PATROZOU, M.D.
Research Associate
Alpert Medical School
Brown University
Providence, Rhode Island
Attending Physician
Infectious Diseases Consultant
Hygeia General Hospital
Athens, Greece

ALISON PATTERSON, M.D.
Resident in Obstetrics and Gynecology
Department of Obstetrics and Gynecology
University of Colorado
Aurora, Colorado

STEVEN PELIGIAN, D.O.

PRANITH PERERA, M.D.
Fellow
Department of Gastroenterology
The Warren Alpert School of Medicine of Brown University
Providence, Rhode Island

KIMBERLY PEREZ, M.D.
Assistant Professor
Attending Physician
Department of Medicine
Division of Hematology and Oncology
Alpert Medical School
Brown University
Providence, Rhode Island

KATHARINE A. PHILLIPS, M.D.
Director
Body Dysmorphic Disorder Program
Rhode Island Hospital
Professor of Psychiatry and Human Behavior
Alpert Medical School
Brown University
Providence, Rhode Island

PAUL A. PIRRAGLIA, M.D., M.P.H.
Assistant Professor of Medicine
Alpert Medical School
Brown University
Rhode Island Hospital
Providence, Rhode Island

WENDY A. PLANTE, Ph.D.
Clinical Assistant Professor of Psychiatry and Human Behavior
Alpert Medical School
Brown University
Rhode Island Hospital
Hasbro Children's Research Center
Providence, Rhode Island

KEVIN PLUMLEY, M.D.
Resident, Internal Medicine
Providence, Rhode Island

SHARON S. HARTMAN POLENSEK, M.D., Ph.D.
Assistant Professor of Neurology
Center for Dizziness and Balance Disorders
Emory University
Atlanta, Georgia
Chief
Audiology and Speech Pathology
Atlanta VA Medical Center
Decatur, Georgia

SAMUEL H. POON, M.D.
Rheumatologist
Department of Internal Medicine
Harrington Memorial Hospital
Southbridge, Massachusetts

DONN POSNER, Ph.D., C.B.S.M.
Director, Clinical Behavioral Medicine
Sleep Disorders Center of Lifespan Hospitals
Clinical Associate Professor
Alpert Medical School
Brown University
Providence, Rhode Island

ARUNDATHI G. PRASAD, M.D.
Clinical Instructor
Department of Obstetrics and Gynecology/Resident Education
State University of New York at Buffalo
Women's and Children's Hospital
Buffalo, New York

AMANDA PRESSMAN, M.D.
Instructor in Medicine
Alpert Medical School
Brown University
Women's Medicine Collaborative
Center for Women's Gastrointestinal Health
Providence, Rhode Island

MICHAEL PRODROMOU, M.D.
Internal Medicine Resident
Warren Alpert Medical School
Brown University
Rhode Island Hospital
Providence, Rhode Island

KITTICHAI PROMRAT, M.D.
Assistant Professor
Division of Gastroenterology
Department of Medicine
Alpert Medical School
Brown University
Chief
Gastroenterology Section
Providence VA Medical Center
Providence, Rhode Island

SHAHNAZ PUNJANI, M.D.
Fellow, Preventive Cardiology
Providence VA Medical Center
Alpert Medical School
Brown University
Providence, Rhode Island

MATTHEW I. QUESENBERRY, M.D.
Assistant Professor
Hematology/Oncology
Alpert Medical School
Brown University
Rhode Island Hospital
Providence, Rhode Island

HEIDI RADLINSKI, M.D., M.P.H.
Clinical Instructor
Department of Family Medicine
Alpert Medical School
Brown University
Providence, Rhode Island
Assistant Director of Maternal Child Health Program Memorial Hospital of Rhode Island
Pawtucket, Rhode Island

RADHIKA A. RAMANAN, M.D., M.P.H.
Assistant Professor of Medicine
University of California, San Francisco
San Francisco, California

SHALINE D. RAO, M.D.
Clinical Fellow in Cardiovascular Medicine
Division of Cardiology
Columbia University Medical Center
New York Presbyterian Hospital
New York, New York

WASIM RASHID, M.D.
Director
Geriatric Psychiatry
Rhode Island Hospital
Providence, Rhode Island

NEHA P. RAUKAR, M.D., M.S., F.A.C.E.P.
CAQ Primary Care Sports Medicine
Assistant Professor
Director, Division of Sports Medicine
Department of Emergency Medicine
The Warren Alpert School of Medicine of Brown University
Providence, Rhode Island

JOHN L. REAGAN, M.D.
Assistant Professor
Department of Hematology/Oncology
Rhode Island Hospital/The Miriam Hospital
Alpert Medical School
Brown University
Providence, Rhode Island

RICHARD REGNANTE, M.D.
Division of Cardiovascular Medicine
Alpert Medical School
Brown University
Providence, Rhode Island

VICTOR I. REUS, M.D.
Professor
Department of Psychiatry
School of Medicine
Langley Porter Psychiatric Institute
University of California, San Francisco
San Francisco, California

HARLAN G. RICH, M.D., F.A.C.P., A.G.A.F.
Director of Endoscopy
Rhode Island Hospital
Associate Professor of Medicine
Alpert Medical School
Brown University
Providence, Rhode Island

ROCCO J. RICHARDS, M.D.
Roger Williams Medical Center
Department of Internal Medicine
Boston University School of Medicine
Boston, Massachusetts

RACHEL ROACH, M.S.N., A.P.R.N.-B.C.
Teaching Associate of Medicine
Geriatrics and Palliative Medicine
Brown University
Consultant, Inpatient Palliative Care
Geriatrics and Palliative Medicine
Rhode Island Hospital
Providence, Rhode Island

LUTHER K. ROBINSON, M.D.
Associate Professor of Pediatrics
Director
Dysmorphology and Clinical Genetics
State University of New York at Buffalo
Buffalo, New York

DOMINIC RODA, D.P.M.
Podiatry Resident
Roger Williams Medical Center
Boston University School of Medicine
Boston, Massachusetts

JAMISON ROGERS, M.D.
Forensic Psychiatry Fellow
Clinical Assistant Professor
Department of Psychiatry and Human Behavior
Alpert Medical School
Brown University
Providence, Rhode Island

ANISHKA S. ROLLE, M.D.
Rheumatologist
Southside Regional Medical Center
HealthSouth Rehabilitation Hospital
Petersburg, Virginia
John Randolph Medical Center
Richmond, Virginia
AMDC Physicians Arthritis and Osteoporosis Clinic
Colonial Heights, Virginia

JULIE L. ROTH, M.D.
Assistant Professor
Department of Neurology
Alpert Medical School
Brown University
Attending Physician
Department of Neurology
Rhode Island Hospital
Providence, Rhode Island

LAUREN ROTH, M.D.
Assistant Professor
Division of Reproductive Endocrinology and Infertility
Department of Obstetrics and Gynecology
University of Colorado
Aurora, Colorado

AMITY RUBEOR, D.O.
Assistant Professor (Clinical)
Department of Family Medicine
The Warren Alpert School of Medicine of Brown University
Providence, Rhode Island
Clinical Team Leader
Department of Family Medicine
Memorial Hospital of Rhode Island
Pawtucket, Rhode Island

PHILLIP RUISI, D.O.
Cardiology Fellow
Rhode Island Hospital
The Miriam Hospital
Providence VA Medical Center
Providence, Rhode Island

IMMAD SADIQ, M.D.
Clinical Assistant Professor of Medicine
Division of Cardiology
Alpert Medical School
Brown University,
Providence, Rhode Island

GAGAN SAHNI, M.D., F.A.C.C., F.A.C.P.
Assistant Professor of Medicine
Cardiovascular Institute
Mount Sinai Hospital
New York, New York

NUHA R. SAID, M.D.
Rheumatologist
Medical Clinic of North Texas
Denton, Texas

HEMANT K. SATPATHY, M.D.
Fellow
Division of Maternal Fetal Medicine
Department of Obstetrics and Gynecology
Emory University
Atlanta, Georgia

RUBY K. SATPATHY, M.D.
Fellow, Cardiology
Department of Internal Medicine
Creighton University
Omaha, Nebraska

JASON M. SATTERFIELD, PH.D.
Director
Behavioral Medicine
Associate Professor of Clinical Medicine
University of California, San Francisco
San Francisco, California

BRIAN SAVOIE, M.D.
Intern
Department of Internal Medicine
Roger Williams Medical Center
Providence, Rhode Island

SYEDA M. SAYEED, M.D.
Clinical Instructor
Department of Medicine
Alpert Medical School
Brown University
The Miriam Hospital
Rhode Island Hospital
Providence, Rhode Island

DAPHNE SCARMANGAS-PLUMLEY, M.D.
Resident of Internal Medicine
Roger Williams Medical Center
Boston University School of Medicine
Providence, Rhode Island

PETER J. SELL, D.O.
Assistant Professor
Department of Pediatrics
University of Massachusetts Medical School
Pediatric Hospitalist
Division of Pediatric Critical Care
University of Massachusetts Memorial Medical Center
Worcester, Massachusetts
Assistant Professor (Clinical)
Department of Family Medicine
Warren Alpert School of Medicine
Brown University
Providence, Rhode Island

CLAUDIA SERRANO-GOMEZ, M.D.
Clinical Assistant Professor, Cardiology
New York University
Faculty
Interventional Cardiology
Tisch Hospital
Bellevue Hospital
New York, New York

CATHERINE SHAFTS, D.O.
Regional Medical Director
Generations Family Health Center, Inc.
Assistant Clinical Professor
Department of Family Medicine
Warren Alpert School of Medicine
Brown University
Providence, Rhode Island

GRACE SHIH, M.D.
Assistant Professor
Department of Family Medicine
University of Washington
Seattle, Washington

ASHA SHRESTHA, M.D.
Fellow
Division of Rheumatology
Albert Einstein College of Medicine
Montefiore Medical Center
Bronx, New York

MARK SIGMAN, M.D.
Professor of Surgery
Division of Urology
Alpert Medical School
Brown University
Providence, Rhode Island

JOANNE M. SILVIA, M.D.
Clinical Assistant Professor,
Department of Family Medicine
Alpert Medical School
Brown University
Providence, Rhode Island

DIVYA SINGHAL, M.D.
Neurologist
Clinical Neurophysiology Fellow
Department of Neurology
Louisiana State University
New Orleans, Louisiana

JON SKALECKI, M.D.
Department of Internal Medicine
Roger Williams Medical Center
Providence, Rhode Island

JOHN SLADKY, M.D.
Staff Neurologist
Associate Program Director
Wilford Hall Medical Center
San Antonio, Texas

JEANETTE G. SMITH, M.D.
Assistant Professor of Medicine
Department of Gastroenterology
Alpert Medical School
Brown University
Providence, Rhode Island

U. SHIVRAJ SOHUR, M.D., PH.D.
Assistant Professor of Neurology
Harvard Medical School
Boston, Massachusetts

SCOTT M. SOUTHER, M.D.
Resident, Internal Medicine
Boston University
Boston, Massachusetts
Roger Williams Medical Center
Providence, Rhode Island

MATTHEW STANISHEWSKI, D.O.
Rheumatology Fellow
Rheumatology and Internal Medicine
Boston University School of Medicine
Boston, Massachusetts
Roger Williams Medical Center
Providence, Rhode Island

JOHANNES STEINER, M.D.
Fellow, Cardiovascular Disease
Brown University Medical School
Providence, Rhode Island

PHILIP STOCKWELL, M.D.
Cardiology
Brown University School of Medicine
Rhode Island Hospital
Providence, Rhode Island

PADMAJA SUDHAKAR, M.B.B.S.
Resident
Neurology Department
University of Kentucky College of Medicine
Lexington, Kentucky

MARY BETH SUTTER, M.D.
Maternal, Child, and Reproductive Health Fellow
Department of Family Medicine
University of New Mexico
Albuquerque, New Mexico

ARUN SWAMINATHAN, M.B.B.S.
Resident
Neurology Department
University of Kentucky College of Medicine
University of Kentucky Hospital
Lexington, Kentucky

ANGELA M. TABER (PLETTE), M.D.
Assistant Professor of Medicine
Department of Hematology and Oncology
Alpert Medical School
Brown University
Providence, Rhode Island

DOMINICK TAMMARO, M.D.
Associate Professor of Medicine
Warren Alpert School of Medicine of Brown University
Internal Medicine Residency Director
Rhode Island Hospital
Providence, Rhode Island

SARAH TAPYRIK, M.D.
Fellow, Pulmonary Diseases
NYU Department of Pulmonary and Critical Care
New York, New York

SHAMAIL TARIQ, M.D.
Cardiology Fellow
Department of Medicine
University of California, Irvine,
Orange, California

TAHIR TELLIOGLU, M.D.
Assistant Professor of Psychiatry and Human Behavior
Alpert Medical School
Brown University
Director
Substance Abuse Division
Department of Psychiatry
Rhode Island Hospital
Providence, Rhode Island

IRIS L. TONG, M.D.
Assistant Professor
Department of Medicine
Alpert Medical School
Brown University
Director, Women's Primary Care
Women's Medicine Collaborative
Providence, Rhode Island

MARGARET TRYFOROS, M.D.
Assistant Professor of Family Medicine (Clinical)
Alpert Medical School
Brown University,
Providence, Rhode Island

JOSEPH R. TUCCI, M.D., F.A.C.P., F.A.C.E.
Professor of Medicine
Boston University School of Medicine
Boston, Massachusetts
Adjunct Professor of Medicine
Alpert Medical School
Brown University
Director
Division of Endocrinology and Metabolism
Roger Williams Medical Center
Providence, Rhode Island

SEAN H. UITERWYK, M.D.
Clinical Assistant Professor of Community and Family Medicine
Geisel School of Medicine at Dartmouth
Hanover, New Hampshire
White River Family Practice
White River Junction, Vermont

NICOLE J. ULLRICH, M.D., PH.D.
Associate Professor of Neurology
Harvard Medical School
Director of Neurologic Neuro-oncology
Boston Children's Hospital
Boston, Massachusetts

EMILY VAN KIRK, M.D.
PGY-2 Internal Medicine Resident
Roger Williams Medical Center
Providence, Rhode Island

MARISA E. VAN POZNAK, M.D.
Attending Physician
Department of Internal Medicine
Women and Infants Hospital
Warren Alpert School of Medicine
Brown University
Providence, Rhode Island

POOJA VERMA, M.D.
Roger Williams Medical Center
Providence, Rhode Island

JORGE A. VILLAFUERTE, M.D.
Clinical Instructor in Orthopedic Surgery
Harvard Medical School
Assistant Professor in Orthopedic Surgery
Boston University Medical School
Associate Chief of Orthopedic Surgery
VA Boston HealthCare System
Boston, Massachusetts

MARC PAUL WAASE, M.D., PH.D.
Cardiology Fellow
Columbia University
New York Presbyterian Hospital
New York, New York

CHARLES WANG, M.D.
Gastroenterology Fellow
Rhode Island Hospital
Warren Alpert School of Medicine
Brown University
Providence, Rhode Island

TARA M. WAYT, D.O.
Emergency Medicine Residency Program
University of Connecticut School of Medicine
Farmington, Connecticut
Hartford Hospital
Hartford, Connecticut

ADAM J. WEINBERG, M.D.
Resident
Internal Medicine
Boston University Medical Center
Boston, Massachusetts

DENNIS M. WEPPNER, M.D., F.A.C.O.G.
Associate Professor of Clinical Gynecology/Obstetrics
State University of New York at Buffalo
Clinical Chief
Department of Gynecology/Obstetrics
Millard Fillmore Hospital
Buffalo, New York

JORDAN WHITE, M.D., M.P.H.
Assistant Professor (Clinical)
Department of Family Medicine
Alpert Medical School
Brown University
Providence, Rhode Island
Staff Physician
Memorial Hospital of Rhode Island
Pawtucket, Rhode Island

LAUREL M. WHITE, M.D.
Clinical Assistant Professor
Department of Obstetrics and Gynecology Division of Maternal Fetal Medicine
State University of New York at Buffalo
Buffalo, New York

HILARY B. WHITLACH, M.D.
Chief of Endocrinology
Providence VA Medical Center
Assistant Professor of Medicine
Alpert Medical School
Brown University
Providence, Rhode Island

MATTHEW P. WICKLUND, M.D., F.A.A.N.
Professor
Department of Neurology
Penn State College of Medicine
Vice-Chair for Education
Department of Neurology
Milton S. Hershey Medical Center
Hershey, Pennsylvania

JEFFREY P. WINCZE, PH.D.
Department of Pyschiatry
Rhode Island Hospital
Clinical Assistant Professor
Department of Psychiatry and Human Behavior
Warren Alpert Medical School of Brown University
Providence, Rhode Island

MARLENE FISHMAN WOLPERT, M.P.H., C.I.C.
Director
Infection Prevention and Control
St. Joseph Health Services of Rhode Island
North Providence, Rhode Island

TZU-CHING (TEDDY) WU, M.D., M.P.H.
Assistant Professor of Neurology
University of Texas Medical School at Houston
Director of Telemedicine
Mischer Neuroscience Institute
Houston, Texas

WEN-CHIH WU, M.D., M.P.H.
Staff Cardiologist
Providence VA Medical Center
Associate Professor of Medicine
Alpert Medical School
Brown University
Providence, Rhode Island

WEN Y. (HELENA) WU-CHEN, M.D.
Department of Neurology
Temple University Hospital
Philadelphia, Pennsylvania

BETH J. WUTZ, M.D.
Clinical Assistant Professor of Medicine
Division of Internal Medicine/Pediatrics
Kajeida Health–Buffalo General Hospital
State University of New York at Buffalo
Buffalo, New York

SARAH L. XAVIER, D.O.
Director of Psychiatric Services
Rhode Island Training School
Director
Child & Adolescent Forensic Psychiatry
Rhode Island Hospital
Clinical Assistant Professor of Psychiatry and Human Behavior
Alpert Medical School
Brown University
Providence, Rhode Island

AUGUSTIN G. YIP, M.D., PH.D.
Clinical Assistant Professor
Butler Hospital
Department of Psychiatry and Human Behavior
Brown University
Providence, Rhode Island

JOHN Q. YOUNG, M.D., M.P.P.
Associate Clinical Professor
University of California, San Francisco
School of Medicine
San Francisco, California

CANDICE YUVIENCO, M.D.
Assistant Clinical Professor of Medicine
Department of Internal Medicine
Division of Rheumatology
University of California, San Francisco-Fresno
Fresno, California

FARIHA ZAHEER, M.D.
Assistant Professor of Neurology
Baylor College of Medicine
Michael. E. DeBakey VA Medical Center
Houston, Texas

TALIA ZENLEA, M.D.
Director of the Center for Inflammatory Diseases
Women's Medicine Collaborative
Assistant Professor
Warren Alpert School of Medicine
Brown University
Providence, Rhode Island

MARK ZIMMERMAN, M.D.
Director
Outpatient Psychiatry, Partial Hospital Program
Rhode Island Hospital/The Miriam Hospital
Professor of Psychiatry and Human Behavior
Alpert Medical School
Brown University
Providence, Rhode Island

BERNARD ZIMMERMANN, M.D.
Director
Division of Rheumatology
Roger Williams Medical Center
Associate Professor of Medicine
Boston University School of Medicine
Providence, Rhode Island

SCOTT J. ZUCCALA, D.O., F.A.C.O.G.
Staff Physician
Mercy Hospital of Buffalo
Buffalo, New York

RYAN W. ZUZEK, M.D.
Fellow, Clinical Cardiology
Division of Cardiology
Alpert Medical School
Brown University
Providence, Rhode Island

To my sons, Dr. Vito F. Ferri and Dr. Christopher A. Ferri, and my daughter-in-law, Dr. Heather A. Ferri, for their help and constant support, and to my wife, Christina, for her patience during manuscript preparation. A special thanks to all the readers who have personally commented on the merits of this book and through their suggestions have helped make this product a best-seller in the medical field.

Fred F. Ferri, M.D.
Clinical Professor
Alpert Medical School
Brown University
Providence, Rhode Island

This book is intended to be a clear and concise reference for physicians and allied health professionals. Its user-friendly format was designed to provide a fast and efficient way to identify important clinical information and to offer practical guidance in patient management. The book is divided into five sections and an appendix, each with emphasis on clinical information.

The tremendous success of the previous editions and the enthusiastic comments from numerous colleagues have brought about several positive changes. Each section has been significantly expanded from prior editions, bringing the total number of medical topics covered in this book to more than 1000. Nearly 500 new illustrations and tables have been added to the edition to enhance recollection of clinically important facts. The expedited claims submission and reimbursement, ICD-10CM codes have been added to all the topics, along with existing ICD-9CM codes. Please note that the implementation of the ICD-10CM codes has been delayed until at least 2015; therefore, for billing purposes please use the ICD-9CM codes until the ICD-10CM codes are officially implemented.

Section I describes in detail more than 800 medical disorders. Twenty-one new topics have been added to the 2015 edition. Each medical topic in this section is arranged alphabetically, and the material in each topic is presented in outline format for ease of retrieval. Topics with an accompanying algorithm in Section III are identified with an algorithm symbol (ALG). Similarly, if topics also have a Patient Teaching Guide (PTG) available online, this has been noted. Throughout the text, key quick-access information is consistently highlighted, clinical photographs are used to further illustrate selected medical conditions, and relevant ICD-10CM codes are listed. Most references focus on current peer-reviewed journal articles rather than outdated textbooks and old review articles. Evidence-based medicine data have been added to relevant topics.

Topics in this section use the following structured approach:

1. Basic Information (Definition, Synonyms, ICD-9CM and ICD-10CM Codes, Epidemiology & Demographics, Physical Findings & Clinical Presentation, Etiology)
2. Diagnosis (Differential Diagnosis, Workup, Laboratory Tests, Imaging Studies)
3. Treatment (Nonpharmacologic Therapy, Acute General Rx, Chronic Rx, Disposition, Referral)
4. Pearls & Considerations (Comments, Suggested Readings)
5. Evidence-Based Data and References

Section II includes the differential diagnosis, etiology, and classification of signs and symptoms. This section has been significantly expanded for the 2015 edition with the addition of 38 new topics. It is a practical section that allows the user investigating a physical complaint or abnormal laboratory value to follow a "workup" leading to a diagnosis. The physician can then easily look up the presumptive diagnosis in Section I for the information specific to that illness.

Section III includes clinical algorithms to guide and expedite the patient's workup and therapy. Twenty new algorithms have been added for the 2015 edition. Many physicians describe this section as particularly valuable in today's managed-care environment.

Section IV includes normal laboratory values and interpretation of results of commonly ordered laboratory tests. By providing interpretation of abnormal results, this section facilitates the diagnosis of medical disorders and further adds to the comprehensive, "one-stop" nature of our text.

Section V focuses on preventive medicine. Information in this section includes recommendations for the periodic health examination, screening for major diseases and disorders, patient counseling, and immunization and chemoprophylaxis recommendations.

The **Appendix** has been divided into six major sections. Section I contains extensive information on complementary and alternative medicine (CAM). With the material in this appendix, we hope to lessen the current scarcity of exposure of allopathic and osteopathic physicians to the diversity of CAM therapies. Section II focuses on nutrition with emphasis on dietary supplements, vitamins, and minerals. Section III deals with diagnosis and treatment of acute poisoning. Section IV is a guide on impairment and disability evaluation. Section V, available online, contains an extensive section on primary care procedures. Section VI contains several patient teaching guides not linked to Section I topics.

As clinicians, we all realize the importance of patient education and the need for clear communication with our patients. Toward that end, practical patient instruction sheets, organized alphabetically and covering the majority of the topics in this book, are available online and can be easily customized and printed from any computer. They represent a valuable addition to patient care and are useful for improving physician-patient communication, patient satisfaction, and quality of care.

I believe that we have produced a state-of-the-art information system with significant differences from existing texts. It contains five sections and patient education guides that could be sold separately based on their content, yet are available under a single cover, offering the reader a tremendous value. I hope that the *Clinical Advisor*'s user-friendly approach, numerous unique features, and yearly updates will make this book a valuable medical reference, not only to primary care physicians but also to physicians in other specialties, medical students, and allied health professionals.

Fred F. Ferri, M.D., F.A.C.P.

Note: Comments from readers are always appreciated and can be forwarded directly to Dr. Ferri at fred_ferri@brown.edu.

EVALUATION OF EVIDENCE

Ferri's Clinical Advisor evaluates all evidence based on a rating system published by the American Academy of Family Physicians. In order to indicate the strength of the supporting evidence, each summary statement is accorded one of three levels:

LEVEL A

- Systematic reviews of randomized controlled trials, including meta-analyses
- Good-quality randomized controlled trials

LEVEL B

- Good-quality nonrandomized clinical trials
- Systematic reviews not in Level A
- Lower-quality randomized controlled trials not in Level A
- Other types of study: case-control studies, clinical cohort studies, cross-sectional studies, retrospective studies, and uncontrolled studies

LEVEL C

- Evidence-based consensus statements and expert guidelines

SOURCES OF EVIDENCE

Evidence is summarized principally from three critically evaluated, very highly regarded sources:

- **Cochrane Systematic Reviews** are respected throughout the world as one of the most rigorous searches of medical journals for randomized controlled trials. They provide highly structured systematic reviews, with evidence included or excluded on the basis of explicit quality-related criteria, and they often use meta-analyses to increase the power of the findings of numerous studies.
- ***Clinical Evidence*** is produced by the BMJ Publishing Group. It provides synopses of the best currently available evidence on the treatment and prevention of many clinical conditions, based on searches and appraisals of the available literature.
- **The National Guideline Clearinghouse™** is a comprehensive database of evidence-based clinical practice guidelines and related documents produced by the Agency for Healthcare Research and Quality in partnership with the American Medical Association and the American Association of Health Plans.

In addition, where evidence exists that has not yet been critically reviewed in one of the three sites above, the evidence is summarized briefly, categorized, and fully referenced. Guidelines are also sourced from government and professional bodies.

Ferri's Clinical Advisor 2015 — How to Use This Book

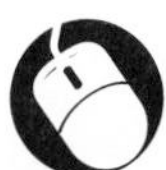 Mouse icon – Indicates content with additional references, figures, or tables available at www.expertconsult.com

PTG — PTG icon – indicates an accompanying Patient Teaching Guide available at www.expertconsult.com There are also many additional PTGs online not linked to a topic in Section I.

ALG — ALG icon – indicates a topic with an accompanying Algorithm in Section III or additional Algorithms available at www.expertconsult.com

EBM — EBM icon – indicates evidence-based medicine data added to relevant topics available at www.expertconsult.com

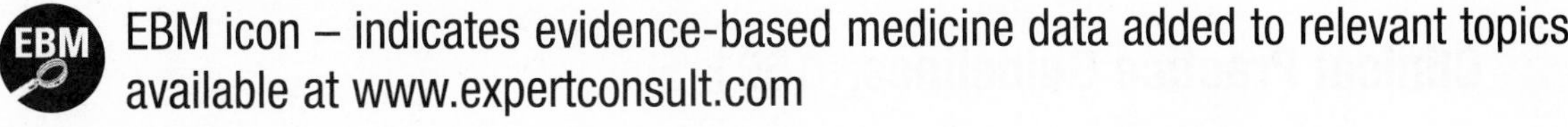

SECTION I **Diseases and Disorders**

PTG indicates that a Patient Teaching Guide is available at www.expertconsult.com.

Additional Topics Available at www.expertconsult.com

SECTION I Figures, Tables, and Boxes Available at www.expertconsult.com

SECTION II **Differential Diagnosis**

SECTION III **Clinical Algorithms**

Additional Algorithms Available at www.expertconsult.com

SECTION IV Laboratory Tests and Interpretation of Results

SECTION V Clinical Practice Guidelines

APPENDIX I Complementary and Alternative Medicine

APPENDIX II Nutrition

APPENDIX III Acute Poisoning

APPENDIX V Primary Care Procedures, available at www.expertconsult.com

APPENDIX VI Patient Teaching Guides, available at www.expertconsult.com

Additional *PTGs* Available at www.expertconsult.com Not Linked to Topics in Section I

2015

Ferri's CLINICAL ADVISOR

5 Books in 1

Diseases and Disorders*

*Please note that the implementation of the ICD-10CM codes has been delayed until at least 2015; therefore, for billing purposes please use the ICD-9CM codes until the ICD-10CM codes are officially implemented.

BASIC INFORMATION

DEFINITION

An abdominal aortic aneurysm (AAA) is a focal dilation of the abdominal aortic artery to at least 1.5 times the diameter measured at the level of the renal arteries, or exceeding the normal diameter of the abdominal aorta by 50%. The normal diameter at the renal arteries is 2 cm (range 1.4-3.0 cm), and a diameter 3 cm or larger is generally considered aneurysmal.

SYNONYMS

AAA

ICD-9CM CODES
441.4 Aneurysm, abdominal (aorta)
441.3 Ruptured abdominal aortic aneurysm
ICD-10CM CODES
I71.4 Abdominal aortic aneurysm, without rupture
I71.3 Abdominal aortic aneurysm, ruptured

EPIDEMIOLOGY & DEMOGRAPHICS

- Approximately 15,000 deaths/year in the United States are attributed to AAA.
- AAA is predominantly a disease of older adults, affecting men more than women (4:1).
- The prevalence rate ranges from 4% to 9% in men older than age 60.
- Clinically important AAAs ≥4 cm are present in 1% of men ages 55 to 64, and the prevalence rate increases by 2% to 4% per decade thereafter.
- The peak incidence is among men approximately 70 years old.
- The frequency is much higher in smokers than in nonsmokers (8:1), and the risk decreases slowly after smoking cessation.
- AAA is 2 to 4 times more common in first-degree male relatives of known AAA patients.
- Risk factors for AAA are similar to other atherosclerotic cardiovascular diseases; they include age, smoking, male sex, family history, hypertension, hyperlipidemia, and peripheral vascular disease. Aneurysm of other large vessels is also a risk factor for AAA.
- Rupture of the AAA occurs in 1% to 3% of men age 65 or older.
  - Rupture is the 10th leading cause of death in men older than age 55.
  - Mortality from rupture is 70% to 95%.
  - Risk factors for rupture include cardiac or renal transplants, severe obstructive lung disease, uncontrolled blood pressure, female sex, and ongoing tobacco use.
- The U.S. Preventive Services Task Force recommends one-time screening for AAA by ultrasonography in men ages 65 to 75 who have a history of smoking and in those 60 years and older with a history of AAA in a parent or sibling. These populations have been shown to have a higher prevalence of AAA, and selectively screening this group has been shown to decrease AAA-specific mortality.
- A recent decline in incidence and prevalence of AAA and related mortality has been attributed to reductions in tobacco use.

PHYSICAL FINDINGS & CLINICAL PRESENTATION

- Most aneurysms are asymptomatic and incidentally discovered on imaging studies; however, symptomatic aneurysms are at an increased risk for rupture.
- Physical examination has a sensitivity of 76% for detecting AAAs >5 cm and only 29% for AAAs 3.0-3.9 cm.
- Symptomatic patients may present with abdominal, back, flank, or groin pain.
- A pulsatile epigastric mass that may or may not be tender may be present.
- Abdominal pain radiating to the back, flank, and groin.
- Abdominal bruits can be present in case of renal or visceral arterial stenosis.
- Common iliac arteries can be aneurysmal and palpable in the lower abdominal quadrants. In addition, prominent femoral and popliteal pulses warrant an abdominal ultrasound and lower extremity ultrasound.
- Early satiety, nausea, and vomiting may be caused by compression of adjacent bowel.
- Venous thrombosis or insufficiency may occur from iliocaval venous compression.
- Thromboembolization can cause lower extremity pain and discoloration.
- Ureteral obstruction and hydronephrosis can cause flank and groin pain and lead to obstructive renal failure.
- Rupture classically presents as a triad of abdominal or back pain, hypotension, and a pulsatile abdominal mass in 50% of patients.
- Acute blood loss may lead to myocardial infarction; arteriovenous fistulas may present as heart failure; aortoenteric fistulas may present as hematemesis or melena associated with abdominal and back pain.

ETIOLOGY

- Exact etiology is unknown and is likely multifactorial. AAA formation and rupture may result from elastin and collagen degradation by proteases such as plasmin, matrix metalloproteinases (MMPs), and cathepsin S and K.
- Degenerative:
  - The most common association is atherosclerosis. It is uncertain if atherosclerosis causes or results from AAAs.
  - Tobacco use: >90% of people who develop an AAA have smoked at some point in their life.
- Inherited: Familial clusters are common. High familial prevalence rate is notable in male individuals. The nature of the genetic disorder is unclear but may be linked to alpha-1-antitrypsin deficiency or X-linked mutation. Connective tissue disorders, such as Marfan's syndrome and Ehlers-Danlos syndrome, have also been strongly associated with AAA.
- Inflammatory, arteritis.
- Infection, mycotic: syphilis, *Salmonella.*

NATURAL HISTORY

- The risk of aneurysmal rupture is largely influenced by aneurysm size, rate of expansion, and sex. Other factors associated with increased risk for rupture include continued smoking, uncontrolled hypertension, and increased wall stress.
- AAAs tend to develop in the infrarenal aorta.
- Higher tension in the abdominal aorta (together with histopathologic changes such as accumulation of foam cells, cholesterol crystals, and matrix metalloproteinases) renders the abdominal aortic wall more susceptible to dilation and subsequent rupture.
- The 5-year rupture rate of asymptomatic AAAs is 25% to 40% for aneurysms >5.0 cm in diameter, 1% to 7% for AAAs 4.0 to 5.0 cm, and nearly 0% for AAAs <4.0 cm. The rate of rupture of aneurysms that were 4.0-5.5 cm in diameter is four times greater in women compared with men.
- Mortality rate after rupture can be as high as 90% because most patients do not reach the hospital in time for surgical repair. Of those who reach the hospital, the mortality rate is still 50%, compared with the 1% to 4% mortality rate for elective repair of a nonruptured AAA.

Dx DIAGNOSIS

DIFFERENTIAL DIAGNOSIS

Almost 75% of patients with AAA are asymptomatic, and the condition is discovered on routine examination or serendipitously when ordering studies for other symptoms. Diagnosis of AAA should be considered in the differential of the following symptoms: abdominal pain, back pain, and/or pulsatile abdominal mass.

LABORATORY TESTS

Not routinely indicated. For suspected infected or inflammatory aneurysms, WBC, ESR/CRP, and blood cultures can be considered. An elevated D-dimer may indicate a thrombus within the aneurysm. Fig 1-1 describes an algorithm for the diagnosis and treatment of abdominal aortic aneurysms.

IMAGING STUDIES

- Plain radiographs may show the outline of an aneurysm in calcified aortas. This is an insensitive test for diagnosing AAA.
- Abdominal ultrasound (Fig. 1-2) is nearly 100% accurate in identifying an aneurysm and estimating the size to within 0.3–0.4 cm. It is not accurate in estimating the extension to the renal arteries or the iliac arteries.
- Computed tomography (CT) (Fig 1-3) scan is recommended for preoperative aneurysm imaging and estimates the size of the AAA to within 0.3 mm. There are no false-negative results, and the scan can localize the extent to renal vessels with more precision than ultrasound. CT can also detect the integrity of the wall and exclude rupture.

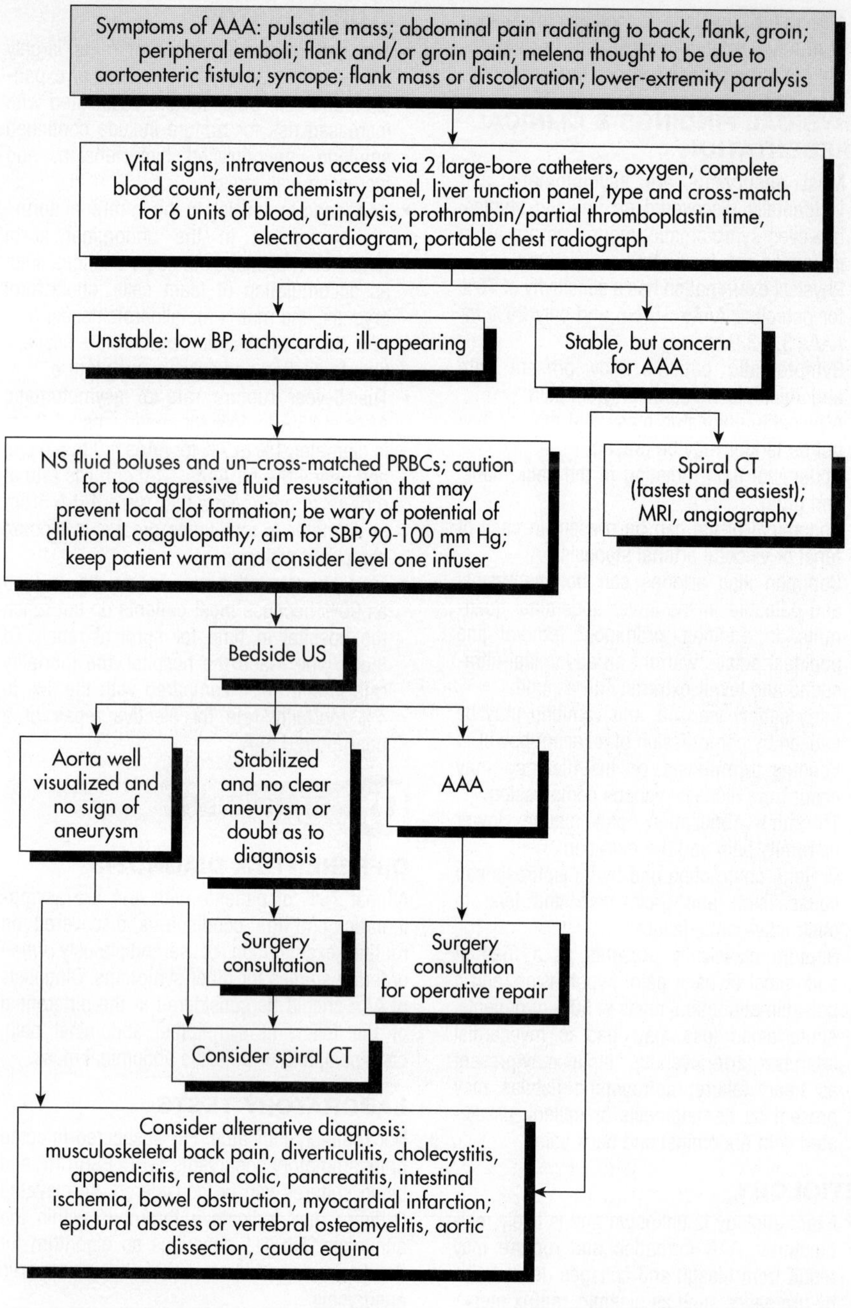

Abdominal Aortic Aneurysm 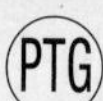 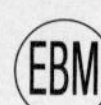 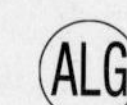

Symptoms of AAA: pulsatile mass; abdominal pain radiating to back, flank, groin; peripheral emboli; flank and/or groin pain; melena thought to be due to aortoenteric fistula; syncope; flank mass or discoloration; lower-extremity paralysis

→ Vital signs, intravenous access via 2 large-bore catheters, oxygen, complete blood count, serum chemistry panel, liver function panel, type and cross-match for 6 units of blood, urinalysis, prothrombin/partial thromboplastin time, electrocardiogram, portable chest radiograph

→ Unstable: low BP, tachycardia, ill-appearing

→ NS fluid boluses and un–cross-matched PRBCs; caution for too aggressive fluid resuscitation that may prevent local clot formation; be wary of potential of dilutional coagulopathy; aim for SBP 90-100 mm Hg; keep patient warm and consider level one infuser

→ Bedside US

- Aorta well visualized and no sign of aneurysm → Consider spiral CT; Consider alternative diagnosis
- Stabilized and no clear aneurysm or doubt as to diagnosis → Surgery consultation → Consider spiral CT
- AAA → Surgery consultation for operative repair

→ Stable, but concern for AAA

→ Spiral CT (fastest and easiest); MRI, angiography → Consider alternative diagnosis

Consider alternative diagnosis: musculoskeletal back pain, diverticulitis, cholecystitis, appendicitis, renal colic, pancreatitis, intestinal ischemia, bowel obstruction, myocardial infarction; epidural abscess or vertebral osteomyelitis, aortic dissection, cauda equina

FIGURE 1-1 Algorithm for the diagnosis and treatment of abdominal aortic aneurysms (AAAs). *BP*, Blood pressure; *CT*, computed tomography; *MRI*, magnetic resonance imaging; *NS*, normal saline; *PRBCs*, packed red blood cells; *SBP*, systolic blood pressure; *US*, ultrasonography. (From Adams JG et al: *Emergency medicine, clinical essentials*, ed 2, Philadelphia, 2013, Elsevier.)

- Magnetic resonance angiography (MRA) may also be used and is at least as accurate as CT.
- Diagnostic aortography has essentially been replaced by other noninvasive imaging modalities such as CT or MR angiography. Intraoperative angiography is still used for determining treatment options and post-procedure efficacy.

Rx TREATMENT

NONPHARMACOLOGIC THERAPY

- Despite lack of data substantiating reduction in expansion rate through treatment of cardiac risk factors, nonpharmacologic treatment continues to focus on risk factor modification (most importantly smoking cessation, diet, and exercise).
- Serial studies have shown that expansion rates are faster in current smokers than in former smokers. Patients with known AAA or a family history of aneurysms should be advised to stop smoking and be offered smoking cessation interventions.
- Definitive treatment depends on the size of the aneurysm (see "Chronic Rx").

ACUTE GENERAL Rx

- Acute symptomatic or ruptured AAA can be treated with open surgical or endovascular aneurysm repair (EVAR). The choice is determined by anatomic considerations, operative risks, and availability of regular patient follow-up for EVAR.
- Emergent open repair has been the traditional method of treatment. However, recent studies report fewer perioperative deaths and shorter hospital stay with EVAR. More centers are increasingly using endovascular repair for patients who fit certain anatomic and physiologic criteria.
- The major limitations for EVAR include anatomical issues such as tortuosity or small caliber iliac arteries and inability to follow up of patients to exclude late failure of stents grafts and development of endoleaks.

CHRONIC Rx

- Blood pressure and fasting lipids should be monitored and controlled as recommended for patients with atherosclerotic disease. Statins are associated with decreased mortality after successful AAA repair, and are recommended for those with known AAA to reduce the progression of atherosclerosis.
- The most commonly used predictor of rupture is the maximum diameter of the AAA.
- Monitoring by ultrasound or CT scan should be performed every 6 to 12 months for patients with AAAs measuring 4.0 to 5.4 cm in diameter and by ultrasound every 2 years for those with AAAs measuring <4 cm.

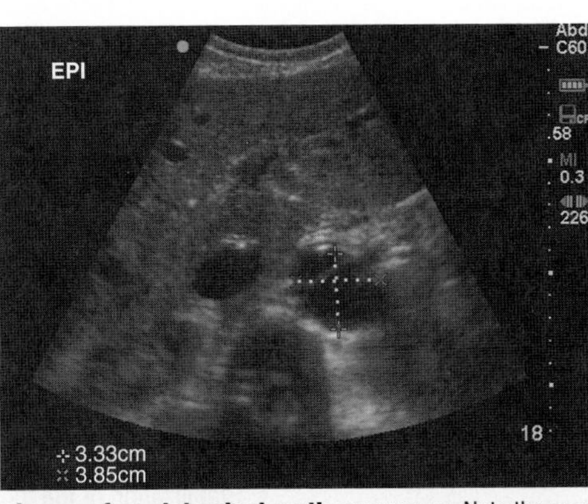

FIGURE 1-2 Transverse image of an abdominal aortic aneurysm. Note the measurements of 3.35 × 3.85 cm. The inferior vena cava is seen to the patient's right of the aorta, and the vertebral body is seen below the two vessels. Note also that there appears to be an echogenic flap within the aorta, possibly representing an aortic dissection. (From Adams JG et al: *Emergency medicine, clinical essentials*, ed 2, Philadelphia, 2013, Elsevier.)

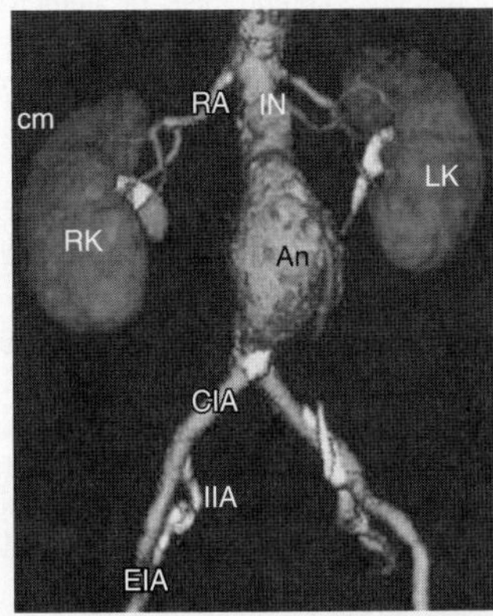

FIGURE 1-3 Three-dimensional CT image illustrates the presence of an infrarenal abdominal aortic aneurysm. *An,* Aneurysm; *CIA,* common iliac artery; *EIA,* external iliac artery; *IIA,* internal iliac artery; *IN,* infrarenal neck; *LK,* left kidney; *RA,* renal artery; *RK,* right kidney. (From Townsend CM et al [eds]: *Sabiston textbook of surgery,* ed 17, Philadelphia, 2004, Saunders.)

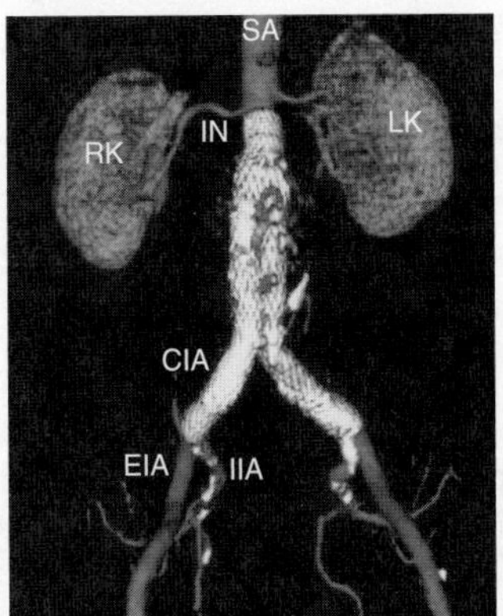

FIGURE 1-4 Endovascular abdominal aortic aneurysm repair involves aneurysm exclusion with an endoluminal aortic stent-graft introduced remotely, usually through the femoral artery. An endovascular graft extends from the infrarenal aorta to both common iliac arteries, preserving the flow to the internal iliac arteries. *CIA,* Common iliac artery; *IIA,* internal iliac artery; *IN,* infrarenal aortic neck; *LK,* left kidney; *RK,* right kidney; *SA,* suprarenal aorta. (From Townsend CM et al [eds]: *Sabiston textbook of surgery,* ed 17, Philadelphia, 2004, Saunders.)

- Long-term beta-blocker therapy has slowed the rate of aortic dilation and decreased the incidence of aortic complications in patients with Marfan's syndrome. Several studies have also suggested that beta-blocker therapy may reduce the rate of expansion and risk of rupture; however, conclusive evidence is lacking. In a Cochrane Database Systematic Review, propranolol was poorly tolerated in all beta-blocker trials and had only minimal, nonsignificant protective benefit.
- Antibiotics such as doxycycline and roxithromycin have shown to limit the expansion of small AAAs.
- Surgical repair to eliminate the risk for rupture should be performed for patients with infrarenal or juxtarenal AAA of approximately 5.5 cm or larger in diameter. All patients who are symptomatic should undergo repair, regardless of size.
- There is no clear advantage to early repair (open or endovascular) for small AAAs (less than 5.5 cm).
- Percutaneous, endovascular, stent-anchored grafts placed with the patient under local anesthesia have provided an alternative approach (Fig. 1-4) for patients with favorable anatomy. In patients who have undergone endovascular repair, long-term surveillance is required to assess for an endoleak, stent migration, change in aneurysm size, and need for re-intervention.
- Randomized trials have shown that endovascular repair of AAA is associated with a significantly lower operative mortality than open surgical repair but it has increased rates of graft-related complications and reintervention, and is more costly. EVAR leads to increased long-term survival among younger patients but not among older patients. There are no differences between endovascular repair and open surgical repair in total mortality or aneurysm-related mortality in the long term.
- Based on current data, less than 1% of endovascular repairs require open conversion and approximately half of all early endoleaks resolve spontaneously within a period of 30 days.
- Endovascular repair in patients who are poor candidates for open repair, as determined by comorbidities, is of uncertain effectiveness.
- In high-risk patients undergoing AAA repair, specifically those with coronary artery disease or those with more than one clinical risk factor based on the American Heart Association (AHA) guidelines, preoperative administration of beta-blockers titrated to a goal heart rate of 60 have been shown to decrease incidence of death from cardiac causes or nonfatal myocardial infarctions.
- Patients with chronic obstructive pulmonary disease (COPD) are at higher risk for major clinical complications, particularly if the COPD is suboptimally managed or if it is present in conjunction with cardiac or renal disease. Smoking cessation for 2 months before surgery has also been shown to decrease pulmonary morbidity.
- Renal dysfunction is a strong predictor of mortality, showing up to as high as 41% mortality in those with impaired renal function compared with 6% in those without renal dysfunction.

REFERRAL

- Vascular surgical referral should be made in asymptomatic patients with AAAs that are approximately 4.5 cm.
- In patients with an expansion rate of 0.6-0.8 cm/year, it is reasonable to offer repair, although small studies have shown that using expansion as a criterion for surgical referral is of unclear benefit.
- It is important to optimize any comorbid conditions before surgical referral.

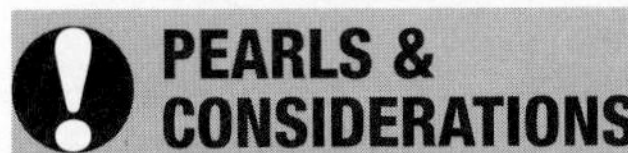

PEARLS & CONSIDERATIONS

- Repairing asymptomatic AAAs smaller than 5.5 cm has not been shown to improve survival because the risk of rupture is lower than the risk of surgery.

COMMENTS

- Most AAAs are infrarenal.
- Surgical risk is increased in patients with coexisting coronary artery disease, pulmonary disease, or chronic renal failure. Evaluation for ischemia and aggressive perioperative hemodynamic monitoring help identify high-risk patients and decrease postoperative complications.
- It is estimated that AAA at <5 cm expand at a rate of 0.4 cm/year.

SUGGESTED READINGS

available at www.expertconsult.com

RELATED CONTENT

Abdominal Aortic Aneurysm (AAA) (Patient Information)

AUTHORS: **JIN KYUNG KIM, M.D., Ph.D., F.A.C.C.,** and **PRANAV M. PATEL, M.D., F.A.C.C., F.S.C.A.I.**

A

Diseases and Disorders

BASIC INFORMATION

DEFINITION

Abruptio placentae is the separation of placenta from the uterine wall before delivery of the fetus. There are three classes of abruption based on maternal and fetal status, including an assessment of uterine contractions, quantity of bleeding, fetal heart rate monitoring, and abnormal coagulation studies (fibrinogen, prothrombin time, partial thromboplastin time).

- Grade I: mild vaginal bleeding, uterine irritability, stable vital signs, reassuring fetal heart rate, normal coagulation profile (fibrinogen 450 mg%)
- Grade II: moderate vaginal bleeding, hypertonic uterine contractions, orthostatic blood pressure measurements, unfavorable fetal status, fibrinogen 150 to 250 mg%
- Grade III: severe bleeding (may be concealed), hypertonic uterine contractions, overt signs of hypovolemic shock, fetal death, thrombocytopenia, fibrinogen <150 mg%

SYNONYMS

Premature separation of placenta

ICD-9CM CODES

641.2	Premature separation of placenta
641.21	Premature separation of placenta, delivered, with or without mention of antepartum condition
641.23	Premature separation of placenta, antepartum condition or complication

ICD-10CM CODES

O45.8X9	Other premature separation of placenta, unspecified trimester
O45.8X1	Other premature separation of placenta, first trimester
O45.8X2	Other premature separation of placenta, second trimester
O45.8X3	Other premature separation of placenta, third trimester
O45.91	Premature separation of placenta, unspecified, first trimester
O45.92	Premature separation of placenta, unspecified, second trimester
O45.93	Premature separation of placenta, unspecified, third trimester

EPIDEMIOLOGY & DEMOGRAPHICS

INCIDENCE (IN U.S.): One in 86 to 206 births; incidence by grade: I = 45%, II = 30%, III = 25%; 80% occur before the onset of labor

RISK FACTORS: Hypertension (greatest association), trauma, polyhydramnios, multifetal gestation, smoking, use of cocaine, chorioamnionitis, preterm premature rupture of membranes

RECURRENCE RATE: 5% to 17%, some studies showing a 5- to 10-fold increase in risk; with two prior episodes, 25%

PHYSICAL FINDINGS & CLINICAL PRESENTATION

- Triad of uterine bleeding (concealed or per vagina), hypertonic uterine contractions or signs of preterm labor, and evidence of fetal compromise exists.
- More than 80% of cases have external bleeding; 20% of cases have no bleeding but have indirect evidence of abruption, such as failed tocolysis for preterm labor.
- Tetanic uterine contractions are found in only 17% of cases unless grade II or III abruption.

ETIOLOGY

- Primary etiology: unknown
- Hypertension: found in 40% to 50% of grade III abruptions
- Rapid decompression of uterine cavity, as can occur in polyhydramnios or multifetal gestation
- Blunt external trauma (motor vehicle accident, spousal abuse)

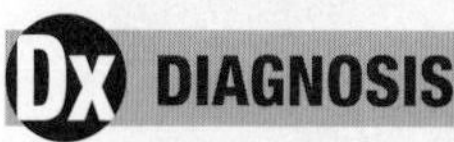

DIAGNOSIS

DIFFERENTIAL DIAGNOSIS

- Placenta previa
- Cervical or vaginal trauma
- Labor
- Cervical cancer
- Rupture of membranes
- The differential diagnosis of vaginal bleeding in pregnancy is described in Section III

WORKUP

- Initial assessment should evaluate for the source of bleeding, ruling out placenta previa that may contraindicate any type of vaginal examination (e.g., pelvic speculum examination).
- Continuous fetal heart monitoring is indicated for all viable gestations (60% incidence of fetal distress in labor); may show early signs of maternal hypovolemia (late decelerations or fetal tachycardia) before overt maternal vital sign changes.
- Actual amount of blood loss is often greater than initially perceived because of the possibility of concealed retroplacental bleeding and apparent "normal" vital signs. The relative hypervolemia of pregnancy initially protects the patient until late in the course of bleeding, when abrupt and sudden cardiovascular collapse can occur.

LABORATORY TESTS

- Baseline hemoglobin helps quantify blood loss and establish baseline values for serial comparisons during expectant management.
- Coagulation profile: platelets, fibrinogen, prothrombin, and partial thromboplastin time. Diffuse intravascular coagulation can develop with severe abruption. If fibrinogen is <150 mg%, estimated blood loss is approximately 2000 ml; if fibrinogen is <100 mg%, consider fresh frozen plasma to prevent further bleeding.
- Type and antibody screen is important to identify Rh-negative patients who may need Rh immune globulin.

IMAGING STUDIES

Ultrasound should include fetal presentation and status, amniotic fluid volume, placental location, as well as any evidence of hematoma (retroplacental, subchorionic, or preplacental).

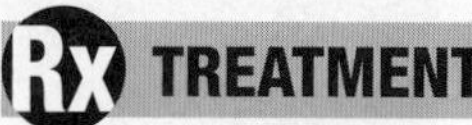

TREATMENT

ACUTE GENERAL Rx

- Stabilization of the mother is the first priority.
- Treatment depends on gestational age of the fetus, severity of the abruption, and maternal status.
- Initial assessment for signs of maternal hemodynamic compromise or hemorrhagic shock; large-bore intravenous access, with crystalloid fluid resuscitation using a replacement of 3 ml lactated Ringer's solution for every 1 ml estimated blood loss.
- Indwelling Foley catheter to monitor urine output and maternal volume status, with a goal of 30 ml/hr urine output.
- Assess fetal status and gestational age by sonogram and continuous fetal heart rate monitoring.
- Because of the unpredictable nature of abruptions, cross-matched blood should be made available during the initial resuscitation period.

CHRONIC Rx

- In the term fetus or when lung maturity has been documented, delivery is indicated.
- In the preterm fetus or a fetus with an immature lung profile, consider betamethasone 12.5 mg IM q24h for two doses and then delivery, depending on the severity of the abruption and the likelihood of fetal complications from preterm birth.
- Cesarean section should be reserved for cases of fetal distress or for standard obstetric indications. While cesarean delivery may be needed to stabilize the fetal and/or maternal status, the mother's coagulation status may complicate the procedure and availability of blood products may be critical.
- In select cases, such as severe prematurity with a stable mother and mild contractions, magnesium sulfate can be used for tocolysis, 6 g IV loading dose then 3 g/hr maintenance, to allow for a course of steroids.

DISPOSITION

Because of the unpredictable nature of abruptions, expectant management should occur only under controlled circumstances and is rarely practiced.

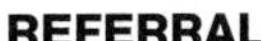

REFERRAL

Abruptio placentae places mother and fetus in a high-risk situation and should be managed by a qualified obstetrician in a facility with capability for neonatal and maternal resuscitation, for supporting a preterm infant if delivery is indicated at an early gestational age, and for performing emergency cesarean sections.

RELATED CONTENT

Premature Labor (Related Key Topic)
Vaginal Bleeding During Pregnancy (Related Key Topic)
Abruptio Placentae (Patient Information)

AUTHOR: **RUBEN ALVERO, M.D.**

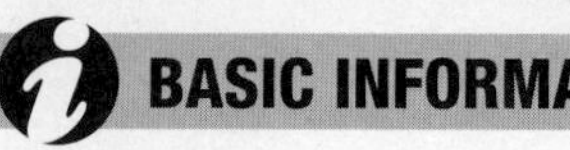

BASIC INFORMATION

DEFINITION

A brain abscess is a focal intracerebral infection that can arise as a complication from a bacterial, fungal, or protozoal infection, surgery, or trauma.

ICD-9CM CODES
324.0 Brain abscess
ICD-10CM CODES
G06.0 Intracranial abscess and granuloma

EPIDEMIOLOGY & DEMOGRAPHICS

INCIDENCE: Uncommon (occurs about 2% as commonly as brain tumors)
PEAK INCIDENCE: Preadolescence and middle age (and depends on predisposing condition)
PREDOMINANT AGE: Occurs at any age
PREDOMINANT SEX:
- Men affected more than women (ratio 2:1 to 3:1)

PHYSICAL FINDINGS & CLINICAL PRESENTATION

- Classic triad: fever, headache, and focal neurologic deficit (present in less than 50% of cases).
- Clinical presentation is often due to the manifestations of the space-occupying lesion rather than to signs of systemic infection.
- Fever is present in only 32% to 79% of patients.
- Headache is usually localized to the side of the abscess; onset can be gradual or severe; present in an average of 70% to 75% of cases.
- Focal neurologic findings (e.g., seizures, hemiparesis, aphasia, ataxia) depend on the location of the abscess and are seen in 23% to 66% of cases.
- Papilledema is present in 9% to 51% of cases.
- Presence of adjacent infections (dental abscess, otitis media, and sinusitis) may be a clue to the underlying diagnosis and should be sought in any suspected case.
- Time course from symptom onset to presentation ranges from hours in fulminant cases to more than 1 month; 75% present in the first 2 weeks.
- The nonspecific presentation of a brain abscess warrants that clinicians maintain a high index of suspicion. Table 1-1 describes common initial features of brain abscess.

TABLE 1-1 Brain Abscess: Initial Features in 123 Cases

Headache	55%
Disturbed consciousness	48%
Fever	58%
Nuchal rigidity	29%
Nausea, vomiting	32%
Seizures	19%
Visual disturbance	15%
Dysarthria	20%
Hemiparesis	48%
Sepsis	17%

From Goldman L, Schafer AI: *Goldman's Cecil medicine,* ed 24, Philadelphia, 2012, Saunders.

ETIOLOGY

- Brain abscesses are classified based on the likely portal of entry and can arise from:
  Contiguous infection
  Hematogenous spread from a remote site
- Likely source of abscess and common organisms involved:
  A. Contiguous focus or primary infection (55% of all brain abscesses):
     1. Paranasal sinus: occur in frontal lobe; streptococci (especially microaerophilic and anaerobic streptococci), *Bacteroides, Haemophilus,* and *Fusobacterium* spp.
     2. Otitis media/mastoiditis: occur in temporal lobe and cerebellum; aerobic and anaerobic streptococci, Enterobacteriaceae, *Bacteroides,* and *Pseudomonas* spp.
     3. Dental sepsis: occur in frontal lobe; mixed *Fusobacterium, Bacteroides,* and *Streptococcus* spp. *(especially S. viridans* and *anaerobic streptococci)*
     4. Penetrating head injury: site of abscess depends on site of wound; *Staphylococcus aureus, aerobic streptococci, Clostridium* spp., Enterobacteriaceae
     5. Postoperative: *Staphylococcus epidermidis* and *S. aureus,* Enterobacteriaceae, and *Pseudomonas aeruginosa*
  B. Hematogenous spread from a distant site of infection (25% of all brain abscesses): abscesses most commonly multiple, especially in middle cerebral artery distribution; infecting organism(s) depend on source.
     1. Congenital heart disease: streptococci, *Haemophilus* spp.
     2. Endocarditis: *S. aureus,* viridans streptococci
     3. Urinary tract: Enterobacteriaceae, Pseudomonadaceae
     4. Intraabdominal: streptococci, Enterobacteriaceae, anaerobes
     5. Lung: streptococci, *Actinomyces* spp., *Fusobacterium* spp.
     6. Immunocompromised host: *Toxoplasma* species, fungi, Enterobacteriaceae, *Nocardia* spp., tuberculosis, listeriosis
  C. Cryptogenic (unknown source): 20% of all brain abscesses

Dx DIAGNOSIS

DIFFERENTIAL DIAGNOSIS

- Other parameningeal infections: subdural empyema, epidural abscess, thrombophlebitis of the major dural venous sinuses and cortical veins
- Embolic strokes in patients with bacterial endocarditis
- Mycotic aneurysms with leakage
- Acute hemorrhagic leukoencephalitis
- Parasitic infections: toxoplasmosis, echinococcosis, cysticercosis
- Metastatic or primary brain tumors
- Cerebral infarction
- CNS vasculitis
- Chronic subdural hematoma
- Table E1-2 summarizes the differential diagnosis of central nervous system infection and tumor

WORKUP

Physical examination, laboratory tests, and imaging studies

LABORATORY TESTS

- White blood cell counts are elevated in 60% of patients.
- Erythrocyte sedimentation rate is usually elevated but may be normal.
- Blood cultures are most often negative (10% positive).
- Lumbar puncture is contraindicated in patients with suspected abscess (20% die or experience neurologic decline).
- The yield of Gram stain and culture of material aspirated at time of surgical drainage is very high.

IMAGING STUDIES

- MRI with and without gadolinium is the diagnostic procedure of choice; provides superior detail compared with CT scan (higher sensitivity and specificity than CT scan, but not always immediately available).
- CT scan (Fig. 1-5) with intravenous contrast is still an excellent test (sensitivity 95%-99%).
- Serial CT or MRI scanning is recommended to follow the response to therapy.

Rx TREATMENT

ACUTE GENERAL Rx

- Effective treatment involves a combination of empiric antibiotic therapy and timely excision or aspiration of the abscess.
- If evidence of edema or mass effect, treatment of elevated intracranial pressure is paramount.
  - Hyperventilation of mechanically ventilated patient.
  - Dexamethasone initially in a dosage of 10 mg IV followed by 4 mg IV q6h until symptoms of cerebral edema subside. Steroids should be discontinued as soon as possible.
  - Mannitol 0.25 to 1 g/kg IV over 20 to 30 min q6 to 8h; maximum of 6 g/kg in 24 hr.
- Medical therapy is never a substitute for surgical intervention to relieve increased intracranial pressure. Neurologic deterioration usually mandates surgery.
- Steroids should be limited to patients with severe cerebral edema or midline shift.

MEDICAL Rx

If abscess <2.5 cm and patient is neurologically stable and conscious, may start antibiotics and observe. Empiric antibiotic therapy guided by:
- Abscess location
- Suspicion of primary source
- Presence of single or multiple abscesses
- Patient's underlying medical conditions (e.g., HIV, immunocompromised)

Selection of empiric antibiotic therapy:
- Primary infection or contiguous source:
  1. Otitis media/mastoiditis, sinusitis, dental infection: third-generation cephalosporin (cefotaxime 2 g q4h IV or ceftriaxone 2 g q12h IV) plus metronidazole 15 mg/kg IV as a loading dose, then 7.5 mg/kg q8h IV, not to exceed 4 g per day
  2. Dental infection: penicillin G (20 million to 24 million units per day IV in six divided doses) plus metronidazole (dose as above)
  3. Head trauma: third-generation cephalosporin (cefotaxime 2 g IV q4h or ceftriaxone 2 g IV q12h) plus nafcillin 2 g IV q4h or vancomycin (30 mg/kg IV in two divided doses adjusted for renal function)
  4. Postoperative neurosurgery: vancomycin (dose as above) plus ceftazidime (2 g IV q8h) or cefepime (2 g IV q8h), or meropenem (1 g IV q8h). Replace vancomycin with nafcillin (2g IV q4h) if susceptibility testing reveals methicillin-sensitive *Staphylococcus aureus.*
- Hematogenous spread (congenital heart disease, endocarditis, urinary tract, lung, intraabdominal): vancomycin (empiric therapy, dose as above) or nafcillin (if susceptibility testing reveals methicillin-sensitive *S. aureus,* dose as above) plus metronidazole plus third-generation cephalosporin (cefotaxime 2 g IV q4h or ceftriaxone 2 g IV q12h)

Duration of antibiotic therapy is guided by the clinical course and whether or not the abscess was surgically aspirated or excised. It is usually prolonged. Surgical therapy may be required for clinical failure if the patient is receiving antibiotics alone. Most recommend parenteral treatment for at least 4 to 6 weeks, with repeated neuroimaging to ensure adequate resolution. (Imaging weekly could be considered for first 2 weeks of therapy, then every 2 weeks until resolution.)

SURGICAL Rx

- Two indications for surgical intervention:
  1. Collect specimens for culture and sensitivity
  2. Reduce mass effect
- Stereotactic biopsy or aspirate of the abscess if surgically feasible
- Essential to selection of targeted antimicrobial coverage
- Timing and choice of surgery depends on:
  - Primary infection source
  - Number and location of the abscesses
  - Whether the procedure is diagnostic or therapeutic
  - Neurologic status of the patient

DISPOSITION

- Prompt diagnostic consideration, early institution of appropriate antimicrobial therapy, and advanced neuroradiologic imaging have reduced the mortality rate from brain abscesses from 40% to 80% in the preantibiotic era to 10% to 20% at present.
- Morbidity is usually manifest as persistent neurologic sequelae (seizures, intellectual or behavioral impairment, motor deficits).

REFERRAL

Consultation with a neurosurgeon is mandatory.

PEARLS & CONSIDERATIONS

COMMENTS

- It is important to maintain a high index of suspicion because a brain abscess often presents with nonspecific symptoms.
- Rapid imaging and early institution of appropriate antimicrobial therapy improve patient morbidity and mortality.
- Neurosurgical consultation is mandatory.

PREVENTION

Because brain abscesses arise from either contiguous infections or hematogenously from a remote site, early and appropriate treatment of predisposing infections is paramount to prevent brain abscess.

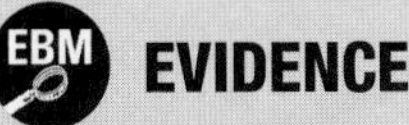

EVIDENCE

available at www.expertconsult.com

SUGGESTED READINGS

available at www.expertconsult.com

RELATED CONTENT

Brain Abscess (Patient Information)

AUTHORS: **ERICA HARDY, M.D., M.M.S.,** and **KELLY A. MCGARRY, M.D.**

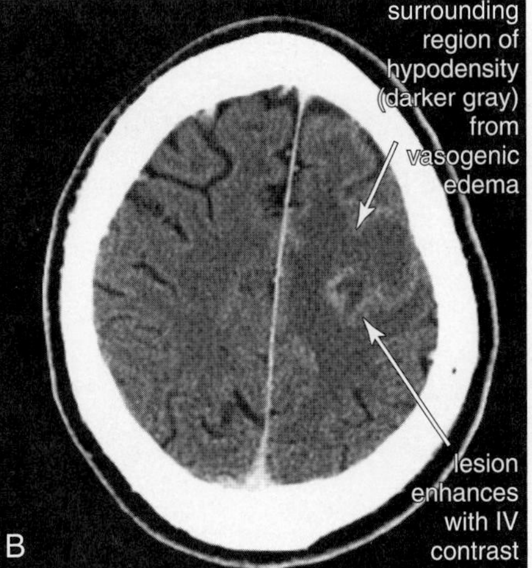

FIGURE 1-5 Brain abscess. This 48-year-old male presented with status epilepticus. Computed tomography (CT) showed a parietal mass, which at brain biopsy was found to be an abscess. Cultures grew mixed gram-positive and gram-negative organisms and anaerobes. The patient was subsequently found to be human immunodeficiency virus positive. **A**, Noncontrast head CT, brain windows. **B**, CT with intravenous (IV) contrast moments later, brain windows. Abscesses and other infectious, inflammatory, or neoplastic lesions typically have surrounding hypodense regions representing vasogenic edema. When IV contrast is administered **(B),** the lesion may enhance peripherally, often referred to as ring enhancement. (From Broder JS: *Diagnostic imaging for the emergency physician,* Philadelphia, 2011, Saunders.)

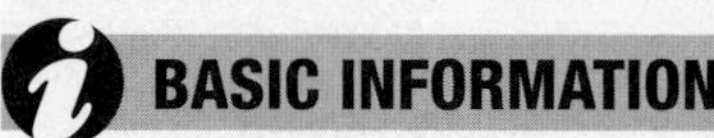

BASIC INFORMATION

DEFINITION

Breast abscess is an acute inflammatory process resulting in the formation of a collection of purulent material in breast tissue. Typically there is painful erythematous mass formation in the breast, occasionally draining through the overlying skin or nipple duct.

SYNONYMS

Subareolar abscess
Lactational or puerperal abscess

ICD-9CM CODES

6.110 Abscess of the breast
675.0 Abscess of the nipple related to childbirth
675.1 Abscess of the breast related to childbirth

ICD-10CM CODES

091.119 Abscess of breast associated with pregnancy, unspecified trimester

EPIDEMIOLOGY & DEMOGRAPHICS

INCIDENCE: 10% to 30% of all breast abscesses are lactational; acute mastitis occurs in 2.5% of nursing mothers, with one in 15 of these women developing abscess. Smoking and diabetes may be risk factors for non-puerperal mastitis with abscess.

PHYSICAL FINDINGS & CLINICAL PRESENTATION

Painful erythematous induration involving breast and leading to fluctuant abscess

ETIOLOGY

- Lactational abscess: milk stasis and bacterial infection leading to mastitis and then abscess, with *Staphylococcus aureus* the most common causative agent
- Subareolar abscess:
    1. Central ducts involved, with obstructive nipple duct changes leading to bacterial infection
    2. Cultured organisms mixed, including anaerobes, staphylococci, streptococci, and others

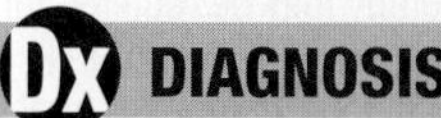

DIAGNOSIS

DIFFERENTIAL DIAGNOSIS

- Inflammatory carcinoma
- Advanced carcinoma with erythema, edema, and/or ulceration
- Tuberculous abscess (rare in the United States)
- Hidradenitis of breast skin
- Sebaceous cyst with infection

WORKUP

- Clinical examination
- If abscess suspected, referral to surgeon for incision, drainage, and biopsy

LABORATORY TESTS

- Perform culture and sensitivity test of abscess contents.
- If mammogram or ultrasound is required but prevented by discomfort, perform after treatment and subsequent resolution of abscess.

Rx TREATMENT

NONPHARMACOLOGIC THERAPY

- Established abscess: incision and drainage
- Biopsy of abscess cavity wall to exclude carcinoma

ACUTE GENERAL RX

- Antibiotics: generally staphylococci in lactational abscess. Recommended initial antibiotic therapy is nafcillin or oxacillin 2 g q4h IV or cefazolin 1 g q8h IV for 10 to 14 days. Alternative includes vancomycin 1 g IV q12h.
- If acute mastitis is identified and treated early without the development of an abscess, resolution without drainage is possible.
- Subareolar abscess: broad-spectrum antibiotic treatment (e.g., cephalexin 500 mg PO qid or cefazolin 1 g q8h IV for 10 to 14 days for more severe infection) and drainage are needed to control acute phase. If abscess is odoriferous, consider anaerobes as most likely etiology and add metronidazole 500 mg PO/IV tid.

CHRONIC RX

Further surgical treatment for recurrences or fistula

DISPOSITION

- Lactational abscess: possible to continue breastfeeding without risk of infection to the infant
- Subareolar abscess:
    1. High risk for recurrence or complication of fistula formation
    2. Patient informed and referred to General Surgery for evaluation and treatment

REFERRAL

- If abscess drainage required
- If subareolar abscess involved, refer to surgery

RELATED CONTENT

Breast Cancer (Related Key Topic)
Mastodynia (Related Key Topic)
Breast Abscess (Patient Information)

SUGGESTED READINGS
available at www.expertconsult.com

AUTHORS: **TAKUMA NEMOTO, M.D.,** and **RUBEN ALVERO, M.D.**

BASIC INFORMATION

DEFINITION

Epidural abscess is a suppurative infection of the central nervous system localized between the dura mater and the overlying skull or vertebral column. There are two types of epidural abscess: spinal epidural abscess (SEA) and intracranial epidural abscess (IEA), depending on the location within the central nervous system.

SYNONYMS

Spinal epidural abscess
Intraspinal abscess

ICD-9CM CODES
324.9 Epidural abscess
324.0 Intracranial abscess

ICD-10CM CODES
G06.2 Extradural and subdural abscess, unspecified

EPIDEMIOLOGY & DEMOGRAPHICS

INCIDENCE: Spinal epidural abscess: 2 to 25 patients per 100,000 admissions; spinal epidural abscess is 9 times more common than intracranial abscess

PEAK INCIDENCE: Median age at onset of spinal epidural abscess: 50 years old

PREVALENCE: Greatest between 50 and 70 years of age

PREDOMINANT SEX: More common in men

RISK FACTORS: Bacteremia, secondary to distant infection; epidural cathether placement (0.5% to 3% risk), paraspinal injections of glucocorticoids or for pain management, contiguous bone or soft tissue infection, intravenous drug abuse, diabetes, immunosuppressive therapy, HIV

PHYSICAL FINDINGS & CLINICAL PRESENTATION

- Initially nonspecific, such as fever and malaise
- Classic triad: fever, spinal pain, and neurologic deficits are not common
- More commonly:
  - Localized and significant back pain is present.
  - Nerve root pain is present ("shooting" or "electrical" from involved nerve root).
  - Motor weakness, sensory changes, and even paralysis can occur.
  - Fever may not be a prominent sign.

ETIOLOGY

- Bacteria enter the epidural space most often secondary to hematogenous spread from foci elsewhere in the body (25% to 50% of cases) or by direct extension from nearby infected tissues such as vertebral body or psoas muscle. A local intervention such as injection can also cause infection.
- Hematogenous foci include furuncles, cellulitis, urinary tract infection, pharyngitis, and pneumonia.
- Microbiology:
  - *Staphylococcus aureus,* including methicillin-resistant *S. aureus* (MRSA), accounts for 50% to 90% of cases.
  - Aerobic and anaerobic streptococci account for 8% to 17% of cases.
  - Aerobic gram-negative rods *(Escherichia coli* and *Pseudomonas)* account for 10% to 17% of cases.
  - Coagulase-negative staphylococci can be seen with spinal procedures.

DIAGNOSIS

DIFFERENTIAL DIAGNOSIS

- Disc and degenerative bone disease
- Metastatic tumors
- Vertebral discitis and osteomyelitis

WORKUP

Includes a combination of physical exam with neurologic evaluation, blood work, and radiographic studies

LABORATORY TESTS

- Blood cultures
- Culture of fluid or pus by CT-guided aspiration if possible
- Erythrocyte sedimentation rate and/or C-reactive protein
- CBC with differential

IMAGING STUDIES

- MRI with gadolinium is the diagnostic test of choice and imperative if diagnosis is considered.
- CT is an alternative but not as good as MRI for visualizing spinal cord and epidural space.
- CT myelography can be performed if MRI is not available.

TREATMENT

NONPHARMACOLOGIC THERAPY

- Immediate surgery is required if neurologic deficits occur or the patient worsens with medical therapy.
- CT-guided aspiration of abscess with antimicrobial therapy is an alternative treatment to surgery for patients without neurologic deficits.

ACUTE GENERAL Rx

- Empiric antibiotic regimen should include antibiotics effective against staphylococci (including MRSA), streptococci, and gram-negative rods.
- Examples are vancomycin (30 to 60 mg/kg daily divided in q12h doses adjusted for creatinine clearance *plus* metronidazole (500 mg IV q8h) *plus* cetriaxone (2 g IV q12h) or ceftazidime (2 g IV q8h) if *Pseudomonas* is suspected.
- If cultures reveal methicillin-sensitive *S. aureus,* use nafcillin 2 g IV q4h

CHRONIC Rx

Antimicrobial therapy tailored to culture results may have to be continued for 4 to 6 weeks depending on whether or not there was surgical or CT-guided drainage. If osteomyelitis is suspected, treat for 6 to 8 weeks.

DISPOSITION

- Mortality rates vary from 5% to 32%. Irreversible paralysis can affect 4% to 22% of patients.
- Complete recovery is more likely if neurologic signs are present less than 24 hours before the start of treatment.
- Final functional capacity may continue to improve for up to 1 year after the end of treatment.

REFERRAL

- Neurosurgery should be involved early when this diagnosis is considered.
- Refer to an interventional radiologist for possible aspiration.
- An infectious diseases evaluation is needed for antimicrobial therapy.

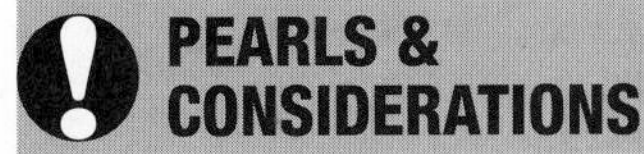

PEARLS & CONSIDERATIONS

COMMENTS

It is important to think of spinal epidural abscess early to permit early treatment and prevent permanent neurologic deficits.

SUGGESTED READINGS

available at www.expertconsult.com

RELATED CONTENT

Abscess, Brain (Related Key Topic)

AUTHOR: **GLENN G. FORT, M.D., M.P.H.**

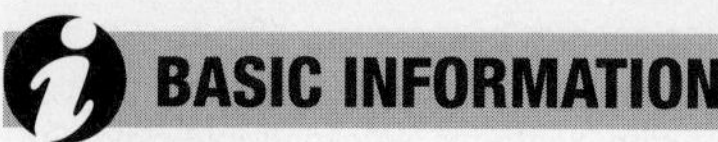

BASIC INFORMATION

DEFINITION

Liver abscess is a necrotic infection of the liver usually classified as pyogenic or amebic.

SYNONYMS

Pyogenic hepatic abscess
Amebic hepatic abscess

ICD-9CM CODES
572.0 Abscess of liver
ICD-10CM CODES
K75.0 Abscess of liver

EPIDEMIOLOGY & DEMOGRAPHICS

INCIDENCE: Incidence of pyogenic liver abscess is 2.3 cases per 100,000 population.

PREVALANCE (WORLDWIDE): Amebic liver abscess is more common than pyogenic liver abscess.

PREVALENCE (IN U.S.): Pyogenic liver abscess is more common than amebic liver abscess.

PREDOMINANT SEX AND AGE: More common in men than women; male/female ratio of 2:1; most common in fourth to sixth decades of life.

PHYSICAL FINDINGS & CLINICAL PRESENTATION

- Fever, chills, and sweats
- Weakness/malaise
- Anorexia with weight loss
- Nausea, vomiting, and diarrhea
- Cough with pleuritic chest pain
- Right upper quadrant abdominal pain
- Hepatomegaly
- Splenomegaly
- Jaundice
- Pleural effusions, rales, and friction rubs may be present
- Most abscesses occur on the right lobe of the liver

ETIOLOGY

- Pyogenic liver abscess is usually polymicrobial (*Klebsiella pneumoniae* [43%], *Escherichia coli* [33%], *Streptococcus* spp. [37%], *Pseudomonas aeruginosa, Proteus* spp., *Bacteroides* spp. [24%], *Fusobacterium* spp., *Actinomyces* spp., gram-positive anaerobes, and *Staphylococcus aureus*).
- Pyogenic liver abscess occurs from:
    1. Biliary disease with cholangitis (accounts for approximately 40% to 60%).
    2. Gallbladder disease with contiguous spread to the liver.
    3. Diverticulitis or appendicitis with spread via the portal circulation.
    4. Hematogenous spread via the hepatic artery, though uncommon; if a solitary organism is isolated, a distant source of hematogenous seeding should be sought.
    5. Penetrating wounds.
    6. Cryptogenic.
    7. Infection by way of portal system (portal pyemia).
    8. No causes found in approximately half of cases.
    9. Incidence increased in patients with diabetes and metastatic cancer.
    10. Table 1-3 summarizes underlying etiology and bacteriology of liver abscesses.
- Amebic hepatic abscess is caused by the parasite *Entamoeba histolytica.* Amebiasis is usually due to fecal-oral contamination and invades the intestinal mucosa, gaining entry into the portal system to reach the liver.

Box 1-1 describes pearls for amebic liver abscesses.

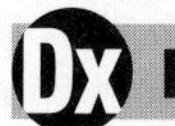

DIAGNOSIS

The diagnosis of liver abscess requires a high index of suspicion after a detailed history and physical examination. Imaging studies and microbiologic, serologic, and percutaneous techniques (e.g., aspiration) confirm the presence of a liver abscess.

DIFFERENTIAL DIAGNOSIS

- Cholangitis
- Cholecystitis
- Diverticulitis
- Appendicitis
- Perforated viscus
- Mesentery ischemia
- Pulmonary embolism
- Pancreatitis

TABLE 1-3 Underlying Etiology and Bacteriology

Etiology	Bacteriology
Biliary, benign	*Escherichia coli* *Klebsiella* spp. *Enterococcus*
Biliary, malignant	*Pseudomonas* spp. Multiply resistant GN aerobes VRE Yeast
Diverticulitis/ appendicitis	GN aerobes *Bacteroides fragilis*
Severe cholecystitis	See Biliary, benign *Clostridium perfringens* *Bacteroides* spp.
Subcutaneous abscess	*Staphylococcus* spp. MRSA
Endocarditis	*Enterococcus* spp. *Staphyloccus* spp.
Cryptogenic	Anaerobes

GN, Gram negative.
From Cameron, JL, Cameron AM: *Current surgical therapy,* ed 10, Philadelphia, 2011, Saunders.

WORKUP

- The workup of a liver abscess should focus on differentiating between amebic and pyogenic causes.
- Features suggesting an amebic cause include travel to an endemic area, single abscess rather than multiple abscesses, subacute onset of symptoms, and absence of conditions predisposing to pyogenic liver abscess, as highlighted under "Etiology."
- Laboratory studies are not specific but are useful as adjunctive tests.
- Imaging studies cannot differentiate between the two, and bacteriologic cultures may be sterile in 50% of the cases.

LABORATORY TESTS

- Complete blood count: leukocytosis
- Liver function tests: alkaline phosphatase is most commonly elevated (95% to 100%); aspartate transaminase (AST) and alanine transaminase (ALT) elevated in 50% of cases; elevated bilirubin (28% to 30%); decreased albumin
- Prothrombin time (INR): prolonged (70%)
- Blood cultures: positive in 50% of cases
- Aspiration (50% sterile)
- Stool samples for *E. histolytica* trophozoites (positive in 10% to 15% of amebic liver abscess cases)
- Serologic testing for *E. histolytica* should be done on all patients, but it is important to remember that it does not differentiate acute from old infections.

IMAGING STUDIES

- Ultrasound (80% to 100% sensitivity in detecting abscesses) shows round or oval hypoechogenic mass (Fig. 1-6, *A*).
- CT scan is more sensitive in detecting hepatic abscesses and contiguous organ extension and is the imaging study of choice (Fig. 1-6, *B*).
- Chest x-ray: abnormal in 50% of the cases, may reveal elevated right hemidiaphragm, subdiaphragmatic air-fluid levels, pleural effusions, and consolidating infiltrates.

BOX 1-1 Pearls for Amebic Liver Abscesses

- Only 10% to 20% of patients with amebic liver abscess have a history of diarrhea.
- Treat the intestinal infection to prevent relapse of amebic liver abscess. Failure to use luminal amebicidal agents after metronidazole in cases of amebic abscess results in a 10% relapse rate.
- Failure to show response to antiamebic medication requires evaluation for polymicrobial infection with bacteria.
- Amebic abscess usually responds clinically to antimicrobial therapy in 3 to 7 days, although imaging takes several months to show resolution.
- Percutaneous drainage is rarely required.

From Cameron, JL, Cameron AM: *Current surgical therapy,* ed 10, Philadelphia, 2011, Saunders.

- Most liver abscesses are single; however, multiple liver abscesses can occur with systemic bacteremia.

Rx TREATMENT

NONPHARMACOLOGIC THERAPY

- The management of pyogenic liver abscess differs from that of amebic liver abscess.
- Medical management is the cornerstone of therapy in amebic liver abscess, whereas early intervention in the form of surgical therapy or catheter drainage and parenteral antibiotics is the rule in pyogenic liver abscess.

ACUTE GENERAL Rx

- Percutaneous drainage under CT or ultrasound guidance is essential in the treatment of pyogenic liver abscesses.
- Aspiration of hepatic amebic abscesses is not required unless there is no response to treatment or a pyogenic cause is being considered.
- Empiric broad-spectrum antibiotics are recommended initially until culture results are available. Common choices include:
  1. Metronidazole (500 mg IV q8h) plus ceftriaxone or cefoxitin or levofloxacin.
  2. Metronidazole plus a beta-lactam/beta-lactamase inhibitor, such as piperacillin/tazobactam (4.5 g q6h), ticarcillin-clavulanate (3.1 g q4h), or ampicillin-sulbactam (3 g q6h).
  3. Metronidazole plus a carbapenem, such as imipenem (500 mg IV q6h), meropenem (1 g q8h), or ertapenem (1 g daily).
  4. In patients with penicillin allergy, clindamycin 600 to 900 mg IV q8h with an aminoglycoside can be considered.
  5. Duration of antibiotic treatment is usually 4 to 6 wk with IV antibiotics used for the first 1 to 2 wk or until a favorable clinical response, followed thereafter with oral antibiotics (e.g., metronidazole 500 mg PO q8h plus ciprofloxacin 500 mg PO q12h).
  6. Third-generation cephalosporins should not be used as single agents for empiric therapy because of risk of the emergence of beta-lactamase-producing bacteria.
- Antibiotic coverage for amebic liver abscesses includes:
  1. Tissue agent: metronidazole 750 mg PO tid for 10 days
  2. Luminal agent: after therapy with tissue agent treatment with any luminal agent is required even if the stool is negative, such as paromomycin for 10 days or diiodohydroxyquin for 20 days.

CHRONIC Rx

- If fever persists for 2 wk despite percutaneous drainage and antibiotic therapy as outlined under "Acute General Rx," or if there is failure of aspiration or failure of percutaneous drainage, surgery is indicated.
- In patients not responding to intravenous antibiotics and percutaneous drainage, hepatic artery antibiotic infusion can be considered.
- In patients with evidence of metastatic disease that is causing biliary obstruction, a gastroenterology consultation for endoscopic retrograde cholangiopancreatography and stenting should be considered.

DISPOSITION

- Most patients with pyogenic liver abscesses defervesce within 2 wk of treatment with antibiotics and drainage.
- No randomized controlled studies have evaluated the optimal duration of antibiotic therapy for pyogenic liver abscess. Typical duration of antibiotic therapy is at least 4 to 6 wk.
- Pyogenic liver abscess cure rates using percutaneous drainage and antibiotics have been reported to be between 88% and 100%.
- Mortality rate of untreated pyogenic liver abscess is nearly 100%.
- Most patients with amebic liver abscesses defervesce within 4 to 5 days of treatment.
- Amebic liver abscess mortality rate is <1% unless complications occur (see "Comments").
- Follow-up imaging should be used to monitor response to therapy; continue treatment until CT scan shows complete or near-complete resolution of cavity.

REFERRAL

Infectious disease, gastroenterology, interventional radiology, and general surgical consultations are recommended in any patient with hepatic abscess.

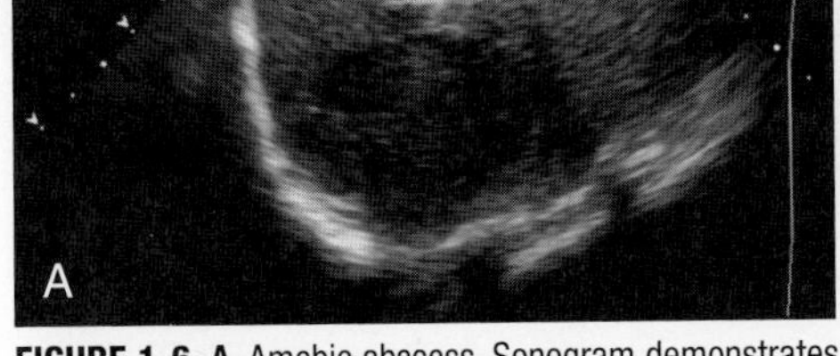
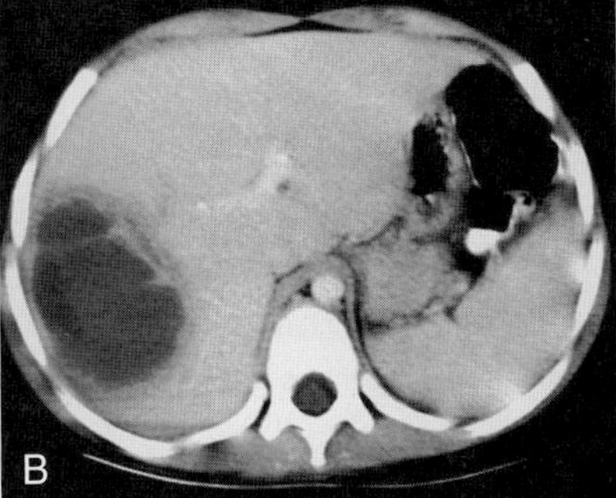

FIGURE 1-6 **A,** Amebic abscess. Sonogram demonstrates a hypoechogenic mass in the right lobe of the liver with a more hypoechoic surrounding rim. **B,** CT scan demonstrates a low-attenuation mass in the right lobe of the liver with a prominent halo. (From Kuhn JP et al: *Caffrey's pediatric diagnostic imaging,* vol 2, ed 10, Philadelphia, 2004, Mosby.)

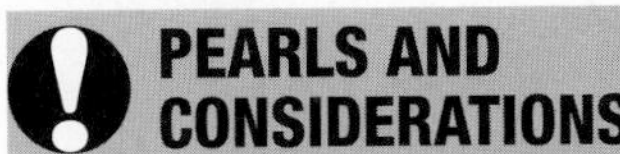

PEARLS AND CONSIDERATIONS

COMMENTS

- Complications of pyogenic and amebic liver abscesses include:
  1. Pleuropulmonary extension, resulting in empyema, abscess, and fistula formation
  2. Peritonitis
  3. Purulent pericarditis
  4. Sepsis
- Amebic liver abscesses complicate amebic colitis in nearly 10% of cases.

SUGGESTED READINGS

available at www.expertconsult.com

RELATED CONTENT

Liver Abscess (Patient Information)

AUTHOR: **TANYA ALI, M.D.**

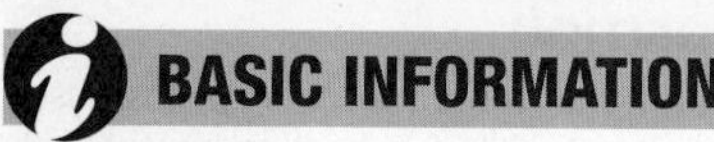

BASIC INFORMATION

DEFINITION

A lung abscess is an infection of the lung parenchyma resulting in a necrotic cavity containing pus.

SYNONYMS

Pulmonary abscess

ICD-9CM CODES
513.0 Abscess of the lung
ICD-10CM CODES
J85.1 Abscess of lung with pneumonia
J85.2 Abscess of lung without pneumonia

EPIDEMIOLOGY & DEMOGRAPHICS

INCIDENCE: Has decreased over the last 30 years as a result of antibiotic therapy.

- Lung abscess in patients age 50 and over is associated with primary lung neoplasia in 30% of the cases.
- Lung abscesses commonly coexist with empyemas.

RISK FACTORS (See Table 1-4):

1. Alcohol-related problems
2. Seizure disorders
3. Cerebrovascular disorders with dysphagia
4. Drug abuse
5. Esophageal disorders (e.g., scleroderma, esophageal carcinoma, etc.)
6. Poor oral hygiene
7. Obstructive malignant lung disease
8. Bronchiectasis

PHYSICAL FINDINGS & CLINICAL PRESENTATION

- Symptoms are generally insidious and prolonged, occurring for weeks to months
- Fever, chills, and sweats
- Cough
- Sputum production (purulent with foul odor)
- Pleuritic chest pain
- Hemoptysis
- Dyspnea
- Malaise, fatigue, and weakness
- Tachycardia and tachypnea
- Dullness to percussion, whispered pectoriloquy, and bronchophony
- Amphoric breath sounds (low-pitched sound of air moving across a large open cavity)

ETIOLOGY

- The most important factor predisposing to lung abscess is aspiration.
- Following aspiration as a major predisposing factor is periodontal disease.
- Lung abscess is rare in an edentulous person.
- Approximately 90% of lung abscesses are caused by anaerobic microorganisms (peptostreptococci, microaerophilic streptococci such as *Streptococcus milleri, Bacteroides* species, *Fusobacterium nucleatum, Prevotella*). Pulmonary actinomycosis will also generate lung abscess.
- In most cases anaerobic infection is mixed with aerobic or facultative anaerobic organisms *(S. aureus, E. coli, K. pneumoniae, P. aeruginosa).*
- Parasitic organisms including *Paragonimus westermani* and *Entamoeba histolytica.*
- Fungi including *Aspergillus, Cryptococcus, Histoplasma, Blastomyces,* and *Coccidioides* spp.
- Immunocompromised hosts may become infected with *Aspergillus,* mycobacteria, *Nocardia, Legionella micdadei,* and *Rhodococcus equi.*
- Lung necrosis caused by community strains of MRSA (USA 300 strain) in young adults or adolescents after acute influenza was initially reported in 2002 and can be quite fulminant.

Dx DIAGNOSIS

Lung abscess may be primary or secondary.

- *Primary lung abscess* refers to infection from normal host organisms within the lung (e.g., aspiration, pneumonia).
- Secondary lung abscess results from other preexisting conditions (e.g., endocarditis, underlying lung cancer, pulmonary emboli).

Lung abscess may be acute or chronic.

- Acute lung abscess is present if symptoms are of less than 4 to 6 wk.
- Chronic lung abscess is present if symptoms last longer than 6 wk.

DIFFERENTIAL DIAGNOSIS

The differential diagnosis is similar to that for cavitary lung lesions:

- Bacterial (anaerobic, aerobic, infected bulla, empyema, actinomycosis, tuberculosis)
- Fungal (histoplasmosis, coccidioidomycosis, blastomycosis, aspergillosis, cryptococcosis, zygomycetes)
- Parasitic (amebiasis, echinococcosis)
- Malignancy (primary lung carcinoma, metastatic lung disease, lymphoma, Hodgkin's disease)
- Granulomatosis with polyangiitis, sarcoidosis, endocarditis, and septic pulmonary emboli

WORKUP

- The workup of a patient with lung abscess attempts to elicit a primary or a secondary cause.
- Blood tests are not specific in diagnosing lung abscesses.
- Most diagnoses are made from imaging studies; however, to diagnose a specific cause bacteriologic studies are needed.

LABORATORY TESTS

- CBC with leukocytosis
- Bacteriologic studies
  1. Sputum Gram stain and culture (commonly contaminated by oral flora)
  2. Percutaneous transtracheal aspiration
  3. Percutaneous transthoracic aspiration
  4. Fiberoptic bronchoscopy using bronchial brushings or bronchoalveolar lavage is the most widely used intervention when trying to obtain diagnostic bacteriologic cultures
- Blood cultures on some occasions (<30%) may be positive
- If an empyema is present, obtaining empyema fluid via thoracentesis may isolate the organism

IMAGING STUDIES

- Chest x-ray makes the diagnosis of lung abscess showing the cavitary lesion with an air-fluid level.
- Lung abscesses are most commonly found in the posterior segment of the right upper lobe.
- Chest CT scan can localize and size the lesion and assist in differentiating lung abscesses from other pathologic processes (e.g., tumor, empyema, infected bulla, etc.) (Fig. 1-7).

Rx TREATMENT

NONPHARMACOLOGIC THERAPY

- Oxygen therapy
- Postural drainage
- Respiratory therapy maneuvers

ACUTE GENERAL Rx

Piperacillin/tazobactam 3.375 g IV q6h in aspiration pneumonia with lung abscess

- Ceftriaxone 1 g IV q24h plus metronidazole 1 g IV q12h
- Clindamycin is more effective for anaerobic lung abscess than penicillin alone. Dose: 600 mg IV q8h until improved, then 300 to 600 mg PO q6h.

TABLE 1-4 Risk Factors for Aspiration Pneumonia and Lung Abscess

Increased bacterial inoculum	Periodontal disease, gingivitis, tonsillar or dental abscess, drugs that decrease gastric acidity
Impairment of consciousness	Drugs, alcohol, general anesthesia, metabolic encephalopathy, coma, shock, cerebrovascular accident, cardiopulmonary arrest, seizures, surgery, trauma
Impaired cough and gag reflexes	Vocal cord paralysis, intratracheal anesthesia, endotracheal tube, tracheostomy, myopathy, myelopathy, other neurologic disorders
Impairment of esophageal function	Diverticula, achalasia, strictures, disorders of gastrointestinal motility, neoplasm, tracheoesophageal fistula, pseudobulbar palsy
Emesis	Nasogastric tube, gastric dilation, ileus, intestinal obstruction

From Cohen J, Powderly WG: *Infectious diseases,* ed 2, St Louis, 2004, Mosby.

- Penicillin 1 to 2 million units IV q4h until improvement (afebrile, decreased phlegm production), followed by penicillin VK 500 mg PO q6h for 2 to 3 weeks but often up to 6 to 8 weeks) can be given with metronidazole doses of 7.5 mg/kg IV q6h followed by PO 500 mg bid to qid dosing as an alternative to clindamycin.
- Penicillin should not be used alone because many mouth flora anaerobes now produce penicillinase enzymes. Metronidazole should not be used alone because it is not active against microaerophilic streptococci and some anaerobic cocci.
- Other alternatives are ampicillin/sulbactam and carbapenems such as ertapenem and meropenem.

CHRONIC Rx

- Bronchoscopy to assist with drainage and/or diagnosis is indicated in patients who fail to respond to antibiotics or if there is suspected underlying malignancy.
- Surgery is indicated on rare occasions (<10%) in patients with complications of lung abscess (see "Comments").

DISPOSITION

- More than 95% of patients are cured with the use of antibiotics alone.
- Complications of lung abscesses include:
  1. Empyema
  2. Massive hemoptysis
  3. Pneumothorax
  4. Bronchopleural fistula
  5. Hepatobronchial fistula
  6. Brain abscess
  7. Bronchiectasis
- Mortality is low in community-acquired lung abscess (2.5%).
- Hospital-acquired lung abscess carries a high mortality rate (65%).

REFERRAL

If lung abscess is present, consultation with pulmonary and infectious disease specialist is recommended.

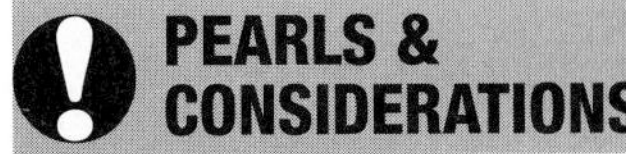

PEARLS & CONSIDERATIONS

COMMENTS

- Refractory cases are usually the result of:
  1. Large cavity size (>6 cm)
  2. Recurrent aspiration
  3. Thick-walled cavities
  4. Underlying lung carcinoma
  5. Empyema formation
- Necrotizing pneumonia is similar to a lung abscess but differs in size (<2 cm in diameter) and number (usually multiple suppurative cavitary lesions).

SUGGESTED READINGS

available at www.expertconsult.com

RELATED CONTENT

Lung Abscess (Patient Information)

AUTHOR: **GLENN G. FORT, M.D., M.P.H.**

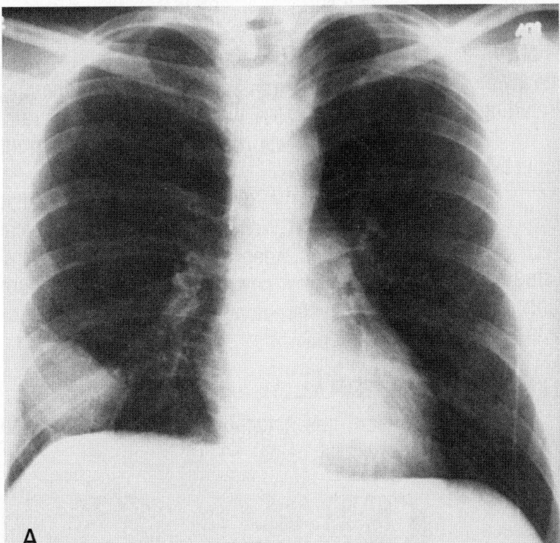

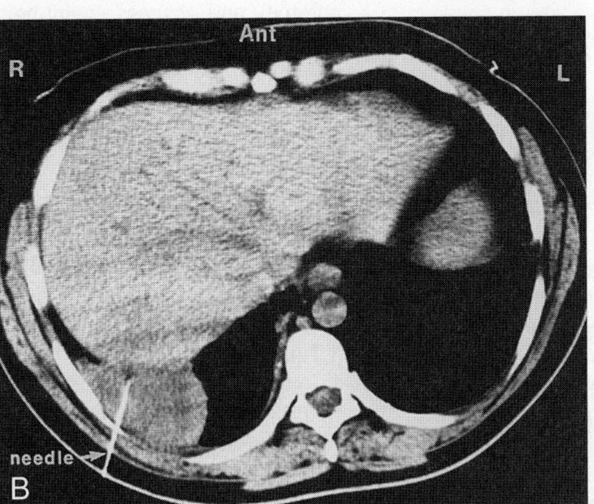

FIGURE 1-7 Lung abscess. On a chest radiograph, a lung abscess may look to be a solid rounded lesion **(A)**, or, if it has a connection with the bronchus, there may be an air-fluid level in a thick-walled cavitary lesion. CT scanning **(B)** can be used to localize the lesion and to place a needle for drainage and aspiration of contents for culture. (From Mettler FA [ed]: *Primary care radiology,* Philadelphia, 2000, Saunders.)

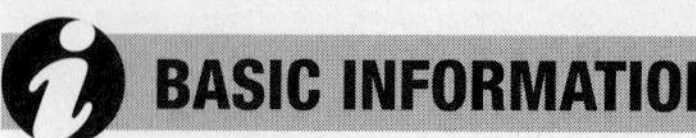

BASIC INFORMATION

DEFINITION

Pelvic abscess is an acute or chronic infection, most commonly involving the pelvic viscera. Treatment and possible cure require directed therapy that will involve antibiotic therapy and, if medical therapy fails, subsequent surgical therapy. There are four categories based on etiologic factors:

- Ascending infection, spreading from cervix through endometrial cavity to adnexa, forming a tuboovarian complex
- Infection occurring in the puerperium, which spreads to the adnexa from the endometrium or myometrium by a hematogenous or lymphatic route
- Abscess complicating pelvic surgery
- Involvement of the pelvic viscera as a result of spread from contiguous organs, such as appendicitis or diverticulitis

SYNONYMS

Tuboovarian abscess (TOA)
Vaginal cuff abscess

ICD-9CM CODES

614.2 Salpingitis and oophoritis not specified as acute, subacute, or chronic

ICD-10CM CODES

N70.93 Salpingitis and oophoritis, unspecified
N70.0 Acute salpingitis and oophoritis
N70.1 Chronic salpingitis and oophoritis

EPIDEMIOLOGY & DEMOGRAPHICS

INCIDENCE:

- 34% of hospitalized patients with pelvic inflammatory disease
- 1% to 2% of patients undergoing hysterectomy, most with vaginal approach
- Peak incidence third to fourth decade

RISK FACTORS: Same risk factors as for pelvic inflammatory disease, although in 30% to 50% of patients there is no prior history of salpingitis before abscess forms.

PHYSICAL FINDINGS & CLINICAL PRESENTATION

- Abdominal or pelvic pain (90%)
- Fever or chills (50%)
- Abnormal bleeding (21%)
- Vaginal discharge (28%)
- Nausea (26%)
- Up to 60% to 80% present in the absence of fever or leukocytosis; absence of these findings should not exclude diagnosis

ETIOLOGY

- Mixed flora of anaerobes, aerobes, and facultative anaerobes, such as *Escherichia coli, Bacteroides fragilis, Prevotella* spp., aerobic streptococci, and *Peptococcus* and *Peptostreptococcus* spp.
- *Neisseria gonorrhoeae* and *Chlamydia* are the major etiologic bacteria in cervicitis and salpingitis but are rarely found in abscess cavity cultures.
- In elderly patients consider diverticular disease.

Dx DIAGNOSIS

DIFFERENTIAL DIAGNOSIS

- Pelvic neoplasms, such as ovarian tumors and leiomyomas.
- Inflammatory masses involving adjacent bowel or omentum, such as ruptured appendicitis or diverticulitis.
- Pelvic hematomas, as may occur after cesarean section or hysterectomy.
- Section III describes the diagnostic approach to patients with a pelvic mass; the differential diagnosis of pelvic mass is described in Section II.
- The differential diagnosis of pelvic pain is described in Section II.
- Sonogram or CT scan: commonly used due to associated pain and guarding, resulting in a suboptimal abdominal or pelvic examination, and to characterize anatomic abnormalities such as an adnexal mass.
- Most common cause of preventable death: physician delay in diagnosis.

LABORATORY TESTS

- CBC with differential
- Aerobic as well as anaerobic cultures of cervix, blood, urine, sputum, peritoneal cavity (if entered), and abscess cavity before starting antibiotics
- Pregnancy test in patients of reproductive age

IMAGING STUDIES

- Sonogram: noninvasive, inexpensive study to confirm diagnosis, estimate size of abscess, and monitor response to therapy; sensitivity >90%
- CT scan: used for both diagnosis and therapy (CT-guided drainage) (Fig. E1-8)
  1. Useful where sonogram provides insufficient information, as with intraabdominal abscesses
  2. Success rate with CT-guided abscess drainage: unilocular, 90%; multilocular, 40%

Rx TREATMENT

Major concerns:

1. Desire for future fertility
2. Likelihood of rupture of abscess, with resulting peritonitis, septic shock, and morbid sequelae

ACUTE GENERAL Rx

- Clinical quandary is whether patient requires immediate surgery (uncertain diagnosis or suspicion of rupture) or management with IV antibiotics, reserving surgery for those with inadequate clinical response (e.g., 48 to 72 hr of therapy, with persistent fever or leukocytosis, increasing size of mass, or suspicion of rupture)
- Surgery indicated in poor response to medical therapy. Early surgery may be needed in those with large adnexal masses (>8 cm), or in immunocompromised patients
- Antibiotic combinations:
  1. Clindamycin 900 mg IV q8h or metronidazole 500 mg IV q6-8h plus gentamicin either 5 to 7 mg/kg q24h or 1.5 mg/kg q8h
  2. Alternatives: ampicillin-sulbactam 3 g IV q6h or cefoxitin 2 g IV q6h or cefotetan 2 g IV q12h plus doxycycline 100 mg IV q12h
- During medical management, high index of suspicion for acute rupture, such as acute worsening of abdominal pain or new-onset tachycardia and hypotension, mandating immediate surgical intervention after patient stabilization
- Surgical options:
  1. Laparoscopy with drainage and irrigation
  2. Transvaginal colpotomy (abscess must be midline, dissect rectovaginal septum, and be adherent to vaginal fornix)
  3. Laparotomy, including total abdominal hysterectomy with bilateral salpingo-oophorectomy or unilateral salpingo-oophorectomy
  4. Evidence of ruptured tuboovarian abscess is a surgical emergency

DISPOSITION

- Of patients treated with medical therapy, response in 75%, with a 50% pregnancy rate. Pregnancy rate decreases with recurrent episodes.
- No response in 30% to 40%; can be treated with either CT-guided drainage or surgical intervention, keeping in mind that unilateral adnexectomy may give equal chance of cure versus hysterectomy, yet preserve reproductive potential.

REFERRAL

If patient has a tuboovarian abscess, refer to gynecologist.

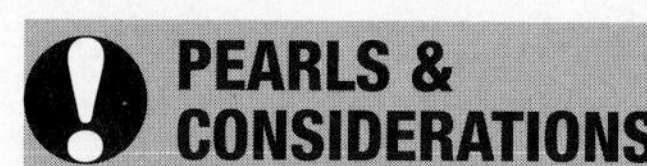

PEARLS & CONSIDERATIONS

COMMENTS

If *Actinomyces* species is isolated from culture, treatment with penicillin is required for an extended period (6 wk to 3 mo).

SUGGESTED READINGS

available at www.expertconsult.com

RELATED CONTENT

Pelvic Inflammatory Disease (Related Key Topic)
Pelvic Abscess (Patient Information)

AUTHORS: **SCOTT J. ZUCCALA, D.O.**, and **RUBEN ALVERO, M.D.**

BASIC INFORMATION

DEFINITION

A perirectal abscess is a localized inflammatory process that can be associated with infections of soft tissue and anal glands based on anatomic location. Perianal and perirectal abscesses may be simple or complex, causing suppuration. Infections in these spaces may be classified as superficial perianal or perirectal with involvement in the following anatomic spaces: ischiorectal, intersphincteric, perianal, and supralevator. The Parks classification of anorectal abscess is subdivided into intersphincteric, transsphincteric, suprasphincteric, and extrasphincteric abscess (Fig. 1-9).

SYNONYMS

Rectal abscess
Perianal abscess
Anorectal abscess

ICD-9CM CODES
566 Perirectal abscess
ICD-10CM CODES
K61.0 Anal abscess
K61.1 Rectal abscess

EPIDEMIOLOGY & DEMOGRAPHICS

INCIDENCE (IN U.S.): Commonly encountered
PREDOMINANT SEX: Male >female
PREDOMINANT AGE: All ages
PEAK INCIDENCE: Not seasonal; common
GENETICS: None known

PHYSICAL FINDINGS & CLINICAL PRESENTATION

- Localized perirectal or anal pain—often worsened with movement or straining
- Perirectal erythema or cellulitis
- Perirectal mass by inspection or palpation
- Fever and signs of sepsis with deep abscess
- Urinary retention

ETIOLOGY

- Polymicrobial aerobic and anaerobic bacteria involving one of the anatomic spaces (see "Definition"), often associated with localized trauma
- Microbiology: most bacteria are polymicrobial, mixed enteric and skin flora
- Predominant anaerobic bacteria:
  1. *Bacteroides fragilis*
  2. *Peptostreptococcus* spp.
  3. *Prevotella* spp.
  4. *Porphyromonas* spp.
  5. *Clostridium* spp.
  6. *Fusobacterium* spp.
- Predominant aerobic bacteria:
  1. *Staphylococcus aureus*
  2. *Streptococcus* spp.
  3. *Escherichia coli*
  4. *Enterococcus* spp.

DIAGNOSIS

Many patients will have predisposing underlying conditions including:

- Malignancy or leukemia
- Immune deficiency
- Diabetes mellitus
- Recent surgery
- Steroid therapy

DIFFERENTIAL DIAGNOSIS

- Neutropenic enterocolitis
- Crohn's disease (inflammatory bowel disease)
- Pilonidal disease
- Hidradenitis suppurativa
- Tuberculosis or actinomycosis; Chagas' disease
- Cancerous lesions
- Chronic anal fistula
- Rectovaginal fistula
- Proctitis—often STD-associated, including: syphilis, gonococcal, chlamydia, chancroid, condylomata acuminata
- AIDS-associated: Kaposi's sarcoma, lymphoma, CMV

WORKUP

- Examination of rectal, perirectal/perineal areas
- Rule out necrotic process and crepitance suggesting deep tissue involvement
- Local aerobic and anaerobic culture
- Blood cultures if toxic, febrile, or compromised
- Possible sigmoidoscopy

IMAGING STUDIES

Usually not indicated unless extensive disease abscess but can include CT. One study showed that CT had only a sensitivity of 77% and was particularly poor in detecting a perirectal abscess in immunocompromised patients.

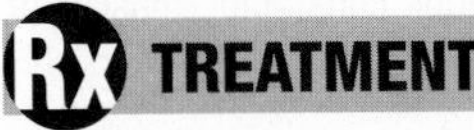

TREATMENT

ACUTE GENERAL Rx

- Incision and drainage of abscess
- Debridement if necrotic tissue
- Rule out need for fistulectomy
- Local wound care—packing
- Sitz baths

Antibiotic treatment: directed toward coverage for mixed skin and enteric flora

OUTPATIENT—ORAL:

- Trimethoprim/sulfamethoxazole DS bid or ciprofloxacin 750 mg bid or levofloxacin 750 mg q24h plus metronidazole 500 mg q6h x 7-10 days
- Amoxicillin/clavulanic acid 875 to 1000 mg 2 tabs bid
- Clindamycin 150 to 300 mg PO q8h ± ciprofloxacin

INPATIENT—INTRAVENOUS:

- Piperacillin/tazobactam 3.375 g IV q6 to 8h
- Ampicillin/sulbactam 1.5 to 3 g IV q6h
- Cefotetan 1 to 2 g IV q8h
- Imipenem or meropenem 500 to 1000 mg IV q8h

DISPOSITION

Follow-up with a general surgeon or infectious disease physician is often warranted.

REFERRAL

- General surgeon or colorectal surgeon for drainage.
- AIDS specialist may be needed for perirectal complications of HIV infection.
- Gastroenterologist follow-up may be warranted in Crohn's disease with perirectal fistula and other complications.

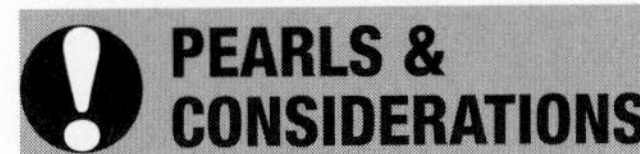

PEARLS & CONSIDERATIONS

Perirectal abscess may be a presenting manifestation of type 2 diabetes mellitus in older adults. Check the blood sugar in patients to exclude the possibility of undiagnosed diabetes mellitus.

SUGGESTED READINGS

available at www.expertconsult.com

RELATED CONTENT

Perirectal Abscess (Patient Information)

AUTHOR: **GLENN G. FORT, M.D., M.P.H.**

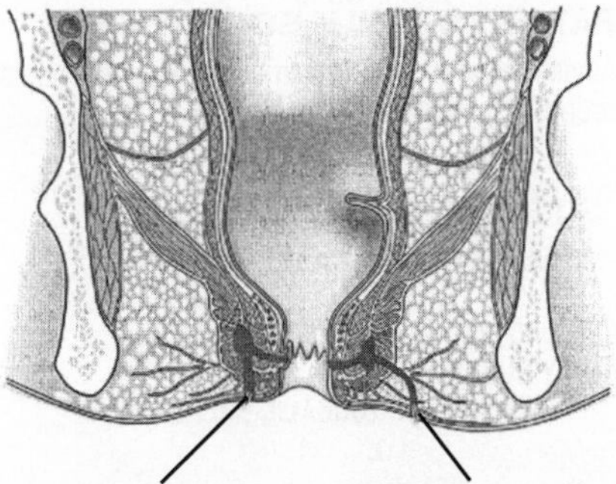

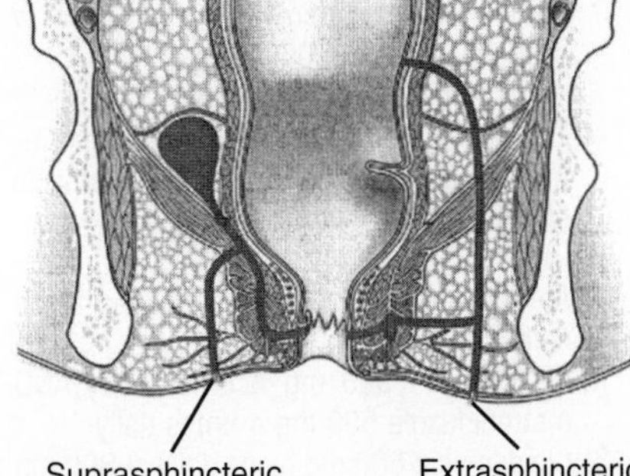

FIGURE 1-9 Parks classification of anorectal abscess. (From Cameron JL, Cameron AM: *Current surgical therapy,* ed 10, Philadelphia, 2011, Saunders.)

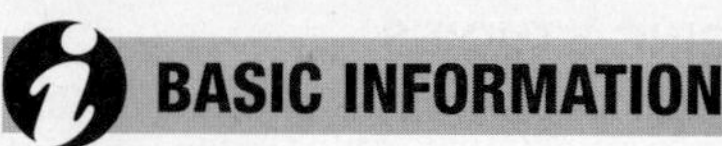

BASIC INFORMATION

DEFINITION

Peritonsillar abscess is an acute infection located between the capsule of the palatine tonsil and the superior constrictor muscle of the pharynx.

SYNONYMS

Quinsy, PTA

ICD-9CM CODES
475.0 Peritonsillar abscess
ICD-10CM CODES
J36 Peritonsillar abscess

EPIDEMIOLOGY & DEMOGRAPHICS

INCIDENCE (IN U.S.): 30:100,000/yr for ages 5-59. For adolescents, the incidence is 40:100,000/yr. It is the most common deep infection of the head and neck in children and adolescents, accounting for at least 50% of cases.

PEAK INCIDENCE: Bimodal frequency during the year, with highest occurrence from November to December and April to May.

PREVALENCE: 45,000 cases/yr in the United States

PREDOMINANT SEX: Male >female

PREDOMINANT AGE: Highest incidence is adults aged 20-40 yr.

RISK FACTORS: Smoking, periodontal disease, oropharyngeal or dental infection, male gender

PHYSICAL FINDINGS & CLINICAL PRESENTATION

- Sore throat, which may be severe and unilateral
- Dysphagia and odynophagia
- Otalgia on the side of abscess
- Foul-smelling breath
- Facial swelling
- Drooling
- Headache
- Fever
- Trismus
- Hoarseness, muffled voice (also called "hot potato voice")
- Tender submandibular and anterior cervical lymph nodes
- Tonsillar hypertrophy with likely peritonsillar edema
- Contralateral deflection of the uvula
- Stridor

ETIOLOGY

- Peritonsillar abscess is usually a complication of tonsillitis or acute bacterial pharyngitis caused by blockage of salivary ducts. Tonsillitis → peritonsillar cellulitis → peritonsillar abscess
- Group A β-hemolytic *Streptococcus* is the most common bacterial cause, accounting for 15% to 30% of cases in children and 5% to 10% of cases in adults.
- Less common aerobic causes are *Staphylococcus aureus, Haemophilus influenzae, Neisseria* species.
- The most common anaerobic organism is *Fusobacterium.*

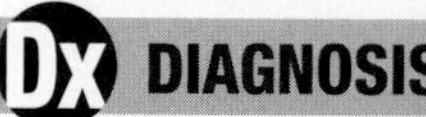

DIAGNOSIS

DIFFERENTIAL DIAGNOSIS

- Tonsillitis
- Infectious mononucleosis
- Peritonsillar cellulitis
- Retropharyngeal abscess
- Epiglottitis
- Dental abscess (retromolar)
- Lymphoma
- Ludwig's angina

WORKUP

- Based on history and physical exam
- Consider additional testing if presentation is less clear.

LABORATORY TESTS

- Consider rapid strep antigen testing and/or pharyngeal culture and sensitivity.
- Aspiration of the abscess for culture and sensitivity (see "Treatment" for role of aspiration in tx)

IMAGING STUDIES

- Consider ultrasound, CT scan (Fig. E1-10), or MRI to help differentiate abscess from cellulitis or mass
- Intraoral ultrasound may improve diagnosis and aspiration of peritonsillar abscess compared with visual inspection in adult patients.
- MRI provides better soft-tissue differentiation than CT

Rx TREATMENT

NONPHARMACOLOGIC THERAPY

- Drainage of the abscess by needle aspiration or by surgical incision and drainage

ACUTE GENERAL Rx

- Aspiration or surgical drainage AND antibiotics for 10 to 14 days
- Initial antibiotics should cover group A *Streptococcus* and anaerobes
  Intravenous
  - Piperacillin/tazobactam or ticarcillin/clavulanate. If penicillin allergic, use IV clindamycin (600-900 mg IV q8h).
  - Ampicillin-sulbactam 3 g q6h
  - Penicillin G 10 million units q6h AND metronidazole 500 mg q6h (may use clindamycin 900 mg q8h if penicillin allergic)

  OR oral
  - Amoxicillin-clavulanic acid 875 mg twice daily
  - Penicillin VK 500 mg 4 times daily AND metronidazole 500 mg 4 times daily
  - Clindamycin 600 mg twice daily or 300 mg 4 times daily
- Then appropriate selection of antibiotics should be guided by culture and sensitivity of the organism. Consulting local antimicrobial guidelines for resistance profiles is also advisable for empiric coverage before culture results are available.

CHRONIC Rx

- Tonsillectomy can be considered 3 to 6 mo after diagnosis of peritonsillar abscess with or without the diagnosis of recurrent tonsillitis.
- Though rare, in adults and children with an acute case of peritonsillar abscess and a history of recurrent pharyngitis or previous peritonsillar abscess, a specialist may recommend a *quinsy or hot tonsillectomy,* an immediate removal of the tonsils after starting IV antibiotics.

DISPOSITION

- Successful treatment is defined by symptomatic improvement in sore throat, fever, and/or tonsillar swelling within 24 hr of intervention.
- Treatment failure is defined by lack of symptomatic improvement or worsening despite 24 hr of antimicrobial therapy (with or without surgical drainage).

REFERRAL

- Consider ENT or diagnostic radiology for drainage of abscess.
- Consider ENT for tonsillectomy if criteria are met.

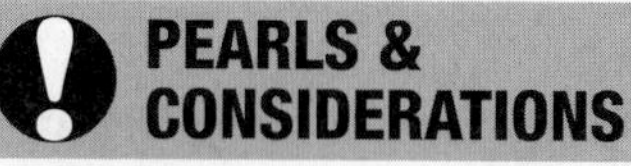

PEARLS & CONSIDERATIONS

COMMENTS

- Risk for a recurrence is immediate (within 4 days) and long term (2 to 3 yr).
- Most recurrences occur shortly after the initial presentation, suggesting continued infection rather than recurrence.
- Overall recurrence rate is 10% to 15%.
- Supportive treatment for pain control and hydration.

PREVENTION

- Adequate treatment of peritonsillar abscess.
- Up to 30% of patients with peritonsillar abscess meet criteria for tonsillectomy.

PATIENT/FAMILY EDUCATION

Advise family members to call with any trouble breathing, swallowing, or talking.

SUGGESTED READINGS
available at www.expertconsult.com

AUTHORS: **PETER J. SELL, D.O.,** and **AMITY RUBEOR, D.O.**

BASIC INFORMATION

DEFINITION

Renal abscess and perinephric abscess are a purulent complication of an underlying urinary infection of the ascending tract with an obstructed pyelonephritis. Predisposing factors include diabetes and renal stones. There is lobar necrosis with renal abscess and perirenal fat necrosis in perinephric abscess.

SYNONYMS

Intrarenal abscess
Perinephric abscess

ICD-9CM CODES
590.2 Renal and perinephric abscess
ICD-10CM CODES
N15.1 Renal and perinephric abscess

EPIDEMIOLOGY & DEMOGRAPHICS

INCIDENCE: Ranges from 1 to 10 per 10,000 hospital admissions
PREDOMINANT SEX AND AGE: In one study median age was 59.8 years
RISK FACTORS: Diabetes and renal stones

PHYSICAL FINDINGS & CLINICAL PRESENTATION

- Symptoms include fever, flank pain, abdominal pain, and urinary frequency or dysuria
- At times renal abscess can present insidiously in the elderly or persons with diabetes.

ETIOLOGY

These infections may be a complication of a urinary tract infection that ascends to the upper tract, usually due to gram-negative bacteria, or a complication of a bacteremia with hematogenous seeding to the kidney, usually secondary to a *Staphylococcus aureus* infection.

Dx DIAGNOSIS

DIFFERENTIAL DIAGNOSIS

- Acute pyelonephritis with papillary necrosis
- Acute lobar nephronia: acute nonsuppurative renal infection
- Renal cell carcinoma
- Malakoplakia: rare granulomatous inflammatory disease seen with *Escherichia coli* infection
- Emphysematous pyelonephritis: gas formation within the renal parenchyma caused by infection by facultative anaerobes or *Candida* spp.

WORKUP

Combination of laboratory tests and imaging

LABORATORY TESTS

- Blood cultures, urine cultures, urinalysis, and CBC are basic tests.
- Elevated ESR or C-reactive protein may be marker for a deep-seated infection.

IMAGING STUDIES

- Ultrasound may show thick-walled fluid-filled cavity in renal parenchyma. A perinephric abscess is confined to the perinephric space by Gerota's fascia.
- CT with contrast is preferred over ultrasound for the diagnosis (Fig. 1-11).
- MRI and nuclear scans are of limited value.

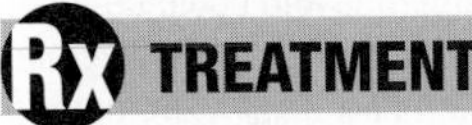

TREATMENT

Antibiotic therapy and, when necessary, interventional radiology or surgical drainage procedure

NONPHARMACOLOGIC THERAPY

- Therapy for a renal abscess greater than 5 cm in diameter should be percutaneous drainage by CT- or US-guided therapy along with intravenous antibiotics.
- A perinephric abscess should be drained percutaneously with CT or US guidance.
- At times a nephrectomy may be required for severe cases, usually in diabetic patients.

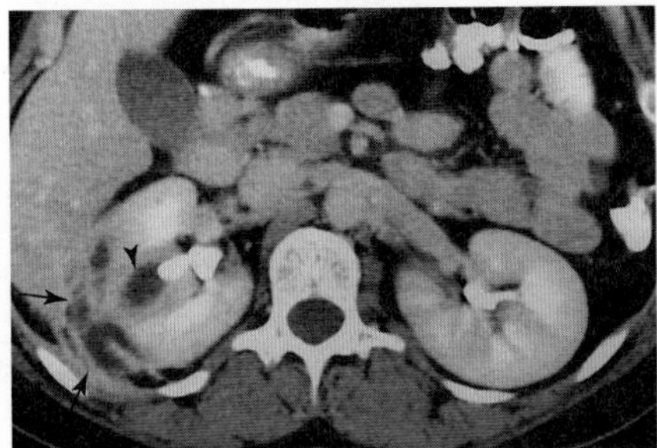

FIGURE 1-11 Renal abscess. Contrast-enhanced CT scan shows an abscess in the medulla of the kidney *(arrowhead)* with penetration and extension into the perinephric space *(arrows)*. (Courtesy L. Towner.)

ACUTE GENERAL Rx

A renal abscess less than 5 cm in diameter can be treated successfully with targeted intravenous therapy (92% success rate for abscess 3 to 5 cm in diameter). Antibiotic choices are based on culture results but initially should target gram-negative bacteria unless infection is secondary to staphylococcal bacteremia. Empiric antibiotic therapy in geographic areas where fluoroquinolone resistance rates are <10% consists of ciprofloxacin 400 mg IV loading dose. In areas with high fluoroquinolone resistance rates, ceftriaxone 1 g IV is appropriate. If perinephric abscess is associated with staphylococcal bacteremia, give IV nafcillin if methicillin-susceptible *Staphylococcus aureus* (MSSA) or vancomycin 1 g IV q12h if methicillin-resistant *S. aureus*.

CHRONIC RX

Antibiotic therapy generally continues for 2 to 3 weeks, some of which can be completed with oral therapy.

DISPOSITION

Antibiotics such as trimethoprim-sulfamethoxazole and quinolone antibiotics penetrate well in the kidney and are ideal oral agents for therapy.

REFERRAL

Interventional radiology, urologic surgeon, and infectious diseases consult

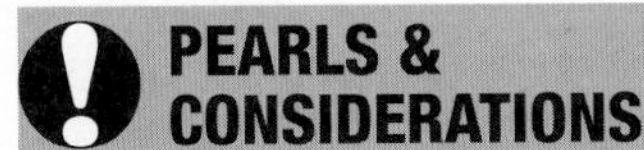

PEARLS & CONSIDERATIONS

COMMENTS

This diagnosis should be considered in patients who are being treated for pyelonephritis with appropriate antibiotics and fail to respond clinically after 5 days.

PREVENTION

Early and targeted therapy for urinary tract infections, especially in diabetic patients

SUGGESTED READINGS

available at www.expertconsult.com

RELATED CONTENT

Pyelonephritis (Related Key Topic)
Urinary Tract Infection (Related Key Topic)

AUTHOR: **GLENN G. FORT, M.D., M.P.H.**

BASIC INFORMATION

DEFINITION

Retropharyngeal abscess is a soft tissue infection of the throat involving retropharyngeal space. The anatomic boundaries of the retropharyngeal space are the middle layer of the deep cervical fascia (abutting the posterior esophageal wall) anteriorly and the deep layer of the deep cervical fascia posteriorly (Fig. 1-12). These two fasciae fuse inferiorly at the level between the first and second thoracic vertebrae.

ICD-9CM CODES
478.79
ICD-10CM CODES
J39.0 Retropharyngeal and parapharyngeal abscess

EPIDEMIOLOGY & DEMOGRAPHICS

Retropharyngeal abscess occurs most commonly in children between the ages of 2 and 4 yr, analogous to suppurative cervical adenitis. This represents the peak age group for numerous viral upper respiratory tract infections and their attendant complications, acute otitis media and sinusitis. Retropharyngeal space infection is less common in older children and adults because the lymph nodes atrophy by the age of 3 to 4 yr.

PHYSICAL FINDINGS & CLINICAL PRESENTATION

- The onset of a retropharyngeal infection may be insidious, with little more than fever, irritability, drooling, a muffled voice (dysphonia), or possibly nuchal rigidity.
- The acute symptoms relate to pressure and inflammation produced by the abscess on either the airway or the upper digestive tract and pharynx. The patient may have intense dysphagia, drooling, and odynophagia, or there may be some element of respiratory distress from edema and inflammation of the airway (stridor, tachypnea, or both).
- Unwillingness to move the neck because of discomfort is often a prominent presenting feature and should lead to consideration of retropharyngeal abscess if the child is febrile and irritable.
- Extension of the neck is usually affected more than flexion. This causes the patient to hold his or her neck stiffly or to present with torticollis.
- Trismus is unusual.
- On physical examination it may be possible to appreciate midline or unilateral swelling of the posterior pharyngeal wall. The mass may be fluctuant to the examining finger, and care must be taken to avoid rupture of the abscess into the upper airway.

Complications are numerous and could be fatal; these include airway obstruction, septicemia, thrombosis of the internal jugular vein, carotid artery rupture, and acute necrotizing mediastinitis. Aspiration with resultant pneumonia may complicate retropharyngeal abscess if rupture of the abscess occurs and empties into the airway. Infection can spread from one space in the neck to another.

The most dreaded complication is jugular vein suppurative thrombophlebitis (Lemierre's syndrome), in which the vessels of the carotid sheath become infected, leading to bacteremia and metastatic spread of infection to the lungs, brain, and mediastinum.

ETIOLOGY

- The retropharyngeal space comprises two chains of lymph nodes that drain the nasopharynx, adenoids, posterior paranasal sinuses, middle ear, and eustachian tube. Accordingly, suppurative infections in these areas may provide the seeds for infection for retropharyngeal abscess.
- The predominant bacterial species are *Streptococcus pyogenes* (group A *Streptococcus*), *Staphylococcus aureus*, and respiratory anaerobes (including *Fusobacteria, Prevotella,* and *Veillonella* species). *Haemophilus* species are also occasionally found.
- In young children, infection usually reaches this space by lymphatic spread from a septic focus in the pharynx or sinuses.
- In adults, infection may reach the retropharyngeal space from either local or distant sites. Penetrating trauma (e.g., from chicken bones or iatrogenic) is the usual source of local spread. More distant sources of infection include odontogenic sepsis and peritonsillar abscess (now a rare cause).

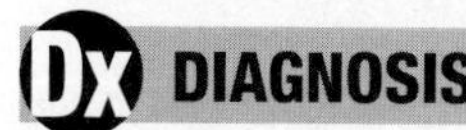

DIAGNOSIS

DIFFERENTIAL DIAGNOSIS

- Cervical osteomyelitis
- Pott's disease
- Meningitis
- Calcific tendonitis of the long muscle of the neck

IMAGING STUDIES

- A lateral neck film may be helpful in delineating the presence of a retropharyngeal abscess and may demonstrate cervical lordosis; the retropharyngeal space is considered widened and pathologic if it is greater than 7 mm at C2 or 14 mm at C6 (Fig. 1-13).
  - There must be attention to technical issues when performing the study, especially in children. The film should be a perfect

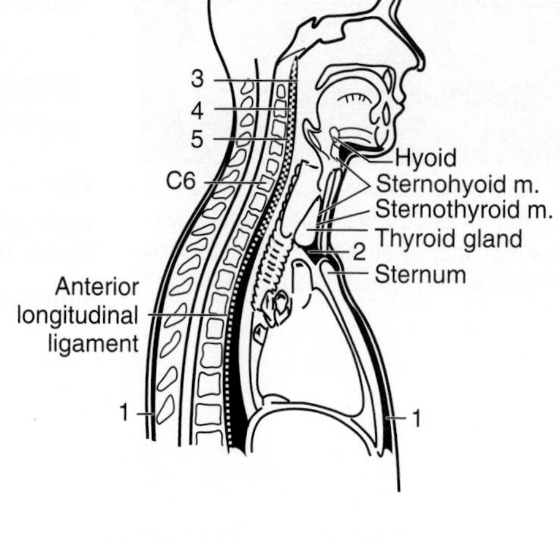

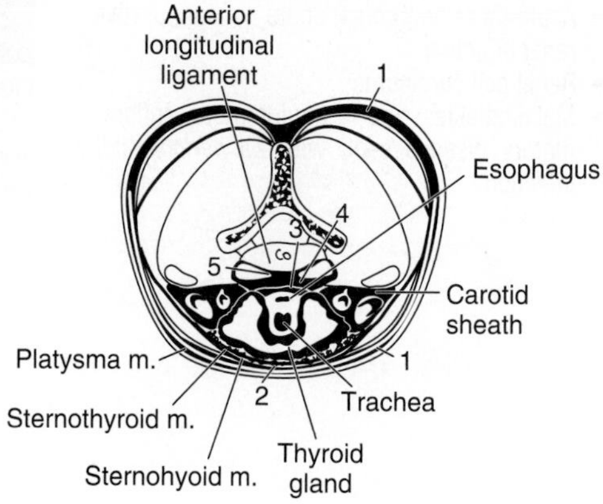

FIGURE 1-12 Relation of various cervical fascial spaces to the superficial and deep layers of the cervical fascia. A, Cross section of the neck at the level of the thyroid isthmus. **B,** Coronal section in the suprahyoid region of the neck. *1,* Superficial space; *2,* pretracheal space; *3,* retropharyngeal space; *4,* "danger" space; *5,* prevertebral space.

lateral, and the child must keep the neck in extension during inspiration to avoid a false thickening of the retropharyngeal space. Crying, particularly in infants, may also cause false thickening of the retropharyngeal space.

- A CT scan of the neck is the best tool to identify abscesses in the retropharyngeal area, but it is not perfect. Both the sensitivity and specificity of the CT scan in predicting the presence of drainable purulent material are quite variable from study to study, ranging between 68% and 100%.
  - The CT scan provides more information than the plain radiograph because it can generally differentiate between retropharyngeal cellulitis and retropharyngeal abscess and can demonstrate extension of the retropharyngeal abscess to contiguous spaces in the neck. Findings on CT common to both cellulitis and abscess are a low-density core, soft tissue swelling, obliterated fat planes, and mass effect. The best differential finding on CT scan is "complete rim enhancement," which is indicative of abscess (Fig. 1-14). The abscess may be seen as a mass impinging on the posterior pharyngeal wall.

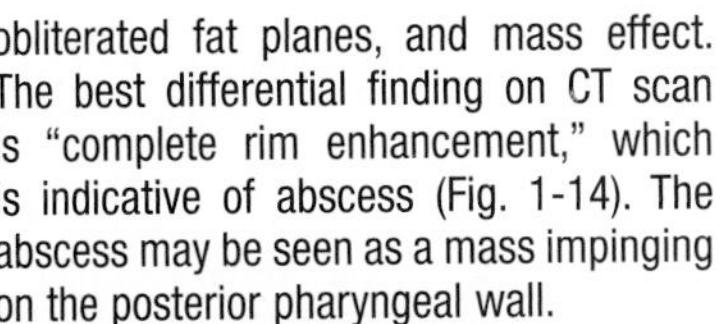

- MRI of the neck is more sensitive than CT, and technetium scanning can be helpful in detecting bone involvement. T2-weighted images may identify and localize areas of pus for drainage or aspiration. Gadolinium enhancement is important to accurately define the soft tissue component. Finally, MRI is useful for imaging vascular lesions, such as jugular thrombophlebitis.

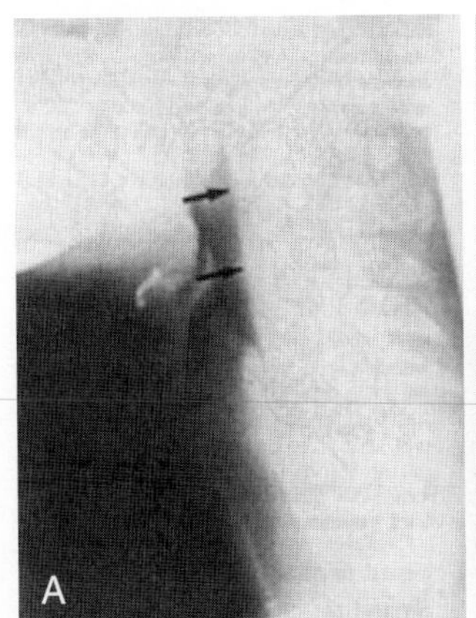

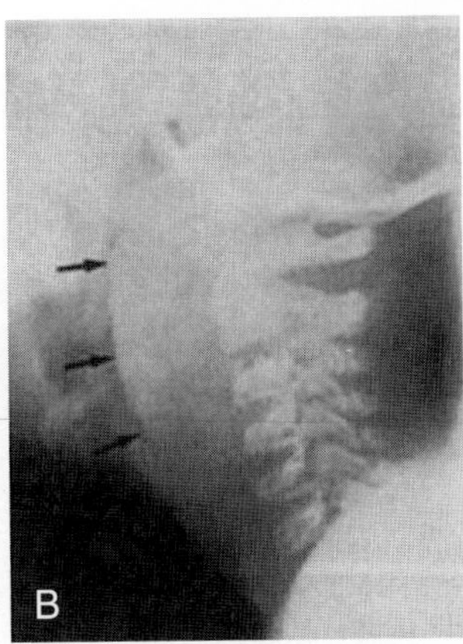

FIGURE 1-13 Lateral radiographs of the neck show normal lateral cervical view **(A)** and expansion of the prevertebral soft tissues by a retropharyngeal abscess **(B).**

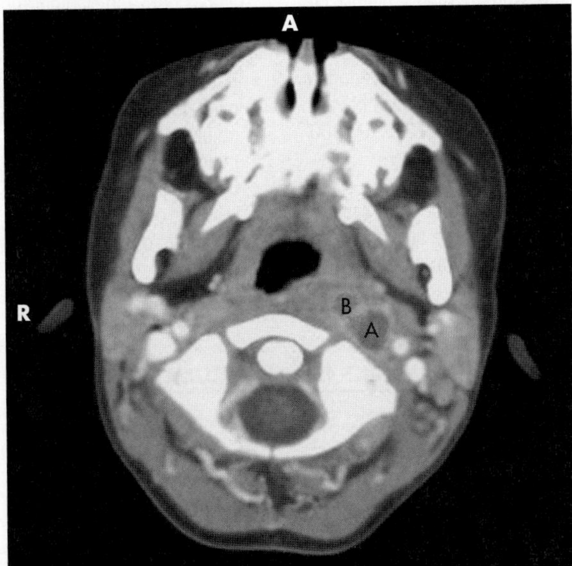

FIGURE 1-14 CT scan of a retropharyngeal abscess (*A* and *B*) demonstrates a low-density core, soft tissue swelling, obliterated fat planes, mass effect, and rim enhancement.

Rx TREATMENT

ACUTE GENERAL & CHRONIC Rx

- High-dose penicillin (2 million to 4 million units IV q4h) plus metronidazole (500 mg IV q8h) or ampicillin-sulbactam (50 mg/kg/dose IV q6h) or clindamycin (13 mg/kg/dose IV q8h) are effective antimicrobial selections. Parenteral treatment is maintained until the patient is afebrile and clinically improved. Antibiotics should be adjusted as culture data become available, and oral therapy is continued to complete at least a 14-day course.
- Surgical intervention has historically played a prominent role in the management of retropharyngeal abscess in conjunction with antibiotic therapy. Drainage is indicated when there is a large hypodense area or when a patient has not responded to parenteral therapy alone.
- When the CT does not demonstrate a large hypodense area, a trial of antibiotic therapy without drainage is appropriate. Some investigators also support a trial of IV antibiotic therapy alone when small abscesses are identified by CT scans as long as there is no compromise of the airway.

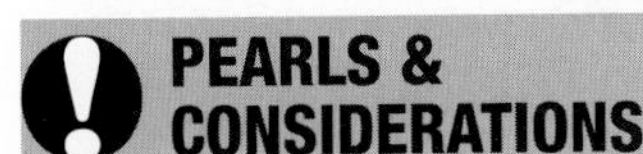

PEARLS & CONSIDERATIONS

PREVENTION

The complications of deep neck infection in any space are numerous and potentially fatal. Early diagnosis, with prompt and appropriate management, is key to avoiding these complications.

AUTHOR: **RUBY K. SATPATHY, M.D.**

BASIC INFORMATION

DEFINITION

Definition from the Federal Child Abuse Prevention and Treatment Act (CAPTA): any recent act or failure to act on the part of a parent or caretaker that results in death, serious physical or emotional harm, sexual abuse or exploitation of a child; or an act or failure to act which presents an imminent risk of serious harm to a child.

- Neglect: failure to provide for the basic needs of a child
  1. Physical neglect: failure to provide necessary food, shelter, and supervision
  2. Medical neglect: failure to provide necessary medical or mental health care
  3. Educational neglect: failure to meet educational needs
  4. Emotional neglect: failure to attend to emotional needs, exposure to domestic violence
- Physical abuse: physical injury inflicted by a parent or caregiver intentionally or in the course of excessive discipline
- Sexual abuse: sexual act inflicted by parent or caretaker; includes exploitation and pornography
- Emotional/psychological abuse: pattern of behavior of caretaker toward a child that impairs emotional development. This includes verbal abuse, cruelty, and threats. Difficult to prove. Almost always present when other forms of abuse occur.
- Abandonment: child left and parents' whereabouts unknown.
- Substance abuse: includes: prenatal exposure to mother's use of illicit drugs; manufacture of methamphetamine in the presence of a child; selling or giving drugs to a child; use of mood-altering substance by caregivers that impairs their ability to provide care for their child.

SYNONYMS

Child maltreatment syndrome
Physical abuse
Sexual abuse
Battered child syndrome
Shaken baby syndrome
Shaken impact syndrome
Abusive head trauma

Complex coding categorized as physical, psychological, sexual

ICD-9-CM and DSM-5 CODES

995.51-995.54

ICD-10CM CODES

T74.9 Maltreatment syndrome, unspecified
T74.3 Psychological abuse
T74.2 Sexual abuse

EPIDEMIOLOGY & DEMOGRAPHICS

INCIDENCE (IN U.S.): Any reports of incidence are underestimates because many cases are not recognized or reported. The following data are based on Child Protective Services (CPS) state aggregate as reported in *Child Maltreatment 2011*. In 2011, roughly 676,569 unique children were determined to be victims of abuse or neglect. This is a rate of 9.1 unduplicated victims per 1000 children.

- Types of abuse by percentage (note the total is greater than 100% since children are often victims of more than one type of abuse).
  1. Neglect: 78.5%
  2. Physical abuse: 17.6%
  3. Sexual abuse: 9.1%
  4. Psychological abuse: 9%
  5. Medical neglect: 2.2%
  6. Other: 10.1% (e.g., abandonment, threats of harm, congenital drug addiction)
- For 2011, an estimated 1570 child deaths were caused by abuse or neglect.
  - Overall annual death rate resulting from abuse or neglect is estimated to be 2.1 deaths/100,000 children.
  - 71% of these deaths were due to neglect alone or in combination with other forms of abuse; 48% were due to physical abuse; alone or in combination.
  - 81.6% of these children were younger than 4 yr of age with 42% less than 1 yr old.
  - Most fatalities were directly caused by one or both parents (78%).
  - Many child abuse fatalities are underreported because of misdiagnosis or variations in state definitions and coding.
- 80% of abused children were victimized by one or both of their parents.
- One fifth of adult women report history of molestation or sexual assault as a child or adolescent.

PREDOMINANT SEX: There is a slight predominance of girls as victims. However, boys have a higher child fatality rate than girls (2.5/100,000 for boys and 1.8/100,000 for girls)

PREDOMINANT AGE: Youngest children (0 to 3 yr old) have the highest rates of victimization with 27% being younger than the age of 3.

GENETICS: No known genetic factors.

ETIOLOGY

Multiple factors contribute to the incidence. No factor or combination of factors can definitively predict which children will be victimized. Factors contributing to risk of abuse or neglect include the following:

- Parent
  1. Substance abuse
  2. Mental illness
  3. Intellectual impairment
  4. Parental history of being abused as a child
- Child
  1. Low birth weight or prematurity
  2. Chronic physical disability
- Family
  1. Social isolation
  2. Poor parent-child bonding
  3. Stress: unemployment, chronic illness, eviction, arrest, poverty
  4. Domestic violence
- Community/society
  1. Limited transportation
  2. Limited day care
  3. Unsafe neighborhoods
  4. Poverty

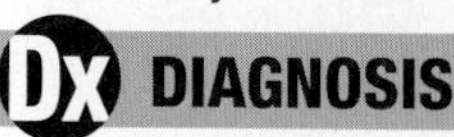

DIAGNOSIS

Careful history and physical examination are the most important aspects of the evaluation. Careful documentation of any statements regarding origin of injuries or history of abuse is crucial. Chart and photographic documentation of injuries is also essential. The following are keys to the final diagnosis:

- Patterned bruising (e.g., loop-shaped, square, oval) is indicative of being struck with an object (Fig. 1-15).
- Injury observed is incompatible with the history provided.
- History of injury provided is incompatible with the developmental capabilities of the child.

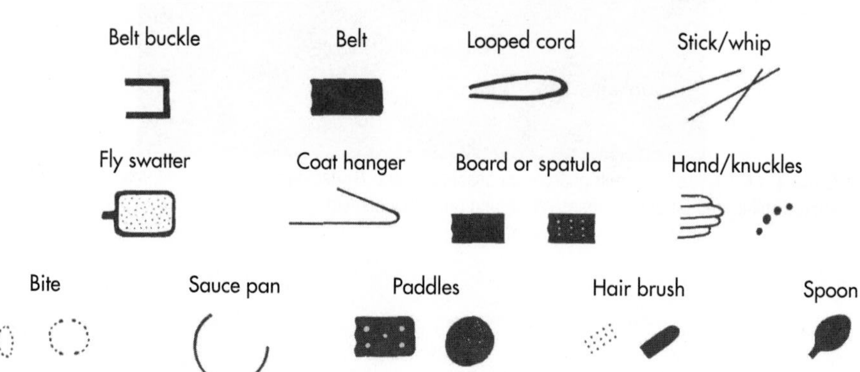

FIGURE 1-15 A variety of instruments may be used to inflict injury on a child. Often the choice of an instrument is a matter of convenience. Marks tend to silhouette or outline the shape of the instrument. The possibility of intentional trauma should prompt a high degree of suspicion when injuries to a child are geometric, paired, mirrored, of various ages or types, or on relatively protected parts of the body. Early recognition of intentional trauma is important to provide therapy and prevent escalation to more serious injury. (From Kliegman RM et al: *Nelson textbook of pediatrics,* ed 19, Philadelphia, 2011, Saunders.)

A

Diseases and Disorders I

- Delay in seeking care for a significant injury (e.g., callus formation on a fracture, eschar formation on a burn).
- Bruising is rare in healthy preambulatory infants and warrants further investigation.
- Multiple significant injuries of different ages.
- Infant with clinically significant head trauma attributed to a trivial cause (e.g., a short fall). Often associated with retinal hemorrhages and skeletal fractures, which are indicative of shaken baby syndrome or abusive head trauma.
- Certain fractures in infants without a history of significant trauma (e.g., motor vehicle accident) are characteristic of abuse: metaphyseal, rib, sternum, scapula, vertebral body.
- Inflicted contact burns are indicated by an impression of the burning object: lighter, iron, cigarette (Fig. 1-16).
- Inflicted immersion burns are indicated by "stocking" burns of the feet or "glove" burns of the hands. Stocking burns are often associated with buttocks/perineal burns from immersion of a minor in a flexed position.
- Most sexual abuse victims will have a normal or nonspecific genital examination. A normal genital examination does not mean the child was not abused. History is the most important part of the diagnosis. Forensic interview by a trained professional is recommended, as is an examination by a health care provider experienced in child sexual abuse evaluations for child and adolescent victims of sexual abuse.
- The identification of a sexually transmitted disease in a prepubertal child who is beyond the neonatal period is suggestive of sexual abuse. Reporting and further careful investigation are warranted. Consult current CDC guidelines and a child sexual abuse expert for further guidance.

DIFFERENTIAL DIAGNOSIS

In all categories, accidental injury is the most common entity to be distinguished from abuse. Accidental injuries are most common over bony prominences: forehead, elbows, knees, shins; soft, fleshy areas are more common for inflicted injury: buttocks, thighs, upper arms. Table 1-5 describes patterns of injury.

BRUISING

- Bleeding disorder (idiopathic thrombocytopenic purpura, hemophilia, leukemia, hemorrhagic disease of the newborn, von Willebrand's disease)
- Connective tissue disorder (Ehlers-Danlos syndrome, vasculitis)
- Pigments (Mongolian spots)
- Dermatitis (phytophotodermatitis, nickel allergy)
- Folk treatment (coining, cupping)

BURNS

- Chemical burn
- Impetigo
- Folk treatment (moxibustion)
- Dermatitis (phytophotodermatitis)

INTRACRANIAL HEMORRHAGE

- Bleeding disorder
- Perinatal trauma (should resolve by 4 wk)
- Arteriovenous malformation rupture
- Glutaric aciduria

FRACTURES

- Osteogenesis imperfecta
- Rickets
- Congenital syphilis
- Very low birth weight (osteopenia of prematurity)

SEXUAL ABUSE

- Normal variants
- Lichen sclerosis et atrophicus
- Congenital abnormalities
- Urethral prolapse
- Hemangioma
- Nonsexually acquired infection (group A *Streptococcus, Shigella*)

WORKUP (Fig. E1-17)

History and physical examination:

- Careful history from all caretakers and child.
- Scene investigation may be necessary.
- Complete physical examination.
- Sexual abuse: forensic interview and magnified examinations by trained professionals are the standard for evaluation and evidence collection. This is especially important to avoid further psychological or physical trauma to the child.

Laboratory tests to assess for bleeding disorder in the case of children with suspicious bruising. These tests may not be necessary if the abuse was witnessed or if the child has clear patterned bruising or other indicators of physical abuse:

- CBC with differential and platelets.
- Prothrombin time, activated partial thromboplastin time.
- Von Willebrand factor antigen and activity
- Factor VIII and IX levels
- Alanine aminotransferase, amylase, urinalysis should be considered in infants or other children with abdominal bruising to look for evidence of internal injury to the liver, pancreas, or kidneys.

Laboratory tests to assess for bleeding disorder in the case of children with suspicious ICH. These tests may not be necessary if the abuse was witnessed or if the child has clear patterned bruising or other indicators of physical abuse:

- CBC with differential and platelets.
- Prothrombin time, activated partial thromboplastin time.
- Factor VIII and IX levels
- DIC Panel
- Consultation with a child abuse expert physician should be strongly considered to ensure that appropriate medical evaluation is carried out in children with suspicion of abusive head trauma.

Laboratory tests for sexual abuse:

- If within 72 hr of acute sexual assault/abuse, swabs are obtained from the oropharynx, areas of skin exposure (use an alternate light source to ID), genitalia, and rectum to send to the crime lab for DNA and other testing. Also collect samples of foreign hair, blood, saliva, or other tissue if present. A wet mount from cervical/vaginal specimen should be done to look for motile sperm.
- Per current CDC recommendations, adolescent victims of acute assault should have appropriate specimens collected from sites of penetration or attempted penetration for *Neisseria gonorrheae* and *Chlamydia.* Nucleic acid amplification tests (NAATs) may be used and are preferred. In females, wet mount and culture or POC testing of vaginal swab for

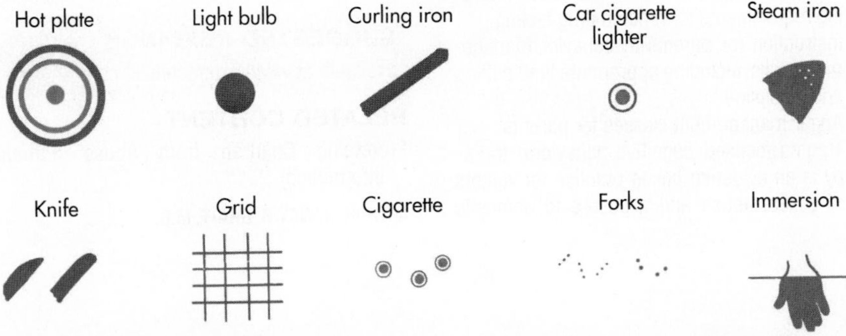

FIGURE 1-16 Marks from heated objects cause burns in a pattern that duplicates that of the object. Familiarity with the common heated objects that are used to traumatize children facilitates recognition of possible intentional injuries. The location of the burn is important in determining its cause. Children tend to explore surfaces with the palmar surface of the hand and rarely touch a heated object repeatedly or for a long time. (From Kliegman RM et al: *Nelson textbook of pediatrics,* ed 19, Philadelphia, 2011, Saunders.)

TABLE 1-5 Patterns of Injury

Accidental	Nonaccidental
Unilateral	Bilateral/symmetrical
Isolated injury	Multiple injuries
Amorphous shape	Well-defined shape
Prominent bone areas	Soft tissue areas
Posterior aspect of body	Anterior aspect of body
One age of injury	Multiple ages of injury

From Fuhrman BP et al: *Pediatric critical care,* ed 4, Philadelphia, 2011, Saunders.

T. vaginalis should also be done. If there is itching, vaginal discharge or malodor present, wet mount for bacterial vaginosis and *Candida* should also be done. Serum should be obtained for HIV, hepatitis B, and syphilis testing acutely. If negative, HIV and syphilis testing should be repeated 6, 12, and 24 wk after the assault.

- Child victims (i.e., prepubertal) should have specimens collected if considered high risk for a sexually transmitted infection (STI) per current CDC recommendations. Cervical specimens are not collected and vaginal specimens must be collected with care by an experienced provider to avoid further trauma to the child. Gonorrhea and *Chlamydia* culture is the gold standard for diagnosis and legal purposes. However, many providers now analyze specimens using urine or vaginal NAAT followed by culture confirmation or 2nd NAAT if any positive results are obtained. Any culture testing positive for *N. gonorrheae* should be confirmed by at least two laboratory tests that are based on different principles. Specimens should be collected for gonorrhea and *Chlamydia,* wet mount, and blood for serologic testing (HIV, hepatitis B, syphilis) in the following cases:
  1. Child has a past or current symptom of an STI, such as vaginal discharge, genital ulcer, or vaginal pain or currently diagnosed STI
  2. Alleged assailant is known to have an STI or be at high risk for an STI
  3. A sibling or adult in the same household has a known STI
  4. Evidence of ejaculation or of oral, genital, and/or anal penetration is present on the examination
  5. Child or parent requests testing

IMAGING STUDIES

Physical abuse:

- Radiographic skeletal survey for all children up to 2 yr; for 2- to 5-yr-olds, done only for severe abuse. Consider repeat skeletal survey in 2 wk if severe physical injury is present.
- Noncontrast head CT scan or MRI for all children <1 yr; for children over 1 yr, clinical judgment should be used.
- Head MRI for children with significant abusive head trauma. This is used as an adjunct a few days after initial head CT.
- Abdominal CT scan if indicated by clinical examination or laboratory evaluation.
- Box E1-2 describes the specificity of radiologic findings for child abuse.

Rx TREATMENT

ACUTE GENERAL Rx

- Stabilize and treat acute medical injuries.
- Report to Child Protective Services. HIPAA allows reports for suspected child abuse without parental authorization.
- Early report to law enforcement for suspected physical abuse or sexual abuse to allow scene investigation.
- Disposition, once medically stable, is dependent on CPS. The child cannot be returned home if the environment is not safe.
- Physician should remain available to discuss with investigators. This is often critical to determining the outcome of the case and placement of the child.
- Because follow-up of adolescent sexual assault victims can be difficult, many experts recommend empiric treatment for STIs: gonorrhea, *Chlamydia, Trichomonas,* and bacterial vaginosis. Pregnancy prophylaxis should also be offered. Hepatitis B immunization should be offered if not previously given. HIV prophylaxis is offered in certain situations depending on local epidemiology and type of assault. Consult local infectious disease experts for current recommendations. Repeat examination should be done in 2 wk for all victims of sexual assault, especially if they declined empiric treatment. If empiric treatment was not done, STI testing should be repeated at the 2-week follow-up visit.
- Empiric treatment of child victims of sexual abuse is generally not recommended. This is especially important if NAATs are used for screening for STIs because confirmation is necessary for any positive results. Careful follow-up within 2 wk and treatment based on culture results are indicated. HIV prophylaxis is offered in certain circumstances according to local epidemiology and risk. Consult with a local infectious disease expert for further recommendations.

CHRONIC Rx

- Often depends on CPS and court-ordered interventions
- Treatment of parental mental illness
- Treatment of parental substance abuse, including requirements for random drug testing
- Instruction for parents in behavior management skills, including appropriate limit setting and discipline
- Anger management classes for parents
- Trauma-focused cognitive-behavioral therapy is an evidence-based practice for victims of sexual abuse and exposure to domestic violence; useful to include nonoffending parent/caregiver
- Ongoing individual and family therapy
  - Parent-child interactive therapy is an evidence-based practice that is used with young children with behavioral problems and parent-child relationship problems
  - Child-parent psychotherapy is an evidence-based practice that is for young children (<5 yr) who have experienced a trauma and their caregivers
- May need long-term placement in foster care before it is safe to return home. In extreme cases of abuse, parental rights may be terminated without offering services.

OUTCOMES

- Victims of chronic abuse and neglect:
  - Have higher rates of mental illness (depression, suicide, posttraumatic stress disorder, eating disorders)
  - Have more cognitive difficulties, often impaired academic performance
  - Are more likely to become aggressive
  - Are more likely as adults to have adverse physical health outcomes (cardiovascular disease, cancer, STDs)
- Victims of abusive head trauma:
  - One third die, one third have severe disability, one third appear normal in the short term.

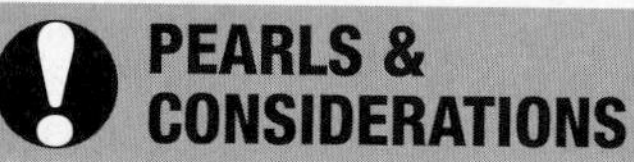

PEARLS & CONSIDERATIONS

PREVENTION

- Home visitation by a specially trained nurse to high-risk families during pregnancy and infancy has shown positive outcomes (Nurse-Family Partnership).
- Anticipatory guidance at health visits to teach normal developmental expectations and appropriate discipline.
- Screening to identify at-risk or abused children.
- Targeted education in the newborn nursery for shaken baby prevention has been shown to be effective.
- Substance abuse prevention and treatment.
- Identification and intervention for domestic violence before children are born.

SUGGESTED READINGS

available at www.expertconsult.com

RELATED CONTENT

Protecting Children from Abuse (Patient Information)

AUTHOR: **NANCY R. GRAFF, M.D.**

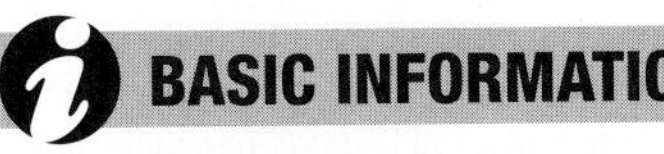

BASIC INFORMATION

DEFINITION

Drug abuse is a recurring pattern of harmful use of a substance despite adverse consequences to work, school, relationships, the legal system, or physical health. This may occur concurrently with or independently from *substance dependence,* in which the impairment or distress is more pervasive and often (though not necessarily) includes physical dependence and withdrawal symptoms (Table 1-6).

SYNONYMS

Substance use disorder
Substance abuse
Addiction

> **ICD-9CM and DSM-5 codes are defined by specific substance.**
> **ICD-10CM CODES**
> F19.129 Other psychoactive substance abuse, unspecified
> F10-F19 Defined by specific substance
> The new term *substance use disorder* in the fifth edition of the *Diagnostic and Statistical Manual of Mental Disorders* (DSM-5) combines the categories of substance abuse and substance dependence into a single disorder measured on a continuum from mild to severe.

EPIDEMIOLOGY & DEMOGRAPHICS

INCIDENCE (IN U.S.): Alcohol or drug dependence: 5% to 10% of population
PREVALENCE (IN U.S.): Approximately 15% of patients in primary care practice have an at-risk pattern of drug and/or alcohol use; lifetime prevalence of any alcohol use disorder: 30%; prescription drug misuse is on the rise with 5% past-year prevalence.
PREDOMINANT SEX: Males >females
PREDOMINANT AGE:
- Problematic use of substances may begin in early life (8 to 10 yr).
- Mean age of onset of problem drinking is approximately 25 yr for men and 30 yr for women.

PEAK INCIDENCE: For most substances: age 15 to 30 yr

TABLE 1-6 Key Features of Substance Abuse

1. The substance is often taken in larger amounts over a longer period than intended
2. Unsuccessful efforts to cut down
3. A great deal of time spent obtaining the substance or recovering from its effects
4. Craving
5. Social, occupational, or recreational
6. Recurrent despite hazards
7. Tolerance or withdrawal

Reprinted from Goldman L, Bennett JC (eds): *Cecil textbook of medicine,* ed 22, Philadelphia, 2004, Saunders.

DURATION OF CONDITION:
- Men: average >20 yr of heavy drinking
- Women: average 15 yr of heavy drinking
- In general, substance use disorders are chronic and relapsing and often progressive

GENETICS: There is evidence of nonspecific genetic factors. Addiction may result in part from underlying, inherited abnormalities in brain structure that impair behavior control and encourage impulsive behavior.

PHYSICAL FINDINGS & CLINICAL PRESENTATION

- Polysubstance use and comorbidity with psychiatric disorders are common.
- History often reveals recurring behavioral problems, such as relationship, work, or legal problems; violence and traumatic injuries; and anxiety, depression, insomnia, and cognitive and memory dysfunction.
- Repeated requests for early refills of controlled substances and obtaining prescriptions from multiple providers should raise concern for prescription drug abuse (Table 1-7).
- Physical findings may include injection marks, nasal lesions or recurrent epistaxis, poor dentition, scars or bruises from falls or trauma, and poor nutritional status; signs/symptoms of intoxication or withdrawal are highly suggestive of substance use disorder.

ETIOLOGY

Several models of addiction have been proposed:
1. Disease model: Addiction is a mental illness, which occurs as a result of the impairment of healthy neurochemical or behavioral processes.
2. Genetic model: Genetic predisposition is often a factor in dependency and certain addictive behaviors.
3. Social model: Person–environment interactions (i.e., socialization, imitation of observable behavior, and the influence of modeling) shape addictive behavior.

Dx DIAGNOSIS

DIFFERENTIAL DIAGNOSIS

- Psychiatric disorders such as depression, mania, psychosis, and anxiety disorders may coexist or occur as a consequence of substance use.
- Rule out seizure disorder and underlying illness.

WORKUP

- A thorough history is crucial for diagnosis.
- The physician's history-taking style and techniques strongly affect patient's willingness to report use and participate in future treatment activities.
- A structured, nonjudgmental approach is generally preferable:
  1. Ask about quantity and frequency of alcohol or drug use. For example, the National Institute on Alcohol Abuse and Alcoholism (NIAAA) declares that *problem drinking* is defined as more than 2 drinks per day for men and more than 1 drink per day for women or anyone older than 65 yr.
  2. Use a short screening instrument such as the CAGE questionnaire ("1. Have you ever felt you need to Cut down on your alcohol or drug use? 2. Have people Annoyed you by criticizing your alcohol or drug use? 3. Have you ever felt Guilty about alcohol or drug use? 4. Have you ever felt you need to drink first thing in the morning [Eye opener] to stop shakiness?").

TABLE 1-7 "Red Flags" for Abuse Behavior and Opioid Addiction

Potential Abuse/Addiction Behaviors*

1. Patient displays an overwhelming focus on opioid issues during clinic visits that occupies a significant proportion of the clinic visit and impedes progress with other pain issues or medical problems.
2. Patient has a pattern of early refills (three or more) or escalating drug use in the absence of acute change or progression of his or her medical condition.
3. Patient generates multiple telephone calls or unscheduled visits to request more opioids, early refills, or problems associated with the opioid prescription that often creates a disturbance of the clinic staff.
4. There is a pattern of prescription problems with reports of medications lost, spilled, or stolen.
5. Patient has supplemental sources of opioids from multiple providers, emergency departments, or illegal sources.

Additional "Red Flag" Abuse Behavior

1. Selling prescribed medications
2. Prescription forgery
3. Stealing another patient's medications
4. Injecting or snorting oral medication
5. Concurrent use of illicit drug(s)
6. Appears intoxicated or oversedated
7. Insists on obtaining a specific opioid medication

*Adapted from Chabal criteria for opioid abuse.
From Hochberg MC et al: *Rheumatology,* ed 5, St Louis, 2011, Mosby.

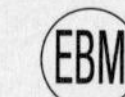

- Problematic behavior during intoxication or withdrawal is diagnostic.
- Because self-report of substance use and its consequences can be unreliable, obtaining corroborating information, such as from family members, past detoxifications, or drug rehabilitations is often helpful.
- Adolescent drug abuse detection and treatment is extremely challenging. Stages of adolescent substance use are described in Table 1-8. An assessment for evaluating the seriousness of adolescent drug abuse is described in Table 1-9.

LABORATORY TESTS

- Blood alcohol content (BAC) measured on the breath is practical to define intoxication and provides a rough measure of impairment.
- Obtain toxicology screen in urine or blood samples.
- Biologic markers such as elevated mean corpuscular volume (MCV), g-glutamyltransferase (GGT), liver function tests (AST and ALT), and carbohydrate deficient transferrin (CDT) may also be used to diagnose and monitor.

TABLE 1-8 Stages of Adolescent Substance Abuse

Stage	Description
1	Potential for abuse • Decreased impulse control • Need for immediate gratification • Available drugs, alcohol, inhalants • Need for peer acceptance
2	Experimentation: learning the euphoria • Use of inhalants, tobacco, marijuana, and alcohol with friends • Few, if any, consequences • Use may increase to weekends regularly • Little change in behavior
3	Regular use: seeking the euphoria • Use of other drugs, e.g., stimulants, LSD, sedatives • Behavioral changes and some consequences • Increased frequency of use; use alone • Buying or stealing drugs
4	Regular use: preoccupation with the "high" • Daily use of drugs • Loss of control • Multiple consequences and risk-taking • Estrangement from family and "straight" friends
5	Burnout: use of drugs to feel normal • Polysubstance use/cross-addiction • Guilt, withdrawal, shame, remorse, depression • Physical and mental deterioration • Increased risk-taking, self-destructive, suicidal

From Kliegman RM et al: *Nelson textbook of pediatrics,* ed 19, Philadelphia, 2011, Saunders.

IMAGING STUDIES

Not helpful in routine diagnosis and management of substance abuse, but possibly useful in the management of sequelae of substance abuse (e.g., brain imaging to evaluate the alcohol abuse–associated increased risk of subdural hematomas or increased evidence of cerebral atrophy).

Rx TREATMENT

NONPHARMACOLOGIC THERAPY

- First assess readiness for change; if precontemplative or contemplative, counsel about risks of use and benefits of abstinence; a motivational interviewing approach has been shown to be effective.
- Nonpharmacologic strategies have the greatest documented efficacy: advice, feedback, goal setting, problem solving, and additional contacts for further assistance.
- Opiate contracts, prohibiting a patient from getting early refills or obtaining opiates from multiple prescribers, should be considered for all patients with chronic pain receiving opioid painkillers, especially for patients with a history of substance abuse or medication abuse.
- Relapse prevention facilitated by avoidance of trigger stimuli or by uncoupling trigger stimuli from substance ingestion.
- Self-help and support groups such as Alcoholics Anonymous and Narcotics Anonymous are helpful in achieving and maintaining sobriety.
- Residential or inpatient treatment programs should be a consideration for any individual with continued or escalating use despite outpatient treatment.

ACUTE GENERAL Rx

- Detoxification is an important first step in substance abuse treatment. Its goals are to facilitate withdrawal and reduce symptoms, initiate abstinence, and refer the patient to ongoing treatment.
- Benzodiazepines are effective in acute alcohol withdrawal for the management of symptoms as well as the prevention of seizures. One strategy is to give the patient a loading dose of a long-acting benzodiazepine (e.g., 20 mg of diazepam) and then continue the benzodiazepine as scheduled while tapering down the dose gradually. An alternative "symptom-driven" strategy is to follow the patient closely with serial assessments, such as the Clinical Institute Withdrawal Assessment for Alcohol (CIWA) scale, and to dose with 1 to 2 mg of lorazepam as needed to treat withdrawal symptoms.
- The prophylactic administration of thiamine and folic acid (first intravenously or intramuscularly followed by supplemental oral doses) in alcohol withdrawal is recommended before starting any carbohydrate-containing fluids or food to prevent Wernicke-Korsakaff syndrome (alcoholic encephalopathy and psychosis). Magnesium appears to be effective in the treatment of alcohol withdrawal–related cardiac arrhythmias, but not other symptoms of alcohol withdrawal.
- Beta-blockers and clonidine generally should be avoided in alcohol withdrawal; they may mask markers of the severity of the withdrawal (blood pressure and pulse rate).
- Unlike withdrawal from alcohol or benzodiazepines, opioid withdrawal is not life threatening.
- Clonidine alleviates the discomfort of opiate withdrawal. Clonidine tablets, 0.1 mg q4-6h as needed, can be used while monitoring patient's blood pressure. Clonidine transdermal patch, 0.1 mg/24 hr, can be used to treat autonomic hyperactivity symptoms; however, it has a very slow onset and may take 2-3 days to achieve therapeutic levels. Antidiarrheals, ibuprofen, and dicyclomine can be used as adjuncts to treat opiate withdrawal symptoms.
- Methadone taper is an effective approach for detoxification in opioid dependence.
- Buprenorphine is a partial μ-opioid receptor agonist that may be used for detoxification and maintenance in treatment of opioid dependence (see dosing in next section).

TABLE 1-9 Assessing the Seriousness of Adolescent Drug Abuse

Variable	0	+1	+2
Age (yr)	>15	<15	
Sex	Male	Female	
Family history of drug abuse		Yes	
Setting of drug use	In group		Alone
Affect before drug use	Happy	Always poor	Sad
School performance	Good, improving		Recently poor
Use before driving	None		Yes
History of accidents	None		Yes
Time of week	Weekend	Weekdays	
Time of day		After school	Before or during school
Type of drug	Marijuana, beer, wine	Hallucinogens, amphetamines	Whiskey, opiates, cocaine, barbiturates

Total score: 0-3, less worrisome; 3-8, serious; 8-18, very serious.
From Kliegman RM et al: *Nelson textbook of pediatrics,* ed 19, Philadelphia, 2011, Saunders.

CHRONIC Rx

- Naltrexone helps reduce craving for alcohol. Naltrexone 50 mg once daily for 12 wk can be a useful adjunct to substance abuse counseling or rehabilitation programs. Randomized treatment studies are equivocal for long-term outcomes. Naltrexone reduces relapse and the intensity or frequency of any drinking that does occur. It can be hepatotoxic and is contraindicated in opiate users. Intramuscular naltrexone (380 mg monthly) may be considered if adherence is an issue.
- Acamprosate also helps reduce craving for alcohol. Acamprosate 666 mg three times daily may be an effective adjunct to counseling. A recent meta-analysis showed overall benefit with increase in the number of abstinent days.
- Disulfiram provokes acetaldehyde accumulation after alcohol ingestion, producing a toxic state manifested by nausea, headache, flushing, and respiratory distress. Studies have shown limited efficacy mostly due to noncompliance.
- Topiramate may be an alternative treatment for alcoholism. In a 12-wk randomized trial topiramate up to 300 mg daily significantly reduced the number of heavy drinking days.
- Methadone maintenance for opiate addiction is effective and involves once-daily dosing of methadone in a controlled setting via methadone clinics.
- Buprenorphine is as effective as low-dose methadone and may be prescribed by physicians who have completed approved training. For induction, initiate 12 to 24 hr after short-acting opioid use and 24 to 48 hr after long-acting opioid use. Use buprenorphine/naloxone tablets in most patients, since buprenorphine-only tablets have risk of abuse. Maximum first-day dosage is 4 to 8 mg of buprenorphine. Titrate buprenorphine dose up to 12 mg on day 2 for signs of withdrawal. Then adjust dosage in frequent outpatient visits (weekly) to minimum needed for maintenance (up to 32 mg daily).
- Naltrexone (oral or injectable) may also be used for maintenance in opioid dependence treatment, though evidence of effectiveness is limited.
- Always combine pharmacotherapy with counseling.
- Treatment of comorbid psychiatric disorders improves outcomes.
- Intervention may be used to break through **denial** of a person with a serious addictive disorder to help the person acknowledge that he or she suffers from a disorder and agree to treatment.

DISPOSITION

- Substance abuse is a chronic relapsing illness, so relapses are best approached as part of the course of the illness, as opposed to as treatment failure.
- The goal of treatment is always abstinence, but success of treatment is measured by return of function, increasing duration between relapses, and prevention of sequelae of use.

REFERRAL

Physicians should refer patients who do not make progress on changing substance use patterns to addiction specialists and/or specialized substance abuse programs. Patients with comorbid psychiatric illness should be referred for mental health care.

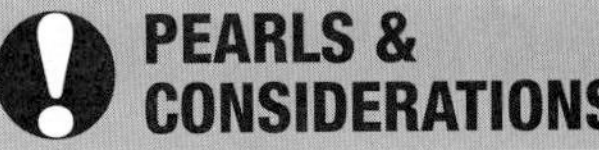

PEARLS & CONSIDERATIONS

- Acute withdrawal from alcohol can become life threatening.
- Withdrawal from opioids can resemble a severe case of the flu.
- A brief intervention (providing information and advising the patient to reduce consumption of alcohol) by the primary care doctor has been demonstrated in randomized trials to reduce drinking in at-risk patients.
- Treatment rates for alcohol use disorders remain low despite available effective treatments.

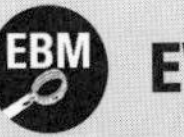

EVIDENCE

available at www.expertconsult.com

SUGGESTED READINGS

available at www.expertconsult.com

RELATED CONTENT

Drug Abuse (Patient Information)
Alcoholism (Related Key Topic)

AUTHORS: **TAHIR TELLIOGLU, M.D., OMRI BERGER, M.D.,** and **RADHIKA A. RAMANAN, M.D., M.P.H.**

BASIC INFORMATION

DEFINITION

Elder abuse includes abuse committed by someone in a trust relation whether in the community or institutional setting.

- Physical abuse: inflicting physical pain or injury
- Sexual abuse: inflicting nonconsensual sexual activity
- Psychological abuse: inflicting mental anguish, including intimidation, humiliation, or threats
- Financial abuse: improper use of resources, property, or assets without the person's consent
- Neglect: abandonment, failure to fulfill a care-taking obligation, including provision of food, safe shelter, physical health and mental health care, or basic custodial care

SYNONYMS

Battered elder syndrome
Elder mistreatment
Domestic violence in the elderly
Diogenes syndrome

Adult maltreatment and neglect problems cover a range of diagnostic codes depending on whether the issue is confirmed or suspected and whether the problem is physical, psychological, or sexual.
Core Codes:
ICD-9-CM and DSM-5 CODES
995.81/82/83
ICD-10CM CODES

T74	Maltreatment syndrome
T74.0	Neglect or abandonment
T74.1	Physical abuse
T74.2	Sexual abuse
T74.3	Psychological abuse
T74.8	Other maltreatment syndromes
T74.9	Maltreatment syndromes, unspecified

EPIDEMIOLOGY & DEMOGRAPHICS

INCIDENCE: According to the National Center on Elder Abuse, between 1 and 2 million Americans aged 65 yr and older have been injured, exploited, or mistreated by someone whom they depend on for care.
PEAK INCIDENCE: >75 yr; more recent studies now suggest <75 yr
PREVALENCE:

- About 10% of those 60 years or older
- Emotional followed by financial abuse are the most common forms.
- 12-month U.S. prevalence rates: emotional abuse 9.0% and 4.6%; physical abuse 0.2% and 1.6%; sexual abuse 0.6%; neglect 0.5%; and financial abuse 3.5% and 5.2%.
- Family members reported 21% of nursing home residents were neglected on one or more occasion in the past 12 months, and over 24% had been subjected to physical abuse during their entire stay.
- Among caregivers of patients with dementia in the U.K., one half reported behaving abusively at least some of the time, and one third reported "important" levels of abuse. Verbal abuse was common and physical abuse was rare.
- Elder abuse is associated with increased risk of mortality, functional impairment, and greater emotional distress, including depression, anxiety, and posttraumatic stress.
- Adult intimate partner violence perpetrators are significantly more likely to have witnessed intimate partner violence as a child than nonperpetrators.

RISK FACTORS (VICTIM):

- Impaired cognition
- Shared living situation and premorbid relationship with abuser
- Social isolation and poor social support
- Mental or physical dependence
- Female
- Low household income
- ADL assistance

RISK FACTORS (PERPETRATOR):

- Relationship conflict with the victim
- Substance abuse, mental illness, particularly depression
- Dependence on the victim and unemployment
- Being an involuntary caregiver, overwhelmed or resentful
- History of being abused as a child

PHYSICAL FINDINGS & CLINICAL PRESENTATION

- Physical abuse with multiple injuries at various stages with implausible descriptions of their origins.
- Fear, hypervigilance, or withdrawal.
- Evidence of poor nutrition, dehydration, poor hygiene, multiple or neglected pressure ulcers, genital or anal pain, neglected medical conditions, or evidence of restraint use (bruises around wrists or ankles).
- Toxicologic evidence of unprescribed medications.
- Poor adherence, frequent no-shows, or little contact with health care system.
- Caregiver not allowing interviewing the patient alone.

Dx DIAGNOSIS

DIFFERENTIAL DIAGNOSIS

- Dementia
- Depression, substance misuse, or other psychiatric disorder
- Malnutrition from intrinsic causes
- Nonadherence to medical treatment
- Relationship distress
- Falling

WORKUP

1. Ask direct specific questions such as:
   - "Has anyone close to you called you names or put you down recently?"
   - "Are you afraid of anyone who lives with you or cares for you"
   - "Has anyone at home ever hurt you?"
   - "Has anyone touched you without your consent?"
   - "Has anyone forced you to do things you didn't want to do?"
   - "Has anyone taken things or money that belong to you without your OK?"
   - "Have you signed any documents that you don't understand?"
   - "Are you often alone?"
   - "When you need help has anyone ever failed to help you take care of yourself?"
   - "If appropriate, ask, "Have you been abused?"
2. Interview patient separately from the suspected abuser.
3. Pelvic examination if sexual abuse suspected.
4. Take photographs of physical injuries as legal evidence.

LABORATORY TESTS & IMAGING STUDIES

- Toxicology screens and therapeutic drug monitoring are sometimes helpful.
- Other tests and radiology according to presentation.

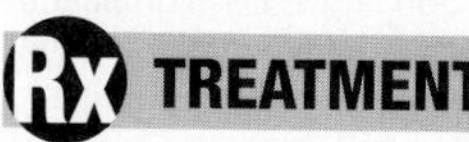

Rx TREATMENT

NONPHARMACOLOGIC THERAPY

- Separate patient and abuser.
- Patient and caregiver may benefit from psychiatric evaluation and treatment for substance abuse, mental illness, or cognitive impairment.
- If appropriate, assess the patient's capacity.
- Fig. 1-18 describes a management algorithm for geriatric abuse.

ACUTE GENERAL Rx

- As indicated for injury or pain relief
- As indicated for mental disorders, dementia, or delirium

DISPOSITION

If the patient's level of disability does not allow independent living, institutionalization may be required. Guidelines vary at the state and county levels regarding guardianship and conservatorship requirements.

REFERRAL

- For outpatients, report to local adult protective services agency. Reporting is mandatory in most states.
- For nursing home patients, report to regional long-term care ombudsman. Reporting is mandatory under federal law.
- Mental health services may be needed

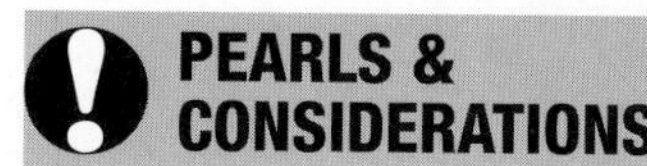

PEARLS & CONSIDERATIONS

COMMENTS

Care should be taken in interacting with the alleged abuser so that access to the victim is not lost.

PREVENTION

- Offer social services (e.g., respite care or homecare) for stressed caregivers.
- Make financial arrangements and arrange durable power of attorney for health care and finances while patient is still cognitively intact.

PATIENT & FAMILY EDUCATION

In the U.S., the elder care help line is 1-800-677-1116.

National Center on Elder Abuse: http://www.ncea.aoa.gov

JAMA Patient Page: Hildreth CJ et al: JAMA patient page. Elder abuse, *JAMA* 302(5):588, 2009

SUGGESTED READINGS

available at www.expertconsult.com

RELATED CONTENT

Elder Abuse (Patient Information)

AUTHOR: **ROBERT KOHN, M.D.**

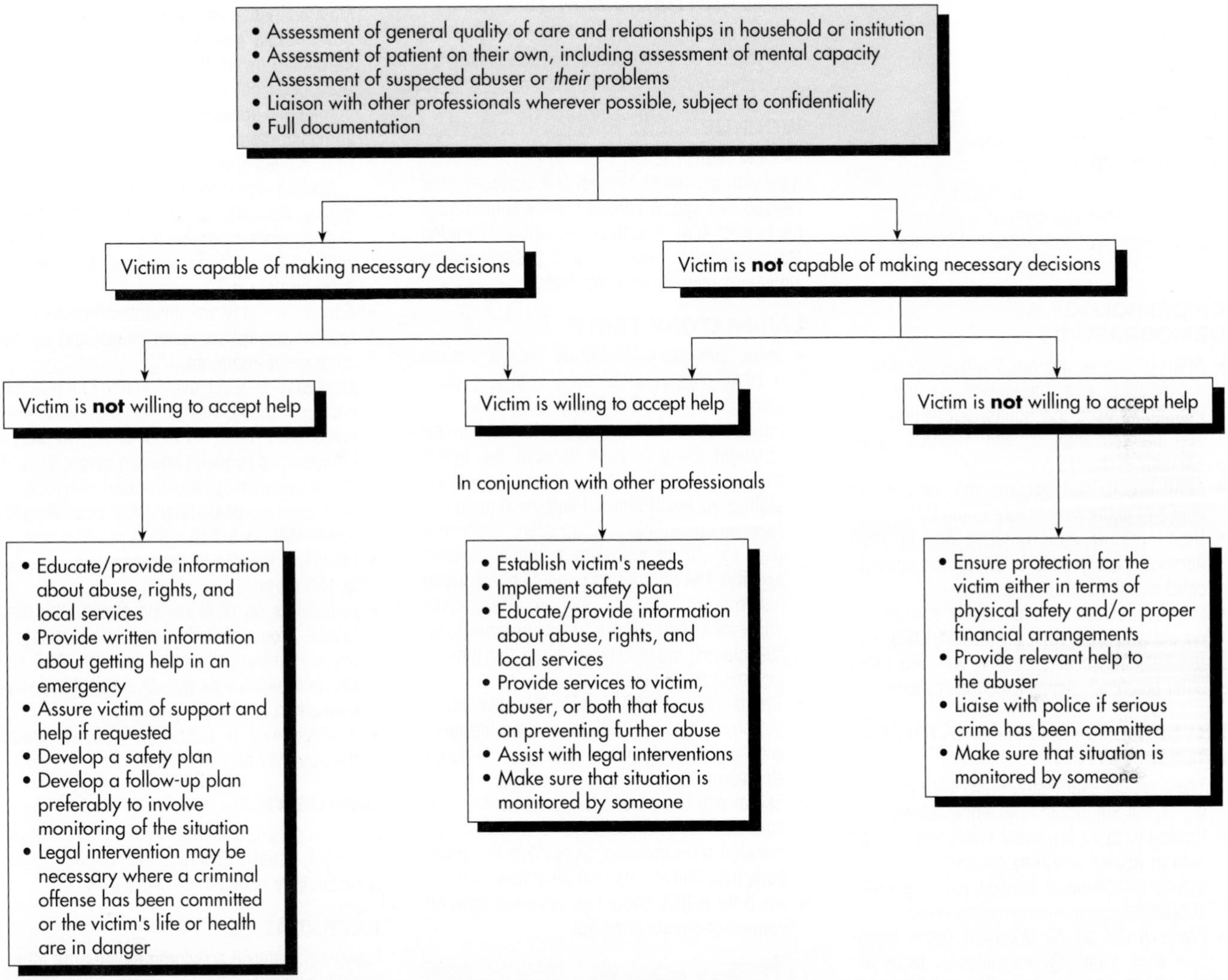

- Assessment of general quality of care and relationships in household or institution
- Assessment of patient on their own, including assessment of mental capacity
- Assessment of suspected abuser or *their* problems
- Liaison with other professionals wherever possible, subject to confidentiality
- Full documentation

→ Victim is capable of making necessary decisions

→→ Victim is **not** willing to accept help

- Educate/provide information about abuse, rights, and local services
- Provide written information about getting help in an emergency
- Assure victim of support and help if requested
- Develop a safety plan
- Develop a follow-up plan preferably to involve monitoring of the situation
- Legal intervention may be necessary where a criminal offense has been committed or the victim's life or health are in danger

→→ Victim is willing to accept help

In conjunction with other professionals

- Establish victim's needs
- Implement safety plan
- Educate/provide information about abuse, rights, and local services
- Provide services to victim, abuser, or both that focus on preventing further abuse
- Assist with legal interventions
- Make sure that situation is monitored by someone

→ Victim is **not** capable of making necessary decisions

→→ Victim is willing to accept help (see above)

→→ Victim is **not** willing to accept help

- Ensure protection for the victim either in terms of physical safety and/or proper financial arrangements
- Provide relevant help to the abuser
- Liaise with police if serious crime has been committed
- Make sure that situation is monitored by someone

FIGURE 1-18 Management of geriatric abuse. (From Tallis RC, Fillit HM [eds]: *Brocklehurst's textbook of geriatric medicine and gerontology,* ed 6, London, 2003, Churchill Livingstone.)

BASIC INFORMATION

DEFINITION

Acetaminophen (APAP) poisoning is a disorder caused by excessive intake of APAP and is manifested by jaundice, nausea, vomiting, and potential death from hepatic necrosis if not treated appropriately.

SYNONYMS

Paracetamol poisoning

ICD-9CM CODES
965.4 Acetaminophen poisoning
ICD-10CM CODES
T39.1 Poisoning by 4-aminophenol derivatives, accidenta
X60 Intentional self-poisoning by 4-aminophenol derivatives

EPIDEMIOLOGY & DEMOGRAPHICS

- APAP is one of the most widely prescribed antipyretics and analgesics in the U.S. Potentially toxic ingestions, both intentional and unintentional, exceed 100,000 cases annually in the U.S.
- APAP toxicity has become the number one cause of acute liver failure in the U.S.
- Death rate is approximately one in 1000 persons. Nearly 50% of exposures occur in children ≤6 yr.
- Hepatic necrosis is most likely to occur in people who are chronically malnourished, who regularly abuse alcohol, and who are using other potentially hepatotoxic medications.

PHYSICAL FINDINGS & CLINICAL PRESENTATION

- The physical examination may vary depending on the amount of time since ingestion.
- Phase I (0 to 24 hr): Initial symptoms may be mild or absent and may consist of anorexia, diaphoresis, malaise, nausea, vomiting, and a subclinical rise in transaminase levels.
- Phase II (24 to 72 hr): right upper quadrant pain, vomiting, somnolence, tachycardia, hypotension, and continued increase in transaminases
- Phase III (72 to 96 hr): hepatic necrosis with abdominal pain, jaundice, hepatic encephalopathy, coagulopathy, hypoglycemia, renal failure, fatality from multiorgan failure
- Phase IV (4 days to 2 wk): complete resolution of symptoms and complete resolution of organ failure
- Table E1-10 summarizes the four phases/stages of acetaminophen poisoning

ETIOLOGY

- The amount of APAP necessary for hepatic toxicity varies with the patient's body size and hepatic function. It is recommended that APAP intake should not exceed 4 g for adults and 90 mg/kg in children within a 24-hr period.
- Using standardized nomograms calculating the APAP plasma level and the number of hours after ingestion, the clinician can determine potential hepatic toxicity. See the APAP ingestion algorithm (Fig. E1-19).

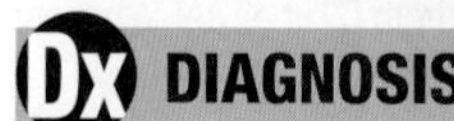

DIAGNOSIS

DIFFERENTIAL DIAGNOSIS

- Liver disease from alcohol abuse or hepatitis
- Ingestion of other hepatotoxic substances
- Bacterial/viral gastroenteritis

WORKUP

Initial workup is aimed at confirming APAP overdose with plasma APAP level and assessment of hepatic damage. A careful history should elicit the time of APAP ingestion, amount, preparation (e.g., extended release) and possibility co-ingestants (see "Laboratory Tests").

LABORATORY TESTS

- Initial laboratory evaluation should include a STAT plasma APAP level with a second level drawn approximately 4 hr after the initial ingestion. Subsequent levels can be obtained every 2 to 4 hr until the levels stabilize or decline. These levels should be plotted on the Rumack-Matthew nomogram (see acetaminophen ingestion algorithm [Fig. E1-19] to calculate potential hepatic toxicity). The nomogram cannot be used with patients who present >24 hr after ingestion, took extended-release preparations, had chronic ingestions, or when the time of ingestion is unknown.
- Transaminases (AST, ALT), bilirubin level, prothrombin time (INR), blood urea nitrogen, and creatinine should be initially obtained on all patients.
- Serum and urine toxicology screen for other potential toxic substances is also recommended on admission. Screening for infectious hepatitis should also be considered.
- Urine for β-hCG should be obtained from all women of childbearing age.

TREATMENT

NONPHARMACOLOGIC THERAPY

Consultation with a Poison Control Center is recommended for patients who have ingested a large amount of APAP and/or other toxic substances. A single toxic dose of APAP usually exceeds 7 g or 150 mg/kg in the adult.

ACUTE GENERAL Rx

- Hepatotoxicity is defined as any increase in alanine aminotransferase (ALT) or aspartate aminotransferase (AST) >1000 IU/L, and hepatic failure is hepatotoxicity with hepatic encephalopathy. For those who cannot be risk stratified using the nomogram, the American College of Emergency Physicians recommends that *N*-acetylcysteine be administered without delay to those >12 yr and >8 hr after ingestion at presentation.
- Administer activated charcoal 1g/kg PO if the patient is seen within 1 hr of ingestion or the clinician suspects polydrug ingestion that delays gastric emptying.
- Determine blood levels 4 hr after ingestion; if in the toxic range, start *N*-acetylcysteine (NAC) either IV (Acetadote) or PO (Mucomyst). Acetylcysteine IV loading dose is 150 mg/kg ×1 diluted in 200 ml D5W over 15 to 60 min. Maintenance dose is 50 mg/kg diluted in 500 ml D5W over 4 hr, followed by 100 mg/kg diluted in 1000 ml D5W over 16 hr. The dose does not require adjustment for renal or hepatic impairment or for dialysis. Total administration time is 21 hours.
- Oral administration is 140 mg/kg PO as a loading dose, followed after 4 hr by 70 mg/kg PO q4h for a total of 17 doses. *N*-acetylcysteine therapy should be started within 24 hr of APAP overdose. Total administration time is 72 hours.
- Advantages of IV administration include more reliable absorption, fewer doses, and shorter duration of treatment.
- Monitor APAP level; use graph to plot possible hepatic toxicity. Repeat AST/ALT and APAP levels after 12 to 14 hr of IV acetylcysteine infusion and continue infusion longer than 16 hr if transaminases are elevated, if APAP concentration is measurable, or if coagulopathy exists (INR >1.5-2.0).
- Provide adequate IV hydration (e.g., D_5½NS at 150 ml/hr).
- In patients on IV *N*-acetylcysteine with liver failure, frequent monitoring of vital signs, oxygen saturation by pulse oximetry, AST, and serum creatinine as well as signs of hypoglycemia and infection is essential.
- If APAP level is nontoxic, *N*-acetylcysteine therapy may be discontinued.

DISPOSITION

Most patients (90%) will recover fully without persisting hepatic abnormalities. Hepatic failure is particularly unusual in children <6 yr.

REFERRAL

Psychiatric referral is recommended after intentional ingestions.

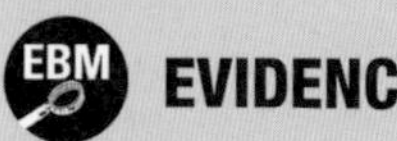

EVIDENCE

available at www.expertconsult.com

SUGGESTED READINGS

available at www.expertconsult.com

RELATED CONTENT

Acetaminophen Overdose (Patient Information)

AUTHOR: **TARA M. WAYT, D.O.**

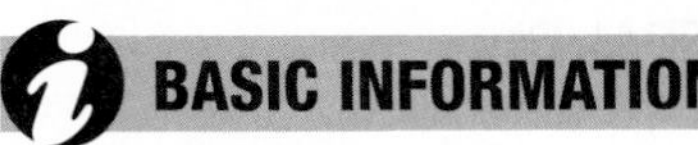

BASIC INFORMATION

DEFINITION

Achalasia is a motility disorder of the esophagus classically characterized by incomplete relaxation of the lower esophageal sphincter (LES) and aperistalsis of esophageal smooth muscle. The result is functional obstruction of the esophagus.

SYNONYMS

Achalasia and cardiospasm
Achalasia (of cardia)
Aperistalsis of esophagus
Megaesophagus
Esophageal achalasia
Esophageal cardiospasm

ICD-9CM CODES
530.0 Achalasia
ICD-10CM CODES
K22.0 Achalasia of cardia

EPIDEMIOLOGY & DEMOGRAPHICS

- Annual incidence is approximately 0.5-1.0 in 100,000 persons.
- Prevalence is <10 per 100,000 persons.
- Although the onset of symptoms may occur at any age, incidence is typically bimodal, 20 to 40 yr, then after 60 yr, with greater incidence in the older group.
- Men and women are affected equally.

PHYSICAL FINDINGS & CLINICAL PRESENTATION

Symptoms:
- Dysphagia (most commonly with both solids and liquids)
- Difficulty belching
- Regurgitation
- Chest pain and/or heartburn
- Globus
- Frequent hiccups
- Vomiting of undigested food
- Symptoms of aspiration such as nocturnal cough; possible dyspnea and pneumonia
- Weight loss

Physical findings:
- Focal lung examination abnormalities and wheezing also possible

ETIOLOGY

- Etiology is poorly understood.
- Loss of myenteric nerve fibers in the LES and smooth muscle portion of the esophagus. This has been associated with lymphocytic and eosinophilic infiltrates and fibrosis in later stages of disease.
- Loss of intrinsic inhibitory neurons in the myenteric plexus as well as depletion of networks of interstitial cells of Cajal of the LES, leads to incomplete relaxation secondary to loss of inhibitory neurotransmitters nitric oxide and vasoactive intestinal polypeptide.
- This motility disorder may be caused by autoimmune degeneration of the esophageal myenteric plexus because association with the HLA class II antigen DQw1 has been noted. Antimyenteric plexus and other antineural autoantibodies have also been described.
- Abnormal immune reactions to neurotropic viruses such as varicella zoster, herpes simplex type 1, and measles viruses have been implicated, but the association has not been confirmed. A host T cell–mediated response may lead to neuronal injury.
- Achalasia is also seen in the rare autosomal recessive disorder Allgrove syndrome (achalasia, alacrima, autonomic disturbance, and acetylcholine insensitivity), which has been linked to a gene mutation on chromosome 12q13. Neurons in this syndrome may be susceptible to oxidative injury.

Dx DIAGNOSIS

DIFFERENTIAL DIAGNOSIS

- Primary achalasia:
  - Idiopathic
- Secondary achalasia:
  - Chagas disease
  - Vagal injury or surgery, including fundoplication
  - Achalasia-like esophageal dilation has been described after laparoscopic gastric banding
- Pseudoachalasia:
  - Esophageal cancer
  - Infiltrating gastric cancer
  - Oat cell and bronchogenic lung cancer
  - Lymphoma
  - Amyloidosis
  - Paraneoplastic syndrome
- Angina
- Bulimia
- Anorexia nervosa
- Gastric bezoar
- Gastritis
- Peptic ulcer disease
- Postvagotomy dysmotility
- Esophageal disease (Table 1-11):
  - Gastroesophageal reflux disease
  - Sarcoidosis
  - Amyloidosis
  - Esophageal stricture
  - Esophageal webs and rings
  - Scleroderma
  - Barrett's esophagus
  - Esophagitis
  - Diffuse esophageal spasm

WORKUP

- Physical examination and laboratory analyses to rule out other causes and assess complications
- Imaging studies, manometry, and endoscopy (may be complementary)

LABORATORY TESTS

- Assessment of nutritional status
- Complete blood count, ECG, stress test if diagnosis is in doubt
- Serologic assays for *Trypanosoma cruzi* (Chagas disease) in appropriate individuals

IMAGING STUDIES

Barium swallow with fluoroscopy may demonstrate:
- Uncoordinated or absent esophageal contractions (loss of peristalsis)
- An acutely tapered contrast column ("bird's beak"; Fig. 1-20)

TABLE 1-11 Esophageal Motor Disorders

	Achalasia	Scleroderma	Diffuse Esophageal Spasm
Symptoms	Dysphagia Regurgitation of nonacidic material	Gastroesophageal reflux disease Dysphagia	Substernal chest pain (angina-like) Dysphagia with pain
Radiographic appearance	Dilated, fluid-filled esophagus Distal *bird-beak* stricture	Aperistaltic esophagus Free reflux Peptic stricture	Simultaneous noncoordinated contractions
Manometric findings			
Lower esophageal sphincter	High resting pressure Incomplete or abnormal relaxation with swallow	Low resting pressure	Normal pressure
Body	Low-amplitude, simultaneous contractions after swallowing	Low-amplitude peristaltic contractions or no peristalsis	Some peristalsis Diffuse and simultaneous nonperistaltic contractions, occasionally high amplitude

From Andreoli TE et al: *Andreoli and Carpenter's Cecil essentials of medicine,* ed 8, Philadelphia, 2010, Saunders.

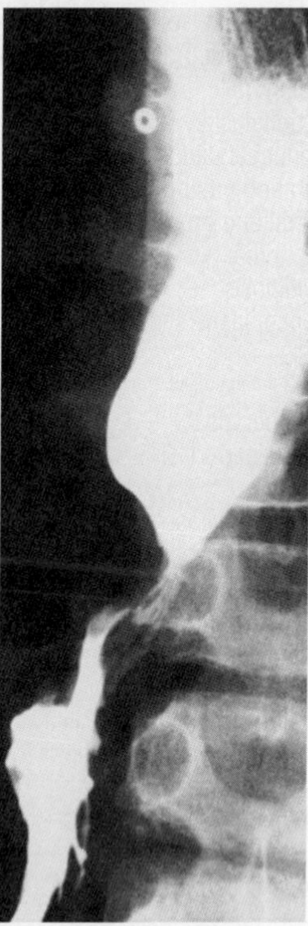

FIGURE 1-20 Classic appearance of achalasia of the esophagus. The dilated esophagus ends in a narrow segment. (From Hoekelman R [ed]: *Primary pediatric care,* ed 3, St Louis, 1997, Mosby.)

- Dilation of the distal (smooth muscle portion) esophagus
- Esophageal air-fluid level with evidence of poor esophageal emptying

Manometry is generally considered to be the "gold standard" test to confirm the diagnosis. In classic achalasia, abnormalities are as follows:

- Low-amplitude disorganized contractions/aperistalsis
- Incomplete or absent LES relaxation after swallow
- High LES pressure
- A subset of patients with "vigorous achalasia" may have high-amplitude, long-duration, simultaneous esophageal contractions. This term is now felt to be imprecise because of a newer classification of the disease.
- High-resolution manometry (HRM), or high-resolution esophageal pressure topography (HREPT), has recently defined subsets of patients with achalasia who may have different responses to medical or surgical therapies. Unlike classic achalasia (type I), type II achalasia shows panesophageal pressurization to greater than 30 mm Hg with ≥20% of test swallows, and type III achalasia shows spastic lumen-obliterating contractions of the distal esophagus with ≥20% of swallows.
- HREPT has also defined an achalasia variant described as esophagogastric junction outflow obstruction.
- Direct visualization by endoscopy, including careful visualization of the esophagogastric junction and cardia, should be performed to exclude other causes of dysphagia, including "functional esophagogastric junction obstruction," strictures, secondary causes of achalasia (including infiltrating cancers), and pseudoachalasia.

Rx TREATMENT

NONPHARMACOLOGIC THERAPY

- The goals of therapy are to decrease LES pressure, relieve symptoms, and prevent progression to a dilated or megaesophagus.
- Pneumatic dilation may benefit 65% to 90% of patients. Multiple sessions may be required, and most protocols use a graded dilation approach, starting with a 30-mm balloon, and repeating if required with a 35-mm or 40-mm balloon. Some studies suggest this may be more effective in women or older patients. Esophageal rupture or perforation is a rare complication (2% to 4%) that may be managed conservatively in some stable patients with a small perforation.
- Surgical: laparoscopic, or now less commonly open, (Heller's) esophagomyotomy is effective (90%). Approximately 35% of patients undergoing surgery will develop reflux disease. As a result, some surgeons will perform a "loose" antireflux repair as part of the surgical procedure. Some studies suggest this may be more effective in men and younger patients. An observational study has suggested that those who have had prior endoscopic treatment before myotomy may not do as well as those who have a primary myotomy.
- Studies suggest that type I and type II patients have better treatment responses to these therapies compared with type III patients.
- A large European study suggested that in experienced hands, patients may expect similar medium-term outcomes from myotomy and balloon dilation. A meta-analysis suggests better long-term durability of myotomy. Balloon dilation may be the more cost-effective treatment.
- Assessment of esophagogastric junction distensibility by an endoscopic functional luminal imaging probe may help to better evaluate the efficacy of treatment.
- Endoscopic submucosal myotomy (POEM [per oral endoscopic myotomy]) has been reported in several series and is being explored as another option for treatment.
- Esophagectomy has been performed in patients with end-stage achalasia with a sigmoid or mega-esophagus who have failed myotomy or pneumatic dilation.

GENERAL Rx

- Medications may be useful for short-term symptom relief and in patients with refractory chest pain. They should only be considered in patients unable to receive, or who are scheduled for, more definitive procedures. LES pressure may be lowered by 50% through sublingual use of long-acting nitrates (e.g., isosorbide dinitrate 5 to 20 mg) or calcium channel blockers (e.g., nifedipine 10 to 30 mg). Side effects are common and duration of relief tends to be short. Sildenafil was shown to be effective in a few small, short-term studies, but it is generally not recommended.
- Botulinum toxin injection will benefit up to 85% of patients by inhibiting acetylcholine release from cholinergic nerve endings, blocking the unopposed cholinergic stimulation of the LES, but having no impact on the myogenic tone; up to half of these patients will require repeat injections by 6 months. A few studies have suggested that repeated injections can lead to fibrosis, which may complicate subsequent attempts at surgical therapy.

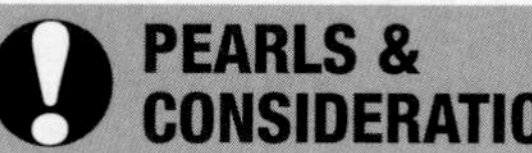

PEARLS & CONSIDERATIONS

COMMENTS

- Medication has a limited role in treatment.
- Botulinum toxin is transiently effective in improving symptoms. Pneumatic dilation and surgical myotomy provide more durable long-term responses and are the treatment of choice for most patients. Botulinum toxin should be considered primarily in patients too elderly or ill to be considered for these other therapies.
- Patients with achalasia may be at long-term risk of squamous cell carcinoma of the esophagus and non–reflux-associated esophagitis. Treated patients may be at long-term risk for reflux esophagitis, Barrett's esophagus, and adenocarcinoma.

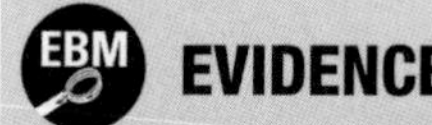

EVIDENCE

available at www.expertconsult.com

SUGGESTED READINGS

available at www.expertconsult.com

RELATED CONTENT

Dysphagia (Related Key Topic)
Achalasia (Patient Information)

AUTHOR: **HARLAN G. RICH, M.D., F.A.C.P., A.G.A.F.**

BASIC INFORMATION

DEFINITION

Achilles tendon rupture is a disruption of the continuity of the Achilles tendon that most often results from the combination of mechanical stress and intratendinous degeneration.

ICD-9CM CODES
727.67 Nontraumatic rupture of Achilles tendon
ICD-10CM CODES
M66.27 Spontaneous rupture of extensor tendons, ankle and foot

EPIDEMIOLOGY & DEMOGRAPHICS

INCIDENCE: 1 in 10,000/year (third most frequent tendon disruption in the body)
PEAK INCIDENCE: 30 to 39 yr age group
PREDOMINANT AGE: 30 to 55 yr age group
RISK FACTORS: General risk factors include the recreational athlete, advancing age, previous tear or rupture, extreme change in training level, or participation in a new activity. Other risk factors can be categorized into intrinsic and extrinsic.

- **Intrinsic:** Achilles tendinitis/tendinosis, tight musculature, poor vascularity, tibial varum, overpronation, cavus foot, systemic lupus erythematosus, rheumatoid arthritis, gout
- **Extrinsic:** Inadequate training equipment/training techniques, recent steroid or fluoroquinolone therapy

PHYSICAL FINDINGS & CLINICAL PRESENTATION

The typical patient is a middle-aged man who gives a history of recent physical activity with a sudden push-off, jump, or misstep that causes a snap sensation or audible pop in the back of the leg, followed by the onset of acute pain, swelling, and weakened plantarflexion power. Patients commonly relate feeling as though they were "hit in the back of the leg with a bat." Most often patients have sedentary occupations and indulge occasionally in strenuous activity.

- Depending on the severity of the rupture, initial pain may not be severe.
- Several hours after injury, diffuse pain, swelling, and ecchymosis are usually evident.
- The patient has difficulty walking, with a weakened plantarflexion power and inability to perform a single heel raise on the injured extremity.
- Referred stabbing pain in the posterior leg and ankle from muscle spasm is common.
  - A palpable gap within the Achilles tendon, which increases with dorsiflexion of the ankle, is present.

ETIOLOGY

Although a history of direct trauma is uncommon, it may include blunt trauma to the posterior ankle, crushing injury, and laceration. Indirect injury as a cause of rupture is more common. Etiologic factors of indirect injury are of three types: mechanical, vascular, and related to poor tissue quality.

- Mechanical: involves variations of a rapid loading process on an already tensed tendon such as a sudden dorsiflexion of the ankle with the knee extended while an eccentric load is applied
  - Tripping on a curb
  - Lunging for a tennis shot
  - Jumping from a height
- Vascular: factors include the known watershed area located 2 to 6 cm proximal to the insertion, an area of poor blood supply.
- Poor tissue quality: refers to the common notion that prior tendon degeneration is required to weaken the tendon before it is ruptured. This often occurs in the form of repetitive microtrauma from improper training techniques.

DIAGNOSIS

DIFFERENTIAL DIAGNOSIS

- Achilles tendinopathy
- Retrocalcaneal bursitis
- Ankle sprain
- Calcaneal avulsion fracture
- Partial rupture of gastrocnemius
- Plantaris rupture
- Rupture of Baker's cyst
- Os trigonum syndrome
- Plantaris rupture

WORKUP

Approximately 25% of Achilles tendon ruptures are misdiagnosed initially. A thorough history and physical exam, coupled with high clinical suspicion, can prevent this from happening. The clinical history in most presentations is very specific, and the physical exam is usually diagnostic. Below is a list of specific clinical tests and imaging modalities. Please see section "Physical Findings & Clinical Presentation" for more information.

- Thompson's test: The patient is placed in a prone position with the knees flexed. The examiner squeezes the calf musculature, which should produce plantarflexion of the ankle. If no plantarflexion is obtained, this indicates an Achilles tendon rupture (a positive test). (See Fig. 1-21.)
- Matles' test: The patient is placed in the prone position with the knees flexed to 90 degrees. If the injured foot falls to neutral or a dorsiflexed position, the Achilles tendon is ruptured (a positive test).
- MRI and ultrasound may be useful when clinical suspicion is high, but clinical tests are inconclusive.

TREATMENT

Controversy exists over conservative versus surgical repair of the ruptured Achilles tendon, but most evidence shows that early treatment has a far better prognosis than later repair. Conservative treatment is associated with a higher re-rupture rate. Surgical repair often facilitates earlier return to full activity. In general, older, more sedentary patients should be treated conservatively and younger athletic patients should receive surgical repair.

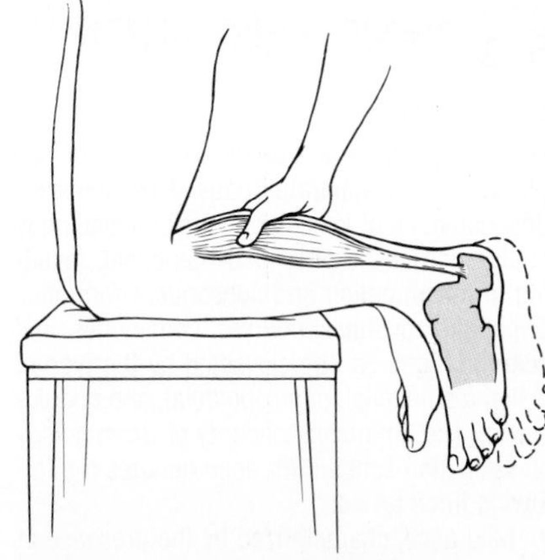

FIGURE 1-21 Thompson's test. Compression of the calf muscles normally produces plantarflexion of the ankle. If the Achilles tendon is ruptured, this reponse is greatly diminished or absent. (From Browner BD et al: *Skeletal trauma: basic science, management, and reconstruction,* ed 3, Philadelphia, 2003, Saunders.)

- *Conservative treatment:* A long leg cast is applied with the foot in approximately 20 degrees equinovarus, ensuring that the knee is bent during the casting process. The cast is removed at 8 weeks, with gradual reduction in equinovarus with a short leg cast. After removal of the cast, physical therapy should be instituted to regain dorsiflexion of the ankle. This gradual process may take up to 12 weeks. The total conservative rehabilitation period may last 6-9 months.
- *Surgical treatment:* Several surgical techniques exist to repair the ruptured Achilles tendon. Many involve lengthening and flap down methods to bridge the gap in the tendon. Multiple biologic grafts are available that may be used to augment and reinforce the rupture site. After surgery, 10 to 12 weeks of immobilization followed by rehabilitation is recommended.

DISPOSITION

- Conservative care carries a 20%-30% chance of re-rupture.
- Re-rupture rates are very low with surgical repair
- A physical therapist should work closely with the patient in the rehabilitation period regardless of whether surgical or conservative care is used.
- Early treatment, whether conservative or surgical, has far better results than treatment of neglected cases

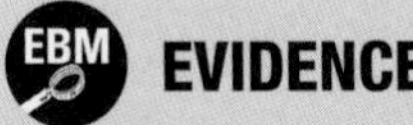

EVIDENCE

available at www.expertconsult.com

SUGGESTED READINGS

available at www.expertconsult.com

RELATED CONTENT

Achilles Tendon Rupture (Patient Information)

AUTHOR: **DOMINIC RODA, D.P.M.**

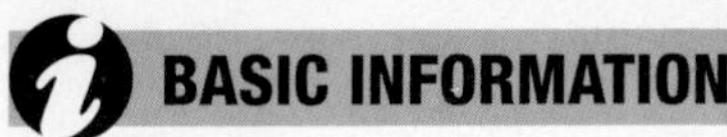

BASIC INFORMATION

DEFINITION

Acne vulgaris is a chronic disorder of the pilosebaceous apparatus caused by abnormal desquamation of follicular epithelium leading to obstruction of the pilosebaceous canal, resulting in inflammation and subsequent formation of papules, pustules, nodules, comedones, and scarring. Acne can be classified by the type of lesion (comedonal, papulopustular, and nodulocystic). The American Academy of Dermatology classification scheme for acne denotes the following three levels:

1. Mild acne: characterized by the presence of comedones (noninflammatory lesions), few papules and pustules (generally <10), but no nodules.
2. Moderate acne: presence of several to many papules and pustules (10 to 40) along with comedones (10 to 40). The presence of >40 papules and pustules along with larger, deeper nodular inflamed lesions (up to five) denotes moderately severe acne (Fig. 1-22).
3. Severe acne (Fig. 1-23): presence of numerous or extensive papules and pustules as well as many nodular lesions.

SYNONYMS

Acne

ICD-9CM CODES
706.1 Acne vulgaris
ICD-10CM CODES
L70.0 Acne vulgaris

EPIDEMIOLOGY & DEMOGRAPHICS

- Acne is the most common skin disease in the U.S.
- It is most common in teenagers (highest incidence between ages of 16 and 18 yr).

PHYSICAL FINDINGS & CLINICAL PRESENTATION

- Open comedones (blackheads), closed comedones (whiteheads)
- Greasiness (oily skin)
- Presence of scars from prior acne cysts
- Various stages of development and severity may be present concomitantly
- Common distribution of acne: face, back, and upper chest
- Inflammatory papules, pustules, and ectatic pores

ETIOLOGY

- Overactivity of the sebaceous glands and blockage in the ducts. The obstruction leads to the formation of comedones, which can become inflamed because of overgrowth of *Propionibacterium acnes.*
- Exacerbated by environmental factors (hot, humid, tropical climate), medications (e.g., iodine in cough mixtures, hair greases), industrial exposure to halogenated hydrocarbons.

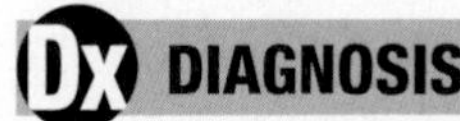

DIAGNOSIS

DIFFERENTIAL DIAGNOSIS

- Gram-negative folliculitis
- Staphylococcal pyoderma
- Acne rosacea
- Drug eruption
- Sebaceous hyperplasia
- Angiofibromas, basal cell carcinomas, osteoma cutis
- Occupational exposures to oils or grease
- Steroid acne
- Hidradenitis suppurativa
- Perioral dermatitis
- Pseudofolliculitis barbae
- Miliaria
- Seborrheic dermatitis

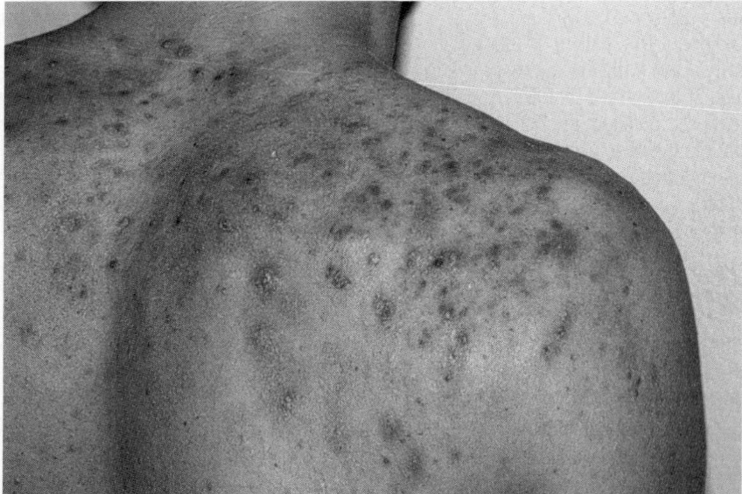

FIGURE 1-22 Acne on back and shoulders. This acne is typically inflammatory and usually needs oral antibiotics or possibly isotretinoin, but the patient may apply topical medication as well. Heat and sweat may aggravate the condition. (From White GM, Cox NH [eds]: *Diseases of the skin*, ed 2, St Louis, 2006, Mosby.)

WORKUP

History and physical examination:

- Inquire about previous treatment
- Careful drug history
- Family history, history of cyclic menstrual flares
- History of use of cosmetics and cleansers
- Oral contraceptive use

LABORATORY TESTS

- Laboratory evaluation is generally not helpful.
- Patients who are candidates for therapy with isotretinoin should have baseline liver enzymes, cholesterol, and triglycerides checked because this medication may result in elevation of lipids and liver enzymes.
- A negative serum pregnancy test or two negative urine pregnancy tests should also be obtained in females 1 wk before initiation of isotretinoin; it is also imperative to maintain effective contraception during and 1 mo after therapy with isotretinoin ends because of its teratogenic effects. Pregnancy status should be rechecked at monthly visits.
- If hyperandrogenism is suspected in female patients, levels of dehydroepiandrosterone sulfate, testosterone (total and free), and androstenedione should be measured. For women with regular menstrual cycles, serum androgen measurements generally are not necessary.

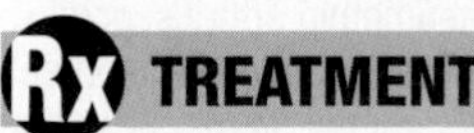

TREATMENT

NONPHARMACOLOGIC THERAPY

Blue light (ClearLight therapy system) can be used for treatment of moderate inflammatory acne vulgaris. Light in the violet/blue range can cause bacterial death by a photoreaction in which porphyrins react with oxygen to generate reactive oxygen species, which damage the cell membranes of *P. acnes.* Treatment usually consists of 15-min exposures twice weekly for 4 wk.

ACUTE GENERAL Rx

Treatment generally varies with the type of lesions (comedones, papules, pustules, cystic lesions) and the severity of acne.

- Comedones (noninflammatory acne) can be treated with retinoids or retinoid analogs. Topical retinoids are comedolytic and work by normalizing follicular keratinization. Commonly available agents are Adapalene (Differin, 0.1% gel or cream, applied once or twice daily), tazarotene (Tazorac 0.1% cream or gel applied daily), tretinoin (Retin-A 0.1% cream or 0.025 gel applied once daily), tretinoin microsphere (Retin-A Micro, 0.1% gel, applied at bedtime). Tretinoin is inactivated by ultraviolet light and oxidized by benzoyl peroxide; therefore it should only be applied at night and not used concomitantly with benzoyl peroxide.
- Tretinoin is pregnancy category C and tazarotene is pregnancy category X. Salicylic acid preparations (e.g., Neutrogena 2% wash) have keratolytic and anti-inflammatory properties and are also useful in the treatment of comedones. Large, open comedones (blackheads) should be expressed.

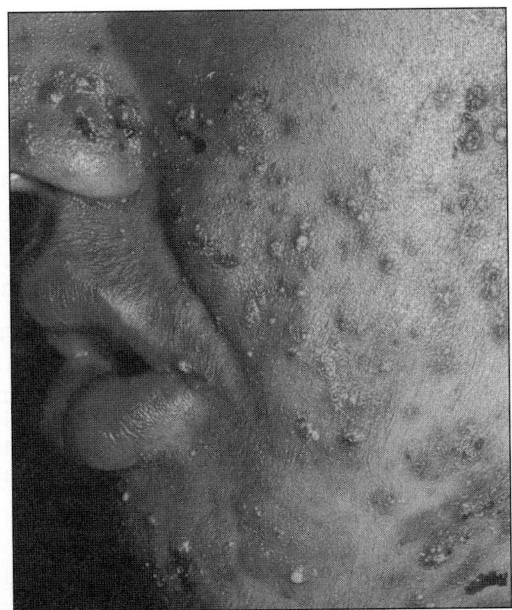

FIGURE 1-23 Severe acne. Acne this severe on presentation should prompt the consideration of early use of isotretinoin. The dose should be low initially to prevent a severe flare. An oral tetracycline or erythromycin may be helpful to calm the acne before isotretinoin. (From White GM, Cox NH [eds]: *Diseases of the skin,* ed 2, St Louis, 2006, Mosby.)

- Patients should be reevaluated after 4 to 6 wk. Benzoyl peroxide gel (2.5% or 5%) may be added if the comedones become inflamed or form pustules. The most common adverse effects are dryness, erythema, and peeling. Topical antibiotics (erythromycin, clindamycin lotions or pads) can also be used in patients with significant inflammation. They reduce *P. acnes* in the pilosebaceous follicle and have some anti-inflammatory effects. The combination of 5% benzoyl peroxide and 3% erythromycin (Benzamycin) or 1% clindamycin with 5% benzoyl peroxide (BenzaClin) is highly effective in patients who have a mixture of comedonal and inflammatory acne lesions.
- Fixed-dose combinations of clindamycin phosphate 1.2% and tretinoin 0.025% are available (Veltin gel, Ziana) and are more effective than either product used alone; however, they are much more expensive than the individual generic components.
- Pustular acne can be treated with tretinoin and benzoyl peroxide gel applied on alternate evenings; drying agents (sulfacetamide-sulfa lotions [Novacet, Sulfacet]) are also effective when used in combination with benzoyl peroxide; oral antibiotics (doxycycline 100 mg qd or erythromycin 1 g qd given in 2 to 3 divided doses) are effective in patients with moderate to severe pustular acne. Patients not responding well to these antibiotics can be switched to minocycline 50 to 100 mg bid; however, this medication is more expensive.
- Patients with nodular cystic acne can be treated with systemic agents: antibiotics (erythromycin, tetracycline, doxycycline, minocycline), isotretinoin (available on restricted basis), or oral contraceptives. Periodic intralesional triamcinolone (Kenalog) injections by a dermatologist are also effective. The possibility of endocrinopathy should be considered in patients responding poorly to therapy.
- Isotretinoin is indicated for acne resistant to antibiotic therapy and severe acne. It is available only on a restricted basis. Dosage is 0.5 to 1 mg/kg/day in 2 divided doses (maximum of 2 mg/kg/day); duration of therapy is generally 20 wk for a cumulative dose ≥120 mg/kg for severe cystic acne. Before using this medication patients should undergo baseline laboratory evaluation (see "Laboratory Tests"). This drug is absolutely contraindicated during pregnancy because of its teratogenicity. It should be used with caution in patients with history of depression. Physicians, distributors, pharmacies, and patients must register in the iPLEDGE program (http://www.ipledgeprogram.com) before using isotretinoin.
- Azelaic acid is a bacteriostatic dicarboxylic acid used to normalize keratinization and reduce inflammation. It can be used in pregnant women.
- Oral contraceptives reduce androgen levels and therefore sebum production. They represent a useful adjunctive therapy for all types of acne in women and adolescent girls. Commonly used agents are norgestimate/ethinyl estradiol (Ortho Tri-Cyclen) and drosperinone/ethinyl estradiol (Yasmin).

REFERRAL

Referral for intralesional injection and dermabrasion should be considered in patients with severe acne unresponsive to conventional therapy.

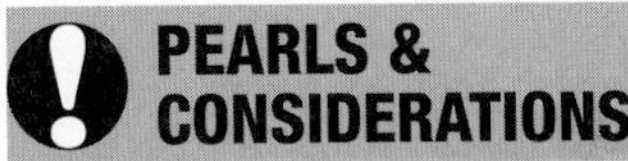

PEARLS & CONSIDERATIONS

- Gram-negative folliculitis should be suspected if inflammatory acne worsens after several months of oral antibiotic therapy.
- Acne may worsen during the first 3 to 4 wk of retinoid therapy before improving.

COMMENTS

Indications for systemic therapy of acne are:

- Painful deep papules or nodules
- Extensive lesions
- Active acne with severe scarring or hyperpigmentation
- Patient's morale

Patients should be educated that in most cases acne can be controlled but not cured and that at least 4 to 6 wk of initial therapy should be required before significant improvement is noted.

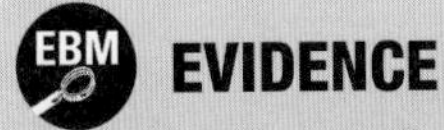

EVIDENCE

available at www.expertconsult.com

SUGGESTED READINGS

available at www.expertconsult.com

AUTHOR: **FRED F. FERRI, M.D.**

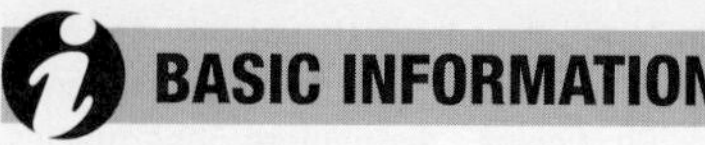

BASIC INFORMATION

DEFINITION

Acoustic neuroma is a benign proliferation of the Schwann cells that cover the vestibular branch of the eighth cranial nerve (CN VIII). Symptoms are commonly a result of compression of the acoustic branch of CN VIII, the facial nerve (CN VII), and the trigeminal nerve (CN V). The glossopharyngeal nerve (CN IX) and vagus nerve (CN X) are less commonly involved. In extreme cases compression of the brain stem may lead to obstruction of cerebrospinal fluid (CSF) outflow and elevated intracranial pressure (ICP).

SYNONYMS

Vestibular schwannoma

ICD-9CM CODES
225.1 Acoustic neuroma
ICD-10CM CODES
D33.3 Benign neoplasm of cranial nerves

EPIDEMIOLOGY & DEMOGRAPHICS

Annual incidence is approximately one in 80,000 patients per year, with a higher incidence in patients with neurofibromatosis type 2 (NF2). There may be a slight female predominance. The tumor most commonly presents in the fifth and sixth decades.

PHYSICAL FINDINGS & CLINICAL PRESENTATION

- Most frequently unilateral hearing loss and/or tinnitus. Also balance problems, vertigo, facial pain (trigeminal neuralgia) and weakness, difficulty swallowing, fullness or pain of the involved ear. Headache may occur.
- With elevated ICP, patients may also have vomiting, fever, and visual changes.
- Hearing loss is the most common presenting complaint and is usually high frequency.

ETIOLOGY

The etiology is incompletely understood, but long-term exposure to acoustic trauma has been implicated. Bilateral acoustic neuromas may be inherited in an autosomal-dominant manner as part of NF2. This disease is associated with a defect on chromosome 22q1. Childhood exposure to low-dose radiation for benign head and neck conditions may increase risk for acoustic neuromas. There is inconclusive evidence to link chronic exposure to radiofrequency radiation from cellular telephone use and the risk for developing brain tumors.

Dx DIAGNOSIS

DIFFERENTIAL DIAGNOSIS

- Benign positional vertigo
- Menière's disease
- Trigeminal neuralgia
- Cerebellar disease
- Normal-pressure hydrocephalus
- Presbycusis
- Glomus tumors
- Vertebrobasilar insufficiency
- Ototoxicity from medications
- Other tumors:
  - Meningioma, glioma
  - Facial nerve schwannoma
  - Cavernous hemangioma
  - Metastatic tumors

WORKUP

- A detailed neurologic examination with special attention to the cranial nerves is crucial.
- Otoscopic evaluation may help rule out other causes of hearing loss.

LABORATORY TESTS

- Audiometry is useful, often showing asymmetric, sensorineural, high-frequency hearing loss.
- CSF protein may be elevated.

IMAGING STUDIES

- MRI with gadolinium (Fig. 1-24) is the preferred test. It can detect tumors as small as 2 mm in diameter.
- High-resolution CT scan with and without contrast can detect tumors 1 cm in diameter or larger.
- Treatment decisions should be based on the size of the tumor, rate of growth (older patients tend to have slower-growing tumors), degree of neurologic deficit, desire to preserve hearing, life expectancy, age of the patient, and surgical risk. A combination of treatments can also be used.

Rx TREATMENT

NONPHARMACOLOGIC THERAPY

- Surgery is the definitive treatment. Choice of approach (middle cranial fossa, translabyrinthine, or retromastoid suboccipital) may vary depending on the size of the tumor, amount of residual hearing desired, and degree of surgical risk that can be tolerated. Partial resection is sometimes undertaken to minimize the risk of injury to nearby structures. Intraoperative facial nerve monitoring is recommended.
- Radiation therapy (stereotactic radiotherapy, stereotactic radiosurgery, or proton beam radiotherapy) is useful for tumors <3 cm in diameter or for those in whom surgery is not an option. Radiotherapy after partial resection has also been used to minimize complications.
- Age alone is not a contraindication to surgery.

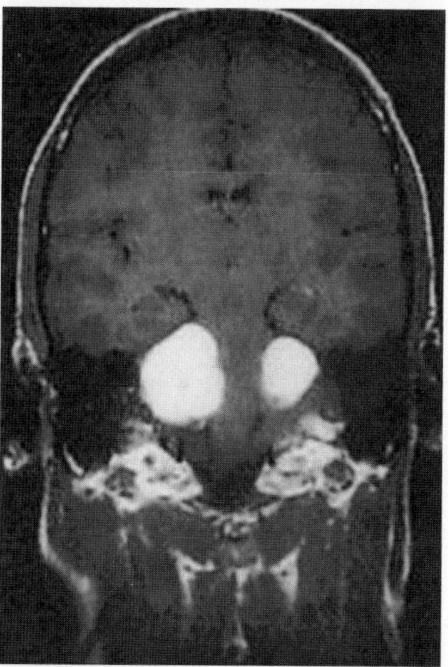

FIGURE 1-24 MR with enhancement shows bilateral acoustic neuromas. Coronal view. (From Kanski JJ, Bowling B: *Clinical ophthalmology, a systematic approach,* ed 7, Philadelphia, 2011, Saunders.)

ACUTE GENERAL Rx

Bevacizumab, an antivascular endothelial growth factor (VEGF) monoclonal antibody, has been shown to improve hearing and reduce the volume of growing acoustic neuromas in some neurofibromatosis type 2 patients.

CHRONIC Rx

Observation with MRI every 6 to 12 mo may be appropriate for frail patients with small tumors, but risk of unrecoverable hearing loss may increase if surgery is delayed. Also, progressive hearing loss may occur despite absence of growth on subsequent imaging.

DISPOSITION

Hearing can be preserved at near-preoperative levels in more than two thirds of patients with small- to medium-sized tumors. Occurrence of secondary radiation-related tumors following radiosurgery is rare. There are no standard posttreatment follow-up recommendations. Therefore, an individualized approach to follow-up imaging and audiometry is recommended.

REFERRAL

Prompt referral to an ear-nose-throat specialist or neurosurgeon who is facile with all three surgical approaches is recommended.

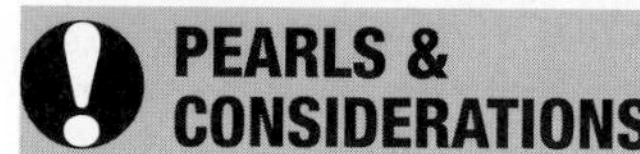

PEARLS & CONSIDERATIONS

COMMENTS

- Presents most commonly as unilateral, sensorineural hearing loss.
- Treatment outcomes are generally good, with cure rates approaching 90% at 5 years.
- Of those who are managed with observation only, approximately half have continued enlargement and approximately one fifth eventually have a surgical intervention.

PATIENT/FAMILY EDUCATION

Acoustic Neuroma Association: http://anausa.org.

SUGGESTED READINGS

available at www.expertconsult.com

RELATED CONTENT

Tinnitus (Related Key Topic)
Acoustic Neuroma (Patient Information)

AUTHORS: **SRIVIDYA ANANDAN, M.D.,** and **COURTNEY CLARK BILODEAU, M.D.**

BASIC INFORMATION

DEFINITION

Acquired immunodeficiency syndrome (AIDS) is a disorder caused by infection with the human immunodeficiency virus (HIV) and marked by progressive deterioration of the cellular immune system, leading to secondary (opportunistic) infections or malignancies.

SYNONYMS

AIDS

ICD-9CM CODES
042 AIDS, unspecified
ICD-10CM CODES
B20 Human immunodeficiency virus [HIV] disease

EPIDEMIOLOGY & DEMOGRAPHICS

INCIDENCE (IN U.S.):
- In 2011, the estimated number of persons diagnosed with AIDS was 32.052.
- In 2010, the estimated number of deaths of persons with an AIDS diagnosis was 15,529.
- In 2009, about 48% of new AIDS cases were in black/African Americans, almost 20% in Hispanics, and about 27% in white Americans.
- Over 50% of the AIDS cases in 2011 were among gay, bisexual, or other men who have sex with men (MSM).

PREVALENCE (IN U.S.):
- At the end of 2010, the estimated number of persons living with an AIDS diagnosis was 487692.
- The cumulative number of AIDS diagnoses through 2010 in the U.S. was 1,155,792.

PREDOMINANT SEX: Over 50% of AIDS diagnoses occur in men who have sex with men (MSM).
PREDOMINANT AGE: The predominant age group diagnosed with AIDS is 30-49 years of age.
PEAK INCIDENCE: Ages 45-49
GENETICS:
- Familial disposition: Although there is no proven genetic predisposition, individuals with deletions in the *CCR5* gene are immune from infection with macrophage tropic virus (the predominant virus in sexual transmission).
- Congenital infection:
  1. Transmittable from an infected mother to the fetus in utero in as many as 30% of pregnancies.
  2. No specific congenital malformations associated with infection; low birth weight and spontaneous abortion are possible.
- Neonatal infection: transmission possible to the neonate intrapartum or postpartum through breastfeeding.

PHYSICAL FINDINGS & CLINICAL PRESENTATION

- Nonspecific findings: fever, weight loss, anorexia.
- Specific syndromes:
  1. Seen in association with opportunistic infection and malignancies, so-called indicator diseases; these include:
     a. Opportunistic infections:
        Disseminated strongyloidiasis
        Disseminated toxoplasmosis, cryptococcosis, histoplasmosis, cytomegalovirus (CMV), herpes simplex, or mycobacterial disease
        Candida esophagitis or bronchopulmonary disease
        Chronic *Cryptosporidia* spp. diarrhea
        Pneumocystis jiroveci pneumonia (PJP)
        Extensive pulmonary and extra-pulmonary tuberculosis
        Recurrent bacterial pneumonia
        Progressive multifocal leukoencephalopathy (PML)
     b. AIDS-related neoplasms:
        Kaposi's sarcoma
        Primary brain lymphoma
        Invasive cervical carcinoma
        High-grade B-cell non-Hodgkin's lymphoma, Burkitt's lymphoma, undifferentiated non-Hodgkin's lymphoma, or immunoblastic lymphoma
  2. Most common:
     Respiratory infections (*Pneumocystis jiroveci* [formerly known as *Pneumocystis carinii*] pneumonia, TB, bacterial pneumonia, fungal infection)
     CNS infections (toxoplasmosis, cryptococcal meningitis, TB)
     GI (cryptosporidiosis, isosporiasis, CMV); Sections II and III describe organisms associated with diarrhea in patients with AIDS
     Eye infections (CMV, toxoplasmosis)
     Kaposi's sarcoma (cutaneous or visceral) or lymphoma (nodal or extranodal)
- Possibly asymptomatic.
- Diagnosis of AIDS if T-lymphocyte subset analysis demonstrating CD4 cell count <200 or <14% of total lymphocyte in the presence of proven HIV infection even in the absence of other infections.
- The various manifestations of HIV infection are described in Section II.

ETIOLOGY

- Caused by infection with HIV-1 or HIV-2.
- Transmitted by heterosexual or male homosexual contact, needle-sharing (during IV drug use), transfusion of contaminated blood or blood products, and from infected mother to fetus or neonate as described previously.

DIAGNOSIS

DIFFERENTIAL DIAGNOSIS

- Other wasting illnesses mimicking the nonspecific features of AIDS:
  1. TB
  2. Neoplasms
  3. Disseminated fungal infection
  4. Malabsorption syndromes
  5. Depression
- Other disorders associated with dementia or demyelination producing encephalopathy, myelopathy, or neuropathy.

WORKUP

Prompt evaluation of respiratory, CNS, and GI complaints

LABORATORY TESTS

- HIV antibody testing. See "Human Immunodeficiency Virus" topic for the 2014 revised surveillance case definition for HIV infection.
- T-lymphocyte subset analysis: performed to determine the degree of immunodeficiency (i.e., CD4 cell count).
- Viral load assay: to plan long-term antiviral therapy and to follow progression and success of treatment (i.e., HIV RNA PCR).
- CSF examination: for meningitis (if indicated).
- Serologic tests for syphilis, hepatitis B, hepatitis C, and toxoplasmosis.
- Genotypic resistance testing: used to assess for primary resistance in naïve patients and secondary resistance in patients failing a regimen.
- Eye exam: to evaluate for CMV retinitis in patients with CD4 counts <50 cells/mm^3.
- Cryptococcal antigen: part of the evaluation in AIDS patients with CD4 counts <100 cells/mm^3 who have fever, diffuse pneumonia, or symptoms of meningitis.
- Evaluation for infection with mycobacterium (TB or MAI) including PPD, sputum cultures, chest radiograph, and blood cultures for acid-fast bacteria, depending on clinical presentation.

IMAGING STUDIES

- MRI or CT of head for encephalopathy or focal CNS complications (e.g., toxoplasmosis, lymphoma).
- Pulmonary gallium scanning to aid in the diagnosis of *Pneumocystis jiroveci* (*P. carinii*) pneumonia.
- Baseline chest radiograph.

TREATMENT

NONPHARMACOLOGIC THERAPY

- Maintain adequate caloric intake.
- Encourage good oral hygiene and regular dental care.
- Avoid high-risk behaviors that increase the risk of repeated exposure to HIV and other potential pathogens—safer sexual practices, avoid sharing needles, etc.
- Update vaccines—particularly the pneumococcal and hepatitis B vaccine along with annual influenza vaccines.
- Avoid administration of any live attenuated vaccines that may be a risk to these immunocompromised patients (i.e., MMR, varicella).
- When feasible, avoid activities that might increase risk of exposure to opportunistic infections (i.e., cleaning out a cat litter box [toxoplasmosis], getting scratched by a cat [*Bartonella* infections], exposure to pet

reptiles [salmonellosis], traveling to developing countries [cryptosporidiosis, tuberculosis], eating undercooked foods and drinking from unsafe water supplies, etc.).

ACUTE GENERAL Rx

Acute management of opportunistic infections and malignancies is reviewed elsewhere in this text under specific AIDS-related disorders.

CHRONIC Rx

For all HIV-infected patients, particularly those meeting the case definition of AIDS:

- Preventive therapy for *Pneumocystis jiroveci* pneumonia and TB (see specific chapters elsewhere in this text). With the advent of modern antiretroviral therapy many patients have experienced substantial restoration of cellular immune function. It has become clear that preventive therapy for *Pneumocystis jiroveci* and *Mycobacterium avium* complex as well as suppressive therapy for CMV and cryptococcal infection can often be safely withdrawn if the CD4 cell count rises above 200 for at least 6 months.
- Based on the Department of Health and Human Services (DHHS) Guidelines of 2013, active antiretroviral therapy (ART) should be started regardless of CD4 cell count. Individuals with CD4 cell counts <350 and especially CD4 cell counts <200 should be strongly encouraged to start ART in a timely fashion.
- ART usually includes three-drug combinations of:
  1. Nucleoside reverse transcriptase inhibitors (NRTI): tenofovir (TDF), zidovudine (AZT), didanosine (DDI), lamivudine (3TC), emtricitabine (FTC), stavudine (D4T), and abacavir (ABC).
  2. Protease inhibitors (PI): saquinavir, amprenavir, indinavir, nelfinavir, agenerase, lopinavir/ritonavir, atazanavir, and darunavir.
  3. Nonnucleoside reverse transcriptase inhibitors (NNRTI): nevirapine, delavirdine, efavirenz (EFV), etravirine, and rilpivirine.
  4. Integrase inhibitors: raltegravir, elvitegravir, and dolutegravir.
  5. Others: maraviroc and enfuvirtide.

The protease inhibitor ritonavir should be used in low dose (100 mg) in combination with other protease inhibitors to obtain more sustained drug levels. Usual initial dosing regimens include two NRTIs and an NNRTI (or a PI or raltegravir). Examples of initial regimens recommended by the guidelines:

1. Atripla (EFV/TDF/FTC) in a single combination pill taken once a day
2. Truvada (TDF/FTC) plus either atazanavir (with ritonavir), darunavir (with ritonavir), or raltegravir
3. Truvada (TDF/FTC) may be substituted with either epzicom (ABC/3TC) or combivir (AZT/3TC). Before using ABC, individuals should be tested for the presence of HLA-B*5701 to check for hypersensitivity to this drug.

All these drugs have unique and class-specific side effects and require careful and expert follow-up to achieve optimal antiviral effects, ensure compliance, and maintain efficacy. Antiviral response should be monitored by baseline HIV viral load and CD4 count and repeat measurement at 2 weeks and 4 weeks into treatment and then periodically (every 3 months) to ensure viral suppression.

- An approach to evaluating chronic diarrhea in patients with HIV infection is described in Fig. E1-25, the approach to the acutely ill HIV-infected patient is outlined in Fig. E1-26, and the evaluation of HIV-positive patients with respiratory complaints is described in Figs. E1-27 and E1-28. The approach to a patient with a suspected CNS lesion is described in Figs. E1-29 and E1-30. Fig. E1-31 presents an approach to cardiac dysfunction.
- Genotypic resistance testing is strongly encouraged for all patients initiating treatment and for any patient failing antiretroviral therapy. Poor adherence to therapy, however, often underlies virologic failure.

DISPOSITION

The outlook for AIDS has changed radically since the advent of ART therapy from an essentially fatal disease to a chronic medical illness compatible with long-term survival and remarkably good quality of life. Patients should be aggressively treated for severe illnesses as outcomes following ICU admissions remain good. This is accomplished through expert and continuous follow-up, use of ART, and careful detail to compliance to medications and lifestyle modification.

REFERRAL

All patients with AIDS: to a physician knowledgeable and experienced in the management of the disease and its complications

SUGGESTED READINGS

available at www.expertconsult.com

RELATED CONTENT

Acquired Immunodeficiency Syndrome (AIDS) (Patient Information)

AUTHOR: **PHILIP A. CHAN, M.D., M.S.**

BASIC INFORMATION

DEFINITION

Actinic keratoses (AKs) are common skin lesions usually presenting as multiple, erythematous or yellow-brown, dry, scaly lesions in the middle aged or elderly.

SYNONYMS

Solar keratosis
Senile keratosis
AK

ICD-9CM CODES
702.0 Actinic keratosis
ICD-10CM CODES
L57.0 Actinic keratosis

EPIDEMIOLOGY & DEMOGRAPHICS

INCIDENCE: In regions of the northern hemisphere, 11%-25% of adults have a minimum of one AK. In regions closer to the equator, 40%-60% of adults have a minimum of one AK.

PEAK INCIDENCE: The risk of squamous cell carcinoma in patients with AK is 6%-10%. Incidence increases with age, and mortality from nonmelanoma skin cancers increases significantly in the sixth decade. The rate of mortality is approximately 0.1% of the incidence rate (Table 1-12).

PREVALENCE:
- In the United States, 58.08 million per year.
- Highest prevalence in those with fair complexions with high sun exposure.
- Approximately 60% of predisposed individuals older than 40 years will have one AK.
- Caucasians' risk increases with age: at age 20-29 prevalence is <10%; at age 80-89, prevalence is approximately 75%.

PREDOMINANT SEX AND AGE: Males > females, age 65-74. Occurs most in those with fair complexions who burn rather than tan following sun exposure.

GENETICS: There is increased frequency of non-melanoma skin cancers connected to squamous cell cancers with the genetic conditions xeroderma pigmentosum, oculocutaneous albinism, epidermodysplasia verruciformis, dystrophic epidermolysis bullosa, Ferguson-Smith syndrome, and Muir-Torre syndrome.

RISK FACTORS:
- Immunosuppression, exposure to ultraviolet (UV) light, ionizing radiation, arsenic, human papillomavirus, cigarette smoke, chronic ulcers, thermal burns, chronic discoid lupus erythematosus, and nonhealing wounds.
- Lichen planus, lichen sclerosis, linear and classic porokeratosis, and disseminated superficial actinic porokeratosis.
- Age, gender, skin color, and mutations in p53 tumor suppressor gene.

PHYSICAL FINDINGS & CLINICAL PRESENTATION

- Typical lesions occur on sun-damaged skin, usually on the face and neck and the dorsal aspects of hands (Fig. 1-33) and forearms.
- Advanced lesions are characterized by a hard, spiky scale (Fig. 1-34) and usually measure 1 cm in diameter or less. Early lesions manifest with redness and minimal scale. With progression, scales become thicker and yellow and may resemble a small squamous cell carcinoma. On examinations, lesions are rough and gritty (Fig. 1-35).
- The surrounding skin frequently shows additional features of sun damage, including atrophy (Fig. 1-36), pigment changes, and telangiectasia.
- Classifications
  - Hypertrophic AK with a cutaneous horn: Biopsy is necessary to distinguish the cutaneous horn from squamous cell carcinoma, seborrheic keratosis, verruca, and trichilemmoma and basal cell carcinoma. Hypertrophic AK has appearance of thick, scaling skin elevations.
  - Lichenoid AK: Most commonly found on the torso and upper extremities. Must be distinguished from BCC due to pink and pearly characteristics.
  - Proliferative AK: Often reappear after treatment and are characterized by a diameter >1 cm. Often occurs in same differential as Bowen's disease or SCC.
  - Spreading pigmented AK: Must be biopsied to distinguish from lentigo maligna–type melanoma in situ as well as solar lentigo.
  - Actinic cheilitis: Characterized by red and sometimes abrasive lesions around the border of the lips and skin.

ETIOLOGY

- Sun exposure, ionizing radiation.
- Arsenic, polycyclic hydrocarbon exposure.

DIAGNOSIS

DIFFERENTIAL DIAGNOSIS

- Heavily pigmented variants may be clinically mistaken for lentigo maligna.
- Basal cell or squamous cell carcinoma.
- Seborrheic keratosis.
- Eczema.
- Bowen disease (intraepithelial carcinoma).
- Wart.
- Lichenoid keratosis.
- Cutaneous lupus.

TABLE 1-12 Incidence Rates Per Year (Per 100,000) of BCC and SCC by Geographic Location

Geographic Location	BCC (Men/Women)	SCC (Men/Women)
Finland	49/45	9/5
Switzerland	52/38	16/8
The Netherlands	53/38	—
United Kingdom	112/54	32/6
New Hampshire	159/87	32/8
Rochester, Minnesota	175/124	63/23
United States	247/150	65/24
Hawaii	576/298	153/92
Nambour, Australia	2074/1579	1035/472

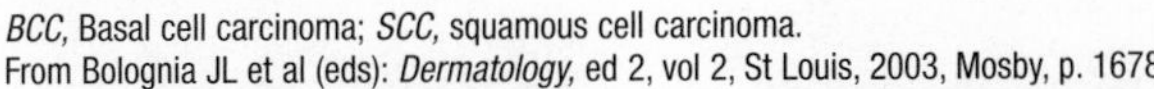

BCC, Basal cell carcinoma; *SCC,* squamous cell carcinoma.
From Bolognia JL et al (eds): *Dermatology,* ed 2, vol 2, St Louis, 2003, Mosby, p. 1678.

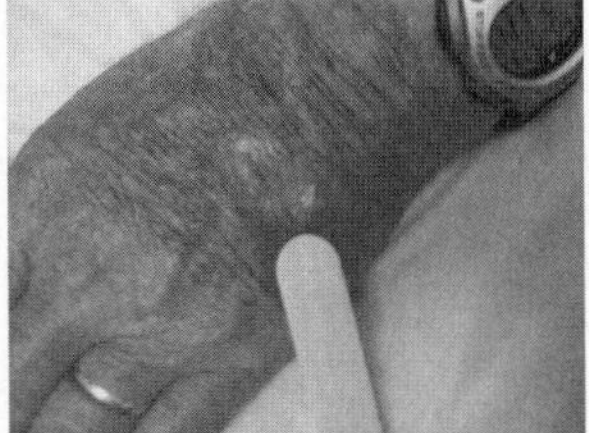

FIGURE 1-33 Several scaly, adherent, yellow-brown lesions on the sun-exposed dorsum of the hand. (From Ferri F et al: *Ferri's fast facts in dermatology,* Philadelphia, 2010, Saunders.)

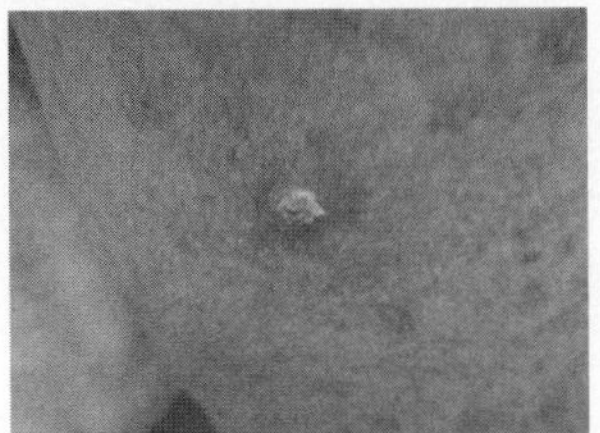

FIGURE 1-34 Scaly, raised lesion on sun-exposed back. Pain was elicited when scraping this lesion. (From Ferri F et al: *Ferri's fast facts in dermatology,* Philadelphia, 2010, Saunders.)

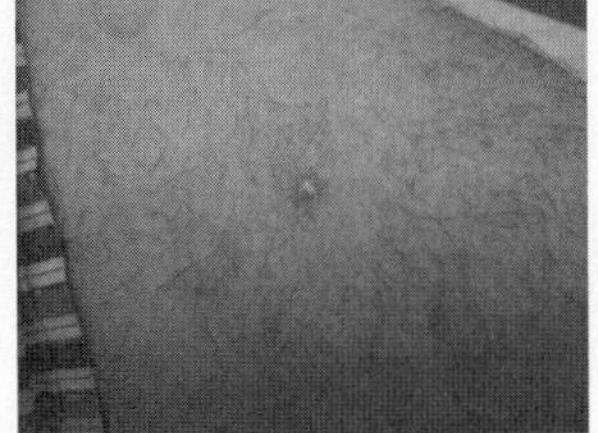

FIGURE 1-35 Raised, rough, gritty actinic keratosis on the anterior thigh of an outdoorsman. (From Ferri F et al: *Ferri's fast facts in dermatology,* Philadelphia, 2010, Saunders.)

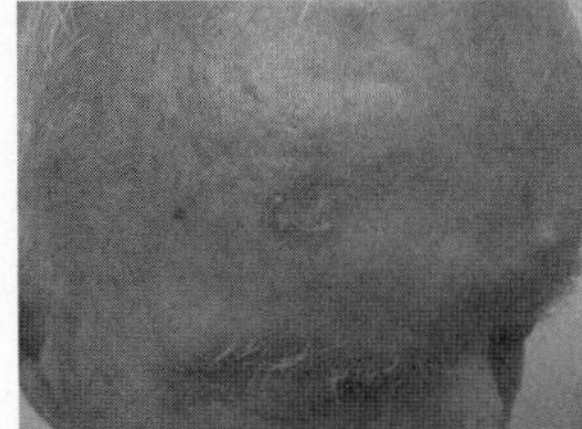

FIGURE 1-36 Actinic keratosis (shown here on a patient's forehead) is often best appreciated by its rough, tactile quality, similar to that of sandpaper. (From Ferri F et al: *Ferri's fast facts in dermatology,* Philadelphia, 2010, Saunders.)

WORKUP

- History, physical, and lesion biopsy. Include risk assessment and family or personal history of skin cancers or previous skin lesions.

LABORATORY TESTS

- Skin biopsy in recurrent lesions or when diagnosis is unclear to rule out squamous cell or basal cell carcinoma.
- Microscopy reveals atypical keratinocytes in the lower epidermis basal layers. They are enlarged and often lack normal polarity. The thickness of the epidermis can be compromised with a distribution of atrophic to hyperplastic. Abnormal keratinocytes can cause parakeratosis of the overlying stratum corneum. Visible signs of an alternating orthohyperkeratosis can overlie the spared epithelium, causing the signature "flag sign." Additionally, there is a distinct margin between normal epidermis and the region of AK at lateral edges. Histologic subtypes are hypertrophic, acantholytic, lichenoid, and bowenoid, which are characterized by a thick stratum corneum, lack of intracellular cohesion, presence of lymphocytic infiltrate in papillary dermis, and either lack of association of adnexal epithelium or full epithelial thickness with pleomorphic kertinocytes, respectively.

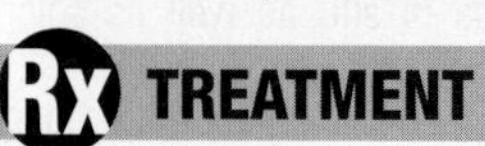

TREATMENT

NONPHARMACOLOGIC THERAPY

- Cryosurgery with liquid nitrogen.
- Carbon dioxide laser.
- Dermabrasion.
- Chemical peel.
- Curettage.
- Excision.
- Photodynamic therapy with 5-aminolevulinic acid and blue light (16 minutes) or methyl aminolevulinate and red light (7-10 minutes).

ACUTE GENERAL Rx

- Topical 5-fluorouracil bid for 4 weeks.
- Topical diclofenac sodium 3% gel bid for 60-90 days.
- Topical imiquimod 5% cream bid for 3-4 months.
- Oral retinoids.
- Topical Ingenol mebutate 0.05% gel applied for 2 days with exception of face—or 0.015% for 3 days. Combination medication therapy or nonpharmacologic therapy with pharmacologic therapy is common (especially in refractory AK).

REFERRAL

- To a dermatologist for biopsy of suspicious lesions, then follow up minimum annually or semiannually.

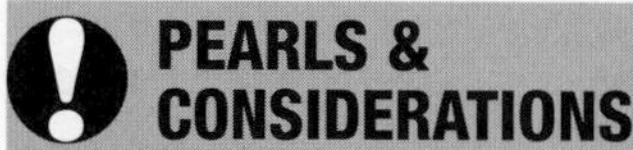

PEARLS & CONSIDERATIONS

COMMENTS

- AKs are of particular importance because they are a sensitive indicator of exposure to UV light and strongly predict the likelihood of developing cutaneous squamous cell carcinoma.
- The cumulative probability of development of invasive squamous cell carcinoma in patients with 10 or more AKs has been estimated at 14% in a 5-year period.
- It is estimated that up to 10% of AKs tend to progress to invasive carcinoma.

PREVENTION

- Avoidance of sun exposure or sunless tanning booths, use of sunscreens.
- Routine self-skin examinations.
- Pharmaceutical prevention:
  - Mild to moderate reduction of AK formation has been documented with the use of topical tretinoin, isotretinoin, and arotinoid methysulfone.
  - Nicotinamide as preventative rx has been documented to have a possible 30% relative reduction in AK.
  - Decreased AK development has been documented with the use of high-SPF sunscreens.
  - Decreased AK development has been seen in patients with xeroderma pigmentosum who used DNA repair enzymes.
  - Decreased AK formation has been documented in high-risk patients (specifically those with xeroderma pigmentosum, nevoid basal cell carcinoma syndrome, and organ transplantation recipients) with the use of oral retinoids.

SUGGESTED READINGS

available at www.expertconsult.com

AUTHORS: **FRED F. FERRI, M.D.,** and **HEATHER FERRI, D.O.**

BASIC INFORMATION

DEFINITION

Actinomycosis is an indolent, slowly progressive infection caused by anaerobic or microaerophilic bacteria, mostly from the genus *Actinomyces,* that normally colonize the mouth, vagina, and colon. Actinomycosis is characterized by the formation of painful abscesses, soft tissue infiltration, and draining sinuses.

SYNONYMS

Actinomyces infection
Lumpy jaw

ICD-9CM CODES
039.9 Actinomycosis
ICD-10CM CODES
A42.9 Actinomycosis, unspecified

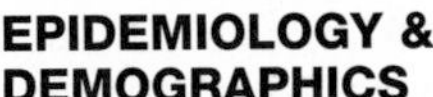

EPIDEMIOLOGY & DEMOGRAPHICS

Geographic distribution:

- Actinomycosis is worldwide in distribution.
- Commonly found as normal flora of the oral cavity (within gingival crevices, tonsillar crypts, periodontal pockets, dental plaques, and carious teeth), pharynx, tracheobronchial tree, gastrointestinal tract, and female urogenital tract.

Incidence and prevalence:

- Incidence 1:300,000 in 1970s but now less with better oral hygiene and antibiotic use.
- Males infected more often than females 3:1.
- Can occur at any age but commonly seen in midlife.

PHYSICAL FINDINGS & CLINICAL PRESENTATION

Actinomycosis can affect any organ. Although not typically considered as opportunistic pathogens, *Actinomyces* species capitalize on tissue injury or mucosal breach to invade adjacent structures in the head and neck regions. As a result, dental infections and oromaxillofacial trauma are common antecedent events. Characteristic manifestations include:

- Cervicofacial disease (most common site):
  1. Occurs in the setting of poor dental hygiene, recent dental surgery, or minor oral trauma
  2. Painful soft tissue swelling (Fig. 1-37) commonly seen at the angle of the mandible
  3. Fever, chills, and weight loss
  4. Trismus
  5. Soft tissue facial infection with sinus tract or fistula formation
- Thoracic disease:
  1. Can involve the lungs, pleura, mediastinum, or chest wall.
  2. Presumed secondary to aspiration of *Actinomyces* organisms in patients with poor oral hygiene.
  3. Fever, cough, weight loss, and pleuritic chest pains are common symptoms.
  4. Signs of pneumonia or pleural effusion may be present.
  5. With extension beyond the lungs to mediastinal structures and the chest wall, signs and symptoms of pericarditis, empyema, chest wall sinus drainage, and tracheoesophageal fistula can all occur (Fig. 1-38).
- Abdominal disease:
  1. Occurs most commonly after appendectomy, perforated bowel, diverticulitis, or surgery to the gastrointestinal tract.
  2. Lesions develop most commonly in the ileocecal valve, causing abdominal pain, fever, weight loss, and a palpable mass.
  3. Extension may occur to the liver, causing jaundice and abscess formation.
  4. Sinus tracts to the abdominal wall can occur.

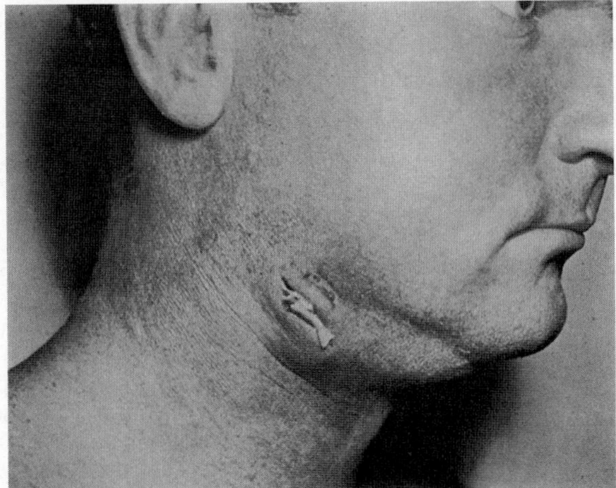

FIGURE 1-37 Actinomycosis of the jaw, observed at Letterman General Hospital, San Francisco, Calif., in a sergeant who had punctured the floor of his mouth while picking his teeth. (Office of Medical History, Office of the Surgeon General, U.S. Army; from Goldman L, Schaefer AI: *Goldman's Cecil medicine,* ed 24, Philadelphia, 2012, Saunders.)

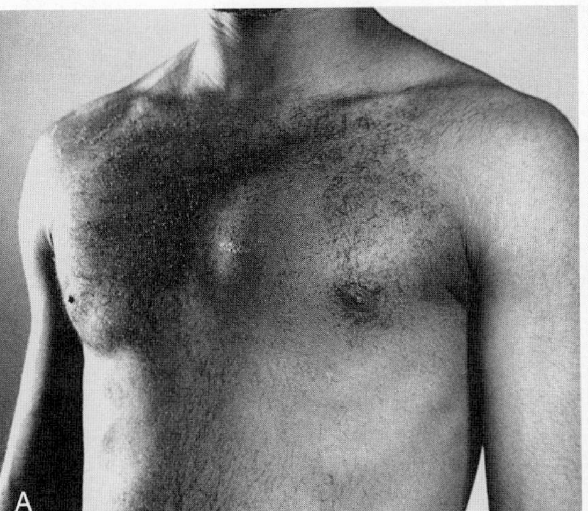

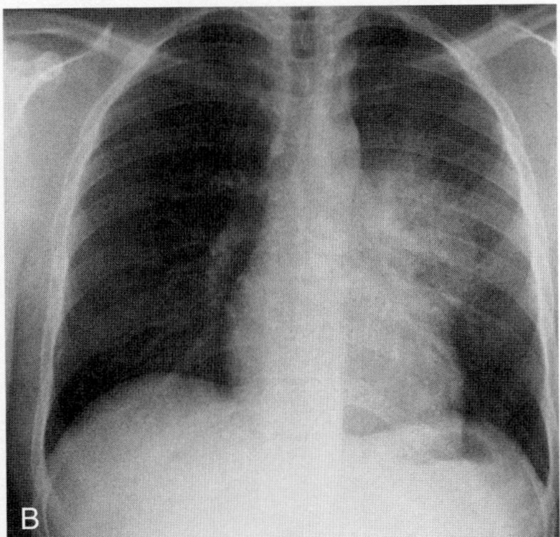

FIGURE 1-38 Thoracic actinomycosis. A, Initial presentation with a bulging mass lesion in the chest wall with a central sinus tract. **B,** The chest radiograph with the associated pulmonary infiltrate. (From Gorbach SL: *Infectious diseases,* ed 2, Philadelphia, 1998, Saunders.)

- Pelvic disease:
  1. Commonly occurs by extension from abdominal disease of the ileocecal valve to the right adnexa (80% of cases).
  2. Endometritis.

ETIOLOGY

- Actinomycosis is most commonly caused by *Actinomyces israelii.* Other causes are *A. naeslundii, A. odontolyticus, A. viscosus,* and *A. meyeri.*
- *Actinomyces* are gram-positive, non–spore-forming, filamentous, anaerobic or microaerophilic rods.
- Actinomycosis infections are polymicrobial, usually associated with *Streptococcus, Bacteroides, Eikenella corrodens, Enterococcus,* and *Fusobacterium* spp.
- Infects individuals only after entry into disrupted mucosa or tissue injury.
- Predisposing conditions include diabetes mellitus, malnutrition, and immunosuppression.

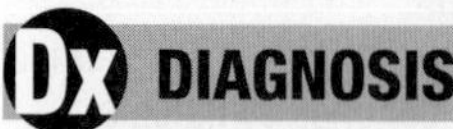

DIAGNOSIS

Isolating the bacteria in the proper clinical setting makes the diagnosis of actinomycosis.

DIFFERENTIAL DIAGNOSIS

- Cervicofacial disease: odontogenic abscesses, brachial cleft cyst
- Pulmonary disease: nocardiosis, botryomycosis, chromomycosis, fungal disease of the lung, tuberculosis
- Intestinal disease: intestinal tuberculosis, ameboma, Crohn's disease, colon cancer
- Pelvic disease: chronic pelvic inflammatory disease, Crohn's disease
- CNS disease: other forms of brain abscess, brain tumors, toxoplasmosis, intracranial hematoma

WORKUP

The workup includes obtaining specimens either by aspirating abscesses, excising sinus tracts, or tissue biopsies. All specimens should be set up to culture anaerobic bacteria and held at least 5 to 7 days.

LABORATORY TESTS

- Isolating "sulfur granules" from tissue specimens or draining sinuses confirms the diagnosis of actinomycosis. *Actinomyces* are noted for forming characteristic sulfur granules in infected tissue but not in vitro. The term *sulfur granule* is a misnomer, reflecting only the yellow color of the granule in pus, because the granules are not composed of any sulfur at all.
  1. Sulfur granules are nests of *Actinomyces* species. Sulfur granules may be macroscopic or microscopic.
  2. Sulfur granules are crushed and stained for identification of *Actinomyces* organisms and may take up to 3 wk to grow in culture media.

IMAGING STUDIES

Imaging studies are useful adjunctive tests in localizing the site and spread of infection.

1. Chest x-ray examination
2. CT scan of the head, chest, abdomen, and pelvic areas is useful

Rx TREATMENT

NONPHARMACOLOGIC THERAPY

- Incision and drainage of abscesses
- Excision of sinus tract

ACUTE GENERAL Rx

- Ampicillin 50 mg/kg/day in 3-4 divided doses x 4-6 wk, then Pen VK 2-4 g/day PO x 4-6 wk. In place of ampicillin, can also use penicillin 3-4 million units IV q4h for 4-6 wk.
- In penicillin-allergic patients, erythromycin (500-1000 mg IV q6h), tetracycline or doxycycline (100 mg IV q12h), and clindamycin (900 mg IV q8h) are reasonable alternatives. Other alternatives include cetriaxone, imipenem, and piperacillin/tazobactam.
- Avoid use of metronidazole, aminoglycosides, oxacillin, and cephalexin.

CHRONIC Rx

- Following 4 to 6 wk IV amoxicillin or penicillin, oral penicillin V 500 mg PO qid for 4 to 6 wk. Longer treatment may be necessary in selected cases.
- Other available oral agents are erythromycin, doxycycline, and clindamycin.
- Treatment of associated microorganisms is not needed.

DISPOSITION

- Clinical actinomycosis, if not treated, spreads to contiguous tissues and structures ignoring tissue planes. Hematogenous spread, although possible, is rare.
- Actinomycosis is very sensitive to antibiotics but requires chronic long-term treatment to prevent relapse.

REFERRAL

If the diagnosis of actinomycosis is suspected, consultation with an infectious disease specialist is suggested. General surgical consultation for excision of sinus tracts and abscess incision and drainage is recommended.

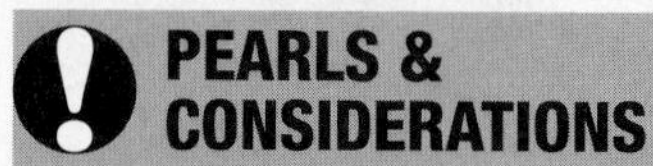

PEARLS & CONSIDERATIONS

COMMENTS

- There is no person-to-person transmission of *Actinomyces.*
- Isolation of the organism in an asymptomatic individual does not mean the person has actinomycosis. Active symptoms must be present to make the diagnosis.
- Pelvic actinomycosis has been associated with use of an intrauterine device (IUD).
- Actinomycosis can also involve the CNS, causing multiple brain abscesses.

SUGGESTED READINGS

available at www.expertconsult.com

AUTHOR: **GLENN G. FORT, M.D., M.P.H.**

BASIC INFORMATION

DEFINITION

Acute bronchitis is a self-limited inflammation of trachea and bronchi.

SYNONYMS

Chest cold

ICD-9CM CODES
466.0 Acute bronchitis
ICD-10CM CODES
J20.9 Acute bronchitis, unspecified

EPIDEMIOLOGY & DEMOGRAPHICS

- Highest incidence in smokers, older adults, and young children and during winter months.
- In the U.S. there are nearly 30 million ambulatory visits annually for cough, leading to more than 12 million diagnoses of "bronchitis."
- Acute lower respiratory tract infection is the most common condition treated in primary care.

PHYSICAL FINDINGS & CLINICAL PRESENTATION

- Cough, usually worse in the morning, often productive; mainly caused by transient bronchial hyperresponsiveness
- Low-grade fever
- Substernal discomfort worsened by coughing
- Postnasal drip, pharyngeal injection
- Rhonchi that may clear after cough, occasional wheezing

ETIOLOGY

- Viral infections are the leading cause of bronchitis (rhinovirus, influenza virus, adenovirus, respiratory syncytial virus)
- Atypical organisms *(Mycoplasma, Chlamydia pneumoniae)*
- Bacterial infections *(Bordetella pertussis, Haemophilus influenzae, Moraxella, Streptococcus pneumoniae)*

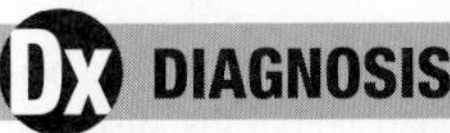

DIAGNOSIS

DIFFERENTIAL DIAGNOSIS

- Pneumonia
- Asthma
- Sinusitis
- Bronchiolitis
- Aspiration
- Cystic fibrosis
- Pharyngitis
- Cough secondary to medications
- Neoplasm (elderly patients)
- Influenza
- Allergic aspergillosis
- Gastroesophageal reflux disease
- Congestive heart failure (in elderly patients)
- Bronchogenic neoplasm

WORKUP

Seldom necessary (e.g., to rule out pneumonia, neoplasm)

LABORATORY TESTS

Laboratory tests are generally not necessary.

IMAGING STUDIES

Chest x-ray examination is usually reserved for patients with suspected pneumonia, influenza, or underlying chronic obstructive pulmonary disease (COPD) and no improvement with therapy.

Rx TREATMENT

NONPHARMACOLOGIC THERAPY

- Avoidance of tobacco and other pulmonary irritants
- Increased fluid intake
- Use of vaporizer to increase room humidity

ACUTE GENERAL Rx

- Inhaled bronchodilators (e.g., albuterol, metaproterenol) prn for 1 to 2 wk in patients with wheezing or troublesome cough. Inhaled albuterol has been proven effective in reducing the duration of cough in adults with uncomplicated acute bronchitis.
- Cough suppression with dextromethorphan and guaifenesin is commonly recommended; addition of codeine for cough suppression if cough is severe and is significantly interrupting patient's sleep pattern.
- Use of antibiotics (TMP-SMX, amoxicillin, doxycycline, cefuroxime) for acute bronchitis is generally not indicated; should be considered only in patients with concomitant COPD and purulent sputum or in patients with suspected pertussis. In the few cases of acute bronchitis caused by *B. pertussis* or atypical bacteria such as *C. pneumoniae* or *Mycoplasma pneumoniae,* early use of macrolide antibiotics is reasonable.
- Antibiotics are overused in patients with acute bronchitis (70% to 90% of office visits for acute bronchitis result in treatment with antibiotics); this practice pattern is contributing to increases in resistant organisms.

CHRONIC Rx

Avoidance of tobacco and other pulmonary irritants

DISPOSITION

- Complete recovery within 7 to 10 days in most patients.
- Patients should be informed to expect to have a cough for 10 to 14 days after the visit.

REFERRAL

For pulmonary function testing only in patients with recurrent bronchitis and suspected underlying pulmonary disease

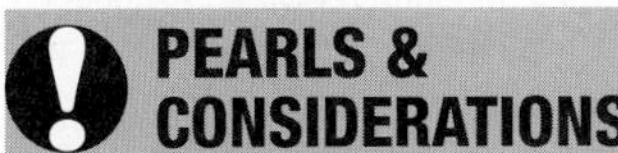

PEARLS & CONSIDERATIONS

COMMENTS

- Intervention studies reveal that patient and physician education are effective in reducing the use of antibiotic therapy. No offer or delayed offer of antibiotics for acute uncomplicated lower respiratory tract infection is acceptable, is associated with little difference in symptom resolution, and is likely to reduce antibiotic use and beliefs in the effectiveness of antibiotics.
- It is helpful to refer to acute bronchitis as a "chest cold." Patients should be informed that antibiotics are probably not going to be beneficial and may result in significant side effects.

SUGGESTED READINGS

available at www.expertconsult.com

RELATED CONTENT

Acute Bronchitis (Patient Information)

AUTHOR: **FRED F. FERRI, M.D.**

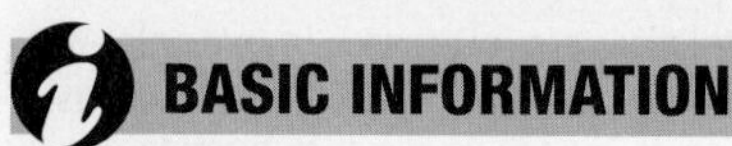

BASIC INFORMATION

DEFINITION

Acute coronary syndrome (ACS) represents a spectrum of clinical disorders that include unstable angina (UA), non–ST-elevation myocardial infarction (NSTEMI), and ST-elevation myocardial infarction (STEMI). Although the severity of disease will vary between the three subsets of ACS, they share a common clinical presentation and pathophysiology. This syndrome is typically caused by atherosclerotic coronary artery disease (CAD). In this spectrum, UA and NSTEMI are represented electrocardiographically by ST-segment depression and T-wave inversion in the appropriate clinical setting (i.e., chest discomfort). NSTEMI is represented by the addition of positive cardiac biomarkers. STEMI is represented by ST-segment elevation or presumed new left bundle branch block on electrocardiogram (ECG). ACS should be thought of as a continuous spectrum as UA will often progress to a myocardial infarction if left untreated (Table 1-13).

SYNONYMS

Unstable angina
NSTEMI
STEMI
Acute myocardial infarction

ICD-9CM CODES
410.0 Acute Myocardial Infarction
411.1 Intermediate Coronary Syndrome
ICD-10CM CODES
I20.0 Unstable angina
I21.0-I21.3 ST elevation (STEMI)
I21.4 non-ST elevation (NSTEMI) myocardial infarction
I24.9 Acute ischemic heart disease, unspecified

EPIDEMIOLOGY & DEMOGRAPHICS

INCIDENCE: In the United States there are 1.56 million hospitalizations for ACS yearly; 0.89 million are listed as myocardial infarction, and the remainder are UA. Approximately two thirds of myocardial infarctions are listed as NSTEMI, with the remainder being listed as STEMI. The underlying etiology, atherosclerotic CAD, is the number one cause of mortality.

PREDOMINANT SEX AND AGE: In evaluating chest pain, male gender and older age are important clinical factors that can identify ACS as a potential cause. The 2007 overall death rate from cardiovascular disease was 126 per 100,000. The rates were 165.6 per 100,000 for white males, 191.6 per 100,000 for African-American males, 94.2 per 100,000 for white females, and 121.5 per 100,000 for African-American females.

RISK FACTORS: Hypertension, diabetes mellitus, dyslipidemia, tobacco use, family history of premature CAD (CAD in a male first-degree relative younger than 55 years or a female younger than 65 years). Presence of these risk factors causes damage to the vascular endothelium and progression of atherosclerotic coronary artery plaques.

PHYSICAL FINDINGS & CLINICAL PRESENTATION

- Symptoms often, but not always, include chest discomfort described as a pressure that may radiate to the left arm, neck, jaw, or back. Typical angina is substernal in location, brought on by emotional or physical stress, and relieved with rest and/or nitroglycerin.
- Women, diabetics, and the elderly often have an atypical presentation for ACS.
- Angina is considered unstable if it is new onset (<2 months), increasing in frequency (crescendo pattern), or occurring at rest (typically lasting >20 minutes).
- "Anginal equivalents" may include dyspnea, nausea, vomiting, and fatigue.
- ECG for UA and NSTEMI may reveal ST-segment depression and/or T-wave inversion. ECG for definition of STEMI will reveal at least 1-mm ST-segment elevation in two contiguous leads or new left bundle branch block in the appropriate clinical setting.
- Physical exam findings alone are insufficient for the diagnosis of ACS. It is, however, important to assess the patient's hemodynamic stability and volume status. The patient may be diaphoretic and tachycardic. Signs of heart failure may be present, which include elevated jugular venous pressure (JVP), presence of an S3 gallop, and peripheral edema.

ETIOLOGY

Atherosclerotic CAD is the underlying etiology. The hallmark of ACS is the vulnerable atherosclerotic plaque, which typically has a thin fibrous cap and a large lipid core. This vulnerable plaque ultimately ruptures, which leads to platelet activation and aggregation, leading to thrombus formation. STEMI typically results from complete thrombotic occlusion of a coronary artery, whereas UA and NSTEMI often have partial occlusion. Angiographically, it is often the intermediate coronary artery lesions (30% to 50% diameter vessel stenosis) that lead to subtotal or total vessel occlusion in two thirds of STEMI cases.

Dx DIAGNOSIS

DIFFERENTIAL DIAGNOSIS

Chest pain mimicking ACS may be the result of various underlying disorders, some of which are also accompanied by ECG changes and/or cardiac biomarker release. Examples include acute pulmonary embolism, acute aortic dissection, pericarditis, myocarditis, costochondritis, pneumonia, tension pneumothorax, perforating ulcer, or Boerhaave syndrome.

WORKUP

Focused history and physical exam, 12-lead ECG, cardiac biomarkers, and chest radiograph (CXR). Initial biomarkers may not be positive. Often serial biomarkers are drawn every 6 to 8 hours for a total of three sets for the purposes of ruling out myocardial infarction (MI), or until peak to determine the severity of an established MI. Echocardiogram may reveal new regional wall motion abnormalities. Figure 1-39 summarizes the evaluation of patients for acute coronary syndrome.

LABORATORY TESTS

- Cardiac biomarkers, which include creatine kinase (CK), its MB isoenzyme, myoglobin, and troponin I or T, will be positive in the setting of NSTEMI or STEMI. See Fig. 1-40*A* for timing of release of each biomarker.Troponin I is the most sensitive biomarker for cardiac myocyte damage and also predicts 42-day mortality in ACS (Fig. 1-40*B*)
- Testing for B-type natriuretic peptide (BNP) levels may also be helpful in patients with heart failure.
- A complete fasting lipid panel should be obtained during the hospital admission.

RISK MODELS AND RISK SCORES

Risk models and scores such as TIMI , PURSUIT, and GRACE based on clinical, ECG, and laboratory data at presentation help to discriminate patients at high risk versus low risk for short- and intermediate-term adverse outcomes (Fig.1-40*C*).

IMAGING STUDIES

- CXR to assist in evaluating for volume status and for other possible causes of chest discomfort.
- In patients for whom ECG and cardiac biomarkers are nondiagnostic but the suspicion for ACS is high given the history, an echocardiogram may be helpful to assess left ventricular (LV) function and regional wall motion abnormalities.

TABLE 1-13 Acute Coronary Syndromes

	SPECTRUM OF ACUTE CORONARY SYNDROME		
	Unstable Angina	**NSTEMI**	**STEMI**
Chest discomfort	+	+	+
Cardiac biomarkers	–	+	+
ECG changes	TWI and/or ST depression	TWI and/or ST depression	ST elevation or presumed new left bundle branch block
Pathophysiology	Partial/transient thrombotic occlusion	Partial/transient thrombotic occlusion	Complete thrombotic occlusion

NSTEMI, Non–ST-segment elevation myocardial infarction; *STEMI,* ST-segment myocardial infarction; *TWI,* T-wave inversion; *ECG,* electrocardiogram.

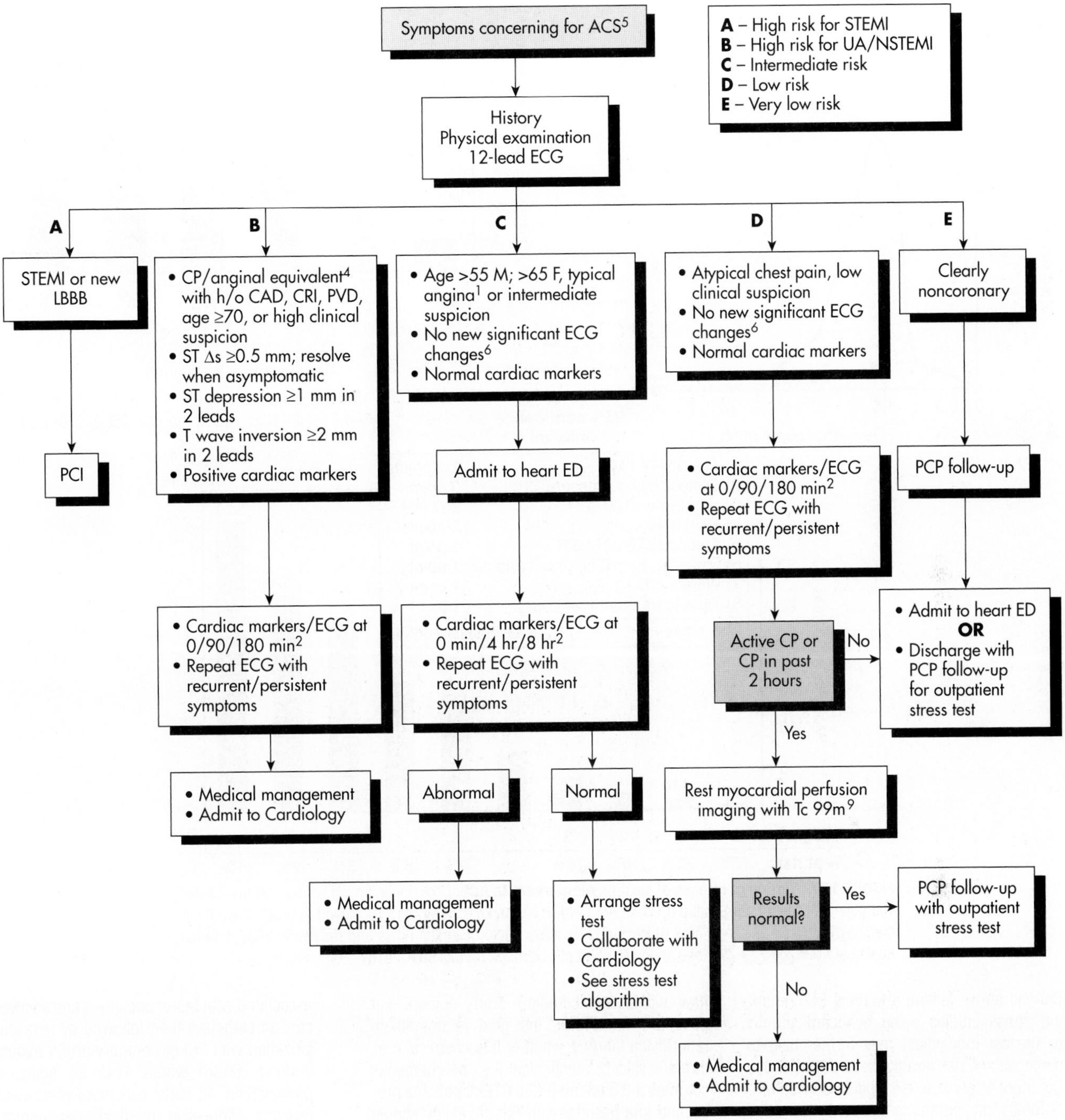

DEFINITIONS:

[1]**Typical angina:**
1) Substernal chest pain or discomfort that is 2) provoked by exertion or emotional stress and 3) relieved by rest and/or nitroglycerin

[2]**Cardiac marker timing:** based on symptom onset; in cases of uncertainty assume symptom onset at ED arrival

[3]**ECG normal:** no significant ST depression/T wave inversions, BBB, LVH with repolarization, conduction defect, digoxin effect

[4]**Anginal equivalent:**
- Any symptoms that the physician feels may represent ACS
- Exertional dyspnea—most common anginal equivalent symptom

[5]**ACS:**
- STE-ACS—1 mm ST elevation in 2 leads
- NSTE-ACS
  - NSTEMI—positive cardiac biomarkers
  - Unstable angina—ischemia with negative biomarkers

[6]**New significant ECG changes:**
- ST Δs ≥0.5 mm; resolve when asymptomatic
- ST depression ≥1 mm in 2 leads
- T wave inversion ≥2 mm in 2 leads

[7]**Regadenoson** is preferred agent for chemical nuclear stress test. Technetium Tc-99m tetrofosmin is the preferred tracer.

FIGURE 1-39 Evaluation of patients for acute coronary syndrome (ACS). *CAD,* Coronary artery disease; *CP,* chest pain; *CRI,* chronic renal insufficiency; *ECG,* electrocardiogram; *ED,* emergency department; *h/o,* history of; *LBBB,* left bundle branch block; *NSTE,* non–ST-segment elevation; *NSTEMI,* non–ST-segment elevation myocardial infarction; *PCP,* primary care physician; *PVD,* peripheral vascular disease; *STE,* ST-segment elevation; *STEMI,* ST-segment elevation myocardial infarction; *UA,* unstable angina. (From Adams JG et al: *Emergency medicine, clinical essentials,* ed 2, Philadelphia, 2013, Elsevier.)

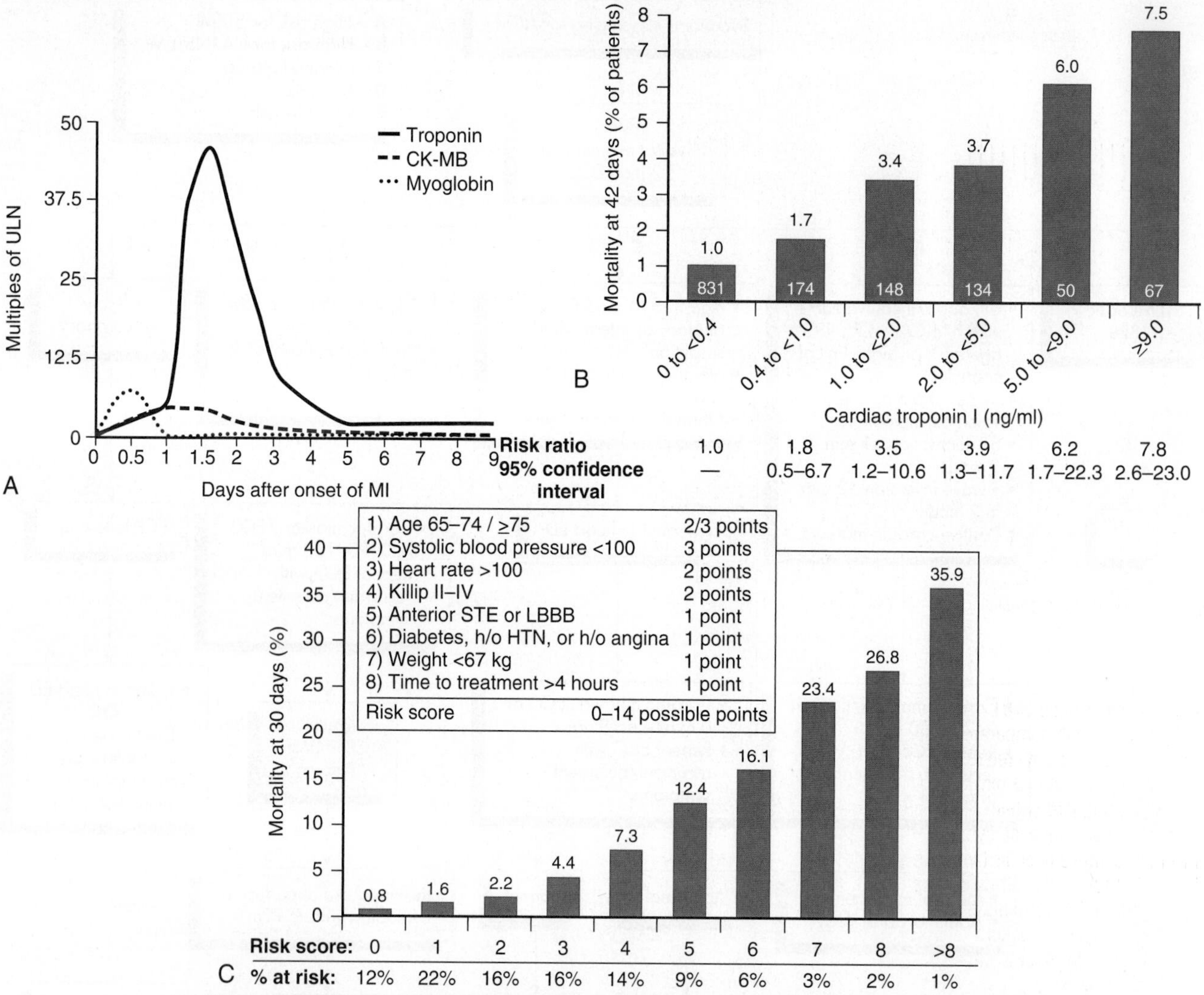

A

Multiples of ULN (0, 12.5, 25, 37.5, 50)

— Troponin
-- CK-MB
··· Myoglobin

Days after onset of MI (0, 0.5, 1, 1.5, 2, 3, 4, 5, 6, 7, 8, 9)

B

Mortality at 42 days (% of patients)

Cardiac troponin I (ng/ml)	0 to <0.4	0.4 to <1.0	1.0 to <2.0	2.0 to <5.0	5.0 to <9.0	≥9.0
Mortality (%)	1.0	1.7	3.4	3.7	6.0	7.5
n	831	174	148	134	50	67
Risk ratio	1.0	1.8	3.5	3.9	6.2	7.8
95% confidence interval	—	0.5–6.7	1.2–10.6	1.3–11.7	1.7–22.3	2.6–23.0

C

1) Age 65–74 / ≥75	2/3 points
2) Systolic blood pressure <100	3 points
3) Heart rate >100	2 points
4) Killip II–IV	2 points
5) Anterior STE or LBBB	1 point
6) Diabetes, h/o HTN, or h/o angina	1 point
7) Weight <67 kg	1 point
8) Time to treatment >4 hours	1 point
Risk score	0–14 possible points

Mortality at 30 days (%)

Risk score:	0	1	2	3	4	5	6	7	8	>8
Mortality (%)	0.8	1.6	2.2	4.4	7.3	12.4	16.1	23.4	26.8	35.9
% at risk:	12%	22%	16%	16%	14%	9%	6%	3%	2%	1%

FIGURE 1-40 Timing of release of cardiac biomarkers in ACS. *ULN,* Upper limit of normal; *MI,* myocardial infarction. (Modified from Shapiro BP, Jaffe AS: Cardiac biomarkers. In Murphy JG, Lloyd MA [eds]: *Mayo Clinic cardiology: concise textbook*, ed 3, Rochester, MN: Mayo Clinic Scientific Press and New York, 2007, Informa Healthcare USA, pp 773-780; and Anderson JL et al: *J Am Coll Cardiol* 50:e1-e157, 2007, Fig. 5.)

- Cardiac stress testing (treadmill ECG, imaging stress studies using echocardiography or nuclear modalities) may further help to diagnose and risk stratify these patients.(See Coronary Artery Disease topic in Section I.)
- Coronary angiogram/cardiac catheterization will reveal coronary artery luminal irregularities/stenotic lesions. In patients with ACS who undergo coronary angiography, approximately 25% will have one vessel disease, 25% will have two vessel disease, 25% will have three vessel diease, 10% will have left main disease, and 15% will have coronary stenosis of <50% or normal coronaries.

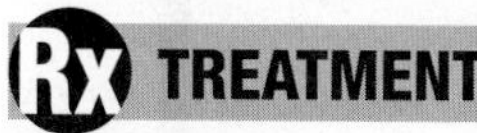 TREATMENT

The overall goal for patients with UA and NSTEMI is to relieve myocardial ischemia and to prevent recurrent cardiovascular events. Antithrombotic therapy is needed to reduce thrombus burden, prevent further thrombosis, and improve coronary artery flow. Revascularization is typically needed to prevent further events and improve flow within the coronary artery lumen. For patients with STEMI, the goal is immediate reperfusion therapy, whether it is chemical (i.e., thrombolysis) or mechanical (i.e., percutaneous coronary intervention [PCI]). STEMI patients presenting to a hospital with PCI capability should be treated with primary PCI within 90 minutes of first medical contact (Figs. 1-41 and 1-42). Thrombolytic therapy should not be administered 24 hours after initial diagnosis of STEMI.

NONPHARMACOLOGIC THERAPY

- STEMI is a medical emergency and requires immediate reperfusion therapy; the best outcomes are seen with cardiac catheterization with primary PCI. Guidelines call for a goal door-to-balloon time of ≤90 minutes.
- Patients with UA or NSTEMI should be risk stratified in conjunction with the cardiology consult service. Risk scores such as the TIMI and GRACE scores can be used to decide between an early invasive strategy and an initial conservative management strategy. Overall, an early invasive strategy is associated with better outcomes and involves cardiac catheterization followed by revascularization with PCI or coronary artery bypass grafting (CABG) within 4 to 24 hours of presentation. An initial conservative strategy involves aggressive medical management and revascularization only if ischemia recurs or is documented on noninvasive testing. This should only be reserved for selected patients with low-risk scores (TIMI score 0-2).
- Bed rest and continuous ECG monitoring is recommended for all ACS patients. Supplemental oxygen should be administered to patients with signs of hypoxia or respiratory distress. Finger pulse oximetry should be utilized to assess arterial oxygen saturation.

ACUTE GENERAL Rx

- All patients with ACS should receive full-dose aspirin with the first dose chewed to establish a high blood level for its antiplatelet effects. Thereafter, daily dose of 75 to 325 mg are prescribed and continued indefinitely,

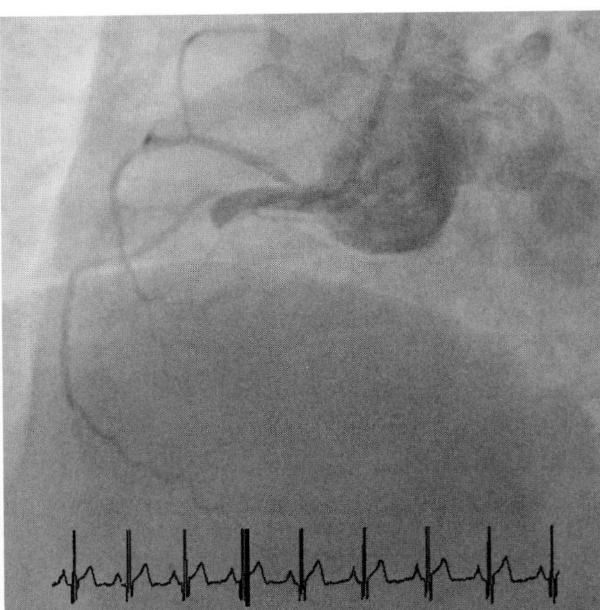

FIGURE 1-41 Right coronary artery totally occluded proximally during STEMI.

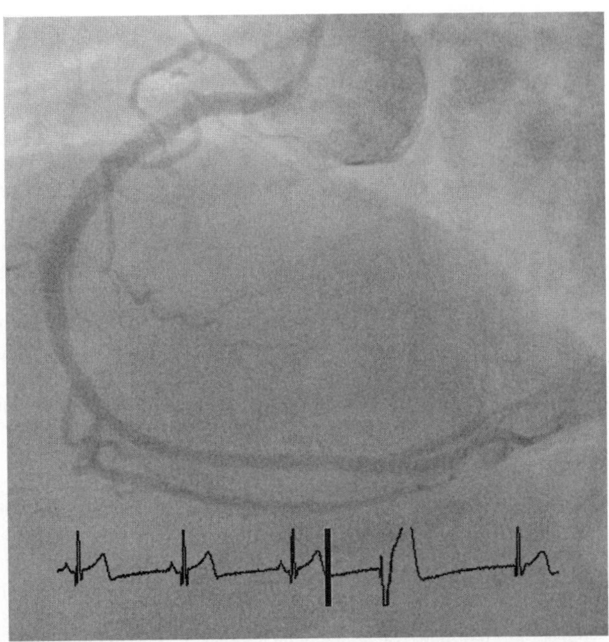

FIGURE 1-42 Right coronary artery after successful percutaneous coronary artery stenting during STEMI.

with the lower dose of 81 mg showing lower bleeding risk with comparable efficacy.

- Beta-blocker therapy reduces ischemia by decreasing myocardial oxygen demand and should be initiated within 24 hours of onset of ACS unless signs or symptoms of heart failure are present or arrhythmias preclude its use. Oral administration, titrated to a heart rate of 50-60 beats/min, is preferred. Intravenous beta-blockers should not be administered to STEMI patients who have any of the following:
  1. Signs of heart failure,
  2. Evidence of a low output state,
  3. Increased risk for cardiogenic shock, or
  4. Other relative contraindications to beta-blockade (PR interval >0.24 second, second- or third-degree heart block, active asthma, or reactive airway disease).
- Nitroglycerin is a vasodilator that should be administered to relieve chest discomfort in all ACS patients. It can be administered sublingually at first, up to 3 doses, followed by intravenous administration if symptoms persist. In the setting of an inferior STEMI, it is wise to rule out a right ventricular (RV) infarct with a right-sided ECG before the administration of nitroglycerin. This is because RV infarcts are preload dependent and nitroglycerin decreases preload through venodilation, which leads to hypotension in this setting. This can be corrected by discontinuing nitroglycerin and starting intravenous fluids. Nitroglycerin provides no mortality benefit in ACS patients.
- Oxygen should be administered to patients with shortness of breath, signs of acute heart failure, cardiogenic shock, or an arterial oxyhemoglobin saturation of less than 94%. The 2011 American College of Cardiology/American Heart Association (ACC/AHA) guidelines recommend against the routine usage of oxygen therapy beyond 6 hours without compelling evidence of benefit.
- The 2012 ACC/AHA Guidelines for unstable angina/NSTEMI has downgraded the recommendation for morphine use for uncontrolled ischemic chest discomfort from a Class I to a Class IIa recommendation due to reports linked to increased mortality.
- Calcium channel blockers (nondihydropyridine) may be used in patients with persisting or recurrent symptoms, despite treatment with beta-blockers and nitroglycerin. They work by causing coronary vasodilation and decreasing myocardial oxygen demand. They are useful when beta-blockers are contraindicated and in patients with Prinzmetal variant angina. Calcium channel blockers should not be used in cases of severe LV dysfunction or pulmonary edema.
- Patients routinely taking nonsteroidal antiinflammatory drugs (NSAIDs) (except for aspirin), both nonselective as well as COX-2 selective agents, before STEMI should discontinue those agents at the time of presentation with STEMI because of the increased risks of mortality, reinfarction, hypertension, heart failure, and myocardial rupture associated with their use.
- Angiotensin-converting enzyme (ACE) inhibitors may be added and should be used within 24 hours of onset of ACS in all patients with depressed LV function (ejection fraction [EF] <40%) or pulmonary vascular congestion. Angiotensin receptor blockers (ARBs) should be used in patients who are ACE inhibitor intolerant.
- Antithrombotic therapy is critical in treating the underlying pathophysiology of ACS. This consists of administering antiplatelet and anticoagulant agents.
- Antiplatelet agents inhibit platelet activation and aggregation. Aspirin is a cyclooxygenase inhibitor that blocks platelet aggregation and should be administered to all ACS patients without contraindications at an initial dose of 162 mg to 325 mg. Clopidogrel is a thienopyridine agent that inhibits platelet activation and aggregation. It should be administered in all ACS patients, with the timing dependent on the clinical scenario and management strategy. It requires a loading dose of 300 mg to 600 mg followed by 75 mg daily. It should be discontinued at least 5 days before CABG. Other antiplatelet agents that can be substituted instead of clopidogrel include prasugrel, ticlopidine, and ticagrelor. However, maintenance doses of aspirin above 100 mg reduce the effectiveness of ticagrelor and should be avoided after any initial dose; use with aspirin 75-100 mg per day. Prasugrel is not recommended in STEMI patients with stroke or transient ischemic attack (TIA), or those patients managed with fibrinolysis. As a rule, all ACS patients should have two antiplatelet agents initiated and should be continued up to 12 months regardless of conservative vs invasive strategy.
- GP IIB/III a inhibitors may be considered as an intravenous antiplatelet therapy in addition to aspirin for
  - Medium- or high-risk patients with UA/NSTEMI in whom an invasive strategy is planned (Class I). Eptifibatide or tirofiban may be used prior to PCI and any GP IIB/IIIa inhibitor, including abciximab, may be used during PCI.
  - Patients in whom an initial conservative strategy is selected, if recurrent symptoms/ischemia, heart failure, or serious arrhythmias subsequently appear, then prior to diagnostic angiography an IV GP

IIb/IIIa inhibitor (Eptifibatide or tirofiban) may be started (Class I).

- Anticoagulant agents should be administered to all ACS patients. Options include either unfractionated heparin (UFH), or low-molecular-weight heparin (enoxaparin), or factor Xa inhibitors such as fondaparinux, or direct thrombin inhibitors such as bivalirudin.
- In the most recent guidelines, enoxaparin and UFH have both received Class I recommendations for use among ACS patients managed conservatively or invasively, but enoxaparin is preferred for conservatively managed patients.
- For STEMI, fondaparinux can be used for anticoagulation. It has been shown to decrease bleeding complications as compared with either UFH or LMWH. However, it has a long half-life (15 hours), and thrombosis on catheters has been noted when using only fondaparinux in the cath lab.
- Bivalirudin is a reversible direct thrombin inhibitor and may be considered as an alternative to UFH and GP IIb/IIIa inhibitors in patients with STEMI (HORIZONS AMI trial) who are undergoing primary PCI (PPCI). When bivalirudin was compared to UFH plus a glycoprotein inhibitor in patients with STEMI and PPCI, less bleeding and a short- and long-term reduction in cardiac events and overall mortality was observed. With bivalirudin, there is no risk of heparin-induced thrombocytopenia, less bleeding is observed, and no anticoagulant monitoring is needed. Similar results were reported in the use of bivalirudin alone in patients with UA/NSTEMI in the ACUITY trial when compared to enoxaparin/UFH with GP IIb/IIIa arms.

CHRONIC Rx

- Post-ACS medical therapy involves aspirin, statin, beta-blocker, and a second anti-platelet agent such as clopidogrel, ticagrelor, or prasugrel.
- Lipid lowering with statins has been evaluated in trials such as the MIRACL study, in which high-dose atorvastatin 80 mg reduced death, MI, and cardiac events at 16 weeks when administered early, within 24-96 hours after an ACS. The A-Z trial and PROVE IT trials demonstrated benefit of early statin therapy with LDL targets <70 mg/dl in ACS.
- ACE inhibitors may be added to treat hypertension and should be used in all patients with depressed LV function (EF <40%) or pulmonary vascular congestion. ARBs should be used in patients who are ACE inhibitor intolerant.
- Eplerenone, an aldosterone receptor blocker, should be considered in post-MI patients with LV EF ≤40% and evidence of congestive heart failure.
- Cardiac rehabilitation and a monitored exercise program should be recommended.
- Aggressive risk factor management, including smoking cessation, weight loss, diet and exercise, diabetes control, and so on, for secondary prevention of future events is crucial.

REFERRAL

- All ACS patients should be cared for in conjunction with the cardiology consult service.
- When appropriate, referral to a cardiac surgeon may be necessary for CABG.

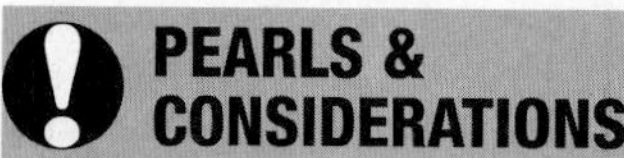

PEARLS & CONSIDERATIONS

COMMENTS

- ACS is common and a leading cause of mortality in the United States.
- The diagnosis hinges on the basics—history and physical, ECG, biomarkers, and CXR.
- Remember the potentially fatal non-ACS causes of chest discomfort, which include acute pulmonary embolism and acute ascending aortic dissection.
- STEMI patients presenting to a hospital with PCI capability should be treated with primary PCI within 90 minutes of first medical contact.
- STEMI patients presenting to a hospital without PCI capability and who cannot be transferred to a PCI center and undergo PCI within 90 minutes of first medical contact should be treated with fibrinolytic therapy within 30 minutes of hospital presentation unless fibrinolytic therapy is contraindicated.

PREVENTION

- Primary prevention of ACS is based on recognizing the major risk factors for CAD and treating them as appropriate.
- Patients with depressed LV function (ejection fraction <35%) at least 40 days after an acute MI benefit from an implantable cardioverter defibrillator (ICD) for the prevention of sudden cardiac death.

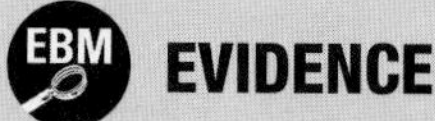

EVIDENCE

available at www.expertconsult.com

SUGGESTED READINGS

available at www.expertconsult.com

RELATED CONTENT

Acute Coronary Syndrome (Patient Information)
Angina (Related Key Topic)
Myocardial Infarction (Related Key Topic)

AUTHORS: **SHAMAIL TARIQ, M.D.**, and **PRANAV M. PATEL, M.D., F.A.C.C., F.S.C.A.I.**

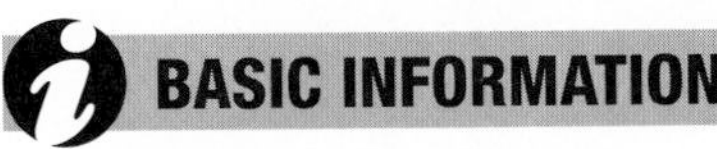

BASIC INFORMATION

DEFINITION

Acute kidney injury (AKI) is the rapid (<48 hr) impairment in renal function resulting in retention of products in the blood that are normally excreted by the kidneys and thus volume and acid-base dysregulation in the body. Criteria and classifications of AKI are described in Table 1-14.

SYNONYMS

ARF
Acute renal insufficiency syndrome
Acute renal failure
AKI

ICD-9CM CODES
584.9 Acute renal failure, unspecified
ICD-10CM CODES
N17.9 Acute kidney failure, unspecified

EPIDEMIOLOGY & DEMOGRAPHICS

- Incidence of AKI is 3 cases/1000 persons. AKI requiring dialysis develops in five in 100,000 persons annually.
- >10% of intensive care unit patients develop ALL.
- >40% of hospital AKI is iatrogenic.
- The most common cause of AKI in hospitalized patients is intrinsic renal failure caused by acute tubular necrosis (ATN) and prerenal disease.
- AKI occurs in 20% of patients with moderate sepsis and more than 50% of patients with septic shock and positive blood cultures.
- Can occur at any age; however, various underlying causes occur in certain age groups.

PHYSICAL FINDINGS & CLINICAL PRESENTATION

- The physical examination should focus on volume status. The physical findings noted below vary with the duration and rapidity of onset of renal failure.
- Peripheral edema resulting from volume overload, heart failure, liver failure, or nephrotic syndrome
- Skin pallor, ecchymoses
- Arrhythmias due to electrolyte imbalances and acidosis
- Oliguria (i.e., <400 to 500 ml urine/24 hr; however, patients can have nonoliguric renal failure), anuria
- Change in mental status, delirium, lethargy, myoclonus, seizures
- Uremic odor, pruritus
- Flank pain, fasciculations, muscle cramps
- Tachypnea, tachycardia
- Weakness, anorexia, generalized malaise, nausea
- Pulmonary rales due to volume overload
- Flapping tremors
- Pericardial effusion
- Hypotension or hypertension can occur, suggesting volume depletion and overload, respectively

ETIOLOGY

- Prerenal: inadequate perfusion caused by hypovolemia, congestive heart failure, cirrhosis, sepsis. Sixty percent of community-acquired cases of AKI are from prerenal conditions.
- Postrenal: outlet obstruction from prostatic enlargement, fibrosis, ureteral obstruction (stones), bilateral renal vein occlusion. Postrenal causes account for 5% to 15% of community-acquired AKI.
- Intrinsic renal: glomerulonephritis, ATN, rhabdomyolysis, systemic hypotension, sepsis, drug toxicity, contrast nephropathy. Contrast-induced nephropathy (increase in serum creatinine >25% within 3 days of intravascular contrast administration in absence of an alternative cause) is the third most common cause of new AKI in hospitalized patients.
- Causes of AKI are described in Table 1-15.

TABLE 1-14 RIFLE and AKIN Criteria for Diagnosis of Acute Kidney Injury

RIFLE CLASSIFICATION		
	GFR Criteria	**Urine Output Criteria**
Risk	S_{Cr} >1.5 × baseline or ΔGFR >25% reduction	UO <0.5 ml/kg/h × 6 h
Injury	S_{Cr} >2.0 × baseline or ΔGFR >50% reduction	UO <0.5 ml/kg/h × 12 h
Failure	S_{Cr} >3.0 × baseline or ΔGFR >75% reduction or S_{Cr} >4.0 mg/dl	UO <0.3 ml/kg/h × 24 h or anuria × 12 h
Loss	Persistent acute kidney injury = Complete loss of function for >4 wk	
ESRD	End-stage renal disease >3 mo	
AKIN CLASSIFICATION		
Stage	**Serum Creatinine Criteria**	**Urine Output Criteria**
1	ΔS_{Cr} ≥0.3 mg/dl (30 μmol/L) or S_{Cr} ≥1.5, ≤2.0 × baseline	UO <0.5 ml/kg/h × 6 h
2	S_{Cr} >2.0, ≤3.0 × baseline	UO <0.5 ml/kg/h × 12 h
3	S_{Cr} >3.0 × baseline or S_{Cr} ≥4.0 mg/dl with an acute rise ≥0.5 mg/dl (50 μmol/L) or on renal replacement therapy	UO <0.3 ml/kg/h × 24 h or anuria × 12 h

AKIN, Acute Kidney Injury Network; *GFR,* glomerular filtration rate; *RIFLE,* risk, injury, failure, loss, ESRD; *SCr,* serum creatinine; *UO,* urinary output.
From Floege J et al: *Comprehensive clinical nephrology,* ed 4, Philadelphia, 2010, Saunders.

DIAGNOSIS

DIFFERENTIAL DIAGNOSIS

Refer to "Etiology." Diagnostic tests to distinguish prerenal and renal AKI are described in Table 1-16. A diagnostic approach to patients with suspected AKI is described in Fig. 1-43.

LABORATORY TESTS

- Elevated serum creatinine: the rate of rise is approximately 1 mg/dl/day in complete renal failure.
- Elevated blood urea nitrogen (BUN): BUN/creatinine ratio is >20:1 in prerenal azotemia, postrenal azotemia, and acute glomerulonephritis; it is <20:1 in acute interstitial nephritis and ATN (Table 1-17).
- Electrolytes (potassium, phosphate) are elevated; bicarbonate level, sodium, and calcium are decreased; metabolic acidosis is noted
- Close monitoring of 24-hr urinary volume.
- Complete blood count may reveal anemia because of decreased erythropoietin production, hemoconcentration, hemolysis, or leuckocytosis, suggesting infection.
- Urinalysis may reveal the presence of hematuria (glomerulonephritis), proteinuria (nephrotic syndrome), casts (e.g., granular casts in ATN, red blood cell casts in acute glomerulonephritis, white blood cell casts in acute interstitial nephritis), eosinophiluria (acute interstitial nephritis). However, these urinary findings may be absent in less severe disease.
- Urinary sodium and urinary creatinine should also be obtained to calculate the fractional excretion of sodium (FENa) (FENa = Urine sodium/Plasma sodium × Plasma creatinine/Urine creatinine × 100). FENa is <1 in prerenal failure and >1 in intrinsic renal failure in patients with urine output <400 ml/day. The FENa can be falsely high in patients taking diuretics. It can also be falsely low in several intrinsic renal conditions such as acute glomerulonephritis, contrast-induced nephropathy, and rhabdomyolysis.
- Urinary osmolarity is 250 to 300 mOsm/kg in ATN, <400 mOsm/kg in postrenal azotemia, and >500 mOsm/kg in prerenal azotemia and acute glomerulonephritis (Table 1-18).
- Combined use of cystatin C, a protein that is freely filtered by the glomerulus, and serum creatinine has been shown to improve estimates of GFR in AKI.

 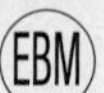

TABLE 1-15 Etiologies of Acute Kidney Injury

Prerenal Causes (Decreased Renal Blood Flow)	Intrinsic Renal Causes	Postrenal Causes
Hypovolemia Renal losses (diuretics, osmotic agents, polyuria) Gastrointestinal losses (vomiting, diarrhea) Cutaneous losses (burns, exfoliative syndromes) Hemorrhage Pancreatitis **Decreased Cardiac Output** Congestive heart failure Pulmonary embolism Acute myocardial infarction Severe valvular heart disease Abdominal compartment syndrome Renal artery obstruction (stenosis, embolism, thrombosis, dissection) **Systemic Vasodilation** Sepsis Anaphylaxis Anesthetics Drug overdose **Afferent Arteriolar Vasoconstriction** Hypercalcemia Drugs (NSAIDs, amphotericin B, calcineurin inhibitors, norepinephrine, radiocontrast agents, aminoglycosides) Hepatorenal syndrome Efferent arteriolar vasodilation (angiotensin converting enzyme inhibitors, aldosterone receptor blockers)	**Vascular: Large and Small Vessels** Trauma Renal vein obstruction (thrombosis, ventilation with high-level PEEP, abdominal compartment syndrome) Microangiopathy (thrombotic thrombocytopenic purpura, hemolytic-uremic syndrome, disseminated intravascular coagulation, preeclampsia) Malignant hypertension Scleroderma renal crisis Transplant rejection Atheroembolic disease **Glomerular** Antiglomerular basement membrane disease (Goodpasture syndrome) Antineutrophil cytoplasmic antibody-associated glomerulonephritis (Wegener granulomatosis) Immune complex glomerulonephritis, systemic lupus erythematosus, postinfectious cryoglobulinemia, primary membranoproliferative glomerulonephritis **Tubular** Ischemic Cytotoxic Heme pigment (rhabdomyolysis, intravascular hemolysis) Crystals (tumor lysis syndrome, seizures, ethylene glycol poisoning, vitamin C megadose, acyclovir, indinavir, methotrexate) Drugs (aminoglycosides, lithium, amphotericin B, pentamidine, cisplatin, ifosfamide, radiocontrast agents), synthetic cannabinoid use **Interstitial** Drugs (penicillins, cephalosporins, NSAIDs, proton pump inhibitors, allopurinol, rifampin, indinavir, mesalamine, sulfonamides) Infection (pyelonephritis, viral infection) **Systemic Disease** Sjögren syndrome, sarcoidosis, systemic lupus erythematosus, lymphoma, leukemia, tubulonephritis, uveitis	**Ureteral Obstruction** Calculus Tumor (intrinsic or extrinsic) Fibrosis Ligation during pelvic surgery **Bladder Neck Obstruction** Benign prostatic hypertrophy Prostate cancer Neurogenic bladder Tricyclic antidepressants Ganglionic blockers Bladder tumor Calculus Hemorrhage/clot **Urethral Obstruction** Strictures Tumor Phimosis Renal calcinosis Obstructed urinary catheter, ureteral stent, or ileal conduit Pelvic trauma, retroperitoneal hematoma

NSAIDs, Nonsteroidal anti-inflammatory drugs; *PEEP,* positive end-expiratory pressure.
Modified from Cameron JL, Cameron AM: *Current surgical therapy,* ed 10, Philadelphia, 2011, Saunders.

TABLE 1-16 Diagnostic Tests to Distinguish Between Prerenal and Renal Acute Kidney Injury

Index	Prerenal Causes	Renal Causes
FENa	<1%	>2%
Urine sodium	<10 mmol/L	>40 mmol/L
Urine/plasma osmolality	>1.5	1 to 1.5
Renal failure index	<1	>2
BUN/creatinine ratio	>20	<10

BUN, Blood urea nitrogen; *FENa,* fractional excretion of sodium. Calculation of FENa: (Urine sodium × Plasma creatinine)/(Plasma sodium × Serum creatinine) × 100. Renal failure index: (Urine sodium × Urine creatinine)/Plasma creatinine.
From Cameron JL, Cameron AM: *Current surgical therapy,* ed 10, Philadelphia, 2011, Saunders.

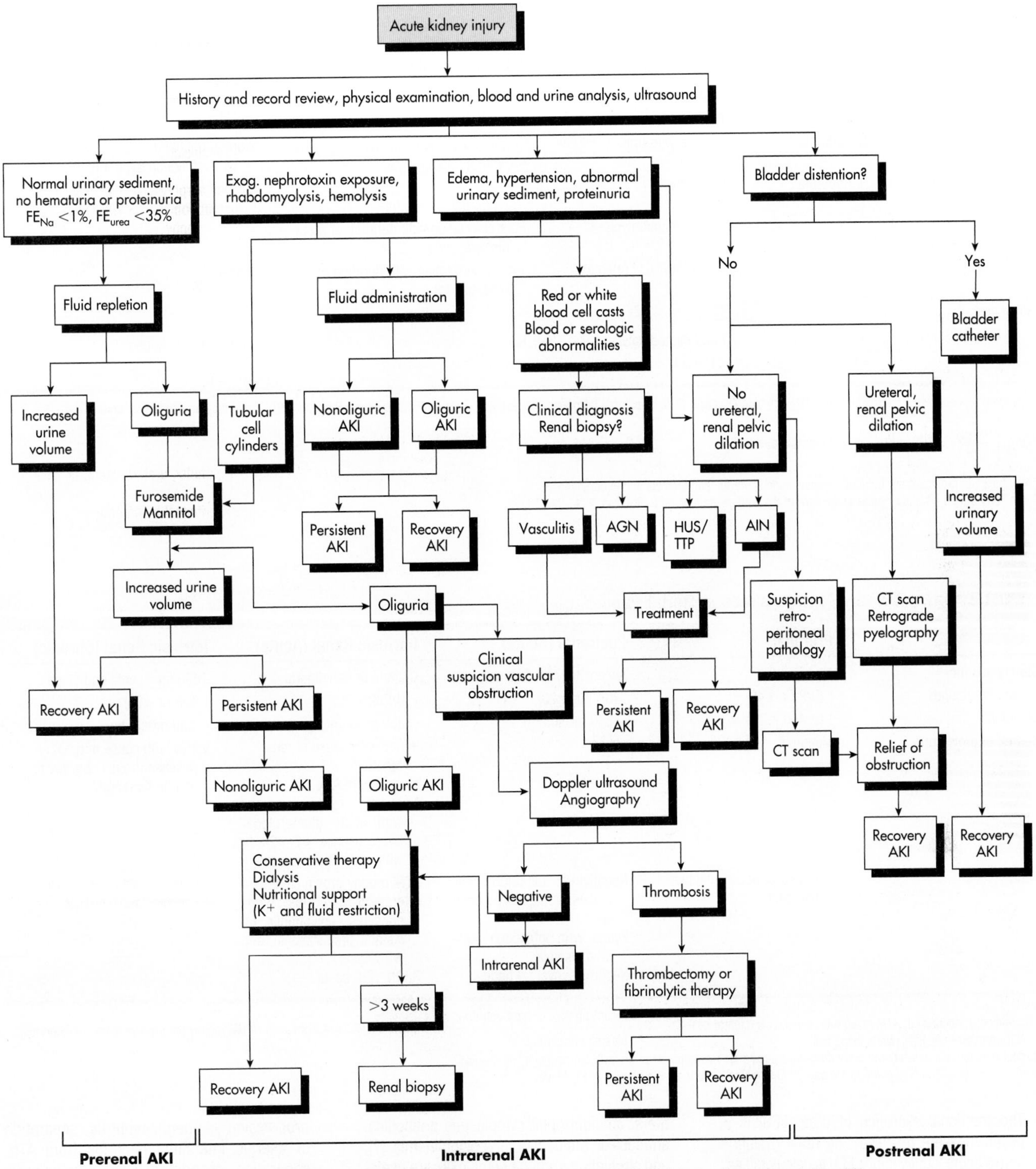

Acute kidney injury

History and record review, physical examination, blood and urine analysis, ultrasound

Normal urinary sediment, no hematuria or proteinuria FE_{Na} <1%, FE_{urea} <35%

Exog. nephrotoxin exposure, rhabdomyolysis, hemolysis

Edema, hypertension, abnormal urinary sediment, proteinuria

Bladder distention?

No

Yes

Fluid repletion

Fluid administration

Red or white blood cell casts Blood or serologic abnormalities

Bladder catheter

Increased urine volume

Oliguria

Tubular cell cylinders

Nonoliguric AKI

Oliguric AKI

Clinical diagnosis Renal biopsy?

No ureteral, renal pelvic dilation

Ureteral, renal pelvic dilation

Furosemide Mannitol

Persistent AKI

Recovery AKI

Vasculitis

AGN

HUS/TTP

AIN

Increased urinary volume

Increased urine volume

Oliguria

Treatment

Suspicion retro-peritoneal pathology

CT scan Retrograde pyelography

Clinical suspicion vascular obstruction

Recovery AKI

Persistent AKI

Persistent AKI

Recovery AKI

CT scan

Relief of obstruction

Nonoliguric AKI

Oliguric AKI

Doppler ultrasound Angiography

Recovery AKI

Recovery AKI

Conservative therapy
Dialysis
Nutritional support
(K^+ and fluid restriction)

Negative

Thrombosis

Intrarenal AKI

Thrombectomy or fibrinolytic therapy

>3 weeks

Recovery AKI

Renal biopsy

Persistent AKI

Recovery AKI

Prerenal AKI | **Intrarenal AKI** | **Postrenal AKI**

FIGURE 1-43 Diagnostic approach to patients with suspected AKI. *AGN,* Acute glomerulonephritis; *AIN,* acute interstitial nephritis; *CT,* computed tomography; *Exog.,* exogenous; *HUS/TTP,* hemolytic-uremic syndrome/thrombotic thrombocytopenic purpura. (From Floege J et al: *Comprehensive clinical nephrology,* ed 4, Philadelphia, 2010, Saunders.)

TABLE 1-17 Serum and Radiographic Abnormalities in Renal Failure

	Prerenal	Postrenal (Acute)	Intrinsic Renal (Acute)	Intrinsic Renal (Chronic)
BUN	↑ 10:1 > Cr	↑ 20-40/day	↑ 20-40/day	Stable; ↑ varies with protein intake
Serum creatinine	N/moderate ↑	↑ 2-4/day	↑ 2-4/day	Stable ↑ (production equals excretion)
Serum potassium	N/moderate ↑	↑ varies with urinary volume	↑↑ (particularly when patient is oliguric) ↑↑↑ with rhabdomyolysis	Normal until end stage, unless tubular dysfunction (type 4 RTA)
Serum phosphate	N/moderate ↑	Moderate ↑	↑	Becomes significantly elevated when serum creatinine surpasses 3 mg/dl
		↑↑ with rhabdomyolysis	Poor correlation with duration of renal disease	
Serum calcium	N	N/-↓ with PO_4^{-3} retention	↓ (poor correlation with duration of renal failure)	Usually ↓
Renal size				
By ultrasonography	N/↑	↑ and dilated calyces	N/↑	↓ and with ↑ echogenicity
FE_{Na}*	<1	<1 → >1	>1†	1

↑, Increase; ↓, decrease; ↑↑, large increase; ↑↑↑, very high increase; *BUN,* blood urea nitrogen; *Cr,* creatinine; *N,* normal; *Na,* sodium; *P,* plasma; *RTA,* renal tubular acidosis; *U,* urine.

*$FE_{Na}\left[\dfrac{U/P_{Na^+}}{U/P_{Cr}} \times 100\right]$ (useful only in oliguric patient).

†May be ≤1 in radiocontrast-induced myoglobinuric acute tubular necrosis and in early sepsis.
From Ferri FF (ed): *Practical guide to the care of the medical patient,* ed 8, St Louis, 2011, Mosby.

TABLE 1-18 Urinary Abnormalities in Renal Failure

	Prerenal	Postrenal (Acute)	Intrinsic Renal (Acute)	Intrinsic Renal (Chronic)
Urinary volume	↓	Absent-to-wide fluctuation	Oliguric or nonoliguric	1000 ml + until end stage
Urinary creatinine	↑ (U/P Cr ±40)	↓ (U/P Cr ±20)	↓ (U/P Cr <20)	↓ (U/P Cr <20)
Osmolarity	↑ (±400 mOsm/kg)	(<350 mOsm/kg)	(<350 mOsm/kg)	(<350 mOsm/kg)
Degree of proteinuria	Minimum	Absent	Varies with cause of renal failure: Modest with ATN Nephrotic range common with acute glomerulopathies, usually <2 g/24 hr with interstitial disease*	Varies with cause of renal disease (from 1-2 g/day to nephrotic range)
Urinary sediment	Negative, or occasional hyaline cast	Negative or hematuria with stones or papillary necrosis Pyuria with infectious prostatic disease Nephrosis: oval fat bodies	ATN: muddy brown casts Interstitial nephritis: lymphocytes, eosinophils (in stained preparations), and WBC casts RPGN: RBC casts	Broad casts with variable renal "residual" acute findings

↑, Increased; ↓, decreased; *ATN,* acute tubular necrosis; clearance = $\dfrac{\text{urinary concentration} \times \text{urinary voluume}}{\text{plasma concentration}}$; *Cr,* creatinine; *RBC,* red blood cell; *RPGN,* rapidly progressive glomerulonephritis; *U/P,* urine/plasma; *WBC,* white blood cell.
*Except nonsteroidal anti-inflammatory drug-induced allergic interstitial nephritis with concomitant "nil disease."
From Ferri FF (ed): *Practical guide to the care of the medical patient,* ed 8, St Louis, 2011, Mosby.

- The fractional excretion of urea (FEU) is a useful measure for assessing renal dysfunction in acute kidney injury. FEU is calculated as:

  $$\frac{\text{serum creatinine} \times \text{urinary urea}}{\text{serum urea} \times \text{urinary creatinine}}$$

  An FEU of less than 35% suggests a prerenal cause of acute kidney injury, whereas a value over 50% indicates an intrinsic cause. FEU is more useful than FENa in patients on diuretics.
- Blood cultures for patients suspected of sepsis
- Liver function tests, immunoglobulins, and protein electrophoresis in patients suspected of myeloma
- Decreased complement levels and elevated anti–glomerular basement membrane antibody titers, antineutrophil cytoplasmic antibodies, antinuclear antibodies, cryoglobulinemia [?], and circulating immune complexes are useful diagnostic tools for diagnosing glomerulonephritis or vasculitis.
- Creatinine kinase in patients with suspected rhabdomyolysis.
- Renal biopsy may be indicated in patients with intrinsic renal failure when considering specific therapy; major uses of renal biopsy are differential diagnosis of nephrotic syndrome, separation of lupus vasculitis from other vasculitis and lupus membranous from idiopathic membranous, confirmation of hereditary nephropathies on the basis of the ultrastructure, diagnosis of rapidly progressing glomerulonephritis, separation of allergic interstitial nephritis from ATN, separation of primary glomerulonephritis syndromes.
- Tubular enzymes are studied as biomarkers for renal failure. Among them are proximal renal tubular epithelial antigen (HRTE-1), N-acetyl-beta-glucosaminidase (NAG), alpha-glutathione S-transferase (alpha-GST), gamma-glutamyltranspeptidase (gamma-GT), and lactate dehydrogenase (LDH). The majority of them are released before an increase in serum creatinine; however, they do not provide any clear parameters to differentiate ATN from prerenal failure.

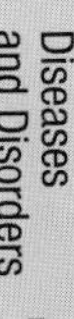

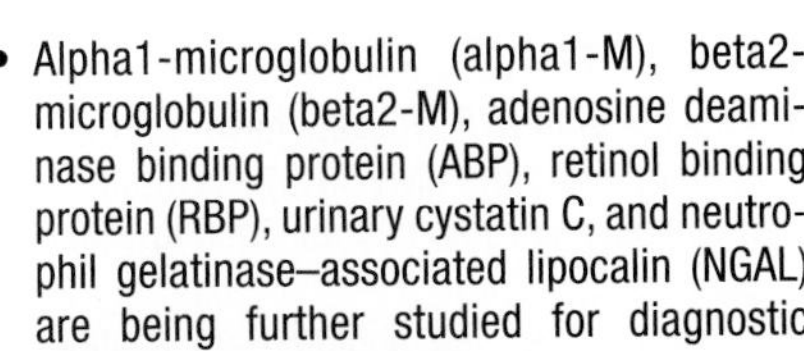

- Alpha1-microglobulin (alpha1-M), beta2-microglobulin (beta2-M), adenosine deaminase binding protein (ABP), retinol binding protein (RBP), urinary cystatin C, and neutrophil gelatinase–associated lipocalin (NGAL) are being further studied for diagnostic evaluation.

IMAGING STUDIES

- ECG is done to evaluate changes especially in hyperkalemia.
- Chest x-ray is useful to evaluate for congestive heart failure and for pulmonary renal syndromes (Goodpasture's syndrome, Wegener's granulomatosis).
- Abdominal x-rays when suspecting renal or ureteric calculi.
- Ultrasound of kidneys is used to evaluate kidney size (useful to distinguish acute from chronic renal failure), evaluate for the presence of obstruction, and evaluate renal vascular status (with Doppler evaluation).
- Computed tomography (CT) with radiocontrast agent administration is usually avoided in AKI; however, unenhanced CT scans are useful for the identification of obstructing ureteral stones.

Rx TREATMENT

NONPHARMACOLOGIC THERAPY

- Stop all nephrotoxic medications.
- Dietary modification to supply adequate calories while minimizing accumulation of toxins; appropriate control of fluid balance. Physicians should recommend a nutrition program with an energy prescription of 120 to 150 KJ/kg/day and restriction of potassium (60 mEq/day), sodium (90 mEq/day), and phosphorus (800 mg/day). Ideal protein supplementation ranges from 0.6 to 1.4 g/kg depending on whether dialysis is required.
- Daily weight.
- Modifications of dosage of renally excreted drugs.

ACUTE GENERAL Rx

- Correction of electrolyte abnormalities
- Loop diuretics in patients with volume overload and, if needed, pressors or vasodilators in patients with congestive heart failure

Specific treatment is variable with etiology of AKI:

- Prerenal: IV volume expansion in hypovolemic patients.
- Intrinsic renal: discontinuation of any potential toxins and treatment of condition causing the renal failure. In severe cases of acute interstitial nephritis, a trial of steroids is also given to improve clinical course.
- Postrenal: removal of obstruction. Immediate insertion of catheter for lower urinary tract obstruction and nephrostomy or ureteral stents are required in patients with upper urinary tract obstruction.
- IV insulin and glucose for patients with hyperkalemia-related ECG changes who could not be admitted to the hospital immediately.
- Intermittent hemodialysis and continuous renal replacement therapy have similar outcomes for patients with AKI.

CHRONIC Rx

- Monitoring of renal function and electrolytes.
- Doses of medications that are renally excreted should be adjusted according to creatinine clearance to prevent further damage to the kidneys.
- Prevention of further insults to the kidneys with proper hydration, especially before contrast studies, and avoidance of nephrotoxic agents. Hydration with sodium bicarbonate (addition of 154 ml of 1000 mEq/L sodium bicarbonate to 846 ml of 5% dextrose in water) before contrast exposure is more effective than hydration with sodium chloride for prophylaxis of contrast-induced renal failure. Administration of N-acetylcysteine prophylaxis has shown conflicting results regarding its ability to reduce the risk of contrast-induced nephropathy. In high-risk patients having angiography or angioplasty, the RenalGuard System using saline plus N-acetylcysteine and furosemide has been shown to be better than sodium bicarbonate plus N-acetylcysteine for preventing contrast-induced AKI.
- See "Chronic Kidney Disease" entry for indications for initiation of dialysis. Daily hemodialysis is superior to every-other-day hemodialysis in patients with ATN and ARF.

DISPOSITION

- General indications for initiation of dialysis are:
  1. Florid symptoms of uremia (encephalopathy, pericarditis)
  2. Severe volume overload
  3. Severe acid-base imbalance
  4. Significant derangement in electrolyte concentrations (e.g., hyperkalemia, hyponatremia)
- Intermittent hemodialysis and continuous renal replacement therapy have similar outcomes for patients with AKI.
- Renal function recovery (ability to discontinue dialysis) varies from 50% to 75% in survivors of AKI.
- Overall mortality rate in AKI is nearly 50%, varying from 60% in patients with ATN to 35% in patients with prerenal or postrenal AKI.
- The combination of AKI and sepsis is associated with a 70% mortality rate.

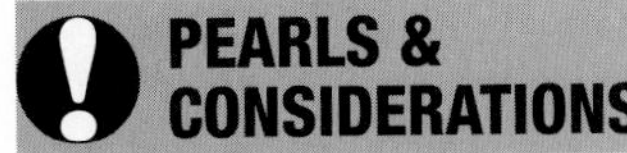

PEARLS & CONSIDERATIONS

- Patients with AKI are susceptible to infections and sepsis.
- Dosing of certain drugs needs to be modified in patients with AKI.

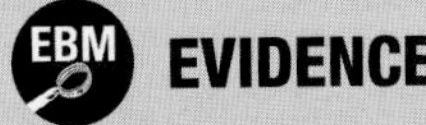

EVIDENCE

available at www.expertconsult.com

SUGGESTED READINGS

available at www.expertconsult.com

RELATED CONTENT

Acute Renal Failure (Patient Information)
Chronic Renal Failure (Patient Information)

AUTHORS: **SYEDA M. SAYEED, M.D.,** and **FRED F. FERRI, M.D.**

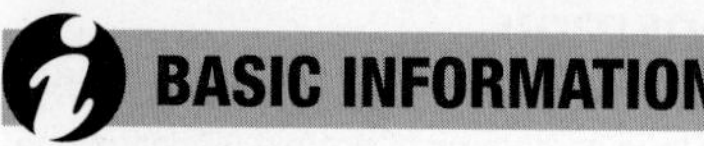

BASIC INFORMATION

DEFINITION

Acute liver failure (ALF) is defined as rapid development (<26 wk) of severe hepatic injury, coagulation abnormalities (international normalized ratio [INR] >1.5), and encephalopathy in a patient without preexisting liver disease, in the absence of acute alcoholic hepatitis.

SYNONYMS

Fulminant hepatic failure
Fulminant hepatitis
Fulminant hepatic necrosis
Acute hepatic necrosis
Acute and subacute necrosis of liver

ICD-9CM CODES
070.9 Unspecified viral hepatitis without mention of hepatic coma
573.3 Hepatitis, unspecified
ICD-10CM CODES
72.00 Acute liver failure w/o coma
72.01 Acute liver failure w/ coma

EPIDEMIOLOGY & DEMOGRAPHICS

INCIDENCE (IN U.S.): Affects approximately 2000 people/yr

PREDOMINANT SEX AND AGE: Seen more in women than men (73% vs. 27%)

RISK FACTORS: Intentional drug overdose, intravenous drug use, alcohol use, occupational exposure to blood or body fluids, taking hepatotoxic medications

PHYSICAL FINDINGS & CLINICAL PRESENTATION

- Symptoms of ALF include mental status changes, nausea, vomiting, easy bleeding or bruising. Abdominal pain and jaundice are often present.
- Physical findings include some degree of encephalopathy (see Table 1-19) and may include icteric sclera, jaundice, asterixis, hepatomegaly, decreased hepatic mass on percussion, and ascites. Multisystem organ failure can ensue. In rare cases, cerebral edema and increased intracranial pressure can occur, with abnormal pupillary exam, hypertension, bradycardia, seizures, and loss of brainstem reflexes.

TABLE 1-19 Grades of Encephalopathy

Grade	Description
I	Changes in behavior with minimal change in level of consciousness
II	Gross disorientation, drowsiness, possibly asterixis, inappropriate behavior
III	Marked confusion, incoherent speech, sleeping most of the time but arousable to vocal stimuli
IV	Comatose, unresponsiveness to pain, decorticate or decerebrate posturing

- Vesicular skin lesions are suggestive of herpes simplex virus (HSV).
- Family history of unexplained liver disease/cirrhosis should prompt ocular exam to look for Kayser-Fleischer rings (copper rings around the iris seen in Wilson disease).

ETIOLOGY

- Common causes include:
  1. Acetaminophen toxicity (46%)
  2. Indeterminate (14%)
  3. Idiosyncratic drug reaction (12%)
  4. Viral hepatitis (A, B) (10%)

Rarer causes include alcoholic hepatitis, autoimmune hepatitis, Wilson disease, ischemic hepatopathy, Budd-Chiari syndrome, acute fatty liver of pregnancy, venoocclusive disease, toxin ingestion (e.g., mushroom poisoning *[Amanita phalloides]*), sepsis, infiltrative malignancy (breast cancer, lymphoma, myeloma, melanoma, small cell lung cancer), and other viruses (adenovirus, hepatitis E, HSV).

DIAGNOSIS

DIFFERENTIAL DIAGNOSIS

- Severe acute hepatitis (including alcoholic hepatitis) —jaundice and coagulopathy without encephalopathy
- Cirrhosis (includes decompensated cirrhosis)
- Hepatocellular carcinoma

WORKUP (Box 1-3)

- Clinical history is critical and should include medication use (prescriptions, over-the-counter medications, herbal supplements), alcohol use, recreational drug use, prior symptoms of jaundice, onset of symptoms, history of suicide attempts, recent travel to endemic areas of viral hepatitis, and family history of liver failure/disease.
- Laboratory evaluation: complete blood count, liver function tests (LFTs) (AST, ALT, alkaline phosphatase, GGT, total and direct bilirubin, PT/INR, albumin), chemistry panel (sodium, potassium, chloride, bicarbonate, BUN, creatinine, glucose, magnesium, phosphate, calcium), arterial blood gas, arterial lactate, blood type and screen, acetaminophen level, ethanol level, toxicology screen, viral hepatitis serologies (anti–hepatitis A IgM, hepatitis B surface antigen, anti–hepatitis B core IgM, anti–hepatitis C antibody, hepatitis C viral load, anti–hepatitis E Ab, HSV-1 IgM, varicella zoster virus, ceruloplasmin level, pregnancy test, arterial ammonia level, autoimmune markers (ANA, ASMA, total IgG levels), HIV-1, HIV-2, amylase, lipase, ceruloplasmin.
- Abdominal ultrasound with Dopplers, CT/MRI of the head
- Prompt liver biopsy (via transjugular approach to decrease risk of bleeding) should be performed in cases where:
  1. the etiology remains unknown after initial workup or
  2. it is thought to be secondary to autoimmune hepatitis or malignancy.

LABORATORY TESTS

- Patients with ALF typically have a prolonged prothrombin time (INR >1.5), elevated transaminases, elevated bilirubin, and low platelet count (<150,000).
- Other possible lab findings can include an elevated BUN/creatinine (studies show 30%-50% also have acute kidney injury), hypoglycemia (impairment of gluconeogenesis), hypophosphatemia, hypomagnesemia, hypokalemia, acidosis or alkalosis, elevated LDH, and elevated ammonia.

IMAGING STUDIES

- Abdominal ultrasound with Dopplers should be ordered to evaluate for Budd-Chiari syndrome, cirrhosis, portal hypertension, hepatic congestion, and hepatic steatosis.
- CT or MRI scan of the head should be obtained to ensure no other causes for altered mental status.

BOX 1-3 Investigations in Fulminant Hepatic Failure

Baseline essential investigations
Biochemistry
- Bilirubin, transaminases
- Alkaline phosphatase
- Albumin
- Urea and electrolytes
- Creatinine
- Calcium, phosphate
- Ammonia
- Acid-base, lactate
- Glucose

Hematology
- Full blood count, platelets
- PT, PTT
- Factors V or VII
- Blood group cross-match

Septic screen
Omitting lumbar puncture
- Radiology
- Chest radiograph
- Abdominal ultrasound
- Head CT scan or MRI

Neurophysiology
- Electroencephalogram

Diagnostic investigations
Serum
- Acetaminophen levels
- Cu, ceruloplasmin (>3 yr)
- Autoantibodies
- Immunoglobulins
- Amino acids
- Lactate
- Pyruvate
- Hepatitis A, B, C, E
- EBV, CMV, HSV
- Other viruses

Urine
- Toxic metabolites
- Amino acids, succinylacetone
- Organic acids
- Reducing sugars

CMV, Cytomegalovirus; *EBV,* Epstein-Barr virus; *HSV,* herpes simplex virus; *PT,* prothrombin time; *PTT,* partial thromboplastin time.

From Fuhrman BP, Zimmerman JJ: Fuhrman and Zimmerman's pediatric critical care, ed 4, Philadelphia, 2011, Mosby.

Rx TREATMENT (Boxes 1-4 and 1-5)

NONPHARMACOLOGIC THERAPY

- Initial treatment should focus on the patient's mental status.
- A liver specialist should be notified urgently, and arrangements should be made for imminent transfer to a transplant center.
- Patients with suspected acetaminophen toxicity should have LFTs monitored every 12 hr. Otherwise, LFTs can be monitored daily.
- Chemistry panels and PT/INR should be monitored every 8-12 hr.
- Glucose finger sticks should be checked every 6 hr initially to evaluate for hypoglycemia.
- Because of the increased risk of infection, daily urine, sputum, and blood cultures should be checked in the absence of signs or symptoms of infection.
- Patients with Grade I encephalopathy or greater should be admitted to a monitored setting (e.g., intensive care unit [ICU]) given rapidity of mental status deterioration and need for close neurologic monitoring. Sedating medications should be avoided as it may worsen hepatic encephalopathy. If necessary short acting medications should be used given decreased hepatic clearance.
- Patients with grade III/IV encephalopathy should be intubated for airway protection, and transfer to a transplant center should be made a priority once the patient is stabilized. Placement of ICP monitoring devices should be considered to evaluate for ICH.
- Hypotension can occur due to decreased oral intake as well as extravasation of fluid into extravascular space. Care must taken to maintain cerebral perfusion pressures (MAP goal is >70 mm Hg and CPP 60-80 mm Hg) in order to optimize neurologic recovery from ALF. Patients can be resuscitated with normal saline; acidotic patients can be resuscitated with ½ normal saline with 75 meq/L sodium bicarbonate.
- Norepinephrine is the initial vasopressor of choice; vasopressin can be added as a second pressor. Persistent hypotension despite fluid resuscitation and pressor support should prompt concern for adrenal insufficiency.
- Nutritional support should be initiated early. A daily intake goal of 60 g of protein is recommended to prevent catabolism of protein stores.
- For acetaminophen ingestions (known or suspected), refer to Acute General Rx.

ACUTE GENERAL Rx

- Correction of coagulopathy should be avoided because it can interfere with assessment of liver function.
- In the setting of life-threatening bleeding, FFP and recombinant factor VIIa can be considered.
- Patient should be placed on stress ulcer prophylaxis given risk of gastrointestinal bleeding.
- Antibiotics should be started immediately if infection is suspected. Sources usually include respiratory, urinary, and blood; there is no evidence for empiric antibiotic treatment.
- If acetaminophen is the known or suspected cause, an IV acetylcysteine protocol must be initiated (there are few studies on oral *N*-acetylcysteine [NAC] treatment). NAC is not harmful and dramatically alters the course in acetaminophen toxicity, so there should be a low threshold to start it, particularly in young patients or those with no known cause of ALF.
  The 20-hr protocol is:
  1. Initial loading dose of 150 mg/kg IV given over 60 min followed by
  2. 12.5 mg/kg IV/hr over 4 hr followed by
  3. 6.25 mg/kg IV/hr for 16 hr

A repeat acetaminophen level and ALT should be checked at hour 18 of treatment. If either acetaminophen level or ALT is elevated, the 16-hour portion of treatment (6.25 mg/kg) should be extended and another ALT, INR, or acetaminophen level should be checked every 12 hr. The acetylcysteine can be stopped once the acetaminophen level is undetectable, INR < 2, or ALT is shown to be either normal or decreasing.

BOX 1-4 Management of Fulminant Hepatic Failure

No sedation except for procedures
Minimal handling
Enteric precautions until infection ruled out
Monitor:
- Heart and respiratory rate
- Arterial BP, CVP
- Core/toe temperature
- Neurologic observations
- Gastric pH (>5.0)
- Blood glucose (>4 mmol/L)
- Acid-base
- Electrolytes
- PT, PTT

Fluid balance
- 75% maintenance
- Dextrose 10%-50% (provide 6-10 mg/kg/min)
- Sodium (0.5-1 mmol/L)
- Potassium (2-4 mmol/L)

Maintain circulating volume with colloid/FFP
Coagulation support only if required
Drugs
- Vitamin K
- H_2 antagonist
- Antacids
- Lactulose
- *N*-acetylcysteine for acetaminophen toxicity
- Broad-spectrum antibiotics
- Antifungals

Nutrition
- Enteral feeding (1-2 g protein/kg/day)
- PN if ventilated

BP, Blood pressure; *CVP,* central venous pressure; *FFP,* fresh frozen plasma; *PN,* parenteral nutrition; *PT,* prothrombin time; *PTT,* partial thromboplastin time.
From Fuhrman BP, Zimmerman JJ: *Fuhrman and Zimmerman's pediatric critical care,* ed 4, Philadelphia, 2011, Mosby.

DISPOSITION

- Because of the potential for rapid deterioration of mental status and progression to multiorgan dysfunction, these patients should be managed in an ICU.
- Given the tenuous state, potential for rapid deterioration, and overall poor prognosis of these patients, they should be transferred to a liver transplant center once stabilized. A liver specialist should be consulted upon presentation. The King's College Criteria remains the most useful assessment tool to assess need for liver transplantation (see Table 1-20).
- Overall mortality from ALF is 30%-40%.
- Transplant-free survival in ALF in the setting of acetaminophen, hepatitis A, shock liver, and pregnancy-related disease is >50%; for all other causes of ALF, transplant-free survival is <25%.

BOX 1-5 Hepatic Replacement Therapeutic Options Available to Patients with Fulminant Hepatic Failure

Liver Transplantation
Cadaveric transplantation
Whole liver
Reduced-size liver
Split liver
Auxiliary partial liver
Orthotopic position
Heterotopic position
Auxiliary whole liver
Heterotopic position
Living-related transplantation
Left lateral segment
Left lobe
Extended left lobe
Right lobe

Artificial Liver Assist Devices
Non–cell-based systems
Charcoal hemoperfusion
High-volume plasmapheresis
Continuous high-frequency hemodiafiltration
Molecular adsorbent recirculating system (MARS)
Cell-based systems (bioartificial liver assist devices)
Primary porcine hepatocytes
Human hepatoblastoma cells
Extracorporeal liver assist device (ELAD)

Hepatocyte Transplantation

From Vincent JL, Abraham E, Moore FA, et al: *Textbook of critical care,* ed 6, Philadelphia, 2011, Saunders.

TABLE 1-20 King's College Hospital Criteria for Liver Transplantation in Acute Liver Failure

Acetaminophen-Induced Acute Liver Failure	Non–Acetaminophen Induced Acute Liver Failure
Arterial pH <7.3 (irrespective of grade of encephalopathy) *OR* Grade III or IV encephalopathy *and* Prothrombin time >100 sec *and* Serum creatinine >3.4 mg/dL	Prothrombin time >100 seconds (irrespective of grade of encephalopathy *OR* Any of three of the following variables (irrespective of grade of encephalopathy): 1. Age <10 yr or >40 yr 2. Etiology: non–A hepatitis, non–B hepatitis, halothane hepatitis, idiosyncratic drug reactions 3. Duration of jaundice before onset of encephalopathy >7 days 4. Prothrombin time >50 sec 5. Serum bilirubin >18 mg/dL

PEARLS & CONSIDERATIONS

- ALF is severe hepatic injury with INR >1.5 and hepatic encephalopathy from a disease process that started <26 wk before presentation in a patient with no prior history of liver disease.
- Close to ½ of acute liver is due to drug ingestion, usually acetaminophen.
- Rapidity of deterioration referral must be made as soon as possible to a liver transplant center.
- There should be a low threshold to start NAC.
- Do not correct coagulopathy unless life-threatening bleeding occurs or it is recommended by the liver transplant hepatologist.

SUGGESTED READINGS

available at www.expertconsult.com

RELATED CONTENT

Hepatorenal Syndrome (Related Key Topic)
Encephalopathy (Related Key Topic)
Hepatopulmonary Syndrome (Related Key Topic)
Ascites (Related Key Topic)
Acetaminophen Poisoning (Related Key Topic)

AUTHORS: **PRANITH PERERA, M.D.**, and **TALIA ZENLEA, M.D.**

BASIC INFORMATION

DEFINITION

Acute respiratory distress syndrome (ARDS) is a form of noncardiogenic pulmonary edema that results from acute damage to the alveoli. It is characterized by acute diffuse infiltrative lung lesions with resulting interstitial and alveolar edema, severe hypoxemia, and respiratory failure. The cardinal feature of ARDS, refractory hypoxemia, is caused by formation of protein-rich alveolar edema after damage to the integrity of the lung's alveolar-capillary barrier.

The definition of ARDS based on the American–European Consensus Conference (AECC) from 1994 included the following components:

1. The syndrome must present acutely
2. A ratio of Pao_2 to Fio_2 ≤200 regardless of the level of positive end expiratory pressure (PEEP)
3. The detection of bilateral pulmonary infiltrates on frontal chest radiograph
4. Absence of congestive heart failure (pulmonary artery wedge pressure [PAWP] ≤18 mm Hg or no clinical evidence of elevated left atrial pressure on the basis of chest radiograph or other clinical data)

The Berlin definition of ARDS adopted in 2011 addresses some of the limitations of the AECC definition and establishes the following criteria for ARDS:

- Timing: Within 1 week of a known clinical insult or new or worsening respiratory symptoms
- Chest imaging (chest x-ray or CT scan): Bilateral opacities, not fully explained by effusions, lobar/lung collapse, or nodules
- Origin of edema: Respiratory failure not fully explained by cardiac failure or fluid overload. Need objective assessment (e.g., echocardiography) to exclude hydrostatic edema if no risk factor present
- Oxygenation (if altitude is higher than 1000 m, the correction factor should be calculated as follows: [Pao_2/Fio_2 × {barometric pressure/760}]

1. Mild: 200 mm Hg <Pao_2/Fio_2 ≤300 mm Hg with PEEP or CPAP ≥5 cm H_2O (this may be delivered noninvasively in the mild ARDS group)
2. Moderate: 100 mm Hg <Pao_2/Fio_2 ≤200 mm Hg with PEEP or CPAP ≥5 cm H_2O
3. Severe; Pao_2/Fio_2 ≤100 mm Hg with PEEP or CPAP ≥5 cm H_2O

SYNONYMS

ARDS
Adult respiratory distress syndrome

ICD-9CM CODES
518.82 Acute respiratory distress syndrome
ICD-10CM CODES
J80 Acute respiratory distress syndrome

EPIDEMIOLOGY & DEMOGRAPHICS

- More than 150,000 ARDS cases per year in the U.S. 7.1% of all patients admitted to an ICU and 16.1% of all patients on mechanical ventilation develop ARDS.
- Incidence is 1.5 to 8.3 cases per 100,000 per year.
- Approximately 50% of patients who develop ARDS do so within 24 hours of the inciting event. Mortality rate is 40% to 50%.

PHYSICAL FINDINGS & CLINICAL PRESENTATION

- Signs and symptoms
  1. Dyspnea
  2. Chest discomfort
  3. Cough
  4. Anxiety
- Physical examination
  1. Tachypnea
  2. Tachycardia
  3. Hypertension
  4. Coarse crepitations of both lungs
  5. Fever may be present if infection is the underlying etiology

ETIOLOGY

- Sepsis (>40% of cases)
- Aspiration: near-drowning, aspiration of gastric contents (>30% of cases)
- Trauma (>20% of cases)
- Multiple transfusions, blood products
- Drugs (e.g., overdose of morphine, methadone, heroin; reaction to nitrofurantoin)
- Noxious inhalation (e.g., chlorine gas, high O_2 concentration)
- Postresuscitation
- Cardiopulmonary bypass
- Pneumonia
- Burns
- Pancreatitis
- A history of chronic alcohol abuse significantly increases the risk of developing ARDS in critically ill patients
- Table 1-21 describes risk factors associated with development of ARDS.

TABLE 1-21 Risk Factors Associated with Development of Acute Lung Injury and Acute Respiratory Distress Syndrome

Direct Lung Injury	Indirect Lung Injury
Pneumonia	Sepsis
Aspiration of gastric contents	Multiple trauma
Pulmonary contusion	Cardiopulmonary bypass
Fat, amniotic fluid, or air emboli	Drug overdose
Near-drowning	Acute pancreatitis
Inhalational injury	Transfusion of blood products
Reperfusion pulmonary edema	

From Vincent JL et al: *Textbook of critical care,* ed 6, Philadelphia, 2011, Saunders.

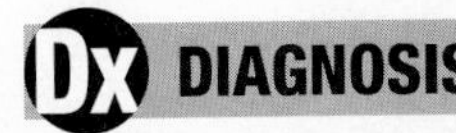

DIAGNOSIS

DIFFERENTIAL DIAGNOSIS

- Cardiogenic pulmonary edema
- Viral pneumonitis
- Lymphangitic carcinomatosis

WORKUP

The search for an underlying cause should focus on treatable causes (e.g., infections such as sepsis or pneumonia)

- Arterial blood gases (ABGs)
- Hemodynamic monitoring
- Bronchoalveolar lavage (selected patients)

LABORATORY TESTS

- ABGs:
  1. Initially: varying degrees of hypoxemia, generally resistant to supplemental oxygen
  2. Respiratory alkalosis, decreased Pco_2
  3. Widened alveolar-arterial gradient
  4. Hypercapnia as the disease progresses
- Bronchoalveolar lavage:
  1. The most prominent finding is an increased number of polymorphonucleocytes.
  2. The presence of eosinophilia has therapeutic implications because these patients respond to corticosteroids.
- Blood and urine cultures

IMAGING STUDIES

Chest radiograph (Fig. 1-44).

- The initial chest radiograph might be normal in the initial hours after the precipitating event.
- Bilateral interstitial infiltrates are usually seen within 24 hr; they often are more prominent in the bases and periphery.
- "White out" of both lung fields can be seen in advanced stages.
- CT scan of chest: diffuse consolidation with air bronchograms, bullae, pleural effusions. Pneumomediastinum and pneumothoraces may also be present.

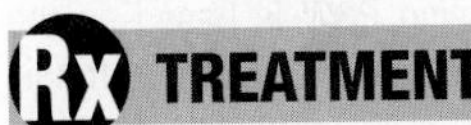

TREATMENT

NONPHARMACOLOGIC THERAPY

Treatment of ARDS is supportive.
Hemodynamic monitoring:

- Can be used for the initial evaluation of ARDS (in ruling out cardiogenic pulmonary edema) and its subsequent management. However, a pulmonary catheter is not indicated in the routine management of ARDS and trials have shown that clinical management involving the early use of pulmonary artery catheters in patients with ARDS did not significantly affect mortality and morbidity rates and may result

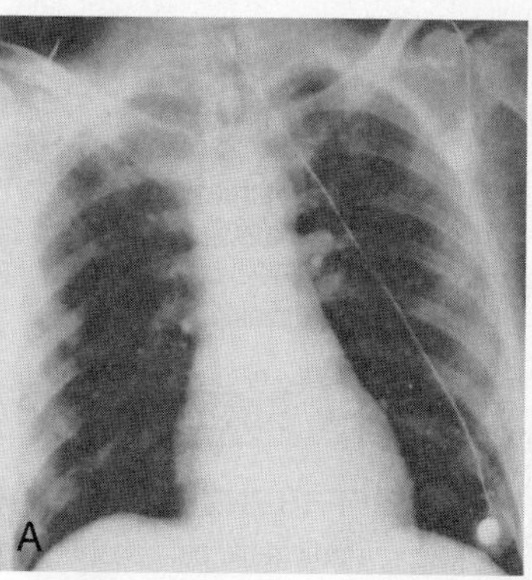

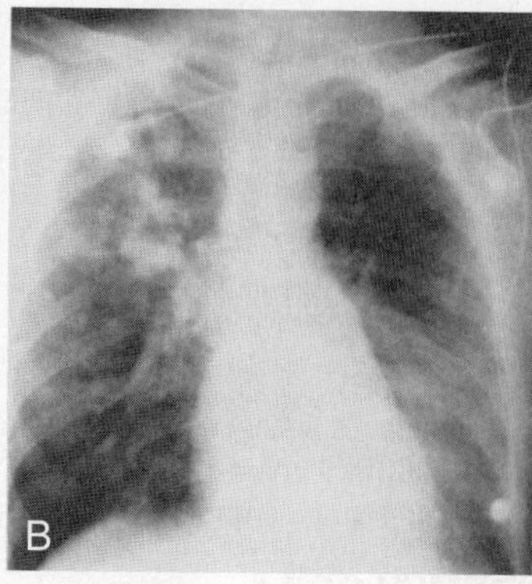

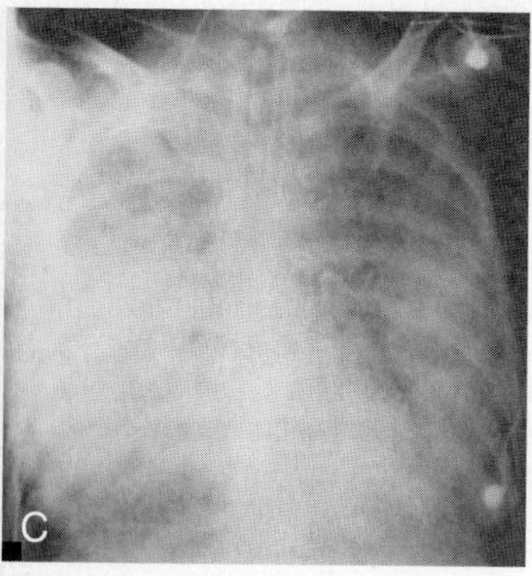

FIGURE 1-44 Acute respiratory distress syndrome. X-ray of a young man who had sustained severe trauma and blood loss in a road traffic accident; the limbs cover a period of 5 days from a relatively normal x-ray **(A),** to bilateral infiltrates **(B),** to bilateral "white out"'**(C),** accompanied by severe hypoxemia. A Swan-Ganz catheter for measurement of pulmonary artery "wedge" pressure (as a reflection of left atrial pressure) can be seen in situ on the x-ray in **C.** The patient died shortly after the last film. (From Souhami RL, Moxham J: *Textbook of medicine,* ed 4, London, 2002, Churchill Livingstone.)

in more complications as compared with a central venous catheter.

- Although no dynamic profile is diagnostic of ARDS, the presence of pulmonary edema, a high cardiac output, and a low pulmonary capillary wedge pressure (PCWP) is characteristic of ARDS.
- It is important to remember that partially treated intravascular volume overload and flash pulmonary edema can have the hemodynamic features of ARDS; filling pressures can also be elevated by increased intrathoracic pressures or with fluid administration; cardiac function can be depressed by acidosis, hypoxemia, or other factors associated with sepsis.

Ventilatory support: mechanical ventilation is generally necessary to maintain adequate gas exchange (Table E1-22). General recommendations for ventilator settings in ARDS are described in Table 1-23. A low tidal volume and low plateau pressure ventilator strategy are recommended to avoid ventilator-induced injury. Assist-control is generally preferred initially with the following ventilator settings:

- Fio_2 1.0 (until a lower value can be used to achieve adequate oxygenation). When possible, minimize oxygen toxicity by maintaining Fio_2 at <60%.
- Tidal volume: Set initial tidal volume at 6 ml/kg of predicted body weight (PBW = 50.0 + 0.91 [height: 152.4 cm] for men, PBW = 45.5 + 0.91 [height: 152.4 cm] for women). The concept of using PBW is based on the fact that lung size depends most strongly on height and sex; PBW normalizes the tidal volume to lung size. Aim to maintain plateau pressure (Pplat) at <30 mm Hg.
- PEEP 5 cm H_2O or greater (to increase lung volume and keep alveoli open). PEEP should be applied in small increments of 3 to 5 cm H_2O (see Table E1-22) to achieve acceptable arterial saturation (>0.9) with nontoxic Fio_2 values (<0.6) and acceptable airway plateau pressures (>30 to 35 cm H_2O). It is important to remember that an increase in PEEP may lower cardiac output and, despite improvement in Pao_2, may actually have a negative effect on tissue oxygenation (the major determinants of tissue oxygenation are hemoglobin, percent saturation, and cardiac output). The optimal level of PEEP remains unestablished. Although higher levels of PEEP may help prevent life-threatening hypoxemia and be associated with lower hospital mortality in patients meeting criteria for ARDS, such benefit is unlikely in patients with less severe lung injury and a strategy of treating such patients with high PEEP levels may be harmful.
- Inspiratory flow: 60 L/min.
- Ventilatory rate: high ventilatory rates of 18 to 24 breaths/min are often necessary in patients with ARDS because of their increased physiologic dead space and smaller lung volumes. Patients must be monitored for excessive intrathoracic gas trapping (auto-PEEP or intrinsic PEEP) that can depress cardiac output.
- Sedation: GABA receptor agonists (including propofol and benzodiazepines such as midazolam) have traditionally been the most commonly administered sedative drugs for ICU patients. Recent trials indicate that the alpha-2 agonist dexmedetomidine (Precedex) may have distinct advantages. At comparable sedation levels, dexmedetomidine-treated patients spent less time on ventilator, experienced less delirium, and developed less tachycardia and hypertension. The most notable adverse effect of dexmedetomidine was bradycardia. Preliminary trials involving early administration of the neuromuscular blocking agent cisatracurium in patients with severe ARDS have shown improvement in the adjusted 90-day survival and increase in the time off the ventilator without increase in muscle weakness. However, patients who receive continuous infusions of sedatives generally need to be on mechanical ventilation longer than those who receive intermittent dosing. Paralysis of patients with neuromuscular blockade (NMB) to facilitate controlled ventilation is associated with protracted mechanical ventilation and postparalysis weakness. It should ideally be conducted for a brief period, and limited to patients with severe ARDS. Daily interruption of sedation (daily awakening) in mechanically ventilated patients is safe and is associated with a shorter length of mechanical ventilation.
- The management of sedation and delirium can have important effects on the outcomes of patients in ICUs. The best outcomes are achieved with the use of a protocol in which the depth of sedation and the presence of pain and delirium are routinely monitored, pain is treated promptly and effectively, sedation is kept to the necessary minimum for the comfort and safety of the patient, and early mobilization is achieved whenever possible (Reade, Finfer, 2014).

ACUTE GENERAL Rx

Identify and treat precipitating conditions:

- Blood and urine cultures and trial of antibiotics in presumed sepsis (routine administration of antibiotics in all cases of ARDS is not recommended).
- Prompt repair of bone fractures in patients with major trauma.
- Bowel rest and crystalloid resuscitation in pancreatitis.
- Fluid management: In most patients with ARDS, fluid restriction is associated with better outcomes than a liberal fluid policy. Optimal fluid and hemodynamic management of patients with ARDS should be patient specific; in general, administration of crystalloids is recommended if a downward trend in PCWP is associated with diminished cardiac index, resulting in prerenal azotemia, oliguria, and relative tachycardia. On the other hand, if PCWP increases with little or no change in cardiac index, one should consider diuretic therapy and use of low-dose dopamine (2 to 4 μg/kg/min) to maintain natriuresis and support adequate renal flow.
- Positioning the patient: changes in position can improve oxygenation by improving the distribution of perfusion to ventilated lung regions; repositioning (lateral decubitus positioning) should be attempted in patients with hypoxemia that is not responsive to other medical interventions. Placing patients with moderate and severe hypoxemia in a prone position may improve their oxygenation. Recent trials (Guerin et al) have shown that in patients with severe ARDS, early application of prolonged prone-positioning sessions significantly decreases 28-day and 90-day mortality.

TABLE 1-23 Recommendations for Ventilator Settings in ARDS

Conventional Mechanical Ventilation		
Mode		Volume- or pressure-controlled "Airway pressure release ventilation" preferred when preservation of spontaneous ventilation is desired
Tidal volume	6-10 ml/kg	Permissive hypercapnia (increase <5 mm Hg/h) $PaCO_2$ 65-85 mm Hg well tolerated unless increased ICP Arterial pH >7.15
End-inspiratory plateau pressure	<30 cm H_2O	Above this limit, increased risks of barotrauma and air leaks
Positive end-expiratory pressure	10-15 cm H_2O	Lower PEEP levels, if heterogeneous lung injury Higher PEEP levels, if diffuse lung injury Consider early prone positioning (6-12 h)
Respiratory rate	20-60 beats/min	Adjusted to age; higher than normal may limit hypercapnia
Inspiratory/expiratory ratio	1:2 to 1:1	Check for inadvertent PEEP
FiO_2	<60%-80%	Depends on how the diseased lung may be recruited PaO_2 40-60 mm Hg, SpO_2 85%-95%
High-Frequency Oscillatory Ventilation		
Amplitude pressure	30-50 cm H_2O	To achieve visible chest vibrations
Mean airway pressure	15-30 cm H_2O	To achieve adequate chest recruitment (7 to 9 ribs)
Respiratory rate	3-10 Hz	Decrease to increase tidal volume (usually not measured)
Inspiratory/expiratory ratio	1:3 to 1:1	1:1 more appropriate in diffuse lung injury
FiO_2	<60%-80%	Depends on whether the lung may be recruited

ICP, Intracranial pressure.
From Fuhrman BP et al: *Pediatric critical care,* ed 4, Philadelphia, 2011, Saunders.

- Corticosteroids: routine use of corticosteroids in ARDS is not recommended; corticosteroids may be beneficial in patients with many eosinophils in the bronchoalveolar lavage fluid. Systemic infections should be ruled out or adequately treated before administration of corticosteroids. Use of methylprednisolone has not been shown to increase the rate of infectious complications but is associated with a higher rate of neuromuscular weakness. In addition, starting methylprednisolone therapy more than 2 wk after the onset of ARDS may increase the risk of death.
- Nutritional support: nutritional support, preferably administered by the enteral route, is necessary to maintain adequate colloid oncotic pressure and intravascular volume. The inclusion of eicosapentaenoic acid from fish oil may be beneficial in improving ventilation requirements and length of stay in patients with ARDS.
- Tracheostomy: tracheostomy is warranted in patients requiring >2 wk of mechanical ventilation; discussion regarding tracheostomy should begin with patient (if alert and oriented) and family members/legal guardian after 5 to 7 days of ventilatory support. Early tracheostomy (within 4 days of admission to critical care) does not limit mortality and results in many unneeded procedures (Young et al, 2013).
- Some form of deep vein thrombosis prophylaxis is indicated in all patients with ARDS.
- Stress ulcer prophylaxis with sucralfate suspension (by nasogastric tube), or IV proton pump inhibitors or H_2 blockers.
- The use of surfactant remains controversial. Patients who receive surfactant have a greater improvement in gas exchange in the initial 24-hour period than patients who receive standard therapy alone; however, the use of exogenous surfactant does not improve survival.

DISPOSITION

- Patients who survive ARDS are at risk of diminished functional capacity, mental illness, and decreased quality of life. Prognosis for ARDS varies with the underlying cause. Prognosis is worse in patients with chronic liver disease, nonpulmonary organ dysfunction, sepsis, and advanced age.
- Elevated values of dead space fraction ($[Paco_2 - Peco_2]/Paco_2$; normal is <0.3) is associated with an increased risk of death.
- In ARDS, the percentage of potentially recruitable lung is variable and associated with the response to PEEP.
- Overall mortality rate varies between 32% and 45%. Most deaths are attributable to sepsis or multiorgan dysfunction rather than primary respiratory causes.
- Recent trials have shown that as compared with the current standard of care, a ventilator strategy using esophageal measures to estimate the transpulmonary pressure significantly improves oxygenation and compliance. Further trials will determine if this approach should be widely adapted.
- Strategies for treatment of life-threatening refractory hypoxemia (prone positioning, inhaled nitric acid, extracorporeal membrane oxygenation (ECMO), high-frequency oscillatory ventilation, recruitment maneuvers) may improve oxygenation, but their impact on mortality remains unproven. Use of ECMO in combination with lung protective ventilation was found to be beneficial as a treatment strategy early in the course of ARDS related to H1N1 infection. Extracorporeal gas exchange may allow the use of low tidal volumes and lower levels of inspired oxygen and use of higher PEEP if desired. ECMO is costly and labor-intensive. The role and proper use of ECMO for patients with ARDS have not been clearly defined. General indications for venovenous ECMO in severe cases of ARDS are:
  - Severe hypoxemia (e.g., ratio of PaO_2 to FiO_2 <80 despite the application of high levels of PEEP [typically 15 to 20 cm H_2O]) for at least 6 hr in patients with potentially reversible respiratory failure
  - Uncompensated hypercapnia with acidemia (pH <7.15) despite the best accepted standard of care for management with a ventilator
  - Excessively high end-inspiratory plateau pressure (>35 to 45 cm H_2O, according to the patient's body size) despite the best accepted standard of care for management with a ventilator

REFERRAL

Surgical referral for tracheostomy (see "Acute General Rx").

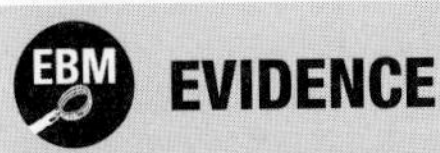

EVIDENCE

available at www.expertconsult.com

SUGGESTED READINGS

available at www.expertconsult.com

RELATED CONTENT

Acute Respiratory Distress Syndrome (ARDS) (Patient Information)

AUTHOR: **FRED F. FERRI, M.D.**

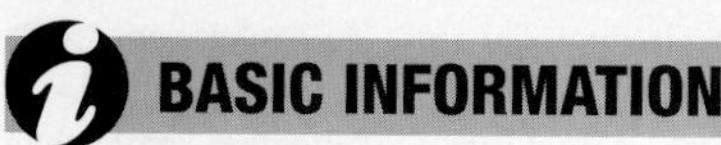

BASIC INFORMATION

DEFINITION

Acute stress disorder (ASD) includes severe acute stress reactions (ASRs) that occur between 3 days to one month after exposure to a traumatic event.

SYNONYMS

ASD, ASR

ICD-9CM and DSM-5 CODES
308.3 Other acute reactions to stress
ICD-10CM CODES
F43.0 Acute stress reaction

EPIDEMIOLOGY & DEMOGRAPHICS

PREVALENCE:
Prevalence varies according to the nature of the traumatic event. Prevalence is estimated at less than 20% in cases that do not involve assault, and at 20%-50% in cases of interpersonal trauma (e.g., rape, assault, witnessing a mass shooting)

PREDOMINANT AGE:
Diagnosed among individuals of all ages. It should be noted that children may manifest symptoms differently (e.g., may report frightening dreams that do not directly reflect the trauma). Young children may also not report fear at the time of the trauma or when re-experiencing the trauma

PREDOMINANT SEX:
Females more than males

GENETICS:
Differential function of the serotonin transporter may mediate differential responses to trauma. The 5-HTTLPR may constitute a genetic candidate region. Higher rates of ASD among women may be attributable to higher rates of violence against women and sex-linked neurobiological differences in the stress response.

RISK FACTORS:
- Greater perceived severity of the trauma (i.e., catastrophic interpretations of the event, exaggerated appraisals of future harm, hopelessness), high levels of negative affect, avoidant coping style, history of prior trauma, lack of social support, premorbid mental disorder (e.g., preexisting anxiety or depressive disorders)

PHYSICAL FINDINGS & CLINICAL PRESENTATION

DSM-5 criteria are met when the following criteria are satisfied:

A. Exposure to actual or threatened serious injury, death, or sexual violation in one or more of the following ways:
- Directly experiencing a traumatic event
- Witnessing a traumatic event as it occurred
- Learning that a traumatic event occurred to a family member or close friend
- Repeated or extreme exposure to traumatic details of an event

B. Presence of nine or more of the following symptoms from any of the following five categories: 1) Intrusion; 2) negative mood; 3) dissociation; 4) avoidance; and 5) arousal
- Recurrent, distressing, involuntary memories of the trauma (intrusion)
- Recurrent distressing dreams relating to the trauma (intrusion)
- Flashbacks to the event, in which the individual feels/acts as if the event is recurring (intrusion)
- Intense or prolonged psychological distress or physiological reaction in response to cues that are reminiscent of the trauma (intrusion)
- Continual inability to experience positive emotions (negative mood)
- Altered sense of reality (dissociation)
- Inability to remember components of the trauma (dissociation)
- Avoidance of memories, thoughts, or feelings associated with the event (avoidance)
- Avoidance of external reminders of the event (avoidance)
- Sleep disturbance (arousal)
- Irritability and anger outbursts (arousal)
- Hypervigilance (arousal)
- Difficulties concentrating (arousal)
- Exaggerated startle response (arousal)

Symptoms typically begin immediately after the trauma and must persist for at least 3 days (up to one month) and result in clinically significant impairment in functioning. If symptoms persist for greater than 1 month, a diagnosis of post-traumatic stress disorder (PTSD) may be considered. Symptoms must not be attributable to a medical condition or substance use.

ETIOLOGY

Factors predicting the development of ASD have not been established; however, multiple theoretical models have been proposed. Dissociative models propose that individuals minimize the emotional consequences of trauma by restricting awareness of the event to reduce fear. Cognitive perspectives propose that intentional cognitive processes (e.g., avoidance, distraction, dysfunctional appraisals, attribution of responsibility) result in pathological reactions to trauma. Biological theories focus on the immediate effects of trauma on neuronal function, including cortisol, catecholamines, glucocorticoids, serotonin, and endogenous opioids as mediating factors of the trauma response.

Dx DIAGNOSIS

DIFFERENTIAL DIAGNOSIS

- Adjustment disorder
- Panic disorder
- Dissociative disorders
- PTSD
- Obsessive-compulsive disorder
- Psychotic disorders
- Traumatic brain injury

WORKUP

- Diagnosis is made based on individual interviews, including a history of past trauma, age at the time of the trauma, and duration of the trauma. Structured clinical interviews may be used, and may be supplemented with standardized self-report measures. It should be noted that dissociative symptoms may prevent individuals from remembering components of the trauma, as well as remembering feelings of fear, helplessness or horror. Collateral data from other sources (family members, close friends, medical providers, therapists, etc.) may be useful.

LABORATORY TESTS

- None indicated

IMAGING STUDIES

- None indicated

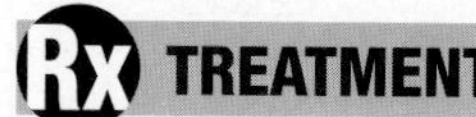

TREATMENT

Early treatment should focus on establishing a therapeutic alliance and acknowledging fears about reexposure. Resilience-focused psychosocial interventions may focus on better tolerating the distress of trauma-related memories, reducing re-experiencing and reactivity to reminders of the trauma, reducing trauma-related avoidance and sleep disturbances and nightmares, increasing social support, decreasing behaviors that interfere with daily life, limiting generalization of the danger experienced, and altering maladaptive attributions and appraisals. In cases of interpersonal trauma, safety planning is necessary for individuals who remain in unsafe situations or relationships. Pharmacological treatment is typically reserved for individuals who have already received psychotherapy. There are few controlled pharmacological treatment trials for ASD. There are currently no medications approved by the FDA for treatment of ASD. Clinicians may consider FDA-approved medications for PTSD, such as paroxetine and sertraline.

NONPHARMACOLOGIC THERAPY

- Cognitive behavioral therapy
- Prolonged exposure
- Cognitive processing therapy
- Relaxation and mindfulness

ACUTE GENERAL Rx

- Acute medication may be necessary when the individual is dangerous, agitated, or psychotic. In emergencies, short-acting benzodiazepines or neuroleptics with minimal side effects may be effective.
- Antiadrenergic agents may be useful for treatment of arousal.
- Brief, time-limited treatment using benzodiazepines may be useful for treating arousal, insomnia, and anxiety. It should be noted that prolonged use of benzodiazepines has been associated with higher rates of PTSD.
- Prazosin is recommended for treatment of nightmares.
- SSRIs and other antidepressants may be useful for re-experiencing symptoms, avoidance, and hyperarousal.

COMPLEMENTARY & ALTERNATIVE MEDICINE

Patients may find activities that increase relaxation (i.e., yoga, mindfulness, meditation) useful.

DISPOSITION

Treatment should be delivered in the least restrictive environment that can ensure patient safety. Most patients with ASD can be managed in an outpatient setting. Partial or inpatient hospitalization may be necessary for crisis management, and may be considered for patients who have comorbid psychiatric/medical diagnoses; who are experiencing suicidal or homicidal ideation, plans, or intention; or who are severely ill.

REFERRAL

Patients are treated by a mental health clinician.

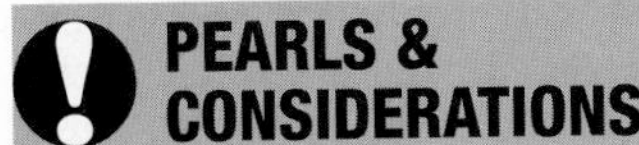

PEARLS & CONSIDERATIONS

COMMENTS

- Although many individuals with ASD go on to develop PTSD, many with ASD do not go on to develop PTSD. Available data at this time suggest that ASD criteria are not adequate for identifying individuals at risk for developing PTSD.
- Standardized assessment tools, such as the Structured Clinical Interview for DSM-5 Dissociative Disorders (SCID-D), the Acute Stress Disorder Interview (ASDI), the Stanford Acute Stress Reaction Questionnaire (SASRQ), and the Acute Stress Disorder Scale (ASDS) may be helpful in the diagnosis of ASD and/or treatment monitoring.

PREVENTION

Critical incident stress debriefing (CISD) following a trauma is typically administered in one two-to three-hour group session within 72 hours of the trauma, with the goals of allowing survivors to "vent." There is some evidence that CISD does not prevent PTSD and may contribute to poor recovery. Psychological first aid (PFA) is designed to improve outcomes following trauma by fostering safety, calmness, social connectedness, and optimism. Although PFA has received some empirical support, questions remain regarding the optimal format of administration.

PATIENT & FAMILY EDUCATION

National Center for PTSD, Public Section, Information on Trauma and PTSD for Veterans, the General Public and Families: Acute Stress Disorder. (http://www.ptsd.va.gov/public/pages/acute-stress-disorder.asp)

SUGGESTED READINGS

Available at www.expertconsult.com

RELATED CONTENT

Post-traumatic Stress Disorder (Related Key Topic)

AUTHOR: **LINDSAY M. ORCHOWSKI, PH.D.**

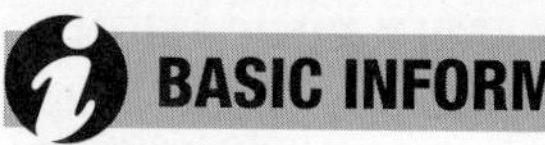

BASIC INFORMATION

DEFINITION

The acute cessation of urinary flow; inability to void.

SYNONYMS

Inability to urinate

ICD-9CM CODES
788.20 Retention of urine, unspecified
ICD-10CM CODES
R33.9 Retention of urine, unspecified

EPIDEMIOLOGY & DEMOGRAPHICS

INCIDENCE: Can occur in any age group and both sexes. It is the most common urologic emergency.
PEAK INCIDENCE: Males older than age 60. Over a 5-year period, AUR will occur in 10% of men older than 70 and one third of men older than 80.
PREVALENCE: Increased longevity has caused an increase in prevalence.
PREDOMINANT SEX AND AGE: Men older than 60 years.
GENETICS: None known.
RISK FACTORS: Obstructive risk factors include benign prostatic hypertrophy (BPH) and bladder, pelvic, and urethral masses. Acute trauma, surgery, medications (especially over-the-counter [OTC] antihistamines), neurologic disease, and infection can be contributing or precipitating factors, particularly when superimposed on obstructive risk factors.

PHYSICAL FINDINGS & CLINICAL PRESENTATION

- Patients will present with the acute inability to pass urine.
- Pain in the lower abdomen and suprapubic region is typical (this is not typically present with chronic urinary retention due to the more gradual onset).
- The bladder may be palpable on abdominal or rectal exam. There may be tenderness with deep palpation.
- Patients with cognitive deficits may present with restlessness, discomfort, worsened confusion, or delirium but may not be able to give the history of urinary retention.

ETIOLOGY

- Most commonly the result of obstruction from various causes, including BPH and bladder and pelvic masses.
- Nonobstructive causes include medications, surgery, trauma, neurologic disease, and infection.
- In older patients, cause is frequently multifactorial, with an underlying obstructive risk factor and an acute precipitant.
- In women, AUR may be caused by benign tumors (especially fibroids); malignant tumors of pelvic, urethral, or vaginal origin; postpartum vulvar edema; or labial fusion.
- Infection such as prostatitis, urethritis, and genital herpes and herpes zoster can also cause AUR.

Dx DIAGNOSIS

DIFFERENTIAL DIAGNOSIS

- AUR is typically self-evident to the cognitively intact patient, and to the physician. Differential diagnosis focuses on the underlying cause of the problem.

WORKUP

- History should focus on urologic symptoms, including dysuria, hematuria, history of retention, and urologic cancer.
- Review of symptoms (ROS) should include fever, back pain, neurologic symptoms, and rash.
- History should include a complete list of prescribed and OTC medications.
- Rectal exam for masses, fecal impaction, perineal sensation, and sphincter tone.
- Pelvic exam for female patients.
- Neurologic exam to rule out an underlying neurologic cause.

LABORATORY TESTS

- Creatinine level. Note that in acute retention this may not be elevated above baseline.
- Urinalysis and culture (which will be obtained via catheterization).
- BUN, electrolytes
- Prostate-specific antigen (PSA) testing is not helpful in the acute situation, as it is expected to be elevated during an episode of retention.

IMAGING STUDIES

- Imaging may not be necessary when AUR is felt to be due to reversible causes.
- Ultrasound may be valuable, particularly if there is suspicion of a pelvic mass.
- Pelvic computed tomography (CT) scan is done if, on physical exam or ultrasound, masses are found requiring further evaluation.
- Magnetic resonance imaging (MRI) is used when symptoms suggest spinal cord problems.
- Evaluation of bladder function may be considered after initial management, particularly in women with no evidence of anatomic obstruction.

Rx TREATMENT

NONPHARMACOLOGIC THERAPY

- Given that AUR recurs 68% of the time when caused by BPH, consider surgical treatment for this issue. Transurethral resection of the prostate (TURP) should be delayed until at least 30 days after the episode of AUR, to minimize surgical complications.

ACUTE GENERAL Rx

- Prompt bladder decompression and drainage is the initial management of AUR.
- Urethral catheterization should be promptly initiated if the patient has no history of recent genitourinary (GU) surgery.
- If there is a history of recent surgery, suprapubic catheterization is indicated.
- Partial drainage and clamping of catheter is not necessary and may increase the risk of urinary tract infection (UTI).
- Clean intermittent catheterization (CIC) may be considered, although in the acute setting it may be limited by patient acceptance and the time required for teaching this technique. Use of CIC may improve the rate of spontaneous voiding.

CHRONIC Rx

- Consider catheter removal in 2 to 3 days, particularly in patients younger than 65 years old, when the catheterized volume is less than 1 L, and when a precipitating event can be identified.
- Otherwise 1 to 2 weeks of catheterization should be considered before voiding trial.
- Alpha blockers are effective in treatment of the symptoms of BPH and may increase the success of trials of early removal of catheter.
- 5-Alpha reductase inhibitors are not effective for acute management when AUR is caused by BPH, due to slow onset of the decrease of prostate volume.

COMPLEMENTARY & ALTERNATIVE MEDICINE

- None noted.

DISPOSITION

- Patients may be sent home if close follow-up can be assured.
- Hospital admission may be needed, particularly in patients with urosepsis or when retention is due to malignancy or spinal cord compression.

REFERRAL

- To urology, particularly in cases where the underlying cause cannot be addressed acutely or is not self-limited.
- To gynecology when gynecologic masses are the underlying cause of AUR.

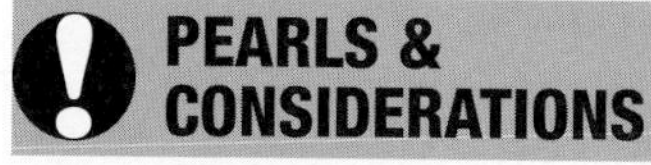

PEARLS & CONSIDERATIONS

PREVENTION

Patients with BPH should avoid the use of antihistamines, sedatives, and other medications that can precipitate acute retention. Inhaled anticholinergic agents may increase the risk of AUR and should be used cautiously in patients with risk factors, especially BPH.

PATIENT/FAMILY EDUCATION

Education regarding catheter use and care is helpful in patients who are discharged to home.

SUGGESTED READINGS

available at www.expertconsult.com

AUTHOR: **MARGARET TRYFOROS, M.D.**

BASIC INFORMATION

DEFINITION

Adrenal insufficiency is characterized by inadequate secretion of corticosteroids resulting from partial or complete destruction of the adrenal glands.

SYNONYMS

Primary adrenocortical insufficiency
Addison disease

ICD-9CM CODES
255.4 Addison disease
ICD-10CM CODES
E27.1 Primary adrenocortical insufficiency
E27.2 Addisonian crisis
E27.3 Drug-induced andrenocortical insufficiency
E23.3 Hypopituitarism

EPIDEMIOLOGY & DEMOGRAPHICS

PREVALENCE: Five cases/100,000 persons
PREDOMINANT SEX: Female/male ratio of 2:1

PHYSICAL FINDINGS & CLINICAL PRESENTATION

- Adrenal insufficiency may present insidiously with nonspecific symptoms. A high index of suspicion is required for diagnosis. About half of patients may present acutely with adrenal crises. Table 1-24 summarizes the clinical features of primary adrenal insufficiency.
- Hyperpigmentation of skin (Fig. E1-45) and mucous membranes is a cardinal sign of adrenal insufficiency: more prominent in palmar creases, buccal mucosa, pressure points (elbows, knees, knuckles), perianal mucosa, and around areolas of nipples
- Hypotension, postural dizziness
- Generalized weakness, chronic fatigue, malaise, anorexia
- Amenorrhea and loss of axillary hair in females

ETIOLOGY

- Autoimmune destruction of the adrenal glands (80% of cases)
- Tuberculosis (TB) (15% of cases)
- Carcinomatous destruction of the adrenal glands, lymphoma
- Adrenal hemorrhage (anticoagulants, trauma, coagulopathies, pregnancy, sepsis)
- Adrenal infarction (antiphospholipid syndrome, arteritis, thrombosis)
- AIDS (adrenal insufficiency develops in 30% of patients with AIDS, often cytomegalovirus [CMV] adrenalitis)
- Other: sarcoidosis, amyloidosis, hemochromatosis, Wegener's granulomatosis, postoperative, fungal infections (candidiasis, histoplasmosis)

TABLE 1-24 Clinical Features of Primary Adrenal Insufficiency

Feature	Frequency (%)
Symptoms	
Weakness, tiredness, fatigue	100
Anorexia	100
Gastrointestinal symptoms	92
Nausea	86
Vomiting	75
Constipation	33
Abdominal pain	31
Diarrhea	16
Salt craving	16
Postural dizziness	12
Muscle or joint pains	13
Signs	
Weight loss	100
Hyperpigmentation	94
Hypotension (<110 mm Hg systolic)	88-94
Vitiligo	10-20
Auricular calcification	5
Laboratory Findings	
Electrolyte disturbances	92
Hyponatremia	88
Hyperkalemia	64
Hypercalcemia	6
Azotemia	55
Anemia	40
Eosinophilia	17

From Melmed S, Polonsky KS, Larsen PR, Kronenberg HM: *Williams textbook of endocrinology*, ed 12, Philadelphia, 2011, Saunders.

DIAGNOSIS

DIFFERENTIAL DIAGNOSIS

Sepsis, hypovolemic shock, acute abdomen, apathetic hyperthyroidism in the elderly, myopathies, gastrointestinal malignancy, major depression, anorexia nervosa, hemochromatosis, salt-losing nephritis, chronic infection

WORKUP

- If the clinical picture is highly suggestive of adrenocortical insufficiency, the diagnosis can be made with the rapid adrenocorticotropic hormone (ACTH) test (Fig. E1-46):
  1. Give 250 mcg ACTH (Sinachten, tetracosatrin) by IV push and measure cortisol levels at 0, 30, and 60 min.
  2. An increase in serum cortisol level to peak concentration >500 nmol/L (18 mcg/dl) indicates a normal response. Cortisol level <18 mcg/dl at 30 or 60 min is suggestive of adrenal insufficiency.
  3. Measure plasma ACTH. A high ACTH level confirms primary adrenal insufficiency.
- Critical illness-related corticosteroid insufficiency (e.g., in sepsis) is best established with the 1-mcg ACTH stimulation test in which cortisol levels are measured at baseline and 30 min after administration of ACTH. A level <25 mcg/dl (690 nmol/L) or an increment over baseline of <9 mcg (250 nmol/L) represents an inadequate adrenal response.
- Secondary adrenocortical insufficiency (caused by pituitary dysfunction) can be distinguished from primary adrenal insufficiency by the following:
  1. Normal or low plasma ACTH level after rapid ACTH
  2. Absence of hyperpigmentation
  3. No significant impairment of aldosterone secretion (because aldosterone secretion is under control of the renin-angiotensin system)
  4. Additional evidence of hypopituitarism (e.g., hypogonadism, hypothyroidism)

LABORATORY TESTS

- Hyponatremia, hyperkalemia
- Decreased glucose
- Increased BUN/creatinine ratio (prerenal azotemia)
- Mild normocytic, normochromic anemia, neutropenia, lymphocytosis, eosinophilia (significant dehydration may mask hyponatremia and anemia), hypercalcemia, metabolic acidosis
- A morning cortisol level >500 mmol/L (18 mcg/dl) generally excludes the diagnosis whereas a level <165 mmol/L (6 mcg/dl) is suggestive of Addison disease and requires further evaluation (see "Workup")
- Useful tests in evaluating the cause of adrenal insufficiency are: PPD (rule out TB), adrenal cortex antibodies and 21-hydroxylase antibodies (rule out autoimmune Addison disease),

 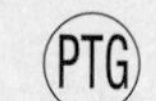

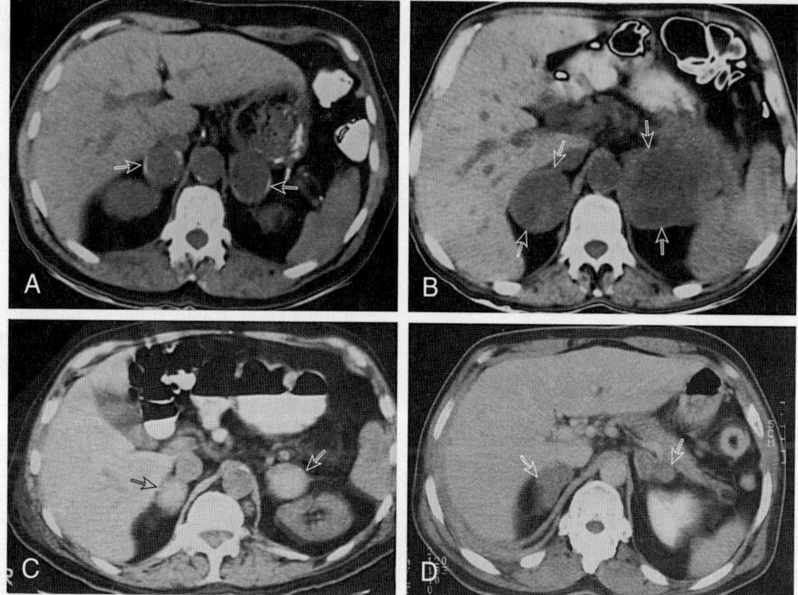

FIGURE 1-48 Computed tomographic (CT) scans of patients with primary adrenal insufficiency. The affected adrenal glands are indicated by arrows. **A,** CT scan of a 59-year-old man with histoplasmosis. Notice the subcapsular calcium in both glands. **B,** CT scan of a 59-year-old man with metastatic melanoma. **C,** CT scan of an 80-year-old man with bilateral adrenal hemorrhage resulting from anticoagulation for pulmonary emboli. **D,** Bilateral adrenal tuberculomas in a 79-year-old man with tuberculosis affecting the urogenital tract. (**A** and **B** courtesy of Dr. William D. Salmon, Jr.; **C,** courtesy of Dr. Craig R. Sussman.) (From Melmed S, Polonsky KS, Larsen PR, Kronenberg HM: *Williams textbook of endocrinology,* ed 12, Philadelphia, 2011, Saunders.)

plasma very-long-chain fatty acids (rule out adrenoleukodystrophy)

IMAGING STUDIES

- Chest radiograph may reveal a small heart (Fig. E1-47).
- Abdominal radiograph: adrenal calcifications may be noted if the adrenocortical insufficiency is secondary to TB or fungal infection.
- Abdominal CT scan (Fig. 1-48): small adrenal glands generally indicate either idiopathic atrophy or longstanding TB, whereas enlarged glands are suggestive of early TB or potentially treatable diseases.

Rx TREATMENT

NONPHARMACOLOGIC THERAPY

- Perform periodic monitoring of serum electrolytes, vital signs, and body weight; liberal sodium intake is suggested.
- Periodic measurement of bone density may be helpful in identifying patients at risk for the development of osteoporosis.
- Patients should carry a MedicAlert bracelet and an emergency pack containing hydrocortisone 100-mg ampule, syringe, and needle.
- Patients and partners should be educated on how to give IM injection in case of vomiting or coma.

ACUTE GENERAL Rx

- Addisonian crisis is an acute complication of adrenal insufficiency characterized by circulatory collapse, dehydration, nausea, vomiting, hypoglycemia, and hyperkalemia.
  1. Draw plasma cortisol level; do not delay therapy while waiting for confirming laboratory results.
  2. Administer hydrocortisone 100 mg IV immediately, followed by 100 to 200 mg of hydrocortisone every 24 hours divided into 3 or 4 doses; if patient shows good clinical response, gradually taper dosage and change to oral maintenance dose (usually prednisone 7.5 mg/day).
  3. Provide adequate volume replacement with D_5NS solution until hypotension, dehydration, and hypoglycemia are completely corrected. Large volumes (2 to 3 L) under continuous cardiac monitoring may be necessary in the first 2 to 3 hr to correct the volume deficit and hypoglycemia and to avoid further hyponatremia.
- Identify and correct any precipitating factor (e.g., sepsis, hemorrhage).

CHRONIC Rx

- Give hydrocortisone 15 to 20 mg PO every morning and 5 to 10 mg in late afternoon or prednisone 5 mg in morning and 2.5 mg hs.
- Give oral fludrocortisone 0.05 mg/day to 0.20 mg/day: this mineralocorticoid is necessary if the patient has primary adrenocortical insufficiency. The dose is adjusted based on the serum sodium level and the presence of postural hypotension or marked orthostasis.
- Instruct patients to increase glucocorticoid replacement in times of stress and to receive parenteral glucocorticoids if diarrhea or vomiting occurs. Typical supplementation varies from 25 mg PO qd of hydrocortisone for minor medical and surgical stress to 50 to 100 mg IV hydrocortisone q8h for sepsis-induced hypotension or shock.
- The administration of dehydroepiandrosterone 50 mg PO qd improves well-being and sexuality in women with adrenal insufficiency.

SUGGESTED READINGS

available at www.expertconsult.com

RELATED CONTENT

Addison's Disease (Patient Information)

AUTHOR: **FRED F. FERRI, M.D.**

BASIC INFORMATION

DEFINITION

Adult-onset Still's disease (AOSD) is a rare systemic autoinflammatory disorder of unknown etiology characterized by high spiking quotidian fever >102° F, arthralgia or arthritis, evanescent skin rash, and leukocytosis with neutrophilic predominance. Temperature often returns to normal between fever spikes. Articular symptoms may be absent or mild initially, but most patients develop a persistent destructive arthropathy.

SYNONYMS

Adult Still's disease, Wissler's syndrome, Wissler-Fanconi syndrome

ICD-9CM CODES
714.2 Other rheumatoid arthritis with visceral or systemic involvement
ICD-10CM CODES
M06.1 Adult-onset Still disease

EPIDEMIOLOGY & DEMOGRAPHICS

INCIDENCE: 0.22/100,000 in men, 0.34/100,000 in women
PEAK INCIDENCE: Age 16-35
PREVALENCE: Unknown
PREDOMINANT SEX AND AGE: Slightly women > men, bimodal 15-25 and 36-46
GENETICS: Relative risk ranging from 2.1 to 2.9 associated with HLA B17, B18, B35, and DR2. Cytokine production also implicated in the pathogenesis: IL6, IL2, interferon gamma, and tumor necrosis factor alpha (TNF-alpha)
RISK FACTORS: Stress has been proved to be the only known risk factor.

PHYSICAL FINDINGS & CLINICAL PRESENTATION

- Triad: High spiking fevers, characteristic rash, and arthritis/arthralgias
- Fever is >102° F, transient, quotidian in pattern, usually in the late afternoon or early evening
- Nonspecific symptoms: myalgias, serositis including pleuritis and pericarditis, sore throat
- Rash is typically an evanescent, salmon pink, and maculopapular located on the trunk and proximal extremities and accompanies the fever. Often resolves when patient is afebrile.
- Arthritis is symmetric and destructive, involving the wrists, knees, and ankles. Extensive carpal involvement distinguishes this from rheumatoid arthritis (Figs. 1-49 and 1-50).

ETIOLOGY

- None identified

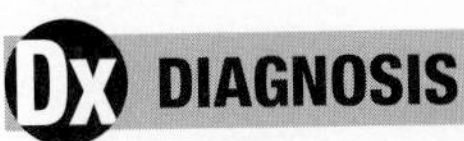

DIAGNOSIS

DIFFERENTIAL DIAGNOSIS

- Infection, malignancy, or autoimmune disorders
  1. Infection: Rubella, CMV, EBV, mumps, coxsackievirus, adenovirus
  2. Neoplasms: Leukemia, lymphoma, angioblastic lymphadenopathy
  3. Autoimmune: Reactive arthritis, spondyloarthropathies, dermatomyositis, vasculitis
  4. Periodic fever syndromes: Familial Mediterranean fever (FMF), TNF receptor–associated periodic syndrome (TRAPS)

DIAGNOSTIC CRITERIA

Multiple potential diagnostic criteria have been proposed in the evaluation of patients suspected of having adult-onset Still's disease.

1. Yamaguchi et al. (93.5% sensitivity)

MAJOR CRITERIA
- Arthralgia >2 weeks
- Fever > 102° F; intermittent >1 week
- Typical rash
- WBC >10,000

MINOR CRITERIA
- Sore throat
- Lymphadenopathy and/or splenomegaly
- LFT abnormalities
- Negative ANA and RF

Exclusion criteria: infections, malignancies, and rheumatic diseases

Diagnosis: 4 criteria with at least 2 major criteria

2. Cush (80.6% sensitivity)

MAJOR CRITERIA
- Quotidian fever >102° F
- Evanescent rash
- WBC >12 + ESR >40
- Negative ANA and RF
- Carpal ankylosis

MINOR CRITERIA
- Onset age <35 years
- Arthritis
- Prodromal sore throat
- Reticuloendothelial system involvement
- Abnormal LFTs
- Serositis
- Cervical or tarsal ankylosis

Probable AOSD: 10 points with 12 weeks of observation

Definite AOSD: 10 points with 6 months observation

3. Fautrel et al. (80.6% sensitivity, 98.5% specificity)

MAJOR
- Spiking fever >102° F
- Arthralgia
- Transient erythema
- Pharyngitis
- PMN >80%
- Glycosylated ferritin <20%

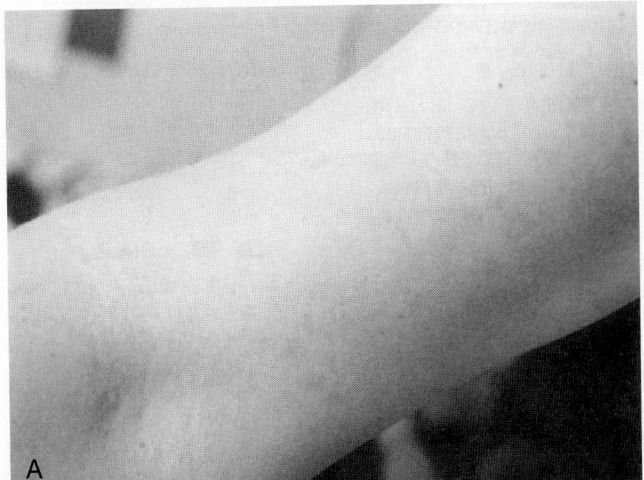

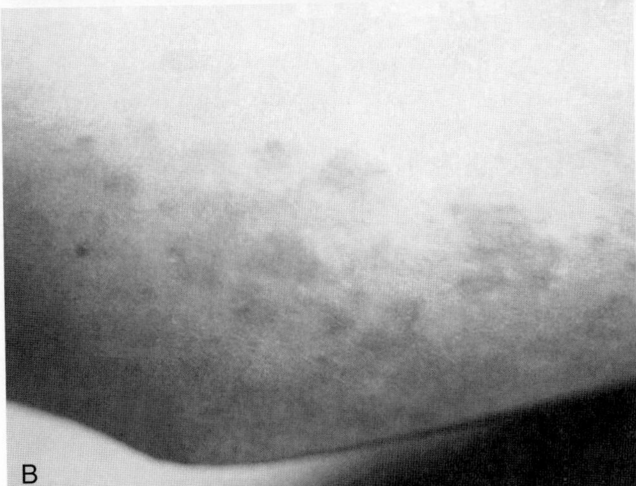

FIGURE 1-49 Typical salmon-colored rash. (From: Figure 3 and 4 page 778, borrowed from Fautrel B: Adult-onset still disease, *Best Practice & Research Clinical Rheumatology* 22;5:773-92, 2008.)

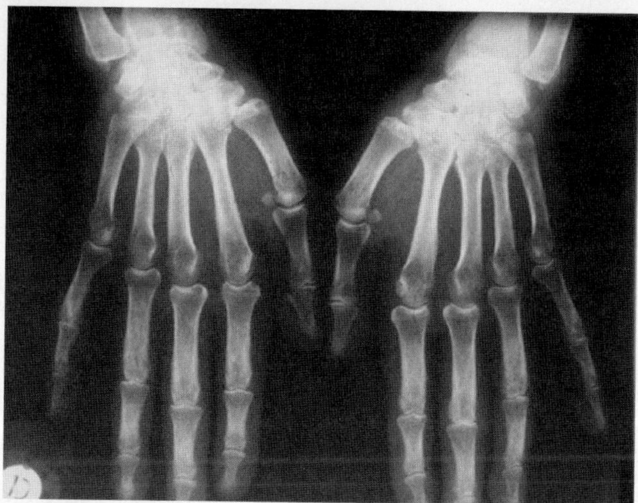

FIGURE 1-50 Ankylosing carpal arthritis. (From Figure 2 page 777, borrowed from Fautrel B: Adult-onset Still disease, *Best Practice & Research Clinical Rheumatology* 22;5:773-92, 2008.)

MINOR

- Maculopapular rash
- Leukocytosis >10

Diagnosis: 4 major criteria or 3 major + 2 minor criteria

WORKUP

- According to differential diagnosis

LABORATORY TESTS

- CBC generally demonstrates leukocytosis with a predominance of polymorphonuclear leukocytes.
- ANA and RF are generally negative in AOSD, whereas inflammatory markers are generally markedly elevated.
- Liver transaminases are often elevated.
- Ferritin can be markedly elevated beyond the level expected for a typical inflammatory process.
- Glycosylated ferritin (if available)

IMAGING STUDIES

- Radiographs are not helpful at early onset of symptoms; helpful if chronic.
- Radionuclide bone scan and MRI with gadolinium may be used for early diagnosis.

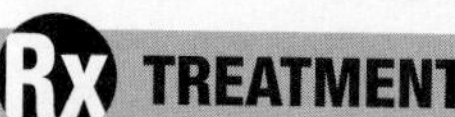

TREATMENT

NSAIDs, corticosteroids, and disease-modifying antirheumatic drugs are generally used to control symptoms.

NONPHARMACOLOGIC THERAPY

- Control of stress factors

ACUTE GENERAL Rx

- NSAIDs at full doses
- Systemic glucocorticoids are often required to control systemic inflammation.

CHRONIC Rx

- In patients with persistent symptoms, steroid-sparing immunomodulatory disease–modifying agents are often required.
- Oral or injectable methotrexate is often added to control chronic disease.
- TNF-inhibitors including etanercept and infliximab can be effective at controlling symptoms.
- Anti-IL6 and IL1 blockade may also be effective in controlling disease activity.

DISPOSITION

- Three distinct patterns of its clinical course
  1. Self-limited/monocyclic pattern: systemic symptoms of fever, rash, serositis, organomegaly; remission in 1 year
  2. Intermittent/polycyclic pattern: recurrent fevers with or without articular symptoms; may have complete remission between flares that could be years apart
  3. Chronic articular pattern: severe articular presentation leading to joint destruction; more disability, worst prognosis

REFERRAL

- Rheumatology for diagnosis and treatment
- Dermatology for evaluation and possible biopsy of rash

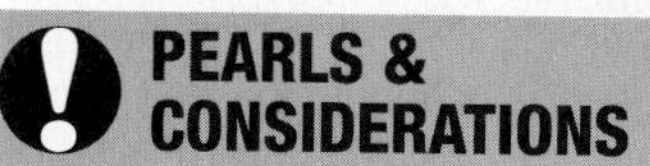

PEARLS & CONSIDERATIONS

COMMENTS

- Evanescent rash often dissipates when the patient is afebrile; it is therefore important to do a skin exam while the patient is febrile.
- Fever may present before arthritis, complicating accurate diagnosis.

PREVENTION

None

AUTHOR: **CRISOSTOMO BALIOG, Jr., M.D.**, and **HARALD A. HALL, M.D.**

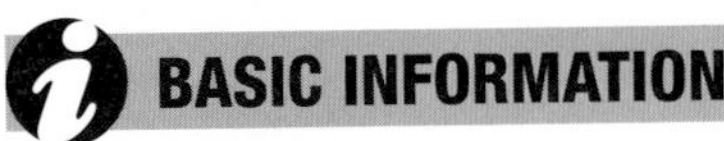

DEFINITION

Alcoholic hepatitis is a severe, progressive, inflammatory, and cholestatic liver disease occurring in patients with long-term ethanol abuse.

ICD-9CM CODES
571.1 Acute alcoholic hepatitis
ICD-10CM CODES
K70.10 Alcoholic hepatitis without ascites
K70.9 Alcoholic liver disease, unspecified

EPIDEMIOLOGY & DEMOGRAPHICS

- Approximately 2 million people in the U.S. (about 1% of the population) are affected by alcoholic liver disease.
- Typical presentation age: 40 to 50 yr. Majority occurs before age 60.

PREVALENCE: Approximately 25% to 30%

PREDOMINANT SEX AND AGE: The majority of patients are males. Males are two times as likely as women to abuse alcohol. However, women develop alcoholic hepatitis after a shorter time and smaller amount of alcoholic exposure than men.

GENETICS: No genetic predilection for any one race. In the U.S., however, there is increased incidence in minority groups.

RISK FACTORS: Drinking multiple alcohol types, drinking alcohol between meal times, poor nutrition, female gender, obesity, Hispanic ethnicity, long-term ingestion of >10 to 20 g/day of alcohol in women and >20 to 40 g/day in men

PHYSICAL FINDINGS & CLINICAL PRESENTATION

Common presenting symptoms include:

- Nausea /vomiting
- Malaise
- Low-grade fever
- Anorexia
- Abdominal distention/pain
- Weight loss
- Complications of liver impairment (GI bleed; confusion, lethargy, ascites)

Findings on physical examination include:

- Fever
- Tachycardia
- Hepatomegaly
- Jaundice
- Splenomegaly
- Asterixis (a flapping tremor)
- Peripheral edema
- Abdominal distention with shifting dullness (ascites)
- Hepatic bruit
- With coexistent cirrhosis look for:
  - Gynecomastia
  - Proximal muscles wasting
  - Spider angiomata
  - Altered hair distribution

Dx DIAGNOSIS

DIFFERENTIAL DIAGNOSIS

- Hepatitis B
- Hepatitis C
- Nonalcoholic steatohepatitis (NASH)
- Chronic pancreatitis
- Drug-induced liver injury
- Hemochromatosis
- Cholangitis

WORK-UP

- A thorough and detailed history is needed.
- Relevant questions may include:
  - When patients started drinking
  - Number of times patient drinks per day
  - How many years of regular/daily drinking
  - Types of alcohol
  - Home or bar drinking?
  - Rehabilitation for drinking?
  - Social problems (e.g., arrest for public intoxication or driving under the influence, marital discord due to alcoholism)

LABORATORY TESTS

- Elevated C-reactive protein
- Electrolyte disorder
- Hypophosphatemia
- Hypomagnesemia
- CBC (may reveal leukocytosis with bandemia or anemia)
- Elevated transaminase (AST >45 U/L but <300 U/L; AST:ALT ratio >1.5)
- S-bilirubin >2 mg/dl
- Increased prothrombin time (PT)
- Decreased gamma glutamyltransferase (GGT)
- Carbohydrate-deficient transferrin (CDT) is a reliable marker for chronic alcoholism
- Screening tests to rule out other conditions include checking:
  - Hepatitis B surface antigen (HBsAg)
  - Anti–hepatic C
  - Ferritin-transferrin saturation
  - Alpha-fetoprotein
  - Alkaline phosphatase

IMAGING STUDIES

Ultrasonography is the preferred imaging study.

LIVER BIOPSY

- Liver biopsy is rarely needed.
- Useful to:
  - Confirm the diagnosis.
  - Evaluate the effect of coexisting disease.
  - Rule out cirrhosis.
  - Exclude other diagnosis (especially other causes of liver diseases).
- Typical finding include:
  - Macrovascular steatosis
  - Hepatocyte injury (ballooning and necrosis)
  - Mallory's bodies (characteristic of alcoholic hepatitis)
  - Perivenular fibrosis
  - Portal and lobular inflammation

Rx TREATMENT

Treatment can be divided into three main components:

1 Lifestyle modifications
2 Nutritional support
3 Pharmacologic therapy

LIFESTYLE MODIFICATIONS

- Abstinence from alcohol (this improves both short- and long-term survival)
- Smoking cessation (to decrease oxidative stress)
- Treatment of substance abuse

NUTRITIONAL SUPPORT

- Good nutrition is an essential part of treatment because many patients with alcoholic hepatitis are usually in a catabolic state.
- Nutritional support includes:
  - Liberal vitamin supplementation (especially thiamine, folic acid, vitamin K)
  - Minerals supplementation (**but not iron**)
  - Calorie counting is essential. A high calorie intake (1.2 to 1.4 times the normal resting intake) may be required.
  - Protein intake of 1.2 to 1.5 g/kg of ideal body weight per day will provide adequate support. **Exception: in patients with severe encephalopathy, protein restriction may be required.**

PHARMACOLOGIC THERAPY

Severe alcoholic hepatitis may require treatment. Severity can be assessed by calculating the Model for End-Stage Liver Disease (MELD) score or Maddrey's Discriminant Function (DF) or the Glasgow score.

- Maddrey's DF = 4.6 × PT in sec prolonged + serum bilirubin (mg/dl)
  - DF >32 indicates significant or severe alcoholic hepatitis (30 day mortality of 50%).
- MELD score can easily be calculated (visit http://www.unos.org/resources/meldpeldcalculator.asp?index=98). This score predicts short-term survival in patients with cirrhosis. A score ≥20 predicts increased short-term mortality.
- Glasgow score: contains four variables (BUN, PT, WBC count, and bilirubin). A score ≥9 indicates increased mortality.

Indications for initiating therapy include:

- DF >30
- MELD >20
- Glasgow score >8
- Hepatic encephalopathy

Patients with severe alcoholic hepatitis may be treated with glucocorticosteroids (prednisolone 40 mg/day for 28 days with a 2-wk taper). Glucocorticosteroids reduce hepatic injury, suppress inflammation, and promote liver regeneration. There are various other treatments, but these are mainly experimental.

LIVER TRANSPLANTATION

- Its role in the management of alcohol hepatitis is unknown.
- Usually reserved for patients with end-stage liver disease.
- Patients with alcoholic hepatitis must be sober for at least 6 mo before they can be eligible for consideration for liver transplantation.

REFERRAL

Severe acute alcoholic hepatitis may require ICU care and referral to different subspecialists:

- GI/hepatology
- Nutritional services
- Nephrology (for acute renal failure, hepatorenal syndrome)
- Neurology (for change in mental status, seizures)
- Infectious disease (for fever/leukocytosis)

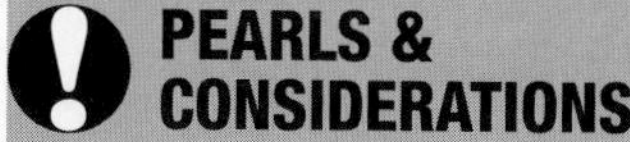

PEARLS & CONSIDERATIONS

COMMENTS

- Referral to substance abuse treatment programs may be helpful.
- Periodic follow-up to monitor patient's response to check BMP and LFTs.
- Encourage alcohol abstinence.
- If patient develops liver cirrhosis, check serum alpha-fetoprotein every 6 mo and liver ultrasound annually to rule out hepatocellular carcinoma.
- Vaccinate patient against hepatitis A and B viruses, pneumococci, and influenza A virus.

SUGGESTED READINGS

available at www.expertconsult.com

RELATED CONTENT

Alcoholic Hepatitis (Patient Information)

AUTHOR: **DANIEL K. ASIEDU, M.D., PH.D., F.A.C.P.**

BASIC INFORMATION

DEFINITION

Moderate drinking has been defined as two standard drinks (e.g., 12 oz of beer) per day and one drink per day for women and persons older than 65 yr. Although not generally included under the alcoholism topic, hazardous or at-risk drinking should also be considered. For men, *at-risk drinking* is defined as more than 14 drinks/wk or more than 4 drinks/occasion. For women, at-risk drinking is defined as approximately half that given for men.

The American Psychiatric Association defines diagnostic criteria for *alcohol withdrawal* as follows:

A. Cessation of (or reduction in) alcohol use that has been heavy and prolonged.

B. Two (or more) of the following, developing within several hours to a few days after criterion A:

1. Autonomic hyperactivity (e.g., sweating or pulse rate >100 beats/min)
2. Increased hand tremor
3. Insomnia
4. Nausea and vomiting
5. Transient visual, tactile, or auditory hallucinations or illusions
6. Psychomotor agitation
7. Anxiety
8. Grand mal seizures

C. The symptoms in criterion B cause clinically significant distress or impairment in social, occupational, or other important areas of functioning.

The symptoms are not attributable to a general medical condition and are not better accounted for by another mental disorder.

SYNONYMS

Alcohol abuse
Substance abuse

ICD-9CM CODES
303.9 Alcoholism
ICD-10CM CODES
F10 Mental and behavioral disorders due to use of alcohol
F10.1 Mental and behavioral disorders due to use of alcohol: harmful use
F10.2 Mental and behavioral disorders due to use of alcohol: dependence syndrome
F10.3 Mental and behavioral disorders due to use of alcohol: withdrawal state
F10.4 Mental and behavioral disorders due to use of alcohol: withdrawal state with delirium
F10.5 Mental and behavioral disorders due to use of alcohol: psychotic disorder
F10.6 Mental and behavioral disorders due to use of alcohol: amnesic syndrome

EPIDEMIOLOGY & DEMOGRAPHICS

INCIDENCE (IN U.S.):

- The clinical history suggests alcohol problems in 15% to 20% of patients in primary care and hospitalized patients. In the U.S., alcohol abuse generates nearly $223 billion in annual economic costs. An estimated 9% of adults in the U.S. have alcohol dependence.
- 20% achieve abstinence without help; 70% achieve sobriety for 1 yr.

PREVALENCE (IN U.S.): 7% of population ≥18 yr

PREDOMINANT SEX:

- Lifetime risk for males 8% to 10%
- Lifetime risk for females 3% to 5%

PEAK INCIDENCE: 20 to 40 yr. The most common age range for initial treatment of alcohol dependence is 35 to 45 yr. However, the peak period for meeting alcohol dependence criteria is ≥10 years earlier.

GENETICS: More common with a family history of alcoholism and in patients of Irish, Scandinavian, and Native American descent

PHYSICAL FINDINGS & CLINICAL PRESENTATION

- Recurring minor trauma
- Gastrointestinal bleeding from gastritis and/or varices
- Pancreatitis (acute and chronic)
- Liver disease
- Odor of alcohol on breath
- Tremulousness
- Tachycardia
- Peripheral neuropathy
- Recent memory loss

ETIOLOGY

- Social and genetic factors important
- Risk factors:
  1. Broken homes
  2. Unemployment
  3. Divorce
  4. Recurrent depression
  5. Addiction to another substance, including tobacco

Dx DIAGNOSIS

WORKUP

- The USPSTF recommends that clinicians screen adults 18 years and older for alcohol misuse and provide persons engaged in risky or hazardous drinking with brief behavioral counseling interventions to reduce alcohol misuse. Several screening tests (CAGE, TWEAK, CRAFFT, AUDIT-C) are available. The four-item CAGE (feeling need to Cut down, Annoyed by criticism, Guilty about drinking, and need for an Eye-opener in the morning) is the most popular screening test in primary care (Fig. E1-51). A positive response should lead to further questioning. The sensitivity of the CAGE ranges from 43% to 94% and its specificity ranges from 70% to 97%. The five-item TWEAK scale (Tolerance, Worry, Eye-openers, Amnesia, [K] cut down) and the TACE questionnaire (Tolerance, Annoyance, Cut down, Eye-opener) are designed to screen pregnant women for alcohol misuse. They detect lower levels of alcohol consumption that may pose risks during pregnancy. The CRAFFT questionnaire (riding in Car with someone who was drinking, using alcohol to Relax, using alcohol while Alone, Forgetfulness, criticism from Friends and Family, Trouble) is useful as a screening tool for adolescents. Its sensitivity is 92% and specificity 64% for alcohol abuse. Single-question screening about alcohol consumption in a day ("When was the last time you had more than X drinks in a day?" [where X = 5 for men and 4 for women]) with the threshold set at "in the past 3 months" is 85% sensitive and 70% specific in men and 82% and 70% in women for unhealthy alcohol use. The 3-question AUDIT-C is a shorter form of the 10-item AUDIT, and the questions center on the quantity and frequency of alcohol use. It asks how often someone has had a drink containing alcohol, how many standard drinks containing alcohol one consumes on a typical day when one is drinking, and how often one has six or more drinks on one occasion. Scoring ranges from 0-4 on each question with a total score range of 0-12. A total score of 3 or higher for women and 4 or higher for men indicates alcohol use disorder and need for further assessment. Its sensitivity ranges from 85% in Hispanic women to 95% in white men.
- Laboratory evaluation (see below).

LABORATORY TESTS:

- Lab tests alone do not accurately detect alcohol problems but can help identify medical complications related to alcohol use, such as pancreatitis or cirrhosis.
- Gamma-glutamyltransferase (GGTP), generally elevated
- Liver transaminases (alanine aminotransferase [ALT], aspartate aminotransferase [AST]), often elevated, may be normal or low in advanced liver disease.
- Low albumin level, hypophosphatemia, hypomagnesemia from malnutrition
- Complete blood count (CBC) reveals elevated mean corpuscular volume from toxic effect of alcohol on erythrocyte development in nutritional deficiencies.
- Stool for occult blood may be positive as a result of gastritis or variceal bleeding
- RBC folate, vitamin B_{12} level, vitamin B_6, vitamin B_1 level

IMAGING STUDIES

Indicated only with a history of trauma. CT or ultrasound of abdomen may reveal fatty liver or cirrhosis in advanced stages.

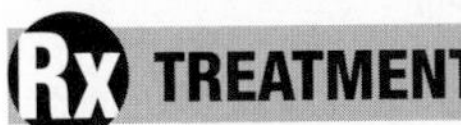

TREATMENT

NONPHARMACOLOGIC THERAPY

- Twelve-step facilitation, cognitive behavioral therapy, and motivational enhancement therapy improve the chances of recovery in patients with alcohol abuse and dependence.
- Depression, if present, should be treated at same time alcohol is withdrawn.

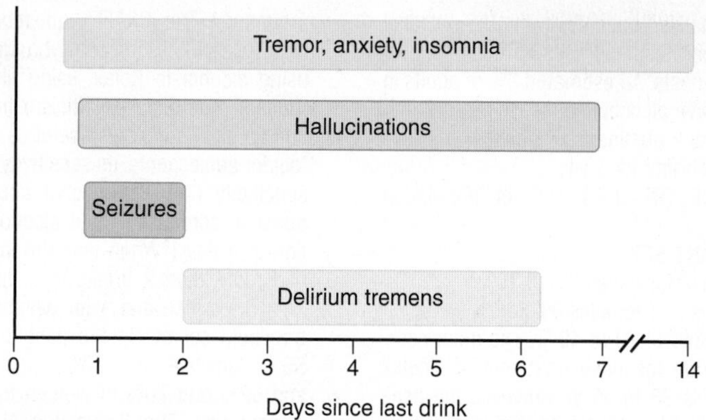

FIGURE 1-52 Time course of alcohol withdrawal. (From Goldman L, Schafer AI: *Goldman's Cecil medicine,* ed 24, Philadelphia, 2012, Saunders.)

ACUTE GENERAL Rx

Alcohol withdrawal syndrome (AWS) occurs when a person stops ingesting alcohol after prolonged consumption. It can result in four possible clinical patterns depending on the severity of the patient's alcohol abuse and the time from the patient's previous alcohol ingestion. Fig. 1-52 illustrates typical symptoms depending on time course of alcohol withdrawal. Blood ethanol level decreases by ~20 mg/dl/hr (Fig. E1-53) in a normal person. Although discussed separately, these withdrawal states blend together in real life. Table E1-25 summarizes medications for the treatment of alcohol dependence.

1. **Tremulous state** (early alcohol withdrawal, "impending DTs," "shakes," "jitters").
   a. Time interval: usually occurs 6 to 8 hr after the last drink or 12 to 48 hr after reduction of alcohol intake; becomes most pronounced at 24 to 36 hr.
   b. Manifestation: tremors, mild agitation, insomnia, tachycardia; symptoms are relieved by alcohol.
   c. Detoxification can be in the outpatient (ambulatory) or inpatient setting. Candidates for outpatient detoxification should have a reasonable support system (e.g., reliable contact person) who can monitor progress and lack of any significant comorbid conditions (e.g., suicide risk, seizure disorder, coexisting benzodiazepine dependence, prior unsuccessful outpatient detoxification, pregnancy, cirrhosis) or risk factors for severe withdrawal (age >40 yr, drinking >100 g of ethanol daily [e.g., 1 pint of liquor or eight 12-oz cans of beer, random blood alcohol concentration >200 mg/dl]).
   d. Inpatient treatment:
      (1) Admit to medical floor (private room); monitor vital signs q4h; institute seizure precautions; maintain adequate sedation.
      (2) Administer lorazepam as follows:
         (a) Day 1: 2 mg PO q4h while awake and not lethargic.
         (b) Day 2: 1 mg PO q4h while awake and not lethargic.
         (c) Day 3: 0.5 mg PO q4h while awake and not lethargic.
         (d) NOTE: Hold sedation for lethargy or abnormal vital or neurologic signs. The preceding doses are only guidelines; it is best to titrate the dose case by case.
      (3) In patients with mild to moderate withdrawal and without history of seizures, individualized benzodiazepine administration (rather than a fixed-dose regimen) results in lower benzodiazepine administration and avoids unnecessary sedation. The Clinical Institute Withdrawal Assessment Scale for Alcohol, Revised (CIWA-Ar) scale (Box E1-6) can be used to measure the severity of alcohol withdrawal. It consists of 10 items: nausea; tremor; autonomic hyperactivity; anxiety; agitation; tactile, visual, and auditory disturbances; headache; and disorientation. Each item is assigned a score from 0 to 7. For example, in the "agitation" category 0 indicates normal activity, and 7 indicates that the patient constantly thrashes about. For the category of "tremor," 0 indicates that tremor is not present and 7 that tremor is severe, even with arms not extended. The maximum total score is 67. Patients with mild AWS symptoms (CIWA-Ar score <8 to 10 can be monitored on an outpatient basis. Benzodiazepines are recommended in patients with substantial withdrawal symptoms (CIWA-Ar score >12). Patients with CIWA-Ar score of ≥15 should be admitted to detox unit. In-patient treatment is also recommended for patients with history of withdrawal seizures and for those with suicidal ideation and significant comorbidities.
      (4) Beta-adrenergic blockers: beta-blockers are useful for controlling blood pressure and tachyarrhythmias. However, they do not prevent progression to more serious symptoms of withdrawal and, if used, should not be administered alone but in conjunction with benzodiazepines. Beta-blockers should be avoided in patients with contraindications to their use (e.g., bronchospasm, bradycardia, or severe congestive heart failure). Centrally acting alpha-adrenergic agonists such as clonidine ameliorate symptoms in patients with mild to moderate withdrawal but do not reduce delirium or seizures.
      (5) Vitamin replacement: thiamine 100 mg IV or IM for at least 5 days plus oral multivitamins. The IV administration of glucose can precipitate Wernicke's encephalopathy in alcoholics with thiamine deficiency; therefore thiamine administration should precede IV dextrose.
      (6) Hydration PO or IV (high-caloric solution): if IV, glucose with Na^+, K^+, Mg^{2+}, and phosphate replacement prn.
      (7) Laboratory studies.
         (a) CBC, platelet count, INR.
         (b) Electrolytes, glucose, blood urea nitrogen, creatinine.
         (c) GGTP, ALT, AST.
         (d) Phosphorus and magnesium.
         (e) Serum vitamin B_{12} and folic acid (if megaloblastic features in blood smear).
      (8) Diagnostic imaging: generally not necessary; if subdural hematoma is suspected (evidence of trauma, persistent lethargy), a CT scan should be ordered.
      (9) Social rehabilitation: group therapy such as Alcoholics Anonymous; identification and treatment of social and family problems should be initiated during the patient's hospital stay.
2. Alcoholic hallucinosis:
   a. Manifestations: hallucinations usually are auditory, but hallucinations occasionally are visual, tactile, or olfactory; usually there is no clouding of sensorium as in delirium (clinical presentation may be mistaken for an acute schizophrenic episode). Disordered perceptions become most pronounced after 24 to 36 hr of abstinence.
   b. Treatment: same as for DTs (see "withdrawal seizures").
3. Withdrawal seizures ("rum fits"):
   a. Time interval: usually occurs 7 to 30 hr after cessation of drinking, with a peak incidence between 13 and 24 hr.
   b. Manifestations: generalized convulsions with loss of consciousness; focal signs are usually absent; consider further investigation with CT scan of head and electroencephalography if clearly indicated (e.g., presence of focal neurologic deficits, prolonged postictal confusion state). In addition, in a febrile patient who is having a seizure or altered mental state, a lumbar puncture is necessary.
   c. Treatment:
      (1) Diazepam 2.5 mg/min IV until seizure is controlled (check for respiratory depression or hypotension) may be

beneficial for prolonged seizure activity; IV lorazepam 1 to 2 mg q2h can be used in place of diazepam. Withdrawal seizures generally are self-limited and treatment is not required; the use of phenytoin or other anticonvulsants for short-term treatment of alcohol withdrawal seizures is not recommended.

(2) Thiamine 100 mg IV, followed by IV dextrose, should also be administered.

(3) Electrolyte imbalances (increased Mg^{2+}, decreased K^+, increased or decreased Na^+, decreased PO_4^{3-}) that may exacerbate seizures should be corrected.

4. DTs:
   a. Time interval: variable; usually occurs within 1 wk after reduction or cessation of heavy alcohol intake and persists for 1 to 3 days. Peak incidence is 72 hr and 96 hr after the cessation of alcohol consumption.
   b. Manifestations: profound confusion, tremors, vivid visual and tactile hallucinations, autonomic hyperactivity; this is the most serious clinical presentation of alcohol withdrawal (mortality rate is approximately 15% in untreated patients).
   c. Treatment
      (1) Admission to a detoxification unit where patient can be observed closely.
      (2) Vital signs q30min (neurologic signs, if necessary).
      (3) Use of lateral decubitus or prone position if restraints are necessary
      (4) NPO: nasogastric tube for abdominal distention may be necessary but should not be routinely used.
      (5) Laboratory studies: same as for early alcohol withdrawal.
      (6) Vigorous hydration (4 to 6 L/day): IV with glucose (Na^+, K^+, PO_4^{3-} and Mg^{2+} replacement).
      (7) Vitamins: thiamine 100 mg IV qd. The initial dose of thiamine should precede the administration of IV dextrose; multivitamins (may be added to the hydrating solution).
      (8) Sedation: control of agitation should be achieved with rapid-acting sedative-hypnotic agents in adequate doses to maintain light somnolence for the duration of delirium.
         (a) Initially: lorazepam 2 to 5 mg IM/IV repeated prn.
         (b) Maintenance (individualized dosage): chlordiazepoxide, 50 to 100 mg PO q4-6h, lorazepam 2 mg PO q4h, or diazepam 5 to 10 mg PO tid; withhold doses or decrease subsequent doses if signs of oversedation are apparent.
         (c) Midazolam is also effective for managing DTs. Its rapid onset (sedation within 2 to 4 min of IV injection) and short duration of action (approximately 30 min) make it an ideal agent for titration in continuous infusion.
      (9) Treatment of seizures (as previously described).
      (10) Diagnosis and treatment of concomitant medical, surgical, or psychiatric conditions.

CHRONIC Rx

- See "Referral."
- Pharmacotherapies for alcoholism include:
  - Acamprosate is a synthetic compound with a chemical structure similar to the neurotransmitter gamma-aminobutyric acid and the amino acid neuromodulator taurine. Its mechanism of action is not completely understood. It is indicated for the maintenance of abstinence from alcohol in patients with alcohol dependence who are abstinent at treatment initiation. It should be used only as part of a comprehensive psychosocial treatment program. It does not cause a disulfiram-like reaction as a result of ethanol ingestion. Dose is two 333-mg tablets tid. Treatment should be initiated as soon as possible after the period of alcohol withdrawal, when the patient has achieved abstinence, and should be maintained if the patient relapses.
  - The long-acting opiate antagonist naltrexone inhibits the rewarding effects of alcohol. The starting dose is 25 mg/day, increased to 50 mg PO qd after 1 wk. An extended-release, once-monthly injection of naltrexone is also available and can be used along with psychosocial support to maintain alcohol abstinence. In patients with opioid dependence, naltrexone can precipitate acute withdrawal syndrome and should not be used at least 7 days from last opioid use. There are no established guidelines on the appropriate length of naltrexone treatment for alcohol dependence. One study recommends at least 3 mo of treatment.
  - In a recent study, gabapentin showed a significant dose-response effect, and estimates of effect sizes were larger than those seen for naltrexone and acamprosate.[1]
  - Disulfiram (Antabuse). Dosage is 500 mg max qd for 1 to 2 wk, then 125 to 500 mg qd. It interferes with the metabolism of alcohol by inhibiting aldehyde dehydrogenase, causing an accumulation of acetaldehyde. It produces unpleasant symptoms (nausea, flushing, elevated blood pressure, headache, weakness) when alcohol is ingested. It is an older drug that is now rarely used.

DISPOSITION

See "Referral."

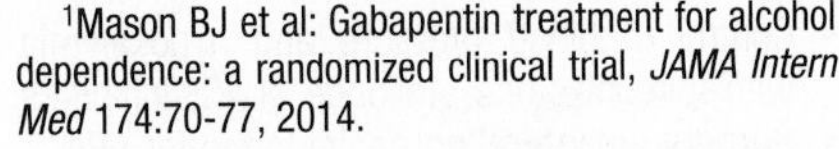

[1]Mason BJ et al: Gabapentin treatment for alcohol dependence: a randomized clinical trial, *JAMA Intern Med* 174:70-77, 2014.

REFERRAL

- To Alcoholics Anonymous or Adult Children of Alcoholics
- Family members to Al-Anon or Al-A-Teen
- Many cities have Salvation Army Adult Rehabilitation centers; all patients accepted, regardless of ability to pay

PEARLS & CONSIDERATIONS

COMMENTS

- Relative indications for inpatient alcohol detoxification are as follows: history of DTs or withdrawal seizures, severe withdrawal symptoms, concomitant psychiatric or medical illness, pregnancy, multiple previous detoxifications, recent high levels of alcohol consumption, and lack of reliable support network.
- Detoxification is not a stand-alone treatment but should serve as a bridge to a formal treatment program for alcohol dependence.
- The cure rate for alcoholism is highly disappointing, regardless of the modality. Only those who want to be helped will be helped. An effective strategy for the primary care physician is a prominently displayed sign in the office that states, "If you think you consume too many alcoholic beverages, please discuss it with me." Those who do open up the discussion can be given the facts in a nonjudgmental way and often can be helped. All too often problem drinkers lie on the questionnaire until they face a life-threatening health issue—and even then denial often reigns supreme.
- In a recent clinical trial, patients receiving medical management with naltrexone (100 mg/day), combined behavioral intervention (CBI), or both fared better on drinking outcomes, whereas acamprosate showed no evidence of efficacy, with or without CBI. No combination produced better efficacy than naltrexone or CBI alone in the presence of medical management.

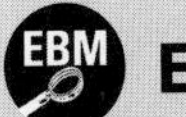

EVIDENCE

available at www.expertconsult.com

SUGGESTED READINGS

available at www.expertconsult.com

RELATED CONTENT

Alcohol Addiction (Patient Information)
Alcoholic Hepatitis (Related Key Topic)
Abuse, Drug (Related Key Topic)
Wernicke Syndrome (Related Key Topic)

AUTHOR: **FRED F. FERRI, M.D.**

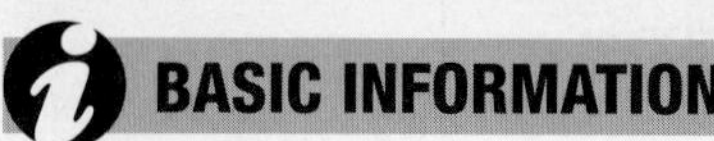

BASIC INFORMATION

DEFINITION

Primary hyperaldosteronism is a clinical syndrome characterized by hypokalemia, hypertension, low plasma renin activity (PRA), and excessive aldosterone secretion.

SYNONYMS

Hyperaldosteronism
Primary aldosteronism
Conn's syndrome

ICD-9CM CODES
255.1 Primary aldosteronism
ICD-10CM CODES
E26.0 Primary hyperaldosteronism
E26.1 Secondary hyperaldosteronism
E26.8 Other hyperaldosteronism
E26.9 Hyperaldosteronism, unspecified

EPIDEMIOLOGY & DEMOGRAPHICS

INCIDENCE: 1% to 2% of patients with hypertension
PREVALENCE: More common in females

PHYSICAL FINDINGS & CLINICAL PRESENTATION

- Generally asymptomatic
- If significant hypokalemia is present, possible muscle cramping, weakness, paresthesias
- Hypertension
- Polyuria, polydipsia

ETIOLOGY

- Aldosterone-producing adenoma (>60%)
- Idiopathic hyperaldosteronism (>30%)
- Glucocorticoid-suppressible hyperaldosteronism (<1%)
- Aldosterone-producing carcinoma (<1%)

Dx DIAGNOSIS

DIFFERENTIAL DIAGNOSIS

- Diuretic use
- Hypokalemia from vomiting, diarrhea
- Renovascular hypertension
- Other endocrine neoplasm (pheochromocytoma, deoxycorticosterone-producing tumor, renin-secreting tumor)

WORKUP

Fig. E1-54 provides guidance on when to consider testing for primary aldosteronism. Fig. E1-55 describes a diagnostic approach to patients with suspected primary aldosteronism. CT, MRI, and adrenal vein sampling (AVS) are used to distinguish unilateral from bilateral increased aldosterone secretion. This distinction will dictate treatment options since unilateral primary aldosteronism is treated surgically rather than medically. In patients with hypokalemia and a low PRA, confirming tests for primary hyperaldosteronism include the following:

- 24-hr urine test for aldosterone and potassium levels (potassium >40 mEq and aldosterone >15 mcg).
- Captopril test: administer 25 to 50 mg of captopril (an angiotensin-converting enzyme [ACE] inhibitor) and measure plasma renin and aldosterone levels 1 to 2 hr later. A plasma aldosterone level >15 ng/dl confirms the diagnosis of primary aldosteronism. This test is more expensive and is best reserved for situations in which the 24-hr urine test for aldosterone is ambiguous.
- 24-hr urinary tetrahydroaldosterone (<65 mcg/24 hr) and saline infusion test (plasma aldosterone >10 ng/dl) can also be used in ambiguous cases.
- The renin-aldosterone stimulation test (posture test) is helpful in differentiating idiopathic hyperaldosteronism (IHA) from aldosterone-producing adenoma (APA). Patients with APA have a decrease in aldosterone levels at 4 hr, whereas patients with IHA have an increase in aldosterone levels.
- As a screening test for primary aldosteronism, an elevated plasma aldosterone-renin ratio (ARR), drawn randomly from patients taking hypertensive drugs, is predictive of primary aldosteronism (positive predictive value 100% in a recent study). ARR is calculated by dividing plasma aldosterone (mg/dl) by PRA (mg/ml/hr). ARR >100 is considered elevated.
- Bilateral AVS may be done to localize APA when adrenal CT scan is equivocal. In APA, ipsilateral/contralateral aldosterone level is >10:1, and ipsilateral venous aldosterone concentration is very high (>1000 ng/dl).
- A diagnostic evaluation of hypertensive patients with suspected aldosteronism is described in the online version of Section III.

LABORATORY TESTS

Routine laboratory tests can be suggestive but are not diagnostic of primary aldosteronism. Common abnormalities are:

- Spontaneous hypokalemia or moderately severe hypokalemia while receiving conventional doses of diuretics
- Possible alkalosis and hypernatremia

IMAGING STUDIES

- Adrenal CT scans (with 3-mm cuts) or MRI may be used to localize neoplasm.
- Adrenal scanning with iodocholesterol (NP-59) or 6-beta-iodomethyl-19-norcholesterol after dexamethasone suppression. The uptake of tracer is increased in those with aldosteronoma and absent in those with IHA and adrenal carcinoma.

Rx TREATMENT

NONPHARMACOLOGIC THERAPY

- Regular monitoring and control of blood pressure
- Low-sodium diet, tobacco avoidance, maintenance of ideal body weight, and regular exercise

ACUTE GENERAL Rx

- Control of blood pressure and hypokalemia with spironolactone, amiloride, or ACE inhibitors
- Surgery (unilateral adrenalectomy) for APA

CHRONIC Rx

Chronic medical therapy with spironolactone, eplerenone, amiloride, or ACE inhibitors to control blood pressure and hypokalemia is necessary in all patients with bilateral IHA.

DISPOSITION

- Unilateral adrenalectomy normalizes hypertension and hypokalemia in 70% of patients with APA after 1 yr. After 5 yr, 50% of patients remain normotensive.
- Experimental animal studies have suggested that long-term exposure to increased aldosterone levels in untreated aldosteronism may result in renal structural damage. However, clinical trials have shown that primary aldosteronism is characterized by partially reversible renal dysfunction in which elevated albuminuria is a marker of a dynamic rather than structural renal defect.

REFERRAL

Surgical referral for unilateral adrenalectomy after confirmation of unilateral APA or carcinoma

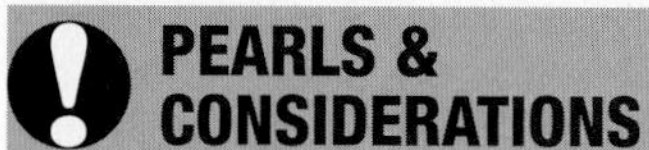

PEARLS & CONSIDERATIONS

- Frequent monitoring of blood pressure and electrolytes postoperatively is necessary because normotension after unilateral adrenalectomy may take up to 4 mo.
- Recent investigations regarding serum aldosterone and the incidence of hypertension in nonhypertensive persons indicate that increased aldosterone levels within the physiologic range predispose to the development of hypertension.

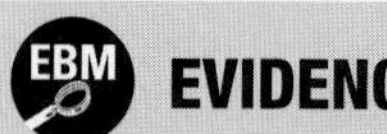

EVIDENCE

available at www.expertconsult.com

SUGGESTED READINGS

available at www.expertconsult.com

RELATED CONTENT

Aldosteronism (Patient Information)

AUTHOR: **FRED F. FERRI, M.D.**

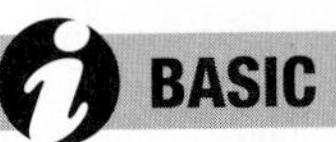

BASIC INFORMATION

DEFINITION

Allergic rhinitis is an IgE-mediated hypersensitivity response to nasally inhaled allergens that causes sneezing, rhinorrhea, nasal pruritus, and congestion. It may be seasonal or perennial.

SYNONYMS

Hay fever
IgE-mediated rhinitis
Seasonal allergic rhinitis
SAR

ICD-9CM CODES
477.9 Allergic rhinitis
ICD-10CM CODES
J30.1 Allergic rhinitis due to pollen
J30.2 Other seasonal allergic rhinitis
J30.3 Other allergic rhinitis
J30.4 Allergic rhinitis, unspecified

EPIDEMIOLOGY & DEMOGRAPHICS

- Allergic rhinitis affects approximately 10% to 20% of the U.S. population and 40% of children.
- Mean age of onset is 8 to 12 yr.
- The prevalence of allergic rhinitis in patients presenting to their primary care provider with nasal symptoms is estimated to be 30% to 60%.

PHYSICAL FINDINGS & CLINICAL PRESENTATION

- Pale or violaceous mucosa of the turbinates caused by venous engorgement (this can distinguish it from erythema present in viral rhinitis)
- Nasal polyps
- Lymphoid hyperplasia in the posterior oropharynx with cobblestone appearance
- Erythema of the throat, conjunctival and scleral injection
- Clear nasal discharge
- Clinical presentation: usually consists of sneezing, nasal congestion, cough, postnasal drip, loss of or alteration of smell, and sensation of plugged ears

ETIOLOGY

- Pollens in the springtime, ragweed in fall, grasses in the summer
- Dust, mites, animal allergens
- Smoke or any irritants
- Perfumes, detergents, soaps
- Emotion, changes in atmospheric pressure or temperature

Dx DIAGNOSIS

DIFFERENTIAL DIAGNOSIS

- Infections (sinusitis; viral, bacterial, or fungal rhinitis)
- Rhinitis medicamentosa (cocaine, sympathomimetic nasal drops)
- Vasomotor rhinitis (e.g., secondary to air pollutants)
- Septal obstruction (e.g., deviated septum), nasal polyps, nasal neoplasms
- Systemic diseases (e.g., Wegener's granulomatosis, hypothyroidism [rare])

WORKUP

- The initial strategy should be to determine whether patients should undergo diagnostic testing or receive empirical treatment.
- Workup is often unnecessary if the diagnosis is apparent. A detailed medical history is useful in identifying the culprit allergen.
- Selected patients with allergic rhinitis that is not controlled with standard therapy may benefit from allergy testing to target allergen avoidance measures or guide immunotherapy. Allergy testing can be performed using skin testing or radioallergosorbent (RAST) testing. Immunoglobulin E (IgE) testing using newest generation assays is also an excellent tool for diagnosing the cause of symptoms related to rhinitis. Allergy testing with skin or blood testing is most useful as confirmatory tests when the patient's history is compatible with an IgE-mediated reaction and should generally be reserved for ambiguous or complicated cases.
- Examination of nasal smears for the presence of neutrophils to rule out infectious causes and the presence of eosinophils (suggestive of allergy) may be useful in selected patients.
- Peripheral blood eosinophil counts are not useful in allergy diagnosis.

Rx TREATMENT

NONPHARMACOLOGIC THERAPY

- Maintain allergen-free environment by covering mattresses and pillows with allergen-proof casings, eliminating carpeting, eliminating animal products, and removing dust-collecting fixtures.
- Use of air purifiers and dust filters is helpful.
- Maintain humidity in the environment below 50% to prevent dust mites and mold.
- Use air conditioners, especially in the bedroom.
- Remove pets from homes of patients with suspected sensitivity to animal allergens.
- Use of acupuncture to treat seasonal allergic rhinitis is controversial. A recent trial showed that acupuncture led to statistically significant improvement in disease-specific quality of life and antihistamine use measures after 8 weeks of treatment compared with sham acupuncture and with rescue medication alone.

ACUTE GENERAL Rx

- Determine if the patient is troubled by swollen turbinates (best treated with decongestants) or blockages secondary to mucus (effectively treated by antihistamines).
- Topical nasal steroids are very effective and are preferred by many as first-line treatment for allergic rhinitis in adults. Patients should be instructed on proper use and informed that improvement might not occur for at least 1 wk after initiation of therapy. Commonly available inhalers follow.
  - Beclomethasone dipropionate: one to two sprays in each nostril bid
  - Fluticasone: initially two sprays in each nostril qd or one spray in each nostril bid, decreasing to one spray in each nostril qd based on response
  - Flunisolide: initially two sprays in each nostril bid
  - Budesonide: two sprays in each nostril bid or four sprays in each nostril qam
- Most first-generation antihistamines can cause considerable sedation and anticholinergic symptoms. The second-generation antihistamines (loratadine, fexofenadine, cetirizine, levocetirizine, desloratadine) are preferred because they do not have any significant anticholinergic or sedative effects.
- Montelukast, a leukotriene receptor antagonist commonly used for asthma, is also effective for allergic rhinitis. Usual adult dose is 10 mg qd.
- Azelastine is an antihistamine nasal spray effective for seasonal allergic rhinitis. Olopatadine is an intranasal H_1-antihistamine alternative to azestaline in mild to moderate seasonal allergic rhinitis.

CHRONIC Rx

- Cromolyn sodium: one spray to each nostril three to four times daily can be used for prophylaxis (mast cell stabilizer).
- Immunotherapy is generally reserved for patients responding poorly to the above treatments.

DISPOSITION

Most patients experience significant relief with avoidance of allergens and proper use of medications.

REFERRAL

Allergy testing in patients with severe symptoms who are unresponsive to therapy or when the diagnosis is uncertain

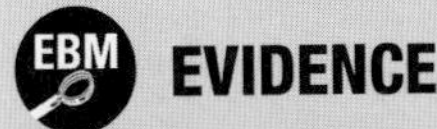

EVIDENCE

available at www.expertconsult.com

SUGGESTED READINGS

available at www.expertconsult.com

RELATED CONTENT

Allergic Rhinitis (Patient Information)

AUTHOR: **FRED F. FERRI, M.D.**

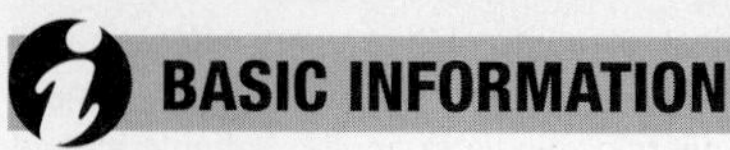

BASIC INFORMATION

DEFINITION

Alopecia is the term used to describe involuntary hair loss, typically on the scalp but can occur anywhere over the body. *Nonscarring alopecia* is hair loss without clinically apparent scarring, inflammation, or skin atrophy. *Scarring alopecia* is characterized by permanent hair loss accompanied by tissue destruction in the form of scarring, inflammation, and/or skin atrophy.

SYNONYMS

Hair loss
Balding

ICD-9CM CODES

704.0	Alopecia
704.01	Alopecia Areata
704.02	Telogen Effluvium

ICD-10CM CODES

L63	Alopecia aerata
L63.0	Alopecia (capitis) totalis
L64	Androgenic alopecia
L64.0	Drug-induced androgenic alopecia
L64.8	Other androgenic alopecia
L64.9	Androgenic alopecia, unspecified
L65	Other nonscarring hair loss
L66	Cicatricial alopecia
L65.9	Nonscarring hair loss, unspecified
L63.8	Other alopecia areata
L65.0	Telogen effluvium

EPIDEMIOLOGY & DEMOGRAPHICS

INCIDENCE: Depends on etiology, for example:

- Alopecia areata affects 1% of the U.S. population by age 50 yr. There is a higher incidence at a younger age and both sexes are affected equally.
- Androgenetic alopecia affects males > females with 50% of Caucasian men affected by age 50 yr. Less common in Asians and African-American men, and often has later onset. By age 70, 40% of females are affected with incidence increasing after menopause.

GENETICS: Depends on etiology, for example:

- Androgenetic alopecia is polygenic with variable penetrance and can be inherited from one or both parents
- Certain scarring alopecias are more predominant in people with coarser hair.

ETIOLOGY

NONSCARRING

- Failure of follicle production
- Hair shaft abnormality
- Pattern hair loss, i.e., androgenetic alopecia
- Hair breakage, i.e., trichotillomania, traction alopecia, cosmetic overprocessing
- Problem with cycling (excess shedding), i.e., telogen effluvium, anagen effluvium, loose anagen syndrome, alopecia areata, syphilis

SCARRING

- Infectious: tinea capitis with inflammation (kerion), bacterial folliculitis as in dissecting folliculitis and folliculitis decalvans
- Neoplasm: alopecia mucinosa in cutaneous T-cell lymphoma or alopecia neoplastica due to metastatic carcinoma (breast cancer)
- Autoimmune: chronic cutaneous lupus erythematosus
- Congenital

CLINICAL FEATURES

HISTORY: A careful history must be taken and should include time course for hair loss, the pattern of hair loss, any recent change in life situation/stresses, any associated medical conditions, new medications, any family history of hair loss, diet, hair care practices, and other skin/nail symptoms.

PHYSICAL EXAMINATION:

- General: patient's emotional response to hair loss
- Hair/skin:
  - Hair thinning/loss
  - May have fine downy hairs also referred to as vellous hairs
  - Skin may show changes consistent with inflammation, infection, and/or atrophy
  - Women may show virilization (e.g., hirsutism)
  - Exclamation point hairs can be seen in alopecia areata
  - Broken hairs of different length may be seen in traumatic alopecia
  - Hairs that crack or crumble with palpation most often signify shaft damage due to overprocessing

Dx DIAGNOSIS

WORKUP

- Pull test—no shower for 24 hr, 60 hairs are gently pulled from the scalp, removal of 6 or more hairs is considered positive result and indicated telogen effluvium (active shedding). Look for telogen bulbs on recovered hairs to differentiate from breaking (blunt ends)
- Punch biopsy—Mandatory when suspecting scarring alopecia. Send two punches: one for vertical and one for horizontal sectioning for histopathologic analysis preferably by a dermatopathologist
- Trichogram—quantifies hair loss. Pull 25-50 hairs and measure proportion of anagen to catagen and telogen hairs under light microscopy. Ten to twenty percent telogen hairs is normal, >35% is highly suspicious for telogen effluvium.
- Fig. E1-56 describes the evaluation and treatment of alopecia in females.

LABORATORY TESTS

Initiate laboratory studies if not clear based on clinical presentation:

- CBC—rule out Fe deficiency
- Total Fe/ferritin—rule out subclinical Fe deficiency
- TSH—rule out underlying thyroid disease
- ANA—screen for autoimmune disease
- RPR—rule out cutaneous syphilis if history suggestive of increased risk

DIFFERENTIAL DIAGNOSIS

NONSCARRING

- *Telogen effluvium:* This type of alopecia is usually diffuse thinning that follows significant life stress (death of loved one, high fever, severe infection, crash dieting) or change in hormones (postpartum, change in or cessation of oral contraceptives). Patient often presents with a bag of hair that has fallen out. This is caused by a large number of anagen (growing) hairs entering telogen (dying phase) simultaneously. Telogen effluvium is more common in women.
- *Androgenetic alopecia:* Gradual thinning of hair and a trend toward finer hair, which in men has a typical pattern of receding anterior bitemporal hairline resulting in an M-shaped pattern and hair loss at the vertex and in women has a typical pattern of thinning along vertex with or without frontotemporal thinning. This type of thinning is due to a combination of genetic predisposition and androgenic conversion of hair follicles into vellus-like follicles.
- *Alopecia areata:* Patches of acute hair loss (Fig. 1-57, A), typically 2-5 cm in diameter, with normal-appearing skin, black dots

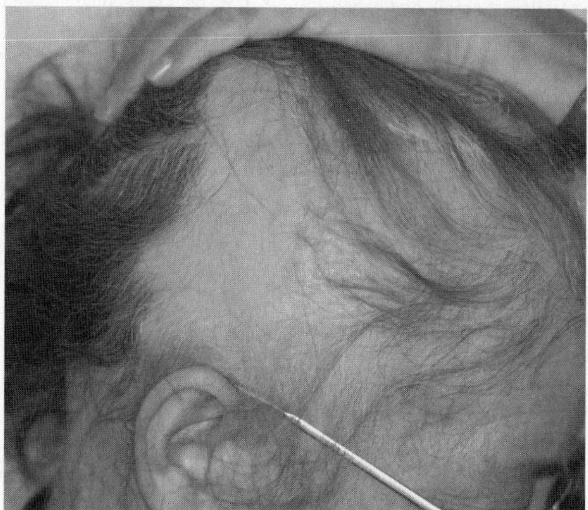

FIGURE 1-57 A, Alopecia areata: patchy hair loss. The alopecic area is devoid of hairs, and the scalp does not present inflammatory changes. (From Goldman L, Schafer AI: *Goldman's Cecil medicine,* ed 24, Philadelphia, 2012, Saunders.)

(cadaver hairs, point noir) from hair that breaks before reaching the skin's surface, and occasional "exclamation point hairs," which are evidence of hair breaking off as they are pushed from the follicle. Fingernails may show fine pitting. On biopsy, lymphocytes surround the hair bulb and resemble a "swarm of bees," evidence of the autoimmune etiology. Patients often have positive family history.

AA Universalis (AAU)—generalized loss of body hair

AA Totalis (AAT)—complete loss of scalp hair

- *Tinea:* This type of hair loss is evident in round patches, possibly with scarring, erythema, and lymphadenopathy. This is the most common type of hair loss in children. Diagnosis can be made by scraping the erythematous edge and placing the scraping with KOH under a microscope to check for hyphae. Wood's lamp only fluoresces if tinea is caused by *Microsporum* spp.; however, the most common (in the U.S.) *Trichophyton* spp. does not fluoresce. If a kerion (severe alopecia associated with bogginess) is present, it may cause scarring.
- *Traumatic alopecia:* This type of hair loss is in a pattern consistent with breaking off of hairs due to traction (hair pulling) or chemical or heating agents (hair straightening or permanent). Etiology usually becomes apparent with careful history taking and visualizing the pattern of hair loss. In trichotillomania (Fig. 1-57, B) the alopecia area has an irregular shape, scalp excoriations may present, and hairs are broken at different lengths.

SCARRING

- *Lichen planus:* The hair loss associated with LP is typically associated with scaling and atrophy of pruritic, painful skin underlying the hair loss. This hair loss is more common in middle-aged women. While there are numerous variations in clinical presentation, the general clinical picture is one of a chronic inflammatory condition of the skin, nails, mucous membranes, and/or hair. The typical skin lesions are flat topped, violaceous lesions with white lines (Wickham's striae), while the typical oral lesions are milky white.
- *Chronic cutaneous (discoid) lupus erthematosus:* This type of hair loss frequently is evident in well-demarcated, erythematous plaques in chronically sun-exposed areas of skin. Lesions exhibit hypopigmentations or hyperpigmentations, atrophy, erythema, and scaling. It may be present concurrently with SLE or be the first presenting symptom of SLE, but in most cases it is a purely cutaneous condition.
- *Tinea with kerion:* A kerion represents an exuberant delayed-type hypersensitivity reaction to the tinea capitis, resulting in one (or many) inflamed boggy plaque(s) on the scalp depending on the severity of the infection.

Rx TREATMENT

- *Telogen effluvium:* Stop insulting stress/medication and in 3-4 months anagen recurs. Hair density should be normalized by 12 months. Multiple medications have been shown to be an inciting factor and one should consider stopping them (these include, but are not limited to, enalapril, colchicine, levodopa, metoprolol, propranolol, oral contraceptives, and lithium). Full regrowth is expected in most cases.
- *Androgenetic alopecia:* For men, the most likely first-line treatment is oral finasteride (type II 5α-reductase inhibitor) which leads to lower levels of dihydrotestosterone. This leads to hair regrowth in about 6 months, but with cessation, hair returns to pattern of loss within 6–9 months. Topical minoxidil has shown similar results to finasteride and can be useful in partially restoring lost hair in both men and women. Discontinuation of minoxidil will result in loss of regrown hair often over several months. In women with elevated androgens, antiandrogens such as spironolactone, flutamide, and cimetidine may be considered. Other options include surgical intervention with hair transplantation or hair flaps, camouflaging agents, the use of a hairpiece, or low-level light therapy.
- *Alopecia areata:* Spontaneous remission occurs in patchy AA, but less commonly in AAT or AAU. Glucocorticoids (GCs) are the mainstay of treatment but have little effect on the long-term outcome of hair loss—topical GC for small patches, intralesional injection of high-potency GC, and even systemic steroids can all be temporarily effective but at the cost of glucocorticoid exposure. Induction of allergic contact dermatitis using short-contact anthralin therapy or squaric acid sensitization can be effective but tends to have significant local discomfort, thereby limiting its use. Photochemotherapy has shown some beneficial outcomes, although there is a high relapse rate after discontinuation.
- *Tinea capitis:* To effectively treat tinea capitis, oral antifungal agents must be used. Griseofulvin is considered the drug of choice in the U.S., and the recommended time course is 6 weeks to several months. Other oral agents to consider include terbinafine, itraconazole, fluconazole, and ketaconazole. If there is a kerion (area of boggy, purulent inflammation underlying the area of hair loss), the patient is at increased risk for scarring alopecia due to bacterial superinfection and a short course of oral steroids and oral antibiotic must be considered.
- *Traumatic alopecia:* First priority is stopping inciting activity/agent, ideally leading to gradual resolution of hair loss and hair regrowth.
- *Lichen planus:* Associated hair loss is often permanent; however, for symptomatic control of itching and pain, topical or oral glucocorticoids may be considered.
- *Chronic cutaneous discoid erythematosus:* The best prevention is sun protection, with SPF lotion. Treatment options center around the cautious use of topical or intralesional glucocorticoids. Hydroxychloroquinone and retinoids are also used with caution.

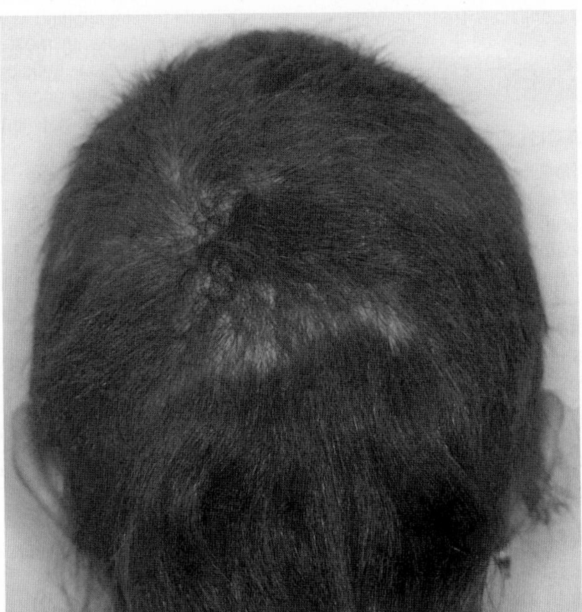

FIGURE 1-57 B, Trichotillomania: patchy hair loss. The alopecic area has an irregular shape and present hairs are broken at different lengths. Also note scalp excoriations. (From Goldman L, Schafer AI: *Goldman's Cecil medicine,* ed 24, Philadelphia, 2012, Saunders.)

REFERRAL

Dermatology

PATIENT/FAMILY EDUCATION

Alopecia areata: www.naaf.org

SUGGESTED READINGS

available at www.expertconsult.com

RELATED CONTENT

Alopecia (Patient Information)

AUTHOR: **JON SKALECKI, M.D.**

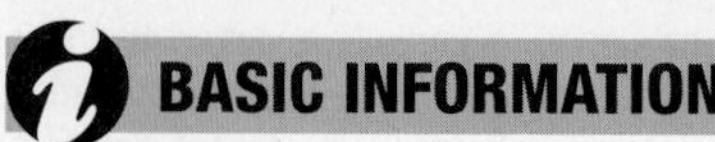

BASIC INFORMATION

DEFINITION

Alpha-1-antitrypsin deficiency is a genetic deficiency of the protease inhibitor alpha-1-antitrypsin that results in a predisposition to pulmonary emphysema and hepatic cirrhosis.

SYNONYMS

AATD

ICD-9CM CODES
277.6 Alpha-1-antitrypsin deficiency
ICD-10CM CODES
E88.01 Alpha-1-antitrypsin deficiency

EPIDEMIOLOGY & DEMOGRAPHICS

- Underrecognized by clinicians, but accounts for approximately 2%-5% of chronic obstructive pulmonary disease (COPD) cases in Americans
- Prevalence is about 1 per 3000 to 5000 people in North America
- Inherited as an autosomal codominant disorder
- Most frequent mutation is in the *SERPINA 1* gene (previously known as *PI* gene)
- Most common alleles are:
  - normal "M" allele (95% frequency in the U.S.)
  - deficient variant "Z" allele (1% to 2%)
  - deficient variant "S" allele (2% to 3%)
- Severe deficiency is most commonly due to homozygotes ZZ
- Risk of lung disease is uncertain with MZ genotype, but increased with SZ genotype (especially in smokers)
- One in 10 individuals of European descent carries one of two mutations that may result in partial alpha-1-antitrypsin deficiency

PHYSICAL FINDINGS & CLINICAL PRESENTATION

- Physical findings and clinical presentation are varied and depend on phenotype (see "Etiology")
- Most often affects the lungs but can also involve liver and skin
- Classically associated with early-onset, severe, lower-lobe predominant panacinar emphysema; bronchiectasis may also be seen
- Symptoms are similar to "typical" COPD presentation (dyspnea, cough, sputum production)
- Liver involvement includes neonatal cholestasis, cirrhosis in children and adults, and primary carcinoma of the liver
- Panniculitis is the major dermatologic manifestation

ETIOLOGY

- Degree of alpha-1-antitrypsin deficiency depends on phenotype.
- "MM" represents the normal genotype and is associated with alpha-1-antitrypsin levels in the normal range.
- Mutation most commonly associated with emphysema is Z, with homozygote (ZZ) resulting in approximately 85% deficit in plasma alpha-1-antitrypsin concentrations.
- Development of emphysema is believed to result from an imbalance between the proteolytic enzyme elastase, produced by neutrophils, and alpha-1-antitrypsin, which normally protects lung elastin by inhibiting elastase.
- Deficiency of alpha-1-antitrypsin increases risk of early-onset emphysema, but not all alpha-1-antitrypsin deficient individuals will develop lung disease.
- Smoking increases risk and accelerates onset of COPD.
- Liver disease is caused by pathologic accumulation of alpha-1-antitrypsin in hepatocytes.
- Similar to lung disease, skin involvement is thought to be attributable to unopposed proteolysis in skin.

Dx DIAGNOSIS

DIFFERENTIAL DIAGNOSIS

See "Chronic Obstructive Pulmonary Disease."
See "Cirrhosis."

WORKUP

- Suspicion for alpha-1-antitrypsin deficiency usually results from emphysema developing at an early age and with basilar predominance of disease.

LABORATORY TESTS

- Serum level of alpha-1-antitrypsin can confirm or reject suspicion of deficiency.
- Investigate possibility of abnormal alleles with genotyping.
- Pulmonary function testing is generally consistent with "typical" COPD.

IMAGING STUDIES

- Chest x-ray shows characteristic emphysematous changes at lung bases.
- High-resolution chest CT usually confirms the lower-lobe predominant emphysema and may also show significant bronchiectasis.

Rx TREATMENT

NONPHARMACOLOGIC THERAPY

- Avoidance of smoking is paramount.
- Avoidance of other environmental and occupational exposures that may increase risk of COPD. Routine vaccinations are also recommended.

ACUTE GENERAL Rx

Acute exacerbations of COPD from alpha-1-antitrypsin deficiency are treated in a similar fashion to "typical" COPD exacerbations.

CHRONIC Rx

- The goal of treatment in alpha-1-antitrypsin deficiency is to increase serum alpha-1-antitrypsin levels above a minimum, "protective" threshold of 50 mg/dL.
- Although several therapeutic options are under investigation, IV administration of pooled human alpha-1-antitrypsin is currently the only approved method to raise serum alpha-1-antitrypsin levels. AAT augmentation therapy has been approved by the FDA for patients with AAT deficiency who have COPD. Augmentation therapy is expensive ($60,000 to $100,000/year) and requires lifelong treatment. However, given the cost and a lack of evidence of clinical benefit, a 2010 Cochrane Collaboration review noted that augmentation therapy with alpha-1-antitrypsin cannot be recommended.
- Organ transplantation for patients with end-stage lung or liver disease is also an option.

DISPOSITION

- Prognosis of patients with alpha-1-antitrypsin deficiency will depend on phenotype and level of deficiency.
- Among patients with severe alpha-1-antitrypsin deficiency, the most common underlying causes of death are emphysema (72%) and cirrhosis (10%).

REFERRAL

- Referral to specialists with experience in AAT deficiency is preferred
- Pulmonary and hepatology referrals for advanced lung and liver disease, or if replacement therapy is contemplated (e.g., moderate-severe lung disease)
- Lung and liver transplantation in suitable cases

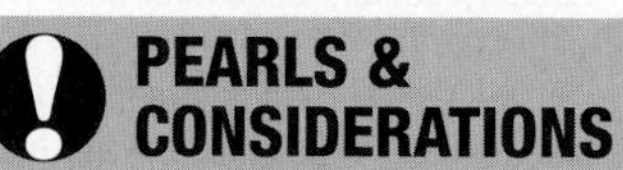

PEARLS & CONSIDERATIONS

- The liver damage arising from the mutation is not from a deficiency in alpha-1-antitrypsin but from a pathologic accumulation of alpha-1-antitrypsin in hepatocytes.
- Strong association between PI*ZZ phenotypes and liver disease has prompted recommendations for AATD testing in individuals with unexplained liver disease.
- Consider alpha-1-antitrypsin deficiency in patients presenting with lower-lobe predominant emphysema; in most smokers without alpha-1-antitrypsin deficiency, emphysema predominates in the upper lobes.
- Alpha-1-antitrypsin deficiency is believed to be under-recognized.
- The American Thoracic Society and the European Respiratory Society recommend testing for AAT deficiency in all patients with COPD, emphysema, or asthma with irreversible obstruction, whereas the Global Initiative for Chronic Obstructive Lung Disease only recommends testing for those with early-onset COPD (age <45 yr) or a strong family history of COPD.

SUGGESTED READINGS
available at www.expertconsult.com

RELATED CONTENT

Chronic Obstructive Pulmonary Disease (Related Key Topic)
Cirrhosis (Related Key Topic)
Alpha-1-Antitrypsin Deficiency (Patient Information)

AUTHORS: **JOSEPH A. DIAZ, M.D., M.P.H.**, and **MOHAMMAD ASHKIANI, M.D.**

BASIC INFORMATION

DEFINITION

Dementia is a syndrome characterized by progressive loss of previously acquired cognitive skills including memory, language, insight, and judgment. Alzheimer's disease (AD) is believed to account for the majority (50% to 75%) of all cases of dementia.

ICD-9CM CODES
331.0 Alzheimer's disease
290.0 Senile dementia, uncomplicated
ICD-10CM CODES
G30.9 Alzheimer's disease, unspecified
F03.90 Unspecified dementia without behavioral disturbance

EPIDEMIOLOGY & DEMOGRAPHICS

INCIDENCE: Risk doubles every 5 yr after the age of 65; above the age of 85 the incidence is about 8%.
PREVALENCE: Currently an estimated 5.2 million Americans have AD; 6% between the ages of 65 and 74, 44% between 75 and 84, and 46% at 85 years and older.
PREDOMINANT SEX: Female

PHYSICAL FINDINGS & CLINICAL PRESENTATION

- Spouse or other family member, usually not the patient, notes insidious memory impairment.
- Patients have difficulties learning and retaining new information and handling complex tasks (e.g., balancing the checkbook), and have impairments in reasoning, judgment, spatial ability, and orientation (e.g., difficulty driving, getting lost away from home).
- Behavioral changes, such as mood changes and apathy, may accompany memory impairment. In later stages patients may develop agitation and psychosis.
- Atypical presentations include early and severe behavioral changes, focal findings on examination, parkinsonism, hallucinations, falls, or onset of symptoms younger than the age of 65.

Dx DIAGNOSIS

There is no definitive imaging or laboratory test for the diagnosis of AD. Diagnosis is commonly made based on clinical history, a thorough physical and neurologic examination, and use of reliable and valid diagnostic criteria (i.e., DSM-IV or NINDCS-ADRDA) such as the following:
- Loss of memory and one or more additional cognitive abilities (aphasia, apraxia, agnosia, or other disturbance in executive functioning)
- Impairment in social or occupational functioning that represents a decline from a previous level of functioning and results in significant disability
- Deficits that do not occur exclusively during the course of delirium
- Insidious onset and gradual progression of symptoms
- Cognitive loss documented by neuropsychologic tests
- No physical signs, neuroimaging, or laboratory evidence of other diseases that can cause dementia (i.e., metabolic abnormalities, medication or toxin effects, infection, stroke, Parkinson's disease, subdural hematoma, or tumors)

The National Institute on Aging (NIA) and the Alzheimer's Association recommended new diagnostic criteria and guidelines for AD in 2011. These differ from prior DSM-IV or NINDCS-ADRDA criteria in that they now recommend that AD be considered a disease well before the onset of symptoms, they incorporate the use of biomarkers in diagnosis, and they define three distinct stages of AD: (1) *preclinical* AD, in which there is measurable biologic evidence of AD pathology but no symptoms; (2) *mild cognitive impairment* (MCI) due to AD, in which there is mild memory loss but no functional impairment at home or work; and (3) *dementia due to AD.*

DIFFERENTIAL DIAGNOSIS

- Cancer (brain tumor, meningeal neoplasia)
- Infection (AIDS, neurosyphilis, PML)
- Toxic/metabolic (EtOH, hypothyroidism, vitamin B_{12} deficiency, mercury exposure, drug effects)
- Organ failure (dialysis dementia, Wilson's disease)
- Vascular disorder (multiple strokes, severe small vessel changes, chronic vasculitides, or chronic subdural hematoma)
- Depression (pseudodementia)

WORKUP

HISTORY & GENERAL PHYSICAL EXAMINATION:
- Medication lists should always be reviewed for drugs or home remedies that may cause mental status changes.
- Patients should be screened for depression, because it can sometimes mimic dementia but also often occurs as a coexisting condition and should be treated.
- On examination, look for signs of metabolic disturbance, presence of psychiatric features, or focal neurologic deficits.

MENTAL STATUS TESTING: Brief mental status testing can be done easily and quickly in the office. For detecting mild cognitive impairment and dementia, the Montreal Cognitive Assessment (MoCA, http://www.mocatest.org/) is a highly sensitive 30-point test that takes approximately 10 minutes to administer. Cognitive domains tested include visual-spatial, attention, verbal recall, language, abstraction and orientation. A score of 25 points or less (26 points if the patient has less than 12 years of education) indicates cognitive impairment. The test is available in over 35 languages and dialects, and multiple forms in English allow for repeated assessments over time.

Mental status testing should include tests that assess the following cognitive functions:
- Orientation: ask the patient to give the day, date, month, year, and place and to name the current president.
- Attention: ask the patient to recite the months of the year forward and in reverse.
- Verbal recall: ask the patient to remember three items; test for recall after a 1- and 5-min delay.
- Language: ask the patient to write and then read a sentence; have the patient name both common and less common objects.
- Visual-spatial: ask the patient to draw a clock and to set the hands of the clock at 11:10.

Patients with AD typically have trouble with verbal recall, plus visual-spatial or language deficits. Attention is usually preserved until the late stages of AD, so consider alternate diagnoses in patients who perform poorly on tests of attention.

LABORATORY TESTS

- CBC
- Serum electrolytes
- Glucose
- BUN/creatinine
- Liver and thyroid function tests
- Serum vitamin B_{12}
- Syphilis serology (RPR), if supported by clinical history
- HIV screening as appropriate
- Lumbar puncture if history or signs of cancer, infectious process, or when the clinical presentation is unusual (i.e., rapid progression of symptoms)
- EEG if there is history of seizures, episodic confusion, rapid clinical decline, or suspicion of Creutzfeldt-Jakob disease
- Measurement of apolipoprotein E genotyping, CSF tau and amyloid, and functional imaging including positron emission tomography (PET) or single proton emission computed tomography (SPECT) are not yet routinely indicated
- Brain biopsy (usually reserved for diagnoses such as prion disease, certain vasculitides). Generally performed post mortem.

IMAGING STUDIES

- CT scan or MRI to rule out hydrocephalus and mass lesions, including subdural hematoma
- Florbetapir-PET imaging of the brain correlates with the presence and density of beta-amyloid

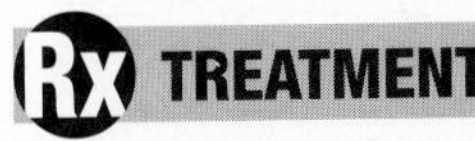

TREATMENT

NONPHARMACOLOGIC THERAPY

- Patient safety, including risks associated with impaired driving, wandering behavior, leaving stoves unattended, and accidents, must be addressed with the patient and family early and appropriate measures implemented.
- Wandering, hoarding or hiding objects, repetitive questioning, withdrawal, and social inappropriateness often respond to behavioral therapies.

ACUTE GENERAL Rx

None

CHRONIC RX

1. Symptomatic treatment of memory disturbance (Table 1-26):
   a. Cholinesterase inhibitors (ChEIs):
   FDA approved for the treatment of mild to moderate AD. Common side effects include nausea, diarrhea, and anorexia and may be bothersome enough to require a slower escalation of dosage or switching to another agent.
   b. NMDA receptor antagonist: memantine (Namenda)
   FDA approved for the treatment of moderate to severe AD. Common side effects include constipation, dizziness, or headache. Memantine is contraindicated in patients with renal insufficiency or history of seizures.
2. Symptomatic treatment of neuropsychiatric and behavioral disturbances (Table 1-27).
   Depression, agitation, delusions, or hallucinations may respond to medications.

DISPOSITION & REFERRAL

- Patients with complex or atypical presentations or challenging management issues should be referred to a neurologist or another specialist with expertise in dementia.
- Approximately 1 in 8 hospitalized patients with AD who develop delirium will have at least one adverse outcome (e.g., institutionalization, cognitive decline, death) associated with delirium.
- Family education and support may help reduce need for skilled nursing facility, and reduce caregiver stress, depression, and burnout.

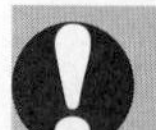

PEARLS & CONSIDERATIONS

The physician should make a thorough search for the treatable causes of dementia. Current American Academy of Neurology practice parameters recommend:
- Treat cognitive symptoms of AD with ChEIs.
- Treat agitation, psychosis, and depression.
- Encourage caregivers to participate in educational programs and support groups.

COMMENTS

- Ginkgo biloba is marketed widely as effective in delaying cognitive impairment; however, trials have shown that it is not effective in reducing the incidence of Alzheirmer dementia or dementia overall.
- Higher midlife fitness levels seem to be associated with lower hazards of developing all-cause dementia later in life independent of cerebrovascular disease.
- Lower plasma beta-amyloid 42/40 is associated with greater cognitive decline among elderly persons without dementia over 9 yr, and this association is stronger among those with low measures of cognitive reserve.
- The *APOE* genotype provides information on the risk for AD, but the genotyping of patients raises ethical and emotional concerns. Because the benefits of genetic testing are often modest, and the tests themselves often imprecise in identifying risk, the test is generally discouraged. Recent trials, however, reveal that the disclosure of *APOE* genotyping results to adult children of patients with AD did not result in significant short-term psychological risks. Test-related distress was reduced among those who learned that they were *APOE*4 negative. Persons with high levels of emotional distress before undergoing genetic testing are more likely to have emotional difficulties after disclosure.

For additional information for patients, families, and clinicians, contact the following organizations:
- Alzheimer's Association (www.alz.org; 800-272-3900)
- Alzheimer's Disease Education and Referral Center (http://www.nia.nih.gov/Alzheimers; 800-438-4380)

TABLE 1-26 Symptomatic Treatment of Memory Disturbance

	Initial Dose	Target Dose
Donepezil	5 mg qd for 4-6 weeks	10 mg qd
Rivastigmine	1.5 mg bid with food, increase by 1.5 mg bid weekly	3-6 mg bid
Galantamine	4 mg bid with food, increase by 4 mg bid every 4 weeks	8-12 mg bid
Memantine	5 mg qd, increase by 5 mg weekly	10 mg bid

TABLE 1-27 Treatment of Behavioral and Neuropsychiatric Symptoms

	Initial Dose	Maximum Dose
Atypical Antipsychotics		
Olanzapine	2.5 mg qd to bid, may increase by 2.5 mg as needed	7.5 mg bid
Quetiapine	25 mg bid, may increase by 25 mg every 2 days	250 mg tid
Antidepressants		
Sertraline	25-50 mg qd, may increase by 25 mg every week	200 mg qd
Citalopram	10 mg qd, may increase after 1 week	20 mg qd

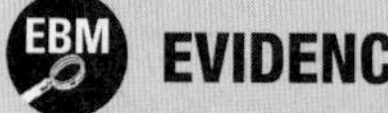

EVIDENCE

available at www.expertconsult.com

SUGGESTED READINGS

available at www.expertconsult.com

RELATED CONTENT

Table E3-10, Screening Tests for Diagnosis of Dementia
Alzheimer's Disease (Patient Information)
Mild Cognitive Impairment (Related Key Topic)

AUTHOR: **TAMARA G. FONG, M.D., PH.D.**

BASIC INFORMATION

DEFINITION

Amaurosis fugax is a temporary loss of monocular vision caused by transient retinal ischemia.

ICD-9CM CODES
362.34 Amaurosis fugax
ICD-10CM CODES
G45.3 Amaurosis fugax

EPIDEMIOLOGY & DEMOGRAPHICS

INCIDENCE (IN U.S.): An uncommon but important presentation of carotid artery disease
PEAK INCIDENCE: Approximately 55 yr

PHYSICAL FINDINGS & CLINICAL PRESENTATION

- Onset is sudden, typically lasting seconds to minutes, and often accompanied by scotomas such as a shade or curtain being pulled over the front of the eye (usually downward).
- Vision loss can be complete, hemianopic, or quadrantic.
- Acute stage: cholesterol emboli may be seen in retinal artery (*Hollenhorst plaque*): carotid bruits or other evidence of generalized atherosclerosis.
- If embolus is cardiac in origin, atrial fibrillation is often present.

ETIOLOGY

- Usually embolic from the internal carotid artery or the heart
- Giant cell arteritis causing inflammation of retinal arteries
- Hyperviscosity syndromes, such as sickle cell disease, which causes ischemia in the vascular territory of the ophthalmic artery
- Hypercoagulability states
- Transient vasospasm often associated with exercise

Dx DIAGNOSIS

DIFFERENTIAL DIAGNOSIS

- Retinal migraine: in contrast to amaurosis, the onset of visual loss develops more slowly, usually over 15 to 20 min.
- Transient visual obscurations occur in the setting of papilledema; intermittent rises in intracranial pressure briefly compromise optic disc perfusion and cause transient visual loss lasting 1 to 2 seconds. The episodes may be binocular. If the visual loss persists at the time of evaluation (i.e., vision has not yet recovered), then the differential diagnosis should be broadened to include:
  - Anterior ischemic optic neuropathy: arteritic (classically GCA) or nonarteritic
  - Central retinal vein occlusion

WORKUP

- Workup should focus on embolic sources, but GCA should always be considered.
- Careful examination of retina; embolus may be visible and confirm the diagnosis (Fig. 1-58).
- Auscultation of arteries for carotid bruits.
- Examination of all pulses and for temporal artery tenderness.
- Inquire about symptoms of GCA (scalp tenderness, headache, fever, jaw claudication).
- Examine for signs of hemispheric stroke resulting from intracranial aneurysm (contralateral limb and facial weakness or sensory loss, aphasia, etc.).

LABORATORY TESTS

- Complete blood count with erythrocyte sedimentation rate and C-reactive protein.
- Serum chemistries, including lipid profile.
- Cardiac enzymes and ECG.
- Hypercoagulable workup is discretionary based on younger age and history.

IMAGING STUDIES

- Carotid Doppler imaging followed by MR or CT angiography as indicated.
- Transthoracic echocardiography is indicated to screen for sources of emboli in patients with evidence of heart disease and in patients without an evident source for transient neurologic deficit. Transesophageal echocardiography is more sensitive for detecting cardiac sources of emboli (ventricular mural thrombus, atrial appendage, patent foramen ovale, aortic arch).
- MRI of the brain with diffusion-weighted imaging to look for infarcts, especially those presenting with focal neurologic disturbances.

Rx TREATMENT

NONPHARMACOLOGIC THERAPY

- Diet (decrease saturated fatty acids and high-cholesterol foods)
- Exercise
- Cessation of tobacco use

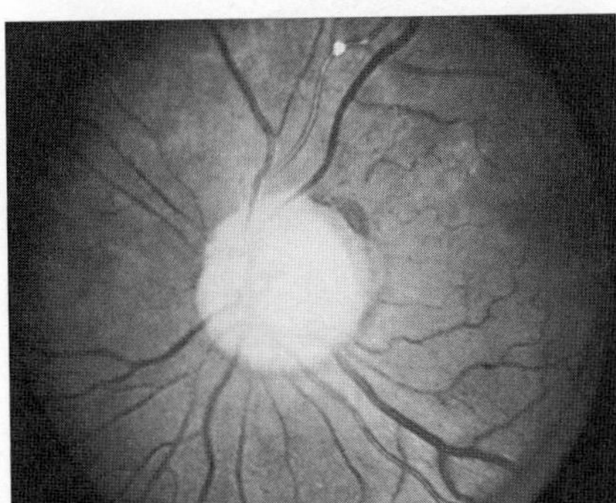

FIGURE 1-58 A cholesterol crystal embolus lodged at an arterial bifurcation. (From Stein JH [ed]: *Internal medicine,* ed 5, St Louis, 1998, Mosby.)

ACUTE GENERAL Rx

- Investigate as an emergency.
- Aspirin if etiology is presumed embolic.
- If GCA is suspected, start prednisone and refer for temporal artery biopsy within 48 hr (see "Giant Cell Arteritis" in Section I).

CHRONIC Rx

- Reduce risks by carotid endarterectomy or carotid stenting if stenosis >70%. Stenting may be performed in high-risk surgical candidates.
- Control hypertension and manage vascular risk factors.
- Antiplatelet therapy.
- Consider starting an HMG-CoA reductase inhibitor.

DISPOSITION

Among patients with >50% carotid stenosis who do not undergo carotid endarterectomy, those who present with transient monocular blindness have an approximate 10% risk of stroke in 3 yr compared with an approximate 20% risk in patients who present with a hemispheric transient ischemic attack (TIA).

REFERRAL

- Recommend referral to a neurologist for evaluation and workup.
- If significant carotid stenosis, consider carotid endarterectomy or carotid stenting for the following:
  1. High-grade (≥70%) stenosis
  2. Multiple TIAs despite medical therapy in the setting of high-grade or ulcerative disease

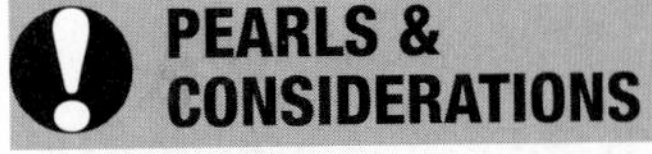

PEARLS & CONSIDERATIONS

- Cholesterol emboli in retinal arteries on funduscopy confirm the diagnosis.
- Recognize that transient visual loss has multiple other causes.

SUGGESTED READINGS
available at www.expertconsult.com

RELATED CONTENT

Carotid Stenosis (Related Key Topic)
Giant Cell Arteritis (Related Key Topic)
Transient Ischemic Attack (Related Key Topic)
Amaurosis Fugax (Patient Information)

AUTHOR: **TZU-CHING (TEDDY) WU, M.D., M.P.H.**

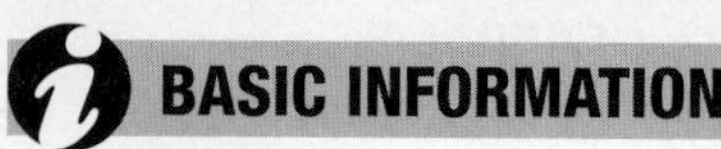

BASIC INFORMATION

DEFINITION

Amblyopia refers to a decrease in vision in one or both eyes in the presence of an otherwise normal ophthalmologic examination. The major types of amblyopia are strabismic, anisometropic (refractive), and combined strabismic and refractive. Less common types are ametropic and deprivation (rare).

SYNONYMS

Deprivation amblyopia
Occlusion amblyopia
Strabismus amblyopia
Refractive amblyopia
Organic or toxic amblyopias
Lazy eye

ICD-9CM CODES
368.00 Amblyopia
ICD-10CM CODES
H53.00 Unspecified amblyopia, unspecified eye

EPIDEMIOLOGY & DEMOGRAPHICS

INCIDENCE (IN U.S.): 1% to 5% of the general population. Amblyopia is the leading cause of vision loss in children. It is also the cause of permanent vision loss in 2.9% of adults.
PREVALENCE (IN U.S.): High incidence in premature infants with drug-dependent mothers and in neurologically impaired children. Children with a family history of strabismus or amblyopia are at increased risk.
PREDOMINANT SEX: None
PREDOMINANT AGE: Childhood
PEAK INCIDENCE: Childhood

PHYSICAL FINDINGS & CLINICAL PRESENTATION

Decreased vision using best refraction in the presence of normal corneal, lens, retinal, and optic nerve appearance (Fig. 1-59).

ETIOLOGY

- Visual deprivation
- Strabismus
- Occlusion with patching
- Refractive error organic lesions in the nervous system
- Toxins

DIAGNOSIS

DIFFERENTIAL DIAGNOSIS

- Central nervous system (CNS) disease (brainstem)
- Optic nerve disorders
- Corneal or other eye diseases
- Retinal disorders

WORKUP

- Complete eye examination to find cause of amblyopia or deprivation of vision. Referral to an ophthalmologist is recommended for any child with a visual acuity in either eye of ≤20/40 at age 3 to 5 yr or worse at age ≥6 yr or a two-line difference in acuity between eyes.
- Motility evaluation.

LABORATORY TESTS

Usually none

IMAGING STUDIES

Usually not necessary unless central nervous system (CNS) lesion suspected

TREATMENT

NONPHARMACOLOGIC THERAPY

- Treatment depends on the age of the patient, severity of amblyopia, and compliance with patching or atropine.
- Glasses or prisms to align eyes with minor deviations and improve vision.
- Patching and atropine are both effective. Atropine 1% is used daily for 6 mo; patching is used 2 to 6 hr/day for 6 mo. Patching may be more effective; 50% get best vision improvement by 16 wk.
- Removal of the cause of the amblyopia if possible.
- Surgery to align the eyes or remove obstruction to vision.

CHRONIC Rx

- Patching or optics, including prisms and atropine, most effective in 3- to 7-yr-olds; although treatment ideally should begin before age 5, a recent trial demonstrated that children may benefit even at an older age.

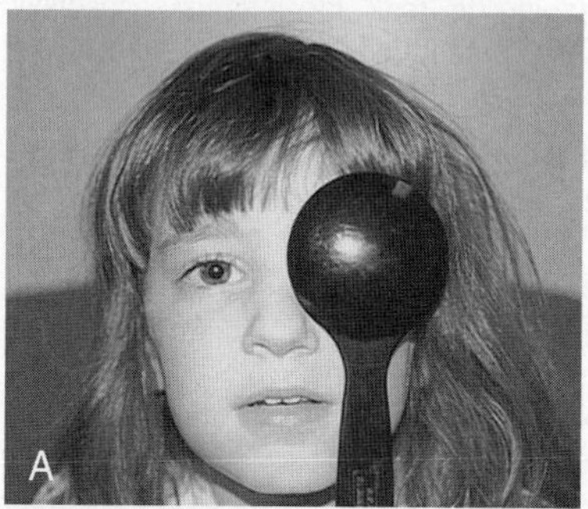

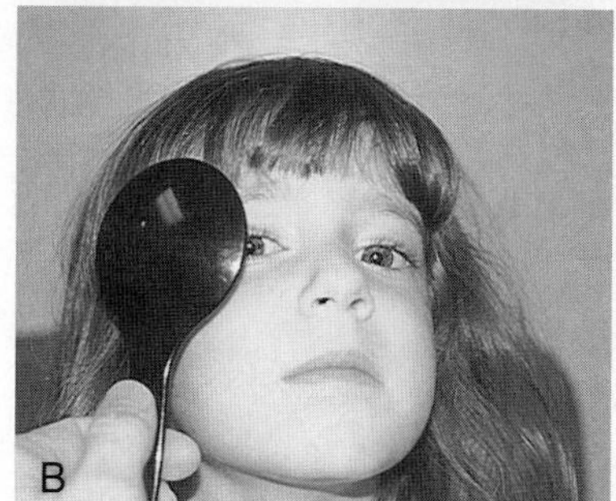

FIGURE 1-59 A, This child happily fixes with her right eye and does not object if the left eye is covered. **B,** When the right eye is covered she moves her head away and tries to remove the cover, demonstrating a fixation preference for the right eye and amblyopia of the left eye. (From Hoekelman R [ed]: *Primary pediatric care,* ed 3, St Louis, 1997, Mosby.)

- Tapering the amount of time a patch is worn each day at the end of treatment reduces the risk of recurrence.

DISPOSITION

Immediate patching, alternating eyes daily

REFERRAL

To ophthalmologist if vision is compromised

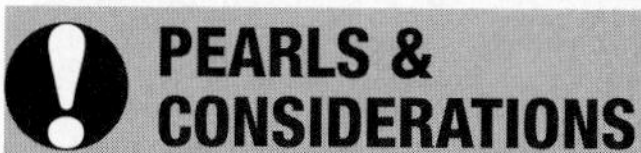

PEARLS & CONSIDERATIONS

COMMENTS

- The earlier the referral, the better the outcome. Amblyopia is more responsive to treatment among children younger than 7 years of age. Although the average treatment response is smaller in children 7 to less than 13 years of age, some children show a marked response to treatment.
- The success of therapy is highly dependent on treatment compliance.
- Amblyopia recurs in 25% of children after patching is discontinued.

SUGGESTED READINGS

available at www.expertconsult.com

AUTHORS: **MELVYN KOBY, M.D.,** and **R. SCOTT HOFFMAN, M.D.**

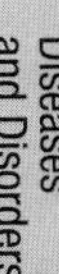

BASIC INFORMATION

DEFINITION

Amebiasis is an infection caused by the protozoal parasite *Entamoeba histolytica.* Although primarily an infection of the colon, amebiasis may cause extraintestinal disease, particularly liver abscess.

SYNONYMS

Amebic dysentery (when severe intestinal infection)

ICD-9CM CODES
006.9 Amebiasis
ICD-10CM CODES
A06.9 Amebiasis, unspecified

EPIDEMIOLOGY & DEMOGRAPHICS

INCIDENCE (IN U.S.): 1.2 cases per 100,000 U.S. population. Highest in institutionalized patients, and travelers to/immigrants from developing nations.
PREVALENCE (IN U.S.): 4% (80% of infections asymptomatic)
PREDOMINANT SEX:
- Equal sex distribution in general
- Striking male predominance of liver abscess

PREDOMINANT AGE: 2nd through 6th decades
PEAK INCIDENCE: Peaks at age 2 to 3 yr and >40 yr

PHYSICAL FINDINGS & CLINICAL PRESENTATION

- Often nonspecific
- Approximately 20% of cases symptomatic
  1. Diarrhea, which may be bloody
  2. Abdominal and back pain
- Abdominal tenderness in 83% of severe cases
- Fever in 38% of severe cases
- Hepatomegaly, right upper quadrant tenderness, and fever in almost all patients with liver abscess (may be absent in fulminant cases)

ETIOLOGY

- Caused by the protozoal parasite *E. histolytica. E. dispar* and *E. moshkovskii* are 10 times more common but nonpathogenic and difficult to distinguish from *E. histolytica.*
- Transmission by the fecal-oral route
- Infection usually localized to the large bowel, particularly the cecum where a localized mass lesion (ameboma) may form
- Extraintestinal infection in which the organism invades the bowel mucosa and gains access to the portal circulation

DIAGNOSIS

DIFFERENTIAL DIAGNOSIS

- Severe intestinal infection possibly confused with ulcerative colitis or other infectious enterocolitis syndromes, such as those caused by *Shigella, Salmonella, Campylobacter,* or invasive *Escherichia coli*
- In elderly patients: ischemic bowel possibly producing a similar picture

WORKUP

- Three stool specimens over a period of 7 to 10 days to search for cysts or trophozoites has a sensitivity of 85% to 95%, but microscopy cannot differentiate between the species
- Concentration and staining the specimen with Lugol's iodine or methylene blue to increase the diagnostic yield
- Fecal leukocytes not always present

LABORATORY TESTS

- Fecal ELISA antigen detection is specific for *E. histolytica* (87% percent sensitive) and also useful for diagnosis of liver abscess.
- Mucosal biopsy is occasionally necessary to look for cysts or trophozoites.
- Serum antibody assays specific for *E. histolytica* are available and are particularly sensitive and specific for extraintestinal infection or severe intestinal disease.
- Aspiration of abscess fluid is used to distinguish amebic from bacterial abscesses.

IMAGING STUDIES

Abdominal imaging studies (sonography or CT scan) to diagnose liver abscess

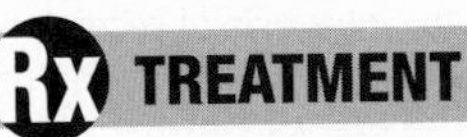

TREATMENT

ACUTE GENERAL Rx

- Table 1-28 summarizes drug treatment options for amebiasis in adults and children.
- Liver abscess is generally responsive to medical management but surgical intervention indicated for extension of liver abscess into pericardium or for toxic megacolon.

DISPOSITION

Host immunity incomplete and reinfection rate high for patients remaining at risk

REFERRAL

- For consultation with infectious diseases specialist for extraintestinal infection or persistent or relapsing intestinal infection
- For surgical consultation:
  1. For toxic megacolon
  2. For impending rupture of or extension of liver abscess into adjacent structures

TABLE 1-28 Drug Treatment for Amebiasis

Medication	Adult Dosage (Oral)	Pediatric Dosage (Oral)*
Invasive Disease		
Metronidazole	Colitis or liver abscess: 750 mg tid for 7-10 days	Colitis or liver abscess: 35-50 mg/kg/day in 3 divided doses for 7-10 days
or		
Tinidazole	Colitis: 2 g once daily for 3 days Liver abscess: 2 g once daily for 3-5 days	Colitis: 50 mg/kg/day once daily for 3 days Liver abscess: 50 mg/kg/day once daily for 3-5 days
Followed by:		
Paromomycin (preferred)	500 mg tid for 7 days	25-35 mg/kg/day in 3 divided doses for 7 days
or		
Diloxanide furoate† or	500 mg tid for 10 days	20 mg/kg/day in 3 divided doses for 7 days
Iodoquinol	650 mg tid for 20 days	30-40 mg/kg/day in 3 divided doses for 20 days
Asymptomatic Intestinal Colonization		
Paromomycin (preferred) or Diloxanide furoate† or Iodoquinol	As for invasive disease	As for invasive disease

*All pediatric dosages are up to a maximum of the adult dose.
†Not available in the United States.
From Kliegman RM et al: *Nelson textbook of pediatrics,* ed 19, Philadelphia, 2011, Saunders.

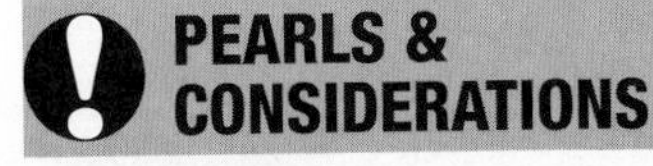

PEARLS & CONSIDERATIONS

COMMENTS

- Infection with other intestinal parasites, particularly *Giardia lamblia,* may coexist with amebiasis.
- There is a high prevalence of *E. dispar* in homosexual males, which is nonpathogenic but may be difficult to distinguish from the pathogen *E. histolytica.*

SUGGESTED READINGS

available at www.expertconsult.com

RELATED CONTENT

Amebiasis (Patient Information)

AUTHOR: **GLENN G. FORT, M.D., M.P.H.**

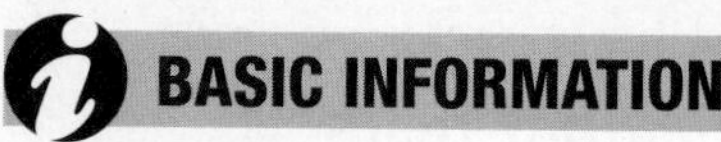

BASIC INFORMATION

DESCRIPTION

Amenorrhea means absence of menstruation. It is classified as either primary or secondary depending on whether the patient has had previous menstrual cycles.

- Primary amenorrhea is defined as the absence of menses by age 16 in the presence of secondary sexual characteristics. However, in the absence of these secondary sexual features by the age of 14 years, one should begin the workup for primary amenorrhea.
- Secondary amenorrhea is the absence of menses for more than six months in a patient who has had previous normal progesterone withdrawal cycles. The duration of amenorrhea required for the diagnosis of secondary amenorrhea varies somewhat depending on the source.

ICD-9CM CODES
626.0 Absence of menstruation
ICD-10CM CODES
N91.2 Amenorrhea, unspecified

EPIDEMIOLOGY & DEMOGRAPHICS

- Incidence of primary amenorrhea and secondary amenorrhea in the U.S. is <1% and 5% to 7%, respectively.
- There is no racial or ethnic predilection.

ETIOLOGY

- Physiologic amenorrhea
  1. Pregnancy
  2. Lactation
  3. Menopause
- Pathologic amenorrhea
  A. Primary amenorrhea
    1. Hypergonadotropic hypogonadism
      a. Turner's syndrome
      b. Pure gonadal dysgenesis
      c. Autoimmune oophoritis
      d. 17,20-desmolase deficiency or 17-hydroxylase deficiency
      e. Galactosemia
    2. Eugonadism (Table 1-29)
      a. Müllerian agenesis
      b. Transverse vaginal septum
      c. Imperforate hymen
      d. Androgen insensitivity syndrome (AIS) (1%)
      e. 5-alpha reductase deficiency
      f. Polycystic ovarian syndrome (PCOS)
      g. Adult-onset congenital adrenal hyperplasia (CAH)
      h. Cushing's syndrome
      i. Hypothyroidism
    3. Hypogonadotropic hypogonadism
      a. Constitutional delay
      b. Hypothalamic disorders
      c. Pituitary diseases
      d. Other CNS diseases
  B. Secondary amenorrhea
    1. Ovarian diseases
      a. PCOS
      b. Iatrogenic (oophorectomy, S/P radiation, chemotherapy)
      c. Primary ovarian insufficiency (previously premature ovarian failure [POF])
      d. Ovarian tumors
    2. Hypothalamic dysfunction
      a. Functional (eating disorders, exercise, stress)
      b. Congenital GnRH deficiency
      c. Infiltrative diseases (sarcoidosis, histiocytosis, lymphoma)
    3. Pituitary diseases
      a. Hyperprolactinemia (drug induced, hypothyroidism, prolactinoma)
      b. Craniopharyngiomas
      c. Empty sella syndrome
      d. Sheehan's syndrome
      e. S/P radiation
      f. Infiltrative diseases
    4. Asherman's syndrome
    5. Others
       Hypothyroidism, Cushing's syndrome, adult-onset congenital adrenal hyperplasia, drug induced (Lupron Depot, Depo-Provera, levonorgestrel IUD, Danazol, etc.), chronic illnesses

PHYSICAL FINDINGS & CLINICAL PRESENTATION

- Turner's syndrome
  - Usually presents with primary amenorrhea unless mosaic
  - Short stature
  - Epicanthic folds
  - Low-set ears
  - High-arched palate
  - Micrognathia
  - Sensorineural hearing loss
  - Otitis media
  - Webbing of the neck
  - Pigmented nevi
  - Square/shield chest
  - Widely spaced nipples
  - Absent breast development
  - Bicuspid aortic valve
  - Coarctation of aorta
  - Cubit valgus
  - Short fourth metacarpal
  - Hyperconvex nails
  - Leg edema
  - Renal abnormalities
  - Autoimmune disorders including thyroiditis
  - Diabetes mellitus
- Pure gonadal dysgenesis
  - Unlike Turner's syndrome has no dysmorphic features
- Müllerian agenesis
  - Sporadic inheritance
  - Primary amenorrhea
  - Normal breast development
  - Normal pubic and axillary hair
  - Normal female external genitalia
  - Absent uterus and upper part of vagina
  - Ovaries present
  - Renal and vertebral anomalies in some patients; renal agenesis should be evaluated
- Transverse vaginal septum and imperforate hymen
  - Primary amenorrhea
  - Progressive cyclic lower abdominal pain
  - Imperforate hymen or transverse vaginal septum on pelvic examination
  - Perirectal fullness from hematocolpos
  - Imaging with MRI identifies level of obstruction
- Androgen insensitivity syndrome
  - Primary amenorrhea
  - X-linked recessive inheritance in some patients
  - Normal breast development
  - Absent pubic and axillary hair
  - Testis may be present in the groin or inguinal canal
  - Uterus and vagina absent
  - No associated renal or vertebral anomalies
- Adult-onset congenital adrenal hyperplasia
  - Commonly seen in Ashkenazi Jewish, Inuit Native American, French Canadian, Mexican population
  - Mimics the presentation of PCOS
  - Features of hyperandrogenism (virilization, hirsutism, acne)
  - Hypertension
- 5-alpha reductase deficiency
  - Primary amenorrhea
  - Undergo striking virilization at puberty
- PCOS
  - Usually presents with secondary amenorrhea and oligomenorrhea
  - Features of hyperandrogenism
  - Obesity (60% to 80% of PCOS patients)
  - Infertility
  - Insulin resistance, predisposition to type II diabetes mellitus
  - Association with the metabolic syndrome
- Cushing's syndrome (rare disorder, prevalence 1/1,000,000)
  - Secondary amenorrhea
  - Features of hyperandrogenism
  - Abnormal fat distribution (dorsocervical fat pad [buffalo hump], spider legs, significant central obesity)
  - Abdominal striae due to weakening of skin integument
  - Easy bruising
  - Hypertension
  - Proximal muscle weakness
- Hypothyroidism
  - Secondary amenorrhea
  - Lethargy
  - Constipation
  - Decreased appetite
  - Weight gain
  - Cold intolerance
  - Hair loss
  - Dry skin
  - Hypotension
  - Bradycardia
- Primary ovarian insufficiency (previously premature ovarian failure)
  - Secondary amenorrhea prior to the age of 40
  - History of oophorectomy or pelvic radiation or chemotherapy
  - Vasomotor symptoms

- Dry, thin vaginal mucosa without rugosity
    - Associated autoimmune or karyotypic abnormalities possible
- Hyperprolactinemia
    - Usually presents with secondary amenorrhea
    - History of use of drugs such as antipsychotics, oral contraceptive (OC) pills, antidepressants, antihypertensives, H_2 blockers, opioids, etc.
    - Pituitary adenomas may be associated with headache, vomiting, vision changes
    - Galactorrhea
- Sheehan's syndrome
    - History of secondary amenorrhea following postpartum hemorrhage
    - Failure of lactation
    - Other features of hypopituitarism
- Asherman's syndrome
    - History of D&C
    - Secondary amenorrhea
    - Recurrent miscarriage/infertility
- Functional hypothalamic disorders
    - Usually presents with secondary amenorrhea
    - History of eating disorders, severe exercise or stress
    - Use of street drugs
- Kallmann's syndrome
    - Usually presents with anosmia, congenital defect of development of both the GnRH neurons and olfactory placode

Dx DIAGNOSIS

- First step in the workup of amenorrhea is to rule out pregnancy by serum/urine pregnancy test.
- Diagnostic workup depends on history and physical.
- Primary amenorrhea (Fig. E1-60 and Box E1-7):
    - Pelvic ultrasonography or MRI to detect any anatomic abnormalities of uterus, cervix, ovaries, or vagina. At times examination under anesthesia is needed to assess the pelvic organs.
    - Karyotyping (46,XX in Müllerian agenesis; 46,XY in AIS; 45,XO in Turner's syndrome) is done when uterus is absent or Turner's syndrome is suspected.
    - Serum FSH, TSH/FT4, prolactin, estradiol: FSH 40 mIU/ml along with estradiol <20 pg/ml is indicative of ovarian insufficiency. Prolactin >200 ng/ml is suggestive of prolactinoma. Lower levels may also be associated with prolactinoma. Threshold levels may vary by laboratory, and providers are advised to become familiar with their institution's normal range.
    - Check serum testosterone (male range in AIS; female range in Müllerian agenesis) when uterus is absent or in presence of features of hyperandrogenism.
    - 17-alpha hydroxyprogesterone level in presence of features of hyperandrogenism to rule out CAH. In addition to high level of 17 alpha hydroxyprogesterone due to compromised 21-hydroxylase activity, these patients have elevated level of serum progesterone and deoxycorticosterone, hypernatremia, and hypokalemia.
    - MRI of head in presence of:
- Primary hypogonadotrophic hypogonadism.
    - Hyperprolactinemia.
    - Visual field defects.
    - Headaches.
    - Signs of hypothalamic-pituitary dysfunction.
- Secondary amenorrhea (Fig. E1-61):
    - Serum FSH, TSH/FT4, prolactin, estradiol:

TABLE 1-29 Congenital Anatomic Causes of Primary Amenorrhea with Normal Breast Development*

Diagnosis	Müllerian Agenesis	Androgen Insensitivity (AI)	Transverse Vaginal Septum	Imperforate Hymen
Patients with primary amenorrhea†	15%	1%	3%	1%
Patients with primary amenorrhea and apparent obstruction or absence of vagina†	75%	5%	15%	5%
Chromosomes‡	46,XX	46,XY	46,XX	46,XX
Gonads	Ovaries	Testes	Ovaries	Ovaries
Serum testosterone‡	Normal female level	Normal male level (high)	Normal female level	Normal female level
Vagina	Absent or shallow	Absent or shallow	Obstructed by septum which may be thick or thin, high or low	Obstructed by thin membrane, which may look blue from hematocolpos
Axillary/pubic hair	+	Absent unless AI is incomplete	+	+
Cyclic pain	±	−	+	+
Uterus	Absent or rudimentary	−	+	+
Mass	−	−	+ Can present with acute urinary retention as hematocolpos mass obstructs urethra	+ Can present with acute urinary retention
Introitus bulges with Valsalva maneuver	−	−	−	+
Associated anomalies	Urinary tract and skeletal	Inguinal hernias; gonadal malignancy in adulthood	Major urinary tract abnormalities in 15%	Possibly some increase in urinary tract abnormalities
Treatment	Vaginal dilation or surgical neovagina	Gonadectomy after age 16-18 yr Vaginal dilation or surgical neovagina	Surgical approach depends on extent and location of septum; may be extensive; should be done as soon as possible	Excision of hymen as soon as possible; diagnostic needle aspiration contraindicated because of risk of infection
Fertility	Advanced reproductive technology required; in vitro fertilization surrogate with uterus to gestate pregnancy	Not fertile	Variable, low septa have a better prognosis than do high septa	Usually fertile

+, Present; −, absent; ±, may be present or absent.
*Cervix not visible on pelvic examination. Short vagina; may be absent or obstructed.
†Data from Reindollar RH, Byrd JR, McDonough PG: Delayed sexual development: a study of 252 patients, *Am J Obstet Gynecol* 140:371, 1981.
‡Sometimes useful in differentiating Müllerian agenesis from androgen insensitivity.
From Kliegman RM et al: *Practical strategies in pediatric diagnosis and therapy,* ed 2, Philadelphia, 2004, Elsevier.

- Low serum FSH with low estradiol indicates secondary (hypogonadotropic) hypogonadism.
- High serum FSH with low estradiol suggests primary (hypergonadotropic) hypogonadism.
- Progesterone withdrawal bleeding.
    - 10 mg medroxyprogesterone is given for 10 days.
    - Withdrawal bleeding suggests euestrogenic anovulation in presence of normal end organ (outflow tract) and ovarian function.
- Estrogen-progesterone withdrawal bleeding:
    - In the absence of progesterone withdrawal bleeding, the patients are exposed to 25 to 35 days of estrogen (0.625-2.5 mg Premarin daily) followed by 10 days of medroxyprogesterone.
    - Withdrawal bleeding indicates hypogonadism.
    - Absence of bleeding suggests defects with end organ (e.g., Asherman's syndrome).
- Serum LH, testosterone and DHEA-S:
    - When features of hyperandrogenism seen these tests are ordered.
    - Serum testosterone >200 ng/ml suggests androgen-producing adrenal or ovarian tumors (high index of suspicion with moderate elevation; threshold value not required in cases of ovarian or adrenal tumors). This level may be mildly elevated in patients with PCOS.
    - DHEA-S >700 mcg/dl suggests adrenal origin over ovarian (high index of suspicion with moderate elevation; threshold value not required in cases of ovarian or adrenal tumors).
    - LH/FSH ratio >2 in patient with PCOS.
- Pelvic ultrasound when PCOS or ovarian tumor suspected.
- Abdominal CT when adrenal tumor suspected.
- MRI of head when indicated.
- HSG, sonohysterography, or diagnostic hysteroscopy in patients with suspected Asherman's syndrome.
- Karyotyping is indicated when POF occurs before the age of 30.
- Other tests which are rarely needed:
    - Serum transferrin when hemochromatosis is suspected.
    - Serum ACE when sarcoidosis is suspected.

Rx TREATMENT

- The treatment of amenorrhea depends on the etiology, as well as the aims of the patient, such as a desire to treat hirsutism or to become pregnant.
- In the absence of pregnancy, withdrawal bleeding may be induced in the majority of patients with amenorrhea using 5 to 10 mg of medroxyprogesterone for 10 days.
- Estrogen replacement along with calcium and vitamin D should be instituted in essentially every patient with hypogonadism to avoid osteoporosis. Women with a uterus require continuous or intermittent progesterone administration to protect against endometrial hyperplasia or cancer. Frequently, it is easiest to prescribe combination OC pills. For most patients, continuation until ~50 years, the usual age of menopause, seems reasonable. Young women in whom secondary sex characteristics have failed to develop fully should be exposed initially to very low dose estrogen (0.3 mg of conjugated equine estrogen or equivalent) given unopposed daily for 6 mo with incremental dose increases at 6-mo intervals until the required maintenance dose is achieved. Cyclic progesterone therapy, 12 to 14 days per month, should be instituted once vaginal bleeding ensues.
- Most patients with anatomic abnormalities will require surgical correction. Creation of a new vagina for patients with Müllerian agenesis is usually delayed until the woman is emotionally mature and ready to participate in the postoperative care required to maintain vaginal patency. However, if adequate correction is impossible, pregnancy will often require a surrogate to carry a gestation. One should not forget to look for the associated urogenital anomalies in these patients and, when present, treat them appropriately.
- In patients with androgen insensitivity syndrome, the incidence of gonadal malignancy is 22%. However, it rarely occurs before the age of 20. Gonadectomy is performed by laparoscopy following breast development and the attainment of adult stature. In the absence of a uterus these individuals only need estrogen replacement without progesterone.
- Women with adult-onset CAH may be treated with low-dose corticosteroids in addition to sex steroids to partially block ACTH stimulation of adrenal function and thereby decrease overproduction of adrenal androgens.
- Patients with primary ovarian insufficiency (POI) will need estrogen and progesterone replacement. These patients will require in vitro fertilization using donor oocytes to conceive. These patients have an increased risk of osteoporosis and heart disease. It can also be associated with autoimmune disorders such as hypothyroidism, Addison's disease, and diabetes mellitus. Therefore, fasting blood glucose, TSH, and, if clinically appropriate, morning cortisol should be measured. In the presence of a Y chromosome, removal of gonadal tissue is recommended at the time of diagnosis to avoid gonadal tumors.
- Hypothyroidism should be treated with thyroid replacement.
- Hyperprolactinemia is treated by avoiding the culprit drugs or by giving dopamine agonists, such as bromocriptine or cabergoline. Pituitary adenomas rarely require surgery but may be performed if secondary deficits such as visual changes are observed, when they are resistant to medical therapy, or the lesion is rapidly growing.
- Treatment of hypothalamic amenorrhea depends on the etiology. Patients with eating disorders or who exercise excessively will require behavioral modification and nutritional counseling. Elite athletes may choose not to alter their exercise regimens and will therefore require estrogen treatment and prevention of osteoporosis. When associated with infertility, ovulation induction with clomiphene citrate, exogenous gonadotropins, or pulsatile GnRH therapy should be offered.
- The primary treatment of PCOS is weight loss through diet and exercise. Other treatment options include:
    1. Use of OC pills or cyclic progestational agents to help maintain a normal endometrium.
    2. Insulin-sensitizing agents such as metformin to reduce insulin resistance and improve ovulatory function. Recent studies suggest that insulin-sensitizing agents may not be as effective in improving ovulatory effort.
    3. Oral contraceptives and/or spironolactone to treat hyperandrogenism.
    4. Clomiphene citrate or an aromatase inhibitor such as letrozole to induce ovulation.
- In patients with Asherman's syndrome, hysteroscopic lysis of intrauterine adhesions is followed by administration of long-term exogenous estrogen to stimulate regrowth of endometrial tissue.
- Geneticist consult is given in patients with hereditary causes of amenorrhea.
- Psychiatrist consult is needed in patients with major depression, anorexia nervosa, bulimia nervosa, or other major psychiatric disorders.

COMPLICATIONS

- Osteoporosis
- Endometrial hyperplasia and uterine cancer
- Infertility

PROGNOSIS

Depends on the primary cause of amenorrhea

PATIENT EDUCATION

- Patients with amenorrhea should be reassured that this is, in and of itself, not a concern.
- All women with an intact endometrium should understand the risks of unopposed estrogen action, whether the estrogen is exogenous such as through hormone therapy, or endogenous such as PCOS.
- Hypoestrogenic women should be counseled about the importance of estrogen replacement to protect against bone loss.
- Potential for future childbearing should be discussed.

SUGGESTED READINGS

available at www.expertconsult.com

RELATED CONTENT

Infertility (Related Key Topic)
Pituitary Adenoma (Related Key Topic)
Polycystic Ovary Syndrome (Related Key Topic)
Sheehan's Syndrome (Related Key Topic)
Amenorrhea (Patient Information)

AUTHOR: **HEMANT K. SATPATHY, M.D.**

BASIC INFORMATION

The word "amnesia" is derived from the Greek word *amnéstia* meaning "forgetfulness."

DEFINITION

The acquired inability to learn new, or recall previously learned information. The impairment compromises social and occupational functioning. It is caused by an identifiable medical condition or by persisting effects of a substance. Disorder is not caused by delirium or dementia. It may be transient or chronic.

SOME WELL-KNOWN AMNESTIC DISORDERS

Korsakoff syndrome
Transient global amnesia

Dementia, delirium, and amnestic disorders have been subsumed under the category, "Neurocognitive Disorders" in DSM-5.
With behavioral disturbance:
ICD-9CM and DSM-5 CODES
294.11
ICD-10CM CODES
F02.81
Without behavioral disturbance:
ICD-9CM and DSM-5 CODES
294.10
ICD-10CM CODES
F02.80

EPIDEMIOLOGY & DEMOGRAPHICS

INCIDENCE: Data not available on true incidence or lifetime risk of most amnestic disorders. Transient global amnesia has an incidence in the general population of 23 to 50 per 100,000 population over age 50.
PREDOMINANT AGE: Variable, depending on causative pathology. Transient global amnesia onset usually after age 50 years. Korsakoff syndrome usually presents in patients after the age of 40.
GENETICS: Genetic defect for thiamine metabolism has been described in Korsakoff syndrome.

PHYSICAL FINDINGS & CLINICAL PRESENTATION

HISTORY
- Diagnosis depends on history.
- The inability to learn new or recall previously learned information is the key feature of this disorder.
- The Mini-Mental State Examination is useful. Patients unable to recall events that transpire during the interview but may have a normal digit span and be able to attend to the conversation.
- Neuropsychiatric testing demonstrates specific memory impairments in absence of other cognitive deficits
- Patients are unable to recall events subsequent to the onset of the amnesia.
- Individuals may learn new motor tasks but are unable to recall those learning experiences.
- Amnesia generally is both anterograde and retrograde.
- Commonly, patients are disoriented to time and place. Most lack insight while others may have insight but appear indifferent. Some present with personality change or confabulation.
- Table 1-30 describes memory systems. Clinico-anatomic correlations of memory disorders are described in Table 1-31.

ETIOLOGY (MEDICAL CONDITIONS AND PERSISTENT EFFECTS OF DRUGS)

The etiology can be either medical or due to the persistent effects of a substance/chemical.
- Traumatic brain injury
- Focal tumors or infarction
- Herpes simplex encephalitis
- Cerebral anoxia
- Korsakoff syndrome (thiamine deficiency)
- Carbon monoxide poisoning
- Transient amnesia may arise from concussion, acute intoxication, anesthesia, medications, seizures, transient global amnesia, and electroconvulsive therapy
- Persistent effects of drugs (note that this must not be because of acute effects of intoxication or withdrawl)

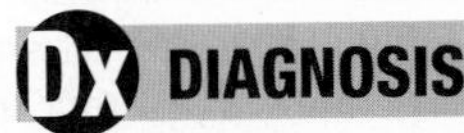

DIAGNOSIS

DIFFERENTIAL DIAGNOSIS

- Dementia
- Delirium
- Major depression
- Minimal cognitive impairment
- Dissociative amnesia
- Memory impairment in substance intoxication or withdrawal
- Malingering
- Factitious disorder

WORKUP

- Complete medical history and mental status testing, with emphasis on identifying underlying medical condition and/or history of drug use
- Neuropsychological testing

LABORATORY TESTS

Tests to determine potential underlying medical condition (e.g., B_{12} levels, TSH, brain imaging).

IMAGING STUDIES

- No specific or diagnostic features of amnestic disorder are detectable on imaging.
- Brain MRI indicates specific atrophy in diencephalic structures in Korsakoff syndrome and in the hippocampus in hypoxic amnesia.
- Neuroradiologic examination with MRI is valuable in the diagnosis of acute Wernicke's encephalopathy.

TABLE 1-30 Description of Memory Systems

Type of Memory Function	Regional Localization	Learning Efficiency	Time Span until Effective Retrieval	Capacity	Clinical Testing Techniques	Examples in Daily Life
Declarative episodic memory	Hippocampus, medial thalamus	Single exposure	Decades	Very large, with rehearsal and elaboration	Recall of 3-4 words after 5 min	Recall of recent events and conversations
Declarative semantic memory	Temporal-parietal association cortices	Capable of single exposure; enhanced with repetition	Decades	Very large, perhaps limitless	Confrontation naming, general knowledge	Vocabulary, knowledge of life events from remote past
Attention span, "immediate memory"	Primary auditory or visual cortex	Single exposure only	Seconds	Very small: 7 ± 2 digits (auditory)	Digit span	Dialing a telephone number after hearing it or reading it
Working memory	Lateral frontal cortex	Single exposure only	Seconds	Small	Digits backward	Supporting many mental activities, such as mental arithmetic, abstract reasoning
Procedural memory	Basal ganglia, probably association neocortices	Requires extensive training	Decades	Moderate	Experimental laboratory methods only	Retention of motor skills, e.g., riding a bicycle or typing

From Goldman L, Schafer AI: *Goldman's Cecil medicine*, ed 24, Philadelphia, 2012, Saunders.

TABLE 1-31 Clinico-Anatomic Correlations of Memory Disorders

Anatomic Site of Damage	Memory Finding	Other Neurologic and Medical Findings
Frontal lobe	Lateralized deficits in working memory—right: spatial defects, left: verbal defects, impaired recall with spared recognition	Personality change Perseveration Chorea, dystonia Bradykinesia, tremor, rigidity
Basal forebrain	Domain-independent declarative memory deficits	
Ventromedial cortex	Frontal lobe-type declarative memory deficits	Upper visual field defects
Hippocampus and parahippocampal cortex	Bilateral lesions yield global amnesia, unilateral lesions show lateralization of deficits—left: verbal deficits; right: spatial deficits	Myoclonus Depressed level of consciousness Cortical blindness Autonomations
Fornix	Global amnesia	
Mammillary bodies	Declarative memory deficits	Confabulation, ataxia, nystagmus, signs of alcohol withdrawal
Dorsal and medial dorsal nucleus thalamus	Declarative memory deficits	Confabulation
Anterior thalamus	Declarative memory deficits	
Lateral temporal cortex	Deficits in autobiographical memory	

From Goetz CG, Pappert EJ: *Textbook of clinical neurology*, Philadelphia, 1999, Saunders.

- Brain MR diffusion-weighted imaging may show hippocampal lesions in transient global amnesia.

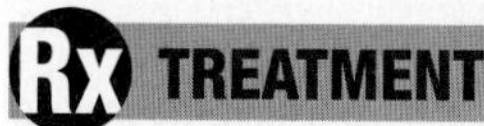

TREATMENT

Treatment is as diverse as the medical conditions causing it.

NONPHARMACOLOGIC THERAPY

- Cognitive rehabilitation to promote recovery from brain injury may be helpful.
- Supervised living to ensure appropriate long-term care.

ACUTE GENERAL Rx

Initial treatment directed to the underlying etiology. Generally, transient global amnesia has full remission of symptoms. Korsakoff, on the other hand, is not usually improved significantly, even after administration of thiamine.

CHRONIC Rx

No known effective treatments to reverse or ameliorate memory deficits.

DISPOSITION

Amnesias may be chronic or transient depending upon etiology.

REFERRAL

Refer for neuropsychological testing.

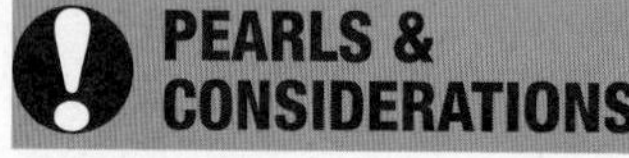

PEARLS & CONSIDERATIONS

COMMENTS

In Korsakoff syndrome, anterograde amnesia (disturbance in acquisition of new information) is more prominent than retrograde amnesia (problems remembering old information).

PREVENTION

Cases of amnestic disorder due to trauma are usually not preventable. Refraining from abuse of alcohol and other drugs prevents substance-induced amnestic disorder, and high-dose thiamine has been shown to prevent Korsakoff syndrome.

PATIENT & FAMILY EDUCATION

Respite care and in-home services for family caregivers

SUGGESTED READINGS

available at www.expertconsult.com

AUTHOR: **WASIM RASHID, M.D.**

BASIC INFORMATION

DEFINITION

Amyotrophic lateral sclerosis (ALS) is a progressive, degenerative neuromuscular condition of undetermined etiology affecting corticospinal tracts and anterior horn cells, resulting in dysfunction of both upper motor neurons (UMN) and lower motor neurons (LMN), respectively.

SYNONYMS

Lou Gehrig's disease

ICD-9CM CODES
335.20 Amyotrophic lateral sclerosis
ICD-10CM CODES
G12.21 Amyotrophic lateral sclerosis

EPIDEMIOLOGY & DEMOGRAPHICS

INCIDENCE:
- 0.5 to 2 cases per 100,000 persons.
- Onset is usually between the ages of 50 and 70 yr.
- Male/female ratio is 2:1.

PREVALENCE: Five in 100,000 persons

PHYSICAL FINDINGS & CLINICAL PRESENTATION

- LMN signs (weakness, hypotonia, wasting, fasciculations, hypoflexia or areflexia).
- UMN signs (loss of fine motor dexterity, spasticity, extensor plantar responses, hyperreflexia, clonus).
- Preservation of extraocular movements, sensation, bowel and bladder function.
- Dysarthria, dysphagia, pseudobulbar affect, frontal lobe dysfunction.
- Respiratory insufficiency typically occurs late in the disease.
- ALS comprises approximately 90% of adult-onset motor neuron diseases. Other presentations of motor neuron disease include progressive muscular atrophy, primary lateral sclerosis, progressive bulbar palsy, progressive pseudobulbar palsy, and ALS-parkinsonism-dementia complex.

ETIOLOGY

- 90% to 95% of all cases are sporadic; of the familial cases, 10% to 20% are associated with a genetic defect in the copper-zinc superoxide dismutase enzyme.

Dx DIAGNOSIS

DIFFERENTIAL DIAGNOSIS

- Multifocal motor neuropathy with conduction block
- Cervical spondylotic myelopathy with polyradiculopathy
- Spinal stenosis with compression of lumbosacral nerve roots
- Chronic inflammatory demyelinating polyneuropathy with central nervous system lesions
- Syringomyelia
- Syringobulbia
- Foramen magnum tumor
- Meningeal carcinomatosis
- Spinal muscular atrophy
- Polyglucosan body disease
- Bulbospinal muscular atrophy (Kennedy disease)
- Monomelic amyotrophy
- ALS-like syndromes have been reported in the setting of lead intoxication, HIV, hyperparathyroidism, hyperthyroidism, lymphoma, and vitamin B_{12} deficiency.

WORKUP

- Electromyography and nerve conduction studies (El Escorial criteria; see Table E1-35)
- Assessment of respiratory function (forced vital capacity [FVC], negative inspiratory force)

LABORATORY TESTS

- Vitamin B_{12}, thyroid function, parathyroid hormone, HIV may be considered.
- Serum protein and immunofixation electrophoresis.
- DNA studies for SMA or bulbospinal atrophy, hexosaminidase levels in pure LMN syndrome.
- 24-hour urine for heavy metals if indicated.

IMAGING STUDIES

- Craniospinal neuroimaging contingent on clinical scenario
- Modified barium swallow to evaluate aspiration risk

Rx TREATMENT

NONPHARMACOLOGIC THERAPY

- Noninvasive positive-pressure ventilation may improve quality of life and may increase tracheostomy-free survival in patients with respiratory difficulty (defined by orthopnea or FVC 50% of predicted).
- Percutaneous endoscopic gastrostomy (PEG) tube placement improves nutritional intake, promotes weight stabilization, and eases medication administration. Some studies suggest PEG placement may prolong life 1 to 4 mo, particularly when placed before FVC falls to ≤50% of predicted value.
- Nutrition, speech therapy, physical and occupational therapy services.
- Suction device for sialorrhea.
- Communication may be eased with computerized assistive devices.
- Early discussion of living will, resuscitation orders, desire for PEG and tracheostomy, potential long-term care options.
- Encourage contact with local support groups.

ACUTE GENERAL Rx

Riluzole (Rilutek), a glutamate antagonist, is the only FDA-approved medication known to extend tracheostomy-free survival in patients with ALS. Dosage is 50 mg q12h, at least 1 hr before or 2 hr after meals. It is shown to prolong survival by 2 to 3 months. Manufacturer recommends checking alanine aminotransferase (ALT) once a month for 3 months initially, followed by once every 3 months until the first year of therapy is completed. ALT should be checked periodically thereafter.

CHRONIC Rx

- Sialorrhea may respond to either glycopyrrolate or amitriptyline (consider either propranolol or metoprolol if secretions are thick). Botulinum toxin may be effective in medically refractory cases.
- Spasticity may be treated pharmacologically with baclofen, tizanidine, clonazepam.
- Pseudobulbar affect may improve with amitriptyline, sertraline (Zoloft), or dextromethorphan/quinine.

DISPOSITION

- Mean duration of symptoms is 3 to 5 yr.
- Approximately 20% of patients survive >5 yr.

REFERRAL

- Referral to a neurologist experienced in neuromuscular disease is recommended to confirm the diagnosis. One prospective, population-based study suggested improved survival in subjects treated in a multidisciplinary clinic.
- Gastrointestinal referral for PEG placement is recommended while FVC remains >50% to minimize morbidity attributable to risks inherent to the procedure.

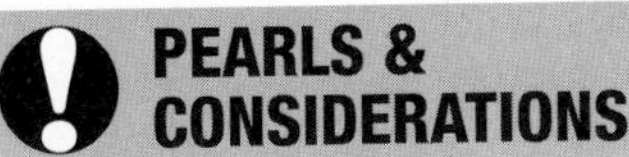

PEARLS & CONSIDERATIONS

- Patient-physician communication is an integral and essential part in both the initial diagnosis and subsequent treatment of ALS.
- A multidisciplinary approach to supportive care may lead to an improved level of daily functioning and foster an increased sense of independence.

SUGGESTED READINGS

available at www.expertconsult.com

RELATED CONTENT

Amyotrophic Lateral Sclerosis (Patient Information)

AUTHOR: **TAYLOR HARRISON, M.D.**

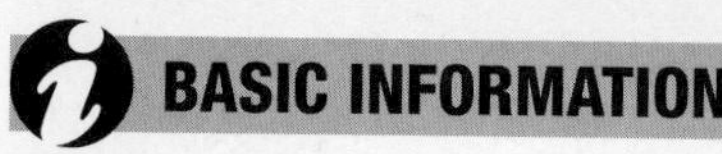

BASIC INFORMATION

DEFINITION

An anaerobic infection is caused by one of a group of bacteria that requires a reduced oxygen tension for growth.

ICD-9CM CODES
See specific condition

ICD-10CM CODES
A41.4 Sepsis, anaerobic
A48 Cellulitis, anaerobic

PHYSICAL FINDINGS & CLINICAL PRESENTATION

- May occur at any site, but most are anatomically related to mucosal surfaces
- Should be suspected when there is foul-smelling tissue, soft tissue gas, necrotic tissue, or abscesses
- Head and neck
  1. Odontogenic infections from dental or soft tissue possibly progressing to periapical abscesses, at times extending to bone
  2. Both anaerobic and aerobic pathogens in chronic sinusitis, chronic mastoiditis, peritonsillar abscess, and chronic otitis media
  3. Complications: deep neck space infections, brain abscesses, mediastinitis
  4. Specific examples of anaerobic infections in head and neck:
     a. Ludwig's angina: bilateral infection of sublingual and submandibular spaces that causes swelling of the base of the tongue with potential airway compromise. Usually mixed aerobic and anaerobic flora
     b. Lemierre's syndrome: jugular vein suppurative thrombophlebitis caused by anaerobic bacteria: *Fusobacterium necrophorum*
- Pleuropulmonary
  1. May involve anaerobes present in the oropharynx
  2. Aspiration more common in persons with altered mental status or seizures
  3. Anaerobic bacteria more likely in those with gingivitis or periodontitis
  4. Manifestations: necrotizing pneumonia, empyema, lung abscess
- Intraabdominal
  1. Disruption of intestinal integrity leading to infection involving anaerobic bacteria
  2. Bacteria from colonic neoplasm, perforated appendicitis, diverticulitis, or bowel surgery, causing bacteremia, peritonitis, at times intraabdominal abscesses
  3. Resulting infections usually mixed, containing both anaerobes and aerobes
- Female genital tract
  1. Anaerobes in bacterial vaginosis, salpingitis, endometritis, pelvic abscesses, septic abortion; infections tend to be mixed
  2. Possible pelvic thrombophlebitis when resolving pelvic infection is accompanied by new or persistent fever
- Other anaerobic infections
  1. Skin and soft tissue infection at any site
  2. More commonly associated infections: synergistic gangrene, bite wound infections, infected decubitus ulcers
  3. Clinical significance of anaerobes in diabetic foot infections unclear
  4. Anaerobic bacteremia uncommon with source usually intraabdominal, followed by female genital tract, pleuropulmonary, and head and neck infections
  5. Osteomyelitis especially when associated with decubitus ulcers or vascular insufficiency
  6. Facial bone osteomyelitis from adjacent infections of the teeth or sinuses

ETIOLOGY

- Most commonly endogenous, arising from bacteria that normally line mucosal surfaces
- Disruption of mucosal barriers resulting from various conditions (trauma, ischemia, surgery, perforation), with infection occurring when organisms gain access to normally sterile sites, causing tissue destruction and abscess formation
- Synergy between different anaerobes or between anaerobes and aerobes important
- Examples of anaerobic bacteria include gram-negative bacteria such as *Bacterioides* species, *Fusobacterium* and *Prevotella* species; and gram-positive bacteria such as *Peptostreptococcus, Clostridium* species, and *Actinomyces* species

Dx DIAGNOSIS

DIFFERENTIAL DIAGNOSIS

- Primary differential possibility is an aerobic bacterial infection without the presence of anaerobic bacteria.
- Ischemic necrosis without accompanying anaerobic infection (or "dry" gangrene [noninfected necrosis] vs. "wet" gangrene [infected tissue with anaerobic infection]).

WORKUP

- Specimens submitted for anaerobic culture should be processed within 30 min and may take up to 5 to 7 days to grow
- Large volume of material more likely to have significant growth; swabs less efficient for transporting infected material
- Blood cultures—preferably before antibiotic administration

LABORATORY TESTS

- Elevated WBC count, with extremely high WBC counts sometimes seen with pseudomembranous colitis
- Positive stool *C. difficile* toxin A and B assay
- Increased lactate levels in ischemia or perforation
- Possible positive blood or wound cultures, but failure to grow anaerobes in culture may be common, attributed to inadequate culturing techniques or fastidious organisms

IMAGING STUDIES

- Plain film of an affected area to show gas in tissues, free air resulting from a perforated viscus, or an air/fluid level inside an abscess
- Ultrasound, CT scan, or MRI to reveal abscesses or tissue destruction

Rx TREATMENT

NONPHARMACOLOGIC THERAPY

- Removal of necrotic tissue
- Drainage of abscesses (accomplished by CT scan–guided percutaneous drainage)

ACUTE GENERAL Rx

Oral antibiotics with anaerobic activity: clindamycin, metronidazole, and chloramphenicol

- Broader spectrum of activity with amoxicillin/clavulanate
- Penicillin VK in odontogenic infections
- Oral metronidazole for *C. difficile*–associated diarrhea, with oral vancomycin used for severe, recurrent, or recalcitrant infections

Parenteral antibiotics for more serious illness

- IV clindamycin, metronidazole, and chloramphenicol
- Cephalosporins (anaerobic or mixed infections): cefoxitin and cefotetan
- Extended-spectrum penicillins (e.g., piperacillin) and combination beta-lactamase plus beta-lactamase inhibitor drugs (e.g., clavulanic acid, sulbactam, tazobactam)
  1. Significant anaerobic activity, plus various degrees of broad-spectrum coverage
  2. Include ampicillin/sulbactam, ticarcillin/clavulanate, and piperacillin/tazobactam
- Imipenem or other carbapenems, such as meropenem, doripenem, or ertapenem, which are broad-spectrum agents with extensive anaerobic activity
- Actinomycosis treated with penicillin for 6 to 12 mo
- SMX/TMP and fluoroquinolones are generally ineffective, but some newer quinolones (e.g., moxifloxacin) have inhibitory activity against anaerobes

DISPOSITION

It is essential that all necrotic debris be removed when treating an anaerobic infection or it will recur; follow-up is critically important to ensure resolution of the process.

REFERRAL

Refer to a surgeon if drainage is required; infectious disease consultation may be useful in complicated patients or if treatment regimen is failing or slow to respond.

SUGGESTED READINGS
available at www.expertconsult.com

AUTHOR: **GLENN G. FORT, M.D., M.P.H.**

BASIC INFORMATION

DEFINITION

A fissure is a tear in the epithelial lining of the anal canal (i.e., from the dentate line to the anal verge).

SYNONYMS

Anorectal fissure
Anal ulcer

ICD-9CM CODES
565.0 Anal fissure
ICD-10CM CODES
K60.2 Anal fissure, unspecified

EPIDEMIOLOGY & DEMOGRAPHICS

PREDOMINANT SEX: Occurs in men more than women. Women are more likely to have anterior fissure than men (10% vs. 1%, respectively). Common in women before and after childbirth.
PREDOMINANT AGE: Can occur at any age. Most common in young and middle-aged adults. Most common cause of rectal bleeding in infants.

PHYSICAL FINDINGS & CLINICAL PRESENTATION

With separation of the buttocks will see a tear in the posterior midline or, less frequently, in the anterior midline (Fig. 1-65)

- Acute anal fissure:
  1. Sharp burning or tearing pain exacerbated by bowel movements
  2. Bright-red blood on toilet paper, a streak of blood on the stool or in the water
- Chronic anal fissure:
  1. Pruritus ani
  2. Pain seldom present
  3. Intermittent bleeding
  4. Sentinel tag at the caudal aspect of the fissure, hypertrophied anal papilla at the proximal end
- Underlying disease possible if the fissure:
  1. Is ectopically located
  2. Extends proximal to the dentate line
  3. Is broad-based or deep
  4. Is especially purulent

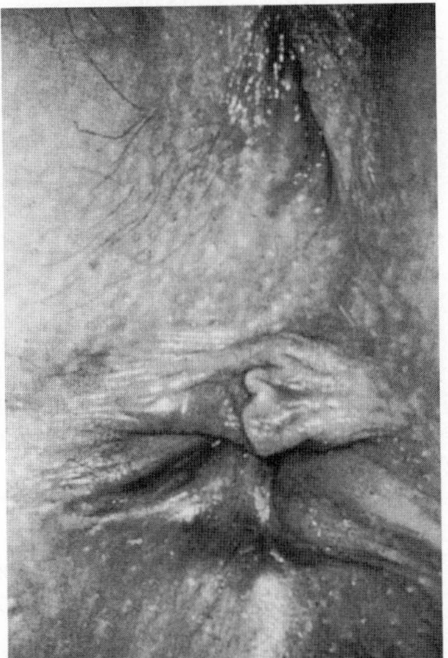

FIGURE 1-65 Lateral anal fissure. (From Seidel HM et al: *Mosby's guide to physical examination,* ed 3, St Louis, 1995, Mosby. Courtesy Gershon Efron, MD, Sinai Hospital of Baltimore.)

ETIOLOGY

- Most initiated after passage of a large, hard stool
- May result from frequent defecation and diarrhea
- Bacterial infections: tuberculosis (TB), syphilis, gonorrhea, chancroid, lymphogranuloma venereum
- Viral infections: herpes simplex virus, cytomegalovirus, human immunodeficiency virus
- Inflammatory bowel disease (IBD): Crohn's disease, ulcerative colitis
- Trauma: surgery (hemorrhoidectomy), foreign bodies, anal intercourse
- Malignancy: carcinoma, lymphoma, Kaposi sarcoma

DIAGNOSIS

DIFFERENTIAL DIAGNOSIS

- Proctalgia fugax
- Thrombosed hemorrhoid
- Carcinoma

WORKUP

- Digital rectal examination after lubricating the entire anus with anesthetic jelly (i.e., 2% lidocaine) and waiting 5 to 10 min
- Anoscopy
- Proctosigmoidoscopy to exclude inflammatory or neoplastic disease
- Biopsy if doubt exists about the etiology of the condition
- All studies done under adequate anesthesia

IMAGING STUDIES

- Colonoscopy if diagnosis of IBD or malignancy is suspected
- Small-bowel series occasionally obtained for similar reasons

TREATMENT

NONPHARMACOLOGIC THERAPY

- Sitz baths
- High-fiber diet
- Increased oral fluid intake

ACUTE GENERAL Rx

- Bulk-producing agent (e.g., Metamucil) or stool softener
- Local anesthetic jelly (may exacerbate pruritus ani)
- Nitroglycerin ointment (0.4%): apply 1 inch of ointment (equivalent to 1.5 mg of nitroglycerin) intraanally every 12 hours for up to 3 weeks. This medication (Reactiv) is expensive (over $400 for 30-g tube) and can cause headaches. Topical Diltiazem (compounded by pharmacist) is also effective and much less expensive.
- Suppositories *not* recommended
- Surgery

CHRONIC Rx

- Surgery: lateral internal anal sphincterotomy. It is a more durable treatment for chronic anal fissure compared with topical nitroglycerin therapy and does not compromise long-term fecal continence
- Topical glyceryl trinitrate ointment
- Injection of botulinum toxin (an injection into each side of the internal anal sphincter) is effective in healing chronic anal fissures in more than 90% of patients

DISPOSITION

Outpatient surgery

REFERRAL

- If fissure does not resolve with conservative therapy in 4 to 6 wk
- If patient prefers surgery for acute fissure
- If patient has chronic fissure

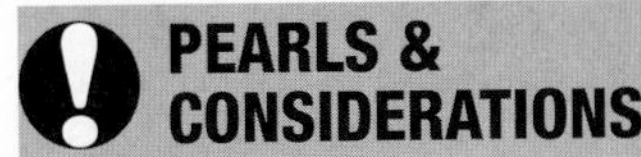

PEARLS & CONSIDERATIONS

COMMENTS

HIV-positive patients should be referred to clinicians who are well versed in the myriad infectious and neoplastic conditions that masquerade as anal ulcers in these patients.

SUGGESTED READINGS

available at www.expertconsult.com

RELATED CONTENT

Anorectal Fistula (Related Key Topic)
Hemorrhoids (Related Key Topic)
Anal Fissure (Patient Information)

AUTHOR: **RUBEN ALVERO, M.D.**

BASIC INFORMATION

DEFINITION

Anaphylaxis is a sudden-onset, life-threatening event characterized by respiratory, cardiovascular, gastrointestinal, and cutaneous manifestations, as well as vasodilatory hemodynamic changes in response to a particular allergen. Anaphylactoid reaction is closely related to anaphylaxis. It is caused by release of mast cells and basophil mediators triggered by non–IgE–mediated events.

SYNONYMS

Anaphylactoid reaction.

ICD-9CM CODES

995.0	Anaphylactic shock
995.60	Anaphylaxis due to food
999.4	Anaphylaxis due to immunization
977.9	Anaphylaxis due to drugs
989.5	Anaphylaxis following stings

ICD-10CM CODES

T78.2	Anaphylactic shock, unspecified, initial encounter
T78.00XA	Anaphylactic reaction due to unspecified food, initial encounter
T80.52XA	Anaphylactic reaction due to vaccination, initial encounter
T50.904A	Poisoning by unspecified drugs, medicaments, and biologic substances, undetermined, initial encounter
T63.94XA	Toxic effect of contact with unspecified venomous animal, undetermined, initial encounter

EPIDEMIOLOGY & DEMOGRAPHICS

INCIDENCE: The incidence of anaphylaxis in the U.S. is 58.9 cases per 100,000 person-years. Lifetime prevalence is 0.05% to 2%, with a mortality rate of 1%. Anaphylaxis rates are 0.0004% for food, 0.7% to 10% for penicillin, 0.22% to 1% for radiocontrast media, and 0.5% to 5% after insect stings. Annual mortality is 500 to 1000 persons per year in the U.S.

PHYSICAL FINDINGS & CLINICAL PRESENTATION

- Urticaria, pruritus, skin flushing, angioedema
- Dyspnea, cough, wheezing, shortness of breath
- Nausea, vomiting, diarrhea, difficulty swallowing
- Hypotension, tachycardia, weakness, dizziness, malaise, vascular collapse

ETIOLOGY

Anaphylaxis results from sudden systematic release of histamine and other inflammatory mediators from basophils and mast cells. This causes swelling of the mucus membranes and the urticarial rash on the skin. Virtually any substance may induce anaphylaxis.

- Foods and food additives: peanuts, tree nuts, eggs, shellfish, fish, cow's milk, fruits, soy
- Medications: antibiotics, especially penicillins, insulin, allergen extracts, opiates, vaccines, NSAIDs, contrast media, streptokinase
- Bee or wasp sting, snake venom, fire ant venom
- Blood products, plasma, immunoglobulin, cryoprecipitate, whole blood
- Latex

Dx DIAGNOSIS

DIFFERENTIAL DIAGNOSIS

- Endocrine disorders (carcinoid, pheochromocytoma)
- Globus hystericus, anxiety disorder
- Systemic mastocytosis
- Pulmonary embolism, serum sickness, vasovagal reactions
- Severe asthma (the key clinical difference is the abrupt onset of symptoms in anaphylaxis versus a history of progressive worsening of symptoms)
- Septic shock or other form of vasodilatory shock
- Airway foreign body

WORKUP

Workup is aimed at ruling out other conditions that may mimic anaphylaxis (e.g., vasovagal syncope may be differentiated by presence of bradycardia as opposed to tachycardia seen in anaphylaxis; the absence of hypoxemia in arterial blood gas [ABG] analysis may be useful to exclude pulmonary embolism or foreign body aspiration).

LABORATORY TESTS

- Laboratory evaluation is generally not helpful because anaphylaxis is typically diagnosed clinically.
- ABG analysis may be useful to exclude pulmonary embolism, status asthmaticus, and foreign body aspiration.
- Elevated serum and urine histamine levels and serum tryptase levels can be useful for diagnosis of anaphylaxis, but these tests are not commonly available in the emergency setting.

IMAGING STUDIES

Generally not helpful.

- Chest radiography for evaluation of foreign body aspiration or pulmonary pathology is indicated in patients with acute respiratory compromise.
- Consider ECG in all patients with sudden loss of consciousness or reports of chest pains or dyspnea and in any elderly patient. ECG in anaphylaxis usually reveals sinus tachycardia.

Rx TREATMENT

NONPHARMACOLOGIC THERAPY

- Establish and protect airway. Provide supplemental O_2 if indicated.
- IV access should be rapidly established, and IV fluids (i.e., normal saline) should be administered. The patient should be placed supine or in Trendelenburg position if hemodynamically unstable.
- Cardiac monitoring is recommended.

ACUTE GENERAL Rx

- Epinephrine should be rapidly administered as an IM injection at a dose of 0.3 mg of aqueous epinephrine for adults and children >30 kg. Epinephrine 0.15 mg should be given for children <30 kg (1:1000 concentration). Intramuscular administration is preferred because it provides more reliable and quicker rise to effective plasma levels. The dose may be repeated after approximately 5-15 min if symptoms persist.
- Adjunct therapies include H_1 and H_2 receptor antagonists, diphenhydramine 25-50 mg IV or IM, or PO in mild cases, and famotidine 20-40 mg IV, or PO in mild cases. Although useful to improve cutaneous erythema and pruritus, H_1 antagonists are not as effective as epinephrine, since onset of action is 1 to 2 hours and they are not effective in reversing upper airway obstruction or improving hypotension.
- Corticosteroids are not useful in the acute episode because of their slow onset of action; however, they should be administered in most cases to prevent prolonged or recurrent anaphylaxis. Commonly used agents are prednisone, methylprednisolone 40 to 250 mg IV in adults (1 to 2 mg/kg in children), or longer-acting dexamethasone.
- Aerosolized β-agonists (e.g., albuterol, 2.5 mg, repeat prn 20 min) are useful to control bronchospasm.
- Vasopressor therapy with epinephrine (1:10,000), or dopamine is indicated in patients with refractory hypotension after crystalloid resuscitation.

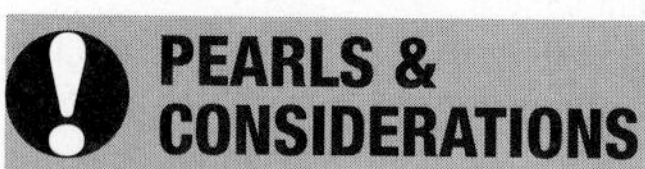

PEARLS & CONSIDERATIONS

COMMENTS

- Patient education regarding the nature of the illness and preventive measures is recommended. A documented history of previous anaphylactic episodes or known anaphylaxis triggers is the most reliable method of identifying individuals at risk.
- Prescription for prefilled epinephrine syringe (EpiPen or EpiPen Jr.) should be given, and the patient should be instructed on the use of this emergency kit, and to carry it on his/her person at all times. School-aged children should keep an additional EpiPen at school with the appropriate staff.
- Patients should also be advised to carry or wear a MedicAlert ID describing substances that have caused anaphylaxis.
- Avoidance of radiologic contrast is also recommended in those who have had a prior reaction. However, pretreatment regimens with methylprednisolone and diphenhydramine exist for those who have had contrast reactions in the past.
- Venom immunotherapy immediately after a sting is effective and recommended for up to 5 yr after the anaphylactic incident.

SUGGESTED READINGS

available at www.expertconsult.com

AUTHOR: **TARA M. WAYT, D.O.**

BASIC INFORMATION

DEFINITION

Aplastic anemia is a bone marrow failure syndrome defined by peripheral blood pancytopenia and hypocellular bone marrow.

SYNONYMS

Refractory anemia
Hypoplastic anemia

ICD-9CM CODES
284.9 Aplastic anemia
284.8 Acquired aplastic anemia
284.0 Congenital aplastic anemia
ICD-10CM CODES
D61.9 Aplastic anemia, unspecified
D60.9 Acquired pure red cell aplasia, unspecified
D60.8 Other acquired pure red cell aplasias

EPIDEMIOLOGY & DEMOGRAPHICS

INCIDENCE: The annual incidence of aplastic anemia is 2 cases per million.
PREDOMINANT SEX AND AGE: The incidence has two peaks, with most patients presenting between ages 15 and 25 or after 60 yr.

PHYSICAL FINDINGS & CLINICAL PRESENTATION

- Mucosal bleeding, easy bruising, petechiae or heavy menstrual bleeding is seen secondary to thrombocytopenia.
- Fatigue, lassitude, skin pallor, exertional dyspnea, or palpitations are seen secondary to anemia.
- Infection is an uncommon presentation, but neutropenia may lead to fever and sore throat.
- Various physical manifestations like short stature, skeletal or nail changes may be seen in congenital forms of aplastic anemia.

ETIOLOGY

- In most patients with idiopathic aplastic anemia, bone marrow failure results from immunologically mediated, active destruction of blood-forming cells by lymphocytes.
- Mutations in *TERT,* the gene for the RNA component of telomerase, cause short telomerases in congenital aplastic anemia and in some cases of apparently acquired hematopoietic failure. In patients with severe aplastic anemia receiving immunosuppressive therapy, telomere length is unrelated to response but is associated with risk of relapse, clonal evolution, and overall survival.
- Common etiologic factors in acquired aplastic anemia include:
  - Toxins (e.g., benzene, insecticides)
  - Drugs (e.g., felbamate [Felbatol], cimetidine, NSAIDs, antiepileptics, gold salts, chloramphenicol, sulfonamides, trimethadione, quinacrine, phenylbutazone)
  - Ionizing irradiation
  - Infections (e.g., hepatitis C, HIV, Epstein-Barr virus, parvovirus B19)
- Inherited aplastic anemia
  - Fanconi's anemia
  - Reticular dysgenesis
  - Dyskeratosis congenita
  - Nonhematologic syndromes (Down syndrome, etc.)
  - Shwachman-Diamond syndrome
- Pregnancy
- Idiopathic

DIAGNOSIS

DIFFERENTIAL DIAGNOSIS

- Bone marrow infiltration from lymphoma, carcinoma, myelofibrosis
- Severe infection
- Hypoplastic myelodysplastic syndrome or hypoplastic acute myeloid leukemia in adults
- Hypersplenism
- Hairy cell leukemia

WORKUP

- Diagnostic workup (Fig. E1-66) consists primarily of bone marrow aspiration and biopsy, and laboratory evaluation (CBC and examination of blood film).
- Bone marrow examination generally shows paucity or absence of erythropoietic and myelopoietic precursor cells (Fig. E1-67, *B* and *C*); patients with pure red cell aplasia demonstrate only absence of red blood cell (RBC) precursors in the marrow.

LABORATORY TESTS

- CBC reveals pancytopenia (Fig. E1-68, *A*). Macrocytosis and toxic granulation of neutrophils may also be present. Isolated cytopenias may occur in the early stages.
- Reticulocyte count reveals reticulocytopenia.
- Additional initial laboratory evaluation should include Ham test and/or peripheral blood flow cytometry to exclude paroxysmal nocturnal hemoglobinuria and testing for hepatitis C.

IMAGING STUDIES

MRI with spin-echo sequence is helpful in the study of bone marrow disease, and the high fat content of an aplastic marrow can be easily seen on MRI.

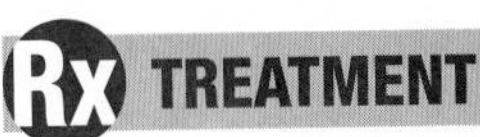

TREATMENT

NONPHARMACOLOGIC THERAPY

Discontinue any offending drugs or agents.

ACUTE GENERAL Rx

- Aggressive treatment of neutropenic fevers with parenteral broad-spectrum antibiotics.
- Administer platelet and RBC transfusions as needed; however, it is important to avoid transfusions in patients who are candidates for bone marrow transplantation.
- Fig. E1-69 describes a treatment algorithm for aplastic anemia.

CHRONIC Rx

- Allogenic bone marrow transplantation (ABMT) from a human leukocyte antigen (HLA)–matched sibling donor is curative.
- Patients who do not have a matched sibling can be treated with a matched unrelated transplant, but the mortality rate is higher.
- Immunosuppressive therapy with antithymocyte globulin (ATG) is an effective alternate treatment for patients who are not candidates for ABMT.
- Other immunosuppressive agents such as cyclosporin, cyclophosphamide, or corticosteroids also have a role in the treatment of aplastic anemia.
- Androgens such as danazol are effective second-line agents.
- The oral thrombopoietin mimetic eltrombopag can improve hematopoiesis in refractory severe aplastic anemia.

DISPOSITION

- The most recent update of the European Group for Bone Marrow Transplantation long-term survival rate has been reported to be 80%.
- Graft rejection and graft-versus-host disease are the major complications of ABMT.

REFERRAL

Hematology referral is indicated in all patients with aplastic anemia.

SUGGESTED READINGS
available at www.expertconsult.com

RELATED CONTENT

Fig. 3-12 Algorithm for Diagnosis of Anemias

AUTHORS: **BILAL H. NAQVI, M.D.,** and **FRED F. FERRI, M.D.**

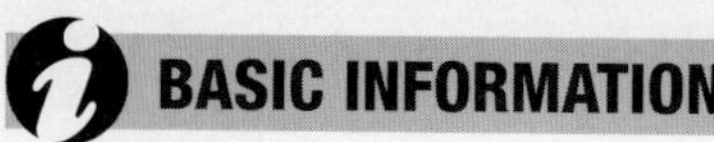

BASIC INFORMATION

DEFINITION

Autoimmune hemolytic anemia (AIHA) is anemia secondary to premature destruction of red blood cells (RBCs) caused by the binding of autoantibodies and/or complement to RBCs. A classification of the hemolytic anemias is described in Table 1-36.

ICD-9CM CODES
283.0 Autoimmune hemolytic anemia
ICD-10CM CODES
D58.9 Drug-induced autoimmune hemolytic anemia

EPIDEMIOLOGY & DEMOGRAPHICS

Predominant sex and age: most common in women <50 yr.

PHYSICAL FINDINGS & CLINICAL PRESENTATION

- Pallor, jaundice.
- Tachycardia with a flow murmur may be present if anemia is pronounced.
- Most common presentation is dyspnea and fatigue.
- Patients with intravascular hemolysis may present with dark urine and back pain.
- The presence of hepatomegaly and/or lymphadenopathy suggests an underlying lymphoproliferative disorder or malignancy; splenomegaly may indicate hypersplenism as a cause of hemolysis.

ETIOLOGY

- Warm antibody mediated: immunoglobulin (Ig) G (often idiopathic or associated with leukemia, lymphoma, thymoma, myeloma, viral infections, and collagen-vascular disease)
- Cold antibody mediated: IgM and complement in majority of cases (often idiopathic; at times associated with infections, lymphoma, or cold agglutinin disease)
- Drug induced: three major mechanisms:
  1. Antibody directed against Rh complex (e.g., methyldopa)
  2. Antibody directed against RBC-drug complex (hapten induced; e.g., penicillin)
  3. Antibody directed against complex formed by drug and plasma proteins; the drug-plasma protein-antibody complex causes destruction of RBCs (innocent bystander; e.g., quinidine)

TABLE 1-36 Classification of the Hemolytic Anemias

Acquired
Environmental factors
Antibody: immunohemolytic anemias
Mechanical trauma: TTP, HUS, heart valve
Toxins, infectious agents: malaria, etc.
Membrane defects
Paroxysmal nocturnal hemoglobinuria
Spur cell anemia
Hereditary spherocytosis, etc.
Congenital
Defects of cell interior
Hemoglobinopathies: sickle cell, thalassemia
Enzymopathies: G6PD deficiency, etc.

G6PD, Glucose-6-phosphate dehydrogenase; *HUS*, hemolytic-uremic syndrome; *TTP*, thrombotic thrombocytopenic purpura.
From Goldman L, Schafer AI: *Goldman's Cecil medicine*, ed 24, Philadelphia, 2012, Saunders.

Dx DIAGNOSIS

DIFFERENTIAL DIAGNOSIS

- Hemolytic anemia caused by membrane defects (paroxysmal nocturnal hemoglobinuria, spur cell anemia, Wilson disease)
- Non–immune mediated (microangiopathic hemolytic anemia, hypersplenism, cardiac valve prosthesis, giant cavernous hemangiomas, march hemoglobinuria, physical agents, infections, heavy metals, certain drugs [nitrofurantoin, sulfonamides, ribavarin])

WORKUP

Evaluation consists primarily of laboratory evaluation to confirm hemolysis and exclude other causes of the anemia. Although most cases of AIHA are idiopathic, potential causes should always be sought. Section III describes an algorithm for evaluation of suspected hemolytic anemia.

LABORATORY TESTS

- Initial laboratory tests: complete blood count (anemia), reticulocyte count (elevated; Fig. E1-70 describes the evaluation of anemia with elevated reticulocyte count), liver function studies (elevated indirect bilirubin, lactate dehydrogenase), evaluation of peripheral smear (Fig. E1-71), Coombs test (positive direct Coombs test indicates presence of antibodies or complement on the surface of RBCs [Fig. E1-72]; positive indirect Coombs test implies presence of anti-RBC antibodies freely circulating in the patient's serum [Fig. E1-73]), haptoglobin level (decreased)
- IgG antibody and IgM antibody
- Hepatitis serology, antinuclear antibody
- Urinary tests may reveal hemosiderinuria or hemoglobinuria

IMAGING STUDIES

- Chest x-ray
- CT scan of chest and abdomen to rule out lymphoma should be considered

Rx TREATMENT

NONPHARMACOLOGIC THERAPY

- Discontinuation of any potentially offensive drugs
- Plasmapheresis exchange transfusion for severe life-threatening cases only
- Avoid cold exposure in patients with cold antibody

ACUTE GENERAL RX

- Prednisone 1 to 2 mg/kg/day in divided doses initially in warm antibody AIHA. Corticosteroids are generally ineffective in cold antibody AIHA.
- Splenectomy in patients responding inadequately to corticosteroids when RBC sequestration studies indicate splenic sequestration.
- Immunosuppressive drugs and/or immunoglobulins only after both corticosteroids and splenectomy (unless surgery is contraindicated) have failed to produce an adequate remission.
- Danazol, typically used in conjunction with corticosteroids (may be useful in warm antibody AIHA).
- Immunosuppressive drugs (azathioprine, cyclophosphamide) may be useful in warm antibody AIHA but are indicated only after both corticosteroids and splenectomy (unless surgery is contraindicated) have failed to produce an adequate remission.

DISPOSITION

Prognosis is generally good unless anemia is associated with underlying disorder with a poor prognosis (e.g., leukemia, myeloma).

REFERRAL

- Hematology referral in all cases of AIHA
- Surgical referral for splenectomy in refractory cases

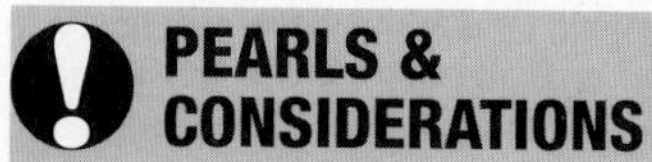

PEARLS & CONSIDERATIONS

COMMENTS

- The direct Coombs test (also known as the direct antiglobulin test) demonstrates the presence of antibodies or complement on the surface of RBCs and is the hallmark of autoimmune hemolysis.
- Warm AIHA is often associated with autoimmune diseases, whereas cold AIHA often follows viral infections (e.g., mononucleosis) and *Mycoplasma pneumoniae* infections.
- HIV can induce both warm and cold AIHA.

SUGGESTED READINGS

available at www.expertconsult.com

RELATED CONTENT

Fig. E3-16 Anemia with reticulocytosis (Algorithm)

AUTHOR: **FRED F. FERRI, M.D.**

BASIC INFORMATION

DEFINITION

Inflammatory anemia refers to mild to moderately severe anemia (with hemoglobin [Hb] ranging from 7-12 g/dl), associated with chronic infections, inflammatory disorders, and some malignancies. Inflammatory anemia is also commonly referred to as anemia of chronic disease (ACD). The anemia is typically normocytic, normochromic, and hypoproliferative.

SYNONYMS

Anemia of chronic disease
Anemia of inflammation
ACD

ICD-9CM CODES
285.21 Anemia in chronic kidney disease
285.22 Anemia in neoplastic disease
285.29 Anemia of other chronic illness
ICD-10CM CODES
D63.8 Anemia in chronic diseases classified elsewhere
D63.0 Anemia in neoplastic disease
D64.8 Anemia, unspecified

EPIDEMIOLOGY & DEMOGRAPHICS

PREVALENCE: The prevalence rate in the elderly ranges from 8% to 44%, with the greatest prevalence in men 85 yr and older.
- Second-most prevalent anemia after iron deficiency anemia
- Perhaps one third of elderly adults with anemia suffer from anemia of chronic disease, anemia of chronic renal failure, or both
  - 11% of men and 10.2% of women age 65 to 85 yr
  - >20% of adults older than 85 yr

PREDOMINANT SEX AND AGE: Male sex >85 yr of age

RISK FACTORS:
- Chronic inflammatory conditions like autoimmune disorders (e.g., rheumatoid arthritis, systemic lupus erythematosus, vasculitis and sarcoidosis, inflammatory bowel disease [Crohn's disease/ulcerative colitis])
- Neoplasia (both hematologic cancer and solid tumors)
- Chronic kidney disease
- Infection (acute/chronic—viral, bacterial, parasitic, and fungal)
- Chronic rejection after solid-organ transplantation

PHYSICAL FINDINGS & CLINICAL PRESENTATION

Most patients are asymptomatic but may have general findings like skin pallor and conjunctival pallor.

ETIOLOGY

It is caused by several mechanisms
- Altered iron homeostasis: Increased uptake and retention of iron within the cells of reticuloendothelial system (RES). Increase in Hepcidin (decreases duodenal iron absorption and blocks iron release from RES)
- Reduced erythrocyte survival
- Reduced erythropoietin production (EPO levels can be elevated in ACD, but are relatively low to the level of anemia)
- Impaired erythropoiesis due to iron restriction and suppressed bone marrow erythroid response to EPO.

DIAGNOSIS

DIFFERENTIAL DIAGNOSIS

Iron deficiency anemia
Other causes of normocytic anemia
- Red blood cell loss or destruction
  - Acute blood loss
  - Hypersplenism
  - Hemolysis
- Decreased red blood cell production
  - Primary causes
    - Marrow hypoplasia or aplasia
    - Myelopathies
    - Myeloproliferative disease
    - Pure red blood cell aplasia
  - Secondary causes
    - Chronic renal failure
    - Liver disease
    - Endocrine deficiency states
    - Sideroblastic anemia

WORKUP

Detailed history and physical examination

LABORATORY TESTS

CBC, reticulocyte count, reticulocyte index and peripheral smear, Serum iron levels, total iron-binding capacity, transferrin saturation, and ferritin and erythropoietin level. Sometimes a bone marrow biopsy is needed. Table E1-37 describes laboratory characteristics of inflammatory anemia. Usual findings are as follows:
- Hb levels (typically): 8 to 9.5 g/dl
- Low reticulocyte count (reflecting ineffective erythropoiesis)
- Low serum iron concentration (also low in iron deficiency anemia)
- Low transferrin saturation (also low in iron deficiency anemia)
- Serum ferritin (marker of iron storage and acute phase reactant) normal or increased (Fig. E1-74).
  - Acute inflammatory states may mimic the hematologic profile of anemia of chronic disease
- Soluble transferrin receptor (sTfR) levels remain within normal limits (elevated in iron deficiency anemia)
  - TfR index (sTfR/log Ferritin): in patients with normal to high ferritin, it helps to differentiate combined ACD/IDA (>2) from ACD (<1) (Fig. E1-74).
- Hepcidin: low in IDA, elevated in ACD and normal in ACD/IDA.
- Erythropoietin level not very useful. Expected to be low in CKD and doesn't alter the management or ESA dose. In other causes of ACD, EPO levels will start to increase whenever Hb <10g/dl.
- Peripheral smear usually reveals hypochromic normocytic RBCs (Fig. E1-75, *A*). Bone marrow shows that erythroid precursors are present in normal numbers (Fig. E1-75, *B*) and iron stores are increased in stromal histiocytes (Fig. E1-76).

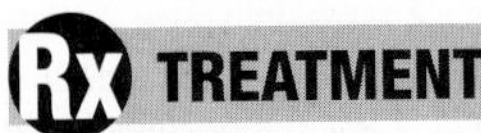

TREATMENT

Treat the underlying disorder/disease.

ACUTE GENERAL Rx

Blood transfusion is usually reserved for severe anemia (with Hb level <7 g/dl or <8 g/dl in patients with cardiac disease) especially if complicated with ongoing bleeding.

CHRONIC Rx

- Erythropoiesis-stimulating agents (ESA) (epoetin alfa and darbepoetin alfa) are FDA approved for use in patients with anemia resulting from:
  - CKD
  - Chemotherapy
  - Zidovudine therapy.

  In June 2011, FDA released modified recommendations for more conservative dosing of (ESA) when used to treat patients with CKD (TREAT trial. Hb target >11g/dl resulted in increase in cardiovascular events and stroke).

  ESA dose should be individualized for each patient and the lowest sufficient dose to reduce blood transfusions should be used (Hb target: not clearly defined!? the lowest possible, 9-10g/dl in most situations)
- Supplemental iron: Before initiation of erythropoietin therapy, iron deficiency needs to be ruled out. After starting ESA therapy, ASH/ASCO guidelines (Rizzo et al, 2010) recommend periodic monitoring of iron status. When no response to oral therapy, parental iron therapy is to be considered before stating that patient is non-responsive to iron therapy (? hepcidin effect). Maintain a transferrin saturation of >20% and a Ferritin ≥100ng/ml.

REFERRAL

Hematology and oncology

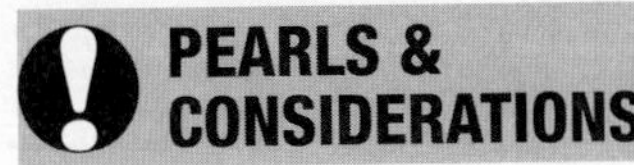

PEARLS & CONSIDERATIONS

COMMENTS

The anemia of inflammation, which also includes anemia of critical illness, is a condition that presents similarly to anemia of chronic disease but develops within days of the onset of illness (major surgery, myocardial infarction, sepsis, major trauma). An anemia similar to anemia of inflammation is seen in some elderly patients in the absence of identifiable chronic disease.

SUGGESTED READINGS

available at www.expertconsult.com

AUTHOR: **TONY ABDO, M.D.**

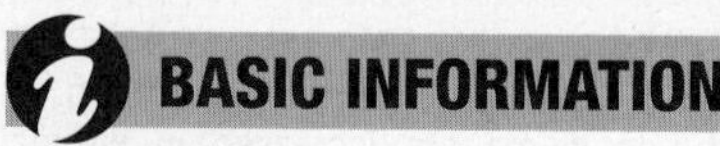

BASIC INFORMATION

DEFINITION

Anemia is defined as a hemoglobin level 2 standard deviations below normal for age and sex. Iron deficiency anemia is anemia resulting from inadequate iron supplementation or excessive blood loss.

ICD-9CM CODES
280.9 Iron deficiency anemia
648.2 Iron deficiency anemia complicating pregnancy

ICD-10CM CODES
D50.9 Iron deficiency anemia, unspecified
O99.019 Anemia complicating pregnancy, unspecified trimester

EPIDEMIOLOGY & DEMOGRAPHICS

- Dietary iron deficiency occurs often in infants as a result of unsupplemented milk diets. It is also commonly seen in women during their reproductive years, as a result of heavy menstrual periods, and during pregnancy (increased demand).
- Iron deficiency is the most common nutritional deficiency worldwide.
- The prevalence of iron deficiency is greatest among toddlers ages 1 to 2 yr (7%) from inadequate intake and female individuals ages 12 to 49 yr (9% to 16%) from menstrual losses.
- The prevalence of iron deficiency is 2% in adult men, 9% to 12% in non-Hispanic white women, and 20% in black and Mexican American women.
- GI cancer is diagnosed in 10% of elderly patients with iron deficiency anemia.

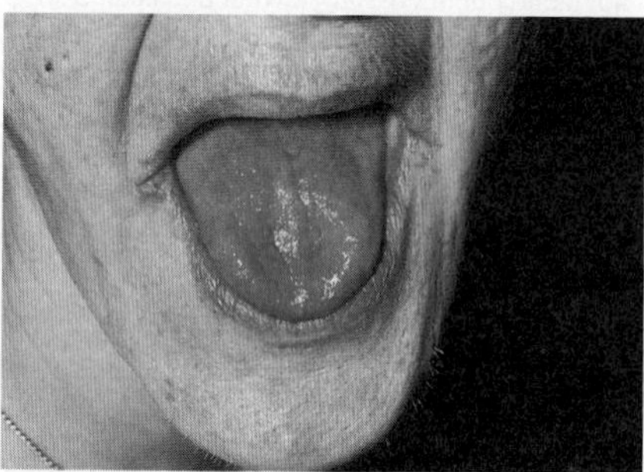

FIGURE 1-77 Iron deficiency. (From White GM, Cox NH [eds]: *Diseases of the skin, a color atlas and text*, ed 2, St. Louis, 2006, Mosby.)

PHYSICAL FINDINGS & CLINICAL PRESENTATION

- Most patients have normal examination results.
- Skin pallor and conjunctival pallor may be present.
- Signs and symptoms specific for iron deficiency are koilonychias, pica, pagophagia, blue sclera, glossitis, and angular stomatitis (Fig. 1-77).
- Patients with severe anemia can have palpitations, headache, weakness, dizziness, and easy fatigability.

ETIOLOGY

- Blood loss from GI or menstrual bleeding (genitourinary blood loss less often the cause)
- Dietary iron deficiency (rare in adults)
- Poor iron absorption in patients with gastric or small-bowel surgery
- Repeated phlebotomy
- Increased requirements (e.g., during pregnancy)
- Other: traumatic hemolysis (abnormally functioning cardiac valves), idiopathic pulmonary hemosiderosis (iron sequestration in pulmonary macrophages), paroxysmal nocturnal hemoglobinuria (intravascular hemolysis)
- The most common cause worldwide is hookworm infection

Dx DIAGNOSIS

DIFFERENTIAL DIAGNOSIS

- Anemia of chronic disease
- Sideroblastic anemia
- Thalassemia trait
- Lead poisoning

WORKUP

Diagnostic workup consists primarily of laboratory evaluation. Table 1-38 describes laboratory studies differentiating the most common microcytic anemias. Most patients with iron deficiency anemia are asymptomatic in the early stages. With progressive anemia, the major symptoms are fatigue, dizziness, exertional dyspnea, pagophagia (ice eating), and pica. Patient history may also suggest GI blood loss (melena, hematochezia, hemoptysis).

LABORATORY TESTS

- Laboratory results vary with the stage of deficiency.
- Absent iron marrow stores and decreased serum ferritin are the initial abnormalities.
- Decreased serum iron and increased total iron-binding capacity (TIBC) are the next abnormalities.
- Hypochromic microcytic anemia is present with significant iron deficiency.
- Peripheral smear in patients with iron deficiency generally reveals microcytic hypochromic red blood cells (Fig. 1-78) with a wide area of central pallor, anisocytosis, and poikilocytosis when severe.
- Laboratory abnormalities consistent with iron deficiency are low serum ferritin level, increased RBC distribution width with values generally >15, low mean corpuscular volume, low mean corpuscular hemoglobin, increased TIBC, and low serum iron.
- In patients diagnosed with iron deficiency anemia, a GI workup including an upper endoscopy and colonoscopy is recommended to look for source of iron loss.

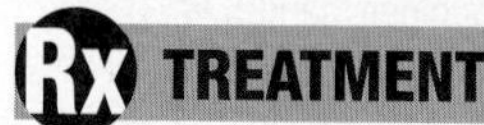

Rx TREATMENT

The goal of therapy is to supply sufficient iron to correct the low hemoglobin and replenish iron stores.

NONPHARMACOLOGIC THERAPY

Patients should be instructed to consume foods that contain large amounts of iron, such as liver, red meat, and legumes.

ACUTE GENERAL Rx

- Treatment consists of ferrous sulfate 325 mg PO daily for at least 6 mo. Doses higher than 325 mg/day are poorly tolerated. Calcium supplements can decrease iron absorption; therefore, these two medications should be staggered.
- Parenteral iron therapy is reserved for patients with poor tolerance, noncompliance with oral preparations, or malabsorption.
- Transfusion of packed RBCs is indicated in patients with severe symptomatic anemia.

CHRONIC Rx

Patients should be instructed to continue their iron supplements for at least 6 mo or longer to correct depleted body iron stores.

TABLE 1-38 Laboratory Studies Differentiating the Most Common Microcytic Anemias

Study	Iron Deficiency Anemia	α or β Thalassemia	Anemia of Chronic Disease
Hemoglobin	Decreased	Decreased	Decreased
MCV	Decreased	Decreased	Normal-decreased
RDW	Increased	Normal	Normal-increased
RBC	Decreased	Normal-increased	Normal-decreased
Serum ferritin	Decreased	Normal	Increased
Total Fe binding capacity	Increased	Normal	Decreased
Transferrin saturation	Decreased	Normal	Decreased
FEP	Increased	Normal	Increased
Transferrin receptor	Increased	Normal	Increased
Reticulocyte hemoglobin concentration	Decreased	Normal	Normal-decreased

Fe, Ferritin; *FEP*, free erythrocyte protoporphyrin; *MCV*, mean corpuscular volume; *RBC*, red blood cell; *RDW*, red cell distribution width.
From Kliegman RM et al: *Nelson textbook of pediatrics*, ed 19, Philadelphia, 2011, Saunders.

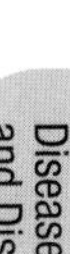

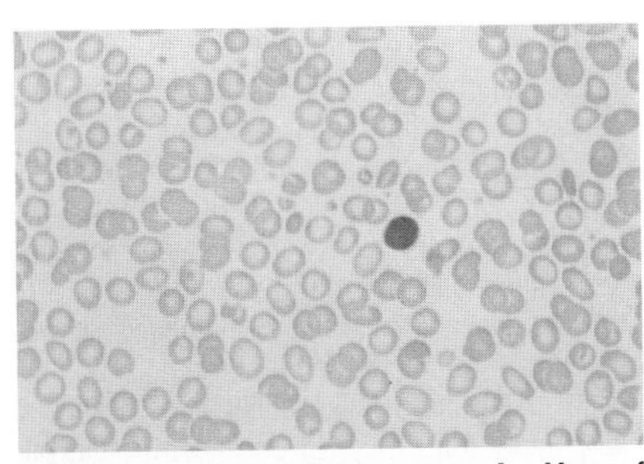

FIGURE 1-78 Iron deficiency anemia. Many of these red blood cells are microcytic (smaller than the nucleus of the normal lymphocyte near the center of the field) and hypochromic (with central areas of pallor that exceed half the diameter of the cells). (From Goldman L, Schafer AI: *Goldman's Cecil medicine,* ed 24, Philadelphia, 2012, Saunders.)

DISPOSITION

- Most patients respond rapidly to iron supplementation with improvement in CBC and general well-being (Table 1-39). GI side effects from oral iron therapy are common and may require decreased dosage to once every other day or to change to parenteral iron.
- A differential diagnosis of microcytic anemia that fails to respond to oral iron is described in Table 1-40.

REFERRAL

GI referral for evaluation of GI malignancy is recommended in all patients with iron deficiency and suspected GI blood loss.

PEARLS & CONSIDERATIONS

COMMENTS

- Iron deficiency may impair aerobic performance and worsen symptoms in patients with heart failure. Treatment with IV iron in patients with chronic heart failure and iron deficiency has been shown to improve symptoms, quality of life, and functional capacity.
- If the diagnosis of iron deficiency anemia is made, locating the suspected site of iron loss is mandatory.

SUGGESTED READINGS

available at www.expertconsult.com

RELATED CONTENT

Fig. 3-12 Algorithm for diagnosis of anemias
Iron Deficiency Anemia (Patient Information)

AUTHORS: **BILAL H. NAQVI, M.D.,** and **FRED F. FERRI, M.D.**

TABLE 1-39 Responses to Iron Therapy in Iron-Deficiency Anemia

Time after Iron Administration	Response
12-24 hr	Replacement of intracellular iron enzymes; subjective improvement; decreased irritability; increased appetite
36-48 hr	Initial bone marrow response; erythroid hyperplasia
48-72 hr	Reticulocytosis, peaking at 5–7 days
4-30 days	Increase in hemoglobin level
1-3 mo	Repletion of stores

From Kliegman RM et al: *Nelson textbook of pediatrics,* ed 19, Philadelphia, 2011, Saunders.

TABLE 1-40 Differential Diagnosis of Microcytic Anemia That Fails to Respond to Oral Iron

Poor compliance (true intolerance of iron is uncommon)
Incorrect dose or medication
Malabsorption of administered iron
Ongoing blood loss including gastrointestinal, menstrual, and pulmonary
Concurrent infection or inflammatory disorder inhibiting the response to iron
Concurrent vitamin B_{12} or folate deficiency
Diagnosis other than iron deficiency

- Thalassemias
- Hemoglobin C and E disorders
- Anemia of chronic disease
- Lead poisoning
- Sickle thalassemias, hemoglobin SC disease
- Rare microcytic anemias

From Kliegman RM et al: *Nelson textbook of pediatrics,* ed 19, Philadelphia, 2011, Saunders.

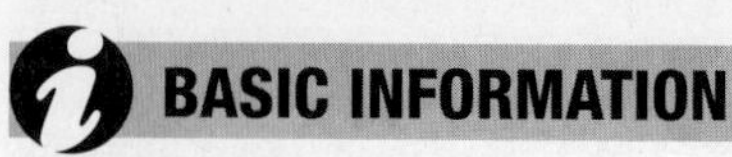

BASIC INFORMATION

DEFINITION

Pernicious anemia (PA) is an autoimmune disease resulting from antibodies against intrinsic factor and gastric parietal cells.

SYNONYMS

Megaloblastic anemia resulting from vitamin B_{12} deficiency

ICD-9CM CODES
281.0 Pernicious anemia
ICD-10CM CODES
D51 Vitamin B_{12} deficiency anemia due to intrinsic factor deficiency

EPIDEMIOLOGY & DEMOGRAPHICS

- Increased incidence in females and older adults (diagnosis is unusual before age 35 yr)
- The overall prevalence of undiagnosed PA after age 60 yr is 1.9%
- Prevalence is highest in women (2.7%), particularly in black women (4.3%)
- Increased incidence of autoimmune disease (e.g., type 1 diabetes mellitus, Graves disease, Addison disease), *Helicobacter pylori* infection

PHYSICAL FINDINGS & CLINICAL PRESENTATION

- Mucosal pallor, glossitis
- Peripheral sensory neuropathy with paresthesias initially and absent reflexes in advanced cases
- Loss of joint position sense, pyramidal or long tract signs
- Possible splenomegaly and mild hepatomegaly
- Generalized weakness and delirium/dementia

ETIOLOGY

- Gastric/antiparietal cell antibodies in >70% of patients; antiintrinsic factor antibodies in >50% of patients
- Atrophic gastric mucosa
- Inborn errors of cobalamin-cofactor synthesis are rare. The cobalamin gene *(cblD)* is localized to human chromosome 2q23.2. Mutations in the gene designated MMADHC (methylmalonic aciduria, cblD type, and homocystinuria) are responsible for the cblD defect in vitamin B_{12} metabolism.
- Fig. E1-79 illustrates the components and mechanism of cobalamin absorption. An etiopathophysiologic classification of cobalamin deficiency is described in Section II.

Dx DIAGNOSIS

DIFFERENTIAL DIAGNOSIS

- Nutritional vitamin B_{12} deficiency
- Malabsorption
- Chronic alcoholism (multifactorial)
- Chronic gastritis related to *H. pylori* infection
- Folic acid deficiency
- Myelodysplasia

WORKUP

- The clinical presentation of PA varies with the stage. Initially, patients may be asymptomatic. In advanced stages patients may have impaired memory, depression, gait disturbances, paresthesias, and reports of generalized weakness.
- Investigation consists primarily of laboratory evaluation.
- Endoscopy and biopsy for atrophic gastritis may be performed in selected cases.
- Diagnosis is crucial because failure to treat may result in irreversible neurologic deficits.

LABORATORY TESTS

- Complete blood count generally reveals macrocytic anemia and leukopenia with hypersegmented neutrophils (Fig. E1-80).
- Mean corpuscular volume (MCV) is generally significantly elevated in the advanced stages.
- Reticulocyte count is low to normal.
- Falsely low serum cobalamin levels can occur in patients with severe folate deficiency, in patients using high doses of ascorbic acid, and when cobalamin levels are measured after nuclear medicine studies (radioactivity interferes with cobalamin radioimmunoassay measurement).
- Falsely high normal levels in patients with cobalamin deficiency can occur in severe liver disease or chronic granulocytic leukemia.
- The absence of anemia or macrocytosis does not exclude the diagnosis of cobalamin deficiency. Anemia is absent in 20% of patients with cobalamin deficiency, and macrocytosis is absent in >30% of patients at the time of diagnosis. It can be blocked by concurrent iron deficiency or anemia of chronic disease and may be masked by thalassemia trait.
- Schilling test is abnormal in part I; part II corrects to normal after administration of intrinsic factor.
- Laboratory tests used for detecting cobalamin deficiency in patients with normal vitamin B_{12} levels include serum and urinary methylmalonic acid level (elevated), total homocysteine level (elevated), intrinsic factor antibody (positive).
- An increased concentration of plasma methylmalonic acid does not predict clinical manifestations of vitamin B_{12} deficiency and should not be used as the only marker for diagnosis of B_{12} deficiency.
- Additional laboratory abnormalities can include elevated lactate dehydrogenase, direct hyperbilirubinemia, and decreased haptoglobin.
- Bone marrow aspirate may show giant C-shaped neutrophil bands and megaloblastic normoblasts (Fig. E1-81).

Rx TREATMENT

NONPHARMACOLOGIC THERAPY

Avoid folic acid supplementation without proper vitamin B_{12} supplementation.

ACUTE GENERAL Rx

Traditional therapy of a cobalamin deficiency consists of IM injections of vitamin B_{12} 1000 mcg/wk for the initial 4 to 6 wk followed by 1000 mcg/mo IM indefinitely. In patients who have no nervous system involvement, intranasal cyanocobalamin may be used in place of IM cyanocobalamin when hematologic parameters have returned to normal range. The initial dose of intranasal cyanocobalamin (Nascobal) is 1 spray (500 mcg) in one nostril once per week. Cost generally exceeds $120/mo. Monitor response and increase dose if serum B_{12} levels decline. Consider return to intramuscular vitamin B_{12} supplementation if decline recurs.

CHRONIC Rx

- Parenteral vitamin B_{12} 1000 mcg/mo or intranasal cyanocobalamin 500 mcg/wk (see "Acute General Rx") for the remainder of life.
- Oral cobalamin (1000 to 2000 mcg/day) has been reported as also being effective in mild cases of pernicious anemia because approximately 1% of an oral dose is absorbed by passive diffusion, a pathway that does not require intrinsic factor. Cost for 1 mo of therapy is approximately $5.

DISPOSITION

Anemia generally resolves with appropriate treatment. Neurologic deficits, if present at diagnosis, may be permanent.

REFERRAL

Gastrointestinal referral for endoscopy on diagnosis of PA and surveillance endoscopy every 5 yr to rule out gastric carcinoma.

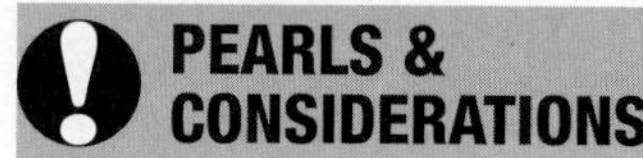

PEARLS & CONSIDERATIONS

COMMENTS

- Patients must understand that therapy is lifelong.
- Self-injection of vitamin B_{12} may be taught in selected patients. Cost of monthly injection is less than $5.

SUGGESTED READINGS
available at www.expertconsult.com

RELATED CONTENT

Fig. 3-12 Algorithm for diagnosis of anemias
Pernicious Anemia (Patient Information)

AUTHOR: **FRED F. FERRI, M.D.**

BASIC INFORMATION

DEFINITION

Sideroblastic anemia is a heterogeneous group of blood disorders whose two distinctive features are ring sideroblasts in the bone marrow (abnormal erythroblasts with excessive iron accumulation in the mitochondria) and impaired heme biosynthesis. They are classified as hereditary, acquired, and reversible.

SYNONYMS

Hereditary sideroblastic anemias
Acquired idiopathic sideroblastic anemia (AISA)
Reversible sideroblastic anemias

ICD-9CM CODES
285.0 Sideroblastic anemia
ICD-10CM CODES
D64.0 Hereditary sideroblastic anemia
D64.1 Secondary sideroblastic anemia due to disease
D64.3 Other sideroblastic anemias

EPIDEMIOLOGY & DEMOGRAPHICS

- Sex-linked; primarily affects males.
- AISA affects middle-aged and older adults.

PHYSICAL FINDINGS & CLINICAL PRESENTATION

The symptoms for sideroblastic anemia are the same for any anemia and iron overload:

- Fatigue, weakness, palpitations, shortness of breath, headaches, and irritability.
- Physical findings may include pallor, tachycardia, hepatosplenomegaly, S3 gallop, jugular vein distention, and rales.

ETIOLOGY

- The hereditary forms can be X-linked, autosomal dominant or autosomal recessive.
- Acquired forms may be associated with chemotherapy or irradiation.
- Refractory anemia with ringed sideroblast develops as a subtype of myelodysplasia.
- Reversible sideroblastic anemia can be caused by alcohol, isoniazid, pyrazinamide, cycloserine, chloramphenicol, or copper deficiency.

DIAGNOSIS

The principal feature is indolent and progressive, mild, lifelong anemia that goes unnoticed. Symptoms of iron overload may lead to discovery of the underlying disorder. The history and clinical findings, together with typical laboratory findings, usually permit accurate diagnosis of each type of sideroblastic anemia. The molecular defects can be identified in several hereditary forms and in some patients with AISA.

DIFFERENTIAL DIAGNOSIS

- Sideroblastic anemia must be differentiated from other causes of microcytic hypochromic anemia: iron deficiency anemia, thalassemia, anemia of chronic disease, and lead poisoning.
- Tissue iron overload from sideroblastic anemia may act similar to hereditary hemochromatosis with liver cirrhosis, diabetes, congestive heart failure, or cardiac arrhythmias.

WORKUP

Laboratory evaluation: CBC, iron studies, free erythrocyte protoporphyrin level, MRI, bone marrow aspiration, and liver biopsy.

LABORATORY TESTS

- Hypochromic microcytic anemia for the hereditary type and normo- or macrocytic anemia for AISA.
- High serum iron levels, low transferrin along with increased transferrin saturation and high serum ferritin.
- Peripheral smear: dimorphic large and small cells (Fig. E1-82) revealing Pappenheimer bodies or siderocytes when stained for iron.
- Bone marrow shows increased iron stores (Fig. E1-83) and the classic ringed sideroblasts not seen in normal bone marrow tissue (Fig. 1-84). The ringed sideroblasts represent iron storage in the mitochondria of normoblasts.
- In transfusion-dependent anemias, monitoring of ferritin and transferrin saturation levels is recommended despite minimal transfusion needs to avoid iron overload.
- Features of ineffective erythropoiesis like increase in indirect bilirubin concentration, decrease in haptoglobin, increase in LDH, and normal or increase in reticulocyte number is seen.

TREATMENT

Treatment is directed at controlling symptoms of anemia and preventing organ damage from iron overload.

NONPHARMACOLOGIC THERAPY

Avoid alcohol

ACUTE GENERAL Rx

- A trial of pyridoxine (100-200 mg) is indicated for all patients with hereditary sideroblastic anemia.
- 25% to 50% may show full or partial response to pyridoxine.
- Patients who do not respond will need to be treated with blood transfusion.
- Chelation therapy is needed for patients with transfusion-dependent anemia to prevent complications of iron overload.

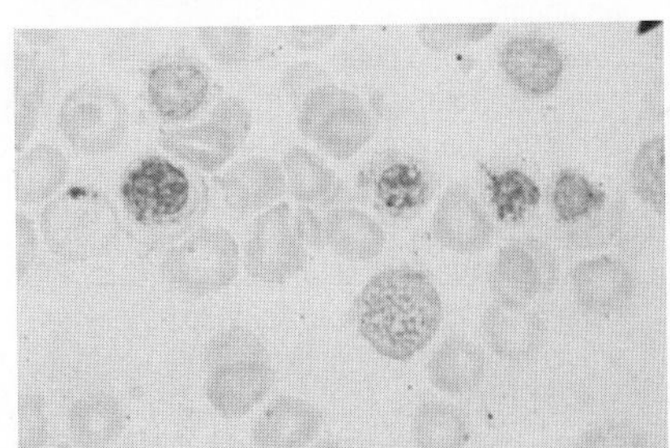

FIGURE 1-84 Prussian blue iron stain of the bone marrow shows ringed sideroblasts. (From Goldman L, Ausiello D [eds]: *Cecil textbook of medicine,* ed 24, Philadelphia, 2012, Saunders.)

- Erythropoietin and granulocyte colony-stimulating factor may show some success in treating MDS-associated refractory anemia with ringed sideroblast.
- Secondary sideroblastic anemia caused by medication can be reversed by withdrawing the medication and administering vitamin B_6 (50 to 200 mg/day).

CHRONIC Rx

- Organ dysfunction resulting from iron overload will require periodic phlebotomy to keep serum ferritin level <300 ng/ml.
- Iron chelating therapy for patients with moderately severe anemia in those who require regular red cell transfusion: deferoxamine continuous infusion or the oral agent deferasirox (EXJADE).
- Splenectomy should be avoided at all costs.

DISPOSITION

In patients with anemia alone, life expectancy is normal. In patients dependent on blood transfusions, morbidity from iron overload can be expected. There are two types of AISA:

1. Pure sideroblastic anemia: with dysplasia confined to the erythroid cell lineage; survival similar to age-matched controls; no incidence of leukemic transformation.
2. Refractory anemia with ringed sideroblasts: dysplastic features involving the red cell lineage, granulopoiesis, and/or megakaryopoiesis; approximately 5% will develop acute leukemia. Erythropoietin and granulocyte colony-stimulating factor therapy do not change survival.

REFERRAL

- Hematology.
- Families with severe forms of hereditary sideroblastic anemia should receive genetic counseling.

PEARLS & CONSIDERATIONS

- Sideroblastic anemia can be thought of as an iron-loading anemia secondary to defective heme synthesis.
- A predisposition to leukemia evolution has not been observed in patients with hereditary forms.
- Symptoms rather than an absolute hemoglobin level or hematocrit should guide transfusion therapy.

COMMENTS

Vitamin B_6, or pyridoxal phosphate, is a required cofactor in heme synthesis, and drugs such as isoniazid, cycloserine, and pyrazinamide can inhibit its function.

SUGGESTED READINGS

available at www.expertconsult.com

RELATED CONTENT

Fig. 3-12 Algorithm for Diagnosis of Anemias

AUTHOR: **BILAL H. NAQVI, M.D.**

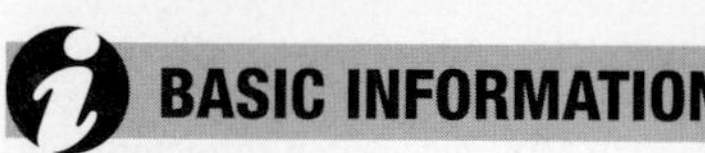

BASIC INFORMATION

DEFINITION

Angina pectoris is a term used to describe a clinical syndrome, typically characterized by chest, jaw, shoulder, back or arm discomfort, that is caused by myocardial ischemia. This is most commonly related to atheromatous plaque in more than 1 large epicardial coronary arteries; however, myocardial ischemia may occur in the absence of obstructive coronary artery disease (CAD), such as uncontrolled hypertension, valvular heart disease, hypertrophic cardiomyopathy, coronary spasm, or endothelial dysfunction. Any situation that causes an imbalance in myocardial oxygen supply and demand can cause an angina syndrome. Angina can be classified as follows:

1. Chronic stable ischemic heart disease (ISHD):
   - Predictable. Usually follows a precipitating event (e.g., climbing stairs, sexual intercourse, a heavy meal, emotional stress, cold weather).
   - Generally same severity as previous attacks; relieved by rest or by the customary dose of nitroglycerin.
   - Caused by a fixed coronary artery obstruction secondary to atherosclerosis. The presence of one or more obstructions in major coronary arteries is likely; the severity of stenosis is usually >70%.
2. Unstable (rest or crescendo, acute coronary syndrome; will be reviewed under Acute Coronary Syndrome):
   - Recent onset. Less than 2 months after the onset of the symptoms.
   - Increasing severity, duration, or frequency of chronic angina.
   - Occurs at rest or with minimal exertion.
3. Prinzmetal's variant:
   - Occurs at rest.
   - Manifests electrocardiographically as episodic ST-segment elevations.
   - Caused by coronary artery spasms with or without superimposed CAD.
   - Patients also more likely to develop ventricular arrhythmias.
4. Microvascular angina (syndrome X):
   - Refers to patients with angina symptoms, positive exercise test, normal coronary angiograms and no coronary spasm. Defective endothelium-dependent dilation in the coronary microcirculation contributes to the altered regulation of myocardial perfusion and the ischemic manifestations in these patients.
   - Patients with chest pain and normal or nonobstructive coronary angiograms are predominantly women, and many have a prognosis that is not as benign as commonly thought (2% risk of death or myocardial infarction [MI] at 30 days of follow-up).
5. Refractory angina:
   - Refers to patients who, despite optimal medical therapy, have both angina and objective evidence of ischemia and are not considered candidates for revascularization.
6. Other:
   - Angina due to aortic stenosis and idiopathic hypertrophic subaortic stenosis, cocaine-induced coronary vasoconstriction.

FUNCTIONAL CLASSIFICATION

Stable angina should be classified using a grading system. The most commonly adopted is that of the Canadian Cardiovascular Society:

- Class I: Ordinary physical activity, such as walking or climbing stairs, does not cause angina. Angina occurs with strenuous, rapid, or prolonged exertion at work or recreation.
- Class II: Slight limitation of ordinary activity. Angina occurs on walking or climbing stairs rapidly; walking uphill; walking or stair climbing after meals, in cold, in wind, or under emotional stress; or only during the few hours after awakening. Angina occurs on walking more than two level blocks and climbing more than one flight of ordinary stairs at a normal pace and in normal conditions.
- Class III: Marked limitations of ordinary physical activity. Angina occurs on walking one to two level blocks and climbing one flight of stairs in normal conditions and at a normal pace.
- Class IV: Inability to carry on any physical activity without discomfort; anginal symptoms may be present at rest.

ICD-9CM CODES
411.1 Angina, stable
413 Angina pectoris
413.1 Prinzmetal's angina
413.9 Angina, unspecified
ICD-10CM CODES
I20.8 Other forms of angina pectoris
I20.9 Angina pectoris, unspecified
I20.1 Angina pectoris with documented spasm
I20.8 Other forms of angina pectoris

EPIDEMIOLOGY & DEMOGRAPHICS

- Based on the NHANES survey 2007-2010, an estimated of 15.4 million have coronary heart disease of which 7.8 million have angina.
- Angina is most common in middle-aged and elderly men
- Women are usually affected after menopause
- The initial manifestation of ischemic heart disease is angina pectoris in 50%, and about 50% of patients presenting to the hospital with acute coronary syndrome have preceding angina.
- Two older population-based studies from Olmstead County, MN, and Framingham, MA showed annual rated of myocardial infarction in patients with symptomatic angina of 3-3.5%/year
- Within 12 months of initial diagnosis, 10% to 20% of patients with diagnosis of stable angina progress to MI or unstable angina

PHYSICAL FINDINGS & CLINICAL PRESENTATION

- Although there is significant individual variation, most patients report substernal chest pain (pressure, tightness, heaviness, sharp pain, sensation similar to intestinal gas or dysphagia).
- Pain is of short duration (typically <10 minutes); nonpleuritic; and often accompanied by shortness of breath, nausea, diaphoresis, and numbness or pain in the left arm, jaw, or shoulder. Ischemic pain of more than 30 minutes' duration should raise concern for possible MI.
- Women are more likely than men to report atypical chest pain or discomfort (65% reported on Women's Ischemic Syndrome Evaluation [WISE] study).
- Elderly and diabetics may report symptoms other than chest pain, such as dyspnea, fatigue, or diaphoresis.

ETIOLOGY

RISK FACTORS:

- Advanced age
- Male sex
- Genetic predisposition, family history of premature coronary artery disease (CAD) in first degree relatives (men younger than 55 years of age, and women younger than 65 years of age).
- Smoking (risk is almost double)
- Hypertension (risk is double if systolic blood pressure is >180 mm Hg)
- Hyperlipidemia
- Impaired glucose tolerance or diabetes mellitus
- History of stroke or peripheral arterial disease
- Chronic kidney disease (CKD)
- Metabolic syndrome
- Physical inactivity
- Obesity (weight >30% over ideal). A higher body mass index during childhood is also associated with an increased risk of coronary heart disease (CHD) in adulthood
- Hypothyroidism
- Left ventricular hypertrophy
- Aortic stenosis or idiopathic subaortic stenosis
- Oral contraceptive use
- Cocaine use (used by >5 million Americans regularly and is responsible for >64,000 emergency department [ED] evaluations yearly to rule out myocardial ischemia)
- Coronary artery calcium is associated with an increased risk of MI
- Long-term use of nonsteroidal anti-inflammatory drugs (NSAIDs)
- Exposure to air pollution from traffic (dilute diesel exhaust) promotes myocardial ischemia and is associated with adverse cardiovascular events
- Low serum folate levels required for conversion of homocysteine to methionine are associated with an increased risk of fatal CHD. Hyperhomocysteinemia has a toxic effect on vascular endothelium and interferes with proliferation of arterial wall smooth muscle cells.
- Elevated plasma homocysteine level is a strong and independent risk factor for CHD events, especially in patients with type 2 diabetes mellitus.

- Elevated levels of highly sensitive C-reactive protein (hs-CRP, cardio CRP), suggesting that diseases associated with systemic inflammation can lead to accelerated atherosclerosis
- Depression
- Vasculitis
- Elevated levels of lipoprotein-associated phospholipase A_2
- Elevated fibrinogen levels
- Low level of red blood cell glutathione peroxidase-1 activity
- Radiation therapy

Dx DIAGNOSIS

DIFFERENTIAL DIAGNOSIS

Nonischemic Cardiovascular: Aortic dissection, pericarditis

Pulmonary: Pulmonary embolism, pneumothorax, pneumonia, pleuritis

Gastrointestinal: Esophageal, esophagitis, spasm, reflux, biliary colic, cholecystitis, choledocholithiasis, cholangitis, peptic ulcer, pancreatitis

Chest Wall: Costochondritis, fibrositis, rib fracture, sternoclavicular arthritis, Herpes zoster (before the rash)

Psychiatric: Anxiety disorders, hyperventilation, panic disorder, primary anxiety, affective disorders (i.e., depression), somatiform disorders, thought disorders (i.e., fixed delusions)

WORKUP

- In patients with chest pain, the probability of CAD should be estimated on the basis of patient age, sex, cardiovascular risk factors, and pain characteristics
- The most important diagnostic factor is the history. Chest pain or left arm pain or discomfort occurring with exertion and relieved by rest in a patient with cardiovascular risk factors is consistent with a high likelihood of CAD
- In assessing the likelihood of underlying ISHD it is helpful to classify the chest pain as typical angina, atypical angina, and or noncardiac chest pain.
- Typical angina, (definite) will have the following three features: (1) substernal chest discomfort with a characteristic, quality and duration, (2) provoked by exertion or emotional stress, and (3) relieved by rest and/or nitroglycerin (NTG).
- Atypical angina, (probable) will have two of these above three features.
- Noncardiac chest pain will have one of these above features.
- Physical examination may be completely normal in many patients; however, certain findings may be helpful in the assessment of the patient with suspected ISHD. Some findings may identify consequences of ischemia or possible causes of the anginal syndrome other than CAD. The presence of hypertension, arcus senilis, xanthelasma, carotid or peripheral bruits, and a prominent S4 are all physical signs that could raise concern for the presence of CAD. A murmur of mitral regurgitation may be a marker of an ischemic cardiomyopathy or transient ischemia. A murmur suggestive of hypertrophic cardiomyopathy or aortic stenosis may suggest a cause of angina other than CAD

LABORATORY TESTS

- Initial laboratory tests in patients with chronic ISHD should include a hemoglobin, fasting glucose, and fasting lipid panel
- Cardiovascular screening: Measurement of total cholesterol, low-density lipoprotein cholesterol (LDL-C), high-density lipoprotein cholesterol (HDL-C), and fasting serum triglycerides. Also, measurement of Non–HDL-C, the ratio of total cholesterol to HDL-C, and apolipoprotein fractions (e.g., apolipoprotein B100, apolipoprotein A1)
- Electrocardiogram should be obtained during pain and when the patient is free of any discomfort. A normal resting electrocardiogram is not unusual in patients with ISHD; in patients who present with chest pain, 1%-6% who have an acute MI will have a normal or nondiagnostic electrocardiogram. Chest X Ray PA and lateral, to rule out heart failure, valvular disease, pericardial disease, aortic aneurysm/dissection.
- Cardio-CRP (hs-CRP): Its elevation is a relatively moderate predictor of CHD, and it adds prognostic information to that conveyed by the Framingham risk score.

EXERCISE TESTING AND IMAGING STUDIES

- The value of further testing is greatest in patients who have an intermediate risk of CAD. Exercise testing is used for the purpose of diagnosis as well as prognosis. If the patient is physically capable to perform at least moderate physical exercise, exercise stress testing (Fig. 1-85) is useful because of the important prognostic information obtained from exercise performance and the hemodynamic response. Patients who have an intermediate risk of CAD, as patients in a low-risk or high-risk category are more likely to have a false-positive or false-negative result, respectively. Risk assessment is also indicated in patients with ISHD who are being considered for revascularization of known coronary stenosis of unclear physiological significance. Stress echocardiography or stress testing with myocardial perfusion imaging may be employed when baseline electrocardiographic abnormalities are present that render the electrocardiographic response to exercise uninterpretable, such as >1 mm ST segment depression, LBBB, WPW, paced ventricular rhythm, digoxin treatment with ST segment changes. Stress echocardiography has the advantage of higher specificity and a lower cost. Stress radionuclide perfusion imaging has a higher sensitivity, particularly for single-vessel coronary disease, and has a higher technical success rate. When the patient is unable to exercise adequately, pharmacological testing (i.e., dobutamine, adenosine, regadenoson) may be used with these imaging modalities
- A very good predictor of risk for a patient with stable angina is the Duke treadmill score, which incorporates the patient's functional status (METS or time in minutes during the Bruce protocol), ST-segment depression, and an angina index. Patients with favorable Duke scores have a 5-year survival rate of >97%; this is independent of other factors such as coronary anatomy and LV function
- Echocardiography is indicated in patients with systolic murmur suggestive of aortic stenosis, hypertrophic cardiomyopathy, mitral valve prolapse, previous MI, pathological Q waves, complex ventricular arrhythmias, heart failure, hypertension, diabetes, and abnormal EKG.

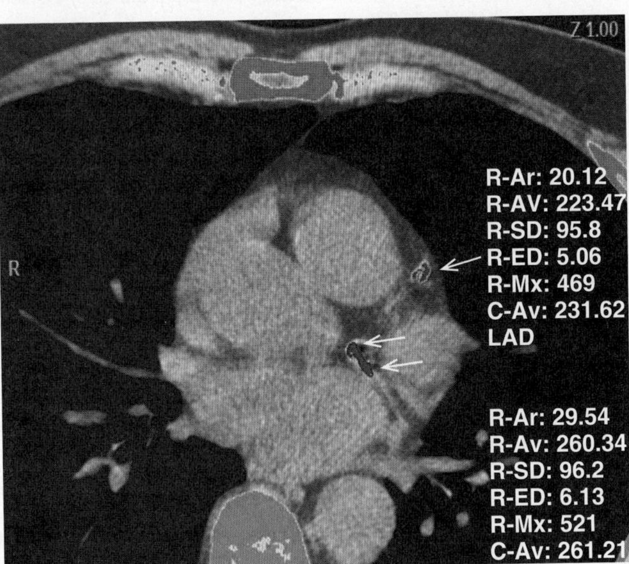

FIGURE 1-85 Example of coronary artery calcium scoring in which calcified foci are identified within the left anterior descending (orange; single arrow) and left circumflex (pink outlined in blue; double arrow) coronary arteries. The region's area (R-Ar) and its average density in Hounsfield units (R-Av) are displayed and used in the area-density calcium scoring calculation. (From Bonow RO et al: *Heart disease,* ed 9, Philadelphia, 2012, Saunders.)

- Cardiac computed tomography (CCTA; Fig 1-86) is useful for the detection of subclinical CAD in asymptomatic patients with an intermediate Framingham 10-year risk estimate of 10% to 20%. Detects and quantifies coronary calcium and evaluates the lumen and wall of the coronary artery. CCTA can be useful as a first-line test for risk assessment in patients with ISHD who are unable to exercise to an adequate workload regardless of interpretability of ECG. Also can be used when a functional test has an indeterminate result. CCTA CT cost and radiation exposure are limiting factors to recommending widespread routine use of this marker
- Coronary artery calcium (CAC) score is a strong predictor of incidence of CAD and provides predictive information beyond that provided by standard risk factors. A below 100 indicates low risk, and a score above 300 high risk.
- Cardiac magnetic resonance imaging (CMRA), in addition to its use for diagnosis of arrhythmogenic right ventricular dysplasia, can also be used to assess myocardial perfusion and viability as well as function. Additional studies are needed to determine the cost effectiveness of these studies in patients with ischemic cardiomyopathy
- Coronary angiography, invasive, remains the gold standard for the identification of clinically significant CAD. Angiography is performed to define the location and extent of coronary disease; indicated in selected patients who are candidates for coronary revascularization (either coronary artery bypass graft [CABG] surgery or angioplasty).

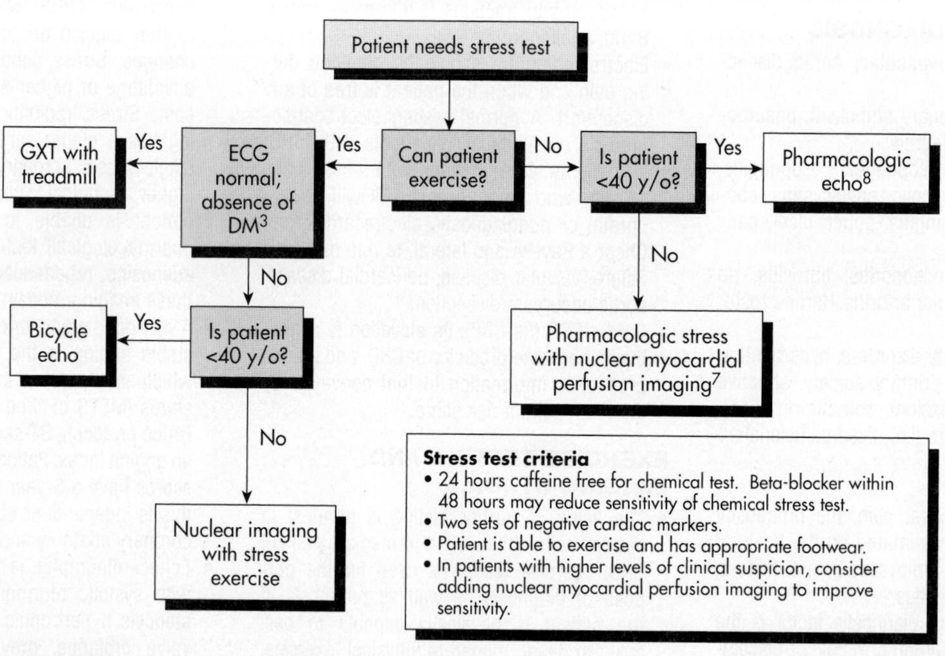

DEFINITIONS:

1 Typical angina:
1) Substernal chest pain or discomfort that is 2) provoked by exertion or emotional stress and 3) relieved by rest and/or nitroglycerin

2 Cardiac marker timing: based on symptom onset; in cases of uncertainty assume symptom onset at ED arrival

3 ECG normal: no significant ST depression/T wave inversions, BBB, LVH with repolarization, conduction defect, digoxin effect

4 Anginal equivalent:
- Any symptoms that the physician feels may represent ACS
- Exertional dyspnea—most common anginal equivalent symptom

5 ACS:
- STE-ACS—1 mm ST elevation in 2 leads
- NSTE-ACS
  - NSTEMI—positive cardiac biomarkers
  - Unstable angina—ischemia with negative biomarkers

6 New significant ECG changes:
- ST Δs ≥ 0.5 mm; resolve when asymptomatic
- ST depression ≥ 1 mm in 2 leads
- T wave inversion ≥ 2 mm in 2 leads

7 Regadenoson is preferred agent for chemical nuclear stress test. Technitium Tc 99m tetrofosmin is the preferred tarcer.

FIGURE 1-86 Stress test algorithm. *ACS*, Acute coronary syndrome; *BBB*, bundle branch block; *DM*, diabetes mellitus; *ECG*, electrocardiogram; echo, echocardiography; *ED*, emergency department; *GTX*, graded exercise test; *LVH*, left ventricular hypertrophy; *NSTE*, non–ST-segment elevation; *NSTEMI*, NSTE myocardial infarction; *STE*, ST-segment elevation; *y/o*, years old. (From Adams JG et al: *Emergency medicine: clinical essentials,* ed 2, Philadelphia, 2013, Saunders.)

Rx TREATMENT

NONPHARMACOLOGIC THERAPY

- Aggressive modification of preventable risk factors through patient education on weight reduction in obese patients, regular aerobic exercise program (at least 30-60 min/day), correction of folate deficiency, reduced intake of saturated fats (to <7% of total calories), trans fatty acids (to <1% of total calories), cholesterol (to <200 mg/day), low-sodium diet (<2 g/day), cessation of tobacco use, and teaching importance of medication adherence). Whole grains as the main form of carbohydrates, an abundance of fruits and vegetables, and adequate omega-3 fatty acids are optimal for prevention of ISHD.
- Correction of possible aggravating factors (e.g., anemia, hypertension, diabetes mellitus, hyperlipidemia, thyrotoxicosis). Use caution regarding the routine use of blood transfusions to maintain arbitrary hematocrit levels in stable patients with IHD.

PHARMACOLOGIC THERAPY

Treatment can be classified based on medications that prevent MI and death.

- Aspirin reduces cardiovascular mortality and morbidity rates by 20%-25% among patients with CAD. Initial dose is at least 160 mg/day followed by 75-162 mg/day. It inhibits the enzyme cyclooxygenase and synthesis of thromboxane A2 and reduces the risk of adverse cardiovascular events by 33% in patients with unstable angina. Patients intolerant to aspirin can be treated with the other antiplatelet agents (see below).
- Clopidogrel is a thienopyridine, which acts by irreversibly blocking the P2Y12 adenosine diphosphate receptor on the platelet surface, thereby interrupting platelet activation and aggregation. Patients are now commonly being tested to see if clopidogrel is effectively inhibiting platelets, although the usefulness of these tests in vivo has not yet demonstrated clinical utility. The hepatic enzyme CYP2C19 is competitively inhibited by most proton pump inhibitors (PPIs), and earlier studies had suggested an increased risk of clopidogrel failure, leading to concerns of stent thrombosis. Recent studies have not demonstrated clinically significant increased risk of adverse cardiovascular events due to interference with clopidogrel's efficacy. Clopidogrel can be combined with ASA in high-risk patients with ISHD.
- Prasugrel, a newer P2Y12 receptor inhibitor, and ticagrelor, the newest CTPT inhibitor are faster, more potent, more predictable, and have less patient intervariability antiplatelet agents than clopidogrel. These have been studied in patients with acute coronary syndromes (ACSs). Studies in patients with ISHD are undergoing. However, they are associated with a slight increased risk of bleeding when compared with clopidogrel.
- Beta-adrenergic blockers, which prevent MI and death, are first-line therapy in the management of angina pectoris. They achieve their major antianginal effect by decreasing myocardial oxygen demand by reducing heart rate and systolic blood pressure product, AV nodal conduction, and myocardial contractility contributing to a reduction in angina onset, with improvement in the ischemic threshold during exercise and in symptoms. Absent contraindications, they should be regarded as initial therapy for stable angina for all patients. Their dose should generally be adjusted to reduce the resting heart rate to 55-60 beats/min.
- Nitrates cause venodilation and relaxation of vascular smooth muscle; the decreased venous return from venodilation decreases diastolic ventricular wall tension (preload) and thereby reduces mechanical activity (and myocardial oxygen consumption) during systole. Relaxation of vascular smooth muscle increases coronary blood flow and reduces systemic pressure. Dilatation of the artery wall not affected by plaque, but independent of an intact endothelium, leading to reduced resistance across the obstructed lumen. Nitroglycerin contributes to coronary blood flow redistribution by augmenting collateral flow and lowering ventricular diastolic pressure from areas of normal perfusion to ischemic zones. Nitroglycerin also has demonstrated antithrombotic and antiplatelet effects. Sublingual nitroglycerin should be prescribed to all patients with ISHD for angina relief. Tolerance to nitrates can be minimized by avoiding sustained blood levels with a daily nitrate-free period (e.g., omission of bedtime dose of oral isosorbide dinitrate or 12 hr on/12 hr off transdermal nitroglycerin therapy). Nitrates are relatively contraindicated in patients with hypertrophic obstructive cardiomyopathy, and should also be avoided in patients with severe aortic stenosis. Nitrates should not be used within 24 hr of sildenafil (Viagra) or vardenafil (Levitra) or within 48 hr of tadalafil (Cialis) because of the potential for hypotension.
- Calcium channel blockers are antiischemic medications that have no proven mortality benefit in ISHD. They improve myocardial oxygen supply by decreasing coronary vascular resistance and augmenting epicardial conduit vessel and systemic arterial blood flow. Myocardial demand is decreased by a reduction in myocardial contractility, systemic vascular resistance, and arterial pressure. They are first-line treatment when beta-blockers are contraindicated. They play a major role in preventing and terminating myocardial ischemia induced by coronary artery spasm. They are particularly effective in treating microvascular angina. All classes of calcium channel blockers reduce anginal episodes, increase exercise duration, and reduce use of sublingual nitroglycerin in patients with effort-induced angina. Short-acting calcium channel blockers should be avoided. Calcium channel blockers (particularly non-dihydropyridine) should generally also be avoided in patients with CHF secondary to systolic dysfunction due to its negative inotropic effect.
- Ranolazine inhibits the late inward sodium current, indirectly reducing the sodium-dependent calcium current during ischemic conditions and leading to improvement in ventricular diastolic tension and oxygen consumption. It seems to increase the efficiency of energy production in the heart, maintaining cardiac function. Its antianginal and antiischemic effects do not depend on reductions in heart rate or blood pressure. It is indicated for treatment of chronic angina that is inadequately controlled with other antianginals. It represents a new class of drugs known as metabolic modulators and is labeled for use in combination with beta-blockers, amlodipine, or nitrates in patients without an adequate antianginal response to those agents. Side effects include prolongation of QT interval. Low doses of diltiazem and verapamil should be used with ranolazine. The extended-release preparation reduces the frequency of angina, improves exercise performance, and delays the development of exercise-induced angina and ST-segment depression.
- Angiotensin-converting enzyme (ACE) inhibition through changes in the physiological balance between angiotensin II and bradykinin could contribute to the reductions in LV and vascular hypertrophy, atherosclerosis progression, plaque rupture, and thrombosis; the favorable changes in cardiac hemodynamics; and the improved myocardial oxygen supply/demand. It has been shown to be effective in reducing cardiovascular death, MI, and stroke in patients who are at risk for or who had vascular disease. They are indicated in patients with hypertension, diabetes, LVEF <40%, and CKD.
- Use of lipid-lowering drugs is recommended in patients with CAD and in patients with hyperlipidemia refractory to diet and exercise. Among patients who have recently had an acute coronary syndrome, an intensive lipid-lowering statin regimen to reduce LDL cholesterol to <70 mg/dl is a reasonable treatment objective. Statins also decrease the level of the inflammatory marker hs-CRP independently of the magnitude of change in lipid parameters.

REFERRAL

Revascularization (see Table 1-41):

- Revascularization methods should be formulated when taking into consideration to improve survival or improve symptoms. Revascularization includes either percutaneous coronary intervention (balloon angioplasty and stenting) or CABG.
- **To improve survival:**
  - Perform CABG for patients with significant (>50% diameter stenosis) left main coronary artery stenosis. More than 70% diameter stenosis in three main epicardial vessels, >70% diameter stenosis in two major coronary arteries with severe or extensive myocardial ischemia, and in patients with mild to moderate LV systolic dysfunction (EF 35%-50%) and significant multivessel CAD. Left internal mammary

artery (LIMA) graft improves survival when used to bypass a proximal left anterior descending (LAD) artery stenosis.
 - Percutaneous coronary intervention (PCI) is reasonable as an alternative to CABG in selected stable patients with unprotected left main CAD, low risk of PCI procedural complications, and a high likelihood of good long-term outcome *and* clinical characteristics that predict a significantly increased risk of adverse surgical outcomes (e.g., STS-predicted risk of operative mortality >5).
- **To improve symptoms:**
 - CABG or PCI to improve symptoms is beneficial in patients with one or more significant (>70% diameter) coronary artery stenoses amenable to revascularization and unacceptable angina despite maximal medical treatment, or in whom increasing medical therapy cannot be implemented because of medication contraindications, adverse effects, or patient preferences.
 - Hybrid coronary revascularization: LIMA-to-LAD artery grafting and of >1 non-LAD coronary artery can be used in patients who have an unfavorable aorta, have poor target vessels for CABG, are unsuitable graft conduits, or have unfavorable LAD for PCI.
- Surgical therapy improves prognosis, particularly in diabetic patients with multivessel disease. Compared with percutaneous coronary intervention (PCI), CABG is more effective in relieving angina and leads to fewer repeated revascularizations but has a higher risk for procedural stroke. Survival to 10 years is similar for both procedures.

Angioplasty and coronary stents (Fig. E1-87):
- PCI has an established place in treating angina but is not superior to intensive medical therapy to prevent MI and death in symptomatic or asymptomatic patients. Patients selected for PCI should also be candidates for CABG. Approximately 80% of patients show immediate benefit after PCI. The development of coronary stents has increased the number of patients who can be treated in the cardiac laboratory. Cardiac stents (Fig. E1-88) are currently used in nearly 95% of all patients with PCI lesions. The rate of restenosis is reduced by placing a stent electively in primary atheromatous lesions. The major limitations of stenting are subacute thrombosis, restenosis within the stent, bleeding complications when anticoagulants are used after stenting, and higher cost. The combination of aspirin and thienopyrimidines (P2Y12 antagonists) is effective in preventing coronary stent thrombosis and the duration of therapy depends on whether bare metal stents (BMS) or drug-eluting stents (DES) are used. Duration of dual antiplatelet therapy can be as short as 4 weeks for BMS, but 12 months of therapy is generally required for DES. This difference in duration is due to the lack of endothelium proliferation in DES initially, which confers a higher risk of stent thrombosis than with BMS. New drug-eluting stents with thin struts releasing Limus-family analogs from durable polymers have lowered the risk of stent thrombosis compared with early-generation stents releasing sirolimus or pallitaxel. Current evidence supports the use of drug-eluting stents in most clinical settings without safety concerns (unless there are contraindications to use of dual antiplatelet therapy). Recent data has shown that extending clopidogrel therapy beyond 6 months after stent placement does not reduce death or ischemic events, and it increases the risk of bleeding complications.
- Provide alternative therapies for relief of symptoms in patients with refractory angina. Although some of these therapies may improve symptoms and quality of life, they have not been shown to improve mortality rate.

1. Enhanced external counterpulsation (EECP)
2. Spinal cord stimulation
3. Transmyocardial revascularization (TMR)

The following treatments have not shown to be beneficial in reducing cardiovascular risk or improve clinical outcomes: estrogen therapy, vitamin C, vitamin E, and beta-carotene supplementation; treatment of elevated homocysteine with folate or vitamins B_6 and B_{12}; chelation therapy; garlic; coenzyme Q10; selenium; or chromium.

TABLE 1-41 Current Recommendations for Myocardial Revascularization in Patients with Chronic Stable Angina

CABG Surgery versus Medical Therapy
Among patients with medically refractory angina pectoris, CABG surgery is indicated for symptom improvement.
Among patients with medically stable angina pectoris, CABG surgery is indicated to prolong life in left main coronary artery disease or three-vessel disease (regardless of left ventricular function) and, possibly, to help symptoms.
CABG surgery may be indicated for prolongation of life if the proximal left anterior descending coronary artery is involved (regardless of the number of diseased vessels).
CABG surgery may reduce the composite end point of death, myocardial infarction, or stroke in diabetic patients with extensive multivessel (two- to three-vessel) coronary artery disease compared with medical therapy.
PCI versus Medical Therapy
For the initial management of patients with stable ischemic heart disease, PCI does not reduce the risk of death, myocardial infarction, or other major cardiovascular events when added to optimal medical therapy.
Among patients with medically refractory angina pectoris, PCI is indicated for symptom improvement.
PCI may be indicated in the presence of severe myocardial ischemia, regardless of symptoms. PCI does not appear to improve survival compared with medical treatment among patients with one- or two-vessel disease.
In the absence of symptoms or myocardial ischemia, PCI is not indicated (merely for the presence of an anatomic stenosis).
PCI versus CABG Surgery
For single-vessel disease, PCI and CABG surgery provide excellent symptom relief, but repeated revascularization procedures are required more frequently after PCI. Intracoronary stenting is preferred to regular PCI, but direct comparison with CABG surgery is limited.
For treated diabetic patients with two- or three-vessel disease, CABG surgery is the treatment of choice.
For nondiabetic patients, multivessel PCI and CABG surgery are acceptable alternatives. The choice of PCI or CABG surgery for initial treatment depends primarily on local expertise and the patient's and physician's preferences.
In general, PCI is preferred for patients at low risk and CABG surgery for patients at high risk.

CABG, Coronary artery bypass graft; *PCI*, percutaneous coronary intervention.
From Goldman L, Schafer AI: *Goldman's Cecil medicine*, ed 24, Philadelphia, 2012, Saunders.

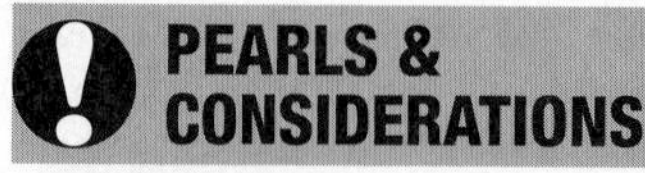

PEARLS & CONSIDERATIONS

COMMENTS

- Although nitrate responsiveness is usually an integral part of a diagnostic strategy for ISHD, recent reports question its value and conclude that in a general population admitted for chest pain, relief of pain after nitroglycerin treatment does not predict active CAD and should not be used to guide diagnosis in the acute care setting.
- CABG is associated with higher long-term survival rates and lower rates of repeat revascularization than PCI and stenting; however, patients often prefer stenting because it is less invasive, involves a shorter hospital stay, and has a lower in-hospital mortality rate.

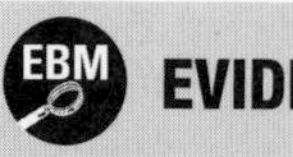

EVIDENCE

available at www.expertconsult.com

SUGGESTED READINGS

available at www.expertconsult.com

RELATED CONTENT

Acute Coronary Syndrome (Related Key Topic)
Angina (Patient Information)

AUTHOR: **CLAUDIA SERRANO-GOMEZ, M.D.**

BASIC INFORMATION

DEFINITION

- The mucocutaneous swelling caused by the release of vasoactive mediators is called urticaria and angioedema.
- Urticaria causes edema of the superficial dermis.
- Angioedema involves the deep layers of the dermis and the subcutaneous tissue.

SYNONYMS

Angioneurotic edema
HAE (hereditary angiodema)

ICD-9CM CODES
995.1 Angioedema (allergic)
277.6 Angioedema (hereditary)
ICD-10CM CODES
T78.3 Angioedema
D84.1 Angioedema, hereditary

EPIDEMIOLOGY & DEMOGRAPHICS

INCIDENCE: 100 to 3000/100,000 persons (for urticaria and angioedema)

LIFETIME PREVALENCE: Approximately 20% of the population experiences urticaria and/or angioedema at some time during life. The prevalence of hereditary angioedema is 1 case per 50,000 persons.

DEMOGRAPHICS:

Race: Slightly more common among African Americans.

Sex: More occurrences in women than men.

Angioedema commonly occurs after adolescence in the third decade of life.

Angioedema can occur together with urticaria (40%) or alone (20%); the remaining 40% have urticaria alone.

PHYSICAL FINDINGS & CLINICAL PRESENTATION

- Angioedema may be acute or chronic.
  1. Acute angioedema is defined as symptoms lasting 6 wk.
  2. Chronic angioedema is defined as symptoms lasting >6 wk.
- Urticaria is commonly known as "hives" and is:
  1. Pruritic
  2. Palpable and well demarcated
  3. Erythematous
  4. Millimeters to centimeters in size
  5. Multiple in number
  6. Fades within 12 to 24 hr
  7. Reappears at other sites
- Angioedema is characterized by the following:
  1. Nonpruritic
  2. Burning
  3. Not well demarcated
  4. Involves eyelids (Fig. 1-89), lips, tongue, and extremities
  5. Can involve the upper airway, causing respiratory distress
  6. Can involve the gastrointestinal tract, leading to cyclic abdominal pain, nausea, vomiting, and diarrhea
  7. Resolves slowly

ETIOLOGY

- Angioedema, with or without urticaria, is classified as acquired (allergic or idiopathic) or hereditary.
- Angioedema is primarily caused by mast cell activation and degranulation with release of vasoactive mediators (e.g., histamine, serotonin, bradykinins), resulting in postcapillary venule inflammation, vascular leakage, and edema in the deep layers of the dermis and subcutaneous tissue.
- Pathologically, angioedema has both immunologic- and nonimmunologic-mediated mechanisms.
  1. Immunoglobulin E–mediated angioedema may result from antigen exposure (e.g., foods [milk, eggs, peanuts, shellfish, tomatoes, chocolate, sulfites] or drugs [penicillin, aspirin, nonsteroidal anti-inflammatory drugs, phenytoin, sulfonamides, recombinant tissue plasminogen activator]).
  2. Complement-mediated angioedema involving immune complex mechanisms can also lead to mast cell activation that manifests as serum sickness.
  3. Hereditary angioedema is an autosomal-dominant disease caused by a deficiency of or mutation in C1 esterase inhibitor (C1-INH). C1-INH is a protease inhibitor normally present in high concentrations in the plasma. C1-INH serves many functions, one of which is to inhibit plasma kallikrein, a protease that cleaves kininogen and releases bradykinin. Deficient C1-INH activity results in excess concentration of kininogen and the subsequent release of kinin mediators.
  4. Acquired angioedema is usually associated with other diseases, most commonly B-cell lymphoproliferative disorders, but may also result from the formation of autoantibodies directed against C1 inhibitor protein.
  5. Other causes of angioedema include infection (e.g., herpes simplex, hepatitis B, Coxsackie A and B, *Streptococcus, Candida, Ascaris,* and *Strongyloides*), insect bites and stings, stress, physical factors (e.g., cold, exercise, pressure, and vibration), connective tissue diseases (e.g., systemic lupus erythematosus, Henoch-Schönlein purpura), and idiopathic causes. Angiotensin-converting enzyme (ACE) inhibitors can increase kinin activity and lead to angioedema.

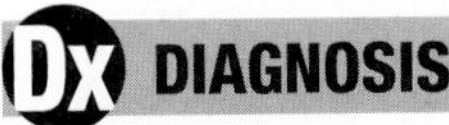

DIAGNOSIS

A detailed history and physical examination usually establish the diagnosis of angioedema. Extensive laboratory testing is of limited value.

DIFFERENTIAL DIAGNOSIS

- Cellulitis
- Arthropod bite
- Hypothyroidism
- Contact dermatitis
- Atopic dermatitis
- Mastocytosis
- Granulomatous cheilitis
- Bullous pemphigoid
- Urticaria pigmentosa
- Anaphylaxis
- Erythema multiforme
- Epiglottitis
- Peritonsillar abscess

WORKUP

- An extensive workup searching for the cause of angioedema is often unrevealing (90%).
- Workup, including diagnostic blood tests and allergy testing, is performed according to results of the history and physical examination.

LABORATORY TESTS

- Complete blood count, erythrocyte sedimentation rate, and urinalysis are sometimes helpful as part of the initial evaluation.
- Stools for ova and parasites.
- Serology testing.
- C4 levels are usually reduced in acquired and hereditary angioedema (occurring without urticaria). If C4 levels are low, C1-INH levels and activity should be obtained. There are isolated reports of hereditary angioedema with normal C4 levels but reduced C1-INH levels.

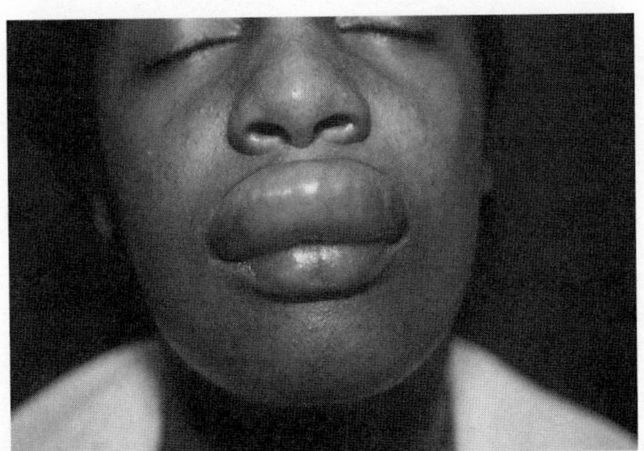

FIGURE 1-89 Angioedema of the upper lip, with severe swelling of deeper tissues. (From Goldstein BG, Goldstein AO: *Practical dermatology,* ed 2, St Louis, 1997, Mosby.)

- Skin and radioallergosorbent testing may be done if food allergies are suspected.
- Skin biopsy is usually done in patients with chronic angioedema refractory to corticosteroid treatment.

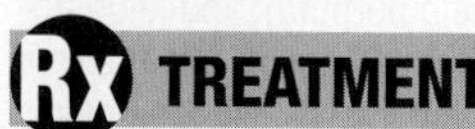

TREATMENT

NONPHARMACOLOGIC THERAPY

- Eliminate the offending agent
- Avoid triggering factors (e.g., cold, stress)
- Cold compresses to affected areas

ACUTE GENERAL Rx

- Acute life-threatening angioedema involving the larynx is treated with:
  1. Epinephrine 0.3 mg in a solution of 1:1000 given SC
  2. Diphenhydramine 25 to 50 mg IV or IM
  3. Cimetidine 300 mg IV or ranitidine 50 mg IV
  4. Methylprednisolone 125 mg IV
- Mainstay therapy in nonhereditary angioedema is H_1 antihistamines
  1. Diphenhydramine 25 to 50 mg q6h
  2. Chlorpheniramine 4 mg q6h
  3. Hydroxyzine 10 to 25 mg q6h
  4. Cetirizine 5 to 10 mg qd
  5. Loratadine 10 mg qd
  6. Fexofenadine 60 mg qd
- H_2 antihistamines can be added to H_1 antihistamines
  1. Ranitidine 150 mg bid
  2. Cimetidine 400 mg bid
  3. Famotidine 20 mg bid
- Tricyclic antidepressants
  1. Doxepin 25 to 50 mg qd
- Corticosteroids are rarely required for symptomatic relief of acute angioedema.
- Antihistamines are probably ineffective in acute hereditary angioedema.
- Purified plasma-derived C1-INH replacement therapy is effective and safe in treating acute attacks of hereditary angioedema caused by C1 inhibitor deficiency. Cost is a limiting factor. Acute attacks can be managed with plasma-derived or recombinant preparations of C1 inhibitor, with ecallantide, a specific plasma kallikrein inhibitor, or with the use of the B2 bradykinin-receptor antagonist icatibant.

CHRONIC Rx

- Chronic angioedema is treated as described under "Acute General Rx."
- Corticosteroids are used more often in chronic nonhereditary angioedema.
- Prednisone 1 mg/kg/day for 5 days and then tapered over a period of weeks.
- Androgens (danazol, stanozolol, oxandrolone, methyltestosterone) and antifibrinolytic agents can be used for the treatment of chronic hereditary angioedema, which does not respond to antihistamines or corticosteroids but are associated with many adverse effects. Long-term prophylaxis with plasma-derived C1 inhibitor is safe and effective and may be used in patients who have frequent or severe attacks. Cost is a limiting factor. C1-INH replacement therapy was approved by the FDA in 2008. Available agents are Cinryze and Berinert. Icatibant is a new bradykinin-receptor antagonist in hereditary angioedema currently undergoing trials.

DISPOSITION

- Antihistamines achieve symptomatic relief in more than 80% of patients with nonhereditary acute angioedema.
- In chronic nonhereditary angioedema, corticosteroids are given in addition to antihistamines.
- A small percentage of people will have recurrence of symptoms after steroid treatment.
- Chronic angioedema can last for months and even years.

REFERRAL

Dermatology consultation is recommended in patients with chronic angioedema, hereditary angioedema, and recurring angioedema.

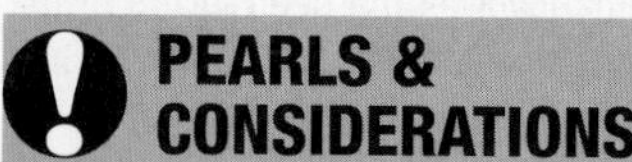

PEARLS & CONSIDERATIONS

ACE inhibitors can cause angioedema up to many months after initiation. There are multiple case reports and case series of angiotensin receptor blocker (ARB)–induced angioedema, although the risk is substantially less than that of ACE inhibitors. (Incidence rates per 1000 person-years are 4.38 cases for ACE inhibitors, 1.66 cases for ARBs.) The incidence rate is also very high for the direct renin inhibitor aliskiren (4.67).

COMMENTS

- Identifying a cause for angioedema in patients is often difficult and met with frustration.
- Chronic angioedema, unlike acute angioedema, is rarely caused by an allergic reaction.

SUGGESTED READINGS

available at www.expertconsult.com

RELATED CONTENT

Angioedema (Patient Information)

AUTHOR: **MEL L. ANDERSON, M.D.**

BASIC INFORMATION

DEFINITION

Ankle fractures involve the lateral, medial, or posterior malleolus of the ankle and may occur either alone or in some combination. Associated ligamentous injuries are included.

CLASSIFICATION

The Danis-Weber (Fig. 1-90) and Lauge-Hensen classifications of ankle fratures are described in Table 1-42.

ICD-9CM CODES
824.8 Ankle fracture (malleolus) (closed)
824.2 Lateral malleolus fracture (fibular)
824.0 Medial malleolus fracture (tibial)
ICD-10CM CODES
S82.899A Other fracture of unspecified lower leg, initial encounter for closed fracture
S82.63XA Displaced fracture of lateral malleolus of unspecified fibula, initial encounter for closed fracture
S82.53XA Displaced fracture of medial malleolus of unspecified tibia, initial encounter for closed fracture

PHYSICAL FINDINGS & CLINICAL PRESENTATION

- Deformity usually depends on extent of displacement
- Pain, tenderness, and hemorrhage at the site of injury
- Gentle palpation of ligamentous structures (especially deltoid ligament) to determine the extent of soft tissue injury
- Evaluation of distal neurovascular status; results recorded

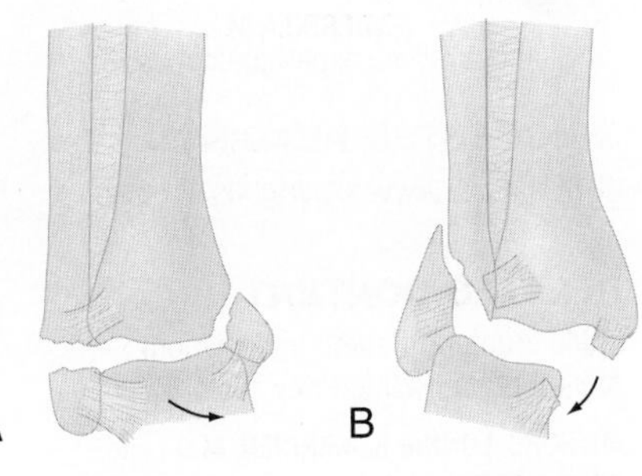

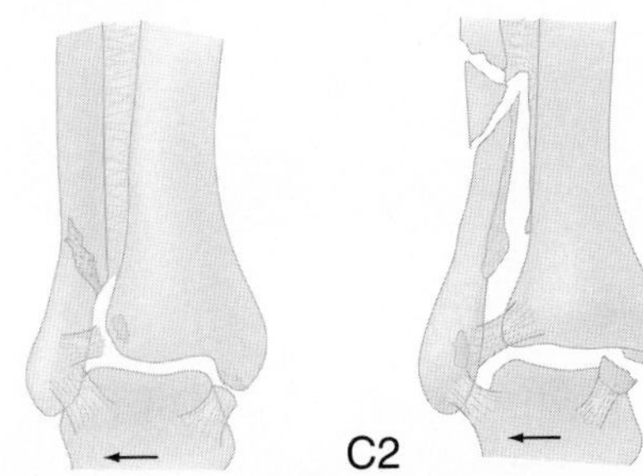

FIGURE 1-90 The Danis-Weber classification of ankle fractures focuses on the location of the fibular fracture in relation to the tibiotalar joint. (From Wilson FC: The pathogenesis and treatment of ankle fractures: classification. In Green WB [ed]: *Instructional course lectures,* ed 39, Easton, PA, 1990, American Academy of Orthopedic Surgeons.)

ETIOLOGY

- The ankle depends on its ligamentous and bony support for stability. The joint, or *mortise,* is an inverted U with the dome of the talus fitting into the medial and lateral malleoli. The posterior margin of the tibia is often called the *third* or *posterior malleolus.*
- Most common ankle fractures are the result of eversion or lateral rotation forces on the talus (in contrast with common sprains, which are usually caused by inversion).

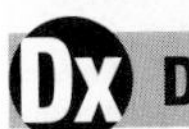

DIAGNOSIS

The diagnosis is usually established on the basis of the nature of the injury, the presence of typical findings of bony tenderness with swelling, and abnormal imaging studies.

DIFFERENTIAL DIAGNOSIS

- Ankle sprain
- Avulsion fracture of hindfoot or metatarsal

IMAGING STUDIES

Standard AP and lateral views (Fig. 1-91) accompanied by an AP taken 15 degrees internally rotated. The last view is taken to properly visualize the mortise.

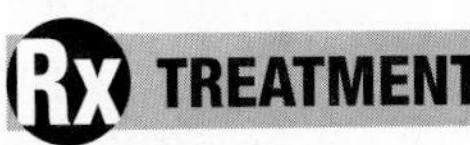

TREATMENT

All fractures: elevation and ice to control swelling for 48 to 72 hr.

ACUTE GENERAL Rx

- Clinical and roentgenographic assessment of the status of the ankle mortise and stability of the injury is mandatory to determine treatment.
- There is potential for displacement if both sides of the joint are significantly injured (e.g., fracture of the lateral malleolus with deltoid ligament injury).
- Deviation of the position of the talus in the mortise could lead to traumatic arthritis.
- If there is no widening of the ankle mortise, many injuries can be safely treated with simple casting without reduction:
  1. Undisplaced or avulsion fractures of either malleolus below the ankle joint line:
     a. Stability of the joint is not compromised and a short leg walking cast or ankle support is sufficient.

TABLE 1-42 Classifications and Treatment of Ankle Fractures

	Normal	Abnormal
Talocrural angle—angle formed by parallel line to distal tibial articular surface and line connecting malleolar tips	**8-15 degrees** (or 83 degrees ± 4 degrees if perpendicular used)	> 2-3 degrees difference from contralateral = **fibular shortening**
Medial clear space—distance between lateral border of medial malleolus and lateral border of talus	< **4 mm** and equal to superior clear space	> 4 mm = lateral talar shift and **instability**
Tibiofibular clear space—distance between medial wall of fibula and tibial incisura	< **6 mm** on AP and mortise views	> 6 mm = **syndesmotic disruption (instability)**
Talar tilt—difference between medial and lateral superior clear space measurements	< **2 mm**	> 2 mm = **instability**

Classification:

1. **Danis-Weber**—based on location of fibular fracture A. Below syndesmosis B. At level of syndesmosis C. Above syndesmosis	2. **Lauge-Hansen**—based on position of foot and deforming force Supination external rotation—most common Supination adduction Pronation external rotation Pronation abduction

Treatment: Surgical decisions mostly based on stability.

Stable	Unstable
Isolated lateral malleolar fractions if:	**Lateral malleolus fractures** if:
Below syndesmosis	Medial injury/tenderness (bimalleolar equivalent)
No medial ligament injury or talar shift	Talar shift
Displacement < 5 mm	Above syndesmosis
No shortening	Shortened or displaced > 5 mm
Isolated medial malleolus fractures (although 5%-15% nonunion rates have been reported)	**Bimalleolar fractures** **Trimalleolar fractures** (fix posterior if > 25% of articular surface) **Maisonneuve fractures**

From Parvizi J: *High-yield orthopedics,* Philadelphia, 2010, Saunders.

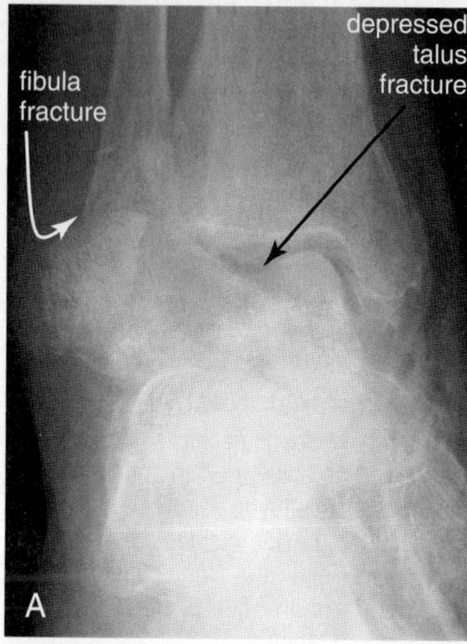

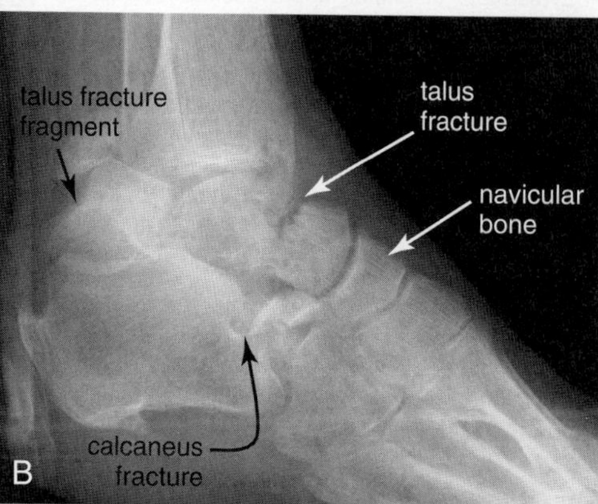

FIGURE 1-91 **A,** Anterior-posterior view. **B,** Lateral view. A depressed talus fracture is visible. In **B,** this fracture is seen to run through the midbody of the talus. **A** also demonstrates a distal fibula fracture, whereas in **B,** a calcaneal fracture is seen. The patient underwent CT to characterize these fractures further. (From Broder JS: *Diagnostic imaging for the emergency physician,* Philadelphia, 2011, Saunders.)

 b. Weight bearing is allowed as tolerated.
 c. In 4 to 6 wk, protection may be discontinued.
2. Isolated undisplaced fractures of the medial, lateral, or posterior malleolus:
 a. Usually stable and require only the application of a short leg walking cast with the ankle in the neutral position or fracture cast boot.
 b. Immobilization should be continued for 8 wk.
 c. Fracture line of lateral malleolus may persist roentgenographically for several months, but immobilization beyond 8 wk is usually unnecessary.
 d. Undisplaced bimalleolar fractures are treated with a long leg cast flexed 30 degrees at the knee to prevent motion and displacement of the fracture fragments. In 4 wk, a short leg walking cast may be applied for an additional 4 wk.
3. Isolated fractures of the lateral malleolus that are slightly displaced:
 a. May be treated with casting if no medial injury is present.
 b. A below-knee walking cast is applied with ankle in the neutral position; weight bearing is allowed as tolerated.
 c. Six wk of immobilization is sufficient.
 d. If medial tenderness is present, suggesting deltoid ligament rupture, a carefully molded cast may suffice if weight bearing is not allowed and the patient is followed up closely for signs of instability, especially after swelling recedes. If significant widening of the medial ankle mortise (increase in the "medial clear space") develops as a result of lateral displacement of the talus, referral for possible reduction is indicated.
 e. If signs of instability are already present at initial examination (widening of the medial clear space with medial tenderness), referral is indicated.
4. Undisplaced fracture of the distal fibular epiphysis:
 a. Often diagnosed clinically.
 b. There is tenderness over the epiphyseal plate.
 c. Roentgenographic findings are often negative.
 d. A short leg walking cast or fracture boot is applied for 4 wk.
 e. Growth disturbance is rare.
5. Isolated posterior malleolar fractures involving less than 25% of the joint surface on the lateral roentgenogram:
 Safely treated by applying a short leg walking cast or fracture brace. (Fractures involving >25% of the weight-bearing surface should be referred because of the potential for instability and subsequent traumatic arthritis.)

CHRONIC Rx

- Early motion is encouraged through a home exercise program.
- Protection from reinjury is appropriate for 4 to 6 wk after cast or brace removal.
- Temporary increase in lower extremity swelling that frequently occurs after short leg cast removal may benefit from the use of support hose.

DISPOSITION

Significant factors involved in the development of traumatic arthritis:
- Amount of joint trauma at the time of injury
- Eventual position of the talus in the mortise

Fracture nonunion is uncommon unless displacement is significant.

REFERRAL

Orthopedic consultation for:
- Unstable ankle joint
- Widened ankle mortise
- Posterior malleolar fracture over 25% of joint with incongruity
- Marked displacement of fracture fragment

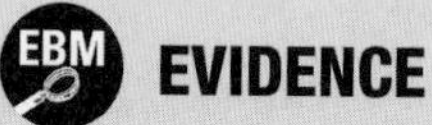

EVIDENCE

available at www.expertconsult.com

SUGGESTED READINGS

available at www.expertconsult.com

RELATED CONTENT

Ankle Fracture (Patient Information)
Ankle Sprain (Related Key Topic)

AUTHORS: **LONNIE R. MERCIER, M.D.,** and **FRED F. FERRI, M.D.**

BASIC INFORMATION

DEFINITION

An ankle sprain is an injury to the ligamentous support of the ankle. Most (85%) involve the lateral ligament complex (Fig. 1-92). The anterior inferior tibiofibular (AITF) ligament, deltoid ligament, and interosseous membrane may also be injured. Damage to the tibiofibular syndesmosis is sometimes called a *high sprain* because of pain above the ankle. Lateral ankle sprains classically are graded I, II, or III, representing no, partial, or complete rupture of the lateral ligaments, respectively. Table 1-43 describes a classification of ankle sprains

ICD-9CM CODES
845.00 Sprain, ankle or foot
ICD-10CM CODES
S93.409A Sprain of unspecified ligament of unspecified ankle, initial encounter

EPIDEMIOLOGY & DEMOGRAPHICS

PREVALENCE: One case/10,000 people each day
PREDOMINANT SEX: Varies according to age and level of physical activity

PHYSICAL FINDINGS & CLINICAL PRESENTATION

- Often a history of a "pop"
- Variable amounts of tenderness and hemorrhage
- Possible abnormal anterior drawer test (pulling the plantar flexed foot forward to determine if there is any abnormal increase in forward movement of the talus in the ankle mortise) (Fig. 1-93)
- Inversion sprains: tender laterally; syndesmotic injuries: area of tenderness is more anterior and proximal
- Evaluation of motor function (Fig. 1-94)

ETIOLOGY

- Lateral injuries usually result from inversion and plantar flexion injuries.
- Eversion and rotational forces may injure the deltoid or AITF ligament or the interosseous membrane.

DIAGNOSIS

DIFFERENTIAL DIAGNOSIS

- Fracture of the ankle or foot, particularly involving the distal fibular growth plate in the immature patient
- Avulsion fracture of the fifth metatarsal base

WORKUP

- History and clinical examination are usually sufficient to establish the diagnosis.
- Plain radiographs are always needed.

IMAGING STUDIES

Roentgenographic evaluation (Fig. 1-95): According to the Ottawa criteria, radiography is indicated if there is pain in the malleolar or midfoot zone, and either bone tenderness over an area of potential fracture or an inability to bear weight for four steps immediately after the injury and in the physician's office.

TREATMENT

ACUTE GENERAL Rx

- The first line of treatment is described by the mnemonic *RICE:*
  - ***R**est*
  - ***I**ce* (3 to 7 days)
  - ***C**ompression*
  - ***E**levation*
- Pain control with NSAIDs, acetaminophen, mild opioids
- In 48 to 72 hr, active range of motion and weight bearing as tolerated
- Compression, support, and bracing is best achieved with an Air-Stirrup brace combined with an elastic compression wrap, or lace-up support alone.
- In 4 to 5 days, exercise against resistance added
- Possible cast immobilization for some patients who require early independent walking; short leg orthoses also available for the same purpose
- Surgery is rarely recommended, even for grade III sprains; reports of equally satisfactory outcomes with nonsurgical treatment

CHRONIC Rx

- Lateral heel and sole wedge to prevent inversion
- Protective taping or bracing during vigorous activities (Fig. 1-96)
- Strengthening exercises

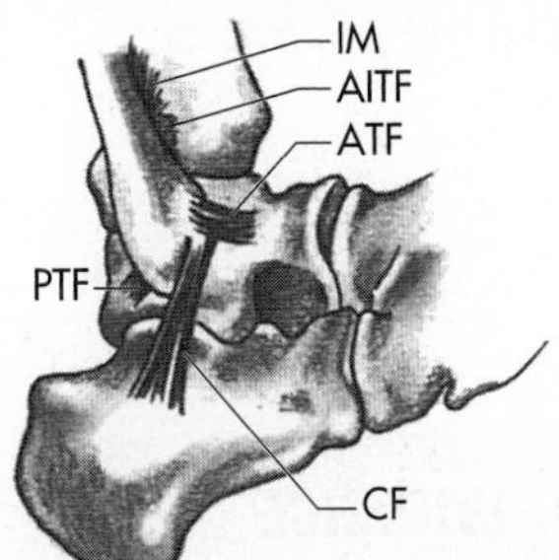

FIGURE 1-92 The lateral ankle ligaments, anterior and posterior talofibular *(ATF, PTF)* and calcaneofibular *(CF).* Also shown are the anterior inferior tibiofibular ligament *(AITF)* and the beginning of the interosseous membrane *(IM).* (From Mercier LR [ed]: *Practical orthopaedics,* ed 4, St Louis, 1995, Mosby.)

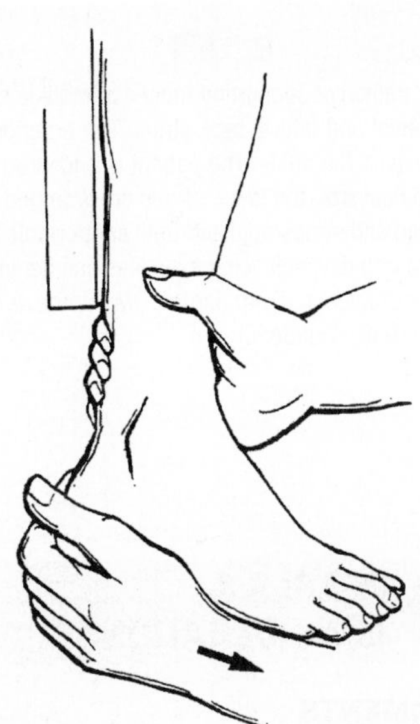

FIGURE 1-93 Anterior drawer test of the ankle (tests the integrity of the anterior talofibular ligament). (From Brinker MR, Miller MD: *Fundamentals of orthopaedics,* Philadelphia, 1999, Saunders.)

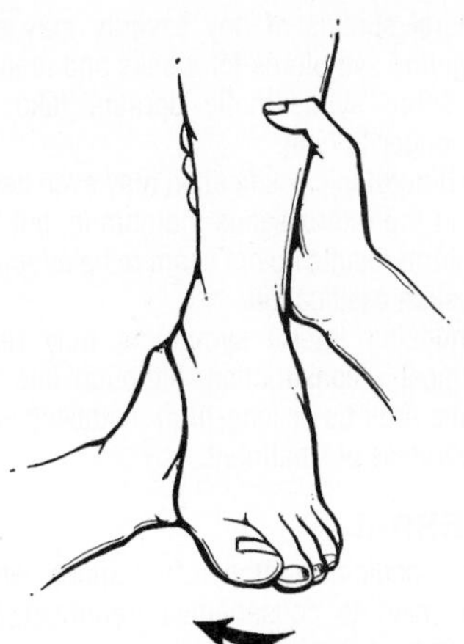

FIGURE 1-94 Talar tilt test (inversion stress) of the ankle (tests the integrity of the anterior talofibular ligament and the calcaneofibular ligament). (From Brinker MR, Miller MD: *Fundamentals of orthopaedics,* Philadelphia, 1999, Saunders.)

TABLE 1-43 Classification of Ankle Sprains

TYPE OF INJURY	EXTENT OF INJURY	PHYSICAL FINDINGS
Grade I	Stretch of the ligament with microscopic but not macroscopic tearing	Minor swelling but no joint instability
Grade II	Involves partial tearing of the particular ligament	Minor to moderate swelling and some instability of the affected ankle
Grade III	Involves complete rupture of the ligament	Significant swelling, tenderness, and ecchymosis; instability of the joint and inability to bear weight

From Adams JG et al: *Emergency medicine, clinical essentials,* ed 2, Philadelphia, 2013, Elsevier.

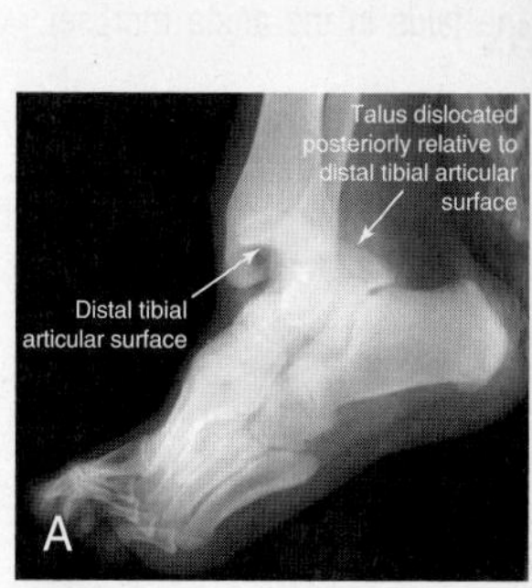

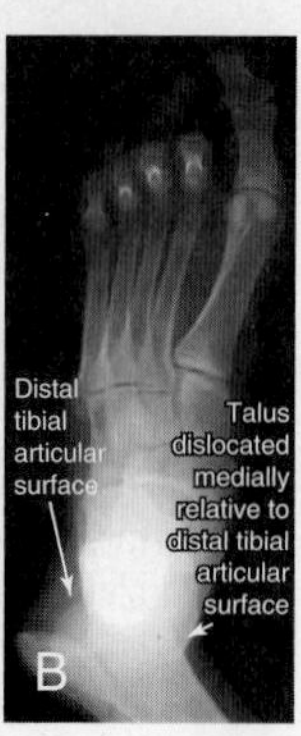

FIGURE 1-95 Tibiotalar dislocation. This 17-year-old male landed on his left ankle after dunking a basketball, sustaining a deformity. His tibiotalar joint is dislocated, with the talus dislocated posteriorly (visible on the lateral view, **A**) and medially (visible on the anterior-posterior view, **B**). No fractures are present in this case, although fractures are commonly associated with this injury because of the amount of force required to dislocate the ankle. This was an open injury, and the patient underwent exploration, irrigation, and debridement with primary closure. (From Broder JS: *Diagnostic imaging for the emergency physician,* Philadelphia, 2011, Saunders.)

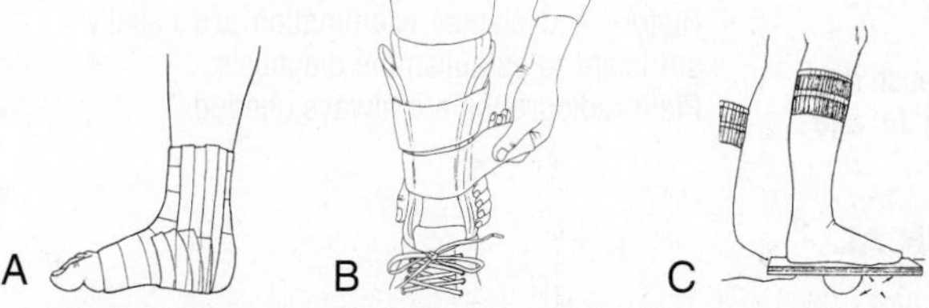

FIGURE 1-96 A, The most effective method of supporting most acute ankle sprains is by using an ACE wrap (BD, Franklin Lakes, NJ) reinforced with 1-inch medial and lateral tape strips. The anterior and posterior aspects of the ankle are left free to allow the patient to flex and extend the ankle. The patient is encouraged to bear weight with crutches. **B,** Diagram of an air splint. Straps are adjusted to heel size, the lower straps are wrapped about the ankle, and the side extensions are centered. The splint is then pressurized and straps adjusted until comfortable support and pressure are attained. **C,** As the ankle pain subsides, about the third to fifth day, balancing exercises can begin to allow the patient to regain ankle proprioception and avoid recurrent instability problems. (From Jardon OM, Mathews MS: Orthopedics. In Rakel RE [ed]: *Textbook of family practice,* ed 5, Philadelphia, 1995, Saunders.)

DISPOSITION

- Lateral sprains of any severity may cause lingering symptoms for weeks and months.
  1. Some syndesmotic sprains take even longer to heal.
  2. Heterotopic ossification may even develop in the interosseous membrane, but long-term results do not seem to be affected by such ossification.
- Continuing lateral symptoms may require surgical reconstruction, although late traumatic arthritis or long-term instability is rare regardless of treatment.

REFERRAL

For orthopedic consultation for patients who do not respond to conservative treatment. Most ankle sprains resolve in 2-6 wk.

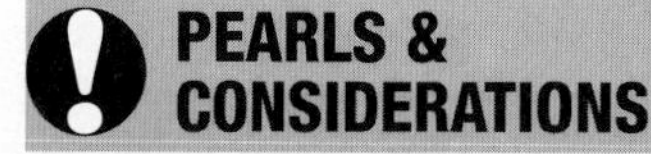

PEARLS & CONSIDERATIONS

COMMENTS

If healing seems delayed (more than 6 wk), the following conditions should be considered:

1. Talar dome fracture
2. Reflex sympathetic dystrophy
3. Chronic tendinitis
4. Peroneal tendon subluxation
5. Other occult fracture
6. Peroneal weakness (poor rehabilitation)
7. A "high" (syndesmotic) sprain

Repeat plain roentgenograms, bone scan, or MRI may be indicated.

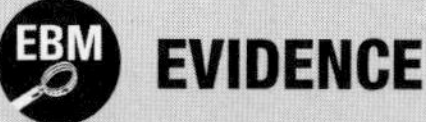

EVIDENCE

available at www.expertconsult.com

SUGGESTED READINGS

available at www.expertconsult.com

RELATED CONTENT

Ankle Sprain (Patient Information)
Ankle Fracture (Related Key Topic)

AUTHOR: **LONNIE R. MERCIER, M.D.**

BASIC INFORMATION

DEFINITION

Ankylosing spondylitis is a type of inflammatory arthritis involving the sacroiliac joints and axial skeleton characterized by ankylosis and enthesitis (inflammation at tendon insertions). It is one of a family of overlapping syndromes called seronegative spondyloarthropathies that includes reactive arthritis (Reiter syndrome), psoriatic spondylitis, and enteropathic arthritis.

SYNONYMS

Marie-Strümpell disease

ICD-9CM CODES
720.0 Ankylosing spondylitis
ICD-10CM CODES
M45.9 Ankylosing spondylitis of unspecified sites in spine

EPIDEMIOLOGY & DEMOGRAPHICS

PREVALENCE: Between 0.1% and 1% of the population
PREDOMINANT AGE AT ONSET: 15 to 35 yr
PREDOMINANT SEX: Male/female ratio 2 to 3:1

PHYSICAL FINDINGS & CLINICAL PRESENTATION

- Prolonged morning back stiffness of insidious onset lasting more than 3 mo
- Bilateral sacroiliac tenderness (sacroiliitis)
- Limited lumbar spine motion (Fig. 1-97)
- Tenderness at tendon insertion sites, especially the Achilles tendons and plantar fascia
- Loss of chest expansion reflecting rib cage involvement
- Occasionally, peripheral joint arthritis, usually involving the large joints of the lower extremities
- In advanced cases the typical posture consists of compensatory hyperextension of neck, fixed flexion of hips, and compensatory flexion of knees (Fig. 1-98)
- Extraskeletal manifestations may affect the cardiovascular system (aortic insufficiency), lungs (pulmonary fibrosis), and eye (uveitis)

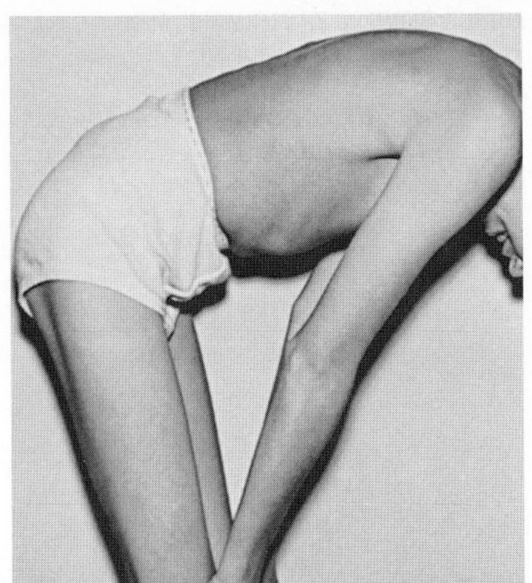

FIGURE 1-97 Loss of lumbodorsal spine mobility in a boy with ankylosing spondylitis. The lower spine remains straight when the patient bends forward. (From Behrman RE: *Nelson textbook of pediatrics,* ed 17, Philadelphia, 2005, Saunders.)

ETIOLOGY

Genetic factors, particularly *HLA-B27,* play an important role in susceptibility to the spondyloarthropathies. Infectious triggers have been implicated in some cases. Tumor necrosis factor is important in the inflammatory response.

DIAGNOSIS

DIFFERENTIAL DIAGNOSIS

- Diffuse idiopathic skeletal hyperostosis (Forestier disease)
- Noninflammatory back pain (A clinical algorithm for the evaluation of back pain is described in Section III.)
- Table 1-44 compares ankylosing spondylitis and related disorders.

LABORATORY TESTS

- Elevated sedimentation rate, C-reactive protein
- Mild hyperchromic anemia
- Demonstration of inflammatory sacroiliitis by radiography or MRI is essential for diagnosis
- HLA/B27 antigen is not useful in the evaluation of noninflammatory back pain because it is present in up to 8% to 10% of the normal population.

IMAGING STUDIES

- Classic features are those of bilateral sacroiliitis on radiographs of the pelvis
- Vertebral bodies lose anterior concave shape and become square
- With progression, calcification of the annulus fibrosus and paravertebral ligaments develop, giving rise to the so-called *bamboo spine* and a "trolley track" appearance (Fig. 1-99).
- MRI (Fig 1-100) may be useful in detecting early inflammatory lesions and is especially helpful when the history is suggestive but radiographs are equivocal.

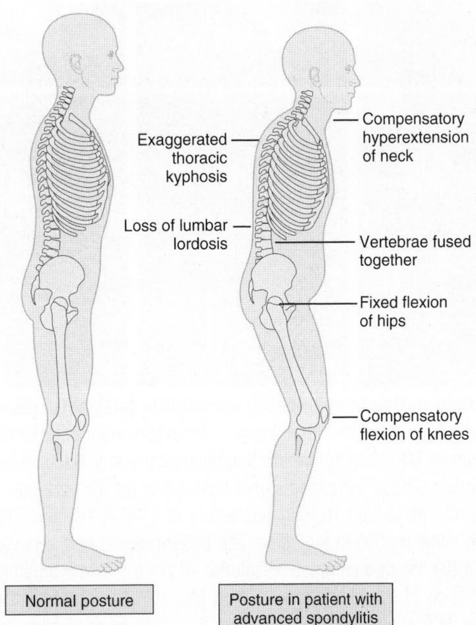

FIGURE 1-98 Ankylosing spondylitis. Typical posture in advanced cases compared with normal posture. (From Ballinger A: *Kumar & Clark's essentials of clinical medicine,* ed 6, Edinburgh, 2012, Saunders.)

TABLE 1-44 Comparison of Ankylosing Spondylitis and Related Disorders

Feature	Ankylosing Spondylitis	Psoriatic Arthritis	Reactive Arthritis	Enteropathic Arthropathy
Gender (M:F)	2-3:1	1:1	8:1 (GU) [1:1 (GI)]	1:1
Age at onset	<40	35-55	20-40	Young adult
Sacroiliitis or spondylitis	100%	~20%	~40%	<20%
Symmetry of sacroiliitis	Symmetric	Asymmetric	Asymmetric	Symmetric
Peripheral arthritis	~25%	95%	90%	15%-20%
Distribution	Axial and lower limbs	Any joint	Lower limbs	Variable
HLA-B27	85%-95%	25%	30%-80%	7%
Uveitis	25%-40%	25%	25%	10%-36%

From Hochberg MC et al: *Rheumatology,* ed 5, St Louis, 2011, Mosby.

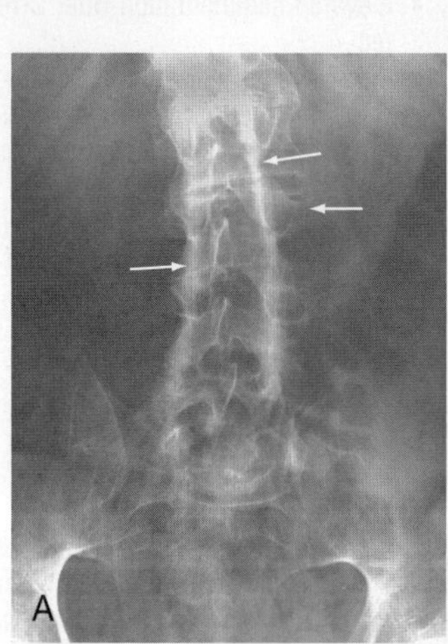

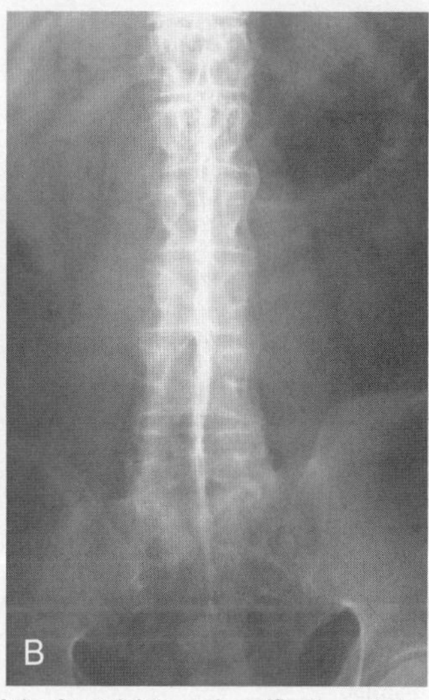

FIGURE 1-99 Ankylosing spondylitis. A, Fusion of the facet joints and ossification of the adjacent soft tissue have produced a "trolley track" appearance *(arrows)*. The sacroiliac joints are fused. Syndesmophytes are present. **B,** In another patient, there is a prominent fusion of the interspinous ligaments producing a "saber sheath" appearance. (From Harris ED: *Kelley's textbook of rheumatology,* ed 7, Philadelphia, 2005, Saunders.)

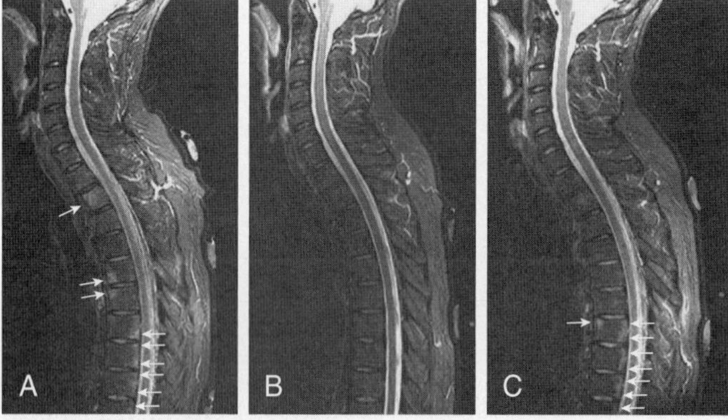

FIGURE 1-100 Spine inflammation in ankylosing spondylitis (magnetic resonance imaging [MRI]). A 43-year-old man with HLA-B27–positive ankylosing spondylitis with deteriorating symptoms, including inflammatory back pain, had an MRI scan before starting biologic therapy. Baseline sagittal short tau inversion recovery (STIR) MRI **(A)** shows diffuse increased signal (edema) in the T2 vertebral body and multiple foci of corner inflammation anteriorly at T5 and T6, and posteriorly at T7, T8, T9, and T10 *(arrows)*. Other images confirmed extensive active inflammation in the spine. The patient responded very well, and after 6 months of therapy, a repeat STIR MRI **(B)** showed complete resolution of bone marrow inflammation. Subsequently, the patient experienced recurrence of symptoms, and a third MRI **(C)** was performed (2 months after anti-TNF therapy was stopped). This MRI shows no edema at T5-T6, a conspicuous new lesion anteriorly at T7, and recurrent inflammation posteriorly in the lower thoracic spine *(arrows)*. (From Firestein GS, et al: *Kelly's textbook of rheumatology*, ed 9, Philadelphia, 2013, Saunders.)

Rx TREATMENT

NONPHARMACOLOGIC THERAPY

- Exercises primarily to maintain on flexibility and aerobic activity are important
- Postural training
  1. Patients must be instructed on spinal extension exercises to avoid fusion in a flexed position
  2. Sleeping should be in the supine position on a firm mattress; pillows should not be placed under the head or knees.

CHRONIC Rx

- NSAIDs: Patients with ankylosing spondylitis should be prescribed full-dose continuous NSAID therapy. There is anecdotal evidence suggesting that indomethacin may be more effective than other NSAIDs, but other NSAIDs are efficacious and may be better tolerated. One study suggested that continuous NSAID therapy may retard the radiographic progression of ankylosing spondylitis.
- Sulfasalazine may be efficacious in some patients, especially for peripheral arthritis
- Tumor necrosis factor (TNF) antagonists such as etanercept, infliximab, and adalimumab have been shown to be very effective for relieving symptoms of spinal inflammatory arthritis in numerous controlled studies. Anti-TNF therapy should be recommended for patients whose symptoms are not completely controlled with NSAIDs, and it sometimes results in dramatic improvement in symptoms, range of motion of the spine, and quality of life for these patients.

DISPOSITION

Most patients have a normal life span but many suffer significant disability from loss of spinal mobility

REFERRAL

All patients with seronegative spondyloarthropathy should be referred to a rheumatologist for consideration of anti-TNF therapy

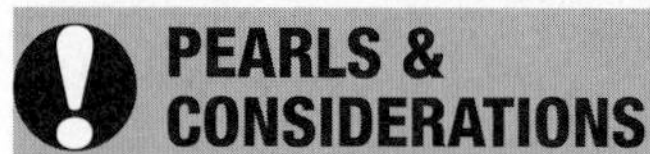

PEARLS & CONSIDERATIONS

A family history of seronegative spondyloarthropathy increases the specificity of testing for *HLA-B27.*

SUGGESTED READINGS

available at www.expertconsult.com

RELATED CONTENT

Fig. 3-180 Spondyloarthropathy, diagnosis (Algorithm)
Fig. 3-181 Spondyloarthropathy, treatment (Algorithm)
Ankylosing Spondylitis (Patient Information)

AUTHOR: **BERNARD ZIMMERMANN, M.D.**

BASIC INFORMATION

DEFINITION

A fistula is an inflammatory tract with a secondary (external) opening in the perianal skin and a primary (internal) opening in the anal canal at the dentate line. It originates in an abscess in the intersphincteric space of the anal canal. Fistulas can be classified as follows:

1. Intersphincteric: fistula track passes within the intersphincteric plane to the perianal skin (most common)
2. Transsphincteric: fistula track passes from the internal opening, through the internal and external sphincter, and into the ischiorectal fossa to the perianal skin (frequent)
3. Suprasphincteric: after passing through the internal sphincter, fistula tract passes above the puborectalis and then tracts downward, lateral to the external sphincter, into the ischiorectal space to the perianal skin (uncommon); if abscess cavity extends cephalad, a supralevator abscess possibly palpable on rectal examination
4. Extrasphincteric: fistula tract passes from the rectum, above the levators, through the levator muscles to the ischiorectal space and perianal skin (rare)

With a horseshoe fistula, the tract passes from one ischiorectal fossa to the other behind the rectum.

SYNONYMS

Fistula-in-ano

ICD-9CM CODES
565.1 Anal fistula
ICD-10CM CODES
K60.3 Anal fistula

EPIDEMIOLOGY & DEMOGRAPHICS

- Common in all ages
- Occurs equally in men and women
- Associated with constipation
- Pediatric age group: more common in infants; boys more than girls

PHYSICAL FINDINGS & CLINICAL PRESENTATION

- Acute stage: perianal swelling, pain, and fever
- Chronic stage: history of rectal drainage or bleeding; previous abscess with drainage
- Tender external fistulous opening, within 2 to 3 cm of the anal verge, with purulent or serosanguineous drainage on compression; the greater the distance from the anal margin, the greater the probability of a complicated upward extension
- Goodsall's rule:
  1. Location of the internal opening related to the location of the external opening.
  2. With external opening anterior to an imaginary line drawn horizontally across the midpoint of the anus: fistulous tract runs radially into the anal canal.
  3. With opening posterior to the transanal line: tract is usually curvilinear, entering the anal canal in the posterior midline.
  4. Exception to this rule: an external, anterior opening that is >3 cm from the anus. In this case the tract may curve posteriorly and end in the posterior midline.
- If perianal abscess recurs, presence of a fistula is suggested

ETIOLOGY

- Most common: nonspecific cryptoglandular infection (skin or intestinal flora)
- Fistulas more common when intestinal microorganisms are cultured from the anorectal abscess
- Tuberculosis
- Lymphogranuloma venereum
- Actinomycosis
- Inflammatory bowel disease (IBD): Crohn's disease, ulcerative colitis
- Trauma: surgery (episiotomy, prostatectomy), foreign bodies, anal intercourse
- Malignancy: carcinoma, leukemia, lymphoma
- Treatment of malignancy: surgery, radiation

DIAGNOSIS

DIFFERENTIAL DIAGNOSIS

- Hidradenitis suppurativa
- Pilonidal sinus
- Bartholin's gland abscess or sinus
- Infected perianal sebaceous cysts

WORKUP

- Digital rectal examination:
  1. Assess sphincter tone and voluntary squeeze pressure
  2. Determine the presence of an extraluminal mass
  3. Identify an indurated track
  4. Palpate an internal opening or pit
- Gentle probing of external orifice to avoid creating a false tract; 50% do not have clinically detectable opening
- Anoscopy
- Proctosigmoidoscopy to exclude inflammatory or neoplastic disease
- All studies done under adequate anesthesia

LABORATORY TESTS

- Complete blood count
- Rectal biopsy if diagnosis of IBD or malignancy suspected; biopsy of external orifice is useless

IMAGING STUDIES

- Colonoscopy or barium enema if:
  1. Diagnosis of IBD or malignancy is suspected
  2. History of recurrent or multiple fistulas
  3. Patient <25 yr
- Small bowel series: occasionally obtained for reasons similar to above
- Fistulography: unreliable but may be helpful in complicated fistulas

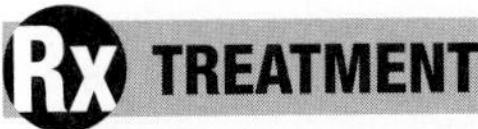

TREATMENT

NONPHARMACOLOGIC THERAPY

Sitz baths

ACUTE GENERAL Rx

- Treatment of choice: surgery
- Broad-spectrum antibiotic given if:
  1. Cellulitis present
  2. Patient is immunocompromised
  3. Valvular heart disease present
  4. Prosthetic devices present
- Stool softener/laxative

CHRONIC Rx

- Surgery
- Surgical goals are as follows:
  1. Cure the fistula
  2. Prevent recurrence
  3. Preserve sphincter function
  4. Minimize healing time
- Methods for the management of anal fistulas: fistulotomy, setons (maintains fistula patent for drainage while spontaneous healing occurs), rectal advancement flaps, colostomy

DISPOSITION

Outpatient surgery

REFERRAL

Refer to a surgeon with expertise in this area

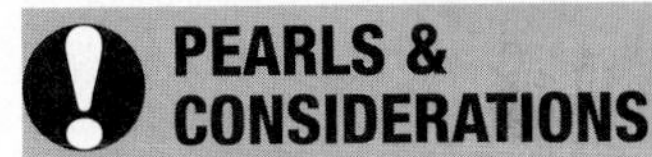

PEARLS & CONSIDERATIONS

COMMENTS

- HIV-positive and diabetic patients with perirectal abscesses/fistulas are true surgical emergencies.
- Risk of septicemia, Fournier's gangrene, and other septic complications make immediate drainage imperative.

SUGGESTED READINGS

available at www.expertconsult.com

RELATED CONTENT

Anal Fissure (Related Key Topic)
Hemorrhoids (Related Key Topic)

AUTHOR: **RUBEN ALVERO, M.D.**

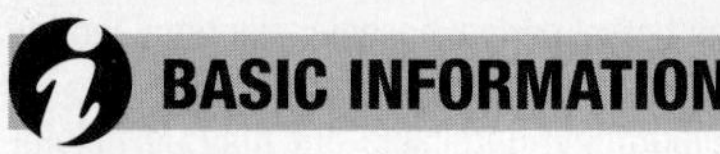

DEFINITION

Anorexia nervosa is a psychiatric disorder characterized by abnormal eating behavior, severe self-induced weight loss, and a specific psychopathology (see "Workup").

ICD-9CM CODES
307.1 Anorexia nervosa
ICD-10CM CODES
F50.00 Anorexia nervosa, unspecified
F50.01 Restricting type
F50.02 Binge-eating/purging type

EPIDEMIOLOGY & DEMOGRAPHICS

INCIDENCE/PREVALENCE (IN U.S.):

- Anorexia nervosa occurs in 0.2% to 1.3% of the general population, with an annual incidence of 5 to 10 cases per 100,000 persons.
- Participation in activities that promote thinness (athletics, modeling) is associated with a higher incidence of anorexia nervosa.

PREDOMINANT SEX: Female/male ratio is 9:1. Approximately 0.5% to 1% of women between the ages of 15 and 30 yr have anorexia nervosa.

PREDOMINANT AGE: Adolescence to young adulthood is the predominant age. Mean age of onset is 17 yr. Approximately 0.5% to 1% of college-aged women have anorexia nervosa.

PHYSICAL FINDINGS & CLINICAL PRESENTATION

Eating disorders can affect every organ system. Primary care physicians must be skilled at recognizing this disorder because patients with mild cases usually present with nonspecific symptoms such as asthenia, cold intolerance, lack of energy, or dizziness. Children and adolescents are at particular risk due to their active phase of growth and development. The physical examination may be normal in the early stages or in mild cases. Patients with moderate to severe anorexia have the following physical characteristics:

- Patient is emaciated and bundled in clothing.
- Skin is dry and has excessive growth of lanugo. Skin may also be yellow-tinged from carotenodermia.
- Brittle nails, thinning scalp hair are present.
- Bradycardia, hypotension, hypothermia, and bradypnea are common.
- Female fat distribution pattern is no longer evident.
- Axillary and pubic hair is preserved.
- Peripheral edema may be present.

ETIOLOGY

- Etiology is unknown, but probably multifactorial (sociocultural, psychological, familial, and genetic factors).
- A history of sexual abuse has been reported in as many as 50% of patients with anorexia nervosa.
- Psychological factors: anorexics often have an incompletely developed personal identity. They struggle to maintain a sense of control over their environment, they usually have a low self-esteem, and they lack the sense that they are valued and loved for themselves.

Dx DIAGNOSIS

DIFFERENTIAL DIAGNOSIS

- Other eating disorders (see Table 1-45)
- Substance abuse
- Depression with loss of appetite
- Obsessive compulsive disorder
- Schizophrenia
- Conversion disorder
- Occult carcinoma, lymphoma
- Endocrine disorders: Addison disease, diabetes mellitus, hypothyroidism or hyperthyroidism, panhypopituitarism
- Gastrointestinal disorders: celiac disease, Crohn's disease, intestinal parasitosis
- Infectious disorders: AIDS, tuberculosis
- A clinical algorithm for the evaluation of anorexia is described in Section III

WORKUP

- A diagnosis can be made by using the following DSM-5 diagnostic criteria for anorexia nervosa.
  A. Restriction of energy intake relative to requirements, leading to a significantly low body weight in the context of age, sex, developmental trajectory, and physical health. Significantly low weight is defined as a weight that is less than minimally normal or, for children or adolescents, less than that minimally expected.
  B. Intense fear of gaining weight or becoming fat, or persistent behavior that interferes with weight gain, even though at a significantly low weight.
  C. Disturbance in the way in which one's body or shape is experience, undue influence of body weight or shape on self-evaluation, or persistent lack of recognition of the seriousness of the current low body weight.

TABLE 1-45 Diagnostic Features of Eating Disorders

Anorexia nervosa	Body weight willfully maintained below normal level Abnormal perception of body morphology Intense fear of weight gain Amenorrhea
Bulimia nervosa	Large uncontrolled eating binges at least twice weekly Inappropriate compensatory behavior (e.g., vomiting, purging)
Binge eating disorder	Large uncontrolled eating binges at least twice weekly No regular inappropriate compensatory disorders Marked distress about binges

From Besser CM, Thorner MO: *Comprehensive clinical endocrinology,* ed 3, St Louis, 2002, Mosby.

Specify type:

Restricting type: During the last 3 mo, the individual has not engaged in recurrent episodes of binge eating or purging behavior (i.e., self-induced vomiting or the misuse of laxatives, diuretics, or enemas). This subtype describes presentations in which weight loss is accomplished primarily through dieting, fasting, and/or excessive exercise.

Binge-eating/purging type: During the last 3 mo, the individual has engaged in recurrent episodes of binge eating or purging behavior (i.e., self-induced vomiting or the misuse of laxatives, diuretics, or enemas).

Severity level: see "Acute General Rx" section

- The SCOFF questionnaire is a screening tool for eating disorders used in England. It consists of the following five questions:
  1. Do you make yourself ***s***ick because you feel full?
  2. Have you lost ***c***ontrol over how much you eat?
  3. Have you lost more than ***o***ne stone (approximately 6 kg) recently?
  4. Do you believe yourself to be ***f***at when others say you are thin?
  5. Does ***f***ood dominate your life?
- A positive response to two or more questions has a reported sensitivity of 100% for anorexia and bulimia and an overall specificity of 87.5%.
- In college-aged women a positive response to any of the following screening questions also warrants further evaluation:
  1. How many diets have you been on in the past year?
  2. Do you think you should be dieting?
  3. Are you dissatisfied with your body size?
  4. Does your weight affect the way you think about yourself?
- Baseline ECG should be performed on all patients with anorexia nervosa. Routine monitoring of patients with prolonged QT interval is necessary; sudden death in these patients is often caused by ventricular arrhythmias related to QT interval prolongation.
- A dual-energy x-ray absorptiometry (DEXA) scan to screen for osteopenia should be considered after 6 mo of amenorrhea in patients suspected of anorexia nervosa.

LABORATORY TESTS

- In mild cases, laboratory findings may be completely normal.
- Endocrine abnormalities:
  1. Decreased follicle-stimulating hormone, luteinizing hormone, T_4, T_3, estrogens, urinary 17-OH steroids, estrone, and estradiol
  2. Normal free T_4, thyroid-stimulating hormone
  3. Increased cortisol, growth hormone, rT_3, T_3RU
  4. Absence of cyclic surge of luteinizing hormone
- Leukopenia, thrombocytopenia, anemia, reduced erythrocyte sedimentation rate, reduced complement levels, and reduced CD4 and CD8 cells may be present.

- Metabolic alkalosis, hypocalcemia, hypokalemia, hypomagnesemia, hypercholesterolemia, and hypophosphatemia may be present.
- Increased plasma b-carotene levels are useful to distinguish these patients from others on starvation diets.

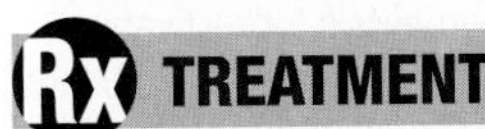

TREATMENT

NONPHARMACOLOGIC THERAPY

- A multidisciplinary approach with psychological, medical, and nutritional support is necessary.
- A goal weight should be set and the patient should be initially monitored at least once a week in the office setting. The target weight is 100% of ideal BW for teenagers and 90% to 100% for older patients.
- Weight gain should be gradual (1 to 3 lb/wk) to prevent gastric dilation. Begin with 800 to 1200 kcal in frequent small meals (to avoid bloating sensation), then increase calories to 1500 to 3000 depending on height and age.
- Add, as necessary, vitamin and mineral supplements.
- In severe cases, total parenteral nutrition must be used (starting at 800 to 1200 kcal/day).
- Electrolyte levels should be strictly monitored.
- Mealtime should be a time for social interaction, not confrontation.
- Postprandially, sedentary activities are recommended. The patient's access to a bathroom should be monitored to prevent purging.

ACUTE GENERAL Rx

- Criteria to decide on the appropriate initial course of treatment for patients with anorexia nervosa are usually based on the presence of complications, percentage of ideal BW, and severity of body image distortion. According to DSM-5,[1] the minimum level of severity is based, for adults, on current body mass index (BMI; see below) or, for children and adolescents, on BMI percentile. The level of severity may be increased to reflect clinical symptoms, the degree of functional disability, and need for supervision.
  - Mild: BMI ≥17 kg/m^2
  - Moderate: BMI 16-16.99 kg/m^2
  - Severe: BMI 15-15.99 kg/m^2
  - Extreme: BMI <15 kg/m^2

[1] American Psychiatric Association: *Desk Reference to the Diagnostic Criteria from DSM-5*, Arlington, VA, 2013, American Psychiatric Association.

- Outpatient treatment is adequate for most patients.
- Indications for hospitalization are described under "Referral" section and summarized in Table 1-46.
- Medically stable patients who are within 85% of ideal BW can be followed up by the primary care physician at 3- or 4-wk intervals, which can be lengthened as the patient improves.
- Pharmacologic treatment generally has no role in anorexia nervosa unless major depression or another psychiatric disorder is present. SSRIs can be used to alleviate the depressed mood and moderate obsessive-compulsive behavior in some individuals.

CHRONIC Rx

- Psychotherapy continued for years and focused specifically on self-image, family and peer interactions, and relapse prevention is an integral part of a successful recovery.
- Family therapy is also recommended, especially in younger patients.

TABLE 1-46 Indications for In-Patient Medical Hospitalization of Patients with Anorexia Nervosa

Physical and Laboratory
Heart rate <45 beats/min
Other cardiac rhythm disturbances
Blood pressure <80/50 mm Hg
Postural hypotension resulting in a >10 mm Hg drop or a >20 beats/min increase
Hypokalemia
Hypophosphatemia
Hypoglycemia
Dehydration
Body temperature <97°F
<80% healthy body weight
Hepatic, cardiac, or renal compromise
Psychiatric
Suicidal intent and plan
Very poor motivation to recover (in family and patient)
Preoccupation with ego-syntonic thoughts
Coexisting psychiatric disorders
Miscellaneous
Requires supervision after meals and while using the restroom
Failed day treatment

From Kliegman RM et al: *Nelson textbook of pediatrics*, ed 19, Philadelphia, 2011, Saunders.

DISPOSITION

- The long-term prognosis is generally poor and marked by recurrent exacerbations. The percentage of patients with anorexia nervosa who fully recover is modest. Most patients continue to have a distorted body image, disordered eating habits, and psychic difficulties.
- Most patients with anorexia nervosa will recover menses within 6 mo of reaching 90% of their ideal BW. It is important to note that patients with anorexia nervosa can become pregnant despite amenorrhea.
- Mortality rates vary from 5% to 20% and are six times that of peers without anorexia. Frequent causes of death are electrolyte abnormalities, starvation, or suicide.
- Factors that predict improved outcome in patients with eating disorders include early age at diagnosis, brief interval before initiation of treatment, good parent-child relationships, and having other healthy relationships with friends or therapists.
- A prolonged QT interval is a marker for risk of sudden death.

REFERRAL

Hospitalization should be considered in the following situations:

1. Severe dehydration or electrolyte imbalance
2. ECG abnormalities (prolonged QT interval, arrhythmias)
3. Significant physiologic instability (hypotension, orthostatic changes)
4. Intractable vomiting, purging, or bingeing
5. Suicidal thoughts
6. Weight loss exceeding 30% of ideal BW and unresponsiveness to outpatient treatment
7. Rapidly progressing weight loss (>2 lb in a week)
8. Failure to progress in nutritional rehabilitation in outpatient treatment

SUGGESTED READINGS

available at www.expertconsult.com

RELATED CONTENT

Fig. 3-20 Evaluation of anorexia (Algorithm)
Anorexia Nervosa (Patient Information)

AUTHOR: **FRED F. FERRI, M.D.**

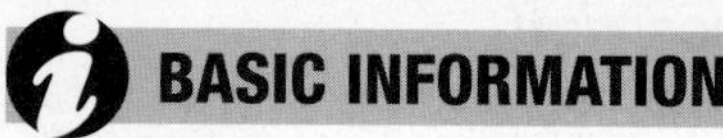

BASIC INFORMATION

DEFINITION

Anoxic brain injury is cerebral ischemic injury due to decreased oxygen or blood flow to the brain typically caused by interruption of cardiac circulation or respiratory failure.

SYNONYMS

Hypoxic-ischemic injury

ICD-9CM CODES
348.1 Anoxic brain damage
ICD-10CM CODES
G93.1 Anoxic brain damage, not elsewhere classified

EPIDEMIOLOGY & DEMOGRAPHICS

INCIDENCE:

- Variable based on diagnostic criteria
- 492,000 out-of-hospital cardiac arrests per year in the U.S.

PREVALENCE:

- Vegetative state varies from 40 to 168 per 1 million population, depending on definition used.
- Recovery is rare after 3 months with life expectancy lasting 2 to 5 years.

RISK FACTORS: Same as risk factors for cardiorespiratory arrest: HTN, hyperlipidemia, tobacco use, and physical inactivity.

PHYSICAL FINDINGS & CLINICAL PRESENTATION

- Variable depending on degree of insult
- Minimally conscious state: altered consciousness with normal sleep-wake cycles and intermittent interaction with the environment: intermittently follows simple commands, and maintains visual tracking
- Vegetative state: able to maintain normal sleep-wake cycles; there is loss of cognitive awareness and ability to interact with environment
- Coma: pathologic loss of awareness and ability to interact with the environment; loss of sleep-wake cycles
- Brain death: irreversible loss of cortical and brainstem function manifesting as loss of awareness, cranial reflexes, and motor response, isoelectric EEG

ETIOLOGY

- Ischemia (decreased cerebral perfusion): myocardial infarction, hemorrhage, shock
- Hypoxia (decreased oxygenation): drowning, strangulation, aspiration, carbon monoxide poisoning

Dx DIAGNOSIS

DIFFERENTIAL DIAGNOSIS

- Other causes of encephalopathy, including toxic, metabolic, infectious, or neoplastic causes; nonconvulsive status epilepticus; hypothermia

WORKUP

- Neurologic examination (coma examination) to ascertain level of encephalopathy
- Systemic evaluation for causes of cardiorespiratory failure
- Laboratory studies (listed below) to evaluate alternate causes of encephalopathy
- Imaging studies: MRI of brain or CT of head (if MRI cannot be obtained)

LABORATORY TESTS

Urine drug screen, serum metabolic profile, ammonia, complete blood count, coagulation panel, finger stick glucose, arterial blood gas, blood alcohol panel, serum neuron-specific enolase (if available)

IMAGING STUDIES

- Imaging is usually not revealing within first 24 hr of an anoxic event.
- Head CT without contrast (Fig. 1-101): obtain 24 hr after anoxic event to evaluate for stroke, trauma, or hemorrhage
- MRI of brain (Fig. 1-102): obtain if head CT scan unrevealing; may show cortical necrosis and infarcts of the basal ganglia
- EEG: to assess for nonconvulsive status epilepticus
- SSEP (somatosensory evoked potentials): obtain 48 hr after anoxic event; poor bilateral cortical response is associated with poor prognosis

OTHER STUDIES

- EEG: to assess for nonconvulsive status epilepticus
- Somatosensory evoked potentials (SSEP): obtain 48 hr after anoxic event; poor bilateral cortical response is associated with poor prognosis

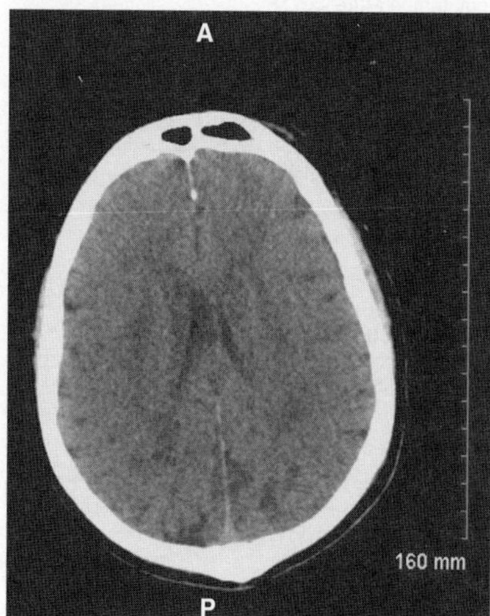

FIGURE 1-101 CT without contrast of a patient 1 day after pulseless electrical activity showing diffuse sulci effacement and loss of gray-white matter differentiation indicating cerebral edema. Diffuse white and gray matter hypodensities are also present. The patient remained comatose and life support was eventually withdrawn.

Rx TREATMENT

NONPHARMACOLOGIC THERAPY

- Hypothermia: evidence suggests that inducing hypothermia 32°-34° C for 24 hr following anoxic brain injury reduces metabolic need and may improve prognosis for recovery.
- Complications from hypothermia include bradycardia, hemodynamic instability, coagulopathy, infection, hyperglycemia, and hypokalemia.
- Contraindications for hypothermia: active hemorrhage, hemodynamic instability, sepsis, or trauma
- Indication for hypothermia: patients who have been resuscitated from a cardiac arrest with VF/VT as the presenting rhythm
- Hyperbaric oxygen is used in carbon monoxide poisoning.

ACUTE GENERAL Rx

- Supportive care: ABCs, secure airway, cardiopulmonary support in the critical care unit
- Control seizures with antiepileptic medications (may need midazolam or propofol drip if severe uncontrolled seizures).
- Treat myoclonus with clonazepam 8-12 mg daily in divided doses; levetiracetam and divalproate may be used for myoclonic status epilpeticus.

CHRONIC Rx

- Maintain adequate nutrition, infection precautions; provide DVT and gastric ulceration prophylaxis.
- Physical, occupational, and speech therapy as indicated per prognosis and patient ability
- May consider withdrawal of treatment per prognosis, family consultation, and respect for autonomy and dignity of the patient

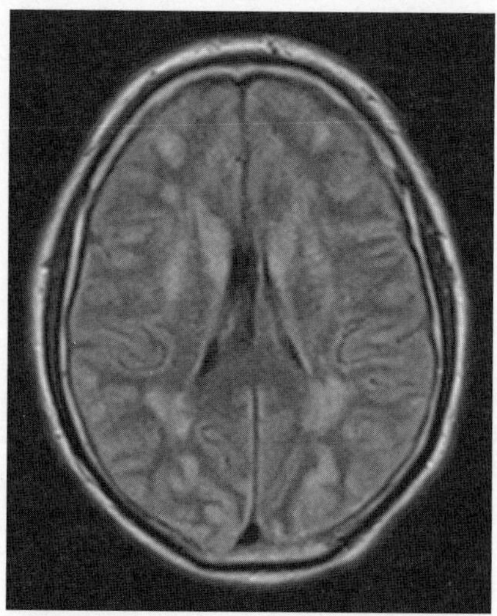

FIGURE 1-102 MRI FLAIR (fluid attenuated inversion recovery) of a patient 1 day after pulseless electrical activity showing bilateral multiple cortical, subcortical, gray and white hyperintensities. The patient remained comatose and life support was eventually withdrawn.

TABLE 1-47 Predictors of Poor Prognosis

Time from Onset of Anoxic Event	Clinical Exam
Initial exam	Pupils do not react to light (reflex absent)
24 hr	Eye movements are not roving conjugate or orienting and motor response is not better than flexor
72 hr	Motor response is not better than flexor
1 wk	Eye movements are not roving conjugate or orienting, no spontaneous eye opening, no following of commands
2 wk	No normal oculocephalic response, no following of commands, no spontaneous eye opening, and eye opening not improved by at least two grades

Composed from data presented in Levy DE et al: Predicting outcome from hypoxic-ischemic coma, *JAMA* 253(10):1420-1426, 1985.

TABLE 1-48 Predictors of Good Prognosis

Time from Onset of Anoxic Event	Clinical Exam
Initial exam	Pupils react to light (reflex present), motor response flexor or extensor, and eye movements spontaneous roving conjugate or orienting
24 hr	Motor response withdrawal or better, and eye opening improved at least 2 grades
72 hr	Motor response withdrawal or better and normal spontaneous eye movements present
1 wk	Follows commands
2 wk	Normal oculocephalic response

Composed from data presented in Levy DE et al: Predicting outcome from hypoxic-ischemic coma, *JAMA* 253(10):1420-1426, 1985.

DISPOSITION

Varies per extent of insult from acute rehabilitation to long-term care facility to return to home

REFERRAL

Referral to a neurologist is appropriate for definitive prognostication.

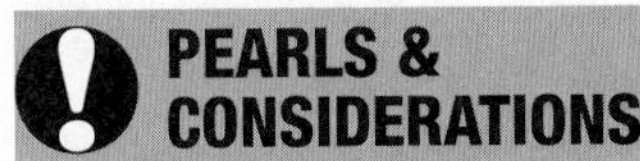

PEARLS & CONSIDERATIONS

COMMENTS

When assessing prognosis, use caution if patient is being treated with anesthetic agents or depressants including anticonvulsants. Refer to Tables 1-47 and 1-48 for indicators of prognosis.

PREVENTION

CPR, risk factor modification, induced hypothermia

PATIENT/FAMILY EDUCATION

Consult with family members regularly and provide accurate assessment of prognosis.

SUGGESTED READINGS

available at www.expertconsult.com

AUTHOR: **ALEXANDRA BOSKE, M.D.**

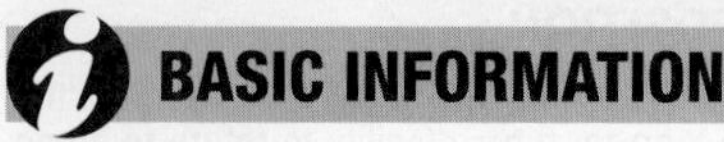

DEFINITION

Antiphospholipid antibody syndrome (APS), the most common acquired thrombophilia, is characterized by clinical features of arterial or venous thrombosis and/or pregnancy morbidity *and* the presence of at least one type of antiphospholipid autoantibody (aPL). aPLs are antibodies directed against serum proteins bound to anionic phospholipids. Autoantibodies bind to antigenic anticoagulants which activate endothelial cells, monocytes, and platelets resulting in complement-mediated thrombosis.

Three types of aPL have been characterized:

- Anticardiolipin antibodies—the most common
- Lupus anticoagulants
- Anti-beta$_2$-glycoprotein-1 antibodies

Primary APS occurs alone; and secondary APS occurs in association with systemic lupus erythematosus (SLE), other rheumatic disorders, or certain infections or medications. APS can affect all organ systems and includes venous and arterial thrombosis, recurrent fetal losses, and thrombocytopenia.

ICD-9CM CODES
795.79 Antiphospholipid antibody syndrome
ICD-10CM CODES
D68.61 Antiphospholipid syndrome

EPIDEMIOLOGY & DEMOGRAPHICS

PREVALENCE:

- Less than 1% of healthy individuals have positive aPLs
- Approximately 10% if patients with a deep venous thrombosis have aPLs
- Nearly 20% of women under 50 who have a cerebrovascular accident (CVA) test positive for aPLs
- 10% to 15% of women with recurrent miscarriages have aPLs
- Rule of 40s with systemic lupus erythematosus; 40% of patients with SLE have aPLs but only 40% of patients with antibodies will have thrombosis

PREDOMINANT AGE: Young to middle-age adults

RISK FACTORS:

- Underlying SLE and collagen-vascular diseases; other autoimmune disorders, including rheumatoid arthritis, Sjögren's syndrome, Behçet's syndrome, primary immune thrombocytopenia (also known as idiopathic thrombocytopenic purpura); AIDS; hypertension (HTN).
- Most individuals are otherwise healthy and have no underlying medical condition.

GENETICS: Some APS-positive families exist, and human leukocyte antigen (HLA) studies have suggested associations with HLA DR7, DR4, and Dqw7+Drw53.

PHYSICAL FINDINGS & CLINICAL PRESENTATION

No pathognomonic findings on examination; Table 1-50 summarizes other features suggesting the presence of antiphospholipid antibodies; abnormal findings consistent with ischemia or infarction.

- Thrombosis:
  - Patients with APS are at risk for both venous and arterial thromboses. Venous thromboses are more common, occurring as the initial manifestation of APS in approximately ~30% of APS patients. Of all patients with deep venous thrombosis, approximately 10% have aPL. The most common site for deep vein thrombosis is the calf, but thromboses may also occur in the renal, hepatic, axillary, subclavian, vena cava, and retinal veins. The most common site of arterial thrombosis is the cerebral vessels, followed by the coronary, renal, mesenteric, and bypass arteries. Recurrent thrombosis is common with APS.
- Commonly involved organ systems include:
  - Central nervous system: stroke, transient ischemic attack, migraine, multi-infarct dementia, epilepsy, movement disorders, transverse myelopathy, depression, Guillain-Barré syndrome, and migraine.
  - Pulmonary: pulmonary embolism and infarction; pulmonary hypertension; acute respiratory distress syndrome; intraalveolar pulmonary hemorrhage; a postpartum syndrome characterized by fever, pleuritic chest pain, dyspnea, and patchy infiltrates with pleural effusion on chest radiograph.
  - Cardiology: Libman-Sacks endocarditis, intracardiac thrombosis, coronary artery disease, myocardial infarction.
  - Gastrointestinal: abdominal pain, gastrointestinal bleed secondary to ischemia, splenic or pancreatic infarction, hepatic vein thrombosis, Budd-Chiari syndrome (second most common cause of syndrome).
  - Renal: proteinuria, acute renal failure, hypertension, renal infarct, renal artery or vein thrombosis, postpartum hemolytic-uremic syndrome.
  - Hematology: thrombocytopenia, hemolytic anemia.
  - Endocrine: Addison's disease secondary to adrenal hemorrhage and, less frequently, thrombosis.
  - Cutaneous: livedo reticularis, cutaneous necrosis, skin ulcerations, gangrene of digits (Fig. 1-106).
  - Obstetrics: recurrent spontaneous abortion, premature delivery or fetal growth retardation.
- Catastrophic APS (CAPS) (Table 1-51): CAPS is a rapidly progressive multiorgan thrombotic disease. Approximately 1% of APS is CAPS; approximately ~45% of CAPS do not present as APS initially. A 50% mortality rate is seen in patients with CAPS. To make the diagnosis of catastrophic APS, four criteria must be satisfied:
  1. Evidence of involvement of three or more organs, systems, and/or tissues. The most common symptoms are abdominal pain, dyspnea, neurologic symptoms, chest pain, and skin rash.
  2. Development of manifestations simultaneously or in ≤1 week.

Table 1-50 Other Features Suggesting the Presence of Antiphospholipid Antibodies

Clinical
Livedo reticularis
Thrombocytopenia (usually 50,000-100,000 platelets/mm^3)
Autoimmune hemolytic anemia
Cardiac valve disease (vegetations or thickening)
Multiple sclerosis–like syndrome, chorea, or other myelopathy
Laboratory
IgA anticardiolipin antibody
IgA anti–β_2-glycoprotein I

From Firestein GS, et al: *Kelly's textbook of rheumatology*, ed 9, Philadelphia, 2013, Saunders.

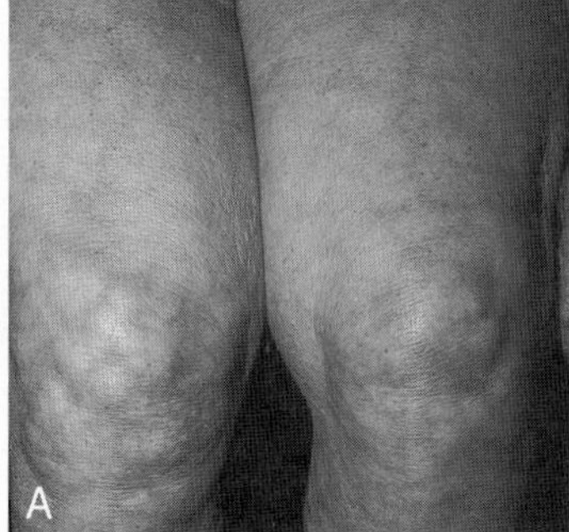

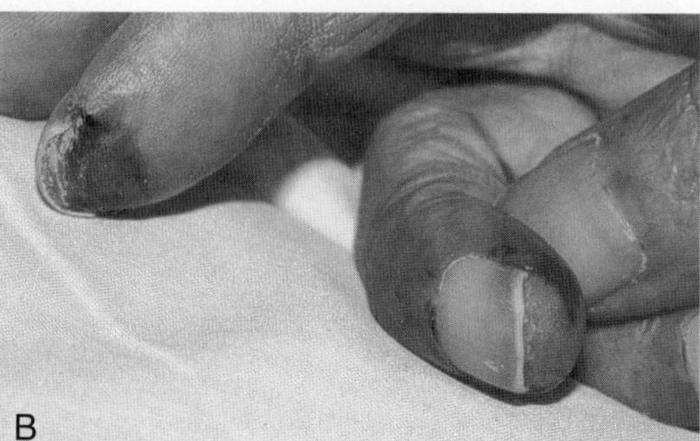

FIGURE 1-106 Antiphospholipid syndrome. The clinical presentations of this disorder are protean and include those shown here. **A,** Broad bands of livedo around the knees in a patient with anticardiolipin antibodies. Physiologic livedo has a finer patterning and less obvious lesions. **B,** Digital infarcts, a nonspecific feature of several vascular occlusion disorders. (From White GM, Cox NH [eds]: *Diseases of the skin, a color atlas and text*, ed 2, St Louis, 2006, Mosby.)

3. Confirmation by histopathology of small-vessel occlusion in at least one organ or tissue.
4. Laboratory confirmation of the presence of aPL.

ETIOLOGY

- aPLs react with negatively charged phospholipids.
- Possible mechanisms of thrombosis include effects of aPL on platelet membranes, endothelial cells, and clotting components such as prothrombin, protein C, or protein S.
- Studies have recently shown that prephospholipids are not immunogenic and that a binding protein (β_2-glycoprotein I) may be the key immunogen in the APS.

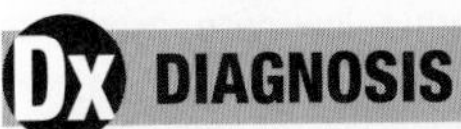

DIAGNOSIS

DIFFERENTIAL DIAGNOSIS

Other hypercoagulable states (inherited or acquired):

- Inherited: ATIII, protein C and protein, S deficiencies, factor V Leiden, prothrombin gene mutation.
- Acquired: heparin-induced thrombocytopenia, myeloproliferative syndromes, cancer
- Nephrotic syndrome.

TABLE 1-51 Differential Diagnosis of Catastrophic Antiphospholipid Syndrome (CAPS)

Laboratory Abnormalities	CAPS	TTP	DIC
Microangiopathic hemolytic anemia	−	+	+
Thrombocytopenia	+	+	+
Fibrinogen/FDP	Normal/ Normal	Normal/ Increased	Decreased/ Increased
Anticardiolipin antibody	+	−	−
Lupus anticoagulant	+	−	−

WORKUP

Diagnostic criteria of APS include at least one clinical criterion and at least one laboratory criterion. A single clot may not be sufficient, especially with other thrombotic risk factors.

- Clinical:
  1. Venous, arterial, or small vessel thrombosis *or*
  2. Morbidity with pregnancy, defined as:
     - Fetal death at ≥10 weeks' gestation *or*
     - ≥1 premature births before 34 weeks' gestation secondary to eclampsia, preeclampsia, or severe placental insufficiency *or*
     - ≥3 unexplained spontaneous abortions at 10 weeks' gestation.
- Laboratory (see Table 1-52):
- Screening tests
  - Partial thromboplastin time (PTT): Elevated, indicating either the presence of a clotting factor deficiency, or the presence of an inhibitor such as a lupus anticoagulant.
  - Mixing study: Elevated. Normal plasma is incubated with the patient's plasma. In cases of clotting factor deficiencies the PTT will correct. If an inhibitor is present the PTT WILL NOT correct.
  - Dilute Russell viper venom time: Elevated. Laboratory clotting requires the addition of phospholipids and calcium to plasma samples. Anti-phospholipid antibodies bind the phospholipids in the test tube, thereby preventing clot formation. The addition of Russell viper venom to plasma results in immediate activation of Factor X (common pathway). It, therefore, will not be prolonged in intrinsic or extrinsic factor deficiencies but will be prolonged in the presence of an antiphospholipid antibody. The Lupus Anticoagulant screen is the addition of Russell viper venom to plasma. In the Lupus Anticoagulant confirmatory testing massive doses of phospholipids are added to saturate the antiphospholipid antibody thereby correcting the prolonged PTT.
- Initial testing for presence of aPL:
  - ELISA anticardiolpin antibody aCL antibody in medium or high titers *or*
  - Lupus anticoagulant activity found *or*
  - Anti-beta$_2$-glycoprotein (anti-b2GPI)-ELISA antibodies no more than 5 years from the clinical event.

Confirmatory aPL testing: repeat after 12 weeks to confirm persistence of aCL, anti-β2GPI or LA test. Transient elevations of aCL can occur. Traditional aPL tests include aCL and B2GPI. Newer aPL tests include aps/PT and β2GPI.

LABORATORY TESTS

Diagnostic evaluation of aCL and LA antibodies is indicated in:

- Patient with underlying SLE or collagen-vascular disease with thrombosis.
- Patient with recurrent, familial, or juvenile deep vein thrombosis (DVT) or thrombosis in an unusual location (mesenteric or cerebral).
- One or more unexplained thrombotic events. Do not test in those at low risk, e.g., the elderly with clot and other risk factors.
- One or more specific pregnancy events.
- Unexplained thrombocytopenia.
- Patients with an elevated PTT.

Abnormal tests include:

- False-positive test for syphilis (RPR/VDRL).
- Lupus anticoagulant activity.
- Presence of anticardiolipin antibodies (ELISA for anticardiolipin is the most sensitive and specific test [>80%]).
- Presence of anti-b$_2$-glycoprotein I antibody.

Rx TREATMENT

ACUTE Rx

Treatment includes use of heparin, low-molecular-weight heparin (LMWH), warfarin, antiplatelet agents, acetylsalicylic acid (aspirin), clopidogrel, hydroxychloroquine.

- For a patient with positive aPL and venous or arterial thrombosis: Treat as would any other thrombosis.
  - Anticoagulation with heparin or LMWH, then followed by indefinite warfarin treatment, with a target international normalized ratio (INR) of 2.0 to 3.0.
  - There is some evidence to support a higher INR target or the addition of other agents in patients with arterial clots, especially if they have recurrent events while taking warfarin.
- Length of treatment needed is unknown, but likely indefinite barring no contraindication to anticoagulation, as the lifelong recurrence rate is 11% to 29%.
- Unfractionated heparin (UFH) is preferred if quick reversibility is needed.

PRIMARY PREVENTION

- Aspirin is of no benefit for prevention in patients with a prior clot.

TABLE 1-52 Assays Used to Confirm Diagnosis of Antiphospholipid Syndrome

Assay	Methodology
"Criteria" aPL Assays	
aCL	ELISA
Anti-β_2-GPI	ELISA
LAC	Clotting/functional assays
"Noncriteria" aPL Assays	
Assays to detect antibodies to other phospholipids (i.e., phosphatidylserine, phosphatidylinositol, phosphatidic acid, phosphatidylglycerol, phosphatidylethanolamine, phosphatidylcholine)	ELISA
Annexin A5 resistance assay	Clotting/mechanistic assay
Assays to detect antibodies to prothrombin or prothrombin/phosphatidylserine	ELISA
Assays to detect antibodies to clotting proteins (i.e., protein C, protein S)	ELISA

aCL, Anticardiolipin; *aPL,* antiphospholipid antibody; *ELISA,* enzyme-linked immunosorbent assay; *LAC,* lupus anticoagulant.
From Hochberg MC et al: *Rheumatology,* ed 5, St Louis, 2011, Mosby.

- Aspirin may help patients without a history of clot.
- Hydroxychloroquine may be useful in those patients with SLE and aPL.
- Avoid oral contraceptive pills; modifiable risk factors for thrombosis such as smoking and immobility should be addressed.
- For pregnant women with a positive test for aPL antibodies without a history of DVT or pregnancy loss, consider low-dose subcutaneous UFH or LMWH SC, aspirin 81 mg, or surveillance.

SECONDARY PREVENTION

- For pregnant women with previously diagnosed APS:
  - Warfarin should be discontinued in early pregnancy secondary to its teratogenic effects.
  - Aspirin 81 mg, and subcutaneous UFH or LMWH to therapeutic partial thromboplastin time (PTT) or factor Xa levels, respectively.
  - Pregnant patients taking LMWH should be transitioned to unfractionated heparin before delivery due to reversibility.
  - Intravenous immunoglobulin (IVIG), plasmapheresis, hydroxychloroquine, statins, clopidogrel, dipyridamole, and rituximab have been used when other treatments have failed.
- For pregnant women with a postive test for aPL antibodies and a history of fewer than three spontaneous abortions:
  - Low-dose aspirin at conception, followed by UFH, prophylactically or an intermediate dose at 7 weeks, continuing until 6 weeks' postpartum.
  - A mid-interval PTT should be checked and should be normal or similar to baseline before therapy.
  - LMWH can be used in place of unfractionated heparin and should be titrated to factor Xa levels in the recommended prophylactic range. The combination aspirin (75 mg daily) plus LMWH has been associated with a higher live birth rate when compared with IVIG.

FOR CATASTROPHIC ANTIPHOSPHOLIPID ANTIBODY SYNDROME

- Highest survival rates are achieved with the combination of anticoagulation, corticosteroids, and IVIG or plasma exchange.
- Case reports have shown rituximab to be a successful therapy for patients with life-threatening thrombosis refractory to anticoagulation.

CHRONIC Rx

- Anticoagulation with warfarin therapy.
- Immunosuppressive agents such as corticosteroids and cyclophosphamide have not been shown to be effective.
- Limited data suggest that hydroxychloroquine may be effective in patients with APS and SLE.

DISPOSITION

- APS patients have a 20% to 70% risk for recurrent thrombosis.
- Initial arterial thrombosis tends to be followed by arterial events, and initial venous thrombosis tends to be followed by venous events.
- Catastrophic APS is associated with a high mortality rate, approaching 50%.
- Incidence of developing catastrophic APS is approximately 0.8% among APS patients.

REFERRAL

To hematology or rheumatology and/or obstetric medicine when diagnosis is made.

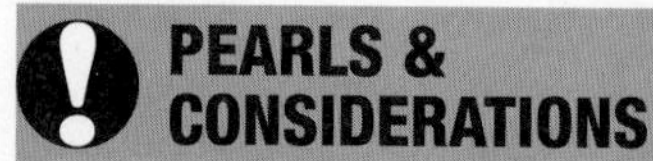

PEARLS & CONSIDERATIONS

COMMENTS

Cerebral features of SLE may be more related to thrombosis than inflammation and may respond better to anticoagulants than immunosuppression.

PREVENTION

Prophylaxis for asymptomatic patients with positive aPL tests without previous thrombosis:

- No routine prophylaxis is recommended.
- Questionable whether low-dose aspirin is effective.
- Antithrombotic prophylaxis for major surgery, prolonged immobilization, and pregnancy.
- Avoid oral contraceptive pills in women with positive aPL test.

SUGGESTED READINGS

available at www.expertconsult.com

RELATED CONTENT

Hypercoagulable States (Related Key Topic)
Deep Vein Thrombosis (Related Key Topic)
Pulmonary Embolism (Related Key Topic)
Antiphospholipid Antibody Syndrome (Patient Information)

AUTHORS: **LYNN BOWLBY, M.D.**, and **JOHN L. REAGAN, M.D.**

BASIC INFORMATION

DEFINITION

Generalized anxiety disorder (GAD) is most likely to present in combination with other psychiatric and medical conditions. Individuals with GAD commonly present with excessive and disproportionately high levels of anxiety, fear, or worry for most days over at least a 6-mo period. The worrying must be greater than would be expected given the situation, and it must cause significant interference in functioning. The subjective anxiety must be accompanied by at least three somatic symptoms (e.g., restlessness, irritability, sleep disturbance, muscle tension, difficulty concentrating, or fatigue). GAD cannot be diagnosed if it occurs only in the context of an active mood disorder, such as depression, or in the context of another active anxiety disorder, such as PTSD or panic disorder.

SYNONYMS

Anxiety neurosis (former name for a subset of anxiety disorders)
Chronic anxiety
GAD

ICD-9CM CODE
300.02
ICD-10CM CODES
F41.1 Generalized anxiety disorder
DSM-IV CODE
300.02

EPIDEMIOLOGY & DEMOGRAPHICS

INCIDENCE (IN U.S.): 6% to 9% per year in adult primary care clinics; 1-yr incident rate per 100 person-yr of 1.12

PEAK INCIDENCE: Peak incidence tends to occur later relative to other anxiety disorders, such as phobias; cumulative incidence of 4.3% by age 34 in a German community sample

PREVALENCE (IN U.S.):
- In general population: lifetime morbid risk of 9%; 12-month prevalence of 2%
- In primary care setting: 3% (the most common anxiety disorder in this setting)

PREDOMINANT SEX: Women are more frequently affected (2:1 ratio) but may present for treatment less often (3:2 female/male).

PREDOMINANT AGE:
- 30% report onset before age 11
- 50% have onset before age 18
- Median age of onset: 30 years

GENETICS: Concordance rates in dizygotic twins and monozygotic twins are not different (0% to 5%)

PHYSICAL FINDINGS & CLINICAL PRESENTATION

- Report of being "anxious" all of their lives.
- Excessive worry, usually regarding family, finances, work, or health.
- Sleep disturbance, particularly early insomnia.
- Muscle tension (typically in the muscles of neck and shoulders) or headache.
- Difficulty concentrating.
- Daytime fatigue.
- GI symptoms compatible with IBS (one third of patients).
- Physical symptoms are the usual reason for seeking medical attention.
- Comorbid psychiatric illness (e.g., dysthymia or major depression) and substance abuse (e.g., alcohol abuse) are frequent.

ETIOLOGY

- Hypotheses include models based on neurotransmitters (catecholamines, indolamines) and developmental psychology (e.g., behavioral inhibition, neuroticism, and harm avoidance).
- Prevalence increased with a family history, increase in stress, history of physical or emotional trauma, and medical illness.

Dx DIAGNOSIS

DIFFERENTIAL DIAGNOSIS

- Wide range of psychiatric and medical conditions:
  - Cardiovascular and pulmonary disease, such as cardiac arrhythmias or COPD
  - Hyperthyroidism, hypoglycemia
  - Substance abuse (e.g., cocaine, amphetamines, and PCP) or withdrawal (e.g., alcohol or benzodiazepines)
  - Other anxiety disorders (e.g., social anxiety disorder), mood disorder

WORKUP

- Screening tests may enhance detection. A screening tool often used in primary care is the GAD-2. It asks, "During the past month, have you been bothered a lot by: (1) Nerves or feeling anxious or on edge? (2) Worrying about a lot of different things?" The response to each question is given a score of 0 (not at all), 1 (several days), 2 (more than half of the days), 3 (nearly every day). A score of ≥3 has a sensitivity of 86% and a specificity of 83% for detecting GAD. A simple 7-item in-office case finding instrument, the GAD-7, includes additional questions to assess symptom severity and can be used to monitor symptoms.
- Physical examination: additional laboratory and radiologic workup depend on presenting symptoms.
- Iatrogenic cause should be suspected if anxiety follows recent changes in medication.

Rx TREATMENT

NONPHARMACOLOGIC THERAPY

- Cognitive-behavioral therapy
- Acceptance and commitment therapy
- Relaxation training
- Biofeedback
- Psychodynamic psychotherapy

PHARMACOLOGIC THERAPY

- SSRIs/SNRIs
- Azapirones (e.g., buspirone)
- Benzodiazepines (less favored)

ACUTE GENERAL Rx

- Acute treatment is rarely indicated because GAD is a chronic condition.
- If patients are in acute distress, the possibility of another cause, including another anxiety disorder such as panic disorder, should be considered.
- Caution in prescribing benzodiazepines because of the propensity for misuse and dependence. If used, the patient should be educated about the options and the risks.

CHRONIC Rx

- SSRIs and SNRIs (e.g., venlafaxine and duloxetine) are effective typical first-line treatment. Particularly useful if comorbid depression present.
- Buspirone can be effective with minimal potential for tolerance or abuse. May be less effective in patients with previous benzodiazepine exposure and may require a high-dose titration.
- Benzodiazepines can be effective under close supervision; however, they have fallen out of favor as a first-line treatment given their potential for functional impairment, abuse, and dependence.
- Sedating antidepressants, such as mirtazapine, may also be useful for initial insomnia secondary to anxious ruminations.

DISPOSITION

- GAD is chronic with periodic exacerbations.
- Treatment is given to reduce level of symptoms and improve functioning. Suicide risk is higher than in the general population.

REFERRAL

- For refractory symptoms.
- For comorbid psychiatric conditions.

SUGGESTED READINGS

available at www.expertconsult.com

RELATED CONTENT

Social Anxiety Disorder (Related Key Topic)
Anxiety (Patient Information)
Panic Disorder (Related Key Topic)

AUTHOR: **KRISTY L. DALRYMPLE, PH.D.**

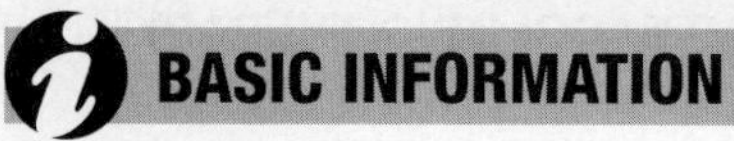

BASIC INFORMATION

DEFINITION

Aortic dissection is part of a spectrum of aortic pathologies (acute aortic syndromes) that include intramural hematomas and penetrating atherosclerotic ulcers. Aortic dissection occurs when blood passes through an intimal tear, separating the intima from the medial layers and creating a false lumen. Intramural hematoma (IMH) occurs when the vasa vasorum ruptures within the medial wall. IMH does not involve an intimal tearing unless a dissection develops. Seventeen percent of IMH will transform into aortic dissection. Penetrating atherosclerotic ulcers destroy the aortic intima and dissect into the aortic media. Unlike aortic dissection, penetrating ulcers occur on the basis of extensive atherosclerosis in the aortic intima. Fig. 1-107 illustrates acute aortic syndromes.

SYNONYMS

Dissecting aortic aneurysm

ICD-9CM CODES
441.00 Aortic dissection
444.01 Aortic dissection, thoracic
ICD-10CM CODES
I71.00 Dissection of unspecified site of aorta

EPIDEMIOLOGY & DEMOGRAPHICS

PREDOMINANT SEX AND AGE: Males (65%) females (35%), ages 60 to 80 yr; mean, 63 yr

INCIDENCE: 2.6-3.5 per 100,000 person-years

RISK FACTORS:
- Hypertension (found in up to 72% of patients with aortic dissection).
- Atherosclerosis (found in up to 31% of patients with aortic dissection)
- Age
- Family history of aortic aneurysms/dissection
- History of cardiac surgery, intraaortic catheterization
- Disorders of collagen (Marfan's syndrome, Ehlers-Danlos syndrome)
- Vascular inflammation (giant cell arteritis, Takayasu arteritis, rheumatoid arthritis, syphilitic aortitis)
- Aortic coarctation, bicuspid aortic valve
- Turner's syndrome
- Cocaine abuse (usually within 12 hours of last use of cocaine)
- Trauma

CLASSIFICATION

Aortic dissection is generally classified according to anatomic location (Fig. 1-108):
- Stanford (more commonly used classification system): type A ascending aorta (proximal), type B descending aorta (distal) (Fig. 1-109)
- DeBakey: type I ascending and descending aorta, type II ascending aorta, type III descending aorta

Aortic dissection can also be classified by acuity of presentation (acute or chronic), based on the time of onset.

PHYSICAL FINDINGS & CLINICAL PRESENTATION

- Sudden onset of severe sharp, tearing, or ripping chest pain
- Anterior chest pain (ascending dissection)
- Back pain, abdominal pain (descending dissection)
- Syncope (secondary to cardiac tamponade or stroke), congestive heart failure (CHF)
- May present with hypertension (70% in type B dissection, 36% for type A), 25% with hypotension (systolic blood pressure <100 mm Hg), which can indicate bleeding, cardiac tamponade, or severe aortic regurgitation
- Pulse and blood pressure differentials (>20 mm Hg between arms) in 9% to 30% of cases, caused by partial compression of subclavian arteries
- Aortic regurgitation in 18% to 50% of cases of proximal dissection, often with diastolic decrescendo murmur
- Myocardial ischemia caused by coronary artery occlusion, most commonly involving the right coronary artery
- Stroke in 5% to 10% of patients
- Horner syndrome (ptosis, miosis, anhidrosis)
- Vocal cord paralysis/hoarse voice

ETIOLOGY

Genetics, in addition to other risk factors listed above, contribute to the development of aortic dissection.

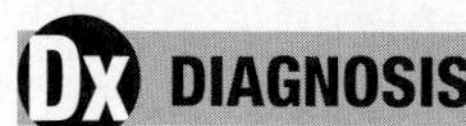

DIAGNOSIS

DIFFERENTIAL DIAGNOSIS

- Known as the great imitator: Pulmonary embolism, acute coronary syndrome, aortic stenosis/insufficiency, nondissecting aneurysm, pericarditis, cholecystitis, peptic ulcer disease, pancreatitis, musculoskeletal pain
- Consider aortic dissection in patients with unexplained stroke, chest pain, syncope, acute-onset CHF, abdominal pain, back pain, and malperfusion of extremities or internal organs.

LABORATORY TESTS

- ECG: helpful to rule out MI, although dissection can lead to coronary ischemia

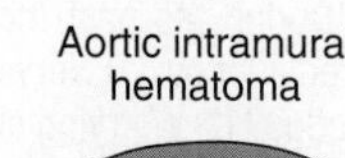

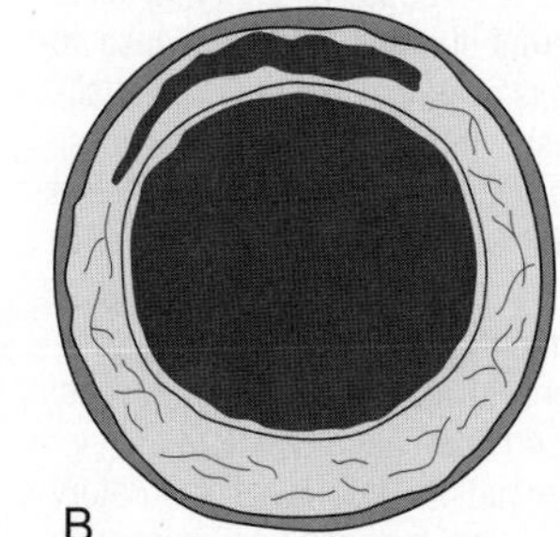

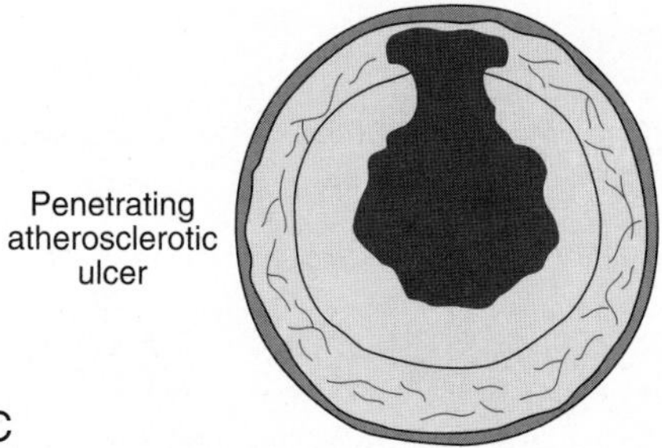

FIGURE 1-107 Acute aortic syndromes. A, Classic aortic dissection. **B,** Aortic intramural hematoma. **C,** Penetrating atherosclerotic aortic ulcer. From Bonow RO, et al: *Heart disease*, ed 9, 2012, Saunders.

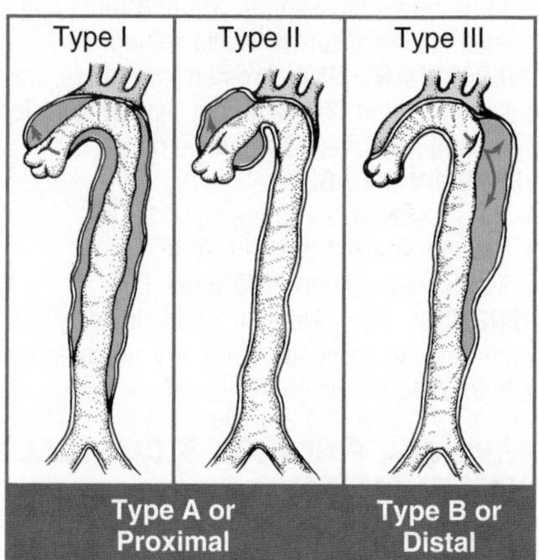

FIGURE 1-108 Classification systems for aortic dissection. (From Isselbacher EM et al: Disease of the aorta. In Braunwald E [ed]: *Heart disease: a textbook of cardiovascular medicine*, ed 5, Philadelphia, 1997, Saunders.)

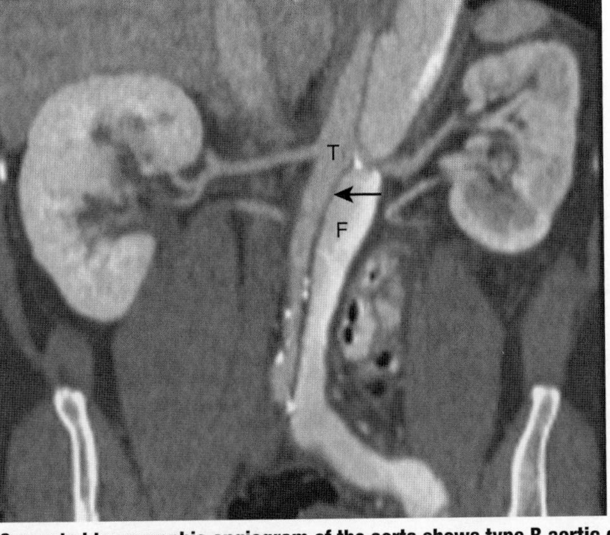

FIGURE 1-109 Computed tomographic angiogram of the aorta shows type B aortic dissection. The intimal flap *(arrow)* separates the two lumen *(T)* from the false lumen *(F)* and compromises blood flow to the right kidney, causing renal atrophy and cortical thinning. (Image courtesy of Bart Domatch, M.D., Radiology Department, University of Texas Southwestern Medical Center, Dallas, TX; from Andreoli TE et al: *Andreoli and Carpenter's Cecil essentials of medicine,* ed 8, Philadelphia, 2010, Saunders.)

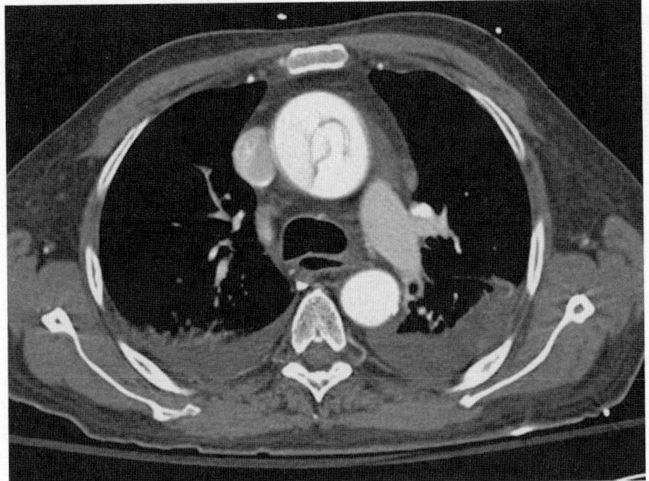

FIGURE 1-110 Thin-slice CT image of a classic ascending dissection with aneurysmal dilation. (From Cameron JL, Cameron AM: *Current surgical therapy,* ed 10, Philadelphia, 2011, Saunders.)

- D-dimer has a 100% negative predictive value but lacks specificity in the setting of acute aortic dissection.
- Three biomarkers with different diagnostic windows can be used in the diagnosis of aortic dissection.
- Smooth muscle myosin heavy chain protein (released from damaged medial smooth muscle) can be used to detect proximal aortic dissections (91% sensitivity and 93% specificity). Myosin heavy chains will peak within 3 hr of dissection and clear within 24 hr of aortic injury.
- CK-BB isoenzyme also peaks within 6 hr of dissection.
- Calponin, a smooth muscle troponin counterpart, increases in aortic dissection with a wider diagnostic window when compared to smooth muscle myosin heavy chain and CK-BB.
- C-reactive protein, fibrinogen, and elastin fragments are under investigation

IMAGING STUDIES

- Multidetector CT is considered the gold standard; but its use may be limited in patients with renal failure as it involves the use of IV contrast. Fig. 1-110 shows a thin-slice CT image of a classic ascending dissection with aneurysmal dilation.
- TEE, multidetector CT, and MRI are all highly sensitive (98% to 100%) and specific (95% to 98%). Test of choice depends on clinical circumstances and hospital availability.
- Transesophageal echocardiography (TEE) is study of choice in unstable patients with type A dissection but is operator dependent.
- MRI has high sensitivity and specificity but limited availability; not suitable for unstable patients; contraindicated with pacemakers, metal devices.
- With medium or high pretest probability, a second diagnostic test should be done if the first is negative.
- Coronary computed tomographic angiography (CTA) may be an alternative and useful diagnostic study when evaluating for pulmonary embolism, acute coronary syndrome, and aortic dissection.
- Aortography rarely done now.
- Chest radiograph may show widened mediastinum (62%) and displacement of aortic intimal calcium. It is negative in 11% to 16% of patients with aortic dissection.
- Although the diagnostic sensitivity of transthoracic echocardiography is suboptimal, it is useful in assessing potential high-risk features or complications, such as pericardial effusion, and making other potential diagnoses. A negative transthoracic echocardiography, however, does not exclude aortic dissection.

Rx TREATMENT

- Proximal dissections (acute type A) require emergent surgery to prevent rupture or pericardial effusion.
- Distal dissections (Stanford type B) are usually treated medically unless distal organ involvement or impending rutpure occurs.
  - Surgical intervention for distal dissections is reserved for patients who have a complicated course, including occlusion of a major aortic branch, dissection, presence within an aortic aneurysm, and evidence of aortic rupture.
  - Fig. 1-111 describes an algorithm for the diagnosis and treatment of aortic dissection.

ACUTE GENERAL Rx

- Admit to ICU for monitoring.
- Target SBP 100 to 120 mm Hg or as low as tolerated; heart rate <60 beats/min to reduce aortic wall stress.
- IV beta-blockers are cornerstones of treatment, but multiple medications may be needed.
  - Propanolol 1 mg every 3 to 5 min; metoprolol 5 mg IV every 5 min; or labetalol 20 mg IV, then 20 to 80 mg every 10 min, followed by nitroprusside 0.3 to 10 mg/kg/min.
  - Nitroprusside should not be used without beta-blockade because vasodilation can induce reflex sympathetic stimulation and increased aortic sheer stress.
  - IV calcium channel blockers with negative inotropy may be used if beta-blockers are contraindicated.
- Pain control, often with morphine.
- Endovascular repair is a feasible, less invasive option for type B aortic dissections, but data are limited. Literature has shown favorable short- and mid-term outcomes. However, long-term outcome data are still under investigation.

CHRONIC Rx

- Chronic aortic dissection (>2 wk) managed with aggressive blood pressure control: target <120/80 mm Hg in most patients.
- Target low-density lipoprotein <70 mg/dl.
- Minimize strenuous physical activity such as heavy lifting.

  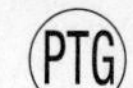

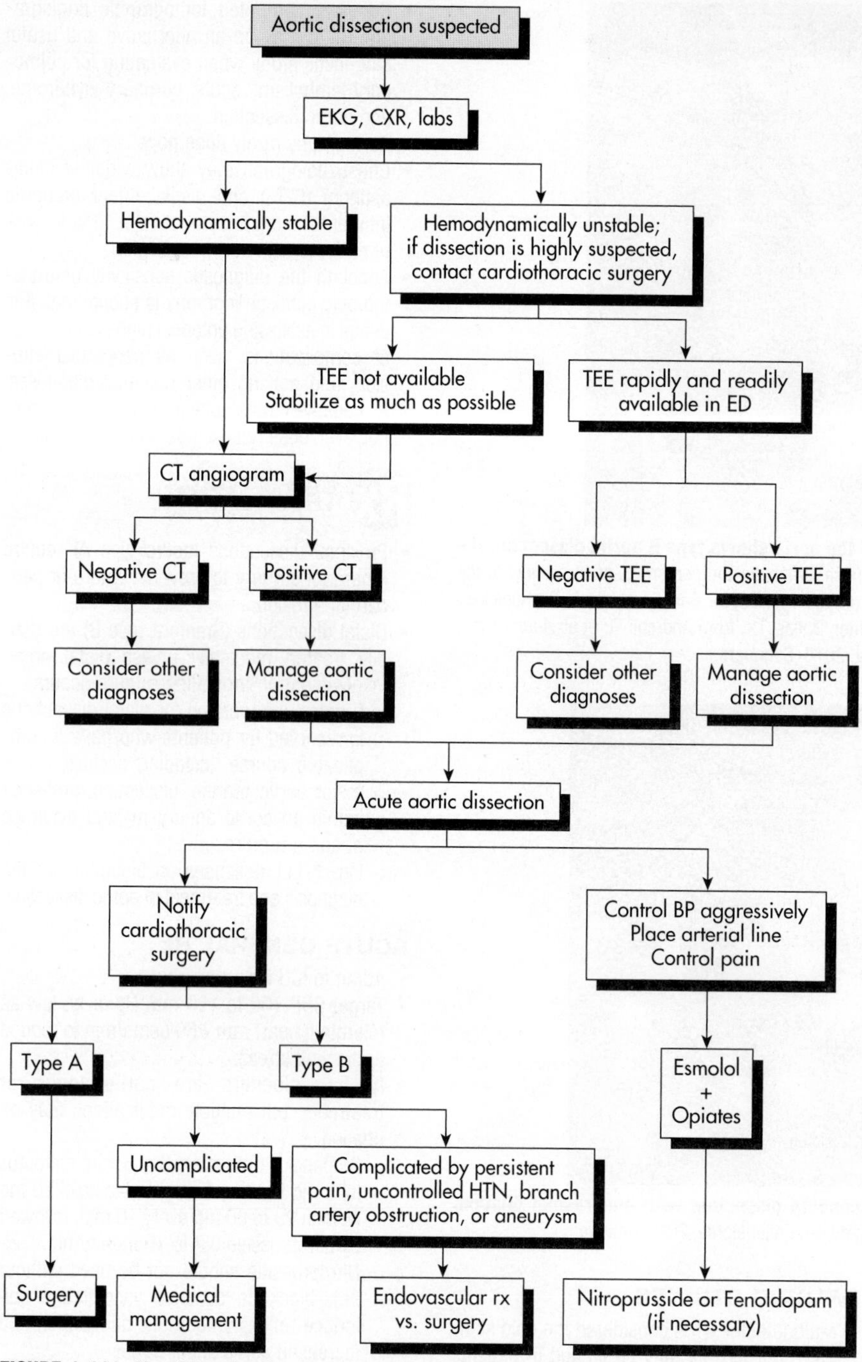

Aortic dissection suspected

EKG, CXR, labs

Hemodynamically stable

Hemodynamically unstable; if dissection is highly suspected, contact cardiothoracic surgery

TEE not available Stabilize as much as possible

TEE rapidly and readily available in ED

CT angiogram

Negative CT

Positive CT

Negative TEE

Positive TEE

Consider other diagnoses

Manage aortic dissection

Consider other diagnoses

Manage aortic dissection

Acute aortic dissection

Notify cardiothoracic surgery

Control BP aggressively Place arterial line Control pain

Type A

Type B

Esmolol + Opiates

Uncomplicated

Complicated by persistent pain, uncontrolled HTN, branch artery obstruction, or aneurysm

Surgery

Medical management

Endovascular rx vs. surgery

Nitroprusside or Fenoldopam (if necessary)

FIGURE 1-111 Algorithm for the diagnosis and treatment of aortic dissection. *BP*, Blood pressure; *CT*, computed tomography; *CXR*, chest radiograph; *ECG*, electrocardiography; *ED*, emergency department; *HTN*, hypertension; *labs*, laboratory tests; *TEE*, transesophageal echocardiography. (Adams JG et al: *Emergency medicine, clinical essentials*, ed 2, Philadelphia, 2013, Elsevier.)

- Serial imaging of the aorta, usually with contrast CT.
- Endovascular repair in chronic type B dissection should be considered when the aortic diameter exceeds 5.5-6.0 cm, when there is uncontrolled pain or blood pressure, or when there is rapid growth of the dissecting aneurysm (>1 cm per year).

DISPOSITION

- 85% mortality rate within 2 weeks for an untreated type A dissection.
- Proximal dissection is a surgical emergency. Time is critical; mortality rate is 1% to 3% per hour.
- Overall, in-hospital mortality rate is 30% with proximal dissections and 10% with distal dissections.

REFERRAL

For ICU management and surgical intervention

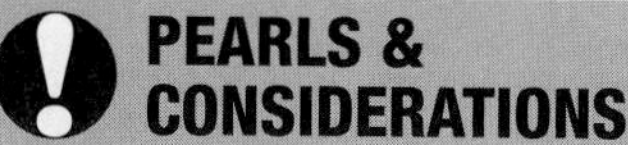

PEARLS & CONSIDERATIONS

- Blood pressure control is essential; beta-blocker is first-line medication.
- Proximal dissection is a surgical emergency.
- Cardiac tamponade is not uncommon in patients with acute type A aortic dissection. Syncope, altered mental status, and a widened mediastinum on chest radiograph on presentation suggest tamponade which warrants urgent operative therapy.
- Surgery for acute type A aortic dissection in patients ≥70 years old can be performed with acceptable outcomes.

SUGGESTED READINGS

available at www.expertconsult.com

RELATED CONTENT

Aortic Dissection (Patient Information)
Abdominal Aortic Aneurysm (Related Key Topic)

AUTHORS: **AHMAD M. ISMAIL, M.D., SUNIT-PREET CHAUDHRY, M.D.,** and **PHILIP STOCKWELL, M.D.**

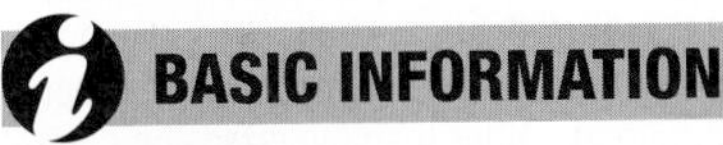

BASIC INFORMATION

DEFINITION

Aortic regurgitation (AR) is retrograde blood flow into the left ventricle from the aorta as a result of an incompetent aortic valve.

SYNONYMS

Aortic insufficiency
AI
AR

ICD-9CM CODES
424.1 Aortic valve disorders
ICD-10CM CODES
I35.1 Aortic valve insufficiency
I35.2 Aortic value stenosis with insufficiency
I35.9 Aortic valve disorder, unspecified
I35.8 Other nonrheumatic aortic valve disorders

EPIDEMIOLOGY & DEMOGRAPHICS

- Prevalence ranges from 4.9% to 10% and increases with age.
- The most common cause of isolated severe AR is aortic root dilation.
- Infectious endocarditis is the most frequent cause of acute AR.

PHYSICAL FINDINGS & CLINICAL PRESENTATION

The pathophysiology of AR is described in Fig. 1-112. The clinical presentation varies depending on whether aortic insufficiency is acute or chronic. Chronic aortic insufficiency is well tolerated (except when secondary to infective endocarditis), and the patients remain asymptomatic for years. Common manifestations after significant deterioration of left ventricular function are dyspnea on exertion, syncope, chest pain, and congestive heart failure (CHF). Acute aortic insufficiency manifests primarily with hypotension caused by a sudden fall in cardiac output and resultant cardiogenic shock. In addition, a rapid rise in left ventricular diastolic pressure results in a further decrease in coronary blood flow.

Physical findings in chronic aortic insufficiency include the following:

- Widened pulse pressure (markedly increased systolic blood pressure, decreased diastolic blood pressure).
- Findings associated with the widened pulse pressure:
  - Bounding pulses, "water hammer" or collapsing pulse (***Corrigan's pulse***), can be palpated at the wrist or on the femoral arteries artery and is caused by rapid rise and sudden collapse of the arterial pressure during late systole.
  - Head "bobbing" with each systole (***de Musset's sign***).
  - "Pistol shot femorals" (***Traube's sign***) is a term used to describe a loud sound over the femoral artery
  - Capillary pulsations (***Quincke's sign***) may occur at the base of the nail beds.
- A to-and-fro Duroziez murmur may be heard over femoral arteries with slight compression.
- Popliteal systolic pressure is increased more than 20 mm Hg over brachial systolic pressure (***Hill's sign***), with a 40 to 60 mm difference representing moderate AR and > 60 mm difference severe AR.
- Other findings associated with AR, which are more of historical than practical interest, include:
  - ***Mueller's sign***—Systolic pulsations of the uvula.
  - ***Becker's sign***—Visible pulsations of the retinal arteries and pupils.
  - ***Mayne's sign***—More than a 15 mm Hg decrease in diastolic blood pressure with arm elevation from the value obtained with the arm in the standard position.
  - ***Rosenbach's sign***—Systolic pulsations of the liver.
  - ***Gerhard's sign***—Systolic pulsations of the spleen.
- Cardiac auscultation reveals:
  1. Displacement of cardiac impulse downward and to the patient's left
  2. S_3 heard over the apex
  3. Decrescendo, blowing diastolic murmur heard along left sternal border
  4. Low-pitched apical diastolic rumble (***Austin-Flint murmur***)—the precise etiology of the murmur is uncertain, but it is generally believed to be related to increased velocity of mitral inflow consequent to the AR.
  5. Early systolic ejection sound and systolic ejection murmur.

In patients with acute aortic insufficiency both the wide pulse pressure and the large stroke volume are absent. A short, blowing diastolic murmur may be the only finding on physical examination.

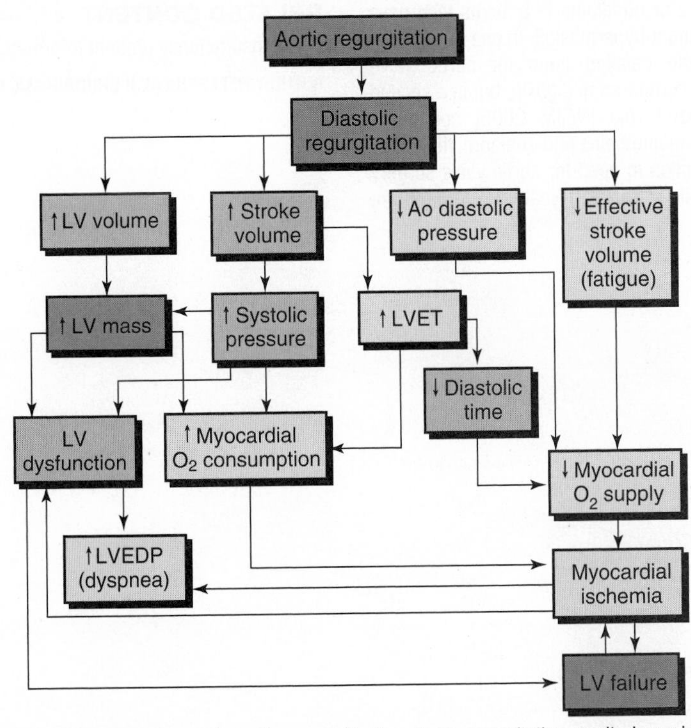

FIGURE 1-112 Pathophysiology of aortic regurgitation. Aortic regurgitation results in an increased left ventricular *(LV)* volume, increased stroke volume, increased aortic *(Ao)* systolic pressure, and decreased effective stroke volume. Increased LV volume results in an increased LV mass, which may lead to LV dysfunction and failure. Increased LV stroke volume increases systolic pressure and prolongation of LV ejection time *(LVET)*. Increased LV systolic pressure results in a decrease in diastolic time. Decreased diastolic time (myocardial perfusion time), diastolic aortic pressure, and effective stroke volume reduce myocardial O_1 supply. Increased myocardial O_2 consumption and decreased myocardial O_2 supply produce myocardial ischemia, which further deteriorates LV function. *LVEDP,* LV end-diastolic pressure. (From Boudoulas H, Gravanis MB: Valvular heart disease. In Gravanis MB [ed]: *Cardiovascular disorders: pathogenesis and pathophysiology,* St Louis, 1993, Mosby.)

ETIOLOGY

- Leaflet abnormalities:
  - Infective endocarditis
  - Rheumatic fibrosis (most common cause in developing countries)
  - Trauma with valvular rupture
  - Congenital bicuspid aortic valve (most common cause in the United States)
  - Myxomatous degeneration
  - Fenfluramine, dexfenfluramine, pergolide, cabergoline
  - Ankylosing spondylitis
- Aortic root or ascending aorta abnormalities:
  - Annuloaortic ectasia
  - Ehlers-Danlos syndrome
  - Marfan's syndrome
  - Trauma: ankylosing spondylitis
  - Syphilitic aortitis
  - Systemic hypertension
  - Aortic dissection

 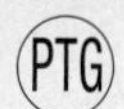

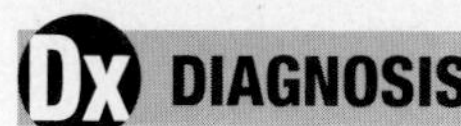

DIAGNOSIS

DIFFERENTIAL DIAGNOSIS

- Patent ductus arteriosus, pulmonary regurgitation, and other valvular abnormalities.
- The differential diagnosis of cardiac murmurs is described in Section II.

WORKUP

- Echocardiogram, chest radiograph, electrocardiogram (ECG), and cardiac catheterization (selected patients).
- Medical history and physical examination focused on the following clinical manifestations:
  1. Dyspnea on exertion.
  2. Syncope.
  3. Chest pain.
  4. CHF.

IMAGING STUDIES

- Chest radiography:
  1. Left ventricular hypertrophy (LVH) (chronic AR).
  2. Aortic dilation.
  3. Normal cardiac silhouette with pulmonary edema: possible in patients with acute AR.
- ECG: LVH.
- Echocardiography (Fig. E1-113) is the main imaging modality to diagnose AR and assess left ventricular size and function. Quantification of the severity of regurgitation can be made either qualitatively by Doppler vena contracta width (severe if >0.6 cm) or quantitatively by effective regurgitant orifice area (severe if >0.30 cm^2) and/or regurgitant volume (severe if >60 mL per/beat).
- Cardiac catheterization is indicated in selected patients to assess the degree of left ventricular dysfunction, to assess the degree of AR when echocardiographic parameters are inconclusive, and to determine if there is coexistent coronary artery disease.

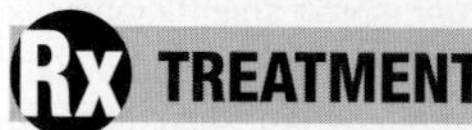

TREATMENT

NONPHARMACOLOGIC THERAPY

- Avoidance of competitive sports and heavy weight lifting if the AR is severe and associated with aortic root dilatation.
- Salt restriction.
- In 2007, the American Heart Association (AHA) guidelines for prevention of infectious endocarditis were revised; and routine antibiotic prophylaxis to undergo dental or other invasive procedures is no longer recommended, unless the patient has a prior history of endocarditis.

MEDICAL:

ACUTE GENERAL Rx:

- Afterload reduction: angiotensin-converting enzyme (ACE) inhibitors and vasodilators (i.e., nitroprusside) in acute AR; diuretics for pulmonary edema.
- Avoid beta-blockers that can prolong diastole.
- Emergent surgical referral for cardiogenic shock.

CHRONIC Rx:

- Long-term vasodilator therapy with ACE inhibitors or nifedipine in patients who have concomitant hypertension. In one 1994 study nifedepine delayed need for aortic valve surgery compared to digoxin, but in a second randomized trial [NEJM 2005] comparing placebo to nifedipine and enalapril, there was no reduction in need for aortic valve surgery when followed up to 7 years. Therefore there is no current definitive indication of medical therapy with afterload reduction for aortic regurgitation other than hypertension control
- Diuretics and sodium restriction for CHF.

SURGICAL RESERVED FOR: REFERRAL

Reserved for:

- Patients with acute severe AR (i.e., infective endocarditis) and cardiogenic shock.
- Patients with hemodynamically stable severe AR undergoing CABG or surgery on the aorta or other heart valves.
- Symptomatic patients with chronic, severe AR.
- Evidence of systolic dysfunction with left ventricular ejection fraction of 50% or less.
- Asymptomatic patients with severe AR and left ventricular ejection fraction >50%, but with left ventricular dilation:
  1. Echocardiographic end- systolic dimension >55 mm *or*
  2. Echocardiographic end- diastolic dimension >75 mm.

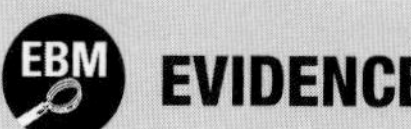

EVIDENCE

available at www.expertconsult.com

SUGGESTED READINGS

Available at www.expertconsult.com

RELATED CONTENT

Aortic Insufficiency (Patient Information)

AUTHOR: **NEELESH LALJI CHUDASAMA, M.D.**

BASIC INFORMATION

DEFINITION

Aortic stenosis (AS) is obstruction to left ventricular systolic outflow across the aortic valve. Symptoms typically appear when the valve orifice decreases to <1 cm^2 (normal orifice is 3 to 4 cm^2). Criteria for severe AS include a valve area <1.0 cm^2, a mean gradient > 40 mm Hg, or a peak gradient > 4 m/s.

SYNONYMS

Aortic valvular stenosis
AS

ICD-9CM CODES
424.1 Aortic valvular stenosis
ICD-10CM CODE
I35.0 Nonrheumatic aortic (valve) stenosis
I35.2 Aortic valve stenosis with insufficiency
I35.8 Other aortic valve disorders
I35.9 Aortic valve disorder, unspecified

EPIDEMIOLOGY & DEMOGRAPHICS

- Aortic stenosis is the most common valve lesion in adults in Western countries.
- Calcific stenosis (most common cause in patients >70 yr) occurs in 75% of patients.

PHYSICAL FINDINGS & CLINICAL PRESENTATION

- Harsh midsystolic, crescendo-decrescendo murmur (Fig. 1-114) best heard at base of heart and radiating into neck vessels; often associated with a thrill or ejection click; may also be heard well at the apex.
- Signs of severe AS include absent or diminished intensity of the second heart sound and/or late rising carotid upstroke with delayed amplitude (pulsus parvus et tardus), presence of S4, and a reverse splitting of the second heart sound.
- Classic symptoms include angina, syncope, and heart failure.
- Acquired von Willebrand disease is seen in approximately 20% of severe AS, which can lead to GI bleeding from angiodysplasia (Heyde's syndrome) that resolves after aortic valve replacement.

ETIOLOGY

- Idiopathic calcification of the aortic valve (most common cause, presents at ages 40 to 60)
- Progressive stenosis of congenital bicuspid valve (found in 1% to 2% of the population, presents at ages 40 to 60)
- Rheumatic heart disease
- Less common causes include congenital (major cause of AS in patients < 30 yr), radiation, and obstructive vegetations (endocarditis)
- Genetic variation in the LPA locus, mediated by Lp(2) levels, is associated with aortic valve calcification across multiple ethnic groups and with incidental clinical aortic stenosis.

DIAGNOSIS

DIFFERENTIAL DIAGNOSIS

- Hypertrophic cardiomyopathy
- Mitral regurgitation
- Ventricular septal defect
- Aortic sclerosis. Aortic stenosis is distinguished from aortic sclerosis by the degree of valve impairment. In aortic sclerosis, the valve leaflets are abnormally thickened but obstruction to outflow is absent or minimal.
- Subvalvular membrane or supravalvular AS

WORKUP

- ECG: may demonstrate left ventricular hypertrophy and/or left atrial abnormality (Fig. 1-115).
- Chest radiograph: may demonstrate cardiomegaly. Poststenotic dilation of the ascending aorta may also be evident.
- Echocardiography (see "Imaging Studies")
- Cardiac catheterization in selected patients (see "Imaging Studies")
- Dobutamine challenge (for low-gradient, low-flow AS)
- Figs. E1-116 and E1-117 describe algorithms for evaluation and treatment of AS.

IMAGING STUDIES

- Chest x-ray:
  1. Poststenotic dilation of the ascending aorta
  2. Calcification of aortic cusps
  3. Rounding of left ventricle (LV) apex
- ECG:
  1. Left ventricular hypertrophy (found in 80% of patients)
  2. Left atrial enlargement
  3. Atrial fibrillation (in late disease)

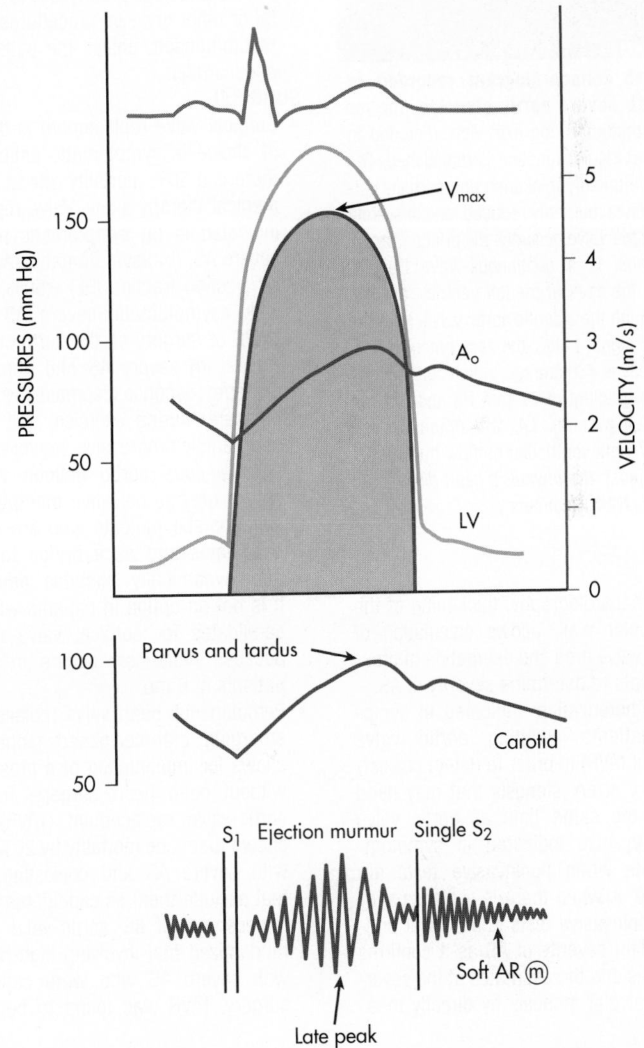

FIGURE 1-114 Relationship between left ventricle (LV) and aortic (Ao) pressures and the Doppler aortic stenosis velocity curve (in red). The pressure difference between the LV and aorta in systole is four times the velocity squared (the Bernoulli equation). Thus, a maximum velocity (Vmax) of 4.3 m/sec corresponds to a maximum LV to Ao pressure difference of 74 mm Hg and a mean systolic gradient of 44 mm Hg. On physical examination, the slow rate of rise and delayed peak in the carotid pulse (or parvus and tardus) matches the contour of the aortic pressure waveform. The murmur corresponds to the Doppler velocity curve with a harsh crescendo-decrescendo late-peaking systolic murmur, best heard at the aortic region (upper right sternal border). Often, a soft, high-pitched diastolic decrescendo murmur of aortic regurgitation also is appreciated. (From Bonow et al [eds]: Braunwald's heart disease, ed 9, Philadelphia, 2012, Saunders.)

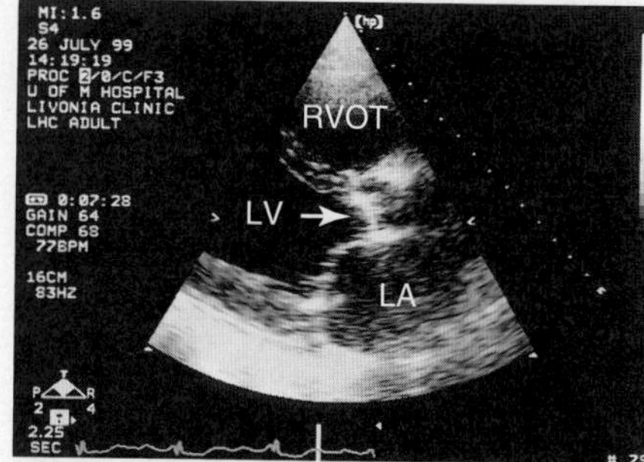

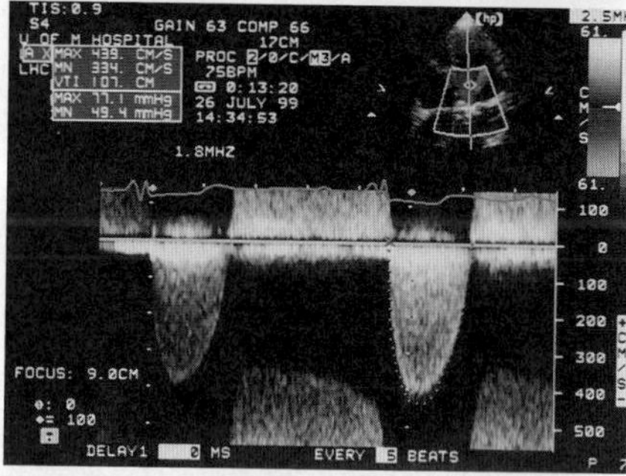

FIGURE 1-115 Echocardiogram recorded in a patient with severe aortic stenosis. The *top panel* is a parasternal long-axis view recorded in systole. Left ventricular function is diminished. The aortic valve is markedly thickened and partially calcified. Its motion is markedly reduced, and in systole it appears that the valve occludes the orifice *(arrow)*. The *lower panel* is a continuous-wave Doppler recorded from the apex of the left ventricle along a line aimed through the stenotic aortic valve. Note the aortic stenosis signal below the zero crossing line. The peak velocity is 430 cm/sec, which corresponds to a maximum gradient of 77 mm Hg and a mean gradient of 49.4 mm Hg. *LA,* left atrium; *LV,* left ventricle; *RVOT,* right ventricular outflow tract. (From Zipes DP et al [eds]: *Braunwauld's heart disease,* ed 7, Philadelphia, 2005, Saunders.)

- Doppler echocardiography: thickening of the left ventricular wall; allows calculation of both aortic valve area and estimation of pressure gradients to determine severity of AS.
- Cardiac catheterization: indicated in symptomatic patients awaiting aortic valve replacement (AVR) in order to detect coexisting coronary artery stenosis that may need bypass at the same time as aortic valve replacement; also indicated in symptomatic patients when noninvasive tests are inconclusive or when there is a discrepancy between noninvasive tests and clinical findings regarding severity of AS as it confirms the diagnosis and the estimates of the severity of the valvular stenosis by directly measuring the gradient across the valve, allowing calculation of the valve area.

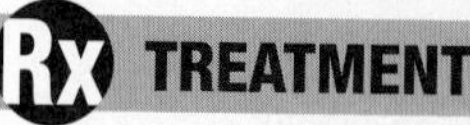

TREATMENT

NONPHARMACOLOGIC THERAPY

- Strenuous activity should be avoided in patients with moderate to severe AS
- Sodium restriction if CHF is present

GENERAL Rx

MEDICAL

- Once symptomatic, AS is a surgical disease.
- Gentle diuresis for volume overload as preload dependent; control hypertension (HTN) but avoid vasodilators (nitrates), maintain sinus rhythm
- In 2007, the AHA guidelines for prevention of infectious endocarditis were revised and routine antibiotic prophylaxis to undergo dental or other invasive procedures is no longer recommended, unless the patient has prior endocarditis.

SURGICAL

- Surgical valve replacement is the treatment of choice in symptomatic patients because there is a 50% mortality rate at 2 years with medical therapy alone. Valve replacement is indicated in (a) symptomatic patients with severe AS, (b) asymptomatic severe AS with LV ejection fraction (EF) <50%, (c) patients with asymptomatic severe AS undergoing CABG or surgery on the aorta or other heart valves, (d) severe AS and abnormal blood pressure response (decrease in systolic blood pressure) during exercise, and (e) patients with rapidly progressive stenosis.
- Percutaneous aortic balloon valvuloplasty serves best as palliative therapy in severely symptomatic patients who are not surgical candidates and as a bridge to surgery in hemodynamically unstable adult patients. It is not an option in patients who are good candidates for surgical valve replacement because restenosis occurs in most adult patients at 6 mo.
- Percutaneous heart valve replacement is an emerging catheter-based technology that allows for implantation of a prosthetic valve without open heart surgery. Transcatheter aortic-valve replacement (TAVR) has been shown to reduce mortality by 20% in patients with severe AS and coexisting conditions that exclude them as candidates for surgical replacement of the aortic valve. In another randomized trial involving high-risk patients with severe AS who were candidates for surgery, TAVR was found to be noninferior to surgical valve replacement for short-term efficacy with similar all-cause mortality at 2 yr. The surgical group had double the incidence of new-onset atrial fibrillation and major bleeding, but the TAVR group had a higher rate of paravalvular regurgitation, major stroke, and vascular complications.

DISPOSITION

- The presence of even mild symptoms is an indicator of poor survival for patients with AS. With the average duration of symptoms before death is angina, 5 yr; syncope, 3 yr; CHF, 2 yr.
- Approximately 75% of patients with symptomatic AS will die within 3 yr of symptom onset unless the aortic valve is replaced.

REFERRAL

- Surgical referral for valve replacement in all symptomatic AS patients. The risk of aortic valve replacement is greater than any potential benefit for truly asymptomatic patients. There are studies that are examining the presence of moderate or severe valvular calcification, together with a rapid increase in aortic jet velocity and elevated BNP, to identify patients with a very poor prognosis who should be considered for early valve replacement rather than have surgery delayed until symptoms develop.
- Surgical mortality rate for valve replacement is 3% to 5%; however, it varies with patient's age (>8% in patients >75 yr).
- Balloon valvuloplasty is useful in infants and children or poor surgical candidates who do not have calcified valve apparatus; it can be done as an intermediate procedure to stabilize high-risk patients before surgery.
- Patients who are considered high risk for cardiac surgery or have contraindications (porcelain aorta) should be referred to a center with a transcatheter program for TAVR evaluation.

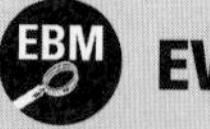

EVIDENCE

available at www.expertconsult.com

SUGGESTED READINGS

available at www.expertconsult.com

RELATED CONTENT

Aortic Stenosis (Patient Information)

AUTHORS: **DEEPA KUMARAIAH, M.D., M.B.A.,** and **VEERANNA MERLA, M.D.**

BASIC INFORMATION

DEFINITION

Appendicitis is the acute inflammation of the appendix.

ICD-9CM CODES
540.9 Appendicitis
540.0 Appendicitis with generalized peritonitis

ICD-10CM CODES
K35.80 Unspecified acute appendicitis
K35.89 Other acute appendicitis
K35.2 Acute appendicitis with generalized peritonitis

EPIDEMIOLOGY & DEMOGRAPHICS

- Appendicitis occurs in 10% of the population, most commonly between the ages of 10 and 30 yr. Median age is 22 years. Lifetime risk is 7%.
- More than 250,000 appendectomies are performed in the U.S. each year.
- It is the most common abdominal surgical emergency.
- Incidence of appendicitis has declined over the past 30 yr.
- Male/female ratio is 3:2 until mid-20s; it equalizes after age 30 yr.

PHYSICAL FINDINGS & CLINICAL PRESENTATION

- In children with abdominal pain, fever is the single most useful sign associated with appendicitis. Vomiting, rectal tenderness, and rebound tenderness along with fever are more indicative of appendicitis in children than in adults.
- Abdominal pain: initially the pain may be epigastric or periumbilical in nearly 50% of patients; it subsequently localizes to the right lower quadrant within 12 to 18 hr. Pain can be found in back or right flank if appendix is retrocecal or in other abdominal locations if there is malrotation of the appendix.
- Pain with right thigh extension *(psoas sign)*, low-grade fever: temperature may be >38° C if there is appendiceal perforation.
- Pain with internal rotation of the flexed right thigh *(obturator sign)* is present.
- Right lower quadrant (RLQ) pain on palpation of the left lower quadrant (LLQ) *(Rovsing's sign)*: physical examination may reveal right-sided tenderness in patients with pelvic appendix.
- Point of maximum tenderness is in the RLQ *(McBurney's point)*.
- Nausea, vomiting, tachycardia, cutaneous hyperesthesias at the level of T12 can be present.

ETIOLOGY

Obstruction of the appendiceal lumen with subsequent vascular congestion, inflammation, and edema; common causes of obstruction are:

- Fecaliths: 30% to 35% of cases (most common in adults)
- Foreign body: 4% (fruit seeds, pinworms, tapeworms, roundworms, calculi)
- Inflammation: 50% to 60% of cases (submucosal lymphoid hyperplasia [most common etiology in children, teens])
- Neoplasms: 1% (carcinoids, metastatic disease, carcinoma)

Dx DIAGNOSIS

DIFFERENTIAL DIAGNOSIS

- Intestinal: regional cecal enteritis, incarcerated hernia, cecal diverticulitis, intestinal obstruction, perforated ulcer, perforated cecum, Meckel's diverticulitis
- Reproductive: ectopic pregnancy, ovarian cyst, torsion of ovarian cyst, salpingitis, tubo-ovarian abscess, mittelschmerz, endometriosis, seminal vesiculitis
- Renal: renal and ureteral calculi, neoplasms, pyelonephritis
- Vascular: leaking aortic aneurysm
- Psoas abscess
- Trauma
- Cholecystitis
- Mesenteric adenitis

WORKUP

Patients with RLQ pain, nausea, vomiting, anorexia, and RLQ rebound tenderness should undergo prompt clinical and laboratory evaluation. Imaging studies are generally not necessary in typical appendicitis and generally reserved for patients with an equivocal likelihood of appendicitis. They are useful when the diagnosis is uncertain. Laparoscopy may be useful as both a diagnostic and a therapeutic modality.

LABORATORY TESTS

- Complete blood count with differential reveals leukocytosis with a left shift in 90% of patients with appendicitis. Total white blood cell (WBC) count is generally lower than 20,000/mm^3. Higher counts may be indicative of perforation. Less than 4% have a normal WBC and differential. A WBC count <10,000/mm^3 decreases the likelihood of appendicitis. Low hemoglobin and hematocrit levels in an older patient should raise suspicion for GI tract carcinoma.
- Microscopic hematuria and pyuria may occur in <20% of patients.
- HCG to rule out pregnancy in females of reproductive age

IMAGING STUDIES

- Multidetector computed tomography (Fig. 1-118) is a useful test for routine evaluation of suspected appendicitis in adults. CT of the abdomen/pelvis without contrast has a sensitivity of >90% and an accuracy >94% for acute appendicitis. A distended appendix, periappendiceal inflammation, and a thickened appendiceal wall are indicative of appendicitis. Table 1-53 describes CT findings of appendicitis. In children and young adults, exposure to CT radiation is of particular concern. Trials with low-dose CT (116 mGy · cm) have shown that low-dose CT is not inferior to standard-dose CT (521 mGy · cm) with respect to negative (unnecessary) appendectomy rates in young adults with suspected appendicitis.
- Ultrasonography (Fig. 1-119) has a sensitivity of 75% to 90% for the diagnosis of acute

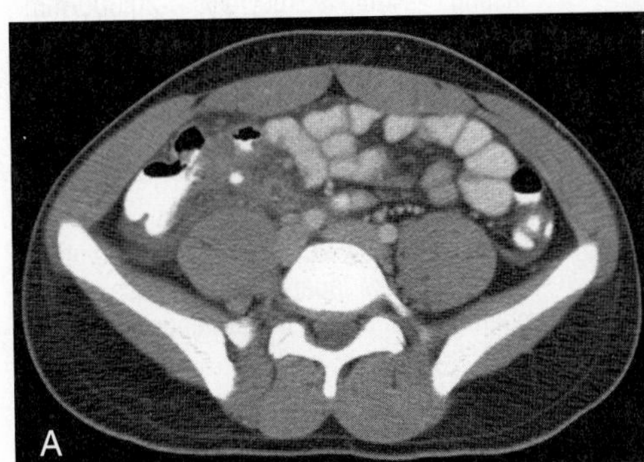

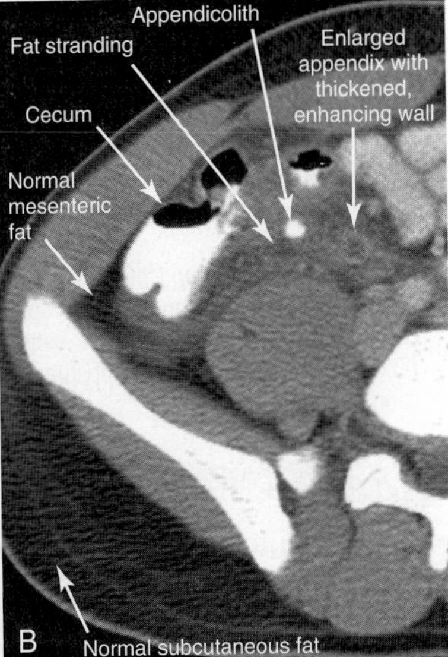

FIGURE 1-118 Appendicitis, CT with IV and oral contrast. This CT demonstrates classic findings of appendicitis in an 18-year-old male with right lower quadrant pain, as seen with CT with IV and oral contrast. Studies suggest that CT without contrast has similar sensitivity and specificity. An enlarged appendix is seen near the cecum as a right lower quadrant tubular structure in short-axis cross section, giving it a circular appearance. The surrounding fat shows stranding, a smoky appearance indicating inflammation (compare with normal mesenteric and subcutaneous fat, which is nearly black). The appendiceal wall shows enhancement, a brightening after administration of IV contrast. This slice also shows an appendicolith, an occasional finding of appendicitis. It does not appear to be within the appendix in this slice, because the appendix bends in and out of the plane of this slice. An appendicolith usually appears as a calcified (white) rounded structure, visible without any contrast. **A,** Axial CT image. **B,** Close-up. (From Broder JS: *Diagnostic imaging for the emergency physician,* Philadelphia, 2011, Saunders.)

 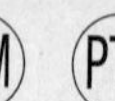 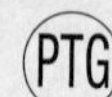

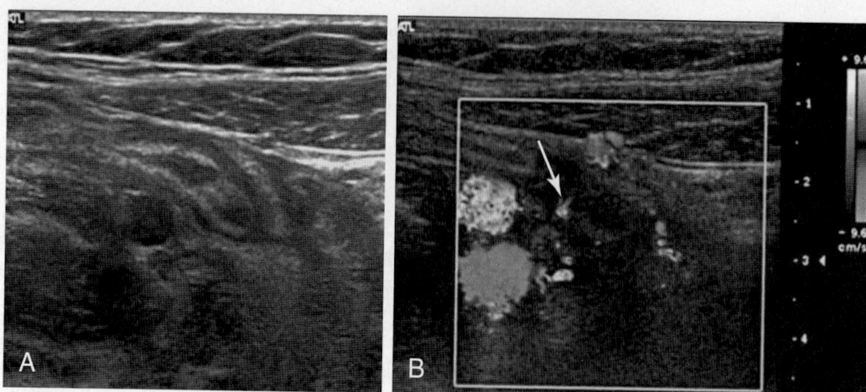

FIGURE 1-119 Appendicitis. A, Transabdominal ultrasound using a linear transducer demonstrates a thick, tubular, noncompressible structure. **B,** Same imaging method with addition of color Doppler ultrasound shows increased vascularity within the luminal wall consistent with inflammation *(arrow).* (From Fielding JR et al: *Gynecologic imaging,* Philadelphia, 2011, Saunders.)

TABLE 1-53 CT Findings of Appendicitis: SCALPEL Mnemonic

Term	Description
Stranding	Fat stranding suggests regional inflammation, possibly because of appendicitis.
Cecum	The appendix originates from the cecum, which should be identified first to help localize the appendix. The cecum may show wall thickening, suggesting appendicitis.
Air	Air outside of the lumen of the appendix is pathologic and suggests perforation. Air within the appendiceal wall is also abnormal.
Large	The normal appendix is <6 mm; an enlarged appendix >6 mm suggests appendicitis. Wall thickening >1 mm also suggests appendicitis.
Phlegmon	Inflammatory changes surrounding the appendix suggest a perforated appendix. A heterogeneous collection called a phlegmon may be seen. If the appendix has ruptured, a pericecal phlegmon may be the only remaining evidence, because the appendix itself may not be seen.
Enhancement	The wall of an abnormal appendix enhances with IV contrast and appears brighter than the normal bowel or the normal psoas muscle.
Lith	An appendicolith is a calcified stone sometimes found in the lumen of an inflamed appendix.

From Broder JS: *Diagnostic imaging for the emergency physician,* Philadelphia, 2011, Saunders.

appendicitis, although it is highly operator dependent and difficult in patients with large body habitus. Ultrasound is useful, especially in pregnancy and in younger women when diagnosis is unclear. Normal ultrasonographic findings should not deter surgery if the history and physical examination are indicative of appendicitis.

- MRI of the abdomen and pelvis can also be used to accurately diagnose acute appendicitis in pregnant patients (100% sensitivity, 93.6% specificity) without exposure to ionizing radiation.

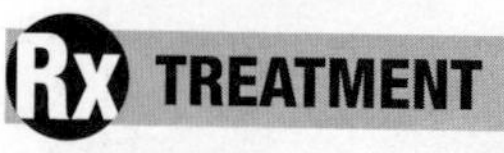

TREATMENT

NONPHARMACOLOGIC THERAPY

- Nothing by mouth
- Do not administer analgesics or antibiotics until the diagnosis is made (may mask signs of peritonitis)

ACUTE GENERAL Rx

- Urgent appendectomy (laparoscopic or open), correction of fluid and electrolyte imbalance with vigorous IV hydration and electrolyte replacement
- IV antibiotic prophylaxis to cover gram-negative bacilli and anaerobes (ampicillin/sulbactam 3 g IV q6h or piperacillin/tazobactam 4.5 g IV q8h in adults)

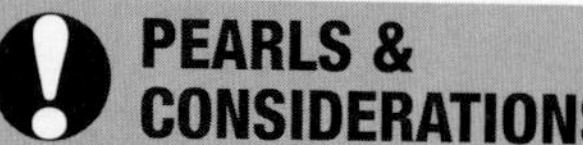

PEARLS & CONSIDERATIONS

COMMENTS

- Perforation is common (20% in adult patients). Indicators of perforation are pain lasting >24 hr, leukocytosis >20,000/mm^3, temperature >102° F, palpable abdominal mass, and peritoneal findings.
- In general, prognosis is excellent. Mortality rate is <1% in young adults without complications; however, it exceeds 10% in elderly patients with ruptured appendix.
- In approximately 20% of patients who undergo exploratory laparotomy because of suspected appendicitis, the appendix is normal.
- Trials comparing antibiotic treatment with emergency appendectomy have shown that amoxicillin plus clavulanic acid is not inferior to emergency appendectomy for acute appendicitis. Researchers have shown that over 60% of patients with uncomplicated appendicitis assigned to the antibiotic group do not need appendectomy. However, the need to remove the appendix in patients with acute appendicitis is so entrenched in the minds of physicians that nonsurgical options are only rarely considered.

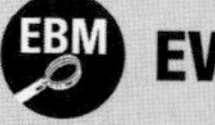

EVIDENCE

available at www.expertconsult.com

SUGGESTED READINGS

available at www.expertconsult.com

RELATED CONTENT

Appendicitis (Patient Information)

AUTHOR: **FRED F. FERRI, M.D.**

BASIC INFORMATION

DEFINITION

Arrhythmogenic right ventricular dysplasia (ARVD) is a disorder characterized by replacement of the normal myocardium by fibrofatty tissue, RV myocyte loss, and RV wall thinning, and represents a kind of cardiomyopathy. It is defined clinically by life-threatening ventricular arrhythmias in otherwise healthy young people.

SYNONYMS

Arrhythmogenic right ventricular cardiomyopathy

ICD-9CM CODES
427.1 Paroxysmal ventricular tachycardia
425.4 Other primary cardiomyopathies
427.89 Other specified cardiac dysrhythmias

ICD-10CM CODES
I42.8 Arrhythmogenic ventricular dysplasia

EPIDEMIOLOGY & DEMOGRAPHICS

INCIDENCE: ARVD comprises 2% of sudden cardiac arrest cases.
PREVALENCE: 1:5000 persons
PREDOMINANT SEX AND AGE: Men <35 yr old
RISK FACTORS: Family history of ARVD
GENETICS:
- Autosomal dominant with variable penetrance, and polymorphic phenotypic expression
- Desmosomal dysfunction (desmosome gene mutations)
- 11 subtypes of ARVD are identified based on the involved genes.

PHYSICAL FINDINGS & CLINICAL PRESENTATION

- Suspect when young males present with syncope, sudden cardiac arrest, ventricular tachycardia, premature ventricular beats originating from the right ventricle, or, less commonly, signs and symptoms of right heart failure. Symptoms vary and range from palpitations, dizziness, and syncope to atypical chest pain, dyspnea, and fatigue.
- Cardiac arrest after physical exertion may be the initial presentation.
- Physical examination will be normal in most patients. Widely split S2 is an important diagnostic clue.

ETIOLOGY

ARVD is characterized by progressive replacement of the right ventricular myocardium with fibrofatty tissue after apoptotic myocardial cell death

DIAGNOSIS

- Diagnosis is made when two major criteria, one major and two minor, or four minor criteria are met.
- See Table 1-54 for diagnostic criteria.

DIFFERENTIAL DIAGNOSIS

- Cardiomyopathy with involvement of the right ventricle
- Uhl's anomaly: rare anomaly that presents mainly in childhood with signs and symptoms and right heart failure. Uhl's anomaly is characterized by a paper-thin right ventricle resulting from death of the myocytes throughout the right ventricle
- Idiopathic RV tachycardia
- Left dominant arrhythmogenic cardiomyopathy

WORKUP

- Resting ECG will have diagnostic findings in 50% to 90% of patients with ARVD. These changes include T-wave inversions in anterior precordial leads V_1-V_6, epsilon waves (Fig. 1-120A), and *ventricular tachycardia* (VT) with left bundle branch block pattern.
- Endomyocardial biopsy is the preferred method for diagnosis of ARVD. It has specificity of 92%, but it lacks sensitivity (<20%).

TABLE 1-54 Criteria for the Diagnosis of Arrhythmogenic Right Ventricular Dysplasia

Global and/or Regional Dysfunction and Structural Alterations
Major
Severe dilation and reduction of right ventricular ejection fraction with no (or only mild) left ventricular impairment Localized right ventricular aneurysms Severe segmental dilation of the right ventricle
Minor
Mild global right ventricular dilation and/or ejection fraction with a normal left ventricle Mild segmental dilation of the right ventricle Regional right ventricular hypokinesis
Tissue Characterization of the Walls
Major
Fibrofatty replacement of myocardium on endomyocardial biopsy
ECG Repolarization Abnormalities
Minor
Inverted T waves in the right precordial leads (V_2 and V_3) in patients older than 12 yr and in the absence of right bundle branch block
ECG Depolarization/Conduction Abnormalities
Major
Epsilon waves or localized prolongation (greater than 110 ms) of the QRS complex in right precordial leads (V_1 through V_3)
Minor
Late potentials visible on signal-averaged ECG
Arrhythmias
Minor
Sustained or nonsustained left bundle branch block type VT documented on ECG, Holter monitoring, or during exercise stress testing Frequent ventricular extrasystoles (more than 1000 per 24 hr on Holter monitoring)
Family History
Major
Familial disease confirmed at autopsy or surgery
Minor
Family history of premature sudden death (younger than 35 yr) caused by suspected ARVD/C Family history (clinical diagnosis based on present criteria)

The diagnosis of arrhythmogenic right ventricular dysplasia is made if one of the following is met: two major criteria, one major and two minor criteria, or four minor criteria.
ARVD/C, Arrhythmogenic right ventricular dysplasia/cardiomyopathy; *ECG,* electrocardiography; *VT,* ventricular tachycardia.
From Anderson EL: Arrhythmogenic right ventricular dysplasia, *Am Fam Physician* 73[8]:1391-1398, 2006.

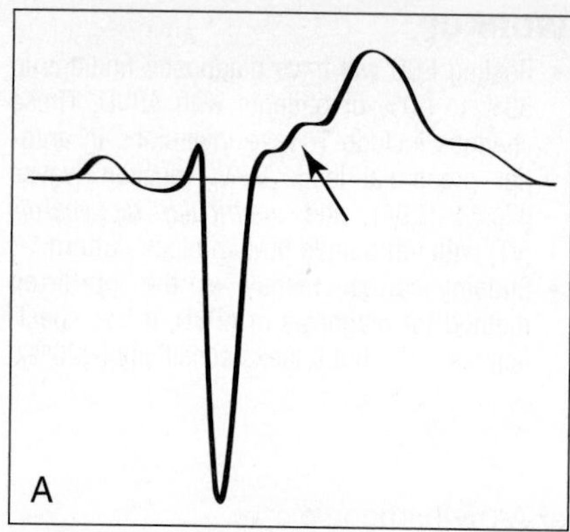

FIGURE 1-120A Epsilon waves are small deflections just beyond the QRS complex. Best visualized in leads V_1-V_3. Any potential in leads V_1-V_3 that exceeds the QRS in leads V6 by more than 25 millisecond should be considered epsilon wave. (From Anderson EL: Arrhythmogenic right ventricular dysplasia, *Am Fam Physician* 73(8):1391-1398, 2006.)

- Electrophysiologic study is important to identify delayed potentials that can lead to tachycardiac events.
- Routine immunohistochemical analysis of a conventional endomyocardial-biopsy sample appears to be a highly sensitive and specific diagnostic test for arrhythmogenic right ventricular cardiomyopathy.

IMAGING STUDIES

- MRI is a noninvasive method to detect structural changes and regional dysfunction. Cardiac MRI (CMR) is the most sensitive method to detect ARVD, but has high false-positive rates. Cardiac CT angiogram (Fig. 1-120B) will reveal thinning and aneurysmal dilation of the RV anterior wall and outflow tract.
- Echocardiography will show right ventricular dilation with regional wall motion abnormalities that varied with the severity of the disease.
- Other imaging modalities used for evaluation of suspected ARVD include signal averaged ECG, Holter monitor, stress test, and radionuclide ventriculography

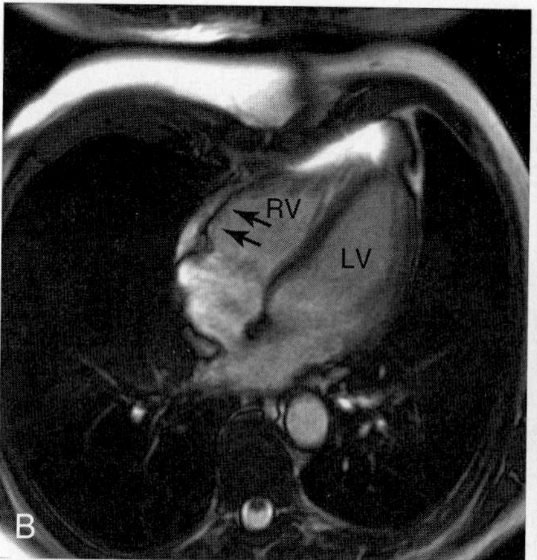

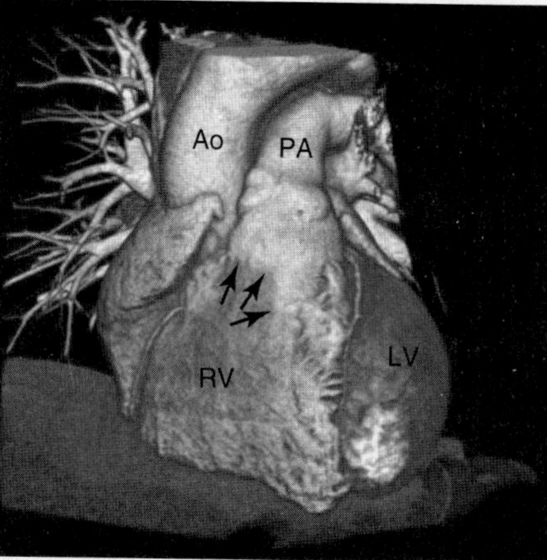

FIGURE 1-120B Right ventricular aneurysm. This cardiac computed tomography angiogram shows thinning and aneurysmal dilation of the RV anterior wall and outflow tract *(arrows)* in a patient with arrhythmogenic right ventricular dysplasia, cardiomyopathy, and ventricular tachycardia. *Ao,* Aorta; *LV,* left ventricle; *PA,* pulmonary artery. (Courtesy of Dr. Nasar Nallamothu, Prairie Cardiovascular Consultants, Springfield, Ill. From Issa Z et al: *Clinical arrhythmology and electrophysiology,* ed 2, Philadelphia, 2012, Saunders.)

Rx TREATMENT

No definitive therapy is available. Treatment goal is to prevent sudden cardiac death. Placement of an automatic implantable cardioverter defibrillator (AICD) may be used to avoid sudden cardiac death in patients with severe symptoms. It is worth noting that complications related to AICD can make this treatment option undesirable in some patients, but with an experienced cardiologist/cardiac center, this can be a great option.

NONPHARMACOLOGIC THERAPY

- Avoidance of activity that may trigger tachycardia
- Right ventriculotomy
- Cardiac transplantation

ACUTE GENERAL Rx

Intravenous amiodarone has been proved to be effective in terminating VT.

CHRONIC Rx

- Antiarrhythmic therapy with sotalol, amiodarone, propafenone, beta-blocker alone or in combination can be used
- Radiofrequency ablation is used in cases of refractory VT, frequent tachycardia after defibrillator placement, or localized arrhythmia sites
- Implantable cardioverted defibrillators hold promise

REFERRAL

- Early cardiology and electrophysiology referral
- Consider referring for genetic counseling

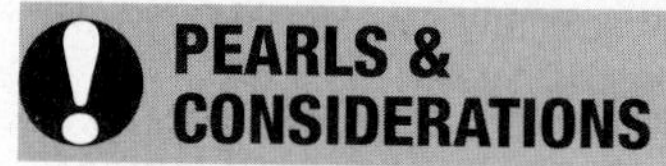

PEARLS & CONSIDERATIONS

PREVENTION

Test first-degree relatives if there is a positive history of sudden cardiac death or death at an early age.

EDUCATION

Patient handout can be found in *American Family Physician* (American Academy of Family Physicians: Information from your family doctor. Arrhythmogenic right ventricular dysplasia: what you should know. *Am Fam Physician* 73(8):1401, 2006).

SUGGESTED READINGS

available at www.expertconsult.com

AUTHORS: **ABDULRAHMAN ABDULBAKI, M.D., NADIA MUJAHID, M.D.,** and **PATRICK NSEREKO, M.D.**

BASIC INFORMATION

DEFINITION

Asbestosis is a slowly progressive diffuse interstitial fibrosis resulting from dose-related inhalation exposure to fibers of asbestos.

ICD-9CM CODES
501 Asbestosis
ICD-10CM CODES
J61 Pneumoconiosis due to asbestos and other mineral fibers

EPIDEMIOLOGY & DEMOGRAPHICS

- Five to 10 new cases per 100,000 persons per year in U.S.
- Prolonged interval (20 to 30 yr) between exposures to inhaled fibers and clinical manifestations of disease
- Most common in workers involved in the primary extraction of asbestos from rock deposits and in those involved in the fabrication and installation of products containing asbestos (e.g., naval shipyards in World War II; installation of floor tiles, ceiling tiles, acoustic ceiling coverings, wall insulation, and pipe coverings in public buildings)

PHYSICAL FINDINGS & CLINICAL PRESENTATION

- Insidious onset of shortness of breath with exertion is usually the first sign of asbestosis.
- Dyspnea becomes more severe as the disease advances; with time, progressively less exertion is tolerated.
- Cough is frequent and usually paroxysmal, dry, and nonproductive.
- Scant mucoid sputum may accompany the cough in the later stages of the disease.
- Fine end-respiratory crackles (rales, crepitations) are heard more predominantly in the lung bases.
- Digital clubbing, edema, jugular venous distention are present.

ETIOLOGY

Inhalation of asbestos fibers

DIAGNOSIS

DIFFERENTIAL DIAGNOSIS

- Silicosis
- Siderosis, other pneumonoconioses
- Lung cancer
- Atelectasis

WORKUP

Documentation of exposure history, diagnostic imaging, pulmonary function testing

LABORATORY TESTS

- Generally not helpful
- Possible mild elevation of erythrocyte sedimentation rate (ESR), positive antinuclear antibody (ANA), and rheumatoid factor (RF) (these tests are nonspecific and do not correlate with disease severity or activity)
- Pulmonary function testing: decreased vital capacity, decreased total lung capacity, decreased carbon monoxide gas transfer
- Arterial blood gases: hypoxemia, hypercarbia in advanced stages

IMAGING STUDIES

Chest radiograph (Fig. 1-121):

- Small, irregular shadows in lower lung zones.
- Thickened pleura, calcified plaques (present under diaphragm and lateral chest wall).
- CT scan of chest confirms diagnosis. Typical findings on high-resolution CT of the chest include increased interstitial markings found mainly at the bases. As the disease progresses, honeycombing is noted.

TREATMENT

NONPHARMACOLOGIC THERAPY

- Smoking cessation, proper nutrition, exercise program to maximize available lung function
- Home oxygen therapy prn
- Removal of patient from further asbestos fiber exposure

GENERAL Rx

- Prompt identification and treatment of respiratory infections
- Supplemental oxygen on a prn basis
- Annual influenza vaccination, pneumococcal vaccination

DISPOSITION

- There is no specific treatment for asbestosis.
- Death is usually from respiratory failure from cor pulmonale.
- Patients with asbestosis have increased risk for mesotheliomas, lung cancer, and tuberculosis. Recent reports indicate that the risk of asbestos-induced lung cancer may be overestimated.
- Survival in patients after development of mesothelioma is 4 to 6 yr.

REFERRAL

To pulmonologist initially

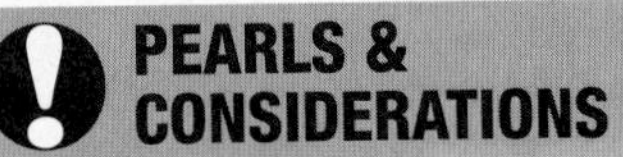

PEARLS & CONSIDERATIONS

COMMENTS

Patient information on asbestosis can be obtained from the American Lung Association, 1740 Broadway, New York, NY 10019.

SUGGESTED READINGS
available at www.expertconsult.com

RELATED CONTENT

Asbestosis (Patient Information)

AUTHOR: **FRED F. FERRI, M.D.**

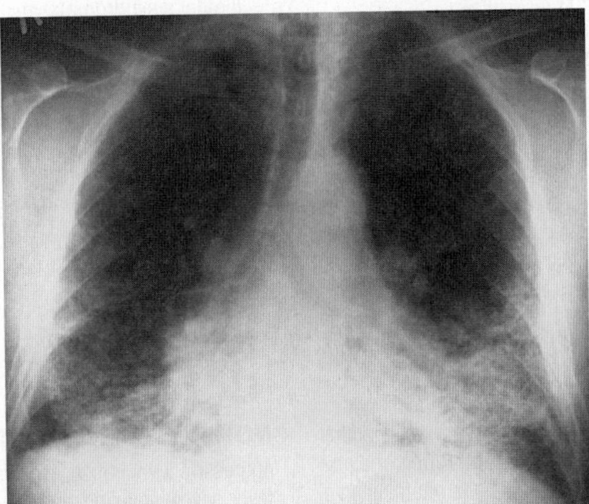

FIGURE 1-121 Asbestosis. Posteroanterior radiograph shows coarse linear opacities at both lung bases obscuring the cardiac borders. (From McLoud TC: *Thoracic radiology: the requisites,* St Louis, 1998, Mosby.)

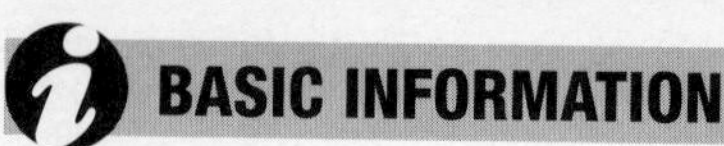

BASIC INFORMATION

DEFINITION

Ascariasis is a parasitic infection caused by the nematode *Ascaris lumbricoides.* The majority of those infected are asymptomatic; however, clinical disease may arise from pulmonary hypersensitivity, intestinal obstruction, and secondary complications.

SYNONYMS

Round worms
Worms

ICD-9CM CODES
127.0 Ascariasis
ICD-10CM CODES
B77.9 Ascariasis, unspecified
B77.81 Ascariasis pneumonia

EPIDEMIOLOGY & DEMOGRAPHICS

INCIDENCE (IN U.S.):
- Unknown
- Three times the infection rates found in blacks as in whites

PEAK INCIDENCE: Unknown
PREVALENCE (IN U.S.): Estimated at 4 million, the majority of which live in the rural southeastern part of the country; ascariasis is associated with poor sanitation
PREDOMINANT SEX: Both sexes probably equally affected, with a possible slight female preponderance
PREDOMINANT AGE: Most common in children from ages 2 to 10 years old and decreases after age 15; infections tend to cluster in families
NEONATAL INFECTION: Probable transmission, though not specifically studied

PHYSICAL FINDINGS & CLINICAL PRESENTATION

- Occurs approximately 9 to 12 days after ingestion of eggs (corresponding to the larva migration through the lungs)
- Nonproductive cough
- Substernal chest discomfort
- Fever
- In patients with large worm burdens, especially children, intestinal obstruction associated with perforation, volvulus, and intussusception
- Migration of worms into the biliary tree giving clinical appearance of biliary colic and pancreatitis as well as acute appendicitis with movement into that appendage
- Rarely, infection with *A. lumbricoides* producing interstitial nephritis and acute renal failure
- In endemic areas in Asia and Africa, malabsorption of dietary proteins and vitamins as a consequence of chronic worm intestinal carriage; 1 billion people worldwide are infected with this nematode

ETIOLOGY

- Transmission is usually hand to mouth, but eggs may be ingested via transported vegetables grown in contaminated soil.
- Eggs are hatched in the small intestine, with larvae penetrating intestinal mucosa and migrating via the circulation to the lungs.
- Larval forms proceed through the alveoli, ascend the bronchial tree, and return to the intestines after swallowing, where they mature into adult worms.
- Estimated time until the female adult worm begins producing eggs is 2 to 3 mo.
- Eggs are passed out of the intestines with feces and can survive for years in warm, moist, shaded soil.
- Within human host, adult worm lifespan is 1 to 2 yr.

Dx DIAGNOSIS

DIFFERENTIAL DIAGNOSIS

Radiologic manifestations and eosinophilia to be distinguished from drug hypersensitivity and Löffler's syndrome

LABORATORY TESTS

- Examination of the stool for *Ascaris* ova (Fig. E1-122)
- Expectoration or fecal passage of adult worm
- Adult male worms: 10 to 30 cm long; adult female worms: larger than male, up to 40 cm
- Eosinophilia: most prominent early in the infection and subsides as the adult worm infestation established in the intestines; usually in 5% to 12% range but can be up to 50%
- Serology: patients develop IgG antibodies, but they cross react with antigens from other helminths and are not protective; thus serology is used more for epidemiologic purposes than for individual diagnosis

IMAGING STUDIES

- Chest x-ray examination to reveal bilateral oval or round infiltrates of varying size (Löffler's syndrome); NOTE: infiltrates are transient and eventually resolve.
- Plain films of the abdomen and contrast studies to reveal worm masses in loops of bowel.
- Ultrasonography and endoscopic retrograde cholangiopancreatography (ERCP) to identify worms in the pancreaticobiliary tract.
- CT scan with oral contrast can also assist in the detection of GI foreign bodies such as parasites.

Rx TREATMENT

NONPHARMACOLOGIC THERAPY

Aggressive IV hydration, especially in children with fever, severe vomiting, and resultant dehydration

ACUTE GENERAL Rx

- All infected patients, including asymptomatic ones, should be treated
  1. Albendazole: 400 mg PO × 3 days is the first-line agent for intestinal infection with *A. lumbricoides*
  2. Mebendazole 100 mg daily × 3 days
- Cure rate with these agents is 95% to 100%, but they are contraindicated in pregnancy.
- Side effects: GI discomfort, headache, and rarely leukopenia
- Alternative agent or for use in pregnancy: pyrantel pamoate (Antiminth)
  1. Given at a dose of 11 mg/kg PO (maximum dose of 1 g/day)
  2. Considered safe for use in pregnant women
- Other alternative agents:
  1. Ivermectin: 150 to 200 mcg/kg orally once
  2. Nitazoxanide: cure rates in heavy worm burden are only 50% to 80%
  3. Piperazine citrate: no longer first-line agent due to toxicity but still used in cases of intestinal or biliary obstruction, as drug paralyzes the worm, helping its expulsion. Dose: 50 to 75 mg/kg once daily up to maximum of 3.5 g for 2 days.
  4. Levamisole: 2.5 mg/kg once orally is recommended by the WHO as alternative therapy, but not available in the U.S.
- Complete obstruction should be managed surgically

DISPOSITION

Overall prognosis is good. Patients should be reevaluated in 2 to 3 months. Reinfection is common.

REFERRAL

- To gastroenterologist in cases of visualized pancreaticobiliary tract or appendiceal obstruction
- To surgeon in cases of complete obstruction or suspected secondary complication (e.g., perforation or volvulus)

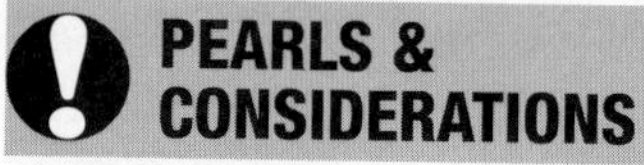

PEARLS & CONSIDERATIONS

COMMENTS

- Hepatic abscess, containing both viable and dead worms, complicating *Ascaris*-induced biliary duct disease has been documented.
- Given the known transmission of the parasite, routine hand washing with soap and proper disposal of human waste would significantly decrease the prevalence of this disease.
- Other protective measures to avoid ingestion of worm eggs:
  1. Peel or cook food.
  2. Boil drinking water.
  3. Do not place small children directly on soil.

SUGGESTED READINGS

available at www.expertconsult.com

RELATED CONTENT

Ascariasis (Patient Information)

AUTHOR: **GLENN G. FORT, M.D., M.P.H.**

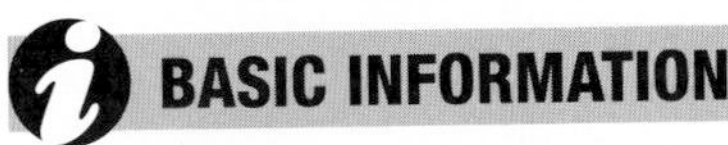

BASIC INFORMATION

DEFINITION

Ascites is the accumulation of excess fluid in the peritoneal cavity, most commonly caused by liver cirrhosis.

SYNONYMS

Fluid in peritoneal cavity
Hydroperitoneum
Hydroperitonia
Hydrops abdominis

ICD-9CM CODES
789.5 Ascites
568.82 Peritoneal effusion (chronic)
ICD-10CM CODES
R18 Ascites
C78.6 Malignant ascites

EPIDEMIOLOGY & DEMOGRAPHICS

Ascites is the most common complication of cirrhosis. Ascites occurs in 50% of individuals with cirrhosis within 10 yr of diagnosis. Cirrhosis is the cause of 75% of cases of ascites. Other causes include malignancy, heart failure, tuberculosis, pancreatitis, nephrotic syndrome, and Budd-Chiari syndrome.

CLINICAL PRESENTATION

- Important information to elicit within history:
  - Viral hepatitis
  - Alcoholism
  - Increasing abdominal girth
  - Increasing lower extremity edema
  - Intravenous drug use
  - Sexual history (i.e., men who have sex with men)
  - History of transfusions
- Important physical exam findings:
  - Bulging flanks
  - Flank dullness to percussion
  - Fluid wave on abdominal exam
  - Lower extremity edema
  - Shifting dullness on abdominal exam
  - Physical signs associated with liver cirrhosis: spider angiomas, jaundice, loss of body hair, Dupuytren's contracture, muscle wasting, bruising, palmar erythema, gynecomastia, testicular atrophy, hemorrhoids, and caput medusae (Fig. 1-123)

FIGURE 1-123 Ascites in a patient with alcoholic cirrhosis showing distended abdomen; dilated superficial collateral veins; hemorrhagic scratch marks due to pruritus and coagulopathy; umbilical varices; and plaster in left iliac fossa indicating diagnostic paracentesis. (From Forbes A et al [eds]: *Atlas of clinical gastroenterology,* ed 3, Oxford, 2005, Mosby.)

ETIOLOGY

Pathophysiology of ascites (Fig. E1-124): increased hepatic resistance to portal flow leads to portal hypertension. The splanchnic vessels respond by increased secretion of nitric oxide, causing splanchnic artery vasodilation. Early in the disease increased plasma volume and increased cardiac output compensate for this vasodilation. However, as disease progresses the effective arterial blood volume decreases, causing sodium and fluid retention through activation of the renin-angiotensin system. The change in capillary pressure causes increased permeability and retention of fluid in the abdomen.

DIAGNOSIS

DIFFERENTIAL DIAGNOSIS

- Chronic parenchymal liver disease, leading to portal hypertension
- Peritoneal carcinomatosis
- Congestive heart failure
- Peritoneal tuberculosis
- Nephrotic syndrome
- Pancreatitis

LABORATORY TESTS

- Initial evaluation should always include:
  - Diagnostic paracentesis (Fig. E1-125). Laboratory tests on this fluid should include a CBC with differential, albumin, total protein, culture and Gram stain. A serum-ascites albumin gradient (SAAG) should be calculated in all patients. If the SAAG is greater than 1.1, the cause of ascites can be attributed to portal hypertension. If SAAG is less than 1.1, a nonportal hypertension etiology of ascites must be sought (see Table 1-55). Optional tests on paracentesis fluid include amylase, LDH, acid-fast bacilli, and glucose levels.
  - AST, ALT, total and direct bilirubin, albumin, alkaline phosphatase, GGTP
  - CBC, coagulation studies
  - Electrolytes, BUN, creatinine

IMAGING STUDIES

- Abdominal ultrasound (Fig. 1-126) is the most sensitive measure for detecting ascitic fluid; a CT or MRI scan is a viable alternative.
- Endoscopy of the upper GI tract to evaluate for esophageal varices if ascites is secondary to portal hypertension.

TREATMENT

NONPHARMACOLOGIC THERAPY

- Sodium-restricted diet (<2 g/day).
- Fluid restriction to 1 L/day in patients with hyponatremia (sodium <130 mEq/L).

ACUTE GENERAL Rx

- Patients with moderate-volume ascites causing only moderate discomfort may be treated on an outpatient basis with the following diuretic regimen: spironolactone 50 to 200 mg qd or amiloride 5 to 10 mg qd. Add furosemide 20 to 40 mg/day in the first several days of treatment, monitoring renal functions carefully for signs of prerenal azotemia (in patients without edema, goal weight loss is 300 to 500 g/day; in patients with edema it is 800 to 1000 g/day).
- Patients with large-volume ascites causing marked discomfort or decrease in activities of daily living may also be treated as outpatients if there are no complications. There are two options for treatment in these patients: (1) large-volume paracentesis or (2) diuretic therapy until loss of fluid is noted (maximum spironolactone 400 mg qd and furosemide 160 mg qd). No difference in long-term mortality rate was found; however, paracentesis is faster, more effective, and associated with fewer adverse effects.
- Table 1-56 summarizes primary medical therapy and adjunctive medications used to increase the efficacy of primary therapy in the treatment of ascites.

CHRONIC Rx

5% to 10% of patients with large-volume ascites will be refractory to high-dose diuretic

TABLE 1-55 Using the Serum-Ascites Albumin Gradient and the Ascites Total Protein Level to Diagnose the Cause of Ascites

Condition	Serum-Ascites Albumin Gradient*	Ascites Total Protein Level†
Cirrhosis	High	Low
Malignant ascites	Low	High
Cardiac ascites	High	High

*High is greater than 1.1 g/dL; low is less than 1.1 g/dL.
†High is greater than 2.5 g/dL; low is less than 2.5 g/dL.
From Goldman L, Schafer AI: *Goldman's Cecil medicine,* ed 24, Philadelphia, 2012, Saunders.

 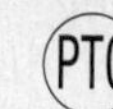

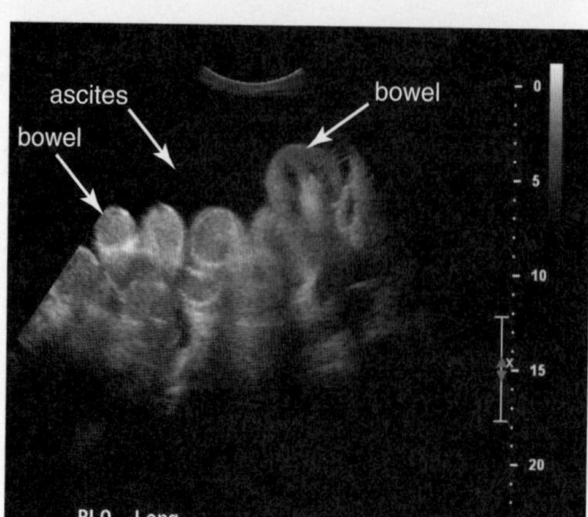

FIGURE 1-126 Ascites, ultrasound. Ultrasound is useful for detection of ascites. Simple fluids such as ascites are excellent sound transmission media, reflecting almost no sound waves. As a consequence, they appear quite hypoechoic *(black)* on ultrasound. This view of the right lower quadrant shows loops of bowel surrounded by fluid. During the ultrasound, the bowel loops would be seen to undergo peristalsis and drift back and forth in the ascitic fluid with patient movement. Ultrasound cannot distinguish the composition of the fluid; ascites, liquid blood, liquid bile, urine, and infectious fluids have a similar appearance, with a few exceptions. Blood may coagulate and form septations within the fluid collection. Infectious fluids also frequently form loculated fluid collections that may be recognized on ultrasound, although the exact composition cannot be determined. (From Broder JS: *Diagnostic imaging for the emergency physician,* Philadelphia, 2011, Saunders.)

TABLE 1-56 Primary Medical Therapy and Adjunctive Medications Used to Increase the Efficacy of Primary Therapy in the Treatment of Ascites

Class	Medication	Dosing	Relevant Action	Notes
Diuretics	Spironolactone	400 mg + qd*	Aldosterone receptor antagonist	Primary therapy
	Furosemide	160 mg + qd*	Inhibits Na-K-2Cl symporter	Primary therapy
	Mannitol	20%*	Osmotic diuresis	Give dose just prior to furosemide and spironolactone
Vasoconstrictors	Octreotide	300 mcg bid*	Splanchnic vasoconstriction, inhibits RAAS	Also used in combination with midodrine to treat hepatorenal syndrome; given for first 5 days following variceal bleeding to decrease recurrence
	Midodrine	7.5 mg tid*	Inhibits RAAS	Also used in combination with octreotide and albumin to treat hepatorenal syndrome
α2-Agonist	Clonidine	0.075 mg bid*	Inhibits sympathetic outflow, inhibits RAAS	Increases sensitivity to spironolactone
Colloid	Albumin	25 g*	Increased oncotic pressure	Also utilized with LVP and in the treatment of hepatorenal syndrome
Aquaretics	None are FDA approved	?	Vasopressin receptor antagonist	May also treat hyponatremia

*The above doses have been derived from various studies and may not be suitable for all patients. Titration is always recommended.
From Cameron JL, Cameron AM: *Current surgical therapy,* ed 10, Philadelphia, 2011, Saunders.

treatment. Treatment strategies include repeated large-volume paracentesis with infusion of albumin every 2 to 4 wk or placement of a transjugular intrahepatic portosystemic shunt (TIPS). A treatment approach to patients with malignant ascites is decribed in Fig. E1-127.

DISPOSITION

Monitor closely for worsening liver function, development of spontaneous bacterial peritonitis (SBP).

REFERRAL

Referral to gastroenterology with ascites

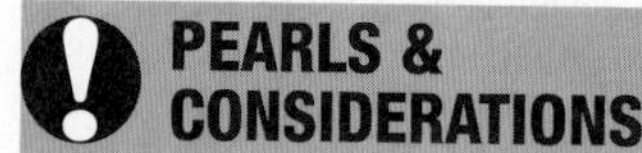

PEARLS & CONSIDERATIONS

COMMENTS

Prevalence of SBP in patients with ascites ranges between 10% and 30%. Presence of at least 250 neutrophils per cubic millimeter of ascitic fluid is diagnostic. Gram negatives such as *E. coli* are the most common isolates. Third-generation cephalosporins are the treatment of choice. By 1 year, 70% of patients have recurrence of SBP and may be prophylaxed with trimethoprim/sulfamethoxazole DS 1 tab PO bid 5 days/wk or ciprofloxacin 750 mg PO once/wk.

PREVENTION

Prevention of liver cirrhosis through avoidance of long-term use of alcohol, immunization against hepatitis A and B, and treatment of hepatitis C

SUGGESTED READINGS

available at www.expertconsult.com

RELATED CONTENT

Ascites (Patient Information)
Cirrhosis (Related Key Topic)

AUTHORS: **JOANNE M. SILVIA, M.D.,** and **PAUL F. GEORGE, M.D.**

BASIC INFORMATION

DEFINITION

Aspergillosis refers to several forms of a broad range of illnesses caused by infection with *Aspergillus* species.

ICD-9CM CODES
117.3 Aspergillosis
117.3 Aspergillosis with pneumonia
117.3 *Aspergillus* infection (A. *flavus, fumigatus, terreus*)
ICD-10CM CODES
B44.9 Aspergillosis, unspecified
B44.89 Other forms of aspergillosis

EPIDEMIOLOGY & DEMOGRAPHICS

INCIDENCE & PREVALENCE:

- *Aspergillus* species are ubiquitous in the environment internationally and occur as a mold found in soil.
- Cause a variety of illness from hypersensitivity pneumonitis to disseminated overwhelming infection in immunosuppressed patients.
- Frequently cultured from hospital wards from unfiltered outside air circulating through open windows as well as water sources.
- Reach the patient by airborne conidia (spores) that are small enough (2.5 to 3 μm) to reach the alveoli on inhalation.
- Can invade the nose, paranasal sinuses, external ear, or traumatized skin.

RISK FACTORS:

- The clinical syndrome depends on the underlying lung architecture, the host's immune response, and the degree of inoculum.
- Incidence of invasive aspergillosis is increasing with advances in the treatment of life-threatening diseases, such as aggressive chemotherapy or bone marrow and organ transplantation. It also can rarely occur in normal hosts, especially associated with influenza A. Liver and lung transplant recipients are at highest risk for pulmonary disease. Genetic deficiency of the soluble-pattern-recognition receptor known as long pentraxin 3 (PTX3) affects the antifungal capacity of neutrophils and may contribute to the risk of invasive aspergillosis in patients treated with hematopoietic stem-cell transplantation (HSCT).
- Patients with AIDS and a CD4 count <50/mm^3 have an increased susceptibility to invasive aspergillosis.
- Pandemic influenza A (H1N1) infection may predispose immunocompromised patients to invasive aspergillosis.

ETIOLOGY

- *A. fumigatus* is the usual cause.
- *A. flavus* is the second most important species, particularly in invasive disease of immunosuppressed patients and in lesions beginning in the nose and paranasal sinuses. *A. niger* can also cause invasive human infection.

ALLERGIC ASPERGILLOSIS

- Is a hypersensitivity pneumonitis.
- Presents as cough, dyspnea, fever, chills, and malaise typically 4 to 8 hr after exposure.
- Repeated attacks can lead to granulomatous disease and pulmonary fibrosis.

ALLERGIC BRONCHOPULMONARY ASPERGILLOSIS (ABPA):

- Symptoms occur most commonly in atopic individuals during the third and fourth decades of life.
- Hypersensitivity reaction to *Aspergillus* fungal antigens present in the bronchial tree.
- Results from an initial type I (immediate hypersensitivity) and type III reactions (immune complexes).
- Underdiagnosed pulmonary disorder in patients with asthma and cystic fibrosis (reported prevalence in asthmatic patients varies from 6% to 28% and in cystic fibrosis 6% to 25%).

ASPERGILLOMAS ("FUNGUS BALLS"):

- In the absence of invasion or significant immune response, *Aspergillus* can colonize a preexisting cavity, causing pulmonary aspergilloma.
- Forms masses of tangled hyphal elements, fibrin, and mucus.
- Patients typically have a history of chronic lung disease, tuberculosis, sarcoidosis, or emphysema.
- Manifests commonly as hemoptysis.
- Many are asymptomatic.

INVASIVE ASPERGILLOSIS:

- Patients with prolonged and profound granulocytopenia or impaired phagocytic function are predisposed to rapidly progressive *Aspergillus* pneumonia.
- Typically a necrotizing bronchopneumonia, ranging from small areas of infiltrate to intensive bilateral hemorrhagic infarction.
- Most common presentation: unremitting fever and a new pulmonary infiltrate despite broad-spectrum antibiotic therapy in an immunosuppressed patient.
- Dyspnea and nonproductive cough are common; sudden pleuritic pain and tachycardia, sometimes with a pleural rub, may mimic pulmonary embolism; hemoptysis is uncommon.
- Chest radiograph (CXR) may reveal patchy bronchopneumonic, nodular densities, consolidation, or cavitation. High-resolution CT scan is more sensitive and specific than CXR in neutropenic patients.
- Immunocompromised patients: invasive pulmonary *Aspergillus* (IPA) generally is acute and evolves over days to weeks; less commonly, patients with normal or only mild abnormalities of the immune system may develop a more chronic, slowly progressive form of IPA.

EXTRAPULMONARY DISSEMINATION:

- Cerebral infarction from hematogenous dissemination may occur in immunosuppressed individuals.
- Abscess formation from direct extension or invasive disease in the sinuses.
- Esophageal or gastrointestinal ulcerations may occur in the immunosuppressed host.
- Fatal perforation of the viscus or bowel infarction may occur.
- Necrotizing skin ulcers involving the extremities (Fig. 1-128).
- Osteomyelitis.
- Endocarditis in patients who have recently undergone open heart surgery.
- Infection of an implantable cardioverter-defibrillator has been reported.

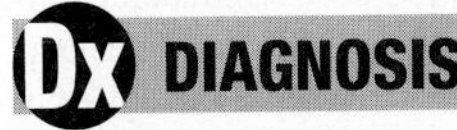

DIAGNOSIS

DIFFERENTIAL DIAGNOSIS

- Tuberculosis
- Cystic fibrosis
- Carcinoma of the lung
- Eosinophilic pneumonia
- Bronchiectasis
- Sarcoidosis
- Lung abscess

WORKUP

Physical examination and laboratory data

LABORATORY TESTS

ABPA:

- Peripheral blood eosinophilia and an elevated total serum immunoglobulin E (IgE) level.
- Skin test with *Aspergillus* antigenic extract is usually positive but nonspecific.
- *Aspergillus* serum precipitating antibody is present in 70% to 100% of cases.
- Sputum cultures may be positive for *Aspergillus* spp. but are nonspecific.

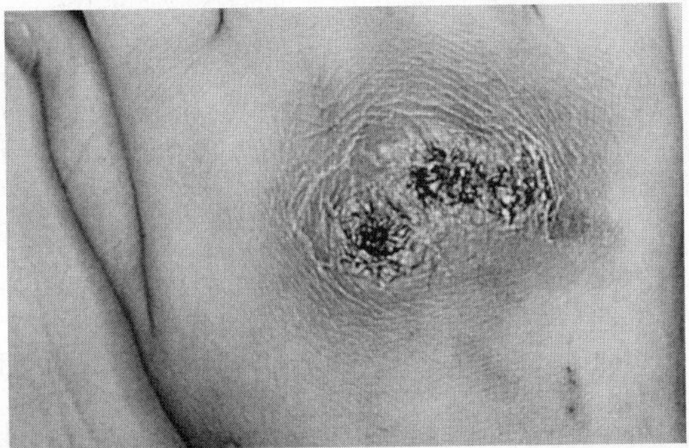

FIGURE 1-128 Cutaneous aspergillosis in a patient with acute leukemia and marked neutropenia. The lesion developed at the site where a steel needle had been left for several days of intravenous infusion. (From Mandell GL [ed]: *Mandell, Douglas, and Bennett's principles and practice of infectious diseases,* ed 6, New York, 2005, Churchill Livingstone.)

 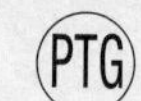

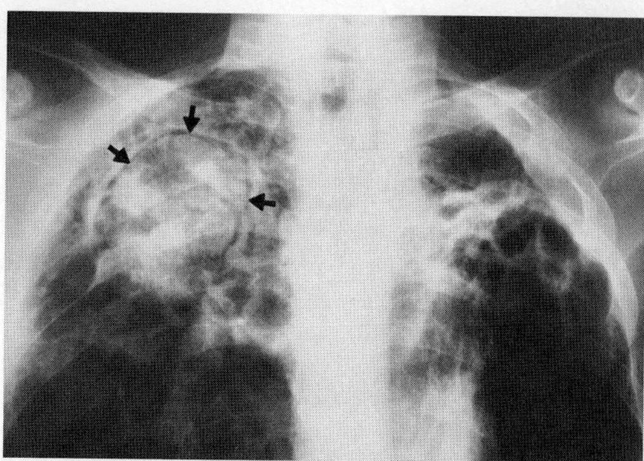

FIGURE 1-129 Fungus ball or mycetoma caused by *Aspergillus*. Coned-down posteroanterior view of the chest of a patient with biapical fibrocavitary tuberculosis accompanied by volume loss. There is a mass in a large right upper-lobe cavity with air dissecting into the cavity producing "air crescents" *(arrows)*. (From McLoud TC: *Thoracic radiology: the requisites*, St Louis, 1998, Mosby.)

ASPERGILLOMAS:

- Sputum culture
- Serum precipitating antibody

Invasive aspergillosis: definitive diagnosis requires the demonstration of tissue invasion (i.e., septate, acute angle branching hyphae) or a positive culture from the tissue obtained by an invasive procedure such as transbronchial biopsy.

- Sputum and nasal cultures: in high-risk patients a positive culture is strongly suggestive of invasive aspergillosis.
- Serology: the *Platelia Aspergillus* ELISA assay detects a circulating fungal antigen, galactomannan, and is used in some centers in neutropenic patients and for those undergoing stem cell transplantation.
- Blood cultures: usually negative.
- Lung biopsy is necessary for definitive diagnosis.
- Biopsy and culture of extrapulmonary lesions.
- Real-time polymerase chain reaction tests are investigational.

IMAGING STUDIES

ABPA:

- CXRs show a variety of abnormalities, from small, patchy, fleeting infiltrates (commonly in the upper lobes) to lobar consolidation or cavitation.
- A majority of patients eventually develop central bronchiectasis.

ASPERGILLOMAS: CXR or CT scans usually show the characteristic intracavity mass partially surrounded by a crescent of air (Fig. 1-129).

INVASIVE ASPERGILLOSIS: CXR and CT scanning may reveal cavity formation.

Rx TREATMENT

ACUTE GENERAL Rx

ABPA:

- Prednisone (0.5 to 1 mg/kg PO) until the CXR has cleared, followed by alternate-day therapy at 0.5 mg/kg PO (3 to 6 mo).
- If a patient is corticosteroid dependent, prophylaxis for the prevention of *Pneumocystis jiroveci* infection and maintenance of bone mineralization should be considered.
- Bronchodilators and physiotherapy.
- Serial CXR and serum IgE useful in guiding treatment.
- Itraconazole 200 mg PO bid for 4 to 6 mo, then taper over 4 to 6 mo may be considered as a steroid-sparing agent or if steroids are ineffective.

ASPERGILLOMAS:

- Controversial and problematic; the optimal treatment strategy is unknown.
- Up to 10% of aspergillomas may resolve clinically without overt pharmacologic or surgical intervention.
- Observation for asymptomatic patients.
- Surgical resection/arterial embolization for those patients with severe hemoptysis or life-threatening hemorrhage.
- For those patients at risk for marked hemoptysis with inadequate pulmonary reserve, consider itraconazole 200 to 400 mg/day PO.

INVASIVE ASPERGILLOSIS:

- The guidelines of the Infectious Diseases Society of America recommend the use of voriconazole as the primary therapy for invasive aspergillosis. Voriconazole dose is 6 mg/kg IV bid followed by 4 mg/kg IV q12h or 200 mg PO q12h for body weight >40 kg but 100 mg PO q12h for body weight <40 kg.
- Amphotericin B 0.8 to 1.2 mg/kg IV qd to total dose of 2 to 2.5 g; itraconazole 200 to 400 mg/d PO × 1 yr.
- Amphotericin B lipid complex (ABLC) 5 mg/kg IV qd in those intolerant of or refractory to amphotericin B.
- Amphotericin B colloidal dispersion (ABCD) 3 to 6 mg/kg IV qd; stepwise approach in those who have not responded to amphotericin B.
- Liposomal amphotericin B (L-AMB) 3 to 5 mg/kg IV qd; stepwise approach is indicated as empiric therapy for presumed fungal infection in febrile neutropenic patients who are refractory to or intolerant of amphotericin B.
- Itraconazole 200 mg IV bid × 4 doses followed by 200 mg IV qd or 200 mg tid for 4 days, then 200 mg PO bid—first-line therapy if not taking p450 inducers. Levels may be obtained to ensure compliance and adequate absorption. Approved only for salvage therapy in the United States at this time.
- Posaconazole 200 mg PO 4x/day followed by 400 mg PO bid after stabilization of disease with food or liquid nutritional supplement to enhance absorption is approved in the European Union, but in the United States is approved only for prophylaxis in leukemic neutropenic patients, those with myelodysplasia, or those who have undergone allogeneic hematopoietic stem cell transplantation; ravuconazole is currently under investigation.
- Caspofungin (Candigas) is the first of a new class of antifungals, the echinocandins, approved for the treatment of invasive aspergillosis in patients who do not respond to or are unable to tolerate other antifungal drugs. Starting dose 70 mg IV over 1 hr on day 1, then 50 mg IV qd thereafter (reduce to 35 mg IV qd in cases with moderate hepatic insufficiency). Can switch to oral voriconazole after 2 to 3 wk if the response is favorable. Micafungin 150 mg IV qd is another alternative.
- Because azoles and echinocandins target different cellular sites, combination therapy may have additive activity against *Aspergillus* species. Although still under investigation, some bone marrow transplant units use caspofungin and voriconazole as the preferred initial treatment, especially in patients receiving high-dose corticosteroids.
- Cytokine therapy may offer future treatment options in conjunction with the currently available antifungals.

REFERRAL

To an infectious diseases specialist

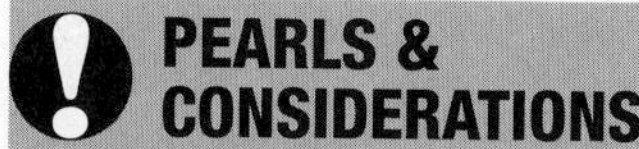

PEARLS & CONSIDERATIONS

- Unlike fluconazole, the potential for drug-drug interactions with voriconazole is high. Azoles may interact with drugs used for chemotherapy by increasing toxicity and/or by reducing efficacy.
- Agitation of hospital buildings by renovations or repairs may increase the incidence of *Aspergillus* infections in immunosuppressed individuals.
- Breakthrough zygomycosis infection may occur with voriconazole treatment.
- *A. terreus* is clinically resistant to amphotericin B.

SUGGESTED READINGS

available at www.expertconsult.com

RELATED CONTENT

Aspergillosis (Patient Information)

AUTHOR: **SAJEEV HANDA, M.D., S.F.H.M.**

BASIC INFORMATION

DEFINITION

The National Asthma Education and Prevention Program (NAEPP) guidelines define asthma as "a chronic inflammatory disease of the airways in which many cells and cellular elements play a role: in particular mast cells, neutrophils, eosinophils, T lymphocytes, macrophages, and epithelial cells. In susceptible individuals, this inflammation causes recurrent episodes of coughing (particularly at night or early in the morning), wheezing, breathlessness, and chest tightness. The episodes are usually associated with widespread but variable airflow obstruction that is reversible either spontaneously or as a result of treatment." *Status asthmaticus* can be defined as a severe continuous bronchospasm.

SYNONYMS

Bronchospasm
Reactive airway disease
Bronchial asthma

ICD-9CM CODES

493.9	Asthma, unspecified
493.1	Intrinsic asthma
493.0	Extrinsic asthma

ICD-10CM CODES

J45	Asthma
J46	Status asthmaticus
J45.0	Predominantly allergic asthma
J45.1	Non-allergic asthma
J45.8	Mixed asthma
J45.9	Asthma, unspecified
J45.909	Unspecified asthma, uncomplicated
J45.20	Mild intermittent asthma, uncomplicated

EPIDEMIOLOGY & DEMOGRAPHICS

- Asthma affects 5% to 12% of the population and accounts for more than 450,000 hospitalizations and nearly 2 million emergency department visits yearly in the U.S.
- It is more common in children (10% of children, 5% of adults).
- 50% to 80% of children with asthma develop symptoms before 5 yr of age. Early childhood risk factors for asthma are described in Table 1-57.
- Overall asthma mortality rate in the U.S. is 20 per 1 million persons.
- The population of seniors with asthma is increasing rapidly in the U.S. These patients have a high level of morbidity and mortality from their asthma.

PHYSICAL FINDINGS & CLINICAL PRESENTATION

Physical examination varies with the stage and severity of asthma and may reveal only increased inspiratory and expiratory phases of respiration. Physical examination during status asthmaticus may reveal:

- Tachycardia and tachypnea
- Use of accessory respiratory muscles
- Pulsus paradoxus (inspiratory decline in systolic blood pressure >10 mm Hg)
- Wheezing: absence of wheezing (silent chest) or decreased wheezing can indicate worsening obstruction
- Mental status changes: generally secondary to hypoxia and hypercapnia and constitute an indication for urgent intubation
- Paradoxic abdominal and diaphragmatic movement on inspiration (detected by palpation over the upper part of the abdomen in a semirecumbent position): important sign of impending respiratory crisis, indicates diaphragmatic fatigue
- The following abnormalities in vital signs are indicative of severe asthma:
  1. Pulsus paradoxus >18 mm Hg
  2. Respiratory rate >30 breaths/min
  3. Tachycardia with heart rate >120 beats/min

ETIOLOGY

- Symptoms are more commonly due to specific (aeroallergens) or nonspecific (dust, cigarette smoke, fumes, cold air, exercise, etc.) exposures.
- Traditionally, intrinsic asthma was described as occurring in patients who have no history of allergies possibly triggered by upper respiratory infections or psychological stress and extrinsic asthma (allergic asthma) brought on by exposure to allergens (e.g., dust mites, cat allergen, industrial chemicals).
- Exercise-induced asthma: seen most frequently in adolescents; manifests with bronchospasm after beginning exercise and improves with discontinuation of exercise.
- Drug-induced asthma: often associated with use of NSAIDs, b-blockers, sulfites, and certain foods and beverages.
- There is a strong association of the *ADAM 33* gene with asthma and bronchial hyperresponsiveness.
- Experimental, genetic, and clinical studies support an important role for Th2 immune pathways in the pathogenesis of severe asthma.

TABLE 1-57 Early Childhood Risk Factors for Persistent Asthma

Parental asthma
Allergy:
Atopic dermatitis (eczema)
Allergic rhinitis
Food allergy
Inhalant allergen sensitization
Food allergen sensitization
Severe lower respiratory tract infection:
Pneumonia
Bronchiolitis requiring hospitalization
Wheezing apart from colds
Male gender
Low birthweight
Environmental tobacco smoke exposure
Possible use of acetaminophen (paracetamol)
Exposure to chlorinated swimming pools
Reduced lung function at birth

From Kliegman RM et al: *Nelson textbook of pediatrics*, ed 19, Philadelphia, 2011, Saunders.

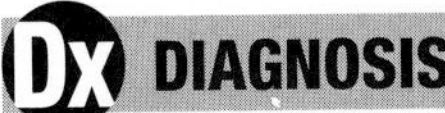

DIAGNOSIS

DIFFERENTIAL DIAGNOSIS

- CHF
- COPD
- Pulmonary embolism (in adult and elderly patients)
- Foreign body aspiration (most frequent in younger patients)
- Pneumonia and other upper respiratory infections
- Rhinitis with postnasal drip
- TB
- Hypersensitivity pneumonitis
- Anxiety disorder
- Wegener's granulomatosis
- Diffuse interstitial lung disease

WORKUP

- The clinician should evaluate for environmental causes (e.g., house dust mites, indoor pets) and exposure to other allergens such as tobacco smoke. For symptomatic adults and children aged >5 yr who can perform spirometry, asthma can be diagnosed after a medical history and physical examination documenting an episodic pattern of respiratory symptoms and from spirometry that indicates partially reversible airflow obstruction (>12% increase and 200 ml in forced expiratory volume in 1 sec [FEV_1] after inhaling a short bronchodilator or receiving a short [2 to 3 wk] course of oral corticosteroids). For children aged <5 yr, spirometry is generally not feasible. Young children with asthma symptoms should be treated as having suspected asthma once alternative diagnoses are ruled out.
- The degree of reversibility measured by spirometry correlates with airway obstruction, and patients with a high degree of reversibility have a greater risk of irreversible airflow obstruction in subsequent years.
- Fig. E1-130 describes an algorithm for diagnosing asthma.
- After diagnosis, severity of asthma should be classified during the initial assessment before initiating therapy. The following questions from Asthma Control and endorsed by the American Lung Association are important in assessing patients with asthma:
  1. Has your asthma prevented normal activities at home or work?
  2. Have you had shortness of breath in the past 4 wk?
  3. Has your asthma kept you awake at night?
  4. How often have you used your asthma inhaler in the last 4 weeks?
  5. Overall, how have you kept your asthma in control in the last 4 weeks?
- Once therapy is initiated, the emphasis for clinical management is changed to the assessment of asthma control. The level of asthma control should be used to guide decisions either to maintain or adjust therapy.
- Schedule visits at 2- to 6-wk intervals for patients who are just starting therapy or who require a step up in therapy to achieve or regain asthma control. Schedule visits at

 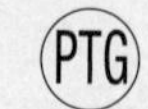

TABLE 1-58 Relative Severity of an Asthmatic Attack as Indicated by PEFR, FEV_1, and MMEFR

Test	Predicted Value (%)	Severity of Asthma
PEFR	>80	
FEV_1	>80	No spirometric abnormalities
MMEFR	>80	
PEFR	>80	
FEV_1	>70	Mild asthma
MMEFR	55-75	
PEFR	>60	
FEV_1	45-70	Moderate asthma
MMEFR	30-50	
PEFR	<50	
FEV_1	<50	Severe asthma
MMEFR	10-30	

FEV_1, Forced expiratory volume in the first second; *MMEFR*, maximal mid-expiratory flow rate; *PEFR*, peak expiratory flow rate.

From Goldman L, Schafer AI: *Goldman's Cecil medicine*, ed 24, Philadelphia, 2012, Saunders.

1- to 6-mo intervals, after asthma control is achieved, to monitor whether asthma control is maintained. The interval will depend on factors such as the duration of asthma control or the level of treatment required. Consider scheduling visits at 3-mo intervals if step-down therapy is anticipated.

LABORATORY TESTS

Laboratory tests are usually not necessary and the results can be normal if obtained during a stable period.

- Arterial blood gases (ABGs) can be used during acute bronchospasm in staging the severity of an asthmatic attack:
  - Mild: decreased Pao_2 and $Paco_2$, increased pH
  - Moderate: decreased Pao_2, normal $Paco_2$, normal pH
  - Severe: marked decreased Pao_2, increased $Paco_2$, and decreased pH
- Complete blood count: leukocytosis with left shift may indicate the existence of bacterial infection.
- Spirometry is recommended at the initial assessment and at least every 1 to 2 yr after treatment is initiated and when the symptoms and peak expiratory flow have stabilized. Spirometry as a monitoring measure may be performed more frequently, if indicated, based on severity of symptoms and the disease's lack of response to treatment.
- Pulmonary function studies: during acute severe bronchospasm, FEV_1 is <1 L and peak expiratory flow rate (PEFR) <80 L/min. Table 1-58 describes the relative severity of an asthma attack as indicated by PEFR, FEV_1 and MMEFR.

IMAGING STUDIES

- Chest x-ray: usually normal, may show evidence of thoracic hyperinflation (e.g., flattening of the diaphragm, increased volume over the retrosternal air space).
- ECG: tachycardia, nonspecific ST-T wave changes are common during an asthma attack; may also show cor pulmonale, right bundle branch block, right axial deviation, counterclockwise rotation.

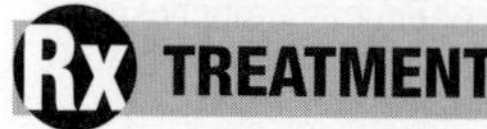

TREATMENT

NONPHARMACOLOGIC THERAPY

- Avoidance of triggering factors (e.g., salicylates, sulfites), environmental or occupational triggers
- Encouragement of regular exercise (e.g., swimming)
- Patient education regarding warning signs of an attack and proper use of medications (e.g., correct use of inhalers)

TABLE 1-59 Classifying Asthma Severity and Initiating Treatment in Youths ≥12 Yr and Adults (Assessing severity and initiating treatment for patients who are not currently taking long-term control medications)

Components of Severity		Classification of Asthma Severity (≥12 yr): Intermittent	Persistent: Mild	Persistent: Moderate	Persistent: Severe
Impairment Normal FEV_1/FVC: 8-19 yr 85% 20-39 yr 80% 40-59 yr 75% 60-80 yr 70%	Symptoms	≤2 days/wk	>2 days/wk but not daily	Daily	Throughout the day
	Nighttime awakenings	≤2x/mo	3-4x/mo	>1x/wk but not nightly	Often 7x/wk
	Short-acting $beta_2$-agonist use for symptom control (not prevention of EIB)	≤2 days/wk	>2 days/wk but not daily, and not more than 1x on any day	Daily	Several times per day
	Interference with normal activity	None	Minor limitation	Some limitation	Extremely limited
	Lung function	Normal FEV_1 between exacerbations			
		FEV_1>80% predicted	FEV_1>80% predicted	FEV_1>60% but <80% predicted	FEV_1<60% predicted
		FEV_1/FVC normal	FEV_1/FVC normal	FEV_1/FVC reduced 5%	FEV_1/FVC reduced>5%
Risk	Exacerbations requiring oral systemic corticosteroids	0-1 per yr	≥2 per yr →		
		← Consider severity and interval since last exacerbation. Frequency and severity may fluctuate over time for patients in any severity category. → Relative annual risk of exacerbations may be related to FEV1.			
Recommended Step for Initiating Therapy		Step 1	Step 2	Step 3	Step 4 or 5
				and consider short course of oral systemic corticosteroids	
		In 2-6 wk, evaluate level of asthma control that is achieved and adjust therapy accordingly.			

The stepwise approach is meant to assist, not replace, the clinical decision-making required to meet individual patient needs.

Level of severity is determined by assessment of both impairment and risk. Assess impairment domain by patient's/caregiver's recall of previous 2-4 wk and spirometry. Assign severity to the most severe category in which any feature occurs.

At present, there are inadequate data to correspond frequencies of exacerbations with different levels of asthma severity. In general, more frequent and intense exacerbations (e.g., requiring urgent, unscheduled care, hospitalization, or ICU admission) indicate greater underlying disease severity. For treatment purposes, patients who had ≥2 exacerbations requiring oral systemic corticosteroids in the past year may be considered the same as patients who have persistent asthma, even in the absence of impairment levels consistent with persistent asthma.

To access the complete *Expert Panel Report 3: Guidelines for the Diagnosis and Management of Asthma*, go to www.nhlbi.nih.gov/guidelines/asthma/asthgdln.pdf.

EIB, Exercise-induced bronchospasm; *FEV_1*, forced expiratory volume in 1 second; *FVC*, forced vital capacity; *ICU*, intensive care unit.

From National Asthma Education and Prevention Program: *Expert panel report 3: Guidelines for diagnosis and management of asthma*, National Institutes of Health, National Heart, Lung, and Blood Institute, August 2007, NIH publication 08-4051.

GENERAL Rx

- The 2007 NAEPP guidelines (see Tables 1-59 to 1-67) broadly classify treatment options by age: 0 to 4 yr, 5 to 11 yr, and >12 yr. An approach to home management of acute asthma is described in Fig. E1-131. When asthma symptoms are mild, short-lived, or infrequent, use of short-acting beta-selective adrenergic agonists (SABAs) administered by inhalation is the most effective therapy for quick relief of asthmatic symptoms. They are recommended for use only as needed for relief of symptoms or before anticipated exposure to known triggers such as exercise. When symptoms become more frequent or more severe, step-up treatment includes use of an inhaled steroid or leukotriene receptor antagonist (LTRA). If symptoms persist, recommendations include use of long-acting beta-agonist (LABA) or LTRA plus inhaled steroid. There are currently several corticosteroid/LABA combination inhalers available (fluticasone/salmeterol [Advair], budesonide/formoterol [Symbicort], mometasone/formoterol [Dulera]). None of these combinations is indicated for the initial treatment of asthma or for acute therapy of asthma symptoms. There is no evidence that one product is more effective than the others. If asthma control remains inadequate, additional treatment consists of inhaled steroid plus LABA plus long-term medication. The addition of omalizumab, an anti-IgE monoclonal antibody, is indicated for the treatment of moderate and severe persistent asthma refractory to other treatment noted earlier. It is administered subcutaneously every 2 or 4 wk. This medicine is expensive ($10,000 to $30,000/yr). Patients should be closely monitored in the first month because omalizumab can result in allergic reactions (anaphylaxis) in 1 to 2 patients/1000. The NIH guidelines recommend considering omalizumab only after consultation with an asthma specialist. Recent trials (Wenzel et al) have also shown that in patients with persistent, moderate to severe asthma and elevated eosinophil levels who used inhaled glucocorticoids and LABAs, therapy with the human monoclonal antibody dupilumab, as compared with placebo, was associated with fewer asthma exacerbations when LABAs and inhaled glucocorticoids were withdrawn, with improved lung function and reduced levels of Th2-associated inflammatory markers.

Treatment of *status asthmaticus* is as follows:

- Oxygen generally started at 2 to 4 L/min by nasal cannula or Venti-Mask at 40% Fio_2; further adjustments are made according to the ABGs.
- Bronchodilators: Initiate treatment with high-dose SABA plus ipratropium bromide administered by means of a nebulizer every 20 min. Use of a metered-dose inhaler with valved holding chamber may be acceptable for patients with mild-to-moderate exacerbations.
- Albuterol nebulizer solution (0.63 mg/3 ml, 1.25 mg/3 ml, 2.5 mg/3 ml, or 5.0 mg/ml): 2.5 to 5 mg every 20 min over the first hr, then 2.5-10 mg every 1-4 hr as needed or 10-15

TABLE 1-60 Assessing Asthma Control and Adjusting Therapy in Youths ≥12 Yr and Adults

Components of Control		Well Controlled	Not Well Controlled	Very Poorly Controlled
		CLASSIFICATION OF ASTHMA CONTROL (≥12 yr)		
Impairment	Symptoms	≤2 days/wk	>2 days/wk	Throughout the day
	Nighttime awakenings	≤2x/mo	1-3x/wk	≥4/wk
	Interference with normal activity	None	Some limitation	Extremely limited
	Short-acting $beta_2$-agonist use for symptom control (not prevention of EIB)	≤2 days/wk	>2 days/wk	Several times per day
	FEV_1 or peak flow	>80% predicted/personal best	60%-80% predicted/personal best	<60% predicted/personal best
	Validated questionnaires			
	ATAQ	0	1-2	3-4
	ACQ	≤0.75*	≥1.5	N/A
	ACT™	≥20	16-19	≤15
Risk	Exacerbations requiring oral systemic corticosteroids	0-1 per yr	≥2 per yr	
		Consider severity and interval since last exacerbation		
	Progressive loss of lung function	Evaluation requires long-term follow-up care		
	Treatment-related adverse effects	Medication side effects can vary in intensity from none to very troublesome and worrisome. The level of intensity does not correlate to specific levels of control but should be considered in the overall assessment of risk.		
Recommended Action for Treatment		Maintain current step. Regular follow-up every 1-6 mo to maintain control. Consider step down if well controlled for at least 3 mo.	Step up 1 step and Reevaluate in 2-6 wk. For side effects, consider alternative treatment options.	Consider short course of oral systemic corticosteroids. Step up 1-2 steps. Reevaluate in 2 wk. For side effects, consider alternative treatment options.

The stepwise approach is meant to assist, not replace, the clinical decision-making required to meet individual patient needs.

The level of control is based on the most severe impairment or risk category. Assess impairment domain by patient's recall of previous 2-4 wk and by spirometry or peak flow measures. Symptom assessment for longer periods should reflect a global assessment, such as inquiring whether the patient's asthma is better or worse since the last visit.

At present, there are inadequate data to correspond frequencies of exacerbations with different levels of asthma control. In general, more frequent and intense exacerbations (e.g., requiring urgent, unscheduled care, hospitalization, or ICU admission) indicate poorer disease control. For treatment purposes, patients who had ≥2 exacerbations requiring oral systemic corticosteroids in the past year may be considered the same as patients who have not-well-controlled asthma, even in the absence of impairment levels consistent with not-well-controlled asthma.

Validated questionnaires for the impairment domain (the questionnaires do not assess lung function or the risk domain)
- ATAQ = Asthma Therapy Assessment Questionnaire
- ACQ = Asthma Control Questionnaire (user package may be obtained at www.qoltech.co.uk or juniper@qoltech.co.uk)
- ACT = Asthma Control Test™
- Minimal Important Difference: 1.0 for the ATAQ; 0.5 for the ACQ; not determined for the ACT

Before step up in therapy:
- Review adherence to medication, inhaler technique, environmental control, and comorbid conditions
- If an alternative treatment option was used in a step, discontinue and use the preferred treatment for that step

*ACQ values of 0.76-1.4 are indeterminate regarding well-controlled asthma.

EIB, Exercise-induced bronchospasm; *FEV_1,* forced expiratory volume in 1 second; *ICU,* intensive care unit.

The Asthma Control Test is a trademark of QualityMetric Incorporated.

From National Asthma Education and Prevention Program: *Expert panel report 3: Guidelines for diagnosis and management of asthma,* National Institutes of Health, National Heart, Lung, and Blood Institute, August 2007, NIH publication 08-4051.

mg/hr continuously. Other useful medications are levalbuterol nebulizer solution (0.31 mg/3 ml, 0.63 mg/3 ml, 1.25 mg/3 ml), and ipratropium nebulizer solution (0.25/ml [0.025%]).

- Corticosteroids:
  1. Early administration is advised, particularly in patients using steroids at home.
  2. Patients may be started on systemic corticosteroids: methylprednisolone, prednisone, or prednisolone may be used. Dose range is from 40-80 mg/day in one or two divided doses, generally given until peak expiratory flow reaches 70% of predicted value.
  3. Generally for corticosteroid courses <1 week there is no need to taper the dose
- IV hydration: judicious use is necessary to avoid congestive heart failure in elderly patients. Aggressive IV hydration is not recommended
- IV antibiotics are indicated when there is suspicion of bacterial infection (e.g., infiltrate on chest radiograph, fever, or leukocytosis).
- Intubation and mechanical ventilation are indicated when previous measures fail to produce significant improvement (Fig. E1-132).
- Discharge home from the emergency department is appropriate if the FEV_1 or PEF after treatment is 70% or greater of the personal best or predicted value and if there is sustained improvement in lung function and symptoms for at least 1 hr.

REFERRAL

Box 1-8 describes indications for referral to an asthma specialist.

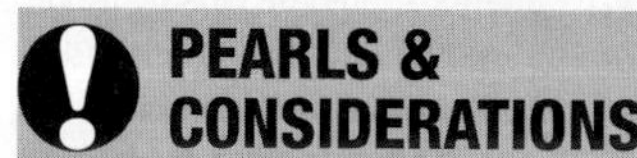

PEARLS & CONSIDERATIONS

COMMENTS

- The differentiation of asthma from COPD can be challenging. A history of atopy and intermittent, reactive symptoms points toward a diagnosis of asthma, whereas smoking and advanced age are more indicative of COPD. Spirometry is useful in distinguishing asthma from COPD.
- In all asthma patients it is important to treat or prevent comorbid conditions (e.g., rhinosinusitis, vocal cord dysfunction, gastroesophageal reflux disease). However, despite the presumed association between asthma and GERD, trials of PPIs in patients with poorly controlled asthma did not reveal any beneficial effects.
- Inhaled low-dose corticosteroids are the single most effective therapy for adult patients with asthma who require more than an occasional use of SABAs to control their asthma.
- Leukotriene modifiers/receptor agonists represent a reasonable alternative in adults unable or unwilling to use corticosteroids; however, these agents are less effective than monotherapy with inhaled corticosteroids.

TABLE 1-61 Stepwise Approach for Managing Asthma in Youths ≥12 Yr and Adults

Intermittent Asthma	Persistent Asthma: Daily Medication Consult with asthma specialist if step 4 care or higher is required. Consider consultation at step 3.					
Step 1 *Preferred:* SABA prn	**Step 2** *Preferred:* Low-dose ICS *Alternative:* Cromolyn, LTRA, nedocromil, or theophylline	**Step 3** *Preferred:* Low-dose ICS + LABA OR Medium-dose ICS *Alternative:* Low-dose ICS + either LTRA, theophylline, or zileuton	**Step 4** *Preferred:* Medium-dose ICS + LABA *Alternative:* Medium-dose ICS + either LTRA, theophylline, or zileuton	**Step 5** *Preferred:* High-dose ICS + LABA AND Consider omalizumab for patients who have allergies	**Step 6** *Preferred:* High-dose ICS + LABA + oral corticosteroid AND Consider omalizumab for patients who have allergies	↑ Step up if needed (first, check adherence, environmental control, and comorbid conditions) **Assess control** Step down if possible (and asthma is well controlled at least 3 months) ↓
Each step: Patient education, environmental control, and management of comorbidities Steps 2-4: Consider subcutaneous allergen immunotherapy for patients who have allergic asthma						
Quick-Relief Medication for All Patients • SABA as needed for symptoms. Intensity of treatment depends on severity of symptoms: up to 3 treatments at 20-minute intervals as needed. Short course of oral systemic corticosteroids may be needed. • Use of SABA >2 days a week for symptom relief (not prevention of EIB) generally indicates inadequate control and the need to step up treatment.						

The stepwise approach is meant to assist, not replace, the clinical decision-making required to meet individual patient needs.
If alternative treatment is used and response is inadequate, discontinue it and use the preferred treatment before stepping up.
Zileuton is a less desirable alternative due to limited studies as adjunctive therapy and the need to monitor liver function. Theophylline requires monitoring of serum concentration levels.
In step 6, before oral systemic corticosteroids are introduced, a trial of high-dose ICS + LABA + either LTRA, theophylline, or zileuton may be considered, although this approach has not been studied in clinical trials.
Steps 1, 2, and 3 preferred therapies are based on Evidence A; step 3 alternative therapy is based on Evidence A for LTRA, Evidence B for theophylline, and Evidence D for zileuton. Step 5 preferred therapy is based on Evidence B. Step 6 preferred therapy is based on (EPR-2 1997) and Evidence B for omalizumab.
Immunotherapy for steps 2-4 is based on Evidence B for house-dust mites, animal danders, and pollens; evidence is weak or lacking for molds and cockroaches. Evidence is strongest for immunotherapy with single allergens. The role of allergy in asthma is greater in children than in adults.
Clinicians who administer immunotherapy or omalizumab should be prepared and equipped to identify and treat anaphylaxis that may occur.
This information is directly abstracted from the 2007 NAEPP *Expert Panel Report 3: Guidelines for the Diagnosis and Management of Asthma* and is not intended to promote or endorse any of the listed products.
To access the complete *Expert Panel Report 3: Guidelines for the Diagnosis and Management of Asthma,* go to www.nhlbi.nih.gov/guidelines/asthma/asthgdln.pdf.
EIB, Exercise-induced bronchospasm; *ICS,* inhaled corticosteroid; *LABA,* inhaled long-acting $beta_2$-agonist; *LTRA,* leukotriene receptor antagonist; *SABA,* inhaled short-acting $beta_2$-agonist.
From National Asthma Education and Prevention Program: *Expert panel report 3: Guidelines for diagnosis and management of asthma,* National Institutes of Health, National Heart, Lung, and Blood Institute, August 2007, NIH publication 08-4051.

TABLE 1-62 Classifying Asthma Severity and Initiating Treatment in Children 5-11 Yr (Assessing severity and initiating treatment in children who are not currently taking long-term control medications)

Components of Severity		CLASSIFICATION OF ASTHMA SEVERITY (5-11 yr of age)			
			PERSISTENT		
		Intermittent	Mild	Moderate	Severe
Impairment	Symptoms	≤2 days/wk	>2 days/wk but not daily	Daily	Throughout the day
	Nighttime awakenings	≤23/mo	3-4x/mo	>1x/wk but not nightly	Often 7x/wk
	Short-acting $beta_2$-agonist use for symptom control (not prevention of EIB)	≤2 days/wk	>2 days/wk but not daily	Daily	Several times per day
	Interference with normal activity	None	Minor limitation	Some limitation	Extremely limited
	Lung function	Normal FEV_1 between exacerbations			
		FEV_1>80% predicted	FEV_1 = >80% predicted	FEV_1 - 60%-80% predicted	FEV_1 <60% predicted
		FEV_1/FVC>85%	FEV_1/FVC>80%	FEV_1/FVC - 75%-80%	FEV_1/FVC <75%
Risk	Exacerbations requiring oral systemic corticosteroids	0-1 per yr	≥2 per yr →		
		← Consider severity and interval since last exacerbation. Frequency and severity may fluctuate over time for patients in any severity category. →			
		Relative annual risk of exacerbations may be related to FEV_1.			
Recommended Step for Initiating Therapy		Step 1	Step 2	Step 3, medium-dose ICS option	Step 3, medium-dose ICS option, or Step 4
				and consider short course of oral systemic corticosteroids	
		In 2-6 wk, evaluate level of asthma control that is achieved and adjust therapy accordingly.			

The stepwise approach is meant to assist, not replace, the clinical decision-making required to meet individual patient needs.
Level of severity is determined by both impairment and risk. Assess impairment domain by patient's/caregiver's recall of previous 2-4 wk and spirometry. Assign severity to the most severe category in which any feature occurs.
At present, there are inadequate data to correspond frequencies of exacerbations with different levels of asthma severity. In general, more frequent and intense exacerbations (e.g., requiring urgent, unscheduled care, hospitalization, or ICU admission) indicate greater underlying disease severity. For treatment purposes, patients who had ≥2 exacerbations requiring oral systemic corticosteroids in the past year may be considered the same as patients who have persistent asthma, even in the absence of impairment levels consistent with persistent asthma.
EIB, Exercise-induced bronchospasm; *FEV_1,* forced expiratory volume in 1 second; *FVC,* forced vital capacity; *ICU,* intensive care unit.
From National Asthma Education and Prevention Program: *Expert panel report 3: Guidelines for diagnosis and management of asthma,* National Institutes of Health, National Heart, Lung, and Blood Institute, August 2007, NIH publication 08-4051.

TABLE 1-63 Assessing Asthma Control and Adjusting Therapy in Children 5-11 Yr

Components of Control		CLASSIFICATION OF ASTHMA CONTROL (5-11 yr of age)		
		Well Controlled	Not Well Controlled	Very Poorly Controlled
Impairment	Symptoms	≤2 days/wk but not more than once on each day	>2 days/wk or multiple times on ≤2 days/wk	Throughout the day
	Nighttime awakenings	≤1x/mo	≥2x/mo	≥2x/wk
	Interference with normal activity	None	Some limitation	Extremely limited
	Short-acting $beta_2$-agonist use for symptom control (not prevention of EIB)	≤2 days/wk	>2 days/wk	Several times per day
	Lung function			
	FEV_1 or peak flow	>80% predicted/personal best	60%-80% predicted/personal best	<60% predicted/personal best
	FEV_1/FVC	>80% predicted	75%-80%	<75% predicted
Risk	Exacerbations requiring oral systemic corticosteroids	0-1 per yr	≥2 per yr	
		Consider severity and interval since last exacerbation		
	Reduction in lung growth	Evaluation requires long-term follow-up care		
	Treatment-related adverse effects	Medication side effects can vary in intensity from none to very troublesome and worrisome. The level of intensity does not correlate to specific levels of control but should be considered in the overall assessment of risk.		
Recommended Action for Treatment		Maintain current step. Regular follow-up every 1-6 mo. Consider step down if well controlled for at least 3 mo.	Step up 1 step and Reevaluate in 2-6 wk. For side effects, consider alternative treatment options.	Consider short course of oral systemic corticosteroids. Step up 1-2 steps. Reevaluate in 2 wk. For side effects, consider alternative treatment options.

The stepwise approach is meant to assist, not replace, the clinical decision-making required to meet individual patient needs.
The level of control is based on the most severe impairment or risk category. Assess impairment domain by patient's/caregiver's recall of previous 2-4 wk and by spirometry or peak flow measures. Symptom assessment for longer periods should reflect a global assessment such as inquiring whether the patient's asthma is better or worse since the last visit.
At present, there are inadequate data to correspond frequencies of exacerbations with different levels of asthma control. In general, more frequent and intense exacerbations (e.g., requiring urgent, unscheduled care, hospitalization, or ICU admission) indicate poorer disease control. For treatment purposes, patients who had ≥2 exacerbations requiring oral systemic corticosteroids in the past year may be considered the same as patients who have persistent asthma, even in the absence of impairment levels consistent with persistent asthma.
Before step up in therapy:
– Review adherence to medications, inhaler technique, environmental control, and comorbid conditions.
– If an alternative treatment option was used in a step, discontinue it and use preferred treatment for that step.
EIB, Exercise-induced bronchospasm; *FEV_1,* forced expiratory volume in 1 second; *ICU,* intensive care unit.
From National Asthma Education and Prevention Program: *Expert panel report 3: Guidelines for diagnosis and management of asthma,* National Institutes of Health, National Heart, Lung, and Blood Institute, August 2007, NIH publication 08-4051.

- Use of LABAs alone without use of a long-term asthma medication, such as an inhaled corticosteroid, is contraindicated. LABAs should also not be used in patients whose asthma is adequately controlled on low- or medium-dose inhaled corticosteroids. Continued use of LABAs may cause down-regulation of the beta-2 receptor with loss of the bronchoprotective effect from rescue therapy with a SABA.
- Patients who remain symptomatic despite inhaled corticosteroids benefit from the addition of LABAs. Trials in patients with poorly controlled asthma despite the use of inhaled glucocorticoids and LABAs have shown that the addition of tiotropium, a long-acting anticholinergic bronchodilator approved for treatment of COPD, increased the time to the first severe exacerbation and provided modest sustained bronchodilation.
- Therapy with with systemic corticosteroids accelerates the resolution of acute asthma and reduces the risk of relapse. There is no evidence that doses >50-100 mg prednisone equivalent are beneficial.
- In patients with allergies and elevated serum immunoglobulin (Ig) E levels, use of anti-IgE therapy is beneficial.
- Bronchial thermoplasty (Alair System) may be used to reduce airway smooth muscle mass and widen the airway in adult patients with severe persistent asthma not well controlled with inhaled corticosteroids and LABAs. It requires the insertion of a catheter via bronchoscopy and use of a radiofrequency controller.
- Biologic modifiers of the Th2 immune pathways (neutralizing monoclonal antibodies, receptor antagonists, soluble receptors) are potential options for the development of new treatments of severe asthma.
- The response to treatment for asthma is characterized by wide individual variability. A functional glucocorticoid-induced transcript 1 gene (GLCCI1) variant is associated with substantial decrements in the response to inhaled glucocorticoids in patients with asthma. Another potential cause of the variability in response to treatment is heterogeneity in the role of interleukin-13 expression in the clinical asthma phenotype. Patients with asthma who have a certain biochemical signature are more likely to respond to an anti–interleukin-13 monoclonal antibody than those without such a signature. Identification of genetic variants can eventually lead to personalized asthma treatment.

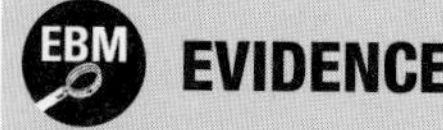

EVIDENCE

available at www.expertconsult.com

SUGGESTED READINGS

available at www.expertconsult.com

RELATED CONTENT

Asthma (Patient Information)

AUTHOR: **FRED F. FERRI, M.D.**

TABLE 1-64 Stepwise Approach for Managing Asthma in Children 5-11 Yr

Intermittent Asthma	**Persistent Asthma: Daily Medication** Consult with asthma specialist if step 4 care or higher is required. Consider consultation at step 3.					
Step 1	**Step 2**	**Step 3**	**Step 4**	**Step 5**	**Step 6**	↑ Step up if needed (first, check adherence, inhaler technique, environmental control, and comorbid conditions)
Preferred: SABA prn	*Preferred:* Low-dose ICS *Alternative:* Cromolyn, LTRA, nedocromil, or theophylline	*Preferred:* Low-dose ICS + either LABA, LTRA, or theophylline OR Medium-dose ICS	*Preferred:* Medium-dose ICS + LABA *Alternative:* Medium-dose ICS + either LTRA or theophylline	*Preferred:* High-dose ICS + LABA *Alternative:* High-dose ICS + either LTRA or theophylline	*Preferred:* High-dose ICS + LABA + oral corticosteroid *Alternative:* High-dose ICS + either LTRA or theophylline + oral systemic corticosteroid	**Assess control**
Each step: Patient education, environmental control, and management of comorbidities Steps 2-4: Consider subcutaneous allergen immunotherapy for patients who have allergic asthma						Step down if possible (and asthma is well controlled at least 3 months) ↓
Quick-Relief Medication for All Patients • SABA as needed for symptoms. Intensity of treatment depends on severity of symptoms: up to 3 treatments at 20-minute intervals as needed. Short course of oral systemic corticosteroids may be needed. • Caution: Increasing use of SABA or use >2 days a week for symptom relief (not prevention of EIB) generally indicates inadequate control and the need to step up treatment.						

The stepwise approach is meant to assist, not replace, the clinical decision-making required to meet individual patient needs.

If alternative treatment is used and response is inadequate, discontinue it and use the preferred treatment before stepping up.

Theophylline is a less desirable alternative due to the need to monitor serum concentration levels.

Step 1 and step 2 medications are based on Evidence A. Step 3 ICS 1 adjunctive therapy and ICS are based on Evidence B for efficacy of each treatment and extrapolation from comparator trials in older children and adults–comparator trials are not available for this age group; steps 4-6 are based on expert opinion and extrapolation from studies in older children and adults.

Immunotherapy for steps 2-4 is based on Evidence B for house-dust mites, animal danders, and pollens; evidence is weak or lacking for molds and cockroaches. Evidence is strongest for immunotherapy with single allergens. The role of allergy in asthma is greater in children than in adults. Clinicians who administer immunotherapy should be prepared and equipped to identify and treat anaphylaxis that may occur.

This information is directly abstracted from the 2007 NAEPP *Expert Panel Report 3: Guidelines for the Diagnosis and Management of Asthma* and is not intended to promote or endorse any of the listed products.

ICS, Inhaled corticosteroid; *LABA*, inhaled long-acting beta$_2$-agonist; *LTRA*, leukotriene receptor antagonist; *SABA*, inhaled short-acting beta$_2$-agonist.

From National Asthma Education and Prevention Program: *Expert panel report 3: Guidelines for diagnosis and management of asthma*, National Institutes of Health, National Heart, Lung, and Blood Institute, August 2007, NIH publication 08-4051.

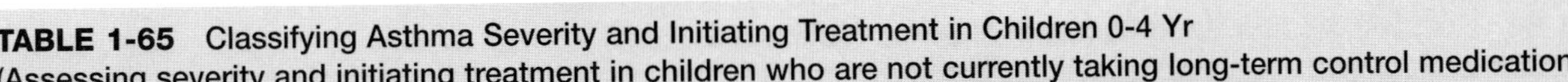

TABLE 1-65 Classifying Asthma Severity and Initiating Treatment in Children 0-4 Yr (Assessing severity and initiating treatment in children who are not currently taking long-term control medications)

		CLASSIFICATION OF ASTHMA SEVERITY (0-4 yr of age)			
			PERSISTENT		
Components of Severity		**Intermittent**	**Mild**	**Moderate**	**Severe**
Impairment	Symptoms	≤2 days/wk	>2 days/wk but not daily	Daily	Throughout the day
	Nighttime awakenings	0	1-2x/mo	3-4x/mo	>1x/wk
	Short-acting $beta_2$-agonist use for symptom control (not prevention of EIB)	≤2 days/wk	>2 days/wk but not daily	Daily	Several times per day
	Interference with normal activity	None	Minor limitation	Some limitation	Extremely limited
Risk	Exacerbations requiring oral systemic corticosteroids	0-1 per yr	≥2 exacerbations in 6 mo requiring oral systemic corticosteroids, or ≥4 wheezing episodes/1 yr lasting >1 day AND risk factors for persistent asthma.		
		← Consider severity and interval since last exacerbation. → Frequency and severity may fluctuate over time. Exacerbations of any severity may occur in patients in any severity category.			
Recommended Step for Initiating Therapy		Step 1	Step 2	Step 3 and consider short course of oral systemic corticosteroids	
		In 2-6 wk, depending on severity, evaluate level of asthma control that is achieved. If no clear benefit is observed in 4-6 wk, consider adjusting therapy or alternative diagnoses.			

The stepwise approach is meant to assist, not replace, the clinical decision-making required to meet individual patient needs.

Level of severity is determined by assessment of both impairment and risk. Assess impairment domain by patient's/caregiver's recall of previous 2-4 wk. Symptom assessment for longer periods should reflect a global assessment such as inquiring whether the patient's asthma is better or worse since the last visit. Assign severity to the most severe category in which any feature occurs.

At present, there are inadequate data to correspond frequencies of exacerbations with different levels of asthma severity. For treatment purposes, patients who had ≥2 exacerbations requiring oral systemic corticosteroids in the past six months, or ≥4 wheezing episodes in the past year, and who have risk factors for persistent asthma may be considered the same as patients who have persistent asthma, even in the absence of impairment levels consistent with persistent asthma.

To access the complete Expert Panel Report 3: Guidelines for the Diagnosis and Management of Asthma, go to www.nhlbi.nih.gov/guidelines/asthma/asthgdln.pdf.

EIB, Exercise-induced bronchospasm.

From National Asthma Education and Prevention Program: *Expert panel report 3: Guidelines for diagnosis and management of asthma,* National Institutes of Health, National Heart, Lung, and Blood Institute, August 2007, NIH publication 08-4051.

TABLE 1-66 Assessing Asthma Control and Adjusting Therapy in Children 0-4 Yr of Age

		CLASSIFICATION OF ASTHMA CONTROL (0-4 yr of age)		
Components of Control		**Well Controlled**	**Not Well Controlled**	**Very Poorly Controlled**
Impairment	Symptoms	≤2 days/wk	>2 days/wk	Throughout the day
	Nighttime awakenings	≤13/mo	>1x/mo	>1x/wk
	Interference with normal activity	None	Some limitation	Extremely limited
	Short-acting $beta_2$-agonist use for symptom control (not prevention of EIB)	≤2 days/wk	>2 days/wk	Several times per day
Risk	Exacerbations requiring oral systemic corticosteroids	0-1 per yr	2-3 per yr	>3 per yr
	Treatment-related adverse effects	Medication side effects can vary in intensity from none to very troublesome and worrisome. The level of intensity does not correlate to specific levels of control but should be considered in the overall assessment of risk.		
Recommended Action for Treatment		Maintain current step. Regular follow-up every 1-6 mo. Consider step down if well controlled for at least 3 mo.	Step up 1 step. Reevaluate in 2-6 wk. If no clear benefit in 4-6 wk, consider alternative diagnoses or adjusting therapy. For side effects, consider alternative treatment options.	Consider short course of oral systemic corticosteroids. Step up 1-2 steps. Reevaluate in 2 wk. If no clear benefit in 4-6 wk, consider alternative diagnoses or adjusting therapy. For side effects, consider alternative treatment options.

The stepwise approach is meant to assist, not replace, the clinical decision-making required to meet individual patient needs.

The level of control is based on the most severe impairment or risk category. Assess impairment domain by caregiver's recall of previous 2-4 wk. Symptom assessment for longer periods should reflect a global assessment such as inquiring whether the patient's asthma is better or worse since the last visit.

At present, there are inadequate data to correspond frequencies of exacerbations with different levels of asthma control. In general, more frequent and intense exacerbations (e.g., requiring urgent, unscheduled care, hospitalization, or ICU admission) indicate poorer disease control. For treatment purposes, patients who had ≥2 exacerbations requiring oral systemic corticosteroids in the past year may be considered the same as patients who have not-well-controlled asthma, even in the absence of impairment levels consistent with not-well-controlled asthma.

Before step up in therapy:

- Review adherence to medications, inhaler technique, and environmental control.
- If an alternative treatment option was used in a step, discontinue it and use preferred treatment for that step.

EIB, Exercise-induced bronchospasm; *ICU,* intensive care unit.

From National Asthma Education and Prevention Program: *Expert panel report 3: Guidelines for diagnosis and management of asthma,* National Institutes of Health, National Heart, Lung, and Blood Institute, August 2007, NIH publication 08-4051.

TABLE 1-67 Stepwise Approach for Managing Asthma in Children 0-4 Yr

Intermittent Asthma	**Persistent Asthma: Daily Medication** Consult with asthma specialist if step 3 care or higher is required. Consider consultation at step 2.					↑
Step 1 *Preferred:* SABA prn	**Step 2** *Preferred:* Low-dose ICS *Alternative:* Cromolyn or montelukast	**Step 3** *Preferred:* Medium-dose ICS	**Step 4** *Preferred:* Medium-dose ICS + either LABA or montelukast	**Step 5** *Preferred:* High-dose ICS + either LABA or montelukast	**Step 6** *Preferred:* High-dose ICS + either LABA or montelukast Oral systemic corticosteroid	Step up if needed (first, check adherence, inhaler technique, and environmental control) **Assess control** Step down if possible (and asthma is well controlled at least 3 months)
Patient Education and Environmental Control at Each Step						
Quick-Relief Medication for All Patients • SABA as needed for symptoms. Intensity of treatment depends on severity of symptoms. • With viral respiratory infection: SABA q 4-6 hours up to 24 hours (longer with physician consult). Consider short course of oral systemic corticosteroids if exacerbation is severe or patient has history of previous severe exacerbations. • Caution: Frequent use of SABA may indicate the need to step up treatment. See text for recommendations on initiating daily long-term-control therapy.						↓

The stepwise approach is meant to assist, not replace, the clinical decision-making required to meet individual patient needs.
If alternative treatment is used and response is inadequate, discontinue it and use the preferred treatment before stepping up.
If clear benefit is not observed within 4-6 wk and patient/family medication technique and adherence are satisfactory, consider adjusting therapy or alternative diagnosis.
Studies on children 0-4 yr are limited. Step 2 preferred therapy is based on Evidence A. All other recommendations are based on expert opinion and extrapolation from studies in other children.
This information is directly abstracted from the 2007 NAEPP *Expert Panel Report 3: Guidelines for the Diagnosis and Management of Asthma* and is not intended to promote or endorse any of the listed products.
ICS, Inhaled corticosteroid; *LABA,* inhaled long-acting beta$_2$-agonist; *SABA,* inhaled short-acting beta$_2$-agonist.
From National Asthma Education and Prevention Program: *Expert panel report 3: Guidelines for diagnosis and management of asthma,* National Institutes of Health, National Heart, Lung, and Blood Institute, August 2007, NIH publication 08-4051.

BOX 1-8 Possible Indications for Referral to an Asthma Specialist

- Severe, acute asthma that has caused loss of consciousness, hypoxia, respiratory failure, convulsions, or near death
- Poorly controlled asthma as indicated by admission to a hospital, frequent need for emergency care, need for oral corticosteroids, absence from school or work, disruption of sleep, interference with quality of life
- Severe, persistent asthma requiring step 4 care (consider for patients who require step 3 care)
- Patient <3 yr who requires step 3 or 4 care (consider for patient <3 yr who requires step 2 care)
- Requirement for continuous oral corticosteroids or high-dose inhaled corticosteroids or more than two short courses of oral corticosteroids within 1 yr
- Need for additional diagnostic testing such as allergy skin testing, rhinoscopy, provocative challenge, complete pulmonary function testing, bronchoscopy
- Consideration for immunotherapy
- Need for additional education regarding asthma, complications of asthma and treatment of asthma, problems with adherence to management recommendations, or allergen avoidance
- Uncertainty of diagnosis
- Complications of asthma, including sinusitis, nasal polyposis, aspergillosis, severe rhinitis, vocal cord dysfunction, gastroesophageal reflux

Modified from National Asthma Education and Prevention Program, National Heart, Lung, and Blood Institute: *Expert Panel Report 2: guidelines for the diagnosis and management of asthma,* Bethesda, MD, 1997, National Institutes of Health, NIH publication No 97-4051.

BASIC INFORMATION

DEFINITION

Astrocytoma is a type of neuroepithelial tumor that arises from glial precursor cells (astrocytes, oligodendrocytes, ependymal cells, epithelial cells of the choroid plexus, and others). Astrocytoma arises from astrocytes within the central nervous system (CNS). They are commonly graded by the World Health Organization (WHO) or the Saint Anne–Mayo grading system.

The WHO grades astrocytomas as follows:

- Grade I: pilocytic astrocytoma
- Grade II: low-grade astrocytoma (LGA), fibrillary infiltrating astrocytoma
- Grade III: anaplastic astrocytoma
- Grade IV: glioblastoma multiforme (GBM)
- Grades III and IV are considered high-grade astrocytomas (HGAs) or malignant.

Kernohan system grades astrocytomas based on histologic features: cellularity, mitoses, pleomorphism, vascularity, and necrosis. It has proved to be of prognostic value.

- Grade I: increased cellularity
- Grade II: greater cellularity than grade I plus pleomorphism
- Grade III: greater cellularity and pleomorphism than grade II plus vascular proliferation
- Grade IV: all the above, plus necrosis and pseudopalisading

SYNONYMS

Astroglial neoplasms

ICD-9CM CODES
191.9 Astrocytoma, unspecified site
ICD-10CM CODES
C71.9 Malignant neoplasm of brain, unspecified

EPIDEMIOLOGY & DEMOGRAPHICS

- According to SEER registry, the incidence of primary CNS tumor is 2.2 to 8.3/100,000 persons and about 30% of these tumors are astrocytomas.
- Astrocytomas can be found at all ages, with an early peak from birth to 4 yr, followed by a trough between the ages of 15 and 24 yr, and then a steady increase in incidence.
- Male/female ratio is 2:1.
- In adults, glioblastoma is the most common brain tumor.
- In children, astrocytomas are the second most common primary brain tumor and medulloblastoma is the most common.
- Low-grade astrocytomas represent approximately 25% of all CNS gliomas in children.
- Peak age of incidence for juvenile pilocytic astrocytomas is 5 to 14 yr.
- Peak age of incidence for glioblastoma is 45 to 70 yr.

GENETICS:

- Alteration of *p53,* a tumor-suppressor gene encoded by the *TP53* gene on chromosome 17, plays a key role in the development of a large number of adult astrocytomas.
- Genetic abnormalities occur in a stepwise manner with accumulation of multiple abnormalities leading to dedifferentiation and transformation into higher grade.
- Abnormalities of the cell cycle regulatory complex that includes p16, cdk6/cyclinD1, cdk4/cyclinD1, and loss of chromosome 9P that targets the CDKN2A locus is thought to play an important role in progression to grade III astrocytoma.
- Transformation to GBM is the result of multiple mitogenic effects, with deregulation of p16-CDK4D1-pRb pathway being an important component. Loss of chromosome 10, which targets the PTEN tumor-suppressor gene, is also a frequent finding.

PHYSICAL FINDINGS & CLINICAL PRESENTATION

The presenting symptoms of astrocytoma depend, in part, on the location of the lesion and its rate of growth. Astrocytomas classically present with any one or more of the following features:

- Headache (less frequent)
- New-onset partial or generalized seizures (>50%)
- Nausea and vomiting
- Focal neurologic deficit (cranial nerve palsy, hemiplegia, ataxia)
- Change in mental status
- Papilledema (rare)

ETIOLOGY

- The specific etiology of astrocytoma is unknown.
- The only proven risk factor for development of astrocytoma has been significant exposure to ionizing radiation.
- Other risk factors, such as increased exposure to certain chemicals (petroleum, solvents, lead, pesticides and herbicides), have been proposed but not proved.

DIAGNOSIS

A provisional diagnosis of astrocytoma is made on clinical grounds and radiographic imaging studies. Tissue pathology is needed to establish the diagnosis and to grade the astrocytoma.

DIFFERENTIAL DIAGNOSIS

The differential diagnosis is vast and includes any cause of headache, seizures, change in mental status, and focal neurologic deficits.

WORKUP

- A CT scan or MRI of the head makes the diagnosis of an intracranial brain tumor. However, tissue is needed to establish a diagnosis of astrocytoma.
- Stereotactic biopsy under CT or MRI guidance has been shown to be a relatively safe and accurate method for diagnosis of LGA.
- In the presence of mass effect, either clinically or radiologically, craniotomy with open biopsy and tumor debulking is more appropriate than stereotactic biopsy to establish a tissue diagnosis.

LABORATORY TESTS

There are no diagnostic or supportive blood tests for astrocytoma.

IMAGING STUDIES

- MRI (Fig. 1-133) is the diagnostic imaging study of choice. MRI with contrast and magnetic resonance angiography are used to locate the margins of the tumor, distinguish vascular masses from tumors, detect LGAs not seen by CT scan, and provide clear views of the posterior fossa.
- Newer imaging modalities like magnetic resonance spectroscopy, dynamic enhanced MRI, diffusion perfusion MRI, and functional MRI may lead to improved tumor delineation and functional mapping, and provide information to facilitate resection.

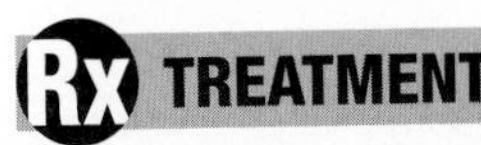

ACUTE GENERAL Rx

- Once a clinical diagnosis is made on imaging and there is evidence of edema, patients

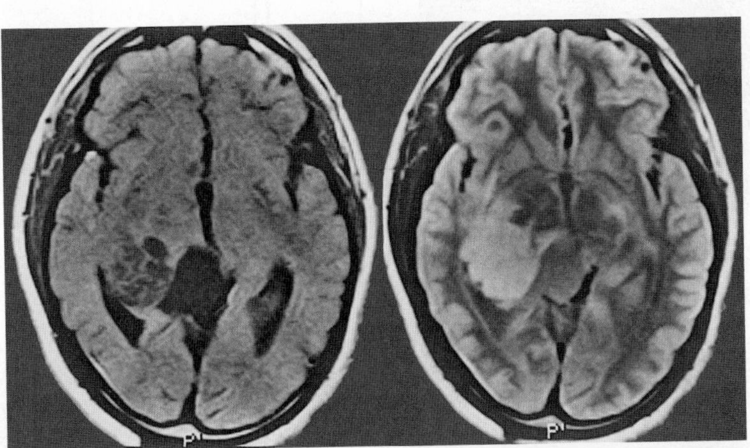

FIGURE 1-133 MR image of a low-grade astrocytoma, demonstrating a hypointense right temporal lesion without contrast enhancement on T1 and hyperintense signal on T2. (From Goetz CG, Pappert EJ: *Textbook of clinical neurology,* Philadelphia, 1999, Saunders.)

 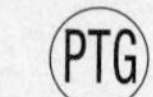

should be started on dexamethasone 10 mg intravenously (IV) followed by 4 mg IV q6h.

- If there is increased intracranial pressure and impending herniation, patient should be started on IV mannitol, and mechanical ventilation with hyperventilation should be considered if there is depressed consciousness.
- Surgery remains the initial treatment of almost all astrocytomas, particularly if the tumor is in an anatomically accessible location. Surgery helps in the following ways:
  1. Establishing a pathologic diagnosis and providing information on grade
  2. Debulking the tumor
  3. Alleviating intracranial pressure
- Grade I astrocytomas are usually circumscribed, and complete resection is possible with a high likelihood of long-term remission.
- In grade II astrocytomas, the extent of surgical resection and amount of postoperative residual disease is an important variable for time to first relapse. Randomized trials have shown that postoperative radiotherapy in grade II astrocytoma increases progression-free survival (PFS), but no increase in median survival occurs.
- In grade III and grade IV astrocytomas, gross total resection is the initial treatment of choice. Patients with no residual enhancing tumor have a longer median survival (17.9 vs 12.9 mo; $P<0.001$) than patients with residual tumor.
- Use of radiation after surgery in high-grade astrocytomas has shown a clear benefit in overall survival.
- In a randomized trial of patients with GBM, radiation with concurrent temozolomide versus radiation alone followed by six cycles of adjuvant temozolomide increases median and overall survival, and this is considered the standard of care for patients with GBM.

CHRONIC Rx

- Attempt at reresection again should be considered in all types of astrocytomas on relapse if possible and in grade I astrocytomas can lead to long-term remissions.
- Radiation therapy can be considered in the relapsed setting in grade II astrocytomas if not given in the adjuvant setting. Chemotherapy has been tried but has no proven role in these tumors.
- Chemotherapy in anaplastic astrocytomas that have relapsed after radiation (Fig. 1-134) does have a role, and the active agents are nitrosourea-based regimen and temozolomide. Grade III anaplastic astrocytomas that have 1p and 19q deletions are especially sensitive to chemotherapy.
- Bevacizumab alone or more commonly in combination with irinotecan is an effective regimen in relapsed GBM, with a response rate of 30% to 50% on the basis of at least two prospective phase II trials.
- Patients presenting with seizures should be treated with anticonvulsants.

DISPOSITION

- Approximately 10% to 35% of astrocytomas (usually grade I pilocytic astrocytomas) are amenable to complete surgical excision and cure. WHO grade I astrocytomas usually do not progress to higher grade tumors.
- Grade II astrocytomas have a median survival of 7.7 yr if they are low risk and 3.2 yr if they are high risk.
- Grade III astrocytomas have a 3-yr survival rate of 55%.
- Median survival for patients with GBM is about 1 yr. Median survival of patients with GBM treated with supportive care is approximately 14 wk. This increases to 20 wk with surgical resection alone, 36 wk with surgery plus x-ray therapy, and 40 to 50 wk with the addition of adjuvant chemotherapy.

REFERRAL

A team of specialty consultations is indicated in patients diagnosed with astrocytoma. A neurosurgeon, radiation oncologist, and neurooncologist are all needed to assist in establishing the diagnosis and to provide immediate and follow-up treatment.

SUGGESTED READINGS

available at www.expertconsult.com

RELATED CONTENT

Brain Cancer (Patient Information)

AUTHOR: **BILAL H. NAQVI, M.D.**

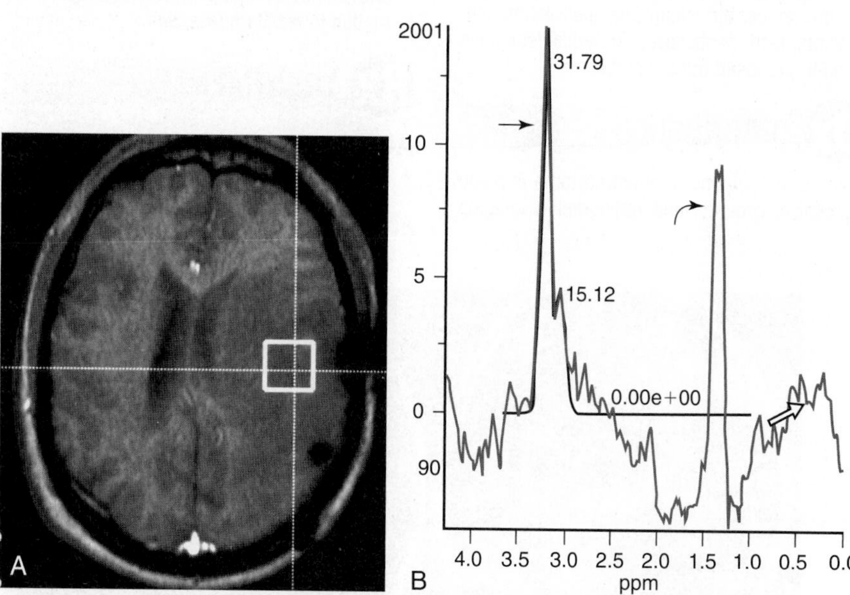

FIGURE 1-134 Recurrent high-grade astrocytoma. Study performed after radiation therapy (not shown) showed increased edema and mass effect; differential diagnosis included recurrent tumor and radiation necrosis. **A,** Axial MRI scan shows volume of tissue *(box)* selected for spectroscopy. **B,** Proton spectroscopy reveals increase in choline peak *(arrow),* decrease in *N*-acetyl aspartate peak *(curved arrow),* and appearance of a lactate peak *(open arrow).* This appearance is consistent with recurrent tumor, which was verified with repeat surgery and biopsy. (From Vincent JL et al: *Textbook of critical care,* ed 6, Philadelphia, 2011, Saunders.)

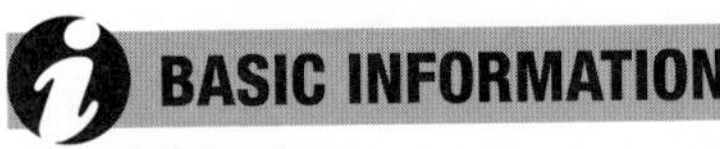

BASIC INFORMATION

DEFINITION

Ataxia refers to a general incoordination of movement and a disturbance of speech; it is a dysfunction of coordination, force, and tone. It can affect the limbs, structures involved in swallowing, and vision.

SYNONYMS

Gait instability
Loss of balance
Functional impairment

ICD-9CM CODES

334.3	Other cerebral ataxia
334.4	Cerebellar ataxia in diseases classified elsewhere
438.84	Effects of cerebrovascular disease ataxia
334.0	Friedreich's ataxia

ICD-10CM CODES

R27.0	Ataxia, unspecified

EPIDEMIOLOGY & DEMOGRAPHICS

INCIDENCE:
Hereditary ataxia can affect 1 in 50,000 people in the United States.

PEAK INCIDENCE:
Can affect all age groups. Hereditary ataxias peak in young adulthood.

PREVALENCE:
13.9 per 10,000.

PREDOMINANT SEX AND AGE:
Ataxia can affect both sexes in equal proportions.

GENETICS:
The most common type of inherited ataxia in the United States is Friedreich ataxia (FA) which is autosomal recessive. The second most inherited ataxia is autosomal dominant spinocerebellar ataxia (SCA) type 3.

RISK FACTORS:
- A positive family history of ataxia
- Excessive alcohol use
- Hypothyroidism
- Anticonvulsant use
- A history of celiac disease
- A history of cerebrovascular disease

PHYSICAL FINDINGS & CLINICAL PRESENTATION

- Most individuals will complain of double vision or a sense of the environment moving and then a sense of unsteadiness and eventually frequent falls. Speech may become unintelligible, and they are frequently asked to repeat themselves. A history of difficulty cycling or performing physical activities may be present.
- Physical exam findings include slurred speech, nystagmus, square wave jerks, dysconjugate gaze, and ocular bobbing. Dysmetria and past pointing may be noted in the finger to nose and heel to shin testing. Finger chase may be abnormal. Dysdiadochokinesia may be noted on exam.
- Gait is notable for wide-based and difficulty turning and possible easy falling to one side. Tandem gait is abnormal.

ETIOLOGY

- Ataxia can be caused by hereditary, structural, and metabolic factors.
- Hereditary factors include mitochondrial diseases such as MELAS (mitochondrial encephalopathy, lactic acidosis, stroke-like episodes) and MIRAS (mitochondrial recessive ataxic syndrome).
- Structural causes may be due to lesions of the cerebellum such as stroke, masses, Arnold-Chiari malformation, and multiple sclerosis.
- Metabolic causes include hypothyroidism and vitamin E, B1, and B12 deficiency, alcohol, and celiac disease.

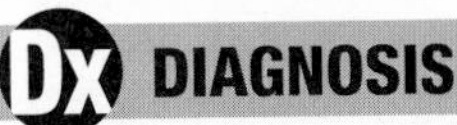

DIAGNOSIS

DIFFERENTIAL DIAGNOSIS

- Ataxia
- Vitamin (B12, B1, B6, or E) deficiency
- Alcoholism
- Anticonvulsant use, such as phenytoin.
- Inherited metabolic disorder, such as Alexander's disease
- Severe neuropathy
- Epilepsy
- Celiac sprue disease
- Wilson's disease
- Cerebral anoxia
- Cerebral tumors
- Stroke
- Cerebellitis
- Conversion disorder

WORK-UP

- The work up for ataxia should be systematic and should always look for easily reversible disorders.
- Always start with a family history and investigate for any family members that were affected. This may guide genetic testing.
- Head imaging, preferably magnetic resonance imaging (MRI), is highly recommended
- A lumbar puncture may be necessary if infection is suspected.

LABORATORY TESTS

- Complete metabolic panel including liver function tests
- Complete blood count and a manual differential
- Thyroid function tests
- HIV and RPR
- Vitamin B12, B1, B6, and E.
- Anti-endomysial antibodies
- Anti-tissue transglutaminase
- Deamidated gliadin peptide
- Serum copper and ceruloplasmin

IMAGING STUDIES

- MRI with contrast is preferable.
- Computed tomography (CT) scan of the head if MRI is not feasible.
- Cardiac echocardiogram is recommended for the inherited ataxias.

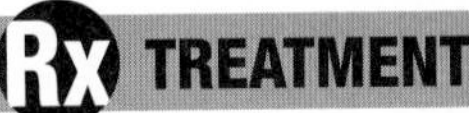

TREATMENT

Treatment of ataxia is highly variable. The best way to treat ataxia is to investigate the cause and, if treatable, then treat the underlying condition. For example, if there is a vitamin deficiency, then vitamin replacement is recommended.

However, sometimes the cause is genetic or unknown, and treatment is directed at minimizing complications, such as neuropathy or cardiac disease, and rehabilitative therapy for the ataxia and motor complications.

NONPHARMACOLOGIC THERAPY

- Rehabilitative services such as physical, occupational, and speech therapy are a necessary part of the treatment of all ataxias, and evidence suggests it does improve functional status for individuals affected by ataxia.

ACUTE GENERAL Rx

- Abrupt and sudden ataxia should always be subjected to a stroke workup, which includes a CT of the head within minutes of presenting.

CHRONIC Rx

- Search for the underlying cause and focus on symptomatic management to prevent future disabilities. Rehabilitative services are integral to long-term care. Always evaluate cardiac and renal function and check for signs of developing neuropathy.

COMPLEMENTARY AND ALTERNATIVE MEDICINE

- There is currently no widely accepted or evidence-based forms of complementary medicine for ataxia.

DISPOSITION

- Reversible causes of ataxia may see rapid improvement in symptoms. Genetic ataxias tend to be progressive.

REFERRAL

- Always refer to a neurologist

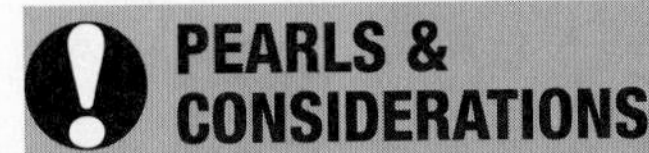

PEARLS & CONSIDERATIONS

COMMENTS

Look for reversible causes.

PREVENTION

A gluten-free diet would be preferable for people with celiac sprue disease.

PATIENT/FAMILY EDUCATION

Educate families on the need to be supportive and make the home environment safe.

RELATED TOPICS

Friedreich's Ataxia (Related Key Topic)

AUTHOR: **NAWAZ HACK, M.D.**

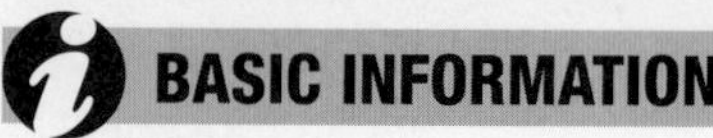

BASIC INFORMATION

DEFINITION

Atelectasis is the collapse of lung volume.

ICD-9CM CODES
518.0 Atelectasis
ICD-10CM CODES
J98.11 Atelectasis

EPIDEMIOLOGY & DEMOGRAPHICS

- Occurs frequently in patients receiving mechanical ventilation with higher Fio_2
- Dependent regions of the lung are more prone to atelectasis: they are partially compressed, they are not as well ventilated, and there is no spontaneous drainage of secretions with gravity

PHYSICAL FINDINGS & CLINICAL PRESENTATION

- Decreased or absent breath sounds
- Abnormal chest percussion
- Cough, dyspnea, decreased vocal fremitus and vocal resonance
- Diminished chest expansion, tachypnea, tachycardia

ETIOLOGY

- Mechanical ventilation with higher Fio_2
- Chronic bronchitis
- Cystic fibrosis
- Endobronchial neoplasms
- Foreign bodies
- Infections (e.g., TB, histoplasmosis)
- Extrinsic bronchial compression from neoplasms, aneurysms of ascending aorta, enlarged left atrium
- Sarcoidosis
- Silicosis
- Anterior chest wall injury, pneumothorax
- Alveolar injury (e.g., toxic fumes, aspiration of gastric contents)
- Pleural effusion, expanding bullae
- Chest wall deformity (e.g., scoliosis)
- Muscular weaknesses or abnormalities (e.g., neuromuscular disease)
- Mucus plugs from asthma, allergic bronchopulmonary aspergillosis, postoperative state

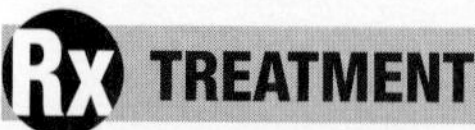

DIAGNOSIS

DIFFERENTIAL DIAGNOSIS

- Neoplasm
- Pneumonia
- Encapsulated pleural effusion
- Abnormalities of brachiocephalic vein and the left pulmonary ligament

WORKUP

- Chest radiograph (Fig. 1-136)
- CT scan and fiberoptic bronchoscopy (selected patients)

IMAGING STUDIES

- Chest radiograph will confirm diagnosis.
- CT scan is useful in patients with suspected endobronchial neoplasm or extrinsic bronchial compression.
- Fiberoptic bronchoscopy (selected patients) is useful for removal of foreign body or evaluation of endobronchial and peribronchial lesions.

Rx TREATMENT

NONPHARMACOLOGIC THERAPY

- Deep breathing, mobilization of the patient
- Incentive spirometry
- Tracheal suctioning
- Humidification
- Chest physiotherapy with percussion and postural drainage

ACUTE GENERAL Rx

- Positive-pressure breathing (continuous positive airway pressure by face mask, positive end-expiratory pressure for patients on mechanical ventilation)
- Use of mucolytic agents (e.g., acetylcysteine [Mucomyst])
- Recombinant human DNase (dornase alpha) in patients with cystic fibrosis
- Bronchodilator therapy in selected patients

CHRONIC Rx

- Chest physiotherapy
- Humidification of inspired air
- Frequent nasotracheal suctioning

DISPOSITION

Prognosis varies with the underlying etiology

REFERRAL

- Bronchoscopy for removal of foreign body or plugs unresponsive to conservative treatment
- Surgical referral for removal of obstructing neoplasms

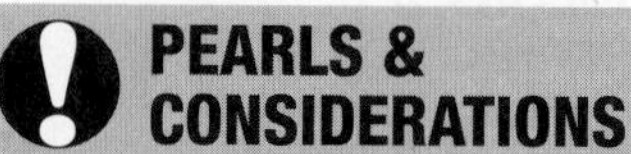

PEARLS & CONSIDERATIONS

COMMENTS

Patients should be educated that frequent changes of position are helpful in clearing secretions. Sitting the patient upright in a chair is recommended to increase both volume and vital capacity relative to the supine position.

RELATED CONTENT

Atelectasis (Patient Information)

AUTHOR: **FRED F. FERRI, M.D.**

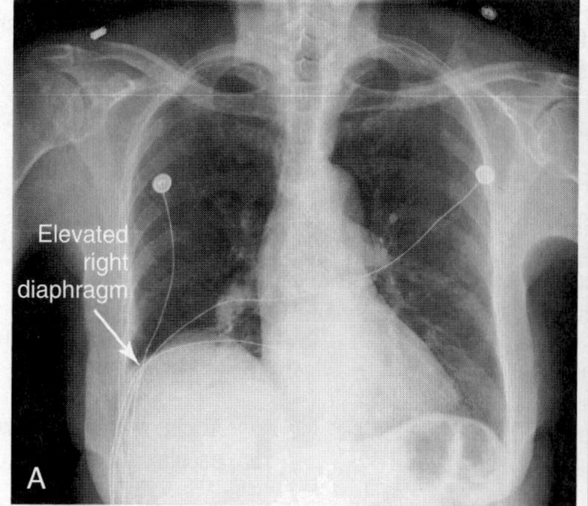

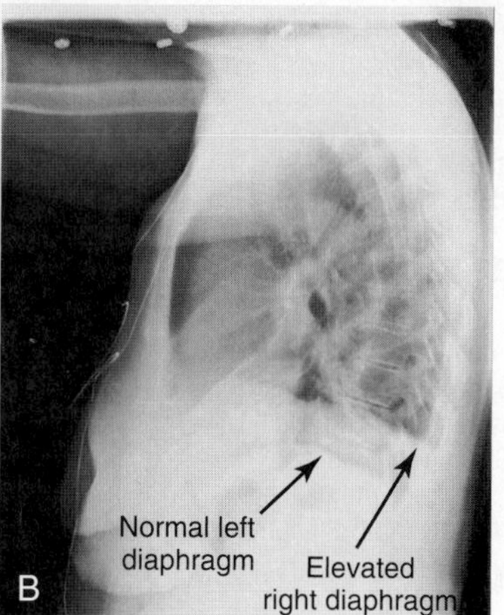

FIGURE 1-136 Atelectasis with elevated diaphragm: an example of volume loss. The right hemidiaphragm in this patient appears elevated on both the posterior-anterior **(A)** and the lateral **(B)** views. Is this the correct interpretation of the x-ray, and if so, what is the cause? Consider the alternative interpretations. A subpulmonic pleural effusion would appear similar, as it would have the same density as liver, heart, and diaphragm and would layer over the diaphragm with the patient upright. This appears less likely in that a meniscus might be seen along the lateral chest wall with a pleural effusion but is not present here. In addition, a pleural effusion occupies space and might be expected to push the heart to the left, whereas in this case the heart may be slightly deviated to the right. Atelectasis of the lower right lung would result in volume loss, pulling the heart and hemidiaphragm into the space normally occupied by lung. This is consistent with the observed features. An infiltrate in this location could explain the x-ray findings but appears less likely for similar reasons to those cited for effusion. Some simple maneuvers could narrow the differential diagnosis. Chest ultrasound, decubitus x-ray views, or CT could identify an effusion. (From Broder JS: *Diagnostic imaging for the emergency physician,* Philadelphia, 2011, Saunders.)

BASIC INFORMATION

DEFINITION

Atopic dermatitis is a genetically determined eczematous eruption that is pruritic, symmetric, and associated with personal family history of allergic manifestations (atopy).

SYNONYMS

Eczema
Atopic neurodermatitis
Atopic eczema

ICD-9CM CODES
691.8 Atopic dermatitis
ICD-10CM CODES
L20.89 Other atopic dermatitis

EPIDEMIOLOGY & DEMOGRAPHICS

- Incidence is between 5 and 25 cases/1000 persons.
- Highest incidence is among children (10% to 20%). It accounts for 4% of acute care pediatric visits. It affects 1% to 3% of the adult population.
- Onset of disease before age 5 yr in 85% of patients.
- More than 50% of children with generalized atopic dermatitis develop asthma and allergic rhinitis by age 13 yr.
- Concordance in monozygotic twins is 77%.

PHYSICAL FINDINGS & CLINICAL PRESENTATION

- Atopic dermatitis presentation can be subdivided into three phases:
  - Acute: vesicular, crusting, weeping eruption
  - Subacute: dry, scaly, erythematous papules and plaques
  - Chronic: lichenification from repeated scratching
- The lesions are typically on the neck, face, upper trunk, and bends of elbows and knees (symmetric on flexural surfaces of extremities) (Fig. E1-137). Atopic dermatitis lesions are usually discrete but vaguely delineated, scaly, and erythematous.
- There is dryness, thickening of the involved areas, discoloration, blistering, and oozing.
- Papular lesions are frequently found in the antecubital and popliteal fossae.
- In children, red scaling plaques are often confined to the cheeks and the perioral and perinasal areas.
- Inflammation in the flexural areas and lichenified skin is a very common presentation in children.
- Constant scratching may result in areas of hypopigmentation or hyperpigmentation (more common in blacks).
- In adults, redness and scaling in the dorsal aspect of the hands or about the fingers are the most common expression of atopic dermatitis; oozing and crusting may be present.
- Secondary skin infections may be present (*Staphylococcus aureus,* dermatophytosis, herpes simplex).

ETIOLOGY

Unknown; elevated T-lymphocyte activation, defective cell immunity, and B-cell IgE overproduction may play a significant role.

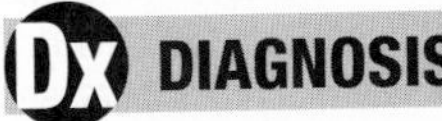

DIAGNOSIS

DIFFERENTIAL DIAGNOSIS

- Scabies
- Psoriasis
- Dermatitis herpetiform
- Contact dermatitis
- Photosensitivity
- Seborrheic dermatitis
- Candidiasis, tinea
- Lichen simplex chronicus
- Other: xerosis, impetigo, Wiskott-Aldrich syndrome, PKU, ichthyosis, HIV dermatitis, nonnummular eczema, histiocytosis X, malignancies (T-cell lymphoma/Mycosis fungoides, Letterer-Siwe disease), graft-versus-host disease, metabolic and nutritional deficiences (zinc, niacin, pyridoxine deficiences)

WORKUP

Diagnosis is based on the presence of three of the following major features and three minor features.

MAJOR FEATURES:
- Pruritus
- Personal or family history of atopy: asthma, allergic rhinitis, atopic dermatitis
- Facial and extensor involvement in infants and children
- Flexural lichenification in adults

MINOR FEATURES:
- Elevated IgE
- Eczema-perifollicular accentuation
- Recurrent conjunctivitis
- Ichthyosis
- Nipple dermatitis
- Wool intolerance
- Cutaneous *S. aureus* infections or herpes simplex infections
- Food intolerance
- Hand dermatitis (nonallergic irritant)
- Facial pallor, facial erythema
- Cheilitis
- White dermographism
- Early age of onset (after 2 mo of age)

LABORATORY TESTS

- Lab tests are generally not helpful.
- Elevated IgE levels are found in 80% to 90% of atopic dermatitis.
- Consider skin biopsy only in cases unresponsive to treatment.

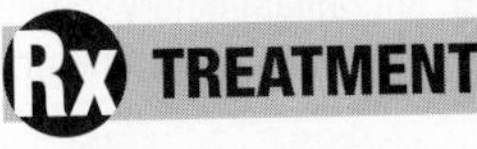

TREATMENT

NONPHARMACOLOGIC THERAPY

- Clip nails to decrease abrasion of skin

Avoidance of triggering factors:
- Sudden temperature changes, sweating, low humidity in the winter
- Contact with irritating substance (e.g., wool, cosmetics, some soaps and detergents, tobacco)
- Foods that provoke exacerbations (e.g., eggs, peanuts, fish, soy, wheat, milk)
- Stressful situations
- Allergens and dust
- Excessive hand washing

GENERAL Rx

- Emollients can be used to prevent dryness. Severely affected skin can be optimally hydrated by occlusion in addition to application of emollients.
- Low-potency topical corticosteroids (e.g., 1% to 2.5% hydrocortisone) may be helpful and are generally considered first-line therapy. Use intermediate-potency steroids (e.g., triamcinolone, fluocinolone) for more severe cases and limit potent corticosteroids (e.g., betamethasone, desoximetasone, clobetasol) to severe cases.
- Oral antihistamines (e.g., hydroxyzine, diphenhydramine) are effective in controlling pruritus and inducing sedation, restful sleep, and prevention of scratching during sleep. Doxepin and other tricyclic antidepressants also have antihistamine effect, induce sleep, and reduce pruritus.
- The topical immunomodulators pimecrolimus and tacrolimus are especially useful for treatment of the face and intertriginous sites, where steroid-induced atrophy may occur. However, due to concerns about carcinogenic potential, the FDA recommends limiting their use for short periods in patients who are intolerant or unresponsive to other treatments. Pimecrolimus cream 1% is applied bid and has antiinflammatory effects secondary to blockage of activated T-cell cytokine production. Tacrolimus ointment (0.03% or 0.1%) applied bid is a macrolide that suppresses humoral and cell-mediated immune responses.
- Oral prednisone, IM triamcinolone, Goeckerman regimen, PUVA are generally reserved for severe cases.
- Cyclosporine, azathioprine, mycophenolate, and interferon gamma are sometimes tried for recalcitrant disease in adults by physicians who specialize in severe inflammatory skin conditions.

DISPOSITION

- Resolution occurs in approximately 70% of patients by adulthood.
- Most patients have a course characterized by remissions and intermittent flares.

SUGGESTED READINGS
available at www.expertconsult.com

RELATED CONTENT

Dermatitis (Patient Information)

AUTHOR: **FRED F. FERRI, M.D.**

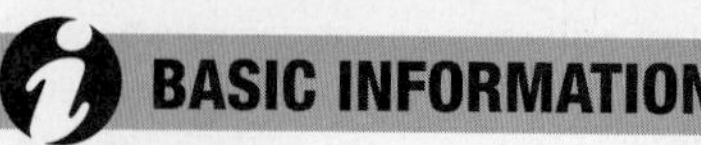

BASIC INFORMATION

DEFINITION

Atrial fibrillation (AF) is a supraventricular tachyarrhythmia characterized by disorganized and rapid atrial activation and uncoordinated atrial contraction. The ventricular rate is dependent on the conduction properties of the atrioventricular node, which can be influenced by vagal/sympathetic tone, medications, or disease of the atrioventricular node.

Multiple classification schemes have been used in the past to characterize AF. The current classification scheme (divided into three major types) used by the ACC/AHA guideline committee is as follows:

- Paroxysmal AF—more than one episode of AF that terminate spontaneously within 7 days (most episodes last less than 24 hr)
- Persistent AF—episodes of AF that last longer than 7 days and may require either pharmacologic or electrical intervention to terminate
- Permanent AF—AF that has persisted for longer than 1 yr, either because cardioversion has failed or because cardioversion has not been attempted
- In addition to the previous AF categories, which are mainly defined by episode timing and termination, the ACC/AHA/ESC guidelines describe additional AF categories in terms of other characteristics of the patient:
- Lone atrial fibrillation (LAF)—generally refers to AF in younger patients (<60 yr old) who have normal echocardiographic findings
- Nonvalvular AF—absence of rheumatic mitral valve disease, a prosthetic heart valve, or mitral valve repair
- Secondary AF—occurs in the setting of a primary condition that may be the cause of the AF, such as acute myocardial infarction, cardiac surgery, pericarditis, myocarditis, hyperthyroidism, pulmonary embolism, pneumonia, or other acute disease. It is considered separately because AF is less likely to recur once the precipitating condition has resolved.

SYNONYMS

AF
PAF

ICD-9CM CODES
427.31 Atrial fibrillation
ICD-10CM CODES
I48 Atrial fibrillation and flutter

EPIDEMIOLOGY & DEMOGRAPHICS

- The prevalence of AF increases with age, from 0.1% in adults >55 yr old to 9% of those >80 yr old.
- AF affects 2.7 million people in the U.S. AF is uncommon in infants and children and, when present, almost always occurs in association with structural heart disease.
- The incidence of AF is significantly higher in men than in women in all age groups (1.1% versus 0.8%). AF appears to be more common in whites than in blacks, who may have lower awareness of the disease.
- Stroke due to thromboembolism is the most common and dreaded complication of AF. The rate of ischemic stroke in patients with nonrheumatic AF averages 5% a year, which is somewhere between two and seven times the rate of stroke in patients without AF. The risk of stroke is not due solely to AF; it increases substantially in the presence of other cardiovascular diseases. The attributable risk of stroke from AF is estimated to be 1.5% for those aged 50 to 59 yr old, and it approaches 36% for those aged 80 to 89 yr old.

PHYSICAL FINDINGS & CLINICAL PRESENTATION

Clinical presentation is variable:

- Palpitations, dizziness, or lightheadedness
- Fatigue, weakness, or impaired exercise tolerance
- Angina
- Dyspnea
- Some patients are asymptomatic
- Cardiac auscultation revealing irregularly irregular rhythm
- Thromboembolic phenomenon such as stroke

ETIOLOGY

- The most frequent change in AF is the loss of atrial muscle mass and atrial fibrosis.
- Fibrillation is caused by multiple wandering wavelets, usually originating from the pulmonary veins. Both reentrant and focal mechanisms have been proposed.
- Vascular causes: hypertensive heart disease
- Valvular heart disease
- Pulmonary causes: pulmonary embolism, chronic obstructive pulmonary disease, obstructive sleep apnea, carbon monoxide poisoning
- Structural cardiac disease: cardiomyopathy, congestive heart failure, coronary artery disease, myocardial infarction, congenital heart disease (especially those that lead to atrial enlargement such as atrial septal defect)
- Pericarditis and myocarditis
- Arrhythmias: atrial tachycardias and atrial flutters have been associated with atrial fibrillation, as has Wolff-Parkinson-White syndrome
- Endocrine: thyrotoxicosis, hyperthyroidism or subclinical hyperthyroidism, pheochromocytoma, obesity
- Surgery: both cardiac and noncardiac
- Electrolytes: hypokalemia, hypomagnesemia
- Systemic stress: fever, anemia, hypoxia, sepsis, infections (e.g., pneumonia)
- Medications/toxins: digitalis, adenosine, theophylline, amphetamines, cocaine, antihistamines, alcohol abuse and/or withdrawal, caffeine, steroidal anti-inflammatory drugs (SAIDs), nonsteroidal anti-inflammatory drugs (NSAIDs)
- Frequency of vigorous exercise is associated with an increased risk of developing AF in young men and joggers
- Porphyrias have been associated with autonomic dysfunction and increased risk of AF
- Patients with metabolic syndrome, excessive vitamin D intake, or excessive niacin intake have a higher risk of AF

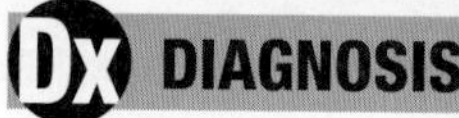

DIAGNOSIS

DIFFERENTIAL DIAGNOSIS

- Multifocal atrial tachycardia
- Atrial flutter
- Frequent atrial premature beats
- Atrial tachycardia
- Atrioventricular nodal reentry tachycardia (AVNRT)
- Wolff-Parkinson-White syndrome

WORKUP

The evaluation of atrial fibrillation involves diagnosis, determination of the etiology, and classification of the arrhythmia. A minimal evaluation includes a history and physical examination, ECG, transthoracic echocardiogram, and case-specific laboratory work to rule out secondary AF.

LABORATORY TESTS

- Thyroid-stimulating hormone, free T_4
- Serum electrolytes
- Toxicity screen
- CBC count (looking for anemia, infection)
- Cardiac enzymes—CK and/or troponin level (to investigate cardiomyopathies or myocarditis and myocardial infarction)
- BNP (to evaluate for CHF)
- D-dimer/CT scan of chest PE protocol (if the patient has risk factors to merit a pulmonary embolism workup)

IMAGING STUDIES

- ECG (Fig. 1-138)
- Absence of P waves
- Fibrillatory or f waves at the isoelectric baseline with varying amplitude, morphology, and intervals
- Irregular ventricular rate
- Echocardiography to rule out structural heart disease (evaluate ventricular size, thickness, and function, atrial size, pericardial disease, and valve function)
- Holter monitor: useful only in selected patients to evaluate paroxysmal AF
- Transesophageal echocardiography (TEE): helpful to evaluate for left atrial thrombus (particularly in the LA appendage) to guide cardioversion or ablation (if thrombus is seen, cardioversion should be delayed)
- CT and MRI: in patients with a positive D-dimer result, chest CT angiogram may be necessary to rule out pulmonary embolus. Three-dimensional imaging technologies (CT scan or MRI) are often helpful to evaluate atrial anatomy if AF ablation is planned
- Six-minute walk test or exercise test: six-minute walk or exercise testing can help assess the adequacy of rate control. Exercise testing can also exclude ischemia prior to treatment of patients with class Ic antiarrhythmic drugs and can be used to reproduce exercise-induced AF
- Holter monitor or event recorder if the diagnosis of AF is in question, such as in paroxysmal cases
- Electrophysiologic study to clarify the mechanism of wide QRS tachycardia with AF, such as in suspected Wolff-Parkinson-White syndrome

Rx TREATMENT

NONPHARMACOLOGIC THERAPY

- Avoidance of alcohol in patients with suspected excessive alcohol use
- Avoidance of caffeine and nicotine
- Treatment of underlying source/cause, if any found
- The Cox-Maze III surgical procedure, with its recent modifications creating electrical barriers to the macroreentrant circuits that are believed to underlie AF, is being performed with good results in several medical centers (preservation of sinus rhythm in 70% to 95% of patients without the use of long-term antiarrhythmic medication). Success rates are higher in paroxysmal than in persistent or permanent atrial fibrillation. It is important to understand that ablation therapy will not eliminate the need to take anticoagulant drugs. Even after ablation, patients with AF face increased risk of thromboembolic events and most electrophysiologists suggest lifelong anticoagulation. Although catheter-based radiofrequency ablation is no longer considered experimental, it is not the first-line treatment for most patients. Clear indications for catheter ablation remain undefined. In general, surgery is reserved for patients with rapid heart rate refractory to pharmacologic therapy or those who cannot tolerate pharmacologic therapy.
- Pulmonary vein ablation for chronic AF: Sinus rhythm can be maintained long term in the majority of patients with chronic AF by circumferential pulmonary vein ablation performed in experienced centers. The American College of Cardiology/American Heart Association/European Society of Cardiology (ACC/AHA/ESC) 2011 updated guidelines state that catheter ablation done in experienced centers is useful in maintaining sinus rhythm in selected patients with significantly symptomatic, paroxysmal AF who have not responded to treatment with an antiarrhythmic drug and have normal or mildly dilated left atria, normal or mildly reduced LV function, and no severe pulmonary disease. Established centers have reported success rates of 70% to 85% in patients with paroxysmal AF, but most patients may require more than one ablation to achieve success. Success with persistent AF is much lower.
- Pulmonary vein isolation is being increasingly used to treat AF in patients with heart failure. Trials have shown that pulmonary vein isolation is superior to AV node ablation with biventricular pacing in patients with heart failure who have drug-refractory AF.

ACUTE GENERAL Rx

New-onset AF:

- If the patient is hemodynamically unstable (hypotension, congestive heart failure or angina), perform synchronized cardioversion after immediate conscious sedation with a rapid short-acting sedative (e.g., midazolam). The likelihood of cardioversion-related clinical thromboembolism is low in patients with AF lasting <48 hr. Patients with AF lasting >2 days have a 5% to 7% risk for clinical thromboembolism if cardioversion is not preceded by several weeks of warfarin therapy. However, if transesophageal echocardiography reveals no atrial thrombus, cardioversion may be performed safely after anticoagulation has been achieved. Alternatively, patients can be safely anticoagulated for approximately 1 mo and then undergo cardioversion without transesophageal echocardiogram. Anticoagulant therapy should be continued for at least 1 mo after cardioversion to minimize the incidence of adverse thromboembolic events. It can be stopped after 1 mo as long as AF has not recurred.
- If the patient is hemodynamically stable, a rate-control strategy is typically pursued initially.
  Treatment options for rate control include the following:
  1. Diltiazem 0.25 mg/kg (maximum of 25 mg) given intravenously (IV) over 2 min followed by a second dose of 0.35 mg/kg (maximum of 25 mg) 15 min later if the rate is not slowed to <100 beats/min. May then follow with IV infusion 10 mg/hr (range, 5 to 15 mg/hr) to achieve a resting heart rate of <100 beats/min. Onset of action after IV administration is usually within 3 min, with peak effect most often occurring within 10 min. After the ventricular rate is slowed, the patient can be changed to oral diltiazem 60 to 90 mg q4 to 6h. High doses of calcium channel blockers can exacerbate heart failure and thus should be used with caution in patients presenting with symptoms of heart failure and/or depressed ejection fraction.
  2. Verapamil 2.5 to 5 mg IV initially, then 5 to 10 mg IV 10 min later if the rate is still not slowed to <100 beats/min. After the ventricular rate is slowed, the patient can be changed to oral verapamil 80 to 120 mg q6 to 8h. Main concern is hypotension and heart failure with this medication. Due to its poor safety profile, it is infrequently used.
  3. Esmolol, metoprolol, and atenolol are beta-blockers available in IV preparations that can be used in AF. High doses of β-blockers can have negative inotropic effects in heart failure and should be used with caution.
  4. Digoxin is not a potent atrioventricular nodal blocking agent, has a potential for toxicity and, therefore, cannot be relied on for acute control of the ventricular response but may be used in conjunction with β-blockers and calcium channel blockers. However, it is very useful in the hypotensive or heart failure patient, which is not infrequent. When used, give 0.5 mg IV loading dose (slow), then 0.25 mg IV 6 hr later. A third dose may be needed after 6 to 8 hr; daily dose varies from 0.125 to 0.25 mg (decrease dosage in patients with renal insuf-

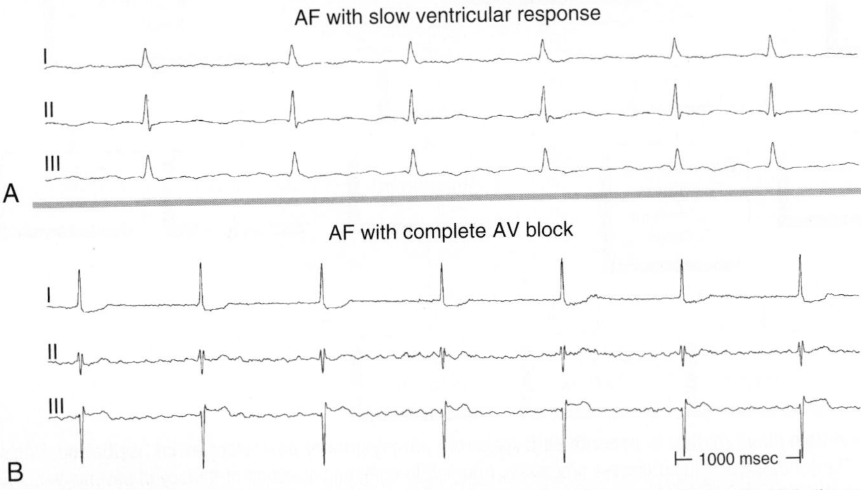

FIGURE 1-138 Atrial fibrillation (AF) with slow ventricular rate. A, The ventricular rhythm is irregular, indicating that it is the result of conducted atrial beats. B, The ventricular rhythm is regular, consistent with the presence of complete atrioventricular *(AV)* block and a regular junctional escape rhythm. (From Issa Z et al: *Clinical arrhythmology and electrophysiology,* ed 2, Philadelphia, 2012, Saunders.)

ficiency and elderly patients) depending on the heart rate and signs/symptoms of digoxin toxicity.

5. Amiodarone has a class IIa recommendation from the ACC/AHA/ESC for use as a rate-controlling agent for patients who are intolerant of or unresponsive to other agents, such as patients with heart failure who may otherwise not tolerate diltiazem or metoprolol. Caution should be exercised in those who are not receiving anticoagulation because amiodarone can promote cardioversion, thereby posing a thromboembolic risk.

- All atrioventricular nodal blocking agents should be avoided in patients with Wolff-Parkinson-White syndrome and AF because, by blocking the AV node, AF impulses may be transmitted exclusively down the accessory pathway, which can result in ventricular fibrillation. If this happens, the patient will require immediate defibrillation. Procainamide, flecainide, or amiodarone can be used instead if Wolff-Parkinson-White syndrome is suspected.
- In the acute setting, pharmacologic cardioversion (e.g., ibutilide, dofetilide) is less commonly used than electrical cardioversion. A major disadvantage with pharmacologic cardioversion is the risk of development of ventricular tachycardia and other serious arrhythmias, especially due to acute prolongation of the QT interval.

CHRONIC Rx

- Per the AFFIRM and RACE trials, either rate control or rhythm control strategies show no difference in composite cardiovascular end points of death, CHF, bleeding, drug side effects, or thromboembolism. Both approaches have similar outcomes as long as appropriate anticoagulation is maintained based on the individual's stroke risk.
- For patients without symptomatic AF, rate-control strategy with calcium channel blockers, beta-blockers, or digoxin is a reasonable option. RACE 2 trial indicates that a lenient rate control strategy, with a target resting heart rate of <110 beats/min is noninferior for a composite primary end point that included CV death, heart-failure hospitalization, stroke, and other major events over a median 3-yr follow-up as compared to a strict control strategy, with a target resting heart rate of <80 beats/min and an exercise heart rate of <110 beats/min.
- AV nodal ablation with permanent pacemaker implantation may become necessary in some patients in whom rate is difficult to control despite drugs and cardioversion.
- In patients with symptomatic AF, younger patients, or those with difficult to control heart rate, attempt should be made to maintain sinus rhythm with antiarrhythmic agents. Options of antiarrhythmic agents include amiodarone, dronedarone, (paroxysmal atrial fibrillation only without heart failure), dofetilide, flecainide, propafenone (contraindicated with structural heart disease), procainamide, or sotalol. The decision of which strategy to follow should be best made in consultation with cardiology. Use of dronedarone should be avoided in patients with persistent and/or permanent atrial fibrillation due to worsened cardiovascular outcomes, especially in those with concomitant symptomatic heart failure (See Fig. 1-139 for proposed algorithm to guide maintenance of sinus rhythm).
- The decision whether to pursue long-term anticoagulation must be made in light of the patient's risk for a cardioembolic event versus risk for a bleeding event. The CHA2DS2-VASc has largely superseded the CHADS2 scoring system (C = congestive heart failure; H = hypertension; A = age (>75 years is 2 points); D= diabetes; S= stroke, transient ischemic attack, or thromboembolic disease (2 points); V = vascular disease, A = age 65-74 years; and Sc = sex category, with females getting 1 extra point). Patients with a CHA2DS2-VASc score of 0 are considered low risk, 1 to 2 are considered moderate risk, and >2 are considered high risk and would benefit from long-term anticoagulation (e.g., warfarin).
- Anticoagulation with warfarin is generally not recommended in patients with CHADS-VASc score of >1 (other than for female), there is mounting evidence of benefit for anticoagulation. Increasing amounts of evidence now show that aspirin likely does not protect a person from stroke in AF and has recently been dropped from the European Atrial Fibrillation guidelines. Target INR for patients with a CHADS-VASc score of >2 is 2 to 3 and should be diligently monitored to avoid risk of stroke versus bleeding. Patients with

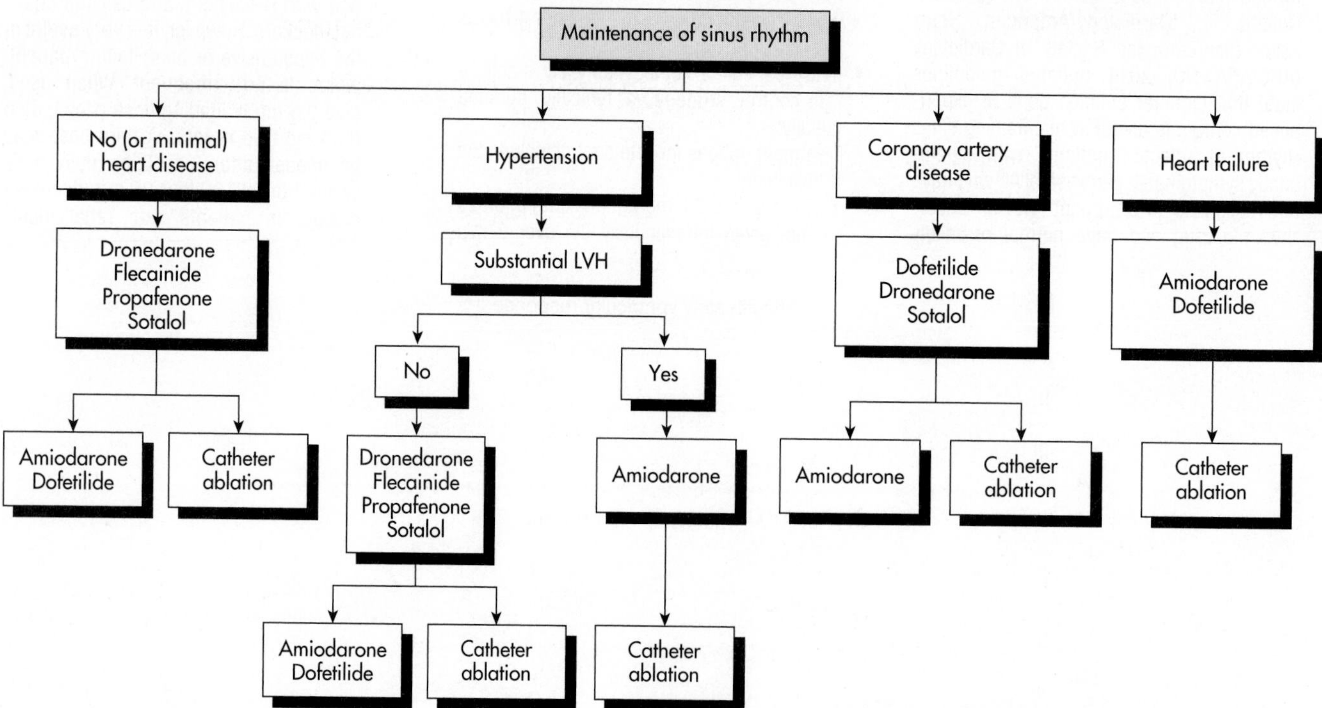

FIGURE 1-139 Therapy to maintain sinus rhythm in patients with recurrent paroxysmal or persistent atrial fibrillation. Drugs are listed alphabetically and not in order of suggested use. The seriousness of heart disease progresses from left to right, and selection of therapy in patients with multiple conditions depends on the most serious condition present. *LVH,* Left ventricular hypertrophy. (From 2011 ACCF/AHA/HRS Focused Update on the Management of Patients With Atrial Fibrillation [Updating the 2006 Guideline]: A Report of the American College of Cardiology Foundation/American Heart Association Task Force on Practice Guidelines, *J Am Coll Cardiol* 57[2]:223-242, 2011.)

hypertrophic cardiomyopathy or thyrotoxicosis with AF also have a high risk of stroke and should be anticoagulated irrespective of their CHADS-VASc score.

- Alternatives to warfarin now include several factor Xa inhibitors and a direct thrombin inhibitor.
  - Dabigatran is an FDA-approved direct thrombin inhibitor indicated to reduce the risk of stroke and systemic embolism in patients with nonvalvular atrial fibrillation. In the RE-LY trial, 18,113 patients with nonvalvular AF and at least one risk factor for stroke (mean CHADS2 score 2.1) were randomly assigned to receive oral dabigatran at one of two doses (110 or 150 mg) twice daily, or adjusted-dose warfarin. After a median follow-up of 2 yr, the rate of the primary efficacy outcome of stroke (including hemorrhagic stroke) or systemic embolism was 1.54%, 1.11%, and 1.71% per year in the dabigatran 110 mg, dabigatran 150 mg, and warfarin groups, respectively. Dabigatran 110 mg was noninferior compared to adjusted-dose warfarin, whereas dabigatran 150 mg was significantly more effective than warfarin. In patients <75 yr, lower risks of both intracranial and extracranial bleeding were found in both doses of dabigatran compared with warfarin. In patients >75 yr, intracranial bleeding risk is lower, but extracranial bleeding risk is similar or higher with both doses of dabigatran when compared with warfarin. No monitoring is generally required for dabigatran unless risk of renal insufficiency exists where dose adjustment is needed. Disadvantages include twice-daily dosing, the need for consistent timing of doses because its effects wear off quickly compared to warfarin.
- Factor Xa inhibitors (apixaban, rivaroxaban) are also effective in reducing stroke and systemic embolism in patients with atrial fibrillation. The ARISTOTLE trial in patients at high risk for stroke (mean CHADS2 score 2.1) using apixaban and the ROCKET AF trial using rivaroxaban in patients with CHADS2 score 3.5 showed that these anticoagulants reduce the risk of stroke, systemic embolism, and serious bleeding compared with warfarin. Rivaroxaban showed noninferior efficacy to warfarin and apixaban showed superior stroke reduction and an overall mortality benefit. Rivaroxaban is dosed once a day and apixaban is dosed twice a day. Edoxaban is a fourth agent that has not been approved yet, although clinical trials appear promising for its higher daily dosed regimen.
- For patients in whom anticoagulation with warfarin or other anticoagulants is contraindicated due to high bleeding risk, left atrial appendage closure should be considered (Watchman device).

PROGNOSIS

- AF is associated with a 1.5- to 1.9-fold higher risk of death, which is in part due to the strong association between AF and thromboembolic events.
- AF is also independently associated with an increased risk of incident MI, especially in women and blacks.[1]
- Development of AF predicts heart failure and is associated with a worse New York Heart Association Heart Failure classification. AF may also worsen heart failure in individuals who are dependent on the atrial component of the cardiac output.
- AF in the setting of acute myocardial infarction was associated with a 40% increase in mortality compared to patients in sinus rhythm.

DISPOSITION

Factors associated with maintenance of sinus rhythm after cardioversion include:

- Left atrium diameter <60 mm
- Absence of mitral valve disease
- Short duration of AF

REFERRAL

Refer to a cardiologist those patients in whom antiarrhythmic therapy or catheter-based/surgical intervention is being considered.

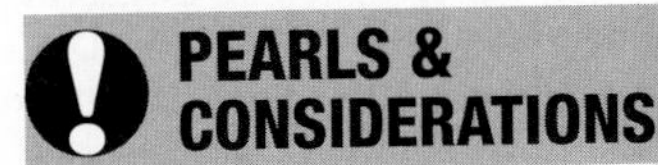

COMMENTS

The number of patients anticoagulated in the U.S. is approximately half the amount that should be anticoagulated for AF, resulting in a large burden of stroke. The exact burden of AF needed to trigger the need for anticoagulation is not known. Reversal agents for the new class of anticoagulation are in development.

The American Academy of Family Physicians and the American College of Physicians provide the following recommendations for the management of newly detected AF:

- Rate control with chronic anticoagulation is the recommended strategy for the majority of asymptomatic patients with chronic AF. Rhythm control has not been shown to be superior to rate control (with chronic anticoagulation) in reducing morbidity and mortality, and may be inferior in some patient subgroups to rate control. Rhythm control is appropriate when based on other special considerations, such as patient symptoms, exercise tolerance, and patient preference.
- Patients with AF should receive chronic anticoagulation, unless they are at low risk for stroke as stated earlier or have specific contraindications.
- For patients with AF, the following drugs are recommended for their demonstrated efficacy in rate control during exercise and while at rest: atenolol, metoprolol, diltiazem, and verapamil (drugs listed alphabetically by class). Digoxin is effective only for rate control at rest and, therefore, should be used only as a second-line agent for rate control in AF.
- For patients who elect to undergo acute cardioversion to achieve sinus rhythm in AF, both direct-current cardioversion and pharmacologic conversion are appropriate options in an otherwise healthy patient.
- Both transesophageal echocardiography with short-term prior anticoagulation followed by early acute cardioversion (in absence of intracardiac thrombus) with post-cardioversion anticoagulation vs. delayed cardioversion with preanticoagulation and postanticoagulation are appropriate management strategies for patients who elect to undergo cardioversion.
- Among patients with paroxysmal AF without previous antiarrhythmic drug treatment, radiofrequency ablation compared with antiarrhythmic drugs resulted in a lower rate of recurrent atrial tachyarrhythmias at 2 years. However, recurrence was frequent in both groups.[2]

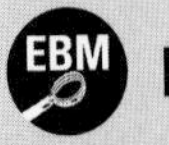

EVIDENCE

available at www.expertconsult.com

SUGGESTED READINGS

available at www.expertconsult.com

RELATED CONTENT

Atrial Fibrillation (Patient Information)

AUTHORS: **BARRY FINE, M.D., Ph.D.**, and **VEERANNA MERLA, M.D.**

[1]Soliman EZ et al: Atrial fibrillation and the risk of myocardial infarction, *JAMA Int Med* 174(1):107-113, 2014.

[2]Morillo CA et al: Radiofrequency ablation vs antiarrhythmic drugs as first-line treatment of paroxysmal atrial fibrillation (RAAFT-2), a randomized trial, *JAMA* 311(7):692-699, 2014.

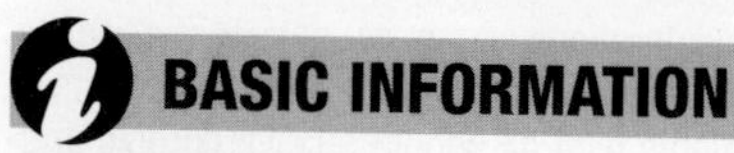

BASIC INFORMATION

DEFINITION

Atrial flutter is characterized by an atrial macroreentrant circuit (typically in the right atrium) leading to regular atrial depolarizations, typically at a rate of 250 to 350 beats/min. There is typically 2:1 conduction through the atrioventricular node, resulting in heart rates close to 150 beats/min. Higher degrees of atrioventricular (AV) block can occur in patients with AV nodal disease, with increased vagal tone, or when certain drugs such as AV-blocking agents are used. The atrial impulses may be conducted at a constant rate through the atrioventricular node, resulting in a regular rhythm, or the atrial impulses may be conducted at a variable rate, resulting in an irregular rhythm.

ICD-9CM CODES
427.32 Atrial flutter
ICD-10CM CODES
I48.92 Unspecified atrial flutter

EPIDEMIOLOGY & DEMOGRAPHICS

- Atrial flutter is the second most common atrial tachyarrhythmia after atrial fibrillation, with an estimated 200,000 new cases annually in the United States.
- Atrial flutter is common during the first week after open-heart surgery.
- Atrial flutter occurs 2.5 times more frequently in men than in women.
- Patients taking antiarrhythmics for chronic suppression of atrial fibrillation may convert to atrial flutter.
- Atrial flutter is typically seen in patients with underlying structural heart disease and is uncommon in children or young adults.

CLASSIFICATION

The Wells classification remains the most commonly used. There are two types of atrial flutter, the common type I and rarer type II. They can only manifest as one type at a time.

TYPE I: Type I atrial flutter, also known as common atrial flutter or typical atrial flutter, has an atrial rate of 240 to 350 beats/min. The reentrant loop circles the right atrium, passing through the cavo-tricuspid isthmus—a body of fibrous tissue in the lower atrium between the inferior vena cava, and the tricuspid valve.

Type I flutter is further divided into two subtypes, known as counterclockwise atrial flutter and clockwise atrial flutter, depending on the direction of the current passing through the loop.

- Counterclockwise atrial flutter (also known as cephalad-directed atrial flutter or typical atrial flutter) is the most common type. The flutter waves are inverted in electrocardiogram (ECG) leads II, III, and aVF.
- Clockwise atrial flutter (atypical): The reentry loop cycles in the opposite direction; thus, the flutter waves are upright in leads II, III, and aVF.

TYPE II: Type II atrial flutter is considered to result from an intraatrial reentrant circuit that is much shorter than type I, at an atrial rate of usually 340 to 440 beats/min. Left atrial flutter type II is common after incomplete left atrial ablation procedures.

Type I is distinguished from type II by:

1. The flutter rate (240-340 beats/min compared to 340-440 beats/min in type II).
2. The observation that type II can change in a "stepwise" manner to type I.
3. The existence of an excitable gap in type I, defined as a period after the wave of depolarization that has recovered its excitability and can be reactivated. After a depolarizing stimulus excites an area of the atrium in type I atrial flutter, it travels slowly in a long pathway with sufficient time for an "excitable gap." In contrast, type II lacks excitable gaps, likely due to short intraatrial reentrant circuits.

PHYSICAL FINDINGS & CLINICAL PRESENTATION

- Palpitations
- Dizziness, lightheadedness, syncope, or near syncope
- Angina
- Congestive heart failure
- Embolic phenomena from intracardiac thrombus

ETIOLOGY

- Rheumatic heart disease
- Congenital heart disease
- Left ventricular dysfunction
- Acute myocardial infarction (rarely)
- Thyrotoxicosis
- Pulmonary embolism
- Mitral valve disease
- Cardiac surgery
- Chronic obstructive pulmonary disease
- Obesity
- Pericarditis
- Pulmonary hypertension
- Atrial flutter can also occur spontaneously or as a result of organization of atrial fibrillation from antiarrhythmic therapy

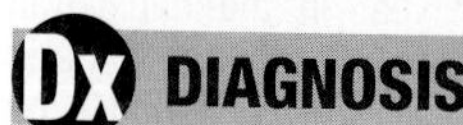

DIAGNOSIS

DIFFERENTIAL DIAGNOSIS

- Atrial fibrillation
- Paroxysmal atrial tachycardia:
  Supraventricular tachycardia, atrioventricular node reentry
  Supraventricular tachycardia, junctional ectopic tachycardia
  Supraventricular tachycardia, Wolff-Parkinson-White syndrome

WORKUP

- ECG
- Laboratory evaluation

LABORATORY TESTS

- Thyroid function studies
- Serum electrolytes

IMAGING STUDIES

- ECG (Fig. 1-140):
  - Absence of P waves.

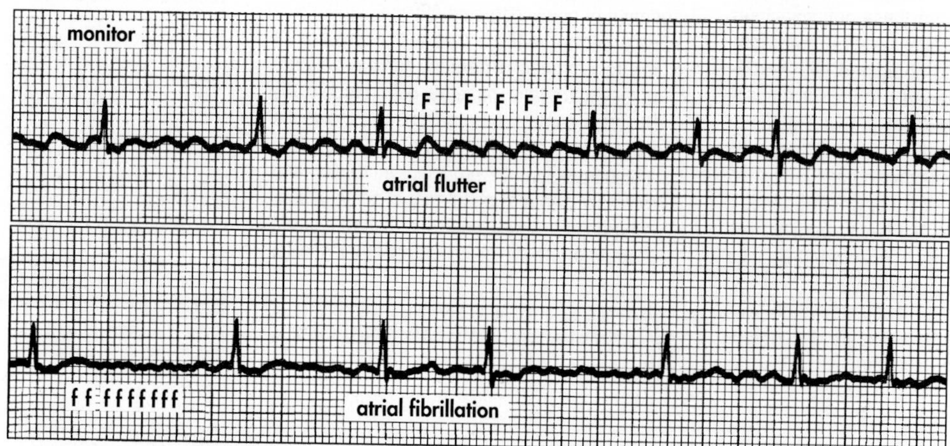

FIGURE 1-140 Atrial flutter and fibrillation. Notice the sawtooth waves with atrial flutter *(F)* and the irregular fibrillatory waves with atrial fibrillation *(f)*. (From Goldberger AL [ed]: *Clinical electrocardiography,* ed 5, St Louis, 1994, Mosby.)

- Regular, "sawtooth," or "F" (flutter)" wave pattern in the isoelectric baseline, best seen in leads II, III, and AVF.
- There is rarely 1:1 atrioventricular (AV) conduction in atrial flutter (unless pre-excitation is present). Rather, AV conduction is usually in a 2:1, 3:1, or 4:1 fashion, with corresponding usual ventricular rates of 150, 100, or 75 beats/min, respectively (assuming an atrial rate of 300 beats/min).

- Echocardiography to evaluate for structural heart disease (ventricular size, thickness, and function; atrial size, and valve function).
- Transesophageal echocardiography: consider in patients with associated structural or functional heart disease to ascertain the presence of intracardiac thrombi, in the absence of an appropriate duration of anticoagulation.
- Holter monitoring or event recorder to assess for paroxysmal atrial flutter or rate control or to identify the arrhythmia if symptoms are nonspecific or to identify triggering events.
- Electrophysiologic studies: required for a precise diagnosis, for mapping pathway, and for ablation.

Rx TREATMENT

NONPHARMACOLOGIC THERAPY

- Valsalva maneuver or carotid sinus massage usually slows the ventricular rate (increases grade of AV block) and may make flutter waves more evident. Adenosine may be similarly helpful.
- Direct current cardioversion is the treatment of choice for acute management of atrial flutter associated with hemodynamic instability or debilitating symptoms such as angina, congestive heart failure, or poor perfusion. Electrical cardioversion may be successful with energies as low as 25 joules, but since 100 joules is virtually always successful, this may be a reasonable initial shock strength. If the electrical shock results in atrial fibrillation, a second shock at a higher energy level is used to restore normal sinus rhythm. Sedation of a conscious patient is highly recommended before cardioversion is performed. The use of external defibrillators with biphasic waveforms decreases the amount of energy required for cardioversion and improves cardioversion success rate.
- Overdrive pacing in the atrium may also terminate atrial flutter. This method is especially useful in patients who have recently undergone cardiac surgery and still have temporary atrial pacing wires.
- Radiofrequency ablation to interrupt the atrial flutter is highly effective for patients with chronic or recurring atrial flutter and is generally considered first-line therapy in those with recurrent episodes of atrial flutter. It has been shown to improve health-related quality of life. However, there remains an increased risk of subsequent atrial fibrillation and stroke.

ACUTE Rx

- Treatment choices are based on clinical circumstances. If the patient is unstable, proceed directly to electrical cardioversion.
- In the hemodynamically stable patient, proceed with rate control or rhythm control strategy.
- AV blocking agents such as calcium channel blockers, beta-blockers, and digitalis may all be used for rate control. Atrial flutter may spontaneously convert to normal sinus rhythm with this strategy.
- In general, atrial flutter is more difficult to rate-control than atrial fibrillation.
- The rate of recurrence of atrial flutter is difficult to determine because most published data combine atrial flutter with atrial fibrillation. However, the recurrence rate is substantial, perhaps 50% at 1 yr.
- Ibutilide is the first-line medication for chemical cardioversion of atrial flutter in patients with normal systolic function and QT intervals. Success rate is approximately 60% to revert atrial flutter to a sinus mechanism and it is more effective than procainamide, sotalol, or amiodarone.

CHRONIC Rx

- Fewer data exist to decide on the choice of rate control versus rhythm control in patients with atrial flutter. There are several options to help maintain sinus rhythm after cardioversion of atrial flutter, such as dofetilide, amiodarone, flecainide, propafenone, or sotalol. The choice of antiarrhythmic therapy is, in part, dictated by the presence or absence of underlying structural heart disease. In patients who have chronic atrial flutter, rate control (to rates as physiologic as possible) can be achieved using AV blocking agents, to prevent occurrence of tachycardia-mediated cardiomyopathy.
- Although data are much less convincing than in atrial fibrillation, current consensus is to treat atrial flutter similar to atrial fibrillation in terms of the risk for thromboembolic events and the need for anticoagulation. In this case, the CHADS2 scoring system (see "Atrial Fibrillation" entry) can be used to risk-stratify patients for their need to stay on long-term anticoagulation.

DISPOSITION

More than 85% of patients convert to regular sinus rhythm after cardioversion with as little as 25 to 50 joules.

REFERRAL

Refer patients who are considered for rhythm control of atrial flutter to cardiologists, especially patients who are candidates for radiofrequency ablation.

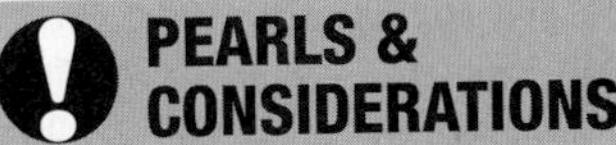

PEARLS & CONSIDERATIONS

COMMENTS

- Patients with atrial flutter have a stroke risk at least as high as those with atrial fibrillation and carry a greater risk for subsequent development of atrial fibrillation than in the general population.
- Anticoagulation should be considered for all patients whose CHA2DS2-VASc score is ≥2.
- Anticoagulation with warfarin is generally not recommended in patients with a CHA2DS2-VASc score of zero. For patients with a CHA2DS2-VASc score of 1 who do not want to undergo anticoagulation, low-dose aspirin is an appropriate alternative.

SUGGESTED READINGS

available at www.expertconsult.com

RELATED CONTENT

Fig. 3-138 Palpitations, dizziness, and/or syncope (Algorithm)
Fig. 3-185 Tachycardia, diagnostic approach (Algorithm)
Fig. 3-186 Tachycardia, narrow complex (Algorithm)
Atrial Flutter (Patient Information)

AUTHORS: **SAURAV CHATTERJEE, M.D., FRED F. FERRI, M.D.,** and **WEN-CHIH WU, M.D., M.P.H.**

A

Diseases and Disorders I

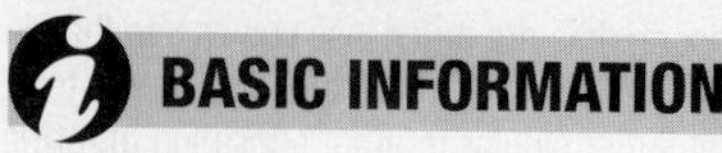

DEFINITION

Atrial myxoma is a benign neoplasm of mesenchymal origin and is the most common primary tumor of the heart.

SYNONYMS

Cardiac myxoma

ICD-9CM CODES
212.7 Benign neoplasm, heart
ICD-10CM CODES
D15.1 Benign neoplasm of heart

EPIDEMIOLOGY & DEMOGRAPHICS

- Primary cardiac tumors are extremely rare, with an autopsy frequency of 0.001% to 0.03%. The most frequent cardiac tumors are metastases, occurring 30 times more frequently than primary tumors.
- Myxomas account for 30% to 50% of all primary tumors of the heart.
- 65% of cardiac myxomas occur in females. 4.5% to 10% of cardiac myxomas are familial (Carney syndrome).
- Average age of incidence of sporadic cases is 30 to 50 yr but can occur at any age.
- Average age of incidence of familial cases is 25 yr.
- Most arise in the left atrium (75%), but myxomas can also be found in the right atrium (18%), right ventricle (4%), and left ventricle (3%).

PHYSICAL FINDINGS & CLINICAL PRESENTATION

Patients with atrial myxomas, when symptomatic, characteristically present in one of three ways:

1. Atrioventricular valve obstruction (e.g., mitral or tricuspid valve): may present with dyspnea, orthopnea, paroxysmal nocturnal dyspnea, edema, dizziness, syncope, chest pain, atrial fibrillation, and sudden death (rare). A marked change in the severity of any symptom caused by a change in position of the patient, especially if recumbency relieves dyspnea, is suggestive of myxoma
2. Systemic embolization: leading to cerebrovascular accidents, pulmonary embolism, paradoxical embolism
3. Constitutional symptoms: fever, weight loss, arthralgias, Raynaud's phenomenon

On exam there may be widely split loud S1, secondary pulmonary hypertension, murmurs of regurgitation (holosystolic) or stenosis (rumbles), an early diastolic sound 80-120 milliseconds after A2 called "tumor plop" which may resemble an opening snap,

ETIOLOGY

- Most cases (90%) of atrial myxomas are sporadic with no known cause
- Carney complex, transmitted in an autosomal dominant pattern, accounts for the majority of familial myxomas and as much as 7% of cardiac myxomas. Carney syndrome manifests as cardiac and extracardiac myxomas, pigmented skin discoloration, endocrine hyperactivity, and other tumors, such as schwannomas. There at least three different genetic loci with two identified genes for this complex

Dx DIAGNOSIS

DIFFERENTIAL DIAGNOSIS

- Primary valvular diseases: mitral stenosis, mitral regurgitation, tricuspid stenosis, tricuspid regurgitation
- Pulmonary hypertension
- Endocarditis
- Vasculitis
- Atrial thrombus
- Pulmonary embolism
- Cerebrovascular accidents
- Collagen-vascular disease
- Carcinoid heart disease
- Benign tumors of the heart (papillary fibroelastoma, rhabdomyoma, fibroma, teratoma, and lipoma)
- Malignant tumors of the heart (angiosarcoma, rhabdosarcoma, fibrosarcoma, and leiomyosarcoma)
- Metastatic tumors to the heart (melanoma, lung, breast, renal, esophageal, and sarcomas)

WORKUP

A high index of suspicion is needed because the clinical manifestations are nonspecific and similar to many common cardiovascular and pulmonary diseases.

LABORATORY TESTS

Although not very specific, the following laboratory findings may be abnormal in patients with atrial myxomas:

- Complete blood count: anemia, polycythemia, thrombocytopenia may occur
- Erythrocyte sedimentation rate, C-reactive protein, and serum immunoglobulins are commonly elevated
- Electrocardiogram: left or right atrial enlargement, atrial fibrillation, premature ventricular depolarizations, or ventricular tachycardia

IMAGING STUDIES

- Echocardiography: initial test of choice in suspected cases of atrial myxoma
- Chest radiograph: about one third of patients have normal findings. Evidence of altered cardiac contour, pulmonary edema, and chamber enlargement may be present.
- Transesophageal echocardiography: is the recommended measure for initial assessment and may better define cardiac masses not clearly visualized by transthoracic echocardiography
- CT: often used for diagnosis; defines tumor extension and evaluates adjacent cardiac structures
- MRI (Fig. E1-141): delineates size, shape, and tissue characteristics, helping distinguish thrombus from tumor
- Cardiac catheterization: will show neovascularization in 50% of the cases and may be required to rule out concomitant coronary artery disease in anticipation of surgical excision

Rx TREATMENT

ACUTE GENERAL THERAPY

- Surgical excision is the treatment of choice
- Surgery should be done promptly because systemic embolization and/or sudden death can occur while waiting for the procedure

CHRONIC Rx

Postoperative arrhythmias and conduction abnormalities were present in 26% of patients and can be treated accordingly.

DISPOSITION

- Surgical results have reported a 95% survival rate after a follow-up of 3 yr.
- Careful follow-up is necessary because up to 5% of sporadic cases and 20% of familial cases of atrial myxoma may recur within the first 6 yr after surgery.
- Sudden death in untreated patients may occur in up to 15%, resulting from coronary or systemic embolization or obstruction of the mitral or tricuspid valve.

REFERRAL

- Consultation with a cardiologist is recommended.
- Once the presence of cardiac tumor is confirmed, consultation with a cardiovascular surgeon is needed for prompt surgical excision.

PEARLS & CONSIDERATIONS

- Approximately two thirds of patients present with cardiovascular symptoms, specifically dyspnea, often suggestive of valvular obstruction.
- Nearly one third of patients have evidence of systemic embolization.

COMMENTS

Annual echocardiograms should be performed to monitor for recurrence of atrial myxomas after surgical excision.

SUGGESTED READINGS
available at www.expertconsult.com

RELATED CONTENT

Atrial Myxoma (Patient Information)

AUTHORS: **BARRY FINE, M.D., Ph.D,** and **VEERANNA MERLA, M.D.**

BASIC INFORMATION

DEFINITION

Atrial septal defect (ASD) is an abnormal communication within the atrial septum that allows blood flow between the atria. It should be distinguished from patent foramen ovale, which is a persistent patency of the flaplike communication in which the septum primum covering the fossa ovalis overlaps the superior limbic band of the septum secundum. Fig. 1-142 illustrates the physiology of ASD. There are several forms of ASD (Fig. 1-143):

- Primum: This type of ASD occurs when there is failure of fusion of endocardial cushion with the septum primum. The inferior location of the defect on the septum frequently results in involvement of the atrioventricular valves, with resultant cleft anterior mitral leaflet.
- Secundum: The most common form of ASD; it represents a deficiency of the septum primum or a septum secundum, or both. This defect most often occurs in the region of the fossa ovalis.
- Sinus venosus defect: This defect is located at the junction of the right atrium and superior vena cava, and is not a "true ASD" as it does not involve the true atrial septum. In a sinus venosus defect, the wall separating the pulmonary veins and the right atrium is deficient, causing a left-to-right shunt. Most commonly this defect involves the right upper pulmonary vein, which is still connected to the left atrium, but the drainage is anomalous. Less commonly, the right lower pulmonary vein is involved.
- Coronary sinus septal defect (unroofed coronary sinus): This defect results when the wall separating the coronary sinus from the left atrium is deficient, causing a right-to-left shunt. This is not a "true ASD" because it is not a defect in the atrial septum. This defect is often associated with a persistent left superior vena cava.

SYNONYMS

ASD
Interatrial septal defect

ICD-9CM CODES
429.71 Atrial septal defect
745.60 Endocardial cushion defect, unspecified type
745.61 Ostium primum defect
745.5 Ostium secundum type atrial septal defect
745.6 Endocardial cushion defects

ICD-10CM CODES
Q21.1 Atrial septal defect

EPIDEMIOLOGY & DEMOGRAPHICS

- Secundum, 75%; primum, 15%-20%; sinus venosus, 5%-10%; coronary sinus, <1%
- Incidence is greater in female sex and in patients with Down syndrome
- Accounts for 8% to 10% of congenital heart abnormalities
- Prevalence is 1.6 per 1000 live births
- Holt-Oram syndrome is an autosomal dominant disorder that involves skeletal anomalies, such as absent radial bones in both arms, as well as ASD and cardiac conduction disease, such as AV blocks.

PHYSICAL FINDINGS & CLINICAL PRESENTATION

- Pansystolic murmur best heard at apex secondary to mitral regurgitation (ostium primum defect)
- Wide fixed split of S_2
- Visible and palpable pulmonary artery pulsations
- Ejection systolic flow murmur (pulmonary valve flow murmur)
- Diastolic rumble (atrioventricular valve flow murmur)
- Prominent right ventricular (RV) impulse
- Increased jugular venous pressure (with RV failure)
- Cyanosis and clubbing (severe cases)
- Exertional dyspnea and fatigue
- Infants with large ASDs: recurrent respiratory infections, heart failure, and failure to thrive
- Patients with small defects: generally asymptomatic

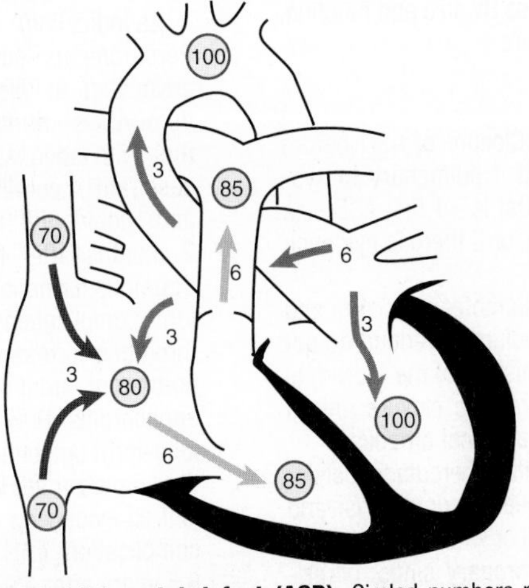

FIGURE 1-142 Physiology of atrial septal defect (ASD). Circled numbers represent oxygen saturation values. The numbers next to the arrows represent volumes of blood flow (in L/min/m²). This illustration shows a hypothetical patient with a pulmonary-to-systemic blood flow ratio (Qp:Qs) of 2:1. Desaturated blood enters the right atrium from the venae cavae at a volume of 3 L/min/m² and mixes with an additional 3 L of fully saturated blood shunting left to right across the ASD; the result is an increase in oxygen saturation in the right atrium. Six liters of blood flow through the tricuspid valve and cause a mid-diastolic flow rumble. Oxygen saturation may be slightly higher in the right ventricle because of incomplete mixing at the atrial level. The full 6 L flows across the right ventricuar outflow tract and causes a systolic ejection flow murmur. Six liters return to the left atrium, with 3 L shunting left to right across the defect and 3 L crossing the mitral valve to be ejected by the left ventricle into the ascending aorta (normal cardiac output). (From Kliegman RM et al: *Nelson textbook of pediatrics,* ed 19, Philadephia, 2011, Saunders.)

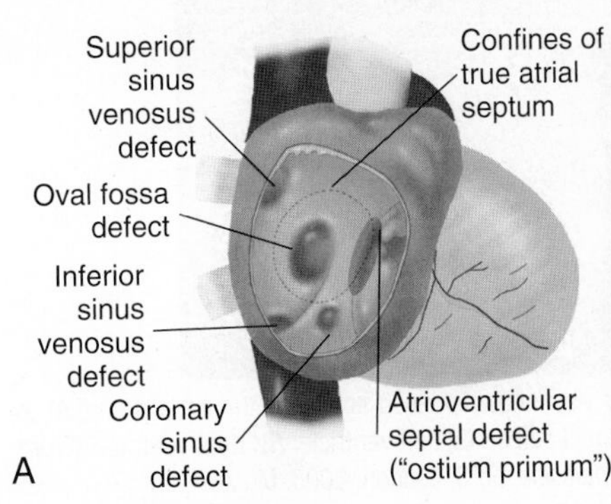

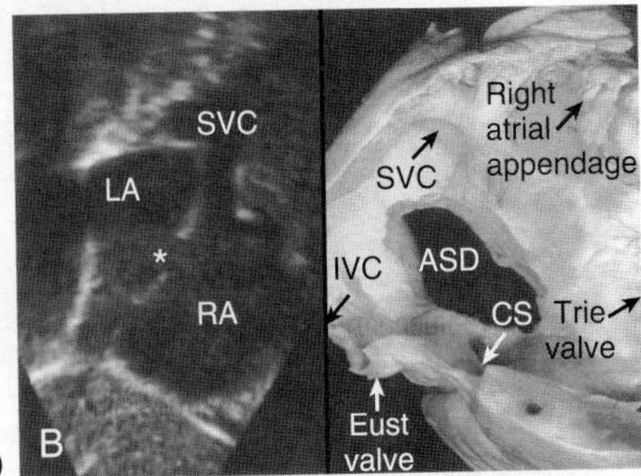

FIGURE 1-143 A, Schematic diagram outlining the different types of interatrial shunting that can be encountered. Note that only the central defect is suitable for device closure. **B,** Subcostal right anterior oblique view of a secundum atrial septal defect *(ASD) (asterisk)* that is suitable for device closure. The right panel is a specimen as seen in a similar view, outlining the landmarks of defect. *CS,* Coronary sinus; *IVC,* inferior vena cava; *LA,* left atrium; *RA,* right atrium; *SVC,* superior vena cava. (From Zipes DP et al [eds]: *Braunwauld's heart disease,* ed 7, Philadelphia, 2005, Saunders.)

Dx DIAGNOSIS

DIFFERENTIAL DIAGNOSIS

- Primary pulmonary hypertension
- Pulmonary stenosis
- Rheumatic heart disease
- Mitral valve prolapse
- Cor pulmonale

WORKUP

- ECG:
  - Ostium primum defect: left axis deviation, incomplete or total right bundle branch block, prolongation of PR interval
  - Sinus venosus defect: left axis deviation, abnormal P axis
  - Ostium secundum defect: right axis deviation, incomplete or total right bundle branch block, right atrial enlargement
- Chest x-ray examination
- Echocardiography (Fig. 1-144)
- Cardiac catheterization
- Cardiac magnetic resonance imaging (MRI), CT, or both

IMAGING STUDIES

- Chest x-ray: cardiomegaly, right heart enlargement, increased pulmonary vascular pattern
- Echocardiography with saline bubble contrast and Doppler flow studies: may demonstrate the size of the defect, the direction of shunting, presence of anomalous pulmonary return (in sinus venosus ASD), right heart volume overload, and elevated pulmonary artery pressures
- Transesophageal echocardiography is much more sensitive than transthoracic echocardiography in identifying sinus venosus defects and is preferred by some for the initial diagnostic evaluation
- Cardiac catheterization: Left heart catheterization is not usually a diagnostic necessity; it is only useful when the coronary arteries need to be assessed before surgery. Right heart catheterization may be necessary to assess shunt size, extent of pulmonary hypertension, and pulmonary vascular resistance (PVR), and to assess pulmonary artery vasoreactivity in response to vasodilators.
- Cardiac MRI and CT: may be useful if echo is not diagnostic; MRI is gold standard for assessing RV size and function, and it can determine whether the right-sided chambers are, in fact, enlarged. MRI is also good to assess pulmonary venous return; cardiac CT can offer similar information

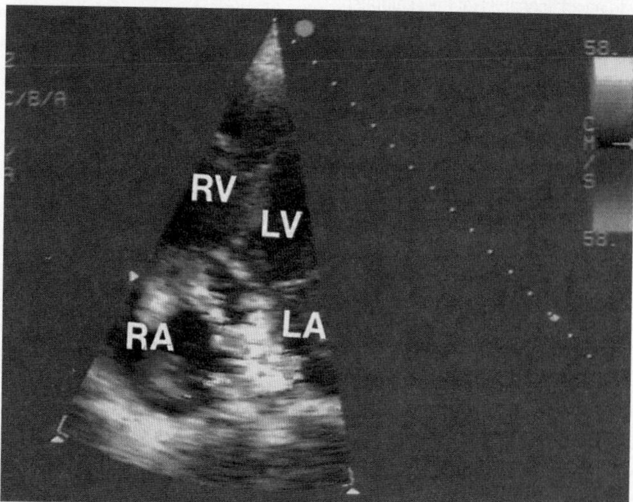

FIGURE 1-144 Color flow Doppler apical four-chamber view showing blood flow from the left atrium (LA) to the right atrium (RA) through a moderately sized atrial septal defect. *LV,* Left ventricle; *RV,* right ventricle. (From Forbes CD, Jackson WF: *Color atlas and text of clinical medicine,* ed 3, London, 2003, Mosby.

Rx TREATMENT

NONPHARMACOLOGIC THERAPY

- Symptomatic patients should avoid strenuous activity.
- Patients with small shunts (<10 mm) without pulmonary artery hypertension (PAH) and normal RV size are generally asymptomatic and require no medical therapy. Routine assessment of these patients includes symptoms, arrhythmias, and embolic events.
- A repeat echocardiogram should be obtained every 2 to 3 yr to assess RV size and function, and pulmonary pressure.

GENERAL Rx

- Children and infants: Closure of ASD before age 10 yr is indicated if pulmonary to systemic flow ratio [Qp/Qs] is >1.5:1, ASD size is significantly >5 mm, or if there is evidence of RV dilatation.
  - Small ASDs with a diameter of <5 mm and no evidence of RV volume overload do not impact the natural history of the individual and thus may not require closure unless associated with paradoxical embolism.
  - Closure of an ASD either percutaneously or surgically is indicated for right atrial and RV enlargement with or without symptoms.
  - A sinus venosus, coronary sinus, or primum ASD should be repaired surgically rather than by percutaneous closure.
  - Surgical closure of secundum ASD is reasonable when concomitant surgical repair/replacement of a tricuspid valve is considered or when the anatomy of the defect precludes the use of a percutaneous device.
- Adults: Closure of an ASD, either percutaneously or surgically, may be considered in the presence of net left-to-right shunting with Qp/Qs >1.5:1, pulmonary hypertension with pulmonary artery pressure less than two-thirds systemic levels, PVR less than two-thirds systemic vascular resistance, or when responsive to either pulmonary vasodilator therapy or test occlusion of the defect (patients should be treated in conjunction with providers who have expertise in the management of pulmonary hypertensive syndromes).
- Patients with severe irreversible PAH and no evidence of a left-to-right shunt should not undergo ASD closure.
- Closure of an ASD, either percutaneously or surgically, is reasonable in the presence of:
  - Paradoxical embolism (Class 2a indication)
  - Documented orthodeoxia-platypnea (Class 2a indication)
- Percutaneous catheter device closure is advocated in many patients with secundum ASDs (if stretched diameter is <41 mm with adequate rims), with >95% success rate. A combination of low-dose aspirin and clopidogrel is usually prescribed for 6 months after the procedure to prevent thrombus formation. Potential mid- and long-term complications of device closure include thrombus formation, device erosion into the aortic root, atrial dysrhythmias, and infective endocarditis. However, in recent studies the long-term outcomes of device closures using the Amplatzer septal occlude had been excellent as evidenced by no deaths and minimal complication in 151 patients followed for 6.5 years after ASD closure. In October 2013 The Food and Drug Administration (FDA) began alerting health care providers and patients that in very rare instances, tissue surrounding the Amplatzer ASO can break down (erode) and result in life-threatening emergencies that require immediate surgery. According to published estimates, these events occur in approximately 1 to 3 of every 1,000 patients implanted with the Amplatzer. Close clinical follow up and an echocardiogram is recommended predischarge, at 1 week, at 6 months, and at 12 months after implant.
- Percutaneous closure is contraindicated in those with sinus venous, primum, or secundum defects with unsuitable anatomy (too large; too small; too close to coronary sinus, AV valves, or pulmonary veins; or inadequate rims), presence of sepis, bleeding disorder, or intracardiac thrombi.
- In adult patients undergoing surgical closure, the surgical mortality should be <1%. Surgical closure of ASD improves function status, exercise capacity, and patient survival; however, it does not prevent atrial

fibrillation or stroke, especially if patients are operated on after age 40. Concomitant maze procedure may be considered for intermittent or chronic atrial tachyarrhythmias in adults with ASDs who are undergoing surgical repair.

DISPOSITION

- Mortality rate is high in patients with significant ostium primum defect if left untreated, with complications like RV failure, cerebral abscess, and PAH leading to permanent right-to-left shunting (Eisenmenger syndrome).
- Patients with small shunts (<10 mm) have a normal life expectancy.
- Basic preoperative assessment for adult congenital heart disease (ACHD) patients should include systemic arterial oximetry, an ECG, chest radiograph, TTE, and blood tests for full blood count and coagulation screen.
- Intracardiac shunts are considered moderate risk for preoperative evaluation for noncardiac procedure. High-risk features include severe systolic dysfunction (EF <35%), severe pulmonary hypertension whether primary or secondary, cyanotic heart disease, or severe left-side outlet obstruction.
- Annual clinical follow-up is recommended for patients postoperatively if their ASD was repaired as an adult to monitor for PAH, atrial arrhythmias, RV or LV dysfunction, and coexisting valvular lesions.
- Preoperative atrial fibrillation is a risk factor for immediate postoperative and long-term atrial fibrillation. Patients with a repaired ASD still have an increased risk for development of atrial fibrillation that directly correlates with the age at which the defect is corrected (later correction poses greater risk).
    - After closure, anticipated benefits include improved functional status and exercise capacity, improved survival after closure as a child, improved quality of life, prevention of right-heart failure, and prevention of PAH.
    - Potential mid- to long-term complications after ASD closure in adulthood include tachyarrhythmias (atrial fibrillation or atrial flutter), bradyarrhythmias (sinus node dysfunction or heart block), stroke (greater risk in older patients), residual ASDs (small usually close spontaneously, large may be because of patch dehiscence), right-heart failure or pulmonary artery hypertension (risk is inversely related to age at time of closure), mitral valve regurgitation or subaortic stenosis (usually in patients with primum ASDs), device migration/erosion, and pulmonary venous congestion (uncommon).
    - Pregnancy is usually well tolerated in women with ASDs. Follow-up is recommended because of small risk for paradoxical embolus, stroke, arrhythmia, and heart failure. If known, ASDs should be closed before pregnancy if indicated. The sole contraindication to pregnancy in women with an ASD is severe PAH.
    - Scuba diving is generally contraindicated in patients with small ASDs who are medically managed for such risks as paradoxical emboli. In addition, high-altitude climbing should be avoided because it can cause oxygen desaturation from right-to-left shunting in these patients.
- In regard to infective endocarditis prophylaxis for dental procedures,
    - Prophylaxis is not indicated for an ASD.
    - Prophylaxis is indicated for a completely repaired ASD, or any congenital heart disease with prosthetic material during the first 6 mo after the procedure.
    - Prophylaxis is indicated for a repaired ASD, or any congenital heart defect with residual defects at the site or adjacent to the site of a prosthetic patch or prosthetic device (both of which inhibit endothelialization).

The estrogen-containing oral contraceptive pill is not recommended in ACHD patients at risk of thromboembolism, such as those with cyanosis related to an intracardiac shunt, atrial fibrillation, severe PAH, or Fontan repair.

SUGGESTED READINGS

available at www.expertconsult.com

RELATED CONTENT

Atrial Septal Defect (ASD) (Patient Information)

AUTHOR: **SYEDA M. SAYEED, M.D.**

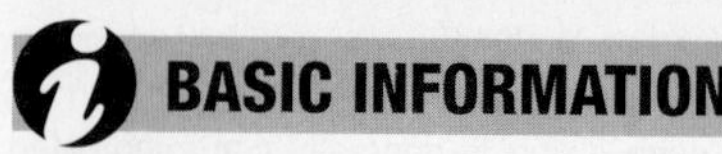

DEFINITION

Attention deficit hyperactivity disorder (ADHD) is a chronic disorder of attention and/or hyperactivity-impulsivity. Symptoms must be present before 7 yr of age, last at least 6 mo, and cause functional impairment in multiple settings. The diagnostic keys for ADHD are described in Table 1-68.

SYNONYMS

Hyperactivity
Hyperkinetic disorder
Attention deficit disorder (ADD)

ICD-9CM CODES
314.00 Attention deficit hyperactivity disorder
ICD-10CM CODES
F90.0 predominantly inattention
F90.1 predominantly hyperactivity
F90.2 combined
DSM-V CODES
314.00

EPIDEMIOLOGY & DEMOGRAPHICS

PEAK INCIDENCE: Diagnosis is usually first made in school-aged children (6 to 9 yr).
PREVALENCE: 8% to 10% of school-aged children and 2% to 5% of adults
PREDOMINANT SEX: Among children, male predominance with ratio of 2:1 to 4:1. Among adults, ratio is closer to 1:1 (sex difference may reflect referral bias).
PREDOMINANT AGE: Some symptoms must occur before age 7 yr. Symptoms (especially hyperactivity) tend to diminish with age. Up to 70% continue to meet criteria in adolescence, and an estimated 40% to 65% have some symptoms in adulthood.
GENETICS: Strong polygenetic component. First-degree relatives of ADHD patients have 5 times greater risk of ADHD relative to controls. Studies suggest potential involvement of several genes, including those associated with serotonin and glutamate transporters as well as dopamine metabolism.
RISK FACTORS: Possible environmental and epidemiologic risk factors include in utero tobacco/drug exposure or hypoxia, low birth weight, prematurity, pregnancy, lead exposure (though most children with elevated lead levels do not develop ADHD), head trauma in young children, family dysfunction, low socioeconomic status. Evidence does not support a clear association between dietary factors (e.g., refined sugar, food additives) and ADHD.

TABLE 1-68 Diagnostic Keys for Attention Deficit Hyperactivity Disorder

1. Inattention
   a. Careless mistakes in schoolwork, work, or other activities
   b. Seems not to listen when spoken to directly
   c. Poor follow through on schoolwork or chores
   d. Difficulty organizing
   e. Easily distracted by extraneous stimuli and is forgetful
2. Hyperactivity
   a. Trouble sitting still
   b. May act as if "driven by a motor"
   c. May talk excessively
3. Impulsivity
   a. Trouble holding back in class
   b. Trouble taking turns
   c. Interrupts

PHYSICAL FINDINGS & CLINICAL PRESENTATION

- Three types:
  1. Predominantly inattentive: difficulty organizing, planning, remembering, concentrating, starting/completing tasks; symptoms may not be present during preferred activities.
  2. Predominantly hyperactive-impulsive: edgy/restless, talkative, disruptive/intrusive, disinhibited, impatient.
  3. Combined.
- Usually diagnosed in elementary school when achievement is compromised and behavioral problems are not tolerated. Children with academic underproductivity, problems with peer and family relations, or discipline issues are often referred for evaluation. Of the more than 4 million children in the U.S. who have ADHD, most have comorbid conditions (see below) and nearly half use special education and mental health services.
- Up to 50% may have associated disorders such as psychiatric diagnoses (oppositional defiant disorder, conduct disorder, depression, anxiety), learning disabilities, or substance abuse.
- In adults, hyperactivity is less common, but restlessness, edginess, and difficulty relaxing are often seen. Disorganization and difficulty completing tasks are other common complaints.

ETIOLOGY

Strongest evidence exists for genetic inheritance. Other theories include abnormal metabolism of brain catecholamines, structural brain abnormalities, reduced activation in the basal ganglia and anterior frontal lobe, as well as environmental factors (see earlier).

Dx DIAGNOSIS

DIFFERENTIAL DIAGNOSIS

- Medical: visual/hearing impairment, seizure disorder, head injury, sleep disorder, medication interactions, mental retardation, developmental delay, thyroid abnormalities, lead toxicity.
- Psychiatric: depression, bipolar disorder, anxiety, obsessive-compulsive disorder, conduct disorder, posttraumatic stress disorder, and substance abuse.
- Psychosocial: mismatch of learning environment with ability, family dysfunction, abuse/neglect.

WORKUP

- Clinical interview should include assessment of symptoms and impact on work/school and relationships; developmental history; personal and family psychiatric history, including substance abuse; social history, including family dysfunction; medical history.
- Physical examination should be performed to investigate medical causes for symptoms, coexisting conditions, and contraindications to treatment. Special focus should be paid to evaluation of dysmorphic features; neurologic examination, including assessment for neurocutaneous findings; and assessment of hearing and vision.
- Information from collateral sources (parents, partners, teachers) is crucial to diagnosis. Many patients will not display symptoms during an office visit and may underreport or overreport symptoms.
- Self-rating scales and standardized symptom-specific questionnaires from collateral sources can help diagnose and assess response to treatment. The use of ADHD-specific rating scales over broadband behavioral scale is associated with improved sensitivity and specificity.
- Laboratory or imaging studies should be undertaken only if indicated by history or physical examination.
- Ancillary testing (e.g., IQ/achievement testing, language evaluation, and mental health assessment) may be indicated based on clinical findings and may require referral.

Rx TREATMENT

NONPHARMACOLOGIC THERAPY

- The majority of studies comparing the efficacy of pharmacologic vs nonpharmacologic interventions demonstrate the superiority of pharmacologic treatments.
- Studies on combined treatments have not shown significant improvements in core ADHD symptoms when behavioral treatments are added to stimulant medications. However, improvements in related areas of concern such as parent-child relations, aggressiveness, teacher-rated social skills, and reaching achievement have been seen in combined treatment groups.
- Prevailing opinion favors a multimodal approach in which nonpharmacologic behavioral therapies including parent-child behavioral therapy and social skills training can be used to target comorbid conditions or behaviors that have not responded to medication.
- Behavioral therapy alone is often considered when symptoms and impairment are mild, if parents are opposed to or patients cannot tolerate medications, or if there is uncertainty or disagreement about the diagnosis (e.g., between parents and teachers).

- Educational interventions are recommended, particularly in the setting of learning disabilities. Children with ADHD are entitled to reasonable educational accommodations under a 504 Plan or the Individuals with Disabilities Education Act.
- Behavioral interventions (e.g., goal setting and rewards systems) show short-term efficacy and are endorsed by most national organizations (e.g., American Academy of Pediatrics, American Medical Association). Time management and organizational skills appear useful. Social skills training may also be useful.
- Psychotherapy such as cognitive therapy, play therapy, or insight-oriented therapy are unlikely to be useful in addressing the core symptoms of ADHD. However, it may be beneficial in treating comorbid psychiatric conditions.
- Elimination diets are not routinely recommended.
- Many support and advocacy groups provide education and other resources (e.g., Children and Adolescents with ADHD, National ADD Association, American Academy of Child and Adolescent Psychiatry).

ACUTE GENERAL Rx

- Most studies on treatment of ADHD are performed in children; limited data available on adults.
- Mainstay of treatment is stimulant medications. Second-line therapies include antidepressants and alpha-agonists.
- Stimulants:
  1. Release or block uptake of dopamine and norepinephrine.
  2. Include short- and long-acting methylphenidate, dextroamphetamine, and dextroamphetamine/amphetamine combinations (mixed amphetamine salts). A methylphenidate patch is available, as is a pro-drug form of dextroamphetamine, lisdexamfetamine (Vyvanse), which is designed to limit the abuse potential.
  3. All stimulants equally effective; however, not all patients improve with stimulants. Patients who do not respond well to one stimulant may respond to another.
  4. Do not cause euphoria or lead to addiction when taken as directed.
  5. Improve cognition, inattention, impulsiveness/hyperactivity, and driving skills. Limited impact on academic performance, learning, and emotional problems.
  6. Side effects are usually mild, reversible, and dose dependent, including anorexia, weight loss, sleep disturbances, increased heart rate and blood pressure, irritability, moodiness, headache, onset or worsening of motor tics, reduction of growth velocity (but not adult height). Do not worsen seizures in patients on adequate anticonvulsant therapy. Rebound of symptoms can occur with withdrawal of medication.
  7. Stimulants have generally been associated with cardiovascular events and death. Patients should be carefully evaluated for cardiovascular disease before beginning therapy and be periodically monitored, including blood pressure checks, while they are treated. However, despite concerns regarding cardiovascular risk, these medications are generally safe. Recent studies have shown that among young and middle-aged adults, current or new use of ADHD medications, compared with nonuse or remote use, is not associated with an increased risk of serious cardiovascular events. Routine, pre-treatment screening with ECGs is not currently recommended by the American Academy of Pediatrics or the American Academy of Child and Adolescent Psychiatry.
- Atomoxetine (Strattera):
  1. Selective norepinephrine reuptake inhibitor.
  2. Generally felt to be less effective than stimulants, but a useful alternative in patients who have not tolerated or responded to stimulants or in the setting of patient or family substance abuse.
  3. Efficacy and safety of use beyond 2 years of treatment have not been studied. There have been reports of behavioral abnormalities and increased suicidality in children and adolescents.
  4. Side effects: gastrointestinal upset, sleep disturbance, decreased appetite, dizziness, sexual side effects in men. Cardiovascular side effects have also been reported.
  5. There have been rare reports of severe liver injury in adults and children.
- Antidepressants (bupropion, imipramine, desipramine, nortriptyline):
  1. May be useful in patients with coexisting psychiatric disorders.
  2. Studies comparing efficacy versus stimulants are inconclusive.
  3. Side effects: arrhythmias, anticholinergic effects, lowering of seizure threshold.
- Alpha-2-adrenergic agonists (clonidine, guanfacine)
  1. Appear to be less effective than stimulants, but may be particularly useful as an adjunctive treatment to stimulants, particularly in patients with a partial stimulant response or who experience side effects such as sleep disturbance or concurrent symptoms of overarousal, irritability, or aggression.
  2. Extended-release formulations of guanfacine (Intuniv) and clonidine (Kapray) have been approved by the FDA for treatment of ADHD in children ages 6 to 17 yr. A transdermal clonidine patch is also available.
  3. Potential side effects include sedation, fatigue, headache, bradycardia, hypotension, and depression.
- Use of medications, particularly stimulants (which are monitored under the Controlled Substance Act), requires frequent monitoring.

DISPOSITION

- Although symptoms may change over time, for many patients ADHD represents a chronic condition that requires lifelong management.
- Patients are at higher risk for academic underachievement, lower socioeconomic status, work and relationship difficulties, high-risk behavior, and psychiatric comorbidities.

REFERRAL

- Diagnosis complicated by difficult-to-treat comorbid psychiatric conditions, developmental disorders, or mental retardation
- Lack of adequate response to stimulants/atomoxetine

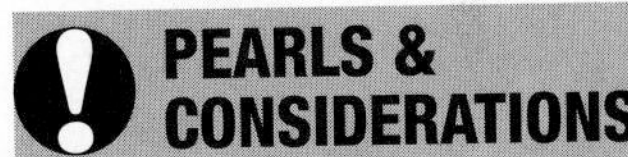

- The World Health Organization's Adult Self-Report Scale (ASRS) v1.1 has good sensitivity and adaptability to the primary care setting.
- Among adults with persistent ADHD symptoms treated with medication, trials have shown that the use of cognitive behavioral therapy compared with relaxation with educational support resulted in improved ADHD symptoms, which were maintained at 12 mo.
- ADHD has been associated with criminal behavior in some studies. Data analysis has shown that among patients with ADHD, rates of criminality are lower during periods when they receive ADHD medication.
- Recommendations for the diagnosis and management of ADHD have been published by the Centers for Disease Control and Prevention (www.cdc.gov/ncbddd/adhd/treatment/treatment.html).

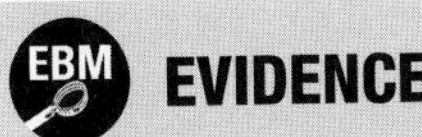

available at www.expertconsult.com

SUGGESTED READINGS

available at www.expertconsult.com

RELATED CONTENT

Attention Deficit Hyperactivity Disorder (ADHD) (Patient Information)

AUTHORS: **EMILY R. KATZ, M.D.**

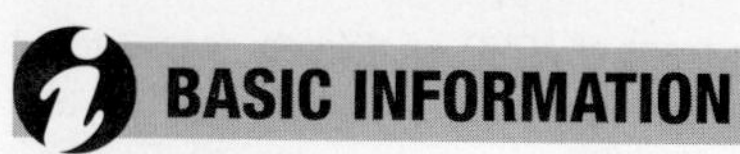

BASIC INFORMATION

DEFINITION

Autism spectrum disorders encompass a continuum of developmental disorders characterized by marked social impairment. Table 1-69 describes the diagnostic keys for autistic disorder. There is usually impairment in several additional domains, integral to social functioning, including language and communication. Stereotypic behavior and sensory issues (i.e., hypersensitivity, hyposensitivity) also are prominent. Onset is typically before age 3 yr. and may be diagnosed as early as 15-18 mo of age. In rare cases, a child may be observed to develop normally to 18-24 mo and be diagnosed with autism at 30-36 mo. The diagnosis of Asperger's syndrome is typically made at a later age with 50% of affected children first diagnosed in kindergarten or 1st grade. DSM-5 criteria will no longer differentiate autism and Asperger's as separate disorders. Instead, an overarching diagnosis of autism spectrum disorder will be applied to both syndromes using severity levels to identify the magnitude of social and behavioral impairment.

SYNONYMS

ASD
Autism
Autistic disorder
Early infantile autism
Childhood autism
Kanner's autism
Asperger disorder
Pervasive developmental disorder PDD NOS

ICD-9CM CODES
299.00 Autism spectrum disorder
ICD-10CM CODES
F84.0 Autism spectrum disorder
DSM-5 CODE
299.00 Autism spectrum disorder

EPIDEMIOLOGY & DEMOGRAPHICS

INCIDENCE (IN U.S.): Autism spectrum disorder afflicts less than 1% of children in the U.S.
PREVALENCE: 1:88 (1:54 for boys)
PREDOMINANT SEX: Male/female ratio of 2.1 to 6.5:1.0

TABLE 1-69 Diagnostic Keys for Autistic Disorder

1. Impairment in social interaction
   a. Uses nonverbal behaviors
   b. Poor peer relationships
   c. Lack of interest in shared activities
   d. Lack of social or emotional reciprocity
2. Impairments in communication
   a. Delay in language
   b. Stereotyped or repetitive language
   c. Lack of age-appropriate social play
3. Repetitive behaviors
   a. Inflexibility
   b. Preoccupation with parts of objects

PREDOMINANT AGE: Lifelong
PEAK INCIDENCE: Before age 3 yr
GENETICS:
- Autism spectrum disorder is highly heritable with a heritability index of 82 to 90.
- De novo mutations account for 10% to 20% of autism spectrum disorder cases. Active research into common biologic mechanisms underlying autism spectrum disorders (including defective synaptic function) has identified chromosomal abnormalities in 6 major genes with as many as 20-30 additional genes in contributory roles, including glutamate-related genes.
- 5% risk rate for siblings of an affected individual, unless fragile X syndrome is determined as the pathway, increasing the risk rate to 50%.
- 70% to 95% concordance for autism spectrum disorder in monozygotic twins and 5% for dizygotic pairs.
- Clinical signs of autism spectrum disorder correlate with abnormal brain development. Overgrowth and neural dysfunction are evidence at young ages and involve an abnormal excess number of neurons in the prefrontal cortex (PFC). This entirely neurobiologic signal of abnormal development has been reported to begin at 9 to 18 months of age.

PHYSICAL FINDINGS & CLINICAL PRESENTATION

- Common triad of marked impairment in social interactions, impaired and atypical verbal and nonverbal communication, and repetitive and usual behavior or play
- Marked impairment in the understanding and use of both verbal and nonverbal communication, including unchanging facial expression and lack of gestures during interactions
- Stereotypic behavior or language (i.e., echolalia, palilalia)
- Perceptual hypersensitivity (i.e., auditory, tactile, olfactory, gustatory) and avoidance of novel stimuli; or perceptual hyposensitivity (e.g., abnormally high threshold for pain)

ETIOLOGY

- Majority of cases are not associated with a comorbid medical condition. However, 2/3 of cases have a comorbid psychiatric feature (ADHD 29%, Anxiety 22%, Bipolar 20%, Depression 20%).
- Significant increase in comorbid seizure disorder (25%) and developmental delay (75%).
- Autism spectrum disorder is sometimes associated with other neurologic conditions (e.g., encephalitis, cytomegalovirus, toxoplasmosis, tuberous sclerosis, phenylketonuria [PKU], fragile X syndrome), suggesting that it also may result from nonspecific neuronal injury.
- Several studies have shown that there is no association between immunizations (specifically MMR vaccine) or thimerosal-containing vaccines (i.e., DPT) and autism spectrum disorder.
- Maternal use of valproate during pregnancy has been associated with increased risk for autism spectrum disorder and childhood autism in offspring.[1]
- Studies have raised concern about an association between the use of selective serotonin uptake inhibitors (SSRIs) during pregnancy, and an increased risk of autism. A recent study,[2] however, did not detect a significant association between maternal use of SSRIs during pregnancy and autism spectrum disorder in the offspring.
- Current research on the Shank family of proteins (SHANK3 [SH3 and multiple ankyrin repeat domains 3]) suggest that the systematic effects of alterations in Shank3 might contribute to the systematic features of autism spectrum disorders found in many patients.

Dx DIAGNOSIS

DIFFERENTIAL DIAGNOSIS

- Rett's syndrome: occurs in females; follows a brief period of normal development (i.e., 12-15 mo; characterized by severe neurodevelopmental regression including head growth deceleration, loss of purposeful use of hands, hyperventilation (risk of aerophagia), and motor incoordination
- Childhood disintegration disorder: normal development until age 4 yr, followed by marked neurodevelopmental and behavioral regression beginning with loss of bladder and bowel control
- Childhood-onset schizophrenia: follows period of normal development
- Asperger's syndrome: lacks the language and cognitive deficits characteristic of autism
- Isolated symptoms of autism spectrum disorder: when occurring in isolation, defined as disorders (i.e., Phelan-Mcdermid syndrome, Aciardi syndrome, selective mutism, expressive language disorder, mixed receptive-expressive language disorder, stereotypic movement disorder, severe-to-profound intellectual disability [aka mental retardation])

WORKUP

- Rule out underlying medical condition including genetic intellectual disability syndromes
- Administer age-appropriate diagnostic instruments based on questionnaires and observation noting scales. Validated autism spectrum disorder–specific screening tools are available for children age ≥18 mo (e.g., Modified Checklist for Autism in Toddlers, Childhood Autism Rating Scale; Autism Diagnostic Observation Scale; Autism Diagnostic Interview-Revised; PDDST-III; Asperger's Syndrome Diagnostic Scale; Gilliam Asperger's Diagnostic Scale) and

---

[1]Christensen J et al: Prenatal valproate exposure and risk of autism spectrum disorders and childhood autism, *JAMA* 309:1696-1703, 2013.

[2]Hviid A et al: Use of selective serotonin reuptake inhibitors during pregnancy and risk of autism, *N Engl J Med* 369:2406-2415, 2013.

are being developed for younger children. General developmental screening tools are currently used in children <18 mo.

LABORATORY TESTS

- PKU screen (usually done at birth in the U.S.)
- Lead exposure screening
- Audiology testing for young children with autism spectrum disorders; school-based hearing screening may be sufficient in older children with autism spectrum disorders and without significant language or learning deficits
- Karyotype, microarray analysis, and DNA testing for fragile X syndrome in both boys and girls

IMAGING STUDIES

- EEG to diagnose coexisting seizure disorder if seizure is suspected or if language regression is present (i.e., Landau-Kleffner syndrome)
- Brain MRI if tuberous sclerosis or Aicardi syndrome (callosal agenesis) is suspected

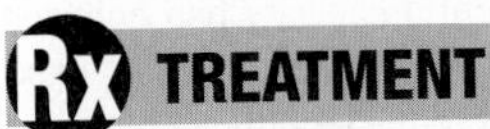

TREATMENT

NONPHARMACOLOGIC THERAPY

- Consistent behavioral training program in both the home and school environments
- A number of programs are currently used; many are based on applied behavioral analysis (ABA), others include Pivotal Response Training (PRT), Floortime, and the Early Start Denver Model for Young Children with Autism.
- Special educational program focused on language and communication skills, social and life skills development
- Highly structured home environment
- Education for families and teachers; the Autism Speaks™ website may be helpful in this regard: http://www.autismspeaks.org/about_us.php

ACUTE GENERAL Rx

- Obsessive or ritualistic behaviors: selective serotonin reuptake inhibitors (SSRIs), atypical antipsychotics, valproic acid
- Aggression, irritability, self-injury: atypical antipsychotic agents (e.g., risperidone), α-agonists, anticonvulsant mood stabilizers, SSRIs, beta-blockers, opiate antagonist (self-injury only)
- Hyperactivity, impulsivity, inattention: stimulants, alpha-agonists, atypical antipsychotics
- Anxiety: SSRIs, buspirone, mirtazapine
- Bipolar, mood lability: valproic acid, carbamazepine, lithium, aripiprazole
- Depression: SSRIs, mirtazapine

CHRONIC Rx

- Extended use of medications used for acute management of comorbid psychiatric disorder.
- Pharmacotherapy is palliative, not curative of autism spectrum disorder

DISPOSITION

- Most children will require some degree of assistance as adults.
- DSM-5 identifies 3 severity levels based on social communication and restricted, repetitive behaviors: Level 1 (requiring support), Level 2 (requiring substantial support), and Level 3 (requiring very substantial support).
- With early diagnosis and proper treatment/support, the prognosis for children without language and intellectual impairment (aka Asperger's syndrome) is fair to very good despite ongoing symptoms.
- Poorer outcomes include a lack of joint attention by age 4 yr, a lack of functional speech by age 5 yr, intellectual disability, seizures, comorbid medical or psychiatric syndromes, and a pervasive lack of social relatedness.
- Best outcomes are associated with early identification and treatment, the development of oral communication skills, and the cognitive and behavioral capacity for inclusion in regular education settings with typically developing peers.

REFERRAL

Assistance may be needed in diagnosis (child psychiatrist, clinical psychologist, geneticist, pediatric neurologist, developmental pediatrician), management (speech language pathologist, occupational therapist), parental teaching (psychiatric social worker), or intervention with the school system (educational advocate, attorney).

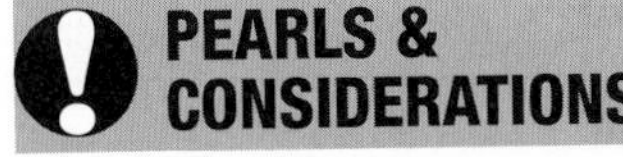

PEARLS & CONSIDERATIONS

- There is no scientific evidence of a relation between childhood vaccination and the development of autism.
- Preliminary evidence suggests that a disproportionate number of children with autism spectrum disorder suffer from sleep difficulties, including obstructive sleep apnea, with sequelae mimicking ADHD.
- The Center for Autism & Developmental Disabilities at Bradley Hospital, an affiliate of the Brown Medical School, is the largest and most comprehensive treatment program in the U.S. for children with autism spectrum disorder and comorbid psychiatric illness (www.bradleyhospital.org).
- University of California Davis M.I.N.D. Institute is devoted to the study of autism (http://www.ucdmc.ucdavis.edu/mindinstitute).

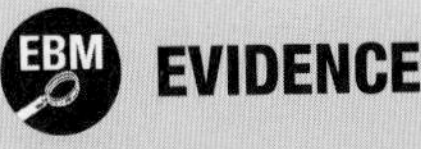

EVIDENCE

available at www.expertconsult.com

SUGGESTED READINGS

available at www.expertconsult.com

RELATED CONTENT

Autism (Patient Information)

AUTHORS: **ROWLAND P. BARRETT, PH.D.**

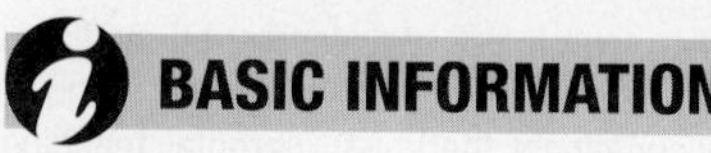

BASIC INFORMATION

DEFINITION

Cerebral arteriovenous malformations (AVMs) are congenital vascular lesions that are characterized by blood flow from high-pressure arterial vessels directly into thin-walled veins without passing through an intervening capillary/venule system (Fig. 1-145A).

SYNONYMS

AVM

ICD-9CM CODES
Q28.2 Arteriovenous malformation of cerebral vessels
I60.8 Ruptured cerebral arteriovenous malformation
ICD-10CM CODES
Q28.2 Arteriovenous malformations of cerebral vessels

EPIDEMIOLOGY & DEMOGRAPHICS

INCIDENCE:

- Detection rates in large prospective studies range from 1.1 to 1.4 per 100,000 person-years.
- Incidence of hemorrhage, the most common and often most clinically dangerous presentation, is estimated to be 2% to 4% per year.

PREVALENCE: Estimated about 1.3 per 100,000

PREDOMINANT SEX AND AGE:

- There is a slight male preponderance; studies of varying populations show 1.04:1 to 1.2:1 M:F ratio.
- Peak age at time of hemorrhage occurrence is about 20 years, but it can occur in younger and older patients.

GENETICS:

- Cerebral AVMs are sporadic in most cases.
- AVMs are present in about 20% of cases of Osler-Weber-Rendu syndrome (also known as hereditary hemorrhagic telangiectasia [HHT]), an autosomal dominant disorder that results in abnormal blood vessel formation in the skin, lungs, liver, brain, and other organs.

RISK FACTORS:

- Male sex and presence of HHT are risk factors for AVM.
- The risk of hemorrhage is increased with prior hemorrhage, presence of a single draining vein, and diffuse nidus morphology.

PHYSICAL FINDINGS & CLINICAL PRESENTATION

- The most common presentation is hemorrhage; symptoms vary based on location and magnitude of hemorrhage.
- Patients may present with seizures or neurologic deficits related to mass effect of the AVM nidus.
- Headache and pulsatile tinnitus may be present.
- In infants, AVM may present as cyanotic heart failure, macrocephaly, or hydrocephalus.
- A bruit may be auscultated through the scalp or orbit.
- AVMs may also present with associated intracranial aneurysms that occur on distant, unrelated vessels, on a proximal artery that feeds the aneurysm (flow-related aneurysm), or within the AVM nidus itself (intranidal aneurysm). Patients may present with a subarachnoid hemorrhage related to the aneurysm rather than to the AVM.

ETIOLOGY

AVMs are congenital abnormalities caused by failure of formation of a capillary bed between embryonic arterial and venous vascular plexuses during the first trimester of gestation.

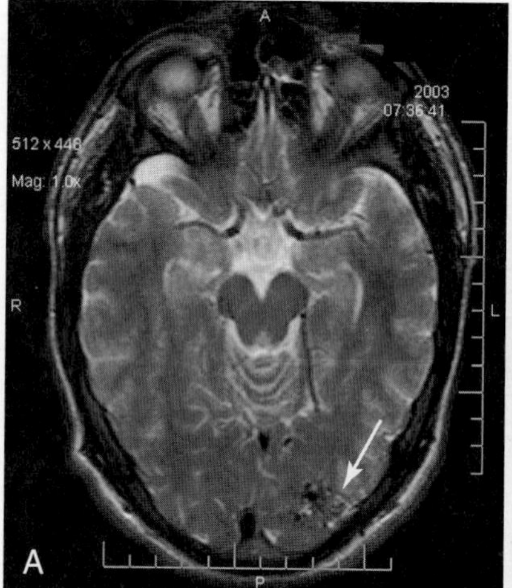

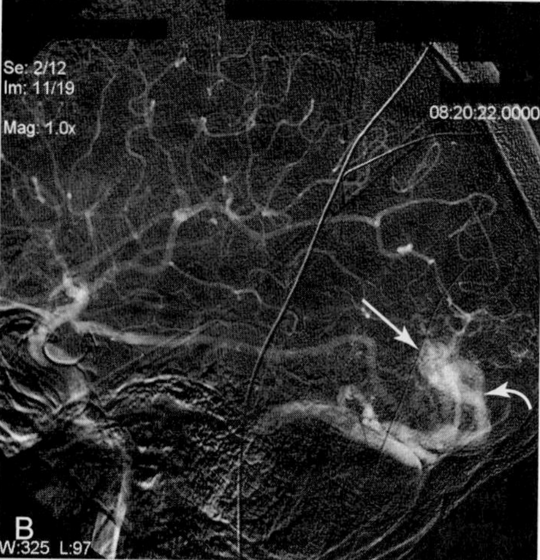

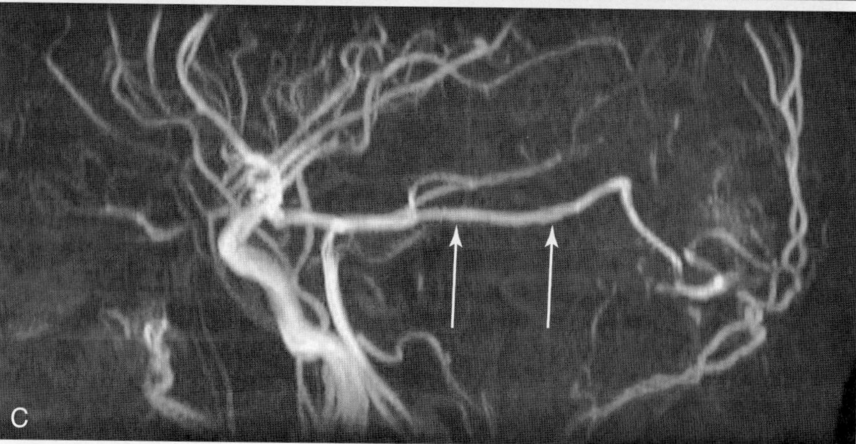

FIGURE 1-145A A 14-year-old child with a left occipital arteriovenous malformation (AVM). A, MRI shows multiple flow voids in the left occipital lobe *(arrow).* **B,** Lateral view from catheter angiogram confirms the presence of an AVM *(arrow)* and early draining veins *(curved arrow).* **C,** Lateral maximum intensity projection image from an MR angiogram shows an enlarged posterior cerebral artery branch *(arrows),* which feeds the tangle of abnormal vessels. (From Fuhrman BP et al: *Pediatric critical care,* ed 4, Philadelphia, 2011, Saunders.)

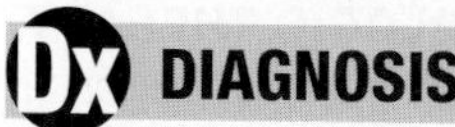

DIAGNOSIS

DIFFERENTIAL DIAGNOSIS

The differential diagnosis of cerebral AVMs includes other vascular lesions such as cavernous malformations, dural arteriovenous fistulas, and intracranial aneurysms. Table E1-70 compares vascular malformations, and Table E1-71 describes major differences between hemangiomas and vascular malformations.

LABORATORY TESTS

- CBC and BMP with renal function panel prior to contrast dye administration with CT angiography/cerebral angiogram.
- PT/INR/PTT should be drawn and corrected in the case of bleeding diathesis.

IMAGING STUDIES

- In the acute setting, a CT scan of the head to check for hemorrhage and a CT angiogram of the head for characterization of the lesion may be helpful (although calcification may be present and potentially pose as small acute blood).
- MRI of the brain delineates the nidus and its relationship to surrounding soft tissue structures better than a CT scan; however, in the setting of an acute hemorrhage these details will be obscured.
- Four-vessel cerebral angiogram (arteriogram) is the best study to evaluate AVM. Angiography in multiple projections helps identify the number and location of feeding and draining vessels for treatment planning (Fig. 1-145B). High-resolution images of the nidus may also reveal other irregularities such as aneurysms that often arise given the abnormal histology of the vessel walls and the high-pressure blood flow traversing them.

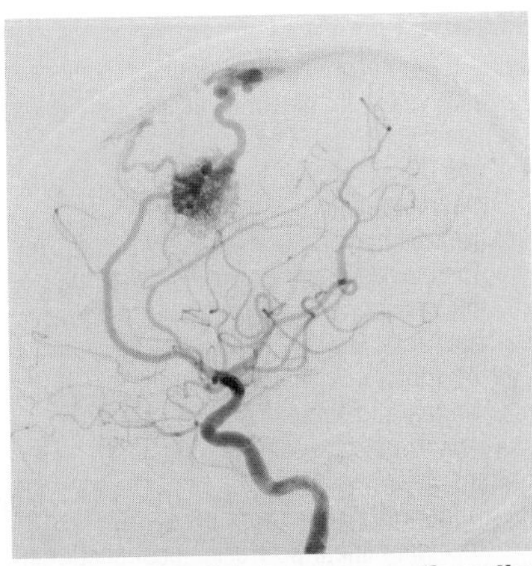

FIGURE 1-145B Arteriovenous malformation of the frontal lobe. The anterior cerebral artery provides primary arterial supply with venous drainage superficially into the superior sagittal sinus.

Rx TREATMENT

Pharmacologic management of seizures with antiepilepsy drugs and of headaches with oral analgesics can provide symptomatic relief.

NONPHARMACOLOGIC THERAPY

- Nonemergent outpatient setting: cerebral angiogram provides characterization of the lesion. Based on angiographic characteristics, the Spetzler-Martin AVM grading system may be used to help guide treatment (Table 1-72). In general, grade 5 AVMs are considered unresectable; they are not treated because the risks of treatment likely outweigh the risk of hemorrhage. Current tools for the treatment of AVMs include surgical resection, radiosurgery, and endovascular embolization (with liquid glues or embolic agents).
- Surgical resection: in low-grade lesions by an experienced neurosurgeon yields a high cure rate (~95% in published studies). Resection should include removal of all of the nidus of the AVM; failure to remove the complete nidus may increase the risk of recurrence. An increasing Spetzler-Martin grading scale increases risk of neurologic complications. Intraoperative imaging techniques such as indocyanine-green in-field angiography and conventional digital subtraction angiography are used to verify complete resection.
- Radiosurgery: alternative definitive treatment for AVMs. Traditionally employed to treat AVMs in eloquent areas (e.g., brainstem); sterotactic radiosurgery is increasingly used for higher Spetzler-Martin grade AVM. Reported rates of confirmed radiographic obliteration after AVM radiosurgery range from 47%-90%.

TABLE 1-72 Spetzler-Martin Arteriovenous Malformation (AVM) Grading Scale*

Characteristic	Points Assigned
AVM Size	
Less than 3 cm	1
3-6 cm	2
Greater than 6 cm	3
Location	
Eloquent	1
Noneloquent	2
Venous Drainage Pattern	
Deep	1
Superficial	0

*The grade is the sum of the points from all three categories. Eloquent brain is defined as sensorimotor, language, or visual cortex, internal capsule, brainstem, diencephalon, cerebellar peduncles, and deep cerebellar nuclei. Venous drainage is considered deep if any of the venous drainage is by deep veins (as opposed to exclusively cortical venous drainage).

From Spetzler RF, Martin NA: A proposed grading system for arteriovenous malformations, *J Neurosurg* 65:476-483, 1986.

- Endovascular embolization involves transarterial superselective blockage of the AVM. It has become an important adjunctive tool. Currently recommended and approved for use before resection, preoperative embolization can reduce arterial flow and pressure within the AVM, assisting in speed and safety of surgical resection. In addition, embolization may often be used to treat intranidal or flow-related aneurysms in coordination with either resection or radiosurgery. Embolization alone in obliterating an AVM is not routinely recommended.
- Treatment decisions should take into consideration the morbidity associated with the treatment modality versus the risk of future hemorrhage or neurologic deterioration. Disability stemming from intractable seizures or severe headaches may make invasive definitive treatment a more attractive option.

Acute cerebral hemorrhage: In the case of an acute hemorrhage, airway and breathing must be maintained, with intubation if necessary. Acute neurosurgical intervention for clot evacuation may be warranted. Microsurgical resection of the AVM may or may not be feasible in the acute setting and is controversial.

DISPOSITION

Whether the patient is receiving elective treatment of a known lesion or presenting with an acute hemorrhage, the patient should receive care in a progressive or intensive care unit with experience dealing with cerebrovascular disease. Once the patient is stabilized, appropriate rehabilitation should be arranged.

REFERRAL

- Cerebral AVMs should be managed by a qualified neurosurgeon.
- Referral to radiation medicine for adjuvant radiosurgery should be made when indicated.
- Referral to an interventional radiologist for endovascular treatment may be warranted.
- Treatment in a primary stroke center or other specialized center that offers all treatment modalities is recommended.

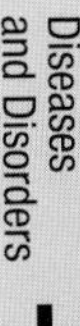

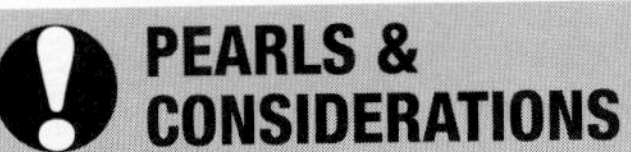

PEARLS & CONSIDERATIONS

COMMENTS

No two AVMs are exactly the same; individualization of treatment decisions is the mainstay. Additionally, many AVMs could be effectively treated through one of several modalities or a combination thereof. Factors such as patient age, overall health status, radiographic characteristics, route of surgical access, and potential morbidities of each treatment modality are vital variables in consideration for treatment. The advisability of intervention for unruptured AVMs remains controversial. In a recent randomized trial comparing medical management with specific interventions to obliterate AVMs (neurosurgery, embolization, radiotherapy, or a combination) the rates of neurological disability were much higher in the intervention group than with conservative treatment.[1]

PATIENT/FAMILY EDUCATION

If a patient with a known AVM suffers from acute-onset neurologic deficits or strokelike symptoms, emergency medical attention is warranted for potential hemorrhage. Presence of AVMs, cerebral or otherwise, in family members should be disclosed to the patient's primary care physician because the presence of a genetic condition predisposing to cerebral AVMs should be considered.

SUGGESTED READINGS

available at www.expertconsult.com

AUTHORS: **STEPHEN L. GRUPKE, M.D., M.S.,** and **JUSTIN F. FRASER, M.D.**

[1]Mohr JP et al: Medical management with or without interventional therapy for unruptured brain arteriovenous malformations (ARUBA): a multicentre non-blinded, randomized trial, *Lancet* 383:614-621, 2014.

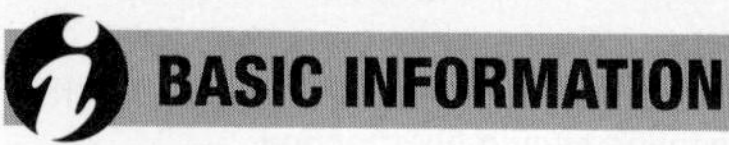

BASIC INFORMATION

DEFINITION

Avascular necrosis (AVN) is ischemic death of bone due to insufficient blood supply. Osteonecrosis is not a specific disease entity but a final common pathway to several disorders that impair blood supply to the femoral head and other locations.

SYNONYMS

AVN
Osteonecrosis
Aseptic necrosis

ICD-9CM CODES
733.40 Aseptic necrosis
733.43 Aseptic necrosis of femoral condyle
733.42 Aseptic necrosis of femoral head
733.41 Aseptic necrosis of humeral head
733.44 Aseptic necrosis of talus

ICD-10CM CODES
M87 Idiopathic aseptic necrosis of bone
M87.1 Osteonecrosis due to drugs
M87.2 Osteonecrosis due to previous trauma
M87.3 Other secondary osteonecrosis
M87.9 Osteonecrosis, unspecified

EPIDEMIOLOGY & DEMOGRAPHICS

- 15,000 new cases per year in the U.S. It is most commonly associated with the hip and accounts for 10% of total hip replacements in the U.S.
- Usually occurs in middle age and is more frequent in males than females
- Associated conditions:
  1. Corticosteroid treatment: 35%
  2. Alcohol abuse: 22%
  3. Idiopathic and other: 43%
  4. Hemoglobinopathies, pancreatitis, chronic renal failure, SLE, chemotherapy, decompression sickness
- Common sites involved
  1. Femoral head
  2. Femoral condyle
  3. Humeral head
  4. Navicular and lunate wrist bones
  5. Talus

PHYSICAL FINDINGS & CLINICAL PRESENTATION

- May be asymptomatic in early stages
- Pain in the involved area exacerbated by movement or weight bearing in later stages
- Decreased range of motion as the disease progresses
- Functional limitation

ETIOLOGY

Final common pathway of conditions that lead to impairment of the blood supply to the involved bone. Trauma disrupting the blood supply is the most common cause of AVN. Arterial factors are considered the most common cause of AVN. Table 1-73 describes proposed mechanism of disease of common conditions associated with osteonecrosis.

TABLE 1-74 Modified Steinberg Staging System for Osteonecrosis

Stage	Radiographic Appearance	Reversible
I	Normal radiographs, but abnormal bone scan or magnetic resonance image	Yes
II	Lucent and sclerotic changes	Yes
III	Subchondral fracture without flattening	No
IV	Subchondral fracture with flattening or segmental depression of femoral head	No
V	Joint space narrowing or acetabular changes	No
VI	Advanced degenerative changes	No

(From Firestein GS, Budd RC, Gabriel SE, et al: *Kelly's textbook of rheumatology*, ed 9, Philadelphia, 2013, Saunders.)

STAGING

Table 1-74 describes the Modified Steinberg Staging System for osteonecrosis.

Stages:

- Stage 0
  - Asymptomatic
  - Normal imaging
  - Histologic findings only (i.e., silent osteonecrosis)
- Stage 1
  - Asymptomatic or symptomatic
  - Normal radiographs and CT scan
  - Abnormal bone scan or MRI
- Stage 2
  - Abnormal radiographs or CT scan, including linear sclerosis, focal bead mineralization, cysts; however, the overall architecture of the involved bone is normal
- Stage 3
  - Early evidence of mechanical bone failure (subchondral fracture), but the overall shape of the bone is still intact
- Stage 4
  - Flattening or collapse of the bone
- Stage 5
  - Joint space narrowing
- Stage 6
  - Extensive joint destruction

Dx DIAGNOSIS

DIFFERENTIAL DIAGNOSIS

- None in late stages
- Early: any condition causing focal musculoskeletal pain, including arthritis, bursitis, tendinitis, myopathy, neoplastic bone and joint diseases, traumatic injuries, pathologic fractures

WORK-UP

Fig. 1-146 describes a diagnostic algorithm for osteonecrosis.

IMAGING STUDIES (Fig. 1-147)

1. MRI: the most sensitive technology to diagnose early aseptic necrosis. The first sign is a margin of low signal. An inner border of high signal associated with a low-signal line

TABLE 1-73 Proposed Mechanism of Disease of Common Conditions Associated with Osteonecrosis

	MECHANISM OF OSTEONECROSIS							
Associated Condition	Apoptosis	Osteoblast/ Osteoclast Homeostasis	Lipid Abnormalities	Coagulation Abnormalities	Oxidative Stress	Parathyroid/ Calcium Imbalance	Vascular Plugging	Vasoactive Substances
Corticosteroids	X	X	X	X	X			X
Bisphosphonates	X	X	X					
Alcohol abuse	X	X	X	X	X			
Trauma	X	X						X
Renal transplantation	X	X		X		X		
Dialysis						X		
Sickle cell disease							X	

(From Firestein GS, Budd RC, Gabriel SE, et al: *Kelly's textbook of rheumatology*, ed 9, Philadelphia, 2013, Saunders.)

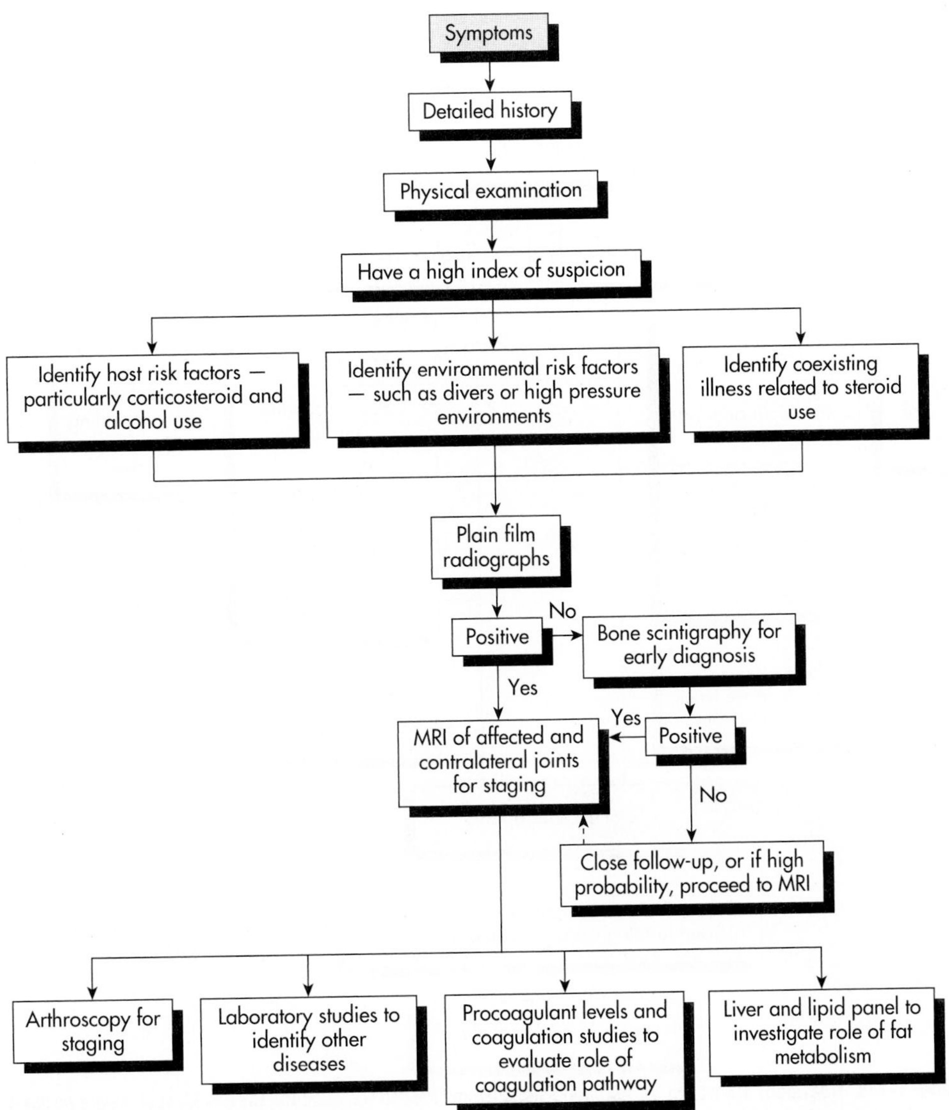

FIGURE 1-146 Diagnostic algorithm for osteonecrosis. *MRI*, Magnetic resonance image. (From Firestein GS, Budd RC, Gabriel SE, et al: *Kelly's textbook of rheumatology*, ed 9, Philadelphia, 2013, Saunders.)

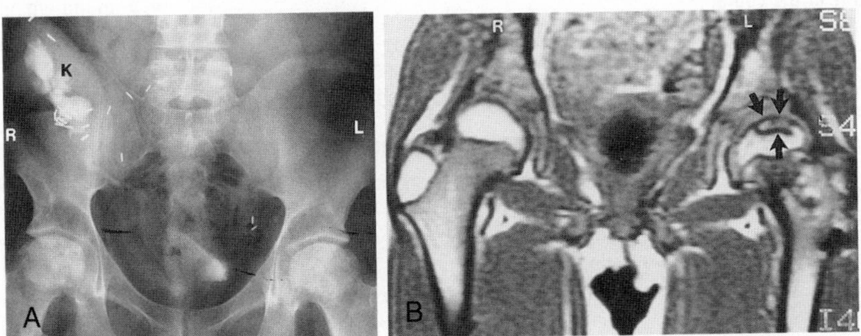

FIGURE 1-147 Aseptic necrosis of the hips. A, Aseptic necrosis can occur from a number of causes, including trauma and steroid use. In this patient, an anteroposterior view of the pelvis shows a transplanted kidney (K) in the right iliac fossa. Use of steroids has caused this patient to have bilateral aseptic necrosis. The femoral heads are somewhat flattened, irregular, and increased in density. **B,** Aseptic necrosis in a different patient is demonstrated on an MRI scan as an area of decreased signal *(arrows)* in the left femoral head. This is the most sensitive method for detection of early aseptic necrosis. (From Mettler FA [ed]: *Primary care radiology,* Philadelphia, 2000, Saunders.)

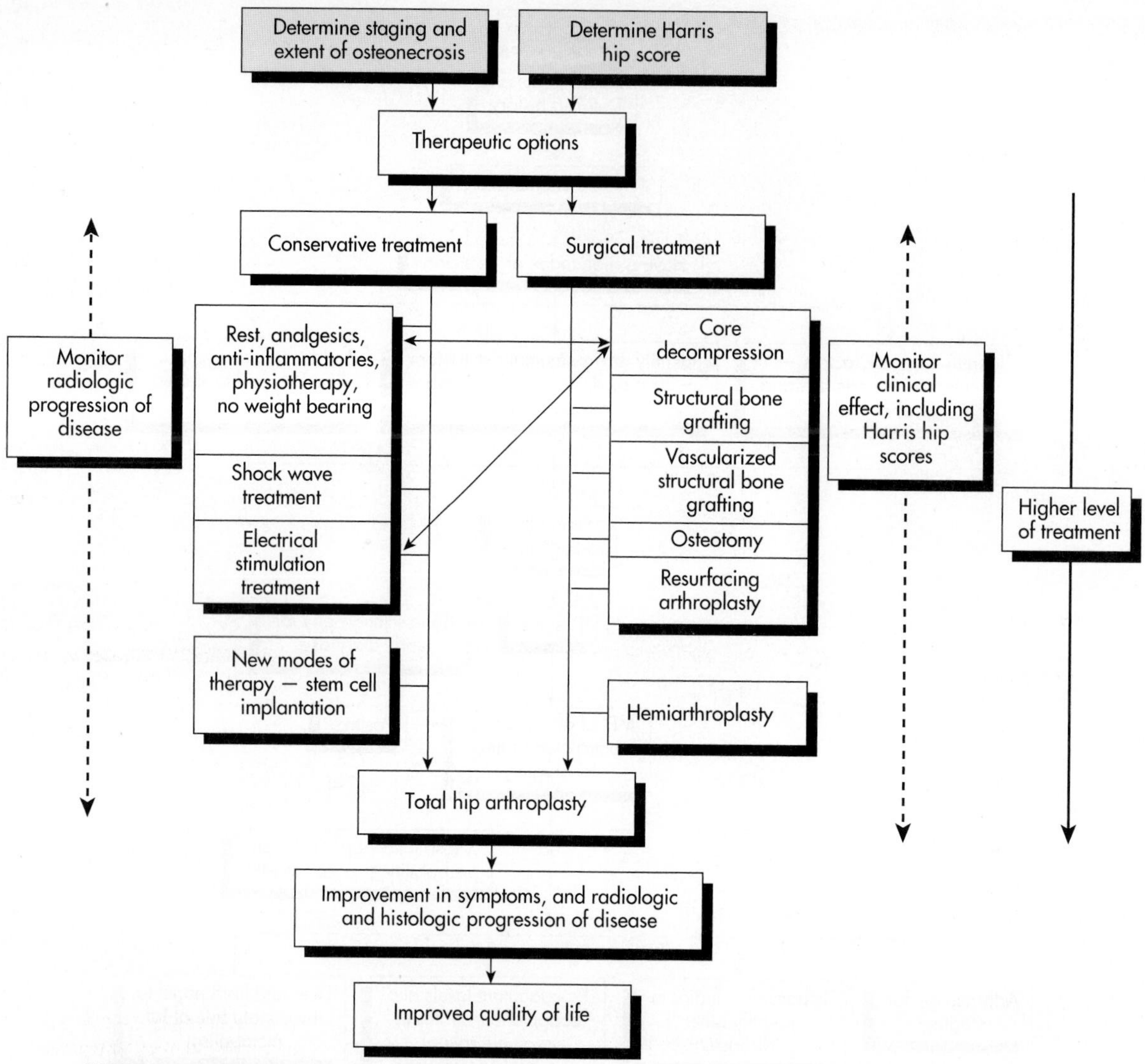

Determine staging and extent of osteonecrosis
Determine Harris hip score
Therapeutic options
Conservative treatment
Surgical treatment
Monitor radiologic progression of disease
Rest, analgesics, anti-inflammatories, physiotherapy, no weight bearing
Shock wave treatment
Electrical stimulation treatment
New modes of therapy — stem cell implantation
Core decompression
Structural bone grafting
Vascularized structural bone grafting
Osteotomy
Resurfacing arthroplasty
Hemiarthroplasty
Monitor clinical effect, including Harris hip scores
Higher level of treatment
Total hip arthroplasty
Improvement in symptoms, and radiologic and histologic progression of disease
Improved quality of life

FIGURE 1-148 Treatment algorithm for osteonecrosis. (From Firestein GS, Budd RC, Gabriel SE, et al: *Kelly's textbook of rheumatology*, ed 9, Philadelphia, 2013, Saunders.)

is specific for aseptic necrosis ("double line sign"). Sensitivity is 75% to 100%.

2. Radiography: insensitive early in the course. The earliest changes include diffuse osteopenia, areas of radiolucency with sclerotic border, and linear sclerosis. Later, a subchondral lucency (crescent sign) indicates subchondral fracture. More advanced cases reveal flattening, collapsed bone, and abnormal bone contour. In late disease, osteoarthritic changes are seen.
3. Bone scan:
   - Early: "cold" area.
   - Later: increased radionuclide uptake as a result of remodeling.
   - Sensitivity in early disease is only 70% and specificity is poor.
4. CT scan: may reveal central necrosis and area of collapse before those are visible on radiographs.

Rx TREATMENT

PREVENTION

- Manage etiologic conditions
- Minimize corticosteroid use

NONPHARMACOLOGIC THERAPY

- Core decompression: effectiveness 35% to 95% in early phases
- Bone grafting
- Osteotomies
- Joint replacement

ACUTE GENERAL Rx

- Decrease weight bearing of affected area.
- Pulsing electromagnetic fields applied externally (still experimental).
- Peripheral vasodilators (e.g., dihydroergotamine) (unproven).

- Late-stage AVN is most often treated by total joint arthroplasty.
- A treatment algorithm for osteonecrosis is described in Fig. 1-148.

PROGNOSIS

- When diagnosed at an early stage treatment is appropriate in all cases because 85% to 90% can be expected to progress to a more advanced stage.
- Contralateral joint involvement is common (30% to 70%).

SUGGESTED READINGS

available at www.expertconsult.com

RELATED CONTENT

Avascular Necrosis (Patient Information)

AUTHOR: **FRED F. FERRI, M.D.**

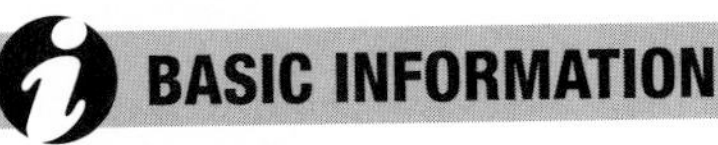

BASIC INFORMATION

DEFINITION

Babesiosis is a tick-transmitted protozoan disease of animals, caused by intraerythrocytic parasites of the genus *Babesia.* Humans are incidentally infected, resulting in a nonspecific febrile illness. The disease can be severe in immunocompromised hosts.

ICD-9CM CODES
088.82 Babesiosis
ICD-10CM CODES
B60.0 Babesiosis

EPIDEMIOLOGY & DEMOGRAPHICS

INCIDENCE (IN U.S.): Unknown
PREVALENCE (IN U.S.):

- In areas of high endemicity, seropositivity ranging from 9% (Rhode Island) to 21% (Connecticut)
- Highest number of reported cases in New York

PREDOMINANT SEX: Males (most likely through increased exposure to vectors during recreational or occupational activities)
PREDOMINANT AGE: Severity apparently increasing with age greater than 60 yr
PEAK INCIDENCE: Spring and summer months, May through September
GENETICS: None known
CONGENITAL INFECTION: At least one case of probable vertical transmission
NEONATAL INFECTION: At least two cases of perinatal transmission
BLOOD TRANSFUSION: Many instances

PHYSICAL FINDINGS & CLINICAL PRESENTATION

- Incubation period 1 to 4 wk, or 6 to 9 wk in transfusion-associated disease
- Gradual onset of irregular fever, chills, diaphoresis, headache, myalgia, arthralgia, fatigue, and dark urine
- On physical examination: petechiae, frank or mild hepatosplenomegaly, and jaundice. Most patients have a normal physical exam.
- Infection with *B. divergens* (Europe) producing a more severe illness with a rapid onset of symptoms and increasing parasitemia progressing to massive intravascular hemolysis and renal failure

ETIOLOGY

- Vector: Deer tick, *Ixodes scapularis* (also known as *I. dammini*)
    1. Feeds on rodents during the spring and summer while in its larval and nymphal stages and on deer as an adult
    2. Requires a blood meal to mature to each stage, hence human infection
    3. During the warmer months in endemic areas, humans are readily infected while engaging in outdoor activities
- *B. microti* and *B. divergens* account for most human infections.
- In the U.S., cases caused by *B. microti* are acquired on offshore islands of the northeastern coast, including Nantucket Island, Cape Cod, and Martha's Vineyard in Massachusetts; Block Island in Rhode Island; and Long Island, Fire Island, and Shelter Island in New York; as well as the nearby mainland including Connecticut and New Jersey.
- Sporadic cases reported from California, Georgia, Maryland, Minnesota, Virginia, Wisconsin, and most recently the WA-1 strain from Washington State and the MO-1 strain from Missouri.
- *B. divergens* is implicated in human disease in Europe, where the disease remains rare and predominantly associated with asplenia.
- Majority of cases are asymptomatic.
- May be transmissible by transfusion, through platelets and erythrocytes.
- Mixed infections (*B. microti* and *Borrelia burgdorferi,* the causative agent of Lyme disease) are estimated to occur in 10% (Rhode Island and Connecticut) to 60% (New York) of cases.

Dx DIAGNOSIS

DIFFERENTIAL DIAGNOSIS

- Amebiasis
- Ehrlichiosis
- Hepatic abscess
- Leptospirosis
- Malaria
- Salmonellosis, including typhoid fever
- Acute viral hepatitis
- Hemorrhagic fevers
- Subacute bacterial endocarditis

WORKUP

Should be suspected in any febrile patient living or traveling in an endemic area, irrespective of exposure history to ticks or tick bites, especially if asplenic

LABORATORY TESTS

- The preferred method for diagnosing babesiosis is PCR using whole blood specimens.
- Babesial DNA by polymerase chain reaction (PCR) has comparable sensitivity and specificity to microscopic analysis of thin blood smears. PCR is more sensitive than smears at the onset of infection when parasite load may be minimal.
- Diagnosis achieved serologically by indirect immunofluorescence assay (IFA) is specific for *B. microti.*
    1. Assay is hampered by the inability to distinguish between exposed patients and those who are actively infected.
    2. IGG titer of ≥1:64 is indicative of seropositivity, whereas one ≥1:1024 is considered diagnostic of acute infection. IGM titer of 1:64 is considered indicative of acute infection.
    3. Immunoglobulin M indirect immunofluorescent-antibody test may be highly sensitive and specific for diagnosis. IGM titer of 1:64 is considered indicative of acute infection.
- CBC to reveal mild to moderate pancytopenia
- Abnormally elevated serum chemistries, including creatinine, liver function profile, lactate dehydrogenase, and indirect and total bilirubin levels; hepatoglobin is low.
- Urinalysis to reveal proteinuria and hemoglobinuria
- Examination of Giemsa- or Wright-stained thin blood films for intraerythrocytic parasites
    1. In its classic, though infrequently seen, form a "tetrad" or "Maltese cross" composed of four daughter cells attached by cytoplasmic strands is observed (Fig. 1-149).
    2. More commonly, smaller forms composed of a single chromatin dot are eccentrically located within bluish cytoplasm.
    3. Parasitized erythrocytes may be multiply infected but not enlarged.
    4. Extra-erythrocytic forms may be seen.

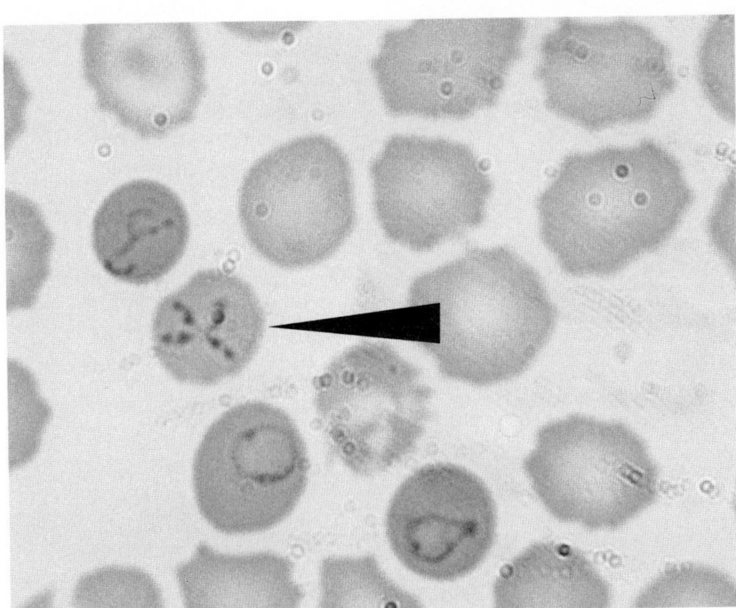

FIGURE 1-149 Babesia spp. Single and multiple intraerythrocytic parasites can be seen. The *arrow* marks a typical Maltese cross. (From Cohen J, Powderly WG: *Infectious diseases,* ed 2, St Louis, 2004, Mosby.)

 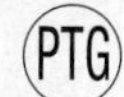

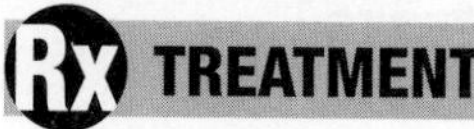

TREATMENT

NONPHARMACOLOGIC THERAPY

Supportive care with adequate hydration

ACUTE GENERAL Rx

- In patients with intact spleens: predominantly asymptomatic or if symptomatic, generally self-limited
- Therapy reserved for the severely ill patient, especially if asplenic, elderly, or immunosuppressed. Therapy may be offered to any symptomatic patient.
- Combination of atovaquone 750 mg q12h and azithromycin 500 mg on day 1 and 250 mg per day thereafter for 7 to 10 days appears to be as effective as a regimen of clindamycin and quinine with fewer adverse reactions. This is the preferred regimen for mild disease.
- Combination of quinine sulfate 650 mg PO tid plus clindamycin 600 mg PO tid (600 mg parenterally qid) taken for 7 to 10 days: effective but may not eliminate parasites
- Severely ill patients are hospitalized and treated with clindamycin and quinine
- Exchange transfusions in addition to antimicrobial therapy: successful treatment for severe infections in asplenic patients associated with high levels of *B. microti* or *B. divergens* parasitemia. Exchange transfusion is recommended for patients with >10% parasitemia, but may be considered for any severely ill patient.
- Relapsed and immunocompromised patients may require a longer duration of therapy.

DISPOSITION

Prognosis is usually good and fatal outcomes are rare.

REFERRAL

- For prompt consultation with an infectious disease specialist if the diagnosis is acutely suspected, especially in the asplenic, elderly, or immunocompromised patient
- For hospitalization for the severely ill patient who may require exchange transfusions in addition to antibiotic therapy

PEARLS & CONSIDERATIONS

COMMENTS

- Prevention of babesiosis in asplenic or immunocompromised hosts is best achieved by avoidance of areas where the vector is endemic, especially May through September.
- If residence or travel in endemic areas is unavoidable, advise patients to perform daily cutaneous self-examination, wear light-colored clothing (to facilitate removal of ticks), tuck pants into socks, and apply tick repellent (diethyltoluamide and dimethylphthalate) to skin or clothing.
- Advise a daily inspection for ticks in family pets (e.g., cats and dogs).
- Infection with *B. divergens,* especially in the asplenic patient, is often fatal.
- Concurrent cases of babesiosis and Lyme disease have been documented—check for combined infection in severely ill patients.
- A combination of clindamycin and quinine has been successfully used to treat babesiosis during the third trimester of pregnancy without incurring apparent adverse effect on the fetus.
- In 2011 the CDC added babesiosis to the list of nationally notifiable diseases.

SUGGESTED READINGS

available at www.expertconsult.com

RELATED CONTENT

Babesiosis (Patient Information)

AUTHOR: **PATRICIA CRISTOFARO, M.D.**

BASIC INFORMATION

DEFINITION

Baker's cyst is a fluid-filled popliteal bursa located along the medial border of the popliteal fossa. It is an extension of the semimembranosus bursa posteriorly (see Fig. 1-150).

SYNONYMS

Popliteal synovial cyst

ICD-9CM CODES
727.51 Baker's cyst (knee)

ICD-10CM CODES
M71.2 Synovial cyst of popliteal space [Baker], unspecified knee

EPIDEMIOLOGY & DEMOGRAPHICS

- Most are asymptomatic and incidentally found on imaging exams.
- Occurs at all ages, most commonly between age 35-70, increasing with age.
- The prevalence of popliteal cysts varies based on the imaging technique used and the age of the patient population.
- Between 2% and 6% of all patients believed to have clinical deep venous thrombosis (DVT) have symptomatic Baker's cysts.
- Approximately 5% to 40% of MRIs performed for osteoarthritis or internal derangement reveal popliteal cysts.

PHYSICAL FINDINGS & CLINICAL PRESENTATION

- Symptoms associated with associated joint pathology (knee swelling or stiffness)
- Pain in the popliteal space
- Leg edema
- Prominence of the popliteal fossa
- Decreased range of motion of the knee
- Locking of the knee
- Foucher's sign: The cyst becomes hard with knee extension and soft with knee flexion.
- Neuropathic lancinating pains radiating from the knee down the back of the leg
- Pain/discomfort with prolonged standing and hyperflexion of the knee
- Presence of associated DVT

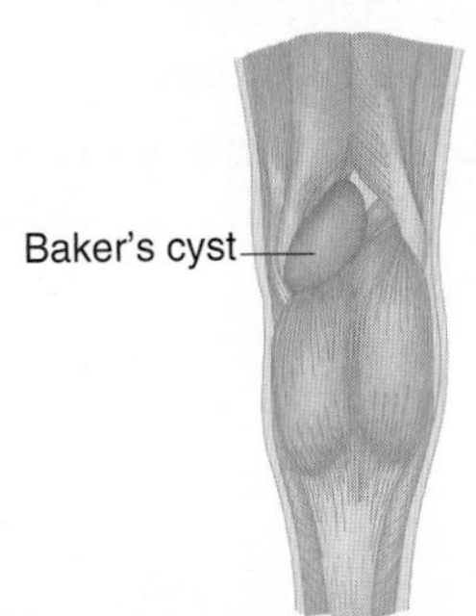

FIGURE 1-150 Baker's cyst is an extension of the semimembranosus bursa posteriorly. This bursa is often connected with a joint cavity. (From Marx J: *Rosen's emergency medicine: concepts and clinical practice,* ed 6, Philadelphia, 2006, Saunders.)

ETIOLOGY

- Believed to be fluid distention of bursal sac separating semimembranous tendon from medial head of gastrocnemius.
- May represent a true cyst but more often a degenerative or inflammatory joint disease or injury; they usually communicate with adjacent knee joint space. Thus a Baker's cyst usually denotes increased intraarticular pressure from underlying joint disease. Sequestration of synovial fluid in the popliteal fossa can result from a valve-like effect between joint space and cyst controlled by gastrocnemius-semimembranosus muscle changes with knee flexion and extension.
- In children, popliteal cysts are usually a primary process arising from the gastrocnemius-semimembranosus bursa without direct communication with the joint space.
- In adults, Baker's cysts are usually associated with pathologic changes of the knee joint, such as the following:
    - Rheumatoid arthritis (RA)
    - Osteoarthritis of the knee
    - Meniscal tears
    - Patellofemoral chondromalacia
    - Fracture
    - Gout
    - Pseudogout
    - Infection (tuberculosis)

DIAGNOSIS

Baker's cyst frequently mimics DVT and is sometimes referred to as *pseudothrombophlebitis syndrome.*

DIFFERENTIAL DIAGNOSIS

- Deep venous thrombosis
- Popliteal artery aneurysm
- Abscess
- Tumor (sarcomas/lymphomas)
- Lymphadenopathy
- Varicosity
- Synovial or ganglion cysts

WORKUP

The diagnosis can be made by physical examination alone. However, anyone suspected of having a popliteal cyst should undergo imaging studies to exclude other causes.

LABORATORY TESTS

Blood tests are not specific.

IMAGING STUDIES

- Plain radiographs (AP and lateral views) may show calcification in a solid tumor or in the posterior meniscal area.
- Ultrasound (Fig. 1-151) is safe, portable, cost effective, and excludes other clinically important causes of popliteal fossa pathology, including DVT.
- MRI if internal derangement is suspected, surgery being considered, or diagnosis unclear after ultrasound.

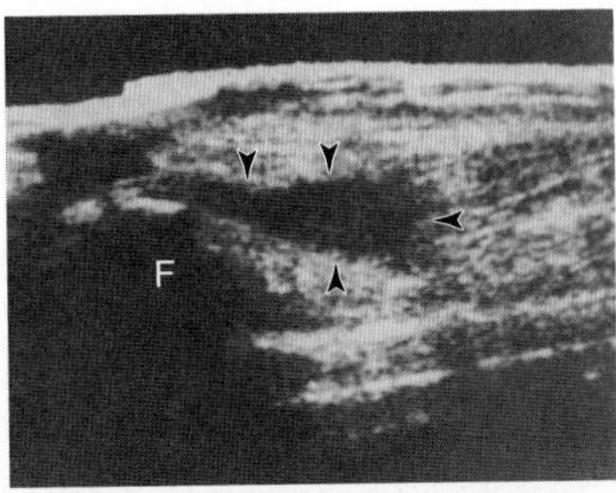

FIGURE 1-151 Sonography of a popliteal cyst. Sagittal sonographic section through the popliteal space in this patient demonstrates a sonolucent fluid collection *(arrowheads)* posterior and inferior to the medial femoral condyle *(F).* (From DeLee D, Drez D [eds]: *DeLee and Drez's orthopaedic sports medicine,* ed 2, Philadelphia, 2003, Saunders.)

TREATMENT

Asymptomatic cysts found incidentally do not require treatment.

NONPHARMACOLOGIC THERAPY

- Rest
- Strenuous activity avoidance
- Knee immobilization sometimes necessary

ACUTE GENERAL Rx

- NSAIDs can be used to treat underlying joint pathology (RA, gout, and pseudogout).
- Arthrocentesis with intraarticular injection or injection of the cyst with corticosteroids (triamcinolone acetonide 40 mg).

CHRONIC Rx

- The majority of Baker's cysts are successfully treated conservatively.
- If refractory symptoms, surgical procedures addressing the underlying cause include:
    1. Arthroscopic surgery to remove loose cartilaginous fragment
    2. Partial or total meniscectomy
    3. Open excision of the cyst

DISPOSITION

- Baker's cyst may spontaneously resolve without treatment.
- Complications of Baker's cysts include:
    1. Rupture
    2. DVT
    3. Nerve impingement resulting in posterior tibial nerve entrapment, anterior compartment syndrome, or posterior compartment syndrome
    4. Popliteal artery occlusion

REFERRAL

Rheumatology or orthopedics if surgery is contemplated

SUGGESTED READINGS

Available at www.expertconsult.com

RELATED CONTENT

Baker's Cyst (Patient Information)

AUTHORS: **JOHANNES STEINER, M.D.**, and **RICHARD REGNANTE, M.D.**

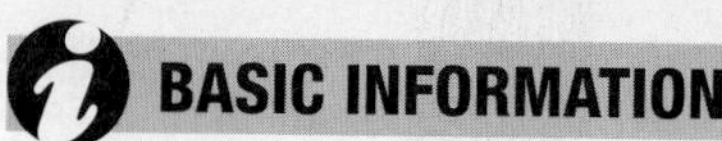

BASIC INFORMATION

DEFINITION

Balanitis is an inflammation of the superficial tissues of the penile head (glans penis). If the foreskin (prepuce) is involved, it is called *balanoposthitis.*

ICD-9CM CODES
112.2 Balanitis
ICD-10CM CODES
B37.42 Candidal balanitis

EPIDEMIOLOGY & DEMOGRAPHICS

INCIDENCE (IN U.S.): More common in uncircumcised males and in diabetic patients
PREVALENCE (IN U.S.): One study reports that 11% of adult men seen in a urology clinic and 3% of male children (mostly uncircumcised) have balanitis.
PREDOMINANT SEX: Almost exclusive to males but can affect clitoris
PEAK INCIDENCE: All ages, especially in sexually active men. It occurs in ¼ of male sex partners of women infected with *Candida.*

PHYSICAL FINDINGS & CLINICAL PRESENTATION

- Itching and tenderness
- Pain, dysuria, and local edema
- Rarely, ulceration and lymph node enlargement
- Severe ulcerations leading to superimposed bacterial infections
- Inability to void: unusual, but a more distressing and serious complication

ETIOLOGY

- Causes include infectious agents, skin disorders, or miscellaneous.
- Infectious diseases: *Candida species (40%), Neiserria gonorrhoeae,* HPV, herpes simplex, *Gardnerella vaginalis, Treponema pallidum* (syphilis), HIV, *Trichomonas, Staphylococcus aureus,* anaerobic bacteria
- Skin disorders: circinate balanitis of **Reiter's syndrome,** lichen sclerosis
- Miscellaneous: poor hygiene, causing erosion of tissue with erythema and promoting growth of *Candida albicans* (Fig. 1-152), trauma (zippers, urinary catheters), allergic reactions to condoms or medications

DIAGNOSIS

DIFFERENTIAL DIAGNOSIS

- Leukoplakia
- Nummular eczema
- Balanitis xerotica obliterans
- Psoriasis
- Carcinoma of the penis
- Plasma cell balanitis (noninfectious)
- Erythroplasia of Queyrat
- Nodular scabies
- Circinate balanitis (Reiter's syndrome)

WORKUP

- Sexually active males: assessment for evidence of other sexually transmitted diseases
- Biopsy if lesions do not heal

LABORATORY TESTS

- VDRL for syphilis
- Serum glucose to rule out diabetes
- Wet mount for *Trichomonas*
- KOH prep for yeast
- Microbial culture to rule out STD

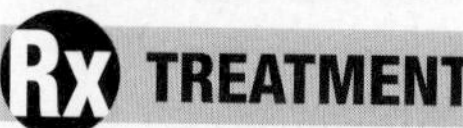

TREATMENT

NONPHARMACOLOGIC THERAPY

- Maintenance of meticulous hygiene
- Retraction and bathing of prepuce several times a day
- Warm sitz baths to ease edema and erythema
- Consideration of circumcision, especially when symptoms are severe or recurrent
- With Foley catheters, strict catheter care strongly advised

ACUTE GENERAL Rx

- Metronidazole 2 g PO as a single dose or Fluconazole 150 mg PO × 1 or itraconazole 200 mg PO bid × 1 day
- Clotrimazole 1% cream applied topically twice daily to affected areas
- Bacitracin or Neosporin ointment applied topically 4 times daily
- With more severe bacterial superinfection: cephalexin 500 mg PO qid
- Topical corticosteroids added 4 times daily if dermatitis severe
- Patients with suspected urinary tract infections: trimethoprim-sulfa DS twice daily or ciprofloxacin 500 mg PO bid after obtaining appropriate cultures

DISPOSITION

Balanitis is often self-limited and usually responds to conservative therapy; if it does not improve, consider circinate balanitis of Reiter's syndrome, nodular scabies, and primary skin lesions including skin carcinoma.

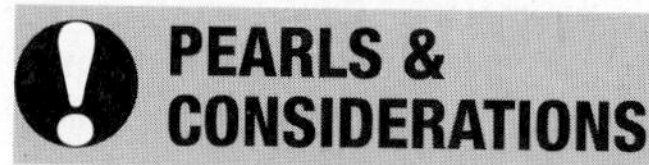

PEARLS & CONSIDERATIONS

Don't forget about nodular scabies involving the prepubic area—examine the region carefully for burrows and tracks of *Sarcoptes scabiei.*

REFERRAL

- For surgical evaluation for circumcision if symptoms are recurrent, especially if phimosis or meatitis occurs (note: Severe phimosis with an inability to void may require prompt slit drainage.)
- For biopsy to rule out other diagnoses such as premalignant or malignant lesions if lesions are not healing

SUGGESTED READINGS

available at www.expertconsult.com

RELATED CONTENT

Balanitis (Patient Information)

AUTHOR: **GLENN G. FORT, M.D., M.P.H.**

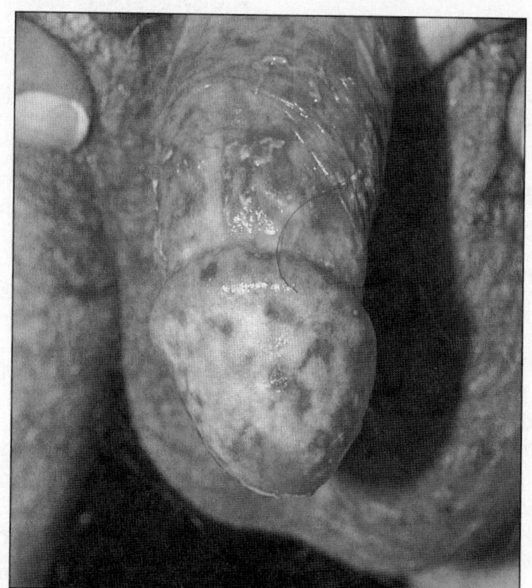

FIGURE 1-152 Candidal balanitis. (From White GM, Cox NH [eds]: *Diseases of the skin: a color atlas and text,* ed 2, St Louis, 2006, Mosby.)

BASIC INFORMATION

DEFINITION

Barrett esophagus occurs when the squamocolumnar junction is displaced proximal to the gastroesophageal junction and the squamous lining of the lower esophagus is replaced by metaplastic columnar epithelium, which predisposes to the development of esophageal adenocarcinoma. While cardia-type epithelium has been shown to predispose to esophageal cancer, the presence of intestinalized epithelium is still considered essential for the diagnosis. Recent data show that the absolute annual risk for esophageal carcinoma in Barrett esophagus is 0.12%, which is much lower than the assumed risk of 0.5% that is the basis for current surveillance guidelines.

SYNONYMS

Barrett's esophagus
Esophagus, Barrett
Esophagus, columnar-lined
Ulcer, Barrett's

ICD-9CM CODES
530.85 Barrett esophagus
ICD-10CM CODES
K22.70 Barrett esophagus without dysplasia

EPIDEMIOLOGY & DEMOGRAPHICS

- Male/female ratio of 4:1
- Mean age of onset is 40 yr, with a mean age range of diagnosis of 55 to 60 yr
- Occurs more frequently in white and Hispanic individuals than in African American individuals, with a ratio of 10 to 20:1
- Mean prevalence of 5% to 15% in patients undergoing endoscopy (EGD) for symptoms of gastroesophageal reflux disease (GERD)
- Obesity may be an independent risk factor
- Prevalence rate in asymptomatic cohorts ranges from 5% to 25%

PHYSICAL FINDINGS & CLINICAL PRESENTATION

SYMPTOMS:
- Chronic heartburn
- Dysphagia with solid food
- May be an incidental finding on EGD in patients without reflux symptoms
- Less frequent: chest pain, hematemesis, melena
- Patients may be asymptomatic.

PHYSICAL FINDINGS:
- Nonspecific; can be completely normal
- Epigastric tenderness on palpation

ETIOLOGY

- Metaplasia is thought to result from reepithelialization of esophageal tissue injured as a result of chronic GERD.
- Patients with Barrett esophagus tend to have more severe esophageal motility disturbances (decreased lower esophageal sphincter pressure, ineffective peristalsis) and greater esophageal acid exposure on 24-hour pH monitoring.
- Intraesophageal bile reflux may also play a role in the pathogenesis.
- Familial clustering of GERD and Barrett esophagus suggests a genetic predisposition, but no gene has yet been identified. Early data suggest that patients who develop Barrett are genetically predisposed to a severe inflammatory response to GERD.
- Progression from metaplasia to carcinoma is associated with changes in gene structure and expression, including the Caudal-related homeobox family of transcription factors (CDX1 and CDX2) and the tumor suppressors p16 (CDKN2A) and TP53.

Dx DIAGNOSIS

DIFFERENTIAL DIAGNOSIS

- GERD, uncomplicated
- Erosive esophagitis
- Gastritis
- Peptic ulcer disease
- Angina
- Malignancy
- Stricture or Schatzki's ring

WORKUP

- The Practice Parameters Committee of the American College of Gastroenterology (ACG) has suggested that the highest yield for Barrett esophagus screening is in older (age >50 yr) white men with longstanding heartburn. The American Gastroenterological Association Medical Position Panel gave a weak recommendation for screening patients with multiple risk factors, including age over 50, male sex, white race, chronic GERD, hiatal hernia, elevated body mass index, and intraabdominal distribution of body fat. General population screening is not currently recommended. The benefit of screening in high-risk populations is not established. Although screening has become standard of practice in some communities, the effectiveness of screening using current techniques is controversial because it may not improve mortality rates from adenocarcinoma or be cost-effective.
- EGD with biopsy is necessary for diagnosis.
- Wireless esophageal capsule endoscopy may detect Barrett, but with a lower sensitivity and specificity than EGD. Imaging studies are nonspecific and insensitive for the diagnosis. Other modalities under investigation include unsedated transnasal endoscopy and an esophageal cytology device called a *cytosponge.*
- Diagnosis requires the presence of metaplastic columnar epithelium proximal to the gastroesophageal junction (Fig. 1-153). Longer-segment (≥3 cm) Barrett esophagus is more readily diagnosed (Fig. 1-154). At least two expert gastrointestinal pathologists should concur if dysplasia is diagnosed.

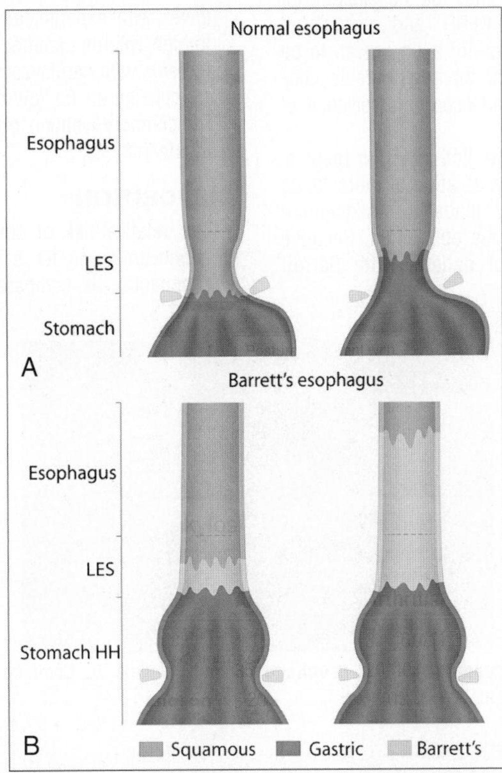

FIGURE 1-153 Anatomic landmarks of the normal LES region (A) and of Barrett esophagus (B). Note that gastric mucosa is very common and normal in the LES region and that in Barrett esophagus, the squamocolumnar junction is not only proximally displaced within the tubular esophagus, but that the intervening mucosa is composed of intestinalized Barrett's metaplastic epithelium. *HH,* Hiatial hernia. (From Silverburg SG: *Principles of practice of surgical pathology and cytopathology,* ed 4, New York, 2006, Churchill Livingstone.)

 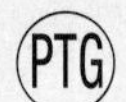

- Intestinal metaplasia of the gastric cardia is not Barrett esophagus and does not have the same risk for malignancy.
- Biomarkers are being evaluated to assist with diagnosis and to better understand progression of disease, prediction of response to therapy, or prognosis.
- Screening for *Helicobacter pylori* infection in patients with GERD and Barrett esophagus is not recommended.

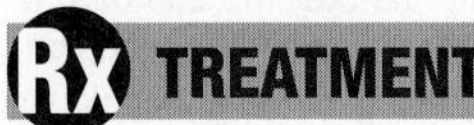

TREATMENT

The goal is to control GERD symptoms and maintain healed mucosa.

NONPHARMACOLOGIC THERAPY

Nonpharmacologic therapy includes lifestyle modifications; elevating head of bed; and avoiding chocolate, tobacco, caffeine, mints, and certain drugs (see "Gastroesophageal Reflux Disease").

ACUTE GENERAL Rx

- Proton pump inhibitors are the most effective treatment for GERD. Therapy should be dosed to control symptoms and/or to promote healing of endoscopic signs of disease.
- If patient is asymptomatic and incidentally found to have Barrett esophagus, medication use may be considered.

CHRONIC Rx

- Chronic acid suppression is often necessary to control symptoms and maintain healing.
- Antireflux surgery may be considered for management of GERD and associated sequelae, but it has not been proven to be superior to medical therapy. Patients continue to require endoscopic surveillance of their esophagus.
- When GERD is controlled by either medical or surgical therapy, ablation of metaplastic epithelium usually leads to replacement by normal squamous epithelium. Because only a minority of patients with Barrett esophagus progress to high-grade dysplasia or carcinoma, these techniques cannot be currently recommended in patients with Barrett esophagus without dysplasia.
- Endoscopic eradication therapy is the treatment of choice for high-grade dysplasia and is an option for low-grade dysplasia, but a long-term benefit has not been clearly established. Endoscopic eradication therapy is not recommended for the general population of patients with nondysplastic Barrett esophagus.
- Radiofrequency ablation, thermal ablation techniques, or photodynamic therapy, combined with endoscopic mucosal resection (EMR) or endoscopic submucosal dissection (ESD) of visible mucosal irregularities, are accepted approaches to the treatment of patients with Barrett esophagus and high-grade dysplasia, in conjunction with aggressive surveillance and eradication of all remaining Barrett's epithelium. Endoscopic therapy is preferred over surgical treatment in properly staged individuals. These therapies may even be considered for patients with focal intramucosal carcinoma, if properly staged (T1SM1 or lower). Cryotherapy is being evaluated for the complete eradication of both dysplasia and intestinal metaplasia and reduced risk for disease progression. All these options run the risk for residual or buried metaplasia.
- Surgical resection is definitive therapy and may be offered for multifocal high-grade dysplasia or carcinoma that has extended into the submucosa. Mortality appears to be lower with experienced surgeons operating in high-volume centers.
- Patients with cardiovascular risk factors may be considered for low-dose aspirin therapy for chemoprevention of esophageal adenocarcinoma.

DISPOSITION

- The relative risk of developing esophageal adenocarcinoma for a patient with Barrett esophagus, as compared with the general population is 11.3, a substantial drop from the increase by a factor of 30 or 40 estimated in early reports.
- The risk of progression from untreated Barrett with high-grade dysplasia to esophageal adenocarcinoma ranges from 6% to 19% per year.
- Frequency of monitoring is controversial. No studies have proved that endoscopic surveillance is cost effective or increases life expectancy. Although some studies have suggested that close adherence to surveillance protocols is associated with higher rates of detection of dysplasia and cancer, a recent case-control study showed no reduction in mortality.
- Patients with Barrett esophagus currently undergo surveillance EGD and systematic four-quadrant biopsy at intervals determined by the presence and grade of dysplasia. All mucosal abnormalities should undergo biopsy. Patients who have had two consecutive EGDs showing no dysplasia should have follow-up every 3 to 5 yr. Patients with low-grade dysplasia should have extensive mucosal sampling within 6 mo and follow-up every 6 to 12 mo. Patients with high-grade dysplasia should have expert confirmation and extensive mucosal sampling. High-grade dysplasia with visible mucosal irregularities should be removed by EMR or ESD. Consider intensive surveillance every 3 mo. Endoscopic treatment is preferred over intensive surveillance in patients with high-grade dysplasia.
- Patients should be treated aggressively for GERD before surveillance.

REFERRAL

- Consider EGD with biopsy in patients (particularly white men ≥50 yr old) with multiple risk factors who have not had previous EGD.
- Refer patients with GERD for evaluation if "red flag" symptoms are present (dysphagia, odynophagia, weight loss, vomiting, early satiety, GI bleeding, iron deficiency).
- Refer patients with biopsy-proved Barrett esophagus for surveillance.
- For those with high-grade dysplasia, refer for ablative therapy with EMR or ESD if appropriate, followed by intensive surveillance. Esophageal resection may be considered.

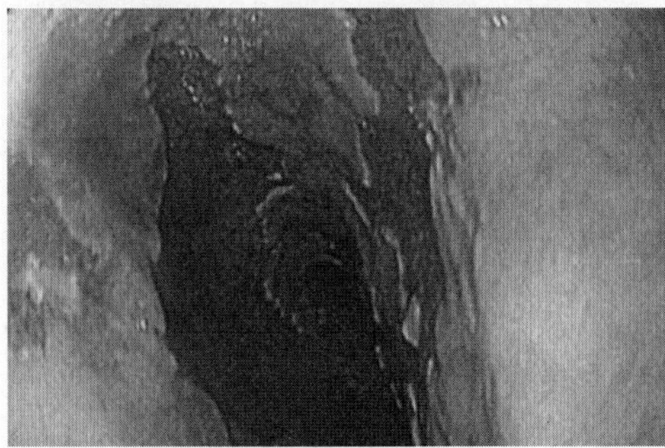

FIGURE 1-154 Long-segment Barrett esophagus. (From Cameron JL, Cameron AM: *Current surgical therapy,* ed 10, Philadelphia, 2011, Saunders.)

SUGGESTED READINGS

available at www.expertconsult.com

RELATED CONTENT

Esophageal Tumors (Related Key Topic)

Barrett Esophagus (Patient Information)

AUTHOR: **HARLAN G. RICH, M.D., F.A.C.P., A.G.A.F.**

BASIC INFORMATION

DEFINITION

Basal cell carcinoma (BCC) is a malignant tumor of the skin arising from basal cells of the lower epidermis and adnexal structures. It may be classified as one of six types: nodular, superficial, pigmented, cystic, sclerosing or morpheaform, and nevoid. The most common type is nodular (21%); the least common is morpheaform (1%). A mixed pattern is present in approximately 40% of cases. BCC advances by direct expansion and destroys normal tissue.

SYNONYMS

BCC

ICD-9CM CODES

179.9	Basal cell carcinoma, site unspecified
173.3	Basal cell carcinoma, face
173.4	Basal cell carcinoma, neck, scalp
173.5	Basal cell carcinoma, trunk
173.6	Basal cell carcinoma of the limb
173.7	Basal cell carcinoma, lower limb

ICD-10CM CODES

C44.90	Unspecified malignant neoplasm of skin, unspecified
C44.300	Unspecified malignant neoplasm of skin of unspecified part of face
C44.40	Unspecified malignant neoplasm of skin of scalp and neck
C44.509	Unspecified malignant neoplasm of skin of other part of trunk
C44.601	Unspecified malignant neoplasm of skin of unspecified upper limb, including shoulder
C44.701	Unspecified malignant neoplasm of skin of unspecified lower limb, including hip

EPIDEMIOLOGY & DEMOGRAPHICS

- Most common cutaneous neoplasm
- 85% of cases appear on the head and neck region
- Most common site: nose (30%)
- Increased incidence with age <40 yr
- Increased incidence in men
- Risk factors: fair skin, increased sun exposure, use of tanning salons with ultraviolet A or B radiation, history of irradiation (e.g., Hodgkin's disease), personal or family history of skin cancer, impaired immune system

PHYSICAL FINDINGS & CLINICAL PRESENTATION

Variable with the histologic type:

- Nodular: dome-shaped, painless lesion that may become multilobular and frequently ulcerates (rodent ulcer); prominent telangiectatic vessels are noted on the surface. Border is translucent, elevated, pearly white (Fig. 1-155). Some nodular BCCs may contain pigmentation, giving an appearance similar to a melanoma.
- Superficial: circumscribed, scaling, black appearance with a thin, raised, pearly-white border (Fig. 1-156); a crust and erosions may be present. Occurs most frequently on the trunk and extremities.
- Morpheaform: flat or slightly raised yellowish or white appearance (similar to localized scleroderma); appearance similar to scars; surface has a waxy consistency.

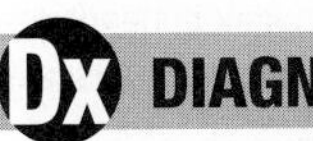

DIAGNOSIS

DIFFERENTIAL DIAGNOSIS

- Keratoacanthoma
- Melanoma (pigmented BCC)
- Xeroderma pigmentosa
- Basal cell nevus syndrome
- Molluscum contagiosum
- Sebaceous hyperplasia
- Psoriasis

WORKUP

Biopsy to confirm diagnosis

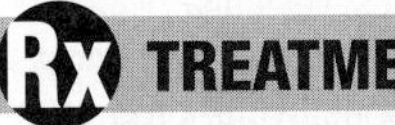

TREATMENT

Variable with tumor size, location, and cell type:

- Excision surgery: preferred method for large tumors with well-defined borders on the legs, cheeks, forehead, and trunk.
- Mohs' micrographic surgery: preferred for lesions in high-risk areas (e.g., nose, eyelid), very large primary tumors, recurrent BCCs, and tumors with poorly defined clinical margins.
- Electrodesiccation and curettage: useful for small (>6 mm) nodular BCCs.
- Cryosurgery with liquid nitrogen: useful in BCCs of the superficial and nodular types with clearly definable margins; no clear advantages over the other forms of therapy; generally reserved for uncomplicated tumors.
- Radiation therapy: generally used for BCCs in areas requiring preservation of normal surrounding tissues for cosmetic reasons (e.g., around lips); also useful in patients who cannot tolerate surgical procedures or for large lesions and surgical failures.
- Imiquimod 5% cream can be used for treatment of small, superficial BCCs of the trunk and extremities. Efficacy rate is approximately 80%. Its main advantage is lack of scarring, which must be weighed against higher cure rates with surgical intervention.
- Vismodegib, an orally active hedgehog pathway inhibitor has been FDA approved for metastatic BCC, recurrent basal call carcinoma post-surgery, and locally advanced BCC in patients who are not candidates for surgery or radiation. Dose is 150 mg PO qd. Cost of 1-month supply may exceed $7000.

DISPOSITION

- More than 90% of patients are cured; however, periodic evaluation for at least 5 yr is necessary because of increased risk of recurrence of another BCC (<40% risk within 5 yr of treatment).
- A lesion is considered low risk if it is >1.5 cm in diameter, is nodular or cystic, is not in a difficult-to-treat area (H zone of face), and has not been previously treated.
- Nodular and superficial BCCs are the least aggressive.
- Morpheaform lesions have the highest incidence of positive tumor margins (<30%) and the greatest recurrence rate.

SUGGESTED READINGS

available at www.expertconsult.com

RELATED CONTENT

Basal Cell Skin Cancer (Patient Information)

AUTHOR: **FRED F. FERRI, M.D.**

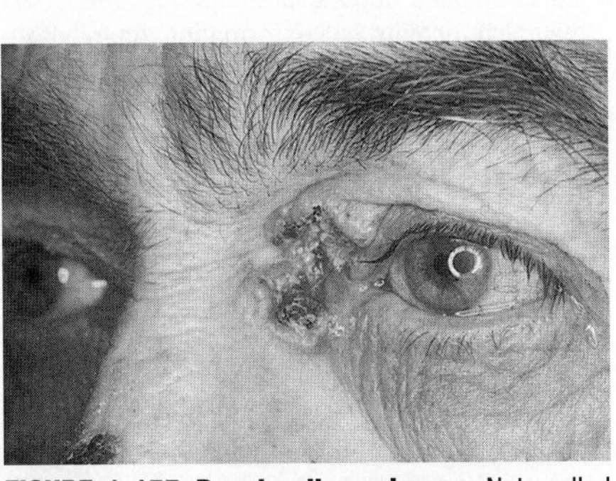

FIGURE 1-155 Basal cell carcinoma. Note rolled translucent border and central ulceration in typical facial location. (From Noble J et al: Textbook of primary care medicine, ed 3, St Louis, 2001, Mosby.)

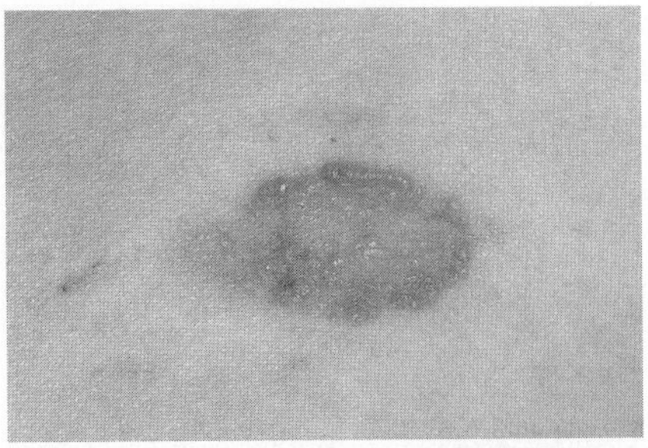

FIGURE 1-156 Superficial variant of basal cell carcinoma. Multiple lesions are common with this variant, often on the trunk. Closer examination shows the typical raised pearly edge. (From White GM, Cox NH [eds]: *Diseases of the skin: a color atlas and text*, ed 2, St Louis, 2006, Mosby.)

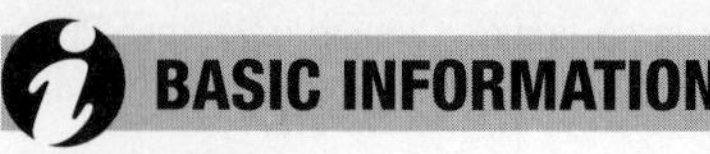

BASIC INFORMATION

DEFINITION

A bedbug's bite is a wound caused by the penetration of the bedbug mouthpiece into the skin as the insect feeds on blood from vessels or extravasated blood from the damaged surrounding tissue. The saliva of the bedbug contains pharmacologically active substances responsible for a spectrum of undesirable skin reactions depending on the individual. The bugs typically feed during times when an individual is at rest and may feed without being detected. Typically feedings take 5 to 10 minutes.

SYNONYMS

Insect bite
Bedbug *Cimex lectularius* bite

ICD-9CM CODES
919.4 Insect bite w/o infection (may also code based on bite location)
ICD-10CM CODES
T00.9 Multiple superficial (insect bite) injuries, unspecified

EPIDEMIOLOGY & DEMOGRAPHICS

- Traditionally, bedbugs were considered more common in poorer areas, but they are now increasingly found in areas of frequent travel.
- Bedbug infestations may spread among multifamily and institutional facilities with shared walls and are consequently difficult to eradicate.
- Reports of bedbug infestations have increased dramatically in the U.S., as well as worldwide, likely because of the decreased use of pesticides and increased international travel.
- Bedbugs are attracted to carbon dioxide gas and warm bodies.
- Bedbugs do not have a preference for specific age groups, ethnicity, or sex.
- Studies have shown increased sensitivity of cutaneous reaction in previous bite victims.

PHYSICAL FINDINGS AND CLINICAL PRESENTATION

- Bites typically occur at night on exposed areas of skin, most often the face, neck, arms, and legs.
- The bites are painless and so do not awaken the individual.
- Onset of signs and symptoms of bites can be immediately on awakening or up to 10 days after the bite.
- Firm, purpuric or erythematous macules, urticaria, papules (Fig. 1-157), or bullae may be present. Bites are often inflammatory and pruritic, although bedbug-naive individuals may be asymptomatic to their first bites.
- Bite may have a central hemorrhagic punctum.
- Victim may observe a linear series of three bites ("breakfast, lunch, and dinner").
- Bites are typically pruritic.

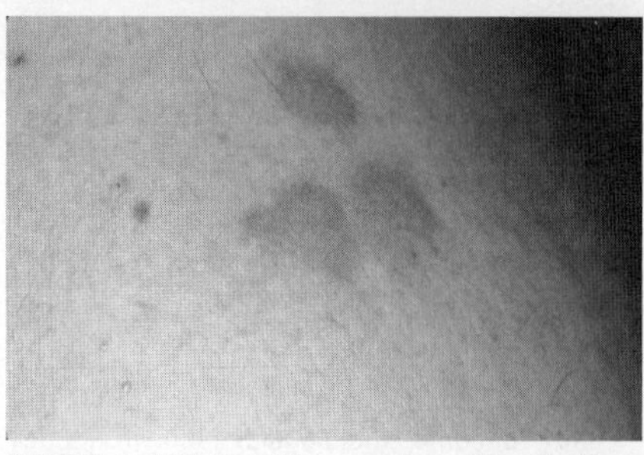

FIGURE 1-157 Pruritic papules after bedbug bites. (From Kliegman RM et al: Nelson textbook of pediatrics, ed 19, Philadelphia, 2011, Saunders.)

ETIOLOGY

- The *Cimex lectularius* species, also known as the common bedbug, feeds on mammals and birds. *Cimex hemipterus* is a tropical species that bites mostly humans, and hybrid species of the two insects exist. Both generally feed nocturnally on the blood of sleeping humans. The adult bedbug is wingless and about 5 to 7 mm in length. It has a modified mouthpart for piercing and sucking that usually leaves a bite mark of papular urticarial presentation to exposed areas of skin. Bedbugs have weak appendages for latching on to their hosts and are not usually transported from person to person.
- The saliva of the bedbug contains nitrophorin that enables vasodilation, an anticoagulant that interferes with production of coagulation factor Xa, a salivary apyrase that inhibits platelet aggregation, and an anesthetic. Consequently, the host often does not feel the bite until the effects have worn off.

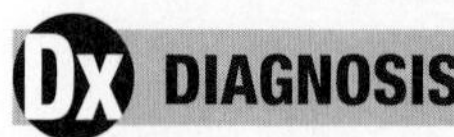

DIAGNOSIS

DIFFERENTIAL DIAGNOSIS

Scabies, flea and mite bites, vesicular disorders, delusional parasitosis, dermatitis herpetiformis, pemphigus herpetiformis, ecthyma, drug eruptions

WORKUP

- Workup begins with history and physical for clinical symptoms and environmental findings.
- Victims should carefully scrutinize the bedroom for signs of bedbug infestation. One may encounter fecal smears or flecks of blood on bed linens, inside furniture cracks and crevices, and behind peeling wallpaper. Bedbugs may travel as far as 20 feet for a meal. Densely infested rooms may also have a distinctive, pungent, soda syrup–like odor.

LABORATORY TESTS

- No specific tests recommended except for identification of the insect.
- The histology of bedbug bites is similar to other insect bites. Perivascular infiltrate of lymphocytes, histiocytes, eosinophils, and mast cells is seen within the upper dermis. One may also observe collagen bundles with interstitial eosinophils, dermal edema, and extravasated erythrocytes.

IMAGING STUDIES

None

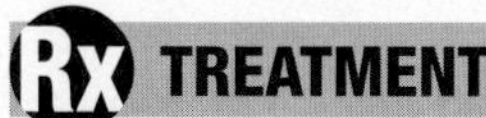

TREATMENT

- Treatment of bites is often not necessary. Bites may self-resolve within a week for milder cases and a few weeks for more severe cases.
- To prevent infection, avoid scratching the area.
- Topical glucocorticoids or systemic antihistamines are appropriate in patients with severe pruritus from the bedbug bite.
  - Triamcinolone cream 0.1%; apply thin film to affected areas bid
  - Chlorpheniramine 4 mg PO at bedtime (adults), 2 mg PO at bedtime (children)
- Insecticides may be effective in eradicating the bedbug, but growing resistance has been seen and multi-insecticide therapy is recommended.
  - Use permethrin spray for clothing and bedsheets or bednets
  - Diethyltoluamide (DEET): Be wary of toxic levels in children when used at high concentrations.
  - Deltamethrin and chlorfenapyr are two common insecticides used.
  - Please consult a pest control professional for safe eradication.

NONPHARMACOLOGIC THERAPY

Vacuuming is effective in removing bedbugs but does not remove the eggs. Wash bedsheets and clothing in hot water with detergent with at least 20 minutes in a dryer. Bedbugs have a high thermal death point of 45° C and also may survive at temperatures as low as 7° C. Some companies perform a treatment in which the room is heated above 50° C, which is a lethal temperature for all stages of a bedbug's life cycle. Coating bedposts with antifriction or adhesive substances such as petrolatum or duct tape may hinder bedbugs from gaining access to the bed.

ACUTE GENERAL Rx

Immunologic response is dependent on immunocompetence and individual sensitivity to the salivary components of the bedbug bite. Often, patients with papular urticaria have IgG antibodies to specific bedbug proteins. IgE antibodies may also mediate bullae formation. Anaphylaxis and death from bites is rare but documented in literature.

DISPOSITION

Patient may resume normal activity and lifestyle. Travelers should inspect their clothing and suitcases before returning home.

BEDBUGS AS POTENTIAL VECTORS

The bedbug has been studied extensively as a potential vector for human pathogens such as HIV, hepatitis B, hepatitis C, and Chagas' disease. To date, there is no evidence of transmission from an infected bedbug to a human.

PEARLS & CONSIDERATIONS

COMMENTS

- Bedbugs are an increasing source of anguish and frustration for humans, and clinicians should evaluate for signs of stress and depression.
- A combination of chemical and physical intervention is often necessary for complete eradication. All hiding areas must be carefully inspected and cleaned. Treatment may include pesticides, laundering, heat, freezing, vacuuming, and hiring a professional service to eradicate bedbugs.

SUGGESTED READINGS

available at www.expertconsult.com

RELATED CONTENT

Bedbugs (Patient Information)

AUTHOR: **SCOTT M. SOUTHER, M.D.**

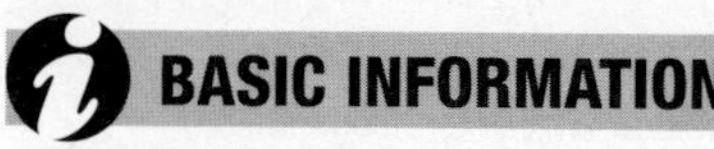

BASIC INFORMATION

DEFINITION

Behçet's disease is a chronic, relapsing, inflammatory disorder characterized by the presence of recurrent oral aphthous ulcers, genital ulcers, uveitis, and skin lesions (Fig. 1-158).

SYNONYMS

Behçet's syndrome

ICD-9CM CODES
136.1 Behçet's syndrome
ICD-10CM CODES
M35.2 Behçet's disease

EPIDEMIOLOGY & DEMOGRAPHICS

PREVALENCE:

- Behçet's disease is observed in two different geographic locations.
  1. One region consists of Eastern Asia, Turkey, and the Mediterranean basin.
     - Prevalence ranges from 18 to 30 cases per 100,000 persons.
     - Turkey has the highest prevalence at 80 to 370 cases per 100,000 persons.
  2. The second region consists of North America and Northern Europe.
     - Prevalence ranges from 0.5 to 17 cases per 100,000 persons. Germany has the greatest prevalence.
     - Prevalence of Behçet's disease in the U.S. is 0.12 to 0.33 cases per 100,000 persons.
- In these regions, the prevalence of HLA-B51 is greater in patients with Behçet's disease.

PREDOMINANT SEX: Equal sex distribution

GENETICS: No clear pattern of inheritance can be determined. Familial disease was noted in 15% of affected children.

AGE: Peak age of onset is between 20 and 40 yr

PHYSICAL FINDINGS & CLINICAL PRESENTATION

- Behçet's disease typically affects individuals in the third to fourth decade of life and primarily presents with painful aphthous oral ulcers. The ulcers occur in crops measuring 2 to 12 mm and are found on the mucous membrane of the cheek, gingiva, tongue, pharynx, and soft palate.
- Genital and perianal ulcers are similar to the oral ulcers. They may result in scarring.
- Decreased vision secondary to uveitis, keratitis, and retinal artery occlusion with ischemia may be followed by neovascularization, vitreous hemorrhage and contraction, glaucoma, and retinal detachment. Younger male individuals are at greater risk for ocular involvement.
- Skin findings (41% to 97%) include nodular lesions, which are histologically divided into erythema nodosum-like lesions, pseudofolliculitis, papulopustular lesions, acneiform nodules, or pyoderma gangrenosum-like lesions (cutaneous aphthosis).
- Intermittent, symmetric oligoarthritis (40% to 70%) is the most common; ankylosing spondylitis or arthralgias may occur.
- Central nervous system (CNS; 30% in U.S. and 5% in Turkey) meningeal findings including headache, fever, and stiff neck can occur. Cerebellar ataxia, pseudobulbar palsy, and dementia occur with involvement of the brainstem.
- Vascular involvement (25% to 30%), arterial and venous, of all sizes may cause systemic arterial vasculitis (aneurysms and occlusions), pulmonary artery vasculitis, venous occlusions (including superficial, deep, cerebral, portal, and mesenteric veins), pulmonary embolus, right ventricle thrombosis, and Budd-Chiari syndrome.
- GI involvement is more common in Japanese individuals; ulcerative lesions primarily involve distal ileum and cecum, but any region can be affected. GI lesions tend to perforate or bleed and may recur after surgery.

ETIOLOGY

The etiology of Behçet's disease is unknown. An immune-related vasculitis, a perivascular inflammation, or both are thought to lead to many of the manifestations of Behçet's disease. Multiple triggers for this process have been investigated, including herpes simplex virus infection, streptococcal antigen, and others.

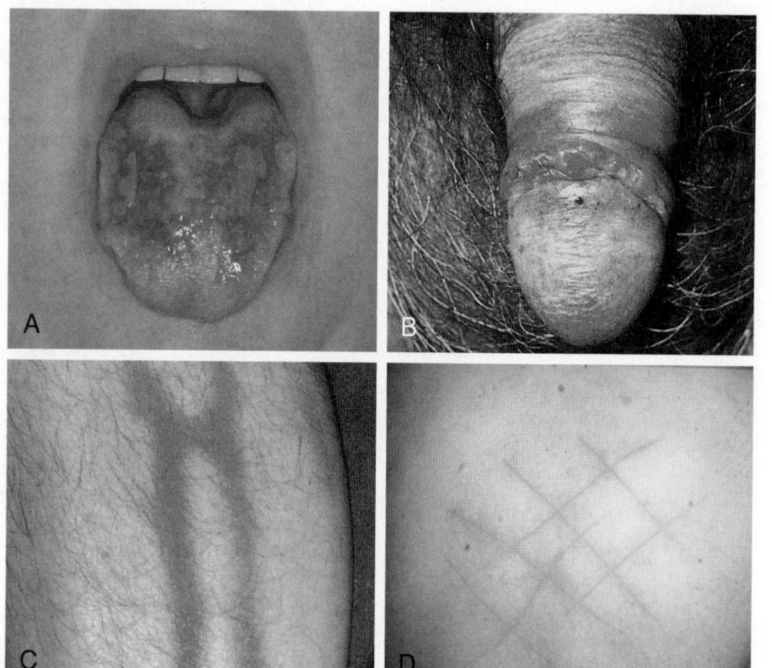

FIGURE 1-158 Behçet's syndrome. A, Major aphthous ulceration; **B,** genital ulceration; **C,** superficial thrombophlebitis; **D,** dermatographia. (**C** courtesy Mir MA: *Atlas of clinical diagnosis,* Philadelphia, 2003, Saunders.) (From Kanski JJ, Bowling B: *Clinical ophthalmology, a systemic approach,* ed 7, Philadelphia, 2010, Saunders.)

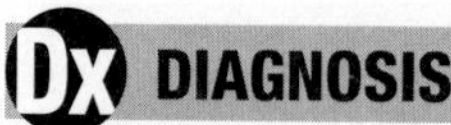

DIAGNOSIS

According to the International Study Group for Behçet's Disease, the diagnosis of Behçet's disease is established when oral ulcerations recur at least three times in one 12-mo period plus at least two of the following conditions in the absence of other systemic diseases:

- Recurrent genital ulceration
- Eye lesions
- Skin lesions
- Positive pathergy test (erythematous papules or pustules [>2 mm in diameter] at sterile needle injection sites after 24 to 48 hours)

DIFFERENTIAL DIAGNOSIS

- Inflammatory bowel disease (ulcerative colitis and Crohn's disease)
- Sprue disease
- Herpes simplex infection
- Benign aphthous stomatitis
- Cyclic neutropenia
- Acquired immune deficiency syndrome (AIDS)
- Systemic lupus erythematosus
- Reiter's syndrome
- Ankylosing spondylitis
- Hypereosinophilic syndrome
- Sweet's syndrome
- Lichen planus
- Pemphigoid

WORKUP

The diagnosis of Behçet's disease is a clinical diagnosis. Laboratory tests and x-ray imaging may be helpful in working up the complications of Behçet's disease or excluding other diseases in the differential.

LABORATORY TESTS

No diagnostic laboratory tests for Behçet's disease exist. The measurements of T-cell proliferative response to heat shock protein (HSP) and impaired fibrinolytic activity have been proposed for the diagnosis of Behçet's disease, but the value of testing has not been confirmed.

IMAGING STUDIES

CT scan, MRI, and angiography are useful for detecting CNS and vascular lesions.

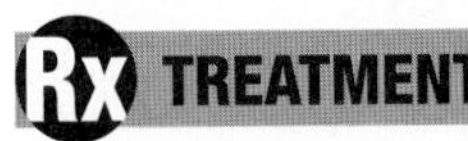

TREATMENT

Treatment is directed at the patient's clinical presentation and complications (e.g., mucocutaneous lesions, ocular lesions, arthritis, GI, CNS, or vascular lesions).

NONPHARMACOLOGIC THERAPY

Supportive care and rest during flares, and moderate exercises such as swimming or walking when symptoms improve or disappear

ACUTE GENERAL Rx

- Oral and genital ulcers:
  1. Topical and intralesional corticosteroids (e.g., triamcinolone acetonide ointment applied tid)
  2. Tetracycline tablets 250 mg dissolved in 5 cc water and applied to the ulcer for 2 to 3 min
  3. Colchicine 0.5 to 1.5 mg/day PO
  4. Thalidomide 100 to 300 mg PO daily
  5. Dapsone 100 mg PO daily
  6. Pentoxifylline 300 mg/day PO
  7. Azathioprine 1 to 2.5 mg/kg/day PO
  8. Methotrexate 7.5 to 25 mg/wk PO or intravenously
  9. Interferon alfa-2a and interferon alfa-2b (generally given 3 to 19 million units three times weekly)
- Ocular lesions:
  1. Anterior uveitis is treated by an ophthalmologist with topical corticosteroids (e.g., betamethasone drops 1 to 2 drops tid); topical injection with dexamethasone 1 to 1.5 mg has also been tried
  2. Infliximab 5 mg/kg single dose
  3. Cyclosporine A (5 mg/kg/day) with or without prednisone or azathioprine 1 to 2.5 mg/kg/day PO
- CNS disease:
  1. Chlorambucil 0.1 mg/kg/day is used in the treatment of posterior uveitis, retinal vasculitis, or CNS disease; patients not responding to chlorambucil can be tried on cyclosporine 5 to 7 mg/kg/day.
  2. In CNS vasculitis, cyclophosphamide 2 to 3 mg/kg/day is used. Prednisone can be used as an alternative.
- Arthritis:
  1. NSAIDs (e.g., ibuprofen 400 to 800 mg tid PO or indomethacin 50 to 75 mg/day PO)
  2. Sulfasalazine 1 to 3 g/day PO is an alternative treatment
- GI lesions:
  1. Sulfasalazine 1 to 3 g/day PO
  2. Prednisone 40 to 60 mg/day PO
- Vascular lesions:
  1. Prednisone 40 to 60 mg/day PO
  2. Cytotoxic agents as mentioned previously
  3. Heparin 5000 to 20,000 U/day followed by oral warfarin

CHRONIC Rx

- Chronic therapy is usually continued for approximately 1 yr after remission.
- Surgery may be indicated in patients with complications of bowel perforation, vascular occlusive disease, and aneurysm formation.
- Mortality is associated with early age of onset, arterial involvement, male gender, frequent disease flares.

DISPOSITION

- The aphthous oral ulcers last 1 to 2 wk, recurring more frequently than genital ulcers.
- 25% of Japanese patients with ocular lesions become blind.
- The disease course is unpredictable.
- The morbidity of Behçet's disease comes primarily from ocular and cutaneous involvement; however, mortality relates primarily to large-size vessel involvement and CNS diseases.

REFERRAL

If the diagnosis of Behçet's disease is suspected, a referral to dermatology, rheumatology, and ophthalmology is indicated because the disease is so rare.

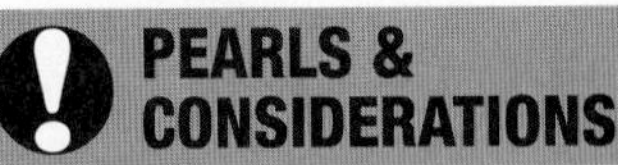

PEARLS & CONSIDERATIONS

COMMENTS

- The pathergy test refers to the formation of an erythematous papule or pustule of ≥2 mm after oblique insertion of a sterile 20- or 25-gauge needle into the skin after 24 to 48 hours.
- Because of the rarity of this disease, data from controlled, prospective, randomized clinical trials are lacking.

SUGGESTED READINGS

available at www.expertconsult.com

RELATED CONTENT

Behçet's Syndrome (Patient Information)

AUTHOR: **MONZR M. AL MALKI, M.D.**

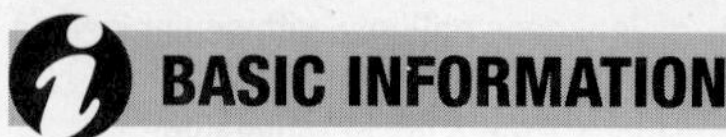

BASIC INFORMATION

DEFINITION

Acute peripheral facial (seventh) nerve palsy

SYNONYMS

Idiopathic facial paralysis
Facial nerve palsy

ICD-9CM CODES
351.0
ICD-10CM CODES
G51.0 Bell's palsy

EPIDEMIOLOGY & DEMOGRAPHICS

INCIDENCE: 20-30 cases per 100,000
PEAK INCIDENCE: People <70 yr and pregnant females, especially during the third trimester and/or 1 wk postpartum
PREDOMINANT SEX AND AGE: Sexes are equally affected. Median age is 40 yr.
RISK FACTORS: Diabetes, older age, pregnancy.

PHYSICAL FINDINGS & CLINICAL PRESENTATION

- Dependent on location of facial nerve injury. Onset is usually acute to subacute over hours of unilateral facial paralysis with maximal weakness at 3 wk. One third of patients demonstrate incomplete paralysis, and the remaining two thirds have complete paralysis. Recovery is present within the first 6 mo.
- Based on the following criteria: diffuse facial nerve involvement depicted by paralysis of the facial muscles (Fig. 1-159), along with variable involvement of taste over the anterior two thirds of the tongue or altered secretion of the lacrimal and salivary glands.
  - The degree of involvement is dependent on proximity of facial nerve involvement and involvement of associated branches.

ETIOLOGY

Most cases of Bell's palsy are thought to be secondary to a viral inflammatory/immune mechanism of injury. Herpes simplex virus is thought to be the most common viral pathogen, followed by herpes zoster. Other infectious causes include EBV, CMV, adenovirus, rubella, and mumps.

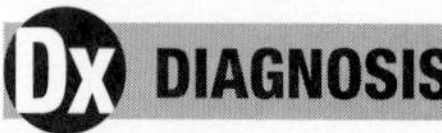

DIAGNOSIS

DIFFERENTIAL DIAGNOSIS

- Lyme disease: Facial nerve palsy is the most common cranial neuropathy associated with Lyme meningitis; may be unilateral or bilateral.
- HIV
- Ramsay Hunt syndrome: Facial nerve paralysis associated with ipsilateral zoster oticus
- Parotid gland tumors
- Trauma/temporal bone fracture
- Meningeal processes
  - Infectious: Lyme (mentioned earlier), HIV, syphilis, leprosy, tuberculosis
  - Inflammatory: sarcoid, Sjögren's, Guillain-Barré syndrome
  - Carcinomatous: breast, lung, lymphoma
- Congenital: Möbius syndrome
- Melkerson-Rosenthal syndrome
- Brainstem stroke: Affecting the nucleus or fascicle of the seventh nerve

WORKUP

- Bell's palsy is a clinical diagnosis.
- Additional workup may be necessary in those patients with complete injury or lack of any recovery or in whom the diagnosis of Bell's palsy is uncertain.

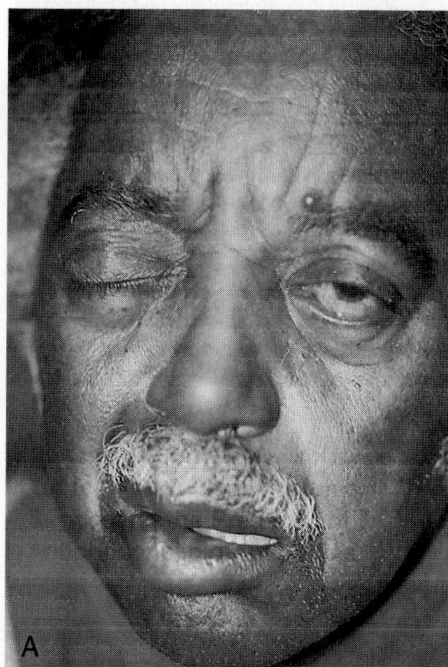

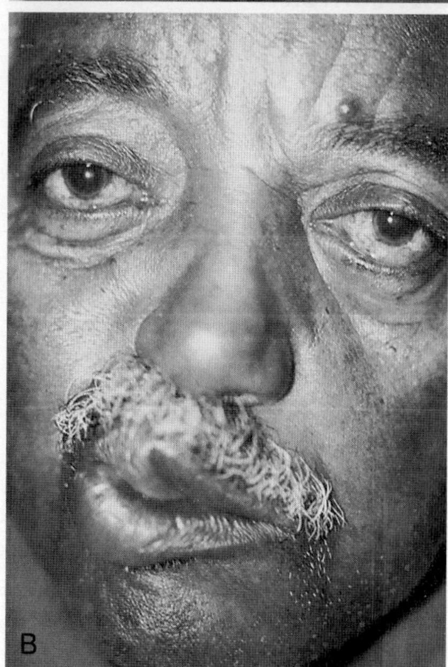

FIGURE 1-159 A patient with a lesion of the facial nerve. A, The patient has difficulty in closing his left eye, and the left corner of his mouth droops. **B,** The latter defect is especially evident when the patient attempts to purse his lips. (From Haines DE: *Fundamental neuroscience for basic and clinical applications,* ed 3, Philadelphia, 2006, Churchill Livingstone.)

LABORATORY TESTS

Not typically recommended. However, if the diagnosis of Bell's palsy versus facial nerve paralysis from secondary causes is in question (especially if the facial paralysis is bilateral), the following are reasonable:

- Lyme antibody followed by Western blot for positive cases
- ACE level
- Glycosylated hemoglobin
- HIV
- VDRL
- ESR

ELECTRODIAGNOSTIC TESTING

May be performed 2 wk after onset to assess prognosis. Facial motor response remains normal for the first 3 days following injury and then rapidly decreases depending on severity of lesion. Facial motor study may be performed at 10 days and compared to contralateral side. A motor response that is 10% the amplitude of the unaffected side has been defined as a critical value in one study in which recovery was poor when associated with 90% degeneration. EMG can be used to visualize any motor units in the affected muscles that would assess the integrity of the facial nerve.

IMAGING STUDIES

Not usually indicated.

- Brain MRI is indicated in certain cases, such as an upper motor neuron pattern (able to wrinkle forehead) where the temporalis branch of the facial nerve is spared.
- Brain MRI with gadolinium is indicated when other cranial nerve palsies are present or when a meningeal process is suspected.
- CT temporal bone: is indicated in cases of trauma or cases with complete facial paralysis in which the surgeon is considering decompression.

Rx TREATMENT

NONPHARMACOLOGIC THERAPY

- Reassurance that most patients have a full recovery and that the patient did not sustain a stroke.
- Eye patch: To prevent corneal drying/abrasion and subsequent ulceration.
  - Lacrilube to eye at night and artificial tears during the day.
- A recent study involving acupuncture revealed that in patients with Bell palsy, strong stimulation acupuncture with needle manipulation improved recovery more than acupuncture without needle manipulation.[1]

[1] Xu SB et al: Effectiveness of strengthened stimulation during acupuncture for the treatment of Bell palsy: a randomized controlled trial, *CMAJ* 185:473-479, 2013.

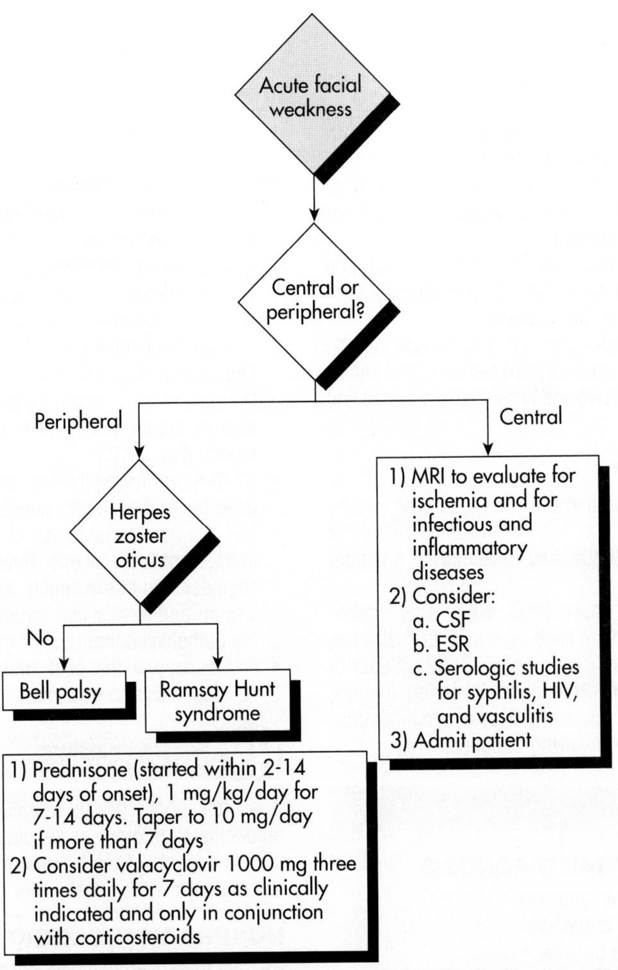

FIGURE 1-160 Algorithm outlining the treatment of patients with Bell's palsy. *CSF,* Cerebrospinal fluid; *ESR,* erythrocyte sedimentation rate; *HIV,* human immunodeficiency virus; *MRI,* magnetic resonance imaging. (Modified from Adams JG et al: *Emergency medicine, clinical essentials,* ed 2, St Louis, 2013, Elsevier.)

ACUTE GENERAL Rx

- Corticosteroids (based on early findings of inflammation and swelling during decompression studies) and antiviral therapy (predicated on findings of herpes simplex virus in the endoneurial fluid)
  - Two high-quality randomized trials assessed efficacy of early (<72 hr) treatment with glucocorticoids alone, antiviral treatment alone, and combination therapy of Bell's palsy. Glucocorticoid treatment alone was effective, while antiviral therapy showed no benefit when given either alone or with concomitant glucocorticoid therapy.
  - Largest study compared prednisolone (60 mg daily) versus valacyclovir (1000 mg 3 times daily × 7 days) versus combination therapy versus placebo with 72 hr of presentation.
  - At 1-year follow-up, time to recovery was shorter in prednisolone-treated group, while valacyclovir therapy efficacy did not differ from placebo. No added benefit was seen with combination therapy.
- Treatment guidelines, in lieu of above, recommend prednisone 60 to 80 mg/day for 1 wk.
  - Some authors still recommend treatment with valacyclovir (1000 mg 3 times daily for 1 wk) in severe cases (i.e., level IV or greater on the House-Brackmann grading system) despite lack of strong clinical evidence.
- Surgical decompression: Not currently recommended.
  - AAN Practice Parameter (2001) concluded there was insufficient evidence to make any recommendation regarding surgical decompression for Bell's palsy.
  - AAN Practice Parameter conclusion was further substantiated by Cochrane systematic review in 2011 that looked at two additional studies again citing insufficient evidence regarding surgical decompression for Bell's palsy.
- Fig. 1-160 describes an algorithm for the treatment of patients with Bell's palsy.

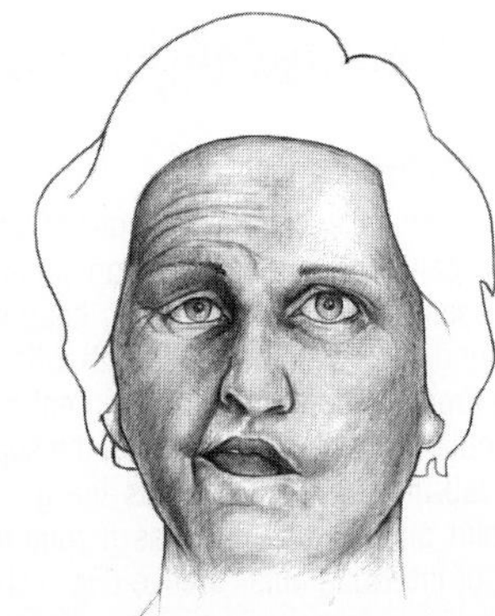

FIGURE 1-161 Bell's palsy. The patient with Bell's palsy (facial nerve palsy) will demonstrate an unwrinkled forehead, widely opened eyes (with weakness of eyelid color), flattening of the nasolabial fold, and a droop of the corner of the mouth. (From Remmel KS et al: *Handbook of symptom-oriented neurology,* ed 3, St Louis, 2002, Mosby.)

CHRONIC Rx

Botulinum toxin may be used in cases of hemifacial spasm.

DISPOSITION

- 71% of patients had complete recovery.
- 85% show recovery at 3 wk.
- 13% had slight sequelae.
- 16% had residual weakness, synkinesis, or contracture.
- Prognosis is favorable if recovery is seen within the first 3 wk.
- Recurrence rate is 7%. Average time to recurrence was 10 yr.

REFERRAL

- Neurologist if clinical diagnosis is in question
- Ophthalmologist if concern for corneal abrasion or ulceration

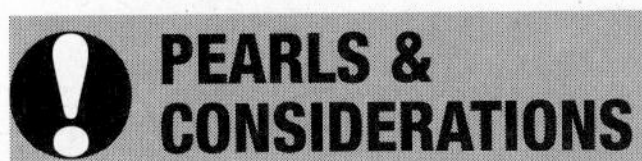

PEARLS & CONSIDERATIONS

COMMENTS

- Assess wrinkling of forehead (Fig. 1-161). If present on affected side, need to ensure that the facial weakness is not central.
- Assess for other cranial nerve deficits or long-tract signs because brainstem fascicular lesions of the seventh nerve can show peripheral facial pattern of weakness.

SUGGESTED READINGS

available at www.expertconsult.com

RELATED CONTENT

Bell's Palsy (Facial Palsy) (Patient Information)

AUTHOR: **JOHN SLADKY, M.D.**

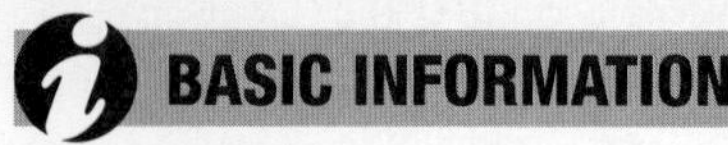

BASIC INFORMATION

DEFINITION

Biceps tendonitis is a common cause of anterior shoulder pain characterized by an inflammatory process that involves the long head of the biceps tendon as well as its sheath within the bicipital groove. The tendon involvement can be intraarticular from its attachment to the superior glenoid labrum as it runs across the glenohumeral joint and extraarticular as it runs in the bicipital or intertubercular groove (Fig. 1-162).

SYNONYMS

Bicipital tendonitis
Bicipital tenosynovitis
Biceps tendinosis

ICD-9CM CODES
726.12 Bicipital tenosynovitis
ICD-10CM CODES
M75.20 Bicipital tendinitis, unspecified shoulder

EPIDEMIOLOGY & DEMOGRAPHICS

INCIDENCE: 41% of complete rotator cuff tears have concomitant biceps tendonitis
PREVALENCE: Common but prevalence uncertain
PREDOMINANT AGE: 18 to 35 yr old
RISK FACTORS: Athletes involved in throwing sports, swimming, contact sports, weight lifting, gymnastics, martial arts; repetitive overhead movements among carpenters, electricians, mechanical wheelchair users

PHYSICAL FINDINGS & CLINICAL PRESENTATION

- Pain referred to the anterior shoulder
- Pain that worsens at night
- A history of trauma may or may not be present
- Pain on lifting, pulling, and repetitive overhead reaching
- Most common physical exam finding is tenderness over bicipital groove by palpating the biceps tendon 3 to 6 cm below the anterior acromion and felt most easily in 10 degrees of internal rotation
- Yergason's test—pain on biceps tendon area on resisted supination of pronated forearm with elbow at 90 degrees
- Speed's test—pain on the biceps tendon area on resisted forward flexion of the shoulder with elbows and arms fully supinated and extended

ETIOLOGY

- Primary—of unknown cause and the inflammation is specific to the intertubercular groove without any associated shoulder pathology
- Secondary—associated with other pathologic conditions such as rotator cuff disease, impingement syndrome, SLAP (Superior Labrum from Anterior to Posterior) injuries, presence of spurs or any systemic inflammatory disease involving the shoulders

DIAGNOSIS

DIFFERENTIAL DIAGNOSIS

- Impingement syndrome
- Rotator cuff tendonitis
- Subacromial bursitis
- Rotator cuff tears
- SLAP injuries
- Adhesive capsulitis
- Acromioclavicular joint arthritis
- Glenohumeral joint arthritis
- Cervical radiculopathy
- Coracoid impingement
- Brachial plexus neuritis

WORKUP

May proceed to imaging modalities

IMAGING STUDIES

- X-ray plain films are usually normal in primary tendinopathy; special views of the bicipital groove may demonstrate presence of spurs
- Musculoskeletal ultrasound evaluates dynamic movements of the biceps tendon; it is 49% sensitive but 91% to 97% specific; use in both diagnosis and treatment
- Ultrasound may reveal the presence of effusion in the long head of the biceps tendon sheath (Fig. 1-163)
- CT/MRI arthrography are early techniques used to reliably identify shoulder pathology
- MRI is a non-invasive way of getting detailed images of the biceps tendon and other shoulder structures such as the superior labrum and rotator cuff structures and identify pathologies that may or may not coexist
- Arthroscopy is the gold standard technique for diagnosis and treatment.

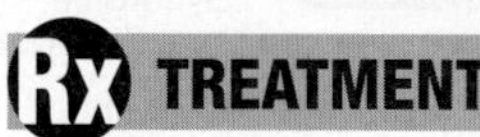

TREATMENT

It is often necessary to establish whether the tendonitis is primary or secondary to address certain aspects of the treatment. Initial conservative treatment is usually very successful.

NONPHARMACOLOGIC THERAPY

Ice, rest from overhead physical activities, physical therapy after acute phase

ACUTE GENERAL Rx

Nonsteroidal anti-inflammatory drugs (NSAIDs) are good adjuncts to treatment that expedites the recovery process by decreasing edema, inflammation, and pain.

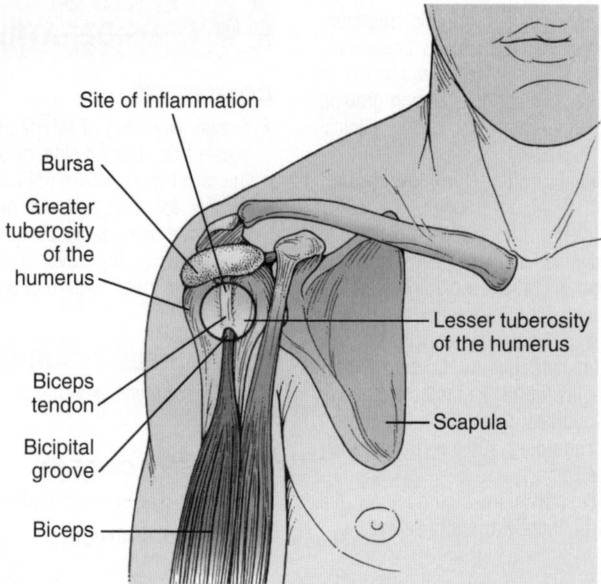

FIGURE 1-162 Anatomic location of the long head of the biceps tendon with surrounding structures of the shoulder. (From Roberts JR et al: *Clinical procedures in emergency medicine,* ed 5, Philadelphia, 2009, Saunders.)

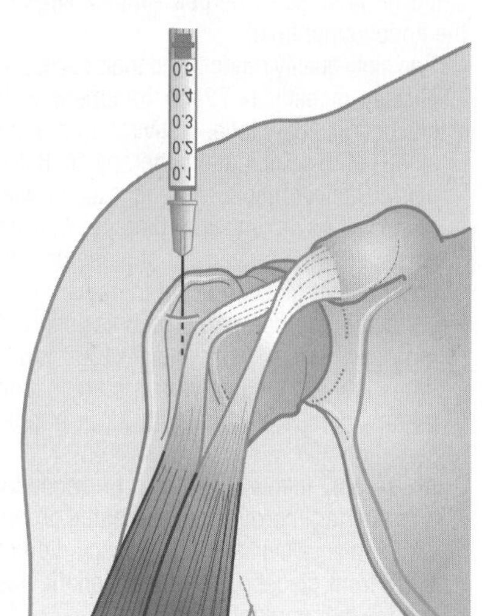

FIGURE 1-163 Injection of the long head of the biceps tendon in the bicipital groove. (From Adams JG et al: *Emergency medicine, clinical essentials,* ed 2, St Louis, 2013, Elsevier.)

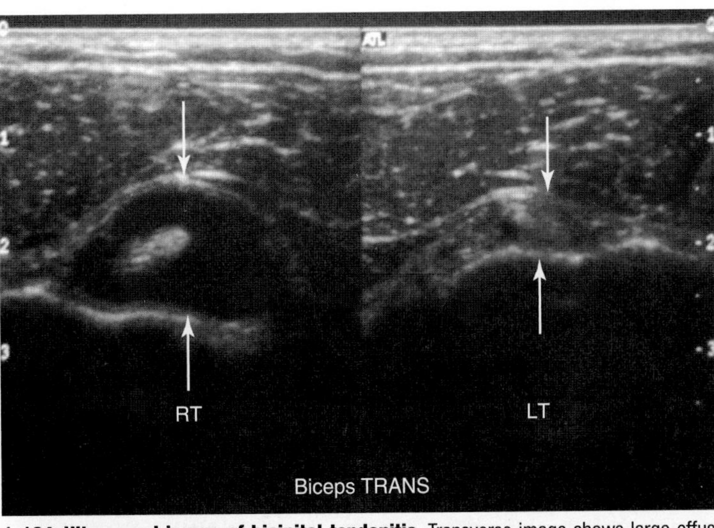

FIGURE 1-164 Ultrasound image of bicipital tendonitis. Transverse image shows large effusion in the long head of biceps tendon sheath. (From Hoechberg MC et al: *Rheumatology,* ed 5, St Louis, 2011, Mosby.)

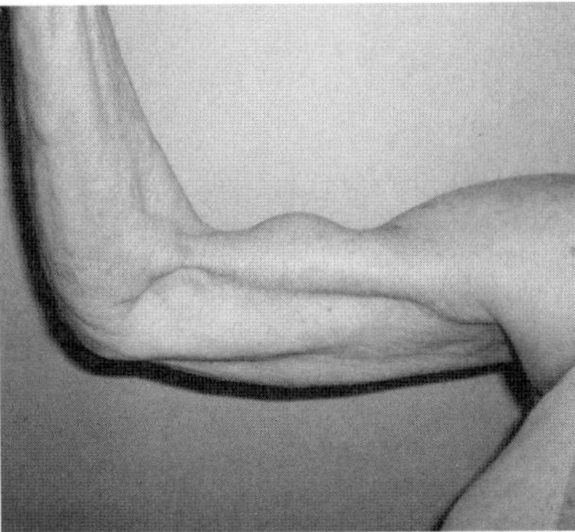

FIGURE 1-165 Popeye deformity after a biceps tendon rupture. (Illustration borrowed from Fernandez et al FIGURE 4, PAGE 7. Seminarios de la Fundación Española de Reumatologia Maniobras exploratorias del hombro doloros martes, 13 jul 2010, Elsevier.)

CHRONIC Rx

- If with persistent pain or severe night symptoms that fail to resolve after 6 to 8 wk of conservative treatment, corticosteroid injections may be considered
- Injection into the tendon sheath (Fig. 1-164), with care not to inject into the biceps tendon, may have good to excellent results; best done under ultrasound guidance
- Subacromial steroid injections can address tendonitis secondary to impingement
- Glenohumeral joint injection delivers the steroids directly to the intraarticular portion of the biceps that is often irritated
- Gradual biceps and rotator cuff strengthening with physical therapy if symptoms have decreased
- Low-power laser therapy has reported beneficial effects but disputes exist

DISPOSITION

- Usually self-limited with conservative measures
- If pain persists after 3 mo, referral to orthopedic surgery
- Surgical options are tendon debridement, release of constricted synovial sheath, tenodesis, or tenotomy.
- Tenodesis is done by moving the attachment to relieve pressure of the irritated tendon; results in better strength and cosmesis but requires longer rehab; consider for younger, active patients
- Tenotomy consists of cutting the long head of the biceps tendon prior to its intraarticular superior labral insertion; technically simple procedure with short rehabilitation but deformity, weakness, and cramping may occur; consider for older patients
- Can progress to tendon rupture resulting in a "Popeye deformity" (Fig. 1-165)

REFERRAL

- Refer to physical therapy early in the phase of conservative treatment
- Refer to orthopedics if symptoms persist beyond 3 to 4 mo

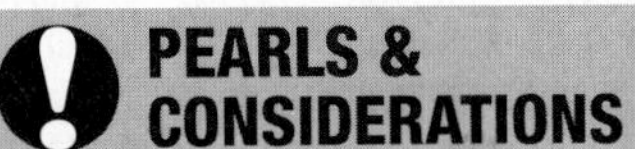

PEARLS & CONSIDERATIONS

COMMENTS

A complete rotator cuff tear almost always involves the biceps tendon as its intraarticular portion gets exposed to the overlying acromion, which causes further impingement and pain.

PREVENTION

After corticosteroid injection, patient should not return immediately to vigorous physical activities that could potentially progress into a biceps tendon complete tear.

SUGGESTED READINGS

available at www.expertconsult.com

AUTHOR: **CRISOSTOMO R. BALIOG, JR., M.D.**

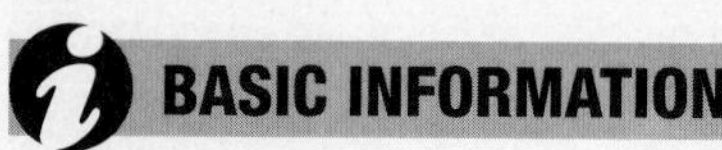

BASIC INFORMATION

DEFINITION

Bipolar disorder is an episodic, recurrent, and frequently progressive condition in which the afflicted individual experiences at least one episode of mania, characterized by at least 1 wk of continuous symptoms of elevated, expansive, or irritable mood, in association with three or more of the following symptoms (four if irritability is the presenting mood):

- Decreased need for sleep
- Grandiosity or inflated self-esteem
- Pressured speech
- Flight of ideas or subjective sense of racing thoughts
- Distractibility
- Increased level of goal-directed activity
- Problematic behavior with a high potential for painful consequences

Most individuals with bipolar disorder also experience one or more episodes of major depression over their lifetimes or have symptoms of a depressive episode commingled with those of mania (mixed episode). Hypomanic episodes may also occur.

SYNONYMS

Manic-depression
Cycloid psychosis

BIPOLAR I

ICD-9CM and DSM-5 CODES

296.4-296.7 Depression symptoms

ICD-10CM CODES

F42.0 Bipolar affective disorder, current episode hypomanic
F31.1 Bipolar affective disorder, current episode manic without psychotic symptoms
F31.2 Bipolar affective disorder, current episode manic with psychotic symptoms
F31.3 Bipolar affective disorder, current episode mild or moderate depression
F31.4 Bipolar affective disorder, current episode severe depression without psychotic symptoms
F31.5 Bipolar affective disorder, current episode severe depression with psychotic symptoms
F31.6 Bipolar affective disorder, current episode mixed
F31.8 Bipolar II disorder

EPIDEMIOLOGY & DEMOGRAPHICS

INCIDENCE: 0.016% to 0.021%

PREVALENCE (IN U.S.): 0.4% to 1.6% (lifetime); bipolar spectrum disorders: 2.8%

PREDOMINANT SEX: Equal distribution among male and female

PREDOMINANT AGE: Lifelong condition with age of onset 14 to 30 yr

PEAK INCIDENCE: Onset in 20s

GENETICS:

- Concordance rates for monozygotic twins: 0.7 to 0.8; for dizygotic twins: 0.2
- Risk of affective disorder in offspring with one affected parent with bipolar disorder: 27% to 29%; with two affected parents: 50% to 74%
- Heritability estimate of 0.85
- No specific causal mutations have been identified. Genome-wide association analyses have suggested a role for *CACNA1C, ODZ4,* and *NCAN,* among others, and implicated ion channelopathies in pathogenesis of bipolar disorder. It remains unclear whether the high heritability is the result of the additive effect of many common risk variants or a fewer higher-risk rare variants.

PHYSICAL FINDINGS & CLINICAL PRESENTATION

- Mania associated with:
  - Psychomotor activation that is usually goal directed but not necessarily productive
  - Increase in goal-directed activity and excessive involvement in activities leading to unexpected adverse outcomes
  - Elevated, euphoric, and frequently labile mood
  - Decreased need for sleep
  - Flight of ideas with rapid, loud, pressured speech
- Psychosis may occur, with delusions, hallucinations, and formal thought disorder
- Depressive episodes resembling major depressive disorder (see "Depression, Major"); however, atypical features (hypersomnia, weight gain) may be present
- Mixed states, characterized by activation, irritability, and dysphoria, also possible

KEY DIAGNOSTIC CRITERIA DISTINGUISHING BIPOLAR I DISORDER FROM BIPOLAR II DISORDER*:

Manic episode (Bipolar I Disorder)

- Distinct period during which there is an abnormally and persistently elevated, expansive, or irritable mood lasting at least 1 wk (or less if hospitalization is required)
- Must be accompanied by at least three of the following symptoms (four if mood is only irritable): inflated self-esteem or grandiosity, decreased need for sleep, pressured speech, racing thoughts, distractibility, increased involvement in goal-directed activity or psychomotor agitation, excessive involvement in pleasurable activities with a high potential for painful consequences
- Symptoms do not meet criteria for a mixed episode
- Disturbance must be sufficiently severe to cause marked impairment in social or occupational functioning or to require hospitalization, or it is characterized by the presence of psychotic features
- Symptoms not due to direct physiologic effect of medication, general medication condition, or substance abuse

*Criteria are from the American Psychiatric Association: *Diagnostic and statistic manual of mental disorders, fifth edition,* Washington, DC, 2013, American Psychiatric Association.

Hypomanic episode (Bipolar II Disorder)

- Distinct period during which there is an abnormally and persistently elevated, expansive, or irritable mood lasting at least 4 days
- Must be accompanied by at least three of the following symptoms (four if mood is only irritable): inflated self-esteem or grandiosity, decreased need for sleep, pressured speech, racing thoughts, distractibility, increased involvement in goal-directed activity or psychomotor agitation, excessive involvement in pleasurable activities with a high potential for painful consequences
- Hypomanic episodes must be clearly different from the person's usual nondepressed mood, and there must be a clear change in functioning that is not characteristic of the person's usual functioning
- Changes in mood and functioning must be observable by others. In contrast to a manic episode, a hypomanic episode is not severe enough to cause marked impairment in social or occupational functioning or to require hospitalization, and there are no psychotic features
- Symptoms not due to direct physiologic effect of medication, general medication condition, or substance abuse

ETIOLOGY

Hypotheses:

1. Abnormalities of receptor and membrane function, calcium dysregulation
2. Alteration of cAMP, MAP kinase, protein kinase C, arachidonic acid cascade, and glycogen synthase kinase-3 signal transduction pathways; mitochondrial dysfunction
3. Alteration in cell survival pathways, glial and neuronal death and loss of neuroplasticity

Dx DIAGNOSIS

DIFFERENTIAL DIAGNOSIS

- Secondary manias caused by medical disorders (e.g., hyperthyroidism, AIDS, stroke, Cushing syndrome) or pharmacologic treatment (e.g., steroids, stimulants).
- First onset of mania after age 50 yr suggestive of secondary mania.
- Less severe, and possibly distinct, conditions of bipolar type II and cyclothymia
- Comorbid substance abuse or dependency may confound diagnosis and treatment.
- Presentation can be confused with schizophrenia or paranoid psychosis.

WORKUP

- History
- Physical examination
- Mental status examination
- Mood Disorder Questionnaire (MDQ)

LABORATORY TESTS

Because of high rate of secondary manias, initial evaluation to confirm health of all major organ systems (routine chemistries, complete blood count, urinalysis, sedimentation rate)

IMAGING STUDIES

- Consider brain imaging if late onset or if neurologic examination is abnormal.
- Neuroimaging may show evidence of ventricular enlargement or increased white matter hyperintensities; decrements in prefrontal and temporal lobe cortical thickness also reported.

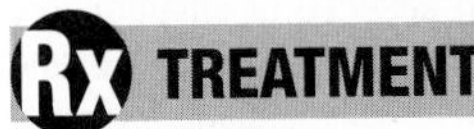

TREATMENT

NONPHARMACOLOGIC THERAPY

- Cognitive-behavioral and family-focused psychoeducational psychotherapy to help patients cope with consequences of the disease, improve adherence with medications, and identify possible environmental triggers
- Bright light therapy in the northern latitudes in individuals exhibiting a seasonal pattern of winter depression
- Lifestyle "regularization"

ACUTE GENERAL Rx

- First-line agents for acute mania and mixed states: lithium 1500 to 1800 mg/day (0.8 to 1.2 mEq/L), valproate 1000 to 1500 mg/day (50 to 125 ng/ml), carbamazepine 600 to 800 mg/day (4 to 12 micrograms/ml), oxcarbazepine 900 to 2400 mg/day, olanzapine 10 to 20 mg/day, risperidone 2 to 4 mg/day, quetiapine 350 to 800 mg/day, ziprasidone 80 to 120 mg/day, asenapine 10-20 mg/day, or aripiprazole 10 to 30 mg/day.
- Useful adjuncts to acute treatment of mania: benzodiazepines: lorazepam 1 to 2 mg q4h, clonazepam 1 to 2 mg q4h.
- Traditional antidepressants can induce manic episodes and exacerbate mania in mixed episodes.
- Lamotrigine can have acute antidepressant benefit, but appears more effective in prophylaxis of future episodes.
- Although best evidence data are limited, first-line options for bipolar depression include lithium, quetiapine, lamotrigine, lurasidone, and olanzapine/fluoxetine combination. Bupropion may have a lower risk for triggering mania, and MAOIs or ECT may be efficacious in treatment-resistant cases.

CHRONIC Rx

- Goal of long-term treatment: prevention of relapse or episode recurrence
- Best agents for prophylaxis of mania: lithium, valproate, and olanzapine (carbamazepine/oxcarbazepine possibly beneficial)
- Best agents for prophylaxis of depression: lamotrigine and lithium
- Risk/benefit of atypical antipsychotics in maintenance unclear
- Long-term use of antidepressants: frequently destabilizes patient and leads to more frequent relapses; depression outweighs mania as the most debilitating dimension over the life span.

DISPOSITION

- Course is variable.
- More than 90% of patients having a single manic episode are likely to experience others.
- Uncontrolled manic or depressive episodes can lead to additional episodes.
- Lithium shown to specifically decrease suicidal risk.
- Psychosocioeconomic consequences of both mania and depression can be severe and disabling.

REFERRAL

- If use of antidepressant contemplated
- If patient is severely manic, rapid cycling, or suicidal or is in a bipolar, mixed episode

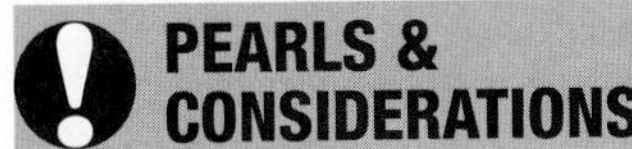

PEARLS & CONSIDERATIONS

COMMENTS

- All patients presenting with depression should be asked about past personal and family history of mania and hypomania; 70% of bipolar patients have previously been misdiagnosed.
- Prompt recognition of the earliest signs of mania in a given individual (e.g., decreased need for sleep, increased rate of speech) allows earlier intervention and a better likelihood of preventing a full episode.
- Bipolar disorder in children frequently manifests as behavioral disinhibition and temper dysregulation, but current consensus indicates that the condition is overdiagnosed in this age group.
- Patients treated with atypical antipsychotic agents should be carefully monitored for development of metabolic syndrome.
- Despite some variation in prevalence, the severity, impact, and patterns of comorbidity of bipolar disorder are similar in different countries in world health surveys.
- Bipolar disorder often co-occurs with anxiety disorders, and attention deficit hyperactivity disorder (ADHD), making attribution of specific symptoms difficult.
- Patients receiving anticonvulsants or antidepressants should be monitored for a possible increase in suicidal thoughts or behavior.
- There is preliminary evidence that nutraceutical agents like omega-3 fatty acids and N-acetyl cysteine (NAC) may have efficacy in the treatment of bipolar disorder.

PATIENT/FAMILY EDUCATION

Information available at www.NMHA.org/ and www.dbsalliance.org/.

SUGGESTED READINGS

available at www.expertconsult.com

RELATED CONTENT

Depression, Major (Related Key Topic)
Bipolar Disorder (Patient Information)

AUTHOR: **VICTOR I. REUS, M.D.**

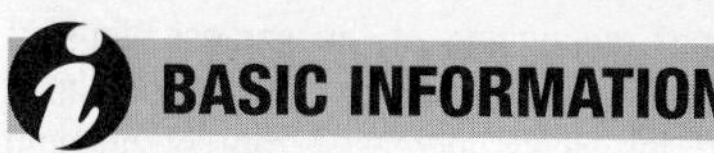

BASIC INFORMATION

DEFINITION

Bone cell death in the jaw observed with therapeutic dosages of bisphosphonates (BPs). Osteoclast apoptosis may occur due to the antiresorptive effects of BPs preventing the release of bone regenerative proteins and thus preventing bone renewal. This results in tissue loss and exposed bone. BPs are not believed to be toxic to osteoblasts, although evidence suggests some antiangiogenic effects.

Bisphosphonate-related osteonecrosis of the jaw (BRONJ) primarily involves the jawbone due to its higher risk for complications from minor injury and infection when the healing potential or vascular supply is compromised. BPs may accumulate more in bones with higher turnover rates, such as the maxilla and mandible. BRONJ is more likely to occur with use of nitrogen-containing BPs due to their greater potency.

Cases of ONJ have been reported in patients with malignancy treated with high doses of denosumab. Therefore, the American Dental Association now uses the term "antiresorptive agent-induced osteonecrosis of the jaw" (ARONJ).

SYNONYMS

Bisphosphonate-induced osteonecrosis of the jaw (BIONJ)

ICD-9CM CODES
Not applicable
ICD-10CM CODES
M87.180 Osteonecrosis due to drugs, jaw

EPIDEMIOLOGY & DEMOGRAPHICS

INCIDENCE
- The incidence with alendronate has been estimated to be 0.7 per 100,000 persons per year by the original manufacturer.
- The incidence after tooth extraction has ranged from 8.3% to 40% in the medical literature.
  - Incidence at 42 months after tooth extraction has been estimated at 3.9% with oral BPs and 14.8% with IV BPs.

PEAK INCIDENCE: BRONJ has been identified as early as 7 months after the use of IV BPs in patients with cancer, and as early as 13 months in patients with osteoporosis and absence of malignant disease. Incidence may depend on when dentoalveolar surgery occurs.

PREVALENCE
- Prevalence in 2008 estimated at 13.3% of patients with cancer who received an IV BP
- Most prevalent in patients with multiple myeloma or breast cancer vs. other cancers or osteoporosis

PREDOMINANT SEX AND AGE
- Sex not statistically associated with BRONJ
- Age greater than or equal to 65

GENETICS: Single nucleotide polymorphisms (SNPs) have been identified in the *CYP2C8* gene among patients with multiple myeloma and exposure to IV BPs.

RISK FACTORS: The 2009 American Association of Oral and Maxillofacial Surgeons (AAOMS) position paper indicated that dentoalveolar surgery such as tooth extraction or root canal and use of IV BPs are the greatest risk factors for development of BRONJ.
- Patients with cancer exposed to IV BPs who undergo dentoalveolar surgery have an estimated 5- to 21-fold increased risk for BRONJ than similar patients who do not undergo this surgery.
- IV formulations such as zoledronic acid: risk ratio for developing BRONJ is 14.6 with IV versus oral products. The risk of developing BRONJ with oral forms may increase when duration is greater than 3 years and may be potentiated by concomitant use of chronic corticosteroids.
- Patients with cancer who are exposed to IV BPs have a 2.7- to 4.2-fold increased risk versus similar patients not exposed to IV BPs.
- Longer duration of BP therapy
- Age greater than or equal to 65 with risk ratio estimated to be 200.2 in those exposed to IV BPs vs. similar patients not exposed
- Malignancy
- Chemotherapeutic agents and corticosteroids
- History of periodontal and dental abscesses
- Bacterial infection

PHYSICAL FINDINGS & CLINICAL PRESENTATION

- Exposed bone in the maxilla or mandible, with 65% of cases involving the mandible. Multifocal or bilateral involvement may be present.
- Pain in the maxillofacial region, although one third of lesions may be painless
- Tooth mobility/spontaneous tooth loss
- Mucosal swelling, erythema, ulceration, altered sensation
- Infection

ETIOLOGY

- Exposure to IV or oral BPs

Dx DIAGNOSIS

The AAOMS considers a diagnosis of BRONJ if the following three characteristics are present:
1. Current or previous treatment with a BP
2. Exposed bone in the maxillofacial region persisting for more than 8 weeks
3. No history of radiation therapy to the maxillofacial region

DIFFERENTIAL DIAGNOSIS

- Suppurative osteomyelitis of the jaw (SOJ)
- Osteoradionecrosis of the jaw (ORNJ)
- Alveolar osteitis, gingivitis, periodontitis, dental caries, and temporomandibular joint disorders.

WORKUP

- Treatment history, including medications and radiation therapy
- Past medical history, including malignancy

LABORATORY TESTS

A validated diagnostic test is not available to identify patients at an increased risk of BRONJ. Tissue biopsy should only be performed if metastatic disease is strongly suspected and its detection would change the management of BRONJ. Histopathology of BRONJ shows empty osteocytic lacunae, empty Haversian and Volkmann canals, an absence of inflammatory cells or blood vessels in the marrow space, and absence of extracellular collagenase.

IMAGING STUDIES

Panoramic and periapical radiographs

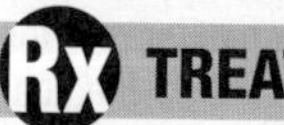

TREATMENT

Goals of treatment for BRONJ include:
- Control and/or reduce pain.
- Control secondary infection.
- Minimize progression or occurrence of bone necrosis.

NONPHARMACOLOGIC THERAPY

Surgery for BRONJ should be deferred if possible as a surgical margin with viable bone is difficult to obtain. The entire jawbone likely has been exposed to accumulation of BPs, and therefore successful eradication of necrotic bone is often not possible. Those areas of necrosis that consistently irritate soft tissues should undergo debridement as necessary. Limited evidence supports the use of hyperbaric oxygen as adjunct to surgery and antibiotics to slow progression and improve pain.

The AAOMS recommends the following surgical strategies based on BRONJ staging:
- Stage 0 (no clinical evidence of necrotic bone): no surgery
- Stage I (exposed and necrotic bone, asymptomatic): no surgery
- Stage II (exposed and necrotic bone with pain and/or infection): superficial debridement
- Stage III (exposed and necrotic bone with pain, infection, **and** one of the following features: necrosis extending beyond alveolar bone, pathologic fracture, extraoral fistula, oral antral or nasal communication, osteolysis extending to mandible of sinus floor): surgical debridement or resection for palliation of infection and pain

ACUTE GENERAL Rx

Both chlorhexidine mouth rinse and antibiotics for 1 to 3 weeks have been found useful for stage reduction.
- Chlorhexidine 0.12% antibacterial mouth rinse daily for Stages I to III
- Oral antibiotics for symptomatic Stage II, and oral or IV antibiotics for Stage III
- Analgesics for Stages II or III

CHRONIC Rx

- Determine whether discontinuation of BPs is appropriate.
  - Evaluate potential benefit of continuing BP, such as relief of bone pain in malignancy, or prevention of fractures with high morbidity and mortality.

- BPs have a prolonged half-life, so return to normal osteoclast function and bone turnover may be too gradual.
- Consider other risks of BPs such as spontaneous atypical fractures.
- If discontinuing BP therapy, consider other alternative treatments for osteoporosis or bone pain.
- Anecdotal case reports exist for using teriparatide or pentoxifylline with tocopherol to heal BRONJ.

DISPOSITION

- Patients with involvement of the maxilla appear to have a greater likelihood of repeat surgery.
- Patients on oral BPs may have less severe complications and may have a better response.
- Treatment with antibiotics and chlorhexidine mouth rinse, withdrawal of BPs, and surgical removal of loose sequestra may possibly reduce pain and lesions of osteonecrosis.

REFERRAL

Oral and maxillofacial surgeon

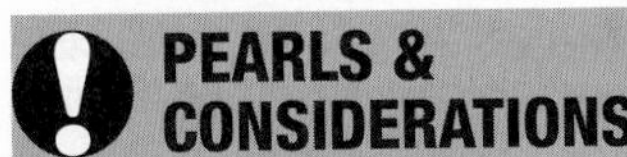

PEARLS & CONSIDERATIONS

COMMENTS

- Patients may be asymptomatic for weeks to years before BRONJ is apparent. Radiographic changes may not be observed until significant disease has developed.
- Tooth extraction may be difficult to avoid in patients at high risk of BRONJ if an underlying bacterial infection is present.
- Patients with cancer are at highest risk as the dosage of BPs are much greater for osteoporosis.
- A statement regarding the unknown optimal duration of bisphosphonates was recently added to product labeling by the FDA. Discontinuation of bisphosphonates after 3-5 years of use for patients at low risk of fractures should be considered. Patients at low-risk include those without history of fracture and those initially prescribed bisphosphonates for treatment of osteopenia or prevention of osteoporosis.
  - Results from the FLEX trial suggest that women with postmenopausal osteoporosis who have taken alendronate for 5 years and are at low risk of vertebral fractures may discontinue the drug for up to 5 years.
- Results from the HORIZON-PFT extension trial suggest that women with postmenopausal osteoporosis who have taken IV zoledronic acid for 3 years and are at low risk of vertebral fractures may discontinue for up to 3 years.

PREVENTION

- Regular dental hygiene and routine dental examinations
- Assessment of patients for other risk factors of BRONJ
- Completion of any anticipated dental procedures before beginning BP therapy
- Consideration of appropriateness of oral BP instead of IV formulations
- After dentoalveolar surgery, initiation of BPs delayed by 2 to 3 weeks to allow for osseous healing
- Careful monitoring of patients after dentoalveolar surgery
- Examination of mucosa in patients with full or partial dentures
- In asymptomatic patients receiving IV BPs, limiting dental surgery to removal of nonrestorable teeth and avoiding dental implants in patients who also have cancer
- In asymptomatic patients exposed to less than 3 years of oral BPs with concomitant corticosteroids 3 months before dental surgery, consider a drug holiday
- In asymptomatic patients exposed to more than 3 years of oral BPs, consider a drug holiday before dental surgery

PATIENT/FAMILY EDUCATION

- All healthcare providers should be aware of past and current BP use
- Contact a healthcare provider if any of the following are noticed:
  - Presence of exposed bone in the maxillofacial area
  - Persisting pain in the maxillofacial area
  - Signs of infection such as fever, pus, and swelling
- Practice good dental hygiene and keep regular dental appointments

SUGGESTED READINGS

available at www.expertconsult.com

AUTHORS: **CHRISTINE EISENHOWER, PHARM.D.**, and **ANNE L. HUME, PHARM.D.**

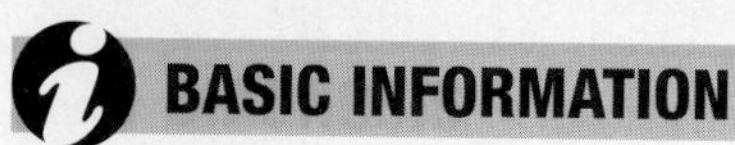

BASIC INFORMATION

DEFINITION

A bite wound can be animal or human, accidental or intentional.

ICD-9CM CODES
879.8 Bite wound, unspecified site
ICD-10CM CODES
T14.1 Open wound of unspecified body region
T01.9 Multiple open wounds, unspecified
S31.000A Unspecified open wound of lower back and pelvis without penetration into retroperitoneum, initial encounter

EPIDEMIOLOGY & DEMOGRAPHICS

- Bite wounds account for 1% of emergency department visits.
- More than 1 million bites occur in human beings annually in the U.S.
- Dog bites account for 85% to 90% of all bites and result in 10 to 20 fatalities yearly in the U.S.; cat bites account for 10% to 20%. The animal typically is owned by the victim.
- Infection rates are highest for cat bites (30% to 50%), followed by human bites (15% to 30%) and dog bites (5%).
- The extremities are involved in 75% of bites.

PHYSICAL FINDINGS & CLINICAL PRESENTATION

- The appearance of the bite wound is variable (e.g., puncture wound, tear, avulsion).
- Cellulitis, lymphangitis, and focal adenopathy may be present in infected bite wounds.
- Patient may have fever and chills.

ETIOLOGY

- Increased risk of infection: human and cat bites, closed-fist injuries, wounds involving joints, puncture wounds, face and lip bites, bites with skull penetration, bites in immunocompromised hosts
- Most frequent infecting organisms:
  1. *Pasteurella* spp.: responsible for majority of infections within 24 hr of dog *(P. canis)* and cat *(P. multocida, P. septica)* bites
  2. *Capnocytophaga canimorsus* (formerly DF-2 bacillus): a gram-negative organism responsible for late infection, usually after dog bites
  3. Gram-negative organisms *(Pseudomonas, Haemophilus)*: often found in human bites
  4. *Streptococcus* spp., *Staphylococcus aureus*
  5. *Eikenella corrodens* in human bites

Dx DIAGNOSIS

DIFFERENTIAL DIAGNOSIS

- Bite from a rabid animal (often the attack is unprovoked)
- Factitious injury

WORKUP

- Determination of the time elapsed since the patient was bitten, status of rabies immunization of the animal, and underlying medical conditions that might predispose the patient to infection (e.g., DM, immunodeficiency)
- Documentation of bite site, notification of appropriate authorities (e.g., police department, animal officer)

LABORATORY TESTS

- Generally not necessary
- Hct if there has been significant blood loss
- Wound cultures (aerobic and anaerobic) if there is evidence of sepsis or victim is immunocompromised; cultures should be obtained before irrigation of the wound but after superficial cleaning

IMAGING STUDIES

Radiographs are indicated when bony penetration is suspected or if there is suspicion of fracture or significant trauma; they are also useful for detecting foreign bodies (when suspected).

Rx TREATMENT

NONPHARMACOLOGIC THERAPY

- Local care with debridement, vigorous cleansing, and saline irrigation of the wound; debridement of devitalized tissue
- High-pressure irrigation to clean bite wound and ensure removal of contaminants (e.g., use saline solution with a 30- to 35-ml syringe equipped with a 20-gauge needle or catheter with tip of syringe placed 2 to 3 cm above the wound)
- Avoid blunt probing of wounds (increased risk of infection)
- If the animal is suspected to be rabid: infiltrate wound edges with 1% procaine hydrochloride, swab wound surface vigorously with cotton swabs and 1% benzalcuronium solution or other soap, and rinse wound with normal saline

ACUTE GENERAL Rx

- Avoid suturing of hand wounds and any wounds that appear infected
- Puncture wounds should be left open
- Give antirabies therapy and tetanus immune globulin (250 to 500 units IM in limb contralateral to toxoid) and toxoid (adult or child older than 5 yr: 0.5 ml DT given IM, child <5 yr 0.5 ml DPT IM) as needed
- Use empiric antibiotic therapy in high-risk wounds (e.g., cat bite, hand bites, face bites, genital area bites, bites with joint or bone penetration, human bites, immunocompromised host): amoxicillin-clavulanate 875 to 1000 mg bid for 7 days or cefuroxime 500 mg bid for 7 days
- In hospitalized patients, IV antibiotics of choice are cefoxitin 1-2 g q6h, ampicillin-sulbactam 1.5-3 g q6h, ticarcillin-clavulanate 3 g q6h, cefoxitin 2 g IV q8h, or ceftriaxone 1-2 g q24h
- Penicillin allergy: animal bite (doxycycline or moxifloxacin or trimethoprim/sulfamethoxazole with either clindamycin or metronidazole); human bite (moxifloxacin plus clindamycin, trimethoprim/sulfamethoxazole plus metronidazole)
- Prophylactic therapy for persons bitten by others with HIV and hepatitis B (see Section V)
- Table 1-76 summarizes the treatment of mammalian bites

DISPOSITION

- Prognosis is favorable with proper treatment.
- Important prognostic factors are type and depth of wound, which compartments are entered, and pathogenicity of inoculated bacteria.
- Punctures that are difficult to irrigate adequately, carnivore bites over vital structures (arteries, nerves, joints), and tissue crushing that cannot be debrided have a worse prognosis.
- In general, human bites have a higher complication and infection rate than do animal bites.
- Nearly 50% of the anaerobic gram-negative bacilli isolated from human bite wounds may be penicillin resistant and beta-lactamase positive.

PREVENTION

- Box 1-9 provides advice for avoiding the bites and attacks of common pets.

REFERRAL

- Hospitalization and IV antibiotic therapy for infected human bites; bites with injury to joints, nerves, or tendons; or any animal bites unresponsive to oral therapy.
- Human bites with tendon involvement should go to operating room for washout.
- In the outpatient setting, bite wounds should be reevaluated within 48 hr to assess for signs of infection.

SUGGESTED READINGS

available at www.expertconsult.com

RELATED CONTENT

Animal and Human Bites (Patient Information)

AUTHOR: **FRED F. FERRI, M.D.**

TABLE 1-76 Treatment of Mammalian Bites

Type	Wound Care	Antibiotic PR.	Tetanus PR.	Rabies PR.	HIV PR.	Hepatitis PR.
Human	High-pressure irrigation of the wound with normal saline or dilute (<1%) povidone-iodine solution; débride devitalized tissue or ragged edges	Amoxicillin-clavulanate, second-generation cephalosporin with anaerobic activity, penicillin plus dicloxacillin, clindamycin plus ciprofloxacin or trimethoprim-sulfamethoxazole	Tetanus immunoglobulin (250 units IM) and tetanus toxoid (0.5 mg IM) if never had a tetanus vaccine or have not had 3 doses of tetanus toxoid; tetanus toxoid (0.5 mg IM) if >5 yr since previous tetanus booster	None	ART therapy started within the first 48-72 hr and continued for 28 days or bite source tested HIV negative; refer to the hospital for the specific drugs used in ART therapy	HBIG (0.06 ml/kg IM); HBV given at separate site from HBIG
Cat	High-pressure irrigation of the wound with normal saline or dilute (<1%) povidone-iodine solution; débride devitalized tissue or ragged edges	Amoxicillin-clavulanate, second-generation cephalosporin with anaerobic activity, penicillin plus a first-generation cephalosporin, clindamycin plus a fluoroquinolone or trimethoprim-sulfamethoxazole	Tetanus immune globulin (250 units IM) and tetanus toxoid (0.5 mg IM) if never had a tetanus vaccine or have not had 3 doses of tetanus toxoid; tetanus toxoid (0.5 mg IM) if >5 yr since previous tetanus booster	HRIG (20 IU/kg) injected IM and/or around the bite site; rabies vaccine (1 ml IM) given in the deltoid in adults and in the thigh in children, on days 0, 3, 7, 14, and 28	None	None
Dog	High-pressure irrigation of the wound with normal saline or dilute (<1%) povidone-iodine solution; débride devitalized tissue or ragged edges	Amoxicillin-clavulanate, second-generation cephalosporin with anaerobic activity, penicillin plus a first-generation cephalosporin, clindamycin plus a fluoroquinolone or trimethoprim-sulfamethoxazole	Tetanus immune globulin (250 units IM) and tetanus toxoid (0.5 mg IM) if never had a tetanus vaccine or have not had 3 doses of tetanus toxoid; tetanus toxoid (0.5 mg IM) if >5 yr since previous tetanus booster	HRIG (20 IU/kg) injected IM and/or around the bite site; rabies vaccine (1 ml IM) given in the deltoid in adults and in the thigh in children, on days 0, 3, 7, 14, and 28	None	None

ART, Antiretroviral therapy; *HBIG*, hepatitis B immune globulin; *HBV*, hepatitis B vaccine; *HIV*, human immunodeficiency virus; *HRIG*, human rabies immune globulin; *IM*, intramuscularly; *PR.*, prophylaxis.
From Adams JG et al: *Emergency medicine: clinical essentials*, ed 2, Philadelphia, 2013, Elsevier.

BOX 1-9 Advice for Avoiding the Bites and Attacks of Common Pets*

Dogs
- Do not leave a young child alone with a dog.
- Never approach or try to pet an unfamiliar dog, especially if it is tied up or confined.
- Always ask the dog's owners if you can pet the dog.
- Do not lean over a dog or pet it directly on the head.
- Do not kiss a dog.
- Avoid quick or sudden movements that may startle a dog.
- Never pet or step over a sleeping dog.
- Never try to take a bone or toy away from a dog (other than your own dog).
- Know the appearance of an angry dog: barking, growling, snarling with teeth showing, ears laid flat, legs stiff, tail up, and hair on the back standing up.
- Never step between two fighting dogs; if you need to separate them, use a bucket of water or a hose.
- Do not approach a female dog that is nursing her pups.
- Teach injury prevention advice to children from an early age.

Cats
- Be aware that some cats do not like prolonged petting.
- Know warning signs of an impending bite: twitching of the tail, restlessness, and "intention" bites (i.e., the cat moves to bite but does not bite).

Ferrets
- Do not sell or adopt a ferret that is known to bite.
- Do not push your fingers through the wires of a ferret cage.
- Reach for a ferret from the side with the palm upward rather than from above.
- Do not handle food and then handle young ferrets without washing your hands first.
- Do not poke a ferret or pull on its tail or ears.
- Never leave a ferret alone with a child or infant.
- If a ferret bites and locks on very tightly, pour cold and fast-running water over its face.

*The prevention of bites and injuries from other animals is addressed in the appropriate sections of this chapter.
From Auerbach P: *Wilderness medicine, expert consult*, premium edition—Enhanced online features and print, Philadelphia, 2012, Elsevier.)

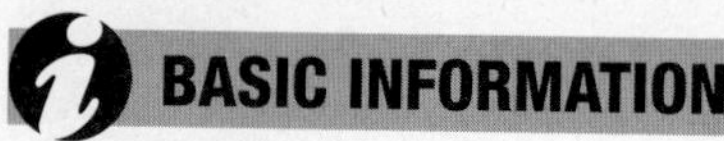

DEFINITION

There are two major classes of arthropods: insects and arachnida. This chapter focuses on the class arachnida. Arachnid bites consist of bites caused by:

- Spiders
- Scorpions
- Ticks

ICD-9CM CODES

E905.1 Venomous spiders (black widow spider, brown spider, tarantula)
E905.2 Scorpion
989.5 Bites of venomous snakes, lizards, and spiders; tick paralysis
E906.4 Bite of nonvenomous arthropod; insect bite NOS

ICD-10CM CODES

T63.301A Toxic effect of unspecified spider venom, accidental (unintentional), initial encounter
T63.2X1A Toxic effect of venom of scorpion, accidental (unintentional), initial encounter
E906 Bite of nonvenomous arthropod; insect bite NOS

EPIDEMIOLOGY & DEMOGRAPHICS

- Spiders—ubiquitous; only three types potentially significantly harmful:
  1. Sydney funnel web spider—Australia
  2. Black widow (Fig. E1-166)—worldwide (excluding Alaska)
  3. Brown recluse (Fig. E1-167)—most common (South Central U.S.)
- Scorpions—various warm climates: Africa, Central South America, Middle East, India; Texas, New Mexico, California, and Nevada in the U.S.
- Ticks—woodlands

PHYSICAL FINDINGS & CLINICAL PRESENTATION

Spiders:

- Sydney funnel web—natracotoxin toxin
  1. Piloerection, muscle spasms leading to tachycardia, hypertension, increased intracranial pressure, coma
- Black widow—females toxic
  1. Initial reaction: local swelling, redness (two fang marks) leading to local piloerection, edema, urticaria, diaphoresis, lymphangitis
  2. Pain in limb leading to rest of body (chest pain, abdominal pain), compartment syndrome
- Brown recluse
  1. Minor sting or burn.
  2. Wound may become pruritic and red with a blanched center with vesicle (Fig. E1-168). Can necrose, especially in fatty areas (Fig. E1-169). Leaves eschar, which sloughs and leaves ulcer; can take months to heal.
  3. Systemic symptoms: headache, fever, chills, gastrointestinal upset, hemolysis, renal tubular necrosis, disseminated intravascular coagulation possible.

Scorpions:

- Sting leading to sympathetic and parasympathetic stimulation: hypertension, bradycardia, vasoconstriction, pulmonary edema, reduced coronary blood flow, priapism, inhibition of insulin
- Also possible: tachycardia, arrhythmia, vasodilation, bronchial relaxation, excessive salivation, vomiting, sweating, bronchoconstriction, pancreatitis.
- Clinically significant scorpion envenomation by *Centruroides sculpturatus* produces a severe neuromotor syndrome and respiratory insufficiency that often requires ICU admission.

Ticks: U.S., Europe, Asia

- Very small (<1 mm). Must be attached >36 hr to transmit disease.
- Lyme disease—most common
  1. Early: erythema migrans in 60% to 80% of cases
  2. 7 to 10 days: mild to moderate constitutional symptoms—disseminated—secondary skin lesions, fever, adenopathy, constitutional symptoms, facial palsy, peripheral neuropathy, lymphocytic meningitis, meningoencephalitis, cardiac manifestations (heart block)
  3. Late: chronic arthritis, dermatitis, neuropathy, keratitis
- Babesiosis (see "Babesiosis")
- Ehrlichiosis/Anaplasmosis (see "Babesiosis" and "Lyme Disease")

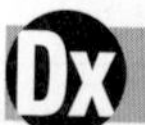

DIAGNOSIS

DIFFERENTIAL DIAGNOSIS

- Cellulitis
- Urticaria

Other tick-borne illnesses:

- Babesiosis
- Tick-borne relapsing fever
- Tularemia
- Rocky Mountain spotted fever
- Ehrlichiosis/anaplasmosis
- Colorado tick fever
- Tick paralysis
- Community-acquired cutaneous methicillin-resistant *Staphylococcus aureus*

WORKUP

Physical examination: thorough skin examination may reveal fang marks, attached ticks, black eschar.

Rx TREATMENT

ACUTE GENERAL Rx

Spiders:

- Sydney funnel web
  1. Pressure, immediate immobilization, supportive care, antivenin.
- Black widow
  1. Treatment based on severity of symptoms; bite is rarely fatal.
  2. All should receive oxygen, IV, cardiac monitor, tetanus prophylaxis.
  3. Symptomatic/supportive therapy.
  4. 10% calcium gluconate for muscle cramps (controversial).
  5. Antivenin only for more severe reactions; it carries a risk of anaphylaxis.
     - Dose: one vial in 100 ml 0.9% saline over 20 to 30 min.
     - Skin test before use.
     - Give antihistamines with use.
- Brown recluse
  1. Pain management, tetanus, supportive treatment.
  2. No consensus regarding best treatment; some evidence for hyperbaric oxygen.

Scorpions:

- Fluids, supportive care, species-specific antivenin (equine based, risk of serum sickness) is controversial.
- IV administration of scorpion-specific F(ab')2 antivenom has been reported effective in resolving the clinical syndrome within 4 hours and reducing the need for concomitant sedation with midazolam and reducing the levels of circulating unbound venom.

Ticks:

- Prophylactic: tick >36 hr: single dose of doxycycline 200 mg
- Early localized disease
  1. Treatment of choice in children: amoxicillin for 14 days.
  2. Doxycycline preferred in patients with possible concurrent ehrlichiosis.
  3. Early disseminated: treatment depends on manifestation.
  4. Late disease: may require longer term or IV therapy; controversial for neurologic disease (see "Lyme Disease").

DISPOSITION

- For patients with systemic reactions, send home with emergency epinephrine kit.
- If severe or anaphylactic reaction, admit and observe for 48 hr for cardiac, renal, or neurologic problems.

REFERRAL

For patients with systemic reactions, refer to allergist for immunotherapy; 95% to 98% effective in preventing anaphylaxis.

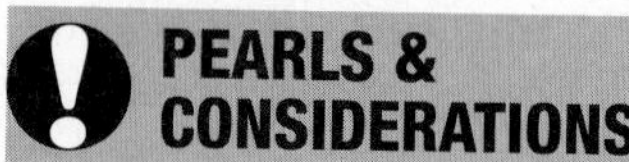

Actual spider bites rare, need witnessed bite, patient should bring spider if possible for confirmation. Bites usually occur in settings of unusually close contact with spider. Bedbugs becoming more prevalent, repeated exposure increases severity of reaction.

SUGGESTED READINGS

available at www.expertconsult.com

RELATED CONTENT

Bites and Stings, Insect (Related Key Topic)
Bites and Stings (Patient Information)

AUTHOR: **GAIL M. O'BRIEN, M.D.**

BASIC INFORMATION

DEFINITION

Most stinging insects belong to the Hymenoptera order and include yellow jackets (most common cause of reactions), hornets, bumblebees, sweat bees, wasps, harvester ants, fire ants, and the Africanized honey bee ("killer bee"). Brown recluse spiders, although not insects, are another common cause of bites (see "Bites and Stings, Arachnids"). The usual effect of a sting is intense local pain, some immediate erythema, and often a small area of edema from the injecting venom. Allergic reactions can be either local or generalized, leading to anaphylactic shock. The majority of reactions occur within the first 6 hr after the sting or bite, but a delayed presentation may occur up to 24 hr.

SYNONYMS Venom allergy

ICD-9CM CODES
989.5 Stings (bees, wasps)
989.5 Bites (fire ant, brown recluse spider)

ICD-10CM CODES
T63.444A Toxic effect of venom of bees, undetermined, initial encounter
T63.464A Toxic effect of venom of wasps, undetermined, initial encounter
T63.424A Toxic effect of venom of ants, undetermined, initial encounter

EPIDEMIOLOGY & DEMOGRAPHICS

PREVALENCE (OF BEE STINGS AND INSECT BITES):
- Unknown.
- Account for 2.3% of ED visits.
- Greater than 5% of the population is allergic, systemically or an excessive local reaction, to the venom of one or more stinging insects.
- Most anaphylactic reactions occur during summer months in those most likely to be exposed, including children, males, outdoor workers. There are no tests to accurately predict reaction; the reaction to a prior sting is still the best predictor.
- Approximately half of fatal reactions occur without prior allergic response.
- Bites by fire ants and brown recluse spiders are less likely to cause systemic disease.

INCIDENCE (IN U.S.): Forty to 100 people die each year from insect sting anaphylaxis; anaphylaxis occurs more often within 10 to 30 min of a sting. Delayed reactions are rare, occurring only in <0.3% of stings.

PHYSICAL FINDINGS & CLINICAL PRESENTATION

Stings:
- Cutaneous: the skin is the most common site of a local allergic reaction. Manifestations include flushing, urticaria, pruritus, and angioedema. Local reactions may last several days.
- Respiratory: Symptoms of upper and lower airway obstruction including hoarseness, choking, throat tightness or tingling may progress to stridor, laryngeal edema, laryngospasm, and bronchoconstriction. This is the leading cause of anaphylactic death.
- Cardiovascular: most common reaction is hypotension which can progress to profound hypovolemic shock. Tachycardia and arrhythmia may occur. Myocardial infarction is rare. Cardiac manifestations are the second leading cause of death from anaphylaxis.
- Other symptoms: abdominal pain, nausea, vomiting, and diarrhea.

Fire ant bites:
- Initial wheal and flare response.
- Subsequent development of circularly arrayed blisters within 24 hr (Fig. 1-170).
- Blisters may develop appearance of pustules, but they are not infected.

ETIOLOGY

Stings:
- Most systemic reactions to insect stings are classic immunoglobin E (IgE)–mediated reactions. Anaphylaxis can be the presenting sign of indolent mastocytosis.
- Reactions occur in previously sensitized patients who have produced high titers of IgE antibody to insect venom antigens.
- Sensitization to wasp venom requires only a few stings and can occur after a single sting.
- Sensitization to bee venom occurs mainly in people who have been stung frequently by bees.
- Fig. 1-171 illustrates representative venomous hymenoptera

Bites:
- Fire ant venom contains proteins toxic to the skin.

Dx DIAGNOSIS

DIFFERENTIAL DIAGNOSIS

- Stings: cellulitis, bites
- Bites: stings, cellulitis

WORKUP

History is essential for accurate diagnosis including timing of sting or bite and type of insect (bee, wasp, spider, or ant) if known.

LABORATORY TESTS

- Skin test: either skin prick test or intradermal method with fire ant or hymenoptera venom.
- Venom skin tests and occasionally radioallergosorbent tests (RAST) to provide additional information, only for those with history of a systemic reaction.
- Venom-specific IgE tests are of limited use.

Rx TREATMENT

ACUTE GENERAL Rx

Sting:
- Local Poison Control Center can be contacted
- Removal of the stinger most easily performed with a flat tool such as a credit card, followed by cleansing and application of ice.
- Avoid squeezing, which may push venom out of the venom sac and into the tissue.
- Consider treatment with oral antihistamines and nonsteroidal antiinflammatory medications and topical corticosteroids for limited reactions.
- Patients with previous reactions or multiple stings to the mouth or neck should be evaluated in an emergency department.
- Larger swellings may benefit from oral steroids.
- Generalized reactions should be treated with epinephrine. Antihistamines, oxygen, IV corticosteroids, beta-agonists, pressors, and IV fluids may also be beneficial for anaphylaxis.

Bite:
- Supportive care—wash with soap and water
- Application of ice or cooling. Calamine lotion may be helpful.
- Surveillance for secondary infection

DISPOSITION

Sting:
- Prognosis for a limited reaction is excellent.
- Subsequent anaphylaxis may occur in 35% to 65% of patients stung again with history of prior systemic reaction. Large local reaction does not predict a systemic reaction.
- There is no evidence that the next sting will necessarily cause a more severe reaction. Variable outcome is due to the patient's age, comorbidities, time elapsed since prior exposure, dose of venom injected, and site of sting.
- Watch for secondary cellulitis.
- Patients who have a history of a severe allergic reaction or a systemic reaction:
  - Should be educated in avoidance of stinging insects
  - Carry syringes preloaded with epinephrine for self-administration
  - Undergo testing for IgE antibodies to stinging insects
  - Be considered for immunotherapy, reduces chance of serious allergic reaction by 90%
  - Consider carrying medical identification for stinging insect hypersensitivity

Bite:
- Prognosis for fire ant bite is excellent.
- Large lesions from brown recluse spider bites may take months to heal.
- Watch for secondary cellulitis.

REFERRAL

- Consider a referral to an allergist for venom immunotherapy (VIT).
- Risk of subsequent anaphylaxis with immunotherapy falls to <3%.
- VIT for 3 to 5 yr induces long-term protection in most patients.

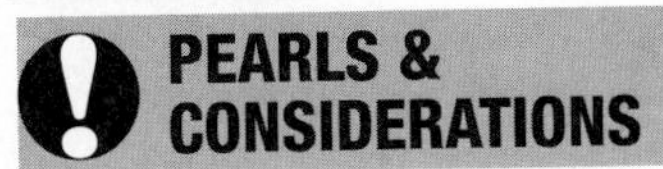

PEARLS & CONSIDERATIONS

Hypersensitivity to stings is common. Reactions range from local nonallergic reaction to venom to life-threatening anaphylaxis. Venom-specific immunotherapy is highly effective in decreasing subsequent anaphylaxis. Although venom immunotherapy is currently indicated only for systemic reactions, investigation is under way to assess efficacy for prevention of large local reactions, which can result in significant morbidity.

 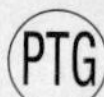

SUGGESTED READINGS
available at www.expertconsult.com

RELATED CONTENT

Bites and Stings, Arachnids (Related Key Topic)
Bites and Stings (Patient Information)

AUTHORS: **LYNN BOWLBY, M.D.** and **JENNIFER JEREMIAH, M.D.**

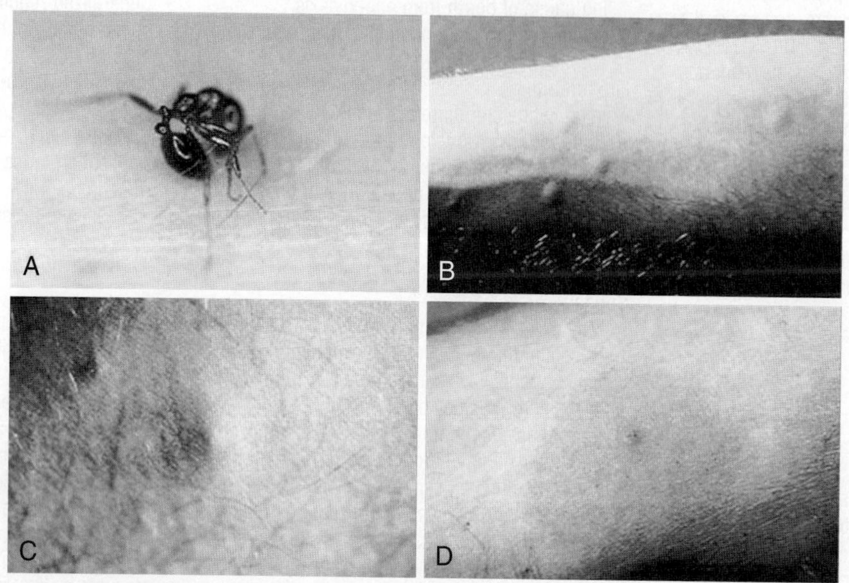

FIGURE 1-170 **A,** Stinging fire ant (*S. invicta*). **B,** Wheal-and-flare reactions 5 minutes after multiple fire ant stings. **C,** Sterile pustule 24 hours after fire ant sting. **D,** Cutaneous late-phase allergic reaction 24 hours after fire ant sting. Excoriated sterile pustule in center of lesion. (From Kemp SF et al: Expanding habitat of the imported fire ant (*Solenopsis invicta*): a public health concern, *J Allergy Clin Immunol* 105(4):683-691, 2000.)

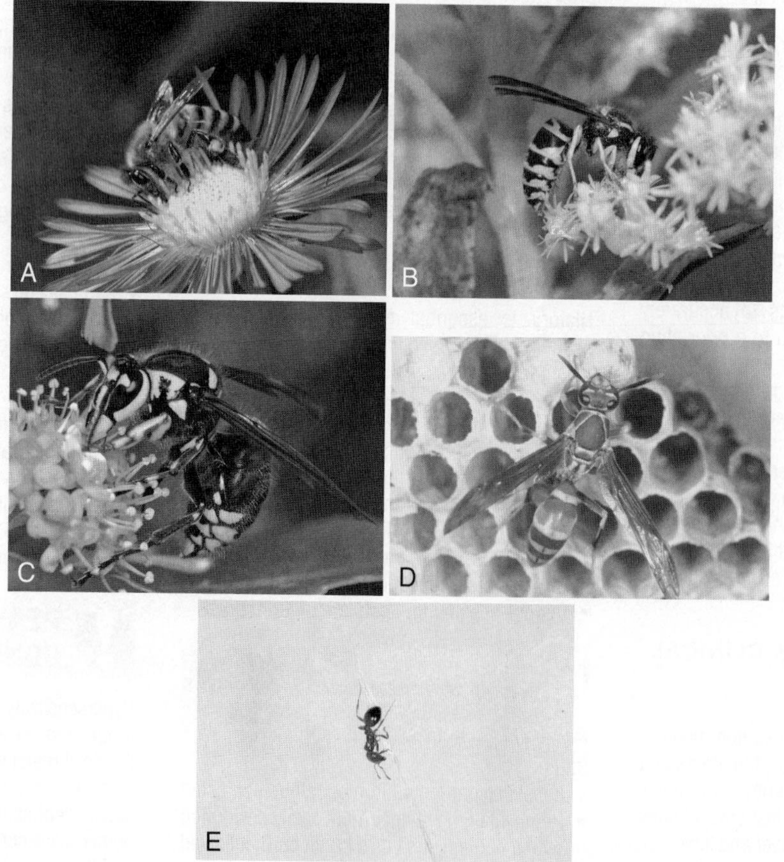

FIGURE 1-171 Stinging insects of the order Hymenoptera: A, Honeybee (*Apis mellifera*). **B,** Yellow jacket (*Vespula maculifrons*). **C,** White-faced hornet (*Dolichovesupla maculata*). **D,** Paper wasp (*Polistes exclamans*). **E,** Imported fire ant (*Solenopsis invicta*). (Reproduced by permission of ALK-Abelló A/S, Hørsholm, Denmark.)

BASIC INFORMATION

DEFINITION

Injury resulting from snake biting a human.

ICD-9CM CODES
989.5 Venomous poisoning
ICD-10CM CODES
T63.001A Toxic effect of unspecified snake venom, accidental (unintentional), initial encounter

EPIDEMIOLOGY & DEMOGRAPHICS

- 45,000 snakebites occur annually in the U.S. Of the 5000 to 7000 caused by poisonous snakes, approximately 5 to 12 result in fatality (i.e., <1%-2%). Children, the elderly, and those in whom treatment has been delayed are at highest risk.
- In the U.S., at least one species of poisonous snake (Fig. 1-172) has been identified in every state except Alaska, Hawaii, and Maine. Table 1-77 summarizes medically important snake families. The Crotalidae family, which includes rattlesnakes, copperheads, and cottonmouths, is responsible for the vast majority of venomous snakebites. The Elapidae family includes the mambas and cobras internationally, but in the U.S. includes only the coral snake. Coral snakes are not only much less common in the U.S., than Crotalids, but they also tend to be less aggressive and account for only 1% of venomous snakebites in the U.S.

PHYSICAL FINDINGS & CLINICAL PRESENTATION

In addition to local tissue injury, envenomation may affect the renal, neurologic, gastrointestinal, vascular, and coagulation systems. Symptoms vary widely depending on type of envenomation. Not all snakebites are poisonous and not all bites lead to envenomation. Species-specific signs and symptoms following envenomation are discussed.

CROTALIDAE (PIT VIPERS): Local signs and symptoms
- Pain within 5 min
- Edema within 30 min
- Erythema of site and adjacent tissues/serous or hemorrhagic bullae, ecchymosis, and/or lymphangitis over the ensuing hours (Fig. 1-173)

If no edema or erythema is manifested within 8 hr after a confirmed Crotalid snakebite, it is safe to assume envenomation did not occur. (Roughly 25% of cases do not involve envenomation.) In general, rattlesnake bites are more severe than those of the other snakes in the Crotalid family.

Systemic manifestations may include:
- Mild to moderate nausea/vomiting, perioral paresthesias, metallic taste, tingling of fingers or toes (especially with rattlesnake bites), and/or fasciculations (local or generalized)
- Severe hypotension (due to increased vascular permeability), mental status change, respiratory distress, tachycardia, acute renal failure, rhabdomyolysis, and coagulopathies including intravascular hemolysis and disseminated intravascular coagulation

ELAPIDAE (CORAL SNAKES): Signs and symptoms:
- Local symptoms are far less pronounced (little or no pain/swelling immediately after the bite).
- Neurologic symptoms are more common due to neurotoxins in Elapid venom.
- Systemic symptoms predominate, but onset may be delayed for up to 12 hr. Examples include:
  - Altered mental status and cranial nerve palsies featuring ptosis, dysphagia, or dysarthria
  - Tremors

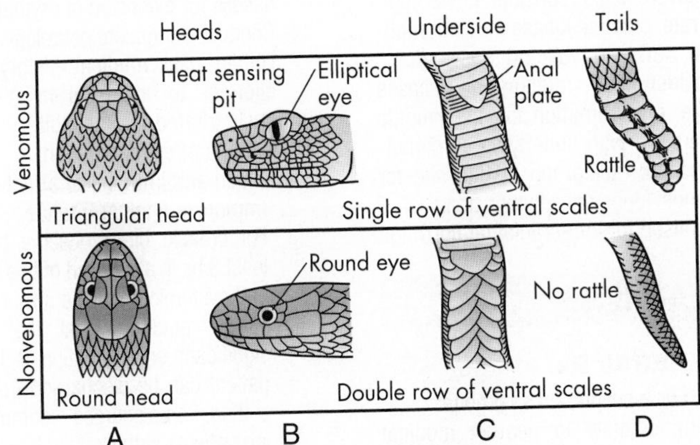

FIGURE 1-172 Comparison of pit vipers and nonvenomous snakes. Rattle in **D** (*top*) applies to rattlesnakes only. (**A** to **D**, From Sullivan JB et al: North American venomous reptile bites. In Auerbach PS [ed]: *Wilderness medicine: management of wilderness and environmental emergencies,* ed 3, p. 684, St Louis, 1995, Mosby.)

TABLE 1-77 Medically Important Snake Families

Family	Venomous?	Location	Examples	Toxin Effects/Other Comments
Colubridae	Some species	Most parts of the world	Garter snakes (*Thamnophis* spp), king snakes and milk snakes (*Lampropeltis* spp)	Largest family of snakes; most are considered harmless to humans; a few species are dangerously toxic (e.g., African boomslang [*Dispholidus typus*])
Boidae	None	Most parts of the world	*Boa* sp, *Python* sp	Constrictors; unsupervised children should not be allowed access to large constrictors
Viperidae				
Subfamily Crotalinae (pit vipers)	All	Americas, Asia	Rattlesnakes (*Crotalus* spp), cottonmouths and copperheads (*Agkistrodon* spp), Lancehead pit vipers (*Bothrops* spp)	Heat-sensing "pit" between each eye and nostril
Subfamily Viperinae (true vipers)	All	Europe, Africa, Middle East, Asia	Puff adder (*Bitis arietans*), Gaboon viper (*Bitis gabonica*)	No heat-sensing pits
Elapidae	All	Americas, Africa, Middle East, Asia	Cobras (*Naja* spp), mambas (*Dendroaspis* spp), kraits (*Bungarus* spp), coral snakes (*Micrurus* spp), and the venomous snakes of Australia	Highly variable venom effects—some largely neurotoxic, others causing severe local tissue damage
Hydrophiidae	All	Warm waters of the Pacific Ocean, Indian Ocean, and Oceania (none in the Atlantic Ocean)	Sea snakes including the pelagic sea snake (*Pelamis platurus*)	Neurotoxins and myotoxins; rarely bite humans unless provoked

From Kliegman RM et al: *Nelson textbook of pediatrics,* ed 19, Philadelphia, 2011, Saunders.

- Intense salivation, nausea, vomiting, or abdominal pain
- Loss of DTRs and respiratory depression (late manifestations)

ETIOLOGY

- Farm workers and other people working or doing recreational activities in the outdoors are the most common victims of snake bites, because they are in the snakes' natural habitat.
- Intoxication and intentional provocation also contribute to many of the cases of snake bites in the U.S.

Dx DIAGNOSIS

DIFFERENTIAL DIAGNOSIS

- Harmless snakebite
- Scorpion bite
- "Dry bite"
- Insect bite
- Cellulitis
- Laceration or puncture wound
- Necrotizing fasciitis

NOTE: Harmless snakebites are usually characterized by four rows of small scratches (teeth in upper jaw) separated from two rows of scratches (teeth in lower jaw). This is in distinction to venomous snakebites, which should have paired puncture wounds produced by the snake's fangs, whether other teeth marks are noted. A "dry bite" is a bite with puncture wounds but no evidence of swelling, erythema, or lab abnormalities.

WORKUP

An estimated 25% of venomous snakebites do not result in envenomation, but all cases of suspected envenomation should be observed for 8 hr or longer:

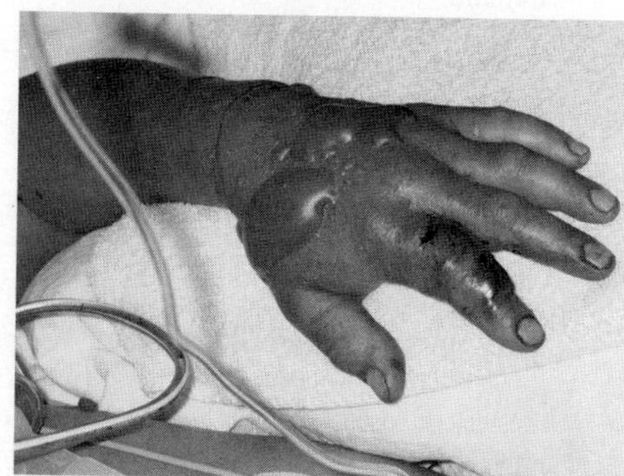

FIGURE 1-173 Southern Pacific rattlesnake *(Crotalus helleri)* bite wounds. (Courtesy Sean Bush, M.D.)

- Check for signs of envenomation.
  - Swelling, tenderness, redness, ecchymosis, or blebs at the bite site
  - Elevated protime, decreased fibrinogen or platelets
  - Systemic signs such as hypotension, bleeding complications, vomiting, diarrhea, angioedema, or neurotoxicity
- Determine if patient has indications for antivenom (Table 1-78). Continual reassessment is indicated throughout the observation period because severity of symptoms may change.

LABORATORY TESTS

- For all suspected envenomations, obtain CBC (with peripheral smear and platelet count), DIC screen (PT/INR, PTT, fibrinogen, fibrin degradation products, d-dimer), ECG, serum electrolytes, BUN, Cr, and urinalysis. Serial measurements of hemoglobin, platelets, protime, and fibrinogen are needed to monitor for acute and delayed hematologic complications.
- For more severe bites, consider LFTs, sedimentation rate, creatine kinase (rule out rhabdomyolysis), ABG, and type and crossmatch.
- Other: consider chest radiograph in cases with severe envenomation or in patients over 40 years old with underlying cardiopulmonary disease; radiograph of bite site for retained fangs (poor sensitivity); head CT if concern is raised for intracranial hemorrhage

Rx TREATMENT

ACUTE GENERAL Rx

IN THE FIELD: For a suspected snakebite:

- Transport immediately to nearest medical facility. No treatments in the field should delay travel to the nearest facility where an antivenom agent can be given if necessary.
- Immobilize affected part.
- Remove any constricting items. Applying tourniquets, incising, and applying suction to the wound is discouraged. Tourniquets cause more local tissue damage due to tissue necrosing venom seen in Crotalid bites and should not delay transport to a medical facility.
- Do not apply ice; keep victim warm.
- Avoid alcohol, stimulants (caffeine), or agents that can suppress mental status.

IN THE HOSPITAL:

- Record vital signs: BP, HR, T, RR, and O_2 sat.
- Establish intravenous access and initiate IV hydration with crystalloid if the patient is hypotensive.
- Obtain time of bite and description of snake if possible. Crotalids have a triangle-shaped head, nostril holes (pits), and elliptical pupils. The most dangerous of the crotalids is the rattlesnake, distinguished by its telltale rattle. Elapids, like the western and eastern coral snakes of the U.S., have brightly colored red, black, and yellow stripes.
- Obtain and initiate reconstitution of appropriate antivenom. (Antivenoms are typically supplied in powder form and must be reconstituted before administration. If using older antivenoms, this process can take up to 1 hr, so it is recommended that it be initiated as soon as the patient arrives in the ED.)
  - Inspect site of bite for fang marks and local symptoms.
  - Delineate margins of erythema/edema with a marker.
  - Measure circumference of bitten part at two or more proximal sites and compare with unaffected limb; repeat every 15 to 20 min; assess for extension of erythema/edema.
  - Conduct a complete neurologic examination.
  - Obtain past medical history; ask about allergies to horse serum in those previously treated for snakebite.
- If no signs of envenomation:
  1. Clean and immobilize affected part.
  2. Immunize against tetanus.
  3. For crotalid bites, observe patient for at least 8 hr. If, at the end of this interval, local and systemic sequelae are absent and lab values remain normal, the likelihood of significant envenomation is low, and the patient can be discharged from the acute setting. Some sources recommend observing patients with Crotalid bites to the lower extremities for at least 24 hours because swelling in the larger compartments of the legs could be slower and less easily recognizable. All definitive elapid bites should be treated. If elapid bite is only suspected, the patient must be monitored for up to 18 hr as symptoms can be delayed.
- Patients who have progressive local symptoms or any systemic symptoms should be considered for antivenom. Crotalid envenomations without any progressive local or any systemic symptoms can be monitored for 12 to 24 hours, with repeat labs obtained 4 to 6 hours prior to discharge. If they have no new symptoms during that period of observation, they may be safely discharged. Specifically, copperhead bites often need no further interventions.
- Contact Poison Control: 1-800-222-1222; they can provide guidance and track snake bite incidence

Once the decision is made to use antivenom:

- Prepare epinephrine 0.5 to 1.0 mg (0.5-1 ml of a 1:1000 solution) to be administered subcutaneously (SQ) in case of a hypersensitivity reaction to the antivenom. The incidence of hypersensitivity reaction with sheep-based antivenom, now standard for crotalid envenomations, is estimated to be less than 1 in 7. This is much lower than that with horse serum antivenom previously used for crotalid and currently the standard for elapidad envenomations.

TABLE 1-78 Indications for Snake Antivenom Administration

Evidence of systemic toxicity:	
Hemodynamic or respiratory instability	Hypotension, respiratory distress
Hemotoxicity	Clinically significant bleeding or abnormal coagulation studies
Neurotoxicity	Any evidence of toxicity: usually beginning with cranial nerve abnormalities and progressing to descending paralysis including the diaphragm
Evidence of local toxicity	*Progressive* soft tissue swelling

From Kliegman RM et al: *Nelson textbook of pediatrics,* ed 19, Philadelphia, 2011, Saunders.

Empiric prophylactic antihistamines or epinephrine have not been proved to prevent reactions.

ANTIVENOM TREATMENT OF CROTALID (RATTLESNAKE, PIT VIPER, COPPERHEAD, COTTONMOUTH) ENVENOMATIONS

- For patients with mild to moderate symptoms:
  - An initial IV loading dose of 4 to 6 vials (depending on the size and age of the patient and the severity of the bite) is infused over 60 min. The infusion should be given very slowly for the first 10 min to watch for allergic reaction. For patients with shock or serious active bleeding, use an intial dose of 8 to 12 vials.
  - If the patient has not responded after 1 hr, repeat the initial dose.
- Relapse is seen in up to two thirds of patients after an initial response. Consequently, it is recommended that three maintenance doses—each consisting of 2 vials—be given at 6, 12, and 18 hr following the patient's initial response to the loading dose.
- The manufacturer of Crofab maintains a 24/7 hotline: 877-377-3784
- Antivenin Crotalidae Polyvalent horse serum is no longer produced but may still be available at some pharmacies. It should be given as follows:
  - Progressive local or any systemic symptoms: 5 to 10 vials
  - Severe symptoms: 15 vials
  - Shock: 20 vials

ANTIVENOM TREATMENT OF ELAPIDAE (CORAL SNAKE) ENVENOMATIONS:

- Production of horse serum–based coral snake antivenom was discontinued in 2006 (horse serum–based antivenoms are being phased out due to much higher risk of hypersensitivity). All stock is expired as of October 31, 2008, except for lot 4030026, which received a 3-yr extension until October 31, 2013, and there has been no update at the time of this submission. After that date, one option will be to seek compassionate release of expired stock in conjunction with your local Poison Control Center. A potent, safe, sheep-based antivenom for elapid bites exists and is being used internationally but is not yet approved in the U.S. Another option is to contact a zoo that cares for exotic snakes and obtain Mexican coral snake or Australian Tiger snake antivenom, although efficacy for North American coral snake envenomation is unproved.
- For confirmed coral snake bites, antivenom should be administered immediately if available.
- If there are no systemic symptoms at the time of administration, start with 3 vials. If symptoms progress, repeat with 5 vials.
- If systemic symptoms are already present, an initial dose of 6 to 10 vials is recommended.

TREATMENT OF NONNATIVE (EXOTIC) SNAKEBITES

- For bites by exotic or nonnative snakes, contact a Poison Control Center or your local zoo. (Zoos with exotic snakes are required to maintain a supply of snake-specific antivenom on their premises.)

DISPOSITION

Prognosis is good with prompt evaluation and treatment. All patients who receive antivenom should be monitored in an ICU setting. Patients should be monitored for 18 to 24 hours after initial control of progression of symptoms. If at that time they have no progression of symptoms and labs prior to discharge are normal, patients can be safely discharged home. Give instructions to return for worsening nondependent swelling, abnormal bleeding, or signs of serum sickness and to follow bleeding precautions (no contact sports, elective surgery, etc.) for 2 weeks. Patients who received antivenom need follow-up in 2 to 3 days and in 5 to 7 days to evaluate for delayed hematologic complications and serum sickness.

REFERRAL

Refer to a medical facility with ICU for administration of antivenom. The approach to snakebites should be multidisciplinary and should include medical toxicology or other physican snakebite specialist, as well as hematology or nephrology consultations if needed. All cases of snake bites should also be reported to Poison Control and the local health department as data are limited.

PEARLS & CONSIDERATIONS

OTHER CONSIDERATIONS

- Dosage of antivenom is based on typical envenomation rather than age or weight, so dose is the same for children and adults.
- Pregnancy is not a contraindication to antivenom. The rate of miscarriage is significantly lower in pregnant patients treated with antivenom.
- Immunize against tetanus if no booster within past 5 yr; if never immunized, give immunoglobulin as well as toxoid.
- Manage pain as needed (narcotic preferred to NSAIDs due to theoretical bleeding complications).
- Avoid sedation in Mojave rattlesnake, Eastern diamondback rattlesnake, and coral snake bites as all can have more systemic and neurologic than local effects.
- Antibiotics rarely needed; reserve for moderate to severe contamination or definite infection; broad-spectrum coverage to include gram negatives preferred (i.e., ampicillin-sulbactam or quinolone derivatives).
- Antivenom is most effective when given within 4 hr of the bite and least effective if delayed beyond 12 hr. Systemic symptoms (coagulopathy, CNS effects, etc.) respond better to treatment than do local symptoms (erythema/edema, bullae, etc.).
- Although local wound effects can be severe, wound management should not take precedence over antivenom administration. Some studies suggest that even in the case of compartment syndrome, antivenom may be more effective than fasciotomy, although both may be necessary.

COMPLICATIONS

- Allergic reactions were very frequent with horse serum antivenoms. Cro-fab from sheep serum should be preferentially used over equine serum if available.
- Anaphylaxis occurs within 30 min and should be treated by immediately stopping the infusion to managing the symptoms of anaphylaxis, including epinephrine SQ or IM initially and IV if needed, diphenhydramine IV, and hydrocortisone IV. If the anaphylactic symptoms can be managed and the envenomation is severe, the infusion can then be resumed.
- Delayed hematologic complications are common and can manifest up to 4 days post treatment. Most bleeding is self-limited but can rarely be severe, necessitating close follow-up.
- Serum sickness occurs 7 to 14 days after antivenom administration and is characterized by fever, rash, arthralgias, and lymphadenopathy. It can be treated with prednisone 60 mg/d PO, tapered over 7 to 10 days.
- Injuries also result from:
  - Tourniquet placement on the field, which should be avoided
  - Ice application (cryotherapy), which can worsen tissue damage
- National Poison Control hotline: 800-222-1222

SUGGESTED READINGS

available at www.expertconsult.com

RELATED CONTENT

Snake Bites (Patient Information)

AUTHORS: **ROBERT BUTLER, M.D.,** and **NEHA P. RAUKAR, M.D., M.S.**

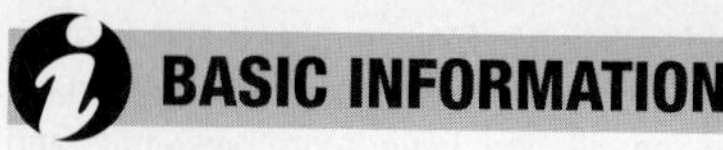

BASIC INFORMATION

DEFINITION

Bladder cancer is a heterogeneous spectrum of neoplasms ranging from non–life-threatening, low-grade, superficial papillary lesions to high-grade invasive tumors, which often have metastasized at the time of presentation. It is a field change disease in which the entire urothelium from the renal pelvis to the urethra may be susceptible to malignant transformation. The three types of bladder cancer are transitional cell carcinoma (TCCa), squamous cell carcinoma, and adenocarcinoma.

ICD-9CM CODES

Primary:	188.9
Secondary:	198.1
CIS:	233.7
Benign:	223.3
Uncertain behavior:	236.7
Unspecified:	239.4

ICD-10CM CODES

C67.9	Malignant neoplasm of bladder, unspecified
C79.11	Secondary malignant neoplasm of bladder
D09.0	Carcinoma in situ of bladder
D30.3	Benign neoplasm of bladder
D41.4	Neoplasm of uncertain behavior of bladder
D49.4	Neoplasm of unspecified behavior of bladder

EPIDEMIOLOGY & DEMOGRAPHICS

Each year over 70,000 new cases are diagnosed and more than 14,000 deaths are attributed to bladder cancer. Overall, bladder cancer is the sixth most prevalent malignancy in the U.S. and the seventh leading cause of solid-cancer–related death.

Until 1990, the incidence of bladder cancer in the U.S. was rising. Since 1990, the incidence of bladder cancer is decreasing at a rate of 0.8% per year (1.2% among men and 0.4% among women).

PREDOMINANT SEX: In males, it is the fourth most common cancer, accounting for 10% of all cancers. In females, it is the eighth most common cancer, accounting for 4% of all cancers.

RISK: The lifetime risk of developing bladder cancer is 2.8% in white males, 0.9% in black males, 1% in white females, and 0.6% in black females.

Smoking:

- Users of "black" tobacco in place of "blond" tobacco have a twofold to threefold increase in developing bladder cancer.
- Smoking risk is based on consumption:
  - A twofold to threefold increase for subjects smoking at least 10 cigarettes per day
  - The risk increases again when the daily consumption rises above 40 to 60 cigarettes per day
- Smokers of low-tar and nicotine cigarettes have a lower risk when compared with higher tar and nicotine cigarettes.
- Those who smoke unfiltered cigarettes have a 50% increased risk of bladder cancer compared with those who smoke filtered cigarettes.
- Pipe smokers have a lower risk of bladder cancer compared with cigarette smokers.
- Cigars, snuff, and chewing tobacco, although implicated in nonurologic cancers, are not believed to influence bladder cancer risk.

Diet:

- Diets rich in beef, pork, and animal fat increase risk of bladder cancer.
- There is no indication that consumption of non-beer alcoholic drinks contributes to bladder cancer development.
- Beer consumption has been linked to bladder cancer development as a result of the presence of nitrosamines in the beer. Nitrosamines have also been implicated in the development of rectal cancer.
- Drinking coffee is not believed to contribute to bladder cancer risk. There is additional evidence that coffee consumption is protective for colorectal cancers, possibly by diminishing fecal transit time.
- Medications: Long-term (>1 yr) use of pioglitazone and rosiglitazone

PEAK INCIDENCE: Incidence increases with age: higher after age 60 yr, uncommon younger than 40 yr.

GENETICS: It is thought to be multifactorial in etiology, involving both genetic and environmental interactions. Overall, approximately 20% to 25% of the male population in the U.S. with bladder cancer is estimated to have the disease as a result of occupational exposure.

DISTRIBUTION: In North America, transitional cell carcinomas comprise 93%, squamous cell carcinomas comprise 6%, and adenocarcinomas account for 1% of bladder cancers.

PATHOGENESIS: Two pathways exist for bladder cancer (TCCa):

1. Papillary superficial disease occasionally leading to invasive cancer (75%)
2. Carcinoma in situ (CIS) and solid invasive cancer with high risk of disease progression (25%)

Two distinct forms of "superficial cancer" exist:

1. T_a: Papillary low-grade tumor with a high rate of recurrence; disease progression occurs in 5%.
2. T_1: Higher grade papillary tumor that infiltrates the lamina propria; often associated with flat CIS that may involve the urothelium diffusely. Disease progression occurs in 30% to 50%.

Subdivided into:

- T_{1a}: Penetration of tumor up to the muscularis mucosa; disease progression in 5.3%
- T_{1b}: Penetration of tumor through the muscularis mucosa; disease progression 53%

Flat CIS:

- Entirely different and separate pathway of cancer development whose mechanism is manifested by dysplasia, which leads to the occurrence of poorly differentiated malignant cells that replace or undermine the normal urothelium and extend along the plane of the bladder wall. It penetrates the basement membrane and lamina propria in 20% to 30% of cases and is associated with the development of solid tumor growth. A defect in chromosome 17p53 occurs in 50% of the cases.

At presentation, 72% of cancers are localized to the bladder, 20% of the cancers extend to the regional lymph nodes, and 3% present with distant metastases. Eighty percent of superficial TCCa recur, with up to 30% progressing to a higher stage or grade. Younger patients most commonly develop low-grade papillary noninvasive TCCa and are less likely to have recurrences when compared with older patients with similar lesions. Involvement of the upper tracts with tumor occurs in 25% to 50% of the cases.

STAGING (BASED ON THE TNM SYSTEM):

T_0	No tumor in specimen
T_{is}	CIS
T_a	Papillary TCCa noninvasive
T_1	Papillary TCCa into lamina propria
T_2	TCCa invasive of superficial muscle
T_{3a}	Invasive of deep muscle
T_{3b}	Invasive of perivesical fat
T_{4a}	Invasive of adjacent pelvic organ
T_{4b}	Invasive of pelvic wall with fixation

Invasive of nodal status

N_0	No nodal involvement
N_{1-3}	Pelvic nodes
N_4	Nodes above bifurcation
N_x	Unknown

Invasive of metastatic status

M_0	No distant metastases
M_1	Distant metastases
M_x	Unknown

MOLECULAR EPIDEMIOLOGY: TCCa is usually a field change disease with tumors arising at different times and sites in the urothelium, suggesting a polyclonal etiology of bladder cancer. Bladder cancers have been associated with abnormalities on chromosomes 1, 4, 11, 5, 7, 3, 9, 21, 18, 13, 8; with alterations in suppressor genes *P53,* retinoblastoma gene, and *P16;* and with alterations in oncogenes H-ras and epidermal growth factor receptor.

PHYSICAL FINDINGS & CLINICAL PRESENTATION

- Gross, painless hematuria
- Microhematuria
- Frequency, urgency, occasional dysuria
- With locally invasive to distant metastatic disease, the presentation can include:
  - Abdominal pain
  - Flank pain
  - Lymphedema
  - Renal failure
  - Anorexia
  - Bone pain

ETIOLOGY

Bladder cancer is a potentially preventable disease associated with specific etiologic factors:

- Cigarette smoking is associated with 25% to 65% of cases. The risk of developing a TCCa is two to four times higher in smokers than in nonsmokers, and that risk persists for many years, being equal to nonsmokers only after 12 to 15 yr of smoking abstinence. Smoking tobacco is associated with tumors that are characterized by higher histologic grade, increased tumor stage, increase in the numbers of tumor present, and increased tumor size.

- Occupational exposures: dye workers, textile workers, tire and rubber workers, petroleum workers.
- Chemical exposure: O-toluidine, 2-naphthylamine, benzidine, 4-amino-biphenyl, and nitrosamines.
- Exposure to herpes papilloma virus type 16.

Squamous carcinomas are associated with:

- Schistosomiasis
- Urinary calculi
- Indwelling catheters
- Bladder diverticula

Miscellaneous causes:

- Phenacetin abuse
- Cyclophosphamide
- Pelvic irradiation
- Tuberculosis

Adenocarcinomas are associated with:

- Exstrophy
- Endometriosis
- Neurogenic bladder
- Urachal abnormalities
- As a secondary site for distant metastases from other organs (e.g., colon cancer)

Dx DIAGNOSIS

- History and physical examination.
- Urinalysis.
- Cystoscopy with bladder barbotage and biopsy. Fluorescence cystoscopy offers improvement in the detection of flat neoplastic lesions such as carcinoma in situ.
- Transurethral resection of bladder tumor(s).
- There is insufficient evidence to determine whether a decrease in mortality rate from bladder cancer occurs with hematuria testing, urinary cytology, or a variety of other tests on exfoliated urinary cells or other substances.
- In addition to urinary cytology and bladder barbotage, BTA, NMP22, and fibrin degradation products have been approved by the FDA as bladder cancer tumor markers. No marker has general, widespread acceptance because the results are affected by the presence of stents, recent urologic manipulation, stones, infection, bowel interposition, and prostatitis, creating false-positive results.

DIFFERENTIAL DIAGNOSIS

- Urinary tract infection
- Frequency-urgency syndrome
- Interstitial cystitis
- Stone disease
- Endometriosis
- Neurogenic bladder

LABORATORY TESTS

- Urine cytology.
- Urine telomerase: telomerase activity in voided urine or bladder washings determined by the telomeric repeat amplification protocol (TRAP) assay. This test has been reported to accurately detect the presence of bladder tumors in men. It represents a potentially useful noninvasive diagnostic innovation for bladder cancer detection in high-risk groups such as habitual smokers or in symptomatic patients.

RADIOLOGIC TESTS

- IVP, renal ultrasound, retrograde pyelography, CT scan, and MRI.
- One or a combination of studies can be used. In the absence of skeletal symptoms, bone scan is not recommended.

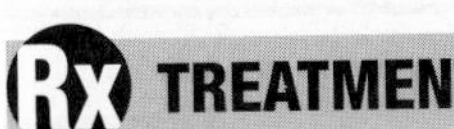

Rx TREATMENT

NONPHARMACOLOGIC THERAPY

- Initially, transurethral resection of bladder tumor (TURBT) (Fig. 1-174)
- Loop biopsy of the prostatic urethra if high-grade TCCa is suspected
- If superficial disease, follow-up protocol with repeat TURBT and/or the use of intravesical agents is recommended
- For advanced bladder cancer, radical cystectomy with urethrectomy (unless orthotopic diversion is planned) and either ileal loop conduit or orthotopic diversion

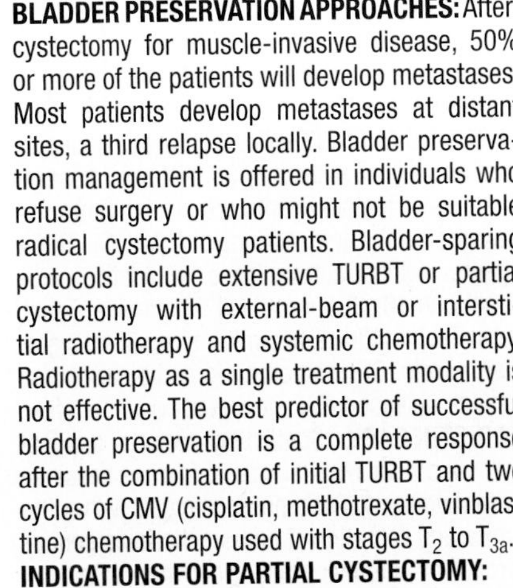

BLADDER PRESERVATION APPROACHES: After cystectomy for muscle-invasive disease, 50% or more of the patients will develop metastases. Most patients develop metastases at distant sites, a third relapse locally. Bladder preservation management is offered in individuals who refuse surgery or who might not be suitable radical cystectomy patients. Bladder-sparing protocols include extensive TURBT or partial cystectomy with external-beam or interstitial radiotherapy and systemic chemotherapy. Radiotherapy as a single treatment modality is not effective. The best predictor of successful bladder preservation is a complete response after the combination of initial TURBT and two cycles of CMV (cisplatin, methotrexate, vinblastine) chemotherapy used with stages T_2 to T_{3a}.

INDICATIONS FOR PARTIAL CYSTECTOMY:

- Tumor within a bladder diverticulum
- Solitary, primary, and muscle-invasive or high-grade lesion of a region of the bladder that allows complete excision with adequate surgical margins
- Inability to adequately resect tumor by TURBT alone because of size or location
- Tumor overlying a ureteral orifice requiring ureteral reimplantation
- Biopsy of a radiation-induced ulceration
- Palliation of severe local symptoms
- Patient refusal of urinary diversion
- Poor-risk patient who is not a diversion candidate

CONTRAINDICATIONS:

- Multiple tumors
- CIS
- Cellular atypia on biopsy
- Prostatic invasion
- Invasion of the trigone
- Inability to achieve adequate surgical margins
- Prior radiotherapy
- Inability to maintain adequate bladder volume after resection
- Evidence of extravesical tumor extension
- Poor surgical risk

ACUTE GENERAL Rx

INDICATIONS FOR INTRAVESICAL CHEMOTHERAPY:

- High-grade tumor
- Tumor size >5 cm
- Tumor multiplicity
- Presence of CIS
- Positive urinary cytologic findings after a resection
- Incomplete tumor resection

Intravesical agents: thiotepa, Adriamycin, mitomycin C, AD-32, BCG, interferon, bropirimine, Epodyl, interleukin-2, and keyhole-limpet hemocyanin. Photodynamic therapy with hematoporphyrin derivatives has also been used.

INDICATIONS FOR CYSTECTOMY:

- Large tumors not amenable to complete TURBT
- High-grade tumor
- Multiple tumors with frequent recurrences
- Diffuse CIS not responsive to intravesical chemotherapy
- Prostatic urethra involvement

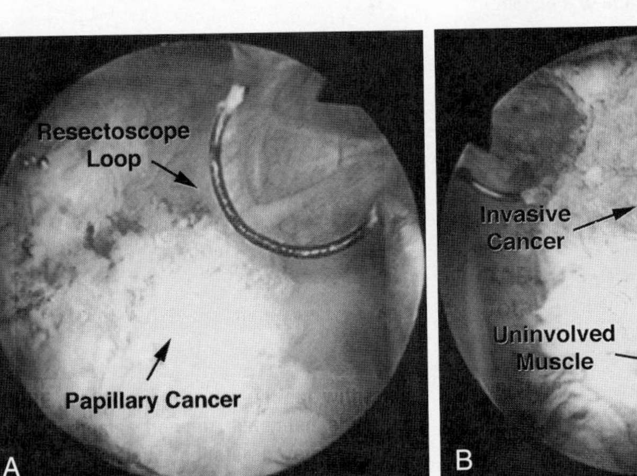

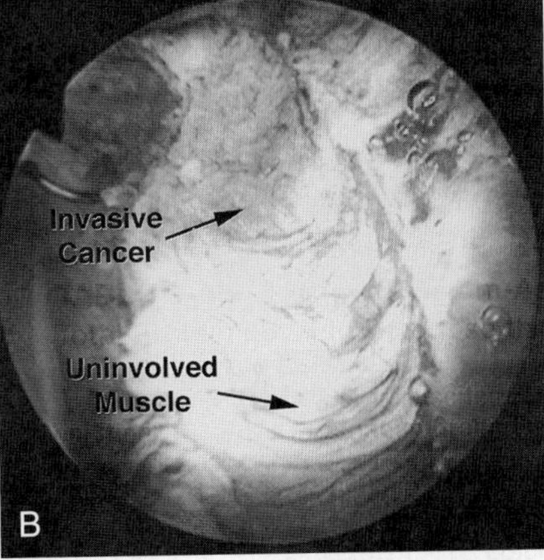

FIGURE 1-174 A, Papillary bladder cancer in right lower aspect of photo with resection loop poised to begin transurethral resection. **B,** Demonstration of grossly uninvolved muscularis propria *(bottom)* and cancer grossly invading the bladder wall *(top)*. (From Abeloff MD: *Clinical oncology*, ed 3, Philadelphia, 2004, Churchill Livingstone.)

- Irritative bladder symptoms with upper tract deterioration
- Muscle-invasive disease
- Disease outside the bladder

SYSTEMIC CHEMOTHERAPY: Used as neoadjuvant and adjuvant therapy for systemic disease. The most effective agents are cisplatin, methotrexate, vinblastine, Adriamycin (MVAC). Other agents include mitoxantrone, vincristine, etoposide (VP16), 5-fluorouracil, ifosfamide, Taxol, gemcitabine, Piritrexim, mitomycin C, and gallium nitrate. Chemotherapy in combination can provide palliation and modest survival benefit.

RADIOTHERAPY: Conflicting reports suggest that superficial bladder cancer is more sensitive to radiotherapy. Squamous changes within the tumor and secretion of human chorionic gonadotropin by the lesion are associated with poor response to radiotherapy. Only 20% to 30% of patients with invasive bladder cancer can be cured by external-beam radiation therapy alone. It is used in combination with surgery or with systemic agents to treat bladder cancer primarily in patients who are not surgical candidates or who refuse surgery. Trials with synchronous chemotherapy with fluorouracil and mitomycin C combined with radiotherapy have shown significant improved locoregional control of bladder cancer, as compared with radiotherapy alone in patients with muscle-invasive bladder cancer.

CHRONIC Rx

FOLLOW-UP RECOMMENDATIONS FOR SUPERFICIAL BLADDER CANCER:

- Cystoscopy, bladder barbotage, and bimanual examination every 3 mo for 2 yr, then every 6 mo for 2 yr, and annually thereafter.
- Upper tract studies are based on the risk of upper tract tumor development, generally every 2 to 5 yr.

FOLLOW-UP RECOMMENDATIONS FOR ADVANCED DISEASE:

Bladder preservation:

- Cystoscopy, barbotage, bimanual examination, biopsy (when indicated), every 3 mo for 2 yr, then every 6 mo for 2 yr, yearly thereafter
- CT scan of abdomen and pelvis every 6 mo for 2 yr in addition to chest x-ray examination, liver function testing, and serum creatinine

Cystectomy with ileal loop/orthotopic bladder:

- Neobladder endoscopy and IVP yearly
- CT scan of abdomen and pelvis every 6 mo for 2 yr in addition to chest x-ray examination, liver function tests, and serum creatinine
- Loopogram every 6 mo for 2 yr, then annually

PEARLS & CONSIDERATIONS

COMMENTS

- The most useful prognostic parameters for bladder tumor recurrence and subsequent cancer progression are tumor grade, depth of tumor penetration, multifocal tumors, frequency of recurrence, tumor size, CIS, lymphatic invasion, papillary or solid tumor configuration.
- Box 1-10 describes the American Urological Association Guideline Recommendations for bladder cancer.

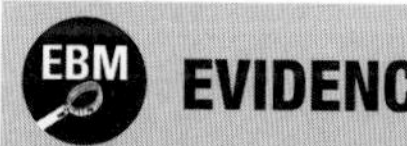

EVIDENCE

available at www.expertconsult.com

SUGGESTED READINGS

available at www.expertconsult.com

RELATED CONTENT

Bladder Cancer (Patient Information)

AUTHORS: **PHILIP J. ALIOTTA, M.D., M.S.H.A.**, and **RUBEN ALVERO, M.D.**

BOX 1-10 American Urological Association Guideline Recommendations

For all index patients:

- Standard: Physicians should discuss with the patient the treatment options and the benefits and harms, including side effects, of intravesical treatment.

For a patient who presents with an abnormal growth on the urothelium but who has not yet been diagnosed with bladder cancer:

- Standard: If the patient does not have an established histologic diagnosis, a biopsy should be obtained for pathologic analysis.
- Standard: Under most circumstances, complete eradication of all visible tumors should be performed.
- Standard: If bladder cancer is confirmed, periodic surveillance cystoscopy should be performed.
- Option: An initial single dose of intravesical chemotherapy may be administered immediately postoperatively.

For a patient with small volume, low-grade Ta bladder cancer:

- Recommendation: An initial single dose of intravesical chemotherapy may be administered immediately postoperatively.

For a patient with multifocal and/or large volume, histologically confirmed, low-grade Ta or a patient with recurrent low-grade Ta bladder cancer:

- Recommendation: An induction course of intravesical therapy with bacillus Calmette-Guérin or mitomycin C is recommended for the treatment of these patients with the goal of preventing or delaying recurrence.
- Option: Maintenance bacillus Calmette-Guérin or mitomycin C may be considered.

For a patient with initial histologically confirmed high-grade Ta, T1, and/or carcinoma in situ bladder cancer:

- Standard: For patients with lamina propria invasion (T1) but without muscularis propria in the specimen, repeat resection should be performed prior to additional intravesical therapy.
- Recommendation: An induction course of bacillus Calmette-Guérin followed by maintenance therapy is recommended for treatment of these patients.
- Option: Cystectomy should be considered for initial therapy in select patients.

For a patient with high-grade Ta, T1, and/or carcinoma in situ bladder cancer that has recurred after prior intravesical therapy:

- Standard: For patients with lamina propria invasion (T1) but without muscularis propria in the specimen, repeat resection should be performed prior to additional intravesical therapy.
- Recommendation: Cystectomy should be considered as a therapeutic alternative for these patients.
- Option: Further intravesical therapy may be considered for these patients.

From the American Urological Association, Guideline Division, http://www.auanet.org.

BASIC INFORMATION

DEFINITION

Blepharitis is a chronic inflammation of the eyelid margins that is often refractory to treatment with infectious and noninfectious etiologies.

SYNONYMS

Eyelid infection or inflammation
Eczema of the eyelids
Dermatoblepharitis
Angular blepharitis

ICD-9CM CODES
373.0 Blepharitis

ICD-10CM CODES
H01.009 Unspecified blepharitis unspecified eye, unspecified eyelid

EPIDEMIOLOGY & DEMOGRAPHICS

- Common in children, particularly those with atopic dermatitis and eczema
- Adults with seborrhea involving the eyelids

PHYSICAL FINDINGS & CLINICAL PRESENTATION

- Common symptoms: red eyes, burning sensation, excessive tearing, blurred vision, pruritic eyelids
- Chronically infected lids are usually diffusely erythematous, with collarettes (fibrin exudate) at the base of the lashes (Fig. 1-179)
- Lid margins thicken over time, with associated loss of eyelashes (madarosis), misdirected growth of lashes (trichiasis), and overflow or inspissation of the meibomian glands.
- Associated conjunctivitis with erythema, edema but no discharge.
- Chalazion: chronic sterile inflammation of an oil gland of the eyelid
- Superficial punctate erosions of the inferior corneal epithelium are common.
- More severe findings, such as corneal pannus, ulcerative keratitis, or lid ectropion, are less common.

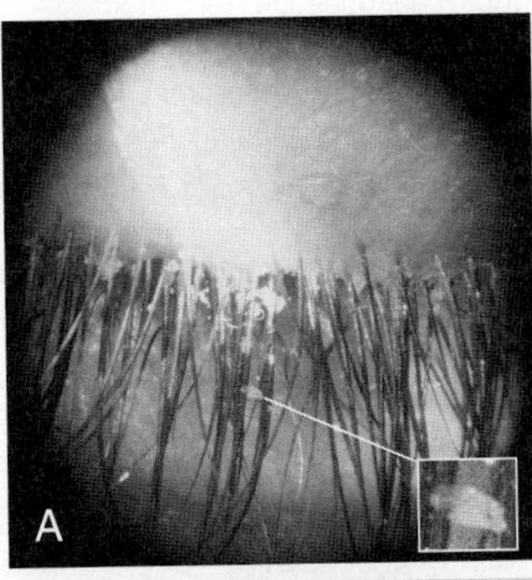

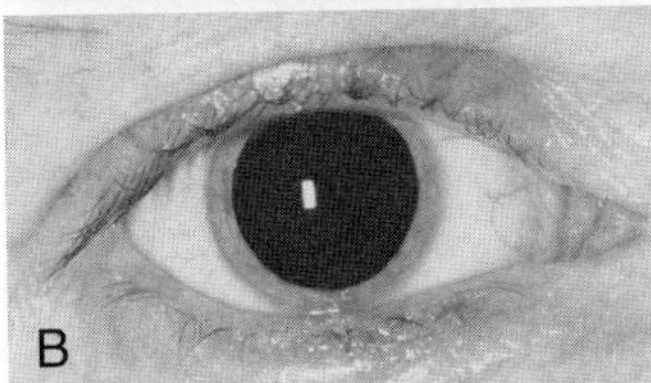

FIGURE 1-179 A, Seborrheic blepharitis. The typical scales (scurf) are translucent and easily removed. **B,** Staphylococcal blepharitis showing the typical lid margin erythema and discharge. (From Palay D [ed]: *Ophthalmology for the primary care physician,* St Louis, 1997, Mosby.)

ETIOLOGY

Multiple: bacterial and nonbacterial causes

- Staphylococcal infection most common but streptococcal, Moraxella, and other bacterial infections; viral infections (e.g., herpes simplex, herpes zoster, *Molluscum contagiosum*); and a number of ecoparasites, including pediculosis, may cause blepharitis
- Seborrheic dermatitis
- Rosacea
- Dry eye (keratoconjunctivitis sicca): decrease in tear volume
- Meibomian gland dysfunction
- Contact lens intolerance
- Two categories of blepharitis:
  1. Anterior blepharitis, most often associated with staphylococcal infection
  2. Posterior blepharitis, associated with meibomian gland dysfunction and seborrheic dermatitis or rosacea

NOTE: Blepharitis patients have normal skin microflora in greater amounts (mostly *S. epidermidis* and *Propionibacterium acnes*). (*S. aureus* and *S. epidermidis* can be cultured in 10% to 35% and 90% to 95% of healthy persons, respectively.)

DIAGNOSIS

DIFFERENTIAL DIAGNOSIS

- Keratoconjunctivitis sicca
- Eyelid malignancies
- Herpes simplex blepharitis
- Molluscum contagiosum
- Phthiriasis palpebrarum
- *Phthirus pubis* (pubic lice)
- Demodex folliculorum (transparent mites)
- Allergic blepharitis

WORKUP

Scrapings of the eyelids to show polymorphonuclear leukocytes and gram-positive cocci

LABORATORY TESTS

Eyelid cultures and antibiotic sensitivity testing (usually not done unless patient fails to respond to initial treatment regimen)

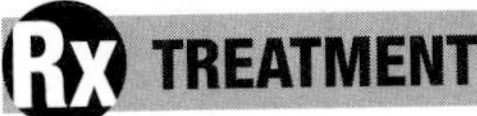

TREATMENT

NONPHARMACOLOGIC THERAPY

- Alkaline soaps may be beneficial; alcohol and some detergents remove surface lipids and microflora.
- Hot compresses applied to closed lids for 5 to 10 min: heat loosens debris from lid margins and increases meibomian gland fluidity.
- Firm massage of the lid margins to enhance the flow of secretions from glands, followed by cleansing of the lids with cotton-tipped applicators dipped in a 50:50 mixture of baby shampoo and water.
- Lashes and lid margins scrubbed vigorously while the eyelids are closed, followed by thorough rinsing.
- Following local massage and cleansing, the mainstay of treatment is application of topical antibiotic ointment to the eyelid margins.
  1. Most effective topical antibiotics include bacitracin, erythromycin or 1% azithromycin solution, aminoglycoside and fluoroquinolone ophthalmic ointments.
  2. Ointment is applied 1 to 4 times daily, depending on the severity, for 1 to 2 wk, followed by once daily, at bedtime, for another 4 to 8 wk until all signs of inflammation have disappeared.
- Oral antibiotics: long-term use of doxycycline or tetracycline in a tapering dose may be helpful in severe cases for patients older than 8 years of age.
- Topical glucocorticoids: short-term use in acute exacerbations of blepharitis

For patients with rosacea:

1. Tetracycline 250 mg orally 4 times daily or doxycycline 100 mg orally bid along with local treatment for several months

Recalcitrant cases with antibiotic resistance:

1. Vancomycin eye drops 1%
2. Ciprofloxacin or ofloxacin eye drops

CHRONIC Rx

By definition, this is a chronic condition for which there is frequently no cure.

Some newer agents being evaluated are topical cyclosporine 0.05% eye drops, thermal pulsation systems to break up material in meibomian glands, topical metronidazole and topical tacrolimus, and tear lipid substitutes.

DISPOSITION

This condition may be refractory to treatment.

REFERRAL

To an ophthalmologist if patient fails to respond to local therapy.

SUGGESTED READINGS
available at www.expertconsult.com

AUTHOR: **GLENN G. FORT, M.D., M.P.H.**

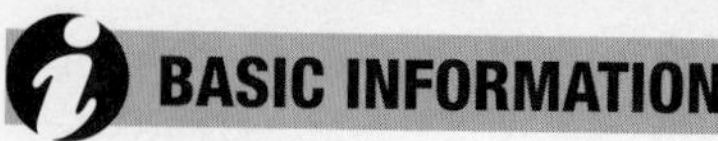

BASIC INFORMATION

DEFINITION

Body dysmorphic disorder (BDD) is classified as an obsessive-compulsive and related disorder. It is characterized by preoccupation with one or more perceived defects or flaws in physical appearance that are not observable or appear slight to others, as well as repetitive behaviors (e.g., excessive grooming, mirror checking) in response to the appearance concerns. The preoccupations cause clinically significant distress or impairment in social, occupational, or other important areas of functioning. The appearance preoccupations are not better explained by concerns with body fat or weight in a person whose symptoms meet diagnostic criteria for an eating disorder.

SYNONYMS

Dysmorphophobia
BDD

ICD-9CM and DSM-5 CODES
300.7
ICD-10CM CODES
F45.22 Body dysmorphic disorder

EPIDEMIOLOGY & DEMOGRAPHICS

- Affects 1.7% to 2.4% of the general population (in nationwide epidemiologic studies)
- Prevalence among cosmetic surgery patients (in most studies) is 7% to 15%.
- Prevalence among dermatology patients is 9% to 14%.
- Slightly higher prevalence among females
- Onset most commonly in adolescence

PHYSICAL FINDINGS & CLINICAL PRESENTATION

- Excessive preoccupation (obsession) with one or more perceived defects in appearance that are not observable or appear slight to others. Any part of the body may be a focus of concern; skin, hair, and nose concerns are most common. Most patients are preoccupied with multiple body areas.
- The body areas with which the patient is concerned appear physically normal; if a physical defect is present, it is slight, and the patient's reaction to it is excessive.
- Most patients have poor insight or are delusional (i.e., completely convinced) regarding the accuracy of their belief about the appearance of the perceived defects.
- Over the course of the disorder, all patients engage in repetitive behaviors such as frequent mirror checking, excessive grooming, camouflaging (trying to hide the perceived flaws—e.g., with makeup, a hat, hair), skin picking, reassurance seeking, and repeatedly measuring or feeling the perceived defect. The intent of these behaviors is to check, try to improve, or be reassured about the appearance of the perceived flaws.
- Nearly all experience impairment in psychosocial functioning and quality of life; impairment is usually substantial.
- Suicidal ideation, suicide attempts, and completed suicide appear common.
- Commonly co-occurring mental disorders are major depressive disorder, substance use disorders, social anxiety disorder, obsessive-compulsive disorder (OCD), and personality disorder.

ETIOLOGY

Likely multifactorial, with both genetic and environmental risk factors (e.g., teasing). Neuropsychological and fMRI studies indicate abnormalities in visual processing consisting of excessive focus on details rather than larger configural elements of visual stimuli.

Dx DIAGNOSIS

Psychiatric interview
- Ask:
  1. Are you very worried about your appearance in any way? *OR:* Are you unhappy with how you look?
  2. Does this concern with your appearance preoccupy you?
  3. How much distress does this concern cause you?
  4. What effect does this concern have on your life?
  5. Is there anything you feel an urge to do over and over again in response to your appearance concerns? (Give examples, such as mirror checking, comparing with others, skin picking)

DIFFERENTIAL DIAGNOSIS

- Often undiagnosed because of patient's reluctance to divulge symptoms due to shame and fear of being misunderstood (e.g., considered vain)
- OCD
- Eating disorder
- Social anxiety disorder
- Major depressive disorder

WORKUP

Clinical evaluation focused on BDD symptoms and associated impairment in functioning.

Rx TREATMENT

NONPHARMACOLOGIC THERAPY

- CBT, with a focus on cognitive restructuring, exposure and response prevention; CBT must be specifically tailored to BDD's unique symptoms.
- Do not try to talk patients out of their concern; it is ineffective.
- Avoid cosmetic procedures.

ACUTE GENERAL Rx

Precautions/hospitalization if actively suicidal

CHRONIC Rx

- SRIs are medication of choice; relatively high doses often needed.
- Other agents (e.g., neuroleptics, tricyclic antidepressants other than clomipramine) do not appear as beneficial.
- CBT tailored specifically to BDD is recommended with or without an SRI.
- Support groups if available.

DISPOSITION

- Untreated BDD tends to be chronic and can lead to social isolation; school dropout; major depression; unnecessary surgery, dermatologic treatment, or other cosmetic treatment; and even suicide.
- With correct diagnosis and treatment, a majority improve.

REFERRAL

Refer for psychiatric evaluation and treatment if diagnosis is suspected.

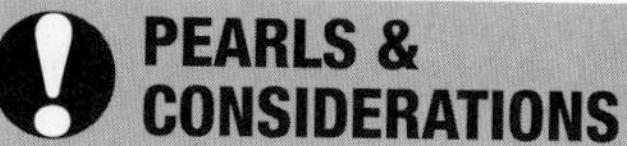

PEARLS & CONSIDERATIONS

- In clinical settings, more than 60% have co-occurring major depressive disorder.
- Reassurance is rarely helpful.
- Patients often have an unrealistic expectation of improvement with plastic surgery, dermatologic treatment, and other cosmetic procedures; these treatments do not appear to be effective.
- All patients should be screened for suicidality.

PATIENT/FAMILY EDUCATION

- Patients and family members usually benefit from psychoeducation.
- Family support and encouragement of appropriate treatment is important.
- Phillips KA: *Understanding Body Dysmorphic Disorder: An Essential Guide.* Oxford University Press, 2009
- http://www.BDDProgram.com (http://www.rhodeislandhospital.org/RIH/Services/MentalHealth/BodyImage/default.htm)

SUGGESTED READINGS

Available at www.expertconsult.com

RELATED CONTENT

Obsessive Compulsive Disorder (Related Key Topic)
Body Dysmorphic Disorder (Patient Information)

AUTHOR: **KATHARINE A. PHILLIPS, M.D.**

BASIC INFORMATION

DEFINITION

Primary malignant bone tumors are invasive and anaplastic and have the ability to metastasize. Most arise from the marrow (myeloma), but tumors may develop from bone, cartilage, fat, and fibrous tissues. Leukemia and lymphoma are excluded from this discussion.

FIBROSARCOMA AND LIPOSARCOMA: Extremely rare. They are similar to tumors arising in soft tissue.

OSTEOSARCOMA: A rare primary malignant tumor of bone characterized by malignant tumor cells that produce osteoid or bone. Several variants have been described: parosteal sarcoma, periosteal sarcoma, multicentric, and telangiectatic forms.

CHONDROSARCOMA: A malignant cartilage tumor that may develop primarily or secondarily from transformation of a benign osteocartilaginous exostosis or enchondroma.

EWING'S SARCOMA: A malignant tumor of unknown histogenesis.

MULTIPLE MYELOMA: A neoplastic proliferation of plasma cells.

SYNONYMS

Multiple myeloma:

1. Plasma cell myeloma
2. Plasmacytoma

ICD-9CM CODES

203.0 Multiple myeloma
170.9 Neoplasm, bone (periosteum), primary malignant
M9180/3 Osteosarcoma
N9220/3 Chondrosarcoma
M9260/3 Ewing's sarcoma

ICD-10CM CODES

C90.00 Multiple myeloma not having achieved remission
C41.9 Malignant neoplasm of bone and articular cartilage, unspecified

EPIDEMIOLOGY & DEMOGRAPHICS

MULTIPLE MYELOMA:

- The most common tumor in bone
- Age at onset: usually >40 yr
- Male/female ratio of 2:1

OSTEOGENIC SARCOMA:

- Average age at onset: 10 to 20 yr
- Males afflicted more often than females
- Parosteal sarcoma in older patients

CHONDROSARCOMA:

- Age at onset: 40 to 60 yr
- Male/female ratio of 2:1

EWING'S SARCOMA: Age at onset: 10 to 15 yr

PHYSICAL FINDINGS & CLINICAL PRESENTATION

MULTIPLE MYELOMA:

- May present as a systemic process or, less commonly, as a "solitary" lesion
- Early manifestations: anorexia, weight loss, and bone pain; majority of cases present initially with back pain that often leads to the detection of a destructive skeletal lesion
- Other organ systems eventually become involved, resulting in more bone pain, anemia, renal insufficiency, and/or bacterial infections, usually as a result of the dysproteinemia typical of this disorder
- Possible secondary amyloidosis, leading to cardiac failure or nephrotic syndrome

OSTEOSARCOMA:

- Most originating in the metaphysis
- 50% to 60% around the knee
- Possible pain and swelling, but otherwise healthy patient
- Osteosarcoma in conjunction with Paget's disease, manifested primarily as a sudden increase in bone pain

CHONDROSARCOMA:

- Tumor most commonly involving the pelvis, upper femur, and shoulder girdle
- Painful swelling

EWING'S SARCOMA:

- Painful soft tissue mass often present
- Possibly increased local heat
- Midshaft of a long bone usually affected (in contrast to other tumors)
- Weight loss, fever, and lethargy

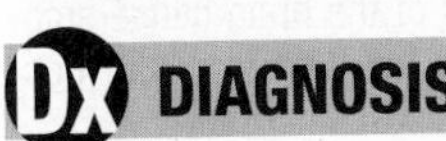

DIAGNOSIS

DIFFERENTIAL DIAGNOSIS

- Osteomyelitis
- Metastatic bone disease

LABORATORY TESTS

- Slightly elevated alkaline phosphatase in osteosarcoma
- In Ewing's sarcoma: reflective of systemic reaction; include anemia, an increase in white blood cell count, and an elevated sedimentation rate
- In multiple myeloma:
  1. Bence Jones protein in the urine
  2. Anemia and elevated sedimentation rate
  3. Characteristic dysproteinemia on serum protein electrophoresis
  4. Diagnostic feature: peak in the electrophoretic pattern suggestive of a monoclonal gammopathy
  5. Rouleaux formation in the peripheral blood smear
  6. Often presence of hypercalcemia, but alkaline phosphatase levels usually normal

IMAGING STUDIES

- Classic osteogenic sarcoma penetrates the cortex early in many cases.
  1. A blastic (dense), lytic (lucent), or mixed response may be seen in the affected bone (Fig. E1-180).
  2. An aggressive perpendicular sunburst pattern may be present as a result of periosteal reaction, and peripheral Codman's triangles are often noted.
  3. Margins of the tumor are poorly defined.
- Speckled calcifications in a destructive radiolucent lesion are usually suggestive of chondrosarcoma.
- Ewing's sarcoma is characterized radiographically by mottled, irregular destructive changes with periosteal new bone formation. The latter may be multilayered, producing the typical "onion skin" appearance.
- Typical roentgenographic finding in multiple myeloma is the "punched out" lesion with sharply demarcated edges.
  1. Multiple lesions are usual.
  2. Diffuse osteoporosis may be the only finding in many cases.
  3. Pathologic fractures are common.

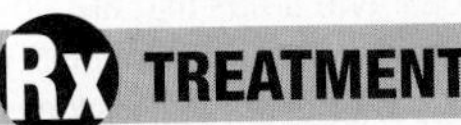

TREATMENT

The evaluation and treatment of malignant bone tumors are complicated. Diagnostic studies and treatment should be supervised by an orthopedic cancer specialist and oncologist.

DISPOSITION

- In the past 20 yr, dramatic improvements have been made in the treatment protocols for osteosarcoma with the use of adjuvant multidrug regimens and limb-sparing surgery.
- Prognosis of multiple myeloma remains poor despite new therapies.
- Prognosis for Ewing's sarcoma has improved with a combination of chemotherapy, local resection, and radiation therapy.
- Chondrosarcomas are not sensitive to chemotherapy or radiation, and prognosis depends on the grade of the tumor and the ability to obtain an adequate resection.

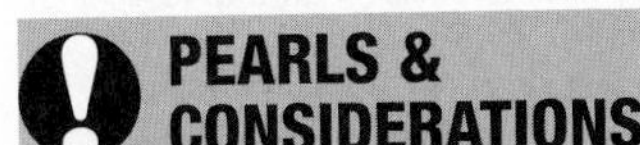

PEARLS & CONSIDERATIONS

Early diagnosis is important because most tumors have not metastasized at the time of initial presentation.

SUGGESTED READINGS

available at www.expertconsult.com

RELATED CONTENT

Multiple Myeloma (Related Key Topic)
Multiple Myeloma (Patient Information)

AUTHORS: **LONNIE R. MERCIER, M.D**, and **FRED F. FERRI, M.D.**

BASIC INFORMATION

DEFINITION

Borderline personality disorder (BPD) is characterized by a pervasive pattern of instability in interpersonal relationships, self-image, affect regulation, and impulse control that causes significant subjective distress or impairment of functioning. The individual must meet five or more of the following criteria:

1. Frantic efforts to avoid real or imagined abandonment
2. Unstable and intense personal relationships characterized by alternating between extremes of idealization and devaluation
3. Identity disturbance characterized by an unstable self-image
4. Impulsivity in at least two areas that are potentially self-damaging (e.g., overspending, sex, substance abuse, binge eating, reckless driving)
5. Recurrent suicidal behavior, gestures, threats, or self-mutilating behavior
6. Affective instability due to a marked reactivity of mood
7. Chronic feelings of emptiness
8. Inappropriate, intense anger or difficulty controlling anger
9. Transient, stress-related paranoid ideation or severe dissociative symptoms

ICD-9CM and DSM-5 CODES
301.83
ICD-10CM CODES
F60.3 Emotionally unstable personality disorder

EPIDEMIOLOGY & DEMOGRAPHICS

PREVALENCE: Affects approximately 1% to 2% of the general population and up to 10% of psychiatric outpatients
PREDOMINANT SEX: Female (3:1)
PREDOMINANT AGE: 20s
GENETICS: BPD is five times as likely if disorder is present in a first-degree relative. Increased prevalence of mood disorders and substance abuse disorders also found in first-degree relatives.
RISK FACTORS: Association with childhood physical, sexual, or emotional abuse and/or neglect

PHYSICAL FINDINGS & CLINICAL PRESENTATION

- No specific associated physical findings.
- Mental status examination may reveal affective lability.
- Clinical presentation may reveal the following:
  - A pervasive sense of loneliness and emptiness.
  - Underlying negative affect with dysphoria.
  - High frequency of multiple psychiatric disorders, especially posttraumatic stress disorder (PTSD), mood disorders, attention-deficit/hyperactivity disorder, and substance use disorders. Intense emotions with difficulty returning to emotional baseline.
  - All-or-nothing, either/or cognitive style that is represented by a phenomenon known as "splitting," in which patient sees situations or people as all good or all bad.
  - Difficulty in maintaining commitment to long-term goals; history of numerous stormy relationships and multiple jobs.
  - Reports a high number of sexual partners due to either/both impulsivity and victimization.
  - Reacts with rage, panic, despair to actual or perceived abandonment; may present with suicidality or self-mutilating behavior in response to recent stressor.
  - Attempts to block the experience of pain, which may induce feelings of derealization, depersonalization, changes in consciousness, and/or brief psychotic reactions with delusions and hallucinations.
  - Substance use, gambling, overspending, eating binges, and/or self-mutilation as a way to escape intensely painful affect.
- Some patients may display psychotic symptoms.

ETIOLOGY

- Interaction of psychosocial adversity plus genetic factors
- Hypotheses:
  1. Genetic: increased risk if first-degree relative with BPD.
  2. Biologic: abnormalities in limbic system and other areas of the brain cause emotional dysregulation. Serotonergic functioning appears to be disturbed.
  3. Environmental: history of childhood abuse (most commonly sexual) or neglect.

DIAGNOSIS

DIFFERENTIAL DIAGNOSIS

- Histrionic and narcissistic personality disorders share some common features.
- Dysthymia and other depressive disorders: requires a stability of affective symptoms not seen in BPD.
- Bipolar disorder: mood changes in BPD often triggered by stressors and less sustained than in bipolar disorder. Many patients with BPD are incorrectly diagnosed with bipolar disorder.
- Substance abuse or dependence: often induces impulsive, emotionally labile behavior.
- Posttraumatic stress disorder (PTSD): individuals with BPD often have history of trauma but do not avoid the feared stimulus or reexperience the trauma, as with PTSD.
- Mild cases of schizophrenia may superficially resemble BPD.

WORKUP

- History (helpful to gather collateral information from family and friends)
- Physical examination
- Mental status examination

LABORATORY TESTS

- Toxicology screen; substance use is common and can mimic features of personality disorders.
- Screen for HIV and other sexually transmitted illnesses.

IMAGING STUDIES

Structural and functional MRI demonstrate amygdala hyperactivity, reduced hippocampus and amygdala volume, greater activation within the insula and posterior cingulate cortex, and less activation in regions extending from the amygdala to the cingulate and prefrontal cortex. PET scans reveal reduced metabolism in prefrontal cortex. Recent PET research reveals dysregulation of endogenous opioid function. Imaging is not recommended as part of routine evaluation.

TREATMENT

NONPHARMACOLOGIC THERAPY

Dialectical behavior therapy (DBT), mentalization-based therapy, variations of cognitive behavior therapy (CBT), and transference-focused psychotherapy, a type of psychodynamic therapy, have the most empirical support from randomized trials. The goal of DBT and most CBT variations is to help patients improve mindfulness, control impulsive behaviors and angry outbursts, and develop social skills. The emphasis of mentalization treatment is to teach patients to stand outside of their feelings and observe emotions in oneself and others. The focus of transference-focused psychotherapy is on examining the affect-laden themes that emerge in the relationship between patient and therapist. Effective therapeutic treatments typically combine weekly group and individual therapy meetings.

ACUTE GENERAL Rx

Low-dose antipsychotics to control impulsivity, brief psychotic episodes.

CHRONIC Rx

- Medications have low-to-moderate effectiveness and are most effective in improving symptoms of impulsivity, mood instability, and self-destructive behavior. Effectiveness only studied for the first 3 mo of treatment.
- SSRIs if concurrent mood disorder. Higher doses may be required than for major depression.
- Low-dose antipsychotics.
- Mood stabilizers (lithium, valproate, carbamazepine, topiramate).
- In preliminary studies, omega-3 fatty acids improve irritability.

DISPOSITION

- Course is variable. The most unstable period is typically in early adulthood; the majority achieve greater stability in social/occupational functioning later in life but often continue with difficulty maintaining intimate relationships.
- Clinically salient features such as alcohol/substance use and self-injury may be less common in older adults.
- No evidence of progression to schizophrenia, but there is a high incidence of concurrent major depression and other Axis I disorders.
- Patients with high pre-treatment symptom severity who report a strong therapeutic alliance with their providers report highest treatment benefits.

REFERRAL

- Referral to mental health specialist:
    - For diagnosis and management.
    - Use of pharmacotherapy
    - Patient is severely impaired or suicidal

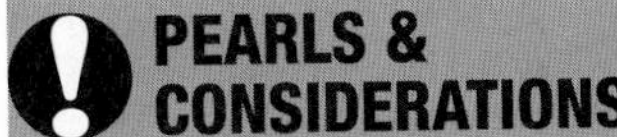

PEARLS & CONSIDERATIONS

COMMENTS

- Consider frequent, brief, scheduled visits for needy, demanding, or somaticizing patients with BPD.
- Validate the patient's feelings while stating the expectation of behavior control.
- Be matter-of-fact; avoid expressing extreme emotions.
- Be alert to the risk of suicide and assess suicide risk often.
- Be alert to the risk of nonsuicidal self-harm, such as cutting
- Convey a demeanor of competence but openly acknowledge minor errors.
- Have a low threshold for seeking psychiatric consultation.
- An alternative model of diagnosing borderline personality disorder exists in the DSM-5 section III, consisting of: (1) impairment in personality functioning (identity, self-direction, empathy, or intimacy) and (2) four or more of seven maladaptive personality traits (emotional lability, anxiousness, separation insecurity, depressivity, impulsivity, risk-taking, and hostility).

PREVENTION

- There are no known ways to prevent BPD (or other personality disorders).
- Suicidality should be actively and consistently monitored.
- Benzodiazepines, narcotic analgesics, and other drugs with potential for dependency should be used rarely and with great caution, due to impaired impulse control and risk of addictive behavior.
- Patients should be asked frequently and in detail about parenting practices. Low frustration tolerance, externalization of blame for psychological distress, and impaired impulse control put children at risk for neglect or abuse.

PATIENT & FAMILY EDUCATION

National Alliance for the Mentally Ill (NAMI; http://www.nami.org) provides patient information, online chat groups, and information on support groups throughout the U.S. for people with BPD and their families.

Additional, local support groups for BPD are common and should be investigated.

SUGGESTED READINGS

available at www.expertconsult.com

RELATED CONTENT

Borderline Personality Disorder (Patient Information)

AUTHORS: **MARK ZIMMERMAN, M.D.** and **THERESA A. MORGAN, PH.D, M. PHIL**

BASIC INFORMATION

DEFINITION

Botulism is an illness caused by a neurotoxin produced primarily by *Clostridium botulinum.* Five types of disease can occur: foodborne botulism, wound botulism, infant intestinal botulism, adult enteric botulism (similar to infant botulism), and inhalational botulism. Of note, inhalational botulism is exceedingly rare, but could occur as a result of bioterrorism.

SYNONYMS

Clostridium botulinum food poisoning
Botulinum toxin food poisoning
Wound botulism
Infantile botulism

ICD-9CM CODES
005.1 Botulism
ICD-10CM CODES
A05.1 Botulism food poisoning

EPIDEMIOLOGY & DEMOGRAPHICS

INCIDENCE (IN U.S.): Approximately 24 cases/yr of foodborne illness, 29 cases/yr of wound botulism, and 94 cases/yr of infant botulism

PHYSICAL FINDINGS & CLINICAL PRESENTATION

- Symptoms usually begin 12 to 36 hr following ingestion.
- Severity of illness is related to the quantity of toxin ingested.
- Significant findings:
  1. Acute, bilateral cranial nerve palsies, with ocular and bulbar manifestations being most frequent (diplopia, ophthalmoplegia, ptosis, dysphagia, dysarthria, fixed and dilated pupils, and dry mouth)
  2. Usually bilateral nerve involvement that may progress to a descending flaccid paralysis
  3. No sensory deficits, aside from possible blurred vision
  4. GI symptoms (dry mouth, nausea, vomiting, diarrhea, or cramps)
  5. Generally an absence of fever
  6. Normal heart rate to mild bradycardia with patient remaining normotensive
- Wound botulism
  1. Occurs primarily in injecting drug users (subcutaneous "black tar" heroin injection—"skin popping") or with traumatic injury.
  2. Presentation is similar to that of foodborne disease, except for a longer incubation period (4-14 days) and absence of GI symptoms.
  3. Fever is uncommon and if present may be due to wound infection, which is not always apparent

ETIOLOGY

- Cause is one of several types of neurotoxins (usually A, B, E, or F) produced by *C. botulinum,* an anaerobic, gram-positive bacillus. Spore production guarantees survival of the organism in extreme conditions, and they are found in the environment worldwide. Botulinum toxin is the most powerful neurotoxin known.
- Disease results from absorption of toxin into the circulation from a mucosal surface or wound. Botulinum toxin does not penetrate intact skin.
- In foodborne variety, disease is caused by ingestion of preformed toxin. Although rapidly inactivated by heat, the toxin can survive the proteolytic environment of the stomach.
- In wound botulism, toxin is elaborated by organisms that contaminate a wound.
- In infant botulism (and probably adult botulism of unknown etiology), toxin is produced by organisms in the GI tract. Antibiotic use and achlorhydria can predispose to colonization by *C. botulinum* and elaboration of toxin.
- Inhalational botulism has been demonstrated experimentally in primates. Rare case reports of inhalational botulism from snorting contaminated cocaine have been reported, and there is concern for the potential use of manufactured aerosolized toxin as a bioterrorism agent.

Dx DIAGNOSIS

DIFFERENTIAL DIAGNOSIS

- Myasthenia gravis, Lambert-Eaton myasthenic syndrome
- Guillain-Barré syndrome or other acute inflammatory demyelinating polyneuropathy
- Tick paralysis
- CVA
- Other: polio, heavy metal intoxication, and shellfish poisoning

LABORATORY TESTS

- Anaerobic cultures of serum, of food, and/or stool
- Food, serum, and stool are sent for toxin assay.
- Public health laboratories may perform mouse bioassay testing, which confirms toxin type in 75% of cases.

Rx TREATMENT

NONPHARMACOLOGIC THERAPY

- Supportive care with intubation if respiratory failure occurs
- Debridement of the wound in wound botulism

ACUTE GENERAL Rx

- **For non-infants:** Give equine heptavalent botulinum antitoxin (HBAT), which contains antibodies for seven known botulism types (A through G), as early as possible. Once a clinical diagnosis is made, antitoxin should be administered before laboratory confirmation.
  1. The antitoxin is available from the Centers for Disease Control and Prevention (1-404-639-2206 Monday-Friday or 1-404-639-2888 evenings/weekends); it is derived from horse serum, so there is a significant incidence of serum sickness.
  2. Skin testing (conjunctival instillation and observation for 15 min), and possible desensitization, is recommended before treatment. Reported hypersensitivity rates range from 9-20%
- Give wound botulism patients penicillin 2 million U IV q4h after antitoxin has been given. Use metronidazole 500 million U IV q8h as alternative for penicillin allergic patients. Avoid aminoglycosides and tetracyclines, as they are ineffective and can worsen neuromuscular blockade.
- **For infants:** Give human botulinum immunoglobulin (Baby BIG) IV, single dose. Call 1-510-540-2646. Do not use equine antitoxin. Babies with infantile intestinal botulism may benefit from a cathartic to mechanically clear the number of *C. botulinum* vegetative forms and spores residing in the gastrointestinal tract. Avoid antibiotics in infant botulism because antimicrobials may lyse *C. botulinum* in the gut and increase toxin load.

DISPOSITION

- Highest mortality in the first cases in an outbreak, with subsequent cases receiving rapid treatment
- Complete recovery for most individuals (may take up to 1 year)

REFERRAL

Immediate for all cases to an ER and an infectious disease consultant

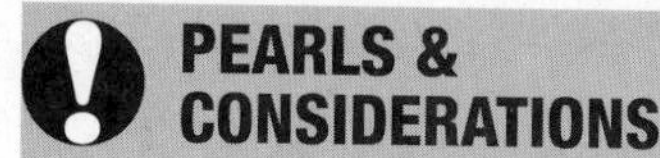

PEARLS & CONSIDERATIONS

COMMENTS

- Routine cooking inactivates the toxin, but spores are resistant to environmental factors. At room temperature, spores can germinate and produce toxin. Pressure cooking can kill spores as well, however.
- Most outbreaks are associated with home-canned foods, including fruits, vegetables, and fish.
- Patients must be closely monitored for progression to respiratory paralysis.
- Notify public health authorities immediately to alert other health care services of possible additional cases and to initiate investigation into cause and scope of outbreak.
- Immunity to botulism does not occur after toxin exposure/infection, and repeated botulism can occur.

SUGGESTED READINGS

available at www.expertconsult.com

RELATED CONTENT

Botulism (Patient Information)

AUTHOR: **RUSSELL J. MCCULLOH, M.D.**

BASIC INFORMATION

DEFINITION

Brain metastases result from a spread of cancers originating in other organs to the brain. Brain metastases are the most common intracranial tumors in adults and account for more than one half of brain tumors.

SYNONYMS

ICD-9CM CODES

198 Secondary neoplasm of other specified sites

ICD-10CM CODES

C80.0 Malignant neoplasm, primary site unknown
C80.9 Malignant neoplasm, unspecified
C79.89 Secondary malignant neoplasm of other specified sites

EPIDEMIOLOGY & DEMOGRAPHICS

INCIDENCE:

- In the United States, an estimated 98,000 to 170,000 new cases occur each year, which represents 24% to 45% of all cancer patients. The increased incidence is likely due to improved detection and better control of extracerebral disease. The incidence is higher in autopsy series, where 20% of patients with systemic disease have brain metastases.
- The prevalence is thought to be 120,000 to 140,000/yr.

PREDOMINANT SEX AND AGE:

- In patients with systemic malignancies, brain metastases occur in 10% to 30% of adults and 6% to 10% of children. Of these, about 60% of patients are between the ages of 50 to 70.
- There is no gender predilection.

RISK FACTORS:

- In adults, the most common primary tumors accounting for brain metastases are carcinomas, including lung (16% to 20%), breast (5%), kidney (7% to 10%), and colorectal cancers (1% to 2%), and melanoma (7%).
- In children, the most common primary tumors are sarcomas, neuroblastoma, and germ cell tumors.

PHYSICAL FINDINGS & CLINICAL PRESENTATION

- Brain metastases should be suspected in any cancer patient who develops acute neurologic signs or symptoms. Neurologic symptoms, however, are common in patients with systemic cancer. In an analysis of more than 800 patients with neurologic symptoms, brain metastases were found in only 16%.
- Symptoms:
    - Headache occurs in 40% to 50% of patients with brain metastases. Frequency is higher with metastases located in the posterior fossa, which may result in obstructive hydrocephalus. The headache is often accompanied by nausea, vomiting, focal neurologic signs, and postural variation.
    - Focal neurologic signs/symptoms are the presenting symptom in 20% to 40% of patients. Hemiparesis is the most frequent complaint.
    - Cognitive dysfunction, including memory problems and/or mood/personality changes, is the presenting problem in 30% to 45% of patients.
    - The frequency of seizures in patients with metastatic brain tumor is 30% to 40%.
    - Acute stroke secondary to hemorrhage into a metastasis, hypercoagulability, or local vascular invasion accounts for 5% to 10% of patients.

ETIOLOGY

The most common mechanism of metastasis to the brain is by hematogenous spread. The most common location is at the junction of the gray and white matter. The blood vessels decrease in diameter in these regions, which is thought to act like a trap for clumps of tumor cells. Different tumor types have a tendency to metastasize to different regions of the brain. For example, metastases of small cell lung carcinoma are equally distributed in all regions, whereas pelvic (prostate and uterine) and gastrointestinal tumors more commonly metastasize to the posterior fossa.

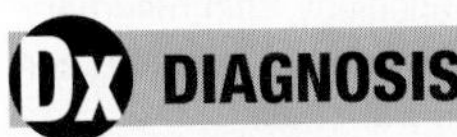

DIAGNOSIS

DIFFERENTIAL DIAGNOSIS

- Primary brain tumor
- Infection: abscess/fungal disease
- Progressive multifocal leukoencephalopathy
- Demyelinating disease: multiple sclerosis, postinfectious encephalomyelitis
- Cerebral infarction/bleeding
- Effects of treatment, such as radiation necrosis

LABORATORY TESTS

- Routine laboratory studies are not typically helpful.
- Lumbar puncture is generally contraindicated due to increased intracranial pressure and risk of herniation.
- Brain biopsy is necessary in some cases for a definitive diagnosis, particularly in the case of unknown primary tumor.

IMAGING STUDIES

- MRI (Fig. 1-181) with and without contrast is the imaging study of choice. Important features on MRI that suggest brain metastases include: presence of multiple lesions, localization at the junction of the gray and white matter, circumscribed margins, large amounts of vasogenic edema. CT of head with contrast (Fig. 1-182) can be used when MRI is contraindicated.
- MR spectroscopy and PET are useful to delineate tumor from other space-occupying lesions or from radiation necrosis.
- Newer experimental imaging studies, such as receptor-targeted and ligand-based molecular imaging, are on the horizon.
- Patients without a known primary tumor. In about 80% of patients, brain metastases develop after the diagnosis of systemic cancer. In the remaining patients, brain metastases are diagnosed simultaneously or before the primary tumor is found. In patients without a known primary tumor, the lung should be the primary focus of evaluation. Other frequent sites include melanoma, colon cancer, and breast cancer. PET scan may be useful in these patients to help identify the primary tumor or to identify other sites of metastatic disease—these latter sites might also be more amenable to biopsy.

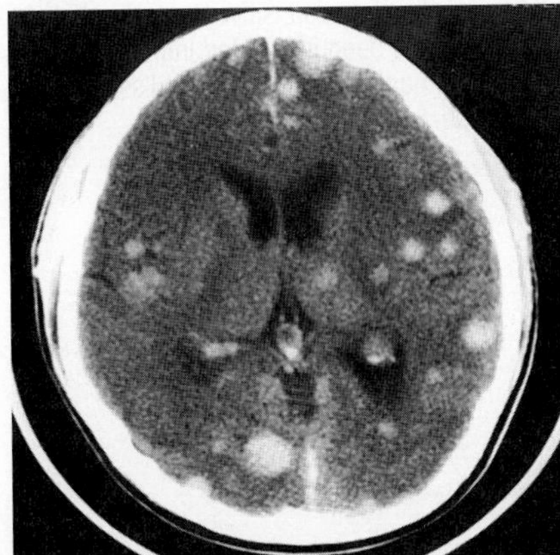

FIGURE 1-182 Intracranial metastatic disease. Axial contrast-enhanced CT scan of head reveals multiple enhancing nodules throughout gray and white matter structures consistent with metastatic disease. (From Vincent JL et al [eds]: *Textbook of critical care*, ed 6, Philadelphia, 2011, Saunders.)

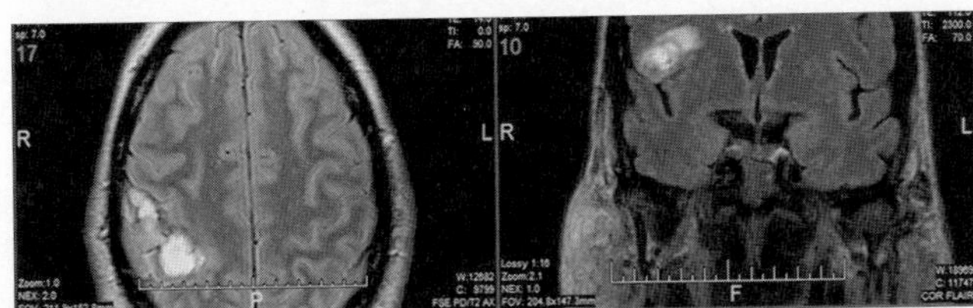

FIGURE 1-181 Brain magnetic resonance imaging (axial and coronal fluid-attenuated inversion recovery sequences) showing hemorrhagic metastatic deposition in the inferior right frontoparietal lobe (lobulated high signal focus) in a 40-year-old woman with metastatic choriocarcinoma to the brain. (From Fielding JR et al: *Gynecologic imaging*, Philadelphia, 2011, Saunders.)

 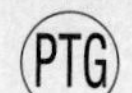

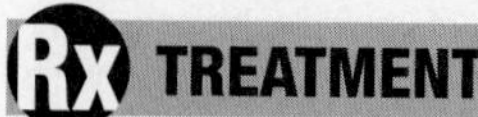

TREATMENT

- Management of patients with brain metastases is influenced by the overall prognosis and may include treatments targeted at the metastases, management and prevention of complications (seizures, edema), and treatment of systemic malignancy, where appropriate.
- In patients considered to have a favorable prognosis, treatment focuses on eradication or control of the brain metastases. Approaches include surgical resection and radiation therapy.
- In patients with poor prognosis, treatment focuses on symptom control.

ACUTE GENERAL Rx

- Steroids are used to reduce peritumoral edema and intracranial pressure.
- Antiepileptics are started for patients who present with seizures. Prophylactic treatment for seizure is not necessary in patients with no prior history of seizure.
- Anticoagulants are sometimes used to prevent venous thromboembolic disease.

CHRONIC Rx

- Radiation therapy has become the mainstay of treatment for brain metastases, including whole brain radiation therapy and stereotactic radiosurgery (SRS).
- For highly chemosensitive tumors, chemotherapy has been integrated into the primary management of patients with disseminated disease.
- For other tumors (e.g., small cell and non-small cell lung cancers, breast cancer, melanoma) systemic chemotherapy or molecularly targeted agents may be of palliative value when surgery, whole brain radiation therapy, and SRS have failed or are inappropriate. In most cases, two to three agents in combination and in conjunction with whole brain radiation therapy are used.

DISPOSITION

- The median survival of patients who receive supportive care and are treated with corticosteroids only is approximately 1 to 2 months.
- Key prognostic factors are performance status, extent of systemic disease, and age. Most favorable outcome is found in patients with Karnofsky performance score ≥70, age younger than 70 years, no systemic disease or local control of primary tumor without extracranial metastases, and female gender. In this group, median survival is estimated at 7.1 months.

REFERRAL

Treatment involves a multispecialty team. Consultations from oncology, neurosurgery, neurology, radiation oncology, psychiatry, and physical therapy are all warranted.

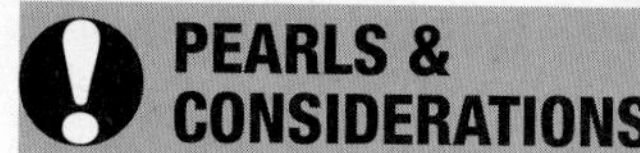

PEARLS & CONSIDERATIONS

COMMENTS

- Brain metastases are the most common intracranial tumors in adults, accounting for more than half of all brain tumors.
- Lung cancer, melanoma, renal cell carcinoma, and breast cancer are the most common primary tumors that metastasize to the brain.
- MRI is the most reliable imaging modality.
- Patient treatment depends upon the overall prognosis.

PATIENT/FAMILY EDUCATION

American Brain Tumor Association (http://www.abta.org)

National Brain Tumor Society (http://www.braintumor.org)

SUGGESTED READINGS

available at www.expertconsult.com

RELATED CONTENT

Brain Cancer (Patient Information)

AUTHOR: **NICOLE J. ULLRICH, M.D., PH.D.**

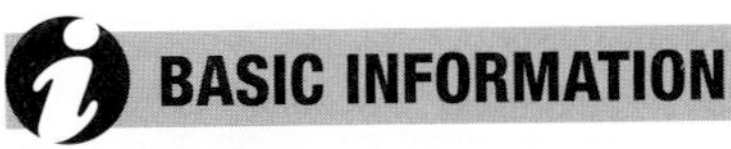

BASIC INFORMATION

DEFINITION

Brain neoplasms are a diverse group of primary (nonmetastatic) tumors arising from one of many different cell types within the central nervous system (CNS). Specific tumor subtypes and prognosis depend on the tumor cell of origin and pattern of growth. The diffuse low-grade gliomas (LGGs) include World Health Organization Grade II astrocytomas, oligodendrogliomas, and oligoastrocytomas.

SYNONYMS

Low-grade glioma (LGG)
Glioneuronal tumor
Meningioma
Primary brain tumor

ICD-9CM CODES
225.0 Brain neoplasm (benign)
239.2 Brain neoplasm (unspecified)
ICD 10-CM CODES
D33.2 Benign neoplasm of brain, unspecified

EPIDEMIOLOGY & DEMOGRAPHICS

INCIDENCE: U.S. incidence rate is approximately 24.6 cases/100,000 persons per yr for all primary brain tumors (Table 1-79). One third of these are considered malignant and the remainder benign or borderline malignant. The incidence rate in children aged 0 to 19 years is lower (48.6/1,000,000 children). Primary brain neoplasms account for ~2% of all cancers, with a disproportionate share of cancer morbidity and mortality. It is the most common cause of cancer death in children up to 15 yr.
PEAK INCIDENCE: Depends on histology, though highest peak at ~age 50 yr
PREDOMINANT SEX AND AGE: Slight male preponderance (8.0 vs. 5.5/100,000 person/yr)
GENETICS: Most primary CNS neoplasms are sporadic; 5% is associated with hereditary syndromes that predispose to neoplasia. The most common of these include:

- Li-Fraumeni syndrome: *p53* mutation on chromosome 17q13, gliomas
- Von Hippel-Lindau: VHL, chromosome 3p25, hemangioblastoma
- Tuberous sclerosis: TSC1/TSC2 (chromosome 9q34/16p13), subependymal giant cell astrocytoma
- Neurofibromatosis type 1: NF1, chromosome 17q11, neurofibroma, optic nerve glioma, low-grade glioma
- Neurofibromatosis type 2: NF2, chromosome 22q12, schwannoma, meningioma, ependymoma
- Retinoblastoma: pRB, chromosome 13q, retinoblastoma
- Gorlin's syndrome: chromosome 9q31, desmoplastic medulloblastoma

RISK FACTORS: Exposure to ionizing radiation has been implicated in meningiomas, gliomas, and nerve sheath tumors. No convincing evidence has shown a link with trauma, occupation, cellular phone use, diet, or electromagnetic fields.

PHYSICAL FINDINGS & CLINICAL PRESENTATION

- In general, the location, size, and rate of growth will determine the symptoms and signs of a brain tumor.
- Headache is common and is the worst symptom in nearly half of all patients. Symptoms of intracranial pressure may also be present, including nausea and vomiting. Headache may be localizing. Papilledema is suggestive of obstructive hydrocephalus.
- Seizures occur in 33% of patients and are among the most common symptoms, particularly with brain metastases and low-grade gliomas. The type of seizure and clinical presentation depends on location. Seizures are more common in low-grade compared with high-grade gliomas. It is thought that patients with seizures typically have smaller tumors at time of diagnosis compared with those with other symptoms, because the onset of seizures prompts an imaging study, leading to an earlier diagnosis.
- Focal neurologic signs and symptoms, including muscle weakness, sensory changes, or visual disturbances are also quite frequent. In addition, cognitive dysfunction, accompanied by changes in memory or personality change, may be recounted, often in retrospect.

ETIOLOGY

Most cases are idiopathic, though specific chromosomal abnormalities have been implicated in some tumor types.

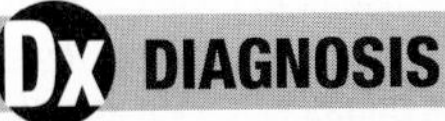

DIAGNOSIS

- Diagnosis is typically based on clinical presentation and imaging characteristics.
- Tumors are best seen on MRI; calcifications are sometimes present.
- Benign and low-grade tumors, typically in the glioma family, are heterogeneous. Recent results have implicated molecular pathway alterations in a subset of patients.

LABORATORY

- Ultimately, only histologic examination can provide the exact diagnosis. Information may also be gleaned from additional features such as proliferative index, immunohistochemical stains, and electron microscopy.
- The current classification schema for gliomas is based on pathologic and microscopic criteria. Tumor histology/histologic diagnosis (World Health Organization [WHO] grading system), includes number of mitoses, capillary endothelial proliferation, and necrosis (*Note:* There can be a high degree of morbidity based on tumor location, even with more benign histology.)
- Genetic analysis of tumors is rapidly becoming important for genetic classification, stratification of treatments, and predicting outcome. Different subtypes of gliomas have distinct gene-expression profiles, which can be distinguished from one another and from normal tissue; these differences typically involve pathways of cell proliferation, energy metabolism, and signal transduction. In adults, global expression profiling identified differences in 360 genes between low-grade and high-grade tumors.

DIFFERENTIAL DIAGNOSIS

- Stroke/cerebral hemorrhage
- Abscess/parasitic cyst
- Demyelinating disease: multiple sclerosis, postinfectious encephalomyelitis
- Metastatic tumors
- Primary CNS lymphoma

WORKUP

- Neuroimaging studies and pathologic sampling are the most important diagnostic

TABLE 1-79 Frequency of Primary CNS Tumors

CHILDREN (0-14 YEARS)		ADULTS (≥15 YEARS)	
Type	Percentage	Type	Percentage
Glioblastoma	20	Glioblastoma	50
Astrocytoma	21	Astrocytoma	10
Ependymoma	7	Ependymoma	2
Oligodendroglioma	1	Oligodendroglioma	3
Medulloblastoma	24	Medulloblastoma	2
Neuroblastoma	3	Neurilemmoma	2
Neurilemmoma	1	Pituitary adenoma	4
Craniopharyngioma	5	Craniopharyngioma	1
Meningioma	5	Meningioma	17
Teratoma	2	Pinealoma	1
Pinealoma	2	Hemangioma	2
Hemangioma	3	Sarcoma	1
Sarcoma	1	Others	5
Others	5	Total	100
Total	100		

From Goetz CG, Pappert EJ: *Textbook of clinical neurology,* Philadelphia, 1999, Saunders.

modalities in evaluation of brain tumors and may be critical for preoperative planning.

IMAGING STUDIES

- MRI with gadolinium enhancement is highly sensitive, though CT scanning is useful if calcification or hemorrhage suspected. MRI permits visualization of the tumor, as well as the relation to the surrounding tissue. Enhancing tumor can be distinguished from surrounding edema. Low-grade tumors often present as an infiltrating lesion without mass effect. MRI is superior to CT scanning to evaluate the meninges, subarachnoid space, and posterior fossa, and for defining relation to major intracranial vessels.
- Magnetic resonance spectroscopy is increasingly being used as a diagnostic tool to define metabolic composition of an area of interest and may be useful to contrast areas of tumor progression from radiation necrosis. N-acetylaspartate is often decreased in brain tumors, whereas choline, a component of cell membranes, is increased because of high cellular turnover.
- PET scan is helpful to distinguish neoplastic lesions (with high rate of metabolism) from other lesions such as demyelination or radiation necrosis (with a much lower metabolic rate). Such lesions take up greater amounts of glucose than surrounding tissues or tumors with slower metabolic rates. May be useful to help map functional areas of the brain before surgery or radiation.
- Functional MRI is now used as an adjunct in perioperative planning for patients whose lesion is in vital regions, such as those responsible for speech, language, and motor control.

Rx TREATMENT

NONPHARMACOLOGIC THERAPY

- Maximal surgical removal or debulking is the initial treatment of choice and provides tissue for diagnosis and molecular characterization. Maximal safe resection is often favored with a trend toward improved survival with this approach.
- Biopsy alone is performed if the tumor is located in eloquent regions of brain or is inaccessible; this is essential for histopathologic diagnosis. Biopsy can be performed under CT or MRI guidance using stereotactic localization.
- If the tumor is benign (e.g., meningioma, acoustic neuroma), often no further therapy is required.

ACUTE GENERAL Rx

Antiseizure medications have been used perioperatively and to control seizures resulting from focal lesions. Prophylactic use of anticonvulsants is not typically recommended without clear history of seizures.

CHRONIC Rx

- Chemotherapy (combination or single agent) may be used before, during, or after surgery and radiation therapy. (In children, chemotherapy is often used to delay radiation therapy.) Radiosensitizers may help increase the therapeutic effect of radiation therapy.
- Radiation is useful for certain types of tumors and is often used if there is residual tumor after surgery; conventional radiation uses external beams over a period of weeks, whereas stereotactic radiosurgery delivers a single, high dose of radiation to a well-defined area (usually <1 cm). Long-term effects of radiation therapy include radiation necrosis (particularly of white matter), blood vessel hyalinization, and secondary tumors (usually meningiomas, sarcomas, and malignant astrocytomas).
- Experimental therapies are continually in development and are typically based on molecular characterization of tumors and small molecule blockers of signal transduction cascades. Some of these therapies involve antisense molecules, biologic agents, immunotherapies, or angiogenesis inhibitors. Intratumoral drug infusions and convection-enhanced delivery of novel agents are currently under study.

DISPOSITION

In general, younger age, high performance status, and lower pathologic grade have more favorable prognosis. For all histologic subtypes of brain tumors, pediatric and young adult patients have a better survival rate.

REFERRAL

- All cases warrant evaluation by an oncologist and neurosurgeon.
- Patients should be evaluated for physical and occupational therapy.
- Children should undergo neuropsychologic evaluations and screening for learning disabilities.

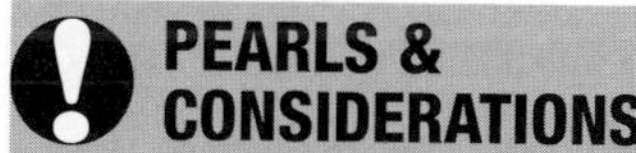

PEARLS & CONSIDERATIONS

COMMENTS

In general, younger age, high performance status, and lower pathologic grade have more favorable prognosis. For all histologic subtypes of brain tumors, pediatric and young adult patients have a better survival.

PATIENT/FAMILY EDUCATION

American Brain Tumor Association (http://www.abta.org)

National Brain Tumor Society (http://www.braintumor.org)

Pediatric Low Grade Astrocytoma (PLGA) (http://fightplga.org)

SUGGESTED READINGS

available at www.expertconsult.com

RELATED CONTENT

Brain Cancer (Patient Information)

AUTHOR: **NICOLE J. ULLRICH, M.D., PH.D.**

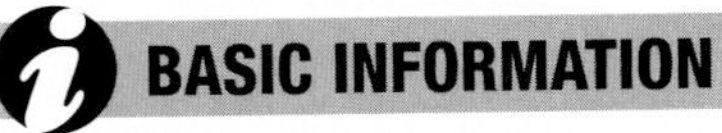

BASIC INFORMATION

DEFINITION

Brain neoplasms are a diverse group of primary (nonmetastatic) tumors arising from one of the many different cell types within the central nervous system. Malignant brain tumors are defined by histopathologic features and a rapidly progressive pattern of growth. Glioblastoma is the most common primary brain tumor in adults, accounting for 50% to 60% of primary brain tumors.

SYNONYMS

Glioblastoma
GBM

ICD-9CM CODES
191.9
ICD-10CM CODES
C71.9 Malignant neoplasm of brain, unspecified

EPIDEMIOLOGY & DEMOGRAPHICS

INCIDENCE: Annual incidence rate of glioblastoma is approximately 2 to 3 cases/100,000 persons in Europe and North America. High-grade/malignant astrocytomas are slightly more common in whites than in blacks, Latinos, and Asians.

PREDOMINANT SEX AND AGE: Glioblastoma is slightly more common in men than women with a male/female ratio of 3:2. Peak incidence is between 45 and 70 yr. Approximately 10% of glioblastomas occur in children.

PEAK INCIDENCE: High-grade gliomas, such as anaplastic astrocytoma and glioblastoma, tend to originate in the fourth to fifth decade of life and beyond.

RISK FACTORS: Prior radiation may increase risk for primary brain tumor. Glioblastomas are more common in individuals who have a heritable cancer predisposition syndrome, such as Li-Fraumeni syndrome and Turcot syndrome. Prior history of a low-grade astrocytoma, which may progress into a higher grade tumor.

GENETICS: Malignant progression is associated with inactivation of *PTEN* tumor-suppressor gene and amplification of epidermal growth factor receptor *(EGFR)* gene. Overexpression of *EGFR* gene occurs in 40% to 50% of primary glioblastoma cases. Loss of heterozygosity on chromosome 10q occurs in 60% to 90% of both primary and secondary glioblastoma cases and is associated with poor prognosis. The pathway involving mutations of the tumor-suppressor gene *p53* is typically associated with secondary glioblastoma. Other genetic mutations have also been recognized as potential contributors in the pathogenesis of glioblastoma, including *PTEN* and *MDM2*. Deletion of *NFKBIA* has an effect that is similar to the effect of *EGFR* amplification in the pathogenesis of glioblastoma and is associated with comparatively short survival.

PHYSICAL FINDINGS & CLINICAL PRESENTATION

- In general, the location, size, and rate of growth will determine the symptoms and signs. Clinical history of patients with glioblastoma is typically brief, <3 mo in the majority of patients with primary glioblastoma.
- Most frequent symptoms include:
  - Headache occurs in the majority of cases. The headache can be localizing or may result from increased intracranial pressure.
  - Seizures occur in 30% to 60% depending on tumor location and grade.
  - Symptoms and signs of hydrocephalus and raised intracranial pressure (headache, vomiting, clouding of consciousness, papilledema).
  - Other symptoms seen in 20% or more of patients include memory loss, focal motor weakness, visual changes, language deficits, and cognitive disturbances or memory changes due to involvement of the temporal and frontal lobes.

ETIOLOGY

- Glioblastomas are classified as primary or secondary. Primary glioblastoma constitutes the majority of cases (60%) in adults older than 50 yr and are considered de novo tumors. Secondary glioblastoma typically involves malignant progression from a lower grade (grade II or III) glioma.

Dx DIAGNOSIS

DIFFERENTIAL DIAGNOSIS

- Stroke
- Arteriovenous malformations
- Abscess/parasitic cyst (neurocysticercosis)
- Demyelinating disease: tumefactive multiple sclerosis, postinfectious encephalomyelitis
- Metastases
- Primary central nervous system lymphoma

LABORATORY TESTS

- Routine laboratory studies are not typically helpful.
- Lumbar puncture is generally contraindicated; cerebrospinal fluid studies do not add much specific additional information for the diagnosis for glioblastoma.
- Ultimately, only a histologic examination can provide the exact diagnosis. Information may also be gleaned from additional features such as proliferative index, immunohistochemical stains, and electron microscopy, as well as molecular markers.

IMAGING STUDIES (Fig. 1-183)

- MRI with and without contrast is the imaging study of choice, though CT scanning is useful if calcification or hemorrhage is suspected. MRI permits visualization of the tumor, as well as the relation to the surrounding tissue. Enhancing tumor can be distinguished from surrounding edema. MRI is superior to CT scanning to evaluate the meninges, subarachnoid space, and posterior fossa, and for defining relation to major intracranial vessels.
- Magnetic resonance spectroscopy (MRS) is increasingly being used as a diagnostic tool to define metabolic composition of an area of interest and may be useful to contrast areas of tumor progression from radiation necrosis. N-acetylaspartate, a marker of neurons, is often decreased in brain tumors, whereas choline, a component of cell membranes, is increased because of high cellular turnover.
- PET scan is helpful to distinguish neoplastic lesions (with high rate of metabolism) from other lesions such as demyelination or radiation necrosis (with a much lower metabolic rate). Such lesions take up greater amounts of glucose than surrounding tissues or tumors with slower metabolic rates. PET imaging also aids in preoperative planning to increase diagnostic yield and to help map functional areas of the brain before surgery.
- Functional MRI is now used as an adjunct modality in perioperative planning for patients whose lesion is in vital regions (eloquent regions), such as those responsible for speech, language, and motor control.

Rx TREATMENT

- Current standard-of-care therapies include surgery, radiation, and palliative chemotherapy,

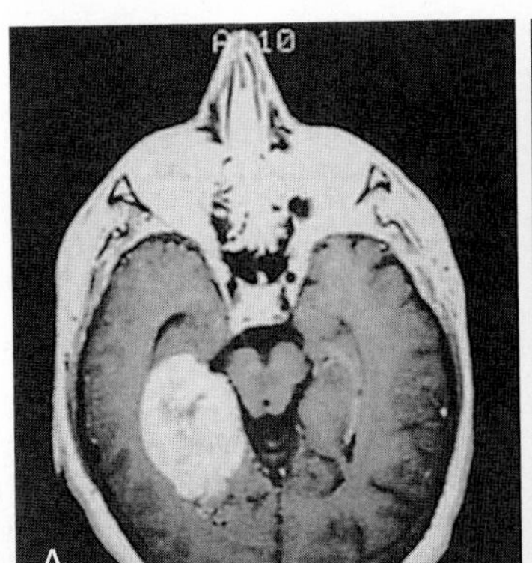

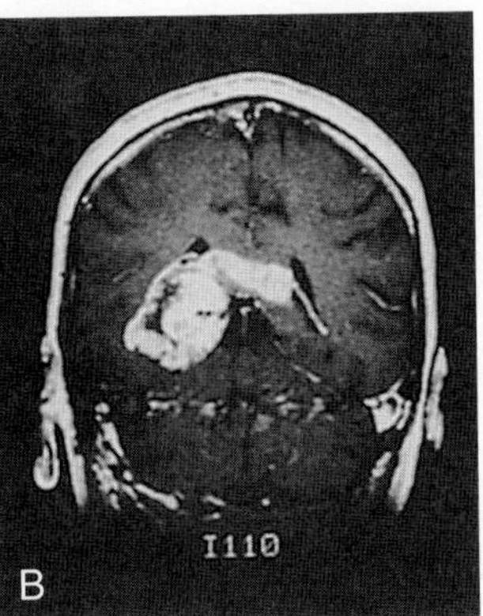

FIGURE 1-183 Glioblastoma multiforme. Axial **(A)** and coronal **(B)** postcontrast enhanced T1-weighted image showing a large homogeneously contrast-enhancing mass in the right medial temporal lobe with extension across the midline. (From Specht N [ed]: *Practical guide to diagnostic imaging,* St Louis, 1998, Mosby.)

all of which have significant adverse effects and limited efficacy. Median time to recurrence after standard therapy is 6.9 mo.

PHARMACOLOGIC AND NONPHARMACOLOGIC THERAPY

- Maximal surgical removal or debulking is the initial treatment of choice and is the first stage in treatment. Removal of 98% or more of the tumor is associated with a significantly longer event-free survival.
- Biopsy alone is performed if the tumor is located in eloquent regions of brain or is inaccessible; this is essential for histopathologic diagnosis. Biopsy can be performed with CT or MRI guidance using stereotactic localization.
- Radiation therapy is the mainstay of treatment for individuals with glioblastoma and improves local control and overall survival after surgery. Even patients with a gross total resection of tumor have a high recurrence rate.
- Chemotherapy (combination or single agent) may be used before, during, or after surgery and radiation therapy. (In children, chemotherapy is often used to delay radiation therapy.) Radiosensitizers may help increase the therapeutic effect of radiation therapy. Conventional treatment includes radiation in combination with temozolomide. Bevacizumab is used to treat patients with glioblastoma at progression after standard therapy.
- Experimental therapies in development are typically based on molecular characterization of tumors and small molecule blockers of signal transduction cascades. Some of these therapies involve antisense molecules, biologic agents, immunotherapies, or angiogenesis inhibitors. Intratumoral drug infusions and convection-enhanced delivery of novel agents are currently under study. In addition, delivery systems such as the use of a vector to permit gene transfer with the goal to selectively kill cancer cells are being investigated.

ACUTE GENERAL Rx

- Steroids are used to reduce edema and may also be used perioperatively or during radiation therapy.
- Antiepileptic medications have been used perioperatively and to control seizures resulting from focal lesions. Prophylactic use of anticonvulsants is not typically recommended without clear history of seizures.

DISPOSITION

- Glioblastoma multiforme is the most aggressive form of primary brain tumor. The important prognostic factors include the extent of resection, patient age, tumor grade/histology, and performance status. In general, younger age, high performance status, and lower pathologic grade have more favorable prognosis. For all histologic subtypes of brain tumors, pediatric and young adult patients have a better survival.
- Terminal events typically result from increased intracranial pressure.

REFERRAL

Treatment should involve a multispecialty team with consultations from oncology, neurosurgery, neurology, radiation oncology, psychiatry, and physical therapy.

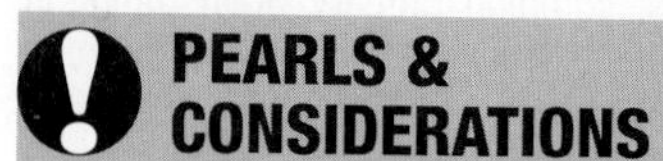

PEARLS & CONSIDERATIONS

COMMENTS

Glioblastoma is distinguished pathologically by the presence of vascular proliferation and necrosis.

PATIENT/FAMILY EDUCATION

American Brain Tumor Association

National Brain Tumor Society (http://www.braintumor.org)

SUGGESTED READINGS

available at www.expertconsult.com

RELATED CONTENT

Brain Cancer (Patient Information)

AUTHOR: **NICOLE J. ULLRICH, M.D., PH.D.**

BASIC INFORMATION

DEFINITION

The term *breast cancer* refers to invasive carcinoma of the breast, whether ductal or lobular.

SYNONYMS

Carcinoma of the breast

ICD-9CM CODES
174.9 Malignant neoplasm female breast

ICD-10CM CODES
C50.919 Malignant neoplasm of unspecified site of unspecified female breast

EPIDEMIOLOGY & DEMOGRAPHICS

- Nearly exclusively the disease of women, with only 1% of breast cancers in males
- Steady increase in its incidence in the U.S., with approximately 210,000 new patients annually; more than 50,000 are Stage 0 ductal carcinoma in situ (DCIS).
- Annual mortality of approximately 40,000
- Risk steadily increases with age. Table 1-80 describes risk factors for breast cancer.

TABLE 1-80 Risk Factors for Breast Cancer

Risk Factor	Relative Risk
Any benign breast disease	1.5
Postmenopausal hormone replacement (estrogen with or without progestin)	1.5
Menarche at <12 yr	1.1-1.9
Moderate alcohol intake (two to three drinks/day)	1.1-1.9
Menopause at >55 yr	1.1-1.9
Increased bone density	1.1-1.9
Sedentary lifestyle and lack of exercise	1.1-1.9
Proliferative breast disease without atypia	2
Age at first birth >30 yr or nulliparous	2-4
First-degree relative with breast cancer	2-4
Postmenopausal obesity	2-4
Upper socioeconomic class	2-4
Personal history of endometrial or ovarian cancer	2-4
Significant radiation to chest	2-4
Increased breast density on mammogram	2-4
Older age	>4
Personal history of breast cancer (in situ or invasive)	>4
Proliferative breast disease with atypia	>4
Two first-degree relatives with breast cancer	5
Atypical hyperplasia and first-degree relative with breast cancer	10

From Goldman L, Schafer AI: *Goldman's Cecil medicine*, ed 24, Philadelphia, 2012, Saunders.

- Genetically defined group of women with *BRCA-1* or *BRCA-2* genes identified to carry lifetime risk as high as 85%

PHYSICAL FINDINGS & CLINICAL PRESENTATION

- Increasing number of small breast cancers found by mammograms
- Patients usually completely free of physical findings
- Palpable tumors possibly as small as 1 cm or even smaller
- Size of the mass and its location measured and documented
- Skin and/or nipple retraction and skin edema, erythema, ulcer, satellite nodule
- Nodal enlargement in axilla and supraclavicular areas
- Advanced disease: clinical signs of pleural effusion and/or hepatomegaly
- Rare instances: clear, serous, or bloody discharge only symptom
- Nipple evaluation (see "Paget's Disease of the Breast")

ETIOLOGY

- Precise mechanism of carcinogenesis not understood. Gene expression analysis has altered the way breast cancer is perceived in that it is no longer regarded as a single disease. Estrogen receptor (ER)-positive and ER-negative cancers are clinically distinct diseases. So-called triple negative breast cancers constitute approximately 20% of all breast cancers but have different behavior than non-triple negative. The term refers to absence of the estrogen, progesterone, and HER2/neu receptors. Absence of these receptors removes an important target for non-surgical treatment. Stage for stage, long-term prognosis is similar when compared to receptor-positive tumors, but the overall treatment approach will need to be more aggressive. Relapse rates are also different, with an initially elevated rate up to five years but subsequently with substantial decrease in the rate of cancer relapse.
- Approximately 10% of all women with breast cancer have a germline mutation of *BRCA-1, BRCA-2, P53,* or other mutations.
- Possibly interaction of ovarian estrogen, nonovarian estrogen, estrogens of exogenous origin with breast tissue of varied carcinogenic susceptibility to develop cancer
- Other known or suspected variables: childbearing, breastfeeding practice, diet, physical activities, body mass, alcohol intake
- *BRCA-1* and *BRCA-2* genes are responsible for 90% of hereditary breast cancer

Dx DIAGNOSIS

DIFFERENTIAL DIAGNOSIS

The following nonmalignant breast lesions can simulate breast cancer on both physical and mammogram examinations:

- Fibrocystic changes
- Fibroadenoma
- Hamartoma

WORKUP

- Physical examination:
  1. Mass detected by patient or medical professional: workup required
  2. Negative mammogram: breast cancer not ruled out
  3. Sonogram: to demonstrate mass to be cyst, usually eliminating need for further workup
  4. Screening with both MRI and mammography might rule out cancerous lesions better than mammography alone in women who are known or likely to have an inherited predisposition to breast cancer
- To establish diagnosis:
  1. Positive aspiration cytology on a clinically and mammographically malignant mass—highly accurate but still requires open biopsy confirmation
  2. Stereotactic core needle biopsy diagnosis: Stereotactic- and ultrasonography-guided core-needle biopsy procedures seem to be almost as accurate as open surgical biopsy with lower complication rates. They are reliable with invasive carcinoma identified, but negative or equivocal results require careful evaluation
  3. Atypical hyperplasia or in situ carcinoma found by core needle biopsy: open surgical biopsy confirmation still required
  4. Excisional or incisional biopsy: establishes diagnosis

NOTE: Do not rely on negative mammogram or negative aspiration cytology findings to exclude malignancy. Make appropriate referral. Obtain imaging studies such as bone scan, chest x-ray, CT scan of abdomen, or CT scan of liver.

- Breast radiologic evaluation and an algorithm for breast cancer screening and evaluation are described in Section III. The differential diagnosis of breast lumps is described in Section II.

IMAGING STUDIES

Mammograms (Fig. 1-184): 30% to 50% of breast cancers detected by screening mammograms only as a spiculated mass, a mass with or without microcalcifications, or a cluster of microcalcifications. MRI is an excellent modality that is particularly useful in patients with breast implants and when there is a strong family history of breast cancer. MRI is also better than other methods of assessing the response to neoadjuvant chemotherapy and is useful in identifying the primary tumor in patients who present with axillary adenopathy.

Rx TREATMENT

NONPHARMACOLOGIC THERAPY

- Early breast cancer: primarily surgical or surgical and radiotherapeutic. Table 1-81 compares ductal versus lobular carcinoma in situ. Adjuvant treatment guidelines for patients with early-stage invasive breast cancer are described in Table 1-82.
- Choice in 60% to 70% of women between modified mastectomy and breast-conserving treatment, which consists of lumpectomy, axillary staging with sentinel node biopsy or axillary dissection, and breast irradiation

 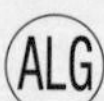 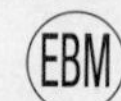

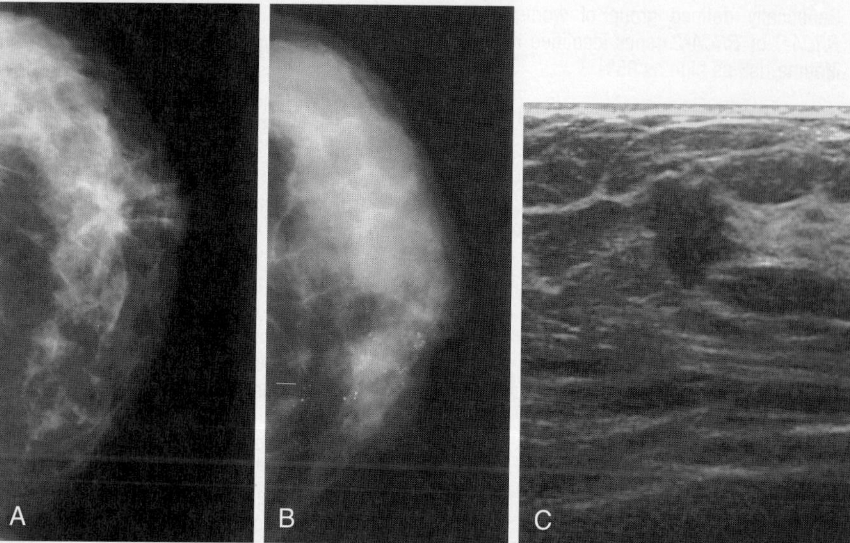

FIGURE 1-184 Mammogram and ultrasound findings of breast disease. A, A stellate mass in the breast. The combination of a density with spiculated borders and distortion of surrounding breast architecture suggests a malignancy. **B,** Clustered microcalcification. Fine, pleomorphic, and linear calcifications that cluster together suggest the diagnosis of ductal carcinoma in situ (DCIS). **C,** An ultrasound image of breast cancer. The mass is solid, containing internal echoes, and displaying an irregular border. Most maligant lesions are taller than they are wide. (From Townsend CM et al [eds]: *Sabiston textbook of surgery*, ed 17, Philadelphia, 2004, Saunders.)

TABLE 1-81 Carcinoma in Situ: Lobular Versus Ductal

Feature	Lobular Carcinoma in Situ	Ductal Carcinoma in Situ
Age	Younger	Older
Palpable mass	No	Uncommon
Mammographic appearance	Not detected on mammography	Microcalcifications, mass
Immunophenotype	E-cadherin negative	E-cadherin positive
Usual manifestation	Incidental finding on breast biopsy	Microcalcifications on mammography or breast mass
Bilateral involvement	Common	Uncertain
Risk and site of subsequent breast cancer	25% risk for invasive breast cancer in either breast over remaining lifespan	At site of initial lesion; 0.5% risk/yr of invasive breast cancer in opposite breast
Prevention	Consider tamoxifen or raloxifene	Consider tamoxifen or raloxifene if estrogen-receptor positive
Treatment	Yearly mammography and breast examination	Lumpectomy ± radiation; mastectomy for large or multifocal lesions

From Goldman L, Schafer AI: *Goldman's Cecil medicine*, ed 24, Philadelphia, 2012, Saunders.

- Recent trials reveal that among patients with limited sentinel lymph nodes (SNL), metastatic breast cancer treated with breast conservation and systematic therapy, the use of sentinel lymph node dissection (SNLD) alone compared with axillary lymph node dissection (ALND) did not result in inferior survival

ACUTE GENERAL Rx

DCIS: Local breast-conserving therapy (lumpectomy plus radiation therapy) or mastectomy followed by tamoxifen therapy in estrogen receptor-positive cases

- Invasive breast cancer: Mastectomy and sentinel lymph node evaluation *or* lumpectomy and sentinel lymph node evaluation plus whole breast radiation therapy
- Invasive breast cancer may require adjuvant chemotherapy or endocrine therapy. Standard chemotherapy consists of either cyclophosphamide, methotrexate, and fluorouracil or cyclophosphamide plus doxorubicin. Endocrine therapy is recommended after chemotherapy in patients with hormone-receptor positive tumors. Adjuvant hormone therapy with anti-estrogen drugs reduces disease recurrence and mortality in these postmenopausal women with breast cancer. Aromatase inhibitors decrease the agonist effect of estrogen by inhibiting estrogen synthesis and have become preferred first-line hormonal treatment agents over the selective estrogen receptor modulator tamoxifen.
- Table 1-83 describes intrinsic molecular subtypes of breast cancer. Molecular targets in clinical breast cancer management are described in Table 1-84. Clinicopathologic considerations for patients with ER-positive and human epidermal growth factor receptor 2 (HER2)-negative disease are summarized in Table 1-85.
- Weekly paclitaxel after standard adjuvant chemotherapy with doxorubicin and cyclophosphamide improves disease-free and overall survival in women with breast cancer. However, patients with *HER2*-negative, estrogen-receptor–positive, node-positive breast cancer may gain little benefit from administration of paclitaxel after adjuvant chemotherapy with doxorubicin plus cyclophosphamide.
- Fig. 1-185 illustrates considerations for adjuvant chemotherapy in the management of recurrent and metastatic breast cancer.
- The combination of the aromatase inhibitor anastrozole and fulvestrant is superior to anastrozole alone or sequential anastrozole and fulvestrant for the treatment of HR-positive metastatic breast cancer.
- Trastuzumab emtansine (T-DM1), an antibody-drug conjugate incorporating HER2-targeted antitumor properties of trastuzumab with the cytotoxic activity of the microtubule inhibitor agent DM1, has been shown to significantly prolong progression-free and overall survival with less toxicity than lapatinib plus capecitabine in patients with HER2-positive advanced breast cancer.

CHRONIC Rx

Follow-up required after proper treatment of primary breast cancer includes:

- Periodic clinical evaluations as delineated by medical oncologist or surgeon
- Annual mammograms/MRI
- Other tests as indicated
- Patient instruction in monthly breast self-examination technique

DISPOSITION

- Prognosis after curative therapy: depends on size of tumor, extent of nodal metastasis, and pathologic grade of tumor
    1. Patient with 1-cm tumor with no axillary node metastasis: 10-yr disease-free survival rate of 90%
    2. Patient with 3-cm tumor with metastasis in four nodes: 10-yr disease-free survival rate of 15% if no systemic adjuvant therapy given
    3. Outlook for most patients is between these extremes
- Systemic adjuvant therapy: improves prognosis significantly. Women who take tamoxifen for 10 yr lower their risk of recurrence by 25% and dying of breast cancer by 27% compared with those who took the pills for just 5 yr.
- Isolated tumor cells or micrometastases in regional lymph nodes is associated with a reduced 5-yr rate of disease-free survival among women with favorable early-stage breast cancer who do not receive adjuvant therapy. Survival is improved in patients with isolated tumor cells or micrometastases who received adjuvant therapy.
- Retrospective analyses suggest that occult lymph-node metastases are an important prognostic factor for disease recurrence of survival among patients with breast cancer; however, recent trials indicate that the magnitude of the difference in outcome at 5 yrs

TABLE 1-82 Adjuvant Treatment Guidelines for Patients with Early-Stage Invasive Breast Cancer*

Patient Group*	Treatment
Favorable Histology (Tubular or Colloid)	
ER- and/or PR-Positive Breast Cancer	
<1 cm	No adjuvant therapy
1-2.9 cm	Consider adjuvant hormonal therapy†
≥3 cm or node-positive	Adjuvant hormonal therapy ± adjuvant chemotherapy†
ER- and PR-Negative Breast Cancer	
<1 cm	No adjuvant therapy
1-2.9 cm	Consider adjuvant chemotherapy
≥3 cm or node-positive	Adjuvant chemotherapy
Hormone Receptor-Positive (ER- and/or PR-Positive) Breast Cancer	
Lymph Nodes Negative	
≤0.5 cm	No adjuvant therapy
0.6-1.0 cm well differentiated and no unfavorable features‡	Consider adjuvant hormonal therapy
0.6-1.0 cm moderate or poorly differentiated or unfavorable features	Adjuvant hormonal therapy ± adjuvant chemotherapy
>1 cm	Adjuvant hormonal therapy ± adjuvant chemotherapy
Lymph Nodes Positive	
	Adjuvant hormonal therapy + adjuvant chemotherapy
Hormone Receptor-Negative (ER- and PR-Negative) Breast Cancer	
≤0.5 cm	No adjuvant therapy
0.6-1.0 cm	Consider chemotherapy
>1 cm or lymph-node positive	Adjuvant chemotherapy
HER2 Positive	
	Trastuzumab should be added to the suggested treatment above for all node-positive patients; trastuzumab not recommended for tumors ≤1 cm for most node-negative patients; for tumors >1 cm, trastuzumab should be considered for most patients

*Data are insufficient to make chemotherapy recommendations for patients ≥70 yr. Treatment should be individualized for these patients based on life expectancy and comorbidity.
†In ER-positive or PR-positive patients, decisions regarding the added value of chemotherapy in addition to hormonal therapy alone can be aided by accurately assessing the added value of chemotherapy in individual patients using a web-based model: www.adjuvantonline.com or Oncotype Dx assay.
‡Unfavorable characteristics include high-grade tumor, blood vessel or lymphatic invasion by tumor, and high tumor proliferation rate (high S phase by flow cytometry or high Ki-67 value by immunohistochemistry) or HER2-positive status.
ER, Estrogen receptor; *HER2,* human epidermal growth factor receptor 2; *PR,* progesterone receptor.
Modified from National Comprehensive Cancer Network Guidelines. Available at www.nccn.org.

TABLE 1-83 Intrinsic Molecular Subtypes of Breast Cancer

Type	Characteristics	Markers
Luminal A	Low grade, high ER, 50% of breast cancer	ER+, PR+, HER2−, CK8+, CK18+
Luminal B	Higher grade, lower ER, 10% of breast cancer	ER+, PR+/−, HER2+/−
HER2	High grade, p53 mutations, 5% to 10% of breast cancer	ER−, PR−, HER2+
Basal	High proliferation CK5+, CK14+, CK17+, EGFR+,30% of breast cancer	ER−, PR−, HER2−

CK, Cytokeratin.
From Cameron JL, Cameron AM: *Current surgical therapy,* ed 10, Philadelphia, 2011, Saunders.

is small (1.2 percentage points). These data do not favor a clinical benefit of additional evaluation (including immunohistochemical analysis) of initially negative sentinel nodes in patients with breast cancer.

- The addition of zoledronic acid to adjuvant endocrine therapy improves disease-free survival in premenopausal patients with estrogen-responsive early breast cancer.

REFERRAL

Referral is necessary as soon as breast cancer is suspected.

PEARLS & CONSIDERATIONS

Breast cancer in pregnancy and lactation:

1. Frequency in women 40 yr or younger reported to be 15%
2. May carry worse prognosis because disease discovery delayed by engorged and nodular breast changes and/or because disease progression more rapid in pregnancy
3. Survival rates similar to those for nonpregnant early-stage breast cancer patients in same age group
4. Mass usually found by patient or obstetrician
5. Expedient workup recommended, including mammography and sonography
6. Diagnosis to be made without delay
7. Choice of mastectomy or lumpectomy with axillary dissection for treatment
8. Adjuvant chemotherapy delayed until third trimester or after delivery
9. Irradiation to breast after lumpectomy delayed until after delivery

Ductal carcinoma in situ (DCIS, intraductal carcinoma) (see Table 1-81):

1. Discovered by mammogram as cluster of microcalcifications and/or density
2. Presents less often as a palpable mass or nipple discharge
3. Before mammogram screening, DCIS accounted for 1% of all breast cancers
4. Now 15% to 20% or even higher proportion have DCIS
5. Formerly treated with mastectomy, now lumpectomy
6. Cure rates 98% to 99%
7. No axillary dissection required
8. With radiation, breast recurrences reduced
9. Mastectomy possibly required with extensive and/or high-grade DCIS
10. Systemic adjuvant treatment is not indicated

Inflammatory carcinoma:

1. Rare but rapidly progressive and often lethal form of breast cancer
2. Presents as erythematous and edematous breast resembling mastitis
3. Biopsy required, including skin
4. Treatment with combination chemotherapy followed by surgery and radiation therapy
5. Prognosis once dismal, now 5-yr disease-free survival in 50% of patients

COMMENTS

- The U.S. Preventive Services Task Force (USPSTF) now recommends against automatic "routine" screening of younger women (age range 40 to 49). The task force recommends biennial screening mammography for all middle-aged women (age range 50 to 74). It also states that current evidence is insufficient to assess the benefits and harms of screening mammography in older women (aged 75 and older). The task force also discourages women from performing breast self-examination. Several other U.S. organizations, such as the American Congress of Obstetricians and Gynecologists, however, still recommend annual screening beginning at age 40. This has created confusion

 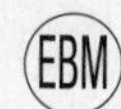 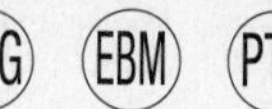

TABLE 1-84 Molecular Targets in Clinical Breast Cancer Management

Target	Drug	Status
ER	Tamoxifen	Survival benefit, adjuvant treatment, and metastatic disease, premenopausal and postmenopausal women
	Aromatase inhibitors (anastrozole, letrozole, exemestane)	Survival benefit, adjuvant and metastatic disease, postmenopausal women
	Fulvestrant	Second-line therapy, metastatic disease in postmenopausal women
HER2	Trastuzumab	Survival benefit, adjuvant and metastatic disease
HER1+ HER2	Lapatinib	Second-line therapy, metastatic disease; phase II adjuvant trials ongoing
HER1 (EGFR)	Gefitinib, erlotinib	Benefit unclear after phase II trials
	Cetuximab	In trial
VEGF	Bevacizumab	Progression-free survival benefit, metastatic disease; phase III adjuvant trials ongoing
PARP1/PARP2	PARP1 inhibitor	Improved PFS, OS in phase II trial, phase III initiated

OS, Overall survival; *PFS,* progression-free survival.
From Cameron JL, Cameron AM: *Current surgical therapy*, ed 10, Philadelphia, 2011, Saunders.

TABLE 1-85 Clinicopathologic Considerations for Patients with ER-Positive, HER2-Negative Disease

Clinicopathologic Features	Consider Adding Chemotherapy	Factors Not Useful for Decision	Consider Endocrine Therapy Only
ER and PR	Lower ER/PR levels		Higher ER/PR levels
Grade	Grade 3	Grade 2	Grade 1
Proliferation	Ki-67 >30%	Ki-67 16% to 30%	Ki-67 ≤15%
Nodes	Node positive (four or more nodes)	Node positive (one to three nodes)	Node negative
Peritumoral vascular invasion	Extensive PVI		Absence of PVI
Tumor size	>5 cm	2.1-5 cm	≤2cm
Patient preference	Favors using all possible treatments		Favors avoiding side effects of chemotherapy

Adapted from highlights of the St. Gallen consensus panel. From Cameron JL, Cameron AM: *Current surgical therapy*, ed 10, Philadelphia, 2011, Saunders.

among both physicians and the general public. Physicians should be familiar with the risks and benefits of various competing recommendations in order to better counsel patients.

- Breast radiologic evaluation, evaluation of nipple discharge, and evaluation of palpable mass are described in Section III.
- Exposure of the heart to ionizing radiation during breast cancer radiotherapy increases risk of ischemic heart disease. The increased rate of ischemic heart disease begins within a few years of exposure and continues for at least 20 yr. The increase is proportional to the mean radiation dose to the heart.

RISK REDUCTION STRATEGIES:

- Prophylactic bilateral mastectomy reduces the risk for invasive breast cancer by >90%.
- Selective estrogen receptor modulators (SERM) reduce the incidence of hormone receptor-positive invasive breast cancer by 50%.

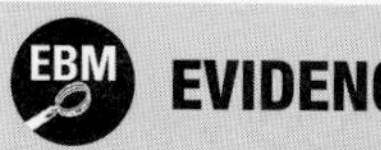

EVIDENCE

available at www.expertconsult.com

SUGGESTED READINGS

available at www.expertconsult.com

RELATED CONTENT

Abscess, Breast (Related Key Topic)
Fibrocystic Breast Disease (Related Key Topic)
Fig. 3-37, Breast, nipple discharge evaluation (Algorithm)
Fig. E3-38, Breast, radiologic evaluation (Algorithm)
Fig. 3-39, Breast, routine screen or palpable mass evaluation (Algorithm)
Breast Cancer (Patient Information)
Breast Cancer: For Men (Patient Information)

AUTHORS: **TAKUMA NEMOTO, M.D.**, and **RUBEN ALVERO, M.D.**

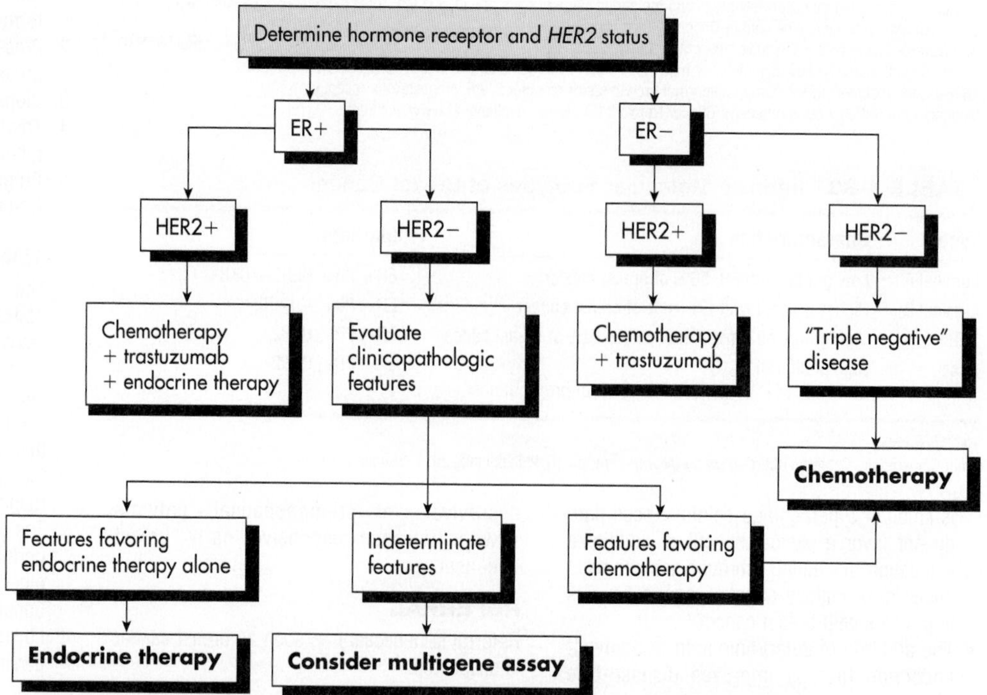

FIGURE 1-185 Management of recurrent and metastatic breast cancer. Considerations for adjuvant chemotherapy. (From Cameron JL, Cameron AM: *Current surgical therapy,* ed 10, Philadelphia, 2011, Saunders.)

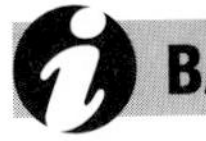

BASIC INFORMATION

DEFINITION

Breech presentation occurs when fetal longitudinal axis is such that the cephalic pole occupies the uterine fundus (Fig. 1-186). Three types exist: frank (48% to 73%, flexed hips, extended knees), complete (4.6% to 11.5%, flexed hips and knees), and footling (12% to 38%, hips extended).

ICD-9CM CODES

652.2 Breech presentation without mention of version

763.0 Breech delivery and extraction affecting fetus or newborn

ICD-10CM CODES

083 Breech extraction

032.1 Maternal care for breech extraction

EPIDEMIOLOGY & DEMOGRAPHICS

INCIDENCE: Gestational age dependent: 3%-4% overall, 14% at 29-32 wk, 33% at 21-24 wk

PERINATAL MORTALITY: 3-5 times increase over vertex presentation at term, regardless of delivery route. When corrected for associated increase in congenital anomalies and complications of prematurity, morbidity and mortality rates approach those of vertex presentation at term regardless of delivery route.

PHYSICAL FINDINGS & CLINICAL PRESENTATION

- Lack of presenting part on vaginal examination
- Fetal heart tones heard above the umbilicus
- Leopold maneuvers revealing mobile fetal part in the uterine fundus

ETIOLOGY

- Abnormal placentation (fundal), uterine anomalies (fibroids, septa), pelvic or adnexal masses, alterations in fetal muscular tone, or fetal malformations
- Associated conditions: trisomy 13, 18, 21; Potter syndrome; myotonic dystrophy; prematurity

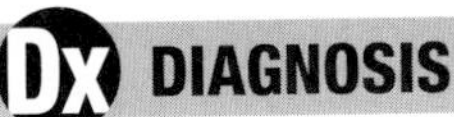

DIAGNOSIS

DIFFERENTIAL DIAGNOSIS

Vertex, oblique, or transverse lie

WORKUP

- Determine reason for breech presentation, history of uterine anomalies, gestational age, or associated fetal congenital anomalies
- Assess fetal status by continuous FHR monitoring or ultrasound
- Assess pelvis to determine feasibility of vaginal delivery
- Assess risk for safety of vaginal versus abdominal delivery

IMAGING STUDIES

Ultrasound to evaluate for:

- Fetal anomalies, such as hydrocephalus
- Placental location
- Position of fetal head relative to spine (check for hyperextension)
- Estimated fetal weight (2500 to 3800 g for attempt of vaginal delivery)
- Type of breech (frank, complete, footling)

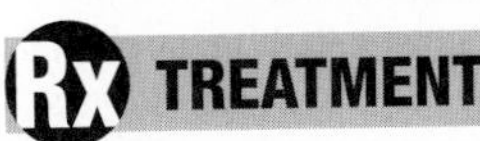

TREATMENT

ACUTE GENERAL Rx

- Vaginal delivery in selected patients (see "Comments" section): allow maternal expulsive forces to deliver fetus until scapula visible (avoiding traction); with flexion and/or Piper forceps, deliver fetal head
- Perform Cesarean section (see "Comments")
- External cephalic version: success 60% to 75% after 37 wk, contraindicated with placental abruption, low-lying placenta, maternal hypertension, previous uterine incision, multiple gestation, non-reassuring fetal status
- Adequate pelvic/cervical relaxation essential (i.e., anesthesia in-room during delivery with uterine relaxants on hand [nitroglycerin, terbutaline])

COMPLICATIONS

- Head entrapment: leading cause of death (with the exception of anomalous fetuses), 88 cases per 1000 deliveries; avoid by maintaining flexion of fetal head, use of Piper forceps or Dührssen's incisions. Avoid hyperextension of head during delivery.
- Cord prolapse: usually occurs late in labor. Incidence depends on type of breech: frank (0.5%), complete (4%-5%), footling (10%).
- Nuchal arm: arm extended above fetal head, occurs when there is undue traction before delivery of fetal scapulas. Treatment: bring trapped arm across infant's face.

DISPOSITION

If confounding variables are corrected for (prematurity, associated congenital anomalies [6.3% of breeches vs. 2.4% in general population]), route of delivery plays less important role in fetal outcome than previously believed, if the obstetrician performing the delivery is experienced in breech delivery. As fewer providers perform breech deliveries and seasoned obstetricians retire, fewer new physicians learn the technique of breech delivery.

REFERRAL

An obstetrician trained in vaginal breech delivery is prerequisite for attempt; explain to the patient that with cesarean section certain risks (i.e., hyperextension of the fetal head with resultant spinal cord injury) may be minimized but not eliminated.

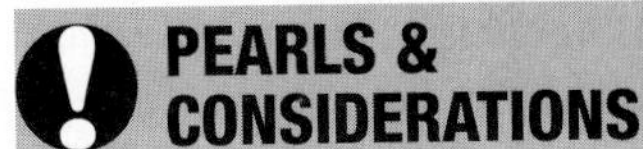

PEARLS & CONSIDERATIONS

COMMENTS

For breech presentation, mortality rate increased 13-fold and morbidity 7-fold, mainly due to an increase in congenital anomalies, perinatal hypoxia, birth injury, prematurity.

No contraindication to induction of labor in breech presentation; labor not prohibited in primigravida.

CRITERIA FOR TRIAL OF LABOR:

- Estimated fetal weight 2500 to 3800 g (recognizing inherent error in estimated fetal weight approximations: actual fetal weight may be substantially smaller)
- Frank breech
- Adequate pelvis
- Flexed fetal head
- Continuous fetal monitoring
- Normal progress of labor
- Bedside availability of anesthesia and capability for immediate cesarean section
- Informed consent
- Obstetrician trained in vaginal breech delivery

CRITERIA FOR CESAREAN SECTION:

- Estimated fetal weight <1500 g or >4000 g
- Footling presentation (20% risk of cord prolapse, usually late in course of labor)
- Inadequate pelvis
- Hyperextended fetal head (21% risk of spinal cord injury)
- Nonreassuring fetal status
- Abnormal progress of labor
- Lack of trained obstetrician

RELATED CONTENT

Premature Labor (Related Key Topic)
Breech Birth (Patient Information)

AUTHOR: **RUBEN ALVERO, M.D.**

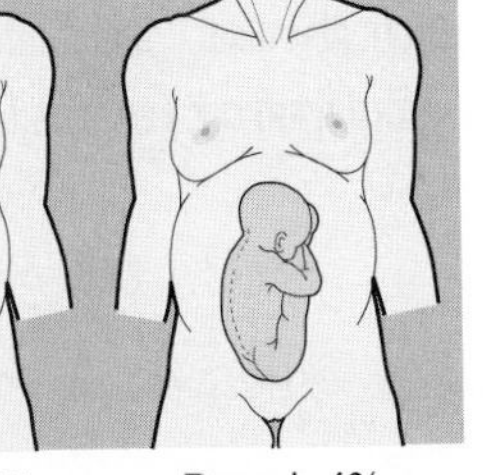

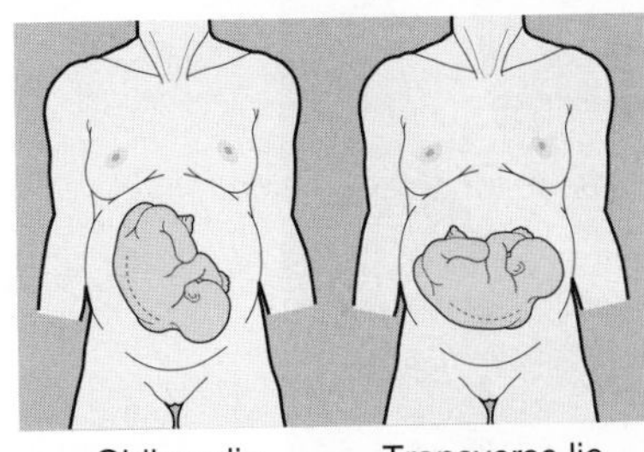

FIGURE 1-186 Fetal lie at term. (From Drife J, Magowan B: *Clinical obstetrics and gynecology*, Philadelphia, 2004, Saunders.)

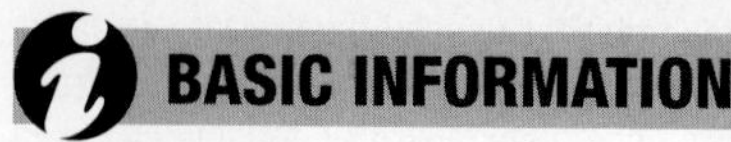

BASIC INFORMATION

DEFINITION

Bronchiectasis is the abnormal dilation and destruction of bronchial walls, which may be congenital or acquired.

ICD-9CM CODES
494.0 Bronchiectasis
ICD-10CM CODES
J47.9 Bronchiectasis, uncomplicated

EPIDEMIOLOGY & DEMOGRAPHICS

- Cystic fibrosis is responsible for nearly 50% of all cases of bronchiectasis.
- Acquired primary bronchiectasis is uncommon because of rapid diagnosis of pulmonary infections and frequent use of antibiotics.
- Effective childhood immunizations have led to a significant decrease in the incidence of bronchiectasis resulting from pertussis.

PHYSICAL FINDINGS & CLINICAL PRESENTATION

- Moist crackles at lung bases
- Cough with expectoration of large amount of purulent sputum
- Fever, night sweats, generalized malaise, weight loss
- Hemoptysis
- Halitosis, skin pallor
- Clubbing (infrequent)

ETIOLOGY

- Cystic fibrosis
- Lung infections (pneumonia, lung abscess, TB, fungal infections, viral infections)
- Abnormal host defense (panhypogammaglobulinemia, Kartagener's syndrome, AIDS, chemotherapy)
- Localized airway obstruction (congenital structural defects, foreign bodies, neoplasms)
- Inflammation (inflammatory pneumonitis, granulomatous lung disease, allergic aspergillosis)

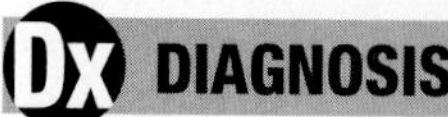

DIAGNOSIS

DIFFERENTIAL DIAGNOSIS

- TB
- Asthma
- Chronic bronchitis or chronic sinusitis
- Interstitial fibrosis
- Chronic lung abscess
- Foreign body aspiration
- Cystic fibrosis
- Lung carcinoma

LABORATORY TESTS

- Sputum for Gram stain, culture and sensitivity, and acid-fast bacteria
- Complete blood count with differential (leukocytosis with left shift, anemia)
- Serum protein electrophoresis to evaluate for hypogammaglobulinemia
- Antibody test for aspergillosis
- Sweat test in patients with suspected cystic fibrosis

IMAGING STUDIES

- Chest radiograph: hyperinflation, crowded lung markings, small cystic spaces at the base of the lungs.
- High-resolution CT scan of the chest (Fig. 1-187) has become the best tool to detect cystic lesions and exclude underlying obstruction from neoplasm. The CT study should be a noncontrast study with the use of 1- to 1.5-mm window every 1 cm with acquisition time of 1 sec. Typical findings on CT include dilation of airway lumen, lack of tapering of an airway toward periphery, ballooned cysts at the end of bronchus, and varicose constrictions along airways.
- Bronchoscopy may be helpful to evaluate hemoptysis, rule out obstructive lesions, and remove mucus plugs.

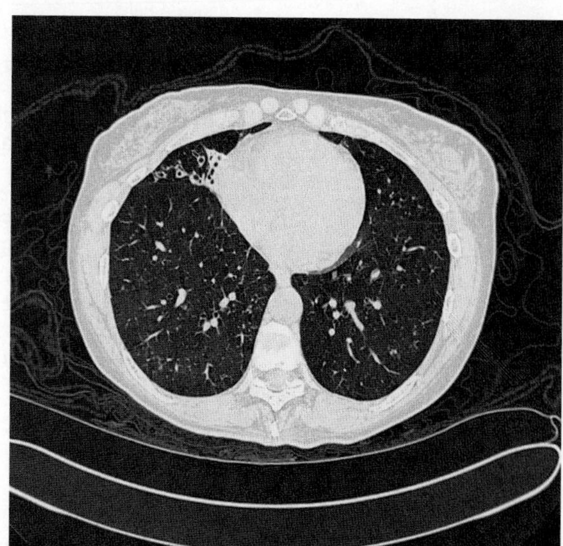

FIGURE 1-187 High-resolution computed tomographic image of nodular bronchiectasis due to nontuberculous mycobacterium infection. (From Goldman L, Schafer AI: *Goldman's Cecil medicine,* ed 24, Philadelphia, 2012, Saunders.)

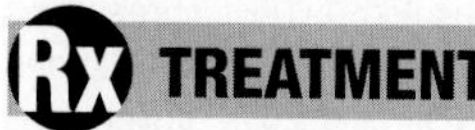

TREATMENT

NONPHARMACOLOGIC THERAPY

- Postural drainage (reclining prone on a bed with the head down on the side) and chest percussion with use of inflatable vests or mechanical vibrators applied to the chest may enhance removal of respiratory secretions.
- Adequate hydration.
- Supplemental oxygen for hypoxemia.

ACUTE GENERAL Rx

- Antibiotic therapy is based on the results of sputum, Gram stain, and culture and sensitivity; in patients with inadequate or inconclusive results, empiric therapy with amoxicillin/clavulanate 500 to 875 mg q12h, TMP-SMX q12h, doxycycline 100 mg bid, or cefuroxime 250 mg bid for 10 to 14 days is recommended.
- Bronchodilators are useful in patients with demonstrable airflow obstruction.

CHRONIC Rx

- Avoidance of tobacco
- Maintenance of proper nutrition and hydration
- Prompt identification and treatment of infections
- Pneumococcal vaccination and annual influenza vaccination

DISPOSITION

Prognosis is variable with severity of the disease and underlying etiology of bronchiectasis.

REFERRAL

Surgical referral for partial lung resection in patients with localized severe disease unresponsive to medical therapy or in patients with massive hemoptysis

SUGGESTED READINGS

Available at www.expertconsult.com

RELATED CONTENT

Bronchiectasis (Patient Information)

AUTHOR: **FRED F. FERRI, M.D.**

BASIC INFORMATION

DEFINITION

Brugada syndrome (BRS) is a genetically determined channelopathy characterized by typical electrocardiographic abnormalities. No other features are needed for diagnosis. BRS predisposes one to sudden cardiac death (SCD) secondary to polymorphic ventricular tachycardia (PVT)/ventricular fibrillation (VF) in the absence of structural heart disease.

SYNONYMS

BRS

ICD-9CM CODES
746.89 Other specified congenital anomalies of heart
ICD-10CM CODES
I49.9 Cardial arrhythmia, unspecified
I47.2 Ventricular tachycardia

EPIDEMIOLOGY & DEMOGRAPHICS

INCIDENCE: The incidence ranges from 1 to 5:10,000 people in Europe and 12:10,000 in Southeast Asia.
PREVALENCE: It comprises 4% of SCD and 20% of SCD in structurally normal hearts. Although found in every population, the prevalence is much higher in Asian and Southeast Asian countries; in fact in some Southeast Asian countries, such as Laos and Thailand, it may be the most common form of natural death in younger males.
PREDOMINANT SEX AND AGE: BS is more common in males (80% of patients). Mean age at presentation is 40 to 45.
GENETICS: The disease is autosomal dominant with variable expression.

- Twelve culprit genes have been identified so far.
- *SCN5A,* the gene that encodes for the alpha subunit of the cardiac sodium channel, accounts for about 20% to 25% of cases of BRS.
- Genetic abnormalities are only found in ⅓ of patients; thus the impact of genetic testing is limited. When available, it may be useful in identifying silent carriers.
- In all genotypes, the basic abnormality is either a decrease in the inward sodium or calcium current, or an increase in the outward potassium current.

RISK FACTORS

- First-degree relatives with the disease

PHYSICAL FINDINGS & CLINICAL PRESENTATION

- Physical exam is usually benign.
- Classic ECG finding is a pattern of right bundle branch block (RBBB) with persistent ST elevation of cove-like morphology and T-wave inversion in the anterior leads (V_1-V_3)
- Often an incidental finding diagnosed from a typical ECG pattern
- Palpitations
- Nocturnal agonal respirations
- Syncope
- Sudden cardiac arrest (SCA)/SCD secondary to rapid PVT that frequently degenerates into VF more often at night
- Three ECG patterns were described. Type 1 is the most common and characteristic (Fig. 1-190A).
- Type 1 ECG pattern can be transient and may be provoked (sodium channel blockers, vagal maneuvers, increased alpha-adrenergic tone, beta-blockers, tricyclic or tetracyclic antidepressants, fever, hypokalemia, hyperkalemia, hypercalcemia, and alcohol and cocaine toxicity). Types 2 and 3 can change to type 1 pattern with these triggers as well. Table E1-87 describes drugs used to unmask Brugada ECG pattern.

ETIOLOGY

- Autosomal dominant inheritance with varying penetration
- Mutations in SCN5A16 gene leading to a loss of function of the cardiac sodium (Na^+) channel by different mechanisms is the most common genotype found among BS patients. Table E1-88 describes the molecular basis of BS.

DIAGNOSIS

Diagnosis is made by ECG alone.

- ST segment elevation with type 1 morphology ≥2 mm in one or more right-sided leads (V_1-V_2), occurring either spontaneously or after provocative drug testing
- Type II or III ECG that converts into type 1 following sodium channel blocker (procainamide/flecainide/ajmaline) challenge (Fig. 1-190A)

DIFFERENTIAL DIAGNOSIS

A number of diseases can lead to a BRS-like abnormality on the surface ECG, including the following:

- Atypical RBBB
- Early repolarization
- Acute pericarditis
- Acute myocardial infarction or ischemia
- Pulmonary embolism
- Various central and autonomic system abnormalities
- Duchenne's muscular dystrophy
- Electrolyte abnormalities such as hyperkalemia and hypercalcemia
- Arrhythmogenic right ventricular cardiomyopathy
- Pectus excavatum

WORKUP

- Cardiology consult is strongly recommended if BRS is suspected.
- Clinical history with special emphasis on syncope, palpitations, nocturnal agonal respirations, and family history
- Echocardiography to rule out structural heart disease. While no structural heart disease is usually apparent, there are some recent reports indicating mild abnormalities in the right ventricle (RV) and left ventricle (LV).
- MRI, especially to rule out ARVC (arrhythmogenic right ventricular cardiomyopathy)
- Electrophysiology study. No consensus exists on the value of arrhythmia induction in predicting future clinical events in individual patients. However, findings such as HV (His ventricular) conduction interval >60 ms and VERP (ventricular effective refractory period) <200 ms during electrophysiology study can help in confirming a diagnosis.

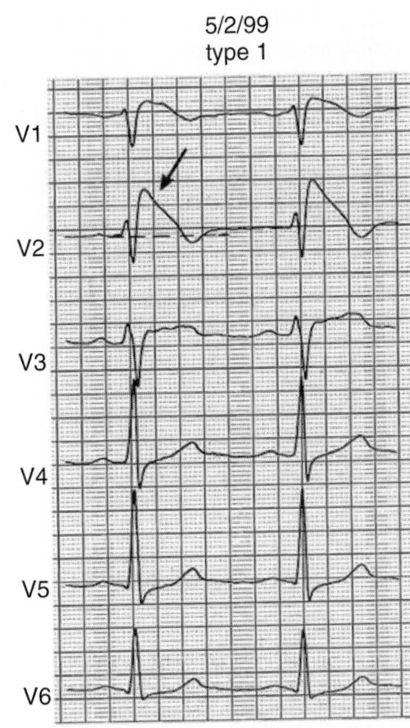

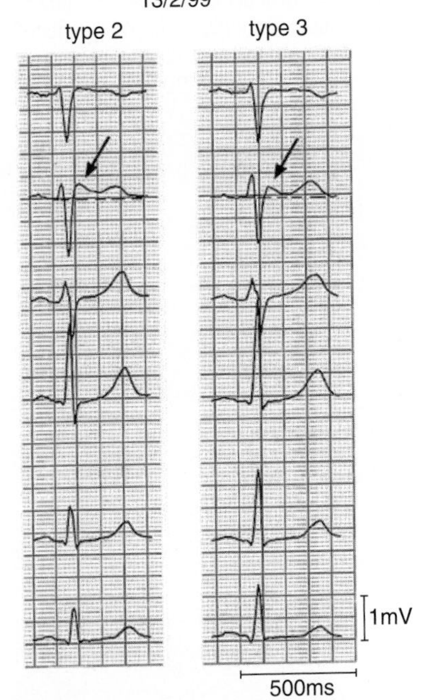

FIGURE 1-190A ECG changes in Brugada syndrome. ST elevation occurs in the anterior precordial leads, leads V1 and V2. Type 1 (coved) ECGs with 1 mV of ST elevation have the most prognostic significance. (From Strickberger SA et al: AHA/ACCF scientific statement on the evaluation of syncope, *J Am Coll Cardiol* 47:473-484, 2006.)

- Laboratory tests are unhelpful. Genetic testing may be helpful but not necessary for diagnostic purposes.
- First-degree relatives should obtain ECG and be evaluated for symptoms.

Risk stratification in the asymptomatic patient

- The following are considered indicators of high risk
  - Spontaneous type 1 ECG at baseline
  - Presence of fragmented QRS on ECG
  - RVERP (right ventricular effective refractory period) < 200 ms on EPS
  - Male sex
  - Spontaneous atrial fibrillation

Note that family history of sudden death is not considered a high risk feature in BRS.

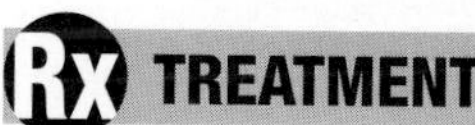

TREATMENT

NONPHARMACOLOGIC THERAPY

- The only effective strategy that prevents sudden cardiac death in BRS is implantable cardioverter-defibrillator (ICD). Currently there are no class I recommendations for primary prevention because clinical events are extremely rare, even in high-risk patients. Fig. E1-190B depicts the algorithm for clinical decision making regarding recommendation of an ICD.
- Definitive candidates for ICD (class I) are patients who survived SCD or have had sustained VT (secondary prevention).
- ICD can be useful (class IIa) for patients who have type 1 ECG pattern in the absence of class IC drug test associated with history of syncope.
- ICD may be considered (class IIb) if there is inducible VF on electrophysiologic (EP) study.
- Patients with spontaneous type 1 ECG without syncope or inducible VF on EP study or asymptomatic patients with drug-induced type 1 ECG pattern are considered a lower risk group for SCD, and ICD is not indicated in these patients.

ACUTE GENERAL Rx

- Isoproterenol (class IIa) is also used for electrical strom.
- Quinidine, which blocks both Ito and IKr currents in the RV epicardium, is used in patients with a history of multiple appropriate ICD shocks, as well as for electrical storms and treatment of supraventricular tachycardia (SVT) in these patients. It is also useful in cases where the patient refuses an ICD implant or when an ICD implant is contraindicated.
- Radiofrequency ablation: There are a few published case reports of radiofrequency ablation of premature ventricular contractions (PVCs) leading to reduced clinical events. These have been performed in patients already implanted with an ICD. In addition, epicardial substrate ablation in the right ventricular outflow tract (RVOT) has been shown to prevent VF inducibility.

REFERRAL

Consultation with cardiology is strongly recommended if BRS is suspected.

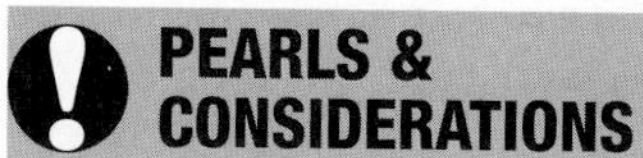

PEARLS & CONSIDERATIONS

COMMENTS

- The clinical manifestations, such as syncope and SCD, are rare in the pediatric group, but fever can acutely predispose to cardiac arrest. Mean age of presentation is 40 to 45 years.
- Cardiac events may occur during sleep, at rest, or after a large meal.
- BRS patients should be advised to avoid all drugs that may induce a type 1 ECG pattern and/or be known to trigger ventricular arrhythmias, and avoid unnecessary use of drugs (a drug that is not yet identified as potentially dangerous for these patients does not make its use safe). For up-to-date information on this matter, the following website has been developed: www.brugadadrugs.org.
- Fever may induce the appearance of a type 1 BRS ECG pattern and may trigger episodes of PVT/VF in BRS patients. In the case of fever, close ECG monitoring is appropriate in combination with lowering of the body temperature.
- The classic ECG changes in BRS can be transient with patients having normal ECGs in between highly abnormal ones.
- The appearance of syncope, seizures, or nocturnal agonal respiration must lead to prompt medical evaluation.
- Family screening of BS in first-degree relatives is strongly recommended.
- Although participation in sports is not strictly prohibited, competitive training can lead to development of strong vagal tone and subsequent higher risk of clinical events. Hence, participation in sports at a competitive or professional level is not advised.
- Once diagnosed initially by an ECG pattern, all patients must be followed up on a regular basis by an electrophysiologist.

PREVENTION

Identification of patients with BRS, risk stratification, and appropriate screening of family members is paramount to the prevention of SCD.

PATIENT/FAMILY EDUCATION

Immediate family members should be notified and be screened for BRS.

SUGGESTED READINGS

available at www.expertconsult.com

AUTHOR: **JOYDEEP GHOSH, M.D., F.A.C.C.**

BASIC INFORMATION

DEFINITION

Forcible clenching or grinding of the teeth during sleep or wakefulness, often leading to damage of the teeth.

ICD-9CM CODES
306.8 Bruxism
ICD-10CM CODES
F45.8 Other somatoform disorders

EPIDEMIOLOGY & DEMOGRAPHICS

- Occurs in 15% of children and 75% of adults
- Familial cases have occasionally been described.
- Bruxism often presents between age 10 and 20 yr but may persist throughout life.
- Nocturnal bruxism is noted most often during stages I and II NREM sleep and REM sleep.

PHYSICAL FINDINGS & CLINICAL PRESENTATION

Complaints of grinding of teeth from a sleep partner or members of the family are common. In many cases the masticatory system will adapt to the phenomenon, but in severe cases nearly every part of the masticatory system may be damaged. Excessive wearing of dentition is the most common physical finding. Tender or hypoatrophied masticatory muscles may also be observed.

ETIOLOGY

- Cause is controversial.
- Possible causes include occlusal discrepancies, anatomy of the bony structures of the orofacial region, part of the sleep arousal response, disturbances of the central dopaminergic system, smoking, alcohol, drugs, stress, and personality.

DIAGNOSIS

DIFFERENTIAL DIAGNOSIS

- Dental compression syndrome
- Temporomandibular joint disorders
- Chronic orofacial pain disorders
- Oral motor disorders
- Malocclusion

WORKUP

- History should have an emphasis on sleep habits, including excessive snoring, pain in the temporal mandibular region, interview with close family members, health habits, personality quirks.
- Physical examination of the teeth and masticatory muscles is mandatory.
- Sleep studies in selected cases may be helpful.

LABORATORY TESTS

None indicated unless a systemic disease is suspected (e.g., infection, autoimmune disorder)

IMAGING STUDIES

X-ray studies of teeth and temporomandibular joints

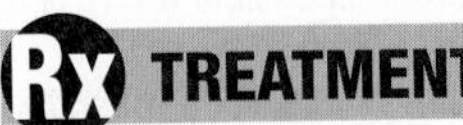

TREATMENT

NONPHARMACOLOGIC THERAPY

Biofeedback, psychological counseling, and elimination of harmful health habits have been used with limited success.

GENERAL Rx

- Oral splints (Fig. 1-191); nightguard to protect teeth may be useful
- Correction of malocclusion
- Pain management (e.g., gabapentin, ibuprofen)
- Medication to relieve anxiety and improve sleep (e.g., benzodiazepine or trazodone at bedtime)
- Local injections of botulinum toxin into masseter muscles to prevent dental and temporomandibular joint complications

DISPOSITION

Referral to dentist mandatory if damage to teeth evident

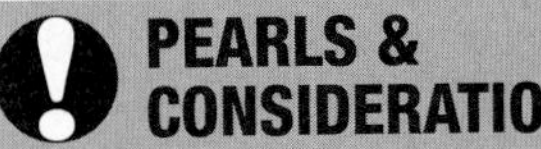

PEARLS & CONSIDERATIONS

- Like any poorly understood disease, treatment is often unsatisfactory and subject to quackery.
- Both diurnal and nocturnal bruxism may be associated with various movement and degenerative disorders (e.g., Huntington disease, oromandibular dystonia) and are quite common in children with cerebral palsy and mental retardation.

SUGGESTED READINGS

available at www.expertconsult.com

RELATED CONTENT

Bruxism (Tooth Grinding) (Patient Information)

AUTHOR: **FRED F. FERRI, M.D.**

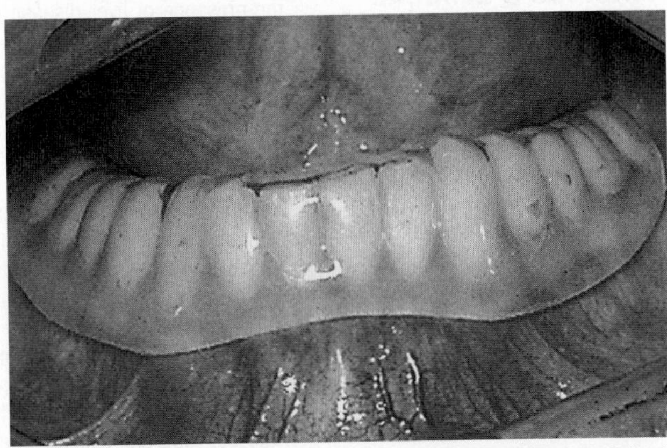

FIGURE 1-191 Occlusal splint. (From Hochberg MC et al [eds]: *Rheumatology,* ed 3, St Louis, 2003, Mosby.)

BASIC INFORMATION

DEFINITION

Budd-Chiari syndrome (BCS) is a rare disease defined by the obstruction of hepatic venous outflow anywhere from the small hepatic veins to the junction of the inferior vena cava (IVC) and the right atrium. Primary BCS is defined by endoluminal obstruction as seen in thromboses or webs. Secondary BCS occurs when the obstruction is caused by compression or invasion by a lesion originating outside the veins (tumor, abscess, cyst, etc.). It can also be a postoperative complication of orthotopic liver transplantation.

SYNONYMS

Hepatic vein thrombosis
Obliterative endophlebitis of the hepatic veins
IVC thrombosis (obliterative hepatocavopathy)

ICD-9CM CODES
453.0 Budd-Chiari syndrome
ICD-10CM CODES
I82.0 Budd-Chiari syndrome

EPIDEMIOLOGY & DEMOGRAPHICS

INCIDENCE: 1/2.5 million persons per yr
PREDOMINANT SEX: In Western countries, women are more commonly affected (approximately 2/3 of cases)
PREDOMINANT AGE: Presentation is usually in the third and fourth decades of life, with the median age being 35

PHYSICAL FINDINGS & CLINICAL PRESENTATION

Clinical presentation and characteristics vary with geography. In Africa and South Asia, intravascular webs are more often associated with IVC thrombosis with a stronger association with subsequent hepatocellular carcinoma. In the U.S., BCS is more commonly associated with primary myeloproliferative disorders and underlying hypercoagulable states. Underlying factors that contribute to BCS can be identified in ~85% of cases; multiple causative factors are identified in 50% of cases.

- Clinical manifestations can be caused by complete or partial occlusion of any or all of the three major hepatic veins, or inferior vena cava.
- Presentation is variable according to the degree, location, acuity of obstruction, and presence of collateral circulation:
  - Fulminant/acute (20%): severe right upper quadrant abdominal pain, fever, nausea, vomiting, jaundice, hepatomegaly, transudative ascites, marked elevation in serum aminotransferases (ALT >5 times the upper limit of normal), elevation of alkaline phosphatase to 300 to 400 IU/L, decrease in coagulation factors, variceal bleeding, encephalopathy within 8 wk of onset of jaundice; biospy, if performed, would reveal liver cell loss; early recognition and treatment are essential for survival; a slow decrease in ALT is associated with poor survival.
  - Subacute/chronic (60%): vague abdominal discomfort, gradual progression to caudate lobe hypertrophy with atrophy of the rest of the liver, portal hypertension with or without cirrhosis and its sequelae, transudative ascites, lower-extremity edema, esophageal varices, splenomegaly, coagulopathy, hepatorenal syndrome in up to half of patients, hepatopulmonary syndrome in up to 28% of patients, and rarely, encephalopathy
  - Asymptomatic (5% to 20%): usually discovered incidentally by abnormal liver function tests

ETIOLOGY

- Primary myeloproliferative diseases: 20% to 53%
  - Polycythemia vera, responsible for 10% to 40% of cases
  - Essential thrombocythemia and idiopathic myelofibrosis are less common causes
  - *JAK2* mutations are implicated in cases of idiopathic BCS (identified in 26% to 59% of cases)
  - Rare but recently reported: idiopathic hypereosinophilia syndrome
- Hypercoagulable states (inherited and acquired): often coexist with other causes, 30% to 65%
  - Factor V Leiden (25%)
  - Factor II gene mutation (5%)
  - Anticardiolipin antibodies (25%)
  - Hyperhomocysteinemia (22%)
  - Paroxysmal nocturnal hemoglobinuria (19%)
- Protein C, protein S, and antithrombin III deficiency are difficult to interpret because the presence of liver disease may confound results.
- Heterozygosity for G20210A prothrombin gene mutation or methylene-tetrahydrofolate reductase (MTHFR) mutation may be seen in BCS
- Pregnancy and oral contraceptive pills (cases reported after <2 wk of use)
- Malignancy (up to 10% of cases, causing external compression or invasions of vascular structures)
  - Most commonly due to hepatocellular carcinoma but also can be due to neoplasms of the kidney, adrenal gland, pancreas, stomach, and sarcomas of the right atrium, inferior vena cava, and hepatic veins
- Rare but reported: sickle cell anemia, infections with liver abscess, hydatid cyst (echinococcosis), schistosomiasis, sarcoidosis, Behçet's disease (<5%), membranous webs of IVC or hepatic veins (more common in Africa and South Asia, can be congenital or acquired secondary to underlying myeloproliferative disorder), abdominal trauma, liver torsion, ulcerative colitis, celiac disease, idiopathic (10% to 20%)

Dx DIAGNOSIS

DIFFERENTIAL DIAGNOSIS

- Hepatitis from ischemia, viral infection, toxin, alcohol
- Cholecystitis
- Hepatic venoocclusive disease (sinusoidal obstruction syndrome)
- Congestive hepatopathy, also known as *cardiac cirrhosis,* from tricuspid regurgitation, right atrial myxoma, constrictive pericarditis
- Cirrhosis from any etiology

LABORATORY TESTS

- Assessment of liver injury and function: serum aminotransferases, alkaline phosphatase, prothrombin time (PT), albumin, bilirubin
- Exclusion of another form of liver disease: viral hepatitis panel, autoantibodies (antinuclear antibody, anti–smooth muscle antibody, anti-mitochondrial antibody), serum iron, transferrin saturation, ferritin, ceruloplasmin, and α-1 antitrypsin
- Ascites protein content >3.0 g/dl and serum ascites albumin gradient ≥1.1 g/dl are suggestive of transudative ascites from BCS, cardiac or pericardial disease
- Evaluation for underlying myeloproliferative disorder and hypercoagulable state: CBC, bone marrow biopsy, tests for hypercoagulable states (Factor V Leiden, prothrombin gene G20210A mutation, protein C, protein S, and antithrombin deficiencies, antiphospholipid antibodies, hyperhomocystinemia, paroxysmal nocturnal hemoglobinuria, and MTHFR C677T mutation); protein C, protein S, and antithrombin deficiencies may be difficult to interpret in the setting of liver dysfunction, but levels <20% of normal are suggestive of a true deficiency; thrombophilia screening for the JAK2 V617F mutation may be useful if no other cause for myeloproliferative disorders/hypercoagulable states identified

IMAGING STUDIES

- Diagnosis of BCS is made by radiographic imaging.
- Ultrasound and color and pulsed Doppler are the first-line tests. Diagnostic sensitivity and specificity are 85% to 90%. Findings include large hepatic vein with an absent flow signal, or with reversed or turbulent flow; large intrahepatic collateral vessels;

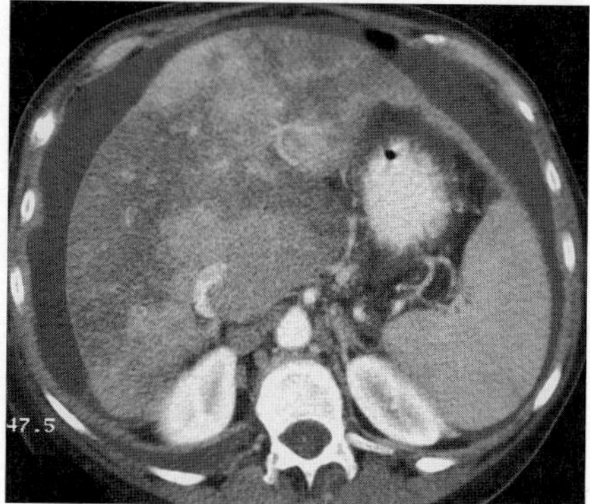

FIGURE 1-192 CT scan of Budd-Chiari syndrome. The appearances are not immediately diagnostic for the nonexpert, and infiltrative disease is sometimes suspected. (From Forbes A et al [eds]: *Atlas of clinical gastroenterology,* ed 3, 2005, Mosby.)

enlarged, stenotic, thickened, or tortuous hepatic veins; and caudate lobe hypertrophy (as the caudate lobe has an alternate blood supply through anastomoses).

- MRI with gadolinium contrast—better than contrast-enhanced CT (Fig. 1-192), with a sensitivity and specificity of approximately 90%—is the second-line test. Findings include obstructed hepatic veins or IVC; large, intrahepatic or subcapsular collaterals; and caudate lobe hypertrophy. Three-dimensional contrast-enhanced magnetic resonance angiography (MRA, see Fig. E1-193) rivals hepatic venography in sensitivity.
- Contrast-enhanced CT may reveal similar findings as Doppler ultrasound, as well as delayed or absent filling of the hepatic veins, parenchymal opacification of the liver, and narrowing of the inferior vena cava.
- CT image reconstruction of vasculature is becoming available.
- Venography: This is not essential for diagnosis; it should be performed when other noninvasive imaging tests are nondiagnostic in the setting of strong clinical suspicion for BCS, measurement of pressure gradients can help predict success of percutaneous or surgical shunt intervention and plan surgical intervention. Confirms the pathognomonic web pattern caused by collateral venous flow.
- Liver biopsy: This is not necessary to diagnose BCS but may be helpful in patients with cirrhosis in whom the diagnosis remains uncertain and critical for differentiating from hepatic venoocclusive disease. Findings include hepatic congestion, hepatocyte necrosis and fibrosis in centrilobular areas, and compensatory nodular regenerative hyperplasia with progression to fibrosis and cirrhosis. In advanced BCS, may also see infarction caused by concomitant thrombosis of the intrahepatic, extrahepatic, and portal veins. There are conflicting studies regarding the association of histologic findings and prognosis.

Rx TREATMENT

NONPHARMACOLOGIC THERAPY

- Goal of therapy is decompression of hepatic congestion.
- In general, therapeutic procedures should be introduced by order of increasing invasiveness based on response/failure to therapy rather than disease severity.
- Hypercoagulable states should be investigated in all patients.

ACUTE GENERAL Rx

- Anticoagulation, first with low-molecular-weight heparin (LMWH), followed by warfarin, even in the absence of an underlying hypercoagulable disorder
- In situ thrombolysis: can be successful when performed in recently thrombosed veins (clot less than 3 to 4 wk old) that are well defined on venography and do not involve the inferior vena cava; mature clots are nonresponsive to thrombolysis, and bleeding risk is high if portal hypertension has developed
- Balloon angioplasty: complicated by 50% restenosis rate; effective when membranous webs are the etiology
- Stenting: may improve long-term patency rates to 90%, but if placed above the intrahepatic IVC, may complicate future liver transplantation
- Transjugular intrahepatic portosystemic shunt (TIPS) has been increasingly used in recent years; usually performed in patients with no improvement on anticoagulation therapy or when a dilatable lesion cannot be found; TIPS has replaced surgical shunting as the most common invasive therapeutic procedure; recently polytetrafluoroethylene (ePTFE)-coated stents have improved TIPS-patency rates, especially in patients with underlying hypercoaguable defects.
- Surgical portal systemic shunts: feasibility depends on technical factors, long-term patency of the stent, the extent of liver damage before surgery, as well as on locating a center with well-trained surgeons
- Liver transplant may be indicated in patients with fulminant hepatic failure and in patients who fail to respond to TIPS; 10-year survival reported to range between 69% and 84%.
- Supportive measures

CHRONIC Rx

- Lifelong anticoagulation: Warfarin therapy with a target international normalized ratio (INR) of 2 to 3 lessens, but does not completely prevent, recurrence. This should be continued permanently unless the patient has an adverse event to anticoagulation.
- In patients with an underlying myeloproliferative disorder, treatment with hydroxyurea and aspirin, or anagrelide, may be given instead of traditional anticoagulation.
- Treat liver dysfunction and complications related to portal hypertension, such as ascites (diuretics and low-sodium diet).
- Invasive interventions should be reserved for symptomatic patients who do not improve with medical therapy.
- Manage shunt thrombosis, which is a common complication.
- Liver transplantation is another treatment option; up to 10% recurrence of BCS after transplant has been recognized
- Monitor for development of hepatocellular carcinoma and transformation of myeloproliferative disease in patients with longstanding, well-controlled BCS.

DISPOSITION

Prognosis is variable and depends on multiple factors, including time to recognition and treatment, etiology, acuity, the type of intervention, and the condition of the patient at the time of treatment. Overall mortality rates are decreasing with the use of anticoagulation and early diagnosis of asymptomatic cases. Survival rates have been reported as 77%, 65%, and 57% at 1, 5, and 10 yr from diagnosis. A prognostic index called the *Rotterdam BCS Index* has been described: 1.27 × Encephalopathy + 1.04 × Ascites + 0.72 × PT + 0.004 × Bilirubin. Encephalopathy and ascites are scored as 1 for present or 0 as absent, and PT is scored as greater (1) or less than (0) an INR of 2.3. An index of >1.1 correlates to low risk (5-yr survival rate, 89%), 1.1 to 1.5 with intermediate risk (5-yr survival rate, 74%), and <1.5 with high risk (5-yr survival rate, 42%).

REFERRAL

Fulminant presentations should immediately be referred to a center capable of liver transplantation. All cases benefit from referral to a hepatologist, a hematologist, an interventional radiologist, and a surgeon specializing in hepatobiliary disease.

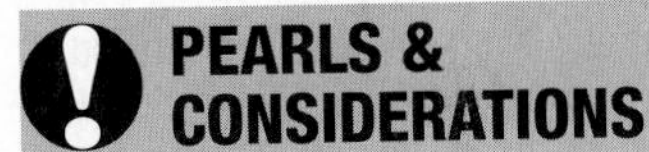

PEARLS & CONSIDERATIONS

COMMENTS

- Look for one or more underlying causes, especially hypercoagulable or hematologic disorders, and malignancies or space-occupying lesions that may compress or invade the hepatic outflow tract.
- Myeloproliferative disorders are most common.
- Diagnosis relies on imaging, beginning with Doppler ultrasound.
- Treatment with anticoagulation comes first, followed by invasive interventions as needed. Prophylaxis of portal hypertension can reduce the risk of major bleeding associated with anticoagulation therapy.
- Referral for liver transplantation may be necessary.
- Prognosis depends on presence of ascites, encephalopathy, PT, and serum bilirubin levels.

PREVENTION

In the setting of known risk factors, such as a hypercoagulable state or myeloproliferative disorder, any additional risks, such as smoking or oral contraceptive therapy, should be avoided.

SUGGESTED READINGS

available at www.expertconsult.com

RELATED CONTENT

Hypercoagulable States (Related Key Topic)
Budd-Chiari Syndrome (Patient Information)

AUTHORS: **MICHAEL PRODROMOU, M.D.** and **JEANETTE G. SMITH, M.D.**

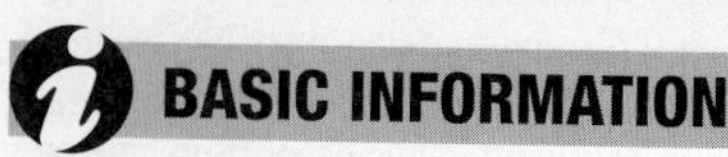

BASIC INFORMATION

DEFINITION

Bulimia nervosa is a prolonged illness characterized by a specific psychopathology. According to the *Diagnostic and Statistical Manual of Mental Disorders,* 5th edition. Bulimia nervosa can be diagnosed by: (A) recurrent episodes of binge eating. An episode of binge eating is characterized by both of the following:

1. Eating, in a discrete period of time, an amount of food that is definitely larger than what most individuals would eat in a similar period of time under similar circumstances.
2. A sense of lack of control over gating during the episode.

(B) Recurrent inappropriate compensators/behaviors in order to prevent weight gain, such as self-induced vomiting; misuse of laxatives, diuretics, or other medications; fasting, or excessive exercise. (C) The binge eating and inappropriate compensatory behaviors both occur, on average, at least once a week for 3 mo. (D) Self-evaluation is unduly influenced by body shape and weight. (E) The disturbance does not occur exclusively during episodes of anorexia nervosa.

ICD-9CM CODES
783.6 Bulimia
ICD-10CM CODES
F50.2 Polyphagia, bulimia nervosa

EPIDEMIOLOGY & DEMOGRAPHICS

INCIDENCE/PREVALENCE: Affects 1% to 3% of female adolescents and young adults
PREDOMINANT SEX: Female/male ratio of 10:1
PREDOMINANT AGE: Adolescence to young adulthood; mean age of onset: 17 yr

PHYSICAL FINDINGS & CLINICAL PRESENTATION

- Parotid and salivary gland swelling
- Scars on the back of the hand and knuckles (Russell sign) from rubbing against the upper incisors when inducing vomiting
- Eroded enamel, particularly on the lingual surface of the upper teeth; pyorrhea and other gum disorders possible
- Petechial hemorrhages of the cornea, soft palate, or face possibly noted after vomiting
- Loss of gag reflex, well-developed abdominal musculature
- Often no emaciation; normal physical examination possible

ETIOLOGY

- Etiology is unknown but likely multifactorial (sociocultural, psychological, familial factors).
- Bulimia is much more common in Western societies, where there is a strong cultural pressure to be slender.
- According to the American Psychiatric Association, patients with eating disorders display a broad range of symptoms that occur along a continuum between those of anorexia nervosa and bulimia.

Dx DIAGNOSIS

DIFFERENTIAL DIAGNOSIS

- Schizophrenia
- Gastrointestinal disorders
- Neurologic disorders (seizures, Kleine-Levin syndrome, Klüver-Bucy syndrome)
- Brain neoplasms
- Psychogenic vomiting

WORKUP

- The following questions are useful to screen patients for bulimia:
  1. "Are you satisfied with your eating habits?"
  2. "Do you ever eat in secret?"
- Answering "no" to the first question and/or "yes" to the second question has 100% sensitivity and 90% specificity for bulimia. The SCOFF questionnaire can also be used as a screening tool for eating disorders (see "Anorexia Nervosa").
- According to DSM-5, the level of severity is based on the frequency of inappropriate compensatory behaviors and may be increased to reflect other symptoms and degree of functional disability, as noted below:
  Mild: An average of 1-3 episodes of inappropriate compensatory behaviors per week.
  Moderate: An average of 4-7 episodes of inappropriate compensatory behaviors per week
  Severe: An average of 8-13 episodes of inappropriate compensatory behaviors per week
  Extreme: An average of ≥14 inappropriate compensatory behaviors per week
- Table 1-89 describes eating and weight control habits commonly found in children and adolescents with an eating disorder.

LABORATORY TESTS

- Electrolyte abnormalities from vomiting (hypokalemia and metabolic alkalosis) or diarrhea from laxative abuse (hypokalemia and hyperchloremic metabolic acidosis)
- Hyponatremia, hypocalcemia, hypomagnesemia (caused by laxative abuse)
- Elevated cortisol, decreased luteinizing hormone, decreased follicle-stimulating hormone

Rx TREATMENT

NONPHARMACOLOGIC THERAPY

- Cognitive behavioral therapy, particularly interpersonal therapy to control abnormal behaviors
- Use of food diaries, nutritional counseling, and planning meals at least 1 day in advance are useful measures to counter abnormal eating behaviors
- Correction of electrolyte abnormalities

ACUTE GENERAL Rx

- Selective serotonin reuptake inhibitors are generally considered to be the safest medication option in these patients. They are useful in severely depressed patients and in those who do not benefit from cognitive behavioral therapy.
- Prompt recognition and treatment of complications:
  1. Ipecac cardiotoxicity from laxative abuse
  2. Electrolyte abnormalities (see "Laboratory Tests")
  3. Esophagitis and Mallory-Weiss tears; esophageal rupture from repeated vomiting
  4. Aspiration pneumonia and pneumomediastinum
  5. Menstrual irregularities (including amenorrhea)
  6. Gastrointestinal abnormalities: acute gastric dilation, pancreatitis, abdominal pain, constipation

CHRONIC Rx

- Psychotherapy continued for years and focused specifically on self-image and family and peer interactions is an integral part of successful recovery.
- Family therapy is also recommended, especially in younger patients.

DISPOSITION

Course is variable and marked by frequent recurrence of exacerbations.

REFERRAL

- In addition to the primary care physician, the multidisciplinary team should include a dietician, a psychiatrist, and a family therapist.
- Hospitalization should be considered for patients with severe electrolyte abnormalities or those with suicidal thoughts.

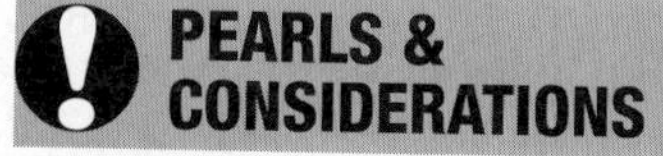

PEARLS & CONSIDERATIONS

COMMENTS

- Bulimia has a close association with depression, bipolar disorder, obsessive-compulsive disorder, alcoholism, and substance abuse.
- Bulimia should be considered in all patients (especially adolescents) with unexplained hypokalemia and metabolic alkalosis.

SUGGESTED READINGS

available at www.expertconsult.com

RELATED CONTENT

Bulimia (Patient Information)

AUTHOR: **FRED F. FERRI, M.D.**

TABLE 1-89 Eating and Weight Control Habits Commonly Found in Children and Adolescents with an Eating Disorder

	PROMINENT FEATURES		CLINICAL COMMENTS REGARDING EATING DISORDER HABITS	
Habit	**Anorexia Nervosa**	**Bulimia Nervosa**	**Anorexia Nervosa**	**Bulimia Nervosa**
Overall intake	Inadequate energy (calories), although volume of food and beverages may be high due to very low caloric density of intake due to "diet" and nonfat choices	Variable, but calories normal to high; intake in binges often "forbidden" food or drink that differs from intake at meals	Consistent inadequate caloric intake leading to wasting of the body	Inconsistent balance of intake, exercise and vomiting, but severe caloric restriction is short-lived
Food	Counts and limits calories, especially from fat; emphasis on "healthy food choices" with reduced caloric density Monotonous, limited "good" food choices, often leading to vegetarian or vegan diet Strong feelings of guilt after eating more than planned leads to exercise and renewed dieting	Aware of calories and fat, but less regimented in avoidance than AN Frequent dieting interspersed with overeating, often triggered by depression, isolation, or anger	Obsessive-compulsive attention to nutritional data on food labels and may have "logical" reasons for food choices in highly regimented pattern, such as sports participation or family history of lipid disorder	Choices less structured, with more frequent diets
Beverages	Water or other low- or no-calorie drinks; nonfat milk	Variable, diet soda common; may drink alcohol to excess	Fluids often restricted to avoid weight gain	Fluids ingested to aid vomiting or replace losses
Meals	Consistent schedule and structure to meal plan Reduced or eliminated caloric content, often starting with breakfast, then lunch, then dinner Volume can increase with fresh fruits, vegetables, and salads as primary food sources	Meals less regimented and planned than in AN; more likely impulsive and unregulated, often eliminated following a binge-purge episode	Rigid adherence to "rules" governing eating leads to sense of control, confidence, and mastery	Elimination of a meal following a binge-purge only reinforces the drive for binge later in the day
Snacks	Reduced or eliminated from meal plan	Often avoided in meal plans, but then impulsively eaten	Snack foods removed early because "unhealthy"	Snack "comfort foods" can trigger a binge
Dieting	Initial habit that becomes progressively restrictive, although often appearing superficially "healthy" Beliefs and "rules" about the patient's idiosyncratic nutritional requirements and response to foods are strongly held	Initial dieting gives way to chaotic eating, often interpreted by the patient as evidence of being "weak" or "lazy"	Distinguishing between healthy meal planning with reduced calories and dieting in ED may be difficult	Dieting tends to be impulsive and short-lived, with "diets" often resulting in unintended weight gain
Binge eating	None in restrictive subtype, but an essential feature in binge-purge subtype	Essential feature, often secretive Shame and guilt prominent afterward	Often "subjective" (more than planned but not large)	Relieves emotional distress, may be planned
Exercise	Characteristically obsessive-compulsive, ritualistic, and progressive May excel in dance, long-distance running	Less predictable May be athletic, or may avoid exercise entirely	May be difficult to distinguish active thin vs. ED	Males often use exercise as means of "purging"
Vomiting	Characteristic of binge-purge subtype May chew then spit out, rather than swallow, food as a variant	Most common habit intended to reduce effects of overeating Can occur after meal as well as a binge	Physiologic and emotional instability prominent	Strongly "addictive" and self-punishing, but does not eliminate calories ingested—many still absorbed
Laxatives	If used, generally to relieve constipation in restrictive subtype, but as a cathartic in binge-purge subtype	Second most common habit used to reduce or avoid weight gain, often used in increasing doses for cathartic effect	Physiologic and emotional instability prominent	Strongly "addictive," self-punishing, but ineffective means to reduce weight (calories are absorbed in the small intestine, but laxatives work in the colon)
Diet pills	Very rare, if used; more common in binge-purge subtype	Used to either reduce appetite or increase metabolism	Use of diet pills implies inability to control eating	Control over eating may be sought by any means

AN, Anorexia nervosa; *BN,* bulimia nervosa; *ED,* eating disorder.
From Kliegman RM et al: *Nelson textbook of pediatrics,* ed 19, Philadelphia, 2011, Saunders.

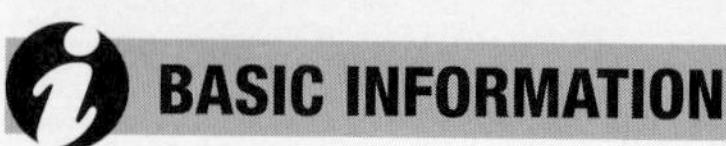

BASIC INFORMATION

DEFINITION

Bullous pemphigoid is an autoimmune, subepidermal blistering disease commonly seen in the elderly. A related entity is cicatricial pemphigoid, which predominantly affects the mucous membranes.

SYNONYMS

Pemphigoid

ICD-9CM CODES
694.5 Pemphigoid
ICD-10CM CODES
L12.0 Bullous pemphigoid

EPIDEMIOLOGY & DEMOGRAPHICS

- Occurs most commonly in people older than 60 yr, with peak incidence in those aged ≥80 yr
- Incidence is approximately 10 cases per 1 million persons
- No gender or racial predilection
- Most common of the autoimmune bullous dermatoses

PHYSICAL FINDINGS & CLINICAL PRESENTATION

HISTORY:

- Skin lesions typically start as eczematous or urticarial plaques on the extremities and are often very pruritic
- Taut blisters can form within 1 wk to several months

PHYSICAL FINDINGS:

- Anatomic distribution
    1. Flexor surfaces of the arms and legs, groin, axilla, chest, and abdomen; generally spares the head and neck
    2. Rare involvement of mucous membranes
- Lesion configuration
    1. May be localized to the extremities or generalized
    2. Lesions irregularly grouped but may sometimes be serpiginous (Fig. 1-194)
- Lesion morphology
    1. Taut blisters (bullae) measuring 5 mm to 2 cm in diameter filled with clear or bloody fluid on either normal or erythematous skin are characteristic
    2. Heal without scarring but may leave postinflammatory hyperpigmentation

ETIOLOGY

- Autoimmune disease with immunoglobulin (Ig) G and/or C3 complement targeting hemidesmosomal antigens located in the epidermal basement membrane zone
- Drug-induced pemphigoid, although rare, can occur in patients taking penicillamine, furosemide, captopril, penicillin, or sulfasalazine

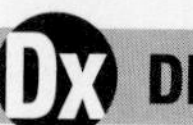

DIAGNOSIS

Skin biopsy aids in the diagnosis, and specimens should be sent for routine histochemical staining and direct immunofluorescence.

DIFFERENTIAL DIAGNOSIS

- Cicatricial pemphigoid
- Epidermolysis bullosa acquisita
- Pemphigus
- Linear IgA disease

LABORATORY TESTS

- Histology of lesional skin shows a subepidermal blister with a superficial inflammatory infiltrate, often with numerous eosinophils
- Indirect immunofluorescence detects anti–basement membrane antibodies in 70% of patients with bullous pemphigoid.
- Direct immunofluorescence of perilesional skin shows C3 and IgG linearly arranged along the epidermal basement membrane.
- Approximately half of patients will have a peripheral blood eosinophilia.

Rx TREATMENT

Bullous pemphigoid may be a self-limited disease, but its course may last from months to years. Treatment is based on the degree of disease involvement and the rate of disease progression.

NONPHARMACOLOGIC THERAPY

- Mild soaps with emollients to wet skin after bathing
- Topical antipruritic creams

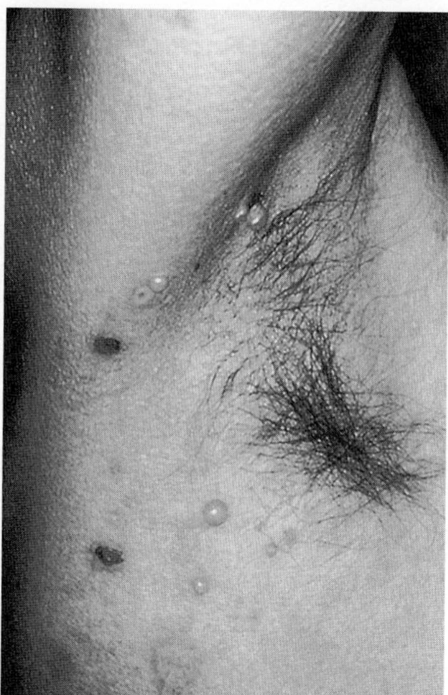

FIGURE 1-194 Bullous pemphigoid. Note intact bullae with erosions in a flexural distribution. (From Goldstein BG, Goldstein AO: *Practical dermatology,* ed 2, St Louis, 1997, Mosby.)

ACUTE GENERAL RX

Localized disease:

- Potent topical steroids (e.g., clobetasol) until blistering ceases with gradual tapering over several weeks
- Oral antihistamines to control pruritus

Generalized disease:

- Mainstay of therapy is prednisone, usually beginning with a minimal dose of 1 mg/kg/day
- Steroid-sparing agents, such as azathioprine or mycophenolate mofetil, may be started with prednisone or shortly after prednisone therapy is initiated and may be continued once prednisone is discontinued
- Tetracyclines
- Low-dose methotrexate has recently been suggested to be an optimal therapy in the elderly
- Rituximab, a monoclonal antibody to CD20, has been used for treatment-refractory bullous pemphigoid

CHRONIC Rx

- Prednisone combined with steroid-sparing agents with the goal of limiting oral corticosteroid intake
- Other immunosuppressive agents, such as cyclophosphamide or cyclosporine, are occasionally used

DISPOSITION

Mortality rates are estimated at between 10% and 40% after 1 yr. Patients with widespread disease requiring immunosuppressive therapy and with other comorbidities are at highest risk for complications from the disease. Approximately 50% of treated patients experience remission within 2 to 6 yr.

REFERRAL

Dermatology

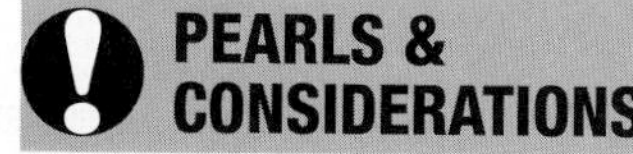

PEARLS & CONSIDERATIONS

COMMENTS

- Bullous pemphigoid is mainly a disease of elderly persons and should be suspected in older persons with chronic pruritic eruptions and in those patients who have new-onset taut vesicles and bullae
- Not believed to represent a paraneoplastic process.

RELATED CONTENT

Bullous Pemphigoid (Patient Information)

AUTHORS: **JESSICA CORWIN, M.D., M.P.H.**, and **KACHIU LEE, B.A.**

BASIC INFORMATION

DEFINITION

- Cutaneous burns can be classified by type of injury (e.g., thermal vs. chemical), burn depth (e.g., 1st, 2nd, 3rd degree), extent of burn (total burn surface area [TBSA]), and burn severity (e.g., minor vs. major). Types of burn injury include thermal (flames, scalds, hot contactants), chemical, electrical, and radiation burns. This chapter will focus on thermal and electrical burns.
- Burns can affect skin and respiratory, ocular, oral, and genital mucosa.

SYNONYMS

Thermal injury
Chemical injury
Electrical injury
Radiation injury

ICD-9CM CODES
942-949 (by region, % burn)
ICD-10CM CODES
T29.0 Burns of multiple regions, unspecified degree
T30.0 Burn of unspecified body region, unspecified degree
T30.1 Burn of first degree, body region unspecified
T30.2 Burn of second degree, body region unspecified
T30.3 Burn of third degree, body region unspecified
T31.0 Burns involving less than 10% of body surface
T31.1 Burns involving 10-19% of body surface
T31.2 Burns involving 20-29% of body surface
T31.3 Burns involving 30-39% of body surface
T31.4 Burns involving 40-49% of body surface
T31.5 Burns involving 50-59% of body surface

EPIDEMIOLOGY & DEMOGRAPHICS

PREVALENCE (IN U.S.):
- More than 1.2 million individuals experience burns in the U.S., and burn injuries account for approximately 500,000 emergency department visits, with 9% (45,000) requiring hospitalization, with 0.8% (4,000) resulting in death annually.
- Of thermal injury, scald burn from liquid is most common—followed by flame, flash burn, then contact burn.

PREDOMINANT AGE & SEX:
- Children ages 2-4 years have the greatest frequency of burns (most commonly scald burns), with male adolescent and young adults ages 17-25 with second greatest frequency (most commonly from flammable liquids).

PHYSICAL FINDINGS & CLINICAL PRESENTATION

- It is important to note that burns occur unevenly—often with various depths (Table 1-90).
- 1st-degree (superficial) burns—penetrate epidermis only (minimal barrier loss)
  - Very painful, intact, erythematous skin with minimal to no edema and no blistering.
- 2nd-degree (partial-thickness) burns—epidermis and part of dermis is affected.
  - Moist, very painful skin with edema and blistering/blebs
  - Superficial partial-thickness burns—cherry red with two-point discrimination intact, incredibly painful.
  - Deep partial-thickness burns—mottled white and cherry red; only the sensation of pressure is intact in these areas
- 3rd-degree (full-thickness) burns—entire epidermis and dermis are affected, with destruction of hair follicles and sweat glands.
  - The skin is dry, charred, pale, painless, and leathery. Charred vessels may be visible beneath, little or no pain, and hair pulls out easily.

DIAGNOSIS

CLASSIFICATION

- Burns are classified by (1) depth of injury, (2) extent of injury, and (3) severity, according to the American Burn Association.
- Depth of injury (see Table 1-90)
  - Indicates how the wound will heal and whether grafting will be needed
- Extent of TBSA
  - The TBSA is best classified by using age-specific burn charts and the "rule of nines"(Fig. 1-195).
  - For scattered burns, utilizing patient's palm including fingers to equate 1% body surface area can be helpful.
  - TBSA indicates how aggressively the patient will need to be resuscitated
- Severity—determined by burn depth, TBSA, age, location, type of injury, and presence/absence of coexisiting conditions. Severity classification helps triage patients to outpatient, inpatient, or burn unit care (see Table 1-91).
  - Minor burns—outpatient management.
  - Moderate burns—admission to hospital with experience managing burns or burn center referral.
  - Major burns—referral to burn center

LABORATORY STUDIES (MODERATE OR MAJOR BURNS)

- CBC, electrolytes, BUN, creatinine, glucose, liver function tests, venous blood gas, blood coagulation, and type and screen in anticipation of blood transfusion
- *If smoke inhalation expected:* serial ABG carboxyhemoglobin, and continuous ECG
- *If electrical burn or if concern for rhabdomyolysis:* urinalysis, urine myoglobin, and CPK levels
- *If severe lactic acidosis:* consider checking cyanide level.

IMAGING STUDIES

- If smoke inhalation suspected: chest radiograph and bronchoscopy
- If high-voltage electrical burn: cardiac monitoring 1st 24 hours

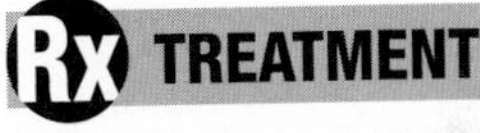

TREATMENT

DIFFERENTIAL DIAGNOSIS

Cultural practices leading to burnlike lesions in distinctive patterns (e.g., cupping, coining, moxibustion), cellulitis, Stevens-Johnson syndrome/toxic epidermolytic necrolysis

ACUTE GENERAL Rx

MINOR BURNS (1ST DEGREE BURNS AND 2ND/3RD DEGREE BURNS OF LIMITED TBSA)
- Outpatient management—"6 Cs"

TABLE 1-90 Categorization of Burn by Depth

Burn Type	Histologic Depth	Clinical Presentation	Treatment	Healing Time/Prognosis
1st degree	Epidermis	Erythematous but intact skin, no blisters, pain may range in severity	Topical salves, cold compresses, NSAIDs for pain control	2-5 days with no scarring
Superficial 2nd degree (partial thickness)	Papillary dermis	Erythematous with superficial blisters, intense pain	Topical antimicrobials with gauze dressing or biosynthetic dressing (if widespread), pain control	5-21 days with no grafting
Deep 2nd degree (partial thickness)	Reticular dermis	Erythematous with superficial/deep blisters, range of pain depending on nerve involvement	Same	21-35 days with no infection; if infected, converts to full-thickness burn
3rd degree (full thickness)	Through dermis to subcutaneous tissue. Can involve fascia, muscle and bone.	White or black, possible eschar, may or may not be painful depending on nerve damage	Usually requires grafting, may require resuscitation depending on TBSA affected, pain control	Large areas require grafting, but small areas may heal from the edges after weeks

From Kliegman RM et al: *Nelson textbook of pediatrics,* ed 19, Phildelphia, 2011, Saunders; and Kessides MC, Skelsey MK: Management of acute partial-thickness burns, *Cutis* 86:249-257, 2010.

- Clothing: Remove hot or burned clothing
- Cooling: Cool (approximately 54° F) for 10-30 minutes (under faucet or compress) to reduce edema/pain by conducting heat away from skin. Not recommended with extensive burns due to theoretical risk of hypothermia and shock. No ice packs.
- Cleaning: Wash gently with mild alcohol-free soap, then normal saline daily. Remove all old ointment and any loose skin. Blot dry. No evidence supports vigorous cleansing with antiseptic solutions. Embedded materials should be removed by copious irrigation using a large-gauge syringe.
- Chemoprophylaxis: Tetanus immunization (all deep 2nd and 3rd degree burns). Routine skin cultures are NOT recommended except when wound infection suspected, and prophylactic systemic antibiotics are NOT recommended. All 2nd and 3rd degree burns are treated with topical antimicrobial agent. This may include silver sulfadiazine, bacitracin, bismuth-impregnated Vaseline gauze, or silver-impregnated synthetic dressings.
- Covering: All 2nd and 3rd degree burns should be covered with sterile dressing. If financial resources are limited, instead of gauze can purchase cotton gloves, T-shirts, or similar at discount stores, wash, and reuse.
- Comfort: Analgesics around the clock are recommended. Tylenol and NSAIDs—alone or in combination with opioids. Additional "rescue" analgesics before dressing changes and physical activity recommended.

Moderate and Major Burns (2nd/3rd degree burns of extensive TBSA)

- Patients with moderate/major burns should be admitted to the hospital or referred to a burn center. Indications for hospitalization for burns are described in Table 1-91.
- Resuscitation (in addition to above)
  - Assessment of ABCs: Establish airway and assess breathing (inspect for inhalation injury and intubate for suspected airway edema, often seen 12-24 hr later; O_2; establish circulation (place two large-bore peripheral IV lines, ECG).
  - IV fluid resuscitation—Parkland formula (Ringer's lactate at 2-4 ml/kg per % TBSA per 24 hr with half the calculated fluid given in the first 8 hr is an effective modality in severe burns).
  - Baseline neurologic and vascular assessment
  - Foley catheter and NG tube (20% of patients develop an ileus)—urine output 30 ml/hr
  - Optimize nutritional support: Mayes equations to calculate energy requirements after burn (Box 1-11)
- Frequent reassessment in the first 24-72 hours, as wound depth can change significantly
- The four phases of burn care, with physiologic changes and objectives are described in Table E1-92. Box 1-12 describes the modified Brooke resuscitation formula.

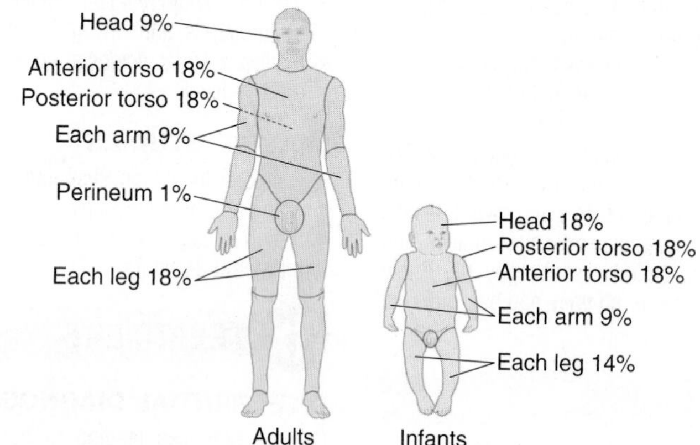

FIGURE 1-195 The "rule of nines" for estimating second-degree and third-degree burns. Because infants have significantly larger heads and smaller legs than do adults, different rules must be used in evaluating these patients. A simple, practical rule is that the palm of the patient's hand, with fingers, equals 1% of the total body area. (From Ferri F: *Practical guide to the care of the medical patient,* ed 9, St Louis, 2014, Elsevier.)

BURN WOUND CARE BY BURN DEPTH Rx

General

- Vigilant wound care with dressings to prevent evaporation and minimize threat of wound colonization and infection of nonintact skin.
- Daily activity necessary to maintain function of burned extremity, decrease pain and swelling, and promote healing

1st-degree burns (skin intact):

- *Dressing:* None required (except to protect from injury); topical antibacterial agents not recommended
- *Other:* Emollients, cool compresses (avoid ice), if pruritic, trial of antihistamines
- *Prognosis:* Heals within 1 week without scarring. May heal with pigmentary changes (limit by sunscreen and sun avoidance of area for 1 year).

2nd degree (superficial partial-thickness) burns without adherent exudate or eschar:

- *Blisters:* Sharp debridement of ruptured blisters; leave intact blisters. Quicker healing and reduced infections when intact blisters are not disturbed. Consider unroofing blisters that show no sign of resorption over several weeks, or contain cloudy fluid.

TABLE 1-91 Classification of Burns by Severity and Indications for Hospitalization or Burn Center Referral

Criteria	Minor Burn	Moderate Burn	Major Burn
Total body surface area (%)	• All 1st degree burns <10% adults <5% children or elderly • <2% for 3rd degree	• 2nd degree burns 10%-20% adults 5%-10% in children or elderly • 2%-5% 3rd degree	• All 1st degree burns >20% adults >10% children and elderly • >5% 3rd degree
Type of burn injury		• Low-voltage burn • Suspected inhalation injury	• High-voltage burn • Chemical burn • Known
Location		Circumferential burn	• Clinically significant burn to face, eyes, ears, genitalia, over joints
Coexisting conditions		• Concomitant medical problem predisposing to infection (e.g., diabetes, sickle cell anemia)	• Significant associated injuries (e.g., fracture, other major trauma)
	Outpatient management	Inpatient management—consider referral to burn center*	Referral to burn center

*Per the American Burn Association (ABA), any partial-thickness burn >10% total body surface area, or any factors listed in moderate or major burn category warrant referral to burn center. Additional factors per the ABA include burned children in a hospital without qualified personnel or equipment for the care of children and burn injury in a patient who will require special social, emotional, or rehabilitative intervention (including suspected child abuse).

Modified from Singer AJ, Dagum AB: Current management of acute cutaneous wounds, *N Engl J Med 359* (10):1037-1046, 2008; www.ameriburn.org.

BOX 1-11 Mayes Equations to Calculate Energy Requirement After a Burn

Mayes equation for a 5- to 10-year-old burn patient with injury <50% TBSA:

$$818 + 37.4\,(\text{weight in kilograms}) + 9.3 \times \%\ \text{TBSA burn}$$

Mayes equation for a 5.5-year-old patient with a 45% TBSA scald burn weighing 20 kg:

$$818 + 37.4\ (20\ \text{kg}) + 9.3 \times 45\,\%\ \text{TBSA scald}$$

$$818 + 748 + 481.5 = 2047.5\ \text{calories/day}$$

From Fuhrman BP et al: *Pediatric critical care,* ed 4, Philadelphia, 2011, Saunders.

BOX 1-12 Modified Brooke Resuscitation Formula

0-24 Hours

Adults and Children >10 kg

Lactated Ringer's: 2-4 mL/kg/% burn/24 hr (first half in first 8 hr)

Colloid: none*

Children <10 kg

Lactated Ringer's: 2-3 mL/kg/% burn/24 hr (first half in first 8 hr)

Lactated Ringer's with 5% dextrose: 4 mL/kg/hr

Colloid: none

24-48 Hours

All Patients

Crystalloid: to maintain urine output. If silver nitrate is used, sodium leaching will mandate continued isotonic crystalloid. If other topical is used, free water requirement is significant. Serum sodium should be monitored closely. Nutritional support should begin, ideally by the enteral route.

Colloid: (5% albumin in lactated Ringer's):

0%-30% burn: none

30%-50% burn: 0.3 mL/kg/% burn/24 hr

50%-70% burn: 0.4 mL/kg/% burn/24 hr

>70% burn: 0.5 mL/kg/% burn/24 hr. *Note:* The Modified Brooke formula is a common consensus formula that is only useful in individual patients if adjusted to physiologic endpoints. Like all resuscitative formulas, it is a helpful starting point, but optimum-quality resuscitation requires the bedside presence of a physician capable of regularly evaluating resuscitation endpoints.

*Increasingly, early colloid infusion (generally 5% albumin) is being used in patients with very large burns, particularly if they are young or resuscitation is not going smoothly.

From Vincent JL et al: *Textbook of critical care,* ed 6, Philadelphia, 2011, Saunders.

- *Dressing:* Topical antimicrobial ointment (bacitracin) or A&D ointment with nonadherent dressing twice a day. Alternate: biosynthetic dressing (alginates, hydrofibers, or foam dressings)—many with silver as antimicrobial (absorb exudates, maintain moist environment, require fewer dressing changes, which reduces pain/anxiety)
- *Prognosis:* heal with minimal scarring in 10-14 days. May heal with pigmentary changes (reduced with sunscreen and sun avoidance of area x 1 year)

2nd degree (deep partial-thickness) burns with adherent exudates; localized 3rd degree burns; cellulitic wounds:

- *Dressing:* silver sulfadiazine 1%: broader spectrum, better penetration of necrotic tissue than bacitracin, but inhibits epithelialization. Must stop use once exudates and eschar have separated from wound. Alternative: enzymatic debrider (e.g., Santyl or Accuzyme)—chemically debrides devitalized tissue without harming healthy tissue.
- *Referral:* Burn specialist for consultation regarding need for excision and grafting.
- *Prognosis:* Deep 2nd degree burns heal with significant scarring, often take 3-4 weeks to heal. If infected, converts to 3rd degree burn. 3rd degree burns typically require skin graft, but small areas may heal from edges after weeks.

DISPOSITION/FOLLOW-UP CARE

- Outpatient: Evaluate next day to assess level of injury, level of pain, and ability to manage dressing changes on own. If insufficient, daily evaluation until complete wound epithelialization recommended. Epithelialization = tiny islands of epithelialization throughout wound. If no epithelialization after 2 weeks, or subsequent evaluation reveals 3rd degree burn, referral to burn surgeon recommended. Box E1-13 describes common complications in burn patients.
- Following re-epithelialization, visits every 4-6 weeks to monitor for hypertrophic scar formation (early referral to burn/scar specialist if occurs).
- Mortality rates higher in patients >60 yr of age, with burns >40% TBSA, or with inhalation injury. Long-term risk of developing squamous cell carcinoma of the skin within burn injury. Long-term monitoring necessary.

REFERRAL

Consultation of burn specialist or burn center referral per Table 1-91.

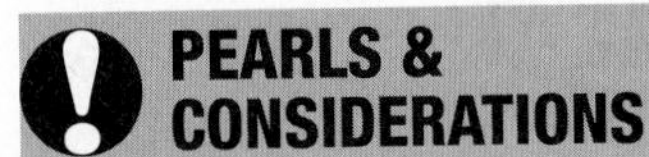

COMMENTS

- In circumferential skin burns, look for compartment syndrome of limbs (e.g., tightening, progressive deterioration of peripheral motor and sensory exam findings, severe pain, and loss of arterial Doppler signals). Escharotomy may be necessary.
- If child abuse is suspected, social services at the hospital or child protective services must be contacted.
- Fig. E1-196 describes an algorithm for the treatment of chemical burns.

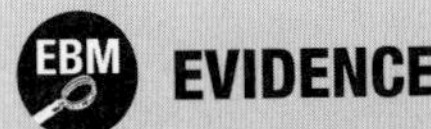

available at www.expertconsult.com

SUGGESTED READINGS

available at www.expertconsult.com

RELATED CONTENT

Burns (Patient Information)

AUTHOR: **LISA PAPPAS-TAFFER, M.D.**

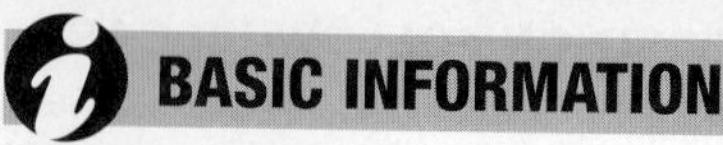

BASIC INFORMATION

DEFINITION

Bursitis is an inflammation of bursa, a thin-walled sac lined with synovial tissue. Bursae facilitate movement of tendons and muscles over bony prominences.

SYNONYMS

Student's elbow (olecranon bursitis)
Housemaid's knee (prepatellar bursitis)
Weaver's bottom (ischial gluteal bursitis)
Baker's cyst (gastrocnemius-semimembranosus bursa)

ICD-9CM CODES

726.19 Subacromial bursitis
726.33 Olecranon bursitis
726.5 Ischiogluteal bursitis (hip)
726.5 Iliopsoas bursitis (hip)
726.61 Anserine bursitis
726.5 Trochanteric bursitis
726.65 Prepatellar bursitis
727.51 Baker's cyst
726.79 Retrocalcaneal bursitis

ICD-10CM CODES

M75.80 Other shoulder lesions, unspecified shoulder
M70.20 Olecranon bursitis, unspecified elbow
M70.60 Trochanteric bursitis, unspecified hip
M70.70 Other bursitis of hip, unspecified hip
M76.899 Other specified enthesopathies of unspecified lower limb, excluding foot
M70.40 Prepatellar bursitis, unspecified knee
M71.20 Synovial cyst of popliteal space [Baker], unspecified knee
M77.50 Other enthesopathy of unspecified foot

PHYSICAL FINDINGS & CLINICAL PRESENTATION

- Local swelling, tenderness, erythema, warmth over the site of bursa
- Pain with active joint movement greater than passive range of motion or at rest
- Range of motion less painful and restricted in septic bursitis than in septic arthritis
- Referred pain

ETIOLOGY

- Direct trauma or repetitive injury
- Infection (septic bursitis)—from hematogenous seeding or spread from contiguous infection (*Staphylococcus aureus* >80%)
- Crystal diseases (e.g., gout, pseudogout)
- Systemic inflammatory arthritis RA
- Bleeding

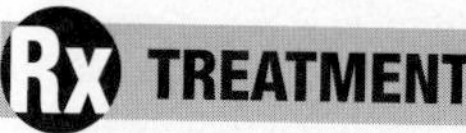

DIAGNOSIS

DIFFERENTIAL DIAGNOSIS

- Acute monoarthritis due to septic arthritis or crystal arthritis (gout, pseudogout)
- Tendinitis, tenosynovitis (occasionally)
- Cellulitis

WORKUP

- Bursal fluid aspiration: send for Gram stain; culture and sensitivity; cell count; and crystal analysis

IMAGING STUDIES

- Plain radiography can rule out foreign body penetration and other potential or coexisting bone or joint problems such as fracture (Fig. 1-197)
- MRI to define soft tissue involvement
- Musculoskeletal US for visualizing superficial and deep bursae and aspiration/injection

TREATMENT

NONPHARMACOLOGIC THERAPY

- Avoid direct pressure or repetitive irritation
- Joint protection (e.g., kneeling pads)
- Rest, ice, elevation for acute phase
- Physical therapy

ACUTE GENERAL Rx

- Septic:
  1. Appropriate antibiotic coverage and drainage. If MSSA, use nafcillin or oxacillin 2 g IV q4h or dicloxacillin 500 mg PO qid. If MRSA, use vancomycin 15-20 mg/kg IV q8-12h or linezolid 600 mg PO bid.
  2. Serial aspirations of purulent fluid or surgical drainage may be indicated.
- Nonseptic:
  1. Aspiration of bursal fluid or blood from acute trauma
  2. Nonpharmacologic therapy
  3. Traumatic bursitis may respond well to aspiration and corticosteroid injection.
  4. Crystal-related bursitis: systemic antiinflammatories or injection of corticosteroid

CHRONIC Rx

- Aspiration of fluid, followed by compression dressing to prevent fluid reaccumulation (repeat aspiration may be required)
- Steroid injection into bursa (40 mg triamcinolone mixed with 1-3 ml lidocaine, depending on size of bursa)
- NSAIDs, although steroid injection may be more effective in certain types of bursitis

DISPOSITION

- Nonsurgical treatment is effective in most cases. Surgical drainage may be indicated for loculated bursitis. Recurrent bursitis may require open bursectomy.

REFERRAL

Orthopedic consultation may be needed to assist in treatment of septic bursitis or for excision of chronic enlarged bursa when indicated.

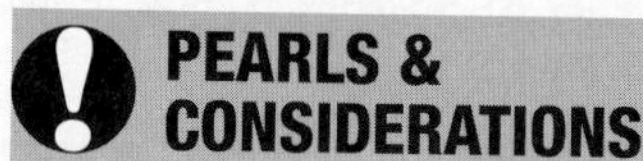

PEARLS & CONSIDERATIONS

- Bursae in patients with RA are not usually the sole site of active flare. Therefore, in patients with RA, acute bursitis should be considered septic bursitis until proven otherwise.

COMMENTS

- Scapulothoracic bursitis is underrecognized and undertreated. It results from friction between superomedial angle of scapula and adjacent second and third ribs. Crepitus, snapping, and tenderness are suggestive findings; it can also cause chest wall pain.
- Do not incise and drain sterile bursae because chronic draining sinus tract may develop.
- In bursitis caused by infectious or systemic inflammatory disorders, the leukocytosis in bursal fluid may be substantially less intense than the elevations in the joint fluid.
- Investigate crystal-induced bursitis for underlying metabolic or hematologic diseases (hemochromatosis, hyperparathyroidism [calcium pyrophosphate deposition disease]), and for hyperuricemia (gout).

SUGGESTED READINGS

available at www.expertconsult.com

RELATED CONTENT

Bursitis (Patient Information)

AUTHOR: **CANDICE YUVIENCO, M.D.**

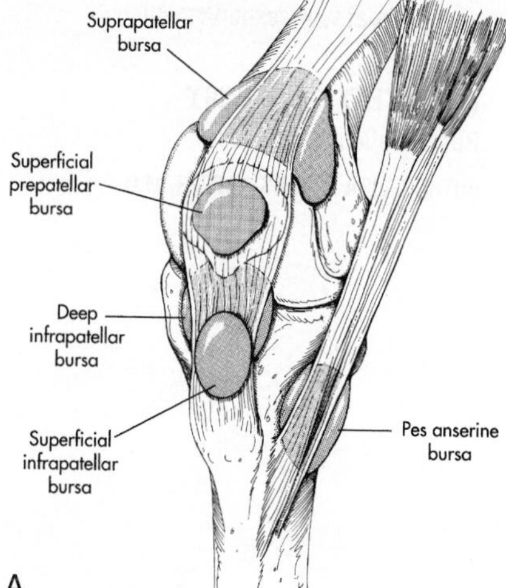

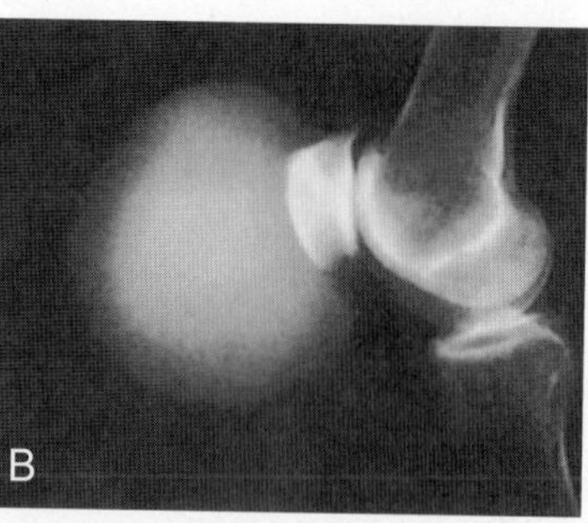

FIGURE 1-197 A, Bursae around the knee. **B,** Markedly swollen prepatellar bursa. (From Scudieri G [ed]: *Sports medicine principles of primary care,* St Louis, 1997, Mosby.)

BASIC INFORMATION

DEFINITION

Calcium pyrophosphate dihydrate crystal deposition disease, commonly known as pseudogout, refers to an acute synovitis caused by calcium pyrophosphate dihydrate (CPPD) crystals. CPPD deposition diseases comprise a spectrum of clinical syndromes including pseudogout, chondrocalcinosis, and pyrophosphate arthropathy. *Chondrocalcinosis* (CC) refers to the presence of calcification in cartilage by radiograph and does not confirm the diagnosis of pseudogout as it can be present in other types of crystal deposition diseases or asymptomatic. Pyrophosphate arthropathy is the term used for a chronic structural arthropathy related to CPPD deposition.

SYNONYMS

Pseudogout
CPPD crystal deposition disease
Chondrocalcinosis
Pyrophosphate arthropathy

ICD-9CM CODES
275.4 Chondrocalcinosis
ICD-10CM CODES
M11.2 Other chondrocarcinosis
M11.9 Crystal arthropathy, unspecified
M11.8 Other specified crystal arthropathies
M11.1 Familial chondrocalcinosis

EPIDEMIOLOGY & DEMOGRAPHICS

PREVALENCE:

- The epidemiology of CPPD crystal deposition is described in Table 1-93.
- Most linked with advancing age (average age of 70)

GENETICS: Associated with *ANKH* (ankylosis human) gene, which functions to transport inorganic pyrophosphate (PPi) out of cells. Familial mutations can increase extracellular PPi and lead to onset of CPPD disease in third or fourth decade of life.

PHYSICAL FINDINGS & CLINICAL PRESENTATION

- Acute pseudogout: monoarticular attacks most commonly involve the knee but can be polyarticular. Patients, especially the elderly, can have systemic manifestations such as fever and altered mental status. Situations that may trigger acute CPPD crystal arthritis are described in Box 1-14.
- Asymptomatic CC
- Pyrophosphate arthropathy: chronic arthritis with osteoarthritic features
- "Pseudo–polymyalgia rheumatica (pseudo-PMR)": pain and stiffness in the neck and shoulder girdle mimicking PMR
- "Pseudo–rheumatoid arthritis (pseudo-RA)": symmetric polyarthritis
- Crowned-dens syndrome caused by crystal deposition in the ligamentum flavum of the cervical spine either asymptomatic or causing acute neck pain

TABLE 1-93 Epidemiology of Calcium Pyrophosphate Dihydrate Crystal Deposition

Age association	Rises with age
Sex distribution	(F:M) 1:1
Chondrocalcinosis prevalence	8.1% (age range 63-93)
Pyrophosphate arthropathy prevalence	3.4% (age range 40-89)
Geography	Appears ubiquitous
Genetic associations	Mutations of *ANKH* gene on chromosome 5p (CCAL2) and unknown genes on chromosome 8q (CCAL1)

From Hochberg MC et al: *Rheumatology,* ed 5, St Louis, 2011, Mosby.

ETIOLOGY

- Idiopathic
- Metabolic: hyperparathyroidism, hypophosphatasia, hypomagnesemia, hemochromatosis, ochronosis, familial hypocalciuric hypercalcemia, X-linked hypophosphatemic rickets

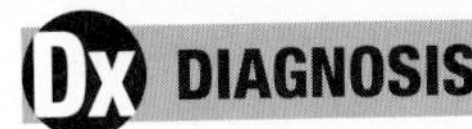

DIAGNOSIS

BOX 1-14 Situations That May Trigger Acute Calcium Pyrophosphate Dihydrate Crystal Arthritis

Definite
Direct trauma to joint
Intercurrent medical illness (e.g., chest infection, myocardial infarction)
Surgery (especially parathyroidectomy)
Blood transfusion, parenteral fluid administration
Joint lavage

Possible
Institution of thyroxine replacement therapy
Intra-articular injection of hyaluronan
Bisphosphonate treatment

Note: Most cases of pseudogout develop spontaneously.

From Hochberg MC et al: *Rheumatology,* ed 5, St Louis, 2011, Mosby.

DIFFERENTIAL DIAGNOSIS

- Gouty arthritis
- Septic arthritis
- RA
- PMR

Table 1-94 describes metabolic diseases predisposing to CPPD disposition. Section II describes the differential diagnosis of acute monoarticular and oligoarticular arthritis and crystal-induced arthritides. An algorithm for evaluation and treatment of CPPD is shown in Fig. 1-198.

LABORATORY TESTS

- Arthrocentesis with presence of weakly positive birefringent rhomboid-shaped crystals (yellow perpendicular and blue parallel to polarizer axis) (Fig. E1-199)
- Synovial fluid should always be analyzed for cell count with differential, crystals, Gram stain, and culture because gout and septic arthritis can coexist with pseudogout.
- Evaluate for possible metabolic cause, especially in younger patients aged <55 yr or patients with florid polyarticular disease. Box 1-15 describes screening blood tests for metabolic diseases associated with CPPD crystal deposition.

IMAGING STUDIES

Plain radiographs often reveal CC located parallel to subchondral bone.

- Classic locations for CC include knee menisci (Fig. E1-200), wrist triangular fibrocartilage, and symphysis pubis (Fig. 1-201).

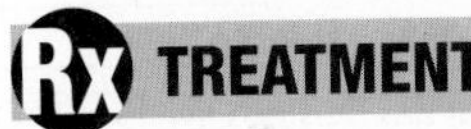

TREATMENT

NONPHARMACOLOGIC THERAPY

General measures such as immobilization of inflamed joint

ACUTE GENERAL Rx

- Monoarticular pseudogout:
  - Aspiration with corticosteroid injection (often superior to systemic treatment in the elderly)
- Polyarticular pseudogout:
  - Oral corticosteroids or NSAIDs if not contraindicated

TABLE 1-94 Metabolic Diseases Predisposing to Calcium Pyrophosphate Dihydrate Deposition

	CC	Pseudogout	Chronic PA
Hemochromatosis	Yes	Yes	Yes
Hyperparathyroidism	Yes	Yes	No
Hypophosphatasia	Yes	Yes	No
Hypomagnesemia	Yes	Yes	No
Hypothyroidism	No	No	No
Gout	Possibly	Possibly	No
Acromegaly	Possibly	No	No
Ochronosis	Yes	Yes	No
Familial hypocalciuric hypercalcemia	Possibly	No	No
X-linked hypophosphatemic rickets	Possibly	Possibly	Possibly

CC, Chondrocalcinosis; *PA,* pyrophosphate arthropathy.

CHRONIC GENERAL Rx

Prophylaxis: daily low-dose colchicine 0.6 mg twice daily or once daily as tolerated

- Pseudo-RA or refractory disease: hydroxychloroquine or methotrexate
- Treat underlying metabolic disease

DISPOSITION

Structural joint damage may occasionally occur, requiring arthroplasty in rare cases.

REFERRAL

Rheumatology

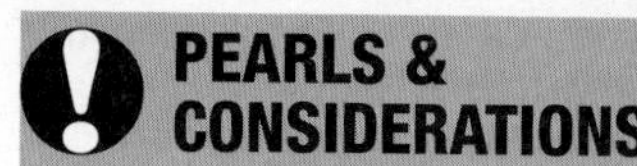

PEARLS & CONSIDERATIONS

COMMENTS

Acute pseudogout attacks have been reported to occur in the setting of surgical procedures, diuresis, bisphosphonate administration, and hyaluronate joint injections.

SUGGESTED READINGS

available at www.expertconsult.com

RELATED CONTENT

Gout (Related Key Topic)
Pseudogout (Patient Information)

AUTHOR: **ELISABETH B. MATSON, D.O.**

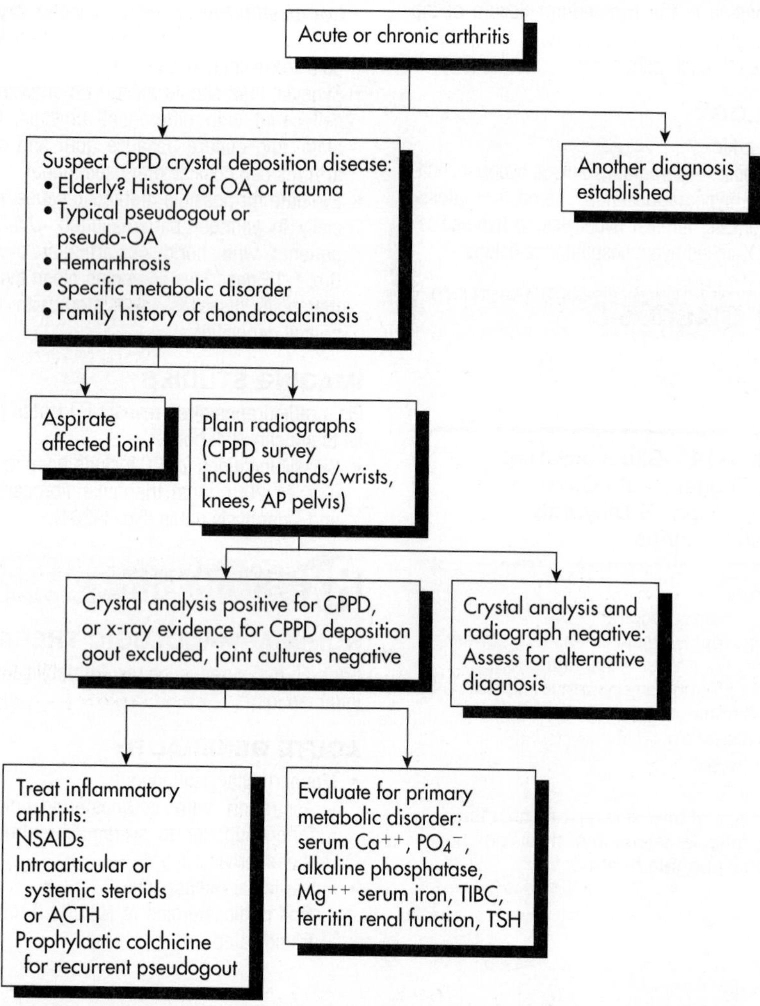

FIGURE 1-198 Algorithm for evaluation and treatment of calcium pyrophosphate dihydrate disease. *ACTH,* Adrenocorticotropic hormone; *AP,* anteroposterior; *CPPD,* calcium pyrophosphate deposition; *NSAIDs,* nonsteroidal anti-inflammatory drugs; *OA,* osteoarthritis; *TIBC,* total iron-binding capacity; *TSH,* thyroid-stimulating hormone. (From Harris ED et al: *Kelley's textbook of rheumatology,* ed 7, Philadelphia, 2005, Saunders.)

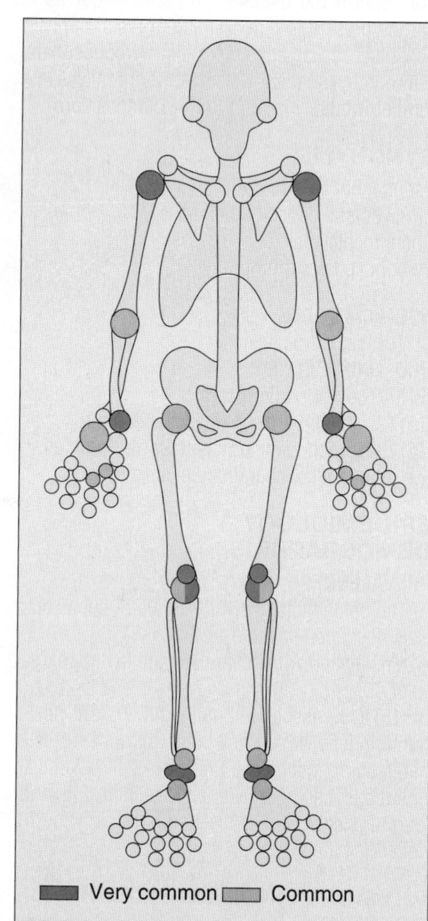

FIGURE 1-201 Chronic arthropathy. Common sites of involvement of chronic pyrophosphate. (From Hochberg MC et al: *Rheumatology,* ed 5, St Louis, 2011, Mosby.)

BOX 1-15 Screening Blood Tests for Metabolic Diseases Associated with Calcium Pyrophosphate Dihydrate Crystal Deposition

Calcium
Alkaline phosphatase
Magnesium
Ferritin
Liver function
Thyroid-stimulating hormone

From Hochberg MC et al: *Rheumatology,* ed 5, St. Louis, 2011, Mosby.

BASIC INFORMATION

DEFINITION

Infection caused by the species of the genus *Candida,* mainly *Candida albicans. Candida* species are ubiquitous. They are the most common fungal pathogens affecting mankind. Cutaneous candidiasis comprises superficial *Candida* infections of the skin and mucosal membranes.

Cutaneous candidiasis can be classified into two subgroups: cutaneous candidiasis syndromes and chronic mucocutaneous syndromes. Cutaneous candidiasis syndromes include:
- Generalized cutaneous candidias
- Intertrigo
- *Candida* folliculitis
- Paronychia/onychomycosis
- Perianal candidiasis
- Erosio interdigitalis blastomycetica
- Balanitis

Chronic mucocutaneous syndromes include:
- Oropharyngeal candidiasis
- Esophageal candidiasis
- Vulvovaginal candidiasis
- GI candidiasis (gastric/intestines/perianal)
- *Candida* cystitis

SYNONYMS

Yeast infection
Candidosis
Moniliasis
Oidiomycosis

ICD-9CM CODES
112 Candidiasis
ICD-10CM CODES
B37.2 Candidiasis of skin and nail
B37.8 Candidiasis, unspecified
B37.89 Other sites of candidiasis

EPIDEMIOLOGY & DEMOGRAPHICS

- *Candida* species: it is the most common fungal infection in immunocompromised people.
- Most females (75%) experience an episode of vulvovaginal candidiasis in their lifetime.

INCIDENCE: Estimated to be 50 cases per 100,000 persons

PREVALENCE: Colonizes more than 50% of U.S. population

PREDOMINANT SEX AND AGE
- Female >male
- No predominant age, but neonates and the elderly (adults >65 yr) are susceptible to *Candida* colonization and to getting nucocutaneous candidiasis.

RISK FACTORS:
Risk factors that allow *Candida* infection include:
- Age >65 yr
- Females in the third trimester
- Defects in the mucocutaneous barrier (e.g., wounds, burns, ulcerations)
- Decreased/defective granulocytes/monocytes
- Diseases of white blood cells (e.g., chronic granulomatous disease)
- Complement deficiency
- Certain diseases associated with cell-mediated immunity (e.g., HIV, DM)
- Use of certain medications (e.g., broad-spectrum antibiotics, high doses of corticosteroids)
- Increased skin pH due to panty liners and occlusive attire
- **Chronic mucocutaneous candidiasis** (CMC) is characterized by susceptibility to *Candida* infection of skin, nails, and mucous membranes. Patients with recessive CMC and autoimmunity have mutations in the autoimmune regulator *AIRE.* Mutations in the CC domain of *STAT1* underlie autosomal dominant CMC and lead to defective Th1 and Th17 responses which may explain the increased susceptibility to fungal infections (van de Veerdonk et al).

Anatomical sites predisposed to *Candida* infection include:
- Axilla
- Beneath the breast, abdominal fold, intertriginous areas
- Periungual creases
- Inguinal creases
- Back and buttocks of bedridden persons

PHYSICAL FINDINGS & CLINICAL PRESENTATION

There are several clinical presentations of cutaneous candidiasis. A few are presented here.

A. Cutaneous candidiasis
   1. Presents as erythematous, sometimes shiny with flakes and fluid lesions at the edge of the redness (satellite pustules). It is itchy and the skin becomes inflamed. Pustules may be present in candidiasis of the scrotal and perineal skin.

B. Gastrointestinal tract candidiasis
   1. Oropharyngeal candidiasis
      - Usually seen in diabetics, after exposure to inhaled steroids or broad-spectrum antibiotics and in immunosuppressed individuals (e.g., patients with a history of HIV infection). Symptoms include:
         - White thick patches on the oral mucosa
         - Dysphagia, mouth soreness, and pain
         - Tongue burning
      - Physical examination shows:
         - Erythema of the buccal mucosa
         - White patches on buccal cavity surfaces
         - Transverse fissuring
   2. Esophageal candidiasis:
      - History of oropharyngeal candidiasis
      - Symptoms include:
         - Dysphagia
         - Odynophagia
         - Epigastric pain
         - Retrosternal pain
      - Physical examination shows:
         - Affects mainly the distal one third of the esophagus
         - Endoscopy shows areas of the erythema and edema; scattered white patches or ulcers.
   3. Perianal candidiasis
      - Skin maceration
      - Itching
      - Frequently extends to the perineum

C. Paronychia/onychomycosis
   - Fungal infection of the nail and surrounding tissues
   - Associated with diabetes mellitus and immersion of hands or feet in water
   - History: pain and redness around and beneath the nail and nail bed
   - Physical exam: inflammation around the toe nail. There may also be nail thickening and discoloration (dystrophic nails). Nail loss may also occur.

D. Respiratory tract candidiasis
   1. Usually seen in hospitalized patients
   2. About 25% of outpatients have their respiratory tract colonized by *Candida* species
      - Genitourinary tract candidiasis
      - Vulvovaginal candidiasis
         - It causes itching, curdy white discharge, and occasionally dysuria and dyspareunia.
         - On examination the mucosa may be inflamed.
         - Painful erythema or itchy penile inflammation may occur in male sexual partners of affected females.
      - *Candida* balanitis
         - Usually acquired through sexual contact with a partner who has vulvovaginal candidiasis.
         - Symptoms include penile pruritus and white patches on penis.
         - Physical exam: dry, erythematous, and scaly patches on penis.

E. Others
   1. Erosio interdigitalis blastomycetica: Denudating/macerating area commonly seen in third web space
   2. *Candida* folliculitis: Pustulous nodules in hairy areas
   3. Intertrigo: This occurs in folds of the skin and creases (Fig. 1-202). It is characterized by erosions, exudation, oozing, and maceration.

ETIOLOGY

The most common cause of cutaneous candidiasis is *Candida albicans.*

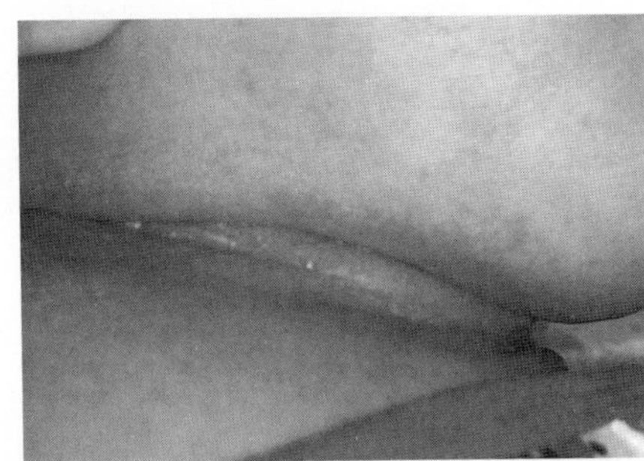

FIGURE 1-202 Intertriginous candidosis of the neck. (From Kliegman RM et al: *Nelson textbook of pediatrics,* ed 19, Philadelphia, 2011, Saunders.)

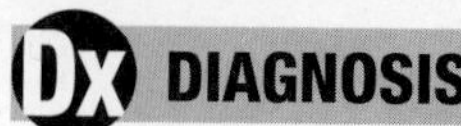

DIFFERENTIAL DIAGNOSIS

Intertrigo

WORKUP

Mucocutaneous and cutaneous candidiasis

- Obtain scrapings from the skin, oral, and vaginal mucosa or nails.
- The presence of hyphae/pseudohyphae or budding yeast cells on wet smear, as well as confirmation by culture, is the recommended procedure to diagnose cutaneous candidiasis.
- KOH smears are helpful.

Respiratory candidiasis

- Sputum Gram stain: shows yeast cells
- Sputum cultures
- Lung biopsy: establishes the diagnosis (Fig. 1-202)

Gastrointestinal candidiasis

- Upper endoscopy with or without biopsy (Fig. 1-203)

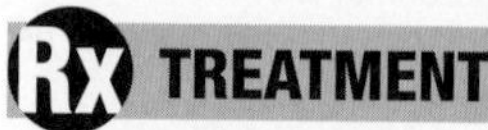

PHARMACOLOGIC THERAPY

A. Cutaneous candidiasis
   1. Decrease/prevent moisture in area
   2. Apply antifungal agents (nystatin powder or cream with an azole or ciclopirox [e.g., clotrimazole, econazole, miconazole])

B. Gastrointestinal candidiasis
   1. Oropharyngeal candidiasis
      - Treat with either
        - Oral topical antifungal agent (e.g., nystatin swish and swallow) OR
        - Systemic oral azoles (e.g., fluconazole)

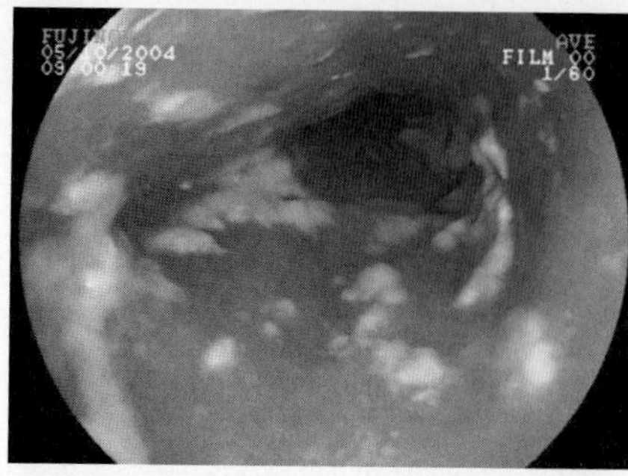

FIGURE 1-203 Endoscopic appearance of esophageal candidiasis. (Courtsey Dr. B. Rembacken, Leeds, U.K.)

      - In HIV-positive patients, use high doses of fluconazole (100-200 mg PO qd for 7-14 days), itraconazole, or posaconazole.
   2. *Candida* esophagitis
      - Treat with systemic fluconazole for 2 to 3 wk.
      - Treat with IV fluconazole if patient is unable to take oral medication.

C. Genitourinary tract candidiasis
   - Vulvovaginal candidiasis: Treatment options for acute cases include:
     - A single dose of oral fluconazole (fluconazole 150 mg PO × 1 dose) OR
     - Topical antifungal agent
   - For chronic or recurrent cases, treat with fluconazole 150 mg qod × 3 doses and then 150 mg/wk for 6 mo.

D. Chronic mucocutaneous candidiasis
   - Treatment with azoles is effective (e.g., fluconazole 100-400 mg daily).
   - When patient improves, follow with maintenance treatment with same azole for life.

FOLLOW-UP CARE

Mucocutaneous candidiasis

- Patient should be instructed to call or follow up if symptoms persist, recur, or worsen.
- For recurrent infections:
  - Check HIV antibodies.
  - Check FBS, HbA_{1c}.
  - Rule out hematologic malignancy or solid organ malignancy.
  - Refer to linfectious disease specialist if no etiology is found.

PREVENTION

- Maintaining dry environment (e.g., by wearing cotton underwear)
- Decreased use of antibiotic
- No douching

SUGGESTED READINGS

available at www.expertconsult.com

RELATED CONTENT

Candidiasis (Patient Information)

AUTHOR: **DANIEL K. ASIEDU, M.D., Ph.D., F.A.C.P.**

BASIC INFORMATION

DEFINITION

Severe and invasive diseases are caused by *Candida* infection. Invasive candidiasis embodies a variety of diseases including candidemia, disseminated candidiasis, meningitis, and endophthalmitis.

SYNONYMS

Systemic candidiasis

ICD-9CM CODES
112.5 Disseminated candidiasis
ICD-10CM CODES
B37.89 Other sites of candidiasis
B37.1 Pulmonary candidiasis
B37.2 Candidiasis of skin and nail
B37.5 Candidal meningitis
B37.6 Candidal endocarditis
B37.7 Candidal sepsis
B37.9 Candidiasis unspecified

EPIDEMIOLOGY & DEMOGRAPHICS

INCIDENCE: Estimated to be 22 to 24 cases per 100,000 persons per year
PREVALENCE: No data available
PREDOMINANT SEX AND AGE: Equal between males and females; all ages are susceptible.
RISK FACTORS: Prolonged hospitalization and ICU stay, use of broad-spectrum antibiotics, prolonged indwelling of catheters (especially central venous catheters), acute and chronic renal failure, surgery requiring general anesthesia, cancer (e.g., solid neoplasms), transplantation (bone marrow or solid organ), recent chemotherapy/radiation therapy, use of immunosuppressive drugs, parenteral alimentation, use of internal prosthetic devices

PHYSICAL FINDINGS & CLINICAL PRESENTATION

1. History
   - Fever unresponsive to broad-spectrum antibiotics
   - History of prolonged indwelling IV catheter
   - A personal history of any of the risk factors listed earlier
2. Physical findings (general)
   - Fever
   - Hypotension
   - Generalized malaise
   - Tachycardia
   - Change in mental status
3. Specific diseases
   - Candidemia
     - *Candida* species are isolated from at least one blood culture.
     - Most common form of invasive candidiasis
     - Physical exam may include fever, macronodular skin lesions, septic shock, *Candida* endophthalmitis.
   - Disseminated candidiasis
     - Seen in patients with neutropenia
     - Associated with multiple deep-organ infections or failure
     - Blood culture negative
     - Fever not responding to broad-spectrum antibiotics
     - Physical exam: discrete erythematous or palpable rash, sepsis/septic shock
   - Endophthalmitis
     - Iatrogenic/accidental fungal infection of the eye (exogenous) or hematogenous seeding of the eye (endogenous)
     - Starts as choroidal lesion, progresses to vitreitis and endophthalmitis and eventually blindness
     - Physical exam shows fever. Funduscopic examination shows large and off-white cottonball-like lesions with indistinct borders.
   - *Candida* infection of the CNS
     - Exogenous and endogenous forms
     - Commonly found in long-term ICU patient
     - May present as meningitis, mycotic aneurysms, change in mental status
     - Physical examination reveals fever, neck rigidity, confusion, and coma.
   - Candidal musculoskeletal infections
     - Previously uncommon; now relatively common probably due to increased frequency of candidemia and disseminated candidiasis
     - Knee and vertebral column (especially lumbosacral vertebral disks and vertebral bodies) are involved.
     - Physical exam is usually unremarkable but may show tenderness over involved area, fever, erythema, bone deformity, weight loss, and sometimes a draining fistulous tract.
   - Candidal infections of the heart
     - May present as infective endocarditis, myocarditis, or pericarditis.
     - Physical examination reveals fever, hypotension, tachycardia, new or changing murmur.
   - Hepatosplenic candidiasis (chronic systemic candidiasis)
     - Seen in patients with hematologic malignancy and neutropenia; usually develops during recovery from a neutropenic state (normally after undergoing myeloablative chemotherapy)
     - On examination, patients have low-grade fever, right upper quadrant pain, palpable/tender liver, splenomegaly, and rarely jaundice.
   - *Candida* peritonitis
     - Associated with GI surgery, peritoneal dialysis
     - Clinical manifestations include fever, chills, abdominal pain; nausea, vomiting, constipation.
     - Physical examination reveals abdominal distention, abdominal pain, absent bowel sounds.
   - Other forms of invasive candidiasis
     - *Candida* splenic abscess
     - *Candida* cholecystitis
     - Renal candidiasis

ETIOLOGY

- Several species of *Candida* exist in nature
- Medically significant include:
  - *C. albicans:* together with *C. glabrata,* they account for 70% to 80% of *Candida* in invasive candidiasis.
  - *C. glabrata:* together with *C. albicans,* they account for 70% to 80% of *Candida* in invasive candidiasis.
  - *C. parapsilosis:* associated with indwelling vascular catheters and prosthetic devices
  - *C. tropicalis:* especially in leukemic patients
  - *C. krusei:* resistant to fluconazole and ketoconazole

DIAGNOSIS

DIFFERENTIAL DIAGNOSIS

- Sepsis (bacterial)
- Septic shock
- Cryptococcosis
- Aspergillosis

WORKUP

LABORATORY TESTS

- Laboratory studies are nonspecific.
- High index of suspicion is needed.
- Candidemia/disseminated candidiasis
  - Blood cultures: helpful but low positive yield
  - Serum (1,3) beta-D-glucan detection assay: high specificity and high positive predictive value
- Hepatosplenic candidiasis (focal)
  - Elevated serum alkaline phosphatase

IMAGING STUDIES

- Imaging studies are generally not required or useful.
- Ultrasound is useful for diagnosing hepatosplenic abscess. "Bull's eye or target lesions" are observed in the liver and spleen.
- CT scanning may be used to diagnose hepatosplenic candidiasis, as well as intraabdominal/renal abscesses.
- ECHO is useful to rule in or rule out *Candida* endocarditis.

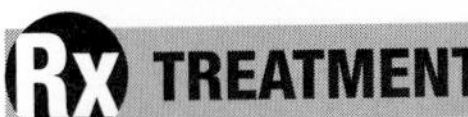

TREATMENT

- To successfully treat invasive *Candida* infection, it is important to start antifungal medication as early as possible.
- Antifungals available include:
  - Azoles (e.g., fluconazole, posaconazole, itraconazole, voriconazole). They inhibit the synthesis of ergosterol, a fungal cell component.
  - Echinocandins (e.g., caspofungin, micafungin, anidulafungin). These are glucan synthesis inhibitors. Glucan is an important component of fungal cell walls.
  - Polyenes (e.g., amphotericin B, lipid formulation of amphotericin, nystatin). Broad spectrum. Their mechanism of action is to increase cytoplasmic permeability.

- Antimetabolites (e.g., flucytosine). Flucytosine is deaminated to 5-fluorouracil in fungal cell. 5-Fluorouracil inhibits RNA and protein synthesis.

TREATMENT PLANS

CANDIDEMIA:
- Treatment depends on whether the patient is neutropenic or not.
  - Nonneutropenic adult patients: drug of choice is fluconazole; 800 mg as loading dose then 400 mg/day for at least 2 wk after clinical improvement or negative blood culture. Amphotericin B is equally efficacious.
  - Neutropenic adult patients: an echinocandin is the drug of choice (e.g., caspofungin 70 mg IV loading dose then 50 mg/day IV or micafungin 100 mg/day IV or anidulafungin 200 mg IV loading dose then 100 mg IV all for at least 2 wk after clear blood culture and after clinical improvement.

DISSEMINATED CANDIDIASIS

Fluconazole is the drug of choice.

DISSEMINATED CANDIDIASIS WITH END-ORGAN INFECTION
- Treatment is the same as for candidemia of nonneutropenic patients. In most cases, therapy is prolonged for at least 4 to 6 wk.
- The echinocandins are the first-line therapy.

OSTEOMYELITIS OR SEPTIC ARTHRITIS
- Fluconazole 400 mg IV or PO *or*
- Lipid-based amphotericin B 3-5 mg/kg qd

ENDOCARDITIS
- Caspofungin 50-150 mg/day or
- Micafungin 100-150 mg/day or
- Anidulafungin 100-200 mg/day

MYOCARDITIS
- Lipid-based amphotericin B 3-5 mg/kg daily *or*
- Fluconazole 400-800 mg daily IV or PO

ESOPHAGITIS
- Fluconazole 200-400 mg/day or
- Caspofungin 50 mg IV daily

PERICARDITIS
- Lipid-based amphotericin B 3-5 mg/kg daily *or*
- Fluconazole 400-800 mg PO qd IV or PO

SURGICAL CARE

Include:
- Drainage
- Removal of any foreign bodies
- Surgical debridement
- Organ-specific care (e.g., valve replacement for endocarditis, splenectomy for splenic abscess, or vitrectomy for fungal endophthalmitis)

DISPOSITION
- Several factors affect prognosis: infection site, degree of immune suppression, and how quickly diagnosis and therapy is initiated
- Overall mortality rate: 30% to 40%

REFERRAL
- Always involve an infectious disease specialist.
- Referral to specialist will depend on the organ involved. For example:
  - Endocarditis will require a cardiothoracic surgeon.
  - Endophthalmitis will require an ophthalmologist.

FOLLOW-UP CARE
- Prolonged periods, mainly in the hospital, of antifungal treatment may be necessary.
- Closely monitor patients on amphotericin B because of the high incidence of side effects. Check basic metabolic panel, magnesium, and CBC at least twice a week.

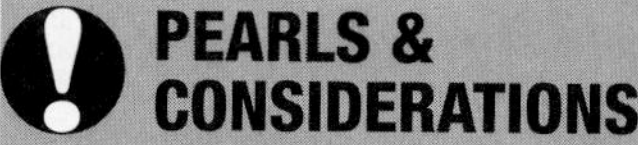

PREVENTION

Basic preventive measures are similar to those used for nosocomial infections. This includes:
- Maximizing hand hygiene recommendations:
  - Hand washing
  - Using alcohol/chlorhexidine solution
- Adhering strictly to recommendations for placement and care of central lines and catheters.
- Judicious use of antimicrobials

PROPHYLAXIS

Antifungal prophylaxis recommended for:
- Solid organ transplant recipients
- Stem cell transplant recipients

PATIENT/FAMILY EDUCATION
- Inform them about the risk factors for invasive candidiasis.
- Inform them of the seriousness of the disease and the associated high morbidity/mortality rates, thus requiring aggressive treatment.
- Side effects and toxicities associated with treatment

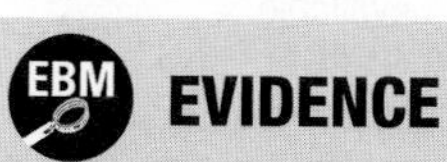

available at www.expertconsult.com

SUGGESTED READINGS

available at www.expertconsult.com

RELATED CONTENT

Candidiasis (Patient Information)

AUTHOR: **DANIEL K. ASIEDU, M.D., PH.D., F.A.C.P**

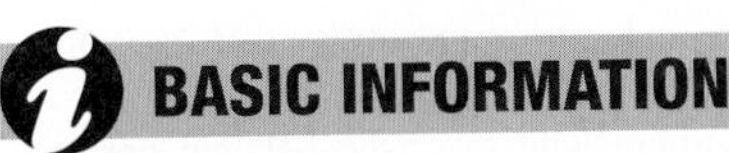

DEFINITION

Carbon monoxide (CO) is a colorless, odorless, tasteless, nonirritating gas. When inhaled it produces toxicity by causing cellular hypoxia and damage.

ICD-9CM CODES
986 Carbon monoxide poisoning
ICD-10CM CODES
T68 Toxic effect of carbon monoxide
T58.01 Toxic effect of carbon monoxide from motor vehicle exhaust, accidental (unintentional), initial encounter

EPIDEMIOLOGY & DEMOGRAPHICS

- A leading cause of accidental and intentional poisoning in the U.S.
- CO poisoning is seen more frequently during the fall and winter months in cold climates. Frequently seen after storm-related power outages, mostly due to the use of portable gasoline-powered electrical generators.
- In adults, 20% of CO poisonings occur in occupational settings.

PHYSICAL FINDINGS & CLINICAL PRESENTATION

- Depends on the severity and duration of exposure. The brain and heart are most sensitive to CO poisoning.
- Presentation is often nonspecific and may be mistaken for a flulike illness.
- Severity of poisoning does not correlate with carboxyhemoglobin (COHb) levels.
- Mild to moderate poisoning may present with headache, malaise, dizziness, nausea, dyspnea, difficulty concentrating, confusion, and blurred vision. Patients may have tachypnea and tachycardia.
- Severe poisoning may present with hypotension, arrhythmias, myocardial ischemia, pulmonary edema, lethargy, ataxia, loss of consciousness, seizure, coma, or rarely, cherry-red skin.
- Delayed neurologic sequelae may develop days to weeks after apparent recovery from acute poisoning. Patients may present with neurologic or psychiatric symptoms (cognitive deficits, memory loss, personality changes, movement disorders, Parkinson's, psychosis, neurologic deficits).

ETIOLOGY

- CO results from the incomplete combustion of carbon-containing compounds. CO poisoning occurs from inhaling smoke from fires, motor vehicle exhaust, or the burning of fuel (oil, wood, coal, gasoline, natural gas) in poorly functioning or improperly ventilated devices (heating systems, stoves/grills, portable generators, etc.). Methylene chloride (paint stripper) fumes are converted to CO by the liver.
- CO toxicity results from tissue hypoxia and direct CO-mediated damage at the cellular level. This may explain why COHb levels alone are not predictive of clinical toxicity. The mechanisms of CO toxicity are not completely understood.
- CO impairs oxygen delivery. CO reversibly binds hemoglobin with an affinity 250 times greater than oxygen, displacing oxygen from hemoglobin and decreasing the oxygen-carrying capacity of blood. By binding to hemoglobin, CO changes the structure of the hemoglobin molecule and decreases oxygen release to tissue.
- CO also interferes with peripheral oxygen utilization. It binds to other heme-containing proteins including cytochromes and myoglobin. Cellular respiration is depressed by inhibition of the mitochondrial cytochrome oxidase system. By binding to myoglobin, CO decreases its ability to use and store oxygen.
- Neurologic toxicity is not explained by hypoxia alone and is related to the complex intracellular actions of CO. CO precipitates an inflammatory cascade that results in oxidative damage and brain lipid peroxidation.

Dx DIAGNOSIS

DIFFERENTIAL DIAGNOSIS

- Viral syndromes
- Cyanide, hydrogen sulfide
- Methemoglobinemia
- Amphetamines and derivatives
- Cocaine, phencyclidine (PCP)
- Cyclic antidepressants
- Phenothiazines
- Theophylline

WORKUP

History (duration and source of CO exposure, loss of consciousness), physical examination (detailed neurologic examination), laboratory and imaging tests

LABORATORY TESTS

- COHb level (measured by CO-oximetry on arterial blood; venous blood may be used to screen large populations exposed to CO or monitor change in COHb with treatment). COHb level >3% in nonsmokers confirms exposure. Table 1-95 describes the half-life of COHb. Heavy smokers may have baseline levels of up to 10%. Levels may be low if the patient has already received supplemental oxygen or if delay occurs between exposure and testing.

TABLE 1-95 Half-Life of COHb

Oxygen Concentration	Half-Life
21% (room air)	4-5 hr
100% (mask or endotracheal)	60-90 min
100% (hyperbaric molecular oxygen)	20-30 min

From Fuhrman BP et al: *Pediatric critical care*, ed 4, Philadelphia, 2011, Saunders.

- Direct measurement of arterial carboxyhemoglobin (by CO-oximetry): Pulse oximetry and arterial blood gas (ABG) may be falsely normal because neither measures oxygen saturation of hemoglobin directly. Pulse oximetry is inaccurate because of the similar absorption characteristics of oxyhemoglobin and COHb. An ABG is inaccurate because it measures oxygen dissolved in plasma (which is not affected by CO) and then calculates oxygen saturation of hemoglobin.
- Electrolytes, glucose, BUN, creatinine, cardiac biomarkers, ABG (lactic acidosis and rhabdomyolysis may develop), CBC (polycythemia from hypoxia in chronic CO poisoning).
- ECG (ischemia, arrhythmia).
- Pregnancy test (fetus at high risk).
- Consider toxicology screen.

IMAGING STUDIES

- Chest x-ray (noncardiogenic edema)
- Brain CT, MRI if neurologic abnormalities are present

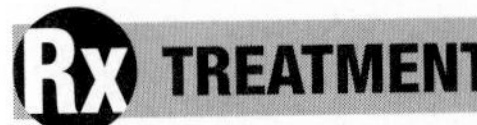

ACUTE GENERAL Rx

- Remove from site of CO exposure.
- Ensure adequate airway.
- Continuous ECG monitor.
- Fetal monitoring if pregnant.
- 100% oxygen by nonrebreather mask or endotracheal tube (decreases half-life of COHb from 4 to 6 hr to 60 to 90 min) until COHb level is <10% and patient is asymptomatic.
- Hyperbaric oxygen (2.5 to 3 atm).
  - Questionable beneficial effect over normobaric oxygen. Disparate findings in various studies: some suggest hyperbaric oxygen treatment reduces the incidence of neurologic sequelae, and others have found it worsens neurologic outcomes compared to normobaric oxygen treatment.
  - Decreases half-life of COHb to 20 to 30 min; increases amount of oxygen dissolved in plasma. It also reduces CO binding to other heme-containing proteins.
  - Consider for:
    1. Severe intoxication (COHb >25%, history of loss of consciousness, neurologic symptoms or signs, cardiovascular compromise, severe metabolic acidosis)
    2. Pregnant women with COHb >20% or signs of fetal distress. CO elimination is slower in fetus than mother, fetal Hgb has greater affinity for CO than adult Hgb
  - Should be instituted quickly if deemed necessary
- Consider concomitant poisoning with other toxic/irritant gases that may be present in smoke (e.g., cyanide) or thermal injury to airway. Toxic effects of CO and cyanide are synergistic.
- Identify source of exposure and determine if poisoning was accidental.

DISPOSITION

- Patients with mild accidental poisoning can be treated in an ambulatory setting. Those with moderate/severe poisoning or coexisting illness require hospitalization.
- Survivors of severe poisoning are at 14% to 40% risk for neurologic sequelae.
  - Deficits are usually apparent within 3 wk of poisoning but may present months later.
  - Risk of developing sequelae is greater if patient lost consciousness during acute poisoning and with older age.
  - Brain MRI and functional CT may reveal changes; damage is seen most often in the globus pallidus and deep white matter.
  - Recovery may occur over months to years.
- CO-mediated cardiac damage is associated with increased long-term mortality.
- High risk of fetal demise

REFERRAL

- American Association of Poison Control Centers: 1-800-222-1222
- Hyperbaric unit; accredited facilities are listed on the Undersea & Hyperbaric Medical Society website (www.uhms.org)
- Psychiatric evaluation if intentional poisoning

PEARLS & CONSIDERATIONS

- Severity of poisoning and prognosis do not correlate with COHb levels.
- Neuropsychometric testing is an objective measure of cognitive function but is not universally used.
- Imaging techniques and biomarkers to allow for early prediction of CNS damage are being studied but are not ready for application.
- Pulse oximeter measurement of CO saturation has limited clinical use.
- Treatment with hydroxocobalamin (for cyanide toxicity) may make subsequent COHb testing unreliable.
- Contact local Fire Department to assess environment and identify source of CO.

SUGGESTED READINGS

available at www.expertconsult.com

RELATED CONTENT

Carbon Monoxide Poisoning (Patient Information)

AUTHOR: **SUDEEP KAUR AULAKH, M.D.**

BASIC INFORMATION

DEFINITION

Carcinoid syndrome is a symptom complex characterized by paroxysmal vasomotor disturbances, diarrhea, and bronchospasm. It is caused by the action of amines and peptides (serotonin, bradykinin, histamine) produced by tumors arising from neuroendocrine cells.

SYNONYMS

Flush syndrome
Argentaffinoma syndrome

ICD-9CM CODES
259.2 Carcinoid syndrome
ICD-10CM CODES
E34.0 Carcinoid syndrome

EPIDEMIOLOGY & DEMOGRAPHICS

INCIDENCE:

- Carcinoid tumors are found incidentally in 0.5% to 0.75% of autopsies.
- Carcinoid tumors are principally found in the following organs: appendix (40%); small bowel (20%; 15% in the ileum); rectum (15%); bronchi (12%); esophagus, stomach, and colon (10%); and ovary, biliary tract, and pancreas (3%).
- The incidence of carcinoids is 2.47 to 4.48/100,000, depending on race and sex, and is highest in black men. The overall incidence has increased over the last 30 years due in part to improved diagnostic modalities.
- Carcinoid tumors can be classified using the WHO classification as follows:
  - WHO I: Well-differentiated, <2 cm diameter, low proliferation index (<2%), confined to mucosa and submucosa
  - WHO II: Differentiated, >2 cm diameter, invasive growth, high proliferation index (2%-15%)
  - WHO III: Poorly differentiated carcinomas with metastases and proliferation index >15%

PHYSICAL FINDINGS & CLINICAL PRESENTATION

- Cutaneous flushing (75% to 90%)
  1. The patient usually has red-purple flushes starting in the face, then spreading to the neck and upper trunk (Fig. E1-204).
  2. The flushing episodes last from a few minutes to hours (longer-lasting flushes may be associated with bronchial carcinoids).
  3. Flushing may be triggered by emotion, alcohol, or foods or may occur spontaneously.
  4. Dizziness, tachycardia, and hypotension may be associated with the cutaneous flushing.
- Diarrhea (>70%): often associated with abdominal bloating and audible peristaltic rushes
- Intermittent bronchospasm (25%): characterized by severe dyspnea and wheezing
- Facial telangiectasia
- Tricuspid insufficiency, pulmonic stenosis from carcinoid heart lesions

ETIOLOGY

- Carcinoid syndrome is caused by neoplasms originating from neuroendocrine cells.
- Carcinoid tumors do not usually produce the syndrome unless liver metastases are present or the primary tumor does not involve the gastrointestinal tract.

DIAGNOSIS (Fig. 1-205)

DIFFERENTIAL DIAGNOSIS

- Flushing: Carcinoid syndrome must be distinguished from idiopathic flushing (IF); patients with IF more often are female, are younger, and have a longer duration of symptoms; palpitations, syncope, and hypotension occur primarily in patients with IF. Additional causes of flushing that need to be ruled out are menopause, medications (niacin, nitrates), alcohol, renal cell carcinoma, medullary cancer of thyroid, VIPoma, mastocytosis, and chronic use of food additives (nitrites, sulfites)
- Diarrhea: IBD, IBS, laxative abuse, infectious colitis
- Bronchospasm: asthma, foreign body, GERD, lung neoplasm

LABORATORY TESTS

- The biochemical marker for carcinoid syndrome is increased 24-hr urinary 5-hydroxyindoleacetic acid, a metabolite of serotonin (5-hydroxytryptamine).
- False elevations can be seen with ingestion of certain foods (bananas, pineapples, eggplant, avocados, walnuts) and certain medications (acetaminophen, caffeine, guaifenesin, reserpine); therefore patients should be on a restricted diet and avoid these medications when the test is ordered.
- Falsely low results can occur with use of alcohol, aspirin, MAO inhibitors, and St. John's wort.
- Liver function studies are an unreliable indicator of liver involvement.

IMAGING STUDIES

- CT scan of chest is useful to detect bronchial carcinoids.
- CT scan or MRI of abdomen or a liver and spleen radionuclide scan is useful to detect liver metastases (palpable in >50% of cases).
- Iodine-123–labeled somatostatin can detect carcinoid endocrine tumors with somatostatin receptors.
- Scanning with radiolabeled octreotide (Fig. E1-206) can visualize previously undetected or metastatic lesions.
- PET scan.

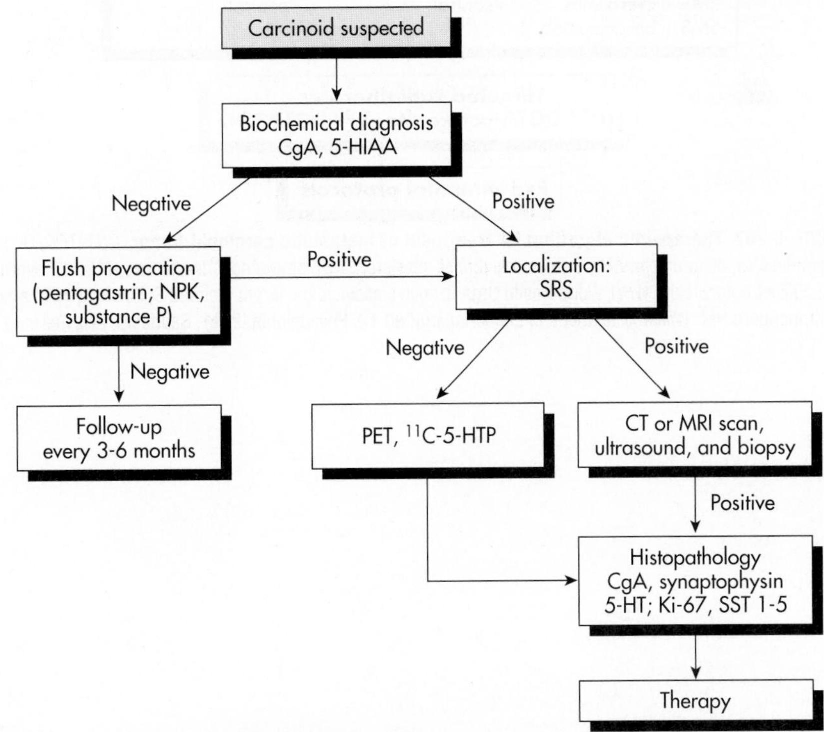

FIGURE 1-205 Diagnostic algorithm for patients with carcinoid tumors. *CgA,* Chromogranin A; *C-5-HTP,* C-5-hydroxytryptophan; *CT,* computed tomography; *5-HIAA,* 5-hydroxyindoleacetic acid; *5-HT,* 5-hydroxytryptamine; *MRI,* magnetic resonance imaging; *NPK,* neuropeptide K; *PET,* positron emission tomography; *SRS,* somatostatin receptor scintigraphy; *SST 1-5,* somatostatin receptor subtypes 1 through 5. (From Melmed S, Polonsky KS, Larsen PR, Kronenberg HM: *Williams textbook of endocrinology,* ed 12, Philadelphia, 2011, Saunders.)

 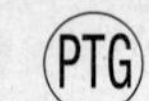

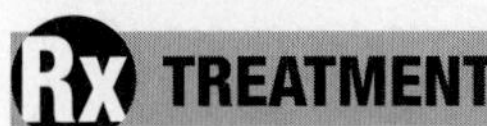

NONPHARMACOLOGIC THERAPY

Avoidance of ethanol ingestion (may precipitate flushing)

GENERAL Rx

- Surgical resection of the tumor can be curative if the tumor is localized or palliative and results in prolonged asymptomatic periods if metastases are present. Surgical manipulation of the tumor can, however, cause severe vasomotor abnormalities and bronchospasm (carcinoid crisis).
- Percutaneous embolization and ligation of the hepatic artery can decrease the bulk of the tumor in the liver and provide palliative treatment of tumors with hepatic metastases.
- Cytotoxic chemotherapy: combination chemotherapy with 5-fluorouracil and streptozocin can be used in patients with unresectable or recurrent carcinoid tumors; however, it has only limited success. Fig. 1-207 describes a therapeutic algorithm for treatment of metastatic carcinoid tumor.

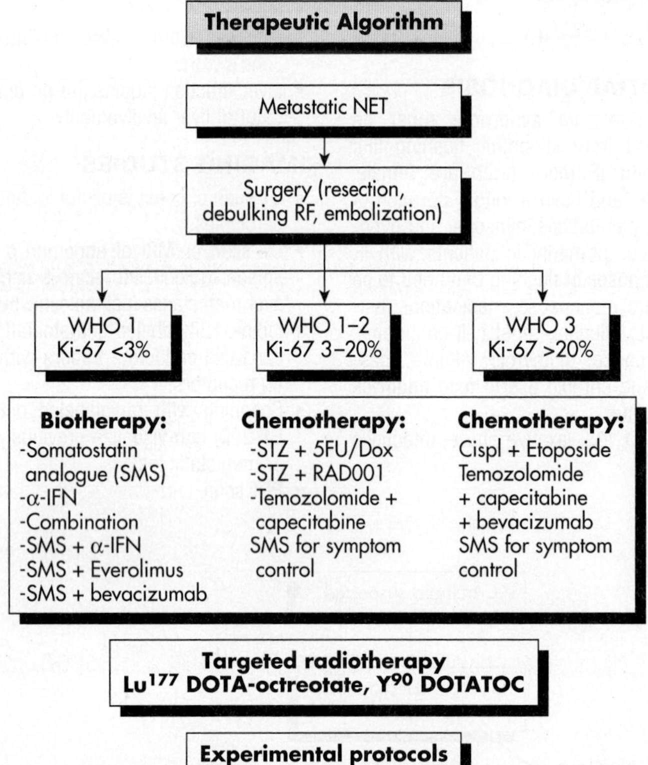

FIGURE 1-207 Therapeutic algorithm for treatment of metastatic carcinoid tumor. *DOTATOC,* DOTA-octreotide; *Dox,* doxorubicin; *5FU,* 5-fluorouracil; *IFN,* interferon; *NET,* neuroendocrine tumor; *RAD001,* everolimus; *STZ,* streptozotocin; *WHO,* World Health Organization classification. (From Melmed S, Polonsky KS, Larsen PR, Kronenberg HM: *Williams Textbook of Endocrinology,* ed 12, Philadelphia, 2011, Saunders, Elsevier Inc.)

- Control of clinical manifestations:
  1. Somatostatin analogues (octreotide and lanreotide) are effective for both flushing and diarrhea in most patients. Interferon alfa may be useful as an additive therapy for persistent symptoms despite use of somatostatin analogues; however, data remain inconclusive.
  2. Flushing may be controlled by the combination of H_1- and H_2-receptor antagonists (e.g., diphenhydramine 25 to 50 mg PO q6h and ranitidine 150 mg bid).
  3. Diarrhea may respond to diphenoxylate with atropine (Lomotil).
  4. Bronchospasm can be treated with aminophylline and/or albuterol.
- Nutritional support: supplemental niacin therapy may be useful to prevent pellagra because the tumor uses dietary tryptophan for serotonin synthesis, resulting in a nutritional deficiency in some patients.
- Interferon alfa may be useful as an additive to control symptoms unresponsive to somatostatin analogues.
- Echocardiography and monitoring for right-sided congestive heart failure are recommended for patients with unresectable disease because endocardial fibrosis, involving predominantly the endocardium, chordae, and valves of the right side of the heart, can occur.

DISPOSITION

Carcinoids of the appendix and rectum have a low malignancy potential and rarely produce the clinical syndrome; metastases are also uncommon if the size of the primary lesion is <2 cm in diameter.

RELATED CONTENT

Carcinoid Syndrome (Patient Information)

AUTHOR: **FRED F. FERRI, M.D.**

BASIC INFORMATION

DEFINITION

Cardiac tamponade is a life-threatening condition where an accumulation of fluid within the pericardial sac causes equal elevation of atrial and pericardial pressures, an exaggerated inspiratory decrease in arterial systolic pressure (pulsus paradoxus), and arterial hypotension.

ICD-9CM CODES
423.3 Cardiac tamponade
ICD-10CM CODES
I31.9 Disease of pericardium, unspecified

PHYSICAL FINDINGS & CLINICAL PRESENTATION

- Chest pain
- Tachypnea/dyspnea
- Beck's triad
  1. Absolute or relative hypotension
  2. Elevated jugular venous pressure (with prominent *x* descent and blunted *y* descent)
  3. Muffled heart sounds
- Tachycardia (except in uremia or hypothyroid patients)
- Pulsus paradoxus (decrease in systolic arterial pressure of 10 mm Hg or more during normal inspiration while in normal sinus rhythm)
- Pericardial friction rub may be present
- Reduced or absent apical cardiac impulse

ETIOLOGY

Acute (rapidly accumulating pericardial effusion leading to cardiac tamponade): does not need a large amount of effusion to cause tamponade
- Penetrating trauma
- Aortic dissection
- Post-infarction myocardial rupture and/or hemorrhagic pericarditis
- Iatrogenic (central line and pacemaker insertions, post–coronary bypass surgery or post–percutaneous coronary intervention)

Subacute or chronic (effusion is usually large):
- Malignancy (e.g., lung, breast, lymphoma)
- Viral pericarditis (e.g., Coxsackie, human immunodeficiency virus)
- Bacterial, fungal, or tuberculous pericarditis
- Uremia
- Hypothyroidism/myxedema (rare)
- Collagen vascular disease (e.g., lupus, rheumatoid arthritis, scleroderma)
- Radiation
- Idiopathic

DIAGNOSIS

Cardiac tamponade is a clinical diagnosis made at the bedside from history and physical examination. The echocardiogram will help confirm or reject the clinical diagnosis. Tamponade can be confirmed invasively by the measurement of elevated intrapericardial pressures with an intrapericardial catheter and right-sided heart catheterization. Typical findings are diastolic equalization of pressures, usually ranging from 10 to 30 mm Hg (diastolic pulmonary artery pressure = right ventricular diastolic pressure = right atrial pressure = intrapericardial pressure) and lowering of the intrapericardial pressure with fluid drainage. Thereafter, the underlying etiology must be determined with specific laboratory work (see "Laboratory Tests" below).

DIFFERENTIAL DIAGNOSIS

Other conditions that can also lead to elevated jugular venous pressure, decreased systemic pressure, and pulsus paradoxus include:
- Chronic obstructive pulmonary disease
- Constrictive pericarditis (Table 1-96)
- Restrictive cardiomyopathy
- Right ventricular infarction
- Pulmonary embolism
- Chronic biventricular heart failure

LABORATORY TESTS

- Electrolytes, blood urea nitrogen, creatinine, erythrocyte sedimentation rate, thyroid function tests, antinuclear antibody, rheumatoid factor, PPD, blood cultures, viral titers, and pericardial fluid analysis and cultures
- Possible 12-lead ECG findings:
  - Sinus tachycardia
  - PR depression and/or diffuse ST elevations if acute pericarditis is present
  - Electrical alternans (beat to beat alternations in the QRS complex) (Fig. 1-208)
  - Low voltage if massive effusion is present. (QRS complex <0.5 mV in the limb leads and <1.0 mV in precordial leads)

IMAGING STUDIES

- Chest radiograph (enlarged cardiac silhouette with clear lung fields) (Fig. 1-209)
- Chest CT (may overestimate size of the effusion) (Fig. 1-210)
- Echocardiogram findings (Fig. E1-211):
  - Pericardial effusion
  - Diastolic collapse of the right atrium (late diastole) is virtually 100% sensitive but has low specificity.
  - Diastolic collapse of the right ventricle (early diastole) is pathognomic.
  - >25% mitral and tricuspid valve inflow variation with respiration
  - Plethoric inferior vena cava (IVC dilation and <50% decrease in the diameter of the IVC during inspiration)
  - Left atrial collapse (high specificity)
- Cardiac catheterization as discussed earlier will see equalization of intracardiac diastolic pressures and increase of right-sided pressures and reduction of left-sided pressures, which subsequently causes pulsus paradoxus

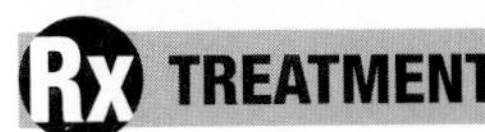

TREATMENT

NONPHARMACOLOGIC THERAPY

- Cardiac tamponade should be treated emergently.
- Avoid drugs that reduce preload (e.g., nitrates, diuretics).
- Large pericardial effusions without hemodynamic compromise (tamponade) can be managed conservatively with careful monitoring, treatment of the underlying cause,

TABLE 1-96 Hemodynamics in Cardiac Tamponade and Constrictive Pericarditis

	Tamponade	Constriction
Paradoxical pulse	Usually present	Present in ~1/3
Equal left- and right-sided filling pressures	Present	Present
Systemic venous wave morphology	Absent *y* descent	Prominent *y* descent (M or W shape)
Inspiratory change in systemic venous pressure	Decrease (normal)	Increase or no change (Kussmaul sign)
"Square root" sign in ventricular pressure	Absent	Present

From Bonow RO: *Heart disease*, ed 9, Philadelphia, 2012, Saunders.

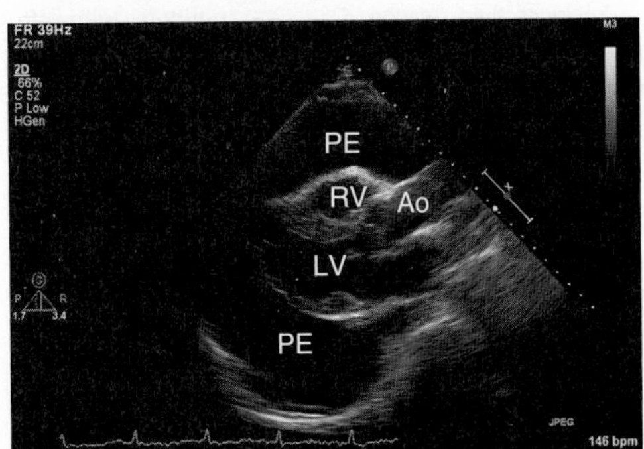

FIGURE 1-208 Two-dimensional echocardiogram of a large, circumferential pericardial effusion (PE). Ao, Aorta; LV, left ventricle; RV, right ventricle. (From Kabbani SS, LeWinter M: Cardiac constriction and restriction. In Crawford MH, DiMarco JP [eds]: *Cardiology*, St Louis, 2001, Mosby.)

 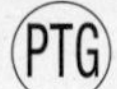

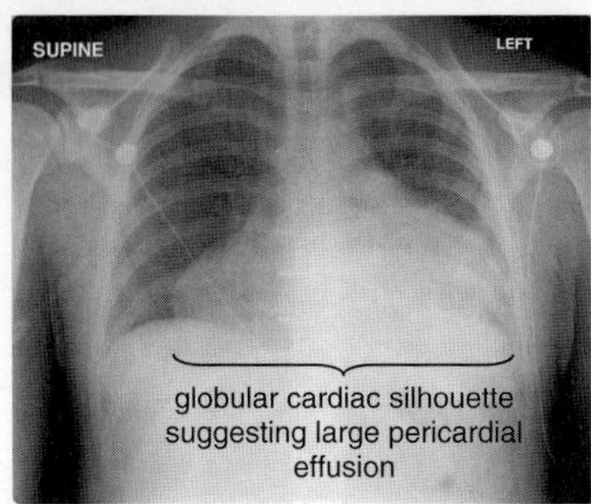

FIGURE 1-209 Massive pericardial effusion and tamponade. This 23-year-old male has a history of aortic valve replacement for infective endocarditis. He presented with increased chest pain and dyspnea. His chest x-ray shows a globular cardiac silhouette, suggesting a large pericardial effusion. The lung fields and right costophrenic angle appear clear, although the left costophrenic angle is hidden behind the heart and cannot be assessed. The patient underwent chest computed tomography to evaluate his aorta, as he complained of severe interscapular pain as well (see Fig. 1-210). (From Broder JS: *Diagnostic imaging for the emergency physician,* Philadelphia, 2011, Saunders.)

clinical follow-up, and frequent serial surveillance echocardiography.

ACUTE GENERAL Rx

- Aggressive intravascular volume expansion (saline or blood)
- Emergency pericardial fluid removal by pericardiocentesis or surgical pericardiotomy by way of the subxiphoid pericardial window
- Pericardiocentesis should be performed under fluoroscopic or echocardiographic guidance when available
- Pericardiocentesis is an absolute contraindication if the etiology of the pericardial effusion is aortic dissection.
- Inotropic or vasopressor support if above measures cannot be performed immediately

CHRONIC Rx

- Depends on etiology.
- Pericardiocentesis with draining catheter: the catheter can be left inside the pericardium to allow continued drainage for 24 to 48 hr. If residual fluid still persists with hemodynamic compromise, surgical drainage should be sought. In the absence of hemodynamic compromise or significant residual fluid, discontinuation of the draining catheter can be done with periodic postprocedure echocardiographic monitoring of reaccumulation (e.g., 24 hr, 7 days, 30 days, 3 mo, 6 mo, 12 mo) depending on the etiology and rate of reaccumulation.
- Other surgical drainage procedures include:
  1. Subxiphoid pericardiotomy drainage
  2. Limited pericardiectomy draining the pericardial fluid into the left hemithorax
  3. Pericardial window
  4. Complete pericardiectomy, especially in patients with effusive-constrictive pericarditis or bacterial pericarditis (see "Pearls & Considerations" below).

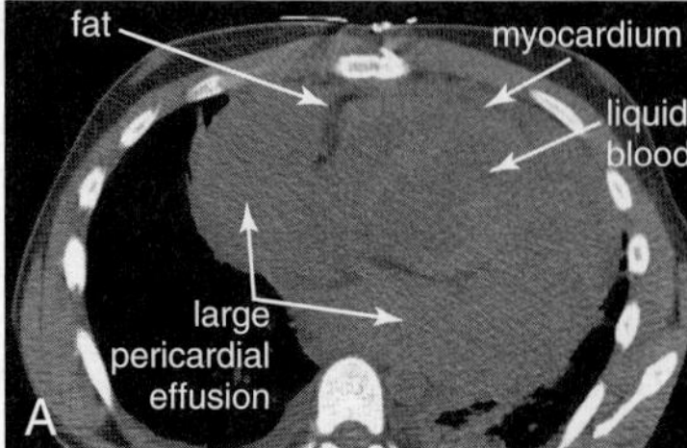

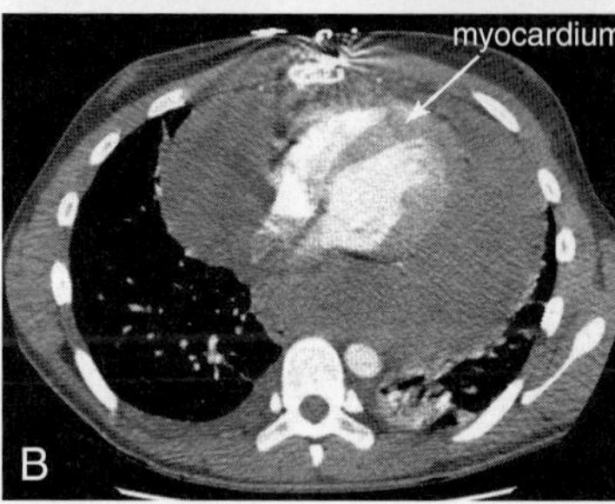

FIGURE 1-210 Massive pericardial effusion. Same patient as Fig. 1-209. The patient underwent chest computed tomography (CT) without **(A)** and then with **(B)** intravenous contrast to evaluate his aorta, which was normal. However, the CT confirmed a massive pericardial effusion surrounding a normal-appearing heart. Without contrast, note that fluid blood within the chambers of the heart has a slightly lower density than the pericardial effusion, which has a density more similar to that of myocardium. When contrast is administered, the ventricular chambers fill completely, and the myocardium enhances and becomes somewhat brighter than the surrounding pericardial effusion. The heart itself is outlined by a thin stripe of fat, which appears nearly black on soft tissue windows. The patient developed hypotension, suggesting cardiac tamponade, and pericardial window was performed for drainage of the effusion. In the operating room, the effusion was found to be coagulated blood. (From Broder JS: *Diagnostic imaging for the emergency physician,* Philadelphia, 2011, Saunders.)

DISPOSITION

The prognosis of cardiac tamponade depends on the underlying cause.

REFERRAL

- Emergent cardiology consultation should be made if cardiac tamponade is suspected.
- Cardiothoracic surgery consultation should also be considered if surgical pericardial drainage is indicated.

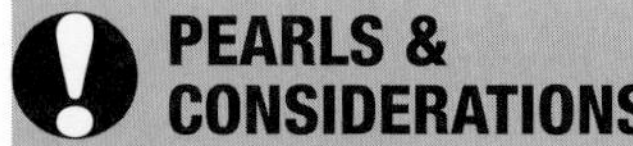

PEARLS & CONSIDERATIONS

- Cardiac tamponade should always be considered during pulseless electrical activity arrest and may require emergent pericardiocentesis.
- Evaluation for pulsus paradoxus should always be performed during normal respiration because deep inspiration may render a false-positive finding.
- Strong consideration should be given to performing early pericardiocentesis in patients who have pericardial effusion associated with bacterial pneumonia or empyema because the incidence of bacterial pericarditis is especially high in this clinical situation and the subsequent development of cardiac tamponade and severe chronic constrictive pericarditis occurs frequently.
- Pericardiocentesis is an absolute contraindication if the etiology of the pericardial effusion is due to aortic dissection extending into the pericardial sac.
- As little as 100 ml of fluid can lead to acute cardiac tamponade if the rate of accumulation is rapid, whereas with gradual accumulation, the pericardial sac can hold up to 5 L of fluid before tamponade occurs.

SUGGESTED READINGS

available at www.expertconsult.com

RELATED CONTENT

Cardiac Tamponade (Patient Information)

AUTHORS: **JENNIFER JANTZ, M.D.,** and **ARAVIND RAO KOKKIRALA, M.D.**

DEFINITION

Cardiomyopathy, chemical-induced (CMc) is the changes of cardiac structure and function caused by chemical compounds, either medically prescribed or not medically prescribed. The common chemicals available in the U.S. include alcohol, cocaine, amphetamine, doxorubicin, 5-fluorouracil (5-FU), zidovudine, and trastuzumab.

SYNONYMS

Alcoholic cardiomyopathy (ACM)
Cocaine-induced CM
Anabolic steroid–induced CM
Anthracycline-induced CM

ICD-10CM CODES

I42.7 Cardiomyopathy due to drug and external agent

EPIDEMIOLOGY & DEMOGRAPHICS

- ACM occurs in about 10% of alcoholics. The prevalence ranges from 23% to 40% of nonischemic cardiomyopathy.
- Doxorubicin-induced cardiomyopathy is dose dependent-based on cumulative doses. The incidence is reported as 0.14% at doses less than 300 mg/m^2, 5% at doses less than 450 mg/m^2, 7% at 550 mg/m^2, and as great as 18% at 700 mg/m^2.
- Significant cardiotoxicity is also caused by the chemotherapeutic agents trastuzumab, used commonly in breast cancer, which can cause cardiomyopathy in >8% cases but is a reversible cardiomyopathy. However, the incidence of cardiomyopathy can be as high as 27% when given in conjunction or following anthracycline therapy.
- Other chemotherapeutic agents known to cause cardiomyopathy include epirubicin, docetaxel, mitomycin, cyclophosphamide, bortezomib, sunitinib, 5-fluorouracil [5-FU], and emerging reports of carfilzomib.

PREDOMINANT SEX AND AGE: Among ACM cases, men represent more than 80% and have higher mortality. In all races, blacks have higher death rates compared to whites. Anthracycline- and trastuzumab-induced cardiomyopathy is predominantly more common in those age >60 years.

GENETICS

- In patients with ACM, deletion (DD) genotype of ACE is more common than insertion (II) and deletion insertion (DI) genotypes.
- Anthracycline-induced cardiomyopathy is linked to an increase in cardiac oxidative stress, via the pathways of mitochondria, nitric oxide synthesis, and nicotinamide adenine dinucleotide phosphate reduced.
- One study suggests that polymorphisms in the carbonyl reductase genes could be related to anthracycline-induced CM.

RISK FACTORS

- Consumption of more than 90 gm/day of alcohol for more than 5 years is necessary to develop ACM.
- The occurrence of chronic anthracycline-induced CM is correlated to cumulative dose (ranging from 7% to 26% of patients who received >550 mg/m^2), age, preexisting heart disease, concomitant chemotherapy, and history of mediastinal radiation therapy. Children are more susceptible to anthracycline-induced CM.
- Continuous infusions of chemotherapy pose a higher risk for cardiotoxicity, compared to bolus regimens.

PHYSICAL FINDINGS & CLINICAL PRESENTATION

The majority of clinical characteristics of CMc are similar to the dilated cardiomyopathy of other etiologies. Symptoms may develop either insidiously or acute in onset.

- The acute anthracycline-induced cardiotoxicity can start at anytime after the first dose and presents with arrhythmias, most commonly supraventricular tachycardia, ventricular dysfunction, and pericardial diseases. The sub-acute and chronic symptoms occur from 3 months after the last dose to 10 years later. Patients usually present with congestive heart failure (CHF). More recently, mortality has improved as a result of medical treatment with ACE inhibitors and beta-blockers.
- Cardiac symptoms after 5-FU treatment include angina (most common), myocardial infarction, arrhythmia, acute pulmonary edema, cardiac arrest, and pericarditis. The mortality of 5-FU–induced cardiotoxicity is 2% to 13%.
- The presentation of CHF may occur over 15 years of heavy drinking. In the presentation of arrhythmia, atrial fibrillation is most common and ventricular tachycardia is also experienced frequently.
- Patients with cocaine CM may present with adrenergic symptoms (palpitations, pallor, diaphoresis, and anxiety), hypertension, angina, atrial and ventricular arrhythmia, and heart failure.
- Anabolic steroids can cause left ventricular hypertrophy and dilation, and can lead to heart failure, arrhythmia, myocardial infarction, hypertension, and sudden death.

ETIOLOGY

The underlying mechanism of chemotherapy is not well established. Several pathways have been proposed, including an increase in oxidative stress, free radical production, apoptosis, disturbance of DNA, RNA and protein synthesis, and vasospasm. Nutritional deficiency also plays a role in ACM.

Dx DIAGNOSIS

DIFFERENTIAL DIAGNOSIS

- Ischemic cardiomyopathy
- Dilated cardiomyopathy, related to valvular disease, hypertension, and causes other than chemicals
- Cirrhotic cardiomyopathy

WORKUP

- The diagnosis is based on the history of chemical exposure and the clinical presentation of heart failure, arrhythmia, and angina pectoris.
- Electrocardiogram (ECG) and serum electrolytes, renal function, and liver function
- Serum troponin and brain natriuretic peptide (BNP) levels
- Transthoracic echocardiogram for the evaluation of heart structure and function
- Rule out the diagnosis of coronary artery disease by coronary angiography.

LABORATORY TESTS

- There are no specific diagnostic tests to help differentiate CMc from other forms of CM, but the following laboratory tests are generally helpful.
- Serum electrolytes, renal function, liver function, thyroid-stimulating hormone, iron profile, and inflammatory factors
- Serum troponin and BNP (nonspecific) Recent studies have suggested that early elevation of troponin I levels within 72 hours of chemotherapy infusion may be an early predictor of future development of cardiomyopathy.

IMAGING STUDIES

- ECG
  - ST deviation and atrial and ventricular arrhythmia in 5-FU toxicity
    - Sinus tachycardia
    - Nonspecific ST-T change
    - Decreased QRS voltage
    - Prolonged QT interval
- Echocardiogram
  - Asymptomatic alcoholics may present with mild left ventricular (LV) hypertrophy, diastolic dysfunction, LV dilation, and decrease in left ventricular ejection fraction (LVEF).
  - Baseline LVEF should be performed before initiation of doxorubicin-based chemotherapy with either serial echocardiograms or MUGA (multigated acquisition) scan.
    - If baseline LVEF is >55%, then subsequent evaluation should be at the end of treatment if anthracycline dose is <200 mg/m^2 or serially at 200, 300, 350, and 400 mg/m^2 dose completion. Doxorubicin therapy should be discontinued if there is a >15% absolute drop or >10% drop below normal or symptomatic congestive heart failure develops.
- Radionuclide imaging (Figure 1-212).
  - If baseline LVEF ≤55%, the cardiac risks vs. oncological benefits should be discussed with the patient, cardiologist, and oncologist before initiating therapy. Cardioprotective agents such as ACE inhibitors and beta blockers should be initiated and serial LVEF measurements done after each dose. Starting doxorubicin for LVEF <30% is absolutely contraindicated.
  - Even after chemotherapy is completed, annual LVEF measurements with echocardiograms or MUGA scans should be done for 5 years to detect late anthracycline cardiotoxicity.

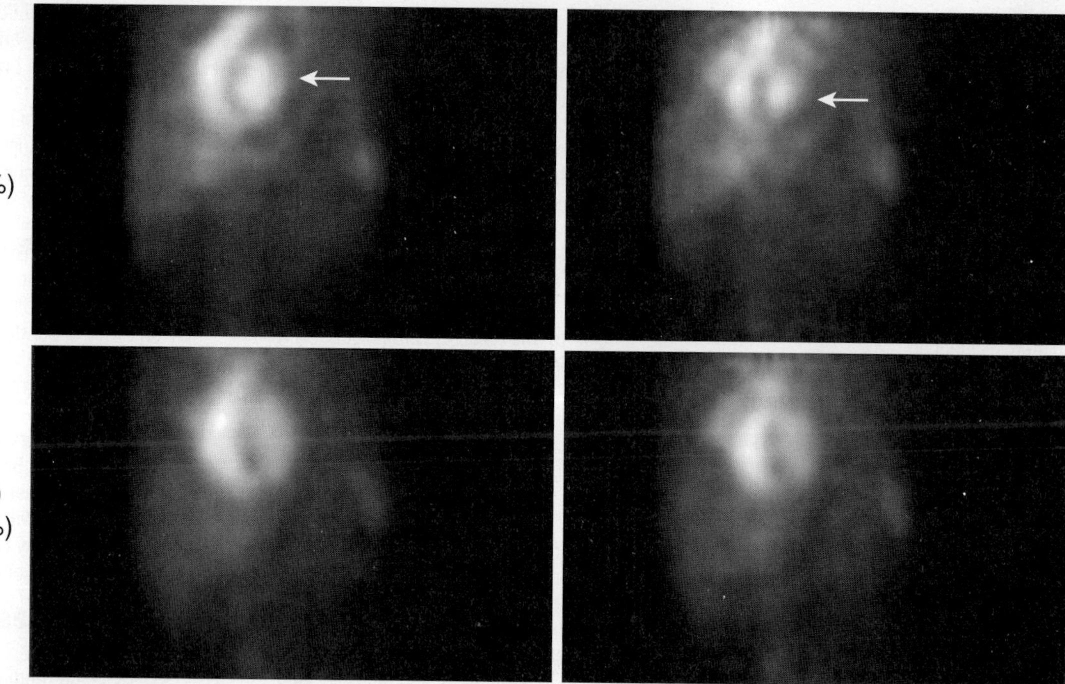

FIGURE 1-212 Technetium-99m-pertechnetate multigated acquisition scans in a 47-year-old woman with breast cancer treated with doxorubicin. The top scan was taken before initiation of doxorubicin and cyclophosphamide therapy in September 2009. The left ventricular ejection fraction (left ventricular end-diastolic counts minus left ventricular end-systolic counts/left ventricular end-diastolic counts 100) was calculated at 60%. The bottom scan was taken in March 2010 after treatment with a total doxorubicin dose of 451 mg/m^2. Left ventricular ejection fraction was calculated at 28%. Left ventricle (*white arrows*) during end-diastole and end-systole. (From Figuerado VM: Chemical cardiomyopathies: the negative effects of medications and nonprescribed drugs on the heart, *Am J Med* 124:480-488, 2011.)

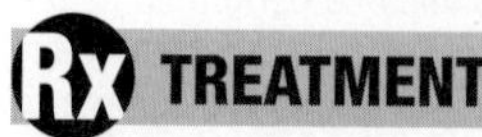

TREATMENT

NONPHARMACOLOGIC THERAPY

- The noninvasive assessment of LV function before, during, and after anthracycline-containing chemotherapy by means of echocardiograms and MUGA scan.
- To reduce the risk of anthracycline-induced cardiotoxicity, the lifetime cumulative dosage should be limited to 450 mg/m^2 in adults.
- Other approaches include the use of infusion other than bolus, liposome encapsulation of doxorubicin, less cardiotoxic analogs of doxorubicin such as epirubicin, and co-administration of dexrazoxane.
- Termination of 5-FU treatment if presenting cardiac symptoms and re-administration is not recommended
- In patients with ACM, abstinence can significantly reverse LV systolic dysfunction.

ACUTE GENERAL Rx

- Treat decompensated CHF with diuresis, and vasopressors if low cardiac output.
- For angina in acute cocaine intoxication, benzodiazepines, nitrites, and calcium channel blockers are the first line of therapy. Once myocardial infarction is indicated by ECG and serum troponin, patients should be evaluated by cardiac catheterization.

CHRONIC Rx

- Nitrites, beta-blockers, and calcium channel blockers angina caused by 5-FU
- Dexrazoxane is an ethylenediaminetetraacetic acid–like chelator that acts by binding to iron, which prevents anthracycline cardiotoxicity. American Society of Clinical Oncology 2008 guideline suggests a 10:1 ratio of dexrazoxane to anthracycline, administered 15 to 30 minutes prior to doxorubicin administration. However, the routine use of the drug is not recommended except in the case of a cumulative dose of doxorubicin of 300 mg/m^2 or greater.
- Beta-blocker: In one study, carvedilol preserves LV diastolic function and chamber size after doxorubicin treatment, compared to placebo.
- ACE inhibitor: Enalapril and ramipril can improve myocardial contractility after doxorubicin or epirubicin treatment.
- Thiamine, folic acid, and multivitamins are adjunctive treatment of ACM.

DISPOSITION

Prognosis depends on the dosage of chemicals and the severity of LV dysfunction.

REFERRAL

Closely follow up with cardiologist.

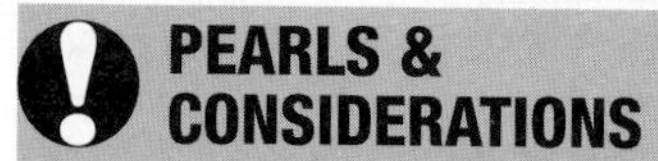

PEARLS & CONSIDERATIONS

Routine follow up is not recommended. Acute cardiotoxicity of chemotherapy is uncommon and not life-threatening. The presentation of chronic toxicity ranges from asymptomatic decline in LVEF to heart failure. The incidence is dose-limited.

SUGGESTED READINGS

available at www.expertconsult.com

AUTHORS: **SADDAM SALEH ABISSE, M.D.**, and **ARAVIND RAO KOKKIRALA, M.D.**

BASIC INFORMATION

DEFINITION

Dilated cardiomyopathy describes a group of diseases involving the myocardium and characterized by myocardial dysfunction that is not wholly the result of hypertension, coronary atherosclerosis, valvular dysfunction, or congenital or other structural heart disease. As a result, the heart is enlarged and the ventricles are dilated with impaired systolic function.

SYNONYMS

Congestive cardiomyopathy

ICD-9CM CODES
425.4 Other primary cardiomyopathies
425.5 Alcoholic cardiomyopathy
425.8 Cardiomyopathy in other diseases classified elsewhere
425.9 Secondary cardiomyopathy, unspecified

ICD-10 CODES
I42.5 Other restrictive cardiomyopathy
I42.6 Alcoholic cardiomyopathy
I43 Cardiomyopathy in diseases classified elsewhere
I42.7 Cardiomyopathy due to drug and external agent

EPIDEMIOLOGY & DEMOGRAPHICS

- The estimated prevalence of dilated cardiomyopathy in the general adult population is approximately 1:2500. The incidence is approximately 4 to 8 per 100,000 persons per yr.
- The incidence of dilated cardiomyopathy is greatest in middle age and among men.
- It is the most common cardiomyopathy and accounts for 25% of cases of congestive heart failure.

PHYSICAL FINDINGS & CLINICAL PRESENTATION

The patient will present the common symptoms of congestive heart failure, which may be of insidious or more sudden onset. The patient may also be asymptomatic and the diagnosis made by the unexpected finding of cardiomegaly on a chest x-ray. The history should focus also on information that could help determine the etiology. Classical signs of heart failure may be absent. When present, findings are indistinguishable from other heart failure syndromes, including:

- Increased jugular venous pressure
- Narrow pulse pressure
- Pulmonary rales, hepatomegaly, peripheral edema
- S3, S4
- Mitral regurgitation, tricuspid regurgitation (less common)

ETIOLOGY

In approximate order of occurrence:

- Idiopathic (often a viral infection that cannot be confirmed)
- Infections (viral [Coxsackie B, adenovirus, parvovirus, HIV], rickettsial, mycobacterial, toxoplasmosis, trichinosis, Chagas' disease)
- Alcoholism (15% to 40% of all cases in Western countries)
- Uncontrolled tachyarrhythmia ("tachycardia-mediated")
- Peripartum (greatest risk from last trimester of pregnancy to 6 mo postpartum)
- Chemotherapeutic (anthracycline, doxorubicin, daunorubicin) or pharmacologic agents (antiretrovirals, phenothiazines)
- Substance abuse (cocaine, heroin, organic solvents "glue-sniffer's heart")
- Postmyocarditis
- Toxins (cobalt, lead, phosphorus, carbon monoxide, mercury)
- Collagen-vascular disease (systemic lupus, rheumatoid arthritis, polyarteritis, dermatomyositis, sarcoidosis)
- Heredofamilial neuromuscular disease (e.g., muscular dystrophy)
- Excess hormones (acromegaly, osteogenesis imperfecta, myxedema, thyrotoxicosis, diabetes)
- Hematologic (e.g., sickle cell anemia, hemochromatosis)
- Stress-induced (i.e., takotsubo or broken heart syndrome)
- TTN truncating mutations (mutations in TTN, the gene encoding the sarcome protein titin) are a common cause of dilated cardiomyopathy, occurring in approximately 25% of familial cases of idiopathic dilated cardiomyopathy and in 18% of sporadic cases.

Dx DIAGNOSIS

Dilated cardiomyopathy is a diagnosis of exclusion, made after ruling out other potential causes of myocardial dysfunction.

DIFFERENTIAL DIAGNOSIS

- Coronary atherosclerosis, that is, left ventricular dysfunction secondary to ischemia and/or myocardial infarction
- Valvular dysfunction (especially aortic and mitral regurgitation)
- Other cardiomyopathies (restrictive, hypertrophic)
- Pulmonary disease (embolism, obstructive, restrictive)
- Pericardial abnormalities (constrictive pericarditis, tamponade)
- Hypothyroidism/myxedema

WORKUP

- Medical history: emphasis on symptoms of dyspnea, orthopnea, paroxysmal nocturnal dyspnea, weight gain, palpitations, or signs of systemic and pulmonary embolism
- Physical exam (see "Physical Findings & Clinical Presentation")
- Testing (see "Laboratory Tests" and "Imaging Studies" for more detail): laboratory, chest x-ray, ECG, echocardiogram, cardiac catheterization; myocardial biopsy is not routinely recommended, unless acute myocarditis requiring immunosuppressive therapy is considered (e.g., giant cell myocarditis)

LABORATORY TESTS

- Chemistries/metabolites (deficiencies), renal function tests (renal dysfunction)
- Cardiac biomarkers (elevation of cardiac troponin or BNP)
  - Persistently increased cardiac troponin T levels are a marker of poor outcome in cardiomyopathy patients
- Endocrine (particularly thyroid)
- Iron studies (hemochromatosis, deficiency)
- Rheumatologic and Inflammatory (ANA, ESR, CRP)
- Others as indicated (HIV, Lyme, neurohormonal)

IMAGING STUDIES

Chest x-ray:

- Cardiac silhouette enlargement (particularly left ventricle)
- Pulmonary vascular redistribuition and congestion (Kerley B lines, cephalization of vasculature), pleural effusion (may appear as unilateral, most often on the right side)

ECG:

- ECG findings are typically nonspecific, and sinus tachycardia is usually a reflection of underlying heart failure
- Intraventricular conduction defects and left bundle branch block
- Arrhythmias (atrial fibrillation, premature ventricular or atrial contractions, ventricular tachycardia)

Echocardiogram (Fig. E1-213):

- Low ejection fraction with global hypokinesis
- Four-chamber enlargement (LV enlargement usually predominates)
- Mitral or tricuspid regurgitation (due to incomplete leaflet closure caused by ventricular dilation)

Cardiac catheterization:

- On initial presentation to exclude obstructive epicardial coronary artery disease

Cardiac magnetic resonance imaging (CMRI):

- Particularly if infiltrative or inflammatory etiology suspected

Rx TREATMENT

NONPHARMACOLOGIC THERAPY

- Treatment of underlying disease (systemic lupus, alcoholism)
- Dietary sodium restriction (<2 g/day).
- Exercise training has been shown to be associated with reduced risk for hospitalization and death in patients with history of heart failure in limited trials; enrollment in a formal cardiac rehabilitation program may be beneficial in improving patient's functional status

ACUTE GENERAL Rx

- Diuretics are indicated for all patients with current symptoms or history of heart failure and reduced left ventricular ejection fraction (LVEF) with evidence of volume overload (peripheral edema, orthopnea, paroxysmal nocturnal dyspnea).

- ACE inhibitors (and angiotensin receptor blockers) have been shown to have favorable effects on ventricular remodeling in patients with cardiomyopathy and a demonstrable mortality benefit in these patients. Therefore they are recommended in all patients with reduced LV systolic function, regardless of symptoms, unless specific contraindications exist.
- Beta-blockers (in particular, carvedilol, long-acting metoprolol, and bisoprolol) work by inhibiting the adverse effects of the sympathetic nervous system in patients with ventricular systolic dysfunction, and have likewise shown a mortality benefit in patients with LV systolic dysfunction; unless specifically contraindicated, they should be started once the acute exacerbation has resolved.
- Aldosterone antagonists have shown mortality benefit along with decreased rate of hospitalization for heart failure in patients with symptomatic heart failure and reduced LV systolic function. They should be used following label guidelines and with close monitoring of renal function and potassium.
- Additional medical therapies (direct renin inhibitors, hydralazine/nitrates, digitalis) can be considered in certain patient subpopulations with persistent symptoms on otherwise optimal medical management.
- Patients with associated coronary atherosclerosis (angina, ECG changes, reversible defects on myocardial perfusion imaging) may benefit from percutaneous or surgical revascularization.

CHRONIC Rx

- As above in "Acute General Rx."

DISPOSITION

- Annual mortality rate is 20% in patients with moderate heart failure, and it exceeds 50% in patients with severe heart failure. Once symptomatic, hospitalizations are frequent and readmission rates are high (>50% at 3 mo). A multispecialty treatment approach (e.g., primary care, cardiology, nutrition, cardiac rehabilitation) is recommended.
- Factors associated with an adverse outcome in dilated cardiomyopathy are described in Table 1-97.

REFERRAL

- Patients with dilated cardiomyopathy are at increased risk for ventricular arrhythmias and sudden cardiac death. Implantation of a cardiac defibrillator for primary prevention of sudden cardiac death can be considered for patients with LVEF <35% on optimal medical therapy regardless of symptom status.
- Patients with LVEF <35%, bundle branch block on ECG (QRS ≥0.12 sec), and persistent heart failure symptoms may benefit from cardiac resynchronization therapy via a biventricular pacemaker.
- Consider heart transplantation for relatively young patients (there is no precise age threshold) free of other significant comorbid conditions who are unresponsive to medical therapy. Dilated cardiomyopathy is the reason for 45% of all heart transplantations in the U.S.

TABLE 1-97 Factors Associated with an Adverse Outcome in Dilated Cardiomyopathy

Clinical	Noninvasive	Invasive
NYHA Class III/IV	Low LV ejection fraction	High LV filling pressures
Increasing age	Marked LV dilation	
Low exercise peak oxygen consumption	Low LV mass	
Marked intraventricular conduction delay	≥Moderate mitral regurgitation	
Complex ventricular arrhythmias	Abnormal diastolic function	
Abnormal signal-averaged ECG	Abnormal contractile reserve	
Evidence of excessive sympathetic stimulation	Right ventricular dilation or dysfunction	
Protodiastolic gallop (S_3)		
Elevated serum BNP		
Elevated uric acid		
Decreased serum sodium		

BNP, Brain natriuretic peptide; *ECG,* electrocardiogram; *LV,* left ventricular; *NYHA,* New York Heart Association.
From Hare JM: The dilated, restrictive, and infiltrative cardiomyopathies. In Bonow RO et al (eds): *Braunwald's heart disease—a textbook of cardiovascular medicine,* ed 9, St Louis, 2011, Saunders.

PEARLS & CONSIDERATIONS

COMMENTS

- Patients should be encouraged to restrict or eliminate alcohol and reduce sodium intake (<2 g daily).
- Patients may benefit from daily weight checks as a means of early detection of volume overload and decompensated heart failure.
- Vulnerability to cardiomyopathy among chronic alcohol abusers is partially genetic and related to the presence of the ACE DD genotype.
- Idiopathic dilated cardiomyopathy is often familial, and apparently healthy relatives may have latent, early, or undiagnosed disease. Echocardiographic evaluation of family members is recommended.
- Incorporation of sequencing approaches that detect TTN truncations into genetic testing for dilated cardiomyopathy may substantially increase test sensitivity and allow earlier diagnosis of dilated cardiomyopathy.

SUGGESTED READINGS

available at www.expertconsult.com

RELATED CONTENT

Fig. 3-43 Initial approach to classification of cardiomyopathy (Algorithm)
Table 3-2 Profiles of Myocardial Disease
Dilated Cardiomyopathy (Patient Information)

AUTHORS: **ATIZAZUL H. MANSOOR, M.D., DAVID J. FORTUNATO, M.D., F.A.C.C.,** and **FRED F. FERRI, M.D.**

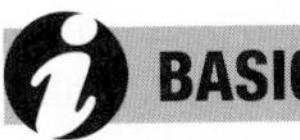

BASIC INFORMATION

DEFINITION

Hypertrophic cardiomyopathy (HCM) is an autosomal dominant myocardial disorder characterized by disorganized myocyte architecture and marked thickening (hypertrophy) of the left ventricular wall (>15 mm), without dilation, not explained by another cardiac or systemic disorder. The interventricular septum is the most common site of enlargement, though hypertrophy may involve other focal regions or may be concentric. HCM may result in hemodynamically significant obstruction within the left ventricular outflow tract (LVOT) and/or impairment of the diastolic function of the left ventricle.

SYNONYMS

HCM
Hypertrophic cardiomyopathy
Idiopathic hypertrophic subaortic stenosis (IHSS)
Hypertrophic obstructive cardiomyopathy (HOCM)
Asymmetric septal hypertrophy (ASH)

ICD-9CM CODES

425.1 Hypertrophic obstructive cardiomyopathy
425.4 Other primary cardiomyopathies
746.84 Congenital obstructive anomalies of the heart not elsewhere classified

ICD-10 CODES

I42.1 Obstructive hypertrophic cardiomyopathy

EPIDEMIOLOGY & DEMOGRAPHICS

- Prevalence in the general population is 1 in 500 (the most common genetically transmitted cardiovascular disease).
- HCM is the most common cause of sudden cardiac death in young athletes (more commonly among blacks).
- There is equal prevalence in men and women (probably underdiagnosed in women).
- It occurs across ethnicities, perhaps underdiagnosed among blacks.
- Mortality rate is approximately 1%/yr, as high as to 2%/yr in children.
- The most common form of the disease is familial (60% to 70% of cases), and it follows an autosomal dominant inheritance pattern with variable expression.
- Spontaneous mutations can also occur, accounting for approximately 20% of cases. It is otherwise indistinguishable from the familial form.
- A variant form seen in the elderly (5% to 10% of cases) has a better prognosis, and it is not typically associated with sudden cardiac death.
- The familial form is usually diagnosed in young patients. It is most often caused by a mutation in one of the contractile protein genes of the cardiac sarcomere. 1400 mutations with variable phenotype, expressivity, and penetrance have been identified thus far. Most of the affected genes include β-myosin heavy chain, myosin-binding protein C, cardiac troponin T and I, α-tropomyosin, actin, titin, and myosin light chains.
- Nonsarcomeric genetic mutations that cause storage disease (e.g., Fabry disease) have a very similar clinical presentation.
- Apical HCM is a variant more common among Asians: as many as 41% of Chinese HCM and 15% of Japanese HCM patients. Clinically there is no LVOT obstruction.

PHYSICAL FINDINGS & CLINICAL PRESENTATION

Patients may have subtle symptoms of progressive congestive heart failure (CHF). At time of diagnosis, most patients are asymptomatic, referred and diagnosed based on family history. HCM may be suspected on the basis of abnormalities found on physical examination. Classic findings include:

- Harsh, systolic, crescendo–decrescendo murmur at the left sternal border or apex. The murmur increases with maneuvers that decrease venous return or LV size (Valsalva, standing), and decreases with those that increase venous return or afterload (squatting, hand grip, post-Valsalva release).
- Paradoxic splitting of S2 (if left ventricular obstruction is present).
- S4 may be present.
- Double or triple LV apical impulse ("triple ripple": atrial contraction, early rapid ejection, and late slow ejection).
- Pulsus bisferens (double pulsation on palpation of the carotid pulse).

Increased obstruction can occur with:

- Drugs: digitalis, β-adrenergic stimulators (isoproterenol, dopamine, epinephrine), nitroglycerin, vasodilators, diuretics, alcohol
- Hypovolemia
- Tachycardia
- Valsalva maneuver
- Standing position

Decreased obstruction is seen with:

- Drugs: β-adrenergic blockers, calcium channel blockers, disopyramide, α-adrenergic stimulators
- Volume expansion
- Bradycardia
- Hand-grip exercise
- Squatting position
- Release phase of the Valsalva maneuver

Clinical manifestations are as follows:

- Dyspnea
- Syncope (usually seen with exercise)
- Angina
- Palpitations
- Sudden cardiac death

ETIOLOGY

- Genetic: Autosomal dominant trait with variable penetrance caused by mutations in multiple genes encoding proteins of the cardiac sarcomere and calcium regulation. To date, >1400 mutations have been identified among at least 13 genes.
- Sporadic occurrence.

Dx DIAGNOSIS

DIFFERENTIAL DIAGNOSIS

- Hypertensive heart disease
- Valvular disease, especially aortic stenosis
- Cardiac amyloidosis
- Fabry disease
- Non–sarcomeric protein mutations: gamma 2 regulatory subunit of AMP-activated protein kinase (PRKAG2) mutation
- Lysosome-associated membrane protein 2 (LAMP2) mutation: Danon disease
- Athlete's heart

WORKUP

- Medical history: focus on signs and symptoms of CHF (dyspnea, orthopnea, paroxysmal nocturnal dyspnea), palpitations, any history of syncope or presyncope, chest pain, and family history of sudden death.
- Physical exam: see "Physical Findings & Clinical Presentation."
- Genetic counseling with or without testing.
- ECG is abnormal in 75% to 95% of patients, although there are no pathognomonic findings. Typical findings include:
    - LV hypertrophy (abnormally tall R waves in the precordial leads) in up to 80% of patients
    - Abnormal Q waves in lateral and inferior leads (Fig. 1-214)
    - T wave inversions (associated with the apical hypertrophy predominant variant)
- Echocardiography (Fig. 1-215) is usually diagnostic as the majority of patients have significant LV hypertrophy. (See "Imaging Studies" for details.)
- 24-hour Holter monitor to screen for potentially lethal ventricular arrhythmias (principal cause of syncope or sudden death in obstructive cardiomyopathy) should be performed at diagnosis and annually afterward as part of routine follow-up regardless of symptoms.
- In the absence of significant LVOT obstruction, exercise testing is indicated at diagnosis and annually afterward to evaluate for symptoms and response to exercise. A drop in systolic blood pressure or failure to augment with exercise is a marker of poor prognosis and it is one of the indicators for referral for myotomy/myomectomy.
- Biomarkers of myocardial fibrosis in HCM include BNP and high-sensitivity cardiac troponin T and I.
- Screening for sarcomere protein gene mutations in family members of patients with HCM can identify a broad subgroup of patients with increased propensity toward long-term impairment of left ventricular function and adverse outcome, irrespective of the myofilament (thick, intermediate, or thin) involvement.

IMAGING STUDIES

- Chest x-ray may be normal or show cardiomegaly.
- Two-dimensional echocardiography is used to establish the diagnosis and assess the severity of obstruction when present. LV wall thickness will usually be >15 mm (although some may be genetically positive but phenotype negative), and most patients (up to 95%) will have asymmetric (ratio of septum thickness to left ventricular wall thickness >1.3:1) LV wall hypertrophy. Symmetric LV hypertrophy

 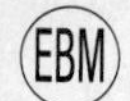

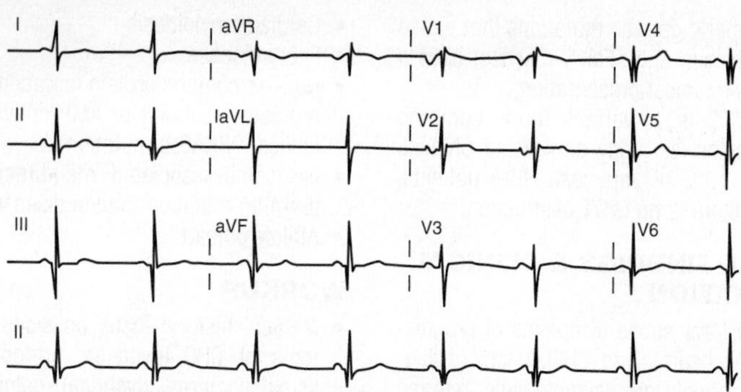

FIGURE 1-214 Surface ECG in a patient with hypertrophic cardiomyopathy. Note the deep narrow Q waves in the inferolateral leads. (From Issa Z et al: *Clinical arrhythmology and electrophysiology,* ed 2, Philadelphia, 2012, Saunders.)

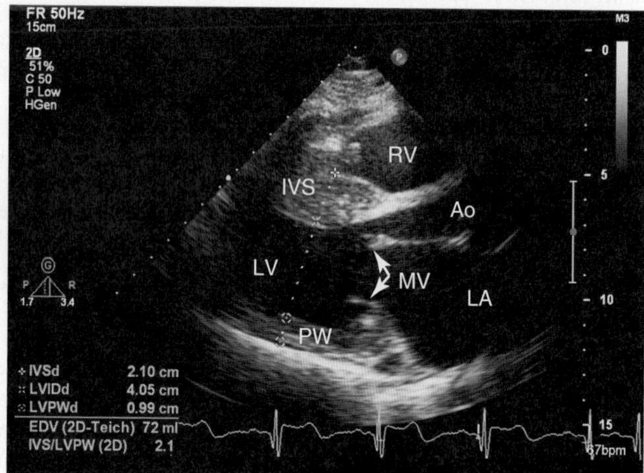

FIGURE 1-215 Echocardiographic appearance of hypertrophic cardiomyopathy. Parasternal long-axis view from a patient with hypertrophic cardiomyopathy demonstrating asymmetrical septal hypertrophy. The interventricular septum (marked by *arrow*) measures 2.1 cm; the posterior wall measures 0.99 cm. *Ao,* Aorta; *IVS,* interventricular septum; *LA,* left atrium; *LV,* left ventricle; *MV,* mitral valve; *PW,* posterior wall; *RV,* right ventricle. (From Issa Z et al: *Clinical arrhythmology and electrophysiology,* ed 2, Philadelphia, 2012, Saunders.)

is less common. The septum is most often affected, followed by the left ventricular midcavity and apex. In addition, 25% to 30% of patients will manifest systolic anterior motion of the anterior leaflet of the mitral valve, causing obstruction of the LVOT and mitral regurgitation. Two-dimensional strain imaging echocardiography is useful for differentiation of HCM and cardiac amyloidosis from other causes of ventricular wall thickening. Up to 80% of HCM patients will also have diastolic dysfunction as evidenced by pulsed mitral valve inflow pattern and tissue Doppler.

- Cardiac MRI or cardiac CT may be of diagnostic value when echocardiographic studies are technically inadequate. MRI is also useful in identifying unusual segmental hypertrophy undetectable by standard echocardiography and can detect myocardial replacement fibrosis (an independent predictor of adverse cardiac outcomes and ventricular arrhythmias) using late gadolinium enhancement.

TREATMENT

NONPHARMACOLOGIC THERAPY

- Avoid volume depletion: HCM patients experience decrease in stroke volume and consequent increase in left ventricular outflow gradient with exercise. This may lead to hypotension, dizziness, and syncope.
- Exercise restriction: the risk of sudden cardiac death is increased by exercise in HCM patients. Participation in competitive sports and intense physical activity should be avoided. As a part of a healthy lifestyle, low-intensity aerobic exercise is reasonable.
- Advise avoidance of alcohol: alcohol use (even in small amounts) may result in increased obstruction of the left ventricular outflow tract.

GENERAL Rx

- Therapy for HCM is directed at blocking the effect of catecholamines that can exacerbate the dynamic left ventricular outflow tract obstruction and avoiding vasodilator or diuretic agents that can also worsen the obstruction.
- Beta-blockers: The beneficial effects of beta-blockers on symptoms (principally dyspnea and chest pain) and exercise tolerance appear to be largely a result of a decrease in the heart rate with consequent prolongation of diastole and increased passive ventricular filling. By reducing the inotropic response, beta-blockers may also reduce myocardial oxygen demand and decrease the outflow gradient during exercise, when sympathetic tone is increased.
- The nondihydropyridine calcium channel blockers (verapamil, diltiazem) can also decrease left ventricular outflow obstruction through a mechanism similar to beta-blockers. However, they are mainly second-line agents used in patients who cannot tolerate beta-blockers as they have theoretic vasodilatory properties as well that may worsen severe outflow tract gradients.
- Disopyramide is an antiarrhythmic that is also a negative inotrope, resulting in further decrease in outflow gradient. It is sometimes used in combination with beta-blockers.
- Prophylactic antibiotics before dental, GI, and genitourinary procedures are no longer recommended according to the 2007 American Heart Association (AHA) guidelines.
- Avoid use of digitalis, intravenous inotropes, dihydropyridine calcium channel blockers, nitrates, and vasodilators.
- Diuretics, angiotensin-converting enzyme inhibitors, and angiotensin receptor blockers should be used with caution.
- Implantable cardiac defibrillators (ICDs) are a safe and effective therapy in HCM patients prone to ventricular arrhythmias. In their practice guidelines, the major cardiology societies (AHA/ACC/HRS) give a strong recommendation (Class I) for ICD implantation in all patients with HCM who have had an episode of sustained ventricular tachycardia or fibrillation. In addition, they endorse the prophylactic placement of an ICD (Class IIa recommendation) for patients with one or more of the major risk factors for sudden cardiac death (outlined in "Disposition").
- Dual-chamber pacing may provide symptomatic relief, particularly in those who are over 65 yrs of age.
- HCM patients are at an increased risk of atrial fibrillation (AF) as well as systemic thromboembolization. AF occurs in over 20% of the HCM population. AF is an important source of symptoms, morbidity, and mortality and correlates to a worse prognosis. AF therapy should aim for thromboembolic risk mitigation with a vitamin K antagonist (unless contraindicated) and symptom alleviation via rate or rhythm control.
- Fig E1-216 describes management strategies for subgroups of patients within the broad HCM clinical spectrum.

DISPOSITION

HCM is not a static disease. Some adults may experience subtle regression in wall thickness, whereas others (~5% to 10%) paradoxically evolve into an end-stage cardiomyopathy resembling dilated cardiomyopathy, characterized by cavity enlargement, left ventricular wall thinning, and systolic dysfunction. Patients with HCM are at increased risk for sudden death, especially if onset of symptoms began during childhood. Severe left ventricular outflow obstruction at rest is also a strong, independent predictor of severe symptoms of heart failure and death. ICD

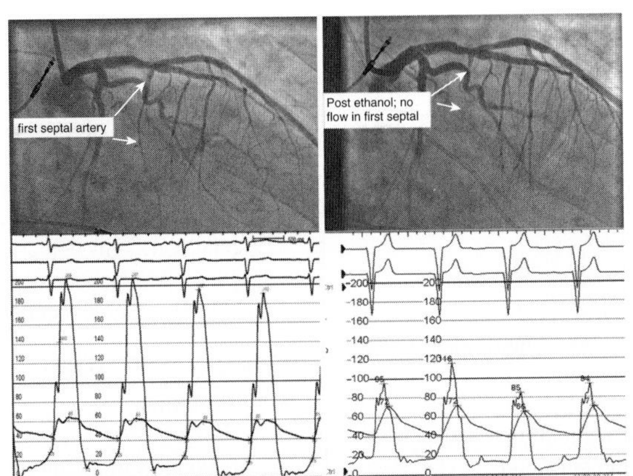

FIGURE 1-217 Septal ablation for obstructive hypertrophic cardiomyopathy. *Left,* Large pressure gradient between the left ventricle and aorta. A large proximal septal perforating artery is identified. *Right,* Following selective injection of ethanol, there is no flow within the septal artery and the gradient is dramatically reduced. (From Bonow RO et al: *Braunwald's heart disease—a textbook of cardiovascular medicine,* ed 9, St Louis, 2011, Saunders.)

implantation for primary prevention should be considered if patients (particularly the young) have any of the following high risk features:

- Personal history of sudden cardiac death or out of hospital cardiac arrest (major risk factor)
- Spontaneous sustained ventricular tachycardia or ventricular fibrillation (major risk factor)
- Family history of premature death caused by HCM
- Unexplained syncope
- Nonsustained ventricular tachycardia during Holter monitoring
- A marked outflow tract gradient (≥50 mm Hg)
- Substantial hypertrophy (>30 mm)
- Marked left atrial enlargement
- Abnormal blood pressure response during exercise
- Delayed gadolinium enhancement on cardiac magnetic resonance imaging

REFERRAL

- Surgical treatment (septal myectomy involving resection of the basal septum) is now the gold standard for relieving outflow tract obstruction in patients with large outflow gradient (≥50 mm Hg) and severe symptoms unresponsive to medical therapy. The risk for sudden death from arrhythmias is not altered by surgery. When this operation is performed by experienced surgeons in tertiary referral centers, the operative mortality rate is <1%, and many patients are able to achieve near-normal exercise capacity after surgery. Mitral valvuloplasty or plication in combination with myectomy may be necessary in <5% of patients.
- Septal ablation: As an alternative, nonsurgical reduction of the interventricular septum can be done in patients with HCM refractory to pharmacologic treatment, particularly in those who are not candidates for myectomy due to high surgical risk. This technique involves the injection of ethanol in a septal perforator branch of the left anterior descending coronary artery (Fig. 1-217), producing a controlled myocardial infarction of the interventricular septum, and thereby reducing septal mass and consequently the left ventricular outflow tract gradient. This method may lead to improvement in both subjective and objective measures of exercise capacity, but results are not as effective as surgery and are associated with a high incidence of heart block, requiring permanent pacing in approximately one fourth of patients and/or recurrence of obstruction and symptoms.

PEARLS & CONSIDERATIONS

COMMENTS

- Clinical screening of first-degree relatives with two-dimensional echocardiography and ECG is indicated. Starting at the age of 12, periodic screening at 12-18 month intervals is recommended for children of patients with HCM and in competetive athletes. Periodic screening of first-degree adult family members not in competitive athletics is recommended at 5-yr intervals because hypertrophy may not be detected until the sixth decade of life. Genetic testing is not indicated in relatives of index patients who do not have a definite pathogenic mutation.
- Genetic counseling and screening is recommended in first-degree relatives of patients with HCM. Genetic screening of first-degree relatives can refine or eliminate the need for periodic clinical screening. At least 13 genes are known to cause HCM, among them: cardiac myosin binding protein-C, beta-myosin heavy chain, troponin T, troponin I, alpha tropomyosin, actin regulatory light chain, and essential light chain. Clinical predictors of positive genotype, such as the presence of ventricular arrhythmias, age at diagnosis, degree of left ventricular wall hypertrophy, and family history of HCM, may aid in patient selection for genetic testing and increase the yield of cardiac sarcomere gene screening. Currently a mutation can be identified in 40% to 60% of all cases, sporadic or familial.
- All HCM patients who wish to become pregnant should be given prenatal counseling about the risk of transmission (about 50%) to their offspring and should be followed at a tertiary care center that specializes in high-risk pregnancies. Most patients with HCM tolerate pregnancy well due to the higher circulating blood volume.
- The mortality rate in HCM is approximately 1% to 2% per yr.
- About one third of HCM patients will not have a resting or labile outflow gradient (i.e., nonobstructive form of HCM), and lethal ventricular arrhythmias can occur in the absence of obstruction or symptoms.
- Myocardial fibrosis is a hallmark of hypertrophic cardiomyopathy. Biomarkers of collagen metabolism such as serum C-terminal propeptide of type I procollagen (PICP) are significantly higher in mutation carriers without left ventricular hypertrophy and in subjects with overt hypertrophic cardiomyopathy than in controls, indicating that a probiotic state precedes the development of hypertrophy of fibrosis identifiable with cardiac MRI.

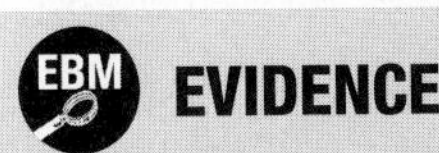

EVIDENCE

available at www.expertconsult.com

SUGGESTED READINGS

available at www.expertconsult.com

AUTHORS: **MARC PAUL WAASE, M.D., Ph.D.,** and **VEERANNA MERLA, M.D.**

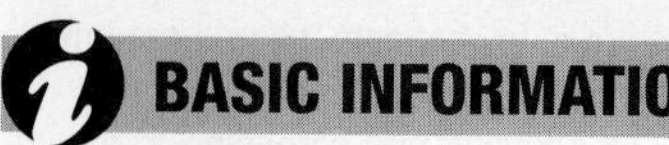

BASIC INFORMATION

DEFINITION

Restrictive cardiomyopathy refers to either an idiopathic or a systemic myocardial disorder (in the absence of ischemic, hypertensive, valvular, and congenital heart disease) characterized by restrictive filling, normal or reduced left ventricular (LV) and right ventricular (RV) volumes, and normal or near normal systolic LV and RV function. Except for primary nonhypertrophic cardiomyopathy and a few infiltrative diseases, restrictive cardiomyopathies are secondary.

ICD-9CM CODES

425.4 Other primary cardiomyopathies
425.9 Secondary cardiomyopathy, unspecified
277.39 Restrictive cardiomyopathy secondary to amyloidosis

ICD-10CM CODES

I42.5 Other restrictive cardiomyopathy
I42.8 Other cardiomyopathies
I43.1 Cardiomyopathy in metabolic diseases
I42.9 Cardiomyopathy, unspecified

EPIDEMIOLOGY & DEMOGRAPHICS

- Relatively uncommon cardiomyopathy, accounting for 5% of all primary myocardial diseases
- Most frequently caused by amyloidosis, myocardial fibrosis (following open heart surgery, transplantation or radiation).
- Patients classified as having "idiopathic" restrictive cardiomyopathy may have mutations in the gene for cardiac troponin I, and restrictive cardiomyopathy may represent an overlap with hypertrophic cardiomyopathy in many familial cases.

PHYSICAL FINDINGS & CLINICAL PRESENTATION

Restrictive cardiomyopathy presents with symptoms of progressive left-sided and right-sided heart failure:

- Fatigue, weakness (caused by low output as patients are unable to augment cardiac output by increasing heart rate without compromising ventricular filling).
- Progressively worsening exercise intolerance and dyspnea.
- Anginal chest pain can be seen (particularly in patients with amyloidosis) from myocardial compression of small coronaries.
- Palpitations (atrial fibrillation is common), dizziness or syncope (from orthostasis, heart block, or malignant arrhythmia).
- Edema, ascites, hepatomegaly, distended neck veins (from elevated heart pressures).
- Kussmaul's sign may be present (rise, or failure to fall, of the jugular venous on inspiration).
- On auscultation: murmurs of mitral or tricuspid regurgitation may be heard; an S3 may be present.
- Apical impulse may be palpable (can help distinguish it from constrictive pericarditis) and nondisplaced.

ETIOLOGY

Disease may be classified according to pathophysiologic processes:

Infiltrative:
- Amyloidosis (most common overall)
- Sarcoidosis (usually results in a dilated cardiomyopathy with regional wall motion abnormalities)

Noninfiltrative:
- Idiopathic (familial subtypes may have genetic overlap with hypertrophic cardiomyopathy)
- Scleroderma
- Diabetic cardiomyopathy
- Pseudoxanthoma elasticum

Storage diseases:
- Hemochromatosis (unusual as it is commonly associated with a dilated cardiomyopathy)
- Glycogen or other storage diseases (Gaucher, Hurler, Fabry—all rare)

Endomyocardial:
- Endomyocardial fibrosis
- Hypereosinophilic syndrome (Loeffler's)

- Carcinoid heart disease
- Radiation
- Metastatic cancers
- Drug related (anthracyclines, serotonin, ergotamine, busulfan, methylsergide)

DIAGNOSIS

DIFFERENTIAL DIAGNOSIS

- Constrictive pericarditis (see Table E1-98)
- Valvular dysfunction (especially aortic stenosis)
- Hypertrophic cardiomyopathy
- Hypertensive heart disease

WORKUP

- Blood count (to identify eosinophilia), iron studies, serum renal function studies, chest x-ray, ECG, echocardiogram.
- Cardiac catheterization, magnetic resonance imaging, and computed tomography (selected cases)
- Aspiration biopsy of subcutaneous fat to detect amyloidosis.
- Endomyocardial biopsy if diagnostic confirmation needed.
- Brain natriuretic peptide (BNP) serum levels: there is data suggesting that BNP levels are markedly elevated in restrictive cardiomyopathy but near normal in patients with constrictive pericarditis, despite nearly identical clinical and hemodynamic features, most likely resulting from the lack of myocardial stretching in constriction that is required for BNP release.

IMAGING STUDIES

- Chest x-ray:
  - Ranges from normal cardiomediastinal silhouette to moderate cardiomegaly (primarily because of biatrial enlargement).
  - Evidence of heart failure may be present.
  - Presence of pericardial calcification favors alternate diagnosis of constrictive pericarditis.
- ECG:
  - Nonspecific ST-T wave abnormalities are the most common finding. Voltage may be low in infiltrative etiologies such as amyloidosis.
  - Frequent atrial and ventricular ectopy are often present. Atrial fibrillation may be present.
  - High-degree atrioventricular block, intraventricular conduction delay may be seen in advanced cases.
- Echocardiogram (Fig. 1-218):
  - Biatrial enlargement almost always present.
  - Wall thickness depends on etiology; often thickened in infiltrative disease such as amyloidosis.
  - Myocardial appearance may be altered (speckled pattern suggestive of infiltration).
  - Ventricular chamber sizes and systolic function are often normal or reduced.
  - Echo Doppler shows evidence of diastolic dysfunction. Tissue Doppler demonstrates low mitral annular velocities.
- Cardiac catheterization:
  - Characteristic hemodynamic finding is a dip and plateau, or square-root sign in the left ventricular tracing, where deep and rapid decline in ventricular pressure at the

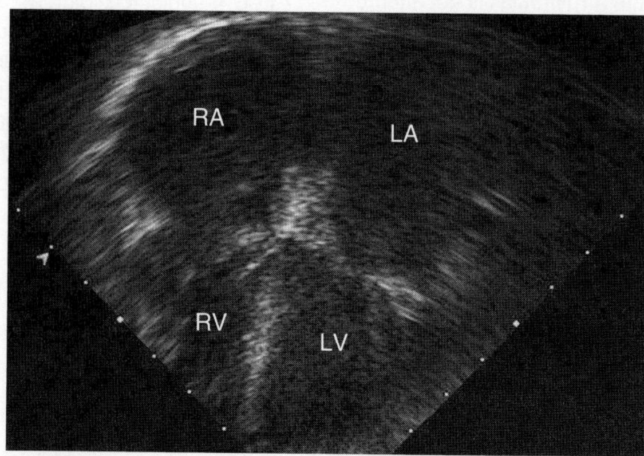

FIGURE 1-218 Echocardiogram of a patient with restrictive cardiomyopathy. The optical four-chamber view shows the markedly enlarged right and left atria, compared to the normal-sized left and right ventricular chambers. *LA,* Left atrium; *LV,* left ventricle; *RA,* right atrium; *RV,* right ventricle. (From Kliegman RM et al: *Nelson textbook of pediatrics,* ed 19, Philadelphia, 2011, Saunders.)

onset of diastole is immediately followed by rapid rise and plateau in early diastolic phase. To distinguish restrictive cardiomyopathy from constrictive pericarditis:

Constrictive pericarditis: Usually involves both ventricles and leads to equalization of diastolic pressures between all four cardiac chambers to within 5 mm Hg. There is a discordance in RV and LV pressures generated during inspiration, which is due to increased ventricular interdependence and decreased left atrial filling (caused by a decreased gradient in inspiration between the pulmonary veins, which are outside the constrictive process and the left atrium).

Restrictive cardiomyopathy: Impairs the left ventricle more than the right, often with left-sided end-diastolic pressures of 5 mm Hg greater than the right. The presence of increased pulmonary arterial systolic pressures is also suggestive of restrictive disease.

- Cardiac computed tomographic scan may be helpful to identify a thickened and calcified pericardium, consistent with constrictive pericarditis.
- Cardiac magnetic resonance imaging (CMRI) may also be useful to distinguish restrictive cardiomyopathy from constrictive pericarditis (thickness of the pericardium greater than 4 mm in the latter). CMRI is particularly helpful in the diagnosis of the amyloid or sarcoid variants and may have value in other variants as well. Late gadolinium enhancement can be seen with infiltrative diseases.

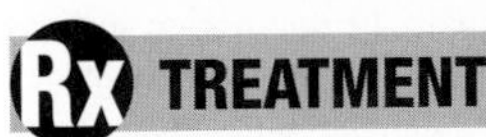

TREATMENT

NONPHARMACOLOGIC THERAPY

Congestive symptoms may respond to dietary sodium restriction (<2 g/day).

ACUTE GENERAL Rx

Treatment of volume overload and heart failure symptoms with diuretic therapy.

CHRONIC Rx

- Treatment involves management of the underlying disease if it exists:
  - Hemochromatosis may respond to repeated phlebotomy and iron chelators to decrease iron deposition in the heart.
  - Sarcoidosis may respond to corticosteroid therapy.
  - Primary amyloidosis may respond to anti-plasma cell therapy with chemotherapeutics (usually melphalan) and steroids. Autologous bone marrow biopsy, if EF is >40%, may also be indicated.
  - Eosinophilic cardiomyopathy may respond to corticosteroid and cytotoxic drugs.
  - There is no effective therapy for other causes of restrictive cardiomyopathy.
- Overall, the goal of treatment is to reduce symptoms by decreasing filling pressures while preserving cardiac output. Since there is currently no drug available to specifically act on myocardial relaxation, therapy centers on low-dose diuretics to lower the preload.
- Beta-blockers or calcium channel blockers have not been demonstrated to improve symptoms or alter the course of disease.
- ACE inhibitors (or angiotensin receptor blockers [ARBs]) and vasodilators should be avoided in patients with amyloidosis as they are poorly tolerated. Even small doses can trigger profound hypotension (probably due to associated autonomic neuropathy).
- Atrial fibrillation is common and patients with it or with a history of embolization should be anticoagulated. Tachycardia (of any cause) is poorly tolerated and a common cause of decompensation. Rate control is of paramount importance. Cardioversion in case of rapid atrial fibrillation should be considered. Of note, digoxin should be used with caution as it is potentially arrhythmogenic (particularly in patients with amyloidosis).
- Fibrosis of the cardiac conduction system may result in complete heart block presenting as dizziness or syncope (especially in amyloidosis) and pacemaker implantation may be required. The course of restrictive cardiomyopathy is variable and depends on the underlying etiology. Death usually results from heart failure or arrhythmias, and interventions aimed at addressing these are recommended.
  - For the amyloid variant, an implantable cardiac defibrillator offers little prophylactic benefit as the cause of sudden cardiac death is usually electromechanical disassociation.

DISPOSITION

Prognosis varies with the etiology of the cardiomyopathy but is poor overall as disease is rarely detected before advanced stages.

REFERRAL

Cardiac transplantation can be considered in patients with refractory symptoms and idiopathic or familial restrictive cardiomyopathies.

SUGGESTED READINGS

available at www.expertconsult.com

RELATED CONTENT

Fig. 3-43 Initial approach to classification of cardiomyopathy (Algorithm)
Restrictive Cardiomyopathy (Patient Information)

AUTHOR: **BARRY FINE, M.D., Ph.D**

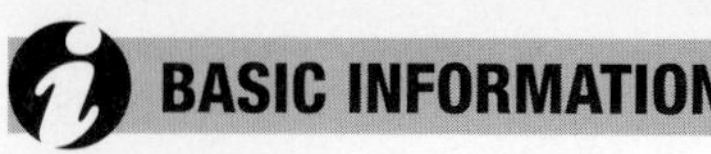

BASIC INFORMATION

DEFINITION

Stress cardiomyopathy (SC) is a syndrome characterized by transient systolic dysfunction and ballooning of the apical and/or mid segments of the left ventricle (LV) that mimics acute myocardial infarction (MI) but in the absence of obstructive coronary artery disease with acute ECG changes including ST segment elevation or depression, in the absence of recent head trauma, intracranial hemorrhage, pheochromocytoma, myocarditis, or hypertrophic cardiomyopathy. Typically, but not always, it is preceded by severe illness or intense emotional, physical, or psychological stress. Initially described in the 1990s in Japan, on left ventriculography this irreversible cardiomyopathy has a distinctive shape similar to a tako-tsubo pot with a narrow neck and round bottom, used by fishermen to trap octopi.

SYNONYMS

Takotsubo cardiomyopathy (TTC)
Left ventricular apical ballooning syndrome (LVABS)
Broken heart syndrome

ICD-9CM CODES
429.83
ICD-10CM CODES
I51.81 Takotsubo syndrome

EPIDEMIOLOGY & DEMOGRAPHICS

INCIDENCE: Uncertain, although increasingly reported. The recurrence rate is 11.4% over 4 yr after initial presentation. Occurs mostly in summer; fewest cases in winter.
PREVALENCE: Studies suggest that it comprises 0.7% to 2.5% of cases presenting with acute coronary syndrome (ACS).
PREDOMINANT SEX AND AGE: Postmenopausal women (90%) are predominantly affected.
RISK FACTORS: Frequently, but not always, triggered by severe medical illness or intense emotional or physical stress (death of loved ones, domestic abuse, fierce arguments, financial hardships, etc.)

PHYSICAL FINDINGS & CLINICAL PRESENTATION

- Acute substernal chest pain, dyspnea, syncope, shock, electrocardiographic (ECG) changes, or elevated cardiac biomarkers; similar to an acute MI.
- Heart failure, a frequent complication (30%) of takotsubo, is seen mostly in patients with other comorbidities and poor functional class. Recovery of function within a few days or weeks after admission is typical. In one experimental study, resolution was described as immediate after injection of adenosine.
- Overall prognosis is benign, but even short-term LV dysfunction can lead to thromboembolic phenomena. Anticoagulation is recommended for certain patients.

ETIOLOGY

Not well understood. Hypotheses include excessive catecholamine release, coronary artery spasm, and/or microvascular disease. Unknown why women are more commonly affected or why the apex and/or mid cavity are affected.

Several mechanisms have been advocated for acute and reversible coronary microvascular dysfunction:

- Acute microvascular spasm.
- Excessive sympathetic stimulation may induce myocardial metabolic impairment and stunning. Neurogenic stunned myocardium caused by an acute cardiac autonomic dysfunction.
- Coronary artery disease with aborted myocardial infarction transient coronary occlusion by a fast-dissolving clot spontaneous reperfusion
- Occurrence in postmenopausal women may support the hypothesis of stress-mediated vasoconstriction enhanced by estrogen depletion
- Studies have documented elevated plasma norepinephrine and epinephrine levels in Takotsubo cardiomyopathy.
- Increased serum concentrations of catecholamines have been shown to generate direct myocyte injury. Oxidation of catecholamines results in the formation of highly toxic substances and free radicals, causing intracellular calcium overload and myocardial cell damage. The typical histologic signs of catecholamine toxicity, which are described as focal, mononuclear, inflammatory areas of fibrotic response and characteristic contraction bands, are also reported to be present in takotsubo cardiomyopathy.
- Several studies have indicated that beta-adrenoceptor stimulation is associated with alteration in gene expression of Ca(2+)-regulatory proteins, which are crucial for contractile function.

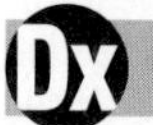

DIAGNOSIS

Mayo Clinic proposed criteria (2008): All 4 criteria required to make diagnosis.

- Transient hypokinesis, akinesis, or dyskinesis in the left ventricular mid segments with or without apical involvement (Fig. 1-219); regional wall motion abnormalities (RWMA) that extend beyond a single epicardial vascular distribution; and frequently, but not always, a stressful trigger.
- Absence of obstructive coronary disease or angiographic evidence of acute plaque rupture.
- New ECG abnormalities (ST-segment elevation and/or T-wave inversion) or modest elevation in cardiac troponins. Ogura and associates reported that the absence of reciprocal changes, the absence of abnormal Q wave, and the sum of ST-segment elevation in leads V4–6 more than the sum of ST-segment elevation in leads V1-3 identified takotsubo cardiomyopathy with a high sensitivity and specificity. Kosuge and associates recently reported that the combination of the presence of ST-segment depression in lead aVR and the absence of ST-segment elevation in lead V1 also showed a high sensitivity and specificity for diagnosing takotsubo cardiomyopathy. Q-T dispersion is more common in Takotsubo.
- Absence of pheochromocytoma or myocarditis.
- An inverted takotsubo pattern—mid ventricular ballooning with sparing of the basal and apical segments—atypical variant.
- The RWMA of the right ventricle is present in 30% of patients who tend to develop CHF and who have a poor outcome.

DIFFERENTIAL DIAGNOSIS

- Acute MI
- Cardiac syndrome X
- Prinzmetal's angina
- Myocarditis
- Cocaine abuse

WORK-UP

- This should be suspected in postmenopausal women who present with ACS after intense stress.
- Cardiology consult should be immediately obtained
- Significant CAD should be ruled out as an etiology of the cardiomyoapthy, usually by coronary catheterization.

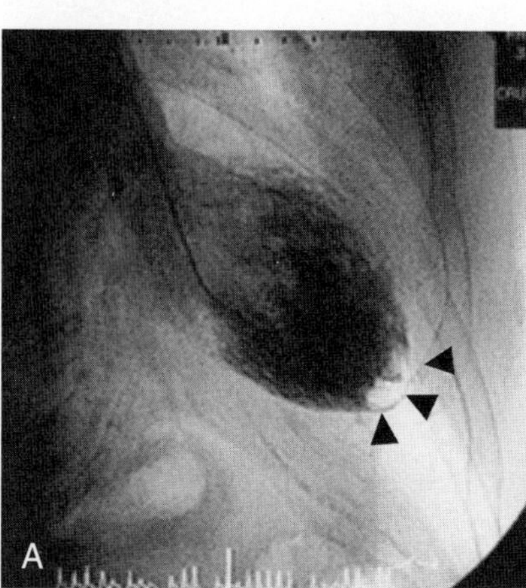

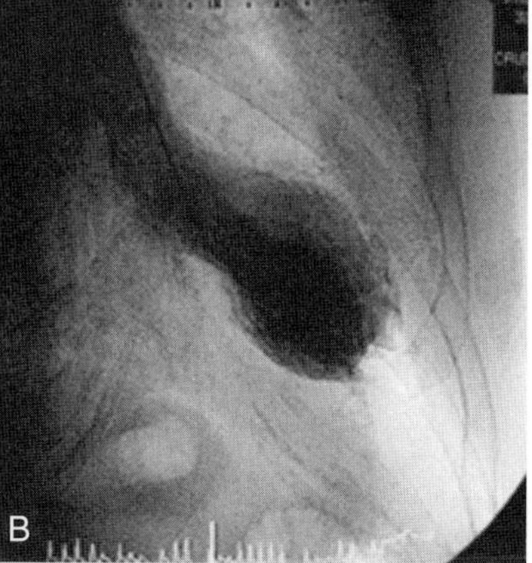

FIGURE 1-219 A and **B,** Left ventriculogram showing apical ballooning characteristic of stress-induced cardiomyopathy. (From Mitsuma W et al: *JACC* 51(1): cover, 2008.)

LABORATORY TESTS

Cardiac biomarkers are often elevated, but typically less than MI. Beta natriuretic peptide (BNP) levels are also commonly elevated.

IMAGING STUDIES

- Typically diagnosed in the catheterization lab during left ventriculography, although echocardiography (ECHO) can also show the characteristic apical ballooning. Contrast ECHO is quite useful to exclude apical thrombus. Cardiovascular MRI at the time of initial clinical presentation may provide relevant functional and tissue information that might aid in the establishment of the diagnosis of SC.
- Cardiac magnetic imaging (CMR) features helpful in diagnosis: absence of late gadolinium enhancement (LGE) in contrast to MI and consistent with myocardial viability.

COMPLICATIONS

- Approximately 20% include cardiogenic shock, heart failure, arrhythmias, intraventricular thrombus formation (incidence 2.5%), acute clinically significant mitral regurgitation, LV outflow tract (LVOT) obstruction, free wall rupture, and even death. An LV apical thrombus carries a great risk of cerebrovascular accident and distant embolization during the recovery phase.
- Risk score to predict likelihood of acute HF based on three variables: age >70 years, presence of physical stressor, and LV ejection fraction <40%.

Rx TREATMENT

There are no randomized data or established consensus. In most cases, supportive care is sufficient without specific therapy, due to a favorable prognosis. Standard treatment for systolic dysfunction including beta blockers, ACE inhibitors, and diuretics for volume overload. Patients who are in shock should get urgent ECHO to determine presence of LVOT obstruction.

NONPHARMACOLOGIC THERAPY

Patients in shock without significant LVOT obstruction may benefit from an intraaortic balloon pump (IABP).

ACUTE GENERAL Rx

- Patients who are hemodynamically stable should be started on a beta-blocker, ACE inhibitor, and diuretic if needed.
- Patients who are in shock and with significant LVOT obstruction may benefit from cautious fluid resuscitation (if no significant pulmonary congestion), and use of beta-blockers (can improve hemodynamics by resolution of the obstruction). The use of IABP in this case is controversial due to the potential worsening of LVOT obstruction.
- Patients with systolic anterior motion (SAM) of the anterior mitral valve leaflet or LVOT obstruction should not be exposed to inotropic agents even if they are in shock.

CHRONIC Rx

- Continued medical therapy and repeat ECHO (in 4 to 6 wk) to ensure normalization of systolic function (most patients normalize by this time).
- Duration of medical therapy is debatable.
- Three months of anticoagulation is suggested if an intraventricular thrombus is detected.

Recently published data could not find the protective effect of beta blockers in preventing the occurrence or recurrence of stress-induced cardiomyopathy.

DISPOSITION

Carries a favorable prognosis compared to STEMI or NSTEMI; in-hospital mortality is approximately 2%.

REFERRAL

Follow-up with a cardiologist is suggested.

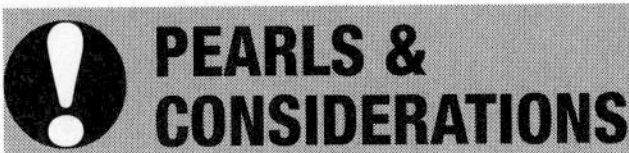

PEARLS & CONSIDERATIONS

COMMENTS

The term *takotsubo* is the Japanese name for an octopus trap (*tako-tsubo*), which has a similar shape of the LV in systole during a left ventriculogram (see Fig. 1-219).

PREVENTION

Minimizing stress may reduce incidence but no data to support this.

SUGGESTED READINGS

available at www.expertconsult.com

AUTHOR: **RABIA ARSHAD, M.D.**

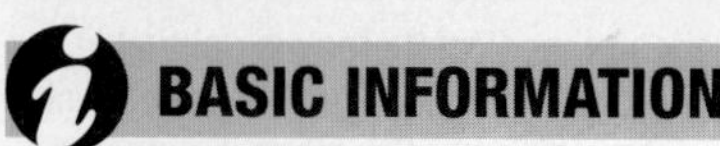

BASIC INFORMATION

DEFINITION

Cardiorenal syndrome (CRS) is a pathophysiologic disorder in which acute or chronic dysfunction of the heart or kidneys can induce acute or chronic dysfunction of the other organ. Another definition proposed by the National Heart, Lung, and Blood Institute (NHLBI) is one in which therapy to relieve congestive symptoms of heart failure is limited by progressive renal insufficiency. There are five types of CRS:

Type 1: Acute cardiac dysfunction leading to acute kidney injury

Type 2: Chronic heart failure leading to renal dysfunction

Type 3: Acute kidney injury leading to or resulting in acute cardiac dysfunction

Type 4: Chronic kidney disease (CKD) leading to cardiac dysfunction

Type 5: Systemic conditions that cause both cardiac and renal dysfunction

This section will focus on CRS types 1 and 2.

ICD-9CM CODES

404 Cardiorenal syndrome

ICD-10CM CODES

I13 Hypertensive heart and renal disease

I13.0 Hypertensive heart and renal disease with (congestive) heart failure

I13.2 Hypertensive heart and renal disease with both (congestive) heart failure and renal failure

I17.8 Other renal failure

EPIDEMIOLOGY & DEMOGRAPHICS

- CKD is present in 20% to 67% of patients with congestive heart failure (CHF).
  - Women, the elderly, whites, and patients with diabetes or systolic blood pressure >160 mm Hg have an increased incidence.
  - In general terms, mortality is increased in patients with heart failure who have a reduced glomerular filtration rate (GFR)
  - Patients with chronic kidney disease have an increased risk of both atherosclerotic heart disease and heart failure.
  - Cardiovascular disease is responsible for about 50% of deaths in patients with CKD
- 20%-30% of patients who are treated for acute or chronic CHF will develop acute kidney injury.
  - In patients with acute CHF, the severity of acute kidney injury is increased with decreased left ventricular systolic function and baseline CKD.
  - Only 9% of patients with acute heart failure in the ADHERE trial had normal renal function with GFR >90 ml/min/1.73 m^2.

PHYSICAL FINDINGS & CLINICAL PRESENTATION

- Acute/subacute decompensated heart failure (ADHF)
  - Clinical symptoms:
    - Dyspnea with exertion or at rest
    - Orthopnea
    - Paroxysmal nocturnal dyspnea
    - Right upper quadrant pain
  - Vital signs:
    - Sinus tachycardia
    - Hypertension
    - Elevated respiratory rate
    - Narrow pulse pressure
    - Pulsus alternans
  - Physical exam findings:
    - Elevated jugular venous pressures in the neck
    - Peripheral edema
    - Third heart sound (S3)
    - Respiratory crackles
    - Abdominal ascites
    - Hepato- and splenomegaly
    - Scrotal edema
- Chronic heart failure
  - Clinical symptoms:
    - Dyspnea
    - Fatigue
    - Anorexia
  - Vital signs:
    - Similar to ADHF, but may not have sinus tachycardia, and may have hypotension associated with a low cardiac output state.
  - Physical exam findings:
    - Similar to ADHF, but may lack respiratory crackles because crackles are more a sign of the rapidity of the collection of fluid within the alveoli rather than the total volume of fluid
- These findings of heart failure will be associated with laboratory findings of kidney disease (discussed later) or in extreme cases physical exam findings of severe kidney disease such as asterixis, uremic frost, or uremic smell, and uremic pericarditis, etc.

ETIOLOGY

The etiology of CRS can be divided into four mechanisms:

- Reduced renal perfusion
  - Is a common cause of CRS type 1 (acute CHF resulting in acute kidney injury)
  - Loop diuretic therapy can lead to reduced ventricular preload, which can result in as much as 20% reduction in cardiac output.
- Increased renal venous pressure
  - Can occur secondary to elevated central venous pressure or elevated intraabdominal pressure
  - The frequency of worsening kidney function is lowest in patients who have a CVP less than 8 mm Hg.
  - An increase in GFR can occur following diuretic therapy, which is most likely mediated by a reduction in renal venous pressure and/or a reduction in right ventricular dilatation.
- Right ventricular dilatation and dysfunction
  - May result in increased central venous pressures, which results in increased renal venous pressures and therefore a reduced GFR.
  - Right ventricular dilatation and dysfunction begets reduced left ventricular filling and therefore poor forward flow to the kidneys.
- Neurohormonal
  - Caused by activation of the renin-angiotensin-aldosterone system, sympathetic nervous system, antidiuretic hormone, and endothelin-1, which results in both increased salt and water retention and systemic vasoconstriction leading to decreased renal perfusion
  - The activation of the above systems overwhelm the vasodilatory effects of natriuretic peptides, nitric oxide, prostaglandins, and bradykinin.

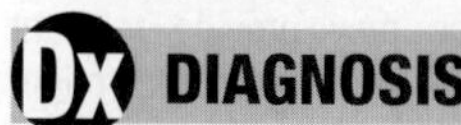

DIAGNOSIS

DIFFERENTIAL DIAGNOSIS

- Before making the diagnosis of CRS, it is necessary to rule out other causes of renal failure such as:
  - Prerenal causes
    - Volume depletion (overdiuresis, gastrointestinal losses, or vomiting)
    - Fluid overload states besides CHF (cirrhosis, nephrotic syndrome)
  - Intrinsic renal disease
    - Acute tubular necrosis
    - Glomerular disease
      - Nephrotic and nephritic syndromes
  - Postrenal causes
    - Obstruction

WORKUP

- The medical history will be consistent with symptoms of CHF and may include dyspnea, orthopnea, paroxysmal nocturnal dyspnea, edema, increasing abdominal girth, or weight gain. Additionally, laboratory results will show signs of kidney injury.
- Diagnostic workup includes chest radiograph, echocardiogram, renal ultrasound, and laboratory tests (see next section)

LABORATORY TESTS

- Serum creatinine
  - Patients with CRS whose creatinine levels were elevated at least 0.3 to 0.5 mg/dl had an odds ratio of 1.48 for mortality compared with those whose creatinine levels were elevated less than 0.3 mg/dl.
    - If creatinine levels increased by >0.5 mg/dl, the odds ratio of mortality increased to 3.22.
- Estimated glomerular filtration rate (eGFR)
  - Similar results to that of creatinine, but is more accurate for diagnosing elderly patients with less muscle mass
- Blood urea nitrogen
  - Admission levels >43 mg/dl are associated with a higher in-hospital mortality rate in patients with CRS
- Cystatin C
  - Better correlation to GFR than serum creatinine
- Beta natriuretic peptide (BNP)
  - Patients with initial admission values exceeding 480 pg/ml had a 51% chance of death, hospital readmission, or emergency room visit within 6 months compared with patients whose levels were <230 pg/ml.

- It can be difficult to distinguish between CKD and impaired kidney function due to cardiorenal syndrome. Some patients have both underlying CKD and CRS. Findings that support underlying CKD include significant proteinuria (>1000 mg/day), urine sediment with hematuria and/or pyuria and cellular casts, and/or small kidneys on ultrasound.

IMAGING STUDIES

- Chest radiograph
  - May show signs of fluid overload, such as pulmonary edema, pulmonary effusions, or fluid in the fissure
- Echocardiogram
  - Will help to determine if there is underlying systolic or diastolic dysfunction
- Renal ultrasound
  - Can help to distinguish between acute and chronic kidney disease, and can help rule out obstruction as a cause of worsening renal function

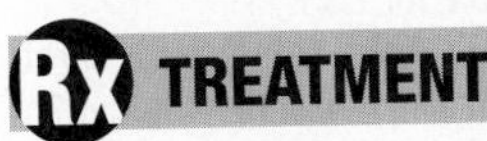

TREATMENT

NONPHARMACOLOGIC THERAPY

- Fluid restriction
- Hemodialysis/ultrafiltration
  - Can be used if there is no response to pharmacologic treatment or if the use of pharmacologic agents is limited secondary to hemodynamics or worsening laboratory values
- Left ventricular assist device/cardiac resynchronization therapy (CRT)
  - Can be used to improve forward flow and cardiac dyssynchrony. Use of CRT has been proven to improve ejection fraction by 7% and improve CHF symptoms in patients who have NYHA class II heart failure and above with ejection fractions less than 35% with a left bundle branch block morphology QRS duration greater than 150 ms.

ACUTE GENERAL Rx

There is no treatment that directly improves eGFR/serum creatinine level, but an increase in cardiac output can reduce the incidence of the four mechanisms of CRS listed previously.

- Diuretics
  - Fluid off-loading helps patients return to their ideal position on the Frank-Starling curve.
  - Removal of fluid will improve renal perfusion pressure by decreasing central venous pressure, therefore decreasing renal venous pressure and reducing right ventricular dilation along with improvement in right ventricular systolic function that will then lead to improved left ventricular performance.
  - May need high doses to achieve success because of decreased diuretic responsiveness as eGFR decreases
- Inhibitors of the renin-angiotensin-aldosterone system
  - Includes angiotensin converting enzyme (ACE) inhibitors, angiotensin receptor blockers, and aldosterone antagonists, along with newer renin inhibitors
    - Use is limited by worsening renal function, especially when serum creatinine is above 2.5
    - Allows for decreasing use of diuretic therapy
- Vasodilators
  - Includes nitroglycerin, nitroprusside, and nesiritide
    - Work by increasing renal perfusion pressure by putting patients back on the Starling curve and improving forward flow
- Ionotropic agents
  - Includes dobutamine, dopamine, and milrinone
  - Are used in treatment of cardiogenic shock as well as in low cardiac output states with normal blood pressures, and work by improving cardiac output, resulting in better renal perfusion pressures
  - Caution: dobutamine and milrinone can lower blood pressures.
- The use of mechanical methods of fluid removal such as extracorporeal ultrafiltration (UF) may be needed to achieve control of fluid retention, particularly in patients who become resistant and/or refractory to diuretic therapy. UF removes salt and water isotonically by driving the patient's blood through a highly permeable filter via an extracorporeal circuit in an arteriovenous or venovenous mode. With slow continuous UF, the patient's intravascular fluid volume remains stable as fluid shifts from the extravascular to intravascular space without affecting cardiac hemodynamics.

DISPOSITION

Is based upon improvement of patient's volume status as creatinine levels return to baseline

REFERRAL

Consultation by a cardiologist and nephrologist are recommended.

SUGGESTED READINGS

available at www.expertconsult.com

RELATED CONTENT

Acute Kidney Injury (Related Key Topic)
Heart Failure (Related Key Topic)

AUTHORS: **PHILLIP RUISI, D.O.,** and **ARAVIND RAO KOKKIRALA, M.D.**

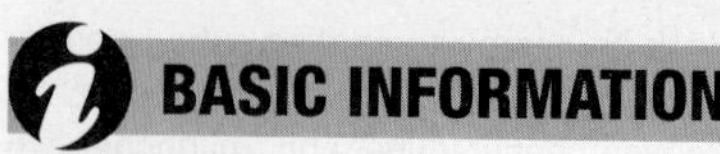

BASIC INFORMATION

DEFINITION

Light-headedness, dizziness, presyncope, or syncope in a patient with carotid sinus hypersensitivity is defined as carotid sinus syndrome (CSS). Carotid sinus hypersensitivity is the exaggerated response to carotid stimulation resulting in bradycardia, hypotension, or both. CSS is often considered a variant of neurocardiogenic syncope.

SYNONYMS

Carotid sinus syncope
CSS
Carotid sinus hypersensitivity

ICD-9CM CODES

337.0 Idiopathic peripheral autonomic neuropathy
780.2 Syncope or collapse

ICD-10CM CODES

G90.01 Carotid sinus syncope
R55 Syncope and collapse

EPIDEMIOLOGY & DEMOGRAPHICS

- Carotid sinus hypersensitivity accounts for 1% of syncopal episodes.
- Carotid sinus hypersensitivity is frequently associated with atherosclerosis and diabetes mellitus.
- Incidence increases with age, with an average age of onset at 61 to 74 yr.
- Men are affected more often than women (2:1).
- CSS is rarely found in patients younger than 50 yr.

MECHANISM

- The carotid sinus is located in the internal carotid artery.
- There is a reflex loop between the mechanoreceptors of the carotid sinus and the vagal nucleus in the midbrain.
- There is an exaggerated cardioinhibitory and vasodepressor reaction caused by decreased sympathetic and increased parasympathetic outflow to the heart and vasculature, respectively.

PHYSICAL FINDINGS & CLINICAL PRESENTATION

- Usually associated with sudden neck movements, neck palpation, shaving, or tight-fitting collars
- Usually associated with prodrome of nausea, warmth, pallor, or diaphoresis
- Light-headedness or presyncopal symptoms
- Syncope

Properly performed carotid sinus massage (CSM) at the bedside is diagnostic. European Society of Cardiology recommends carotid sinus massage as part of the exam in patients with syncope of unknown etiology and age over 40. This maneuver can elicit three types of responses in patients with carotid sinus hypersensitivity (see "Diagnosis").

1. CSM should be performed with the patient in the supine and upright position while monitoring the patient's blood pressure by cuff and heart rate by ECG.
2. CSM should be performed on only one carotid artery at a time.
3. Vigorous circular pressure is applied over one carotid artery at the level of the cricoid cartilage for 10 seconds and repeated on the opposite side if no effect is produced.
4. Contraindications to CSM include the presence of carotid artery bruits, documented carotid artery stenosis >70%, history of stroke or transient ischemic attack <3 mo, history of myocardial infarction <6 mo, history of serious ventricular arrhythmia, or prior carotid endarterectomy.
5. Complications of transient visual disturbance or transient paresis occur in <1% of patients.
6. False-positive results with carotid sinus massage may be relatively common in the elderly population. Thus alternative explanation for syncope should be investigated prior to attribution of symptoms to carotid sinus hypersensitivity.

ETIOLOGY

- Idiopathic
- Head and neck tumors (e.g., thyroid)
- Significant lymphadenopathy
- Carotid body tumors
- Prior neck surgery

DIAGNOSIS

- The diagnosis of CSS is made when carotid sinus hypersensitivity is demonstrated by CSM and no other cause of syncope is identified.
- CSM can elicit three types of responses diagnostic of carotid sinus hypersensitivity:
  1. Cardioinhibitory type: CSM producing (1) asystole for at least 3 sec in the absence of symptoms or (2) reproduction of symptoms occurring with a decline in heart rate of 30% to 40% or asystole of up to 2 sec in duration. Symptoms should not recur when CSM is repeated after atropine infusion.
  2. Vasodepressor type: CSM producing (1) a decrease in systolic blood pressure of 50 mm Hg in the absence of symptoms or 30 mm Hg in the presence of neurologic symptoms; (2) no evidence of asystole; or (3) neurologic symptoms that persist after infusion of atropine.
  3. Mixed type: CSM producing both types of responses.

DIFFERENTIAL DIAGNOSIS

All causes of syncope

WORKUP

- CSS is a diagnosis of exclusion.
- Exclude other causes of syncope or presyncope: detailed history, physical examination including orthostatic vital signs, ECG. Other tests should be considered depending on the clinical setting.

TREATMENT

NONPHARMACOLOGIC THERAPY

Reassurance and education are important. Avoid applying neck pressure from tight collars, shaving, or rapid head turning.

ACUTE GENERAL Rx

Treatment will vary according to the type of carotid hypersensitivity response and symptoms present (see "Chronic Rx").

CHRONIC Rx

Therapy is divided into three classes: medical, surgical (carotid denervation), and cardiac pacing.

- Surgical therapy has been largely abandoned except in cases of compressing tumors or masses responsible for CSS.
- For infrequent and mildly symptomatic carotid sinus hypersensitivity of either the cardioinhibitory or vasodepressor type, treatment is generally not necessary.
- Cardiac pacing: 2008 ACC/AHA/HRS device guidelines recommend pacing in patients with recurrent syncope in spontaneous occurring carotid sinus stimulation, in whom carotid sinus pressure induces ventricular asystole of more than 3 seconds.

Permanent pacing may be considered in patients with recurrent syncope of unexplained origin, and a hypersensitive cardioinhibitory response of 3 seconds or more.

Permanent pacing is not indicated for carotid sinus hypersensitivity with no, or only vague, symptoms.

For symptomatic patients with a vasodepressor response to CSM:

- No medical treatment is proven to be effective
- Drugs, such as vasodilators, that would worsen the response should be discontinued or reduced if feasible
- Sympathomimetics: midodrine 2.5 to 10 mg tid
- Serotonin-specific reuptake inhibitors
- Fludrocortisone
- Elastic knee-high or thigh-high stockings
- Carotid sinus denervation

For symptomatic patients with CSS with a mixed response to CSM:

- Combination of dual-chamber permanent pacemaker and agents used to treat vasodepressor response

DISPOSITION

- Up to 50% of the patients have recurrent symptoms.
- No increased mortality rate in patients with idiopathic CSS compared with the general population.

REFERRAL

Cardiology referral is indicated if cardiac testing, such as tilt-table test, or pacemaker placement is being considered.

Neurology referral is indicated if neurologic causes of syncope are suggested by history or physical examination findings.

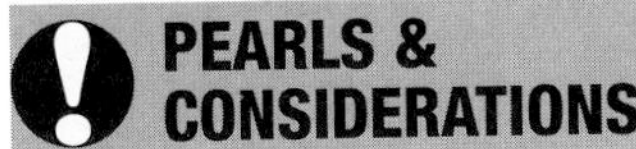

PEARLS & CONSIDERATIONS

The most common type of CSS is cardioinhibitory, followed by mixed and vasodepressor responses.

Driving restrictions in the 2009 ESC syncope update and 1996 AHA/NASPE statement are stratified according to whether patients have mild or severe syncope.

Mild syncope is defined as infrequent mild symptoms (usually without syncope), clear precipitating causes (usually standing), warning signs, and infrequent occurrence. For patients with mild sinus hypersensitivity, no driving restrictions are recommended for private or commercial driving.

Severe syncope is classified as severe symptoms (with syncope), without warning and in any position, no clear precipitating causes, and/or frequent occurrence. For patients with severe hypersensitivity, all driving is prohibited. If symptoms are controlled, driving is permitted 1 to 6 months after, based on the modality of treatment.

COMMENTS

Prognosis depends on the underlying cause.

SUGGESTED READINGS

available at www.expertconsult.com

RELATED CONTENT

Fig. E1-904 Syncope (Algorithm)
Fig. 3-96 Hypotension (Algorithm)
Syncope (Patient Information)

AUTHOR: **BARRY FINE, M.D., Ph.D.**

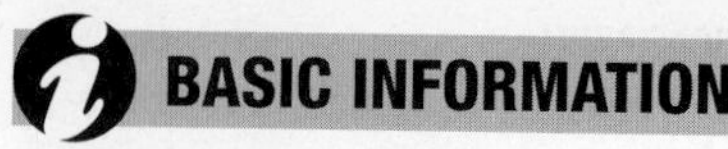

BASIC INFORMATION

DEFINITION

Carotid stenosis is narrowing of the arterial lumen within the carotid artery that is typically a result of atherosclerosis.

SYNONYMS

Atherosclerotic disease of the carotid artery

ICD-9CM CODES
433.1 Carotid stenosis
ICD10-CM CODES
I65.29 Occlusion and stenosis of unspecified carotid artery

EPIDEMIOLOGY & DEMOGRAPHICS

INCIDENCE: 2.2 to 8/1000 persons per yr
PREVALENCE: 1.1 to 77/100,000 persons; it is estimated that 5/1000 persons aged 50 to 60 yr and 100/1000 persons >80 yr have carotid stenosis >50%. (*Note:* The incidence of carotid stenosis is unknown as screening is not routine. However, the incidence of transient ischemic attack [TIA], a common presenting symptom of carotid stenosis, is well known.)
PREDOMINANT SEX AND AGE: Male/female ratio of 2:1; more common in whites than African Americans and Asians
PEAK INCIDENCE: Peak incidence is between 50 and 60 yr of age.
GENETICS: Multifactorial; twin studies (monozygous vs. dizygous) suggest a familial influence
RISK FACTORS: Hypertension, dyslipidemia, diabetes mellitus, and smoking are the four major risk factors.

PHYSICAL FINDINGS & CLINICAL PRESENTATION

Patients with carotid stenosis are often asymptomatic, but many have the presence of a carotid bruit or TIA.

- Carotid bruit: In general, the presence of a carotid bruit is a better indicator of generalized atherosclerosis and as such, is a better predictor of ischemic heart disease than future stroke.
- TIA: Carotid stenosis is classically heralded by ipsilateral transient monocular blindness (amaurosis fugax), contralateral numbness or weakness, contralateral homonymous hemianopsia, aphasia, or *syncope (if bilateral disease is present).*

ETIOLOGY

- Atherosclerosis (most common by far)
- Aneurysm
- Arteritis
- Carotid dissection
- Fibromuscular dysplasia
- Postradiation necrosis
- Vasospasm

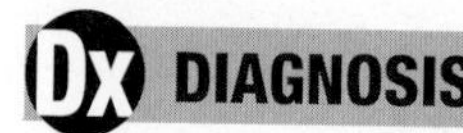

DIAGNOSIS

DIFFERENTIAL DIAGNOSIS

Aneurysm, arteritis, and carotid dissection

WORKUP

Systematic history, examination, and diagnostic studies to assess for carotid stenosis and other risk factors of TIA

LABORATORY TESTS

CBC, basic metabolic panel, fasting lipid profile, PT/international normalized ratio, APTT, CRP

IMAGING STUDIES

- Four imaging modalities are available for the evaluation of carotid stenosis (Table 1-99).
- Patients who have neurologic sequelae suggestive of carotid stenosis should be screened via carotid duplex. If carotid stenosis is suspected on carotid duplex, but inconclusive, magnetic resonance angiography, computed tomography angiography, or conventional angiography should be obtained to confirm the degree of stenosis (Fig. 1-220).

Rx TREATMENT

NONPHARMACOLOGIC THERAPY

Carotid endarterectomy (CEA) and carotid angioplasty and stenting (CAS) are available.

CEA—several studies have proved the efficacy of this procedure. The selection of surgical candidates should be guided primarily by the presence or absence of symptoms and the degree of stenosis.

Asymptomatic patients: Four major trials have investigated the benefit of CEA in an asymptomatic patient with carotid stenosis: Carotid Artery Surgery Asymptomatic Narrowing Operation vs Aspirin (CASANOVA), Veterans Affairs Cooperative Study Group, Asymptomatic Carotid Atherosclerosis Study (ACAS), and Asymptomatic Carotid Surgery Trial (ACST). In addition, a meta-analysis was subsequently performed.

Pearls:

Most studies have shown that a benefit from CEA in asymptomatic patients is not seen until 2 yr after surgery.

CEA should be considered in asymptomatic patients only if the perioperative risk for stroke and death at the given surgical institution is less than 3%.

The studies failed to show a benefit in the presence of contralateral carotid occlusion.

Recommendations for asymptomatic patients with carotid stenosis:

CEA should be considered in patients between the ages of 40 and 75 yr with asymptomatic 60% to 99% stenosis if their life expectancy is greater than 5 yr and the perioperative stroke and mortality rates are <3%. However, medical therapy has improved since early trials comparing medical management and revascularization. Stroke rates have fallen to about 1% in medically treated patients over the past decade, and many experts are

TABLE 1-99 Imaging Modalities for Carotid Stenosis

Imaging Modality	Benefit	Drawback
Cerebral angiography	• Gold standard • Assesses plaque morphology • Assesses presence of collaterals	• Invasive • High cost • 4% incidence rate of complications • 1% incidence rate of serious complications or death
Carotid duplex	• Sensitive in detecting high-grade stenosis (>70%) • Less invasive • Lower cost	• Can be limited by body habitus • Technician dependent • Overestimates degree of stenosis
Magnetic resonance angiography (MRA)	• Sensitive in detecting high-grade stenosis (>70%) • Less operator dependent	• Overestimates degree of stenosis • Cannot be performed in patients who are critically ill, unable to tolerate supine positioning, have pacemaker or other ferromagnetic hardware, or are claustrophobic* • Expensive • Takes much longer to obtain compared with other modalities
Computed tomography angiography (CTA)	• Sensitive for high-grade stenosis	• Contraindicated in patients with serum creatinine concentration >1.5 mg/dl

*One study revealed that ~17% of patients are unable to tolerate MRA secondary to claustrophobia or are unable to lie still for procedure.

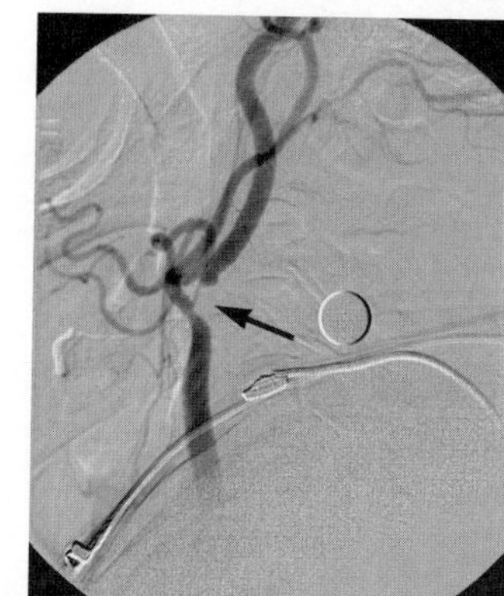

FIGURE 1-220 Conventional angiography demonstrating severe stenosis of the internal carotid artery at the bifurcation.

favoring intensified medical management rather than revascularization procedures in patients with ACS.

All patients undergoing CEA should be started on aspirin (ASA; 81 or 325 mg daily) before surgery and should be continued indefinitely. Although variations exist among surgeons, ASA is typically continued during the perioperative period.

Symptomatic patients: Two major trials (North American Symptomatic Carotid Endarterectomy Trial [NASCET] and European Carotid Surgery Trial [ECST]) and subsequent pooled analysis have shown the benefit of CEA in patients with symptomatic carotid stenosis.

Pearls:

There is improved outcome in patients with mild stroke or TIA for surgical treatment within 2 wk of the symptomatic event.

Men seem to benefit more when compared with women.

CEA does not appear to be beneficial in women with 50% to 69% stenosis.

Despite increased perioperative risk, patients with contralateral carotid occlusion who undergo CEA have benefit in terms of stroke and death rate when compared with patients undergoing medical management alone.

Recommendations:

CEA is recommended for recently symptomatic patients with 70% to 99% stenosis if their life expectancy is >5 yr and perioperative risk for mortality is <6%. Number needed to treat (NNT) at 5 yr = 6.3.

CEA is beneficial for recently symptomatic men with 50% to 69% stenosis if their life expectancy is >5 yr and perioperative risk of mortality is <6%. NNT at 5 yr 5=22.

Medical management is recommended for patients with stenosis <50%.

ASA (81 or 325 mg daily) should be initiated before CEA and continued after surgery.

CAS (stenting) is a less invasive alternative to CEA. Five major studies have compared stenting and CEA (Stent-Protected Angioplasty vs. Carotid Endarterectomy [SPACE], endarterectomy vs. stenting in patients with symptomatic severe carotid stenosis [EVA-3S], Stenting and Angioplasty with Protection in Patients at High Risk for Endarterectomy [SAPPHIRE]), Carotid Revascularization Endarterectomy Versus Stenting [CREST] and the International Carotid Stenting Study [ICSS].

Recommendations:

CAS may be considered for symptomatic patients with >70% carotid stenosis who have either difficult surgical access, intracranial stenosis, or medical risk that increases the risk of surgery (those with severe cardiac or pulmonary disease, contralateral carotid occlusion, prior neck surgery, prior neck irradiation, contralateral laryngeal nerve palsy, recurrent stenosis after prior CEA, age >0 yr).

CAS should be considered only if operators have periprocedural morbidity and mortality rates between 4% and 6%.

ASA should be given before procedure and indefinitely after procedure.

Clopidogrel should be given for 6 mo to 2 yr after stent placement or continued indefinitely depending on individual circumstances.

Risk for CAS:

Minor or major stroke related to hyperperfusion syndrome, periprocedural bradycardia, hypotension, and restenosis.

Hyperperfusion syndrome: 1.1%

Restenosis: 0.5% to 2%

Stenting vs. Endarterectomy for Treatment of Carotid Artery Stenosis

The large CREST study, published in 2010, demonstrated no difference in primary outcomes (stroke, myocardial infarction or death in the periprocedural period or ipsilateral stroke within 4 years following randomization).

Results from ICSS, a large, multicenter, international study comparing CEA and CAS, were recently released. This study showed an increased risk of stroke, periprocedural complication, and death in those patients undergoing stenting compared to those undergoing CEA. Additionally, a study on MRI findings following the procedure revealed an increased occurrence of "silent strokes" in those patients undergoing CAS. Long-term follow-up is still ongoing.

Despite the recent reports from ICSS, individual results may depend on factors such as the surgeon's experience and skill, and age of the patient with older patients (>70 yr) possibly doing better with CEA.

Results from SPACE, a multicenter European trial designed to test the hypothesis that CAS is not inferior to CEA, failed to demonstrate a higher incidence of periprocedural complications at 2 yr when CAS was compared to CEA. In addition, the study failed to demonstrate a significant difference in primary outcomes (ipsilateral stroke or death). However, the study failed to demonstrate CAS was noninferior to CEA.

ACUTE GENERAL Rx

- General medical therapy should be aimed at risk factor reduction. As stated earlier, the major risk factors for carotid stenosis are hypertension, diabetes mellitus, dyslipidemia, and smoking (see "Stroke, Secondary Prevention").
- Antiplatelet therapy: Three antiplatelet options are available for patients with carotid stenosis: ASA, ASA plus dipyridamole, and clopidogrel.

DISPOSITION

Disposition and prognosis depend on several variables (Table 1-100): the degree of stenosis, the presence of symptoms, medication compliance, and the type of intervention (if any).

TABLE 1-100 Carotid Stenosis Management

Degree of Carotid Stenosis	<50%	50%-69%	70%-99%
Asymptomatic	• Medical management	• Men: CEA if stenosis >60% and age <75 yr; otherwise, medical management • Women: medical management	• Men <75 yr: CEA • Women: medical management
Symptomatic	• Medical management	• Men: CEA • Women: medical management	• Men: CEA • Women: CEA

CEA, Carotid endarterectomy.

PEARLS & CONSIDERATIONS

There are ongoing studies concerning the best treatment of patients with carotid artery stenosis. Based on the results of these studies, guidelines may change rapidly.

SPECIAL CONSIDERATION

Some studies have shown that in patients with bilateral hemodynamically significant stenosis (>70%), reduction of blood pressure resulted in worse outcome in terms of stroke. These patients would likely be candidates for CEA.

Carotid artery occlusion (100% blockage), for which there is no routine treatment, is being reexamined in the national Carotid Occlusion Surgery Study (http://www.cosstrial.org). Consider referring symptomatic carotid occlusion patients for consideration of this study.

PREVENTION

Prevention of carotid stenosis should be guided at pursuing a healthy lifestyle and management of risk factors for development of atherosclerosis.

PATIENT/FAMILY EDUCATION

Patients should be counseled on pursuing a healthy lifestyle to include exercise and smoking cessation. In addition, patients should take an active role in controlling blood pressure and blood glucose. Further educational materials can be found online at: http://www.strokecenter.org/education.

EVIDENCE

available at www.expertconsult.com

SUGGESTED READINGS

available at www.expertconsult.com

RELATED CONTENT

Carotid Stenosis (Patient Information)

AUTHOR: **JOSEPH R. OWENS, M.D.**

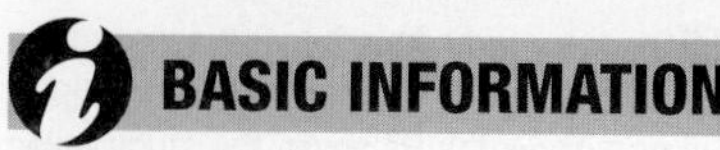

BASIC INFORMATION

DEFINITION

Carpal tunnel syndrome is a compressive neuropathy of the median nerve as it passes under the transverse carpal ligament at the wrist (Fig. E1-221). It is the most common entrapment neuropathy.

SYNONYMS

CTS

ICD-9CM CODES
354.0 Carpal tunnel syndrome
ICD-10CM CODES
G56.0 Carpal tunnel syndrome, unspecified upper limb

EPIDEMIOLOGY & DEMOGRAPHICS

PREVALENT AGE: 30 to 60 yr
PREVALENT SEX: Females are affected two to five times as often as males.

PHYSICAL FINDINGS & CLINICAL PRESENTATION

- Pain, paresthesia in 1st, 2nd, 3rd, and lateral ½ of 4th fingers, worse at night
- Tinel's sign at wrist (Fig. 1-222): tapping lightly over the median nerve on the volar surface of the wrist produces a tingling sensation radiating from the wrist to the hand
- Phalen's sign (Fig. 1-223): reproduction of symptoms after 1 min of gentle, unforced wrist flexion
- Carpal compression test: direct pressure over the patient's carpal tunnel for 30 sec elicits symptoms
- Findings may be bilateral in up to 65% of patients
- Thenar atrophy in longstanding cases with weakness of thumb abduction and opposition

ETIOLOGY

- Idiopathic in most cases
  - Increased intracarpal tunnel pressure
  - Ischemia, friction, or angulation of median nerve
- Space-occupying lesions in carpal tunnel (tenosynovitis, ganglia, aberrant muscles)
- Can be associated with diabetes, hypothyroidism, pregnancy, connective tissue diseases, acromegaly, amyloidosis
- Repetitive strain or job-related mechanical overuse may be a risk factor
- Crystal-induced rheumatic disorders

Dx DIAGNOSIS

DIFFERENTIAL DIAGNOSIS

- Cervical radiculopathy
- Chronic tendinitis
- Other arthritides
- Complex regional pain syndrome
- Brachial plexopathy, thoracic outlet syndrome
- Polyneuropathy
- Other entrapment neuropathies
- Traumatic wrist injuries

IMAGING STUDIES

Carpal tunnel syndrome is a clinical diagnosis but imaging may assist workup in uncertain situations. High-resolution ultrasound has been very effective in supporting the diagnosis. Roentgenograms or MRI may be helpful in ruling out other conditions.

ELECTRODIAGNOSTIC STUDIES

Nerve conduction velocity tests demonstrate impaired sensory conduction across the carpal tunnel. Electromyography may show active denervation muscle potentials.

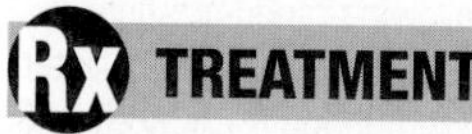

TREATMENT

ACUTE GENERAL Rx

- Activity modification
- Nocturnal wrist splint
- No evidence for effectiveness of NSAIDs
- Corticosteroid injection of carpal canal on ulnar side of palmaris longus tendon proximal to wrist crease (Figs. E1-224 and E1-225): can be done with palpation guidance or under ultrasound guidance. A recent trial[1] has shown that methylprednisolone injections for CTS have significant benefits in relieving symptoms at 10 wk and reducing the rate of surgery 1 yr after treatment, but 3 out of 4 patients had surgery within 1 yr.
- Low-dose oral corticosteroids can be considered.
- Short-term benefit from ultrasound therapy (physical therapy modality)
- Ergonomic keyboards

DISPOSITION

Clinical course may have remissions and exacerbations. Some may progress from intermittent to persistent sensory complaints (numbness, tingling, paresthesias), then later to develop motor symptoms. In pregnancy, symptoms usually resolve spontaneously weeks after delivery.

REFERRAL

Surgical referral is needed if conservative treatment fails. It is usually reserved for severe symptoms or presence of weakness/thenar atrophy. Surgery (sectioning of transverse carpal ligament) to release pressure on the median nerve is done by open or endoscopic approach, with good long-term results.

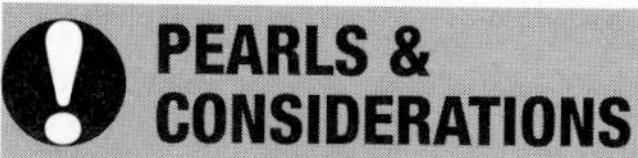

PEARLS & CONSIDERATIONS

- The sensory changes of carpal tunnel syndrome spare the thenar eminence. This distinctive pattern occurs because the palmar sensory cutaneous branch of the median nerve arises proximal to the wrist, passing over, rather than through the tunnel.
- Role of repetitive hand or wrist use and workplace factors in the development of carpal tunnel syndrome remains controversial.

SUGGESTED READINGS

available at www.expertconsult.com

RELATED CONTENT

Carpal Tunnel Syndrome (Patient Information)

AUTHOR: **CANDICE YUVIENCO, M.D.**

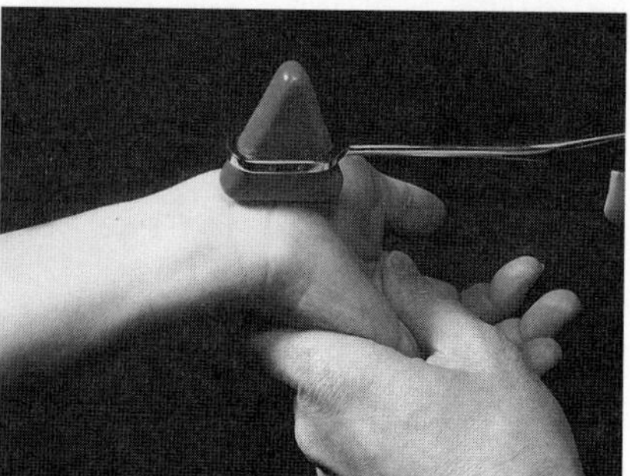

FIGURE 1-222 Tinel's sign. The wrist is held in extension while gentle percussion is performed over and just proximal to the transverse carpal ligament. (From Hochberg MC et al: *Rheumatology,* ed 5, St Louis, 2011, Mosby.)

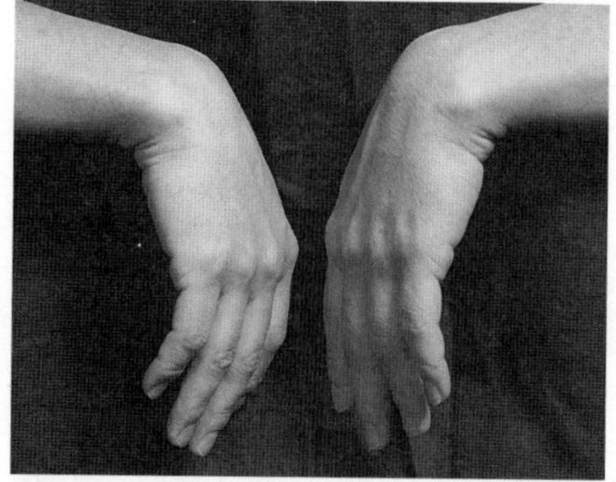

FIGURE 1-223 Phalen's (wrist flexion) test. With the wrists held in unforced flexion for 30 to 60 seconds, a positive test reproduces or worsens the patient's symptoms. (From Hochberg MC et al: *Rheumatology,* ed 5, St Louis, 2011, Mosby.)

[1]Methylprednisolone injections for the carpal tunnel syndrome: a randomized, placebo-controlled trials, *Ann Int Med* 159:309-317, 2013.

BASIC INFORMATION

DEFINITION

Cataracts are the clouding and opacification of the normally clear crystalline lens of the eye. The opacity may occur in the cortex, the nucleus of the lens, or the posterior subcapsular region, but it is usually in a combination of areas.

SYNONYMS

Congenital cataracts (e.g., from rubella)
Metabolic cataracts (e.g., caused by diabetes)
Hereditary cataracts
Age-related senile cataracts (nuclear sclerotic and cortical cataracts)
Traumatic cataracts
Toxic or drug-induced cataracts (e.g., caused by steroids)
Lenticular opacities

ICD-9CM CODES
366 Cataract
ICD-10CM CODES
H26.9 Cataract, unspecified
H25.0 Senile incipient cataract
H25.1 Senile nuclear cataract
H26.0 Infantile, juvenile and presenile cataract

EPIDEMIOLOGY & DEMOGRAPHICS

INCIDENCE (IN U.S.): Most common cause of treatable blindness; cataract removal is the most frequent surgical procedure in patients >65 yr (1.3 million operations per year, with an annual cost of approximately $3 billion). By year 2020 more than 30 million Americans will have cataracts. Of Americans >40 yr, 20.5 million (17.2%) have cataracts. Of these, 5% have had surgery.

PEAK INCIDENCE:
- In early life: congenital and hereditary causes predominant; consider drug related, diabetes, and trauma
- In older age group: senile cataracts (after 40 yr)

PREDOMINANT AGE: Elderly; some stage of cataract development is present in >50% of persons 65 to 74 yr and in 65% of those >75 yr. Lens clouding begins at 39 to 40 yr and then usually progresses either slowly or rapidly depending on individual and health.

GENETICS: Hereditary with syndromes such as galactosemia, homocystinuria, diabetes

PHYSICAL FINDINGS & CLINICAL PRESENTATION

- Cloudiness and opacification of the crystalline lens of the eye (Figs. 1-226 and E1-227)
- Decrease or absence of the red reflex (important in pediatric ages, since visual acuity is more difficult to assess)
- Painless decreased visual acuity
- Glare and decreased night vision (early symptom: difficulty with night driving)

ETIOLOGY

- Heredity
- Trauma
- Toxins
- Age related
- Drug related (e.g., corticosteroids, statin use)
- Congenital
- Inflammatory (e.g., history of uveitis)
- Diabetes
- Collagen vascular disease
- Statin use

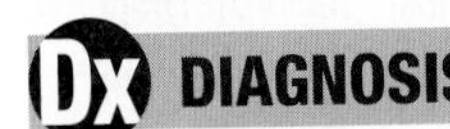

DIAGNOSIS

DIFFERENTIAL DIAGNOSIS

- Corneal lesions
- Retinal lesions, detached retina, tumors
- Vitreous disease, chronic inflammation

WORKUP

- Complete eye examination, including visual acuity and measurement of refractive error, slit lamp examination, dilated funduscopic examination, and brightness acuity testing
- Complete physical examination for other underlying causes

LABORATORY TESTS

- Rarely, urinary amino acid screening and central nervous system imaging studies with congenital cataracts
- Fasting glucose in young adults with cataracts
- Diabetes, collagen vascular disease, other metabolic diseases in younger patients
- Genetic and hereditary evaluation

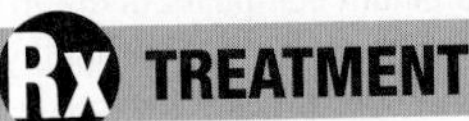

TREATMENT

There is no evidence that antioxidants or drugs will slow or treat cataracts.

NONPHARMACOLOGIC THERAPY

- Wait until vision is compromised before doing surgery.
- Plan cataract removal with intraocular lens implantation when vision is compromised and limiting activities of daily living, such as driving at night or reading. Removal of the cataract should be expected to improve the ability of the patient to perform these activities. Another indication to remove cataracts might be to improve the examination view for treatment and assessment of retinal diseases.
- Decision for timing of surgery depends upon patient complaints, best corrected visual acuity (e.g., 20/50), and glare measurements (brightness acuity test decreases vision significantly).

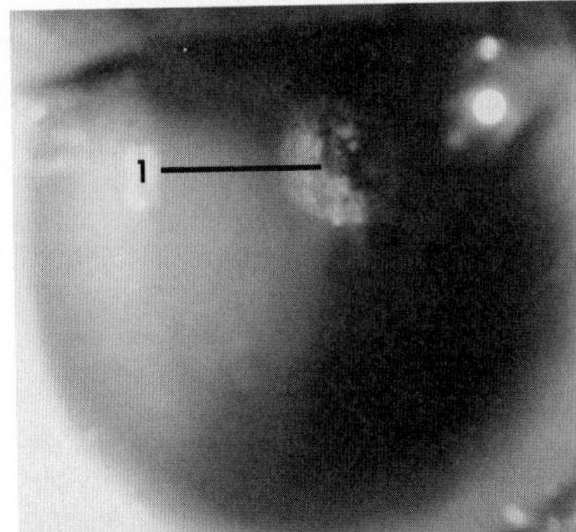

FIGURE 1-226 The central location of a posterior subcapsular cataract *(1)*. (From Palay D [ed]: *Ophthalmology for the primary care physician,* St Louis, 1997, Mosby.)

ACUTE GENERAL Rx

None necessary except when acute glaucoma or inflammation occurs

CHRONIC Rx

- Change glasses as cataracts develop.
- Myopia is common, and glasses can be adjusted until surgery is contemplated.

DISPOSITION

Refer if sight is compromised or the eye is red or inflamed.

REFERRAL

Refer to ophthalmologist for evaluation for extraction when vision is compromised (see "Nonpharmacologic Therapy").

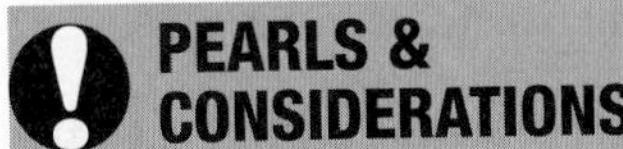

PEARLS & CONSIDERATIONS

- Patients want to know five things about cataracts:
  1. Chance for vision improvement
  2. When vision will improve
  3. Risk from surgery (such as infection, hemorrhage, retinal detachment, corneal problems)
  4. Effect of surgery, including reduction of refractive errors
  5. Types of complications
- Men planning cataract surgery should, if feasible, delay the use of alpha blockers until after surgery has been completed. The risk of intraoperative floppy iris syndrome is substantial among men taking tamsulosin. This is often unavoidable, and discontinuation of alpha blockers does not help, although intraoperative techniques have improved to make floppy iris syndrome less complicated.

SUGGESTED READINGS

available at www.expertconsult.com

RELATED CONTENT

Cataracts (Patient Information)

AUTHORS: **MELVYN KOBY, M.D., and R. SCOTT HOFFMAN, M.D.**

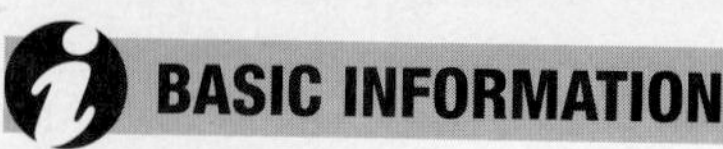

BASIC INFORMATION

DEFINITION

Cat-scratch disease (CSD) is an infectious disease consisting of gradually enlarging regional lymphadenopathy occurring after contact with a feline. Atypical presentations are characterized by a variety of neurologic manifestations as well as granulomatous involvement of the eye, liver, spleen, and bone. The disease is usually self-limiting, and recovery is complete; however, patients with atypical presentations, especially if immunocompromised, may suffer significant morbidity and mortality.

SYNONYMS

Cat-scratch fever
Benign inoculation lymphoreticulosis
Nonbacterial regional lymphadenitis

ICD-9CM CODES
078.3 Cat-scratch disease
ICD-10CM CODES
A28.1 Cat-scratch disease

EPIDEMIOLOGY & DEMOGRAPHICS

PREVALENCE: Unknown
INCIDENCE (IN U.S.):
- 9 to 10 cases per 100,000 persons per year (22,000 cases per year)
- Majority of reported cases occur in persons <21 yrs

PEAK INCIDENCE: August through January

PHYSICAL FINDINGS & CLINICAL PRESENTATION

- Classic, most common finding: regional lymphadenopathy occurring within 2 wk of a scratch or contact with felines; usually a new kitten in the household
- Tender, swollen lymph nodes most commonly found in the head and neck (Fig. E1-228), followed by the axilla and the epitrochlear, inguinal, and femoral areas
- Erythematous overlying skin, showing signs of suppuration from involved lymph nodes
- On careful examination; evidence of cutaneous inoculation in the form of a nonpruritic, slightly tender pustule or papule
- Fever in most patients
- Malaise and headache in fewer than a third of patients
- Atypical presentations in fewer than 15% of cases
  1. Usually in association with lymphadenopathy and a low-grade or frank fever (>101° F, >38.3° C)
  2. Include granulomatous involvement of the conjunctiva (Parinaud's oculoglandular syndrome) and focal masses in the liver, spleen, and mesenteric nodes
- CNS involvement: neuroretinitis, encephalopathy, encephalitis, transverse myelitis, seizure activity, and coma
- Osteomyelitis in adults and children
- Can be a cause of culture-negative endocarditis
- In HIV-infected and other immunocompromised patients, B. *henselae* is the cause of bacillary angiomatous and peliosis hepatis

ETIOLOGY

- Major cause: *Bartonella henselae,* possibly *Afipia felis* and *Bartonella clarrigeiae*
- Mode of transmission: predominantly by direct inoculation through the scratch, bite, or lick of a cat, especially a kitten
- Also can be transmitted by flea bite (with the flea obtaining the bacteria from a bacteremic cat); rarely after exposure to a dog, probably secondary to flea bites
- Approximately 2 wk after introduction of the bacteria into the host, regional lymphatic tissues displaying granulomatous infiltration associated with gradual hypertrophy
- Possible dissemination to distant sites (e.g., liver, spleen, and bone), usually characterized by focal masses or discrete parenchymal lesions

DIAGNOSIS

DIFFERENTIAL DIAGNOSIS

Granulomas of this syndrome must be differentiated from those associated with:
- Tularemia
- Tuberculosis or other myobacterial infections
- Brucellosis
- Sarcoidosis
- Sporotrichosis or other fungal diseases
- Toxoplasmosis
- Lymphogranuloma venereum
- Benign and malignant tumors such as lymphoma

WORKUP

Diagnosis should be considered in patients who present with a predominant complaint of gradually enlarging regional (focal) lymphadenopathy, often with fever and a recent history of having contact with a cat. A primary ulcer at the site of the cat scratch may or may not be present at the time lymphadenopathy becomes manifest.

LABORATORY TESTS

- Serologies: An IFA or EIA *Bartonella* serology (titer ≥1:64) is diagnostic. A PCR assay on tissue or blood is also available.
- Lymph node biopsy: granulomatous inflammation consistent with CSD.
- Warthin-Starry silver stain on biopsy can identify the bacteria.
- Histopathologically, Warthin-Starry silver stain has been used to identify the bacillus.
- Culture: *B. henselae* is a fastidious, slow-growing, gram-negative rod that requires specific culture techniques for tissue or blood.
- Routine laboratory findings:
  1. Mild leukocytosis or leukopenia
  2. Infrequent eosinophilia
  3. Elevated ESR or CRP
- Abnormalities of bilirubin excretion and elevated hepatic transaminases are usually secondary to hepatic obstruction by granuloma, mass, or lymph node.
- In patients with neurologic manifestations, lumbar puncture usually reveals normal CSF, although there may be a mild pleocytosis and modest elevation in protein.
- CSD skin test is no longer used for clinical purposes.

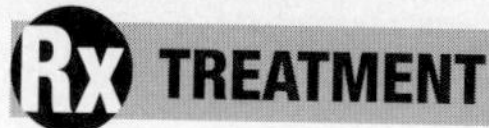

TREATMENT

NONPHARMACOLOGIC THERAPY

- Warm compresses to the affected nodes
- In cases of encephalitis or coma: supportive care

ACUTE GENERAL Rx

- This disease is typically self-limited and generally resolves within 2 to 6 months. Most studies show no additional benefit from antibiotic therapy.
- It would be prudent to treat severely ill patients, especially if immunocompromised, with antibiotic therapy, because these patients tend to suffer dissemination of infection and increased morbidity.
- *Bartonella* is usually sensitive to a 5-day course of azithromycin, or alternatively tetracycline, sulfa, and the quinolones can be used for 7 to 10 days.
- When the isolate is proven by culture, the patient should receive antibiotic therapy as directed by the obtained susceptibilities.
- Antipyretics and NSAIDs may also be used.

DISPOSITION

Overall prognosis is good.

REFERRAL

- To an appropriate subspecialist to evaluate specific lesions
- For diagnostic aspiration or excision in presence of regional lymphadenopathy, bone lesions, and mesenteric lymph nodes and organs
- To ophthalmologist for ocular granulomas
  1. Usually diagnosed clinically
  2. Rarely require excision

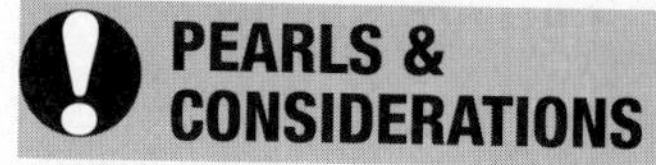

PEARLS & CONSIDERATIONS

COMMENTS

- A presentation of this syndrome, especially in patients with HIV infection or impaired cellular immunity, may be fever of unknown origin.
- Hepatic and splenic granulomas, coronary valve infections may offer few physical clues to diagnosis, emphasizing the need for a complete history.
- CSD should be considered in the differential diagnosis of school-aged children presenting with status epilepticus.
- Chronically immunocompromised patients considering the acquisition of a young feline should be made aware of the possible risk of infection.
- No signs of illness may be apparent in bacteremic kittens.

SUGGESTED READINGS

available at www.expertconsult.com

RELATED CONTENT

Cat-Scratch Disease (Patient Information)

AUTHOR: **GLENN G. FORT, M.D., M.P.H.**

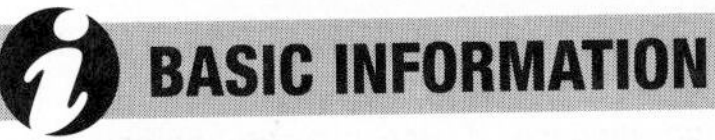

BASIC INFORMATION

DEFINITION

Celiac disease is a chronic autoimmune disease characterized by malabsorption and diarrhea precipitated by ingestion of food products containing gluten. Gluten is a protein complex found in wheat, rye, and barley.

SYNONYMS

Gluten-sensitive enteropathy
Celiac sprue
Nontropical sprue

ICD-9CM CODES
579.0 Celiac disease
ICD-10CM CODES
K90.0 Celiac disease

EPIDEMIOLOGY & DEMOGRAPHICS

- The prevalence of celiac disease is 1% in the general population in North America and Western Europe and 5% in high-risk groups such as first-degree relatives of persons with the disease. The prevalence of celiac disease in the U.S. has increased fourfold over the past three decades. Worldwide celiac disease affects 0.6% to 1% of the population.
- Incidence is highest during infancy and the first 36 mo of life (after introduction of foods containing gluten), in the third decade (frequently associated with pregnancy and severe anemia during pregnancy), and in the seventh decade.
- There is a slight female predominance.
- The average age of diagnosis is in the fifth decade of life.
- The risk for celiac disease is 5% to 10% in newborn children of parents with the disease and nearly 20% in siblings.
- It is estimated that only 10% to 15% of persons with celiac disease in the U.S. have been diagnosed.

PHYSICAL FINDINGS & CLINICAL PRESENTATION

- Physical examination may be entirely within normal limits.
- Weight loss, dyspepsia, short stature, and failure to thrive may be noted in children and infants (Fig. 1-229).
- Weight loss, fatigue, and diarrhea are common in adults.
- Abdominal pain, nausea, and vomiting are unusual.
- Pallor as a result of iron-deficiency anemia is common.
- Atypical forms of the disease are being increasingly recognized and include osteoporosis, short stature, anemia, infertility, and neurologic problems. Manifestations of calcium deficiency, such as tetany and seizures, are rare and can be exacerbated by coexistent magnesium deficiency.
- Angular cheilitis, aphthous ulcers, atopic dermatitis, and dermatitis herpetiformis are frequently associated with celiac disease.

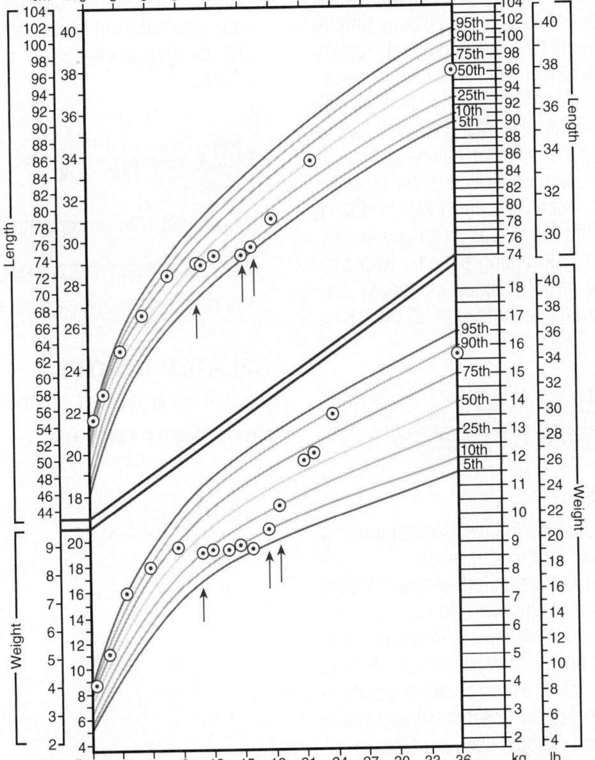

FIGURE 1-229 Gluten-sensitive enteropathy. Growth curve demonstrates initial normal growth from 0 to 9 mo, followed by onset of poor appetite with intermittent vomiting and diarrhea after initiation of gluten-containing diet *(single arrow).* After biopsy-confirmed diagnosis and treatment with gluten-free diet *(double arrow),* growth improves. (From Kliegman RM et al: *Nelson textbook of pediatrics,* ed 19, Philadelphia, 2011, Saunders.)

- Table 1-101 summarizes the clinical spectrum of celiac disease.

ETIOLOGY

- Celiac sprue is considered an autoimmune-type disease, with tissue transglutaminase (tTG) suggested as a major autoantigen. It results from an inappropriate T-cell–mediated immune response against ingested gluten in genetically predisposed individuals who carry either HLA-DQ2 or HLA-DQ8 genes. There is sensitivity to gliadin, a protein fraction of gluten found in wheat, rye, and barley. In patients with celiac disease, immune responses to gliadin fractions promote an inflammatory reaction, mainly in the upper small intestine, manifested by infiltration of the lamina propria and the epithelium with chronic inflammatory cells and villous atrophy.
- Seroconversion to celiac autoimmunity may occur at any time.
- Timing of introduction of gluten into the infant diet is associated with the appearance of celiac disease in children at risk. Children initially exposed to gluten in the first 3 mo of life have a fivefold increased risk. Current recommendations are to delay introduction of gluten into the diet of a genetically susceptible infant until 4 to 6 mo of age while the mother continues to breastfeed.

Dx Diagnosis

Diagnostic criteria for celiac disease require at least four out of five or three out of four if the HLA genotype is not performed:

1. Typical symptoms of celiac disease
2. Positivity of serum celiac disease Ig A class autoantibodies at high titer
3. *HLA-DQ2* or *HLA-DQ8* genotypes

TABLE 1-101 Clinical Spectrum of Celiac Disease

Symptomatic
Frank malabsorption symptoms: chronic diarrhea, failure to thrive, weight loss
Extraintestinal manifestations: anemia, fatigue, hypertransaminasemia, neurologic disorders, short stature, dental enamel defects, arthralgia, aphthous stomatitis
Silent
No apparent symptoms in spite of histologic evidence of villous atrophy
In most cases identified by serologic screening in at-risk groups (see laboratory tests)
Latent
Subjects who have a normal histology, but at some other time, before or after, have shown a gluten-dependent enteropathy
Potential
Subjects with positive celiac disease serology but without evidence of altered jejunal histology
It might or might not be symptomatic

From Kliegman RM et al: *Nelson textbook of pediatrics,* ed 19, Philadelphia, 2011, Saunders.

 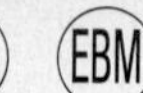

4. Celiac enteropathy at the small intestinal biopsy
5. Response to gluten-free diet

DIFFERENTIAL DIAGNOSIS

- Inflammatory bowel disease
- Laxative abuse
- Intestinal parasitic infestations
- Lactose intolerance
- Other: irritable bowel syndrome, tropical sprue, chronic pancreatitis, Zollinger-Ellison syndrome, cystic fibrosis (children), lymphoma, eosinophilic gastroenteritis, short bowel syndrome, Whipple's disease
- Intestinal lymphoma, tuberculosis, radiation enteritis, HIV enteropathy

LABORATORY TESTS

- IgA anti-tTG antibody by enzyme-linked immunosorbent assay (tissue transglutaminase [tTG] test) is the best screening serologic test for celiac disease. IgA antiendomysial antibodies (EMA) test is also a good screening test for celiac disease but is best used as a confirmatory test in cases of borderline positive results. In patients with IgA deficiency, the IgG DPG test (deamidated gliadin peptides) can be used for diagnosis. Screening of close relatives is initially done with PCR testing for HLA DQ2 or HLA DQ8. Those that are positive should then have serum tTG IgA screening
- CBC, ferritin level: Iron-deficiency anemia (microcytic anemia, low ferritin level) may be present.
- Celiac disease can lead to malabsorption: Screen for vitamin B_{12} level, folate level, vitamin D level, serum calcium, albumin, magnesium; vitamin B_{12} deficiency, vitamin D deficiency, hypomagnesemia, and hypocalcemia are not uncommon in celiac disease.
- Biopsy of the small bowel, considered the gold standard, has been questioned as a reliable and conclusive test in all cases. It may be reasonable in children with significant elevations of tTG levels (>100 U) to first try a gluten-free diet and consider biopsy in those who do not improve with diet.
- The HLA-DQ2 allele is identified in >90% of patients with celiac disease, and HLA-DQ8 is identified in most of the remaining patients. These genes occur in only 30% to 40% of the general population. Their greatest diagnostic value is in their negative predictive value, making them useful when negative in ruling out the disease.

IMAGING STUDIES

- Consider bone density in newly diagnosed adult patients.
- Capsule endoscopy can be used to evaluate mucosa of the small intestine, especially if future innovations will allow mucosal biopsy.

Rx TREATMENT

NONPHARMACOLOGIC THERAPY

Patients should be instructed on a gluten-free diet (avoidance of wheat, rye, and barley). Safe grains (gluten-free) include rice, corn, oats, buckwheat, millet, amaranth, quinoa, sorghum, and teff (an Ethiopian cereal grain). The lowest amount of daily gluten that causes damage to the celiac intestinal mucosa is 10-15 mg/day. One slice of bread contains 1.6 g of gluten.

GENERAL Rx

- Correct nutritional deficiencies with iron, folic acid, calcium, vitamin D, and vitamin B12 as needed.
- Prednisone 20 to 60 mg qd gradually tapered is useful in refractory cases.
- Lifelong gluten-free diet is necessary. A referral to a nutritionist experienced in celiac disease and gluten-free diet is recommended at initial diagnosis.

DISPOSITION

- Prognosis is good with adherence to a gluten-free diet. Rapid improvement is usually seen within a few days of treatment. Healing of the intestinal damage typically occurs within 6-24 mo after initiation of the diet. Lack of response to gluten-free diet occurs in 5% of patients and is due to unintentional ingestion of gluten or presence of coexisting GI disorders such as IBD, lactose or other carbohydrate intolerance, and pancreatic insufficiency.
- Serial antigliadin or antiendomysial antibody tests can be used to monitor the patient's adherence to a gluten-free diet.
- Repeat small-bowel biopsy after treatment generally reveals significant improvement. It is also useful to evaluate for increased risk of small-bowel T-cell lymphoma in these patients, especially untreated patients. Some experts recommend a repeat biopsy only in selected patients who have an unsatisfactory response to a strict gluten-free diet; however, recent data (Lebwohl et al) show that the risk for lymphoproliferative malignancy (LPM) is affected by the results of follow-up intestinal biopsy performed to document mucosal healing. Increased risk for LPM in CD is associated with the follow-up biopsy results, with a higher risk among patients with persistent villous atrophy. Follow-up biopsy may effectively stratify patients with CD by risk for subsequent LPM.

PEARLS & CONSIDERATIONS

COMMENTS

- The presence of dermatitis herpetiformis is pathognomonic for celiac disease.
- In close relatives, repeated serum tTG IgA testing may be useful in those with positive HLA DQ2 or HLA DQ8 tests because celiac disease may not manifest until later in life, and initial negative results do not preclude the possibility of future onset of celiac disease
- Celiac disease should be considered in patients with unexplained metabolic bone disease, osteoporosis, or hypocalcemia, because gastrointestinal symptoms are absent or mild. Clinicians should also consider testing children and young adults for celiac disease if unexplained weight loss, abdominal pain or distention, or chronic diarrhea present.
- Screening for celiac disease is recommended in first-degree relatives. It should also be considered in patients with type 1 diabetes mellitus and in those with certain autoimmune disorders such as primary biliary cirrhosis, primary sclerosing cholangitis, autoimmune hepatitis, IBD, thyroid disease (hypothyroidism occurs in up to 15% of patients with celiac disease), SLE, RA, and Sjogren's syndrome due to increased risk of celiac disease in these populations. Screening persons with Down syndrome or Turner syndrome has also been recommended.
- The prevalence of celiac disease in patients with dyspepsia is twice that of the general population. Screening for celiac disease should be considered in all patients with persistent dyspepsia.
- Patients with celiac disease have an overall risk of cancer that is almost twice that of the general population. The risk of adenocarcinoma of the small intestine is increased manifold compared with the risk in the general population. Celiac disease is also associated with an increased risk for non-Hodgkin's lymphoma, especially of T-cell type and primarily localized in the gut. Lymphoma is 4 to 40 times more common, and death from lymphoma is 11 to 70 times more common in patients with celiac disease.
- Patients with celiac disease who have followed a gluten-free diet for prolonged periods may not experience relapse of symptoms for several months after gluten is reintroduced.

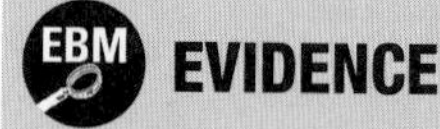

EVIDENCE

Available at www.expertconsult.com

SUGGESTED READINGS

Available at www.expertconsult.com

RELATED CONTENT

Celiac Disease (Patient Information)

AUTHOR: **FRED F. FERRI, M.D.**

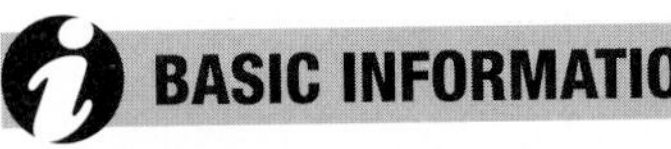

DEFINITION

Cellulitis is a superficial inflammatory condition of the skin and underlying tissues characterized by erythema, warmth, and tenderness of the involved area.

SYNONYMS

Erysipelas (cellulitis generally caused by group A β-hemolytic streptococci)
SSSIs (skin and skin structure infections)
ABSSSIs (acute bacterial skin and skin structure infections)

ICD-9CM CODES
682.9 Cellulitis
ICD-10CM CODES
L03.90 Cellulitis, unspecified

EPIDEMIOLOGY & DEMOGRAPHICS

- Occurs most frequently in diabetics, immunocompromised hosts, and patients with venous and lymphatic compromise.
- Frequently found near skin breaks (trauma, surgical wounds [surgical site infections develop in 2% to 5% of all surgical procedures], ulcerations, tinea infections). Edema, animal or human bites, subadjacent osteomyelitis, and bacteremia are potential sources of cellulitis.
- Skin and soft-tissue infections account for >14 million outpatient visits in the U.S./yr.

PHYSICAL FINDINGS & CLINICAL PRESENTATION

Variable with the causative organism:

- Erysipelas (Fig. E1-230): superficial-spreading, warm, erythematous lesion distinguished by indurated, elevated margin; lymphatic involvement, vesicle formation common.
- Staphylococcal cellulitis: area involved is erythematous, hot, and swollen; differentiated from erysipelas by nonelevated, poorly demarcated margin; local tenderness and regional adenopathy are common; up to 85% of cases occur on the legs and feet.
- *Haemophilus influenzae* cellulitis: area involved is a blue-red/purple-red color; occurs mainly in children; generally involves the face in children and the neck or upper chest in adults.
- *Vibrio vulnificus:* larger hemorrhagic bullae, cellulitis, lymphadenitis, myositis; often found in critically ill patients in septic shock.

ETIOLOGY

- Group A β-hemolytic streptococci (may follow a streptococcal infection of the upper respiratory tract). β-hemolytic streptococci are implicated in most cases of non-traumatic cellulitis.
- Staphylococcal cellulitis: Diabetics, athletes, men who have sex with men, people living in public housing, and incarcerated men are at greater risk for methicillin-resistant *S. aureus* (MRSA) infection. A community-acquired MRSA strain, USA 300, is replacing nosocomial strains of MRSA in hospitals.
- IV drug use: MRSA, *P. aeruginosa*.
- *V. vulnificus:* higher incidence in patients with liver disease (75%) and in immunocompromised hosts. *V. vulnificus* infection is the leading cause of death related to seafood consumption in the U.S.
- *Erysipelothrix rhusiopathiae:* common in people handling poultry, fish, or meat.
- *Aeromonas hydrophila:* generally occurs in contaminated open wounds in fresh water.
- Fungi *(Cryptococcus neoformans):* in immunocompromised granulopenic patients.
- Gram-negative rods *(Serratia, Enterobacter, Proteus, Pseudomonas):* may be present in immunocompromised or granulopenic patients.
- Hot tub exposure: *P. aeruginosa*; fish tank exposure: *Mycobacterium marinum.*
- Bites: Human *(Eikenella corrodens),* dog *(Pasteurella multocida, C. canimorsus),* cat *(P. multocida),* rat *(Streptobacillus moniliformis).*

Dx DIAGNOSIS

DIFFERENTIAL DIAGNOSIS:

- Necrotizing fasciitis (reddish-purple discoloration of skin, rapid increase in size, woody induration and pale appearance rather than erythema, violaceous bullae, pain out of proportion to appearance, sepsis)
- Deep vein thrombosis
- Peripheral vascular insufficiency
- Paget disease of the breast
- Thrombophlebitis
- Acute gout
- Psoriasis
- *Candida* intertrigo
- Pseudogout
- Osteomyelitis
- Insect bite
- Fixed drug eruption
- Lymphedema
- Contact dermatitis
- Olecranon bursa infection
- Herpetic whitlow, early herpes zoster (before blisters)
- Erythema migrans (Lyme disease)
- Rare: *Vaccinia* vaccination, Kawasaki disease, pyoderma gangrenosum, Sweet syndrome, carcinoma erysipeloides, anaerobic myonecrosis, erythromelalgia, eosinophilic cellulitis (Well's syndrome), familial Mediterranean fever

LABORATORY TESTS:

- Gram stain, culture (aerobic and anaerobic):
  1. Aspirated material from:
     a. Advancing edge of cellulitis
     b. Any vesicles
  2. Swab of any drainage material
  3. Punch biopsy (in selected patients)
- Blood cultures in hospitalized patients, patients with cellulitis superimposed on lymphedema, patients with buccal or periorbital cellulitis, and patients suspected of having a salt- or fresh-water source of infection. Bacteremia uncommon in cellulitis (positive blood cultures in 4% of patients).
- Anti-streptolysin O (ASLO) titer (in suspected streptococcal disease)

The cause of cellulitis remains unidentified in most patients. Patients with recurrent lower-extremity cellulitis should be inspected for tinea pedis. If found it should be treated.

IMAGING STUDIES

CT or MRI in patients with suspected necrotizing fasciitis (deep-seated infection of the subcutaneous tissue that results in the progressive destruction of fascia and fat).

Rx TREATMENT

NONPHARMACOLOGIC THERAPY

Immobilization and elevation of the involved limb. Cool sterile saline dressings to remove purulence from any open lesion. Support stockings in patients with peripheral edema.

ACUTE GENERAL RX

Erysipelas:

- PO: dicloxacillin 500 mg PO q6h
- IV: cefazolin 1 g q6 to 8h or nafcillin 1.0 or 1.5 g IV q4 to 6h

NOTE: Use vancomycin 1 g IV q12h in patients allergic to penicillin.

Staphylococcal cellulitis:

- PO: dicloxacillin 250 to 500 mg qid
- IV: nafcillin 1 to 2 g q4 to 6h
- Cephalosporins (cephalothin, cephalexin, cephradine) also provide adequate antistaphylococcal coverage, except for MRSA.
- Trimethoprim-sulfamethoxazole (160 mg/800 mg 1 PO bid) may be appropriate in mild MRSA infections. Use vancomycin 1.0 to 2.0 g IV qd or linezolid 0.6 g IV q12h in patients allergic to penicillin or cephalosporins and in patients with moderate/severe MRSA. Daptomycin (Cubicin), a cyclic lipopeptide, can be used as an alternative to vancomycin for complicated skin and skin structure infections. Usual dose is 4 mg/kg IV given over 30 min every 24 hr. Telavancin is a new glycopeptide derivative of vancomycin effective for gram-positive skin and skin structure infections, including those caused by MRSA. Tedizolid is an oxazolidinone effective in ABSSSI as an alternative to linezolid. Ceftaroline fosamil (Teflaro) is a new IV cephalosporin also effective against MRSA.

H. influenzae cellulitis:

- PO: cefixime or cefuroxime
- IV: cefuroxime or ceftriaxone

Vibrio vulnificus:

- Doxycycline 100 mg IV bid + ceftazidime 2 g IV q8h or IV ciprofloxacin 400 mg bid. Mild cases treated with oral antibiotics (doxycycline 100 mg bid + ciprofloxacin 750 mg bid).
- IV support and admission into intensive care unit (mortality rate >50% in septic shock).

E. rhusiopathiae:

- Penicillin

A. hydrophila:

- Aminoglycosides
- Chloramphenicol
- Complicated skin and skin structure infections in hospitalized patients can be treated with daptomycin (Cubicin) 4 mg/kg IV q24h

SUGGESTED READINGS

available at www.expertconsult.com

RELATED CONTENT

Cellulitis (Patient Information)

AUTHOR: **FRED F. FERRI, M.D.**

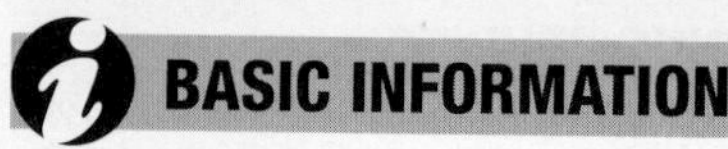

BASIC INFORMATION

DEFINITION

Cerebral palsy (CP) is a group of disorders of the central nervous system characterized by aberrant control of movement or posture, present since early in life and not the result of a progressive or degenerative disease. Fig. 1-231 provides a classification of CP.

SYNONYMS

Little's disease
Congenital static encephalopathy
Congenital spastic paralysis
CP

ICD-9CM CODES
343 Infantile cerebral palsy
342 Hemiplegia and hemiparesis
344 Quadriplegia and quadriparesiss
ICD-10CM CODES
M41.40 Neuromuscular scoliosis, site unspecified

EPIDEMIOLOGY & DEMOGRAPHICS

INCIDENCE (IN U.S.): 2 to 2.5 persons per 1000 live births

PREDOMINANT SEX: Males and females affected equally

PREDOMINANT AGE: Diagnosis typically made at 3 to 5 years of age

PHYSICAL FINDINGS & CLINICAL PRESENTATION

- Monoplegia, diplegia, quadriplegia, hemiplegia
- Often hypotonic in newborn period, followed by development of hypertonia
- Spasticity
- Athetosis
- Delay in motor milestones
- Hyperreflexia
- Seizures
- Mental retardation in many individuals

ETIOLOGY

Multifactorial, including low birth weight, congenital malformation, asphyxia, multiple gestation, intrauterine exposure to infection, neonatal stroke, hyperbilirubinemia, and maternal thyroid malfunction

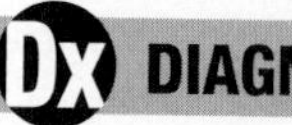

DIAGNOSIS

A motor deficit is always present. The usual presenting complaint is that child is not reaching motor milestones at the appropriate age. Medical history establishes that the child is not losing function (i.e., that deficit is static and not progressive). This history, combined with a neurologic examination establishing that motor deficit is due to a cerebral abnormality, establishes the diagnosis of CP. Serial examinations may be necessary.

DIFFERENTIAL DIAGNOSIS

Other causes of neonatal hypotonia include muscular dystrophies, spinal muscular atrophy, Down syndrome, and spinal cord injuries. Causes of progressive spasticity in children include metabolic diseases involving white matter (e.g., leukodystrophy).

WORKUP

- Laboratory tests are not necessary to establish the diagnosis.
- Workup is helpful for assessment of recurrence risk, implementation of prevention programs, and medicolegal purposes.

LABORATORY TESTS

- Metabolic and genetic testing should be considered if on follow-up the child has (1) evidence of deterioration or episodes of metabolic decompensation, (2) no etiology determined by neuroimaging, (3) family history of childhood neurologic disorder associated with CP, or (4) developmental malformation on neuroimaging. Hypercoagulability workup should be considered if neuroimaging is suggestive of a remote stroke.
- EEG should be obtained when a child with CP has a history suggestive of seizures.
- Children with CP should be screened for ophthalmologic and hearing impairments, as well as speech and language disorders. Nutrition, growth, and swallowing function should be monitored.

IMAGING STUDIES

- Neuroimaging is recommended if the etiology has not been established previously, for example by perinatal imaging.
- MRI, when available, is preferred to CT scanning because of higher yield in determining an etiology and timing of the insult leading to CP.

FIGURE 1-231 Classification of cerebral palsy. Although overlaps in terminology exist, cerebral palsy can be classified according to distribution (regional versus global involvement, hemiplegic, diplegic, quadriplegic), physiologic type (spastic, dyskinetic/dystonic, dyskinetic/athetoid, ataxic), or presumed neurologic substrate (pyramidal, extrapyramidal). (From Canale ST, Beaty JH: *Campbell's operative orthopaedics,* ed 11, Philadelphia, 2007, Mosby.)

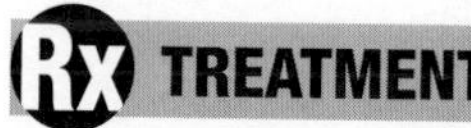

TREATMENT

NONPHARMACOLOGIC THERAPY

- Physical therapy, occupational therapy, and speech therapy.
- Orthotics and casting are used to increase musculotendinous length.

ACUTE GENERAL Rx

If present, treatment of seizures

CHRONIC Rx

- Treatment of seizures, as directed by seizure type.
- Medical treatment of spasticity includes baclofen (oral and intrathecal), as well as botulinum toxin A.
- Surgical treatments of spasticity include dorsal rhizotomy, tendon lengthening, and osteotomy.

DISPOSITION

Most children with CP live at home. Those children with severely impaired mobility or other disabilities may live in chronic-care nursing facilities.

REFERRAL

If the child has difficulty with spasticity, physical medicine and rehabilitation referrals are especially helpful.

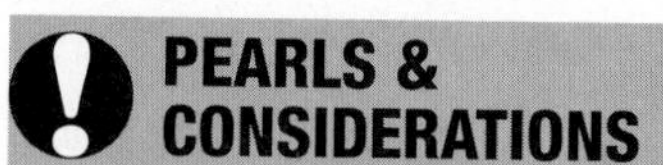

PEARLS & CONSIDERATIONS

- In full-term infants, there is usually no history of traumatic delivery.
- Compared with delivery at 40 wks' gestation, delivery at 37 or 38 wks or at 42 wks or later was associated with an increased risk of CP.

SUGGESTED READINGS

available at www.expertconsult.com

RELATED CONTENT

Cerebral Palsy (Patient Information)

AUTHOR: **MAITREYI MAZUMDAR, M.D., M.P.H., M.SC.**

BASIC INFORMATION

DEFINITION

Cerebral vasculitis refers to a group of heterogenous disorders characterized by pathologic inflammation and leukocytoclastic changes in the blood vessel walls.

SYNONYMS

Central nervous system angiitis
Cerebral arteritis

ICD-9CM CODES
437.4 Cerebral arteritis
ICD-10CM CODES
I67.7 Cerebral arteritis, not elsewhere classified

EPIDEMIOLOGY & DEMOGRAPHICS

INCIDENCE: Average annual incidence rate is 2.4 cases per 1,000,000 person-yr.
PEAK INCIDENCE: Fourth decade of life
PREDOMINANT SEX: Males are affected twice as often as females.
PREDOMINANT AGE: Usual age of presentation is in the third and fourth decades of life, but can present in age ranging from 17 to 70 yr.
GENETICS: Multifactorial
RISK FACTORS: Infections, connective tissue disorders, systemic vasculitis, and substance abuse are the prominent risk factors for secondary cerebral vasculitis.
CLASSIFICATION:
- Primary cerebral vasculitis or primary angiitis of the central nervous system (CNS): involvement of the blood vessels in brain or spinal cord without involvement of blood vessels or organs beyond the CNS.
- Secondary CNS vasculitis (Table 1-102): involvement of the brain or spinal cord blood vessels by a systemic disorder such as systemic vasculitis, connective tissue disorders, infections, malignancy, or substance abuse.

PHYSICAL FINDINGS & CLINICAL PRESENTATION

- Presentation of cerebral vasculitis is diverse and includes the following:
  - Nonspecific symptoms such as weight loss, lethargy, vomiting, headache, and confusion in the early course of the disease.
  - Neurologic manifestations: seen in 80% of patients during course of illness; may mimic multiple sclerosis, with a relapsing and remitting course.
  - Stroke can occur in 40% of the patients; transient ischemic attacks have been reported in 30%-50% of patients.
  - Seizures occur in 25% of patients.
  - Other common presentations include intracerebral hemorrhage (11%) and intracranial space-occupying lesions (15%).
- Secondary vasculitis often presents with stroke-like symptoms. Sjögren's syndrome and Behçet's disease can have varied presentations that mimic multiple sclerosis, seizures, movement disorders, encephalopathy, dementia, and aseptic meningitis.

ETIOLOGY

The exact etiology of primary cerebral vasculitis is unknown. It has been associated with various infectious agents such as herpes zoster, mycoplasma, HIV, and unknown viruses. Amyloid angiopathy has been described with primary cerebral vasculitis.

DIAGNOSIS

DIFFERENTIAL DIAGNOSIS

- Reversible cerebral vasoconstriction syndromes
- Intracranial vessels atherosclerosis
- Cerebral emboli
- Intravascular lymphoma
- Sarcoidosis
- Cerebral autosomal dominant arteriopathy with subcortical infarcts and leukoencephalopathy (CADASIL)

WORKUP

- Brain biopsy (usually nondominant temporal lobe tip along with overlying leptomeninges) is the gold standard for diagnosis of cerebral vasculitis.
- Cerebral angiography supports the diagnosis of CNS vasculitis but has low sensitivity and specificity (Fig. 1-232).

TABLE 1-102 Common Causes of Secondary Cerebral Vasculitis and Associated Features

Giant cell arteritis/Takayasu's arteritis	"Pulseless disease," fever, weight loss, syncope, visual field defects
Polyarteritis nodosa	Fever, weight loss, arthralgia, renal failure, myocardial infarction
Churg-Strauss syndrome	Asthma-like features followed by multiple-organ system involvement including GI, skin, kidneys, CNS, heart
Wegener's granulomatosis	Rhinitis, epistaxis, hemoptysis, hematuria, chronic renal failure
Behçet's disease	Oral ulcers, genital ulcers, skin lesions, uveitis, iritis
Systemic lupus erythematosus	Malar rash, oral ulcers, photosensitivity, arthralgia, renal failure, anemia, ANA positive
Rheumatoid arthritis	Arthritis involving hand joints, radiologic evidence of joint erosion, rheumatoid factor positive
Sjögren's syndrome	Dry mouth, dry eyes, involvement of lung, liver, pancreas, joints
Lymphoma	Fever, weight loss, night sweats, lymph node enlargement, hepatosplenomegaly

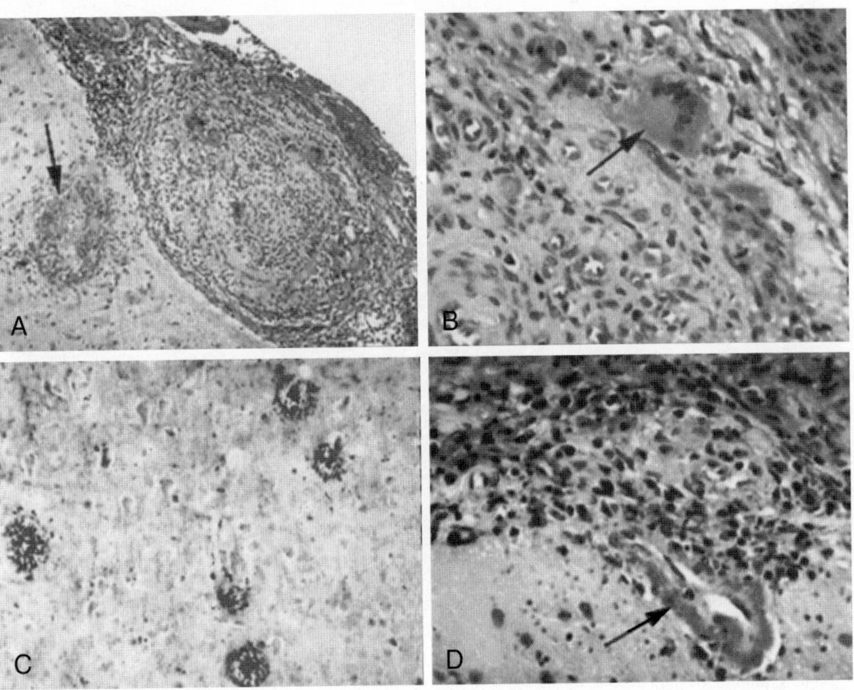

FIGURE 1-232 **A,** Low-power hematoxylin and eosin stain (10×) demonstrates diffuse inflammation in the leptomeninges with infiltration of lymphocytes, eosinophils, and macrophages with destruction of the vessel wall. **B,** A multinucleated giant cell *(arrow)*. **C,** Multiple neuritic plaques are seen on this silver stain. **D,** Congo red stain demonstrating the presence of amyloid within a vessel wall *(arrow)*. (From Jacobs DA et al: Primary central nervous system angiitis, amyloid angiopathy and Alzheimer's pathology presenting with Balint's syndrome, *Surv Ophthalmol* 49[4]:454-459, 2004.)

LABORATORY TESTS

- Lumbar puncture: may show elevated cerebrospinal fluid opening pressure, elevated protein, lymphocytic pleocytosis, and negative microbial cultures.
- Basic laboratory testing: should include CBC with differential, blood urea nitrogen and serum creatinine, hepatic functions and enzymes, erythrocyte sedimentation rate, RPR (for syphilis), C-reactive protein, and urine analysis.
- Specific serologic tests to evaluate autoimmune causes: ANA, rheumatoid factor, anti–double-stranded DNA, anti SS-A, anti SS-B, anti–neutrophil cytoplasmic antibody (ANCA), complement 3 and 4, cryoglobulins, serum immunoglobulins, and HIV testing.

IMAGING STUDIES

Magnetic resonance imaging (MRI) is the neuroimaging of choice. Abnormal findings are seen in 90% to 100% of the patients. Cerebral cortex, deep white and gray matter changes are commonly reported (Fig. 1-233).

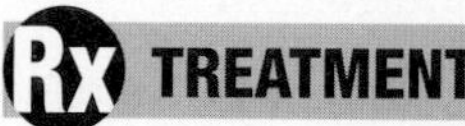

TREATMENT

There are no randomized controlled trials evaluating treatment of cerebral vasculitis. Treatment strategies are similar to other systemic vasculitis.

NONPHARMACOLOGIC THERAPY

Patients with permanent deficits are provided with physical and occupational therapy.

ACUTE GENERAL Rx

- Steroids: For suspected cases, empiric therapy with glucocorticoids is started after exclusion of infectious causes. Intravenous methylprednisolone 1 g daily for 3 days is preferred for patients with severe disease; otherwise, oral prednisone is started at 1 mg/kg/day.

CHRONIC Rx

- Steroids: Oral prednisone is continued at high dose (1 mg/kg/day) for 4 to 6 wk and then tapered over 12 mo.
- Immunosuppressive treatment: cyclophosphamide orally for 3 to 6 months for remission induction. Once stable, milder and relatively safer immunosuppressants such as azathioprine, methotrexate, or mycophenolate are used for 2 to 3 years.

DISPOSITION

Course and prognosis of the disease is variable. It depends on the extent of neurologic involvement, severity of deficits, and response to treatment. Neurologic deficits may resolve acutely, slowly, or not at all. Some patients have symptomatic improvement with resolution of headache or altered mental status. Some have improvement in laboratory values, and others have improved MRI scans.

REFERRAL

- Neurology: referral to neurology is indicated in patients with neurologic deficits of uncertain etiology, younger age, intractable headaches, or uncertain diagnosis.
- Neurosurgical consult for brain biopsy.

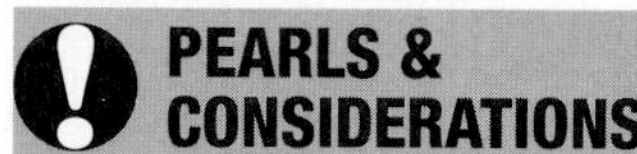

PEARLS & CONSIDERATIONS

COMMENTS

- Cerebral vasculitis is a rare disorder that is difficult to diagnose because of variable presentation.
- Early recognition of the clinical symptoms and signs is important to prevent long-term morbidity and mortality.
- Systemic causes should be excluded.
- Patients may need chronic immunosuppressive treatment.

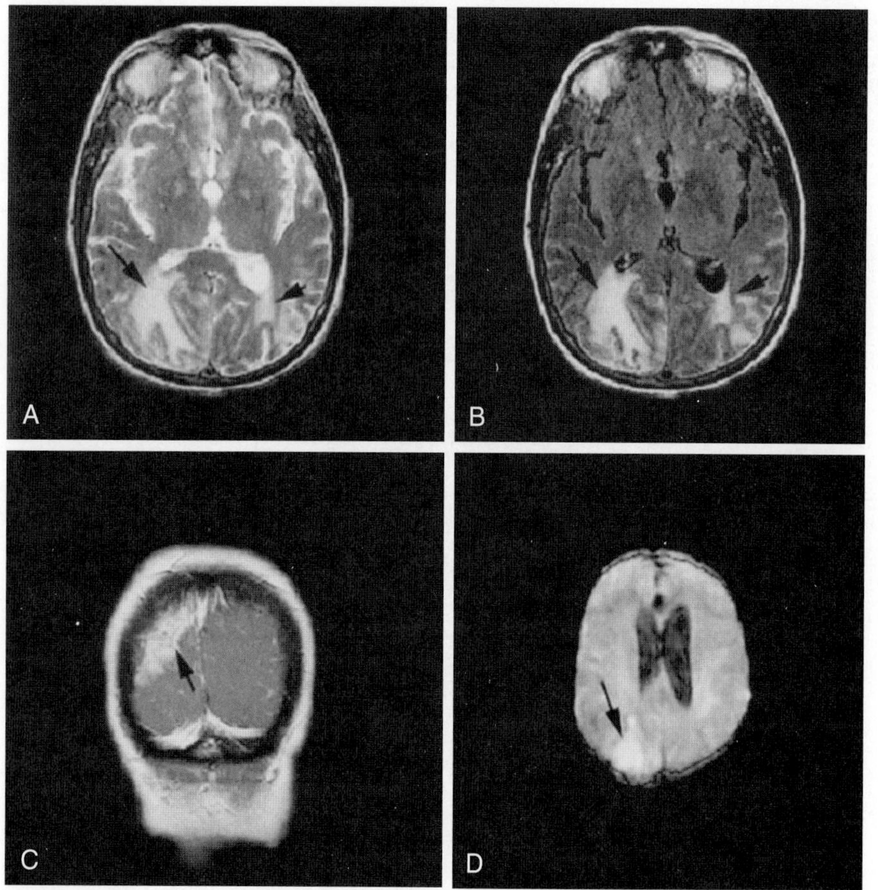

FIGURE 1-233 **A,** Axial T2-weighted image shows abnormal signal in bilateral parietooccipital lobes, greater on the right than left *(arrows).* **B,** Axial fluid attenuated inversion recovery image further delineating the extent of bilateral parietooccipital lesions *(arrow).* **C,** Coronal T1-gadolinium study demonstrating nodular leptomeningeal enhancement in the lesion *(arrow).* **D,** Diffusion-weighted magnetic resonance imaging shows bright signal in the right parietooccipital region, suggesting ischemic changes *(arrow).* (From Jacobs DA et al: Primary central nervous system angiitis, amyloid angiopathy and Alzheimer's pathology presenting with Balint's syndrome, *Surv Ophthalmol* 49[4]:454-459, 2004.)

SUGGESTED READINGS

available at www.expertconsult.com

RELATED CONTENT

Vasculitis (Related Key Topic)

AUTHOR: **FARIHA ZAHEER, M.D.**

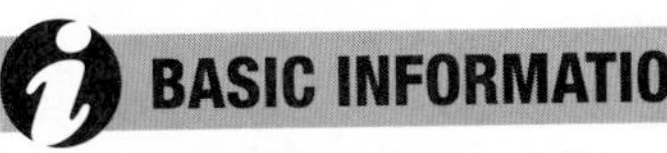

BASIC INFORMATION

DEFINITION

Cervical cancer is the penetration of the basement membrane and infiltration of the stroma of the uterine cervix by malignant cells.

ICD-9CM CODES
180 Malignant neoplasm of cervix uteri
ICD-10CM CODES
C53.9 Malignant neoplasm of cervix uteri, unspecified

EPIDEMIOLOGY & DEMOGRAPHICS

INCIDENCE: Approximately 15,000 new cases annually, with 4000 to 5000 associated deaths. U.S. has age-adjusted mortality rate of 2.6 per 100,000 persons.

PREDOMINANCE: Higher incidence rates occur in developing countries. Among the U.S. population, Hispanics have a higher incidence than African Americans, who likewise have a higher incidence than whites. Worldwide, cervical cancer is the third most common cancer in women.

RISK FACTORS: Smoking, early age at first intercourse, multiple sexual partners, immunocompromised state, nonbarrier methods of birth control, infection with high-risk human papillomavirus (HPV; types 16 and 18), and multiparity.

PHYSICAL FINDINGS & CLINICAL PRESENTATION

- Unusual vaginal bleeding, particularly postcoital
- Vaginal discharge and/or odor
- Advanced cases may present with lower-extremity edema or renal failure
- Early stages, may be little or no obvious cervical lesion; more advanced cases may have large, bulky, friable lesions encompassing majority of vagina

ETIOLOGY

- Infection with high-risk HPV types is necessary, although not sufficient, cause of almost all cases of cervical cancer. Persistent HPV infection leads to precancerous changes of cervix (cervical intraepithelial neoplasia [CIN]). CIN can progress to invasive cervical cancer.
- More than 40 HPV types can infect cervix. Most cases are believed to be linked to presence of HPV 16, 18, 45, and 56 by interaction of E6 oncoprotein on p53 gene product.
- There may be an association with past infection with *Chlamydia trachomatis.*

DIAGNOSIS

DIFFERENTIAL DIAGNOSIS

- Cervical polyp or prolapsed uterine fibroid
- Preinvasive cervical lesions
- Neoplasia metastatic from a separate primary neoplasia

WORKUP

- Thorough history and physical examination.
- Pelvic examination with careful rectovaginal examination.
- Compared with Pap testing, HPV testing has greater sensitivity for detection of CIN. Addition of HPV test for high-risk types to Pap test to screen women in mid-30s for cervical cancer reduces incidence of grade 2 or 3 CIN or cancer detected by subsequent screening examinations.
- Colposcopy with directed biopsy and endocervical curettage.
- FIGO staging described in Table 1-103.

LABORATORY TESTS

- Complete blood count, chemistry profile
- SCC antigen in research setting
- Carcinoembryonic antigen

IMAGING STUDIES

- Chest x-ray
- Depending on stage, may need cystoscopy, sigmoidoscopy or barium enema, CT scan or MRI (Fig. E1-234), lymphangiography
- Intravenous pyelogram

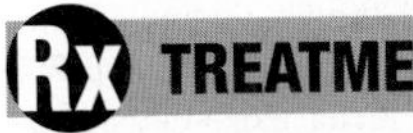

TREATMENT

NONPHARMACOLOGIC THERAPY

- FIGO stage IA: cone biopsy or simple hysterectomy
- FIGO stage IB or IIA: type III radical hysterectomy and pelvic lymphadenectomy or pelvic radiation therapy
- Advanced or bulky disease: multimodality therapy (radiation, chemotherapy, and/or surgery); platinum use before radiation therapy

ACUTE GENERAL Rx

Table 1-103 summarizes treatment according to tumor stage. Chemotherapy is cisplatin-based. In advanced cases, cervical cancer may present with massive and acute vaginal bleeding requiring volume and blood replacement, vaginal packing or other hemostatic modalities, and/or high-dose local radiotherapy.

CHRONIC Rx

- Physical examination with Pap smear every 3 mo for 2 yr, every 6 mo for 3-5 yr, annually thereafter
- Chest x-ray examination annually

DISPOSITION

Five-year survival varies by stage:

- Stage I: 60% to 90%
- Stage II: 40% to 80%
- Stage III: <60%
- Stage IV: <15%

Early detection by Pap smear is imperative to long-term improvements in survival.

REFERRAL

Gynecologic oncologist for all invasive disease

TABLE 1-103 FIGO Staging of Cervical Cancer

Stage	Invasion	Prognosis 5-yr Survival	Treatment
1_{A1}	Depth of invasion up to 3 mm and width up to 7 mm (includes early stromal invasion of up to 1 mm)	84%-90% if tumor < 3 cm; 85% will have negative pelvic nodes and 95% of these patients will be 'cured'	Local excision; if margins of cone clear (i.e., no residual tumor or CIN) then conization is adequate, with no need for pelvic lymphadenectomy
1_{A2}	Depth of invasion between 3 and 5 mm (i.e., 3.1-5 mm) and width up to 7 mm	66% if tumor > 3 cm	Simple hysterectomy and pelvic lymphadenectomy
1_{B1}	Tumor confined to cervix and diameter less than 4 cm		Radical hysterectomy or radiotherapy
1_{B2}	Tumor confined to cervix and diameter more than 4 cm		Radical hysterectomy or radiotherapy
II_A	Upper 1/3 vagina	62%	Radical hysterectomy or radiotherapy
II_B	Upper 2/3 of vagina plus parametrial disease		Radiotherapy ± chemotherapy
III_A	Lower 1/3 vagina	40%	Radiotherapy ± chemotherapy
III_B	Pelvic sidewall and/or hydronephrosis		Radiotherapy ± chemotherapy
IV_A	Bladder, rectum	15%	Radiotherapy ± chemotherapy
IV_B	Beyond pelvis		Radiotherapy ± chemotherapy

From Drife J, Magowan B: *Clinical obstetrics and gynecology,* Philadelphia, 2004, Saunders.

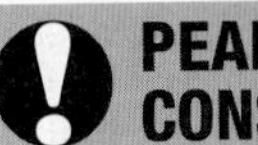

PEARLS & CONSIDERATIONS

- Gardasil is a vaccine indicated in males and females age 9-26 yr for the prevention of cervical cancer caused by HPV types 6, 11, 16, and 18.
- Available evidence supports discontinuation of cervical cancer screening among women aged 65 yrs or older who have had adequate screening and are not otherwise at high risk.

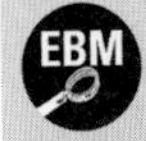

EVIDENCE

Available at www.expertconsult.com

SUGGESTED READINGS

Available at www.expertconsult.com

RELATED CONTENT

Cervical Dysplasia (Related Key Topic)
Cervical Cancer (Patient Information)

AUTHOR: **RUBEN ALVERO, M.D.**

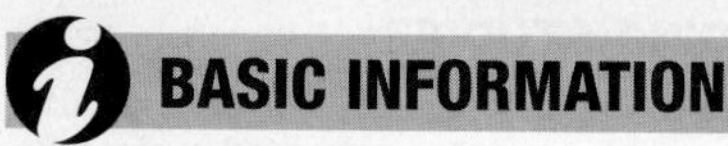

BASIC INFORMATION

DEFINITION

Cervical disk syndromes refer to diseases of the cervical spine resulting from disk disorder, either herniation or degenerative change (spondylosis). When posterior osteophytes compress the anterior spinal cord, lower extremity symptoms may result, a condition called *cervical spondylotic myelopathy.*

ICD-9CM CODES

722.4 Degenerative intervertebral cervical disk

722.71 Degenerative cervical disk with myelopathy

ICD-10CM CODES

M50.00 Cervical disk disorder with myelopathy, unspecified cervical region

M50.30 Other cervical disk degeneration, unspecified cervical region

EPIDEMIOLOGY & DEMOGRAPHICS

PREVALENCE: 10% of general adult population (symptoms in 50% of population at some time in their life)

PREDOMINANT SEX: Males and females affected equally

PREDOMINANT AGE: 30 to 60 yr

PHYSICAL FINDINGS & CLINICAL PRESENTATION

- Neck pain, radicular symptoms, or myelopathy, either alone or in combination
- Limited neck movement
- Pain with neck motion, especially extension
- Referred unilateral interscapular pain, resulting in a local trigger point
- Radicular arm pain (usually unilateral), numbness, and tingling possible, most commonly involving the C6 (C5-C6 disk) or C7 (C6-C7 disk) nerve root
- Weakness and reflex changes (C6, biceps; C7, triceps)
- Myelopathy, possibly resulting in gait disturbance, weakness, and even spasticity
- Sensory examination usually not helpful

ETIOLOGY

Unknown

DIAGNOSIS

DIFFERENTIAL DIAGNOSIS

- Rotator cuff tendinitis
- Carpal tunnel syndrome
- Thoracic outlet syndrome
- Brachial neuritis

A differential diagnosis for evaluation of neck pain is described in Section II.

WORKUP

- In most cases, the diagnosis can be established on a clinical basis alone.
- Fig. E1-235 describes an algorithm for a workup of suspected cases.

IMAGING STUDIES

- Plain roentgenograms within the first few weeks
  1. Usually normal in soft disk herniation
  2. With chronic degenerative disk disease, usually loss of height of the disk space, anterior and posterior osteophyte formation, and encroachment on the intervertebral foramen by osteophytes
- Myelography, CT scanning, and MRI indicated in patients whose symptoms do not resolve or when other spinal pathology suspected
- Electrodiagnostic studies to confirm the diagnosis or rule out peripheral nerve disorders

TREATMENT

NONPHARMACOLOGIC THERAPY

- Rest and cervical collar if needed
- Local modalities such as heat
- Physical therapy (Fig. 1-236)
- Avoid extreme range-of-motion exercises in degenerative disk disease

ACUTE GENERAL Rx

- Nonsteroidal anti-inflammatory drugs
- "Muscle relaxants" for their sedative effect
- Analgesics as needed
- Epidural steroid injection for radicular pain

DISPOSITION

- Usually improves with time
- Surgical intervention in >5%

REFERRAL

Orthopedic or neurosurgical consultation for intractable pain or neurologic deficit

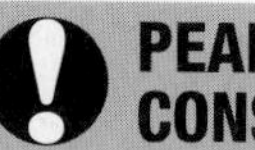

PEARLS & CONSIDERATIONS

Myelopathy from cervical spondylosis is the most common cause of acquired spastic paralysis in the adult and is usually progressive. Whether to intervene surgically is a complicated decision in these patients.

COMMENTS

- Pain relief with physical therapy seems anecdotal and short lived; any overall improvement usually parallels what would have probably occurred naturally.
- Sometimes carpal tunnel syndrome and cervical radiculopathy occur together; this is called *double-crush syndrome* and results from nerve compression at two separate levels. Proximal compression may decrease the ability of the nerve to tolerate a second, more distal compression.
- Surgical intervention is indicated primarily for relief of radicular pain caused by nerve root compression or for the treatment of myelopathy; it is generally not helpful when the chief complaint is neck pain alone.
- In many cases of cervical spondylosis with myelopathy, the lower-extremity symptoms are much more disabling than the neck symptoms, a situation that can cause some difficulty in determining their etiology.

SUGGESTED READINGS

available at www.expertconsult.com

RELATED CONTENT

Cervical Disc Syndrome (Patient Information)

AUTHOR: **LONNIE R. MERCIER, M.D.**

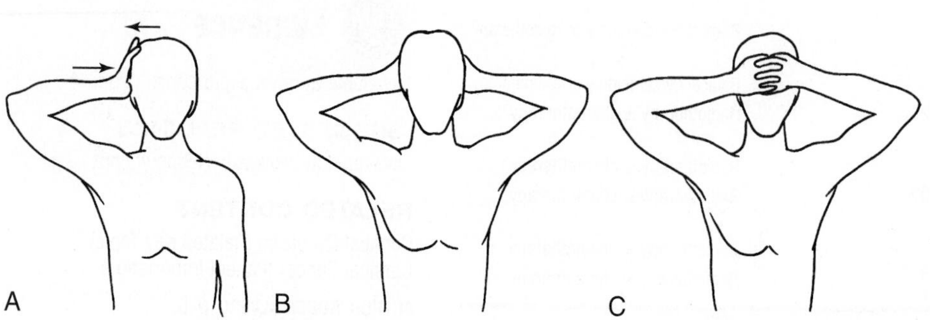

FIGURE 1-236 Isometric neck exercises. **A,** The hand is placed against the side of the head slightly above the ear, and pressure is gradually increased while resisting with the neck muscles and keeping the head in the same position. The position is held 5 sec, relaxed, and repeated five times. **B,** The exercise is performed on the other side and then from the back and front **(C).** The exercise should be performed three to four times daily. (From Mercier LR [ed]: *Practical orthopedics,* ed 4, St Louis, 1995, Mosby.)

BASIC INFORMATION

DEFINITION

Cervical dysplasia refers to atypical development of immature squamous epithelium that does not penetrate the basement epithelial membrane. Characteristics include increased cellularity, nuclear abnormalities, and increased nuclear:cytoplasmic ratio. A progressive loss of squamous differentiation exists beginning adjacent to the basement membrane and progressing to the most advanced stage (severe dysplasia), which encompasses the complete squamous epithelial layer thickness. The revised 2001 Bethesda System terminology was used in a National Institutes of Health consensus conference, sponsored by the American Society for Colposcopy and Cervical Pathology (ASCCP) and its partner professional organizations in 2006. The conference updated therapeutic options for women based on studies such as the **A**SC-US (atypical squamous cells of undetermined significance)/**LS**IL (low-grade squamous intraepithelial lesions) **T**riage **S**tudy (ALTS) that appeared after revision of the Bethesda classification.

In 2012, the American Cancer Society (ACS), American Society for Colposcopy and Cervical Pathology (ASCCP), and the American Society for Clinical Pathology (ASCP) published a new set of recommendations for lifetime assessment and early diagnosis of cervical dysplasia and cancer. The overall purpose of the study is to reduce the number of lifetime assessments, thereby reducing the possible morbidity associated with excess testing and also optimizing the co-evaluation with Pap smear and HPV testing. In brief, women younger than 21 years of age should not have any screening. Women 21–29 years of age should have testing every three years with only cytology. With negative cytology or HPV-negative ASC-US, patients can repeat every three years. For HPV-positive ASC-US or cytology with LG-SIL, follow-up is as per the 2006 guidelines (essentially a colposcopic examination as the initial step with follow-up steps depending on the findings). Women between the ages of 30–65 should have co-testing every 5 years with both Pap cytology and HPV testing. Alternatively, it is also acceptable to perform cytology alone, but then the testing interval should be every three years. With negative cytology or HPV-negative ASC-US, patients can repeat with co-testing every five years. For HPV-positive ASC-US or cytology with LG-SIL, follow-up is as per the 2006 guidelines, as previously documented. For patients with positive HPV but negative cytology, the patient can repeat testing 12 months later with co-testing; patients can also specifically test for HPV 16 or HPV 16/18 genotypes and, if positive, should be referred for colposcopy. Patients with positive HPV but negative 16 and/or 18 should be retested in 12 months with co-testing.

Women over the age of 65 and those with a history of hysterectomy (including removal of cervix) should no longer be tested unless they had previous diagnosis of CIN 2 or more severe; these women should be tested for at least 20 years. Women who have been vaccinated for HPV should still use age-specific recommendations for screening.

BETHESDA 2001 UPDATED CLASSIFICATION: The Bethesda 2001 System was the result of a year-long iterative process held to update the original 1991 system and to broaden participation in the consensus process, clarify reporting of abnormalities, and incorporate data that had been collected since the initial system was created.

The reporting system includes the following areas:

Specimen adequacy: The system defines the specimen as either satisfactory for evaluation or unsatisfactory and then specifies the reason for inadequacy if necessary.

General categorization (optional): This serves to triage the specimen into normal finding (negative for intraepithelial lesion or malignancy) or identifies it as an "epithelial abnormality." The descriptions are meant to be mutually exclusive.

Interpretation/result: Makes a distinction between "interpretation" and "diagnosis" of the specimen so that the interpretation may be incorporated into the overall clinical context for the particular patient being evaluated.

Negative for intraepithelial lesion or malignancy: In this screening test, no intraepithelial lesion or malignancy is identified. Non-neoplastic findings such as organisms or reactive cellular findings may be specified but are still considered to be a negative result.

- Epithelial cell abnormalities:
  - Squamous cell:
    - Atypical squamous cell (ASC) of undetermined significance (ASC-US) emphasizing the unusual but still possible association with underlying cervical intraepithelial neoplasia (CIN) II/III and extremely rare possibility of squamous cell carcinoma
    - ASC cannot exclude high-grade squamous intraepithelial lesion (HSIL) (ASC-H), suggesting a risk for CIN II/III that is intermediate between ASC-US and HSIL
    - Low-grade squamous intraepithelial lesion (LSIL) suggests a transient viral infection with a greater likelihood for regression, more likely to encompass human papillomavirus (HPV) infection and CIN I histologically
    - HSIL suggestive of a more persistent viral infection and with a greater risk for progressive disease, more likely to encompass CIN II/III and carcinoma in situ (CIS) histologically
    - Squamous cell carcinoma
  - Glandular cell
    - Atypical glandular cells (should specify endocervical, endometrial, or not otherwise specified)
    - Atypical glandular cell, favor neoplasia (should specify endocervical or not otherwise specified)
    - Endocervical adenocarcinoma in situ (AIS)
    - Adenocarcinoma

Other: Endometrial cells in a woman ≥40 yr of age. Because menopausal status is sometimes uncertain, age was chosen to discriminate women who might, with the findings of endometrial cells on cytology, warrant further evaluation with endometrial sampling

KEY POINTS:

1. The cytologic distinction of low grade (LSIL) and high grade (HSIL) do not necessarily equate to the histologic classifications CIN I and CIN II/III.
2. The 2006 conference notes that one cytologic abnormality can have different histologic risk in different women and highlights "special populations" such as adolescent and young women, and those women who are pregnant. In young women, spontaneous HPV clearance rates are exceptionally high. The new testing recommendations essentially remove the possibility of testing women younger than 21 years of age.
3. DNA testing for high-risk HPV types is incorporated into the evaluation and treatment algorithms for women with cytologic cervical abnormalities.

Histologically, a two-tiered system is developed in this guideline that distinguishes between the lower-risk CIN I and higher-risk CIN II/III diagnoses.

ICD-9CM CODES
622.1 Dysplasia of cervix (uteri)
ICD-10CM CODES
N87.9 Dysplasia of cervix uteri, unspecified

EPIDEMIOLOGY & DEMOGRAPHICS

PREDOMINANT AGE:

- Dysplasia: peak age, 26 yr (3600 cases/100,000 persons)
- CIS: peak age, 32 yr (1100 cases/100,000 persons)
- Invasive cancer: peak age <60 yr (800 cases/100,000 persons)

PEAK INCIDENCE:

- Age 35 yr
- Abnormal Pap smear rate revealing dysplasia approximates 2% to 5% depending on population risk factors and false-negative rate variance
- False-negative rate approaching 40%
- Average age-adjusted incidence of severe dysplasia is 35 cases/100,000 persons
- Approximately half of the cases of new cervical cancer had never been screened, and another 10% had not been screened in over 5 years. Many of these women come from underserved or underresourced communities. The single biggest impact in reducing the morbidity and mortality from cervical cancer would come from appropriately addressing these health disparities.

PHYSICAL FINDINGS & CLINICAL PRESENTATION

- Cervical lesions associated with dysplasia often are not visible to the naked eye; therefore, physical findings are best viewed by colposcopy of a 3% acetic acid–prepared cervix.
- Patients evaluated by colposcopy are identified by abnormal cervical cytology screening from Pap smear screening.
- Colposcopic findings:
    1. Leukoplakia (white lesion seen by the unaided eye that may represent condyloma, dysplasia, or cancer)
    2. Acetowhite epithelium with or without associated punctation, mosaicism, abnormal vessels
    3. Abnormal transformation zone (abnormal iodine uptake, "cuffed" gland openings)

ETIOLOGY

- Strongly associated and initiated by oncogenic HPV infection (high-risk HPV types are 16, 18, 31, 33, 35, 45, 51, 52, 56, and 58; low-risk HPV types are 6, 11, 42, 43, and 44)
- Risk factors:
    - HPV
    - Any heterosexual coitus
    - Coitus during puberty (transformation-zone metaplasia peak)
    - Diethylstilbestrol exposure
    - Multiple sexual partners
    - Lack of prior Pap smear screening
    - History of STD
    - Other genital tract neoplasia
    - HIV
    - Tuberculosis
    - Substance abuse
    - "High-risk" male partner (HPV)
    - Low socioeconomic status
    - Early first pregnancy
    - Tobacco use

Dx DIAGNOSIS

DIFFERENTIAL DIAGNOSIS

- Metaplasia
- Hyperkeratosis
- Condyloma
- Microinvasive carcinoma
- Glandular epithelial abnormalities
- Vulvar intraepithelial neoplasm
- Vaginal intraepithelial neoplasm
- Metastatic tumor involvement of the cervix

WORKUP

- Periodic history and physical examination (including cytologic screening) depending on age, risk factors, and history of preinvasive cervical lesions
- Consider screening for sexually transmitted disease (gonorrhea, *Chlamydia*, herpes, HIV, HPV)
- Abnormal cytology (HSIL/LSIL, initial ASC/ASC-US/ASC-H in high-risk patients, recurrent in low-risk/postmenopausal patients) and grossly evident suspicious lesions; refer for colposcopy and possible directed biopsy/endocervical curettage (ECC) (examination should include cervix, vagina, vulva, and anus)
- For glandular cell abnormalities (AGCs): refer for colposcopy and possible directed biopsy/ECC, and consider endometrial sampling
- In pregnancy: abnormal cytology followed by colposcopy in the first trimester and at 28 to 32 wk; only high-grade lesions suspect for cancer biopsied; ECC contraindicated

LABORATORY TESTS

- Gonorrhea, chlamydia to rule out STD
- Pap cytology screening (requires appropriate sampling, preparation, cytologist interpretation, and reporting)
- Colposcopy and directed biopsy, ECC for indications (see "Workup")
- HPV DNA typing if identified abnormal cytology
- As compared with Pap testing, HPV testing has greater sensitivity for the detection of intraepithelial neoplasia

IMAGING STUDIES

- Cervicography
- Computer-enhanced Pap cytology screening (e.g., PAPNET)

MANAGEMENT

Refer to the literature for a more comprehensive approach. The following treatment paradigms in Table 1-104 give a general outline for care.

DISPOSITION

- Because of the large number of women in high-risk groups, the prevalence of HPV, and the high false-negative Pap smear rate, routine Pap smear screening should be strongly encouraged for all women, especially those with a history of cervical dysplasia. The addition of an HPV test to the Pap test reduces the incidence of CIN II or III, or cancer detected by subsequent screening.
- Success rates for treatment approach 80% to 90%.
- Detection of persistence of recurrence requires careful follow-up.
- Cervical treatment possibly results in infertility (cervical stenosis or incompetence), which requires careful consideration and discretion for use of LEEP and cone biopsy.
- Appropriate counseling and informed consent are needed when considering any form of management of cervical dysplasia.

REFERRAL

- Patients with abnormal Pap cytology should be referred to a provider, likely a trained obstetric gynecologist, who can appropriately treat the patient in an age-specific manner and also perform a colposcopy if indicated as part of the new recommendations. Given the morbidity associated with both underevaluating and treating as well as reacting excessively to cytologic findings, a provider who is intimately familiar with American Society for Colposcopy and Cervical Pathology guidelines should be sought.
- Patients with identified abnormal cytology should be evaluated by a skilled colposcopist (defined as documented didactic and preceptorship training, including 50 cases of identified pathology, ongoing colposcopy activity with a minimum of 2 cases/wk, quality-assurance log, and periodic continuing medical education).
- If treatment is required, patient should be referred to a gynecologist or gynecologic oncologist skilled in the diagnosis and treatment of preinvasive cervical disease.

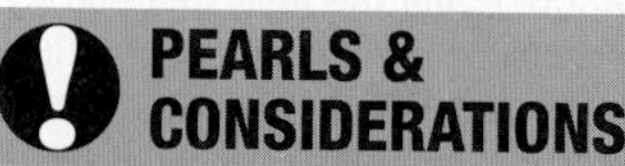

PEARLS & CONSIDERATIONS

COMMENTS

- Testing for human papillomavirus by Hybrid capture 2 DNA test will identify 91% of the small proportion of women with post-treatment residual or recurrent disease, but 30% of all women who are tested will test positive and need colposcopy.
- Gardasil is a vaccine indicated in girls and women aged 9 to 26 yr for the prevention of CIN caused by HPV types 6, 11, 16, and 18. Food and Drug Administration approval for boys and men 9 to 26 yr was given in 2009.

SUGGESTED READINGS

available at www.expertconsult.com

RELATED CONTENT

Cervical Cancer (Related Key Topic)
Cervical Polyps (Related Key Topic)
Cervical Dysplasia (Patient Information)

AUTHORS: **DENNIS M. WEPPNER, M.D.**, and **RUBEN ALVERO, M.D.**

TABLE 1-104 Summary of Recommendations

Population	Page Number	Recommended Screening Method	Management of Screen Results	Comments
<21 yr	183	No screening		
21-29 yr	183-185	Cytology alone every 3 yr	HPV-positive ASC-US or cytology of LSIL or more severe: Refer to ASCCP Guidelines Cytology Negative or HPV-Negative ASC-US Re-screen with cytology in 3 yr	
30-65 yr	185-191	HPV and cytology "cotesting" every 5 yr (preferred)	HPV-positive ASC-US or cytology of LSIL or more severe: Refer to ASCCP guidelines HPV positive, cytology negative: Option 1 Y 12-month follow-up with cotesting Option 2 Y test for HPV16 or HPV16/18 genotypes If HPV16 or HPV16/18 positive, refer to colposcopy If HPV16 or HPV16/18 negative, 12-mo follow-up with cotesting Cotest negative or HPV-negative ASC-US: Rescreen with cotesting in 5 yr	Screening by HPV testing alone is not recommended for most clinical settings.
		Cytology alone every 3 yr (acceptable)	HPV-positive ASC-US or cytology of LSIL or more severe: Refer to ASCCP guidelines Cytology negative or HPV-negative ASC-US: Rescreen with cytology in 3 yr	
>65 yr	191-192	No screening following adequate negative prior screening		Women with a history of CIN2 or a more severe diagnosis should continue routine screening for at least 20 yr
After hysterectomy	192-193	No screening		Applies to women without a cervix and without a history of CIN2 or a more severe diagnosis in the past 20 yr or cervical cancer ever.
HPV vaccinated	193-195	Follow age-specific recommendations (same as unvaccinated women)		

From Saslow D et al: American Cancer Society, American Society for Colposcopy and Cervical Pathology, and American Society for Clinical Pathology screening guidelines for the prevention and early detection of cervical cancer, *J Low Gen Tract Dis* 16(3):175-204, 2012.

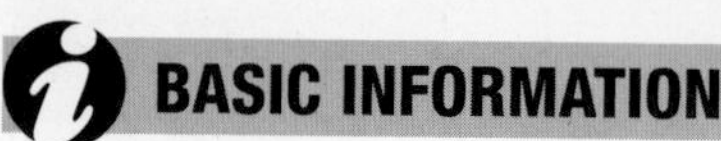

BASIC INFORMATION

DEFINITION

A cervical polyp is a growth protruding from the cervix or endocervical canal. Polyps that arise from the endocervical canal are called *endocervical polyps*. If they arise from the ectocervix, they are called *cervical polyps*.

ICD-9CM CODES
622.7 Mucous polyp of cervix
ICD-10CM CODES
N84.1 Polyp of cervix uteri

EPIDEMIOLOGY & DEMOGRAPHICS

Cervical polyps are found in approximately 4% of all gynecologic patients. They most commonly present in perimenopausal and multigravida women between the ages of 30 and 50 yr. Endocervical polyps are more common than cervical polyps and are almost always benign (Fig. 1-237). Malignant degeneration is extremely rare.

PHYSICAL FINDINGS & CLINICAL PRESENTATION

Polyps may be single or multiple and vary in size from being extremely small (a few mm) to large (4 cm). They are soft, smooth, and reddish-purple to cherry-red in color. They bleed easily when touched. Very large polyps can cause some cervical dilation. There may be vaginal discharge associated with cervical polyps if the polyp has become infected.

ETIOLOGY

- Most unknown
- Inflammatory
- Traumatic
- Pregnancy

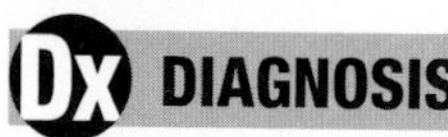

DIAGNOSIS

DIFFERENTIAL DIAGNOSIS

- Endometrial polyp
- Prolapsed myoma
- Retained products of conception
- Squamous papilloma
- Sarcoma
- Cervical malignancy

WORKUP

Polyps are most commonly asymptomatic and are usually found at the time of annual gynecologic pelvic examination. Polyps are also found in women who present for evaluation of intermenstrual or postcoital bleeding and for profuse vaginal discharge. Polyps are generally painless. Unless a patient has a bleeding abnormality that necessitates evaluation by a physician, polyps would go undiagnosed until the next Pap smear was obtained.

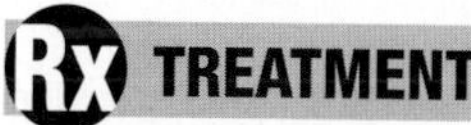

TREATMENT

NONPHARMACOLOGIC THERAPY

Simple surgical excision can be done in the office. The physician should be prepared for bleeding, which can easily be controlled with silver nitrate or Monsel's solution. Most commonly a polyp is excised by grasping it at the stalk with a sponge forceps or similar device and twisting it off. Polyps can also be excised by electrocautery or, in the case of very large polyps, in an outpatient surgical suite. Sexual intercourse and tampon use are to be avoided until the patient's follow-up visit. Douching is not to be performed. Although cervical polyps are overwhelmingly benign, they should be sent to pathology for definitive histologic diagnosis.

ACUTE GENERAL Rx

Generally no medication is needed.

CHRONIC Rx

Patient is followed up in 2 wk for recheck of the surgical excision site unless there is active bleeding, in which case she would be seen immediately. The cervix should be checked at the patient's routine gynecologic visits.

DISPOSITION

Because these are almost always benign, no further treatment is usually needed. Annual gynecologic examinations should be performed to check for any regrowths.

REFERRAL

To a gynecologist for removal of polyps

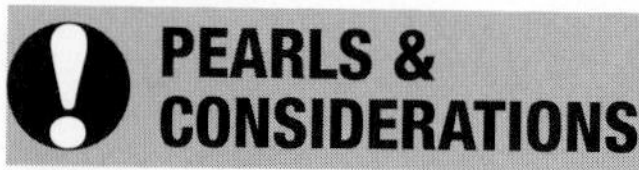

PEARLS & CONSIDERATIONS

COMMENTS

A Pap smear should be obtained before removing the polyp. If an abnormal Pap smear is obtained, it is possible that the cause will be the polyp. If a colposcopic evaluation is needed, this should also be performed. During pregnancy the cervix is highly vascularized. If the polyps are stable and benign appearing, they should be observed during the pregnancy and removed only if they cause bleeding.

SUGGESTED READINGS

available at www.expertconsult.com

RELATED CONTENT

Cervical Dysplasia (Related Key Topic)
Cervical Polyps (Patient Information)

AUTHOR: **RUBEN ALVERO, M.D.**

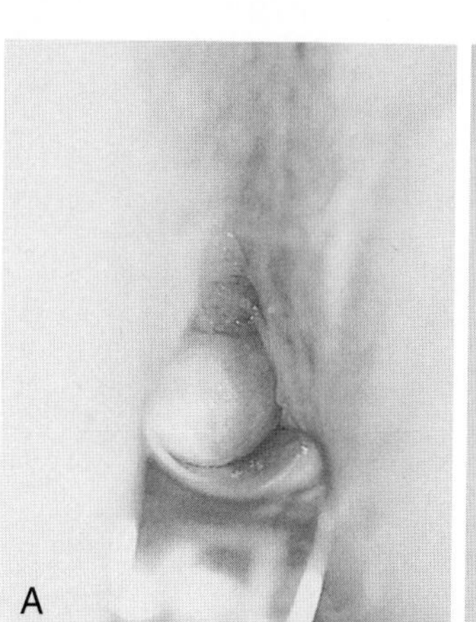

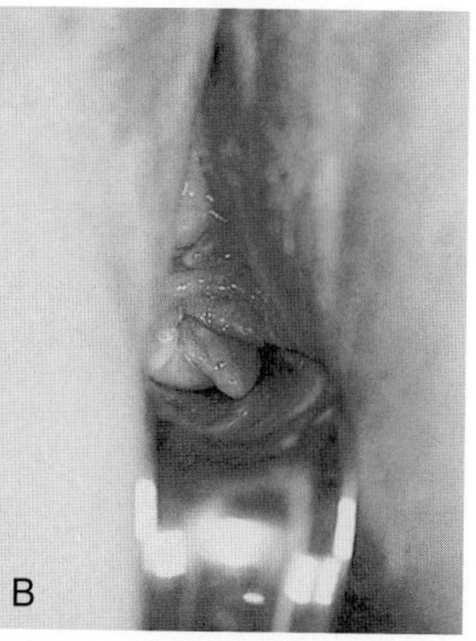

FIGURE 1-237 **A,** Fibroid polyp protruding through the external cervical os. **B,** Small endocervical polyp. (From Symonds EM, Macpherson MBA: *Color atlas of obstetrics and gynecology,* St Louis, 1994, Mosby.)

BASIC INFORMATION

DEFINITION

Cervicitis is an infection of the cervix. It may result from direct infection of the cervix, or it may be secondary to uterine or vaginal infection.

SYNONYMS

Endocervicitis
Ectocervicitis
Mucopurulent cervicitis

ICD-9CM CODES

616.0	Cervicitis
098.15	Acute gonococcal cervicitis
079.8	*Chlamydia* infection

ICD-10CM CODES

N72	Inflammatory disease of cervix uteri
A54.03	Gonococcal cervicitis, unspecified
A74.89	Other chlamydial diseases

EPIDEMIOLOGY & DEMOGRAPHICS

Cervicitis accounts for 20% to 25% of patients with abnormal vaginal discharge. It is most common in adolescents, but it can be found in any sexually active woman. Practicing unsafe sex with multiple partners increases the risk of developing cervicitis as well as other sexually transmitted diseases.

PHYSICAL FINDINGS & CLINICAL PRESENTATION

Cervicitis is usually asymptomatic or associated with mild symptoms. Copious purulent or mucopurulent vaginal discharge (Fig. 1-238), pelvic pain, and dyspareunia may be present if cervicitis is severe. The cervix can be erythematous and tender on palpation during bimanual examination. The cervix may also bleed easily when obtaining cultures or a Pap smear. Patients may have postcoital bleeding.

ETIOLOGY

- *Chlamydia trachomatis*
- *Trichomonas*
- *Neisseria gonorrhoeae*
- Herpes simplex
- *Trichomonas vaginalis*
- Human papillomavirus

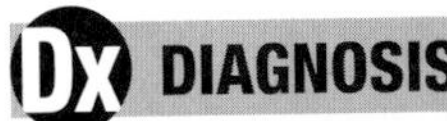

DIAGNOSIS

DIFFERENTIAL DIAGNOSIS

- Carcinoma of the cervix
- Cervical erosion
- Cervical metaplasia
- Cervical ectropion

WORKUP

The patient usually presents with a vaginal discharge or history of postcoital bleeding. Otherwise the patient is asymptomatic and diagnosed during routine examination. On examination there is gross visualization of yellow, mucopurulent material on the cotton swab.

LABORATORY TESTS

A finding of leukorrhea (>10 WBC per high-power field on microscopic examination of vaginal fluid) has been associated with chlamydial and gonococcal infection of the cervix. Positive Gram stain is found. Nucleic acid amplification tests (NAAT) should be used for diagnosing *C. trachomatis* and *N. gonorrhoeae* in women with cervicitis; this testing can be performed in either vaginal, cervical, or uterine samples. Use a wet mount to look for trichomonads, but because the sensitivity of microscopy to detect *T. vaginalis* is relatively low (~50%), symptomatic women with cervicitis and negative microscopy for trichomonads should receive further testing with culture. Obtain a Pap smear. HIV testing is recommended in all patients with supposed cervicitis. Although HSV-2 infection has been associated with cervicitis, the utility of specific testing (i.e., culture or serologic testing) for HSV-2 in this setting is unknown.

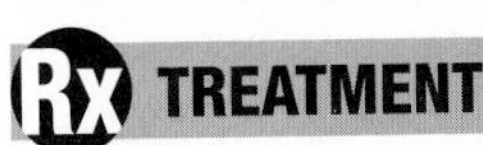

TREATMENT

NONPHARMACOLOGIC THERAPY

- Cervicitis is treated in an outpatient setting. Safe sex should be practiced with the use of condoms.
- Partners should be treated in all cases of infection proven by culture.

ACUTE GENERAL Rx

Because *Chlamydia* and *N. gonorrhoeae* cause 50% of cases of infectious cervicitis, if it is suspected treat without waiting for test results. Administer ceftriaxone 125-mg IM single dose followed by azithromycin 1-g single dose or doxycycline 100 mg PO bid for 7 days. If the patient is pregnant, treat with azithromycin 1-g single dose instead of using doxycycline, which is contraindicated in pregnant or nursing mothers. If *Trichomonas* is the etiologic agent, treat with metronidazole 2-g single dose. For herpes, treat with acyclovir 200 mg PO five times daily for 7 days.

DISPOSITION

Cervicitis responds well to antibiotics. Possible complications to watch for are a subsequent pelvic inflammatory disease (PID) and infertility (found in 5% to 10% of patients with increasing rates with repeat episodes of PID). Repeat cultures should be performed after treatment. Sexual relations can be resumed after negative cultures.

REFERRAL

If subsequent PID develops, consider hospital admission for IV antibiotics.

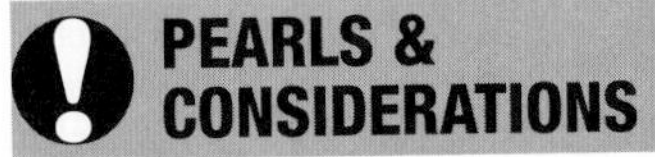

PEARLS & CONSIDERATIONS

COMMENTS

- Management of sex partners of women tested for cervicitis should be appropriate for the identified or suspected STD.
- Repeat testing 3-6 mo after treatment is recommended for all women diagnosed with chlamydia or gonorrhea,[1] and all sex partners in the preceding 60 days should be evaluated and treated for the STDs for which the index patient received treatment.

SUGGESTED READINGS

available at www.expertconsult.com

RELATED CONTENT

Chlamydia Genital Infections (Related Key Topic)
Gonorrhea (Related Key Topic)
Urethritis, Nongonococcal (Related Key Topic)
Cervicitis (Patient Information)

AUTHORS: **GEORGE T. DANAKAS, M.D.**, and **RUBEN ALVERO, M.D.**

FIGURE 1-238 Colposcopy of a woman with mucopurulent cervicitis and purulent discharge from endocervical os. (Courtesy Dr. David Soper, Richmond, VA. From Mandell GL [ed]: *Mandell, Douglas, and Bennett's principles and practice of infectious diseases,* ed 6, New York, 2005, Churchill Livingstone.)

[1]Hosenfeld CB et al: Repeat infection with chlamydia and gonorrhea among females: a symptomatic review of the literature, *Sex Transm Dis* 36:478-488, 2009.

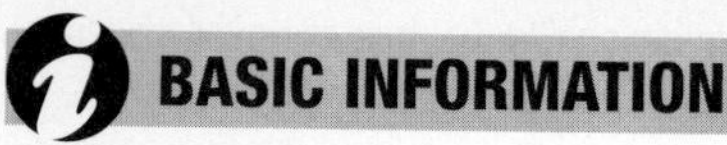

BASIC INFORMATION

DEFINITION

Chagas' disease is an infection caused by the protozoan parasite *Trypanosoma cruzi.* This is a vector-borne disease transmitted by reduviid bugs from multiple wild and domesticated animal reservoirs. The disease is characterized by an acute nonspecific febrile illness that may be followed, after a variable latency period, by chronic cardiac, GI, and neurologic sequelae. Globally, Chagas' disease affects 8 to 11 million persons; vector-borne disease (as opposed to congenital infection) occurs only in the Americas.

SYNONYMS

American trypanosomiasis

ICD-9CM CODES
086.2 Chagas' disease
ICD-10CM CODES
B57.0 Acute Chagas' disease with heart involvement
B57.2 Chagas' disease (chronic) with heart involvement

EPIDEMIOLOGY & DEMOGRAPHICS

INCIDENCE (IN U.S.):
- Seven cases of autochthonous transmission in California, Texas, Tennessee, Louisiana
- In the last 2 decades, six cases of laboratory-acquired infection, three cases of transfusion-associated transmission, and nine cases of imported disease reported to the Centers for Disease Control and Prevention (none of the imported cases involved returning tourists)
- Infection has been transmitted by organ transplantation
- Infection has been transmitted congenitally from mother to fetus over more than one generation

PREVALENCE (IN U.S.): Based on regional seroprevalence studies in Hispanic blood donors, it is estimated that between 300,000 and 300,500 persons infected with *T. cruzi* are currently residing in the U.S.

In the Americas, 8 to 10 million people are believed to be infected.

PREDOMINANT SEX: Male = female

PREDOMINANT AGE:
- In highly endemic areas, mean age of acute infection: approximately 4 yr
- Variable age distribution for both types of chronic disease, depending on geography
- Mean age of onset of chronic disease: usually between 35 and 45 yr

PEAK INCIDENCE: Unknown

GENETICS:

Congenital infection: Congenital transmission has been documented with attendant high fetal mortality and morbidity in surviving infants.

Neonatal infection: In rural areas, within substandard housing, transmission is likely to occur.

PHYSICAL FINDINGS & CLINICAL PRESENTATION

- Inflammatory lesion that develops about 1 wk after contamination of a break in the skin with infected insect feces (chagoma)
  1. Area of induration and erythema
  2. Usually accompanied by local lymphadenopathy
- Presence of Romaña's sign, which consists of unilateral painless palpebral and periocular edema, when conjunctiva is portal of entry
- Constitutional symptoms of fever, fatigue, and anorexia, along with edema of the face and lower extremities, generalized lymphadenopathy, and mild hepatosplenomegaly after the appearance of local signs of disease
- Myocarditis in a small portion of patients, sometimes with resultant CHF
- Uncommonly, CNS disease, such as meningoencephalitis, which carries a poor prognosis
- Symptoms and signs of disease persisting for weeks to months, followed by spontaneous resolution of the acute illness; patient then in the indeterminate phase of the disease (asymptomatic with attendant subpatent parasitemia and reactive antibodies to *T. cruzi* antigens)
- Chronic disease may become manifest years to decades after the initial infection:
  1. Most common organ involved: heart, followed by GI tract, and to a much lesser extent the CNS
     a. Cardiac involvement takes the form of arrhythmias or cardiomyopathy, but rarely both.
     b. Cardiomyopathy is bilateral but predominantly affects the right ventricle and is often accompanied by apical aneurysms and mural thrombi.
     c. Arrhythmias are a consequence of involvement of the bundle of His and have been implicated as the leading cause of sudden death in adults in highly endemic areas.
     d. Right-sided heart failure, thromboembolization, and rhythm disturbances associated with symptoms of dizziness and syncope are characteristic.
  2. Patients with megaesophagus: dysphagia, odynophagia, chronic cough, and regurgitation, frequently resulting in aspiration pneumonitis
  3. Megacolon: abdominal pain and chronic constipation, which, when severe, may lead to obstruction and perforation
  4. CNS symptoms: most often secondary to embolization from the heart
  5. Varying degrees of peripheral neuropathy

ETIOLOGY

- *T. cruzi*
  1. Found only in the Americas, ranging from the southern U.S. to southern Argentina
  2. Transmitted to humans by various species of bloodsucking reduviid ("kissing") insects, primarily those of the genera *Triatoma, Panstrongylus,* and *Rhodnius*
  3. Usually found in burrows and trees where infected insects transmit the parasite to natural reservoirs (e.g., opossums and armadillos)
  4. Intrusion into enzootic areas for farmland, allowing insects to take up residence in rural dwellings, thus including humans and domestic animals in the cycle of transmission
  5. Initial infection of insects by ingesting blood from animals or humans that have circulating flagellated trypanosomes (trypomastigotes)
  6. Multiplication in the insect midgut as epimastigotes, then differentiation into metacyclic trypomastigotes discharged with the feces during subsequent blood meals (Fig. 1-239)
  7. Transmission to the second mammalian host through contamination of mucous membranes, conjunctivae, or wounds with insect feces containing infected forms
- In the vertebrate host
  1. Movement of parasites into various cell types, intracellular transformation into amastigotes, and thereafter differentiation into trypomastigotes
  2. Following rupture of the cell membrane, parasitic invasion of local tissues or hematogenous spread to distant sites, maintaining a parasitemia infective for vectors
- In addition to insect vectors, *T. cruzi* is transmitted through blood transfusions, transplacentally,

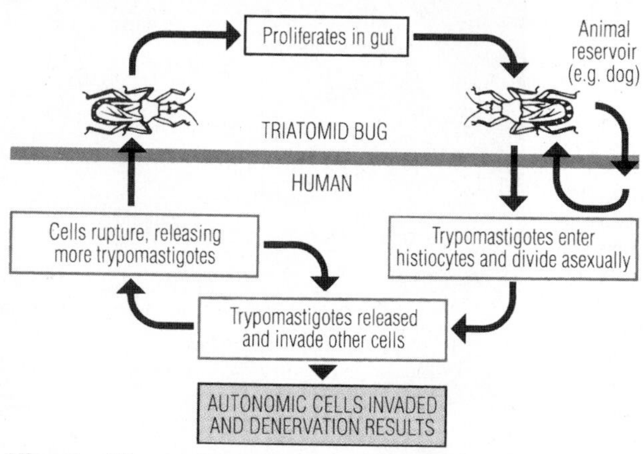

FIGURE 1-239 Lifecycle of *Trypanosoma* cruzi. (From Souhami RL, Mozham J: *Textbook of medicine,* ed 4, London, 2002, Churchill Livingstone.)

and, occasionally, secondary to laboratory accidents or ingestion, including breast milk
- In 2007, voluntary screening was initiated in the U.S. blood supply; it is estimated to cover 75% to 90% of the blood supply.
- Platelet transfusions appear to be more infective than packed red blood cells.

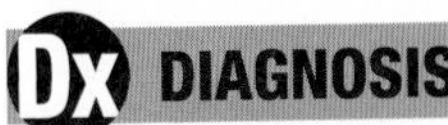

DIAGNOSIS

DIFFERENTIAL DIAGNOSIS

Acute disease
- Early African trypanosomiasis
- New World cutaneous and mucocutaneous leishmaniasis

Chronic disease
- Idiopathic cardiomyopathy
- Idiopathic achalasia
- Congenital or acquired megacolon

WORKUP

Principal considerations in diagnosis:
- A history of residence where transmission is known to occur
- Recent receipt of a blood product while in an endemic area
- Occupational exposure in a laboratory

LABORATORY TESTS

For acute diagnosis:
- Demonstration of *T. cruzi* in wet preparations of blood (Fig. 1-240), buffy coat, or Giemsa-stained smears
- Xenodiagnosis, a technique involving laboratory-reared insect vectors fed on subjects with suspected infection thereafter examined for parasites, and culture of body fluids in liquid media to establish diagnosis
  1. Hampered by the length of time required for completion
  2. Of limited use in clinical decision making with regard to drug therapy
  3. Although xenodiagnosis and broth culture are considered to be more sensitive than microscopic examination of body fluids, sensitivities may not exceed 50%
- Recent advances in serologic testing include immunoblot assay, in situ indirect fluorescent antibody, PCR-based techniques, and an immunochromatographic assay (Chagas Stat Pak)
- Response to treatment in acute, reactivated, or congenital infection can be assessed by quantitative PCR.

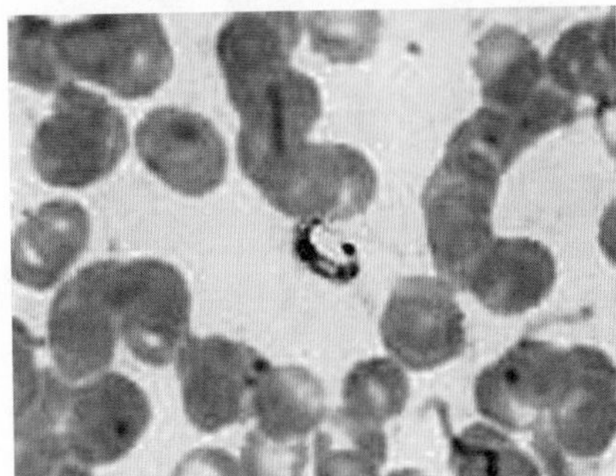

FIGURE 1-240 *T. cruzi* in human blood film. The causative agent occurs in blood films characteristically as short C-shaped or S-shaped trypomastigotes with a prominent kinetoplast. It is otherwise monomorphic *(Giemsa × 950)*. (From Hoffmann R et al: *Hematology: basic principles and practice*, ed 5, Philadelphia, 2009, Churchill Livingstone.)

For chronic *T. cruzi* infection:
- Traditional serologic tests including: complement fixation (CF), indirect immunofluorescence (IIF), indirect hemagglutination, and enzyme-linked immunosorbent assay (ELISA)
- Serologic tests have variable sensitivity and specificity and frequent false-positive results
- Saliva ELISA may be useful as a screening diagnostic test in epidemiologic studies of chronic trypanosomiasis infection in endemic areas
- Confirmation requires at least two different tests, and if discordant, three tests.

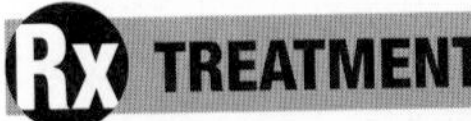

TREATMENT

NONPHARMACOLOGIC THERAPY

- Chronic chagasic heart disease: mainly supportive
- Megaesophagus: symptoms usually amenable to dietary measures or pneumonic dilation of the esophagogastric junction
- Chagasic megacolon: in its early stages responsive to a high-fiber diet, laxatives, and enemas

ACUTE GENERAL Rx

It is now recommended that all patients—acute, indeterminant, and chronic—be treated with antiparasitic therapy. Treatment for individuals older than 50 years requires consideration of risk/benefit as the treatment appears to be more toxic at this age.

A single course of each of the medications below is thought to offer an approximately 50% cure rate. Neither drug is approved by the FDA but both can be obtained free of charge from the CDC and used under investigational protocol. Consultations and requests for drugs can be made to: Parasitic Diseases Public Inquiries Line (770-448-7775), parasites.cdc.gov, www.cdc.gov/parasites/chagas, CDC Drug Service (404-639-3670).

Benznidazole, a nitroimidazole derivative:
- Has demonstrated similar efficacy as nifurtimox in limited trials, is usually better tolerated and is viewed by most experts as first-line treatment
- Recommended oral dosage: 5 to 7 mg/kg/day for 30 to 90 days

Nifurtimox:
- Recommended oral dosage for adults: 8 to 10 mg/kg/day given in 3 to 4 divided daily doses and continued for 90 to 120 days
- Parasitologic cure in approximately 50% of those treated; should be begun as early as possible

- Neither drug can be used during pregnancy.
- Do not use in cases of severe renal or hepatic dysfunction.
- Triazoles offer a new class of therapy. Case reports have had success with posaconazole.

CHRONIC Rx

- In patients with indeterminate phase or chronic disease: Some evidence of benefit in a recent uncontrolled trial with benznidazole in patients with chagasic cardiomyopathy
- In patients exhibiting bradyarrhythmias: pacemakers
- In individuals with congestive heart failure:
  1. Treat with standard modalities for dilated, right-sided, cardiomyopathic disease.
  2. Cardiac transplant is an option for end-stage cardiomyopathy; moreover, reactivation rate found to be low and amenable to therapy without subsequent infection of the allograft.
  3. Myotomy or esophageal resection is reserved for patients with advanced disease.
- In advanced chagasic megacolon associated with chronic fecal impaction, perforation, or, less commonly, volvulus: surgical resection

DISPOSITION

Based on a few prospective studies, most patients infected with *T. cruzi* will not develop symptomatic Chagas' disease.

REFERRAL

- For consultation with an infectious disease specialist or communication with the Centers for Disease Control and Prevention when the disease is acutely suspected
- To a cardiologist for pacemaker implantation for patients with bradyarrhythmias
- To a surgeon for symptomatic disease with chagasic megaesophagus or megacolon

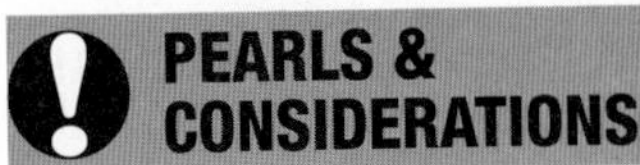

PEARLS & CONSIDERATIONS

COMMENTS:
- All children of an infected mother should be screened for Chagas; household members should also be screened.
- In recipients of solid organ or bone marrow transplants, patients with AIDS, or those receiving chemotherapy, there may be reactivation of indeterminate phase disease.
- Mortality predictors associated with chagasic cardiomyopathy include CHF, QT-interval dispersion, left ventricular (LV) end-systolic dimension, the presence of pathologic Q waves, frequent PVCs, and isolated LAFB on ECG.
- Chagasic esophageal disease has an increased incidence of esophageal malignancy.
- The use of pyrethroid-impregnated curtains may represent an option for the reduction or elimination of Chagas' disease transmission in certain endemic areas.

SUGGESTED READINGS

available at www.expertconsult.com

AUTHOR: **PATRICIA CRISTOFARO, M.D.**

BASIC INFORMATION

DEFINITION

Charcot-Marie-Tooth disease (CMT) is a heterogeneous group of noninflammatory inherited peripheral neuropathies characterized by chronic motor and sensory polyneuropathy. It is the most common inherited neuromuscular disorder (see also "Neuropathy, Hereditary").

SYNONYMS

Peroneal muscular atrophy
Hereditary motor and sensory neuropathy (HMSN)
CMT

ICD-9CM CODES

356.1 Charcot-Marie-Tooth disease, paralysis, or syndrome

ICD-10CM CODES

G60.0 Hereditary motor and sensory neuropathy

EPIDEMIOLOGY & DEMOGRAPHICS

PREVALENCE: 1:2500; CMT type 1 and type 2 are the major divisions with an estimated prevalence of 40 per 100,000

PREDOMINANT AGE: Onset usually 10 to 20 yr, and infants may be symptomatic.

GENETICS: Transmission may be autosomal dominant, autosomal recessive, or X-linked, with some sporadic cases reported. Duplication of *peripheral myelin protein 22* (PMP22) is the most common cause of CMT. CMT is classified into types 1 through 7 and is genetically heterogeneous with at least 43 CMT genes known.

PHYSICAL FINDINGS & CLINICAL PRESENTATION

- Wide variation in clinical presentation, but affected individuals in a family tend to have similar symptoms
- Symmetric, slowly progressive distal motor neuropathy resulting in weakness and atrophy in legs, often progresses to involve hands
- High-arched feet (pes cavus), claw toe deformities (Fig. 1-242), and hammer toes
- Atrophy of the lower legs producing a stork-like appearance (muscle wasting does not involve the upper legs) (Fig. 1-243)
- Nerve enlargement
- Mild to moderate distal sensory loss; uncommonly can have painful paresthesias
- Decreased proprioception and weakness of ankle dorsiflexors often interfere with balance and gait (steppage gait)
- Depressed or absent deep tendon reflexes in many cases
- Hearing loss and hip dysplasia are under-recognized manifestations
- Ambulation usually maintained throughout life
- CMT has been reported to be associated with renal diseases, mostly focal segmental glomerulosclerosis (FSGS)

ETIOLOGY

Genetic abnormalities cause defects in either peripheral nerve myelination, or result in axonal degeneration. Mutations in one of several myelin genes result in defects in myelin structure, maintenance, and formation. Duplication of the PMP22 gene causes CMT1A, the most common type of hereditary motor sensory neuropathy (~40% overall). INF_2 mutations appear to cause many cases of FSGS-associated CMT.

Dx DIAGNOSIS

DIFFERENTIAL DIAGNOSIS

- Other inherited neuropathies
- Acquired peripheral neuropathies such as toxic, metabolic, infectious, endocrine, inflammatory, immune-mediated, and nutritional polyneuropathies

WORKUP

- Clinical diagnosis is based on family history, characteristic presentation, and findings on detailed physical and neurologic examination.
- Electrophysiologic studies are often diagnostic and may help define various subtypes of CMT.
- Occasionally, sural nerve biopsy is helpful in establishing diagnosis.

Rx TREATMENT

ACUTE GENERAL Rx

- Symptomatic and supportive, managed by multidisciplinary team including physical and occupational therapy
- Special shoes with good ankle support, ankle/foot orthoses.
- Some require crutches/cane for gait stability; <5% need wheelchair.
- Daily heel cord stretching exercises and hand grip exercises.
- Musculoskeletal pain may respond to acetaminophen or NSAIDs; neuropathic pain may respond to tricyclic antidepressants or drugs such as carbamazepine or gabapentin.

CHRONIC Rx

Occasionally, orthopedic surgery is required to correct severe pes cavus deformity or hip dysplasia. Avoiding obesity is essential as this makes walking difficult; avoiding potentially neurotoxic medications is also important, particularly *Vinca* alkaloids.

DISPOSITION

- Disability is usually compatible with a long life.
- 10% to 20% of patients are asymptomatic.

REFERRAL

- Orthopedic consultation for bracing and surgical treatment of deformity
- Genetic counseling and family planning

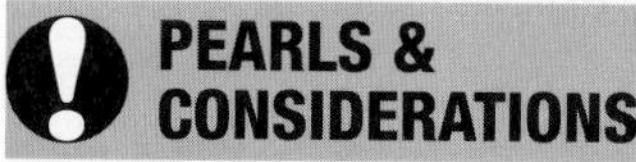

PEARLS & CONSIDERATIONS

COMMENTS

Patient information on CMT disease is available from the Muscular Dystrophy Association, 3300 East Sunrise Drive, Tucson, AZ 85718; (520) 529-2000.

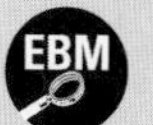

EVIDENCE

available at www.expertconsult.com

SUGGESTED READINGS

available at www.expertconsult.com

RELATED CONTENT

Charcot-Marie-Tooth Disease (Patient Information)

AUTHOR: **CANDICE YUVIENCO, M.D.**

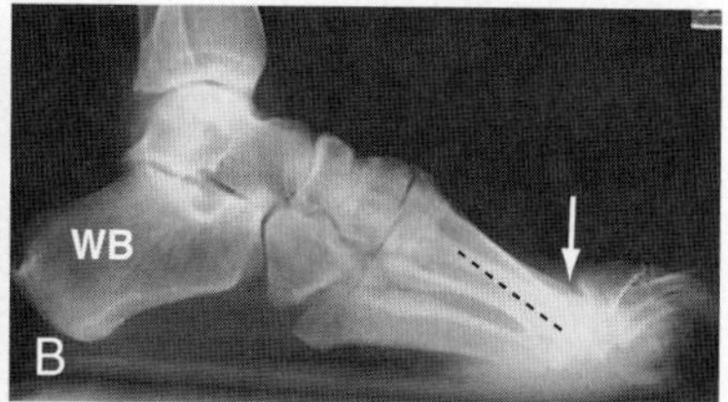

FIGURE 1-242 A, Non–weight-bearing view of cavus and claw toe deformities in a patient with Charcot-Marie-Tooth disease. **B,** On weight-bearing view, plantar flexion of first ray is less noticeable, but clawed hallux remains, indicating fixed extension contracture at first metatarsophalangeal joint. (From Canale ST, Beaty JH: *Campbell's operative orthopedics,* ed 11, Philadelphia, 2007, Mosby.)

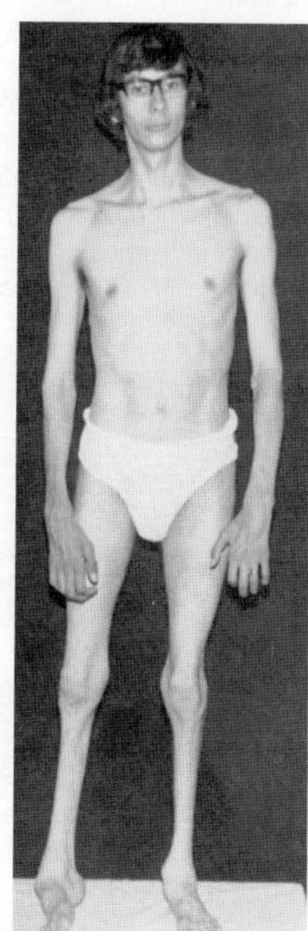

FIGURE 1-243 Patient with Charcot-Marie-Tooth disease showing marked wasting of calf muscles and intrinsic foot muscles. (From Dubowitz V: *Muscle disorders in childhood,* London, 1995, Saunders.)

BASIC INFORMATION

DEFINITION

Charcot's joint was first described by Jean Martin Charcot in reports of patients with tabes dorsalis. The term now describes a chronic progressive arthropathy that is associated with peripheral neuropathy and commonly results in destruction of the bone and soft tissues at peripheral weight-bearing joints. It is characterized early on by acute inflammation that often leads to joint degeneration, instability from joint dislocation and pathologic fractures, and gross deformities.

SYNONYMS

Neuropathic arthropathy
Charcot osteoarthropathy
Charcot neuroosteoarthropathy

ICD-9CM CODES
094.0 Charcot's arthropathy
ICD-10CM CODES
A52.16 Charcot's arthropathy

EPIDEMIOLOGY & DEMOGRAPHICS

PREVALENCE:

- Estimated as 0.08% to 13% in patients with diabetes mellitus.
- 5 cases per 100 of those with peripheral neuropathy, primarily affecting the foot.
- 20% to 40% of patients with syringomyelia (shoulder, elbow, and wrist are most commonly involved).
- 5% to 10% of patients with tabes dorsalis (spine, hip, knee, and ankle are most commonly involved).
- Average age of onset is 50 to 60 years.
- No definite sex predilection, and ethnic variance is unknown.

PHYSICAL FINDINGS & CLINICAL PRESENTATION

- Initial presentation is with a diffusely warm, erythematous, and swollen joint with or without associated pain. Continual attacks may occur, or there could be progressive arthropathy and insidious swelling over months to years.
- Pain is typically less than expected based on the severity of clinical and radiographic findings.
- It commonly affects the mid-foot (tarsus and tarsometatarsal joints), but the forefoot and hind foot can also be involved.
- Joint instability, osseous debris around the joint, and crepitus may be seen with progressive disease.
- Frank dislocation, fracture, and subsequent bony deformity may occur over time. Additionally, plantar ulcers may affect neuropathic foot joints.

ETIOLOGY

The most common identifiable risk factors for Charcot osteoarthropathy include any condition that causes a peripheral or autonomic neuropathy. Diabetes mellitus with peripheral neuropathy is the most common cause (Fig. 1-244). Less common associations include renal dialysis, syringomyelia, tabes dorsalis, Charcot-Marie-Tooth disease, congenital indifference to pain, chronic alcoholism, poliomyelitis, syphilis, leprosy, familial amyloid neuropathy, spinal or peripheral nerve surgery, and spinal dysraphism. Two theories contribute to the underlying processes involved in the disease:

1. Neurotraumatic theory:
   - Impairment or loss of protective joint sensation with continued weight bearing and repetitive stress.
   - Rapid and extensive bone destruction leads to joint subluxation, dislocation, and possible deformity.
   - Chronic inflammation eventually contributes to joint instability and incongruity.
2. Neurovascular theory:
   - Autonomic neuropathy leads to increased blood flow to the affected joints.
   - Enhanced osteoclastic bone resorption contributes to osteopenia and further susceptibililty to bone destruction.

DIAGNOSIS

DIFFERENTIAL DIAGNOSIS

- Osteomyelitis
- Cellulitis
- Inflammatory arthritides, particularly gout or pseudogout
- Deep vein thrombosis
- Infectious arthritis/septic joint
- Osteoarthritis
- Complex regional pain syndrome

WORKUP

History and physical examination findings are important to establishing the diagnosis.

Early diagnosis, before radiographic changes are evident, requires a high index of suspicion because the acute phase is characterized by the classical signs of an acute inflammatory process.

- Patients should be tested for an underlying peripheral neuropathy.
- It may be helpful to diagnose or rule out a previously unrecognized contributing condition or risk factor for the above.

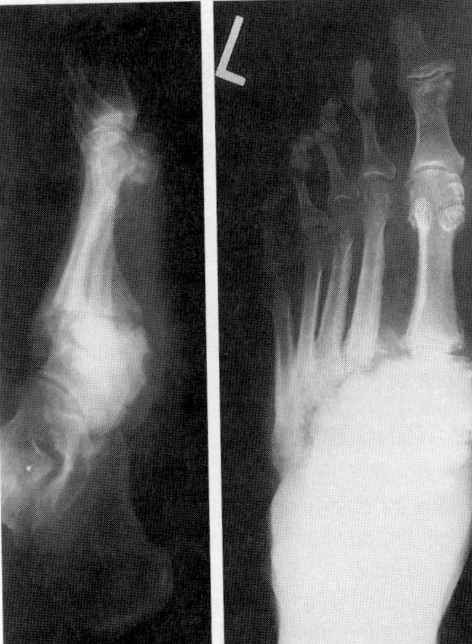

FIGURE 1-244 Diabetes mellitus and neuropathic arthritis. Note lateral displacement of metatarsals *(left)* and fragmentation and osseous debris *(right)*. (From Goldman L, Ausiello D [eds]: *Cecil textbook of medicine,* ed 22, Philadelphia, 2004, Saunders.)

LABORATORY TESTS

- A complete blood count and metabolic panel, and additional testing to determine a possible underlying cause may include vitamin B_{12}, folate, RPR, ALP, and PTH
- In questionable cases, aspiration, sometimes including biopsy, to rule out soft tissue or bone infection and a septic joint

IMAGING STUDIES

Plain x-rays

- May reveal variable degrees of destruction and joint disruption. This is usually sufficient to establish the diagnosis in most cases.
- Three radiographic stages correspond to clinical progression of the disease: fragmentation, coalescence, and reconstruction.
- A technetium diphosphate bone scan or MRI can provide more detail when the clinical picture is not too clear.

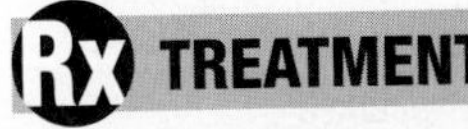

TREATMENT

ACUTE GENERAL Rx

The cornerstone of therapy involves offloading, which is best achieved with total contact casts (or, alternatively, removable cast walkers) and cessation of weight-bearing activities. The average use of a cast is 12 to 18 wk. In some instances, surgical correction of a joint might be necessary, but this should be avoided in most instances because it is associated with a relatively high failure rate.

PHARMACOLOGIC THERAPY

Antiresorptives such as bisphosphonates and calcitonin have shown improved symptom control and decreased bone turnover markers in controlled trials.

DISPOSITION

Early diagnosis of Charcot's joint is imperative to avoid compromise of bone and joint integrity. In general, it typically takes 1 to 2 yr for complete healing of a Charcot's joint. Once bony changes set in they are very difficult if not impossible to reverse. Timely, appropriate treatment can greatly reduce the risk of irreversible damage and future morbidity.

REFERRAL

Patient should be referred to a high-risk foot clinic.

SUGGESTED READINGS

available at www.expertconsult.com

RELATED CONTENT

Charcot Joint (Patient Information)

AUTHOR: **ANISHKA S. ROLLE, M.D.**

BASIC INFORMATION

DEFINITION

Chemotherapy-induced nausea and vomiting (CINV) refers to adverse effects of drugs used to treat cancer. There are three recognized subtypes: acute-phase CINV, where nausea and vomiting begin minutes to hours after initiation of chemotherapy; delayed-phase CINV, where symptoms begin or return 24 hours or more after administration of therapy(s); and anticipatory CINV, where nausea and vomiting begin before receiving therapy.

SYNONYMS

Drug-induced nausea and vomiting
Chemotherapy-induced emesis

ICD-9CM CODES
787.01 Nausea with vomiting
787.02 Nausea alone
787.03 Vomiting alone
E933.1 Adverse effect of antineoplastic and immunosuppressive drugs
V58.11-V58.12 Encounter for antineoplastic chemotherapy and immunotherapy

ICD-10CM CODES
R11.2 Nausea with vomiting, unspecified
R11.0 Nausea
R11.10 Vomiting, unspecified
V58.11-V58.12 Encounter for antineoplastic chemotherapy and immunotherapy

EPIDEMIOLOGY & DEMOGRAPHICS

- The patient's risk for development of nausea and vomiting is most strongly dependent on the chemotherapy agent used.
- With certain chemotherapy regimens, nausea and vomiting will occur in almost 100% of patients. However, patients' tolerance may vary, and symptoms can be as low as 10%.
- Symptoms may be dose dependent (the higher the dose, the greater the risk for symptoms).
- CINV is more likely to affect female and younger patients.
- Patients expecting CINV before receiving therapy are at greater risk of experiencing symptoms (anticipatory emesis).
- Patients with a history of alcohol consumption are at lower risk.
- Patients with a history of motion sickness are at greater risk.

PHYSICAL FINDINGS & CLINICAL PRESENTATION

- For acute-phase CINV, nausea and vomiting start within minutes to hours after receiving chemotherapy.
- For delayed-phase CINV, nausea and vomiting begin or return 24 hours or more after receiving chemotherapy.
- With anticipatory CINV, symptoms begin before receiving therapy.
- Other symptoms may include anxiety and lightheadedness.
- The most common physical findings are elevated pulse and abnormal blood pressure (elevated if the person is highly anxious, reduced if the patient is dehydrated).
- Symptoms such as diarrhea, fever, headache, and abdominal pain may suggest an alternative diagnosis; physical examination findings such as increased blood pressure, abdominal tenderness, or focal neurologic deficits may suggest symptoms caused by cancer progression or other acute illness such as infection.

ETIOLOGY

CINV is probably the result of chemotherapy drugs acting in two places: in the gastrointestinal tract directly and in the vomiting center of the brain. In both areas, nausea and vomiting are mediated by the actions of certain neurotransmitters, with serotonin, dopamine, and neurokinin being the most important.

Dx DIAGNOSIS

DIFFERENTIAL DIAGNOSIS

- The two main considerations are progression of cancer and infection
- Intestinal/gastric: obstruction or partial obstruction of the digestive tract from tumor
- Neurologic: metastases to the brain causing vomiting; metastatic infiltration of nerves affecting the digestive tract
- Infectious: acute bacterial, viral, or parasitic infections of the digestive tract causing symptoms (usually diarrhea will be present)
- Renal: dehydration leading to acute kidney injury and failure, causing a worsening of nausea and vomiting

WORKUP

No workup is indicated if patient's symptoms and onset of nausea and vomiting fit the usual presentation for CINV. If other symptoms or unexpected physical examination findings are present, then other causes need to be ruled out. A combination of blood work and imaging may be helpful.

LABORATORY TESTS

- If the onset of symptoms is not typical for CINV, then blood tests such as a CBC, liver function tests, and kidney function tests may be indicated.
- Stool studies looking for infections from bacteria or parasites may be ordered if diarrhea is also present.

IMAGING STUDIES

- Abdominal radiographs may be ordered to look for obstruction of the digestive tract but will not provide any information about tumor progression.
- Abdominal CT scan will provide more detailed information about local cancer progression/invasion in the proximity of the digestive tract and whether obstruction of the digestive tract is present.
- Brain CT scan or magnetic resonance imaging (MRI) will provide information about possible metastases to the brain.

Rx TREATMENT

- Treatment depends on the likelihood of a given drug or drug regimen to cause CINV and is preventive in nature.
- For chemotherapy agents with a high probability of causing CINV, adding antinausea medications has proven to be highly effective in symptom prevention.
- Drug of choice and its duration of use is highly dependent on the chemotherapy regimen used.
- The most common treatment combination includes a serotonin-receptor antagonist (ondansetron, granisetron, dolasetron, tropisetron, or palonosetron), a corticosteroid (methylprednisolone or dexamethasone), and a neurokinin-1 receptor antagonist (aprepitant).
- Many other drugs are available, such as prochlorperazine, metochlopramide, haloperidol, and marinol, but they are less effective and have greater potential for adverse effects.
- Benzodiazepines (usually lorazepam) may help in patients with significant anxiety levels that lead to anticipatory CINV.
- Patients with uncontrolled symptoms may require hospitalization for supportive care including intravenous fluids.

NONPHARMACOLOGIC THERAPY

For those patients with a significant anxiety component to their CINV, cognitive behavioral therapy may help.

DISPOSITION

Although CINV is one of the most feared complications of cancer therapy, its treatment has been revolutionized in the last 20 years, with most patients achieving adequate symptom control.

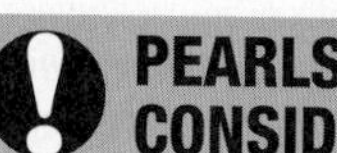

PEARLS & CONSIDERATIONS

COMMENTS

- Aggressive symptom control in the acute phase of CINV is the key initial therapeutic approach. Prevention of the acute phase has led to much improved control of the delayed phase, which, in turn, has greatly decreased the incidence of anticipatory CINV.
- Prevention of symptoms is much easier to achieve than controlling or treating symptoms once they have begun.

SUGGESTED READINGS

available at www.expertconsult.com

AUTHOR: **BYUNG KIM, M.D.**

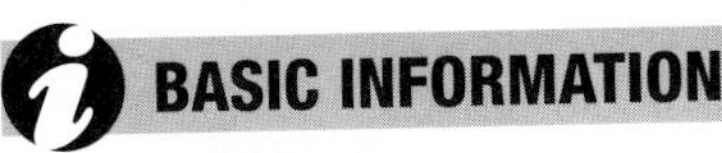

BASIC INFORMATION

DEFINITION

Genital infection with *Chlamydia trachomatis* may result in urethritis, epididymitis, cervicitis, and acute salpingitis, but often it is asymptomatic in women (see "Pelvic Inflammatory Disease"). In men, urethritis, mucopurulent discharge, dysuria, and urethral pruritus are noted.

ICD-9CM CODES
597.80 Urethritis
604.0 Epididymitis
616.0 Cervicitis
381.51 Acute salpingitis
ICD-10CM CODES
N34.1 Nonspecific urethritis
N45.4 Abscess of epididymis or testis
N72 Inflammatory disease of cervix uteri

EPIDEMIOLOGY & DEMOGRAPHICS

- *Chlamydia trachomatis* is the most common sexually transmitted disease in the U.S. More than 4 million infections occur annually, although the exact number is unknown because reporting is not required in all states. Occurrence is common worldwide and has been increasing steadily over the last 2 decades in the U.S., Canada, Australia, and Europe.
- Most women with endocervical or urethral infections are asymptomatic.
- Up to 45% of cases of gonococcal infection may have concomitant chlamydial infection.
- Infertility or ectopic pregnancy can result as a complication from symptomatic or asymptomatic chronic infections of the endometrium and fallopian tubes.
- Conjunctival and pneumonic infection of the newborn may result from infection in pregnancy.
- In men 15% to 55% of cases are caused by *C. trachomatis.* Complications of nongonococcal urethritis in men infected with *C. trachomatis* include epididymitis and Reiter's syndrome.

PHYSICAL FINDINGS & CLINICAL PRESENTATION

Clinical manifestations may be similar to those of gonorrhea: mucopurulent endocervical discharge, with edema, erythema, and easily induced endocervical bleeding caused by inflammation of endocervical columnar epithelium. Less-frequent manifestations may include bartholinitis, urethral syndrome with dysuria and pyuria, and perihepatitis (Fitz-Hugh–Curtis syndrome).

ETIOLOGY

- *Chlamydia trachomatis,* serotypes D through K
- Obligate, intracellular bacteria

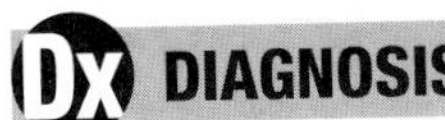

DIAGNOSIS

DIFFERENTIAL DIAGNOSIS

Gonorrhea, nongonococcal urethritis (nonchlamydial etiologies)

WORKUP

Diagnosis based on laboratory demonstration of evidence of infection in intraurethral or endocervical swab by various tests. The intracellular organism is less readily recovered from the discharge.

LABORATORY TESTS

- Cell culture is the reference method for diagnosis (single culture sensitivity 80% to 90%), but it is labor intensive and takes 48 to 96 hr; it is not suited for large screening programs.
- Nonculture methods:
  - NAATs are very sensitive tests for cervical and male urethral specimens and are FDA-approved for use with urine.
  - Direct fluorescent antibody tests
  - Enzyme immunoassay
  - DNA probes
  - Polymerase chain reaction (PCR)
- With the exception of PCR, the other tests are probably less specific than cell culture and may yield false-positive results.
- Because this is an intracellular organism, purulent discharge is not an appropriate specimen. An adequate sample of infected cells must be obtained.
- Ten white blood cells per high-power field.

Rx TREATMENT

ACUTE GENERAL Rx

Nongonococcal urethritis, urethritis, cervicitis, conjunctivitis (except for lymphogranuloma venereum):

- Azithromycin 1 g PO × 1 *or*
- Doxycycline 100 mg PO bid for 7 days
- Alternatives
  1. Erythromycin base 500 mg PO qid for 7 days *or*
  2. Erythromycin ethylsuccinate 800 mg PO qid for 7 days *or*
  3. Ofloxacin 300 mg PO bid for 7 days
  4. Levofloxacin 500 mg PO qd for 7 days

Infection in pregnancy:

- Erythromycin base 500 mg PO qid for 7 days *or*
- Amoxicillin 500 mg PO tid for 7 days

Alternatives:

1. Erythromycin base 250 mg PO qid for 7 days *or*
2. Erythromycin ethylsuccinate 800 mg PO qid for 7 days *or*
3. Erythromycin ethylsuccinate 400 mg PO qid for 14 days *or*
4. Azithromycin 1 g PO (single dose)

NOTE: Doxycycline and ofloxacin are contraindicated in pregnancy. Safety and efficacy of azithromycin are not established in pregnancy and lactation, although preliminary data indicate that it may be safe and effective. Erythromycin estolate is contraindicated in pregnancy because of drug-related hepatotoxicity.

FOLLOW-UP: Reculture after therapy completion and refer partners for evaluation and treatment.

RECURRENT AND PERSISTENT URETHRITIS: Retreat noncompliant patients with the above regimens. If patient was initially compliant, recommended regimens: metronidazole 2 g PO in single dose plus erythromycin base 500 mg PO qid for 7 days or erythromycin ethylsuccinate 800 mg PO qid for 7 days.

CLINICAL PEARL

When treating *Chlamydia,* it is best to assume concomitant gonorrhea because co-infection is common. Combination of cetriaxone 125 mg IM single dose plus azithromycin 1 g PO single dose will treat both.

REFERRAL

Refer to infectious disease specialist if persistent infection or gynecologist if salpingitis is suspected.

SUGGESTED READINGS

available at www.expertconsult.com

RELATED CONTENT

Cervicitis (Related Key Topic)
Gonorrhea (Related Key Topic)
Pelvic Inflammatory Disease (Related Key Topic)
Urethritis, Gonococcal (Related Key Topic)
Urethritis, Nongonococcal (Related Key Topic)

AUTHOR: **RUBEN ALVERO, M.D.**

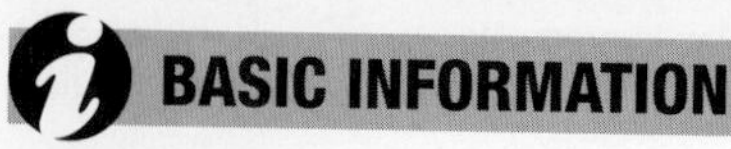

BASIC INFORMATION

DEFINITION

Cholangitis refers to an inflammation and/or infection of the hepatic and common bile ducts associated with obstruction of the common bile duct.

SYNONYMS

Biliary sepsis
Ascending cholangitis
Suppurative cholangitis

ICD-9CM CODES
576.1 Cholangitis
ICD-10CM CODES
K83.0 Cholangitis

EPIDEMIOLOGY & DEMOGRAPHICS

INCIDENCE (IN U.S.): Complicates approximately 1% of cases of cholelithiasis
PEAK INCIDENCE: Seventh decade
PREVALENCE (IN U.S.): 2 cases/1000 hospital admissions
PREDOMINANT SEX:
- Females, for cholangitis secondary to gallstones
- Males, for cholangitis secondary to malignant obstruction and HIV infection

PREDOMINANT AGE: Seventh decade and older; unusual <50 yr of age

PHYSICAL FINDINGS & CLINICAL PRESENTATION

- Usually acute onset of fever, abdominal pain (RUQ), and jaundice (Charcot's triad)
- All signs and symptoms in only 50% to 85% of patients
- Often, dark coloration of the urine resulting from bilirubinuria
- Complications:
  1. Bacteremia (50%) and septic shock
  2. Hepatic abscess and pancreatitis

ETIOLOGY

Obstruction of the common bile duct causing rapid proliferation of bacteria in the biliary tree
- Most common cause of common bile duct obstruction: stones, usually migrated from the gallbladder
- Other causes: prior biliary tract surgery with secondary stenosis, tumor (usually arising from the pancreas or biliary tree), and parasitic infections from *Ascaris lumbricoides* or *Fasciola hepatica*
- Iatrogenic after contamination of an obstructed biliary tree by endoscopic retrograde cholangiopancreatoscopy (ERCP) or percutaneous transhepatic cholangiography (PTC)
- Primary sclerosing cholangitis (PSC)
- HIV-associated sclerosing cholangitis: associated with infection by CMV, *Cryptosporidium,* Microsporidia, and *Mycobacterium avium* complex

Dx DIAGNOSIS

DIFFERENTIAL DIAGNOSIS

- Biliary colic
- Acute cholecystitis
- Liver abscess
- Peptic ulcer disease (PUD)
- Pancreatitis
- Intestinal obstruction
- Right kidney stone
- Hepatitis
- Pyelonephritis

WORKUP

- Blood cultures
- CBC
- Liver function tests

LABORATORY TESTS

- Usually, elevated WBC count with a predominance of polymorphonuclear forms
- Elevated alkaline phosphatase and bilirubin in chronic obstruction
- Elevated transaminases in acute obstruction
- Positive blood cultures in 50% of cases, typically with enteric gram-negative aerobes (e.g., *E. coli, Klebsiella pneumoniae*), enterococci, or anaerobes

IMAGING STUDIES

- Ultrasound:
  1. Allows visualization of the gallbladder and bile ducts to differentiate extrahepatic obstruction from intrahepatic cholestasis
  2. Insensitive but specific for visualization of common duct stones
- CT scan:
  1. Less accurate for gallstones
  2. More sensitive than ultrasound for visualization of the distal part of the common bile duct
  3. Also allows better definition of neoplasm
- ERCP:
  1. Confirms obstruction and its level
  2. Allows collection of specimens for culture and cytology
  3. Indicated for diagnosis if ultrasound and CT scan are inconclusive
  4. May be indicated in therapy (see "Treatment")

Rx TREATMENT

NONPHARMACOLOGIC THERAPY

Biliary decompression
- May be urgent in severely ill patients or those unresponsive to medical therapy within 12 to 24 hr
- May also be performed semielectively in patients who respond
- Options:
  1. ERCP with or without sphincterotomy or placement of a draining stent
  2. Percutaneous transhepatic biliary drainage for the acutely ill patient who is a poor surgical candidate
  3. Surgical exploration of the common bile duct

ACUTE GENERAL Rx

- Nothing by mouth
- Intravenous hydration
- Broad-spectrum antibiotics directed at gram-negative enteric organisms, anaerobes, and enterococcus such as carbapenems (meropenem: 1 g q8h or imipenem: 500 mg IV q6h if life threatening), piperacillin/tazobactam: 3.375 or 4.5 g IV q6h, or ampicillin-sulbactam, or ticarcillin-clavulanate; if infection is nosocomial, post-ERCP, or the patient is in shock, broaden antibiotic coverage.

CHRONIC Rx

Repeated decompression may be necessary, particularly when obstruction is related to neoplasm.

DISPOSITION

Excellent prognosis if obstruction is amenable to definitive surgical therapy; otherwise relapses are common.

REFERRAL

- To biliary endoscopist if obstruction is from stones or a stent needs to be placed
- To interventional radiologist if external drainage is necessary
- To a general surgeon in all other cases
- To an infectious disease specialist if blood cultures are positive or the patient is in shock or otherwise severely ill

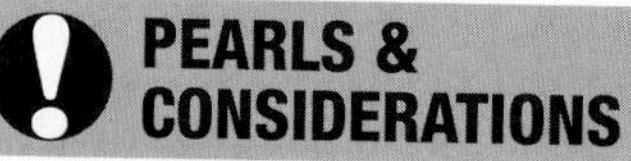

PEARLS & CONSIDERATIONS

- Cholangitis is a life-threatening form of intra-abdominal sepsis, though it may appear to be rather innocuous at its onset.
- Antibiotics alone will not resolve cholangitis in the presence of biliary obstruction because high intrabiliary pressures prevent antibiotic delivery. Decompression and drainage of the biliary tract to alleviate the obstruction with antimicrobial therapy is the therapy of choice.

SUGGESTED READINGS

available at www.expertconsult.com

AUTHOR: **GLENN G. FORT, M.D., M.P.H.**

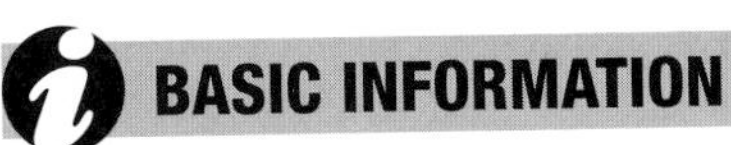

BASIC INFORMATION

DEFINITION

Cholecystitis is acute or chronic inflammation of the gallbladder generally caused by gallstones (>95% of cases).

SYNONYMS

Gallbladder attack

ICD-9CM CODES

575.0 Acute cholecystitis
574.0 Calculus of the gallbladder with acute cholecystitis
575.1 Cholecystitis without mention of calculus

ICD-10CM CODES

K81.9 Acute cholecystitis
K80.00 Calculus of gallbladder with acute cholecystitis without obstruction
K81.9 Cholecystitis, unspecified

EPIDEMIOLOGY & DEMOGRAPHICS

- Acute cholecystitis occurs most commonly in women during the fifth and sixth decades. Approximately 120,000 cholecystectomies are performed for acute cholecystitis annually in the U.S.
- The incidence of gallstones is 0.6% in the general population and much higher in certain ethnic groups (>75% of Native Americans by age 60 yr). Most patients with gallstones are asymptomatic. Of such patients, biliary colic develops in 1% to 4% annually.

PHYSICAL FINDINGS & CLINICAL PRESENTATION

- Pain and tenderness in the right hypochondrium or epigastrium; pain possibly radiating to the infrascapular region
- Palpation of the right upper quadrant (RUQ) eliciting marked tenderness and stoppage of inspired breath (Murphy's sign)
- Guarding
- Fever (33%)
- Jaundice (25% to 50% of patients)
- Palpable gallbladder (20% of cases)
- Nausea and vomiting (>70% of patients)
- Fever and chills (>25% of patients)
- Medical history often revealing ingestion of large, fatty meals before onset of pain in the epigastrium and RUQ

ETIOLOGY

- Gallstones (>95% of cases)
- Ischemic damage to the gallbladder, critically ill patient (acalculous cholecystitis)
- Infectious agents, especially in patients with AIDS (cytomegalovirus, *Cryptosporidium*)
- Strictures of the bile duct
- Neoplasms, primary or metastatic
- Risk factors for cholelithiasis include age, obesity, female sex, rapid weight loss, ethnicity/race (Native American), use of contraceptives, pregnancy, diabetes mellitus, hemolysis, total parenteral nutrition, biliary parasites

Dx DIAGNOSIS

DIFFERENTIAL DIAGNOSIS

- Hepatic: hepatitis, abscess, hepatic congestion, neoplasm, trauma
- Biliary: neoplasm, stricture, sphincter of Oddi dysfunction
- Gastric: pelvic ulcer disease, neoplasm, alcoholic gastritis, hiatal hernia, non-ulcer dyspepsia
- Pancreatic: pancreatitis, neoplasm, stone in the pancreatic duct or ampulla
- Renal: calculi, infection, inflammation, neoplasm, ruptured kidney
- Pulmonary: pneumonia, pulmonary infarction, right-sided pleurisy
- Intestinal: retrocecal appendicitis, intestinal obstruction, high fecal impaction, irritable bowel syndrome (IBS), inflammatory bowel disease (IBD)
- Cardiac: myocardial ischemia (particularly involving the inferior wall), pericarditis
- Cutaneous: herpes zoster
- Trauma
- Fitz-Hugh-Curtis syndrome (perihepatitis), ruptured ectopic pregnancy
- Subphrenic abscess
- Dissecting aneurysm
- Nerve root irritation caused by osteoarthritis of the spine

WORKUP

Workup consists of detailed history and physical examination coupled with laboratory evaluation and imaging studies. No single clinical finding or laboratory test is sufficient to establish or exclude cholecystitis without further testing.

LABORATORY TESTS

- Leukocytosis (12,000 to 20,000) is present in >70% of patients.
- Elevated alkaline phosphatase, ALT, AST, bilirubin; bilirubin elevation >4 mg/dl is unusual and suggests presence of choledocholithiasis.
- Elevated amylase may be present (consider pancreatitis if serum amylase elevation exceeds 500 U).

IMAGING STUDIES

- Ultrasound of the gallbladder (Fig. E1-245) is the preferred initial test; it will demonstrate the presence of stones and also dilated gallbladder with thickened wall and surrounding edema in patients with acute cholecystitis.
- Nuclear imaging (HIDA scan) (Fig. E1-246) is useful for diagnosis of cholecystitis when sonogram is inconclusive: sensitivity and specificity exceed 90% for acute cholecystitis. This test is only reliable when bilirubin is <5 mg/dl. A positive test result (absence of gallbladder filling within 60 min after the administration of tracer) will demonstrate obstruction of the cystic or common hepatic duct; the test will not demonstrate the presence of stones.
- CT scan of abdomen is useful in cases of suspected abscess, neoplasm, or pancreatitis.
- Plain radiograph of the abdomen generally is not useful because <25% of stones are radiopaque.

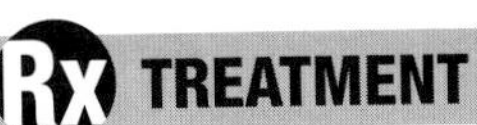

Rx TREATMENT

NONPHARMACOLOGIC THERAPY

Provide IV hydration; withhold oral feedings.

ACUTE GENERAL Rx

- Laparoscopic (percutaneous) cholecystectomy (PC) is considered the treatment of choice for most patients. The rate of conversion to open cholecystectomy is higher when laparoscopic cholecystectomy (CCY) is performed for acute cholecystitis rather than for uncomplicated cholelithiasis; conservative management with IV fluids and antibiotics (ampicillin-sulbactam 3 g IV q6h or piperacillin-tazobactam 4.5 g IV q8h) may be justified in some high-risk patients to convert an emergency procedure into an elective one with a lower mortality rate.
- Endoscopic retrograde cholangiopancreatography with sphincterectomy and stone extraction can be performed in conjunction with laparoscopic cholecystectomy for patients with choledochal lithiasis; approximately 7% to 15% of patients with cholelithiasis also have stones in the common bile duct.

DISPOSITION

- Prognosis is good; elective laparoscopic cholecystectomy can be performed as outpatient procedure.
- Hospital stay (when necessary) varies from overnight with laparoscopic cholecystectomy to 4 to 7 days with open cholecystectomy.
- Complication rate is approximately 1% (hemorrhage and bile leak) for laparoscopic cholecystectomy and <0.5% (infection) with open cholecystectomy.

REFERRAL

Surgical referral in all patients with acute cholecystitis

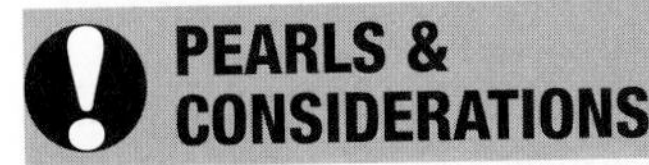

PEARLS & CONSIDERATIONS

COMMENTS

- Patients should be instructed that stones may recur in bile ducts.
- Gallbladder aspiration, in which all fluid visualized by ultrasound is aspirated, represents a nonsurgical treatment when patients who are at high operative risk develop acute cholecystitis. Salvage cholecystectomy is reserved for nonresponders.

SUGGESTED READINGS

available at www.expertconsult.com

RELATED CONTENT

Gallbladder Attack (Cholecystitis) (Patient Information)
Cholelithiasis (Related Key Topic)

AUTHOR: **FRED F. FERRI, M.D.**

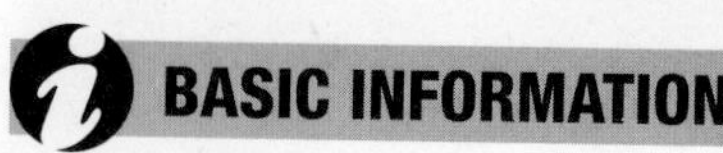

BASIC INFORMATION

DEFINITION

Cholelithiasis is the presence of stones in the gallbladder.

SYNONYMS

Gallstones

ICD-9CM CODES
574.2 Calculus of the gallbladder without mention of cholecystitis
574.0 Calculus of the gallbladder with acute cholecystitis

ICD-10CM CODES
K80.2 Calculus of gallbladder without cholecystitis
K80.5 Calculus of bile duct without cholangitis or cholecystitis

EPIDEMIOLOGY & DEMOGRAPHICS

- Gallstone disease can be found in 12% of the U.S. population. Of these, 2% to 3% (500,000 to 600,000) are treated with cholecystectomies each year.
- Annual medical expenditures for gallbladder surgeries in the U.S. exceed $5 billion.
- Incidence of gallbladder disease increases with age. Highest incidence is in the fifth and sixth decades. Predisposing factors for gallstones are female sex, pregnancy, age >40 yr, family history of gallstones, obesity, ileal disease, oral contraceptives, diabetes mellitus, rapid weight loss, estrogen replacement therapy. Risk factors for the development of cholelithiasis are described in Table E1-105.
- Patients with gallstones have a 20% chance of developing biliary colic or its complications at the end of a 20-yr period.

PHYSICAL FINDINGS & CLINICAL PRESENTATION

- Physical examination is entirely normal unless patient is having biliary colic; 80% of gallstones are asymptomatic.
- Typical symptoms of obstruction of the cystic duct include intermittent, severe, cramping pain affecting the right upper quadrant.
- Pain occurs mostly at night and may radiate to the back or right shoulder. It can last from a few minutes to several hours.

ETIOLOGY

- 75% of gallstones contain cholesterol and are usually associated with obesity, female sex, and diabetes mellitus; mixed stones are most common (80%); pure cholesterol stones account for only 10% of stones.
- 25% of gallstones are pigment stones (bilirubin, calcium, and variable organic material) associated with hemolysis and cirrhosis. These tend to be black-pigmented stones that are refractory to medical therapy.
- 50% of mixed-type stones are radiopaque.

Dx DIAGNOSIS

DIFFERENTIAL DIAGNOSIS

- Peptic ulcer disease
- Gastroesophageal reflux disease
- Irritable bowel disease
- Pancreatitis
- Neoplasms
- Nonnuclear dyspepsia
- Inferior wall myocardial infarction
- Hepatic abscess

LABORATORY TESTS

Generally normal unless patient has biliary obstruction (elevated alkaline phosphatase, bilirubin).

IMAGING STUDIES

- Ultrasound of the gallbladder (Fig. E1-247) will detect small stones and biliary sludge (sensitivity, 95%; specificity, 90%); the presence of dilated gallbladder with thickened wall is suggestive of acute cholecystitis.
- Nuclear imaging (HIDA scan) can confirm acute cholecystitis ($>90\%$ accuracy) if gallbladder does not visualize within 4 hr of injection and the radioisotope is excreted in the common bile duct.
- Common bile duct stones can be detected noninvasively by magnetic resonance cholangiopancreatography or invasively by endoscopic retrograde cholangiopancreatography (ERCP) and intraoperative cholangiography.

Rx TREATMENT

NONPHARMACOLOGIC THERAPY

Lifestyle changes (avoidance of diets high in polyunsaturated fats, weight loss in obese patients; however, avoid rapid weight loss)

ACUTE GENERAL Rx

- The management of gallstones is affected by the clinical presentation.
- Asymptomatic patients do not require therapeutic intervention. Proposed criteria for prophylactic cholecystectomy are described in Table 1-106.

TABLE 1-106 Proposed Criteria for Prophylactic Cholecystectomy

Life expectancy >20 years
Calculi >2 cm in diameter
Calculi >3 mm and patent cystic duct
Radiopaque calculi
Gallbladder polyps >15 mm
Nonfunctioning or calcified gallbladder ("porcelain" gallbladder)
Women <60 years
Patients in areas with high prevalence of gallbladder cancer

From Cameron JL, Cameron AM: *Current surgical therapy,* ed 10, Philadelphia, 2011, Saunders.

- Surgical intervention is generally the ideal approach for symptomatic patients. Laparoscopic cholecystectomy is generally preferred over open cholecystectomy because of the shorter recovery period and lower mortality rate. Between 5% and 26% of patients undergoing elective laparoscopic cholecystectomy will require conversion to an open procedure. Most common reason is the inability to clearly identify the biliary anatomy.
- Laparoscopic cholecystectomy after endoscopic sphincterectomy is recommended for patients with common bile duct stones and residual gallbladder stones. Where possible, single-stage laparoscopic treatments with removal of duct stones and cholecystectomy during the same procedure are preferable.
- Patients who are not appropriate candidates for surgery because of coexisting illness or patients who refuse surgery can be treated with oral bile salts: ursodiol or chenodiol. Candidates for oral bile salts are patients with cholesterol stones (radiolucent, noncalcified stones), with a diameter of ≤ 15 mm and having three or fewer stones. Candidates for medical therapy must have a functioning gallbladder and must have absence of calcifications on CT scans.
- Extracorporeal shock wave lithotripsy (ESWL) is another form of medical therapy. It can be used in patients with stone diameter of ≤ 3 cm and having three or fewer stones.

DISPOSITION

- Recurrence rate after bile acid treatment is approximately 50% in 5 yr. Periodic ultrasound is necessary to assess the effectiveness of treatment.
- After ESWL, stones recur in approximately 20% of patients after 4 yr.
- Patients with at least one gallstone <5 mm in diameter have a greater than fourfold increased risk of presenting with acute biliary pancreatitis. A policy of watchful waiting in such cases is generally unwarranted.
- A potential serious complication of gallstones is acute cholangitis. ERCP and endoscopic sphincterectomy followed by interval laparoscopic cholecystectomy are effective in acute cholangitis.

SUGGESTED READINGS

available at www.expertconsult.com

RELATED CONTENT

Gallstones (Patient Information)
Cholecystitis (Related Key Topic)

AUTHOR: **FRED F. FERRI, M.D.**

BASIC INFORMATION

DEFINITION

Chorea is the term used to describe brief movements that involve contiguous muscle groups. It comes from the Greek word meaning "dance."

SYNONYMS

Sydenham's chorea
Saint Vitus dance

ICD-9CM CODES
333.4 Huntington's chorea
333.5 Other choreas
392 Rheumatic chorea
ICD-10CM CODES
G25.4 Drug-induced chorea
G25.5 Other chorea

EPIDEMIOLOGY & DEMOGRAPHICS

INCIDENCE:
No published data exist on the incidence of chorea in the United States.
PREDOMINANT SEX AND AGE:
Can affect any age and sex depending on the cause.
RISK FACTORS:
The most important risk factors are a family history of Huntington's disease, exposure to rheumatic fever as a child, or being pregnant with a history of rheumatic fever.

PHYSICAL FINDINGS & CLINICAL PRESENTATION

Presentation depends on the underlying cause. Huntington's disease typically presents with neuropsychiatric symptoms that predate choreiform movements. In the case of Sydenham's and drug-induced chorea or chorea gravidarum, the hyperkinetic movements involving the hands and face may be noticed first. Brief contiguous movement that is not rhythmic and facial grimacing can be clues.

ETIOLOGY

- Genetic causes include Huntington's disease, neuroacanthocytosis, and Wilson's disease.
- Infectious causes include rheumatic fever causing Sydenham's chorea, chorea gravidarum during pregnancy, and spongiform encephalopathy (e.g., prion disease).
- Drug-induced causes include oral contraceptives, tricyclic antidepressants, cimetidine, digoxin, verapamil, baclofen, steroids, and antiepileptics.
- Strokes in the thalamic area of the brain can also cause choreiform movements.

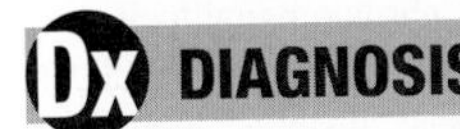

DIAGNOSIS

DIFFERENTIAL DIAGNOSIS

- Huntington's disease
- Stroke
- Prion disease
- Rheumatic fever
- Conversion disorder

LABORATORY TESTS

- Complete metabolic panel
- CBC with manual smear looking for acanthocytes
- Serum copper and ceruloplasmin levels
- Thyroid function tests
- Streptolysin O antibodies
- Erythrocyte sedimentation rate

IMAGING STUDIES

- MRI of the brain
- Echocardiogram if rheumatic fever is suspected

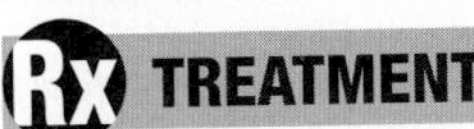

TREATMENT

- Depending on the cause, treatment must be tailored.
- Huntington's disease can be treated with tetrabenazine.
- Drug-induced chorea can be treated by withdrawing the offending drug.

NONPHARMACOLOGIC THERAPY

Rehabilitative services such as physical therapy, occupational therapy, and speech therapy are important for genetic forms of chorea.

ACUTE GENERAL Rx

Sudden-onset chorea warrants head imaging.

CHRONIC Rx

Tetrabenazine as medical therapy for the chorea and a multidisciplinary approach are useful for Huntington's chorea.

COMPLEMENTARY MEDICINE

There are case reports showing some efficacy in acupuncture for the treatment of temporomandibular chorea in a patient with Sydenham's chorea.

DISPOSITION

Sydenham's chorea and chorea gravidarum tend to resolve in a few weeks.

Huntington's disease is a progressive neurodegenerative disorder.

REFERRAL

Refer to a neurologist.

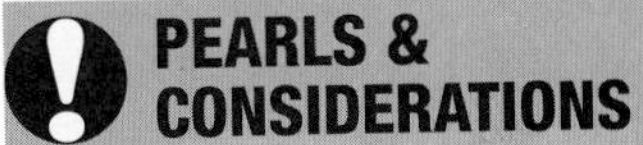

PEARLS & CONSIDERATIONS

COMMENTS

Chorea is a symptom of an underlying disorder. Investigations are targeted toward identifying reversible causes.

PREVENTION

Treat streptococcal throat infection early to prevent future complications.

PATIENT/FAMILY EDUCATION

For Huntington's disease or other genetic forms of chorea, it is important to provide support and refer to support groups.

SUGGESTED READINGS

Available at www.expertconsult.com

RELATED CONTENT

Rheumatic Fever (Related Key Topic)

AUTHOR: **NAWAZ HACK, M.D.**

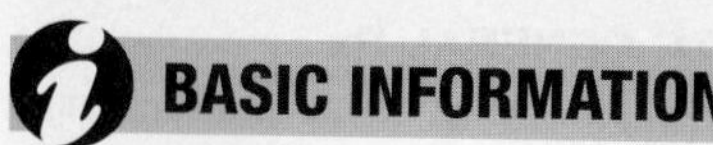

BASIC INFORMATION

DEFINITION

Chronic fatigue syndrome (CFS) is characterized by four or more of the following symptoms, present concurrently for at least 6 mo:

- Impaired memory or concentration
- Sore throat
- Tender cervical or axillary lymph nodes
- Muscle pain
- Multijoint pain
- New headaches
- Unrefreshing sleep
- Postexertion malaise for longer than 24 hr

SYNONYMS

Yuppie flu
CFS
Chronic Epstein-Barr syndrome

ICD-9CM CODES
780.7 Chronic fatigue syndrome
300.8 Neurasthenia
ICD-10CM CODES
R53.82 Chronic fatigue, unspecified
F45.8 Other somatoform disorders

EPIDEMIOLOGY & DEMOGRAPHICS

PREVALENCE IN U.S.: 10 to 300 cases per 100,000 persons
PREDOMINANT AGE: Young adulthood and middle age
PREDOMINANT SEX: Females affected more often than males
ECONOMICS: The estimated annual cost of lost productivity exceeds $10 billion.

PHYSICAL FINDINGS & CLINICAL PRESENTATION

- There are no physical findings specific for CFS.
- The physical examination may be useful to identify fibromyalgia and other rheumatologic conditions that may coexist with CFS.

ETIOLOGY

- The etiology of CFS is unknown.
- Some theorize that a viral illness may trigger certain immune responses that lead to the various symptoms. Most patients often report the onset of their symptoms with a flulike illness.
- The presence of numerous psychiatric comorbidities in CFS have led some experts to question the existence of any organic etiology.

Dx DIAGNOSIS

DIFFERENTIAL DIAGNOSIS

- Psychosocial depression, dysthymia, anxiety-related disorders, and other psychiatric diseases
- Sleep apnea
- Infectious diseases (subacute bacterial endocarditis, Lyme disease, fungal diseases, mononucleosis, HIV, chronic hepatitis B or C, tuberculosis (TB), chronic parasitic infections)
- Autoimmune diseases: systemic lupus erythematosus, myasthenia gravis, multiple sclerosis, thyroiditis, rheumatoid arthritis
- Endocrine abnormalities: hypothyroidism, hypopituitarism, adrenal insufficiency, Cushing's syndrome, diabetes mellitus, hyperparathyroidism, pregnancy, reactive hypoglycemia
- Occult malignant disease
- Substance abuse
- Systemic disorders: chronic renal failure, chronic obstructive pulmonary disease, cardiovascular disease, anemia, electrolyte abnormalities, liver disease
- Other: inadequate rest, sleep apnea, narcolepsy, fibromyalgia, sarcoidosis, medications, toxic agent exposure, Wegener's granulomatosis, vitamin deficiency

LABORATORY TESTS

- No specific laboratory tests exist for diagnosing CFS. Initial laboratory tests are useful to exclude other conditions that may mimic or may be associated with CFS.
  1. Screening laboratory tests: CBC, ESR, ALT, total protein, albumin, globulin, alkaline phosphatase, calcium, phosphorus, glucose, BUN, creatinine, electrolytes, TSH, and urinalysis are useful.
  2. Serologic tests for Epstein-Barr virus, *Candida albicans,* human herpesvirus 6, and other studies for immune cellular abnormalities are not useful; these tests are expensive and generally not recommended.
- Other tests may be indicated depending on the history and physical examination (e.g., ANA, RF in patients presenting with joint complaints or abnormalities on physical examination, Lyme titer in areas where Lyme disease is endemic).

IMAGING STUDIES

Generally not recommended unless history and physical examination indicate specific abnormalities (e.g., chest radiography in any patient suspected of TB or sarcoidosis)

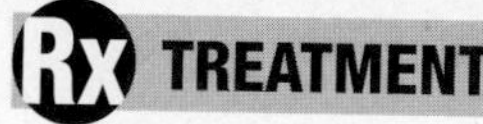

TREATMENT

NONPHARMACOLOGIC THERAPY

- Patients should be reassured that the illness is not fatal and that most patients improve over time.
- An initially supervised exercise program to preserve and increase strength is beneficial for most patients and can improve symptoms.
- Cognitive behavioral therapy trials have shown positive effects on fatigue levels, work, depression/anxiety, and social adjustment.

GENERAL Rx

Therapy is generally palliative. The following medications may be helpful; however, evidence is conflicting:

- Antidepressants: The choice of antidepressant varies with the desired side effects. Patients with difficulty sleeping or fibromyalgia-like symptoms may benefit from low-dose tricyclics (doxepin 10 mg hs or amitriptyline 25 mg qhs). When sedation is not desirable, low-dose SSRIs (paroxetine 20 mg qd) often help alleviate fatigue and associated symptoms.
- NSAIDs can be used to relieve muscle and joint pain and headaches.

"Alternative" medications (herbs, multivitamins, nutritional supplements) are very popular with many CFS patients but are generally not very helpful.

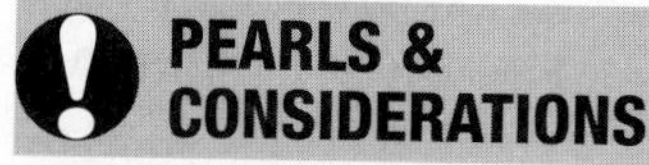

PEARLS & CONSIDERATIONS

COMMENTS

- In CFS the symptoms are serious enough to reduce daily activities by >50% in the absence of any other medically identifiable disorders.
- Moderate to complete recovery at 1 yr occurs in 22% to 60% of patients with CFS.

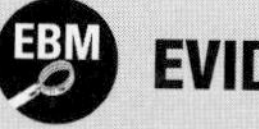

EVIDENCE

available at www.expertconsult.com

SUGGESTED READINGS

available at www.expertconsult.com

RELATED CONTENT

Fig. 3-74 Evaluation of Fatigue (Algorithm)
Chronic Fatigue Syndrome (Patient Information)

AUTHOR: **FRED F. FERRI, M.D.**

BASIC INFORMATION

DEFINITION

Symmetric proximal and distal weakness with associated sensory loss along with reduced or absent reflexes for >2 mo

SYNONYMS

Chronic inflammatory demyelinating polyneuropathy
Chronic inflammatory demyelinating polyradiculoneuropathy

ICD-9CM CODES
357.81 Chronic inflammatory demyelinating polyneuritis
ICD-10CM CODES
G61.81 Chronic inflammatory demyelinating polyneuritis

EPIDEMIOLOGY & DEMOGRAPHICS

PREVALENCE: 0.5/100,000 children; 1 to 2/100,000 adults
PREDOMINANT SEX AND AGE: Slightly higher in males
RISK FACTORS: Association with certain systemic medical conditions (see under "Differential Diagnosis" below), but association is unclear

PHYSICAL FINDINGS & CLINICAL PRESENTATION

- Occurrence of symmetrical weakness in both proximal and distal muscles that progressively increases over 2 mo
- Associated with impaired sensation, postural instability, reduced or absent deep tendon reflexes, and variable craniofacial-bulbar involvement

ETIOLOGY

Immune-mediated disorder emerging from interplay of both cell-mediated and humoral immune responses directed against incompletely characterized peripheral nerve antigens. May also be associated with various concurrent illnesses (Table 1-108), although the pathogenetic significance is unclear.

DIAGNOSIS

There is no universal consensus regarding diagnostic criteria for CIDP. The three most widely used are the American Academy of Neurology (AAN), Saperstein, and Inflammatory Neuropathy Cause and Treatment (INCAT) criteria.
- The AAN and INCAT criteria are the least stringent regarding clinical criteria and require motor and sensory function in one limb, whereas the Saperstein criteria are more stringent, requiring both symmetrical proximal and distal weakness.
  - Therefore, a patient with DADS (distal acquired demyelinating symmetric neuropathy) could fulfill AAN and INCAT criteria for CIDP.
- All require cerebral spinal fluid analysis to assess for albuminocytologic dissociation.
- Nerve conduction study (NCS): All require some features of demyelination including prolonged distal latencies and F-waves, slowed velocities, and at least one nerve demonstrating partial conduction block (feature of acquired demyelination).
- INCAT criteria do not require a nerve biopsy.
- See Table 1-108 for complete review of differences.

DIFFERENTIAL DIAGNOSIS

- Other demyelinating neuropathies such as:
  - Distal acquired demyelinating symmetric neuropathy (DADS)
  - Multifocal motor neuropathy (MMN)
  - Multifocal acquired demyelinating sensory and motor neuropathy (MADSAM; Lewis-Sumner syndrome)
- Inherited neuropathies: family history, genetic testing, and lack of acquired demyelinating features on NCS will help differentiate it from CIDP
- Metabolic neuropathies: diabetes, uremia
- Paraneoplastic neuropathy: associated with lymphoma or carcinoma
- Neuropathy associated with monoclonal gammopathy: associated with osteosclerotic myeloma, MGUS, and Waldenström's macroglobulinemia.
- Neuropathy associated with infectious diseases: HIV and leprosy
- Neuropathy associated with systemic inflammatory or immune-mediated diseases:
  - Sarcoidosis
  - Amyloidosis
  - Vasculitis: PAN, Behçet's, Sjögren's, cryoglobulinemia, lupus, Castleman's disease, granulomatosis with polyangiitis, Churg-Strauss
- Toxic neuropathies: ETOH, acrylamide, drugs (platinum-based agents, amiodarone, tacrolimus, perhexilene)

WORKUP

Nerve conduction studies and EMG to assess for demyelinating polyneuropathy with features of acquired demyelination (temporal dispersion) and conduction block (Fig. 1-249)

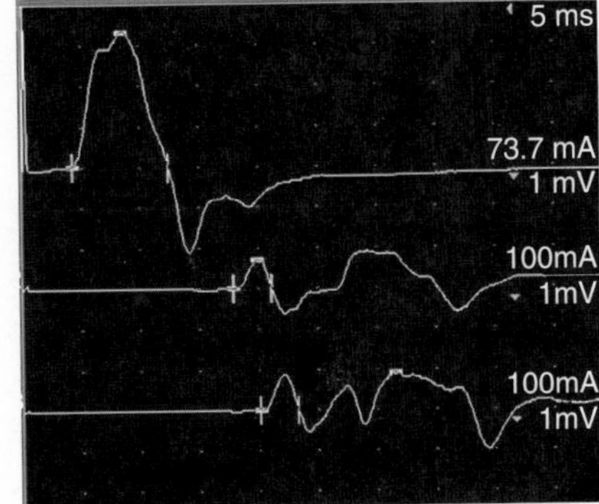

FIGURE 1-249 Conduction block.

TABLE 1-108 Diagnostic Criteria

Feature	American Academy of Neurology (AAN) Criteria	Saperstein Criteria	Inflammatory Neuropathy Cause and Treatment Criteria
Clinical involvement	Motor dysfunction, sensory dysfunction of >1 limb or both	Major: Symmetric proximal and distal weakness; minor: exclusively symmetrical distal weakness or sensory loss	Progressive or relapsing motor and sensory dysfunction of >1 limb
Time course	≥2 mo	≥2 mo	≥2 mo
Reflexes	Reduced or absent	Reduced or absent	Reduced or absent
Electrodiagnostics	Any 3 of the following 4 criteria: partial conduction block of ≥1 motor nerve, reduced velocity of ≥2 motor nerves, prolonged distal latency of ≥2 motor nerves, or prolonged F-waves of ≥2 motor nerves	2 of the 4 AAN electrodiagnostic criteria	Partial conduction block of ≥2 motor nerves and abnormal conduction velocity or distal latency or F-wave latency in 1 other nerve; or, in the absence of partial conduction block, abnormal conduction velocity, distal latency, or F-wave latency in 3 motor nerves; or electrodiagnostic abnormalities indicating demyelination in 2 nerves and histologic evidence of demyelination
CSF analysis	WBC count <10, negative CSF VDRL, and elevated protein (supportive)	Protein >45, WBC <10 (supportive)	CSF recommended but not mandatory
Biopsy findings	Evidence of demyelination and remyelination	Predominant features of demyelination; inflammation (not required)	Not mandatory (except in cases with electrodiagnostic abnormalities in only 2 motor nerves)

LABORATORY TESTS

- CSF analysis to assess for albumin-cytologic dissociation (i.e., elevated protein with normal cell count), along with appropriate laboratory studies to exclude associated conditions.
- Nerve biopsy specimens (rarely done now) also reveal signs of demyelination with variable degrees of inflammation and secondary axonal loss.

IMAGING STUDIES

MRI with/without gadolinium may show enlargement and enhancement of the proximal nerve root segments, respectively (Figs. 1-250 and 1-251)

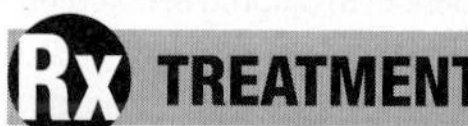

TREATMENT

Therapies are directed at blocking the underlying immune processes to arrest demyelination and inflammation and to prevent secondary axonal degeneration. The most widely used forms of immunomodulatory therapy are IV immunoglobulin (IVIg), plasmapheresis/plasma exchange (PE), and corticosteroids. There is no difference in efficacy between these three modalities of treatment. Azathioprine, myocophenylate mofetil, cyclophosphamide, rituximab, and cyclosporine may be used as secondary agents.

NONPHARMACOLOGIC THERAPY

Orthotics/braces for significant distal weakness

ACUTE GENERAL Rx

IVIg 2 g/kg divided over 2 to 5 days; plasmapheresis (5 to 6 exchanges)

CHRONIC Rx

- Oral prednisone (1 mg/kg daily starting dose). Typically changed to every other day after 1 mo or when strength plateaus. Reduce by 10 mg every month until 20 mg every other day. Then reduce by 5 mg/mo. Get tuberculin skin test prior to administration. Treat with calcium and vitamin D; low-sodium/high-protein diet, routine ophthalmologic evaluation for cataract and glaucoma screening, and surveillance for diabetes and GERD symptoms/signs.
- PREDICT study: Compared decadron 40 mg daily x4 days per month with prednisone 60 mg daily x2 months and then tapered over 27 wk. No difference in efficacy was found between the two groups. Less weight gain and cushingoid features occurred with pulsed steroids but possibly more sleep and psychological disturbances.
- Pulsed solumedrol: No standard regimen. However, 1000 mg x3 days can be used, followed by 1000 mg wk with the goal of reduced frequency to every 2 to 12 wk.
- IVIg: 0.4 to 1 g/kg administered monthly. Check baseline IgA level. Check renal function panel and survey for hypercoagulable states and development of headache.
- Mycophenylate mofetil: Start 500 mg bid and increase in 2 to 4 wk to 1 g bid (check CBC, LFTs, and CBC monthly for first 3 mo, then every 3 mo thereafter). May cause GI upset.
- Imuran: Start 25 to 50 mg bid and increase in 4 wk to 100 mg bid (check baseline LFTs and CBC for first 3 mo, then every 3 mo thereafter). Watch for idiosyncratic reaction of fever, GI upset. If occurs, cannot re-challenge patient.
- Cytoxan: Used for severe cases. 1000 mg/m^2 monthly for 6 months (moderate dose) or 50 mg/kg daily × 4 days (high dose).
- Other treatments used (case reports/anecdotal evidence): etanercept, rituximab, tacrolimus, interferon beta-1a.

DISPOSITION

- In one series, 90% of patients with CIDP improved. However, relapse rate was approximately 50%. In Mayo Clinic series, 64% of the patients were either improved or in remission and able to work, 8% were ambulatory but unable to work, 11% were bedridden or wheelchair bound, and 11% died from the disease.
- Patients with CIDP associated with IgM monoclonal gammopathy often respond poorly to treatment.
- Younger age, female gender, and relapsing-remitting course may portend a more favorable prognosis.

REFERRAL

- Neurologist, physical therapy/occupational therapy, orthotics

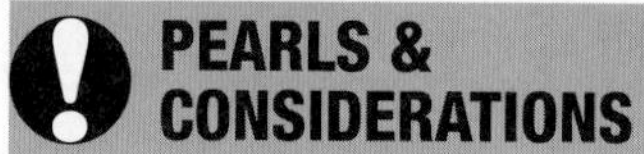

PEARLS & CONSIDERATIONS

- Patients are compliant with Imuran treatment if MCV >100.
- Always place PPD prior to initiation of steroid treatment.
- Consider Bactrim 3 times weekly in patients concomitant with steroids and other immunosuppressant agent for *Pneumocystis* pneumonia prophylaxis (especially in patients with coexisting lung disease).
- NCS: Look for acquired features of demyelination
  - Conduction block
  - Temporal dispersion
- CSF: Albuminocytologic dissociation; high CSF protein with normal cell count.

PATIENT/FAMILY EDUCATION

CIDP is a chronic illness usually characterized by a relapsing-remitting course that typically responds well to treatment. Early referral to a neurologist is important, and education on steroid side effects and mitigating factors is paramount.

SUGGESTED READINGS

available at www.expertconsult.com

AUTHOR: **JOHN SLADKY, M.D.**

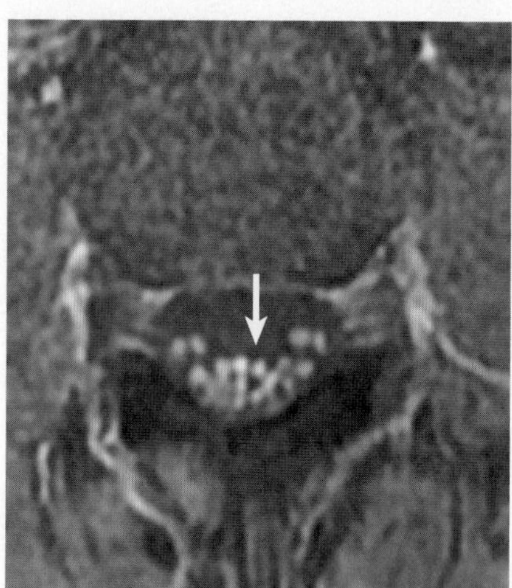

FIGURE 1-250 Contrast-enhanced MRI shows enhancement of nerve roots.

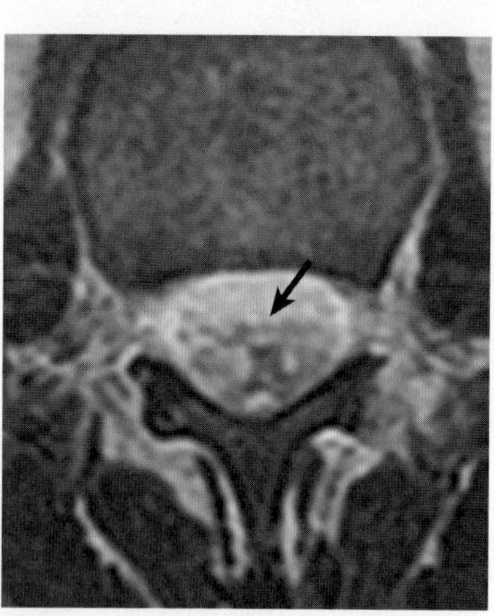

FIGURE 1-251 T2-weighted axial MRI shows enlarged nerve roots.

BASIC INFORMATION

DEFINITION

Chronic kidney disease (CKD) is a progressive decrease in renal function (glomerular filtration rate [GFR] <60 ml/min for >3 mo) with subsequent accumulation of waste products in the blood, electrolyte abnormalities, and anemia. The mechanisms and manifestations of CKD are summarized in Table 1-109. The National Kidney Foundation Disease Outcomes Quality Initiative defines CKD as follows, regardless of clinical diagnosis (Table 1-110): kidney damage (usually defined as an albumin-creatinine ratio [ACR] ≥30 mg/g) or a glomerular filtration rate (GFR) <60 ml/min per 1.73 m^2 (usually estimated from the serum creatinine level) for at least 3 mo. Table 1-111 describes standardized terminology for stages of chronic renal failure.

Table E1-112 describes the risk, injury, failure, and end-stage kidney disease (RIFLE) classification.

SYNONYMS

CKD
CRF
Chronic kidney disease
Chronic renal failure
End-stage renal disease

ICD-9CM CODES
585 Chronic renal failure
IC-10CM CODES
N18.9 Chronic kidney disease, unspecified

EPIDEMIOLOGY & DEMOGRAPHICS

- The prevalence of patients with CKD in the U.S. is approximately 11%.
- The number of patients with end-stage renal disease (ESRD) is increasing at the rate of 7% to 9% per year in the U.S. The increases are partially explained by the increasing prevalence of diabetes mellitus and hypertension, the leading risk factors for CKD. Each year two in 10,000 persons develop end-stage CKD.
- In the U.S., >250,000 people per year receive dialysis treatment for ESRD.
- Although kidney transplantation is considered the best choice for renal replacement therapy, many patients are not eligible for transplantation and more than 100,000 patients start dialysis each year.

TABLE 1-109 Pathophysiology of Chronic Kidney Disease

Manifestation	Mechanisms
Accumulation of nitrogenous waste products	Decrease in glomerular filtration rate
Acidosis	Decreased ammonia synthesis Impaired bicarbonate reabsorption Decreased net acid excretion
Sodium retention	Excessive renin production Oliguria
Sodium wasting	Solute diuresis Tubular damage
Urinary concentrating defect	Solute diuresis Tubular damage
Hyperkalemia	Decrease in glomerular filtration rate Metabolic acidosis Excessive potassium intake Hyporeninemic hypoaldosteronism
Renal osteodystrophy	Impaired renal production of 1,25-dihydroxycholecalciferol Hyperphosphatemia Hypocalcemia Secondary hyperparathyroidism
Growth retardation	Inadequate caloric intake Renal osteodystrophy Metabolic acidosis Anemia Growth hormone resistance
Anemia	Decreased erythropoietin production Iron deficiency Folate deficiency Vitamin B_{12} deficiency Decreased erythrocyte survival
Bleeding tendency	Defective platelet function
Infection	Defective granulocyte function Impaired cellular immune functions Indwelling dialysis catheters
Neurologic symptoms (fatigue, poor concentration, headache, drowsiness, memory loss, seizures, peripheral neuropathy)	Uremic factor(s) Aluminum toxicity Hypertension
Gastrointestinal symptoms (feeding intolerance, abdominal pain)	Gastroesophageal reflux Decreased gastrointestinal motility
Hypertension	Volume overload Excessive renin production
Hyperlipidemia	Decreased plasma lipoprotein lipase activity
Pericarditis, cardiomyopathy	Uremic factor(s) Hypertension Fluid overload
Glucose intolerance	Tissue insulin resistance

From Kliegman RM et al: *Nelson textbook of pediatrics,* ed 19, Philadelphia, 2011, Saunders.

PHYSICAL FINDINGS & CLINICAL PRESENTATION

- Skin pallor, ecchymoses.
- Edema, leg cramps, restless legs, peripheral neuropathy.
- Hypertension.
- Emotional lability and depression, decreased mental acuity.
- The clinical presentation varies with the degree of renal failure and its underlying etiology. Common symptoms are generalized fatigue, nausea, anorexia, pruritus (Fig. E1-252), sleep disturbances, smell and taste disturbances, hiccups, and seizures.
- Clinical manifestations of uremic encephalopathy are described in Table 1-109.

ETIOLOGY

- Diabetes (37%), hypertension (30%), chronic glomerulonephritis (12%)
- Polycystic kidney disease
- Tubular interstitial nephritis (e.g., drug hypersensitivity, analgesic nephropathy), obstructive nephropathies (e.g., nephrolithiasis, prostatic disease)
- Vascular diseases (renal artery stenosis, hypertensive nephrosclerosis)
- Autoimmune diseases

DIAGNOSIS

- CKD is primarily distinguished from acute RF by the duration (progression over several months).

TABLE 1-110 Criteria for Definition of Chronic Kidney Disease

Kidney damage for ≥3 months, as defined by structural or functional abnormalities of the kidney, with or without decreased GFR, that can lead to decreased GFR, manifest by either:
- Pathologic abnormalities
- Markers of kidney damage, including abnormalities in the composition of blood or urine, or abnormalities in imaging tests
- GFR <60 ml/min/1.73 m^2 for ≥3 months, with or without kidney damage

GFR, Glomerular filtration rate.
From Floege J et al: *Comprehensive clinical nephrology,* ed 4, Philadelphia, 2010, Saunders.

WORKUP

- Laboratory evaluation and imaging studies should be aimed at identifying reversible causes of acute decrements in GFR (e.g., volume depletion, urinary tract obstruction, heart failure) superimposed on chronic renal disease.
- Sonographic evaluation of the kidneys reveals smaller kidneys with increased echogenicity in CKD.
- Kidney biopsy: generally not performed in patients with small kidneys or with advanced disease.

LABORATORY TESTS

- Elevated blood urea nitrogen (BUN), creatinine, creatinine clearance. GFR is the best overall indicator of kidney function. It can be estimated by using prediction equations that take into account the serum creatinine level and some or all specific variables (body size, age, sex, race). GFR calculators are available on the National Kidney Foundation website (http://www.kidney.org/kls/professionals/gfr_calculator.cfm).
- Urinalysis: may reveal proteinuria, red blood cell casts.
- Serum chemistry: elevated BUN and creatinine, hyperkalemia, hyperuricemia, hypocalcemia, hyperphosphatemia, hyperglycemia, decreased bicarbonate. Measure urinary protein excretion. The finding of a protein/creatinine ratio of >1000 mg/g suggests the presence of glomerular disease.
- Special studies: serum and urine immunoelectrophoresis (in suspected multiple myeloma), antinuclear antibody (in suspected systemic lupus erythematosus).
- Cystatin C is a cysteine proteinase inhibitor produced by all nucleated cells, freely filtered at the glomerulus but not secreted by tubular cells. Given these characteristics, it may be superior to creatinine concentration both in kidney disease and as a marker of acute kidney injury. It is a better index of kidney function in elderly patients and a better predictor of outcomes than creatinine. The association of cystatin C is stronger than the association of measured GFR with all-cause and cardiovascular mortality in patients with advanced CKD.

IMAGING STUDIES

- Ultrasound of kidneys to measure kidney size and rule out obstruction
- Plain x-rays done for other reasons may reveal extraskeletal calcifications (Fig. E1-253).

CLASSIFICATION

A classification of CKD based on GFR is described in Table 1-113.

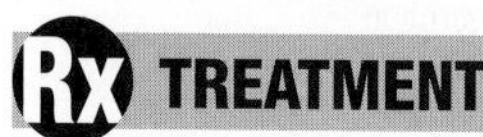

TREATMENT

The management plan for patients with CKD varies according to stage (Table 1-114)

TABLE 1-111 Standardized Terminology for Stages of Chronic Kidney Disease

Stage	Description	GFR (ml/min/1.73 m^2)
1	Kidney damage with normal or increased GFR	>90
2	Kidney damage with mild decrease in GFR	60-89
3	Moderate decrease in GFR	30-59
4	Severe decrease in GFR	5-29
5	Kidney failure	<15 or on dialysis

GFR, Glomerular filtration rate.
From Kliegman RM et al: *Nelson textbook of pediatrics,* ed 19, Philadelphia, 2011, Saunders.

TABLE 1-113 Classification of Chronic Kidney Disease Based on GFR

CKD Stage	Definition
1	Normal or increased GFR; some evidence of kidney damage reflected by microalbuminuria, proteinuria, and hematuria as well as radiologic or histologic changes
2	Mild decrease in GFR (89-60 ml/min per 1.73 m^2) with some evidence of kidney damage reflected by microalbuminuria, proteinuria, and hematuria as well as radiologic or histologic changes
3	GFR 59 to 30 ml/min per 1.73 m^2
3A	GFR 59 to 45 ml/min per 1.73 m^2
3B	GFR 44-30 ml/min per 1.73 m^2
4	GFR 29-15 ml/min per 1.73 m^2
5	GFR <15 ml/min per 1.73 m^2; when renal replacement therapy in the form of dialysis or transplantation has to be considered to sustain life

GFR, Glomerular filtration rate.
The suffix p to be added to the stage in proteinuric patients (proteinuria >0.5 g/24h)
Classification of CKD based on GFR as proposed by the Kidney Disease Outcomes Quality Initiative (KDOQI) guidelines and modified by NICE in 2008.
From Floege J et al: *Comprehensive clinical nephrology,* ed 4, Philadelphia, 2010, Saunders.

NONPHARMACOLOGIC THERAPY

- Provide adequate nutrition and calories (147 to 168 kJ/kg/day in energy intake, chiefly from carbohydrate and polyunsaturated fats). Table 1-115 describes nutritional recommendations in renal disease. Referral to a dietitian for nutritional therapy for patients with GFR <50 ml/1.73 m^2 is recommended and is now a covered service by Medicare.
- Restrict sodium (approximately 100 mmol/day), potassium (≤60 mmol/day), and phosphate (<800 mg/day).
- Blood pressure: The optimal blood pressure target in patients with CKD is unclear. Available evidence is inconclusive but does not prove that a blood pressure target of <130/80 mm Hg improves clinical outcomes more than a target of <140/90 mm Hg in adults with CKD. Whether a lower target benefits patients with proteinuria >300 to 1000 mg/dl requires further evaluation.
- Adjust drug doses to correct for prolonged half-lives.
- Restrict fluid if significant edema is present.
- Resistance exercise training can preserve lean body mass, nutritional status, and muscle function in patients with moderate CKD.
- Avoid radiocontrast agents. Hydration with sodium bicarbonate before contrast exposure is more effective than hydration with sodium chloride for prophylaxis of contrast-induced renal failure.
- Smoking cessation.
- Initiate hemodialysis, usually performed in center three times per week, or peritoneal dialysis, usually done by the patient at home (see "General Rx"). Prompt referral to nephrologist is helpful. Late evaluation of patients with chronic renal disease is associated with greater burden and severity of comorbid disease and shorter survival. Suggested criteria for referral to a nephrologist is described in Table 1-116.
- Kidney transplantation in selected patients.

GENERAL Rx

- Angiotensin-converting enzyme (ACE) inhibitors and angiotensin receptor blockers (ARBs) are useful in reducing proteinuria and slowing the progression of chronic renal disease, especially in hypertensive diabetic patients. The combination of ACEi and ARBs is not recommended and should be used only with great caution in patients with CKD due to increased risk of hyperkalemia, hypotension, and worsening renal failure. A systolic blood pressure between 110 and 129 mm Hg may be beneficial in patients with urine protein excretion >1.0 g/day. Systolic blood pressure <110 mm Hg may be associated with a higher risk for kidney disease progression.
- Initiation of dialysis:
    1. Urgent indications: uremic pericarditis, neuropathy, neuromuscular abnormalities, CHF, hyperkalemia, seizures.
    2. Judgmental indications: creatinine clearance 10 to 15 ml/min; progressive

anorexia, weight loss, reversal of sleep pattern, pruritus, uncontrolled fluid gain with hypertension and signs of CHF.

3. General indications for initiation of dialysis are summarized in Table 1-117. Suggested steps for resolving conflict in the shared decision about starting dialysis are described in Fig. E1-254. Recent trials have shown that early initiation of dialysis in patients with stage 5 CKD is not associated with increased survival. Initiation of dialysis when the GFR is 10 to 14 ml/min per 1.73 m^2 does not enhance survival compared with a strategy of symptom-driven initiation or initiation of dialysis at eGFR <7 ml/min per 173 m^2.

- Erythropoiesis-stimulating agents epoetin-alpha and darbepoetin-alpha can be used to reduce the need for transfusions in patients with anemia. Anemia should not be fully corrected in patients with CKD. Maintaining a target hemoglobin of 10 g/dl or hematocrit 30% to 33% is satisfactory. Targeting higher hemoglobin levels in CKD may increase risks for stroke, hypertension, and serious cardiovascular events.
- Diuretics for significant fluid overload (loop diuretics are preferred).
- Correction of hypertension to at least 130/85 mm Hg with ACE inhibitors (avoid in patients with significant hyperkalemia), ARBs, and/or nondihydropyridine calcium channel blockers (verapamil, diltiazem) can be used in patients intolerant to ACE inhibitors or when other agents are needed to control blood pressure.
- Correction of electrolyte abnormalities (e.g., calcium chloride, glucose, sodium polystyrene sulfonate for hyperkalemia), sodium bicarbonate in patients with severe metabolic acidosis.
- Lipid management[1]: The Kidney Disease Improving Global Outcomes (KDIGO) 2013 guidelines for lipid management in CKD does not use LDL cholesterol to identify patients with CKD who should receive lipid lowering

[1] Tonelli M et al: Lipid management in chronic kidney disease: synopsis of the kidney disease: improving global outcomes 2013 clinical practice guideline, *Ann Int Med* 160:182-189, 2014.

C

Diseases and Disorders

TABLE 1-114 Management Plan for Patients with Chronic Kidney Disease, According to Stage

KDOQI Classification	GFR (ml/min)	Typical Serum Creatinine in 65-kg Subject	Consequences	Actions to Consider
3	30-59	2 mg/dl (170 μmol/L)	Hypertension, secondary hyperparathyroidism	6-monthly eGFR initially 12-monthly eGFR if stable Annual Hb, K, Ca, P Treat hypertension Immunize against hepatitis B
4	15-29	4 mg/dl (350 μmol/L)	*Plus* anemia, hyperphosphatemia	3-monthly eGFR initially 6-monthly eGFR if stable 6-monthly Hb, K, Ca, P, and PTH Start phosphate-restricted diet and phosphate binders Correct vitamin D deficiency Start vitamin D analogue Plan renal replacement therapy, including vascular access
5	<15	8 mg/dl (700 μmol/L)	*Plus* sodium and water retention, anorexia, vomiting, reduced higher mental function	Plan elective start of dialysis or preemptive renal transplant
5	<5	17 mg/dl (1500 μmol/L)	*Plus* pulmonary edema, coma, fits, metabolic acidosis, hyperkalemia, death	Start dialysis or provide palliative care

The table gives a rough guide to the level of serum creatinine corresponding to each stage of CKD in a typical 65-kg subject and shows the approximate timing of the anticipated clinical problems and interventions required as CKD progresses. At each stage, the action plan for the previous CKD stage should be followed if it has not already been initiated.
eGFR, Estimated glomerular filtration rate; *PTH*, parathyroid hormone.
From Floege J et al: *Comprehensive clinical nephrology*, ed 4, Philadelphia, 2010, Saunders

TABLE 1-115 Nutritional Recommendations in Renal Disease

Daily Intake	Predialysis CRF	Hemodialysis	Peritoneal Dialysis
Protein (g/kg ideal BW) (see KDOQI[24] for estimation of adjusted edema-free body weight)	0.6-1.0 Level depends on the view of the nephrologist 1.0 for nephrotic syndrome	1.1-1.2 This is a broad recommendation as protein intake would be individualized for the patient's nutritional status, serum phosphate levels, and dialysis adequacy	1.0-1.3
Energy (kcal/kg BW)	35 (<60 yr) 30-35 (>60 yr)	35 (<60 yr) 30-35 (>60 yr)	35 including dialysate calories (<60 yr) 30-35 including dialysate calories (<60 yr)
Sodium (mmol)	<100 (more if salt wasting)	<100	<100
Potassium	Reduce if hyperkalemic	Reduce if hyperkalemic	Reduce if hyperkalemic; potassium restriction is generally not required
	If hyperkalemic, advice will take the form of decreasing certain foods (e.g., some fruits and vegetables) and giving information about cooking methods		
Phosphorus	Reduce; level dependent on protein intake Advice will take the form of reducing certain foods (e.g., dairy, offal, some shellfish) and giving information about the timing of binders with high-phosphorus meals and snacks		
Calcium	In CKD stages 3-5, total intake of elemental calcium (including dietary calcium) should not exceed 2000 mg/day	Total intake of elemental calcium (including dietary calcium) should not exceed 2000 mg/day	Total intake of elemental calcium (including dietary calcium) should not exceed 2000 mg/day

Recommendations are for typical patients but should always be individualized on the basis of clinical, biochemical, and anthropometric indices.
BW, Body weight; *CKD*, chronic kidney disease; *CRF*, chronic renal failure; *KDOQI*, Kidney Disease Outcomes Quality Initiative.
From Floege J et al: *Comprehensive clinical nephrology*, ed 4, Philadelphia, 2010, Saunders.

TABLE 1-116 Suggested Criteria for Referral of Patients with Chronic Kidney Disease to a Nephrologist

New Diagnosis	Stage 3	Stage 4
eGFR <30 ml/min/per 173 m²	eGFR falling by >4 ml/min per year	eGFR <20 ml/min per 173 m²
Hemoglobin <11 g/dl	eGFR <50 ml/min in patient younger than 50 years	eGFR falling by >4 ml/min per year
K^+ >6 mmol/L	Hemoglobin <11 g/dl	Hemoglobin <11 g/dl
Ca <2.1 mmol/L	K^+ >6 mmol/L	K^+ >6 mmol/L
Pi >1.5 mmol/L	Ca <2.1 mmol/L	Ca <2.1 mmol/L
PTH >3× upper limit normal	Pi >1.5 mmol/L	Pi >1.5 mmol/L
Hematuria		PTH >3× upper limit normal
Urine ACR >30 mg/mmol		
Suspected renovascular disease		

ACR, Albumin to creatinine ratio; *eGFR,* estimated glomerular filtration rate; *PTH,* parathyroid hormone.
Modified from NICE CKD guideline. From Floege J et al: *Comprehensive clinical nephrology,* ed 4, Philadelphia, 2010, Saunders.

TABLE 1-117 When to Initiate Dialysis

Indications for early start on dialysis
- Intractable fluid overload
- Intractable hyperkalemia
- Malnutrition due to uremia
- Uremic neurologic dysfunction
- Uremic serositis
- Functional deterioration otherwise unexplained

Uremic cognitive dysfunction can affect learning
Therefore, home-based self-dialysis may need to start earlier than center-assisted dialysis.

Start of dialysis may be delayed if patient is
asymptomatic, awaiting imminent kidney transplant, awaiting imminent placement of permanent HD or PD access, or, after appropriate education, has chosen conservative therapy.

If start of dialysis is delayed,
patient should be re-evaluated regularly to see if dialysis has become necessary.

Patients who choose PD
should not be required to have HD access placed, but venous sites for possible future HD access in arms should be preserved since HD may be required in the future.
Incremental start on PD may be considered if there is significant residual renal function.

Nephrologists should consider conservative (non-dialysis) treatment of kidney failure an integral part of their clinical practice.

HD, hemodialysis; *PD,* peritoneal dialysis.
Modified from NKF KDOQI Clinical Practice Guideline for initiation of dialysis. http://www.kidney.org/professional/Kdoqi/guideline_upHD_PD_VA/pd_rec1.htm. From Floege J et al: *Comprehensive clinical nephrology,* ed 4, Philadelphia, 2010, Saunders.

therapy and suggests focusing on the absolute risk for coronary events and evidence that such treatment is beneficial. They recommend treatment with a statin or statin/ezetimibe combination in adults aged ≥50 yr with eGFR <60 ml/min/1.73 m² but not treated with chronic dialysis or kidney transplantation.
- Control of renal osteodystrophy with calcium supplementation and vitamin D. Starting dose of calcium carbonate is 0.5 g with each meal, increased until the serum phosphorus concentration is normalized (most patients require 5 to 10 g/day). Calcitriol 0.125 to 0.25 mcg/day PO is effective in increasing serum calcium concentration. Paricalcitol, a new vitamin D analogue, has been reported to be more effective than calcitriol in lessening the elevations in serum calcium and phosphorus levels.
- Dietary phosphate restriction effectively reduces serum phosphate levels and is recommended in all patients with ESRD. For additional management of hyperphosphatemia, calcium-based agents are inexpensive, well tolerated, and should be the first-line phosphate binders for patients undergoing dialysis. Sevelamer and lanthanum are also effective as phosphate binders, but are much more expensive.
- General considerations in the continuing assessment of the CKD patient are described in Table 1-118.
- A sequential approach to the uremic patient with pruritus is described in Fig. E1-255.

DISPOSITION

- Prognosis is influenced by comorbidity of multisystem diseases. Late referral of patients to a nephrologist is associated with higher mortality and morbidity rates and higher costs. Despite recommendations for early referral, up to 64% of patients with CKD are still referred late.
- Lower predialysis serum sodium concentration is associated with an increased risk of death.
- Apolipoprotein E variation predicts CKD progression, independent of diabetes, race, lipid, and nonlipid factors. The e2 allele moderately increases risk of kidney disease progression, whereas allele e4 decreases the risk.
- The use of cystatin C alone or in combination with creatinine strengthens the association between the eGFR and the risks of death and end-stage renal disease across diverse populations (Shlipak et al).
- Kidney transplantation in selected patients improves survival. The 2-yr kidney graft survival rate for living related donor transplantations is >80%, whereas the 2-yr graft survival rate for cadaveric donor transplantation is approximately 70%.
- Principles underlying withdrawal of dialysis are described in Table 1-119.

TABLE 1-118 Continuing Assessment of the Chronic Kidney Disease Patient

Kidney Function

Has kidney function declined?
Has kidney function declined at the predicted rate?
If not, are there exacerbating factors?
Should dialysis be started?
Are there life-threatening complications?
- Pericarditis
- Fluid overload
- Resistant hypertension
- Hyperkalemia
- Uncompensated metabolic acidosis

Should access be created or transplantation planned?

Supportive Treatment

Can salt, potassium, and fluid balance be improved by diet or diuretics?
Is the phosphate controlled?
Is the dose of vitamin D compound appropriate?
Should erythropoietin (EPO) be prescribed?
Are nutritional supplements needed?
Does the patient need counseling?

Questions to be posed in evaluation of the patient.
From Floege J et al: *Comprehensive clinical nephrology,* ed 4, Philadelphia, 2010, Saunders.

TABLE 1-119 Principles Underlying Withdrawal of Dialysis

The ultimate responsibility for the decision rests with the physician, not the relative.
The patient's interests and dignity should be protected at all times.
The process should not be rushed. If there is any doubt about the correctness of the decision, treatment should continue.
There should be an open discussion among the multidisciplinary team to avoid any damaging disagreements.
The psychological needs of the health care team should not be overlooked.
Palliative care must be given in the most appropriate environment, e.g., a hospice or, ideally, the patient's own home.

From Floege J et al: *Comprehensive clinical nephrology,* ed 4, Philadelphia, 2010, Saunders.

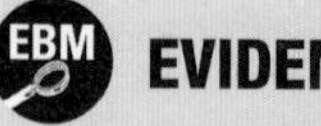

EVIDENCE

available at www.expertconsult.com

SUGGESTED READINGS

available at www.expertconsult.com

AUTHOR: **FRED F. FERRI, M.D.**

BASIC INFORMATION

DEFINITION

Chronic obstructive pulmonary disease (COPD) is an inflammatory respiratory disease usually caused by exposure to tobacco smoke. It is characterized by the presence of airflow limitation that is not fully reversible. The pathophysiology of COPD is related to chronic airway irritation, mucus production, and pulmonary scarring. Traditionally, COPD was described as encompassing *emphysema*, characterized by loss of lung elasticity and destruction of lung parenchyma with enlargement of air spaces, and *chronic bronchitis*, characterized by obstruction of small airways and productive cough >3 mo for more than 2 successive yr. These terms are no longer included in the formal definition of COPD, although they are still used clinically. Although emphysema and chronic bronchitis are commonly associated with COPD, neither is required to make the diagnosis.

SYNONYMS

COPD
Emphysema
Chronic bronchitis

ICD-9CM CODES
496 COPD
492.8 Emphysema
ICD-10CM CODES
J44.9 Chronic obstructive pulmonary disease, unspecified
J43.9 Emphysema, unspecified

EPIDEMIOLOGY & DEMOGRAPHICS

- COPD affects more than 5% of adults in the U.S.
- Between 10% and 20% of COPD in the U.S. is due to occupational or other exposure to chemical vapors, irritants, and fumes; 80% to 90% is due to cigarette smoking.
- COPD is the third leading cause of death in the U.S.
- Highest incidence is in males >40 yr.
- 16 million office visits, 500,000 hospitalizations, 120,000 deaths annually, and >$18 billion in direct health care costs annually can be attributed to COPD.
- Patients with COPD living in isolated rural areas of the U.S. are at greater risk for COPD exacerbation-related mortality than those living in urban areas, independent of hospital rurality and volume.

PHYSICAL FINDINGS & CLINICAL PRESENTATION

- Patients with COPD have historically been classically subdivided in two major groups based on their appearance:
  1. *Blue bloaters* are patients with chronic bronchitis; the name is derived from the bluish tinge of the skin (as a result of chronic hypoxemia and hypercapnia) and from the frequent presence of peripheral edema (from cor pulmonale); chronic cough with production of large amounts of sputum is characteristic.
  2. *Pink puffers* are patients with emphysema; they have a cachectic appearance but pink skin color (adequate oxygen saturation); shortness of breath is manifested by pursed-lip breathing and use of accessory muscles of respiration.
- COPD may present with combinations of the following manifestations:
  1. Cyanosis, chronic cough (usually productive but may be intermittent and may be unproductive), tachypnea, tachycardia.
  2. Dyspnea (persistent, progressive), pursed-lip breathing with use of accessory muscles for respiration, decreased breath sounds, wheezing.
  3. Chronic sputum production.
  4. Chest wall abnormalities (hyperinflation, "barrel chest," protruding abdomen).
  5. Flattening of diaphragm.
- Acute exacerbation of COPD is mainly a clinical diagnosis and generally manifests with worsening dyspnea, increase in sputum purulence, and increase in sputum volume. However, respiratory symptom status is not a reliable indicator of the presence of airflow obstruction. Individuals with normal spirometric values may report respiratory symptoms, whereas individuals who have severe to very severe airflow obstruction by spirometry may report no symptoms.

ETIOLOGY

- Tobacco exposure
- Occupational exposure to pulmonary toxins (e.g., dust, noxious gases, vapors, fumes, cadmium, coal, silica). The industries with the highest exposure risk are plastics, leather, rubber, and textiles.
- Atmospheric pollution.
- Alpha-1-antitrypsin deficiency (rare; <1% of COPD patients).

DIAGNOSIS

DIFFERENTIAL DIAGNOSIS

- Heart failure (HF)
- Asthma
- Tuberculosis, other respiratory infections
- Bronchiectasis
- Cystic fibrosis
- Neoplasm
- Pulmonary embolism
- Obliterative bronchiolitis
- Diffuse panbronchiolitis
- Sleep apnea, obstructive
- Hypothyroidism <50% predicted

WORKUP

Chest x-ray (seldom diagnostic but useful to exclude alternative diagnosis [CHF, TB]), pulmonary function testing (spirometry), oxygen saturation, blood gases (useful in selected patients with FEV_1 <50% predicted or with acute exacerbation). Alpha-1-antitrypsin deficiency screening may be useful in Caucasians with suspected COPD and no clear risk factors.

LABORATORY TESTS

- CBC: generally not helpful, may reveal leukocytosis with left shift during acute exacerbation. Recent trials have shown that eosinophilia in COPD patients predicts response to corticosteroids.
- Sputum may be purulent with bacterial respiratory tract infections. Sputum staining and cultures are usually reserved for cases refractory to antibiotic therapy.
- Arterial blood gases: normocapnia, mild to moderate hypoxemia may be present. ABGs and pulse oximetry are usually used to determine if a patient is a candidate for long-term oxygen therapy or if hypercapnia is present (ABGs).
- Spirometry pulmonary function testing (PFT) with measurement of forced vital capacity (FVC) and forced expiratory volume in 1 s (FEV_1). Spirometry should be obtained to diagnose airflow obstruction in clinically stable patients with respiratory symptoms. It should not be used to screen for airflow obstruction in individuals without respiratory symptoms. Spirometry reveals that the primary physiologic abnormality in COPD is an accelerated decline in FEV_1 from the normal rate in adults >30 yr of approximately 30 ml/yr to nearly 60 ml/yr. PFT results in COPD reveal abnormal diffusing capacity, increased total lung capacity and/or residual volume, and fixed reduction in FEV_1 in patients with emphysema; normal diffusing capacity and reduced FEV_1 are found in patients with chronic bronchitis. Stage and severity of COPD according to postbronchodilator spirometry are described in Table 1-120. It is important to note that FEV_1 does not correlate well with individual patients' severity of dyspnea, exercise limitations, or health status.

TABLE 1-120 Stage and Severity of COPD According to Postbronchodilator Spirometry

Stage and Severity	Definition
I: Mild	FEV_1/FVC <0.70, FEV_1 ≥80% of predicted
II: Moderate	FEV_1/FVC <0.70, 50%≤FEV_1 <80% of predicted
III: Severe	FEV_1/FVC <0.70, 30%≤FEV_1 <50% of predicted
IV: Very severe	FEV_1/FVC <0.70, FEV_1 <30% of predicted or FEV_1 <50% of predicted plus chronic respiratory failure

Data from the Global Initiative for Chronic Obstructive Lung Disease. http://www.goldcopd.com.<ce:br/>From Goldman L, Schafer AI: *Goldman's Cecil medicine*, ed 24, Philadelphia, 2012, Saunders.

Evaluation of patients should also focus on symptom control and risk for adverse events in addition to FEV_1.

- Patients with COPD can generally be distinguished from asthmatics by their incomplete response to albuterol (change in FEV_1 <200 ml and 12%) and absence of an abnormal bronchoconstrictor response to methacholine or other stimuli. However, nearly 40% of patients with COPD respond to bronchodilators.

ASSESSMENT

- The global initiative for chronic obstructive lung disease (COLD) assigns patients with COPD into four groups (A, B, C, D) based on on (1) the degree of airflow restriction (Table 1-120), (2) a patient symptom score using one of two symptom questionnaires (CAT or mMRC), or (3) the number of COPD exacerbations in one year.[1]

IMAGING STUDIES

Chest x-ray:

- Hyperinflation with flattened diaphragm, tenting of the diaphragm at the rib, and increased retrosternal chest space (Fig. 1-256)
- Decreased vascular markings and bullae in patients with emphysema
- Thickened bronchial markings and enlarged right side of the heart in patients with chronic bronchitis

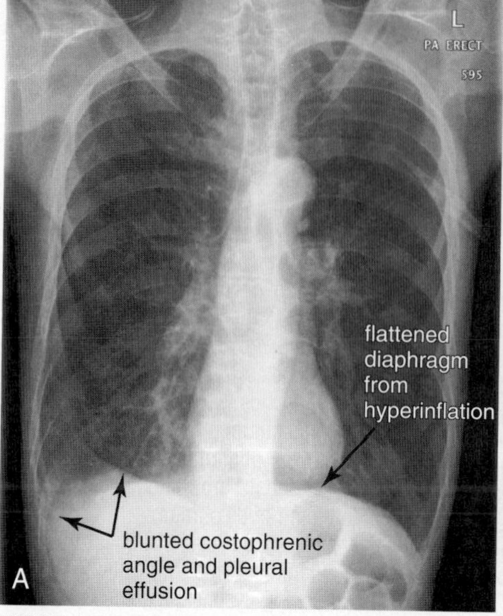

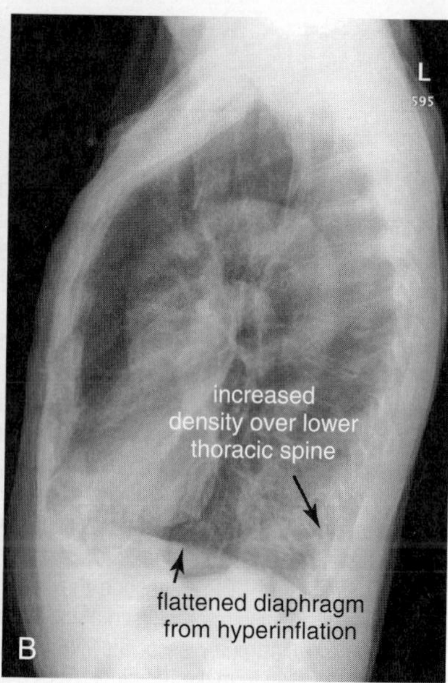

FIGURE 1-256 Chronic obstructive pulmonary disease (COPD). A, Posterior-anterior (PA) upright chest x-ray. **B,** Lateral upright chest x-ray. This 63-year-old man with a history of COPD presented with 2 weeks of worsening cough with yellow sputum and dyspnea. His oxygen saturation was 87% in the emergency room. He has evidence of hyperinflation with flat diaphragms (particularly evident on the lateral x-ray, **B**). The patient also has a blunted right costophrenic angle with an apparent effusion and increased densities in both the right and the left lung base **(A).** The lateral x-ray also shows increased density overlying the inferior thoracic spine, an abnormal spine sign. (From Broder JS: *Diagnostic imaging for the emergency physician,* Philadelphia, 2011, Saunders.)

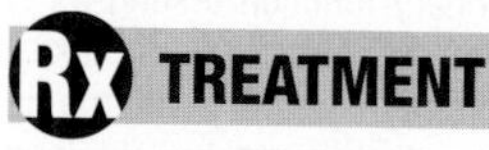

TREATMENT

NONPHARMACOLOGIC THERAPY

- Avoidance of tobacco and elimination of air pollutants.
- Supplemental oxygen, usually through a face mask, to ensure oxygen saturation >90% as measured by pulse oximetry. Continuous oxygen therapy should be prescribed for patients with COPD who have arterial partial pressure of oxygen 55 mm Hg or less, or oxygen saturation 88% or less as measured by pulse oximetry.
- Pulmonary clearing: careful nasotracheal suction is indicated only in patients with excessive secretions and an inability to expectorate. Mechanical percussion of the chest as applied by a physical or respiratory therapist is ineffective with acute exacerbations of COPD.
- Pulmonary rehabilitation should be considered in COPD patients who remain symptomatic despite optimal medical management. Medicare will cover up to 36 sessions of pulmonary rehabilitation in COPD patients.
- Weight loss in obese patients.

GENERAL Rx

- Pharmacologic treatment should be administered in a stepwise approach according to the severity of disease and patient's tolerance for specific drugs. Fig. E1-257 describes general management approaches for COPD. When using the COLD assessment criteria, pulmonary rehabilitation is recommended for patients in groups B, C, and D. Those in group A should receive a short-acting anticholinergic or short-acting β_2-agonist for mild intermittent symptoms. For patients in group B, long-acting anticholinergics or long-acting β_2-agonists should be added. Patients in group C or D are at high risk of exacerbations and should receive a long-acting anticholinergic or a combination of an inhaled corticosteroid and a long-acting β_2-agonist.
  - Bronchodilators improve symptoms, quality of life, and exercise tolerance, and decrease incidence of exacerbations. Inhaled bronchodilators *may be used* for stable COPD patients with respiratory symptoms and FEV_1 between 60% and 80% of predicted. They are *recommended* for stable COPD patients with respiratory symptoms and FEV_1 <60% of predicted. Recent guidelines from ACP, ACCP, ATS, and ERS recommend that clinicians prescribe monotherapy using either long-acting inhaled anticholinergics or long-acting inhaled beta-agonists for symptomatic patients with COPD and FEV_1 <60% of predicted. Clinicians should base the choice of specific monotherapy on patient preference, cost, and adverse effect profile.
  - Short-acting beta-2 agonists (e.g., albuterol metered-dose inhaler 1 to 2 puffs q4 to 6h prn) or short-acting anticholinergic agents (e.g., ipratropium inhaler 2 puffs qid) are acceptable in patients with mild, variable symptoms. Anticholinergics are also effective and are available in combination with albuterol (Combivent). Long-acting inhaled agents are preferred in patients with mild to moderate or continuous symptoms. Tiotropium is an excellent long-acting bronchodilator. It is very effective for long-term, once-a-day use. It has been shown to be superior to salmeterol, an inhaled long-acting beta-agonist (LABA) in patients with moderate to severe COPD; however, recent trials have shown higher hospitalization rates and mortality with tiotropium compared to LABAs. Aclidinium is another orally inhaled long-acting anticholinergic for long-term maintenance treatment of bronchospasm associated with COPD. Unlike tiotropium, which is predominantly renally excreted, it can be used safely in renal impairment.
  - Addition of inhaled steroids (fluticasone, budesonide, triamcinolone) is used to reduce exacerbations in patients with moderate to severe COPD. Inhaled steroids are reserved for patients with either ≥2 exacerbations annually or FEV_1 <50% of predicted. The role of inhaled corticosteroids (ICS) in COPD is controversial. Although some trials have demonstrated mild improvement in patients' symptoms and decreased frequency of exacerbations, most pulmonologists believe that these drugs are ineffective in most patients with COPD but should be considered for patients with moderate to severe airflow limitation who have persistent symptoms despite optimal bronchodilator

[1]Lee H, Kim J, Tagmazyan K: Treatment of stable chronic obstructive pulmonary disease: the GOLD guidelines, *Am Fam Physician* 88(10):655-663, 2013.

TABLE 1-121 Guideline Recommendations for Hospital Management of COPD Exacerbations

	Global Initiative for Chronic Obstructive Lung Disease*	American Thoracic Society/ European Respiratory Society†	National Institute for Clinical Excellence‡
Date of statement	2010	2004	2010
Diagnostic testing	Chest radiograph, oximetry, ABGs, and ECG. Other testing as warranted by clinical indication.	Chest radiograph, oxygen saturation, ABGs, ECG, sputum Gram stain and culture.	Chest radiograph, ABG, ECG, complete blood count, sputum smear and culture, blood cultures if febrile.
Bronchodilator therapy	Inhaled short-acting β_2-agonist is recommended. Consider ipratropium if inadequate clinical response. Consider theophylline or aminophylline as second-line intravenous therapy.	Inhaled short-acting β_2-agonist and/or ipratropium with spacer or nebulizer, as needed.	Administer inhaled drugs by nebulizer or handheld inhaler. Specific agents and dosing regimens not specified. Consider theophylline if inadequate response to inhaled bronchodilators.
Antibiotics	Recommended if (1) increases in dyspnea, sputum volume, and sputum purulence all are present; (2) increase in sputum purulence along with increase in either dyspnea or sputum volume; or (3) need for assisted ventilation. See original document for complex treatment algorithm.	Base choice on local bacterial resistance patterns. Consider amoxicillin/clavulanate or respiratory fluoroquinolones. If *Pseudomonas* species and/or other Enterobacteriaceae are suspected, consider combination therapy.	Administer only if history of purulent sputum. Initiate with an aminopenicillin, a macrolide, or a tetracycline, taking into account local bacterial resistance patterns. Adjust therapy according to sputum and blood cultures.
Systemic corticosteroids	Daily prednisolone 30-40 mg (or its equivalent) orally for 7-10 days.	Daily prednisone 30-40 mg orally for 10-14 days. Equivalent dose intravenously if unable to tolerate oral intake. Consider inhaled corticosteroids.	Daily prednisolone 30 mg (or its equivalent) orally for 7-14 days.
Supplemental oxygen	Maintain oxygen saturation >90%. Monitor ABGs for hypercapnia and acidosis.	Maintain oxygen saturation >90%. Monitor ABGs for hypercapnia and acidosis.	Maintain oxygen saturation within the individualized target range. Monitor ABGs.
Assisted ventilation	Indications for NPPV include severe dyspnea, acidosis (pH ≤7.35) and/or hypercapnia (PCO_2 >45 mm Hg), and respiratory rate >25 breaths/min. Contraindications to NPPV include respiratory arrest, hemodynamic instability, impaired mental status, copious bronchial secretions, and extreme obesity. Intubate if contraindication to NPPV or failure of NPPV (worsening ABGs or clinical status). Consider likelihood of recovery and patient's wishes and expectations before intubation.	Consider with pH <7.35 and PCO_2 >45-60 mm Hg and respiratory rate >24 breaths/min. Institute NPPV in a controlled environment, unless there are contraindications (e.g., respiratory arrest, hemodynamic instability, impaired mental status, copious bronchial secretions, and extreme obesity). Intubate if contraindication to NPPV or failure of NPPV (worsening ABGs or clinical status).	NPPV treatment of choice for persistent hypercapnic respiratory failure. Consider functional status, body mass index, home oxygen, comorbidities, prior ICU admissions, age, and FEV_1 when assessing suitability for intubation and ventilation.

*Data from http://www.goldcopd.com.
†Data from MacNee W. Standards for the diagnosis and treatment of patients with COPD: a summary of the ATS/ERS position paper. *Eur Respir J* 23:932-946, 2004.
‡Data from http://www.nice.org.uk.
ABGs, Arterial blood gases; *ECG,* electrocardiogram; *ICU,* intensive care unit; *NPPV,* noninvasive positive pressure ventilation.
From Goldman L, Schafer AI: *Goldman's Cecil medicine,* ed 24, Philadelphia, 2012, Saunders.

therapy. ICS therapy does not affect 1-yr all-cause mortality among patients with COPD and is associated with a higher risk of pneumonia.

- Roflumilast is a selective oral PDE4 inhibitor useful to reduce the risk of COPD exacerbations in patients with severe COPD associated with chronic bronchitis and a history of exacerbations. It is not a bronchodilator and is not indicated for the relief of acute bronchospasm.
- Recent guidelines from ACP (American College of Physicians), ACCP (American College of Chest Physicians), ATS (American Thoracic Society), and ERS (European Respiratory Society) suggest that clinicians may administer combination inhaled therapies for symptomatic patients with stable COPD and FEV_1 <60% predicted. They also recommend that clinicians should prescribe pulmonary rehabilitation for symptomatic patients with an FEV_1 <50% predicted and continuous oxygen therapy in patients with COPD who have resting hypoxemia (Pao_2 <55 mm Hg or Spo_2 <88%).

• Acute exacerbation of COPD (increase in sputum volume and purulence, worsening dyspnea) can be treated with:

- Aerosolized beta-2 agonists (e.g., metaproterenol nebulizer solution 5% 0.3 ml or albuterol nebulized 5% solution 2.5 to 5 mg).
- Anticholinergic agents, which have equivalent efficacy to inhaled beta-adrenergic agonists. Inhalant solution of ipratropium bromide 0.5 mg can be administered every 4 to 8 hr.
- Short courses of systemic corticosteroids have been shown to improve spirometric and clinical outcomes. Treatment failure occurs less often in patients who receive low-dose steroids than in those receiving high-dose parenteral steroids. Oral prednisone 40 mg/day for 5 to 14 days is generally effective. Courses of treatment that are extended for >14 days confer no added benefit and increase the risk of adverse events. Recent trials[2] have shown that in patients with acute COPD exacerbations, systemic glucocorticoid treatment for 5 days is not inferior to treatment for 14 days.
- Use of noninvasive positive pressure ventilation (NIPPV) decreases the risk of endotracheal intubation and decreases intensive care unit admission rates. Contraindications to its use are uncooperative patient, decreased level of consciousness, hemodynamic instability, inadequate mask fit, and severe respiratory acidosis. Increased airway pressure can be delivered by using inspiratory positive airway pressure, continuous positive airway pressure, or bilevel positive airway pressure, which combines the other modalities. When using NIPPV, the nasal mask is usually tolerated the best; however, patients must be instructed to keep their mouths closed while breathing with the nasal apparatus. Oxygen can be delivered at 10 to 15 L/min and started in spontaneous ventilation mode with an initial expiratory positive airway pressure setting of 3 to 5 cm H_2O and an inspiratory positive airway pressure setting of up to 10 cm H_2O. Adjustments in these settings should be made in 2-cm H_2O increments. It is important to monitor patients with frequent vital signs measurements, arterial blood gases, or pulse oximetry. Intubation

[2]Leuppi JD et al: Short-term vs conventional glucocorticoid therapy in acute exacerbations of chronic obstructive pumonary disease: the REDUCE randomized clinical trial, *JAMA* 309:2223-2231, 2013.

 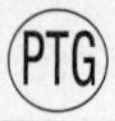 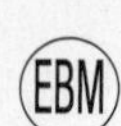 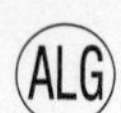

BOX 1-16 Indications for Invasive Mechanical Ventilation

Severe dyspnea, with use of accessory muscles and paradoxical abdominal motion
Respiratory frequency >35 breaths/min
Life-threatening hypoxemia (Pao_2 <40 mm Hg or Pao_2/Fio_2 <200 mm Hg)
Severe acidosis (pH <7.25) and hypercapnia ($Paco_2$ >60 mm Hg)
Respiratory arrest
Somnolence, impaired mental status
Cardiovascular complications (hypotension, shock, heart failure)
Other complications: metabolic abnormalities, sepsis, pneumonia, pulmonary embolism, barotrauma, massive pleural effusion
Noninvasive positive-pressure ventilation failure (or exclusion criteria)

Fio_2, inspired oxygen fraction; *Pao_2,* partial pressure of carbon dioxide in arterial blood; *Pao_2,* partial pressure of oxygen in arterial blood.
From Vincent JL et al: *Textbook of critical care,* ed 6, Philadelphia, 2011, Saunders.

and mechanical ventilation may be necessary if previous measures fail to provide improvement.
  - IV aminophylline administration is controversial and generally not recommended. When used in patients with refractory symptoms, serum levels should be closely monitored (keep level 8 to 12 mcg/ml) to minimize risks of tachyarrhythmias.
- Approximately 50% of COPD exacerbations are caused by bacterial infection. Antibiotics are indicated in suspected bacterial respiratory infection (e.g., increased purulence and volume of phlegm).
  - *Haemophilus influenzae* and *Streptococcus pneumoniae* are frequent causes of acute bronchitis.
  - Oral antibiotics of choice are azithromycin, levofloxacin, amoxicillin-clavulanate, trimethoprim-sulfamethoxazole, doxycycline, and cefuroxime.
  - The two best predictors of potential benefit from antibiotics are purulent sputum and C-reactive protein (CRP) level >40 mg/L.[3]
- Guaifenesin may improve cough symptoms and mucus clearance; however, mucolytic medications are generally ineffective. Their benefits may be greatest in patients with more advanced disease.
- Guideline recommendations for hospital management of COPD exacerbations are described in Table 1-121. Indications for invasive mechanical ventilation are described in Box 1-16.

Lung volume reduction surgery has been proposed as a palliative treatment for severe emphysema. Overall it increases the chance of improved exercise capacity but does not confer a survival advantage over medical therapy. It is most beneficial in patients with both predominantly upper-lobe emphysema and low baseline exercise capacity.

- In patients with end-stage emphysema who have an FEV_1 <25% of predicted normal value after administration of bronchodilator and additional complications such as severe hypoxemia, hypercapnia, and pulmonary hypertension, single-lung transplantation should be considered a surgical option.
- Trials involving endobronchial valves that allow air to escape from a pulmonary lobe but not to enter it have been done to improve lung function by reducing lobar volume in patients with advanced heterogeneous emphysema. Results have shown modest improvements in lung function, symptoms, and exercise tolerance, but more frequent exacerbations of COPD. Other complications included pneumonia and hemoptysis postimplantation.

DISPOSITION

- After the initial episode of respiratory failure, 5-yr survival is approximately 25%.
- Development of cor pulmonale or hypercapnia and persistent tachycardia are poor prognostic indicators.

PEARLS & CONSIDERATIONS

COMMENTS

- All patients with COPD should receive pneumococcal vaccine and yearly influenza vaccine.
- Early antibiotic administration is associated with improved outcomes among patients hospitalized for acute exacerbations of COPD regardless of the risk of treatment failure.
- In assessing the severity of COPD, the FEV_1 is limited by the fact that it does not take into account the systemic manifestations of COPD. The BODE index (body mass index, degree of obstruction, dyspnea, and exercise capacity) has been proposed as a multidimensional scale to better assess the morbidity and mortality associated with COPD. It is better than the FEV_1 alone at predicting the risk of death from any cause and from respiratory causes among patients with COPD. In the BODE index, obstruction is measured by FEV_1 and dyspnea is measured by the modified Medical Research Council (MMRC) dyspnea questionnaire in a 6-minute walk test. A score of 0 on the MMRC indicates that the individual is not troubled with breathlessness except with strenuous exercise, 1 indicates shortness of breath when hurrying or walking up a slight hill, and 2 means the individual walks slower than people of the same age due to breathlessness or has to stop for breath when walking at own pace on level ground. A score of 3 means severe dyspnea because the person has to stop for breath after walking approximately 100 meters or after a few minutes on level ground, and a score of 4 indicates very severe dyspnea and is given when the individual is too breathless to leave the house or is breathless when dressing or undressing.
- Pulmonary artery enlargement as determined by a ratio of the diameter of the pulmonary artery to the diameter of the aorta [PA:A ratio] of >1 detected by CT is associated with severe exacerbations of COPD.
- The average person with COPD has one or two acute exacerbations each year. Prophylactic use of macrolide antibiotics (azithromycin 250 mg/day) has been shown to decrease the frequency of exacerbations and improve quality of life among selected patients with COPD; however, it leads to hearing decrements in a small percentage of patients and increased prevalence of macrolide-resistant bacteria colonizing the airway and is therefore not recommended.

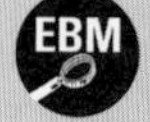

EVIDENCE

available at www.expertconsult.com

SUGGESTED READINGS

available at www.expertconsult.com

RELATED CONTENT

Chronic Obstructive Pulmonary Disease (Patient Information)
Emphysema (Patient Information)

AUTHOR: **FRED F. FERRI, M.D.**

[3]Miravilles M et al: Is it possible to identify exacerbations of mild to moderate COPD that do not require antibiotic treament? *Chest* 144:1571, 2013.

BASIC INFORMATION

DEFINITION

Churg-Strauss syndrome (CSS) refers to a systemic granulomatous vasculitis accompanied by severe asthma (core clinical feature) and hypereosinophilia. Classification criteria and definition for CSS are described in Table 1-122.

SYNONYMS

Allergic angiitis
Allergic granulomatosis

ICD-9CM CODES
446.4 Angiitis, allergic granulomatous
ICD-10CM CODES
M31.30 Wegener's granulomatosis without renal involvement

EPIDEMIOLOGY & DEMOGRAPHICS

- Overall incidence of 2.4 cases per 1 million persons in the U.S. Among asthma patients, the annual incidence of CSS is estimated to average 34.6 per 1 million patients.
- Usually occurs at a mean age of 50 yr but may present as young as 4 yr or in the elderly
- Slight male/female predominance (1.3:1).
- With treatment, 1-year survival is approximately 90% and 5-year survival is 62%.

PHYSICAL FINDINGS & CLINICAL PRESENTATION

The clinical picture of CSS typically consists of three partially overlapping phases, which may or may not be sequential:

1. Prodromal phase:
   - Severe adult-onset asthma, with or without allergic rhinitis, sinusitis, headache, cough, and wheezing
   - Precedes development of systemic vasculitis by several years
2. Eosinophilic/tissue infiltration phase:
   - Peripheral eosinophilia and eosinophilic infiltration of the lungs, myocardium, and gastrointestinal (GI) tract, with or without granulomas
   - Signs and symptoms of cough, fever, anorexia, weight loss, sweats, malaise, nausea, vomiting, abdominal pain, and diarrhea
3. Systemic vasculitic phase:
   - Development of necrotizing vasculitis that is clinically apparent primarily in peripheral nerves, skin, and kidneys
   - Any organ can be affected, with skin involvement present in 50% to 67% of patients

Skin involvement is divided into three categories:

1. Erythematous maculopapules (can resemble erythema multiforme)
2. Hemorrhagic lesions (associated with wheals)
3. Cutaneous and subcutaneous nodules

ETIOLOGY

- Etiology unknown, but believed to be an autoimmune-mediated process
- Triggering factors implicated in CSS include inhaled allergens, vaccinations, infections, and drugs such as macrolides (see "Comments").

Dx DIAGNOSIS

- Clinical findings and biopsy showing eosinophilic vasculitis
- The American College of Rheumatology (ACR) has established the criteria for CSS diagnosis in patients without vasculitis:
  - Asthma
  - Eosinophilia >10% of white blood cell count
  - Mononeuropathy or polyneuropathy
  - Migratory pulmonary infiltrates
  - Paranasal sinus abnormalities
  - Extravascular eosinophils on biopsy

The presence of any four or more of the six criteria yields a sensitivity of 85% and a specificity of 99.7%. For patients with vasculitis, the presence of asthma and eosinophilia was 90% sensitive and 99% specific for CSS.

DIFFERENTIAL DIAGNOSIS

- Polyarteritis nodosa (PAN)
- Wegener's granulomatosis (WG)
- Goodpasture syndrome
- Loeffler syndrome
- Hypereosinophilia syndrome
- Rheumatoid arthritis
- Leukocytoclastic vasculitis

Although similar and at times grouped with patients with PAN or WG, CSS differs in that:

- CSS vasculitis involves small-sized arteries, veins, and venules
- CSS, unlike PAN, predominantly involves the lung. Other organs affected include heart, GI system, central nervous system, kidney, and skin
- Kidney involvement is much less common in CSS than in WG. Pulmonary lesions in WG usually involve the upper respiratory tract rather than the peripheral lung parenchyma in CSS
- CSS shows necrotizing vasculitis along with eosinophilic granulomas

LABORATORY TESTS

- Complete blood count with differential: eosinophilia >10% is an American College of Rheumatology (ACR) diagnostic criterion
- Blood urea nitrogen and creatinine may be mildly elevated, suggesting renal involvement
- Urinalysis may show mild hematuria and proteinuria.
- 24-hour urine for protein; greater than 1 g/day is a poor prognostic factor
- Perinuclear antineutrophilic cytoplasmic antibody (P-ANCA) is found in 13% to 70% of patients. Negative ANCA does not rule out CSS
- Stools may be positive for occult blood (enteric involvement during eosinophilic phase)
- Elevation of aspartate aminotransferase, alanine aminotransferase, and creatine phosphokinase may indicate liver or muscle (skeletal or cardiac) involvement
- Rheumatoid factor and antinuclear antibody may be positive. Erythrocyte sedimentation rate is usually elevated
- Biopsy helps confirm the diagnosis. Surgical lung biopsy is the gold standard. Transbronchial biopsy is rarely helpful. Necrotizing vasculitis and extravascular necrotizing granulomas, usually with eosinophilic infiltrates, are suggestive of CSS. The presence of eosinophils in extravascular tissues is most specific for CSS

IMAGING STUDIES

- Chest radiograph is abnormal in eosinophilic and vasculitic phases: asymmetrical bilateral patchy migratory infiltrates, interstitial lung disease, or nodular infiltrates (Fig. 1-258). Small pleural effusions are found in 29% of cases
- Lung lesions in CSS are noncavitating, as opposed to those in WG
- Paranasal sinus films may reveal sinus opacification, which is an ACR diagnostic criterion
- Angiography is sometimes done in patients with mesenteric ischemia or renal involvement

TABLE 1-122 Classification Criteria and Definition for Churg-Strauss Syndrome

CLASSIFICATION CRITERIA		DEFINITION
Lanham (Requires 2 of 3)	**American College of Rheumatology (Requires 4 of 6)**	**Chapel Hill Consensus Conference**
Asthma Eosinophilia (>10% WBC count or >1.5 · 10^9) Systemic vasculitis affecting at least two extrapulmonary sites	Asthma Eosinophilia (>10% total WBC count) Neuropathy (mono or polyneuropathy) Pulmonary infiltrates (migratory or transitory) Paranasal sinus abnormality (pain, tenderness or radiologic abnormality) Extravascular eosinophils (in a biopsy including an artery, arteriole, or venule)	Eosinophil-rich and granulomatous inflammation involving the respiratory tract, necrotizing vasculitis affecting small to medium-sized vessels, and associated with asthma and eosinophilia

WBC, White blood cell.
From Hochberg MC et al: *Rheumatology,* ed 5, St Louis, 2011, Mosby.

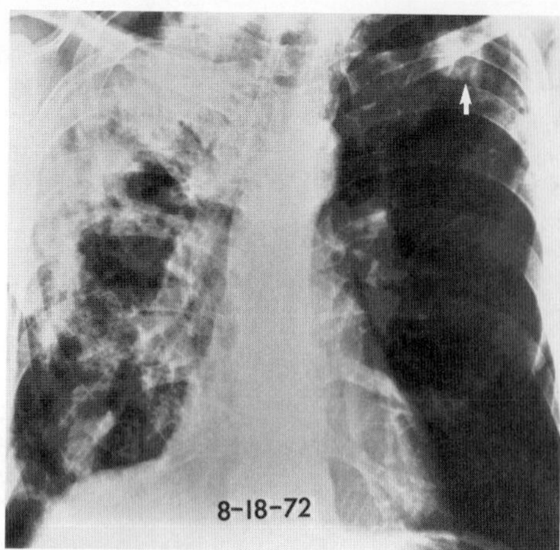

FIGURE 1-258 Allergic angiitis and granulomatosis. Posteroanterior chest radiograph demonstrates peripheral air space consolidation in the right lung and a nodule *(arrow)* in the left upper lobe in this asthmatic patient. (From McLoud TC [ed]: *Thoracic radiology: the requisites,* St Louis, 1998, Mosby.)

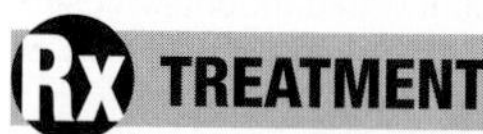

TREATMENT

NONPHARMACOLOGIC THERAPY

Oxygen therapy in severe asthmatic exacerbations

PHARMACOLOGIC THERAPY

The following five factors suggest poor prognosis (five-factor score) and determine the aggressiveness of the immune suppressive therapy:

1. Proteinuria >1 g/day
2. Creatinine >1.58 mg/dl
3. Cardiomyopathy
4. GI tract involvement
5. Central nervous system involvement

ACUTE GENERAL Rx

- Corticosteroids are the treatment of choice if no poor prognostic factors are present. Prednisone 1 mg/kg/day is the starting dose and is continued for 6 to 12 wk and then tapered to 10 mg/day at 1 yr as clinical disease resolves. Response to steroids may be dramatic. Patients with extensive disease may require IV corticosteroids.
- A drop in the patient's eosinophil count and the erythrocyte sedimentation rate indicates a response to treatment. ANCA does not reliably correspond with disease activity.

CHRONIC Rx

- In patients with one or more poor prognostic factors, immunosuppressant agents (cyclophosphamide 1 to 2 mg/kg/day) are used with corticosteroids as first-line therapy. Limit duration of cyclophosphamide to a maximum of 6 mo.
- In patients who do not respond to corticosteroid treatment or in CSS relapse, cyclophosphamide therapy is indicated as a second-line therapy.
- Azathioprine (2 mg/kg/day) or high-dose intravenous immunoglobulin has shown benefit in patients with severe disease and in patients unresponsive to corticosteroids.
- Corticosteroids, in combination with interferon-alpha, have also been used in refractory cases but may be difficult to tolerate.
- Patients with persistent symptoms of asthma will require long-term corticosteroids even if vasculitis is no longer present.
- Maintenance therapy using methotrexate (15 to 25 mg/wk) or azathioprine (2 mg/kg/day) is an alternative to cyclophosphamide.

DISPOSITION

- Clinical remission is obtained in more than 90% of patients after treatment. Relapse is common on cessation of therapy (approximately 26%).
- 5-yr survival rate with treatment is between 60% and 90% and decreases to 50% at 7 yr. Asthma generally remains persistent, and ischemic damage to peripheral nerves can be permanent.
- The 5-yr survival rate of untreated CSS is 25%.
- Death usually occurs from progressive refractory vasculitis, myocardial involvement (approximately 50% of deaths), or severe GI involvement (mesenteric ischemia, pancreatitis).

REFERRAL

- A pulmonary referral for diagnosis and management is appropriate.
- Patients should be followed up closely by rheumatology. Patients usually need long-term immunosuppressive medications.

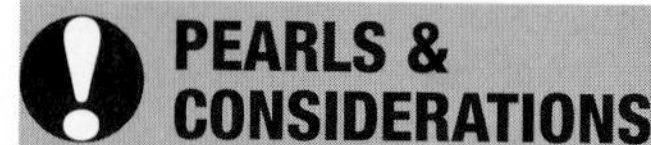

PEARLS & CONSIDERATIONS

COMMENTS

- CSS is a rare disease that is less common than other ANCA-associated vasculitides
- CSS is distinguished from other vasculitides by the nearly universal presence of adult-onset asthma that typically precedes all other symptoms. Family history is often negative for allergies or asthma
- Up to 77% of patients in the prodromal phase of CSS require oral steroids for asthma control
- Patients often have constitutional symptoms of weight loss, fever, and malaise before specific organ involvement is clinically evident
- Peripheral nerve involvement from vasculitis of the vasa vasorum commonly manifests as mononeuritis multiplex. Patients may present with sudden foot or wrist drop, along with sensory deficits in the distribution of one or more distal nerves
- Most patients with GI involvement are symptomatic. Gastroenteritis, acute abdomen, cholecystitis, hemorrhage, bowel perforation, and mesenteric ischemia have all been reported in patients with CSS
- Most patients with CSS respond to corticosteroid treatment and do not require cytotoxic therapy
- Symptoms of CSS typically appear as oral corticosteroids are being decreased or discontinued for the treatment of asthma and not triggered by leukotriene receptor-1 antagonists, as previously reported
- Compared to WG, patients more often present with history of atopy, asthma, or allergic rhinitis. When present, eosinophilia in CSS is often >1000 eosinophils/mm^3 compared with WG, where eosinophilia is much milder (<500 eosinophils/mm^3)
- The heart is involved in up to 60% of patients with CSS and represents a major cause of mortality

SUGGESTED READINGS

available at www.expertconsult.com

AUTHORS: **KACHIU LEE, B.A.,** and **JESSICA CORWIN, M.D., M.P.H.**

BASIC INFORMATION

DEFINITION

Cirrhosis is defined histologically as the presence of fibrosis and regenerative nodules in the liver. It can be classified as micronodular, macronodular, or mixed; however, each form may be seen in the same patient at different stages of the disease. Cirrhosis manifests clinically with portal hypertension, hepatic encephalopathy, and variceal bleeding.

ICD-9CM CODES
571.5 Cirrhosis of the liver
571.2 Cirrhosis of the liver secondary to alcohol

ICD-10CM CODES
K74.60 Hepatic fibrosis and cirrhosis
K70.30 Alcoholic cirrhosis of liver without ascites
K74.6 Other and unspecified cirrhosis of liver

EPIDEMIOLOGY & DEMOGRAPHICS

- Cirrhosis is the eleventh leading cause of death in the U.S. (9 per 100,000 persons annually).
- Alcohol abuse and viral hepatitis are the major causes of cirrhosis in the U.S.

PHYSICAL FINDINGS & CLINICAL PRESENTATION

SKIN: Jaundice, palmar erythema (alcohol abuse), spider angiomata, ecchymosis (thrombocytopenia or coagulation factor deficiency), dilated superficial periumbilical vein (caput medusae), increased pigmentation (hemochromatosis), xanthomas (primary biliary cirrhosis), and needle tracks (viral hepatitis). Cutaneous lesions often accompany cirrhosis and can be found in >40% of people with chronic alcoholism.
EYES: Kayser-Fleischer rings (corneal copper deposition seen in Wilson's disease; best diagnosed with slit lamp examination), scleral icterus
BREATH: Fetor hepaticus (musty odor of breath and urine found in cirrhosis with hepatic failure)
CHEST: Possible gynecomastia in men
ABDOMEN: Tender hepatomegaly (congestive hepatomegaly), small, nodular liver (cirrhosis), palpable, nontender gallbladder (neoplastic extrahepatic biliary obstruction), palpable spleen (portal hypertension), venous hum auscultated over periumbilical veins (portal hypertension), ascites (portal hypertension, hypoalbuminemia)
RECTAL EXAMINATION: Hemorrhoids (portal hypertension), guaiac-positive stools (alcoholic gastritis, bleeding esophageal varices, peptic ulcer disease, bleeding hemorrhoids)
GENITALIA: Testicular atrophy in males (chronic liver disease, hemochromatosis)
EXTREMITIES: Pedal edema (hypoalbuminemia, failure of right side of the heart), arthropathy (hemochromatosis)
NEUROLOGIC: Flapping tremor, asterixis (hepatic encephalopathy), choreoathetosis, dysarthria (Wilson's disease)

ETIOLOGY

- Alcohol abuse
- Secondary biliary cirrhosis, obstruction of the common bile duct (stone, stricture, pancreatitis, neoplasm, sclerosing cholangitis)
- Drugs (e.g., acetaminophen, isoniazid, methotrexate, methyldopa)
- Hepatic congestion (e.g., CHF, constrictive pericarditis, tricuspid insufficiency, thrombosis of the hepatic vein, obstruction of the vena cava)
- Primary biliary cirrhosis
- Hemochromatosis
- Chronic hepatitis B or C
- Wilson's disease
- Alpha-1-antitrypsin deficiency
- Infiltrative diseases (amyloidosis, glycogen storage diseases, hemochromatosis)
- Nutritional: jejunoileal bypass
- Others: parasitic infections (schistosomiasis), idiopathic portal hypertension, congenital hepatic fibrosis, systemic mastocytosis, autoimmune hepatitis, hepatic steatosis, inflammatory bowel disease (IBD)

DIAGNOSIS

WORKUP

In addition to an assessment of liver function, the evaluation of patients with cirrhosis should also include an assessment of renal and circulatory function. Diagnostic workup is aimed primarily at identifying the most likely cause of cirrhosis. The history is extremely important:

- Alcohol abuse: alcoholic liver disease
- History of hepatitis B (chronic active hepatitis, primary hepatic neoplasm, or hepatitis C)
- History of IBD (primary sclerosing cholangitis)
- History of pruritus, hyperlipoproteinemia, and xanthomas in a middle-aged or elderly woman (primary biliary cirrhosis)
- Impotence, diabetes mellitus, hyperpigmentation, arthritis (hemochromatosis)
- Neurologic disturbances (Wilson's disease, hepatolenticular degeneration)
- Family history of "liver disease" (hemochromatosis [positive family history in 25% of patients], alpha-1-antitrypsin deficiency)
- History of recurrent episodes of right upper quadrant pain (biliary tract disease)
- History of blood transfusions, IV drug abuse (hepatitis C)
- History of hepatotoxic drug exposure
- Coexistence of other diseases with immune or autoimmune features (immune thrombocytopenic purpura, myasthenia gravis, thyroiditis, autoimmune hepatitis)

LABORATORY TESTS

- Decreased hemoglobin and hematocrit, elevated mean corpuscular volume, increased blood urea nitrogen (BUN) and creatinine (the BUN may also be "normal" or low if the patient has severely diminished liver function), decreased sodium (dilutional hyponatremia), and decreased potassium (as a result of secondary aldosteronism or urinary losses). Evaluation of renal function should also include measurement of urinary sodium and urinary protein from 24-hr urine collection.
- Decreased glucose in a patient with liver disease, indicating severe liver damage.
- Other laboratory abnormalities:
    - Alcoholic hepatitis and cirrhosis: possible mild elevation of alanine aminotransferase (ALT) and aspartate aminotransferase (AST), usually <500 IU; AST >ALT (ratio >2:3).
    - Extrahepatic obstruction: possible moderate elevations of ALT and AST to levels <500 IU.
    - Viral, toxic, or ischemic hepatitis: extreme elevations (>500 IU) of ALT and AST.
    - Transaminases may be normal despite significant liver disease in patients with jejunoileal bypass operations or hemochromatosis or after methotrexate administration.
    - Alkaline phosphatase elevation can occur with extrahepatic obstruction, primary biliary cirrhosis, and primary sclerosing cholangitis.
    - Serum lactate dehydrogenase is significantly elevated in metastatic disease of the liver; lesser elevations are seen with hepatitis, cirrhosis, extrahepatic obstruction, and congestive hepatomegaly.
    - Serum gamma-glutamyl transpeptidase is elevated in alcoholic liver disease and may also be elevated with cholestatic disease (primary biliary cirrhosis, primary sclerosing cholangitis).
    - Serum bilirubin may be elevated; urinary bilirubin can be present in hepatitis, hepatocellular jaundice, and biliary obstruction.
    - Serum albumin: significant liver disease results in hypoalbuminemia.
    - Prothrombin time/INR: elevation in patients with liver disease indicates severe liver damage and poor prognosis.
    - Presence of hepatitis B surface antigen implies acute or chronic hepatitis B.
    - Presence of antimitochondrial antibody suggests primary biliary cirrhosis, chronic hepatitis.
    - Elevated serum copper, decreased serum ceruloplasmin, and elevated 24-hr urine may be diagnostic of Wilson's disease.
    - Protein immunoelectrophoresis may reveal decreased α-1 globulins (alpha-1-antitrypsin deficiency), increased IgA (alcoholic cirrhosis), increased IgM (primary biliary cirrhosis), increased IgG (chronic hepatitis, cryptogenic cirrhosis).
    - An elevated serum ferritin and increased transferrin saturation are suggestive of hemochromatosis.
    - An elevated blood ammonia suggests hepatocellular dysfunction; serial values, however, are generally not useful in monitoring patients with hepatic encephalopathy because there is poor correlation between blood ammonia level and degree of hepatic encephalopathy.
    - Serum cholesterol is elevated in cholestatic disorders.
    - Antinuclear antibodies (ANA) may be found in autoimmune hepatitis.
    - Alpha fetoprotein: levels >1000 pg/ml are highly suggestive of primary liver cell carcinoma.

 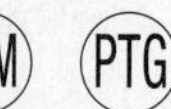

- Hepatitis C viral testing identifies patients with chronic hepatitis C infection.
- Elevated level of serum globulin (especially gamma-globulins) and positive ANA test may occur with autoimmune hepatitis.
- End-stage liver disease is characterized by decreased levels of most procoagulant factors with the notable exceptions of factor VIII and von Willebrand factor, which are elevated.

IMAGING STUDIES

- Ultrasonography is the procedure of choice for detecting gallstones and dilation of common bile ducts. The use of sonography on a periodic basis to screen for hepatocellular carcinoma in patients with cirrhosis has been questioned and should be avoided until additional data are available.
- CT scan is useful for detecting mass lesions in liver and pancreas, assessing hepatic fat content, identifying idiopathic hemochromatosis, diagnosing Budd-Chiari syndrome early, assessing dilation of intrahepatic bile ducts, and detecting varices and splenomegaly.
- MRI can be used to identify hemangiomas.
- Technetium-99m sulfur colloid scanning is rarely used but can be useful for diagnosing cirrhosis (there is a shift of colloid uptake to the spleen and bone marrow), identifying hepatic adenomas (cold defect is noted), and diagnosing Budd-Chiari syndrome (there is increased uptake by the caudate lobe).
- Endoscopic retrograde cholangiopancreatography can be used for diagnosing periampullary carcinoma and common duct stones; it is also useful in diagnosing primary sclerosing cholangitis.
- Percutaneous transhepatic cholangiography is useful when evaluating patients with cholestatic jaundice and dilated intrahepatic ducts by ultrasonography; presence of intrahepatic strictures and focal dilation is suggestive of primary sclerosing cholangitis.
- Percutaneous liver biopsy is useful in evaluating hepatic filling defects; diagnosing hepatocellular disease or hepatomegaly; evaluating persistently abnormal liver function tests; and diagnosing hemachromatosis, primary biliary cirrhosis, Wilson's disease, glycogen storage diseases, chronic hepatitis, autoimmune hepatitis, infiltrative diseases, alcoholic liver disease, drug-induced liver disease, and primary or secondary carcinoma.

Rx TREATMENT

NONPHARMACOLOGIC THERAPY

- Avoid any hepatotoxins (e.g., ethanol, acetaminophen), improve nutritional status
- Transjugular intrahepatic portosystemic shunt (TIPS) in patients with recurrent variceal hemorrhage despite optical medical therapy (Fig. E1-259). Early use of TIPS is associated with significant reductions in treatment failure and in mortality in patients with cirrhosis who are hospitalized for acute variceal bleeding and are at high risk for treatment failure.

GENERAL Rx

- Beta-blockers with or without nitrates in patients with cirrhosis and variceal hemorrhage.
- Pruritus due to liver disease may be treated with cholestyramine 4 g/day initially. Dose can be increased to 24 g/day as needed
- Remove excess body iron with phlebotomy and deferoxamine in patients with hemochromatosis.
- Remove copper deposits with D-penicillamine in patients with Wilson's disease.
- Long-term ursodiol therapy will slow the progression of primary biliary cirrhosis. It is, however, ineffective in primary sclerosing cholangitis.
- Glucocorticoids (prednisone 20 to 30 mg/day initially or combination therapy or prednisone and azathioprine) is useful in autoimmune hepatitis.
- Liver transplantation may be indicated in otherwise healthy patients (age <65 yr) with sclerosing cholangitis, chronic hepatitis cirrhosis, or primary biliary cirrhosis with prognostic information suggesting <20% chance of survival without transplantation. Contraindications to liver transplantation are AIDS, most metastatic malignancies, active substance abuse, uncontrolled sepsis, and uncontrolled cardiac or pulmonary disease.
- Treatment of complications of portal hypertension (ascites, esophagogastric varices, hepatic encephalopathy, and hepatorenal syndrome; refer to these individual topics in Section I).

DISPOSITION

- Prognosis varies with the etiology of the patient's cirrhosis and whether there is ongoing hepatic injury. Regression of cirrhosis has been demonstrated after antiviral therapy in some patients with chronic hepatitis C. Regression is associated with decreased disease-related morbidity and improved survival. Mortality rate exceeds 80% in patients with hepatorenal syndrome.
- If advanced cirrhosis is present and transplantation is not feasible, survival is 1 to 2 yr.
- Cirrhosis is associated with an increased risk for hepatocellular carcinoma. However, the risk is low (1% 5-year cumulative risk in alcoholic cirrhosis).

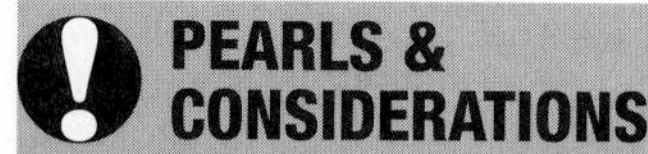

PEARLS & CONSIDERATIONS

COMMENTS

- Thrombocytopenia and advanced Child-Pugh cases (Table 1-123) are associated with the presence of varices. These factors are useful to identify cirrhotic patients who benefit most from referral for endoscopic screening for varices.
- A combination of endoscopic and drug therapy reduces overall and variceal rebleeding in cirrhosis more than either therapy alone.
- PPI use, but not H_2RA use, is associated with risk for serious infections in patients with decompensated cirrhosis.

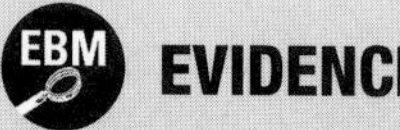

EVIDENCE

available at www.expertconsult.com

SUGGESTED READINGS

available at www.expertconsult.com

RELATED CONTENT

Ascites (Related Key Topic)
Cirrhosis (Patient Information)
Esophageal Varices (Related Key Topic)
Encephalopathy (Related Key Topic)
Hepatorenal Syndrome (Related Key Topic)
Primary Biliary Cirrhosis (Related Key Topic)

AUTHOR: **FRED F. FERRI, M.D.**

TABLE 1-123 Child-Pugh Staging Criteria

	CHILD-PUGH SCORE		
Criteria	**1 Point**	**2 Points**	**3 Points**
Total serum bilirubin (mg/dl)	<2	2-3	>3
Serum albumin (g/dl)	>3.5	2.8-3.5	<2.8
INR	<1.70	1.71-2.20	>2.20
Ascites	No ascites	Ascites controlled	Ascites not controlled
Encephalopathy	No encephalopathy	Encephalopathy controlled	Encephalopathy not controlled
	INTERPRETATION OF CHILD-PUGH SCORES		
	Points	**Life Expectancy**	**Perioperative Mortality**
Child Class A	5-6	15-20 yr	10%
Child Class B	7-9	Candidate for liver transplant	30%
Child Class C	10-15	1-3 yr	82%

BASIC INFORMATION

DEFINITION

Claudication refers to reproducible discomfort of muscles brought on by exertion and relieved with rest. This disorder results from a supply and demand imbalance in blood flow that is due to peripheral arterial disease (PAD). Intermittent vascular claudication is most common in the muscle groups of the lower extremities but it can also affect the upper extremities.

SYNONYMS

Intermittent claudication

ICD-9CM CODES
443.9 Peripheral vascular disease, unspecified
440.21 Intermittent claudication due to atherosclerosis

ICD-10CM CODES
I74 Arterial embolism and thrombosis
I74.5 Embolism and thrombosis of iliac artery
I73.9 Peripheral vascular disease, unspecified
I73.89 Other specified peripheral vascular diseases

EPIDEMIOLOGY & DEMOGRAPHICS

- The prevalence of PAD in the United States is approximately 12% to 21% of individuals 65 yrs or older and affects about 10 million Americans.
- Risk factors associated with development of PAD are similar to coronary atherosclerosis (CAD) and include increasing age, cigarette smoking, hypertension, diabetes mellitus, and dyslipidemia. In addition, chronic kidney disease, metabolic syndrome, and patients with elevated levels of C-reactive protein, lipoprotein(a), and homocysteine are at increased risk. Nontraditional risk factors include race/ethnicity, with African American patients being at higher risk.
- A strong correlation exists between PAD, CAD, carotid artery stenosis, and generalized cerebrovascular disease.
- The American College of Cardiology/American Heart Association (ACC/AHA) guidelines suggested the following distribution of clinical presentation of PAD in patients 50 yrs of age:
  - Asymptomatic: 20% to 50%
  - Atypical leg pain: 40% to 50%
  - Classic claudication: 10% to 35%
  - Critical limb ischemia: 1% to 2%

PHYSICAL FINDINGS & CLINICAL PRESENTATION

- The severity of symptoms varies with degree of PAD, collateral blood supply, and exertional demands.
- Classic symptoms include exertional calf pain, which causes the patient to cease exertion and the pain generally resolves within 10 min. Claudication can also classically present in the buttock and hip, thigh, calf, or foot, with one or more of the following signs or symptoms, depending on the level and degree of peripheral stenosis:
  - Diminished or absent pedal pulses
  - Bruit over the distal aorta, iliac, or femoral arteries
  - Pallor of the distal extremities on elevation with cooling to the touch
  - Rubor with prolonged capillary refill on dependency
  - Trophic changes, including hair/nail loss and muscle atrophy
  - Nonhealing ulcers, necrotic tissue, and gangrene
  - Weakness, numbness, or heaviness in the lower extremities
- True vascular claudication must be distinguished from "pseudoclaudication" which can be caused by severe venous obstruction or insufficiency, chronic compartment syndrome, spinal stenosis, osteoarthritis, and inflammatory muscle diseases. The characteristic features of pseudoclaudication that distinguish it from claudication are summarized in Table 1-124.
- Location of pain usually corresponds to analogous anatomy:
  - Buttock and hip: Aortic or iliac disease
  - Thigh: Aorta, iliac or common femoral artery
  - Upper two thirds of calf: Superficial femoral artery
  - Lower one third of calf: Popliteal artery
  - Foot: Tibial or peroneal artery
- Asymptomatic PAD is typically diagnosed by screening studies (exercise ankle brachial index, lower extremity ultrasound) or incidentally on physical exam. Symptoms of intermittent claudication classically start distally within a muscle group (below the stenosis) and then ascend with continued activity. Rest pain that occurs with leg elevation and is relieved paradoxically by walking may suggest severe PAD. Critical limb ischemia may present as tissue ulceration and gangrene, which requires prompt intervention.

ETIOLOGY

The primary cause of claudication is peripheral atherosclerosis, resulting in inability to supply enough blood to meet the metabolic demand of limb muscles first with activity then ultimately at rest.

TABLE 1-124 Characteristic Features of Pseudoclaudication That Distinguish It from Claudication

	Claudication	Pseudoclaudication
Characteristics	Limb cramping, tightness, fatigue	Similar to claudication with numbness
Location of discomfort	Lower extremity involving buttock, hip, thigh, calf, foot	Similar to claudication
Induced by exercise	Yes	Variable
Reproducible with distance walked	Consistent	Variable
Occurs with standing	No	Yes
Actions which provide relief	Stand	Sit
Time to relief	<5 min	≥30 min

Dx DIAGNOSIS

DIFFERENTIAL DIAGNOSIS

- Spinal stenosis (neurogenic or pseudoclaudication)
- Musculoskeletal disorders: Arthritis or myositis
- Degenerative osteoarthritic joint disease, predominantly of the lumbar spine and hips
- Compartment or popliteal artery entrapment syndrome
- Peripheral neuropathy
- Atheromatous embolization and deep venous thrombosis
- Vasculitis: Thromboangiitis obliterans, Takayasu, or giant cell arteritis

WORKUP

History and physical findings suggest the diagnosis of claudication and noninvasive studies help confirm the diagnosis.

- Measurement of resting ankle–brachial index (ABI) should be performed in all patients at risk for PAD and repeated at least once every 5 yrs. At-risk patients include:
  - Patients 18 yrs or older with walking impairment, claudication, or non-healing lower-extremity wounds
  - Asymptomatic patients 50 to 69 yrs old with a history of smoking or diabetes
  - All patients 70 yrs or older
- An ABI is the ratio of highest ankle systolic pressure to the highest brachial systolic pressure of either arm. A normal ABI is 1.00 to 1.40. A low ABI has been shown to be an independent predictor of mortality.
- The severity of PAD is based on the resting ABI. The value of the ABI correlates with the severity of the perfusion mismatch but does not define the level of obstructive disease.
  - Borderline disease: ABI at rest 0.91 to 0.99
  - Mild disease: ABI at rest 0.71 to 0.90
  - Moderate disease: ABI at rest 0.41 to 0.70
  - Severe disease: ABI at rest <0.40
- Segmental systolic pressures are measured at the level of the thigh, calf, ankle, metatarsal, and toes. Normally, there should be <20 mm Hg difference in pressures between adjacent segments. If the gradient is >20 mm Hg, a

significant stenosis is suspected in the interval vascular segment.

- Both ABI and segmental pressures can be taken before and after exercise by walking 1 to 2 mi/hr (5 min, or symptom-limited) to quantify severity of symptoms objectively. An ABI that decreases by at least 15% following exercise indicates significant PAD.
- ABI >1.3 may represent significant PAD. In such cases, measuring a toe–brachial index can increase the sensitivity of testing, as highly calcified arteries are incompressible and may have a normal or increased ABI. A toe–brachial index <0.7 is considered abnormal.

IMAGING STUDIES

- Duplex ultrasound can be used to assess occlusion location, length, and patency of the distal arterial system or prior grafts. Ultrasound is an excellent noninvasive modality for surveillance monitoring after revascularization.
- In patients with prior infrainguinal bypass grafts, the long-term patency should be evaluated at regular intervals using a duplex ultrasound. The 2011 ACC guidelines recommends routine surveillance using a duplex ultrasound at approximately 3, 6, and 12 mo after graft placement and then yearly.
- Magnetic resonance angiography (MRA) and CT angiography (CTA) are effective for imaging of the aorta and peripheral lower-extremity arteries above the knee. MRA has almost replaced catheter-based angiography, with 90% sensitivity and 97% specificity in identification of hemodynamically significant stenosis in the lower extremities.
- MRA and CTA are useful to delineate the anatomy and help plan percutaneous and surgical revascularization.
- Angiography (Fig. 1-260) remains the gold standard for diagnosing PAD, especially below the knee, and is needed before revascularization.

Rx TREATMENT

NONPHARMACOLOGIC THERAPY

- Smoking cessation is vital.
- Aggressive risk factor modification for hypertension, dyslipidemia, and diabetes mellitus, including diet and weight loss counseling, is recommended.
- Supervised exercise training should be performed for a minimum of 30 to 45 minutes, in sessions performed at least 3 times per week for a minimum of 12 weeks.
- Lifestyle therapy in conjunction with exercise can be as or more effective than pharmacologic therapy and in some cases even better than stent revascularization, as shown by the CLEVER Study.
- New prospective data point to intermittent pneumatic compression as a promising adjunctive therapy.

ACUTE GENERAL Rx

Revascularization by an endovascular or surgical approach is usually reserved for patients with symptoms refractory to medical therapy or impending critical limb ischemia.

CHRONIC Rx

- Aspirin 81 to 325 mg daily is standard therapy. Thienopyridines (clopidogrel and ticlodipine) can be considered as alternatives, especially for those intolerant of aspirin. There is no current data to support combination treatment (CHARISMA trial).
- Hydroxymethyl glutaryl (HMG) coenzyme-A reductase inhibitor (statin) medication is indicated for all patients with PAD.
  - LDL cholesterol level of less than 100 mg/dl is recommended.
  - Patients with concomitant high risk for ischemic events should be treated to a goal LDL cholesterol level of less than 70 mg/dl.
- Antihypertensive therapy with beta-adrenergic blocking drugs and/or ACE inhibitors should be administered to all hypertensive patients with PAD to reduce the risk of MI, stroke, congestive heart failure, and cardiovascular death.
  - In non-diabetics, the target blood pressure is <140 mm Hg systolic over 90 mm Hg diastolic.
  - In diabetics or patients with chronic renal disease, the target blood pressure is <130 mm Hg systolic over 80 mm Hg diastolic.
- Cilostazol 100 mg bid may be used in conjunction with aspirin or clopidogrel. It has been shown to increase walking distance by 50% to 67% in symptomatic patients.
- Pentoxifylline 400 mg three times per day may be considered as second-line alternative therapy to cilostazol to improve walking. However, the clinical effectiveness of pentoxifylline as therapy for claudication is not well established.
- In those patients with type II diabetes, a recent secondary analysis of the BARI 2D trial showed that an insulin-sensitizing approach (Metformin, Glitizones) reduces the risk of developing PAD when compared to insulin-providing therapy (Glipizide, Insulin). These patients also have lower rates of revascularization and amputation.
- Individuals with intermittent claudication who are offered the option of endovascular or surgical intervention should:
  - Be provided information regarding supervised claudication exercise therapy and pharmacotherapy
  - Receive comprehensive risk factor modification and antiplatelet therapy
  - Have a significant disability, either being unable to perform normal work or having serious impairment of other activities important to the patient
  - Have lower-extremity PAD lesion anatomy such that the revascularization procedure would have a low risk and a high probability of initial and long-term success
- Revascularization is indicated in patients with refractory rest pain or claudication that limits their lifestyle. It is also indicated in those with non-healing ulcers or gangrene, and in a select group of patients with functional disability. Common procedures include:
  - Aorto-iliofemoral reconstruction or bypass or infrainguinal bypass (e.g., femoropopliteal, femorotibial).
  - Angioplasty, often with stenting, is used primarily on short, discrete stenotic lesions in the iliac or femoropopliteal arteries
  - Endovascular intervention is recommended as the preferred revascularization for iliac and femoropopliteal arterial lesions.

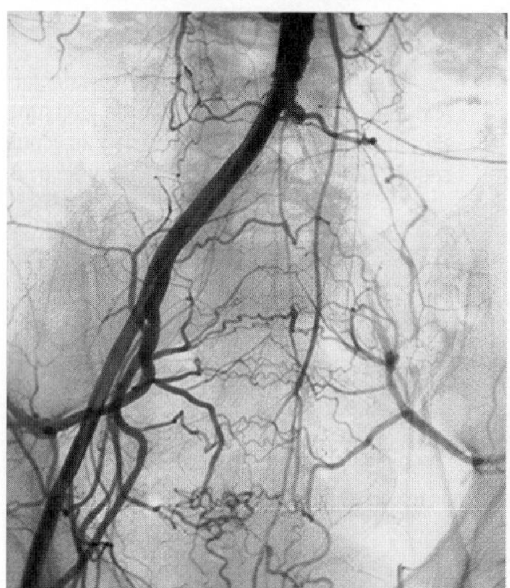

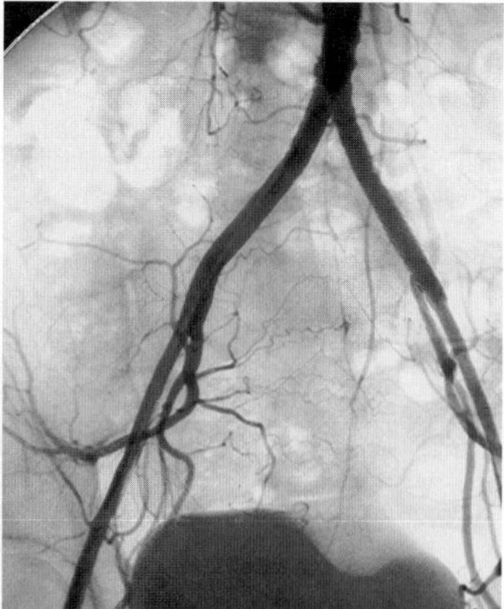

FIGURE 1-260 Angiogram of the distal abdominal aorta and iliac arteries demonstrates an occluded left common iliac artery with extensive collateral circulation from contralateral internal iliac artery *(left panel),* which resolved after successful stent implantation *(right panel).* (Images courtesy of Bart Domatch, MD, Radiology Department, University of Texas Southwestern Medical Center, Dallas, Texas. From Andreoli TE et al: *Andreoli and Carpenter's Cecil essentials of medicine,* ed 8, Philadelphia, 2010, Saunders.)

- Stenting is effective primary therapy for common iliac artery and external iliac artery stenosis and occlusions. However, it is not recommended in the femoral, popliteal, or tibial arteries due to a low success rate.

COMPLEMENTARY & ALTERNATIVE MEDICINE

- A meta-analysis found that over 12 to 24 wk, *Ginkgo biloba* increased pain-free walking distance by 34 m compared with placebo, although the benefit is not well established according to ACC/AHA guidelines.
- Naftidrofuryl, a serotonin receptor inhibitor, available in Europe, has shown some efficacy in improving claudication symptoms.
- Estrogen replacement therapy, propionyl-L-carnitine, L-arginine, oral vasodilators, prostaglandins, and chelation therapy are ineffective in the treatment of intermittent claudication.

DISPOSITION

- Intermittent claudication progressing to an ischemic leg or limb loss is unusual, especially with aggressive use of conservative treatments, risk factor modification, exercise, and smoking cessation.
- The 5-yr risk for development of ischemic ulceration in patients treated for diabetes and with ABI <0.5 was 30% compared with only 5% in patients with neither characteristic.

REFERRAL

Consultation with physicians specializing in vascular medicine is recommended for the patient with threatened limb loss, rest pain, non-healing ulcers, functional disability from pain, and gangrene.

PEARLS & CONSIDERATIONS

- Approximately 70% of patients with peripheral vascular disease will have concomitant coronary artery disease.
- Beta-blockers may worsen claudication symptoms in some patients, although their underuse is associated with excess cardiovascular death. Patients with intermittent claudication are less likely to receive beta-blocker therapy after an initial myocardial infarction. Those who do not receive post-MI beta-blockers have at least a threefold higher mortality.
- Patients with peripheral vascular disease may benefit from secondary cardiovascular prevention with clopidogrel versus aspirin more so than other high-risk patients (CAPRIE trial).

COMMENTS

- Claudication is a marker for generalized atherosclerosis. This group of patients has a higher risk of death from cardiovascular events than from limb loss. Patients with claudication experience diminished overall quality of life similar to patients with diagnosed coronary artery or cerebrovascular disease.
- The ABI is more closely associated with exercise tolerance and severity of disease in persons with peripheral arterial disease more than intermittent claudication or other leg symptoms.

SUGGESTED READINGS

available at www.expertconsult.com

RELATED CONTENT

Peripheral Arterial Disease [PAD] (Related Key Topic)

Poor Circulation (Claudication) (Patient Information)

AUTHORS: **ELLIOT M. GROVES, M.D., M.ENG.,** and **PRANAV M. PATEL, M.D., F.A.C.C., F.S.C.A.I.**

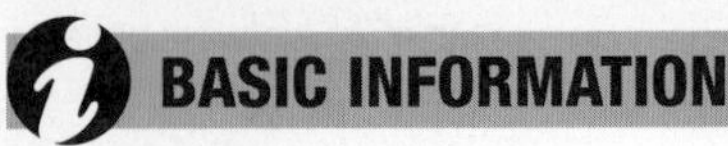

BASIC INFORMATION

DEFINITION

Clostridium difficile infection (CDI) is the occurrence of diarrhea and bowel inflammation associated with antibiotic use. CDI can manifest clinically in several forms ranging from fulminant diarrhea and leukocytosis associated with pseudomembranous colitis, mild to severe acute diarrhea, short-term colonization seen typically in health care facilities, and recurrent CDI with 60 days after initial treatment occurring in 20% to 30% of cases.

SYNONYMS

Antibiotic-induced colitis
Pseudomembranous colitis
CDI

ICD-9CM CODES
008.45 *Clostridium difficile,* pseudomembranous colitis
ICD-10CM CODES
A04.7 Enterocolitis due to *Clostridium difficile*

EPIDEMIOLOGY & DEMOGRAPHICS

- Cephalosporins are the most frequent offending agent in CDI because of their high rates of use.
- The antibiotic with the highest incidence is clindamycin (10% incidence of CDI with its use).
- Since 1996, the incidence of CDI has more than doubled. Severity of CDI has also increased due to the emergence of an epidemic virulent strain (NAP1/BI/027). CDI is the most common infectious cause of healthcare-associated diarrhea in adults and is responsible for approximately 3 million cases of diarrhea and colitis in the U.S. every year.

PHYSICAL FINDINGS & CLINICAL PRESENTATION

- Abdominal tenderness (generalized or lower abdominal)
- Fever
- In patients with prolonged diarrhea, poor skin turgor, dry mucous membranes, and other signs of dehydration may be present

ETIOLOGY

The NAP1 strain is predominant among patients with *C. difficile* infection, whereas asymptomatic patients are more likely to be colonized with other strains. Risk factors for *C. difficile* (the major identifiable agent of antibiotic-induced diarrhea and colitis):

- Administration of antibiotics: can occur with any antibiotic, but occurs most frequently with clindamycin, ampicillin, cephalosporins, and fluoroquinolone
- Prolonged hospitalization
- Advanced age
- Abdominal surgery
- Underlying disease (malignancy, renal failure, debilitated status)
- Hospitalized, tube-fed patients are at risk for *C. difficile*–associated diarrhea. Clinicians should consider testing for *C. difficile* in tube-fed patients with diarrhea unrelated to the feeding solution.
- PPI and H_2 blocker therapy increases risk of CDI and recurrent CDI. Risk is 1.7-fold higher with PPIs.

Dx DIAGNOSIS

The clinical signs of CDI generally include diarrhea, fever, and abdominal cramps after use of antibiotics.

DIFFERENTIAL DIAGNOSIS

- Gastrointestinal bacterial infections (e.g., *Salmonella, Shigella, Campylobacter, Yersinia*)
- Enteric parasites (e.g., *Cryptosporidium, Entamoeba histolytica*)
- Inflammatory bowel disease
- Celiac sprue
- Irritable bowel syndrome
- Ischemic colitis
- Antibiotic intolerance

WORKUP

- All patients with diarrhea accompanied by current or recent antibiotic use should be tested for *C. difficile* (see later discussion). Testing and treatment for CDI is not recommended in asymptomatic individuals.
- Sigmoidoscopy (without cleansing enema) may be necessary when the clinical and laboratory diagnosis is inconclusive and the diarrhea persists.
- In antibiotic-induced pseudomembranous colitis, the sigmoidoscopy often reveals raised white-yellow exudative plaques adherent to the colonic mucosa (Fig. 1-261).

LABORATORY TESTS

- Stool test for *C. difficile* toxin: enzyme-linked immunosorbent assay for *C. difficile* toxins A and B. The latter is used most widely in the clinical setting. It has a sensitivity of 85% and a specificity of 100%.
- *C. difficile* toxin can be detected by cytotoxin tissue-culture assay (cytotoxin assay, gold standard for identifying *C. difficile* toxin in stool specimen). This test is difficult to perform and results are not available for 24 to 48 hr.
- Fecal leukocytes (assessed by microscopy or lactoferrin assay) are generally present in stool samples.
- Complete blood count usually reveals leukocytosis. A sudden increase in white blood cells to >30,000/mm^3 may be indicative of fulminant colitis.

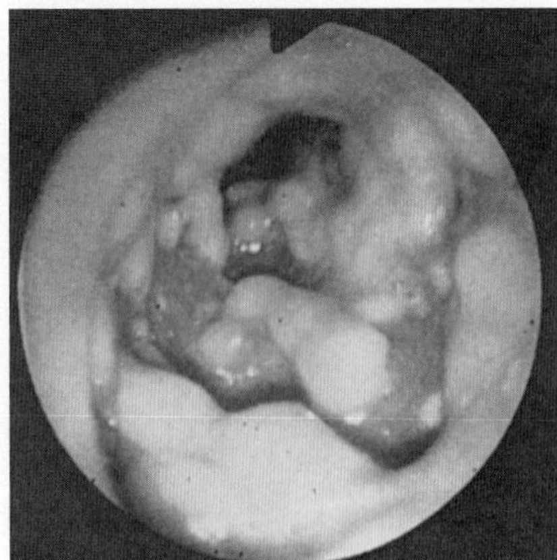

FIGURE 1-261 Pseudomembranous plaques seen with colonoscopy in a patient with *Clostridium difficile*–associated pseudomembranous colitis. (From Gorbach SL: *Infectious diseases,* ed 2, Philadelphia, 1998, Saunders.)

IMAGING STUDIES

Abdominal film (flat plate and upright) is useful in patients with abdominal pain or evidence of obstruction on physical examination.

Rx TREATMENT

NONPHARMACOLOGIC THERAPY

- Discontinue offending antibiotic.
- Fluid hydration and correction of electrolyte abnormalities
- Probiotics to restore natural defense mechanisms may be useful as adjuvant therapy; however, evidence is limited.
- Fecal microbiota transplantation is an excellent treatment modality for recurrent CDI. Trials have shown that it is more effective than vancomycin and may become standard treatment for recurrent CDI.

ACUTE GENERAL Rx

- Metronidazole 500 mg PO qid for 10 to 14 days.
- Vancomycin 125 mg PO qid for 10 to 14 days in cases resistant to metronidazole. However, vancomycin may be considered as first-line therapy in hospitalized patients who are seriously ill.
- When parenteral therapy is necessary (e.g., patient with paralytic ileus), IV metronidazole 500 mg qid can be used. It can also be supplemented with vancomycin 500 mg by nasogastric tube with intermittent clamping or retention enema.
- IV tigecycline (a broad-spectrum antibiotic used for skin or soft-tissue infection) can be used as adjunctive or alternative therapy for severe refractory *C. difficile* toxin infection.
- The addition of monoclonal antibodies against *C. difficile* toxins to antibiotic agents has been shown to reduce the recurrence of *C. difficile* infection.
- Fidaxomicin, a newer antibiotic, has shown non-inferiority to vancomycin and a lower rate of CDI recurrence.
- Fecal transplantation: When standard treatment has failed, intestinal microbiota transplantation (IMT) is an effective alternative therapy (eradication rate is 94%). It involves infusing intestinal microorganisms (in a suspension of healthy donor stool) into the intestine of a

sick patient via enema, gastroscope/colonoscope, or nasojejunal tube to restore the microbiota.

SURGICAL MANAGEMENT OF CDI

- Indications: CDI unresponsive to medical therapy, fulminant colitis
- Clinical features: colonic distention, severe abdominal pain/tenderness, systemic inflammatory response syndrome. Diarrhea may be absent because of ileus.
- Surgical approaches:
  - Traditional (subtotal or total colectomy), high mortality (50%)
  - Colon-sparing (loop ileostomy with intraoperative colonic lavage using warmed polyethylene glycol solution via the ileostomy and instillations of postoperative vancomycin flushes via the ileostomy); lower mortality compared to traditional approach

CHRONIC Rx

Judicious future use of antibiotics to prevent recurrences (e.g., avoid prolonged antibiotic therapy)

DISPOSITION

- Most patients recover completely with appropriate therapy. Fever resolves within 48 hr and diarrhea within 4 to 5 days. Overall mortality rate is 1% to 2.5% but exceeds 10% in untreated patients. CDI recurrence after an initial episode is 20% to 25% regardless of initial treatment with metronidazole or vancomycin. Each recurrence increases risk of repeat episodes (65% chance of recurrence after 3 CDI episodes). Recurrent CDI usually represents relapse rather than reinfection, no matter how long between episodes. Recurrent episodes are best treated with a prolonged course of oral vancomycin tapered off over several weeks to months.
- Hospital-acquired CDI is independently associated with an increased risk of in-hospital death.

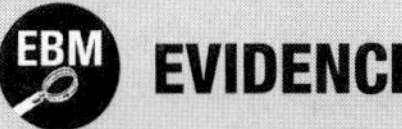

EVIDENCE

available at www.expertconsult.com

SUGGESTED READINGS

available at www.expertconsult.com

RELATED CONTENT

Pseudomembranous Colitis (Patient Information)

AUTHOR: **FRED F. FERRI, M.D.**

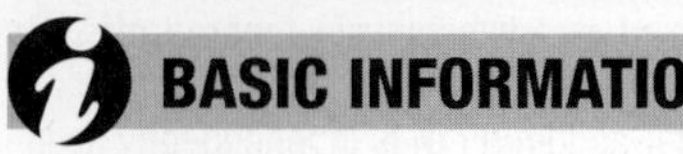

BASIC INFORMATION

DEFINITION

Cocaine is an alkaloid derived from the coca plant *Erythroxylum coca,* native to South America, which contains approximately 0.5% to 1% cocaine. The drug produces physiologic and behavioral effects when administered orally, intranasally, intravenously, or by inhalation after smoking. Cocaine has potent pharmacologic effects on dopamine, norepinephrine, and serotonin neurons in the central nervous system (CNS) involving alteration and blockade of cellular membrane transport and prevention of reuptake. Cocaine's second action involves the blockage of voltage-gated sodium ion membrane channels, which is responsible for its anesthetic effect. The mechanisms by which cocaine may induce myocardial ischemia or infarction are described in Fig. E1-262. Table 1-125 describes the pharmacokinetics of cocaine according to route of administration.

SYNONYMS

Cocaine hydrochloride: topical solution (FDA approved as a topical anesthetic)
Crack: this is produced when the hydrochloride molecule is removed by ether extraction, which frees the basic cocaine molecule or "free base." Heating does not destroy the free base; rather, it melts at 98° F and vaporizes at higher temperatures allowing it to be smoked.
Freebase: aqueous solution of cocaine hydrochloride converted to a more volatile base state by the addition of alkali, thereby extracting the cocaine base in a residue or precipitate
Street names include Bernice, Blow, C, Carrie, Cecil, Charlie, Coke, Dust, Dynamite, Flake, Gin, Girl, Gold dust, Green gold, Jet, Powder, Star dust, Paradise, Pimp's drug, Snow, Stardust, White girl, Yay, Yayo
Liquid lady = alcohol + cocaine
Speedball = heroin + cocaine
Street measures: hit (2 to 200 mg), snort, line, dose, spoon (approximately 1 g)

ICD-9CM CODES
304.2 Cocainism
ICD-10CM CODES
T40.5 Poisoning, cocaine
F14.20 Cocaine dependence, uncomplicated

EPIDEMIOLOGY & DEMOGRAPHICS

- The 1993 National Household Survey on Drug Abuse estimated that 4.5 million Americans used cocaine in 1992, with 1.3 million reporting use at least monthly. When reviewed in 1998, this had not changed significantly.
- Of note between 1993 and 1994, intravenous cocaine and heroin abusers accounted for a major new group of persons with HIV in several metropolitan areas.
- In 1999 an estimated 25 million Americans admitted that they used cocaine at least once—3.7 million the previous year and 1.5 million currently.
- The 2010 National Survey on Drug Use and Health indicates that there were 1 million individuals aged 12 yr. or older who had dependence or abuse of cocaine in the preceding year. This compares with 1.1 million in 2009, 1.4 million in 2008, and 1.6 million in 2007.
- The most recent National Survey on Drug Use and Health (2012) reports that there were 1.6 million individuals aged 12 yr or older who had dependence or had abuse of cocaine in the preceding year compared with 1.4 million in 2011.

PHYSICAL FINDINGS & CLINICAL PRESENTATION

PHASE I:
- CNS: euphoria, agitation, headache, vertigo, twitching, bruxism, unintentional tremor
- Nausea, vomiting, fever, hypertension, tachycardia

PHASE II:
- CNS: lethargy, hyperreactive deep tendon reflexes, seizures (status epilepticus)
- Sympathetic overdrive: tachycardia, hypertension, hyperthermia
- Incontinence

PHASE III:
- CNS: flaccid paralysis, coma, fixed dilated pupils, loss of reflexes
- Pulmonary edema
- Cardiopulmonary arrest

Psychological dependence manifests with habituation, paranoia, and hallucinations (cocaine "bugs"):
CNS: Cerebral ischemia and infarction, cerebral arterial spasm, cerebral vasculitis, cerebral vascular thrombosis, subarachnoid hemorrhage, intraparenchymal hemorrhage, seizures, cerebral atrophy, movement disorders, and hyperthermia
Cardiac: Acute myocardial ischemia and infarction (Table 1-126), arrhythmias (Table 1-127), and sudden death, dilated cardiomyopathy and myocarditis, infective endocarditis, aortic rupture, acceleration of coronary atherosclerosis
Pulmonary: Inhalation injuries (secondary to smoking crack cocaine): cartilage and nasal septal perforation, oropharyngeal ulcers; immunologically mediated diseases: hypersensitivity pneumonitis, bronchiolitis obliterans; pulmonary vascular lesions and hemorrhage, pulmonary infarction, pulmonary edema secondary to left ventricular failure, pneumomediastinum, and pneumothorax
Gastrointestinal: Gastroduodenal ulceration and perforation; intestinal infarction or perforation, colitis
Renal: Acute renal failure secondary to rhabdomyolysis and myoglobinuria; renal infarction; focal segmental glomerulosclerosis

TABLE 1-126 Characteristics of Patients with Cocaine-Induced Myocardial Infarction

Dose of Cocaine
Five or six lines (150 mg), up to 2 g
Serum concentration, 0.01 to 1.02 mg/liter
Frequency of Use
Reported in chronic, recreational, and first-time users
Route of Administration
Occurs with all routes of administration
75% of reported MIs occurred after intranasal use
Age
Mean, 34 yr (range, 17-71 yr)
20% younger than 25 yr
Sex
80% to 90% male
Timing
Often within minutes of cocaine use
Reported as late as 5 to 15 hr after use

From Bonow RO et al: *Heart disease,* ed 9, Philadelphia, 2012, Saunders.

TABLE 1-127 Cardiac Dysrhythmias and Conduction Disturbances Reported with Cocaine Use

Sinus tachycardia
Sinus bradycardia
Supraventricular tachycardia
Bundle branch block
Complete heart block
Accelerated idioventricular rhythm
Ventricular tachycardia
Ventricular fibrillation
Asystole
Torsades de pointes
Brugada pattern (right bundle branch block with ST-segment elevation in leads V_1, V_2, and V_3)

From Bonow RO et al: *Heart disease,* ed 9, Philadelphia, 2012, Saunders.

TABLE 1-125 Pharmacokinetics of Cocaine According to Route of Administration

Route of Administration	Onset of Action	Peak Effect	Duration of Action
Inhalation (smoking)	3-5 sec	1-3 min	5-15 min
Intravenous	10-60 sec	3-5 min	20-60 min
Intranasal or other mucosal	1-5 min	15-20 min	60-90 min

From Bonow RO et al: *Heart Disease,* ed 9, Philadelphia, 2012, Saunders.

Obstetric: Placental abruption, low infant weight, prematurity, microcephaly
Psychiatric: Anxiety, depression, paranoia, delirium, psychosis, suicide

ETIOLOGY

Cocaine may be absorbed through different routes with varying degrees of speed:
- Nasal insufflation/snorting: 2.5 min
- Smoking: <30 sec
- Oral: 2 to 5 min
- Mucosal: <20 min
- Intravenous injection: <30 sec

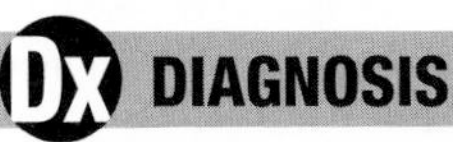

DIAGNOSIS

DIFFERENTIAL DIAGNOSIS

- Methamphetamine ("speed") abuse
- Methylenedioxyamphetamine ("ecstasy") abuse
- Cathione ("khat") abuse
- Lysergic acid diethylamide (LSD) abuse

WORKUP

Physical examination and laboratory evaluation

LABORATORY TESTS

- Toxicology screen (urine): cocaine is metabolized within 2 hr by the liver to major metabolites, benzoylecgonine and ecgonine methyl ester, which are excreted in the urine. Metabolites can be identified in urine within 5 min of IV use and up to 48 hr after oral ingestion.
- Blood: CBC, electrolytes, glucose, BUN, creatinine, calcium.
- Arterial blood gas analysis.
- ECG.
- Serum creatinine kinase and troponin concentration.

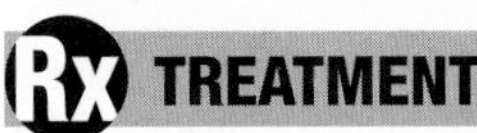

TREATMENT

There is no specific antidote and, at present, no drug therapy is uniquely effective in treating cocaine abuse and dependence. In addition, adulterants, contaminants, and other drugs may be admixed with street cocaine. Amantadine may provide effective treatment for cocaine-dependent patients with severe cocaine withdrawal symptoms, as well as the other dopamine agonist bromocriptine (1.5 mg PO tid), which may alleviate some of the symptoms of craving associated with acute cocaine withdrawal.

ACUTE GENERAL Rx

Acute cocaine toxicity requires following advanced poisoning treatment and life support. A suspected "body packer" should have an abdominal radiograph to detect the continued presence of cocaine-containing condoms in the intestinal tract. If present, gentle catharsis with charcoal and mineral oil should be performed with ICU admission and monitoring.

SPECIFIC TREATMENT

INHALATION: Wash nasal passages
AGITATION:
- Check STAT glucose
- Diazepam 15 to 20 mg PO or 2 to 10 mg IM or IV for severe agitation

HYPERTHERMIA:
- Check rectal temperature, creatine kinase, electrolytes
- Monitor with continuous rectal probe; bring temperature down to 101° F within 30 to 45 min

RHABDOMYOLYSIS:
- Vigorous hydration with urine output at least 2 ml/kg
- Mannitol or bicarbonate for rhabdomyolysis resistant to hydration

SEIZURE MANAGEMENT (STATUS EPILEPTICUS):
- Diazepam 5 to 10 mg IV over 2 to 3 min; may be repeated every 10 to 15 min.
- Lorazepam 2 to 3 mg IV over 2 to 3 min; may be repeated.
- Phenytoin loading dose 15 to 18 mg/kg IV at a rate not to exceed 25 to 50 mg/min under cardiac monitoring.
- Phenobarbital loading dose 10 to 15 mg/kg IV at a rate of 25 mg/min; an additional 5 mg/kg may be given in 30 to 45 min if seizures are not controlled.
- For refractory seizures, consider:
  1. Pancuronium 0.1 mg/kg IV
  2. Halothane general anesthesia
  3. Both require EEG monitoring to determine brain seizure activity.

HYPERTENSION: Cocaine-induced hypertension usually responds to benzodiazepines. If this fails:
- Consider arterial line for continuous blood pressure monitoring
- Avoid the use of calcium channel blockers because they may potentiate the incidence of seizures and death, especially in body packers.
- The use of beta-blockers may exacerbate cocaine-induced vasoconstriction.
- Phentolamine (unopposed adrenergic effects) or nitroglycerin may be required.
- If diastolic pressure >120 mm Hg: hydralazine hydrochloride 25 mg IM or IV; may repeat q1h.
- If hypertension is uncontrolled or hypertensive encephalopathy is present: sodium nitroprusside initially at 0.5 μg/kg/min not to exceed 10 μg/kg/min.

CHEST PAIN:
- Chest radiograph, ECG, cardiac enzymes.
- Benzodiazepines for agitation.
- Acetylsalicylic acid and nitroglycerin for ischemic pain. (Aspirin is contraindicated if dissection is suspected.)
- Percutaneous transluminal coronary angioplasty possibly better than thrombolysis for cocaine-associated myocardial infarction.
- Phentolamine will reverse cocaine-induced vasoconstriction and may be administered 5 to 10 mg every 5 to 10 minutes.
- The use of beta-adrenergic blockers remains controversial because of the unopposed alpha-adrenergic effects of cocaine.
- If beta-blockers are to be used, this should be preceded by administration of phentolamine to prevent unopposed alpha adrenergic stimulation. Many authors recommend not using beta-blockers until the cocaine has been systemically eliminated.

VENTRICULAR ARRHYTHMIAS (CONSIDERATIONS):
- Antiarrhythmic agents should be used with caution during the early period after cocaine exposure as a result of their proarrhythmic and proconvulsant effects.
- Lidocaine 1.5 mg/kg IV bolus followed by IV infusion (controversial: may be proarrhythmic and proconvulsant).
- Termination of ventricular arrhythmias may be resistant to lidocaine and even cardioversion.
- $NaHCO_3^-$ is under investigation in cocaine-mediated conduction abnormalities and rhythm disturbances.
- In a cardiac arrest situation secondary to cocaine toxicity, vasopressin offers a theoretical advantage over epinephrine as it increases coronary blood flow and myocardial oxygen availability.

DISPOSITION

Although many patients who use cocaine may not require treatment because of the short half-life of the drug, others may require specific treatment for possible cocaine-related complications.

REFERRAL

Consider psychotherapy or behavioral therapy once stable. There is some evidence that topiramate 300 mg orally daily added to cognitive behavioral therapy may be beneficial in patients with severe withdrawal symptoms.

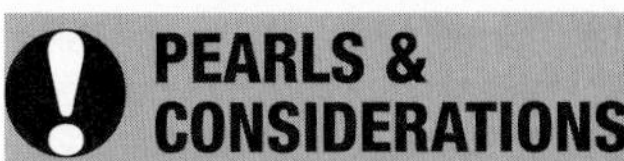

PEARLS & CONSIDERATIONS

- Cocaine-induced vasoconstriction may be exacerbated by the use of selective and nonselective beta-adrenergic blocking agents.
- The use of lidocaine in treating ventricular arrhythmias may precipitate seizures and further arrhythmias.

SUGGESTED READINGS

available at www.expertconsult.com

RELATED CONTENT

Abuse, Drug (Related Key Topic)
Cocaine Abuse and Dependence (Patient Information)
Drug Abuse (Patient Information)

AUTHOR: **SAJEEV HANDA, M.D., S.F.H.M.**

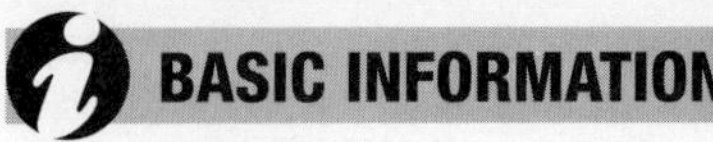

BASIC INFORMATION

DEFINITION

Coccidioidomycosis is an infectious disease caused by inhaling the spores of the fungus *Coccidioides immitis.* Clinical syndromes range from subclinical pulmonary disease to pneumonia and disseminated disease mostly in immunocompromised hosts. Most cases occur in the southwest part of the U.S.

SYNONYMS

San Joaquin Valley fever

ICD-9CM CODES

114.0 *Coccidioides* pneumonia
114.1 Cutaneous or extrapulmonary (primary) coccidioidomycosis
114.3 Disseminated or prostate coccidioidomycosis
114.5 Pulmonary coccidioidomycosis
114.2 Coccidioidal meningitis
114.4 Chronic coccidioidomycosis

ICD-10CM CODES

B38.9 Acute pulmonary coccidioidomycosis
B38.3 Cutaneous coccidioidomycosis
B38.89 Other forms of coccidioidomycosis
B38.2 Pulmonary coccidioidomycosis, unspecified
B38.4 Coccidioidomycosis meningitis
B38.1 Chronic pulmonary coccidioidomycosis

EPIDEMIOLOGY & DEMOGRAPHICS

INCIDENCE (IN U.S.): Estimated annual infection rate 150,000 persons, predominantly in southwest U.S. and appears to be rising due to increased population and construction in the area.
PEAK INCIDENCE: Seasonal in endemic areas with the higest risk being in the dry season after a rainy season as the mold lies a few inches below desert surface in soil and can become aerosolized.
PREVALENCE: 28.65 cases per 1 million population in the southwest U.S. in 2002 based on patients requiring hospital admission.
PREDOMINANT SEX: Males, between the ages of 25 and 55 yr
Clinical disease more severe in older children and adults

PHYSICAL FINDINGS & CLINICAL PRESENTATION

- The clinical manifestations vary widely according to the host, the severity of the illness, and location of dissemination.
- Asymptomatic infections or illness consistent with a nonspecific upper respiratory tract infection in at least 60%.
- Symptoms of primary infection—cough, malaise, fever, chills, night sweats, anorexia, weakness, and arthralgias (desert rheumatism)—in remaining 40% within 3 wk of exposure.
- Erythema nodosum and erythema multiforme more common in women.
- Scattered rales and dullness on percussion.
- Spontaneous improvement within 2 wk of illness, with complete recovery usual.
- Pulmonary nodules and cavities in <10% of those patients with primary infection; half of these patients asymptomatic.
- In a small portion of these patients: a progressive pneumonitis, often with a fatal outcome.
- Immunocompromised or diabetic patients may progress to chronic pulmonary disease.
- Over many years, granulomas rupture, leading to new cavity formation and continued fibrosis, often accompanied by hemoptysis.
- Disseminated or extrapulmonary disease in approximately 0.5% of acutely infected patients.
  1. Early signs of probable dissemination: fever, malaise, hilar adenopathy, and elevated ESR persisting in the setting of primary infection.
  2. Most organs are susceptible to dissemination, with heart and GI tract generally spared.
- Musculoskeletal involvement: bone lesions often unifocal, ribs, long bones, and vertebral lesions are common.
  1. Joint lesions predominantly unifocal, most commonly involving the ankle and knee, and often accompanying adjacent sites of osteomyelitis.
- Meningeal involvement: headache, fever, weakness, confusion, lethargy, cranial nerve defects, seizures; meningeal signs often minimal or absent.
- Cutaneous involvement: variable lesions—pustules, papules, plaques, nodules, ulcers, abscesses, or verrucous proliferative lesions.
  1. Dissemination and fatal outcomes most common in men, pregnant women, neonates, immunocompromised hosts, and individuals of dark-skinned races, especially those of African, Filipino, Mexican, and Native American ancestry.

ETIOLOGY

- *Coccidioides immitis* is endemic to North and South America.
- In the U.S., endemic areas coincide with the Lower Sonoran Life Zone, with semiarid climate, sparse flora, and alkaline soil in Arizona, California, New Mexico, and Texas.
- Fungus exists in the mycelial phase in soil, having barrel-shaped hyphae (arthroconidia). Arthrospores are aerosolized and deposit in the alveoli, then fungus converts to thick-walled spherule.
- Internal spherical spores (endospores) are released through spherule rupture and mature into new spherules (parasitic cycle).
- Fungus incites a granulomatous reaction in host tissue, usually with caseation necrosis.

Dx DIAGNOSIS

DIFFERENTIAL DIAGNOSIS

- Acute pulmonary coccidioidomycoses:
  1. Community-acquired pneumonias caused by *Mycoplasma* and *Chlamydia*
  2. Granulomatous diseases, such as *Mycobacterium tuberculosis* and sarcoidosis
  3. Other fungal diseases, such as *Blastomyces dermatitidis* and *Histoplasma capsulatum*
- Coccidioidomas: true neoplasms

WORKUP

Suspected in patients with a history of residence or travel in an endemic area, especially during periods favorable to spore dispersion (e.g., dust storms and drought followed by heavy rains)

LABORATORY TESTS

- CBC to reveal eosinophilia, especially with erythema nodosum
- Routine chemistries: usually normal but may reveal hyponatremia
- Elevated serum levels of IgE; associated with progressive disease
- CSF cell counts and chemistry: pleocytosis with mononuclear cell predominance associated with hypoglycorrhachia and elevated protein level
- Definitive diagnosis based on demonstration of the organism by culture from body fluids or tissues
  1. Greatest yield with pus, sputum, synovial fluid, and soft tissue aspirations, varying with the degree of dissemination
  2. Possible positive cultures of blood, gastric aspirate, pleural effusion, peritoneal fluid, and CSF, but less frequently obtained
  3. Lab personnel are at risk of infection by inhalation on opening culture plates so lab should be notified the disease is suspected, but it is not contagious from person to person.
- Serologic evaluations
  1. Latex agglutination and complement fixation
  2. Elevated serum complement-fixing antibody (CFA) titers ≥1:32 strongly correlated with disseminated disease, except with meningitis where lower titers seen
  3. In meningeal disease: CFA detected in CSF except with high serum CFA titers secondary to concurrent extraneural disease
  4. Enzyme-linked immunosorbent assay (ELISA) against a 33-kDa spherule antigen to detect and monitor CNS disease
- PCR
- Skin test: currently not available, and its use was limited as patients with severe disease may be anergic. Skin testing may still have use in epidemiologic surveys.

IMAGING STUDIES

Chest x-ray:

- Reveals unilateral infiltrates, hilar adenopathy, or pleural effusion in primary infection
- Shows areas of fibrosis containing usually solitary, thin-walled cavities that persist as residua of primary infection
- Possible coccidioidoma, a coinlike lesion representing a healed area of previous pneumonitis

Rx TREATMENT

NONPHARMACOLOGIC THERAPY

- Supportive care in mild symptomatic disease
- In patients with extrapulmonary manifestations involving draining skin, joint, and soft tissue infection: local wound care to avoid possible bacterial superinfection

ACUTE GENERAL Rx

- In general, drug therapy is not required for patients with asymptomatic pulmonary disease and most patients with mild symptomatic primary infection.
- Chemotherapy is indicated under the following circumstances:
  1. Severe symptomatic primary infection
  2. High serum CFA titers
  3. Persistent symptoms >6 wk
  4. Prostration
  5. Progressive pulmonary involvement
  6. Pregnancy
  7. Infancy
  8. Debilitation
  9. Concurrent illness (e.g., diabetes, asthma, COPD, malignancy)
  10. Acquired or induced immunosuppression
  11. Racial group with known predisposition for disseminated disease
- Fluconazole
  1. Most commonly, oral therapy with 400 mg/day up to 1.2 g/day appears to be the drug of choice for meningeal and deep-seated mycotic infections.
  2. In patients with AIDS, fluconazole may be considered the drug of choice for initial and maintenance therapy.
  3. All patients with coccidioidal meningitis should continue azole therapy indefinitely.
- Itraconazole
  1. 400 to 600 mg/day achieves 90% response rate in bone, joint, soft tissue, lymphatic, and genitourinary infections.
  2. Itraconazole may be more efficacious than fluconazole in the treatment of skeletal (bone) infections.
- Posaconazole is a new triazole that has recently been approved for use for systemic mycoses such as coccidioidomycosis; its relative efficacy compared to other agents will need additional clinical study.
- For pulmonary infections, treatment with either fluconazole or itraconazole, given for 6 to 12 wk, appears to be equal in efficacy.
- Amphotericin B is the classic therapy for disseminated extraneural disease, dose 0.6 to 1 mg/kg/day, qd for the first week then 0.8 mg/kg every other day, for a total dose of 1 to 2.5 g or until clinical and serologic remission is accomplished.
  1. Local instillation into body cavities such as sinuses, fistulae, and abscesses has been adjunct to therapy.
  2. Liposomal amphotericin B is probably equally effective.
  3. Duration of therapy for extraneural disease is undefined but probably about 1 yr.
- With meningeal disease: fluconazole 400 to 1000 mg PO q24h indefinitely
  1. Intrathecal amphotericin B is the alternate treatment modality, given alone or preceding the use of oral agents.
  2. Begin in doses of 0.01 to 0.025 mg/day, gradually increasing the dose as tolerated, to 0.5 mg/day with the patient in Trendelenburg's position.
  3. If given via Ommaya reservoir, as in ventriculitis, dose may be increased to 1.5 mg/day if tolerated.
  4. Concomitant parenteral therapy with amphotericin B is used for simultaneous extraneural disease as standard doses and with purely meningeal disease in smaller doses, although not strictly indicated.
  5. Intrathecal therapy is usually given three times a week for at least 3 mo, then discontinued or gradually tapered until once every 6 wk through 1 yr of therapy.
  6. Patients need routine monitoring of CSF, CFA, cell count, and chemistries for at least 2 yr following cessation of therapy.
- For osteomyelitis, soft tissue closed-space infections, and pulmonary fibrocavitary disease: surgical debridement, drainage, or resection, respectively, in addition to oral azole therapy or parenteral administration of amphotericin B.

CHRONIC Rx

For chronically immunocompromised patients, lifelong therapy with oral azoles or amphotericin B

DISPOSITION

- Prognosis for primary symptomatic infection is good.
- Immunocompromised patients are most likely to have disseminated disease and higher morbidity and mortality.
- Risk factors for poor outcome in patients with active coccidioidomycosis are described in Table 1-128.

TABLE 1-128 Risk Factors for Poor Outcome in Young Patients with Active Coccidioidomycosis

Primary Infections
Severe, prolonged (≥6 wk), or progressive infection
Risk Factors for Extrapulmonary Dissemination
Primary or acquired cellular immune dysfunction (including patients receiving tumor necrosis factor inhibitors)
Neonates, infants, the elderly
Male sex (adult)
Filipino, African, Native American, or Latin American ethnicity
Late-stage pregnancy and early postpartum period
Standardized complement fixation antibody titer >1:16 or increasing titer with persisting symptoms
Blood group B
HLA class II allele-DRBI*1301

From Kliegman RM et al: *Nelson textbook of pediatrics,* ed 19, Philadelphia, 2011, Saunders.

REFERRAL

- To surgeon for the evaluation of chronic hemoptysis, enlarging cavitary lesions despite chemotherapy and intrapleural rupture, osteomyelitis, and other synovial or soft tissue closed space infections
- For neurosurgical consultation in patients with meningeal disease to establish the delivery route of intrathecal drug therapy

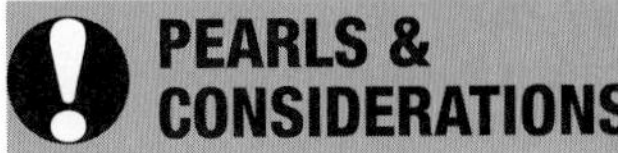

PEARLS & CONSIDERATIONS

COMMENTS

- Although coccidioidomycosis is a great imitator, a diagnosis will become apparent if a high degree of suspicion is maintained and appropriate testing (serologic testing, cultures, and histology) is performed.
- Infected body fluids contained within a closed moist environment (e.g., sputum in a specimen cup) provide the opportunity for the fungus to revert to its hyphal form whereby spores may be made airborne on opening of the container. This is a biohazard for laboratory personnel. Purulent drainage into a cast, allowing conversion of fungus to the saprophytic phase, has been responsible for acute disease when the cast was opened and the spores were unintentionally made airborne.
- Patients with a remote history of exposure, especially if immunosuppressed by medication or disease, may reactivate primary disease and suffer rapid dissemination.
- Although cardiac disease is rare, constrictive pericarditis in the setting of disseminated coccidioidomycosis has been documented and is potentially fatal.
- Organ transplant recipients may develop disease if the transplant donor has unrecognized active coccidioidomycosis at the time of death.

SUGGESTED READINGS

available at www.expertconsult.com

RELATED CONTENT

Coccidioidomycosis (Patient Information)

AUTHOR: **GLENN G. FORT, M.D., M.P.H.**

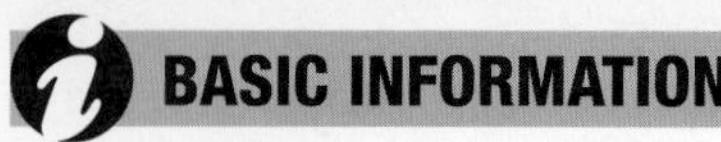

BASIC INFORMATION

DEFINITION

Colorectal cancer (CRC) is a neoplasm arising from the luminal surface of the large bowel; locations include descending colon (40% to 42%), rectosigmoid and rectum (30% to 33%), cecum and ascending colon (25% to 30%), and transverse colon (10% to 13%).

ICD-9CM CODES
154.0 Colorectal cancer

ICD-10CM CODES

C18	Malignant neoplasm of colon
C18.2	Malignant neoplasm of colon, ascending colon
C18.4	Malignant neoplasm of colon, transverse colon
C18.6	Malignant neoplasm of colon, descending colon
C18.7	Malignant neoplasm of colon, sigmoid colon
C19	Malignant neoplasm of rectosigmoid junction

EPIDEMIOLOGY & DEMOGRAPHICS

- CRC is the third most common cancer and the second leading cause of cancer deaths in the U.S. (>160,000 new cases and >55,000 deaths/yr).
- Peak incidence is in the seventh decade of life. The lifetime risk for development of CRC is 1 in 17, with 90% of cases occurring after age 50 yr.
- 50% of rectal cancers are within reach of the examiner's finger, and 50% of colon cancers are within reach of the flexible sigmoidoscope.
- CRC accounts for 14% of all cases of cancer (excluding skin malignancies) and 14% of all yearly cancer deaths.
- Risk factors:
  - Hereditary polyposis syndromes
  - Familial polyposis (high risk)
  - Gardner's syndrome (high risk)
  - Turcot's syndrome (high risk)
  - Peutz-Jeghers syndrome (low to moderate risk)
  - Inflammatory bowel disease (IBD), both ulcerative colitis and Crohn's disease
  - Family history of "cancer family syndrome"
  - Heredofamilial breast cancer and colon carcinoma
  - History of previous colorectal carcinoma
  - Women undergoing irradiation for gynecologic cancer
  - First-degree relatives with colorectal carcinoma
  - Age >40 yr
  - Possible dietary factors (diet high in fat or meat, beer drinking, reduced vegetable consumption); prolonged high consumption of red and processed meat may increase the risk for cancer of the large intestine
  - Hereditary nonpolyposis colon cancer (HNPCC): autosomal dominant disorder characterized by early age of onset (mean age, 44 yr) and right-sided or proximal colon cancers, synchronous and metachronous colon cancers, mucinous and poorly differentiated colon cancers; accounts for 1% to 5% of all cases of CRC
  - Previous endometrial or ovarian cancer, particularly when diagnosed at an early age
  - The gut bacterium *Fusobacterium nucleatum* has been linked to CRC. Researchers have shown that it contains a unique receptor that binds to the colorectal cells, stimulating inflammation and carcinogenesis.

PHYSICAL FINDINGS & CLINICAL PRESENTATION

- Physical examination may be completely unremarkable.
- Digital rectal examination can detect approximately 50% of rectal cancers.
- Palpable abdominal masses may indicate metastasis or complications of colorectal carcinoma (abscess, intussusception, volvulus).
- Abdominal distention and tenderness are suggestive of colonic obstruction.
- Hepatomegaly may be indicative of hepatic metastasis.

ETIOLOGY

CRC can arise through two mutational pathways: microsatellite instability or chromosomal instability. Germline genetic mutations are the basis of inherited colon cancer syndromes; an accumulation of somatic mutations in a cell is the basis of sporadic colon cancer.

Dx DIAGNOSIS

DIFFERENTIAL DIAGNOSIS

- Diverticular disease
- Strictures
- IBD
- Infectious or inflammatory lesions
- Adhesions
- Arteriovenous malformations
- Metastatic carcinoma (prostate, sarcoma)
- Extrinsic masses (cysts, abscesses)

WORKUP

The clinical presentation of colorectal malignancies is initially vague and nonspecific (weight loss, anorexia, malaise). It is useful to divide colon cancer symptoms into those usually associated with the right side of the colon and those commonly associated with the left side of the colon because the clinical presentation varies with the location of the carcinoma.

- Right side of colon:
  - Anemia (iron deficiency from chronic blood loss).
  - Dull, vague, and uncharacteristic abdominal pain may be present, or patient may be completely asymptomatic.
  - Rectal bleeding is often missed because blood is mixed with feces.
  - Obstruction and constipation are unusual because of large lumen and more liquid stools.
- Left side of colon:
  - Change in bowel habits (constipation, diarrhea, tenesmus, pencil-thin stools).
  - Rectal bleeding (bright red blood coating the surface of the stool).
  - Intestinal obstruction is frequent because of small lumen.

Early diagnosis of patients with surgically curable disease (Dukes A/B) is necessary because survival time is directly related to the stage of the carcinoma at the time of diagnosis. Appropriate screening recommendations are discussed in Section V.

CLASSIFICATION AND STAGING

Dukes and UICC classification for CRC:

A. Confined to the mucosa-submucosa (stage I)
B. Invasion of muscularis propria (stage II)
C. Local node involvement (stage III)
D. Distant metastasis (stage IV)

TNM Classification:

Stage	TNM Classification
I	T1-2, N0, M0
IIA	T3, N0, M0
IIB	T4, N0, M0
IIIA	T1-2, N1, M0
IIIB	T3-4, N1, M0
IIIC	T(any), N2, M0
IV	T(any), N(any), M1

LABORATORY TESTS

- Positive fecal occult blood test (FOBT): Many primary care physicians use single digital FOBT as their primary screening test for CRC. Single FOBT has low specificity for detecting human hemoglobin, is a poor screening method for CRC (sensitivity, 4.9%), and is inappropriate as the only test because negative results do not decrease the odds of advanced neoplasia. The American College of Gastroenterology recommends fecal immunochemical test as a replacement for guaiac-based FOBT for CRC detection. Annual Hemoccult SENSA and fecal DNA testing every 3 yr are alternative cancer detection tests.
- Microcytic anemia on CBC may be indicative of chronic blood loss.
- Increased plasma carcinoembryonic antigen (CEA) level: CEA should not be used as a screening test for CRC because it can be increased in patients with many other conditions (smoking, IBD, alcoholic liver disease). A normal CEA result does not exclude the diagnosis of CRC.
- Liver function tests should be ordered.

IMAGING STUDIES

- Colonoscopy with biopsy (primary assessment tool): The American College of Physicians (ACP) recommends that patients should be offered a colonoscopy beginning at age 50 yr and repeated every 10 yr in average-risk patients. Screening is recommended in African Americans beginning at 45 yr of age. Persons with only one first-degree relative with CRC or advanced adenomas diagnosed at 60 yr or older may be screened as at average risk. A family history of small tubular adenomas in first-degree relatives is not considered to increase the risk for CRC. The U.S. Preventive Services Task Force guidelines state that screening should not be routinely recommended in persons older than 75 yr, and it should not be recommended at all in persons older than 85 yr. If persons between the ages of 75 and 85 yr have never undergone screening, the decision about screening should be individualized according to health status. The ACP recommends that clinicians stop screening for colorectal cancer in adults over age 75 yr or in adults with a life expectancy of <10 yr. Table 1-130 describes CRC screening and surveillance recommendations.

- Computed tomography colonoscopy (CTC) virtual colonoscopy (VC) uses helical (spiral) CT scanning to generate a two- or three-dimensional virtual colorectal image (Fig. E1-264). CTC does not require sedation; but, like optical colonoscopy, it requires some bowel preparation (either bowel cathartics or ingestion of iodinated contrast medium with meals during the 48 hr before CT) and air insufflation. It also involves substantial exposure to radiation. In addition, patients with lesions detected by VC will require traditional colonoscopy. Compared with colonoscopy, CTC sensitivity for detection of polyps >10 mm ranges from 70% to 96%, and specificity ranges from 72% to 96%. CTC has replaced double-contrast barium enema as the radiographic screening alternative when patients decline colonoscopy.
- Capsule endoscopy allows visualization of the colonic mucosa but is not recommended as a screening procedure because its sensitivity for detecting colonic lesions is low compared with colonoscopy.
- CT scanning of the abdomen, pelvis, and chest assists in preoperative staging.
- PET scanning can display functional information and is accurate in the detection of CRC and its distant metastases. Combined PET/CT scanners are increasingly more available, and are useful to detect and characterize malignant lesions. Colonography composed of a combined modality of PET and CT is a newer diagnostic modality that can provide whole-body tumor staging in a single session.

Rx TREATMENT

GENERAL Rx

- Surgical resection: 70% of CRCs are resectable for cure at presentation; 45% of patients are cured by primary resection. Stage I and II tumors are curable by surgical resection, and up to 73% of cases of stage III can be cured by surgery combined with adjuvant chemotherapy.
- The backbone of chemotherapy treatment of CRC is fluorouracil (FU). Leucovorin (folinic acid) enhances the effect of FU and is given concomitantly. Adjuvant chemotherapy with combination of 5-FU and levamisole substantially increases cure rates for patients with stage III colon cancer and should be considered standard treatment for all such patients and selected patients with high-risk stage II colon cancer (adherence of tumor to an adjacent organ, bowel perforation, or obstruction).
- Radiation therapy is a useful adjunct to FU and leucovorin therapy for stage II or III rectal cancers.
- When given as adjuvant therapy after a complete resection in stage III disease, FU increases overall 5-yr survival rate from 51% to 64%. The use of adjuvant FU in stage II disease (no involvement of regional nodes) is controversial because 5-yr overall survival is 80% for treated or untreated patients, and the addition of FU only increases the probability of a 5-yr disease-free interval from 72% to 76%. For patients with standard-risk stage III tumors (e.g., involvement of one to three regional lymph nodes), both FU alone and FU with oxaliplatin (Eloxatin, an inhibitor of DNA synthesis) are reasonable choices. In general, reversible peripheral neuropathy is the main side effect of FU plus oxaliplatin. The oral fluoropyrimidine capecitabine (Xeloda) is a prodrug that undergoes enzymatic conversion to FU. It is an effective alternative to IV FU as adjuvant treatment for stage III colon cancer because it has a lower incidence of mouth sores and bone marrow suppression. It does, however, have an increased incidence of palmar-plantar erythrodysesthesia (hand-foot syndrome).
- Irinotecan (Camptosar), a potent inhibitor of topoisomerase I, a nuclear enzyme involved in the unwinding of DNA during replication, can be used to treat metastatic CRC refractory to other drugs, including 5-FU; it may offer a few months of palliation but is expensive and is associated with significant toxicity.
- Oxaliplatin (Eloxatin), a third-generation platinum derivative, can be used in combination with FU and leucovorin (FL) for patients with metastatic CRC whose disease has recurred or progressed despite treatment with FL plus irinotecan. FL plus oxaliplatin should be considered for high-risk patients with stage III cancers (e.g., more than three involved regional nodes [N2] or tumor invasion beyond the serosa [T4 lesion]).
- Laboratory studies have identified molecular sites in tumor tissue that may serve as specific targets for treatment by using epidermal growth factor receptor (EGFR) antagonists and angiogenesis inhibitors. The monoclonal antibodies cetuximab (Erbitux), panitumumab (Vectibix), and bevacizumab (Avastin) have been approved by the FDA for advanced CRC. Bevacizumab is an angiogenesis inhibitor that binds and inhibits the activity of human vascular endothelial growth factor. Cetuximab and panitumumab are EGFR blockers that inhibit the growth and survival of tumor cells that overexpress EGFR. Cetuximab has synergism with irinotecan, and its addition to irinotecan in patients with advanced disease resistant to irinotecan increases the response rate from 10% when cetuximab is used alone to 22% with combination of cetuximab and irinotecan. The addition of bevacizumab to FL in patients with advanced CRC has been reported to increase the response rate from

TABLE 1-130 Colorectal Cancer (CRC) Screening and Surveillance Recommendations

Indication	Recommendations
Average risk	Beginning at age 50 yr: Colonoscopy every 10 yr Computed tomographic colonography every 5 yr Flexible sigmoidoscopy every 5 yr Double-contrast barium enema every 5 yr (Stool blood testing annually or stool DNA testing acceptable but not preferred)
One or two first-degree relatives with CRC at any age or adenoma at age < 60 yr	Colonoscopy every 5 yr beginning at age 40 yr, or 10 yr younger than earliest diagnosis, whichever comes first
Hereditary nonpolyposis CRC	Genetic counseling and screening† Colonoscopy every 1 to 2 years beginning at age 25 yr and then yearly after age 40 yr‡
Familial adenomatous polyposis and variants	Genetic counseling and testing† Flexible sigmoidoscopy yearly beginning at puberty‡
Personal history of CRC	Colonoscopy within 1 yr of curative resection; repeat at 3 yr and then every 5 yr if normal
Personal history of colorectal adenoma	Colonoscopy every 3 to 5 yr after removal of all index polyps
Inflammatory bowel disease	Colonoscopy every 1 to 2 yr beginning after 8 yr of pancolitis or after 15 yr if only left-sided disease

*Recommendations proposed by the American Cancer Society and U.S. Multi-Society Task Force on Colorectal Cancer; recommendations for average-risk patients also endorsed by the American College of Radiology.
†Whenever possible, affected relatives should be tested first because of potential false-negative results.
‡Screening recommendation for individuals with positive or indeterminate tests as well as for those who refuse genetic testing.
From Andreoli TE et al: *Andreoli and Carpenter's Cecil essentials of medicine,* ed 8, Philadelphia, 2010, Saunders.

17% to 40%. Severe dermatologic toxicity can occur with both cetuximab and panitumumab.
- The liver is generally the initial and most common site of CRC metastases. Resection of metastases limited to the liver is curative in more than 30% of selected patients. In patients who undergo resection of liver metastases, postoperative treatment with a combination of hepatic arterial infusion of floxuridine and IV FU improves the outcome at 2 yr. Trials comparing hepatic resection (HR) and radiofrequency ablation (RFA) in the treatment of solitary colorectal liver metastases reveal that HR has better outcome; however, in tumors <3 cm, RFA can be recommended in patients who are not surgical candidates due to comorbidities or when the liver met is poorly localized anatomically.

CHRONIC Rx

Follow-up is indicated with:
- Physician visits with a focus on the clinical and disease-related history, directed physical examination guided by this history, coordination of follow-up, and counseling every 3 to 6 mo for the first 3 yr, then decreased frequency thereafter for 2 yr
- Colonoscopy yearly for the initial 2 yr, then every 3 yr
- Baseline CEA level can be obtained; if elevated, it can be used after surgery as a measure of completeness of tumor resection or to monitor tumor recurrence. If used to monitor tumor recurrence, CEA should be obtained every 3 to 6 mo for up to 5 yr. The role of CEA for monitoring patients with resected colon cancer has been questioned because of the small number of cures attributed to CEA monitoring despite the substantial cost in dollars and physical and emotional stress associated with monitoring.

DISPOSITION

The 5-yr survival rate varies with the stage of the carcinoma:
- Dukes:
  - Dukes A 5-yr survival rate >80%
  - Dukes B 5-yr survival rate 60%
  - Dukes C 5-yr survival rate 20%
  - Dukes D 5-yr survival rate 3%
- TNM classification:

Stage	TNM Classification	5-yr Survival Rate
I	T1-2, N0, M0	>90%
IIA	T3, N0, M0	60-85%
IIB	T4, N0, M0	60-85%
IIIA	T1-2, N1, M0	25-65%
IIIB	T3-4, N1, M0	25-65%
IIIC	T(any), N2, M0	25-65%
IV	T(any), N(any), M1	5-7%

- Overall 5-yr disease-free survival rate has increased from 50% to 63% during the past two decades.
- High-frequency microsatellite instability in CRC is independently predictive of a relatively favorable outcome and reduces the likelihood of metastases.
- In patients with Dukes C (stage III) CRC, there is improved 5-yr survival among women treated with adjuvant chemotherapy (53% with chemotherapy vs. 33% without) and among patients with right-sided tumors treated with adjuvant chemotherapy.
- Retention of 19q alleles in microsatellite-stable cancers and mutation of the gene for the type I receptor for tumor growth factor B1 in cancers with high levels of microsatellite instability point to a favorable outcome after adjuvant chemotherapy with FU-based regimens for stage II colon cancer.
- Expression patterns of microRNA are systemically altered in colon adenocarcinomas. High miR-21 expression is associated with poor survival and poor therapeutic outcome.
- Guanylyl cyclase 2 C (GUCY2C) has been identified as a marker expressed by colorectal tumors that could reveal occult metastases in lymph nodes. Expression of GUCY2C in histologically negative lymph nodes appears to be independently associated with time to recurrence and disease-free survival in patients with lymph nodes free of tumor cells by histopathology (pN0) in CRC.
- The optimal timing from surgery to initiation of adjuvant chemotherapy is unknown. Meta-analysis of available literature suggests that longer time to adjuvant chemotherapy is associated with worse survival rates among patients with resected CRC.
- Regular aspirin use after the diagnosis of CRC has been reported to be associated with lower risk for CRC-specific and overall mortality, especially among individuals with tumors that overexpress cyclooxygenase-2. Regular aspirin use is associated with lower BRAF-wild type colorectal cancer but not with BRAF-mutated cancer risk. All aspirin doses starting with 75 mg daily had similar effects on CRC incidence and mortality.

REFERRAL

- Surgical referral for resection
- Oncology referral for adjuvant chemotherapy in selected patients
- Radiation oncology referral for patients with stage II or III rectal cancers

PEARLS & CONSIDERATIONS

COMMENTS

- Metastases of tumor cells to regional lymph nodes is the single most important prognostic factor in patients with colon cancer.
- Decreased fat intake to 30% of total energy intake, increased fiber, and fruit and vegetable consumption may reduce CRC risk. Recent literature reports, however, do not support a protective effect from dietary fiber against CRC in women.
- Chemoprophylaxis with aspirin (81 mg/day) reduces the incidence of colorectal adenomas in persons at risk.
- Statins inhibit the growth of colon cancer lines. Use of statins is associated with a 47% relative reduction in the risk for CRC. Additional trials are necessary to investigate the overall benefits of statins in preventing CRC.
- The National Cancer Institute has published consensus guidelines for universal screening for HNPCC in patients with newly diagnosed CRC. Tumors in mutation carriers of HNPCC typically exhibit microsatellite instability, a characteristic phenotype caused by expansion or contraction of short nucleotide repeat sequences. These guidelines (Bethesda Guidelines) are useful for selective patients for microsatellite instability testing. Screening patients with newly diagnosed CRC for HNPCC is cost effective, especially if the benefits to their immediate relatives are considered.
- Expression of guanylyl cyclase C mRNA in lymph nodes is associated with recurrence of CRC in patients with stage II disease. Analysis of guanylyl cyclase mRNA expression by reverse transcription polymerase chain reaction may be useful for CRC staging.
- The use of either annual or biennial FOBT significantly reduces the incidence of CRC.
- The detection of mutations in the *APC* gene from stool samples is a promising new modality for early detection of colorectal neoplasms.
- KRAS mutations are consistently associated with reduced overall and progression-free survival and increased treatment failure.

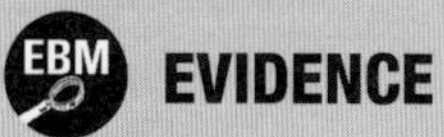

EVIDENCE

available at www.expertconsult.com

SUGGESTED READINGS

available at www.expertconsult.com

RELATED CONTENT

Colon Cancer (Patient Information)

AUTHOR: **FRED F. FERRI, M.D.**

BASIC INFORMATION

DEFINITION

Compartment syndrome is a condition that occurs when elevated pressure within a limited space compromises the circulation, with increased risk of irreversible damage to its contents and their function. Acute compartment syndrome is a surgical emergency.

SYNONYMS

None

ICD-10CM CODES

958.90	Compartment syndrome unspecified
958.90	Compartment syndrome, not otherwise specified
T79.A0	Compartment syndrome, unspecified, initial encounter

EPIDEMIOLOGY & DEMOGRAPHICS

- Occurs most commonly after acute trauma, especially with long bone fractures, comprising 75% of cases.
- It usually occurs in persons <35 yr.
- Incidence is higher in males.
- It can occur in other parts, such as the foot, thigh, gluteal region, and abdomen.
- Supracondylar fractures in children can commonly lead to compartment syndrome.
- 6%-9% of open tibial fractures are complicated by compartment syndrome.
- It is seen in all races and ethnicities.

PATHOPHYSIOLOGY

Compartment syndrome occurs when the blood flow is less than the tissue metabolic demands, causing tissue injury. It occurs when the intracompartmental pressure increases limiting venous outflow with rising venous pressure, resulting in compromise of the local circulation and tissue hypoxia with decreased arteriovenous pressure gradient. Venous congestion additionally leads to tissue edema and interstitial pressure, and the compartment pressure continues to increase. Compartment pressure able to cause the condition ranges between 10 and 30 mm Hg of diastolic pressure.

Different conditions are known to cause compartment syndrome:

- Conditions that limit compartment volume, such as when patients have fracture casts, when sedated or comatose patients lie on a limb for a prolonged period, or when patients have tight dressings that are applied externally
- Conditions that cause increased compartment content, such as bleeding from vascular injury or diathesis, fractures or finger injuries, reperfusion after ischemic injury such as embolectomy and arterial bypass grafting, and thermal or electrical burn injuries
- Other injuries, such as extravasation of IV fluids, injection of recreational drugs, and snake bites.

PHYSICAL FINDINGS & CLINICAL PRESENTATION

Signs and symptoms are usually apparent but can be unreliable and can lead to delayed diagnosis. Acute compartment syndrome can worsen within hours; therefore serial examination is important in a patient with suspected compartment syndrome. Patients with tense painful limbs are considered to have acute compartment syndrome; however, diagnosis is confirmed with the assessment of elevated compartment pressure. Clinical signs and symptoms include the following:

- Pain disproportional to injury (the earliest sign)
- Constant deep pain and pain that is referred to the compartment on passive stretching of the muscles of the affected compartment (Fig. 1-265A)
- Reduced sense of touch or sensation (hypesthesia) within the territory of the nerve passing the compartment (in acute anterior compartment syndrome, the patient may have hypesthesia in the territory of the first webspace)
- Tense and swollen compartment (Figs. 1-265B and 1-265C)
- Muscle weakness
- Paresis (late finding) that suggests permanent muscle damage
- Capillary refill can be slow but normal.
- Peripheral pulses that are normally palpable even in severe conditions
- Tingling and numbness in the affected limb. Hypesthesia or paresthesia should be evaluated with pinprick, light touch, and two-point discrimination tests.

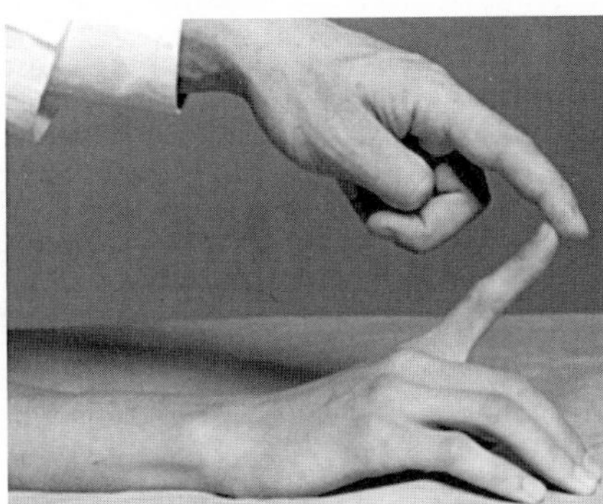

FIGURE 1-265A Passive extension of the digit causes pain referred to the compartment. (From Browner BD et al [eds]: *Skeletal trauma,* ed 4, Philadelphia, 2009, Saunders.)

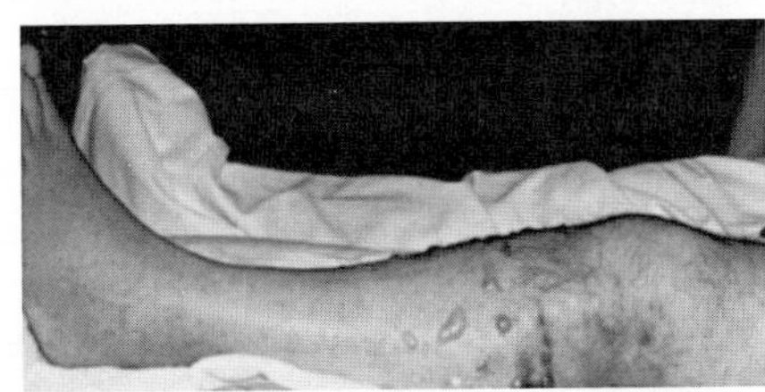

FIGURE 1-265B Acute compartment syndrome of the leg. (From Browner BD et al [eds]: *Skeletal trauma,* ed 4, Philadelphia, 2009, Saunders.)

DIAGNOSIS

Diagnosis is based on clinical signs and symptoms along with compartment pressure. Compartment pressure testing may be unnecessary if the diagnosis is clinically obvious.

DIFFERENTIAL DIAGNOSIS

- Muscle strains
- Cellulitis
- Gangrene
- Peripheral vascular injury
- Necrotizing fasciitis
- Stress fractures
- Deep vein thrombosis and thrombophlebitis
- Tendinitis
- Muscle contusion
- Tarsal tunnel syndrome
- Posterior ankle syndrome
- Popliteal artery impingement
- Claudication
- Tumor
- Venous insufficiency

LABORATORY TESTS

Diagnosis is based on clinical findings and the measurement of compartment pressures. Laboratory values are not useful in the diagnosis of compartment syndrome. Laboratory studies are important, though, for other diagnoses or associated conditions.

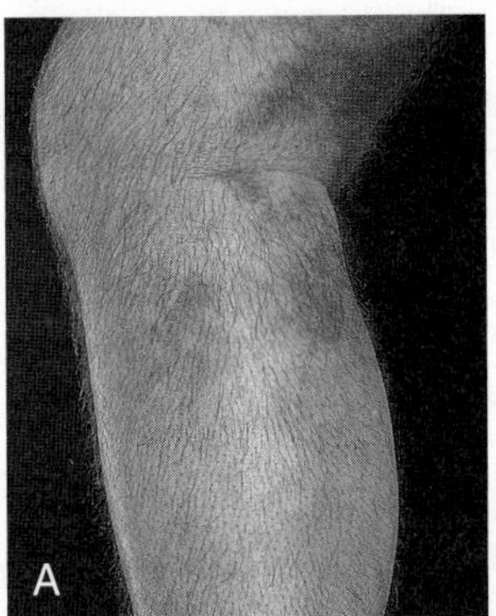

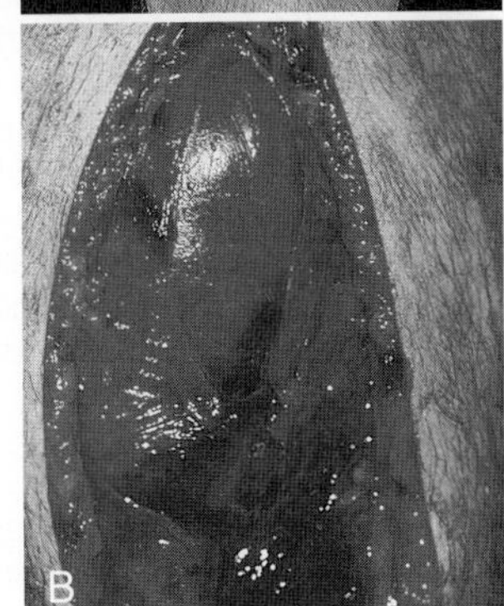

FIGURE 1-265C A, Severe calf swelling due to anterior and posterior compartment syndromes after ischemia-reperfusion. **B,** Appearance after emergency fasciotomy. Note edematous muscle and hematoma. (Courtesy Michael J. Allen, FRCS, Leicester, UK. From Floege J et al: *Comprehensive clinical nephrology,* ed 4, Philadelphia, 2010, Saunders.)

- CBC with differential for evaluation of infection
- Creatine phosphokinase (CK) levels, which can rise as muscle injury develops
- Metabolic panel for the assessment of electrolytes and renal function
- Coagulation profile for bleeding diathesis
- Urinalysis for rhabdomyolysis
- Urine and serum myoglobin levels

IMAGING STUDIES

- Direct intracompartmental pressure measurement can be done by handheld manometer, wick or slit catheter technique, and simple needle manometer system. Compartment syndrome is diagnosed when the difference between diastolic blood pressure and compartment pressure (Δ pressure) is $\leq$30 mm Hg.
- Ultrasonography can be used to rule out deep vein thrombosis, or Doppler ultrasonography can be used to evaluate blood flow to the extremity. Arteriography should be used to evaluate the adequate blood flow through a compartment.
- Near-infrared spectroscopy and technetium-99m methoxyisobutylisonitrile scintigraphy can also be used.
- Radiography can be used on the affected limb for fracture or foreign body evaluation.

Rx TREATMENT

Treatment goal is to keep intracompartmental pressure low and prevent tissue injury (Fig. 1-265D).

NONPHARMACOLOGIC THERAPY

- Immediate relieving of all external pressure on the affected compartment
- Removal of casts, splints, and dressings
- Placing limb at heart level to avoid decreased or increased blood flow

ACUTE GENERAL RX

- Analgesics for pain
- Hyperbaric oxygen
- Hypotension can worsen tissue ischemia and thus should be treated with IV isotonic saline.
- Fasciotomy of the affected compartment is indicated if there has been >6 hr of limb ischemia, or immediate decompression should be performed when the compartment pressure > 30-35 mm Hg.
- When compartment pressures are trending downward, it is often safe to hold fasciotomy emergently, provided the Δ pressure is also improving.

CHRONIC RX

- Aftercare of fasciotomy wound: Wound is inspected after 48 hours and dead tissue is removed.
- Wounds are left open, requiring later skin grafting or delayed wound closure.
- Opsite sheet and boot lace techniques are also used for closing fasciotomy wounds.
- Concomitant fractured bones should also be stabilized with plating, external fixation, or intramedullary nailing.

DISPOSITION

With early diagnosis and treatment, the prognosis is excellent for recovery of the muscles and nerves inside the compartment. The following conditions can be prevented:

- Permanent nerve damage/paralysis
- Muscle contracture
- Gangrene
- Amputation
- Muscle necrosis
- Fracture nonunion
- Rhabdomyolysis that leads to renal failure
- Compartment syndrome that can occur in open fractures
- Permanent nerve injury, which can occur after 12-24 hr of compression; mortality rates in patients who need fasciotomy is ≈15%.

REFERRAL

Patients with suspected compartment syndrome should be referred promptly to orthopaedic and general surgery.

PEARLS & CONSIDERATIONS

- Universal precautions and aseptic measures are necessary for patients undergoing fasciotomy because the risk of local and systemic infection is high with the procedure.
- Invasive monitoring techniques should be undertaken with adequate analgesia so that patient immobility is ensured while the pressure is measured.
- Injection of local anesthetics into the compartment can increase the pressure and pain and therefore should be avoided.
- Patients with fracture casts should be informed about the risks of swelling, and patients should also be encouraged to wear appropriate equipment while playing sports.
- A history of coagulation disorders and the use of anticoagulants should be mentioned in a patient's medical history.

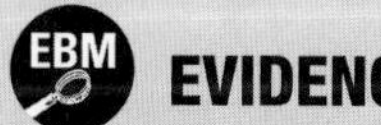

EVIDENCE

available at www.expertconsult.com

SUGGESTED READINGS

available at www.expertconsult.com

RELATED CONTENT

Compartment Syndrome (Patient Information)

AUTHOR: **SYEDA M. SAYEED, M.D.**

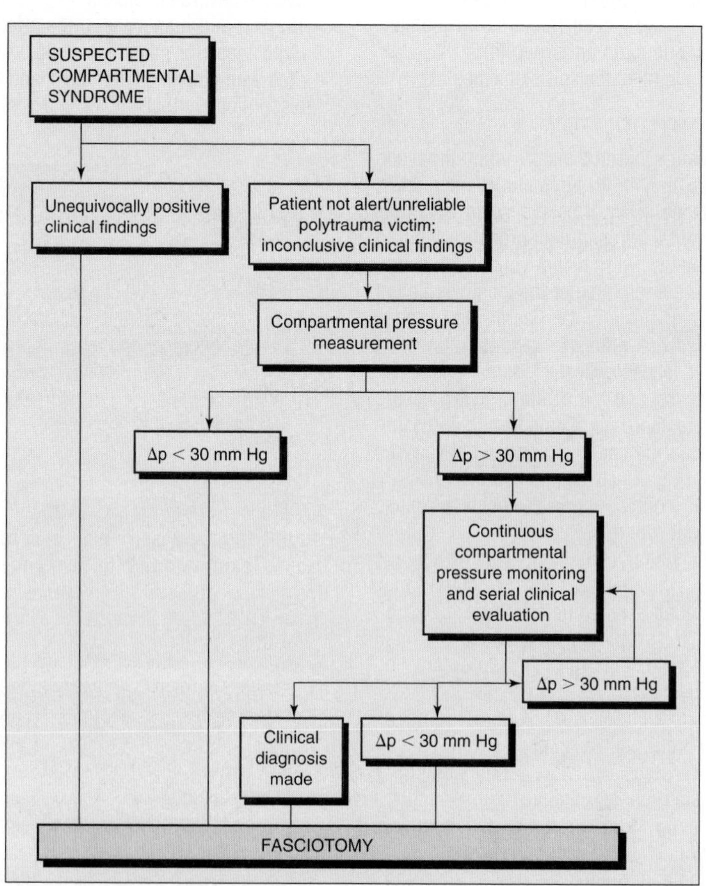

FIGURE 1-265D Algorithm for management for a patient with suspected compartment syndrome. Δp is defined as the difference between the diastolic pressure and the measured compartment pressure in mm Hg as documented by McQueen and Court-Brown. (From Browner BD et al [eds]: *Skeletal trauma,* ed 4, Philadelphia, 2009, Saunders.)

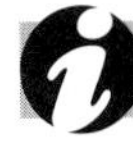

BASIC INFORMATION

DEFINITION

Complex regional pain syndrome (CRPS) is a pain disorder characterized by constant and intense limb pain associated with vasomotor and neurosensory abnormalities, skin changes, and demineralization of bone. CRPS has been divided into type I, in which there is usually an initiating noxious event but no distinct nerve lesion, and type II, in which a definable (usually traumatic) nerve lesion exists. CRPS type I generally correlates with the syndrome formerly known as reflex sympathetic dystrophy (RSD) and CRPS type II equates with what was previously termed causalgia. The term *shoulder-hand syndrome* has been used to describe CRPS in the setting of myocardial infarction or ischemia.

SYNONYMS

Reflex sympathetic dystrophy
Shoulder hand syndrome
CRPS

ICD-9CM CODES
337.20 Dystrophy, sympathetic (posttraumatic) (reflex)
ICD-10CM CODES
M89.0 Algoneurodystrophy
G90.59 Complex regional pain syndrome I of other specified site

EPIDEMIOLOGY & DEMOGRAPHICS

The incidence and prevalence of CRPS are not known. It occurs in adults and children. Common situations in which CRPS is seen include extremity trauma, burns, stroke, and orthopedic and podiatric procedures. Immobilization of the limb often precedes the development of symptoms. CRPS in the setting of myocardial infarction seems to be decreasing, presumably due to early mobilization and more effective pain control.

PHYSICAL FINDINGS & CLINICAL PRESENTATION

CRPS is divided into three stages:

1. Acute stage (occurring within hours to days after the injury).
   - Burning or aching pain occurring over the injured extremity.
   - Hyperalgesia (exaggerated response to nociceptive stimuli).
   - Edema.
   - Dysthermia.
   - Increased hair and nail growth.
2. Dystrophic stage (3-6 months after injury).
   - Burning pain radiating both distally and proximally from the site of injury.
   - Brawny edema (Fig. E1-266).
   - Hyperhidrosis.
   - Hypothermia and cyanosis.
   - Muscle tremors and spasms.
   - Increased muscle tone and reflexes.
3. Atrophic stage (6 months after injury).
   - Spread of pain proximally.
   - Alllodynia (pain response to stimuli that are not normally painful).
   - Cold, pale, cyanotic skin.
   - Tropic skin changes with subcutaneous atrophy.
   - Contractures.

ETIOLOGY

The exact pathogenetic mechanisms underlying CRPS have not been fully elucidated, but most theories include the formation of an abnormal reflex arc in the sympathetic nervous system that is modulated by cortical centers to produce peripheral vascular disturbances. Persistent pain in the peripheral nervous system is modulated by inflammatory neuropeptides including substance P, which has been shown to be elevated in the serum of patients with CRPS-I. Increased concentrations of tumor necrosis factor and IL-6 have been demonstrated in the skin of patients with CRPS-I, and immune abnormalities such as reduced numbers of CD8-positive T lymphocytes have also been seen.

Dx DIAGNOSIS

Criteria proposed for the diagnosis of CRPS type I include:

- An initiating noxious event, spontaneous pain or alloying/hyperalgesia disproportionate to the inciting event.
- Evidence of edema, skin blood flow, or sweating abnormality in the region of the pain.
- Absence of other conditions that could explain the symptoms.

Tests such as nuclear medicine bone scanning, nerve conduction testing, and plain radiographs are often indicated to confirm the diagnosis and rule out other possibilities.

DIFFERENTIAL DIAGNOSIS

The differential diagnosis includes nerve entrapment syndromes such as cervical radiculopathy, myofascial pain syndromes, and fibromyalgia.

WORKUP

- Bone scintigraphy (Fig. E1-267) shows decreased perfusion of the affected areas if done soon after the onset of symptoms. If done after 6 weeks of symptoms, bone scan may show increased uptake in the region of the peripheral joints of the involved extremity.
- Electrophysiologic testing is useful to identify nerve injury in patients with type II CRPS.
- Plain radiographs show diffuse patchy osteopenia.
- Skin temperature measurements can be used as a diagnostic test.
- Autonomic testing, although not commonly done, has been proposed.
  1. Measuring resting sweat output.
  2. Measuring resting skin temperature.
  3. Quantitative sudomotor axon reflex test.

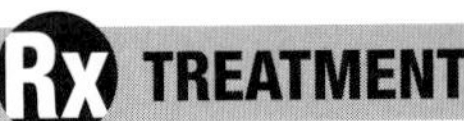

TREATMENT

Treatment of CRPS is largely empiric, based mostly on anecdotal reports, extrapolation from drug trials for other painful conditions, and clinical experience. Therapy should be tailored to stage of disease progression and severity of symptoms.

NONPHARMACOLOGIC THERAPY

- Physical therapy.
- Patient education.

PHARMACOLOGIC THERAPY

Suggested regimens:

Stage 1
- Tricyclic antidepressants (amitriptyline 25-150 mg or doxepin 5-20 mg).
- Prednisone 1 mg/kg for 2 weeks, then taper by 10 mg every 2 weeks.
- Alendronate 70 mg PO weekly.

Stage II
- Topical capsaicin.
- Gabapentin 300 mg tid.
- Regional nerve blocks.

Stage III
- Sympathetic ganglion blocks.
- Refer to multidisciplinary pain center.

NOTE: High-dose vitamin C may decrease the incidence of CRPS following wrist fracture and foot and ankle surgery or trauma.

DISPOSITION

Spontaneous remission can occur after several weeks to months.

REFERRAL

Cases in which the diagnosis is not clear or there is suboptimal response to therapy should promptly be referred to a multidisciplinary pain clinic.

PEARLS & CONSIDERATIONS

COMMENTS

- CRPS is a common clinical entity without clear definition, pathophysiologic features, or treatment.
- Early mobilization in high-risk situations is important for prevention of CRPS.
- Prompt diagnosis and aggressive physical and pharmacologic therapy may prevent progression to chronic, intractable pain.

SUGGESTED READINGS
available at www.expertconsult.com

AUTHOR: **BERNARD ZIMMERMANN, M.D.**

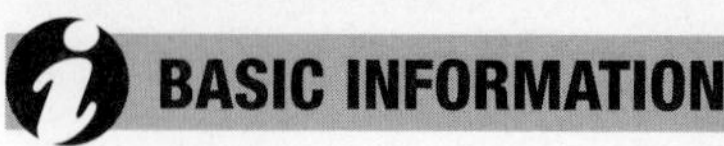

BASIC INFORMATION

DEFINITION

- Concussion is a mild traumatic brain injury that manifests with self-limited symptoms at the less severe end of the brain injury spectrum.
- It is a complex pathophysiologic process affecting the brain, induced by traumatic biomechanical forces. It may be caused by a direct blow to the head, face, neck, or elsewhere on the body with an "impulsive" force transmitted to the head.
- Concussion typically results in the rapid onset of short-lived impairment of neurologic function that resolves spontaneously. It may result in neuropathologic changes, but the acute clinical symptoms largely reflect a functional disturbance rather than a structural injury.

SYNONYMS

Sports-related mild traumatic brain injury (mTBI)

ICD-9CM CODES

850.0 Concussion (no loss of consciousness)

850.11 Concussion (loss of consciousness of ≤30 min)

850.9 Concussion unspecified

ICD-10CM CODES

S06.0 Concussion

EPIDEMIOLOGY & DEMOGRAPHICS

INCIDENCE: 3.8 million sports- and recreation-related concussions occur each year in the U.S. It is estimated that as many as 50% of concussions go unreported.

PREVALENCE: Each year, U.S. emergency departments treat an estimated 135,000 sports- and recreation-related TBIs, including concussions, among children ages 5 to 18.

PREDOMINANT SEX AND AGE: Children and teens are more likely to get a concussion and take longer to recover than adults. Limited studies have shown that in sports that are played by both men and women, women are at more risk of sustaining a concussion.

RISK FACTORS: High-impact sports and recreation; six times more likely in organized sports than leisure physical activity. Individuals who have sustained a concussion previously are at a higher risk of sustaining another concussion. Athletes with a body mass index (BMI) >27 kg/m^2 and those who train <3 hr/wk are also at greater risk.

PHYSICAL FINDINGS & CLINICAL PRESENTATION

See Table 1-131.

ETIOLOGY

- Concussion occurs when rotational or angular acceleration forces are applied to the brain, resulting in shear strain of the underlying neural elements.
- This may be associated with a blow to the skull; however, direct impact to the head is not required.

Dx DIAGNOSIS

DIFFERENTIAL DIAGNOSIS

See "Postconcussive Syndrome"

TABLE 1-131 Symptoms and Signs of Concussion

Mental Status Changes
Amnesia
Confusion
Disorientation
Easily distracted
Excessive drowsiness
Feeling dinged, stunned, or foggy
Impaired level of consciousness
Inappropriate play behaviors
Poor concentration and attention
Seeing stars or flashing lights
Slow to answer questions or to follow directions
Physical or Somatic
Ataxia or loss of balance
Blurry vision
Decreased performance or playing ability
Dizziness
Double vision
Fatigue
Headache
Lightheadedness
Nausea, vomiting
Poor coordination
Ringing in the ears
Seizures
Slurred, incoherent speech
Vacant stare/glassy-eyed
Vertigo
Behavior or Psychosomatic
Emotional lability
Irritability
Low frustration tolerance
Personality changes
Nervousness, anxiety
Sadness, depressed mood

From Patel DR et al: Sports related concussions in adolescents, *Pediatr Clin N Am* 57:652, 2010.

WORKUP

- Sideline assessment:
  - No athlete with a suspected concussion should return to play that day.
  - Neurologic assessment using a standardized tool, such as s SCAT3 (Sports Concussion Assessment Tool), which includes the BESS (Balance Error Scoring System) and Maddocks Questions or SAC (Standardized Assessment of Concussion)
  - Monitor for deterioration; no athlete should be left alone
- Neurocognitive testing:
  - Computer-based programs, such as ImPACT, ANAM, CogSport
  - Neuropsychiatric testing administered by a neuropsychologist
- Gait/balance testing with a tool such as the Balance Error Scoring System (BESS)
- When used in combination, symptom assessment, balance assessment, and neurocognitive testing provide a sensitivity of >90% for the identification of concussion.

IMAGING STUDIES

- CT imaging is indicated in any athlete with a Glasgow Coma Scale score of ≤15 or a rapidly changing neurologic exam.
- Imaging should be reserved for athletes in whom intracerebral bleeding is suspected; PECARN guidelines

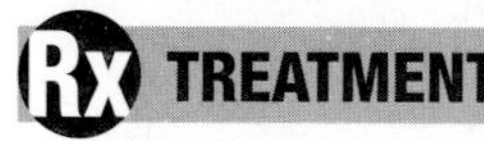

TREATMENT

ACUTE GENERAL Rx

- Removal from game
- Physical rest
  - No return to play until asymptomatic for 24 hr
  - Follow return-to-play guidelines (Table 1-132)
- Cognitive rest to limit symptoms
  - Modifications at school
  - Modifications at home/recreation
  - Encourage sleep

CHRONIC Rx

See "Postconcussive Syndrome"

TABLE 1-132 Graduated Return to Play Protocol

Rehabilitation Stage	Functional Exercise at Each Stage of Rehabilitation	Objective of Each Stage
1. No activity	Complete physical and cognitive rest	Recovery
2. Light aerobic exercise	Walking, swimming, or stationary cycling, keeping intensity <70% maximum predicted heart rate No resistance training	Increase heart rate
3. Sport-specific exercise	Skating drills in ice hockey, running drills in soccer No head impact activities	Add movement
4. Noncontact training drills	Progression to more complex training drills, e.g., passing drills in football and ice hockey May start progressive resistance training	Exercise, coordination, and cognitive load
5. Full contact practice	After medical clearance, participate in normal training activities	Restore confidence and assess functional skills by coaching staff
6. Return to play	Normal game play	

From Putukian M: The acute symptoms of sports-related concussion: diagnosis and on-field management, *Clin Sports Med* 30(58), 2011.

DISPOSITION

- Table 1-132 summarizes the American Academy of Neurology, American Medical Society for Sports Medicine, and International Conference on Concussion recommendations on returning to play after a concussion.
- If concussion symptoms occur with activity at one level, the athlete should stop the activity, rest until symptoms resolve, and then restart his or her progression at the level that did not elicit symptoms
- There are no evidence-based guidelines for disqualifying or retiring an athlete from sport after a concussion. Each case should be individually considered.

REFERRAL

Sports-medicine physician, neuropsychology or concussion center

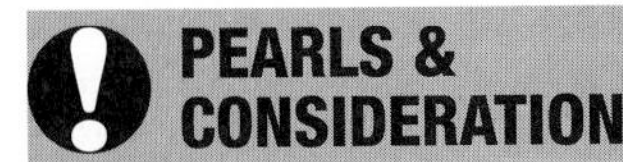

PEARLS & CONSIDERATIONS

PREVENTION

- Preparticipation evaluations for all athletes
- Preparticipation neurocognitive and balance testing to establish a baseline
- There is currently no evidence to support the use of concussion prevention head bands or mouth guards.

PATIENT/FAMILY EDUCATION

Centers for Disease Control and Prevention: http://www.cdc.gov/concussion/support.html

SUGGESTED READINGS

available at www.expertconsult.com

RELATED CONTENT

Concussion (Patient Information)

AUTHORS: **PETER J. SELL, D.O.**, and **AMITY RUBEOR, D.O.**

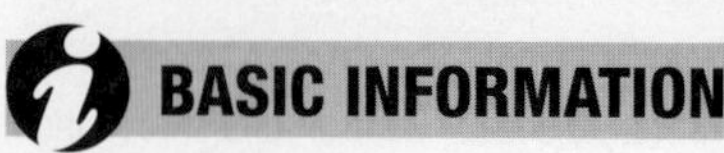

BASIC INFORMATION

DEFINITION

Conduct disorder (CD) is a repetitive and persistent pattern of behaviors in which either the basic rights of others are violated and/or major age-appropriate societal rules are violated. Classified under the DSM-5 category "disruptive, impulse control, and conduct disorders."

For childhood onset:
ICD-9CM and DSM-5 CODES
312.81
ICD-10CM CODES
F91.1
For adolescent onset:
ICD-9CM and DSM-5 CODES
312.32
ICD-10CM CODES
F91.2

EPIDEMIOLOGY & DEMOGRAPHICS

INCIDENCE: 1% (12-mo span, National Comorbidity Survey-Replication [NCS-R])
PREVALENCE: Approximately 2% to 10%; NCS-R: 9%. Disruptive behavior disorders are considered the most common reason for referral of children to mental health providers.
PREDOMINANT SEX: More common in males (4:1 preadolescence and 2:1 postadolescence). It is unclear if CD females are underrepresented, as diagnostic criteria were validated on male samples. Nonconfrontational aggression and promiscuity are examples of possible gender-specific criteria that, at this time, have unknown predictive validity.
PREDOMINANT AGE: Most common onset in early adolescence. Median age of onset is 11 yr.
GENETICS: Risk increased if parent or sibling with disorder.
RISK FACTORS: There are various temperamental (including lower-than-average intelligence, especially verbal), family-level (including parental rejection or neglect, early institutional living, frequent caregiver changes, large family size, parental criminality or substance use), and community-level (including peer rejection, association with delinquent peer group, exposure to violence) risk factors.

PHYSICAL FINDINGS & CLINICAL PRESENTATION

- The DSM-5 lists 15 possible behavioral manifestations of CD, grouped into four categories: aggression to people and animals, destruction of property, deceitfulness or theft, and serious violations of rules. Three of the 15 behaviors are required to have occurred in the last 12 mo, and one behavior must have occurred in the last 6 mo.
- Specifiers describe the age of onset and the severity of the disorder.
- New to the DSM-5 is an additional specifier addressing issues relating to intent and reaction to the behaviors, including the following options: "With limited prosocial emotions," "lack of remorse or guilt," "callous-lack of empathy," "unconcerned about performance," and "shallow or deficient affect."
- CD represents a heterogeneous group with respect to presentation, etiology, severity, and course.
- Symptom severity often progresses over time with age (i.e., lying and truancy to sexual assault and robbery).
- Aggressive youth are more likely to interpret as negative or hostile the intent of neutral others and are more likely to believe that conflict can be adequately resolved via aggression.
- Poor frustration tolerance, irritability, temper outbursts, and recklessness are often associated with CD.
- Slow resting heart rate associated with reduced autonomic response to fear is the most replicated of all biologic markers for conduct problems.

ETIOLOGY

Estimated population variance in antisocial behavior accounted for by:
- Genes: 50%
- Environmental factors shared among family members: 20%
- Environmental factors unshared among family members: 20% to 30%

DIAGNOSIS

DIFFERENTIAL DIAGNOSIS

- Oppositional defiant disorder
- ADHD
- Mood disorder
- Adjustment disorder
- Substance abuse, dependence, intoxication, or withdrawal
- Post-traumatic stress disorder
- Antisocial personality disorder (for those >18 yr)
- Adaptive behavior or subcultural delinquency

WORKUP

Diagnosis is made based on history, including individual and family interviews as well as collateral data from additional sources (e.g., parents, teachers, other medical providers, therapist).

LABORATORY TESTS

Consider urine toxicology for possible substance use comorbidity.

IMAGING STUDIES

None indicated; however, both structural and functional differences have been noted in certain areas of the brain in individuals with CD.

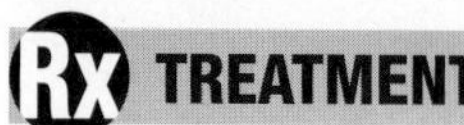

TREATMENT

Initial treatment of CD should include psychosocial and environmental interventions aimed at decreasing the frequency and severity of delinquent behaviors. If the interventions listed here are not effective, or if serious concerns exist regarding safety or impairment in functioning, pharmacologic interventions targeting specific symptoms (e.g., aggression) or comorbid disorders (e.g., ADHD, anxiety disorders, or mood disorders) may help. There are currently no medications approved by the FDA for the treatment of CD.

NONPHARMACOLOGIC THERAPY

- Parent management training
- Cognitive problem-solving skills training (including elements of social skills, conflict resolution, anger management, impulse control, and vocational training)
- Multisystemic therapy (MST)
- Social skills training
- Individual psychotherapy
- Family psychotherapy
- Higher levels of care such as a hospital or acute residential setting may be required for stabilization if acute safety concerns develop in the context of CD, such as severe aggression.
- Legal involvement and/or out-of-home-placements may be necessary to monitor safety of both the patient and the community.

PHARMACOLOGIC THERAPY

Medication may be considered as an adjunct to behavioral treatment or in cases where comorbidity is a factor. There is some evidence for symptom improvement with trials of several classes of psychotropic medications—including stimulants, mood stabilizers, atypical antipsychotics, antidepressants, and alpha-2 agonists—all of which seem to target aggressive symptoms in particular; medication, however, should never be used alone or as first-line treatment for CD.

DISPOSITION

- Approximately half of those with early onset of CD persist with antisocial behaviors into adulthood. There is no reliable way to predict which 50% will persist.
- Approximately half of those with early onset of CD do not develop antisocial personality disorder in adulthood. This subgroup is at higher risk for depression, anxiety, and social isolation as adults.
- Approximately 85% of those with adolescent onset of CD do not demonstrate lifetime persistent violence, convictions, and incarcerations. However, adult prognosis may often include substance abuse and crimes that go largely undetected.

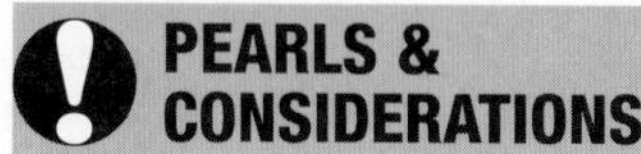

PEARLS & CONSIDERATIONS

COMMENTS

- Treatment noncompliance is common.
- Expect 30% treatment noncompliance rate.

SUGGESTED READINGS

available at www.expertconsult.com

AUTHORS: **ELIZABETH A. LOWENHAUPT, M.D.,** and **SARAH L. XAVIER, D.O.**

BASIC INFORMATION

DEFINITION

Condyloma acuminatum is a sexually transmitted viral disease of the vulva, vagina, and cervix caused by the human papillomavirus (HPV). 90% of genital warts are caused by HPV 6 or 11.

SYNONYMS

Genital warts
Venereal warts
Anogenital warts

ICD-9CM CODES
078.11 Condyloma acuminatum
ICD-10CM CODES
A63.0 Anogenital (venereal) warts

EPIDEMIOLOGY & DEMOGRAPHICS

- Seen mostly in young adults, with peak age of onset of 16 to 25 yr
- A sexually transmitted disease spread by skin-to-skin contact
- Highly contagious, with 25% to 65% of sexual partners developing it
- Virus shed from both macroscopic and microscopic lesions
- Average incubation time is 2 mo (range, 1 to 8 mo)
- Predisposing conditions: diabetes, pregnancy, local trauma, and immunosuppression (e.g., transplant recipients, those with HIV infection)

PHYSICAL FINDINGS & CLINICAL PRESENTATION

- Usually found in genital area but can be present elsewhere
- Lesions usually in similar positions on both sides of perineum
- Initial lesions pedunculated, soft papules about 2 to 3 mm in diameter, 10 to 20 mm long; may occur as single papule or in clusters
- Size of lesions varies from pinhead to large cauliflower-like masses (Fig. E1-268)
- Usually asymptomatic, but if infected can cause pain, odor, or bleeding
- Vulvar condyloma more common than vaginal and cervical
- Four morphologic types: condylomatous, keratotic, papular, and flat warts
- Intraanal anal warts are observed predominantly in persons who have had receptive anal intercourse.

ETIOLOGY

- HPV DNA types 6 and 11 usually found in exophytic warts and have no malignant potential
- HPV types 16 and 18 usually found in flat warts and are associated with increased risk of malignancy
- Recurrence associated with persisting viral infection of adjacent normal skin in 25% to 50% of cases

Dx DIAGNOSIS

DIFFERENTIAL DIAGNOSIS

- Abnormal anatomic variants or skin tags around labia minora and introitus
- Dysplastic warts

WORKUP

- Colposcopic examination of lower genital tract from cervix to perianal skin with 3% to 5% acetic acid
- Biopsy of vulvar lesions that lack the classic appearance of warts and that become ulcerated or do not respond to treatment
- Biopsy of flat, white, or ulcerated cervical lesions

LABORATORY TESTS

- Pap smear
- Cervical cultures for *Neisseria gonorrhoeae* and *Chlamydia*
- Serologic test for syphilis
- HIV testing offered
- Wet mount for trichomoniasis, *Candida albicans,* and *Gardnerella vaginalis*
- Testing for diabetes (blood glucose)

Rx TREATMENT

NONPHARMACOLOGIC THERAPY

- Keep genital area dry and clean.
- If present, keep diabetes well controlled.
- Advise use of condoms to prevent spread of infection to sexual partner.

ACUTE GENERAL Rx

Factors that influence selection of treatment include wart size, wart number, anatomic site of wart, wart morphology, patient preference, cost of treatment, convenience, adverse effects, and provider experience.
Keratolytic agents:

- Podophyllin (Podofilox 0.5% solution or gel)
  - Acts by poisoning mitotic spindle and causing intense vasospasm
  - Applied directly to lesion weekly and washed off in 6 hr
  - Used in minimal vulvar or anal disease
  - Applied cautiously to nonkeratinized epithelial surfaces
  - Contraindicated in pregnancy
  - Discontinued if lesions do not disappear in 6 wk; switch to other treatment
- Sinecatechin 15% ointment
  - Applied tid (0.5 cm strand of ointment to each wart)
  - Should not be continued longer than 16 wk
- Trichloroacetic acid (30% to 80% solution)
  - Acts by precipitation of surface proteins
  - Applied twice monthly to lesion
  - Indicated for vulvar, anal, and vaginal lesions; can be used for cervical lesions
  - Less painful and irritating to normal tissue than podophyllin
- 5-Fluorouracil
  - Causes necrosis and sloughing of growing tissue
  - Can be used intravaginally or for vulvar, anal, or urethral lesions
  - Better tolerated; 3 g (two thirds of vaginal applicator) applied weekly for 12 wk
  - Possible vaginal ulceration and erythema
  - Patient's vagina examined after four to six applications
  - 80% cure rate

Physical agents:

- Cryotherapy with liquid nitrogen or cryoprobe
  - Can be used weekly for 3 to 6 wk
  - 62% to 79% success rate
  - Not suitable for large warts
- Laser therapy
  - Done by physician with necessary expertise and equipment
  - Painful; requires anesthesia
- Electrocautery or excision
  - For recurrent, very large lesions
  - Local anesthesia needed

Immunotherapy:

- Interferon
  - Injected intralesionally at a dose of 3 million U/m^2 three times weekly for 8 wk
  - Side effects: fever, chills, malaise, headache
- Imiquimod 5% cream at night, 3× per wk up to 16 wk increases wart clearance after 3 mo
- Interferon, topical: increases wart clearance at 4 wk

DISPOSITION

- Follow-up exam every 6 to 12 mo, as needed.
- Correct and consistent male condom use might lower the chances of giving or getting genital HPV, but such use is not fully protective because HPV can infect areas that are not covered by a condom.

PREVENTION

- Routine vaccination of females at age 11 or 12 through age 26.
- Routine vaccination of males at age 11 or 12 through age 21 (up to age 26 for men who have sex with men or are immunocompromised patients).

SUGGESTED READINGS

available at www.expertconsult.com

RELATED CONTENT

Chancroid (Related Key Topic)
Lymphogranuloma Venereum (Related Key Topic)
Syphilis (Related Key Topic)
Genital Warts (Patient Information)
Warts (Related Key Topic)

AUTHORS: **GEORGE T. DANAKAS, M.D.,** and **RUBEN ALVERO, M.D.**

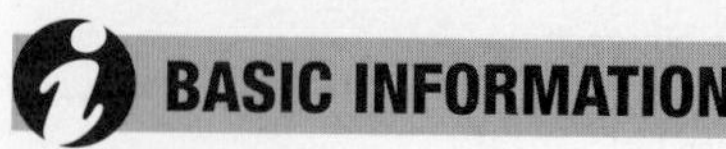

BASIC INFORMATION

DEFINITION

The term *conjunctivitis* refers to an inflammation of the conjunctiva resulting from a variety of causes, including allergies and bacterial, viral, and chlamydial infections.

SYNONYMS

"Red eye"
Pink eye
Acute conjunctivitis
Subacute conjunctivitis
Chronic conjunctivitis
Purulent conjunctivitis
Pseudomembranous conjunctivitis
Papillary conjunctivitis
Follicular conjunctivitis
Newborn conjunctivitis

ICD-9CM CODES
372.30 Conjunctivitis, unspecified
ICD-10CM CODES
H10.9 Unspecified conjunctivitis
B30 Viral conjunctivitis
H10.0 Mucopurulent conjunctivitis
H10.1 Acute atopic conjunctivitis
H10.4 Chronic conjunctivitis

EPIDEMIOLOGY & DEMOGRAPHICS

INCIDENCE (IN U.S.): 1.6% to 12% in *newborns*
PREVALENCE (IN U.S.):

- Allergic conjunctivitis (Fig. E1-270), the most common form of ocular allergy, is usually associated with allergic rhinitis and may be seasonal or perennial.
- Bacterial or viral conjunctivitis is often seasonal and can be extremely contagious.

PREDOMINANT AGE: Occurs at *any* age. Most cases in adults are due to viral infection. Children are more prone to develop bacterial conjunctivitis than viral forms.
PEAK INCIDENCE: More common in the spring and fall, when *viral* infections and pollens increase

PHYSICAL FINDINGS & CLINICAL PRESENTATION

- Infection and chemosis of conjunctivae with discharge. Gluing of the eyelids and no itching is more indicative of a bacterial cause (Fig. 1-271).
- Cornea is clear or can be involved.
- Vision is often normal but can be blurred.

ETIOLOGY

- Bacterial: *Haemophilus influenzae*, *Streptococcus pneumoniae*, and *Moraxella catarrhalis* in children; *Staphylococcus* species in adults. Gram-negative infections are more common in contact lens wearers. Gonococcal ophthalmia neonatorum is caused by *Neisseria gonorrhoeae* acquired by exposure of the neonatal conjunctivae to infected cervicovaginal secretions during delivery.
- Viral: Most common overall cause of infectious conjunctivitis
- Chlamydial.

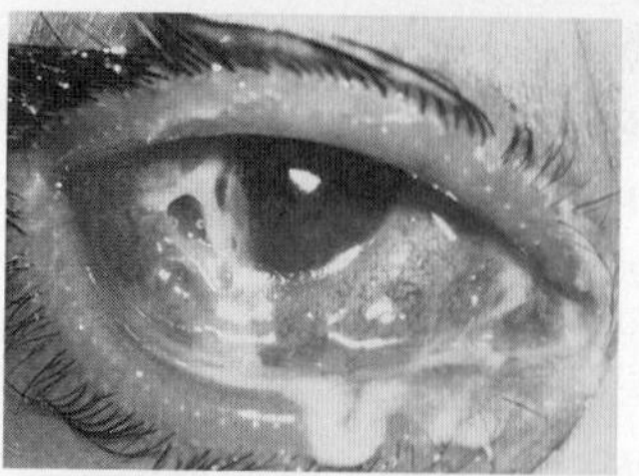

FIGURE 1-271 Bacterial conjunctivitis. Purulent discharge and conjunctiva hyperemia suggest bacterial conjunctivitis. Viral conjunctivitis produces watery discharge, foreign body sensation, preauricular lymphadenopathy, and conjunctival follicles seen on slit lamp examination. (Reproduced with permission from the American Academy of Ophthalmology. From Goldman L, Schafer AI: *Goldman's Cecil medicine,* ed 24, Philadelphia, 2012, Saunders.)

- Allergic.
- Traumatic.

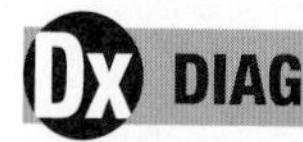

DIAGNOSIS

DIFFERENTIAL DIAGNOSIS

- Acute glaucoma
- Corneal lesions
- Acute iritis
- Episcleritis
- Scleritis
- Uveitis
- Canalicular obstruction

WORKUP

- History and physical examination
- Reports of itching, pain, and visual changes

LABORATORY TESTS

Cultures are useful if not *successfully* treated with antibiotics; initial culture is usually not necessary, since normal conjunctival flora interferes with helpful culture results.

TREATMENT

NONPHARMACOLOGIC THERAPY

- Warm compresses if infective conjunctivitis.
- Cold compresses if irritative or allergic conjunctivitis.
- Contact lenses should be taken out until an infection is completely resolved. Nondisposable lenses should be cleaned thoroughly as recommended by the manufacturer, and a new lens case should be used. Disposable contact lenses should be thrown away.

ACUTE GENERAL Rx

- The majority of cases of bacterial conjunctivitis are self-limiting and no treatment is necessary in uncomplicated cases.[1] Antibiotic drops (e.g., levofloxacin, ofloxacin, ciprofloxacin, tobramycin, gentamicin ophthalmic solution, 1 or 2 drops q2 to 4h) are indicated for complicated bacterial conjunctivitis, in conjunctivitis caused by gonorrhea or chlamydia, and in bacterial conjunctivitis in contact lens wearers.
- Caution: be careful with ophthalmic corticosteroid treatment and avoid unless sure of diagnosis; corticosteroids can exacerbate infections and have been associated with increased intraocular pressure and cataract formation.
- An oral antihistamine (cetirizine, loratadine, desloratadine, or fexofenadine) is effective in relieving itching.
- Mast cell stabilizers (e.g., ketotifen, olopatadine, azelastine bid) are effective for allergic conjunctivitis. Others include Elestat, Optivar, and Patanol.
- Bepotastine, alcaftadine, azelastine, epinastine, and ketotifen are H1-antihistamines and mast cell stabilizers effective for topical treatment of itching associated with allergic conjunctivitis. The topical NSAID ketorolac (0.5%, 1 drop qd) is also useful in allergic conjunctivitis. Table E1-134 describes topical ophthalmic medications for allergic conjunctivitis.
- Antihistamine/decongestant combinations such as pheniramine/naphazoline (Visine A), available over the counter, are more effective than either agent alone but have a short duration and can result in rebound vasodilatation with prolonged use. Others include Naphcon-A, Albacon-A, and Opcon-A.

CHRONIC Rx

- Depends on cause.
- If allergic, nonsteroidals such as Voltaren, Acular, and Xibrom ophthalmic solution; mast cell stabilizers such as Elestat, Alocril, Patanol, and Zaditor are useful for improving ocular itching in patients with allergic conjunctivitis.
- If an infection, use antibiotic drops (see "Acute General Rx").
- Dry eyes need artificial tears (Restasis) or lacrimal duct plugs when indicated.

DISPOSITION

Follow carefully for the first 2 wk to ensure secondary complications do not occur. Otitis media can develop in 25% of children with *Haemophilus influenzae* conjunctivitis. Bacterial keratitis occurs in 30/1000 contact lens wearers.

REFERRAL

To ophthalmologist if symptoms are refractory to initial treatment. Indications for urgent referral are severe eye pain or headache, photophobia, decreased vision, and contact lens use.

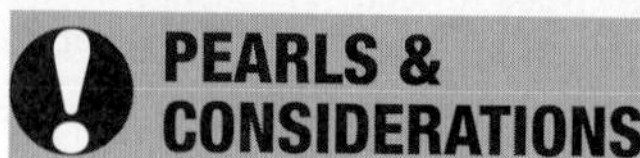

PEARLS & CONSIDERATIONS

COMMENTS

- Red eyes are not simply conjunctivitis when the patient has significant pain or loss of sight. However, it is usually safe to treat pain-free eyes and the normal-seeing red eye with lid hygiene and topical treatment.

[1]Azari AA, Barney NP: Conjunctivitis, a systematic review of diagnosis and treatment, *JAMA* 310(16):1721-1729, 2013.

- Use caution with patients wearing soft contact lenses, infants, and the elderly.
- Do not use steroids indiscriminately; use only when the diagnosis is certain.
- Bacterial conjunctivitis is generally self-limiting. Over 60% of persons will improve with placebo within 2 to 5 days.

RELATED CONTENT

Conjunctivitis (Patient Information)

AUTHOR: **R. SCOTT HOFFMAN, M.D.**

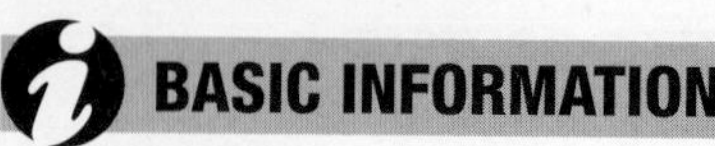

BASIC INFORMATION

DEFINITION

Contact dermatitis is an acute or chronic skin inflammation, usually eczematous dermatitis resulting from exposure to substances in the environment. It can be subdivided into "irritant" contact dermatitis (nonimmunologic physical and chemical alteration of the epidermis) and "allergic" contact dermatitis (delayed hypersensitivity reaction).

SYNONYMS

Irritant contact dermatitis
Allergic contact dermatitis

ICD-9CM CODES
692 Contact dermatitis and other eczema
ICD-10CM CODES
L23 Allergic contact dermatitis
L23.0 Allergic contact dermatitis due to metals
L23.1 Allergic contact dermatitis due to adhesives
L23.2 Allergic contact dermatitis due to cosmetics
L23.3 Allergic contact dermatitis due to drugs in contact with skin
L23.4 Allergic contact dermatitis due to dyes
L23.5 Allergic contact dermatitis due to other chemical products
L25.9 Unspecified contact dermatitis, unspecified cause

EPIDEMIOLOGY & DEMOGRAPHICS

- 20% of all cases of dermatitis in children are caused by allergic contact dermatitis.
- Rhus dermatitis (poison ivy, poison oak, and poison sumac) is responsible for most cases of contact dermatitis.
- Frequent causes of irritant contact dermatitis are soaps, detergents, and organic solvents.
- Chemical irritants (e.g., cutting fluids used in machining, solvents) account for most cases of irritant contact dermatitis. Occupational skin diseases are second only to traumatic injuries as the most common types of occupational disease.

PHYSICAL FINDINGS & CLINICAL PRESENTATION

Clinical presentation varies with the responsible agent and affected area of skin.

IRRITANT CONTACT DERMATITIS:

- Mild exposure may result in dryness, erythema, and fissuring of the affected area (e.g., hand involvement in irritant dermatitis caused by exposure to soap (Fig. E1-272), genital area involvement in irritant dermatitis caused by prolonged exposure to wet diapers).
- Eczematous inflammation may result from chronic exposure.

ALLERGIC CONTACT DERMATITIS:

- Poison ivy dermatitis can present with vesicles and blisters; linear lesions (as a result of dragging of the resins over the surface of the skin by scratching) are a classic presentation.
- The pattern of lesions is asymmetric; itching, burning, and stinging may be present.
- The involved areas are erythematous, warm to touch, swollen, and may be confused with cellulitis.

ETIOLOGY

- Irritant contact dermatitis: cement (construction workers), rubber, ragweed, malathion (farmers), orange and lemon peels (chefs, bartenders), hair tints, shampoos (beauticians), rubber gloves (medical, surgical personnel)
- Allergic contact dermatitis: poison ivy, poison oak, poison sumac, rubber (shoe dermatitis), nickel (jewelry), balsam of Peru (hand and face dermatitis), neomycin, formaldehyde (cosmetics)

Dx DIAGNOSIS

DIFFERENTIAL DIAGNOSIS

- Impetigo
- Lichen simplex chronicus
- Atopic dermatitis
- Nummular eczema, dyshidrotic eczema
- Seborrheic dermatitis
- Inverse psoriasis, palmoplantar psoriasis
- Scabies
- Tinea pedis

WORKUP

- Medical history: gradual onset versus rapid onset, number of exposures, clinical presentation, occupational history.
- Physical examination: contact dermatitis in the neck may be caused by necklaces, perfumes (Fig. E1-273), after-shave lotion. Involvement of the axillae is often secondary to deodorants, clothing. Face involvement can occur with cosmetics, airborne allergens, aftershave lotion.

LABORATORY TESTS

- Patch testing has a sensitivity and specificity of 70% to 80%. It is useful to confirm the diagnosis of contact dermatitis; it is indicated only when inflammation persists despite appropriate topical therapy and avoidance of suspected causative agent; patch testing should not be used for irritant contact dermatitis because this is a nonimmunologic-mediated inflammatory reaction.
- Dermoscopy and microscopy when suspecting scabies and mites.
- A potassium hydroxide (KOH) preparation may be useful if suspecting tinea or *Candida* infection.

Rx TREATMENT

NONPHARMACOLOGIC THERAPY

Avoidance of suspected allergens

ACUTE GENERAL Rx

- Removal of the irritant substance by washing the skin with plain water or mild soap within 15 min of exposure is helpful in patients with poison ivy, poison oak, or poison sumac dermatitis.
- Cold or cool water compresses for 20 to 30 min 5 to 6 times a day for the initial 72 hr are effective during the acute blistering stage.
- Topical steroids (clobetasol 0.05%, triamcinolone 0.1%) are effective for acute localized allergic contact dermatitis lesions. Lower-potency topical steroids are preferred on face, anogenital regions, and flexural surfaces to minimize risk of skin atrophy. Oral corticosteroids (e.g., prednisone 20 mg bid for 6 to 10 days) are generally reserved for severe, widespread dermatitis.
- IM steroids (e.g., Kenalog) are used for severe reactions and in patients requiring oral corticosteroids but unable to tolerate PO.
- Oral antihistamines (e.g., hydroxyzine 25 mg q6h) will control pruritus, especially at night; calamine lotion is also useful for pruritus; however, it can lead to excessive drying.
- Colloidal oatmeal (Aveeno) baths can also provide symptomatic relief.
- Patients with mild to moderate erythema may respond to topical steroid gels or creams.
- Patients with shoe allergy should change their socks at least once a day; use of aluminum chloride hexahydrate in a 20% solution (Drysol) qhs will also help control perspiration.
- Use hypoallergenic surgical gloves in patients with rubber and surgical glove allergy.

DISPOSITION

Allergic contact dermatitis generally resolves within 2 to 4 wk if reexposure to allergen is prevented.

REFERRAL

For patch testing in selected patients, see "Laboratory Tests."

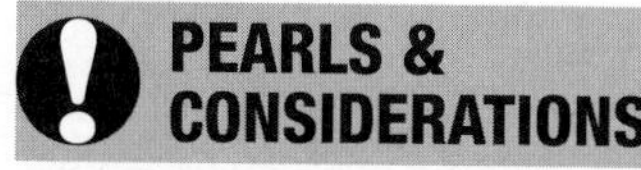

PEARLS & CONSIDERATIONS

COMMENTS

Commercially available corticosteroid dose packs should be avoided, because they generally provide an inadequate amount of medication.

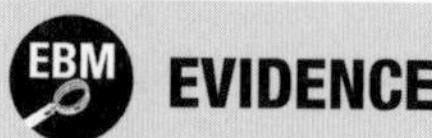

EVIDENCE

available at www.expertconsult.com

SUGGESTED READINGS

available at www.expertconsult.com

RELATED CONTENT

Contact Dermatitis (Patient Information)

AUTHOR: **FRED F. FERRI, M.D.**

BASIC INFORMATION

DEFINITION

Contraception refers to the various modalities that a sexually active couple use to prevent pregnancy. These options can be either medical or nonmedical and used by men or women or both. An algorithm for helping couples select a contraceptive method is described in Fig. E1-274. The options are as follows:

- No contraception (unprotected intercourse) failure rate 85% both typical use and perfect use
- Abstinence
  - 12.4% of unmarried men
  - 13.2% of unmarried women
  - More frequently practiced before age 17 yr
  - No intercourse experienced by 13% of women ages 30 to 34 yr
  - Failure rate 0%
- Withdrawal
  - Used in only 2% of sexually active women
  - Failure rate with perfect use, 4%; with typical use, 19%
- Rhythm method (natural family planning)
  - Failure rate with perfect use, 1% to 9%; with typical use, 20%
  - Symptothermal type: mucus method and ovulation pain combined with basal body temperature
  - Ovulation (Billings' method): takes into account mucus quality
  - Basal body temperature method: uses biphasic temperature chart
  - Lactation amenorrhea method: effective in fully breastfeeding women, especially 70 to 100 days after delivery; depends on number of feedings per day
- Barriers
  - Diaphragm and cervical cap: failure rate 5% to 9% in nulliparous women, 20% in multiparous women
  - Female condom: failure rate with perfect use, 5.1%; with typical use, 12.4%; FDA labeling states 25% failure rate
  - Male condom: failure rate with perfect use, 3%; with typical use, 12%
  - Spermicides (aerosols, foam, jellies, creams, tabs): failure rate with perfect use, 3%; with typical use, 21%
- Oral contraceptives (Fig. E1-275)
  - Failure rate with perfect use, <1%; with typical use, 3%
  - Come in combinations of estrogen/progestin or as progestin only
- Hormonal implants and injectables
  - Implanon (etonogestrel) implant 2-yr cumulative pregnancy rate 0.05%. Nexplanon is essentially the same as Implanon but with a barium sulfate core for easier radiologic detection and a preloaded applicator to facilitate insertion.
  - Depo-Provera: failure rate 0.3% in first year of use
  - Lunelle failure rate 0.2% in first year
  - Nestorone-releasing single implant: not yet available
  - Jadelle implant: Succesor to the Norplant implant, which has been discontinued in the U.S. The Jadelle implant is not available in the U.S.
- Mini pill (progesterone only pill)
  - Failure rate with typical use, 1.1% to 13.2%
  - With perfect use, 5 pregnancies per 1000 women
- Emergency postcoital contraception
  - Decreases pregnancy rate by 75% with women treated immediately postcoitally
  - Involves dedicated hormonal (Plan B, which contains levonorgestrel) use or intrauterine device (IUD) insertion
- IUD (available over the counter in some states)
  - Progestasert: failure rate with perfect use, 2%; with typical use, 3%
  - Copper T (30-A): failure rate with perfect use, 0.8%; with typical use, 3%
  - Levonorgestrel Intrauterine System (Mirena)
    - 1-yr failure rate, 1%
    - 5-yr cumulative failure rate, 0.71 per 100 women
- Female sterilization (tubal ligation): failure rate with perfect use, 0.2%; with typical use, 3%
- Male sterilization (vasectomy): failure rate of 0.1% in first year
- Vaginal ring (Nuva ring): failure rate pearl index 0.77
- Contraceptive patch (Ortho Evra): failure rate 0.4% to 0.7%

SYNONYMS

Birth control
Family planning

ICD-9CM CODES

V25.01	Oral contraceptives
V25.02	Other contraceptive measures
V25.09	Family planning
V25.1	IUD
V25.2	Sterilization

ICD-10CM CODES

Z30.011	Encounter for initial prescription of contraceptive pills
Z30.018	Encounter for initial prescription of other contraceptives
Z30.09	Encounter for other general counseling and advice on contraception
Z30.430	Encounter for insertion of intrauterine contraceptive device
Z30.2	Encounter for sterilization

Dx DIAGNOSIS

WORKUP

- Thorough medical history
- Thorough surgical history
- Obstetric history (was fertility desired with conception?)
- Gynecologic history, including:
  - History of previous sexually transmitted diseases
  - Number of partners
  - Previous difficulties with contraception
  - Frequency of intercourse
- Family history

LABORATORY TESTS

- Pap smear
- Cultures, aerobic and *Chlamydia*
- Pregnancy test if suspected pregnancy
- Lipid profile if family history of premature vascular event

Rx TREATMENT

NONPHARMACOLOGIC THERAPY

- Male condoms
  - 95% latex (rubber), 5% skin or natural membrane
  - Proper use: place on an erect penis and leave ½-inch empty space at the tip of the condom; use with non–oil-based lubricants
  - Effectiveness increased when used with spermicides
- Female condoms
  - Composed of polyurethane, with one end open and one end closed
  - Proper use: place closed end over cervix, open end hanging out of vagina to cover penis and scrotum
  - Highly effective against HIV
- Spermicides
  - Types: nonoxynol, octoxynol
  - Forms: jellies, creams, foams, suppositories, tablets, soluble films
  - Proper use: put in immediately before intercourse; may be used with other barrier methods
- Diaphragm and cervical cap
  - Must be fitted by practitioner, used with contraceptive gels, and refitted with weight gain or loss of 4.5 kg. Must also be refit after pregnancy.
  - Diaphragm sizes: 50 to 105 mm; cervical cap sizes 26, 28, and 30 mm
  - The correct fit allows the woman to remain ambulatory without feeling the device
  - Proper use of diaphragm: put in immediately before intercourse and keep in for 6 hr after intercourse; must not remain in the vagina for longer than 24 hr
  - Proper use of cervical cap: fit over the cervix exactly; must not remain in place for longer than 48 hr
- Lactation amenorrhea method
  - Depends on number of feedings per day; effective as birth control for 6 mo if 15 or more feedings, lasting 10 min each, are accomplished daily. If woman meets criteria (e.g., breastfeeding only source of infant feeding) 0.5%-2.0% failure rate in the first 6 months after delivery.
  - Not a common practice in the U.S.
- Withdrawal
  - Withdrawal of the penis from the vagina before ejaculation
  - Depends on self-control
- Rhythm method
  - Depends on awareness of physiology of male and female reproductive tracts
  - Sperm viable in vagina for 2 to 7 days
  - Ovum life span 24 hr

- Sterilization
  - Male:
    - Vasectomy to interrupt vas deferens and block passage of sperm to seminal ejaculate
    - Scalpel and nonscalpel techniques available
    - More easily performed procedure than female sterilization and does not require general anesthesia
  - Female:
    - Leading method of birth control in U.S. in women older than 30 yr
    - Interrupts fallopian tubes, blocking passage of ovum proximally and sperm distally through tube
    - Several types; modified Pomeroy done during cesarean section or interval laparoscopic using clips (Filshie, Hulka) or banding
    - Essure-tubal occlusion through hysteroscopic placement of micro-inserts into the fallopian tubes.

ACUTE GENERAL Rx

- Combination oral contraceptives
  - Taken daily for 21 days, pill-free interval of 7 days
  - Less than 50 mcg ethinyl estradiol in most common combination oral contraceptives; progestins most commonly used in combination pills are norethindrone, levonorgestrel, norgestrel, norethindrone acetate, ethynodiol diacetate, norgestimate, or desogestrel; triphasic combination oral contraceptives (give varying doses of progestin and estrogens throughout cycle); monophasic oral contraceptives: offer same dose of progestin and estrogen throughout cycle, taken daily at same time; estrophasic pill (constant progesterone with variation of estrogen throughout the cycle)
  - If pill taken with antibiotics, efficacy affected by inadequate gastrointestinal absorption in most cases; only rifampin truly reduces pill's effectiveness
  - Increased body weight decreases effectiveness
  - Table E1-135 describes oral contraceptive formulations available in the United States. Guidelines for use of combination estrogen-progestin contraceptives in women 35 years of age and older are described in Table E1-136
- Mini pill
  - Progestin only; taken without a break
  - Causes much irregular bleeding because of the lack of estrogen effect on the lining of the uterus
  - Table E1-137 provides a summary and recommendations for progestin-only oral contraceptive use
- Hormonal implants and injectables
  - Implanon/Nexplanon
    - Single etonogestrol-secreting device that is inserted underneath the skin
    - Among the most effective contraceptive available
    - Approved by FDA in 2006 and effective over 3-yr period
  - Depo-Provera
    - Medroxyprogesterone acetate given every 3 mo in IM injection form
    - Major side effect: irregular bleeding
    - Fertility return possibly delayed up to 1 year or longer after last injection
    - Table E1-138 provides a summary and recommendations for depot medroxyprogesterone acetate (DMPA) use
  - Lunelle: monthly injectable administered intramuscularly. Contains 0.5 ml aqueous, 5 mg estradiol cypionate, and 25 mg medroxyprogesterone acetate
- Postcoital contraception
  - Done on emergency basis, usually as a result of noncompliance with birth control or failure of birth control (e.g., condom breakage) at the time of ovulation
  - Methods:
    - Hormonal methods
      - Levonorgestrel is available either as two 0.75 mg tablets taken 12 hr apart (next choice) or as a 1.5 mg tablet taken once (Plan B, one step). It is indicated for emergency contraception to be used within 72 hr after unexpected intercourse. It can be obtained OTC by women >15 yr of age and by prescription by younger patients
      - Ulipristal (ELLA) is a progesterone-receptor agonist/antagonist available by prescription only. It is a 30-mg, single-dose tablet and can be taken up to 5 days after unexpected intercourse
    - Copper IUD insertion within 5 days of coitus
- IUD
  - Device inserted into uterus to prevent sperm and ovum from uniting in fallopian tube
  - Types available in the U.S.:
    - ParaGard (Copper T/30-A): a polyethylene T wrapped with a fine copper wire effective for 10 yr
    - Mirena Levonorgestrel Intrauterine System: a T-shaped system with a chamber that contains levonorgestrel. Releases 20 mcg/day; is effective for 5 yr
- Vaginal ring (NuvaRing)
  - Provides daily dose of 120 mcg of etonogestrel and 15 mcg ethinyl estradiol
  - Stays in vagina 3 wk and is removed the fourth for a contraceptive-free interval analogous to the placebo pills in oral contraceptive pills
  - Increased body weight decreases effectiveness
- Contraceptive patch (Ortho-Evra)
  - Provides low daily dose of steroids
  - Releases a progestin and estrogen (ethinyl estradiol)
  - Patch size 20 cm^2
  - Each patch contains 6 mg norelgestromin and delivers an estimated continuous systemic dose of 150 mcg norelgestromin and 20 mcg of ethinyl estradiol; common dose 250 mcg/day progestin and 25 mcg/day estrogen
  - Worn 3 out of 4 wk
  - Increased body weight decreases effectiveness
  - Concern for increased risk of thromboembolic events

CHRONIC Rx

- With all the previously mentioned types of birth control, patient is followed up at least yearly, or as necessary, if problems arise.
- Full history, physical examination, and Pap smear, including cultures when needed, are performed yearly.
- Patients with medical problems are followed up approximately every 6 mo when taking hormonal therapy.

DISPOSITION

- Follow yearly or more frequently according to patient's side effects.
- Tailor birth control to patient according to different needs or side effects present at different times in life. Effective counseling also requires an understanding of a woman's preference and medical risks, benefits, side effects, and contraindications of each contraceptive method.

COMMENTS

- With hormonal contraception, if neurologic or cardiac symptoms arise, stop method immediately, evaluate, and refer to internist when appropriate.
- The effectiveness of long-actiing reversible contraception (IUDs and implants) is superior to that of contraceptive pills, patch, or ring and is not altered in adolescents and young women.

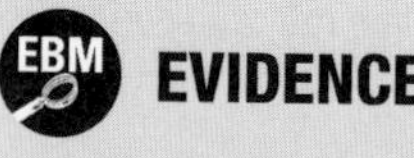

EVIDENCE

available at www.expertconsult.com

SUGGESTED READINGS

available at www.expertconsult.com

RELATED CONTENT

Contraception (Patient Information)

AUTHOR: **RUBEN ALVERO, M.D.**

BASIC INFORMATION

DEFINITION

Conversion disorder (functional neurologic symptom disorder) is a diagnosis of exclusion that presents with one or more symptoms of altered voluntary motor or sensory function that cannot be explained by medical evaluation or a culturally sanctioned behavior or experience. The symptom or deficit is not intentionally produced, distinguishing conversion disorder from factitious disorder or malingering. Conversion disorder is usually characterized by a single symptom that is sporadic, such as paralysis, blindness, numbness, or the inability to speak. Symptoms are preceded by a psychological conflict or stressor that may or may not be remembered and may have happened recently or in the distant past. The conversion symptom is presumed to express and manage the psychological distress, or "convert" the distress into a neurologic symptom. There is no well-validated physiologic model for conversion disorder, but advances in neuroscience and neuroimaging may reveal new etiologies.

SYNONYMS

Dissociative conversion
Hysterical neurosis
Medically unexplained symptom
Psychogenic, nonorganic, or functional symptom

ICD-9CM and DSM-5 CODES
300.01
ICD-10CM CODES

F44-F44.7	(depending on symptoms)
F44.9	Dissociative (conversion) disorder, unspecified

EPIDEMIOLOGY & DEMOGRAPHICS

- Incidence ~5-10/100,000 in general population, 20-100/100,000 in hospital inpatients
- All ages, including early childhood
- Associated with axis I (depression more than anxiety) and axis II disorders (most commonly histrionic, passive dependent, and passive aggressive)

PHYSICAL FINDINGS & CLINICAL PRESENTATION

- Presents with a motor symptom (e.g., paralysis, aphonia, difficulty swallowing), a sensory symptom (loss of sensation, double vision, blindness, deafness), a psychogenic seizure, or "mixed" (symptoms from >1 category).
- Physical exam findings that are incompatible with neurologic diseases, such as Hoover sign (weakness of hip extension returns to normal strength with contralateral hip flexion against resistance), weakness of plantar flexion on the exam table in an individual able to walk on tiptoes, positive tremor entrainment test, normal EEG or closed eyes with resistance to opening during non-epileptic seizure, or tunnel vision.
- Symptoms tend to occur in isolation (compared with multisystem involvement in somatization disorder).
- The symptoms or signs persist whether the patient is observed or unobserved, though are typically worse when the patient is attentive to them.
- May last from hr to yr and usually sporadic.
- May occur in the context of documented medical illness (e.g., a patient with epileptic seizure may also have psychogenic seizure).
- May have comorbid axis I or axis II disorders, commonly depression, panic attacks, generalized anxiety, and PTSD.

ETIOLOGY

- Complex interplay of neurologic and psychologic factors is not well-understood.
- Presumed to be preceded by psychological conflict or stressor that is completely or partially unconscious.
- Functional brain imaging studies suggest alterations in processing of sensory and motor signals.

DIAGNOSIS

Diagnosis is specific to symptom type:
- Weakness or paralysis
- Abnormal movement (tremor, dystonic movement, myoclonus, gait disorder)
- Swallowing symptom
- Speech symptom (e.g., dysphonia, slurred speech)
- Seizure
- Anesthesia or sensory loss
- Special sensory symptom (e.g., visual, olfactory, auditory)
- Mixed symptoms

DIFFERENTIAL DIAGNOSIS

Broad differential diagnosis depending on presenting signs and symptoms, including neurologic disease (e.g., multiple sclerosis, CNS neoplasm, myasthenia gravis, Guillain-Barré syndrome, amyotrophic lateral sclerosis, Parkinson's disease, seizure disorder, systemic lupus erythematosus, spinal cord compression, intracerebral infarct, drug-induced dystonia, and HIV); somatic symptom disorder; factitious disorder and malingering; dissociative disorders; body dysmorphic disorders; depressive disorders; panic disorders.

LABORATORY TESTS

- No gold standard diagnostic tests exist; no single finding is pathognomonic.
- Laboratory tests or procedures may be needed to rule out other medical conditions (e.g., EEG for seizures, EMG for lower motor neuron paralysis, optokinetic drum test in blindness).

TREATMENT

NONPHARMACOLOGIC THERAPY

- Cognitive behavioral therapy is often the treatment of choice, although evidence is mixed.
- A long tradition of psychodynamic therapy exists but has not been validated by controlled trials.
- Treatment success has been associated with a caring, long-term relationship between patient and physician and a safe, nonconfrontational approach, with the exception of psychogenic seizure for which empathic confrontation and acceptance of disease is advocated as a foundation of treatment.
- Physical and occupational therapy can help "retrain" the patient in normal behaviors and is important for maintaining strength and function in extended cases of paralysis.
- Studies have shown no additional benefit to hypnosis, although case records describe successful treatment with hypnosis.

GENERAL Rx

- Antidepressants may be helpful for underlying mood or anxiety disorders.
- Longstanding symptoms may require inpatient treatment.

DISPOSITION

Long-term follow-up essential for recurrent conversion symptoms and underlying mood disorders.

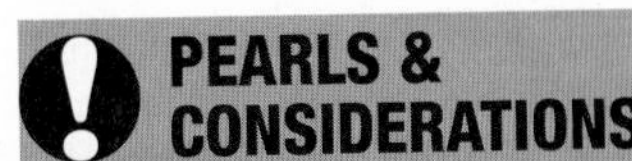

PEARLS & CONSIDERATIONS

COMMENTS

- Good prognostic factors: sudden onset, presence of psychological stressors at onset, short duration between diagnosis and treatment, high level of intelligence, absence of other psychiatric or medical disorders.
- Poor prognostic factors: severe disability, long duration of symptoms, age >40 yr at onset, and convulsions or paralysis as presenting symptoms.
- Differentiation between conversion, somatization, dissociative, factitious, and malingering disorders, as well as organic versus functional etiologies, may be challenging.
- Studies show an association between sexual trauma and conversion symptoms, although evidence does not support causality because of confounding and methodologic factors.
- Although not well demonstrated, some argue that conversion and somatized symptoms are more prevalent in cultures without an articulated concept of affective disorder or in which mental illness is highly stigmatized.

SUGGESTED READINGS

available at www.expertconsult.com

RELATED CONTENT

Conversion Disorder (Patient Information)

AUTHOR: **KAILA COMPTON, M.D., PH.D.**

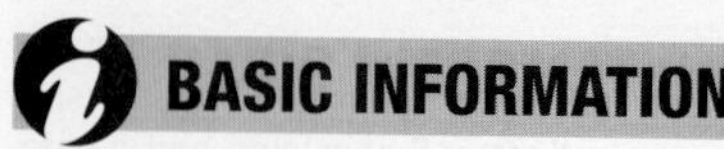

BASIC INFORMATION

DEFINITION

Cor pulmonale is an alteration in the structure and function of the right ventricle (RV) from pulmonary hypertension caused by diseases of the upper or lower airways, lungs, or pulmonary vasculature. It is a state of cardiopulmonary dysfunction that may result from multiple etiologies rather than a specific disease state. Right-sided heart failure resulting from primary disease of the left heart and congenital heart disease are not considered in this disorder.

SYNONYMS

Acute cor pulmonale
Chronic cor pulmonale

ICD-9CM CODES
415.0 Cor pulmonale, acute
416.9 Cor pulmonale, chronic
ICD-10CM CODES
I26.0 Pulmonary embolism with acute cor pulmonale
I27.81 Cor pulmonale (chronic)

ETIOLOGY

Acute cor pulmonale is a disorder in which the right ventricle (RV) is dilated and the muscular wall is stretched thin, usually as a result of acute pulmonary embolism. This may present with often life-threatening cardiogenic shock, or death, but if the patient survives the initial event, then the RV often recovers and cor pulmonale no longer exists after several weeks.

Chronic cor pulmonale is hypertrophy of the right ventricle caused by increased afterload in the pulmonary circuit, resulting in either acute or chronic right ventricular failure depending on the time course of the elevation in pulmonary vascular resistance. Mechanisms leading to pulmonary hypertension and thus predisposing to the development of cor pulmonale include:

- Pulmonary vasoconstriction leading to increased RV afterload, often resulting from conditions causing alveolar hypoxia and/or respiratory acidosis (e.g., high altitude/hypobaric hypoxia, obstructive sleep apnea/obesity-hypoventilation syndrome, chronic obstructive pulmonary disease). In pulmonary arterial hypertension (PAH), pulmonary vasoconstriction may occur in the absence of a primary cause of hypoxemia, due to imbalances between vasoconstrictor and vasodilator expression in the pulmonary circulation.
- Anatomic reduction or remodeling of the pulmonary vascular bed leading to increased RV afterload (e.g., emphysema, interstitial lung disease, pulmonary emboli, pulmonary arterial hypertension)
- Increased blood viscosity leading to increased RV afterload (e.g., polycythemia related to chronic hypoxemia, polycythemia vera, Waldenström's macroglobulinemia)
- Chronic thrombotic and/or embolic disease

PHYSICAL FINDINGS & CLINICAL PRESENTATION

No symptoms are specific for cor pulmonale. Typically, the symptoms depend on the underlying disease process. The symptoms are most often a result of right ventricular failure:

- Dyspnea, fatigue, chest pain, or syncope with exertion (from pulmonary hypertension, RV ischemia, and impaired cardiac output)
- Right upper quadrant abdominal pain and anorexia (from passive hepatic congestion)
- Hoarseness (caused by compression of the left recurrent laryngeal nerve by dilation of the main pulmonary artery; known as *Ortner's syndrome*)
- Signs of right ventricular failure: jugular venous distention, peripheral edema, hepatic congestion, ascites, and a right ventricular third heart sound
- Signs of associated tricuspid regurgitation: holosystolic murmur heard best along the left parasternal border (augments during inspiration), prominent V-wave on jugular venous pulse, and pulsatile hepatomegaly (in severe tricuspid regurgitation)
- Pulmonary hypertension will increase the intensity of the pulmonic component of S2, which may be narrowly split
- Rarely, cough and hemoptysis

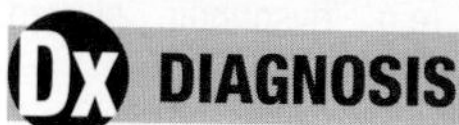

DIAGNOSIS

WORKUP

Search for an underlying pulmonary process resulting in pulmonary hypertension:

- Left ventricular dysfunction should be excluded in initial assessment with an echocardiogram.
- Worldwide, chronic mountain sickness is an important cause of cor pulmonale.
- 80% to 90% of cor pulmonale cases are attributable to chronic obstructive pulmonary disease (COPD) and should include complete pulmonary function tests (PFTs).
- Consideration of obstructive sleep apnea, chronic thromboembolic disease, pulmonary arterial hypertension, and musculoskeletal disease should be given in the absence of parenchymal lung disease.

LABORATORY TESTS

- Complete blood count may show erythrocytosis from chronic hypoxia.
- Arterial blood gas levels confirm hypoxemia and acidosis or hypercapnia.
- BNP may be elevated from RV dilation.
- Connective tissue disorder workup to exclude scleroderma, lupus, rheumatoid arthritis
- HIV testing

IMAGING STUDIES

- Chest radiograph may show underlying pulmonary disease and evidence of pulmonary hypertension (e.g., enlargement of the pulmonary arteries or right atrium and right ventricular dilation or "pruning" of the peripheral vasculature) (Fig. 1-276).
- ECG may reveal right ventricular hypertrophy with R/S ratio >1 in leads V_1 and R/S ratio <1 in leads V_5,V_6, right atrial enlargement (P-pulmonale), right-axis deviation, or the triad of $S_1Q_3T_3$ indicative of RV strain.
- Echocardiogram to detect right ventricular enlargement and/or hypertrophy and estimate pulmonary artery pressure.
- Perfusion scintigraphy (VQ scan) to rule out chronic thromboembolic pulmonary hypertension (CTEPH)
- Cardiac MRI can accurately measure right ventricular dimensions and function.
- Right-sided heart catheterization measures pulmonary artery pressures and pulmonary vascular resistance. It can also determine response to oxygen or vasodilators.

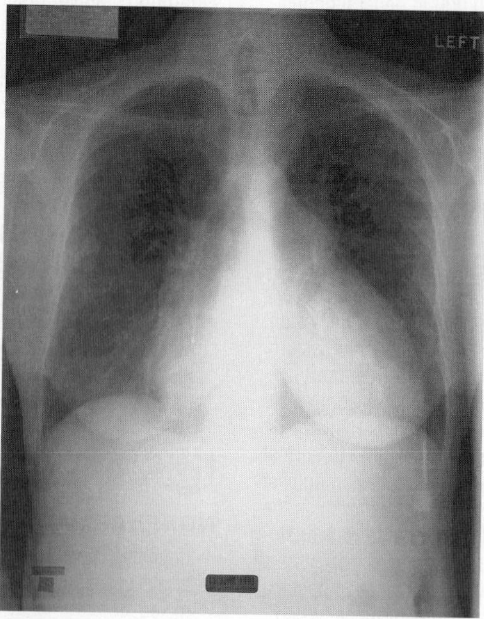

FIGURE 1-276 Chest radiography in a patient with severe intrinsic pulmonary vascular disease demonstrating enlargement of the main pulmonary artery, right ventricle, and right atrium. (From Crawford MH et al [eds]: *Cardiology,* ed 2, St Louis, 2004, Mosby.)

Importantly, right heart catheterization allows assessment of pulmonary capillary wedge pressure, allowing right heart failure from pulmonary venous hypertension due to left heart disease to be ruled out.

- Chest CT can assess for pulmonary parenchymal disease and embolus in the pulmonary vasculature.

Rx TREATMENT

The treatment of cor pulmonale is directed toward the underlying etiology while also reversing hypoxemia, improving right ventricular contractility, decreasing pulmonary artery vascular resistance, and improving pulmonary hypertension

NONPHARMACOLOGIC THERAPY

- Supplemental oxygen to correct hypoxemia is an important management step in the treatment of cor pulmonale related to hypoxemia. Goal O_2 sat of more than 90% is recommended.
- Continuous positive airway pressure is used in patients with obstructive sleep apnea.
- Sodium and fluid restriction in setting of edema from RV failure
- Phlebotomy is reserved as adjunctive therapy in patients with polycythemia (hematocrit >55%) who have acute decompensation of cor pulmonale or remain polycythemic despite long-term oxygen therapy. Phlebotomy has been shown to decrease mean pulmonary artery pressure and pulmonary vascular resistance.
- Low-level aerobic exercise, avoiding heavy physical exercise, or isometric exercises that may cause syncope

ACUTE GENERAL Rx

- Pulmonary embolism is the most common cause of acute cor pulmonale (see "Pulmonary Embolism"). The treatment is anticoagulation, hemodynamic support, and consideration of thrombolytics. Catheter-based thrombectomy or surgical embolectomy are potential salvage therapies in patients who cannot receive anticoagulation or thrombolysis, or whose condition continues to deteriorate despite thrombolytics and anticoagulation.
- Acute cor pulmonale may also be seen in cases of acute respiratory distress syndrome (ARDS), related to hypercapnia/acidosis, hypoxic pulmonary vasoconstriction, and the effects of mechanical ventilation. The treatment is supportive care for ARDS with low tidal volume ventilation. Extracorporeal membrane oxygen support (ECMO) while awaiting lung recovery from ARDS may also be helpful in maintaining blood oxygenation. Venoarterial ECMO can provide hemodynamic support as well as blood oxygenation.
- In patients with preexisting cor pulmonale, acute pulmonary illnesses or hypoxia can increase pulmonary hypertension and worsen right ventricular function. The underlying exacerbating conditions should be treated.
- Careful attention to fluid balance is important in the management of acute decompensated right heart failure. Both overhydration and overdiuresis should be avoided, with careful monitoring of intake and output, electrolytes and creatinine, and hemodynamics.
- Intravenous inotropes may be employed to support right heart contractility in decompensated right heart failure.
- In acutely decompensated right heart failure due to pulmonary arterial hypertension, IV prostanoid medications are the treatment of choice. Oral pulmonary vasodilators may also be added to the IV prostanoids, but should not be initiated as monotherapy in patients with advanced right heart failure from PAH.

CHRONIC RX

- Long-term oxygen supplementation improves survival in hypoxemic patients with COPD. Indications for oxygen in COPD patients include the following:
  1. Resting PaO_2 ≤55 mm Hg on arterial blood gas
  2. Resting PaO 56–59 mm Hg if clinical presence of right heart failure with dependent edema, P pulmonale on EKG
  3. Desaturation to SpO_2 ≤88% on oximetry with activity or at night
- Right ventricular volume overload should be treated with loop diuretics (e.g., furosemide) and potassium-sparing diuretics such as spironolactone.
- Anticoagulation with warfarin has been shown to have a proven survival benefit in patients with idiopathic pulmonary arterial hypertension and is recommended in other causes of cor pulmonale as well, with a target international normalized ratio (INR) of 1.5-2.5, unlike the target for thromboembolic disease, provided there are no obvious contraindications to long-term anticoagulation but can cause toxicity and arrhythmias.
- Digoxin, though controversial, may be employed as an oral inotropic agent to improve right heart contractility and control atrial arrhythmias.
- Selective oral or parenteral pulmonary vasodilators such as oral calcium channel blockers (CCBs), prostanoids, and endothelin receptor blockers may be used after a right heart catheterization that establishes pulmonary hypertension. If vasoreactivity to calcium channel blockers is established, CCBs may be used to combat pulmonary hypertension. However, if there is no vasoreactivity, prostanoids such as epoprostenol or treprostinil or endothelin receptor blockers such as bosentan may be tried. However, such agents have been shown to be beneficial in the treatment of idiopathic PAH, PAH related to connective tissue disease, and PAH due to congenital heart disease. Pulmonary vasodilators are sometimes considered in other forms of PAH when primary disease management strategies have failed to improve right heart failure.
- Phosphodiesterase inhibitors such as sildenafil and tadalafil are newer vasodilators that improve symptoms, functional class, and mean pulmonary artery pressures as alternatives or in addition to prostanoids.
- Pulmonary thrombendarterectomy may be curative in the special case of cor pulmonale due to chronic thromboembolic pulmonary hypertension.
- Atrial septostomy is a salvage option for patients with ongoing decompensated right heart failure from PAH despite pulmonary vasodilators. Such patients should undergo rapid assessment for possible transplantation.
- Lung transplantation or heart-lung transplantation should be considered in the setting of cor pulmonale from lung diseases or from pulmonary vascular disease.

DISPOSITION

Patients with cor pulmonale should have regular assessment of their functional class (e.g., NYHA or WHO functional class); worse functional class indicates a poorer prognosis. Other poor prognostic features include high right atrial pressure, impaired cardiac output, presence of hyponatremia, elevated BNP levels, low systemic blood pressure, and poor exercise tolerance as demonstrated by a 6-minute walk test.

REFERRAL

Patients with pulmonary disease who have progressed to cor pulmonale should be followed up by a pulmonologist and a tertiary care center that specializes in treatment of advanced pulmonary hypertension.

PEARLS & CONSIDERATIONS

- Identification and treatment of the underlying cause of cor pulmonale is key
- Prognosis and treatment are related to the underlying cause, whereas the presence of cor pulmonale is merely a marker of the underlying disease severity.
- Right heart catheterization is the gold standard to establish diagnosis and to determine treatment, including response to calcium channel blockers, prostanoids, and endothelin endothelin receptor blockers.

COMMENTS

There is increasing interest in selective pulmonary vasodilators to improve right ventricular heart function in patients with cor pulmonale outside of the setting of idiopathic PAH, PAH related to connective tissue disease, and PAH related to congenital heart disease. However, more data on the safety and efficacy of these agents, especially in the setting of hypoxemic lung disease, is needed.

The importance of maintaining or improving right heart function, rather than solely lowering pulmonary pressures, is becoming increasingly apparent in the therapeutic management of patients with pulmonary hypertension and right heart failure.

SUGGESTED READINGS

available at www.expertconsult.com

AUTHOR: **RABIA ARSHAD, M.D.**

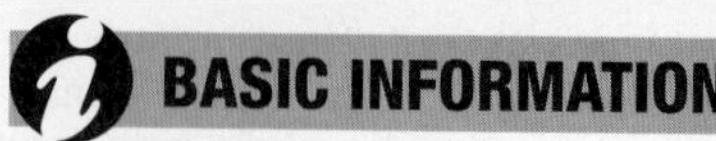

BASIC INFORMATION

DEFINITION

A corneal abrasion is a loss of surface epithelial tissue of the cornea caused by trauma.

SYNONYMS

Corneal erosion
Corneal contusion

ICD-9CM CODES
918.1 Corneal abrasion
ICD-10CM CODES
S05.00XA Injury of conjunctiva and corneal abrasion without foreign body, unspecified eye, initial encounter

EPIDEMIOLOGY & DEMOGRAPHICS

INCIDENCE (IN U.S.): A universal problem. Corneal abrasions comprise 8% of all eye presentations in primary care.
PEAK INCIDENCE: Childhood through active adulthood and older and debilitated patients
PREDOMINANT AGE: Any age

PHYSICAL FINDINGS & CLINICAL PRESENTATION

- Haziness of the cornea
- Disruption of the corneal surface (Fig. 1-277)
- Redness and injection of the conjunctiva
- Pain
- Light sensitivity
- Tearing
- Gritty feeling
- Pain on opening or closing eyes
- Sensation of a foreign body

ETIOLOGY

- Trauma (direct mechanical event)
- Foreign body
- Contact lenses
- Chemical or flash ultraviolet burns

Dx DIAGNOSIS

DIFFERENTIAL DIAGNOSIS

- Acute-angle glaucoma
- Herpes ulcers and other corneal ulcers
- Foreign body in the cornea (be certain it is not a keratitis)
- Infective keratitis

WORKUP

- Fluorescein staining, slit lamp evaluation. After fluorescein staining of the cornea, an abrasion will appear yellow under normal light and green in cobalt blue light.
- Assessment of visual acuity. Vision loss of more than 20/40 requires referral.
- Intraocular pressure
- Rule out corneal laceration
- Rule out other eye pathology. Inspect anterior chamber for blood (hyphema) or pus (hypopyon). If present, refer immediately to ophthalmologist.
- Examine for foreign bodies and remove them if present.
- Confirm red reflex to rule out significant globe injury.

Rx TREATMENT

NONPHARMACOLOGIC THERAPY

- Bandage contact lens can help to speed healing for large epithelial abrasions.
- Warm compresses.
- Pressure dressing (patching) is controversial. Although eye patching traditionally has been recommended in the treatment of corneal abrasions, several studies show that patching does not help and may hinder healing.
- Removal of any foreign particles if present.

ACUTE GENERAL Rx

- Topical antibiotics such as 10% sulfacetamide or ofloxacin 0.3% solution 2 drops qid are commonly prescribed to prevent bacterial superinfection, but evidence for their use is lacking. Ointment forms are often used (e.g., erythromycin, bacitracin ophthalmic QID) to also improve corneal surface lubrication. Antipseudomonal topical antibiotics are, however, recommended for contact lens–related abrasions.
- Pressure patching of eye with eyelid closed is no longer recommended because it can result in decreased oxygen delivery, increased moisture, and a higher chance of infection.
- Cycloplegics such as 5% homatropine are often prescribed to relieve ciliary muscle spasm; however, their benefit has been questioned and they are no longer routinely recommended.
- Topical nonsteroidal anti-inflammatory drugs (NSAIDs) (e.g., diclofenac 0.1% or ketorolac 0.5%) 1 drop qid may be used for pain relief.
- Oral NSAIDs may be used for severe pain.

DISPOSITION

Follow-up in 24 hr and then every 3 days until abrasion has cleared and vision has returned to normal. Less frequent follow-up is appropriate for abrasions ≤4 mm or for uncomplicated abrasions.

REFERRAL

To ophthalmologist if patient has no relief within 24 hr or for patients with deep eye injuries, foreign bodies that cannot be removed, or suspected recurrent corneal erosion.

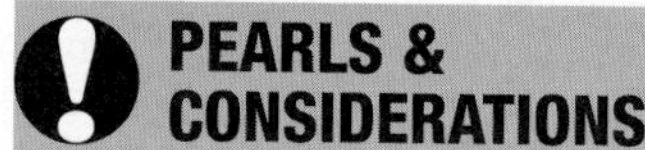

PEARLS & CONSIDERATIONS

COMMENTS

- Never give the patient topical anesthetic to use at home because these can cause decompensation of the cornea, severe delay of epithelial healing, and permanent damage.
- Corticosteroid drops (e.g., dexamethasone, prednisolone) should be avoided, since they can delay healing and exacerbate some corneal infections (herpes viral keratitis, pseudomonas, and fungal ulcers)
- Most corneal abrasions heal in 24 to 48 hr and rarely progress to corneal erosion or infection.
- Improvement in pain is a good indication of corneal epithelial healing. Severe worsening of pain could indicate corneal bacterial infection (keratitis) and should be evaluated urgently.

SUGGESTED READINGS

available at www.expertconsult.com

RELATED CONTENT

Fig. E3-51 Approach to the patient with corneal disorders (Algorithm)
Corneal Foreign Body or Abrasion (Patient Information)

AUTHOR: **MELVYN KOBY, M.D.,** and **R. SCOTT HOFFMAN, M.D.**

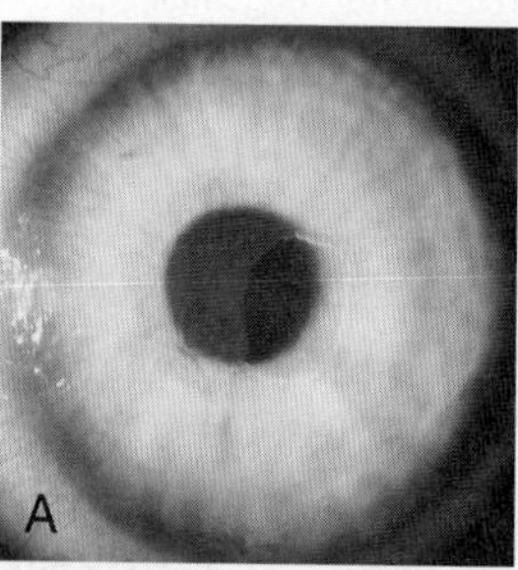

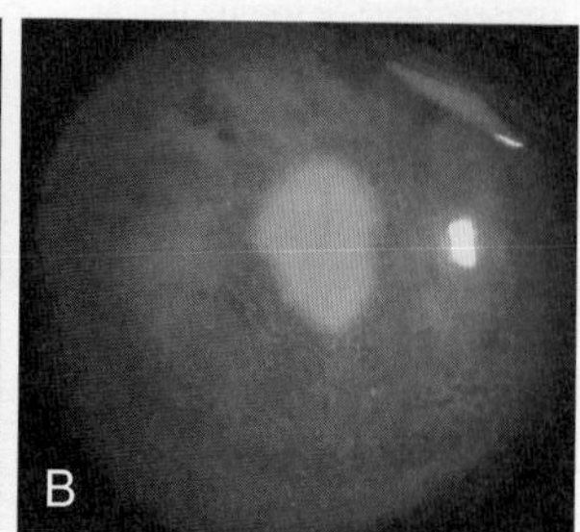

FIGURE 1-277 Corneal epithelial abrasion. A, Epithelial defect without fluorescein highlighting the defect. An irregularity in the otherwise smooth corneal surface is the key to identifying the defect if no fluorescein is available. **B,** Classic fluorescein staining of an epithelial defect. (From Palay D [ed]: *Ophthalmology for the primary care physician,* St Louis, 1997, Mosby.)

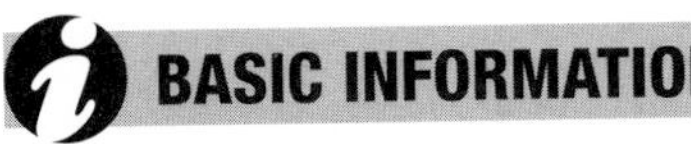

BASIC INFORMATION

DEFINITION

Corneal ulceration refers to the disruption of the corneal surface and/or deeper layers caused by trauma, contact lenses infection, degeneration, or other means.

SYNONYMS

Infectious keratitis with ulceration
Bacterial keratitis with ulceration
Viral keratitis with ulceration
Fungal keratitis with ulceration

ICD-9CM CODES
370.0 Corneal ulcer NOS
ICD-10CM CODES
H16.009 Unspecified corneal ulcer, unspecified eye

EPIDEMIOLOGY & DEMOGRAPHICS

INCIDENCE (IN U.S.): Four to six cases per month seen by an average general ophthalmologist
PREVALENCE (IN U.S.): Common
PREDOMINANT SEX: Either
PREDOMINANT AGE: All ages

PHYSICAL FINDINGS & CLINICAL PRESENTATION

- Localized, well-demarcated, infiltrative lesion with corresponding focal ulcer (Fig. 1-278) or oval, yellow-white stromal suppuration with thick mucopurulent exudate and edema. Usually red, angry-looking eye with infiltration in surrounding area of cornea.
- Eye possibly painful, with conjunctival edema and infection (pain is a helpful indicator of progression or improvement in infectious keratitis).
- Sterile neurotrophic ulcers with tissue breakdown and no pain.

ETIOLOGY

- Complication of contact lens wear, trauma, or diseases such as herpes simplex keratitis or keratoconjunctivitis sicca. Often associated with collagen vascular disease and severe exophthalmus and thyroid disease.
- Viral causes often contagious.

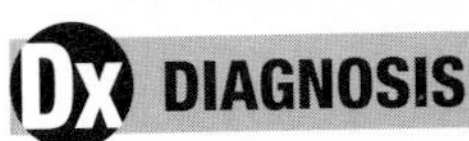

DIAGNOSIS

DIFFERENTIAL DIAGNOSIS

- *Pseudomonas* and pneumococcus and other bacterial infection—virulent
- *Moraxella, Staphylococcus, α-Streptococcus* infection—less virulent
- Herpes simplex infection or disease caused by other viruses
- Contact lens ulcers differ
- Autoimmune keratitis (e.g., peripheral ulceration with RA, SLE)
- Acute angle closure glaucoma

WORKUP

- Fluorescein staining, slit lamp
- Appearance often typical
- Differentiate carefully with contact lens wearers
- Note previous eye surgery or laser vision correction

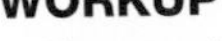

LABORATORY TESTS

Microscopic examination and culture of scrapings are indicated for vision-threatening keratitis (lesions are large or central location in the cornea)

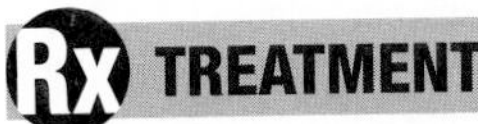

TREATMENT

NONPHARMACOLOGIC THERAPY

- Warm compresses for blepharitis, eyelid hygiene
- Bandage contact lenses
- Patching
- Stop contact lens wearing

ACUTE GENERAL Rx

- An ophthalmic emergency, refer to ophthalmologist same day
- Intense antibiotic and antiviral therapy may be needed for infectious keratitis
- Topical antibiotics (often broad coverage, new generation fluoroquinolones)
- Nonsteroidal anti-inflammatory drugs and cycloplegic may help with comfort
- Bacterial infection: subconjunctival cefazolin or gentamicin (topical Zymar, Vigomax, etc.)
- Fungal infection: hospitalization and topical application of antifungal agents
- Herpes: viral keratitis can have similar symptoms, should avoid steroid drops unless diagnosis is near certain and showing improvement, since viral keratitis can worsen with steroid

DISPOSITION

Ideally treated by an ophthalmologist if the patient does not rapidly respond to antibiotics (within 24 hr)

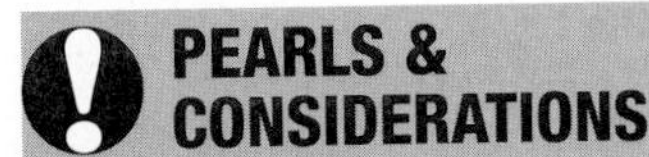

PEARLS & CONSIDERATIONS

- Always stop contact lens wearing.
- Always refer ulcers to ophthalmologist.
- Never treat with topical anesthetics or steroids.

COMMENTS

Do not use topical steroids because herpes, fungal, or other ulcers may be aggravated, leading to perforation of the cornea. Antibiotics may delay response and result in overgrowth of nonbacterial (fungal and amoebic) pathogens.

SUGGESTED READINGS

available at www.expertconsult.com

RELATED CONTENT

Fig. E3-51 Approach to the patient with corneal disorders (Algorithm)

AUTHORS: **MELVYN KOBY, M.D.,** and **R. SCOTT HOFFMAN, M.D.**

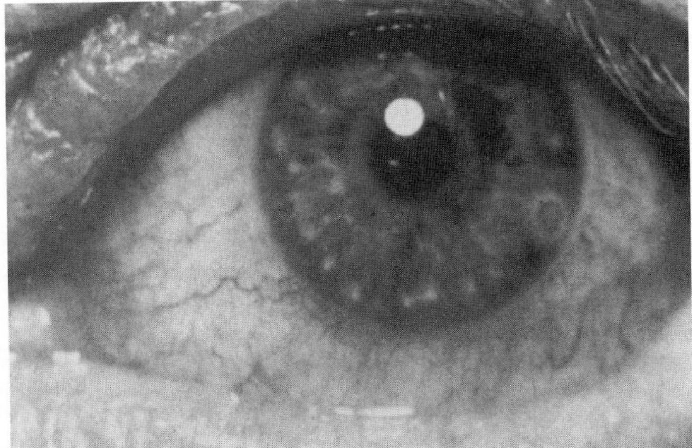

FIGURE 1-278 Peripherally located corneal ulcer. (From Marx JA [ed]: *Rosen's emergency medicine,* ed 5, St Louis, 2002, Mosby.)

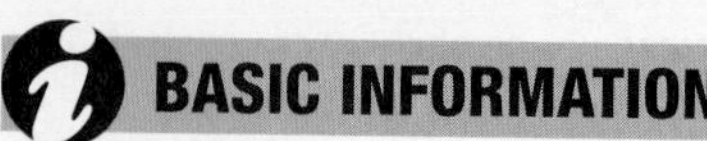

BASIC INFORMATION

DEFINITION

Coronary artery disease (CAD) is a clinical syndrome that suggests limitation of coronary blood flow to the myocardium as a result of flow-limiting atherosclerotic lesions. It is characterized by exertional symptoms as described below.

This topic addresses only stable CAD. Acute coronary syndromes (ACS), angina pectoris, and myocardial infarction are addressed as separate topics elsewhere.

SYNONYMS

Atherosclerotic heart disease
CAD
Chronic stable angina
Stable ischemic heart disease

ICD-9CM CODE
414.01 Coronary atherosclerosis of native coronary artery
ICD-10CM CODE
I25.1 Atherosclerotic heart disease
I25.0 Atherosclerotic cardiovascular disease

EPIDEMIOLOGY & DEMOGRAPHICS

INCIDENCE: Increases with age
PEAK INCIDENCE: Increases in age in women but peaks in men between the ages of 55 and 65 years
PREVALENCE: 1 in 3 adults in the United States have some form of cardiovascular disease. There were 380,000 deaths in the United States in 2010.
PREDOMINANT SEX AND AGE: Male predominance, no predominant age
GENETICS: Not applicable
RISK FACTORS: Age, male sex, hypertension, hyperlipidemia, diabetes mellitus, obesity, tobacco use, family history, claudication

PHYSICAL FINDINGS & CLINICAL PRESENTATION

- Left anterior chest discomfort often described as squeezing, choking, heavy, and occasionally hot or cold sensations
- Associated symptoms include fatigue, dyspnea, weakness, lightheadedness, nausea, diaphoresis, altered mental status, and syncope.
- Typically lasts 3 to 5 minutes but usually does not last more than 30 minutes
- Women and diabetics may not present with classic symptoms.
- Elicited by physical exertion, emotional stress, cold exposure, consumption of heavy meal, smoking
- Radiation to the neck, shoulder, arm, jaws, epigastrium, or back

ETIOLOGY

- Myocardial ischemia caused by the impairment of coronary blood flow secondary to coronary atherosclerosis that has built up over decades

Dx DIAGNOSIS

DIFFERENTIAL DIAGNOSIS

- Cardiovascular causes
  - Aortic dissection
  - Pericarditis
  - Pulmonary embolism
- Pulmonary causes
  - Pneumothorax
  - Pneumonia
  - Pleuritis
- Gastrointestinal causes
  - Esophageal spasm
  - Esophagitis
  - GERD
  - Cholecystitis
  - Choledocholithiasis
  - Cholangitis
  - Peptic ulcer
  - Pancreatitis
  - Costochondritis
- Chest wall causes
  - Rib fracture
  - Sternoclavicular arthritis
  - Herpes zoster
- Psychiatric causes
  - Anxiety disorders

WORKUP

- See Fig. 1-279

LABORATORY TESTS

- Basic metabolic panel is helpful to rule out noncardiac causes.
- Complete blood count can help rule out anemia-related chest discomfort.
- Fasting cholesterol panel is important in assessment of control of lipid-related risk factors.
- Hemoglobin A1c is important to follow glycemic control.

IMAGING STUDIES

- Electrocardiogram is important for assessing for prior cardiac injury.
- Exercise treadmill stress test is the gold standard to assess physiologic cardiac stress response.
- Stress tests combined with imaging is the next best option if ETT cannot be performed due to physical limitation or if baseline ECG is abnormal.
- Echocardiogram to assess left ventricular ejection fraction (LVEF)
- Those with high-risk features (Box 1-17) should undergo coronary angiography to assess coronary anatomy for revascularization.
- Cardiac computed tomography angiography is an emerging imaging modality that can be considered as an alternative to stress testing.
- Coronary angiography is useful for both diagnostic and therapeutic interventions if symptoms change or cardiac injury is evident.

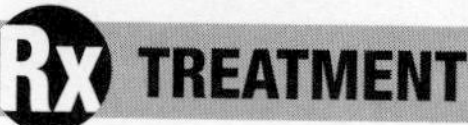

Rx TREATMENT

- See Fig. 1-280
- Successful treatment of CAD entails minimizing the likelihood of death while maximizing health and function.

NONPHARMACOLOGIC THERAPY

- 20-30 minutes of aerobic exercise most days of the week
- Mediterranean diet has been studied and has demonstrated benefit in outcomes.
- Smoking cessation
- Weight reduction can reduce various risk factors with improved lipid and glycemic control.
- Enhanced external counterpulsation is used for refractory cases.
- Transmyocardial laser revascularization (TMLR) may relieve symptoms in refractory angina. The mechanics by which TMLR reduces angina is not well understood.
- Coronary angiography with PCI or CABG for patients on optimal medical therapy with persistent symptoms

ACUTE GENERAL Rx

- Rest
- Sublingual nitroglycerin if rest does not provide adequate relief

CHRONIC Rx

- Antianginal therapy
  - Nitrates (isosorbide mononitrate and isosorbide dinitrate). These medications treat ischemia by venodilation to decrease preload, dilate epicardial coronary arteries, and recruit coronary collaterals. Furthermore, they attenuate platelet aggregation. Although they do not influence survival or decrease cardiovascular death in patients with chronic CAD, they do lower the rate of angina frequency and increase time to ischemic ECG findings on treadmill testing.
  - Beta-adrenergic antagonists (metoprolol, atenolol, carvedilol, or any other beta-blockers with the exception of those with intrinsic sympathomimetic activity). Drugs should be titrated to a heart rate of ≤60 beats/min at rest and ≤75 beats/min with exertion.
  - Calcium channel blockers (CCBs; amlodipine or verapamil). The antianginal efficacy of CCBs is comparable to beta-blockers; however, the efficacy of monotherapy for reducing MI or cardiac death has not been demonstrated.
  - Ranolazine. This is a selective inhibitor of late sodium influx into myocytes, which leads to decreased myocardial contractility. It can be used in combination with beta-blockers and significantly reduced time to onset of angina and exercise performance (CARISA trial). Although it rarely may cause QT prolongation, it has not been linked to any clinically important arrhythmias.
  - May benefit from combination therapy of the above

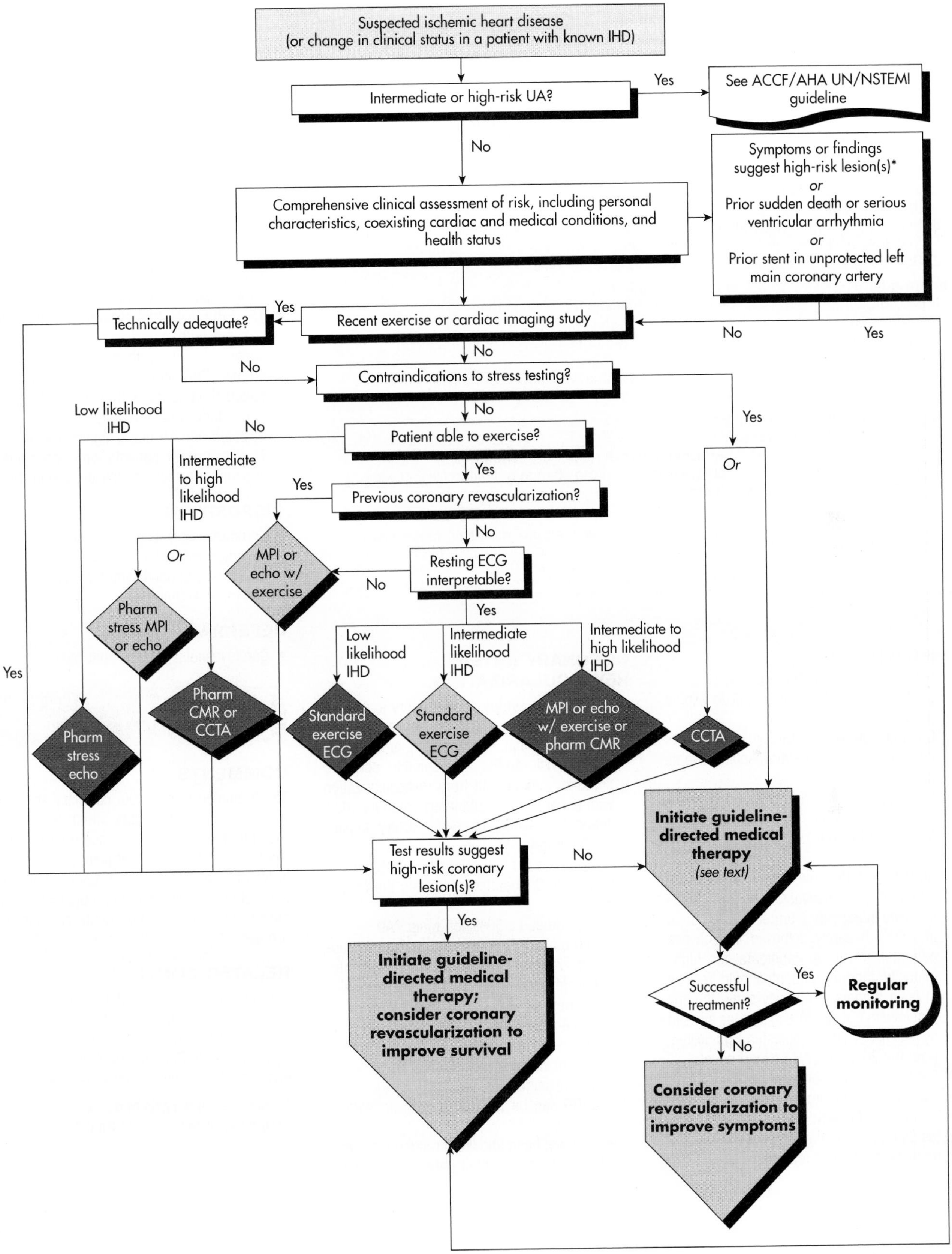

Suspected ischemic heart disease (or change in clinical status in a patient with known IHD)

Intermediate or high-risk UA?

Yes

See ACCF/AHA UN/NSTEMI guideline

No

Comprehensive clinical assessment of risk, including personal characteristics, coexisting cardiac and medical conditions, and health status

Symptoms or findings suggest high-risk lesion(s)*
or
Prior sudden death or serious ventricular arrhythmia
or
Prior stent in unprotected left main coronary artery

No

Yes

Recent exercise or cardiac imaging study

Yes

Technically adequate?

Yes

No

No

Contraindications to stress testing?

Yes

Or

No

Patient able to exercise?

Low likelihood IHD

No

Intermediate to high likelihood IHD

Or

Yes

Previous coronary revascularization?

Yes

No

Resting ECG interpretable?

No

MPI or echo w/ exercise

Pharm stress MPI or echo

Pharm CMR or CCTA

Pharm stress echo

Yes

Low likelihood IHD

Intermediate likelihood IHD

Intermediate to high likelihood IHD

Standard exercise ECG

Standard exercise ECG

MPI or echo w/ exercise or pharm CMR

CCTA

Test results suggest high-risk coronary lesion(s)?

No

Initiate guideline-directed medical therapy (see text)

Yes

Initiate guideline-directed medical therapy; consider coronary revascularization to improve survival

Successful treatment?

Yes

Regular monitoring

No

Consider coronary revascularization to improve symptoms

FIGURE 1-279 Diagnosis of patients with suspected ischemic heart disease.

*CCTA is reasonable only for patients with intermediate probability of IHD. CCTA, Computed coronary tomography angiography; CMR, cardiac magnetic resonance; ECG, electrocardiogram; Echo, echocardiography; IHD, ischemic heart disease; MI, myocardial infarction; MPI, myocardial perfusion imaging; Pharm, pharmacologic; UA, unstable angina; and UA/NSTEMI, unstable angina/non–ST-elevation myocardial infarction. (From 2012 ACCF/AHA/ACP/AATS/PCNA/SCAI/STS Guideline for the Diagnosis and Management of Patients With Stable Ischemic Heart Disease: A report of the American College of Cardiology Foundation/American Heart Association Task Force on Practice Guidelines, and the American College of Physicians, American Association for Thoracic Surgery, Preventive Cardiovascular Nurses Association, Society for Cardiovascular Angiography and Interventions, and Society of Thoracic Surgeons, *J Am Coll Cardiol* 60:e44-e164, 2012.)

 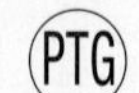

BOX 1-17 Noninvasive Risk Stratification

High risk (>3% annual mortality rate)
1. Severe resting left ventricular dysfunction (LVEF<35%)
2. High-risk treadmill score (≤-11)
3. Severe exercise left ventricular dysfunction (exercise LVEF <35%)
4. Stress-induced large perfusion defect (particularly if anterior)
5. Stress-induced multiple perfusion defects of moderate size
6. Large, fixed perfusion defect with LV dilation or increased lung uptake (thallium-201)
7. Stress-induced moderate perfusion defect with LV dilation or increased lung uptake (thallium-201)
8. Echocardiographic wall motion abnormality (involving >2 segments) developing at low dose of dobutamine (≤10 mg/kg/min) or at a low heart rate (<120 beats/min)
9. Stress echocardiographic evidence of extensive ischemia

Intermediate risk (1% to 3% annual mortality rate)
1. Mild/moderate resting left ventricular dysfunction (LVEF 35% to 49%)
2. Intermediate-risk treadmill score (score between -11 and <5)
3. Stress-induced moderate perfusion defect without LV dilation or increased lung intake (thallium-201)
4. Limited stress echocardiographic ischemia with a wall motion abnormality only at doses of dobutamine involving ≤2 segments

Low risk (<1% annual mortality rate)
1. Low-risk treadmill score (≥5)
2. Normal or small myocardial perfusion defect at rest or with stress
3. Normal stress echocardiographic wall motion or no change of limited resting wall motion abnormalities during stress

From ACCF/SCAI/STS/AATS/AHA/ASNC/HFSA/SCCT 2012: Appropriate use criteria for coronary revascularization focused update: A report of the American College of Cardiology Foundation Appropriate Use Criteria Task Force, Society for Cardiovascular Angiography and Interventions, Society of Thoracic Surgeons, American Association for Thoracic Surgery, American Heart Association, American Society of Nuclear Cardiology, and the Society of Cardiovascular Computed Tomography, *J Am Coll Cardiol* 59:857-881, 2012.

- Antiplatelet therapy
  - Aspirin therapy (71-162 mg/day)
  - Clopidogrel for those intolerant to aspirin therapy
  - Combination of aspirin and clopidogrel does not reduce cardiovascular events (CHARISMA trial).
  - Newer antiplatelet drugs such as prasugrel and ticagrelor have been studied in ACS but not in stable CAD.
- Statins
  - HMG-CoA reductase inhibitors (statins) (atorvastatin, rosuvastatin) with high-intensity therapy for a target LDL reduction of >50% if safely achieved in high-risk patients; if not a candidate for high-intensity therapy, patient should receive at least moderate-intensity statin therapy that lowers LDL by 30% to 50% as advised by the new ATP IV cholesterol guidelines from the 2013 ACC/AHA expert panel.
- ACE-inhibitors (captopril, enalapril, lisinopril) are a class I recommendation for patients with chronic CAD with LV dysfunction or diabetes and a class II recommendation for CAD patients without these features.

CORONARY ARTERY REVASCULARIZATION

- Patients with symptoms refractory to optimal medical therapy (OMT) as above or those with high clinical, stress testing, or an angiographic risk profile and suitable coronary anatomy may benefit from revascularization with either PCI (percutaneous coronary intervention) or CABG (coronary artery bypass graft) surgery.
- ACC/AHA class I indications for CABG surgery in chronic CAD patients includes the following:
  - High grade (>50%) left main CAD
  - Left main CAD-equivalent anatomy including >70% luminal stenosis in the left anterior descending artery and left circumflex arteries
  - Three-vessel disease with LVEF <50%
  - Single- or two-vessel CAD with a large area of viable myocardium at risk
  - Severe angina despite medical therapy if CABG can be performed with acceptable risk
- PCI has not been shown to reduce long-term rates of MI and death in patients with stable chronic CAD and therefore has no class I indications. PCI is suitable in patients with suitable anatomy with refractory or lifestyle-limiting angina who have failed OMT. Recent trials such as the Courage Trial have demonstrated no significant difference between OMT and PCI in overall survival, MI, and ACS over 5 years in patients with chronic stable CAD.
- The SYNTAX trial, which used a numerical score based on qualitative plaque features on angiography, showed that surgical revascularization was associated with a lesser risk of stroke and major cardiac events if the SYNTAX score was high (>33).
- The FREEDOM trial showed that in diabetic patients with multivessel disease, CABG is superior to PCI with drug-eluting stents in chronic CAD and should remain the revascularization strategy of choice in this patient population. CABG resulted in lower rates of death and MI but a higher risk of stroke. This is true for patients with either insulin-dependent or non–insulin-dependent DM.

DISPOSITION

- Coronary artery disease is a common chronic condition with which many patients can live for years with good symptom control on optimal medical therapy.

REFERRAL

- Cardiovascular disease specialist

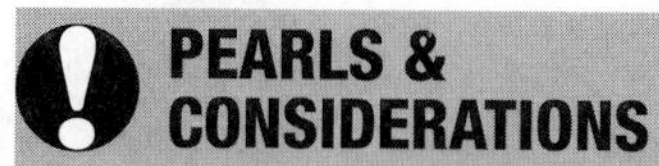

COMMENTS

The transition from stable coronary artery disease to unstable angina must be carefully monitored. Symptoms of concern include more frequent episodes of chest pain, chest pain that is less responsive to nitroglycerin, or first episode of chest pain. Regarding unstable angina, please refer to section on Acute coronary syndromes.

RELATED CONTENT

Coronary Artery Disease (Patient Information)
Acute Coronary Syndrome (Related Key Topic)
Angina Pectoris (Related Key Topic)
Hyperlipidemia (Related Key Topic)
Myocardial Infarction (Related Key Topic)

AUTHORS: **SYED R. LATIF, M.D.**, and
GAGAN SAHNI, M.D. F.A.C.C., F.A.C.P.

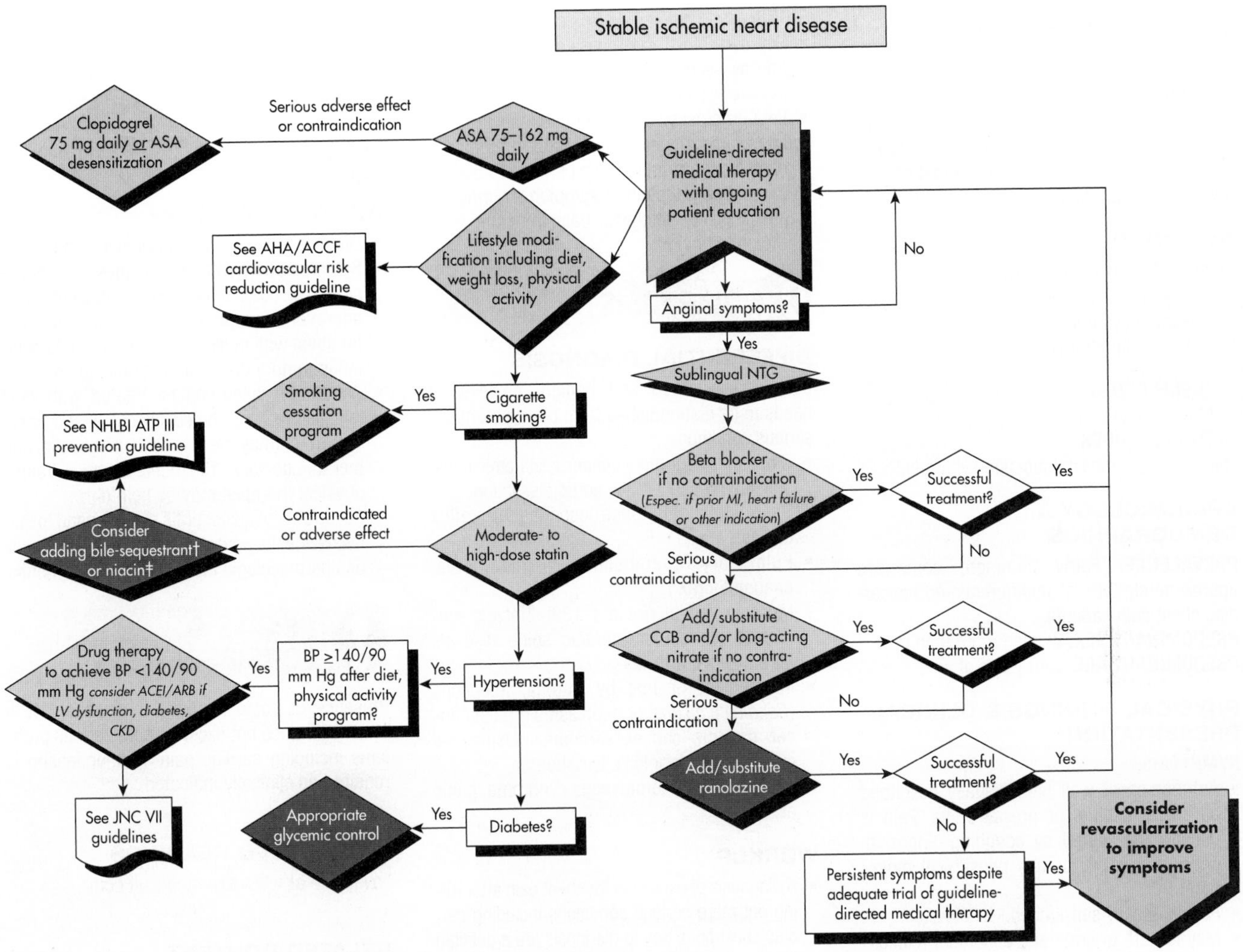

Stable ischemic heart disease

Guideline-directed medical therapy with ongoing patient education

ASA 75–162 mg daily

Serious adverse effect or contraindication

Clopidogrel 75 mg daily *or* ASA desensitization

Lifestyle modification including diet, weight loss, physical activity

See AHA/ACCF cardiovascular risk reduction guideline

Cigarette smoking?

Yes

Smoking cessation program

Moderate- to high-dose statin

Contraindicated or adverse effect

Consider adding bile-sequestrant† or niacin‡

See NHLBI ATP III prevention guideline

Hypertension?

Yes

BP ≥140/90 mm Hg after diet, physical activity program?

Yes

Drug therapy to achieve BP <140/90 mm Hg *consider ACEI/ARB if LV dysfunction, diabetes, CKD*

See JNC VII guidelines

Diabetes?

Yes

Appropriate glycemic control

Anginal symptoms?

No

Yes

Sublingual NTG

Beta blocker if no contraindication (*Espec. if prior MI, heart failure or other indication*)

Yes

Successful treatment?

Yes

No

Serious contraindication

Add/substitute CCB and/or long-acting nitrate if no contraindication

Yes

Successful treatment?

Yes

No

Serious contraindication

Add/substitute ranolazine

Yes

Successful treatment?

Yes

No

Persistent symptoms despite adequate trial of guideline-directed medical therapy

Yes

Consider revascularization to improve symptoms

FIGURE 1-280 Algorithm for guideline-directed medical therapy for patients with SIHD.*

*The algorithms do not represent a comprehensive list of recommendations (see text for all recommendations).

†The use of bile acid sequestrant is relatively contraindicated when triglycerides are ≥200 mg/dL and is contraindicated when triglycerides are ≥500 mg/dL.

‡Dietary supplement niacin must not be used as a substitute for prescription niacin. ACCF, American College of Cardiology Foundation; ACEI, angiotensin-converting enzyme inhibitor; AHA, American Heart Association; ARB, angiotensin-receptor blocker; ASA, aspirin; ATP III; Adult Treatment Panel 3; BP, blood pressure; CCB, calcium channel blocker; CKD, chronic kidney disease; HDL-C, high-density lipoprotein cholesterol; JNC VII, Seventh Report of the Joint National Committee on Prevention, Detection, Evaluation, and Treatment of High Blood Pressure; LDL-C, low-density lipoprotein cholesterol; LV, left ventricular; MI, myocardial infarction; NHLBI, National Heart, Lung, and Blood Institute; and NTG, nitroglycerin. (From 2012 ACCF/AHA/ACP/AATS/PCNA/SCAI/STS Guideline for the Diagnosis and Management of Patients With Stable Ischemic Heart Disease: A report of the American College of Cardiology Foundation/American Heart Association Task Force on Practice Guidelines, and the American College of Physicians, American Association for Thoracic Surgery, Preventive Cardiovascular Nurses Association, Society for Cardiovascular Angiography and Interventions, and Society of Thoracic Surgeons, *J Am Coll Cardiol* 60:e44-e164, 2012.)

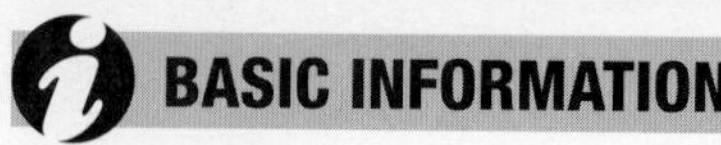

BASIC INFORMATION

DEFINITION

Clinical condition characterized by pain and tenderness at costochondral or chondrosternal joints of the anterior chest wall without obvious swelling or induration.

SYNONYMS

Anterior chest wall syndrome
Chest wall pain syndrome
Costosternal syndrome
Parasternal chondrodynia

ICD-9CM CODES
733.6 Costochondritis
ICD-10CM CODES
M94.0 Chondrocostal junction syndrome

EPIDEMIOLOGY & DEMOGRAPHICS

PREVALENCE: Fairly common, comprises approximately 28% of undifferentiated noncardiac chest pain patients.
PREDOMINANT SEX: Women more than men
PREDOMINANT AGE: >40 years of age

PHYSICAL FINDINGS & CLINICAL PRESENTATION

SYMPTOMS:

- Anterior chest wall pain, usually described as sharp, aching, or pressure-like. Pain is usually aggravated by coughing, sneezing, deep inspiration, or any chest wall movement.
- Pain is usually self-limited.
- May radiate to arms and shoulders mimicking cardiac pain.

SIGNS:

- Reproducible tenderness of costochondral (mostly second through fifth) or costosternal junction without localized swelling or induration.
- Pain on crossed-chest adduction of arm and backward extension of arm from 90 degrees of abduction signifies pain of musculoskeletal origin. Reproduction of symptoms during dry needling also suggests pain from musculoskeletal origin.

Dx DIAGNOSIS

DIFFERENTIAL DIAGNOSIS

Usually self-limited and benign; however, it needs to be distinguished from other potentially serious conditions.

- Cardiac pain: primary concern; ischemic chest pain, acute pericarditis, aortic dissection
- Gastrointestinal: gastroesophageal reflux disease
- Pulmonary embolism, pneumonia, pneumothorax
- Musculoskeletal (Table 1-139): Tietze's syndrome, cervical or thoracic spine disease, fibromyalgia, arthritis
- Involvement of ribs by trauma, infections (*Candida albicans*) or neoplasms (breast cancer, prostate cancer, sarcoma, plasma cell cytoma, non-Hodgkin's lymphoma)
- Miscellaneous: fibromyalgia syndrome, panic attack

WORKUP

- A diagnosis of exclusion for chest pain after ruling out more serious conditions including cardiac chest pain. Key to diagnosis are a detailed history, a meticulous physical examination, and a few rationally selected diagnostic studies, including electrocardiogram and chest x-ray to rule out cardiopulmonary causes. Usefulness of nuclear scanning with technetium99 scintigraphy, gallium, or bone scanning to assist diagnosis of costochondritis is not clear.

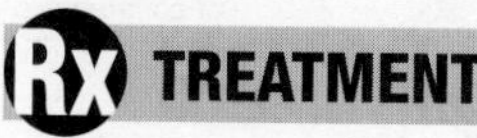

Rx TREATMENT

ACUTE GENERAL Rx

- Often self-limiting, so reassurance is important.
- Symptomatic treatment includes local application of heat, minimizing of activities that aggravate symptoms, stretching exercises for chest wall muscles, and nonsteroidal anti-inflammatory drugs or acetaminophen.
- Refractory cases can be treated with local injections of combined lidocaine and corticosteroid (may be a useful diagnostic and therapeutic tool). Dry needling by a trained physical therapist may be helpful.
- Recurrent costochondritis may respond to sulfasalazine; however, there are no clinical trials on pharmacologic therapy for costochondritis.

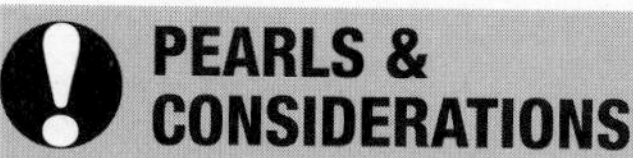

PEARLS & CONSIDERATIONS

Presence of costochondritis in a patient with chest pain does not exclude more serious problems including cardiac pain. Further testing is required as clinically indicated.

SUGGESTED READINGS

available at www.expertconsult.com

RELATED CONTENT

Costochondritis (Patient Information)

AUTHOR: **ASHA SHRESTHA, M.D.**

TABLE 1-139 Musculoskeletal Chest Pain

Disorder	Clinical Features	Comments
Tietze's syndrome	Painful swelling of usually 2nd or 3rd costochondral junctions.	Less common than costochondritis; commonly affects young people of either sex. Exact cause is unknown, but a traumatic pathogenesis has been associated. The disease course is mostly self-limited. Non-Hodgkin's lymphoma of medial clavicular head has been reported to mimic Tietze syndrome.
Costochondritis	Pain and tenderness at the costochondral or chondrosternal junctions without a notable swelling. The 2nd-5th costal cartilages are most commonly involved.	Certain maneuvers like "crowing rooster" maneuver (extension of the cervical spine and traction on the posteriorly extended arm) and traction on the adducted arm with head rotated to ipsilateral side may reproduce the pain.
Slipping rib syndrome	Pain at the lower costal cartilages, associated with increased mobility of the anterior end of a costal cartilage. Most commonly affects 10th rib and occasionally 8th and 9th ribs.	Maneuver such as hooking the fingers under the anterior costal margin and pulling the rib cage anteriorly may produce a palpable click of the cartilages slipping over one another.
Cervical, thoracic disc disease	Referred regional pain from affected areas. Often aggravated by spine motion and may be accompanied by radicular pain into arm if cervical origin or along intercostal nerve if thoracic origin. Symptoms reproduced by Spurling's maneuver (steady pressure to head causing increased axial loading on the nerve root).	May mimic chest disease if spinal complaints are minimal and referred or radicular symptoms predominate.
Fibromyalgia	Widespread pain with multiple other peripheral tender points.	Female/male ratio of 9:1. Prevalent age 30-50 yr. Frequently associated with tension headache, irritable bowel syndrome, and psychiatric symptoms.
Sternoclavicular or manubriosternal joint involvement in osteoarthritis, inflammatory conditions (rheumatoid arthritis, ankylosing spondylitis, psoriatic arthritis), and infection	Dull, aching local pain with tenderness. Occasional bony joint enlargement with soft tissue swelling.	Crepitus may rarely be present.

BASIC INFORMATION

DEFINITION

Craniopharyngiomas are tumors arising from squamous cell remnants of Rathke's pouch, located in the infundibulum or upper anterior hypophysis.

SYNONYMS

Subset of nonadenomatous pituitary tumors

ICD-9CM CODES
237.0 Craniopharyngioma
ICD-10CM CODES
D44.3 Neoplasm of uncertain behavior of pituitary gland

EPIDEMIOLOGY & DEMOGRAPHICS

PEAK INCIDENCE: Occurs at all ages; peak during the first 2 decades of life, with a second small peak occurring in the sixth decade.
PREDOMINANT SEX:
- Both sexes are usually equally affected.
- Craniopharyngiomas are the most common nonglial tumors in children and account for 3% to 5% of all pediatric brain tumors.

PHYSICAL FINDINGS & CLINICAL PRESENTATION

- The typical onset is insidious and a 1- to 2-year history of slowly progressive symptoms is common.
- Presenting symptoms are usually related to the effects of a sella turcica mass. Approximately 75% of patients report headache and have visual disturbances.
- The usual visual defect is bitemporal hemianopsia. Optic nerve involvement with decreased visual acuity and scotomas and homonymous hemianopsia from optic tract involvement may also occur.
- Other symptoms include mental changes, nausea, vomiting, somnolence, or symptoms of pituitary failure. In adults, sexual dysfunction is the most common endocrine complaint, with impotence in men and primary or secondary amenorrhea in women. Diabetes insipidus is found in 25% of cases. In children, craniopharyngiomas may present with dwarfism.
- More than 70% of children at the time of diagnosis present with growth hormone deficiency, obstructive hydrocephalus, short-term memory deficits, and psychomotor slowing.

ETIOLOGY

Craniopharyngiomas are believed to arise from nests of squamous epithelial cells that are commonly found in the suprasellar area surrounding the pars tuberalis of the adult pituitary.

DIAGNOSIS

DIFFERENTIAL DIAGNOSIS

- Pituitary adenoma
- Empty sella syndrome
- Pituitary failure of any cause
- Primary brain tumors (e.g., meningiomas, astrocytomas)
- Metastatic brain tumors
- Other brain tumors
- Cerebral aneurysm

LABORATORY TESTS

- Hypothyroidism (low FT_4, FT_3 with high thyroid-stimulating hormone).
- Hypercortisolism (low cortisol) with low adrenocorticotropic hormone.
- Low sex hormones (testosterone, estriol) with low follicle-stimulating hormone and luteinizing hormone.
- Diabetes insipidus (hypernatremia, low urine osmolarity, high plasma osmolarity).
- Prolactin may be normal or slightly elevated.
- Pituitary stimulation tests may be required in some cases.

IMAGING STUDIES

- MRI (Fig. 1-281) or head CT if MRI is contraindicated. MRI features include a multicystic and solid enhancing suprasellar mass. Hydrocephalus may also be present if the mass is large. CT usually reveals intratumoral calcifications.
- Visual field testing for bitemporal hemianopsia.
- Skull film may show:
  - Enlarged or eroded sella turcica (50%)
  - Suprasellar calcification (50%)

TREATMENT

GENERAL Rx

- Traditionally, surgery has been the main treatment for craniopharyngioma. However, radiation treatment instead of surgery may be an option in selected cases.
- Surgical resection (curative or palliative).
  - Transsphenoidal surgery for small intrasellar tumors
  - Subfrontal craniotomy for most patients
- Overall prognosis is good with 80%-90% chance of permanent cure.
- Postoperative radiation.
- Intralesional ^{32}P irradiation or bleomycin for unresectable tumors. Long-term complications of radiation include secondary malignancies, optic neuropathy, and vascular injury.

PROGNOSIS

- Overall prognosis is good with 80%-90% chance of permanent cure.
- Operative mortality rate: 3% to 16% (higher with large tumors).
- Postoperative recurrence rate: <20% of cases after total resection and 60% of cases after subtotal resection. Most recurrences occur within the first 2 yr after surgery.
- 5-yr and 10-yr survival: 88% and 76%, respectively, with surgery and radiation.
- The most important factors that correlate with prognosis are the extent of resection and postoperative radiation.
- Long-term post-treatment hormonal, visual, and neurological problems occur in a significant percentage of patients.

RELATED CONTENT

Craniopharyngioma (Patient Information)

AUTHOR: **FRED F. FERRI, M.D.**

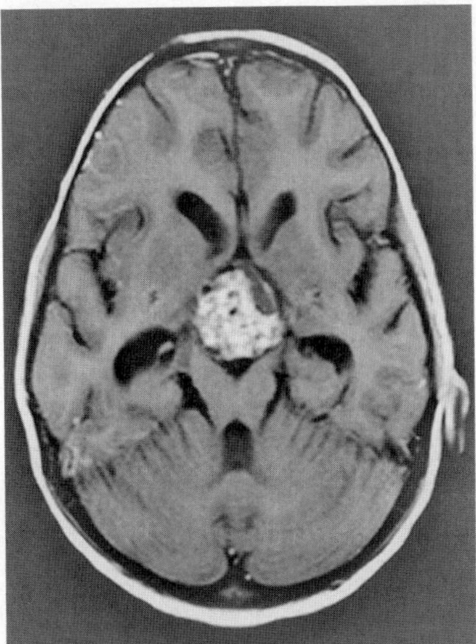

FIGURE 1-281 MRI scan of a craniopharyngioma, demonstrating a cystic contrast-enhancing mass in the suprasellar area extending upward and compressing the hypothalamus. (From Goetz CG: *Textbook of clinical neurology,* Philadelphia, 1999, Saunders.)

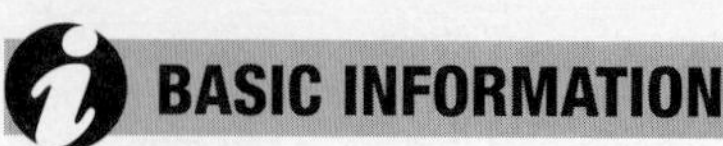

DEFINITION

Creutzfeldt-Jakob disease (CJD) is a progressive, fatal, dementing neurologic illness caused by an infectious protein agent known as a *prion.*

SYNONYMS

Transmissible spongiform encephalopathy
Mad cow disease
Prion disease
Bovine spongiform encephalopathy

OTHER PRION DISEASES

Fatal familial insomnia
Kuru
Gerstmann-Sträussler-Scheinker syndrome (GSS)

ICD-9CM CODES
046.1 Creutzfeldt-Jakob disease
ICD-10CM CODES
A81.00 Creutzfeldt-Jakob disease, unspecified

EPIDEMIOLOGY & DEMOGRAPHICS

- Incidence of one per 1 million population per year
- Peak age 60 yr (range, 16 to 82 yr)—sporadic cases are seen in an older population while the variant subtype is commonly seen in younger patients
- 5% to 10% familial, remaining cases are sporadic; iatrogenic cases (corneal transplants, dura mater allograft, human pituitary extract, blood or blood product transfusion, reused medical equipment such as EEG depth electrodes) are very rare—about 1%; variant CJD is caused by ingestion of meat from cows with prion disease and is more commonly seen in Great Britain

PHYSICAL FINDINGS & CLINICAL PRESENTATION

- Cognitive deficits: Patients present with cognitive deficits (dementing illness—memory loss, behavioral abnormalities, higher cortical function impairment), usually a subacute rapid progressive encephalopathy or dementia. Prodromal symptoms such as fatigue, depression, weight loss, and disorders of sleep and appetite may be seen in about one third of patients. Early stages are characterized by confusion with hallucinations, delusions, and agitation.
- More than 80% will have myoclonus—generalized and exaggerated by startle.
- Pyramidal tract signs (weakness), cerebellar signs (clumsiness), and extrapyramidal signs (parkinsonian features) are seen in more than 50% of the cases.
- Less common features include cortical visual abnormalities, abnormal eye movements, vestibular dysfunction, sensory disturbances, autonomic dysfunction, lower motor neuron signs, and seizures.

ETIOLOGY

Small proteinaceous infectious particle (prion): Noninfectious prion protein (PrP) is a cellular protein found on the surfaces of neurons. Normal function is not known. This normal protein is converted to a protease-resistant infectious agent by the infectious prion protein.

- Normal prion protein (PRNP) gene is found on human chromosome 20.
- Methionine and valine distribution on codon 129 of the PRNP determines the six clinical phenotypes of CJD.

Dx DIAGNOSIS

- Definite CJD: Neuropathologically confirmed spongiform encephalopathy in a case of progressive dementia.
- Probable CJD: History of rapidly progressive dementia (<2 yr) with typical EEG and with at least two of the following clinical features: myoclonus, visual or cerebellar dysfunction, pyramidal or extrapyramidal features, akinetic mutism.
- Possible CJD: Same as probable CJD without EEG findings.

DIFFERENTIAL DIAGNOSIS

- Other progressive dementias (Alzheimer's disease, frontotemporal dementia, Lewy body dementia, and vascular dementia)
- Infectious (viral, HIV, fungal, TB, Whipple's disease)
- Inflammatory/autoimmune (CNS vasculitis, Hashimoto's encephalopathy, SSPE)
- Metabolic (vitamin deficiency, endocrine)
- Cancers (CNS lymphoma, gliomatosis cerebri, paraneoplastic)
- Other conditions, toxic (heavy metal poisoning)

A clinical algorithm for the evaluation of dementia is described in Section III, "Dementia."

WORKUP

- Evaluate for treatable causes of dementia (see "Alzheimer's Disease").
- Brain biopsy is gold standard for diagnosis, but it is usually not performed because there is no treatment or cure.
- Lumbar puncture with spinal fluid analysis for presence of 14-3-3 protein or human prion protein (PrP^{Sc}).
- Recent guidelines issued by the American Academy of Neurology states that clinicians should order assays for 14-3-3 in patients with rapidly progressive dementia, strong suspicion of sporadic CJD and an uncertain diagnosis (pretest probability 20% to 90%). The test has a high false-positive and false-negative rate due to its presence in other chronic noninflammatory dementing diseases.

LABORATORY TESTS

- Presence of periodic sharp wave complexes on EEG in cases of rapidly progressive dementia has a sensitivity of 67% and a specificity of 86%.
- In cases of probable or possible CJD, presence of the 14,3,3 protein in CSF has a 95% positive predictive value with its absence having a 92% negative predictive value. Test for presence of human prion protein (PrP^{Sc}) in CSF has been reported to be 83% sensitive and 100% specific. Repeated testing for 14.3.3 protein increases the probability of a positive result. Enolase and neopterin in CSF are the other nonspecific markers that may have adjunct diagnostic value.
- The National Prion Disease Pathology Surveillance Center at Case Western Reserve University performs specific diagnostic tests free of charge.

IMAGING STUDIES

MRI scan can show areas of restricted diffusion in the basal ganglia and cerebral cortex. MRI diffusion-weighted imaging has a sensitivity of 92.3% and a specificity of 93.8% only in cases of rapidly progressive dementia. T2-weighted imaging may also show subtle hyperintensities in the lenticular nuclei in about 82% of cases.

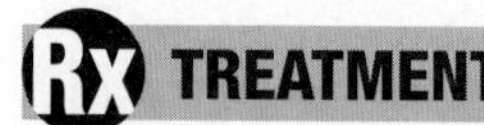

NONPHARMACOLOGIC THERAPY

Full-time caregiver and/or nursing home: Social work can be helpful with end-of-life discussions, family counseling, and optimizing appropriate home services. Proper disposal of medical equipment and avoidance of organ transplants from these patients prevent transmission of the disease.

ACUTE GENERAL Rx

No known therapy

CHRONIC Rx

No known therapy

DISPOSITION

The disease is fatal. Mean duration of illness is 8 mo (range, 1 to 130 mo). One in 7 survives to 1 yr, and 1 in 30 survives to 2 yr. Better survival found in younger age at onset of disease and female gender. Increased survival may be falsely reported due to coexisting dementias such as Alzheimer's with earlier onset of dementia than CJD.

REFERRAL

- Neurology for evaluation of any rapidly progressive dementia
- Social work

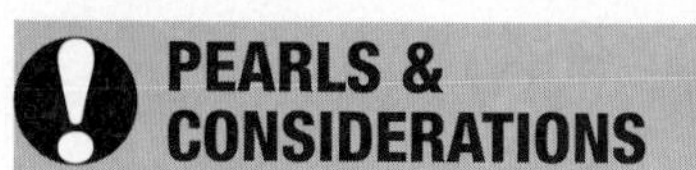

COMMENTS

- A diagnosis of CJD should be considered in patients with rapid progression of dementia from unknown causes.
- Exposure to human or animal nervous tissues increases the odds of CJD in patients presenting with progressive dementia.

- Related diseases in human beings: kuru, fatal familial insomnia, Gerstmann-Sträussler-Scheinker syndrome, new-variant CJD.
- Related diseases in animals: scrapie, bovine spongiform encephalopathy (mad cow disease).

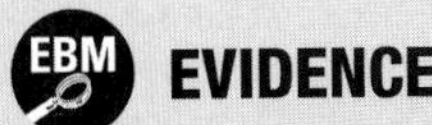

EVIDENCE

available at www.expertconsult.com

SUGGESTED READINGS

available at www.expertconsult.com

AUTHOR: **ARUN SWAMINATHAN, M.B.B.S.,** and **SACHIN KEDAR, M.B.B.S., M.D.**

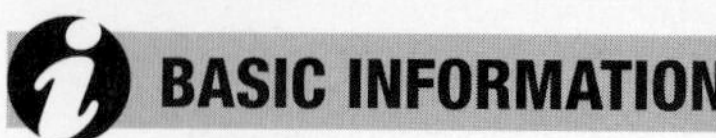

BASIC INFORMATION

DEFINITION

Crohn's disease is an inflammatory disease of the bowel of unknown etiology, most commonly involving the terminal ileum and manifesting primarily with diarrhea, abdominal pain, fatigue, and weight loss.

SYNONYMS

Regional enteritis
Inflammatory bowel disease (IBD)

ICD-9CM CODES
555.9 Crohn's disease, unspecified site
555.0 Crohn's disease, small intestine
555.1 Crohn's disease involving large intestine

ICD-10CM CODES
K50.90 Crohn's disease, unspecified, without complications
K50.00 Crohn's disease of small intestine without complications
K50.10 Crohn's disease of large intestine without complications

EPIDEMIOLOGY & DEMOGRAPHICS

PREVALENCE:

- One case per 1000 persons; most common in whites and Jews
- Crohn's disease affects approximately 380,000 to 480,000 persons in the U.S.
- Incidence: bimodal with a peak in the third decade of life and another in the fifth decade

PHYSICAL FINDINGS & CLINICAL PRESENTATION

- Abdominal tenderness, mass, or distention
- Chronic or nocturnal diarrhea
- Weight loss, fever, night sweats
- Hyperactive bowel sounds in patients with partial obstruction, bloody diarrhea
- Delayed growth and failure of normal development in children
- Perianal and rectal abscesses, multiple sinuses and scarring (Fig. E1-282), mouth ulcers, cobblestone appearance of oral mucosa (Fig. E1-283) and atrophic glossitis
- Extraintestinal manifestations (Table E1-140): joint swelling and tenderness, hepatosplenomegaly, erythema nodosum, clubbing, tenderness to palpation of the sacroiliac joints
- Symptoms may be intermittent with varying periods of remission

ETIOLOGY

Unknown. Pathophysiologically, Crohn's disease involves an immune system dysfunction.

Dx DIAGNOSIS

DIFFERENTIAL DIAGNOSIS

- Ulcerative colitis (see Table 1-141)
- Infectious diseases (tuberculosis, *Yersinia, Salmonella, Shigella, Campylobacter*)
- Parasitic infections (amebic infection)
- Pseudomembranous colitis
- Ischemic colitis in elderly patients
- Lymphoma
- Colon carcinoma
- Diverticulitis
- Radiation enteritis
- Collagenous colitis
- Fungal infections *(Histoplasma, Actinomyces)*
- Gay bowel syndrome (in homosexual patient)
- Carcinoid tumors
- Celiac sprue
- Mesenteric adenitis

LABORATORY TESTS

- Decreased hemoglobin and hematocrit from chronic blood loss, effect of inflammation on bone marrow, and malabsorption of vitamin B_{12}
- Hypokalemia, hypomagnesemia, hypocalcemia, and low albumin in patients with chronic diarrhea
- Vitamin B12 and folate deficiency
- Elevated erythrocyte sedimentation rate
- Positive anti–*Saccharomyces cerevisiae* antibodies
- Elevated INR (due to vitamin K malabsorption)
- Fecal calprotectin has been reported as useful in screening of patients with suspected IBD. Based on a pretest probability of 32% in adults, an abnormal calprotectin test result increases the posttest probability to 91%, and a normal result reduces the probability of IBD to 3%. False elevations may occur with other gastrointestinal diseases such as bacterial, viral, and protozoal causes of infective diarrhea

ENDOSCOPIC EVALUATION

Endoscopic features of Crohn's disease include asymmetric and discontinued disease, deep longitudinal fissures, cobblestone appearance, and presence of strictures. Crypt distortion and inflammation are also present. Granulomas may be present.

IMAGING STUDIES

- Barium imaging studies are essentially outdated examinations. When performed, they reveal deep ulcerations (often longitudinal and transverse) and segmental lesions (skip lesions, strictures, fistulas, cobblestone appearance of mucosa caused by submucosal inflammation); "thumbprinting" is common, and "string sign" in terminal ileum may be noted. Although the diagnosis may be suggested by radiographic studies, it should be confirmed by endoscopy and biopsy when possible.
- CT of abdomen may show thickening of the terminal ileum (Fig. 1-284) and is helpful in identifying abscesses and other complications.
- Magnetic resonance enterography (MRe) is superior to other imaging modalities in its ability to distinguish active from chronic fibrotic disease. It is, however, more expensive.

TABLE 1-141 Differentiating Features

	Ulcerative Colitis	Crohn's Disease
Site of involvement	Only involves colon Rectum almost always involved	Any area of the gastrointestinal tract Rectum usually spared
Pattern of involvement	Continuous	Skip lesions
Diarrhea	Bloody	Usually nonbloody
Severe abdominal pain	Rare	Frequent
Perianal disease	No	In 30% of patients
Fistula	No	Yes
Endoscopic findings	Erythematous and friable Superficial ulceration	Aphthoid and deep ulcers Cobblestoning
Radiologic findings	Tubular appearance resulting from loss of haustral folds	String sign of terminal ileum RLQ mass, fistulas, abscesses
Histologic features	Mucosa only Crypt abscesses	Transmural Crypt abscesses, granulomas (about 30%)
Smoking	Protective	Worsens course
Serology	p-ANCA more common	ASCA more common

ASCA, Anti–*Saccharomyces cerevisiae* antibodies; *p-ANCA,* perinuclear antineutrophil cytoplasmic antibody; *RLQ,* right lower quadrant.
From Andreoli TE et al: *Andreoli and Carpenter's Cecil essentials of medicine,* ed 8, Philadelphia, 2010, Saunders.

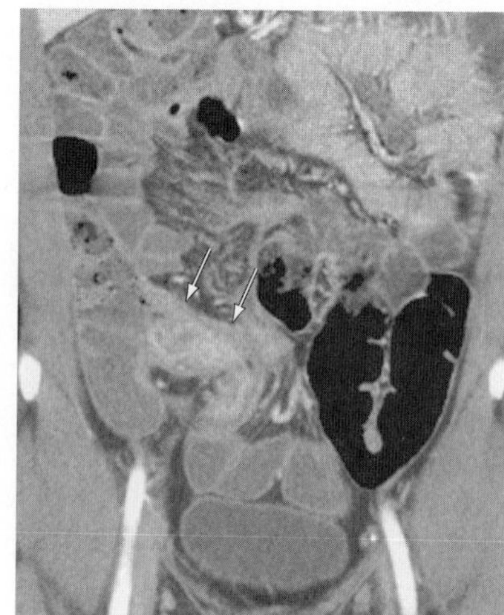

FIGURE 1-284 Coronal reformat from a contrast-enhanced computed tomographic scan shows thickening in the terminal ileum with enhancement (arrows) suggestive of Crohn's disease. (From Fielding JR et al: *Gynecologic imaging,* Philadelphia, 2011, Saunders.)

- In 5% to 10% of patients with IBD, a clear distinction between ulcerative colitis and Crohn's disease cannot be made. In general, Crohn's disease can be distinguished from ulcerative colitis by the presence of transmural involvement and the frequent presence of noncaseating granulomas and lymphoid aggregates on biopsy.

Rx TREATMENT

The medical management of Crohn's disease is based on disease activity. According to Hanauer and Sanborn, disease activity can be defined as follows:

- Mild to moderate disease: The patient is ambulatory and able to take oral alimentation. There is no dehydration, high fever, abdominal tenderness, painful mass, obstruction, or weight loss of >10%.
- Moderate to severe disease: Either the patient has not responded to treatment for mild to moderate disease or has more pronounced symptoms, including fever, significant weight loss, abdominal pain or tenderness, intermittent nausea and vomiting, or significant anemia.
- Severe fulminant disease: Either the patient has persistent symptoms despite outpatient steroid therapy or has high fever, persistent vomiting, evidence of intestinal obstruction, rebound tenderness, cachexia, or evidence of an abscess.
- Remission: The patient is asymptomatic or without inflammatory sequelae, including patients responding to acute medical intervention.

NONPHARMACOLOGIC THERAPY

- Nutritional supplementation is needed in patients with advanced disease. Total parenteral nutrition may be necessary in selected patients.
- Low-residue diet is necessary when obstructive symptoms are present.
- If diarrhea is prominent, increased dietary fiber and decreased fat in the diet are sometimes helpful.
- Psychotherapy is useful for situational adjustment crises. A trusting and mutually understanding relationship and referral to self-help groups are very important because of the chronicity of the disease and the relatively young age of the patients.
- Avoid oral feedings during acute exacerbation to decrease colonic activity: a low-roughage diet may be helpful in early relapse.

ACUTE GENERAL Rx

- Traditionally, initial treatment consists of 5-aminosalicylate drugs (sulfasalazine, olsalazine, balsalazide, mesalamine: oral or rectal). Sulfasalazine, 500 mg PO qid initially, increased qd or qod by 1 g until therapeutic dosages of 4 to 6 g/day are achieved, is often initially used. Individuals with sulfa allergies should avoid sulfasalazine. Folate supplementation is recommended because sulfasalazine inhibits folate absorption. Oral salicylates, such as mesalamine (Asacol, Rowasa), are as effective as sulfasalazine and better tolerated and have become preferred agents despite their higher cost.
- Corticosteroids have been the mainstay for treating moderate to severe active Crohn's disease. Prednisone 40 to 60 mg/day is useful for acute exacerbation. Steroids are usually tapered over approximately 2 to 3 mo. Some patients require a low dose for a prolonged period of maintenance.
- Steroid analogues are locally active corticosteroids that target specific areas of inflammation in the gastrointestinal tract. Budesonide is available as a controlled-release formulation and is approved for mild to moderate active Crohn's disease involving the ileum and/or ascending colon. The adult dose is 9 mg qd for a maximum of 8 wk.
- Immunosuppressants such as azathioprine 150 mg/day, methotrexate, or cyclosporine can be used for severe, progressive disease. In patients with Crohn's disease who enter remission after treatment with methotrexate, a low dose of methotrexate maintains remission.
- Metronidazole 500 mg qid may be useful for colonic fistulas and treatment of mild to moderate active Crohn's disease. Ciprofloxacin 1 g qd has also been found to be effective in decreasing disease activity.
- TNF inhibitors: Infliximab, a chimeric monoclonal antibody targeting tumor necrosis factor-α, is effective in the treatment of enterocutaneous fistulas. This medication can induce clinical improvement in 80% of patients with Crohn's disease refractory to other agents. It can be used in combination with other medications such as azathioprine in patients with severe Crohn's disease. A PPD test should be done before using this medication. Adalimumab and certolizumab are other TNF inhibitors also effective in inducing remissions and may be useful in adult patients with Crohn's disease who cannot tolerate infliximab or have symptoms despite receiving infliximab therapy.
- Natalizumab, a selective adhesion-molecule inhibitor, has been reported to be effective in increasing the rate of remission and response in patients with active Crohn's disease. It is effective for patients in whom anti-TNF therapy has been unsuccessful. Recent trials with pegylated antibody fragments in patients with moderate to severe Crohn's disease involving certolizumab pegol revealed a modest improvement in response rates but no significant improvement in remission rates.
- Hydrocortisone enema bid or tid is useful for proctitis.
- Most patients who have anemia associated with Crohn's disease respond to iron supplementation. Erythropoietin is useful in patients with anemia refractory to treatment with iron and vitamins.

CHRONIC Rx

- Monitor disease activity with symptom review and laboratory evaluation (complete blood count and sedimentation rate)
- Liver tests and vitamin B_{12} levels monitored on a yearly basis

DISPOSITION

One tenth of patients have prolonged remission, three quarters have a chronic intermittent disease course, and one eighth have an unremitting course.

REFERRAL

- Surgical referral is needed for complications such as abscess formation, obstruction, fistulas, toxic megacolon, refractory disease, or severe hemorrhage. Approximately 40% to 50% of patients will require some type of bowel surgery within the first 5 years of Crohn's disease. A conservative surgical approach is necessary because surgery is not curative. Multiple surgeries may also result in short bowel syndrome.

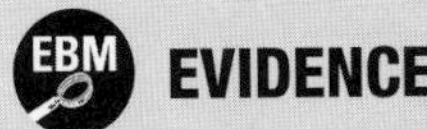

EVIDENCE

available at www.expertconsult.com

SUGGESTED READINGS

available at www.expertconsult.com

RELATED CONTENT

Crohn's Disease (Patient Information)

AUTHOR: **FRED F. FERRI, M.D.**

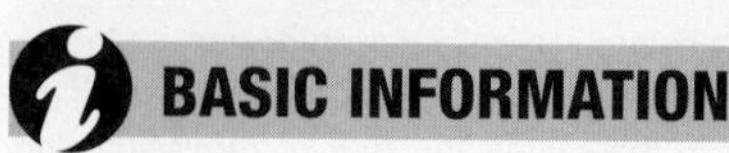

BASIC INFORMATION

DEFINITION

Cryoglobulins are serum immunoglobulins that precipitate when cooled and redissolve when heated. A classification of cryoglobulins is described in Table E1-142. Cryoglobulinemia is a clinical syndrome that results from systemic inflammation caused by cryoglobulin-containing immune complexes. Mixed cryoglobulinemia is a vasculitis of small and medium-sized arteries and veins due to the deposition of complexes of antigen, cryoglobulin, and complement in the vessel walls.

SYNONYMS

Cryoglobulinemic vasculitis
Cryoproteinemia
Mixed cryoglobulinemia
Essential cryoglobulinemia

ICD-9CM CODES
273.2 Cryoglobulinemia, cryoglobulinemic vasculitis (CV), mixed cryoglobulinemia (MC)
ICD-10CM CODES
D89.1 Cryoglobulinemia

EPIDEMIOLOGY & DEMOGRAPHICS

PREVALENCE:

- Prevalence of mixed cryoglobulinemia is approximately 1:100,000
- More than 50% of patients with HCV are found to have mixed cryoglobulinemia
- Three types: I (monoclonal), II (IgM monoclonal and IgG polyclonal), and III (polyclonal)

PREDOMINANT SEX AND AGE: Female:male ratio of 3:1

PREDOMINANT AGE: Mean age reported is 42 to 52 yr

RISK FACTORS: Hepatitis C virus (HCV) infection, connective tissue disorders, lymphoproliferative disorders

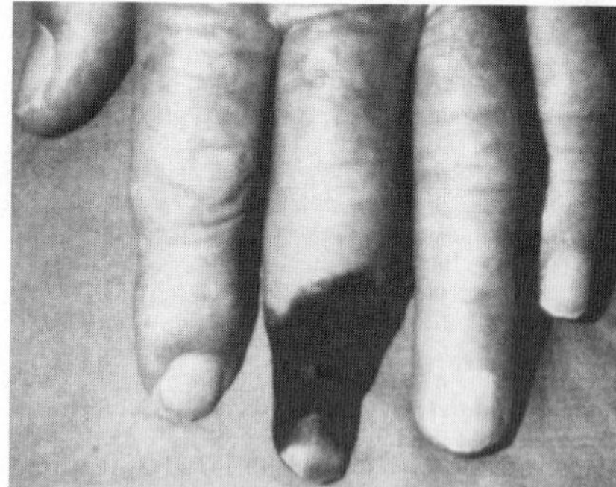

FIGURE 1-285 Cryoglobulinemia. (From Hoffman R et al: *Hematology, basic principles and practice*, ed 6, New York, 2013, Elsevier.)

PHYSICAL FINDINGS & CLINICAL PRESENTATION

- ***Meltzer triad*** of purpura, arthralgias/myalgia, and weakness
- Other symptoms include dyspnea, cough, numbness, abdominal pain, acrocyanosis
- Hypertension, hepatosplenomegaly, Raynaud's phenomenon, and in severe cases, distal necrosis and ulcerations of lower limbs (Fig. 1-285)

ETIOLOGY

- Intravascular deposition of cryoglobulins leads to ischemic insults in territory supplied by vasa nervorum
- Necrotizing vasculitis caused by cryoglobulin precipitation
- Infections: HCV, mycosis fungoides, HBV, Epstein-Barr virus, cytomegalovirus, *Treponema pallidum, Mycobacterium leprae,* and in post-streptococcal glomerulonephritis
- Lymphoproliferative disorders: chronic lymphocytic leukemia, Waldenström's macroglobulinemia, multiple myeloma
- Connective tissue disorders: rheumatoid arthritis, systemic lupus erythematosus (SLE), scleroderma, Sjögren's syndrome, vasculitis
- Renal diseases including proliferative glomerulonephritis

DIAGNOSIS

DIFFERENTIAL DIAGNOSIS

Antiphospholipid syndrome, SLE, lupus, Churg-Strauss syndrome, cirrhosis, glomerulonephritis, Goodpasture syndrome, hemolytic uremic syndrome, hepatitis, lymphoma, sarcoidosis, Waldenström's hypergammaglobulinemia

WORKUP

History and physical examination; laboratory tests; imaging tests depending on patients' presentations

LABORATORY TESTS

- Serum cryoglobulins, rheumatoid factor, serum complement, hepatitis C titers, urinalysis, CBC, ALT, AST, BUN, creatinine
- Electromyogram/nerve conduction studies may demonstrate axonal changes and distal muscle denervation
- Sural nerve and skin biopsy

IMAGING STUDIES

Chest x-ray for pulmonary involvement, CT to study for malignancy, and angiography for vasculitis

TREATMENT

- Immunosuppressive therapies such as corticosteroids are the mainstay treatment for mixed cryoglobulinemia.
- In patients with HCV, IFN-α can be added. The treatment of HCV-related mixed cryoglobulinemia is difficult due to the multifactorial origin and polymorphism of the syndrome. Therapy is aimed at eradicating the HCV infection, suppressing B-cell clonal expansion and cryoglobulin production and ameliorating symptoms
- Combination of pegylated IFN-α with ribavirin results in 77% remission.
- Variable success rate with plasma exchange, intravenous immunoglobulin, and anti-CD20 (rituximab) treatments

NONPHARMACOLOGIC THERAPY

Avoidance of cold exposure

ACUTE GENERAL Rx

NSAIDs in those with general fatigue and arthralgia; see "Treatment" for further management

DISPOSITION

Overall prognosis is worse with concomitant renal disease. Mean survival rate is ~50% at 10 yr.

REFERRAL

Consider referring to a nephrologist if there is renal involvement; hematologist in those with lymphoproliferative disorders; gastroenterologist/hepatologist in hepatitis; rheumatologist in connective tissue disease cases; and consider clinical immunologist in severe cases.

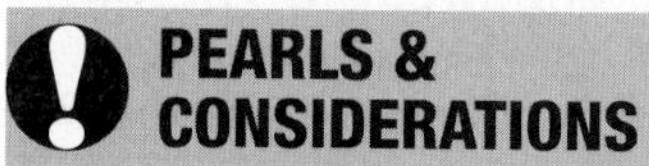

PEARLS & CONSIDERATIONS

COMMENTS

Always look for underlying causes for cryoglobulinemia.

PREVENTION

Avoidance of cold exposure, avoidance of late complications

PATIENT/FAMILY EDUCATION

Inform patients about early signs/symptoms of cryoglobulinemia so that treatments can be rendered before the development of complications.

SUGGESTED READINGS

available at www.expertconsult.com

AUTHOR: **QUANG P. LE, M.D., M.P.H.**

BASIC INFORMATION

DEFINITION

Cryptococcosis is an infection caused by the fungal organism *Cryptococcus neoformans.*

SYNONYMS

C. neoformans var. *neoformans* infection
C. neoformans var. *gatti* infection
C. neoformans var. *grubii* infection

ICD-9CM CODES
117.5 Cryptococcosis
ICD-10CM CODES
B45.9 Pulmonary cryptococcosis
B45.1 Cerebral cryptococcosis
B45.2 Cutaneous cryptococcosis
B45.3 Osseous cryptococcosis
B45.7 Disseminated cyrptococcosis
B45.9 Cryptococcosis, unspecified

EPIDEMIOLOGY & DEMOGRAPHICS

INCIDENCE (IN U.S.)

- 0.8 cases/million persons/year
- 6% to 7% in HIV-infected persons with AIDS

PEAK INCIDENCE: 20 to 40 yr (parallel to AIDS epidemic)
PREDOMINANT SEX: Equal sex distribution when corrected for HIV status
PREDOMINANT AGE: Less than 2 yr of age; 20 to 40 yr of age
NEONATAL INFECTION: Very uncommon

PHYSICAL FINDINGS & CLINICAL PRESENTATION

- More than 90% present with meningitis; almost all have fever and headache.
- Meningismus, photophobia, mental status changes are seen in approximately 25%.
- Increased intracranial pressure.
- Most common infections outside the CNS:
  1. In the lungs (fever, cough, dyspnea)
  2. In the skin (cellulitis, papular eruption)
  3. In the lymph nodes (lymphadenitis)
  4. Potential involvement of virtually any organ

ETIOLOGY

- Caused by the fungal organism *C. neoformans*

There are 3 varieties of *Cryptococcus spp.* and 4 capsular serotypes: Serotype A is *Cryptococcus neoformans* var. *grubii* and Serotype D is known as *Cryptococcus neoformans* var. *neoformans.* Both cause disease primarily in immunocompromised patients. Serotype B and C are known as *C. neoformans* var. *gatti.* This organism causes disease primarily in normal hosts.

- Infection originates by inhalation into the respiratory tract followed by dissemination to the CNS in most cases, usually without recognizable lung involvement
- Almost always in the setting of AIDS or other disorders of cellular immune function
- Neutropenia alone poses a much lower risk of significant cryptococcal infection

DIAGNOSIS

DIFFERENTIAL DIAGNOSIS

- Subacute meningitis (caused by *Listeria monocytogenes, Mycobacterium tuberculosis, Histoplasma capsulatum,* viruses)
- Intracranial mass lesion (neoplasms, toxoplasmosis, TB)
- Pulmonary involvement confused with *Pneumocystis jiroveci* pneumonia when diffuse or confused with TB or bacterial pneumonia when focal or involving the pleura
- Skin lesions confused with bacterial cellulitis or molluscum contagiosum

WORKUP

- Lumbar puncture to exclude cryptococcal meningitis.
- CT scan of the head when focal lesion or increased intracranial pressure is suspected.
- Biopsy of enlarged lymph nodes and skin lesions if feasible.

LABORATORY TESTS

- Culture and India ink stain (60% to 80% sensitive in culture-proven cases [Fig. 1-286]) examination of the CSF in all cases when CNS involvement is suspected
- Blood and serum cryptococcal antigen assay (>90% sensitivity and specificity)
- Culture and histologic examination of biopsy material
- HIV

IMAGING STUDIES

- CT scan or MRI of the head if focal neurologic involvement is suspected
- Chest x-ray examination to exclude pulmonary involvement

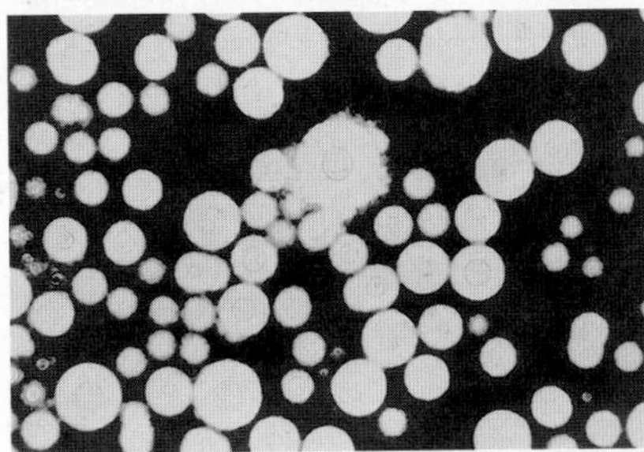

FIGURE 1-286 India ink preparation of cerebrospinal fluid revealing encapsulated cryptococci. Note the large capsules surrounding the smaller organisms. (From Andreoli TE [ed]: *Cecil essentials of medicine,* ed 4, Philadelphia, 1997, Saunders.)

TREATMENT

ACUTE GENERAL Rx

- Induction therapy for CNS disease (meningitis) is initiated with IV amphotericin B (0.5 to 0.8 mg/kg/day) with flucytosine 37.5 mg/kg PO q6h until afebrile and cultures negative (≈6 wk), then stop amphotericin B/flucytosine and start fluconazole 200 mg PO q24h or fluconazole 400 mg PO q24h for 8-10 wk or longer (up to 2 yr) to reduce relapse rate.
- Alternative: IV fluconazole for initial therapy in patients unable to tolerate amphotericin B.
- If symptomatic increased intracranial pressure, consider multiple therapeutic lumbar taps or intraventricular shunt.

CHRONIC Rx

- Fluconazole (200 to 400 mg PO qd) is highly effective in preventing a relapse in HIV-infected patients; development of resistance may occur. Itraconazole is an alternative agent.
- Immune reconstitution syndrome following the institution of HAART can cause transient worsening of meningitis and necessitate the use of a short course of corticosteroids.

DISPOSITION

Without maintenance therapy, relapse rate is >50% among AIDS patients.

REFERRAL

- For consultation with infectious diseases specialist in all cases
- For neurologic consultation if level of consciousness is depressed or focal lesion is present

PEARLS & CONSIDERATIONS

Cryptococcal meningitis can be remarkably insidious in nonimmunocompromised patients.

COMMENTS

Cryptococcosis is considered an AIDS-defining infection; thus all patients should be HIV tested.

SUGGESTED READINGS

available at www.expertconsult.com

RELATED CONTENT

Cryptococcosis (Patient Information)

AUTHORS: **PHILIP A. CHAN, M.D., M.S.,** and **GLENN G. FORT, M.D., M.P.H.**

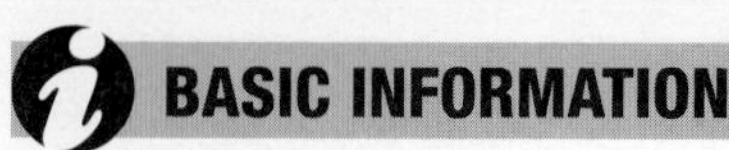

BASIC INFORMATION

DEFINITION

The intracellular protozoan parasite *Cryptosporidium parvum* is associated with gastrointestinal disease and diarrhea, especially in AIDS patients or immunocompromised hosts. It is also associated with sporadic infections and waterborne outbreaks in immunocompetent hosts.

Other species, including *C. hominis, C. felis, C. muris,* and *C. meleagridis,* are now described to be pathogens as well.

SYNONYMS

Cryptosporidiosis

ICD-9CM CODES
007.4 Cryptosporidia infection
ICD-10CM CODES
A07.2 Cryptosporidiosis

EPIDEMIOLOGY & DEMOGRAPHICS

INCIDENCE (IN U.S.):

- Approximately 2% in industrial countries, 5% to 10% in developing countries
- 10% to 20% of HIV patients in U.S. may excrete cyst

PREVALENCE: Worldwide, especially third world countries; associated with poor hygiene as a waterborne pathogen

PREDOMINANT SEX: Male = female

TRANSMISSION:

- Person to person (daycare, family members)
- Animal to person (pets, farm animals)
- Environmental (water-associated outbreaks, including travel associated with swimming in or drinking contaminated water or eating contaminated food)
- May be significant pathogen causing diarrhea in AIDS

PHYSICAL FINDINGS & CLINICAL PRESENTATION

- Spectrum of illness ranging from asymptomatic to severe enteritis
- Usually limited to gastrointestinal tract
- Diarrhea, severe abdominal pain (2 to 28 days)
- Impaired digestion, dehydration
- Fever, malaise, fatigue, nausea, vomiting
- Pneumonia if aspirated

ETIOLOGY

Cryptosporidium hominis, C. parvum, C. felis, C. muris, C. meleagridis

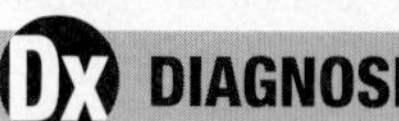

DIAGNOSIS

Clinical presentation of acute gastrointestinal illness, especially associated with HIV or with travel and waterborne outbreaks.

DIFFERENTIAL DIAGNOSIS

- *Campylobacter*
- *Clostridium difficile*
- *Entamoeba histolytica*
- *Giardia lamblia*
- *Salmonella*
- *Shigella*
- Microsporidia
- Cytomegalovirus
- *Mycobacterium avium*

Disease may cause cholecystitis, reactive arthritis, hepatitis, pancreatitis, pneumonia in immunocompromised or HIV-infected patients.

WORKUP

- Stool evaluation looking for characteristic oocyst by modified acid-fast stain (Fig. 1-288).
- Direct immunofluorescence using monoclonal antibodies is the gold standard for stool exams.
- HIV

TREATMENT

- May be self-limited in normal host over several weeks. Antidiarrhea agents Pepto-Bismol, Kaopectate, or loperamide may give symptomatic relief.
- Pharmacologic treatment with antibiotics has been largely unsatisfactory in AIDS patients. Antiviral therapy is the treatment of choice to restore the immune system. Oocyst excretion reduction has been shown with nitazoxanide 500 mg PO bid for 3 days in immunocompetent patients. If treatment fails, consider a trial of paromomycin, metronidazole, or trimethoprim/sulfamethoxazole. However, these medications have not been approved for treatment of *Cryptosporidium.*
- Nitazoxanide elixir has been approved for the treatment of cryptosporidiosis in children ages 1 to 11 yr.
- Biliary cryptosporidiosis can be treated with antiretroviral therapy in the HIV setting.

DISPOSITION

- A self-limited disease in immunocompetent patients with complete recovery over 2 to 3 weeks.
- Chronic arthralgia, headache, malaise, and weakness may persist after cryptosporidial infection even in immunologically normal people.
- If severe and prolonged disease (>30 days), testing for HIV and other immunocompromised states is appropriate along with a referral to an infectious disease specialist or gastroenterologist.

REFERRAL

- To an infectious disease specialist if symptoms persist and if HIV infection is found
- To a gastroenterologist if chronic malabsorption, or biliary or pancreatic complications occur

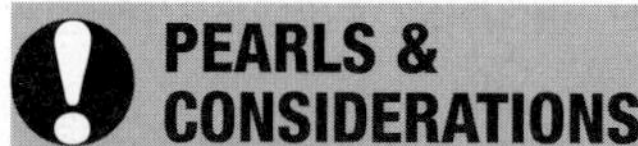

PEARLS & CONSIDERATIONS

- Chronic cryptosporidiosis (>30 days of diarrhea from *Cryptosporidium* spp. infection) in a patient with HIV is an AIDS-qualifying opportunistic infection.
- *Cryptosporidium hominis* has a limited host range (humans), whereas *Cryptosporidium parvum* has a wide host range including humans, horses, cattle, other domesticated animals, and wild animals; both species present a similar illness in humans.

SUGGESTED READINGS

available at www.expertconsult.com

AUTHORS: **PHILIP A. CHAN, M.D., M.S.,** and **GLENN G. FORT, M.D., M.P.H.**

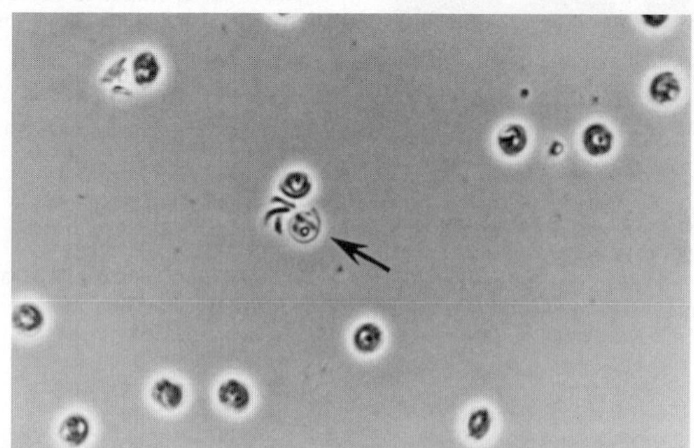

FIGURE 1-288 Human stool-derived *Cryptosporidium* oocysts. Excysting oocyst *(arrow)* is releasing three of its four sporozoites. (Phase-control microscopy ×630.) (From Gorbach SL: *Infectious diseases,* ed 2, Philadelphia, 1998, Saunders.)

BASIC INFORMATION

DEFINITION

Cubital Tunnel Syndrome is a compression neuropathy of the ulnar nerve as it traverses the cubital tunnel at the elbow (Fig. 1-289). It is the second most common entrapment neuropathy of the upper extremity.

ICD-9CM CODES
354.2 Cubital tunnel syndrome
ICD-10CM CODES
G56.2 Lesion of ulnar nerve, unspecified upper limb

EPIDEMIOLOGY & DEMOGRAPHICS

Males and females equally affected. Cubital tunnel syndrome is, after carpal tunnel syndrome, the second most common compression neuropathy of the upper extremity.

PHYSICAL FINDINGS & CLINICAL PRESENTATION

- Paresthesias, numbness along distribution of ulnar nerve (little finger and medial half of ring finger); pain is less common
- Positive Tinel's sign at elbow over the ulnar groove—highest negative predictive value
- Positive elbow flexion test (flexion of elbow with wrist extended for 30 sec may reproduce symptoms)
- Pressure provocation test (direct pressure over cubital tunnel for 60 sec elicits symptoms)
- "Scratch collapse" test—positive if temporary loss of external rotation resistance after examiner scratches over the compressed ulnar nerve; due to allodynia
- Signs of old trauma or elbow instability (valgus stress)
- Ulnar nerve may be subluxable over medial epicondyle with elbow motion
- Weakness/atrophy of intrinsic musculature of hand in longstanding cases (Fig. 1-290)
- "Intrinsic minus" or claw hand; due to paralysis of lumbricals and interossei (clawing usually worse in ring and small fingers)
- Masse's sign—hand appears flattened due to hypothenar muscle paralysis
- Wartenberg's sign—due to weakness of interossei: weak adduction of small finger
- Froment's sign—compensation by thumb flexor (flexor pollicis longus, median-nerve innervated) for diminished thumb pinch strength (paralysis of adductor pollicis, which is innervated by ulnar nerve)

Ulnar nerve
Medial epicondyle
Flexor carpi ulnaris
Ulnar collateral ligament

FIGURE 1-289 The cubital tunnel. The fibro-osseous canal is formed by the medial epicondyle, ulnar collateral ligament, and flexor carpi ulnaris muscle. Elbow flexion decreases the volume of the channel. (From Hochberg MC et al: *Rheumatology*, ed 5, St Louis, 2011, Mosby.)

ETIOLOGY

- Previous trauma, fractures
- Chronic pressure over ulnar groove from occupational stress, unusual elbow positioning
- Cubitus valgus deformity
- Subluxation of ulnar nerve
- Repeated stretching during throwing motion
- Elbow synovitis, osteophytes
- Local muscular hypertrophy
- Increased cubital tunnel pressure, particularly in elbow flexion
- Symptoms develop due to local nerve ischemia

DIAGNOSIS

DIFFERENTIAL DIAGNOSIS

- Tardy ulnar palsy
- Medial epicondylitis
- Other peripheral neuropathies
- Carpal tunnel syndrome
- Cervical radiculopathy
- Ulnar nerve compression at wrist (Guyon's canal)

WORKUP

Diagnosis can usually be established clinically. Provocative tests have either inadequate or inconsistent sensitivity and specificity. These tests are operator dependent and may have substantial inter-rater variation.

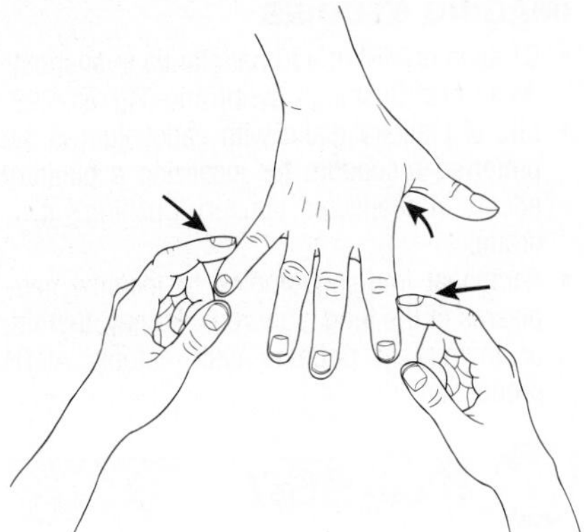

FIGURE 1-290 Testing for intrinsic (ulnar) motor weakness (fanning the fingers against resistance). Always look for atrophy of the first dorsal interosseus *(curved arrow)* when ulnar nerve lesions are suspected. (From Mercier LR: *Practical orthopedics*, ed 5, St Louis, 2000, Mosby.)

IMAGING STUDIES

- Routine roentgenograms may be helpful in ruling out other conditions.
- Electrodiagnostic studies: nerve conduction tests and electromyography are useful to confirm the clinical diagnosis and can help localize site of compression.
- High-resolution ultrasound may be a valuable adjunct to diagnosis.
- On ultrasound, there was strong correlation found between greater ulnar nerve cross-sectional area at the elbow and presence of cubital tunnel syndrome, using electrodiagnostic criteria as the reference standard.

TREATMENT

ACUTE GENERAL Rx

- Activity modification, avoiding prolonged/repetitive flexion
- Elbow pads to relieve pressure, splints limiting flexion
- Physical therapy

DISPOSITION

- There is tendency toward spontaneous recovery with mild/moderate or intermittent symptoms if provocative causes are avoided.
- If muscle atrophy has developed, recovery of strength may be incomplete despite treatment.

REFERRAL

Surgical referral needed in cases of failed medical management. Patients with constant symptoms or muscle atrophy usually require surgical treatment. Surgical treatment can consist of ulnar nerve in situ decompression, partial medical epicondylectomy and endoscopic ulnar nerve decompression, or anterior transposition of the ulnar nerve (subcutaneous, intramuscular, or submuscular).

PEARLS & CONSIDERATIONS

Patients with cubital tunnel syndrome are 4 times more likely to present with atrophy than those with carpal tunnel syndrome. Surgical decompression has been shown to be successful and may be adequate in most cases. More recently, endoscopic decompression techniques have been described. Ulnar nerve transposition and medial epicondylectomy are other surgical options.

SUGGESTED READINGS

available at www.expertconsult.com

RELATED CONTENT

Cubital Tunnel Syndrome (Patient Information)

AUTHOR: **CANDICE YUVIENCO, M.D.**

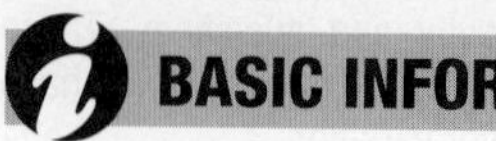

BASIC INFORMATION

DEFINITION

- Cushing's syndrome is the occurrence of clinical abnormalities associated with glucocorticoid excess as a result of exaggerated adrenal cortisol production or long-term glucocorticoid therapy.
- Cushing's disease is Cushing's syndrome caused by pituitary adrenocorticotropic hormone (ACTH) excess.

ICD-9CM CODES
255.0 Cushing's disease or syndrome
ICD-10CM CODES
E24 Cushing syndrome
E24.2 Drug-induced Cushing syndrome
E24.3 Ectopic ACTH syndrome
E24.8 Other Cushing syndrome
E24.9 Cushing syndrome, unspecified
E24.9 Pituitary-dependent Cushing's disease

PHYSICAL FINDINGS & CLINICAL PRESENTATION

- Hypertension
- Central obesity with rounding of the facies (moon facies); thin extremities
- Hirsutism, menstrual irregularities, hypogonadism
- Skin fragility, ecchymoses, red-purple abdominal striae (Fig. E1-291), acne, poor wound healing, hair loss, facial plethora, hyperpigmentation (with ACTH excess)
- Psychosis, emotional lability, paranoia
- Muscle wasting with proximal myopathy

NOTE: The previous characteristics are not commonly present in Cushing's syndrome caused by ectopic ACTH production. Many of these tumors secrete a biologically inactive ACTH that does not activate adrenal steroid synthesis. These patients may have only weight loss and weakness.

ETIOLOGY

- Iatrogenic from long-term glucocorticoid therapy (common)
- Pituitary ACTH excess (Cushing's disease; 60%)
- Adrenal neoplasms (30%)
- Ectopic ACTH production (neoplasms of lung, pancreas, kidney, thyroid, thymus; 10%)
- Table E1-143 summarizes the incidence of tumors associated with the ectopic adrenocorticotropic hormone syndrome
- A classification of causes of Cushing's syndrome is described in Table E1-144

DIAGNOSIS

DIFFERENTIAL DIAGNOSIS

- Alcoholic pseudo-Cushing's syndrome (endogenous cortisol overproduction)
- Obesity associated with diabetes mellitus
- Adrenogenital syndrome

WORKUP (Table E1-145)

- In patients with a clinical diagnosis of Cushing's syndrome the initial screening test is the overnight dexamethasone suppression test:
  1. Dexamethasone 1 mg PO given at 11 PM
  2. Plasma cortisol level measured 9 hr later (8 AM)
  3. Plasma cortisol level <5 mcg/100 ml excludes Cushing's syndrome
- Serial measurements (two or three consecutive measurements) of 24-hr urinary free cortisol and creatinine (to ensure adequacy of collection) are undertaken if overnight dexamethasone test is suggestive of Cushing's syndrome. Persistent elevated cortisol excretion (>300 mcg/24 hr) indicates Cushing's syndrome.
- The low-dose (2 mg) dexamethasone suppression test is useful to exclude pseudo-Cushing's syndrome if the previous results are equivocal. Corticotropic-releasing hormone (CRH) stimulation after low-dose dexamethasone administration (dexamethasone-CRH test) is also used to distinguish patients with suspected Cushing's syndrome from those who have mildly elevated urinary free cortisol level and equivocal findings.
- The high-dose (8 mg) dexamethasone test and measurement of ACTH by radioimmunoassay are useful to determine the etiology of Cushing's syndrome.
  1. ACTH undetectable or decreased and lack of suppression indicate adrenal cause of Cushing's syndrome.
  2. ACTH normal or increased and lack of suppression indicate ectopic ACTH production.
  3. ACTH normal or increased and partial suppression suggest pituitary excess (Cushing's disease).

Bilateral inferior petrosal sinus sampling (BIPSS) can be used to distinguish pituitary Cushing's disease from the ectopic ACTH syndrome (Fig. E1-292).

LABORATORY TESTS

- Hypokalemia, hypochloremia, metabolic alkalosis, hyperglycemia, hypercholesterolemia
- Increased 24-hr urinary free cortisol (>100 mcg/24 hr)

IMAGING STUDIES

- CT scan or MRI of adrenal glands in suspected adrenal Cushing's syndrome (Fig. E1-293)
- MRI of pituitary gland with gadolinium is the preferred procedure for localizing a pituitary edema in suspected pituitary Cushing's syndrome
- Additional imaging studies to localize neoplasms of the lung, pancreas, kidney, thyroid, or thymus in patients with ectopic ACTH production

TREATMENT

GENERAL Rx

The definitive treatment of Cushing's syndrome is surgical removal of the tumor causing excessive production of cortisol:

- Pituitary adenoma: transsphenoidal microadenomectomy is the therapy of choice in adults. Pituitary irradiation is reserved for patients not cured by transsphenoidal surgery. In children, pituitary irradiation may be considered as initial therapy because 85% of children are cured by radiation. Stereotactic radiotherapy (photon knife or gamma knife) is effective and exposes the surrounding neuronal tissues to less irradiation than conventional radiotherapy. Total bilateral adrenalectomy is reserved for patients not cured by transsphenoidal surgery or pituitary irradiation.
- Adrenal neoplasm:
  1. Surgical resection of the affected adrenal
  2. Glucocorticoid replacement for approximately 9 to 12 mo after the surgery to allow time for the contralateral adrenal gland to recover from its prolonged suppression
  3. In nonsurgical candidates, suppression of adrenal steroid production can be accomplished with ketoconazole. Mifepristone, an antiprogestin, can also be used for control of hyperglycemia secondary to hypercortisolism in adults with endogenous Cushing's syndrome. It should be avoided in women who are or who could become pregnant.
- Bilateral micronodular or macronodular adrenal hyperplasia: bilateral total adrenalectomy
- Ectopic ACTH:
  1. Surgical resection of the ACTH-secreting neoplasm
  2. Control of cortisol excess with metyrapone, aminoglutethimide, mifepristone, or ketoconazole
  3. Control of the mineralocorticoid effects of cortisol and 11-deoxycorticosteroid with spironolactone
  4. Bilateral adrenalectomy: a rational approach to patients with indolent, unresectable tumors

DISPOSITION

Prognosis is favorable in patients with surgically amenable disease.

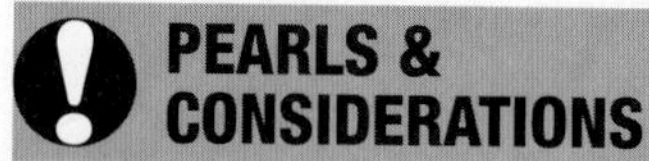

PEARLS & CONSIDERATIONS

COMMENTS

- A single midnight serum cortisol level (normal diurnal variation leads to a nadir around midnight) >7.5 mcg/dl has been reported as 96% sensitive and 100% specific for the diagnosis of Cushing's syndrome.
- Screening for multiple endocrine neoplasia type I should be considered in patients with Cushing's disease.

SUGGESTED READINGS

available at www.expertconsult.com

RELATED CONTENT

Cushing's Syndrome (Patient Information)

AUTHOR: **FRED F. FERRI, M.D.**

BASIC INFORMATION

DEFINITION

Cystic fibrosis (CF) is an autosomal recessive disorder characterized by dysfunction of exocrine glands.

ICD-9CM CODES
277.0 Cystic fibrosis
ICD-10CM CODES
E84.9 Cystic fibrosis, unspecified

EPIDEMIOLOGY & DEMOGRAPHICS

- CF is the most common fatal hereditary disorder of whites in the U.S. (one case per 2500 whites) and second most common life-shortening childhood-onset inherited disorder in the U.S., behind sickle cell disease.
- Median age at diagnosis is 5.3 mo. Median survival is 30 yr.
- Carrier screening is associated with a decrease in incidence of CF.

PHYSICAL FINDINGS & CLINICAL PRESENTATION

- Failure to thrive in children
- Increased anterior/posterior chest diameter
- Basilar crackles and hyperresonance to percussion
- Digital clubbing
- Chronic cough
- Abdominal distention
- Greasy, smelly feces

ETIOLOGY

Chromosome 7 gene mutation (*CFTR* gene) resulting in abnormalities in chloride transport and water flux across the surface of epithelial cells; the abnormal secretions cause obstruction of glands and ducts in various organs and subsequent damage to exocrine tissue (recurrent pneumonia, atelectasis, bronchiectasis, diabetes mellitus, biliary cirrhosis, cholelithiasis, intestinal obstruction, increased risk of gastrointestinal malignancies).

TABLE 1-147 Diagnostic Criteria for Cystic Fibrosis (CF)

Presence of typical clinical features (respiratory, gastrointestinal, or genitourinary)
OR
A history of CF in a sibling
OR
A positive newborn screening test
PLUS
Laboratory evidence for CFTR (CF transmembrane regulator) dysfunction:
Two elevated sweat chloride concentrations obtained on separate days
OR
Identification of two CF mutations
OR
An abnormal nasal potential difference measurement

From Kliegman RM et al: *Nelson textbook of pediatrics*, ed 19, Philadelphia, 2011, Saunders.

DIAGNOSIS

DIFFERENTIAL DIAGNOSIS

- Immunodeficiency states
- Celiac disease
- Asthma
- Recurrent pneumonia

WORKUP

A diagnosis of CF requires a positive quantitative pilocarpine iontophoresis test with one or more phenotypic features consistent with CF (e.g., chronic suppurative obstructive lung disease, pancreatic insufficiency) or documented CF in a sibling or first cousin. Table 1-147 describes diagnostic criteria for CF. Conditions suggesting the diagnosis of CF in adults and recommended diagnostic studies are described in Table 1-148.

LABORATORY TESTS

- Pilocarpine iontophoresis (sweat test): diagnostic of CF in children if sweat chloride is >60 mmol/L (>80 mmol/L in adults) on two separate tests on consecutive days. Repeat testing may be necessary because not all infants have sufficient quantities of sweat for reliable testing. Table 1-149 describes conditions associated with false-positive and false-negative sweat test results.
- DNA testing may be useful for confirming the diagnosis and providing genetic information for family members.
- Sputum culture and sensitivity and Gram stain (frequent bacterial infections with *Staphylococcus aureus, Pseudomonas aeruginosa* [most common virulent respiratory pathogen], *Haemophilus influenzae*). Bronchoalveolar lavage (BAL) is used at times to aid in the early diagnosis of pulmonary infection in non-expectorating patients. However, evidence for its clinical benefit is lacking. Trials have shown that among infants diagnosed with CF, BAL-directed therapy did not result in a lower prevalence of *P. aeruginosa* infection or lower total CF-CT score when compared with standard therapy at age 5 years.
- Low albumin level, increased 72-hr fecal fat excretion.
- Pulse oximetry or arterial blood gases: hypoxemia.
- Pulmonary function studies: decreased total lung capacity, forced vital capacity, pulmonary diffusing capacity.

TABLE 1-148 Approach to Diagnosis of Cystic Fibrosis in Adult Patients

Conditions Suggesting the Diagnosis of Cystic Fibrosis in Adults
Recurrent pancreatitis
Male infertility
Chronic sinusitis
Nasal polyposis
Nontuberculous mycobacterial infection
Allergic bronchopulmonary mycosis
Bronchiectasis
Recommended Diagnostic Studies
Sweat electrolyte determination
Extended CFTR mutation analysis
Nasal potential difference
High-resolution CT scan to identify bronchiectasis
CT scan of sinuses for polyposis
Sputum induction or bronchoalveolar lavage to identify bacterial and fungal pathogens

CFTR, Cystic fibrosis transmembrane conductance regulator; *CT*, computed tomography.
From Goldman L, Schafer AI: *Goldman's Cecil medicine*, ed 24, Philadelphia, 2012, Saunders.

IMAGING STUDIES

- Chest x-ray (Fig. 1-295): may reveal focal atelectasis, peribronchial cuffing, bronchiectasis, increased interstitial markings, hyperinflation
- High-resolution chest CT scan: bronchial wall thickening, cystic lesions, ring shadows (bronchiectasis)

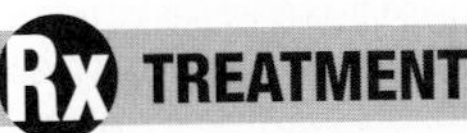

TREATMENT

NONPHARMACOLOGIC THERAPY

- Postural drainage and chest percussion
- Encouragement of regular exercise and proper nutrition
- Psychosocial evaluation and counseling of patient and family members

TABLE 1-149 Conditions Associated with False-Positive and False-Negative Sweat Test Results

With False-Positive Results
Eczema (atopic dermatitis)
Ectodermal dysplasia
Malnutrition/failure to thrive/deprivation
Anorexia nervosa
Congenital adrenal hyperplasia
Adrenal insufficiency
Glucose-6-phosphatase deficiency
Mauriac syndrome
Fucosidosis
Familial hypoparathyroidism
Hypothyroidism
Nephrogenic diabetes insipidus
Pseudohypoaldosteronism
Klinefelter syndrome
Familial cholestasis syndrome
Autonomic dysfunction
Prostaglandin E infusions
Munchausen syndrome by proxy
With False-Negative Results
Dilution
Malnutrition
Edema
Insufficient sweat quantity
Hyponatremia
Cystic fibrosis transmembrane conductance regulator (CFTR) mutations with preserved sweat duct function

From Kliegman RM et al: *Nelson textbook of pediatrics*, ed 19, Philadelphia, 2011, Saunders.

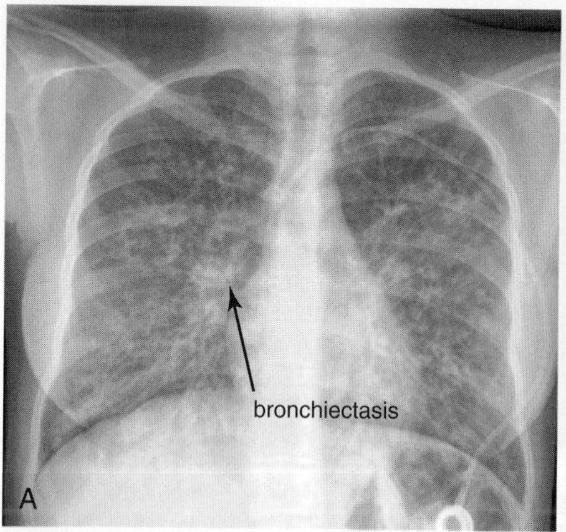

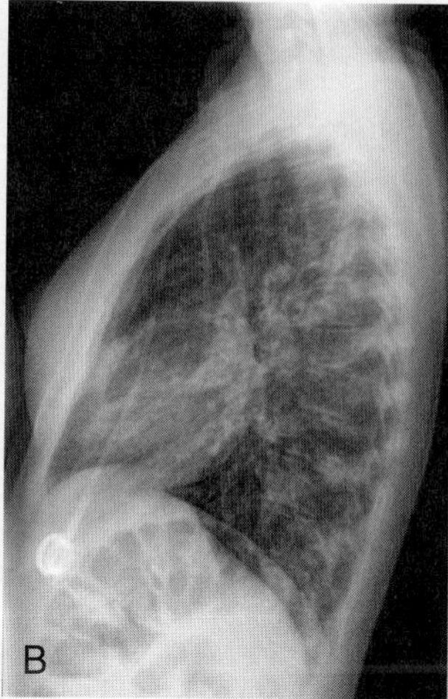

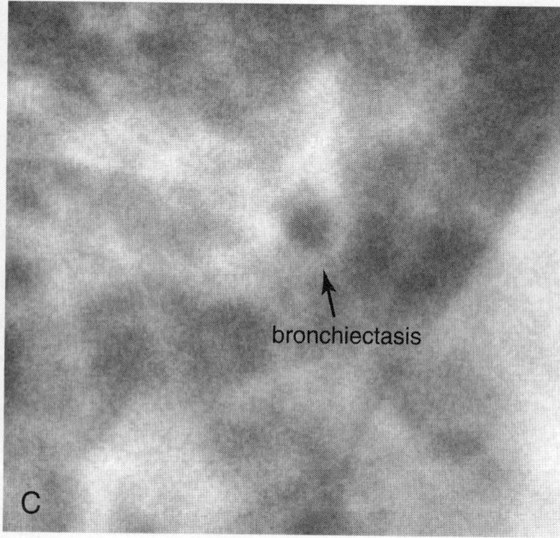

FIGURE 1-295 Cystic fibrosis. Cystic fibrosis is aptly named. Chest x-ray findings include increased interstitial density of fibrosis and cystic changes of lung parenchyma similar to chronic obstructive pulmonary disease. Bronchiectasis (dilation of bronchi, potentially eroding into bronchial arteries and presenting with hemoptysis) may be visible on chest x-ray as large and thickened bronchioles particularly when viewed in short axis (when bronchioles are oriented perpendicular to the frontal plane). This l5-year-old with cystic fibrosis presented with cough and dyspnea. Does she have pneumonia? Comparison with prior x-rays showed no changes. **A,** Posterior-anterior chest x-ray. **B,** Lateral chest x-ray. **C,** Close-up from **A** showing bronchiectasis. (From Broder JS: *Diagnostic imaging for the emergency physician,* Philadelphia, 2011, Saunders.)

ACUTE GENERAL Rx

- Antibiotic therapy based on results of Gram stain and culture and sensitivity of sputum (PO quinolones for *Pseudomonas,* cephalosporins for *S. aureus,* IV aminoglycosides [tobramycin] plus ceftazidime or ticarcillin for life-threatening *Pseudomonas* infections). Inhaled antibiotics (aztreonam or tobramycin) can also be used and can achieve high airway concentration with lower systemic side effects. Macrolides are also active against *Pseudomonas aeruginosa.* For *S. aureus* infection, use oxacillin or nafcillin 2 g IV p4h if MSSA; if dealing with MRSA, use IV vancomycin 1 g q12h. A recent study using azithromycin maintenance in children with CF for 6 mo found less use of additional antibiotics and improvement in some aspects of pulmonary function. Additional studies may be necessary to determine if azithromycin should be used as a primary therapy or rescue treatment.
- Bronchodilators for patients with airflow obstruction.
- Long-term pancreatic enzyme replacement.
- Alternate-day prednisone (2 mg/kg) possibly beneficial in children with CF (decreased hospitalization rate, improved pulmonary function); routine use of corticosteroids not recommended in adults; among children with CF who have received alternate-day treatment with prednisone, boys, but not girls, have persistent growth impairment after treatment is discontinued.
- Proper nutrition and vitamin supplementation.
- Recombinant human deoxyribonuclease (DNase [Dornase alpha]) 2.5 mg qd or bid given by aerosol for patients with viscid sputum. It lowers the viscosity of sputum. It is useful to improve mucociliary clearance by liquefying difficult-to-clear pulmonary secretions. It is, however, very expensive; it is most beneficial in patients with forced vital capacity values >40% of predicted. Its cost can be decreased by using alternate-day rhDNase therapy.
- Intermittent administration of inhaled tobramycin has been reported beneficial in CF.
- Newer treatment modalities involve increasing the activity of CF transmembrane conductance regulator (CFTR) protein. Ivacaftor (a CFTR potentiator) is FDA approved for oral treatment of CF in patients 6 years and older with the G551D mutation (5% of patients with CF). It can decrease the frequency of pulmonary exacerbations and improve lung function. Dose is 150 mg PO BID. Cost is a significant limiting factor.
- Treatment of impaired glucose tolerance and diabetes mellitus.

CHRONIC Rx

Pneumococcal and influenza vaccination

DISPOSITION

- Bronchiectasis develops early in the course of cystic fibrosis, being detectable in infants as young as 10 wk of age, and is persistent and progressive. Recent data[1] reveal that neutrophil elastase activity in BAL fluid in early life is associated with early bronchiectasis in children with cystic fibrosis.
- More than 50% of children with CF live beyond age 20 yr. During the past 2 decades, survival among patients with late-stage CF has lengthened substantially. This is believed due to increased use of NBH DNase.
- Lung transplantation is the only definitive treatment; 3-yr survival after transplantation exceeds 50%.
- Obstructive azoospermia is present in >98% of postpubertal males.
- The SERPINA Z allele is a risk factor for liver disease in CF. Patients that carry the Z allele are at a greater risk of developing severe liver disease with portal hypertension.

REFERRAL

- For lung transplantation in selected patients. Indications for lung transplantation are FEV_1 <30% of predicted, rapidly progressive respiratory deterioration, increasing number of hospital admissions, massive hemoptysis, recurrent pneumothorax, arterial partial pressure of oxygen <55 mm Hg, arterial partial pressure of carbon dioxide >50 mm Hg, multiresistant organisms, wasting. Young female patients should be referred earlier because of overall poor prognosis.
- For screening of family members with DNA analysis.

[1]Sly PD et al: Risk factors for bronchiectasis in children with cystic fibrosis, *N Engl J Med* 368: 1963-1970, 2013.

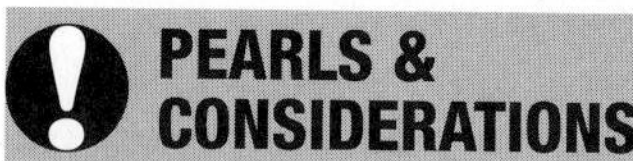

PEARLS & CONSIDERATIONS

COMMENTS

- Clinicians should think of CF in any patient with bronchiectasis plus any of the following: male infertility, recurrent idiopathic pancreatitis, recurrent nasal polyposis.
- Genetic testing for CF should be offered to adults with a positive family history of CF, couples currently planning a pregnancy, and couples seeking prenatal care.
- Inhalation of hypertonic saline (5 ml of 7% sodium chloride qid) has been reported to produce a sustained acceleration of mucus clearance and improved lung function.
- The prevalence of MRSA in the respiratory tract of individuals with CF has increased dramatically over the past decade and is associated with worse survival.

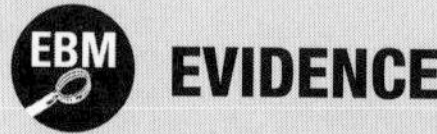

EVIDENCE

available at www.expertconsult.com

SUGGESTED READINGS

available at www.expertconsult.com

RELATED CONTENT

Cystic Fibrosis (Patient Information)
Bronchiectasis (Related Key Topic)

AUTHOR: **FRED F. FERRI, M.D.**

BASIC INFORMATION

DEFINITION

Cysticercosis is an infection caused by the tissue deposition of larval forms of the pork tapeworm *Taenia solium. T. solium* cysts, or cysticerci, may accumulate in any human tissue, including the eyes, spinal cord, skin, muscle, heart, and brain. Central nervous system (CNS) involvement is common and is known as neurocysticercosis. Humans most commonly acquire cysticercosis from human tapeworm carriers, or via ingestion of larval cysts in infected pork or soil tapeworm eggs in contaminated water. Larvae in the gastrointestinal tract migrate hematogenously to tissues, where they encyst, forming cysticerci.

SYNONYMS

Cysticerciasis
Taeniasis
Pork tapeworm

ICD-9CM CODES
123.1 Cysticercosis
ICD-10 CODES
B69 Cysticercosis
B69.0 Cysticercosis of central nervous system
B69.1 Cysticercosis of eye
B69.8 Cysticercosis of other sites
B69.9 Cysticercosis, unspecified

EPIDEMIOLOGY & DEMOGRAPHICS

- *T. solium* infection is worldwide in distribution. Tapeworm infection and cysticercosis are endemic in developing countries where pigs are raised as a food source.
- Serologic studies from endemic areas of Latin America have demonstrated seroprevalences of 4% to 24% in native populations.
- Neurocysticercosis is the most common cause of acquired epilepsy worldwide and has become an important parasitic disease in the U.S., especially in states with large immigrant populations from countries where the disease is endemic.

PHYSICAL FINDINGS & CLINICAL PRESENTATION

- After ingestion of *T. solium* eggs or cysts, human beings may remain asymptomatic for years.
- The symptoms vary and depend on the location of cysticerci. Cysticerci in muscles and skin may form "cold" nodules, which are usually asymptomatic but may calcify and be seen on radiographs.
- Neurocysticercosis, or the presence of cysts within the brain parenchyma, is usually asymptomatic. Symptoms stem from inflammation associated with the degeneration of cysts.
- Seizures are the most common manifestation of neurocysticercosis, occurring in 70% to 90% of symptomatic cases. Headache is also common.
- Inflammation around degenerating cysts may result in focal encephalitis, vasculitis, chronic meningitis, and cranial nerve palsies.
- In 10% to 20% of cases of neurocysticercosis, cysts lodge within the ventricular system and result in obstructive hydrocephalus, causing acute intracranial hypertension. Symptoms are caused by the presence of the parasite itself, ependymal inflammation, and/or fibrosis, each of which block the circulation of cerebrospinal fluid (CSF). Death may occur from progressive hydrocephalus, cerebral edema, or intractable seizures.
- Ocular cysticercosis occurs in less than 5% of infections and is generally asymptomatic. Inflammation in response to degenerating cysticerci may result in chorioretinitis, vasculitis, or retinal detachment, threatening vision.

ETIOLOGY

- *T. solium* has a complex two-host life cycle.
- Human beings are the only definitive host and harbor the adult worm in the intestine (taeniasis). However, both human beings and pigs can serve as intermediate hosts and harbor the larvae or cysticerci.

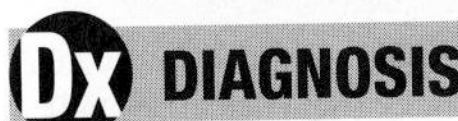

DIAGNOSIS

DIFFERENTIAL DIAGNOSIS

- Idiopathic epilepsy
- Migraine
- CNS vasculitis
- Primary neoplasia of CNS
- Chronic CNS infections, including toxoplasmosis, coccidioidomycosis, tuberculosis, and cryptococcosis
- Brain abscess
- CNS involvement with sarcoidosis or systemic lupus erythematosus

WORKUP

Comprehensive clinical history: obtain information on current and previous travel and residence, including geographic area, sanitary conditions, and dietary habits, most importantly consumption of undercooked pork.

LABORATORY TESTS

- Definitive diagnosis is based on the histopathologic demonstration of cysticerci in the tissue involved.
- Peripheral eosinophilia is usually absent.
- Stool examination for ova and proglottids of *T. solium* is insensitive and not specific for the diagnosis of cysticercosis.
- CSF examination may demonstrate pleocytosis, with lymphocytic or eosinophilic predominance, low glucose, and elevated protein with neurocysticercosis. However, CSF is normal in most cases.
- Serologic testing is supportive of a suspected diagnosis of cysticercosis. Antibody detection by enzyme-linked immunoelectrotransfer blot (EITB) assay is the test of choice for serodiagnosis. It has high sensitivity and specificity in comparison with previous assays and can be performed on serum or CSF. However, the diagnostic performance of the EITB can vary in different patient populations depending on the activity of the cysts and number of lesions. Single calcified lesions are more likely to be associated with a false-negative assay result, with 38% of patients with a single brain lesion testing negative in one study. Antibodies detected by EITB can persist for years after successful therapy limiting the usefulness of this assay in following patients after treatment. In endemic regions, the test is useful in ruling out disease but is positive in a significant proportion of exposed individuals without disease.
- Antigen detection by enzyme-linked immunosorbent assay can predict the presence of viable *Cysticerca* organisms, even in cases where all CNS lesions are calcified and presumed to be inactive. Furthermore, high antigen levels suggest the presence of subarachnoid neurocysticercosis. This method may be particularly useful in monitoring patients following therapy. Parasite antigen levels usually fall within 3 months of successful treatment.
- More recently, amplification of *T. solium* DNA, with the method of polymerase chain reaction, has been achieved (sensitivity 96.7%).

IMAGING STUDIES

- Plain radiographs of the extremities may reveal calcified cysts in patients with soft tissue or muscle involvement.
- For diagnosis of neurocysticercosis, CT and MRI are most commonly used.
- Brain CT (Fig. 1-296) has a sensitivity and specificity of 95% and can identify living cysticerci, which appear as hypodense lesions, as well as degenerating cysts, which appear as isodense or hyperdense lesions with surrounding edema. CT is the best method for detecting calcification associated with prior infection, which suggests inactivity.
- Brain MRI is the most accurate technique to assess the extent of infection, location, and evolutionary stage of the parasites. MRI provides detailed images of living and degenerating cysts, perilesional edema, as well as small cysts or those located in the ventricles, brainstem, and cerebellum. However, MRI has a low sensitivity for detecting calcified lesions, which are the most common neuroimaging finding in endemic populations.

Rx TREATMENT

ACUTE GENERAL Rx

Asymptomatic cysticercosis:

- There is no evidence that administering antiparasitic therapy is beneficial.

Symptomatic neurocysticercosis:

- Treatment decisions in neurocysticercosis should be individualized. Initial measures should focus on the symptomatic management before considering antiparasitic therapy when appropriate.
- Patients with active lesions, with evidence of surrounding edema and/or inflammation, generally warrant treatment with antiparasitics, corticosteroids, and anticonvulsants.

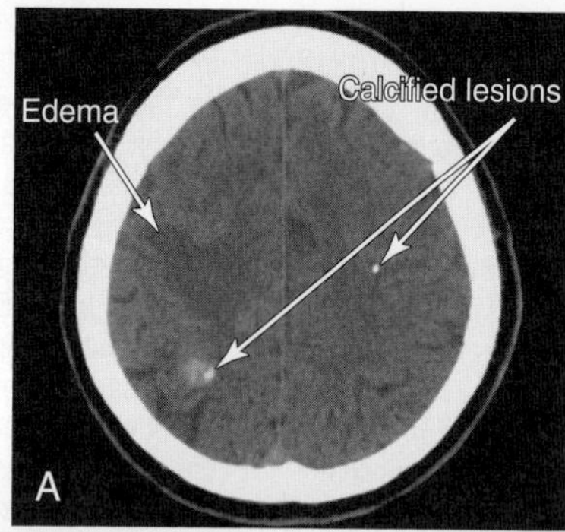

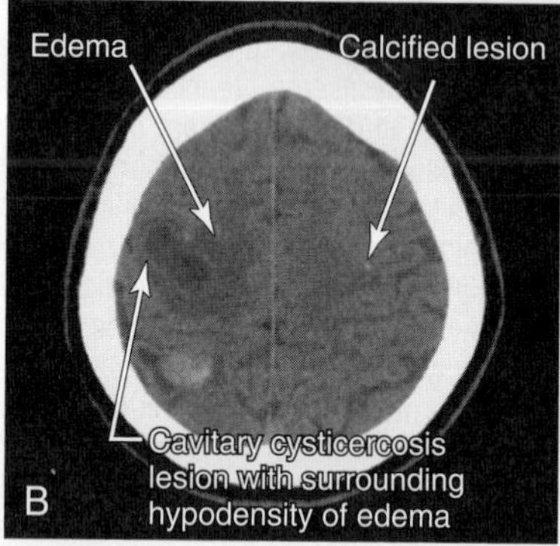

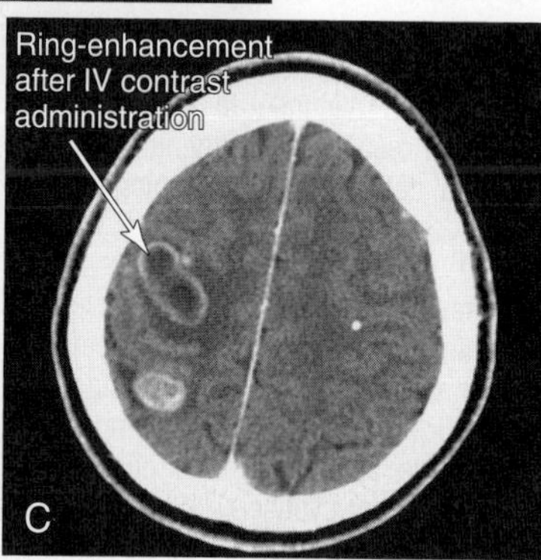

FIGURE 1-296 Neurocysticercosis. This 40-year-old Bolivian male presented with left-hand weakness. **A-B,** Noncontrast head CT, brain windows. **C,** CT with contrast moments later—compare this with image **B.** A slice through the same level of the brain before contrast administration. Hypodense lesions are present, with surrounding hypodensity *(dark gray)* representing edema. Scattered calcifications are also seen, which are a common feature of old neurocysticercosis lesions. Administration of IV contrast leads to ring enhancement, a feature of many infectious and inflammatory conditions, including neurocysticercosis, brain abscess, and toxoplasmosis. (From Broder JS: *Diagnostic imaging for the emergency physician,* Philadelphia, 2011, Saunders.)

- Anticonvulsant therapy:
- Patients who have seizures or are considered at risk for recurrent seizures based on imaging should be treated with anticonvulsants.
- Antiparasitic therapy:
  - Pharmacologic therapy is indicated in the treatment of symptomatic patients with multiple viable brain parenchymal cysticerci. However, despite treatment, only 30% to 50% of lesions resolve within 6 months.
  - Calcified cysticerci are inactive and do not warrant antiparasitic treatment.
  - Antiparasitic therapy is often unnecessary in patients with single cysts, which are usually self-limited and resolve within 6 months.
- Cysticidal therapy:
  - Antiparasitic therapy hastens the disappearance of cysts and should initially be given in conjunction with corticosteroids to control the inflammation associated with dying organisms.
  - Patients with viable parenchymal or subarachnoid cysts should be treated with albendazole 15 mg/kg/day PO divided BID for 7 days or praziquantel 50 mg/kg/day divided TID for 28 days. Albendazole is preferred since praziquantel management is more complicated due to an interaction with corticosteroids. Patients should be medicated with prednisolone 2 mg/kg/day or 0.15 mg/kg/day oral dexamethasone, either concurrent with albendazole, or starting albendazole on the third day of corticosteroids. Antiparasitics should be used cautiously in patients with massive cysticercal infection of the brain parenchyma (≥50 cysts) or cysticercal encephalitis. These patients should be managed initially with corticosteroids, and perhaps mannitol, to control intracranial hypertension. Once the inflammation and the edema have resolved by MRI, antiparasitics can be administered.
  - Praziquantel may cause drug interactions with other agents metabolized by the cytochrome p450 systems, including phenytoin and phenobarbital. Furthermore, praziquantel serum levels are decreased by concomitant use of corticosteroids.
  - Albendazole has no significant drug interactions with anticonvulsants.
  - Albendazole is considered to be the drug of choice due to slightly better efficacy, greater availability, and lower cost.
  - The combined use of albendazole and praziquantel for neurocysticercosis has been reported.
- Surgical therapy:
  - Surgery may be indicated in patients with obstructive hydrocephalus or giant cysts with associated intracranial hypertension.
  - Minimally invasive neurosurgery (neuroendoscopy) for cyst removal and ventricular shunt formation has greatly improved the management of intraventricular neurocysticercosis.
  - Extraparenchymal cysticercosis, including ocular, subarachnoid, and intraventricular disease, carries a poor prognosis and requires a more aggressive approach. When feasible, complete surgical excision of lesions remains the definitive therapy.

CHRONIC Rx

- A recently published study suggests that prolonged antiparasitic therapy does not improve outcomes in patients with neurocysticercosis and seizures. Antiparasitic therapy, in fact, delayed calcification of lesions. Antiepileptic medications may need to be continued indefinitely.
- Rare patients with neurocysticercosis develop chronic or recurrent perilesional inflammation, requiring long-term, high-dose steroid therapy. Methotrexate has been reported to be of use as a steroid-sparing agent in this setting.

DISPOSITION

- In seizure-free, stable neurocysticercosis, outpatient management is appropriate.
- Patients with seizures should be restricted from driving.

REFERRAL

- Infectious diseases consultation
- Neurology consultation in patients with seizures
- Neurosurgical consultation if extraparenchymal neurocysticercosis or obstructive hydrocephalus is present

PREVENTION

- Eradication of taeniasis/cysticercosis is possible with implementation of meat inspection, improvement of pig husbandry, and improvement of socioeconomic conditions in endemic areas.
- A porcine vaccine against *T. solium* has been developed and successfully implemented in Peru, Mexico, and Australia.
- There is currently no human vaccine to prevent tapeworm infection or cysticercosis.

PATIENT & FAMILY EDUCATION

- Pork should be inspected for the presence of cysticerci, which are visible in raw meat.
- Pork must be well cooked.
- Proper disposal of human excreta and handwashing are of utmost importance to break the transmission cycle in households.

SUGGESTED READINGS

available at www.expertconsult.com

RELATED CONTENT

Cysticercosis (Patient Information)

AUTHORS: **ELENI PATROZOU, M.D.,** and **STACI A. FISCHER, M.D.**

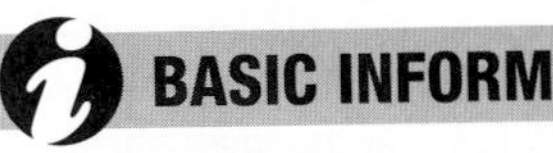

BASIC INFORMATION

DEFINITION

Infection with cytomegalovirus (CMV), a herpes virus, is common in the general population, with multiple mechanisms for transmission, often during childhood and adolescence. CMV is associated with pregnancy and can be a congenital disease. CMV is also associated with immunocompromised states and may be life threatening.

SYNONYMS

CMV
Heterophil-negative mononucleosis
Cytomegalic inclusion disease virus

ICD-9CM CODES

078.5	CMV infection
771.1	Congenital or perinatal CMV infection
V01.7	Exposure to CMV

ICD-10CM CODES

B25.9	Cytomegaloviral disease, unspecified
P35.1	Congenital cytomegalovirus infection
Z20.820	Contact with and (suspected) exposure to varicella

EPIDEMIOLOGY & DEMOGRAPHICS

- Seroprevalence is widespread: 40% to 100% antibody positivity in adults.
- Increased infection develops perinatally, in day care exposure, and then during reproductive age, related to sexual activity.

ROUTES OF TRANSMISSION

- Blood transfusions
- Sexually (STDs) via uterus, cervix, and semen
- Perinatally via breast milk
- Transplant of organs—bone marrow, kidneys, liver, heart, or lung

PHYSICAL FINDINGS & CLINICAL PRESENTATION

CHILDREN: Congenital—25% of infected children with symptoms if congenital:
- Petechial rash
- Jaundice and/or hepatosplenomegaly
- Lethargy
- Respiratory distress
- CNS involvement, seizures

Postnatal acquisition:
- CMV mononucleosis
- Pharyngitis, croup, bronchitis, pneumonia

HEALTHY ADULTS:

Common
- May be asymptomatic
- CMV mononucleosis similar to EBV mononucleosis
- Fever—lasting 9 to 30 days—mean of 19 days

Less common
- Exudative pharyngitis
- Lymphadenopathy, hepatitis, splenomegaly
- Interstitial pneumonia (rare)
- Nonspecific rash
- Thrombocytopenia/hemolytic anemia

Rare
- Guillain-Barré syndrome
- Meningoencephalitis
- Myocarditis

IMMUNOSUPPRESSED PATIENTS:
- Febrile mononucleosis
- GI ulcerations, hepatitis, pneumonitis, retinitis, encephalopathy, meningoencephalopathy
- HIV associated—dementia, demyelination, retinitis, acalculous cholecystitis, adrenalitis, diarrhea, enterocolitis, esophagitis
- Diabetes associated with pancreatitis
- Adrenalitis associated with HIV

ETIOLOGY

CMV infection can remain latent, reactive with immunosuppression.

Dx DIAGNOSIS

DIFFERENTIAL DIAGNOSIS

Congenital:
- Acute viral, bacterial, parasitic infections including other congenitally transmitted agents (toxoplasmosis, rubella, syphilis, pertussis, croup, bronchitis)

Acquired:
- EBV mononucleosis
- Viral hepatitis—A, B, C
- Cryptosporidiosis
- Toxoplasmosis
- *Mycobacterium avium* infections
- Human herpesvirus 6
- Acute HIV infection

WORKUP

- Laboratory confirmation combined with clinical findings often with leukopenia, thrombocytopenia, lymphocytosis
- Serology:
  1. Detection of CMV-IgM antibodies suggests recent infection. CMV-IgG antibodies usually appear 2 to 3 weeks after infection.
  2. Molecular amplification tests: options include PCR assays on plasma, leukocytes and whole blood, nucleic acid sequence based amplification (NASBA), and Hybrid Capture System CMV DNA test. These tests are used in immunocompromised patients, AIDS and transplant patients.
- Cultures: using human fibroblast cultures of blood, CSF, urine, BAL, and biopsy specimens but can take 1 to 6 weeks
- Funduscopic—necrotic patches with white granular component of retina
- Biopsy—"owl's eye" inclusion bodies on tissue sample
- HIV

IMAGING STUDIES

- Chest radiograph—if pneumonitis suspected, consider bronchoscopy
- Endoscopy—if GI involvement
- CT scan/MRI—if CNS involvement

Rx TREATMENT

NONPHARMACOLOGIC THERAPY

- Strict hand washing and standard precautions limit CMV transmission in health care facilities.
- Antiretroviral therapy (ART) in patients with CD4 count <50/mm^3 for the goal of CD4 >100/mm^3 for a 3- to 6-mo period

ACUTE GENERAL Rx

For compromised hosts with CMV retinitis or pneumonitis:
- Ganciclovir 5 mg/kg q12h IV x 14 to 21 days, then valganciclovir: 900 mg PO q24h or alternative regimen
- Ganciclovir intraocular implant plus valganciclovir 900 mg PO q24h or alternative regimen
- Foscarnet 90 mg/kg q12h x 14 to 21 days, then 90 mg to 120 mg/kg IV q24h or alternative regimen
- Cidofovir 5 mg/kg IV q day x 14 days, then 5 mg/kg IV q 2 weeks
- Fomivirsen-salvage therapy for CMV retinitis 300 μg injected into vitreous

DISPOSITION

- CMV infection in patients who are immunocompromised (especially those with AIDS, bone marrow and solid organ transplant recipients, and disorders of cell-mediated immune function) will need expert, long-term follow-up by an infectious disease specialist or immunologist familiar with the care of such patients.
- CMV mononucleosis, hepatitis, pharyngitis, etc. in immunologically normal hosts are usually self-limiting infections requiring no special follow-up plans.

REFERRAL

- To an ophthalmologist if CMV retinitis is present
- To an infectious disease specialist or AIDS specialist for patients who are HIV-positive with CMV disease
- To a cellular immunologist or transplant specialist in the case of CMV infection in a transplant recipient
- To a pediatric infectious disease specialist for congenital CMV infection

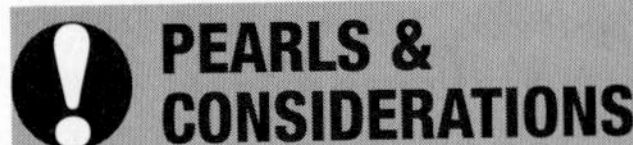

PEARLS & CONSIDERATIONS

CMV is ubiquitous in the environment and is asymptomatically shed by latently infected persons with CMV infection, making it difficult to protect patients who are immunocompromised from acquiring this infection.

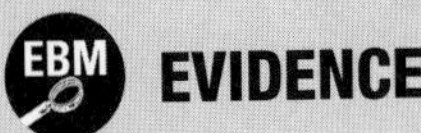

EVIDENCE

available at www.expertconsult.com

SUGGESTED READINGS

available at www.expertconsult.com

AUTHOR: **GLENN G. FORT, M.D., M.P.H.**

BASIC INFORMATION

DEFINITION

Venous thromboembolism is any thromboembolic event occurring within the venous system. Deep vein thrombosis (DVT) is the development of thrombi in the deep veins of the extremities or pelvis.

SYNONYMS

DVT
Venous thromboembolism (VTE) (VTE includes DVT and pulmonary embolism [PE])
Deep venous thrombosis

ICD-9CM CODES

451.1	Thrombosis of deep vessels of lower extremities
451.83	Thrombosis of deep veins of upper extremities
541.9	Deep vein thrombosis of unspecified site

ICD-10CM CODES

I80.29	Phlebitis and thrombophlebitis of other deep vessels of lower extremities
I80.293	Phlebitis and thrombophlebitis of other deep vessels of lower extremity, bilateral
I80.8	Phlebitis and thrombophlebitis of other sites
I80.9	Phlebitis and thrombophlebitis of unspecified site

EPIDEMIOLOGY & DEMOGRAPHICS

- Annual incidence of VTE is 0.1% to 0.27%, affecting up to 5% of the population during their lifetimes.
- The risk of recurrent thromboembolism is higher among men than women.
- About 5% to 15% of persons with untreated DVT die from pulmonary embolism.

PHYSICAL FINDINGS & CLINICAL PRESENTATION

- Pain and swelling of the affected extremity
- In lower extremity DVT: leg pain on dorsiflexion of the foot (***Homans' sign***)
- Physical examination may be unremarkable in early DVT

ETIOLOGY

The etiology is often multifactorial (prolonged stasis, coagulation abnormalities, vessel wall trauma). The following are risk factors for DVT:

- Prolonged immobilization (>3 days)
- Postoperative state
- Trauma to pelvis and lower extremities for lower extremity DVT; central line placement for upper extremity DVT
- Birth control pills, high-dose estrogen therapy; conjugated equine estrogen but not esterified estrogen is associated with increased risk of DVT; estrogen plus progestin is associated with doubling the risk of venous thrombosis. The use of bevacizumab is also significantly associated with an increased risk of developing DVT in cancer patients receiving this drug.
- Visceral cancer (lung, pancreas, alimentary tract, genitourinary tract)
- Age >60 yr
- History of thromboembolic disease
- Hematologic disorders (e.g., factor V Leiden mutation [FVL], antithrombin III deficiency, protein C deficiency, protein S deficiency, heparin cofactor II deficiency, sticky platelet syndrome, G20210A prothrombin mutation, lupus anticoagulant, dysfibrinogenemias, anticardiolipin antibody, hyperhomocystinemia, concurrent homocystinuria, high levels of factors VIII, XI, and single nucleotide polymorphisms [SNPs] such as CYP4V2)
- Pregnancy and early puerperium
- Obesity (BMI >30)
- Congestive heart failure
- Surgery, fracture, or injury involving lower leg or pelvis
- Plaster cast immobilization
- Surgery requiring >30 min of anesthesia
- Gynecologic surgery (particularly gynecologic cancer surgery)
- Recent travel (within 2 wk, lasting ≥2 hr). Every 2 hr spent traveling increases VTE risk by 18%.
- Smoking and abdominal obesity
- Central venous catheter or pacemaker insertion
- Superficial vein thrombosis (10% risk of DVT within 3 mo), varicose veins
- Collagen vascular disease
- Nephrotic syndrome
- Myeloproliferative disorders
- Long-term exposure to particulate air pollution is also associated with altered coagulation function and DVT risk.

Dx DIAGNOSIS

DIFFERENTIAL DIAGNOSIS

- Postphlebitic syndrome
- Superficial thrombophlebitis
- Ruptured Baker's cyst
- Cellulitis, lymphangitis, Achilles tendinitis
- Hematoma
- Muscle or soft tissue injury, stress fracture
- Varicose veins, lymphedema
- Arterial insufficiency
- Abscess
- Claudication
- Venous stasis

WORKUP

- The clinical diagnosis of DVT is inaccurate. Pain, tenderness, swelling, or color changes are not specific for DVT.
- Clinical prediction rules can be used to establish pretest probability of DVT. The Wells prediction rules for DVT and for pulmonary embolism are described in Box 1-18. These rules perform better in younger patients without a history of DVT and in those without comorbidities. In younger patients without associated comorbidities and a low pretest probability using Wells criteria and a negative high-sensitivity D-dimer test, the diagnosis of DVT can be reasonably excluded.
- Compression ultrasonography (CUS; Fig. E1-297) is preferred as the initial study to diagnose DVT in patients with intermediate to high pretest probability. An initial negative test limited to the proximal leg should be repeated after 5 days (if the clinical suspicion of DVT persists) to exclude DVT that is propagating proximally from the calf. Comprehensive ultrasonography (whole-leg CUS) is a more extensive test that examines the deep veins from the inguinal ligament to the level of the malleolus. Literature reports indicate that it may be safe to withhold anticoagulation after negative results on comprehensive duplex ultrasonography in nonpregnant patients with a suspected first episode of symptomatic DVT of the leg.

LABORATORY TESTS

- Laboratory tests are not specific for DVT. Baseline prothrombin time (INR), partial thromboplastin time, and platelet count should be obtained on all patients before starting anticoagulation. D-dimer testing is sensitive but not specific for DVT. A negative

BOX 1-18 Wells Prediction Rule for Diagnosing Deep Venous Thrombosis: Clinical Evaluation Table for Predicting Pretest Probability of Deep Venous Thrombosis*

Clinical Characteristic	Score
Active cancer (treatment ongoing, within previous 6 mo, or palliative)	1
Paralysis, paresis, or recent plaster immobilization of the lower extremities	1
Recently bedridden >3 days or major surgery within 12 wk requiring general or regional anesthesia	1
Localized tenderness along the distribution of the deep venous system	1
Entire leg swollen	1
Calf swelling 3 cm larger than asymptomatic side (measured 10 cm below tibial tuberosity)	1
Pitting edema confined to the symptomatic leg	1
Collateral superficial veins (nonvaricose)	1
Alternative diagnosis at least as likely as deep venous thrombosis	22

*Clinical probability: low, ≤0; intermediate, 1-2; high, ≥3. In patients with symptoms in both legs, the more symptomatic leg is used.

Reprinted from Wells PS et al: Value assessment of pretest probability of deep-vein thrombosis in clinical management, *Lancet* 351:1795-1798, 1997.

result (D-dimer <0.5 mcg/ml) can exclude the diagnosis, but a positive result (≥0.5 mcg/ml) mandates additional testing with venous ultrasonography.

- Use of D-dimer assay by ELISA is useful in the management of suspected DVT. The combination of a normal d-dimer study on presentation together with a normal compression venous ultrasound is useful to exclude DVT. DVT can be ruled out in patients who are clinically unlikely to have DVT and who have a negative d-dimer test. Compressive ultrasonography can be safely omitted in such patients. Fig. E1-298 is an algorithm for the diagnosis of DVT.
- Laboratory evaluation of young patients with DVT, patients with recurrent thrombosis without obvious causes, and those with a family history of thrombosis should include protein S (both total and free PS), protein C, fibrinogen, antithrombin III level, lupus anticoagulant, anticardiolipin antibodies, anti-β2 glycoprotein1, factor V Leiden, factor VIII, factor IX, and fasting plasma homocysteine levels. HIT antibody may also be useful in the correct context (heparin exposure and abrupt onset of unexplained decrease in platelet count, whether thrombocytopenic or not). It is important to remember that the lupus anticoagulant assay and antithrombin, protein C, protein S, and dysfibrinogenemia testing cannot be properly interpreted if the patient is already on warfarin, whereas anticardiolipin antibody test, prothrombin G20210A factor VII:C, factor V Leiden, and PT polymorphism can be performed when the patient is on warfarin.

IMAGING STUDIES

- Compression ultrasonography (CUS) is generally preferred as the initial study because it is noninvasive and can be repeated serially (useful to monitor suspected acute DVT); it offers good sensitivity for detecting proximal vein thrombosis (in the popliteal or femoral vein) (see Fig. E1-297). Its disadvantages are poor visualization of deep iliac and pelvic veins and poor sensitivity in isolated or nonocclusive calf vein thrombi. Whole-leg compression ultrasound can generally exclude proximal and distal DVT in a single evaluation. Withholding anticoagulation following a single negative whole-leg CUS is associated with a relatively low risk of venous thromboembolism (3.5% of inpatients will develop DVT) during a 3-mo follow-up.
- Contrast venography is the gold standard for evaluation of DVT of the lower extremity. It is, however, invasive and painful. Additional disadvantages are the increased risk of phlebitis, new thrombosis, renal failure, and hypersensitivity reaction to contrast media; it also gives poor visualization of the deep femoral vein in the thigh and the internal iliac vein and its tributaries.
- Magnetic resonance direct thrombus imaging (MRDTI) is an accurate noninvasive test for diagnosis of DVT. It is particularly useful in suspected DVT patients with leg casts, which prevent CUS and in pregnant patients with positive D-dimer and negative CUS (Fig. E1-299). Current limitations are its cost and lack of widespread availability.

Rx TREATMENT

NONPHARMACOLOGIC THERAPY

- Gradual resumption of normal activity. Immobility promotes stasis and propagation of DVT. Patients should get up and walk as tolerated. The theoretical risk that ambulation may dislodge thrombi in the legs, precipitating PE, is unfounded.
- Patient education on anticoagulant therapy and associated risks.

ACUTE GENERAL Rx

- Initial treatment of DVT requires therapeutic doses of heparin (low-molecular-weight heparin [LMWH] or unfractionated). LMWH is preferred due to ease of administration, less hemorrhage, and significantly fewer deaths. Unfractionated heparin is recommended in patients with renal insufficiency because LMWH is predominantly excreted in the urine.
- LMWH is generally administered for 5 to 7 days. Recommended dose of enoxaparin is 1 mg/kg q12h SC. Once-daily fondaparinux, a synthetic analog of heparin, is also as effective and safe as twice-daily enoxaparin in the initial treatment of patients with symptomatic DVT. Once systemic anticoagulation is initiated, vitamin K antagonist warfarin is initiated. For most patients, warfarin is started on the same day as heparin and is titrated to maintain an INR between 2 and 3. After ≥5 days, heparin is stopped and warfarin is continued as monotherapy. Long-term LMWH may be preferable to warfarin in patients with cancer or those whose INR is difficult to control. Other possible alternatives to warfarin may include the oral factor Xa inhibitors rivaroxaban, apixaban, or edoxaban, or dabigatran, a direct oral thrombin inhibitor. These new anticoagulants are noninferior to warfarin, do not require periodic lab monitoring, and have a relatively low bleeding risk. They may eventually become preferred agents for extended treatment of venous thromboembolism.
- Outpatient treatment of DVT is appropriate for patients without prior DVT, thrombophilic conditions, or substantial comorbidity, but not for those who are pregnant or likely not to adhere to therapy.
- Exclusions from outpatient treatment of DVT include patients with potential high complication risk (e.g., hemoglobin <7, platelet count <75,000, guaiac-positive stool, recent cerebrovascular accident or noncutaneous surgery, noncompliance).
- Compression stockings are effective in reducing the incidence of postthrombotic syndrome and should be used starting within 1 mo of proximal DVT and continued for at least 1 yr after diagnosis.
- Insertion of an inferior vena cava filter to prevent pulmonary embolism is recommended in patients with contraindications to anticoagulation (e.g., hemorrhagic stroke, active internal bleeding, pregnancy), HIT in a patient with an active VTE/PE, recurrent PE despite adequate anticoagulant therapy, emergent surgery in patient with DVT, presence of free-floating iliofemoral thrombus, lower IVC thrombosis (incipient embolization), and chronic pulmonary (thromboembolic) hypertension with limited pulmonary reserve.
- Thrombolytic therapy (streptokinase) can be used in rare cases (unless contraindicated) in patients with extensive iliofemoral venous thrombosis and a low risk of bleeding. There are concerns about hemorrhagic complications related to the large doses of thrombolytics required in systemic thrombolysis for DVT (2% to 10% risk of major hemorrhagic complications).
- Other treatment modalities for DVT include surgical thrombectomy and catheter-directed thrombolysis (CDT). Thromboreduction by surgical thrombectomy is effective but invasive and expensive. CDT is also invasive, carries a bleeding risk, and will require ICU admission.

CHRONIC Rx

- The optimal duration of anticoagulant therapy varies with the cause of DVT and the patient's risk factors. The risk of recurrence is low if VTE is provoked by surgery, intermediate if provoked by a nonsurgical risk factor, and high if unprovoked. These risks should determine whether patients with VTE should undergo short-term vs. indefinite treatment.
- Therapy for 3 mo is generally satisfactory in patients with reversible risk factors (low-risk group). A high d-dimer level measured after 3 mo of anticoagulation in patients with unprovoked DVT should favor a longer duration of therapy.
- Anticoagulation for 6 mo is recommended for patients with idiopathic venous thrombosis or medical risk factors for DVT (intermediate-risk group). About 20% of patients with unprovoked venous thromboembolism have a recurrence within 2 yr after the withdrawal of oral anticoagulant therapy. Use of daily low-dose aspirin after discontinuation of anticoagulant treatment may provide a modest reduction in DVT risk.
- Indefinite anticoagulation is necessary in patients with DVT associated with active cancer; long-term anticoagulation is also indicated in patients with inherited thrombophilia (e.g., deficiency of antithrombin III, protein C or S antibody), high factor VIII levels, antiphospholipid antibody, and those with recurrent episodes of idiopathic DVT (high-risk group). Long-term anticoagulation should also be considered in the presence of comorbidities such as paroxysmal nocturnal hemoglobinuria (PNH), SLE (especially with nephrotic syndrome), some myoproliferative disorders, IBD, and Cushing's syndrome.

- Measurement of D-dimer after withdrawal of oral anticoagulation may be useful to estimate the risk of recurrence in selected patients. In patients with a first unprovoked DVT, positive d-dimer test results after cessation of anticoagulation predict recurrence, regardless of test timing or patient's age. Patients with a first spontaneous DVT and a d-dimer level <250 mg/ml after withdrawal of oral anticoagulation have a low risk of DVT recurrence. Recent trials show that in patients who have completed at least 3 mo of anticoagulation for a first episode of unprovoked DVT and after approximately 2 yr of follow-up, a negative D-dimer result is associated with a 3.5% annual risk of recurrent disease, whereas a positive D-dimer result is associated with an 8.9% annual risk for recurrence. Hence, elevated d-dimer levels would be an indication for prolonged therapy (for 1 or 2 more yr at a minimum).
- The presence of residual thrombosis on ultrasonography when warfarin therapy is discontinued is also associated with an increased risk for subsequent recurrent DVT; a recent trial showed that tailoring the duration of anticoagulation on the basis of the persistence of residual thrombi on ultrasonography may reduce the rate of recurrent DVT. Additional trials are needed before this approach can be adapted for all patients.
- Patients with DVT and pulmonary embolism are at high risk of recurrence whenever anticoagulation is discontinued; therefore, many experts recommend prolonged anticoagulation in this population group, especially if other risk factors for recurrence are present.

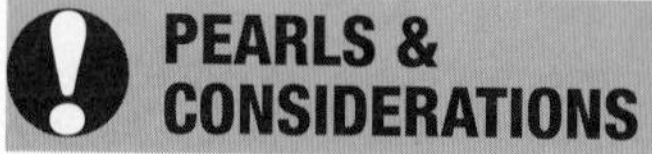

PEARLS & CONSIDERATIONS

COMMENTS

- When using heparin, there is a risk of heparin-induced thrombocytopenia (HIT) (with unfractionated more so than with LMWH). Platelet count should be obtained initially and repeated every 3 days while on heparin.
- ***PROPHYLAXIS OF DVT:*** Recommended in all patients at risk (e.g., low-molecular-weight heparin [enoxaparin 30 mg SC bid or fondaparinux 2.5 mg SC daily] after major trauma, post surgery of hip and knee; enoxaparin 40 mg SC qd post-abdominal surgery in patients with moderate to high DVT risk; gradient elastic stockings alone or in combination with intermittent pneumatic compression [IPC] boots following neurosurgery). Graduated compression stockings (GCSs) are effective for preventing air-travel-related DVT and in reducing the risk of DVT in patients hospitalized for conditions other than stroke. The type of GCSs is also important because proximal DVT occurs more often in patients with stroke who wear below-knee stockings than in those who wear high-length stockings. The new oral anticoagulants (rivaroxaban, apixaban, etc.) are effective for thromboprophylaxis after THR and TKR. However, their clinical benefits over LMWH are marginal, they are more expensive, and they lack antidotes for timely reversal in case of bleeding.
- ***RECURRENT THROMBOEMBOLISM:*** The risk of recurrent venous thromboembolism in heterozygous carriers of factor V Leiden and a first spontaneous venous thromboembolism is similar to that of non-carriers of factor V Leiden; therefore, heterozygous patients should receive secondary thromboprophylaxis for a similar length of time as patients without factor V Leiden.
- ***POST-THROMBOTIC SYNDROME:*** Approximately 20% to 50% of patients with DVT develop postthrombotic syndrome characterized by leg edema, pain, venous ectasia, skin induration, and ulceration. Patients with extensive DVT and those with more severe postthrombotic manifestations 1 month after DVT have poorer long-term outcomes. Recent trials have shown that compression stockings after DVT do not prevent post-thrombotic syndrome.
- Exercise following DVT is reasonable because it improves flexibility of the affected leg and does not increase symptoms in patients with postthrombotic syndrome.
- Previously undiagnosed cancer is frequent in patients with newly diagnosed DVT. A cancer screening strategy should be considered in all patients with unprovoked venous thromboembolism.
- ***UPPER EXTREMITY DVT:*** It is less common than lower extremity DVT and is seen more frequently in patients requiring central venous catheters or wires. It confers risk for mortality, recurrent thromboembolic events, and post-thrombotic syndrome similar to that of lower extremity DVT. It is classified as primary upper extremity DVT (***Paget-Schroetter syndrome***) defined as a thrombus in the axillary and subclavian veins in absence of identifiable thrombosis risk factors. It accounts for 20% of upper extremity DVT cases and may be due to an underlying anatomic abnormality at the thoracic outlet in combination with local hypercoagulability due to venous stretching or perivascular fibrosis from recurrent venous compression. Secondary upper extremity DVT is defined as any DVT related to a predisposing factor (e.g., insertion of central venous catheter, wires, or other devices, malignancy). In patients with secondary upper extremity DVT removal of the catheter is not routinely recommended but is warranted if there is a catheter malfunction or infection, if anticoagulation therapy is contraindicated or has failed, or if the catheter is no longer needed. Anticoagulation therapy in upper extremity DVT consists of use of vitamin K antagonists except in patients with cancer, for whom low-molecular-weight heparin is preferred. Optimal duration of anticoagulation treatment in upper extremity DVT is 3 to 6 mo (including in those in whom a central catheter has been removed)
- ***REVERSAL OF ANTICOAGULATION:*** Vitamin K (1 mg PO or 2 mg IV) can be used to reverse elevated INR (3 to 6) when elective or urgent procedures are needed. The administration of vitamin K can take more than 24 hr to fully restore vitamin K dependent coagulation factors II, VII, IX, and X. The American College of Chest Physicians recommends the following guidelines for managing elevated INRs or bleeding in patients receiving vitamin A antagonist therapy:
  - INR 5 to <9 and no significant bleeding: omit dose and give vitamin K (1 to 2.5 mg orally). Monitor the next day and use additional vitamin K if necessary.
  - INR >9 and no significant bleeding: hold vitamin K antagonist, give 5 to 10 mg orally of vitamin K. Monitor the next day and use additional vitamin K if necessary. Resume therapy at lower dose when INR therapeutic.
  - Serious bleeding at any elevation of INR: hold vitamin K antagonist and supplement with prothrombin complex concentrates (PCC). Give vitamin K (10 mg by slow IV infusion over 30 min to reduce the risk of anaphylaxis). Vitamin K1 can be repeated every 12 hr. PCC composition in the U.S. (3-factor PCC) includes clotting factors II, IX, and X but minimal amounts of factor VII (unlike PCC products available outside of the U.S. [4-factor PCC], which have a significant amount of factor VII). In order to replace the low factor VII some clinicians in the U.S. will also give fresh frozen plasma (FFP) in addition to vitamin K and PCC in patients with life-threatening warfarin-related bleeding.

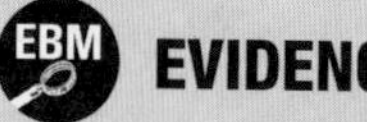

EVIDENCE

available at www.expertconsult.com

SUGGESTED READINGS

available at www.expertconsult.com

RELATED CONTENT

Deep Vein Thrombosis (DVT) (Patient Information)
Hypercoagulable State (Related Key Topic)
Antiphospholipid Antibody Syndrome (Related Key Topic)
Pulmonary Embolism (Related Key Topic)

AUTHOR: **FRED F. FERRI, M.D.**

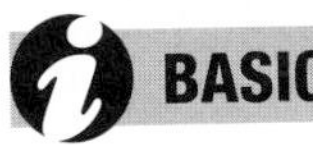

BASIC INFORMATION

DEFINITION

Delayed puberty is clinically defined as the lack or incomplete development of secondary sex characteristics by an age at which 95% of the population start to mature sexually. For girls, a delay is defined as no breast development by age 13 or primary amenorrhea by age 16. For boys, a delay is classified as no testicular enlargement by age 14.

SYNONYMS

Pubertal delay

ICD-9CM CODES
259.0 Delay in sexual development and puberty, not elsewhere classified
ICD-10CM CODES
E30.0 Delayed puberty

EPIDEMIOLOGY & DEMOGRAPHICS

PREVALENCE: Prevalence and incidence for children presenting with delayed puberty are unknown. However, delayed puberty is more common in boys.

GENETICS: Constitutional pubertal delay (CPD) often runs in families. Although specific gene mutations have yet to be identified, studies have shown that 50% to 75% of patients with CPD have at least one parent who experienced a delay in puberty. The inheritance pattern for CPD is thought to be autosomal dominant.

PHYSICAL FINDINGS & CLINICAL PRESENTATION

- Girls with pubertal delay have an absence of breast development by age 13, absence of menarche by age 16, or absence of menarche within 3 years of thelarche. Boys with pubertal delay show no evidence of testicular enlargement, further defined as testes <2.5 cm, by age 14. Absence of pubic and/or axillary hair is common, as is lack of growth spurt.
- Patients with a constitutional delay in puberty are short in stature with a normal growth rate and otherwise good health.
- Boys often fall below the 10th percentile on a height chart with normal rate of growth between 4 and 6 cm per yr.

ETIOLOGY

Causes for pubertal delay can be separated into four categories (from most to least common):

1. Constitutional delay, which is a temporary delay in puberty seen mostly in boys and tends to run in families. Patients are typically short in stature with normal growth rate and appropriate skeletal age.
2. Functional hypogonadotropic hypogonadism secondary to malnutrition or chronic disease. Celiac sprue, inflammatory bowel disease (IBD), hypothyroidism, diabetes mellitus, cystic fibrosis, and eating disorders such as anorexia nervosa are examples of illnesses that can cause a temporary yet reversible delay in puberty. Clinical suspicion is warranted when underweight children present with pubertal delay.
3. Hypergonadotropic hypogonadism caused by primary gonadal failure. Congenital disorders such as cryptorchidism; chromosomal disorders such as gonadal dysgenesis, Klinefelter's syndrome, and Turner's syndrome; and acquired causes secondary to chemotherapy, pelvic radiation, and gonadal surgery are organic dysfunctions that result in gonadal failure despite adequate hypothalamic-pituitary function. In this group of disorders, luteinizing hormone (LH) and follicle-stimulating hormone (FSH) levels are elevated yet cannot stimulate ovaries and testicles to produce estrogen and testosterone, respectively, leading to hypogonadism and absence of secondary sex characteristics.
4. Permanent hypogonadotropic hypogonadism secondary to genetic or acquired defects along the hypothalamic-pituitary-gonadal (HPG) axis. Kallmann's syndrome is a genetic mutation in *KAL1* found on the X chromosome and responsible for migration of gonadotropin-releasing hormone and olfactory neurons into the hypothalamus. Children with Kallmann's syndrome present with pubertal delay and anosmia. Other mutations such as *FGFR1* and *DAX1* have been linked to congenital gonadotropin deficiencies and pubertal delay. Acquired defects such as hemochromatosis, sickle cell anemia, and pituitary tumors can cause delayed puberty and other hypothalamic syndromes, including Prader-Willi. Table E1-150 provides a classification of puberty and sexual infantilism.

DIAGNOSIS

DIFFERENTIAL DIAGNOSIS

Normal or low serum LH, FSH

- Constitutional pubertal delay
- Functional hypogonadotropic hypogonadism
  - Malnutrition or eating disorder
  - Strenuous exercise
  - Chronic illness (hypothyroidism, celiac disease, IBD, cystic fibrosis, and so on)
- Hypopituitarism
  - Panhypopituitarism
  - Isolated gonadotropin deficiency
  - Kallmann's syndrome (associated with anosmia)
  - Prader-Willi syndrome
- Hyperprolactinemia
  - Pituitary adenoma
  - Drug-associated (cannabis, cocaine)

Increased serum gonadotropins

- Hypergonadotropic hypogonadism
  - Turner's syndrome (gonadal dysgenesis)
  - Klinefelter's syndrome
  - Gonadal dysgenesis
  - Noonan syndrome
  - Bilateral gonadal failure
    - Primary testicular failure
    - Anorchia
    - Premature ovarian failure
    - Resistant ovary syndrome
    - Radiation, chemotherapy
    - Trauma
    - Infections (e.g., mumps, orchitis)

Other conditions

- Androgen sensitivity syndrome
- Steroidogenic enzyme defects

WORKUP

- Given the extensive differential diagnosis for pubertal delay, a systematic and focused approach is necessary. Table E1-151 describes differential diagnostic features of delayed puberty and sexual infantilism. A careful history, including family history and social history, can identify eating and exercise habits, chronic illnesses, weight loss, poor weight gain, changes in bowel habits, and parental history of pubertal delay. Figs. 1-300 and 1-301 describe an algorithm for the evaluation of delayed puberty in males and females.
- Growth measurement should include height and weight, a growth chart to assess rate of growth, and calculation of the sex-adjusted midparental height that represents the statistically most probable adult height for the child.
  - For boys, add 2.5 inches (6.5 cm) from the mean of the parents' heights. For girls, subtract 2.5 inches (6.5 cm) from the mean of the parents' heights.
  - Physical exam can reveal signs of sexual maturation, stigmata of congenital syndromes, and nutritional status. Include neurologic exam (visual fields, ophthalmologic), thyroid, chest, heart, abdomen, and Tanner staging.

LABORATORY TESTS

- Serum LH, FSH, testosterone, and estradiol can help distinguish disorders of congenital or acquired gonadal failure from other causes. By age 10 to 12 yr gonadal failure produces elevated levels of serum LH and FSH. If levels are low or normal, constitutional delay is the most common diagnosis.
- Chromosomal analysis if there is a suspicion of gonadal dysgenesis or Klinefelter's syndrome.
- Screening studies include complete blood count, erythrocyte sedimentation rate, serum prolactin, serum thyroid-stimulating hormone, and free T4.
- Endocrinologist may do further studies such as IGF-1 to screen for growth hormone disorders and GnRH stimulation testing.

IMAGING STUDIES

Bone age skeletal radiograph of the left hand and wrist determines skeletal age, which is delayed in constitutional delay and GnRH deficiency. MRI of the head should be considered if there is high clinical suspicion for tumors of pituitary or hypothalamic origin. Pelvic ultrasound can be helpful in detecting intraabdominal testes and to evaluating müllerian anatomy.

TABLE 1-150 Differential Diagnostic Features of Delayed Puberty and Sexual Infantilism

Condition	Stature	Plasma Gonadotropins	GnRH Test LH Response	Plasma Gonadal Steroids	Plasma DHEAS	Karyotype	Olfaction
Constitutional delay in growth and adolescence	Short for chron. age, usually appropriate for bone age	Prepubertal, later pubertal	Prepubertal, later pubertal	Low, later normal	Low for chron. age, appropriate for bone age	Normal	Normal
Hypogonadotropic Hypogonadism							
Isolated gonadotropin deficiency	Normal, absent pubertal growth spurt	Low	Prepubertal or no response	Low	Appropriate for chron. age	Normal	Normal
Kallmann's syndrome	Normal, absent	Low	Prepubertal or no response	Low	Appropriate for chron. age	Normal	Anosmia; pubertal growth spurt or hyposmia
Idiopathic multiple pituitary hormone deficiencies	Short stature and poor growth since early childhood	Low	Prepubertal or no response	Low	Usually low	Normal	Normal
Hypothalamic-pituitary tumors	Late-onset decrease in growth velocity	Low	Prepubertal or no response	Low	Normal or low for chron. age	Normal	Normal
Primary Gonadal Failure							
Syndrome of gonadal dysgenesis (Turner's syndrome) and variants	Short stature since childhood	High	Hyperresponse for age	Low	Normal for chron. age	45,X or variant	Normal
Klinefelter's syndrome and variants	Normal to tall	High	Hyperresponse at puberty	Low or normal	Normal for chron. age	47,XXY or variant	Normal
Familial XX or XY gonadal dysgenesis	Normal for age	High	Hyperresponse	Low	Normal for chron. age	46,XX or 46,XY	Normal

chron., chronologic; *DHEAS*, dehydroepiandrosterone sulfate; *GnRH*, gonadotropin-releasing hormone; *LH*, luteinizing hormone.
From Melmed S, Polonsky KS, Larsen PR, Kronenberg HM: *Williams' textbook of endocrinology*, ed 12, Philadelphia, 2011, Saunders.

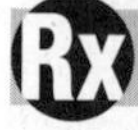

TREATMENT

- Treat underlying cause if identified.
- Constitutional delay can be managed with reassurance that the delay will have no effect on final adult height or development. Short-term hormonal therapy can be used to hasten puberty if the delay is causing severe psychosocial difficulties. PO oxandrolone can be given daily or IM depot testosterone q6wk for 3-6 mo for boys to improve velocity of growth. Girls can receive oral estradiol once daily for 3-6 mo.
- Malnutrition and chronic disease can best be treated by correcting the underlying etiology. A short (3-6 mo) treatment course, as described above, may be indicated for children with psychosocial difficulties.
- Permanent causes of pubertal delay can be treated by inducing puberty with testosterone for boys and estrogen plus progesterone for girls.
- Patients with Turner's syndrome will need adjunct growth hormone with or without oxandrolone.
- Gonadotropin deficiency or hypogonadism may require lifelong sex steroid replacement.
- Psychosocial evaluation, support, and treatment as needed.
- Table E1-152 summarizes the management and treatment of delayed puberty.

REFERRAL

Pediatric endocrinology

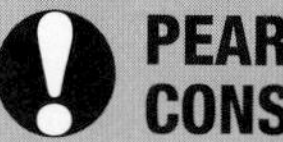

PEARLS & CONSIDERATIONS

COMMENTS

- Constitutional delay is the most common cause of pubertal delay and is often associated with a positive family history in parents and/or siblings, but it is a diagnosis of exclusion, so other causes, such as Turner's syndrome and systemic disorders, should be ruled out first.
- Bone age demonstrates more clearly than chronologic age how far an individual has progressed toward maturity and predicts the potential for further growth.
- No studies reliably differentiate constitutional delay from gonadotropin deficiency.

PATIENT & FAMILY EDUCATION

- The Magic Foundation, a support group for patients and their families (http://www.magicfoundation.org)
- The American Academy of Family Physicians (http://www.aafp.org)
- American Academy of Pediatrics (http://www.aap.org)
- Pediatric Endocrine Society (http://www.lwpes.org)
- Nemours Foundation (kiddshealth.rog/teen/sexual_health/changing_body/puberty)
- www.noonansyndrome.org

SUGGESTED READINGS

available at www.expertconsult.com

RELATED CONTENT

Delayed Puberty (Patient Information)

AUTHORS: **STEPHANIE A. CURRY, M.D.**, and **RACHAEL M. BIANCUZZO, MSIV**

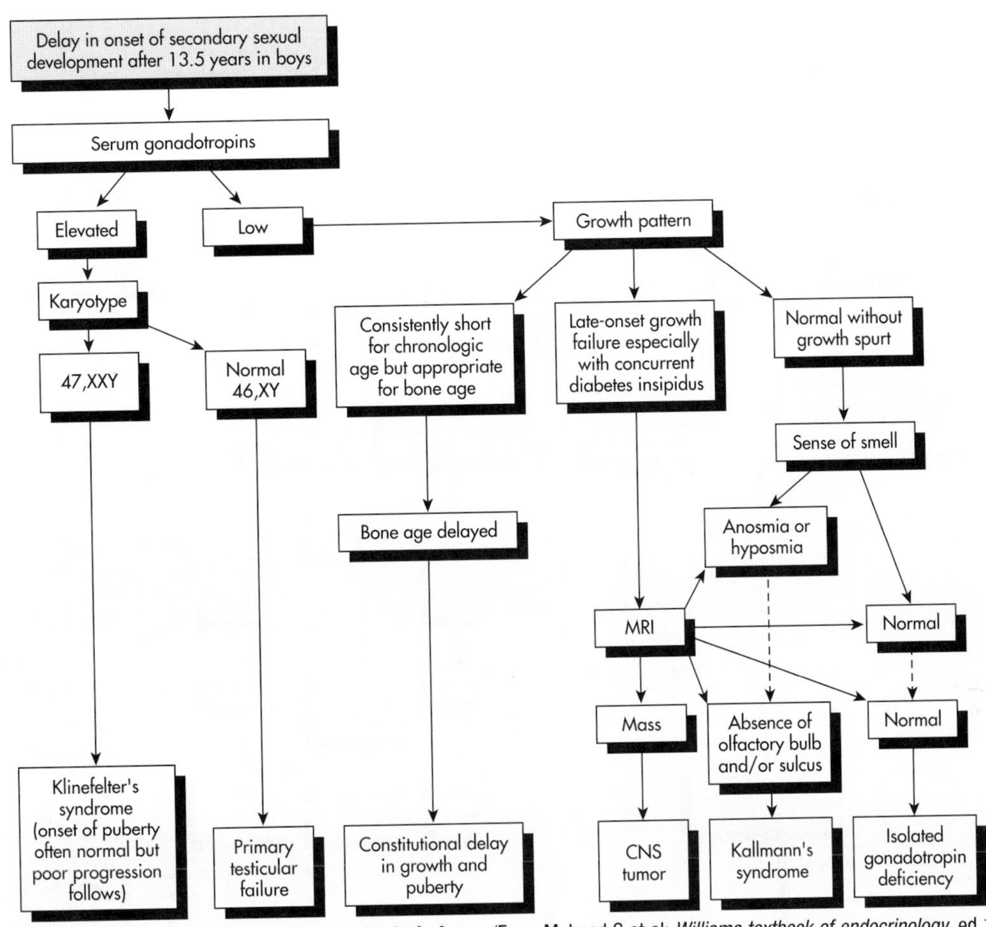

FIGURE 1-300 Flow chart for the evaluation of delayed puberty in boys. (From Melmed S et al: *Williams textbook of endocrinology*, ed 12, Philadelphia, 2011, Saunders)

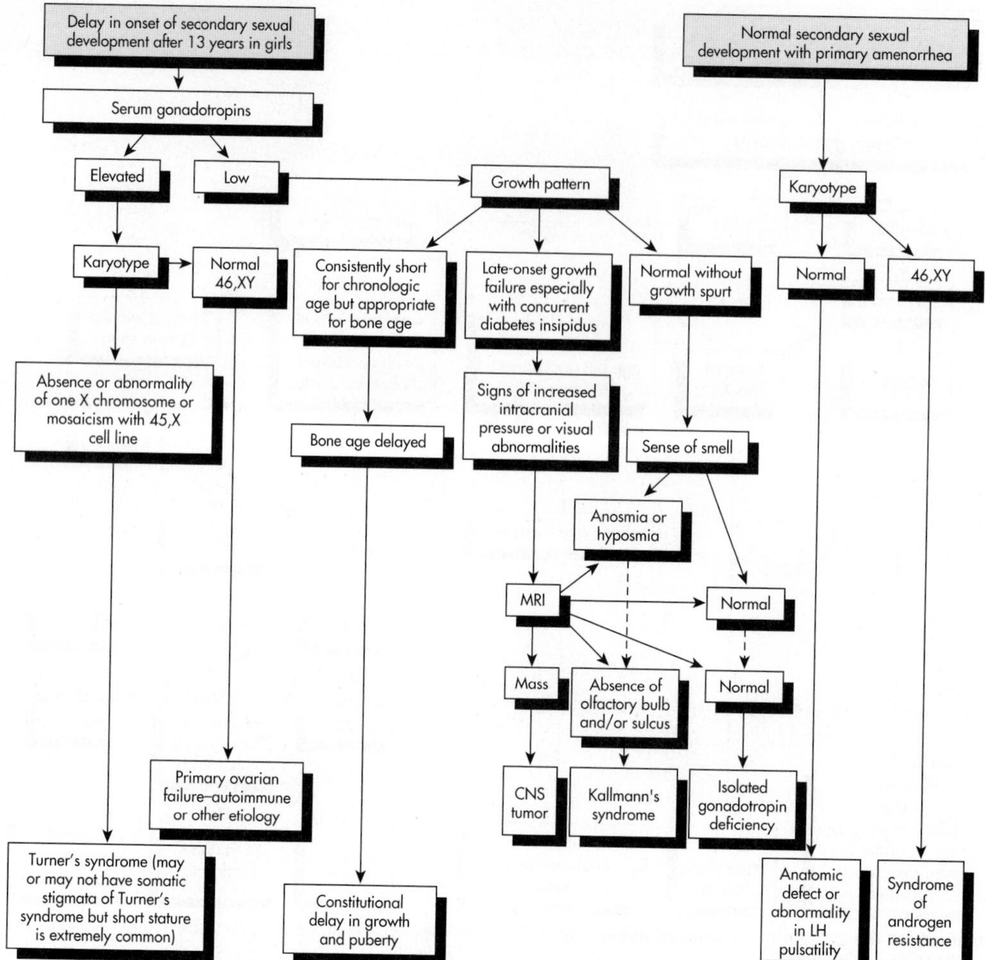

FIGURE 1-301 Flow chart for the evaluation of delayed puberty in girls. (From Melmed S et al: *Williams textbook of endocrinology*, ed 12, Philadelphia, 2011, Saunders)

BASIC INFORMATION

DEFINITION

The key to delirium is that it has an acute/subacute onset and is the most common mental disorder in patients with medical illness. The American Psychiatric Association's *Diagnostic and Statistical Manual*, 5th edition (DSM-5) defines delirium as:

- Disturbance of consciousness with reduced ability to focus, sustain, or shift attention.
- The disturbance develops over a short period of time (usually hours to days) and tends to fluctuate during the course of a day.
- An additional disturbance in cognition (e.g., memory deficit, disorganization, language, visuospatial ability, or perception).
- A change in cognition or development of a perceptual disturbance that is not better accounted for by a preexisting, established, or evolving dementia.
- There is evidence from history, physical exam, or lab findings that the disturbance is caused by medical condition, substance intoxication or withdrawal (i.e., due to a drug of abuse or to a medication), or exposure to a toxin, or is due to multiple etiologies.

SYNONYMS

Acute confusional state
Acute brain syndrome
Toxic or metabolic encephalopathy

THEORIES REGARDING PATHOPHYSIOLOGY

- Neuroinflammation, with increased permeability of the blood-brain barrier
- Acetylcholine deficiency
- Other neurotransmitter imbalances, including excesses of norepinephrine, serotonin (which may actually exert a beneficial effect on the stress of illness), and, most important, dopamine

CLASSIFICATION

Hyperactive, hypoactive, and mixed subtype

ICD-9CM CODES
780.09 Delirium
ICD-10CM CODES
F05 Delirium, not induced by alcohol and other psychoactive substances
F05.9 Delirium, unspecified
F06.0 Organic hallucinosis
F05.8 Other delirium
F05.0 Delirium not superimposed on dementia
F05.1 Delirium superimposed on dementia

EPIDEMIOLOGY & DEMOGRAPHICS

Hypoactive is more common (20% to 86% prevalence vs. 6% to 31% for hyperactive). It is often overlooked and seems to portend a worse prognosis. Any age, race, or gender can be affected. Pediatric delirium is often missed but remains important because delirium is associated with longer hospital stays, decreased cognitive performance, and increased mortality. Risk factors include extremes of age, severe pain, illicit substance use, surgery, dementia, and kidney or liver failure (Tables E1-153 and 1-154).

PHYSICAL FINDINGS & CLINICAL PRESENTATION

- Symptoms may differ both among and within one patient. Thus history from various caregivers may conflict because delirium implies a mental status that is frequently in flux. Family members or caregivers report that the patient "isn't acting quite right." Symptoms may include poor attention, sleepiness, agitation, or psychosis.
- Change in cognition, perceptual problems (such as visual, auditory, or somatosensory hallucination usually with lack of insight), memory loss, disorientation, difficulty with speech and language. It is important to ascertain from family member or caregivers the patient's level of functioning before onset of delirium.
- Elderly patients with delirium often do not look sick.
- Physical examination should be performed, focusing on signs of infection, dehydration, or chronic disease that may be exacerbated. Vital signs are key. Consider using the Mini-Mental Status Exam or the Montreal Cognitive Assessment.
- Fig. E1-302 describes an algorithm for evaluation of mental status changes in an older patient.

ETIOLOGY

Can be multifactorial; often falls into one of the following categories:

- Drugs: benzodiazepines are the worst offenders, but other drugs such as narcotics, anticholinergics, beta-blockers, steroids, nonsteroidal anti-inflammatory drugs, digoxin, cimetidine, can cause delirium; also, withdrawal states such as alcohol withdrawal or benzodiazepine withdrawal can cause delirium
- Infection or inflammation
- Metabolic: kidney or liver failure, thyroid, adrenal or glucose dysregulation, anemia, vitamin deficiency such as Wernicke's encephalopathy or vitamin B_{12} deficiency, inborn metabolic errors such as porphyrias or Wilson's disease
- Stress: surgery, sleep problems, pain, fever, hypoxia, anesthesia, environmental changes, fecal or urinary retention, burns
- Fluids, electrolytes, nutrition (FEN): dysregulation of calcium, magnesium, potassium, or sodium; dehydration; volume overload; altered pH
- Brain disorder: CNS infection, head injury, hypertensive encephalopathy

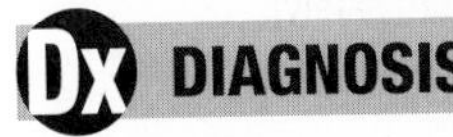

DIAGNOSIS

DIFFERENTIAL DIAGNOSIS

- Primary psychiatric illness
- Dementia
- Sundowning
- Nonconvulsive status epilepticus

Remember, delirium may coexist with any of the above. Table 1-155 describes clinical factors that help differentiate delirium and dementia from psychiatric disease.

LABORATORY TESTS

- Complete blood count, blood urea nitrogen, creatinine, electrolytes, liver function tests, ammonia, drug levels (digoxin, lithium)
- Toxicology screen, urinalysis, urine culture
- Thyroid function tests, vitamin B_{12}, and folate levels
- Rapid plasma reagin for syphilis, blood, urine, and spinal fluid culture
- Arterial blood gas

IMAGING STUDIES

- Consider head CT (to look for bleed, trauma, tumor, atrophy, dementia, stroke)
- Chest radiograph (to look for tumor, infection)

ELECTROENCEPHALOGRAM

- To exclude seizure, confirm diagnosis of metabolic encephalopathy

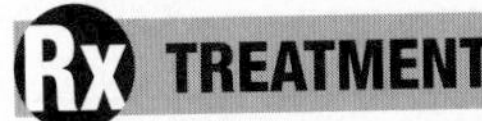

TREATMENT

NONPHARMACOLOGIC THERAPY

- The most important consideration is to keep the patient safe by using a variety of methods, including frequent reorientation.

TABLE 1-154 Mnemonic for Risk Factors for Delirium and Agitation

IWATCHDEATH	DELIRIUM
Infection	**D**rugs
Withdrawal	**E**lectrolyte and physiologic abnormalities
Acute metabolic	**L**ack of drugs (withdrawal)
Trauma/pain	**I**nfection
Central nervous system pathology	**R**educed sensory input (blindness, deafness)
Hypoxia	**I**ntracranial problems (CVA, meningitis, seizure)
Deficiencies (vitamin B_{12}, thiamine)	**U**rinary retention and fecal impaction
Endocrinopathies (thyroid, adrenal)	**M**yocardial problems (MI, arrhythmia, CHF)
Acute vascular (hypertension, shock)	
Toxins/drugs	
Heavy metals	

CHF, Congestive heart failure; *CVA,* cerebrovascular accident; *MI,* myocardial infarction.
From Vincent JL et al: *Textbook of critical care,* ed 6, Philadelphia, 2011, Saunders.

- A quiet, restful, simplified environment with cues to time and location such as clock or calendar are helpful, as well as consistent staff providing both personal and medical care. If possible, encourage familiar family members and friends to keep the patient company.
- Early mobilization and minimized use of physical restraints (use of physical restraints if necessary to ensure safety).
- Visual and hearing aids for patients with these impairments.

ACUTE GENERAL Rx

- Reverse any treatable cause, such as volume repletion for patients with dehydration, antibiotics for urinary tract infection.
- Haloperidol can be used with caution to control agitation, with doses ranging from 0.25 to 2 mg IM/IV twice daily, repeating the dose every 20 to 30 min until patient has calmed and using lower doses for the elderly.
- Risperidone 0.5 mg twice daily (off-label use, non-FDA approved) can also be used with caution with a slow increase to desired dose, not to exceed 1.0 to 2.0 mg.
- Avoid benzodiazepines and meperidine.

CHRONIC Rx

Delirium is not a chronic condition;if assessing a more long-term mental status change, consider other diagnoses.

DISPOSITION

Requires frequent monitoring often necessitating hospital level of care to ensure safety and assess etiology.

REFERRAL

Consider neurologic or psychiatric consultation if not improved in several days or in complicated cases.

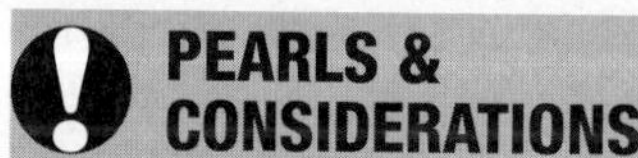

PEARLS & CONSIDERATIONS

COMMENTS

Although benzodiazepines are frequently used in hospitalized patients for sedation and are the mainstay of therapy for alcohol withdrawal, they must be used with caution in the elderly because they can have a paradoxical effect on agitation.

PREVENTION

- Avoid polypharmacy as much as possible.
- Optimize chronic medical conditions.
- Provide frequent reorientation and a soothing environment for high-risk patients (e.g., lights on during the day, off at night; open curtains during the day so patient can see the weather).
- In patients over 70 without dementia, regular exercise has been associated with lower risk for developing delirium, and early return to physical activity can improve outcomes in ill patients.

PATIENT & FAMILY EDUCATION

Inform about the above preventive techniques, especially polypharmacy risks.

SUGGESTED READINGS

available at www.expertconsult.com

RELATED CONTENT

Delirium Tremens (Related Key Topic)

AUTHORS: **CRISTINA ANTONIO PACHECO, M.D.**, and **POOJA VERMA, M.D.**

TABLE 1-155 Clinical Factors That Help Differentiate Delirium and Dementia from Psychiatric Disease

Characteristic	Delirium	Dementia	Psychiatric Illness
Symptoms			
Age at onset	<12 or >40 yr	Usually elderly, >50 yr	13-40 yr
Onset	Acute	Gradual or insidious	Gradual
Symptom course	Rapid, fluctuating	Stable and progressive	Stable
Duration	Days to weeks	Months to years	Months to years
Reversibility	Usually	Rarely	Rarely
History			
Past medical history	Substance abuse, medical illness	Comorbid conditions of aging	Previous psychiatric history
Family history	Unusual	History of dementia	History of psychiatric illness
Physical Examination			
Vital signs	Usually abnormal	Usually normal	Usually normal
Involuntary activity	May have tremors, asterixis, etc.	None unless coexistent disease	None
Mental Status			
Affect	Emotional lability	Flat affect with advanced disease	Flat affect
Orientation	Usually impaired	Impaired with advanced disease	Rarely impaired
Attention	Impaired	Slow to focus	Disorganized
Hallucinations	Primarily visual	Rare	Primarily auditory
Speech	Slow, incoherent, dysarthric	Usually coherent	Usually coherent
Consciousness	Decreased to impaired	Normal (clear)	Alert
Intellectual function	Usually impaired	Impaired	Intact

From Adams JG et al: *Emergency medicine, clinical essentials*, ed 2, Philadelphia, 2013, Elsevier .

BASIC INFORMATION

DEFINITION

Delirium tremens is overactivity of the central nervous system after cessation of alcohol intake. The time interval is variable; it usually occurs within 1 wk after reduction or cessation of heavy alcohol intake and persists for 1 to 3 days.

SYNONYMS

Alcohol withdrawal syndrome
DTs
Alcoholic delirium

ICD-9CM CODES
291.00 Alcohol withdrawal delirium
ICD-10CM CODES
F10.231 Alcohol dependence with withdrawal delirium

EPIDEMIOLOGY & DEMOGRAPHICS

INCIDENCE (IN U.S.): Up to 500,000 cases annually
PEAK INCIDENCE: 30 yr and older
PREDOMINANT SEX: Male
PEAK AGE: Teenage years and older
GENETICS: More common with patients who have relatives who are alcoholics

PHYSICAL FINDINGS & CLINICAL PRESENTATION

- Initially: anxiety, insomnia, tremulousness
- Early: tachycardia, sweating, anorexia, agitation, headache, gastrointestinal distress
- Late: seizures, visual hallucinations, delirium

ETIOLOGY

Alcoholism

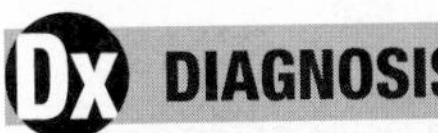

DIAGNOSIS

DIFFERENTIAL DIAGNOSIS

- Coexisting illness
- Trauma
- Drug use

WORKUP

- Frequent rating of symptoms (hallucinations, tremor, sweating, agitation, orientation).
- The Clinical Institute Withdrawal Assessment-Alcohol (CIWA-A) scale can be used to measure the severity of alcohol withdrawal. It consists of the 10 following items:
  1. Nausea
  2. Tremor
  3. Autonomic hyperactivity
  4. Anxiety
  5. Agitation
  6. Tactile disturbances
  7. Visual disturbances
  8. Auditory disturbances
  9. Headache
  10. Disorientation

  The maximum score is 67.

LABORATORY TESTS

- Electrolytes (including magnesium, phosphate)
- Close monitoring of glucose levels
- Drug screen (blood and urine)

IMAGING STUDIES

CT scan of head if there is a history of head trauma.

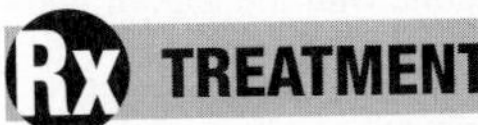

TREATMENT

NONPHARMACOLOGIC THERAPY

Refer to drug rehabilitation program after patient recovers.

ACUTE GENERAL Rx

- Admission to a detoxification unit where patient can be observed closely.
- Vital signs q30min initially (neurologic signs, if necessary).
- Use of lateral decubitus or prone position if restraints are necessary.
- Nothing by mouth: nasogastric tube for abdominal distention may be necessary but should not be routinely used.
- Vigorous hydration (4 to 6 L/day): IV with glucose (Na^+, K^+, PO_4^{-3}, and Mg^{2+} replacement). Use with caution in patients with CHF.
- Vitamins: thiamine 100 mg IV qd. The initial dose of thiamine should precede the administration of IV dextrose; multivitamins (may be added to the hydrating solution).
- Sedation (sedation can be achieved using fixed-dose regimen or individualized benzodiazepine administration [see CIWA-Ar score] in Alcohol-Related Disorders):
  - Initially: lorazepam 2 to 5 mg IM/IV repeated prn
  - Maintenance (individualized dosage): chlordiazepoxide, 50 to 100 mg PO q4 to 6h, lorazepam 2 mg PO q4h, or diazepam 5 to 10 mg PO tid; withhold doses or decrease subsequent doses if signs of oversedation are apparent.
  - Midazolam is also effective for managing DTs. Its rapid onset (sedation within 2 to 4 min of IV injection) and short duration of action (approximately 30 min) make it an ideal agent for titration in continuous infusion.
- Treatment of seizures: diazepam 2.5 mg/min IV until seizure is controlled (check for respiratory depression or hypotension) may be beneficial for prolonged seizure activity; IV lorazepam 1 to 2 mg q2h can be used in place of diazepam. In general, withdrawal seizures are self-limited and treatment is not required; the use of phenytoin or other anticonvulsants for short-term treatment of alcohol withdrawal seizures is not recommended.
- Diagnosis and treatment of concomitant medical, surgical, or psychiatric conditions.

CHRONIC Rx

Alcoholics Anonymous has the best record in breaking addiction, but the results are still disappointing.

DISPOSITION

Refer to drug rehabilitation program.

REFERRAL

If cardiac arrhythmias are prominent or respiratory distress develops

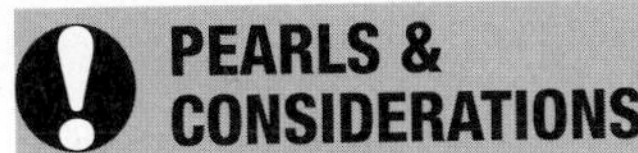

PEARLS & CONSIDERATIONS

COMMENTS

This is a potentially lethal disease if not carefully treated. Mortality rate is 15% in untreated patients.

SUGGESTED READINGS

available at www.expertconsult.com

RELATED CONTENT

Alcohol-Related Disorders (Related Key Topic)
Delirium Tremens (Patient Information)
Delirium (Related Key Topic)

AUTHOR: **FRED F. FERRI, M.D.**

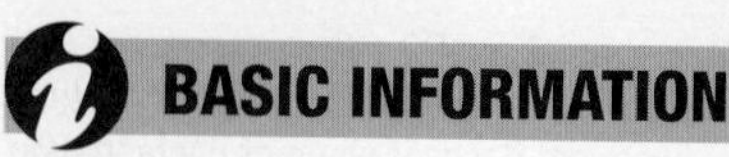

BASIC INFORMATION

DEFINITION

A fixed belief characterized by a person's preoccupation that his or her skin is infested by insects, worms, or other living organisms.

SYNONYMS

Morgellon's disease

ICD-9CM and DSM-5 CODES
297.1
ICD-10CM CODES
F22.0 Delusional disorder

EPIDEMIOLOGY & DEMOGRAPHICS

INCIDENCE: Unknown
PEAK INCIDENCE: Occurs more often later in life
PREVALENCE: Unknown
PREDOMINANT SEX AND AGE: For patients less than age 50, the male/female ratio is 1:1; for patients older than 50, females predominate by a ratio of 3:1
GENETICS: Unknown
RISK FACTORS: None known

PHYSICAL FINDINGS & CLINICAL PRESENTATION

- Patients complain of living organisms infesting their skin, sometimes including mucosal tissues.
- Patients have often been to specialists, including dermatologists, allergists, and infectious disease specialists.
- Patients may bring in samples of skin or hair, stating that they have looked at tissue under a microscope and have seen organisms. These samples are often brought in a matchbox ("matchbox sign") or wrapped in plastic wrap ("Saran sign").
- Skin may show areas of excoriation.

ETIOLOGY

Unknown: Thought to be mediated through dopaminergic pathways in the brain given the known etiology of other psychotic disorders and the ability of cocaine use to create symptoms of formication (see below).

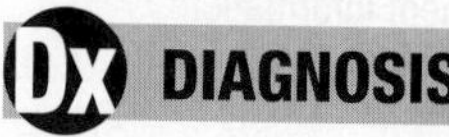

DIAGNOSIS

DIFFERENTIAL DIAGNOSIS

- Primary psychiatric disorders include formication, in which patients experience crawling and biting sensations on their skin, although they are not delusional about the cause.
- Substance abuse should be considered: case reports exist of cocaine and amphetamine use leading to these delusions.
- Neuropsychiatrically, B_{12} deficiency, diabetic neuropathy, cardiovascular disease, multiple sclerosis, hyperthyroidism, and brain lesions can all cause similar delusions.
- Other medical causes that deserve workup include primary skin lesions, systemic diseases that may present with skin lesions, and disorders of infestation.

WORKUP

- Skin biopsy may exclude dermatitis herpetiformis (although many patients have already been to their primary care doctor and dermatologist and have had a skin biopsy done, likely many times).
- Mineral oil preparation may exclude scabies, and a microscopic examination may exclude louse infestation.
- Thorough history is likely to yield the very fixed nature of the belief and an unwillingness to come to terms with the lack of findings on the exam.

LABORATORY TESTS

- Pruritus workup: iron studies, LFTs, CBC, UA, TSH, Chem 7, Folate, B_{12}
- Lumbar puncture (especially when multiple sclerosis is highly suspected)
- CRP (especially when an infectious etiology is suspected)
- Urine toxicology screen to evaluate substance use

IMAGING STUDIES

- Head CT, without contrast
- MRI

TREATMENT

- Antipsychotics have been shown to lead to full to partial remission in 60% to 100% of cases.
- Classically, Orap was the treatment of choice, although it has been associated with QTc prolongation.
- Multiple studies describe the use of second-generation antipsychotics, but these have been shown to cause weight gain and metabolic syndrome.
- Numerous antipsychotics have a black box warning about the risk of sudden death in the elderly and must be administered carefully for patients who have issues with QTc.
- Given all of these issues, a careful risk/benefit analysis is needed, including the assistance of family members of elderly patients.

NONPHARMACOLOGIC THERAPY

- Given the fixed nature of the belief, patients often refuse referral to a mental health specialist.
- A treatment (e.g., Permethrin) should not be recommended "just in case" because it may reinforce the patient's belief.
- Repeat visits with medical providers may be helpful to provide assurance and prevent harm from further workup.

ACUTE GENERAL Rx

Antipsychotics (Table 1-156)

COMPLEMENTARY & ALTERNATIVE MEDICINE

There is no evidence on the use of complementary or alternative medicine for this disorder.

REFERRAL

Referral to an outpatient psychiatrist may be helpful, but patients are often resistant.

PREVENTION

No preventive measures have been identified.

PATIENT/FAMILY EDUCATION

Psychoeducation may be helpful for the patient and family, although resistance from the patient can be expected.

SUGGESTED READINGS

available at www.expertconsult.com

RELATED CONTENT

Schizophrenia (Related Key Topic)
Alcohol-Related Disorders (Related Key Topic)
Cocaine Overdose (Related Key Topic)
Delirium (Related Key Topic)

AUTHOR: **ANTHONY GALLO, M.D.**

TABLE 1-156 Antipsychotics

Antipsychotic Drug	Dosage
Haloperidol	0.5-10 mg PO bid
Pimozide	2-12 mg PO qam
Perphenazine	4-16 mg PO tid
Olanzapine	2.5-10 mg PO bid
Aripiprazole	2.5-20 mg PO qam
Quetiapine	12.5-200 mg PO bid
Ziprasidone	20-80 mg PO bid
Risperidone	0.5-3 mg PO bid

BASIC INFORMATION

DEFINITION

A neurodegenerative disease characterized by dementia concurrent with or preceding parkinsonian symptoms typically by 1 yr with other core features including fluctuations in attention and alertness and recurrent visual hallucinations. Diagnostic criteria for dementia syndrome associated with Lewy body pathology are described in Box 1-19. The disease characteristically responds to cholinesterase inhibitors, is relatively unresponsive to L-dopa, and is very sensitive to neuroleptics.

SYNONYMS

Lewy body dementia
Diffuse Lewy body disease
Lewy body type senile dementia
Cortical Lewy body disease

ICD-9CM CODES
Lewy bodies
331.82 [294.11] with behavioral disturbance
331.82 [294.10] without behavioral disturbance
ICD-10CM CODES
G31.83 Dementia with Lewy bodies

EPIDEMIOLOGY & DEMOGRAPHICS

INCIDENCE: Accounts for 10% to 22% of all dementias.
PEAK INCIDENCE: Affects individuals in their sixth decade or older.
PREVALENCE: Estimated 0.7% of individuals older than age 65.
PREDOMINANT SEX AND AGE:
- Sex: Male predominance
- Mean age of onset: 75 yr. On average, 10 yr greater for dementia with Lewy bodies (DLB) than Parkinson's disease (PD).

GENETICS:
- Most cases are sporadic with a discordance among monozygotic twins, which suggests that environment or other epigenetics play a major role in the incidence of DLB.
- Multiplication of alpha-synuclein gene (SNCA) has been reported in families with DLB.
- Other factors include glucocerebrosidase genetic mutations, high prevalence of Lewy bodies with presenilin-1 mutations, and polymorphisms of the coding region for the synuclein genes.

RISK FACTORS:
- Male sex
- Advanced age

PHYSICAL FINDINGS & CLINICAL PRESENTATION

- Importance of recognizing DLB relates to its pharmacologic management, including responsiveness to cholinesterase inhibitors, sensitivity to side effects of neuroleptics, and relative unresponsiveness to L-dopa.
- Insidious onset of dementia with core features of fluctuations in cognition, recurrent visual hallucinations, and extrapyramidal motor symptoms, along with other features either suggestive or supportive of the clinical diagnosis. Refer to "Revised Criteria for the Clinical Diagnosis of Dementia with Lewy Bodies" (McKeith I et al, *Neurology,* 2005).
- Detailed neuropsychological assessment demonstrates a characteristic profile of impairments in visuoperceptual, attentional, and executive functions, which reflects a combination of cortical and subcortical damage.

ETIOLOGY

- SNCA is a protein normally found at the synapse with a role in vesicle production. In its insoluble form, SNCA aggregates into Lewy bodies found at the cortical and subcortical levels.
- Lewy bodies are round, eosinophilic, intracytoplasmic inclusions in the nuclei of neurons.
- Cortical Lewy bodies are found in deep cortical layers of the anterior frontal and temporal lobes, the cingulate gyrus, and insula.
- As in PD, Lewy bodies aggregate in the following structures: substantia nigra, locus coeruleus, raphe nuclei, nucleus basalis of Meynert, and brain stem nuclei.

Dx DIAGNOSIS

DIFFERENTIAL DIAGNOSIS

- Similar to Parkinson's disease with dementia, including fluctuation in neuropsychological function, neuropsychiatric features, and extrapyramidal motor features
- Diagnosis of DLB when dementia occurs before or concurrently with extrapyramidal features—arbitrarily set as the "1-yr rule" vs. Parkinson's disease with dementia, which occurs after 1 yr
- Dementia: Alzheimer's disease (AD), vascular dementia
- Parkinsonian features: progressive supranuclear palsy, multisystem atrophy, corticobasal degeneration
- Rapidly progressive form: Creutzfeldt-Jakob disease. Lack of cerebellar signs may help distinguish DLB from classic CJD (but not variant form of CJD)
- Psychiatric features: late-onset psychosis or depression with psychotic features
- Hallucinations with fluctuations in consciousness: temporal lobe epilepsy (TLE)

WORKUP

- Lumbar puncture to rule out underlying chronic infections. Protein 14-3-3 may be present in both DLB and CJD.
- EEG to rule out potential TLE. However, either DLB or TLE may show nonspecific slowing or periodic complexes.

LABORATORY TESTS

- Rule out other potential reversible causes for dementia including:
  - Hormonal dysregulation: thyroid stimulating hormone, free thyroxine
  - Vitamin deficiency: thiamine, cyanocobalamin, folate
  - Vascular risk factors: lipid profile, Hgb A_{1c}, homocysteine, syphilis (FTA-ABS), or ApoE genetype

IMAGING STUDIES

- MRI typically shows a relative preservation of the hippocampi and medial temporal lobe volumes (as found in AD) but generalized atrophy and white matter changes.
- Functional imaging including single photon emission computed tomography (SPECT) demonstrates hypoperfusion of the occipital region.

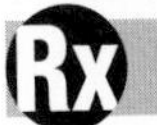

TREATMENT

Patient and caregiver education on benefits, side effects, and limitations of treatment is very important. Based on the preference of the patient and caregiver, a fine balance between psychosis and Parkinsonism features confounds the treatment choices.

NONPHARMACOLOGIC THERAPY

- Social interaction and environmental novelty may improve cognitive dysfunction and psychiatric features often exacerbated by low levels of arousal and attention.
- Behavioral methods, such as avoiding previously exposed environmental triggers known to cause anxiety, agitation, or aggression.
- Physical therapy, mobility aids, and daily exercise.

BOX 1-19 Diagnostic Criteria for the Dementia Syndrome Associated with Lewy Body Pathology

The cognitive disturbance is of insidious onset and is progressive, based on evidence from the history or serial cognitive examination
The presence of at least two of the following:
- Parkinsonism (rigidity, resting tremor, bradykinesia, postural instability, parkinsonian gait disorder)
- Prominent, fully formed visual hallucinations
- Substantial fluctuations in alertness or cognition
- Rapid eye movement sleep behavior disorder
- Severe worsening of parkinsonism by antipsychotic drugs

The disturbance is not better accounted for by a systemic disease or another brain disease

From Goldman L, Schafer AI: *Goldman's Cecil medicine,* ed 24, Philadelphia, 2012, Saunders.

ACUTE GENERAL Rx

Neuroleptic for disabling, persistent psychotic features despite initiation of a cholinesterase inhibitor. A very low dose of an atypical antipsychotic (quetiapine 12.5 mg daily) may be started after patient/caregiver education regarding the sensitivity to neuroleptics.

CHRONIC Rx

- Cholinesterase inhibitors for cognitive and behavioral symptoms. Rivastigmine (6 to 12 mg per day orally or 9.5 mg per day by transdermal patch) has shown in RCT a significant reduction in anxiety, delusions, and hallucinations, as well as significantly improved performance on neuropsychological testing.
- Antiparkinson medications for disabling parkinsonian features. L-Dopa is reported to be more effective with fewer side effects than dopamine agonists. Begin at a low dose of l-dopa (25/100 mg tid), and slowly titrate over several weeks as tolerated and according to response.
- Selective serotonin reuptake inhibitors are commonly used for depression.
- If REM sleep disorder remains disabling (or patient has not responded to an atypical antipsychotic initiated for psychosis), a trial of low-dose clonazepam (0.25 to 0.5 mg) or melatonin (3 mg) at bedtime remains an option.
- Orthostatic hypotension may be aided by nonpharmacologic therapy, such as supportive stockings, or pharmacologically by midodrine and/or fludrocortisone.
- Memantine demonstrated an improvement in clinical global measure and remains well-tolerated but may worsen hallucinations or delusions.
- Avoid anticholinergics (including tricyclic antidepressants) and benzodiazepines.

DISPOSITION

- Survival resembles the progression of AD, but a minority of cases may have a rapid disease course.
- Progression in cognitive decline, similar to AD, by an approximate 10% per year on cognitive testing.

REFERRAL

DLB requires a multidisciplinary approach including the general practitioner, neurologist, neuropsychologist, and/or neuropsychiatrist.

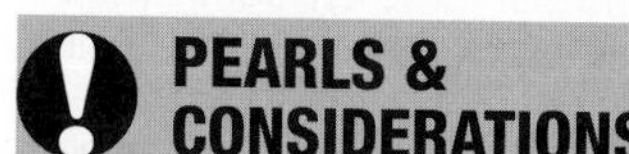

PEARLS & CONSIDERATIONS

COMMENTS

- Clinical presentation helps differentiate DLB from AD. AD presents with early signs of anterograde episodic memory loss without the benefit of recognition on neuropsychological testing due to cortical atrophy at the medial temporal lobe region.
- Vascular dementia may also present with evidence of frontal-subcortical features but typically without the core features listed in the criteria above.
- Bed partners may report that individuals with DLB "act out their dreams," sometimes violently, leading to sleeping in separate beds. A history of REM sleep behavior may precede the diagnosis by many years.

PATIENT/FAMILY EDUCATION

- Visual hallucinations (VH) typically consist of innocuous, well-formed, detailed images of animate figures. Unless VH lead to a potential threat to self or others, avoid antipsychotics due to the sensitivity of neuroleptics. Family/friends are often more alarmed by the VH than the patient with DLB.
- Apathy is a common clinical feature of DLB and mimics changes in mood, including depression, or excessive daytime somnolence. These features are often noticed by family/friends.

SUGGESTED READINGS

available at www.expertconsult.com

AUTHORS: **D. BRANDON BURTIS, D.O.,** and **GLEN FINNEY, M.D.**

BASIC INFORMATION

DEFINITION

Dependent personality disorder (DPD) is characterized by a pervasive and excessive need to be taken care of that leads to submissive and clinging behavior and fears of separation. DPD begins by early adulthood and causes significant distress or impairment in multiple domains of functioning. Individuals must meet five or more of the following criteria:

1. Difficulty making routine decisions without an excessive amount of advice and reassurance from others.
2. Need others to assume responsibility for most major areas of their life.
3. Difficulty expressing disagreement with others because of fear of loss of support or approval.
4. Difficulty initiating or completing projects on own because of a lack of self-confidence in abilities rather than lack of motivation or energy.
5. Excessive attempts to obtain nurturance and support from others.
6. Feel uncomfortable or helpless when alone because of exaggerated fears of being unable to care for self.
7. Urgently seek another relationship when a close relationship ends.
8. Unrealistically preoccupied with being left to take care of self.

SYNONYMS

None

ICD-9CM and DSM-5 CODES
301.6
ICD-10CM
F60.7 Dependent personality disorder

EPIDEMIOLOGY & DEMOGRAPHICS

PREVALENCE: 0.5% in general population. Dependent traits, as opposed to the disorder itself, are among the most frequently reported in outpatient mental health clinics.

PREDOMINANT SEX: Female (2:1) in clinical settings.

CLINICAL PRESENTATION

- Early onset and chronic course. Impairment is frequently mild.
- On interview, will defer excessively to partner or parent.
- Indecision in routine decisions.
- Depend on a parent or spouse to decide where they should live, work, and recreate and who they should befriend.
- Need for others to function for them goes beyond age-appropriate and situation-appropriate requests for assistance.
- Will agree with objectionable opinions, submit to unreasonable requests, and not express appropriate anger or disappointment for fear of alienating the person without whom they believe they cannot function.
- Convinced that they are not capable of independent function and present themselves as inept.
- Often do not develop independent living skills, perpetuating their dependency.
- Social relations tend to be limited to those few people on whom the person depends.

ETIOLOGY

Chronic physical illness or separation anxiety disorder may predispose for DPD.

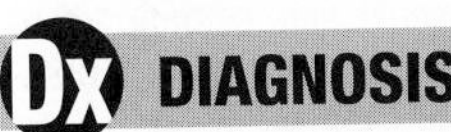

DIAGNOSIS

DIFFERENTIAL DIAGNOSIS

- Dependency and personality changes arising as a consequence of an Axis I disorder.
- Dependency arising as a consequence of a general medical condition.
- Most common comorbid Axis I conditions are major depressive and other mood disorders, anxiety disorders, including social phobia, and adjustment disorder.
- Most common comorbid personality disorders are histrionic, avoidant, and borderline. Each of these disorders is characterized by dependent features. DPD is distinguished by its predominantly submissive, reactive, and clinging behavior.

WORKUP

- History: collateral information is essential to establishing the presence of longstanding interpersonal pattern in multiple domains of the patient's life.
- Physical examination.
- Mental status examination.

LABORATORY TESTS

Tests necessary to rule out medical causes of personality changes

IMAGING STUDIES

Tests necessary to rule out medical causes of personality changes

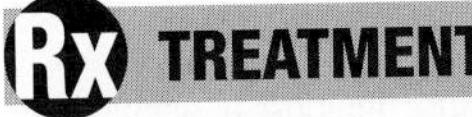

TREATMENT

NONPHARMACOLOGIC THERAPY

- Cognitive-behavioral and psychodynamic psychotherapy to diminish and better contain anxiety and to help patients develop sense of self as competent and requisite assertiveness skills
- Psychodynamic psychotherapy to help develop improved self-concept and interpersonal functioning

ACUTE GENERAL Rx

Benzodiazepines to control highly anxious states

CHRONIC Rx

Selective serotonin reuptake inhibitors (SSRIs) and selective serotonin-norepinephrine reuptake inhibitors (SNRIs) for comorbid depression, social phobia, other anxiety disorders, and agoraphobia

DISPOSITION

- Chronic course; severity is variable
- Impairments often mild
- At increased risk for major depression, social phobia, and other anxiety disorders, including panic and agoraphobia

REFERRAL

- If pharmacotherapy or psychotherapy is contemplated
- If patient's functioning is impaired

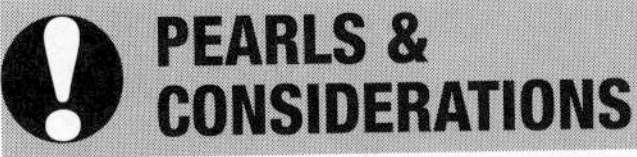

PEARLS & CONSIDERATIONS

COMMENTS

- DPD patients fear illness will lead to abandonment by others.
- This fear of simultaneous helplessness and abandonment intensifies neediness and may lead to dramatic demands for urgent medical attention.
- When physicians do not respond as wanted, angry outbursts may ensue.
- Medical care can also become a means by which dependency needs are met. As a result, some of these patients may unconsciously or consciously prolong their illness for primary gain.
- Physicians often react to the extreme neediness with avoidance or overengagement, leading to burnout.
- Management guidelines:
  1. Overall strategy is to provide reassurance and allay fear of abandonment.
  2. Specific strategies include scheduling frequent visits, noncontingent care (i.e., scheduling visits regardless of whether ill or not).
  3. Establish firm and realistic limits to availability as early as possible in treatment.
  4. Enlist other members of health care team for support.
  5. Encourage patient to develop additional "outside" support systems.

SUGGESTED READINGS

available at www.expertconsult.com

AUTHOR: **JOHN Q. YOUNG, M.D., M.P.P.**

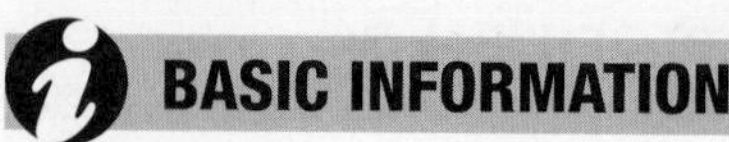

BASIC INFORMATION

DEFINITION

Major depression is an episodic, frequently recurring syndrome. The diagnosis requires that five of nine criteria be present for 2 wk. One of these nine criteria must be either a persistent depressed mood or pervasive anhedonia (loss of interest or pleasure in all, or almost all, usual interests or activities). Other symptoms include sleep disturbance (insomnia or hypersomnia), appetite loss/gain or weight loss/gain, fatigue, psychomotor retardation or agitation, difficulty concentrating or indecisiveness, feelings of guilt or worthlessness, and recurrent thoughts of death or suicidal ideation.

SYNONYMS

Unipolar affective disorder
Clinical depression
Melancholia
Manic-depressive illness, depressed type
Depressive episode

Codes depend on whether the episode is single or recurrent, and also on clinical severity.

ICD-9CM and DSM-5 CODES
296.2x-296.3x

ICD-10CM CODES

F32.9 Depressive episode, unspecified
F33.0 Recurrent depressive episode, current episode mild
F33.1 Recurrent depressive disorder, current episode moderate
F33.2 Recurrent depressive disorder, current episode severe without psychotic symptoms
F33.3 Recurrent depressive disorder, current episode severe with psychotic symptoms
F33.4 Recurrent depressive disorder, currently in remission
F33.9 Recurrent depressive disorder, unspecified

EPIDEMIOLOGY & DEMOGRAPHICS

LIFETIME RISK (IN U.S.): 10% of men, 20% of women

PREVALENCE (IN U.S.): Point prevalence in a community sample is 3% of men, 4.5% to 9.3% of women, and 1% of children. Prevalence of 20% to 40% in patients with comorbid medical conditions.

PREDOMINANT SEX: Female/male ratio 2:1

PREDOMINANT AGE: 25 to 44 yr; 5% of adolescents

PEAK INCIDENCE: 30 to 40 yr; 13% of postpartum women

GENETICS:

- Clear evidence of familial predominance
- Prevalence is 2 to 3 times greater among first-degree relatives.
- Concordance among monozygotic twins approximately 50%
- No established pattern of inheritance

PHYSICAL FINDINGS & CLINICAL PRESENTATION

- Clinical evaluation facilitated by organizing the major symptoms into four hallmarks: (1) depressed mood, (2) anhedonia, (3) physical symptoms (sleep disturbance, appetite problem, fatigue, psychomotor changes), and (4) psychological symptoms (difficulty concentrating or indecisiveness, guilt or worthlessness, and suicidal ideation).
- A stressful life event, typically a serious loss, may trigger a depressive episode. DSM-5 recommends that clinical judgment be used to determine if depression in the context of a loss should be used to determine if a diagnosis of a disorder is warranted.
- Patients often present with somatic complaints such as pain, fatigue, insomnia, dizziness, headache, or gastrointestinal problems.
- May be associated with mood-congruent delusional thinking (paranoid and melancholic themes).
- May be associated with active or passive suicidal ideation.
- Serious misconduct may appear in adolescents.
- May be underdiagnosed in elderly patients, with signs and symptoms attributed to normal aging.
- May be underdiagnosed in medically ill patients, with signs and symptoms attributed to medical illness or considered appropriate reaction to medical condition.

ETIOLOGY

- A heterogeneous group of disorders probably arising from various etiologies.
- Genetic and environmental experiences, and their interaction, each contribute.
- Significant psychosocial stressors, especially loss, often trigger depression, particularly for first episodes.
- Numerous biologic correlates have been identified, though none is considered causative or diagnostic. Genes that influence the production and reuptake of serotonin, norepinephrine, and dopamine, as well as nerve cell growth in brain regions underlying memory and emotional processing, are of greatest interest. Abnormalities in brain regions underlying emotion regulation and reward processing, as well as irregularities in cortisol responding, appear to play a role.
- Cognitive risk factors include a pessimistic style of explaining negative events, a tendency to ruminate, and biases in processing emotional information and events.

Dx DIAGNOSIS

DIFFERENTIAL DIAGNOSIS

- Anxiety disorders (e.g., social phobia, PTSD, obsessive compulsive disorder), substance abuse, and personality disorders often present with depressive symptoms.
- Important to determine if a depressive episode is part of major depression or part of bipolar disorder.
- Important to distinguish from adjustment disorder. Depression in the context of a stressful life event is diagnosed as major depressive disorder if the symptom criteria are met and adjustment disorder if the symptom criteria are not met. There is no evidence that medication is effective for adjustment disorder.
- Approximately 10% to 15% of depression caused by general medical illnesses, such as Alzheimer's disease, Parkinson's disease, stroke, end-stage renal failure, cardiac disease, HIV infection, and cancer.
- Some medical conditions present as depression (e.g., hypothyroidism, hyperthyroidism or neurosyphilis).
- Premenstrual dysphoric disorder.
- In elderly, depression often coexists with dementia.

WORKUP

- Careful medical history is required
- Physical examination reveals no specific diagnostic signs of depression
- Mental status examination
- Self-report scales can assist in screening.
- Commonly used validated screening tools include the 15-item Geriatric Depression Scale in the elderly and the Patient Health Questionnaire (PHQ)-2 and PHQ-9. The PHQ-2 has a 97% sensitivity and 67% specificity in adults. If it is positive for depression, the PHQ-9 should be administered. The PHQ-9 has a 61% sensitivity and 94% specificity for depression in adults.

LABORATORY TESTS

- No laboratory studies are diagnostic.
- The following can assist in ruling out other confounding issues:
  1. Routine blood chemistry evaluation
  2. CBC with differential
  3. Thyroid function studies
  4. Vitamin B_{12} levels

IMAGING STUDIES

With unusual presentations (e.g., associated with new-onset severe headache, focal neurologic signs, a cognitive or sensory disturbance), the following may be performed:

- EEG (diffuse slowing indicates metabolic encephalopathy)
- Anatomic brain imaging (CT scan or MRI)

Rx TREATMENT

NONPHARMACOLOGIC THERAPY

- Good evidence that cognitive-behavioral therapy is as effective as antidepressant medication in achieving significant reduction or remission (Table 1-157).
- Problem solving and interpersonal psychotherapies have efficacy rates of 50% to 60%.
- "New wave" cognitive-behavioral therapies (e.g., acceptance and commitment therapy, mindfulness-based CBT) have demonstrated efficacy, but as of yet it is unknown whether they are superior to traditional CBT.

TABLE 1-157 Treatments of Depression

Name of Psychotherapy	Approach
Cognitive psychotherapy	Identify and correct negativistic patterns of thinking.
Interpersonal psychotherapy	Identify and work through role transitions or interpersonal losses, conflicts, or deficits.
Problem-solving therapy	Identify and prioritize situational problems; plan and implement strategies to deal with top-priority problems.
Psychodynamic psychotherapy	Use therapeutic relationship to maximize use of the healthiest defense mechanisms and coping strategies.

From Goldman L et al: *Goldman's Cecil medicine,* ed 24, Philadelphia, 2012, Saunders.

- By 12 wk, psychotherapy and medication approaches are equally effective.
- Patients with severe symptoms should generally not be treated by psychotherapy alone.
- Evidence, although mixed, that combined psychotherapy and medication may be more effective than either treatment alone.
- Factors, including history of childhood maltreatment, presence of precipitant stressful life events, and depression severity, may affect treatment response and risk of recurrence.

ACUTE GENERAL Rx

- Concurrent medical or psychiatric illnesses, history of prior response, cost, and side effects should be considered when selecting initial treatment. Fig. E1-307 describes guidelines for the treatment of depression in the primary care setting.
- Antidepressants are helpful in approximately 60% to 70% of cases, though sustained remission rates are lower.
- Selective serotonin reuptake inhibitors (SSRIs) generally are first-line.
- According to the STAR-D trial, approximately 30% achieve remission with the first prescribed medication after 3 months of treatment. Another 25% to 30% respond to treatment, but do not achieve remission. Treatment-refractory patients should be switched to another SSRI or to another class of medication, offered adjunctive medication such as bupropion, or referred for evidence-based counseling. Approximately 25% more patients will achieve remission with this secondary intervention.
- Response to antidepressants for many patients is seen as early as 2 wk, and among patients showing little to no response, the odds of later response decrease the longer patients remain unimproved.
- To date no benefit of combining antidepressants as first-line treatment. Also no clear advantage has been identified for switching medications within vs. across different classes, or to switching vs. augmentation.
- Therapy should be continued for 4 to 9 mo after the full remission of symptoms.
- Electroconvulsive therapy is the most effective means available for the treatment of severe, refractory depression. Transcranial magnetic stimulation has also shown evidence of efficacy though effects are modest and to date electroconvulsive therapy has shown superior efficacy.
- Antipsychotic medication should be added for psychotic depression. Antipsychotic medication has also been shown to be helpful in augmenting antidepressants for nonpsychotic depression.
- Ketamine found to be rapidly effective in treatment-resistant depression. However, treatment remains experimental and effects do not persist.

CHRONIC RX

Long-term treatment, in some cases, lifelong recommended for multiple depressive episodes, an episode duration longer than 2 yr, a severe episode or significant suicidality, or a strong family history of severe depression or bipolar disorder.

DISPOSITION

- Major depression is often a relapsing and remitting illness.
- Physical symptoms predict a favorable response to biologic intervention.
- Additional episodes experienced by >50% after one episode, with each additional episode linked to increased risk for subsequent episodes.
- Without treatment, episodes last an average of 6 to 12 mo; risk of recurrence higher without treatment.
- For many depressed individuals, subthreshold residual symptoms are present between episodes and define the majority of an individual's course of depression. Such symptoms may lead to impairment and warrant prolonged treatment.

REFERRAL

- If treatment refractory
- If patient suicidal or psychotic
- For suspected bipolar depression

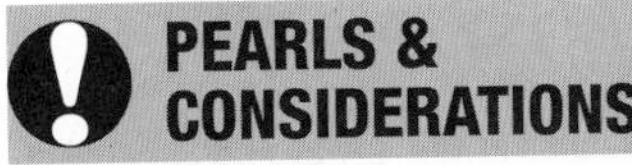

PEARLS & CONSIDERATIONS

COMMENTS

- All threats of suicide should be taken very seriously. Clinicians can use the mnemonic SAL: Is the method specific? Is it available? Is it lethal?
- Rule out bipolar affective disorder before initiating antidepressant medication. Screening scales for bipolar disorder can be helpful in primary care settings to identify patients at increased risk for bipolar disorder, although unclear benefit in mental health settings.
- Many patients and families reluctant to acknowledge depression because of stigma.
- A two-question screener is as effective as longer instruments. A positive answer to either question warrants a full assessment.
  1. Over the past 2 weeks, have you ever felt down, depressed, or hopeless?
  2. Over the past 2 weeks, have you felt little interest or pleasure in doing things?
- Depression screening programs without treatment programs are unlikely to improve depression outcomes.
- Strict monitoring of patients who initiate antidepressant therapy is necessary both for safety and to ensure optimal treatment. Use of self-report scales to measure symptom severity are helpful in monitoring outcome and may result in improved outcomes.

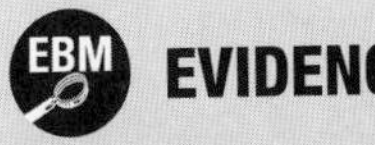

EVIDENCE

available at www.expertconsult.com

SUGGESTED READINGS

available at www.expertconsult.com

RELATED CONTENT

Bipolar Disorder (Related Key Topic)
Depression (Patient Information)

AUTHORS: **MARK ZIMMERMAN, M.D.,** and **CATHERINE D'AVANZATO, M.S.**

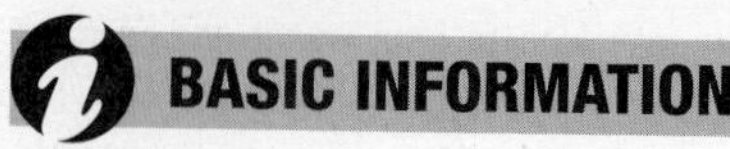

BASIC INFORMATION

DEFINITION

De Quervain's tenosynovitis refers to painful inflammatory process of first dorsal retinacular compartment containing abductor pollicis longus and extensor pollicis brevis tendons.

SYNONYMS

Stenosing tenosynovitis of the radial styloid process
Stenosing tenovaginitis of the first dorsal compartment
De Quervain's disease
De Quervain's tendonitis
De Quervain's stenosinig tenosynovitis
Tendinosis

ICD-9CM CODES

727.04 Radial styloid tenosynovitis, de Quervain disease
727.0 Synovitis and tenosynovitis
727.05 Other tenosynovitis of hand and wrist

ICD-10CM CODES

M65.4 Radial styloid tenosynovitis [de Quervain]
M65.9 Synovitis and tenosynovitis, unspecified
M65.849 Other synovitis and tenosynovitis, unspecified hand

EPIDEMIOLOGY & DEMOGRAPHICS

- More common in women than in men (10:1)
- Usually occurs between the ages of 30 and 50
- Associated with rheumatoid arthritis (RA)
- Can be seen in new mothers or daycare providers due to holding the babies with an outstretched thumb
- Seen more frequently in certain occupations involving repetitive wrist motion (e.g., clerical, assembly, and manual labor)

PHYSICAL FINDINGS & CLINICAL PRESENTATION

- Pain over the styloid process of the radius with grasping and isometric thumb abduction
- Pain may radiate up to the volar aspect of the wrist or to the thumb
- Swelling on the radial styloid
- Tenderness in the anatomic snuffbox
- Positive Finkelstein's test (Fig. 1-308)
- Crepitance
- Rarely, numbness of dorsum of thumb
- Absence of local heat on examination

ETIOLOGY

- Repetitive use or overuse of the hand and thumb involving pinching with the thumb while moving wrist in radial and ulnar directions causing thickening of the fibrous tendon sheath (e.g., typing, writing, nailing, golfing, fly-fishing, etc.).
- Acute trauma to the first extensor dorsal compartment.
- Inflammatory joint conditions like RA and conditions causing calcium apatite deposition.

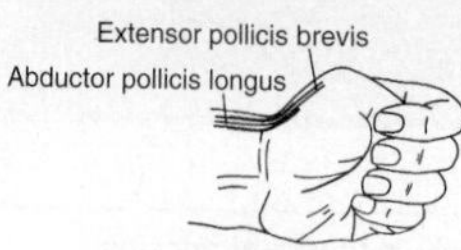

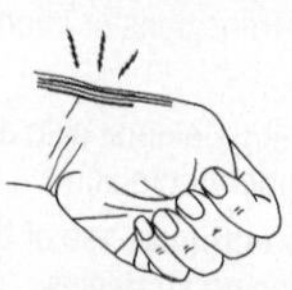

FIGURE 1-308 Finkelstein's test is positive in de Quervain's stenosing synovitis. Ulnar flexion of the wrist produces pain over the dorsal compartment containing the extensor pollicis brevis and abductor pollicis longus. (From Noble J [ed]: *Textbook of primary care medicine,* ed 2, St Louis, 1996, Mosby.)

DIAGNOSIS

- The diagnosis of de Quervain's tenosynovitis is based on the clinical triad of:
  1. Tenderness over the radial styloid
  2. Swelling over the first dorsal retinacular compartment
  3. Pain on ulnar movement of the wrist with the thumb adducted and flexed (Finkelstein's test; see Fig. 1-308).
- Consideration can be given to injecting 1.5 ml of 1% Xylocaine into the tenosynovial sac, and if all three physical signs resolve, the diagnosis is confirmed, allowing for differentiation from carpometacarpal (CMC) osteoarthritis (OA).
- Finkelstein maneuver can also be present in first CMC joint OA; therefore it should also be evaluated if this test is positive.

DIFFERENTIAL DIAGNOSIS

- Carpal tunnel syndrome
- Arthritis (e.g., degenerative OA or RA)
- Gout
- Infiltrative tenosynovitis
- Radiculopathy
- Compression neuropathy (e.g., superficial branch of the radial nerve "bracelet syndrome")
- Ganglia
- Infection (e.g., tuberculosis, bacterial)
- Scaphoid fracture
- Intersection syndrome

LABORATORY TESTS

- ESR is usually normal in patients with de Quervain's tenosynovitis.
- Arthrocentesis to rule out gout (crystals) and infection (Gram stain, culture of aspirate).

IMAGING STUDIES

- Imaging of wrist and thumb not necessary unless fracture or arthritis suspected.

TREATMENT

NONPHARMACOLOGIC THERAPY

- Rest
- Avoid repetitive movements of hand or thumb
- Splinting (thumb spica)
- Icing (4-6 times a day for 15 min)
- Physiotherapy

ACUTE GENERAL Rx

- Corticosteroid injection using 20 to 40 mg triamcinolone acetonide and 1% Xylocaine is effective in relieving pain.
- NSAIDs (ibuprofen 800 mg tid or naproxen 500 mg bid)
- Topical hydrocortisone on the radial styloid for mild conditions

CHRONIC Rx

- Once signs of active inflammation have resolved after 3-4 wk, gentle stretching exercises involving abductor and extensor tendons usually help recovery.
- Surgical release is generally reserved for patients not responding to NSAIDs and corticosteroid injection therapy.

DISPOSITION

- ~90% of patients have relief of symptoms with either single or multiple steroid injections.
- Rarely, steroid injection use can cause infection and tendon rupture.
- Accidental injection of the glucorticoid in the subcutaneous tissue instead of sheath of first extensor (dorsal) compartment should be avoided to prevent fat and dermal atrophy.
- If left untreated, can lead to fibrosis and decrease in mobility (stenosing tenosynovitis).
- Surgical control of symptoms achieved in 90% of referred cases
- Complications of surgery include:
  1. Radial nerve damage
  2. Paresthesia (10%)
  3. Neuroma
  4. Scarring
- Recovery rates are higher with early treatment to ~80% after 6 wk but <40% after 4 yr.

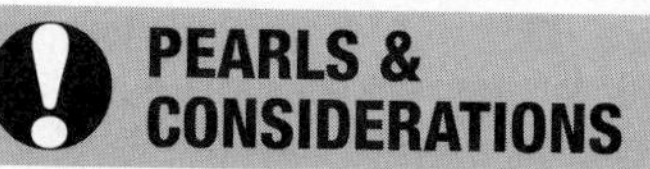

PEARLS & CONSIDERATIONS

- Steroid injection is generally recommended after failure of conservative treatment for 2-6 wk.
- Pain relief usually noted within 48 hr, with patient becoming asymptomatic 1-2 week after corticosteroid injection.
- If no improvement by 6 wk post second corticosteroid injection, refer to orthopedic hand surgeon.
- Without treatment it will not improve and can get worse.
- Condition can recur if triggering activity continues.

SUGGESTED READINGS

available at www.expertconsult.com

RELATED CONTENT

De Quervain's Tenosynovitis (Patient Information)

AUTHORS: **SYEDA M. SAYEED, M.D.**, and **UZMA NASIR, M.D.**

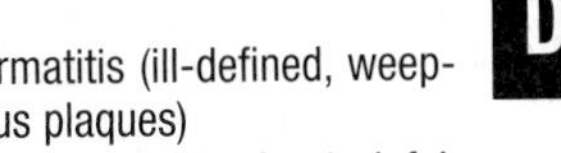

BASIC INFORMATION

DEFINITION

Dermatitis herpetiformis (DH) is an autoimmune blistering disease that is considered to be a cutaneous manifestation of celiac disease (CD). It is associated with gluten-sensitive enteropathy in nearly all cases, although only 20% of patients have gastrointestinal symptoms. Approximately 25% of patients with CD will have DH.

SYNONYMS

Duhring disease

ICD-9CM CODES
694.0 Dermatitis herpetiformis
ICD-10CM CODES
L13.0 Dermatitis herpetiformis

EPIDEMIOLOGY & DEMOGRAPHICS

PREVALENCE (IN U.S.): 11.2 cases per 100,000 persons; prevalence for CD is one in 133 adults
PREDOMINANT SEX: Male predominance (2:1); however, female predominance in children
PREDOMINANT AGE: Fourth decade of life, but can occur at any age
PREDOMINANT RACE: Most common in Caucasians of Northern European ancestry
GENETICS: Both CD and DH have a strong genetic component. Eleven percent of patients with DH have a first-degree relative with either DH or CD. Specific HLA genes (involved in processing gliadin antigen in genetically susceptible individuals) have also been shown to predispose to developing DH (HLA-DQ2 in 90%, DQ8 in the remaining 10%). However, less than 50% of genetic predisposition is attributed to HLA genes.

PHYSICAL FINDINGS & CLINICAL PRESENTATION

- Classically, small fragile clusters ("herpetiform" vesicles) distributed symmetrically on extensor surfaces (elbows, knees, scalp, back, and buttocks) (Fig. 1-309). However, due to intense pruritus, pin-point erosions and excoriations are often the most prominent findings on examination, with intact vesicles rare.
- Spontaneous improvement with cyclic exacerbations is common.
- Celiac-type enamel defects to permanent teeth, oral vesicles, or palmoplantar purpura have been reported as potential associated findings.

PATHOGENESIS

CD and DH are both autoimmune-mediated by IgA class autoantibodies. Dietary gluten is central to the pathogenesis in both. It is hypothesized that gluten byproduct, gliadin, complexes with tissue transglutaminase (tTG) in the gut, binding as an antigen to HLA-DQ2 on T-cells, creating an immune response resulting in anti-tTG IgA antibodies (i.e., anti-endomysial antibodies) in the blood result. However, unlike CD, patients with DH also have high-affinity antibodies against epidermal transglutaminase (eTG). Antigenetic cross-reactivity has been hypothesized.

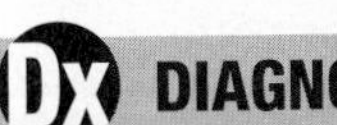

DIAGNOSIS

Physical examination and routine histopathology are often suggestive of DH; however, direct immunofluorescence (DIF) of a perilesional skin biopsy has pathognomonic findings and is the gold standard for diagnosis.

DIFFERENTIAL DIAGNOSIS

- Clinically and histologically, the differential diagnosis includes linear IgA dermatosis, bullous pemphigoid, and bullous lupus. These diagnoses can be differentiated by DIF on perilesional skin biopsy
- Other clinical diagnoses to consider:
  - Scabies (check for interdigital burrows, involvement of genitalia)
  - Arthropod bite (papular urticaria over exposed areas)
  - Eczematous dermatitis (ill-defined, weeping erythematous plaques)
  - Herpes simplex or zoster infection (painful, not symmetric)
  - Generalized pruritus (no blister history)

WORKUP, LABORATORY TESTS

- Evaluation for gastrointestinal symptoms, family history of DH or CD, and pruritus should be sought in patients with suspected DH
- **Lesional skin biopsy:** will demonstrate a neutrophil-rich subepidermal bulla and rule out many conditions.
- **DIF of normal-appearing perilesional skin biopsy:** will demonstrate pathognomonic IgA deposits localized to the dermal papillae and dermal-epidermal junction in a granular pattern.
- Checking for circulating antibodies in the blood (anti-gliadin, anti-endomysial, or anti-reticulin IgA antibodies) is not recommended as part of the diagnostic workup for DH. However, they can be helpful in confirming the diagnosis of DH in cases where linear IgA cannot be excluded on DIF.

TREATMENT

A gluten-free diet (GFD) and dapsone are considered first-line therapy, and are often started in conjunction.

- GFD improves symptoms of both GI and skin disease, with GI responding quicker (skin responds after 2 months).
- Dapsone results in improvement of skin manifestations within days but does not treat GI manifestations. Dapsone is often tapered over time, while lifelong gluten avoidance is often necessary.
- A recent small study demonstrated that a GFD alone was comparable to a gluten-free diet plus dapsone in the treatment of DH; hence GFD is an essential component in the treatment of DH.

NONPHARMACOLOGIC THERAPY

- First line: GFD
  - Avoid barley, rye, wheat (rice, corn, and oats okay)
  - Consultation with a dietitian recommended
  - Most patients need to follow diet indefinitely; however, cases of spontaneous remission have been reported.
- Second line: elemental diet (controversial)
  - Can consider elemental diet (avoidance of whole proteins) in those patients who do not adequately respond to a strict GFD; however, data are limited.

ACUTE GENERAL Rx

- First line: dapsone
  - Initial dose 25-50 mg PO daily with gradual increase to an average maintenance dose of 0.5-1 mg/kg daily (often maintenance dose of 100 mg daily).

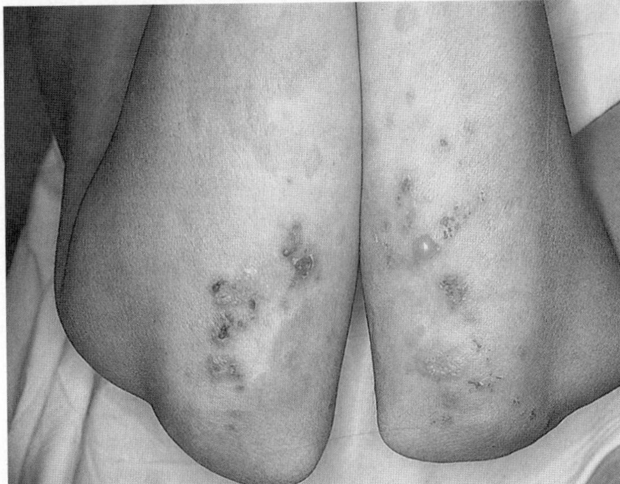

FIGURE 1-309 Dermatitis herpetiformis is an immunologically mediated blistering disease. There is a strong association of dermatitis herpetiformis with HLA-B8, DR3. Gluten-sensitive enteropathy is a common associated finding. The lesions are grouped (herpetiform) and extremely pruritic. (From Callen JP [ed]: *Color atlas of dermatology,* ed 2, Philadelphia, 2000, Saunders.)

 - Clinical monitoring weekly is recommended to optimize dose (optimal dose is when 1-2 new lesions/wk)
 - Caution: dapsone may produce hemolysis (especially if G6PD deficiency), agranulocytosis, methemoglobinemia, systemic drug hypersensitivity reaction (DRESS), and a peripheral neuropathy.
 - Baseline labs: CBC, LFTs, G6PD levels. After the initiation of therapy, monitor CBC every week x1 month, then every other week x2 months, monthly x4 months, then every 3-4 months. Monitor LFTs every 3-4 months.
- Second-line alternatives
 - Sulfapyridine (500-1500 mg/day) or sulfasalazine (500-1000 mg bid) may be substituted in cases of dapsone intolerance.
 - Reported efficacy in uncontrolled studies and case reports have suggested efficacy with tetracyclines, nicotinamide, cyclosporine, colchicine, and heparin
- Symptomatic relief for pruritus
 - Potent and superpotent topical corticosteroids (atrophy with prolonged use, limit to 14 days per month), non-sedating antihistamines twice daily, sedating antihistamines at bedtime, sarna lotion

CHRONIC Rx

- As DH is considered to represent the cutaneous manifestations of CD, lifelong avoidance of gluten is typically recommended. Information about educational resources, such as national and local support groups, should be provided (www.celiac.org).
- Patients with DH and CD have an increased risk of developing Hashimoto's thyroiditis, non-Hodgkin lymphoma, and GI lymphomas. An increased incidence of other autoimmune disorders (type 1 diabetes mellitus, pernicious anemia, Addison's disease, vitiligo, systemic lupus erythematosus, rheumatoid arthritis, and Sjögren's syndrome) and osteoporosis have also been reported.
 - Screening for thyroid disease (TSH, antithyroid peroxidase antibody titers) is typically recommended
 - Screening for autoimmune connective tissue diseases should be considered if suspicious signs or symptoms
 - Routine screening for GI lymphomas is controversial

REFERRAL

- Dermatologist for skin biopsy and management of cutaneous disease
- Gastroenterology for evaluation of CD
- Nutritionist to educate patients about gluten-free diet
- National support groups (www.celiac.org) and local support groups

PEARLS & CONSIDERATIONS

- Classic areas involved are those that are exposed if in a "fetal position."
- Lesions may be worsened by iodides and certain NSAIDs; systemic steroids ineffective.
- Location of biopsies is important! False-negative DIF can result if biopsies are taken from lesional skin (should be taken from normal-appearing skin adjacent to lesion) as diagnostic IgA deposits are usually destroyed by the blistering process.
- GFD results in reduced IgA in skin on DIF (with eventual disappearance) and reduced anti-endomysial antibodies in the blood. Hence, serologies (e.g., anti-endomysial antibodies) can be used to monitor degree of compliance to dietary gluten restriction.
- Some studies have suggested a possible protective effect of GFD against intestinal lymphoma. First-degree relatives do not appear to be at increased risk for GI or systemic lymphomas in the absence of DH or CD.

SUGGESTED READINGS

available at www.expertconsult.com

RELATED CONTENT

Celiac Disease (Related Key Topic)
Celiac Disease (Patient Information)

AUTHORS: **LISA PAPPAS-TAFFER, M.D.,** and **IRIS L. TONG, M.D.**

BASIC INFORMATION

DEFINITION

Diabetes insipidus is a polyuric disorder resulting from insufficient production of vasopressin (pituitary [neurogenic] diabetes insipidus) or unresponsiveness of the renal tubules to vasopressin (nephrogenic diabetes insipidus).

ICD-10CM CODES
253.5 Diabetes insipidus
ICD-10CM CODES
E23.2 Diabetes insipidus

EPIDEMIOLOGY & DEMOGRAPHICS

GENETICS:

- Nephrogenic diabetes insipidus can be inherited as a sex-linked recessive trait.
- There is also a rare autosomal-dominant form of neurogenic diabetes insipidus.

PHYSICAL FINDINGS & CLINICAL PRESENTATION

- Central diabetes insipidus is usually abrupt in onset whereas in compulsive water drinking there is a more vague history of onset
- Nocturia is unusual in compulsive water drinkers and more common in central diabetes insipidus
- Polyuria: urinary volumes ranging from 2.5 to 6 L/day
- Polydipsia (predilection for cold or iced drinks)
- Neurologic manifestations (seizures, headaches, visual field defects)
- Evidence of volume contractions

NOTE: The physical findings and clinical manifestations are generally not evident until vasopressin secretory capacity is reduced to <20% of normal.

ETIOLOGY

Neurogenic diabetes insipidus:

- Idiopathic
- Neoplasms of brain or pituitary fossa (craniopharyngiomas, metastatic neoplasms from breast or lung)
- Posttherapeutic neurosurgical procedures (e.g., hypophysectomy)
- Head trauma (e.g., basal skull fracture)
- Granulomatous disorders (sarcoidosis or tuberculosis)
- Histiocytosis (Hand-Schüller-Christian disease, eosinophilic granuloma)
- Familial (autosomal dominant); some cases autosomal recessive
- Other: interventricular hemorrhage, aneurysms, meningitis, postencephalitis, multiple sclerosis, Guillain-Barré syndrome

Nephrogenic diabetes insipidus:

- Drugs: lithium, aminoglycosides, antivirals amphotericin B, demeclocycline, methoxyflurane anesthesia
- Familial: X-linked
- Metabolic: hypercalcemia or hypokalemia
- Other: sarcoidosis, amyloidosis, pyelonephritis, polycystic disease, sickle cell disease, postobstructive, low-protein diets (protein malnourishment)

Dx DIAGNOSIS

DIFFERENTIAL DIAGNOSIS

- Diabetes mellitus, nephropathies
- Primary polydipsia, medications (e.g., chlorpromazine)
- Osmotic diuresis (glucose, mannitol, anticholinergics)
- Psychogenic polydipsia, electrolyte disturbances

WORKUP

- The diagnostic workup is aimed at showing that polyuria is caused by the inability to concentrate urine and determining whether the problem is the result of decreased vasopressin or insensitivity to vasopressin. This is done with the water deprivation test (Table E1-158):
  - After baseline measurement of weight, vasopressin, plasma sodium, and urine and plasma osmolarity, the patient is deprived of fluids under strict medical supervision.
  - Frequent (q2h) monitoring of plasma and urine osmolarity follows.
  - The test is generally terminated when plasma osmolarity is >295 mOsm/kg or the patient loses ≥3.5% of initial body weight.
  - Diabetes insipidus is confirmed if the plasma osmolarity is >295 mOsm/kg and the urine osmolarity is <500 mOsm/kg.
  - To distinguish nephrogenic from neurogenic diabetes insipidus, the patient is given 5 U of vasopressin and the change in urine osmolarity is measured. A significant increase (>50%) in urine osmolarity after administration of vasopressin is indicative of neurogenic diabetes insipidus.
- A diagnostic algorithm for diabetes insipidus is described in Fig. E1-310.

LABORATORY TESTS

- Decreased urinary specific gravity (≤1.005)
- Baseline plasma osmolality >295 mOsm/kg is suggestive of central diabetes mellitus whereas values below 270 mOsm/kg favor compulsive water drinking. Decreased urinary osmolarity (usually <200 mOsm/kg) even in the presence of high plasma osmolality
- Hypernatremia, increased plasma osmolarity, hypercalcemia, hypokalemia

IMAGING STUDIES

MRI of the pituitary if neurogenic diabetes insipidus is confirmed

TREATMENT

NONPHARMACOLOGIC THERAPY

- Patient education regarding control of fluid balance and prevention of dehydration with adequate fluid intake or IV D_5W
- Daily weight

ACUTE GENERAL Rx

Therapy varies with the degree and type of diabetes insipidus (Table E1-159).

- Neurogenic diabetes insipidus:
  - Desmopressin acetate (DDAVP) 20-40 mcg qd intranasally in 1-3 divided doses or in tablet form 0.1-1.2 mg. Usual oral dose is 0.1 to 1.2 mg/day in 2-3 divided doses. Desmopressin is also available in injectable form given as 2-4 mcg/day SC or IV in 2 divided doses.
  - Vasopressin tannate in oil: 2.5 to 5 U IM q24 to 72h; useful for long-term management because of its long half-life.
  - In mild cases of neurogenic diabetes insipidus, polyuria may be controlled with HCTZ 50 mg qd (decreases urine volume by increasing proximal tubular reabsorption of glomerular infiltrate).
- Nephrogenic diabetes insipidus:
  - Removal of the underlying cause. However, prolonged lithium therapy can lead to irreversible nephrogenic diabetes insipidus even after lithium therapy is withdrawn.
  - Amiloride 5 mg/day for lithium-related disease
  - Low-sodium diet and chlorothiazide to induce mild sodium depletion

CHRONIC Rx

Patients should be aware of the danger of dehydration and the need for liberal water intake.

REFERRAL

Endocrinology consultation for diagnostic testing

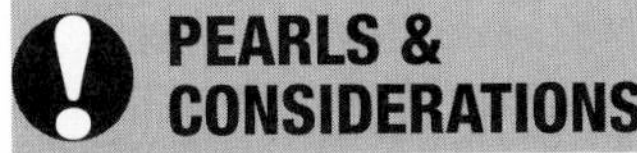

PEARLS & CONSIDERATIONS

COMMENTS

- Patients should be instructed to wear a medical identification tag or bracelet identifying their medical illness.
- In central diabetes insipidus, the use of DDAVP has become the standard of care. Extensive clinical experience has shown it to be both safe and effective in the treatment of this disorder.
- The treatment of nephrogenic diabetes insipidus is more complicated than the central form, and opinion varies among experts in the field. Consultation with a specialist is always recommended in this setting.

SUGGESTED READINGS

available at www.expertconsult.com

RELATED CONTENT

Diabetes Insipidus (Patient Information)

AUTHOR: **FRED F. FERRI, M.D.**

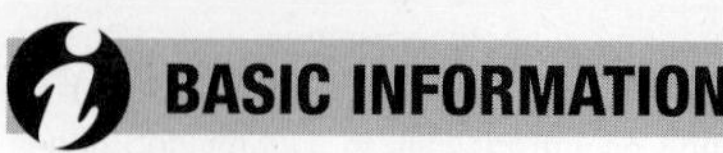

BASIC INFORMATION

DEFINITION

- Diabetes mellitus (DM) refers to a syndrome of hyperglycemia resulting from many different causes (see "Etiology"). It is broadly classified into type 1 and type 2 DM. The terms "insulin-dependent" and "non–insulin-dependent" diabetes are obsolete because when a person with type 2 diabetes needs insulin, he or she remains labeled as type 2 and is not reclassified as type 1. Table 1-160 provides a general comparison of the two types of DM.
- The American Diabetes Association (ADA) defines DM as follows:
  - A fasting plasma glucose (FPG) ≥126 mg/dl, which should be confirmed with repeat testing on a different day. Fasting is defined as no caloric intake for at least 8 hr.
  - Symptoms of hyperglycemia and a casual (random) plasma glucose ≥200 mg/dl. Classic symptoms of hyperglycemia include polyuria, polydipsia, and unexplained weight loss.
  - An oral glucose tolerance test (OGTT) with a plasma glucose ≥200 mg/dl 2 hr after a 75 g (100 g for pregnant women) glucose load.
  - A hemoglobin A_{1c} (HbA1c) value ≥6.5%.
- Individuals with glucose levels higher than normal but not high enough to meet the criteria for diagnosis of DM are considered to have "prediabetes," the diagnosis of which is made as follows:
  - A fasting plasma glucose 100 to 125 mg/dl; this is referred to as impaired fasting glucose.
  - After OGTT, a 2-hr plasma glucose 140 to 199; this is referred to as impaired glucose tolerance.
  - A hemoglobin A_{1c} value 5.7% to 6.4%.
- Table 1-161 describes diagnostic categories for DM and at-risk states.

SYNONYMS

IDDM (insulin-dependent diabetes mellitus)
NIDDM (non–insulin-dependent diabetes mellitus)
Type 1 diabetes mellitus (insulin-dependent diabetes mellitus)
Type 2 diabetes mellitus (non–insulin-dependent diabetes mellitus)

ICD-9CM CODES

250.0 Diabetes mellitus (NIDDM)
250.1 Insulin-dependent diabetes mellitus without complication (IDDM)

ICD-10CM CODES

E11.5 Type 2 diabetes mellitus with peripheral circulatory complications
E11.6 Type 2 diabetes mellitus with other specified complications
E11.7 Type 2 diabetes mellitus with multiple complications
E11.8 Type 2 diabetes mellitus with unspecified complications
E11.9 Type 2 diabetes mellitus without complications

EPIDEMIOLOGY & DEMOGRAPHICS

- DM affects 9% to 10% of the U.S. population. Prevalence rates vary considerably by race/ethnicity.
- Incidence rate increases with age, varying from 2% in persons age 20 to 44 yr to 18% in persons 65 to 74 yr. Type 2 DM can have a long presymptomatic phase, leading to a 4- to 7-yr delay in diagnosis.
- Diabetes accounts for 8% of all legal blindness in the United States and is the leading cause of end-stage renal disease (ESRD).
- Patients with diabetes are 2-4 times more likely than nondiabetic patients to experience development of cardiovascular disease.

PHYSICAL FINDINGS & CLINICAL PRESENTATION

1. Physical examination varies with the presence of complications and may be normal in early stages
2. Diabetic retinopathy:
   a. Nonproliferative (background diabetic retinopathy):
      (1) Initially: microaneurysms, capillary dilation, waxy or hard exudates, dot and flame hemorrhages, atrioventricular shunts
      (2) Advanced stage: microinfarcts with cotton wool exudates, macular edema
   b. Proliferative retinopathy: characterized by formation of new vessels, vitreous hemorrhages, fibrous scarring, and retinal detachment
3. Cataracts and glaucoma occur with increased frequency in patients with diabetes
4. Diabetic neuropathy
   a. Distal sensorimotor polyneuropathy
      (1) Symptoms include paresthesia, hyperesthesia, or burning pain involving bilateral distal extremities, in a "stocking-glove" distribution. This can progress to motor weakness and ataxia.
      (2) Physical examination may reveal decreased pinprick sensation, sensation to light touch, vibration sense, and loss of proprioception. Motor disturbances such as decreased deep tendon reflexes and atrophy of interossei muscles can also be seen.
   b. Autonomic neuropathy:
      (1) GI disturbances: esophageal motility abnormalities, gastroparesis, diarrhea (usually nocturnal)

TABLE 1-160 General Comparison of the Two Types of Diabetes Mellitus

	Type 1	Type 2
Previous terminology	Insulin-dependent diabetes mellitus (IDDM), type I, juvenile-onset diabetes	Non–insulin-dependent diabetes mellitus, type II, adult-onset diabetes
Age of onset	Usually <30 yr, particularly childhood and adolescence, but any age	Usually >40 yr, but any age
Genetic predisposition	Moderate; environmental factors required for expression; 35%-50% concordance in monozygotic twins; several candidate genes proposed	Strong; 60%-90% concordance in monozygotic twins; many candidate genes proposed; some genes identified in maturity-onset diabetes of the young
Human leukocyte antigen associations	Linkage to DQA and DQB, influenced by DRB (3 and 4) (DR2 protective)	None known
Other associations	Autoimmune; Graves' disease, Hashimoto's thyroiditis, vitiligo, Addison's disease, pernicious anemia	Heterogenous group, ongoing subclassification based on identification of specific pathogenic processes and genetic defects
Precipitating and risk factors	Largely unknown; microbial, chemical, dietary, other	Age, obesity (central), sedentary lifestyle, previous gestational diabetes
Findings at diagnosis	85%-90% of patients have one and usually more autoantibodies to ICA512/IA-2/IA-2β, GAD_{65}, insulin (IAA)	Possibly complications (microvascular and macrovascular) caused by significant preceding asymptomatic period
Endogenous insulin levels	Low or absent	Usually present (relative deficiency), early hyperinsulinemia
Insulin resistance	Only with hyperglycemia	Mostly present
Prolonged fast	Hyperglycemia, ketoacidosis	Euglycemia
Stress, withdrawal of insulin	Ketoacidosis	Nonketotic hyperglycemia, occasionally ketoacidosis

GAD, Glutamic acid decarboxylase; *IA-2/IA-2β,* tyrosine phosphatases; *IAA,* insulin autoantibodies; *ICA,* islet cell antibody; *ICA512,* islet cell autoantigen 512 (fragment of IA-2).
From Andreoli TE (ed): *Cecil essentials of medicine,* ed 6, Philadelphia, 2005, Saunders.

TABLE 1-161 Diagnostic Categories*: Diabetes Mellitus and At-Risk States

	2-HOUR (75-g) OGTT RESULT		
Fasting Plasma Glucose Level	**<140 mg/dl**	**140-199 mg/dl**	**≥200 mg/dl**
<100 mg/dl	Normal	IGT†	DM
100-125 mg/dl	IFG†	IGT† *and* IFG†	DM
≥126 mg/dl	DM	DM	DM
HbA_{1c} Level	**<5.7%**	**5.7-6.4%**	**≥6.5%**
	Normal	High-risk†	DM

*These diagnostic categories are based on the combined fasting plasma glucose level and a 2-hour, 75-g oral glucose tolerance test (OGTT) result. Note that a confirmed random plasma glucose level of 200 mg/dl or higher in the appropriate clinical setting is diagnostic of diabetes and precludes the need for further testing.
†May be referred to as prediabetes.
DM, Diabetes mellitus; *IFG,* impaired fasting glucose; *IGT.* impaired glucose tolerance.
From Goldman L, Schafer AI: *Goldman's Cecil medicine,* ed 24, Philadelphia, 2012, Saunders.

(2) Genitourinary (GU) disturbances: neurogenic bladder (hesitancy, weak stream, and dribbling), impotence
(3) Cardiovascular (CV) disturbances: orthostatic hypotension, tachycardia, decreased heart rate variability (HRV). Decreased heart rate variability is associated with increased cardiac mortality, independent of ejection fraction.

c. Polyradiculopathy: painful weakness and atrophy in the distribution of ≥1 contiguous nerve roots.
d. Mononeuropathy involving cranial nerves III, IV, or VI or peripheral nerves can also occur.

5. Diabetic nephropathy: pedal edema, pallor, weakness, uremic appearance
6. Foot ulcers: occur in 15% of individuals with diabetes (annual incidence rate 2%) and are the leading causes of hospitalization; they are usually secondary to a combination of factors, including peripheral vascular insufficiency, repeated trauma (unrecognized because of sensory loss), and superimposed infection.
   a. Patient symptoms are usually less than would be expected from clinical findings, due to loss of sensation related to peripheral neuropathy.
   b. Comprehensive foot exams include visual inspection, assessment of pedal pulses, and assessment of protective sensation using a 10-g monofilament to test sensation.
   c. Prevention of foot ulcers in an individual with diabetes includes strict glucose control, patient education, prescription footwear, intensive podiatric care, and evaluation for surgical interventions
7. Neuropathic arthropathy (Charcot's joints): bone or joint deformities from repeated trauma (secondary to peripheral neuropathy; Fig. E1-311).
8. Necrobiosis lipoidica diabeticorum: plaque-like reddened areas with a central area that fades to white-yellow found on the anterior surfaces of the legs (Fig. E1-312); in these areas, the skin becomes very thin and can ulcerate easily.

ETIOLOGY

IDIOPATHIC DIABETES:

Type 1 DM: results from beta-cell destruction, usually leading to absolute insulin deficiency

- Hereditary factors:
  1. Islet cell antibodies (found in 90% of patients within the first yr of diagnosis)
  2. Higher incidence of human leukocyte antigen (HLA) types DR3, DR4
  3. 50% concordance rate in identical twins
- Environmental factors: viral infection (possibly Coxsackie virus, mumps virus)

Type 2 DM: results from insulin resistance and a progressive defect in insulin secretion.

- Hereditary factors: 90% concordance rate in identical twins
- Environmental factors: obesity, sedentary lifestyle, high carbohydrate content in food

DIABETES SECONDARY TO OTHER FACTORS:

- Hormonal excess: Cushing's syndrome, acromegaly, glucagonoma, pheochromocytoma
- Drugs: glucocorticoids, diuretics, oral contraceptives
- Insulin receptor unavailability (with or without circulating antibodies)
- Pancreatic disease: pancreatitis, pancreatectomy, hemochromatosis, cystic fibrosis
- Genetic syndromes: maturity onset diabetes of the young (MODY, monogenetic diabetes accounting for 2% to 5% of diabetes), familial hyperlipidemias, myotonic dystrophy, lipoatrophy
- Gestational diabetes (GDM): diabetes diagnosed during pregnancy that is due to pregnancy-related insulin resistance

Dx DIAGNOSIS

DIFFERENTIAL DIAGNOSIS

- Diabetes insipidus
- Stress hyperglycemia
- Diabetes secondary to hormonal excess, drugs, pancreatic disease

LABORATORY TESTS

- Diagnosis of DM is made on the basis of the following tests:
  1. Fasting glucose ≥126 mg/dl on two occasions
  2. Non-FPG ≥200 mg/dl and symptoms of DM
  3. OGTT (75-g glucose load for nonpregnant individuals) with 2-hr value >200 mg/dl
  4. Glycosylated hemoglobin (HbA_{1c}) ≥6.5%
- Screening for prediabetes and diabetes in asymptomatic patients (see Table 1-162):
  1. Should be considered in adults of any age who are overweight (body mass index [BMI] >25 kg/m^2) or obese (BMI >30) and who have one or more additional risk factors for diabetes.
  2. In those who are without these risk factors, testing should begin at age 45 yr.
  3. If screen is normal, repeat testing should be carried out at least at 3-yr intervals.
- Detection and diagnosis of gestational diabetes mellitus (GDM)
  1. Screen for GDM using risk factor analysis and use of an OGTT. Pregnant women who are not known to have diabetes should be screened for gestational diabetes at 24 to 48 weeks' gestation with a 75-g oral glucose tolerance test. A diagnosis of GDM is made if any of the following levels of plasma glucose are exceeded: ≥92 mg/dl (5.1 mmol/L) when fasting, ≥80 mg/dl (10 mmol/L) at 1 hour, or ≥153 mg/dl (8.5 mmol/L) at 2 hours.
  2. Women with GDM should be screened for diabetes 6 to 12 wk postpartum and should be followed with subsequent screening for the development of diabetes or prediabetes at least every 3 yr
- Screening for diabetic nephropathy (Fig. E1-313)
  1. Screening should be done at diagnosis and then yearly for type 2 diabetes and 5 yr after diagnosis then yearly in type 2 diabetics.
  2. Screening can be performed using a albumin:creatinine ratio (microalbumin) in a random spot urine collection or by measurement of a 24-hour urine collection for albumin, and creatinine clearance. The urine albumin to creatinine ratio (ACR) is independently associated with mortality at all levels of estimated glomerular filtration rate (eGFR) in older adults with diabetes.
  3. The diagnosis of microalbuminuria (ACR 30-299 mg/24 hr) should be based on 2 to 3 elevated levels within a 3- to 6-mo period because there is a marked variability in day-to-day albumin excretion. Patients with overt macroalbuminuria (>300 mg albumin/24 hr or albumin: creatinine ratio >300) should be followed by urine protein:creatinine ratio.
- A fasting serum lipid panel, serum creatinine, and electrolytes should be obtained yearly on all adult patients with diabetes.
- Self-monitoring of blood glucose (SMBG) is crucial for assessing the effectiveness of the management plan. The frequency and timing of SMBG varies with the needs and goals of each patient. In most patients with type 1 DM and pregnant women taking insulin, SMBG is recommended at least 3 times/day. In patients with type 2 DM not on insulin, recommendations are unclear for SMBG, but testing once or twice/day is acceptable in most patients.

TABLE 1-162 Criteria for Diabetes Screening in Asymptomatic Individuals

1. Testing should be considered in all adults who are overweight (BMI >25 kg/m²*) and have additional risk factors:
   - Physical inactivity
   - A first-degree relative with diabetes
   - High-risk ethnic population (e.g., African American, Hispanic American, Native American, Asian American, Pacific Islander)
   - Delivered a baby weighing more than 9 lb or diagnosed with gestational diabetes mellitus
   - Systemic hypertension (blood pressure >140/90 mm Hg or on antihypertensive therapy)
   - High-density lipoprotein cholesterol level <35 mg/dl or triglyceride level >250 mg/dl
   - Polycystic ovary syndrome
   - Hemoglobin A_{1c} ≥5.7%, impaired glucose tolerance or impaired fasting glucose on prior testing
   - Other clinical conditions associated with insulin resistance (e.g., severe obesity, acanthosis nigricans)
   - History of cardiovascular disease
2. If none of the above criteria are present, screening for diabetes should begin at age 45 yr.
3. If the results are normal, screening should be repeated at least every 3 yr. Depending on initial results and risk status, more frequent testing may need to be considered.

*In some ethnic groups, such as Asians, at-risk body mass index (BMI) may be lower.
Modified from American Diabetes Association, Diagnosis and classification of diabetes mellitus *Diabetes Care* 33(Suppl. 1):S14, 2010. Borrowed from Goldman L, Schafer AI: *Goldman's Cecil medicine*, ed 24, Philadelphia, 2012, Saunders.

- Screening for thyroid dysfunction (TSH level), Vitamin B_{12} deficiency, and celiac disease should be considered in type 1 diabetes due to the increased frequency of other autoimmune diseases in these individuals.

Rx TREATMENT

- Type 1 diabetes requires immediate initiation of insulin therapy.
- The ADA and European Association for the Study of Diabetes recommend lifestyle intervention (diet and exercise) and metformin initiation (unless contraindication such as renal failure) at the time of diagnosis of type 2 diabetes. Therapy should then be augmented with additional agents (including early initiation of insulin therapy) to achieve adequate glycemic control.
- In Type 1 diabetes, intensive glycemic control (HbA1c <7) has been shown in randomized controlled trials (RCT) to reduce the risk of microvascular (neuropathy, retinopathy, nephropathy) and macrovascular (cardiovascular events) complications.
- In Type 2 diabetes, intensive glycemic control (HbA1c <7) has been shown in RCT to reduce the risk of microvascular complications. While intensive glucose control reduced the risk of some cardiovascular disease outcomes (such as nonfatal MI), it did not reduce the risk of cardiovascular death or all cause mortality and increased the risk of severe hypoglycemia.
- It is important to remember that tight glycemic control may burden patients with complex treatment programs, hypoglycemia, weight gain, and costs. Clinicians should individualize HbA1c targets so that they are reasonable and reflect patients' personal and clinical contexts and their informed values and preferences. A target HbA1c >7 is reasonable for motivated new diabetic patients with long life expectancies, whereas less stringent controls (HbA1c 7.5 or higher) may be reasonable in elderly patients with limited life expectancy and elevated risk of hypoglycemia.

NONPHARMACOLOGIC THERAPY

1. Diet
   a. Calories
      (1) The patient with diabetes can be started on 15 calories/lb of ideal body weight; this number can be increased to 20 calories/lb for an active person and 25 calories/lb if the patient does heavy physical labor.
      (2) The calories should be distributed as 45% to 65% carbohydrates, <30% fat, with saturated fat limited to <7% of total calories, and 10% to 30% protein. Daily cholesterol intake should not exceed 300 mg.
      (3) The emphasis should be on complex carbohydrates rather than simple and refined starches, and on polyunsaturated instead of saturated fats in a ratio of 2:1.
   b. Seven food groups
      (1) The exchange diet of the ADA includes bread or starches, meat or proteins, vegetables, fruits, fats, milk, and free foods (e.g., black tea, sugar-free gelatin).
      (2) The name of each exchange is meant to be all-inclusive (e.g., cereal, muffins, spaghetti, potatoes, rice are in the bread group; meats, fish, eggs, cheese, peanut butter are in the protein group).
      (3) The glycemic index compares the increase in blood sugar after the ingestion of simple sugars and complex carbohydrates with the increase that occurs after the absorption of glucose; equal amounts of starches do not give the same increase in plasma glucose (pasta equal in calories to a baked potato causes less of an increase than the potato); thus, it is helpful to know the glycemic index of a particular food product.
      (4) Fiber: Insoluble fiber (bran, celery) and soluble globular fiber (pectin in fruit) delay glucose absorption and attenuate the postprandial serum glucose peak; they also appear to reduce the increased triglyceride level often present in patients with uncontrolled diabetes. A diet high in fiber should be emphasized (20 to 35 g/day of soluble and insoluble fiber).
   c. Other principles
      (1) Modest sodium restriction to 2400 to 3000 mg/day. If hypertension is present, restrict to <2400 mg/day; if nephropathy and hypertension are present, restrict to <2000 mg/day.
      (2) Moderation of alcohol intake recommended (≤2 drinks/day in men, ≤1 drink/day in women).
      (3) Non-nutritive artificial sweeteners are acceptable in moderate amounts.
2. Exercise: increases the cellular glucose uptake by increasing the number of insulin receptors. The following points must be considered:
   a. Exercise program must be individualized and built up slowly. Consider beginning with 15 min of low-impact aerobic exercise 3 times per wk and increasing the frequency and duration to 30 to 45 min of moderate aerobic activity (50% to 70% of maximum age predicted heart rate) to 3 to 5 days/wk.
      (1) In the absence of contraindications, resistance training three times per wk should be encouraged.
   b. Insulin is more rapidly absorbed when injected into a limb that is then exercised, and this can result in hypoglycemia.
   c. Physical activity can result in hypoglycemia if medication dose or carbohydrate consumption is not modified. Ingestion of additional carbohydrates is recommended if pre-exercise glucose levels are <100 mg/dl.
3. Weight loss: to ideal body weight if the patient is overweight. Recent trials have shown that although weight loss has many positive health benefits for people with type 2 DM, such as slower decline in mobility, it does not reduce the number of cardiovascular events.
4. Screening for nephropathy, neuropathy, and retinopathy: annual serum creatinine and urine albumin excretion; initial comprehensive eye examination and at least annually thereafter
5. Diabetes self-management education: could also address psychosocial issues
6. Self-monitoring of blood glucose should occur three to four times per day for patients using multiple insulin injections or on insulin pump therapy
7. Perform HbA1c at least two times a year in patients who are meeting treatment goals and who have stable glycemic control
   - HbA1c quarterly in patients whose therapy has changed or who are not meeting glycemic goals
   - The HbA1c goal for nonpregnant adults in general is <7%
   - In the elderly, those with comorbidities, or those at risk for complications from

hypoglycemia, a more moderate glycemic target (HbA1c 7-8) may be appropriate

GENERAL Rx

- When the previous measures fail to normalize the serum glucose, oral hypoglycemic agents should be added to the regimen in type 2 DM. Tables 1-163 and 1-164 compare therapies for type 2 DM and classes of antihyperglycemic agents.
- The primary mechanism of metformin is to decrease hepatic glucose production and improve insulin sensitivity. Because metformin does not produce hypoglycemia when used as a monotherapy, it is preferred initially for most patients. Metformin reduces mean HbA1c level by 1.1 %. It is contraindicated in patients with severe renal insufficiency with an estimated glomerular filtrate rate <30 ml/min, heart failure, or other clinical states of hypoperfusion, and in patients with significant liver disease.
- Sitagliptin, saxagliptin, vildagliptin, and linagliptin inhibit the enzyme DPP-4, responsible for inactivation and degradation of glucagon-like peptide-1 (GLP-1) and glucose-dependent insulinotropic polypeptide (GIP). These drugs, known as "gliptins," raise blood incretin levels, thereby inhibiting glucagon release and lowering blood glucose levels. When used with metfomin they do not cause hypoglycemia and are preferred over sulfonylureas as second line agents. Cost is a major barrier to their use.
- Exenatide and liraglutide are glucagon-like peptide-1 (GLP-1) agonists. They are incretin mimetics that stimulate release of insulin from pancreatic beta cells and can be used as adjunctive therapy for patients with type 2 DM. GLP-1 agonists are not indicated in type 1 DM and are contraindicated in patients with severe renal impairment. Cost is a barrier to their use.
- Acarbose and miglitol inhibit pancreatic amylase and small intestinal glucosidases, thereby delaying carbohydrate absorption in the gut and reducing associated post-prandial hyperglycemia. The major side effects are flatulence, diarrhea, and abdominal cramps.
- Sulfonylureas increase insulin secretion and work best when given before meals. All sulfonylureas are contraindicated in patients who are allergic to sulfa.
- Pramlintide is a synthetic analog of human amylin, which is synthesized by pancreatic beta cells and cosecreted with insulin in response to food intake. It suppresses glucagon secretion and slows stomach emptying and can be used as an adjunctive treatment for patients with type 1 or type 2 DM who inject insulin at mealtime. Nausea is its major side effect.
- Thiazolidinediones (pioglitazone and rosiglitazone) increase insulin sensitivity and have been used in the therapy of type 2 diabetes. Serum transaminase levels should be obtained before starting therapy and monitored periodically. Thiazolidinediones, in general, result in moderate weight gain and increase the risk for heart failure and osteoporosis/fractures. Rosiglitazone has an FDA black box warning for heart failure exacerbations and myocardial ischemia. Pioglitazone and rosiglitazone cause increased incidence of bladder cancer.
- Sodium-glucose co-transporter 2 ($SGLT_2$) inhibitors (e.g., canagliflozin, dapagliflozin) have recently been approved by the FDA for oral treatment of type 2 DM. By inhibiting $SGLT_2$, these medications decrease glucose re-absorption, increase urinary glucose excretion, and lower blood glucose levels ({down arrow} HbA_{1C} by 0.7%). Side effects include increased risk of genital mycotic infections, UTIs, and volume depletion. Higher cost and limited drug formulary availability are limiting factors.

TABLE 1-163 Comparison of Therapies for Type 2 Diabetes

Property	Lifestyle	Insulins	Sulfonylureas	Metformin	α-Glucosidase Inhibitors	Glitazones	Glinides	Exenatide	Pramlintide
Target tissue	Muscle or fat	Beta cell supplement	Beta cell	Liver	Gut	Muscle	Beta cell	Various	Brain
ΔHbA_{1c} (%) as (monotherapy)	Variable	1->2	1-2	1-2	0.5-1	0.5-2	Re: 1-2 N: 0.5-1	~1	~0.5
Fasting effect	Good	Excellent	Good	Good	Poor	Good	Re: Moderate N: Poor	Poor	Poor
Postprandial effect	Good	Excellent	Good	Good	Excellent	Good	Re: Good N: Excellent	Excellent	Excellent
Severe hypoglycemia	No	Yes	Yes	No	No	No	Re: Yes N: No	No	No
Dosing interval	Continuous	qd to continuous	qd to tid	bid or tid	bid to qid	P: qd Ro: qd or bid	tid to qid with meals	bid	tid
ΔWeight (lb/yr)	+1	+3	+1 to 3	0 to −6	0 to −10	+1 to 13	+1 to 3	−6 to −12	−3 to −6
ΔInsulin	Variable	Increase	Increase	Modest decrease	Modest decrease	Decrease	Increase	Increase	None
ΔLDL	Minimal decrease	Minimal decrease	None	Decrease	Minimal decrease	Increase	None	None	None
ΔHDL	Minimal increase	None	None	Increase	None	Increase	None	Decrease	None
ΔTG	Minimal decrease	Decrease	None	Decrease	Minimal decrease	P: Decrease Ro: None	None	Decrease	None
Common problem	Recidivism, injury	Hypoglycemia, weight gain	Hypoglycemia, weight gain	Transient GI	Flatulence	Weight gain, edema, anemia	Hypoglycemia	GI	GI
Rare problem	—	—	—	Lactic acidosis	—	Hepatotoxicity?	—	—	—
Contraindications	None	None	Allergy	Renal failure, Liver failure, CHF (>80 yr old)	Intestinal disease	Hepatocellular disease	—	None	None
Cost ($/mo)	0-200	30-450	10-15	30-60	40-80	75-180	70-110	170-200	200-400
Maximum effective dose	—	1-2 U/kg per day	maximum or double starting	1000 mg bid	50 mg tid	P: 45 mg qd Ro: 4 mg bid	Re: 2 mg tid N: 120 mg tid	10 μg bid	120 μg ac

Δ, Change; *ac,* before food; *CHF,* congestive heart failure; *GI,* gastrointestinal disturbance; HbA_{1c}, glycosylated hemoglobin; *HDL,* high-density lipoprotein; *LDL,* low-density lipoprotein; *N,* nateglinide; *P,* pioglitazone; *Re,* repaglinide; *Ro,* rosiglitazone; *TG,* triglycerides.
From Melmed S, Polonsky KS, Larsen PR, Kronenberg HM: *Williams textbook of endocrinology,* ed 12, Philadelphia, 2011, Saunders.

TABLE 1-164 Classes of Antihyperglycemic Therapy

Class	Representative Agents	Major Action	HbA_{1c} Lowering (%)	Fasting or Prandial Effect	Usual Dosing Frequency (Doses/Day)	Route	Hypoglycemia	Weight Effect	CVD Risk Factor Benefits	Important Contraindications	Daily Cost ($)
Lifestyle	—	Broad	>1	Both	—	—	No	Loss	Yes	—	—
Biguanide	Metformin	Liver sensitizer	>1	Fasting	1-2	Oral	No	Neutral	Modest	Renal or hepatic failure	<$1
Sulfonylurea	Glimepiride, glipizide	Insulin secretagogue	>1	Fasting	1-2	Oral	Yes	Gain	Negligible	—	<<$1
Meglitinide	Repaglinide	Insulin secretagogue	>1	Both	With meals	Oral	Yes	Gain	Negligible	—	~$5
Benzoic acid–derived	Nateglinide	Insulin secretagogue	<1	Prandial	With meals	Oral	Minimal	Minimal	Negligible	—	~$5
Basal insulin	NPH, glargine, detemir	Insulin supplement/ substitute	>1	Fasting	1	SQ	Yes++	Gain++	Lowers TG	—	~$5
Bolus insulin	R, lispro, aspart, glulisine	Insulin supplement/ substitute	>1	Prandial	With meals	SQ	Yes++	Gain++	Lowers TG	—	~$5
Thiazolidinediones	Pioglitazone, rosi-glitazone	Peripheral sensitizer	>1	Fasting	1	Oral	No	Gain++	Variable (see text)	Heart or liver failure	~$5
α-Glucosidase inhibitors	Acarbose, miglitol	Slow carbohydrate absorption	<1	Prandial	With meals	Oral	No	Neutral	Negligible	—	~$3
Amylinomimetics	Pramlintide	Broad	<1	Prandial	With meals	SQ	No	Loss	Negligible	—	~$10
GLP1 receptor agonists	Exenatide	Broad	~1	Prandial	2	SQ	No	Loss	Modest with weight loss	Pancreatitis, renal failure	~$9
Long-acting GLP1 receptor agonists	Liraglutide	Broad	>1	Both	1	SQ	No	Loss	Lowers BP	Pancreatitis, medul-lary thyroid cancer	~$13
DPP4 inhibitors	Sitagliptin, saxagliptin	Improved insulin/ glucagon secretion	<1	Both	1	Oral	No	Neutral	Negligible	Pancreatitis	~$7
Bile acid sequestrants	Colesevelam	Uncertain	<1	Prandial	1-2	Oral	No	Neutral	Lowers LDL	Hypertriglyceridemia	~$9
Dopamine agonists	Bromocriptine	Uncertain	<1	Fasting	1	Oral	No	Neutral	Modest	—	NA

BP, Blood pressure; *CVD,* cardiovascular disease; *LDL,* low-density lipoprotein; *SQ,* subcutaneous; *TG,* triglyceride.
From Melmed S, Polonsky KS, Larsen PR, Kronenberg HM: *Williams textbook of endocrinology*, ed 12, Philadelphia, 2011, Saunders.

- Combination therapy of various hypoglycemic agents is commonly used when monotherapy results in inadequate glycemic control.
- Insulin is indicated for the treatment of all type 1 DM and for type 2 DM patients whose condition cannot be adequately controlled with diet and oral agents. The American College of Endocrinology and the American Association of Clinical Endocrinologists recommend initiation of insulin therapy in patients with type 2 diabetes and an initial HbA1c level >9%, or if the diabetes is uncontrolled despite optimal oral glycemic therapy. Insulin therapy may be initiated as augmentation, starting at 0.3 unit/kg, or as replacement, starting at 0.6 to 1.0 unit/kg. Table 1-165 describes commonly used types of insulin.
  1. The risks of insulin therapy include weight gain, hypoglycemia, and in rare cases, allergic or cutaneous reactions.
  2. Replacement insulin therapy should mimic normal release patterns.
     a. Approximately 50% to 60% of daily insulin can be given as a long-acting insulin (NPH, ultralente, glargine, detemir) injected once or twice daily
     b. The remaining 40% to 50% can be short-acting (regular) or rapid-acting (lispro, aspart, glulysine) to cover mealtime carbohydrates and correct increased current glucose levels.
- Continuous subcutaneous insulin infusion (CSII, or insulin pump) provides comparable or slightly better control than multiple daily injections. It should be considered for diabetes presenting in childhood or adolescence and during pregnancy. The guidelines for insulin pump therapy from the American Association of Diabetes Educators include "frequent and unpredictable fluctuations in blood glucose" and "patient perceptions that diabetes management impedes the pursuit of personal or professional goals."
- Low-dose aspirin (ASA; 81 mg/day) has been proven to lower the risk of subsequent myocardial infarction, stroke, or vascular death in secondary prevention studies. The ADA recommends low-dose aspirin for primary prevention in diabetic patients with one additional cardiovascular risk factor, including age older than 40 yr, cigarette smoking, hypertension, obesity, albuminuria, hyperlipidemia, and family history of coronary artery disease.
- Measure fasting lipid profile at least annually in adults.
  1. All patients with diabetes with one or more additional risk factors for cardiovascular disease should be on statin therapy together with lifestyle modification regardless of baseline lipid levels.
  2. Diabetic patients aged 40-75 with LDL cholesterol of 70-189 mg/dl and without clinical atherosclerotic cardiovascular disease (ASCVD) should receive at least moderate-intensity statin therapy and consider high-intensity statin therapy if 10-year ASCVD risk is >=7.5%.
- Aggressive antihypertensive therapy is recommended to keep systolic blood pressure (BP) <130 and diastolic BP <80 mm Hg. Use of angiotensin-converting enzyme (ACE) inhibitors or angiotensin receptor blockers (ARBs) to decrease albuminuria and for prevention of progression of kidney disease should be considered regardless of presence of hypertension. Combination therapy with an ACE inhibitor and an ARB should be avoided due to increased risk of adverse effects among patients with diabetic nephropathy.
- Bariatric surgery should be considered in adults with BMI >35 kg/m^2 and type 2 diabetes, especially if the diabetes is difficult to control with lifestyle and pharmacologic therapy.
- Treat hypoglycemia in a conscious person with glucose tab or gel 15 to 20 g, and intramuscular injection of glucagon if unconscious. Patient and family members should be instructed on the administration of glucagon for individuals at significant risk for severe hypoglycemia.

TABLE 1-165 Types of Insulin[a]

Preparation	Brand	Onset (hr)[b]	Peak (hr)	Duration (hr)[c]	Route
Insulin Aspart	NovoLog[d]	<0.25	1-3	3-5	SC, IV, CSII
Insulin Aspart Protamine/Insulin Aspart	NovoLog Mix 70/30[d]	<0.25	1-4	24	SC
Insulin Detemir	Levemire	1	None	24	SC
Insulin Glargine	Lantus[d]	1.1	None	≥24	SC
Insulin Glulisine	Apidra[d]	≤0.25	1	2-4	SC, IV
Insulin Lispro	Humalog[d]	<0.25	1	3.5-4.5	SC
Insulin Lispro Protamine/Insulin Lispro	Humalog Mix 75/25[d]	≤0.25	0.5-1.5	24	SC
	Humalog Mix 50/50[d]	≤0.25	1	16	SC
Insulin Injection Regular (R)	Humulin R[f]	0.5	2-4	6-8	SC, IM, IV
	Novolin N[e]	0.5	2.5-5	8	SC, IM, IV
Insulin Isophane Suspension (NPH)/ Regular Insulin (R)	Humulin 70/30[f]	0.5	2-12	24	SC
	Humulin 50/50[f]	0.5	3-5	24	SC
	Novolin 70/30[e]	0.5	2-12	24	SC
Insulin Isophane Suspension (NPH)	Humulin N[f]	1-2	6-12	18-24	SC
	Novolin N[e]	1.5	4-12	24	SC

[a]Injectable insulins listed are available in a concentration of 100 U/ml; Humulin R, in a concentration of 500 U/ml for SC injection. SC injection only is available by prescription from Lilly for insulin-resistant patients who are hospitalized or in need of medical supervision.
[b]Onset for injectable formulations is always for the subcutaneous (SC) route. All times are approximate.
[c]Maximum effect occurs between these times; actual effect may last longer.
[d]Recombinant human insulin analogue (using *E. coli*).
[e]Recombinant (using *S. cerevisiae*).
[f]Recombinant (using *E. coli*).
CSII, Continuous subcutaneous infusion; *IM,* intramuscularly; *IV,* intravenously.

DISPOSITION

- Diabetic retinopathy occurs in nearly 15% of patients with diabetes after 15 yr of diagnosis and increases 1%/yr after diagnosis. Retinal laser photocoagulation and vitrectomy are effective treatment modalities. Prevention is best accomplished by strict glucose and BP control. Early blockade of the renin-angiotensin system has been shown to slow progression of retinopathy in patients with type 1 diabetes.
- The frequency of neuropathy in patients with type 2 diabetes approaches 70% to 80%. It can be subdivided into sensorimotor neuropathy and autonomic neuropathy. Duloxetine, a selective serotonin and norepinephrine reuptake inhibitor, is effective and FDA approved for relief of diabetic peripheral neuropathy. Pregabalin and gabapentin (900 to 3600 mg/day) are also effective for the symptomatic treatment of peripheral neuropathic pain. Topical capsaicin, 5% lidocaine transdermal patches, amitriptyline, and carbamazepine are also modestly effective.
- Diabetic gastroparesis is most often seen in patients who have had diabetes for at least 10 yr and typically have retinopathy, neuropathy, and nephropathy. Major manifestations are postprandial fullness, nausea, vomiting, and bloating. Pharmacologic therapy involves prokinetic agents (metoclopramide). Endoscopic injection of botulinum toxin into the pylorus and gastric electrical stimulation (using f electrodes placed laparoscopically in the muscle wall of the stomach antrum and connected to a neurostimulator) represent newer approaches to nonpharmacologic therapy.
- Nephropathy: The first sign of renal involvement in patients with DM is most often microalbuminuria, which is classified as incipient nephropathy. Before the current period of intensive glycemic control and blood pressure with ACE inhibitors and angiotensin receptor blockade, it was suggested that 25% to 45% of diabetic patients would develop clinically evident renal disease (pro-

 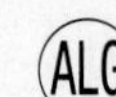

teinuria) and 4% to 17% would pregress to end-stage renal disease. In the current era of intensive glycemic and blood pressure control and ACE/ARB use, clinically evident diabetic nephropathy has declined to 9% and end-stage renal disease 2% to 7%.

- Infections are generally more common in patients with diabetes because of multiple factors, such as impaired leukocyte function, decreased tissue perfusion secondary to vascular disease, repeated trauma because of loss of sensation, and urinary retention secondary to neuropathy.
- Prevention/delay of type 2 diabetes: Patients with prediabetes should achieve weight loss of 5% to 10% of body weight and increase physical activity to at least 150 min/wk of moderate activity such as walking. Metformin therapy may be considered in those at high risk, especially if they have hyperglycemia (HbA1c ≥6) despite lifestyle interventions.

REFERRAL

- Patients with diabetes should be advised to have annual ophthalmologic examinations. In type 1 DM, ophthalmologic visits should begin within 3 to 5 yr of diagnosis, whereas type 2 DM patients should be seen from disease onset.
- Podiatric care can significantly reduce the rate of foot infections and amputations in patients with DM. Noninfected neuropathic foot ulcers require debridement and reduction of pressure.
- Nephrology consultation in all cases of proteinuria, hyperkalemia, uncontrolled BP, and when GFR has decreased to <30 ml/min/1.73 m^2.

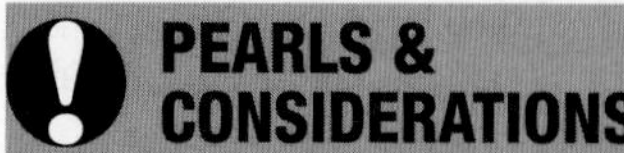

PEARLS & CONSIDERATIONS

COMMENTS

- Because normalization of serum glucose level is the ultimate goal, every patient with diabetes should measure his or her blood glucose with commercially available glucometers unless contraindicated by senility or blindness.
- Underinsured children and those with psychiatric illness are at greater risk for acute complications in type 1 DM and require frequent monitoring and aggressive risk management with diet, exercise, and periodic laboratory evaluation.
- Significant sustained weight loss using bariatric surgery has been reported as effective in achieving remission of type 2 diabetes in morbidly obese patients. Bariatric surgery may be considered for adults with BMI >35 kg/m^2 and type 2 DM, especially if diabetes or associated comorbidities are difficult to control with lifestyle and pharmacologic therapy.
- Cigarette smoking predicts incident type 2 diabetes. For a smoker at risk for diabetes, smoking cessation should be coupled with strategies for diabetes prevention and early detection.
- Glycemic control in hospitalized patients: The American College of Physicans (ACP) recommends against using intensive insulin therapy to strictly control blood glucose in non-surgical intensive care unit (SICU)/medical intensive care unit (MICU) in patients with or without DM. The ACP recommends a target blood glucose level of 140 to 200 mg/dl if insulin therapy is used.

SUGGESTED READINGS

available at www.expertconsult.com

RELATED CONTENT

Diabetic Ketoacidosis (Related Key Topic)
Diabetic Polyneuropathy (Related Key Topic)
Diabetic Retinopathy (Related Key Topic)
Gestational Diabetes Mellitus (Related Key Topic)
Hyperosmolar Hyperglycemic Syndrome (Related Key Topic)
Diabetes Mellitus Type 1 (Patient Information)
Diabetes Mellitus Type 2 (Patient Information)

AUTHORS: **HILARY B. WHITLATCH, M.D., SAINATH GADDAM, M.D.,** and **FRED F. FERRI, M.D.**

BASIC INFORMATION

DEFINITION

Diabetic foot infections (DFIs) are a common and potentially serious problem in persons with diabetes. They usually arise from either a skin ulceration that occurs secondarily to peripheral neuropathy or in a wound caused by some form of trauma. The infection usually involves one or more bacteria and can spread to contiguous tissues including bone causing an osteomyelitis.

SYNONYMS

Diabetic foot ulcer

ICD-9CM CODES
250.80 Diabetes with other specified manifestations, type II or unspecified type, not stated as uncontrolled
707.15 Ulcer of other part of foot

ICD-10CM CODES
E10.5 Diabetes mellitus with peripheral circulatory complications
E10.6 Diabetes mellitus with other specific complications
E11.621 Type 2 diabetes mellitus with foot ulcer

EPIDEMIOLOGY & DEMOGRAPHICS

INCIDENCE
DFIs are the most common cause of hospitalizations for diabetic patients. They account for 20% of all hospital admissions. Nearly one in six patients will die within a year of their infection.

PEAK INCIDENCE
More common in Hispanics, African Americans, and native Americans due to increased rates of diabetes in those populations

PREVALENCE
25 million people in the U.S. have diabetes, of which 15% to 25% will develop a foot ulcer in their lifetime and more than 50% of these will become infected.

PREDOMINANT SEX AND AGE
Females greater than males

RISK FACTORS
- Diabetes greater than 10 years
- Poor glucose control
- Peripheral neuropathy: altered protective sensation and altered pain response
- Diabetic angiopathy: atherosclerotic obstruction of larger vessels leading to peripheral vascular disease
- Evidence of increased local pressure: callus or erythema

PHYSICAL FINDINGS & CLINICAL PRESENTATION

A. Based on guidelines by Infectious Diseases Society of America, infection is present if obvious purulent drainage and/or the presence of two or more signs of inflammation
1. Erythema
2. Pain
3. Tenderness
4. Warmth
5. Induration

B. Systemic signs of infection include:
1. Anorexia, nausea/vomiting
2. Fever, chills, night sweats
3. Change in mental status and recent worsening of glycemic control

C. Various classifications exist but Wagner's Classification is one of most used:
- 0: Pre-ulcerative area without open lesion
- 1: Superficial ulcer (partial/full thickness)
- 2: Ulcer deep to tendon, capsule, bone
- 3: Stage 2 with abscess, osteomyelitis, or joint sepsis
- 4: Localized gangrene
- 5: Global foot gangrene

D. Etiology: most diabetic foot infections are polymicrobial (can involve 5-7 different bacteria) and depend on the extent of involvement
1. Superficial infections are likely due to gram-positive skin bacteria:
   a. *Staphylococcus aureus*, includes methicillin-resistant *S. aureus* (MRSA)
   b. *Streptococcus agalactiae* (group B streptococcus) and *Streptococcus pyogenes* (group A streptococcus)
   c. Coagulase-negative *Staphylococcus*
2. Infections that are deep, chronically infected, or previously treated are likely to be polymicrobial:
   a. Include above bacteria plus enterococci, gram-negative rods including *Pseudomonas aeruginosa* and anaerobes
   b. With gangrene can expect more anaerobic bacteria such as *Clostridia* and *Bacteroides* species
   c. Patients with multiple admissions can have more resistant bacteria such as ESBL-type resistant gram-negative rod bacteria, MRSA, and *Acinetobacter*

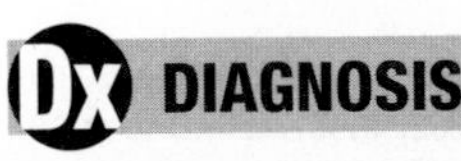

DIAGNOSIS

DIFFERENTIAL DIAGNOSIS

Other inflammatory conditions that can mimic diabetic foot infections include:
- Crystal-associated arthritis such as gout
- Trauma
- Acute Charcot arthropathy from long-standing diabetes
- Venous stasis ulcers
- Deep vein thrombosis

WORKUP

Evaluation of a patient with a DFI involves determining the extent and severity of the infection, identifying the underlying factors that predispose to the infection, and determining the microbiologic etiology.

Physical Examination
- Vital signs: fever, chills, hypotension, tachycardia can be present.
- Detailed wound description: length, width, and depth of wound consistency of drainage character of wound base: granular fibrous necrotic
- Determination of osteomyelitis: highly likely if bone visible. A positive probe test to bone has a sensitivity of 66% and specificity of 85% in diagnosing bone infection.
- Necrotizing infections may present with cutaneous bullae, soft tissue gas, foul odor, and skin discoloration (Fig. 1-314).
- Severe infections may present with gangrene, tissue necrosis, and evidence of tissue ischemia, all of which may be limb threatening.

LABORATORY TESTS

Important to obtain at baseline and to assess response to therapy
- Fewer than 50% of patients have an elevated WBC.
- Determine BUN/Cr, acidosis, hemoglobin A_{1C}, and blood sugar.
- Acute phase reactants: Sed rate and CRP are markers for inflammation.
  - Sed rate >70 increases probability of bone infection.
- Serum prealbumin and albumin are markers for nutritional status and ability to heal.
- An ulcer size larger than 2 cm^2 is indicative of osteomyelitis.
- Gram stains and cultures: superficial cultures should not be obtained as they may contain colonizing bacteria and instead deep tissue cultures (aerobic and anaerobic) should be obtained.

IMAGING STUDIES

- Plain film x-ray evaluates bones and soft issues and can detect presence of tissue gas, which would represent an emergent situation (Fig. 1-315).
- Osteomyelitis appears as radiolucencies, periosteal reaction, and destructive changes. Plain films are 67% specific and 60% sensitive for osteomyelitis.

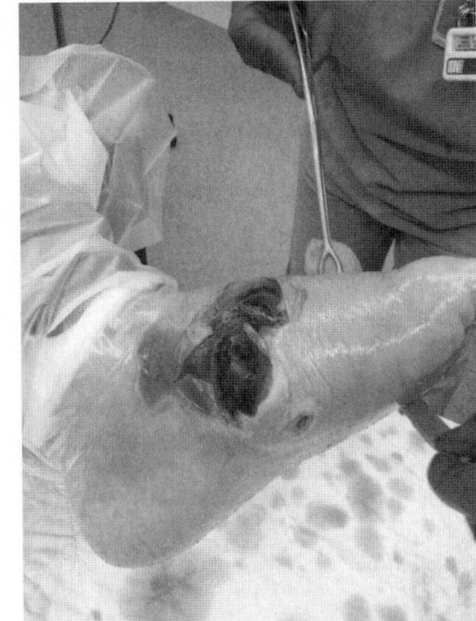

FIGURE 1-314 Foot: Severe diabetic foot infection with significant tissue swelling and necrosis.

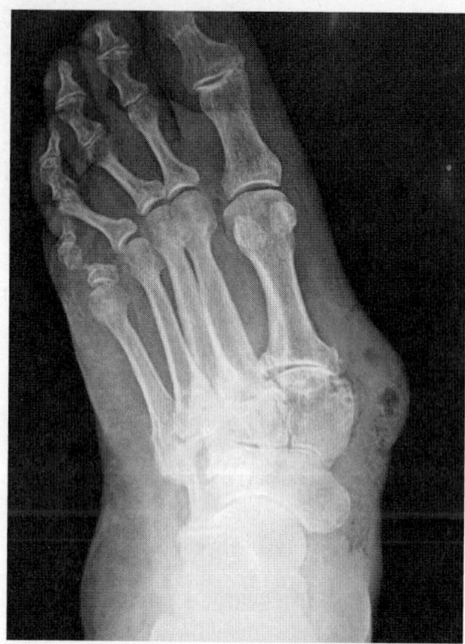

FIGURE 1-315 X-ray: Significant soft tissue swelling in midfoot with numerous gas bubbles seen in the soft tissues.

- Bone scan: Indium-111 or technetium-99 can distinguish acute and chronic infections.
- CT and MRI: MRI is the most sensitive and specific test to detect osteomyelitis and abscess formation.

OTHER DIAGNOSTIC TESTS

- Noninvasive vascular studies: Ankle brachial index (ABI): <0.90 or >1.30 indicates peripheral arterial disease
- Transcutaneous oxygen (TcPO2) tension measurements: predictive of wound healing failure at levels below 25 mm Hg

Rx TREATMENT

Empiric antibiotic regimen should be started based on likely pathogens suspected and severity of disease. Wound management and debridement including surgical consultation are important as well.

NONPHARMACOLOGIC THERAPY

- Good nutrition will promote wound healing.
- Glycemic control will promote healing.
- Fluid and electrolyte balance will improve healing.

ACUTE GENERAL TREATMENT

Wound management

- Debridement of callus and necrotic tissues by wound care specialist or surgeon and at times may require multiple debridements.
- Wound dressing: to absorb exudates and promote healing. Many products are available but none has been proven superior and include:
  - Enzymes
  - Gels
  - Hydrocolloids
  - Antiseptics containing iodine or silver salts
  - Honey
- Relieve pressure on the foot: casts or special shoes.
- Amputation or revascularization procedures such as angioplasty or bypass grafting may be necessary.

Antibiotic management

- Prior to receiving culture results an empiric antibiotic regimen should be started as soon as possible to cover skin bacteria, gram-negative rods, and anaerobes. Options for intravenous therapy include:
- Piperacillin-tazobactam: 3.375 g IV q6h with normal kidney function. Will cover gram-negative rods including *Pseudomonas aeruginosa*, streptococci, anaerobes, and *Staphylococcus aureus*. Adjust dose based on CrCl.
- Meropenem: 1 g IV q8h with normal kidney function has comparable coverage as piperacillin-tazobactam. Similar agents include imipenem and doripenem.
- Third-generation cephalosporin such as cefepime, 2 g IV q8h, or ceftriaxone, 2 g IV qd, have excellent gram-negative coverage and for anaerobic coverage add metronidazole, 500 mg IV q8h, or clindamycin 900 mg IV q8h. Cefepime will cover *Pseudomonas aeruginosa* but ceftriaxone will not.
- For penicillin-allergic patients a combination of ciprofloxacin, 400 mg IV q12h, plus metronidazole or clindamycin is an option. Aztreonam is another option for gram-negative rod coverage, 2 g IV q8h.
- If MRSA suspected need to add IV vancomycin, 15-20 mg/kg IV q8-12h, depending on age and CrCL and follow trough levels to keep above 15. Other options include daptomycin, 4 mg/kg IV qd, which does not have to be adjusted for CrCL or linezolid, 400-600 mg IV q12h.
- If VRE suspected options include tigecycline, 100-mg IV load dose, then 50 mg IV q12h, which also covers MRSA and gram-negative rods but not *Pseudomonas aeruginosa,* or can use daptomycin or linezolid.
- If ESBL gram-negative bacteria are suspected then options include meropenem or ertapenem, 1 g IV qd, or tigecycline.
- Once culture results are known can tailor antibiotics to more specific agent.
- Oral antibiotics used for milder infections include: amoxicillin-clavulanate, 875 mg PO q12h, will cover gram-negative rods, streptococci, and anaerobes, or ciprofloxacin plus metronidazole or clindamycin. Bactrim will cover MRSA and MSSA and some gram-negative rods.

CHRONIC TREATMENT

- Length of therapy: highly variable depending on the severity of the infection. In general 2 to 4 weeks of antibiotics is sufficient. If bone infection suspected or documented may need 4-8 weeks of antibiotics preferably intravenous via a peripherally inserted central line (PICC line).
- Surgical debridement may also be necessary for several weeks.

COMPLEMENTARY MEDICINE

- Hyperbaric oxygen (HBO): Used as an adjunct to antibiotics, debridement, and revascularization in the therapy of chronic, nonhealing wounds associated with diabetes. HBO acts by:
  - Inducing vasoconstriction and reducing vasogenic edema
  - Facilitating fibroblast activity, angiogenesis, and wound healing
  - Killing anaerobic bacteria and augmenting neutrophil bactericidal activity
- Negative pressure wound therapy (wound vac): controlled, subatmospheric pressure applied to an open wound can accelerate healing and closure.
  - An open cell foam insert is cut to fit the open wound and then secured under a clear, vapor-permeable, plastic dressing.
  - Tubing extends from the sponge to a disposable collection canister.
  - A portable pump applies 125 mm Hg of controlled suction to the system. The subatmospheric pressure (suction) is equally distributed across the open wound and evacuates stagnant fluid from the wound.

DISPOSITION

- Following up on sed rates, CRP, BUN/CR, and levels of vancomycin if that antibiotic used.
- Surgical or wound center care follow-up.
- HBO usually involves multiple sessions over several weeks.
- Wound vac is applied for weeks and requires periodic nursing follow-up.

REFERRAL

- Infectious disease consultant for antibiotic management.
- Surgeon or wound care center for surgical treatments.
- Endocrinologist for good diabetes care.
- Vascular surgeon for angioplasty or bypass procedures.

PEARLS & CONSIDERATIONS

- In a meta-analysis of randomized controlled trials on the outcome of DFIs, there was a 22.7% treatment failure rate.
- Patients should be advised to seek prompt medical attention as these infections can progress rapidly to gangrene.

AUTHOR: **GLENN G. FORT, M.D., M.P.H.**

BASIC INFORMATION

DEFINITION

Diabetic ketoacidosis (DKA) is a life-threatening complication of diabetes mellitus resulting from absolute insulin deficiency or insulin resistance with relative insulin deficiency. It is characterized by the presence of an anion gap metabolic acidosis, ketonemia, and hyperglycemia. Patients often present with severe dehydration and altered sensorium.

SYNONYMS

DKA

ICD-9CM CODES
250.1 Diabetic ketoacidosis
ICD-10CM CODES
E10.10 Type 2 diabetes mellitus with other specified complication

EPIDEMIOLOGY & DEMOGRAPHICS

INCIDENCE/PREVALENCE: 6 episodes per 10,000 individuals with diabetes; it accounts for 8% to 29% of all hospital admissions of patients with diabetes

PREDOMINANT AGE: 36% in persons younger than age 30, 27% in persons 30 to 60 years of age, 23% in persons 51 to 70 years of age, and 14% occurring in persons older than 70 years.

PHYSICAL FINDINGS & CLINICAL PRESENTATION

- Evidence of dehydration (tachycardia, hypotension, dry mucous membranes, sunken eyeballs, poor skin turgor)
- Altered mental status
- Tachypnea with air hunger (Kussmaul's respiration)
- Fruity breath odor (caused by acetone)
- Lipemia retinalis in some patients
- Possible evidence of precipitating factors (infected wound, pneumonia)
- Abdominal tenderness in some patients

ETIOLOGY

- Metabolic decompensation in individuals with diabetes is frequently precipitated by an infectious process (up to 40%).
- Poor compliance with insulin therapy and severe medical illness (e.g., pancreatitis, cardiovascular events) are other common causes.
- There is a subgroup of type 2 diabetics who have ketosis-prone diabetes. These persons are often black or Latino, overweight, middle aged, males with a family history of diabetes or newly diagnosed diabetes. This subgroup represents 20% to 50% of persons with DKA.
- Cocaine abuse has been reported as a risk factor for DKA in adult and teenage patients, particularly in patients with multiple admissions.
- Lack of education of primary caregiver (mother, sibling), as well as deficiencies in proper monitoring of blood glucose, correct administration of insulin, supervision of insulin pump maintenance, and monitoring of diabetic caloric restraints are causes of recurrent episodes of DKA.

DIAGNOSIS

DIFFERENTIAL DIAGNOSIS

- Hyperosmolar nonketotic state
- Alcoholic ketoacidosis
- Uremic acidosis
- Metabolic acidosis caused by methyl alcohol or ethylene glycol
- Salicylate poisoning

WORKUP

- Laboratory evaluation (see "Laboratory Tests") to confirm diagnosis and evaluate precipitating factors
- Identification of "trigger," such as infection (blood cultures, urine cultures, chest radiographs), pancreatitis (pancreatic enzymes), or myocardial ischemia (ECG, cardiac enzymes)

LABORATORY TESTS

- Glucose level demonstrates severe hyperglycemia (serum glucose generally >250 mg/dl)
- Arterial blood gases demonstrate metabolic acidosis: arterial pH usually <7.30 with Pco_2 <40 mm Hg
- Serum ketonemia (b-hydroxybutyrate >300 mmol/L), ketonuria, and glycosuria
- Serum electrolytes:
  1. Serum bicarbonate is usually <15 mEq/L.
  2. Serum potassium (K^+) may be low, normal, or elevated. There is always significant total body potassium depletion regardless of the initial potassium level.
  3. Serum sodium is usually decreased as a result of hyperglycemia, dehydration, and lipemia. Assume 1.6-mEq/L decrease in extracellular sodium for each 100-mg/dl increase in glucose concentration.
  4. Calculate the anion gap (AG):

     $$AG = Na^+ - (Cl^- + HCO^-_3)$$

     In DKA, the anion gap is increased (<12) because of high levels of ketones.
  5. Mixed metabolic disturbances demonstrating anion gap metabolic acidosis overlapping with metabolic alkalosis may be present; this is common in patients with DKA with persistent vomiting.
- CBC with differential, urinalysis, and urine and blood cultures to rule out infectious precipitating factor
- Serum calcium, magnesium, and phosphorus; the plasma phosphate and magnesium levels may be significantly depressed and should be rechecked within 12 hr because they may decrease further with correction of DKA
- Blood urea nitrogen and creatinine generally reveal significant dehydration and acute kidney injury.
- A pregnancy test should be performed in all female patients of child-bearing years who present with DKA.
- Amylase, lipase, and liver enzymes should be checked in patients with abdominal pain.

IMAGING STUDIES

- Chest radiographs are helpful to rule out pneumonia. The initial chest film may be negative if the patient has significant dehydration. Repeat chest x-ray after 24 hr if pulmonary infection is strongly suspected.
- Additional imaging, such as CT scanning or abdominal ultrasound, should be considered in the presence of physical exam findings, such as abdominal tenderness.

TREATMENT

NONPHARMACOLOGIC THERAPY

- Monitor mental status, vital signs, and urine output hourly until improved, then monitor every 2 to 4 hours.
- Fingersticks should be checked every 1 to 2 hours while patient is on an insulin drip.
- Basic metabolic panel should be checked every 2 to 4 hours to monitor for anion gap closure (see "Acute General Rx").

ACUTE GENERAL Rx (Fig. E1-316)

Fluid replacement (usual deficit is 6 to 8 L)

1. Do not delay fluid replacement until laboratory results have been received. Fluid deficits are typically 100 ml/kg of body weight. The total fluid administered should not exceed 4 L/m^2/24 hours for fear of causing cerebral edema (CE). One rule of thumb is to deliver fluids (deficit and maintenance) over a period of 48 hours if serum osmolality is >360 mOsm/L.
2. The initial fluid replacement should be with 0.9% normal saline (NS) to expand vascular volume and ensure blood pressure stabilization and organ perfusion. In patients with severe hypernatremia (serum sodium >160 mEq/L), 0.45% normal saline infusion can be used. Careful monitoring for fluid overload is necessary in elderly patients and those with a history of congestive heart failure.
3. The rate of fluid replacement varies with the age of the patient and the presence of significant cardiac or renal disease.
   - The usual rate of infusion is 1 L of 0.9% NS over the first hour, followed by 15 ml/kg/hr 0.9% NS during the second hour. Then change to 0.45% NS at 15 ml/kg/hr to replenish free water.
   - Switch to dextrose D5 0.45% NS when serum glucose is <250 to prevent hypoglycemia and introduce additional glucose substrate (necessary to suppress lipolysis and ketogenesis).

Insulin administration:

1. The patient should be given an initial loading IV bolus of 0.1 U/kg regular insulin followed by a constant infusion at a rate of 0.1 U/kg/hour. Insulin replacement should generally not be started until serum potassium is >3.3 mEq/L to prevent life-threatening hypokalemia.
2. Monitor serum glucose every 1 to 2 hr while patient is on insulin drip, then every 2 to 4 hr.
3. The goal is to decrease serum glucose level by 80 mg/dl/hour (after an initial decline

because of rehydration); if the serum glucose level is not decreasing at the expected rate, double the rate of insulin infusion.

4. When the serum glucose level approaches 250 mg/dl, decrease the rate of insulin infusion to 2 to 3 U/hour and continue this rate until the patient has received adequate fluid replacement, HCO_3^- is close to normal, and ketones have cleared. After target glucose levels are achieved, it usually takes 5 to 7 hr for ketosis to clear. Young children and adolescents have greater levels of human growth hormone, resulting in a prolonged time lag for plasma glucose to reach above levels. Patients with infection and fever have higher metabolic requirements and may need 15% to 20% more insulin than the usual starting dose.
5. Prior to stopping the IV insulin infusion, administer an SC dose of insulin (dose varies with the patient's demonstrated insulin sensitivity). Short (regular) or rapid-acting (aspart, lispro, glulisine) insulins should be administered SC 1 to 2 hr before stopping IV insulin infusion. Intermediate (NPH) or long-acting (glargine, detemir) insulins should be administered 2 to 4 hr before stopping IV insulin infusion.
6. In individuals with newly diagnosed diabetes, the total daily insulin dose to maintain metabolic control ranges from 0.5 to 0.8 U/kg/day. Approximately half of this dose should be given as intermediate or long-acting insulin, and half of this dose should be given as mealtime or prandial insulin, provided the patient is eating.

Electrolyte replacement:

- Potassium replacement: the average total potassium loss in DKA is 300 to 500 mEq.
- K^+ can be supplemented as chloride- and phosphate-containing solutions.
    1. The rate of replacement varies with the patient's serum potassium level, degree of acidosis (decreased pH, increased potassium level), and renal function (potassium replacement should be used with caution in patients with renal failure).
    2. As a rule of thumb, potassium replacement can be guided by presenting serum K level. If K is <3.3, give KCl 20 to 30 mEq/L of intravenous fluid (IVF) until K is >3.3. If K is 3.3 to 5.3, give KCl at 10 to 30 mEq/L IVF to maintain a K of >4. If K is >5.3, hold potassium supplementation until K is <5.3.
    3. Monitor serum potassium level hourly for the first 2 hours, then monitor q2 to 4h.
- Phosphate replacement: If the serum PO_4 is <1.5 mEq/L, give 2.5 mg/kg IV over 6 hours of elemental phosphate. Routine replacement of phosphate (in the absence of laboratory evidence of significant hypophosphatemia) is not indicated. Rapid IV phosphate administration can cause hypocalcemia.
- Magnesium replacement: Replacement is indicated only in the presence of significant hypomagnesemia or refractory hypokalemia/hypocalcemia.

Bicarbonate therapy:

- Routine use of bicarbonate in DKA is contraindicated because it can worsen hypokalemia and can cause cerebral edema. Bicarbonate therapy should be considered only if the arterial pH is <6.9 and HCO_3^- is <5.
- In these patients, 44 to 88 mEq sodium bicarbonate can be added to 1 L of 0.45% NS q2-4h until pH increases to >7.
- Use of bicarbonate therapy is particularly dangerous in the pediatric population. Children with DKA are at increased risk for cerebral edema. Bicarbonate therapy in children with DKA should be limited to those with severe circulatory failure and a high risk for cardiac decompensation resulting from profound acidosis.

PREVENTION

- Provide information/education for teachers, parents, school staff, and caregivers on how to recognize children with undiagnosed diabetes.
- Review sick day management; increase home blood glucose monitoring, education on how to measure urinary or fingerstick ketones, compliance with insulin; and maintain adequate hydration and nutrition.

DISPOSITION

- Average mortality rate in DKA is 5% to 10%.
- In children <10 yr, DKA causes 70% of diabetes-related deaths.
- Cerebral edema (CE) occurs in 1% of episodes of DKA in children and is associated with a mortality rate of 40% to 90%.

REFERRAL

In general, patients with DKA should be admitted to the intensive care unit on an insulin drip. Alert patients who are able to take fluids orally and have mild DKA occasionally can be treated with short-acting insulin analogues under observation and sent home. The American Diabetes Association admission guidelines are a plasma glucose level >250 mg/dl with arterial pH <7.30, serum bicarbonate level <15 mEq/L, and a moderate or greater level of ketones in the serum or urine.

PEARLS & CONSIDERATIONS

COMMENTS

- Although DKA occurs more commonly in type 1 diabetes mellitus, a significant proportion (>20%) occurs in patients with type 2 diabetes, particularly under conditions of extreme stress, severe infection or surgery, and marked hyperglycemia (results in glucose toxicity).
- 30% to 40% of DKA admissions involve patients with newly diagnosed diabetes.
- Potential complications of DKA therapy include hypoglycemia, cerebral edema, cardiac arrhythmias, shock, myocardial infarction, and acute pancreatitis.
- Risk factors for cerebral edema include age <5 yr, high initial BUN, hyperventilation to a $Paco_2$ of <22 mm Hg, and presenting arterial pH of <7.00. It presents 4 to 8 hours after start of rehydration therapy. Presentation may be abrupt with sudden severe headache, vomiting, sudden hypertension, and obtunded sensorium. First management response to CE is to elevate head of the patient to 30-degree angle, IV mannitol, intubation and hyperventilation, and, finally, cutting back of the maintenance fluid to 75%.
- Underinsured children and those with psychiatric illness are at greater risk for DKA.
- Subcutaneous administration of rapid-acting insulin analogues may be reasonable alternatives to IV regular insulin infusion for treating uncomplicated DKA.
- DKA can occur with blood glucose <350 mg/dl in the setting of poor oral intake or pregnancy.
- Ketones can be positive in starvation or with heavy alcohol intake; DKA can coexist with other causes of metabolic acidosis such as lactic acidosis.

SUGGESTED READINGS

available at www.expertconsult.com

RELATED CONTENT

Diabetes Mellitus (Related Key Topic)
Hyperosmolar Hyperglycemic Syndrome (Related Key Topic)

AUTHORS: **HILARY B. WHITLATCH, M.D., SAINATH GADDAM, M.D.,** and **FRED F. FERRI, M.D.**

BASIC INFORMATION

DEFINITION

Diabetic polyneuropathy is a distal symmetric polyneuropathy (DSPN) characterized by numbness, tingling, pain, or weakness that affects the nerves in a stocking-and-glove pattern, beginning in the distal extremities. DSPN leads to substantial pain, morbidity, and impaired quality of life.

SYNONYM(S)

Distal symmetric polyneuropathy (DSPN)
Diabetic peripheral neuropathy

ICD-9-CM CODE(S)
250.6 Diabetes with neurological manifestations
357.2 Polyneuropathy in diabetes
ICD-10-CM CODE(S)
E11.40 Type 2 diabetes mellitus with neurological complications
E11.40 Type 2 diabetes mellitus with diabetic neuropathy, unspecified
E11.41 Type 2 diabetes mellitus with diabetic mononeuropathy
E11.42 Type 2 diabetes mellitus with diabetic polyneuropathy
E11.43 Type 2 diabetes mellitus with diabetic autonomic (poly)neuropathy
E11.44 Type 2 diabetes mellitus with diabetic amyotrophy
E11.49 Type 2 diabetes mellitus with other diabetic neurological complication

EPIDEMIOLOGY & DEMOGRAPHICS

PREVALENCE: The prevalence of diabetic polyneuropathy varies from 10% to 100% in patients with diabetes mellitus in population-based studies. It is the most common form of peripheral neuropathy in the western world.
RISK FACTORS: Patients with poor glycemic control, diabetic nephropathy, or retinopathy are at increased risk.

PHYSICAL FINDINGS & CLINICAL PRESENTATION

- Patients most commonly experience numbness and tingling, but may also experience feelings of tightness or a sensation of heat or cold.
- Pain is not uncommon, is often worst at night, and can be burning, aching, shooting, or lancinating in nature.
- These symptoms begin in the feet and may slowly ascend over months to years. Symptoms in the hands do not generally occur until symptoms in the lower extremities have reached the level of the knees. In more severe cases, the symptoms can spread to the trunk and head.
- Neurologic examination reveals early loss of small-fiber modalities resulting in decreased pinprick and temperature sensation, with later involvement of large-fiber modalities leading to a reduction in vibratory and proprioceptive sensation. Ankle reflexes are usually reduced or absent, and more proximal reflexes may also become involved as the neuropathy progresses. Strength is usually normal, but there can be some motor involvement leading to mild weakness and atrophy, which is usually limited to intrinsic foot muscles and ankle dorsiflexors.

ETIOLOGY

Precise etiology is unknown but most likely involves a complex interaction of metabolic derangements and microvascular insults that occur in the setting of diabetes.

DIAGNOSIS

DIFFERENTIAL DIAGNOSIS

Although diabetes is the leading cause of peripheral neuropathy in developed countries, there are numerous other causes requiring further investigation(s).

WORKUP

- A thorough history and neurologic examination are essential to confirm features consistent with a diabetic polyneuropathy and exclude other features that would suggest alternative diagnoses.
- For some patients, neuropathy may be the presenting feature of previously undiagnosed diabetes.
- Electrodiagnostic evaluation to include nerve conduction studies and electromyography can be helpful in confirming the presence, extent, and severity of a neuropathy.
- Patients with DSPN typically have a reduction of amplitudes and slowing of conduction velocities involving sensory and possibly motor nerves in a length-dependent and symmetric fashion.
- Electromyographic examination of distal muscles may reveal fibrillation potentials, positive sharp waves, and large motor unit action potentials, suggestive of denervation and reinnervation.
- Skin biopsy and nerve biopsy are not necessary in the vast majority of cases.

LABORATORY TESTS

- Fasting blood sugar, hemoglobin A1c, and oral glucose tolerance test should all be considered in patients with peripheral neuropathy without a known history of diabetes.
- A focused laboratory evaluation for other common or potentially treatable causes of neuropathy is also indicated: complete blood cell count, complete metabolic panel to include electrolytes and liver function tests, erythrocyte sedimentation rate, vitamin B12 and folate levels, thyroid function tests, serum protein electrophoresis with immunofixation electrophoresis.
- Additional laboratory tests can be considered based on history or exam findings that may suggest other underlying diagnoses, such as anti-nuclear antibodies, extractable nuclear antigens, and rheumatoid factor.

IMAGING STUDIES

- Imaging is not necessary unless there is concern for an alternate or coexisting process based on the history and examination.

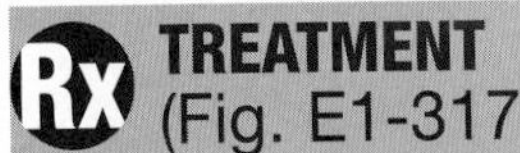

TREATMENT (Fig. E1-317)

CHRONIC Rx

- Table E1-166 summarizes clinical features, diagnosis, and treatment of diabetic autonomic neuropathy
- Glycemic control: The primary treatment for diabetic polyneuropathy is effective glycemic control, as this may improve or at least slow progression of the neuropathy.
- Symptomatic management: Another aspect of treatment is the symptomatic management of pain and paresthesias. The American Academy of Neurology, the American Association of Neuromuscular and Electrodiagnostic Medicine, and the American Academy of Physical Medicine and Rehabilitation have developed an evidence-based guideline for the treatment of painful diabetic neuropathy. Pregabalin, an anticonvulsant, is the only agent in the guideline that has been established as effective for painful diabetic neuropathy. Other probably effective agents are listed below:
    - Topical agents: Lidocaine 5% patch can be applied to painful areas for 12 hours a day, capsaicin 0.075% applied qid.
    - Anticonvulsants: gabapentin (100 to 1200 mg tid) and pregabalin (50 to 100 mg tid)
    - Antidepressants: amitriptyline (10 to 100 mg qhs), nortriptyline (25 to 150 mg qhs), duloxetine (60 to 120 mg daily), and venlafaxine (75 to 225 mg/day).
    - Tramadol (50 mg qid as needed) can be a useful adjunctive analgesic
- Fig. 1-318 describes a treatment algorithm for neuropathic pain after exclusion of nondiabetic etiologies and stabilization of glycemic control

DISPOSITION

The distal sensory loss of diabetic polyneuropathy places patients at increased risk of trauma to the extremities, with the potential for ulceration and infection that could ultimately require amputation if not attended to in a timely fashion.

REFERRAL

- A neurologist can assist in the diagnosis and management of diabetic polyneuropathy.
- Patients with diabetic polyneuropathy should also be evaluated at least annually by a podiatrist and ophthalmologist

 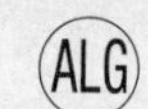

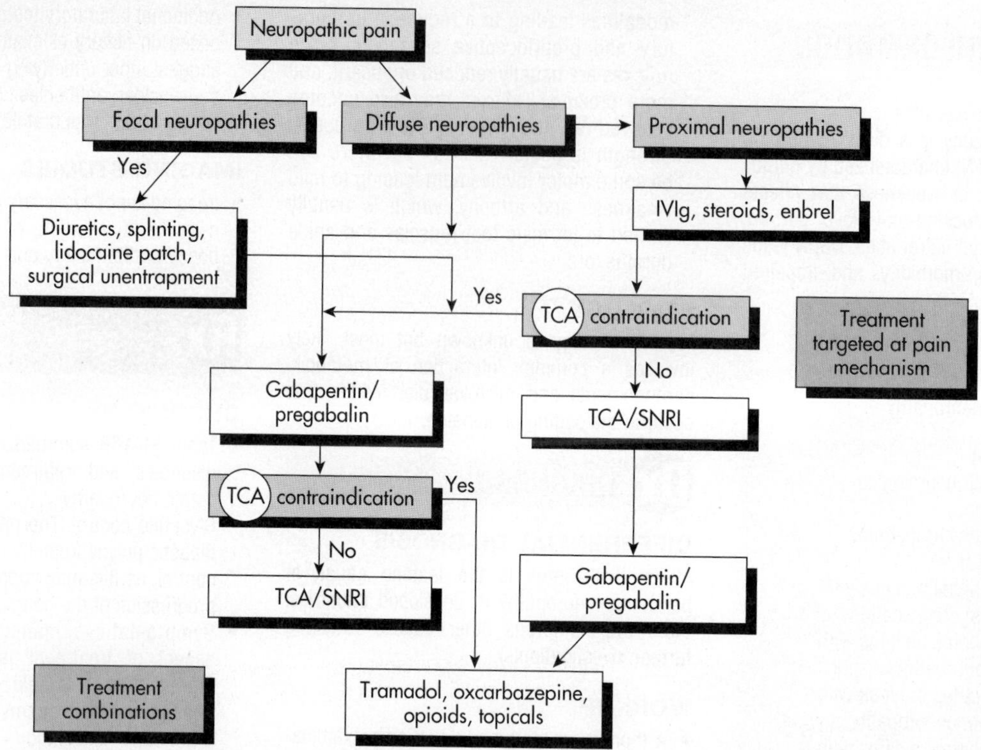

FIGURE 1-318 Treatment algorithm for neuropathic pain after exclusion of nondiabetic etiologies and stabilization of glycemic control. *IVIg*, intravenous immune globulin; *SNRI*, serotonin-norepinephrine reuptake inhibitors; *TCA*, tricyclic antidepressants. (From Melmed S, Polonsky KS, Larsen PR, Kronenberg HM: *Williams textbook of endocrinology*, ed 12, Philadelphia, 2011, Saunders.)

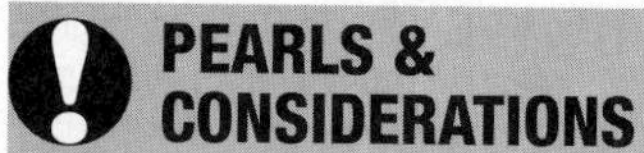

PEARLS & CONSIDERATIONS

COMMENTS

- For many patients, a DSPN or other form of diabetic neuropathy may be the initial presentation of previously undiagnosed diabetes.
- In addition to regular visits with podiatry, patients with diabetic polyneuropathy should be educated on aggressive foot hygiene and the importance of examining their own feet

PATIENT/FAMILY EDUCATION

The following websites are recommended:
http://patienteducationcenter.org/articles/diabetic-neuropathies/
http://www.mayoclinic.com/health/diabetic-neuropathy/DS01045

AUTHOR: **DIVYA SINGHAL, M.D.**

BASIC INFORMATION

DEFINITION

Diabetic retinopathy is an eye abnormality of the retina associated with diabetes and consisting of microaneurysms, punctate hemorrhages, white and yellow exudates, flame hemorrhages, and neovascular vessel growth and can ultimately end in blindness. Diabetic retinopathy can be classified into two stages: nonproliferative and proliferative (Fig. 1-319 and Table 1-167).

SYNONYMS

Nonproliferative diabetic retinopathy (NPDR)
Proliferative (advanced) diabetic retinopathy (PDR)
Diabetic retinopathy (DR)

ICD-9CM CODES

250.5 Diabetes with ophthalmic manifestations
362.1 Retinopathy, diabetic, background
362.02 Retinopathy, diabetic, proliferative

ICD-10CM CODES

E11.319 Type 2 diabetes mellitus with unspecified diabetic retinopathy with macular edema
E11.39 Type 2 diabetes mellitus with other diabetic ophthalmic complication
H35.00 Unspecified background retinopathy
E11.359 Type 2 diabetes mellitus with proliferative diabetic retinopathy without macular edema

EPIDEMIOLOGY & DEMOGRAPHICS

INCIDENCE (IN U.S.):

- Affects 11 million persons. Approximately 40% of patients with diabetes who are over age 40 have retinopathy, including 8.2% who have vision-threatening retinopathy
- A leading cause of blindness in the U.S. between the ages of 20 and 74 yr
- There are 12,000 to 24,000 new cases of diabetic retinopathy-induced blindness each year in the U.S.
- 5000 new cases annually

PEAK INCIDENCE: Begins 10 yr after onset of diabetes

PREVALENCE (IN U.S.): Prevalence of retinopathy increases with duration of diabetes. Found in 18% of people diagnosed with diabetes for 3- to 4-yr duration and in up to 80% of diabetics with a diagnosis of ≥15 yr.

PREDOMINANT SEX: Males and females affected equally

PREDOMINANT AGE: ≥30 yr

GENETICS: Type 1 diabetes: 80% have retinopathy before 30 yr, with 30% having vision-threatening retinopathy.

PHYSICAL FINDINGS & CLINICAL PRESENTATION (Fig. 1-320)

- Microaneurysms
- Hemorrhages
- Exudates
- Macular edema
- Neovascularization
- Retinal detachment
- Hemorrhages in the vitreous
- In early cases, patient may not report a visual disturbance
- Figure E1-321 describes an initial ophthalmic examination flow chart

ETIOLOGY

Vascular endothelial growth factor and erythropoietin have been identified as factors involved in angiogenesis in proliferative diabetic retinopathy. Risk factors for diabetic retinopathy are duration of diabetes, hyperglycemia/glycated hemoglobin value, hypertension, hyperlipidemia, pregnancy, and nephropathy or renal disease. Fig. E1-322 describes a diabetic retinopathy pathogenesis flow chart.

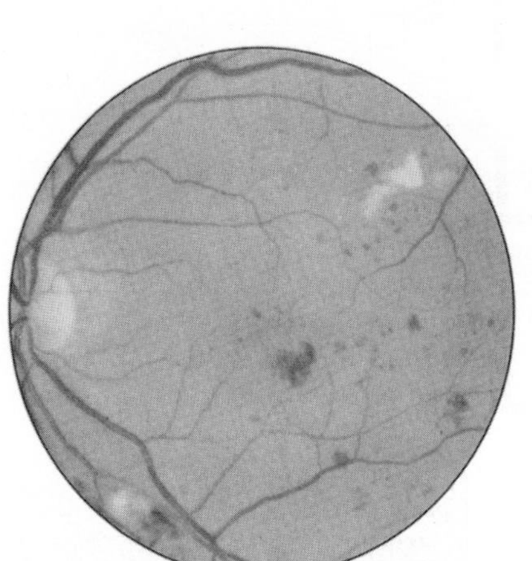

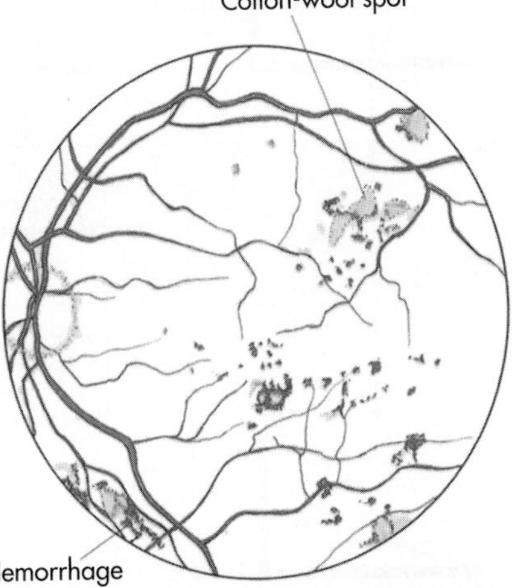

FIGURE 1-319 Background diabetic retinopathy. Note flame-shaped and dot-blot hemorrhages, cotton-wool spots, and microaneurysms. (From Barkaukas VH et al: *Health and physical assessment,* ed 2, St Louis, 1998, Mosby.)

DIAGNOSIS

DIFFERENTIAL DIAGNOSIS

- Retinal examination: look for background retinopathy, microaneurysms, exudate, macular edema, retinal hemorrhage, proliferative neovascular growth on surface of retina
- Retinal inflammatory diseases
- Tumor
- Trauma
- Arteriosclerotic vascular disease
- Hypertension
- Vein or artery occlusion

WORKUP

- Fluorescein angiogram
- Frequent retinal examinations

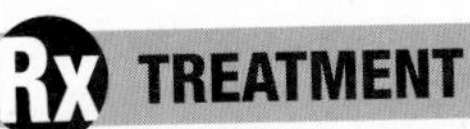

TREATMENT

NONPHARMACOLOGIC THERAPY

- Tight glycemic control remains the cornerstone in the primary prevention of diabetic retinopathy
- Laser treatment when indicated
- Laser treatment with proliferative disease or macular edema
- Photocoagulation of neovascular areas
- Exercise, diet, sugar and lipids control can slow progression of background retinopathy but have no effect on proliferative retinopathy. Trials have shown that glycemic control and combination treatment of dyslipidemia, but not intensive blood-pressure control, reduce the rate of diabetic retinopathy. Intensive glycemic therapy (vs. standard therapy) lowers the incidence of progressive retinopathy (7.3% vs. 10.4%) but not vision loss (16.3% vs. 16.7%) and can result in excess mortality (ACCORD trial)

ACUTE GENERAL Rx

- Laser therapy: pan-retinal and focal retinal laser photocoagulation reduces the risk of visual loss in patients with severe diabetic retinopathy and macular edema
- Vitrectomy
- Repair of retinal detachment
- Medical control of disease and complications and associated diseases (e.g., hypertension)

CHRONIC Rx

- Repeated laser treatments may be necessary
- Diet and exercise; good medical control of disease

DISPOSITION

- Retinal examination should be performed on all routine medical visits. Referral if abnormality seen.
- Routine annual eye examination in all patients with diabetes.
- Prognosis is improved with early diagnosis and treatment.

REFERRAL

Refer to ophthalmologist immediately on finding retinal abnormality to institute early treatment.

 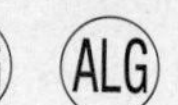

TABLE 1-167 Abbreviated Early Treatment Diabetic Retinopathy Study Classification of Diabetic Retinopathy

Category/Description	Management
Nonproliferative Diabetic Retinopathy (NPDR)	
No DR	Review in 12 mo
Very mild Microaneurysms only	Review most patients in 12 mo
Mild Any or all of: microaneurysms, retinal hemorrhages, exudates, cotton wool spots, up to the level of moderate NPDR. No IRMA or significant beading	Review range 6-12 mo, depending on severity of signs, stability, systemic factors, and patient's personal circumstances
Moderate • Severe retinal hemorrhages (more than ETDRS standard photograph 2A: about 20 medium-large per quadrant) in 1-3 quadrants *or* mild intraretinal microvascular abnormalities (IRMA) • Significant venous beading can be present in no more than 1 quadrant • Cotton-wool spots commonly present	Review in approximately 6 mo PDR in up to 26%, high-risk PDR in up to 8% within a yr
Severe The 4-2-1 rule; one or more of: • Severe hemorrhages in all 4 quadrants • Significant venous beading in 2 or more quadrants • Moderate IRMA in 1 or more quadrants	Review in 4 mo PDR in up to 50%, high-risk PDR in up to 15% within a yr
Very severe Two or more of the criteria for severe	Review in 2-3 mo High-risk PDR in up to 45% within a yr
Proliferative Diabetic Retinopathy (PDR)	
Mild-moderate New vessels on the disc (NVD) or new vessels elsewhere (NVE), but extent insufficient to meet the high-risk criteria	Treatment considered according to severity of signs, stability, systemic factors, and patient's personal circumstances such as reliability of attendance for review. If not treated, review in up to 2 mo
High-risk • New vessels on the disc (NVD) greater than ETDRS standard photograph 10A (about disc area) • Any NVD with vitreous or preretinal hemorrhage • NVE greater than disc area with vitreous or preretinal hemorrhage (or hemorrhage with presumed obscured NVD/E)	Treatment advised—see text Should be performed immediately when possible, and certainly same day if symptomatic presentation with good retinal view

From Kanski JJ, Bowling B: *Clinical ophthalmology, a systematic approach*, ed 7, Philadelphia, 2010, Saunders.

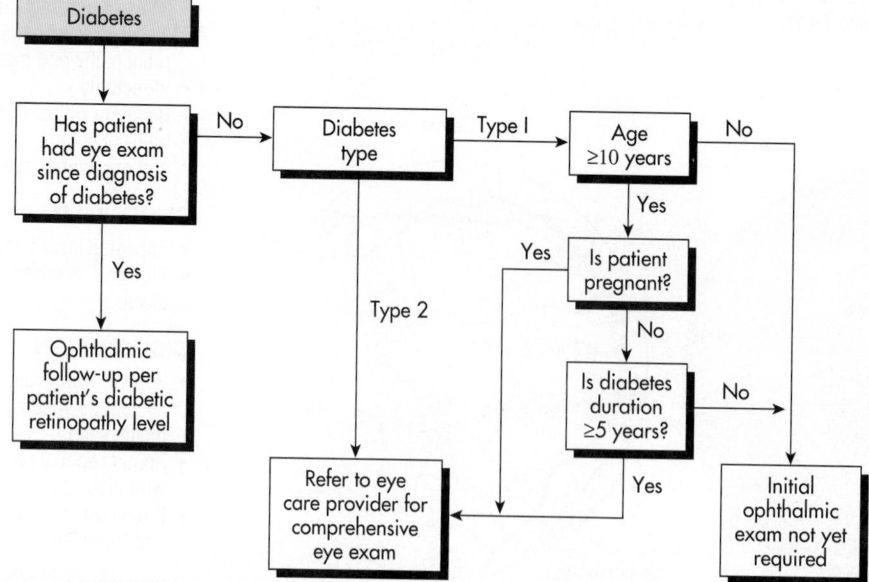

FIGURE 1-320 Initial ophthalmic examination flow chart. Schematic flow chart of major principles involved in determining the timing of initial ophthalmic examination after a diagnosis of diabetes mellitus. These are minimal recommended times. Ocular symptoms, complaints, or other associated medical issues can necessitate earlier evaluation. Guidelines are regularly reevaluated based on new study results. (From Melmed S, Polonsky KS, Larsen PR, Kronenberg HM: *Williams textbook of endocrinology*, ed 12, Philadelphia, 2011, Saunders.)

PEARLS & CONSIDERATIONS

COMMENTS

- Early laser treatment of severe, nonproliferative, and proliferative retinopathy may minimize complications and visual loss.
- Retinopathy is an independent risk marker for cardiovascular disease in patients with type 2 DM.

SUGGESTED READINGS

available at www.expertconsult.com

RELATED CONTENT

Diabetic Retinopathy (Patient Information)
Diabetes Mellitus (Related Key Topic)

AUTHORS: **MELVYN KOBY, M.D.,** and **R. SCOTT HOFFMAN, M.D.**

BASIC INFORMATION

DEFINITION

Discoid lupus erythematosus (DLE) refers to a chronic inflammatory autoimmune skin disorder that can lead to significant disfiguration and scarring. It can be associated with systemic lupus erythematosus (SLE).

SYNONYMS

Chronic cutaneous lupus erythematosus (CLE)

ICD-9CM CODES
695.4 Lupus erythematosus
erythematosus (discoid)
Erythematosus (discoid), not disseminated

ICD-10CM CODES
L93.0 Discoid lupus erythematosus
L93.2 Other local lupus erythematosus

EPIDEMIOLOGY & DEMOGRAPHICS

- Slightly more common in African Americans than in Asians or whites
- CLE is two to three times more likely in women than in men
- Approximately 5% to 10% of patients presenting with DLE will develop SLE; those with widespread, numerous lesions are more likely to progress

PHYSICAL FINDINGS & CLINICAL PRESENTATION

General:
- Early lesions: single or multiple erythematous or violaceous, discrete papules or plaques with scale, often extending into dilated hair follicles (Fig. 1-327)
- Older lesions: peripheral hyperpigmentation with scarring, central depigmentation (Fig. E1-328), and telangiectasia

Anatomic distribution:
- Commonly involves the scalp, face, ears, and extensor surface of the arms
- Mucosal and nail involvement is also possible

Lesion configuration:
- Irregularly grouped, confluent and disfiguring plaques

Lesion morphology:
- Plaque lesions with scale
- Follicular plugging
- Atrophy
- Irreversible, scarring alopecia (34%)
- May be associated with other clinical findings of SLE (e.g., oral ulcers, arthritis, pleuritis, pericarditis)

ETIOLOGY

Unknown, but thought to be an autoimmune-mediated disorder

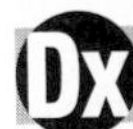

DIAGNOSIS

Clinical findings and skin biopsy are used to establish the diagnosis of DLE

DIFFERENTIAL DIAGNOSIS

Psoriasis, lichen planus or lichen planopilaris, dermatophyte infections, photosensitivity eruption, sarcoidosis, subacute CLE, rosacea, dermatomyositis, cutaneous T-cell lymphoma

LABORATORY TESTS

- Complete blood count is usually normal in isolated DLE, but a small percentage of patients may show low-grade anemia
- Blood urea nitrogen and creatinine are normal in isolated DLE
- Erythrocyte sedimentation rate is elevated in active disease
- Urinalysis may show proteinuria
- Antinuclear antibody positive in 30% to 40% of patients with isolated DLE
- Anti-Ro (SS-A) autoantibodies are present in 1% to 3% of patients
- dsDNA antibodies are uncommon
- Complement levels may be low in rare instances
- Histology of skin reveals hyperkeratosis with follicular plugging, a thickened basement membrane, and a perivascular, interstitial, and appendageal lymphocytic infiltrate

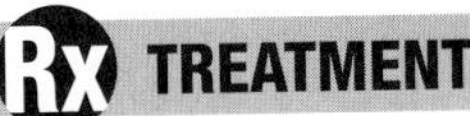

TREATMENT

NONPHARMACOLOGIC THERAPY

Avoid sun exposure by using protective clothing and a broad-spectrum sunscreen of SPF >30

ACUTE GENERAL Rx

1. Topical steroids: intermediate- to high-potency steroids are needed; use caution when applying to the face
2. Intralesional steroids: triamcinolone acetonide 2.5 to 5.0 mg/ml with 1% Xylocaine
3. Topical calcineurin inhibitors: pimecrolimus 1% cream and tacrolimus 0.1% ointment
4. Antimalarial drugs are first-line systemic therapy for cutaneous lupus: hydroxychloroquine sulfate 400 mg PO qd
5. Avoid use of systemic glucocorticoids in patients with isolated DLE because of risks of side effects

CHRONIC Rx

1. Chloroquine 250 to 500 mg PO qd
2. Additional options are methotrexate, mycophenolate mofetil, and cyclosporine.
3. Thalidomide 100 to 300 mg PO before sleep, with water, and >1 hr after meals for refractory CLE
4. Azathioprine 1 mg/kg/day PO for 6 to 8 wk, increase by 5 mg/kg q4 wk until response is seen or dose reaches 2.5 mg/kg/day
5. Dapsone: 100 mg/day

DISPOSITION

If untreated, DLE can lead to significant and permanent atrophy and scarring of the skin.

REFERRAL

Dermatology, rheumatology

PEARLS & CONSIDERATIONS

- Cutaneous lesions account for four of the 11 criteria in the diagnosis of SLE (e.g., malar rash, discoid rash, photosensitivity, and oral ulcers).
- Rarely, patients with DLE may develop nonmelanoma skin cancer in areas of disease.

SUGGESTED READINGS

available at www.expertconsult.com

RELATED CONTENT

Discoid Lupus Erythematosus (Patient Information)
Systemic Lupus Erythematosus (Related Key Topic)

AUTHORS: **KACHIU LEE, B.A.,** and **JESSICA CORWIN, M.D., M.P.H.**

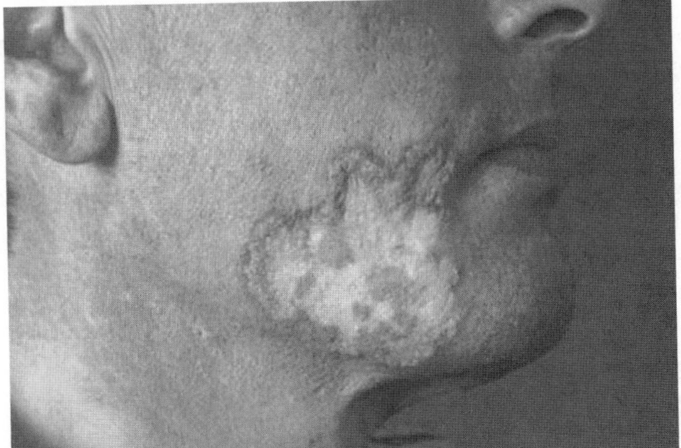

FIGURE 1-327 Classic discoid lupus erythematosus of the face. Note central scarring and erythematous hyperkeratotic borders. (From Hochberg MC et al: *Rheumatology,* ed 5, St Louis, 2011, Mosby.)

BASIC INFORMATION

DEFINITION

Disseminated intravascular coagulation (DIC) is an acquired thromboembolic disorder characterized by generalized activation of the clotting mechanism, which results in the intravascular formation of fibrin and ultimately thrombotic occlusion of small and midsize vessels.

SYNONYMS

Consumptive coagulopathy
DIC
Defibrination syndrome

ICD-9CM CODES
286.6 Disseminated intravascular coagulation
ICD-10CM CODES
D65 Disseminated intravascular coagulation [defibrination syndrome]

EPIDEMIOLOGY & DEMOGRAPHICS

More than 50% of cases are associated with gram-negative sepsis or other septicemic infections.

PHYSICAL FINDINGS & CLINICAL PRESENTATION

- Wound site bleeding, epistaxis, gingival bleeding, hemorrhagic bullae
- Petechiae, ecchymosis, purpura (Fig. E1-329)
- Dyspnea, localized rales, delirium
- Oliguria, anuria, gastrointestinal bleeding, metrorrhagia

ETIOLOGY

- Infections (e.g., gram-negative sepsis, Rocky Mountain spotted fever, malaria, viral or fungal infection)
- Obstetric complications (e.g., dead fetus, amniotic fluid embolism, toxemia, abruptio placentae, septic abortion, eclampsia, placenta previa, uterine atony)
- Tissue trauma (e.g., burns, hypothermia rewarming)
- Neoplasms (e.g., adenocarcinomas [gastrointestinal, prostate, lung, breast], acute promyelocytic leukemia)
- Quinine, cocaine-induced rhabdomyolysis
- Liver failure
- Acute pancreatitis
- Transfusion reactions
- Respiratory distress syndrome
- Toxins (snake bites, amphetamine overdose)
- Other: systemic lupus erythematosus (SLE), vasculitis, aneurysms, polyarteritis, cavernous hemangiomas
- Box E1-21A describes underlying conditions associated with DIC.

Dx DIAGNOSIS

DIFFERENTIAL DIAGNOSIS

- Hepatic necrosis: normal or elevated factor VIII concentrations
- Vitamin K deficiency: normal platelet count
- Hemolytic uremic syndrome
- Thrombotic thrombocytopenic purpura
- Renal failure, SLE, sickle cell crisis, dysfibrinogenemias
- HELLP syndrome (**h**emolysis, **e**levated **l**iver function tests, and **l**ow **p**latelets)
- Fig. E1-330 describes an algorithm for the differential diagnosis of deep vein thrombosis.

WORKUP

Diagnostic workup includes laboratory screening to confirm the diagnosis and exclude conditions noted in the differential diagnosis (Figs. E1-330 and E1-331). Workup is also aimed at distinguishing DIC progression (acute vs. chronic), chief manifestations (thrombotic or hemorrhagic), and extent (localized or systemic). The International Society on Thrombosis and Haemostasis scoring system for DIC is described in Box E1-21B.

LABORATORY TESTS

- Peripheral blood smear generally shows red blood cell fragments (schistocytes) and low platelet count.
- Coagulation factors are consumed at a rate in excess of the capacity of the liver to synthesize them, and platelets are consumed in excess of the capacity of the bone marrow megakaryocytes to release them. Diagnostic characteristics of DIC are decreased fibrinogen level; thrombocytopenia; and increased prothrombin time (PT), partial thromboplastin time (PTT), TT, fibrin split products, bleeding time, and D-dimer.
- Coagulopathy secondary to DIC must be differentiated from that secondary to liver disease or vitamin K deficiency.
  1. Vitamin K deficiency manifests with prolonged PT and normal PTT, TT, platelet, and fibrinogen level; PTT may be elevated in severe cases.
  2. Patients with liver disease have abnormal PT and PTT; TT and fibrinogen are usually normal unless severe disease is present; platelets are usually normal unless splenomegaly is present.
  3. Factors V and VIII are low in DIC, but they are normal in liver disease with coagulopathy.

IMAGING STUDIES

Imaging studies are generally not useful. Chest radiographs may be helpful to exclude infectious processes in patients with pulmonary symptoms such as dyspnea, cough, or hemoptysis.

Rx TREATMENT

NONPHARMACOLOGIC THERAPY

No specific precautions regarding activity level are necessary unless thrombocytopenia is severe.

ACUTE GENERAL Rx

- Correct and eliminate underlying cause (e.g., antimicrobial therapy for infection, removal of necrotic bowel, evacuation of uterus in obstetric emergencies).
- Give replacement therapy with fresh frozen plasma (FFP) and platelets in patients with significant hemorrhage:
  1. FFP 10 to 15 ml/kg can be given with a goal of normalizing international normalized ratio.
  2. Platelet transfusions are given when platelet count is <10,000 (or higher if major bleeding is present).
  3. Cryoprecipitate 1 U/5 kg is reserved for hypofibrinogen states.
  4. Antithrombin III treatment may be considered as a supportive therapeutic option in patients with severe DIC. Its modest results and substantial cost are limiting factors.
- Heparin therapy at a dose lower than that used in venous thrombosis (300 to 500 U/hr) may be useful in selected cases to increase neutralization of thrombin (e.g., DIC associated with acute promyelocytic leukemia, purpura fulminans, acral ischemia).

CHRONIC Rx

Follow-up management includes coagulation screening to assess factor replacement therapy. Laboratory abnormalities generally correct with treatment of the underlying disorder. Long-term laboratory monitoring is not required.

DISPOSITION

Mortality rate in severe DIC exceeds 75%. Death generally results from progression of the underlying disease and complications such as acute renal failure, intracerebral hematoma, shock, or cardiac tamponade.

REFERRAL

Hematology consultation is recommended in all cases of DIC.

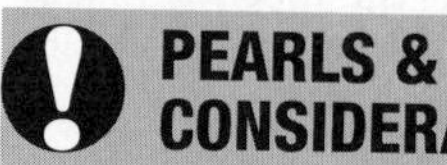

PEARLS & CONSIDERATIONS

COMMENTS

The treatment of chronic DIC is controversial. Low-dose SC heparin and/or combination antiplatelet agents such as aspirin and dipyridamole may be useful.

SUGGESTED READINGS

available at www.expertconsult.com

RELATED CONTENT

Disseminated Intravascular Coagulation (Patient Information)

AUTHOR: **FRED F. FERRI, M.D.**

D

Diseases and Disorders

BASIC INFORMATION

DEFINITION

- Colonic diverticula are herniations of mucosa and submucosa through the muscularis. They are generally found along the colon's mesenteric border at the site where the vasa recta penetrates the muscle wall (anatomic weak point).
- *Diverticulosis* is the asymptomatic presence of multiple colonic diverticula.
- *Diverticulitis* is an inflammatory process or localized perforation of diverticulum.

ICD-9CM CODES
562.10 Diverticulosis of colon
562.11 Diverticulitis of colon
ICD-10CM CODES
K57.30 Diverticulosis of large intestine without perforation or abscess without bleeding
K57.32 Diverticulitis of large intestine without perforation or abscess without bleeding

EPIDEMIOLOGY & DEMOGRAPHICS

- Incidence of diverticulosis in the general population is 35% to 50%.
- Diverticulosis is more common in Western countries, affecting >30% of people >40 yr and >50% of people >70 yr.

PHYSICAL FINDINGS & CLINICAL PRESENTATION

- Physical examination in patients with diverticulosis is generally normal.
- Painful diverticular disease can present with left lower quadrant (LLQ) pain, often relieved by defecation; location of pain may be anywhere in the lower abdomen because of the redundancy of the sigmoid colon.
- Diverticulitis can cause muscle spasm, guarding, and rebound tenderness predominantly affecting the LLQ.

ETIOLOGY

- Diverticular disease is believed to be secondary to low intake of dietary fiber.
- Recent studies indicate a pathogenetic role for inflammation in diverticulitis that may be similar to that of IBS, IBD, or both, based on common histologic findings such as granulomas, infiltrating lymphocytes, TNF, histamine, and matrix metalloproteinases.[1]

DIAGNOSIS

DIFFERENTIAL DIAGNOSIS

- Irritable bowel syndrome
- IBD
- Carcinoma of colon
- Endometriosis
- Ischemic colitis
- Infections (pseudomembranous colitis, appendicitis, pyelonephritis, PID)
- Lactose intolerance
- Celiac disease

LABORATORY TESTS

- WBC count in diverticulitis reveals leukocytosis with left shift.
- Microcytic anemia can be present in patients with chronic bleeding from diverticular disease. MCV may be elevated in acute bleeding secondary to reticulocytosis.

PROCEDURES:
Colonoscopy should be avoided during acute diverticulitis due to the risk of perforation. It can generally be performed after 6 wk to rule out the presence of cancer and IBD.

IMAGING STUDIES

- A CT scan of the abdomen (Fig. E1-332) is recommended as the initial radiologic examination to diagnose acute diverticulitis; It can also diagnose diverticulosis (Fig. E1-333). It has a sensitivity of 93% to 97% and a specificity approaching 100% for diverticulitis. Typical findings are thickening of the bowel wall, fistulas, or abscess formation. CT may also reveal other disease processes (e.g., appendicitis, tubo-ovarian abscess, Crohn's disease) accounting for lower abdominal pain
- Evaluation of suspected diverticular bleeding:
  1. Arteriography if the bleeding is faster than 1 ml/min (advantage: the possible infusion of vasopressin directly into the arteries supplying the bleeding, as well as selective arterial embolization; disadvantages: its cost and invasive nature)
  2. Technetium-99m sulfa colloid
  3. Technetium-99m labeled RBC (can detect bleeding rates as low as 0.12 to 5 ml/min)

TREATMENT

NONPHARMACOLOGIC THERAPY

- Increase in dietary fiber intake and regular exercise to improve bowel function. However, recent studies have challenged the common view that fiber intake protects against diverticulosis
- NPO and IV hydration in severe diverticulitis; NG suction if ileus or small bowel obstruction is present

ACUTE GENERAL Rx

TREATMENT OF DIVERTICULITIS:

- Mild case: broad-spectrum PO antibiotics (e.g., Ciprofloxacin 750 mg bid or levofloxacin 750 mg bid or trimethoprim/sulfamethoxazole DS bid to cover aerobic component of colonic flora *and* metronidazole 500 mg q6h for anaerobes) and liquid diet for 7 to 10 days are commonly prescribed. However, randomized trials and cohort studies have shown that antibiotics are not as beneficial as previously thought and that mesalamine might be useful.[1]
- Severe case: NPO and aggressive IV antibiotic therapy
  a. Ampicillin-sulbactam 3 g IV q6h *or*
  b. Piperacillin-tazobactam 4.5 g IV q8h *or*
  c. Ciprofloxacin 400 mg IV q12h plus metronidazole 500 mg IV q6h *or*
  d. Ticarcillin-clavulanate 3.1 g IV q6h
- Life-threatening case: Imipenem 500 mg IV q6h *or* meropenem 1 g IV q8h
- Surgical treatment (laparoscopic preferred over open colectomy) consisting of resection of involved areas and reanastomosis (if feasible); otherwise a diverting colostomy with reanastomosis performed when infection has been controlled; surgery should be considered in patients with:
  1. Repeated episodes of diverticulitis (two or more)
  2. Poor response to appropriate medical therapy (failure of conservative management)
  3. Abscess or fistula formation
  4. Obstruction
  5. Peritonitis
  6. Immunocompromised patients, first episode in young patient (<40 yr old)
  7. Inability to exclude carcinoma (10% to 20% of patients diagnosed with diverticulosis on clinical grounds are subsequently found to have carcinoma of the colon)

DIVERTICULAR HEMORRHAGE:

1. Bleeding is painless and stops spontaneously in the majority of patients (60%); it is usually caused by erosion of a blood vessel by a fecalith present within the diverticular sac.
2. Medical therapy consists of blood replacement and correction of volume and any clotting abnormalities.
3. Colonoscopic treatment with epinephrine injections, bipolar coagulation, or both may prevent recurrent bleeding and decrease the need for surgery.
4. Surgical resection is necessary if bleeding does not stop spontaneously after administration of 4 to 5 U of PRBCs or recurs with severity within a few days; if attempts at localization are unsuccessful, total abdominal colectomy with ileoproctostomy may be indicated (high incidence of rebleeding if segmental resection is performed without adequate localization).

DISPOSITION

- The risk of recurrence among patients with uncomplicated diverticulitis is 32%-36%. Most patients with diverticulitis respond well to antibiotic management and bowel rest. Up to 30% of patients with diverticulitis will eventually require surgical management.
- Diverticular bleeding can recur in 15% to 20% of patients within 5 yr.

REFERRAL

GI referral for colonoscopy 4-6 wk after resolution of symptoms. In patients who have complications from diverticulitis, colonoscopy is not necessary after radiologically proven uncomplicated diverticulitis. Surgical referral when considering resection.

SUGGESTED READINGS

available at www.expertconsult.com

RELATED CONTENT

Diverticulitis (Patient Information)
Diverticulosis (Patient Information)

AUTHOR: **FRED F. FERRI, M.D.**

[1]Morris AM et al: Sigmoid diverticulitis: a systematic review. *JAMA* 311(3) 287-297, 2014.

BASIC INFORMATION

DEFINITION

Down syndrome is a disorder characterized by mental retardation and multiple organ defects and is caused by a chromosomal abnormality (trisomy 21).

SYNONYMS

Trisomy 21

ICD-9CM CODES
758.0 Down syndrome
ICD-10CM CODES
Q90.9 Down syndrome, unspecified

EPIDEMIOLOGY & DEMOGRAPHICS

INCIDENCE (IN U.S.): 1 in 800 births
PEAK INCIDENCE: Newborn
PREVALENCE (IN U.S.): 300,000 persons
PREDOMINANT SEX: Male/female ratio of 1.3:1.0
PREDOMINANT AGE: Newborn to early adulthood
GENETICS: Nondisjunction causing trisomy 21

PHYSICAL FINDINGS & CLINICAL PRESENTATION

(Fig. 1-334)
- Microcephaly
- Flattening of occiput and face
- Upward slant to eyes with epicanthal folds
- Brushfield spots on iris
- Broad, stocky neck
- Small feet, hands, digits
- Single palmar crease
- Hypotonia
- Short stature
- Associated with congenital heart disease, malformations of the GI tract, cataracts, hypothyroidism, hip dysplasia, obstructive sleep apnea, infantile spasms, moyamoya disease, and myeloproliferative disorders
- About half of children with Down syndrome are born with congenital heart disease, with the most common lesions being atrial septal defect and ventricular septal defect
- Persistent primary congenital hypothyroidism is found in 1 in 141 newborns with Down syndrome, as compared with 1 in 4000 in the general population
- Ophthalmologic disorders increase in frequency with age; >80% of children aged 5 to 12 yr have disorders that need monitoring or intervention, such as refractive errors, strabismus, or cataracts
- Renal and urinary tract abnormalities

FIGURE 1-334 Down syndrome. Note depressed nasal bridge, epicanthal folds, mongoloid slant of eyes, low-set ears, and large tongue. (From Zitelli BJ, Davis HW: *Atlas of pediatric physical diagnosis,* ed 3, St Louis, 1997, Mosby.)

ETIOLOGY

Nondisjunction of chromosome 21

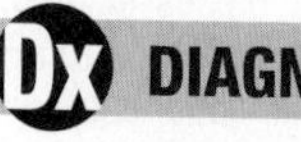

DIAGNOSIS

- The American College of Obstetrics and Gynecology recommends offering fetal chromosomal screening to all pregnant women regardless of age due to improvements in noninvasive screening methods.
- Combined use of serum screening and fetal ultrasound testing for thickened nuchal fold has 85% detection rate with 5% false-positive results. Second-trimester serum screening in combination with maternal age is improved with use of multiple serum markers
- Prenatal cytogenic diagnosis by amniocentesis or chorionic villus sampling
- Postnatal chromosomal karyotype

DIFFERENTIAL DIAGNOSIS

- Congenital hypothyroidism
- Other chromosomal abnormalities

WORKUP

Postnatal chromosomal karyotype

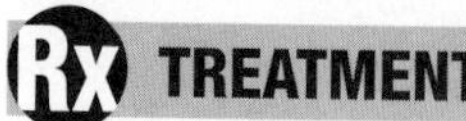

TREATMENT

- Thyroid screen at birth, at age 6 mo, and yearly thereafter
- Echocardiogram in all newborns and cardiac assessment of adolescents for development of mitral valve prolapse
- Treatment consists of vigilant monitoring for comorbid states, such as obesity, hypothyroidism, leukemia, hearing loss, and valvular heart disease
- Prevention of obesity with low-calorie, high-fiber diet
- Auditory brain stem responses in all newborns and aggressive testing for hearing loss in children with chronic otitis media
- Ophthalmologic assessment by age 6 mo for congenital cataracts and annual examinations for monitoring of refractive errors and strabismus
- Regular dental care
- Pelvic examination of women who are sexually active or who have menstrual problems
- Dermatologic issues such as folliculitis can become problematic in adolescents, and require topical antibiotics and careful attention to hygiene

DISPOSITION

Most children with Down syndrome live at home. As these individuals reach adulthood, those with higher functioning sometimes live in supervised settings away from their families.

REFERRAL

Down syndrome clinics use a preventive checklist to anticipate many clinical challenges.

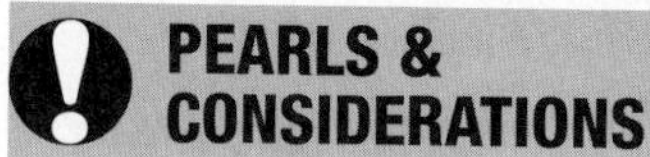

PEARLS & CONSIDERATIONS

COMMENTS

- Screening for atlantoaxial subluxation is controversial.
- Most patients experience neuropathologic changes typical of Alzheimer's disease. Presenting symptoms include seizures, focal neurologic signs, and apathy. If Alzheimer's disease is suspected, screen for treatable diseases such as depression or hypothyroidism.
- This syndrome accounts for approximately one third of moderate-to-severe cases of mental retardation.
- Individuals with Down syndrome have a wide range of function, but all will have decrease in intelligence quotient (IQ) in first decade of life.
- Deficiency of language production relative to other areas of development often causes substantial impairment.
- Though increased maternal age is a risk factor, most children with Down syndrome are born to women younger than 35 yr.

SUGGESTED READINGS

available at www.expertconsult.com

RELATED CONTENT

Down Syndrome (Trisomy, Mongolism) (Patient Information)

AUTHOR: **MAITREYI MAZUMDAR, M.D., M.P.H.**

BASIC INFORMATION

DEFINITION

Dumping syndrome refers to a constellation of postprandial symptoms resulting from rapid delivery of hypertonic stomach contents into the small bowel that is most often caused by gastric surgery, such as procedures for peptic ulcer disease and gastric bypass.

SYNONYMS

Postgastrectomy syndrome
Rapid gastric emptying

ICD-9CM CODES
564.2 Postgastric surgery syndromes
ICD-10CM CODES
K91.1 Postgastric surgery syndromes

EPIDEMIOLOGY & DEMOGRAPHICS

Incidence is 10% of all patients having gastric surgery.

- Vagotomy and pyloroplasty (8.5% to 20%)
- Vagotomy and antrectomy (4% to 27%)
- Subtotal gastrectomy (10% to 40%)
- Parietal cell vagotomy (3% to 5%)
- Gastric bypass surgeries (up to 50%)
- Males and females are affected equally

PHYSICAL FINDINGS & CLINICAL PRESENTATION

1. Early dumping syndrome: symptoms start within 1 hr after eating food:
   - No symptoms in fasting state
   - Nausea, vomiting, and belching
   - Epigastric fullness, cramping, and diarrhea
   - Dizziness, flushing, diaphoresis, and syncope
   - Palpitations and tachycardia
2. Late dumping syndrome: symptoms occurring 1 to 3 hr after eating:
   - Diaphoresis
   - Irritability
   - Difficulty in concentration
   - Tremulousness

ETIOLOGY

Dumping syndrome occurs almost exclusively in patients who have had gastric surgery.

- Systemic symptoms in early dumping syndrome are thought to be partially due to hypovolemia caused by rapid shifts of fluid from the intravascular space into the lumen of the bowel.
- Increase in vasoactive substances related to rapid gastric emptying is thought to play a role in dumping syndrome.
- Late dumping symptoms are thought to be due to reactive hypoglycemia.

DIAGNOSIS

A detailed clinical history and evidence of prior gastric surgery are necessary for the diagnosis.

DIFFERENTIAL DIAGNOSIS

- Pancreatic insufficiency
- Inflammatory bowel disease
- Afferent loop syndromes
- Bile acid reflux after surgery
- Bowel obstruction
- Gastroenteric fistula

WORKUP

Diagnosis is typically made on clinical grounds. In certain clinical settings, where patients exhibit symptoms with no prior history of gastric surgery, oral glucose challenge and imaging studies may be pursued and aid in establishing the diagnosis.

LABORATORY TESTS

Oral glucose challenge test:

- After overnight fasting, oral intake of 50 g of glucose is followed by serial measurements of heart rate, serum glucose, and hydrogen breath test every 15 to 30 min for 3 to 6 hrs. A 30-min hematocrit can also be taken.
- An increase in the heart rate >12 beats/min and a rise in hydrogen breath excretion have a sensitivity of 94% and specificity >92%. An increase of >3% in the 30-min hematocrit is also suggestive of a positive test. A nadir blood glucose <3.3 mmol/L (<59 mg/dl) was present in 75% of late dumpers.

IMAGING STUDIES

- Upper GI series properly defines anatomy.
- Scintigraphic imaging documents rapid gastric emptying and may be useful in patients with dumping syndrome and no prior history of gastric surgery.

TREATMENT

NONPHARMACOLOGIC THERAPY

- Diet modification
  1. Divide caloric intake over six small meals
  2. Limit fluid intake with meals (try to avoid fluids 30 min before meals and following meals)
  3. Decrease carbohydrate intake and avoid simple sugars
  4. Increase/supplement dietary fibers
  5. Avoid milk/milk products

ACUTE GENERAL Rx

- Acarbose 50 mg PO daily can be tried if dietary modification does not help.
- Octreotide 25 to 50 μg SC 30 min before meals is effective in relieving symptoms of dumping syndrome.
- Pectin and guar have been used to increase viscosity of intraluminal contents and relieve symptoms from rapid emptying and absorption.

CHRONIC Rx

- Surgery is considered in patients with severe symptoms refractory to the above-mentioned dietary and acute general treatment.
- Surgical procedures include: reconstruction of the pylorus, converting Billroth II to a Billroth I anastomosis, and a Roux-en-Y reconstruction.
- In severe cases, can consider depot long-acting-release octreotide, given as 10 mg intramuscularly every 4 wks for symptom relief.

DISPOSITION

- Dumping syndrome improves with time. Approximately 1% to 2% of patients will continue to have significant symptoms several months after surgery.
- Dietary modification effectively treats the majority of patients.

REFERRAL

- A gastrointestinal specialist consult is recommended in patients suspected of having dumping syndrome.
- If medical management is unsuccessful, a general surgical consultation is warranted.

PEARLS & CONSIDERATIONS

COMMENTS

- The majority of patients usually manifest with early dumping symptoms or a combination of early and late symptoms. Few have late dumping symptoms alone.
- Octreotide has an inhibitory effect on the release of insulin and other vasoactive substances released by the gut. It also works by decreasing gastric emptying.

SUGGESTED READINGS

available at www.expertconsult.com

AUTHOR: **MARK F. BRADY, M.D., M.P.H., M.M.S.**

BASIC INFORMATION

DEFINITION

Dupuytren's contracture is a disease of the palmar fascia characterized by nodular fibroblastic proliferation that often results in progressive contractures of the fascia and flexion deformity of the fingers.

Dupuytren's diathesis is a more aggressive presentation of the disease. Risk factors include >40 yr, strong family history, bilateral involvement, and ectopic manifestations like plantar and penile fibromatosis.

ICD-9CM CODES
728.6 Dupuytren's contracture
ICD-10CM CODES
M72.0 Palmar fascial fibromatosis [Dupuytren]

EPIDEMIOLOGY & DEMOGRAPHICS

PREVALENCE: Varies depending on ethnicity. The disorder is more common in Scandinavians; some Northern Europeans have a 25% prevalence after the age of 60.
PREVALENT SEX: Male/female ratio of 3.5 to 9:1, becomes 1:1 after age 80 yr.
PREVALENT AGE: 40 to 60 yr
RISK FACTORS: Age >40 yr, positive family history, diabetes mellitus, alcoholism, smoking, HIV infection
GENETICS: Aberrations in genes encoding proteins in the Wnt-signaling pathways are believed to be implicated in the process of fibromatosis in Dupuytren's disease.

PHYSICAL FINDINGS & CLINICAL PRESENTATION

- Usually asymptomatic
- Most common complaints: deformity and interference with the use of the hand by the flexed, contracted fingers (Fig. E1-335)
- Process usually begins on the ulnar side of the hand, often starting at the ring finger; other fingers can be involved
- Isolated, painless nodules that eventually harden and mature into a longitudinal cord that extends into the finger
- Later stages: fibrous cord begins to contract and pull the finger into flexion
- Skin pitting, atrophic grooves
- Tabletop test of Hueston: place hand and fingers prone on a table. Test is positive if hand won't go flat (Fig. 1-336). Surgery is generally not indicated if test is negative
- A staging classification for Dupuytren's contracture is described in Table 1-168.

ETIOLOGY

Unknown.

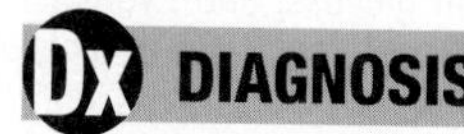

DIAGNOSIS

DIFFERENTIAL DIAGNOSIS

- Soft tissue tumor
- Tendon cyst

WORKUP

The typical case is easily diagnosed clinically. Plain radiographs may be useful to rule out bony abnormalities.

TREATMENT

- Avoidance of repetitive hand trauma; measures include the use of gloves and damping tape to widen grips.
- Stretching exercises.
- Radiotherapy.
- Intralesional corticosteroid injection can be effective in early stages and provide better results in combination with percutaneous needle aponeurotomy.
- Enzymatic fasciotomy by *Clostridium histolyticum* collagenase injection for early, less severe cases: collagenase *C. histolyticum* (Xiaflex) is the first FDA-approved, nonsurgical treatment option for adult Dupuytren's contracture patients with a palpable cord that is highly effective and well tolerated.
- Surgery is usually performed when the metacarpophalangeal joint contracture exceeds 30 degrees or when the proximal interphalangeal joint has any degree of contracture. Another indication for surgery is if there is neurovascular damage of the finger. Percutaneous needle aponeurotomy performed in the office represents an alternative to surgery.

DISPOSITION

Rate of development is variable.

REFERRAL

Evaluation by hand or plastic surgeon if joint contracture begins to develop or for excision of rare nodule that is painful (at any stage)

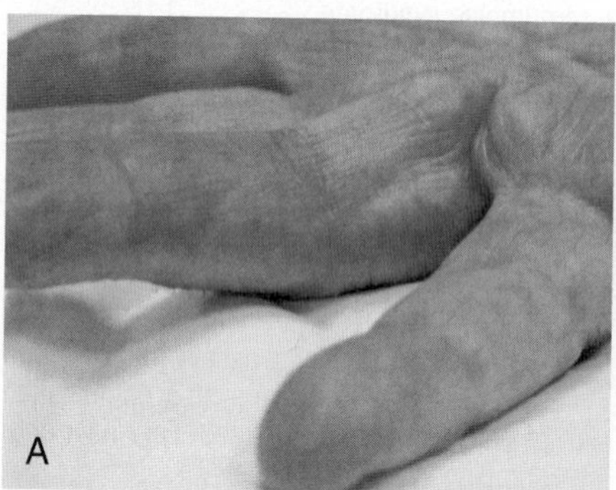

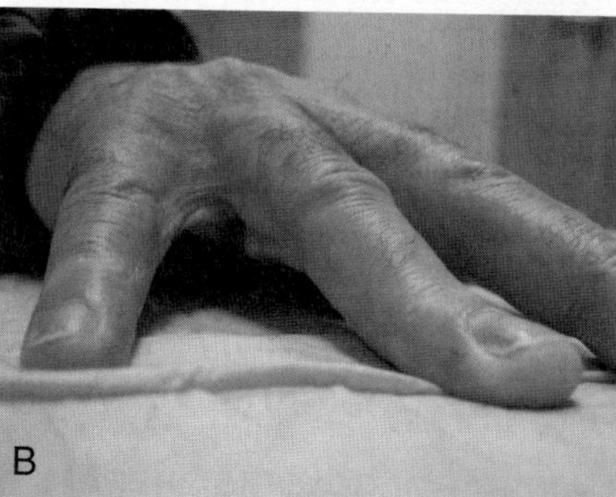

FIGURE 1-336 Dupuytren's contracture of the ring finger. A, Pitting of the skin and a longitudinal cord can be seen causing metacarpophalangeal (MCP) joint flexion. **B**, Contracture/flexion deformity at the MCP joint keeps this patient from flattening his hand against a flat surface. (From Hochberg MC et al: *Rheumatology,* ed 5, St Louis, 2011, Mosby.)

TABLE 1-168 Staging Classification for Dupuytren's Contracture (Woodruff, 1998)

Stage	Description	Management
1	Early palmar disease with no contracture	Leave alone
2	One finger involved, with only metacarpophalangeal joint contracture	Surgery
3	One finger—metacarpophalangeal joint 1 proximal interphalangeal joint	Surgery difficult
4	Stage 3 1 more than one finger involved	Surgery prolonged and only partly successful
5	Finger-in-palm deformity	Consider amputation

From Parvizi J: *High-yield orthopedics,* Philadelphia, 2010, Saunders.

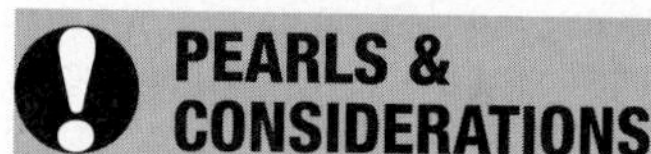

PEARLS & CONSIDERATIONS

COMMENTS

- Dupuytren's contracture develops earlier and more often in certain families.
- Approximately 5% of patients develop a similar condition elsewhere, such as Peyronie's disease or Ledderhose disease (involvement of the plantar fascia).
- Tender knuckle pads (*Garrod's knuckle pad*) over the dorsal aspect of the PIP joints may also be present.
- Individuals with these additional findings are considered to have Dupuytren's diathesis, and their disease is generally more severe and recurrent.

SUGGESTED READINGS
available at www.expertconsult.com

RELATED CONTENT

Dupuytren's Contracture (Patient Information)

AUTHOR: DANIEL E. MENDEZ-ALLWOOD, M.D.

BASIC INFORMATION

DEFINITION

Dysfunctional uterine bleeding (DUB) describes abnormal uterine bleeding in the absence of disease in the pelvis, pregnancy, or medical illness. Parameters of normal menstrual function are described in Box 1-22. Specific types of abnormal bleeding include the following:

- Hypermenorrhea: excessive bleeding amount during normal duration of regular menstrual cycles
- Hypomenorrhea: decreased bleeding amount in regular menstrual cycles
- Menorrhagia: regular normal intervals, excessive flow and duration
- Metrorrhagia: irregular intervals, excessive flow and duration
- Menometrorrhagia: irregular or excessive bleeding during menstruation and between periods
- Oligomenorrhea: intervals >35 days
- Polymenorrhea: intervals <21 days

These terms, while commonly used in practice, increasingly are felt to be confusing. In fact, The FIGO Menstrual Disorders Working Group has been working since 2009 to eliminate many of the confusing and overlapping terms and create simpler definitions that can be intuitively understood by medical professionals and lay people alike. The term *dysfunctional uterine bleeding* was initially used in 1935 but has never been clearly defined and has been used as both a diagnosis and a symptom. It is generally understood to be a term of exclusion when no other cause of bleeding has been established. FIGO recommends that the three diagnoses (disturbances of molecular control of menses, HPO axis abnormalities, and disorders of hemostasis) be grouped under the nonstructural causes of abnormal uterine bleeding. However, these new FIGO terms have not yet made their way into common usage. In addition, the ICD-9 codes have not been updated to reflect this new usage.

SYNONYMS

DUB

ICD-9CM CODES

626	Disorders of menstruation and other abnormal bleeding from female genital tract
626.2	Hypermenorrhea
626.1	Hypomenorrhea
626.2	Menorrhagia
626.6	Metrorrhagia
626.2	Menometrorrhagia
626.1	Oligomenorrhea
626.2	Polymenorrhea

ICD-10CM CODES

N92.5	Other specified irregular menstruation
N92.0	Excessive and frequent menstruation with regular cycle
N91.5	Oligomenorrhea, unspecified
N92.1	Excessive and frequent menstruation with irregular cycle
N94.6	Dysmenorrhea, unspecified

EPIDEMIOLOGY & DEMOGRAPHICS

- Most cases of DUB occur in postmenarchal and perimenopausal age groups.
- During reproductive age, <20% of abnormal bleeding results from anovulatory DUB.

PHYSICAL FINDINGS & CLINICAL PRESENTATION

- A clinical diagnosis of exclusion
- Thorough physical and pelvic examination to exclude the other causes of abnormal bleeding
  1. Includes thyroid, breast, liver, presence or absence of ecchymotic lesions
  2. Patient possibly obese and hirsute (polycystic ovarian disease)
  3. No evidence of any vulvar, vaginal, cervical lesions, uterine (fibroid) or ovarian tumor, urethral caruncle, urethral diverticula, hemorrhoids, anal fissure, colorectal lesions
  4. Bimanual pelvic examination: normal-sized or slightly enlarged uterus

ETIOLOGY

- 90% is caused by anovulation.
- 10% is ovulatory in origin; can be caused by dysfunction of corpus luteum or midcycle bleeding.
- Section II describes the various causes of abnormal uterine bleeding.

Dx DIAGNOSIS

DIFFERENTIAL DIAGNOSIS

- Pregnancy-related cause
- Anatomic uterine causes:
  1. Leiomyomas
  2. Adenomyosis
  3. Polyps
  4. Endometrial hyperplasia
  5. Cancer
  6. Sexually transmitted diseases
  7. Intrauterine contraceptive devices
- Anatomic nonuterine causes:
  1. Cervical neoplasia, cervicitis
  2. Vaginal neoplasia, adhesions, trauma, foreign body, atrophic vaginitis, infections, condyloma
  3. Vulvar trauma, infections, neoplasia, condyloma, dystrophy, varices
  4. Urinary tract: urethral caruncle, diverticulum, hematuria
  5. Gastrointestinal tract: hemorrhoids, anal fissure, colorectal lesions
- Systemic diseases:
  1. Exogenous hormone intake
  2. Coagulopathies: von Willebrand's disease, thrombocytopenia, hepatic failure
  3. Endocrinopathies: thyroid disorder, hypothyroidism and hyperthyroidism, diabetes mellitus
  4. Renal diseases
- Section II describes a differential diagnosis of vaginal bleeding abnormalities.

BOX 1-22 Parameters of Normal Menstrual Function

Cycle interval (days)	21-35
Duration of flow (days)	2-8
Blood loss/cycle (ml)	30-80

From Carlson KJ et al: *Primary care of women*, ed 2, St Louis, 2002, Mosby.

WORKUP

- A detailed history and thorough physical examination, including a pelvic examination to exclude causes mentioned above.
- Clinical algorithms for the evaluation of vaginal bleeding are described in Section III, "Bleeding, Vaginal."

LABORATORY TESTS

- Complete blood count with platelets; possible iron-deficiency anemia or thrombocytopenia
- Prothrombin; partial thromboplastin and bleeding time if coagulopathy is suspected
- Serum human chorionic gonadotropin
- Chemistry profile, including liver function tests
- Thyroid profile
- Stool testing for occult blood
- Urinalysis for hematuria
- Pap smear
- Cultures for gonorrhea and *Chlamydia*
- Serum gonadotropins and prolactin
- Serum androgens
- Endometrial biopsy in women >35 yr or earlier if longstanding history of anovulatory bleeding, such as fewer than 3 menstrual cycles per year
- Hysterogram and hysteroscopy
- Von Willebrand's panel, particularly in perimenarchal women

IMAGING STUDIES

- Pelvic ultrasound, including measurement of endometrial thickness and assessment of myometrial or endometrial defects
- Fluid contrast ultrasound (also called saline sonogram, sonohysterogram, hydrosonogram, and various other names). Distends the uterine cavity so that "filling defects" of the endometrium can be assessed. Such a filling defect may represent an endometrial polyp, uterine fibroid, or neoplasm.

Rx TREATMENT

NONPHARMACOLOGIC THERAPY

Increase iron intake in the form of pills and in a diet rich in iron.

ACUTE GENERAL Rx

- Progestational agents (see Box 1-23)
  1. Progesterone in oil, 100 to 200 mg
  2. Medroxyprogesterone acetate, 20 to 40 mg qd for 15 days
  3. Megestrol acetate, 40 to 120 mg daily in divided doses for 15 days
  4. Oral contraceptives: any oral contraceptive pill, 1 tablet qid for 5 to 7 days,

BOX 1-23 Equivalent Daily Doses of Oral Progestins for the Treatment of Dysfunctional Uterine Bleeding

Medroxyprogesterone acetate (Provera, Cycrin)	10 mg
Micronized progesterone (Prometrium)	400 mg
Norgestrel (Ovrette)	150 μg
Norethindrone acetate (Micronor, Nor-QD)	0.7-1.0 mg

From Carlson KJ et al: *Primary care of women*, ed 2, St Louis, 2002, Mosby.

followed by 1 tablet low-dose estrogen qd for 21 days; causes withdrawal bleeding; should then be on cyclical Provera or continue on oral contraceptives

- Estrogens
  1. Conjugated estrogen (Premarin) 25 mg IV q4h until bleeding is under control (in cases of severe or life-threatening bleeding); maximum three doses
  2. For prolonged bleeding that is not life threatening: Premarin 1.25 mg (Estrace 2 mg) q4h for 24 hr, followed by Provera to bring on withdrawal bleeding; then sequential regimen of estrogen and progestin (Premarin 1.25 mg qd for 24 days, Provera 10 mg for last 10 days) or oral contraceptives
- Surgical treatment
  1. Dilation and curettage (D&C) and hysteroscopy
  2. Endometrial ablation
  3. Hysterectomy

CHRONIC Rx

- Progestational agents
  - Medroxyprogesterone acetate 10 mg qd for 12 days, then cyclically to induce monthly withdrawal bleeding
  - Norethindrone 2.5 to 10 mg qd for 12 days
  - Depo-Provera 150 mg IM and then 150 mg every 3 mo
  - Oral contraceptives, 1 tablet qd
  - Levonorgestrel-releasing intrauterine device (Mirena, currently has an FDA indication for heavy menstrual bleeding in women who use an IUD for contraception)
- Clomiphene citrate: patients with anovulatory bleeding who want to become pregnant. Recent studies suggest that progesterone withdrawal may be counterproductive in patients wishing to start ovulation induction regimen. Pregnancy rates lower when patients undergo withdrawal compared to when random ovulation induction start utilized.
- Others
  - Antiprostaglandins
  - Danazol (rarely used due to side-effect profile)
  - Gonadotropin-releasing hormone analogs (GnRH)
  - Human menopausal gonadotropin (HMG) (desire pregnancy)
  - Tranexamic acid (Lysteda) is an antifibrinolytic agent recently FDA approved for cyclic heavy menstrual bleeding. Dosage in normal renal function is 3900 mg daily (650-mg tablets, 2 tablets tid) for up to 5 days during menses
- Surgical treatment
  1. D&C and hysteroscopy
  2. Endometrial ablation
  3. Hysterectomy

DISPOSITION

Cyclical treatment on birth control pills or Provera for several cycles, then discontinue pill and watch patient for onset of regular menses

REFERRAL

To gynecologist in case of failure of treatment

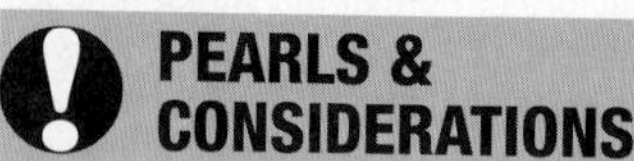

PEARLS & CONSIDERATIONS

COMMENTS

- Table 1-169 describes management options for DUB.
- Patient education material may be obtained from the American College of Obstetricians and Gynecologists, 409 12th Street SW, Washington, DC 20024-2188; phone 202-638-5577.

SUGGESTED READINGS

available at www.expertconsult.com

RELATED CONTENT

Endometrial Cancer (Related Key Topic)
Uterine Fibroids (Related Key Topic)
Fig. 3-32 Evaluation of ovulatory bleeding (Algorithm)
Fig. 3-33 Evaluation of anovulatory bleeding (Algorithm)
Dysfunctional Uterine Bleeding (Patient Information)

AUTHORS: **MANDEEP K. BRAR, M.D.,** and **RUBEN ALVERO, M.D.**

TABLE 1-169 Management of Dysfunctional Uterine Bleeding (DUB)

Bleeding Pattern	Cause	Treatment
Ovulatory DUB		
Heavy menstrual bleeding	Imbalance in endometrial prostacyclins and prostaglandins	Nonsteroidal anti-inflammatory drugs Combination oral contraceptive pill Progestin intrauterine device Endometrial ablation
Midcycle spotting	Periovulatory estrogen decline	None
Delayed menses	Persistent corpus luteum	None (rule out pregnancy)
Anovulatory DUB		
Irregular menses	Unopposed estrogen stimulation of endometrium	Combination oral contraceptive pill Cyclic progestins Endometrial ablation
Postmenopausal bleeding	Endometrial atrophy	Hormone replacement therapy Endometrial ablation

From Carlson KJ, Eisenstat SA et al: *Primary care of women*, ed 2, St Louis, 2002, Mosby.

BASIC INFORMATION

DEFINITION

Dysmenorrhea is pain with menstruation, usually cramping and usually centered in the lower abdomen. It is defined as *primary dysmenorrhea* when there is no associated organic pathology and *secondary dysmenorrhea* when there is demonstrable organic pathology.

SYNONYMS

Menstrual cramps
Painful periods

ICD-9CM CODES
625.3 Dysmenorrhea
ICD-10CM CODES
N94.3 Primary dysmenorrhea
N94.5 Secondary dysmenorrhea
N94.6 Dysmenorrhea, unspecified

EPIDEMIOLOGY & DEMOGRAPHICS

- Approximately 50% of menstruating women are affected by dysmenorrhea, with approximately 10% of them having severe dysmenorrhea with incapacitation for 1 to 3 days/mo.
- Dysmenorrhea is most common in the age group from 20 to 24 yr, and primary dysmenorrhea usually appears within 6 to 12 mo after menarche.
- Dysmenorrhea is more common in women who have menarche at an earlier age, and in those with a longer duration of menstruation.

PHYSICAL FINDINGS & CLINICAL PRESENTATION

- Sharp, crampy, midline, lower abdominal pain without a lower quadrant or adnexal component but possible radiation to the lower back and upper thighs
- Unremarkable pelvic examination in non-menstruating patient
- Accompanying symptoms: nausea, vomiting, headaches, anxiety, fatigue, diarrhea, fainting, and abdominal bloating
- Cramps usually lasting <24 hr and seldom lasting >2 to 3 days
- Secondary dysmenorrhea: dyspareunia is a common complaint, and bimanual pelvic-abdominal examination may demonstrate uterine or adnexal tenderness, fixed uterine retroflexion, uterosacral nodularity, a pelvic mass, or an enlarged, irregular uterus

ETIOLOGY

Prostaglandin $F_2\alpha$ is the agent responsible for dysmenorrhea. It stimulates uterine contractions and cervical stenosis (narrowing) and increases vasopressin release. Behavior and psychological factors have also been implicated in the etiology of primary dysmenorrhea. Primary dysmenorrhea only occurs in ovulatory cycles. Secondary dysmenorrhea is usually caused by endometriosis, adenomyosis, leiomyomas and, less commonly, chronic salpingitis, intrauterine device (IUD) use, or congenital or acquired outflow tract obstruction, including cervical stenosis.

Dx DIAGNOSIS

DIFFERENTIAL DIAGNOSIS

- Adenomyosis
- Adhesions
- Allen-Masters syndrome
- Cervical structures or stenosis
- Congenital malformation of müllerian system
- Ectopic pregnancy
- Endometriosis, endometritis
- Imperforate hymen
- IUD use
- Leiomyomas
- Ovarian cysts
- Pelvic congestion syndrome, pelvic inflammatory disease
- Polyps
- Transverse vaginal septum
- Interstitial cystitis

WORKUP

- Primary dysmenorrhea: characteristic history, physical examination normal with the absence of an identifiable cause of pelvic pain
- Secondary dysmenorrhea: history of onset generally >2 yr after menarche; physical examination may reveal uterine irregularity, cul-de-sac tenderness, or nodularity or pelvic masses

LABORATORY TESTS

- No specific tests diagnostic for dysmenorrhea
- Elevated white blood cell count in the presence of infection
- Human chorionic gonadotropin to rule out ectopic pregnancy

IMAGING STUDIES

- Ultrasound scan of the pelvis to evaluate the presence of leiomyomas, ovarian cysts, or ectopic pregnancy
- Hysterosalpingogram or saline ultrasonography to assess the uterine cavity to rule out endometrial polyps or submucosal or intraluminal leiomyomas. Cystoscopy for evaluation of interstitial cystitis may also be tried.

Rx TREATMENT

NONPHARMACOLOGIC THERAPY

- Applying heat to the lower abdomen with hot compresses, heating pads, or hot water bottles seems to offer some relief.
- Other reassurance that this is a treatable condition.

ACUTE GENERAL Rx

- Nonsteroidal anti-inflammatory drugs such as ibuprofen 400 to 600 mg q4 to 6h or naproxen sodium 500 mg q12h, mefenamic acid 500 mg initial dose followed by 250 mg q6h prn
- Oral contraceptives may be effective at reducing pain in women with primary dysmenorrhea
- Nifedipine 30 mg qd in difficult cases of dysmenorrhea
- Vitamin E supplements may reduce pain compared to placebo
- Magnesium supplements have been found likely to be beneficial
- Thiamine supplements may reduce pain
- The Chinese herbal remedy toki-shakuyakusan may be effective in reducing pain. However, few studies have been of good quality
- Secondary dysmenorrhea: treatment directed to the specific underlying condition; surgery may be indicated if pathology is found on physical examination or by imaging

CHRONIC Rx

Acupuncture and transcutaneous electrical nerve stimulation may be tried. However, there is not enough evidence to support the use of yoga, acupuncture, or massage. In cases in which medical therapy has not worked, laparoscopy or other surgical treatments should be considered depending on the secondary cause of the dysmenorrhea. A directed physical examination, looking for gynecologic masses or nodularity, should be performed. Nontraditional approaches such as acupuncture have been tried with relief in some patients.

DISPOSITION

The majority of patients are satisfactorily treated with good outcomes. Possible chronic complications with primary dysmenorrhea that has not been adequately treated can lead to anxiety and depression. With certain causes of secondary dysmenorrhea, infertility can become a problem.

REFERRAL

If a secondary cause of dysmenorrhea is revealed, refer to the appropriate specialist for further medical or surgical treatment (e.g., gynecologist, urogynecologist, pain management center).

RELATED CONTENT

Dyspareunia (Related Key Topic)
Endometriosis (Related Key Topic)
Premenstrual Syndrome (Related Key Topic)
Dysmenorrhea (Patient Information)

AUTHOR: **RUBEN ALVERO, M.D.**

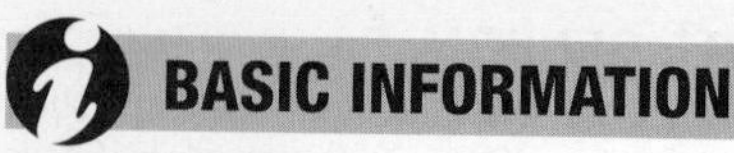

BASIC INFORMATION

DEFINITION

Persistent and/or recurrent pain associated with sexual intercourse

SYNONYMS

Painful intercourse

ICD-9CM CODES

625.0 Pain associated with female genital organs
302.76 Sexual deviations and disorders with functional dyspareunia, psychogenic dyspareunia

ICD-10CM CODES

N94.1 Dyspareunia
F52.6 Dyspareunia not due to a substance or known physiological condition

EPIDEMIOLOGY & DEMOGRAPHICS

PREVALENCE: 7% to 60% depending on definition
PREDOMINANT SEX: Female
AT-RISK POPULATION: No consistent findings regarding:

- Age
- Parity
- Educational status
- Race
- Income
- Marital status

RISK FACTORS:
Lower:

- Frequency of intercourse
- Levels of desire and arousal
- Orgasmic response
- Physical and emotional satisfaction
- General happiness

HISTORICAL FACTORS:

- Pain parameters
  1. Character
  2. Location (Introital, middle, deep)
  3. Onset
  4. Duration
  5. Timing
  6. Chronicity
  7. Cyclicity
  8. Recurrence
- Gynecologic history
  1. History of sexually transmitted disease
  2. History of herpes simplex virus (HSV) or human papillomavirus (HPV)
  3. Other sexual dysfunctions
  4. Prior abdominal or gynecologic surgery
  5. Prior pelvic or abdominal radiation
  6. History of endometriosis, fibroids
  7. History of genital or uterine prolapse
  8. History of gynecologic infection
  9. History of pelvic pain
  10. History of menopausal symptoms
  11. Sexual misinformation
- Obstetric history
  1. Lacerations
  2. Episiotomy
- General medical causes
  1. History of chronic diseases
  2. Gastrointestinal or genitourinary symptoms
  3. Medications
  4. History of psychological disorders
  5. History of dermatologic condition
  6. Religious beliefs
  7. Generalized anxiety

PHYSICAL FINDINGS & CLINICAL PRESENTATION

- Primary versus secondary dyspareunia
  1. Latter with history of pain-free coitus
- Visual inspection of lower genital tract
  1. Discoloration
  2. Ulcerations
  3. Discharge
  4. Prolapse
  5. Dysplastic changes
  6. Infestations
- Physical examination
  1. Sensitivity to light touch
  2. Tenderness to palpation
  3. Genital prolapse
     a. Uterus
     b. Bladder
     c. Cervix
     d. Vagina
     e. Adnexa
     f. Rectum
     g. Bowel
  4. Longitudinal or transverse vaginal septum
  5. Levator muscle tone
  6. Evidence of previous surgery
  7. Vaginal length, depth, caliber constrictions: Assess for shortened or absent vagina

ETIOLOGY

- Pathology or alteration or reduction of genital-associated tissue
- Psychosocial factors
- Marital or relationship discord
- History of sexual abuse

DIAGNOSIS

DIFFERENTIAL DIAGNOSIS

- Congenital deformities (septa/agenesis)
- Imperforate hymen
- Menopausal changes
- Atrophic tissue
- Impaired lubrication
- Psychogenic
- Vaginismus
- Inadequate foreplay
- Endometriosis
- Levator ani myalgia
- Chronic pelvic pain
- Previous surgery (posterior colporrhaphy, perineorrhaphy)
  1. Alteration in vaginal length, depth, caliber
  2. Adhesions
- Infectious
  1. HPV
  2. HSV
  3. Candidiasis
  4. *Tinea cruris*
  5. Acute or chronic salpingitis or endometritis
- Pelvic carcinoma
- Previous radiation
- Adnexal attachment or tubal prolapse
- Pelvic tumor
- Uterine prolapse, malposition, enlargement, or retroversion
- Genital prolapse
- Cystocele, rectocele, enterocele
- Urethral or bladder pathology
- Pelvic congestion (controversial)
- Vulvar vestibulitis
- Postcoital cystitis
- Broad ligament pathology
- Neuroma at the site of previous episiotomy
- Previous sexual abuse
- Vulvodynia
- Contact or allergic dermatitis
- Vitamin A, B, or C deficiency
- Equestrian dyspareunia
- Interstitial cystitis
- Pudendal neuralgia
- Myofascial pain syndrome
- Rectal pathology
- Structural abnormalities or alterations
  1. Muscle
  2. Bone
  3. Ligament

WORKUP

- History and physical examination are key
- If needed:
  1. Colposcopy
  2. Cystoscopy
  3. Consider laparoscopy for unexplained deep dyspareunia

LABORATORY TESTS

- Erythrocyte sedimentation rate
- White blood cell count
- Wet mount
- Cultures
  1. Cervical
     a. Gonorrhea
     b. *Chlamydia*
  2. Vaginal
  3. Lesions
  4. Urine
- Vulva, vaginal, or cervical biopsy
- Pap smear
- HSV antibodies
- Gonadotropin levels

IMAGING STUDIES

Pelvic or abdominal ultrasonography. Transvaginal ultrasonography provides for greater resolution of uterus and ovaries due to proximity to pelvic organs. MRI when diagnosis is unclear with other diagnostic modalities (Fig. 1-337).

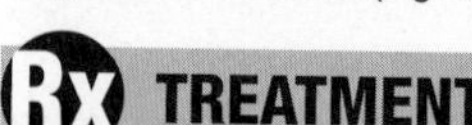

TREATMENT

NONPHARMACOLOGIC THERAPY

- Patient education
- Discontinue exacerbating activity and irritants
- Lubrication with coitus
- Coital position changes to reduce deep thrust discomfort
- Warm or cool soaks

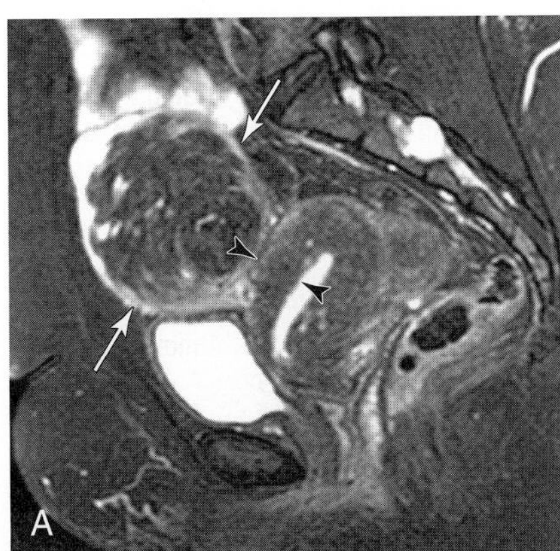

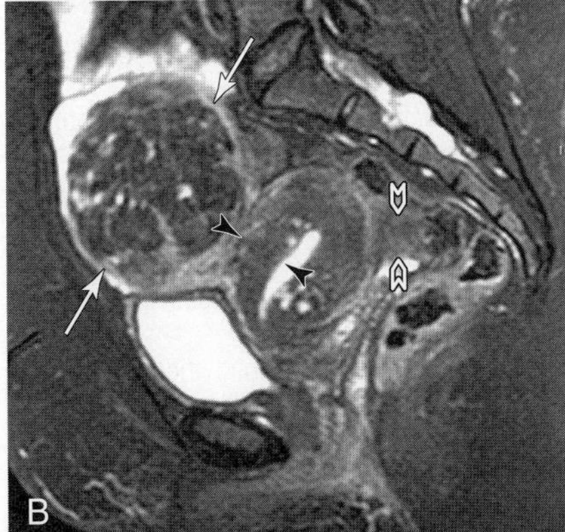

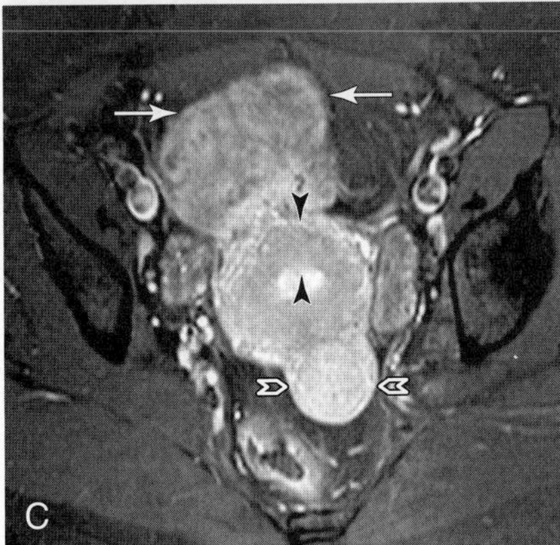

FIGURE 1-337 Adenomyosis and leiomyomata in a 41-year-old woman with pelvic pain, irregular menses, menorrhagia, and dyspareunia. A and **B,** Sagittal T2-weighted fat-suppressed images show a large anterior subserosal fibroid with mixed but predominantly low signal *(arrows),* and a smaller posterior subserosal fibroid with low to intermediate signal *(chevrons).* There is also widening of the junctional zone *(black arrowheads)* with areas of increased T2 signal, indicative of adenomyosis. **C,** Axial three-dimensional gradient echo postcontrast image with fat suppression shows enhancement of the leiomyomata *(white arrowheads and chevrons)* and the thickened junctional zone *(black arrowheads).* (From Fielding JR et al: *Gynecologic imaging,* Philadelphia, 2011, Saunders.)

- Reassurance to patient of nonmalignant condition
- Psychosocial interventions
  1. Systemic desensitization techniques
  2. Behavior modification
- Vaginal dilators
- Vaginal muscle exercises and relaxation techniques
- Excision of pathologic tissue
- Surgical correction of altered, reduced, or deformed tissues

ACUTE GENERAL Rx

- Topical lidocaine, non-hormonal moisturizers and lubricants
- Corticosteroids
- Antiinfective agents if vaginitis found
- Trigger point injections
- Massage/physical therapy
- Acupuncture
- Transcutaneous electrical nerve stimulation
- Stress reduction techniques
- Safe sexual practices
- Hormonal replacement therapy. The FDA has recently approved ospemifene, an oral estrogen agonist/antagonist for treatment of moderate to severe dyspareunia in postmenopausal women with suspected vaginal atrophy.
- Antiviral agents
- Intralesional interferon
- Mild analgesics
- Antidepressants

CHRONIC Rx

All the previous plus:

- Set supportive visits as needed
- Oral contraceptives
- Regular sexual activity
- Balanced diet
- Vitamin supplementation
- Proper hygiene

DISPOSITION

Most patients will have a reduction and/or resolution of their symptoms by using the appropriate therapeutic approaches.

REFERRAL

As with other chronic pain conditions, a multidisciplinary approach using the expertise of psychologists, dermatologists, gynecologic surgeons, infectious disease specialists, or urologists is helpful.

PEARLS & CONSIDERATIONS

- Dyspareunia is a symptom complex resulting from a multitude of etiologies, some of which act simultaneously.
- Uncovering the etiology of dyspareunia is predominantly based on a comprehensive history and physical examination.
- The differential diagnoses can be sorted into superficial, intermediate, and deep dyspareunia categories.
- As with the physical evaluation of any painful condition, attempt—by precise touching (moistened cotton swab), palpation, or applied pressure—to reproduce the patient's chief complaint.
- Performing a one-finger pelvic examination without concurrent abdominal palpation allows a more precise assessment of the source of genital pain.
- Individualize therapy.
- Initiate and maintain an honest diagnosis and compassionate demeanor with the patient and her partner.
- Be open minded, approachable, nonjudgmental, and diligent in your search for a solution to help these often silently suffering patients.

SUGGESTED READINGS

available at www.expertconsult.com

RELATED CONTENT

Painful Intercourse (Patient Information)
Dysmenorrhea (Related Key Topic)
Endometriosis (Related Key Topic)

AUTHORS: **DAVID I. KURSS, M.D.,** and **RUBEN ALVERO, M.D.**

BASIC INFORMATION

DEFINITION

Nonulcerative dyspepsia is a term used to describe signs and symptoms of persistent or recurrent dyspepsia centered in the upper abdomen that have no identifiable organic cause

SYNONYMS

Functional dyspepsia
Idiopathic dyspepsia

ICD-9CM CODES
536.8 Nonulcerative dyspepsia
ICD-10CM CODES
K30 Functional dyspepsia

EPIDEMIOLOGY & DEMOGRAPHICS

- Up to 25% of the general population will experience dyspepsia each year. Of these, 75% will have no evident causative agent.

PHYSICAL FINDINGS & CLINICAL PRESENTATION

Typical clinical presentation is dyspepsia without findings on physical examination to explain the symptoms

ETIOLOGY

The etiology and pathophysiology are still unclear. Research is focused on abnormalities of gastric motor function and visceral hypersensitivity.

- *Helicobacter pylori* infection
- Psychosocial factors—associated with anxiety and depression

RISK FACTORS

Risk factors include:

- Dietary habits such as caffeine, alcohol, or smoking.
- Medications such as NSAIDs, calcium channel blockers, methylxanthines, alendronate, orlistat, acarbose, and potassium supplements.
- Psychological disorders such as anxiety, depression, or personal history of childhood abuse

Dx DIAGNOSIS

DIFFERENTIAL DIAGNOSIS

Nonulcerative dyspepsia is diagnosed when all other organic causes have been excluded, including:

- PUD
- Gastroesophageal reflux
- Gastric/esophageal/other abdominal cancers
- Biliary tract disease
- Gastroparesis, including diabetic gastroparesis
- Pancreatitis
- Medications (i.e., NSAIDs, erythromycin)
- Metabolic disturbances (i.e., hypercalcemia, heavy metals, or hyperkalemia)
- Ischemic bowel disease
- Systemic disorders (i.e., eosinophilic gastritis, Crohn's disease, sarcoidosis, celiac disease, thyroid disorders)

DIAGNOSIS

Developed in 2006 in conjunction with the American Gastroenterological Association, the Rome III criteria lists the following factors, which must be present for the past 3 months and first noticed within 6 months of diagnosis:

- At least one of the following:
  - Postprandial fullness, *or*
  - Early satiety, *or*
  - Epigastric pain, *or*
  - Epigastric burning
- *and* no evidence of structural disease likely to explain the symptoms

WORKUP

The American Gastroenterological Association, as well as the Maastricht III and the IV European consensus, suggest the following:

- The pattern of symptoms overlaps considerably for all types of dyspepsia; therefore, the history and physical should focus on finding specific symptoms that help exclude other causes of dyspepsia.
- Endoscopy should be performed only in patients >55 yr and younger patients with alarming symptoms (e.g., weight loss, progressive dysphagia, recurrent vomiting, evidence of gastrointestinal bleeding, or family history of cancer) presenting with new-onset dyspepsia. Findings consistent with diagnosis of nonulcerative dyspepsia are not conclusive, no presence of *H. pylori*, no signs of gastroesophageal reflux disease, no mucosal inflammation. NOTE: Patients <55 yr and without any alarming symptoms can be treated without endoscopy.

LABORATORY TESTS

H. pylori: Laboratory methods include serologic tests*, monoclonal stool antigen, or urea breath test.

Rx TREATMENT

ACUTE GENERAL Rx

PHARMACOLOGIC THERAPY: Primary treatment is usually initiated with proton pump inhibitors (PPIs), which can be started without performing endoscopy, especially if the patient comes from a population with low prevalence of *H. pylori* infection. If symptoms persist, a trial of antidepressants can be started.

*Serologic testing for *H. pylori* has a low predictive value because colonization is lifelong; it can therefore determine prevalence better than incidence.

Treatment of accompanying symptoms includes:

Predominant Symptom	Possible Etiology	Medication Recommended
Nausea	Motility dysfunction	Prokinetic agent
Bloating	Motility dysfunction	Simethicone and/or prokinetic agent
Pain	Mucosal disease or *H. pylori* infection	Antibiotic trial
Somatic complaints	Psychosocial	Psychotropic medication trial

Medication categories:

- Antacids (i.e., aluminum hydroxide, calcium carbonate)
- Gas-reducing agents, such as those containing simethicone
- H_2-receptor antagonists (i.e., cimetidine)
- PPIs (i.e., omeprazole)
- Prokinetic agents (i.e., metoclopramide)
- Antidepressants (i.e., selective serotonin receptor inhibitors)
- *H. pylori* therapy/antibiotic therapy (various antibiotic regimens, usually 1 PPI)

CHRONIC Rx

Controversy currently exists around the long-term use of PPIs.

COMPLEMENTARY & ALTERNATIVE THERAPIES

Peppermint and caraway oil may be helpful, as well as acupuncture; however, no definitive trials have been performed.

REFERRAL

- Referral to gastroenterology if patient with alarming symptoms (such as GI bleeding, dysphagia, odynophagia, unexplained anemia, change in appetite, and weight loss) or when endoscopy is indicated—although controversy exists about the workup of younger patients.
- Referral to cardiology if cardiac etiology suspected.

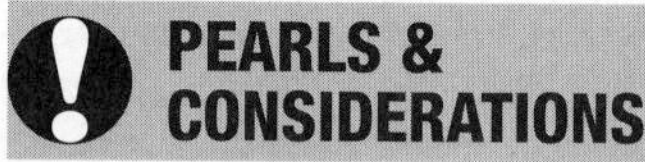

PEARLS & CONSIDERATIONS

PREVENTION

Avoid excessive amounts of caffeine, alcohol, smoking, or long-term use of steroids and NSAIDs.

PATIENT AND FAMILY EDUCATION

http://www.mayoclinic.com/health/stomach-pain/DS00524

SUGGESTED READINGS
available at www.expertconsult.com

RELATED CONTENT

Fig. 3-64 Approach to the patient with dyspepsia (Algorithm)

AUTHORS: **ALVARO MENENDEZ, M.D.,** and **NADINE MBUYI, M.D.**

BASIC INFORMATION

DEFINITION

The term "dysphagia" is derived from the Greek words *dys* (with difficulty) and *phagia* (to eat). It is characterized by abnormal transfer of food from mouth to the stomach, which may involve the oral, pharyngeal, or esophageal stages of swallowing.

ICD-9CM CODES
782.2 Dysphagia
ICD-10CM CODES
R13.10 Dysphagia, unspecified

EPIDEMIOLOGY & DEMOGRAPHICS

- This is seen in 10% of individuals above the age of 50 yr. Its prevalence increases with advancing age.
- Nearly 12% of hospitalized patients have symptoms of dysphagia.
- Up to 30% to 60% of nursing home patients have some form of dysphagia.
- Special populations, including patients with head injury, stroke, or Parkinson's disease, have 30% to 50% prevalence of oropharyngeal dysphagia.

ETIOLOGY

- Oropharyngeal
  1. Neuromuscular causes
     - Stroke
     - Parkinson's disease
     - Multiple sclerosis
     - Myasthenia gravis
     - Amyotrophic lateral sclerosis
     - CNS tumors
     - Muscular dystrophy
     - Thyroid dysfunction
     - Polymyositis and dermatomyositis
     - Sarcoidosis
     - Cerebral palsy
     - Head trauma
     - Metabolic encephalopathy
     - Dementia
     - Bell's palsy
  2. Structural causes
     - Oropharyngeal tumors
     - Zenker's diverticulum
     - Infection of pharynx or neck (mucositis from *Candida,* herpes, and CMV)
     - Thyromegaly
     - Prior surgery or radiotherapy
     - Osteophytes and other spinal disorders
     - Proximal esophageal webs
     - Congenital anomalies (e.g., cleft palate)
     - Poor dentition
- Esophageal
  1. Neuromuscular disorders
     - Achalasia
     - Diffuse esophageal spasm
     - Nutcracker esophagus
     - Hypertensive lower esophageal sphincter
     - Ineffective esophageal motility
     - Scleroderma
     - Reflex-associated dysmotility
  2. Structural disorder
     - Peptic stricture
     - Esophageal rings and webs
     - Diverticuli
     - Carcinoma and benign tumors
     - Foreign bodies
     - Vascular compression
     - Mediastinal masses
     - Spinal osteophytes
     - Mucosal injury (from pills, infection, gastroesophageal reflux disease [GERD], etc.)

PATHOGENESIS

The inability to swallow is caused either by a problem in strength or coordination of the muscles required to move material from the mouth to stomach or by a fixed obstruction somewhere between the mouth and the stomach.

CLINICAL FEATURES

Oropharyngeal dysphagia

- Problem arises within 2 seconds of initiating the voluntary phase of swallowing.
- Typical symptoms include drooling, spillage of food, postnasal regurgitation, difficulty in initiation of swallowing, sialorrhea, sensation of food stuck in the neck, coughing or choking during swallowing, the need to swallow repeatedly to clear food or fluid from the pharynx, dysphonia, nasal speech, hoarseness of voice, and dysarthria.
- A thorough physical examination including that of the nervous system, oral cavity, and the head/neck is very important in patients with oropharyngeal dysphagia.

Esophageal dysphagia

- Problem usually arises several seconds after swallowing.
- Patients often complain of food being stuck in lower substernal area.
- Dysphagia to solids suggests mechanical obstruction.
- Neuromuscular causes result in dysphagia to both solids and liquids. Particularly, patients with achalasia tend to drink a lot of fluids while eating or apply maneuvers such as straightening the back, raising their arms over their heads, or standing to increase intraesophageal pressure to facilitate the emptying of food into the stomach.
- Oftentimes, ingestion of very cold or very hot foods precipitates the dysphagia associated with neuromuscular disorder.
- Delayed regurgitation of food, heartburn, and chest pain are usually present.
- Weight loss is usually associated with malignancy or achalasia.
- Symptoms are intermittent in patients with esophageal dysphagia from benign causes of structural obstruction or diffuse esophageal spasm. However, it is progressive in patients with peptic stricture, esophageal carcinoma, scleroderma, and achalasia.
- In patients with structural obstruction, when the luminal diameter is more than 18 to 20 mm, they are rarely symptomatic, whereas those with a diameter of less than 13 mm are nearly always symptomatic.
- These patients with esophageal dysphagia usually do not have any characteristic physical findings.

Dx DIAGNOSIS

Laboratory evaluation

- CBC
- Thyroid studies
- Nutritional assessment by checking serum protein and albumin levels
- Other studies based on specific clinical conditions

Special studies

- Oropharyngeal dysphagia
  1. Videofluoroscopy is the first test often ordered in evaluation of patients with oropharyngeal dysphagia
  2. Double contrast modified barium swallow study (Fig. E1-338)
  3. Fiberoptic flexible nasopharyngeal laryngoscopy is mandatory in all cases when a structural lesion, particularly malignancy, is suspected.
  4. Pharyngeal and upper esophageal manometry (Fig. E1-339) is occasionally of value to predict which patients will have a favorable outcome from cricopharyngeal myotomy or dilation.
  5. Radiography of head and neck when indicated
- Esophageal dysphagia
  1. Barium esophagography should precede upper endoscopies to identify patients at risk from potential perforation with an endoscopy and to help plan fluoroscopically guided dilation. It is often the first step in evaluating patients with dysphagia, especially if an obstructive lesion is suspected.
  2. EGD
  3. Esophageal manometry is indicated if no abnormality is identified by barium study or EGD.
  4. Esophageal pH monitoring in patients with suspected reflux disease
  5. Endoscopic ultrasonography
  6. Radiograph, CT, and MRI of chest

DIFFERENTIAL DIAGNOSIS

(Fig. 1-340)

- Globus pharyngeus
- Odynophagia
- Phagophobia
- GERD

Rx TREATMENT

- Treatment should be approached with the help of specialists of multiple disciplines (ENT, head and neck surgeon, radiologist, speech pathologist, physical therapist, dietitian, gastroenterologist, physical medicine and rehabilitation specialist, dentist, neurologist, etc.).
- Goal of therapy is airway protection and maintenance of nutrition.
- Alteration of food consistency, volume, and delivery rate plays a major role.

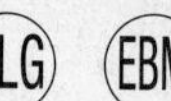

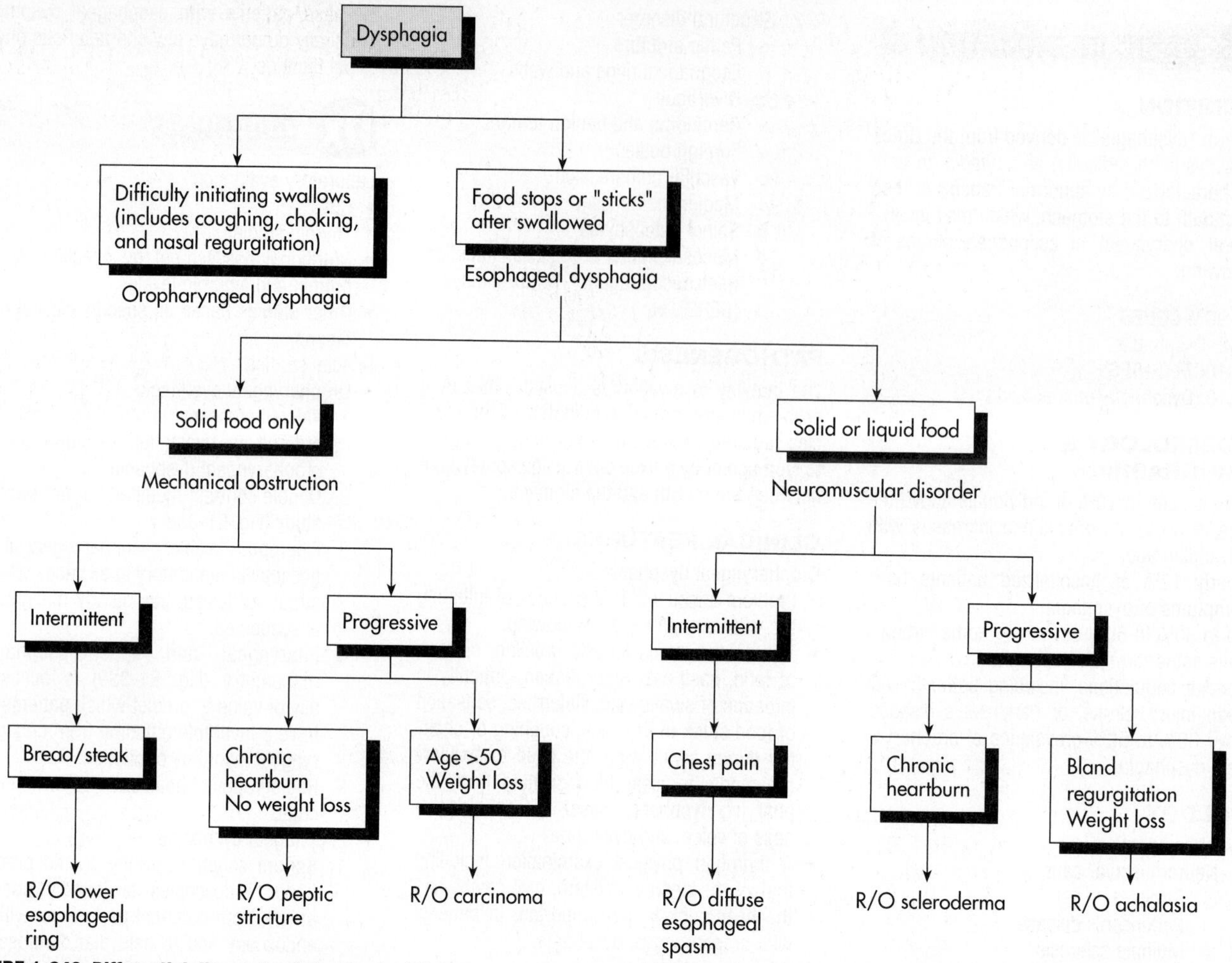

- Dysphagia
  - Difficulty initiating swallows (includes coughing, choking, and nasal regurgitation) — Oropharyngeal dysphagia
  - Food stops or "sticks" after swallowed — Esophageal dysphagia
    - Solid food only — Mechanical obstruction
      - Intermittent
        - Bread/steak → R/O lower esophageal ring
      - Progressive
        - Chronic heartburn No weight loss → R/O peptic stricture
        - Age >50 Weight loss → R/O carcinoma
    - Solid or liquid food — Neuromuscular disorder
      - Intermittent
        - Chest pain → R/O diffuse esophageal spasm
      - Progressive
        - Chronic heartburn → R/O scleroderma
        - Bland regurgitation Weight loss → R/O achalasia

FIGURE 1-340 Differential diagnosis of dysphagia. *RO,* Rule out. (Modified from Andreoli TE [ed]: *Cecil essentials of medicine,* ed 7, Philadelphia, 2008, Saunders.)

- The goal of direct therapy is to change swallowing physiology with medical treatment of primary disease, maxillofacial prosthesis, and cricopharyngeal myotomy
- Indirect therapies include exercise programs for tongue coordination and chewing under the guidance of a speech therapist.
- Maintenance of oral feeding often requires compensatory techniques such as chin-tuck position, rotation of head to the affected side, tilting of head to the strong side, and lying on one's back or on one's side during swallowing.
- Some of the voluntary maneuvers applied include supraglottic swallow, effortful swallow, Mendelson maneuver, Shaker exercise, and the Heimlich maneuver.
- Placement of nasogastric tube, jejunostomy tube, or percutaneous endoscopic gastrotomy (PEG) tube is considered for enteral feeding when other measures fail and the patient remains at significant risk for aspiration or nutrition becomes compromised.
- Treatment of associated GERD should not be forgotten.
- Surgery for chronic aspiration may involve tracheostomy, medialization, laryngeal suspension, laryngeal closure, and/or laryngotracheal separation-diversion.
- Other measures include esophageal dilation removal of foreign body, esophageal resection, chemotherapy, radiotherapy, endoscopic ablation of tumor, photodynamic therapy, esophageal prosthesis/stents, diverticulectomy, intrasphincteric injection of botulinum toxin, surgical myotomy, and others. Smooth muscle relaxants such as nitrates and calcium channel blockers have been used to effectively treat patients with diffuse esophageal spasm and nutcracker esophagus.
- Several scales have been suggested to determine patients' functional outcome. One of them is the "Swallowing Rating Scale."

COMPLICATIONS

- Dehydration
- Malnutrition
- Aspiration pneumonia
- Airway obstruction
- Death resulting from pulmonary complications

PROGNOSIS

- Depends on the etiology.
- Nursing home patients with oropharyngeal dysphagia and a history of aspiration have an approximately 45% mortality rate over 1 yr.
- All patients, especially the elderly, should take their medications with a full glass of water while in upright position well before bedtime.
- Dysphagia should be considered an alarm symptom, indicating the need for immediate evaluation.

PATIENT EDUCATION

Elderly patients with dysphagia should not attribute their symptoms to aging.

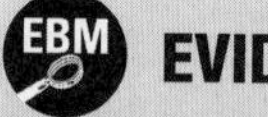

EVIDENCE

available at www.expertconsult.com

SUGGESTED READINGS

available at www.expertconsult.com

RELATED CONTENT

Esophageal Tumors (Related Key Topic)
Gastroesophageal Reflux Disease (Related Key Topic)
Dyspepsia, Nonulcerative (Related Key Topic)

AUTHOR: **HEMANT K. SATPATHY, M.D.**

BASIC INFORMATION

DEFINITION

Dystonia refers to a group of disorders characterized by involuntary muscle contractions (sustained or spasmodic) that lead to abnormal body movements or postures. Dystonia can be generalized or focal, of early (<20 yr) or late onset, and primary or secondary.

SYNONYMS

Blepharospasm
Oromandibular (orofacial) dystonia
Spasmodic (limb or axial) dystonia
Torticollis
Writer's cramp

ICD-10CM CODES

G24	Dystonia
G24.1	Idiopathic familial dystonia
G24.0	Drug induced dystonia
G24.3	Spasmodic torticollis

EPIDEMIOLOGY & DEMOGRAPHICS

PREVALENCE: Estimated at one in 3000 persons.
PREDOMINANT SEX: Cervical dystonia has a 3:2 female preponderance.
PREDOMINANT AGE:
- Onset of focal cervical dystonia is usually in the fifth decade.
- Hereditary forms may have an onset in childhood or adulthood and tend to be more severe.

GENETICS: Autosomal-dominant, autosomal-recessive, and X-linked forms of dystonia have been identified. Ashkenazi Jews are particularly susceptible to primary early-onset dystonia.

CLINICAL PRESENTATION

Focal dystonias produce abnormal sustained muscle contractions in a single region of the body:
- Neck (***torticollis***): most commonly affected site with a tendency for the head to turn to one side
- Eyelids (***blepharospasm***): involuntary closure of the eyelids that leads to excessive eye blinking, sometimes with persistent eye closure and functional blindness
- Mouth (***oromandibular dystonia***): involuntary contraction of muscles of the mouth, tongue, or face
- Hand (***writer's cramp***) (Fig. 1-341)

Generalized dystonia affects multiple areas of the body and can lead to marked joint deformities.
- Isolated foot dystonia is very rare and may suggest an underlying parkinsonian disorder or brain structural abnormality

ETIOLOGY

- Exact pathophysiology of primary dystonia is unknown but believed to involve abnormalities of basal ganglia. Specifically, reduced and abnormal patterns of neuronal activity in the basal ganglia result in disinhibition of the motor thalamus and cortex, leading to abnormal movement.
- Fifteen hereditary forms have been described, including the severe progressive form, dystonia musculorum deformans.
- Secondary dystonia results from central nervous system (CNS) disease of the basal ganglia (stroke, demyelination, hypoxia, trauma), Huntington's disease, Wilson's disease, Parkinson syndromes, and lysosomal storage diseases.
- Acute dystonia can occur with drugs that block dopamine receptors, such as phenothiazines or butyrophenones.
- Tardive dyskinesia can result from long-term treatment with antiemetics (e.g., phenothiazines), antipsychotics (e.g., haloperidol), levodopa, anticonvulsants, or ergots.

DIAGNOSIS

DIFFERENTIAL DIAGNOSIS

- Parkinson's disease
- Progressive supranuclear palsy
- Wilson's disease
- Huntington's disease
- Drug effects
- Table 1-170 describes selected causes of primary and secondary dystonia in childhood

WORKUP

History (family history, birth history, trauma, medication use), physical examination

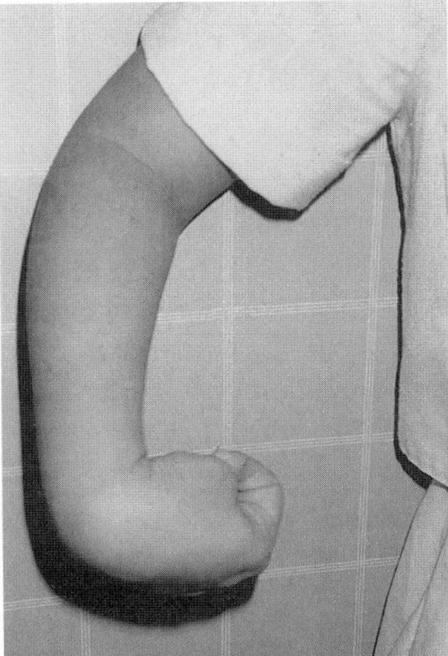

FIGURE 1-341 Focal dystonia of the distal right arm. (From Goldman L, Ausiello D [eds]: *Cecil textbook of medicine,* ed 22, Philadelphia, 2004, Saunders.)

LABORATORY TESTS

- Usually not helpful for diagnosis
- Serum ceruloplasmin if Wilson's disease is suspected

IMAGING STUDIES

- Primary dystonias are generally not associated with structural CNS abnormalities. CT scan or MRI of brain if a CNS lesion is suspected as a cause of secondary dystonia.
- Electrophysiologic testing can provide diagnostic support for the diagnosis.

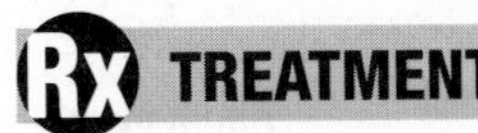

TREATMENT

NONPHARMACOLOGIC THERAPY

- Heat, massage, physical therapy to relieve pain
- Splints to prevent contractures

ACUTE GENERAL Rx

For acute dystonic reactions to phenothiazines/butyrophenones, use diphenhydramine 50 mg IV or benztropine 2 mg IV.

CHRONIC Rx

- Pharmacologic treatment is often ineffective.
- Slowly withdraw offending agents.
- Diazepam, baclofen, or carbamazepine may be helpful.
- Intrathecal baclofen is most useful for spastic or truncal dystonia.
- Trihexyphenidyl or benztropine may be helpful in up to 50% of tardive dystonias.
- For generalized dystonia, a trial of carbidopa/levodopa may be beneficial and diagnostic of dopa-responsive dystonia (DYT5).
- Injections of botulinum toxin into the affected muscles is the standard treatment for focal dystonias. Both type A and type B toxins produced by *Clostridium botulinum* block cholinergic transmission at the neuromuscular junction by inhibiting release of acetylcholine. There are currently several botulinum toxins (Botox, Dysport, Xeomin, Myobloc) FDA approved for cervical dystonia. Botox and Xeomin are also FDA approved for blepharospasm.
- Surgical procedures, including denervation, myectomy, rhizotomy, thalamotomy (pallidotomy), or functional stereotactic surgery, may be helpful for severe, refractory cases.
- Deep brain stimulation is becoming more promising, especially for refractory primary generalized dystonias.

DISPOSITION

Spontaneous remission of focal cervical dystonia can occur, but dystonia is generally progressive and pharmacologic therapy is often ineffective.

REFERRAL

Neurology and/or neurosurgery for severe or refractory cases.
Physical therapy for maintaining flexibility.

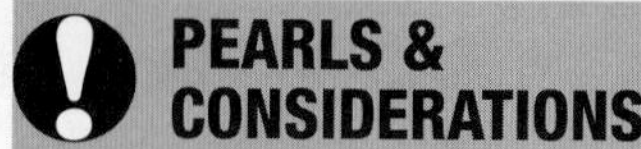

COMMENTS

- Avoid triggers/exacerbating factors.
- Early physical therapy and splinting to prevent contractures.
- Consider botulism injections or deep brain stimulation surgery for severe or refractory dystonia, and for focal dystonias.

SUGGESTED READINGS

available at www.expertconsult.com

AUTHORS: **LYNN MCNICOLL, M.D., F.R.C.P.C.,** and **JULIE L. ROTH, M.D.**

TABLE 1-170 Selected Causes of Primary and Secondary Dystonia in Childhood

Diagnosis	Additional Clinical Features	Diagnosis	Additional Clinical Features
Aicardi-Goutieres syndrome	Encephalopathy, developmental regression Acquired microcephaly Sterile pyrexias Lesions on the digits, ears (chilblain) Epilepsy CT: calcification of the basal ganglia	Leigh syndrome	Motor delays, weakness, hypotonia Ataxia, tremor Elevated lactate MRI: bilateral symmetric hyperintense lesions in the basal ganglia or thalamus
Alternating hemiplegia of childhood	Episodic hemiplegia/quadriplegia Abnormal ocular movements Autonomic symptoms Epilepsy Global developmental impairment Environmental triggers for spells	Lesch-Nyhan syndrome (X-linked)	Male Self-injurious behavior Hypotonia Oromandibular dystonia, inspiratory stridor Oculomotor apraxia Cognitive impairment Elevated uric acid
Aromatic amino acid decarboxylase deficiency (AADC)	Developmental delay Oculogyric crises Autonomic dysfunction Hypotonia	Myoclonus dystonia	Myoclonus Head, upper limb involvement
ARX gene mutation (X-linked)	Male Cognitive impairment Infantile spasms, epilepsy Brain malformation	Niemann-Pick type C	Hepatosplenomegaly Hypotonia Supranuclear gaze palsy Ataxia, dysarthria Epilepsy Psychiatric symptoms
Benign paroxysmal torticollis of infancy	Episodic Cervical dystonia only Family history of migraine	Neuroacanthocytosis	Oromandibular and lingual dystonia
		Neurodegeneration with brain iron accumulation	Cognitive impairment Retinal pigmentary degeneration, optic atrophy
Complex regional pain syndrome	Lower limb involvement Prominent pain	Rapid onset dystonia parkinsonism (DYT12)	Acute onset Distribution face>arm>leg Prominent bulbar signs
Dopa-responsive dystonia (DRD)	Diurnal variation		
Drug-induced dystonia		Rett syndrome	Female Developmental regression following a period of normal development Stereotypic hand movements Acquired microcephaly Epilepsy
Dystonia-deafness optic neuropathy syndrome	Sensorineural hearing loss in early childhood Psychosis Optic atrophy in adolescence		
DYT1 dystonia	Lower limb onset followed by generalization		
Glutaric aciduria type 1	Macrocephaly Encephalopathic crises MRI: striatal necrosis	Spinocerebellar ataxia 17 (SCA17)	Ataxia Dementia, psychiatric symptoms Parkinsonism
GM1 gangliosidosis type 3	Short stature, skeletal dysplasia Orofacial dystonia Speech/swallowing disturbance Parkinsonism MRI: putaminal hyperintensity	Tics	Stereotyped movements Premonitory urge, suppressible
		Tyrosine hydroxylase deficiency	Infantile encephalopathy, hypotonia Oculogyric crises, ptosis Autonomic symptoms Less diurnal fluctuation than DRD
Huntington disease (HD)	Parkinsonism Epilepsy Family history of HD		
Kernicterus	Jaundice in infancy Hearing loss Impaired upgaze Enamel dysplasia MRI: hyperintense lesions in the globus pallidus		

From Kliegman RM et al: *Nelson textbook of pediatrics,* ed 19, Philadelphia, 2011, Saunders.

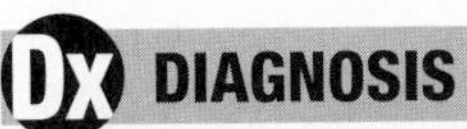

BASIC INFORMATION

DEFINITION

Echinococcosis is a chronic infection caused by the larval stage of several animal cestodes (tapeworms) of the genus *Echinococcus.*

SYNONYMS

Hydatid disease

ICD-9CM CODES
122.9 *Echinococcus* infection
ICD-10CM CODES
B67.90 Echinococcosis, unspecified

EPIDEMIOLOGY & DEMOGRAPHICS

INCIDENCE (IN U.S.): Seen primarily in immigrants, but local transmission can occur in southwestern U.S., California, and Alaska.
PEAK INCIDENCE: Presumed to be acquired in childhood or early adulthood in most cases.
PREVALENCE (IN U.S.): See Incidence
PREDOMINANT SEX: Male = female
PREDOMINANT AGE: 0 to 50 yr of age

PHYSICAL FINDINGS & CLINICAL PRESENTATION

- Signs of an enlarging mass lesion in a visceral site such as the liver, lungs, kidneys, bone, or CNS
- Occasional cyst rupture causing allergic manifestations such as urticaria, angioedema, or anaphylaxis that bring the patient to medical attention
- Incidental discovery of cysts by abdominal or thoracic imaging studies performed for other reasons

ETIOLOGY

- Four species of *Echinococcus: E. granulosus, E. multilocularis, E. oligarthrus,* and *E. vogeli.*
  1. *E. granulosus* is the cause of cystic hydatid disease.
  2. *E. multilocularis* and *E. vogeli* are the causes of alveolar and polycystic disease.
- The disease is transmitted to humans by infected canines (domestic or wild dogs, wolves, foxes), which are the definitive hosts, and seen most commonly in livestock-producing areas of the Middle East, Africa, Australia, New Zealand, Europe, and the Americas, including the southwestern U.S., whereby sheep, goats, camels, or cattle serve as intermediate hosts to humans. Humans are incidental hosts and do not play a role in the transmission cycle.
- The adult tapeworm resides in the small intestine of the canine definitive hosts. Eggs are then shed in the feces of infected canines; human infection occurs by ingestion of viable eggs in contaminated food from intermediate hosts or direct fecal-oral transmission.
- After ingestion of the eggs by intermediate hosts or humans, eggs hatch and release oncospheres, which migrate through intestinal mucosa to definitive organs and develop into enlarging fluid-filled cysts known as hydatid cysts (metacestode).
- It is common in many areas of the world, especially the Middle East.

DIAGNOSIS

DIFFERENTIAL DIAGNOSIS

- Cystic neoplasms (see Table 1-171)
- Abscess (amebic or bacterial)
- Congenital polycystic disease

WORKUP

- Antibody assay
- Imaging study (CT scan [Fig. 1-342], ultrasonography)
- Classification (Fig. 1-343): Table 1-172 describes the World Health Organization Informal Working Group on Echinococcosis classification of hepatic echinococcal cysts.
- Histologic examination of cyst or contents obtained by aspiration or resection (if possible) to confirm diagnosis

LABORATORY TESTS

Antibody assays (ELISA or Western blot) available through CDC: 80% to 100% sensitive and 88% to 96% specific for liver cysts, but less accurate for cysts in other sites, such as lung. A PCR assay is now available for problematic cases. Eosinophilia is not consistently seen and thus not a reliable test.

IMAGING STUDIES

Ultrasonography, CT, and MRI:
- All are extremely sensitive for the detection of cysts, especially in the liver.
- All lack specificity and are inadequate to establish the diagnosis of echinococcosis with certainty.

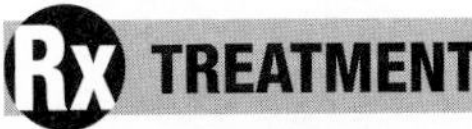

TREATMENT

ACUTE GENERAL Rx

- Albendazole 400 mg PO bid followed by percutaneous aspiration-injection-reaspiration (PAIR) for uncomplicated larval cysts. It consists of puncture (P) and needle aspirate (A) of cyst content followed by inspiration (I) of hypertonic saline (15%-30%) or absolute alcohol, waiting 20 to 30 minutes, then reaspirating (R) with final irrigation. Albendazole is continued for 28 days. Cure rate is 96%.
- Surgical resection: cure rate 90%
- Alternatives to albendazole include mebendazole and praziquantel alone or in combination with mebendazole.

DISPOSITION

- Long-term follow-up is necessary following surgical or medical therapy because of the potential for late relapse.
- Antibody assays and imaging studies are repeated every 6 to 12 mo for several years following successful surgical or medical therapy.

REFERRAL

All patients for evaluation for possible surgical resection of cysts versus PAIR

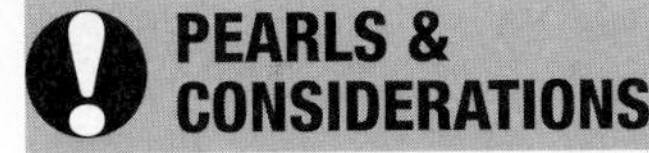

PEARLS & CONSIDERATIONS

COMMENTS

Cyst resection, if indicated, should be performed by surgeons experienced with this procedure.

SUGGESTED READINGS

available at www.expertconsult.com

RELATED CONTENT

Echinococcosis (Patient Information)

AUTHOR: **GLENN G. FORT, M.D., M.P.H.**

TABLE 1-171 Hepatic Cyst Disease: Differential Features on Imaging Studies

Characteristics	Hydatid Cyst	Congenital Cyst	Cystadenoma
Configuration	Cyst within cyst	Single or multiple ± septations	Single ± septations
Wall character	Thick, uniform ± calcification	Thin, uniform	Mural nodules
Cyst contents	Daughter cysts Hydatid sand	Low density	Low density

From Cameron JL, Cameron AM: *Current surgical therapy,* ed 10, Philadelphia, 2011, Saunders.

 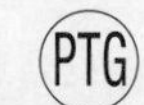

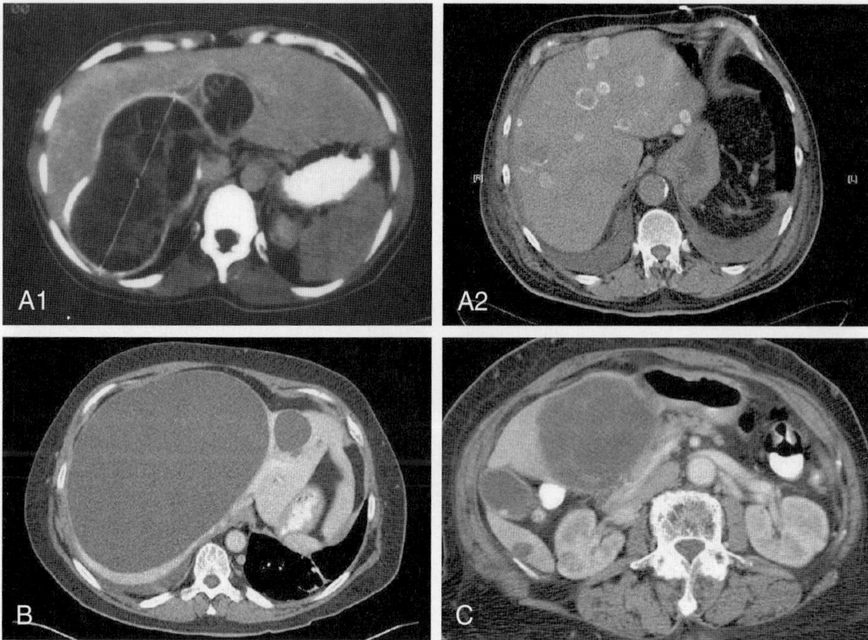

FIGURE 1-342 A comparison of computed tomography scans. A, Hepatic echinococcal cysts. **B,** Congenital cyst. **C,** Cystadenoma. For echinococcal cyst. **A1** demonstrates a single cyst with calcification and daughter cyst caused by *E. granulosa.* **A2** shows multiple small cysts characteristic of *E. multilocularis* infection. (Courtesy Barbara M. Kadell, MD, Professor of Radiology, David Geffen School of Medicine at University of California, Los Angeles. From Cameron JL, Cameron AM: *Current surgical therapy,* ed 10, Philadelphia, 2011, Saunders.)

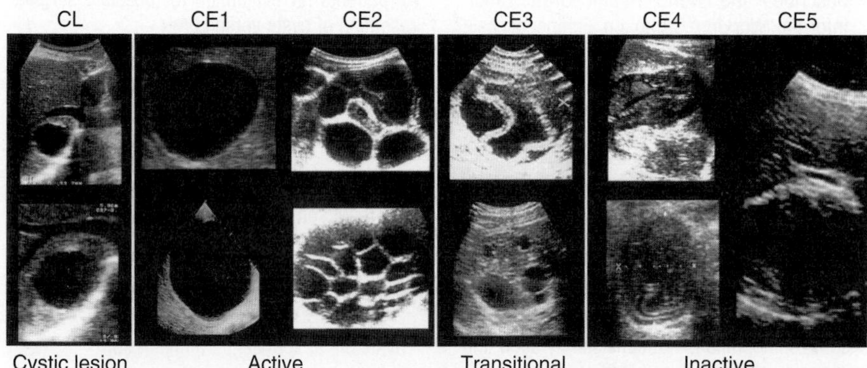

FIGURE 1-343 WHO Informal Working Group on Echinococcosis standardized ultrasound classification of cystic echinococcosis. CL lesions are cystic lesions lacking a distinct wall and may have other diagnoses. CE1 lesions are cystic lesions with a visible wall that may demonstrate protoscolices ("hydatid sand"). CE2 lesions include internal septation. CE3 lesions may be detached from the wall or have daughter cysts with internal thickening. CE4 lesions are heterogeneous lesions with degeneration. CE5 lesions show thick calcification. (From Goldman L, Schafer AI: *Goldman's Cecil medicine*, ed 24, Philadelphia, 2012, Saunders.)

TABLE 1-172 WHO-IWGE Classification of Hepatic Echinococcal Cysts

Type of Cyst	Status	Ultrasound Features	Remarks
CL	Active	Signs not pathognomonic, unilocular, no cyst wall	Usually early stage, not fertile; differential diagnosis necessary
CE 1	Active	Cyst wall, hydatid sand	Usually fertile
CE 2	Active	Multivesicular, cyst wall, rosette-like	Usually fertile
CE 3	Transitional	Detached laminated membrane, "water lily" sign, less round, decreased intracystic pressure	Starting to degenerate, may produce daughter cyst
CE 4	Inactive	Heterogeneous hypoechogenic or hyperechogenic degenerative contents; no daughter cyst	Usually no living protoscolices; differential diagnosis necessary
CE 5	Inactive	Thick, calcified wall, calcification partial to complete; not pathognomonic but highly suggestive of diagnosis	Usually no living protoscolices

WHO-IWGE, World Health Organization Informal Working Group on Echinococcosis.
From Cameron JL, Cameron AM: *Current surgical therapy,* ed 10, Philadelphia, 2011, Saunders.

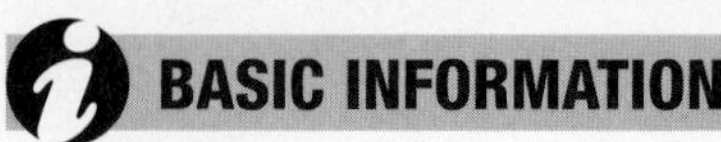

BASIC INFORMATION

DEFINITION

Eclampsia is the occurrence of seizures or coma in a woman with preeclampsia, occurring at >20 wk of gestation or <48 hr postpartum. Atypical eclampsia occurs at <20 wk of gestation or as much as 14 days postpartum.

SYNONYMS

Toxemia
Seizures of pregnancy

ICD-9CM CODES
642.6 Eclampsia
ICD-10CM CODES
O15.9 Eclampsia, unspecified as to time period

EPIDEMIOLOGY & DEMOGRAPHICS

INCIDENCE: One case per 150 to 3000 pregnancies; 2% to 4% of those with preeclampsia
GENETICS: Increased incidence with a first-degree relative (sister or mother) having had eclampsia
RISK FACTORS: Multifetal gestation (3.6% in twin gestation), molar pregnancy, nonimmune hydrops fetalis, uncontrolled hypertension, preexisting hypertension, renal disease

PHYSICAL FINDINGS & CLINICAL PRESENTATION

- Seizure begins as facial twitching, then spreads to generalized clonicotonic state, with cessation of respiration followed by a postictal period of amnesia, agitation, and confusion.
- 40% have severe hypertension, 40% have mild to moderate hypertension, and 20% are normotensive.
- Generalized edema with rapid weight gain (>2 lb/wk) may be one of the earliest signs of eclampsia.
- Persistent occipital headache and hyperreflexia with clonus occur in 80% of patients with eclampsia; epigastric pain occurs in 20% of these patients.

ETIOLOGY

- Exact etiology unknown.
- Common pathway relates to abnormalities in autoregulation of cerebral blood flow. This may involve transient vasospasm, ischemia, cerebral hemorrhage, and edema occurring by a mechanism involving hypertensive encephalopathy, decreased colloid osmotic pressure, and prostaglandin imbalance.

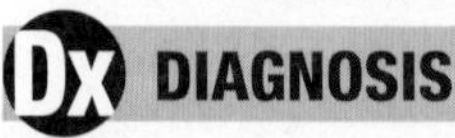

DIAGNOSIS

DIFFERENTIAL DIAGNOSIS

- Preexisting seizure disorder
- Metabolic abnormalities (hypoglycemia, hyponatremia, hypocalcemia)
- Substance abuse
- Head trauma, infection (meningitis, encephalitis)
- Intracerebral bleeding or thrombosis
- Amniotic fluid embolism
- Space-occupying brain lesions or neoplasms
- Pseudoseizure

WORKUP

- Rule out other causes of seizures during pregnancy.
- Atypical presentations such as prolonged postictal state; status epilepticus; gestational age <20 wk or >48 hr postpartum; or signs of meningitis, substance abuse, or severe uncontrolled hypertension should prompt a search for other seizure etiologies.

LABORATORY TESTS

- Proteinuria: severe (49%), mild to moderate (29%), absent (22%)
- HCT: elevated as a result of hemoconcentration
- Platelet count: decreased; LFTs elevated in HELLP syndrome (hemolysis, elevated liver enzymes, and low platelet count)
- BUN and creatinine: elevated with renal involvement
- Serum electrolytes, glucose, calcium, toxicology profile: rule out other causes of seizures
- Hyperuricemia: >6.9 mg/dl found in 70% of eclamptics
- ABG: maternal acidemia and hypoxia

IMAGING STUDIES

- CT scan or MRI indicated in atypical presentation, suspected intracerebral bleeding, or focal neurologic deficit.
- There are abnormal findings, including cerebral edema, hemorrhage, and infarction, in 50% of patients.

Rx TREATMENT

NONPHARMACOLOGIC THERAPY

- Airway protection (risk of aspiration)
- Supportive care during acute event

ACUTE GENERAL Rx

- Maintain airway, adequate oxygenation, and IV access.
- Fetal resuscitation, involving maternal oxygenation, left lateral positioning, and continuous fetal heart rate monitoring, is needed.
- Magnesium sulfate is the drug of choice. Give magnesium sulfate 6 g IV load over 20 min, then 3 g/hr maintenance, for recurrent seizure prophylaxis. If repeated convulsions, may give an additional 2 g IV over 3 to 5 min. Approximately 10% to 15% of patients will have a second seizure after initial loading dose. Check magnesium level 1 hr after loading dose, then q6h (therapeutic range 4 to 6 mg/dl). Antidote for toxicity is calcium gluconate 10 ml of 10% solution. Phenytoin has been used as an alternative in patients in whom magnesium sulfate is contraindicated (renal insufficiency, heart block, myasthenia gravis, hypoparathyroidism).
- Give sodium amobarbital 250 mg IV over 3 min for persistent seizures.
- Treat blood pressure if >160 mm Hg/110 mm Hg with labetalol 20- to 40-mg IV bolus, hydralazine 10 mg IV, or nifedipine 10 to 20 mg sublingual q20min.
- Evaluate patient for delivery.

CHRONIC Rx

- The first priority is stabilization of the mother in terms of adequate oxygenation, hemodynamics, and laboratory abnormalities, such as associated coagulopathies.
- Cervical status and gestational age should be assessed. If unfavorable cervix and <30 wk of gestation, consider C-section; otherwise consider induction.
- Controlled epidural is the anesthesia of choice for labor or C-section.
- Avoid general anesthesia in uncontrolled hypertension to minimize risk of catastrophic cerebral events.

DISPOSITION

The maternal mortality rate for eclampsia averages 5% to 6%. Morbidity rate is 25%, including placental abruption (10%), maternal apnea with fetal asphyxia, aspiration pneumonia, pulmonary edema (4%), renal failure, cardiopulmonary arrest, and coma.

REFERRAL

Because of the potential for serious permanent maternal and fetal sequelae, all cases should be managed by a team approach of obstetrician, neonatologist, and intensivist.

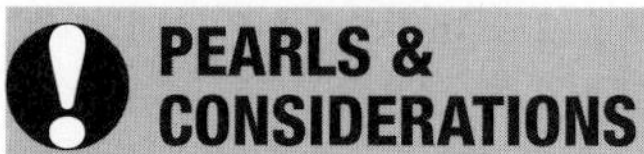

PEARLS & CONSIDERATIONS

COMMENTS

- Eclampsia antepartum, 50%; intrapartum, 20%; and postpartum, 30%.
- Postseizure there is an associated period of fetal bradycardia from 1 to 9 min; if there is evidence of fetal compromise beyond that time, consider alternative etiologies such as placental abruption (23% incidence).

SUGGESTED READINGS

available at www.expertconsult.com

RELATED CONTENT

HELLP Syndrome (Related Key Topic)
Preeclampsia (Related Key Topic)
Eclampsia (Patient Information)

AUTHOR: **RUBEN ALVERO, M.D.**

BASIC INFORMATION

DEFINITION

An ectopic pregnancy (EP) occurs when a fertilized ovum implants outside the endometrial lining of the uterus.

SYNONYMS

Abdominal pregnancy (0.03% to 1%)
Cervical pregnancy (0.5%)
Interstitial pregnancy (1% to 2%)
Ovarian pregnancy (1%)
Tubal pregnancy (97%)

ICD-9CM CODES
633 Ectopic pregnancy
ICD-10CM CODES
000.9 Ectopic pregnancy, unspecified

EPIDEMIOLOGY & DEMOGRAPHICS

- 1% to 2% of pregnancies
- 13% of maternal deaths

PREVALENCE (IN U.S.): Increasing number of EPs; 17,800 reported cases in 1970 and currently over 100,000 reported cases/year.

RISK FACTORS: Previous salpingitis, previous EP, previous tubal ligation, previous tuboplasty, intrauterine device use, progestin-only pill, assisted reproductive techniques

PHYSICAL FINDINGS & CLINICAL PRESENTATION

- Abdominal tenderness: 95%
- Adnexal tenderness: 87% to 99%
- Peritoneal signs: 71% to 76%
- Adnexal mass: 33% to 53%
- Enlarged uterus: 6% to 30%
- Shock: 2% to 17%
- Amenorrhea or abnormal vaginal bleeding: 75%
- Shoulder pain: 10%
- Tissue passage: 6% to 7%

ETIOLOGY

- Anatomic obstruction to zygote passage
- Abnormalities in tubal motility
- Transperitoneal migration of the zygote

DIAGNOSIS

DIFFERENTIAL DIAGNOSIS

- Corpus luteum cyst
- Rupture or torsion of ovarian cyst
- Threatened or incomplete abortion
- Pelvic inflammatory disease
- Appendicitis
- Gastroenteritis
- Dysfunctional uterine bleeding
- Degenerating uterine fibroids
- Endometriosis

WORKUP

1. The classic presentation of EP includes the triad of abnormal vaginal bleeding, pelvic pain, and an adnexal mass. Fig. 1-344 describes a diagnostic approach to suspected EP. Fig. 1-345 *(top)* describes potential sites of ectopic implantations. Consider in all women with abdominopelvic pain and a positive pregnancy test
2. Transvaginal ultrasound
3. Quantitative serum human chorionic gonadotropin level
4. Laparoscopy in equivocal situations and possibly for treatment

LABORATORY TESTS

- Quantitative human chorionic gonadotropin (QhCG): if normal intrauterine pregnancy (IUP), 85% have doubling time of 2 days. If abnormal gestation, will show <66% increase of QhCG within 2 days. However, 13% of ectopic pregnancies have a normal doubling time.
- Progesterone: decreased production in EP; <5 ng/ml strongly predictive of abnormal pregnancy. If >25 ng/ml, strongly predictive of normal IUP.
- Dropping hematocrit associated with tubal rupture, resolving EP, or abnormal intrauterine pregnancy.
- Leukocytosis.

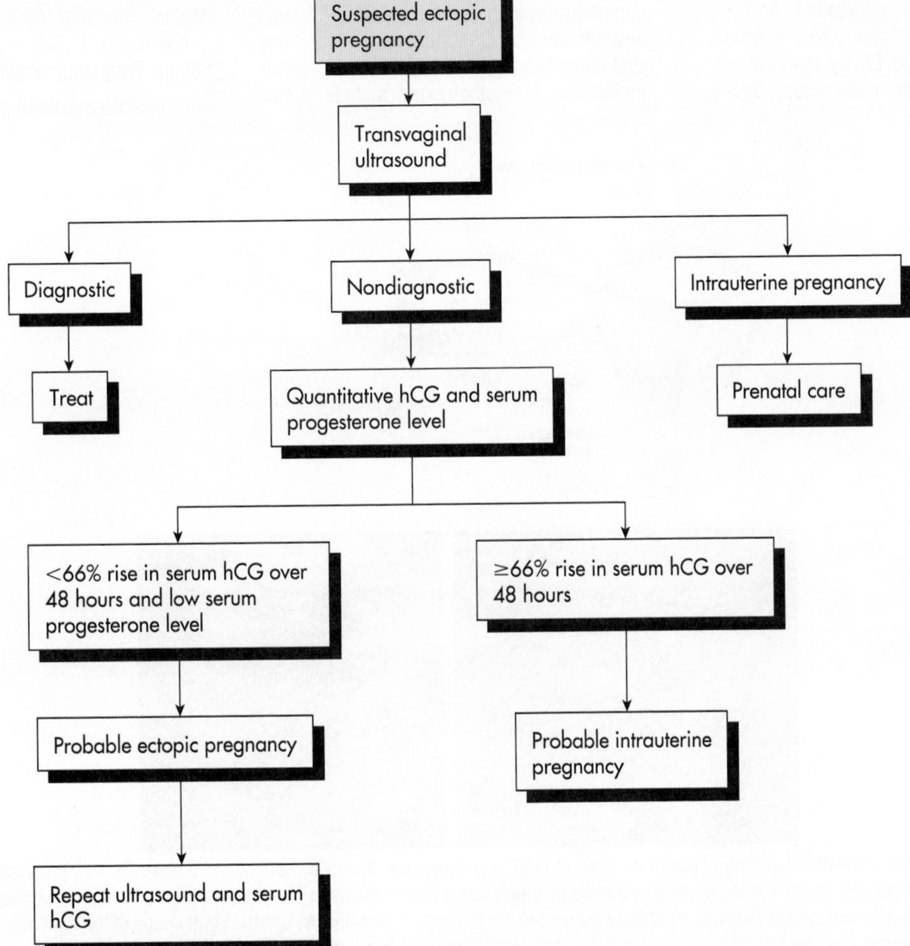

FIGURE 1-344 Ectopic pregnancy. *hCG,* Human chorionic gonadotropin.

IMAGING STUDIES

- Ultrasound: presence of an IUP makes EP extremely unlikely. However, if the patient used assisted reproductive technologies, a heterotopic pregnancy (a pregnancy in the uterus as well as in the fallopian tube) is much more likely to occur (Fig. 1-345, *A* and *B*). A repeat ultrasonographic examination 2 to 7 days after presentation may identify the location of a pregnancy that was not identified on initial ultrasonographic examination.
- If QhCG >6000 mIU/ml, should see IUP on abdominal scan; QhCG >1500 mIU/ml for transvaginal scan. Since transvaginal ultrasonography is overwhelmingly the preferred modality for imaging, the latter value is clearly the discriminatory threshold that is used in diagnosis.
- Findings on ultrasound in EP include:
  1. Empty uterus
  2. Adnexal mass
  3. Cul-de-sac fluid
  4. Fetal sac in tube
  5. Fetal cardiac activity in adnexa

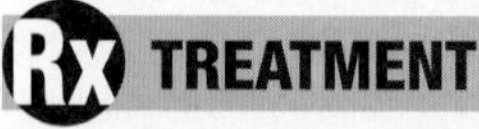

TREATMENT

NONPHARMACOLOGIC THERAPY

Surgery can be performed by laparoscopy if patient is stable or, rarely, by laparotomy if patient is very unstable. Salpingiosis is the direct injection of chemotherapy into the EP by laparoscopy, transvaginal ultrasound, or hysteroscopy. Salpingiosis is the direct injection of chemotherapy into the EP by laparoscopy, transvaginal ultrasound, or hysteroscopy. Direct injection of methotrexate, and possibly KCl if there is active cardiac activity, may be performed when the pregnancy is in a location where there is high morbidity, such as the cervix or cornu.

- Conservative surgery, salpingostomy or segmental resection, depends on tubal location and size of EP.
- Salpingectomy should be considered in the following circumstances:
  1. Ruptured tube
  2. Future fertility not desired
  3. Recurrent EP in the same tube
  4. Uncontrolled hemorrhage

ACUTE GENERAL Rx

- If the patient is stable and compliant, consider medical management with methotrexate. Patient should not have contraindications to methotrexate such as hepatic or renal disease, thrombocytopenia, leukopenia, or significant anemia. There should be no evidence of hemoperitoneum on transvaginal ultrasound. EP should be <3.5 cm mass with QhCG <6,000 to 15,000 mIU/ml, but these are relative contraindications. Presence of cardiac activity in the fetus is also a relative contraindication to methotrexate.
- Most common regimen is methotrexate 50 mg/m^2 of body surface area. May require second dose or surgical intervention if QhCG increases or plateaus (<15% drop) when comparing values from the fourth through seventh day after treatment (day 1 is the day that methotrexate is given). Absolute contraindications to methotrexate include breast feeding, preexisting blood dyscrasias, known sensitivity to methotrexate, active pulmonary disease, chronic liver disease, alcoholism, laboratory evidence of immunodeficiency, renal disease, and peptic ulcer disease.

CHRONIC Rx

Persistent EP results from residual trophoblastic tissue or secondary implantation after conservative surgery. There is a 5% incidence of persistent EP with conservative treatment.

DISPOSITION

If diagnosed and treated early (before rupture), prognosis is excellent for good recovery. Monitor QhCG weekly until negative. Use reliable contraception until hCG is negative. With subsequent pregnancies, follow QhCG and perform early ultrasound to confirm IUP. There is a 12% recurrence rate for EP.

REFERRAL

Should obtain gynecologic consultation if EP is suspected.

SUGGESTED READINGS

available at www.expertconsult.com

RELATED CONTENT

Spontaneous Miscarriage (Related Key Topic)
Vaginal Bleeding during Pregnancy (Related Key Topic)
Ectopic Pregnancy (Patient Information)

AUTHOR: **RUBEN ALVERO, M.D.**

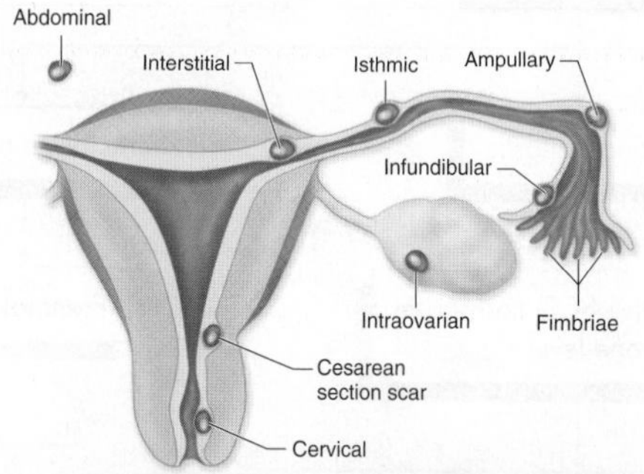

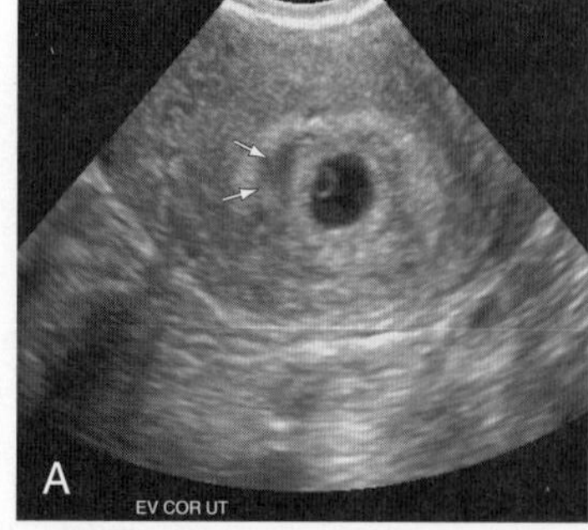

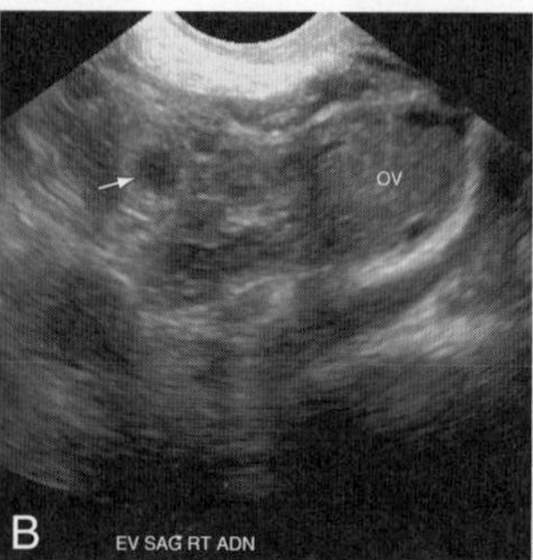

FIGURE 1-345 *Top,* Schematic drawing depicting implantation sites of ectopic pregnancies. **A** and **B,** Heterotopic pregnancy. This pregnant patient presented with vaginal bleeding at 5 to 6 wk of gestational age. **A,** Transverse transvaginal ultrasound (TVUS) image of the uterus reveals an intrauterine gestational sac containing a yolk sac. Note small subchorionic hemorrhage *(arrows),* most likely accounting for the vaginal bleeding. **B,** Sagittal TVUS image of the right adnexa reveals an echogenic tubal ring *(arrow)* clearly separate from the right ovary *(OV),* which was surgically confirmed to be an ectopic pregnancy. (From Fielding JR et al: *Gynecologic imaging,* Philadelphia, 2011, Saunders.)

BASIC INFORMATION

DEFINITION

Human monocytic ehrlichiosis (HME) and human granulocytic anaplasmosis (HGA) are tick-borne rickettsial diseases. HGA was formerly known as human granulocytic ehrlichiosis (HGE). Table 1-174 describes the agent, vector, and geographic prevalence of these diseases.

SYNONYMS

Human granulocytic ehrlichiosis (HGE)
Ehrlichiosis
Human monocytic ehrlichiosis (HME)
Human granulocytic anaplasmosis (HGA)
Anaplasmosis
Ehrlichia phagocytophila
Anaplasma phagocytophilum

ICD-9CM CODES
082.8 Other tick-borne rickettsiosis
ICD-10CM CODES
A77.40 Ehrlichiosis, unspecified

EPIDEMIOLOGY & DEMOGRAPHICS

INCIDENCE (IN U.S.): Highest overall incidence in Rhode Island (36.5 per 1 million), New York, New Jersey, Connecticut, Wisconsin, Minnesota, and northern California; >3000 cases identified in the United States since 2006.
PREDOMINANT SEX: Males outnumber females by 2 to 1.
PREDOMINANT AGE: Most severe disease 50 to 70 yr
PEAK INCIDENCE: Occurs throughout the year, with peak incidence between May and July and again in November.

PHYSICAL FINDINGS & CLINICAL PRESENTATION

- Most common initial symptoms
  1. Fever
  2. Chills, rigor
  3. Headache
  4. Myalgia
- Subsequent symptoms
  1. Anorexia, nausea
  2. Arthralgia
  3. Cough
  4. Confusion (meningoencephalitis in 20% of patients with HME)
  5. Abdominal pain
  6. Rash (erythematous to pustular) <30% in HME, uncommon in HGA
- Complications
  1. Hepatitis
  2. Interstitial pneumonitis; acute respiratory distress syndrome
  3. Renal and respiratory failure
  4. Demyelinating polyneuropathy
  5. Toxic shock–like syndrome
  6. Life-threatening opportunistic infections

ETIOLOGY

- The causative agents are *Ehrlichia chaffeensis* and *Anaplasma phagocytophilum*
- Vector
  1. Almost certainly tick-borne, recently confirmed to be rarely transmitted by infected blood (including nosocomial infection).
  2. Transmitted by *Ixodes scapularis* in the northeastern states and *Amblyomma americanum* in the south central, southeastern, and mid-Atlantic states.
  3. Tick exposure reported in >90% of patients, with ~60% reporting tick bite.
- Mammalian host: deer, horses, dogs, white-footed mice, cattle, sheep, goats, bison
- Host inflammatory and immune responses define final spectrum of disease beyond granulocytes, including hepatitis, interstitial pneumonitis, and nephritis with mild azotemia
- Between 6% and 21% of patients with HGE also have serologic evidence of other *Ixodes* spp. tick-borne diseases: Lyme disease or babesiosis
- Recovery is usual outcome; fatality rate of HGE is about 1%
- ICU care required: 7%

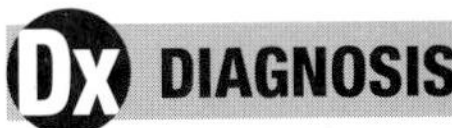

DIAGNOSIS

DIFFERENTIAL DIAGNOSIS

- Rocky Mountain spotted fever, Colorado tick fever, Q fever, relapsing fever
- Babesiosis
- Leptospirosis
- Lyme disease
- Tularemia
- Typhoid fever, paratyphoid fever
- Brucellosis
- Viral hepatitis
- Meningococcemia
- Infectious mononucleosis
- Hematologic malignancy
- TTP (thrombotic thrombocytopenic purpura)
- Table 1-175 describes clinical clues suggesting a diagnosis of a tick-borne illness manifesting as a nonspecific febrile illness

TABLE 1-174 Ehrlichioses and Anaplasmoses

Disease	Agent	Vector	Geographic Repartition
American monocytic ehrlichiosis	*Ehrlichia chaffeensis*	*Amblyomma americanum*	South central, southeastern, mid-Atlantic coastal states
Human granulocytic ehrlichiosis	*Anaplasma phagocytophilum*	*Ixodes ricinus*	Europe, China
		Ixodes scapularis	Northeast, upper Midwest, northern California
E. ewingii	*Ehrlichia ewingii*	*Amblyomma americanum*	South central, southeastern, mid-Atlantic coastal states
Japanese monocytic ehrlichiosis	*Neorickettsia sennetsu*	Helminth of the gray mullet?	Japan
E. canis	*Ehrlichia canis*	*Rhipicephalus sanguineus*	Venezuela

From Goldman L, Schafer AI: *Goldman's Cecil medicine*, ed 24, Philadelphia, 2012, Saunders.

TABLE 1-175 Clinical Clues (History, Physical Examination, or Laboratory) Suggesting the Diagnosis of a Tick-Borne Illness Manifesting as a Nonspecific Febrile Illness*

Disease	Clues
Anaplasmosis	Faint rash possible Low white blood cell or platelet count Elevated hepatic transaminases
Babesiosis	Findings of hemolysis History of splenectomy Presence of faint rash, hepatomegaly, or splenomegaly
Lyme disease	Careful skin examination for any rash consistent with erythema migrans Bradycardia from heart block Associated seventh nerve palsy or lymphocytic meningitis
Colorado tick fever	Saddle-back fever curve
Rocky Mountain spotted fever	Maculopapular or petechial rash Normal white blood cell count or low platelet count Hyponatremia Peripheral edema
Relapsing fever	Recurring episodes of fever with afebrile intervals
Tularemia	Acrally located ulcer Regional lymphadenopathy Possible associated pneumonia

*Apart from an epidemiologic context suggesting a tick-borne disease.
From Adams JG et al: *Emergency medicine, clinical essentials*, ed 2, Philadelphia, 2013, Elsevier.

WORKUP

- Acute blood samples for Giemsa-stained smears
- CBC (leukopenia, thrombocytopenia), liver function (elevated), BUN/creatinine
- Acute serum samples for serology. Antibodies are seldom detected at time of acute infection (they usually appear 2-4 weeks following clinical illness).
- Chest radiograph examination
- Bone marrow rarely needed

LABORATORY TESTS

- Polymerase chain reaction (PCR) to facilitate early diagnosis: detection of *Ehrlichia* DNA in blood or CSF by PCR
- Giemsa-stained smear demonstrating morulae of the organism within granulocytes (sensitivity 20% to 75%) (Fig. 1-347)
- CBC: progressive leukopenia and thrombocytopenia with nadir near day 7
- C-reactive protein concentration is generally elevated
- Liver function tests (LFTs): increase in hepatic transaminases, lactate dehydrogenase, and alkaline phosphatase
- Elevated plasma creatinine concentration may be seen
- Serologic titer (IFA) >80 or fourfold increase in titer to *E. equi* antigen
- Culture on the first 7 days of illness; not readily available in most clinical laboratories

IMAGING STUDIES

- Chest radiograph examination to show interstitial pneumonitis (unusual)
- MRI of the brain

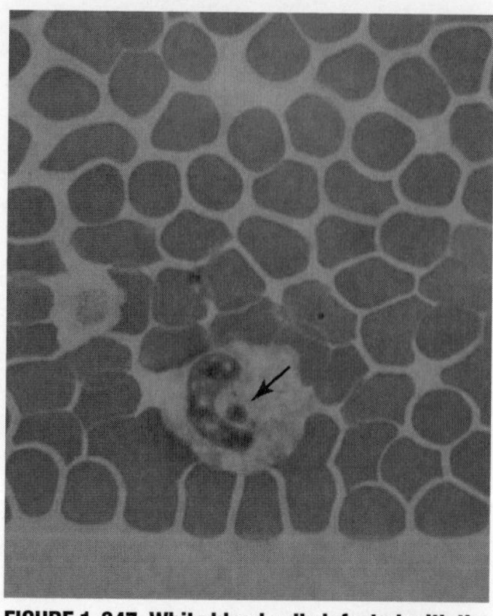

FIGURE 1-347 White blood cells infected with the agent of human granulocytic ehrlichiosis (*Anaplasma phagocytophilum*). (Courtesy Dr. Daniel Caplivski, Division of Infectious Diseases, Mount Sinai School of Medicine.)

Rx TREATMENT

ACUTE GENERAL Rx

- Immediate therapy to limit extent of acute illness and complication
- Doxycycline: 100 mg twice a day for 7 to 14 days is therapy of choice for adults and children >8 yr (4 mg/kg/day in 2 divided doses).
- Rifampin: 300 mg twice a day for 7 to 10 days can be used in pregnancy and for children <8 yr at 10 mg/kg twice per day
- Most patients defervesce within 24 to 48 hr given appropriate treatment.

PROGNOSIS

Poor prognostic indicators include:

- Advanced age
- Concomitant chronic illness (such as diabetes mellitus, collagen-vascular disease)
- Lack of diagnosis recognition
- Delayed onset of specific antibiotic therapy
- Concomitant HIV or organ transplant status

DISPOSITION

- Repeat CBC every 2 to 4 wk until normal.
- A new pathogenic *Ehrlichia* species, close relative of *E. muris* has been identified in Minnesota and Wisconsin. Organism-specific PCR and serologic testing can be used for identification.

REFERRAL

For consultation with infectious diseases specialist in suspected cases

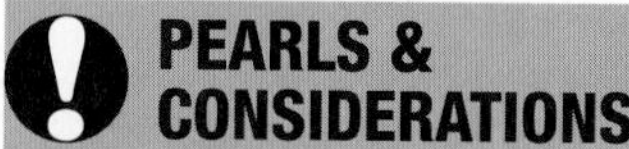

PEARLS & CONSIDERATIONS

COMMENTS

- Duration of time tick must be attached to produce illness as few as 4 hr
- Delay in antibiotic treatment results in poorer outcome. Antibiotic treatment should be initiated as soon as infection is suspected.

SUGGESTED READINGS

available at www.expertconsult.com

RELATED CONTENT

Anaplasmosis (Patient Information)

AUTHOR: **PATRICIA CRISTOFARO, M.D.**

BASIC INFORMATION

DEFINITION

Clinically significant disorders of ejaculation include failure of emission, retrograde ejaculation, premature ejaculation, delayed ejaculation, painful ejaculation, hematospermia, and anorgasmia. Failure of emission occurs when semen is not propulsed into the urethra during orgasm, resulting in a dry ejaculate. Retrograde ejaculation is a backward flow of semen into the bladder. Premature ejaculation refers to ejaculation that occurs sooner than desired, either before or shortly after penetration, causing distress to either one or both partners. Hematospermia is the appearance of blood in the ejaculate. Anorgasmia is the inability to achieve orgasm in a timely manner.

SYNONYMS

Ejaculatory dysfunction
Retarded or delayed ejaculation
Early or rapid ejaculation
Inhibited ejaculation
Anejaculation

ICD-9CM CODES	
608.82	Hematospermia
608.87	Ejaculation, retrograde
608.89	Painful ejaculation
306.59	Ejaculation, psychogenic
302.75	Ejaculation, premature
302.74	Orgasm inhibited male (psychosexual)
ICD-10CM CODES	
N53.14	Retrograde ejaculation
R36.1	Hematospermia
F45.8	Other somatoform disorders
F52.4	Premature ejaculation
F52.32	Male orgasmic disorder

EPIDEMIOLOGY & DEMOGRAPHICS

Men with ejaculatory dysfunction of any type usually indicate higher levels of relationship stress, sexual dissatisfaction, anxiety about sexual performance, and general health issues, compared to sexually functional men. Premature ejaculation is the most prevalent male sexual complaint, affecting 20% to 30% of men, and may be primary (lifelong) or acquired. Retarded or delayed ejaculation is the least common, least studied, and least understood of the male sexual dysfunctions.

CLINICAL PRESENTATION

- Failure of emission: no ejaculate is produced during orgasm. Physical findings may reveal nervous system dysfunction (e.g., spinal cord injury); may present with infertility (e.g., ejaculatory duct obstruction).
- Retrograde ejaculation: little or no ejaculate is expelled out of the urethra at orgasm. Patients may report cloudy postcoital urine. Physical examination is usually normal; may present with infertility.
- Premature ejaculation: ejaculation occurs sooner than desired, either before or shortly after penetration. Physical examination is normal. Up to 30% of patients may report concomitant erectile dysfunction.
- Delayed ejaculation: ejaculation requires prolonged sexual stimulation, often 30 minutes or longer. Physical examination is normal.
- Painful ejaculation: perineal, scrotal, or testicular pain during or shortly after ejaculation. Physical examination may demonstrate pain on examination of external genitalia, or with digital rectal examination; may present with infertility.
- Hematospermia: reddish-brown ejaculate, usually painless. Physical findings are usually unremarkable; not associated with malignancy.
- Anorgasmia: patient is not able to achieve orgasm despite appropriate stimulation.

ETIOLOGY

- Retrograde ejaculation may be caused by anatomic abnormalities of the bladder neck, or nerve injury affecting the bladder neck sphincter.
- Either retrograde ejaculation or failure of emission may result from functional abnormalities, such as spinal cord injury, diabetes mellitus, retroperitoneal surgery, transurethral prostate surgery, urethral strictures, alpha-blocker therapy, antipsychotics, multiple sclerosis, and peripheral neuropathy.
- Premature and delayed ejaculation represent the opposite ends of the spectrum of ejaculatory disorders. The underlying etiology is complex and multifactorial, and includes organic and psychogenic contributions.
- Causes of painful ejaculation may be infectious (e.g., epididymo-orchitis, urethritis, prostatitis), obstructive (e.g., vasectomy, prostatectomy, hernia repair), or psychological.
- Hematospermia may be idiopathic, secondary to prolonged abstinence, or due to infection or inflammation of the genitourinary tract.
- Anorgasmia may be caused by spinal cord injury, psychological factors, dysfunctional sexual techniques, or medications, particularly serotonin re-uptake inhibitors.

DIAGNOSIS

DIFFERENTIAL DIAGNOSIS

- Erectile dysfunction
- Low seminal fluid volume attributable to hypogonadism or ejaculatory duct obstruction
  - Inflammatory disorders of the genitourinary tract
  - Hypoactive sexual desire

LABORATORY TESTS

- For a low-volume ejaculate, post-ejaculate urine should be evaluated for the presence of spermatozoa to differentiate failure of emission from retrograde ejaculation.
- Hematuria, in the setting of hematospermia or painful ejaculation, may signal an underlying inflammatory disorder or a malignancy and should prompt a complete evaluation.
- A fasting blood glucose may be considered if diabetes is suspected as a cause of lack of emission or retrograde ejaculation.
- Urinalysis, urine culture, and screening for sexually transmitted diseases, when indicated, can rule out an infectious etiology of painful ejaculation.

IMAGING STUDIES

Transrectal ultrasonography or pelvic MRI can rule out ejaculatory duct obstruction or absence of the seminal vesicles.

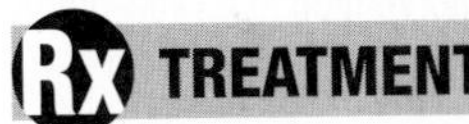

TREATMENT

NONPHARMACOLOGIC THERAPY

- Retrograde ejaculation and failure of emission do not require treatment unless fertility is desired.
- In the setting of retrograde ejaculation, viable sperm can be recovered from the post-ejaculate urine and used for intrauterine insemination or in vitro fertilization.
- Premature ejaculation can improve with psychotherapy and behavioral interventions (e.g., "coronal squeeze" or "start-and-stop" technique) and effective partner communication. These approaches may be more effective when combined with pharmacologic therapy.
- Idiopathic hematospermia may be followed expectantly and is usually self-limited to 10 to 15 ejaculations.
- Anorgasmia caused by serotonin reuptake inhibitors usually improves with withdrawal of the medication. Sexual therapy and counseling can improve anorgasmia caused by dysfunctional sexual techniques or psychological issues. Vibratory or electrical stimulation of emission is helpful in selected cases.

ACUTE GENERAL Rx

- Retrograde ejaculation: pharmacologic therapy is only effective in patients without an anatomic disturbance of the bladder neck. Sympathomimetic medications (phenylpropanolamine, ephedrine, pseudoephedrine) and imipramine may be useful in converting retrograde ejaculation to antegrade ejaculation.
- Failure of emission: may be converted to retrograde ejaculation by oral sympathomimetic therapy, as listed above.
- Premature ejaculation: selective serotonin re-uptake inhibitors (SSRI) (sertraline, fluoxetine) and the tricyclic antidepressant clomipramine can successfully delay ejaculation when taken daily. Recent research has focused on dapoxetine, a short-acting SSRI, which has shown promise as an "on-demand" treatment for premature ejaculation. Topical anesthetics such as lidocaine cream and topical sprays have also been used, with variable success. The use of phosphodiesterase inhibitors (PDE5i) (sildenafil, vardenafil, tadalafil) with SSRIs may be beneficial in men with concomitant erectile dysfunction and premature ejaculation.

 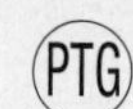

- Antimicrobial treatment (if indicated), NSAIDs, and muscle relaxants may help decrease discomfort associated with painful ejaculation.
- The use of the pharmacologic therapies listed above for the treatment of various disorders of ejaculation is strictly off label and does not carry FDA approval.

SURGICAL THERAPY

There is no role for surgery for the majority of ejaculatory disorders. Rarely, painful ejaculation due to obstructive causes may show improvement with surgical intervention (e.g., vasectomy reversal).

DISPOSITION

Prognosis varies with etiology. Ejaculatory dysfunction attributable to sexual techniques or psychological issues can improve with psychotherapy. Pharmacologic treatment is helpful in treating premature, retrograde, or painful ejaculation.

REFERRAL

All fertility issues and suspected anatomic problems should be referred to a urologist. Professional psychotherapy should be considered for appropriate patients.

SUGGESTED READINGS

available at www.expertconsult.com

RELATED CONTENT

Erectile Dysfunction (Related Key Topic)
Erectile Dysfunction (Patient Information)

AUTHORS: **AKANKSHA MEHTA, M.D.,** and **MARK SIGMAN, M.D.**

BASIC INFORMATION

DEFINITION

Injuries or wounds that occur as a result of contact with an electrical current or lightning.

ICD-9CM CODES
994.8 Electrical shock, nonfatal
ICD-10CM CODES
W87 Exposure to unspecified electric current
W86 Exposure to other specified electric current
W85 Exposure to electric transmission lines
X33 Victim of lightning

EPIDEMIOLOGY & DEMOGRAPHICS

- Causes approximately 1000 deaths annually, with two thirds occurring in persons between ages 15 and 40 yr.
- Most electrical injuries in children occur at home (e.g., oral burns from electrical appliances).
- Most electrical injuries in adults are occupationally related. It ranks fifth as a cause of occupational death.
- Accounts for 4% to 6.5% of all admissions to burn units.
- Lightning strikes kill on average 100 people annually.
  - Eight of every 10 lightning strike victims are male; 75% of lightning deaths in the U.S. occur in the South and Midwest.
  - 25% of lightning deaths are work related.
- Electronic weapons (stun gun and Taser) are capable of causing fatal cardiac arrhythmias.
- Table 1-176 compares lightning injuries with high-voltage electrical injuries.

TABLE 1-176 Lightning Injuries Compared with High-Voltage Electrical Injuries

Factor	Lightning	High Voltage
Energy level	30 million volts, 50,000 Å	Usually much lower*
Time of exposure	Brief, instantaneous	Seconds
Pathway	Flashover, orifice	Deep, internal
Burns	Superficial, minor	Deep, major injury
Renal	Rare myoglobinuria or hemoglobinuria	Myoglobinuric renal failure common
Fasciotomy	Rarely if ever necessary	Common, early, and extensive
Blunt injury	Explosive thunder effect	Falls, being thrown

*Range is 500 V up to millions of volts in transmission lines.
From Auerbach P: *Wilderness medicine, expert consult* Premium Edition—Enhanced Online Features and Print, Philadelphia, 2012, Saunders, Elsevier. 978-1-4377-1678-8.)

PHYSICAL FINDINGS & CLINICAL PRESENTATION

- Cognitive changes: depending on the extent of injury, the patient may be unconscious, seizing, or confused and unable to present a history
- Extensive skin burns (>10% of the body surface)
  1. Located over the entry and exit sites (Fig. 1-348)
  2. Most common entry sites are the hands and skull
  3. Most common exit sites are the heels
  4. "Kissing burns" over the flexor creases
  5. Oral burns are common in children; bleeding from the labial artery may present 7 to 10 days after the injury
  6. Charring at the contact site (Fig. E1-349)
- Asystole or ventricular fibrillation may be the initial cardiac rhythm
- Bone fractures and periosteal burns
- Compartment syndrome from severe muscle tissue damage
- Headaches, memory disturbances
- Weakness and paresthesias
- Otologic injury, conductive hearing loss from tympanic membrane rupture or ossicular disruption
- Rhabdomyolysis and myoglobin-induced acute tubular necrosis
- Vascular injury from coagulation of small vessels or compartment syndrome
- Box 1-24 summarizes the immediate and delayed effects of lightning injuries

ETIOLOGY

- Electricity causes tissue injury by converting electrical energy into heat or by blunt trauma from being thrown from the electrical source or from continuous muscle contraction (tetany).
- The effects of electricity are determined by seven factors: type of current, amount of current, pathway of current, duration, area of contact, resistance of the body, and voltage.
- Tissue damage is greater with higher voltage and longer duration of contact.

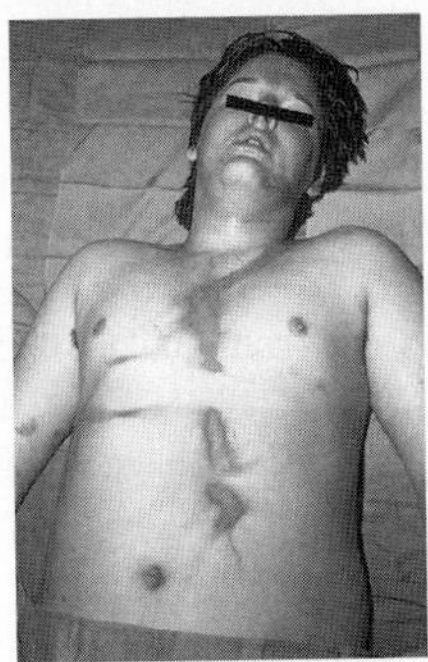

FIGURE 1-348 The arborescent current markings on the face, neck, and anterior trunk of this young patient, which are characteristic of lightning injury, healed without the need for grafting. Note the focal lesions on the right arm, indicating the spread of the current that produced the marks on the right anterolateral aspect of the chest wall. (From Goldman L, Schafer AI: *Goldman's Cecil medicine,* ed 24, Philadelphia, 2012, Saunders.)

- Direct current (DC) contact causes a single muscle contraction, throwing the patient away from the source. Alternating current (AC) contact precipitates a tetanic contraction, not allowing the patient to withdraw from the source and prolonging the duration of contact. AC contact is more ominous than DC contact.
- Electrical injuries are arbitrarily divided into high-voltage (>1000 volts) and low-voltage (<1000 volts) burns. Low-voltage burns involve almost exclusively either the hands or oral cavity. High-voltage injuries have a wide variety of systemic manifestations.
- The entry and exit path of the electrical current determines which tissues are affected.
- Box 1-25 describes the mechanism of lightning injury.

DIAGNOSIS

WORKUP

Physical examination may not reveal the extent of damage that has occurred. Detailed testing to determine the extent of internal organ damage is indicated. In lightning injuries, male victims may have scrotal (on the undersurface of the scrotum) and penile burns, which may often be overlooked. Hemorrhage behind the eardrum with or without perforation is not uncommon. An otoscopic examination is indicated in all lightning strike victims.

LABORATORY TESTS

- Complete blood count
- Blood chemistry profile including electrolytes
- Blood urea nitrogen and creatinine
- Arterial blood gas analysis
- Myoglobin
- Creatinine kinase with isoenzyme fractionation
- Urinalysis, including screening for myoglobinuria
- Liver function tests
- Type and cross-match
- ECG

IMAGING STUDIES

- Radiographs: any suspicious area for bone fractures
- CT scan of the head and cervical spine in patients with suspected head injury, coma, or neurologic deficit

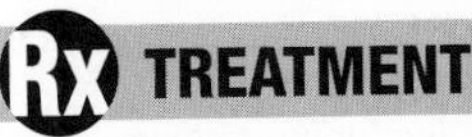

TREATMENT

NONPHARMACOLOGIC THERAPY

- At the scene: ensure the electrical power source of injury is turned off before approaching patients.
- Basic and advanced cardiac life support with cervical spine precautions. Prolonged cardiopulmonary resuscitation should be undertaken regardless of the initial cardiac rhythm.
- Cardiac monitoring.

BOX 1-24 Myths Commonly Cited as Facts in Litigation

These apply to electrical injury as well as lightning injury.

Behavior of Current in the Body

- Current seeks earth.
- Current seeks the path of lowest resistance.
- Nerve tissue is a good conductor, or alternatively, current is preferentially conducted by nerve tissue.
- When a person touches a source of potential, current flows through the skin to other parts of the skin in contact with the same conductor (i.e., current passage is local only).

The Severity of Electric Shock

Myth: If the following are absent, the shock cannot be severe and no deleterious effect can result:

- Being thrown (i.e., if a person is not thrown, the shock is not severe).
- Burns (i.e., if burns are not present, the shock is not severe).
- If the only surface change is a blister, the shock was not severe.
- Entry and exit wounds:
- Must be present
- Demonstrate the current path
- If not present, indicate no shock occurred
- Fuses being blown (i.e., if a fuse does not blow, the shock is not severe enough to harm a victim).
- Low voltage cannot harm.
- Electroconvulsive therapy does not give long-term post–electric-shock symptoms (also false), so any other electric shock cannot be harmful.

Investigations

- If computed tomography (CT) and magnetic resonance imaging (MRI) scans are normal, there are no injuries.
- Negative investigations (e.g., nerve conduction study, electroencephalogram, CT, MRI) mean a victim has not sustained an electric shock.
- Neuropsychological testing is objective and easily interpreted.
- Burns of electrical origin can be distinguished on histologic examination.

Remote Symptoms

- Remote symptoms do not exist.
- Remote symptoms are proportional to the size of the shock.
- Symptoms of the shock that are not present immediately after the shock are not related to it.
- A person getting remote symptoms was psychologically vulnerable all the time.

Miscellaneous

- Litigation increases the potency of the claimed symptoms. Corollary: resolving litigation terminates symptoms.
- Medical specialists understand electricity or lightning.
- Electrical experts can predict lightning or electrical injury.
- A diagnosis of depression, post-traumatic stress disorder, adjustment disorder, and so on, negate an electrical injury causation.
- Residual current devices (RCDs) eliminate the possibility of all shocks. Corollary: a shock occurring when an RCD breaks the circuit cannot be severe.

From Auerbach P: *Wilderness medicine, expert consult* Premium Edition - Enhanced Online Features and Print, Philadelphia, 2012, Saunders, Elsevier. 978-1-4377-1678-8.

BOX 1-25 Mechanisms of Lightning Injury

Electrothermal Effects

1. Direct strike
2. Contact potential
3. Side flash, sometimes called "splash" (1 to 3 may include surface arcs over the body surface)
4. Step voltage (also termed "Earth potential rise" or "ground current")
   a. Transmitted through the ground
   b. Surface arcing
5. Upward streamer current (also called "fifth mechanism")

Blunt Force Trauma Effects

6. Barotrauma
7. Concussive injury
8. Musculoskeletal injury from muscle contraction, falls

From Auerbach P: *Wilderness medicine, expert consult* Premium Edition—Enhanced Online Features and Print, Philadelphia, 2012, Saunders, Elsevier. 978-1-4377-1678-8.)

- Oxygen.
- Tetanus prophylaxis.

ACUTE GENERAL Rx

- IV fluids to maintain urine output of 50 to 100 ml/hr (IV hydration should be reassessed with central nervous system expert in patients at risk of developing cerebral edema).
- Alkalinization of the urine (sodium bicarbonate 50 mEq in 1 L of normal saline) in patients with or at risk of myoglobinuria.
- Furosemide 20 to 40 mg PO or IV and/or mannitol 12.5 g/kg/hr may be used to force diuresis.
- Seizures are treated in the standard fashion.
- Treat burns with sulfadiazine silver dressings.

CHRONIC Rx

- Hospitalization is indicated in patients with high-voltage injuries, extensive burns, central nervous system symptoms, myonecrosis (creatine kinase level more than twice normal, high serum myoglobin levels, or myoglobinuria), new cardiac arrhythmia or ECG changes, or any internal organ damage.
- Ophthalmology consultation at the follow-up to screen for cataract formation (occurs within 1 to 24 mo of a high-voltage electrical injury in 5% to 20% of patients).

DISPOSITION

- Patients with severe burns should be transferred to the regional burn center.
- Complications of electrical injuries include:
  1. Infection
  2. Renal failure from rhabdomyolysis
  3. Seizure disorder
  4. Fasciotomies
  5. Amputation
- Delayed neurologic damage may present as ascending paralysis, amyotrophic lateral sclerosis, or transverse myelitis weeks to years after the injury.
- Vascular damage may also present in a delayed fashion.

REFERRAL

- Referrals to general surgery, burn surgery, trauma surgery, orthopedic surgery, and/or critical care specialists as appropriate in any patient that meets hospitalization criteria. Ophthalmology and ear-nose-throat specialist referral may be indicated.
- Plastic surgery is recommended in children with oral burns.

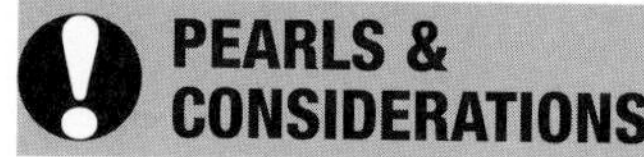

COMMENTS

- The size of external skin burns can often underestimate the degree of internal injury.
- Lightning Strike and Electric Shock Survivors International is a support group that serves people from around the world who have sustained an electric injury (http://www.lightning-strike.org).
- Home safety education provided one to one in a clinical setting or at home, especially with the provision of safety equipment, is effective in increasing the range of safety practices.
- Box E1-26 describes myths regarding electrical and lightning injury commonly cited as facts in litigation.

SUGGESTED READINGS

available at www.expertconsult.com

RELATED CONTENT

Electrical Injury (Patient Information)

AUTHORS: **ROBERT M. KIRCHNER, M.D.,** and **PAUL GORDON, M.D.**

BASIC INFORMATION

DEFINITION

An accumulation of pus in the pleural space, most often caused by bacterial infection.

SYNONYMS

Infected pleuritis
Infected pleural effusion
Purulent pleural effusion

ICD-9CM CODES
510.9 Empyema, lung
ICD-10CM CODES
J86 Pyothorax
A16.5 Empyema due to tuberculosis

EPIDEMIOLOGY & DEMOGRAPHICS

- Empyema is most commonly a complication of bacterial pneumonia, especially in association with pneumococcal or anaerobic infection (40% to 60% of cases of empyema)
- Occur as a complication of thoracic surgery (<20% of cases)
- Penetrating chest trauma (4% to 10% of cases)
- Bronchopleural fistulae resulting from malignancy or lung biopsy

PHYSICAL FINDINGS & CLINICAL PRESENTATION

- May be abrupt or chronic and insidious depending on the etiologic agent and host factors.
- Typically presents as progressive pleuritic chest pain, persistent fever, and other sustained signs and symptoms of infection.
- In anaerobic empyema, particularly that caused by the actinomycetes, the clinical picture is dominated by systemic symptoms and signs: weight loss, malaise, and low grade fever.
- A slowly enlarging chest wall mass.
- As a complication of thoracic trauma or surgery, empyema typically results from contamination of blood within the pleural space several days following the event.
- The physical findings of empyema are those of pleural effusion. Decreased breath sounds and dullness to percussion over the involved part of the thorax is typical. Systemic signs include fever, tachycardia, leukocytosis, and warmth and erythema over the involved area.

ETIOLOGY

Infection of the lung parenchyma spreading to pleural space caused by
- *Streptococcus pneumoniae*
- *Haemophilus influenzae*
- *Staphylococcus aureus*
- *Legionella* species
- *Mycobacterium tuberculosis*
- *Actinomyces* spp.
- A variety of oral anaerobic bacteria have been cultured in 36% to 37% of empyemas: *Bacteroides fragilis, Prevotella* species, *Fusobacterium nucleatum*, and *Peptostreptococcus* are the most common

DIAGNOSIS

DIFFERENTIAL DIAGNOSIS

- Uninfected parapneumonic effusion
- Congestive heart failure
- Malignancy involving the pleura
- Tuberculous pleurisy
- Collagen vascular disease (particularly rheumatoid lung and systemic lupus erythematosus)

LABORATORY TESTS

- Complete blood count; arterial blood gas.
- Blood cultures.
- Pleural fluid analysis in empyema has the characteristics of an exudate with a ratio of pleural fluid to serum protein >0.5 or pleural fluid to serum LDH >0.6. Characteristically, empyema fluid is grossly purulent with visible organisms on Gram stain with glucose <50 mg/dl and pH <7. These findings justify immediate drainage by chest tube or surgery because of the high risk of loculation and progressive systemic infection.

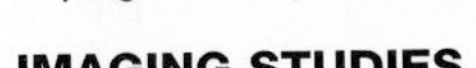

IMAGING STUDIES

- Chest x-ray (Fig. 1-350, *A*)
- Lateral decubitus view to establish the presence of free fluid in the pleural space
- Computed tomography (Fig. 1-350, *B*) to establish the presence of fluid loculation, underlying mass lesions, and other intrathoracic pathology

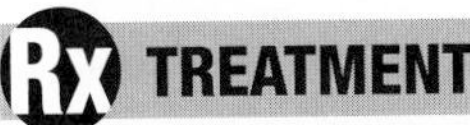

TREATMENT

NONPHARMACOLOGIC THERAPY

Prompt drainage by thoracostomy (chest tube) or open thoracotomy. Video-assisted thoracoscopic surgery (VATS) has greatly improved surgical management of empyemas.

ACUTE GENERAL Rx

- Maintenance of drainage until infection controlled.
- Antibiotics directed at suspected or proven bacterial or fungal pathogens. Initial regimens include cefotaxime or ceftriaxone for suspected *S. pneumoniae* or group A *Streptococcus,* nafcillin or oxacillin for suspected methicillin-sensitive *S. aureus,* vancomycin or linezolid for suspected MRSA, ceftriaxone for suspected *H. influenzae,* and clindamycin plus ceftriaxone when suspecting anaerobes.
- Thoracoscopy or instillation of thrombolytic agents (streptokinase or urokinase) may be considered in refractory, loculated empyema.

CHRONIC Rx

- If thorough drainage cannot be accomplished, open thoracotomy with pleural decortication may be required.
- Lung function should be monitored following completion of therapy.

DISPOSITION

Hospitalization with supplemental oxygen with ventilatory support if necessary

REFERRAL

Consultation by infectious diseases, pulmonary, or thoracic surgery specialists as needed.

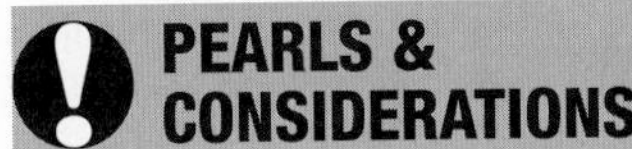

PEARLS & CONSIDERATIONS

COMMENTS

- Empyema caused by actinomycetes may present with erosion through the chest wall and formation of a fistulous tract.
- Nosocomial infection caused by relatively resistant bacterial or fungal pathogens may result in empyema in patients with indwelling thoracostomy tubes.

FIGURE 1-350 Empyema and pneumonia in a teenager. A, Chest radiograph shows opacification of the left thorax. Note shift of mediastinum and trachea (arrowhead) to right. **B,** Thoracic CT scan shows massive left pleural effusion *(asterisk).* Note the compression and atelectasis of the left lung *(arrows)* and shift of the mediastinum to the right. (From Kliegman RM et al: *Nelson textbook of pediatrics,* ed 19, Philadelphia, 2011, Saunders.)

SUGGESTED READINGS

available at www.expertconsult.com

AUTHOR: **GLENN G. FORT, M.D., M.P.H.**

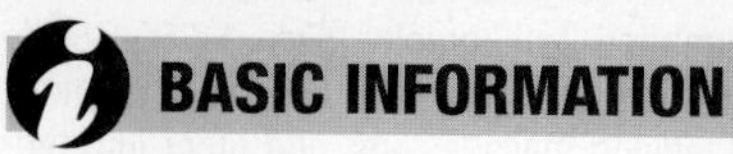

DEFINITION

Acute viral encephalitis is an acute febrile syndrome with evidence of meningeal involvement and of derangement of the function of the cerebrum, cerebellum, or brain stem.

SYNONYMS

Arboviral encephalitis
Brain stem encephalitis
Acute necrotizing encephalitis
Rasmussen encephalitis
Encephalitis lethargica

ICD-9CM CODES
049.9 Viral encephalitis, NOS
ICD-10CM CODES
A86 Unspecified viral encephalitis

EPIDEMIOLOGY & DEMOGRAPHICS

INCIDENCE (IN U.S.): About 20,000 cases/yr are reported to the CDC. In 2012 there was an increase in the number of cases of West Nile virus infection in the U.S.
PEAK INCIDENCE: Any age
PREVALENCE (IN U.S.): Unknown
PREDOMINANT SEX: Male = female
PREDOMINANT AGE: Any age
GENETICS: No specific genetic or congenital predisposition

ETIOLOGY

- Can be caused by a host of viruses, with herpes simplex the most common virus identified.
- Arboviruses transmitted by mosquitoes include Eastern equine encephalitis, Western equine encephalitis, St. Louis encephalitis, Venezuelan equine encephalitis, California virus encephalitis, Japanese B encephalitis, Murray Valley and West Nile encephalitis. Tick-borne diseases include Russian spring-summer encephalitis, Powassan encephalitis, and other lesser known agents.
- Also implicated: rabies-causing agents, CMV, Epstein-Barr, varicella-zoster, echo virus, mumps, adenovirus, coxsackie, rubeola, and herpes viruses.
- Meningoencephalitis: acute retroviral infection
- In the U.S., the most commonly identified etiologies are herpes simplex virus, West Nile virus, and the enteroviruses.

PHYSICAL FINDINGS & CLINICAL PRESENTATION

- Initially, fever and evidence of meningeal irritation
- Headache and stiff neck
- Later, development of signs of cortical dysfunction: lethargy, coma, stupor, weakness, seizures, facial weakness, as well as brainstem findings
- Cerebellar findings: ataxia, nystagmus, hypotonia, myoclonus, cranial nerve palsies, and abnormal tendon reflexes
- Patients with rabies: hydrophobia, anxiety, facial numbness, psychosis, coma, or dysarthria
- Rarely, movement disorders, such as chorea, hemiballismus, or dystonia
- Recall of a prodromal viral-like illness (this finding is not at all uniform)

Dx DIAGNOSIS

DIFFERENTIAL DIAGNOSIS

- Bacterial infections: brain abscess, toxic encephalopathies, TB
- Protozoal infections
- Behçet's disease
- Lupus encephalitis
- Sjögren's syndrome
- Multiple sclerosis
- Syphilis
- Cryptococcus
- Toxoplasmosis
- Brucellosis
- Leukemic or lymphomatous meningitis
- Other metastatic tumors
- Lyme disease
- Cat-scratch disease
- Vogt-Koyanagi-Harada syndrome
- Mollaret's meningitis

WORKUP

- Lumbar puncture to reveal pleocytosis, usually lymphocytic, although neutrophils may be seen early on
- Usually, elevated CSF protein
- Normal or low CSF glucose
- In herpes simplex encephalitis: RBCs and xanthochromia
- Selected tests on CSF fluid in viral encephalitis are described in Table 1-178
- EEG changes showing periodic high-voltage sharp waves in the temporal regions and slow wave complexes suggestive of herpes encephalitis (Fig. 1-351).
- CT scan and MRI to reveal edema and hemorrhage in the frontal and temporal lobes
- Temporal lobe involvement suggests herpes simplex encephalitis
- Basal ganglia and thalami are areas involved as generally seen in Eastern equine encephalitis
- With West Nile infection, MRI changes have shown changes in basal ganglia, thalami, mesial temporal structures, brain stem, and cerebellum
- Arboviral infections suspected during outbreaks in specific areas
- Rising titers of neutralizing antibodies from the acute to the convalescent stage demonstrated but often not helpful in the acutely ill patient
- Polymerase chain reaction (PCR) that amplifies DNA from the CSF for herpes simplex encephalitis

TABLE 1-178 Selected Tests for Viral Encephalitis

Organism/Syndrome	Test	Comment
West Nile Virus		
West Nile encephalitis	IgM in CSF	Diagnostic of CNS invasive disease or acute flaccid paralysis
Herpes Simplex Virus Type 1		
Herpes simplex encephalitis	PCR in CSF	Sensitive and specific in the acute phase
	CSF–serum antibody ratio	Useful 2 weeks to 3 months after onset
Herpes Simplex Virus Type 2		
Neonatal encephalitis	PCR in CSF	Confirmatory, high sensitivity
Relapsing meningitis	PCR in CSF	Sensitive and specific in first 3 days of illness
Varicella-Zoster Virus		
Meningoencephalitis	PCR in CSF	Confirmatory when used with clinical and spinal fluid findings; sensitivity unclear
Epstein-Barr Virus		
EBV encephalitis	PCR in CSF	Suggests CNS invasion by virus
JC Virus		
Progressive multifocal leukoencephalopathy	PCR in CSF	Diagnostic but incompletely (70%) sensitive
Cytomegalovirus		
CMV ventriculitis	PCR in CSF	Sensitive and specific

CMV, Cytomegalovirus; *CNS,* central nervous system; *CSF,* cerebrospinal fluid; *EBV,* Epstein-Barr virus; *PCR,* polymerase chain reaction.
From Goldman L, Schafer AI: *Goldman's Cecil medicine,* ed 24, Philadelphia, 2011, Saunders.

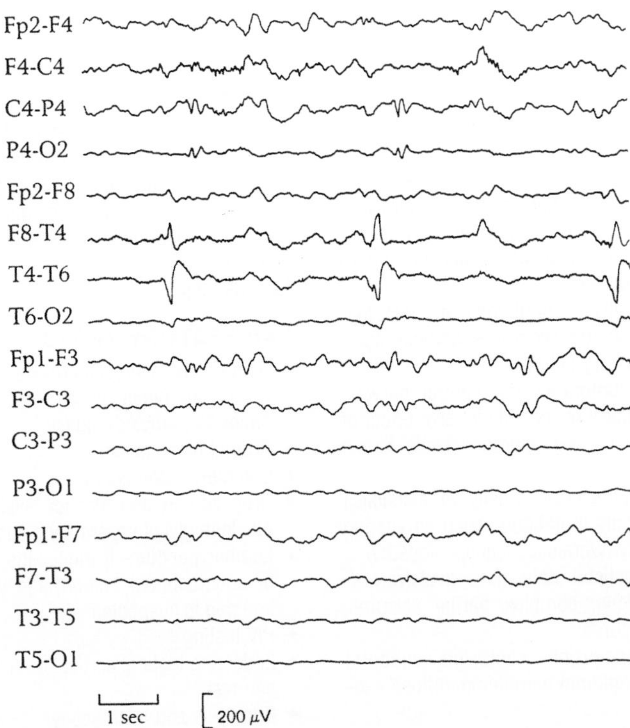

FIGURE 1-351 Repetitive complexes occurring in the right temporal region of a child with herpes simplex encephalitis. (From Goetz CG, Pappert EJ: *Textbook of clinical neurology,* Philadelphia, 1999, Saunders.)

- Rarely, brain biopsy to assist in the diagnosis; viral culture of cerebral tissue obtained if biopsy done
- Classic herpetic skin lesions suggestive of herpes encephalitis
- In diagnosing arboviral encephalitis:
  1. Presence of antiviral IgM within the first few days of symptomatic disease; detected and quantified by ELISA
  2. Unusual to recover an arbovirus from the blood or CSF

LABORATORY TESTS

- Aside from the lumbar puncture, most other laboratory studies are nonspecific.
- Skin lesions and urine may be cultured for herpes simplex and CMV.

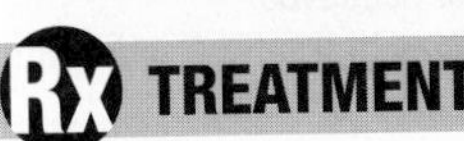

TREATMENT

ACUTE GENERAL Rx

- Supportive care, frequent evaluation, and neurologic examination
- Ventilatory assistance for patients who are moribund or at risk for aspiration
- Avoidance of infusion of hypotonic fluids to minimize the risk of hyponatremia
- For patients who develop seizures: anticonvulsant therapy and follow-up in a critical care setting
- For comatose patients:
  1. Aggressive care to avoid decubitus ulcers, contractures, and DVT
  2. Close attention to weights, input/output, and serum electrolytes
- Acyclovir 30 mg/kg/day IV total dose divided in q8 hour intervals for 14 days for herpes simplex encephalitis
- Short courses of corticosteroids to control brain edema and prevent herniation
- In patients with suspected rabies:
  1. Human rabies immune globulin (HRIG) should be given at a dose of 20 U/kg.
  2. Active immunization may be stimulated by rabies vaccine, which is grown on a human diploid cell line (HDCV) and has reduced the number of doses needed to five.
  3. If suspect animal is a dog or cat and can be found, observe closely for 10 days to detect rabid behavior; any significant illness in the animal should promptly initiate humane sacrifice of the animal with the brain submitted to local or state health departments for pathology and immunologic testing for rabies. Any wild animal suspected of rabies should be humanely sacrificed, if possible, and submitted for rabies testing immediately.
  4. If signs are seen, animal should be euthanized and its brain examined for signs of rabies.
- No specific pharmacologic therapy for most other viral pathogens

CHRONIC Rx

Some patients may develop permanent neurologic sequelae; these patients will benefit from intensive rehabilitation programs, including physical, occupational, and speech therapy.

DISPOSITION

- Patients with suspected encephalitis of any cause should generally be admitted for initial diagnostic workup and specific treatment (if available).
- Long-term management of patients with significant neurologic sequelae from encephalitis (e.g., memory defects, depression, difficulty with organization of thoughts, movement disorders) may benefit from rehabilitation services, home care, or nursing home placement.

REFERRAL

- To a neurologist for initial workup and management
- To an infectious disease specialist for diagnostic and therapeutic plan
- To a rehabilitation service for long-term evaluation and convalescent services

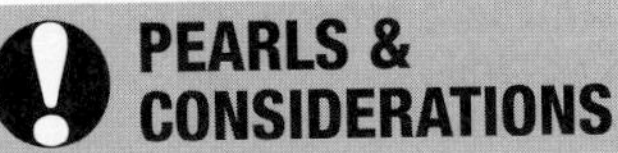

PEARLS & CONSIDERATIONS

- West Nile virus encephalitis occurs primarily in elderly patients >65 years of age.
- Rabies may occur months after contact with the rabid animal, and the exposure (especially bat rabies) may have been seemingly insignificant and even inapparent.
- Experimental therapies are worthy of consideration for some forms of viral encephalitis (e.g., immune plasma, ribavirin, interferons), and expert consultation should be obtained early on for possible treatment interventions with promising experimental therapies (e.g., Milwaukee protocol for rabies).

SUGGESTED READINGS

available at www.expertconsult.com

RELATED CONTENT

Rabies (Related Key Topic)
West Nile Virus Infection (Related Key Topic)

AUTHOR: **GLENN G. FORT, M.D., M.P.H.**

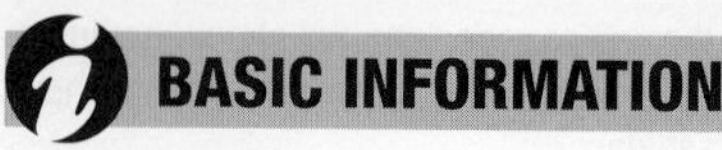

BASIC INFORMATION

DEFINITION

Encephalopathy is a clinical syndrome of global cognitive impairment characterized by impaired arousal, inattention, and disorientation.

SYNONYMS

Delirium, acute confusional state

ICD-9CM CODES	
348.3	Encephalopathy, NOS
348.30	Encephalopathy, unspecified
348.31	Encephalopathy, metabolic
348.39	Encephalopathy, other
349.82	Encephalopathy, toxic
ICD-10 CODES	
G93.40	Encephalopathy, unspecified
G93.41	Metabolic encephalopathy
G93.49	Other encephalopathy
G92	Toxic encephalopathy

EPIDEMIOLOGY & DEMOGRAPHICS

POINT PREVALENCE: 1.1% of adults in the general population >55 yr, 10% to 40% of hospitalized elderly, and 60% of nursing home patients >75 yr; 100,000 to 200,000 cases annually with anoxic encephalopathy

RISK FACTORS: Age, cancer, AIDS, terminal illness, bone marrow transplant, surgery

PHYSICAL FINDINGS & CLINICAL PRESENTATION

- The essential feature of encephalopathy is the patient's inability to maintain a coherent stream of thought or action.
- The history may often suggest a waxing and waning of the level of arousal and general cognitive ability.
- Because toxins and metabolic disturbances are common causes of encephalopathy, the history should focus on exposure to toxins (especially medications) and symptoms suggesting a concurrent illness such as a urinary tract infection or pneumonia.
- Common to all encephalopathies is a fluctuating level of arousal, poor attention, and disorientation.
- Some patients may appear agitated and others lethargic.
- Delusions (fixed false beliefs) and hallucinations are common.
- Asterixis (negative myoclonus) is common.
- Other physical findings may vary depending on the underlying cause of encephalopathy, such as fever, ascites, jaundice, or tachycardia.

ETIOLOGY

The final common pathway of all causes of encephalopathy is widespread, neuronal dysfunction from structural or functional causes. Many conditions are reversible and carry a good prognosis if treated in a timely manner.

- Organ failure (e.g., hepatic encephalopathy, hypoxia, hypercapnia, uremia)
- Infection: systemic (e.g., urinary tract, pneumonia, sepsis) or involving the central nervous system (e.g., meningitis, encephalitis)
- Toxin ingestion or withdrawal (e.g., alcohol, medications [especially psychotropics and neuroleptics], recreational drugs)
- Metabolic disturbances: hyperosmolar states, hypernatremia, hyponatremia, hyperglycemia, hypoglycemia, hypercalcemia, hypophosphatemia, acidosis, alkalosis, inborn errors of metabolism
- Endocrinopathy: hyperthyroidism, hypothyroidism, Cushing's syndrome, adrenal insufficiency, pituitary failure
- Neoplasm: tumors of the central nervous system, primary or metastatic; also effect of distant tumors (e.g., paraneoplastic limbic encephalitis)
- Nutritional deficiency, mostly in alcoholics and chronically ill patients, such as vitamin B_1 deficiency (Wernicke's encephalopathy)
- Seizures: postictal state, nonconvulsive status epilepticus, complex partial seizures, absence seizures
- Trauma: concussion, contusion, subdural hematoma, epidural hematoma, diffuse axonal injury
- Vascular: ischemic and hemorrhagic strokes, vasculitis, venous thrombosis
- Postanoxic encephalopathy
- Psychiatric disease: acute psychosis, depression with psychiatric features
- Acute disease: acute disseminating myelitis, tumefactive multiple sclerosis
- Other: hypertensive encephalopathy, postoperative status, sleep deprivation

Dx DIAGNOSIS

DIFFERENTIAL DIAGNOSIS

Differential diagnosis for encephalopathy is broad. It is typically helpful to distinguish toxic metabolic causes from primary neurologic causes.

- Dementia: distinguished from encephalopathy by a history of slowly progressive cognitive decline over time (fluctuating cognitive function is rare except in diffuse Lewy body disease).
- Hypersomnia
- Aphasia: distinguished from encephalopathy by virtue of it representing a specific disorder of language rather than a global disturbance of cognitive function.
- Depression
- Psychosis: some overlap with encephalopathy because delusions and hallucinations may be common to both.
- Mania
- Vegetative state from cerebral injury; these patients appear awake (eyes are open) but there is no content to their consciousness.
- Akinetic mutism: these patients do not talk and do not move; there is little fluctuation in their state and there is no asterixis or other focal deficit.
- Locked-in syndrome: may be distinguished from encephalopathy by the presence of fixed neurologic deficits (e.g., paralysis of all four limbs); however, the patient is aware of his or her environment.

WORKUP

The best tool in the evaluation of encephalopathy is a good history and physical exam, which will help tailor the remainder of the diagnostic workup. Interview family members and other providers to identify preceding events, medication changes, and medical history. Evaluate focal deficits.

LABORATORY TESTS

- General chemistry: electrolytes, glucose, creatinine, ammonia, blood urea nitrogen, transaminases, amylase, lipase
- Arterial blood gases
- Complete blood count
- Drug screen and alcohol level (must order ethylene glycol separately if suspected)
- Lumbar puncture if meningitis, encephalitis, or subarachnoid hemorrhage with negative imaging is suspected
- HIV testing
- Endocrine testing: cortisol level, thyroid function test
- Urinalysis and microscopy

IMAGING STUDIES

- Chest radiograph to rule out pneumonia
- Head CT to rule out bleeding, hydrocephalus, tumors
- Brain MRI with diffusion-weighted images for suspected encephalitis, tumors, and acute strokes
- Magnetic resonance angiography/venography for strokes, arterial dissection, venous thrombosis
- Conventional angiography for central nervous system (CNS) vasculitis and aneurysms
- EEG: evaluate for subclinical status epilepticus

Rx TREATMENT

The encephalopathy itself is a symptom of these underlying problems. In general, it is best to avoid treating the symptom of encephalopathy with antipsychotics or sedatives.

- The best approach is to treat the underlying toxic or metabolic disturbance.
- Thiamine supplementation
- Glucose for hypoglycemia
- Antibiotics in cases of infections (choose an agent with good CNS penetration in cases of primary CNS infections)
- Insulin in hyperglycemic conditions (e.g., diabetic ketoacidosis, hyperosmolar nonketosis, and sepsis)
- Ensure hemodynamic stability (blood pressure and heart rate)

SUGGESTED READINGS

available at www.expertconsult.com

RELATED CONTENT

Hepatic Encephalopathy (Related Key Topic)

AUTHOR: **JOSHUA CHALKELY, M.S., D.O.**

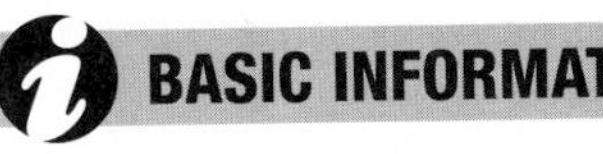

BASIC INFORMATION

DEFINITION/DIAGNOSTIC CRITERIA

DSM-5[1] defines encopresis as:

A. Reverted passage of feces into inappropriate places (e.g., clothing, floor), whether involuntary or intentional

B. At least one such event occurs each month for at least three months

C. The behavior is not attributable to the physiological effects of a substance (e.g., laxatives) or another medical condition except through a mechanism involving constipation

Encopresis may be classified into two types based on published guidelines of the Multinational Working Teams to Develop Criteria for Functional Disorders (Rome III). Definition of functional retentive encopresis requires two of six criteria: 2 or fewer defecations per week, at least 1 episode of incontinence after acquisition of toileting skills, history of excessive fecal retention and or painful or hard bowel movements, presence of large fecal mass in the rectum, history of large diameter stools that may obstruct the toilet. Non-retentive encopresis is fecal incontinence without evidence of constipation or fecal retention in the absence of underlying disease process that explains the symptoms.

SYNONYMS

Stool/fecal incontinence; soiling!

ICD-9CM and DSM-5 CODES
307.7
ICD-10CM CODES
R15 Fecal incontinence
F98.1 Non-organic (psychogenic) encopresis

EPIDEMIOLOGY & DEMOGRAPHICS

PEAK INCIDENCE: Preschool age (though also occurs during school age and adolescence)
PREVALENCE (IN U.S.): 1.5% to 7.5% of children 4 to 12 yr old
PREDOMINANT SEX: More often in males (estimates range from 1.9:1 to 9:1)

PHYSICAL FINDINGS & CLINICAL PRESENTATION

- Most children are toilet-trained for stool by age 4. Traditionally, in primary encopresis, fecal continence is never fully established; in secondary encopresis, soiling is preceded by a period of fecal continence. However, definitions of "primary" vs. "secondary" do not reliably correlate with etiology or outcome.
- Constipation and withholding of stool are significant factors in 80% to 90% of cases ("retentive encopresis"). In 10% to 20%, constipation is not a factor ("nonretentive" encopresis).
- When constipation is longstanding, soft or liquid stool may flow around the retained feces, resulting in overflow incontinence. This may occur several times per day and mistakenly be interpreted as diarrhea.
- Children may report a lack of awareness of stool passage when longstanding constipation/impaction has resulted in loss of rectal tone and sensation. Furthermore, some children habituate to the odor.

ETIOLOGY

- Approximately 96% of children have bowel movements between three times daily to once every other day. When bowel movements are less frequent, stool becomes drier and harder and much more uncomfortable or painful to pass. Children may avoid the discomfort or pain by avoiding elimination, resulting in worsening constipation and overflow incontinence.
- Constipation may begin gradually as a result of a decrease in elimination frequency, or more acutely after an illness or changes in diet.
- Toilet training practices that increase anxiety may also play a role in stool retention, the development of constipation, and eventual encopresis.

Dx DIAGNOSIS

DIFFERENTIAL DIAGNOSIS

- Hirschsprung's disease
- Endocrine disease (hypothyroidism)
- Cerebral palsy
- Myelomeningocele
- Pseudoobstruction
- Anorectal lesions (rectal stenosis)
- Malformations
- Trauma
- Rectal prolapse
- Celiac disease
- Hypothyroidism
- Medications

WORKUP

- History: frequency of elimination, character of the stool, associated pain, and presence of enuresis (with which it is frequently associated).
- Evaluate for other developmental or psychiatric problems.
- Common physical findings in retentive encopresis: abdominal fecal mass, stool-impacted rectum, loose anal sphincter, fecal material in the perianal area, anal tags or fissures.
- Perform a complete neurologic examination to exclude sensorineural or spinal cord abnormalities.

LABORATORY TESTS

- Thyroid function tests, celiac screening tests, electrolytes, calcium, urinalysis, urine culture.
- If concerned about the possibility of Hirschprung's disease, obtain rectal biopsy.

IMAGING STUDIES

- Abdominal imaging to determine extent of obstruction or megacolon
- Anorectal manometric studies or barium enema can support suspicion of Hirschsprung's disease

Rx TREATMENT

ACUTE GENERAL Rx

- Disimpaction is a necessary first step, by oral or rectal route (or combination).
- For oral disimpaction, polyethylene glycol, magnesium citrate, or high doses of mineral oil are effective (avoid use of mineral oil in patients at risk for aspiration).
- Adding stimulant laxatives such as senna or bisacodyl can sometimes make oral disimpaction more effective.
- For rectal disimpaction, phosphate soda, saline, or mineral oil enemas are effective.
- When medical workup determines no constipation ("nonretentive encopresis"), consider toilet-training routines or referral to behavioral health provider.

CHRONIC Rx

- Prevent recurrence of constipation with oral stool softeners (e.g., polyethylene glycol or lactulose) or stool lubricants (mineral oil).
- In immediate postdisimpaction period (1 mo after treatment), stimulant laxatives may be needed if bowel tone remains low; taper use as quickly as possible to avoid dependence.
- Family documentation of stool passage, including location and amount, helps inform medication changes and best times for toilet sitting.
- Praise and other incentives for positive toileting routines and medication can help maintain good bowel habits. Balanced diet and increased fiber intake/supplementation may help.
- Formal behavioral treatment (education, reinforcement of treatment adherence, exercises to improve anal sphincter control) increases treatment success. Biofeedback is advocated by some, with 1-yr results comparable to behavioral treatment. Adjunctive Internet-based interventions that incorporate behavioral therapy and medical management are beginning to show promise.

DISPOSITION

Encopresis may be self-limited or relatively brief in duration; may require prolonged maintenance therapy. Relapses are common.

REFERRAL

Behavioral family therapy should be considered for patients who do not respond to medical treatment within a few months or who have significant contributing psychiatric or family factors.

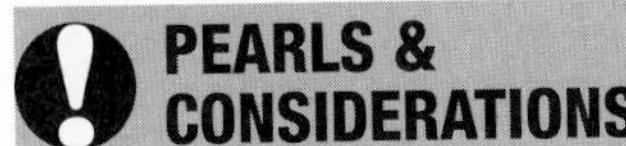

PEARLS & CONSIDERATIONS

- Educate parents and children about constipation and encopresis and defuse negative interactions.
- Emphasize it may need prolonged maintenance therapy and relapses are common.

SUGGESTED READINGS

available at www.expertconsult.com

RELATED CONTENT

Encopresis (Patient Information)

AUTHORS: **CAROLINA S. CEREZO, M.D.,** and **WENDY A. PLANTE, PH.D.**

[1]American Psychiatric Association: *Desk reference to the diagnostic criteria from DSM-5*, Arlington, VA, 2013, American Psychiatric Association.

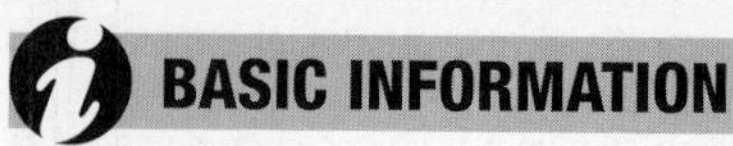

BASIC INFORMATION

DEFINITION

Infective endocarditis is an infection of the endocardial surface of the heart or mural endocardium. Box 1-27 describes the modified Duke criteria for the diagnosis of infective endocarditis.

ACUTE ENDOCARDITIS: Usually caused by *Staphylococcus aureus, Streptococcus pyogenes, Streptococcus pneumoniae,* and *Neisseria* organisms; classic clinical presentation of high fever, positive blood cultures, vascular and immunologic phenomenon

SUBACUTE ENDOCARDITIS: Usually caused by viridans streptococci in the presence of valvular pathology; less toxic, often indolent presentation with lower fevers, night sweats, fatigue

ENDOCARDITIS IN INJECTION DRUG USERS: Often involving *S. aureus* or *Pseudomonas aeruginosa* with variation that may be geographically influenced; tricuspid (Fig. 1-352) or multiple valvular involvement; high mortality rate of 50% to 60%

PROSTHETIC VALVE ENDOCARDITIS (EARLY): Usually caused by *S. aureus* (leading cause of PVE) within 2 mo of valve replacement; other organisms include *S. epidermidis,* gram-negative bacilli, diphtheroids, *Candida* organisms

PROSTHETIC VALVE ENDOCARDITIS (LATE): Typically develops >60 days after valvular replacement; involved organisms similar to early prosthetic valve endocarditis, including viridans streptococci, enterococci, and group D streptococci

NOSOCOMIAL ENDOCARDITIS: Secondary to intravenous catheters, TPN lines, pacemakers; coagulase-negative staphylococci, *S. aureus,* and streptococci most common

Non-HACEK gram-negative bacillus endocarditis is not primarily a disease of injection drug users. More than half of all cases are associated with health care contact

SYNONYMS

Bacterial endocarditis
Subacute bacterial endocarditis (SBE)
Endocarditis

ICD-9CM CODES
421.0 Infective endocarditis
996.61 Prosthetic valve endocarditis

ICD-10CM CODES
I33.0 Acute and subacute infective endocarditis
I33.9 Acute endocarditis, unspecified

EPIDEMIOLOGY & DEMOGRAPHICS

INCIDENCE (IN U.S.): 5 to 7.9 cases/100,000 persons/yr

PEAK INCIDENCE: Females: often <35 yr old; males: 45 to 65 yr old

NOSOCOMIAL ENDOCARDITIS: 14% to 28% of cases

PREVALENCE (IN U.S.): 0.3 to 3 cases/1000 hospital admissions

PREDOMINANT SEX: Male <female

PREDOMINANT AGE: 45 to 65 yr

PHYSICAL FINDINGS & CLINICAL PRESENTATION

- Clinical manifestations of infective endocarditis are described in Table E1-179.
- Fever may be variable in presentation; may be high, hectic, or absent.
- Fever, chills, fatigue, and rigors occur in 25% to 80% of patients.
- Heart murmur may be absent in right-sided endocarditis.
- Embolic phenomenon with peripheral manifestations is found in 50% of patients.
- Skin manifestations include petechiae, Osler nodes (Fig. E1-353), splinter hemorrhages, Janeway lesions (Fig. E1-354).
- Splenomegaly is more common with subacute course.

ETIOLOGY

Staphylococcal infection is now the leading cause of native or prosthetic valve infection. Variation in incidence may occur that is influenced by the patient's risk for developing infection. Risk factors include hemodialysis (8%), IV drug use (10%), mitral regurgitation (43%), aortic regurgitation (26%), and rheumatic heart disease (3.3%).

ACUTE ENDOCARDITIS:
- *S. aureus*
- *S. lugdunensis*
- *S. pneumoniae*
- Streptococcal species and groups A through G
- *Haemophilus influenzae*

SUBACUTE ENDOCARDITIS:
- Viridans streptococci (alpha-hemolytic)
- *S. bovis*
- Enterococci
- *S. aureus*

ENDOCARDITIS IN INJECTION DRUG USERS:
- *S. aureus*
- *P. aeruginosa*
- *Candida* spp.
- Enterococci

PROSTHETIC VALVE ENDOCARDITIS (EARLY):
- *S. epidermidis*
- *S. aureus*
- Gram-negative bacilli
- Group D streptococci

PROSTHETIC VALVE ENDOCARDITIS (LATE):
- *S. epidermidis*
- Viridans streptococci

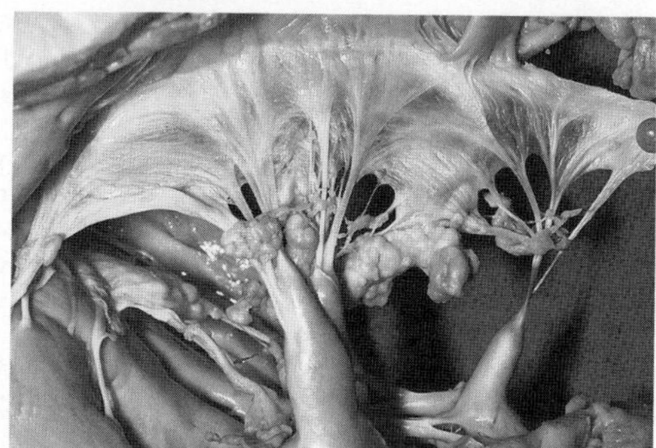

FIGURE 1-352 Tricuspid valve endocarditis. There are large vegetations on the leaflets and the chordae tendineae. (From Crawford MH et al [eds]: *Cardiology,* ed 2, St Louis, 2004, Mosby.)

BOX 1-27 Modified Duke Criteria for the Diagnosis of Infective Endocarditis*

Major Criteria
Positive blood cultures for infective endocarditis
Typical microorganism for infective endocarditis from two separate blood cultures in the absence of a primary focus: *Streptococcus viridans, Streptococcus bovis*
HACEK group: *Haemophilus* species, *Actinobacillus actinomycetemcomitans, Cardiobacterium hominis, Eikenella corrodens,* and *Kingella kingae*
Community-acquired *Staphylococcus aureus* or *enterococci*
Persistently positive blood cultures, defined as recovery of a microorganism consistent with infective endocarditis from blood cultures drawn more than 12 hr apart or all of three or the majority of four or more separate blood cultures, with first and last drawn at least 1 hr apart
Single positive blood culture for *Coxiella burnetii* or antiphase IgG antibody titer >1:800
Evidence for endocardial involvement
TTE (TEE in prosthetic valve) showing oscillating intracardiac mass on a valve or supporting structures, in the path of regurgitant jet or on implanted material, in the absence of an alternative anatomic explanation, *or*
Abscess, *or*
New partial dehiscence of prosthetic valve

Minor Criteria
Predisposition (e.g., prosthetic valve, intravenous drug use)
Fever: 38° C
Vascular phenomena
Immunologic phenomena
Microbiologic evidence: positive blood culture but not meeting major criteria

TEE, Transoesophageal echocardiogram; *TTE,* transthoracic echocardiogram.
From Ballinger A: *Kumar & Clark's essentials of clinical medicine,* ed 6, Edinburgh, 2012, Saunders.
*Adapted from Li JS et al: Proposed modifications to the Duke criteria for the diagnosis of infective endocarditis, *Clin Infect Dis* 30:633-638, 2000.

- *S. aureus*
- Enterococci and group D streptococci

NOSOCOMIAL ENDOCARDITIS:
- Coagulase-negative staphylococci
- *S. aureus*
- Streptococci: viridans, group B, enterococcus

HACEK ORGANISMS:
- Fastidious gram-negative bacilli
- *Haemophilus parainfluenzae*
- *Haemophilus aphrophilus*
- *Actinobacillus actinomycetemcomitans*
- *Cardiobacterium hominis*
- *Eikenella corrodens*
- *Kingella kingae*

RISK FACTORS
- Poor dental hygiene
- Long-term hemodialysis
- Diabetes mellitus
- HIV infection
- Mitral valve prolapse

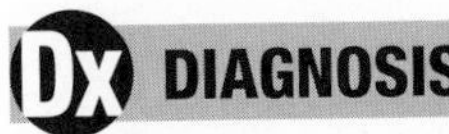

DIAGNOSIS

DIFFERENTIAL DIAGNOSIS
- Brain abscess
- FUO
- Pericarditis
- Meningitis
- Rheumatic fever
- Osteomyelitis
- *Salmonella*
- TB
- Bacteremia
- Pericarditis
- Glomerulonephritis

WORKUP
Physical examination to evaluate for the previous physical findings followed by laboratory testing (see "Laboratory Tests"). Fig. 1-355 describes a diagnostic evaluation of suspected endocarditis. The modified Duke criteria for diagnosis of endocarditis defines "major criteria" as persistently positive blood cultures of organisms typical of endocarditis or endocardial involvement (new valvular regurgitation or positive echocardiogram). "Minor criteria" is defined as presence of predisposing condition or injection drug use, fever, embolic vascular pneumonia (e.g., glomerulonephritis, rheumatoid factor), or positive blood cultures not meeting major criteria. Definite endocarditis is 2 major criteria or 1 major criteria and 3 minor criteria or 5 minor criteria or presence of organisms by culture or histologic examination of a vegetation.

LABORATORY TESTS
- Blood cultures: three sets in first 24 hr
- More culturing if patient has received prior antibiotic
- CBC (anemia possibly present, subacute)
- WBC (leukocytosis is higher in acute endocarditis)
- ESR and C-reactive protein (elevated)
- Positive rheumatoid factor (subacute endocarditis)
- Proteinuria, hematuria, RBC casts

IMAGING STUDIES
- Echocardiogram: two-dimensional. Transthoracic echocardiography (TTE) (Fig. E1-356) is noninvasive and more easily available but has less-than-optimal sensitivity (50%-80%) for endocarditis.
- Transesophageal echocardiography (TEE): more sensitive in detecting vegetations and preferred diagnostic modality. It is especially helpful with prosthetic valves or in detecting perivalvular disease.
- Electrocardiogram: look for cardiac conduction abnormalities, injury pattern, or evidence of pericarditis—any such new findings are suggestive of myocardial abscess

Rx TREATMENT

Initial IV antibiotic therapy (before culture results) is aimed at the most likely organism.

- **Native valve (no history of IV drugs) empiric therapy awaiting cultures:** Pen G 20 million U IV q24h continuous or divided q4h or ampicillin 12 g IV q24h continuous or divided q4h *plus* nafcillin or oxacillin 2 g IV q4h *plus* gentamicin 1 mg/kg IV q8h; other options are vancomycin 15 mg/kg (assuming CrCl ≥80 ml/min) IV q12h *plus* gentamicin 1 mg/kg IM or IV q8h
- **Native valve (IV drug use ± evidence of right-sided endocarditis) empiric therapy:** vancomycin 30-60 mg/kg/day in 2-3 divided doses for trough 15-20 mcg/ml or daptomycin 6 mg/kg IV q24h
- **Native valve (culture positive):** Pen G 12-18 million U/day IV, divided q4h × 2 wk *plus* gentamicin 1 mg/kg q8h IV × 2 wk (target level peak 3 mcg/ml, trough <1 mcg/ml) *or* ceftriaxone 2 g IV q24h × 4 wk
- **Staphylococcal endocarditis (aortic and/or mitral valve)**
  - **MSSA:** nafcillin (or oxacillin) 2 g IV q4h × 4-6 wk *or* cefazolin 2 g IV q8h × 4-6 wk *or* vancomycin 15 mg/kg IV q12h (check level if >2 g/day) × 4-6 wk
  - **MRSA:** vancomycin 30-60 mg/kg/day 2-3 divided doses with trough conc. 15-20 mcg/ml
- **Patients with prosthetic valves or native valves who are allergic to PCN:** vancomycin (1 g IV q12h × 4 wk) *plus* rifampin 600 mg PO qd *and* gentamicin (1 mg/kg IV q8h × 2 wk), assuming normal renal function in adult patients

Antibiotic therapy after identification of the organism should be guided by susceptibility testing, preferably by formal testing by MIC (minimum inhibitory concentration).

DISPOSITION
- The patient may need outpatient IV antibiotic therapy, and arrangements need to be made to ensure safe vascular access and continuity of care with outpatient IV therapy team.
- Long-term follow-up is essential after therapy has ended; relapse of endocarditis may occur.
- Prophylaxis with antibiotics will be needed before dental procedures as a previous episode of endocarditis increases the risk of recurrent endocarditis associated with transient bacteremia from dental procedures.

REFERRAL
- To an infectious disease specialist
- To a cardiologist or a cardiac surgeon if evidence of heart failure, refractory infection, myocardial abscess, valve disruption, or major embolic events occur.
- The timing and indications for surgical intervention to prevent systemic embolism in infective endocarditis remain controversial. Trials have shown that early surgery in patients with infective endocarditis and large vegetations significantly reduced death and embolic events by decreasing the risk of systemic embolism.

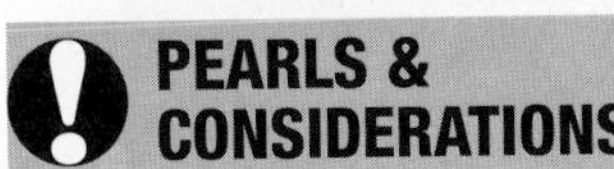

PEARLS & CONSIDERATIONS

COMMENTS
For endocarditis prophylaxis refer to Section V.

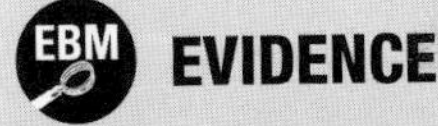

EVIDENCE
available at www.expertconsult.com

SUGGESTED READINGS
available at www.expertconsult.com

RELATED CONTENT
Endocarditis (Patient Information)

AUTHOR: **GLENN G. FORT, M.D., M.P.H.**

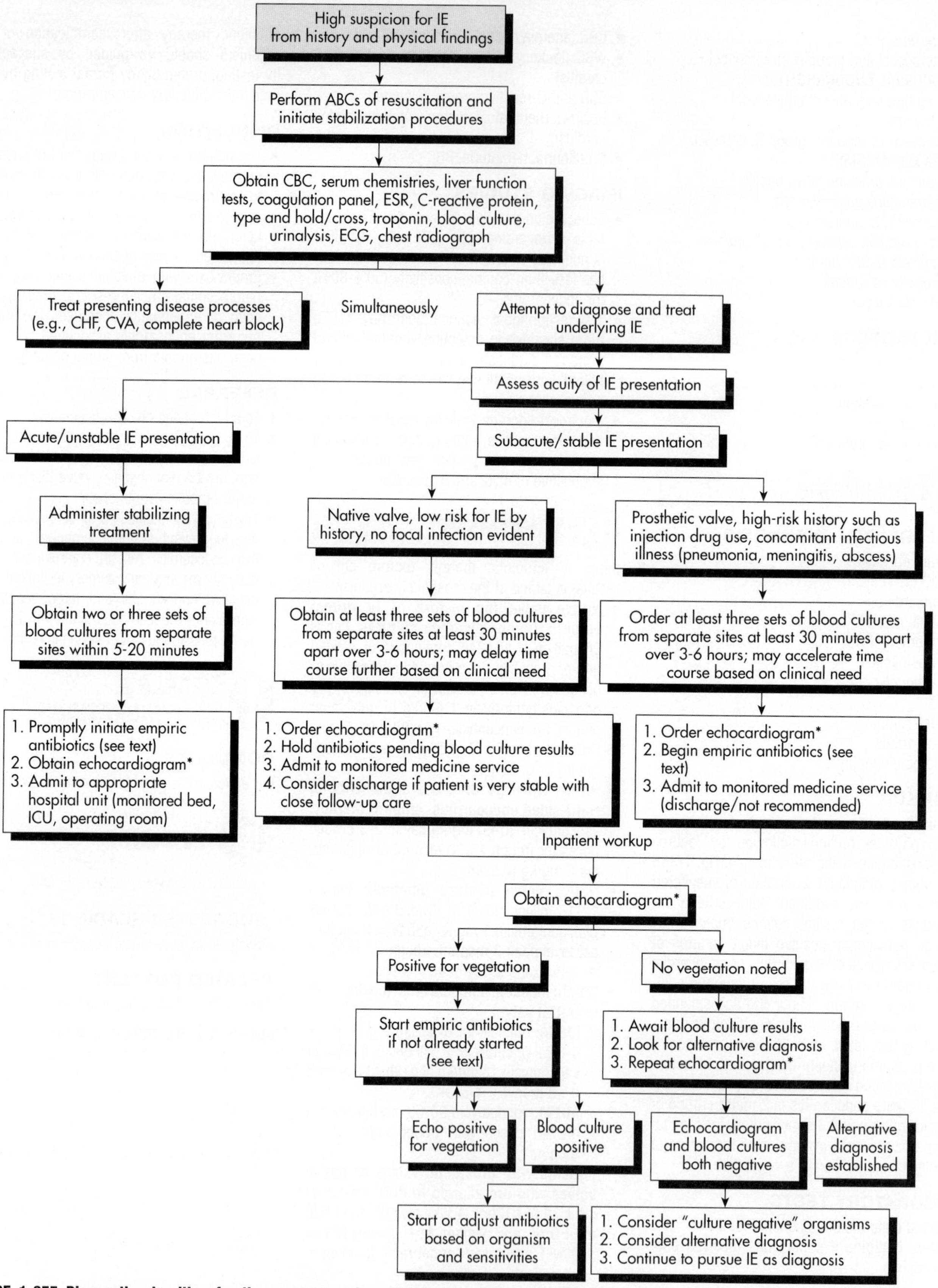

- High suspicion for IE from history and physical findings
- ↓ Perform ABCs of resuscitation and initiate stabilization procedures
- ↓ Obtain CBC, serum chemistries, liver function tests, coagulation panel, ESR, C-reactive protein, type and hold/cross, troponin, blood culture, urinalysis, ECG, chest radiograph
- ↓ Simultaneously:
  - Treat presenting disease processes (e.g., CHF, CVA, complete heart block)
  - Attempt to diagnose and treat underlying IE
    - ↓ Assess acuity of IE presentation
      - **Acute/unstable IE presentation**
        - ↓ Administer stabilizing treatment
        - ↓ Obtain two or three sets of blood cultures from separate sites within 5-20 minutes
        - ↓ 1. Promptly initiate empiric antibiotics (see text) 2. Obtain echocardiogram* 3. Admit to appropriate hospital unit (monitored bed, ICU, operating room)
      - **Subacute/stable IE presentation**
        - Native valve, low risk for IE by history, no focal infection evident
          - ↓ Obtain at least three sets of blood cultures from separate sites at least 30 minutes apart over 3-6 hours; may delay time course further based on clinical need
          - ↓ 1. Order echocardiogram* 2. Hold antibiotics pending blood culture results 3. Admit to monitored medicine service 4. Consider discharge if patient is very stable with close follow-up care
        - Prosthetic valve, high-risk history such as injection drug use, concomitant infectious illness (pneumonia, meningitis, abscess)
          - ↓ Order at least three sets of blood cultures from separate sites at least 30 minutes apart over 3-6 hours; may accelerate time course based on clinical need
          - ↓ 1. Order echocardiogram* 2. Begin empiric antibiotics (see text) 3. Admit to monitored medicine service (discharge/not recommended)
        - Inpatient workup
          - ↓ Obtain echocardiogram*
            - Positive for vegetation → Start empiric antibiotics if not already started (see text)
            - No vegetation noted → 1. Await blood culture results 2. Look for alternative diagnosis 3. Repeat echocardiogram*
              - Echo positive for vegetation → Start empiric antibiotics if not already started (see text)
              - Blood culture positive → Start or adjust antibiotics based on organism and sensitivities
              - Echocardiogram and blood cultures both negative → 1. Consider "culture negative" organisms 2. Consider alternative diagnosis 3. Continue to pursue IE as diagnosis
              - Alternative diagnosis established

FIGURE 1-355 Diagnostic algorithm for the emergency department management of patients in whom infective endocarditis (IE) is suspected. *Echocardiography can be performed via either the transthoracic (TTE) or transesophageal (TEE) technique. TEE is more invasive but is more sensitive for detecting vegetations and complications of IE, such as perivalvular abscesses; it is recommended for prosthetic valves; for situations in which optimal visualization by TTE will be difficult, such as emphysema and morbid obesity; for high suspicion of IE but normal TTE findings; and for high suspicion of a complication of IE, such as perivalvular abscess. Normal findings with either technique do not exclude IE if clinical suspicion is high. Echocardiograms can be repeated in an attempt to identify problems such as vegetations and abscesses that may not be noted initially. *ABCs*, Airway, breathing, and circulation; *CBC*, complete blood count; *CHF*, congestive heart failure; *CVA*, cerebrovascular accident; *ECG*, electrocardiogram; *ESR*, erythrocyte sedimentation rate; *ICU*, intensive care unit. (From Adams JG et al: *Emergency medicine, clinical essentials*, ed 2, Philadelphia, 2013, Elsevier.)

BASIC INFORMATION

DEFINITION

Endometrial cancer (EC) is a malignant transformation of endometrial stroma and/or glands typified by irregular nuclear membranes, nuclear atypia, mitotic activity, loss of glandular pattern, and irregular cell size. The two main histologic subcategories of EC, endometrioid and nonendometrioid EC, show unique molecular aberrations and differing clinical behaviors.

SYNONYMS

Uterine cancer (some forms)

ICD-9CM CODES
182 Malignant neoplasm of body of uterus
ICD-10CM CODES
C54.1 Malignant neoplasm of endometrium
C55 Malignant neoplasm of uterus, part unspecified
C54.9 Malignant neoplasm of corpus uteri, unspecified

EPIDEMIOLOGY & DEMOGRAPHICS

INCIDENCE: 21.2 cases per 100,000 persons; approximately 30,000 new cases annually. It is the most common gynecologic malignancy in the U.S.
PREDOMINANCE: Median age at onset: 60 yr; only 5% occur in women <40 yr
RISK FACTORS: Obesity, diabetes, nulliparity, early menarche and late menopause, unopposed estrogen therapy, tamoxifen use, oligoovulation with chronic unopposed estrogen exposure such as with polycystic ovary syndrome (PCOS), endometrial atypical hyperplasia, endometrial polyps (malignancy is found in 3.6% of endometrial polyps)

PHYSICAL FINDINGS & CLINICAL PRESENTATION

- Abnormal uterine bleeding or postmenopausal bleeding in 90%
- Pyometra or hematometra
- Abnormal Pap smear

ETIOLOGY

Endogenous or exogenous chronic unopposed estrogen stimulation of the endometrium

DIAGNOSIS

DIFFERENTIAL DIAGNOSIS

- Atypical hyperplasia
- Other genital tract malignancy
- Uterine polyps
- Atrophic vaginitis
- Granuloma cell tumor
- Fibroid uterus

WORKUP

- Complete history and physical examination
- Endometrial biopsy or dilation and curettage
- Assessment of operative risk
- Staging (Table 1-180)

LABORATORY TESTS

- Complete blood count
- Chemistry profile including liver function tests
- Consider CA-125 level

IMAGING STUDIES

- Chest x-ray
- CT scan, and/or pelvic ultrasound (Fig. 1-357)
- Endovaginal ultrasound (Fig. 1-358) in postmenopausal women with vaginal bleeding

TREATMENT

NONPHARMACOLOGIC THERAPY

- Surgery is the mainstay of treatment, with or without radiation, depending on tumor stage and grade. Laparoscopic surgery for early-stage EC is as safe and effective as laparotomy. Robotic laparoscopy procedures have increased significantly in recent years for this indication.
- Surgery generally consists of pelvic washings, total abdominal hysterectomy and bilateral salpingo-oophorectomy, omental biopsy, and selective pelvic and periaortic lymphadenectomy, depending on stage and grade.
- Brachytherapy and/or teletherapy are added in an advanced stage.
- Chemotherapy (cisplatin, Adriamycin) or tamoxifen may also be used, especially for advanced or recurrent endometrial cancers.
- Aromatase inhibitors, currently primarily used for breast carcinoma, are being investigated as adjuvant therapy for endometrial cancer.
- Hormonal therapy is an option for some young women with EC who wish to preserve fertility. This choice should be discussed with a gynecologic oncologist.

ACUTE GENERAL Rx

- A thorough workup should be completed before any therapy for EC.
- Surgery is the treatment of choice.

CHRONIC Rx

- Physical and pelvic examination every 3 mo for 2 yr, then every 6 mo for 2 yr, annually thereafter

TABLE 1-180 FIGO Staging of Endometrial Carcinoma

Stage	Definition	Stage at Presentation	Pelvic Nodes	5-Year Survival
I_A	Tumor limited to the endometrium			
I_B	Growth that has invaded <50% of myometrial thickness	73%	>20%	85%
I_C	Growth that has invaded >50% of myometrial thickness			
II_A	Endocervical glandular involvement only	11%	20%	65%
II_B	Cervical stroma involved			
III_A	Invades sero-serosal surface of uterus, ± adnexa, ± positive washings	13%	35%	40%
III_B	Vaginal metastases			
III_C	Metastases to pelvic or para-aortic nodes			
IV_A	Tumor invasion of bladder and/or bowel	3%	50%	10%
IV_B	Distant metastases including intra-abdominal and/or inguinal lymph nodes			

Histopathology: Degree of Differentiation

Uterine adenocarcinoma should be grouped according to the degree of differentiation as follows:
G1 – 5% or less of a solid growth pattern
G2 – 6%-50% of a solid growth pattern
G3 – More than 50% of a solid growth pattern

From Drife J, Magowan B: *Clinical obstetrics and gynecology*, Philadelphia, 2004, Saunders.

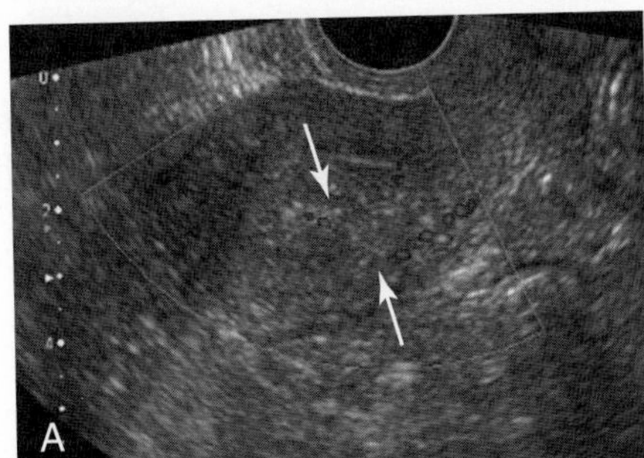

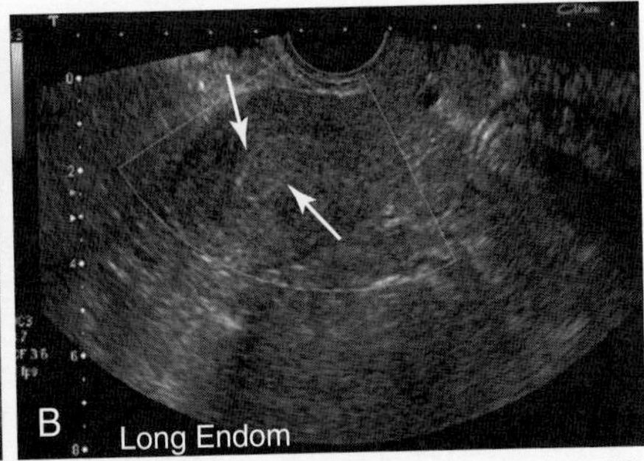

FIGURE 1-357 A 48-year-old woman with endometrial carcinoma. A, Endovaginal ultrasound (US) showing thickened, heterogeneous, cystic, and vascular hyperechoic tissue filling the endometrial cavity *(arrows)*. **B,** Second, sagittal US image showing the same. (From Fielding JR et al: *Gynecologic imaging*, Philadelphia, 2011, Saunders.)

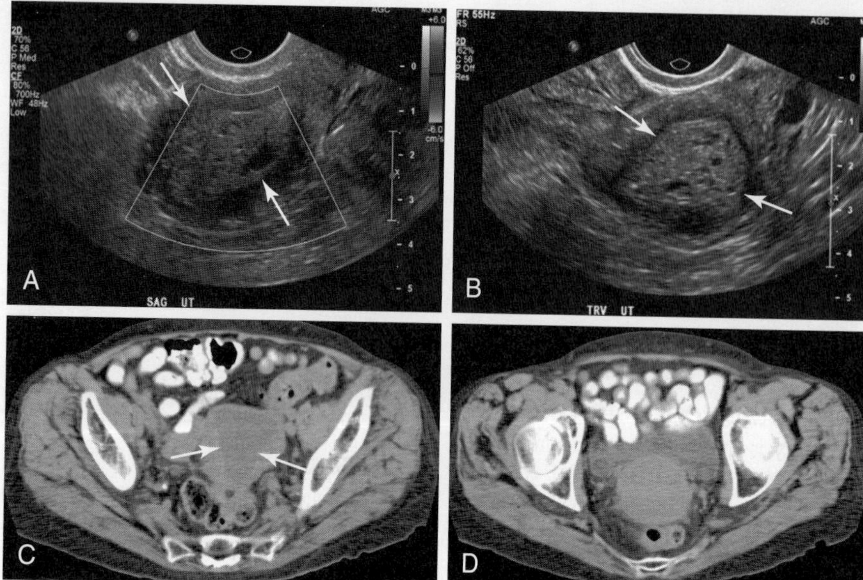

FIGURE 1-358 A 56-year-old woman with endometrial carcinoma. A, Sagittal ultrasound (US) image showing thickened cystic echogenic soft tissue filling the endometrial cavity *(arrows)*. **B,** Axial US image showing thickened cystic echogenic soft tissue filling the endometrial cavity *(arrows)*. **C,** Non–contrast-enhanced axial computed tomographic (CT) image showing low-attenuation tissue filling the endometrial canal *(arrows)* in a postmenopausal patient. Note fundal thinning. **D,** Non–contrast-enhanced axial CT image showing cervical soft tissue fullness. (From Fielding JR et al: *Gynecologic imaging*, Philadelphia, 2011, Saunders.)

- Yearly Pap smear
- Hormone replacement (combination) a consideration in low-risk patients (stage I or early stage II)

DISPOSITION

The majority of cases present early, and the 5-yr survival is generally good:

Stage I	75%-100%
Stage II	65%
Stage III	40%
Stage IV	10%

Some histologic types (clear cell, serous papillary) have worse survival rates.

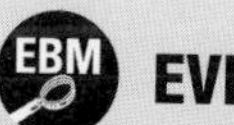

EVIDENCE

available at www.expertconsult.com

SUGGESTED READINGS

available at www.expertconsult.com

RELATED CONTENT

Dysfunctional Uterine Bleeding (Related Key Topic)
Uterine Malignancy (Related Key Topic)
Endometrial Cancer (Patient Information)

AUTHOR: **RUBEN ALVERO, M.D.**

BASIC INFORMATION

DEFINITION

Endometriosis is defined as the presence of functioning endometrial glands and stroma outside the uterine cavity (Fig. 1-359).

ICD-9CM CODES
617.9 Endometriosis
ICD-1-CM CODES
N80.9 Endometriosis, unspecified

EPIDEMIOLOGY & DEMOGRAPHICS

PREVALENCE:
- Endometriosis affects 10% of reproductive-aged women.
- Women with dysmenorrhea: 40% to 60%
- Subfertile women: 20% to 30%
- Incidence peaks at approximately 40 yr

MOST COMMON AGE AT DIAGNOSIS: 25 to 29 yr

GENETICS:
- Multifactorial inheritance pattern
- 6.9% occurrence rate in first-degree female relatives

PHYSICAL FINDINGS & CLINICAL PRESENTATION

- Classic triad is dysmenorrhea, dyspareunia, and infertility.
- Presence of pelvic pain not correlated with the total area of endometriosis, type of lesion, or volume of disease, but is correlated with the depth of infiltration.
- Other symptoms include abnormal bleeding (premenstrual spotting, menorrhagia), cyclic abdominal pain, intermittent constipation/diarrhea, dyschezia, dysuria, hematuria, and urinary frequency.
- Rare manifestations: catamenial hemothorax, bloody pleural effusion, massive ascites occurring during menses.
- Most severe discomfort is associated with lesions >1 cm in depth.
- Bimanual examination may reveal tender uterosacral ligaments, cul-de-sac nodularity, induration of the rectovaginal septum, fixed retroversion of the uterus, adnexal mass, and generalized or localized tenderness.

ETIOLOGY

- Reflux and direct implantation theory: retrograde menstruation with implantation of viable endometrial cells to surrounding pelvic structures (Sampson's theory)
- Coelomic metaplasia theory: transformation of multipotential cells of the coelomic epithelium into endometrium-like cells
- Vascular dissemination theory: transport of endometrial cells to distant sites by the uterine vascular and lymphatic systems
- Autoimmune disease theory: disorder of immune surveillance allows growth of endometrial implants

DIAGNOSIS

DIFFERENTIAL DIAGNOSIS

- Ectopic pregnancy
- Acute appendicitis
- Chronic appendicitis
- Pelvic inflammatory disease (PID)
- Pelvic adhesions
- Hemorrhagic cyst
- Hernia
- Psychologic disorder
- Irritable bowel syndrome
- Uterine leiomyomata
- Adenomyosis
- Nerve entrapment syndrome
- Scoliosis
- Muscular/skeletal strain
- Interstitial cystitis

WORKUP

- Thorough history and physical examination, including inquiry about physical and emotional abuse. Defining diagnosis of endometriosis can be made only by histology of lesions that have been removed surgically
- Laparoscopy for definitive diagnosis
- Revised American Fertility Society (renamed American Society for Reproductive Medicine) scale to classify endometriosis (since 1985):

Stage I	Minimal
Stage II	Mild
Stage III	Moderate
Stage IV	Severe

LABORATORY TESTS

Cancer antigen 125 (CA125): limited overall value in the diagnosis of endometriosis
- Also elevated in ovarian epithelial neoplasm, myomas, adenomyosis, acute PID, ovarian cysts, pancreatitis, chronic liver disease, menstruation, and pregnancy
- CA125 value >35 U/ml: positive predictive value of 0.58 and a negative predictive value of 0.96 for the presence of endometriosis

IMAGING STUDIES

- Ultrasound: for evaluating adnexal mass; ultrasound characteristics may suggest endometriomas versus other benign or malignant ovarian conditions but persistent solid or cystic-solid ovarian masses require definitive tissue diagnosis with laparoscopy.
- MRI:
  1. Highly accurate in detecting endometriomas
  2. Limited sensitivity in detecting diffuse pelvic endometriosis, especially if sessile lesions
- CT scan may show adnexal masses of varying density (Fig. 1-360)

TREATMENT

NONPHARMACOLOGIC THERAPY

Expectant management (observation for 5 to 12 mo) for stage I or stage II endometriosis-associated infertility. Evaluation should take place if the couple meet the diagnostic criteria for infertility.

ACUTE GENERAL Rx

Nonsteroidal anti-inflammatory drugs for symptomatic relief of dysmenorrhea

CHRONIC RX

PHARMACOLOGIC MANAGEMENT:

Estrogen-progesterone:
- State of "pseudopregnancy" created by continuous (discarding pill pack when placebo pills remaining and starting active pills from new pill pack) use of combination oral

FIGURE 1-359 Common sites for endometriotic deposits in the pelvis. (From Drife J, Magowan B: *Clinical obstetrics and gynecology,* Philadelphia, 2004, Saunders.)

contraceptives for minimum of 6 mo and continuing indefinitely
- Breakthrough bleeding treated by administering conjugated estrogens 1.25 mg/day for 2 wk

Progestins:
- Medroxyprogesterone acetate 10 to 30 mg PO qd and occasionally up to 100 mg PO qd
- Alternatively, 100 mg IM q2wk for four doses, followed by 200 mg IM monthly for 4 mo
- Breakthrough bleeding treated with ethinyl estradiol (20 mcg/day) or conjugated estrogens (1.25 mg/day) for 1 to 2 wk
- Comparison with danazol: progestins cost less, have a more tolerable side-effect profile, and have comparable efficacy with regard to pain relief and so are often the first-line drug. Very little justification for the use of danazol.

Gonadotropin-releasing hormone (GnRH) agonists:
- Use usually limited to 6-12 mo due to hypoestrogenic effects such as osteopenia or osteoporosis but can be given longer in certain circumstances, particularly when paired with estrogen add-back therapy. Referral to specialist strongly advised.
- Leuprolide acetate depot 3.75 mg IM monthly or 11.25 mg IM q3mo or nafarelin 200 mcg nasal puffs bid or goserelin 3.6 mg SC monthly
- As effective as danazol for relief of pelvic pain
- Add-back therapy for protection against vasomotor symptoms and bone loss: norethindrone acetate 5 mg PO qd alone or in combination with conjugated estrogen 0.625 mg PO qd
- Add-back therapy allows gonadotropin-releasing hormone (GnRH) agonist use to be extended to 1 yr based on limited studies available

Alternative therapies for inhibition of estrogen action currently under investigation are:
- Aromatase inhibitors: anastrozole, letrozole
- SERM: raloxifene
- Agents enhancing cell-mediated immunity are cytokines (interleukin-12 and interferon-α2b)
- Immunomodulators (loxoribine, levamisole)
- Anti-inflammatory: pentoxifylline

SURGICAL MANAGEMENT:

Conservative:
- Directed at enhancing fertility or treating pain unresponsive to first-line medical treatment
- Usually accomplished through laparoscopy
- Removal or destruction of endometriotic implants by excision, electrocautery, or laser
- Cystectomy for endometrioma; must remove cyst wall to be effective long-term
- Laparoscopic uterosacral nerve ablation for midline pain such as dysmenorrhea or dyspareunia (evidence does not support its use)
- Unless pregnancy is desired, patient is usually started on GnRH agonist therapy or continuous OCP immediately after surgery
- For those desiring pregnancy, surgery alone results in significant increase in fertility

Definitive:
- Directed at relieving endometriosis-associated pain
- Total abdominal hysterectomy with bilateral salpingo-oophorectomy and complete excision or ablation of endometriosis
- Thorough abdominal exploration to ensure removal of all disease
- Must be prepared to manage possible gastrointestinal and urinary tract endometriosis
- 90% effective in pain relief; patient must be counseled that pain relief is not guaranteed
- Estrogen replacement therapy (ERT) to be considered in all women undergoing definitive surgical management; after ERT, recurrence rate is 0% to 5% in women with endometriosis confined to the pelvis but 18% in women with bowel involvement

MANAGEMENT OF ENDOMETRIOSIS-ASSOCIATED INFERTILITY:

Conservative surgery:
- Yields significantly higher pregnancy rate than does expectant management, in part because of correction of mechanical factors such as adhesions

Assisted reproductive technologies:
- Can be used to circumvent unknown mechanism of endometriosis-associated infertility
- Superovulation with clomiphene citrate or human menopausal gonadotropins; clomiphene citrate results in threefold pregnancy rate over either danazol or expectant management
- Further improvement with intrauterine insemination combined with superovulation
- In vitro fertilization if above procedures are unsuccessful

DISPOSITION

Tends to recur unless definitive surgery is performed and should be considered a chronic condition

REFERRAL

To a reproductive endocrinologist for advanced surgical management or infertility management

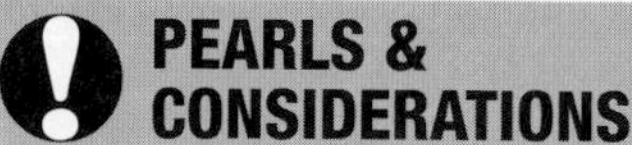

PEARLS & CONSIDERATIONS

COMMENTS

Patient information can be obtained through the following organizations: Endometriosis Association, 8585 North 76th Place, Milwaukee, WI 53223, 414-355-2200 or 800-992-ENDO; Women's Reproductive Health Network, P.O. Box 30167, Portland, OR 97230-9067 or 503-667-7757.

SUGGESTED READINGS

available at www.expertconsult.com

RELATED CONTENT

Dysmenorrhea (Related Key Topic)
Dyspareunia (Related Key Topic)
Endometriosis (Related Key Topic)

AUTHORS: **WAN J. KIM, M.D.,** and **RUBEN ALVERO, M.D.**

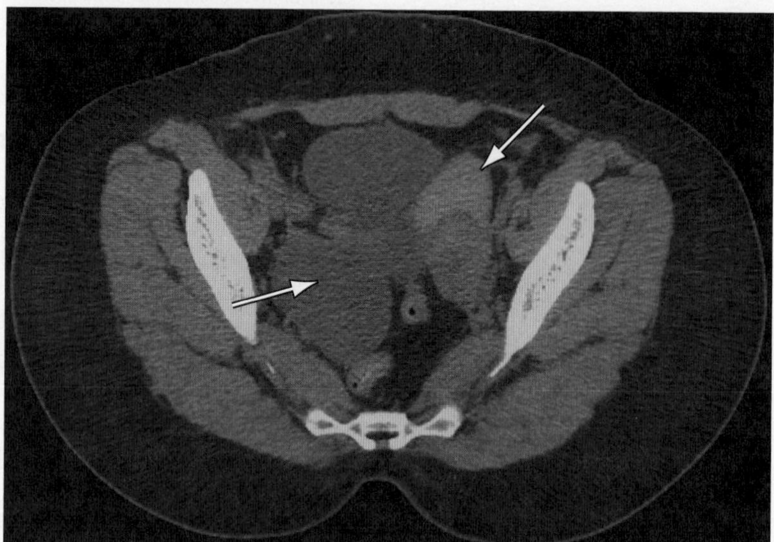

FIGURE 1-360 Computed tomographic scan demonstrates adnexal masses of varying density, subsequently proven to be endometriomas. (From Fielding JR et al: *Gynecologic imaging,* Philadelphia, 2011, Saunders.)

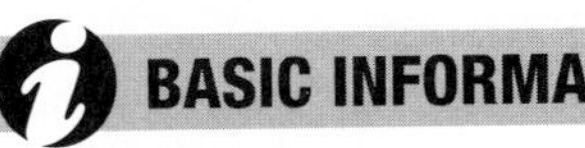

BASIC INFORMATION

DEFINITION

Endometritis is defined as a uterine infection after delivery or abortion.

SYNONYMS

Endomyometritis
Metritis

ICD-9CM CODES
615.9 Endometritis

ICD-10CM CODES
O85 Puerperal sepsis
O86 Other puerperal infections
O86.1 Other infection of genital tract following delivery
O86.8 Other specified puerperal infections

EPIDEMIOLOGY & DEMOGRAPHICS

- Overall rate of postpartum infection: estimated between 1% and 8%
- Most common genital tract infection after delivery
- Usually presents early in postpartum period; more commonly seen after cesarean section than vaginal delivery; also seen with an incomplete abortion (spontaneous abortion, legal abortion, or illegal abortion)
- More common in preterm deliveries
- Possible after any uterine manipulation in the presence of undiagnosed cervicitis or vaginitis

PHYSICAL FINDINGS & CLINICAL PRESENTATION

- Postpartum oral temperature >37.8° C
- Localized uterine tenderness, purulent or foul lochia; physical examination revealing uterine or parametrial tenderness
- Nonspecific signs and symptoms such as malaise, abdominal pain, chills, and tachycardia

ETIOLOGY

Endometritis is usually associated with multiple organisms: group A or B streptococci, *Staphylococcus aureus* and *Bacteroides* species, *Neisseria gonorrhoeae, Chlamydia trachomatis,* enterococci, *Gardnerella vaginalis, E. coli,* and *Mycoplasma.*

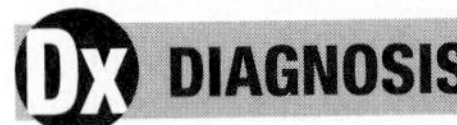

DIAGNOSIS

DIFFERENTIAL DIAGNOSIS

Causes of postoperative or postprocedural infections

WORKUP

Diagnosis based on symptoms of fever, malaise, abdominal pain, uterine tenderness, and purulent, foul vaginal discharge

LABORATORY TESTS

Complete blood count, blood cultures, and uterine culture

IMAGING STUDIES

Ultrasound (Fig. 1-361) may be useful if retained products are considered a possible source of infection.

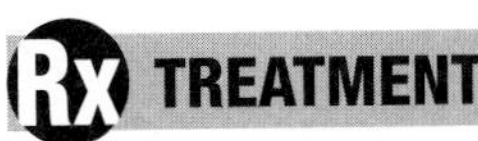

TREATMENT

ACUTE GENERAL Rx

Treatment options include doxycycline plus one of the following:
  - Cefoxitin
  - Ticarcillin-clavulanate
  - Ertapenem
  - Imipenem-cilastatin
  - Meropenem
  - Ampicillin-sulbactam
  - Piperacillin-tazobactam
- An alternative regimen is clindamycin plus aminoglycoside or ceftriaxone.
- Regimen should be continued for at least 48 hr after substantial clinical improvement. If response is not adequate (Table 1-181), check cultures and treat with appropriate antibiotics.

CHRONIC Rx

Watch for recurrent infection.

DISPOSITION

With appropriate antibiotic therapy, 95% to 98% cure rate

REFERRAL

For patients who do not respond within 48 to 72 hr of appropriate antibiotic therapy, obtain an infectious disease consult or gynecologic consultation.

AUTHOR: **RUBEN ALVERO, M.D.**

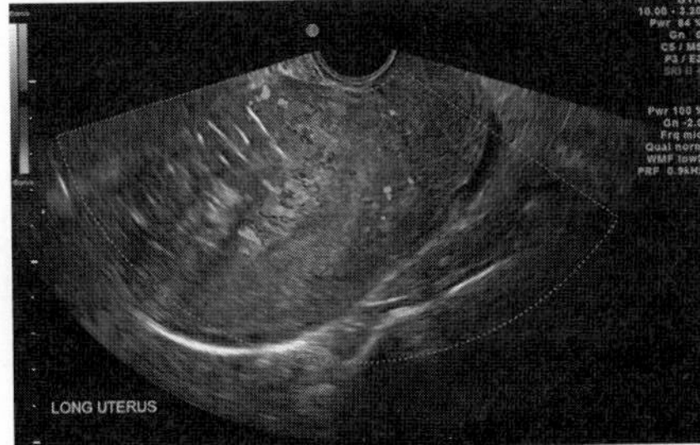

FIGURE 1-361 Endometritis. Patient with uterine tenderness and fever 7 days after classic cesarean section for premature rupture of membranes, chorioamnionitis, and fundic presentation at 27 weeks' gestational age. Sagittal transvaginal ultrasound shows increased vascularity within the endometrium, which can be seen with endometritis. Linear echogenic foci within the anterior myometrium likely represent air and suture material in the vertical uterine incision. Patient's symptoms resolved with antibiotics. (From Fielding JR et al: *Gynecologic imaging*, Philadelphia, 2011, Saunders.)

TABLE 1-181 Identified Causes of Poor Response to Antibiotic Therapy in Patients with Endometritis

Cause	Approximate Prevalence (%)
Infected mass, including abscess, hematoma, septic pelvic thrombophlebitis, pelvic cellulitis, retained placenta	40-50
Resistant organisms, commonly enterococci, in a patient receiving clindamycin-aminoglycoside or a cephalosporin	20
Additional cause, including catheter phlebitis, inadequate dose of antibiotics	10
No cause evident but response to empirical change in antibiotic therapy	20-30

From Gorbach SL: *Infectious diseases,* ed 2, Philadelphia, 1998, Saunders.

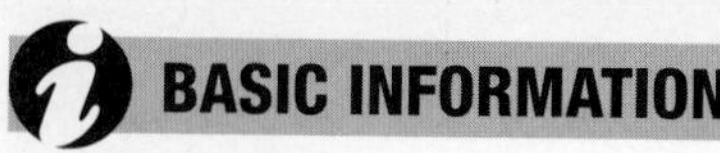

BASIC INFORMATION

DEFINITION

Enuresis refers to the voiding of urine into clothes or in bed that is either voluntary or involuntary in individuals who are expected to be continent (>5 yr of age). The diagnosis is made if voiding occurs at least twice a week for 3 months. Primary enuresis refers to enuresis without a period of continence, whereas secondary enuresis occurs after a period of normal bladder control.

SYNONYMS

Urinary incontinence
Bedwetting

ICD-9CM and DSM-5 CODES
307.6
ICD-10CM CODES
F98.0 Non-organic enuresis

EPIDEMIOLOGY & DEMOGRAPHICS

PEAK INCIDENCE: Ages 5 to 10 yr
PREVALENCE (IN U.S.):
- Age 5 yr: 7% of males and 3% of females
- Age 10 yr: 3% of males and 2% of females
- Ages 15 and older: 1% of males and females

PREDOMINANT SEX: Twice as many males as females at all ages
PREDOMINANT AGE: By definition, enuresis does not begin before age 5 yr, at which time the prevalence is highest, and decreases steadily thereafter at a rate of approximately 12% to 15% per year.
GENETICS:
- Approximately 75% of children with enuresis have a first-degree relative with enuresis.
- Almost twice as common in monozygotic than dizygotic twins.

PHYSICAL FINDINGS & CLINICAL PRESENTATION

Three enuresis subtypes are defined:
- Nocturnal only (also known as monosymptomatic enuresis): occurs in each sleep stage in proportion to the time spent in the particular stage. May occur during transition from deep sleep to REM.
- Diurnal only (also referred to as urinary incontinence): more frequent in girls and rarely after age 9 yr; voiding occurs in early afternoon on school days. Within this subtype, individuals have "urge incontinence" with sudden symptoms of urgency and detrusor instability, or "voiding postponement" where individuals ignore urges until the point of incontinence.
- Combined nocturnal and diurnal (also known as nonmonosymptomatic enuresis).

ETIOLOGY

- Enuresis often correlates with other maturational delays, particularly language, motor skills, and social development.
- May be related to toilet training issues, stress (secondary enuresis), inability to concentrate urine, altered smooth muscle physiology, small bladder capacity, or dysfunction of the arousal system.
- Diurnal enuresis associated with a higher rate of urinary tract infections.

Dx DIAGNOSIS

DIFFERENTIAL DIAGNOSIS

- May be associated with encopresis and sleep disorders such as sleep terrors; much less likely to be a primary psychological disorder.
- Organic causes of enuresis include diabetes mellitus, diabetes insipidus, bladder outlet obstruction, small bladder capacity, detrusor instability, urethral valves, meatal stenosis, cerebral palsy, spina bifida, pelvic mass, impacted stool, sedating medications, nocturnal seizures, and obstructive sleep apnea.

WORKUP

- History and physical examination to rule out anatomic abnormalities. Fluid intake and voiding diaries may be useful.
- Children frequently experience shame, so gentleness and care must be exercised when questioning or examining the child.
- Observation of voiding stream is useful.

LABORATORY TESTS

- Urinalysis with specific gravity and urine culture if white cells or nitrites on analysis.
- Serum studies to rule out diabetes, electrolyte abnormalities, or renal dysfunction.

IMAGING STUDIES

- In complicated cases, or if there is evidence of obstructive sleep apnea, sleep studies may be useful.
- If an anatomic abnormality suspected, urologic imaging, including voiding cystourethrogram and renal sonogram is possibly indicated: an abdominal x-ray may demonstrate stool retention; MRI of the spine if evidence of abnormalities of lower spine or perineum is found on examination.

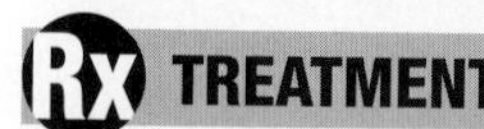

TREATMENT

NONPHARMACOLOGIC THERAPY

Behavioral treatment:
- Alarm and pad technique: up to 80% cure rate, although 30% relapse.
- Scheduled voiding to reduce the frequency of enuretic episodes.
- Motivational therapy including sticker or star charts to reward child for dry nights.
- Punishment for enuresis is not effective.

ACUTE GENERAL Rx

- Desmopressin (DDAVP) administered orally at bedtime significantly reduces the incidence of bedwetting (the intranasal preparation is associated with a greater risk for water intoxication and is not recommended).
- Tricyclic antidepressants (imipramine): efficacy supported by randomized control trials. Use with care in children.
- Serotonin reuptake inhibitors: lack of adequate trials is notable.
- Indomethacin suppositories may reduce normal prostaglandin inhibitory effects on antidiuretic hormone.
- Table 1-182 summarizes medications commonly used for treatment of monosymptomatic nocturnal enuresis. Fig. 1-362 describes an algorithm for management of pediatric enuresis and voiding dysfunction.

DISPOSITION

- After age 5 yr, the rate of spontaneous remissions is approximately 12% to 15% per year.

TABLE 1-182 Medications for Treatment of Monosymptomatic Nocturnal Enuresis

Generic Name (Trade Name)	Dosage Formulation	Dosage Regimen	Mechanisms of Action	Comments
Desmopressin acetate (DDAVP)	Nasal spray pump: 10 μg/0.1 ml spray Tablets: 0.1 mg, 0.2 mg	1 spray (10 μg) per nostril qhs, increasing to 40 μg 0.2 mg PO qhs, increasing up to 0.6 mg	Decreased urine volume Possible effect on sleep arousal through its action as a central nervous system neurotransmitter	Can cause nasal irritation; risk of water intoxication (headache, seizures); hence, restrict fluids 3 hr before the dose
Imipramine hydrochloride (Tofranil)	Tablets: 10 mg, 25 mg, 50 mg; Tofranil PM capsule 75, 100, 125, 150 mg	1.5–2 mg/kg 2 hr before bedtime, not to exceed 2.5 mg/kg or 75 mg max	Anticholinergic effect on bladder Increased resistance of bladder outlet Possible central inhibition of micturition reflex Possible effect on sleep arousal by central noradrenergic facilitation	Can cause sleep disturbance, mood alteration, decreased appetite Risk of cardiac arrhythmia with overdose

Modified from Chandra MM: Enuresis and voiding dysfunction. In Burg FD et al (eds): *Current pediatric therapy,* ed 18, Philadelphia, 2006, Saunders.

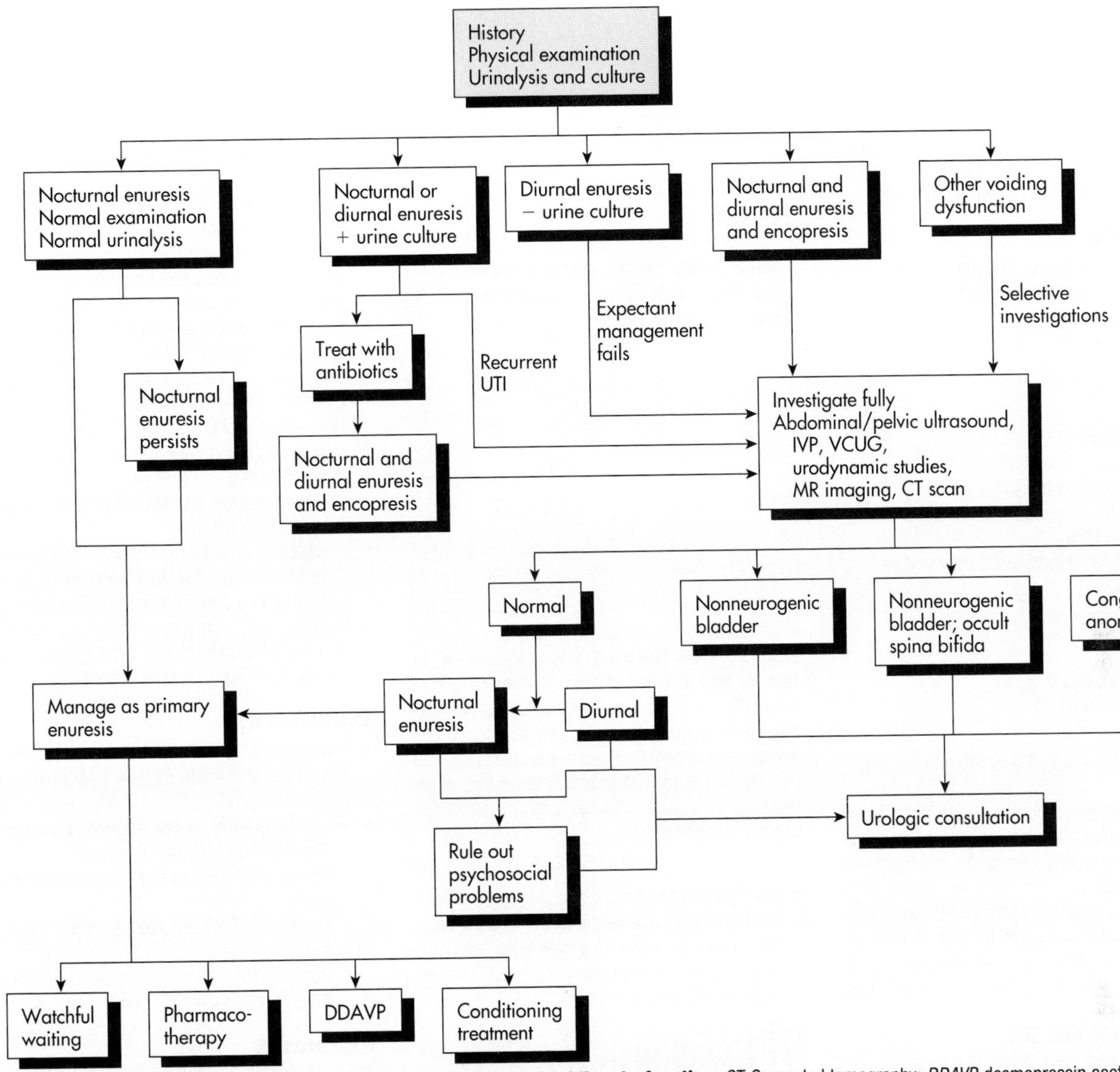

History
Physical examination
Urinalysis and culture

Nocturnal enuresis
Normal examination
Normal urinalysis

Nocturnal or diurnal enuresis + urine culture

Diurnal enuresis − urine culture

Nocturnal and diurnal enuresis and encopresis

Other voiding dysfunction

Treat with antibiotics

Recurrent UTI

Expectant management fails

Selective investigations

Nocturnal enuresis persists

Nocturnal and diurnal enuresis and encopresis

Investigate fully
Abdominal/pelvic ultrasound,
IVP, VCUG,
urodynamic studies,
MR imaging, CT scan

Normal

Nonneurogenic bladder

Nonneurogenic bladder; occult spina bifida

Congenital anomaly

Manage as primary enuresis

Nocturnal enuresis

Diurnal

Urologic consultation

Rule out psychosocial problems

Watchful waiting

Pharmacotherapy

DDAVP

Conditioning treatment

FIGURE 1-362 Algorithm of management of pediatric enuresis and voiding dysfunction. *CT,* Computed tomography; *DDAVP,* desmopressin acetate; *IVP,* intravenous pyelogram; *MR,* magnetic resonance; *UTI,* urinary tract infection; *VCUG,* voiding cystourethrogram. (From Nseyo UO [ed]: *Urology for primary care physicians,* Philadelphia, 1999, Saunders.)

- The disorder usually resolves by adolescence. However, effective treatment spares considerable misery.
- Fewer than 1% will have enuresis as adults.

REFERRAL

If coexisting, a psychiatric condition complicates the course of treatment.

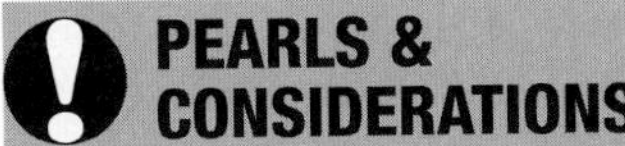

PEARLS & CONSIDERATIONS

Illness, hospitalization, and family stressors may precipitate recurrent enuresis after a period of dryness.

PATIENT & FAMILY EDUCATION

American Academy of Pediatrics www.healthychildren.org/English/ages-stages/toddler/toilet-training/Pages/default.aspx

Kidshealth http://kidshealth.org/parent/general/sleep/enuresis.html

SUGGESTED READINGS

available at www.expertconsult.com

RELATED CONTENT

Bedwetting (Patient Information)

AUTHORS: **CATHLEEN ADAMS, M.D.,** and **MARTA MAJCZAK, M.D.**

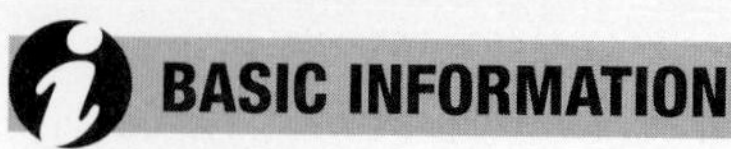

BASIC INFORMATION

DEFINITION

Epicondylitis is inflammation (tendinosis) of the myotendinous junction of the common extensors at the lateral epicondyle or the flexor pronator group at the medial epicondyle of the elbow.

SYNONYMS

Tennis elbow (lateral epicondylitis)
Golfer's elbow (medial epicondylitis)
Elbow tendinosis
Elbow tendinopathy
Epicondylalgia
Elbow tendinitis

ICD-9CM CODES

726.31 Medial epicondylitis
726.32 Lateral epicondylitis
723.4 Radial nerve neuralgia

ICD-10CM CODES

M77.00 Medial epicondylitis, unspecified elbow
M77.10 Lateral epicondylitis, unspecified elbow

EPIDEMIOLOGY & DEMOGRAPHICS

PREVALENCE:

- Prevalence is 1% to 3% in the general population.
  - Tennis players who play >2 hr a day have a two to four times greater risk of developing epicondylitis compared with general population.
  - Smoking, obesity, repetitive movement for at least 2 hrs daily, and forceful activity are also risk factors in the general population.
- The lateral side is involved more often than the medial.

PREVALENT AGE AND SEX:

- Affects women more often than men.
- More common in individuals 40 to 60 years old.

PHYSICAL FINDINGS & CLINICAL PRESENTATION

- Main symptom is of pain in lateral or medial elbow.
  - Pain is typically related to activity.
  - Local tenderness is experienced over the affected epicondyle.
- Pain can be reproduced by administering a forced elbow extension test (Fig. 1-365), offering resistance against wrist extension (Fig. 1-366), or inducing flexion in the affected area.

ETIOLOGY

- Epicondylitis is thought to be secondary to a chronic tendinosis rather than an acute inflammatory process.
- Overuse likely causes tendinous micro-tears, resulting in inflammation, degeneration, immature repair, and tendinosis.

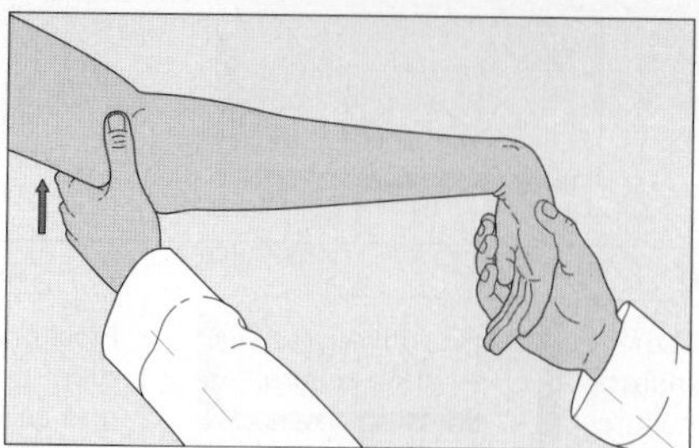

FIGURE 1-365 Forced elbow extension test. (From Hochberg MC et al: *Rheumatology,* ed 5, St Louis, 2011, Mosby.)

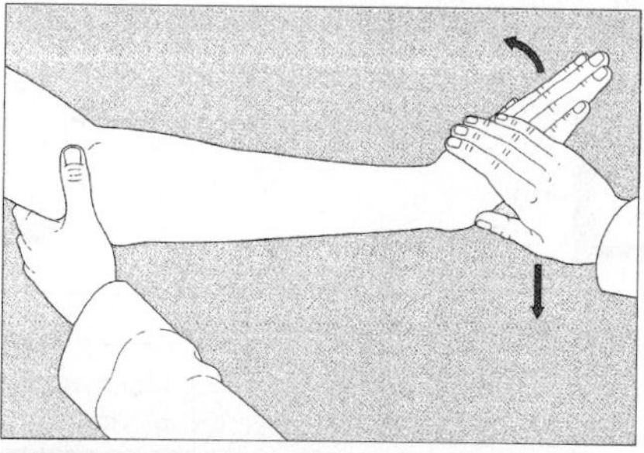

FIGURE 1-366 Resisted wrist extension to test for lateral epicondylitis. The examiner asks the patient to try to extend the wrist but prevents movement by fixing the wrist; this puts tension on the lateral epicondyle without moving the elbow and reproduces the pain of lateral epicondylitis. (From Klippel J et al [eds]: *Primary care rheumatology,* London, 1999, Mosby.)

- Disorganization of normal collagen by invading fibroblasts in association with an immature vascular reparative response and the absence of inflammatory cells is termed angiofibroblastic tendinosis.

Dx DIAGNOSIS

DIFFERENTIAL DIAGNOSIS

- Cervical radiculopathy.
- Intraarticular elbow pathology (osteoarthritis, osteochondritis dissecans, loose body).
- Radial tunnel syndrome (compression of the posterior interosseous nerve).
- Cubital tunnel syndrome (compression of the median nerve).
- Medial collateral ligament instability.
  - Thoracic outlet syndrome.
  - Ulnar neuritis.
  - Valgus extension overload.

IMAGING STUDIES

- Plain radiography is useful to evaluate osteoarthritis, osteochondrosis dissecans, or other bony abnormalities.
- Musculoskeletal (MSK) ultrasonography is not very sensitive; epicondylitis appears as a thickening or thinning of the tendon, as well as decreased echogenecity and poor definition of tendon.
- Magnetic resonance imaging (MRI) is the gold standard in detecting epicondylitis. MRI is the most sensitive test, showing tendon thickening and high T2 signal intensity.

Rx TREATMENT

- Rest, restricted activities, and proper technique during sports activities.
- Nonsteroidal anti-inflammatory drugs (NSAIDs) can be used topically or orally but usually provide only short-term relief.
- Local steroid/lidocaine injection can be considered; however, recent trials have called into question the efficacy of corticosteroid injections for epicondylitis.
- Counterforce brace/wrist orthoses.
- Acupuncture has been found to be beneficial in some cases.
- Physical therapy and eccentric exercise provides short-term relief.
  - Injection of botulinum toxin A at the myotendinous junction has been found to be helpful in a small randomized-control trial.
- Patients with refractory symptoms after 6 months of nonoperative management may benefit from surgical intervention.

DISPOSITION

- Epicondylitis is self-limited in most cases. Resolution of symptoms may take months to years.
- Prognosis is worse in the following conditions:
  - The dominant hand is involved
  - Patient experiences high physical strain at work
  - Duration of symptoms is more than 3 months
  - Patient experiences severe pain at presentation and concomitant neck pain.

REFERRAL

If symptoms do not respond to injections or a 6-month trial of conservative therapy, surgical referral is appropriate.

SUGGESTED READINGS

available at www.expertconsult.com

RELATED CONTENT

Epicondylitis (Tennis Elbow, Golfer's Elbow) (Patient Information)

AUTHOR: **WAFFIYAH AFRIDI, M.D.**

BASIC INFORMATION

DEFINITION

- Epididymitis is an inflammatory reaction of the epididymis caused by either an infectious agent or local trauma. In most cases of acute epididymitis, the testis is also involved (orchitis).
- Epididymitis is considered chronic if lasting ≥6 wk. Chronic epididymitis has been subcategorized into inflammatory chronic epididymitis, obstructive chronic epididymitis, and chronic epididymalgia.

SYNONYMS

Nonspecific bacterial epididymitis
Sexually transmitted epididymitis

ICD-9CM CODES
604 Orchitis and epididymitis
ICD-10CM CODES
N45.1 Epididymitis
A54.00 Gonococcal infection of lower genitourinary tract, unspecified

EPIDEMIOLOGY & DEMOGRAPHICS

INCIDENCE (IN U.S.): Cause of >600,000 visits to physicians per year
PEAK INCIDENCE: Sexually active years
PREDOMINANT SEX: Exclusive to males
PREDOMINANT AGE: All ages affected but usually in sexually active men or older males
CONGENITAL: Congenital urologic structural disorders possibly predisposing to infections

PHYSICAL FINDINGS & CLINICAL PRESENTATION

- Tender swelling of the scrotum with erythema, usually unilateral testicular pain and tenderness
- Dysuria and/or urethral discharge
- Fever and signs of systemic illness (less common)
- Pain and redness on scrotal examination
- Hydrocele or even epididymoorchitis, especially late
- Chronic draining scrotal sinuses with a "beadlike" enlargement of the vas deferens in tuberculous disease

ETIOLOGY

- In young, sexually active men (<35 years of age), the most common infectious agents isolated are *N. gonorrhoeae* and *Chlamydia trachomatis.*
- In older men (>35 years of age) or with underlying urologic disease:
  1. Gram-negative aerobic rods are predominant (i.e., *E. coli*).
  2. Similar organisms are found in men following invasive urologic procedures.
  3. Gram-positive cocci are rarely seen in these groups.
  4. Mycobacteria may also be a cause of epididymitis.
- Young, prepubertal boys may present with epididymitis caused by coliform bacteria; almost always a complication of underlying urologic disease such as reflux.
- In AIDS patients, CMV and *Salmonella* epididymitis have been described. CMV may have a negative urine culture. Toxoplasmosis and *Cryptococcus* should also be considered as a cause of epididymitis in AIDS patients.
- Chronic infectious epididymitis is mostly frequently seen in conditions associated with granulomatous reaction; mycobacterium tuberculosis is the most common granulomatous disease affecting the epididymis.

Dx DIAGNOSIS

DIFFERENTIAL DIAGNOSIS

- Orchitis
- Testicular torsion, trauma, or tumor
- Epididymal cyst
- Hydrocele
- Varicocele
- Spermatocele
- Testicular torsion should be considered in all cases.

WORKUP

- Consideration of a full assessment of the urologic tract in patients with bacterial infection, especially if recurrent
- If discharge is present, cultures and Gram stain smear of urethral exudate. Gram stain will demonstrate ≥5 WBC per oil immersion field.
- In sexually active men: gonococcal cultures of the throat and rectum possibly of value
- If testicular torsion a consideration: radionuclear imaging
- Examination of first void uncentrifuged urine for leukocytes if the urethral Gram stain is negative. Positive leukocyte esterase test on first-void urine or microscopic examination of first-void urine sediment will demonstrate ≥10 WBC per high power field. A culture and Gram-stained smear of this urine specimen should be obtained along with nucleic acid amplification studies (ligase chain reaction [LCR]) from urine samples for gonorrhea and *Chlamydia* spp.
- Imaging with sonogram

LABORATORY TESTS

- Urinalysis and urine culture if dysuria is present or if urinary tract infection is suspected
- Screening test for syphilis, chlamydia, and gonorrhea in sexually active men
- HIV testing and counseling
- PPD placed and chest x-ray viewed if TB suspected (rare cases)
- Rarely, biopsy to ensure the diagnosis of tuberculous epididymitis

Rx TREATMENT

ACUTE GENERAL Rx

- Ice packs and scrotal elevation for relief of pain
- Analgesia with acetaminophen with or without codeine or NSAIDs
- Antibiotics to cover suspected pathogens. Empiric therapy is indicated before laboratory test results are available.
- Recommended regimens are ceftriaxone 250 mg IM in a single dose plus doxycycline 100 mg bid for 10 days. For acute epididymitis most likely caused by enteric organisms, treatment options are levofloxacin 500 mg qd × 10 days or ofloxacin 300 mg bid × 10 days.
- Best treatment for older men with gram-negative bacteriuria: ofloxacin 300 mg PO bid for 10 days or levofloxacin 500 mg PO qd for 10 days
- *Pseudomonas* covered by ciprofloxacin PO or IV or cefepime (2 g IV q12h)
- Consider ampicillin-sulbactam, 3rd-generation cephalosporin, ticarcillin-clavulanate, or piperacillin-tazobactam in toxic-appearing patients.
- Surgical aspiration of local abscesses or even open surgical drainage
- Diabetics: especially prone to develop more extensive scrotal infections, including Fournier's gangrene
- Reinforcement of compliance with antibiotics to avoid partial treatment

CHRONIC Rx

- Repair of underlying structural defects is considered especially if infections are severe or recur.
- Surgical repair of reflux in young boys should be undertaken promptly and at a young age when possible.
- Sex partners of patient should be referred for evaluation and treatment.

DISPOSITION

Usually self-limited (≤6 wk duration in most cases)

REFERRAL

- If abscess or chronic structural problems suspected
- If another diagnosis, such as testicular torsion, is suspected

PEARLS & CONSIDERATIONS

- Recurrent epididymitis in sexually active men is usually related to failure to simultaneously treat sexual partners for STDs.
- Recurrent epididymitis in non-sexually active men is generally related to structural-anatomic defects in the genitourinary system or relapsing disease from inadequate initial treatment or antimicrobial resistance.
- Tuberculous epididymitis fails to respond to seemingly adequate antimicrobial therapy even without characteristic radiographic changes on chest films.

SUGGESTED READINGS

available at www.expertconsult.com

RELATED CONTENT

Epididymitis (Patient Information)

AUTHORS: **PHILIP A. CHAN, M.D., M.S., and GLENN G. FORT, M.D., M.P.H.**

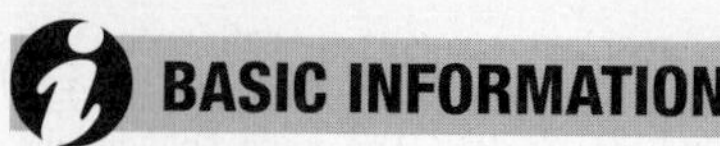

BASIC INFORMATION

DEFINITION

Epidural hematoma (EDH) is the accumulation of blood in the potential space surrounding the brain, between the dura mater and the inner surface of the skull.

SYNONYMS

Extradural hematoma/hemorrhage, EDH

ICD-9CM CODES
432.0 Nontraumatic extradural hemorrhage
852.5 Extradural hemorrhage following injury without intracranial wound
852.5 Extradural hemorrhage following injury with open intracranial wound
ICD-10CM CODES
S06.4 Epidural hemorrhage
I62.1 Now-traumatic extradural hemorrhage

EPIDEMIOLOGY & DEMOGRAPHICS

INCIDENCE: Exact incidence is unknown; however, it is found in 1% to 4% of traumatic head injury cases and 5% to 15% of autopsy series.
PREDOMINANT SEX AND AGE: Male > female
PEAK INCIDENCE: Peak incidence among adolescents and young adults. It is rarely found in patients older than 50-60 years old.
GENETICS: There is a role for genetics in spontaneous (nontraumatic) EDH caused by coagulopathies and vascular malformations.
RISK FACTORS: Head trauma, especially in cases involving skull fracture

PHYSICAL FINDINGS & CLINICAL PRESENTATION

- History of head trauma is present.
- Signs and symptoms vary depending on severity.
- Symptoms: altered mental status, nuchal rigidity, headache, drowsiness, confusion, aphasia, photophobia, and paralysis
- Signs: transient loss of consciousness, followed by a "lucid interval" in 47% of cases, in which the patient is free of any neurologic signs or symptoms. This is followed by clinical deterioration including, vomiting, lethargy, confusion, or seizures. Other signs include focal neurologic deficits such as paralysis of limbs, unequal pupils, and coma. Signs of increased intracranial pressure could be found including the Cushing reflex of hypertension, bradycardia, and respiratory distress. External signs of skull fracture—lacerations, ecchymoses, cerebrospinal fluid (CSF) rhinorrhea or otorrhea—may be observed. Skull fractures can be found in 75%-95% of EDH patients.

ETIOLOGY

- Traumatic: commonly caused by arterial injury (the middle meningeal artery) but may also be injury of the anterior meningeal artery, a dural arteriovenous (AV) fistula at the vertex, or from venous bleeding
- Nontraumatic: caused by an infection/eroding abscess, coagulopathy, hemorrhagic tumors, vascular malformations, postsurgical procedures, and in special populations (e.g., pregnant women, patients receiving hemodialysis)

DIAGNOSIS

DIFFERENTIAL DIAGNOSIS

In the setting of head trauma: subdural hematoma, subarachnoid hemorrhage, cerebral contusion, brain laceration, diffuse brain swelling

WORKUP

- Imaging is the mainstay of diagnosis.
- Serial head CT is the test most commonly used due to its simplicity, widespread use, and availability. Typical appearance is a "lens shaped," or "lentiform" hyperdensity (Fig. 1-367). Box 1-28 describes CT findings of EDH.
- Note: Head CT is not conclusive in 8% of cases possibly due to severe anemia, early scanning (before blood has time to accumulate), and severe hypotension.
- Brain MRI: more sensitive. Indicated in situations in which there is a strong clinical suspicion but no evidence of EDH on head CT (Fig. 1-368).
- Angiography: rarely necessary but may be used to evaluate an underlying vascular lesion.
- NOTE: lumbar puncture (LP) is contraindicated in EDH due to risk of brain stem herniation.

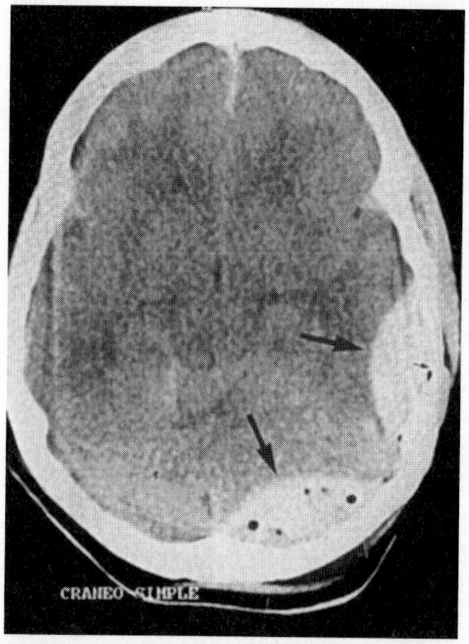

FIGURE 1-367 Head CT showing two epidural hematomas in 23-year-old involved in a motor vehicle accident. Note air bubbles that are a result of linear fracture in the left temporal bone *(short arrow)*.

LABORATORY TESTS

- Laboratory tests are helpful as adjunct to diagnosis but are not the mainstay of diagnosis or treatment.
- CBC may be helpful to evaluate for anemia, although in an acute onset of bleeding, hemoglobin levels can be normal.
- Other tests: renal functions, electrolytes, liver functions, INR may be helpful depending on the case scenario.

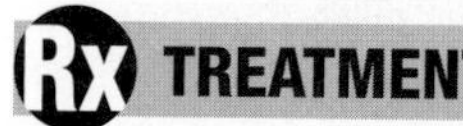

TREATMENT

Acute symptomatic EDH is a neurologic emergency that requires surgical treatment to prevent permanent brain injury.

NONPHARMACOLOGIC THERAPY

- Immediate surgical decompression, ideally within 1-2 hr after traumatic event

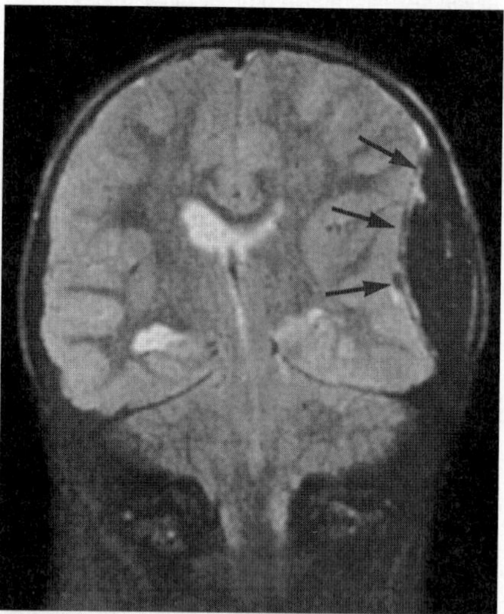

FIGURE 1-368 Epidural hematoma on MRI. Coronal T2-weighted images show hypointense biconvex extraaxial collection in the left temporal region.

BOX 1-28 CT Findings of Epidural Hematoma

- CT appearance: variable white to gray on brain windows
- Location: peripheral to brain, variable but usually temporal region
- Shape: biconvex disc or lens
- Pearl: does not cross suture lines
- White swirl sign means active bleeding
- Significance: may cause mass effect and herniation
- Look for midline shift
- Look for effacement of ventricles and sulci
- Surgical indications: 15-mm thickness or 5-mm midline shift

From Broder JS: *Diagnostic imaging for the emergency physician,* Philadelphia, 2011, Saunders.

- Craniotomy and hematoma evacuation is the treatment of choice. When indicated, identify and ligate the bleeding vessel.
- Burr hole evacuation: this involves drilling a hole in the skull to evacuate the hematoma. It is a lifesaving procedure that is indicated if surgical expertise is limited.

ACUTE GENERAL Rx

- Cardiopulmonary resuscitation and assessment for disability.
- Medical resuscitation maneuvers: head elevation, hyperventilation, monitoring of vital signs and avoidance of hypotension and hyperthermia, sedation if necessary.
- Medications: osmotic diuresis with IV mannitol, cerebrosedating medications, antiepileptics may be used to treat or, in some situations, prevent seizures.
- Reversing anticoagulation should be weighed in terms of advantages versus disadvantages.
- NOTE: glucocorticoid therapy is *not* indicated following head injury and may be related to increased mortality.
- Evaluation for surgery: the best available evidence points toward advantages of decompression procedures. Nonoperative treatment may only be indicated if the patient has no symptoms, no focal neurologic deficit, no coma (Glasgow coma score >8), and EDH volume is less than 30 ml by CT scan, with clot thickness <15 mm and midline shift of less than 5 mm.
- Nonoperative treatment involves close monitoring, hourly neurologic checks, and serial head CT scans.

CHRONIC Rx

- There is a risk of permanent brain damage whether the disorder is treated or not. Most recovery occurs in the first 6 months with some improvement over 2 years.
- Children have a tendency to recover more quickly.
- Patients should be educated on rehabilitative exercises and to alert medical professionals in the event of new neurologic symptoms.
- Support and encouragement to patient and family should always be provided.

REFERRAL

Clinical nurse practitioners, pastoral care staff, and social workers to help patients and families are also appropriate.

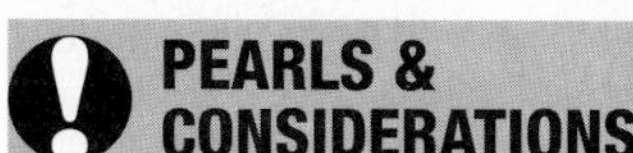

PEARLS & CONSIDERATIONS

- Acute symptomatic EDH is a neurologic emergency.
- EDH should be suspected in any patient with a history of blow to the head leading to a period of loss of consciousness.
- Initial resuscitation is extremely important, but surgery is the mainstay of treatment for acute symptomatic EDH.

PREVENTION

Should be directed toward preventing head trauma: use of appropriate safety equipment (e.g., helmets, hard hats, safe driving, avoiding diving into unknown depths)

PATIENT/FAMILY EDUCATION

Online head injury support groups are helpful: www.headinjury.com/linktbisup.htm, www.headinjury.com/, www.dailystrength.org/c/Brain-Injury/support-group.

SUGGESTED READINGS

available at www.expertconsult.com

AUTHOR: **SCOTT M. SOUTHER, M.D.**

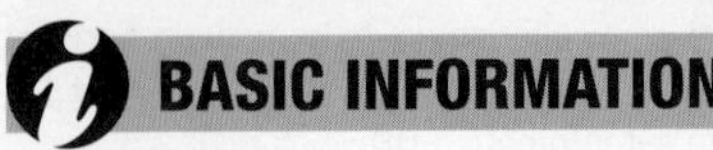

BASIC INFORMATION

DEFINITION

Epiglottitis is a rapidly progressive cellulitis of the epiglottis and adjacent soft tissue structures with the potential to cause abrupt airway obstruction, which can be life-threatening.

SYNONYMS

Supraglottitis
Cherry-red epiglottitis

ICD-9CM CODES
464.30 Epiglottitis
ICD-10CM CODES
J05.1 Acute epiglottis

EPIDEMIOLOGY

INCIDENCE (IN U.S.): due to vaccination against *Haemophilus influenzae* type B, this is a rare infection in children estimated at between 0.6 to 0.8 per 100,000 in one study and for adults at 1.6 per 100,000.
PEAK INCIDENCE: now highest in children ages 6-12
PREDOMINANT SEX: Males

PHYSICAL FINDINGS & CLINICAL PRESENTATION

- Irritability, fever, dysphonia, and dysphagia
- Respiratory distress, with child tending to lean up and forward
- Often, drooling or oral secretions
- Often, presence of tachycardia and tachypnea
- On visualization, edematous and cherry-red epiglottis
- Often, no classic barking cough as seen in croup
- Possibly fulminant course (especially in children), leading to complete airway obstruction

ETIOLOGY

- In children, *Haemophilus influenzae* type b, still most common cause but now rare due to vaccination *Streptococcus pyogenes,* (group A Streptococcus) *Streptococcus pneumoniae, Staphylococcus aureus* (includes MRSA)
- In adults, *Streptococcus pyogenes* (group A Streptococcus), *H. influenzae* (can be isolated from blood and/or epiglottis [about 26% of cases])
- Pneumococci, streptococci, and staphylococci are also implicated.
- Role of viruses in epiglottitis unclear.

DIAGNOSIS

DIFFERENTIAL DIAGNOSIS

- Croup
- Angioedema
- Retropharyngeal or peritonsillar abscess
- Diphtheria
- Foreign body aspiration
- Lingual tonsillitis

WORKUP

- Cultures of blood and urine
- Lateral neck radiograph to show an enlarged epiglottis, ballooning of the hypopharynx, and normal subglottic structures (Fig. 1-369)
  1. Radiographs are of only moderate sensitivity and specificity and take time to perform.
  2. Visualization of the epiglottis may be safer in adults than in children.
- Cultures of the epiglottis

LABORATORY TESTS

- CBC: may reveal a leukocytosis with a shift to the left
- Chest radiograph examination: may reveal evidence of pneumonia in close to 25% of cases
- Cultures of blood, urine, and the epiglottis, as noted previously

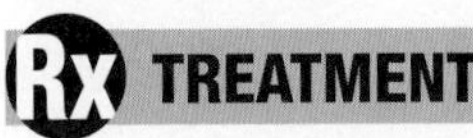

TREATMENT

ACUTE GENERAL Rx

- Maintenance of adequate airway is critical. Fig. E1-370 describes the optimal assessment and management of upper airway obstruction caused by epiglottitis or severe croup. It is crucial to have a tracheostomy set "at bedside."
- Early placement of an endotracheal or nasotracheal tube in a child is advised.
- Closely follow the adult patient, if no signs of airway obstruction, and defer intubation.
- In children, visualization and intubation are best done in the most controlled environment.
- *H. influenzae* in children is much less common in large part due to the HIB vaccine.

Empiric antibiotics:
  - **In children:** use cefotaxime 50 mg/kg IV q8h or ceftriaxone 50 mg/kg IV q24h *plus* vancomycin for its coverage of MRSA. If penicillin allergy, use levofloxacin 10 mg/kg IV q24h *plus* clindamycin 7.5 mg/kg IV q6h.
  - **In adults:** ceftriaxone 2 g IV q24h or cefotaxime *plus vancomycin*
- If possible, obtain cultures before initiating antibiotics.
- If there is an unvaccinated child for *Haemophilus influenzae* at home (or in a day care center) who is >4 yr and living with an index case, give close family contacts of the patient (including adults) rifampin 20 mg/kg/day for 4 days (up to 600 mg/day) for prophylaxis.
- Role of epinephrine or corticosteroids in the management of epiglottitis is not firmly established.

DISPOSITION

Invasive *Haemophilus influenzae* infections and epiglottitis are reportable illnesses; this may be particularly important in recognizing an outbreak in a day care center with unvaccinated children.

REFERRAL

- Close cooperation between the pediatrician or internist, anesthesiologist, and otorhinolaryngologist, especially when epiglottis is visualized and when the patient requires endotracheal intubation
- Best managed in a critical care setting or ICU

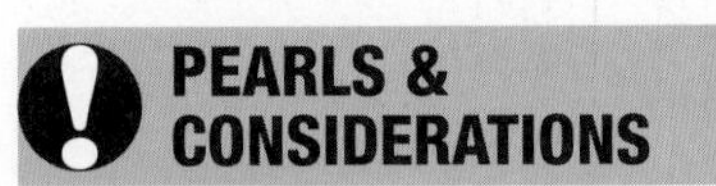

PEARLS & CONSIDERATIONS

The incidence of epiglottitis has diminished markedly since the introduction of the conjugate vaccine against *H. influenzae* serotype B into routine childhood immunization.

SUGGESTED READINGS

available at www.expertconsult.com

RELATED CONTENT

Epiglottitis (Patient Information)

AUTHOR: **GLENN G. FORT, M.D., M.P.H.**

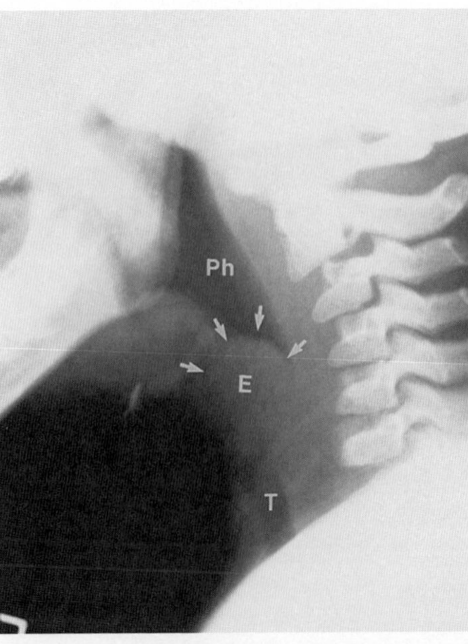

FIGURE 1-369 Epiglottitis. A lateral soft tissue view of the neck shows a ballooned pharynx *(Ph)* with swollen epiglottis *(E)* in the shape of a large thumbprint *(arrows). T,* Trachea. (From Mettler FA [ed]: *Primary care radiology,* Philadelphia, 2000, Saunders.)

BASIC INFORMATION

DEFINITION

Episcleritis is an inflammation of the episclera (Fig. 1-371), the thin layer of vascular elastic tissue between the sclera and conjunctiva.

ICD-9CM CODES
379.0 Scleritis and episcleritis
ICD-10CM CODES
H15.1 Episcleritis

EPIDEMIOLOGY & DEMOGRAPHICS

INCIDENCE (IN U.S.): Relatively rare in an ophthalmologic practice
PEAK INCIDENCE: Most common in middle and old age
PREDOMINANT SEX: None
PREDOMINANT AGE: 40s

PHYSICAL FINDINGS & CLINICAL PRESENTATION

- Red, vascular injection of conjunctiva with engorged and enlarged blood vessels beneath the conjunctions (Fig. 1-372)
- Pain in area of inflammation that is usually localized (severe pain suggests deeper inflammation, see Scleritis)

ETIOLOGY

Associated with collagen-vascular diseases, vasculitis, trauma; often nonspecific

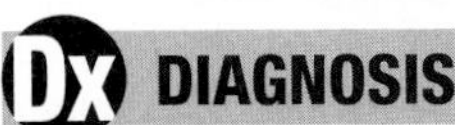

DIAGNOSIS

DIFFERENTIAL DIAGNOSIS

- Acute glaucoma
- Conjunctivitis
- Scleritis
- Subconjunctival hemorrhage
- Congenital or lymphoid masses
- The differential diagnosis of "red eye" is described in Section II

WORKUP

Eye examination, general check-up for collagen-vascular disease or other autoimmune diseases

LABORATORY TESTS

Studies for collagen-vascular disease (e.g., ANA, ESR, RF)

TREATMENT

NONPHARMACOLOGIC THERAPY

Warm compresses

ACUTE GENERAL Rx

- Topical steroids, 1% prednisolone if no glaucoma; nonsteroidal eye drops if there is a tendency for glaucoma
- Nonsteroidal anti-inflammatory drugs (NSAIDs): treat underlying systemic disease

CHRONIC Rx

NSAID eye drops (diclofenac eye drops, ketorolac ophthalmic solution)

DISPOSITION

Close follow-up needed

REFERRAL

To ophthalmologist if patient unresponsive to treatment after a few days

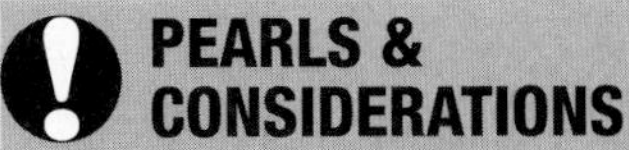

PEARLS & CONSIDERATIONS

COMMENTS

- Can be associated with collagen-vascular disease
- May occur with systemic autoimmune disease. Workup for autoimmune disease is often negative, more likely with scleritis (50%). Ask about other symptoms to find autoimmune disorders, helps to guide workups.

SUGGESTED READINGS
available at www.expertconsult.com

RELATED CONTENT

Episcleritis (Patient Information)

AUTHORS: **MELVYN KOBY, M.D.,** and **R. SCOTT HOFFMAN, M.D.**

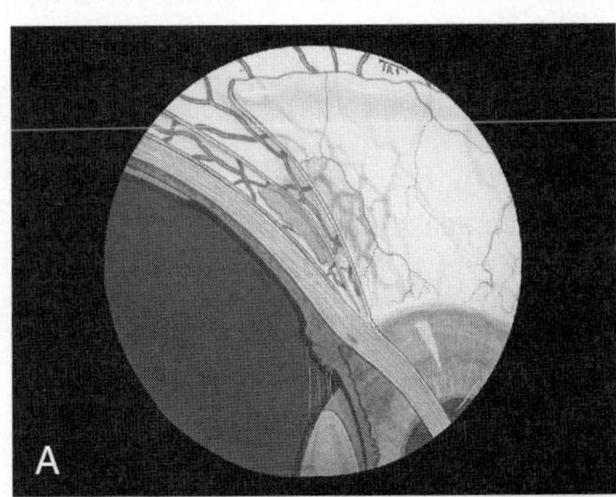

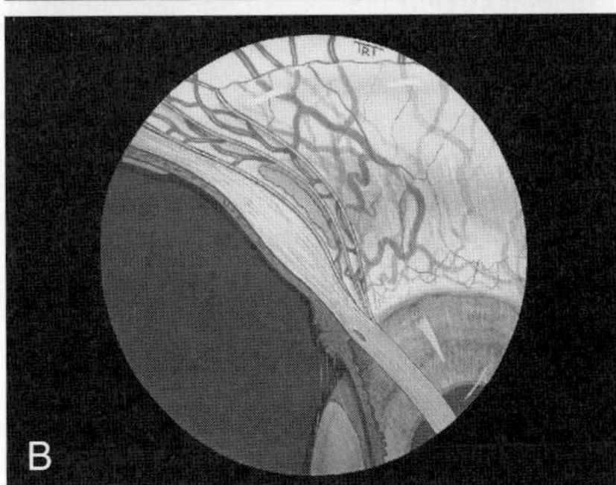

FIGURE 1-371 A, Episcleritis with maximal vascular congestion of the superficial episcleral plexus; **B,** scleritis with scleral thickening and maximal vascular congestion of the deep vascular plexus. (From Kanski JJ, Bowling B: *Clinical ophthalmology, a systematic approach,* ed 7, Philadelphia, 2010, Saunders.)

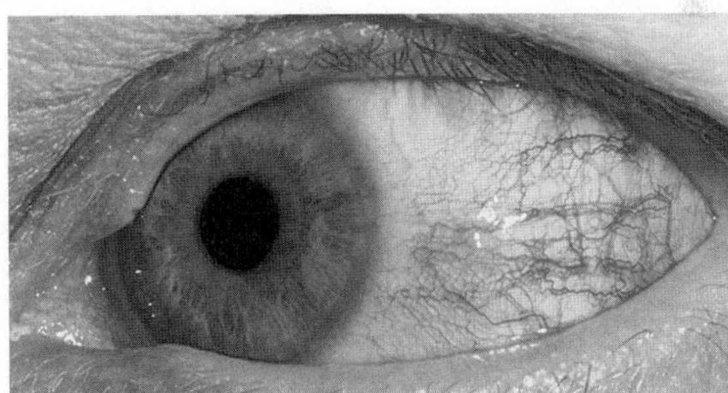

FIGURE 1-372 Nodular episcleritis in a patient with gout. (From Palay D [ed]: *Ophthalmology for the primary care physician,* St Louis, 1997, Mosby.)

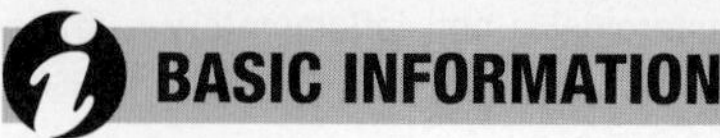

BASIC INFORMATION

DEFINITION

Epistaxis is defined as bleeding from the nose or nasal hemorrhage and is classified as either anterior or posterior.

SYNONYMS

Nosebleed

ICD-9CM CODES
784.7 Epistaxis
ICD-10CM CODES
R04.0 Epistaxis

EPIDEMIOLOGY & DEMOGRAPHICS

- Epistaxis accounts for one of every 200 emergency department visits in the U.S. annually.
- It increases in frequency after age 20 yr and reaches the highest levels among the elderly population.
- More than 80% of cases of epistaxis are anterior in origin (Little's area) and occur from Kiesselbach's plexus.
- Only 5% of patients with epistaxis have posterior bleeds.

PHYSICAL FINDINGS & CLINICAL PRESENTATION

- Nosebleed
- Hypotension and hemodynamic instability with acute, severe epistaxis

ETIOLOGY

- Approximately 90% of epistaxis events are idiopathic.
- Common identifiable causes are:
  1. Cold, dry environment
  2. Trauma (nose picking, accidents, and physical altercations)
  3. Structural deformities (septal deviations or spurs, chronic perforations)
  4. Inflammatory (rhinosinusitis, nasal polyposis)
  5. Allergies
  6. Foreign bodies in the nasal cavity
  7. Tumors (juvenile angiofibroma)
  8. Irritants
  9. Hypertension
  10. Coagulopathy (hemophilia, von Willebrand's disease, thrombocytopenia)
  11. Osler-Weber-Rendu disease
  12. Renal failure
  13. Drugs: aspirin, nonsteroidal antiinflammatory drugs, warfarin, alcohol, sildenafil, and tadalafil
  14. Blood vessel disorders (connective tissue disease, hereditary hemorrhagic telangiectasia)
  15. Pseudoaneurysm and aneurysm of the internal carotid artery might present as epistaxis

Dx DIAGNOSIS

A good attempt should be made to directly visualize the source of bleeding to confirm the diagnosis and determine the best treatment.

DIFFERENTIAL DIAGNOSIS

Pseudoepistaxis must be ruled out. Common extranasal sites of bleeding that can simulate epistaxis include:
1. Pulmonary hemoptysis
2. Bleeding esophageal varices
3. Tumor bleeding from the pharynx, larynx, or trachea

WORKUP

The workup should include laboratory blood testing to exclude obvious causes. Type and cross in anticipation of transfusion if the bleeding is severe.

LABORATORY TESTS

- Hemoglobin and hematocrit
- Platelet count
- Blood urea nitrogen and creatinine
- Coagulation studies (prothrombin time and partial thromboplastin time)
- Type and crossmatching of blood products

IMAGING STUDIES

Radiographic studies are usually not helpful.

Rx TREATMENT

NONPHARMACOLOGIC THERAPY

- Digital compression or pinching of the lower soft cartilaginous part of the nose for 10 min is the method of choice.
- Use cotton or tissue plug.
- The patient should be sitting and leaning forward, breathing through the mouth, allowing blood to flow out of the nostrils as opposed to bending backward, which would allow the blood to flow down the throat.
- Application of cold compresses to the bridge of the nose to cause a vasoconstrictive effect; the patient may also suck on ice to achieve this effect.

ACUTE GENERAL Rx

Anterior epistaxis:
- Local vasoconstriction is performed by moistening a cotton pledget with either:
  1. 4% lidocaine with 1:1000 epinephrine
  2. 4% lidocaine with 1% phenylephrine (Neo-Synephrine)
  3. 4% lidocaine with 0.05% oxymetazoline (Afrin)
  4. 4% cocaine or cocaine 25% in paraffin base ointment and inserting the pledget into the nasal cavity with bayonet forceps.
- Cauterization with silver nitrate or trichloroacetic acid is performed once hemostasis is achieved.
- Anterior nasal packing is needed when local measures are unsuccessful. Nasal packing is performed under local anesthesia and is done by inserting Vaseline gauze strips in layers from the floor of the nasal cavity to the front entrance of the nasal orifice. Enough pressure is placed to tamponade the epistaxis.
- Other commercially available nasal packing uses sponge packs that expand when exposed to blood or moisture and can be used for anterior epistaxis.

Posterior epistaxis:
- Posterior nasal packing
  1. Commercially available nasal sponge packing can be applied
  2. Rolled gauze technique
- Foley catheter balloon insertion into the nasopharynx can be tried in patients with posterior epistaxis.

Newer agents in the treatment of epistaxis:
- Quick clot hemostatic agent, available OTC. When it comes in contact with blood in and around a wound, it absorbs the smaller water molecules from the blood to promote rapid clotting
- Floseal hemostatic matrix, a combination of human thrombin, gelatin matrix, and calcium chloride, which are mixed together and placed at bleeding site
- Recombinant factor VIIa, generally reserved for uncontrolled epistaxis

CHRONIC Rx

- If acute treatment fails to stop the bleeding or the site of bleeding cannot be located, electrocautery or endoscopic cauterization can be used.
- Electrocautery is performed after suitable anesthesia, such as application of a topical anesthetic followed by local anesthetic injection. Only one side of the nasal septum should be cauterized at a time because perforation can result from bilateral cauterization.
- Arterial ligation or embolization has been used in refractory posterior epistaxis.
- For cases involving irritated or inflamed mucosa, a conservative regimen of triamcinolone 0.025%, Nemdyn, Nasalate, or equivalent cream should be applied once a week, combined with nightly application of a small quantity of petroleum jelly to the septum before bedtime.

DISPOSITION

- Most cases of anterior epistaxis from Kiesselbach's plexus can be stopped by nasal compression and local vasoconstriction or cauterization.
- Nasal packing with gauze or sponge can control 90% of anterior epistaxis.
- Anterior and posterior packs are removed in 2 to 3 days. Hospital admission should be considered in patients who cannot be

expected to return for prompt follow-up because prolonged packing increases the risk of pressure necrosis, toxic shock syndrome, sinus infections, and other complications.
- Although rare, epistaxis can lead to death by aspiration of blood, hemodynamic compromise from rapid excessive blood loss, or toxic shock syndrome.

REFERRAL

- If epistaxis cannot be controlled, an ear-nose-throat (ENT) specialist should be called for assistance.
- ENT specialist should be consulted in any patient with posterior epistaxis requiring posterior packing.

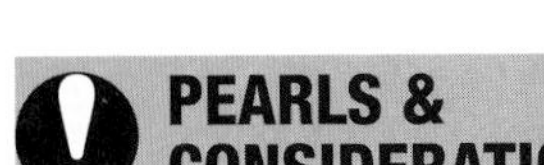

PEARLS & CONSIDERATIONS

COMMENTS

- Silver nitrate cauterization, if done on both sides of the nasal septum, can lead to septal perforation and should be discouraged.
- If anterior nasal packing is done, broad-spectrum antibiotics (e.g., amoxicillin-clavulanate 250 mg PO tid or trimethoprim-sulfamethoxazole 1 tablet PO bid) are used until the anterior packs are removed. Although it is customary to place patients on antibiotics to prevent sinusitis from obstruction, there is no proof that this is effective.
- Complications of nasal packing include:
  1. Aspiration
  2. Dislodged packing
  3. Infection
  4. Nasal trauma

SUGGESTED READINGS

available at www.expertconsult.com

RELATED CONTENT

Nosebleeds (Patient Information)

AUTHOR: **TANYA ALI, M.D.**

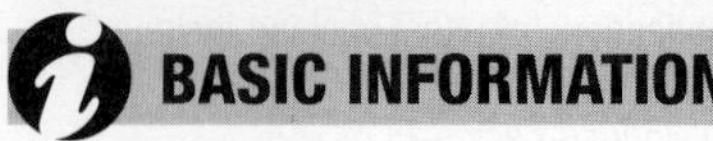

BASIC INFORMATION

DEFINITION

Epstein-Barr virus infection refers to a disease caused by Epstein-Barr virus (EBV), a human herpesvirus.

SYNONYMS

Infectious mononucleosis (IM)
Kissing disease

ICD-9CM CODES
075 Mononucleosis
ICD-10CM CODES
B27.90 Infectious mononucleosis, unspecified without complication

EPIDEMIOLOGY & DEMOGRAPHICS

INCIDENCE (IN U.S.): 5 cases/100,000 persons per yr of IM
PREDOMINANT SEX: Neither, although peak incidence occurs about 2 yr earlier in women
PREDOMINANT AGE:
- Clinical evidence of IM: occurs most commonly at ages 15 to 24 yr
- EBV infection: occurs earlier in life in lower socioeconomic groups

PHYSICAL FINDINGS & CLINICAL PRESENTATION

- Most EBV infections either are asymptomatic or cause a nonspecific viral illness.
- Incubation period is 1 to 2 mo, possibly followed by a prodrome of anorexia, low-grade fever, malaise, headache, and chills; after several days, clinical triad of pharyngitis, moderate to high fever, and adenopathy may appear, accompanied by fatigue and malaise.
- Pharyngitis is usually the most severe symptom; white or necrotic exudates are common.
- Symmetrical lymphadenopathy is most prominent in the posterior more than anterior cervical region but may be diffuse.
- Splenomegaly (50% of cases) is possible, most commonly during the second week of illness.
- Maculopapular or morbilliform rash is uncommon but will occur in patients who receive ampicillin. Patients may have palatal petechiae, periorbital, or palpebral edema. Mucocutaneous oral hairy leukoplakia (OHL), which is associated with intense EBV replication and the action of EBV-encoded proteins such as latent membrane protein-1, may occur.
- Possible IM presentation: fever and adenopathy without pharyngitis.
- Nausea, vomiting, and anorexia are frequent in patients with IM, probably reflecting mild hepatitis encountered in 90% of infected individuals.
- Although complications such as spleen rupture, airway obstruction, and malignancy may be severe and fatal, they are uncommon and tend to resolve completely.
- Hematologic involvement includes hemolytic or aplastic anemia, thrombocytopenia, thrombotic thrombocytopenic purpura/hemolytic-uremic syndrome, and disseminated intravascular coagulation (DIC). Pneumonia, myocarditis, pancreatitis, mesenteric adenitis, myositis, and glomerulonephritis may occur as well. Nervous system involvement includes Guillain-Barré syndrome, facial nerve palsy, meningoencephalitis, aseptic meningitis, transfer myelitis, peripheral neuritis, and optic neuritis.
- IM is usually a self-limited illness. Acute symptoms resolve in 1 to 2 wk, but symptoms of malaise and fatigue often persist for months.
- EBV is related to lymphoproliferative syndromes in transplant recipients and in AIDS patients.
- Increasing evidence showing an association between EBV infection and African Burkitt's, B-cell, T-cell lymphoma, and nasopharyngeal carcinoma. Table E1-183 describes EBV-associated malignancies.

ETIOLOGY

- EBV is a ubiquitous virus.
- Infection during childhood is much less likely to cause significant illness.
- Frequency of IM in late adolescence is attributed to the onset of social contact between the sexes.
- Close personal contact is usually necessary for transmission, although EBV is occasionally transmitted by blood transfusion; transfer via saliva while kissing may be responsible for many cases.

Dx DIAGNOSIS

DIFFERENTIAL DIAGNOSIS

- Heterophile-negative IM caused by cytomegalovirus (CMV)
- Although clinical presentation similar, CMV more frequently follows transfusion
- Bacterial and viral causes of pharyngitis
- Toxoplasmosis
- Acute retroviral syndrome of HIV
- Lymphoma
- Lyme disease

WORKUP

Heterophile antibody and CBC with blood smear. Table E1-184 describes frequently determined EBV-specific antibodies.

LABORATORY TESTS

- Increased WBC common, with a relative lymphocytosis of more than 50% and neutropenia are identified.
- Hallmark of IM: atypical lymphocytes of more than 10% (not pathognomonic) are found.
- Mild thrombocytopenia is present.
- Falling hematocrit signals the possibility of splenic rupture or immune hemolytic anemia.
- Elevated hepatocellular enzymes and cryoglobulins are found in most cases.
- Heterophile antibody:
  - As measured by the monospot test, may be positive at presentation or may appear later in the course of illness.
  - Negative test is repeated in 1 wk if clinical suspicion is high.
  - A positive test has been reported with primary HIV infection.
- Viral capsid antigen (VCA) IgG and IgM are rarely used for diagnosis, but better value in children because heterophile antibody is negative in most of children younger than 8 years.
- PCR DNA for CMV is the test of choice in transplant recipients who develop lymphoproliferative syndromes.

IMAGING STUDIES

Chest radiograph examination:
- May rarely show infiltrates
- Possible elevated left hemidiaphragm with splenic rupture

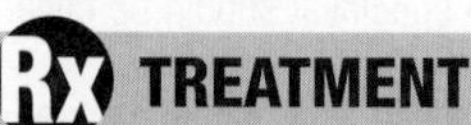

Rx TREATMENT

NONPHARMACOLOGIC THERAPY

- Supportive including rest
- Splenectomy if rupture occurs
- Transfusions for severe anemia or thrombocytopenia

ACUTE GENERAL Rx

- Pharmacologic therapy is not indicated in uncomplicated illness.
- Avoid aspirin due to the risk of Reye's syndrome.
- Avoid ampicillin and amoxicillin as their use can frequently precipitate a nonallergic rash.
- Use of steroids is suggested in patients who have severe thrombocytopenia, hemolytic anemia, impending airway obstruction resulting from enlarged tonsils, or fulminant liver failure. Prednisone 60 to 80 mg PO qd for 3 days, then tapered over 1 to 2 wk.
- Although it may reduce initial viral shedding, there is little evidence to support the use of antiviral agents such as acyclovir in the management of IM.

CHRONIC Rx

An extremely rare, chronic form of IM with persistent fevers and fatigue has been described and should be differentiated from chronic fatigue syndrome, which is not related to EBV.

DISPOSITION

Eventual resolution of all symptoms

REFERRAL

If more than mild illness

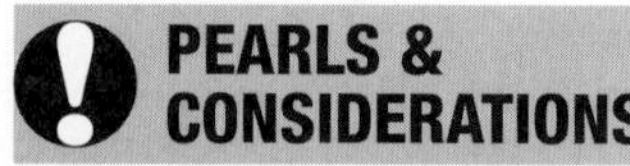

PEARLS & CONSIDERATIONS

COMMENTS

Avoidance of contact sports during the first month of illness because splenic rupture can occur even in the absence of clinically detectable splenomegaly.

SUGGESTED READINGS

available at www.expertconsult.com

RELATED CONTENT

Epstein-Barr Virus Infection (Patient Information)
Mononucleosis (Related Key Topic)

AUTHOR: **MONZR M. AL MALKI, M.D.**

BASIC INFORMATION

DEFINITION

Erectile dysfunction (ED) is the persistent inability to achieve or sustain a penile erection of adequate rigidity to make intercourse possible or satisfactory.

SYNONYMS

ED
Impotence
Male erectile disorder
Sexual dysfunction (a nonspecific term)

ICD-9CM and DSM-5 CODES
307.22
ICD-10CM CODES
N48.4 Impotence of organic origin
F52.2 Failure of genital response
F52.9 Unspecified sexual dysfunction, not caused by organic disorder or disease

EPIDEMIOLOGY & DEMOGRAPHICS

PREVALENCE (IN U.S.):
- Increases with age and presence of vascular comorbidities.
- Approximately 8% in the 20s–30s, 18% in the 50s, 25% in the 60s, 37% in the 70s, 80% in the 80s.

PREDOMINANT SEX: By definition, only in males
PREDOMINANT AGE: Increases with age
RISK FACTORS: Age, coronary artery disease, peripheral vascular disease, hypertension, diabetes mellitus, hypercholesterolemia, prostate surgery, neurologic injury, numerous medications, alcohol, smoking or drug abuse, obesity, obstructive sleep apnea, restless leg syndrome, systemic sclerosis

ETIOLOGY

- Most cases are caused by organic problems related to neurologic, hormonal, or vascular abnormalities or prescription or recreational drugs. In organic ED nocturnal penile tumescence is generally abnormal.
- Psychogenic ED results from mental stress, depression, widower syndrome, and performance anxiety. Characterized by normal nocturnal penile tumescence and otherwise negative test results.
- Vascular disease: History of hypertension (HTN), peripheral vascular disease, ischemic heart disease, diabetes, smoking. In approximately 40% of men >50 yr, the primary cause of ED is related to atherosclerotic disease, diabetes mellitus (DM), neuropathy, or vascular disease.
- Medication side effects: Antihypertensives such as thiazides and clonidine, guanethidine or methyldopa (consider change to ACE inhibitors and calcium channel blockers with lower reported incidence of ED); antiandrogens such as spironolactone, finasteride, ketoconazole; cimetidine (but not ranitidine or famotidine); antidepressants such as selective serotonin reuptake inhibitors [SSRIs]; and antipsychotics.
- Alcohol and nicotine use.
- Recreational drugs, including cocaine, heroin, amphetamines, and marijuana. These may increase libido but impair performance.
- Hormonal dysfunction such as testosterone deficiency (decreases libido and erection), hypothyroidism or hyperthyroidism, hyperprolactinemia, and adrenal insufficiency.
- Neurogenic causes including spinal cord lesions, cortical lesions, and peripheral neuropathies.
- Bicycling has possible, but controversial, association; this may be due to prolonged pressure on the pudendal and cavernosal nerves or compromised blood flow to the cavernosal artery, resulting in penile numbness and impotence.
- Trauma or pelvic surgeries such as radical prostatectomy or cystectomy.

DIAGNOSIS

DIFFERENTIAL DIAGNOSIS

- A useful tool to diagnose/evaluate ED severity is the Sexual Health Inventory for Men.
- Distinguish psychogenic from organic ED.
- Evaluate for underlying etiology of organic ED and comorbid psychiatric condition.

WORKUP

- Clinical history should include time course (abrupt onset may correlate with reversible cause such as medications, psychosocial stress, psychiatric complaint, trauma. Nonsustained erection may be secondary to anxiety or vascular steal syndrome), cause (psychogenic vs. organic), and change in libido.
- Report of spontaneous nocturnal or morning erections indicate intact neurologic reflexes and penile blood flow.
- Decreased libido may indicate endocrinologic or psychogenic cause.
- If possible, interview partner regarding sexual function.
- Medical and social history should address cardiac disease symptoms and risk factors (HTN, DM, hyperlipidemia, smoking, and substance abuse), pelvic surgery, medications, and mental health.
- Physical examination to check blood pressure, visual field defects to evaluate for pituitary tumors; femoral and peripheral pulses, femoral bruits; gynecomastia; neuronal damage (genital sensation, cremasteric reflex); direct penile damage (e.g., plaque formation such as Peyronie's disease); prostate examination; or testicular atrophy and other secondary sexual characteristics.

LABORATORY TESTS

Screen for diabetes mellitus with fasting glucose. Consider lipid panel, thyroid-stimulating hormone, morning serum testosterone (free and total). If decreased testosterone, check prolactin, follicle-stimulating hormone, and luteinizing hormone.

IMAGING STUDIES

Imaging studies are rarely performed except in situations of pelvic trauma or surgery.

OTHER STUDIES

- Nocturnal penile tumescence testing very specific for distinguishing psychogenic versus organic causes.
- Neurogenic etiologies examined by the cremasteric reflex (inner-thigh touch elicits scrotal contraction), the bulbocavernosus reflex, or the pudendal-evoked response.
- Intracorporeal injection of prostaglandin E_1 to distinguish vascular and nonvascular etiologies (erection is achieved in patients with normal vascular systems). If no erection with direct injection of vasoactive substance, consider duplex ultrasound of penile vasculature.
- In patients without an obvious cause of ED, consider screening for cardiovascular disease prior to starting treatment.

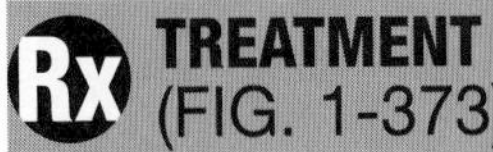

TREATMENT (FIG. 1-373)

NONPHARMACOLOGIC THERAPY

- Various psychotherapeutic approaches: cognitive-behavioral therapy preferred; success rates decrease with advancing age and duration of symptoms.
- Psychosexual therapy (sex therapy and couples therapy) is first line for psychogenic ED. Psychosexual therapy may be used as for adjunctive therapy in ED from any cause to address contributing social and relationship issues.
- Mechanical vacuum devices (function by drawing blood into corpus cavernosum) are 70% to 90% effective but are difficult to use.
- Incorporate vascular risk factor reduction including counsel on diet, exercise, smoking cessation, ETOH intake and screening/treatment for HTN, insulin resistance, and hypercholesterolemia as appropriate. Trials have shown that lifestyle modification and pharmacotherapy for cardiovascular risk factors are effective in improving sexual function in men with ED.

ACUTE GENERAL Rx

- First-line treatment: In setting of sexual stimulation, three selective phosphodiesterase type 5 (PDE5) inhibitors prolong nitric oxide–induced vasodilation by increase of intracavernosal cyclic guanosine monophosphate levels. Sildenafil (Viagra) and vardenafil (Levitra, Staxyn) can be taken 30 to 60 min before sexual activity, and both are effective for about 4 hr. Tadalafil (Cialis) can be taken several hours before sexual activity (although 50% respond within 30 min) and lasts up to 36 hr. All three PDE5 inhibitors have similar efficacy and tolerability, but tadalafil has a longer duration of action and is less affected by high-fat

 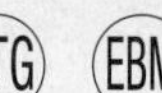

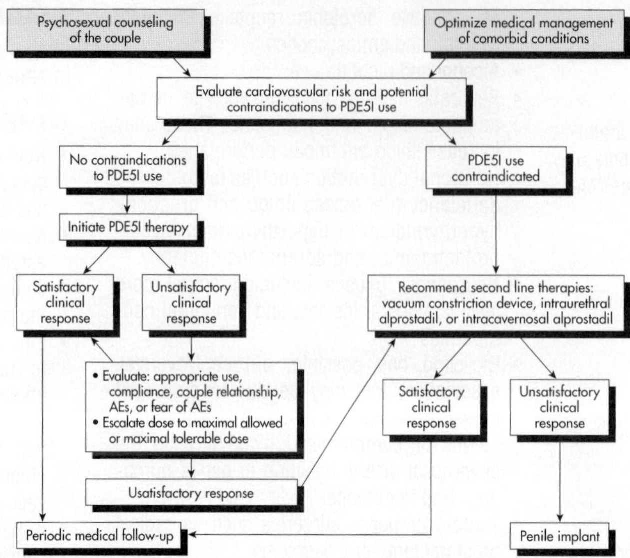

FIGURE 1-373 An algorithmic approach to the treatment of erectile dysfunction in men. *AE,* Adverse effects; *PDE5I,* phosphodiesterase 5 inhibitor. (From Melmed S, Polonsky KS, Larsen PR, Kronenberg HM: *Williams textbook of endocrinology,* ed 12, Philadelphia, 2011, Saunders.)

meals and alcohol. Counsel patients to avoid high-fat meals and excessive alcohol when taking PDE5 inhibitors, as they may impede effectiveness.

- With PDE5 inhibitors, avoid concomitant use of nitrates (absolute contraindication), drugs that inhibit or induce cytochrome P450 CYP3A4, and drugs that prolong the QT interval. Caution in men on alpha-adrenergic blocker therapy because of concern for hypotension; start the lowest dose of PDE5 inhibitor. Caution in men who have had myocardial infarction in the past 6 mo, resting hypotension or uncontrolled hypertension, unstable angina, positive exercise stress test or poor exercise tolerance. Counsel on side effects of headache, flushing, dyspepsia, nasal congestion, changes in color perception (including blue vision for sildenafil and vardenafil but not tadalafil), sudden hearing loss, and priapism (rare). Nonarteritic anterior ischemic optic neuropathy is also a rare association with sildenafil and tadalafil. Consider counseling on safe sexual practices when prescribing PDE5 inhibitors.
- Second-line treatment if PDE5 inhibitors fail: self-injection with intraurethral alprostadil (prostaglandin E_1 [medicated urethral suppository]) applied into meatus of penis before intercourse; or intracavernosal injections of vasodilators (e.g., papaverine or prostaglandin E_1 pellet). Consider combining intraurethral alprostadil with sildenafil. Relatively high success with self-injection, but attrition is high. (Table E1-185)
- Second-line treatment alternative: vacuum constriction pump; has variable satisfaction rate.

CHRONIC Rx

- Psychosexual therapy is helpful as an adjunctive treatment.
- Psychogenic impotence: PDE5 inhibitors are effective in patients with depression because tissues, nerves, hormones, and vasculature are normal. Full psychologic evaluation is recommended before starting treatment. If not responding to other therapies, consider yohimbine (modest efficacy), which acts by blocking presynaptic alpha-2-adrenergic receptors, thereby increasing cholinergic and decreasing adrenergic tone (caution in patients with heart disease due to possible tachycardia and hypertension).
- For men not responding to other approaches: surgical implantation of penile prosthesis.
- Testosterone therapy in men with low testosterone (i.e., hypogonadal); evaluate for prostate cancer before prescribing testosterone.
- Aerobic exercise may improve ED along with pharmacologic treatment.

DISPOSITION

- Psychogenic-acquired ED will remit spontaneously in 15% to 30% of cases.
- Lifelong ED is usually a chronic and unremitting condition.
- Situational ED may remit with changes in social environment but usually recurs.

REFERRAL

- Refer if psychotherapy, sex therapy, or invasive organic treatment required
- Refer to urology if PDE5 inhibitors fail or sudden onset occurs after penile trauma

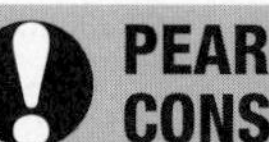

PEARLS & CONSIDERATIONS

- ED is commonly evaluated and treated by primary care physician; refer to urologist if oral therapy fails or surgery is required.
- PDE5 inhibitors are treatment of choice for most causes of ED. Main contraindications are nitrate use and decompensated cardiac disease. Caution in patients on alpha-adrenergic blockers and with blood pressures at extreme ends (significant hypotension or hypertension).
- For optimal response, patients should be appropriately informed of proper use, precautions, and adverse effects of PDE5 inhibitors. Try six to eight times at optimal doses before declaring PDE5 inhibitors a failure. Consider switching among the three PDE5 inhibitors if one fails.
- Men with ED are at increased risk of coronary, cerebrovascular, and peripheral vascular diseases. Screen for cardiovascular risk factors in these patients.

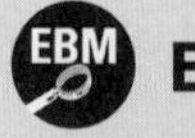

EVIDENCE

available at www.expertconsult.com

SUGGESTED READINGS

available at www.expertconsult.com

RELATED CONTENT

Erectile Dysfunction (Patient Information)

AUTHORS: **CINDY LAI, M.D.,** and **HEMALI PATEL, M.D.**

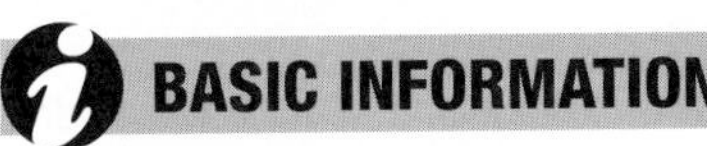

BASIC INFORMATION

DEFINITION

Erysipelas is a type of cellulitis caused by infection of the superficial layers of the skin and cutaneous lymphatics. Erysipelas is characterized by redness, induration, and a sharply demarcated, raised border.

SYNONYMS

St. Anthony's fire

ICD-9CM CODES
035 Erysipelas
ICD-10CM CODES
A46 Erysipelas

EPIDEMIOLOGY & DEMOGRAPHICS

PREDOMINANT AGE: Occurs most often in the young or old

RISK FACTORS: Patients with impaired lymphatic or venous drainage (mastectomy, saphenous vein harvesting) and immunocompromised patients. Athlete's foot is a common portal of entry.

RECURRENCE RATE: Relatively common

PHYSICAL FINDINGS & CLINICAL PRESENTATION

- Distinctive red, warm, tender skin lesion with induration and a sharply defined, advancing, raised border (Fig. 1-374).
- Most common sites are lower extremities and face.
- Systemic signs of infection (fever) are often present.
- Vesicles or bullae may develop.
- After several days lesions may appear ecchymotic.
- After 7 to 10 days desquamation of affected area may occur.

FIGURE 1-374 Erysipelas. Note well-demarcated erythematous plaque on arm. (From Goldstein B [ed]: *Practical dermatology,* ed 2, St Louis, 1997, Mosby. Courtesy Department of Dermatology, University of North Carolina at Chapel Hill.)

ETIOLOGY

- Usually group A β-hemolytic streptococci
- Less often group B, C, or G streptococci
- Rarely *Staphylococcus aureus*

COMPLICATIONS

- Abscess
- Necrotizing fasciitis
- Thrombophlebitis
- Gangrene
- Metastatic infection

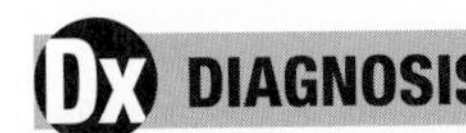

DIAGNOSIS

DIFFERENTIAL DIAGNOSIS

- Other types of cellulitis
- Necrotizing fasciitis
- Deep vein thrombosis
- Contact dermatitis
- Erythema migrans (Lyme disease)
- Insect bite
- Herpes zoster
- Erysipeloid
- Acute gout
- Pseudogout

WORKUP

History, physical examination, and laboratory evaluation

LABORATORY TESTS

Diagnosis is usually made by characteristic clinical setting and appearance.

- Complete blood count and white blood cell count often elevated
- Blood cultures positive in 5% of patients
- Gram stain and culture of any drainage from skin lesions
- Culture of aspirated fluid from leading edge of skin lesion has low yield

IMAGING STUDIES

- Not routinely indicated
- Duplex ultrasound for patients suspected of having deep vein thrombosis
- CT scan or MRI for patients with suspected necrotizing fasciitis

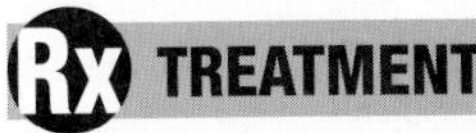

TREATMENT

NONPHARMACOLOGIC THERAPY

- Elevation of the affected limb
- Warm compresses

ACUTE GENERAL Rx

Typical erysipelas of extremity in nondiabetic patient:

- PO: penicillin V 500 mg qid
- IV: penicillin G (aqueous) 1 to 2 million units q6h. Use vancomycin 15 mg/kg IV q12h in penicillin-allergic patients.

NOTE: Use azithromycin in patients allergic to penicillin.

Facial erysipelas (include coverage for *Staphylococcus aureus*):

- PO dicloxacillin 500 mg q6h
- IV nafcillin or oxacillin 2 g q4h
- IV vancomycin 1 g q12h
- Daptomycin 4 mg/kg IV q24h
- Linezolid 600 mg IV q12h

DISPOSITION

Prognosis is good with antibiotic treatment but recurrence is common.

REFERRAL

For surgical debridement for patients with necrotizing fasciitis or for drainage of abscess

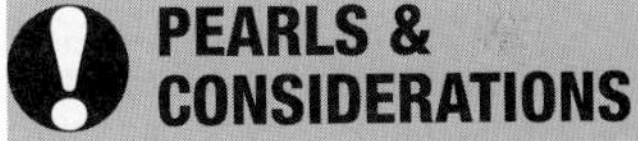

PEARLS & CONSIDERATIONS

- Consider early surgical referral when necrotizing fasciitis suspected. Consider skin biopsy when not responding to appropriate antibiotics.
- Look for tinea pedis as portal of entry in erysipelas of lower extremities. Treat if present.

SUGGESTED READINGS
available at www.expertconsult.com

RELATED CONTENT

Cellulitis (Related Key Topic)
Erysipelas (Patient Information)

AUTHORS: **GAIL M. O'BRIEN, M.D.,** and **MARK J. FAGAN, M.D.**

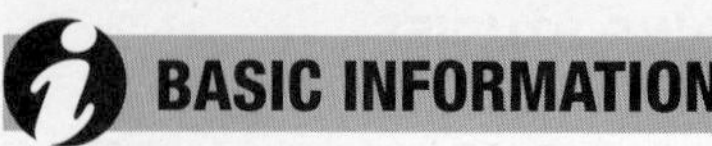

BASIC INFORMATION

DEFINITION

Erythema multiforme is an inflammatory disease characterized by eruption of annular, maculopapular lesions with dark raised, erythematous, or vesiculobullous center surrounded by a pale zone. It is believed to be caused by immune complex formation and subsequent deposition in the skin and mucous membranes. It is considered a hypersensitivity reaction to infection or drugs.

SYNONYMS

EM

ICD-9CM CODES
695.1 Erythema multiforme
ICD-10CM CODES
L51.9 Erythema multiforme, unspecified

EPIDEMIOLOGY & DEMOGRAPHICS

PREDOMINANT AGE: 20 to 40 yr

RISK FACTORS: Often associated with herpes simplex and other infectious agents, drugs, or connective tissue diseases.

PHYSICAL FINDINGS & CLINICAL PRESENTATION

- Prodromal symptoms are mild or absent. Itching or burning at the site of eruption may occur.
- Symmetric skin lesions with a classic "target" appearance (caused by the centrifugal spread of red maculopapules to circumference of 1 to 3 cm with a purpuric, cyanotic, or vesicular center) are present (Fig. 1-375). The papules may enlarge into plaques measuring a few centimeters in diameter with a dark or red central portion. Target lesions may not be apparent for several days.
- Lesions are most common in the back of the hands and feet and extensor aspect of the forearms and legs. Trunk involvement can occur in severe cases.
- Urticarial papules, vesicles, and bullae may also be present and generally indicate a more severe form of the disease.
- Individual lesions heal in 1 to 2 wk without scarring.
- Bullae and erosions may also be present in the oral cavity.

ETIOLOGY

- Immune complex formation and subsequent deposition in the cutaneous microvasculature may play a role in the pathogenesis of erythema multiforme.
- The majority of cases follow outbreaks of herpes simplex virus 1 and 2.
- *Mycoplasma pneumoniae,* fungal infections, medications (bupropion, sulfonamides, penicillins, nonsteroidal anti-inflammatory drugs, barbiturates, phenothiazines, hydantoins).
- In >50% of patients no specific cause is identified.

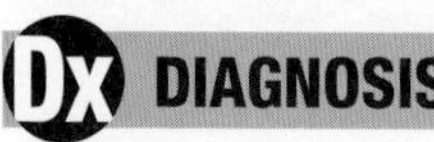

DIAGNOSIS

DIFFERENTIAL DIAGNOSIS

- Chronic urticaria
- Secondary syphilis
- Pityriasis rosea
- Contact dermatitis
- Pemphigus vulgaris
- Lichen planus
- Serum sickness
- Drug eruption
- Granuloma annulare
- Polymorphic light eruption
- Viral exanthem

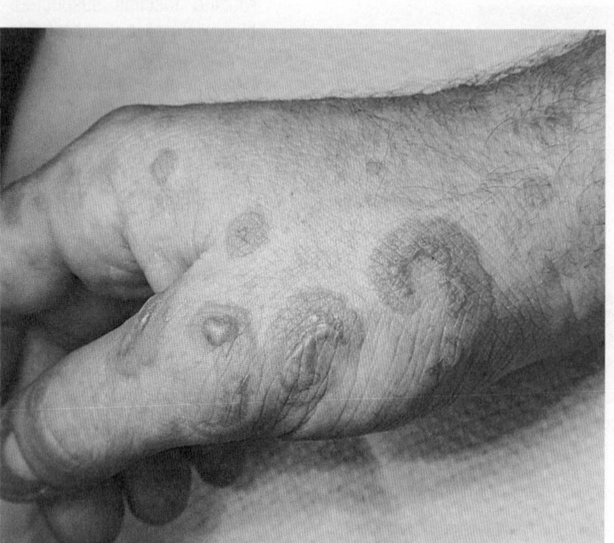

FIGURE 1-375 Iris and arcuate lesions of erythema multiforme. Note erythematous lesions with multiform configurations: target, arcuate, and vesicles. (From Noble J et al: *Textbook of primary care medicine,* ed 2, St Louis, 1995, Mosby.)

WORKUP

- Medical history with emphasis on drug ingestion
- Laboratory evaluation in patients with suspected collagen-vascular diseases
- Skin biopsy when diagnosis is unclear

LABORATORY TESTS

- Complete blood count with differential
- Antinuclear antibody
- Serology for *M. pneumoniae,* HSV-1, HSV-2
- Urinalysis

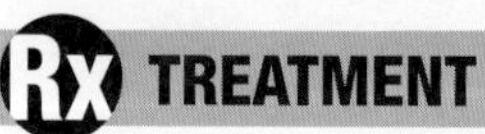

TREATMENT

NONPHARMACOLOGIC THERAPY

- Mild cases generally do not require treatment; lesions resolve spontaneously within 1 mo.
- Potential drug precipitants should be removed.

ACUTE GENERAL Rx

- Treatment of associated diseases (e.g., acyclovir for herpes simplex, erythromycin for *Mycoplasma* infection).
- Prednisone 40 to 80 mg/day for 1 to 3 wk may be tried in patients with many target lesions; however, the role of systemic steroids remains controversial.
- Levamisole, an immunomodulator, may be effective in the treatment of patients with chronic or recurrent oral lesions (dose is 150 mg/day for 3 consecutive days used alone or in combination with prednisone).
- IV immunoglobulins in severe cases.

DISPOSITION

The rash generally evolves over a 2-wk period and resolves within 3 to 4 wk without scarring. A severe bullous form can occur (see entry for "Stevens-Johnson Syndrome").

REFERRAL

Hospital admission in patients with suspected Stevens-Johnson syndrome

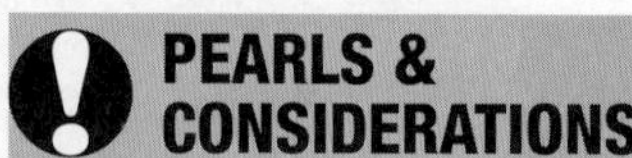

PEARLS & CONSIDERATIONS

COMMENTS

The risk of recurrence of erythema multiforme exceeds 30%. Recurrence may be treated with valacyclovir 500 to 1000 mg/day, famciclovir 125 to 250 mg/day, or acyclovir 400 mg bid. Dapsone, antimalarials, azathioprine, or cyclosporine use is reserved for cases resistant to antivirals.

SUGGESTED READINGS

available at www.expertconsult.com

RELATED CONTENT

Erythema Multiforme (Patient Information)

AUTHOR: **FRED F. FERRI, M.D.**

BASIC INFORMATION

DEFINITION

Erythema nodosum (EN) is an acute, tender, erythematous, nodular skin eruption resulting from inflammation of subcutaneous fat, often associated with bruising. It is the most common form of panniculitis.

ICD-9CM CODES
695.2 Erythema nodosum
ICD-10CM CODES
L52 Erythema nodosum

EPIDEMIOLOGY & DEMOGRAPHICS

INCIDENCE: Two to three cases/100,000 persons per yr
PREDOMINANT SEX: Female/male ratio of 3 to 4:1
PREDOMINANT AGE: 25 to 40 yr

PHYSICAL FINDINGS & CLINICAL PRESENTATION

- Acute onset of tender nodules typically located on the shins (Fig. 1-376) and occasionally seen on the thighs and forearms.
- The nodules are usually ⅛ to 1 inch in diameter but can be as large as 4 inches; they begin as light red lesions, then become darker and often ecchymotic. The nodules heal within 8 wk without ulceration.

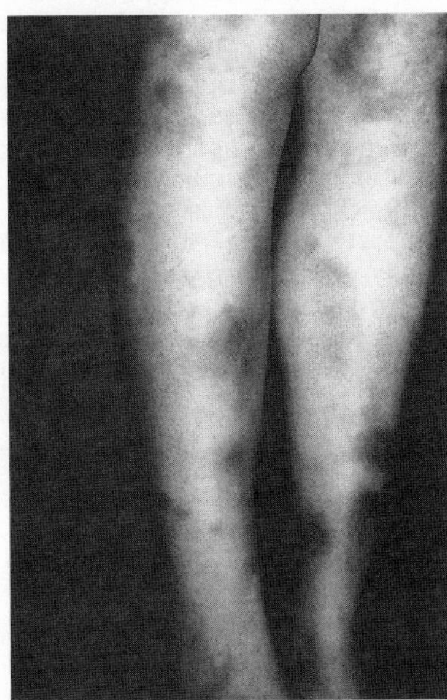

FIGURE 1-376 Erythema nodosum. (From Arndt KA et al: *Cutaneous medicine and surgery, vol 1,* Philadelphia, 1997, Saunders.)

- Associated findings:
  1. Fever
  2. Lymphadenopathy
  3. Arthralgia
  4. Signs of the underlying illness

ETIOLOGY

Cell-mediated hypersensitivity reaction is seen more frequently in persons with human leukocyte antigen (HLA) B8. The lesion results from an exaggerated interaction between an antigen and cell-mediated immune mechanisms leading to granuloma formation. Up to 55% of cases of EN are idiopathic.

Infections:

- Bacteria
  - Streptococcal pharyngitis (28% to 48%)
  - *Salmonella* enteritis
  - *Yersinia* enteritis
  - Psittacosis
  - *Chlamydia pneumoniae* infection
  - *Mycoplasma* pneumonia
  - Meningococcal infection
  - Gonorrhea
  - Syphilis
  - Lymphogranuloma venereum
  - Tularemia
  - Cat-scratch disease
  - Leprosy
  - Tuberculosis
- Fungi
  - Histoplasmosis
  - Coccidioidomycosis
  - Blastomycosis
  - *Trichophyton verrucosum*
- Viruses
  - Cytomegalovirus
  - Hepatitis B
  - Epstein-Barr virus
- Drugs (3% to 10%)
  - Sulfonamides
  - Penicillins
  - Oral contraceptives
  - Gold salts
  - Prazosin
  - Aspirin
  - Bromides
- Sarcoidosis (11% to 25%)
- Inflammatory bowel disease
- Cancer, usually lymphoma
- Ankylosing spondylosis and reactive arthropathies (e.g., associated with inflammatory bowel disease)

DIAGNOSIS

DIFFERENTIAL DIAGNOSIS

- Insect bites
- Posttraumatic ecchymoses
- Vasculitis
- Weber-Christian disease
- Fat necrosis associated with pancreatitis
- Necrobiosis lipoidica
- Scleroderma
- Lupus panniculitis
- Subcutaneous granuloma
- Alpha-1 antitrypsin deficiency

WORKUP

- Physical examination
- Diagnosis of underlying illness by history, physical examination, and laboratory tests as indicated

LABORATORY TESTS

- Erythrocyte sedimentation rate
- Throat culture and antistreptolysin O titer
- PPD
- Others depending on index of suspicion (e.g., stool culture and evaluation for ova and parasites in patients with diarrhea and gastrointestinal symptoms)
- Skin biopsy in doubtful cases:
  1. Early lesion: inflammation and hemorrhage in subcutaneous tissue
  2. Late lesion: giant cells and granulomata

IMAGING STUDIES

Chest radiograph to rule out sarcoidosis and tuberculosis

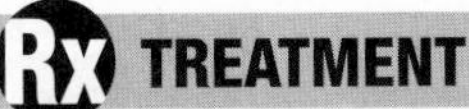

TREATMENT

- The disease is self-limited and treatment is symptomatic. EN nodules develop in pretibial locations and resolve spontaneously over several weeks without scarring or ulceration.
- Treatment of underlying disorders.
- Avoidance of contact irritation of affected areas.
- Nonsteroidal anti-inflammatory drugs for pain.
- Systemic steroids (prednisone 1 mg/kg of body weight/day, tapered over several days) may be useful in severe cases if underlying risk of sepsis and malignancy have been excluded.

PROGNOSIS

Typical case:

- Pain for 2 wk
- Resolution within 8 wk

SUGGESTED READINGS

available at www.expertconsult.com

RELATED CONTENT

Erythema Nodosum (Patient Information)

AUTHOR: **FRED F. FERRI, M.D.**

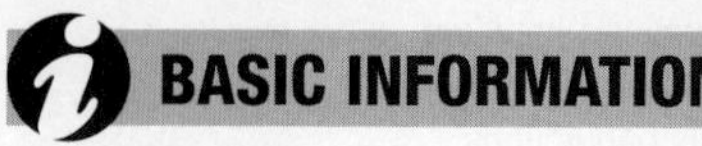

DEFINITION

Esophageal tumors include both benign and malignant neoplasms of the esophageal mucosa and wall. Carcinomas of the esophageal epithelium, both squamous cell and adenocarcinoma, are by far the most common tumors of the esophagus (see Table 1-186). Rare esophageal tumors include both malignant (spindle cell, small cell, sarcoma, lymphoma) and benign neoplasms (leiomyoma, papilloma, and fibrovascular polyps). Approximately 15% of esophageal tumors arise in the proximal esophagus, 50% in the middle third of the esophagus, and 35% in the lower third.

SYNONYMS

Neoplasm of the esophagus
Malignancy of the esophagus

ICD-10CM CODES

C15.X Malignant neoplasm of the esophagus (X defines location)
C15.3 Malignant neoplasm of upper third of esophagus
C15.4 Malignant neoplasm of middle third of esophagus
C15.5 Malignant neoplasm of lower third of esophagus
D00.2 Carcinoma of esophagus, in situ

EPIDEMIOLOGY & DEMOGRAPHICS

INCIDENCE: Varies widely worldwide. It is the eighth most common incident cancer and the seventh leading cause of cancer death worldwide. Rates are increasing every decade and are highest in the Asian esophageal cancer belt, extending from the Caspian Sea to northern China, with certain high-incidence pockets in Finland, Ireland, southeast Africa, and northwest France. Incidence has increased sixfold since 1975. Rates of squamous cell carcinoma are decreasing while rates of adenocarcinomas are dramatically increasing.

PREVALENCE: In the United States, almost 18,000 new cases and more than 15,000 deaths per year, making it the seventh leading cause of death by cancer among men. The majority are diagnosed at an advanced stage (unresectable or metastatic disease).

RACE, AGE, & SEX PREDOMINANCE: In the United States, squamous cell esophageal cancer is more common among blacks than whites, whereas adenocarcinoma is more common in whites than blacks. The overall male/female ratio is 3 to 4:1; the highest male/female ratio is in the Hispanic population. It usually develops in the seventh and eighth decades and is associated with lower socioeconomic status.

GENETICS: Increasing evidence shows that genetics may play a role by increasing susceptibility to esophageal cancer. One well identified disease condition associated with esophageal cancer is tylosis (focal non-epidermolytic palmoplantar keratoderma), linked to loss of heterozygosity on chromosome 17q. Familiar clustering of Barrett's esophagus and the recent identification of germline mutations in affected sibling pairs support a genetic link to esophageal adenocarcinoma.

TABLE 1-186 Classification of Esophageal Cancer

Epithelial
Squamous cell
Ordinary squamous cell
Verrucous squamous cell
Spindle cell (carcinosarcoma)
Adenocarcinoma
Ordinary
Adenoacanthoma
Mucoepidermoid
Adenoid cystic
Small cell
Melanoma
Choriocarcinoma
Metastatic Disease
Lymphoma
Sarcoma

From Abeloff MD: *Clinical oncology,* ed 3, Philadelphia, 2004, Churchill Livingstone.

CLINICAL PRESENTATION

Symptoms and signs:

- Dysphagia (74%): initially occurs with solid foods and gradually progresses to include semisolids and liquids; latter signs usually indicate incurable disease with tumor involving more than 60% of the esophageal circumference. May be felt as chest pain.
- Unintentional weight loss: usually of short duration. Losing >10% of body mass predicts poor outcome.
- Hoarseness: suggests recurrent laryngeal nerve involvement.
- Odynophagia and halitosis: unusual symptoms.
- Cervical adenopathy: usually involving supraclavicular lymph nodes.
- Dry cough: suggests tracheal involvement.
- Aspiration pneumonia: caused by development of a fistula between the esophagus and trachea.
- Iron deficiency anemia, related to chronic GI blood loss.
- Massive hemoptysis or hematemesis: results from the invasion of vascular structures.
- Advanced disease spreads to lymph nodes, liver, lungs, peritoneum, and pleura.
- Hypercalcemia: associated with squamous cell carcinoma from secretion of a parathyroid-like tumor peptide.

Clinical findings:

- Fifty to sixty percent of patients present with locally advanced, regional, or metastatic disease.

ETIOLOGY

Pathogenesis of esophageal cancers is attributable to chronic recurrent oxidative damage from any of the following etiologic agents, which cause inflammation, and esophagitis, increased cell turnover, and, ultimately, initiation of the carcinogenic process.

ETIOLOGIC AGENTS:

- Excess alcohol consumption is strongly associated with squamous cell esophageal cancer in the United States; hard liquor is associated with a higher incidence than wine or beer.
- Tobacco and alcohol synergistically increase risk for squamous cell cancer.
- Smoking may increase the risk of developing adenocarcinoma, particularly in patients with Barrett's.
- Obesity, hiatal hernia, and low-vitamin, high-fat diet.
- Other ingested carcinogens:
  - Nitrates (converted to nitrites): South Asia, China
  - Smoked opiates: Northern Iran
  - Fungal toxins in pickled vegetables
  - Betel nut chewing
- Mucosal damage:
  - Long-term exposure to extremely hot tea (>70° C)
  - Lye ingestion
- Radiation-induced strictures
- Achalasia: incidence of esophageal cancer is seven times greater in this population
- Host susceptibility as a result of precancerous lesions:
  - Plummer-Vinson syndrome (Paterson-Kelly): glossitis with iron deficiency
  - Congenital hyperkeratosis and pitting of palms and soles (tylosis)
- Chronic GERD leading to Barrett's metaplasia and adenocarcinoma via immune cell infiltration and production of inflammatory mediators and reactive oxygen species. The annual rate of transformation from Barrett's to adenocarcinoma is 0.5%.
- Human papillomavirus infection (particularly types 16 and 18) has been variably detected in squamous cell carcinoma of the esophagus, sometimes associated with p53 tumor suppressor gene mutations.
- Possible association with celiac sprue or dietary deficiencies of molybdenum, selenium, zinc, vitamin A.
- Questionable relationship with prolonged bisphosphonate use (≥10 prescriptions, or use <3 yr).

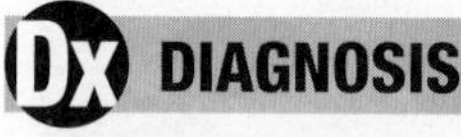

DIFFERENTIAL DIAGNOSIS

- Achalasia
- Scleroderma of the esophagus
- Diffuse esophageal spasm
- Esophageal rings and webs

LABORATORY TESTS

Complete blood cell count, blood chemistry, liver enzymes. No biomarkers are available currently to diagnose, monitor, or predict outcomes.

IMAGING STUDIES

Imaging studies are important not only for diagnosis but for accurate staging (Fig. 1-377):

- Esophagogastroduodenoscopy (EGD) (Fig. 1-378) should be performed initially to visualize smaller tumors, which may be missed by esophagogram, and to allow histopathologic confirmation.

- Endoscopic inspection of the larynx, trachea, and bronchi may identify concomitant cancers of head, neck, and lung ("triple endoscopy").
- Endoscopic ultrasonogram (EUS) (Fig. 1-378) is the most accurate method for locoregional staging: to determine the depth of tumor invasion and to assess for suspicious lymph nodes.
- Double-contrast esophagogram effectively identifies large esophageal lesions (Fig. E1-379).
  - In contrast to benign esophageal leiomyomata, which cause narrowing with preservation of normal mucosal pattern, esophageal carcinomas cause ragged ulcerating mucosal changes in association with deeper infiltration.
- Chest and abdominal CT and/or integrated CT-PET scans can determine tumor spread for preoperative staging.
- Staging laparoscopy may alter treatment plans in 20% to 30% of cases by more accurately staging regional lymph nodes and detecting occult peritoneal metastases.

STAGING

Table 1-187 describes the TNM staging system for cancer of the esophagus from the American Joint Committee on Cancer Criteria.

Rx TREATMENT

ACUTE GENERAL Rx

RESECTION:

- Surgical resection of squamous cell carcinoma and adenocarcinoma of the lower third of the esophagus is indicated for local, resectable disease in the absence of widespread metastasis detected by CT-PET (T1 and T2 tumors). Gastric pull-through or colonic interposition typically is used to provide luminal continuity.
- Endoscopic mucosal resection may replace radical surgical resection in very early tumors with no lymph node involvement (T stage Tis or T1a), but a recent Cochrane review found no studies comparing endoscopic treatment vs. surgery. This may be performed in conjunction with ablative therapies, including radiofrequency ablation, thermal ablation techniques, or photodynamic therapy.
- Complications of surgery:
  - Anatomic fistula (usually with colon interposition, subphrenic abscesses)
  - Respiratory complications
  - Cardiovascular complications are most common, including MI, CVA, and PE
  - Mortality is lower and clinical outcomes are better at high-volume hospitals.

RADIATION THERAPY:

- Squamous cell carcinomas are more radiosensitive than adenocarcinoma. Radiation achieves good local control and is generally only used as monotherapy as a palliative modality for obstructive symptoms in unresectable or advanced cancer. It is best used for cervical esophageal tumors.
- Palliative radiation therapy for bone metastasis is also effective.
- Complications of radiation therapy:
  - Esophageal stricture, radiation-induced pulmonary fibrosis, and transverse myelitis are the most feared.
  - Radiation-induced cardiomyopathy and skin changes are rare.

COMBINATION CHEMOTHERAPY, RADIATION RX, & SURGICAL RX:

- Chemotherapy is most often given with concurrent radiation therapy (chemoradiotherapy). Chemotherapy may sensitize tumor cells to the effects of ionizing radiation, improving the tumoricidal effects of treatment. Two-yr survival is improved with chemoradiotherapy (30%) vs. radiotherapy alone (10%). Trials have shown that preoperative chemoradiotherapy improves survival among patients with potentially curable esophageal or esophagogastric junction cancer.
- Chemoradiotherapy combined with surgery is offered to late Stage I (T2N0 or T3N0), Stage II, and Stage III esophageal cancer patients. In several studies, preoperative chemoradiotherapy plus surgery significantly improved local control, reduced recurrence, and

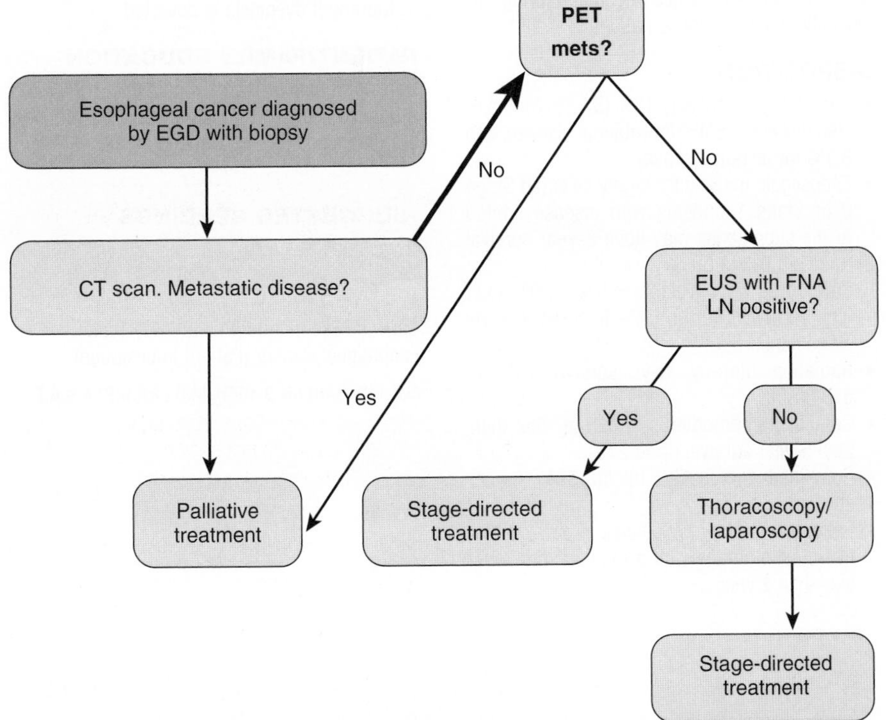

FIGURE 1-377 Algorithm for staging esophageal cancer. *CT,* Computed tomography; *EGD,* esophagogastroduodenoscopy; *mets,* metastases; *PET,* positron emission tomography. (From Cameron JL, Cameron AM: *Current surgical therapy,* ed 10, Philadelphia, 2011, Saunders.)

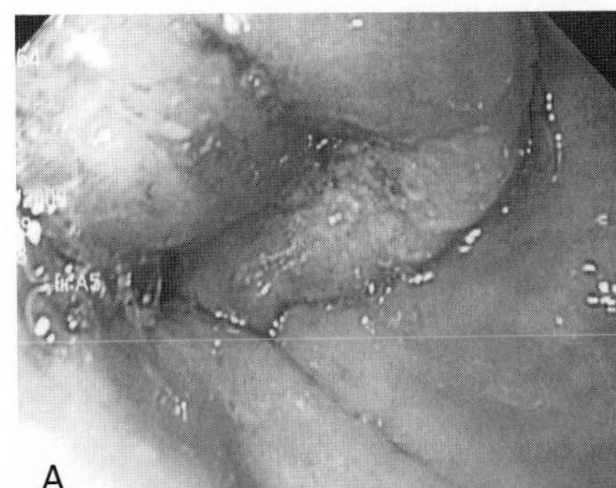

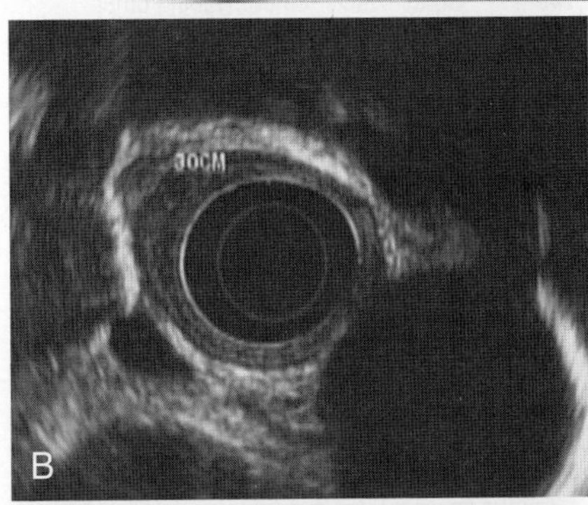

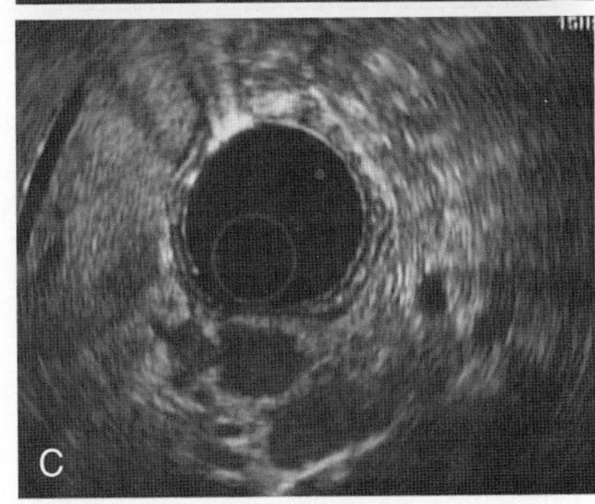

FIGURE 1-378 Esophageal cancer. A, Endoscopic picture of malignant esophageal stricture. **B,** EUS image showing T3 lesion. **C,** Malignant celiac lymphadenopathy. (From Cameron JL, Cameron AM: *Current surgical therapy,* ed 10, Philadelphia, 2011, Saunders.)

reduced mortality compared with surgery alone in patients with resectable esophageal cancer. Trimodal therapy is the preferred treatment for most esophageal cancers.

- Chemoradiotherapy alone may be offered to patients who are not surgical candidates.
- Combination chemotherapy including cisplatin achieved significant tumor reduction in 30% to 60% of patients. Cisplatin is usually given with 5-FU but has also been used in combinations with irinotecan, vinblastine, bleomycin, vindesine, and mitomycin.

TABLE 1-187 TNM Staging System for Cancer of the Esophagus (American Joint Committee on Cancer Criteria)

Primary Tumor (T)*	
TX	Primary tumor cannot be assessed
T0	No evidence of primary tumor
Tis	High-grade dysplasia†
T1	Tumor invades lamina propria, muscularis mucosae, or submucosa
T1a	Tumor invades lamina propria or muscularis mucosae
T1b	Tumor invades submucosa
T2	Tumor invades muscularis propria
T3	Tumor invades adventitia
T4	Tumor invades adjacent structures
T4a	Resectable tumor invading pleura, pericardium, or diaphragm
T4b	Unresectable tumor invading other adjacent structures, such as aorta, vertebral body, trachea, etc.
Lymph Node (N)‡	
NX	Regional lymph nodes cannot be assessed
N0	No regional lymph node metastasis
N1	Metastasis in 1-2 regional lymph nodes
N2	Metastasis in 3-6 regional lymph nodes
N3	Metastasis in 7 or more regional lymph nodes
Distant Metastasis (M)	
MX	Metastasis cannot be assessed
M0	No distant metastasis
M1	Distant metastasis

*(1) At least maximal dimension of the tumor must be recorded and (2) multiple tumors require the T(m) suffix.
†High-grade dysplasia includes all noninvasive neoplastic epithelia that was formerly called carcinoma in situ.
‡Number must be recorded for total number of regional nodes sampled and total number of reported nodes with metastasis.
From Edge S et al (eds): *AJCC cancer staging manual,* ed 7, New York, 2010, Springer.

- Capecitabine and oxaliplatin are as effective as fluorouracil and cisplatin, respectively, in patients with previously untreated esophagogastric cancer.
- Trastuzumab, in combination with more traditional chemotherapy, is being studied for a subset of patients with HER-2 overexpressing esophageal adenocarcinoma.
- Cetuximab, an epidermal growth factor receptor (EGFR) inhibitor, is being studied in combination with more traditional chemotherapy to treat squamous cell carcinomas.
- Complications of chemotherapy include mucositis, GI toxicity, myelosuppression, nephrotoxicity; ototoxicity and neurotoxicity occur with cisplatin.
- Postoperative adjuvant chemotherapy with or without radiation therapy may be offered to node-positive patients who underwent initial surgery alone.

CHRONIC Rx

For patients who have received treatment, the majority of recurrences develop within 12 months. Clinical monitoring, along with lab tests, imaging, and endoscopic evaluation where appropriate (particularly with preoperative Barrett's), are usually performed for postoperative surveillance, without clear benefit in earlier detection or decreased mortality. Palliative procedures such as repeated endoscopic dilation, endoscopic ablation, endoscopic mucosal resection, photodynamic therapy, brachytherapy, feeding tube insertion, or placement of expandable metal stents or polyvinyl prostheses to bypass tumors have been used for unresectable patients. The morbidity and mortality associated with resection in patients with advanced disease and/or for palliation argues against offering this modality to most of these patients.

DISPOSITION

- Overall 5-yr survival is 13% (37.3% for localized disease, 18.4% for regional disease, and 3.1% for distant disease)
- Endoscopic therapy for highly selected Stage 0 or Stage 1 patients with disease limited to the submucosa may have 5-year survival rates of 60% to 90%.
- Surgery: 5-yr survival rate is 5% to 30%, with higher survival (up to 45% to 50%) in early stage cancers
- Radiation therapy: 5-yr survival rate of 6%-20%
- Combined chemotherapy and radiation therapy: 5-year survival up to 27%
- Combined trimodality: up to 39% 5-year survival rate
- Patients with Stage IV disease receive palliative chemotherapy with a median survival of less than 1 year

REFERRAL

- To gastroenterologist for endoscopy for patients with dysphagia, odynophagia, or unexplained weight loss, or for palliative care
- To medical oncologist for evaluation of preoperative chemotherapy
- To radiation oncologist for palliative therapy if tumor is unresectable or obstruction is present
- To hospice if appropriate

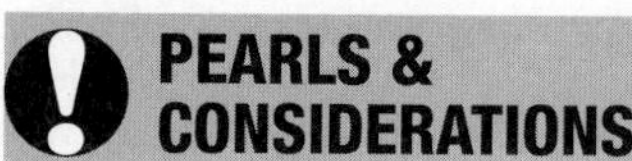

PEARLS & CONSIDERATIONS

COMMENTS

More than 50% of patients with esophageal cancer are diagnosed when the disease is metastatic or unresectable.

PREVENTION

- A diet high in fruits, vegetables, and antioxidants may be associated with lower risk of esophageal cancer.
- Avoid tobacco and excessive alcohol use.
- Avoid ingested toxins known to cause esophageal cancers.
- Aspirin may have a chemopreventative role in Barrett's but is only currently recommended for patients with other (e.g., cardiac) indications.
- There is no evidence that vitamins, Chinese herbal regimens, or green tea prevent esophageal cancer.
- Screening the general population is not recommended. If Barrett's esophagus is detected, regularly scheduled surveillance endoscopies are necessary, with consideration for radiofrequency or other ablation therapy if dysplasia is detected.

PATIENT/FAMILY EDUCATION

Provide education and support about the likely prognosis because most esophageal cancers are diagnosed at an advanced stage.

SUGGESTED READINGS

available at www.expertconsult.com

RELATED CONTENT

Barrett's Esophagus (Related Key Topic)
Esophageal Cancer (Patient Information)

AUTHOR: **HARLAN G. RICH, M.D., F.A.C.P., A.G.A.F.**

BASIC INFORMATION

DEFINITION

Esophageal varices are dilated submucosal veins that occur in patients with underlying portal hypertension, function as a shunt between the portal venous and systemic venous circulation, and can result in severe upper GI hemorrhage.

ICD-10CM CODES
85.00 Esophageal varices without bleeding
I85.01 Esophageal varices with bleeding
I85.10 Secondary esophageal varices without bleeding
I85.11 Secondary esophageal varices with bleeding

ICD-10CM CODES
I85.00 Esophageal varices without bleeding
I85.01 Esophageal varices with bleeding

EPIDEMIOLOGY & DEMOGRAPHICS

INCIDENCE:
- Esophageal varices: 5%-15% per year in patients with cirrhosis
- Hemorrhage:
  - One third of all patients with varices will develop hemorrhage.
  - Variceal hemorrhage occurs in 25%-40% of patients with cirrhosis
  - The risk of bleeding from varices is approximately 15% at 1 year.
  - Survivors of an episode of active bleeding have a 70% risk of recurrent hemorrhage within 1 year.

PREVALENCE: Approximately 50% of patients with cirrhosis have varices at the time of diagnosis.

RISK FACTORS: Cirrhosis, low platelet count and advanced Child-Pugh class, hepatitis C with advanced fibrosis

PHYSICAL FINDINGS & CLINICAL PRESENTATION

- Often asymptomatic until acute upper GI hemorrhage: hematemesis, hypovolemia
- No physical findings specific for esophageal varices
- Stigmata of cirrhosis and portal hypertension may be evident: palmar erythema, telangiectasias, gynecomastia, testicular atrophy, jaundice, caput medusae, lower extremity edema, ascites, splenomegaly, hemorrhoids, asterixis

ETIOLOGY

- Portal hypertension results from obstruction to portal venous outflow, and varices subsequently develop in order to decompress the hypertensive portal vein and return blood to the systemic circulation.
- Varices may appear when portal vein pressures rise above 10-12 mm Hg.
- Cirrhosis is the most common cause of portal hypertension.

DIAGNOSIS

DIFFERENTIAL DIAGNOSIS

- Budd-Chiari syndrome, cirrhosis, portal vein thrombosis, schistosomiasis, Wilson's disease
- Other causes of upper GI bleeding: duodenal or gastric ulcers, gastric cancer, Mallory-Weiss tear

WORKUP

Upper endoscopy, laboratory tests, and imaging

LABORATORY TESTS

- CBC
  - Anemia (blood loss, nutritional deficiencies, alcohol myelosuppression)
  - Thrombocytopenia (hypersplenism, alcohol myelosuppression)
- Renal function panel
  - BUN: often increased in setting of upper GI bleeding
  - Creatinine: often elevated by hypovolemia, monitor for hepatorenal syndrome
  - Sodium: dilutional hyponatremia
- Heme-positive stools
- Type and Crossmatch: in preparation for blood transfusion
- INR/PT and PTT: coagulation factors produced in liver and may be prolonged in liver disease or impairment
- Liver function tests: ALT/AST may be normal in cirrhotic patients due to longstanding fibrosis; elevated alkaline phosphatase and a direct hyperbilirubinemia may be present if cholestatic liver disease is present
- Serum albumin: severe liver disease results in hypoalbuminemia

IMAGING STUDIES

Invasive:
- Esophagogastroduodenoscopy (EGD) (upper endoscopy):
  - In all patients with cirrhosis, screen for the presence or absence of varices and determine subsequent risk for variceal hemorrhage.
  - In patients with compensated cirrhosis who do not have varices, screening is repeated every 2 to 3 years.
  - In patients with decompensated cirrhosis (ascites, hepatic encephalopathy, variceal hemorrhage, or jaundice), it is repeated every year or at the time of first decompensation.
  - Emergently performed if there is evidence of acute upper GI bleeding to diagnose and treat variceal hemorrhage.

Noninvasive:
- Esophagography with barium can diagnose esophageal varices.
- Capsule endoscopy can also diagnose esophageal varices, although sensitivity is not yet established.

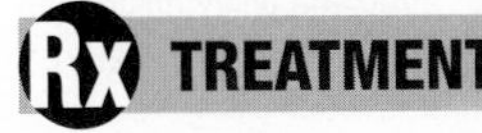

TREATMENT

NONPHARMACOLOGIC THERAPY

- Endoscopic variceal ligation (Fig. 1-380) is an alternative to nonselective beta-blockers for primary prophylaxis against variceal hemorrhage.
  - Typically for patients with medium or large varices at highest risk for hemorrhage (Child-Pugh B/C or red wale markings viewed on endoscopy)
  - Usually 2-4 sessions
  - May not be a permanent solution because varices can recur after initial eradication
  - Associated with significant complications, including hemorrhage from banding-induced ulcerations
    - Therefore should be performed by endoscopists with expertise in prophylactic banding
    - First surveillance endoscopy 1-3 months after obliteration, then every 6-12 months indefinitely

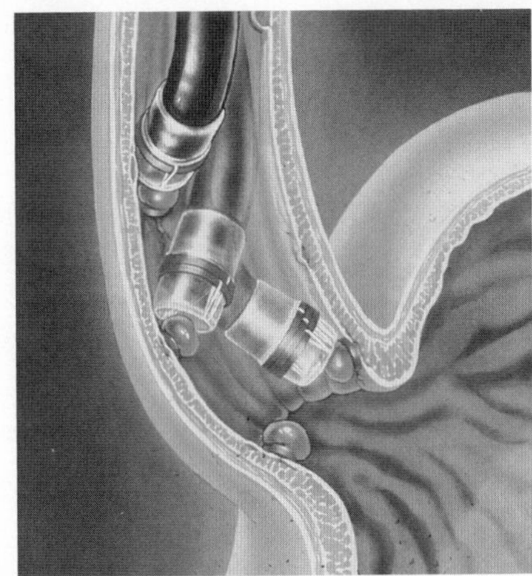

FIGURE 1-380 Esophageal varices. Endoscopic band ligation performed with a multiple-band ligating device. The endoscopist makes circumferential contact between the end of the ligating device and the varix to be ligated. Endoscopic suction draws the varix into the device, after which the elastic band is ejected to ensnare the varix. The ligated tissue sloughs after 3 to 5 days, leaving a shallow ulceration that generally heals within 1 week. (Courtesy Bard Endoscopic Technologies, Billerica, Mass.)

ACUTE GENERAL Rx

- Variceal hemorrhage: acute hemodynamic resuscitation with packed red blood cell transfusion, correct coagulopathy and thrombocytopenia, airway protection and intubation as necessary, antibiotics (ceftriaxone or norfloxacin) for SBP prophylaxis, octreotide maintained for 2-5 days in conjunction with endoscopic therapy
- EGD to treat bleeding esophageal varices by esophageal band ligation or sclerotherapy

CHRONIC Rx

Primary prophylaxis:

- Nonselective beta-blockers such as propranolol (20 mg twice daily) and nadolol (40 mg once daily)
  - Increase as tolerated for goal heart rate of approximately 55 beats/min
  - Blocks the adrenergic dilatory tone in mesenteric arterioles, resulting in unopposed alpha-adrenergic mediated vasoconstriction and therefore a decrease in portal inflow

Secondary prophylaxis:

- All patients with compensated cirrhosis who have bled from esophageal varices should receive esophageal band ligation and beta-blockers, unless beta-blockers are contraindicated.
  - Transjugular intrahepatic portosystemic shunt or surgical shunt may be performed if bleeding from esophageal varices continues or recurs despite this dual therapy.
- For patients with decompensated cirrhosis there is evidence, although limited, against the use of prophylactic beta-blockers due to the risk for increased mortality.

REFERRAL

Consultation with a gastroenterologist is recommended in all patients with cirrhosis or portal hypertension in order to screen for esophageal varices.

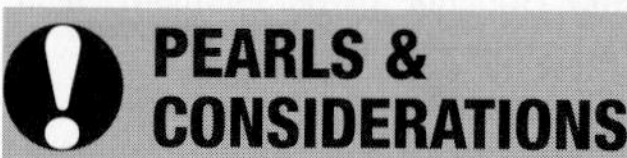

PEARLS & CONSIDERATIONS

Besides variceal size, risk factors for variceal hemorrhage include Child-Pugh class B/C or variceal red wale markings on endoscopy.

PREVENTION

Treatment of the underling liver disease may help to prevent variceal development. However, treatment with nonselective beta-blockers is not recommended because they do not prevent the development of varices.

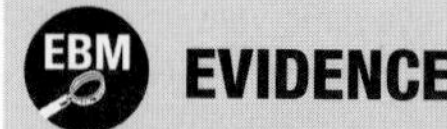

EVIDENCE

available at www.expertconsult.com

SUGGESTED READINGS

available at www.expertconsult.com

RELATED CONTENT

Cirrhosis (Related Key Topic)
Portal Hypertension (Related Key Topic)

AUTHOR: **ADAM J. WEINBERG, M.D.**

BASIC INFORMATION

DEFINITION

A predominantly postural and action tremor that is bilateral and tends to progress slowly over the years in the absence of other neurologic abnormalities.

SYNONYMS

Benign essential tremor
Familial tremor

ICD-9CM CODES
333.1 Essential tremor
ICD-10CM CODES
G25.0 Essential tremor

EPIDEMIOLOGY & DEMOGRAPHICS

Predominant Age: Can begin at any age, but incidence increases after age 40 yr. Prevalence is 6% to 9% for those >60 yr.
Genetics: No gender or racial predominance.

PHYSICAL FINDINGS & CLINICAL PRESENTATION

- Patients complain of tremor that is most bothersome when writing or holding something such as a newspaper or trying to drink from a cup. Worsens under emotional distress.
- Tremor, 4 to 12 Hz, bilateral postural and action tremor of the upper extremities. May also affect the head, voice, trunk, and legs. Typically it is the same amplitude throughout the action, such as bringing a cup to the mouth. No other neurologic abnormalities on examination except difficulty with tandem gait. Patients often note improvement with intake of small amounts of alcohol.

ETIOLOGY

Often an inherited disease, autosomal dominant; sporadic cases without a family history are frequently encountered

DIAGNOSIS

DIFFERENTIAL DIAGNOSIS (see Table 1-188)

- Parkinson's disease—tremor is usually asymmetric, especially early on in the disease, and is predominantly a resting tremor. Patients with Parkinson's disease will often also have increased tone, decreased facial expression, slowness of movement, and shuffling gait.
- Cerebellar tremor—an intention tremor that increases at the end of a goal-directed movement (such as finger to nose testing). Other associated neurologic abnormalities include ataxia, dysarthria, and difficulty with tandem gait.
- Drug-induced—there are many drugs that enhance normal, physiologic tremor. These include caffeine, nicotine, lithium, levothyroxine, β-adrenergic bronchodilators, amiodarone, valproate, and SSRIs.
- Wilson's disease—wing-beating tremor that is most pronounced with shoulders abducted, elbows flexed, and fingers pointing towards each other. Usually there are other neurologic abnormalities including dysarthria, dystonia, and Kayser-Fleischer rings on ophthalmologic examination.
- Physiologic tremor

WORKUP

- Essential tremor is a clinical diagnosis
- All imaging studies (MRI, CT) are unnecessary unless there are other associated neurologic abnormalities
- Obtain TSH (rule out hyperthyroidism)
- In patients younger than 40 yrs with other neurologic abnormalities, send ceruloplasmin, serum Cu, 24-hr urine Cu to rule out Wilson's disease

TREATMENT

Treat essential tremor when it is functionally impairing. Treatments are up to 75% effective.

NONPHARMACOLOGIC THERAPY

- Stress management
- Minimize use of caffeine if consumption is correlated with worsened symptoms.
- Small quantities of alcohol at social functions may be beneficial.

ACUTE GENERAL Rx

Propanolol (20 to 40 mg) may be used in preparation for specific event.

CHRONIC Rx

First-line agents:

- Propranolol/Propranolol LA: Usual starting dose is 30 mg. The usual therapeutic dose is 160 to 320 mg. Although not contraindicated, they must be used with caution in those with asthma, depression, cardiac disease, and diabetes.
- Primidone: Usual starting dose is 12.5 to 25 mg qhs. Usual therapeutic dose is between 62.5 and 750 mg daily (assuming side effects are tolerated). Sedation and nausea are common at treatment initiation.
- Topiramate: 25 mg qhs, may titrate up to about 400 mg

Other agents:

- Gabapentin: 400 mg qhs, usual therapeutic dose is 1200 to 3600 mg
- Alprazolam: 0.75 to 2.75 mg
- Botulinum toxin injected focally may decrease tremor
- Atenonol, sotalol

SURGICAL Rx

Thalamic deep brain stimulation (or possibly thalamotomy) contralateral to side of tremor is reserved for resistant tremor or for patients who do not tolerate drug therapy.

DISPOSITION

Patients should be reassured that the condition is not associated with other neurologic disabilities; however, it can become quite functionally disabling over time.

REFERRAL

This is a condition that usually can be treated by the primary care physician; however, if patient fails first-line therapies then patient should be referred to specialists for other drug trials and other possible surgical options.

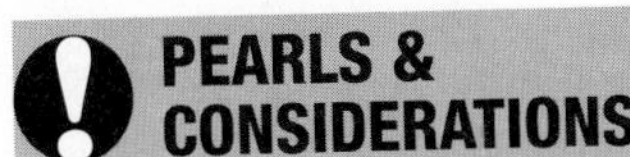

PEARLS & CONSIDERATIONS

- Essential tremor is the most common of all movement disorders.
- In addition to motor dysfunction, essential tremor can cause significant psychological impact on patients in social situations.

SUGGESTED READINGS

available at www.expertconsult.com

RELATED CONTENT

Essential Tremor (Patient Information)

AUTHOR: **U. SHIVRAJ SOHUR, M.D., PH.D.**

TABLE 1-188 Overlapping Features of Various Types of Tremor

Feature	Parkinson's Syndrome	Cerebellar Tremor	Essential Tremor
Present at rest	Yes	No	Yes
Increased tone	Yes	No	No
Decreased tone	No	Yes	No
Postural abnormality	Yes	Yes	No
Head involvement	Yes	Yes	Yes
Intentional component	No	Yes	Yes
Incoordination	No	Yes	No

From Remmel KS et al: *Handbook of symptom-oriented neurology,* ed 3, St Louis, 2002, Mosby.

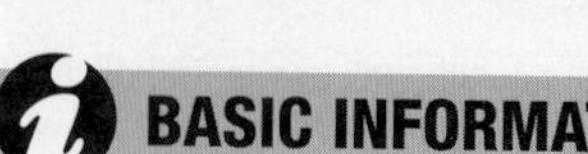

BASIC INFORMATION

DEFINITION

Factitious physical disorder occurs when an individual falsifies physical or psychological signs or symptoms or induces injury or disease with identified deception. The individual presents himself or herself to others as ill, impaired, or injured. The individual may create signs or symptoms by (1) lying, (2) simulating (e.g., putting drops of blood into a urine sample), or (3) actually creating disease (e.g., injecting bacteria or medications). The primary aim is to achieve the patient role, and the behavior persists even in the absence of apparent external rewards. The individual may seek invasive diagnostic testing, surgery, or treatment. Munchausen's syndrome is the most severe variant of factitious physical disorder and is characterized by exaggerated lying (pseudologia fantastica), sociopathy, geographic wandering from hospital to hospital, and a continuous life of patienthood.

SYNONYMS

Factitious disorder
Munchausen's syndrome (the most severe variant of factitious disorder)
Munchausen by proxy (factitious disorder created in another person, usually a child)
Deliberate disability
Hospital addiction syndrome
Artifactual illness
Peregrinating problem patients
Dermatitis artefacta
Surreptitious illness

ICD-9CM and DSM-5 CODES
300.19
ICD-10CM CODES
F68.10 Intentional production or feigning of symptoms or disabilities, either physical or psychological (factitious disorder)

EPIDEMIOLOGY & DEMOGRAPHICS

INCIDENCE (IN U.S.): Unknown
PEAK INCIDENCE: 30 to 40 yr
PREVALENCE (IN U.S.): Unknown but considerable in specific illnesses. For example, 3.3% of patients with fever of unknown origin have a factitious disorder.
PREDOMINANT SEX: Male/female ratio of 2:1 for Munchausen's syndrome but 1:2 for individuals with non-Munchausen type of factitious physical disorder.
PREDOMINANT AGE: 30 to 40 yr
GENETICS: No genetic predisposition known

PHYSICAL FINDINGS & CLINICAL PRESENTATION

- False complaints or self-inflicted injury or symptoms without clear secondary gain. The intentional aspect of the disorder is often evident, such as injecting bacteria to produce infection or taking medication to produce an abnormality.
- Presentation may be acute and dramatic, but the condition can be a chronic, recurring problem.
- Workup is usually negative for naturally occurring organic etiology.
- Clinical picture is atypical for the natural history of disease (e.g., an infection that does not respond to multiple courses of appropriate antibiotics).

ETIOLOGY

- A history of significant childhood illness; physical or sexual abuse are thought to predispose.
- Personality disorders and psychodynamic factors often play a significant role.

DIAGNOSIS

The diagnosis can be made by (1) direct observation of fabrication, (2) the presence of signs or symptoms that contradict laboratory testing, (3) nonphysiologic response to treatment, (4) the presence of physical evidence of fabrication (e.g., syringes at the bedside), and (5) recurrent patterns of illness exacerbation (e.g., just before discharge) or failure to follow the natural history of disease (e.g., a wound that does not heal for no apparent reason).

DIFFERENTIAL DIAGNOSIS

- Malingering: falsifying an illness for a clear secondary gain (e.g., financial gain or avoidance of unwanted duties).
- Somatoform disorders or hypochondriasis: these disorders are produced unconsciously and are not intentionally produced.
- Self-injurious behavior is common in many other psychiatric conditions; in those conditions the patients confess the intentional self-harm and describe motivating factors. The main intent is the self-harm and not to attain the patient role, as occurs in factitious disorder.
- May also present as Munchausen by proxy, in which a mother (86% of time) or other caregiver induces illness in a child (52% between ages of 3 and 13 yr) for the purpose of obtaining medical attention or some other psychological need. Mothers often have a history of somatoform, factitious, or personality disorder themselves.

WORKUP

- Dictated by the presenting complaints.
- No specific tests for Munchausen's syndrome.
- Diagnosis may be made when the patient is caught in the act of lying or inducing an injury. The diagnosis often rests on organic workup failing to reveal a plausible natural organic disease. The failure of usual, or even extensive, treatment to ameliorate a condition is an important clue.

LABORATORY TESTS

- Laboratory testing often reveals inconsistencies.
- Other laboratory abnormalities may reflect the underlying factitious behavior (e.g., hypokalemia in an individual surreptitiously taking furosemide).

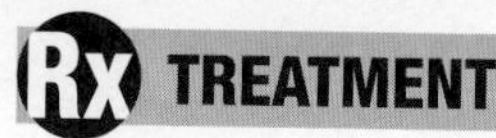

TREATMENT

NONPHARMACOLOGIC THERAPY

Two major approaches:

- Nonpunitive confrontation. Primary physician and psychiatrist conjointly meet with patient and say, "You must be in a lot of distress to be harming yourself as we believe you have been. We would like to help you deal with your distress more adaptively and get you into psychiatric treatment."
- Avoid overt confrontation with patient but provide him or her with a face-saving way to recover. For example, a therapeutic double bind would involve saying, "There are two possibilities here, one is that you have a medical problem that should respond to the next intervention we do, or two, you have a factitious disorder. The outcome will give us the answer."
- Munchausen's syndrome is the most severe variant and may be virtually impossible to treat except to avoid further invasive and iatrogenic disease.

ACUTE GENERAL Rx

Treatment of comorbid psychiatric disorders may be helpful. Treatment with antidepressants or psychotherapy may ameliorate the factitious behavior. Multidisciplinary staff meetings are useful to ventilate feelings and develop cohesive treatment plans.

DISPOSITION

- After being confronted with their behavior, patients may cease factitious behavior, but they more commonly seek other physicians or hospitals, as in the Munchausen variant. Other factitious disorder patients may enter psychotherapy, particularly when they have been given a face-saving approach with avoidance of a humiliating confrontation.
- Extensive medical workups and exploratory surgery are frequent.

REFERRAL

Always obtain psychiatric referral. Risk management attorneys and hospital ethicists may contribute to challenging decision making in these patients.

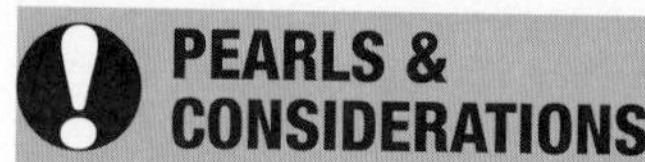

PEARLS & CONSIDERATIONS

Think of factitious disorders whenever there is an unexplained medical course that continues to repeat despite appropriate treatment, particularly in patients associated with the health care field. There is current consideration of whether factitious disorders should be classified in the upcoming DSM-5 as a subset of somatoform disorders. This possibility is related to the challenge of discriminating whether an illness state is being consciously (factitious) or unconsciously (somatoform) produced. Future research will investigate the utility of this possible change in classification.

SUGGESTED READINGS
available at www.expertconsult.com

RELATED CONTENT
Hypochondriasis (Related Key Topic)

AUTHOR: **STUART J. EISENDRATH, M.D.**

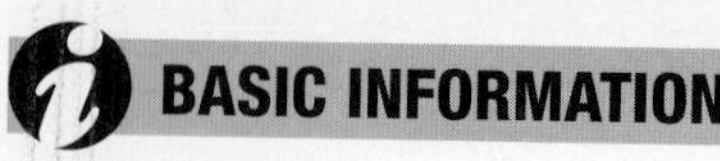

BASIC INFORMATION

DEFINITION

Failure to thrive (FTT) describes a delay in growth and development among children. FTT is a cluster of symptoms rather than a specific disease.

SYNONYMS

Pediatric undernutrition
Faltering growth
Weight faltering
Growth failure

ICD-9CM CODES
263.0 Malnutrition of moderate degree
263.1 Malnutrition of mild degree
263.2 Arrested development following protein-calorie malnutrition
263.8 Other protein-calorie malnutrition
263.9 Unspecified protein-calorie malnutrition
779.34 Failure to thrive in newborn
783.2 Abnormal loss of weight and underweight
783.21 Loss of weight
783.22 Underweight
783.4 Lack of expected normal physiologic development in childhood
783.40 Unspecified lack of normal physiologic development
783.41 Failure to thrive
783.43 Short stature
ICD-10CM CODES
R62.51 Failure to thrive (child)

EPIDEMIOLOGY & DEMOGRAPHICS

INCIDENCE: FTT is a common problem, though its incidence in the community is unclear. A total of 1% to 5% of inpatient pediatric admissions are for evaluation of FTT.
PREDOMINANT SEX AND AGE: FTT most commonly occurs among children ages 6 to 12 months, with 80% presenting before 18 months of age. Most FTT patients present before 3 years of age. Males and females are equally affected.
RISK FACTORS: Poverty is the single greatest risk factor. Nonmedical: poverty, food insecurity, social isolation, neglect, and physical or emotional abuse. Medical: Intrauterine growth restriction (IUGR), prematurity, medical conditions leading to inadequate food intake, food malabsorption, or increased metabolic demand.

PHYSICAL FINDINGS & CLINICAL PRESENTATION

Children have blunted growth in height, weight, head circumference, or any combination of these. Children may have pallid, dry, or cracked skin, sparse hair growth, poorly developed musculature, lack of subcutaneous fat, swollen abdomen, or evidence of vitamin deficiencies.

ETIOLOGY

FTT is the result of inadequate nutrition, which may be due to a wide range of medical or psychosocial causes. FTT can be thought of as stemming from inadequate nutritional intake, malabsorption of nutrients, or increased caloric expenditure, though the actual cause is commonly multifactorial.

Dx DIAGNOSIS

DIFFERENTIAL DIAGNOSIS

- Inadequate nutritional intake: food insecurity, poor parent knowledge of child's needs, formula dilution, excessive juice, breastfeeding difficulties, neglect, behavioral feeding problem, oromotor dysfunction, developmental delay, emesis, gastroesophageal reflux, volvulus, increased intracranial pressure, genetic disease (trisomy 13, 18, 21), and psychiatric conditions
- Malabsorption: cystic fibrosis, celiac disease, food protein insensitivity or intolerance, and inflammatory bowel disease
- Increased metabolic demand: insulin resistance, congenital infection, other infection, genetic syndrome, hyperthyroidism, chronic disease, and malignancy

WORKUP

- Evaluation should include the child's eating habits, caloric intake, parent-child interactions, psychosocial history, and review of systems.
- Height, weight, and weight-to-length measurements are most sensitive, whereas head circumference and body mass index (BMI) may be useful. Common FTT criteria for children younger than 2 years are below, but clinical judgment should be used because normal causes and biologic variants may exist.
  - Length, weight, or BMI below the 3rd or 5th percentile on more than one consecutive visit
  - Weight that drops below two major percentile lines
  - Weight less than 80% of the ideal weight for age
  - Weight-to-length below the 5th percentile or weight-for-length less than 70% to 79% of the median
  - Weight velocity below the 3rd or 5th percentile
  - Weight less than 70% of the 50th percentile; may require hospitalization
- Obtain caliper measurements of skinfold thickness and midarm muscle circumference.
- Observation of a meal being taken to assess potential feeding difficulties.
- A 3-day food diary is helpful, as well as consultation by a nutritionist, to calculate the child's intake of energy, protein, vitamins, and minerals.
- Assess stool frequency, consistency, quantity, as well as fat, blood, or mucus content.
- Routine hospitalization for FTT evaluation is not recommended. Rarely, hospitalization for observed feedings and further workup is warranted.

LABORATORY TESTS

- Laboratory tests have limited utility in screening for FTT unless a specific underlying medical cause is suspected.
- Consider CBC with red blood cell indices, complete chemistry panel, celiac screening, stool examination for fats or reducing substances, or sweat chloride testing. If clinically indicated, thyroid function and growth hormone level can be checked.

IMAGING STUDIES

Imaging tests are not routinely performed but may be warranted depending on underlying medical cause.

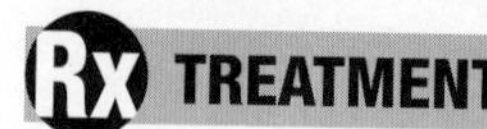

TREATMENT

Identification and management of underlying causes should be implemented. In cases in which there is no underlying medical condition, providing nutrition repletion will, by definition, correct FTT. A multidisciplinary team (including, but not limited to, social workers, occupational/speech therapists, nutritionists/dietitians, nurses, advanced practice nurses, and pediatricians) should be used.

NONPHARMACOLOGIC THERAPY

- Add calorie-dense foods or increase the number of feedings.
- Enteral feeding, percutaneous endoscopic gastrostomy (PEG), and nasogastric feeding tubes can be used to accelerate weight gain, and results should be seen within 2 to 7 days. Caloric intake should be titrated up to goal over 5 to 7 days. Caloric goals by age group: 0 to 6 months: 108 kcal/kg/day, 6 to 12 months: 98 kcal/kg/day, and 1 to 3 years: 102 kcal/kg/day.
- Swift restoration of nutrition can lead to life-threatening refeeding syndrome, where shifts in electrolyte balance (low phosphate, magnesium, potassium), fluid balance (edema), hypoglycemia, and impaired heart function can occur. Calories must therefore be titrated slowly to goal with close monitoring.
- Treat underlying medical conditions, including mental health disorders.
- Assist with family psychosocial stressors.
- Follow up closely, including home nursing visits.
- In cases where economic, psychosocial, or parental issues are suspected and the child's growth is not maintained, state and federal legislation regarding reporting to child protection services must be followed.

ACUTE GENERAL Rx

Multivitamins including iron and zinc

CHRONIC Rx

Nutrient repletion with the goal of accelerated growth should be continued for 4 to 9 months

DISPOSITION

Children with FTT commonly remain small in height and weight. Studies consistently find that children with FTT are more prone to long-term cognitive, learning, and behavioral abnormalities.

REFERRAL

- Indicated based on the cause of FTT
- Hospitalization should be considered in cases of FTT in which a child is less than 70% of predicted weight for length, where outpatient management has failed, when a suspicion of abuse or neglect exists, where signs of traumatic injury are present, or where serious impairment of the child's caregiver is evident.

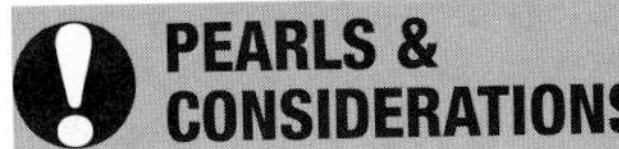

PEARLS & CONSIDERATIONS

COMMENTS

- FTT is a common childhood symptom encountered in the outpatient and inpatient pediatric populations, is caused by undernutrition, and is associated with inadequate nutritional intake, malabsorption, or increased metabolic demand.
- A thorough multidisciplinary approach to assessment, diagnosis, and management should be used to manage nutrient status and any underlying cause(s).
- Child height/length, weight, and weight-for-length measurements with comparison to standard growth curves are useful in the identification of potential cases of FTT.
- FTT treatment should include restoration of nutrition along with treatment of the underlying cause(s), including psychosocial factors.
- Although FTT can usually be managed effectively in the outpatient setting, specific indications for inpatient treatment should be considered.

PREVENTION

Nutritional counseling and anticipatory guidance should be provided at each well-child visit. Enlist dietitians and visiting nurses to provide support to families with children at high risk of FTT.

SUGGESTED READINGS

available at www.expertconsult.com

AUTHOR: **GRAYSON W. ARMSTRONG, B.A.**

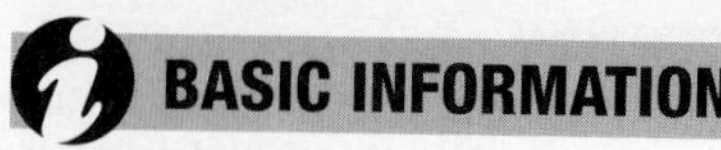

BASIC INFORMATION

DEFINITION

A fall is an "event which results in a person coming to rest inadvertently on the ground and other than a consequence of the following: loss of consciousness, sudden onset of paralysis, or epileptic seizure" (Kellogg International Work Group, *Danish Medical Bulletin,* 34, 1-24).

SYNONYMS

Syncope
Collapse

ICD-9CM CODES
Accidental fall (E880-E888.9)
ICD-10CM CODES
E880-E888.9 Accidental fall

EPIDEMIOLOGY & DEMOGRAPHICS

INCIDENCE:

- Trauma is the fifth leading cause of death in persons older than 65 years of age, and falls are responsible for 70% of accidental deaths in persons 75 years of age and older.
- The incidence of falls among community-dwelling older adults is 30% to 40%. Two thirds of falls in the community are preventable; 6% to 7% of these falls result in fracture.
- The incidence of falls for nursing home and hospitalized older adults is three times the rate of community-dwelling older adults. Over 50% of nursing home residents fall during their stay.
- 20% to 30% of older adults who fall suffer significant injury leading to immobility, dependence, and an increased risk of early death.

PREDOMINANT SEX & AGE:

- Fall-related mortality is highest among older white men followed by white women, black men, and black women.
- The incidence rates of falls increase with advancing age.
- Older adults aged 85 years and over are 10 to 15 times more likely to have a fracture compared with those aged 60 to 65 years.

RISK FACTORS: Three groups of risk factors for falls have been identified (Table 1-189):

1. Intrinsic factors inherent in the older adult who falls
2. Extrinsic factors circumstantial to the older adult who falls
3. Falls in nursing homes
4. Situational or the activity in which the older adult is engaged in when a fall occurs

TABLE 1-189 Risk Factors for Falls in the Elderly

Intrinsic
Aging
Age-related decline in vestibular function might lead to loss of balance, dizziness, and falls. Aging of the vision system (e.g., glaucoma, cataracts, retinopathy) may result in decreased visual acuity, inability to discriminate dark/light, and decreased spatial perception.
Cardiac
Cardiac arrhythmias, carotid sinus hypersensitivity, neurocardiogenic syncope
Neurologic
Parkinson's disease, normal pressure hydrocephalus (NPH), sensory neuropathy, dementia/impaired cognition, cervical myelopathy, senile gait disorder, prior stroke (One third of the elderly have abnormal position sense.)
Musculoskeletal
Lower extremity weakness, impaired knee extension and ankle plantar flexion strength contribute to abnormalities in gait velocity and step length, deconditioning, arthritis, foot abnormalities (such as bunions, calluses, or nail abnormalities)
Vascular
Vertebrobasilar insufficiency, postural hypotension, postprandial hypotension
Metabolic
Hypoglycemia, hypothyroidism, hyponatremia
Psychiatric
Depression
Medications
Use of more than four medications may be associated with an increased risk of falls. Medications that may increase fall risk include benzodiazepines, sleeping medications, neuroleptics, antidepressants, anticonvulsants, class I antiarrhythmics, and antihypertensives (Rao, 2005).
Extrinsic
Environmental
Environmental hazards cause more than 50% of falls in the elderly (cords, furniture, small objects, ill-fitting shoes, slippery surfaces, loose rugs, uneven steps, optical patterns on escalators). Majority occurs with mild-moderate activity (walking, stepping up/down, changing position); 70% occur at home and 10% on stairs (descending > ascending).
Nursing Home Falls
20% have a cardiovascular cause (hypotension: drug induced, postprandial, postural, or bradycardia) 5% are the result of an acute illness such as PNA, febrile illness, UTI, CHF 3% are from an overwhelming intrinsic event such as syncope, seizure, stroke, psychoactive drugs
Situational
Tripping over obstacles, carrying heavy items, descending/ascending stairs, rapid turning, reaching overhead, climbing ladders

CLINICAL PRESENTATION

- Older adults who fall may present with minor soft tissue injuries, such as lacerations or bruising, hip fracture, or head trauma; however, most falls are not reported unless an injury has occurred.
- If an older adult presents for medical attention for a fall or reports recurrent falls in the past year or difficulties in walking or balance, a multifactorial fall risk assessment should be completed.
- The multifactorial fall risk assessment should include:
  - Focused history: A detailed history of events and circumstances surrounding fall, relevant risk factors including review of medications, acute and chronic medical problems (e.g., osteoporosis, urinary incontinence, and cardiovascular disease), and whether the fall was witnessed
  - Physical examination
    - Vital signs including orthostatics
    - Cardiovascular examination assessing for arrhythmias, carotid bruits, or new murmurs
    - Neurologic examination including vision assessment, evaluation of lower extremity strength, peripheral nerves, proprioception, and testing of cortical, extrapyradmidal, and cerebellar function
    - Gait and balance assessment: "Get up and go test" is a rapid assessment that will quickly tell you if the patient needs rehabilitation and what to work on. (Ask patient to stand from a seated position without use of hands, walk 10 feet forward, turn around, and return to chair and sit.)
    - Musculoskeletal exam with attention to joints of lower extremity, feet and footwear.
  - Functional assessment including the older adult's activities of daily living skills, use of adaptive equipment, and fear of falling
  - Environmental assessment of home safety

ETIOLOGY

- Falls are a multifactorial syndrome resulting from the cumulative effects of impaired gait and balance, aging, polypharmacy, depression, cognitive impairment, acute medical illness, or environmental factors (Fig. E1-381).
- Most falls among community-dwelling older adults are due to environmental factors, whereas falls among nursing home residents are a result of confusion, gait impairment, or postural hypotension.

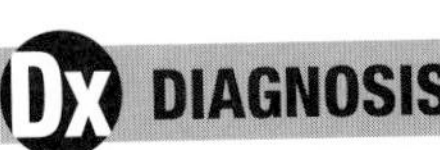

DIAGNOSIS

DIFFERENTIAL DIAGNOSIS

Falls are often a nonspecific symptom of an acute illness (such as delirium, urinary tract infection, acute anemia, or pneumonia) or an exacerbation of a chronic disease (chronic heart failure [CHF] or chronic obstructive pulmonary disease [COPD]). The mnemonic "DELIRIUMS" can be used to assess the differential diagnosis in acute delirium. (**D**rugs, **E**motional [depression], **L**ow PaO_2 [CHF, COPD], **I**nfection, **R**etention [urinary, fecal], **I**ctal status, **U**nder nutrition/hydration, **M**etabolic, **S**ubdural/Sensory [all neurologic causes] workup).

WORKUP

- Older adults presenting with a noninjurious fall need a detailed history and physical exam to identify acute medical illnesses and potential modifiable risk factors. Laboratory and neuroimaging studies may be necessary if the history and physical exam indicate a specific problem. ECG and Holter monitoring may be considered if cardiac arrhythmia is suspected.
- See Fig. E1-381.

LABORATORY TESTS

CBC, stool guaiac, blood chemistries, thyroid function, liver function, vitamin B_{12} level, folate level, erythrocyte sedimentation rate, vitamin D level, drug levels, and urinalysis depending on physical/historical findings

IMAGING STUDIES

- CT or MRI of the brain or cervical spine films in the presence of neurologic or gait impairment.
- Chest x-ray if pulmonary pathology (pneumonia, pulmonary edema) is suspected
- Consider ECG, echocardiography, or Holter monitor if suspicious for structural cardiac abnormality or syncope.

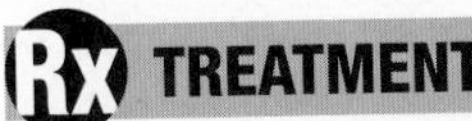

TREATMENT

NONPHARMACOLOGIC THERAPY

- Physical therapy evaluation for gait and balance training, evaluation of appropriate assisted devices (e.g., cane, walker), the use of fall prevention equipment (e.g., low beds, bed alarms).
- Home safety assessment: studies show that 50% of recurrent fallers fell doing the same activity that caused them to fall the first time. This can be prevented by creating a home safety evaluation checklist (preferably done by family member to improve compliance) or arranging for a home safety inspection by a visiting nurse or occupational therapist.
- Minimization or discontinuation of certain medications associated with falls (psychotropics)
- Customized exercise program to improve strength, gait, and balance
- Evaluation of proper footwear, hard sole, and low heel height

ACUTE GENERAL Rx

Hospitalization may be necessary for treatment of hip fracture, subdural hematoma, lacerations, or trauma as well as the treatment of underlying cause of the fall such as infection, metabolic disturbances, cardiovascular (e.g., carotid sinus hypersensitivity, vasovagal syndrome, bradyarrhythmias, and tachyarrhythmias) or neurologic abnormality.

CHRONIC Rx

- Screen and treat for osteoporosis as low bone density increases the risk of hip or other fractures.
- Optimize treatment of chronic illnesses such as CHF, COPD, osteoarthritis, Parkinson's disease, dementia, postural hypotension, and visual problems.
- Vitamin D supplementation of at least 800 IU per day. Epidemiological studies reveal that compared to usual care, short-term intervention with oral nutritional supplementation and dietetic counseling significantly decrease falls in malnourished older adults.

COMPLEMENTARY & ALTERNATIVE MEDICINE

T'ai chi has been shown to reduce the risk of falls in community-dwelling study participants.

DISPOSITION

Falls increase the older adult's risk of hospitalization, institutionalization, and mortality.

REFERRAL

- Referral may be appropriate to cardiologist, ophthalmologist, neurologist, or podiatrist depending on the presence of a specific condition.
- Consider referral to physical therapist for gait and balance training, evaluation for assisted device, or strengthening program.

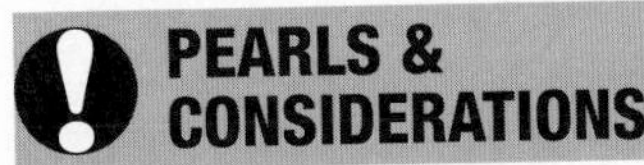

PEARLS & CONSIDERATIONS

COMMENTS

- Fear of falling may lead to restriction of activities, social isolation, and dependence.
- Older adults with four or more risk factors have a 78% chance of falling.
- Mortality from falls has increased by 42% over the past decade.

PREVENTION

The U.S. Preventive Services Task Force recommends exercise or physical therapy and vitamin D supplementation to prevent falls in community-dwelling adults aged 65 or older who are at increased risk for falls. It does not recommend automatically performing an in-depth multifactorial risk assessment in conjunction with comprehensive management of identified risks to prevent falls in community-dwelling adults aged 65 or older because the likelihood of benefit is small. In determining whether this service is appropriate in individual cases, patients and clinicians should consider the balance of benefits and harms on the basis of the circumstances of prior falls, comorbid medical conditions, and patient values.

SCREENING

The "get up and go test" is a quick assessment of balance and gait. A more in-depth screening tool for falls is the Tinetti gait and balance assessment, which evaluates normal and adaptive ability to maintain balance when arising from a chair, standing with eyes closed, turning, and receiving a sternal nudge. It also evaluates several components of gait (step height, postural sway, path deviation). The test is scored on the patient's ability to perform specific tasks. Scoring is done on a 3-point scale with a range of 0 to 2. Individual scores are combined to form three measures: an overall gait assessment score (maximum score = 12), an overall balance assessment score (maximum score = 16), and a gait and balance score (maximum score = 28). In general, patients who score below 19 are at high risk for falls, and those who score 19-24 are at risk for falls.

PATIENT/FAMILY EDUCATION

Providing education and information for the patient and caregiver regarding fall prevention strategies in addition to multifactorial risk reduction strategies

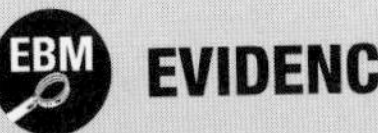

EVIDENCE

available at www.expertconsult.com

SUGGESTED READINGS

available at www.expertconsult.com

AUTHORS: **SEAN H. UITERWYK, M.D., ALICIA J. CURTIN, PH.D., G.N.P.,** and **KEITH BRENNAN, M.D.**

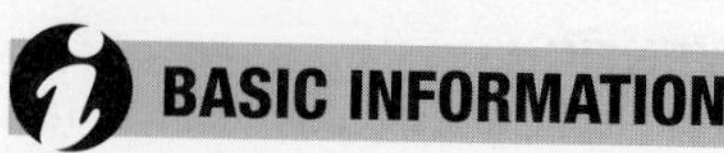

BASIC INFORMATION

DEFINITION

Acute fatty liver of pregnancy (AFLP) is characterized histologically by microvesicular fatty cytoplasmic infiltration of hepatocytes with minimal hepatocellular necrosis.

SYNONYMS

Acute fatty metamorphosis
Acute yellow atrophy

ICD-9CM CODES
646.7 Liver disorders in pregnancy
ICD-10CM CODES
O26.619 Liver and biliary tract disorders in pregnancy, unspecified trimester

EPIDEMIOLOGY & DEMOGRAPHICS

INCIDENCE:
- Approximately one in 10,000 pregnancies
- Equal frequencies in all races and at all maternal ages

AVERAGE GESTATIONAL AGE: 37 wk (range 28 to 42 wk)

RISK FACTORS:
- Primiparity
- Multiple gestation
- Male fetus

GENETICS: Some with a familial deficiency of long-chain 3-hydroxyacyl-coenzyme A dehydrogenase (LCHAD)

PHYSICAL FINDINGS & CLINICAL PRESENTATION

- Initial manifestations:
  1. Nausea and vomiting (70%)
  2. Pain in right upper quadrant or epigastrium (50% to 80%)
  3. Malaise and anorexia
- Jaundice often in 1 to 2 wk
- Late manifestations:
  1. Fulminant hepatic failure
  2. Encephalopathy
  3. Renal failure
  4. Pancreatitis
  5. Gastrointestinal and uterine bleeding
  6. Disseminated intravascular coagulation
  7. Seizures
  8. Coma
- Liver:
  1. Usually small
  2. Normal or enlarged in preeclampsia, eclampsia, HELLP syndrome (hemolysis, elevated liver enzymes, and low platelets), and acute hepatitis
  3. Coexistent preeclampsia in up to 46% of patients

ETIOLOGY

- Postulated that inhibition of mitochondrial oxidation of fatty acids may lead to microvesicular fatty infiltration of liver
- Fatty metamorphosis of preeclamptic liver disease believed to be of different etiology

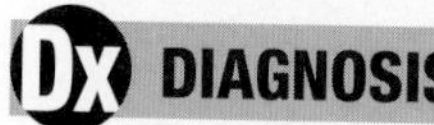

DIAGNOSIS

DIFFERENTIAL DIAGNOSIS

- Acute gastroenteritis
- Preeclampsia or eclampsia with liver involvement
- HELLP syndrome
- Acute viral hepatitis
- Fulminant hepatitis
- Drug-induced hepatitis caused by halothane, phenytoin, methyldopa, isoniazid, hydrochlorothiazide, or tetracycline
- Intrahepatic cholestasis of pregnancy
- Gallbladder disease
- Reye's syndrome
- Hemolytic-uremic syndrome
- Budd-Chiari syndrome
- Systemic lupus erythematosus

WORKUP

- A clinical diagnosis is based predominantly on physical and laboratory findings.
- Most definitive diagnosis is through liver biopsy with oil red O staining and electron microscopy.
- Liver biopsy is reserved for atypical cases only and only after any existing coagulopathy corrected with fresh frozen plasma.

LABORATORY TESTS

Tests to determine the following:
- Hypoglycemia (often profound <60 mg/dl)
- Hyperammonemia
- Elevated aminotransferases (usually <500 U/ml)
- Thrombocytopenia
- Leukocytosis (white blood cell count >15,000)
- Hyperbilirubinemia (usually <10 mg/dl)
- Low albumin
- Hypofibrinogenemia (<300 mg/dl)
- Disseminated intravascular coagulation (DIC) (in 75%)

IMAGING STUDIES

- Ultrasound: best used to rule out other diseases in the differential diagnosis such as gallbladder disease
- CT scan: plays minimal role because of a high false-negative rate

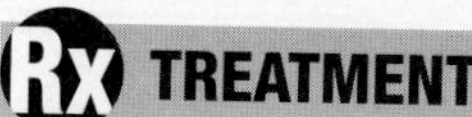

TREATMENT

NONPHARMACOLOGIC THERAPY

- Patient is admitted to intensive care unit for stabilization.
- Fetus is delivered; spontaneous resolution usually follows delivery.
- Mode of delivery is based on obstetric indications and clinical assessment of disease severity.

ACUTE GENERAL Rx

- Decrease in endogenous ammonia through dietary protein restriction; neomycin 6 to 12 g/day PO to decrease presence of ammonia-producing bacteria; magnesium citrate 30 to 50 ml PO or enema to evacuate nitrogenous wastes from colon
- Administration of IV fluids with glucose to keep glucose levels >60 mg/dl
- Coagulopathy corrected with fresh frozen plasma
- Avoidance of drugs metabolized by liver
- Aggressive avoidance and treatment for nosocomial infections; consideration of prophylactic antibiotics
- Monitor closely for development of complications such as hepatic encephalopathy, pulmonary edema, DIC, and respiratory arrest

CHRONIC Rx

Orthotopic liver transplantation is the only treatment for irreversible liver failure.

DISPOSITION

- Before 1980, both maternal and fetal mortality rates were approximately 85%
- Since 1980, both maternal and fetal mortality rates are less than 20%
- Usually rapid return of liver function to normal after delivery
- Minimal risk of recurrence with future pregnancies

REFERRAL

- To tertiary health care facility as soon as diagnosis is suspected.
- Infants of mothers with AFLP should be evaluated for LCHAD deficiency.

SUGGESTED READINGS

available at www.expertconsult.com

RELATED CONTENT

Eclampsia (Related Key Topic)
Preeclampsia (Related Key Topic)

AUTHORS: **ARUNDATHI G. PRASAD, M.D.,** and **RUBEN ALVERO, M.D.**

BASIC INFORMATION

DEFINITION

- Adverse effects of alcohol on developing human represent spectrum of structural anomalies and behavioral and neurocognitive disabilities, most accurately termed fetal alcohol spectrum disorder (FASD) (Table 1-190).
- Children at severe end of spectrum defined as having fetal alcohol syndrome (FAS).

ICD-9CM CODES
760.71 Fetal alcohol syndrome
ICD-10CM CODES
P04.3 Newborn (suspected to be) affected by maternal use of alcohol

EPIDEMIOLOGY & DEMOGRAPHICS

- Alcohol considered to be most common teratogen to which the fetus is liable to be exposed.
- 10% report drinking alcohol during pregnancy and 2% to 4% admit to binge drinking.
- Most common form of mental retardation in U.S.
- Prevalence is 1-2/1000 live births across U.S.
- Each year 40,000 babies are born with FASD.

RISK FACTORS

- Advanced maternal age (>30 yr)
- High parity
- African-American, Alaskan Natives, and Native Indian race
- Binge drinking (>4 drinks per occasion)
- History of prior affected child
- Genetic susceptibility
- Undernutrition
- Low socioeconomic group

PHYSICAL FINDINGS & CLINICAL PRESENTATION

Typical features:

- Growth retardation
  - Prenatal or postnatal
  - Height and/or weight <10%
- Facial dysmorphia
  - Smooth philtrum
  - Thin vermilion border
  - Small palpebral fissure (<10%)
  - Others: epicanthic folds, ptosis of eyelids, flat nasal bridge and midface, upturned nose, railroad track ears, and so forth
- CNS abnormalities
  - Structural
    - Head circumference, 10%
    - Clinically significant brain abnormalities observable through imaging
  - Neurologic
    - Neurologic problems not due to a postnatal insult or fever
  - Functional
    - Intellectual deficit
    - Cognitive or developmental deficits
    - Executive function deficits
    - Motor function delays
    - Problem with attention and hyperactivity
    - Social skills
    - Other problems such as sensory, pragmatic language, and memory

Rare birth defects:

- Cardiac
  - Ventricular septal defect (VSD)
  - Atrial septal defect (ASD)
  - Tetralogy of Fallot
  - Aberrant great vessels
- Skeletal
  - Radioulnar synostosis
  - Hypoplastic nails
  - Clinodactyly
  - Shortened fifth digit
  - Pectus excavatum and carinatum
  - Klippel-Feil syndrome
  - Hemivertebrae
  - Camptodactyly
  - Scoliosis
- Renal
  - Aplastic kidneys
  - Dysplastic kidneys
  - Ureteral duplication
  - Hypoplastic kidneys
  - Hydronephrosis
  - Horseshoe kidneys
- Ocular
  - Strabismus
  - Refractive problems
  - Retinal vascular abnormalities
- Auditory
  - Conductive hearing loss
  - Neurosensory hearing loss
- Others
  - Hockey stick–like palmar crease

ETIOLOGY

- Prenatal damage comes about primarily by direct action of ethanol or its metabolites (e.g., acetaldehyde) on the fetus.
- Exact damaging mechanism is unclear.
- Although the damaging effect of alcohol is different in the various phases of pregnancy, it is by no means limited to first trimester.
- No exact dose-response relationship between alcohol consumed during prenatal period and extent of damage inflicted on infant.
- An occasional drink during pregnancy carries no risk to the fetus, but no level of drinking is known to be safe during pregnancy.
- The least significant effect recognized at 2 drinks/day is smaller birth weight (160 g less than average).
- Until 4-6 drinks/day are consumed, no additional subtle clinical features are evident.
- Most children who have FAS have been born to frankly alcoholic mothers whose intake is ≥8-10 drinks/day, and those who engage in binge drinking.
- The risk of serious problem in the offspring of a chronically alcoholic woman is ~30%-50%; the greatest risk is mental retardation.

SECONDARY DISABILITIES

- Mental health problems
- Dependent living
- Employment problems
- Disruptive school problems
- Trouble with law
- Confinement
- Inappropriate sexual behavior
- Alcohol or drug problems

DIAGNOSIS

- It is a diagnosis of exclusion.
- Diagnosis is difficult prenatally and at birth. Most cases are not diagnosed until school age.

TABLE 1-190 Institute of Medicine's Diagnostic Criteria for Fetal Alcohol–Related Abnormalities

Category 1	
FAS with confirmed maternal alcohol exposure	Presence of classic triad of growth retardation, characteristic facial dysmorphology, and neurodevelopmental abnormalities. This is often defined as full-blown FAS.
Category 2	
FAS without confirmed maternal alcohol exposure	Triad in category 1 is present without confirmed maternal drinking
Category 3	
Partial FAS with confirmed maternal alcohol exposure	Presence of some of the characteristic facial anomalies plus growth retardation or CNS neurodevelopmental abnormalities or behavioral/cognitive abnormalities
Category 4	
FAS with confirmed maternal alcohol exposure and alcohol-related birth defects	Some congenital anomalies as a result of alcohol toxicity
Category 5	
FAS with confirmed maternal alcohol exposure and alcohol-related neurodevelopmental disorder	Evidence of CNS neurodevelopmental abnormalities, a complex pattern of behavioral/cognitive abnormalities, or both, but not necessarily any obvious physical changes

CNS, Central nervous system; *FAS*, fetal alcohol syndrome.

- As the characteristic facial features tend to become decreasingly recognizable as the child reaches adolescence, the diagnosis becomes increasingly difficult with advancing age.
- Prenatal exposure to alcohol is not sufficient to warrant a diagnosis. According to the CDC, diagnosis of FAS requires 3 specific findings and history of prenatal alcohol exposure:
  - Growth restriction (intrauterine or postnatal)
  - CNS involvement
  - Documentation of all three facial abnormalities (smooth philtrum, thin vermilion border, and short palpebral fissure)
- Imaging recommendation during pregnancy with alcohol exposure:
  - High-risk anatomy scan
  - Serial growth scan
  - Fetal echocardiogram at 22 to 24 weeks' intrauterine pregnancy
- Measurement of the ethyl esters of fatty acids in the meconium and hair of the newborn can substantiate maternal alcohol exposure.
- In school-aged children, the diagnostic process should include a through psychological evaluation that assesses multiple domains. Also, supplement the observation by obtaining standardized testing through early intervention programs, public schools, and psychologists in private practice.

DIFFERENTIAL DIAGNOSIS

- Other causes of symmetrical growth retardation including intrauterine infection and aneuploidy
- Aneuploidy (T21, T18, T13)
- Syndromes with overlapping features of FAS:
  - Fetal anticonvulsant syndrome
  - Maternal phenylketonuria
  - Toluene embryopathy
  - Velocardiofacial syndrome (deletion 22q11)
  - Williams syndrome
  - Dubowitz syndrome
  - Cornelia de Lange syndrome

Rx TREATMENT

- As there is no cure for FAS, we need to emphasize prevention.
- For women who are planning pregnancy or who could become pregnant, the U.S. Surgeon General recommends the safest course: to avoid alcohol entirely during pregnancy.
- Women of childbearing age who are not pregnant should drink ≤7 alcoholic drinks/wk and ≤3 drinks on any one occasion.
- Preconception counseling should be offered to women of childbearing age who are at risk for an alcohol-exposed pregnancy.
- Screen all pregnant women for alcohol use.
- The National Institute on Alcohol Abuse and Alcoholism recommends that any woman who reports drinking >7 drinks/wk or >3 drinks on a given day be further assessed for alcohol-related problems.
- The T-ACE (Table 1-191) and TWEAK (Table 1-192) questionnaires are used to identify women drinking enough to potentially damage the fetus. The CAGE questionnaire is less sensitive for screening pregnant women.
- Effective treatment alternatives for women who screen positive for hazardous alcohol use include brief interventions to promote reductions in alcohol use and that facilitate referral to specialized treatment programs.
- Discontinuation or reduction of alcohol consumption at any point in pregnancy may be beneficial.
- The use of alcohol-containing tonics and medications should be avoided. This applies to medications with an alcohol base when the concentration exceeds 10%.
- Alcoholism is one of the few situations in which pregnancy interruption may be discussed with the patient as it may result in FAS.
- Early diagnosis and appropriate treatment may decrease secondary disabilities and recurrence in future pregnancies.
- A child should be referred for full FAS evaluation when substantial prenatal alcohol use by the mother has been confirmed (>7 drinks/wk, >3 drinks on multiple occasions, or both).
- If substantial prenatal exposure is known, with no other positive criteria, the physician should document exposure and closely monitor the child's growth and development.

TABLE 1-191 T-ACE Questions*

T (tolerance)	How many drinks does it take to make you feel high? (3 or more drinks = 2 points)
A (annoyed)	Have people annoyed you by criticizing your drinking? (Yes = 1 point)
C (cut down)	Have you felt you ought to cut down on your drinking? (Yes = 1 point)
E (eye opener)	Have you ever had to drink first thing in the morning to steady your nerves or to get rid of a hangover? (Yes = 1 point)

*A score of 2 or more indicates heavy or problem drinker. Its sensitivity is 70% and specificity is 85%.

TABLE 1-192 TWEAK*

T (tolerance)	How many drinks does it take before you begin to feel the first effects of alcohol? (3 or more drinks = 2 points)
W (worried)	Have close friends or relatives worried about your drinking in the past year? (Yes = 2 points)
E (eye opener)	Do you sometimes take a drink in the morning when you first get up? (Yes = 1 point)
A (amnesia)	Has a friend or family member ever told you about things you said or did while you were drinking that you could not remember? (Yes = 1 point)
K (kut down)	Do you sometimes feel the need to cut down on your drinking? (Yes = 1 point)

*A total of 3 or more points indicates the woman is likely to be a heavy or problem drinker. Its sensitivity is 79% and specificity is 83%.

- When information about prenatal exposure is unknown, a child should be referred for full FAS if any of the following conditions are present: (1) all three dysmorphic facial features (smooth philtrum, thin vermilion border, and small palpebral fissure), (2) one or more of these facial features with growth deficit, (3) one or more facial features with one or more CNS abnormalities, (4) one or more dysmorphic facial features with growth deficit and one or more CNS abnormalities, or (5) any report of concern by a caregiver or parent that a child has or may have FAS.
- Infants and children who are diagnosed with FAS should be evaluated by a physician who is knowledgeable and competent in the evaluation of neurodevelopment and psychosocial problems associated with the diagnosis.
- A multidisciplinary team including a clinical geneticist, developmental pediatrician, mental health professional, social worker, and education specialist is often necessary for management.
- Treatment options include:
  - Medications to help with symptoms
  - Behavior and education therapy
    Friendship training
    Specialized math training
    Executive function training
    Parent-child interaction training
    Parenting and behavior management training
  - Parenting training
    Concentrate on child's strengths and talents
    Accept child's limitations
    Be consistent with everything
    Use concrete language and examples
    Use stable routine that does not change daily
    Keep everything simple
    Be specific (i.e., say exactly what you mean)
    Structure your child's world to provide a foundation for daily living
    Use visualized aids, music, and hands-on activities to help your child learn
    Use positive reinforcement often
    Supervise
    Repeat, repeat, and repeat
  - Emphasis on the following protective factors helps reduce the effects and also assists people with this condition to reach their full potential:
    Diagnosing before 6 yr
    Living in stable nurturing home environment in school years
    Absence of violence
    Involvement in special education and social services
  - Alternative approaches such as biofeedback, auditory training, relaxation therapy, visual imagery, yoga/exercise, acupuncture/acupressure, massage, Reiki, energy healing, animal-assisted therapy, and so forth may play a role.

SUGGESTED READINGS
available at www.expertconsult.com

AUTHOR: **HEMANT K. SATPATHY, M.D.**

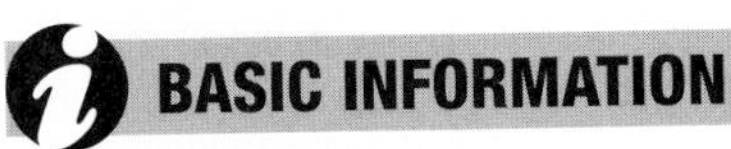

BASIC INFORMATION

DEFINITION

Fever of undetermined origin (FUO) was defined by Petersdorf and Beeson in 1961 as an illness characterized by temperatures >38.3° C (101° F) on several occasions for >3 wk with no known cause despite extensive workup.

- Persistence for >2 wk separates an FUO from an insignificant viral illness.
- Traditionally, diagnosis was made only after a 1-wk inpatient workup. In contemporary practice, much of the workup is performed as an outpatient.

Table 1-193 provides a summary of definitions and major features of subtypes of FUO.

SYNONYMS

Fever of unknown origin

ICD-9CM CODES
780.6 Pyrexia of undetermined origin
ICD-10CM CODES
R50.9 Fever, unspecified

EPIDEMIOLOGY & DEMOGRAPHICS

- The incidence of undiagnosed FUO dropped to <10% in the 1950s but has steadily increased since then.
- True FUOs are uncommon.

CLINICAL PRESENTATION

Fever 38.3° C (101° F or higher) >3 wk

ETIOLOGY

- Infection (16%)
  - Abscess: abdominal, pelvic
  - Tuberculosis
  - HIV infection
  - Nosocomial: urinary tract infection, pneumonia, line-related bacteremia, *Clostridium difficile* colitis, sinusitis
  - Bacterial endocarditis (especially caused by difficult-to-isolate organisms)
  - Biliary tract infection
  - Osteomyelitis, vertebral and mandibular
  - Less common infections: Q fever, leptospirosis, psittacosis, tularemia, secondary syphilis, gonococcemia, chronic meningococcemia, Whipple's disease, yersiniosis, fungal infections
- Malignancy (7%): lymphoma (especially non-Hodgkin's lymphoma), leukemia, renal cell carcinoma, hepatocellular carcinomas, other tumors metastatic to liver
- Noninfectious inflammatory disease (22%)
  - Adult Still's disease (young to middle-aged patients)
  - Temporal arteritis (elderly patients)
  - Other vasculitis: polyarteritis nodosa, Takayasu's arteritis, Wegener's granulomatosis, mixed cryoglobulinemia
- Other (4%)
  - Drug-induced fever
  - Inflammatory bowel disease
  - Sarcoidosis
  - Pulmonary embolism
  - Alcoholic hepatitis
- No diagnosis (51%)

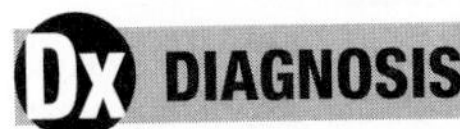

DIAGNOSIS

DIFFERENTIAL DIAGNOSIS

Factitious fever

WORKUP

- Accurate history and careful physical examination are essential. Fig. E1-382 describes an approach to the patient with FUO.
- Laboratory tests and imaging dependent on medical history clues and physical findings.
- When in doubt, perform another complete history and physical examination. Examples of subtle physical findings in patients with FUO are described in Table 1-194.

MEDICAL HISTORY CLUES

- Fever duration, tempo; inciting factors
- Rash, myalgia, weight loss, pain
- Sick contacts
- Past medical history: tuberculosis, HIV, malignancies, surgeries
- Medications

TABLE 1-193 Summary of Definitions and Major Features of the Four Subtypes of Fever of Undetermined Origin

Feature	Classic FUO	Health Care–Associated FUO	Immune-Deficient FUO	HIV-Related FUO
Definition	>38.0°C, >3 wk, >2 visits or 1 wk in hospital	≥38.0°C, >1 wk, not present or incubating on admission	≥38.0°C, >1 wk, negative cultures after 48 hr	≥38.0°C, >3 wk for outpatients, >1 wk for inpatients, HIV infection confirmed
Patient location	Community, clinic, or hospital	Acute care hospital	Hospital or clinic	Community, clinic, or hospital
Leading causes	Cancer, infections, inflammatory conditions, undiagnosed, habitual hyperthermia	Health care–associated infections, postoperative complications, drug fever	Majority due to infections, but cause documented in only 40%-60%	HIV (primary infection), typical and atypical mycobacteria, CMV, lymphomas, toxoplasmosis, cryptococcosis, immune reconstitution inflammatory syndrome (IRIS)
History emphasis	Travel, contacts, animal and insect exposure, medications, immunizations, family history, cardiac valve disorder	Operations and procedures, devices, anatomic considerations, drug treatment	Stage of chemotherapy, drugs administered, underlying immunosuppressive disorder	Drugs, exposures, risk factors, travel, contacts, stage of HIV infection
Examination emphasis	Fundi, oropharynx, temporal artery, abdomen, lymph nodes, spleen, joints, skin, nails, genitalia, rectum or prostate, lower limb deep veins	Wounds, drains, devices, sinuses, urine	Skin folds, IV sites, lungs, perianal area	Mouth, sinuses, skin, lymph nodes, eyes, lungs, perianal area
Investigation emphasis	Imaging, biopsies, sedimentation rate, skin tests	Imaging, bacterial cultures	CXR, bacterial cultures	Blood and lymphocyte count; serologic tests; CXR; stool examination; biopsies of lung, bone marrow, and liver for cultures and cytologic tests; brain imaging
Management	Observation, outpatient temperature chart, investigations, avoidance of empirical drug treatments	Depends on situation	Antimicrobial treatment protocols	Antiviral and antimicrobial protocols, vaccines, revision of treatment regimens, good nutrition
Time course of disease	Months	Weeks	Days	Weeks to months
Tempo of investigation	Weeks	Days	Hours	Days to weeks

CMV, Cytomegalovirus; *CXR,* chest radiograph; *FUO,* fever of undetermined origin.
Adapted from Mandell GL, Bennett JE, Dolin R (eds): *Mandell, Douglas, and Bennett's principles and practice of infectious diseases,* ed 7, Philadelphia, 2010, Churchill Livingstone. Borrowed from Kliegman RM et al: *Nelson textbook of pediatrics,* ed 19, Philadelphia, 2011, Saunders.

- Family history: tuberculosis, malignancies, familial Mediterranean fever
- Social history: daily routine, rural versus urban, pets and animal contacts, arthropod bites, recent and remote travel, socioeconomic status, occupation, military service, sexual history

PHYSICAL FINDINGS

- HEENT (head, ears, eyes, nose, throat): sinus tenderness, dental abscesses, funduscopic lesions
- Neck: adenopathy, palpable thyroid
- Lungs: auscultate for rales
- Heart: murmur
- Abdomen: organomegaly
- Rectal: prostate tenderness
- Pelvic: cervical motion tenderness, fundal or adnexal masses or pain; inguinal adenopathy
- Extremities: clubbing, splinter hemorrhages; tenderness or fluctuance at IV access site
- Musculoskeletal: joint effusions
- Skin: rashes, wounds

LABORATORY TESTS

- Most FUO workups include:
  - Blood cultures (three sets from different sites)
  - Complete blood count with differential
  - Erythrocyte sedimentation rate or C-reactive protein
  - Urinalysis with microscopic exam and culture
  - Transaminases
  - Serum lactate dehydrogenase
  - PPD testing
- Consider
  - HIV antibody testing
  - Creatinine phosphokinase
  - Rheumatoid factor
  - Serum protein electrophoresis
  - Lumbar puncture
  - Thyroid function testing
  - Stool culture and *C. difficile* assay
  - Biopsy (bone marrow, skin, liver lymph nodes, pleural, etc., based on clinical and laboratory findings)
  - Antinuclear antibody testing

May need to repeat tests at regular intervals until diagnosis is established.

IMAGING STUDIES

- Most workups eventually include chest radiograph and abdominal CT scan.
- Further imaging is based on medical history clues and physical findings.
- FDG-PET is very sensitive to detect anatomic sites of inflammation or malignancy. It may help to identify sites requiring further investigation. Further data are needed to evaluate efficacy.

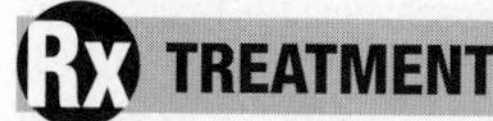

TREATMENT

ACUTE GENERAL Rx

Antibiotics and other treatment indicated only after definitive or highly probable diagnosis is established unless patient is neutropenic, severely ill, or septic.

DISPOSITION

In some cases a diagnosis is not made for years. At 5-yr follow-up, mortality rate among patients with undiagnosed FUO was only 3.2% in one study.

REFERRAL

To an infectious disease specialist, hematologist, or rheumatologist if no diagnosis after thoughtful workup

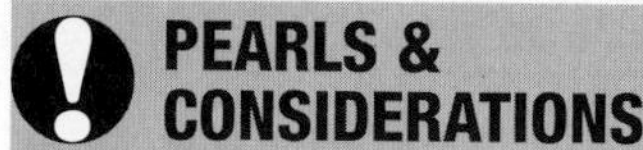

PEARLS & CONSIDERATIONS

COMMENTS

Because of improvements in imaging and laboratory tests, fewer cases of FUO are attributed to infectious causes and more are diagnosed as attributable to tumors and collagen-vascular diseases.

SUGGESTED READINGS

available at www.expertconsult.com

RELATED CONTENT

Fever of Unknown Origin (Patient Information)

AUTHOR: **ETSUKO AOKI, M.D., PH.D.**

TABLE 1-194 Examples of Subtle Physical Findings Having Special Significance in Patients with Fever of Undetermined Origin

Body Site	Physical Finding	Diagnosis
Head	Sinus tenderness	Sinusitis
Temporal artery	Nodules, reduced pulsations	Temporal arteritis
Oropharynx	Ulceration	Disseminated histoplasmosis
	Tender tooth	Periapical abscess
Fundi or conjunctivae	Choroid tubercle	Disseminated granulomatosis*
	Petechiae, Roth's spot	Endocarditis
Thyroid	Enlargement, tenderness	Thyroiditis
Heart	Murmur	Infective or marantic endocarditis
Abdomen	Enlarged iliac crest lymph nodes, splenomegaly	Lymphoma, endocarditis, disseminated granulomatosis*
Rectum	Perirectal fluctuance, tenderness	Abscess
	Prostatic tenderness, fluctuance	Abscess
Genitalia	Testicular nodule	Periarteritis nodosa
	Epididymal nodule	Disseminated granulomatosis
Lower extremities	Deep venous tenderness	Thrombosis or thrombophlebitis
Skin and nails	Petechiae, splinter hemorrhages, subcutaneous nodules, clubbing	Vasculitis, endocarditis

*Includes tuberculosis, histoplasmosis, coccidioidomycosis, sarcoidosis, and syphilis.
From Mandell GL et al (eds): *Mandell, Douglas, and Bennett's principles and practice of infectious diseases*, ed 7, Philadelphia, 2010, Churchill Livingstone.

BASIC INFORMATION

DEFINITION

Fibrocystic breast disease (FCD) is a "nondisease" that includes nonmalignant breast lesions such as microcystic and macrocystic changes, fibrosis, ductal or lobular hyperplasia, adenosis, apocrine metaplasia, fibroadenoma, papilloma, papillomatosis, and other changes. Atypical ductal or lobular hyperplasia is associated with a moderate increase in breast cancer risk.

SYNONYMS

Cystic changes
Chronic cystic mastitis
Mammary dysplasia

ICD-9CM CODES
610.0 Solitary cyst of the breast
610.1 Fibrocystic disease of the breast

ICD-10CM CODES
N60.09 Solitary cyst of unspecified breast
N60.19 Diffuse cystic mastopathy of unspecified breast

EPIDEMIOLOGY & DEMOGRAPHICS

- Ubiquitous in premenopausal women after 20 yr of age
- Palpable nodular changes in the breast termed FCD clinically; such changes observable in more than half of adult women aged 20 to 50 yr

PHYSICAL FINDINGS & CLINICAL PRESENTATION

- Tender breasts
- Nodular areas
- Dominant mass
- Thickening
- Nipple discharge
- Can vary with menstrual cycle

ETIOLOGY

- Although it is frequently seen and diagnosed, mechanism of development is not understood.
- Because it is found in the majority of healthy breasts, it is regarded as a nonpathologic process.
- With hormone replacement therapy, the condition may be carried into menopause.

Dx DIAGNOSIS

DIFFERENTIAL DIAGNOSIS

- If presenting as dominant mass or masses, exclude possible carcinoma.
- Carcinoma: detection is difficult with FCD, particularly among premenopausal women.
- If presenting with nipple discharge, differentiate from discharge of possible malignant origin.

WORKUP

- Exclude breast carcinoma if breast mass, thickening, discharge, and/or pain are present.
- Perform biopsy of suspected area for histologic confirmation.

IMAGING STUDIES

Mammography and ultrasound studies required:

- For mammographic changes (suspicious densities, microcalcifications, architectural distortion): careful evaluation, including possibly biopsy to exclude breast cancer
- Ultrasound study: to establish cystic nature of clinical or mammographic mass lesion

Rx TREATMENT

NONPHARMACOLOGIC THERAPY

- Not considered a "disease" and does not require treatment
- Surgical intervention diagnostic to eliminate possibility of breast cancer
- Periodic physician examination to monitor patients with FCD who have pronounced nodular features
- Aspiration for palpable cysts (NOTE: Cysts often recur; repeat aspiration is not always required unless pain is a problem.)

ACUTE GENERAL Rx

The majority of women require no treatment.

CHRONIC Rx

For breast pain:

- Danocrine (Danazol): limited success reported but significant side effect profile of medication
- Bromocriptine or tamoxifen: used less frequently
- Limited caffeine intake: not as successful in controlling pain or nodularity as originally suggested

DISPOSITION

- Careful evaluation to exclude suspicious changes for breast cancer, then reassurance and periodic reevaluation as required
- Regular self-examination, annual physician examination, and annual mammograms for women with atypical ductal or lobular hyperplasia

REFERRAL

- For further evaluation and/or biopsy if there are suspicious changes that may be associated with FCD (including changing of dominant mass or thickening, persistent or spontaneous discharge, suspicious mammographic changes or lesions)
- To alleviate anxiety associated with breast symptoms or changes

RELATED CONTENT

Breast Cancer (Related Key Topic)
Mastodynia (Related Key Topic)
Fibrocystic Breast Changes (Patient Information)

AUTHOR: **RUBEN ALVERO, M.D.**

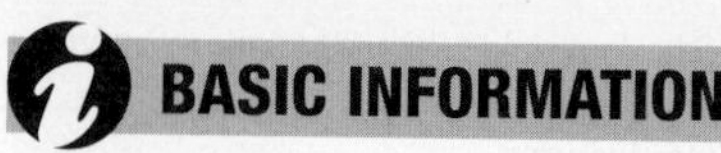

BASIC INFORMATION

DEFINITION

Fibromyalgia (FM) is a disorder of pain processing characterized by chronic, widespread pain, a lack of structural pathology, and the presence of pain augmentation. Central features also include fatigue, sleep disturbance, and tenderness. Rather than being a discrete illness, fibromyalgia is considered by many to be one phenotype of a much larger spectrum of disorders that overlap in individual patients.

ICD-9CM CODES
729.0 Rheumatism, unspecified and fibrositis
729.1 Myalgia and myositis, unspecified
ICD-10CM CODES
M79.7 Fibromyalgia

EPIDEMIOLOGY & DEMOGRAPHICS

PREVALENCE: 2% of U.S. population
PREDOMINANT SEX: Female/male ratio of 7:1
PREDOMINANT AGE: 30 to 50 years

PHYSICAL FINDINGS

Tender points (Fig. 1-383) or generalized tenderness

ETIOLOGY

- Unknown. Genetic and environmental factors predispose individuals to FM. Evidence suggests that both the ascending and descending pain pathways operate abnormally, resulting in central amplification of pain signals, analogous to the "volume control setting" being turned up too high. Familial associations of FM provide strongest evidence that reflect both these factors.
- Once predisposed, FM may be precipitated by events such as abuse, injury from motor vehicle accidents, illness including autoimmune disorders, infections, surgical procedures, and psychological stressors.
- Psychosocial and neuroendocrine factors also influence symptom expression.

PATHOGENESIS

- Augmented pain and sensory processing is a hallmark, resulting in diffuse pain, allodynia (pain brought on by normally nonpainful stimuli), and hyperalgesia (more intense and prolonged pain perception)
- Afflicted persons show altered physiologic responses to painful stimulation at spinal and supraspinal levels.
- Brain neuroimaging studies found differences in brain structure, neurochemical concentrations, and functional brain networks in FM compared with control subjects, with increased pain sensitivity demonstrated in these studies.
- Pain augmentation may also result from a loss of tonic inhibition by descending inhibitory pathways from the brain to the spinal cord.

Dx DIAGNOSIS

DIFFERENTIAL DIAGNOSIS

- Presence of any of the disorders mentioned below does not necessarily exclude a diagnosis of FM because it may occur with many conditions
- Other functional somatic or "central sensitivity" syndromes: myofascial pain, chronic fatigue, irritable bowel, headache/migraines, chronic pelvic and bladder pain disorders, and temporomandibular disorder
- Disorders that can mimic FM (thus must be ruled out clinically) include: hypothyroidism, rheumatic diseases (e.g., rheumatoid arthritis, systemic lupus erythematosus, osteoarthritis, inflammatory myopathies), infection
- Mood and anxiety disorders
- Sleep disorders (e.g., sleep apnea, restless leg syndrome)
- Neurologic disorders
- Medications: statin-induced muscle pain, opioid-induced hyperalgesia

WORKUP

- Thorough history, physical examination, and appropriately selected laboratory studies can usually differentiate FM from connective tissue or other systemic diseases.
- Chronic (>3 mo), widespread pain is the hallmark symptom of FM, but fatigue, tenderness, depression/anxiety, nonrestorative sleep, cognitive difficulties, and functional impairment are other key symptoms.
- The 1990 American College of Rheumatology (ACR) FM Classification Criteria was used for clinical studies:
  1. Chronic, widespread pain in all four quadrants of the body and the axial skeleton.
  2. Pain on digital palpation of at least 11 of 18 tender points (see Fig. 1-383).
- The 2010 ACR preliminary diagnostic criteria for FM do not require a tender point examination; it requires the exclusion of other disorders that would otherwise explain the pain.
- A diagnostic screening tool (Fibromyalgia Diagnostic Screen) developed by Arnold and colleagues was found to accurately screen for FM. This tool includes a patient self-reported questionnaire and an abbreviated physical examination with targeted lab tests.

LABORATORY TESTS

- Selective use of laboratory tests complements the history and physical examination in the diagnosis of FM. Testing should be highly focused on the exclusion of FM mimickers or suspected concurrent diseases.
- Complete blood cell count, routine chemistries, thyroid-stimulating hormone (TSH), erythrocyte sedimentation rate (ESR), and C-reactive protein (CRP) are normal in FM.
- Routine testing for antinuclear antibody (ANA) and/or rheumatoid factor should be avoided unless history and physical examination suggest an autoimmune disease.

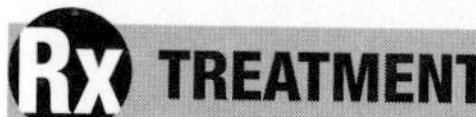

TREATMENT

GENERAL Rx (Fig. 1-384)

- Strong evidence for: low-dose amitriptyline and cyclobenzaprine, serotonin-norepinephrine reuptake inhibitors (milnacipran and duloxetine), and pregabalin.
- The FDA-approved medications for FM are pregabalin, duloxetine, and milnacipran.
- The only analgesic that has demonstrated efficacy in FM has been tramadol, either alone or in combination with acetaminophen.
- Modest evidence exists for gabapentin and SSRIs.
- No evidence that NSAIDs or corticosteroids are effective in FM.
- Avoid narcotic use. There is concern that opioid use and abuse may aggravate chronic widespread pain.
- Nonpharmacologic: strong evidence to support exercise, cognitive behavioral therapy, and patient education.

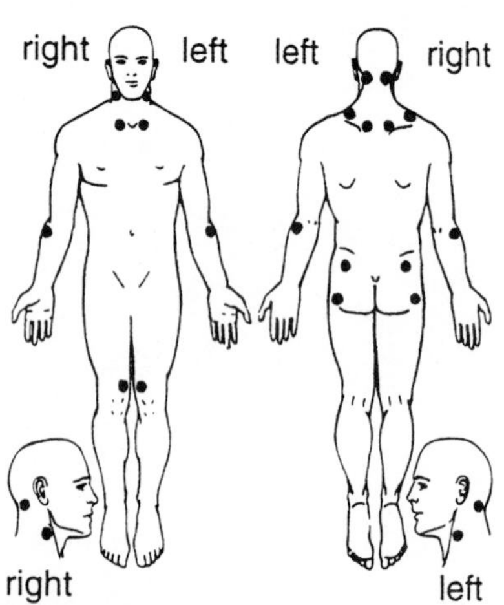

FIGURE 1-383 The sites of the 18 tender points of the 1990 American College of Rheumatology criteria for the classification of fibromyalgia. (From Conn R: *Current diagnosis*, ed 9, Philadelphia, 1997, Saunders.)

DISPOSITION

- The pain and symptoms of FM can wax and wane, vary in physical location and in intensity day to day; many patients continue to have chronic pain and fatigue regardless of therapy.
- Disability rates vary from 9% to 44%.

REFERRAL

Referral to rheumatology, mental health professionals, physical therapy, and rehabilitation may be helpful for a multidisciplinary team approach.

PEARLS & CONSIDERATIONS

Myofascial pain syndrome may represent a localized form of FM. It is associated with trigger points (rather than tender points as seen in FM). Some patients with myofascial pain syndrome may progress to FM.

COMMENTS

FM occurs frequently in patients with some rheumatic diseases such as rheumatoid arthritis, ankylosing spondylitis, and systemic lupus erythematosus, in which prevalence of FM may reach 20%.

EVIDENCE

available at www.expertconsult.com

SUGGESTED READINGS

available at www.expertconsult.com

RELATED CONTENT

Fibromyalgia (Patient Information)

AUTHOR: **CANDICE YUVIENCO, M.D.**

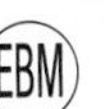

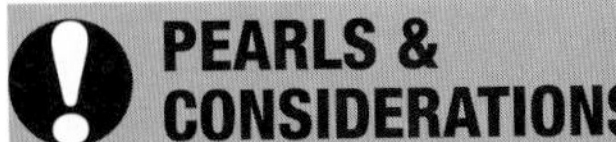

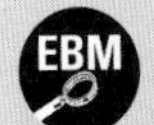

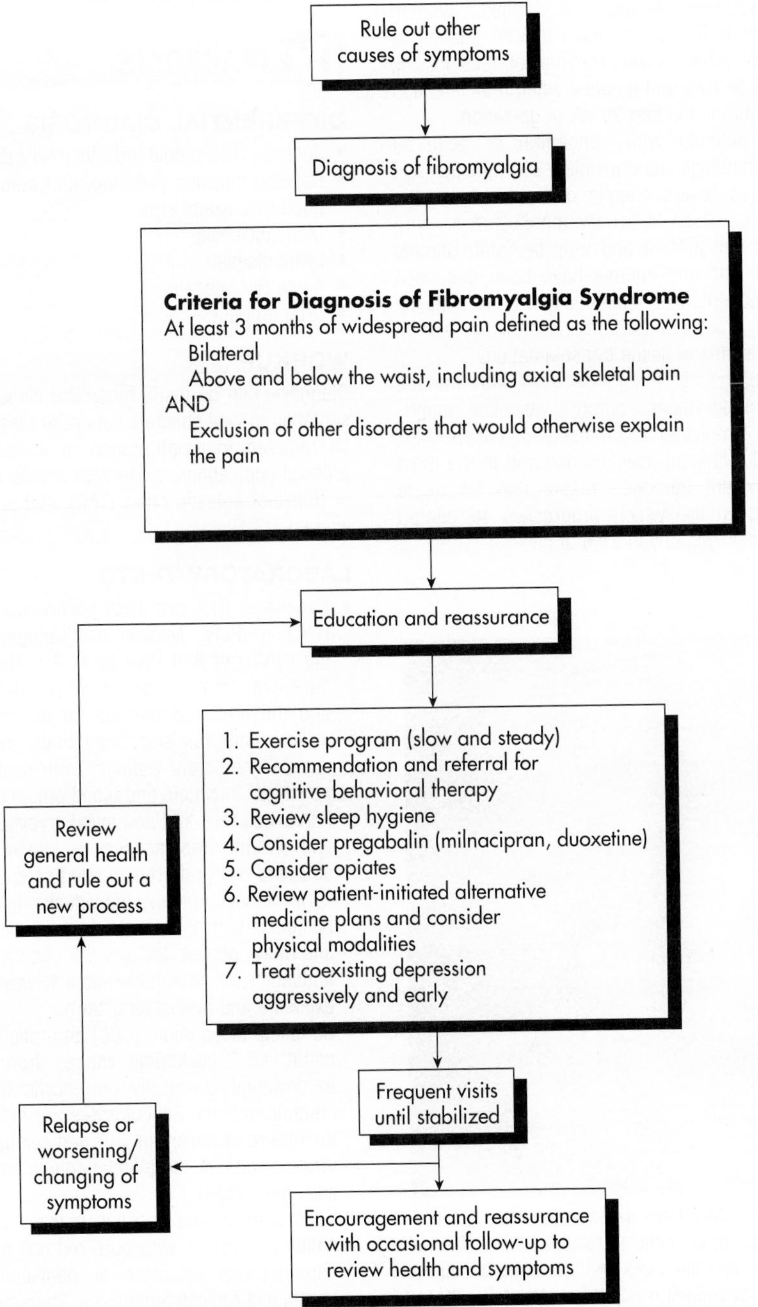

FIGURE 1-384 Treatment algorithm for fibromyalgia. (Modified from Harris ED et al: *Kelley's textbook of rheumatology*, ed 7, Philadelphia, 2005, Saunders.)

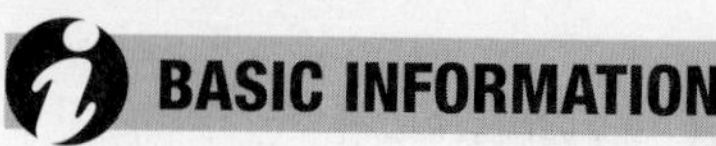

BASIC INFORMATION

DEFINITION

Parvovirus B19 is a small, nonenveloped ssDNA virus that belongs to the *Erythrovirus* genus of the *Parvoviridae* family. It was first discovered in 1975 when units of blood were being screened for hepatitis B and was read as a false positive result (sample 19 in panel B). It causes a spectrum of human disease, from asymptomatic to fatal, depending on the underlying host. Classically, it has been associated with erythema infectiosum (EI), or "fifth disease," the fifth in a series of six viral exanthems that commonly affect school-aged children and are named in order of the dates they were first described. In addition, parvovirus B19 causes a variety of diseases in fetuses, adults, and the immunocompromised.

SYNONYMS

Parvovirus B19
Erythema infectiosum
Fifth disease

ICD-9CM CODES
057.0 Erythema infectiosum (fifth disease)
079.83 Parvovirus B19
ICD-10CM CODES
B08.3 Erythema infectiosum [fifth disease]

EPIDEMIOLOGY & DEMOGRAPHICS

PREDOMINANT AGE: 5 to 18 yr

INCIDENCE: Between 1% and 9% of pregnancies are affected by B19 infection, up to 1 in 200 units of blood are contaminated by B19, 16% of schoolteachers and 9% of daycare workers and homemakers are infected with B19 during epidemics. The infection rate of household contacts may be as high as 50%.

PEAK INCIDENCE: Temperate climates between late winter and early summer, often in cycles of local epidemics that peak every 3 to 10 yr.

PREVALENCE: 15% of school-aged children and 30% to 85% of adults have demonstrated protective IgG antibodies to parvovirus B19.

RISK FACTORS: Exposure to school-aged children, immunosuppression, congenital or acquired hematologic abnormalities, blood transfusion, tissue transplantation.

PHYSICAL FINDINGS & CLINICAL PRESENTATION

- Approximately 25% of those infected are asymptomatic, 50% have nonspecific flulike symptoms, and 25% have the classic symptoms of B19 infection, including rash and/or arthralgias.
- Parvovirus B19 is the most common viral agent associated with rashes in school-aged children. EI is characterized by a bright red, nontender rash most prominent on the cheeks with a circumoral pallor producing the classic "slapped face" appearance (Fig. 1-385), which is often followed by a reticular, lace-like rash on the trunk and extremities. This is typically a transient, self-limited illness that begins with a prodrome of flulike symptoms, such as fever, malaise, myalgias, coryza, headache, nausea, and diarrhea, and ends with the malar rash once viremia has resolved and antibody production has occurred.
- Polyarthralgias and polyarthritis are more commonly seen in adults (especially women) and typically involve symmetric small joints of the extremities. The arthritis is nonerosive. Joint symptoms usually resolve within 3 wk but may rarely become persistent or recurrent. A rash develops in 75% of infected adults, but less than 20% have the classic "slapped face" rash seen in EI. The rash may be exacerbated by changes in temperature, sunlight, exercise, or emotional stress.
- B19 infection during pregnancy can result in fetal anemia, nonimmune hydrops fetalis, miscarriage, or fetal loss. Pregnant women with B19 infection have a 30% chance of fetal transmission. The risk of fetal loss is 5% to 10% and greatest when fetal infection occurs in the first 20 wk of gestation.
- In patients with congenital or acquired hematologic abnormalities, B19 infection can cause severe anemia or transient aplastic crisis, which is usually manifested as pure red cell aplasia and may be fatal. Chronic infection and anemia have been described in patients with leukemia and other cancers, HIV, or congenital immunodeficiency and in recipients of tissue transplantation.
- B19 has also been associated with immune thrombocytopenic purpura, vasculitis, nephritis, lymphadenitis, meningitis, encephalitis, and fulminant liver disease and is the most prevalent pathogen responsible for acute myocarditis, which progresses to dilated cardiomyopathy in 21% of cases.

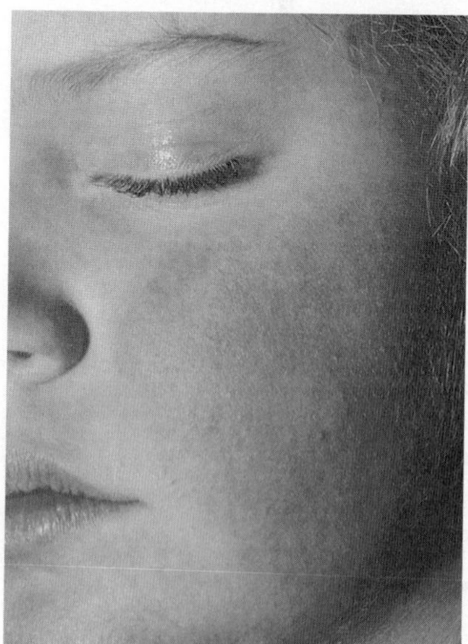

FIGURE 1-385 Fifth disease (erythema infectiosum). Facial erythema "slapped face." The red plaque covers the cheek and spares the nasolabial and the circumoral region. (From Habif TP: *Clinical dermatology: a color guide to diagnosis and therapy,* ed 3, St Louis, 1996, Mosby.)

TROPISM, INCUBATION, INFECTIVITY, & TRANSMISSION

B19 preferentially infects, replicates in, and is directly cytotoxic to erythroid progenitor cells, which may result in profound anemia or pure red cell aplasia. Viremia and the period of greatest infectivity occur 7 to 10 days after exposure and last about 1 wk in immunocompetent individuals, after which time antibody production begins and typical symptoms of rash and arthralgias manifest. Transmission is thought to occur primarily through droplet exposure, as well as person-to-person contact, fomites, vertical transmission, and hematogenous transmission. Because of its nonenveloped capsid, parvovirus B19 is heat stable and difficult to inactivate with solvent detergents, often leading to contamination of blood products.

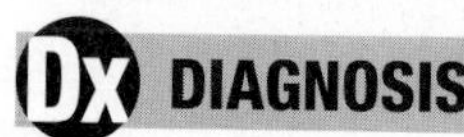

DIAGNOSIS

DIFFERENTIAL DIAGNOSIS

- Juvenile rheumatoid arthritis (Still's disease)
- Rubella, measles (rubeola), and other childhood viral exanthems
- Mononucleosis
- Lyme disease
- Acute HIV infection
- Drug eruption

WORKUP

Diagnosis can be made by typical clinical presentation in well children. Laboratory tests may be required for confirmation in immunosuppressed populations, those with severe anemia or transient aplastic crisis (TAC), and pregnant women.

LABORATORY TESTS

- Parvovirus B19 viral DNA polymerase chain reaction (PCR): Nucleic acid antigen testing (NAAT) of B19 DNA by PCR is the most sensitive method of infection detection and the preferred method for diagnosis in immunocompromised individuals, fetuses, immunocompetent patients with suspected persistent infection, and blood products.
- Parvovirus B19 IgM and IgG: Parvovirus B19 IgM enzyme immunoassay is widely available and the preferred method of diagnosis in immunocompetent individuals. IgM can be found within 7 to 10 days of exposure and may persist for several months. IgG antibodies are detectable about 15 days after exposure and persist long-term.
- Complete blood count (CBC) and reticulocyte count: CBC evaluation ranges from mild to profound classically normocytic normochromic anemia. Reticulocytes are markedly decreased or absent in pure red cell aplasia. White blood cell and platelet counts are typically unchanged.
- Bone marrow biopsy: Bone marrow examination in patients with pure red cell aplasia demonstrates complete or near-complete absence of red cell precursors. Characteristic giant proerythroblasts containing large eosinophilic nuclear inclusions can be seen.

- Prenatal testing: Fetal nuchal translucency measurement and ductus venosus Doppler velocimetry may indicate the presence of severe fetal anemia. Ultrasound may show fetal edema, ascites, pleural effusions, and cardiomegaly in hydrops fetalis.

Rx TREATMENT

ACUTE GENERAL TREATMENT

- No antiviral drug is available.
- Treatment is generally supportive because the majority of B19 infections are asymptomatic or mild and self-limited; nonsteroidal antiinflammatory drugs may be used for relief of joint symptoms.
- Blood transfusion is often required in cases of severe anemia and pure red cell aplasia until red blood cell (RBC) production returns; intrauterine transfusion may be required in fetal infection.
- IV immunoglobulin (IVIG) treatment may be considered for immunocompromised patients with chronic B19 infection and chronic anemia.
- Initiation of highly active antiretroviral therapy (HAART) has been associated with resolution of B19-induced anemia in HIV-infected patients.
- Bone marrow transplantation has been used in individuals with nonresolving aplastic crisis.
- The mainstay of fetal therapy is delivery, which may be followed by resuscitation and ventilation in cases of severe hydrops.

DISPOSITION & PROGNOSIS

- B19 infection is typically self-limited, with symptoms usually resolving within a few weeks and most often requiring only supportive care.
- Children in whom EI develops are no longer contagious and may attend school and daycare.
- Patients in whom persistent arthritis with or without joint erosion develops should be evaluated by a rheumatologist.
- In immunocompetent patients, anemia is typically transient with spontaneous resolution and return of RBC production in days to weeks. In patients with hematologic abnormalities, however, anemia may be severe and may be the result of transient aplastic crisis or pure red cell aplasia, which warrant immediate hematologic evaluation and transfusion.
- Patients with TAC or chronic parvovirus B19 infection pose a risk for nosocomial spread and, when hospitalized, should be isolated with droplet precautions.
- Patients with chronic infection and anemia may require evaluation for possible IVIG treatment.
- Pregnant women with B19 infection have a 30% risk of fetal transmission; they should undergo close monitoring of fetal health and development and may require fetal transfusion or referral to a tertiary care center for delivery in the case of hydrops fetalis.
- Vaccines have not progressed beyond phase I/II clinical trials.

REFERRAL

- To hematologist if signs of marrow suppression
- To rheumatologist if signs of severe or erosive arthritis
- To cardiologist if suspicion of myocarditis

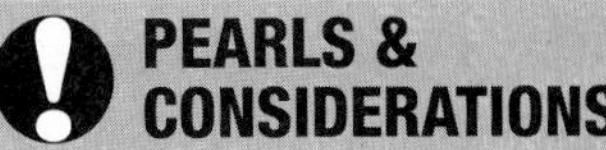

PEARLS & CONSIDERATIONS

- Generally self-limited disease lasting up to 3 wk in immunocompetent individuals
- Symmetric arthritis involving small joints is common in adults, whereas facial rash is common in children
- Can cause severe anemia with or without transient aplastic crisis that may become chronic in patients with hematologic abnormalities, immunocompromise, or malignancy and those after transplantation.
- Infection during pregnancy can cause fetal anemia, hydrops fetalis, or fetal loss.

PREVENTION

- Hand-washing and not sharing food or drinks during epidemics.
- Testing of plasma pools and blood products for B19 contamination.

SUGGESTED READINGS

available at www.expertconsult.com

RELATED CONTENT

Fifth Disease (Patient Information)

AUTHORS: **ANTONELLA FINE, M.D.,** and **DOMINICK TAMMARO, M.D.**

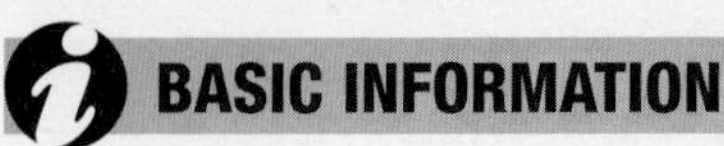

BASIC INFORMATION

DEFINITION

Folliculitis is inflammation of the hair follicle as a result of infection, physical injury, or chemical irritation.

SYNONYMS

Sycosis barbae

ICD-9CM CODES

704.8 Other specified diseases of hair and hair follicles

ICD-10CM CODES

L72.9 Follicular cyst of skin and subcutaneous tissue, unspecified
L73.1 Pseudofolliculitis barbae
L73.8 Other specified follicular disorders
L66.3 Perifolliculitis capitis abscedens

EPIDEMIOLOGY & DEMOGRAPHICS

PREVALENCE: Staphylococcal folliculitis is the most common form of infectious folliculitis; it occurs most commonly in persons with diabetes.

PREDOMINANT SEX: Sycosis barbae occurs most frequently in men who have commenced shaving.

PHYSICAL FINDINGS & CLINICAL PRESENTATION

- The lesions generally consist of painful yellow pustules surrounded by erythema; a central hair is present in the pustules. Furuncles with pus may be present (Fig. 1-388).
- Patients with sycosis barbae may initially present with small follicular papules or pustules that increase in size with continued shaving; deep follicular pustules may occur surrounded by erythema and swelling; the upper lip is frequently involved.
- "Hot tub" folliculitis occurs within 1 to 4 days after the use of a hot tub with poor chlorination. It is characterized by papules and pustules (Fig. 1-389) with surrounding erythema generally affecting the torso, buttocks, and limbs.

ETIOLOGY

- *Staphylococcus* infection (e.g., sycosis barbae), *Pseudomonas aeruginosa* ("hot tub" folliculitis)
- Gram-negative folliculitis *(Klebsiella, Enterobacter, Proteus)* associated with antibiotic treatment of acne
- Chronic irritation of the hair follicle (use of cocoa butter or coconut oil, chronic irritation from workplace)
- Initial use of systemic corticosteroid therapy (steroid acne), eosinophilic folliculitis (AIDS patients), *Candida albicans* (immunocompromised patients)
- *Pityrosporum orbiculare*

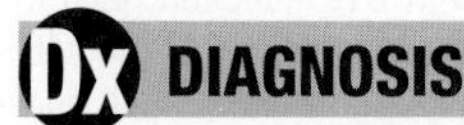

DIAGNOSIS

DIFFERENTIAL DIAGNOSIS

- Pseudofolliculitis barbae (ingrown hairs)
- Acne vulgaris
- Dermatophyte fungal infections
- Keratosis pilaris
- Cutaneous candidiasis
- Superficial fungal infections
- Miliaris

WORKUP

Physical examination and medical history (e.g., use of hot tub: "hot tub" folliculitis; adolescent patients who have started shaving: sycosis barbae; use of occlusive topical steroid therapy: *Staphylococcus* folliculitis).

LABORATORY TESTS

- Generally not necessary.
- Gram stain is useful to identify the infective organisms in infectious folliculitis and to differentiate infectious folliculitis from noninfectious.

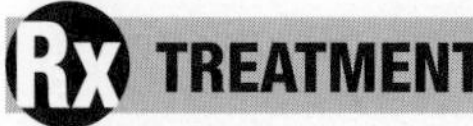

TREATMENT

NONPHARMACOLOGIC THERAPY

- Prevention of chemical or mechanical skin irritation
- Glycemic control in diabetics
- Proper chlorination of hot tubs and spas
- Shaving with a clean razor

ACUTE GENERAL Rx

- Cleansing of the area with chlorhexidine and application of saline compresses to involved area
- Application of 2% mupirocin ointment or 1% Retapamulin ointment for bacterial folliculitis affecting a limited area (e.g., sycosis barbae)
- Treatment of severe cases of *Pseudomonas* folliculitis with ciprofloxacin
- Treatment of *S. aureus* folliculitis with dicloxacillin 250 mg qd for 10 days

CHRONIC Rx

- Chronic nasal or perineal *S. aureus* carriers with frequent folliculitis can be treated with rifampin 300 mg bid for 5 days.
- Mupirocin or Retapamulin ointment applied to nares bid is also effective for nasal carriers.

DISPOSITION

- Most cases of bacterial folliculitis resolve completely with proper treatment.
- Steroid folliculitis responds to discontinuation of steroids.

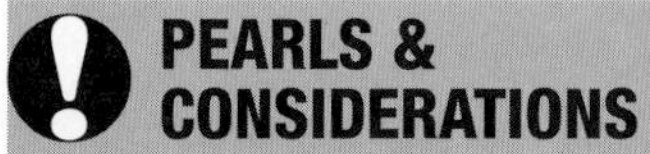

PEARLS & CONSIDERATIONS

COMMENTS

Patients should be instructed in good personal hygiene and avoidance of sharing razors, towels, and washcloths.

RELATED CONTENT

Folliculitis (Patient Information)

AUTHOR: **FRED F. FERRI, M.D.**

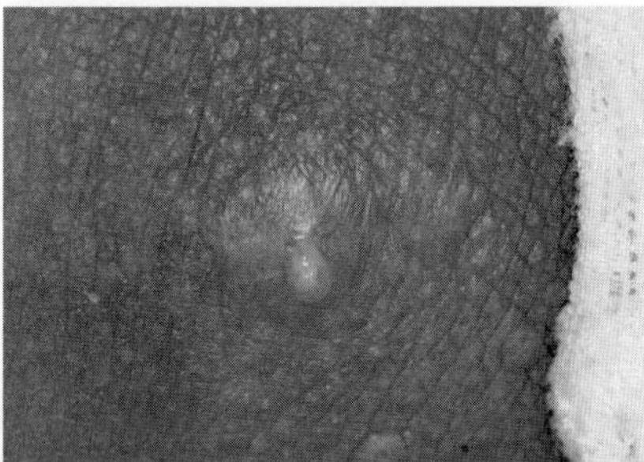

FIGURE 1-388 Rupture and discharge of pus in a furuncle. (From Kliegman RM et al: *Nelson textbook of pediatrics,* ed 19, Philadelphia, 2011, Saunders.)

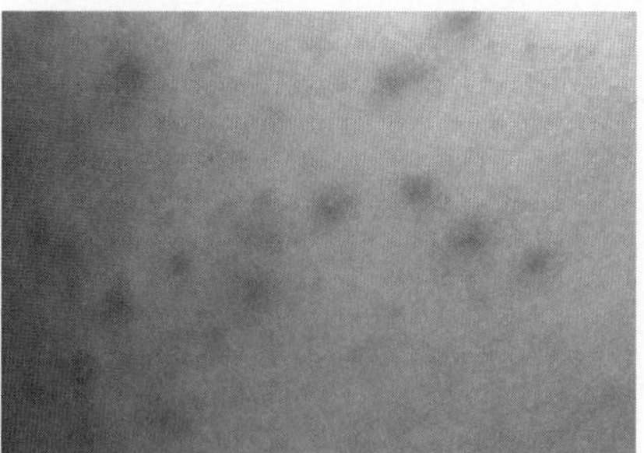

FIGURE 1-389 Papules and pustules in hot tub folliculitis. (From Kliegman RM et al: *Nelson textbook of pediatrics,* ed 19, Philadelphia, 2011, Saunders.)

BASIC INFORMATION

DEFINITION

Food allergies are divided into IgE-mediated and immunologically mediated non-IgE reactions. They include a spectrum of disorders that involve adverse immunologic responses to a dietary antigens.

ICD-9CM CODES
447.1 Allergic rhinitis due to food
558.3 Allergic gastroenteritis and colitis
693.1 Dermatitis due to food taken internally
995.60 Anaphylactic reaction due to unspecified food
995.7 Other adverse food reactions, not elsewhere classified

ICD-10CM CODES
T78.0 Adverse food reaction (including anaphylactic shock)
T78.1 Other adverse food reactions, not elsewhere classified
L27.2 Dermatitis due to ingested food

EPIDEMIOLOGY & DEMOGRAPHICS

INCIDENCE: Food allergies have a cumulative incidence of 6% to 8% for the first 3 yr of life.

PREVALENCE:

- Overall prevalence is 1% to 2% in general population, ~3.9% -8% in children.
- Patient self-reported food allergies have a prevalence of 12% to 13%, demonstrating the importance of objective measures in assessing food allergies.
- Nearly 40% of children with food allergy have a history of severe reactions that, if not treated immediately with proper medication, can lead to hospitalization or even death.[1]
- There is no predilection for race.

PREDOMINANT SEX: Males are more affected than females among children, and among adults, females are more frequently affected.

GENETICS: Children with parents or close relatives with allergies may have a tendency to become allergic to foods.

PHYSICAL FINDINGS & CLINICAL PRESENTATION

- IgE-mediated reactions: (within minutes to a few hours) pruritus, urticaria or angioedema, atopic dermatitis, GI symptoms, conjunctival injection, sneezing, nasal congestion, rhinorrhea, bronchospasm, and anaphylaxis
- Non–IgE-mediated reactions: food-induced enterocolitis, celiac disease, Crohn's disease, dermatitis herpetiformis, and pulmonary reactions such as Heiner syndrome. These illnesses are discussed separately.
- Signs, symptoms, and presentation reflect specific allergic manifestation, but in food allergies there is a reproducible temporal relationship to ingested food allergens.

---

[1]Gupta RS et al: The prevalence, severity, and distribution of childhood food allergy in the United States, *Pediatrics* 128(l):e9-e17, 2011.

ETIOLOGY

Failure to establish tolerance to food antigens. Food proteins not broken down by proteolysis are taken up by intestinal epithelial cells and presented to primed T cells.

DIAGNOSIS

- Thorough history and physical exam should be performed.
- The temporal relationship and reproducibility of the symptoms are most important to establishing the diagnosis.
- A review of ingredient labels may be helpful.
- Confirmatory testing can include skin testing or in vitro testing.
- Skin prick testing (SPT): positive predictive value <50%, but negative predictive value >95%. Thus a negative skin test effectively rules out an IgE-mediated process.
- In vitro testing: RAST testing: Historically it is less sensitive than skin testing, but sensitivity has improved with cut off points indicating a positive predictive value of 95% for allergies to eggs, milk, peanuts, wheat, and fish.
- Neither the size of the wheal in skin prick testing nor the IgE antibody level correlates with severity. However, there may be some increased positive predictive value with larger wheals and higher titers.
- Atopy patch test: used in conjunction with RAST and skin testing in multiallergic children to plan widening the elimination diet. However, it is not recommended in the routine evaluation of food allergies.
- Double-blind, placebo-controlled food challenges are the gold standard test for determining food allergies. These need to be done in a supervised and controlled setting.
- In summary, if the history and lab tests are suggestive of a specific food allergy, that food should be confirmed by SPT, RAST, or food challenge and, once confirmed, eliminated from the diet.

DIFFERENTIAL DIAGNOSIS

- Gastrointestinal disorders
- Irritable bowel syndrome
- Carcinoid syndrome
- Giardiasis
- Structural abnormalities like hiatal hernia, pyloric stenosis, Hirschsprung's disease, tracheoesophageal fistula
- Disaccharidase deficiencies: lactase, sucrase-isomaltase complex, glucose-galactose complex
- Pancreatic insufficiency: cystic fibrosis
- Gallbladder disease
- Peptic ulcer disease
- Malignancy
- Metabolic disorders
- Galactosemia
- Phenylketonuria
- Pharmacologic-related conditions
- Gustatory rhinitis
- Auriculotemporal syndrome (facial flush from tart food)

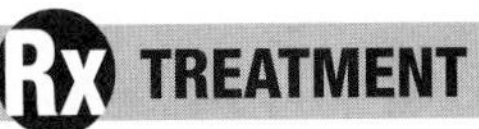

TREATMENT

NONPHARMACOLOGIC THERAPY

- Elimination diet should be used in conjunction with nutritional counseling.
- Formula-fed infants: brief trial of hydrolyzed milk formula as most children with milk allergy induced skin symptoms will respond to the change of formula. Nonresponders may require amino acid–based formula.
- In older children: elimination of one to two suspected foods is appropriate for 2 wk or longer and then reintroducing the foods to determine if symptoms recur.

ACUTE GENERAL Rx

- Antihistamines (both H_1 and H_2 antihistamines), albuterol if wheezing, epinephrine and glucocorticoids in patients with anaphylaxis.
- Patients with documented IgE-mediated reactions should receive and be counseled on the use of epinephrine autoinjector.

NEW TREATMENTS FOR FOOD ALLERGIES

- Oral and sublingual immunotherapy may play a role in management of food allergies, but this is currently under investigation.
- Recombinant vaccines and other immunomodulatory strategies are under development, although monoclonal anti-IgE antibody has shown benefit in adults with peanut allergy.

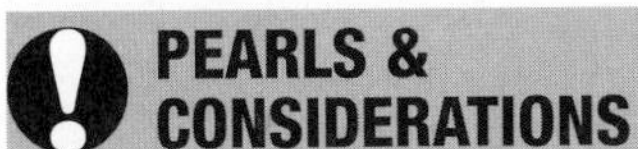

PEARLS & CONSIDERATIONS

- Eczema that develops in first 6 to 12 mo of life is usually the first manifestation of atopy.
- Egg allergy or sensitization is the strongest recognized predictor of respiratory allergies in children and asthma in adults.
- Consultation with trained dietitian is critical to avoid potentially adverse nutritional consequences in children with multiple food allergies.
- Skin testing is the preferred method for identifying food-specific IgE. RAST is useful if there is chance of severe food reaction causing risk to the patient.
- American Academy of Pediatrics recommends avoiding influenza vaccine in patients with severe systemic allergic reactions to egg. Skin prick testing using influenza vaccine containing egg is recommended before vaccination in children with egg allergy and asthma. Skin prick testing not required before MMR vaccine in children with egg allergy.

COMMENTS

- Milk allergy usually resolves by age 5. Risk factors for persistence are early cutaneous manifestations following milk ingestion, development of other atopic conditions, and persistence of milk-specific high IgE titers.

Soy milk is recommended for these children, keeping in mind that about 15% of these children can develop soy allergy.

- Egg allergy has been thought to resolve in 66% of children by 5 yr of age and in 75% of children by 7 yr of age. Trials have shown that oral immunotherapy can desensitize a high proportion of children with egg allergy and induce sustained unresponsiveness in a clinically significant subset.
- Wheat allergy found to resolve by 5 yr of age and soybean allergy by 2 yr of age.

PREVENTION

- There is conflicting evidence regarding the protective effect of breastfeeding on food allergies.
- There is no evidence to suggest that exclusive breastfeeding for 6 mo or more is superior to exclusive breastfeeding for 4 to 6 mo in terms of developing food allergies.
- In high-risk infants who are not exclusively breast fed, there is limited evidence to suggest that feeding with hydrolyzed formula compared to cow's milk formula reduces allergies.
- Currently, there is no evidence to support the use of prebiotics, probiotics, or synbiotics for the prevention of allergic diseases.
- No current evidence exists to support delaying the introduction of solid foods beyond 4 to 6 mo.

PATIENT/FAMILY EDUCATION

Information can be found on American Academy of Allergy, Asthma and Immunology (www.aaaai.org), the Food Allergy and Anaphylaxis Network (www.foodallergy.org), and the Anaphylaxis Campaign (www.anaphylaxis.org.uk).

REFERRAL

Patients may be referred to an allergy/immunology specialist when the diagnosis is uncertain or if avoidance measures are not successful.

SUGGESTED READINGS

available at www.expertconsult.com

RELATED CONTENT

Food Allergies (Patient Information)

AUTHOR: **LUKE BARRÉ, M.D.**

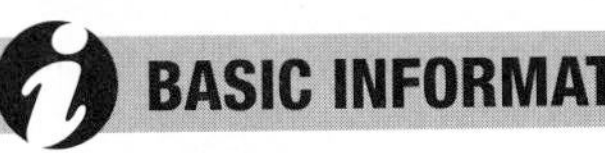

DEFINITION

Food poisoning is an illness caused by ingestion of food contaminated by bacteria and/or bacterial toxins. Table 1-195 describes pathogenic mechanisms in bacterial foodborne disease.

SYNONYMS

Enterotoxin-poisoning
Epidemic vomiting disease

ICD-9CM CODES
See specific illness.

ICD-10CM CODES
A05.9 Bacterial foodborne intoxication, unspecified

EPIDEMIOLOGY & DEMOGRAPHICS

INCIDENCE (IN U.S.):
- Estimated range of 6 to 8 million cases/yr
- Majority of identifiable causes are bacterial, although more than 250 known diseases can be transmitted through food

PEAK INCIDENCE: Varies with specific organism
- Summer: *Staphylococcus aureus, Salmonella, Shigella* spp.
- Summer and fall: *Clostridium botulinum, Vibrio parahaemolyticus*
- Spring and fall: *Campylobacter jejuni*
- Winter: *Clostridium perfringens, Yersinia enterocolitica*

PREDOMINANT AGE: Varies with specific agent
NEONATAL INFECTION: Rare but severe with *Shigella* and *Salmonella* spp.

PHYSICAL FINDINGS & CLINICAL PRESENTATION

- Any combination of GI symptoms and fever
- Specific organisms suspected on the basis of the incubation period and predominant symptoms (Table E1-196), although a great deal of overlap exists
  1. Short incubation period (1 to 6 hr): involve the ingestion of preformed toxin; noninvasive
     a. *S. aureus:* nausea, profuse vomiting, and abdominal cramps common; diarrhea possible, but fever uncommon; usually resolves within 24 hr; foods implicated in outbreaks include meats, mayonnaise, and cream pastries
     b. *B. cereus:* two forms, a short incubation (emetic) form (characterized by vomiting and abdominal cramps in virtually all patients, diarrhea in one third of patients, fever uncommon) and a long incubation (diarrheal) form; illness usually mild, resolves within 12 hr; unrefrigerated rice most often implicated as vehicle
  2. Moderate incubation period (8 to 16 hr): involves the in vivo production of toxin; noninvasive
     a. *C. perfringens:* severe crampy abdominal pain and watery diarrhea common; fever and vomiting unlikely; symptoms usually resolving within 24 hr; outbreaks invariably related to cooked meat or poultry that is allowed to cool without refrigeration; most cases in the fall and winter months. *C. perfringens* is the third most common cause of foodborne illness in the U.S.
     b. *B. cereus:* diarrheal (or long incubation) form most commonly beginning with diarrhea, abdominal cramps, and occasionally vomiting; fever uncommon; usually resolves within 24 hr; the responsible food is usually fried rice
  3. Long incubation period (>16 hr): some toxin-mediated, some invasive
     a. Toxin-producing organisms include:
        (1) *C. botulinum:* should be considered when a diarrheal illness coincides with or precedes paralysis; severity of illness related to the quantity of toxin ingested; characteristic cranial nerve palsies progressing to a descending paralysis; fever usually absent; usually associated with home-canned foods
        (2) Enterotoxigenic *E. coli* (ETEC): most common cause of travelers' diarrhea; after 1- to 2-day incubation period, abdominal cramps and copious diarrhea occur; vomiting and fever uncommon; usually resolves after 3 to 4 days; vehicle usually unbottled water or contaminated salad or ice
        (3) Enterohemorrhagic *E. coli* (EHEC): can cause severe abdominal cramps and watery diarrhea, which may eventually become bloody; bacteria (strain 0157:H7) are noninvasive; no fever; illness may be complicated by hemolytic-uremic syndrome; associated with contaminated beef
        (4) *V. cholerae:* varies from a mild, self-limited illness to life-threatening cholera; diarrhea, nausea, and vomiting, abdominal cramps, and muscle cramps; no fever; severe cases may progress to shock and death within hours of onset; survivors usually have resolution of symptoms in 1 wk; U.S. cases are either imported or result from ingestion of imported food
     b. Invasive organisms include:
        (1) *Salmonella:* associated most often with nontyphoidal strains; incubation period generally 12 to 48 hr; nausea, vomiting, diarrhea, and abdominal cramps typical; fever possible; outbreaks of gastroenteritis related to contaminated poultry, meat, and dairy products
        (2) *Shigella:* asymptomatic infection possible, but some with fever and watery diarrhea that may progress to bloody diarrhea and dysentery; with mild illness, usually self-limited, resolves in a few days; with severe illness, may develop complications; transmission usually from person to person but can occur via contaminated food or water
        (3) *C. jejuni:* the most common foodborne bacterial pathogen; incubation period is about 1 day, then a prodrome of fever, headache, and myalgias; intestinal phase marked by diarrhea associated with fever, malaise, and abdominal pain; diarrhea mild to profuse and bloody; usually resolves in about 7 days, but relapse is possible; associated with undercooked meats and poultry, unpasteurized dairy products, and drinking from freshwater streams
        (4) *Y. enterocolitica* and *Y. pseudotuberculosis:* infrequent causes of enteritis in U.S.; children affected more often than adults; fever, diarrhea, and abdominal pain lasting 1 to 3 wk; some with mesenteric

TABLE 1-195 Pathogenic Mechanisms in Bacterial Foodborne Disease

Preformed Toxin	Toxin Production in Vivo	Tissue Invasion	Toxin Production and/or Tissue Invasion
Staphylococcus aureus	*Clostridium perfringens*	*Campylobacter jejuni*	*Vibrio parahaemolyticus*
Bacillus cereus (short incubation)	*B. cereus* (long incubation)	*Salmonella*	*Yersinia enterocolitica*
Clostridium botulinum	*C. botulinum* (infant botulism)	*Shigella*	
	Enterotoxigenic *Escherichia coli*	Invasive *E. coli*	
	Vibrio cholerae 01 or 0139		
	V. cholerae non-01		
	Shiga toxin–producing *E. coli*		

From Mandell GL et al: *Principles and practice of infectious diseases*, ed 6, Philadelphia, 2005, Churchill Livingstone.

adenitis that mimics acute appendicitis; contaminated food or water is usually responsible

(5) *V. parahaemolyticus:* In U.S., most outbreaks in coastal states or on cruise ships during the summer months; incubation period usually >1 day, followed by explosive watery diarrhea in the majority of cases; nausea, vomiting, abdominal cramps, and headache also common; fever less common; usually resolves by 1 wk; related to ingestion of seafood

(6) Enteroinvasive *E. coli* (EIEC): a rare cause of disease in the U.S.; high incidence of fever and bloody diarrhea; may resemble bacillary dysentery

(7) *V. vulnificus:* may cause serious, often fatal illness in persons with chronic liver disease; GI symptoms usually absent, but fever, chills, hypotension, and hemorrhagic skin lesions possible; patients with liver disease or at increased risk of developing liver disease should avoid eating raw oysters

ETIOLOGY

Classically categorized as either inflammatory (invasive) or noninflammatory:

- Noninflammatory: *B. cereus, S. aureus, C. botulinum, C. perfringens, V. cholerae,* enterotoxigenic *E. coli* (ETEC), and enterohemorrhagic *E. coli* (EHEC); toxin-producing organisms that are noninvasive; fecal leukocytes are not seen.
- Inflammatory: *Campylobacter,* enteroinvasive *E. coli* (EIEC), *Salmonella, Shigella, V. parahaemolyticus,* and *Yersinia;* cause disease by invasion of intestinal tissue; fecal leukocytes are seen.

Dx DIAGNOSIS

DIFFERENTIAL DIAGNOSIS

Gastroenteritis caused by viruses (Norwalk, Noro, or rotavirus), parasites *(Amoeba histolytica, Giardia lamblia),* or toxins (ciguatoxins, mushrooms, heavy metals)

LABORATORY TESTS

- Test stool for fecal leukocytes to help narrow the differential diagnosis:
  1. Send stool for culture and for ova and parasites.
  2. Send stool for *C. difficile* toxin in patients with current or recent antibiotic use.
  3. NOTE: Some pathogens are not identified on routine stool culture; laboratory should be advised if *Yersinia, C. botulinum, Vibrio,* or enterohemorrhagic *E. coli* (0157:H7) are suspected.
  4. Finding *B. cereus, C. perfringens,* or *E. coli* in stool is of little value, because these may be part of the normal bowel flora.
- If botulism suspected, send food, serum, and stool for toxin assay.
- Blood cultures are needed for all febrile patients.

Rx TREATMENT

NONPHARMACOLOGIC THERAPY

Adequate rehydration is the mainstay of therapy.

ACUTE GENERAL Rx

- Gastroenteritis caused by the following organisms requires no antimicrobial treatment: *B. cereus, S. aureus, C. perfringens, V. parahaemolyticus, Yersinia,* and enterohemorrhagic and enteroinvasive *E. coli.*
- The usual cause of traveler's diarrhea is enterotoxigenic *E. coli.* Although usually a self-limited illness, antibiotics can shorten the course.
  1. SMX/TMP one DS tab bid for 3 days
  2. Ciprofloxacin 500 mg PO bid for 3 days
- The mainstay of therapy for cholera is fluid replacement. Antibiotics should be given to decrease shedding and duration of illness.
  1. Doxycycline 100 mg PO bid for 3 days
  2. SMX/TMP one DS tab bid for 3 days
- Treatment is not indicated for *Salmonella* gastroenteritis. Patients who are at high risk of developing bacteremia may be treated for 48 to 72 hr (see "Salmonellosis").
- Although shigellosis tends to be a self-limited illness, antibiotics shorten the course of illness and may limit transmission of the illness (see "Shigellosis").
- Those with moderate or severe *Campylobacter* diarrhea may benefit from treatment.
  1. Erythromycin 500 mg PO qid for 5 days
  2. Ciprofloxacin 500 mg PO bid for 5 days
- *V. vulnificus* sepsis should be treated with:
  1. Doxycycline 100 mg IV bid for 2 wk
  2. Ceftazidime 2 g IV q8h for 2 wk
- For suspected botulism, antitoxin should be administered early (see "Botulism").

CHRONIC Rx

Patients with *Salmonella* infections may become carriers and may require treatment (see "Salmonellosis").

DISPOSITION

- Most infections are self-limited and do not require therapy.
- In immunocompromised host or patient with underlying disease, serious complications are possible.
- Postinfectious syndromes are important with some infections:
  1. Reiter's syndrome: *Salmonella, Shigella, Campylobacter, Yersinia* spp.; more common in genetically susceptible host (HLA-B27+)
  2. Guillain-Barré syndrome: *Campylobacter spp.*

REFERRAL

If more than a mild illness

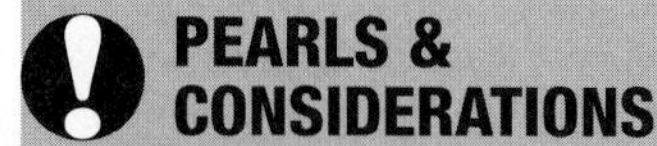

PEARLS & CONSIDERATIONS

COMMENTS

- Grossly underreported and undiagnosed
- All cases to be reported to the local health department

SUGGESTED READINGS

available at www.expertconsult.com

RELATED CONTENT

Bacterial Food Poisoning (Patient Information)
Salmonellosis (Related Key Topic)

AUTHOR: **GLENN G. FORT, M.D., M.P.H.**

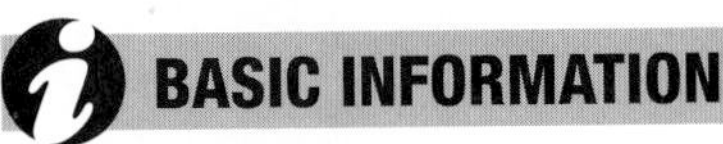

BASIC INFORMATION

DEFINITION

Friedreich's ataxia is the most common hereditary neurodegenerative ataxic disorder, caused by degeneration of dorsal root ganglions, posterior columns, spinocerebellar and corticospinal tracts, and large sensory peripheral neurons.

ICD-9CM CODES
334.0 Friedreich's ataxia
ICD-10CM CODES
G11.1 Early-onset cerebellar ataxia

EPIDEMIOLOGY & DEMOGRAPHICS

INCIDENCE (IN U.S.): Estimated at one in 30,000 whites
PEAK INCIDENCE: 8 to 15 yr
PREVALENCE (IN U.S.): Two to four per 100,000. Carrier rate 1:120 to 1:160; lower prevalence in Asians and people of African descent.
PREDOMINANT SEX: Males and females affected equally
GENETICS: Autosomal recessive; 96% of affected patients are homozygous and 4% are compound heterozygous (two different mutations). Trinucleotide repeat expansion accounts for 94% to 98% of cases, whereas point mutations account for 2% to 6% of cases.

PHYSICAL FINDINGS & CLINICAL PRESENTATION

- Onset of progressive appendicular and gait ataxia, with absent muscle stretch reflexes in the lower extremities.
- With disease progression (within 5 yr): dysarthria, distal loss of position and vibration sense, pyramidal leg weakness, areflexia in all four limbs, and extensor plantar responses.
- Common findings: progressive scoliosis, distal atrophy, pes cavus, and cardiomyopathy (symmetric concentric hypertrophic form in most cases).
- Insulin-requiring diabetes mellitus may occur in 10% of patients, with glucose intolerance occurring in an additional 10% to 20%.

ETIOLOGY

- Genetic: frataxin gene is localized to the centromeric region of chromosome 9q13.
- Normal sequence has six to 27 repeats; abnormal sequence has 120 to 1700 GAA repeats.
- Frataxin deficiency leads to impaired mitochondrial iron homeostasis.

Dx DIAGNOSIS

DIFFERENTIAL DIAGNOSIS

- Charcot-Marie-Tooth disease type 2
- Abetalipoproteinemia
- Severe vitamin E deficiency with malabsorption
- Early-onset cerebellar ataxia with retained reflexes
- Autosomal-dominant cerebellar ataxia (spinocerebellar ataxia)

WORKUP

- Diagnostic criteria include electrophysiologic evidence for a generalized axonal sensory or sensorimotor neuropathy.
- ECG may show widespread T-wave inversion and evidence of left ventricular hypertrophy. ECG abnormalities are present in 65% of patients.
- Sural nerve biopsy shows loss of large myelinated fibers.
- Specific gene testing for the expanded GAA trinucleotide repeat.

LABORATORY TESTS

- Electromyography or nerve conduction study
- ECG and echocardiogram
- Peripheral blood smear for acanthocytes
- Lipid profile
- Two-hour glucose tolerance test
- Vitamin E levels (if necessary)

IMAGING STUDIES

MRI of the spinal cord may demonstrate spinal cord atrophy with essentially normal cerebrum, brainstem, and cerebellum (Fig. 1-390).

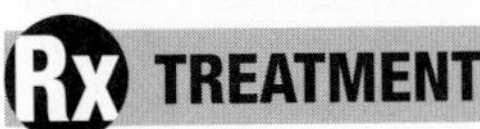

TREATMENT

NONPHARMACOLOGIC THERAPY

- Surgical correction of scoliosis and foot deformities in selected patients

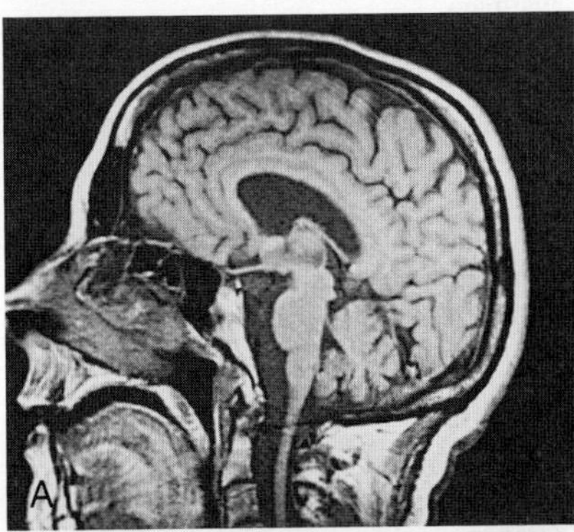

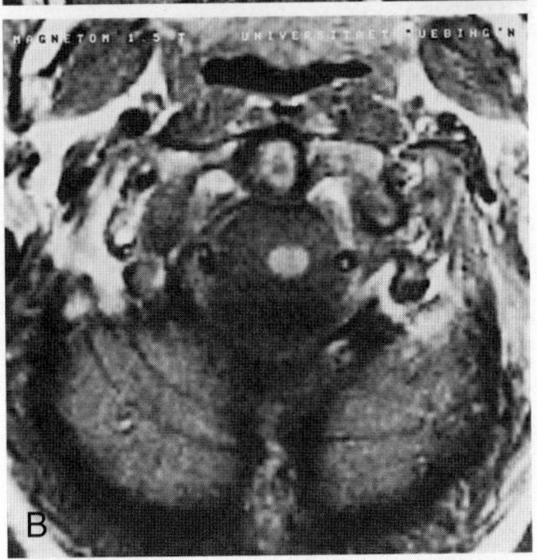

FIGURE 1-390 T1 MRI of the brain (midsagittal section) and spinal cord (axial slice at level of the dens) showing severe shrinkage of the cervical cord, but the cerebellum and brain stem are of normal size. (From Goetz CG: *Textbook of clinical neurology,* Philadelphia, 1999, Saunders.)

- Prosthetic devices as required (e.g., ankle-foot orthosis for foot drop)
- Physical therapy
- Communication devices for patients with severe dysarthria

ACUTE GENERAL Rx

None established.

- An antioxidant, idebenone (short-chain analogue of coenzyme Q10), administered orally at 5 to 20 mg/kg/day with or without vitamin E has demonstrated inconsistent effects on neurologic, cardiac, and psychosocial outcome measures in clinical trials.
- Further research with various antioxidants and iron chelators is ongoing. An open-label pilot study of antioxidants (coenzyme Q10, 400 mg/day, and vitamin E, 2100 U/day) in a small cohort demonstrated slowing in progression of generalized ataxia and kinetic dysfunction and significant improvement in cardiac function with unaltered deterioration in posture, gait, and hand dexterity.

CHRONIC Rx

Chronic management of congestive heart failure is required. Cardiac arrhythmias will warrant pacemaker implantation.

DISPOSITION

- Loss of ambulation typically occurs within 15 yr of symptom onset, and 95% are wheelchair bound by age 45 yr.
- Life expectancy is reduced, particularly if heart disease with or without diabetes mellitus is present.

REFERRAL

- If uncertain about diagnosis
- For genetic counseling (recommended if available)

PEARLS & CONSIDERATIONS

Friedreich's ataxia should be considered in all preadolescent and adolescent children presenting with progressive ataxia. Early recognition of cardiac failure and arrhythmias and institution of appropriate therapy helps prolong survival.

SUGGESTED READINGS

available at www.expertconsult.com

RELATED CONTENT

Friedreich's Ataxia (Patient Information)

AUTHOR: **FARIHA ZAHEER, M.D.**

BASIC INFORMATION

DEFINITION

Frostbite represents tissue injury (or death) from freezing and vasoconstriction induced by severe environmental cold exposure.

SYNONYMS

Cold-induced tissue injury

ICD-9CM CODES
991.3 Frostbite
ICD-10CM CODES

T35.0	Superficial frostbite involving multiple body regions
T34	Frostbite with tissue necrosis
T34.5	Frostbite with tissue necrosis of wrist and hand
T34.8	Frostbite with tissue necrosis of ankle and foot
T34.9	Frostbite with tissue necrosis of other and unspecified sites
T35.4	Superficial frostbite involving multiple body regions
T33.9	Superficial frostbite of unspecified sites, initial encounter

EPIDEMIOLOGY & DEMOGRAPHICS

- Environmental factors include wind chill factor, temperature, duration of exposure, altitude, and degree of wetness. Hands and feet account for 90% of injuries; nose, cheeks, ears, and male genitalia are also more susceptible.
- Host factors include psychiatric illness, neuroleptic and sedative drugs (especially alcohol), immobility, previous frostbite, malnutrition, tobacco use, peripheral neuropathy, peripheral vascular disease, diabetes, exhaustion, and constricting clothing and footwear.

PHYSICAL FINDINGS & CLINICAL PRESENTATION

- Frostbite may be classified into four degrees of injury severity (determined after rewarming) or, more practically, into *superficial* and *deep* groups. This can only be accurately determined after rewarming as initially most frostbite injuries appear similar.
- *Superficial* frostbite involves the skin and subcutaneous tissue. The frozen part is waxy, white (or mottled), and firm but soft and resilient below the surface when gently depressed. After rewarming, there is an initial hyperemia that may be followed by swelling and formation of superficial blisters with clear or milky fluid within 6 to 24 hr (Fig. 1-391). There is no ultimate tissue loss.
- *Deep* frostbite extends into the dermis and may involve muscles, nerves, tendons, or bones. The skin may be hard or wooden, without tissue resilience. Nonblanching cyanosis, hemorrhagic blisters, tissue necrosis (Fig. 1-392), and gangrene may develop. Affected tissue has a poor prognosis and debridement or amputation is generally required.
- Patients initially feel numbness, prickling, and itching. More severe injury can produce paresthesias and stiffness, with burning or throbbing pain on thawing.

ETIOLOGY

Two mechanisms of tissue injury:

1. Freeze-thaw damage. Intracellular ice crystallization leads to cell membrane lysis and cell death followed by thaw-initiated ischemia-reperfusion injury.
2. Vascular stasis and ischemia. Vessels fluctuate between constriction and dilation (the "hunting response") with associated vascular leak and coagulation; ischemia/infarction ensues from a cascade of inflammatory mediators (prostaglandin F, thromboxane A_2, bradykinins, histamine) that contribute to reperfusion injury and thrombus formation and ultimately lead to destruction of the microcirculation and cell death.

DIAGNOSIS

DIFFERENTIAL DIAGNOSIS

- Frostnip: a superficial nonfreezing cold injury associated with intense vasoconstriction and characterized by frost forming on the surface of the skin. Transient numbness, tingling, and pallor resolve quickly with warming.
- Pernio (chilblains): self-limited, cold-induced vasculitis associated with purple plaques or nodules, often affecting dorsum of hands and feet; seen with prolonged cold exposure to above-freezing temperatures
- Cold immersion (trench foot): caused by ischemic injury resulting from sustained, severe vasoconstriction in appendages exposed to wet cold at temperatures above freezing

WORKUP

- Laboratory work is not indicated unless the patient has systemic hypothermia.
- MRI/MRA or triple-phase bone scanning (with technetium) may be used to predict tissue viability in cases of severe frostbite or when thrombolysis is being considered. (MRA has the advantage of showing occluded vessels and viability of surrounding tissues.)

TREATMENT (3 PHASES)

1. FIELD MANAGEMENT

- Prioritize treatment of hypothermia (core body temperature <35° C) with systemic and adjunctive rewarming measures if available (e.g., warmed, humidified oxygen, heated IV saline [45° C], and warming blankets) before thawing frostbitten extremities.
- Remove constricting or wet clothing. Pat dry, insulate, splint, and elevate affected areas.
- Never rub or massage the affected area. Avoid dry heat (e.g., fires and heaters)
- Avoid thawing if there is any risk of refreezing and avoid ambulation on thawed lower extremities (unless only distal toes affected).
- Administer pain medication and topical aloe if available.
- Hydrate.
- Box E1-29 describes the Alaska State Guidelines for prehospital treatment of frostbite.

2. REWARMING

- Rapid rewarming is the key objective.
- Immerse affected area in circulating warm water bath with or without a mild antibacterial agent (e.g., chlorhexidene or povidone-iodine) maintained at 37° to 39° C for at least 30 min, until all tissues are thoroughly rewarmed and pliable with a red-purple color. Water should be continually monitored and warmed to the target temperature. Active motion during rewarming is advisable; massage is not.
- Slow thawing is acceptable when this is not possible. For example, relocating to a warm location and warming with adjacent body heat (e.g., axilla or abdomen) from the patient or caregiver.

3. POST-THAW Rx

- Tetanus prophylaxis and topical antibiotics if potentially contaminated skin wound.
- Consider systemic antibiotics for patients with significant trauma or signs of infection.

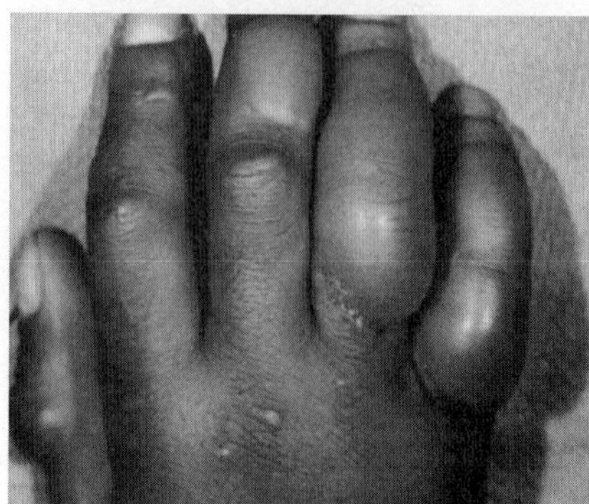

FIGURE 1-391 Large, clear frostbite blisters on the right hand. (From Rosen P [ed]: *Emergency medicine*, ed 4, St Louis, 1998, Mosby.)

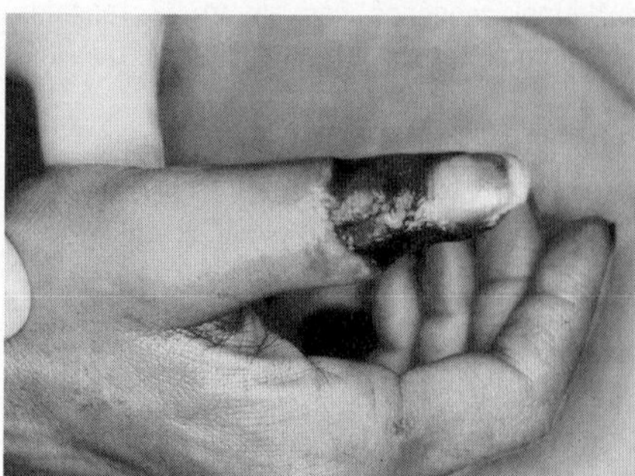

FIGURE 1-392 Third- and fourth-degree frostbite with tissue death. Note demarcation beyond the interphalangeal joint. (From Cameron, JL, Cameron AM: *Current surgical therapy*, ed 10, Philadelphia, 2011, Saunders.)

TABLE 1-197 Frostbite Management: Drugs, Doses, and Modes of Action and Rationale*

Intervention	Dose	Action
Aspirin	75-250 mg orally once daily	Antiplatelet agent, improve rheology
Ibuprofen	400 mg bid or tid orally	Antiprostaglandin effect
Aloe vera gel or cream	With dressing changes every 6 hr	Topical antiprostaglandin effect
Oxygen	2 L/min above 4000 m (13,123 ft) or when Spo_2 is below 90%	Improve tissue oxygenation
Hyperbaric oxygen therapy	2-2.5 atm 1-2 hr daily	Improve tissue oxygenation, improve rheology
Iloprost	2-10 mg/hr IV titrated against side effects	Vasodilator, improve rheology
Nitroglycerin	100 mcg IA single dose	Vasodilator
Papaverine	300 mg over 1hr IA	Vasodilator
Reserpine	0.1 to 0.25 mg once daily	Vasodilator
Buflomedil	400 mg IV **or** 300 mg bid orally	Vasodilator, improve rheology
Pentoxifylline	400 mg tid orally for 2-6 weeks	Vasodilator, improve rheology
10% Dextran 40	20 mL bolus, 20 mL/hr IV	Improve rheology
t-PA	1 mg/hr IA or IV	Thrombolytic agent
LMW heparin	Prophylactic dosage subcutaneously	DVT prevention, anticoagulant
	Therapeutic dosage subcutaneously	Maintain patency of recently thrombolysed vessels
Tetanus prophylaxis		

bid, Twice a day; *DVT,* deep vein thrombosis; *IA,* intra-arterially; *IV,* intravenously; *LMW,* low molecular weight; *Spo_2,* oxygen saturation as measured by pulse oximetry; *tid,* 3 times a day; *t-PA,* tissue plasminogen activator.

*This table is intended to be used as a potential frostbite formulary reference, not as a protocol for treatment. See text for further discussion.

From Auerbach P: *Wilderness medicine, Expert Consult premium edition—enhanced online features and print,* Philadelphia, 2012, Saunders.

- Debride broken clear vesicles and avoid disrupting intact blisters (especially hemorrhagic ones) unless they interfere with mobility.
- Topical aloe vera q6h and ibuprofen 400 to 600 mg bid to tid (or daily aspirin) for several weeks may be beneficial for antiprostaglandin and thromboxane inhibiting effect.
- Thrombolytic therapy. If <24 hr from thawing in a patient with severe frostbite involving an extremity (e.g., extending proximally to PIP joints), imaging (with MR angiography or technetium bone scan) to assess for arterial compromise followed by intra-arterial or intravenous thrombolytic therapy appears to improve reperfusion considerably and reduce subsequent digit amputation.
- Vasodilator therapy. A prospective study of 47 patients comparing prostacyclin and aspirin with or without tPA showed better results with prostacyclin alone; those authors endorse treatment with aspirin plus prostacyclin and consideration of adding tPA for severe frostbite. A direct comparison of prostacyclin vs tPA has not been done.
- Daily dressing changes with dry, sterile, noncompressive, and nonadherent dressings. Splint and elevate hands and feet to reduce edema and separate digits with cotton gauze. Avoid even slightest abrasion to limit risk of infection.
- Whirlpool hydrotherapy with warm water (37-39° C) and an antiseptic for 30 min bid until there is a clear demarcation of necrotic tissues or evidence of tissue healing.
- Gentle, progressive physical therapy after edema resolves.
- Keep site warm, and avoid all vasoconstrictors, including nicotine.
- Dextran, heparin, warfarin, sympathectomy, and hyperbaric oxygen are of potential but unproven benefit.
- Table 1-197 describes drugs used in frostbite management.

DISPOSITION

A majority of patients have long-term residual symptoms, including neuropathic pain, sensory deficits, hyperhidrosis, secondary Raynaud's disease, edema, hair or nail deformities, and (rarely) arthritis. Treatment with tricyclics, calcium channel blockers, and careful protection from further cold exposure may be helpful.

REFERRAL

- Hospitalize for hypothermia or deep frostbite; a burn unit is best.
- Surgical decisions regarding amputation should be deferred until demarcation of viable tissue is clear (1 to 3 mo) unless refractory pain, sepsis, or gangrene occurs.

SUGGESTED READINGS

available at www.expertconsult.com

RELATED CONTENT

Frostbite (Patient Information)

AUTHOR: **MICHAEL P. JOHNSON, M.D.**

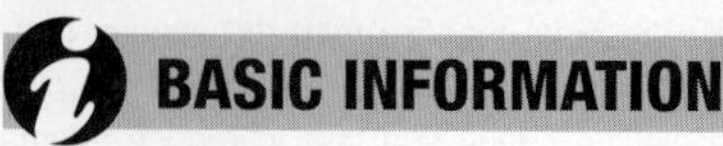

BASIC INFORMATION

DEFINITION

Frozen shoulder is a clinical diagnosis that describes a stiffened glenohumeral (GH) joint characterized by shoulder pain and restricted passive and active range of motion (ROM) (Fig. 1-393). The condition is categorized as primary or idiopathic when there is no underlying cause and secondary when there is an associated precipitating event such as shoulder surgery or identifiable cause such as rotator cuff tears or proximal humerus fractures.

SYNONYMS

Adhesive capsulitis
Periarthritis
Pericapsulitis
Check-rein shoulder
Bursitis Duplay

ICD-9CM CODES
726.0 Adhesive shoulder capsulitis
ICD-10CM CODES
M75.00 Adhesive capsulitis of unspecified shoulder

EPIDEMIOLOGY & DEMOGRAPHICS

- Prevalence of frozen shoulder is 2% to 5% in the general population. There is a higher incidence of up to 10% to 20% in people with diabetes.
- Predominant sex: Females are affected more often than males.
- Most commonly affects patients 40 to 70 years with a peak incidence in the mid-50s.

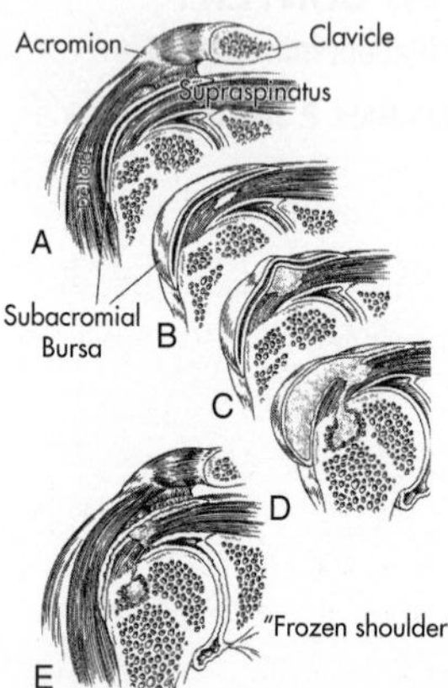

FIGURE 1-393 Sequence of events terminating in frozen shoulder. A, Normal structures of the shoulder. **B,** Supraspinatus tendonitis, sometimes calcific, in the "critical zone." **C,** Spread of inflammation to the tendon sheath and a bulge into the floor of the subacromial bursa. **D,** Rupture into the subacromial bursa and extension of the inflammatory process as an osteitis into the humeral head and greater tuberosity. **E,** Frozen shoulder with involvement of tendons, bursa, capsule, synovium, and muscle with fibrous contracture and markedly diminished volume of the shoulder joint space. (From Noble J [ed]: *Primary care medicine,* ed 2, St Louis, 1996, Mosby.)

PHYSICAL FINDINGS & CLINICAL PRESENTATION

The natural history of frozen shoulder occurs in three phases that usually include full resolution of pain and return of function.

- Painful phase: There is a gradual onset of a painful shoulder that is usually worse at night and difficulty lying on the affected side. This may last from weeks to months.
- Frozen or Intermediate phase: Progressive shoulder stiffness and limitation in range of motion that may last for 1 year. Pain usually is less during this phase. In addition to tenderness on palpation of the GH joint, exam findings may include disuse atrophy of the deltoid and supraspinatus, with the arm held in adduction and internal rotation. There is variable loss in the degrees of restricted active and passive shoulder abduction and external rotation.
- Thawing or Recovery phase: Overall improvement in pain and increase in ROM. This may last for 5-24 months.

ETIOLOGY

- The pathology of frozen shoulder involves a chronic inflammatory response with fibroblastic proliferation.
- Factors that predispose to increased risk for developing a frozen shoulder include:
  1. Prolonged shoulder immobility from trauma (including fracture of the femoral head and neck), surgery, and overuse injuries.
  2. Systemic diseases (diabetes, thyroid disease, stroke, Parkinson's, cardiovascular disease, and inflammatory disease).
- Fig. 1-393 illustrates the sequence of events terminating in frozen shoulder.

DIAGNOSIS

DIFFERENTIAL DIAGNOSIS

- Trauma: shoulder sprain, dislocation, glenoid labrum tear, rotator cuff tear
- Usage, degenerative, and age-related disorders: GH osteoarthritis, avascular necrosis of the humeral head, rotator cuff tendonopathy
- Mechanical: calcific tendonitis, shoulder impingement or derangement
- Neoplasm: Pancoast tumor
- Cervical spondylosis or other cervical disk disease
- Brachial neuritis
- Milwaukee shoulder

WORKUP

- Laboratory studies only contribute to the diagnosis if an underlying condition such as diabetes, cardiovascular disease, or thyroid disease is suspected.
- A subacromial injection test helps to distinguish a frozen shoulder from subacromial disorders.
- Radiographic evaluation of the shoulder with plain x-rays, ultrasound, MRI, or MR arthrography should be considered to rule out other pathologic conditions.
- Characteristic MRI findings can include thickening of the coracohumeral ligament and the joint capsule.
- Musculoskeletal ultrasound can be helpful in demonstrating characteristic soft-tissue findings and limitation in the movement of the supraspinatous tendon during shoulder abduction on dynamic imaging.

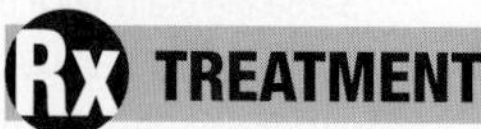

TREATMENT

NONPHARMACOLOGIC THERAPY

Patient education is important in prevention and to improve compliance and outcome expectation.

ACUTE GENERAL Rx

- Initial conservative therapy with heat, analgesics (generally NSAIDs), and physical therapy with passive stretching and ROM exercises
- Course of oral corticosteroids
- Local or intra-articular steroid and lidocaine injection into the subacromial space with or without hydrodilation
- When conservative treatment fails, the following surgical methods may be considered:
  - Shoulder manipulation under anesthesia (rarely needed)
  - Arthroscopic and, rarely, open capsular release

DISPOSITION

- The condition is mostly self-limited. Most patients regain 90% of shoulder motion over time and have improved pain, but symptoms can last from several months to more than 3 years.
- Recurrence in the same shoulder is rare, although it can affect the opposite limb in up to 6% to 17% of patients.

REFERRAL

Rheumatology or orthopedic consultation in patients with resistant disease who fail to respond to conservative treatment

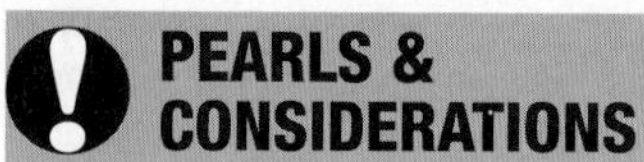

PEARLS & CONSIDERATIONS

COMMENTS

- Arthroscopic shoulder release has been shown to provide beneficial clinical outcome for patients with refractory adhesive capsulitis.

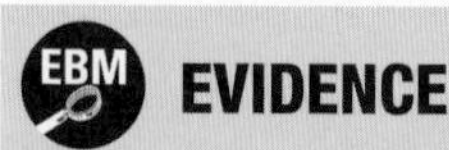

EVIDENCE

available at www.expertconsult.com

SUGGESTED READINGS

available at www.expertconsult.com

RELATED CONTENT

Frozen Shoulder (Patient Information)
Rotator Cuff Syndrome (Related Key Topic)

AUTHOR: **ANISHKA S. ROLLE, M.D.**

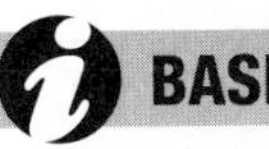

BASIC INFORMATION

DEFINITION

Galactorrhea can be defined as inappropriate lactation (in the absence of pregnancy or postpartum state) as a result of nonphysiologic augmentation of prolactin release.

ICD-9CM CODES
611.6 Galactorrhea
ICD-10CM CODES
N64.3 Galactorrhea not associated with childbirth

PHYSICAL FINDINGS & CLINICAL PRESENTATION

- Milky discharge from nipples (Fig. 1-394) usually occurring bilaterally
- Evidence of chest wall irritation from ill-fitting clothing, herpes zoster, or atopic dermatitis may be present
- Visual field defects (bitemporal hemianopsia) may be present with prolactinomas, particularly if large such as macroadenomas
- Headaches may also occur in cases of large pituitary adenomas
- Evidence of acromegaly, Cushing's disease, or hypothyroidism when galactorrhea is caused by these disorders

ETIOLOGY

- Medications (phenothiazines, metoclopramide, selective serotonin reuptake inhibitors, anxiolytics, buspirone, atenolol, valproic acid, conjugated estrogen and medroxyprogesterone, methyldopa, verapamil, H_2 receptor blockers, octreotide, danazol, tricyclic antidepressants, isoniazid, amphetamine, reserpine, opiates, sumatriptan, rimantadine, oral contraceptive formulations); after infancy, galactorrhea is often medication induced
- Breast stimulation (prolonged suckling), sexual intercourse

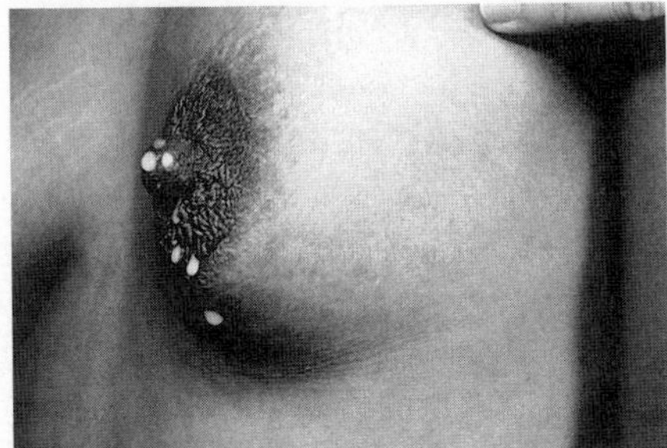

FIGURE 1-394 Galactorrhea. Milk production in a nonpregnant woman resulting from a prolactinoma. (From Haines DE: *Fundamental neuroscience for basic and clinical applications,* ed 3, Philadelphia, 2006, Churchill Livingstone.)

- Pituitary tumors (prolactinomas, craniopharyngiomas)
- Chest wall irritation from ill-fitting clothing, herpes zoster, atopic dermatitis, burns
- Hypothyroidism (diminished feedback inhibition increases thyroid-releasing hormone [TRH], which increases prolactin)
- Increased stress, major trauma
- Chronic renal failure (decreased prolactin clearance)
- Cushing's disease
- Herbs (e.g., fennel, red clover, anise, red raspberry, marshmallow)
- Cannabis
- Spinal cord surgery or injury, or tumors
- Severe gastroesophageal reflux disease, esophagitis (stimulation of thoracic nerves by the cervical and thoracic ganglia)
- Breast surgery
- Idiopathic
- Neonatal ("witch's milk" produced by 2% to 5% of neonates because of precipitous drop in maternal estrogen and progesterone postdelivery)
- Lymphomas, Hodgkin's disease, bronchogenic carcinoma, renal adenocarcinomas
- Sarcoidosis and other infiltrative disorders
- Tuberculosis affecting pituitary gland
- Pituitary stalk resection
- Multiple sclerosis
- Empty sella syndrome
- Acromegaly

DIAGNOSIS

DIFFERENTIAL DIAGNOSIS

- Intraductal papilloma
- Breast cancer
- Paget's disease of breast
- Breast abscess

WORKUP

- Complete history focusing on menstrual irregularity, infertility, previous pregnancies, duration of galactorrhea, medications, visual complaints, fatigue. Age of onset is also significant (e.g., prolactinoma most common between ages 20 and 35 yr; neonatal galactorrhea is usually secondary to transplacental transfer of maternal estrogen)
- Physical examination: hirsutism, acne, obesity, visual field defects, goiter
- Breast examination for presence of nodules, evaluation of discharge (milky versus serosanguineous versus purulent)
- Laboratory testing and imaging studies (see "Laboratory Tests")

LABORATORY TESTS

- Prolactin level (elevated, often <200 ng/ml in prolactinoma but may occur at any prolactin level)
- Human chorionic gonadotropin level (positive in pregnancy)
- TSH (elevated in hypothyroidism)
- Blood urea nitrogen, creatinine (elevated in renal failure), glucose (elevated in Cushing's syndrome)
- Urinalysis (hematuria in renal cell carcinoma)
- Microscopic examination of nipple discharge (scant cellular material, numerous fat globules, can be seen without specific staining)

IMAGING STUDIES

- MRI of brain if prolactin level is elevated, amenorrhea is present, or visual field defects are detected on physical examination.
- High-resolution CT of brain with special coronal cuts through the pituitary region may be helpful in patients with contraindications to MRI; however, it may miss small lesions.

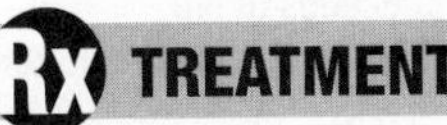

TREATMENT

- Discontinuation of potential offending agents.
- Avoidance of excessive breast stimulation.
- Galactorrhea resulting from prolactinoma can be managed medically or with careful surveillance depending on size and growth of tumor, associated symptoms, and prolactin level. Surgical treatment of prolactinomas is usually reserved for medication failures. Please refer to the topic "Prolactinoma" in Section I for additional information.
- No treatment is necessary for normoprolactinemic patients with idiopathic nonbothersome galactorrhea.
- Normoprolactinemic patients with bothersome galactorrhea may respond to low dose dopamine agonist (e.g., cabergoline 0.25 mg twice weekly).

REFERRAL

Endocrine and surgical consultation if prolactinoma is detected

SUGGESTED READINGS

available at www.expertconsult.com

RELATED CONTENT

Pituitary Adenoma (Related Key Topic)
Prolactinoma (Related Key Topic)
Galactorrhea (Patient Information)

AUTHOR: **FRED F. FERRI, M.D.**

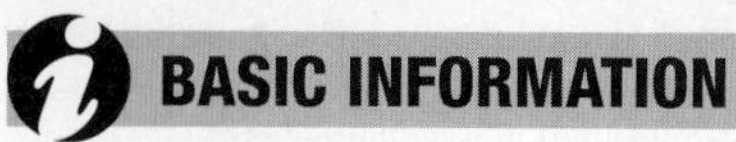

BASIC INFORMATION

DEFINITION

A fluid-filled sac (cyst) overlying a tendon sheath or joint

SYNONYMS

Ganglion

ICD-9CM CODES
727.43 Ganglion
ICD-10CM CODES
M67.4 Ganglion

EPIDEMIOLOGY & DEMOGRAPHICS

- Ganglia are more common in women than men (3:1)
- Can occur at any age, but usually between second and fourth decades of life
- Most common soft tissue tumor of the hand and wrist

PHYSICAL FINDINGS & CLINICAL PRESENTATION

- Most ganglia occur on the dorsum of the wrist (50% to 70%) (Fig. 1-395).
- The volar wrist (18% to 20%) is the next most common site.
- Can also involve the proximal digital flexor tendons and the distal interphalangeal joints.
- Left and right hands are equally affected.
- Ganglia are usually solitary, firm, smooth, round, and fluctuant.
- Pain from mass effect or compression against nearby structure may be present (e.g., median nerve and radial nerve).
- Hand numbness may be present.
- Patient may have hand muscle weakness.
- Ganglia usually develop over a period of months but may arise suddenly.

ETIOLOGY

Ganglia are believed to derive from synovial herniation or expansion from the joint capsule or tendon sheath. Repetitive movement as an etiology is uncertain, although it may cause enlargement of the lesion or worsen symptoms.

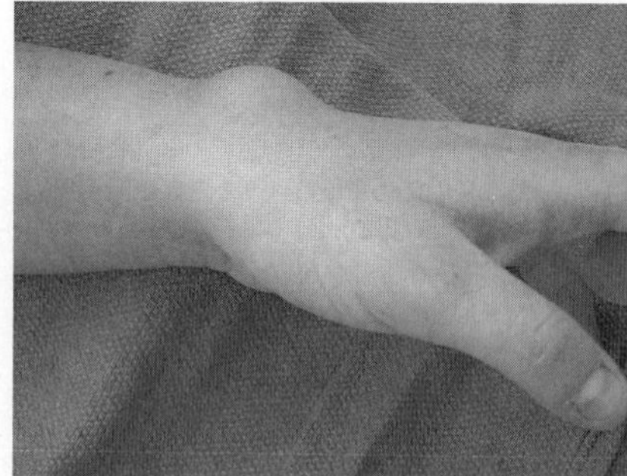

FIGURE 1-395 Dorsal wrist ganglion. (From Hochberg MC et al: *Rheumatology,* ed 5, St Louis, 2011, Mosby.)

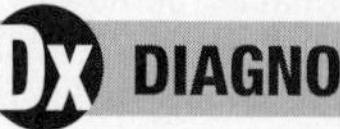

DIAGNOSIS

Direct inspection and localization of the cyst often is enough to make the diagnosis of ganglia. Transillumination is an easy method of differentiating ganglia from solid tumors; ganglia transilluminate while solid tumors do not.

DIFFERENTIAL DIAGNOSIS

- Lipoma
- Fibroma
- Epidermoid inclusion cyst
- Osteochondroma
- Hemangioma
- Infection (tuberculosis, fungi, and secondary syphilis)
- Gout
- Rheumatoid nodule
- Radial artery aneurysm

WORKUP

The workup of ganglia usually consists of history, physical examination, and x-ray imaging.

LABORATORY TESTS

Blood tests are not specific in the diagnosis of ganglia.

IMAGING STUDIES

- Radiographs of the hand and wrist are taken to rule out other bone or joint abnormalities.
- Ultrasound studies are helpful in the diagnosis of ganglia by demonstrating smooth cystic walls that may be septated.
- CT scan can be done if the ultrasound is equivocal.
- MRI helps differentiate malignant bone lesions from cystic structures.
- Arthrography may demonstrate a communication between the joint and ganglia (not commonly done).

Rx TREATMENT

Expectant treatment is appropriate if the mass is not painful or interfering with motor function.

NONPHARMACOLOGIC THERAPY

- Attempts to rupture the cyst by sharp blows with a book or with finger compression are not recommended.
- Aspiration, heat, and sclerotherapy have been tried but have met with high recurrence rates (60%).

ACUTE GENERAL Rx

- Aspiration at the base with a large-bore needle (18-gauge) followed by injection of 20 to 40 mg of triamcinolone acetonide can be tried.
- This may be repeated if the ganglia recurs (35% to 40%).

CHRONIC Rx

Total ganglionectomy and repair of the defect after tracing its connection to the tendon sheath is effective and the surgical procedure of choice.

DISPOSITION

- Ganglia spontaneously resolve in approximately 40% to 50% of cases.
- Aspiration with steroid injection is successful in approximately 65% of cases.
- Surgery provides cure in 85% to 95% of the cases.
- Complications of ganglia include:
  1. Carpal tunnel syndrome with pain and muscle atrophy
  2. Radial nerve impingement
  3. Radial artery compression
- Complications of ganglion surgery include:
  1. Infection
  2. Recurrence (5% to 15%), usually from inadequate excision
  3. Reflex sympathetic dystrophy
  4. Scar formation

REFERRAL

It is best to refer patients with symptomatic ganglia to a hand surgeon.

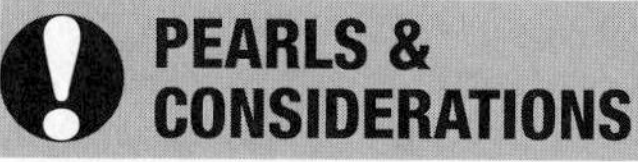

PEARLS & CONSIDERATIONS

- Dorsal ganglia usually originate from the scapholunate ligament.
- Volar ganglia typically originate between the tendons of the flexor carpi radialis and brachioradialis.

COMMENTS

A ganglion's synovial membrane maintains its secretory function. Aspiration of ganglia often demonstrates a viscous, mucinous, clear fluid containing albumin, globulin, and hyaluronic acid.

SUGGESTED READINGS

available at www.expertconsult.com

RELATED CONTENT

Ganglia (Patient Information)

AUTHORS: **RYAN W. ZUZEK, M.D.,** and **IMMAD SADIQ, M.D.**

G

Diseases and Disorders

BASIC INFORMATION

DEFINITION

Gardner's syndrome is a subset of familial adenomatous polyposis (FAP), with prominent extraintestinal manifestations. It is a highly penetrant autosomal-dominant condition characterized by the following:

- Adenomatous intestinal polyps
- Soft tissue tumors
- Osteomas

SYNONYMS

Familial adenomatous polyposis

ICD-9CM CODES
211.3 Familial adenomatous polyposis
ICD-10CM CODES
D12.5 Benign neoplasm of sigmoid colon
D12.4 Benign neoplasm of descending colon
D12.3 Benign neoplasm of transverse colon
D12.2 Benign neoplasm of ascending colon
D12.6 Benign neoplasm of colon, unspecified

EPIDEMIOLOGY & DEMOGRAPHICS

- FAP occurs in approximately 1 in 10,000 births.
- FAP accounts for <1% of all colorectal cancers.
- Individuals develop hundreds to thousands of adenomatous colorectal polyps.
- Polyps usually present in adolescence.
- 100% lifetime risk for colorectal cancer; most diagnosed by 40 yr of age.
- Gastric, duodenal, periampullary, and small bowel polyps occur but have lower malignant potential.
- Increased risk for other tumors: desmoid (15%), duodenal/periampullary (7%), thyroid (2%), brain (1%), childhood hepatoblastoma (1%), nasopharyngeal angiofibroma, pancreatic (2%), adrenal adenoma (10%), and gastric (1%).

PHYSICAL FINDINGS & CLINICAL PRESENTATION

Phenotypic variability is seen in individuals and families with the same mutation. Soft tissue and bone abnormalities may precede intestinal disease. These findings are reported in at least 20% of individuals with FAP.

- Congenital hypertrophy of the retinal pigment epithelium (CHRPE): benign fundus lesions, usually present at birth
- Dental abnormalities: supernumerary or unerupted teeth
- Soft tissue lesions: epidermal or sebaceous cysts, fibromas, lipomas, desmoid tumors (benign, locally invasive, aggressive connective tissue tumor)
- Osteomas (benign bone growths): skull, mandible, long bone
- Anemia, occult blood in stool, bowel obstruction, weight loss

ETIOLOGY

- Caused by mutations of the tumor suppressor gene adenomatous polyposis coli *(APC)* on chromosome 5q21-q22; more than 1000 diseases causing mutations identified. The site of the mutation may explain the prominent extraintestinal lesions found in Gardner's syndrome.
- De novo mutations are responsible for approximately 20% of FAP cases. A subset of these patients have somatic cell mosaicism, which is seen when a new mutation occurs in the APC gene post-fertilization and is present in only a subset of cell types or tissues.

DIAGNOSIS

In individuals with a family history, more than 100 adenomatous colorectal polyps, CHRPE lesions, or genetic testing confirms diagnosis. In those without a family history, more than 100 adenomatous colorectal polyps suggest the diagnosis and genetic testing confirms it.

DIFFERENTIAL DIAGNOSIS

- Turcot's syndrome
- Attenuated FAP
- MUTYH-associated polyposis
- Peutz-Jeghers syndrome
- Juvenile polyposis syndrome
- Hereditary mixed polyposis syndrome
- Hyperplastic polyposis

WORKUP

History, physical examination, laboratory tests, imaging studies

DIAGNOSTIC SCREENING OPTIONS

GENETIC TESTING

NOTE: Genetic counseling should be performed and written informed consent obtained before testing. Refer to a specialized center for counseling and evaluation.

- Should be offered to first-degree relatives of affected individuals (with an identified mutation) at age 10 to 12 yr and clinically suspected individuals.
- Able to identify a mutation in approximately 80% of families. To ensure that the family has a detectable mutation, test an affected family member first.
- If positive in the affected individual, the test can differentiate with 100% accuracy affected and unaffected family members. If negative in the affected individual, screening family members will not be useful in determining disease status.
- If no known family history exists, screening the clinically suspected individual is reasonable. A positive test rules in FAP but a negative test does not rule it out.
- Numerous testing techniques available; may require multiple tests to identify the mutation.

SIGMOIDOSCOPY

- Individuals with a positive genetic test: annual flexible sigmoidoscopy beginning at 10 to 12 yr of age.
- Untested at-risk family members or patients from families with an unidentified *APC* mutation: annual flexible sigmoidoscopy beginning at 10 to 12 yr until 25 yr of age, then decreasing frequency until age 50 yr, when age-appropriate guidelines may be followed.
- Once adenomatous polyps are detected, patients should undergo colonoscopy and evaluation for colectomy.
- Negative genetic test in patients from families with an identified mutation: average risk screening.

CHRPE: Lesions occur in up to 80% of families and are a reliable indicator of affected status in these families.

TREATMENT

- Prophylactic colectomy or proctocolectomy: timing determined by polyp number, size, and degree of dysplasia.
- Consider celecoxib therapy to reduce polyposis.
- Screening of remaining GI tract and screening for extraintestinal manifestations must continue after colectomy.
  - Annual physical examination: history, examination (including thyroid), and blood tests
  - Upper endoscopy to screen for gastric/duodenal polyps: baseline at age 20 yr (earlier if colon polyps detected) and repeated every 1 to 5 yr based on findings
  - Some recommend annual thyroid ultrasound
  - Other possible cancer sites imaged if symptoms occur or if these cancers have occurred in relatives
- Treat soft tissue lesions and osteomas for symptoms or cosmetic concerns. Treat desmoid tumors if they pose a risk to adjacent structures.

DISPOSITION

- 100% chance of colorectal cancer in untreated individuals. Many other neoplasms occur at higher rates.
- Metastatic colorectal cancer is the leading cause of death (58%), followed by desmoid tumors (11%) and duodenal/periampullary adenocarcinoma (8%).

REFERRAL

- Patients should be managed at centers with expertise in FAP, including a gastroenterologist, medical geneticist, and surgeon.
- Genetic counselors can be found at www.nsgc.org.
- Genetic testing sites can be found at www.genetests.org.

PEARLS & CONSIDERATIONS

- Management should be individualized based on genotype, phenotype, and individual preferences.
- Sulindac (NSAID) and celecoxib (COX-2 inhibitor) cause polyp regression in individuals with FAP. Celecoxib is FDA approved for this indication. Cancer risk remains; neither replaces colon resection for cancer prevention. Small studies suggest combination

therapies and dietary supplements may also be effective in reducing polyposis.
- Desmoid tumors frequently occur in the abdomen and are difficult to treat with high rates of recurrence. Growth and recurrence are stimulated by surgery.
- Screen children of affected parents (from infancy to age 10 yr) with alpha-fetoprotein level, liver enzymes, and liver ultrasound to rule out hepatoblastoma.
- Preimplantation and prenatal genetic testing is available.

SUGGESTED READINGS
available at www.expertconsult.com

RELATED CONTENT
Colorectal Cancer (Related Key Topic)

AUTHOR: **SUDEEP KAUR AULAKH, M.D.**

BASIC INFORMATION

DEFINITION

Gastric cancer is an adenocarcinoma arising from the stomach.

SYNONYMS

Stomach cancer
Linitis plastica

ICD-9CM CODES
451 Malignant neoplasm of stomach
ICD-10CM CODES
C16 Malignant neoplasm of stomach
C16.0 Malignant neoplasm of cardia of stomach
C16.1 Malignant neoplasm of stomach
C16.2 Malignant neoplasm of body of stomach
C16.3 Malignant neoplam of pyloric antrum
C16.5 Malignant neoplasm of lesser curvature of stomach, unspecified
C16.6 Malignant neoplasm of greater curvature of stomach, unspecified
C16.8 Malignant neoplasm of overlapping sites of stomach

EPIDEMIOLOGY & DEMOGRAPHICS

- Annual incidence of gastric cancer in the U.S. is seven cases per 100,000 persons. The incidence is much higher in Japan, with rates as high as 80 cases per 100,000 persons.
- Most gastric cancers arise in the antrum (35%).
- The incidence of distal stomach tumors has greatly declined, whereas that of proximal tumors of the cardia and fundus is on the rise.
- Gastric cancer occurs most commonly in male patients >65 yr (70% of patients are >50 yr).
- Incidence of gastric cancer has been declining over the past 30 yr.
- Male/female ratio is 3:2.
- Familiar diffuse gastric cancer is a disease with autosomal-dominant inheritance in which gastric cancer develops at a young age. Germline truncating mutations in the E-cadherin gene *(CDH1)* are found in these families.

PHYSICAL FINDINGS & CLINICAL PRESENTATION

- Medical history may reveal complaints of postprandial fullness with significant weight loss (70% to 80%), nausea/emesis (20% to 40%), dysphagia (20%), and dyspepsia, usually unrelieved by antacids; epigastric discomfort, usually lessened by fasting and exacerbated by food intake, is also common.
- Epigastric or abdominal mass (30% to 50%), epigastric pain.
- Skin pallor from anemia.
- Hard, nodular liver: generally indicates metastatic disease to the liver.
- Hemoccult-positive stools.
- Ascites, lymphadenopathy, or pleural effusions: may indicate metastasis.

ETIOLOGY

Risk factors:

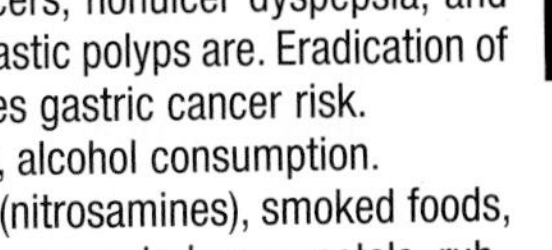

- Chronic *Helicobacter pylori* gastritis. Gastric cancer develops in persons infected with *H. pylori* but not in uninfected persons. Those with histologic findings of severe gastric atrophy, corpus-predominant gastritis, or intestinal metaplasia are at increased risk. Persons with *H. pylori* infection and duodenal ulcer are not at risk, whereas those with gastric ulcers, nonulcer dyspepsia, and gastric hyperplastic polyps are. Eradication of *H. pylori* reduces gastric cancer risk.
- Tobacco abuse, alcohol consumption.
- Food additives (nitrosamines), smoked foods, occupational exposure to heavy metals, rubber, asbestos.
- Chronic atrophic gastritis with intestinal metaplasia, hypertrophic gastritis, and pernicious anemia.

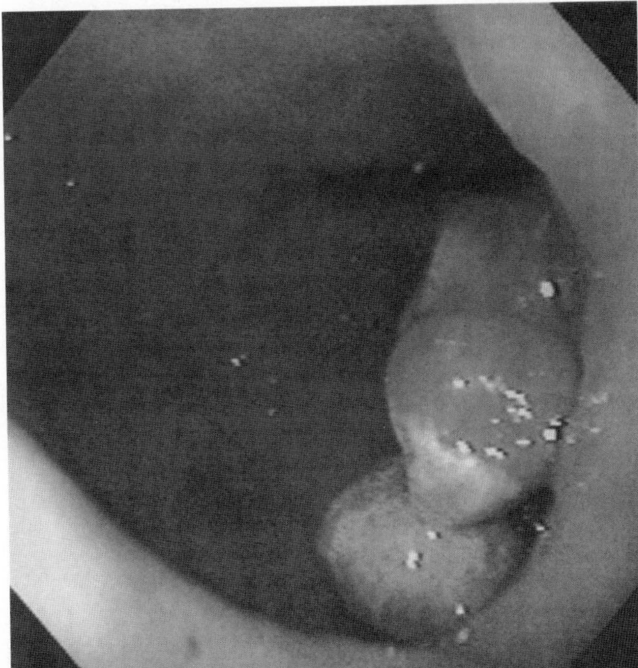

FIGURE 1-396 Polypoid gastric cancer. A trilobed polyp is apparent at the angularis. (From Feldman M, Friedman LS, Brandt LJ [eds]: *Sleisenger & Fordtran's gastrointestinal and liver disease: pathophysiology/diagnosis/management,* ed 8, Philadelphia, 2006, Saunders.)

DIAGNOSIS

DIFFERENTIAL DIAGNOSIS

- Gastric lymphoma (5% of gastric malignancies)
- Hypertrophic gastritis
- Peptic ulcer
- Reflux esophagitis

WORKUP

Upper endoscopy (Fig. 1-396) with biopsy will confirm diagnosis. Endoscopic ultrasonography in combination with CT scanning and operative lymph node dissection can be used in staging of the tumor. Table 1-198 describes staging systems for gastric carcinoma.

LABORATORY TESTS

- Microcytic anemia
- Hemoccult-positive stools
- Hypoalbuminemia
- Abnormal liver enzymes in patients with metastasis to the liver
- Mutation-specific predictive genetic testing by polymerase chain reaction amplification followed by restriction: enzyme digestion and DNA sequencing for truncating mutations in *CDH1* is recommended in families of patients with familial diffuse cancer because gastric cancer develops in three of every four carriers of a mutant *CDH1* gene.

IMAGING STUDIES

Abdominal CT scan (Fig. 1-397) to evaluate for metastasis (70% accurate for regional node metastases)

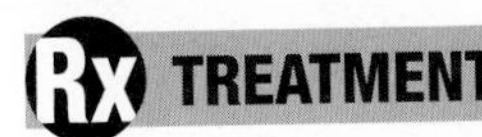

TREATMENT

ACUTE GENERAL Rx

- Gastrectomy with regional lymphadenectomy is performed in patients with curative potential (<30% of patients at time of diagnosis). In patients with operable gastric cancer, a perioperative regimen of epirubicin, cisplatin, and infused fluorouracil decreases tumor size and stage and significantly improves progression-free and overall survival. Postoperative adjuvant chemoradiation therapy using 5-fluorouracil (5-FU) and leucovorin is now the standard of care for resected patients able to tolerate such treatment. Postoperative chemotherapy and radiotherapy, compared with surgical resection alone, can extend

TABLE 1-198 Staging Systems for Gastric Carcinoma*

Modified Astler-Coller	TNM	Characteristics
A	TisN0	Nodes negative; lesion limited to mucosa
B1	T1–2N0	Nodes negative; extension of lesion beyond mucosa but still within gastric wall
B2	T3N0	Nodes negative; extension beyond the entire wall (including serosa if present) without adherence to or invasion of surrounding organs or structures
B3	T4N0	Nodes negative; beyond wall with adherence to or invasion of surrounding organs or structures
C1	Tis–2N1–3	Nodes positive; lesion limited to wall
C2	T3N1–3	Nodes positive; extension of lesion through the entire wall (including serosa)
C3	T4N1–3	Nodes positive; beyond wall with adherence to or invasion of surrounding organs or structures

*Comparison of TNM system with a modification of the Astler-Coller rectal system by Gunderson and Sosin.
From Abeloff MD: *Clinical oncology,* ed 3, Philadelphia, 2004, Elsevier.

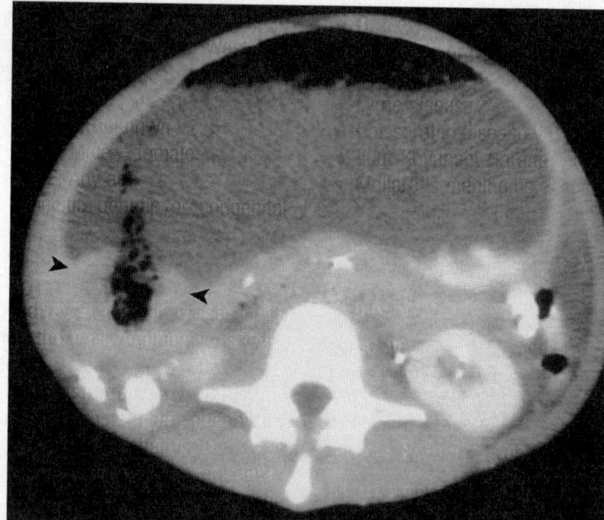

FIGURE 1-397 Gastric outlet obstruction—cancer of the antrum. A markedly distended stomach with an air-fluid level is seen on computed tomography. In this case a mass in the distal end of the antrum is apparent *(arrowheads).* (From Grainger RG, Allison DJ, Dixon AK [eds]. *Grainger & Allison's diagnostic radiology: a textbook of medical imaging,* ed 4, St. Louis, 2001, Churchill Livingstone.)

the survival rate of patients with gastric cancer in those who are able to complete adjuvant therapy.

- When surgical cure is not possible, palliative resection may prolong duration and quality of life.
- Chemotherapy (5-FU, Adriamycin, and mitomycin C) may provide some palliation; however, it generally does not prolong survival. Chemotherapy with docetaxel, cisplatin, and 5-FU can be used for chemotherapy-naive patients with metastatic or locally recurrent gastric cancer. The addition of trastuzumab to cisplatin plus 5-FU or capecitabine may prolong survival in gastric cancer patients expressing HER2.

DISPOSITION

- 5-yr survival rate of gastric carcinoma is 12% overall.
- 5-yr survival for early gastric cancers (usually detected incidentally with endoscopy in populations where screening is recommended) is >35%.

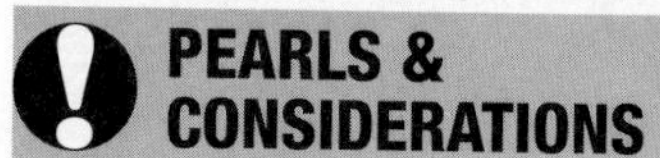

PEARLS & CONSIDERATIONS

COMMENTS

- Gastrectomy patients will need vitamin B_{12} replacement. They are also at risk for dumping syndrome and should be advised to ingest frequent, small meals.
- Prophylactic gastrectomy should be considered in young, asymptomatic carriers of germ-line truncating *CDH1* mutations who belong to families with highly penetrant heredity diffuse gastric cancer.

SUGGESTED READINGS

available at www.expertconsult.com

RELATED CONTENT

Stomach Cancer (Patient Information)

AUTHOR: **FRED F. FERRI, M.D.**

BASIC INFORMATION

DEFINITION

Gastrinoma is a pancreatic or extrapancreatic non-beta islet cell tumor which secretes gastrin. The hypergastrinemic state caused by a gastrinoma results in peptic ulcer disease and is known as Zollinger-Ellison (ZE) syndrome

SYNONYMS

Zollinger-Ellison (ZE) syndrome

ICD-9CM CODES
251.5 Zollinger-Ellison syndrome
ICD-10CM CODES
E16.4 Abnormal secretion of gastrin

EPIDEMIOLOGY & DEMOGRAPHICS

- Incidence is unknown, but 0.1% of all duodenal ulcers are believed to be caused by ZE.
- Occurs in both genders and at any age (most common in ages 30 to 50 yr).
- Two thirds of gastrinomas are sporadic, and one third are associated with multiple endocrine neoplasia type 1 (MEN-1), an autosomal-dominant genetic disorder that also includes hyperparathyroidism and pituitary tumors.
- Approximately 60% of gastrinomas are malignant.
- The incidence and prevalence of pancreatic neuroendocrine tumors are increasing. They represent 1.3% of all cases of pancreatic cancer.

PHYSICAL FINDINGS & CLINICAL PRESENTATION

- The majority of patients (95%) present with symptoms of peptic ulcer (see Section I, "Peptic Ulcer Disease").
- 60% of patients have symptoms related to gastroesophageal reflux disease (see Section I, "Gastroesophageal Reflux Disease").
- One third of patients with ZE have diarrhea and, less commonly, steatorrhea.

The following circumstances warrant suspicion of ZE syndrome:

- Ulcers distal to the first portion of the duodenum
- Multiple peptic ulcers
- Ineffective treatment for peptic ulcer disease with the usual drug doses and schedules
- Peptic ulcer and diarrhea
- Familial history of peptic ulcer
- Patients with a personal or family history suggesting parathyroid or pituitary tumors or dysfunction
- Peptic ulcer and urinary tract calculi
- Patients with peptic ulcer who are negative for *Helicobacter pylori* and do not have a history of nonsteroidal anti-inflammatory drug use

ETIOLOGY

- The pathophysiologic manifestations of ZE syndrome are related to the effects of hypergastrinemia. Gastrin stimulates gastric acid secretion, which in turn is responsible for the development of duodenal ulcers and diarrhea. Gastrin also promotes gastric mucosal epithelial cell growth and resulting parietal cell hyperplasia.
- Gastrinomas are usually small (0.1 to 2 cm) but sometimes large (>20 cm) tumors.
- 60% of gastrinomas are malignant, with liver and regional lymph nodes the most common site of metastases. Histology is not a good predictor of the biology of gastrinomas.
- 60% of patients with MEN-1 have gastrinomas.
- 10% of patients with ZE syndrome have islet cell hyperplasia rather than gastrinomas; in 10% to 20% of patients with gastrinoma the tumors cannot be located because of small size.

Dx DIAGNOSIS

DIFFERENTIAL DIAGNOSIS

- Peptic ulcer disease (see Section I, "Peptic Ulcer Disease")
- Gastroesophageal reflux disease (see Section I, "Gastroesophageal Reflux Disease")
- Diarrhea (see Section III, "Diarrhea, Acute" and "Diarrhea, Chronic")

WORKUP

- Diagnosis of peptic ulcer:
  - Upper gastrointestinal series (may also show prominent gastric rugal folds)
  - Endoscopy
- Gastric acid secretion:
  - Serum gastrin level (fasting) >150 pg/ml (criterion for diagnosis is serum gastrin >1000 pg/ml) (causes of false-positive results: pernicious anemia, renal failure, retained gastric antrum syndrome, diabetes mellitus, rheumatoid arthritis)
- Provocative gastrin level tests:
  - Secretin stimulation
  - Calcium stimulation
  - Standard test meal stimulation
- Gastrinoma localization:
  - Arteriography
  - Abdominal sonography
  - Abdominal CT scan
  - Abdominal MRI/PET scan
  - Selective portal vein branch gastrin level
  - Octreotide scan

Rx TREATMENT

- Surgical resection of the gastrinoma (NOTE: 90% of gastrinomas can be located, resulting in a 40% overall cure rate)
- Total gastrectomy or vagotomy (palliative in some patients)
- Medical treatment
  - Proton pump inhibitors (e.g., omeprazole, lansoprazole)
  - Somatostatin or octreotide
  - Chemotherapy for metastatic gastrinoma with streptozotocin, 5-fluorouracil, and doxorubicin
  - Early trials with everolimus, an oral inhibitor of mammalian target of rapamycin (mTOR) have shown antitumor activity in patients with advanced pancreatic neuroendocrine tumors with significant prolongation of progression-free survival and low rates of severe adverse events
  - Preliminary trials with the tyrosine kinase inhibitor sunitinib have shown encouraging results on prolongation of survival
- Fig. E1-398 describes a treatment algorithm for gastrinoma

PROGNOSIS

Five-year survival:

- Two thirds of all patients
- 20% with liver metastases
- 90% without liver metastases

REFERRAL

To gastroenterologist and surgeon

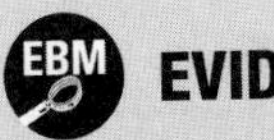

EVIDENCE

available at www.expertconsult.com

SUGGESTED READINGS

available at www.expertconsult.com

RELATED CONTENT

Gastrinoma (Zollinger-Ellison Syndrome) (Patient Information)

AUTHOR: **FRED F. FERRI, M.D.**

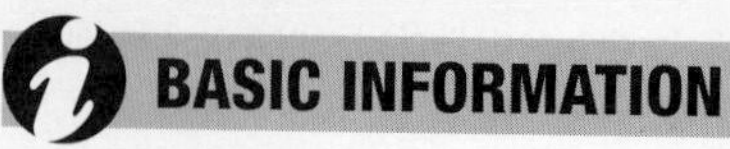

BASIC INFORMATION

DEFINITION

Histologically, *gastritis* refers to inflammation in the stomach. Endoscopically, gastritis refers to a number of abnormal features such as erythema, erosions, and subepithelial hemorrhages. Gastritis can also be subdivided into erosive, nonerosive, and specific types of gastritis with distinctive features both endoscopically and histologically.

SYNONYMS

Erosive gastritis
Hemorrhagic gastritis
Helicobacter pylori gastritis

ICD-9CM CODES
535.5 Gastritis (unless otherwise specified)
535.0 Gastritis, acute
535.3 Alcoholic gastritis
535.1 Atrophic (chronic) gastritis
535.4 Erosive gastritis
535.2 Hypertrophic gastritis

ICD-10CM CODES
K29.70 Gastritis, unspecified, without bleeding
K29.00 Acute gastritis without bleeding
K29.20 Alcoholic gastritis without bleeding
K29.40 Chronic atrophic gastritis without bleeding
K29.60 Other gastritis without bleeding

EPIDEMIOLOGY & DEMOGRAPHICS

- Erosive and hemorrhagic gastritis is most commonly seen in patients taking nonsteroidal anti-inflammatory drugs (NSAIDs), alcoholics, and critically ill patients (usually on ventilator support).
- *H. pylori* infection with gastritis is believed to be present in 30% to 50% of the population; however, the majority are asymptomatic.
- The prevalence of *H. pylori* infection increases with age from <10% in whites <40 yr to >50% in patients >50 yr.

PHYSICAL FINDINGS & CLINICAL PRESENTATION

- Patients with gastritis generally present with nonspecific clinical signs and symptoms (e.g., epigastric pain, abdominal tenderness, bloating, anorexia, nausea [with or without vomiting]). Symptoms may be aggravated by eating.
- Epigastric tenderness in acute alcoholic gastritis (may be absent in chronic gastritis).
- Foul-smelling breath.
- Hematemesis ("coffee grounds" emesis).

ETIOLOGY

- Alcohol, NSAIDs, stress (critically ill patients usually on mechanical respiration), hepatic or renal failure, multiorgan failure
- Infection (bacterial, viral)
- Bile reflux, pancreatic enzyme reflux
- Gastric mucosal atrophy, portal hypertension gastropathy
- Irradiation

Dx DIAGNOSIS

DIFFERENTIAL DIAGNOSIS

- Peptic ulcer disease
- Gastroesophageal reflux disease
- Nonulcer dyspepsia
- Gastric lymphoma or carcinoma
- Pancreatitis
- Gastroparesis

WORKUP

Diagnostic workup includes a comprehensive history and endoscopy with biopsy.

LABORATORY TESTS

- *H. pylori* testing by urea breath test, stool antigen test (*H. pylori* stool antigen), endoscopic biopsy, or specific antibody test is recommended.
  1. The urea breath test documents active infection (sensitivity and specificity >90%). A new card test for ^{14}C urea has recently been developed, providing a testing option in primary care settings. It uses a flat breath card read by a small analyzer.
  2. The stool antigen test is an enzymatic immunoassay (ELISA) that identifies *H. pylori* antigen in a stool specimen with a polyclonal anti–*H. pylori* antibody. It is as accurate as the urea breath test for diagnosis of active infection and follow-up evaluation of patients treated for *H. pylori*. A negative result on the stool antigen test 8 wk after completion of therapy identifies patients in whom eradication of *H. pylori* was unsuccessful.
  3. Histologic evaluation of endoscopic biopsy samples is considered by many the gold standard for accurate diagnosis of *H. pylori* infection. However, detection of *H. pylori* depends on the site and number of biopsy samples, the method of staining, and experience of the pathologist.
  4. Serologic testing for antibodies to *H. pylori* is easy and inexpensive; however, the presence of antibodies demonstrates previous but not necessarily current infection. Antibodies to *H. pylori* can remain elevated for months to years after infection has cleared; therefore antibody levels must be interpreted in light of patient's symptoms and other test results (e.g., peptic ulcer disease (PUD) seen on upper gastrointestinal series).
- Vitamin B_{12} level in patients with atrophic gastritis.
- Hematocrit (low if significant bleeding has occurred).

Rx TREATMENT

NONPHARMACOLOGIC THERAPY

- Avoidance of mucosal irritants such as alcohol and NSAIDs
- Lifestyle modifications with avoidance of tobacco and foods that trigger symptoms

ACUTE GENERAL Rx

Eradication of *H. pylori,* when present, can be accomplished with various regimens:

1. Proton pump inhibitor (PPI) bid *plus* amoxicillin 500 mg bid *plus* metronidazole 500 mg for 10 days.
2. PPI bid *plus* clarithromycin 500 mg bid *and* metronidazole 500 mg bid for 10 days. This regimen is useful in those with penicillin allergy.
3. A 1-day quadruple-therapy regimen may be as effective as a 7-day triple-therapy regimen. The 1-day quadruple-therapy regimen consists of two tablets of 262 mg bismuth subsalicylate qd, one 500-mg metronidazole tablet qd, 2 g of amoxicillin suspension qd, and two capsules of 30 mg of lansoprazole.
4. A 5-day treatment with three antibiotics (amoxicillin 1 g bid, clarithromycin 250 mg bid, and metronidazole 400 mg bid) plus either lansoprazole 30 mg bid or ranitidine 300 mg bid is an efficacious, cost-saving option for patients >55 yr with no history of PUD.
5. A combination of levofloxacin 250 mg bid, amoxicillin 1000 mg bid, and a PPI bid for 10 to 14 days can be used as salvage therapy after unsuccessful attempts to eradicate *H. pylori* using other regimens.
   - A 10-day sequential therapy has been reported to be superior to standard triple therapy for eradication of *H. pylori*. It consists of 5 days of treatment with a PPI and one antibiotic (usually amoxicillin) followed by 5-day treatment with the PPI and two other antibiotics (usually clarithromycin and metronidazole).
6. Prophylaxis and treatment of stress gastritis with sucralfate suspension 1 g orally q4-6h, H_2-receptor antagonists, or PPIs in patients on ventilator support.

CHRONIC Rx

- Omeprazole 20 mg/qd in patients receiving long-term NSAIDs
- Avoidance of alcohol, tobacco, and prolonged NSAID or corticosteroid use

DISPOSITION

- Undetectable stool antigen 4 wk after therapy accurately confirms cure of *H. pylori* infection in initially seropositive healthy subjects with reasonable sensitivity.
- Surveillance gastroscopy in patients with atrophic gastritis (increased risk of gastric cancer).

RELATED CONTENT

Gastritis (Patient Information)
Helicobacter pylori Infection (Related Key Topic)

AUTHOR: **FRED F. FERRI, M.D.**

BASIC INFORMATION

DEFINITION

- Gastroenteritis is a broad term used for various gastrointestinal pathologic states. The main manifestation is diarrhea—often accompanied by nausea, vomiting, malaise, anorexia, fever, abdominal pain, and dehydration.
- Gastroenteritis is a common cause of morbidity/mortality around the world. In the developing world, it is a leading cause of death.

ICD-9CM CODES
009.1 Colitis, enteritis, and gastroenteritis of presumed infectious origin
ICD-10CM CODES
K52.9 Non-infective gastroenteritis and colitis
558.3 Allergic gastroenteritis and coli
K52.1 Infectious gastroenteritis and colitis
K52.0 Gastroenteritis and colitis due to radiation

EPIDEMIOLOGY & DEMOGRAPHICS

- Frequency is difficult to determine.
- It is estimated that there are 1.5 billion cases a year worldwide.
- It is the leading cause of death in many developing countries. Children under the age of 5 yr are most vulnerable.

SEX
Higher mortality seen in women.
AGE
- May occur at any age
- High morbidity and mortality in the very young (younger than 5 yr) and the elderly (people aged 65 or older)

PHYSICAL FINDINGS & CLINICAL PRESENTATION

- A well-taken history is important. This helps to identify the cause of diarrhea and identify patients at risk of complications.
- Patients usually present with:
  - Diarrhea: usually more than 6 stools a day indicates bacterial cause of gastroenteritis
  - Vomiting
  - Abdominal pain
  - Mucus and/or blood in stool: indicating bacterial or parasitic infection
  - Fever
  - Dehydration: this is the main cause of morbidity and mortality. Check for lethargy, dry mucous membrane, poor skin turgor, sunken eyes as signs of dehydration.
  - Malnutrition: this occurs when diarrhea is chronic. There is reduced muscle and fat mass.
  - Abdominal pain: this is a very common symptom in gastroenteritis.
  - Borborygmi: there is significantly increased peristaltic activity, which may cause audible or palpable bowel activity.
  - Perianal erythema: secondary to constantly wet area. Wet buttock and perianal area may result in redness and skin breakdown.

ETIOLOGY

- Bacterial gastroenteritis
  - *Salmonella*
  - *Shigella*
  - *Campylobacter*
  - *Aeromonas* species
  - *Yersinia*
  - Enterohemorrhagic *Escherichia coli*
  - *E. coli*
  - *Clostridium perfringens*
- Viral gastroenteritis (in adults)
  - The caliciviruses such as *Norovirus* genogroup I (e.g., Norwalk), *Norovirus* genogroup II (e.g., South Hampton), *Sapovirus* (e.g., Sapporo).
  - Non-group A *Rotavirus*
  - *Astrovirus*
  - Adenovirus

DIAGNOSIS

DIFFERENTIAL DIAGNOSIS

- Amebiasis
- Appendicitis
- Celiac disease
- Inflammatory bowel disease
- Colon cancer
- Bowel obstruction
- Botulism
- Hemolytic uremic syndrome

WORKUP

- In most cases laboratory tests are not indicated.
- Further workup is indicated in patients who:
  - Have persistent diarrhea
  - Are extremely dehydrated
  - Appear seriously ill
  - Have high fever
  - Present with severe abdominal pain
  - Have bloody diarrhea
  - Have persistent nausea

LABORATORY TESTS

- Routine laboratory tests
  - Tests such as CBC and BMP may not be indicated in making a diagnosis. However, electrolytes and BUN are indicated in patients with severe diarrhea or dehydration.
  - CBC is indicated with severe diarrhea or toxicity. WBC is increased in *Salmonella* infection; eosinophilia is present in parasitic infections.
- Stool studies
  - Presence of blood/leukocytes in stool may indicate inflammatory diarrhea.
  - In *Salmonella* or *Shigella* infections there is an increased fecal leukocyte.
  - Stool leukocytes are absent in viral diarrhea.
- Stool culture
  - Are only useful when positive
  - Usually not necessary in most cases of diarrhea
  - Indications for stool cultures include: bloody stools; prolonged, untreated diarrhea; fever; leukocytes in stool; immunosuppressed patients; immunocompromised patients; and patients who have traveled to remote, exotic, or developing nations. It should also be considered in patients with concurrent or very recent use of antibiotics to rule out *Clostridium difficile* infection as a cause of the diarrhea.
- Examination for ova and parasites (O&P) is indicated in immunosuppressed patients, immunocompromised patients, and patients who have traveled to remote, exotic, or developing nations

IMAGING STUDIES

- In patients with suspected bowel obstruction, perforation, or toxic megacolon, abdominal series is warranted.
- Consider CT scan of the abdomen in older patients with severe abdominal pain.

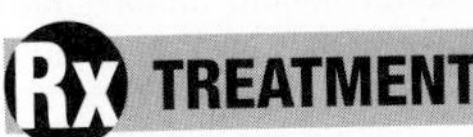

TREATMENT

GENERAL CONSIDERATIONS

- Most infectious diarrhea is self-limited.
- It is important to assess the degree of dehydration by checking BP, pulse, HR, skin turgor, mucous membrane, thirst, urine output, and mental status change.
- Oral rehydration therapy is very important in diarrhea treatment.
- Consider intravenous rehydration when oral rehydration fails. Watch out for potassium depletion.
- Early re-feeding decreases recovery time.

Principles of treatment include:
- Rehydration: orally or intravenously, PRN
- Treatment of symptoms such as fever, abdominal pain, nausea, vomiting as needed
- Identify and treat complications

REHYDRATION
- Oral hydration products include Naturalyte, Rehydralyte.
- Intravenous solutions used include dextrose 5% in 0.5 isotonic NaCl with 50 mEq $NaHCO_3$ and 10-20 mEq KCl.
  - Indications for IV hydration include intractable vomiting, severe dehydration, change in mental status or consciousness, and ileus.
  - Oral hydration is not appropriate due to environmental conditions

TREATMENT OF SYMPTOMS
- Infectious diarrhea sometimes requires empiric treatment with antibiotics. Food-borne toxigenic diarrhea usually does not.
- Traveler's diarrhea: may be treated with ciprofloxacin or TMP/SMZ for 3 days in mild cases and for 5-7 days for moderate to severe cases. Fluoroquinolones are the drug of choice for empirical treatment of infectious gastroenteritis, but they are contraindicated in pregnant women.
- *C. difficile* diarrhea and parasitic infestations with *Giardia* or *Entamoeba* are treated with metronidazole.
- Treat severe nausea and vomiting with antiemetics.
- Antidiarrheal agents may be useful for systematic relief in mild to moderate diarrhea.
- Loperamide (Imodium) or bismuth subsalicylate (Pepto-Bismol) may be used, especially in traveler's or non-bloody diarrhea.

REFERRAL

Referral to infectious disease or gastroenterologist specialist may be indicated in patients:
- With chronic diarrhea
- In whom a parasitic etiology is suspected
- With *C. difficile* resistant to treatment with metronidazole and vancomycin
- With HIV/AIDS
- Who relapse

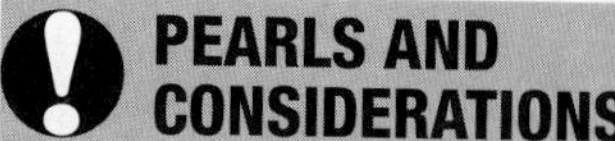

PEARLS AND CONSIDERATIONS

PREVENTION

- Perform proper handwashing before and after eating and after each bowel movement to prevent spread to family members.
- Avoid (raw) shellfish served in certain unregulated places.
- Avoid raw or undercooked eggs and/or poultry.
- Wash all produce before consumption.
- For travelers to high-risk areas:
  - Eat only cooked foods.
  - Drink hot or carbonated beverages.
  - Avoid water, raw peeled fruits/vegetables, green leafy vegetables, and street food sold by street vendors.
  - Vaccines are available for *Salmonella typhi* and *Vibrio cholerae* (the latter provides about 50% protection for 3-6 months).

PATIENT EDUCATION

- Stress the importance of oral rehydration.
- Stress the need for early appropriate feeding.
- Relapse occurs due to dietary noncompliance.
- Travelers to developing areas should be educated on proper avoidance measures and treatment.

RELATED CONTENT

Gastroenteritis (Patient Information)

AUTHOR: **DANIEL K. ASIEDU, M.D., Ph.D, F.A.C.P**

BASIC INFORMATION

DEFINITION

Gastroesophageal reflux disease (GERD) is a motility disorder characterized primarily by heartburn and caused by the reflux of gastric contents into the esophagus. A current definition is a condition that develops when the reflux of stomach contents causes at least two heartburn episodes per week and/or complications.

SYNONYMS

Peptic esophagitis
Reflux esophagitis
GERD

ICD-9CM CODES
530.81 Gastroesophageal reflux disease
530.1 Esophagitis
787.1 Heartburn
ICD-10CM CODES
K21.9 Gastroesophageal reflux disease without esophagitis
R12 Heartburn

EPIDEMIOLOGY & DEMOGRAPHICS

- GERD is one of the most prevalent gastrointestinal disorders. It is the most common GI diagnosis recorded during visits to outpatient clinics. From 14% to 20% of adults are affected.
- Nearly 7% of persons in the U.S. have heartburn daily, 20% have it monthly, and 60% have it intermittently. Incidence in pregnant women exceeds 80%.
- Nearly 20% of adults use antacids or over-the-counter H_2 blockers at least once a week for relief of heartburn.

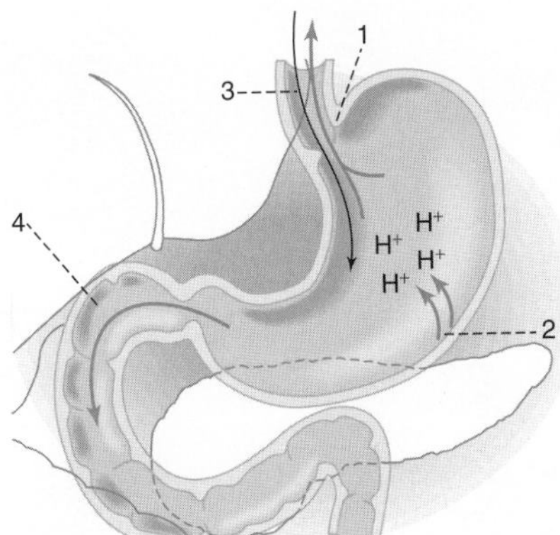

FIGURE 1-399 Pathogenesis of gastroesophageal reflux disease: *(1)* impaired lower esophageal sphincter—low pressures or frequent transient lower esophageal sphincter relaxation; *(2)* hypersecretion of acid; *(3)* decreased acid clearance resulting from impaired peristalsis or abnormal saliva production; *(4)* delayed gastric emptying or duodenogastric reflux of bile salts and pancreatic enzymes. (From Andreoli TE et al: *Andreoli and Carpenter's Cecil essentials of medicine,* ed 8, Philadelphia, 2010, Saunders.)

PHYSICAL FINDINGS & CLINICAL PRESENTATION

- Physical examination: generally unremarkable
- Clinical signs and symptoms: heartburn, dysphagia, sour taste, regurgitation of gastric contents into the mouth
- Chronic cough and bronchospasm
- Chest pain, laryngitis, early satiety, abdominal fullness, and bloating with belching
- Dental erosions in children

ETIOLOGY

- Incompetent lower esophageal sphincter (LES) (see Fig. 1-399)
- Medications that lower LES pressure (calcium channel blockers, alpha-adrenergic antagonists, nitrates, theophylline, anticholinergics, sedatives, prostaglandins)
- Foods that lower LES pressure (chocolate, yellow onions, peppermint)
- Tobacco abuse, alcohol, coffee
- Pregnancy
- Gastric acid hypersecretion
- Hiatal hernia (controversial) present in >70% of patients with GERD; however, most patients with hiatal hernia are asymptomatic
- Obesity is associated with a statistically significant increase in the risk for GERD symptoms, erosive esophagitis, and esophageal carcinoma

DIAGNOSIS

DIFFERENTIAL DIAGNOSIS

- Peptic ulcer disease
- Unstable angina
- Esophagitis (from infections such as herpes, *Candida*), medication induced (doxycycline, potassium chloride)
- Esophageal spasm (nutcracker esophagus)
- Cancer of esophagus

WORKUP

- Aimed at eliminating the conditions noted in the differential diagnosis and documenting the type and extent of tissue damage. Generally, when symptoms of GERD are typical and the patient responds to therapy, there is no need for further diagnostic tests to verify the diagnosis.
- Upper GI endoscopy is useful to document the type and extent of tissue damage in persistent GERD and to exclude potentially malignant conditions such as Barrett's esophagus. The American College of Physicians recommends endoscopy in the setting of GERD in people with heartburn and alarm symptoms (dysphagia, bleeding, anemia, weight loss, and recurrent vomiting). It is also indicated in people with GERD symptoms that persist despite a therapeutic trial of 4 to 8 weeks of bid PPI therapy in patients with severe erosive esophagus after a 2-month course of PPI therapy to assess healing and rule out Barrett's esophagus.
- Fig. E1-400 describes an approach to patients with heartburn.

LABORATORY TESTS

- 24-hr esophageal pH monitoring and Bernstein test are sensitive diagnostic tests; however, they are not practical and generally not done. They are useful in patients with atypical manifestations of GERD, such as chest pain or chronic cough.
- Esophageal manometry is indicated in patients with refractory reflux in whom surgical therapy is planned.

IMAGING STUDIES

An upper GI series is useful in patients unwilling to have endoscopy or with medical contraindications to the procedure. It can identify ulcerations and strictures; however, it may miss mucosal abnormalities. Only one third of patients with GERD have radiographic signs of esophagitis on an upper GI series.

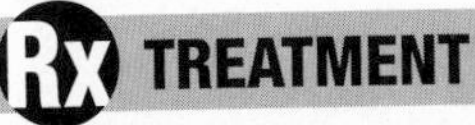

TREATMENT

NONPHARMACOLOGIC THERAPY

- Lifestyle modifications with avoidance of foods (e.g., citrus- and tomato-based products, onions, spicy foods, carbonated beverages, mint, chocolate, fried foods) and drugs that exacerbate reflux (e.g., caffeine, β-blockers, calcium channel blockers, α-adrenergic agonists, theophylline)
- Avoidance of tobacco and alcohol use
- Elevation of head of bed (4 to 8 in) with blocks
- Avoidance of lying down directly after late or large evening meals, consumption of smaller and more frequent meals
- Weight reduction to BMI <25, decreased fat intake
- Avoidance of clothing that is tight around the waist

GENERAL Rx

- Proton pump inhibitors (PPIs) (esomeprazole 40 mg qd, omeprazole 20 mg qd, lansoprazole 30 mg qd, rabeprazole 20 mg qd, or pantoprazole 40 mg qd, or dexlansoprazole 30 mg) are generally safe, tolerated, and highly effective in most patients (Table 1-199).
- H_2 blockers (nizatidine 300 mg qhs, famotidine 40 mg qhs, ranitidine 300 mg qhs, or cimetidine 800 mg qhs) can be used but are generally much less effective than PPIs.
- Antacids (may be useful for relief of mild symptoms; however, they are generally ineffective in severe cases of reflux).
- Prokinetic agents (metoclopramide) are indicated only when PPIs are not fully effective. They can be used in combination therapy; however, side effects limit their use.
- For refractory cases: surgery with Nissen fundoplication. Potential surgical candidates should have reflux esophagitis documented by esophagogastroduodenoscopy and normal esophageal motility as evaluated by manometry. Surgery generally consists of reduction of hiatal hernia when present and placement of a gastric wrap around the gastroesophageal (GE) junction (fundoplication). Although

TABLE 1-199 Drug Therapy for Esophageal Disorders

Agent	Dose
Antacids: Liquid (to Buffer Acid and Increase LESP)	
For example, Mylanta II/Maalox TC (acid-neutralizing capacity, 25 mEq/5 ml)*	15 ml qid 1 hr after meals and at bedtime or as needed
Gaviscon (to Decrease Reflux via a Viscous Mechanical Barrier and Buffer Acid)	
$Al(OH)_3$, $NaHCO_3$, Mg trisilicate, alginic acid	2-4 tablets qid at bedtime or as needed
H_2-Receptor Antagonists (to Decrease Acid Secretion)	
Cimetidine	800 mg bid, 400 mg qid, ≈13 ml bid
Ranitidine	150 mg qid or 10 ml qid; maintenance dose, 150 mg bid, 10 ml bid
Famotidine	20-40 mg bid or 2.5-5 ml bid
Nizatidine	150 mg bid
Proton Pump Inhibitors (to Decrease Acid Secretion and Gastric Volume)†	
Omeprazole	20 mg/day; maintenance dose, 20 mg/day
Lansoprazole	30 mg/day; maintenance dose, 15 mg/day
Pantoprazole	40 mg/day; maintenance dose, 40 mg/day
Rabeprazole	20 mg/day; maintenance dose, 20 mg/day
Esomeprazole	20-40 mg/day; maintenance dose, 20 mg/day
Dexlansoprazole	30-60 mg/day; maintenance dose, 30 mg/day

LESP, Lower esophageal sphinter pressure.
*Patients with reflux are not generally hypersecretors of gastric acid, so the therapeutic doses of antacids are based on their capacity to buffer (normal) basal acid secretion rates of approximately 1 to 7 mEq/hr (mean, 2 mEq/hr) and peak meal-stimulated acid secretion rates of about 10 to 60 mEq/hr (mean, 30 mEq/hr).
†High-dose therapy is a twice-daily administration of the usual daily dose.
From Goldman L, Schafer AI: *Goldman's Cecil medicine,* ed 24, Philadelphia, 2012, Saunders.

laparoscopic fundoplication is now widely used, long-term medical therapy is a better choice for most patients who are willing to remain on daily acid-reduction medication. In patients preferring surgical intervention, surgery should not be advised with the expectation that patients with GERD will no longer need to take antisecretory medications or that the procedure will prevent esophageal cancer among those with GERD and Barrett's esophagus.
- Endoscopic radiofrequency heating of the GE junction (Stretta procedure) is a newer treatment modality for GERD patients unresponsive to traditional therapy. Its mechanism of action remains unclear. Endoscopy gastroplasty (EndoCinch procedure) is also aimed at treating GERD. Initial results appear encouraging; however, long-term studies are needed before recommending these procedures.
- Lifestyle modification must be followed for life because this is generally an irreversible condition.

DISPOSITION

- Recurrence of reflux is common if treatment is discontinued.
- The majority of patients respond well to therapy. In patients with chronic GERD, long-term outcomes are similar between medical therapy with PPIs and anti-reflux surgery. Prolonged use of PPIs is associated with increased risk of fractures of hip, wrist, and spine; increased risk of diarrhea from *Clostridium difficile;* pneumonia; and possible iron deficiency from impaired iron absorption. PPIs also block the effects of clopidogrel by inhibiting cytochrome P450 2C19 isozyme. Therefore all PPIs (other than pantoprazole) should be avoided in patients using clopidogrel. H_2 blockers (e.g., ranitidine) can be used for patients with GERD taking clopidogrel.
- Postsurgical complications occur in nearly 20% of patients (dysphagia, gas, bloating, diarrhea, nausea). Long-term follow-up studies also reveal that within 3 to 5 yr, 52% of patients who had undergone antireflux surgery are taking antireflux medications again.

REFERRAL

- There is a strong and probably causal relation between symptomatic prolonged and untreated GERD, Barrett's esophagus, and esophageal adenocarcinoma. GI referral for upper endoscopy is needed when there are concerns about associated peptic ulcer disease, Barrett's esophagus, or esophageal cancer.
- Patients with Barrett's esophagus should undergo surveillance endoscopy with mucosal biopsy every 2 yr or less because the risk of developing adenocarcinoma of esophagus is at least 30 times greater than that of the general population.
- Testing and treating for *Helicobacter pylori* in patients with GERD has not been shown to improve symptoms.
- All children with dental erosions should be evaluated for GERD.

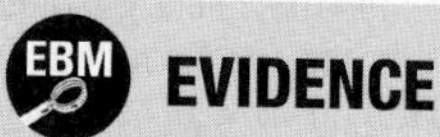

available at www.expertconsult.com

SUGGESTED READINGS

available at www.expertconsult.com

RELATED CONTENT

Gastroesophageal Reflux Disease (GERD) (Patient Information)

AUTHOR: **FRED F. FERRI, M.D.**

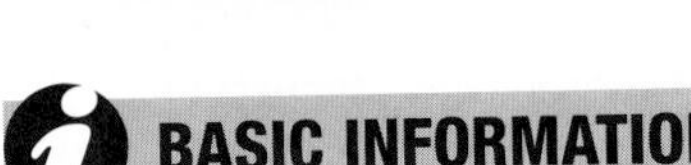

BASIC INFORMATION

DEFINITION

Gender nonconformity or transgender results when a person's natal or biologic gender (chromosomes, hormones, organs, and secondary sexual characteristics) is incongruent with a person's perceived and asserted core gender identity (innate sense of being male or female). Gender dysphoria is often experienced by gender-nonconforming or transgender individuals and implies more than a disconnect or incongruency with physical gender, but a notable discomfort and dislike of one's biologic gender and a desire to be physically different than the gender born into or assigned at birth.

Historically, gender and sexuality are related but separate concepts: gender is who a person is and how they identify as male, female, or somewhere on the continuum; sexuality is about who a person is attracted to or engages with intercourse. Gender and sexuality are evolving concepts within the psychiatric field and may benefit from considering normal developmental perspectives. Gender (natal, identity, and expression) and sexuality (attraction, behaviors, and orientation) are no longer considered binary static descriptors but may be fluid and move along a spectrum of identity and presentation. Although discomfort and dislike of one's biologic and anatomic gender and secondary sexual characteristics are a major component of gender dysphoria disorder, a transgender identity is not limited to dysphoria or psychopathology. When individuals are gender dysphoric, determining their unique perspective may help guide options for care.

SYNONYMS

Gender nonconformity
Transgender
Gender identity disorder
Gender dysphoria in children, adolescents, adults
Unspecified gender dysphoria
Transgender or transsexual

Coding:
Adults and Adolescents
ICD-9CM and DSM-5 CODES
302.85
ICD-10CM CODES
F64.2 Gender identity disorder of childhood
F64.9 Gender identity disorder, unspecified
F64.8 Other gender identity disorder
F64.0 Transsexualism
F64.1 Dual-role transvestism

EPIDEMIOLOGY & DEMOGRAPHICS

DEVELOPMENT & BACKGROUND: Gender development begins as early as 18 months. By age 2 to 4 yr, children understand gender differences and use pronouns such as "him" and "her." Toddlers identify their own gender, and most consider gender a stable personal trait at age 5-6 yr. All children explore and play with gender activities, behaviors, and roles of the opposite gender (called gender play). This stage can last from days to years and does not mean a child is dysphoric or dislikes his or her gender. Many children adopt opposite gender attributes and activities and not want to change to the other gender.

PREDOMINANT AGE

- Gender nonconformity in prepubertal years is more than play; nonconforming prepubertal children exhibit *consistent, persistent, and insistent* play, dress, attributes, and activities of the other gender. Some of these children, but not all, experience dysphoria and mild to intense discomfort and dislike of their biologic gender. In the prepubertal years, males who present to medical providers with this experience outnumber females by 3:1.
- With puberty, attaining a mature and adult gender (who you are) and sexuality (attraction, orientation, behaviors, sexual partner preference) become core developmental tasks of adolescence. At this age, gender nonconforming youth who present for care changes to a ratio of 1:1 male to female.
- Incidence may be heavily associated with cultural expectations. It is generally less acceptable to be a feminized boy than a prepubertal girl who is a "tomboy." A peripubertal spike in gender dysphoria also occurs as pubertal females lose their androgenous appearance, develop breasts, and begin menses.

PREVALENCE: Overall estimates are between 1 in 10,000 to 1 in 100,000 depending on the study and source. Most believe these numbers vastly underestimate prevalence because they originate from adult surgical or gender specialty clinics.

GENETICS: Although data are emerging about sex hormones, the brain, gender identity, and expression, there is no known single or specific genetic basis for gender dysphoria. The disorder has no specific relationships or associations with parent characteristics, socioeconomic status, or race/ethnicity. There may be a link between autism spectrum disorders and gender nonconformity.

RISK FACTORS: There are no proven risk factors for developing gender dysphoria. However, children and teens who are gender nonconforming experience higher rates of child abuse, bullying, mental health concerns (e.g., anxiety, depression, suicidality), and substance use. Transgender adult populations have poorer health outcomes, such as depression, anxiety, self-harm and suicide, substance use, underemployment, homelessness, incarceration, and positive HIV status. Poorer health outcomes are explained by using minority stress theory (chronic stress related to stigma and dysphoria) rather than gender variance as a pathology itself.

PHYSICAL FINDINGS & CLINICAL PRESENTATION

Prepubertal children present with *consistent, persistent, and insistent* interest and expression of other or opposite-gendered activities and behaviors. Boys may be considered more feminine than their same-age peers; they may prefer to wear long hair, nail polish, makeup, girls' jewelry, and clothing. Girls may be considered "tomboys" and reject wearing dresses and skirts, prefer short hair, wear boys' clothing, and participate in traditionally masculine play and activities. During the school-age years, children become sensitive to social expectations and norms. Many gender dysphoric children who do conform in their gender play and expression, however, still experience underlying problems with biology and identity.

Adolescents and adults may present in their natal gender expression as androgenous or as the opposite gender. Many gender dysphoric persons will not present directly with gender dysphoria but present with mood, behavior, or social problems. For many persons, gender dysphoria or the disclosure of gender nonconformity is first elicited as a result of mental health counseling.

For some persons, especially children, social media has provided the initial construct and terminology to understand and then verbalize their feelings. For many adult persons, disclosing or "coming out" socially as transgender is a deeply personal decision and experience that can have an enormous impact on family, social, and economic relationships.

Dx DIAGNOSIS

- Gender dysphoria was an element of gender identity disorder in the DSM IV. Core components included longstanding discomfort with assigned gender; interference with activities of daily living; and no other illness, physical or psychiatric, that would confuse diagnosis.
- Changes to the DSM V begin to remove focus from pathologizing and stigmatization of "disorder." For an individual to be diagnosed with gender dysphoria, marked differences between the individual's natal or assigned gender and expressed/experienced gender must exist for at least six months. This dissonance causes clinically significant distress or impairment in social, occupational, or other important areas of functioning. Children with dysphoria may also express strong and consistent desire to be the other gender. Persons with gender dysphoria can show a range of expression: from a inherent longstanding belief and feeling that one's psyche is more congruent with the opposite gender to strongly believing and desiring not to have or be rid of one's primary and secondary gender's physical characteristics. DSM-5 changes add a post-transition specifier for people who are living full time as the desired gender identity so as to ensure treatment access for hormone therapy, related surgeries, or counseling. Gender dysphoria has a chapter in DSM-5 separate from Sexual Dysfunctions and Paraphilic Disorders. Many gender specialists focus on paradigms using physical or endocrine conditions to avoid stigma and allow for improved access to hormonal and surgical therapies.

- Psychiatric evaluations are no longer considered necessary or essential to "diagnose" gender nonconforming persons. Persons may assert a nonconformity identity without severe self-hatred or significant dysphoric presentation. However, persons with severe dysphoria and sequelae from the mismatch in biology with identity usually benefit from participating in therapy, building skills to create successful transition plans, and/or obtaining treatment for comorbid psychiatric concerns. Persons with significant and active psychosis should be evaluated to determine whether gender issues are separate or integrated within the psychotic experience.

WORKUP

- Clinical interview includes assessment of gender experience from childhood until present; desired name, pronoun, and past and current place on the gender spectrum; past and current attempts to feminize or masculinize with clothing, hair, makeup, hormones, and surgeries; future goals of transitioning, gender identity, and expression. For children, many parents may provide insight as to early childhood gender identity and expression.
- Review for known comorbidities by asking mental health–specific questions about depression, anxiety, self-harm (cutting and suicidal ideation), psychiatric hospitalization, substance use; sexual attraction and behaviors regarding partners, detailed sexual activities, and risk for sexually transmitted infections and pregnancy; social history, experience of bullying, hate crimes, physical or emotional/verbal abuse, homelessness, joblessness, survival sex, and identified social support systems.
- Ideally, this interview is in the context of interviewing the individual as a person and as a holistic health assessment. Persons with experience in behavioral health and gender issues can perform these interviews. Some patients may benefit from therapy or psychiatric evaluation if they have additional mental health concerns, need support to plan transitioning, and would benefit from self-esteem, social skills, and other protective skill building.
- An initial visit may include a physical examination depending on the patient's goals. Many gender dysphoric persons are exquisitely uncomfortable with their genitalia and genital examination. This can often be deferred until the patient is more comfortable and familiar with the provider.
- A general physical examination may be performed, but detailed examination of secondary sexual characteristics (breasts, vulva, penis, testicles) often is deferred. Tanner staging genitalia for peripubertal youth interested in puberty "blockers" or cross-gender hormones is important.
- Laboratory studies may include luteinizing hormone, follicle stimulating hormone, testosterone, or estradiol for peripubertal children wanting to start puberty blockers or gonadotropin-releasing hormone (GnRH) analogues. For youth or adults starting GnRH analogues or cross-gender hormones, baseline laboratory values include CBC, liver panel, liver function tests, and testosterone (or estrogen). Screening for sexually transmitted infections (urine, rectal, and oral *Chlamydia* and gonorrhea; syphilis; herpes simplex virus; HIV; hepatitis B and C), and pregnancy is indicated according to sexual practices. Additional preventive care screening and testing may be deferred. Patients should receive typical preventive and screening tests for both biologic gender and asserted gender.
- Ancillary testing may include various psychiatric screening and diagnostic tools for comorbid depression, anxiety, suicidality, substance use, and interpersonal violence.

Rx TREATMENT

Treatment is determined by patient age and development (including Tanner stage) and desired place on the gender spectrum. Moving from biologic gender to asserted gender identity is known as transition. Transition is typically divided into three stages: reversible, partially reversible, and irreversible.

REVERSIBLE TRANSITION

- Taking on clothes, hair, makeup, name, and pronoun of the identified gender. For prepubertal, androgenous children, "social transition" does not require hormones but does require extensive planning for disclosure, social support, and peer- and school-based activities.
- Puberty blockers or GnRH antagonists are reversible and best when used at very early Tanner stage II breast and testicular development. When used in early puberty, blockers stop puberty with regression to prepubertal hormones and secondary sexual characteristics. This often "buys time" for both a child and a family to determine a safe and supportive social transition plan.
- Puberty blockers can be used for patients who are at Tanner stage III or IV according to genital exam but are still androgenous in regards to other secondary sex characteristics, such as voice, facial and body hair, bone, muscle, and fat deposition. Blockers can also be used to stop penile function or menses, which can be highly distressing to gender dysphoric persons.
- Blockers are *completely reversible*. If stopped, a person can continue into biologic puberty. Most teens who opt to start blockers continue to create a transition plan and eventually move to cross-gender hormones and puberty in their asserted gender. The current literature from the past 30 or more years demonstrates that it is unlikely that an adolescent who is consistently, persistently, and insistently gender nonconforming or transgender will return to his or her natal gender or regret either blockers or cross gender hormones. This can be both of concern and relief to parents as they determine how to best support their child.

PARTIALLY REVERSIBLE TRANSITION

- Cross-gender hormone therapies include testosterone for masculinization and estradiol for feminization. These have many reversible effects on skin changes, fat deposition, and muscle mass. Irreversible effects may include masculine voice changes, areola enlargement with darkening, hair changes and clitoromegaly.
- Estradiol creates softer skin, female body fat deposition (hips/thighs), and breast development. It may impair erectile function, which may or may not be desired because some male-to-female persons still want or depend on penile function for both pleasure and/or for sex work. Estradiol is typically administered sublingually but can be taken orally, intramuscularly, or topically. Topical medicines run the risk of undesired feminization (or masculinization) of sex partners or others in close physical contact.
- Testosterone masculinizes by inducing male hair patterns, deepening the voice, and inducing male-pattern fat and muscle deposition (bulk and abdominal girth) and clitoromegaly. It can lead to vaginal atrophy, resulting in dyspareunia for transgender female-to-male persons who use the vagina for sex. Testosterone comes in a variety of vehicles, including subcutaneous, intramuscular, and topical. Testosterone is teratogenic in pregnancy. Both sex hormones should not be used in lieu of contraception, and future fertility cannot be guaranteed. Persons taking testosterone who are having unprotected penile vaginal sex should be counseled and offered birth control in addition to testosterone.
- Consent to what we know and do not know is an important part of beginning the cross-gender hormone process. Current evidence suggests that estrogen or testosterone are not sufficient to act as contraceptives, nor is future fertility guaranteed, for persons who prioritize having biologic children. For male-to-female persons, sperm banking offers future options for biologic children, although at some expense. For female-to-male persons, oocyte banking is extremely expensive and has not yet demonstrated reliable successful outcomes. For many transgender persons, transition to their asserted identity is more important than creating or carrying genetic children. Many transgender persons would prefer to parent or adopt in their identified or asserted gender.

IRREVERSIBLE TRANSITION

Includes mostly surgical options for masculinization (mastectomy, hystero-oophrectomy, and orchi-peniplasty) or feminization (orchiectomy-penectomy with vulvar reconstruction, breast implants, and other cosmetic surgeries). Many patients opt for partial surgical transition due to expense (surgeries are currently not covered under most insurance plans, or patients are underinsured or uninsured) function (penile implants are typically not sexually functional), and lack of available providers (there are few male-to-female genitoplasty surgeons in the U.S.; many patients travel overseas for surgical care). Most common partial surgical options are mastectomy for female-to-male and breast implants for male-to-female. It is important to ask specific goals for surgery because they vary by individual patient.

ADDITIONAL THERAPIES

Anti-androgens such as spironolactone to prevent male-pattern hair growth and vocal coaching for male-to-female. Individual, family, and marital counseling and therapies can be important for dysphoric individuals with comorbid mental health issues. Reparative therapy is *universally* rejected as *unethical and harmful* by all the national medical and psychological boards and associations. Medications for anxiety, depression, and other mental health concerns may facilitate self-esteem, mood, cognitive function, and social skills building as persons and families negotiate the process of transition. Social support and activity groups may help gender nonconforming persons find community, feel and become less isolated, and improve transition experiences. Support is important to family members who are involved in a patient's transition.

DISPOSITION

- Gender is a physical, emotional, social, and cultural construct across the lifespan that every person experiences. For a gender dysphoric patient or gender nonconforming person, this incongruency may have lifelong implications for physical, emotional, and social well-being.
- Younger patients who begin hormone blockers, are transitioned early both socially and hormonally, and experience puberty in their identified gender may have improved ability to be accepted in their asserted gender, decreased suicidality, and less risk of nonmedical use of street hormones and drugs, and fewer future surgical interventions.
- In addition, evidence suggests that sexual minorities who have early and consistent parental support, despite being gender and sexually nonconforming, have decreased rates of suicide and substance use.
- For persons experiencing some or all of puberty in their biologic but not identified gender, cross-gender hormones and/or gender-affirming surgeries offer the promise of living in their asserted gender. For persons who transition later in life, especially in their 30s and older, physical transition and "passing" are more difficult.
- In addition to minority stress and poorer mental health outcomes, being a visual and visible sexual minority has significant and demonstrated social risks for victimization from hate crimes and interpersonal violence, low socioeconomic status, underemployment, and isolation. Early identification and early transition in a person's identified gender, along with a better likelihood of acceptance, may offer significant psychosocial benefits to many gender dysphoric persons.
- Regardless of timing of transition, safety is a priority in transition planning and important to consider along the lifespan.

REFERRALS

- Providers who are not comfortable with gender or behavioral assessments may want to refer to medical providers with experience and expertise in gender issues and care. This group may include pediatric, family medicine, medicine-pediatrics, and psychiatry providers. Similarly, there are therapists and social workers with expertise in gender dysphoria assessment and management.
- There are few contraindications to transitioning for most gender dysphoric persons. Active psychosis and inability to consent to care would require further psychiatric evaluation but are extremely rare. For older persons, some medical issues involving cardiac, liver, and thromboembolic risks complicate hormone use and need to be taken into consideration.

PEARLS & CONSIDERATIONS

- Periodic assessment of a person's place on the gender spectrum can begin in toddler age children and can continue into adulthood as a potentially effective way of helping identify and support gender dysphoric persons early.
- Early identification and parental support for gender dysphoric and nonconforming persons may lead to improved mental and physical health outcomes.
- Hormone blockers and cross-gender hormones typically offer far more benefit than risk in the treatment of gender dysphoria when a person desires to transition to the opposite gender.

AUTHOR: **MICHELLE FORCIER, M.D., M.P.H.**

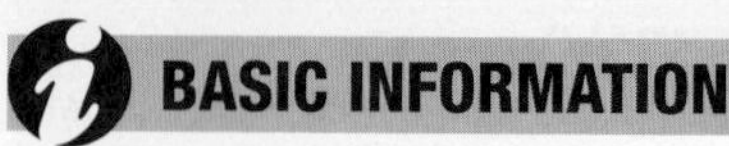

BASIC INFORMATION

DEFINITION

- Glucose intolerance that begins, or is first recognized, during pregnancy.
- In the U.S., the "two-step" approach is commonly used and is currently endorsed by the American College of Obstetricians and Gynecologist (ACOG) and the National Institutes of Health (NIH). Women are first screened with a 1-hr, nonfasting 50-g oral glucose tolerance test. If the result is ≥ 130 mg/dl, a 3-hr, 100-g oral glucose tolerance test is ordered. The diagnosis is made if two or more of the glucose values are met or exceeded:
  Fasting: 95 mg/dl
  1-hr: 180 mg/dl
  2-hr: 155 mg/dl
  3-hr: 140 mg/dl
- The International Association of Diabetes in Pregnancy Study Group has recommended a simplified "one-step" approach to screening and diagnosing gestational DM (GDM). It involves a fasting 75-g, 2-hr oral glucose tolerance test. A diagnosis of GDM is made if any of the following levels of plasma glucose are exceeded: ≥92 mg/dl when fasting, ≥180 mg/dl at 1 hr, or ≥153 mg/dl at 2 hr. Although this approach is endorsed by the American Diabetes Association, the NIH Consensus on GDM did not endorse these guidelines in 2013 because of increases in the prevalence of GDM, along with corresponding costs and interventions without clear evidence of improvement in outcomes.
- Pregnant women with diabetes mellitus (DM) (gestational or preexisting) are classified according to White's classification (Table 1-200).

SYNONYMS

Gestational diabetes
Diet-controlled gestational diabetes (A1)
Insulin-treated gestational diabetes (A2)

ICD-9CM CODES
648.8; if using insulin to treat, add V58.67
ICD-10CM CODES
099.810 Abnormal glucose complicating pregnancy

EPIDEMIOLOGY & DEMOGRAPHICS

INCIDENCE: Approximately 5% to 6% of pregnancies using the two-step approach and 15% to 20% using the one-step approach
PREDOMINANT SEX AND AGE: Women of childbearing age
GENETICS: Higher rate in women with family history of GDM or type 2 diabetes; specific HLA alleles (DR3 or DR4) predispose to the development of DM type 1 after delivery

RISK FACTORS

- Obesity
- Family history of GDM or type 2 diabetes
- Polycystic ovarian syndrome
- Twin gestation
- Hypertension
- Chronic systemic steroid use
- Maternal birth weight >9 lb or <6 lb
- Age >25 y
- Previous infant weighing >9 lb or with shoulder dystocia
- Unexplained perinatal loss or malformation
- Personal history of abnormal glucose tolerance or GDM
- Latin American, Native American, African American, or Asian ethnicity

POTENTIAL RISK FACTORS

- Limited physical activity the year before pregnancy
- Prepregnancy diet low in fiber and high in glycemic load

PHYSICAL FINDINGS & CLINICAL PRESENTATION

Suspect GDM if:
- Fetal size greater than dates
- Macrosomia on ultrasound
- Marked maternal obesity or weight gain

ETIOLOGY

- During normal pregnancy there is increased insulin resistance because of placental secretion of diabetogenic hormones in the late second and third trimesters. Pancreatic beta-cell secretion increases to compensate for the increased insulin resistance. GDM occurs when this need cannot be met.
- Insulin resistance is also exacerbated by an increase in maternal adipose deposition, decreased exercise, and increased caloric intake.

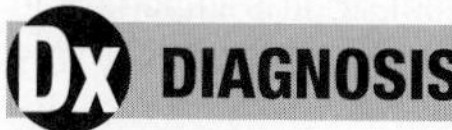

DIAGNOSIS

DIFFERENTIAL DIAGNOSIS

Preexisting type 1 or 2 DM not previously diagnosed

WORKUP

- History with focus on personal medical history, prior pregnancy history, and family history
- Routine prenatal examination
- Laboratory evaluation (see the following)

LABORATORY TESTS

- "Two-step" approach
  - For screening without risk factors, order a 1-hr glucose tolerance test (Nonfasting; 50-g oral glucose load) at 24 to 28 wk
  - For screening with risk factors, order at first prenatal visit, then repeat at 24 to 28 wk if initial screen was normal. If abnormal at intake, consider possibility of undiagnosed preexisting DM and check hemoglobin A1c.
- If 1-hr test result is abnormal (≥130 mg/dl), order 3-hr glucose tolerance test (Fasting: 100-g oral glucose load)
  - Performed after 3 days of unrestricted diet (carbohydrate load is probably not necessary)
  - GDM is diagnosed if two or more of the glucose values are met or exceeded:
    Fasting: ≥95 mg/dl
    1-hr plasma glucose ≥180 mg/dl
    2-hr plasma glucose ≥155 mg/dl
    3-hr plasma glucose ≥140 mg/dl
- If one of four values on 3-hr glucose tolerance test is abnormal, repeat testing in 1 month and consider beginning a diabetic diet
- "One-step" approach
  - Rule out overt diabetes at the initial prenatal visit. A diagnosis of diabetes is made if a woman meets any of the following criteria: fasting plasma glucose >126 mg/dl, A1c >6.5%, random plasma glucose >200 mg/dl
  - Perform a one-step screening at 24 to 28 wk on all pregnant patients who have not already been diagnosed with diabetes or GDM. This is a 2-hr, 75-g oral glucose tolerance test performed after an overnight fast. A diagnosis of GDM is made if one or more of the following values are met or exceeded:
    Fasting: ≥92 mg/dl
    1-hr plasma glucose ≥180 mg/dl
    2-hr plasma glucose ≥153 mg/dl
- The U.S. Preventive Services Task Force (USPSTF) concludes that the evidence is insufficient to recommend for or against routine screening for gestational diabetes. The current evidence is insufficient to assess the balance between the benefits and harms of screening women for GDM either before or

TABLE 1-200 White's Classification for Pregnant Women with Diabetes (Gestational or Preexisting)

Class	Description
A1	DM diagnosed during pregnancy and controlled by diet
A2	DM diagnosed during pregnancy and requiring medication
B	Insulin-requiring DM diagnosed before pregnancy, age >20 yr, lasting <10 yr
C	Insulin-requiring DM, onset at age 10 to 19 yr, with a duration 10 to 19 yr
D	Onset >10 yr or duration >20 yr, or associated with hypertension or background retinopathy
F	DM with renal disease
H	DM with coronary artery disease
R	DM with proliferative retinopathy
T	DM with renal transplant

DM, Diabetes mellitus.

after 24 weeks' gestation. Harms of screening include short-term anxiety in some women with positive screening results and inconvenience to many women and medical practices because most positive screening tests are likely false-positives. Until there is better evidence, clinicians should discuss screening for GDM with their patients and make case-by-case decisions. The discussion should include information about the uncertain benefits and harms as well as the frequency and uncertain meaning of a positive screening test result.

IMAGING STUDIES

Ultrasound for fetal size at least once at 36 to 37 wk; more frequently if macrosomia suspected

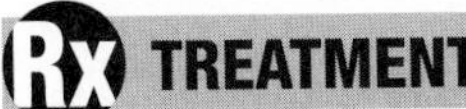

TREATMENT

NONPHARMACOLOGIC THERAPY

- Glucose monitoring:
    - Four times daily: fasting and 2-hr postprandial
    - Goals: fasting <95 mg/dl; 2-hr postprandial <120 mg/dl
    - Can also use 1-hr postprandial goal of <140 mg/dl
- Dietary modifications aimed at glycemic control:
    - Follow a low-fat, high-fiber diet; avoid sugar and concentrated sweets; and eat small, frequent meals.
    - Nutrition counseling for diet that adequately meets the needs of pregnancy but restricts carbohydrates to 35% to 40% of daily calories.
    - For women with a body mass index over 30, restrict calories to 25 kcal/kg actual weight per day.
- Regular moderate exercise

PHARMACOLOGIC Rx

Begin if >20% of glucose values are elevated after trial of diet control:

- Oral hypoglycemics:
    - Oral hypoglycemics are not endorsed by the ACOG or the American Diabetes Association (ADA) but may be considered as initial therapy or used in women who cannot comply with insulin treatment.
    - Glyburide: begin at 2.5 mg qd and titrate up to a maximum of 20 mg qd (10 mg bid). Increase dose as needed by 2.5 to 5 mg/wk.
    - Metformin use in pregnancy remains controversial because it crosses the placenta.
- Insulin:
    - There are no randomized controlled trials on insulin regimens, and therapy is largely guided by expert opinion.
    - Insulin is usually started when initial values are >115 fasting or oral medications have failed to achieve glycemic control.
        1. One commonly used regimen:
            - Insulin 0.7 U/kg/day SQ (based on current pregnant weight), with two thirds of the total daily dose given in the morning and one third of the total daily dose given in the evening
            - One third of each dose is given as short-acting insulin and the remaining two thirds as NPH insulin
        2. Another option:
            - If fasting values are elevated, use NPH at bedtime with initial dose of 0.2 U/kg
            - If postprandial values are elevated, use rapid-acting insulin before meals with initial dose 1.5 U/10 g carbohydrate at breakfast and 1 U/10 g carbohydrate at lunch and dinner
        3. Long-acting insulin such as Lantus does not have sufficient data to determine whether it crosses the placenta; it may be continued in persons with preexisting diabetes who are well controlled but is not recommended in patients with newly diagnosed GDM

ANTENATAL TESTING

Routine blood pressure and urine protein monitoring:

- Class A1: NST/AFI at 40 wk
- Class A2: weekly NST/AFI beginning at 32 wk or when insulin is started
- Poorly controlled diabetes, vascular complications, or hypertension: biweekly NST/AFI beginning at 28 wk and consider admission for initial glycemic control

TIMING AND ROUTE OF DELIVERY

- Class A1 (well controlled): deliver by 41 wk
- Class A2: deliver by 39 completed wk
- Offer elective cesarean section at 39 completed wk if estimated fetal weight is over 4500 g
- Consider delivery by 37 wk if poor control or intrauterine growth retardation after confirmed fetal lung maturity by amniocentesis

INTRAPARTUM MANAGEMENT

- Goal is normoglycemia (80 to 110 mg/dl) using insulin and D5 lactated Ringer's IV fluid
- Monitor glucose hourly
- Preparation for shoulder dystocia
- If on glyburide, discontinue in labor or 12 hr before a scheduled induction

NEONATAL MANAGEMENT

- Check 30- and 60-min glucose
- Watch for signs of hypoglycemia, hypocalcemia, hyperbilirubinemia, and polycythemia

POSTPARTUM MANAGEMENT

- Class A2: check fasting level before discharge; if abnormal, continue checking at home and early follow-up with primary care physician to confirm diagnosis of DM
- 6-wk postpartum visit: screen for diabetes in A1 and A2 women with a 2-hr glucose tolerance test or two fasting values
- If no evidence of DM, screen annually for DM and counsel on risk factor modification

REFERRAL

- Nutritionist
- High-risk obstetrician
- Maternal-fetal medicine
- Diabetes educator

COMPLICATIONS

- Maternal: preeclampsia, future type 2 DM or GDM, operative delivery
- Fetal: polyhydramnios, macrosomia, shoulder dystocia, birth trauma, congenital malformations
- Neonatal: hypoglycemia, hypocalcemia, hyperbilirubinemia, polycythemia, perinatal death, future obesity and DM, impaired fine and gross motor functions; increased rates of inattention and hyperactivity

PEARLS & CONSIDERATIONS

Trials have shown that although treatment of mild gestational DM did not significantly reduce the frequency of a composite outcome that included stillbirth or perinatal death and several neonatal complications, it did reduce the risks of fetal overgrowth, shoulder dystocia, cesarean delivery, and hypertensive disorders.

PREVENTION

Regular exercise, maintenance of ideal body weight, and high-fiber low-glycemic diet

PATIENT & FAMILY EDUCATION

Gestational Diabetes Patient Information
American Academy of Family Physicians
http://www.aafp.org/afp/20031101/1775ph.html

American Dietetic Association
Consumer Nutrition Information and Referrals
http://www.eatright.org
Telephone: 800-366-1655

American Diabetes Association: Gestational Diabetes
http://www.diabetes.org
800-DIABETES (800-342-2383)

NOAH: New York Online Access to Health
http://www.noah-health.org

National Institute of Child Health and Human Development
Managing Gestational Diabetes: A Patient's Guide to a Healthy Pregnancy
http://www.nichd.nih.gov/publications/pubs/gest_diabetes/
800-370-2943

Food and Nutrition Information Center
Food Guide Pyramid
http://www.nal.usda.gov.

SUGGESTED READINGS

available at www.expertconsult.com

RELATED CONTENT

Gestational Diabetes (Patient Information)
Diabetes Mellitus (Related Key Topic)

AUTHORS: **MARY BETH SUTTER M.D., JORDAN WHITE, M.D., M.P.H., NIRALI BORA, M.D., HEIDI RADLINSKI, M.D., M.P.H.,** and **SUSANNA R. MAGEE, M.D., M.P.H.**

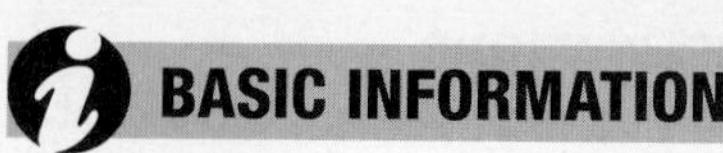

DEFINITION

Giant cell arteritis (GCA) is a segmental systemic granulomatous arteritis affecting medium and large arteries in individuals >50 yr. Inflammation primarily targets extracranial blood vessels, and although the carotid system is usually affected, pathology in the posterior cerebral artery has been reported.

SYNONYMS

Temporal arteritis
Cranial arteritis
GCA
Horton's disease

ICD-9CM CODES
446.5 Temporal arteritis
ICD-10CM CODES
M31.5 Giant cell arteritis with polymyalgia rheumatica
M31.6 Other giant cell arteritis

EPIDEMIOLOGY & DEMOGRAPHICS

INCIDENCE: 17 to 23.3 new cases per 100,000 persons >50 yr; peak incidence is in patients ages 60 to 80 yr
PREVALENCE: 200 cases per 100,000 persons; female/male predominance of twofold to fourfold; more common in Caucasians

PHYSICAL FINDINGS & CLINICAL PRESENTATION

GCA can present with the following clinical manifestations:

- Headache, often associated with marked scalp tenderness—noticed while brushing hair (hair comb allodynia)
- Constitutional symptoms (fever, weight loss, anorexia, fatigue)
- Polymyalgia rheumatica (aching and stiffness of the trunk and proximal muscle groups)
- Visual disturbances (transient or permanent monocular or binocular visual loss)
- Intermittent claudication of jaw and tongue on mastication that is especially prominent when solid food such as steak is chewed
- Table 1-201 describes atypical manifestations of GCA.

Important physical findings in GCA:

- Vascular examination: The temporal artery demonstrates tenderness, decreased pulsation, and nodulation (ropy) (Fig. 1-401); diminished or absent pulses in upper extremities may be seen

TABLE 1-201 Atypical Manifestations of Giant Cell Arteritis

Fever of unknown origin
Respiratory symptoms (especially cough)
Otolaryngeal manifestations
- Glossitis
- Lingual infarction
- Throat pain
- Hearing loss

Large-artery disease
- Aortic aneurysm
- Aortic dissection
- Limb claudication
- Raynaud's phenomenon

Neurologic manifestations
- Peripheral neuropathy
- Transient ischemic attack (TIA) or stroke
- Dementia
- Delirium

Myocardial infarction
Tumorlike lesions
- Breast mass
- Ovarian and uterine mass

Syndrome of inappropriate antidiuretic hormone secretion (SIADH)
Microangiopathic hemolytic anemia

From Harris ED et al: *Kelly's textbook of rheumatology,* ed 7, Philadelphia, 2005, Saunders.

ETIOLOGY

Vasculitis of unknown etiology

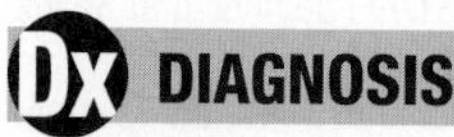

Clinical history and vascular examination remain cornerstones of diagnosis. An algorithm for diagnosing GCA is described in Fig. 1-402. The American College of Rheumatology has proposed the following criteria for the diagnosis of GCA. Presence of three or more of these criteria in a patient with suspected vasculitis is considered to be diagnostic for GCA.

- Age of onset of symptoms >50 yr
- New-onset of or new type of localized headache
- Temporal artery abnormalities including tenderness or decreased pulsation
- Westergren erythrocyte sedimentation rate (ESR) elevated (typically >50 mm/hr)
- Temporal artery biopsy with vasculitis and mononuclear cell infiltrate or granulomatous changes

DIFFERENTIAL DIAGNOSIS

- Other vasculitic syndromes
- Nonarteritic anterior ischemic optic neuropathy (NAION)
- Pituitary apoplexy
- Primary amyloidosis
- Transient ischemic attack, stroke
- Infections
- Occult neoplasm, multiple myeloma

LABORATORY TESTS

- ESR elevated although up to 22.5% of patients with GCA have normal ESR before treatment.
- C-reactive protein (CRP) is typically included in laboratory investigation; it may have greater sensitivity than ESR. CRP typically rises before the ESR.

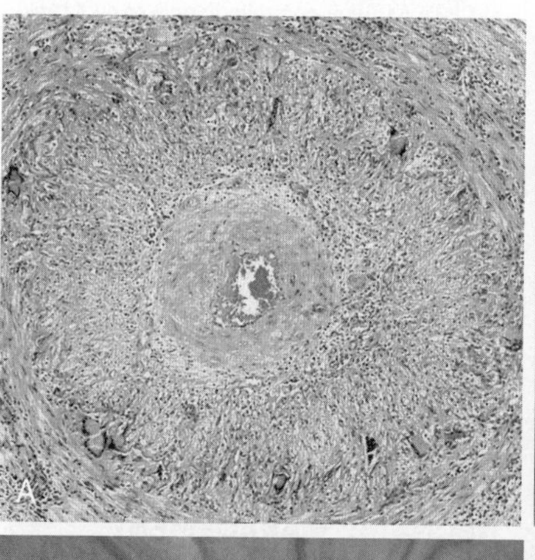

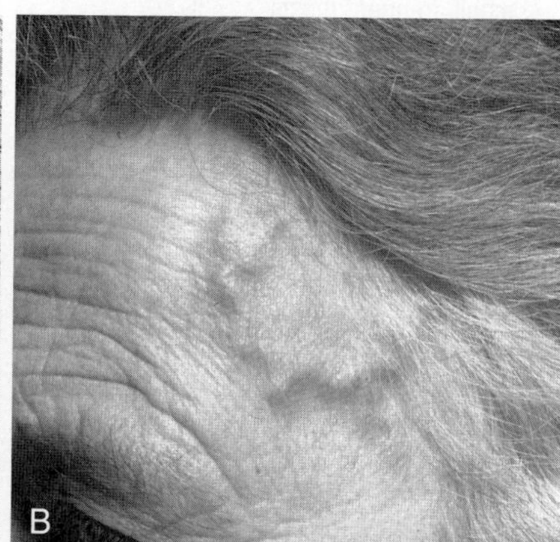

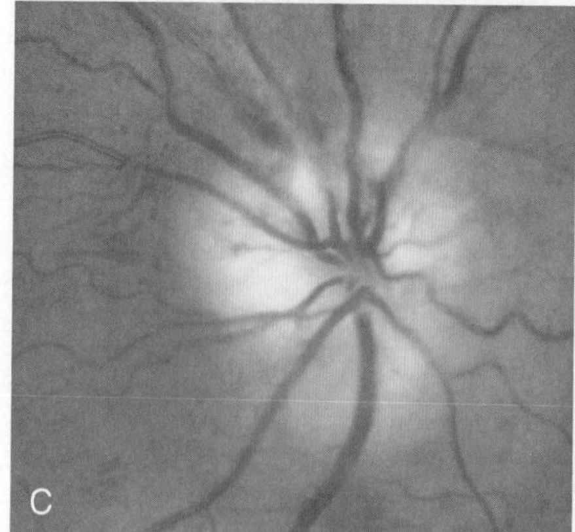

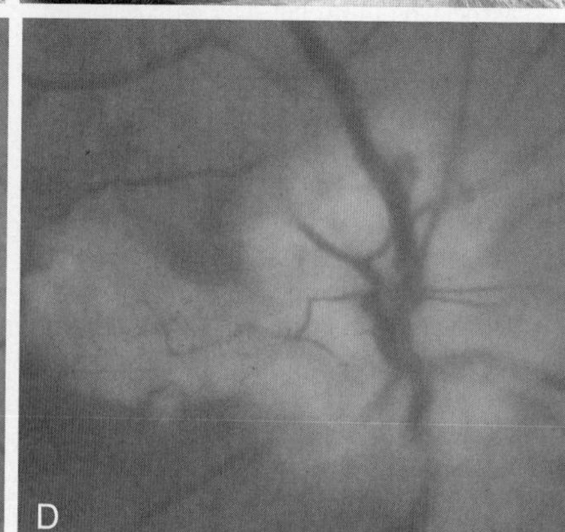

FIGURE 1-401 Giant cell arteritis. A, Histology shows transmural granulomatous inflammation, disruption of the internal elastic lamina, proliferation of the intima, and gross narrowing of the lumen. **B,** The superficial temporal artery is pulseless, nodular, and thickened. **C,** Ischemic optic neuropathy. **D,** Ischemic optic neuropathy and cilioretinal artery occlusion. (From Kanski JJ, Bowling B: *Clinical ophthalmology, a systematic approach,* ed 7, Philadelphia, 2010, Saunders.)

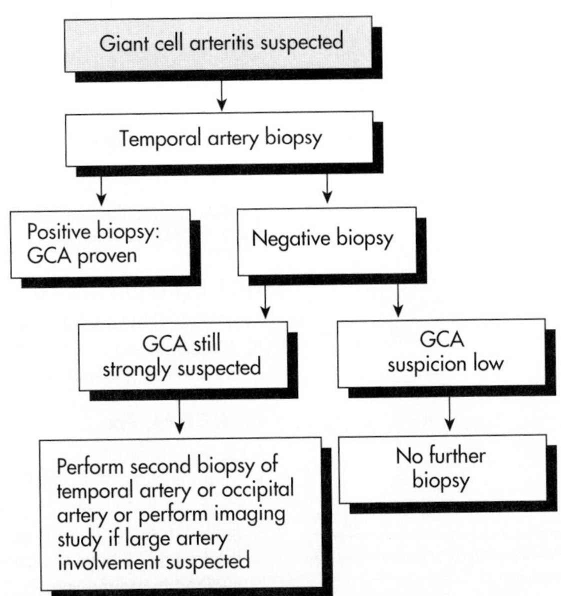

FIGURE 1-402 Algorithm for diagnosing giant cell arteritis (GCA) (From Firestein GS et al: Kelly's textbook of rheumatology, ed 9, Philadelphia, 2013, Saunders.)

- Mild to moderate normochromic normocytic anemia, elevated platelet count.

IMAGING STUDIES

- Color duplex ultrasonography of temporal artery produces three characteristic features—periluminal "halo" over the temporal artery involved, segmental arterial stenosis, and arterial luminal occlusion in severe cases. Clinical utility is not superior to clinical examination with biopsy.
- Contrasted MRI of temporal artery may be performed in patients with contraindications to surgical biopsy of the superficial temporal artery, if treatment with steroids has not been initiated.

Rx TREATMENT

ACUTE GENERAL Rx

- If there is clinical suspicion of GCA, treatment should be initiated without waiting for results of laboratory or imaging studies.
- IV methylprednisolone (250 to 1000 mg for 1 to 3 days) is considered standard of care in patients with severe clinical manifestations such as visual loss from ischemic optic neuropathy.
- Oral prednisone (1 to 1.5 mg/kg/day): high-dose oral regimen should be continued at least until symptoms resolve and ESR returns to normal. Steroid taper is very slow with monitoring of clinical features as well as ESR. Treatment may last up to 2 yr or more.
- Corticosteroids are the treatment of choice. There is no evidence for the role of steroid-sparing agents. Methotrexate may be considered as an adjunct treatment.

DISPOSITION

With steroid therapy there is a dramatic improvement of systemic symptoms but not vision in patients with ischemic optic neuropathy. In one study only 4% of eyes improved in both visual acuity and central visual field.

REFERRAL

- Surgical or ophthalmologic referral for biopsy of temporal artery
- Rheumatology referral for long-term immunosuppressive treatment management

PEARLS & CONSIDERATIONS

- Treatment of GCA should be started if there is clinical suspicion of the disease. Physicians should not wait for laboratory or pathologic confirmation before starting treatment.
- Temporal artery biopsy should be performed as soon as possible but within 2 weeks of initiating treatment with steroids.
- Treatment should not be withheld pending temporal artery biopsy.

COMMENTS

- The relation between polymyalgia rheumatica and GCA is unclear, but the two frequently coexist. They are considered to be different points along the gradient or spectrum of the same disease.
- Clinical picture rather than ESR should be the prime yardstick for continuing prednisone therapy. A rising ESR in a clinically asymptomatic patient with normal hematocrit should raise suspicion for alternate explanations (e.g., infections, neoplasms).
- GCA is associated with a markedly increased risk for the development of aortic aneurysm, which is often a late complication and may cause death. Annual chest radiograph in chronic CGA patients has been suggested, as well as emergent chest CT or MRI for clinical suspicion.
- GCA is also associated with increased risk of myocardial infarction, stroke, and peripheral vascular disease.

SUGGESTED READINGS

available at www.expertconsult.com

RELATED CONTENT

Giant Cell Arteritis (Patient Information)
Temporal Arteritis (Patient Information)

AUTHORS: **ARUN SWAMINATHAN, M.B.B.S.,** and **SACHIN KEDAR, M.B.B.S., M.D.**

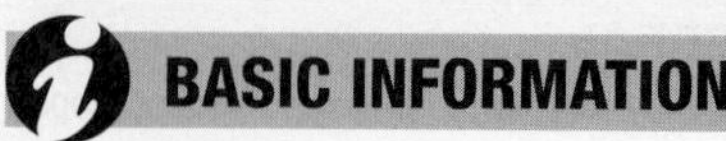

BASIC INFORMATION

DEFINITION

Giardiasis is an intestinal and/or biliary tract infection caused by the protozoal parasite *Giardia lamblia.* The organism is a widespread zoonotic parasite and frequently contaminates fresh water sources worldwide.

SYNONYMS

Giardiasis
Giardia duodenalis
Giardia intestinalis

ICD-9CM CODES
007.1 Giardiasis
ICD-10CM CODES
A07.1 Giardiasis [lambliasis]

EPIDEMIOLOGY & DEMOGRAPHICS

INCIDENCE (IN U.S.):
- Exact incidence unknown. CDC estimates 20,000 cases a year in the U.S.
- Frequently occurs as water-borne outbreaks in international adoptees, travelers, and immunocompromised patients

PREVALENCE (IN U.S.): 4%
PREDOMINANT SEX: Male = female
PREDOMINANT AGE:
- Preschool children, especially if in day care
- 20 to 40 yr of age, especially among sexually active homosexual men

PEAK INCIDENCE:
- Varies with risk factors, outbreaks, but peak onset from early summer through early fall
- All age groups affected

GENETICS: Familial disposition: Patients with common variable immunodeficiency or X-linked agammaglobulinemia are at increased risk of infection.

PHYSICAL FINDINGS & CLINICAL PRESENTATION

- More than 70% with one or more intestinal symptoms (diarrhea, flatulence, cramps, bloating, nausea). Table 1-202 summarizes clinical signs and symptoms of giardiasis
- Incubation period averages 7 to 14 days but can be longer
- Fever in <30%
- Chronic diarrhea, malabsorption, and weight loss, which can be up to 10% of body weight, are common
- GI bleeding is unusual
- Continuous or intermittent symptoms, lasting for 2 to 4 weeks

TABLE 1-202 Clinical Signs and Symptoms of Giardiasis

Symptom	Frequency (%)
Diarrhea	64-100
Malaise, weakness	72-97
Abdominal distention	42-97
Flatulence	35-97
Abdominal cramps	44-81
Nausea	14-79
Foul-smelling, greasy stools	15-79
Anorexia	41-73
Weight loss	53-73
Vomiting	14-35
Fever	0-28
Constipation	0-27

From Kliegman RM et al: *Nelson textbook of pediatrics,* ed 19, Philadelphia, 2011, Saunders.

- Of infected patients, 20% to 25% are asymptomatic and can shed cysts for months

ETIOLOGY

Infection is acquired by ingestion of viable cysts of the organism, typically in contaminated water or food or by fecal-oral contact. *Giardia* cysts are resistant to chlorination and survive well in cold mountain streams.

DIAGNOSIS

DIFFERENTIAL DIAGNOSIS

- Other agents of infective diarrhea (amebae, *Salmonella* sp., *Shigella* sp., *Staphylococcus aureus, Cryptosporidium,* etc.)
- Noninfectious causes of malabsorption

WORKUP

- Stool specimen (three specimens yield 90% sensitivity) as a saline suspension or duodenal aspirate for microscopic examination to establish diagnosis and exclude other pathogens
- Immunoassays for *Giardia* sp. Antigens in stool samples such as the DFA or ELISA are now routinely used in most clinical laboratories. These assays are 85% to 98% sensitive and 90% to 100% specific. They also have a faster turnaround time.

LABORATORY TESTS

Serum albumin, vitamin B_{12} levels, and stool fat test to exclude malabsorption

IMAGING STUDIES

- Not necessary unless biliary obstruction is suspected
- In detection of organism, possible interference by barium in stool from radiographic studies

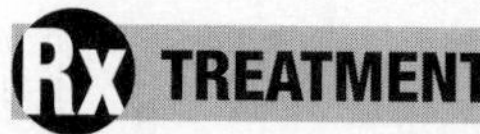

TREATMENT

NONPHARMACOLOGIC THERAPY

Avoidance of milk products to reduce symptoms of transient lactase deficiency that occur in many patients and can last for weeks to months

GENERAL Rx

Adult and pediatric:
- Metronidazole 250 mg PO three times daily for 5 to 7 days is considered the drug of choice in the United States. Pediatric dose: 5 mg/kg tid × 7 days (metronidazole should be avoided in pregnancy).
- Tinidazole: 2 g single dose (50 mg/kg in children over 3 years of age) is a congener of metronidazole
- Nitazoxanide: aged 12 to 47 mo: 100 mg bid × 3 days. Aged 4 to 11 yr: 200 mg bid × 3 days
- Albendazole 400 mg PO qd x 5 days
- Paromomycin 25 to 35 mg/kg/day in three doses for 5 to 10 days
- Can be used in pregnancy

DISPOSITION

Reinfection is possible.

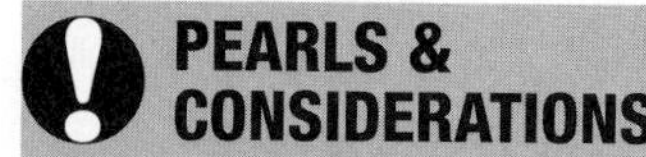

PEARLS & CONSIDERATIONS

COMMENTS

Travelers to endemic areas (developing world, wilderness areas) should be cautioned to boil drinking water or use water purification tablets. Chronic giardiasis as seen in developing nations can cause delays in growth and development in children due to malabsorption and diarrhea.

SUGGESTED READINGS

available at www.expertconsult.com

RELATED CONTENT

Giardiasis (Patient Information)

AUTHOR: **GLENN G. FORT, M.D., M.P.H.**

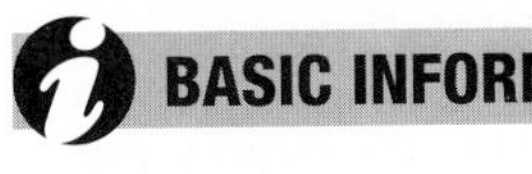

BASIC INFORMATION

DEFINITION

Gilbert's disease is an autosomal-dominant disease characterized by indirect hyperbilirubinemia caused by impaired glucuronyl transferase activity.

SYNONYMS

Gilbert's syndrome

ICD-9CM CODES
277.4 Gilbert's syndrome
ICD-10CM CODES
E80.4 Gilbert's syndrome

EPIDEMIOLOGY & DEMOGRAPHICS

INCIDENCE (IN U.S.): Probable autosomal-dominant disease affecting >5% of the U.S. population
PREDOMINANT SEX: Male/female ratio of 3:1
GENETICS: Most common hereditary hyperbilirubinemia (genotypic prevalence 12%)

PHYSICAL FINDINGS & CLINICAL PRESENTATION

- No abnormalities on physical examination other than mild jaundice when bilirubin exceeds 3 mg/dl.
- A family history of unconjugated hyperbilirubinemia may be present.

ETIOLOGY

- Decreased elimination of bilirubin in bile is caused by inadequate conjugation of bilirubin.
- Alcohol consumption and starvation diet can increase bilirubin level.
- The pathogenesis of Gilbert's syndrome has been linked to a reduction in the bilirubin UGT-1 gene *(HUG-Brl)* transcription, resulting from a mutation in the promoter region.

DIAGNOSIS

DIFFERENTIAL DIAGNOSIS

- Hemolytic anemia
- Liver disease (chronic hepatitis, cirrhosis)
- Crigler-Najjar syndrome

WORKUP

- Most patients are diagnosed during or after adolescence, when isolated hyperbilirubinemia is detected as an incidental finding on routine biochemical testing.
- Laboratory evaluation to exclude hemolysis and liver diseases as a cause of the elevated bilirubin level (Table 1-203).

LABORATORY TESTS

Elevated indirect (unconjugated) bilirubin (rarely exceeds 5 mg/dl)

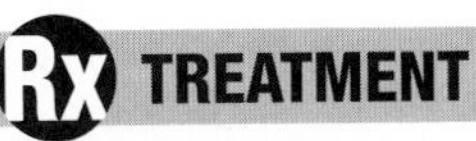

TREATMENT

ACUTE GENERAL Rx

Treatment is generally unnecessary. Phenobarbital (if clinical jaundice is present) can rapidly decrease serum indirect bilirubin level.

DISPOSITION

Prognosis is excellent. Treatment is generally unnecessary.

REFERRAL

Referral is generally not necessary.

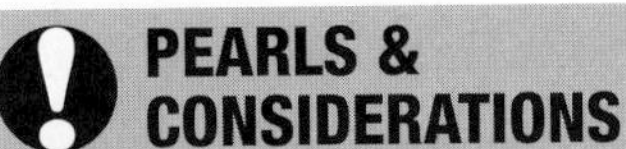

PEARLS & CONSIDERATIONS

COMMENTS

- Patients should be reassured about the benign nature of their condition.
- Fasting for 2 days or significant dehydration may raise the bilirubin level and result in the clinical recognition of jaundice.

AUTHOR: **FRED F. FERRI, M.D.**

TABLE 1-203 Characteristic Patterns of Liver Function Tests

Disorder	Bilirubin	Alkaline Phosphatase	AST	ALT	Prothrombin Time	Albumin
Gilbert's syndrome (abnormal bilirubin metabolism)	↑	NL	NL	NL	NL	NL
Bile duct obstruction (pancreatic cancer)	↑↑↑	↑↑↑	↑	↑	↑-↑↑	NL
Acute hepatocellular damage (toxic, viral hepatitis)	↑-↑↑↑	↑-↑↑	↑↑↑	↑↑↑	NL-↑↑↑	NL-↓↓
Cirrhosis	NL-↑	NL-↑	NL-↑	NL-↑	NL-↑↑	NL-↓↓

ALT, Alanine aminotransferase; *AST,* aspartate aminotransferase; *NL,* normal; ↑ increase; ↓, decrease (arrows indicate extent of change: ↑-↑↑↑, slight to large).
From Andreoli TE (ed): *Cecil essentials of medicine,* ed 6, Philadelphia, 2005, Saunders.

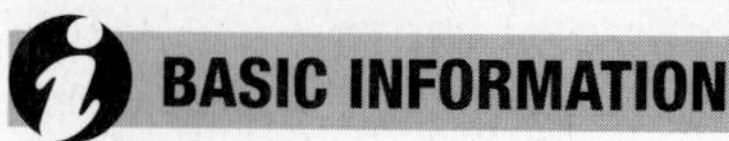

BASIC INFORMATION

DEFINITION

Inflammation of the gums covering the maxilla and mandible

SYNONYMS

None

ICD-9CM CODES
523.1 Chronic gingivitis
523.01 Acute gingivitis
ICD-10CM CODES
K05.0 Acute gingivitis
K05.1 Chronic gingivitis
K05.6 Other disorders of gingivaa and edentulous alveolar ridge

EPIDEMIOLOGY & DEMOGRAPHICS

Gingivitis generally occurs in adults.

PHYSICAL FINDINGS & CLINICAL PRESENTATION

- Inflammation is usually painless. Red velvety gingiva may be present (Fig. 1-403).
- Bleeding may occur with minor trauma such as brushing teeth.
- A bluish discoloration of the gums and halitosis are sometimes present.
- Subgingival plaque may be seen on close examination, and in time, there is detachment of soft tissue from the tooth surface.
- Longstanding infection may lead to destructive periodontal disease, which may involve teeth and bones.
- A dramatic form of gingivitis called acute ulcerative necrotizing gingivitis (ANUG or "trench mouth") can occur. This is manifested by acute, painful inflammation of the gingivae, with bleeding, ulceration, and halitosis. At times this is accompanied by fever and lymphadenopathy.
- Linear gingival erythema ("HIV gingivitis") presents as a brightly inflamed band of marginal gingiva. It may be painful, with easy bleeding and rapid destruction.
- Severe periodontitis can occur in patients with diabetes mellitus or HIV infection and in primary HIV infection (acute retroviral syndrome).
- Pregnancy may be associated with an acute form of gingivitis. Gingivae become inflamed and hypertrophic; this is likely the result of hormonal shifts.

ETIOLOGY

- A variety of organisms may be found in the environment of plaque. Anaerobes play a predominant role in periodontal disease.
- Improper hygiene and poorly fitting dentures may contribute to the development of gingivitis.
- Excessive use of tobacco and alcohol may predispose individuals to gingival disease.
- In patients with HIV infection, gram-negative anaerobes, enteric organisms, and yeast predominate.
- Appropriate oral hygiene, such as flossing and tooth brushing, can prevent the accumulation of bacterial plaque; once dense plaque is present, adequate hygiene becomes more difficult.

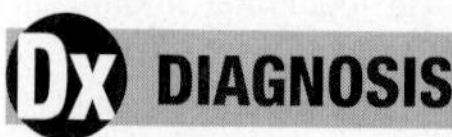

DIAGNOSIS

DIFFERENTIAL DIAGNOSIS

Gingival hyperplasia, which may be caused by long-term use of phenytoin or nifedipine

WORKUP

Oral examination

LABORATORY TESTS

Elevated serum glucose in diabetics

IMAGING STUDIES

Radiographs of the teeth and facial bones may reveal extension of infection to these structures.

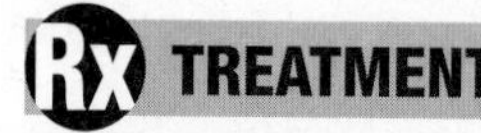

TREATMENT

NONPHARMACOLOGIC THERAPY

Removal of plaque, and at times, debridement of soft tissue

ACUTE GENERAL Rx

- Penicillin VK, 500 mg PO qid for 1 to 2 wk or
- Clindamycin, 300 mg PO qid for 1 to 2 wk
- For linear gingival erythema, chlorhexidine gluconate rinses and nystatin rinses or troches may be used

CHRONIC Rx

Extensive or recurrent infection may require periodic evaluation and debridement.

DISPOSITION

Continued inflammation can eventually lead to destruction of teeth and bone.

REFERRAL

Patients should be referred to a dentist or periodontist.

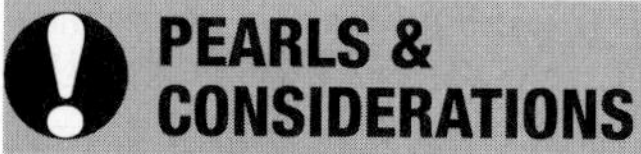

PEARLS & CONSIDERATIONS

COMMENTS

- Presence of periodontal disease is associated with an increased incidence of anaerobic pleuropulmonary infections.
- Existing data support the recommendation to change a toothbrush every 3 mo. Worn brushes seem to be less effective in plaque reduction.

SUGGESTED READINGS

available at www.expertconsult.com

RELATED CONTENT

Gingivitis (Patient Information)
Gingivitis, Necrotizing Ulcerative (Related Key Topic)

AUTHOR: **GLENN G. FORT, M.D., M.P.H.**

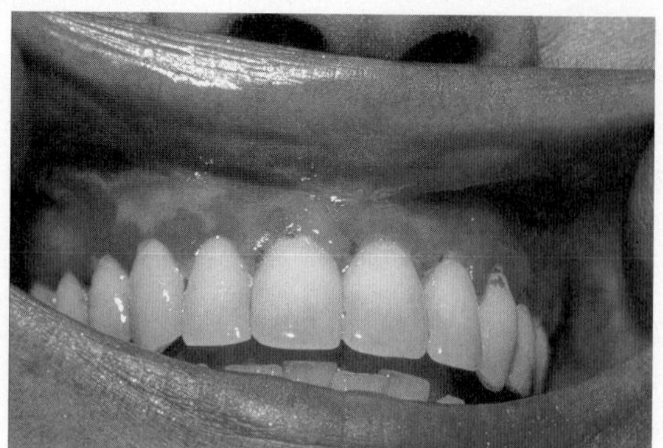

FIGURE 1-403 Gingivitis in a patient with cicatricial pemphigoid. This pattern of periodontal, chronic, red, velvety gingivitis is very suggestive of this disorder but may occur in other blistering diseases. (From White GM, Cox NH [eds]: *Diseases of the skin, a color atlas and text,* ed 2, St Louis, 2006, Mosby.)

BASIC INFORMATION

DEFINITION

Glaucoma is a chronic degenerative optic neuropathy in which the neuro-retinal rim of the optic nerve becomes progressively thinner, thereby enlarging the optic-nerve cup. The classification of glaucomas is based on the appearance of the iridocorneal angle (open angle vs. closed angle) and is further subdivided into primary and secondary types. Primary open-angle glaucoma can occur with or without elevated intraocular pressure (IOP). Normal tension glaucoma refers to primary open-angle glaucoma without elevated intraocular pressure.

SYNONYMS

Chronic simple glaucoma
Primary open-angle glaucoma (POAG)
Open-angle glaucoma (OAG)
Chronic open-angle glaucoma

ICD-9CM CODES
365.1 Open-angle glaucoma
ICD-10CM CODES
H40.1 Primary open-angle glaucoma
H40.8 Glaucoma, unspecified

EPIDEMIOLOGY & DEMOGRAPHICS

INCIDENCE (IN U.S.): Third most common cause of vision loss (75% to 95% of all forms of glaucoma are open angle)

PEAK INCIDENCE:
- Increases after age 40 yr
- Three million cases expected by 2020 because of the rapid increase in aging population

PREVALENCE (IN U.S.):
- Overall prevalence in U.S. population aged >40 yr is estimated to be 1.86%, with 1.57 million white and 398,000 black patients affected.
- 150,000 patients have bilateral blindness.
- Prevalence is higher in diabetics, those with high myopia, and older persons.
- More common in African-American population (three times the age-adjusted prevalence than whites). There is a genetic tendency to OAG; multiple genes have been isolated that are associated with development of high IOP and optic nerve damage.

PREDOMINANT AGE:
- Persons >50 yr
- Can occur in 30s and 40s

PHYSICAL FINDINGS & CLINICAL PRESENTATION

- High intraocular pressures and large optic nerve cup (Ocular Hypertension Treatment Study results very important)
- Corneal edema causes vision loss and blurring (usually no visual symptoms until extremely advanced)
- Abnormal visual fields
- Open anterior chamber angle—evaluated with gonioscopy
- Since early treatable stages of OAG normally have no symptoms, it's important to have routine eye exams, especially patients with family history and patients over 60 yr.
- Secondary forms of OAG may exhibit ocular findings such as pseudo-exfoliation, pigment dispersion, blood in anterior chamber, inflammation

ETIOLOGY

- Uncertain hereditary tendency
- Topical steroids can induce high IOP and cause glaucoma
- Trauma
- Inflammatory (e.g., history of uveitis)
- High-dose oral corticosteroids taken for prolonged periods

Dx DIAGNOSIS

DIFFERENTIAL DIAGNOSIS

- Other optic neuropathies
- Ocular hypertension: IOP is chronically elevated, but not causing optic nerve damage, must monitor closely
- Secondary glaucoma from inflammation and steroid therapy
- Trauma

WORKUP

- Intraocular pressure
- Slit lamp examination
- Visual fields
- Gonioscopy
- Nerve fiber analysis (e.g., GDx, OCT, and HRT)
- Corneal thickness (thick central cornea will result in possible overestimation of the true physiologic IOP, and vice versa, so this is important information in diagnosis and treatment of OAG)

LABORATORY TESTS

Blood sugar

IMAGING STUDIES

- Optic nerve photography—stereo photographs
- Visual field testing
- Laser scan of nerve fiber layer, OCT, HRT. Rarely, MRI of orbits if the glaucoma findings are atypical or suspicious of other causes of optic nerve atrophy

Rx TREATMENT

ACUTE GENERAL Rx

- β-blockers (e.g., Timolol) qd to bid depending on individual response to drug
- Carbonic anhydrase inhibitors (e.g., Diamox 250 mg qid or 500 mg bid)
- Prostaglandin analogs (latanoprost, bimatoprost, travoprost, tafluprost) commonly used as first-line treatment. They lower intraocular pressure by 25%-30% by increasing uveoscleral outflow and reducing aqueous production
- Alpha-2 agonists and cholinergic agonists
- Hyperosmotic agents (mannitol) in acute treatment (IV)
- Laser trabeculoplasty (SLT) as needed

CHRONIC Rx

- At least biannual checks of intraocular pressure and adjustment of medication
- Surgical trabeculectomy and filter valve surgeries can be considered for glaucoma that progresses despite maximal tolerated medical therapies

DISPOSITION

Must be followed by ophthalmologist

REFERRAL

Immediately to ophthalmologist

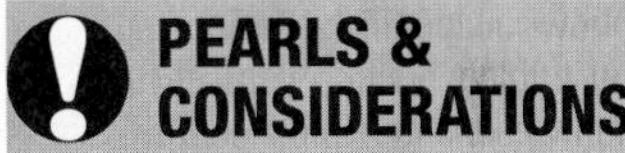

COMMENTS

- Glaucoma is a serious blinding disease that must be monitored professionally by an ophthalmologist. It is mostly asymptomatic until late in the disease when visual problems arise. Even in developed countries half of glaucoma cases are undiagnosed.
- Vision loss from glaucoma cannot be recovered. Early diagnosis and treatment may minimize visual loss.
- Glaucoma is not solely caused by increased intraocular pressure because approximately 20% of patients with glaucoma have normal intraocular pressure. However, high pressure is definitely a risk factor to be considered. Potential sites of increased resistance to aqueous flow are described in Fig. E1-404.

SUGGESTED READINGS

available at www.expertconsult.com

RELATED CONTENT

Glaucoma (Patient Information)

AUTHORS: **MELVYN KOBY, M.D.**, and **R. SCOTT HOFFMAN, M.D.**

BASIC INFORMATION

DEFINITION

Primary angle-closure glaucoma occurs when elevated intraocular pressure is associated with closure of the filtration angle or obstruction in the circulating pathway of the aqueous humor.

SYNONYMS

Acute glaucoma, angle-closure glaucoma (ACG)
Pupillary block glaucoma
Narrow-angle glaucoma
Angle-closure glaucoma

ICD-9CM CODES
365.2 Primary angle-closure glaucoma (PACG)
ICD-10CM CODES
H40.2 Primary angle-closure glaucoma
H40.9 Glaucoma, unspecified

EPIDEMIOLOGY & DEMOGRAPHICS

INCIDENCE (IN U.S.):
- 2% to 8% of all patients with glaucoma
- Higher incidence among those with hyperopia, small eyes, dense cataracts, shallow anterior chambers

PEAK INCIDENCE: Greater >50 yr; high association with hypopia, cataracts, and eye trauma
PREDOMINANT SEX: Females are affected more often than males
PREDOMINANT AGE: 50 to 60 yr
GENETICS: High family history

PHYSICAL FINDINGS & CLINICAL PRESENTATION

- Although angle-closure glaucoma can present with an acute painful crisis associated with blurred vision, more than 75% of patients present with an asymptomatic course with progressive loss of the visual field (similar to that in patients with primary open-angle glaucoma)
- Hazy cornea
- Narrow angle (Fig. E1-405)
- Red eyes
- Pain may be present
- Injection of conjunctiva
- Shallow anterior chamber
- Thick cataract
- Old trauma
- Chronic eye infections

ETIOLOGY

- Narrow angles with acute closure: blockage of circulatory path of the aqueous humor causing increase in intraocular pressure (IOP). ACG occurs more commonly in eyes with shorter axial length (far-sightedness), shallower anterior chamber, and a relatively larger lens (enlarging cataract).
- Secondary angle-closure glaucoma resulting from neovascularization of iris, iris tumors, lens induced, iris scarring, trauma, chronic inflammation with scarring, malignant glaucoma with aqueous misdirection

DIAGNOSIS

DIFFERENTIAL DIAGNOSIS

- Open-angle glaucoma: Angle-closure glaucoma is distinguished from open-angle glaucoma by the closure of the angle between the iris and cornea, obstructing outflow of aqueous humor
- High pressure
- Optic nerve cupping
- Shallow chamber
- Open-angle glaucoma
- Conjunctivitis
- Corneal disease, keratitis
- Uveitis
- Scleritis
- Allergies
- Contact lens wearing with irritation

WORKUP

Comprehensive eye examination: if one suspects narrow angle or angle closure, avoid pupil dilation since this may exacerbate the attack
- Intraocular pressure
- Gonioscopy
- Slit lamp examination
- Visual field examination
- GDx examination (laser scan of nerve fiber layer), OCT
- Optic nerve evaluation
- Anterior chamber depth

LABORATORY TESTS

- Blood sugar and complete blood count (if diabetes or inflammatory disease is suspected)
- Visual field
- GDx nerve fiber analysis, OCT, Heidelberg retinal tomography

IMAGING STUDIES

- Fundus photography
- Fluorescein angiography for neovascular disease such as diabetic retinopathy, retinal vein occlusions
- Ultrasound biomicroscopy and anterior OCT can show relationships of anterior eye structures

TREATMENT

The goal of treatment is to acutely lower pressure on the eye and keep it down.

NONPHARMACOLOGIC THERAPY

Laser iridotomy early in disease process

ACUTE GENERAL Rx

- IV mannitol
- Pilocarpine
- β-blockers
- Diamox
- Laser iridotomy
- Anterior chamber paracentesis (as emergency treatment)

CHRONIC Rx

- Iridotomy
- Trabeculectomy
- Filter valves
- Other laser procedures

DISPOSITION

Refer to ophthalmologist immediately.

REFERRAL

If acute angle-closure episode is suspected, should refer emergently to ophthalmologist.

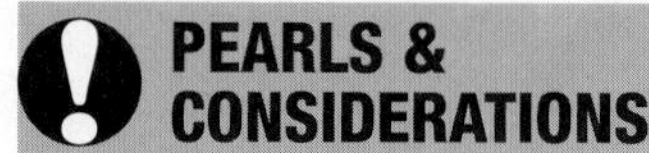

PEARLS & CONSIDERATIONS

COMMENTS

- Do not use antihistamines or vasodilators with narrow-angle glaucoma.
- After iridotomy, the majority of patients will be totally cured and will need no further medication and have no visual loss.
- Lower socioeconomic status and higher levels of social deprivation are risk factors for delayed detection and probable worse outcomes in glaucoma.
- Glaucoma is undiagnosed in 9 out of 10 affected people worldwide and is undiagnosed in 50% of those in developed countries.

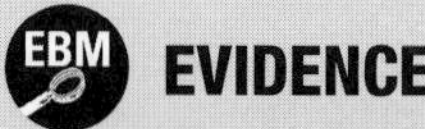

EVIDENCE

available at www.expertconsult.com

SUGGESTED READINGS

available at www.expertconsult.com

RELATED CONTENT

Glaucoma (Patient Information)

AUTHORS: **MELVYN KOBY, M.D.**, and **R. SCOTT HOFFMAN, M.D.**

BASIC INFORMATION

DEFINITION

Glenohumeral dislocation (Fig. 1-406) is complete separation or displacement of the humeral head from the glenoid surface (partial separation is termed *subluxation*). Most often the cause is traumatic, and the humeral head dislocates anteriorly and inferiorly. This may cause a tear of the glenoid labrum (the Bankart lesion). Less commonly the head dislocates posteriorly.

Rarely, multidirectional instability may be present in which dislocation or subluxation, often bilateral, may occur in multiple directions, usually the result of excessive joint laxity and generally without trauma.

ICD-9CM CODES

831.01 Anterior
831.02 Posterior
831.03 Inferior
718.31 Recurrent
718.81 Instability

ICD-10CM CODES

S43.016A Anterior dislocation of unspecified humerus, initial encounter
S43.026A Posterior dislocation of unspecified humerus, initial encounter
S43.036A Inferior dislocation of unspecified humerus, initial encounter
M24.419 Recurrent dislocation, unspecified shoulder
M24.819 Other specific joint derangements of unspecified shoulder, not elsewhere classified

PHYSICAL FINDINGS & CLINICAL PRESENTATION

Traumatic:

- The arm is held in external rotation with anterior dislocation and internal rotation with posterior dislocation.
- Little movement is possible without pain.

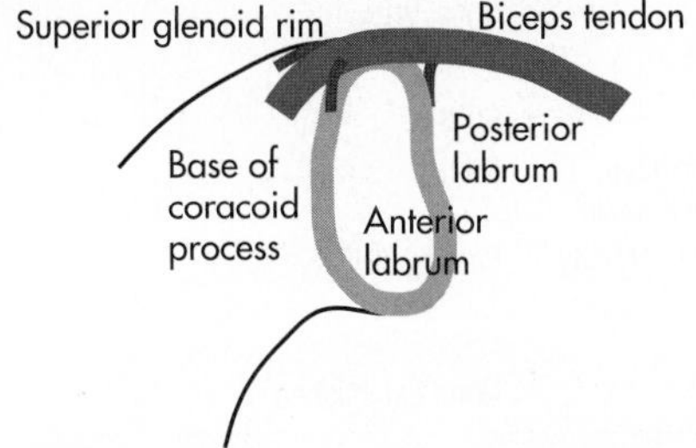

FIGURE 1-406 Glenohumeral dislocation. (From Weissledderer R et al: *Primer of diagnostic imaging*, St Louis, 2007, Mosby.)

- The acromion may appear more prominent, and there is absence of the normal "fullness" beneath the acromion.
- The status of the axillary nerve must always be checked (sensation to the mid-deltoid should be assessed).
- The apprehension test may become positive if anterior instability persists (pain and apprehension that the shoulder will dislocate when the relaxed arm is manually placed in the "throwing position" of external rotation and abduction).
- Recurrent episodes of anterior dislocation may occur with minor movement, such as putting on a coat or turning off a light.

Multidirectional:

- Often difficult to diagnose, especially if only subluxation occurs.
- Recurrent episodes of giving out and weakness, often bilateral and without trauma.
- Sulcus sign is often positive (the arms are pulled downward with the patient standing; a sulcus [indentation] will form between the acromion and humeral head, indicating excessive inferior movement of the head).
- Other signs of generalized joint laxity may be present, such as joint hyperextensibility and the ability of the patient to touch the thumb against the flexor aspect of the forearm.

ETIOLOGY

- Trauma
- Generalized joint laxity (multidirectional)
- Seizures (posterior dislocations)

Dx DIAGNOSIS

DIFFERENTIAL DIAGNOSIS

- Rotator cuff rupture
- Frozen shoulder (posterior dislocation)
- Suprascapular nerve paralysis
- Anterior instability

IMAGING STUDIES

- Acute shoulder injury: true anteroposterior roentgenogram plus lateral view of the glenohumeral joint, either transaxillary or transcapsular
- MRI: to determine soft tissue status, especially the presence of Bankart lesion or rotator cuff tear; may be indicated after a second episode of dislocation

Rx TREATMENT

- Reduction of the acute dislocation by gentle straight traction in the relaxed patient followed by light immobilization
- Gentle limited range-of-motion exercises as pain subsides followed by strengthening exercises at 2 wk

DISPOSITION

- Recurrence of anterior dislocation is common in the young; these patients may have to avoid the arm position associated with dislocation (external rotation with abduction).
- Primary dislocations in patients >40 yr are not generally complicated by recurrence but may result in shoulder stiffness and associated rotator cuff injuries.
- There is an almost 100% recurrence after the third dislocation.

REFERRAL

Surgical reconstruction may be required in the recurrent dislocator.

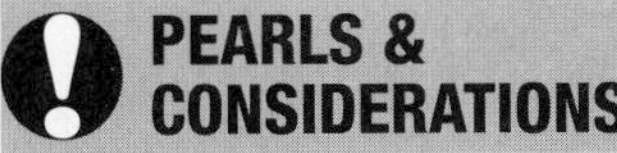

PEARLS & CONSIDERATIONS

COMMENTS

- It is important to know if there was an injury involved in the first episode and if a radiograph was taken to determine direction of the dislocation.
- Up to 50% of posterior dislocations are missed by the first examiner, usually the result of an inadequate lateral radiograph of the glenohumeral joint.
- "Voluntary" posterior dislocators should always be treated nonsurgically.
- Sports activities may be resumed when there is pain-free full flexibility and normal strength.
- Multidirectional instabilities are usually treated nonsurgically with strengthening exercises.
- Dislocations in either direction are occasionally overlooked. If the injury is over 2 to 4 weeks old, enough tissue healing will have occurred to make closed reduction fail. Open reduction or arthroplasty will then be needed in the young. Older patients may improve with therapeutic exercises, and the resultant disability is often acceptable.

SUGGESTED READINGS

available at www.expertconsult.com

AUTHORS: **LONNIE R. MERCIER, M.D., and FRED F. FERRI, M.D.**

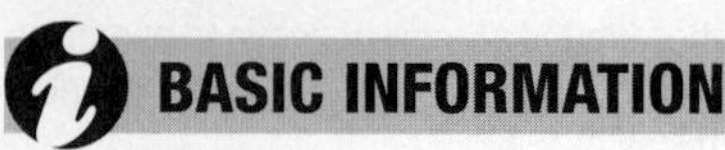

BASIC INFORMATION

DEFINITION

Acute glomerulonephritis is an immunologically mediated inflammation primarily involving the glomerulus that can result in damage to the basement membrane, mesangium, or capillary endothelium.

SYNONYMS

Postinfectious glomerulonephritis
Acute nephritic syndrome

ICD-9CM CODES
583.9 Glomerulonephritis, acute
ICD-10CM CODES
N00.3 Acute nephritic syndrome with diffuse mesangial proliferative glomerulonephritis
N01.3 Rapidly progressive nephritic syndrome with diffuse mesangial proliferative glomerulonephritis

EPIDEMIOLOGY & DEMOGRAPHICS

- More than 50% of cases involve children <13 yr.
- Glomerulonephritis is the most common cause of chronic renal failure (25%).
- Immunoglobulin A (IgA) nephropathy glomerulonephritis (Berger's disease) is the most common glomerulonephritis worldwide.
- Occurs in 4 out of 100,000 cases.

PHYSICAL FINDINGS & CLINICAL PRESENTATION

- Edema (peripheral, periorbital, or pulmonary)
- Joint pains, oral ulcers, malar rash (frequently seen with lupus nephritis)
- Dark urine
- Fatigue, decreased appetite
- Acute onset of hypertension
- Findings of palpable purpura in patients with Henoch-Schönlein purpura
- Heart murmurs may indicate endocarditis
- Impetigo, skin pallor, palpable purpura, tenderness in the abdomen and/or back, pharyngeal erythema may be present

ETIOLOGY

Acute glomerulonephritis may be caused by primary renal disease or a systemic disease. A number of pathogenic processes (e.g., antibody deposition, cell-mediated immune mechanisms, complement activation, hemodynamic alterations) have been implicated in the pathogenesis of glomerular inflammation. Medical disorders generally associated with glomerulonephritis are:

- Group A beta-hemolytic *Streptococcus* infection (other infectious etiologies including endocarditis and visceral abscess)
- Collagen-vascular diseases (systemic lupus erythematosus [SLE])
- Vasculitis (Wegener's granulomatosis, polyarteritis nodosa)
- Idiopathic glomerulonephritis (membranoproliferative, idiopathic, crescentic, IgA nephropathy)
- Goodpasture's syndrome
- Other cryoglobulinemia (Henoch-Schönlein purpura)
- Drug-induced (gold, penicillamine)

Table 1-204 summarizes primary renal diseases that present as acute glomerulonephritis. Diseases associated with rapidly progressive glomerulonephritis and pertinent laboratory findings are described in Table 1-205.

Dx DIAGNOSIS

DIFFERENTIAL DIAGNOSIS

- Cirrhosis with edema and ascites
- Congestive heart failure
- Acute interstitial nephritis
- Acute tubular necrosis
- Severe hypertension
- Hemolytic-uremic syndrome
- SLE, diabetes mellitus, amyloidosis, preeclampsia, sclerodermal renal crisis

WORKUP

Initial evaluation of suspected glomerulonephritis consists of laboratory testing.

LABORATORY TESTS

- Urinalysis (hematuria [dysmorphic erythrocytes and red cell casts], proteinuria)
- Serum creatinine (to estimate glomerular filtration rate [GFR]), blood urea nitrogen
- 24-hr urine for protein excretion and creatinine clearance (to document degree of renal dysfunction and amount of proteinuria).

TABLE 1-204 Summary of Primary Renal Diseases that Manifest as Acute Glomerulonephritis

Diseases	Poststreptococcal Glomerulonephritis	IgA Nephropathy	Goodpasture Syndrome	Idiopathic Rapidly Progressive Glomerulonephritis
Clinical Manifestations				
Age and sex	All ages, mean 7 yr, 2:1 male	10–35 yr, 2:1 male	15–30 yr, 6:1 male	Adults, 2:1 male
Acute nephritic syndrome	90%	50%	90%	90%
Asymptomatic hematuria	Occasionally	50%	Rare	Rare
Nephrotic syndrome	10%–20%	Rare	Rare	10%–20%
Hypertension	70%	30%–50%	Rare	25%
Acute renal failure	50% (transient)	Very rare	50%	60%
Other	Latent period of 1–3 wk	Follows viral syndromes	Pulmonary hemorrhage; iron deficiency anemia	None
Laboratory findings	↑ ASO titers (70%) Positive streptozyme (95%) ↓ C3–C9; normal C1, C4	↑ Serum IgA (50%) IgA in dermal capillaries	Positive anti-GBM antibody	Positive ANCA in some
Immunogenetics	HLA-B12, D "EN" (9)*	HLA-Bw 35, DR4 (4)*	HLA-DR2 (16)*	None established
Renal Pathology				
Light microscopy	Diffuse proliferation	Focal proliferation	Focal → diffuse proliferation with crescents	Crescentic GN
Immunofluorescence	Granular IgG, C3	Diffuse mesangial IgA	Linear IgG, C3	No immune deposits
Electron microscopy	Subepithelial humps	Mesangial deposits	No deposits	No deposits
Prognosis	95% resolve spontaneously 5% RPGN or slowly progressive	Slow progression in 25%–50%	75% stabilize or improve if treated early	75% stabilize or improve if treated early
Treatment	Supportive	Uncertain (options include steroids, fish oil, and ACE inhibitors)	Plasma exchange, steroids, cyclophosphamide	Steroid pulse therapy

*Relative risk.
ACE, Angiotensin-converting enzyme; *ANCA,* antineutrophil cytoplasmic antibody; *ASO,* anti-streptolysin O; *GBM,* glomerular basement membrane; *GN,* glomerulonephritis; *HLA,* human leukocyte antigen; *Ig,* immunoglobulin; *RPGN,* idiopathic rapidly progressive glomerulonephritis.
From Kliegman RM et al: *Practical strategies in pediatric diagnosis and therapy,* ed 2, Philadelphia, 2004, Saunders.

TABLE 1-205 Diseases Associated with Rapidly Progressive Glomerulonephritis and Pertinent Laboratory Studies

Disease	Studies
Renal Limited	
IgA nephropathy	
Postinfectious glomerulonephritis	Low complement, streptococcal serologies, bacterial cultures
ANCA-associated glomerulonephritis (pauci-immune glomerulonephritis)	ANCA titers
Anti-GBM disease (Goodpasture's syndrome)	Anti-GBM antibodies
Systemic Disorders	
Lupus nephritis	Low complement, ANA, dsDNA antibodies
ANCA-associated small-vessel vasculitis	ANCA titers
Anti-GBM disease	Anti-GBM antibodies
Henoch-Schönlein purpura	None
Cryoglobulinemic vasculitis	Low complement, cryoglobulins, hepatitis C serologies

ANCA, Antineutrophil cytoplasmic antibody; *ANA,* antinuclear antibodies; *dsDNA,* double-stranded DNA; *GBM,* glomerular basement membrane; *IgA,* immunoglobulin A.
From Vincent JL et al: *Textbook of critical care,* ed 6, Philadelphia, 2011, Saunders.

TABLE 1-206 Antigens Identified in Glomerulonephritis

Poststreptococcal GN	Streptococcal pyrogenic exotoxin B, plasmin receptor
Anti-GBM disease	α3 type IV collagen (likely induced by molecular mimicry)
IgA nephropathy	Possibly no antigen but rather polymerized polyclonal IgA (?superantigen driven)
Membranous nephropathy	Phospholipase A_2 receptor (idiopathic), neutral endopeptidase in podocyte (congenital), HBeAg (hepatitis associated)
Staphylococcus aureus–associated GN	*Staphylococcus* superantigens induce polyclonal response; not necessarily antigen in glomeruli
Membranoproliferative GN	HCV and HBsAg in hepatitis-associated MPGN
ANCA-associated vasculitis	Proteinase 3 (c-ANCA) and myeloperoxidase (p-ANCA) in neutrophils; antibodies to lysosome-associated membrane protein 2 on endothelial cells (likely induced by molecular mimicry to fimbriated bacterial antigens)

ANCA, Antineutrophil cytoplasmic antibody; *GBM,* glomerular basement membrane; *GN,* glomerulonephritis; *HBeAg,* hepatitis B virus early antigen; *HBsAg,* hepatitis B surface antigen; *HCV,* hepatitis C virus; *IgA,* immuoglobulin A; *MPGN,* membranoproliferative glomerulonephritis.
From Floege J et al: *Comprehensive clinical nephrology,* ed 4, Philadelphia, 2010, Saunders.

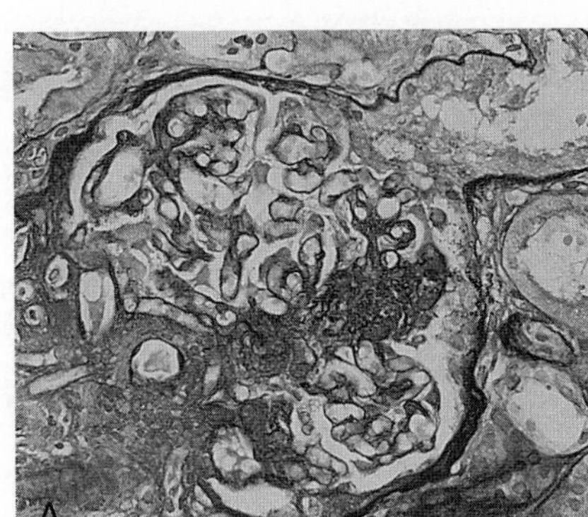

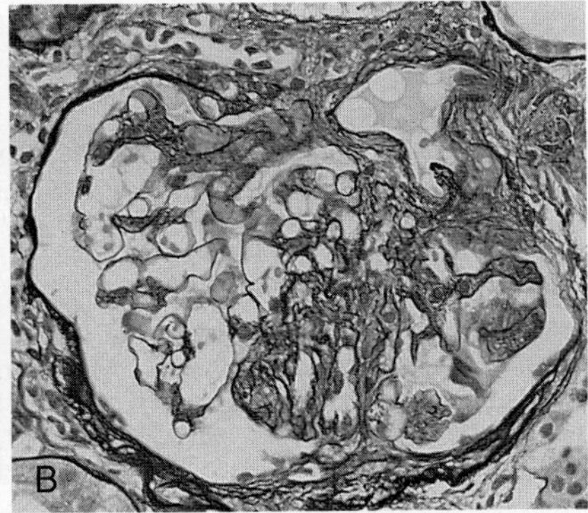

FIGURE 1-407 Light microscopic appearances in focal segmental glomerulosclerosis. Segmental scars with capsular adhesions in otherwise normal glomeruli. A, Periodic acid-Schiff, ×300. **B,** Methenamine silver stain, ×300. (Courtesy Dr. D. Davies. From Johnson RJ, Feehally J: *Comprehensive clinical nephrology,* ed 2, St Louis, 2000, Mosby.)

Proteinuria in acute glomerulonephritis typically ranges from 500 mg/day to 3 g/day, but nephrotic-range proteinuria (>3.5 g/day) may be present.

- Spot urine sodium and creatinine for calculation of fractional excretion of sodium (FENa), which is less than 1% in acute glomerulonephritis.
- Streptococcal tests (Streptozyme), antistreptolysin O (ASO) quantitative titer (highest in 3 to 5 wk); ASO titer, however, is not related to severity of renal disease, duration, or prognosis.
- Additional useful tests depending on the history: anti-DNA antibodies (rule out SLE), CH_{50} level (if elevated, obtain C_3, C_4 levels), triglycerides, cryoglobulins, hepatitis B and C serologies, antineutrophil cytoplasmic antibody (ANCA), c-ANCA (in suspected cases of Wegener's granulomatosis), p-ANCA found in pauciimmune (lack of immune deposits) idiopathic rapidly progressive glomerulonephritis with or without systemic vasculitis, and antiglomerular basement membrane (type alpha[3] IV collagen) antibodies.
- Hematocrit (decrease in glomerulonephritis) and platelet count (thrombocytopenia in cases of lupus nephritis).
- Anti–glomerular basement membrane antibody (in Goodpasture's syndrome).
- Blood cultures are indicated in all febrile patients.
- Antigens identified in glomerulonephritis are described in Table 1-206.

IMAGING STUDIES

- Chest x-ray: pulmonary congestion, Wegener's granulomatosis, and Goodpasture's syndrome.
- Renal ultrasound if GFR is depressed to evaluate renal size and determine extent of fibrosis. A kidney size of <9 cm is suggestive of extensive scarring and low likelihood of reversibility.
- Echocardiogram in patients with new cardiac murmurs or positive blood cultures to rule out endocarditis and pericardial effusion.
- Renal biopsy and light (Fig. 1-407), electron, and immunofluorescent microscopy to confirm diagnosis.
- Kidney biopsy: generally reveals a granular pattern in poststreptococcal glomerulonephritis and a linear pattern in Goodpasture's syndrome; absence of immune deposits suggests vasculitis. It is useful to determine the degree of inflammation and fibrosis. It is also especially important for patients with rapidly progressive glomerulonephritis, in whom prompt diagnosis and treatment are essential.
- Immunofluorescence: generally reveals C_3. Negative immunofluorescence suggests Wegener's granulomatosis, idiopathic crescentic glomerulonephritis, or polyarteritis nodosa.
- Angiography or biopsy of other affected organs if systemic vasculitis is suspected.

 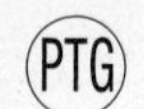

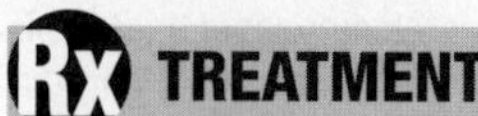

TREATMENT

NONPHARMACOLOGIC THERAPY

- Avoidance of salt if edema or hypertension is present
- Low-protein intake (approximately 0.5 g/kg/day) in patients with renal failure
- Fluid restriction in patients with significant edema
- Avoidance of high-potassium foods

ACUTE GENERAL Rx

- Correction of electrolyte abnormalities (hypocalcemia, hyperkalemia) and acidosis (if present)
- Treatment of streptococcal infection with penicillin (or erythromycin in penicillin-allergic patients)
- Furosemide in patients with significant hypertension and/or edema; hydralazine or nifedipine in patients with hypertension
- Hemodialysis in volume overload, hyperkalemia, uremic symptoms, and encephalopathy
- Immunosuppressive treatment in patients with heavy proteinuria or rapidly decreasing GFR (high-dose steroids, cyclosporin A, cyclophosphamide); corticosteroids generally not useful in poststreptococcal glomerulonephritis
- Fish oil (n-3 fatty acids) 12 g/day; may prevent or slow loss of renal function in patients with IgA nephropathy
- Plasma exchange therapy and immunosuppressive drugs (prednisone and cyclophosphamide); effective in Goodpasture's syndrome
- Short-term therapy with IV cyclophosphamide followed by maintenance therapy with mycophenolate mofetil or azathioprine. Oral mycophenolate mofetil is also effective in induction therapy in patients with lupus nephritis
- Mycophenolate mofetil appears superior to azathioprine in maintaining a renal response to treatment and in preventing relapse in patients with lupus nephritis who responded to induction therapy
- Rituximab and glucocorticoids have been shown to be effective in C3 glomerulonephritis
- Table 1-207 summarizes suggested management of membranoproliferative glomerulonephritis

CHRONIC Rx

- Frequent monitoring of urinalysis, serum creatinine, and blood pressure in the initial 12 mo
- Monitoring for onset of hypertensive retinopathy, encephalopathy
- Angiotensin-converting enzyme (ACE) inhibitors and angiotensin receptor II blockers (ARBs) are used in patients with proteinuria
- Aggressive treatment of infections, particularly streptococcal infections
- Dosage adjustment of all renally excreted medications

DISPOSITION

- Prognosis is generally related to histology, with excellent prognosis in patients with minimal change in glomerulonephritis and focal segmental proliferative glomerulonephritis. Between 25% and 30% of patients with mesangial IgA disease and membranous glomerulonephritis generally progress to chronic renal failure; <70% of patients with mesangial capillary glomerulonephritis will develop chronic renal failure.
- In general, prognosis is worse in patients with heavy proteinuria, severe hypertension, and significant elevations of creatinine.
- Recovery of renal function occurs within 8 to 12 wk in 95% of patients with poststreptococcal glomerulonephritis.

REFERRAL

- Nephrology consultation. The urgency for referral depends on the GFR. Urgent consultation is recommended if GFR is significantly abnormal or rapidly deteriorating or if the patient has systemic symptoms.
- Surgical referral for biopsy in selected cases.

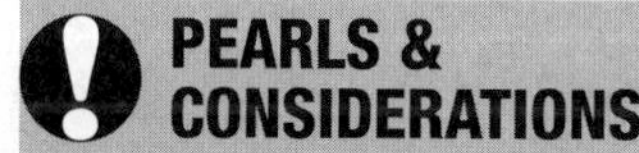

PEARLS & CONSIDERATIONS

COMMENTS

- Anticoagulation to prevent deep vein thrombosis should be considered in patients with a low level of physical activity.
- Monitoring of lipids and aggressive treatment of hyperlipidemias are recommended.
- Close monitoring of side effects of immunosuppressive drugs and complications of corticosteroids is necessary.

SUGGESTED READINGS

available at www.expertconsult.com

RELATED CONTENT

Glomerulonephritis (Patient Information)
Acute Kidney Injury (Related Key Topic)

AUTHORS: **SYEDA M. SAYEED, M.D.**, and **FRED F. FERRI, M.D.**

TABLE 1-207 Suggested Management of Membranoproliferative Glomerulonephritis

Type	Treatment
All types	Supportive therapy following the recommendations discussed in text
Idiopathic MPGN in children	Non-nephrotic proteinuria, normal renal function: follow with 3-month visits Normal renal function and moderate proteinuria (>3 g/day): prednisone 40 mg/m^2 on alternate days for 3 months Nephrotic or impaired renal function: prednisone 40 mg/m^2 on alternate days (80 mg maximum) for 2 years, tapering to 20 mg on alternate days for 3-10 years
Idiopathic MPGN in adults	Non-nephrotic, normal renal function: follow with 3-month visits Nephrotic or impaired renal function: 6-month course of corticosteroid with/without cytotoxic agents (cyclophosphamide) or other drugs used: cyclosporine, tacrolimus, mycophenolate mofetil Rapidly progressive renal failure with diffuse crescents: treat as for idiopathic rapidly progressive glomerulonephritis In the presence of chronic renal failure or nephrotic proteinuria: angiotensin-converting enzyme inhibitors
MPGN associated with hepatitis C virus or cryoglobulinemia	Non-nephrotic, normal renal function: treat with interferon alpha based on severity of liver disease (diagnosed by biopsy) Nephrotic syndrome, reduced renal function, or signs of cryoglobulinemia: pegylated interferon alfa-2b (1 mg/kg weekly) and ribavirin (15 mg/kg/day) for 12 months, followed by a short-term course of low-dose corticosteroids; if relapse occurs, consider high-dose interferon alfa (10 million U daily for 2 weeks, then every other day for 6 more weeks) Rapidly progressive renal failure or severe symptoms of vasculitis (heart failure, pulmonary disease): methylprednisolone 1 g daily for 3 days, followed by oral prednisone 60 mg/daily with slow taper during 2-3 months Cyclophosphamide (2 mg/kg/day with adjustment for renal function) and cryofiltration may be added as adjunctive therapy; when the prednisone is reduced to 20 mg/day and the cyclophosphamide is discontinued, add interferon alfa MPGN in the renal or liver transplant recipient: consider course of oral ribavirin (0.6-1 g/day)

MPGN, Membranoproliferative glomerulonephritis.
From Floege J et al: *Comprehensive clinical nephrology,* ed 4, Philadelphia, 2010, Saunders.

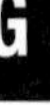

BASIC INFORMATION

DEFINITION

Glossitis is an inflammation of the tongue that can lead to loss of filiform papillae.

ICD-9CM CODES
529.0 Glossitis
ICD-10CM CODES
K14.0 Glossitis

EPIDEMIOLOGY & DEMOGRAPHICS

Glossitis is seen more frequently in patients of lower socioeconomic status, malnourished patients, alcoholics, smokers, elderly patients, immunocompromised patients, and patients with dentures.

PHYSICAL FINDINGS & CLINICAL PRESENTATION

- The appearance of the tongue varies depending on the etiology of the glossitis (Fig. 1-408, *A*). Loss of filiform papillae results in a red, smooth-surfaced tongue.
- The tongue may appear pale in patients with significant anemia.
- Pain and swelling of the tongue may be present when glossitis is associated with infections, trauma, or lichen planus.
- Ulcerations may be present in patients with herpetic glossitis, pemphigus, or streptococcal infection.
- Excessive use of mouthwash may result in a "hairy" appearance of the tongue (Fig. 1-408, *B*)

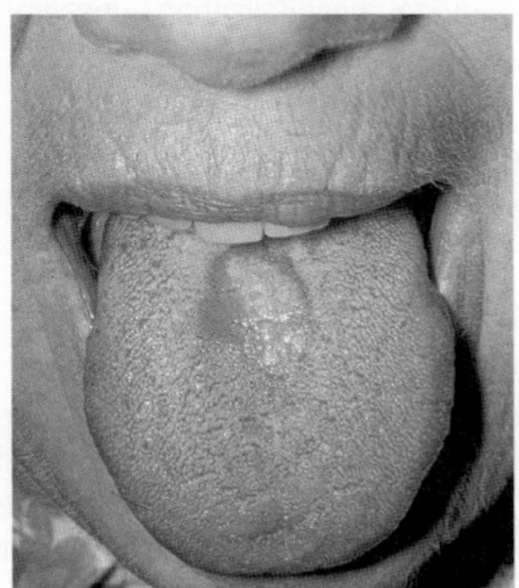

FIGURE 1-408 A, Median rhomboid glossitis. (From White GM, Cox NH [eds]: *Diseases of the skin, a color atlas and text,* ed 2, St Louis, 2006, Mosby.)

ETIOLOGY

- Nutritional deficiencies (vitamin E, riboflavin, niacin, vitamin B_{12}, iron)
- Infections (viral, candidiasis, tuberculosis, syphilis)
- Trauma (generally caused by poorly fitting dentures)
- Irritation of the tongue from toothpaste, medications, alcohol, tobacco, citrus
- Lichen planus, pemphigus vulgaris, erythema multiforme
- Neoplasms

DIAGNOSIS

DIFFERENTIAL DIAGNOSIS

- Infections
- Use of chemical irritants
- Neoplasms
- Skin disorders (e.g., Behçet's syndrome, erythema multiforme)

WORKUP

- Laboratory evaluation to exclude infectious processes, vitamin deficiencies, and systemic disorders
- Biopsy of lesion only when there is no response to treatment

LABORATORY TESTS

- Complete blood count: decreased hemoglobin and hematocrit, low mean corpuscular volume (MCV) (iron-deficiency anemia), elevated MCV (vitamin B_{12} deficiency)
- Vitamin B_{12} level
- 10% KOH scrapings in patients with white patches suspect for candidiasis

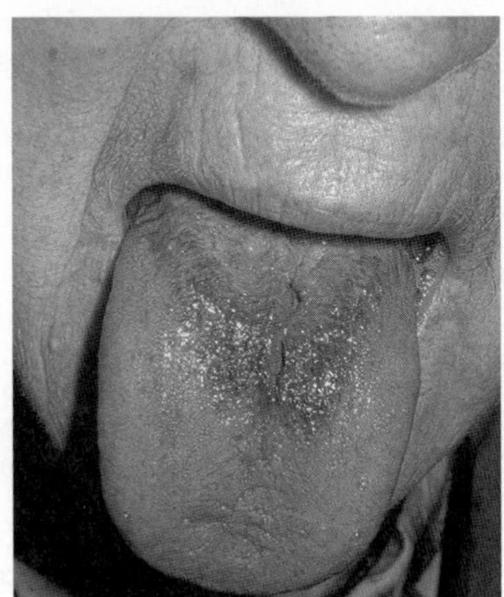

FIGURE 1-408 B, Black hairy tongue. (From White GM, Cox NH [eds]: *Diseases of the skin, a color atlas and text,* ed 2, St Louis, 2006, Mosby.)

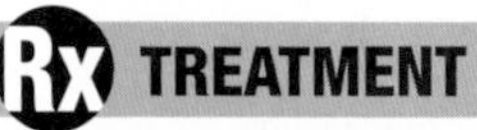

TREATMENT

NONPHARMACOLOGIC THERAPY

Avoidance of primary irritants such as hot foods, spices, tobacco, and alcohol

ACUTE GENERAL Rx

Treatment varies with the etiology of the glossitis.

- Malnutrition with avitaminosis: multivitamins
- Candidiasis: fluconazole 200 mg on day 1, then 100 mg/day for at least 2 wk or nystatin 400,000 U suspension qid for 10 days or 200,000 pastilles dissolved slowly in the mouth four to five times qd for 10 to 14 days
- Painful oral lesions: rinsing of the mouth with 2% lidocaine viscous, 1 to 2 tablespoons q4h prn; triamcinolone 0.1% applied to painful ulcers prn for symptomatic relief

CHRONIC Rx

- Lifestyle changes with elimination of tobacco, alcohol, and other primary irritants
- Dental evaluation for correction of ill-fitting dentures
- Correction of associated metabolic abnormalities such as hyperglycemia from diabetes mellitus

DISPOSITION

Most patients experience prompt improvement with identification and treatment of the cause of the glossitis.

REFERRAL

Surgical referral for biopsy of solitary lesions unresponsive to treatment to rule out neoplasm

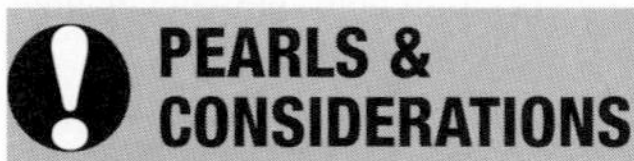

PEARLS & CONSIDERATIONS

COMMENTS

If the primary cause of glossitis is not identified or cannot be corrected, enteric nutritional replacement therapy should be considered in malnourished patients.

RELATED CONTENT

Glossitis (Patient Information)

AUTHOR: **FRED F. FERRI, M.D.**

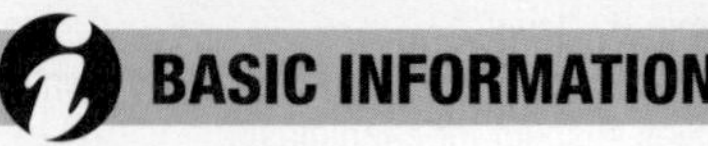

BASIC INFORMATION

DEFINITION

Gonorrhea is a sexually transmitted bacterial infection with a predilection for columnar and transitional epithelial cells. It commonly manifests as urethritis, cervicitis, or salpingitis. Infection may be asymptomatic. It differs between males and females in course, severity, and ease of recognition.

SYNONYMS

Gonococcal urethritis
Gonococcal vulvovaginitis
Gonococcal cervicitis
Gonococcal bartholinitis
Clap
GC

ICD-9CM CODES
098 Gonococcal infections
ICD-10CM CODES
A54.9 Gonococcal infection, unspecified

EPIDEMIOLOGY & DEMOGRAPHICS

- The disease is common worldwide, affects both sexes and all ages, especially younger adults; highest incidence is in inner-city areas, with an estimated 700,000 new cases annually.
- Asymptomatic anterior urethral carriage may occur in 12% to 50% of cases in men.
- Asymptomatic in 50% to 80% of cases in women. Most common dissemination by mucosal passage to fallopian tubes, resulting in pelvic inflammatory disease (PID) in 10% to 15% of infected women. Hematogenous spread may result in septic arthritis and skin lesions. Conjunctivitis rarely occurs but may result in blindness if not rapidly treated. Infection can occur in both men and women in oropharynx and anorectally.
- 700,000 new infections per year (second most commonly reported bacterial STD).

PHYSICAL FINDINGS & CLINICAL PRESENTATION

- Males: purulent discharge from anterior urethra (Fig. E1-409), with dysuria appearing 2 to 7 days after infecting exposure. May have rectal infection causing pruritus, tenesmus, and discharge or may be asymptomatic.
- Females: initial urethritis or cervicitis may occur a few days after exposure, frequently mild. In approximately 20% of cases uterine invasion occurs after menstrual period with signs and symptoms of endometritis, salpingitis, or pelvic peritonitis. The patient may have purulent discharge or inflamed Skene's or Bartholin's glands.
- Classic presentation of acute gonococcal PID is fever, abdominal and adnexal tenderness, and often absence of purulent discharge. Physical examination may be normal if asymptomatic. Disseminated gonococcal infection may manifest with various skin lesions (Fig. E1-410).

ETIOLOGY

- *Neisseria gonorrhoeae* is the gonococcus. Plasmids coding for β-lactamase render some strains resistant to penicillin or tetracycline. There is an increasing frequency of chromosomally mediated resistance to penicillin, tetracycline, fluoroquinolones, and cefoxitin. In the Far East, high-level resistance to spectinomycin is endemic.
- There are a rising number of cases of quinolone-resistant *N. gonorrhoeae* worldwide, with the expected number to rise in the U.S. from importation.
- Men who have sex with men are vulnerable to the emerging threat of antimicrobial-resistant *N. gonorrhoeae.*

Dx DIAGNOSIS

DIFFERENTIAL DIAGNOSIS

- Nongonococcal urethritis (NGU)
- Nongonococcal mucopurulent cervicitis
- *Chlamydia trachomatis*

WORKUP

- Diagnosis depends on bacteriologic investigation.
- Gram-negative intracellular diplococci are diagnostic in male urethral smears (Fig. E1-411). There is a false-negative rate of 60% to 70% in female cervical or urethral smears. Culture, nucleic acid hybridization tests, and nucleic acid amplification tests (NAATs) are available for the detection of genitourinary infection with *N. gonorrhoeae.* Culture and nucleic acid hybridization tests require female endocervical or male urethral swab specimen. NAATs allow testing of the widest variety of specimen types including endocervical swabs, vaginal swabs, urethral swabs (men), and urine (from both men and women).

LABORATORY TESTS

- Gonorrhea culture on Thayer-Martin medium (organism is fastidious; requires aerobic conditions with increased carbon dioxide atmosphere; incubate ASAP). Culture has a sensitivity of 95% or more for urethral specimens from men with symptomatic urethritis and 80% to 90% for endocervical infection in women.
- NAATs: These tests have largely replaced culture in many settings where persons are screened for asymptomatic genital infection. They are not more sensitive than culture for detecting *N. gonorrhoeae* in cervical or urethral specimen; however, they have specificities >99% and retain sensitivity when used to test voided urine or self-collected vaginal swabs.
- Nonamplified DNA probe tests are less sensitive than culture or NAATs and are not useful in the diagnosis of rectal or pharyngeal infection or for testing urine; however, they are inexpensive, readily available and offered in many laboratories in combination assays for *C. trachomatis.*
- Concomitant serologic testing for syphilis on all patients
- Concomitant *Chlamydia* testing on all patients
- Offer of HIV testing and counseling to all patients

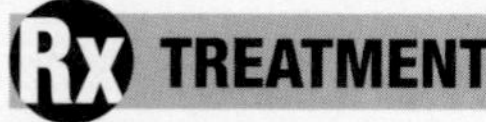

TREATMENT

ACUTE GENERAL Rx

Uncomplicated infections of the cervix, urethra, and rectum:

- Ceftriaxone 250 mg IM × 1 dose *plus* azithromycin 1 g PO single dose *or* doxycycline 100 mg PO bid for 7 days

Alternative regimens:

- Cefixime 400 mg PO x 1 dose *plus* azithromycin 1 g orally single dose *or* doxycycline 100 mg PO bid for 7 days *plus* test of cure in 1 wk
- If the patient has severe cephalosporin allergy, then azithromycin 2 g PO single dose *plus* test of cure in 1 wk

Uncomplicated gonococcal infections of the pharynx:

- Ceftriaxone 250 mg IM x 1 dose *plus* azithromycin 1 g PO single dose *or* doxycycline 100 mg PO bid for 7 days

DISPOSITION

- Pregnant patients require test of cure (as do those treated with regimens other than ceftriaxone/doxycycline); reculture 4 to 7 days after treatment.
- To reduce development of drug resistance, the CDC has recently modified guidelines and recommends reculture of patients who show continued symptoms despite treatment. These patients should be tested with a culture-based gonorrhea test that can detect antibiotic resistance.
- All sexual partners should be identified, examined, tested, and receive presumptive treatment.

REFERRAL

PID requiring hospitalization, disseminated gonococcal infection

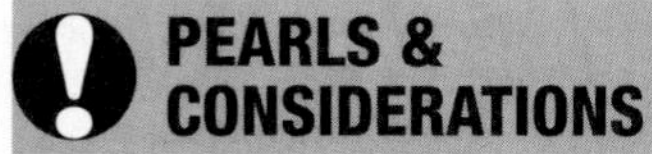

PEARLS & CONSIDERATIONS

COMMENTS

- This is a reportable disease.
- The proportion of gonorrhea cases in heterosexual men who are fluoroquinolone resistant (QRNG) has reached 6.7%, an elevenfold increase from 0.6% in 2001. Fluoroquinolone antibiotics are no longer recommended to treat gonorrhea in the U.S.
- The use of azithromycin as the second antimicrobial is preferred over doxycycline due to the high prevalence of tetracycline resistance.

SUGGESTED READINGS

available at www.expertconsult.com

RELATED CONTENT

Cervicitis (Related Key Topic)
Chlamydia Genital Infections (Related Key Topic)
Pelvic Inflammatory Disease (Related Key Topic)
Gonorrhea (Patient Information)

AUTHOR: **RUBEN ALVERO, M.D.**

BASIC INFORMATION

DEFINITION

Goodpasture's syndrome is an antiglomerular basement membrane antibody involving the lung and kidney. It is characterized by idiopathic recurrence of alveolar hemorrhage and rapidly progressive glomerulonephritis. It can also be defined by the triad of glomerulonephritis, pulmonary hemorrhage, and antibody to basement membrane antigens.

SYNONYMS

Hypersensitivity angiitis

ICD-9CM CODES
446.2 Goodpasture's syndrome
ICD-10CM CODES
M31.0 Hypersensitivity angiitis

EPIDEMIOLOGY & DEMOGRAPHICS

- Goodpasture's syndrome affects predominantly young, white, male smokers.
- Male/female ratio is 6:1.
- Goodpasture's syndrome accounts for 5% of all cases of rapidly progressive glomerulonephritis.
- 80% of patients are HLA-BR2 positive.

PHYSICAL FINDINGS & CLINICAL PRESENTATION

- Dyspnea, cough, hemoptysis
- Skin pallor, fever, arthralgias (may be mild or absent at the time of initial presentation)

ETIOLOGY

Presence of glomerular basement membranes (GBM) antibody deposition in kidneys and lungs with subsequent pulmonary hemorrhage and glomerulonephritis. In the kidneys circulating antibodies bind to the non-collagenous-1 (NC1) domain of type IV collagen in the GBM.

DIAGNOSIS

DIFFERENTIAL DIAGNOSIS

- Wegener's granulomatosis
- Systemic lupus erythematosus
- Systemic necrotizing vasculitis
- Idiopathic rapidly progressive glomerulonephritis
- Drug-induced renal pulmonary disease (e.g., penicillamine)

WORKUP

Laboratory evaluation, diagnostic imaging, immunofluorescence studies of renal biopsy

LABORATORY TESTS

- Presence of circulating serum anti-GBM antibodies
- Absence of circulating immunocomplexes, antineutrophils, cytoplasmic antibodies, and cryoglobulins
- Urinalysis revealing microscopic hematuria and proteinuria
- Elevated blood urea nitrogen and creatinine from rapidly progressive glomerulonephritis
- Immunofluorescence studies of renal biopsy material: linear deposits of anti-GBM antibody, often accompanied by C3 deposition
- Anemia from iron deficiency (from blood loss and iron sequestration in the lungs)

IMAGING STUDIES

Chest radiograph: fluffy alveolar infiltrates, evidence of pulmonary hemorrhage (Fig. 1-412)

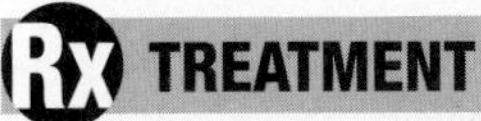

TREATMENT

ACUTE GENERAL Rx

- Combined use of plasmapheresis using albumin replacement for 1-2 wk with immusuppressive therapy with prednisone (1 mg/kg/day) and cyclophosphamide (2 mg/kg/day)
- Dialysis support in patients with renal failure
- Factors influencing decision to treat or not to treat aggressively in Goodpasture's disease are described in Table 1-208

DISPOSITION

Life-threatening pulmonary hemorrhage and irreversible glomerular damage are the major causes of death.

REFERRAL

- Referral for renal biopsy to guide the management
- Consideration for renal transplantation in patients with end-stage renal failure

SUGGESTED READINGS
available at www.expertconsult.com

RELATED CONTENT

Goodpasture's Syndrome (Patient Information)

AUTHOR: **FRED F. FERRI, M.D.**

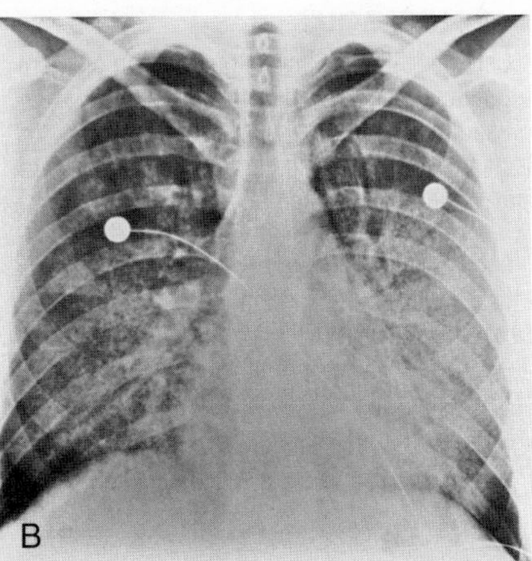

FIGURE 1-412 Goodpasture's syndrome. Posteroanterior chest radiographs several days apart demonstrate consolidation in the left lung **(A)**, which progressed to diffuse alveolar disease (consolidation) **(B)**. (From McLoud TC [ed]: *Thoracic radiology: the requisites,* St Louis, 1998, Mosby.)

TABLE 1-208 Factors Influencing Decision to Treat or Not to Treat Aggressively in Goodpasture's Disease

	Factors Favoring Aggressive Treatment	Factors Against Aggressive Treatment
Pulmonary hemorrhage	Present	Absent
Oliguria	Absent	Present
Creatinine	<5.5 mg/dl (approximately 500 μmol/L)	>5.5-6.5 mg/dl (approximately 500-600 μmol/L) and ANCA negative Severe damage on kidney biopsy No desire for early kidney transplantation
Other factors	Creatinine >5.5-6.5 mg/dl (approximately 500-600 μmol/L) *but* Rapid and recent progression ANCA positive Glomerular damage less severe than expected Crescents recent, nonfibrous Early renal transplantation desired	
Associated disease	Absent	Unusually high risk from immunosuppression

ANCA, Antineutrophil cytoplasmic antibody.
From Floege J et al: *Comprehensive clinical nephrology,* ed 4, Philadelphia, 2010, Saunders.

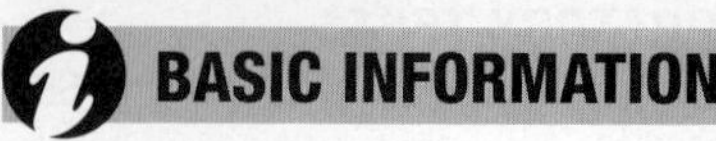

BASIC INFORMATION

DEFINITION

Gout is a term used to refer to a group of disease states caused by tissue deposition of monosodium urate due to prolonged hyperuricemia. Clinical manifestations of gout include acute and chronic arthritis, soft tissue inflammation, tophus formation, gouty nephropathy, and nephrolithiasis. Untreated hyperuricemia in patients with gout may lead to chronic destructive deforming arthritis

ICD-9CM CODES
274.00 Gouty arthritis
274.01 Acute gout
274.02 Chronic gout
274.03 Gout with tophus

ICD-10CM CODES
M10 Gout
M10.0 Idiopathic gout
M10.2 Drug induced gout
M10.3 Gout due to impairment of renal function
M10.4 Other secondary gout
M10.9 Gout, unspecified
M10.1 Lead-induced gout

EPIDEMIOLOGY & DEMOGRAPHICS

PREVALENCE: 5 cases per 1000 persons in the United States. Incidence is rising.

PREDOMINANT SEX: Male/female ratio ~4:1

PREDOMINANT AGE: 30 to 50 yr in men. Older than 60 yr in women

ETIOLOGY

- Gout is induced by inflammation from monosodium urate (MSU) crystal deposition. The primary risk factor for MSU deposition is hyperuricemia.
- Hyperuricemia and gout develop from excessive uric acid production, a decrease in the renal excretion of uric acid, or both.
- Primary hyperuricemia results from an inborn error of metabolism and may be attributed to several biochemical defects.
- Secondary hyperuricemia may develop as a complication of acquired disorders (e.g., leukemia) or as a result of the use of certain drugs (e.g., diuretics). Consumption of alcohol, especially beer, increases the risk of gout, and fructose-rich beverage intake is associated with hyperuricemia.

TABLE 1-209 Key Components of Gout Flares

- Marked tenderness and swelling of affected joint
- Acute onset with maximum pain in 4-12 hr
- Recurrent pattern of similar attacks
- Marked impairment of physical function
- Resolution of symptoms within 3-14 days

From Hochberg MC et al: *Rheumatology,* ed 5, St Louis, 2011, Mosby.

PHYSICAL FINDINGS & CLINICAL PRESENTATION

ACUTE GOUT:
- Rapid onset of pain and swelling and erythema of a distal joint and/or periarticular soft tissue. Table 1-209 summarizes key components of gout flares
- May present as monoarthritis of any joint. Acute gout of the first metatarsophalangeal (MTP) joint (Fig. 1-413) is known as *podagra*
- 10% to 15% of attacks are polyarticular
- Spontaneous resolution occurs over days to weeks

CHRONIC TOPHACEOUS GOUT (Fig. 1-414):
- Insidious onset of painless arthritis and soft tissue swelling
- Distal small joints characteristic
- May be confused with nodal osteoarthritis

Dx DIAGNOSIS

DIFFERENTIAL DIAGNOSIS OF ACUTE GOUT

- Infectious arthritis
- Cellulitis
- Pseudogout
- Trauma

DIFFERENTIAL DIAGNOSIS OF CHRONIC GOUT

- Osteoarthritis (especially nodal OA in women)
- Rheumatoid arthritis
- Psoriatic arthritis

Section II describes the differential diagnosis of acute monoarticular and oligoarticular arthritis.

WORKUP

Arthrocentesis and examination of synovial fluid (Fig. E1-415 and Box E1-30)

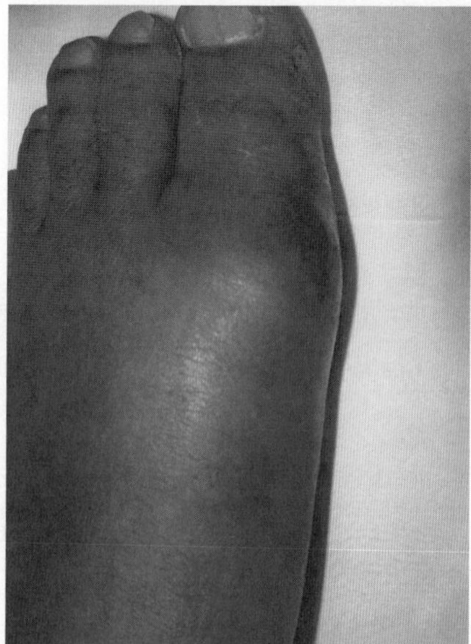

FIGURE 1-413 Podagra or acute gout of the first metatarsophalangeal (MTP) joint is shown. The hyperintense erythema with a dusky hue is characteristic. The area of inflammation usually extends beyond the area of the involved joint. (From Hochberg MC et al: *Rheumatology,* ed 5, St Louis, 2011, Mosby.)

LABORATORY TESTS

- Uric acid: All patients with gout are hyperuricemic at some time, but during an acute attack the serum uric acid may be normal or low.
- Synovial aspirate: usually cloudy and markedly inflammatory in nature. Urate crystals in fluid are needle-shaped and strongly negatively birefringent under polarized microscopy (Fig. E1-416).
- CBC: mild leukocytosis often present
- Inflammatory markers: ESR and CRP often elevated

IMAGING STUDIES

- Plain radiography for diagnosis and evaluation. Not generally indicated in typical gout presentation
- No typical findings in early gouty arthritis but late disease is associated with characteristic punched-out marginal erosions and overhanging edges

Rx TREATMENT OPTIONS FOR ACUTE GOUT

- Nonsteroidal anti-inflammatory medication (see Table 1-210)
  - Indomethacin 75 mg bid
  - Ibuprofen 800 mg tid
  - Naproxen 500 mg bid
  - Celecoxib 800 mg, then 400 mg/day
- Low-dose colchicine (less toxic and as effective as traditional high-dose colchicine): 1.2 mg colchicine PO, followed by 0.6 mg PO 1 hr later.
- Intraarticular corticosteroid injection (treatment of choice for monoarticular large joint attack): Triamcinolone hexacetomide 40 mg or equivalent for knee
- Systemic corticosteroid therapy: Prednisone 40 mg PO for 3 days, then taper over 10 days (effective and safe, but evidence is lacking)

NONPHARMACOLOGIC THERAPY

Lifestyle and dietary modification may be effective in highly motivated patients. Recommendations include reducing ingestion

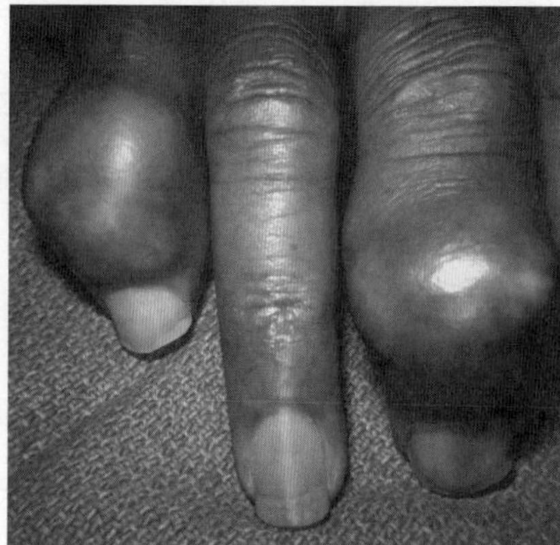

FIGURE 1-414 Large tophi involving the distal interphalangeal joints are commonly seen in gouty patients with preexisting Heberden's nodes. This is particularly characteristic of late-onset gout. (From Hochberg MC et al: *Rheumatology,* ed 5, St Louis, 2011, Mosby.)

of red meat, kidney, liver, yeast extract, shellfish, and overall protein along with restricting alcohol intake. These recommendations should be attempted only in patients with modestly elevated uric acid, as dietary modification can only lower uric acid 1 mg%. Discontinuation of diuretic therapy may help.

PHARMACOLOGIC TREATMENT OF SYMPTOMATIC HYPERURICEMIA

ALLOPURINOL: Allopurinol is very effective and safe when used properly. Correct dosing and patient compliance are essential elements in the prevention of erosive and tophaceous gout. Patients with renal insufficiency are at increased risk for allopurinol hypersensitivity, which manifests as fever, rash, and hepatitis occurring most commonly in the first 3 mo of therapy. The rash may progress to life-threatening toxic epidermal necrolysis if not recognized early.

Traditionally, therapy with allopurinol is initiated several weeks after the acute attack has resolved. However, adding allopurinol at initial presentation may improve long-term compliance without reducing the efficacy of acute treatment. The initial dose should be low (≤100 mg/day depending on creatinine clearance) in patients with renal insufficiency and those with very high uric acid levels. High initial doses are associated with increased incidence of allopurinol hypersensitivity. The serum uric acid should be reevaluated after 4-6 wk of therapy, and the allopurinol dose adjusted to reduce the serum uric acid to less than 6 mg%. The most common therapeutic dosage of allopurinol is 300 mg/day, but dose may be increased by 50-100 mg every two to three weeks until the target serum uric acid level is achieved. There is evidence that increasing allopurinol doses in patients with renal insufficiency does not result in significant toxicity, but concurrent use with statins and colchicine is associated with a higher incidence of adverse effects. Some authors have reported using doses as high as 800 mg daily without excess toxicity.

FEBUXOSTAT: Novel xanthine oxidase inhibitor that has been shown to be more potent than allopurinol 300 mg daily for reducing serum uric acid. The chemical structure of febuxostat is different from allopurinol, making cross-reactive allergy unlikely. The metabolism of febuxostat is primarily hepatic, which obviates the need for dose adjustments due to renal insufficiency. Some cases of hepatic toxicity have been reported, and it is recommended that liver function tests be monitored periodically. Febuxostat may help preserve renal function in patients with chronic kidney disease (CKD) but has not been tested in patients with severe renal failure.

The primary indication for febuxostat is demonstrated allergy to allopurinol. The cost of febuxostat may be as much as 40 times that of allopurinol.

BENEMID AND SULFINPYRAZONE: These uricosuric agents may only be used in patients with good renal function and urinary uric acid less than 600 mg in a 24-hr collection. Compliance is poor due to necessity of taking drugs more often than once daily

PEGLOTICASE: Intravenous pegylated uricase was approved by the FDA in 2010 for treatment of severe refractory tophaceous gout. It is a pegylated recombinant mammalian uricase that rapidly degrades urate when given intravenously. Use is limited by very high cost and significant toxicities including frequent gout flares and anaphylaxis.

PATIENT/FAMILY EDUCATION

It is essential that patients, families, physicians, and other members of the health care team appreciate the importance of compliance with a daily allopurinol regimen if recurrent flares and progression to chronic arthritis and tophi are to be avoided. Allopurinol should be discontinued only for symptoms suggesting the hypersensitivity syndrome. It should be continued during flares, medical illnesses, and surgical procedures.

REFERRAL

- Rheumatologist if diagnosis is not clear or therapy is complicated
- Podiatrist for management of pedal complications

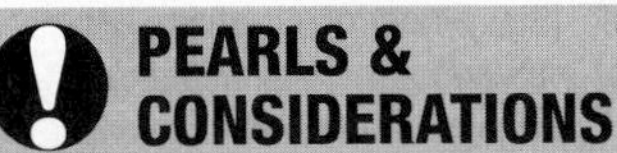

PEARLS & CONSIDERATIONS

Do not stop allopurinol during hospitalizations, surgery, or acute attacks unless there is evidence of drug allergy.

SUGGESTED READINGS

available at www.expertconsult.com

RELATED CONTENT

Gout (Patient Information)

AUTHORS: **BERNARD ZIMMERMANN, M.D.**, and **LUKE BARRÉ, M.D.**

TABLE 1-210 Treatment of Gout

Acute Gout	Interval Gout	Treatment of Hyperuricemia
NSAIDs (preferred): Indomethacin 50 mg qid or ibuprofen 800 mg tid (or other NSAID in full doses). Contraindicated in patients with renal insufficiency and gastrointestinal disorders. *Or* **Colchicine, oral:** 1.2 mg followed by a second dose of 0.6 mg 1 hr later. Contraindicated in patients with renal insufficiency and gastrointestinal disorders *Or* **Intraarticular steroids** (Treatment of choice for large joint monoarthritis): Triamcinolone 40 mg or equivalent for knee *Or* Systemic steroid therapy (for patients in whom NSAIDs and colchicine are contraindicated) Prednisone 30-50 mg PO daily or in divided doses. May use lower dose in diabetic or postsurgical patients.	**Colchicine, oral:** 0.6-1.2 mg/day as prophylaxis against recurrent attacks. **NSAIDs may also be used for prophylaxis.** **Hypouricemic agent:** Indicated for patients with recurrent attacks despite prophylaxis, severe hyperuricemia, presence of tophi, urolithiasis, or gouty arthritis **Other:** Weight loss, reduce alcohol (especially beer), diet low in seafood, red meat, organ meat, and fructose	**Colchicine, oral:** 0.6-1.2 mg/day for 4-6 wk before initiating hypouricemic therapy and for several months afterward to prevent recurrent attacks during initiation of hypouricemic therapy. *And* **Allopurinol:** Initial dose 100 mg/day in patients with renal insufficiency or very high uric acid levels. Increase dose as needed to attain uric acid less than 6 mg/dl. *Or* **Uricosuric agent** (Use only in patients with good renal function and <600 mg uric acid in a 24-hr collection): probenecid, 0.5-1 g bid, or sulfinpyrazone 100 mg tid or qid **Other:** Consider febuxostat for patients allergic to allopurinol. Pegloticase may be useful for selected patients with severe tophaceous gout.

NSAIDs, Nonsteroidal anti-inflammatory drugs.

G

Diseases and Disorders

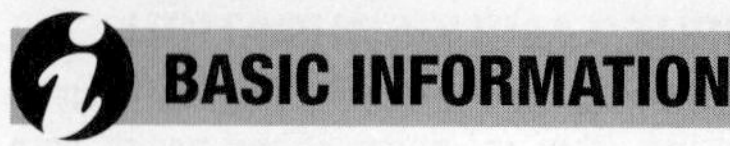

BASIC INFORMATION

DEFINITION

Granuloma annulare (GA) is a chronic, usually self-limited, inflammatory disorder of the dermis that classically presents as arciform to annular plaques located on the extremities.

SYNONYMS

Pseudorheumatoid nodule—subcutaneous granuloma annulare
GA

ICD-9CM CODES
695.89 Granuloma annulare
ICD-10CM CODES
L92.0 Granuloma annulare

EPIDEMIOLOGY & DEMOGRAPHICS

- Most common in children and young adults; most cases of localized GA are diagnosed in patients <30 yr
- Female predominance (2:1)
- Disseminated form associated with diabetes mellitus
- Recurrent in 40% of affected individuals
- A generalized form of GA can occur in up to 15% of patients

PHYSICAL FINDINGS & CLINICAL PRESENTATION

- The four main clinical variants of GA are localized (75%), disseminated (>10 lesions), subcutaneous (occurring primarily in children aged 2 to 5 yr), and perforating (rare form manifesting with 1- to 4-mm papules with a central crust).
- Localized GA starts as a small ring of colored skin or pale erythematous papules.
- Lesions coalesce and evolve into annular plaques over several weeks.
- Plaques undergo central involution and increase in diameter over several months (0.5 to 5 cm) (Fig. 1-417).
- Most frequently found on the lateral and dorsal surfaces of the hands and feet.
- Most lesions resolve spontaneously after several months.
- The generalized form of GA is characterized by hundreds to thousands of small, flesh-colored papules in a symmetric distribution on the trunk and extremities.
- Deep dermal (subcutaneous GA) presents as large, painless, skin-colored nodules that are frequently mistaken for rheumatoid nodules.

ETIOLOGY

Unknown, but may be related to vasculitis, trauma, monocyte activation, or delayed hypersensitivity.

DIAGNOSIS

DIFFERENTIAL DIAGNOSIS

- Tinea corporis
- Lichen planus
- Necrobiosis lipoidica diabeticorum
- Sarcoidosis
- Rheumatoid nodules
- Late secondary or tertiary syphilis
- Arcuate and annular plaques of mycosis fungoides
- Papular GA can simulate insect bites, secondary syphilis, xanthoma
- Annular elastolytic giant cell granuloma

WORKUP

- Diagnosis based on clinical appearance and presentation
- Biopsy when diagnosis is unclear

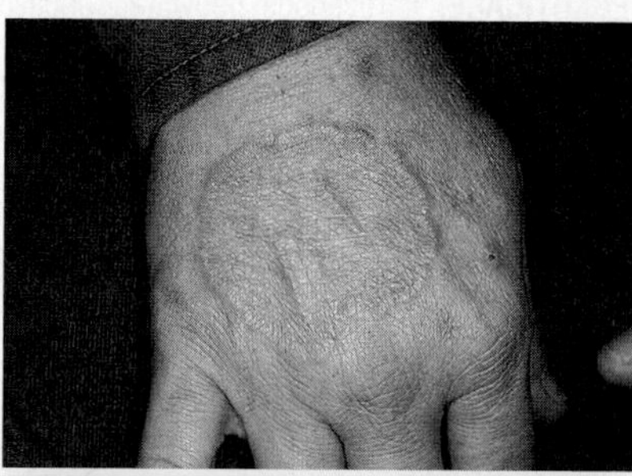

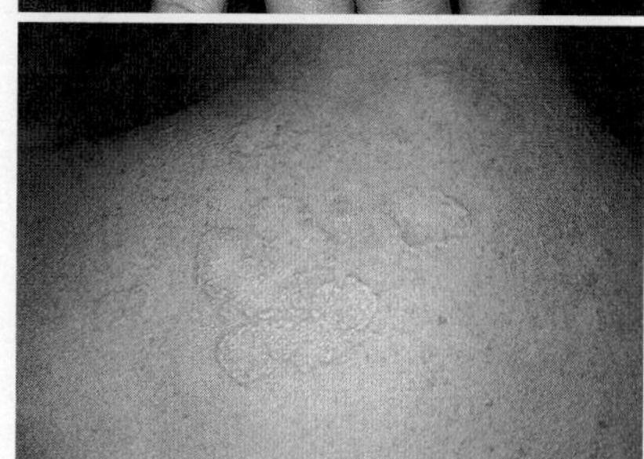

FIGURE 1-417 Granuloma annulare. (From Callen JP [ed]: *Color atlas of dermatology,* ed 2, Philadelphia, 2000, Saunders.)

LABORATORY TESTS

- No laboratory tests will help confirm the diagnosis.
- Biopsy shows focal degeneration of collagen and elastic fibers, mucin deposition, and perivascular and interstitial lymphohistiocytic infiltrate in the upper and middle dermis.

TREATMENT

NONPHARMACOLOGIC THERAPY

Reassurance, given the self-limited and benign nature of GA

CHRONIC Rx

High-potency topical corticosteroids with or without occlusion and intralesional steroid injection into elevated border with triamcinolone 2.5 to 10 mg/ml are useful first-line local therapies.

- Cryosurgery, psoralen ultraviolet-A (UVA) range or UVA-1 therapy, and carbon dioxide laser treatment can also be used.
- Systemic agents (e.g., niacinamide, hydroxychloroquine, chloroquine, cyclosporine, dapsone) are generally reserved for severe cases. Recent case reports indicate positive outcomes with tacrolimus and pimecrolimus and the tumor necrosis factor infliximab.

DISPOSITION

Most lesions resolve spontaneously within 2 yr.

REFERRAL

Dermatology referral recommended for symptomatic, disseminated disease

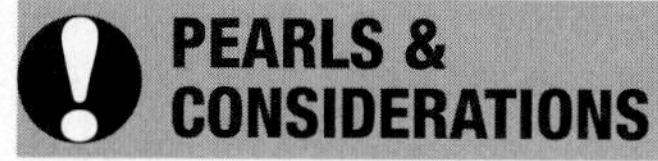

PEARLS & CONSIDERATIONS

COMMENTS

GA has been described as a paraneoplastic granulomatous reaction to Hodgkin's disease, non-Hodgkin's lymphoma, solid organ tumors, and mycosis fungoides.

SUGGESTED READINGS

available at www.expertconsult.com

RELATED CONTENT

Granuloma Annulare (Patient Information)

AUTHOR: **FRED F. FERRI, M.D.**

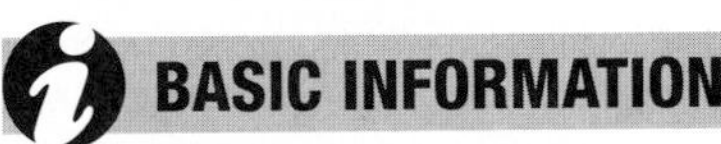

BASIC INFORMATION

DEFINITION

Granulomatosis with polyangiitis (GPA) is multisystem necrotizing vasculitis that generally affects the upper and lower respiratory tracts and the kidneys. It is characterized as an ANCA-associated granulomatous small-vessel vasculitis. Clinical manifestations depend on the tropism of blood vessel involvement and organ systems commonly affected beyond the respiratory tract and kidneys and include neurologic involvement and involvement of the skin and the musculoskeletal systems as well as the gastrointestinal tract.

The disease can also present in a limited form that is generally limited to the upper respiratory tract and can be managed less aggressively that the more diffuse systemic form.

SYNONYMS

Wegener's granulomatosis (WG)

ICD-9CM CODES
446.4 Wegener's granulomatosis
ICD-10CM CODES
M31.3 Wegener's granulomatosis

EPIDEMIOLOGY & DEMOGRAPHICS

INCIDENCE: 3/100,000 in recent U.S. epidemiologic studies, equal in men and women, more common in whites

MEAN AGE AT ONSET: 41 yr

PHYSICAL FINDINGS & CLINICAL PRESENTATION

- Clinical manifestations often vary with the stage of the disease and degree of organ involvement; localized disease often has upper respiratory tract involvement without systemic vasculitis, whereas systemic disease stages include early systemic, generalized, and severe disease.
- Frequent manifestations are:
  1. Upper respiratory tract: chronic sinusitis, chronic otitis media, mastoiditis, nasal crusting, obstruction and epistaxis, nasal septal perforation, nasal lacrimal duct stenosis, saddle nose deformities (resulting from cartilage destruction) (Fig. 1-419). Up to 90% of patients with GPA have one or more of these nasal manifestations.
  2. Ears and eyes: sensorineural and conductive hearing loss, episcleritis, scleritis, ulcerative keratitis, proptosis.
  3. Mouth: chronic ulcerative lesions of the oral mucosa, "mulberry" gingivitis.
  4. Lung: nodules, pulmonary infiltrates, cavitary lesions, and frank hemoptysis (6%-85%).
  5. Kidney: rapidly progressive glomerulonephritis (38%-70%), hematuria.
  6. Skin: cutaneous nodules over extensor surfaces of joints, necrotizing skin lesions, palpable purpura (30%-46%).
  7. Nervous system: mononeuritis multiplex and peripheral neuropathies (15%-40%), meningeal inflammation (pachymeningitis), headaches, and CNS involvement (7%-11%).
  8. Muskuloskeletal: monarthritis or polyarthritis (nondeforming), usually affecting large joints (60%).
  9. Constitutional: fever (23%-30%), weight loss >10% (50%), and fatigue (61%).

ETIOLOGY

Unknown; believed to be initially due to granulomatous inflammation that progresses to systemic vasculitis

Dx DIAGNOSIS

DIFFERENTIAL DIAGNOSIS

- Other granulomatous lung diseases (e.g., sarcoidosis, lymphomatoid granulomatosis, Churg-Strauss syndrome, necrotizing bronchocentric granulomatosis); the differential diagnosis of granulomatous lung disease is described in Section II. Table 1-211 describes differential diagnostic features of ANCA-associated vasculitis.
- Other ANCA-associated vasculitides, including microscopic polyangiitis.
- Goodpasture's syndrome and other causes of glomerulonephritis (e.g., poststreptococcal nephritis).
- Neoplasms (espcially lymphoproliferative disease).
- Bacterial or fungal sinusitis.
- Viral infections
- Cocaine-induced midline destructive lesions and levamisole-induced vasculitis
- Other causes of glomerulonephritis (e.g., poststreptococcal nephritis)

WORKUP

- Granulomatosis with polyangiitis should be suspected in a patient presenting with sinus disease that is unresponsive to conventional treatment and/or pulmonary hemorrhage, glomerulonephritis, mononeuritis multiplex resulting in wrist or foot drop or progressive migratory arthralgias or arthritis.
- Chest x-ray, laboratory evaluation, PFTs, and tissue biopsy for granulomatous lesions.

LABORATORY TESTS

- ANCA serology: positive immunofluorescence test for cytoplasmic pattern of ANCA (c-ANCA, although between 15% and 40% with diagnosis lack these antibodies). In GPA, ANCAs are predominantly directed against proteinase 3 (anti-PR3), which is the confirmatory laboratory test in a patient with positive ANCA staining on immunofluorescence.
- CBC: anemia, leukocytosis.

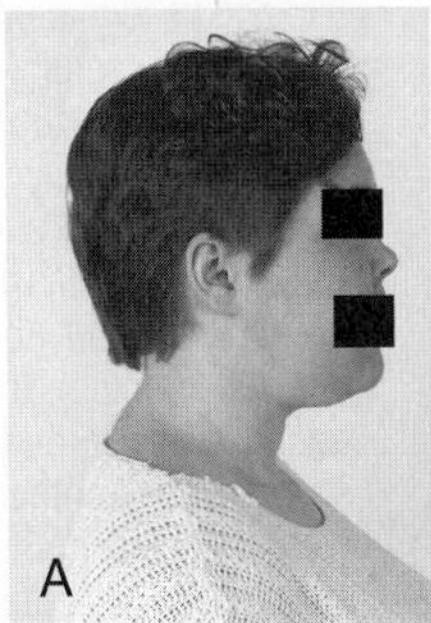

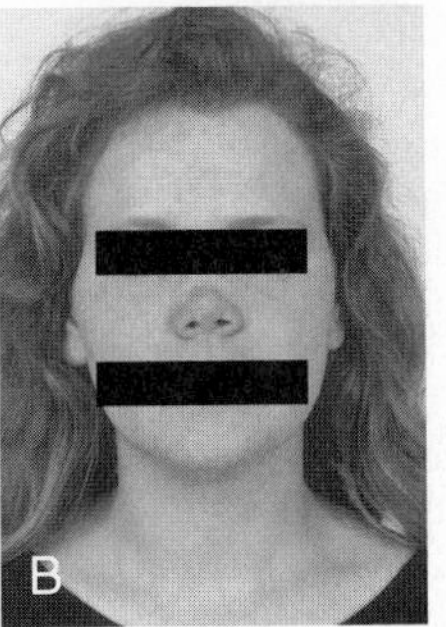

FIGURE 1-419 Saddle-nose deformity in a patient with Wegener's granulomatosis. (From *Kelley's Textbook of Rheumatology*, ed 8, Philadelphia, 2009, Elsevier.)

TABLE 1-211 Differential Diagnostic Features of the Antineutrophil Cytoplasm Antibody–Associated Vasculitides

Feature	Microscopic Polyangiitis	GPA	AGPA	Comments
Glomerulonephritis	+++	+++	+	Progressive renal failure uncommon in AGPA
Pulmonary infiltrates or nodules	++	+++	+++	Asthma and eosinophilia in AGPA
Alveolar hemorrhage	++	++	+	
Upper airway disease	+	+++	++	Ear, nose, and throat disease usually favors GPA
Skin, purpura	+++	+	++	
Peripheral nerve involvement	+	++	+++	Often a prominent feature of AGPA
Central nervous system involvement	+	+	+	

+++, very commonly seen; ++, seen often; +, uncommon finding; *AGPA*, allergic granulomatosis with polyangiitis; *GPA*, granulomatosis with polyangiitis.

From Firestein GS, et al: *Kelly's textbook of rheumatology*, ed 9, Philadelphila, 2013, Saunders

 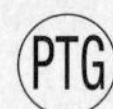

- Chemistry: elevated serum creatinine, decreased creatinine clearance.
- Urinalysis: may reveal hematuria, RBC casts, and proteinuria.
- Inflammatory markers: increased ESR, positive rheumatoid factor, and elevated C-reactive protein may be found.

IMAGING STUDIES

- Chest x-ray: may reveal bilateral multiple nodules, cavitary mass lesions, pleural effusion (20%). Up to one third of patients without pulmonary signs or symptoms have an abnormal chest x-ray (Fig. 1-420).
- Computed tomography (Fig. 1-421) or MRI (Fig. E1-422).
- PFTs: useful in detecting stenosis of the airways.
- Fiberoptic bronchoscopy (endoscopic ENT evaluation): nasal crusting ("golden crusts") are typical on evaluation (Fig. E1-423).
- Biopsy of one or more affected organs should be attempted; the most reliable source for tissue diagnosis is the lung. Lesions in the nasopharynx (if present) can be easily biopsied but biopsy is positive in only 20%. Biopsy of radiographically abnormal pulmonary parenchyma provides the highest yield (>90%).

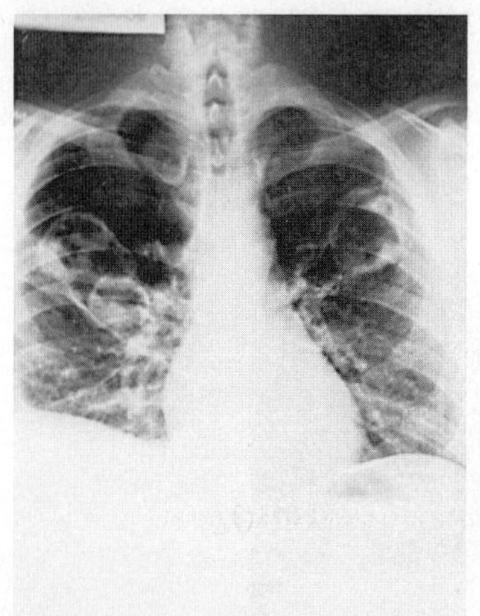

FIGURE 1-420 Chest radiograph shows multiple cavitary pulmonary nodules in patient with Wegener's granulomatosis. (From Weinberg SE et al: *Principles of pulmonary medicine,* ed 5, Philadelphia, 2008, Saunders.)

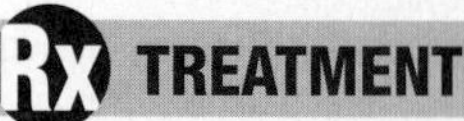

TREATMENT

NONPHARMACOLOGIC THERAPY

- Ensure proper airway drainage.
- Give nutritional counseling.

ACUTE GENERAL Rx

- Based on the RAVE trial, rituximab (375 mg/m^2/wk x4 wk) appears to be more effective than traditional therapy in treating GPA that presents with disease flares and is at least as effective as traditional therapy in treating most ANCA-positive vasculitides for the induction of remission. The RITUXVAS trial concluded that a combined cyclophosphamide-rituximab regimen was noninferior to cyclophosphamide pulsed alone, and rituximab could spare cyclophosphamide pulse dosing and preserve fertility. Both of these studies used concurrent steroid dosing with methylprednisone followed by prednisone.
- Historically, the gold standard for treatment of prednisone 60 to 80 mg/day and cyclophosphamide 20 mg/kg was generally effective and used to control clinical manifestation
- Potentially useful agents for maintenance therapy include rituximab, methotrexate, azathioprine, and mycophenolate mofetil. The MAINRITSAN trial showed that rituximab may be preferable for maintenance therapy, and the CYCAZAREM (for azathioprine) and LEM (for leflunamide) trials showed that these agents can also be used. The WEGENT study showed oral methotrexate and azathioprine were also noninferior for maintenance than intravenous cyclophosphamide.
- Maintenance therapy should generally be continued for 18-24 mo and, if ANCA positivity remains, even as long as 5 years.
- TMP-SMX therapy may represent a useful alternative in patients with lesions limited to the upper or lower respiratory tracts in absence of vasculitis or nephritis. Treatment with TMP-SMX (160 mg/800 mg bid) also reduces the incidence of relapses in patients with granulomatosis with polyangiitis in remission. It is also useful in preventing *Pneumocystis jirovecii* pneumonia (PJP), which occurs in 10% of patients receiving induction therapy. When used for prophylaxis, dose of TMP-SMX (160 mg/800 mg) is 1 tablet three times/wk.
- In patients unable to tolerate TMP-SMX, often because of rash or allergy, PJP prophylaxis can also be achieved with dapsone, atovaquone, or inhaled pentamidine.

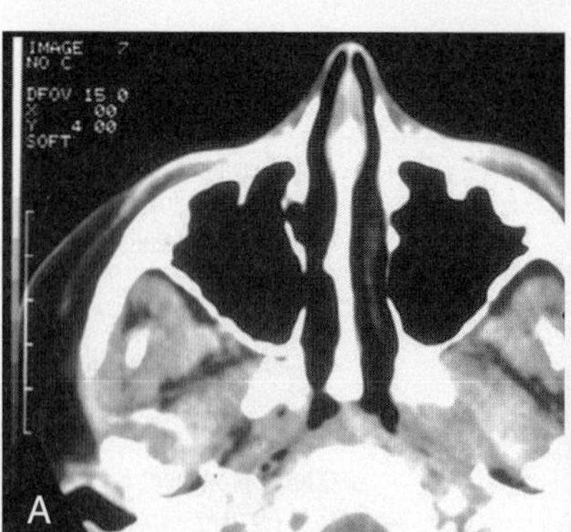

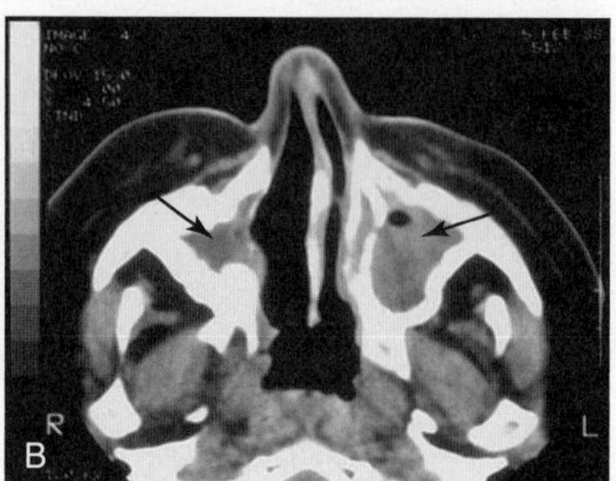

FIGURE 1-421 Computed tomography (CT) scans of the sinuses. A, Normal maxillary sinuses in a recently diagnosed Wegener's granulomatosis (WG) patient. **B,** Sinus CT scan of a patient with long-standing WG: nasal septal deviation to the left, destruction of the medial walls of the right maxillary sinus, opacification of both sinuses with soft tissue densities *(arrows),* and neo-ossification of all maxillary bony structures due to chronic inflammation. (From Hochberg MC et al: *Rheumatology,* ed 5, St Louis, 2011, Mosby.)

DISPOSITION

- Five-year survival with aggressive treatment is approximately 80%; without treatment 2-yr survival is 20%.
- Age >50 yr, impaired renal function, pulmonary involvement at diagnosis, and lack of ENT changes at diagnosis are all associated with worse outcomes and increased mortality rate.
- With standard therapy, remission is achieved by 90%-94% of patients, but relapse is frequent (from 18%-40% at 24 mo).

REFERRAL

- Rheumatology referral for continued treatment.
- ENT, surgical referral for biopsy

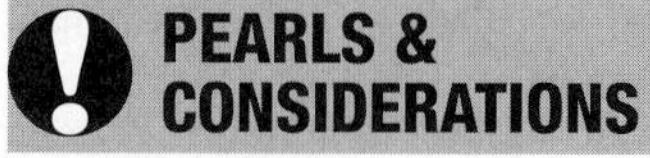

PEARLS & CONSIDERATIONS

COMMENTS

- Granulomatosis with polyangiitis is characterized by granulomatous lesions and vasculitis involving the respiratory tract, lung, and kidneys.
- C-ANCA levels should not dictate changes in therapy, because they correlate erratically with disease activity.
- The incidence of venous thrombotic events in granulomatosis with polyangiitis is significantly higher than the general population. Clinicians should maintain a heightened awareness of the risks of venous thrombosis and a lower threshold for evaluating patients for possible DVT or pulmonary embolism.
- Disease relapse remains a major problem in the course of the disease.

SUGGESTED READINGS

available at www.expertconsult.com

RELATED CONTENT

Wegener's Granulomatosis (Patient Information)

AUTHORS: **AMAR OZA, M.D.,** and **HARALD A. HALL, M.D.**

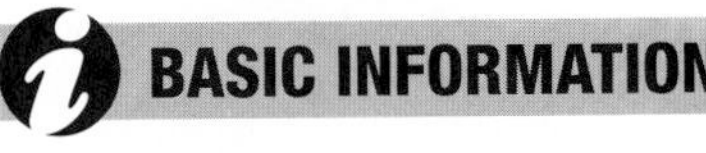

BASIC INFORMATION

DEFINITION

Graves' disease is a hypermetabolic state caused by circulating IgG antibodies that bind to and activate the G-protein–coupled thyrotropin receptor. This activation stimulates follicular hypertrophy and hyperplasia, causing thyroid enlargement as well as increases in thyroid hormone production. It is characterized by thyrotoxicosis, diffuse goiter, and infiltrative ophthalmopathy (edema and inflammation of the extraocular muscles and an increase in orbital connective tissue and fat); infiltrative dermopathy characterized by lymphocytic infiltration of the dermis; accumulation of glycosaminoglycans; and occasionally edema.

SYNONYMS

Thyrotoxicosis

ICD-9CM CODES
242.0 Toxic diffuse goiter
ICD-10CM CODES
E05.00 Thyrotoxicosis with diffuse goiter without thyrotoxic crisis or storm

EPIDEMIOLOGY & DEMOGRAPHICS

INCIDENCE/PREVALENCE: Hyperthyroidism affects 2% of women and 0.2% of men in their lifetimes. More than 80% of these cases are caused by Graves' disease.

PREDOMINANT AGE: Peak incidence is between 40 and 60 yr.

GENETICS: Increased prevalence of HLA-B8 and HLA-DR3 in whites with Graves' disease. Concordance rate is 20% among monozygotic twins.

PHYSICAL FINDINGS & CLINICAL PRESENTATION

- Tachycardia, palpitations, tremor, hyperreflexia
- Goiter, exophthalmos (50% of patients), lid retraction, lid lag
- Nervousness, weight loss, heat intolerance, atrial fibrillation
- Increased sweating, brittle nails, clubbing of fingers
- Localized infiltrative dermopathy (1% to 2% of patients) is most frequent over the anterolateral aspects of the legs, commonly over the pretibial area (pretibial myxedema) (Fig.1-424) but can be found at other sites (especially after trauma)
- Men may have gynecomastia, reduced libido, and erectile dysfunction. Women often have irregular menses

ETIOLOGY

Autoimmune etiology: the activity of the thyroid gland is stimulated by the action of T cells, which induce specific B cells to synthesize antibodies against thyroid-stimulating hormone (TSH) receptors in the follicular cell membrane.

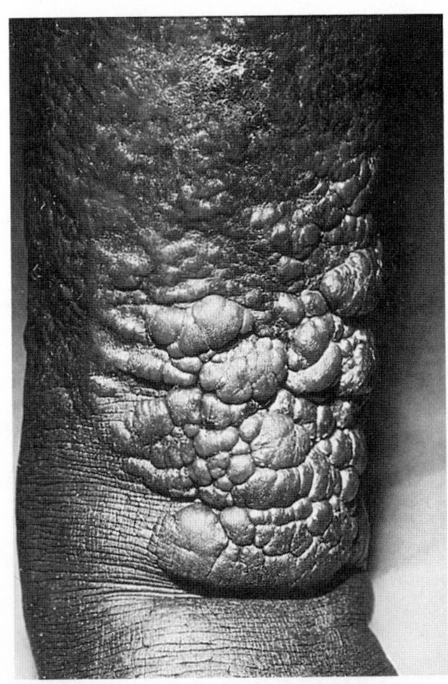

FIGURE 1-424 Chronic pretibial myxedema in a patient with Graves' disease and orbitopathy. The lesions are firm and nonpitting, with a clear edge to feel. (Courtesy of Dr. Andrew Werner, New York, NY.)

Dx DIAGNOSIS

DIFFERENTIAL DIAGNOSIS

- Anxiety disorder
- Premenopausal state
- Thyroiditis
- Other causes of hyperthyroidism (e.g., toxic multinodular goiter, toxic adenoma)
- Other: metastatic neoplasm, diabetes mellitus, pheochromocytoma

WORKUP

- The diagnostic workup includes a detailed medical history followed by laboratory and imaging studies and ECG. Patients often present with anxiety, heat intolerance, menstrual dysfunction, increased appetite, and weight loss. Elderly patients can have an atypical presentation (apathetic hyperparathyroidism). For additional information, refer to the topic "Hyperthyroidism."
- Table 1-212 describes the clinical assessment of the patient with Graves' ophthalmopathy.

LABORATORY TESTS

- Increased free thyroxine (T_4) and free triiodothyronine (T_3)
- Decreased TSH
- Presence of thyroid-stimulating immunoglobulin or thyrotropin-receptor antibodies (useful in selected patients to differentiate Graves' disease from toxic nodular goiter)

IMAGING STUDIES

- 24-hr radioactive iodine uptake (RAIU): increased homogeneous uptake
- CT or MRI of the orbits (Fig. 1-425) is useful if there is uncertainty about the cause of ophthalmopathy

Rx TREATMENT

NONPHARMACOLOGIC THERAPY

- Patient education and discussion of therapeutic options
- Smoking cessation: smoking is associated with an increased risk of progression of Graves' ophthalmopathy.

ACUTE GENERAL Rx

- Antithyroid drugs (ATDs) to inhibit thyroid hormone synthesis or peripheral conversion of T_4 to T_3:
  1. Methimazole or propylthiouracil (PTU) are available. Methimazole is generally preferred because it has a longer half-life, allowing for once-daily dosing. PTU is preferred during pregnancy.
  2. Side effects: skin rash (3% to 5%), arthralgias, myalgias, granulocytopenia (0.5%); rare side effects: aplastic anemia, hepatic necrosis (PTU), cholestatic jaundice.
- Radioactive iodine (RAI):
  1. Treatment of choice for patients >21 yr and younger patients who have not achieved remission after 1 yr of ATD therapy
  2. Contraindicated during pregnancy and lactation
- Surgery: near-total thyroidectomy is rarely performed. Indications: obstructing goiters despite RAI and ATD therapy, patients who refuse RAI and cannot be adequately managed with ATDs, and pregnant women inadequately managed with ATDs.
- Adjunctive therapy: Beta-adrenergic receptor blockers (e.g., atenolol 25 to 100 mg/day) to alleviate the β-adrenergic symptoms of hyperthyroidism (tachycardia, tremor); contraindicated in patients with bronchospasm.

- Graves' ophthalmopathy: methylcellulose eye drops to protect against excessive dryness, sunglasses to decrease photophobia, intraocular and systemic high-dose corticosteroids for severe exophthalmos. Worsening of ophthalmopathy after RAI therapy is often transient and can be prevented by the administration of prednisone. Other treatment options include antiinflammatory and immunosuppressive agents, radiation, and corrective surgical procedures. The administration of the antioxidant selenium (100 μg PO bid) has been recently reported as effective in improving quality of life, reducing ocular involvement, and slowing progression of the disease in patients with mild Graves' orbitopathy. Its mechanism of action is believed to be an effect on the oxygen free radicals and cytokines that play a pathogenic role in Graves' orbitopathy.

CHRONIC Rx

Patients undergoing treatment with ATDs should be seen every 1 to 3 mo until euthyroidism is achieved and every 3 to 4 mo while they are receiving ATDs.

DISPOSITION

- ATDs induce sustained remission in <60% of cases.
- The incidence of hypothyroidism after RAI is >50% within the first year and 2% per year thereafter.
- Complications of surgery include hypothyroidism (28% to 43% after 10 yr), hypoparathyroidism, and vocal cord paralysis (1%).
- Successful treatment of hyperthyroidism requires lifelong monitoring for the onset of hypothyroidism or the recurrence of thyrotoxicosis.
- RAI therapy is followed by the appearance or worsening of ophthalmopathy more often than is therapy with methimazole, particularly in patients who are cigarette smokers. It can be prevented with the administration of prednisone 0.5 mg/kg body weight per day starting 2 to 3 days after RAI, continued for 1 mo, then tapered off over 2 mo.
- Mild to moderate ophthalmopathy often improves spontaneously. Severe cases can be treated with high-dose glucocorticoids, orbital irradiation, or both. Orbital decompression may be used in patients with optic neuropathy and exophthalmos (see "Hyperthyroidism").

TABLE 1-212 Clinical Assessment of the Patient with Graves' Ophthalmopathy

Activity Measures*
Spontaneous retrobulbar pain
Pain on attempted up or down gaze
Redness of the eyelids
Redness of the conjunctiva
Swelling of the eyelids
Inflammation of the caruncle and/or plica
Conjunctival edema
Severity Measures
Lid aperture: distance between lid margins in millimeters with the patient looking in the primary position, sitting relaxed, and with distant fixation
Swelling of the eyelids (absent/equivocal, moderate, severe)
Redness of the eyelids (absent/present)
Redness of the conjunctivae (absent/present)
Conjunctival edema (absent, present)
Inflammation of the caruncle or plica (absent, present)
Exophthalmos: measured in millimeters using the same Hertel exophthalmometer and the same intercanthal distance for an individual patient
Subjective diplopia score†
Eye muscle involvement (ductions in degrees)
Corneal involvement (absent/punctate keratopathy/ulcer)
Optic nerve involvement: best-corrected visual acuity, color vision, optic disk, relative afferent pupillary defect (absent/present), plus visual fields if optic nerve compression is suspected

*Based on the seven classic features of inflammation in Graves' ophthalmopathy. The clinical activity score (CAS) is the total number of items present; a CAS ≥3 indicates active ophthalmopathy.
†Subjective diplopia score: 0 = no diplopia; 1 = intermittent (i.e., diplopia in primary position of gaze, when tired, or when first awakening); 2 = inconstant (i.e., diplopia at extremes of gaze); 3 = constant (i.e., continuous diplopia in primary or reading position).
From Melmed S, Polonsky KS, Larsen PR, Kronenberg HM: *Williams textbook of endocrinology,* ed 12, Philadelphia, 2011, Saunders.

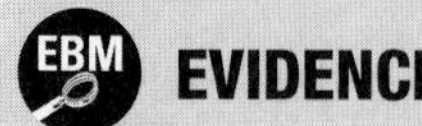

EVIDENCE

available at www.expertconsult.com

SUGGESTED READINGS

available at www.expertconsult.com

RELATED CONTENT

Graves' Disease (Patient Information)
Hyperthyroidism (Related Key Topic)

AUTHOR: **FRED F. FERRI, M.D.**

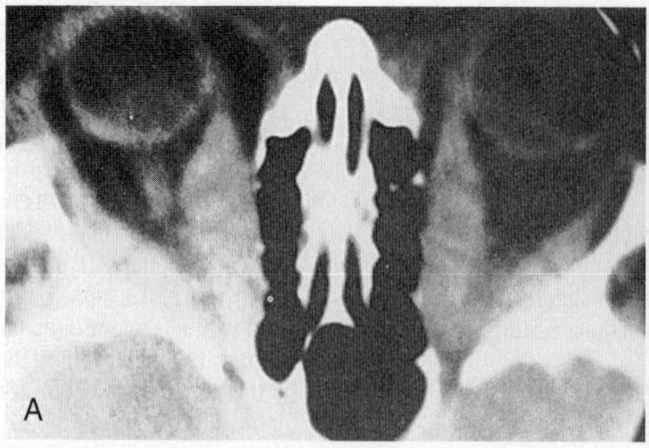

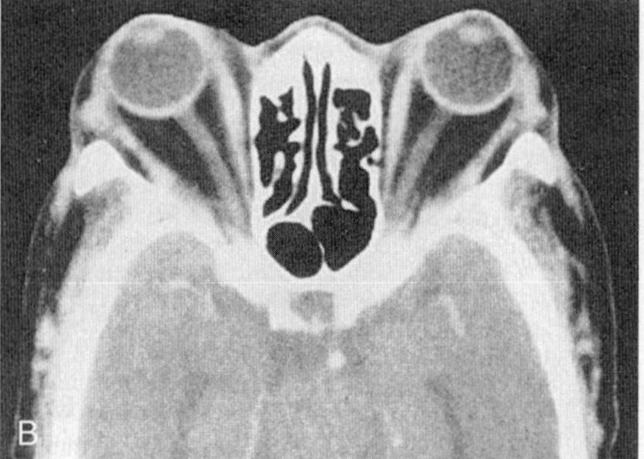

FIGURE 1-425 Computed tomographic scans of orbits in two patients with Graves' orbitopathy. A, Notice the obviously grossly swollen medial rectus extraocular muscles in both orbits and the resulting proptosis. **B**, The patient shows considerable proptosis with only minimal muscle enlargement, suggesting the presence of a large amount of retroorbital fat. (Courtesy of Dr. Peter Som, New York, NY.)

G

Diseases and Disorders

BASIC INFORMATION

DEFINITION

Guillain-Barré syndrome (GBS) is an acute immune-mediated polyradiculoneuropathy (affects nerve roots and peripheral nerves), with predominant motor involvement. It is the most common cause of acute flaccid paralysis in the Western hemisphere and probably worldwide. By definition, maximal clinical weakness occurs within 4 wk of disease onset.

SYNONYMS

AIDP (acute inflammatory demyelinating polyradiculoneuropathy)
Acute polyneuropathy
Ascending paralysis
GBS
Postinfectious polyneuritis

ICD-9CM CODES
357.0 Guillain-Barré syndrome
ICD-10CM CODES
G61.0 Guillain-Barré syndrome

EPIDEMIOLOGY & DEMOGRAPHICS

INCIDENCE: 0.6 to 1.9 cases/100,000 persons annually without geographic variation. Incidence increases with age. A slight peak in incidence occurs between late adolescence and early adulthood. A slight male preponderance (1.25:1) also exists.

PREDISPOSING FACTORS: Viral (HIV, CMV, EBV, influenza) and bacterial *(Campylobacter jejuni, Mycoplasma pneumoniae)* infections; systemic illness (Hodgkin's lymphoma, immunizations). Major antecedents of GBS are described in Box 1-31.

BOX 1-31 Major Antecedents of Guillain-Barré Syndrome

Frequent
Upper respiratory tract infections
Campylobacter jejuni enteritis
Cytomegalovirus infection
Epstein-Barr virus infection
Hepatitis A infection
Hepatitis B infection
Hepatitis C infection
HIV infection

Infrequent
Mycoplasma pneumoniae infection
Haemophilus influenzae infection
Leptospira icterohaemorrhagiae infection
Salmonellosis
Rabies vaccine
Tetanus toxoid
Bacille Calmette-Guérin immunization
Sarcoidosis
Systemic lupus erythematosus
Lymphoma
Trauma
Surgery

Questionable
Hepatitis B vaccine
Influenza vaccine
Hyperthermia
Epidural anesthesia

From Vincent JL et al: *Textbook of critical care*, ed 6, Philadelphia, 2011, Saunders.

ETIOLOGY

- Unknown
- Preceding infectious illness 1 to 4 wk before disease onset has been noted. The most frequent antecedent infection is *C. jejuni* infection (associated with 30% of cases of GBS and 20% of cases of Miller-Fisher syndrome).
- Humoral and cell-mediated immune attack of peripheral nerve myelin, Schwann cells; sometimes with primary axonal involvement

PHYSICAL FINDINGS & CLINICAL PRESENTATION

- Symmetric weakness, most commonly involving proximal muscles initially, subsequently involving both proximal and distal muscles; difficulty in ambulating, getting up from a chair, or climbing stairs.
- Depressed or absent reflexes bilaterally.
- Minimal to moderate glove and stocking paresthesias/dysesthesia/anesthesia or back pain.
- Pain (caused by involvement of posterior nerve roots) may be prominent.
- Autonomic abnormalities (bradyarrhythmias or tachyarrhythmias, hypotension or hypertension).
- Respiratory insufficiency (caused by weakness of bulbar/intercostal muscles).
- Facial paresis, ophthalmoparesis, dysphagia (secondary to cranial nerve involvement).
- GBS consists of several clinical variants based on the pattern of clinical involvement and electrophysiologic findings. These include:
  - AIDP (most common form in Europe and North America)
  - Acute motor axonal neuropathy (AMAN; most prevalent form in China and Japan)
  - Acute motor and sensory axonal neuropathy (AMSAN; has more severe sensory involvement and is associated with more severe clinical course and poorer prognosis)
  - Miller Fisher syndrome (MFS; triad of ophthalmoplegia, ataxia, and areflexia)
  - Acute pandysautonomia (rapid onset of parasympathetic and sympathetic failure without motor or sensory involvement)
  - Regional variants (e.g., pharyngeal-cervical-brachial GBS, pure ataxic GBS)

DIAGNOSIS

DIFFERENTIAL DIAGNOSIS

- Toxic peripheral neuropathies: heavy metal poisoning (lead [microcytic anemia], thallium [alopecia], arsenic [typically accompanied by acute GI illness]), medications (vincristine, disulfiram), organophosphate poisoning, hexacarbon (glue sniffer's neuropathy)
- Nontoxic peripheral neuropathies: acute intermittent porphyria, fulminant vasculitic polyneuropathy, infectious (poliomyelitis, diphtheria, Lyme disease, West Nile virus); tick paralysis
- Neuromuscular junction disorders: myasthenia gravis, botulism, snake envenomations
- Myopathies such as polymyositis, acute necrotizing myopathies caused by drugs
- Metabolic derangements such as hypermagnesemia, hypokalemia, hypophosphatemia
- Acute CNS disorders such as basilar artery thrombosis with brain stem infarction, brain stem encephalomyelitis, transverse myelitis, or spinal cord compression
- Hysterical paralysis or malingering

WORKUP

1. Exclude other causes based on clinical history, examination, and laboratory tests.
2. Lumbar puncture (may be normal in the first 1 to 2 wk of the illness). Typical findings include elevated CSF protein with few mononuclear leukocytes (albuminocytologic dissociation) in 80% to 90% of patients. Elevated CSF cell counts is an expected feature in cases associated with HIV seroconversion.
3. EMG/nerve conduction study (NCS): may be normal in the first 10 to 14 days of the disease. The earliest electrodiagnostic abnormality is prolongation or absence of H-reflexes. NCS evidence of demyelination (prolonged distal latency, conduction velocity slowing, conduction block, temporal dispersion, and prolonged F-waves) in two or more motor nerves confirms diagnosis of AIDP in the appropriate clinical context.

LABORATORY TESTS

- CBC may reveal early leukocytosis with left shift. Electrolytes are tested to exclude metabolic causes.
- Heavy metal testing, urine porphyria screen, creatine kinase, HIV titers, neuroimaging of the brain and spinal cord if diagnosis is uncertain. Nerve root enhancement may be seen on MRI of the lumbosacral spine.
- Antibodies against ganglioside GQ1b may be present in up to 90% of patients with MFS. IgG antibodies against ganglioside GM1 may be associated with AMAN. There are no antiganglioside antibodies commonly associated with AIDP.
- In equivocal cases (especially if peripheral nerve vasculitis is a concern), nerve biopsy may aid in confirming a diagnosis of GBS. Sensory nerve biopsy demonstrates segmental demyelination with infiltration of monocytes and T cells into the endoneurium. Axonal loss is commonly seen in sensory nerve biopsy specimens in GBS.

TREATMENT

NONPHARMACOLOGIC THERAPY

- Close monitoring of respiratory function (frequent measurements of vital capacity, negative inspiratory force, and tidal volume) and pulmonary toilet should be done because respiratory failure is the major complication in GBS.
- Frequent repositioning of patient to minimize formation of pressure sores.

- Prevention of thromboembolism with antithrombotic stockings and SC heparin (5000 U q12h) in nonambulatory patients.
- Emotional support and social counseling for patient and family.

ACUTE GENERAL Rx

- Infusion of IV immunoglobulins (IVIG; 0.4 g/kg/day for 5 days). Always check serum IgA levels before infusion to prevent anaphylaxis in IgA deficient patients.
- Early therapeutic plasma exchange (TPE or plasmapheresis: 200 to 250 ml/kg over five sessions every other day), started within 7 days of onset of symptoms, is beneficial in reducing the need for mechanical ventilation in patients with rapidly progressive disease and results in improved rate of recovery. It is contraindicated in patients with cardiovascular disease (recent MI, unstable angina), active sepsis, and autonomic dysfunction.
- There is no proven benefit from combining IVIG and plasma exchange.
- Mechanical ventilation may be needed if FVC is <12 to 15 ml/kg, vital capacity is rapidly decreasing or is <1000 ml, negative inspiratory force <20 cm H_2O, PaO_2 is <70, the patient is having significant difficulty clearing secretions or is aspirating.

CHRONIC Rx

- Ventilatory support may be necessary in 10% to 20% of patients. Adequate fluid/electrolyte support and nutrition are necessary, especially in patients with dysautonomia or bulbar dysfunction.
- Aggressive nursing care to prevent decubitus, infections, fecal impactions, and pressure nerve palsies.
- Monitoring and treatment of autonomic dysfunction (bradyarrhythmias or tachyarrhythmias, orthostatic hypotension, systemic hypertension).
- Treatment of back pain and dysesthesia with low-dose tricyclics, gabapentin, and so on. Opiate narcotics can be used cautiously in the short term but may compound dysautonomia.
- Stress ulcer prevention in patients receiving ventilator support.
- Physical and occupational therapy rehabilitation, including supportive devices.

DISPOSITION

- Mortality rate is approximately 5% to 10% worldwide. Causes of death include cardiac arrest, pulmonary embolism, and fulminant infections. A recent study showed 62% complete motor recovery, 14% mild weakness, 9% moderate weakness, 4% bed-bound or ventilated, and 8% dead at 1 yr. Another study suggested that about 33% of patients were free from sensory symptoms at 1 yr, with residual sensory loss present in the lower extremities in 67% and 36% in the upper extremities. About 32% had to change their work, 30% were unable to function at home as well as they could before the disease, and 52% had to alter their leisure activities 1 yr after GBS onset. Excessive fatigue is a common complaint in patients during the recovery phase of GBS. This may be treated with exercise therapy (e.g., bicycle exercise training).
- Predictors for poor recovery (inability to walk independently at 1 yr): age >60 yr, preceding diarrheal illness, recent CMV infection, fulminant or rapidly progressing course, ventilatory dependence, reduced motor amplitudes (<20% normal), or inexcitable nerves on NCS. Outcomes may also be influenced by complications of medical therapy.
- GBS is typically a monophasic illness. Recurrence may occur in <5% of patients following full recovery.

REFERRAL

Tracheostomy may be necessary in patients with prolonged ventilatory support. Percutaneous endoscopic gastrostomy may be temporarily required.

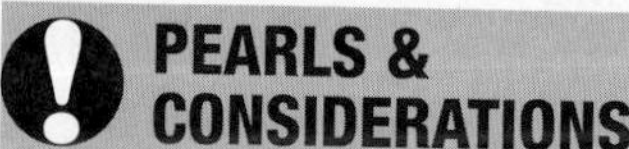

PEARLS & CONSIDERATIONS

- GBS is the most common cause of acute flaccid paralysis.
- Close monitoring of ventilatory function with respiratory mechanics (FVC and NIF) is of paramount importance in all patients with suspected GBS.

PATIENT/FAMILY EDUCATION

Patient education information may be obtained from the Guillain-Barré Foundation International, The Holly Building, 104 1/2 Forrest Avenue, Narberth, PA 19072; phone: (610) 667-0131; fax: (610) 667-7036; toll-free: (866) 224-3301; E-mail: info@gbs-cidp.org

SUGGESTED READINGS

available at www.expertconsult.com

AUTHOR: **DIVYA SINGHAL, M.D.**

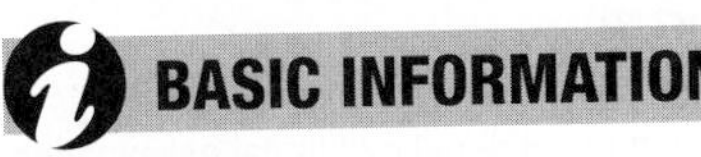

BASIC INFORMATION

DEFINITION

Gynecomastia is a benign enlargement of male breast, resulting from proliferation of glandular breast tissue.

ICD-9CM CODES
611.1 Gynecomastia
ICD-10CM CODES
N62 Hypertrophy of breast

EPIDEMIOLOGY

- Most common reason for male breast evaluation.
- Seen in patients of all age groups.
- 60% to 90% of infants have transient gynecomastia due to high estrogenic state of pregnancy.
- Prevalence during adolescence ranges from 4% to 69%. It results from transient increase of estradiol concentration at the onset of puberty.
- Higher incidence in body builders due to use of anabolic steroids.
- 24% to 65% of older men have gynecomastia. It is secondary to decreased testosterone production with advanced age, increased peripheral conversion of testosterone to estrogen, and at times from side effects of medications.

PATHOPHYSIOLOGY

Altered estrogen-androgen balance, in favor of estrogen.

ETIOLOGY

- Physiologic
  - Infancy
  - Puberty
  - Persistent pubertal gynecomastia seen in 25% of cases
  - Elderly
- Pathologic
  - Idiopathic (25%)
  - Increased estrogen production or action
    - Testicular tumors (3%)
    - Chronic liver disease
    - Malnutrition
    - Hyperthyroidism
    - Adrenal tumors
    - Familial gynecomastia
  - Decreased testosterone production or action (10%)
    - Testicular trauma
    - Testicular torsion
    - Viral orchitis
    - Congenital anorchia
    - Renal failure (1%)
    - Hyperthyroidism (1.5%)
    - Malnutrition
    - Androgen insensitivity syndrome
    - Five-alpha reductase deficiency
    - Pituitary tumors
    - Kallmann syndrome
    - Klinefelter's syndrome
- Medications (10% to 25%)
  Estrogen, gonadotropins, clomiphene, phenytoin, ketoconazole, metronidazole, metoclopramide, alkylating agents, busulfan, methotrexate, cisplatin, cimetidine, ranitidine, omeprazole, flutamide, finasteride, etomidate, HAART therapy, INH, tricyclic antidepressants, phenothiazines, diazepam, haloperidol, calcium channel blocker, ACE inhibitors, spironolactone, digoxin, amiodarone, methyldopa, alcohol, marijuana, heroin, methadone, amphetamine, anabolic steroids
- Table E1-213 summarizes the various causes of gynecomastia.

CLINICAL FEATURES

- Although gynecomastia is usually bilateral, it could be unilateral.
- Characterized by concentric rubbery to firm disk of tissue, which is often mobile and located directly beneath the areola.
- Pain is usually not severe. Varying degree of tenderness and nipple sensitivity are more common than pain, usually in the first 6 mo.

Dx DIAGNOSIS

- Good history and physical examination including review of all medications the patient is taking is helpful.
- Mammogram is recommended for suspected breast cancer.
- Serum concentration of hCG, LH, testosterone, and estradiol should be measured, preferably in the morning, unless the cause is clearly apparent. There is no uniformity of opinion regarding what biochemical evaluation, if any, should be performed in patients with asymptomatic gynecomastia. Fig. E1-426 describes an algorithm for evaluation of gynecomastia.

DIFFERENTIAL DIAGNOSIS

- Breast cancer
  - Mass is usually firm to hard
  - Unilateral
  - Eccentric in location
  - Could be associated with nipple discharge and retraction, lymphadenopathy, and skin dimpling
- Pseudogynecomastia or lipomastia
  - Characterized by fat deposition without glandular proliferation
  - Seen in obese men
  - Bilateral
  - Remain unchanged over time

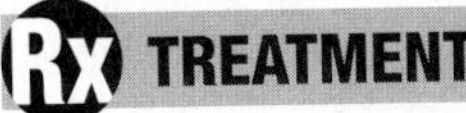

TREATMENT

- Observation is recommended for most patients with physiologic gynecomastia. They often regress spontaneously. Reassurance and follow-up examination in 3 to 6 mo usually suffice.
- Treat the underlying cause, and stop the offending medications.
- Treatment is most effective in the early stages (first 6 mo). Medical therapy often fails when given for longstanding (>12 mo) cases because of the presence of fibrosis.
- Potential indications of early therapy include severe breast enlargement, pain, tenderness, and psychological embarrassment. Consider giving tamoxifen 10 mg orally twice a day to these patients for up to 3 mo. It is not FDA-approved for this purpose. It results in regression of gynecomastia in approximately 80% of patients and, of which, only 60% had complete regression. As far as breast symptoms, such as pain and tenderness, some improvement is usually seen within a month of therapy.
- Surgery is offered for symptomatic gynecomastia that does not respond to medical therapy. However, for adolescents, surgery is deferred until puberty is completed. The different surgical options include subcutaneous mastectomy, ultrasound-guided liposuction, and suction-assisted lipectomy.
- For prevention of gynecomastia in patients with prostate cancer using antiandrogen therapy, one could offer tamoxifen or radiotherapy.

SUGGESTED READINGS
available at www.expertconsult.com

RELATED CONTENT

Gynecomastia (Patient Information)

AUTHOR: **HEMANT K. SATPATHY, M.D.**

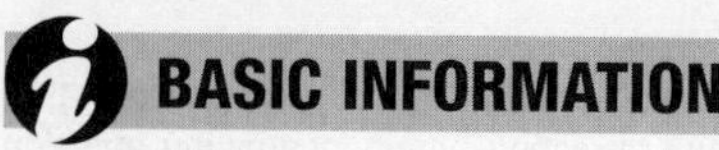

BASIC INFORMATION

DEFINITION

Hand-foot-mouth (HFM) disease is a viral illness characterized by superficial lesions of the oral mucosa and skin of the extremities. HFM is transmitted primarily by respiratory droplet contact in developed countries and feco-oral contact in developing countries. Although children are predominantly affected, adults are also at risk. This disease is usually self-limited and benign, although outbreaks in the Asia Pacific Region have been increasingly complicated by neurological and cardiopulmonary sequelae.

SYNONYMS

Vesicular stomatitis with exanthem
Coxsackie virus infection
Enterovirus infection

ICD-9CM CODES
074.0 Hand-foot-mouth disease
ICD-10CM CODES
B08.4 Enteroviral vesicular stomatits with exanthem

EPIDEMIOLOGY & DEMOGRAPHICS

- Children <5 yr are at the highest risk and have the most severe cases.
- HFM is usually found in children <10 yr.
- HFM is contagious. Close contacts of affected children, including family members and health care workers, are the most commonly affected adults.
- Infection is spread from person to person by direct contact with saliva, respiratory secretions, fluid in vesicles, or stool.
- A person is most contagious during the first week of illness.
- Outbreaks tend to occur during the summer.
- Infection leads to immunity, but a second episode may occur after infection with a different agent.

PHYSICAL FINDINGS & CLINICAL PRESENTATION

Symptoms:
- After a 4- to 6-day incubation period, patients may report odynophagia, sore throat, malaise, and fever (38.3° to 40° C).
- 1 to 2 days later the characteristic oral lesions appear (small red spots that blister and may ulcerate).
- In 75% of cases skin lesions on the extremities accompany these oral manifestations (small flat or raised red bumps, sometimes with blisters).
- 11% of adults have cutaneous findings.
- Lesions appear over the course of 1 or 2 days.

Physical findings:
- Oral lesions, usually between five and ten, are commonly found on the tongue, buccal mucosa, gingivae, and hard palate.
- Oral lesions initially start as 1- to 3-mm erythematous macules and evolve into gray vesicles on an erythematous base.
- Vesicles are frequently broken by the time of presentation and appear as superficial gray ulcers with surrounding erythema.
- Skin lesions of the palms of the hands and soles of the feet start as linear erythematous papules (3 to 10 mm in diameter) that evolve into gray vesicles that may be mildly painful (Fig. 1-427). These vesicles are usually intact at presentation and remain so until they desquamate within 2 wk. Although rare, fingernail or toenail loss after HFM disease has been reported in children. The nail loss was temporary, and nails grew back without intervention.
- Involvement of the buttocks and perineum is present in 31% of cases.
- In rare cases, encephalitis, meningitis, myocarditis, poliomyelitis-like paralysis, and pulmonary edema may develop. Sporadic acute paralysis and long-term neurologic sequelae have been reported with enterovirus 71.
- Although information is limited, there is no clear evidence that pregnancy outcomes are affected.

ETIOLOGY

- Coxsackie virus group A, type 16, was the first and is the most common viral agent isolated.
- Coxsackie viruses A5, A7, A9, A10, B1, B2, B3, B5, and enterovirus 71 have also been implicated.
- Enterovirus 71 is neurotropic with predilection for the brainstem, leading to more severe cases of the disease. Infection rates have been rising in the Asian Pacific region.
- Epidemics have been reported with coxsackie A16 and enterovirus 71.

DIAGNOSIS

DIFFERENTIAL DIAGNOSIS

- Aphthous stomatitis
- Herpes simplex infection
- Herpangina
- Behçet's disease
- Erythema multiforme
- Pemphigus
- Gonorrhea
- Acute leukemia
- Lymphoma
- Allergic contact dermatitis

WORKUP

The diagnosis is usually made on the basis of history and characteristic physical examination.

LABORATORY TESTS

- Not indicated unless the diagnosis is in doubt.
- Throat culture or stool specimen may be obtained for viral testing but may take from 2 to 4 wk for results.

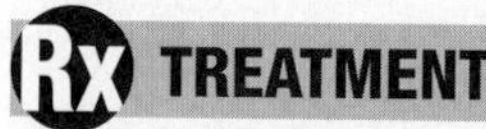

TREATMENT

ACUTE GENERAL Rx

- Symptomatic therapy is given for this usually self-limited disease.
- There are currently no available approved therapies for more severe cases. Antivirals, steroids, and IV immunoglobulin have been tried for enterovirus 71 infections, but these treatments have not been evaluated in randomized, placebo-controlled studies.

DISPOSITION

Prognosis is excellent except in rare cases of central nervous system or cardiac involvement. Most are managed as outpatients.

REFERRAL

Not usually needed

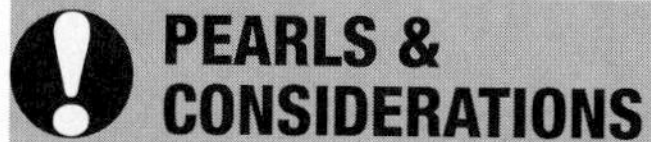

PEARLS & CONSIDERATIONS

- Frequent handwashing, disinfection of contaminated surfaces, and washing of soiled articles of clothing can help reduce transmission.
- HFM has no relation to hoof and mouth disease in cattle.

SUGGESTED READINGS
available at www.expertconsult.com

RELATED CONTENT

Hand, Foot, and Mouth Disease (Patient Information)

AUTHORS: **ERICA J. HARDY, M.D., MMSc.**, and **JENNIFER JEREMIAH, M.D.**

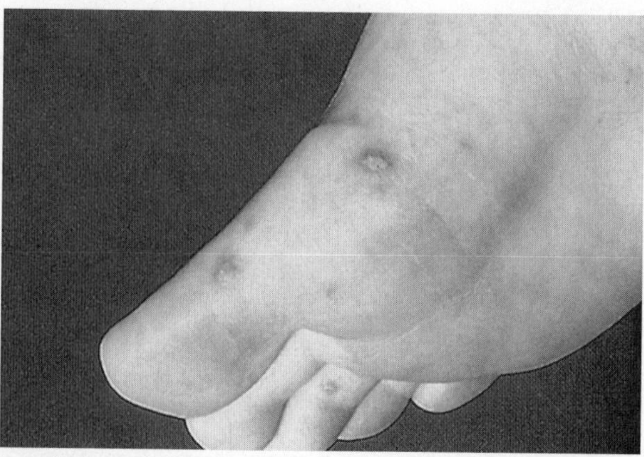

FIGURE 1-427 Hand-foot-mouth disease. Note oval lesions on an erythematous base. (From Goldstein B [ed]: *Practical dermatology,* ed 2, St Louis, 1997, Mosby.)

BASIC INFORMATION

DEFINITION

The term *cluster headache* refers to attacks of severe, unilateral pain that is orbital, supraorbital, temporal, or any combination of these sites, lasting 15 to 180 minutes, and occurring from once every other day to eight times a day. The attacks are associated with one or more of the following, all of which are ipsilateral: conjunctival injection, lacrimation, nasal congestion, rhinorrhea, forehead and facial sweating, miosis, ptosis, and eyelid edema. Most patients are restless or agitated during an attack.

SYNONYMS

Ciliary neuralgia
Erythromelalgia of the head
Erythroprosopalgia of Bing
Horton's headache

ICD-9CM CODES
339.00-339.02 Cluster headache
ICD-10CM CODES
G44.009 Cluster headache syndrome, unspecified, not intractable

EPIDEMIOLOGY & DEMOGRAPHICS

INCIDENCE: Estimated to occur in 0.05% to 1% of the population
PREDOMINANT SEX: Occurs in males at least five times more commonly than in females
PREDOMINANT AGE: Peak age of onset between 20 and 40 yr
GENETICS: May be inherited (autosomal dominant) in approximately 5% of cases

PHYSICAL FINDINGS & CLINICAL PRESENTATION

- During attack: ipsilateral conjunctival injection, lacrimation, nasal congestion, rhinorrhea, facial sweating, Horner's syndrome.
- In contrast to migraine sufferers, patients are agitated and active during an attack.
- Permanent partial Horner's syndrome in 5% of patients; otherwise examination is normal.

ETIOLOGY

Activation of the posterior hypothalamic gray matter resulting in trigeminal activation coupled with parasympathetic activation. The pathophysiology remains controversial.

Dx DIAGNOSIS

- Severe or very severe unilateral orbital, supraorbital, and/or temporal pain lasting 15 to 180 minutes.
- Frequency of every other day to eight per day; they may cluster seasonally or at a certain time in a patient's life.
- Headache is accompanied by at least one of the following (ipsilateral):
  1. Conjunctival injection and/or lacrimation
  2. Nasal congestion and/or rhinorrhea
  3. Eyelid edema
  4. Forehead and facial sweating
  5. Miosis and/or ptosis
  6. Restlessness or agitation

DIFFERENTIAL DIAGNOSIS

- Migraine
- Trigeminal neuralgia
- Temporal arteritis
- Post-herpetic neuralgia
- Venous sinus thrombosis
- Carotid-cavernous fistula or other cavernous sinus lesions
- Other trigeminal autonomic cephalalgias
- Section II describes the differential diagnosis of headaches

WORKUP

Diagnosis is usually established by characteristic history.

IMAGING STUDIES

- None, unless history or examination suggests focal neurologic deficit or headaches change in character or are of new onset.
- MRI of the brain along with vascular imaging may be necessary to exclude secondary headaches at the time of initial diagnosis.

Rx TREATMENT

NONPHARMACOLOGIC THERAPY

Avoidance of alcohol, histamine, nitroglycerin, and tobacco during clusters

ABORTIVE Rx

- Inhalation of 100% oxygen by face mask for 15 min often aborts an attack.
- About 75% of users of triptans (sumatriptan, zolmatriptan) will be pain free within 20 minutes. Only injectable and nasal formulations achieve a rapid response to be efficacious.
- Cafergot, octreotide, intranasal lidocaine, or dihydroergotamine may abort an attack or prevent one if given just before a predictable episode. Acute episode is typically resolved before oral analgesics become effective, although indomethacin and other NSAIDs may also be effective in prolonged attacks.
- Acute episode is typically resolved before oral analgesics become effective, although indomethacin and other NSAIDs may also be effective in prolonged attacks.

PROPHYLAXIS Rx

Various medications have been tried without great success, although good responses may be obtained in up to 50% of cases. Examples include:

- Valproic acid: start at 500 mg/day
- Topiramate: up to 50 mg bid
- Verapamil: up to 480 mg/day as tolerated. Verapamil can be used as first-line prophylactic therapy and can also be used to treat chronic cluster headaches.
- Lithium: 200 mg tid with frequent monitoring and adjustment to maintain therapeutic serum level of 0.4 to 1 mEq/L. Equally effective as verapamil, but with more side effects
- Methysergide: 1 to 2 mg tid; requires familiarity with the potential adverse effects and use of "drug holidays" to decrease risk of fibrosis
- Ergotamine tartrate: 3 to 4 mg/day during clusters
- Prednisone: 60 mg PO daily for 1 wk followed by taper; headaches can return during taper
- Greater and lesser occipital nerve blocks, with the use of local anesthetics including Lidocaine and bupivacaine along with steroids like depomedrol, dexamethasone, or triamcinolone, may be used to shorten the duration of the cluster period. Consensus guidelines from the American Headache Society have been published recently.
- There is emerging evidence for benefit of a sphenopalatine ganglion block that may be available at some centers, for treatment and prophylaxis of cluster attacks.

DISPOSITION

Headache-free periods tend to increase with increasing age.

REFERRAL

Refractory cluster headaches may require referral to a headache specialist.

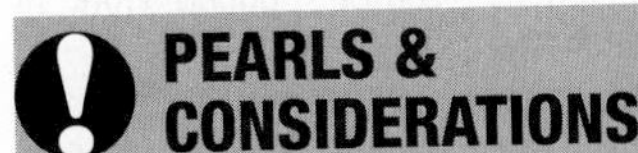

PEARLS & CONSIDERATIONS

COMMENTS

- Cluster headaches are divided into episodic (attacks lasting up to 1 yr with more than 1 mo pain-free periods) and chronic (>1 yr without remission). Episodic cluster headache is six times more common than the chronic form.
- Home oxygen therapy is reasonable for cluster headache sufferers.

SUGGESTED READINGS

available at www.expertconsult.com

RELATED CONTENT

Cluster Headaches (Patient Information)

AUTHOR: **SIDDHARTH KAPOOR, M.D.**

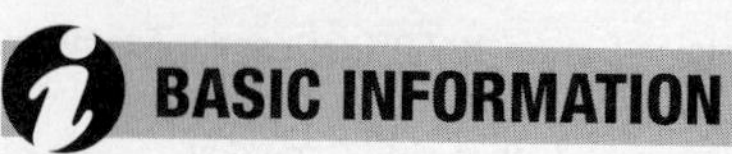

BASIC INFORMATION

DEFINITION

Migraine headaches are recurrent headaches that are either preceded by a focal neurologic symptom (migraine with aura), occur independently without preceding focal neurologic symptoms (migraine without aura), or have atypical presentations (migraine variants). The migraine aura typically is characterized by visual or sensory symptoms that develop over 5 to 60 min. If aura includes motor weakness, the migraine is referred to as hemiplegic. In migraine with and without aura, the headache is typically unilateral, pulsatile, and associated with nausea and vomiting, photophobia, and phonophobia. Migraines that occur ≥15 days every month for ≥3 months are known as chronic; otherwise, they are referred to as episodic.

ICD-9CM CODES

346 Migraine

ICD-10CM CODES

G43.909	Migraine, unspecified, not intractable, without status migrainosus
G43.1	Migraine with aura (classical migraine)
G43.0	Migraine without aura (common migraine)
G43.2	Status migrainosus
G43.3	Complicated migraine

EPIDEMIOLOGY & DEMOGRAPHICS

INCIDENCE: Increases from infancy, peaks during the third decade of life, then decreases

PREVALENCE (IN U.S.): Females: 18%; males: 6%. More than 50% of persons affected by migraine headaches report reduced work or school productivity.

AGE: Peak prevalence between ages of 18 and 49

PREDOMINANT SEX: Female/male ratio of 3:1

GENETICS:
- Familial predisposition: more than 50% of migraine sufferers have an affected family member
- Autosomal-dominant transmission for some rare migraine variants (familial hemiplegic migraine, cerebral autosomal-dominant arteriopathy with subcortical infarcts and leukoencephalopathy [CADASIL]); familial hemiplegic migraines have been associated with calcium channelopathy, sodium channelopathy, and Na^+/K^+- ATPase dysfunction.

PHYSICAL FINDINGS & CLINICAL PRESENTATION

- Normal between episodes
- Normal for migraine without aura.
- Focal motor or sensory abnormalities possible for migraine with aura or migraine variants.
- Common aura types include scintillating scotoma, bright zigzags, homonymous visual disturbance such as paresthesia, speech disturbances, or hemiparesis (familial or sporadic hemiplegic migraine). Other visual phenomena include image distortion or "Alice in Wonderland" effect.

ETIOLOGY

The pathophysiology of migraines is not clearly understood. It is believed that a primary neuronal event results in a trigeminovascular reflex causing neurogenic inflammation. Serotonin, substance P, nitric oxide, and calcitonin gene-related peptide also play a role, but the exact mechanism is unknown. Cortical spreading depression is probably responsible for the aura.

Dx DIAGNOSIS

Migraine without aura:
- Five attacks fulfilling criteria
- Headache attacks lasting 4 to 72 hr
- Headache has at least two of the following characteristics:
  1. Unilateral location
  2. Pulsating quality
  3. Moderate or severe pain intensity
  4. Aggravation or causing avoidance of routine physical activity
- At least one of the following during headache:
  1. Nausea and/or vomiting
  2. Photophobia and phonophobia

Migraine with aura:
- At least two attacks
- Aura consisting of at least one of the following, but no motor weakness:
  1. Fully reversible visual symptoms, including positive and/or negative features
  2. Fully reversible sensory symptoms, including positive and/or negative features
- At least two of the following:
  1. Homonymous visual symptoms and/or unilateral sensory symptoms
  2. At least one aura symptom develops gradually over >5 min and/or different aura symptoms occur in succession over >5 min
- A migraine occurring during or within 60 min of the aura

DIFFERENTIAL DIAGNOSIS

- A diagnosis of migraine is possible only after five recurrent episodes.
- The first or the worst headache should always be investigated and the differential includes headaches from all secondary causes.
- Headache red flags can be remembered by the mnemonic SNOOP:
  - S: systemic symptoms of fever, weight loss
  - S: secondary risk factors of immunosuppression from any cause, cancer
  - N: neurologic deficits, altered consciousness
  - O: onset is sudden, abrupt, or split second
  - O: older, age >50 for new-onset headache should be worked up for giant cell arteritis
  - P: previous headache history is different or there is a change to headache
- Section II describes the differential diagnosis of headaches

WORKUP

- In general, no additional investigation is needed with recurrent, typical attacks with usual age of onset, family history, and a normal physical examination.
- If there is an unusual presentation and/or unexpected findings on examination, investigation for other causes is required.

LABORATORY TESTS

Lumbar puncture for history of abrupt-onset headaches and uncertain diagnosis of migraine

IMAGING STUDIES

- Imaging should be done in patients with headaches and an unexplained abnormal finding on the neurologic examination.
- Imaging should be considered in patients with rapidly increasing headache frequency, history of dizziness or incoordination, headache causing wakening from sleep, or headaches worsening with Valsalva maneuver.

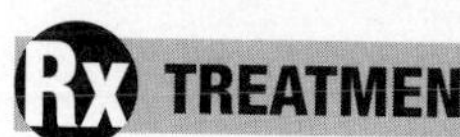

TREATMENT

Consider the use of a headache log/diary to identify triggers of headaches, record efficacy of treatments, and track history of headaches.

NONPHARMACOLOGIC THERAPY

- Avoid any identifiable provoking factors: caffeine, tobacco, and alcohol may trigger attacks, as may dietary or other environmental precipitants (less common)
- Avoid stressors in life and minimize variations in daily routine with regular sleep, meals, and exercise
- Relaxation training, behavioral therapy, and biofeedback. Trials have shown that among young persons with chronic migraine, the use of cognitive behavior therapy (CBT) plus amitriptyline results in greater reductions in days with headaches and migraine-related disability compared with use of headache education plus amitriptyline.[1]

ACUTE ANALGESIC Rx

- Many oral agents are ineffective because of poor absorption from migraine-induced gastric stasis. Non-oral route of administration should be selected in patients with severe nausea or vomiting.
- NSAIDs such as ketorolac, combination analgesics, or barbiturates may be used.

ACUTE ABORTIVE Rx

- IV antiemetic (prochlorperazine, metoclopramide, domperidone): Acute dystonic reactions and akathisia are rare side effects. These are generally not used as monotherapy.
- Ergotamine and ergotamine combinations (PO/PR) and dihydroergotamine (DHE 45) (SC, IV, IM, intranasal) have well-documented efficacy against migraines. DHE is usually administered in combination with an antiemetic drug (Table 1-215).
- Triptans (SC, PO, and intranasal) are now considered the drug class of choice for abortive therapy. Meta-analysis suggests that 10 mg rizatriptan, 40 mg eletriptan, and 12.5 mg almotriptan are most effective.

---

[1]Powers SW et al: Cognitive behavioral therapy plus amitriptyline for chronic migraine in children and adolescents, *JAMA* 310(24):2622-2630, 2013.

TABLE 1-215 Abortive and Analgesic Therapy for Migraine*

Drug	Route	Dose
Triptans (Serotonin Agonists)		
Sumatriptan	Subcutaneous	6 mg, repeat in 2 hr (max 2 doses/day)
Sumatriptan	Oral	25 mg, 50 mg, 100 mg, repeat in 2 hr (max 200 mg/day)
Sumatriptan	Nasal spray	5 mg, 20 mg, repeat in 2 hr (max 40 mg/day)
Zolmitriptan	Oral	1.25, 2.5 mg, 5 mg, repeat in 2 hr (max 10 mg/day)
Zolmitriptan	Nasal spray	5 mg, repeat in 2 hr (max 10 mg/day)
Zolmitriptan	Orally disintegrating tab	2.5, 5 mg, repeat in 2 hr (max 10 mg/day)
Naratriptan	Oral	1 mg, 2.5 mg, repeat in 4 hr (max 5 mg/day)
Rizatriptan	Oral	5 mg, 10 mg, repeat in 2 hr (max 30 mg/day)
Almotriptan	Oral	6.25 mg, 12.5 mg, may repeat in 2 hr (max 25 mg/day)
Eletriptan	Oral	20 mg, 40 mg, may repeat in 2 hr (max 80 mg/day)
Frovatriptan	Oral	2.5 mg, may repeat in 2 hr (max 7.5 mg/day); may also be used for mini prophylaxis
Ergotamine Preparations		
Ergotamine and caffeine	Oral	2 tablets, may repeat 1 tab q30 min (max 6/day)
Ergotamine and caffeine	Rectal	1 suppository, repeat in 1 hr (max 2/day)
Ergotamine	Sublingual	1 tablet, repeat in 1 hr (max 2/day)
Dihydroergotamine	Intramuscular Subcutaneous Intravenous Nasal spray	0.5-1.0 mg, repeat twice at 1-hr intervals (max 3 mg/attack)
Sympathomimetics (with or without Barbiturates or Codeine)		
Isometheptene+ dichloralphenazone+ acetaminophen	Oral	1 to 2 capsules, repeat in 4 hr (max 8/day)
Nonsteroidal Anti-inflammatory Drugs		
Acetaminophen+ (should not be used alone)	Oral	2 tablets, repeat in 6 hr (max 8/day aspirin+caffeine)
Naproxen	Oral	550-750 mg, repeat in 1 hr (max 3 times/wk)
Meclofenamate	Oral	100-200 mg, repeat in 1 hr (max 3 times/wk)
Flurbiprofen	Oral	50-100 mg, repeat in 1 hr (max 3 times/wk)
Ibuprofen	Oral	200-300 mg, repeat in 1 hr (max 3 times/wk)
Antiemetics		
Promethazine	Oral	50-125 mg
	Intramuscular	No clear benefit in migraine, may be used
Prochlorperazine	Oral	1-25 mg
	Rectal	2.5-25 mg (suppository)
	Intramuscular/IV	5-10 mg, good evidence for strong benefit
Chlorpromazine	Oral	10-25 mg
	Rectal	50-100 mg (suppository)
	Intravenous	Up to 35 mg, use with monitoring, some evidence for good benefit
Trimethobenzamide	Oral	250 mg
	Rectal	200 mg
Metoclopramide	Oral	5-10 mg
	Intramuscular	10 mg
	Intravenous	5-10 mg
Dimenhydrinate	Oral	50 mg

*For side effects and contraindications consult the manufacturer's drug insert before prescribing any of these drugs.
Modified from Wiederholt WC: *Neurology for non-neurologists,* ed 4, Philadelphia, 2000, Saunders.

- Early administration improves effectiveness.
- There is an emerging role for the use of IV magnesium (1 g), IV valproate infusions to abort migraine headaches. IV dexamethasone up to 12 mg may be used for headaches lasting more than 72 hours.
- Greater and lesser occipital nerve blocks may also be performed to alleviate pain in the acute setting. This may be combined with auriculotemporal, supraorbital, and supratrochlear nerve block to achieve anesthesia in the area of perceived pain. Steroids should generally be avoided with these nerve blocks because of lack of benefit.

PROPHYLAXIS Rx

- Prophylactic treatment is generally indicated when headaches occur more than once a week or when symptomatic treatments are contraindicated or not effective. They are most effective when initiated during a headache-free period. All prophylaxis should be maintained for at least 3 months before deeming the medication a failure.
- Well-established options for prophylactic treatment include β-blockers (propranolol, timolol, atenolol, metoprolol), tricyclic antidepressants (amitriptyline), and the antiepileptic drugs topiramate and valproic acid.
- Less-established options include calcium channel blockers, selective serotonin reuptake inhibitors, and the antiepileptic drug gabapentin.
- The FDA has approved injection of onabotulinum toxin A (Botox) for prevention of headaches in adult patients with chronic migraines only (≥15 headache days/mo for ≥3 mo). The recommended total dose is 155 total units administered intramuscularly every 12 wk divided among 31 sites in head and neck area (frontalis, corrugator, procerus, occipitalis, temporalis, trapezius, cervical paraspinal muscle group). A maximum of 195 units is allowed.
- Surgical treatment for migraine using nerve decompression has been advocated recently but remains highly controversial, with poorly established results. This should be pursued only in collaboration with a headache specialist.

DISPOSITION

With advancing age, many patients will have sustained reduction of migraine headaches.

REFERRAL

To neurologist if uncertain about diagnosis or treatment not effective

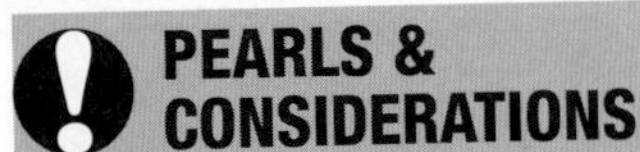

PEARLS & CONSIDERATIONS

- Avoid overuse of narcotics, barbiturates, caffeine, and benzodiazepines because they are habit-forming.
- Long-term use of analgesic medications can result in drug-induced or rebound headaches.

SUGGESTED READINGS

available at www.expertconsult.com

RELATED CONTENT

Migraine Headache (Patient Information)

AUTHOR: **SIDDHARTH KAPOOR, M.D.**

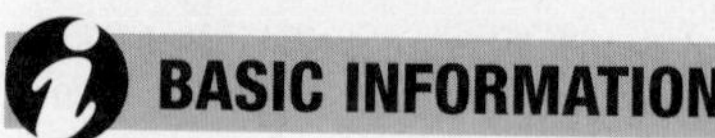

BASIC INFORMATION

DEFINITION

Tension-type headaches (TTH) are recurrent headaches lasting 30 min to 7 days without nausea or vomiting and with at least two of the following characteristics: pressing or tightening quality (nonthrobbing), mild or moderate intensity, bilateral, and not aggravated by routine physical activity.

SYNONYMS

Muscle contraction headache
Tension headache
Stress headache
Essential headache

ICD-9CM CODES
307.81 Tension headache
ICD-10CM CODES
G44.209 Tension-type headache, unspecified, not intractable

EPIDEMIOLOGY & DEMOGRAPHICS

INCIDENCE (IN U.S.): Most common type of headache; as high as 70% of all headaches presenting to primary care physician
PEAK INCIDENCE: Occurs at all ages
PREVALENCE (IN U.S.): Males: 63%/yr; females: 86%/yr
PREDOMINANT SEX: Females are affected more often than males

PHYSICAL FINDINGS & CLINICAL PRESENTATION

Pressure or "bandlike" tightness all around the head; may be worse at the vertex. Cervical, paracervical, and trapezius muscle spasm and/or tenderness on palpation may be present. Scalp tenderness or hypersensitivity to pain also occurs. Symptoms suggestive of migraine are usually not present (e.g., throbbing pain, nausea/vomiting, visual complaints, aura). Either one symptom of photo- or phonophobia does not exclude the diagnosis of TTH.

ETIOLOGY

- Unclear; little data to support postulated muscle contraction component. More likely a multifactorial disorder with several possible concurrent pathophysiologic mechanisms.
- No recent data to support the long-standing belief that these headaches arise from stress or other psychological factors. However, components of stress, sleep deprivation, hunger, and eyestrain may exacerbate symptoms. Stress and poor coping mechanisms may initiate and propagate pain (via activation of second messengers in downstream pain substrates). In episodic TTH, peripheral mechanisms are predominant, whereas central mechanisms are involved in chronic TTH.

Dx DIAGNOSIS

DIFFERENTIAL DIAGNOSIS

- Migraine (would expect associated symptoms; see topic "Headache, Migraine")
- Cervical spine disease
- Intracranial mass (may present with focal neurologic signs, seizures, or headache awakening patient from sleep)
- Idiopathic intracranial hypertension (found more often in obese women of childbearing age, may have papilledema, visual loss, or diplopia)
- Rebound headache from overuse of analgesics
- Secondary headache (e.g., temporomandibular joint syndrome, thyrotoxicosis, polycythemia, drug side effects)
- Migraine and TTH may often coexist and may be difficult to differentiate (suggest headache calendar).
- Section II describes the differential diagnosis of headaches.

WORKUP

- Thorough history and physical examination for any new-onset headache
- Neuroimaging should be performed when unexplained neurologic findings are present on examination or in cases of atypical new-onset sudden and severe headaches.

LABORATORY TESTS

- No routine tests
- Erythrocyte sedimentation rate in elderly patients suspected of having temporal arteritis

IMAGING STUDIES

CT scan and/or MRI may be used to exclude intracranial pathology. MRI is better for imaging the posterior fossa. Contrast should be used if mass lesion is suspected.

Rx TREATMENT

NONPHARMACOLOGIC THERAPY

- Electromyography (EMG) biofeedback has a documented effect, whereas cognitive-behavioral therapy and relaxation training are most likely effective (especially in adolescents and children).
- Physical therapy (including stretching exercises, massage, and ultrasound) and acupuncture may be effective, but there is no robust scientific evidence for efficacy.
- Schultz-type autogenic training (relaxation technique based on passive concentration and body awareness of specific sensations), transcutaneous electrical nerve stimulation, heat

ACUTE GENERAL Rx

Nonnarcotic analgesics (first choice) and combination analgesics containing caffeine (second choice) with limited frequency to prevent drug-induced and/or rebound headache

CHRONIC Rx

- Tricyclic antidepressants (e.g., amitriptyline 10 to 150 mg hs) (first choice); mirtazapine and venlafaxine (second choice); treatment may be limited by side effects.
- Avoid narcotics, limit NSAIDs, consider indomethacin; if related to cervical muscle spasm, may consider trial of muscle relaxants (e.g., Skelaxin 400 to 800 mg tid)
- Botulinum toxin A has been FDA approved for prophylactic treatment of chronic daily headaches. Trials have shown a small-to-modest benefit for chronic headaches but are not associated with fewer tension-type headaches per month.

DISPOSITION

May not respond fully to treatment

REFERRAL

If uncertain about diagnosis or unexplained focal neurologic findings on examination

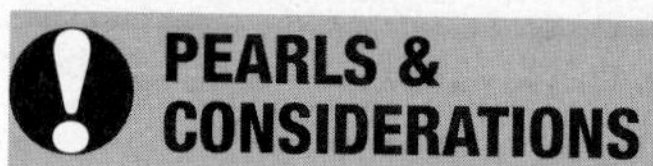

PEARLS & CONSIDERATIONS

It is imperative to avoid overuse of caffeine- and barbiturate-containing medications because of the risk of rebound headaches.

SUGGESTED READINGS

available at www.expertconsult.com

RELATED CONTENT

Tension Headache (Patient Information)

AUTHOR: **RICHARD S. ISAACSON, M.D.**

BASIC INFORMATION

DEFINITION

Healthcare-associated infections (HAIs) are infections associated with healthcare, generally occurring more than 2 calendar days after admission to a hospital. Classification criteria are established by the Centers for Disease Control and Prevention's (CDC) National Healthcare Safety Network (NHSN).

SYNONYMS

Nosocomial infections

ICD-9CM CODES

008.45	*Clostridium difficile*
041.12	MRSA
482.42	MRSA pneumonia
038.12	MRSA septicemia
998.59	Other postoperative infection
999.31	Bloodstream infection due to central venous catheter
997.31	Ventilator-assisted pneumonia
996.31	Due to urethral [indwelling] catheter

ICD-10CM CODES

A04.7	Enterocolitis due to Clostridium difficile
B95.62	Methicillin-resistant Staphylococcus aureus infection as the cause of diseases classified elsewhere
J15.212	Pneumonia due to methicillin-resistant Staphylococcus aureus
A41.02	Sepsis due to methicillin-resistant Staphylococcus aureus
K68.11	Postprocedural retroperitoneal abscess
T80.219A	Unspecified infection due to central venous catheter, initial encounter
J95.851	Ventilator-associated pneumonia
T83.098A	Other mechanical complication of other indwelling urethral catheter, initial encounter

EPIDEMIOLOGY & DEMOGRAPHICS

INCIDENCE (IN U.S.):
- Develop in at least 5% of hospitalized patients; over 1.7 million patients.
- In 2002, HAIs accounted for more than 98,000 deaths.
- In 2002, the annual cost of HAIs in the U.S. was estimated as >$5 billion to $10 billion; adjusts to >$35 billion in 2007 values.
- At least one third of hospital-acquired infections are preventable.
- Leads to increased morbidity and mortality.

PREVALENCE (IN U.S.): 2 million to 4 million cases/yr

PREDOMINANT SEX:
- Overall, approximately equal
- Elderly women: predominantly nosocomial urinary tract infections

PREDOMINANT AGE: Newborns and elderly patients (>60 yr) at highest risk

PEAK INCIDENCE: Varies widely with infection site

RISK FACTORS: Patients with the following conditions can develop HAIs at any age:
- In ICU
- Intubation
- Chronic lung disease
- Renal disease
- Comatose
- Chronic urethral or vascular catheterization
- Malnutrition
- Postoperative state
- Diabetic

PHYSICAL FINDINGS & CLINICAL PRESENTATION

Vary with specific HAIs

ETIOLOGY

- Bacteria (gram-negative bacteria are responsible for >30% of HAIs)
- Fungi
- Viruses

SOURCES AND MODES OF TRANSMISSION:
- Patient's own flora
  - Comprises resistant organisms associated with hospitalization
  - Frequently maintained thereafter by persistent GI colonization
- Unwashed hands of staff
  - Physicians
  - Nurses
- Invasion of protective defenses (intact skin, respiratory cilia, urinary sphincters, and mucosa)
  - IV lines/central lines
  - Catheters
  - Respiratory equipment
  - Surgical wounds
  - Scopes and other imaging devices
- Failure to provide adequate negative pressure, high-volume air flow chambers for airborne infection isolation of patients with TB or disseminated herpes zoster/chickenpox
- Failure to rapidly identify and provide appropriate care (with isolation or precautions) for patients with communicable diseases
- Food
- Fomites
- Personnel attire can become contaminated. Although studies have not yet verified the link between attire contamination and disease transmission, cross-contamination of previously washed hands can occur
- Inattention to safe injection practices has led to outbreaks of hepatitis and fungal meningitis.
  - Do not administer medications from a syringe to multiple patients even if the needle is changed.
  - Use fluid infusion and administration sets (e.g., IV bags/bottles, tubing, connectors) for one patient only and dispose after each use. Do not use bags or bottles as a common source of supply for multiple patients.
  - Use single-dose vials for parenteral medications whenever possible and do not administer medications from single-dose vials to multiple patients or combine leftover contents for later use.
  - Single-dose, single-use vials do not have preservative and should be used for a single patient and a single-case/procedure/injection.
  - When a single dose or single vial is accessed or opened, discard as per manufacturer or at the end of the case or procedure (whichever comes first).
  - Insulin pens should be used for one single designated person only, even if the needle is changed.

RISKS AMPLIFIED:
- Use of broad-spectrum antibiotics
  - Select highly resistant bacteria
  - Establish multidrug-resistant bacteria as endemic flora in microenvironments within the hospital
  - Consider antibiotic stewardship programs to reduce these risks
- Highly vulnerable patients with specific risk factors
  - Immunosuppression (as a result of therapy, transplantation, AIDS)
  - Old age
  - Postsurgery
  - Prolonged surgery
  - Chronic lung disease
  - Ventilator dependence
  - Antacid therapy
  - Vascular lines
  - Hyperalimentation
  - ICU stay
  - Recent antibiotic therapy
- Clustering of seriously ill patients
  - Often with wounds or contaminated drainage
  - Intensifying probability of cross-infection

PREVENTION STRATEGIES: Handwashing/hand hygiene between all patient contacts is the single most important method of decreasing HAI:
- Regular soap and water for at least 15 sec
- Chlorhexidine (particularly good for gram-positive organisms like methicillin-resistant *Staphylococcus aureus* [MRSA]), alcohol handrub or other antiseptic for resistant organisms
- Purpose of soap and water handwash
  - Degrease hand surfaces
  - Flushes away oils and associated bacteria, removal of visible dirt or body fluids
- Procedure
  - Lukewarm water
  - Must include all surfaces
  - Special attention to areas between fingers and to the dirtier dominant hand (most people reflexively wash the cleaner, nondominant hand more vigorously)
- Alcohol handrubs
  - Improve handwashing frequency (less drying to hands, faster, and no need for wash basin and towels for drying)
  - Significantly reduce HAIs
  - Now recommended in essentially all routine healthcare settings
  - Rub hands until dry, approximately 15 sec
- Environmental cleaning
  - New technologies such as hydrogen peroxide vapor or ultraviolet irradiation appear to reduce environmental contamination from *C. difficile* spores, *Norovirus*, and resistant microorganisms.

- Clinical equipment should be properly disinfected or sterilized per manufacturer's instructions.
- High-touch items in patient environment should undergo frequent, thorough disinfection.

METHICILLIN-RESISTANT *STAPHYLOCOCCUS AUREUS* (MRSA):

- Invasive HAIs caused by MRSA decreased 9.4% per year from 2005 through 2008 in the United States.
- Healthcare-associated MRSA strains are typically resistant to many antibiotics, remaining susceptible to vancomycin and trimethoprim/sulfamethoxazole.
- High-risk factors include dialysis, recent stay in acute or long-term care facilities.
- Control measures include hand hygiene, disinfection of equipment, protective attire for isolation, and standard precautions.
- Community-acquired MRSA (CA-MRSA) is associated with soft tissue, presenting as boils, rash, or so-called spider bite, and typically occurs in patients who have no recent healthcare or hospital interaction.
- CA-MRSA often not found in nares.
- CA-MRSA can be sensitive to fluoroquinolones, clindamycin, and/or erythromycin in addition to vancomycin and trimethoprim/sulfamethoxazole.

Refer to Methicillin-Resistant Staphylococcus aureus (MRSA) topic for more information.

VANCOMYCIN-RESISTANT *ENTEROCOCCUS FAECIUM* (VREF):

- The percentage of HAIs caused by VREF increased more than twentyfold between 1989 and 1993, rising from 0% to 9%. By 2005, VREF, vancomycin-resistant *E. faecalis,* and other vancomycin-resistant species of enterococci had become common and endemic nosocomial pathogens accounting for 15% to 40% of all enterococci isolated in the hospital setting.
- A high percentage of VREF isolated, 80%, are also ampicillin resistant.
- Factors predisposing to VREF colonization or infection include a high percentage of hospital days receiving antibiotic therapy, use of IV, underlying disease, immunosuppression, and abdominal surgery.
- Evidence suggests that the vehicle is the hands of healthcare workers (HCWs).
- Control measures:
  - Aggressive isolation of colonized or infected patients
  - Restraint in using broad-spectrum antibiotics
  - Compliance with hand hygiene best practices

Refer to the topic "Vancomycin-Resistant Enterococcus" for more information.

CLOSTRIDIUM DIFFICILE:

- Causes diarrhea as a result of pseudomembranous colitis.
- Accounts for 15% to 25% of healthcare-associated diarrhea.
- Warrants contact precautions and bleach for disinfection.
- Alcohol-based handrub may not eliminate spores of this organism, so can use soap and water to wash hands at sink.
- Spores can be dispersed in the air or room environment surrounding patients.
- Treatment is tiered based on severity.
- Rising incidence of *C. difficile* infection with emerging strains that have up to twentythreefold more toxin production.
- Toxin assays vary widely in ability to detect toxin.
- Only unformed stool specimens should be submitted for laboratory *C. difficile* testing.
- Polymerase chain reaction (PCR) and nucleic acid amplification test/loop mediated isothermal DNA amplification (NAAT/LAMP) are more sensitive test methods than enzyme immunoassay (EIA).
- Antibiotics can predispose persons by altering their normal gut flora.
- Can present in healthy patients with no known risk factors.
- Sometimes causes toxic megacolon or fulminant colitis.

NOROVIRUS:

- Patients present with sudden onset of nausea, vomiting, and/or diarrhea.
- Now considered year-round rather than seasonal.
- Disinfection with bleach.
- Often need to isolate exposed persons for average incubation period, such as 3 days, to prevent outbreak.

SURVEILLANCE

- Crucial for early identification of infections. Enables:
  - Immediate intervention
  - Education
- Prospective, concurrent, hospital surveillance:
  - Electronic data mining provides accurate review
  - Feasible with sophisticated computerized data collection and analysis
- Targeted surveillance addresses high-risk procedures and patient populations
- Routine rate calculations and statistical analyses:
  - Use device-specific days, procedure-specific cases, or patient-days as denominators
  - Enhance early recognition of microclusters of infections by body site and by organism
  - Facilitate proper early control of potential outbreaks
- Active surveillance/screening cultures for multi-drug resistant organisms (MDROs); for example, high-risk populations for MRSA

Dx DIAGNOSIS

MOST COMMON HAI:

- Urinary tract infections (UTIs) (32%)
- Surgical site and other soft tissue infections (22%)
- Pneumonia (15%)
- Bloodstream infections (14%)

HEALTHCARE-ASSOCIATED UTIS:

- General associations:
  - Indwelling urinary (e.g., Foley) catheters
  - Inappropriate catheter care (including opening catheter junctions)
  - Female sex
  - Absence of systemic antibiotics
- Physical findings:
  - Fever
  - Dysuria
  - Leukocytosis
  - Pyuria
  - Flank or costovertebral angle tenderness
- Usual organisms:
  - *E. coli*
  - *Candida*
  - *Enterococcus*
  - *Pseudomonas*
  - *Klebsiella*
  - *Enterobacter*
- Sepsis in 1% to 3% of hospital-associated UTIs
- Prevention bundle to eliminate catheter-associated UTIs (CAUTIs):
  - Use meticulous aseptic technique during insertion and daily perineal care
  - Avoid unnecessary urinary catheters; remove promptly
  - Never open the catheter-collection tubing junction (keep system closed)
  - Obtain all specimens using sterile syringe
  - Remove Foley catheters as soon as possible
  - Substitute intermittent catheterization for Foley catheters

HEALTHCARE-ASSOCIATED BLOODSTREAM INFECTIONS:

- General associations:
  - IV lines
  - Arterial lines
  - Central venous pressure (CVP) lines: lead to catheter-associated bloodstream infection (CLABSI)
  - Phlebitis
  - Hyperalimentation
  - Lack of safe injection best practices
- Fever possibly only presenting sign
- Exit site of all vascular lines carefully evaluated for:
  - Erythema
  - Induration
  - Tenderness
  - Purulent drainage
- Usual organisms for device-associated bacteremia
  - *S. aureus* (including MRSA)
  - *Staphylococcus epidermidis* for long-term IV lines
  - *Enterobacter*
  - *Klebsiella*
  - *Candida* spp.
  - *Pseudomonas aeruginosa* may come from a water source or reflect cutaneous bacteria
- Phlebitis in 1.3 million patients yearly
- Approximately 10,000 annual deaths from IV sepsis
- Prevention bundle to eliminate central line-associated bloodstream infections (CLABSIs):

- ○ Meticulous sterile technique during central catheter line insertion.
- ○ Emphasis should be placed on attention to detail, including handwashing, adherence to guidelines for catheter insertion and maintenance, appropriate use of antiseptic solutions such as chlorhexidine (CHG) to prepare the skin before central line insertion.
- ○ Modified catheter, for example, antiseptic-coated line, may reduce risk for endoluminal colonization and catheter-related sepsis in subclavian lines.
- ○ Decrease use of routine IVs and encourage PO intake.
- ○ Avoid using a femoral vein insertion site. Subclavian central line site is associated with lower infection rate than jugular.
- ○ Bundle to prevent CLABSIs includes hand hygiene, CHG skin prep for insertion of central lines, full barrier protection for insertion of central lines, removal of unnecessary lines, insertion checklist.
- ○ Consider daily CHG baths in ICUs.

HEALTHCARE-ASSOCIATED PNEUMONIAS:

- More common in ICUs
- General associations:
  - Aspiration
  - Intubation: leads to ventilator-associated events (VAE) or ventilator-associated pneumonia (VAP)
  - Altered consciousness
  - Old age
  - Chronic lung disease
  - Postsurgery
  - Antacids
  - Head of bed not elevated
- Signs of pneumonia common among patients on general wards:
  - Cough
  - Sputum
  - Fever
  - Leukocytosis
  - New infiltrate on chest x-ray examination
- Signs more subtle in ICUs, because many patients have purulent sputum because of chronic intubation
  - Change in sputum character or volume
  - Small changes on chest x-ray examination
- Usual organisms:
  - *S. aureus* (including MRSA)
  - *Pseudomonas aeruginosa*
  - *Enterobacter*
  - *Acinetobacter*
  - *Klebsiella*
- Less common organisms:
  - *Stenotrophomonas* spp.
  - *Legionella, Flavobacterium*
  - Respiratory syncytial virus (infants)
  - Adenovirus
- 1% of hospitalized patients affected
- Mortality rate high (40%)
- Prevention bundle:
  - Use meticulous sterile technique during suctioning and handling airway.
  - Do not routinely change ventilator breathing circuits and components. For heat and moisture exchangers, no more frequently than every 48 hr.
  - Drain respirator tubing without allowing fluid to return to respirator.
  - Wash hands routinely to prevent colonization of patients and transfer of organisms among patients.
  - Use of a bundle to prevent VAEs and VAPs to include: elevate the head of bed, provide deep vein thrombosis (DVT) prophylaxis, provide peptic ulcer disease (PUD) prophylaxis, hold sedation, test for ability to extubate, control glucose, gastric decontamination.
  - Consider oral mouth care with CHG for vented patients in ICUs.

SURGICAL AND HEALTHCARE-ASSOCIATED SOFT TISSUE INFECTIONS:

- Associations:
  - Decubitus ulcers
  - Surgical site risks: contaminated or dirty/infected, the American Society of Anesthesiologists' (ASA) physical status classification of ASA 3 or 4, duration of surgery over national average, usually 3 hr
  - Abdominal surgery
  - Presence of drain
  - Preoperative length of stay
  - Surgeon
  - Presence of other infection
- Physical findings:
  - Decubitus ulcer with fluctuance at margin or under firm eschar
  - Erythema extending >2 cm beyond margin of surgical wound
  - Tenderness
  - Induration
  - Erythema
  - Fluctuance
  - Purulent drainage
  - Dehiscence of sutures
- Usual organisms:
  - *S. aureus* (including MRSA)
  - *Enterococcus*
  - *Enterobacter*
  - *Acinetobacter*
  - *E. coli*
- Prevention:
  - Use careful skin care and frequent, proper positioning of patient to prevent decubitus ulcer.
  - Use meticulous sterile surgical technique.
  - Use properly washed and sterilized instruments, processed in accordance with manufacturer's instructions. Minimize immediate-use steam sterilization (formerly known as flash sterilization).
  - Wash hands to decrease colonization when handling postoperative wound.
  - Limit prophylactic antibiotics to 24 hr perioperatively.
  - Double-wrap contaminated dressings (hold in gloved hand and evert gloves over dressings) before disposal.
  - Surgical Care Improvement Project (SCIP) bundle to include antibiotic prophylaxis selection, receipt of antibiotic within 1 hr prior to surgery, discontinuation of antibiotic within 24 hr of surgery end time, cardiac surgery patients with controlled 6 AM postoperative blood glucose, clip rather than shave prep, postoperative normothermia for colorectal surgery patients, removal of Foley catheter by end of postoperative day 2 (except for urologic, gynecologic, or perineal procedures, or on paralytics, vasopressors/inotropics during ICU stay).
  - Preadmission nares MRSA screening often beneficial for open heart and orthopedic implants when time is allowed for decolonization, chlorhexidine showers, and appropriate antibiotic prophylaxis selection.

LABORATORY TESTS

- Appropriate to specific HAI and specific patient's condition
- Cultures generally indicated for proper confirmation of responsible pathogens:
  - Urine
  - Blood
  - Sputum
  - Soft tissue
- Molecular analysis of nosocomial epidemics:
  - Plasmid fingerprinting
  - Restriction endonuclease digestion (plasmid and genomic DNA)
  - Peptide analysis
  - Immunoblotting
  - Ribosomal RNA (rRNA) typing
  - DNA probes
  - Multilocus enzyme electrophoresis
  - Restriction fragment length polymorphism (RFLP)
  - PCR
  - Provide confirmation of point-source or common strains and corroboration of hypotheses reached utilizing classic epidemiology

IMAGING STUDIES

Rarely needed for diagnosis of HAI; helpful for deep surgical site infection.

Rx TREATMENT

ACUTE GENERAL Rx

- Appropriate to etiologic organism:
  - Antibiotic
  - Antifungal
  - Antiviral
- Specific therapy determined after careful consideration of resident flora within the microenvironment in which the patient was hospitalized
  - Empiric therapy
  - Frequently difficult to fashion accurately
  - Often undesirable, unless the patient's clinical condition requires urgent treatment
- Consultation for expert advice regarding antibiotic selection in view of known epidemiologic risks within the hospital (Hospital Epidemiologist or Infectious Disease Specialist)
- Avoid unnecessary treatment for organisms that are colonizing (no signs or symptoms of infection), but not infecting patients

- Prevention of spread of communicable diseases
  - Isolation or precautions (airborne, droplet, contact isolation precautions, and combinations thereof)
  - Classic schema (strict, respiratory isolation and contact [skin and wound] precautions) have been replaced by more streamlined revised guidelines (airborne, droplet, contact isolation precautions, and combinations thereof)
  - Less careful response to some diseases (e.g., hemorrhagic fevers) inadvertently induced by removal of strict isolation category
  - Universal/standard precautions to protect HCWs against splash or splatter of blood or body fluids
  - Tracking roommates of patients with communicable disease, such as Norovirus or influenza and using precautions during the incubation period
- Universal/standard precautions used for all patients during all anticipated contacts with blood, body fluids, or secretions
  - Gloves
  - Goggles/eye shield
  - Gowns that prevent blood or potentially infectious materials from passing through
- Consider aggressive isolation to restrict spread of multidrug-resistant organisms and their plasmids
  - MRSA
  - VREF
  - MDR-GNRs (multidrug-resistant gram-negative rods) can include extended-spectrum β-lactamases (ESBL), carbapenem-resistant Enterobacteriaceae (CRE), some *Acinetobacter baumanni.* New microbiology interpretive criteria (breakpoints) can result in no longer reporting mechanism of resistance.
  - New Delhi metallo-β-lactamase 1 (NDM-1): these are gram-negative Enterobacteriaceae with a new type of carbapenem-resistance gene.

Refer to the topic "Multidrug-Resistant Gram-Negative Rods (MDR-GNRs)" for more information.

DISPOSITION

The Infection Prevention and Control Service and/or Hospital Epidemiologist should be notified when infectious complications occur in the hospital setting; most, but not all, HAIs are potentially avoidable, and every effort should be taken to minimize the risk of infections associated with healthcare. Nationwide success in achieving and sustaining zero CLABSIs, zero CAUIs, and and zero VAPs warrant widespread use of infection prevention bundles to target zero HAIs.

REFERRAL

- To infection preventionist
- To hospital epidemiologist

PEARLS & CONSIDERATIONS

COMMENTS

- Sharp and splash injuries to staff are relatively rare, but nearly all are preventable.
  - Nurses incur most injuries.
  - Usual causes:
    1. Needle sticks
    2. Scalpel and surgical needle injuries
    3. Blood splashes
  - Prevention:
    1. Never recap needles.
    2. Dispose of needles only in rigid, impermeable plastic containers.
    3. Clearly announce instrument passes in the operating room and during procedures. Use passing trays.
    4. Use needleless systems for vascular access and connectors whenever possible to limit HCWs' use of sharp medical devices.
    5. Use gloves, mask, and goggles/eye shield if aerosol or splash is likely.
    6. Never leave needles or other sharp items in beds.
    7. Never dispose of sharp items in regular trash bags.
  - Infection Prevention and Control or Employee Health staff should be consulted immediately after exposure to determine need for prophylaxis for hepatitis B or HIV.
  - All clinical staff should be immune to hepatitis B (natural or vaccine).
- Fungi previously considered to be contaminants are now risks for patients with cancer and organ transplantation.
  - *Candida* spp.
    1. *C. guilliermondii*
    2. *C. krusei*
    3. *C. parapsilosis*
    4. *C. tropicalis*
  - *Aspergillus* spp.
  - *Curvularia* spp.
  - *Bipolaris* spp.
  - *Exserohilum* spp.
  - *Alternaria* spp.
  - *Fusarium* spp.
  - *Scopulariopsis* spp.
  - *Pseudallescheria boydii*
  - *Trichosporon beigelii*
  - *Malassezia furfur*
  - *Hansenula* spp.
  - *Microsporum canis*
- Focused, committed efforts by the entire healthcare staff continuously directed toward prevention:
  - Each HAI addressed as an opportunity to improve the organization and delivery of safe patient care
  - Essential for individual staff members to understand that small risks applied to large populations result in a large number of total events (i.e., HAIs)
- Antibiotic stewardship
  - Choose appropriate antibiotic
  - Minimize vancomycin usage
- The Centers for Medicare & Medicaid Services denies inpatient payments for certain HAIs. Total reimbursement is linked to performance (compare HAI outcome to national benchmark).
- The number of surgical-site *S. aureus* infections acquired in the hospital, particularly cardiac or orthopedic, has been reduced by rapid screening and decolonizing of nasal carriers of *S. aureus* prior to surgery.
- Universal decolonization of ICU patients for MRSA has been advocated without nares screening as a model to reduce bloodstream infection and MRSA clinical isolates.

SUGGESTED READINGS

available at www.expertconsult.com

RELATED CONTENT

Methicillin-Resistant *Staphylococcus aureus* (MRSA) (Related Key Topic)
Multidrug-Resistant Gram-Negative Rods (MDR-GNRs) (Related Key Topic)
Vancomycin-Resistant Enterococcus (VRE) (Related Key Topic)

AUTHOR: **MARLENE FISHMAN WOLPERT, M.P.H., C.I.C.**

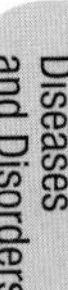

BASIC INFORMATION

DEFINITION

Complete heart block (CHB) is the absence of electrical impulse transmission from the atria to the ventricles when atrioventricular (AV) junction is not physiologically refractory due to functional impairment of the conduction system.

Atria and ventricles are controlled by independent pacemakers; thus, complete AV block is only one cause of complete AV dissociation. It may be acquired or congenital.

SYNONYMS

Third-degree AV block
CHB
Complete AV block

ICD-9CM CODES
426.0 Complete heart block
ICD-10CM CODES
I44.2 Atrioventricular block, complete

EPIDEMIOLOGY & DEMOGRAPHICS

- The prevalence of CHB is 0.04%.
- The prevalence of CHB increases with age.

PHYSICAL FINDINGS & CLINICAL PRESENTATION

Physical examination may be normal. Cannon A waves may appear in the jugular vein periodically due to the right atrium contracting during ventricular systole. Patients may present with the following clinical manifestations:

- Dizziness, palpitations
- Syncope or presyncope (due to reduced cardiac output)
- Fatigue, impaired exercise tolerance
- Mental status changes
- Congestive heart failure
- Angina pectoris
- Some patients may be asymptomatic (e.g., congenital CHB)

ETIOLOGY

- Fibrosis or sclerosis of the conduction system, Lenegre and Lev disease
- Acute myocardial infarction—inferior (14%) or anterior (2%) wall of patients, usually within 24 hours
- Drug effect (digitalis, calcium channel blockers, beta-blockers, amiodarone)
- Cardiomyopathy and myocarditis
- Infiltrative processes of the myocardium (amyloidosis, sarcoidosis, sclerodema, tumor)
- Metabolic abnormalities (hyperkalemia, hypoxia, hypothyroidism)
- Lyme carditis, rheumatoid nodules, polymyositis, Chagas' disease
- Neuromuscular disorders (Becker muscular dystrophy, myotonic muscular dystrophy)
- Congenital (birth from mothers with systemic lupus)
- Hyperkalemia
- Familial: SCN5 sodium channel mutations have been associated with CHB
- Iatrogenic (cardiac surgery, catheter ablation of arrhythmias, percutaneous coronary intervention). Transcatheter aortic valve implantation (TAVI) is shown to be frequently associated with new conduction abnormalities; patients with preexisting right bundle-branch block are at increased risk of CHB (resolves over time in most patients).

Dx DIAGNOSIS

DIFFERENTIAL DIAGNOSIS

- The differential diagnosis includes lesser degree of AV block, automatic junctional rhythms, and nonconducted premature atrial contractions.
- The atrial rate must be faster than the ventricular rate, and episodes of AV dissociation with an accelerated ventricular or junctional pacemaker overtaking the sinus node can often look like heart block on a single electrocardiogram.

WORKUP

- Workup such as routine labs, cardiac biomarkers, and cardiac imaging should be dictated by the clinical circumstances.
- ECG: diagnostic of the disease (Figs. 1-428 and 1-429):
  - P waves are present with a regular atrial rate that is faster than the ventricular rate.
  - P waves are not related to the QRS complexes. The PR intervals are variable.
  - RR intervals are regular.
  - QRS complexes may be normal with rate of 40 to 60 beats/min (block proximal to His bundle) or wide with a rate of <40 beats/min (block distal to His bundle, acquired)—depending on the location of the block in the conduction system.
  - Complete AV block can result from block at the level of AV node (congenital CHB), within the His bundle, or distal to it, in the Pukinje system (acquired).

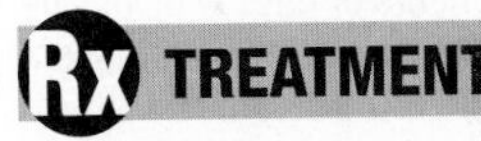

Rx TREATMENT

ACUTE GENERAL Rx

- Initial treatment should focus on the hemodynamic stability and symptoms of the patient.

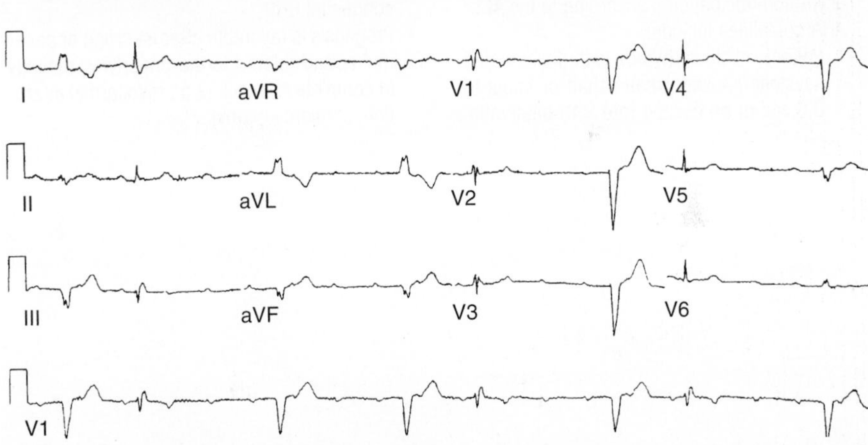

FIGURE 1-429 High-grade atrioventricular block. Note that only three P waves conducted to the ventricle in the whole tracing. Conducted P waves were associated with normal PR intervals and right bundle branch block, a finding suggesting infranodal block. All other P waves were blocked, and ventricular escape rhythm with a left bundle branch block pattern is observed. Note that the block is not caused by retrograde concealment in the atrioventricular node or His-Purkinje system from the ventricular escape complexes because the conducted P waves occurred at a short cycle following the escape complexes. (From Issa Z et al: *Clinical arrhythmology and electrophysiology*, ed 2, Philadelphia, 2012, Saunders.)

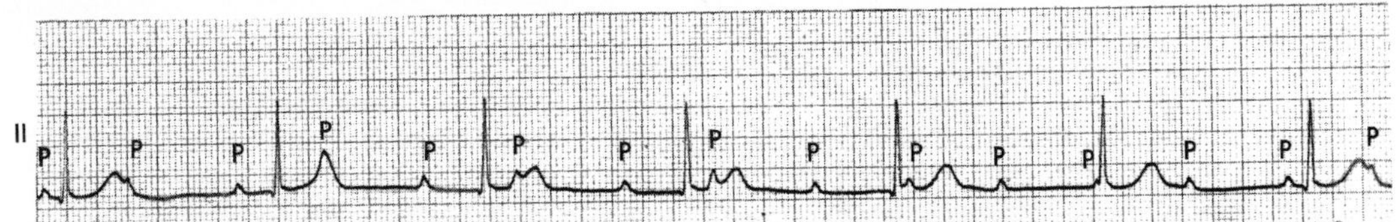

FIGURE 1-428 Third-degree (complete) atrioventricular heart block is characterized by independent atrial (P) and ventricular (QRS) activity. The atrial rate is always faster than the ventricular rate. The PR intervals are completely variable. Some P waves fall on the T wave, distorting its shape. Others may fall in the QRS complex and be "lost." Notice that the QRS complexes are of normal width, indicating that the ventricles are being paced from the atrioventricular junction. (From Goldberger AL [ed]: *Clinical electrocardiography*, ed 5, St Louis, 1994, Mosby.)

- Consider temporary pacemaker insertion if ventricular escape rate is slow (<40 beats/min) and associated with symptoms or hemodynamic compromise.
- CHB as a complication of inferior MI usually only requires temporary pacing; however, a CHB as a result of anterior MI often requires permanent pacing.
- Acquired CHB usually requires pacing, but patients with congenital CHB often have sufficiently rapid escape rhythm to prevent symptoms and avoid permanent pacemaker implantation.
- Withdraw AV-nodal blocking agents if any.
- Short-term therapy (until adequate pacing therapy is established)
  - Vagolytic agents such as atropine may be used to increase the rate of the escape rhythm (for AV nodal level blocks)
  - Catecholamines such as isoproterenol transiently used for a CHB at any site (use with extreme caution or not at all in patients with coronary artery disease).
- Drugs cannot be relied on to increase HR for more than several hours or days without side effects; therefore, temporary or permanent pacemaker insertion is indicated.
- Symptomatic CHB in the absence of a condition that is likely to resolve is an ACC/AHA/HRS Class I indication for permanent pacemaker (PPM) placement.
- Class 1 indications for PPM placement in asymptomatic patients according to the ACC/AHA guidelines include:
  - Patients in sinus rhythm, with documented asystolic pauses greater than or equal to 3.0 sec or an escape rate <40 beats/min, or with an escape rhythm that is below the AV node
  - Patients with atrial fibrillation and bradycardia with one or more pauses of at least 5 sec or longer
  - After catheter ablation of the AV junction
  - If cardiomegaly or LV dysfunction is present with ventricular rates of 40 beats/min or faster
  - Postoperative CHB that is not expected to resolve
  - When it is associated with neuromuscular diseases, such as Erb dystrophy (limb-girdle muscular dystrophy), Kearns-Sayre syndrome, myotonic muscular dystrophy, and peroneal muscular atrophy
  - CHB present during exercise in the absence of myocardial ischemia
- Therapy is directed toward the underlying etiology if there is a reversible source (i.e., IV antibiotics for Lyme disease).
- All patients should be made aware of the high risk of PPM implantation with transcatheter aortic valve implantation (TAVI).

CHRONIC Rx

Patients with PPM need regular follow-up and pacemaker monitoring to ensure proper device functioning.

DISPOSITION

- Mortality is highest in the neonatal period in congenital CHB.
- Prognosis is favorable after insertion of pacemaker and related to the underlying etiology of complete AV block (e.g., myocardial infarction, cardiomyopathy).
- Nonrandomized studies have shown that PPM insertion improves survival in patients with CHB.

REFERRAL

All patients with CHB should be referred to a cardiologist for consideration of temporary and/or PPM implantation.

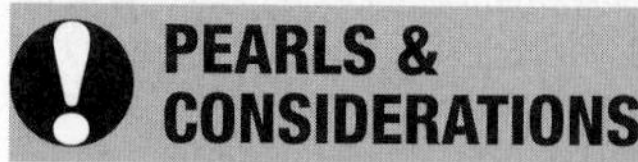

PEARLS & CONSIDERATIONS

COMMENTS

- Patients should be instructed to avoid activities that may damage the pacemaker (e.g., contact sports).
- Pacemaker manufacturers do not recommend any special restrictions regarding proximity to typical household items.
- The presence of a permanent pacemaker is a strong relative contraindication to MRI, although now certain MRI-compatible pacemakers are available.

SUGGESTED READINGS

available at www.expertconsult.com

RELATED CONTENT

Complete Heart Block (Patient Information)

AUTHOR: **BARRY FINE, M.D., Ph.D.**

BASIC INFORMATION

DEFINITION

Second-degree heart block or second-degree atrioventricular (AV) heart block is characterized by a failure of one or more, but not all, atrial impulses to conduct to the ventricles. The block may be at any level of AV conduction system. When more than one atrial impulse is present for each ventricular complex, the rhythm may be described as a ratio of the number of atrial impulses to the number of ventricular complexes. Electrocardiographically there are three types of second-degree block:

- Mobitz type I (Wenckebach):
  - Characterized by a progressive prolongation of the PR interval prior to a blocked nonconducted beat and a shorter PR interval after that blocked beat; the conducted impulse will generally be narrow. The cycle may repeat periodically, leading to "grouped beating."
  - Site of block is usually AV node (proximal to the His bundle).
- Mobitz type II:
  - High-grade AV block (3:1, 4:1, or greater)
  - Characterized by fixed PR intervals before and after blocked beats and is usually associated with a wide QRS morphology (right bundle branch block [RBBB] or left bundle branch block [LBBB] patterns).
  - Site of block is usually infranodal, especially when QRS is wide.
  - It has a greater propensity for progressing to third-degree AV block.
- Pure 2:1 conduction patterns cannot be reliably classified as Mobitz type I or type II

SYNONYMS

Wenckebach block (Mobitz type I block)
Mobitz type II block
AV block

ICD-9CM CODES
426.13 Mobitz type I
426.12 Mobitz type II
ICD-10CM CODES
I44.1 Atrioventricular block, second degree

EPIDEMIOLOGY & DEMOGRAPHICS

Mobitz type I block is more common and may occur in individuals with heightened vagal tone or as a side effect of medications, such as β-blockers or calcium channel blockers.

PHYSICAL FINDINGS & CLINICAL PRESENTATION

- Patients with Mobitz type I are usually asymptomatic. Patients with either type may feel palpitations or the feeling of "missing a beat." Sudden loss of consciousness without warning (Adams-Stokes attack) can occur in patients with Mobitz type II; however, it is much more common in patients with complete heart block.
- Type I block: there is gradual decrease in the intensity of the first heart sound with widening of the a-c interval in the central venous waveform, ending in a pause, and an a wave not followed by a v wave in the neck along with an irregular pulse.
- Type II block: the first heart sound retains a constant intensity, with intermittent ventricular pauses and a waves not followed by v waves in the neck. There is an irregular pulse for most times with intermittent pauses.

ETIOLOGY

- High vagal tone (young patients, athletes at rest)
- Degenerative changes in the AV conduction system
- Ischemia at the AV nodes (type I with inferior wall myocardial infarction [MI] and type II with anterior wall MI)
- Drugs (digitalis, quinidine, procainamide, adenosine, calcium channel blockers [nondihydropyridines], β-blockers)
- Cardiomyopathies, collagen vascular diseases, infiltrative diseases (amyloidosis, sarcoidosis, hematochromatosis)
- Myocarditis/endocarditis (infectious, e.g., Lyme disease, Chagas disease; and noninfectious, e.g., systemic lupus erythematosus)
- Hyperkalemia, hypermagnesemia
- Hypothyroidism
- Prior cardiac valve surgery
- Catheter trauma, catheter ablation for arrhythmias

DIAGNOSIS

DIFFERENTIAL DIAGNOSIS

The ECG easily and reliably distinguishes Mobitz type I from Mobitz type II block and from other conduction abnormalities. It should be distinguished from the less common phenomenon of second-degree sinoatrial node exit block.

Mobitz type I block with a normal QRS complex tends to be benign and usually does not progress to more advanced forms of AV conduction within a short period of time because the disease is mostly confined to within the AV node. Mobitz type II block often precedes the development of Adams-Stokes syncope, symptoms are frequent, prognosis is compromised, and progression to third-degree AV block is common and sudden. Thus, type II second-degree AV block with a wide QRS typically indicates diffuse conduction system disease involving even the infranodal His-Purkinje system.

WORKUP

ECG, ambulatory monitoring (Holter or external loop recorders in selected patients

- Mobitz type I (Fig. 1-430) ECG shows:
  1. Sequential and gradual prolongation of PR interval leading to a nonconducted P wave
  2. Shortened PR interval following the pause as compared to the pre-pause PR interval
  3. Progressive shortening of the R-R interval prior to nonconducted atrial impulse
  4. Usually see "grouped beating" pattern.
- Mobitz type II ECG shows (Fig. 1-431):
  1. Fixed duration of PR interval with constant P-P and R-R intervals
  2. Sudden nonconducted P wave
  3. Abnormal QRS duration or fascicular blocks are common.
- In 2:1 AV block (Fig. 1-432), it cannot be determined based on the 12-lead ECG whether there is Mobitz type I or type II AV block, although a wide QRS complex is suggestive of Mobitz type II.
  1. Administering atropine can improve AV conduction if the AV block is type I or within the AV node; however, if it is infranodal (i.e., tpe II), the increased sinus rate caused by atropine may worsen the ratio of AV conduction, resulting in worsening bradycardia.
  2. Exercise stress testing may function in the same way as atropine above. If the disease is confined to the AV node, it may improve with exercise, but in cases of Mobitz type II AV block, the degree of AV block will worsen.
  3. Carotid sinus stimulation and other vagal maneuvers may worsen the AV block if it is at the level of the AV node (i.e., Mobitz type I) but will paradoxically improve the ratio of AV conduction by slowing down the sinus rate if it is a Mobitz type II or infranodal AV block.

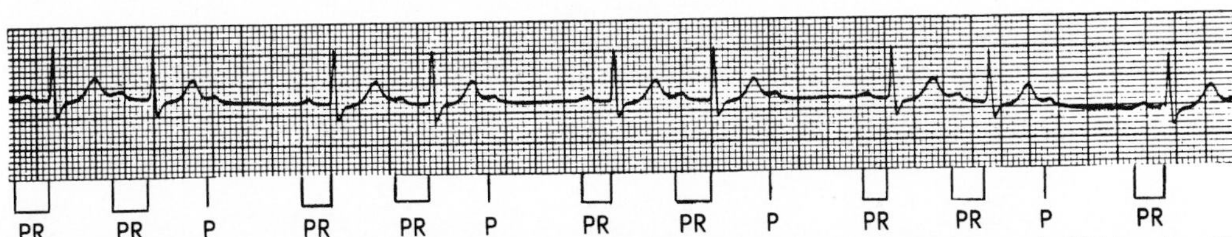

FIGURE 1-430 Wenckebach (Mobitz type I) second-degree atrioventricular block. Notice the progressive increase in PR intervals, with the third P wave in each sequence not followed by a QRS. Wenckebach block produces a characteristically syncopated rhythm with grouping of the QRS complexes (group beating). (From Goldberger AL [ed]: *Clinical electrocardiography,* ed 5, St Louis, 1994, Mosby.)

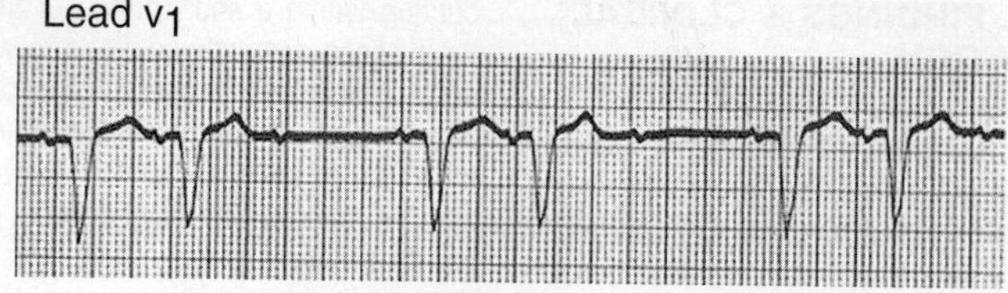

FIGURE 1-431 Mobitz type II AV block with left bundle branch block (LBBB). Note the fixed P-P intervals with no change in PR intervals followed by a sudden nonconducted P wave. The LBBB indicates infranodal disease in the His-Purkinje system that is suggestive of Mobitz type II block.

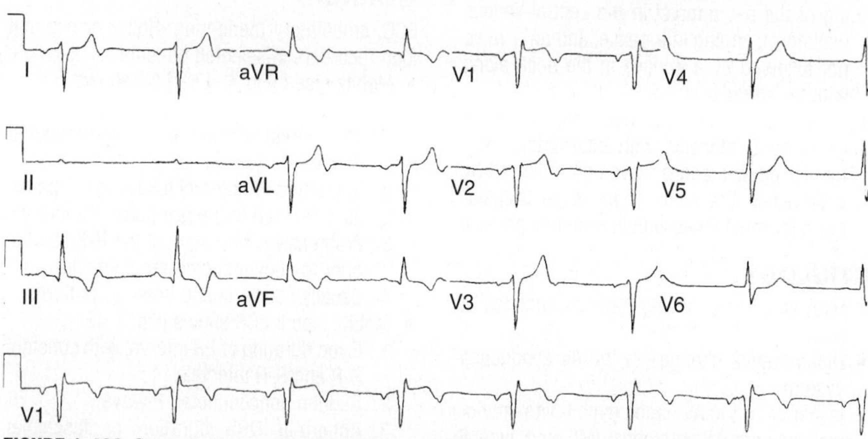

FIGURE 1-432 Second-degree 2:1 atrioventricular block. Notice the short PR interval during conducted complexes and the wide QRS complexes, suggesting block in the His-Purkinje system. (From Issa Z et al: *Clinical arrhythmology and electrophysiology*, ed 2, Philadelphia, 2012, Saunders.)

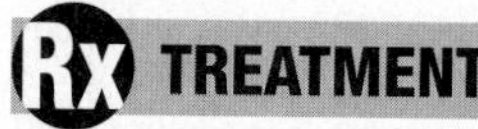

TREATMENT

NONPHARMACOLOGIC THERAPY

Elimination of drugs that may induce AV block such as digoxin, beta-blockers, and calcium channel blockers

ACUTE GENERAL Rx

- Treatment is usually not necessary unless the resting heart rate is <40 beats per min (bpm) while awake.
- If symptomatic (e.g., dizziness), atropine 1 mg (may repeat once after 5 min) may be tried to increase AV conduction; if no response, trial of dobutamine or isoproterenol may be helpful prior to insertion of a pacemaker.
- Atropine
  - Reduces heart block due to hypervagotonia but not due to AV node ischemia
  - Does not increase infranodal conduction (third-degree and second-degree AV block that is below the AV node)
  - Should be used with caution in Mobitz type II AV block due to possible paradoxical decrease in heart rate (as atrial rate increases, AV conduction decreases)
  - Is ineffective in heart transplantation patients
- If associated with anterior wall MI and wide QRS complex, consider insertion of a temporary pacemaker.
- Indications for permanent pacemaker (PPM) implantation by ACC/AHA/HRS 2008 guidelines:
  - Second-degree AV block with associated symptomatic bradycardia regardless of the type or site of the block (class I; level of evidence: B).
  - Second-degree AV block provoked by exercise in the absence of myocardial ischemia (class I; level of evidence: C).
  - Asymptomatic second-degree AV block at intra- or infra-His levels found at electrophysiologic study (class IIa; level of evidence: B).
  - First- or second-degree AV block with symptoms similar to those of pacemaker syndrome or hemodynamic compromise (class IIa; level of evidence: B).
  - Asymptomatic type II second-degree AV block with a wide QRS, including isolated right bundle-branch block (class I; level of evidence: B).
  - PPM is not indicated for asymptomatic type I second-degree AV block at supra-His (AV node) level or that which is not known to be intra- or infra-Hisian (class III; level of evidence: C)

DISPOSITION

Prognosis is good with insertion of a pacemaker.

REFERRAL

Referral for pacemaker insertion (see "Acute General Rx")

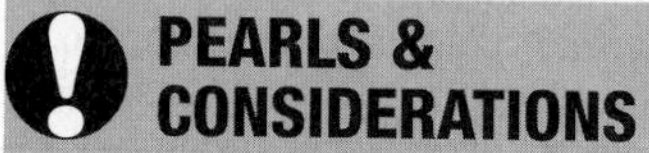

PEARLS & CONSIDERATIONS

COMMENTS

Patients with symptomatic Mobitz type II should be referred for a pacemaker. Asymptomatic patients should be referred if the AV block worsens with exercise and should be followed up routinely for potential development of high-grade AV block.

SUGGESTED READINGS

available at www.expertconsult.com

RELATED CONTENT

Second-Degree Heart Block (Patient Information)

AUTHORS: **AMANDA C. DORAN, M.D., Ph.D.,** and **VEERANNA MERLA, M.D.**

BASIC INFORMATION

DEFINITION

Heart failure (HF) is a complex clinical syndrome that can result from any structural or functional cardiac disorder that impairs the ability of the ventricle to fill with or eject blood. The cardinal manifestations of heart failure are dyspnea and fatigue, which may limit exercise tolerance, and fluid retention, which may lead to pulmonary congestion and peripheral edema. The pathophysiology of HF is related to progressive activation of the neuroendocrine system to compensate for decreased effective circulating volume, leading to total body volume overload and circulatory insufficiency. Specifically, the renin-angiotensin-aldosterone system (RAAS) is implicated as being activated in HF, leading to volume expansion (sodium retention) and cardiac fibrosis (mediated through angiotensin II). Disordered adrenergic stimulation has also been recognized as a key component of progression of disease. The term "congestive heart failure" (CHF) usually denotes a volume-overloaded status as a result of HF. Given that not all patients have volume overload at the time of the evaluation, "congestive heart failure" should be distinguished from the broader term "heart failure."

CLASSIFICATION: The American College of Cardiology/American Heart Association (ACC/AHA) describes the following four stages of HF. This staging model was designed to emphasize the evolution and progression of HF over a continuum and the preventability of HF in at-risk patients.

Stage A: Patients at high risk (e.g., with hypertension, atherosclerotic disease, diabetes mellitus, metabolic syndrome, cytotoxin, family history) for HF but without structural heart disease or symptoms of HF

Stage B: Patients with structural heart disease (e.g., left ventricular [LV] dysfunction) but without symptoms of HF

Stage C: Patients with structural heart disease with prior or current symptoms of HF

Stage D: Patients with refractory HF requiring specialized interventions

In addition to the ACC/AHA stages described above, the New York Heart Association (NYHA) defines four functional classes of HF designed to describe the symptoms of stage C and D HF. The functional classes are intended to assess the symptoms of HF and may fluctuate with therapy. It should be noted that current guidelines employ the functional classes to aid in determination of appropriate treatment.

I. Asymptomatic or symptomatic only at activity levels that would limit normal individuals
II. Symptomatic with ordinary exertion (e.g., 2 city blocks or 1 flight of stairs in a faster than usual pace)
III. Symptomatic with less than ordinary exertion (e.g., less than 2 city blocks or 1 flight of stairs)
IV. Symptomatic at rest

TERMINOLOGY: HF has been traditionally dichotomized as systolic versus diastolic (see Table 1-216). which has now been replaced with the terms HF with preserved ejection fraction (HFpEF) and HF with reduced ejection fraction (HFREF). Other common classifications include right-sided versus left-sided and high-output versus low-output. Systolic HF or HFREF is defined by the presence of impaired contractility of the LV, as measured by ejection fraction (EF) with clinical signs or symptoms of HF. In contrast, HFpEF or diastolic HF has been described as evidence (clinical) of HF with an EF above 50% and evidence of diastolic dysfunction. The term "HF with preserved EF" is preferred over the term "diastolic HF," given that many of the physiologic derangements in this subset of HF are not solely restricted to diastolic function of the heart. Right-sided HF denotes peripheral signs and symptoms of HF without evidence of pulmonary congestion, as opposed to left HF, which typically manifests with pulmonary congestion and subsequent signs and symptoms of right-sided HF. High-output HF involves signs and symptoms of HF but features an elevated cardiac output unable to meet the abnormally high metabolic demands of peripheral tissues, the result of myriad systemic disorders (e.g., systemic arteriovenous fistulas, hyperthyroidism, anemia). The term "acute decompensated HF" (ADHF) refers to worsening of signs or symptoms of HF due to a wide range of causes. Of note, HF is not equivalent to cardiomyopathy or LV dysfunction. These latter terms describe the possible structural or functional reasons for the development of HF, whereas HF is a clinical syndrome characterized by specific symptoms and signs.

SYNONYMS

HF
Congestive heart failure
CHF
Cardiac failure
Cardiogenic shock
Cardiogenic pulmonary edema

ICD-9CM CODES
428.0 Congestive heart failure
ICD-10CM CODES
I50.9 Heart failure, unspecified

TABLE 1-216 Systolic versus Diastolic Heart Failure*

Parameters	Systolic (HFREF)	Diastolic (HFpEF)
History		
Coronary artery disease	+++[†]	++
Hypertension	++	++++
Diabetes	++	++
Valvular heart disease	++++	+
Paroxysmal dyspnea	++	+++
Physical Examination		
Cardiomegaly	+++	+
Soft heart sounds	++++	+
S_3 gallop	+++	+
S_4 gallop	+	+++
Hypertension	++	++++
Mitral regurgitation	+++	+
Rales	++	+
Edema	+++	+
Jugular venous distention	+++	+
Chest Radiograph		
Cardiomegaly	+++	+
Pulmonary congestion	+++	+++
Electrocardiogram		
Left ventricular hypertrophy	++	++++
Q waves	++	+
Low voltage	+++	-
Echocardiogram		
Left ventricular hypertrophy	++	++++
Left ventricular dilation	++	-
Left atrial enlargement	++	++
Reduced ejection fraction	++++	-

*Certain aspects of the history and physical examination, along with clinical measurements, may help to distinguish diastolic from systolic heart failure. For example, patients with hypertensive heart disease and severe left ventricular hypertrophy often experience heart failure because of diastolic dysfunction.
†*Plus signs* indicate "suggestive" (the number reflects relative weight). *Minus signs* indicate "not very suggestive."
HFpEF, Heart failure with preserved ejection fraction; *HFREF,* heart failure with reduced ejection fraction.
From Zipes DP et al (eds): *Braunwald's heart disease*, ed 7, Philadelphia, 2005, Saunders.

EPIDEMIOLOGY & DEMOGRAPHICS

- Of note, there is variability in the reported demographics of HF due to heterogeneous definitions and classifications of HF. Blacks have the highest risk for HF. Incidence rate is lowest among white women and highest among black men, with blacks having a greater 5-yr mortality rate than whites.
- The lifetime risk of developing HF is 20% for Americans ≥40 years of age.
  - In the United States, HF incidence has largely remained stable over the past several decades, with >650,000 new HF cases diagnosed annually.
- HF is primarily a condition of the elderly. Approximately 80% of patients hospitalized with HF are older than 65 yr. HF is the most common inpatient diagnosis in the U.S. for patients aged >65 yr.
- HF incidence increases with age, rising from approximately 20 per 1,000 individuals 65 to 69 yr to >80 per 1,000 individuals among those >85 yr. Before age 75, the incidence of HF is higher in males, but both sexes are equally affected after this age cutoff.
- In the U.S., 1.1 million hospital discharges and 3.2 million hospitalizations/ambulatory care visits were associated with HF in 2007.
- Prevalence: 5.1 million persons in the U.S. and an estimated 23 million persons worldwide. The prevalence of HF is rising, especially in the elderly, particularly due to aging of the population and improved survival from other conditions (e.g., valvular and coronary heart disease).
- In the U.S., more than 550,000 patients annually are diagnosed with HF for the first time. The incidence is higher in the elderly, approaching 1 per 100 persons aged >65 yr per year. Before age 75, the incidence of HF is higher in males but both sexes are equally affected after this age cutoff.
- The estimated (direct and indirect) cost of HF in the U.S. was >$40 billion in 2012, with over half of these costs spent on hospitalizations. The mean cost of HF-related hospitalizations is $23,077 per patient and is higher when HF was a secondary rather than the primary diagnosis.
- HFrEF and HFpEF each make up about half of the overall HF burden.
- Among patients with HF in one large population study, hospitalizations were common after HF diagnosis, with 83% of patients hospitalized at least once and 43% hospitalized at least 4 times. More than half of the hospitalizations were related to noncardiovascular causes.

PHYSICAL FINDINGS & CLINICAL PRESENTATION

Clinical and physical exam findings with HF vary depending on the severity of disease, precipitant factor, comorbid conditions, and whether the failure symptoms are predominantly right-sided or left-sided.

- Common clinical manifestations are:
  - Dyspnea on exertion, progressively worsening to dyspnea at rest, and caused by increasing pulmonary vascular congestion due to inadequate forward flow and subsequent increased pulmonary venous pressure
  - Orthopnea, caused by increased venous return in the recumbent position and further elevated pulmonary venous pressure
  - Paroxysmal nocturnal dyspnea (PND) resulting from multiple factors including increased venous return in the recumbent position, decreased Pao_2 and decreased adrenergic stimulation of myocardial function during sleep
  - Nocturnal angina resulting from increased myocardial oxygen demand (secondary to increased venous return in the recumbent position causing increased preload) in patients with concomitant coronary artery disease (CAD)
  - ***Cheyne-Stokes respiration*** (alternating phases of apnea and hyperventilation) caused by prolonged circulation time from lungs to brain as a result of impaired cardiac output
  - Fatigue, lethargy, and decreased functional capacity resulting from low cardiac output and hypoperfusion of peripheral tissues
- Physical examination:
  - Fine pulmonary crackles, wheezes, tachypnea, hypoxia (due to elevated pulmonary pressures). Crackles may be absent in chronic and longstanding high pulmonary venous pressure because it allows for lymphatic drainage in the lungs to increase.
  - Tachycardia and narrowed pulse pressure (due to increased sympathetic tone)
  - S_3 gallop, paradoxical splitting of S_2, jugular venous distention, peripheral edema in dependent tissues, congestive hepatomegaly, ascites, and hepatojugular reflux (due to volume overload)
  - Perioral and peripheral cyanosis, decreased capillary refill, pulsus alternans, and cool extremities (due to decreased cardiac output)
- Six common clinical presentations identified by European Society of Cardiology of Acute Heart Failure Syndromes:
  1. ADHF presenting with hypertension (SBP >160): the hypertension leads to increased afterload causing pulmonary vascular congestion.
  2. Worsening or decompensation of chronic HF
  3. Flash pulmonary edema
  4. Cardiogenic shock
  5. Acute coronary syndrome (ACS) and ADHF
  6. Isolated RV failure

  Each of these scenarios may require different therapies to effectively stabilize and treat the patient.

Acute precipitants of HF decompensation include noncompliance with salt restriction or medications (most commonly), infection, arrhythmias (e.g., atrial fibrillation), ischemia or infarction, uncontrolled hypertension, new medications (e.g., negative inotropic agents such as calcium channel blockers/antiarrhythmic agents), nonsteroidal anti-inflammatory drugs (NSAIDs), renal dysfunction, toxins (e.g., ethanol and anthracyclines), cardiac surgery, or valvular catastrophe.

ETIOLOGY

LEFT VENTRICULAR FAILURE: The dichotomy of whether HF occurs in the setting of preserved or reduced LV systolic function plays an important role in treatment strategies. Patients with HFpEF may have significant abnormalities in active relaxation and passive stiffness of the LV, renal function, or arterial vasoreactivity.

- Abnormal LV systolic function
  - CAD (acute or chronic ischemia, myocardial infarction [MI], LV aneurysm), which is the most common cause of cardiomyopathy in the U.S., comprising 50%-75% of patients with HF.
  - Increased afterload or pressure overload (severe hypertension, aortic stenosis)
  - Increased preload or volume overload (mitral regurgitation, aortic regurgitation)
  - Cardiomyopathy (dilated cardiomyopathy, dilated phase of hypertrophic cardiomyopathy, ischemic cardiomyopathy)
  - Infectious (Chagas, myocarditis)
  - Infiltrative (amyloidosis, sarcoidosis, hemochromatosis)
  - Toxins (ethanol, cocaine, anthracyclines)
  - Tachycardia induced (e.g., with atrial fibrillation)
- Preserved LV systolic function
  - Impaired relaxation (myocardial ischemia, diabetes mellitus, metabolic syndrome)
  - Tachyarrhythmia (featuring reduced diastolic filling time)
  - Restrictive cardiomyopathy (myocardial stiffness, such as hypereosinophilic syndrome, amyloidosis, hemochromatosis)
  - High cardiac output (thiamine deficiency, anemia, thyrotoxicosis, arteriovenous malformations)
  - Increased afterload (uncontrolled hypertension, aortic stenosis, hypertrophic obstructive cardiomyopathy)
  - Hypervolemia (oliguric renal failure, iatrogenic)

RIGHT VENTRICULAR FAILURE:

- Left-sided HF
- Chronic hypoxemic pulmonary disease
- Valvular heart disease (mitral stenosis or regurgitation)
- Pulmonary embolism
- Primary pulmonary hypertension
- Right-to-left shunts that cause systemic hypoxemia (e.g., large patent foramen ovale and tetralogy of Fallot)
- Left-to-right shunts that cause volume overload (e.g., atrial and ventricular septal defects)
- Bacterial endocarditis (right-sided)
- Right ventricular infarction

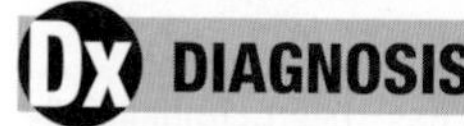

DIAGNOSIS

DIFFERENTIAL DIAGNOSIS

- COPD, asthma
- Cirrhosis

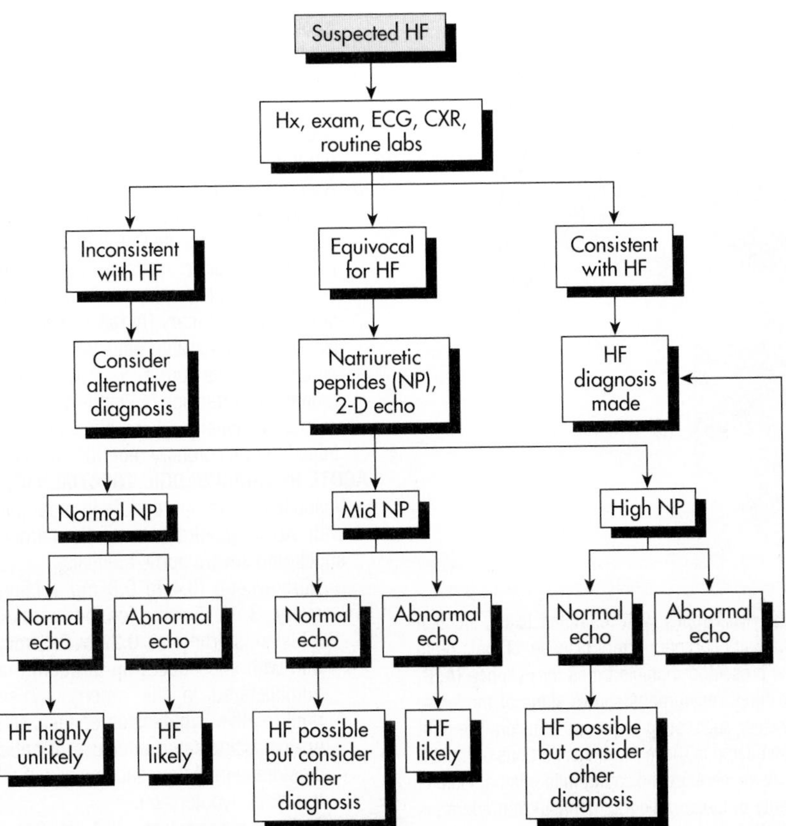

FIGURE 1-433 Flow chart for the evaluation of patients with heart failure. *CXR*, Chest radiograph; *ECG*, electrocardiograph; *echo*, echocardiograph; *HF*, heart failure; *Hx*, history; *NP*, natriuretic peptides. (From Bonow RO et al: *Braunwald's heart disease-a textbook of cardiovascular medicine*, ed 9, St Louis, 2011, Saunders.)

- Nephrotic syndrome
- Venous insufficiency
- Pulmonary embolism
- ARDS (adult respiratory distress syndrome)
- Pneumonia
- Heroin overdose

WORKUP

- A flow chart for the evaluation of patients with heart failure is outlined in Fig. 1-433. Fig. E1-434 describes the stages and treatment options for heart failure.
- Blood work (to diagnose potentially reversible causes, identify comorbidities, and assess disease severity)
  - CBC (to evaluate for anemia, infections), urinalysis, blood urea nitrogen (BUN), creatinine, electrolytes (worsening hyponatremia is a marker of disease severity and is associated with higher mortality rates), liver enzymes (hepatic congestion), thyroid function (especially in the elderly or patients with comorbid atrial fibrillation or known thyroid disease)
  - B-type natriuretic peptide (BNP) is a cardiac neurohormone secreted from the ventricles in response to elevated LV end-diastolic pressure. The sensitivity is low in asymptomatic patients (but elevated BNP levels have been shown to have a negative predictive value up to 90% in symptomatic patients), and BNP elevation generally correlates with severity of disease and parallels closely morbidity and mortality outcome measures. The cleavage remnant n-terminal-pro-BNP (nt-pro-BNP) has a longer half-life and is renally cleared, making it susceptible to alterations in renal function. A level of <300 pg/mL has an age-independent 98% negative predictive value.
  - Cardiac biomarkers may be elevated if ischemia is the precipitant factor. However, slight elevations are very common and may not always be due to obstructive coronary disease. These elevations could be due to subendocardial ischemia (due to increased end-diastolic pressure resulting in decreased perfusion) and necrosis, or cardiomyocyte damage from the inflammatory cytokines or oxidative stress. Impaired renal function is very common, and decreased clearance of the biomarkers can contribute to their elevation. Therefore these elevations should be interpreted in the context of the clinical setting. Despite that, in patients with ADHF, a positive cardiac troponin test (from whatever mechanism) is associated with worse prognosis.
  - Screening for dyslipidemia and glucose intolerance, given that CAD remains the predominant cause of HF.
  - If hemachromatosis is suspected (specifically in Northern European patients), consider checking a transferrin saturation.
  - Consider HIV testing in high-risk patients.
- Electrocardiogram (ECG)
  - Look for signs of prior MI, chamber enlargement, hypertrophy, heart block, arrhythmia, and evidence of pericardial effusion.
  - More than 25% of patients with HF have some form of intraventricular conduction abnormality that is manifest as an increased QRS duration. The most common pattern seen is left bundle-branch block.
- Chest x-ray (Fig. 1-435)
  - Evaluate for pulmonary venous congestion, pulmonary edema, pleural effusion, cardiomegaly, chamber dilation, and Kerley B lines.
- Echocardiography
  - Plays a critical diagnostic role in patients with HF and is useful in assessment of systolic, diastolic, and valvular structure and function
- Exercise stress testing
  - May be useful in evaluating concomitant ischemic etiologies and assessment of degree of disability.
- Cardiac catheterization
  - Left heart catheterization can help to identify coronary artery disease as a cause of heart failure. Right heart catheterization can help to evaluate intracardiac filling pressures, estimates of valvular areas, presence of intracardiac shunts, and calculation of hemodynamic properties such as cardiac output, systemic vascular resistance, and pulmonary artery wedge pressure to further guide management.
- Cardiac MRI
  - Useful modality in accurately estimating EF (with less variability than conventional 2D echocardiography). MRI is also useful in excluding pericardial disease, identifying infiltrative disease, and assessing viability in cases of heart failure caused by underlying ischemic heart disease.

Rx TREATMENT

NONPHARMACOLOGIC GENERAL MEASURES

- Assess the etiology and severity of disease. Educate the patient and family about the nature of the disorder. Assess the home setting and if patient has social support to ensure compliance, especially for patients with dementia.
- Identify and correct precipitating factors (e.g., increased sodium load, medication noncompliance, ischemia, infections, anemia, thyrotoxicosis) and address lifestyle modification (e.g., smoking and alcohol cessation, weight reduction, avoiding use of nonsteroidal antiinflammatory drugs [NSAIDs]). Anemia is common in patients with HF; however, treatment with erythropoiesis-stimulating agents (ESAs) such as darbepoetin alfa have not shown improved clinical outcomes in patients with systolic HF and mild-to-moderate anemia and are not recommended.

 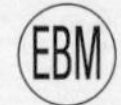 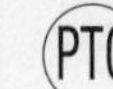

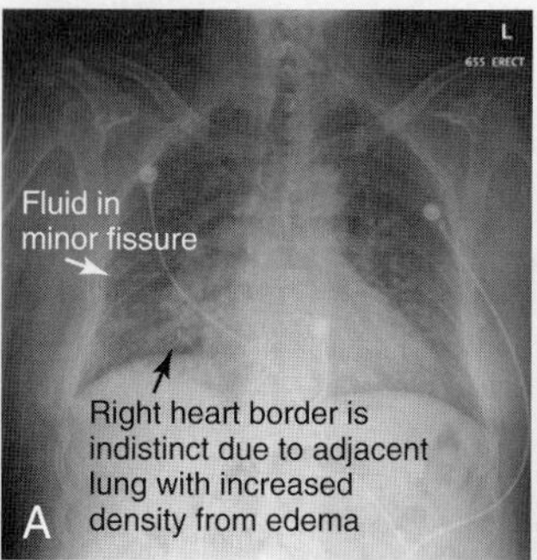

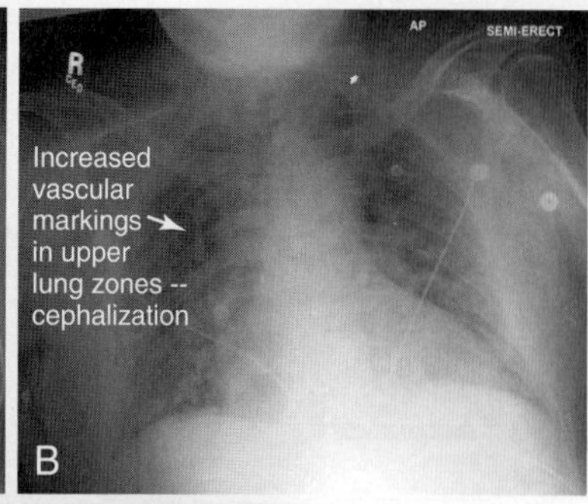

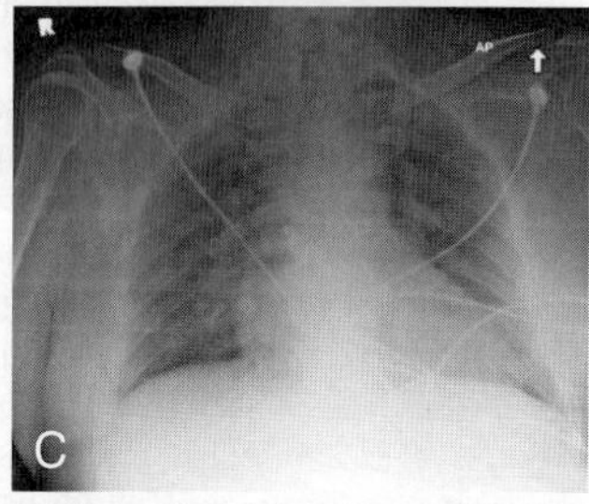

FIGURE 1-435 Congestive heart failure. Mild left ventricular hypertrophy with restricted filling, ejection fraction >55%, and no pericardial effusion. This 63-year-old man with coronary artery disease, chronic renal insufficiency, and diastolic heart failure (ejection fraction >55%) presented multiple times for dyspnea (**A, B,** and **C,** first through third clinical presentations). Each of these three radiographs shows signs of moderate pulmonary edema. The diaphragms and costophrenic angles are clear, suggesting no pleural effusion. The right heart border in all three images is indistinct because of interstitial edema in these locations. Portions of the left heart border are also indistinct. The upper lung fields have a hazy appearance indicating mild edema. Fluid is visible in the minor fissure on all three images. Does the similarity of these radiographs mean that edema is not the cause of the patient's dyspnea? No, he simply presented with pulmonary edema on all three occasions. (From Broder JS: *Diagnostic imaging for the emergency physician,* Philadelphia, 2011, Saunders.)

- Review list of medications and discontinue the ones that can contribute to HF (e.g., NSAIDs, antiarrhythmic drugs, calcium channel blockers, thiazolidinediones)
- Dietary sodium restriction of <2 g/day is commonly recommended to patients with heart failure and is endorsed by many guidelines.
- Restrict fluid intake to <2 L/day in patients with hyponatremia.
- Caloric supplementation should be provided to patients with advanced HF with weight loss and muscle wasting due to cardiac cachexia. Weight loss may reflect cachexia caused by the higher total energy expenditure associated with HF compared with that of healthy sedentary subjects. The diagnosis of cardiac cachexia independently predicts a worse prognosis.
- For patients with coexisting obstructive sleep apnea, continuous positive airway pressure (CPAP) is often recommended after polysomnography, thereby reducing systolic blood pressure and improving LV function.
- Exercise training (or regular physical activity) is recommended as safe and effective for patients with class I to III heart failure who are able to participate to improve functional status. Cardiac rehabilitation is unfortunately an underused preventive measure, although it has been shown to reduce morbidity and mortality.
- Pneumococcal vaccination and annual influenza vaccination.

TREATMENT OF ADHF

- Four phases in treatment of ADHF:
  1st phase: initial stabilization and management
  2nd phase: inpatient hospital care
  3rd phase: early discharge planning and care
  4th phase: early post-discharge care

1st phase: Initial stabilization and management

Short-term goals: hemodynamic stabilization, stabilization of respiratory status, symptom relief, optimization of tissue perfusion, and recognition of more immediately life-threatening conditions (e.g., arrhythmias, valvular catastrophe, MI, cardiac tamponade). Initial therapy of ADHF is contingent on appropriate determination of clinical scenario.

Management as per clinical scenario: (Fig. E1-436)

1. ADHF-associated hypertension: goal is afterload reduction and decrease of systemic hypervolemia. Mode of treatment: diuresis (IV loop diuretics) and vasodilators (acutely nitrates and morphine followed by treatment with ACE inhibitors or angiotensin receptor blockers [ARBs])
2. Worsening or decompensation of chronic HF (HFREF or HFpEF): goal is control of volume status. Treatment is accomplished with vasodilators and diuretics.
3. Flash pulmonary edema: goal is afterload reduction (vasodilators such as nitrates acutely), respiratory status stabilization, and diuresis (IV loop diuretics). May also require careful rate control given that atrial fibrillation or other tachyarrhythmias may decrease cardiac output and result in pulmonary edema.
4. Cardiogenic shock: goal is hemodynamic stabilization. Treatment consists of inotropes + vasopressors ± intraaortic balloon pump ± emergent revascularization if indicated.
5. ACS and ADHF: goal is hemodynamic stabilization + emergent restoration of coronary perfusion. See "Acute Coronary Syndromes."
6. Isolated RV failure: goals are identification of etiology: (1) valvular, (2) pulmonary hypertension, and (3) primary RV failure secondary to ischemia. Treatment: depends on etiology, either corrective surgery vs. treatment of pulmonary hypertension (endothelin antagonists, calcium channel blockers, phosphodiesterase inhibitors) vs. coronary reperfusion therapies.

ACUTE PHARMACOLOGIC TREATMENTS:

- Vasodilators are appropriate in most patients with ADHF (contraindicated in cardiogenic shock and severe aortic stenosis)
  - Nitroglycerin (0.4 to 0.8 mg sublingually every 3 to 5 min, or by intravenous infusion starting at 0.2 to 0.4 mcg/kg/min with subsequent up titration) may be administered in the emergency setting until relative hypotension ensues. Nitrates are contraindicated after use of phosphodiesterase inhibitors such as sildenafil due to risk of hypotension.
  - Sodium nitroprusside (0.1 to 0.2 mcg/kg/min as an intravenous infusion) is a potent vasodilator with balanced venous and arteriolar effects that usually requires hemodynamic monitoring with an arterial line and may precipitate coronary steal and thiocyanate toxicity (elevated risk in renal failure).
  - When given intravenously, loop diuretics have an immediate vasodilator effect that provides clinical relief of symptoms before diuresis begins. Due to gut edema and unpredictable patterns of absorption, oral formulation may become less effective. Therefore intravenous formulation should be used in the acute setting. Studies showed no difference in outcome when using bolus dosing vs. continuous IV infusion. Administration of smaller doses of short-acting loop diuretics multiple times daily is preferable to a single large dose because the kidneys can avidly reabsorb sodium after the initial diuresis. However, if a certain dose is not adequate to force diuresis, the dose, rather than the frequency, should be increased until a single effective dose is reached; more frequent doses can be added as needed. Therefore monitoring of urine output, renal function, and electrolytes is key. The addition of a distal tubule inhibitor such as metolazone 30 min prior to loop diuretic dosing has a synergistic effect and often enhances diuresis because it inhibits sodium reabsorption in the distal segment in the face of increased sodium delivery from the loop. Diuretics should be used with caution in patients with aortic stenosis and

are contraindicated in patients with severe hypotension or cardiogenic shock.

- Inotropic agents are used for temporary hemodynamic support, but have not been shown to improve survival. Many of these agents have serious associated adverse events including myocardial necrosis and malignant arrhythmias.
  - Dobutamine (starting at 2.5 to 5 mcg/kg/min) can be used for inotropic support but is associated with increased myocardial oxygen demand and cardiac arrhythmias and may result in hypotension from decreased systemic vascular resistance.
  - Milrinone (37.5 to 75 mcg/kg loading dose, followed by 0.375 to 0.75 mcg/kg/min) can be used as a vasodilator and inotropic agent, but is associated with increased oxygen demand and cardiac arrhythmias, and may result in hypotension from decreased systemic vascular resistance.
  - Levosimendan is a calcium-sensitizing drug, which also inhibits potassium channels leading to inotropy. However, this agent is not FDA approved for use in the U.S. Currently, this inotrope has been associated with an elevated risk of malignant arrhythmia and higher mortality.
- Renal replacement therapy (can be used as an alternative to pharmacologic diuresis in ADHF when renal function is significantly compromised).
- ACE inhibitors or ARBs, if part of a patient's chronic medication regimen, should be continued in the absence of hypotension, acute renal failure, or hyperkalemia.
- Beta-blockers, if part of a patient's chronic medication regimen, may be continued or reduced in dosage in mild exacerbations of HF but should be discontinued in patients with hypotension or those requiring inotropic support. Beta-blockers should not be initiated in patients who are not on chronic beta-blocker therapy until euvolemia is achieved unless used for rate control.
- Morphine sulfate can cause venodilation and may be used to reduce patient work of breathing and anxiety, but recent retrospective studies have suggested increased incidence of mechanical ventilation and in-hospital mortality in patients who received morphine.
- If ADHF with preserved EF is suspected, therapy is usually aimed at relief of symptoms and correction of any potential precipitating etiologies (e.g., tachycardia, hypertension, ischemia). Treatment generally involves diuretics to reduce pulmonary congestion with caution not to overdiurese given the need for elevated filling pressures in these patients to ensure adequate stroke volume and cardiac output. Nitrates may be useful in providing symptomatic relief but may precipitate hypotension. Ventricular rate should be controlled in the presence of atrial fibrillation, which, at rapid rates, is poorly tolerated in patients with impaired diastolic filling. Negative inotropic agents such as beta-blockers and calcium channel blockers can be used with caution.
- Nesiritide (recombinant brain natriuretic protein) does not reduce morbidity or mortality (ASCEND-HF trial)

2nd phase: Inpatient hospital care

This phase of treatment includes further diuresis and stabilization of volume status. The patient should be carefully brought to euvolemia with daily volume status and electrolyte monitoring. The patient should also be transitioned to oral diuretics when stabilized. Whilst inpatient, the patient should have his/her medical and device management optimized with the therapies discussed later.

3rd phase: Early discharge planning and care

The patient should be transitioned to oral diuretics and be placed on optimum outpatient maintenance therapy, which will be discussed later. If the patient was on IV inotropic therapy, oral regimens should be adjusted while these infusions are tapered off. Prolonged physiologic effects of these IV inotropic agents after their discontinuation before discharge may mask the inadequate diuretic regimen and intolerance to the vasodilator doses. This can result in readmission, especially with milrinone due to its long half-life that can be further prolonged by the common coexisting impaired renal function. Therefore it may be recommended that patients who received inotropic infusions remain hospitalized for at least 48 hours after inotropic agents are discontinued, and optimize the oral regimen.

4th phase: Early post-discharge care

The patient will require re-evaluation and constant monitoring in order to avoid another episode of ADHF. Emphasis should be placed on importance of compliance with instructions regarding dietary restrictions and daily body weight monitoring. Early follow-up should be scheduled as well as outpatient electrolyte monitoring if required after medication adjustments.

CHRONIC TREATMENT OF HF SECONDARY TO SYSTOLIC DYSFUNCTION:

The goals of HF therapy are clinical improvement followed by stabilizing, slowing, or even reversing deterioration in myocardial function, and ultimately a reduction in risk of morbidity (including hospitalization rates) and mortality.

- ACE inhibitors
  - Reduce morbidity and mortality.
  - Produce both venous and arterial vasodilation acutely, thereby reducing both preload and afterload.
  - Potential mechanism of long-term benefit is attenuation of RAAS activation and decreased myocardial remodeling and fibrosis.
  - Used as first-line therapy for asymptomatic LV dysfunction (LVEF <40%) and symptomatic systolic HF (ACC/AHA grades A-D).
  - Therapy should be initiated at low doses to prevent hypotension and rapidly titrated to higher doses as tolerated.
  - Contraindications to the use of ACE inhibitors are renal insufficiency (creatinine clearance <30 ml/min), bilateral renal artery stenosis, hyperkalemia, hypotension, or adverse reactions (e.g., angioedema).
- ARBs
  - Receptor antagonists to the angiotensin II receptor.
  - Clinical trials have not shown any superiority compared to ACE inhibitors in patients with systolic HF (LVEF <40%).
  - Reserved for patients who are ACE inhibitor intolerant.
  - There are conflicting data on the utility of combination therapy with ARBs and ACE inhibitors in addition to beta-blockers for patients who remain symptomatic in the absence of renal dysfunction, hyperkalemia, and outside the post-MI period.
  - Have a similar contraindication profile to ACE inhibitors. Routine combined use of an ACE inhibitor, ARB, and aldosterone antagonist is potentially harmful for patients with HFrEF.
- Beta-adrenergic blockers (beta-blockers)
  - Reduce morbidity and mortality. Such benefits observed with bisoprolol (CIBIS II trial), metoprolol succinate (MERIT-HF trial), and carvedilol (COPERNICUS trial).
  - Benefit is thought to be conferred by blockade of sympathetic effects of neurohormonal stimulation due to HF.
  - Are considered first-line therapy for symptomatic patients with systolic HF (NYHA class ≥II and LVEF <35%).
  - Only carvedilol, bisoprolol, and metoprolol succinate have been approved for the medical treatment of chronic HF; these agents are generally started in patients judged to be euvolemic and dosage is to be slowly uptitrated as tolerated.
  - Adverse effects include worsening HF (due to negative inotropic effects), fatigue, dizziness, bradycardia, hypotension, and bronchospasm.
- Aldosterone receptor antagonists
  - Reduce morbidity and mortality
  - Indicated in patients with NYHA class II-IV HF, with LVEF ≤35%, already treated with ACE inhibitors and beta-blockers without significant renal insufficiency or hyperkalemia. Patients with NYHA class II should have a history of prior cardiovascular hospitalization or elevated plasma natriuretic peptide levels to be considered for aldosterone receptor antagonists. Creatinine should be ≤2.5 mg/dL in men or ≤2.0 mg/dL in women (or estimated glomerular filtration rate >30 mL/min/1.73 m2), and potassium should be <5.0 mEq/L. They are also indicated for post-MI patients with EF ≤40% who have either symptomatic HF or diabetes mellitus.
  - Spironolactone may cause gynecomastia, galactorrhea, and hyperkalemia (especially in patients with baseline renal insufficiency or type 4 renal tubular acidosis). It has been best studied in chronic heart failure with NYHA class III to IV symptoms (RALES study).
  - Eplerenone is associated with fewer endocrine side effects and has especially been studied in postmyocardial infarction left ventricular dysfunction (EPHESUS trial) and

in chronic systolic heart failure with only class II symptoms (EMPHASIS-HF trial).
 - Inappropriate use of aldosterone receptor antagonists is potentially harmful because of life-threatening hyperkalemia or renal insufficiency when serum creatinine is >2.5 mg/dL in men or >2.0 mg/dL in women (or estimated glomerular filtration rate <30 mL/min/1.73 m^2), and/or potassium >5.0 mEq/L.
- Diuretics
 - Are used to maintain euvolemia and to improve symptoms as discussed previously.
 - Although data on diuretic efficacy are limited, a meta-analysis of a few small trials found that they were associated with reduction in mortality as well as reduced hospitalization for HF.
 - Of note, loop diuretics with better bioavailability, such as torsemide and bumetanide, may be used in diuretic-resistant patients but are generally more expensive.
- Combination of isosorbide dinitrate and hydralazine
 - Cause venous (nitrates) and arteriolar (hydralazine) vasodilation resulting in decreased preload and afterload.
 - The combination of hydralazine and isosorbide dinitrate is recommended to reduce morbidity and mortality for patients self-described as African Americans with NYHA class III–IV HFrEF receiving optimal therapy with ACE inhibitors and beta blockers, unless contraindicated.
 - A combination of hydralazine and isosorbide dinitrate can be useful to reduce morbidity or mortality in patients with current or prior symptomatic HFrEF who cannot be given an ACE inhibitor or ARB because of drug intolerance, hypotension, or renal insufficiency, unless contraindicated.
 - Adverse effects of nitrates include hypotension, headaches, and tolerance as well as reflex tachycardial and lupuslike syndrome with hydralazine.
- Digoxin
 - Positive inotropic and negative chronotropic drug that works by inhibition of the sodium-potassium transmembrane exchange pump and through its vagomimetic action
 - Commonly used in patients with concomitant atrial fibrillation
 - Has been shown to reduce HF-related hospitalizations but does NOT confer any mortality benefit (DIG trial). However, there is evidence suggesting that digoxin may actually have an effect on survival that varies with the serum digoxin level; survival was improved when the level was between 0.5 and 0.8 ng/ml (most often in men) and significantly worsened when it was ≥1.2 ng/ml and >0.9 mg/ml in women.
 - Caution must be used in patients with abnormal renal function to avoid digoxin toxicity and life-threatening arrhythmia. Avoid hypokalemia because potassium competes with digoxin on the same site of the Na^+-K^+-ATPase pump.
- Cardiac resynchronization therapy (CRT)
 - Improves morbidity and mortality rates in selected patients.
 - The presence of a bundle-branch block or other intraventricular conduction delay (IVCD) can cause ventricular dyssynchrony, which induces regional loading disparities and reduces the efficiency of ventricular contraction, thereby further impairing the systolic function of a failing ventricle.
 - CRT is indicated for patients who have LVEF ≤35%, sinus rhythm, left bundle-branch block with a QRS duration of 150 ms or greater, and NYHA class II, III, or ambulatory IV symptoms on guideline-directed medical therapy. CRT is NOT indicated in patients whose functional status and life expectancy are limited predominantly by chronic noncardiac conditions. Life expectancy should be >1 yr.
 - In the appropriate subset of patients, CRT in addition to optimal medical therapy has been shown in numerous clinical trials to improve symptoms by at least one NYHA class, improve 6-min walk distance and quality of life, reduce rate of HF-related hospitalization, and reduce rate of all-cause and cardiovascular mortality.
 - Detailed guidelines for CRT are beyond the scope of this chapter. Consultation with cardiology service may be indicated.
- Implantable cardioverter-defibrillators (ICDs)
 - Sudden cardiac death (SCD) is a common cause of death in patients with HF in both ischemic and nonischemic cardiomyopathies. Ventricular tachycardia (VT) degenerating into ventricular fibrillation (VF) is the culprit in the majority of patients with SCD, although bradyarrhythmias do also occur with less frequency.
 - ICD therapy is recommended for primary prevention of SCD to reduce total mortality in selected patients with nonischemic dilated cardiomyopathy or ischemic heart disease at least 40 days post-MI with LVEF ≤35% and NYHA class II or III symptoms on chronic guideline-directed medical therapy, who have reasonable expectation of meaningful survival for >1 year.
 - Patients with HF who survive an episode of sudden cardiac arrest or experience sustained VT in the presence of LVEF <35% are at high risk for future arrhythmic events and SCD and obtain a mortality benefit from ICD placement for secondary prevention, with or without adjunctive therapies such as antiarrhythmic drugs, radiofrequency ablation, surgery, or transplant.
- In the absence of an indication (e.g., atrial fibrillation), routine use of anticoagulation is currently not recommended in patients with HF. Even with the increased risk for LV thrombus formation in dilated cardiomyopathy and subsequent thromboembolization, data are conflicting about benefits of antithrombotic (antiplatelet or anticoagulant) therapy for primary prevention to reduce thromboembolic events or mortality in patients with systolic HF who are in sinus rhythm (SOLVD, V-HeFT, SAVE, HELAS, and WASH trials). It may be reasonable to consider anticoagulation for secondary prevention in patients with HF who had a prior thromboembolic event; however, risks and benefits should be carefully assessed.
- Antiplatelet agents are recommended for patients with concomitant CAD.
- Statins are not beneficial as adjunctive therapy when prescribed solely for the diagnosis of HF in the absence of other indications for their use.
- Calcium channel blocking drugs are not recommended as routine treatment for patients with HFrEF.
- Omega-3 polyunsaturated fatty acid supplementation is reasonable to use as adjunctive therapy in patients with NYHA class II-IV symptoms and HFrEF or HFpEF, unless contraindicated, to reduce mortality and cardiovascular hospitalizations.
- Percutaneous coronary intervention (PCI) or surgical revascularization should be considered in patients with HF and significant CAD who are revascularization candidates.
- In general, the following sequence of drugs is recommended:
 1. Loop diuretics to provide symptom relief and achieve a euvolemic state.
 2. ACE or ARB started at low doses, then increased to a moderate dose in 1-2 weeks.
 3. Beta-blockers after the patient is stable on ACE/ARB treatment. Start a low dose, then uptitrate to goal based on trial data or maximal dose tolerated. Once achieved, uptitration of ACE or ARB to goal doses can be completed.
- The following drugs can be added in selected patients in the absence of contraindications:
 - Aldosterone antagonists improve survival in NYHA class II with LVEF <30% or NYHA class III-IV with EF <35%. Kidney function should be stable with eGFR ≥30 ml/min and potassium <5 mEq/L.
 - Combination of hydralazine with a nitrate in patients (particularly blacks) with a reduced EF.
 - Digoxin reduces hospitalizations for HF and controls HR rate in atrial fibrillation. It can also help control symptoms.

CHRONIC TREATMENT OF HF WITH PRESERVED SYSTOLIC FUNCTION:

- To date, there is a relative dearth of clinical trials examining effective chronic treatment strategies in this subset of patients with HF. Current therapies are mainly for symptomatic relief.
- Therapy centers on relief of volume overload with judicious diuretic use, treatment of ischemia via coronary revascularization, management of atrial fibrillation, controlling

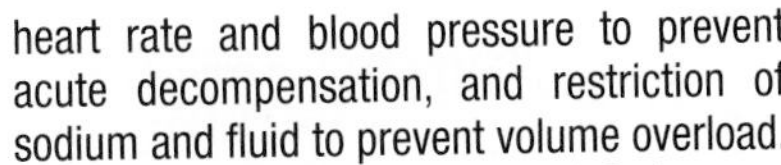

heart rate and blood pressure to prevent acute decompensation, and restriction of sodium and fluid to prevent volume overload.
- Diuretics should be used for relief of symptoms due to volume overload in patients with HFpEF.
- The use of beta-blocking agents, ACE inhibitors, and ARBs in patients with hypertension is reasonable to control blood pressure in patients with HFpEF.
- The use of ARBs might be considered to decrease hospitalizations for patients with HFpEF.
- Omega-3 polyunsaturated fatty acid supplementation is reasonable, unless contraindicated, to reduce mortality and cardiovascular hospitalizations.
- There is no evidence to support routine use of nutritional supplements and they are not recommended for patients with HFpEF.
- Surgical options for contributing critical aortic stenosis, constrictive pericarditis, and hypertrophic cardiomyopathy (HCM) should be entertained in appropriate patients.

DISPOSITION

- Annual mortality of systolic HF ranges from 10% in stable patients with mild symptoms to 50% in patients with NYHA class IV disease (a mortality rate rivaling some malignancies). The Seattle Heart Failure Model provides an accurate estimate of 1-, 2-, and 3-year survival before and after different therapies. This model can be useful to assess the need for LV assist device implantation or urgent transplantation. The calculator is available online at http://depts.washington.edu/shfm/.
- Cardiac transplantation has a 5-yr survival rate of ~70% and represents a viable option in selected patients.
- The use of an LV assist device (LVAD) in patients with advanced HF can result in a clinically meaningful survival benefit and improve quality of life in patients who are not candidates for cardiac transplantation. There are two approved uses of LVADs specifically as a bridge to transplant and as destination therapy. There are two major categories of LVAD pulsatile flow devices vs. continuous flow devices. A recent trial (2008) has indicated that continuous flow devices are associated with increased survival as destination therapy as compared to medically managed controls. Interestingly, more recent trials (2010 and 2011) have shown there was no difference in posttransplantation survival between patients who were bridged with continuous-flow VADs vs. no VADs or even between patients bridged with pulsatile vs. continuous-flow VADs.

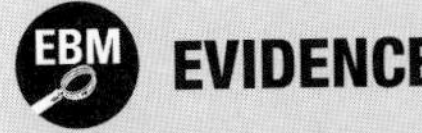

EVIDENCE

available at www.expertconsult.com

SUGGESTED READINGS

available at www.expertconsult.com

RELATED CONTENT

Congestive Heart Failure (CHF) (Patient Information)

AUTHORS: **ALI DAHHAN, M.D.**, and **ARAVIND RAO KOKKIRALA, M.D.**

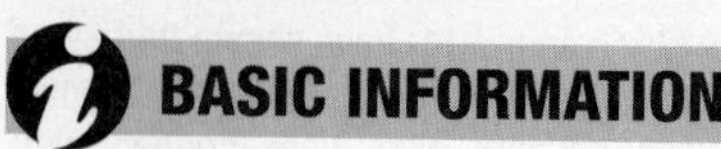

BASIC INFORMATION

DEFINITION

Heat exhaustion and heat stroke are part of a continuum of heat-related illness, and unless factors leading to heat exhaustion are corrected swiftly, affected patients can progress to heat stroke.

- ***Heat exhaustion:*** an illness resulting from prolonged, heavy activity in a hot environment with subsequent dehydration, electrolyte depletion, and rectal temperature >37.8° C but ≤40° C.
- ***Heat stroke:*** a life-threatening heat illness characterized by extreme hyperthermia, dehydration, and neurologic manifestations (core temperature >40° C).

SYNONYMS

Heat illness
Hyperthermia

ICD-9CM CODES
992.0 Heat stroke
992.5 Heat exhaustion
ICD-10CM CODES
T67.5 Heat exhaustion, unspecified
T67.0 Heatstroke and sunstroke
T67.1 Heat syncope
T67.2 Heat cramp
T67.3 Heat exhaustion, anhydrotic
T67.6 Heat fatigue, transient

EPIDEMIOLOGY & DEMOGRAPHICS

INCIDENCE (IN U.S.): Incidence of heat stroke is approximately 20 cases/100,000 population.
PREDOMINANT AGE: Heat exhaustion and stroke occur more frequently in elderly patients, especially those taking diuretics or medications that impair heat dissipation (e.g., phenothiazines, anticholinergics, antihistamines, beta-blockers). Table 1-217 describes factors predisposing to serious heat illness.

PHYSICAL FINDINGS & CLINICAL PRESENTATION

Heat exhaustion:

- Generalized malaise, weakness, headache, muscle and abdominal cramps, nausea, vomiting, hypotension, tachycardia
- Rectal temperature is usually normal
- Sweating is usually present

Heat stroke:

- Neurologic manifestations (seizures, tremor, hemiplegia, coma, psychosis, other bizarre behavior)
- Evidence of dehydration (poor skin turgor, sunken eyeballs)
- Tachycardia, hyperventilation
- Skin is hot, red, and flushed
- Sweating is often (not always) absent, particularly in elderly patients
- Classic heat stroke generally develops slowly over days and occurs predominantly in older persons and in those with chronic illness. Exertional heat stroke is more common in young, healthy persons, has a more rapid onset, and is associated with higher core temperatures. Table 1-218 compares classic and exertional heat stroke. Box 1-33 summarizes organ dysfunction seen in patients with heat stroke.

ETIOLOGY

- Exogenous heat gain (increased ambient temperature)
- Increased heat production (exercise, infection, hyperthyroidism, drugs)
- Impaired heat dissipation (high humidity, heavy clothing, neonatal or elderly patients, drugs [phenothiazines, anticholinergics, antihistamines, butyrophenones, amphetamines, cocaine, alcohol, β-blockers])
- Diuretics, laxatives
- Fig. E1-437 describes an algorithm of the pathophysiology of heat stroke

TABLE 1-217 Factors Predisposing to Serious Heat Illness

Individual Factors
Lack of acclimatization
Low physical fitness
Excessive body weight
Dehydration
Advanced age
Young age
Health Conditions
Inflammation and fever
Viral infection
Cardiovascular disease
Diabetes mellitus
Gastroenteritis
Rash, sunburn, and previous burns to large areas of skin
Seizures
Thyroid storm
Neuroleptic malignant syndrome
Malignant hyperthermia
Sickle cell trait
Cystic fibrosis
Spinal cord injury
Drugs
Anticholinergic properties (atropine)
Antiepileptic (topiramate)
Antihistamines
Glutethimide (Doriden)
Phenothiazines
Tricyclic antidepressants
Amphetamines, cocaine, "Ecstasy"
Ergogenic stimulants (e.g., ephedrine, ephedra)
Lithium
Diuretics
β-Blockers
Ethanol
Environmental Factors
High temperature
High humidity
Little air motion
Lack of shade
Heat wave
Physical exercise
Heavy clothing
Air pollution (nitrogen dioxide)

From Goldman L, Schafer AI: *Goldman's Cecil medicine,* ed 24, Philadelphia, 2012, Saunders.

DIAGNOSIS

DIFFERENTIAL DIAGNOSIS

- Infections (meningitis, encephalitis, sepsis)
- Head trauma
- Epilepsy
- Thyroid storm
- Acute cocaine intoxication
- Malignant hyperthermia
- Heat exhaustion can be differentiated from heat stroke by the following:
  1. Essentially intact mental function and lack of significant fever in heat exhaustion
  2. Mild or absent increases in creatine phosphokinase (CPK), aspartate aminotransferase (AST), lactate dehydrogenase (LDH), and alanine aminotransferase (ALT) in heat exhaustion

WORKUP

- Heat stroke: comprehensive history, physical examination, and laboratory evaluation
- Heat exhaustion: in most cases, laboratory tests are not necessary for diagnosis

LABORATORY TESTS

Laboratory abnormalities may include the following:

- Elevated BUN, creatinine, hematocrit
- Hyponatremia or hypernatremia, hyperkalemia or hypokalemia
- Elevated LDH, AST, ALT, CPK, bilirubin
- Lactic acidosis, respiratory alkalosis (from hyperventilation)
- Myoglobinuria, hypofibrinogenemia, fibrinolysis, hypocalcemia

TREATMENT

- Treatment of heat exhaustion consists primarily of placing the patient in a cool, shaded area and providing rapid hydration and salt replacement.
  1. Fluid intake should be at least 2 L q4h in patients without history of CHF.
  2. Salt replacement can be accomplished by using one-quarter teaspoon of salt or two 10-grain salt tablets dissolved in 1 L of water.

BOX 1-33 Organ Dysfunction Seen in Patients with Heat Stroke

Encephalopathy
Rhabdomyolysis
Acute renal failure
Acute respiratory distress syndrome
Myocardial injury
Hepatocellular injury
Intestinal ischemia and infarction
Pancreatic injury
Hemorrhagic complication (e.g., disseminated intravascular coagulation)

From Adams JG et al: *Emergency medicine, clinical essentials,* ed 2, Philadelphia, 2013, Elsevier.

3. If IV fluid replacement is necessary, young athletes can be given normal saline IV (3 to 4 L over 6 to 8 hr); in elderly patients, consider using D5½NS IV with the rate titrated to cardiovascular status.

- Patients with heat stroke should undergo rapid cooling.
  1. Remove the patient's clothes and place the patient in a cool and well-ventilated room.
  2. If patient is unconscious, position on his or her side and clear the airway. Protect airway and augment oxygenation (e.g., nasal O_2 at 4 L/min to keep oxygen saturation >90%).
  3. Monitor body temperature every 5 min. Measurement of the patient's core temperature with a rectal probe is recommended. The goal is to reduce the body temperature to 39° C (102.2° F) in 30 to 60 min. Advantages, disadvantages, and efficacy of various cooling methods are described in Table E1-219.
  4. Spray the patient with a cool mist and use fans to enhance airflow over the body (rapid evaporation method).
  5. Immersion of the patient in ice water, stomach lavage with iced saline solution, intravenous administration of cooled fluids, and inhalation of cold air are advisable only when the means for rapid evaporation are not available. Immersion in tepid water (15° C, 59° F) is preferred over ice water immersion to minimize risk of shivering.
  6. Use of ice packs on axillae, neck, and groin is controversial because they increase peripheral vasoconstriction and may induce shivering.
  7. Antipyretics are ineffective because the hypothalamic set point during heat stroke is normal despite the increased body temperature.
  8. Intubate a comatose patient, insert a Foley catheter, and start nasal O_2. Continuous ECG monitoring is recommended.
  9. Insert at least two large-bore IV lines and begin IV hydration with NS or Ringer's lactate.
  10. Draw initial laboratory studies: electrolytes, complete blood count, blood urea nitrogen, creatinine, AST, ALT, CPK, LDH, glucose, PT (INR), PTT, platelet count, Ca^{2+}, lactic acid, and arterial blood gases.
  11. Treat complications as follows:
      a. Hypotension: vigorous hydration with normal saline or Ringer's lactate.
      b. Convulsions: diazepam 5 to 10 mg IV (slowly).
      c. Shivering: chlorpromazine 10 to 50 mg IV.
      d. Acidosis: use bicarbonate judiciously (only in severe acidosis).
  12. Observe for evidence of rhabdomyolysis and hepatic, renal, or cardiac failure and treat accordingly.

TABLE 1-218 Comparison of Classic and Exertional Heat Stroke

Patient Characteristics	Classic	Exertional
Age	Young children or elderly	15-55 yr
Health	Chronic illness	Usually healthy
Fever	Unusual	Common
Prevailing weather	Frequent in heat waves	Variable
Activity	Sedentary	Strenuous exercise
Drug use	Diuretics, antidepressants, anticholinergics, phenothiazines	Ergogenic stimulants or cocaine
Sweating	Often absent	Common
Acid-base disturbances	Respiratory alkalosis	Lactic acidosis
Acute renal failure	Uncommon	Common (≈15%)
Rhabdomyolysis	Uncommon	Common (≈25%)
CK	Mildly elevated	Markedly elevated (500-1000 U/L)
ALT, AST	Mildly elevated	Markedly elevated
Hyperkalemia	Uncommon	Common
Hypocalcemia	Uncommon	Common
DIC	Mild	Marked
Hypoglycemia	Uncommon	Common

ALT, Alanine aminotransferase; *AST,* aspartate aminotransferase; *CK,* creatine kinase; *DIC,* disseminated intravascular coagulation.
From Goldman L, Schafer AI: *Goldman's Cecil medicine,* ed 24, Philadelphia, 2012, Saunders.

DISPOSITION

Most patients recover completely within 48 hr. Central nervous system injury is permanent in 20% of cases. Mortality rate can exceed 30% in patients with prolonged and severe hyperthermia. Delayed access to cooling is the leading cause of morbidity and mortality in persons with heat stroke.

SUGGESTED READINGS

available at www.expertconsult.com

RELATED CONTENT

Heat Exhaustion and Heat Stroke (Patient Information)

AUTHOR: **FRED F. FERRI, M.D.**

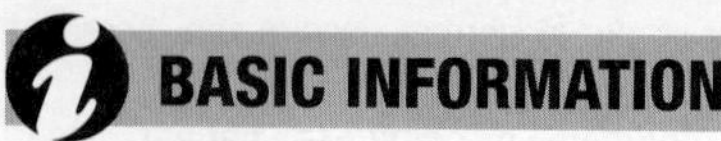

BASIC INFORMATION

DEFINITION

Infection of the human gastric mucosa with the organism *Helicobacter pylori,* a spiral-shaped gram-negative organism with unique features that allow it to survive in the hostile gastric environment.

SYNONYMS

Previously known as *Campylobacter pylori*

ICD-9CM CODES

041.86 *Helicobacter pylori (H. pylori)*

ICD-10CM CODES

B96.81 *Helicobacter pylori (H. pylori)* as the cause of diseases classified elsewhere

EPIDEMIOLOGY & DEMOGRAPHICS

H. pylori is the most common chronic bacterial infection in human beings, probably affecting 50% of the earth's population in all age groups and probably 30% to 40% of the U.S. population. In developing nations, infection is acquired at an earlier age and occurs more frequently.

CLINICAL PRESENTATION

- *H. pylori* causes histologic gastritis in all affected individuals. The majority of cases are asymptomatic and unlikely to proceed to serious consequences.
- *H. pylori* is a causative agent in peptic ulcer disease (PUD), gastric adenocarcinoma, and gastric mucosa-associated lymphoid tissue lymphoma, and may be a risk factor for iron-deficiency anemia and chronic idiopathic thrombocytopenic purpura. It may present with the signs and symptoms of these disorders, including abdominal pain, bloating, anorexia, and early satiety. Fig. 1-438 describes association of *H. pylori* infection and disease states.
- "Alarm symptoms" that should prompt more immediate and aggressive workup include weight loss, dysphagia, protracted nausea or vomiting, anemia, melena, and palpable abdominal mass.

ETIOLOGY

- Route of acquisition is unknown but is presumed to be person to person by oral-oral or fecal-oral exposure.
- The majority of cases are acquired in childhood. Socioeconomic status and living conditions in childhood affect risk of acquisition of infection. These factors include housing density, number of siblings, overcrowding, sharing a bed, and lack of running water.
- *H. pylori* does not invade gastroduodenal tissue, but disrupts the mucous layer, causing the underlying mucosa to be more vulnerable to acid peptic damage.
- What differentiates the subset of patients with *H. pylori* who go on to develop ulcers or cancer remains unclear.

Dx DIAGNOSIS

DIFFERENTIAL DIAGNOSIS

- Infection with *H. pylori* should be considered in the face of PUD, gastric cancer, gastritis, and gastric MALT lymphoma.
- *H. pylori* should be considered in the differential diagnosis of upper gastrointestinal (GI) tract disease, along with non-ulcer dyspepsia, reflux esophagitis, biliary tract disease, gastroparesis, pancreatitis, and ischemic bowel.

Colonization with *Helicobacter pylori*

Primary phenomenon: Tissue response (inflammation)

Secondary phenomenon: Atrophic gastritis | Hyperacidity | Antigenic stimulation | ?

Clinical outcome: Noncardia gastric adenocarcinoma | Duodenal ulceration | B-cell lymphoma | Reflux esophagitis and sequelae

Association with *H. pylori* (odds ratio): 2-8 | 3-6 | 6-20 | 0.2-0.7

FIGURE 1-438 Association of *Helicobacter pylori* colonization and disease states. After *H. pylori* acquisition, virtually all persons develop persistent colonization that lasts for life. Colonization induces tissue responses termed *chronic gastritis.* This process affects gastric physiology, including glandular structure, acid secretion, and antigen processing, which in turn affect disease risk. Colonization with *H. pylori* increases the risk for certain diseases (duodenal ulcer, gastric ulcer, noncardia gastric adenocarcinoma, and B-cell lymphomas) but appears to decrease the risk for gastroesophageal reflux disease and its complications, including Barrett's esophagus, and adenocarcinoma of the esophagus or gastric cardia. (From Mandell GL et al: *Principles and practice of infectious diseases,* ed 7, Philadelphia, 2010, Churchill Livingstone.)

WORKUP

- Workup is indicated in patients with active PUD, a past history of documented peptic ulcer, or gastric MALT lymphoma. The role of routine screening in high-risk populations is not clear. However, numerous studies suggest that *H. pylori* eradication is protective against progression of premalignant lesions. Consider testing for *H. pylori* in patients with idiopathic thrombocytopenic purpura, or with otherwise unexplained iron deficiency anemia. Consider a test-and-treat approach in asymptomatic first-degree relatives of gastric cancer patients.
- Routine identification and treatment of *H. pylori* in cases of non-ulcer dyspepsia, gastroesophageal reflux disease (GERD), nonsteroidal anti-inflammatory drug (NSAID) use, and in asymptomatic individuals in populations at high risk for gastric cancer is considered controversial, although it may be indicated in specific cases. A test-and-treat strategy may be used in patients younger than 55 with uncomplicated dyspepsia who have no alarm symptoms.
- Results of testing must be interpreted in relation to the individual patient's likelihood of *H. pylori* infection based on demographic risk factors. In the U.S. population, increased probability of infection exists in African Americans, Hispanics/Latinos, immigrants from developing nations, patients with poor socioeconomic status, Native Americans from Alaska, and persons >50 yr.
- Routine screening for *H. pylori* is not indicated in asymptomatic patients who are at low risk of infection.
- Infected patients with nonulcer dyspepsia usually benefit from treatment and should be evaluated for *H. pylori.*

LABORATORY TESTS

- Testing may be invasive or noninvasive depending on the need for endoscopy for other indications. There is no indication for endoscopy solely to diagnose *H. pylori.*
- Tests for *H. pylori* are differentiated as active or passive. Active tests provide direct evidence that *H. pylori* infection is currently present and include urea breath testing and stool antigen testing. Passive testing, which includes all serologic testing for *H. pylori,* gives indirect evidence of its presence by detecting the presence of antibodies to the organism. Serologic testing is limited by its inability to distinguish between active current infection and prior infection that has resolved.
- Tests that use urease as a marker (urea breath and stool antigen tests and biopsy for urease activity) may result in false-negative results in patients taking antibiotics, bismuth, or antisecretory therapy, as well as those with active ulcer bleeding. Patients should be off antibiotics for 4 wk and off protein pump inhibitors for 2 wk before urea breath or stool antigen testing.
- When diagnostic endoscopy is indicated (for suspicion or follow-up of PUD or gastric

MALT), antral biopsy should be tested for urease activity. If urease testing is likely to show a false-negative result because of recent proton pump inhibitor (PPI), bismuth, or antibiotic use or active ulcer bleeding, the sample should undergo histologic examination.

- In cases in which biopsy is not indicated, urea breath testing or stool antigen testing are indicated to evaluate for active infection. The sensitivities and specificities of these two tests are similar (>90%). Urea breath testing is slightly more expensive than stool antigen testing, but both costs are in the modest range. Choice can be made based on patient preference and availability.
- In cases in which biopsy is not indicated, consider using serologic testing as the initial approach. However, in individuals with a low pretest probability of infection, positive results should be confirmed with another testing method.

Rx TREATMENT

ACUTE GENERAL Rx

- Test only patients whom you intend to treat if positive (see "Workup" above). At this time, the value of eradicating *H. pylori* infection is proven in patients with PUD or gastric MALT lymphoma.
- The optimal antibiotic regimen has not been defined. In addition to efficacy, side effects, cost, and ease of administration must be considered.
- Due to increasing resistance to clarithromycin, decisions regarding appropriate regimens should take into account local rates of clarithromycin resistance.
- The following regimens may be considered for first-line therapy:
  - PPI twice daily, with twice-daily clarithromycin (500 mg) and amoxicillin (1 g) may be used in areas of low clarithromycin resistance.
  - In cases of penicillin allergy, metronidazole (500 mg bid) may be substituted for amoxicillin.
  - PPI twice daily, combined with bismuth four times daily, as well as tetracycline (500 mg qid) and metronidazole (250 mg) four times daily, is now recommended as first-line therapy in areas of high clarithromycin resistance. Sequential therapy, consisting of 5 days of treatment with a PPI and one antibiotic (usually amoxicillin) followed by 5-day treatment with the PPI and two other antibiotics (usually clarithromycin and metronidazole) may be used in areas of high clarithromycin resistance when bismuth-based therapy is not available.
- Duration of treatment remains controversial. Extending therapy to 10-14 days may improve eradication rates. Use of combination capsules may improve compliance but is likely to be more expensive.
- Prior exposure to a macrolide or metronidazole, for any reason, is associated with increased resistance. A preferable regimen would include medications to which the patient has not been previously exposed.
- Diarrhea and abdominal cramping are commonly observed with many of the regimens. (Probiotics may diminish this effect.) Other side effects may include a metallic taste with metronidazole or clarithromycin, neuropathy, seizures, and disulfiram-like reaction with metronidazole, diarrhea with amoxicillin, photosensitivity with tetracycline, and *Clostridium difficile* infection with any antibiotic exposure. Bismuth may cause black stool and constipation. Tetracycline is contraindicated in pregnant patients.
- 20% of patients may not respond to initial therapy. Optimal retreatment regimens are under investigation. It is important to reinforce compliance. Second-line therapy should be either bismuth-containing quadruple therapy or levofloxacin containing triple therapy (regardless of local clarithromycin resistance patterns). When possible, management of those who do not respond to two courses of therapy should be guided by antimicrobial sensitivity testing.

CHRONIC Rx

- Accepted indications for confirming eradication include *H. pylori*–associated ulcers, MALT lymphoma, and early gastric cancer. It may be considered in those with persistent dyspepsia despite a test-and-treat management strategy (as well as consideration of other causes for the dyspeptic symptoms). Given the increasing prevalence of antibiotic resistance and the decreasing cost of testing, consider confirming eradication of *H. pylori* in all treated patients.
- Serology does not reliably revert to undetectable levels after treatment and should not be used to determine eradication.
- Active tests (urea breath test and stool antigen testing) are preferable. They are equally accurate in confirming eradication, and either may be used depending on availability and patient preference. To reduce the likelihood of false-negative results, testing should be performed at least 4 wk after eradication therapy with PPI and antibiotics or at least 2 wk after the cessation of PPI therapy alone.

DISPOSITION

Consider further evaluation in patients with recurrent symptoms after appropriate treatment.

REFERRAL

- Patients with gastric MALT lymphoma should be followed by a gastroenterologist and oncologist with expertise in the care of lymphoid neoplasms.
- Patients with dyspepsia who have tested positive for *H. pylori* and been treated without resolution should be referred for endoscopy.
- Consider referral for biopsy for culture and sensitivity in patients who have not responded to two attempts at treatment.

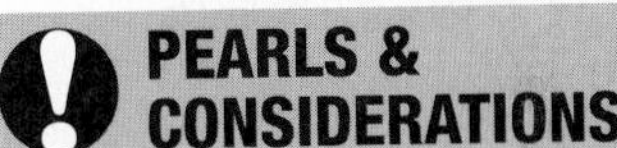

PEARLS & CONSIDERATIONS

- Whether *H. pylori* eradication reduces the risk of gastric cancer is unclear.
- Outcomes in PUD and gastric MALT lymphoma are improved with treatment of associated *H. pylori* infection.
- Tests that provide direct evidence of active *H. pylori* infection (urea breath and stool antigen testing) are preferred but may result in false-negative results in patients taking antibiotics, bismuth, or antisecretory agents.
- Serologic testing does not differentiate active from prior infection. It may be useful when active tests are not indicated, particularly in high-risk patients.
- Be aware of high-risk populations in low-prevalence settings, including immigrants from Mexico, South America, Southeast Asia, and Eastern Europe.

SUGGESTED READINGS

available at www.expertconsult.com

RELATED CONTENT

Helicobacter pylori Infection (Patient Information)
Gastritis (Related Key Topic)
Peptic Ulcer (Related Key Topic)

AUTHOR: **MARGARET TRYFOROS, M.D.**

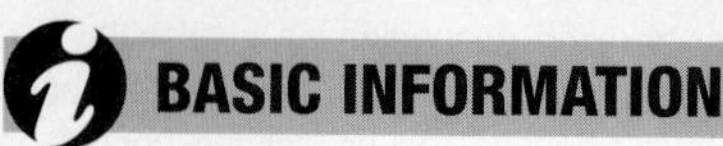

BASIC INFORMATION

DEFINITION

The HELLP syndrome is a serious variant of preeclampsia. HELLP is an acronym for ***h***emolysis, ***e***levated ***l***iver function, and ***l***ow ***p***latelet count. It is the most frequently encountered microangiopathy of pregnancy. There are three classes of the syndrome based on the degree of maternal thrombocytopenia as a primary indicator of disease severity:

Class 1: Platelets ≤50,000/mm^3
Class 2: Platelets >50,000/mm^3 to 100,000/mm^3
Class 3: Platelets >100,000/mm^3

ICD-9CM CODES
642.50 HELLP, episode of care
642.51 HELLP, delivered
642.52 HELLP, delivered with postpartum complications
642.53 HELLP, antepartum complications
642.54 HELLP, postpartum complications
ICD-10CM CODES
O14.2 HELLP syndrome

EPIDEMIOLOGY & DEMOGRAPHICS

- Among women with severe preeclampsia, 6% will manifest with one abnormality suggestive of HELLP syndrome, 12% will develop two abnormalities, and approximately 10% will develop all three.
- The HELLP syndrome, like preeclampsia, is rare before 20 wk of gestation.
- One third of all cases occur postpartum; of these, only 80% are typically diagnosed with preeclampsia before delivery.

RISK FACTORS: Women >35 yr, white, multiparity

RECURRENCE RATE: 3% to 25%

PHYSICAL FINDINGS & CLINICAL PRESENTATION

- Definitive laboratory criteria remain to be validated prospectively.
- Most commonly used criteria include hemolysis defined by the presence of an abnormal peripheral smear with schistocytes, lactate dehydrogenase (LDH) >600 U/L, and total bilirubin >1.2 mg/dl; elevated liver enzymes as serum aspartate aminotransferase (AST) >70 U/L and LDH >600 U/L; low platelet count as less than 100,000/mm^3.
- Although many women with HELLP syndrome are asymptomatic, 80% report right upper quadrant pain and 50% to 60% present with excessive weight gain and worsening edema.

ETIOLOGY

As with other microangiopathies, endothelial dysfunction, with resultant activation of the intravascular coagulation cascade, has been proposed as the central pathogenesis of HELLP syndrome.

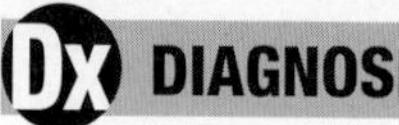

DIAGNOSIS

DIFFERENTIAL DIAGNOSIS

- Appendicitis
- Gallbladder disease
- Peptic ulcer disease
- Enteritis
- Hepatitis
- Pyelonephritis
- Systemic lupus erythematosus
- Thrombotic thrombocytopenic purpura/hemolytic-uremic syndrome
- Acute fatty liver of pregnancy

WORKUP

Because HELLP syndrome is a disease entity based on laboratory values, initial assessment is detailed below.

LABORATORY TESTS

- Initial assessment of suspected HELLP syndrome should include a complete blood count to evaluate platelets, urinalysis, serum creatinine, LDH, uric acid, indirect and total bilirubin levels, and AST/alanine aminotransferase (ALT).
- Tests of prothrombin time, partial thromboplastin time, fibrinogen, and fibrin split products are reserved for women with a platelet count well below 100,000/mm^3.

IMAGING STUDIES

No imaging modalities aid in diagnosis.

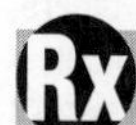

TREATMENT

Treatment depends on gestational age of the fetus, severity of condition, and maternal status. Stabilization of the mother is the first priority.

ACUTE GENERAL Rx

- Assess gestational age thoroughly. Fetal status should be monitored with nonstress tests, contraction stress tests, and/or biophysical profile.
- Maternal status should be evaluated by history, physical examination, and laboratory testing.
- Magnesium sulfate is administered for seizure prophylaxis regardless of blood pressure.
- Blood pressure control is achieved with agents such as hydralazine or labetalol.
- Indwelling Foley catheter to monitor maternal volume status and urine output.

CHRONIC Rx

- In pregnancies of 34 wk or with class 1 HELLP syndrome, delivery, either vaginal or abdominal, within 24 hr is the goal.
- In the preterm fetus corticosteroid therapy to enhance fetal lung maturation is indicated.
- Some reports have shown temporary amelioration of HELLP severity with the administration of high-dose steroids measured by increased urine output, improvement in platelet count, and liver function test.
- Judicious use of blood products, especially in those requiring surgery.
- The patient requires intensive observation for 48 hr postpartum; laboratory levels should begin to improve during this time.

DISPOSITION

The natural history of this disorder is a rapidly deteriorating condition requiring close monitoring of maternal and fetal well-being.

REFERRAL

Preterm patients with HELLP syndrome should be stabilized hemodynamically and transferred to a tertiary care center. Term patients can be treated at a local hospital depending on the availability of obstetric, neonatal, and blood banking services.

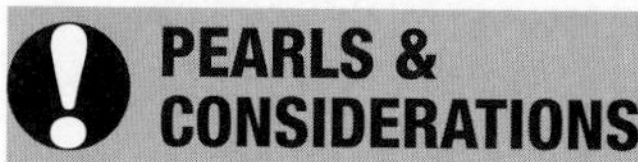

PEARLS & CONSIDERATIONS

- Not all women with HELLP have hypertension or proteinuria.
- Life-threatening hemorrhage is a rare event in HELLP syndrome. Identifiable risk factors predictive of a major hemorrhage are thrombocytopenia (<100,000/mm^3), AST >70 IU/L, and previous gestations.

SUGGESTED READINGS

available at www.expertconsult.com

RELATED CONTENT

Eclampsia (Related Key Topic)
Preeclampsia (Related Key Topic)

AUTHORS: **SONYA S. ABDEL-RAZEQ, M.D.**, and **RUBEN ALVERO, M.D.**

BASIC INFORMATION

DEFINITION

Hemochromatosis is an autosomal-recessive disorder that disrupts the body's regulation of iron and is characterized by increased accumulation of iron in various organs (adrenals, liver, pancreas, heart, testes, kidneys, pituitary) and eventual dysfunction of these organs if not treated appropriately.

SYNONYMS

Bronze diabetes

ICD-9CM CODES
275.0 Hemochromatosis
ICD-10CM CODES
E83.119 Hemochromatosis, unspecified

EPIDEMIOLOGY & DEMOGRAPHICS

INCIDENCE: In whites, approximately 1 in 385 persons

PREDOMINANT SEX AND AGE:

Generally diagnosed in males in their fifth decade. Diagnosis in females is generally not made until 10 to 20 yr after menopause.

GENETICS:

Most common genetic disorder in North European ancestry. Homozygosity for the *C282Y* mutation is now found in approximately 5 of every 1000 persons of European descent.

PHYSICAL FINDINGS & CLINICAL PRESENTATION

- In earlier stages patients completely asymptomatic and diagnosed due to abnormal laboratory tests
- Hepatic dysfunction leading to hepatomegaly, fibrosis, and eventually cirrhosis
- Arthritis
- Gonadal insufficiency leading to loss of libido and testicular atrophy
- Diabetes mellitus: risk greater in patients with family history
- Iron-induced cardiac disease resulting in cardiomyopathy, heart failure, and arrhythmias
- Skin pigmentation

ETIOLOGY

- The majority of the patients diagnosed with hemochromatosis have mutation in the *HFE* gene and are either homozygous for the *C282Y* mutation *(C282Y/C282Y)* or compound heterozygote for the *C282Y* mutation and either the mutation *H63D (C282Y/H63D)* or less commonly the *S65C (C282Y/S65C)*.
- The remainder of the patients are classified as non–*HFE*-associated hemochromatosis.

DIAGNOSIS

DIFFERENTIAL DIAGNOSIS

- Hereditary anemias with defect of erythropoiesis
- Cirrhosis, chronic liver disease, porphyria cutanea tarda
- Repeated blood transfusions
- African dietary iron overload

WORKUP

Medical history, physical examination, and laboratory evaluation should be focused on affected organ systems (see "Physical Findings & Clinical Presentation"). Fig. 1-439 outlines evaluation for possible hereditary hemochromatosis in an individual with negative family history. Liver biopsy is the gold standard for diagnosis; it reveals iron deposition in hepatocytes, bile ducts, and supporting tissues.

LABORATORY TESTS

- Transferrin saturation is the best screening test. Values >45% are an indication for further testing.
- Elevated serum ferritin is good evidence of iron overload, but other causes like chronic inflammatory conditions, malignancy, and so forth need to be ruled out as ferritin is also an acute phase reactant.
- Genotypical screening for *C282Y* and *H63D* mutation in *HFE* gene should be done in patients with high transferrin saturation, elevated ferritin, or both.
- Liver biopsy (Fig. 1-440) is the gold standard but is not needed in somebody who has a persistently elevated transferrin saturation, elevated ferritin, or both.
- Hepatic iron index can help differentiate between various causes of iron overload.
- Elevated aspartate aminotransferase, alanine aminotransferase, and alkaline phosphatase are seen.
- Hyperglycemia is found.
- Endocrine abnormalities (decreased testosterone, luteinizing hormone, follicle-stimulating hormone) are noted.
- Table 1-220 describes laboratory findings in patients with hereditary hemochromatosis.

IMAGING STUDIES

Routine radiologic imaging is not needed.

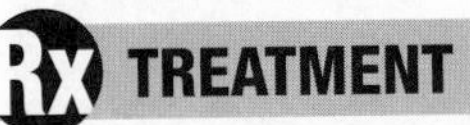

TREATMENT

The goal of therapy is the removal of excess iron and maintaining it at a normal or near-normal level.

NONPHARMACOLOGIC THERAPY

Phlebotomy is the treatment of choice.

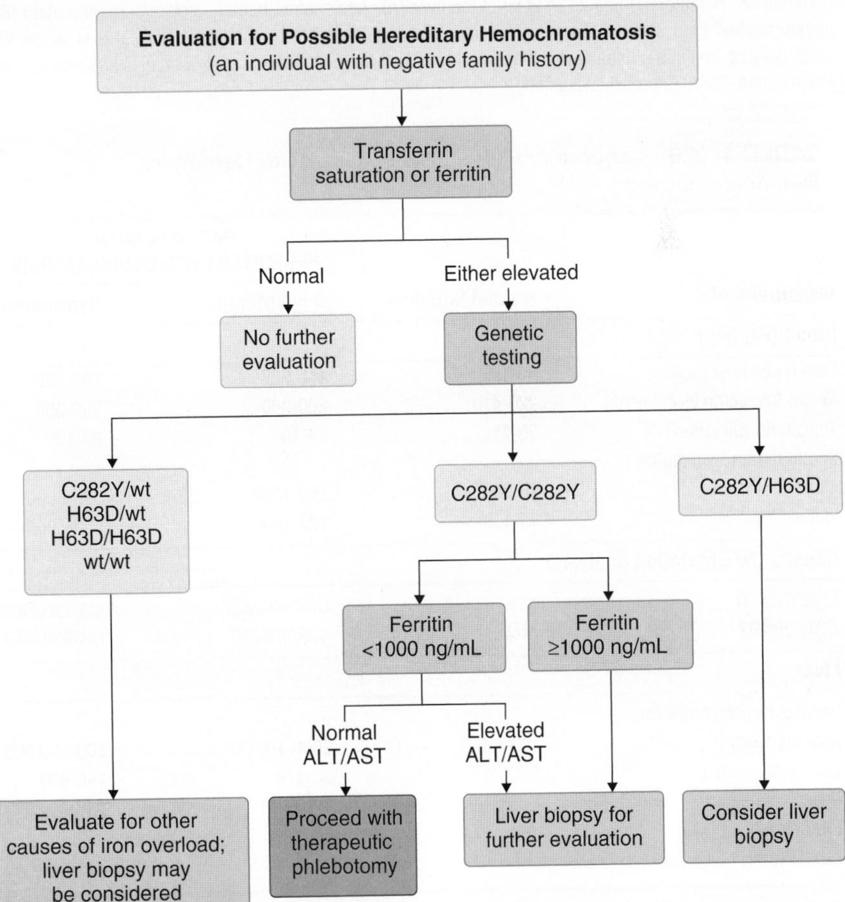

FIGURE 1-439 Algorithm for evaluation of possible hereditary hemochromatosis in a person with a negative family history. *ALT,* Alanine transminase; *AST,* aspartate transminase. (From Goldman L, Schafer AI: *Goldman's Cecil medicine,* ed 24, Philadelphia, 2012, Saunders.)

 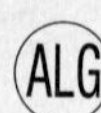 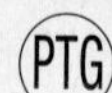

ACUTE GENERAL RX

- The timing and frequency of phlebotomy needs to be individualized for each patient.
- For patients with heavy iron overload twice-weekly phlebotomies should be started. In most patients, weekly phlebotomy is adequate.
- The effectiveness of treatment is monitored by periodic ferritin measurement. The goal is to bring ferritin level below 50 ng/ml.
- Patients with iron overload due to transfusion-dependent anemias may not tolerate phlebotomy. For these patients iron chelation may be needed.
- The chelating agent deferoxamine has to be given daily as a 9- to 12-hr IV or SC infusion and compliance is difficult.
- The oral chelating agent deferasirox (Exjade) is effective but should not be used in patients with high-risk myelodysplastic syndrome because it can cause renal impairment, hepatic impairment, or gastrointestinal hemorrhage, which can be fatal.

CHRONIC RX

After the ferritin has been brought to less than 50 ng/ml, phlebotomy is needed on an as-needed basis to keep the ferritin at that level.

DISPOSITION

- Serum ferritin measurement is the most useful prognostic indicator of disease severity.
- Prognosis is good if phlebotomy is started early (before onset of cirrhosis or diabetes mellitus); women can have the full phenotypic expression of the disease, including cirrhosis, and should also be aggressively treated.

REFERRAL

For liver biopsy if diagnosis is uncertain

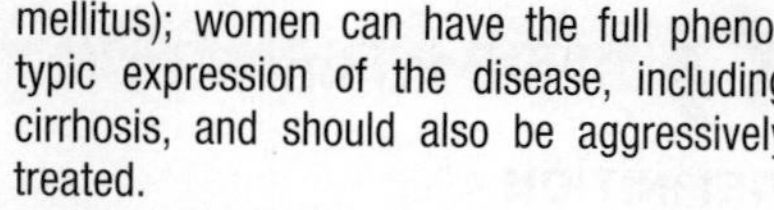
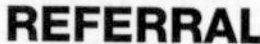
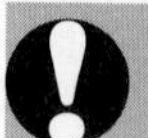

PEARLS & CONSIDERATIONS

COMMENTS

- Persons who are homozygous for the HFE gene mutation *C282Y* comprise 85% to 90% of phenotypically affected individuals.
- Patients with hemochromatosis and serum ferritin levels <1000 ng/ml are unlikely to have cirrhosis. Liver biopsy to screen for cirrhosis may be unnecessary in such patients.
- Cirrhotic patients must be periodically monitored (ultrasound or CT scan) because of their increased risk of hepatocellular carcinoma.
- *HFE* gene testing for *C282Y* mutation is a cost-effective method of screening relatives of patients with hereditary hemochromatosis. The American College of Gastroenterology recommends genotyping persons who have abnormal iron screening tests and first-degree relatives of those identified with *C282Y* homozygosity.
- Established cirrhosis, hypogonadism, destructive arthritis, and insulin-dependent diabetes mellitus secondary to hemochromatosis cannot be reversed with repeated phlebotomy, but their progress can be slowed.
- In patients who are heterozygotes for *C282Y* or *H63D* mutation, clinically meaningful iron overload does not develop.
- Screening for hepatocellular carcinoma is reserved for those with hereditary hemochromatosis and cirrhosis.

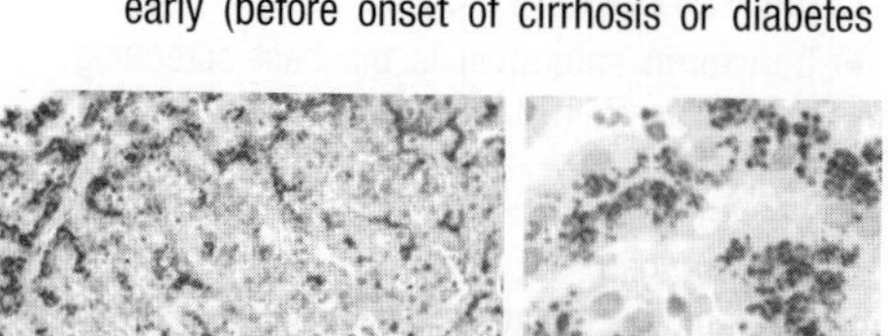
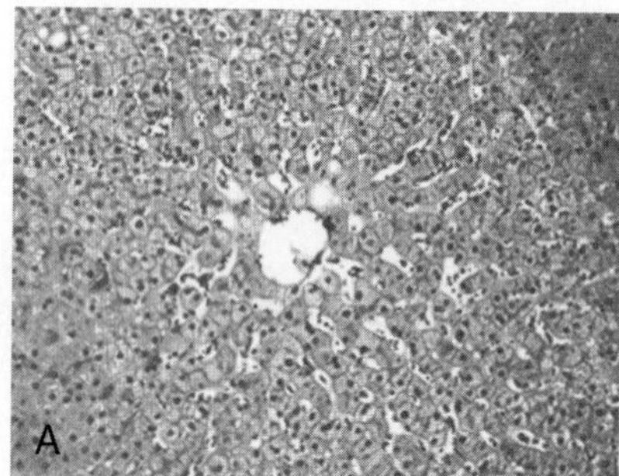
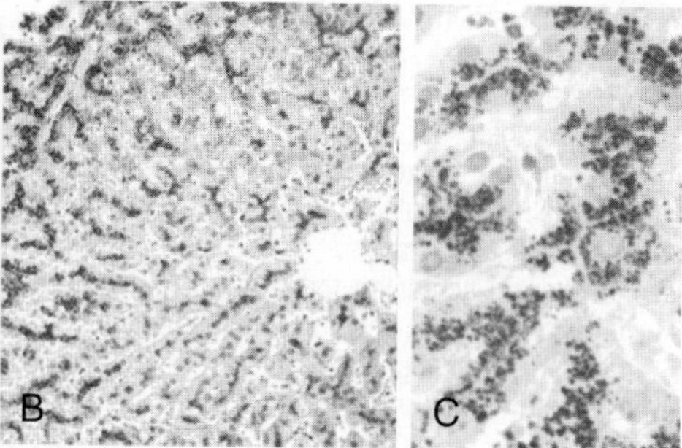

FIGURE 1-440 Hemochromatosis. Liver biopsy sample from a 46-year-old man with homozygous hemochromatosis. Hematoxylin and eosin stain of the liver **(A)** shows intact hepatic architecture. Iron stain **(B, C)** shows marked diffuse iron deposits in the hepatocytes throughout the lobules. A normal liver would show essentially no iron in the hepatocytes. (From Hoffman R et al: *Hematology, basic principles and practice,* ed 5, Philadelphia, 2009, Churchill Livingstone.)

TABLE 1-220 Laboratory Findings in Patients with Hereditary Hemochromatosis

		PATIENTS WITH HEREDITARY HEMOCHROMATOSIS	
Measurements	**Normal Subjects**	**Asymptomatic**	**Symptomatic**
Blood (Fasting)			
Serum iron level (μg/dl)	60-180	150-280	180-300
Serum transferrin level (mg/dl)	220-410	200-280	200-300
Transferrin saturation (%)	20-45	45-100	80-100
Serum ferritin level (ng/ml)			
Men	20-200	150-1000	500-6000
Women	15-150	120-1000	500-6000
Genetic (*HFE* Mutation Analysis)			
C282Y/C282Y	wt/wt[‡]	*C282Y/C282Y*	*C282Y/C282Y*
C282Y/H63D[*]	wt/wt	*C282Y/H63D*	*C282Y/H63D*
Liver			
Hepatic iron concentration			
μg/g dry weight	300-1500	2000-10,000	8000-30,000
μmol/g dry weight	5-27	36-179	140-550
Hepatic iron index[†]	<1	1 to >1.9	>1.9
Liver histology			
Perls' Prussian blue stain	0, 1+	2+ to 4+	3+, 4+

*Compound heterozygote.
†Calculated by dividing the hepatic iron concentration (in μmol/g dry weight) by the age of the patient (in yr). With the increased use of genetic testing in patients with iron overload, the specificity of the hepatic iron index has diminished.
‡wt/wt: wild type (normal).
From Goldman L, Schafer AI: *Goldman's Cecil medicine,* ed 24, Philadelphia, 2012, Saunders.

SUGGESTED READINGS

available at www.expertconsult.com

RELATED CONTENT

Hemochromatosis (Patient Information)

AUTHORS: **BILAL H. NAQVI, M.D.,** and **FRED F. FERRI, M.D.**

BASIC INFORMATION

DEFINITION

Hemolytic-uremic syndrome (HUS) refers to an acute syndrome characterized by microangiopathic hemolytic anemia, thrombocytopenia, and severe renal failure. "Atypical hemolytic-uremic syndrome" is a genetic, life-threatening, chronic disease of complement-mediated thrombotic microangiopathy.

SYNONYMS

HUS

ICD-9CM CODES
283.11 Hemolytic-uremic syndrome
ICD-10CM CODES
D59.3 Hemolytic-uremic syndrome

EPIDEMIOLOGY & DEMOGRAPHICS

- HUS affects mainly children younger than 5 yr with incidence rate of 6.1 cases/100,000.
- Overall incidence is 1 to 2 cases/100,000.
- May be epidemic, most commonly occurring during the summer months in rural populations.
- Most common cause of acute renal failure in children.
- In the U.S., 300 to 700 new cases occur each year.

PHYSICAL FINDINGS & CLINICAL PRESENTATION

- HUS usually preceded by diarrhea in 90% of cases, bloody in 75%
- Abdominal pain, vomiting, and fever
- Neurologic symptoms, principally seizure and somnolence, have been observed in 20% to 25% of cases. Stroke or coma may occur and be associated with significant mortality
- Hypertension
- Hepatomegaly and abnormality in liver function tests
- Anuria or oliguria
- Glucose intolerance and transient diabetes (10%)

ETIOLOGY

Pathologically, it is thought that thrombin generation (probably the result of accelerated thrombogenesis) and inhibition of fibrinolysis lead to renal arteriolar and capillary microthrombi preceding renal injury.
In children:

- *Escherichia coli* serotype 0157:H7 is the leading cause of HUS.
- The infection is acquired by eating undercooked red meat, nonpasteurized milk or milk products, water, fruits, or vegetables. A recent large outbreak of the HUS caused by Shiga-toxin–producing *Escherichia coli* 0104:H4 in Germany was associated with consumption of contaminated sprouts.
- Other causes of HUS in children and adults are:
  - Drugs (cyclosporine, mitomycin, tacrolimus, ticlopidine, clopidogrel, cisplatin, quinine, penicillin, penicillamine, oral contraceptives, and quinine used to treat muscle cramps) and toxins
  - Infection (*Salmonella, Shigella, Yersinia,* Group A streptococci, *Clostridium difficile, Campylobacter,* coxsackie virus, rubella, influenza virus, Epstein-Barr virus)
  - HIV-associated thrombotic microangiopathy
  - Pneumococcal infection
- Complement disorders involving factors H, I, and membrane cofactors protein have been associated with cases of nondiarrhea-associated HUS (atypical HUS).
- Mutations that impair the function of thrombomodulin occur in about 5% of patients with atypical HUS.
- Table 1-221 describes a classification of HUS.

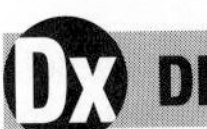

DIAGNOSIS

The triad of thrombocytopenia, acute renal failure, and microangiopathic hemolytic anemia establishes the diagnosis of HUS.

TABLE 1-221 Classification of Hemolytic-Uremic Syndrome

Infection-induced
Verotoxin-producing *Escherichia coli*
Shiga toxin-producing *Shigella dysentereriae* type 1
Neuraminidase-producing *Streptococcus pneumoniae*
Human immunodeficiency virus
Genetic
Von Willebrand factor-cleaving protease (ADAMTS 13) deficiency
Complement factor H (or related proteins) deficiency or mutation
Membrane cofactor protein (MCP) mutations
Thrombomodulin mutations
Complement factor I mutations
Vitamin B_{12} metabolism defects
Familial autosomal recessive of undefined etiology
Familial autosomal dominant of undefined etiology
Sporadic, recurrent, undefined etiology without diarrhea prodrome
Other Diseases Associated with Microvascular Injury
Systemic lupus erythematosus
Antiphospholipid antibody syndrome
Following bone marrow transplantation
Malignant hypertension
Primary glomerulopathy
HELLP (*h*emolytic anemia, *el*evated *l*iver enzymes, *l*ow *p*latelet count) syndrome
Medication-induced
Calcineurin inhibitors (cyclosporine, tacrolimus)
Cytotoxic, chemotherapy agents (mitomycin C, cisplatin, gemcitabine)
Clopidogrel and ticlopidine
Quinine

From Kliegman RM et al: *Nelson textbook of pediatrics,* ed 19, Philadelphia, 2011, Saunders.

DIFFERENTIAL DIAGNOSIS

The differential is vast, including all causes of bloody and nonbloody diarrhea because the GI symptoms usually precede the triad of HUS:

- Thrombotic thrombocytopenic purpura
- Disseminated intravascular coagulation
- Prosthetic valve hemolysis
- Malignant hypertension
- Vasculitis
- Catastrophic antiphospholipid syndrome
- Postpartum acute renal failure
- Scleroderma renal crisis

WORKUP

The workup for suspected HUS patients includes blood tests and stool cultures.

LABORATORY TESTS

- Anemia (hemoglobin <8 g/dl) with peripheral smear shows the hallmark microangiopathic hemolytic anemia with schistocytes, burr cells, and helmet cells (Fig. 1-441)
- Thrombocytopenia (platelet counts usually <60,000/mm^3)
- Reticulocyte count high
- LDH level elevated
- Haptoglobin low
- Indirect bilirubin elevated
- Negative Coombs test
- BUN and creatinine elevated
- Urinalysis: proteinuria, microscopic hematuria, and pyuria
- Stool cultures for *E. coli* 0157:H7 are positive in more than 90% of cases if obtained during the first week of illness. After the first week, only one third are positive.

IMAGING STUDIES

Imaging studies are not very helpful in the diagnosis of HUS.

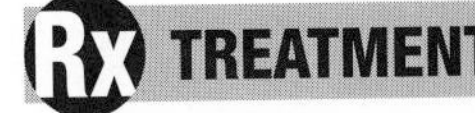

TREATMENT

The treatment of HUS is primarily supportive.

NONPHARMACOLOGIC THERAPY

- Blood transfusions are used for severe anemia.

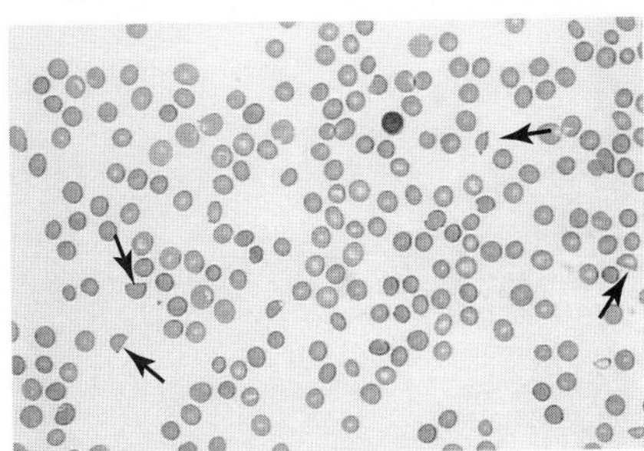

FIGURE 1-441 Hemolytic-uremic syndrome (HUS). Peripheral blood smear from a patient with HUS. The presence of fragmented red blood cells with the appearance of a helmet *(arrows)* is pathognomonic for microangiopathic hemolysis in patients with no evidence of heart valvular disease. (From Floege J et al: *Comprehensive clinical nephrology,* ed 4, Philadelphia, 2010, Saunders.)

- Antibiotics and antimotility agents should be avoided and are not indicated for the treatment of *E. coli* 0157:H7.
- Correction of electrolyte abnormalities and fluid management should be performed.
- Platelet transfusion is preserved only for patients with HUS who have significant bleed or invasive procedure is required.
- Plasma exchange therapy with immunosuppressive agents has been used in patients with severe CNS involvement. Eculizumab, a monoclonal antibody directed toward complement component C_5, has been approved in adults for treatment of atypical HUS. Trials have shown that eculizumab is effective in inhibiting complement-mediated thrombotic microangiopathy in patients with atypical hemolytic-uremic syndrome.[1]
- Tissue-type plasminogen activator (PAI-1) may have a role in improving renal function in recent studies.

ACUTE GENERAL Rx

Hypertension and seizure control

CHRONIC Rx

For anuric or oliguric renal failure, dialysis may be required.

DISPOSITION

- Adults presenting with HUS have a worse prognosis than do children with HUS.

[1]Legendre CM et al: Terminal complement inhibitor eculizumab in atypical hemolytic-uremic syndrome, *N Engl J Med* 368:2164-2181, 2013.

- Mortality rate is less than 5%.
- Morbidity includes:
  - Proteinuria (31%)
  - Renal insufficiency (31%)
  - Hypertension (6%)
- Patients with atypical hemolytic-uremic syndrome ave a lifely risk of systemic clinical complications of thrombotic microangiopathy, including damage to multiple organ systems (e.g., the central nervous system, kidneys, heart, and GI tract). Within 1 yr after a diagnosis of this syndrome, up to 5% of patients treated with plasma exchange or infusion sustain permanent renal damage, have progression to end-stage renal disease, or die.[1]

REFERRAL

- The local health department should be notified if *E. coli* 0157:H7 has been isolated; large food-borne outbreaks have occurred with commercial beef products and asparagus.
- Consultation with hematology and nephrology specialist is recommended for patients with HUS.

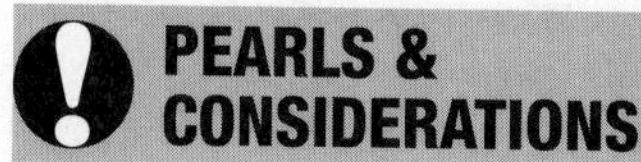

PEARLS & CONSIDERATIONS

COMMENTS

- Children testing positive for the *E. coli* 0157:H7 serotype should not return to school or day care facilities until two consecutive stools test negative for the microorganism.
- *E. coli* 0157:H7 can be transmitted from person to person; therefore universal precautions and handwashing are recommended in preventing the spread of the infection.
- *E. coli* 0111 can also be associated with HUS. In 2008 the largest known U.S. serotype 1 *E. coli* 0111 occurred in Oklahoma, causing 341 illnesses. The HUS attack rate in this *E. coli* 0111 outbreak was comparable to that for *E. coli* 0157-related illness, but most cases occurred among adults. More recently, in May 2011, a large outbreak of diarrhea and HUS caused by an unusual serotype of Shiga-toxin–producing *E. coli* (0104:H4) occurred in Germany, with 908 individuals reported with hemolytic-uremic syndrome, and 34 deaths.

SUGGESTED READINGS

available at www.expertconsult.com

RELATED CONTENT

Hemolytic-Uremic Syndrome (Patient Information)

AUTHORS: **MONZR M. AL MALKI, M.D.**, and **GLENN G. FORT, M.D., M.P.H.**

BASIC INFORMATION

DEFINITION

Hemophilia is a hereditary bleeding disorder caused by low factor VIII coagulant activity (hemophilia A) or low levels of factor IX coagulant activity (hemophilia B).

SYNONYMS

Hemophilia A: Classic hemophilia, factor VIII deficiency hemophilia

Hemophilia B: Christmas disease, factor IX hemophilia

ICD-9CM CODES

286.0 Hemophilia A

286.1 Hemophilia B

ICD-10CM CODES

D66 Hereditary factor VIII deficiency

D67 Hereditary factor IX deficiency

EPIDEMIOLOGY & DEMOGRAPHICS

INCIDENCE/PREVALENCE (IN U.S.): Hemophilia A: 100 cases per 1 million males; hemophilia B: 20 cases per 1 million males. Approximately 400,000 patients have severe hemophilia worldwide.

GENETIC: Both hemophilias have an X-linked recessive pattern of inheritance with only males affected.

PHYSICAL FINDINGS & CLINICAL PRESENTATION

- The clinical features of hemophilia A and B are generally indistinguishable from each other.
- Bleeding is most commonly seen in joints (knees, ankles, elbows), resulting in hot, swollen, painful joints (Fig. 1-442) and subsequent crippling joint deformity. (Fig. 1-443)
- Bleeding can also occur into the muscles and the gastrointestinal tract.
- Compartment syndrome can occur from large hematomas.
- Hematuria may be present.

ETIOLOGY

- Hemophilia A: low factor VIII coagulant (VIII:C) activity; can be classified as mild if factor VIII:C levels are >5%, moderate if levels are 1% to 5%, and severe if levels are <1%.
- Hemophilia B: low levels of factor IX coagulant activity.
- Both disorders are congenital.
- Spontaneous acquisition of factor VIII inhibitors (acquired hemophilia) is rare.

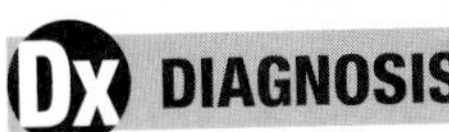

DIAGNOSIS

DIFFERENTIAL DIAGNOSIS

- Other clotting factor deficiencies
- Platelet function disorders
- Vitamin K deficiency

WORKUP

Patients with mild hemophilia bleed only in response to major trauma or surgery and may not be diagnosed until young adulthood. Diagnostic workup includes laboratory evaluation (see "Laboratory Tests").

LABORATORY TESTS

- Partial thromboplastin time (PTT) is prolonged.
- Reduced factor VIII:C level distinguishes hemophilia A from other causes of prolonged PTT.
- Factor VIII antigen, prothrombin time, fibrinogen level, and bleeding time are normal.
- Factor IX coagulant activity levels are reduced in patients with hemophilia B.
- Coagulation factor activity measurement is useful to correlate with disease severity. Normal range is 50 to 150 U/dl; 5 to 20 U/dl indicates mild disease, 2 to 5 U/dl indicates moderate disease, and <2 U/dl indicates severe disease with spontaneous bleeding episodes.

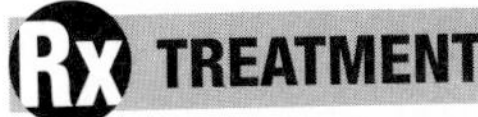

TREATMENT

NONPHARMACOLOGIC THERAPY

- Avoidance of contact sports
- Patient education regarding the disease; promotion of exercises such as swimming
- Avoidance of aspirin or other NSAIDs
- Orthopedic evaluation and physical therapy evaluation in patients with joint involvement
- Hepatitis vaccination

ACUTE GENERAL Rx

(see Table 1-222)

HEMOPHILIA A:

- Reversal and prevention of acute bleeding in hemophilia A and B are based on adequate replacement of deficient or missing factor protein.

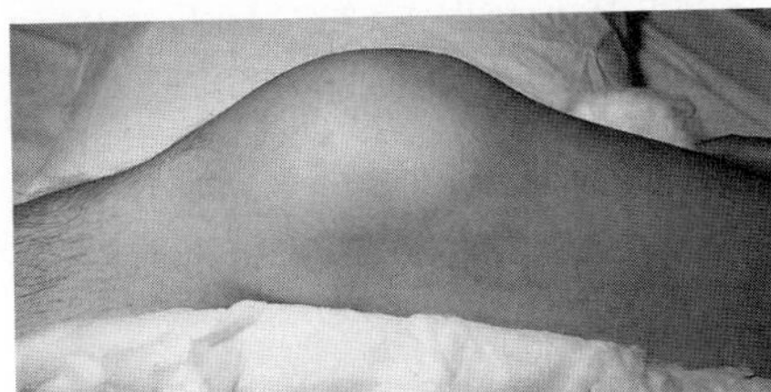

FIGURE 1-442 Acute hemarthrosis of the knee is a common complication of hemophilia. It may be confused with acute infection unless the patient's coagulation disorder is known because the knee is hot, red, swollen, and painful. (From Forbes CD, Jackson WF: *Color atlas and text of clinical medicine,* ed 3, London, 2003, Mosby.)

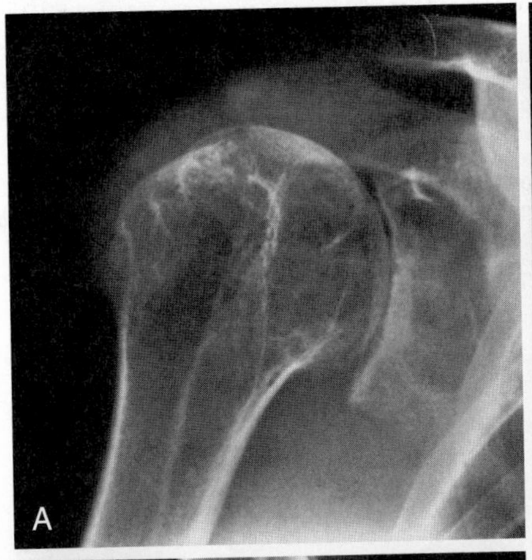

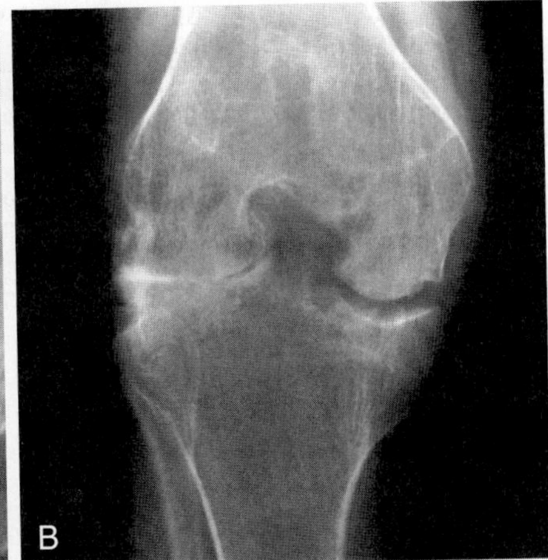

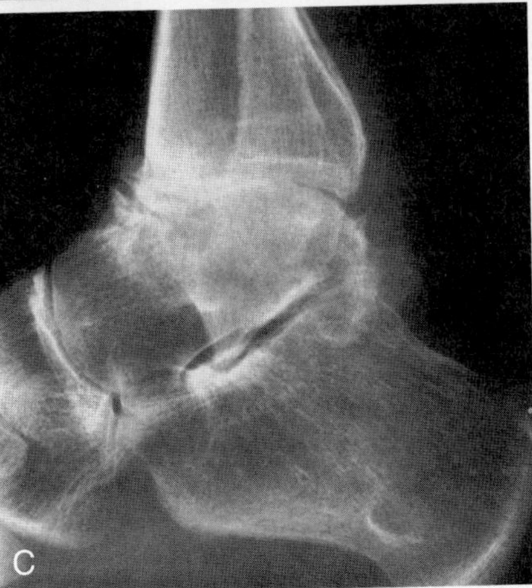

FIGURE 1-443 Radiographic changes associated with hemophilic arthropathy. A, Radiograph of the shoulder showing multiple subchondral cysts in the head of the humerus, an early finding in hemophilic arthropathy. The glenohumeral joint space is fairly well preserved, and range of motion is normal. **B,** Widening of the intercondylar notch and near fusion of the femur and medial tibial condyle in the knee joint affected by hemophilic arthropathy. **C,** Narrowing and fusion of the tibiotalar joint in the ankle. (From Hoffman R et al: *Hematology, basic principles and practice,* ed 5, Philadelphia, 2009, Churchill Livingstone.)

TABLE 1-222 Treatment of Hemophilia

Type of Hemorrhage	Hemophilia A	Hemophilia B
Hemarthrosis*	50 IU/kg factor VIII concentrate† on day 1; then 20 IU/kg on days 2, 3, 5 until joint function is normal or back to baseline. Consider additional treatment every other day for 7-10 days. Consider prophylaxis.	80-100 IU/kg on day 1; then 40 IU/kg on days 2, 4. Consider additional treatment every other day for 7-10 days. Consider prophylaxis.
Muscle or significant subcutaneous hematoma	50 IU/kg factor VIII concentrate; 20 IU/kg every-other-day treatment may be needed until resolved.	80 IU/kg factor IX concentrate‡; treatment every 2-3 days may be needed until resolved.
Mouth, deciduous tooth, or tooth extraction	20 IU/kg factor VIII concentrate; antifibrinolytic therapy; remove loose deciduous tooth.	40 IU/kg factor IX concentrate‡; antifibrinolytic therapy§; remove loose deciduous tooth.
Epistaxis	Apply pressure for 15-20 min; pack with petrolatum gauze; give antifibrinolytic therapy; 20 IU/kg factor VIII concentrate if this treatment fails.ǁ	Apply pressure for 15-20 min; pack with petrolatum gauze; antifibrinolytic therapy; 30 IU/kg factor IX concentrate‡ if this treatment fails.
Major surgery, life-threatening hemorrhage	50-75 IU/kg factor VIII concentrate, then initiate continuous infusion of 2-4 IU/kg/hr to maintain factor VIII >100 IU/dl for 24 hrǁ then give 2-3 IU/kg/hr continuously for 5-7 days to maintain the level at >50 IU/dl and an additional 5-7 days to maintain the level at >30 IU/dl.¶	120 IU/kg factor IX concentrate‡, then 50-60 IU/kg every 12-24 hr to maintain factor IX at >40 IU/dl for 5-7 days, and then at >30 IU/dl for 7 days.
Iliopsoas hemorrhage	50 IU/kg factor VIII concentrate, then 25 IU/kg every 12 hr until asymptomatic, then 20 IU/kg every other day for a total of 10-14 days.**	120 IU/kg factor IX concentrate‡; then 50-60 IU/kg every 12-24 hr to maintain factor IX at >40 IU/dl until patient is asymptomatic; then 40-50 IU every other day for a total of 10-14 days.**††
Hematuria	Bed rest; 1½ × maintenance fluids; if not controlled in 1-2 days, 20 IU/kg factor VIII concentrate; if not controlled, give prednisone (unless patient is HIV-infected).	Bed rest; 1½ × maintenance fluids; if not controlled in 1-2 days, 40 IU/kg factor IX concentrate‡; if not controlled, give prednisone (unless patient is HIV-infected).
Prophylaxis	20-40 IU/kg factor VIII concentrate every other day to achieve a trough level ≥1%.	30-50 IU/kg factor IX concentrate‡ every 2-3 days to achieve a trough level ≥1%.

*For hip hemarthrosis, orthopedic evaluation tor possible aspiration is advisable to prevent avascular necrosis of the femoral head.
†For mild or moderate hemophilia, desmopressin, 0.3 μg/kg, should be used instead of factor VIII concentrate, if the patient is known to respond with a hemostatic level of factor VIII; if repeated doses are given, monitor factor VIII levels for tachyphylaxis.
‡Stated doses apply for recombinant factor IX concentrate; for plasma-derived factor IX concentrate, use 70% of the stated dose.
§Do not give antifibrinolytic therapy until 4-6 hr after a dose of prothrombin complex concentrate.
ǁOver-the-counter coagulation-promoting products may be helpful.
¶Alternatively, give 25 IU/kg every 12 hr to maintain a trough level >50% for 5-7 days followed by 25-30 IU/kg for an additional 5-7 days to maintain trough >25%.
**Repeat radiologic assessment should be performed before discontinuation of therapy.
††If repeated doses of factor IX concentrate are required, use highly purified, specific factor IX concentrate.
Adapted from Montgomery RR et al: Hemophilia and von Willebrand disease. In Nathan DG, Orkin SH (eds): *Nathan and Oski's hematology at infancy and childhood,* ed 5, Philadelphia, 1998, Saunders.

- The choice of the product for replacement therapy is guided by availability, capacity, concerns, and cost. Recombinant factors cost two to three times as much as plasma-derived factors, and the limited capacity to produce recombinant factors often results in periods of shortage. In the U.S., 60% of patients with severe hemophilia use recombinant products.
- Factor VIII concentrates are effective in controlling spontaneous and traumatic hemorrhage in severe hemophilia. The new recombinant factor VIII is stable without added human serum albumin (decreased risk of transmission of infectious agents).
- Alloantibodies (inhibitors) that neutralize factor VIII clotting function occur in nearly 30% of patients with severe hemophilia A after exposure to factor VIII. In these patients, bypassing agents (anti-inhibitor coagulant complex [AICC] and recombinant activated factor VII [rFVIIa]) can be used to treat bleeding. AICC can also be used prophylactically to decrease the frequency of joint and other bleeding events in patients with severe hemophilia A and factor VIII inhibitors.
- Recombinant activated factor VII is useful to stop spontaneous hemorrhages and prevent excessive bleeding during surgery in 75% of patients with inhibitors. Recommended dose is 90 μg/mg of body weight every 2 to 3 hr for treatment of life-threatening hemorrhage. It is, however, very expensive ($1 per μg).
- Desmopressin acetate 0.3 μg/kg q24h (causes release of factor VIII:C) may be used in preparation for minor surgical procedures in mild hemophiliacs.
- Aminocaproic acid (EACA, Amicar) 4 g PO q4h can be given for persistent bleeding that is unresponsive to factor VIII concentrate or desmopressin.

HEMOPHILIA B:

- Infuse factor IX concentrates. It is important to remember that factor IX concentrates contain other proteins that may increase the risk of thrombosis with recurrent use. Therefore factor IX concentrates must be used only when clearly indicated.
- Daily administration of oral cyclophosphamide and prednisone without empirical factor VIII therapy is an effective and well-tolerated treatment for acquired hemophilia.

CHRONIC Rx

- The aim of chronic treatment is to prevent spontaneous bleeding and excessive bleeding during any surgical intervention.
- Prophylaxis with recombinant factor VIII can prevent joint damage and decrease the frequency of joint and other hemorrhages in young boys with severe hemophilia A. The estimated annual cost for treatment of one patient with recombinant factor VIII is $300,000.
- Implantation of genetically altered fibroblasts that produce factor VIII is safe and well tolerated. This form is feasible in patients with severe hemophilia. Hemophilia will likely be the first common, severe genetic disease to be cured by gene therapy.

DISPOSITION

- Despite the advent of virally safe blood products and blood treatment programs, nearly 70% of hemophiliacs are HIV seropositive. Survival is of normal expectancy in HIV-negative patients with mild disease.
- Intracranial bleeds are the second most common cause of death in hemophiliacs after AIDS. They are fatal in 30% of patients, occur in 10% of patients, and are generally the result of trauma.

SUGGESTED READINGS

available at www.expertconsult.com

RELATED CONTENT

Hemophilia (Patient Information)

AUTHOR: **FRED F. FERRI, M.D.**

BASIC INFORMATION

DEFINITION

Hemoptysis is coughing up of blood originating from the lower respiratory tract, ranging from blood-streaked sputum to gross blood. If greater than 100 to 600 ml in 24 hours, considered massive hemoptysis.

ICD-9CM CODES
786.3 Hemoptysis
ICD-10CM CODES
R04.2 Hemoptysis

EPIDEMIOLOGY & DEMOGRAPHICS

INCIDENCE: Unknown, varies based on underlying pathology
RISK FACTORS: Tobacco smoking predisposes to lung cancer, a common cause of hemoptysis. Systemic processes (rheumatologic, renal hematologic) may contribute to alveolar hemorrhage or vasculitis. Anticoagulation can worsen bleeding.

PHYSICAL FINDINGS & CLINICAL PRESENTATION

- Presentation of hemoptysis is variable and can range from minimal blood-tinged sputum to more than 500 ml of gross blood in 24 hr. Other symptoms depend on the underlying etiology and can include cough, sputum production, fever, shortness of breath, weight loss, night sweats, wheezing, and chest pain.
- There are no specific exam findings, but clues to the etiology may be present, for example, focal wheezing, rhonchi or rales on pulmonary exam, murmur of mitral stenosis on cardiac exam.

ETIOLOGY

- There are many potential causes of hemoptysis including airway disease (bronchitis, bronchiectasis, lung neoplasm), infection (necrotizing pneumonia, lung abscess, tuberculosis, fungal infection), inflammatory diseases (Wegener's granulomatosis, Goodpasture's syndrome, lupus), cardiac disease (mitral stenosis after rheumatic heart disease, congenital heart diseases), and others (pulmonary embolism, cocaine use, foreign body, airway trauma, iatrogenic and cryptogenic).

Dx DIAGNOSIS

DIFFERENTIAL DIAGNOSIS

- Various potential causes of lower respiratory tract bleeding
  - Airway disease (bronchitis, bronchiectasis, lung neoplasm)
  - Infection (necrotizing pneumonia, lung abscess, tuberculosis, fungal infection)
  - Inflammatory diseases (Wegener's granulomatosis, Goodpasture's syndrome, lupus)
  - Cardiac disease (mitral stenosis after rheumatic heart disease, congenital heart diseases)
  - Pulmonary embolism
  - Cocaine use
  - Foreign body
  - Airway trauma
- Bleeding from upper respiratory tract
- Hematemesis
- Coagulopathy

WORKUP

Complete history and physical exam may suggest a particular etiology; important to ask about duration and quantity of hemoptysis and smoking history.

LABORATORY TESTS

- Complete blood count
- Coagulation profile
- Serum chemistries including creatinine, urinalysis; if abnormal, consider vasculitis serologies (i.e., ANA, ANCA, anti-GBM)
- Arterial blood gas to assess oxygenation
- Sputum for cultures and cytologic studies

IMAGING STUDIES

- Chest x-ray: all patients with hemoptysis should have a chest x-ray but will likely need additional studies to localize site of bleeding.
- Chest CT: chest CT scan combined with flexible bronchoscopy has the highest yield for localizing the site of bleeding.

Rx TREATMENT

Varies based on underlying etiology and non-massive versus massive hemoptysis

NONPHARMACOLOGIC THERAPY

Massive hemoptysis:
- Arteriographic embolization of bronchial arteries and/or collateral systemic vessels
- Surgical resection of affected lung

ACUTE GENERAL Rx

Massive hemoptysis:
- Stabilize hemodynamic status and oxygenation.
- Reverse any coagulopathy.
- Bronchoscopy can be used to identify cause of hemoptysis (e.g., neoplasm), as well as to help isolate a side/segment of bleeding.
- If site of bleeding is known, place patient with bleeding lung in dependent position to prevent blood from spilling into nonaffected lung.
- Bronchoscopic lavage with iced saline or topical application of epinephrine can be tried as a temporizing measure.
- Bronchoscopic balloon tamponade of bleeding site can be used as temporizing measure.
- Early consultation with interventional radiology and thoracic surgery for definitive intervention is recommended.

Submassive hemoptysis:
For submassive hemoptysis, identify and treat underlying condition. Referral to pulmonologist or hematologist if indicated.

CHRONIC Rx

For patients requiring anticoagulation or antiplatelet therapy for another disorder, consider risks/benefits of continued anticoagulation or antiplatelet therapy.

DISPOSITION

Generally, patients have a good prognosis after an episode of hemoptysis, but those with massive bleeding and/or malignancy tend to have a poorer prognosis.

SUGGESTED READINGS

available at www.expertconsult.com

RELATED CONTENT

Fig. 3-89 Evaluation of hemoptysis (Algorithm)

AUTHORS: **SARAH TAPYRIK, M.D.,** and **MICHAEL BLUNDIN, M.D.**

BASIC INFORMATION

DEFINITION

A hemorrhoid is a varicose dilation of a vein of the superior or inferior hemorrhoidal plexus, resulting from a persistent increase in venous pressure. External hemorrhoids are below the pectinate line (inferior plexus). Internal hemorrhoids are above the pectinate line (superior plexus).

SYNONYMS

Piles

ICD-9CM CODES
455.6 Hemorrhoids
ICD-10CM CODES
K64.9 Unspecified hemorrhoids

EPIDEMIOLOGY & DEMOGRAPHICS

Potential for development of symptomatic hemorrhoids in all adults
PREVALENCE: ~50% of adults in U.S.
PREDOMINANT SEX: Males and females affected equally

PHYSICAL FINDINGS & CLINICAL PRESENTATION

- Painless bleeding with defecation; bleeding is bright red with staining seen on toilet paper
- Perianal irritation
- Mucofecal staining of underclothes
- Acute external hemorrhoids: painful, swollen, and often thrombosed (Fig. 1-444)
- Pain on sitting, standing, or defecating (thrombosed hemorrhoid)
- Prolapse (Fig. 1-445)
- Constipation
- A classification of internal hemorrhoids is described in Table 1-223

ETIOLOGY

- Low-fiber, high-fat diet
- Chronic constipation and straining with defecation
- High resting anal sphincter pressures
- Pregnancy
- Obesity
- Rectal surgery (i.e., episiotomy)
- Prolonged sitting

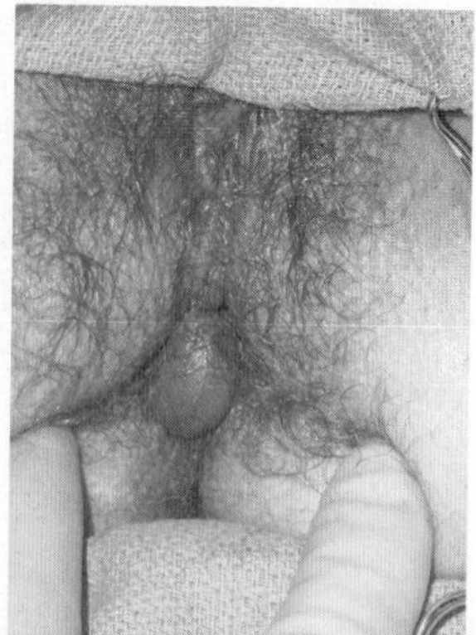

FIGURE 1-444 Thrombosed external hemorrhoid. (From Cameron JL, Cameron AM: *Current surgical therapy,* ed 10, Philadelphia, 2011, Saunders.)

- Anal intercourse

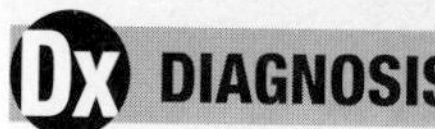

DIAGNOSIS

DIFFERENTIAL DIAGNOSIS

- Fissure
- Abscess
- Anal fistula
- Condylomata acuminata
- Hypertrophied anal papillae
- Rectal prolapse
- Rectal polyp
- Neoplasm (anal cancer, colorectal cancer)
- Inflammatory bowel disease

WORKUP

- Inspection
- Digital rectal examination
- Anoscopy
- Sigmoidoscopy

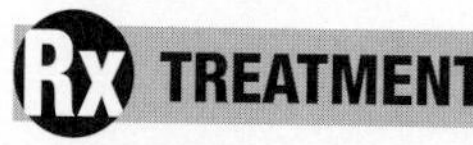

TREATMENT

NONPHARMACOLOGIC THERAPY

- Avoidance of constipation and straining with defecation

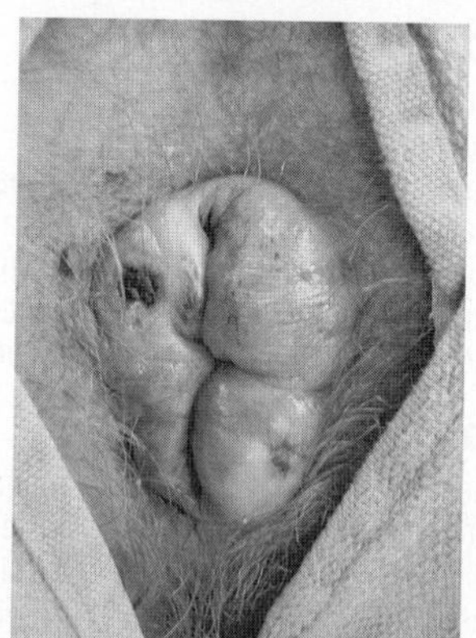

FIGURE 1-445 Prolapsed and thrombosed internal hemorrhoids. (From Cameron JL, Cameron AM: *Current surgical therapy,* ed 10, Philadelphia, 2011, Saunders.)

TABLE 1-223 Classification of Internal Hemorrhoids

SEVERITY (DEGREE)	FINDINGS
First	No prolapse; painless bleeding
Second	Prolapse with straining and spontaneous reduction Mild discomfort and bleeding
Third	Prolapse with straining, which requires manual reduction Some throbbing pain, itching, bleeding, and mucus discharge
Fourth	Permanent prolapse that cannot be reduced Pain and bleeding common Potential for thrombosis and strangulation

From Adams JG et al: *Emergency medicine, clinical essentials,* ed 2, Philadelphia, 2013, Elsevier.

- Avoidance of prolonged sitting on toilet
- High-fiber diet (20 to 30 g/day)
- Increased fluid intake (six to eight glasses of water per day)
- Cleaning with mild soap and water after defecation
- Warm soaks or ice to soothe
- Sitz baths

ACUTE GENERAL Rx

- Fiber supplements to provide bulk (psyllium extracts or mucilloids)
- Medicated compresses with witch hazel
- Topical hydrocortisone (1% to 3% cream or ointment)
- Topical anesthetic spray
- Glycerin suppositories
- Stool softeners
- Surgically remove during first 72 hr after onset

CHRONIC Rx

- Rubber-band ligation
- Injection sclerotherapy
- Photocoagulation
- Cryodestruction
- Hemorrhoidectomy
- Anal dilation
- Laser or cautery hemorrhoidectomy
- Observance for complications: thrombosis, bleeding, infection, anal stenosis or weakness
- Figs. E1-446 and E1-447 illustrate the technique for excision of thrombosed external hemorrhoids

DISPOSITION

Should resolve, but high rate of recurrence

REFERRAL

To colorectal or general surgeon for any hemorrhoid that does not respond to conservative therapy

PEARLS & CONSIDERATIONS

COMMENTS

- Patients need to understand the importance of a healthy diet, regular exercise, and rectal hygiene.
- Stress the importance of avoiding prolonged sitting and straining on the toilet.
- Stress the need not to defer the urge to defecate.

SUGGESTED READINGS

available at www.expertconsult.com

RELATED CONTENT

Anal Fissure (Related Key Topic)
Hemorrhoids (Patient Information)
Hemorrhoids (Primary Care Procedures in Appendix)

AUTHOR: **RUBEN ALVERO, M.D.**

BASIC INFORMATION

DEFINITION

Henoch-Schönlein purpura (HSP) is a systemic, small-vessel, IgA immune complex–mediated leukocytoclastic vasculitis characterized by a tetrad of palpable purpura, abdominal pain, renal disease, and arthritis/arthralgias. It may also present with gastrointestinal (GI) bleeding.

SYNONYMS

Anaphylactoid purpura
Allergic purpura

ICD-9CM CODES
287.0 Henoch-Schönlein purpura
ICD-10CM CODES
D69.0 Allergic purpura

EPIDEMIOLOGY & DEMOGRAPHICS

INCIDENCE: Annual incidence of 20 cases/100,000 population
PEAK INCIDENCE: Majority in spring, rarely in summer
PREVALENCE: Most common vasculitis seen in children and younger age groups; whites and Asians more common than black patients
PREDOMINANT SEX: 2:1 male/female ratio
PREDOMINANT AGE: Seen mostly from ages 4 to 15, although can be seen in older adolescents and young adults

PHYSICAL FINDINGS & CLINICAL PRESENTATION

- Palpable purpura (Fig. 1-448) of dependent areas, especially lower extremities and areas subjected to pressure, such as the beltline in adults or buttocks in toddlers.
- Subcutaneous edema.
- Arthralgias and arthritis in 80%. Typically oligoarticular, affecting lower extremity and large joints. Periarticular swelling and tenderness also noted.
- GI symptoms are seen in approximately one third of patients. Common findings are nausea, vomiting, diarrhea, cramping, abdominal pain, hematochezia, and melena. Complications include GI bleeding (20% to 30%), bowel ischemia, intussusception, and bowel perforation.
- Anecdotally may follow upper respiratory infection.
- Renal involvement is seen in as many as 80% of older children, usually within the first month of illness. Fewer than 5% progress to end-stage renal failure, a major cause of morbidity. Renal manifestations may range from isolated hematuria or proteinuria to acute nephropathy with renal insufficiency.

ETIOLOGY

- Presumptive etiology is exposure to a trigger antigen that causes antibody formation.
- Antigen-antibody (immune) complex deposition then occurs in arteriole and capillary walls of skin, renal mesangium, and GI tract. Immunoglobulin (Ig) A deposition is most common.
- Antigen triggers postulated include drugs, foods, immunization, and upper respiratory and other viral illnesses. Group A streptococcal infection is the most common precipitant in children, seen in up to one third of cases. A recent adult case triggered by pantoprazole has also been reported.
- Serologic and pathologic evidence suggests an association between parvovirus B19 and HSP, which may explain observed cases of HSP that do not respond to corticosteroids or other immunosuppressive therapy.
- Case reports describing development of HSP after treatment with immunosuppressive agents (e.g., etanercept) have been published.
- Recent studies suggest an association with the "Mediterranean fever" (MEFV) gene.

Dx DIAGNOSIS

- Diagnosis is based on the finding of IgA in the affected vessels. Table 1-224 describes common clinical manifestations of HSP.
- Skin manifestations are most common.
- Palpable purpura (see Fig. 1-449) is seen in 70% of adult patients, whereas GI symptoms are more common in children.
- A total of 20% to 54% of children with HSP will have some early renal involvement.
- Skin biopsy shows leukocytoclastic vasculitis. Renal biopsy shows mesangial IgA deposition.
- The presence of two of the following four American College of Rheumatology criteria yields a diagnostic sensitivity of 87.1% and specificity of 87.7%:
  - Palpable purpura unrelated to thrombocytopenia
  - Age <20 yr at onset of first symptoms
  - Bowel angina or ischemia
  - Granulocytic infiltration of arteriole or venule walls on biopsy

TABLE 1-224 Clinical Manifestations of Henoch-Schönlein Purpura

	% at Onset	% during Course
Purpura (nl platelet count)	50	100
Subcutaneous edema	10-20	20-50
Arthritis (large joints)	25	60-85
Gastrointestinal	30	85
Renal	?	10-50
Genitourinary (ddx torsion)	?	2-35
Pulmonary (T_LCO)	?	95
Pulmonary hemorrhage	?	Rare, may be fatal
Central nervous system (headache, organic brain syndrome, seizures)	?	Rare, may be fatal

From Hochberg MC et al: *Rheumatology*, ed 5, St Louis, 2011, Mosby.

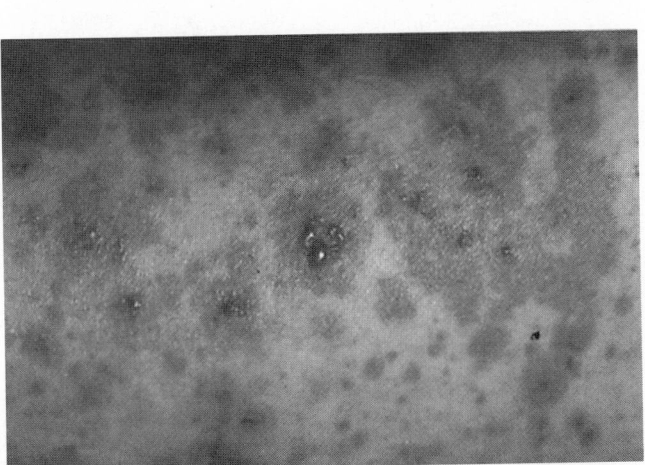

FIGURE 1-448 Palpable purpura in a patient with Henoch-Schönlein purpura. (From Hoffman R et al [eds]: Hematology: basic principles and practice, ed 4, Philadelphia, 2005, Saunders.)

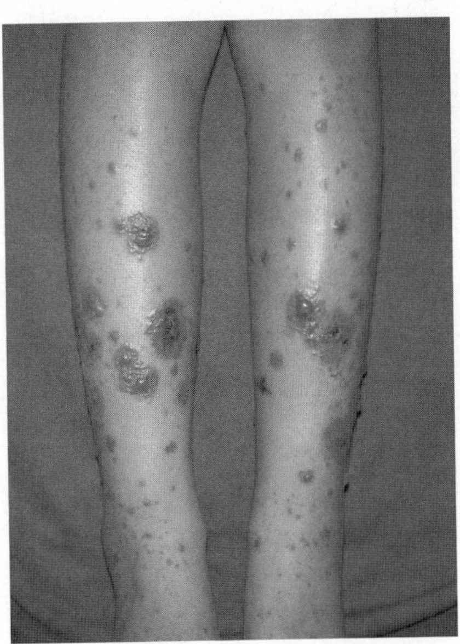

FIGURE 1-449 Extensive palpable purpura over the lower extremities in a 7-yr-old girl with Henoch-Schönlein purpura. (From Hochberg MC et al: *Rheumatology*, ed 5, St Louis, 2011, Mosby.)

 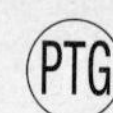

DIFFERENTIAL DIAGNOSIS

- Polyarteritis nodosa
- Meningococcemia
- Thrombocytopenic purpura
- Hypersensitivity vasculitis
- Microscopic polyangiitis
- Wegener granulomatosis

WORKUP

History, physical examination, laboratory testing, skin or renal biopsy

LABORATORY TESTS

- Electrolytes, blood urea nitrogen, and creatinine
- Urinalysis
- Complete blood count
- Prothrombin time, fibrinogen, and fibrin degradation products
- Blood cultures

Laboratory abnormalities are not specific for HSP. Leukocytosis and eosinophilia may be seen. IgA levels are elevated in approximately 50% of patients. Glomerulonephritis may be present (microscopic hematuria, proteinuria, and red blood cell casts). GI involvement may be associated with elevated interleukin (IL) 6 levels. Renal involvement may be associated with elevated IL8 and IgA anticardiolipin antibody levels.

IMAGING STUDIES

Imaging studies are generally not useful in the diagnosis of HSP. Arteriography or magnetic resonance angiography may be helpful in distinguishing from polyarteritis nodosa. Abdominal ultrasound is recommended for patients with severe abdominal pain to detect increased bowel wall thickness, peritoneal fluid, or intussusception.

Rx TREATMENT

- Nonsteroidal anti-inflammatory drugs for arthritis and arthralgias.
- Prednisone 1 mg/kg PO is given if renal or severe GI disease, although clear benefits in renal disease have not been demonstrated according to a recent Cochrane systematic review of pediatric patients.
- A double-blind, randomized, controlled trial found that early treatment with prednisone reduced abdominal pain and joint symptoms but did not prevent development of renal disease. It was effective in the treatment of renal disease once it was established.
- Corticosteroids and azathioprine may be beneficial if rapidly progressive glomerulonephritis is present. Pulse methylprednisolone therapy has also been proposed in patients with glomerulonephritis, mesenteric vasculitis, or pulmonary involvement. Recent reports describe improvement in rapidly progressive glomerulonephritis and nephrotic-range proteinuria after treatment with mycophenolate mofetil. The combination of cyclosporin A with corticosteroids appears to be effective in inducing remission of nephrotic syndrome in adult patients with HSP nephritis.
- Hospitalization for significant GI or renal involvement.

NONPHARMACOLOGIC THERAPY

Supportive care with pain management, adequate hydration, and nutrition

DISPOSITION & PROGNOSIS

- Prognosis excellent, with spontaneous recovery of most patients within 4 wk.
- Increased age of onset generally correlates with morbidity. While end-stage renal disease (ESRD) occurs in 10% to 30% of adult patients with HSP at 15 years, chronic renal insufficiency is the most common long-term morbidity and affects adults more than children.
- GI complications (mesenteric infarction, perforation, and intussusception).
- Recurrences in up to one third of patients, especially within first 4 to 6 mo after initial episode and most commonly in patients with renal involvement. Recurrences less severe than initial episode.

REFERRAL

Nephrologist or gastroenterologist

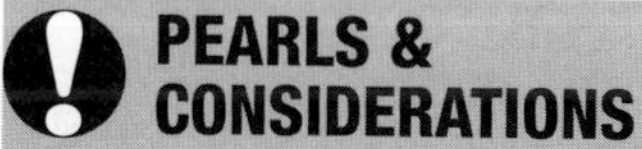

PEARLS & CONSIDERATIONS

- HSP is an IgA-related vasculitis.
- Organ systems involved are skin, joints, GI tract, and kidneys.
- Palpable purpura more common in adults; GI symptoms more common in children.
- Most with spontaneous recovery within 4 wk of onset of symptoms.
- End-stage renal disease occurs in only 5% of patients.
- Steroids and immunosuppressive agents may offer some benefit.

SUGGESTED READINGS

available at www.expertconsult.com

RELATED CONTENT

Henoch-Schönlein Purpura (Patient Information)

AUTHOR: **DOMINICK TAMMARO, M.D.**

BASIC INFORMATION

DEFINITION

There are two forms of heparin-induced thrombocytopenia (HIT). Type 1 HIT is a mild, transient decrease in platelet count that occurs during the first few days of heparin exposure due to platelet agglutination. This form is benign, and the platelet count will return to normal while heparin is continued. This section will refer to Type 2 HIT, an antibody-mediated thrombocytopenia that is associated with a high risk of developing thrombosis.

SYNONYMS

Type II heparin-induced thrombocytopenia
Heparin-induced thrombocytopenia and thrombosis (HITT)
White clot syndrome
Heparin-associated immune thrombocytopenia

ICD-9CM CODES
289.84 Heparin-induced thrombocytopenia (HIT)
ICD-10CM CODES
D75.82 Heparin-induced thrombocytopenia (HIT)

EPIDEMIOLOGY & DEMOGRAPHICS

INCIDENCE: Occurs in 0.2% to 5% of patients exposed to heparin. Unfractionated heparin is associated with a 5 to 10 times higher risk of HIT compared to low-molecular-weight heparin. Initially, there was an overwhelming underdiagnosis of HIT; however, since the introduction of HIT antibody ELISA test, there is a propensity to overdiagnose HIT irrespective of the clinical scenario.
PREDOMINANT SEX AND AGE: Females are at slightly higher risk than males. More common in adults but may also occur in children.
RISK FACTORS: Longer duration of exposure to heparin, type of heparin (unfractionated heparin has a greater risk), type of patient (surgical patients, especially cardiac and orthopedic surgery, are at higher risk than medical patients).

PHYSICAL FINDINGS & CLINICAL PRESENTATION

Suspect in a patient with:
- Exposure to heparin for 4 to 14 days OR who was exposed to heparin in the prior 3 mo
- Unexplained platelet count decrease to 50% below pretreatment baseline
- Onset of thrombocytopenia 5 to 10 days after heparin initiation
- Evidence of acute venous or arterial thrombosis
- Skin lesions/necrosis at heparin injection sites
- Acute anaphylactoid reaction during administration of heparin bolus

ETIOLOGY

Occurs due to the formation of antibodies, directed against heparin in complex with platelet factor 4, which bind to and activate platelets. Activated platelets release platelet factor 4 (leading to more antibody production) and undergo aggregation and premature removal from the circulation (resulting in thrombocytopenia). This platelet activation and antibody formation also can lead to thrombosis. Fig. E1-450 illustrates the mechanism of HIT.

Dx DIAGNOSIS

DIFFERENTIAL DIAGNOSIS

Thrombocytopenia due to other causes including:
- Sepsis
- Disseminated intravascular coagulation
- Thrombocytopenic thrombotic purpura
- Hemolytic uremic syndrome
- Drug-induced thrombocytopenia (other than heparin)
- Antiphospholipid antibody syndrome.

WORKUP

HIT is first and foremost a clinical diagnosis. See Table 1-225 for workup based on pretest probability. If the patient has a low pretest probability score, heparin can be safely continued, and there is no need to send for further testing for HIT. If the patient has a moderate to high pretest probability, HIT testing (Table 1-226), imaging studies for lower-extremity deep venous thrombosis (also consider imaging of upper extremities if swelling is present or venous catheters are in place), cessation of heparin products, and alternative anticoagulation should all be performed. Patients with intermediate

TABLE 1-225 A Diagnostic and Treatment Approach to Heparin-Induced Thrombocytopenia

Suspicion of HIT based upon the "**4 T's**"	Score	Pre-test Probability Score Criteria: 2	1	0
Thrombocytopenia	☐	nadir 20-100, or >50% platelet fall	nadir 10-19, or 30-50% platelet fall	nadir <10, or <30% platelet fall
Timing of onset of platelet fall	☐	day 5-10, or ≤day 1 with recent heparin*	>day 10 or timing unclear (but fits with HIT)	≤day 1 (no recent heparin)
Thrombosis or other sequelae	☐	proven thrombosis, skin necrosis, or ASR†	progressive, recurrent, or silent thrombosis; erythematous skin lesions	none
OTher cause of platelet fall	☐	none evident	possible	definite
Total Pre-test Probability Score	☐	periodic reassessment as new information can change pre-test probability (e.g., positive blood cultures)		

Total Pre-test Probability Score

High	Moderate	Low
8 | 7 | 6	5 | 4	3 | 2 | 1 | 0
Stop heparin‡, give alternative non-heparin anticoagulant argatroban¶ or lepirudin# or danaparoid** (or bivalirudin†† or fondaparinux‡‡)	Physician judgment	Continue (LMW) heparin

HIT Test
- **Positive** test for HIT antibodies: Continue non-heparin anticoagulant until platelet count recovery
- **Negative** test for HIT antibodies: Consider continuing or switching back to (LMW) heparin ##

Imaging studies for lower-limb DVT †††
- **Thrombosis*****: **If HIT,** continue non-heparin anticoagulant until platelet count recovery, then **cautious coumarin overlap¶¶**
- **No Thrombosis**: **If HIT,** consider anticoagulating until platelet count recovery, even if no thrombosis apparent (± coumarin ¶¶)

* recent heparin indicates exposure within the past 30 days (2 points) or past 30-100 days (1 point)
† ASR, acute systemic reaction following *i.v.* heparin bollus (see Table 4)
‡ stop all heparin, including catheter "flushes" and, possibly, heparin-coated catheters
¶ argatroban: approved (U.S., Canada) for isolated HIT and HIT complicated by thrombosis (2 μg/kg/min *i.v.*, adjusted to 1.5-3.0X patient's baseline aPTT or the mean of the laboratory normal range); reduce dose for hepatobiliary compromise: may increase INR more than the other direct thrombin inhibitors, thus requiring care in managing coumarin overlap (see ¶¶ below)
\# lepirudin: approved (U.S., Canada, E.U., elsewhere) for treatment of thrombosis complicating HIT (±0.4 mg/kg *i.v.* bolus, then 0.15 mg/kg/h adjusted to 1.5-2.5X patient's baseline aPTT or mean of the laboratory normal range); used (off-label) also to treat isolated HIT (0.1 mg/kg/h, adjusted by aPTT); to avoid overdosing and anaphylaxis, it may be preferable to omit the bolus, and begin as *i.v.* infusion (except when facing life- or limb-threatening thrombosis); reduce dose for renal insufficiency
** danaparoid: usual *i.v.* bolus, 2,250 U (body weight 60-75 kg) followed by infusion (400 U/hr for 4 h, then 300 U/h for 4 h, then 200 U/h, adjusted by anti-factor Xa levels); this therapeutic-dose regimen is appropriate both for isolated HIT and for HIT complicated by thrombosis (though higher than approved dose in some jurisdictions); withdrawn from U.S. market (2002)
†† bivalirudin: no bolus, *i.v.* infusion 0.15 mg/kg/h adjusted by aPTT; limited experience (off-label)
‡‡ fondaparinux: dosing for HIT not established; limited experience (off-label)
¶¶ delay coumarin pending substantial platelet count recovery (at least >100, preferably >150); begin coumarin in low doses, with at least 4-5 day overlap, stopping alternative anticoagulant when INR therapeutic for 2 days and platelets recovered
\## depending on physician confidence in the laboratory's ability to rule out HIT antibodies (usually, negative PF4-dependent enzyme-immunoassay and/or washed platelet activation assay performed by an experienced laboratory)
*** some thrombi may require special treatment, e.g., thrombectomy for large limb artery thrombosis
††† routine ultrasound of lower-limb veins recommended, since many HIT patients have subclinical deep-vein thrombosis (DVT)

From Warkentin TE et al: Platelet-endothelial interactions: sepsis, HIT, and antiphospholipid syndrome, *Hematology (Am Soc Hematol Educ Prog)* 497-519, 2003.

TABLE 1-226 Laboratory Assays for Heparin-Induced Thrombocytopenia

Assay	Sensitivity (%)	Specificity (%)	Positive Predictive Value (%)	Negative Predictive Value (%)
Functional assay (e.g., serotonin release assay)	88	≈100	≈100	81
PF4/heparin enzyme immunoassay (ELISA)	95-98	86	93	95

ELISA, Enzyme-linked immunosorbent assay; *PF4,* platelet factor 4.
From Goldman L, Schafer AI: *Goldman's Cecil medicine,* ed 24, Philadelphia, 2012, Saunders.

and high pretest probability but no HIT antibodies or intermediate pretest probability and only weakly positive HIT antibodies (based on optical density, see below) can resume heparin use as HIT is unlikely in these scenarios. Patients with high pretest probability and weakly positive antibodies or intermediate/high pretest probability and moderate to strongly positive antibodies likely have HIT and should be treated as such.

LABORATORY TESTS

In the appropriate clinical setting, testing for HIT antibodies with an enzyme-linked immunosorbent assay, or ELISA, can be useful. This test is very sensitive, but not specific. The majority of patients with positive testing for HIT antibodies will not develop clinical HIT. Thus, HIT antibody testing is more effective for ruling out rather than confirming the diagnosis of HIT. More recently, use of the HIT Ab optical density as well as the immunoglobulin subtypes of the HIT antibody have entered the diagnostic realm. Higher optical density levels are associated with increased likelihood of a positive functional assay, higher pretest probability score, and increased risk of thrombosis. Weakly positive optical densities (0.4 to 1.0) are only rarely associated with functional assay positivity. In contrast, optical densities greater than 2.0 almost always show heparin-dependent platelet activation. Optical densities are thus defined as weakly positive (0.4-1.0), moderately positive (1.0-2.0), or strongly positive (>2.0). The HIT Ab IgG subtype is the pathologic antibody for HIT. Hence, use of IgG-specific ELISAs increases the test specificity over the polyspecific (IgA/M/G) antibody. Patients with low pretest probability should not have HIT antibody testing performed, while all patients with intermediate and high pretest probability of HIT benefit from HIT Ab testing.

The gold standard test for HIT is to measure heparin-dependent platelet activation via the serotonin release assay (14C-SRA). Donor platelets are incubated with radiolabeled serotonin. The platelets internalize the serotonin and are then exposed to the patient's serum and heparin at a therapeutic concentration. If antibodies to the platelet factor 4-heparin complex are present in the patient's serum, the platelets react and released radioactive serotonin is then measured. Availability and turn-around time of this test is dependent on the institution, which can influence the test's clinical utility. Cases where there is intermediate pretest probability but only a weakly positive HIT Ab benefit the most from confirmatory SRA testing. Here, a positive SRA test will argue for HIT while negative SRA tests will suggest absence of HIT.

IMAGING STUDIES

Doppler sonography of the extremities in the correct clinical setting

Rx TREATMENT

- For patients with a moderate or high pretest probability, discontinue all heparin exposure. Even if the patient does not have a clinically evident thrombosis, they are at a 50% risk of developing a clot within the subsequent 30 days. Thus, the patient must be started on an alternate anticoagulant.
- Three agents, all direct thrombin inhibitors, are approved for this indication:
  - argatroban (avoid in liver dysfunction)
  - lepirudin (avoid in renal dysfunction)
  - bivalirudin (bivalirudin is approved only for patients with HIT or at risk of HIT who are undergoing PCI).
- These drugs should be continued as a single agent until the platelet count returns to baseline (generally a platelet count of 150 $\times 10^9$/L but it is important to consider the individual patient's baseline), then warfarin can be added at a maximum dose of 5 mg/day. This overlap therapy should continue until the platelet count has reached a stable plateau, the INR has reached the intended target (remember that argatroban artificially elevates the INR), and after a minimum overlap of 5 days of both the direct thrombin inhibitor and warfarin. The length of treatment is controversial, but most clinicians agree that 1 month of alternate anticoagulation is sufficient in the absence of thrombosis, while 3 to 6 months of treatment is required in the presence of thrombosis.
- There is emerging data showing efficacy and lower bleeding risk in HIT for fondaparinux when compared with the direct thrombin inhibitors. Fondaparinux is a synthetic pentasaccharide that binds antithrombin, causing long-acting inhibition of activated factor X, but not thrombin. It is not FDA approved for HIT, but its use in HIT in pregnancy has been reported. It can initiate the formation of anti-PF4 antibodies, but it does not support platelet activation by the newly formed immune complexes.

NONPHARMACOLOGIC THERAPY

All nonpharmacologic therapies including surgical procedures

REFERRAL

Request a hematology consultation.

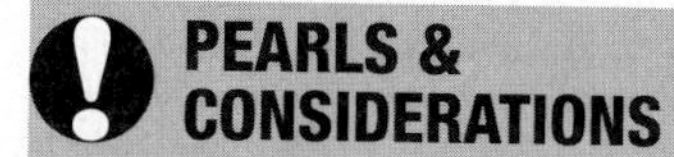

PEARLS & CONSIDERATIONS

COMMENTS

HIT paradoxically causes thrombocytopenia and *clotting,* not bleeding.

PREVENTION

Consider the use of low-molecular-weight heparin (as opposed to unfractionated heparin) as DVT prophylaxis.

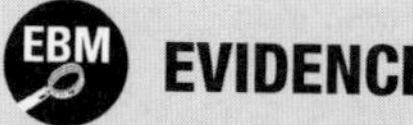

EVIDENCE

available at www.expertconsult.com

SUGGESTED READINGS

available at www.expertconsult.com

AUTHORS: **ANGELA M. TABER, M.D.,** and **JOHN L. REAGAN, M.D.**

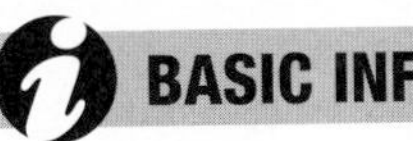

BASIC INFORMATION

DEFINITION

Hepatic encephalopathy is a neuropsychiatric syndrome occurring in patients with severe impairment of liver function and consequent accumulation of toxic products not metabolized by the liver. It is characterized by gradual impairment of the ability to perform mental tasks and to react to external stimuli. ***Minimal hepatic encephalopathy*** refers to patients with hepatic cirrhosis and mild cognitive impairment, but no history of overt encephalopathy.

SYNONYMS

Hepatic coma

ICD-9CM CODES
572.2 Hepatic encephalopathy
ICD-10CM CODES
K72.0 Acute and subacute hepatic failure
K72.1 Chronic hepatic failure
K72.9 Hepatic failure, unspecified

EPIDEMIOLOGY & DEMOGRAPHICS

INCIDENCE/PREVALENCE: Hepatic encephalopathy occurs in >50% of all cases of cirrhosis.

PHYSICAL FINDINGS & CLINICAL PRESENTATION

Hepatic encephalopathy can be classified by clinical stages described in Table 1-227.

The physical examination in hepatic encephalopathy varies with the stage and may reveal the following abnormalities:

- Skin: jaundice, palmar erythema, spider angiomata, ecchymosis, dilated superficial periumbilical veins (caput medusae) in patients with cirrhosis
- Eyes: scleral icterus, Kayser-Fleischer rings (Wilson's disease)
- Breath: fetor hepaticus
- Chest: gynecomastia in men with chronic liver disease
- Abdomen: ascites, small nodular liver (cirrhosis), tender hepatomegaly (congestive hepatomegaly)
- Rectal examination: hemorrhoids (portal hypertension), guaiac-positive stool (alcoholic gastritis, bleeding esophageal varices, peptic ulcer disease, bleeding hemorrhoids)
- Genitalia: testicular atrophy in males with chronic liver disease
- Extremities: pedal edema from hypoalbuminemia
- Neurologic: flapping tremor (asterixis), obtundation, coma with or without decerebrate posturing

ETIOLOGY

- Precipitating factors in patients with underlying cirrhosis (upper gastrointestinal bleeding, hypokalemia, hypomagnesemia, analgesic and sedative drugs, sepsis, alkalosis, increased dietary protein)
- Acute fulminant viral hepatitis
- Drugs and toxins (e.g., isoniazid, acetaminophen, diclofenac and other NSAIDs, statins, methyldopa, loratadine, propylthiouracil, lisinopril, labetalol, halothane, carbon tetrachloride, erythromycin, nitrofurantoin, troglitazone, herbal products, flavocoxid)
- Reye's syndrome
- Shock and/or sepsis
- Fatty liver of pregnancy
- Metastatic carcinoma, hepatocellular carcinoma
- Other: autoimmune hepatitis, ischemic veno-occlusive disease, sclerosing cholangitis, heat stroke, amebic abscesses

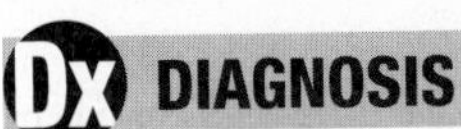

DIAGNOSIS

DIFFERENTIAL DIAGNOSIS

- Delirium caused by medications or illicit drugs
- Cerebrovascular accident, subdural hematoma
- Meningitis, encephalitis
- Hypoglycemia
- Uremia
- Cerebral anoxia
- Hypercalcemia
- Metastatic neoplasm to brain
- Alcohol withdrawal syndrome

WORKUP

Hepatic encephalopathy should be considered in any patient with cirrhosis who presents with neuropsychiatric manifestations. Exclude other etiologies with comprehensive history (obtained from patient, relatives, and others), physical examination, and laboratory and imaging studies. A pertinent history should include exposure to hepatitis, ethanol intake, drug history, exposure to toxins, IV drug abuse, measles or influenza with aspirin use (Reye's syndrome), and history of carcinoma (primary or metastatic). Minimal hepatic encephalopathy may not be obvious on clinical examination, but can be detected with neurophysiologic and neuropsychiatric testing.

LABORATORY TESTS

- Alanine aminotransferase, aspartate aminotransferase, bilirubin, alkaline phosphatase, glucose, calcium, electrolytes, blood urea nitrogen, creatinine, albumin
- Complete blood count, platelet count, prothrombin time, partial thromboplastin time
- Serum and urine toxicology screen in suspected medication or illegal drug use
- Blood and urine cultures, urinalysis
- Venous ammonia level
- Arterial blood gases

IMAGING STUDIES

CT scan or MRI of the brain may be useful in selected patients to exclude other etiologies when diagnosis is unclear.

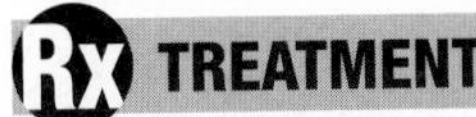

TREATMENT

NONPHARMACOLOGIC THERAPY

- Identification and treatment of precipitating factors
- Restriction of protein intake (30 to 40 g/day) to reduce toxic protein metabolites

ACUTE GENERAL Rx

Table 1-228 summarizes the management of fulminant hepatic failure.

Reduction of colonic ammonia production:

- Lactulose 30 ml of 50% solution qid initially; dose is subsequently adjusted depending on clinical response. Ornithine aspartate 9 g tid is also effective. Lactulose may improve hepatic encephalopathy but may be less effective than antibiotics.
- Neomycin 1 g PO q4 to 6h or given as a 1% retention enema solution (1 g in 100 ml of isotonic saline solution); neomycin should be used with caution in patients with renal insufficiency. Metronidazole 250 mg qid may be as effective as neomycin and is not nephrotoxic; however, long-term use can be associated with neurotoxicity.
- A combination of lactulose and neomycin can be used when either agent is ineffective alone.
- The oral antibiotic rifaximin (550 mg PO bid) is effective in reducing the risk of recurrent hepatic encephalopathy in patients with cirrhosis. It can be taken with lactulose, and the combination of lactulose and rifaximin is superior to lactulose alone in reversing hepatic encephalopathy. Rifamaxin has also been shown to be effective in improving psychometric performance and health-related

TABLE 1-227 Clinical Stages of Hepatic Encephalopathy

Stage	Asterixis	EEG Changes	Clinical Manifestations
I (prodrome)	Slight	Minimal	Mild intellectual impairment, disturbed sleep-wake cycle
II (impending)	Easily elicited	Usually generalized	Drowsiness, confusion, coma/inappropriate behavior, disorientation, mood swings
III (stupor)	Present if patient cooperative	Grossly abnormal slowing of rhythm	Drowsy, unresponsive to verbal commands, markedly confused, delirious, hyperreflexia, positive Babinski sign
IV (coma)	Usually absent	Appearance of delta waves, decreased amplitudes	Unconscious, decerebrate or decorticate response to pain present (stage IVA) or absent (stage IVB)

EEG, Electroencephalogram.
From Fuhrman BP et al: *Pediatric critical care,* ed 4, Philadelphia, 2011, Saunders.

 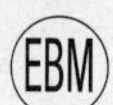 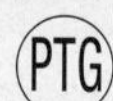

TABLE 1-228 Management of Fulminant Hepatic Failure

No sedation except for procedures
Minimal handling
Enteric precautions until infection ruled out
Monitor:
- Heart and respiratory rate
- Arterial BP, CVP
- Core/toe temperature
- Neurologic observations
- Gastric pH (>5.0)
- Blood glucose (>4 mmol/L)
- Acid-base
- Electrolytes
- PT, PTT

Fluid balance
- 75% maintenance
- Dextrose 10%-50% (provide 6-10 mg/kg/min)
- Sodium (0.5-1 mmol/L)
- Potassium (2-4 mmol/L)

Maintain circulating volume with colloid/FFP
Coagulation support only if required
Drugs
- Vitamin K
- H_2 antagonist
- Antacids
- Lactulose
- *N*-acetylcysteine for acetaminophen toxicity
- Broad-spectrum antibiotics
- Antifungals

Nutrition
- Enteral feeding (1-2 g protein/kg/day)
- PN if ventilated

BP, Blood pressure; *CVP,* central venous pressure; *FFP,* fresh frozen plasma; *PN,* parenteral nutrition; *PT,* prothrombin time; *PTT,* partial thromboplastin time.
From Fuhrman BP et al: *Pediatric critical care,* ed 4, Philadelphia, 2011, Saunders.

quality of life in patients with minimal hepatic encephalopathy. It is well tolerated but expensive.
- Probiotics (e.g., 1 capsule containing 112.5 billion viable lyophilized bacteria tid) might also be beneficial in altering gut flora to reduce ammonia production.

Treatment of cerebral edema:
- Cerebral edema is often present in patients with acute liver failure, and it accounts for nearly 50% of deaths. Monitoring intracranial pressure by epidural, intraparenchymal, or subdural transducers and treatment of cerebral edema with mannitol (100 to 200 ml of 20% solution [0.3 to 0.4 g/kg of body weight]) given by rapid IV infusion are helpful in selected patients (e.g., potential transplantation patients).
- Dexamethasone and hyperventilation (useful in head injury) are of little value in treating cerebral edema from liver failure.

CHRONIC Rx
- Avoidance of any precipitating factors (e.g., high-protein diet, medications)
- Consideration of liver transplantation in selected patients with progressive or recurrent encephalopathy (Box 1-34). Liver transplantation remains the only curative therapeutic option.

DISPOSITION
Prognosis varies with the underlying etiology of the liver failure and the grade of encephalopathy (generally good for grades 1 or 2; poor for grades 3 or 4).

REFERRAL
The early stages of hepatic encephalopathy can be managed in the outpatient setting, whereas stages 3 or 4 require hospital admission.

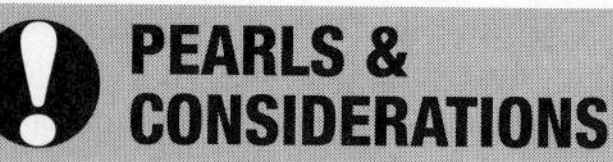
PEARLS & CONSIDERATIONS

COMMENTS
- Long-acting benzodiazepines should not be used to treat anxiety and sleep disorders in patients with cirrhosis, as they may precipitate encephalopathy.
- Patients not responding to supportive therapy should be evaluated for liver transplantation.
- Not all patients with cirrhosis develop hepatic encephalopathy. It has been shown that 40% of persons with cirrhosis and minimal hepatic encephalopathy do not develop overt hepatic encephalopathy in long-term follow-up. There are genetic factors associated with development of hepatic encephalopathy in patients with cirrhosis. Genetic analyses have shown that glutaminase TACC and CACC haplotypes are linked to the risk for overt hepatic encephalopathy.

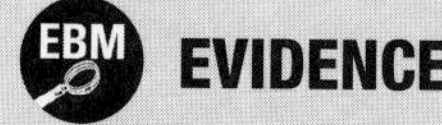
EVIDENCE
available at www.expertconsult.com

SUGGESTED READINGS
available at www.expertconsult.com

RELATED CONTENT
Hepatic Encephalopathy (Patient Information)
Cirrhosis (Related Key Topic)

AUTHOR: **FRED F. FERRI, M.D.**

BOX 1-34 Various Prognostic Criteria Used for Liver Transplantation in Patients with Fulminant Hepatic Failure

King's College Criteria
Acetaminophen overdose:
- Arterial pH <7.3 (irrespective of grade of encephalopathy) or
- PT >100 sec (INR >6.5)
- Serum creatinine >3.4 mg/dl (>300 μmol/L)
- Patients with grade III and IV hepatic encephalopathy

Nonacetaminophen liver injury:
- PT >100 sec (INR >6.5) (irrespective of grade of encephalopathy) or any three of the following variables:
  - Age <10 or >40 years
  - Non-A, non-B hepatitis, halothane hepatitis, idiosyncratic drug reactions
  - Jaundice >7 days before onset of encephalopathy
  - Serum bilirubin 17.4 mg/dl (300 μmol/L)
  - PT >50 sec

Cliché Criteria
Factor V <20% in person <30 years or both of the following:
- Factor V <30% in patients >30 years
- Grade III or IV encephalopathy

Serum Gc Globulin Levels
- Decreasing Gc levels due to dying hepatocytes

Serum α-Fetoprotein Level
- Serial increase from day 1 to day 3 has shown correlation with survival

Liver Biopsy[32]
70% necrosis is discriminant of 90% mortality

Gc, Plasma group-specific component protein; *INR,* international normalized ratio; *PT,* prothrombin time.
From Vincent JL et al: *Textbook of critical care,* ed 6, Philadelphia, 2011, Saunders.

BASIC INFORMATION

DEFINITION

Hepatitis A is generally an acute self-limiting infection of the liver by an enterically transmitted picornavirus, hepatitis A virus (HAV). Infection may range from asymptomatic to fulminant hepatitis.

SYNONYMS

Infectious hepatitis
Short incubation hepatitis
Type A hepatitis
HAV (hepatitis A virus)

ICD-9CM CODES
070.1 Hepatitis A
ICD-10CM CODES
B15.9 Hepatitis A without hepatic coma
B15.0 Hepatitis A with hepatic coma

EPIDEMIOLOGY & DEMOGRAPHICS

INCIDENCE:

- Hepatitis A occurs worldwide, affecting 1.4 million people annually and accounting for 20% to 40% of cases of viral hepatitis in the United States.
- The seroprevalence increases with age, ranging from 10% in individuals aged <5 yr to 74% in those aged >50 yr.
- In the United States, average disease rate was ~15 cases/100,000 persons/yr prior to routine vaccination of all children in certain states. The incidence after 2005 is about 1 case/100,000.
- The incidence is relatively higher in some regions in the United States, including Arizona, Alaska, California, Idaho, Nevada, New Mexico, Oklahoma, Oregon, South Dakota, and Washington.
- At-risk groups include:
  1. Residents and staff of group homes
  2. Children and employees of day care centers
  3. People who engage in oral-anal contact, regardless of sexual orientation
  4. IV drug abusers
  5. Travel to endemic areas
  6. Areas of overcrowding, poor sanitation, inadequate sewage treatment

PREVALENCE:

- Approximately three fourths of the U.S. population has serologic evidence of prior infection.
- Anti-HAV prevalence has an inverse relation to income and household size.

PREDOMINANT SEX: None, except higher infection rates seen in homosexual males who engage in oral-anal contact.

PREDOMINANT AGE/PEAK INCIDENCE:

- In areas of high rates of hepatitis A, virtually all children are infected while younger than 10 yr, but disease is rare.
- In areas of moderate rates of hepatitis A, disease occurs in late childhood and young adults.
- In areas of low rates of hepatitis A, most cases occur in young adults.

INCUBATION PERIOD: Averages 30 days (15 to 50)

PHYSICAL FINDINGS & CLINICAL PRESENTATION

- Infection with HAV may have acute or subacute presentation, icteric or anicteric. Severity of illness seems to increase with age (90% of infection in children aged <5 yr may be subclinical).
- A preicteric, prodromal phase of approximately 1 to 14 days; 15% no apparent prodrome. Symptoms are usually abrupt in onset and may include anorexia, malaise, nausea, vomiting, fever, headache, and abdominal pain.
- Less common symptoms are chills, myalgias, arthralgias, upper respiratory symptoms, constipation, diarrhea, pruritus, urticaria.
- Jaundice occurs in >70% of patients.
- The icteric phase is preceded by dark urine.
- Bilirubinuria is typically followed a few days later by clay-colored stools and icterus.

PHYSICAL EXAMINATION

- Jaundice: Peaks in severity 2 wk after onset
- Hepatomegaly
- Splenomegaly
- Cervical lymphadenopathy
- Evanescent rash
- Petechiae
- Cardiac arrhythmias

COMPLICATIONS

- Cholestasis
- Fulminant hepatitis
- Arthritis
- Myocarditis
- Optic neuritis
- Transverse myelitis
- Thrombocytopenic purpura
- Aplastic anemia
- Red cell aplasia
- Henoch-Schönlein purpura
- IgA dominant glomerulonephritis

ETIOLOGY

- Caused by HAV, a 27-nm, nonenveloped, icosahedral, positive-stranded RNA virus.
- Transmission is fecal-oral route, from person to person. Transmission occurs with close contact or with food- or water-borne outbreaks with inadequately purified water or cooked foods. Recent outbreaks have involved green onions and tomatoes.
- Parenteral transmission is considered rare.
- Vertical transmission has also been reported.

DIAGNOSIS

DIFFERENTIAL DIAGNOSIS

- Other hepatitis virus (B, C, D, E)
- Infectious mononucleosis
- Cytomegalovirus infection
- Herpes simplex virus infection
- Leptospirosis
- Brucellosis
- Drug-induced liver disease
- Ischemic hepatitis
- Autoimmune hepatitis

WORKUP

- IgM antibody specific for HAV
- Liver function tests; ALT and AST elevations are sensitive for liver damage but not specific for HAV
- Elevated ESR
- CBC; may find mild lymphocytosis

LABORATORY TESTS

- Diagnosis confirmed by IgM anti-HAV; it is detectable in almost all infected patients at presentation and remains positive for 3 to 6 mo.
- A fourfold rise in titer of total antibody (IgM and IgG) to HAV confirms acute infection.
- HAV detection in stool and body fluids by electron microscopy.
- HAV RNA detection in stool, body fluids, serum, and liver tissue.
- ALT and AST usually more than 8 times normal in acute infection.
- Bilirubin usually 5 to 15 times normal.
- Alkaline phosphatase minimally elevated but higher level in cholestasis.
- Albumin and prothrombin time are generally normal; if elevated, they may herald hepatic necrosis.
- Fig. 1-451 Illustrates the typical course of hepatis A.

IMAGING STUDIES

- Rarely useful
- Sonogram (fulminant hepatitis)

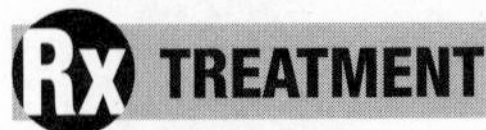

TREATMENT

- Usually self-limited
- Supportive care
- Those with fulminant hepatitis may require hospitalization and treatment of associated complications
- Activity as tolerated
- Advise to avoid alcohol and hepatotoxic drugs
- Patients with fulminant hepatitis should be assessed for liver transplantation

CHRONIC Rx

No chronic HAV and no chronic carrier state

DISPOSITION

- Follow-up as outpatient
- Most patients recover within 2 months of infection, although 10% to 15% of patients will experience a relapse in the first 6 months.
- HAV is a self-limited infection and does not cause chronic hepatitis.

REFERRAL

- To a hepatologist if severe, fulminant hepatitis develops
- To a transplant surgeon if liver transplant becomes a consideration for fulminant hepatitis and liver failure

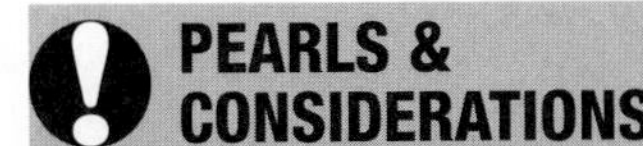

PEARLS & CONSIDERATIONS

- All cases of hepatitis A should be reported to the public heath authorities because food-borne or water-borne outbreaks may occur, and public health efforts (mass vaccination or immunoglobulin therapy) may prevent secondary cases.

- Hepatitis A is a common illness in internationally traveled and developing countries. Pretravel vaccination is strongly recommended for travelers who are HAV susceptible.

PREVENTION

- Improvement in hygiene and sanitation
- Heating food
- Avoidance of water and foods from endemic area

PASSIVE IMMUNIZATION

- Immunoglobulin provides protection against HAV through passive transfer of antibody.
- Preexposure prophylaxis indicated for people traveling to endemic areas (Ig 0.02 or 0.06 ml/kg given IM) and have not received or cannot receive the hepatitis A vaccine prior to departure. The lower dose is effective for up to 3 mo, and the higher dose is effective for up to 5 mo.
- Postexposure prophylaxis (Ig 0.02 ml/kg given IM) is indicated for people with recent exposure (within 2 wk) to HAV and who have not been previously vaccinated. In high-risk patients, vaccine may be administered with immunoglobulin.

ACTIVE IMMUNIZATION

- There are several inactivated and attenuated hepatitis vaccines; only the inactivated vaccines are currently available for use and they have been found to be safe and highly immunogenic: HAVRIX or VAQTA. These can be used in adults and children older than 12 mo. They are given as a two-dose regimen 6 mo to 1 yr apart. A combined hepatitis A and hepatitis B vaccine called TWINRX is also available.
- Protective antibody levels were reached in 94% to 100% of adults 1 mo after the first dose; similar results have been found for children and adolescents.
- Theoretic analyses of antibody levels estimate duration of immunity to be 10 to 20 yr.
- Vaccine should be considered for persons who are at risk: those traveling to or working in endemic areas, homosexual men, illegal drug users, persons with chronic liver disease, children in areas with high rates of hepatitis A infection.
- The Advisory Committee on Immunization Practices recommends routine hepatitis A vaccination for all children beginning at 12 to 23 mo of age.
- Recent data showed equivalency between use of Ig and hepatitis A vaccine for postexposure prophylaxis in preventing symptomatic hepatitis A in healthy persons 2 to 40 yr of age. The Advisory Committee guidelines now provide for the use of Ig or the vaccine for this population. Those patients who are immunocompromised, have chronic liver disease, or are less than 1 yr of age should receive Ig.

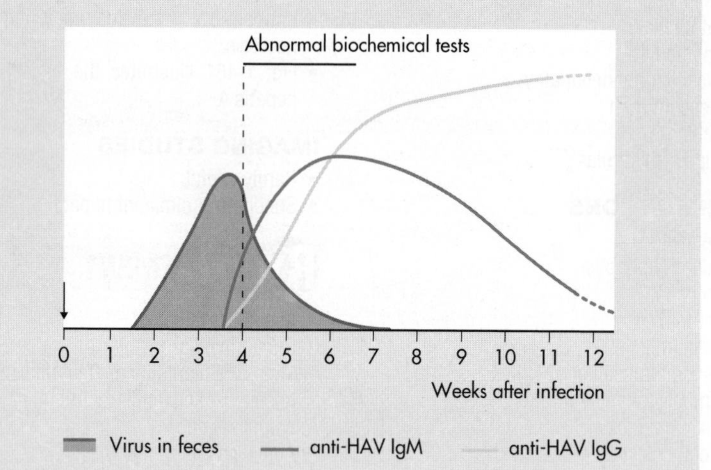

FIGURE 1-451 Course of acute hepatitis A. (From Cohen J, Powderly WG: *Infectious diseases,* ed 2, St Louis, 2004, Mosby.)

SUGGESTED READINGS

available at www.expertconsult.com

RELATED CONTENT

Hepatitis A (Patient Information)

AUTHOR: **GLENN G. FORT, M.D., M.P.H.**

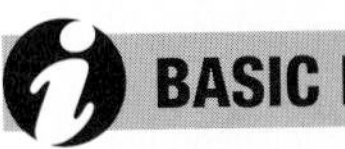

BASIC INFORMATION

DEFINITION

Hepatitis B is an acute infection of the liver parenchymal cells caused by the hepatitis B virus (HBV).

SYNONYMS

Serum hepatitis
Long incubation (30 to 180 days) hepatitis

ICD-9CM CODES
070.3 Hepatitis B
ICD-10CM CODES

B16	Acute hepatitis
B16.9	Acute hepatitis B without delta agent and without hepatic coma
B16.1	Acute hepatitis B with delta agent (coinfection) without hepatic coma
B18.0	Chronic hepatitis B with delta agent
B18.1	Chronic hepatitis B without delta agent
B19.10	Unspecified viral hepatitis B without hepatic coma

EPIDEMIOLOGY & DEMOGRAPHICS

INCIDENCE (IN U.S.):
- ~200,000 to 300,000 infections annually in the United States.
- Much higher incidence in Europe (~1 million new cases annually) and in areas of high endemicity.
- In U.S., transmission is mainly horizontal (percutaneous and mucous membrane exposure to infectious blood and other body fluids [e.g., sexual transmission, either homosexual or heterosexual]); also from needle sharing among drug abusers; occupational exposure to contaminated blood and blood products; persons receiving transfusions of blood and blood products; and hemodialysis patients.

NOTE: Improved screening of blood and blood products has greatly reduced, although not eliminated, the risk of posttransfusion HBV infection.
- In areas of high endemicity, transmission is largely vertical (perinatal): HBV exists in the blood and body fluids. Perinatal transmission from HBsAg-positive mothers is as high as 90% unless immunoprophylaxis is given.

PREVALENCE (IN U.S.):
- The WHO estimates that 400 million people worldwide (6% of the population) are chronic HBV carriers. North America, Western Europe, and Australia are areas of low prevalence, <2%. In the U.S. an estimated 800,000 to 1.4 million people have chronic HBV infection.
- Africa, Asia, and the Western Pacific region are areas of high prevalence, ≥8%.
- Southern and Eastern Europe have intermediate rates, 2% to 7%.
- Chronically infected persons, those with positive HBsAg for >6 mo, represent the major source of infection.
- As many as 95% of infants and children aged <5, who typically have subclinical acute infection, will become chronic HBV carriers.
- Adults are more likely to have clinically evident acute infection, but only 1% to 5% will develop chronic infection.
- ~0.1% of patients with acute infection will develop fulminant acute hepatitis resulting in death.

PREDOMINANT SEX:
- Predominant in males because of increased IV drug abuse, homosexuality
- Females more commonly terminate in chronic carrier state

PREDOMINANT AGE: 20 to 45 yr

PEAK INCIDENCE: 30 to 45 yr of age, at rates of 5% to 20%

GENETICS: Neonatal infection:
- Rare in U.S.
- High (up to 90%) in areas of high endemicity (only 5% to 10% of perinatal infections occur in utero)

PHYSICAL FINDINGS & CLINICAL PRESENTATION (Fig. 1-452)

- Often nonspecific symptoms
- Profound malaise
- Many asymptomatic cases
- Prodrome:
  1. 15% to 20% serum sickness (urticaria, rash, arthralgia) during early HBsAg
  2. HBsAg-Ab complex disease (polyarteritis nodosa–arthritis, arteritis, glomerulonephritis)
- Hepatomegaly (87%) with right upper quadrant (RUQ) tenderness
  1. Hepatic punch tenderness
  2. Splenomegaly: rare (10% to 15%)
- Jaundice, dark urine, with occasional pruritus
- Variable fever (when present, generally precedes jaundice and rapidly declines following onset of icteric phase)
- Spider angiomata: rare; resolves during recovery
- Rare polyarteritis nodosa, cryoglobulinemia

ETIOLOGY

- Caused by HBV (42-nm hepadnavirus with an outer surface coat [HBsAg], inner nucleocapsid core [HBcAg; HBeAg]; DNA polymerase; and partially double-stranded DNA genome). There are eight genotypes (A to H) based on nucleotide sequence. The prevalence of each genotype varies widely.
- Transmission by parenteral route (needle use, tattooing, ear piercing, acupuncture, transfusion of blood and blood products, hemodialysis, sexual contact), perinatal transmission.
- Infection may result from contact of infectious material with mucous membranes and open skin breaks (e.g., HBV is stable and can be transmitted from toothbrushes, utensils, razors, baby toys, assorted medical equipment [respirators, endoscopes]).
- Oral intake of infectious material may result in infection through breaks in the oral mucosa.
- Food or water are virtually never found to be sources of HBV infection.
- Infection occurs primarily in liver, where necrosis probably results from cytotoxic T-cell response, direct cytopathic effect of HBcAg (core antigen), high-level HBsAg (surface antigen) expression, or coinfection with delta (D) hepatitis virus (RNA delta core within HBsAg envelope).
- Recovery (>90%):
  - Fulminant hepatitis occurring in <1% (especially if coinfected with hepatitis D); 80% fatal
  - Unusual (5%) prolonged acute disease for 4 to 12 mo, with recovery
  - Overall fatality increases with age and viral inoculation (e.g., transfusions)
- Chronic infection (1% to 2%):
  - Persistent carrier state without hepatitis (HBsAg positive)
  - Chronic persistent hepatitis (CPH) (clinically well), or chronic active hepatitis (CAH) (HBsAg positive and HBeAg positive)
  - Cirrhosis
  - Hepatocellular carcinoma (especially after neonatal infection)
  - Chronic infection: more common following low-dose exposure and mild acute hepatitis, with earlier age of infection, in males, and in immunosuppressed patients

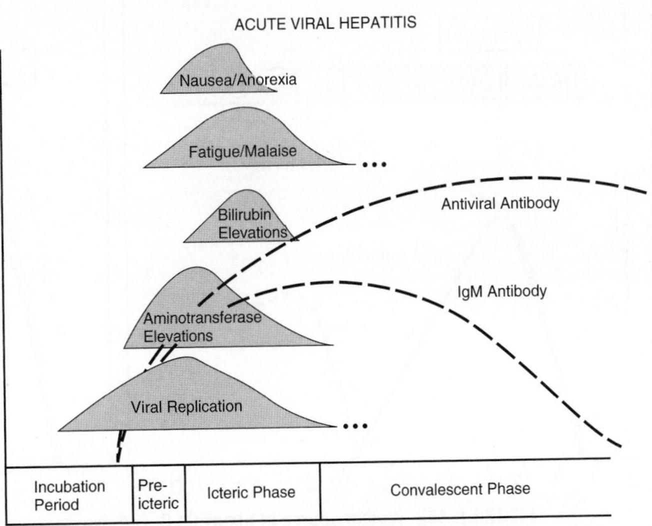

FIGURE 1-452 The typical course of acute viral hepatitis. (From Goldman L, Ausiello D [eds]: *Cecil textbook of medicine*, ed 22, Philadelphia, 2004, Saunders.)

- One third to one quarter of chronically infected will develop progressive liver disease (cirrhosis, hepatocellular carcinoma)

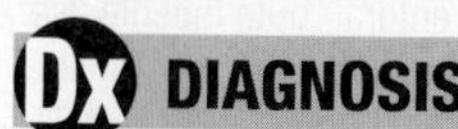

DIAGNOSIS

DIFFERENTIAL DIAGNOSIS

- Acute disease confused with other viral hepatitis infections (A, C, D, E)
- Any viral illness producing systemic disease and hepatitis (e.g., yellow fever, EBV, CMV, HIV, rubella, rubeola, coxsackie B, adenovirus, herpes simplex or zoster)
- Nonviral causes of hepatitis (e.g., leptospirosis, toxoplasmosis, alcoholic hepatitis, drug-induced [e.g., acetaminophen, INH], toxic hepatitis [carbon tetrachloride, benzene])

WORKUP

- Acute serum specimen for hepatitis B serology (HBsAg, HBsAb, HBcAb, HBeAg, HBeAb), HBDNA by PCR
- LFTs
- CBC
- Liver biopsy: rarely indicated for diagnosis of fulminant viral hepatitis, chronic hepatitis, cirrhosis, carcinoma

LABORATORY TESTS

- Diagnosis of acute HBV infection is best confirmed by IgM HBcAb in acute or early convalescent serum or by HBDNA by PCR.
  - Generally, IgM present during onset of jaundice
  - Coexisting HBsAg
- HBsAg and IgG-HBcAb during acute jaundice are strongly suggestive of remote HBV infection and another cause for current illness (Fig. 1-453).
- HBsAb alone is suggestive of immunization response.
- With recovery, HBeAg is rapidly replaced by HBeAb in 2 to 3 mo, and HBsAg is replaced by HBsAb in 5 to 6 mo.
- In chronic HBV hepatitis, HBsAg and HBeAg are persistent without corresponding Ab.
- In chronic carrier state, HBsAg is persistent, but HBeAg is replaced by HBeAb.
- HBcAb develops in all outcomes.
- HBeAg correlation with highest infectivity; appearance of HBeAb heralds recovery.
- LFTs:
  - ALT and AST: usually more than eight times normal (often 1000 U/L) at onset of jaundice (minimal acute ALT/AST rises often followed by chronic hepatitis or hepatocellular carcinoma)
  - Bilirubin: variably elevated in icteric viral hepatitis
  - Alkaline phosphatase: minimally elevated (one to three times normal) acutely
- Albumin and prothrombin time:
  - Generally normal
  - If abnormal, possible harbinger of impending hepatic necrosis (fulminant hepatitis)
- WBC and ESR: generally normal

IMAGING STUDIES

- Rarely useful
- Sonogram to document rapid reduction in liver size during fulminant hepatitis or mass in hepatocellular carcinoma

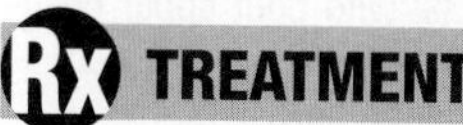

TREATMENT

NONPHARMACOLOGIC THERAPY

- Symptomatic treatment as necessary
- Activity as tolerated
- High-calorie diet preferred; often best tolerated in morning

ACUTE GENERAL Rx

- In most cases of acute HBV infection no treatment necessary; >90% of adults will spontaneously clear infection
- Hospitalization advisable for any patient in danger from dehydration caused by poor oral intake, whose PT is prolonged, who has rising bilirubin level >15 to 20 μg/dl, or who has any clinical evidence of hepatic failure
- IV therapy needed (rarely) for hydration during severe vomiting
- Avoid hepatically metabolized drugs
- No therapeutic measures are beneficial
- Steroids not shown helpful

CHRONIC Rx

- The American Association for the Study of Liver Diseases issued guidelines in 2009 for the evaluation and treatment of hepatitis B.
- The aim of therapy in chronic HBV infection is to eradicate the virus.
- The two modalities of therapy available to achieve this goal have been immune modulators (interferon alfa) and antiviral agents in the form of nucleoside analogues (e.g., lamivudine).
- Pegylated interferon alpha (IFN-α) given as a once-a-week SQ injection for 48 wk is a mainstay of therapy and has largely replaced interferon alpha without pegylation, which required daily or thrice weekly injections. Its mechanism of action is to stimulate the immune system to attack HBV-infected hepatocytes, thus inhibiting viral protein synthesis. Dose: 180 μg SQ weekly.
- A 12-mo course of treatment results in a 30% to 40% response with significant reduction of serum HBV DNA, normalization of ALT, and loss of HBeAg. Seroconversion from HBeAg to HBeAb occurs in 15% to 20%.
- Factors that increase the likelihood of response to IFN-α therapy include:
  - Adult onset of infection
  - High baseline ALT
  - Low baseline HBV DNA
  - Absence of cirrhosis
  - Female
  - HBeAg positive
- Infrequent relapse after successful completion of therapy.
- 80% of patients who lose HBeAg during therapy lose HBsAg in the decade after therapy.

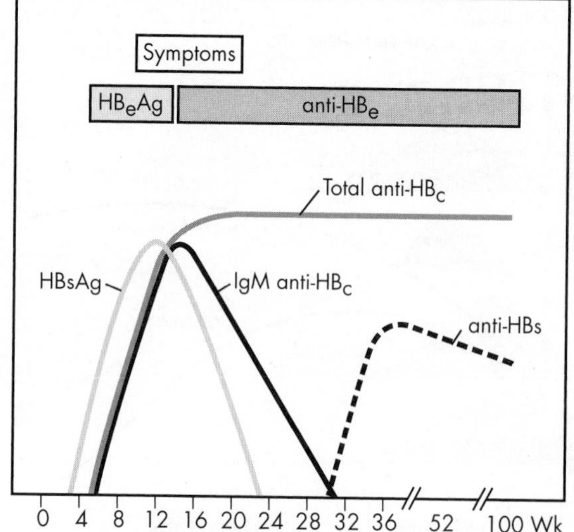

FIGURE 1-453 Typical course of hepatitis B. *Left,* Typical course of acute hepatitis B. *Right,* Chronic hepatitis B. *HBc,* Hepatitis B core; *HBe,* hepatitis B early; *HBsAg,* hepatitis B surface antigen; *IgM,* immunoglobulin M. (From Mandell GL et al: *Principles and practice of infectious diseases,* ed 7, Philadelphia, 2010, Saunders.)

- >50% of patients who do not seroconvert after initial therapy develop a delayed HBeAg seroconversion months to years after therapy.
- Overall incidence of cirrhosis and hepatocellular carcinoma is decreased in those treated with IFN-α.
- IFN-α is successful only in patients with an active immune response; therefore it is not effective in patients with HIV infection and organ transplant patients.
- Asians respond poorly to IFN-α. Patients with genotype A respond well to IFN-α.
- Treatment with IFN-α in general is not well tolerated: side effects include flulike symptoms, injection-site reactions, rash, weight loss, anxiety, depression, alopecia, thrombocytopenia, granulocytopenia, and thyroid dysfunction.
- Nucleoside analogues block viral replication by inhibiting HBV polymerase.
- Lamivudine was the first nucleoside analogue approved for treatment of chronic HBV infection; it has been shown to rapidly reduce HBV replication and suppress HBV DNA to undetectable levels after a few wk of treatment, and treatment for 1 yr is as effective as IFN-α with respect to loss of HBeAg seroconversion to HBeAb and loss of HBV DNA. The high rate of emergence of resistant HBV strains while on therapy has limited the use of lamivudine as a first-line agent (YMDD variants [tyrosine-methionine-aspartate-aspartate]). Dose: 100 mg orally daily with normal kidney function.
- Adefovir dipivoxil: 10 mg orally daily with normal kidney function is a nucleotide reverse transcriptase inhibitor that also has antiviral activity against HBV. It is a prodrug that is converted to the active drug adefovir. It is highly active against HBV and may be useful as a first-line agent or as salvage therapy for patients who are refractory or intolerant to lamivudine. (Nephrotoxicity is a potential side effect, but emergence of resistant strains is less than with lamivudine.)
- Entecavir is a potent nucleoside agent approved for the treatment of hepatitis B, and it appears to be more effective and to present fewer concerns than lamivudine or adefovir regarding the emergence of resistant strains. Dose: 0.5 mg PO dailiy for nucleoside-naïve patients and 1 mg PO daily for lamivudine-resistant patients.
- Telbivudine, a thymidine nucleosidase analogue, has demonstrated greater and more consistent HBV DNA suppression than lamivudine or adefovir after 24 wk of treatment but selects for the same resistant strains as lamivudine. Dose: 600 mg PO daily.
- Tenofovir: more potent than adefovir and suppresses lamivudine, telbiduvine, or entecavir resistant strains. In the U.S. it has become a first-line agent. Dose: 300 mg daily with normal kidney function.
- Combination therapy with two or three nucleoside analogues or combination therapy with IFN-α are currently under investigation.
- Liver transplantation (should be considered for fulminant hepatitis).

DISPOSITION

- Follow-up as outpatient
- Acute disease: usually <6 wk
- Rare fatalities (fulminant hepatitis)
- Possible chronic carrier state, cirrhosis, hepatocellular carcinoma

REFERRAL

To infectious disease specialist and gastroenterologist for consultation regarding fulminant hepatitis or prolonged cholestasis, for cases of uncertain etiology, or for treatment of CAH

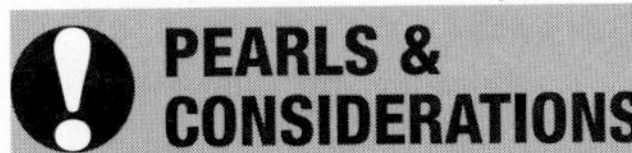

PEARLS & CONSIDERATIONS

COMMENTS

- Virus and HBsAg in high titers in blood for 1 to 7 wk before jaundice and for a variable time thereafter.
- Transmission is possible during entire period of HBsAg (and especially during HBeAg) in serum.
- Universal precautions should be followed for all contacts with blood or secretions/excretions contaminated with blood.
- Preventing before exposure:
  - Lifestyle changes
  - Meticulous testing of blood supply (although some chronically infected, infectious donors are HBsAg negative)
  - Sterilization via steam or hypochlorite
  - Hepatitis B vaccine for high-risk groups given IM in deltoid to induce HBsAb (response should be confirmed) is protective (>90% effective)
  - Recommendation for universal childhood immunization with doses at birth, 1 mo, and 6 mo
- Prevention after exposure:
  - HBV hyperimmune globulin (HBIG) given immediately after needlestick, within 14 days of sexual exposure, or at birth, followed by HBV vaccination
  - Standard immune globulin: nearly as effective as HBIG
- Preventive therapy with lamivudine for patients who test positive for HBsAg and are undergoing chemotherapy may reduce the risk for HBV reactivation and HBV-associated morbidity and mortality,
- Hepatitis B prophylaxis is described in Section V
- Table 1-229 summarizes interpretation of serologic markers and serum DNA in hepatitis B

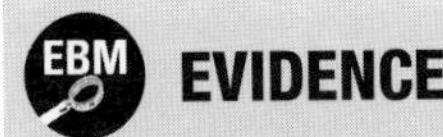

EVIDENCE

available at www.expertconsult.com

SUGGESTED READINGS

available at www.expertconsult.com

RELATED CONTENT

Fig. 3-91 A flow diagram showing the use of specific serologic tests for the diagnosis of acute viral hepatitis in relation to the clinical and epidemiologic setting (Algorithm)
Hepatitis B (Patient Information)

AUTHOR: **GLENN G. FORT, M.D., M.P.H.**

TABLE 1-229 Interpretation of Serologic Markers and Serum DNA in Hepatitis B

	HBsAg	HBeAg	Anti-HBc IgM	Anti-HBc IgG	Anti-HBs	Anti-HBe	HBV DNA*
Acute hepatitis	+	+/−	+				+
Acute hepatitis, window period			+				
Recovery from acute hepatitis			+	+	+	+/−	
Chronic hepatitis	+	+					+
Chronic hepatitis (precore mutant)	+					+	+
Inactive carrier	+					+/−	
Vaccinated					+		

HBsAg, Hepatitis B surface antigen; *HBeAg,* hepatitis Be antigen; *anti-HBc IgM,* hepatitis B core antibody (IgM type); *anti-HBc IgG,* hepatitis B core antibody (IgG type); *anti-HBs,* hepatitis B surface antibody; *anti-HBe,* hepatitis Be antibody; *HBV DNA,* hepatitis B viral DNA.
*HBV DNA >10^5 copies/ml.
From Andreoli TE et al: *Andreoli and Carpenter's Cecil essentials of medicine,* ed 8, Philadelphia, 2010, Saunders.

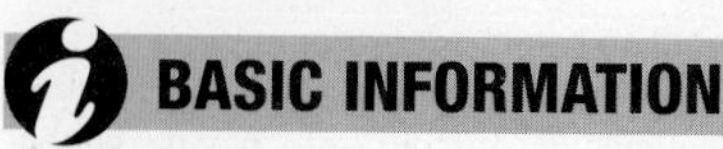

DEFINITION

Hepatitis C is an acute liver parenchymal infection caused by hepatitis C virus (HCV).

SYNONYMS

Transfusion-related non-A, non-B hepatitis (incubation period averages 6 wk, intermediate between hepatitis A and B)

ICD-9CM CODES
070.51 Other viral hepatitis
ICD-10CM CODES
B17.1 Acute hepatitis C
B18.2 Chronic viral hepatitis C
B17.10 Acute hepatitis C without hepatic coma

EPIDEMIOLOGY & DEMOGRAPHICS

Hepatitis C infection is the most common chronic blood-borne infection in the U.S. About 3% of baby boomers test positive for the virus. The CDC now recommends testing for hepatits C for anyone born from 1945 to 1965.

INCIDENCE (IN U.S.):
- 150,000 new cases/yr (37,500 symptomatic; 93,000 later chronic liver disease; 30,700 cirrhosis). The incidence of acute HCV has declined substantially over the past 30 yr (from 7.4/100,000 to 0.7/100,000)
- ~9000 of these ultimately die of HCV infection; most common (40%) cause of nonalcoholic liver disease in the United States

PREVALENCE (IN U.S.):
- Overall prevalence of anti-HCV antibody is 1%-1.2% (an estimated 2.7 million persons nationwide)
- Highest prevalence in hemophiliacs transfused before 1987 and users of injection drugs, 72% to 90%. Over past 30 yr, blood transfusion as a risk factor declined from 15% of cases to 1.9%.
- Among low-risk groups, prevalence 0.6%

PREDOMINANT SEX: Slight male predominance
PREDOMINANT AGE: Highest prevalence in 30- to 49-yr age group (65%)
PEAK INCIDENCE:
- 20 to 39 yr of age
- African Americans and whites have similar incidence of acute disease; Hispanics have higher rates
- Prevalence is substantially higher among non-Hispanic blacks than among non-Hispanic whites

GENETICS: Neonatal infection is rare; increased risk with maternal HIV-1 coinfection

PHYSICAL FINDINGS & CLINICAL PRESENTATION

- Symptoms usually develop 7 to 8 wk after infection (range of 2 to 26 wk), but 70% to 80% of cases are subclinical.
- 10% to 20% report acute illness with jaundice and nonspecific symptoms (abdominal pain, anorexia, malaise).
- Fulminant hepatitis may rarely occur during this period.
- After acute infection, 15% to 25% have complete resolution (absence of HCV RNA in serum, normal ALT).
- Progression to chronic infection is common, 50% to 84%. 74% to 86% have persistent viremia; spontaneous clearance of viremia in chronic infection is rare. 60% to 70% of patients will have persistent or fluctuating ALT levels; 30% to 40% with chronic infection have normal ALT levels.
- 15% to 20% of those with chronic HCV will develop cirrhosis over a period of 20 to 30 yr; in most others, chronic infection leads to hepatitis and varying degrees of fibrosis.
- 0.4% to 2.5% of patients with chronic infection develop hepatocellular carcinoma (HCC).
- 25% of patients with chronic infection continue to have an asymptomatic course with normal LFTs and benign histology.
- In chronic HCV infection, extrahepatic sequelae include a variety of immunologic and lymphoproliferative disorders (e.g., cryoglobulinemia, membranoproliferative glomerulonephritis, and possibly Sjögren's syndrome, autoimmune thyroiditis, polyarteritis nodosa, aplastic anemia, lichen planus, porphyria cutanea tarda, B-cell lymphoma, others).

ETIOLOGY

- Caused by HCV (single-stranded RNA flavivirus).
- Most HCV transmission is parenteral.
- In the United States, advances in screening of blood and blood products in 1990 and 1992 have made transfusion-related HCV infection rare (the risk is estimated to be 0.001% per unit transfused).
- Injecting-drug use accounts for most HCV transmission in the United States (60% of newly acquired cases, 20% to 50% of chronically infected persons).
- Occupational needlestick exposure from an HCV-positive source has a seroconversion rate of 1.8% (range 0% to 7%).
- Nosocomial transmission rates (from surgery and procedures such as colonoscopy and hemodialysis) are extremely low.
- Sexual transmission and maternal-fetal transmission are infrequent (estimated at 5%).
- No identifiable risk in 40% to 50% of community-acquired hepatitis C, but snorting of cocaine by shared use of straw or rolled-up paper has been identified as a risk factor because it causes microscopic bleeding of nasal mucosa.
- HCV infection may stimulate production of cytotoxic T lymphocytes and cytokines (INF-γ), which probably mediate hepatic necrosis.

Dx DIAGNOSIS

DIFFERENTIAL DIAGNOSIS

- Other hepatitis viruses (A, B, D, E)
- Other viral illnesses producing systemic disease (e.g., yellow fever, EBV, CMV, HIV, rubella, rubeola, coxsackie B, adenovirus, HSV, HZV)
- Nonviral hepatitis (e.g., leptospirosis, toxoplasmosis, alcoholic hepatitis, drug-induced hepatitis [acetaminophen, INH], toxic hepatitis)

WORKUP

- Acute hepatitis C antibody
- LFTs; CBC

NOTE: ALT is an easy and inexpensive test to monitor infection and efficacy of therapy. However, ALT levels may fluctuate or even be normal in active or chronic infection and even with cirrhosis, and ALT may remain elevated even after clearance of viremia.

- Liver biopsy with histologic staging is the gold standard for assessing the degree of disease activity and the likelihood of disease progression, and also to help rule out other causes of liver disease

LABORATORY TESTS

- Diagnosis is often by exclusion, because it takes 6 wk to 12 mo to develop anti-HCV antibody (70% positive by 6 wk, 90% positive by 6 mo).
- Diagnostic tests include serologic assays for antibodies and molecular tests for viral particles.
  - Enzyme immunoassay is the test for anti-HCV antibody:
    The current version can detect antibody within 4 to 10 wk after infection.
    False-negative rate in low-risk populations is 0.5% to 1%.
    False negatives also occur in immune-compromised persons, HIV-1, renal failure, HCV-associated essential mixed cryoglobulinemia.
    False positives in autoimmune hepatitis, paraproteinemia, and persons with no risk factors.
  - The recombinant immunoblot assay that was previously recommended as a follow-up to positive antibody test is no longer available. The CDC now recommends that anyone who tests positive for HCV antibodies receive a follow-up HCV RNA test.
  - Qualitative and quantitative HCV RNA tests using PCR:
    Lower limit of detection is <43 IU/ml
    Used to confirm viremia and to assess response to treatment.
    Qualitative polymerase chain reaction (PCR) useful in patients with negative enzyme immunoassay in whom infection is suspected.
    Quantitative tests use either branched-chain DNA or reverse transcription PCR; the latter is more sensitive.
  - Viral genotyping can distinguish among genotypes 1, 2, 3, and 4, which is helpful in choosing therapy; most of these tests use PCR (genotypes 1, 2, 3, and 4 predominate in the U.S. and Europe [1 is especially common in North America]).
  - LFTs:
    ALT and AST may be elevated to more than eight times normal in acute infection; in chronic infection ALT may be normal or fluctuate.
    Bilirubin may be five to 10 times normal.
    Albumin and prothrombin time generally normal; if abnormal, may be harbinger of impending hepatic necrosis.

- WBC and erythrocyte sedimentation rate (ESR) are generally normal.

IMAGING STUDIES

Sonogram: rapid liver size reduction during fulminant hepatitis or mass in HCC

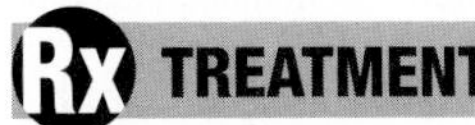

TREATMENT

NONPHARMACOLOGIC THERAPY

Activity and diet as tolerated, avoid saw palmetto and green tea leaf herbs

ACUTE GENERAL Rx

- Supportive care
- Avoid hepatically metabolized drugs.
- Specific Rx for acute HCV infection
- Early treatment with interferon-alpha-2b during acute HCV infection prevents chronic infection. The aim is to decrease viral load early in infection and allow the patient's immune system to control viral replication, thus preventing progression to chronic infection. The primary end point was sustained virologic response (SVR), with absence of HCV RNA in serum 24 wk after completion of therapy.
- Further investigations are in progress.

CHRONIC Rx

- Response to therapy is influenced by HCV genotype. Recent advances in treatment now allow for patients with genotypes 1, 2, and 3 to have SVR and cure rates as high as 75% to 80%. Patients with genotype 4 are more difficult to treat and have cure rates of only 45% to 50%. Fig. E1-454 describes a treatment algorithm in patients with chronic hepatitis C according to HCV genotype.
- Mainstay of therapy currently for patients with genotype 1 is a pegylated interferon-alpha as a weekly SC injection with oral weight-based ribavirin and a protease inhibitor, for a total length of therapy of 12 or 24 wk for most patients. Therapy may go up to 48 wk depending on a history of prior treatment or diagnosis of cirrhosis, and response to therapy measured with viral loads at key intervals during therapy. Two protease inhibitors were approved in 2011: telaprevir and boceprevir and simeprevir was approved in 2013.
  - Telaprevir: 750 mg tid taken with a fatty meal is given from the onset of therapy with the pegylated interferon and ribavirin. Telaprevir's side effects include rashes, pruritus, anemia, hemorrhoids, diarrhea, and anorectal discomfort. Severe rash can occur in 4% of patients.
  - Boceprevir: 800 mg tid starts after a lead-in period of 4 wk of the pegylated interferon and ribavirin. The most common side effects of boceprevir include fatigue, anemia, neutropenia, and thrombocytopenia.
  - Use of telaprevir and boceprevir may dramatically improve the cure rates for genotypes 1 and 4 and require only 12 or 24 wk of therapy. They can be used in a cocktail with a pegylated interferon plus ribavirin.
  - Simeprevir is dosed once-daily and does not exacerbate anemia caused by peginterferon/ribavirin. It can, however, cause rash and photosensitivity reactions. It is as effective as telaprevir and boceprevir except in genotype 1a patients with the NS3 Q80K mutation (>30% of U.S. patients).
- For genotypes 2 and 3 treatment consists of a pegylated interferon and ribavirin at a fixed dose of 800 mg daily (400 mg bid) for 24 weeks. This regimen produces SVR rates as high as 75%. For patients with genotype 4, protease inhibitors are not used and therapy extends for 48 weeks with a pegylated interferon and weight-based ribavirin only. This therapy produces SVR rates of about 45% to 50%.
- Pegylated interferons are interferon-alpha with an attached polyethylene glycol (PEG) molecule. The PEG molecule confers a longer half-life and extended therapeutic activity compared with interferon-alpha and reduced dosing to once a week. A third type of interferon, known as consensus interferon, is also available for treatment of hepatitis C, but it is not a long-acting form like the pegylated interferons.
- Two formulations of PEG interferon are available. Peginterferon alpha-2b (PEG INTRON) uses a weight-based dosage in a once-a-week SC Redipen injection. Peginterferon alpha-2a (Pegasys) uses a fixed dosage in a once-a-week premixed syringe, or Redipen, also SC.
- Both PEG interferon-alpha and ribavirin have numerous contraindications (absolute and relative) to use, and may cause a variety of side effects. Interferon-alpha can cause flulike symptoms, thrombocytopenia, granulocytopenia, rash, alopecia, anorexia, psychiatric disturbances, and other side effects. Ribavirin can cause hemolysis, nausea, anemia, nasal congestion, and pruritus. Ribavirin is contraindicated in pregnancy. Patients should not become pregnant while on therapy and for 6 mo after therapy.
- In patients who fail to respond to interferon-alpha and ribavirin, <10% will respond to retreatment.
- Liver transplantation:
  - Hepatitis C is the main indication for liver transplantation in the United States.
  - It is the only option for patients with deteriorating HCV-related cirrhosis and for some patients with HCC.
  - Recurrent infection occurs in almost all patients with progressive fibrosis and cirrhosis; as many as 20% progress to cirrhosis within 5-yr posttransplant.
- Coinfection with HIV:
  - These patients have a poor response to pegylated interferon-alpha and ribavirin if the immune system is depleted, with a low CD4 count as seen in the AIDS category. It is, however, important to treat patients coinfected with HIV and hepatitis C with antiretroviral therapy. Many coinfected patients are stable from their HIV disease, but have significant morbidity and mortality from their hepatitis C.

DISPOSITION

- Recent trials have shown that SVR rates for genotype 1 infection are higher with triple therapy that includes a protease inhibitor than with standard dual therapy.
- SVR after treatment among HCV-infected persons at any stage of fibrosis is associated with reduced HCC.
- Periodic abdominal ultrasonography for HCC screening.
- Recent guidelines recommend against measurement of alpha-fetoprotein (AFP) to screen for HCC in patients with chronic hepatitis C due to lack of sensitivity, specificity, and predictive values.

REFERRAL

- To a hepatologist or infectious disease specialist for treatment for hepatitis C
- To a transplant surgeon for consideration of liver transplant if indicated

PEARLS & CONSIDERATIONS

- More rapid progression of disease in persons who drink alcohol regularly, persons of advanced age at time of infection, and those coinfected with other viruses (HIV, hepatitis B). All persons with identified HCV infection should receive a brief alcohol screening and intervention as clinically indicated.
- Major depression is a common (20%-40%) side effect of treatment with interferons. Use of the SSRI escitalopram has been found safe and effective for prevention of interferons-associated depression in these patients.
- Regression of cirrhosis has been demonstrated after antiviral therapy in some patients with chronic hepatitis C. Regression is associated with decreased disease-related morbidity and improved survival.
- The presence of interleukin (IL)-28B and HLA class II is independently associated with spontaneous resolution of HCV infection, and single nucleotide polymorphism IL-28B and DQB1*03:01 may explain approximately 15% of spontaneous resolution of HCV infection.

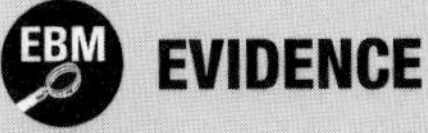

EVIDENCE

available at www.expertconsult.com

SUGGESTED READINGS

available at www.expertconsult.com

RELATED CONTENT

Hepatitis C (Patient Information)

AUTHOR: **GLENN G. FORT, M.D., M.P.H.**

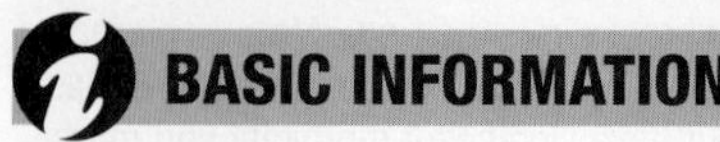

DEFINITION

Autoimmune hepatitis is a chronic inflammatory condition of the liver characterized by elevated serum globulin levels and the presence of circulating autoantibodies. Two types have been described:

- Type 1, or "classic," autoimmune hepatitis is the most predominant form in the U.S. and worldwide (80%); patients are positive for antinuclear antibodies (ANA) and/or antismooth muscle antibodies (SMA). Occurs across all age ranges and may be underdiagnosed in the elderly.
- Type 2 is rare in the U.S. and primarily affects young children. Type 2 is characterized by the presence of antibodies to liver/kidney microsomes (anti-LKM-1) or liver cytosol 1.

This form is generally more advanced at presentation and more difficult to treat.

SYNONYMS

Autoimmune chronic active hepatitis
Chronic active hepatitis
Lupoid hepatitis
Plasma cell hepatitis

ICD-9CM CODES
571.49 Chronic hepatitis
ICD-10CM CODES
K75.4 Autoimmune hepatitis
K73.2 Chronic active hepatitis, not elsewhere classified

EPIDEMIOLOGY & DEMOGRAPHICS

- Annual incidence (estimated): 1.9 cases per 100,000
- Point prevalence (estimated): 16.9 per 100,000
- Type 1: all age groups; type 2: more common in teenagers and young adults
- Female/male ratio is 3.6:1
- Approximately 100,000 to 200,000 persons affected in the U.S.
- Accounts for 3% to 5.9% of liver transplants in U.S.
- Associated with HLA-DRB1*0301 and HLA-DRB1*0401 alleles

CLINICAL PRESENTATION

- Varies from intermittent asymptomatic elevations of liver enzymes to advanced cirrhosis. Cirrhosis is often the presenting stage. AIH can also present initially as a fulminant hepatitis.
- Symptoms may include fatigue, anorexia, nausea, abdominal pain, pruritus, and arthralgia.
- Autoimmune findings may include arthritis, xerostomia, keratoconjunctivitis, cutaneous vasculitis, and erythema nodosum.
- Patients with advanced disease can show hepatosplenomegaly, ascites, peripheral edema, abnormal bleeding, and jaundice.

ETIOLOGY

- Exact etiology is unknown; liver histology demonstrates cell-mediated immune attack against hepatocytes.
- Presence of a variety of autoantibodies suggests an autoimmune mechanism.
- There are likely two components involved: genetic predisposition and an inciting environmental trigger.
- Potential triggering agents such as viruses (hepatitis A, B, C) or drugs (minocycline, nitrofurantoin) likely possess some homology similar to liver-specific antigens.

Dx DIAGNOSIS

- A simplified diagnostic criteria for routine clinical practice has been developed by the International Autoimmune Hepatitis Group (see Table 1-230).
- Histology: Lymphoplasmacytic infiltrate invading the hepatocyte boundary surrounding the portal triad (limiting plate). Also a periportal infiltrate may be seen (interface hepatitis).

DIFFERENTIAL DIAGNOSIS

- Acute viral hepatitis (A, B, C, D, E, cytomegalovirus, Epstein-Barr, herpes)
- Chronic viral hepatitis (B, C)
- Toxic hepatitis (alcohol, drugs)
- Primary biliary cirrhosis
- Primary sclerosing cholangitis
- Hemochromatosis
- Nonalcoholic steatohepatitis
- SLE
- Wilson's disease
- Alpha-1 antitrypsin deficiency

WORKUP

- History and physical examination with attention to the presence of autoimmune abnormalities such as autoimmune thyroiditis, Graves' disease, inflammatory bowel disease, celiac sprue, and rheumatoid arthritis
- Liver function tests and serum gammaglobulins
- Tests for autoantibodies: ANA, SMA, anti-LKM
- Liver biopsy for establishing diagnosis and disease severity

LABORATORY TESTS

- Aminotransferases generally elevated, may fluctuate
- Bilirubin and alkaline phosphatase moderately elevated or normal
- Elevation of gamma globulin (>2.0 g/dl [20 g/L]) and immunoglobulin G
- Circulating autoantibodies often present:
  1. Rheumatoid factor
  2. ANAs
     a. Present in two thirds of patients
     b. Typical pattern is homogeneous or speckled
     c. Titer does not correlate with the stage, activity, or prognosis
  3. SMAs
     a. Present in 87% of patients
     b. Titer does not correlate with course or prognosis
  4. Anti-LKM antibodies
     a. Typically found in patients who are ANA negative and SMA negative
     b. Characterizes type 2 AIH
     c. Present in pediatric population and up to 20% of adults in Europe; also present in patients with drug-induced hepatitis
  5. Autoantibodies against soluble liver antigen and liver-pancreas antigen (anti-SLA/LP)
     a. Present in 10% to 30% of patients
     b. Associated with higher rate of relapse after corticosteroid therapy
     c. Several studies suggest that patients with anti-SLA/LP have a more severe course
  6. Serum p-ANCA levels are useful for diagnosis of the 10% to 15% of patients with negative SMA, ANA, and low gamma globulin levels.
- Hypoalbuminemia and prolonged prothrombin time with advanced disease
- There is a well-described overlap syndrome with primary biliary cirrhosis (7%), primary sclerosing cholangitis (6%), and autoimmune cholangitis (11%). In patients who do not respond to therapy after 3 mo, consider cholangiographic studies to evaluate for primary sclerosing cholangitis.

IMAGING STUDIES

- Ultrasound of liver and biliary tree to rule out obstruction or hepatic mass
- Cirrhosis secondary to AIH is a risk factor for development of hepatocellular carcinoma (although less so than viral hepatitis). Cirrhotics should get ultrasonography and AFP every 6 months.

TABLE 1-230 Simplified Diagnostic Criteria for Autoimmune Hepatitis

Variable	Cutoff	Points	Cutoff	Points
ANA or SMA	≥1:40	1	≥1:80	2
LKM			≥1:40	2
SLA			Positive	2
IgG	≥ULN	1	≥1.1 × ULN	2
Histology	Compatible with AIH	1	Typical of AIH	2
Absence of viral hepatitis			Yes	2

Maximum number of points for all antibodies = 2, total = 8.
Probable AIH ≥6 points, definite AIH ≥7 points.
AIH, Autoimmune hepatitis; *ANA,* antinuclear antibody; *IgG,* immunoglobulin G; *LKM,* liver/kidney microsomes; *SLA,* soluble liver antigen; *SMA,* smooth muscle antibody; *ULN,* upper limit of normal.

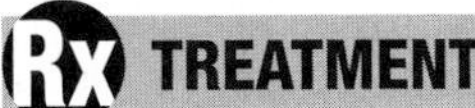

TREATMENT

NONPHARMACOLOGIC THERAPY

- Avoid alcohol and hepatotoxic medications.
- Liver transplantation is an option for end-stage disease or fulminant hepatic failure.

PHARMACOLOGIC THERAPY

- Initial treatment:
  1. Prednisone or prednisolone 60 mg/day PO or combination treatment with prednisone 30 mg/day PO plus azathioprine 50 mg/day PO, with a gradual taper to prednisone 10 mg PO daily over 2 to 3 mo as liver function test (LFT) results normalize. A combination of oral budesonide (6 to 9 mg/day) and azathioprine (1 to 2 mg/kg/day) can be used to induce and maintain remission in patients with non-cirrhotic AIH, with a lower rate of steroid-specific side effects.
  2. Combination therapy allows lower prednisone doses, fewer steroid side effects, and faster normalization of LFTs.
  3. Goal of therapy is remission (normalization of gamma-globulin and bilirubin, reduction of aminotransferases to less than twice the upper limit of normal, resolution of symptoms, and improvement in liver histology).
- Indications for treatment:
  1. Serum aminotransferase >10 times the upper limit of normal
  2. Serum aminotransferase more than five times the upper limit of normal, with serum gamma-globulin level twice the upper limit of normal
  3. Histologic features of bridging necrosis or multiacinar necrosis
  4. Incapacitating symptoms such as fatigue and arthralgia
- Evaluation of treatment response:
  1. Goal is the absence of symptoms, resolution of liver function test abnormalities, and histologic improvement. Generally, this is a steroid-responsive condition, but up to 20% do not respond.
  2. Patients whose transaminase levels normalize may continue to have ongoing active hepatitis involving inflammation and fibrosis. Between 5% and 10% of patients with normal transaminase levels progress to cirrhosis.
  3. Histologic improvement may lag behind clinical and laboratory improvement by as much as 6 mo. Because of this, repeat liver biopsy should be considered after normalization of transaminase levels.
  4. After initial remission is achieved, one may consider tapering medications. Steroid withdrawal should be done only if liver function tests normalize and histologic quiescence is achieved. About 50% to 86% of patients will relapse after this and require long-term maintenance medications.
  5. Complete normalization on biopsy is associated with a 15% to 20% risk of relapse, whereas persistent interface hepatitis is associated with a 90% risk of relapse.

DISPOSITION

- Follow up as outpatient.
- Long-term treatment may be necessary for sustained remission in individuals who continuously relapse and in partial responders.
- Sixty-five percent of patients achieve remission by 18 mo; 80% achieve remission by 3 yr.
- Approximately 10% of patients do not improve with therapy. For these nonresponders, one can try higher dose of combination prednisone/azathioprine. There is limited data pointing toward some success with such agents as cyclosporine and mycophenolate mofetil.
- Patients in whom end-stage liver develops are candidates for liver transplantation. AIH can recur in transplanted livers (18% 5-year probability).

REFERRAL

Patients with advanced cirrhosis or who progress to end-stage liver disease are candidates for liver transplantation and should be referred to appropriate medical centers that provide liver transplantation services.

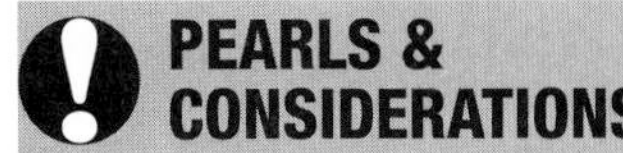

PEARLS & CONSIDERATIONS

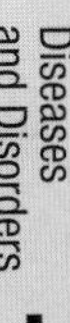

COMMENTS

- ANA and SMA are observed together in 60% of cases. Serum titers >1:40 suggest autoimmune hepatitis.
- A variety of autoimmune conditions can be seen in association with autoimmune hepatitis, including thyroiditis, Graves' disease, ulcerative colitis, rheumatoid arthritis, uveitis, pernicious anemia, Sjögren's syndrome, mixed connective tissue disease, CREST syndrome, and vitiligo.
- Variant forms of autoimmune hepatitis (overlap syndrome) have clinical and serologic findings of autoimmune hepatitis plus features of other forms of chronic liver disease such as primary biliary cirrhosis (PBC) or primary sclerosing cholangitis (PSC).

PREVENTION

None

PATIENT & FAMILY EDUCATION

- American Liver Foundation (ALF): Phone: 800-GO-LIVER (465-4837); Internet: www.liverfoundation.org
- National Digestive Diseases Information clearinghouse: http://digestive.niddk.nih.gov/ddiseases/pubs/autoimmunehep

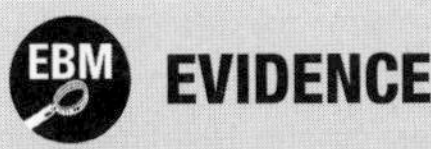

EVIDENCE

available at www.expertconsult.com

SUGGESTED READINGS

available at www.expertconsult.com

RELATED CONTENT

Autoimmune Hepatitis (Patient Information)

AUTHORS: **JUDY NEE, M.D., AMANDA PRESSMAN, M.D.,** and **KITTICHAI PROMRAT, M.D.**

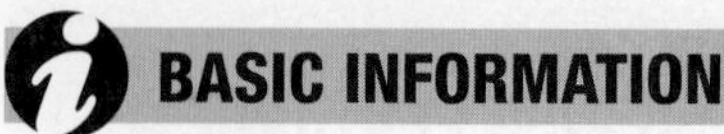

BASIC INFORMATION

DEFINITION

Hepatocellular carcinoma (HCC) is a malignant tumor of the hepatocytes.

SYNONYMS

Hepatoma
HCC

ICD-9CM CODES
155.0 Hepatocellular carcinoma
ICD-10CM CODES
C22.0 Liver cell carcinoma

EPIDEMIOLOGY & DEMOGRAPHICS

Fifth most common cancer worldwide (>500,000 new cases/year) and third most common cause of cancer deaths. Incidence varies worldwide:

- Areas with high rates of hepatitis B and C (Asia, sub-Saharan Africa) have high rates of HCC.
- Males more affected than females, with ratios between 2:1 and 4:1.
- Peak incidence: fifth and sixth decades in Western countries, earlier in areas with perinatal transmission of hepatitis B.
- Incidence rapidly growing in U.S. secondary to chronic hepatitis C infection and obesity leading to nonalcoholic steatohepatitis (NASH).
  - Incidence: during the past two decades, the incidence of HCC in the U.S. has tripled. The greatest proportional increase in cases has been among Hispanics and whites between 45 and 60 years of age
  - Mean age of diagnosis approximately 65 yr
  - HCC is the fastest-rising cause of cancer-related deaths in the United States
- Risk factors:
  - Chronic hepatitis B infection: accounts for 50% of all cases of HCC and virtually all childhood cases
  - Chronic hepatitis C infection: markers of HCV infection are found in 80% to 90% of patients with HCC in Japan, 44% to 66% in Italy, and 30% to 50% in the U.S.
  - Cirrhosis from causes other than viral hepatitis: alcoholic liver disease, nonalcoholic steatohepatitis, primary biliary cirrhosis, hemochromatosis, α1-antitrypsin deficiency, and autoimmune hepatitis
  - Hepatotoxins: alcohol and aflatoxin B1
  - Systemic diseases affecting the liver such as tyrosinemia
  - Obesity and diabetes mellitus

PHYSICAL FINDINGS & CLINICAL PRESENTATION

- One third of patients are asymptomatic. Abdominal pain may be the initial presentation.
- Signs of underlying cirrhosis and portal hypertension are often present.
- Previously compensated cirrhosis with new ascites, encephalopathy, jaundice, or bleeding.
- Paraneoplastic syndromes (hypoglycemia, erythrocytosis, hypercalcemia, severe diarrhea) may be present.

DIAGNOSIS

DIFFERENTIAL DIAGNOSIS

- Metastatic tumor to liver
- Intrahepatic cholangiocarcinoma
- Benign liver tumors such as adenomas, focal nodular hyperplasia, and hemangiomas
- Focal fatty infiltration

WORKUP

- History regarding risk factors
- Physical examination with attention to signs of chronic liver disease
- Laboratory evaluation and imaging studies
- Imaging studies: ultrasound for initial screening; 4-phase multidetector CT scan or dynamic contrast-enhanced MRI for HCC diagnosis

LABORATORY TESTS

- Liver function tests
- α-Fetoprotein (AFP) levels can be elevated in 70% of patients (sensitivity, 40% to 65%; specificity, 80% to 94%). An AFP level of 400 ng/ml or greater is highly suggestive of HCC; however, elevations may not be seen in up to 40% of patients with small HCC lesions (<3 cm).
- Paraneoplastic syndromes associated with HCC may cause hypercalcemia, hypoglycemia, and polycythemia
- Elevated serum HBV DNA level (≥10,000 copies/ml) is a strong risk predictor of HCC independent of HBeAg, serum aminotransferase level, and liver cirrhosis

IMAGING STUDIES

Ultrasound (US), CT scan (Fig. 1-455), or MRI. Ultrasound is most commonly used as a screening test for HCC in high-risk patients every 6 months. The following imaging modalities are recommended based on US findings:

- Hepatic lesion <1 cm needs to be followed with a repeat US every 3 months to ensure the lesion does not change change size. If there is no change in size (remains <1 cm) or characteristics after 24 months, the interval for US surveillance can be increased back to every 6 months
- Hepatic lesion >1 cm needs further imaging to confirm the diagnosis of HCC. Either a 4-phase multidetector CT (MDCT) scan or a dynamic contrast-enhanced MR scan is performed. If the chosen imaging modality shows characteristics typical of HCC (hypervascular in the arterial phase with washout in the portal venous or delayed phase) the diagnosis of HCC is confirmed with no need for additional diagnostic testing or biopsy. If the imaging modality is inconclusive or atypical for HCC then the alternate imaging test must be performed (e.g., if the first modality was MRI then the MDCT scan needs to be performed and vice versa). If the second imaging modality is also inconclusive, a biopsy to confirm diagnosis is recommended.

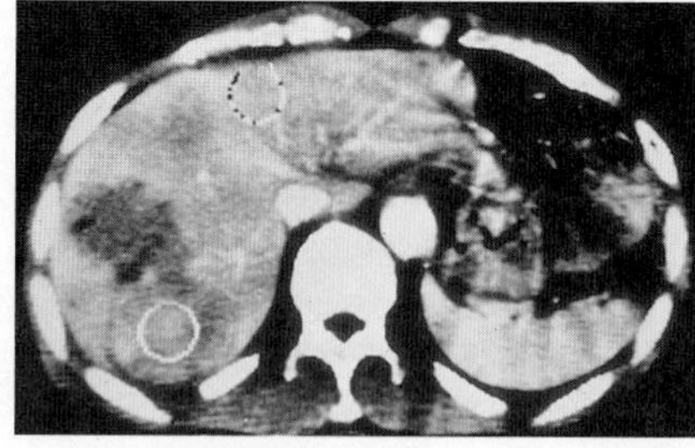

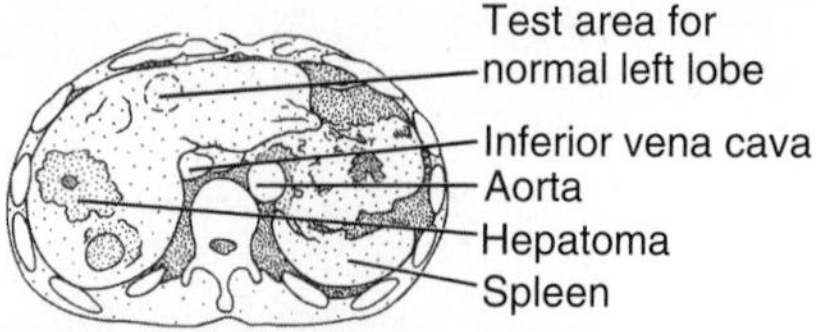

FIGURE 1-455 Hepatoma. CT scan shows a diffuse lesion in the right lobe of an otherwise normal liver. (From Skarin AT: *Atlas of diagnostic oncology,* ed 3, St Louis, 2003, Mosby.)

BIOPSY: Percutaneous biopsy under ultrasound or CT scan is obtained in the event that imaging studies are nondiagnostic or atypical for HCC, or if no cirrhosis is present. Negative biopsy results should be followed and the hepatic nodule reassessed every 3 to 6 months until it is no longer seen, enlarges, or shows diagnostic characteristics.

SCREENING: Screening high-risk patients with US every 6 mo is currently recommended to identify HCC at an early stage. The use of AFP in addition to US is currently under debate; though it does increase detection rate it also increases false-positive results. The use of AFP alone should be discouraged due to limited sensitivity and specificity. Newer tumor markers are currently under investigation, with plasma microRNA expression the most promising. Patients on transplant waiting lists should be regularly screened for HCC because in the U.S. the development of HCC gives increased priority for liver transplantation. Screening for HCC is recommended in the following groups:

- Hepatitis B carriers (HBsAg positive): Asian males >40 yr, Asian females >50 yr, all cirrhotic hepatitis B carriers, family history of HCC and North American blacks/Africans older than age 20 yr
- Cirrhosis (nonhepatitis B): hepatitis C, alcoholic cirrhosis, hemochromatosis, primary biliary cirrhosis, and possibly α1-antitrypsin deficiency, autoimmune hepatitis, and nonalcoholic steatohepatitis

STAGING: According to the Barcelona Clinic Liver Cancer (BCLC) staging classification, treatment is determined according to stage:

- Early stage (A): asymptomatic single tumor 5 cm or 3 nodules, each ≤3 cm (known as Milan criteria)
- Intermediate stage (B): patients with tumors that exceed early criteria but do not yet show cancer-related symptoms, vascular invasion, or metastases
- Advanced stage (C): patients with mild cancer-related symptoms and/or vascular invasion or extrahepatic spread
- End-stage (D): patients with advanced, symptomatic disease

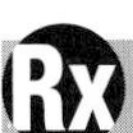

TREATMENT

- Fig. 1-456 describes a treatment algorithm for HCC.
- Early stage: curative treatment (surgical resection or liver transplantation). Patients who have a single lesion can be offered surgical resection if they are noncirrhotic or have cirrhosis but still have well-preserved liver function, normal bilirubin, and no significant portal hypertension. Liver transplantation is an effective option for patients with HCC corresponding to the Milan criteria (Table 1-231). Living donor transplantation can be offered for HCC if the waiting time is expected to be long. Local ablation is safe and effective therapy for patients who cannot undergo resection or as a bridge to transplantation. With these options, survival at 5 yr ranges from 50% to 70%.
- Intermediate stage: Transarterial chemoembolization (TACE) is recommended as first-line noncurative therapy for nonsurgical patients with large/multifocal HCC who do not have vascular invasion or extrahepatic spread. Median survival with this option exceeds 2 yr.
- Advanced stage: sorafenib, an oral multikinase inhibitor of the vascular endothelial growth factor receptor (VEGF), the platelet-derived growth factor (PDGF) receptor, and Raf, a serine-threonine kinase, has been shown to improve survival and delay disease progression. The SHARP trial included patients with advanced HCC in Child-Pugh A cirrhosis and showed increased median survival from 7.9 to 10.7 mo.
- End stage: palliative care.

TABLE 1-231 Milan Criteria of Eligibility for Liver Transplantation

Presence of a tumor ≤5 cm in diameter in patients with single hepatocellular carcinomas
or
≤3 tumor nodules, each 3 cm or less in diameter, in patients with multiple tumors

From Cameron JL, Cameron AM: *Current surgical therapy*, ed 10, Philadelphia, 2011, Saunders.

DISPOSITION

- For unresectable tumors, prognosis is poor; 5-yr survival after surgical resection ranges from 30% to 50%.
- In the U.S. the 5-year overall survival rate for HCC is 10% to 12%.

REFERRAL

To gastroenterologist for treatment planning

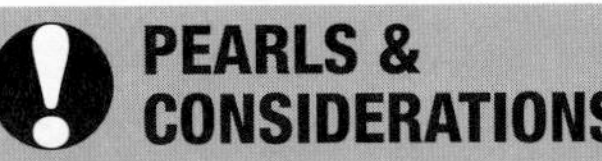

PEARLS & CONSIDERATIONS

PREVENTION

- Universal hepatitis B vaccination in children in endemic areas has been shown to decrease the incidence of HCC.
- Treatment of patients with chronic hepatitis B–associated cirrhosis with lamivudine reduces the incidence of HCC. Treatment with entecavir in chronic hepatitis B-HCC can improve hepatic function and MELD score.
- HCC screening is recommended in high-risk patients because curative therapies are available for small and early HCC.
- The expression patterns of microRNAs in liver tissue in patients with HCC differ between men and women. The miR-26 expression status of such patients is associated with survival and response to adjuvant therapy with interferon alfa.
- Several observational studies have suggested that radiofrequency ablation (RFA) may have survival benefits similar to hepatic resection (HR) in cirrhotic patients affected by HCC who are not candidates for liver transplantation.
- Patients diagnosed with HCC with an AFP >1000 are at increased risk for recurrence after transplantation regardless of tumor size.
- Recent trials have shown that among patients with advanced HCC, treatment with sorafenib plus doxorubicin monotherapy resulted in greater median time to progression-free survival. The degree in which this improvement may represent synergism between sorafenib and doxorubicin remains to be defined.
- There are at least 60 new agents, both TKI (tyrosine kinase inhibitors) and monoclonal antibodies, that are being investigated as targeted therapy for advanced HCC in patients who are intolerant or resistant to sorafenib. The future of therapy for advanced HCC will likely lead to the personalized combination of multiple agents to optimize treatment success.
- SALL4 is a marker for a progenitor subclass of hepatocellular carcinoma with an aggressive phenotype. The absence of SALL4 expression in the healthy adult liver enhances the potential of SALL4 as a treatment target in hepatocellular carcinoma.[1]

[1]Yong KJ et al: Oncofetal gene SALL4 in aggressive hepatocellular carcinoma, *N Engl J Med* 368:2266-2276, 2013.

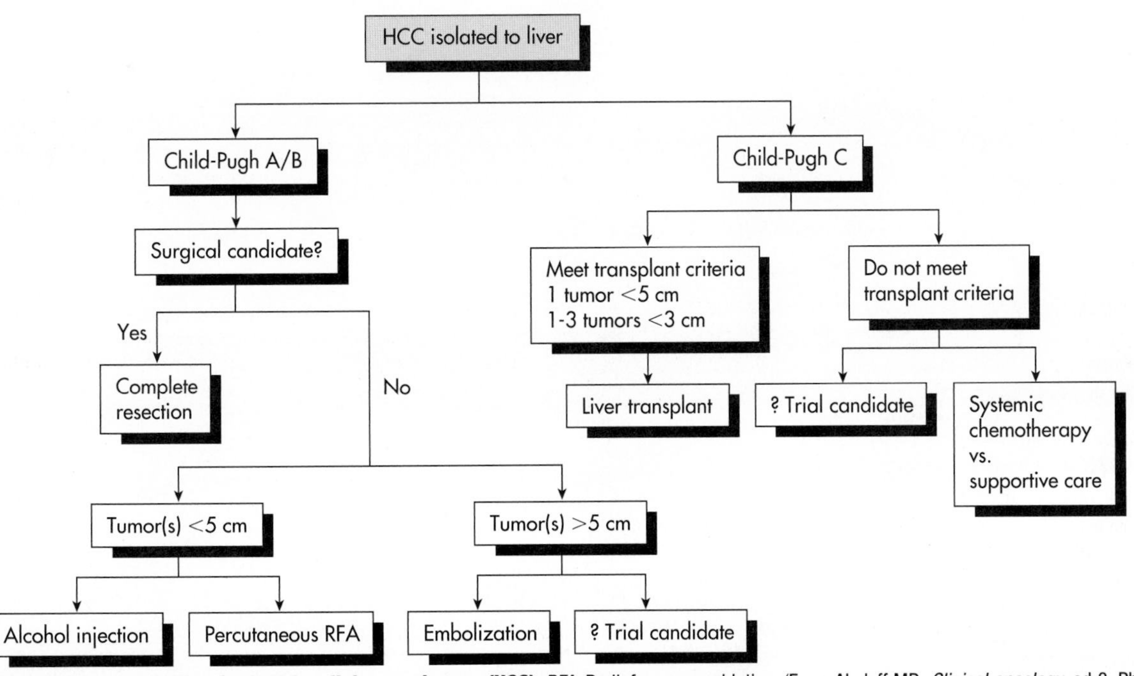

FIGURE 1-456 Treatment algorithm for hepatocellular carcinoma *(HCC).* *RFA,* Radiofrequency ablation. (From Abeloff MD: *Clinical oncology,* ed 3, Philadelphia, 2004, Saunders.)

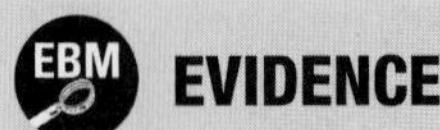

EVIDENCE

available at www.expertconsult.com

SUGGESTED READINGS

available at www.expertconsult.com

RELATED CONTENT

Liver Cancer (Patient Information)

AUTHORS: **PRANITH PERERA, M.D.,** and **JEANETTE G. SMITH, M.D.**

BASIC INFORMATION

DEFINITION

Hepatopulmonary syndrome (HPS) is characterized by intrapulmonary vascular dilation in the setting of liver disease causing an increased alveolar-arterial (A-a) gradient.

SYNONYMS

HPS

ICD-9CM CODES
417.9 Unspecified disease of pulmonary circulation

ICD-10CM CODES
I28.9 Disease of pulmonary vessels, unspecified
K76 Other diseases of liver

EPIDEMIOLOGY & DEMOGRAPHICS

PREVALENCE: Between 5% and 30% of patients with cirrhosis; wide range due to lack of diagnostic criteria

PREDOMINANT SEX AND AGE: There are no data on gender or age prevalence.

RISK FACTORS: Can occur with any degree or etiology of liver disease but is more common in patients with established cirrhosis and portal hypertension. There is no clear relationship between severity of hepatic dysfunction and level of hypoxemia. One recent study suggests that HPS is more common in patients with history of viral hepatitis than in patients with alcoholic cirrhosis.

GENETICS: There are new data suggesting that genes involved in the regulation of angiogenesis are associated with the risk of HPS.

PHYSICAL FINDINGS & CLINICAL PRESENTATION

- Dyspnea
- Platypnea: worsened dyspnea when sitting upright compared to supine position due to further ventilation-perfusion mismatch
- Orthodeoxia: decreased Pao_2 when the patient is sitting upright compared to supine position due to ventilation-perfusion mismatch
- Spider angiomata seen in high number
- Signs of severe hypoxemia (e.g., cyanosis and clubbing of the digits)

ETIOLOGY

Dilation of intrapulmonary arterioles and dilated vascular channels between pulmonary arteries and veins leading to a ventilation-perfusion mismatch and right-to-left shunting (Fig. E1-457). Research shows that nitric oxide plays a role in vasodilation. The relationship of vasodilation to liver disease is unclear. New areas of research include endothelin-1, which is produced by proliferating cholangiocytes, pulmonary angiogenesis, and opiate receptors' influence on NO production.

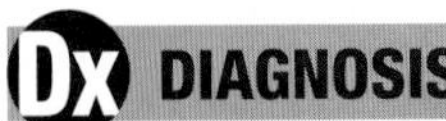

DIAGNOSIS

DIFFERENTIAL DIAGNOSIS

- Portopulmonary hypertension
- Cavopulmonary anastomosis
- Hereditary hemorrhagic telangiectasia (Rendu-Osler-Weber syndrome)
- Chronic lung disease (i.e., COPD or pulmonary fibrosis) with coexisting liver disease

WORKUP

- Diagnosis should be suspected in patients with cirrhosis who develop hypoxemia in absence of other causes (e.g., COPD, thromboembolism).
- Workup includes lab testing and imaging studies (see following), but diagnosis is based on clinical findings.

LABORATORY TESTS

- Arterial blood gas at rest, both supine and erect; Pao_2 <80 mm Hg
- Pulmonary function tests will show nonspecific reduction in DLco.

IMAGING STUDIES

- The most effective screening tool is transthoracic echocardiogram with bubble study to rule out right-to-left cardiac shunt; microbubble opacification in left atrium shows vasodilation of pulmonary vascular bed.
- Chest x-ray may show nonspecific bibasilar interstitial pattern.
- Scintigraphic perfusion scanning: technetium-99m–labeled albumin found in brain or spleen indicates dilated pulmonary vasculature or cardiac right-to-left shunt.
- Pulmonary angiography rarely used unless there is potential to embolize arteriovenous malformation (AVM).

TREATMENT

Ideal treatment would be targeted against pulmonary vasodilation. Most medications have targeted NO production, the activity of NO synthase or endothelin-1, pulmonary angiogenesis, or even bacterial translocation, but no controlled trials exist. Liver transplantation is the only successful treatment, which leads to improvement in gas exchange or compete resolution in gas exchange in the majority of patients. However, severe hypoxemia with Pao_2 <50 has been associated with a high posttransplant mortality. Some studies have shown benefit of transjugular portosystemic shunting, although it is not currently established treatment. Coil embolization in the setting of pulmonary AVMs is another possible area of treatment.

NONPHARMACOLOGIC THERAPY

Oxygen to correct hypoxemia; Pao_2 will partially correct with administration of supplemental O_2.

ACUTE GENERAL Rx

Correct hypoxemia with supplemental O_2.

CHRONIC Rx

Liver transplantation is the only successful treatment; the majority of patients show improvement in oxygenation at 1 year post transplant. There are some data showing worse outcomes for patients with severe HPS (PaO_2 <50%), but mortality appears to be improving.

COMPLEMENTARY & ALTERNATIVE MEDICINE

One study suggested that garlic supplements might decrease A-a gradient in patients with HPS. Studies of diets containing low amount of L-arginine have not shown benefit.

DISPOSITION

The diagnosis of HPS confers a poor prognosis. Patients with HPS have high mortality and shorter median survival than other patients with liver disease, even after adjusting for severity of liver disease. According to one natural history study, compared with patients with similar severity of liver disease and comorbidities whose 5-yr survival was estimated at 63%, those patients with the diagnosis of HPS had a 5-yr survival rate of 23%.

REFERRAL

- Referral to pulmonologist to help in establishing diagnosis
- Referral to a liver transplant center

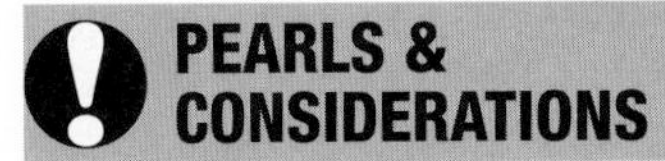

PEARLS & CONSIDERATIONS

COMMENTS

Consider the diagnosis of HPS in patients with cirrhosis who present with dyspnea without signs of pulmonary edema from fluid overload.

SUGGESTED READINGS

available at www.expertconsult.com

RELATED CONTENT

Cirrhosis (Related Key Topic)

AUTHOR: **BEVIN KENNEY, M.D.**

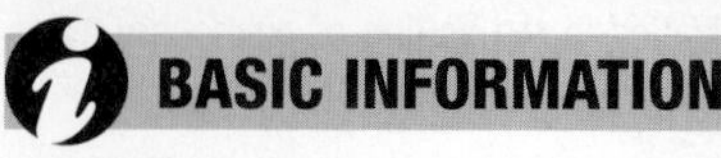

BASIC INFORMATION

DEFINITION

Hepatorenal syndrome (HRS) is a condition of intense renal vasoconstriction (see Fig. 1-458) resulting from loss of renal autoregulation occurring as a complication of severe liver disease. Criteria for HRS are:

1. Serum creatinine concentration >1.5 mg/dl or 24-hr creatinine clearance <40 ml/min
2. Absence of shock, ongoing infection, and fluid loss and no current treatment with nephrotoxic drugs
3. Absence of sustained improvement in renal function (decrease in serum creatinine to <1.5 mg/dl after discontinuation of diuretics and a trial of plasma expansion)
4. Absence of proteinuria (<500 mg/day) or hematuria (<50 red blood cells/high-power field)
5. Absence of ultrasonographic evidence of obstructive uropathy or parenchymal renal disease
6. Urinary sodium concentration <10 mmol/L

Tables 1-232 and 1-233 summarize the classic and the revised diagnostic criteria for HRS.

There are two types of HRS (see Table 1-234):

1. Type 1: progressive impairment in renal function as defined by a doubling of initial serum creatinine >2.5 mg/dl in <2 wk
2. Type 2: stable or slowly progressive impairment of renal function not meeting the above criteria

SYNONYMS

Hepatic nephropathy
Oliguric renal failure of cirrhosis
HRS

ICD-9CM CODES
572.4 Hepatorenal syndrome
ICD-10CM CODES
K76.7 Hepatorenal syndrome

EPIDEMIOLOGY & DEMOGRAPHICS

The probability of HRS in patients with cirrhosis is 18% at 1 yr and 39% at 5 yr.

PHYSICAL FINDINGS & CLINICAL PRESENTATION

- Evidence of cirrhosis is usually present: jaundice, spider angiomas, splenomegaly, ascites, fetor hepaticus, pedal edema

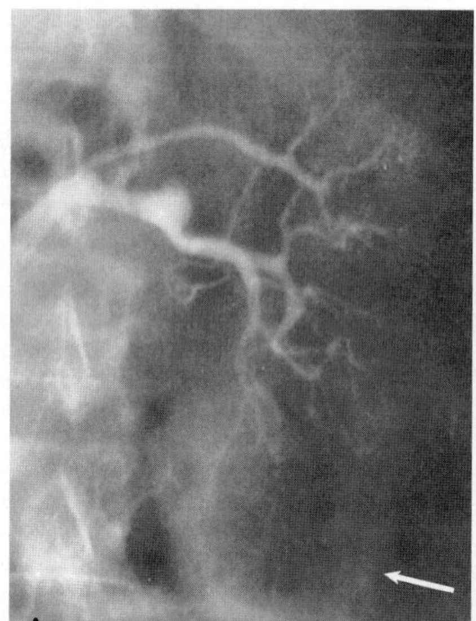

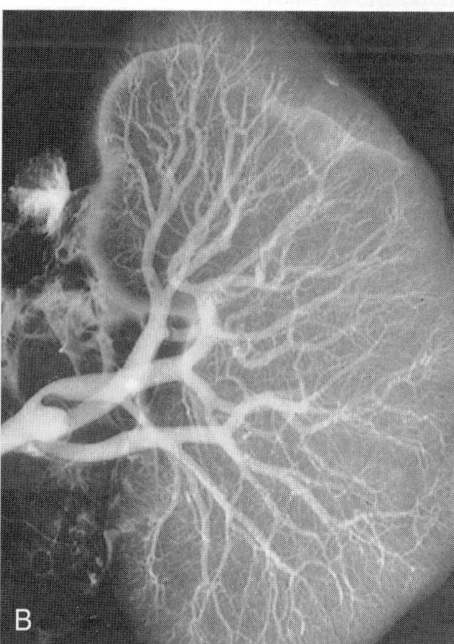

FIGURE 1-458 Hepatorenal syndrome (HRS). A, Renal angiogram (the *arrow* marks the edge of the kidney). **B,** The angiogram carried out in the same kidney at autopsy. Note complete filling of the renal arterial system throughout the vascular bed to the periphery of the cortex. The vascular attenuation and tortuosity seen previously **(A)** are no longer present. The vessels are also histologically normal. This indicates the functional nature of the vascular abnormality in HRS. (From Floege J et al: *Comprehensive clinical nephrology,* ed 4, Philadelphia, 2010, Saunders.)

TABLE 1-232 Diagnostic Criteria for Hepatorenal Syndrome

Major Criteria
Chronic or acute liver disease with advanced hepatic failure and portal hypertension
Low glomerular filtration rate, as indicated by serum creatinine >1.5 mg/dl (135 μmol/L) or 24-hr creatinine clearance <40 ml/min
Absence of shock, ongoing bacterial infection, and current or recent treatment with nephrotoxic drugs
Absence of gastrointestinal fluid losses (repeated vomiting or intense diarrhea)
Absence of renal fluid losses (weight loss >500 g/day for several days in patients with ascites without peripheral edema or 1000 g/day in patients with peripheral edema)
No sustained improvement in renal function (decrease in serum creatinine to 1.5 mg/dl [135 μmol/L] or less or increase in creatinine clearance to 40 ml/min or more) following diuretic withdrawal and expansion of plasma volume with 1.5 liters of isotonic saline
Proteinuria <500 mg/day and no ultrasonographic evidence of obstructive uropathy or parenchymal renal disease
Additional Criteria
Urine volume <500 ml/day
Urine sodium <10 mmol/L
Urine osmolality greater than plasma osmolality
Urine red blood cells <50 per high-power field
Serum sodium concentration <130 mmol/L

From Floege J et al: *Comprehensive clinical nephrology,* ed 4, Philadelphia, 2010, Saunders.

TABLE 1-233 Revised Diagnostic Criteria for Hepatorenal Syndrome

Cirrhosis with ascites
Serum creatinine >1.5 mg/dl (133 μmol/L)
No improvement in serum creatinine (decrease to a level of 1.5 mg/dl) after at least 2 days with diuretic withdrawal and volume expansion with albumin. The recommended dose of albumin is 1 g/kg of body weight per day up to a maximum of 100 g/day.
Absence of shock
No current or recent treatment with nephrotoxic drugs
Absence of parenchymal kidney disease as indicated by proteinuria >500 mg/day, microhematuria (>50 red blood cells per high-power field) and/or abnormal renal ultrasound

From Floege J et al: *Comprehensive clinical nephrology,* ed 4, Philadelphia, 2010, Saunders.

TABLE 1-234 Definition of Hepatorenal Syndrome Type 1 and Type 2

Type 1 Hepatorenal Syndrome
Doubling of serum creatinine >2.5 mg/dl (220 μmol/L) or a 50% reduction in 24-hr creatinine clearance to <20 ml/min <2 weeks
Frequently follows a precipitating event (e.g., infection)
Median survival without treatment: 2 weeks
Type 2 Hepatorenal Syndrome
Less rapid renal functional deterioration than type 1
Mainly presents with refractory ascites
Median survival without treatment: 4–6 months

From Floege J et al: *Comprehensive clinical nephrology,* ed 4, Philadelphia, 2010, Saunders.

- Hepatic encephalopathy: flapping tremor (asterixis), coma
- Tachycardia and bounding pulse
- Oliguria

ETIOLOGY

An exacerbation of end-stage liver disease, HRS may occur after significant reduction of effective blood volume (e.g., paracentesis, GI bleeding, diuretics) or in the absence of any precipitating factors.

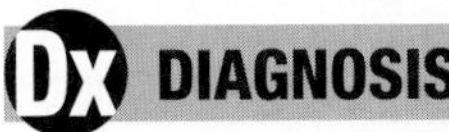

DIAGNOSIS

DIFFERENTIAL DIAGNOSIS

- Prerenal azotemia: response to sustained plasma expansion is good (prompt diuresis with volume expansion). Volume challenge (to increase mean arterial pressure) followed by large-volume paracentesis (to increase cardiac output and decrease renal venous pressure) may be useful to distinguish HRS from prerenal azotemia in patients with FENa <1%. In patients with prerenal azotemia, the increase in renal perfusion pressure and renal blood flow will result in prompt diuresis; the volume challenge can be accomplished by giving a solution of 100 g of albumin in 500 ml of isotonic saline.
- Acute tubular necrosis: urinary sodium >30 mEq/L, fractional excretion of sodium (FENa) >1.5%, urinary/plasma creatinine ratio <30, urine/plasma osmolality ratio = 1, urine sediment reveals casts and cellular debris, no significant response to sustained plasma expansion.

WORKUP

Patients with acute azotemia and oliguria in the setting of liver disease should undergo laboratory evaluation to differentiate HRS from acute tubular necrosis and volume challenge to differentiate HRS from prerenal azotemia if FENa <1%.

LABORATORY TESTS

- Obtain serum electrolytes, blood urea nitrogen, creatinine, osmolality, urinalysis, urinary sodium, urinary creatinine, urine osmolality
- Calculate FENa
- In HRS: urinary sodium <10 mEq/L, FENa <1%, urinary plasma creatinine ratio >30, urinary plasma osmolality ratio >1.5, urine sediment unremarkable

IMAGING STUDIES

Renal ultrasound may be indicated if renal obstruction is suspected.

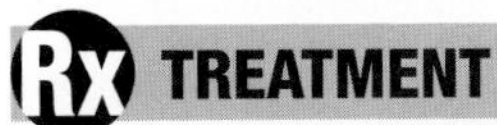

TREATMENT

NONPHARMACOLOGIC THERAPY

- Avoidance of precipitating factors.
- Transjugular intrahepatic portosystemic shunts may be effective in selected patients, but data are limited.
- Dialysis with molecular adsorbent recirculating systems remains investigational until more data are available.

ACUTE GENERAL Rx

- The only effective treatment of HRS is liver transplantation; ornipressin is used in some liver units to avoid further deterioration of renal function in patients awaiting liver transplantation. In general, dopamine and prostaglandins are ineffective in treating patients with HRS.
- The best approach to the management of HRS based on its pathogenesis is the administration of vasoconstrictor drugs (terlipressin, norepinephrine, midodrine). Terlipressin may improve renal perfusion by reversing splanchnic vasodilation, which is the hallmark of HRS. Encouraging results were found in a recent study using continuous IV noradrenalin in combination with albumin and furosemide. In this study, reversal of HRS was achieved in 10 of 12 patients.
- Treatment of HRS with vasoconstrictors for 5 to 15 days in attempt to reduce serum creatinine to <1.5 mg/dl is as follows:
  1. Administration of one of the following drugs or drug combinations:
     a. Norepinephrine (0.5 to 3.0 mg/hr IV)
     b. Midodrine (7.5 mg PO tid, increased to 12.5 mg tid if needed) in combination with octreotide (100 micrograms SC tid, increased to tid prn)
     c. Terlipressin (0.2 to 2.0 mg IV q4 to 12h)
  2. Concomitant administration of albumin (1 g/kg IV on day 1, followed by 20 to 40 g daily)

DISPOSITION

Mortality rate exceeds 80%; liver transplantation is the only curative treatment.

REFERRAL

Referral for liver transplantation when indicated (see "Comments")

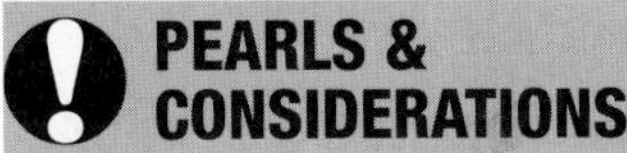

PEARLS & CONSIDERATIONS

COMMENTS

Liver transplantation may be indicated in otherwise healthy patients (age preferably <65 yr) with sclerosing cholangitis, chronic hepatitis with cirrhosis, or primary biliary cirrhosis. Contraindications to liver transplantation are AIDS, most metastatic malignancies, active substance abuse, uncontrolled sepsis, and uncontrolled cardiac or pulmonary disease.

SUGGESTED READINGS

available at www.expertconsult.com

RELATED CONTENT

Hepatorenal Syndrome (Patient Information)

AUTHOR: **FRED F. FERRI, M.D.**

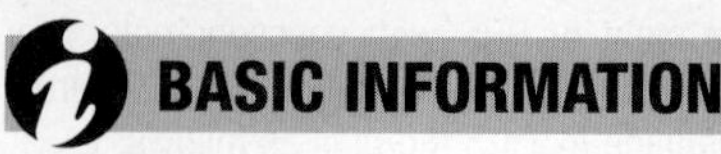

BASIC INFORMATION

DEFINITION

Herpangina is a self-limited upper respiratory tract infection associated with a characteristic vesicular rash on the soft palate.

SYNONYMS

Vesicular stomatitis
Acute lymphonodular pharyngitis

ICD-9CM CODES
074.0 Herpangina
ICD-10CM CODES
B08.5 Enteroviral vesicular pharyngitis

EPIDEMIOLOGY & DEMOGRAPHICS

INCIDENCE (IN U.S.): Unknown
PEAK INCIDENCE: Summer outbreaks common
PREVALENCE (IN U.S.): Unknown
PREDOMINANT SEX: Male = female
PREDOMINANT AGE: 3 to 10 yr

PHYSICAL FINDINGS & CLINICAL PRESENTATION

- Characterized by ulcerating lesions typically located on the soft palate (Fig. 1-459)
- Usually fewer than six lesions that evolve rapidly from a diffuse pharyngitis to erythematous macules and subsequently to vesicles that are moderately painful
- Fever, vomiting, and headache in the first few days of illness but subsiding spontaneously
- Pharyngeal lesions typical for several more days

ETIOLOGY

- Most cases caused by coxsackie A viruses (A2, A4, A5, A6, A10)
- Occasional cases caused by other enteroviruses (echovirus and enterovirus 71)

Dx DIAGNOSIS

DIFFERENTIAL DIAGNOSIS

- Herpes simplex
- Bacterial pharyngitis
- Tonsillitis
- Aphthous stomatitis
- Hand-foot-mouth disease

WORKUP

Diagnosis is typically based on characteristic lesions on the soft palate.

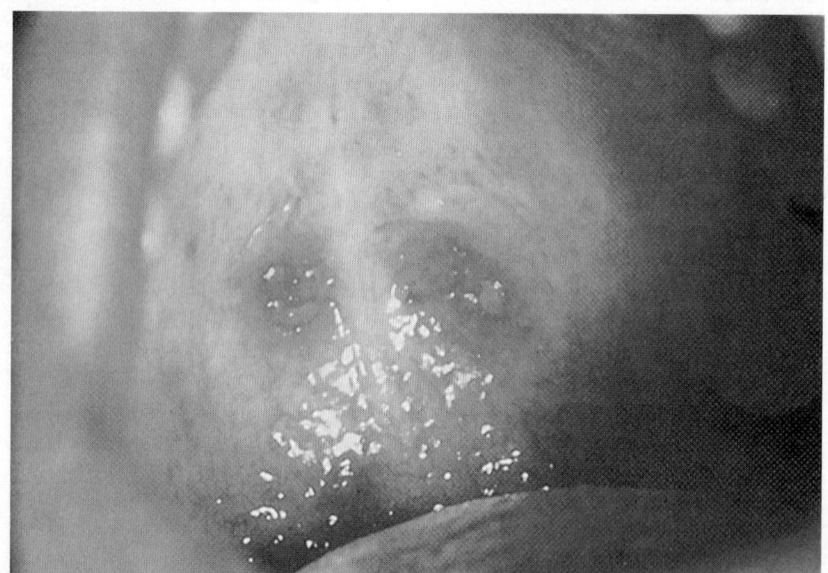

FIGURE 1-459 Herpangina with shallow ulcers in the roof of the mouth. (Courtesy Marshall Guill, M.D. From Goldstein B [ed]: *Practical dermatology,* ed 2, St Louis, 1997, Mosby.)

LABORATORY TESTS

Viral and bacterial cultures of the pharynx to exclude herpes simplex infection and streptococcal pharyngitis if the diagnosis is in doubt

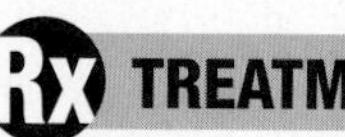

Rx TREATMENT

- Give symptomatic treatment for sore throat: saline gargles and analgesics, and encourage oral fluids.
- No antiviral therapy indicated; avoid antibacterial agents because they are ineffective, increase cost, might result in side effects, and promote antibiotic resistance.

NONPHARMACOLOGIC THERAPY

Analgesic throat lozenges are helpful in some cases.

ACUTE GENERAL Rx

Antipyretics when indicated

CHRONIC Rx

Self-limited infection

DISPOSITION

- Generally, resolution of symptoms within 1 wk
- Persistence of fever or mouth lesions beyond 1 wk suggestive of an alternative diagnosis (see "Differential Diagnosis")

REFERRAL

For consultation with otolaryngologist or infectious disease specialist if the diagnosis is in doubt

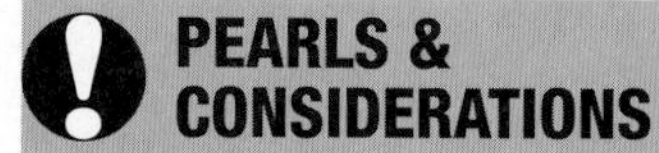

PEARLS & CONSIDERATIONS

COMMENTS

Household outbreaks may occur, especially during the summer months.

SUGGESTED READINGS

available at www.expertconsult.com

RELATED CONTENT

Herpangina (Patient Information)

AUTHOR: **GLENN G. FORT, M.D., M.P.H.**

BASIC INFORMATION

DEFINITION

Herpes simplex is a viral infection caused by the herpes simplex virus (HSV). HSV-1 is associated primarily with oral infections, and HSV-2 causes mainly genital infections. However, either type can infect any site. After the primary infection, the virus enters the nerve endings in the skin directly below the lesions and ascends to the dorsal root ganglia, where it remains in a latent stage until it is reactivated.

SYNONYMS

Genital herpes
Herpes labialis
Herpes gladiatorum
Herpes digitalis

ICD-9CM CODES
054.10 Genital herpes
054.9 Herpes labialis
ICD-10CM CODES
B00.1 Herpesvirus vesicular dermatitis
B00.0 Exzema herpeticum
A60.9 Anogenital herpesviral infection, unspecified
B00.9 Herpesviral infection, unspecified

EPIDEMIOLOGY & DEMOGRAPHICS

- More than 85% of adults have serologic evidence of HSV-1 infection. The seroprevalence of adults with HSV-2 in the U.S. is 25%; however, only approximately 20% of these persons recall having symptoms of HSV infection.
- Most cases of eye or digital herpetic infections are caused by HSV-1.
- Frequency of recurrence of HSV-2 genital herpes is higher than HSV-1 oral labial infection.
- The frequency of recurrence is lowest for oral labial HSV-2 infections.
- The incidence of complications from herpes simplex (e.g., herpes encephalitis) is highest in immunocompromised hosts.
- Male circumcision significantly reduces the incidence of HSV-2.

PHYSICAL FINDINGS & CLINICAL PRESENTATION

Primary infection:

- Symptoms occur from 3 to 7 days after contact (respiratory droplets, direct contact).
- Constitutional symptoms include low-grade fever, headache and myalgias, regional lymphadenopathy, and localized pain.
- Pain, burning, itching, and tingling last several hours.
- Grouped vesicles (Fig. 1-460), usually with surrounding erythema, appear and generally ulcerate or crust within 48 hr.
- The vesicles are uniform in size (differentiating it from herpes zoster vesicles, which vary in size). Scattered erosions covered with exudate may be noted on genitals (Fig. E1-461).
- During the acute eruption the patient is uncomfortable; involvement of lips and inside of mouth may make it unpleasant for the patient to eat; urinary retention may complicate involvement of the genital area.
- Lesions generally last from 2 to 6 wk and heal without scarring.

Recurrent infection:

- Generally caused by alteration in the immune system; fatigue, stress, menses, local skin trauma, and exposure to sunlight are contributing factors.
- The prodromal symptoms (fatigue, burning and tingling of the affected area) last 12 to 24 hr.
- A cluster of lesions generally evolves within 24 hr from a macule to a papule and then vesicles surrounded by erythema; the vesicles coalesce and subsequently rupture within 4 days, revealing erosions covered by crusts.
- The crusts are generally shed within 7 to 10 days, revealing a pink surface.
- The most frequent location of the lesions is on the vermilion border of the lips (HSV-1), the penile shaft or glans penis and the labia (HSV-2), buttocks (seen more frequently in women), fingertips (herpetic whitlow), and trunk (may be confused with herpes zoster).
- Rapid onset of diffuse cutaneous herpes simplex (eczema herpeticum) may occur in certain atopic infants and adults. It is a medical emergency, especially in young infants, and should be promptly treated with acyclovir.
- Herpes encephalitis, meningitis, and ocular herpes can occur in patients with immunocompromised status and occasionally in normal hosts.

ETIOLOGY

HSV-1 and HSV-2 are both DNA viruses.

DIAGNOSIS

DIFFERENTIAL DIAGNOSIS

- Impetigo
- Behçet's syndrome
- Coxsackie virus infection
- Syphilis
- Stevens-Johnson syndrome
- Herpangina
- Aphthous stomatitis
- Varicella
- Herpes zoster

WORKUP

Diagnosis is based on clinical presentation. Laboratory evaluation confirms diagnosis.

LABORATORY TESTS

- Direct immunofluorescent antibody slide tests provide a rapid diagnosis.
- Viral culture is the most definitive method for diagnosis; results are generally available in 1 or 2 days. The lesions should be sampled during the vesicular or early ulcerative stage; cervical samples should be taken from the endocervix with a swab.
- Tzanck smear is a readily available test that will demonstrate multinucleated giant cells. However, it is not a highly sensitive test.
- Pap smear will detect HSV-infected cells in cervical tissue from women without symptoms.
- Serologic tests for HSV: immunoglobulin (Ig) G and IgM serum antibodies. Antibodies to HSV occur in 50% to 90% of adults. The presence of IgM or a fourfold or greater rise in IgG titers indicates a recent infection (convalescent sample should be drawn 2 to 3 wk after the acute specimen is drawn).

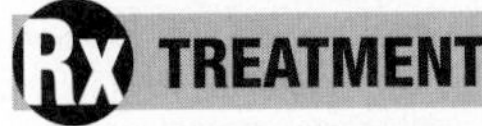

TREATMENT

- Table 1-235 summarizes antiviral chemotherapy for HSV infection.
- Topical acyclovir, penciclovir, and docosanol are optional treatments for recurrent herpes labialis, but they are less effective than oral treatments.

DISPOSITION

Most patients recover from the initial episode or recurrences without complications; immunocompromised hosts are at risk for complications (e.g., disseminated herpes simplex infection, herpes encephalitis).

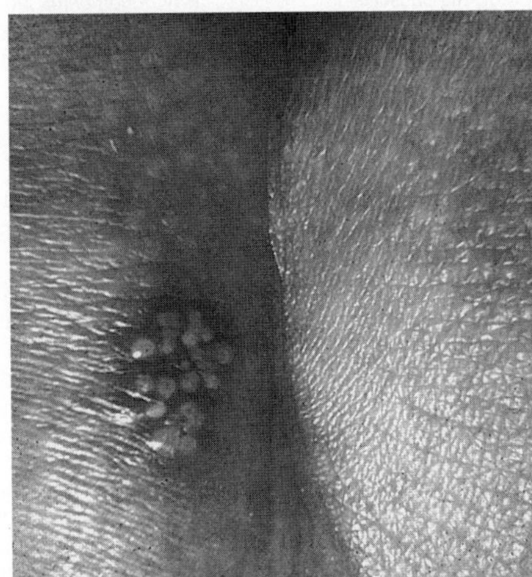

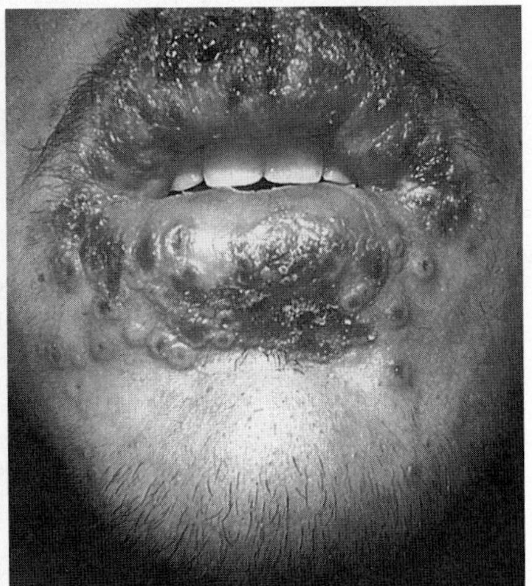

FIGURE 1-460 Herpes simplex. (From Scuderi G [ed]: *Sports medicine: principles of primary care,* St Louis, 1997, Mosby.)

REFERRAL

- Hospital admission in patients with herpes encephalitis or herpes meningitis and in immunocompromised hosts with diffuse herpes simplex infection
- Ophthalmology referral in patients with suspected ocular herpes

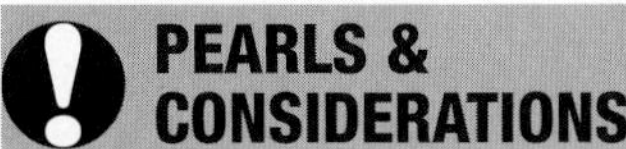

PEARLS & CONSIDERATIONS

COMMENTS

- Provide patient education regarding transmission of HSV.
- Condom use offers significant protection against HSV-1 infection in susceptible women.
- Patients should be instructed on the use of condoms for sexual intercourse and on avoiding kissing or sexual intercourse until lesions are crusted.
- Patients should also avoid contact with immunocompromised hosts or neonates while lesions are present.
- Proper handwashing techniques should be explained.
- Patients with herpes gladiatorum (cutaneous herpes in athletes involved in contact sports) should be excluded from participation in active sports until lesions have resolved.
- Many new HSV-2 infections are asymptomatic. Since HSV-2 antibody tests have become commercially available, an increasing number of persons have learned that they have genital herpes through serologic testing. Persons with asymptomatic HSV-2 infection shed virus in the genital tract less frequently than persons with symptomatic infection, but much of the difference is attributable to less frequent genital lesions because generally lesions are accompanied by frequent viral shedding.
- Suppressive treatment of HSV-2 infection lowers the incidence of genital lesions by 70% to 80%, but cuts the rate of HSV-2 transmission to uninfected partners by only 50%.
- Trials involving investigational herpes simplex vaccine have found it to be effective in preventing HSV-1 genital disease and infection, but not in preventing HSV-2 disease or infection.

SUGGESTED READINGS

available at www.expertconsult.com

RELATED CONTENT

Genital Herpes (Patient Information)

AUTHOR: **FRED F. FERRI, M.D.**

TABLE 1-235 Antiviral Chemotherapy for Herpes Simplex Virus Infection

Mucocutaneous HSV Infections

Infections in Immunosuppressed Patients

Acute symptomatic first or recurrent episodes: IV acyclovir (5 mg/kg q8h) and oral acyclovir (400 mg qid), famciclovir (500 mg PO tid), or valacyclovir (500 mg PO bid) for 7-10 days are effective. Treatment duration may vary from 7-14 days.

Suppression of reactivation disease: IV acyclovir (5 mg/kg q8h), valacyclovir (500 mg PO bid), or oral acyclovir (400-800 mg three to five times per day) prevents recurrences during the immediate 30-day post-transplantation period. Longer-term suppression is often used for persons with continued immunosuppression. In bone marrow and renal transplant recipients, valacyclovir 2 g four times daily is also effective in preventing CMV infection. Valacyclovir 4 g four times daily has been associated with TTP after extended use in HIV-positive persons. In HIV-infected persons, oral famciclovir (500 mg bid) is effective in reducing clinical and subclinical reactivations of HSV-1 and -2.

Genital Herpes

First episodes: Oral acyclovir (200 mg five times per day or 400 mg tid), oral valacyclovir (1000 mg bid), or famciclovir (250 mg bid) for 10-14 days is effective. IV acyclovir (5 mg/kg q8h for 5 days) is given for severe disease or neurologic complications such as aseptic meningitis.

Symptomatic recurrent genital herpes: Oral acyclovir (200 mg five times per day for 5 days, 800 mg PO tid for 2 days), valacyclovir (500 mg bid for 3 or 5 days), or famciclovir (125 mg bid for 5 days). All these therapies are effective in shortening lesion duration.

Suppression of recurrent genital herpes: Oral acyclovir (200-mg capsules bid or tid, 400 mg bid, or 800 mg qd), famciclovir (250 mg bid), or valacyclovir (500 mg or 1000 mg qd or 500 mg bid) prevents symptomatic reactivation. Persons with frequent reactivation (<9 episodes/year) can take 500 mg daily; those with >9 episodes/year should take 1000 mg/daily or 500 mg bid.

Oral-Labial HSV Infections

First episode: Oral acyclovir (200 mg) is given four or five times per day. Famciclovir (250 mg bid) or valacyclovir (1000 mg bid) has been used clinically.

Recurrent episodes: Valacyclovir 1000 mg bid for 1 day or 500 mg bid for 3 days is effective in reducing pain and speeding healing. Self-initiated therapy with six times daily topical 1% penciclovir cream is effective in speeding the healing of oral-labial HSV; topical acyclovir cream has also been shown to speed healing.

Suppression of reactivation of oral-labial HSV: Oral acyclovir (400 mg bid), if started before exposure and continued for the duration of exposure (usually 5-10 days), prevents reactivation of recurrent oral-labial HSV infection associated with severe sun exposure.

Herpetic Whitlow

Oral acyclovir (200 mg) five times daily for 7-10 days.

HSV Proctitis

Oral acyclovir (400 mg five times per day) is useful in shortening the course of infection. In immunosuppressed patients or in patients with severe infection, IV acyclovir (5 mg/kg q8h) may be useful.

Herpetic Eye Infections

In acute keratitis, topical trifluorothymidine, vidarabine, idoxuridine, acyclovir, penciclovir, and interferon are all beneficial. Debridement may be required; topical steroids may worsen disease.

CNS HSV Infections

HSV encephalitis: Intravenous acyclovir (10 mg/kg q8h; 30 mg/kg per day) for 14-21 days is preferred.

HSV aseptic meningitis: No studies of systemic antiviral chemotherapy exist. If therapy is to be given, IV acyclovir (15-30 mg/kg/day) should be used.

Autonomic radiculopathy: No studies are available.

Neonatal HSV infections: Acyclovir (60 mg/kg/day, divided into three doses) is given. The recommended duration of treatment is 21 days. Monitoring for relapse should be undertaken, and some authorities recommend continued suppression with oral acyclovir suspension for 3 to 4 mo.

Visceral HSV Infections

HSV esophagitis: IV acyclovir (15 mg/kg per day). In some patients with milder forms of immunosuppression, oral therapy with valacyclovir or famciclovir is effective.

HSV pneumonitis: No controlled studies exist. IV acyclovir (15 mg/kg per day) should be considered.

Disseminated HSV infections: No controlled studies exist. Intravenous acyclovir (10 mg/kg q8h) nevertheless should be tried. No definite evidence indicates that therapy decreases the risk of death.

Erythema multiforme-associated HSV: Anecdotal observations suggest that oral acyclovir (400 mg bid or tid) or valacyclovir (500 mg bid) suppresses erythema multiforme.

Surgical prophylaxis: Several surgical procedures such as laser skin resurfacing, trigeminal nerve root decompression, and lumbar disk surgery have been associated with HSV reactivation. Intravenous acyclovir (3 mg/kg) and oral acyclovir 800 mg bid, valacyclovir 500 mg bid, or famciclovir 250 mg bid is effective in reducing reactivation. Therapy should be initiated 48 hours before surgery and continued for 3 to 7 days.

Infections with acyclovir-resistant HSV: Foscarnet (40 mg/kg IV q8h) should be given until lesions heal. The optimal duration of therapy and the usefulness of its continuation to suppress lesions are unclear. Some patients may benefit from cutaneous application of trifluorothymidine or 5% cidofovir gel.

CMV, Cytomegalovirus; *CNS,* central nervous system; *HIV,* human immunodeficiency virus; *HSV,* herpes simplex virus; *TTP,* thrombotic thrombocytopenic purpura.

From Mandell GL et al: *Principles and practice of infectious diseases,* ed 6, Philadelphia, 2005, Churchill Livingstone.

BASIC INFORMATION

DEFINITION

Herpes zoster is a disease caused by reactivation of the varicella-zoster virus, with spread of the virus alone from the sensory nerve to the dermatome. After the primary infection (chickenpox), the virus becomes latent in the dorsal root ganglia and reemerges when there is a weakening of the immune system (as a result of disease or advanced age).

SYNONYMS

Shingles
HZ

ICD-9CM CODES	
053.9	Herpes zoster
ICD-10CM CODES	
B02	Herpes zoster
B02.7	Disseminated zoster
B02.8	Zoster with other complications
B02.9	Zoster without complications

EPIDEMIOLOGY & DEMOGRAPHICS

- Herpes zoster occurs during the lifetime of 10% to 20% of the population.
- There is an increased incidence in immunocompromised patients (AIDS, malignancy), the elderly, and children who acquired chickenpox when younger than 2 mo.

PHYSICAL FINDINGS & CLINICAL PRESENTATION

- Pain generally precedes skin manifestation by 3 to 5 days and is generally localized to the dermatome that will be affected by the skin lesions.
- Constitutional symptoms are often present (malaise, fever, headache).
- The initial rash consists of erythematous maculopapules generally affecting one dermatome (thoracic region in majority of cases). Typically the rash does not cross the midline. Some patients (<30%) may have scattered vesicles outside the affected dermatome.
- The initial maculopapules evolve into vesicles and pustules by the third or the fourth day.
- The vesicles have an erythematous base (Fig. E1-462), are cloudy, and have various sizes (a distinguishing characteristic from herpes simplex, in which the vesicles are of uniform size).
- The vesicles subsequently become umbilicated and then form crusts (Fig. E1-463) that generally fall off within 3 wk; scarring may occur.
- Pain during and after the rash is generally significant. Post-herpetic neuralgia occurs after herpes zoster in approximately one third of patients aged 60 years and older and can persist for months or years.
- Secondary bacterial infection with *Staphylococcus aureus* or *Streptococcus pyogenes* may occur.
- Regional lymphadenopathy may occur.
- Herpes zoster may involve the trigeminal nerve (most frequent cranial nerve involved); involvement of the geniculate ganglion can cause facial palsy and a painful ear, with the presence of vesicles on the pinna and external auditory canal (Ramsay Hunt syndrome).

ETIOLOGY

Reactivation of varicella virus (human herpes virus III)

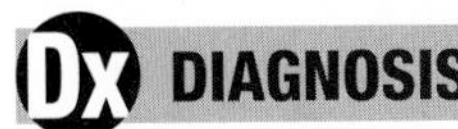

DIAGNOSIS

DIFFERENTIAL DIAGNOSIS

- Rash: herpes simplex and other viral infections
- Pain from herpes zoster: may be confused with acute myocardial infarction, pulmonary embolism, pleuritis, pericarditis, renal colic

LABORATORY TESTS

Laboratory tests are generally not necessary (viral cultures and Tzanck smear will confirm diagnosis in patients with atypical presentation).

TREATMENT

NONPHARMACOLOGIC THERAPY

- Wet compresses (using Burow's solution or cool tap water) applied for 15 to 30 min five to 10 times a day are useful to break vesicles and remove serum and crust.
- Care must be taken to prevent any secondary bacterial infection.

ACUTE GENERAL Rx

- Oral antiviral agents can decrease acute pain, inflammation, and vesicle formation when treatment is begun within 48 hr of onset of rash. Treatment options are:
  1. Valacyclovir 1000 mg tid for 7 days
  2. Famciclovir 500 mg tid for 7 days
  3. Acyclovir 800 mg 5 times daily for 7 to 10 days
- Corticosteroids should be considered in older patients within 72 hr of clinical presentation or if new lesions are still appearing if there are no contraindications. Initial dose is prednisone 40 mg/day decreased by 5 mg/day until finished. When used there is a decrease in the use of analgesics and time to resumption of usual activities, but there is no effect on the incidence and duration of postherpetic neuralgia.
- Immunocompromised patients should be treated with IV acyclovir 500 mg/m^2 or 10 mg/kg q8h in 1-hr infusions for 7 days, with close monitoring of renal function and adequate hydration; vidarabine (continuous 12-hr infusion of 10 mg/kg/day for 7 days) is also effective for treatment of disseminated herpes zoster in immunocompromised hosts.
- Patients with AIDS and transplant recipients may develop acyclovir-resistant varicella-zoster; these patients can be treated with foscarnet (40 mg/kg IV q8h) continued for at least 10 days or until lesions are completely healed.
- Postherpetic neuralgia (Fig. E1-464)
  - Gabapentin 100 to 600 mg tid is effective in the treatment of pain and sleep interference associated with postherpetic neuralgia. Other effective agents are pregabalin, duloxetine, and tricyclic antidepressants.
  - Lidocaine patch 5% is also effective in relieving postherpetic neuralgia. Patches are applied to intact skin after resolution of blisters and crusts to cover the most painful area for up to 12 hr within a 24-hr period.
  - Capsaicin cream can be useful for treatment of postherpetic neuralgia. It is generally applied 3 to 5 times daily for several weeks after the crusts have fallen off. A topical 8% patch formulation of capsaicin is now available by prescription for postherpetic neuralgia.
  - Sympathetic blocks (stellate ganglion or epidural) with 0.25% bupivacaine and rhizotomy are reserved for severe cases unresponsive to conservative treatment.

DISPOSITION

- The incidence of postherpetic neuralgia (defined as pain that persists more than 90 days after onset of rash) increases with age (<30% by age 40 yr, >70% by age 70 yr); antivirals reduce the risk of postherpetic neuralgia.
- Incidence of disseminated herpes zoster is increased in immunocompromised hosts (e.g., 15% to 50% of patients with active Hodgkin's disease).
- Immunocompromised hosts are also more prone to neurologic complications (encephalitis, myelitis, cranial and peripheral nerve palsies, acute retinal necrosis). The mortality rate is 10% to 20% in immunocompromised hosts with disseminated zoster.
- Motor neuropathies occur in 5% of all cases of zoster; complete recovery occurs in >70% of patients.
- Rates of HZ recurrence are more frequently than previously reported and are comparable to rates of first HZ occurrence in immunocompetent individuals.

REFERRAL

- Hospitalization for IV acyclovir in patients with disseminated herpes zoster.
- Patients with herpes zoster ophthalmicus should be referred to an ophthalmologist.
- Vaccination: In the absence of the herpes zoster vaccine, persons who live to 85 yr of age have a 50% risk of herpes zoster. Immunocompetent adults ≥60 yr are appropriate candidates for a single dose of varicella-zoster vaccine (VZV) whether or not they have had a previous episode of herpes zoster. Immunization with VZV (Zostavax) boosts waning immunity in older adults and reduces the severity and duration of pain caused by herpes zoster by 61%. Adults who are VZV

seronegative (never had varicella) should be immunized against varicella with two doses of varicella vaccine (Varivax). Despite its efficacy and safety, use of this vaccine remains low (<8% of potential recipients).

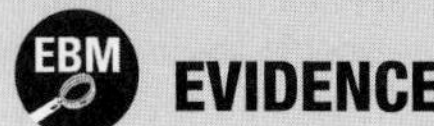

EVIDENCE

available at www.expertconsult.com

SUGGESTED READINGS

available at www.expertconsult.com

RELATED CONTENT

Shingles (Patient Information)

AUTHOR: **FRED F. FERRI, M.D.**

BASIC INFORMATION

DEFINITION

A hiatal hernia is the protrusion of a portion of the stomach into the thoracic cavity through the diaphragmatic esophageal hiatus.

SYNONYMS

Hiatus hernia
Diaphragmatic hernia

ICD-9CM CODES
553.3 Diaphragmatic hernia without obstruction or gangrene
750.6 Congenital hiatal hernia
756.6 Congenital diaphragmatic hernia
ICD-10CM CODES
K44.9 Diaphragmatic hernia without obstruction or gangrene
Q40.1 Congenital hiatus hernia
Q79.0 Congenital diaphragmatic hernia

EPIDEMIOLOGY & DEMOGRAPHICS

- Found in 50% of patients older than 50 yr.
- Prevalence increases with age.
- More prevalent in Western countries than in Africa and Asia.
- Paraesophageal hiatal hernias are more common in women than in men (4:1).
- Associated with diverticulosis (25%), esophagitis (25%), duodenal ulcers (20%), and gallstones (18%).
- More than 90% of patients with endoscopic documentation of esophagitis have hiatal hernias.

PHYSICAL FINDINGS & CLINICAL PRESENTATION

Most patients are asymptomatic. If symptoms are present, they resemble those of gastroesophageal reflux disease (GERD).

- Heartburn
- Dysphagia
- Regurgitation of gastric contents
- Chest pain
- Postprandial fullness
- GI bleed
- Dyspnea
- Hoarseness
- Wheezing with bowel sounds heard over the left lung base

ETIOLOGY

- The repetitive stretching of the gastroesophageal (GE) junction with swallowing and actions (e.g., vomiting) or states (e.g., obesity, pregnancy) that increase intraabdominal pressure may cause widening of the hiatus, rupture of the phrenoesophageal ligament, and onset of the hernia.
- Hiatal hernias are classified as:
  1. Type I: Sliding (Fig. 1-465, *A*), axial, or concentric hiatal hernia (most common type, 99%). Only the GE junction protrudes into the thoracic cavity and the phrenoesophageal ligament remains intact.
  2. Type II: Paraesophageal or rolling hernia (Fig. 1-465, *B*) (1%). The GE junction stays at the level of the diaphragm, but part of the stomach bulges into the thoracic cavity through a defect in the phrenoesophageal ligament.
  3. Type III: Mixed (rare), a combination of type I and type II.
  4. Type IV: Large defect in hiatus that allows other intraabdominal organs to enter the hernia sac.

DIAGNOSIS

DIFFERENTIAL DIAGNOSIS

- Peptic ulcer disease
- Unstable angina
- Esophagitis (caused by *Candida,* herpes, NSAIDs, etc.)
- Esophageal spasm
- Barrett's esophagus
- Schatzki's ring
- Achalasia
- Zenker's diverticulum
- Esophageal cancer

WORKUP

- Exclude conditions noted in the differential diagnosis and document the presence of a hiatal hernia. Upper endoscopy may also be needed to exclude abnormal metaplasia, dysplasia, or neoplasia.

LABORATORY TESTS

- Blood tests are not specific.
- Esophageal manometry, although not commonly done, can be used in establishing a diagnosis (low sensitivity, but high specificity when compared with endoscopy).

IMAGING STUDIES

- Upper gastrointestinal (UGI) barium contrast swallow series: best defines the anatomic abnormality. Demonstration that the gastric cardia is herniated 2 cm above the hiatus is diagnostic. UGI may also reveal a tortuous esophagus (Fig. 1-466). If endoscopy is performed preoperatively, a barium swallow is generally not necessary.
- UGI endoscopy: documents the presence of a hiatal hernia and also excludes commonly associated findings of esophagitis and Barrett's esophagus (recommended at least once during the workup). Greater than 2 cm of gastric rugal fold seen above the margins of the diaphragmatic crura is diagnostic.
- Abdominal ultrasonography: simple, well tolerated. A transdiaphragmatic esophageal diameter of more than or equal to 18 mm is highly suggestive of the presence of a sliding hiatal hernia.

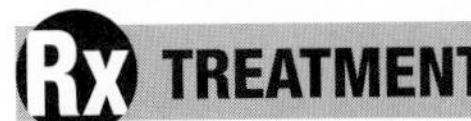

TREATMENT

NONPHARMACOLOGIC THERAPY

- Lifestyle modifications: avoid foods and drugs that decrease lower-esophageal pressure (e.g., caffeine, chocolate, mint, calcium channel blockers, and anticholinergics)
- Weight loss
- Avoid large quantities of food with meals
- Sleep with the head of the bed elevated 6 inches

ACUTE GENERAL Rx

- Antacids may be useful to relieve mild symptoms.
- H_2 antagonists (e.g., cimetidine 400 mg bid, ranitidine 150 mg bid, or famotidine 20 mg bid).
- If significant GERD is present with documented esophagitis, proton pump inhibitors (e.g., omeprazole 20 mg qd or lansoprazole 30 mg qd) are used. Refractory symptoms may require higher doses (e.g., bid dosing).
- Prokinetic agents (e.g., metoclopramide 10 mg taken 30 min before each meal) can be added to an H_2 antagonist or proton pump inhibitor.

CHRONIC Rx

- When indicated, surgery (laparoscopic or open) can be done in patients with refractory symptoms impairing quality of life, or causing intestinal (e.g., recurrent GI bleeds) or extraintestinal complications (e.g., aspiration pneumonia, asthma, or ear-nose-throat complications).

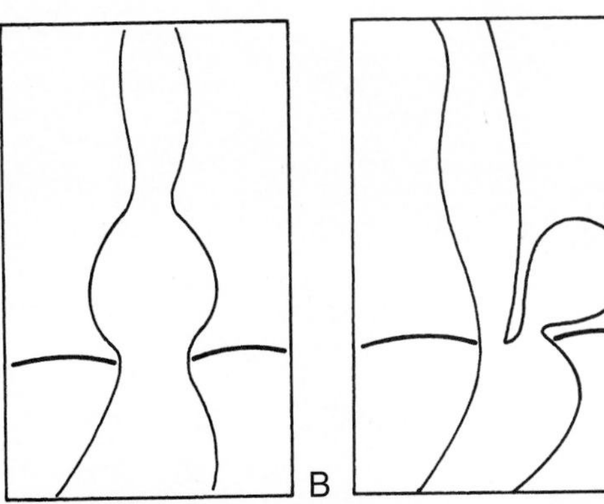

FIGURE 1-465 Types of esophageal hiatal hernia. A, Sliding hiatal hernia, the most common type. **B,** Paraesophageal hiatal hernia. (From Behrman RE: *Nelson textbook of pediatrics,* ed 17, Philadelphia, 2004, Saunders.)

 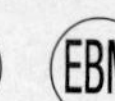 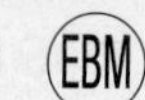

- Prophylactic surgery is a consideration in all paraesophageal hernias because they have a higher incidence of strangulation.

DISPOSITION

- More than 90% of patients having GERD symptoms respond well to medical therapy.
- Complications of hiatal hernias are similar to complications occurring in patients with GERD:
  1. Erosive esophagitis
  2. Ulcerative esophagitis
  3. Barrett's esophagus
  4. Peptic stricture
  5. GI hemorrhage
  6. Extraintestinal complications
  7. Lung collapse or heart failure (severe cases)

REFERRAL

Gastroenterologist: for symptoms refractory to conventional therapy (H_2 antagonists, antacids, and proton pump inhibitors) or having complications previously mentioned.

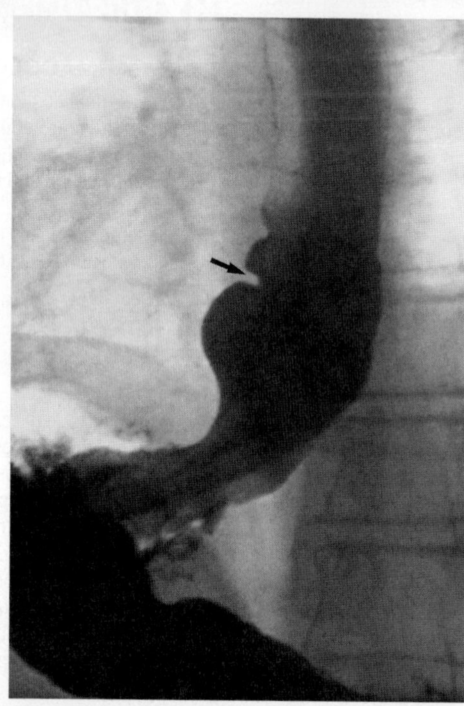

FIGURE 1-466 A sliding hiatal hernia confirmed by the presence of an incisural notch *(arrow)* on the greater curve aspect. (From Grainger RG et al [eds]: *Grainger & Allison's diagnostic radiology,* ed 4, Philadelphia, 2001, Churchill Livingstone.)

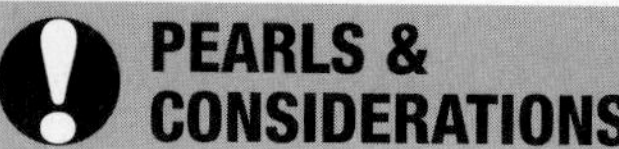

PEARLS & CONSIDERATIONS

COMMENTS

- Gastric ulceration and erosions (***Cameron's lesion***) can occur in the paraesophageal hernia pouch and are an uncommon cause of UGI bleeding.
- May cause iron deficiency anemia.
- Gastric volvulus or torsion can also occur and presents as dysphagia and postprandial pain.
- High incidence of esophagitis even after the eradication of *Helicobacter pylori.*
- The appearance of hiatal hernia may resemble a left atrial mass by echocardiography.

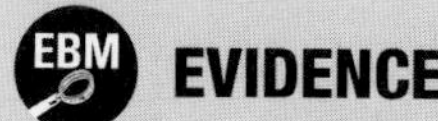

EVIDENCE

available at www.expertconsult.com

SUGGESTED READINGS

available at www.expertconsult.com

RELATED CONTENT

Hiatal Hernia (Patient Information)

AUTHOR: **MARK F. BRADY, M.D., M.P.H., M.M.S.**

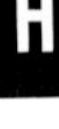

BASIC INFORMATION

DEFINITION

Hidradenitis suppurativa (HS) is a chronic, relapsing suppurative cutaneous disease affecting skin that bears apocrine glands and manifested by abscesses, fistulating sinus tracts, and chronic infection leading to scarring.

SYNONYMS

Acne inversa
Apocrinitis
Verneuil's disease
HS

ICD-9CM CODES
705.83 Hidradenitis
ICD-10CM CODES
L73.2 Hidradenitis suppurativa

EPIDEMIOLOGY & DEMOGRAPHICS

Onset is postpubertal, with an average age of onset of 23 yr; rates decline after age 55 yr.

PREVALENCE: Overall prevalence in the United States is ~1% to 2%.

PREDOMINANT SEX: Female to male ratio is 3:1.

RISK FACTORS:
- Obesity
- Family history (approximately 30%)
- Hyperandrogenism in women
- Cigarette smoking

PHYSICAL FINDINGS & CLINICAL PRESENTATION

The diagnosis is primarily clinical based on the development of typical lesions in a characteristic distribution, with a relapsing nature.

- Early symptoms include pain, itching, burning, erythema, and hyperhidrosis.
- Typical lesions include:
  - Painful erythematous papules and nodules
  - Painful abscesses and inflamed papules or nodules with foul-smelling discharge
  - Dermal contractures and ropelike elevation of the skin
  - Comedones in the apocrine, gland-bearing skin
- Classified into Hurley Stages
  - Stage I: abscesses without sinus tracts or scarring
  - Stage II: multiple abscesses plus sinus tracts and scarring
  - Stage III: diffuse involvement of entire area with abscesses, sinus tracts, and scarring
- The axilla is the most common site (Fig. 1-467).
- Less common sites include the inguinal region, the breasts more often in women, and the perineal or perianal skin more often in men.
- There is a strong tendency toward relapse and recurrence.
- Other characteristics of the disease are:
  - Poor response to conventional antibiotics
  - Often no pathogens from routine cultures of lesions
- The disease is often mistaken for a simple infection and a long delay in diagnosis is common.

ETIOLOGY

- Keratinous materials plug apocrine glands in hair follicles leading to stasis, dilation, rupture, and re-epithelialization of glands.
- Bacteria are trapped and multiply leading to gland rupture with surrounding inflammation and local bacterial infection.
- Over time, repeated nodules and infections cause scarring, which can lead to deep tissue damage and sinus tracts.
- Infectious agents such as *Streptococcus, Staphylococcus,* and *Escherichia coli,* and enteric flora have been identified in cultures, but are likely a secondary cause of the disease.
- There is likely a significant genetic component to the disease. An HS spectrum of different phenotypes has been characterized involving genetic factors that are not yet well described but may be important for future therapy.
- HS has been associated with other endocrine and autoimmune disorders such as diabetes, Cushing's disease, acromegaly, Crohn's disease, and inflammatory arthritis.
- Recent data suggest that the interleukin-12-interleukin-23 pathway and tumor necrosis factor-α (TNF-α) may be involved in the pathogenesis of HS.
- Metabolic syndrome which affects many patients with HS may exacerbate the inflammation associated with HS.

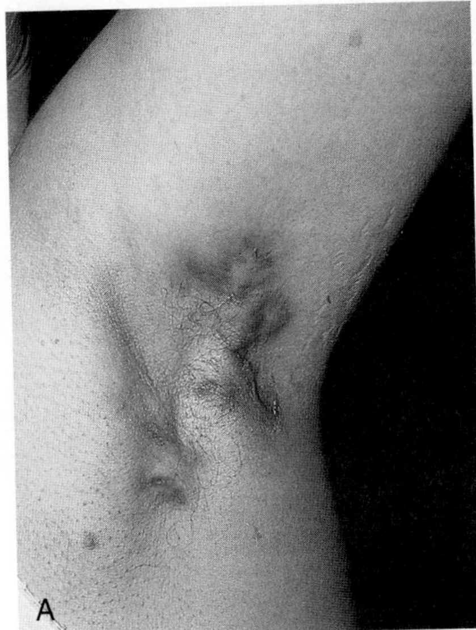

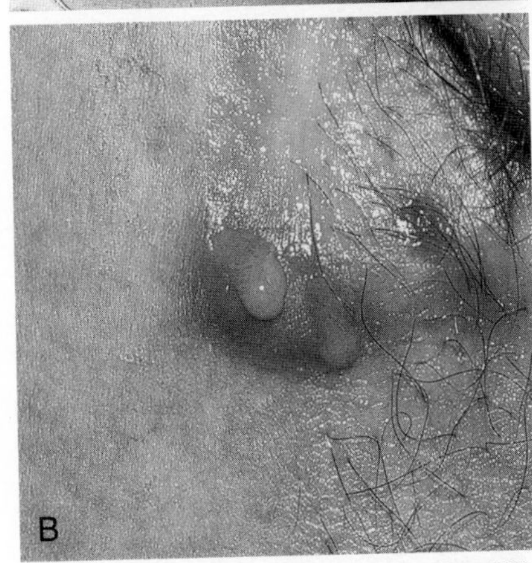

FIGURE 1-467 Hidradenitis suppurativa (HS). A, HS of the axilla. This is the classic appearance with inflammatory nodules and scarred areas. This condition is commonly misdiagnosed as a bacterial infection. **B,** HS of the axilla; a close-up view of the draining pus. When intact, the lesions represent sterile abscesses. Once open, they may become secondarily infected. (From White GM, Cox NH [eds]: *Diseases of the skin: a color atlas and text,* ed 2, St Louis, 2006, Mosby.)

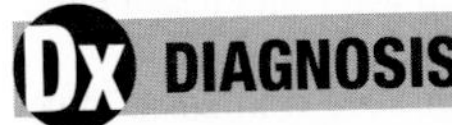

DIAGNOSIS

DIFFERENTIAL DIAGNOSIS

- Follicular pyodermas such as folliculitis, furuncles, carbuncles, and pilonidal cysts
- Granuloma inguinale
- Perianal and vulvar manifestations of Crohn's disease
- Actinomycosis
- Lymphogranuloma venereum
- Dermoid, epidermoid, or Bartholin's cysts
- Tuberculous inflammation of the skin
- Lymphadenitis
- Erysipelas

WORKUP

Primarily a clinical diagnosis based on typical lesion (see "Physical Findings & Clinical Presentation")

LABORATORY TESTS

- Patients with acute lesions may have an elevated erythrocyte sedimentation rate or WBC.
- Febrile and toxic appearing patients should have complete blood count, chemistries, and blood cultures.
- Any pus should be sampled for bacterial culture and sensitivity.

TREATMENT

There is no definitive cure for hidradenitis.

NONPHARMACOLOGIC THERAPY

- Weight loss and control of metabolic syndrome
- Smoking cessation
- Avoidance of shaving, depilatory creams, deodorants
- Warm compresses
- Incision and drainage of nonpurulent lesions is *not* recommended due to recurrence
- Laser therapy, radiotherapy, and cryotherapy currently under study
- Wide local excision for stage III disease

ACUTE AND CHRONIC Rx

- NSAIDs for inflammation and pain.
- Antibiotics never proven to be effective; however, are mainstay of treatment. Can base treatment on the basis of aspirate culture and sensitivities or empirically.
  - Clindamycin is the only topical antibiotic proven to be effective in randomized controlled trial and is appropriate for stage I disease.

- For oral therapy in stage II: consider clindamycin and rifampin in combination. Cephalosporins, dicloxacillin, erythromycin, minocycline, and tetracycline have also been used.
- Severe, recurrent disease can require up to 3 to 6 mo of antibiotics.
- Oral contraceptives with low androgenic progesterone (norgestimate, desogestrel, or gestodene) for women show mixed effectiveness.
- Isotretinoin has been used with mixed effectiveness.
- Metformin has been used with some effectiveness, possibly because of its effects on metabolic syndrome and hyperandrogenism.
- Corticosteroids and other immune suppressants such as cyclosporin, infliximab, and etanercept have been used for stage II disease, with mixed results.
- Adalimumab, an anti–tumor necrosis factor-α antibody given once per week (dose 40 mg/wk) has been used with mixed results, and further studies are needed.

COMPLICATIONS

- Squamous cell carcinoma
- Scarring leading to restricted limb mobility or lymphedema
- Rectal or urethral fistulas

REFERRAL

- Referral to dermatology during stage I to II disease.
- Referral to a surgeon is indicated for stage III disease.

PEARLS & CONSIDERATIONS

COMMENTS

- Patients with hidradenitis are at risk for severe depression, social isolation, and negatively impacted sexuality as a result of their disease.
- There is an average delay in diagnosis of 12 years and most patients are diagnosed in stage II of the disease (recurrent abscesses with scarring and development of sinus tracts).
- It is important to maximize nonmedical treatment, start medical treatment, and refer to a surgeon early in the disease course to ensure the best quality of life for patients.
- The only definitive treatment for hidradenitis is wide excision of the involved skin.

SUGGESTED READINGS

available at www.expertconsult.com

AUTHOR: **MARY BETH SUTTER, M.D.**

BASIC INFORMATION

DEFINITION

High-altitude illness refers to a spectrum of cerebral and pulmonary syndromes related to hypoxemia occurring during rapid ascension to high altitudes. Common acute syndromes include high-altitude pulmonary edema (HAPE), acute mountain sickness (AMS), high-altitude pulmonary edema (HAPE), and high-altitude cerebral edema (HACE). The latter two are thought to represent different points of severity along the same pathophysiologic process in the brain.

SYNONYMS

Altitude sickness
Acute mountain sickness
High-altitude pulmonary edema
High-altitude cerebral edema

ICD-9CM CODES
289 Mountain sickness, acute
993.2 High altitude, effects

ICD-10CM CODES
W94 Exposure to high and low air pressure and changes in air pressure
T70.2 Other and unspecified effects of high altitude

EPIDEMIOLOGY & DEMOGRAPHICS

- More than 30 million people are at risk of developing altitude sickness.
- AMS is the most common of the altitude diseases.
  - Approximately 40% to 50% of people ascending to 14,000 ft (4200 m) from lowland living develop AMS.
- The incidence of HACE is reported to be 0.1 to 2 percent at elevations in excess of 12,000 ft (3000 m). HACE is often complicated by concomitant HAPE.
- Men are five times more likely to develop HAPE than are women.
- AMS and HACE affect men and women equally.

PHYSICAL FINDINGS & CLINICAL PRESENTATION (Table E1-236)

AMS
- Occurs within 6-12 hours after rapid ascent to 8000 ft (2500 m) in 10%-25% of unacclimatized persons.
- Headache is the most common symptom
- Dizziness and lightheadedness
- Nausea, vomiting, and loss of appetite
- Fatigue
- Sleep disturbance from an exaggerated hyperventilatory phase of Cheyne-Stokes respiration in response to hypoxemia and alkalosis
- AMS can evolve into HAPE and HACE.
- Supplemental oxygen may be used to support the clinical diagnosis

HAPE (Fig. 1-468A)
- Typically occurs 2 to 4 days after ascent over 8000 ft (2500 m).
- Dyspnea, loss of stamina
- Dry cough or cough with frothy rust- or pink-tinged sputum
- Chest tightness
- Tachycardia, tachypnea, rales, cyanosis

HACE
- Usually presents several days after AMS
- Confusion, irritability, drowsiness, stupor, hallucinations, mild fever
- Headache, nausea, vomiting
- Truncal ataxia, paralysis, and seizures
- Coma and death from brain herniation may develop within hours of the first symptoms.

ETIOLOGY

- During ascension to altitudes above sea level, the atmospheric pressure decreases. Although the percentage of oxygen in the air remains the same, the partial pressure of oxygen decreases with increased altitude, and can cause hypoxemia. Fig. 1-468B illustrates the effect of altitude on alveolar Pa_{O_2} and oxygen saturation.
- Increased cerebral blood flow and the loss of autoregulation of intracranial pressure may contribute to increased cerebral vascular permeability and subsequent brain edema.
- Hypobaric hypoxia can trigger elevated pulmonary pressures, resulting in protein-rich, hemorrhagic exudates into the lung alveoli due to a breakdown in the pulmonary blood-gas barrier (HAPE).
- The body responds to low oxygen partial pressures through a process of acclimatization (see "Comments").

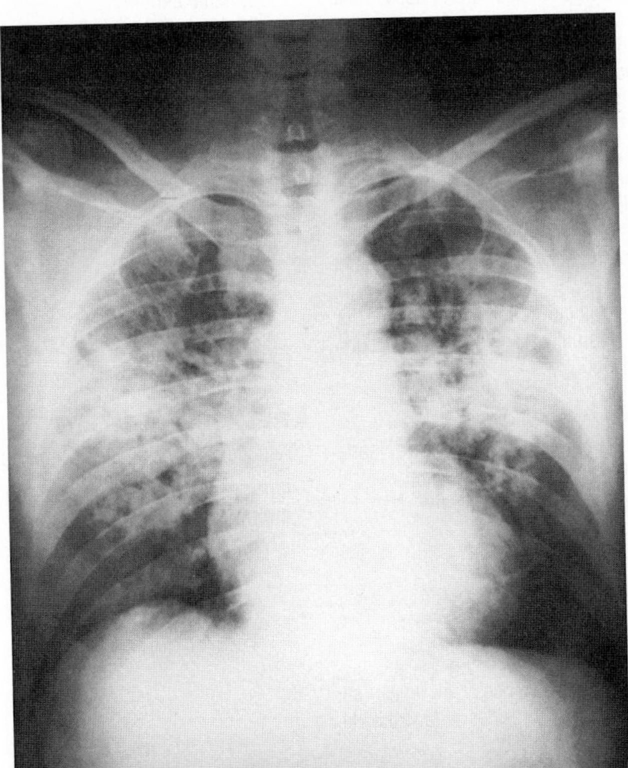

FIGURE 1-468A Chest radiograph showing high-altitude pulmonary edema. (From Strauss RH [ed]: *Sports medicine,* ed 2, Philadelphia, 1991, Saunders.)

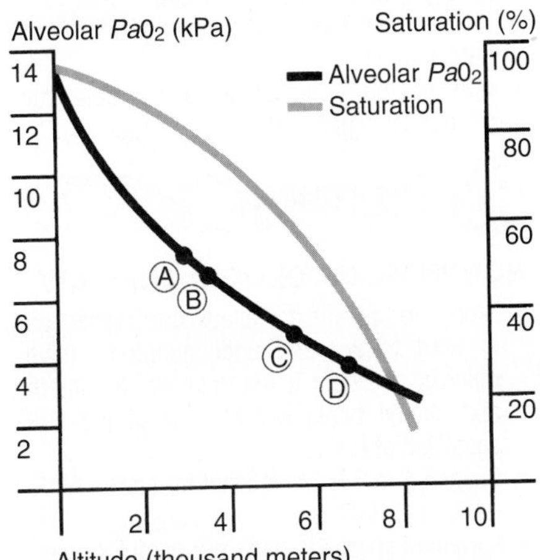

FIGURE 1-468B Effect of altitude on alveolar PaO_2 and oxygen saturation. Because of the steep slope of the oxygen dissociation curve, increasing altitude above 5000 m causes a precipitous fall in saturation. In an unacclimated person, acute change occurs at, *A,* 3000 m (10,000 ft)—slightly impaired memory and judgment, increased heart rate, abdominal cramps and nausea; *B,* 3500 m (12,000 ft)—headache, nausea, diminished visual acuity, and possible pulmonary edema; *C,* 5500 m (18,000 ft)—impaired consciousness after several hours in many people; and *D,* 6750 m (22,000 ft)—loss of consciousness. (From Souhami RL, Moxham J: *Textbook of medicine,* ed 4, London, 2002, Churchill Livingstone.)

DIAGNOSIS

Made by clinical presentation and physical findings.

DIFFERENTIAL DIAGNOSIS

- Dehydration
- Carbon monoxide poisoning
- Hypothermia
- Infection
- Substance abuse
- Congestive heart failure
- Pulmonary embolism
- Cerebrovascular accident
- Box E1-35 summarizes the differential diagnosis of high-altitude illnesses

WORKUP

Typically the diagnosis is self-evident after history and physical examination. Laboratory tests and imaging studies help monitor cardiopulmonary and central nervous system status in patients admitted to the intensive care unit for pulmonary and/or cerebral edema. In patients with HAPE occurring at lower altitudes (<8000 ft), an evaluation of preexisting pulmonary hypertension or a left-to-right shunt should be considered.

LABORATORY TESTS

Not useful, unless to rule out an alternative diagnosis

IMAGING STUDIES

- Chest x-ray showing Kerley B-lines and patchy edema (see Fig. 1-468A)
- CT scan of the head showing diffuse or patchy edema
- MRI of the head showing characteristic intense T2 signal in the white matter

TREATMENT

NONPHARMACOLOGIC THERAPY

- Stop the ascent to allow acclimatization or start to descend until symptoms have resolved. Descent is the definitive treatment and should begin immediately at the first suspicion of HACE.
- Oxygen 4 to 6 L/min is used for severe AMS, HAPE, and HACE.
- Portable hyperbaric bags are useful if available at the site.
- Altitude can cause diuresis that may be mediated by enhanced release of atrial natriuretic peptide. When coupled with the increased fluid loss through increased ventilation, there is a higher risk for dehydration, and adequate hydration should be maintained.

ACUTE PHARMACOLOGIC Rx

- Nonsteroidal anti-inflammatory drugs (e.g., ibuprofen 600 mg every 6 hours, beginning 6 hours before ascending) are effective prophylaxis of traditional altitude sickness and in treating headaches in AMS.
- Acetazolamide 125 to 250 mg PO bid has been effective for both prevention and acute therapy in patients with AMS and HACE.
- Nifedipine 10 mg sublingual followed by long-acting nifedipine 30 mg bid is used for patients with HAPE who cannot descend immediately.
- Dexamethasone 4 mg PO every 6 hr is used in patients with severe AMS, HAPE, or HACE.

CHRONIC Rx

Prevention is the most prudent therapy.

1. Slow, staged ascent to avoid altitude sickness.
2. Start the ascent below 8000 feet.
3. Ascend 1000 feet/day (300 m/day).
4. Spend two nights at the same altitude every 3 days.
5. Sleep at lower heights than the altitude climbed ("climb high, sleep low").
6. Prophylactic therapy with NSAIDs (ibuprofen 600 mg every 6 hours, beginning 6 hours before ascending) or acetazolamide up to 750 mg daily and/or dexamethasone 8 to 16 mg daily decreases the risk of developing AMS (combination may have additive benefit). The drugs should be used until acclimatization occurs.
7. Prophylactic inhalation of a β-adrenergic agonist, salmeterol 125 mcg q12h, or the use of slow-release nifedipine 20 mg bid have both been shown to reduce the risk of HAPE in susceptible individuals.
8. Tadalafil, a long-acting phosphodiesterase inhibitor, has recently been shown to decrease the incidence of HAPE in susceptible individuals.
9. Box E1-36 summarizes field treatment of high-altitude illness.

DISPOSITION

- AMS improves over a period of 2 to 3 days.
- HAPE is the most common cause of death among patients with altitude illnesses.
- More than 60% of patients with HAPE will have recurrence of symptoms on subsequent climbs.
- In HACE, neurologic deficits may persist for weeks but eventually resolve. If coma occurs, prognosis is poor.

REFERRAL

Cardiology and neurology referrals are made in patients with pulmonary edema and central nervous system findings, respectively.

PEARLS & CONSIDERATIONS

COMMENTS

- Acclimatization is the process in which an individual who normally resides at low altitude adapts to hypobaric hypoxia to improve tolerance and performance at higher altitude. These mechanisms include:
  1. An increase in respiratory rates and tidal volume. This hyperventilation allows lowering of arterial carbon dioxide to preserve oxygen delivery, even at extreme altitudes.
  2. An early increase in heart rate and stroke volume to improve oxygen delivery. After 1 wk, both parameters decrease because of diuresis and lower catecholamine levels.
  3. Pulmonary hypertension develops in response to hypoxemia, resulting in improvement of the ventilation-perfusion mismatch but may be maladaptive and lead to the development of HAPE.
  4. Cerebral vasodilation to increase blood flow to the brain.
  5. Rise in hemoglobin and hematocrit. This is a long-term process that takes up to 1 wk to occur in response to the need for improved oxygen delivery.
- Adaptation to altitude is different from acclimatization and refers to physiologic differences in permanent residents at high altitude (e.g., an increased oxygen diffusion capacity).
- High altitude illness can generally be prevented by ascending to 300-500 meters per day at altitudes above 3000 meters and including a rest day every 3-4 day.
- Risk factors for the development of altitude sicknesses are:
  1. Rapid ascent
  2. Previous history of altitude sickness
  3. Strenuous exertion on arrival
  4. Obesity
  5. Male gender
- Physical fitness is not protective against high-altitude illness.
- Both dexamethasone and tadalafil decrease systolic pulmonary artery pressure and may reduce the incidence of HAPE in adults with a history of HAPE. Dexamethasone prophylaxis may also reduce the incidence of AMS in these adults.
- Descent is mandatory for all persons with HACE or HAPE.

SUGGESTED READINGS

available at www.expertconsult.com

RELATED CONTENT

Altitude Sickness (Patient Information)

AUTHORS: **JOHANNES STEINER, M.D.,** and **RICHARD REGNANTE, M.D.,**

BASIC INFORMATION

DEFINITION

Hip fractures are classified as intracapsular or extracapsular. Intracapsular fractures include femoral head and femoral neck fractures (Fig. 1-469). These fractures are further categorized as either displaced or nondisplaced. Extracapsular fractures include intertrochanteric and subtrochanteric fractures, as well as the less common greater and lesser trochanteric fractures. These fractures can be further categorized by the degree of comminution.

SYNONYMS

Hip fracture
Intracapsular fracture
Subcapital fracture
Extracapsular fracture
Intertrochanteric fracture

ICD-9CM CODES

820.8	Femoral neck fracture
820.2	Peritrochanteric fracture

ICD-10CM CODES

S72.0	Fracture of neck of femur
S72.1	Pertrochanteric fracture
S72.2	Subtrochanteric fracture
S72.3	Fracture of shaft of femur
S72.4	Fracture of lower end of femur
S72.7	Multiple fractures of femur
S72.8	Fractures of other parts of femur
S72.009A	Fracture of unspecified part of neck of unspecified femur, initial encounter for closed fracture

EPIDEMIOLOGY & DEMOGRAPHICS

PREVALENCE: Lifetime risk in women ~16%
PREDOMINANT SEX: Female/male ratio of 3:1
PREDOMINANT AGE: 90% >60 yr

PHYSICAL FINDINGS & CLINICAL PRESENTATION

- Hip or groin pain
- Affected limb usually shortened and externally rotated in displaced fractures
- Impacted fractures: possibly no deformity and only mild pain with hip motion
- Mild external bruising

RISK FACTORS

- Osteoporosis
- Age >75
- Gait instability, foot deformities, muscular weakness
- Sensory impairment
- Polypharmacy
- Impaired cognition, depression
- Use of alcohol or benzodiazepines
- Orthostatic hypotension
- Environmental hazards at home (e.g., loose rugs, loose cords)

ETIOLOGY

- Trauma
- Age-related bone weakness, usually caused by osteoporosis
- Increased risk of fractures in elderly (decline in muscle function, use of psychotropic medication, etc.)

DIAGNOSIS

DIFFERENTIAL DIAGNOSIS

- OA of hip, RA of hip
- Hip dislocation
- Pathologic fracture
- Lumbar disk syndrome with radicular pain
- Insufficiency fracture of pelvis
- Trochanteric bursitis
- Septic hip joint
- Pelvic fracture
- Lateral femoral cutaneous nerve entrapment (meralgia paresthetica)
- Osteitis deformans (Paget's disease)

WORKUP

Diagnosis is usually obvious based on clinical and radiographic findings (Figs. 1-470 and 1-471). Fig. E1-472 illustrates the Garden classification of femoral neck fractures.

IMAGING STUDIES

- Standard roentgenograms consisting of an anteroposterior view of the pelvis and a cross-table lateral view of the hip to confirm the diagnosis.
- If initial roentgenograms are negative and diagnosis of an occult femoral neck fracture is suspected, hospital admission and further radiographic assessment with either bone scanning or MRI are recommended.
- Bone scanning is sensitive after 48 to 72 hr.

TREATMENT

- Orthopedic consultation
- Surgery indicated in most cases, usually within 24 hr. Treatment depends on type of fracture:
  - Femoral neck, non-displaced, impacted valgus: cannulated screws
  - Displaced: <50 yr, emergent reduction, cannulated screws; >50 yr: hemiarthroplasty, unipolar vs. bipolar or total hip arthroplasty if preexisting degenerative changes
  - Intertrochanteric: stable, two and three parts, dynamic hip screw (DHS) vs. trochanteric femoral nail (TFN); unstable, four parts, subtrochanteric extension, TFN
  - Reverse obliquity: TFN, blade plate, dynamic condylar screw, not DHS
- Deep vein thrombosis prophylaxis (fondaparinux, LMWH, vitamin K antagonist). Mechanical prophylaxis is contraindicated. Prophylaxis is usually continued for 28-35 days post-op
- Pain management: effective pain management is a primary goal in hip fracture. Opioid analgesics have a high incidence of delirium and constipation. Nerve blockade is effective in reducing acute pain after hip fracture
- Prophylactic antibiotics should be initiated before surgery and continued for 24 hours after surgical repair
- Rehabilitation is a major component of hip fracture treatment and should be initiated on the first postoperative day

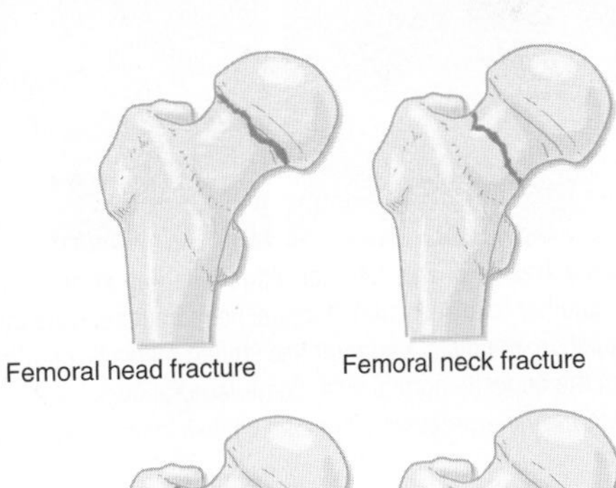

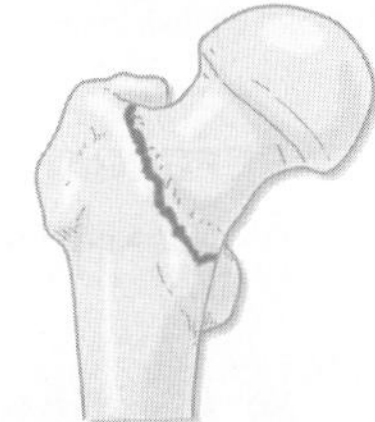

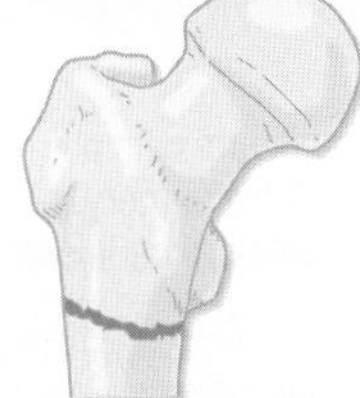

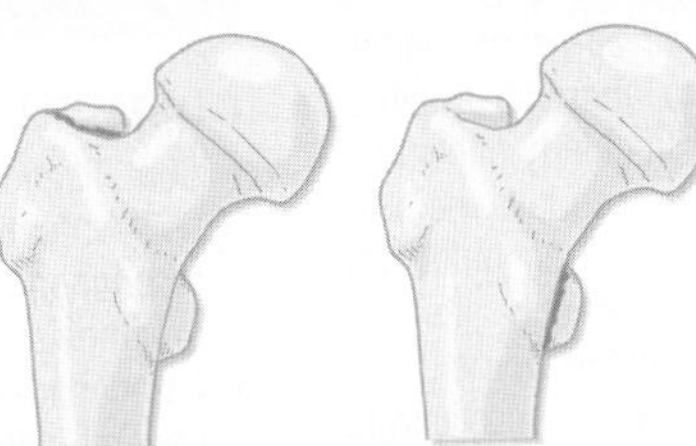

FIGURE 1-469 Types of hip fractures. (From Adams JG et al: *Emergency medicine, clinical essentials,* ed 2, Philadelphia, 2013, Elsevier.)

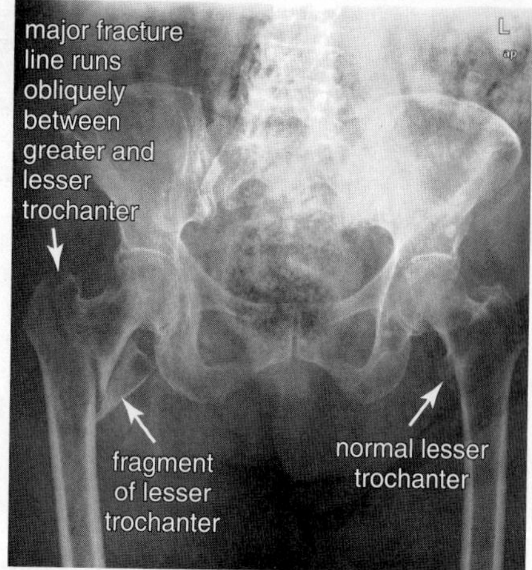

FIGURE 1-470 Intertrochanteric femur fracture: three parts (proximal, distal, and one trochanter). Intertrochanteric femur fractures are common, with the mechanism often being a fall from standing in an elderly patient. The major fracture line usually runs obliquely between the greater and the lesser trochanters. These fractures may have two, three, or four parts classically, although badly comminuted combinations are also possible. Two-part fractures consist of the proximal and distal fragments. Three-part fractures also include a fragment of one trochanter. Four-part fractures include fragments of both trochanters. This 86-year-old female had an unwitnessed fall. She has a typical three-part fracture, with a fragment of the lesser trochanter visible. Note her generalized severe osteopenia. (From Broder JS: *Diagnostic imaging for the emergency physician,* Philadelphia, 2011, Saunders.)

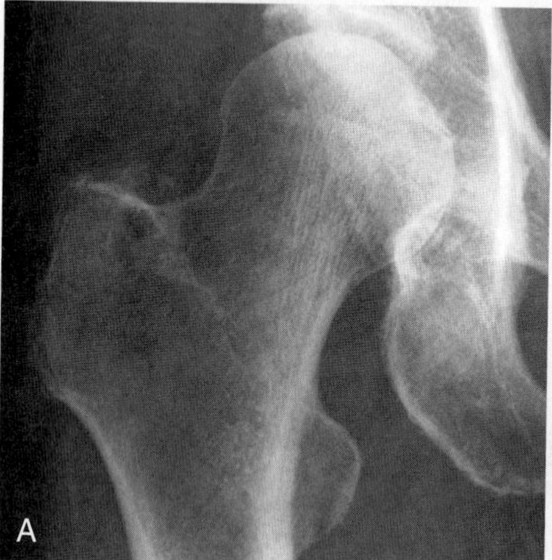

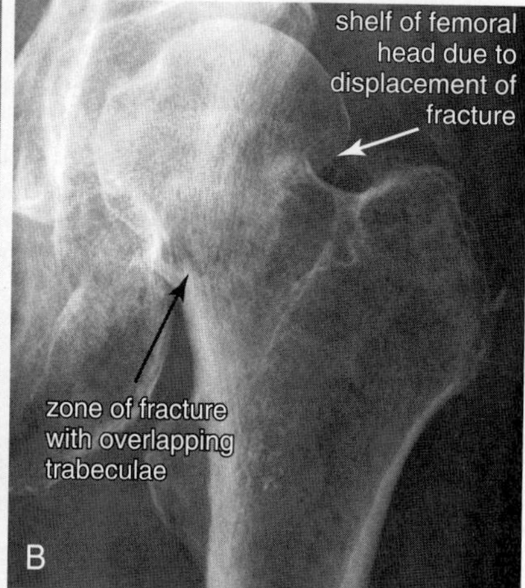

FIGURE 1-471 Femoral neck fracture. This 84-year-old female had an unwitnessed fall. **A,** Normal right hip, osteoporotic. **B,** Left hip, another relatively subtle femoral neck fracture. Note the smudging of the trabeculae of the femoral neck. In addition, the distal fragment has shifted medially, creating an overhanging ledge of the femoral head not seen on the opposite normal side. Some femoral neck fractures are more obvious. (From Broder JS: *Diagnostic imaging for the emergency physician*, Philadelphia, 2011, Saunders.)

- Conservative therapy in patients who are not surgical candidates (too ill for surgery, bed- or wheelchair-bound patients before injury)

DISPOSITION

- Surgical mortality after hip fracture repair is 2% to 3%. Older adults have a five- to eightfold increased risk for all-cause mortality during the first 3 mo after hip fracture. Mortality rate within 1 yr in elderly patients is 25% to 30%. Excess annual mortality persists over time for both women and men, but at any given age, excess annual mortality after hip fracture is higher in men than in women.
- Dementia is a particularly poor prognostic sign.

REFERRAL

For surgical consideration when the diagnosis is made

PEARLS & CONSIDERATIONS

COMMENTS

- Complications: nonunion, avascular necrosis, DVT, infection, delirium, decubitus ulcers, incontinence, persistent pain, loosening of prosthesis
- Intracapsular fractures: occasionally occur in nonambulatory patients
  1. Usually treated nonsurgically, especially in the patient with dementia and limited pain perception
  2. Early bed-to-chair mobilization and vigilant nursing care to avoid skin breakdown
  3. Fracture usually pain free in a short time even if solid bony healing does not occur
- As a result of the increasing life span of the female population, femoral neck fractures are becoming more common. The initial physical examination and roentgenographic studies may be completely negative. Groin pain, sometimes quite severe, may be the only early clue to the diagnosis.
- The rate of hip fracture could be reduced by:
  1. Elimination of environmental hazards (poor lighting, loose rugs)
  2. Regular exercise for balance and strength
  3. Patient education about fall prevention
  4. Medication review to minimize side effects
  5. Prevention and treatment of osteoporosis
- In the U.S., hip fracture rates and subsequent mortality among persons aged 65 yr and older are declining, and comorbidities among patients with hip fractures have increased. Hip fractures are also very expensive ($40,000 in the first year following hip fracture for direct medical costs and $5,000 in subsequent years).
- Fragility (or low-trauma) hip fractures, common in elderly patients with reduced bone density, carry a 1-yr mortality of 26%, while another 58% require long-term care in a nursing facility. Previous fragility hip fracture is associated with a second osteoporotic fracture within the subsequent 5 yr.
- Concurrent prolonged use of proton-pump inhibitors (≥1 yr) is associated with reduced effectiveness of alendronate for preventing hip fractures in older adults.

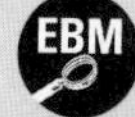

EVIDENCE

available at www.expertconsult.com

SUGGESTED READINGS

available at www.expertconsult.com

RELATED CONTENT

Hip Fracture (Patient Information)

AUTHOR: **LONNIE R. MERCIER, M.D.**

BASIC INFORMATION

DEFINITION

Hirsutism is the development of stiff, pigmented (terminal) facial and body hair (male distribution) in women as a result of excess androgen production.

SYNONYMS

Excessive hair growth

ICD-9CM CODES
704.1 Hirsutism
ICD-10CM CODES
L68.0 Hirsutism

EPIDEMIOLOGY & DEMOGRAPHICS

- Overall prevalence unknown, estimated 5% to 10% in reproductive age women.
- Race and genetics should be considered. Some distinct ethnic populations have minimal body hair and others (Mediterranean, Middle Eastern, South Asian) have moderate to large amounts of body hair while serum androgen levels are similar.
- Social norms and culture also determine how much body hair is cosmetically acceptable.
- Half of all cases of mild hirsutism do not have hyperandrogenemia. "Patient-important hirsutism" refers to hirsutism causing woman sufficient distress to seek care.
- Incidence and presentation of hirsutism is dependent on underlying cause of androgen excess (see "Differential Diagnosis").

PHYSICAL FINDINGS & CLINICAL PRESENTATION

- Timing of symptoms: abrupt onset, short duration, rapid progression, progressive worsening, more severe signs of virilization, or later age of onset suggest androgen-producing tumor, late-onset congenital adrenal hyperplasia, or Cushing's syndrome. Weight increases may produce increased androgen production.
- Menstrual history: menarche, cycle regularity and symptoms of ovulation, fertility, and contraception use. Anovulatory cycles are the most common underlying cause of androgen excess.
- Medication use history: some drugs cause hirsutism or produce androgenic effects (danazol, phenytoin, valproic acid, androgenic progestins (e.g., norgestrel), cyclosporin, minoxidil, metoclopramide, phenothiazines, methyldopa, diazoxide, penicillamine).
- Family history: known or suspected family history of hirsutism, congenital adrenal hyperplasia, insulin resistance, polycystic ovary syndrome (PCOS), infertility, obesity, menstrual irregularity may be found.
- Physical exam reveals deepening voice, body habitus, increased muscle mass, galactorrhea; abdominal and pelvic exam.
- Associated cutaneous manifestations (Fig. 1-473) are acne, acanthosis nigricans, striae, hair distribution, location and quantity, frontotemporal balding, muscle mass, clitoromegaly.
- Ferriman-Gallwey scale, a simple, pictorial system of scoring nine body areas, is the most common method used to quantify hirsutism. It may be unreliable in non-Caucasian women of other ethnicities.

ETIOLOGY

- Presence of hirsutism indicates androgen excess. Total testosterone may be normal, but free testosterone is elevated.
- Androgens induce vellus hair follicles (soft, unpigmented hair) in sex-specific areas (upper lip, chin, midsternum, upper abdomen, back, buttocks) to develop into thicker, more heavily pigmented terminal hairs.
- Anovulatory ovaries are usual source of excess androgens through thecal cell steroidogenesis and conversion of androstenedione to testosterone. The most common cause of hirsutism is polycystic ovary syndrome, which accounts for three out of every four cases.
- Conditions that decrease hepatic production of sex hormone binding globulin (SHBG) decrease protein-bound testosterone and increase free testosterone fraction (e.g., low estrogen, high androgen, and hyperinsulinemic states).
- Late-onset, congenital adrenal hyperplasia enzyme deficiency (most commonly 21-hydroxylase deficiency) produces excess 17 hydroxyprogesterone (17-OHP) and overproduction of androstenedione.
- Rare ovarian tumors primarily derived from Sertoli-Leydig cells, granulosa theca cells, or hilus cells produce excess androgens.
- Rare adrenal tumors produce excess androgens.
- Rare pituitary or hypothalamic tumors produce excess prolactin and can lead to anovulation.
- Box E1-37 summarizes causes of androgen excess in women of reproductive age.

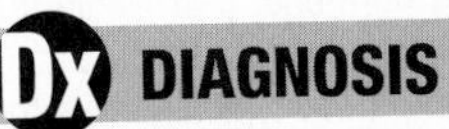

DIAGNOSIS

DIFFERENTIAL DIAGNOSIS

- Androgen-independent vellus hair: soft, unpigmented hair that covers entire body
- Hypertrichosis: diffusely increased total body hair (vellus or lanugo-type) not restricted to androgen-dependent areas often an adverse response to a medication or systemic illness (e.g., anorexia nervosa, porphyria, malnutrition, hypothyroidism)
- PCOS 75%
- Idiopathic 5% to 15%
- Congenital adrenal hyperplasia 1% to 8%
- Insulin resistance syndrome 3% to 4%
- Cushing's syndrome <1%
- Drug induced <1%
- Ovarian tumor <1%
- Adrenal tumor <1%
- Hyperthecosis <1%
- Hyperprolactinemia <1%

WORKUP

- Hirsutism is a clinical diagnosis.
- Management of hirsutism is largely independent of the etiology.
- Workup in selected hirsute women is directed to determine underlying cause of androgen excess.
- See specific conditions for more detailed workup of individual diagnoses.

LABORATORY TESTS

The Endocrine Society Clinical Practice Guideline recommends checking androgen levels in women with moderate or severe hirsutism, sudden onset, rapid progression, or associated menstrual dysfunction, central obesity, clitoromegaly, or acanthosis nigricans.

- Total plasma testosterone (normal range 20-60 ng/dl [0.69-2.1 nmol/L]) or free testosterone: early morning on day 4 to 10 of menstrual cycle to screen for testosterone-secreting tumors. If moderately or markedly elevated (total testosterone >150 ng/dl [5.2 nmol/L], free testosterone >2 ng/dl [0.07 nmol/L]) may image adrenals and ovaries for androgen-secreting tumors.

Other laboratory test considerations if appropriate:

- Prolactin: moderately elevated values should prompt imaging of pituitary-hypothalamic region

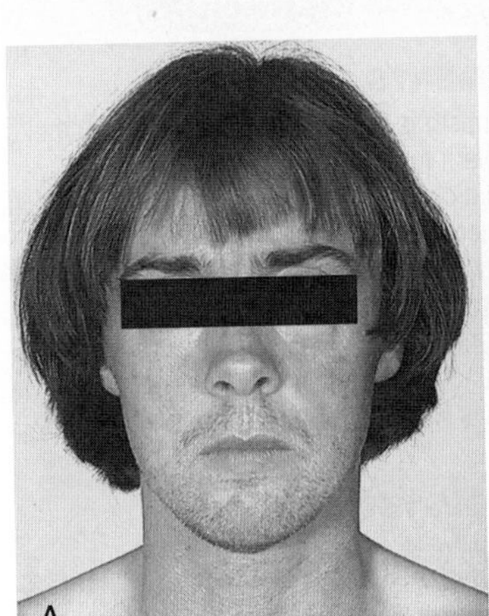

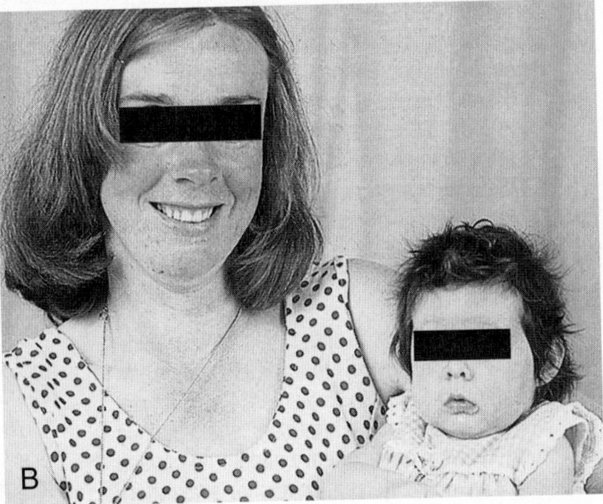

FIGURE 1-473 A patient with an arrhenoblastoma with associated polycystic ovaries before and after treatment. **A,** Before treatment, the patient had marked facial hirsutism. **B,** The patient is shown successfully treated. The tumor was resected and ovulation ensued with clomiphene and human chorionic gonadotropin therapy. (From Besser CM, Thorner MO: *Comprehensive clinical endocrinology,* ed 3, St Louis, 2002, Mosby.)

- 17-OHP (17 α-hydroxyprogesterone): screen for adrenal enzyme deficiencies. Morning value >200 ng/dl in early follicular phase suggests nonclassic (late onset) congenital adrenal hyperplasia due to 21-hydroxylase deficiency and may be confirmed with high-dose (250 mcg) ACTH stimulation test.
- Thyroid-stimulating hormone (TSH): rule out hypothyroidism
- Dehydroepiandrosterone sulfate (DHEA-S): screen for adrenal androgen production as almost entirely produced by adrenals. Levels >700 mcg/dl (13.6 nmol/L) raise suspicion for adrenal androgen-secreting tumor.

Additional laboratory test considerations if appropriate:

- Follicle-stimulating hormone: (FSH): rule out hypoestrogen state (perimenopausal)
- Luteinizing hormone: (LH): typically elevated in PCOS with low or normal FSH
- 24-hour urinary free cortisol: rule out Cushing's syndrome and overproduction of cortisol
- Overnight single-dose dexamethasone suppression test: rule out Cushing's syndrome and adrenal hyperfunction
- Fasting blood sugar (FBS), 2-hr 75-g oral glucose tolerance test, fasting insulin levels: rule out insulin resistance syndrome

IMAGING STUDIES

Imaging study considerations if appropriate:

- Pelvic ultrasound (high resolution, transvaginal): rule out ovarian tumor if total testosterone is elevated
- Abdominal CT/MRI: rule out adrenal tumor if elevated DHEA-S
- Pituitary-hypothalamic region CT/MRI: rule out pituitary tumor if prolactin elevated
- Laparoscopy/laparotomy: rule out small ovarian tumor in cases of elevated testosterone levels without radiologic evidence of adrenal or ovarian pathology

Rx TREATMENT

NONPHARMACOLOGIC THERAPY

- Weight reduction: can reduce androgen production indirectly by reducing insulin-stimulated theca cell androgen production and improve menstrual function, and slow hair growth in obese women.
- Cosmetic: temporary.
  - Shaving: does not stimulate hair growth; lasts days, leaves stubble.
  - Epilation: electronic plucking.
  - Bleaching: removes hair pigment. May cause skin irritation.
  - Mechanical waxing/plucking.
  - Depilatories: gels, lotions, or creams that chemically disrupt sulfide bonds of hair causing dissolution of hair shaft. No stubble.
  - Photoepilation (laser and intense pulsed light [IPL]): hair follicles destroyed by wavelengths of light absorbed by melanin. Good for pigmented hair; laser treatment is more effective than shaving, waxing, and electrolysis. It lasts 3 to 6 months as vellus follicles remain and can be converted to terminal pigmented hair under excess androgens.
- Cosmetic: permanent. Electrolysis: destroys individual hair follicles. May be expensive and time consuming.

ACUTE GENERAL Rx

See "Pharmacologic Therapy."

CHRONIC Rx

See "Pharmacologic Therapy."

PHARMACOLOGIC THERAPY

- Usually second-line treatment following nonpharmacologic, physical methods of hair control, and in consideration of patient's comorbidities and risk factors, patient preferences, area of excess hair amenable to treatment, and access and affordability of treatments.
- Pharmacologic treatments categorized as topical, oral contraceptive pills (OCPs), antiandrogens (potential adverse effects on a developing male fetus, so use with reliable contraception), other treatments directed at specific underlying etiology.
- Topical: Eflornithine topical cream 13.9%: unclear mechanism of action; may inhibit ornithine decarboxylase, retarding hair growth. Temporary cosmetic treatment for facial hair. Applied directly to unwanted facial hair bid with at least 8 hr spaced applications. Does not remove hair, rather slows growth. Slow response over 4 to 8 wk. Hair growth returns upon discontinuation of treatment.
- OCPs: Suppress ovarian steroidogenesis and LH through low-dose estrogen and low androgenic progestational agents. Slow response to treatment. Suppresses new hair growth. Established hair unaffected. Low-dose OCPs with low androgenic progestational agents, for example, desogestrel, drospirenone, norgestimate. Avoid norgestrel and levonorgestrel (higher androgenic progestational agents).
- Antiandrogens: Spironolactone: when OCPs unacceptable or may be added for disappointing results after 6 mo of OCP treatment.
  - Aldosterone-antagonist diuretic inhibits adrenal and ovarian biosynthesis of androgens. May result in ovulation, so consider contraception needs.
  - Slow response usually 6 mo or more.
  - 200 mg PO qd, then decrease to 25 to 50 mg qd maintenance.
  - May cause hyperkalemia.
  - Anovulatory, unopposed estrogen states require progestin management.

REFERRAL

- To endocrinologist if difficulty in determining diagnosis, achieving therapeutic goals, or resistant to first-line therapies. Pre-pubertal and postmenopausal hirsutism is suspicious for neoplastic or secondary endocrine causes and should be referred for further evaluation.
- Consider referral or consultation for following therapies:
  1. Finasteride: antiandrogen, in hair follicle blocks 5α-reductase conversion of testosterone to intranuclearly active 5α-dihydrotestosterone (DHT)
     - Use only with reliable contraception because DHT necessary for normal male fetus urogenital development
     - Not FDA approved for treatment of hirsutism
     - 1 to 5 mg PO qd
  2. Flutamide: inhibits androgen uptake and receptor binding
     - Not recommended by Endocrine Society Clinical Practice Guidelines and not FDA approved for treatment of hirsutism, but used by some European endocrinologists
     - Use only with reliable contraception
     - Reserved for women with severe, resistant hirsutism because of risk of hepatic dysfunction
     - 250 mg PO bid
  3. Cyproterone acetate (not available in U.S.): antiandrogen that competes with DHT for binding androgen receptors. Used as progestin component of OCPs outside U.S.
- Other treatments directed at specific underlying etiology:
  - Metformin/thiazolidinediones: therapy reserved for documented insulin-resistant states.
  - GnRH agonists: recommended only in women with severe hyperandrogenemia (e.g., ovarian hyperthecosis) with suboptimal response to combination low-dose estrogen/progestin pills and antiandrogen treatment. Inhibits gonadotropin and consequently ovarian androgen and estrogen secretion.
  - Dexamethasone: adrenal glucocorticoid suppression is reserved for diagnosis of adrenal enzyme deficiency.
  - Total abdominal hysterectomy/bilateral salpingo-oophorectomy reserved for recalcitrant hirsutism in older female with hyperthecosis and undesired fertility.

PEARLS & CONSIDERATIONS

COMMENTS

- Hirsutism is both an endocrine and cosmetic problem for patients.
- Ovulation induction therapy is indicated in women desiring pregnancy.
- Delay checking serum androgens until oral contraceptives have been discontinued for 2 to 3 mo.
- Evaluation of incidental adrenal mass is always warranted.

SUGGESTED READINGS

available at www.expertconsult.com

RELATED CONTENT

Hirsutism (Patient Information)

AUTHOR: **RICHARD LONG, M.D.**

BASIC INFORMATION

DEFINITION

Histoplasmosis is caused by the fungus *Histoplasma capsulatum* and characterized by a primary pulmonary focus with occasional progression to chronic pulmonary histoplasmosis (CPH) or various forms of dissemination. Progressive disseminated histoplasmosis (PDH) may present with a diverse clinical spectrum, including adrenal necrosis, pulmonary and mediastinal fibrosis, and ulcerations of the oropharynx and GI tract. In those patients coinfected with HIV, it is a defining disease for AIDS.

SYNONYMS

North American histoplasmosis
Ohio Valley fever
Vanderbilt disease

ICD-9CM CODES

115.90 Histoplasmosis
115.94 Histoplasmosis with endocarditis
115.91 Histoplasmosis with meningitis
115.93 Histoplasmosis with pericarditis
115.95 Histoplasmosis with pneumonia
115.92 Histoplasmosis with retinitis

ICD-10CM CODES

B39.9	Histoplasmosis, unspecified
B39.9 with: I39	Endocarditis and heart valve disorders in diseases classified elsewhere
B39.9 with: G02	Meningitis in other infectious and parasitic diseases classified elsewhere
B39.9 with: I32	Pericarditis in diseases classified elsewhere
B39.9 with: J17	Pneumonia in diseases classified elsewhere
B39.9 with: H32	Chorioretinal disorders in diseases classified elsewhere

EPIDEMIOLOGY & DEMOGRAPHICS

INCIDENCE (IN U.S.):

- Unknown for acute pulmonary disease
- For CPH, estimated at 1/100,000 cases in endemic areas
- For PDH in immunocompetent adults, estimated at 1/2000 cases of histoplasmosis

PREVALENCE: Unknown

PREDOMINANT SEX: Clinically evident disease is most common in males; male/female ratio of 4:1

PREDOMINANT AGE:

- CPH is most often seen in males >50 yr old with an associated history of COPD.
- Presumed ocular histoplasmosis syndrome (POHS) is seen between ages of 20 and 40 yr.

PEAK INCIDENCE: Unknown

PHYSICAL FINDINGS & CLINICAL PRESENTATION

- Conidia are deposited in alveoli then converted to yeast forms where they spread to regional lymph nodes and other organs, especially liver and spleen.
- 1 to 2 wk later, a granulomatous inflammatory response begins to contain the yeast in the form of discrete granulomas.
- Delayed-type hypersensitivity to *Histoplasma* antigens occurs 3 to 6 wk after exposure.
- Clinical disease manifests in various forms, depending on host cellular immunity and inoculum size:
  1. Acute primary pulmonary histoplasmosis
     a. An overwhelming number of patients are asymptomatic.
     b. Most clinically apparent infections manifest by complaints of fever, headache, malaise, pleuritic chest pain, nonproductive cough, and weight loss.
     c. Less than 10%, mainly women, complain of arthralgias, myalgias, and skin manifestations such as erythema multiforme or erythema nodosum.
     d. Acute pericarditis presents in a smaller percentage of patients.
     e. Hepatosplenomegaly is most commonly observed in children.
     f. With particularly heavy exposure, there is severe dyspnea, marked hypoxemia, impending respiratory failure.
     g. Most patients are asymptomatic within 6 wk.
  2. CPH
     a. Presents insidiously with low-grade fever, malaise, weight loss, cough, sometimes with blood-streaked sputum or frank hemoptysis.
     b. Most patients with cavitary lesions present with associated COPD or chronic bronchitis, masking underlying fungal disease.
     c. Tends to worsen preexisting pulmonary disease and further contribute to eventual respiratory insufficiency.
  3. PDH
     a. In both acute and subacute forms, constitutional symptoms of fever, fatigue, malaise, and weight loss are common.
     b. Acute form (seen in infants and children) presents with respiratory symptoms, fever ≥101° F (38.3° C), generalized lymphadenopathy, marked hepatosplenomegaly, and fulminant course resembling septic shock associated with a high fatality rate.
     c. Subacute form is more common in adults and associated with lower temperatures, hepatosplenomegaly, oropharyngeal ulceration, focal organ involvement (including adrenal destruction, endocarditis, chronic meningitis, and intracerebral mass lesions).
     d. Course of subacute form is relentless, with untreated patients dying within 2 yr.
     e. Chronic PDH is found in adults and marked by gradual symptoms of weight loss, weakness, easy fatigability; low-grade fever when present; oropharyngeal ulcerations and hepatomegaly and/or splenomegaly in one third of patients.
     f. Less clinical evidence of focal organ involvement in chronic form than in subacute form.
     g. Natural history of chronic form is protracted and intermittent, spanning months to years.
- Histoplasmoma
  1. A healed area of caseation necrosis surrounded by a fibrous capsule
  2. Usually asymptomatic
- Mediastinal fibrosis
  1. A rare consequence of a fibroblastic process that encases caseating mediastinal lymph nodes producing severe retraction, compression, and distortion of mediastinal structures
  2. Constriction of the bronchi resulting in bronchiectasis, also esophageal stenosis associated with dysphagia, and superior vena cava syndrome
- POHS
  1. Diagnosis characterized by distinct clinical features, including atrophic choroidal scars and maculopathy in patients with histories suggestive of exposure to the fungus (e.g., residence in an endemic area)
  2. Patient complains of distortion or loss of central vision without pain, redness, or photophobia
  3. Usually no evidence of infection except for a positive skin reaction to histoplasmin
- In patients with AIDS
  1. Possible presentation as overwhelming infection similar to acute PDH seen in children
  2. Constitutional symptoms: fever, weight loss, malaise, cough, dyspnea
  3. About 10% with cutaneous maculopapular, erythematous eruptions or purpuric lesions on face, trunk, and extremities
  4. Up to 20% with CNS involvement, manifesting as intracerebral mass lesions, chronic meningitis, or encephalopathy

ETIOLOGY

- *H. capsulatum* is a dimorphic fungus present in temperate zones and river valleys worldwide.
- In the U.S., it is highly endemic in southeastern, mid-Atlantic, and central states.
- Exists as mold at ambient temperature and favors soils enriched with bird or bat droppings.

Dx DIAGNOSIS

DIFFERENTIAL DIAGNOSIS

- Acute pulmonary histoplasmosis
  1. *Mycobacterium tuberculosis*
  2. Community-acquired pneumonias caused by *Mycoplasma* and *Chlamydia*
  3. Other fungal diseases, such as *Blastomyces dermatitidis* and *Coccidioides immitis*
- Chronic cavitary pulmonary histoplasmosis: *M. tuberculosis*
- Histoplasmomas: true neoplasms

WORKUP

- Suspect diagnosis in patients who present with a history of residence or travel in an

endemic area, especially if engaged in occupations (e.g., outside construction or street cleaning) or hobbies (e.g., cave exploring) that increase the likelihood of exposure to fungal spores.
- Suspect diagnosis in immunosuppressed patients with remote history of exposure, especially if associated with characteristic calcifications on chest x-ray.

LABORATORY TESTS

- Demonstration of organism on culture from body fluid or tissues to make definitive diagnosis
  1. Especially high yield in patients with AIDS
  2. Characteristic oval yeast cells in neutrophils with Giemsa stain from peripheral smear
  3. Preparations of infected tissue with Gomori's silver methenamine for revealing yeast forms, especially in areas of caseation necrosis
- Serologic tests, including complement-fixing (CF) antibodies and immunodiffusion assays
- Detection of *Histoplasma* antigen in urine: may be influenced by infections with *Blastomyces* and *Coccidioides*
- In PDH
  1. Pancytopenia
  2. Marked elevations in alkaline phosphatase and alanine aminotransferase (ALT) common
- In chronic meningitis (majority of cases)
  1. CSF pleocytosis with either lymphocytes or neutrophils predominating
  2. Elevated CSF protein levels
  3. Hypoglycorrhachia

IMAGING STUDIES

- Chest radiograph examination in acute pulmonary histoplasmosis
  1. Singular or multiple patchy infiltrates, especially in the lower lung fields
  2. Hilar or mediastinal lymphadenopathy with or without pneumonitis
  3. Diffuse nodular or confluent bilateral miliary infiltrates characteristic of heavier exposure
  4. Infrequent pleural effusions, except when associated with pericarditis
- Chest radiograph examination in histoplasmoma: coin lesion displaying central calcification, ranging from 1 to 4 cm in diameter, predominantly located in the subpleural regions
- Chest radiograph examination in CPH:
  1. Upper lobe disease frequently associated with cavities
  2. Preexisting calcifications in the hilum associated with peribronchial streaking extending to the parenchyma
- Chest radiograph examination in acute PDH: hilar adenopathy and/or diffuse nodular infiltrates
- CT scan of adrenals to reveal bilateral enlargement and low-attenuation centers

Rx TREATMENT

NONPHARMACOLOGIC THERAPY

For life-threatening disease seen in acute disseminated disease or infection in patients with AIDS: supportive therapy with IV fluids

ACUTE GENERAL Rx

- No drug therapy is required for asymptomatic pulmonary disease.
- A course of therapy with itraconazole 200 mg PO tid for 3 days, then 200 mg/day PO for 6-12 wk may be beneficial in some patients with acute pulmonary distress. Avoid fluconazole because it is not as active.
- Same therapy appropriate for immunocompetent, mild to moderately symptomatic patients with CPH and subacute and chronic forms of PDH, but duration for 6 to 12 mo.
- Use amphotericin B 0.7 to 1 mg/kg IV for 6 to 12 mo in patients hypersensitive to or intolerant of azole therapy.
- Give amphotericin B for life-threatening disease or continued illness as a result of primary failure or relapse of adequate azole therapy. A lipid formulation of amphotericin B can be used to avoid nephrotoxicity.
  1. For acute pulmonary histoplasmosis associated with acute respiratory distress syndrome (ARDS), acute PDH, and histoplasma meningitis: dose of 0.7 to 1 mg/kg IV q24h
  2. End point of therapy for patient with complicated acute pulmonary disease: total dose of 500 mg
  3. End point for patient with acute PDH: total dose 35 mg/kg or 2.5 g total
  4. For moderately severe or severe acute pulmonary histoplasmosis, add methylprednisolone 0.5-1 mg/kg/day for 1-2 wk to liposomal amphotericin B.
- Chronic cavitary pulmonary histoplasmosis: itraconazole 200 mg PO tid for 3 days, then once or twice daily for at least 12 mo.
- CNS histoplasmosis: liposomal amphotericin B, 5 mg/kg/day for a total of 175 mg/kg over 4-6 wk, then itraconazole 200 mg 2-3×/day for at least 12 mo.
- Endocarditis: surgical treatment with excision of infected valve or graft combined with amphotericin for a total dose of 35 mg/kg or 2.5 g.
- For pericardial disease:
  1. Antifungal therapy: no apparent benefit
  2. Best managed with NSAIDs
- For POHS:
  1. Antifungal therapy: no apparent benefit
  2. May respond to laser therapy

CHRONIC Rx

- In patients with AIDS: lifelong suppressive therapy with either itraconazole, given 200 mg PO qid, or IV amphotericin B at a dose of 50 mg once weekly; a triazole compound posaconazole (400 mg PO bid) may be useful in refractory cases, but clinical experience is limited at this point.
- Prophylaxis in HIV-infected patients with <150 CD4 cells/mm^3: itraconazole 200 mg PO qd

DISPOSITION

For those with chronic or progressive disease, especially if immunocompromised, prognosis is dependent on prompt recognition and timely administration of appropriate antifungal drugs.

REFERRAL

- To an infectious disease specialist in suspected cases of disseminated disease, especially if immunocompromised
- To a pulmonologist for patients with CPH form because of progressive respiratory compromise
- To a thoracic surgeon for decompression procedures for progressive mediastinal fibrosis

PEARLS & CONSIDERATIONS

- *H. capsulatum,* variety *duboisii,* also known as African histoplasmosis, is restricted to Senegal, Nigeria, Zaire, and Uganda.
- Unlike *H. capsulatum,* pulmonary forms of *duboisii* are not seen, and the disease is limited to the skin, soft tissues, and bone.

COMMENTS

- Patients living in endemic areas, especially if immunocompromised, should take appropriate respiratory precautions when disposing of bird waste from rooftop or home aviaries.
- Appropriate respiratory precautions should also be taken when leisure traveling to areas that act as a natural haven for the fungus, such as bat caves.

SUGGESTED READINGS

available at www.expertconsult.com

RELATED CONTENT

Histoplasmosis (Patient Information)

AUTHOR: **GLENN G. FORT, M.D., M.P.H.**

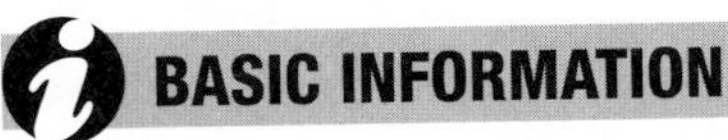

BASIC INFORMATION

DEFINITION

Patients with histrionic personality disorder present with a pervasive pattern of excessive emotionality and attention-seeking behavior that generally begins in early adulthood.

SYNONYMS

Hysterical personality disorder
Psycho-infantile personality disorder
Personality disorder (nonspecific)
Personality disorder (trait specified)

ICD-9CM and DSM-5 CODES
301.50
ICD-10CM CODES
F60.4 Histrionic personality disorder

EPIDEMIOLOGY & DEMOGRAPHICS

PREVALENCE (IN U.S.):

- Diagnosed more often in women (85%); rarely found in men
- Prevalence: 1% to 2%

PREDOMINANT SEX: Female. Cultural factors (e.g., attention-seeking behavior not as acceptable in men) may lead to more common diagnosis in women.

PREDOMINANT AGE: Generally begins in early adulthood

GENETICS: Limited research using interview and self-report methods suggests histrionic personality disorder has a moderate genetic component.

PHYSICAL FINDINGS & CLINICAL PRESENTATION

Features include five or more of the following:

1. Is uncomfortable in situations where he or she is not the center of attention.
2. Interaction with others is often characterized by inappropriate sexually seductive or provocative behavior.
3. Displays rapidly shifting and shallow expression of emotions.
4. Consistently uses physical appearance to draw attention to self.
5. Has a style of speech that is excessively impressionistic and lacking in detail.
6. Shows self-dramatization, theatricality, and exaggerated expression of emotion.
7. Is suggestible (i.e., easily influenced by others or circumstances).
8. Considers relationships to be more intimate than they actually are.

ETIOLOGY

- Unknown
- Hypothesized that childhood events, psychosocial adversity, and genetics are contributory

Dx DIAGNOSIS

DIFFERENTIAL DIAGNOSIS

- Narcissistic and borderline personality disorders share common features.
- Other personality disorders (e.g., antisocial personality disorder, dependent personality disorder)
- Personality change attributable to general medical condition
- Symptoms in association with chronic substance abuse

WORKUP

There is no formal test to establish diagnosis.

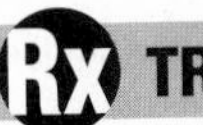

TREATMENT

NONPHARMACOLOGIC THERAPY

- Long-term individual psychotherapy is treatment of choice.
- No controlled psychotherapy studies
- Unlike other people who have personality disorders, these individuals often seek treatment and exaggerate their symptoms and difficulties in functioning.
- Patients tend to be more emotionally needy and are often reluctant to terminate therapy.

ACUTE GENERAL Rx

- No placebo-controlled trials.
- Care should be given when prescribing medications because of the potential for self-destructive or otherwise harmful behaviors.

DISPOSITION

- Therapeutic approaches should not focus on the long-term personality change, but rather short-term alleviation of specific difficulties and deficits within the person's life.
- Therapeutic approaches that emphasize vague somatic, anxious, or depressive symptoms often fail.
- Patients are likely to be intolerant or drop out of treatment approaches that use delayed gratification.
- Symptoms are moderately stable over adulthood and may remit or decrease in intensity with age.

REFERRAL

Primarily treated by mental health professionals

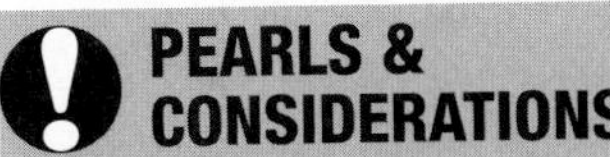

PEARLS & CONSIDERATIONS

- This disorder is difficult to treat.
- Like most personality disorders, patients present for treatment only when stress or other situational factor within their lives has made their ability to function and cope effectively impossible.
- Suicidality should be assessed on a regular basis, and suicidal threats and self-mutilation should not be ignored or dismissed.
- An alternative model in DSM-5 section III reconceptualizes histrionic personality disorder as "Personality Disorder, Trait Specified," which rates: (1) impairment in personality functioning (identity, self-direction, empathy, and/or intimacy) and (2) pathologic trait domains such as attention seeking, grandiosity, and manipulativeness.

PATIENT & FAMILY EDUCATION

Group and family therapy approaches are generally not recommended because individuals with this disorder often try to draw attention to themselves and exaggerate every action and reaction.

SUGGESTED READINGS
available at www.expertconsult.com

AUTHORS: **MARK ZIMMERMAN, M.D.**, and **THERESA A. MORGAN, PH.D., M.PHIL.**

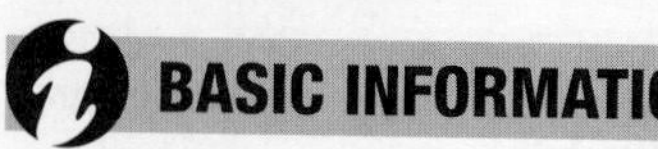

BASIC INFORMATION

- HIV cognitive dysfunction covers a spectrum of disorders ranging from asymptomatic to clinically severe (including AIDS dementia complex or HIV encephalopathy).
- Cognitive, motor, and behavioral abnormalities

SYNONYMS

HIV-associated neurocognitive disorder

ICD-9CM CODES
042 (for diseases related to HIV; no particular code for HIV cognitive dysfunction)
ICD-10CM CODES
B20 Human immunodeficiency virus [HIV] disease
R41.8 Other and unspecified symptoms and signs involving cognitive functions and awareness

EPIDEMIOLOGY

- Presenting complaint in only 3% of cases
- Incidence: reduced from 60% to 1% since introduction of HIV treatment; however, as more HIV-infected patients live longer, prevalence may be increasing.
- Minor cognitive disorders are more common and seen in 20% of patients; not necessarily progressive
- Rarely precedes clinical evidence of HIV infection

CLINICAL FEATURES

- Cognitive changes: forgetfulness, poor attention and concentration, increased difficulty performing complex tasks, slowed psychomotor speed
- Behavioral changes: apathy, lack of initiative, social withdrawal, irritability, occasionally agitation, psychosis or obsessive compulsive disorder
- Motor problems: clumsiness, unsteady gait, poor balance, tremor, leg weakness
- Progressive/later stages: bedbound, severe dementia, bowel/bladder incontinence
- Subcortical dementia (aphasia, apraxia, and agnosia) is uncommon
- Results from inflammation triggered by HIV itself (not related to opportunistic infection) and immune activation of microglia and brain macrophages
- Clinically may resemble Parkinson's disease
- In children: developmental delay, microcephaly, and spasticity are common

RISK FACTORS

- Low CD4 count (less than 200 cells/mm^3)
- High viral load
- Anemia
- Injection drug use
- Hepatitis C
- Female gender
- Older age

Dx DIAGNOSIS

DIAGNOSTIC EVALUATION

- Diagnosis is based on clinical examination and neuropsychometric tests
- MRI head: diffuse, confluent, periventricular white matter lesions on T2 weighted images with normal T1 images
- Lumbar puncture: CSF analysis helps to rule out opportunistic infections. In HIV-related cognitive dysfunction the CSF may show a nonspecific increase in cell count and protein.
- Potential causes for cognitive impairment that must be ruled out include:
  - Opportunistic infections (toxoplasmosis, CNS lymphoma)
  - Vitamin B_{12} deficiency
  - Substance use
  - Organic affective disorder (such as depression and mania)
  - Side effects of prescribed medications

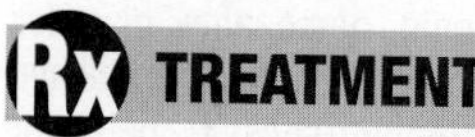

TREATMENT

Early treatment with antiretroviral therapy (ART) leads to clinical improvement.

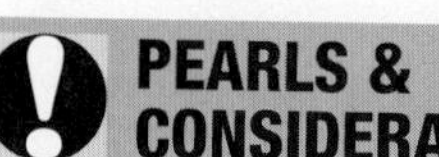

PEARLS & CONSIDERATIONS

- Initiation of ART can lead to rapid improvement in cognitive function in early stages (untreated, life span is typically 4 to 6 mo)
- Most common presenting complaint in children infected with HIV
- Mini-mental status examination (MMSE): baseline scores in HIV patients are very helpful
- Usually cognitive symptoms precede motor abnormalities
- Four HIV-related opportunistic infections that commonly cause cognitive impairment are: toxoplasmosis, cryptococcal meningitis, progressive multifocal leukoencephalopathy, and CNS lymphoma

REFERRALS

- Upon diagnosis/clinical suspicion for HIV associated cognitive dysfunction, referral to neurology is recommended
- Referral to neuropsychology may be considered

SUGGESTED READINGS
available at www.expertconsult.com

AUTHOR: **DIVYA SINGHAL, M.D.**

BASIC INFORMATION

DEFINITION

Hodgkin's lymphoma is a malignant disorder of lymphoreticular origin, characterized histologically by the presence of multinucleated giant cells (Reed-Sternberg cells) usually originating from B lymphocytes in germinal centers of lymphoid tissue.

ICD-9CM CODES

201.9 Hodgkin's lymphoma, unspecified
201.0 Hodgkin's paragranuloma
201.4 Hodgkin's lymphoma, lymphocyte predominance
201.5 Hodgkin's lymphoma, nodular sclerosis
201.6 Hodgkin's lymphoma, mixed cellularity
201.6 Hodgkin's lymphoma, mixed cellularity
201.7 Hodgkin's lymphoma, lymphocyte depletion

ICD-10CM CODES

C81.90 Hodgkin lymphoma, unspecified, unspecified site
C81.00 Nodular lymphocyte predominant Hodgkin lymphoma, unspecified site
C81.10 Nodular sclerosis classical Hodgkin lymphoma, unspecified site
C81.20 Mixed cellularity classical Hodgkin lymphoma, unspecified site
C81.30 Lymphocyte depleted classical Hodgkin lymphoma, unspecified site

EPIDEMIOLOGY & DEMOGRAPHICS

- There is a bimodal age distribution (15 to 34 yr and >50 yr).
- Incidence is 4 in 100,000 cases.
- Concordance for Hodgkin's lymphoma in identical twins suggests that a genetic susceptibility underlies Hodgkin's lymphoma in young adulthood.
- The disease is more common in males (in childhood Hodgkin's lymphoma, >80% occur in males), whites, and higher socioeconomic groups.
- More common in people living in moderate climates.
- There are >8000 new cases of Hodgkin's lymphoma diagnosed annually in the United States.

PHYSICAL FINDINGS & CLINICAL PRESENTATION

- Palpable lymphadenopathy that is generally painless is the most common presenting symptom
- Most common site of involvement: neck region
- Fever and night sweats: fever in a cyclical pattern (days or weeks of fever alternating with afebrile periods) is known as Pel-Epstein fever
- Unexplained weight loss, generalized malaise
- Persistent, nonproductive cough
- Pain associated with alcohol ingestion often because of heavy eosinophil infiltration of the tumor sites is relatively uncommon
- Generalized pruritus
- Hepatosplenomegaly in disease below the diaphragm
- Other: superior vena cava syndrome, spinal cord compression (rare), erythema nodosum, ichthyosis

ETIOLOGY

Unknown; evidence implicating Epstein-Barr virus remains controversial.

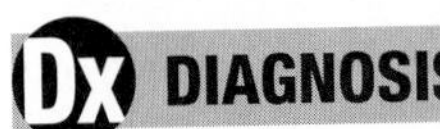

DIAGNOSIS

DIFFERENTIAL DIAGNOSIS

- Non-Hodgkin's lymphoma
- Sarcoidosis
- Infections (e.g., cytomegalovirus, Epstein-Barr virus, toxoplasmosis, HIV, tuberculosis)
- Drug reaction

WORKUP

Diagnosis is confirmed by lymph node biopsy. The World Health Organization classifies Hodgkin's lymphoma into two groups: classical Hodgkin's lymphoma (92% to 97%) and nodular lymphocyte-predominant Hodgkin's lymphoma (3% to 8%). Classic Hodgkin's lymphoma has four main histologic subtypes based on the number of lymphocytes, Reed-Sternberg cells, and the presence of fibrous tissue:

1. Nodular sclerosis (60% to 80%) (Fig. E1-475)
2. Mixed cellularity (15% to 30%) (Fig. E1-476)
3. Lymphocyte predominance (2% to 7%)
4. Lymphocyte depletion (1% to 6%)

Nodular sclerosis occurs mainly in young adulthood, whereas the mixed cellularity type is more prevalent after age 50 yr.

Staging: Table 1-238 describes the Cotswolds staging classification.

Proper staging requires the following:

- Detailed history (with documentation of "B symptoms" and physical examination)
- Surgical biopsy
- Laboratory evaluation (complete blood count, erythrocyte sedimentation rate, blood urea nitrogen, creatinine, alkaline phosphatase, liver function tests, albumin, lactate dehydrogenase, HIV tests, uric acid), immunophenotypic markers (see Table 1-239). Gene-expression profiling for tumor-associated macrophages is a new biomarker for risk stratification
- Chest x-ray (posteroanterior and lateral)
- CT scan of chest, abdomen, pelvis, neck
- Positron emission tomography scan (18-FDG PET scan)
- Bilateral bone marrow biopsy (selected patients)

Box 1-38 summarizes recommended staging procedures for Hodgkin lymphoma.

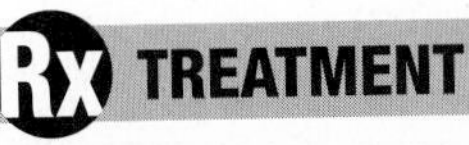

TREATMENT

ACUTE GENERAL Rx

The main therapeutic modalities are radiotherapy and chemotherapy; the indication for which one varies with pathologic stage and other factors. In general, chemotherapy plus involved-field radiotherapy can be used as standard treatment for Hodgkin's lymphoma in early stages with favorable prognostic features. In patients with unfavorable features, four courses of chemotherapy plus involved-field radiotherapy should be the standard treatment. Commonly used therapeutic modalities are:

- Stage I and II: radiation therapy alone (involved-field radiotherapy [35 Gy]) unless a large mediastinal mass is present (mediastinal to thoracic ratio ≥1.3); in the latter case, a combination of chemotherapy and radiation therapy is indicated. Various regimens can be used for combination of chemotherapy. Most oncologists prefer the combination of Adriamycin (doxorubicin), bleomycin, vinblastine, and dacarbazine

TABLE 1-238 Cotswolds Staging Classification for Hodgkin's Lymphoma

Classification	Description
Stage I	Involvement of a single lymph node region or lymphoid structure (e.g., spleen, thymus, Waldeyer ring) or involvement of a single extralymphatic site (IE)
Stage II	Involvement of two or more lymph node regions on the same side of the diaphragm (hilar nodes, when involved on both sides, constitute stage II disease); localized contiguous involvement of only one extranodal organ or site and lymph node regions on the same side of the diaphragm (IIE). The number of anatomic regions involved should be indicated by a subscript (e.g., II3)
III1	With or without involvement of splenic, hilar, celiac, or portal nodes
III2	With involvement of paraaortic, iliac, and mesenteric nodes
Stage IV	Diffuse or disseminated involvement of one or more extranodal organs or tissues, with or without associated lymph node involvement
	Designations applicable to any disease stage
A	No symptoms
B	Fever (temperature, >38° C [100.4° F]), drenching night sweats, unexplained loss of >10% of body weight within the preceding 6 mo
X	Bulky disease (a widening of the mediastinum by more than one third of the presence of a nodal mass with a maximal dimension <10 cm)
E	Involvement of a single extranodal site that is contiguous or proximal to the known nodal site

From Hoffman R et al: *Hematology: basic principles and practice,* ed 5, Philadelphia, 2009, Churchill Livingstone.

 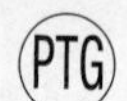

TABLE 1-239 Selected Immunophenotypic Markers and Histologic Characteristics of Use in the Differential Diagnosis of Hodgkin's Lymphoma and Other Lymphoid Neoplasms

Marker	Classical HL	Nodular Lymphocyte Predominant HL	TCRBCL	ALCL
CD30	+	–	–	+
CD15	+	–	–	–
CD20	–/+*	+	+	–
CD45	–	+	+	+/–
CD79a	–	+	+	–
ALK	–	–	–	+/–
EMA	–	+	+	+
Nodular growth protein	+/–†	+	–	–

+, >90% of cases positive; +/–, majority of cases positive; –/+, minority of cases positive; –, <10% of cases positive; *ALCL,* anaplastic large cell lymphoma; *HL,* Hodgkin's lymphoma; *TCRBCL,* T-cell rich B-cell lymphoma.
*CD20 positivity in classical Hodgkin's lymphoma is quite heterogeneous, with a wide range in brightness of staining.
†In classical Hodgkin's lymphoma, a nodular growth pattern is confined to the nodular sclerosing subtype.
From Abeloff MD: *Clinical oncology,* ed 3, Philadelphia, 2004, Saunders.

BOX 1-38 Recommended Staging Procedures for Hodgkin Lymphoma

The following staging procedures are recommended for the initial workup of Hodgkin lymphoma:

1. Adequate surgical biopsy reviewed by an experienced hematopathologist
2. Core-needle biopsy of bone marrow from the posterior iliac crest; needle or surgical biopsy of any suspicious extranodal (e.g., hepatic, osseous, pulmonary, cutaneous) lesions; and cytologic examination of any effusion
3. Detailed history, with attention to the presence or absence of systemic symptoms, and a careful physical examination, emphasizing node chains, size of the liver and spleen, and inspection of Waldeyer ring
4. Routine laboratory tests: complete blood cell count, erythrocyte sedimentation rate, and liver function tests
5. Chest radiographs (posteroanterior and lateral) with measurement of the mass-to-thoracic ratio
6. Neck, chest, and abdominal CT
7. 18-FDG PET scan (Fig. 1-477)

From Hoffman R et al: *Hematology: basic principles and practice,* ed 5, Philadelphia, 2009, Churchill Livingstone.

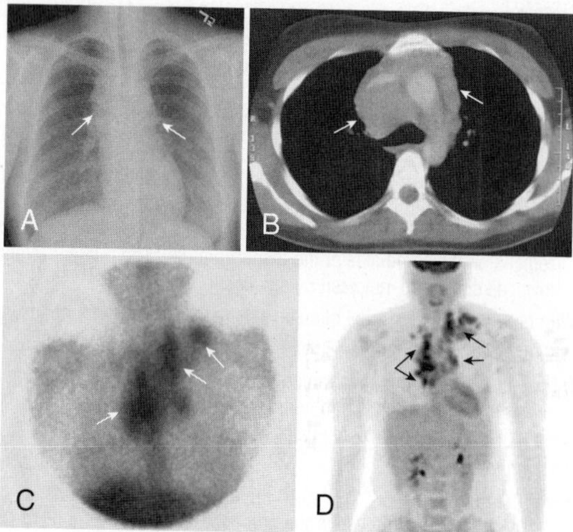

FIGURE 1-477 Imaging of Hodgkin's lymphoma. Bulky Hodgkin's disease as seen on chest radiograph (**A**), computed tomography (CT) of the chest (**B**), gallium scan (**C**), and positron emission tomography (PET) (**D**). The *arrows* indicate sites of disease. Note that the PET and CT scans provide more detailed information than the chest radiograph and gallium scan. (From Goldman L, Schafer AI: *Goldman's Cecil medicine,* ed 24, Philadelphia, 2012, Saunders.)

TABLE 1-240 Characteristics of the ABVD Regimen

Agents: doxorubicin, bleomycin, vinblastine, dacarbazine
All intravenous, total compliance
80% complete response rate
10% primary refractory disease
60%-65% overall disease-free survival
Most relapses occur within the first 4 yr; however, about 10% of all relapses occur beyond 5 yr
Major side effects are nausea, phlebitis, myelosuppression, less cumulative myelotoxicity than MOPP
No infertility
No leukemia

ABVD, Adriamycin (doxorubicin), bleomycin, vinblastine, dacarbazine; *MOPP,* mechlorethamine, Oncovin (vincristine), procarbazine, prednisone.
From Abeloff MD: *Clinical oncology,* ed 3, Philadelphia, 2004, Saunders.

(ABVD). Table 1-240 describes characteristics of the ABVD regimen. Generally, chemotherapy plus radiation treatment is effective in controlling stage IA or IIA nonbulky lymphoma in a high percentage of patients (>85%), but is associated with late treatment-related deaths. Trials have shown that ABVD therapy alone is associated with a higher rate of overall survival (due to lower rate of death from other causes) when compared with treatment that includes ABVD therapy and subtotal nodal radiation therapy.

- Stage IB or IIB: total nodal irradiation is often used, although chemotherapy is performed in many centers.
- Stage IIIA: treatment is controversial. It varies with the anatomic substage after splenectomy.
  1. III$_1$A and minimum splenic involvement: radiation therapy alone may be adequate.
  2. III$_2$ or III$_1$A with extensive splenic involvement: there is disagreement whether chemotherapy alone or a combination of chemotherapy and radiation therapy is the preferred treatment modality.
  3. IIIB and IVB: the treatment of choice is chemotherapy with or without adjuvant radiotherapy.

Recent trials have shown that in patients with early-stage Hodgkin's lymphoma and favorable prognosis, treatment with two cycles of ABVD followed by 20 Gy of involved-field radiation therapy may be as effective as, and less toxic than four cycles of ABVD followed by 30 Gy of involved-field radiation therapy. Long-term effects of this approach need to be fully assessed before it becomes standard of care. BEACOPP, an intensified regimen consisting of bleomycin, etoposide, doxorubicin, cyclophosphamide, vincristine, procarbazine, and prednisone, has been advocated by some as the new standard for treatment of advanced Hodgkin's lymphoma in place of ABVD. Recent trials have shown that treatment with BEACOPP, as compared with ABVD, resulted in better initial tumor control,

TABLE 1-241 Definition of Treatment Groups According to the EORTC/GELA and GHSG

Treatment Group	EORTC/GELA	GHSG	NCIC/ECOG
Early-stage favorable	CS I-II without risk factors (supradiaphragmatic)	CS I-II without risk factors	Standard risk group: favorable CSD I-II (without risk factors)
Early-stage unfavorable (intermediate)	CS I-II with ≥1 risk factors (supradiaphragmatic)	CS I, CSIIA ≥1 risk factors; CS IIB with C/D but without A/B	Standard risk group: unfavorable CS I-II (at least one risk factor)
Advanced stage	CS III-IV	CS IIB with A/B; CS III-IV	High-risk group: CS I or II with bulky disease; intraabdominal disease; CS III, IV
Risk factors (RF)	A large mediastinal mass B age ≥50 yr C elevated ESR* D ≥4 involved regions	A large mediastinal mass B extranodal disease C elevated ESR* D ≥3 involved areas	A ≥40 years B not NLPHL or NS histology C ESR ≥50 mm/h D ≥4 involved nodal regions

*Erythrocyte sedimentation rate (≥50 mm/h without or ≥30 mm/h with B-symptoms).
CS, Clinical stage; *ECOG,* Eastern Cooperative Oncology Group; *EORTC,* European Organization for Research and Treatment of Cancer; *GELA,* Groupe d'Etude des Lymphomes de l'Adulte; *GHSG,* German Hodgkin Study Group; *NCIC,* National Cancer Institute of Canada.
From Hoffman R et al: *Hematology, basic principles and practice,* ed 5, New York, 2009, Churchill Livingstone.

TABLE 1-242 Recommendations for the Primary Treatment of Hodgkin's Lymphoma Outside of Clinical Trials

Group	Stage	Recommendation
Early stages (favorable)	CS I-II A/B, no RFs	2 cycles ABVD; 6 cycles EBVP; *or* VBM ± IF RT (20-30 Gy)
	Early stages (unfavorable, intermediate)	4-6 cycles ABVD; BEACOPP-baseline, Stanford V; *or*
	CS I-II A/B + RFs	MOPP/ABV ± IF RT, 20-30Gy
Advanced stages	CS IIB + RFs, CS III A/B, CS IV A/B	6-8 cycles ABVD; MOPP/ABV; ChlVPP/EVA; BEACOPP-escalated *or* BEACOPP-14 ± RT, 20-30 Gy for residual tumor (PET positive) and/or bulk disease

ABVD regimen, Adriamycin (doxorubicin), vinblastine, bleomycin, and dacarbazine; *BEACOPP-baseline* regimen, bleomycin, etoposide, Adriamycin (doxorubicin), cyclophosphamide, Oncovin (vincristine), procarbazine, and prednisone; *BEACOPP-escalated* regimen, bleomycin, etoposide, Adriamycin (doxorubicin), cyclophosphamide, Oncovin (vincristine), procarbazine, prednisone, and G-CSF; *BEACOPP-14* regimen, bleomycin, etoposide, Adriamycin (doxorubicin), cyclophosphamide, Oncovin (vincristine), procarbazine, prednisone, and G-CSF; *ChlVPP/EVA* regimen, chlorambucil, vinblastine, procarbazine, prednisolone, etoposide, vincristine, Adriamycin (doxorubicin); *CS,* clinical stage; *EBVP* regimen, epirubicin, bleomycin, vinblastine, and prednisone; *IF,* involved field; *MOPP* regimen, mechlorethamine, Oncovin (vincristine), procarbazine, and prednisone; *PET,* positron emission tomography; *RF,* risk factors; *RT,* radiation therapy; *Stanford V* regimen, nitrogen mustard, doxorubicin, vinblastine, bleomycin, vincristine, etoposide, and prednisone; *VBM* regimen, vinblastine, bleomycin, and methotrexate.
From Hoffman R et al: *Hematology, basic principles and practice,* ed 5, New York, 2009, Churchill Livingstone.

TABLE 1-243 Prognostic Factors of Importance in Advanced Hodgkin's Lymphoma*

Gender	male
Age	>45 yr
Stage	IV
Hemoglobin	<105 g/L
White blood cell count	>15 × 10^9/L
Lymphocyte count	<0.6 × 10^9/L or <8% of the white cell differential
Serum albumin	<40 g/L

*Identified by the International Prognostic Factors Project on Advanced Hodgkin's Disease.
From Abeloff MD: *Clinical oncology,* ed 3, Philadelphia, 2004, Saunders.

but the long-term clinical outcome did not differ significantly between the two regimens. In addition, with the use of the escalated BEACOPP regimen, the rate of complications is higher (3% treatment-related death, 20% rate of hospitalization, and 3% rate of secondary leukemia). Thus, if the goal is cure with the least overall toxic effects, especially in elderly population, it is best to favor ABVD therapy, reserving rescue therapy with high-dose chemotherapy and autologous hematopoietic stem-cell transplantation for patients in whom the primary treatment fails. Stanford V (vinblastine, doxorubicin, mechlorethamine, bleomycin, etoposide, vincristine, and prednisone) may be preferred in some cases due to its short administration schedule combining radiation.

- Definitions of treatment groups are described in Table 1-241.
- Recommendations for the primary treatment of Hodgkin's lymphoma outside of clinical trials are described in Table 1-242.

DISPOSITION

- The overall survival at 10 yr is ~60%.
- Cure rates as high as 75% to 80% are now possible with appropriate initial therapy.
- Polyvalent pneumococcal vaccine and other vaccines should be administered especially in patients undergoing splenectomy.
- Poor prognostic features (Table 1-243) include presence of B symptoms, advanced age, advanced stage at initial presentation, mixed cellularity and lymphocyte depletion histology, and increased number of tumor-associated macrophages.
- Chemotherapy significantly increases the risk of leukemia.
- The peak in risk of leukemia is seen approximately 5 yr after the initiation of chemotherapy.
- The risk of leukemia is greater for those who undergo splenectomy and patients with advanced stages of Hodgkin's disease; the risk is unaffected by concomitant radiotherapy.
- Involved-field radiotherapy does not improve the outcome in patients with advanced-stage Hodgkin's lymphoma who have a complete remission after MOPP (mechlorethamine, vincristine, procarbazine, and prednisone)–ABV chemotherapy. Radiotherapy may benefit patients with a partial response after chemotherapy.
- Mediastinal irradiation increases the risk of subsequent death from heart disease caused by sclerosis of the coronary artery from irradiation. Risk increases with high mediastinal doses, minimal protective cardiac blocking, young age at irradiation, and increased duration of follow-up.
- Both chemotherapy and radiation therapy increase the risk of developing secondary solid tumors (Table 1-244).
- Table 1-245 describes potential late complications of Hodgkin's lymphoma treatment and appropriate clinical responses and preventive strategies.

REFERRAL

- To surgery for lymph node biopsy
- Hematology/oncology

TABLE 1-244 Second Neoplasms Seen with Increased Frequency after Successful Hodgkin's Lymphoma Treatment

Acute myelogenous leukemia/myelodysplasia
Non-Hodgkin's lymphoma
Melanoma
Soft tissue sarcoma
Adenocarcinoma
- Breast
- Thyroid
- Lung
- Stomach and esophagus

Squamous cell carcinoma
- Skin
- Uterine cervix
- Head and neck

From Abeloff MD: *Clinical oncology*, ed 3, Philadelphia, 2004, Saunders.

PEARLS & CONSIDERATIONS

COMMENTS

- Young male patients should consider sperm banking before the initiation of therapy.
- Chemotherapy plus involved-field radiotherapy should be the standard treatment for Hodgkin's disease with favorable prognostic features. In patients with unfavorable features, four courses of chemotherapy plus involved-field radiotherapy should be the standard of treatment. After failure of ABVD therapy, more than 60% of patients who have had a relapse and about 30% of patients with initially refractory lymphoma can be reliably cured with high-dose chemotherapy and autologous hematopoietic stem-cell transplantation.

TABLE 1-245 Potential Late Complications of Hodgkin's Lymphoma Treatment and Appropriate Clinical Responses and Preventive Strategies

Risk/Problem	Incidence/Response
Dental caries	Neck or oropharyngeal irradiation can cause decreased salivation. Patients should have careful dental care follow-up and should make their dentist aware of the previous irradiation.
Hypothyroidism	After external beam irradiation that encompasses the thyroid with doses sufficient to cure Hodgkin's lymphoma, at least 50% of patients will eventually become hypothyroid. All patients whose TSH level becomes elevated should be treated with lifelong thyroxine replacement in doses sufficient to suppress TSH levels to low normal. This is also necessary to ensure that the radiation-damaged thyroid is not subjected to long-term stimulation by thyroid-stimulating hormone, which can increase the risk of thyroid neoplasm.
Infertility	ABVD is not known to cause any permanent gonadal toxicity, although oligospermia for 1-2 yr after treatment is common. Direct or scatter radiation to gonadal tissue can cause infertility, amenorrhea, or premature menopause, but this seldom occurs with the current fields used for the treatment of Hodgkin's lymphoma. Thus, with the current chemotherapy regimens and radiation fields used, most patients will not develop these problems. In general, after treatment, women who continue menstruating are fertile, but men require semen analysis to provide a specific answer. High-dose chemoradiotherapy and hematopoietic stem cell transplantation almost always cause permanent infertility in both genders, although some young women occasionally recover fertility.
Impaired immunity to infections	Hodgkin's lymphoma and its treatment can lead to lifelong impairment of full immunity to infection. All patients should be given annual influenza immunization and pneumococcal immunization every 5 years. Patients whose spleen has been irradiated or removed should also be immunized against meningococcal types A and C and *Hemophilus influenza* type B. As for all adults, diphtheria and tetanus immunizations should be kept up-to-date.
Secondary neoplasms	Although uncommon, certain secondary neoplasms occur with increased frequency in patients who have been treated for Hodgkin's lymphoma. These include acute myelogenous leukemia, thyroid, breast, lung, and upper gastrointestinal carcinoma and melanoma, and cervical carcinoma in situ. It is appropriate to screen for these neoplasms for the rest of the patient's life because they might have lengthy induction periods.

ABVD, Adriamycin, bleomycin, vinblastine, dacarbazine; *TSH*, thyroid-stimulating hormone.
From Abeloff MD: *Clinical oncology*, ed 3, Philadelphia, 2004, Saunders.

SUGGESTED READINGS

available at www.expertconsult.com

RELATED CONTENT

Hodgkin's Lymphoma (Patient Information)

AUTHORS: **SYEDA M. SAYEED, M.D.**, and **FRED F. FERRI, M.D.**

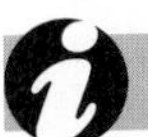

BASIC INFORMATION

DEFINITION

Hookworm is a parasitic infection of the intestine caused by the soil helminths *Necator americanus* and *Ancylostoma duodenale.*

SYNONYMS

Ground itch
Ancylostoma duodenale infection
Necator americanus infection

ICD-9CM CODES
126.35 Hookworm
ICD-10CM CODES
B76.9 Hookworm disease, unspecified

EPIDEMIOLOGY & DEMOGRAPHICS

INCIDENCE (IN U.S.):

- Varies greatly in different areas of the U.S.
- Most common in rural areas of southeastern U.S.
- Poor sanitation and increased rainfall increase incidence

PREVALENCE (IN U.S.): Varies from 10% to 90% in regions where it is found

PREDOMINANT AGE: Schoolchildren

PHYSICAL FINDINGS & CLINICAL PRESENTATION

- Nonspecific abdominal complaints
- Symptoms related to iron deficiency anemia depending on the amount of iron in the diet and worm burden (these organisms consume host's RBCs)
- Fatigue, tachycardia, dyspnea, and high-output failure
- Hypoproteinemia and edema from loss of proteins into the intestinal tract
- Unusual for pulmonary manifestations to occur when the larvae migrate through the lungs
- Skin rash at sites of larval penetration in some individuals without prior exposure: ground itch

ETIOLOGY

Two species can cause this disease: *N. americanus* and *A. duodenale. N. americanus* is the predominant cause of hookworm in the U.S. They are soil nematodes (geohelminthic infections) that are acquired by skin contact (i.e., bare feet) with contaminated soils in moist, warm climate. Worldwide, over 700 million people are infected.

- Infection occurs via penetration of the skin by the larval form, with subsequent migration via the bloodstream to the alveoli, up the respiratory tract, then into the GI tract (Fig. 1-478)
- *Ancylostoma* spp. infection can also occur via the oral route through ingestion of contaminated water supplies
- Sharp mouth parts allow for attachment to intestinal mucosa
- *Ancylostoma* spp. are more likely to cause iron deficiency anemia because they are larger and remove more blood daily from the bowel wall than the other hookworm species, *N. americanus.*

Dx DIAGNOSIS

DIFFERENTIAL DIAGNOSIS

- Strongyloidiasis
- Ascariasis
- Other causes of iron deficiency anemia and malabsorption

WORKUP

Examine stool for hookworm eggs. Shedding of eggs starts around 8 weeks after skin penetration in *N. americanum* infections and longer with *A. duodenale,* but eggs are indistinguishable between the two species.

LABORATORY TESTS

CBC to show hypochromic, microcytic anemia; possible mild eosinophilia and hypoalbuminemia

IMAGING STUDIES

Chest x-ray: generally not helpful, occasionally shows opacities

Rx TREATMENT

NONPHARMACOLOGIC THERAPY

- Prevention of disease by not walking barefoot and by improving sanitary conditions
- Vaccines are in development.

ACUTE GENERAL Rx

- Albendazole 400 mg once PO has become preferred treatment.
- Mebendazole 100 mg PO bid for 3 days or as a 500-mg single dose
- Pyrantel pamoate 11 mg/kg (to max dose of 1 g) PO qd × 3 days
- Iron supplementation may be helpful in patients with iron deficiency.

DISPOSITION

Easily treated

REFERRAL

To gastroenterologist and infectious disease specialist if diagnosis uncertain

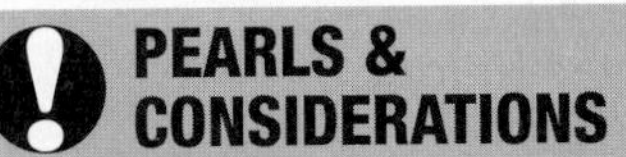

PEARLS & CONSIDERATIONS

COMMENTS

- Appropriate disposal of human wastes is important in controlling the disease in areas with a high prevalence of hookworm infestation.
- Wearing shoes will avoid contact with contaminated soils, and the provision of safe water and sanitation for disposing human excreta is important in control of hookworm.

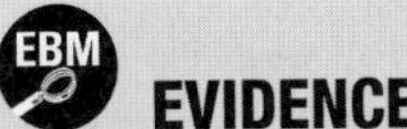

EVIDENCE

available at www.expertconsult.com

SUGGESTED READINGS

available at www.expertconsult.com

RELATED CONTENT

Hookworm Infection (Patient Information)

AUTHOR: **GLENN G. FORT, M.D., M.P.H.**

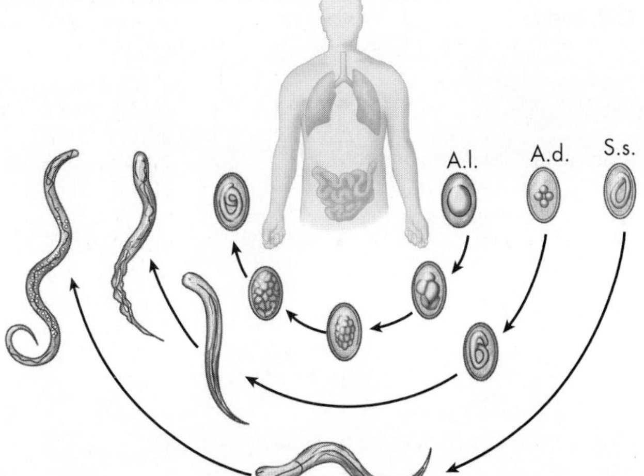

FIGURE 1-478 Life cycle of intestinal nematodes with a migratory phase through the lungs. Eggs are passed with stools in *Ascaris lumbricoides (A.l.), Necator americanus,* or *Ancylostoma duodenale (A.d.),* or they hatch on their way out in *Strongyloides stercoralis (S.s.).* Ascaris eggs mature in soil, and humans are infected upon ingestion of these eggs. With hookworm and strongyloidiasis, humans are infected via skin penetration by filariform larvae. In all three infections, larvae pass through a migratory phase via the lungs before reaching maturity at their final habitat in the small intestine. (From Mandell GL et al: *Principles and practice of infectious diseases,* ed 7, Philadelphia, 2010, Churchill Livingstone.)

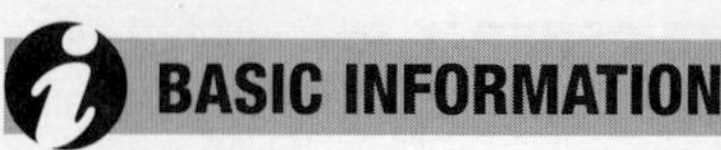

BASIC INFORMATION

DEFINITION

A hordeolum is an acute inflammatory process affecting the eyelid and arising from the meibomian (posterior) or Zeis (anterior) glands. It is most often infectious and usually caused by *Staphylococcus aureus*. When infection involves the meibomian glands, it is called meibomianitis.

SYNONYMS

Stye
Meibomianitis

ICD-9CM CODES
373.11 External hordeolum
373.12 Internal hordeolum
ICD-10CM CODES
H00.019 Hordeolum externum unspecified eye, unspecified eyelid
H00.029 Hordeolum internum unspecified eye, unspecified eyelid

EPIDEMIOLOGY & DEMOGRAPHICS

INCIDENCE (IN U.S.): Unknown
PREVALENCE (IN U.S.): Unknown
PREDOMINANT SEX: No gender predilection
PREDOMINANT AGE: May occur at any age
NEONATAL INFECTION: Rare in the neonatal period
PEAK INCIDENCE: May occur at any age

PHYSICAL FINDINGS & CLINICAL PRESENTATION

- Abrupt onset with pain and erythema of the eyelid
- Localized, tender mass in the eyelid (Fig. 1-479)
- May be associated with blepharitis
- External hordeolum: points toward the skin surface of the lid and may spontaneously drain
- Internal hordeolum: can point toward the conjunctival side of the lid and may cause conjunctival inflammation

ETIOLOGY

- 75% to 95% of cases are caused by *S. aureus.*
- Occasional cases are caused by *Streptococcus pneumoniae*, other streptococci, gram-negative enteric organisms, or mixed bacterial flora.

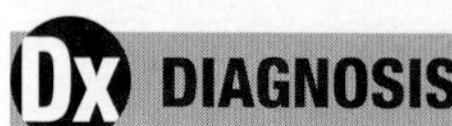

DIAGNOSIS

DIFFERENTIAL DIAGNOSIS

- Eyelid abscess
- Chalazion
- Allergy or contact dermatitis with conjunctival edema
- Acute dacryocystitis
- Herpes simplex infection
- Cellulitis of the eyelid

LABORATORY TESTS

- Generally, none are necessary.
- If incision and drainage are performed, specimens should be sent for bacterial culture.

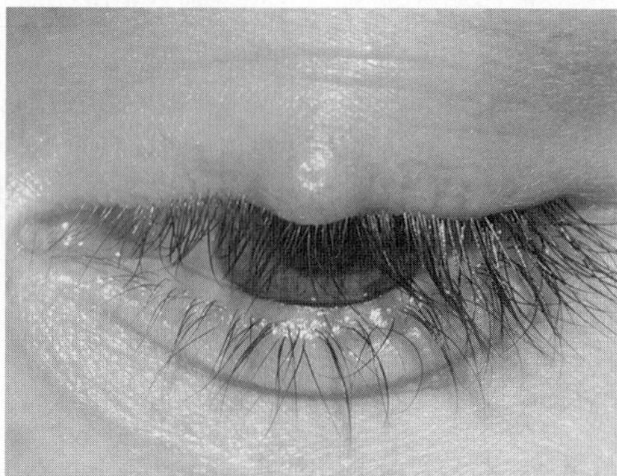

FIGURE 1-479 External stye. (From Palay D [ed]: *Ophthalmology for the primary care physician,* St Louis, 1997, Mosby.)

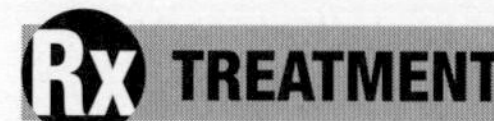

TREATMENT

NONPHARMACOLOGIC THERAPY

External stye (eyelash follicle): Usually responds to warm compresses and will drain spontaneously

ACUTE GENERAL Rx

- Systemic antibiotics generally not necessary
- For internal stye, use hot packs *plus* oral dicloxacillin 500 mg qid x 7 days. If suspecting MRSA, use trimethoprim-sulfamethoxazole DS bid in place of dicloxacillin. In patients with hospital-acquired infection, consider linezolid 600 mg PO bid.
- For external stye, topical erythromycin ophthalmic ointment applied to the lid margins two to four times daily until resolution may be helpful in some cases.
- Incision and drainage: rarely needed but should be considered for progressive infections

DISPOSITION

- Usually sporadic occurrence
- Possible relapse if resolution is not complete

REFERRAL

- For evaluation by an ophthalmologist if visual acuity or ocular movement is affected or if the diagnosis is in doubt
- For surgical drainage if necessary

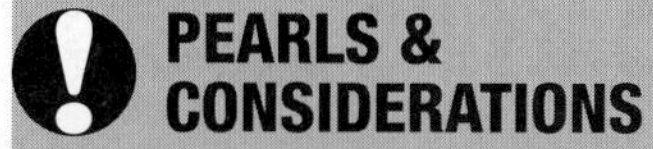

PEARLS & CONSIDERATIONS

COMMENTS

Seborrheic dermatitis may coexist with hordeolum.

SUGGESTED READINGS
available at www.expertconsult.com

RELATED CONTENT

Stye (Hordeolum) (Patient Information)

AUTHOR: **GLENN G. FORT, M.D., M.P.H.**

BASIC INFORMATION

DEFINITION

Horner's syndrome is the clinical triad of ipsilateral ptosis, miosis, and sometimes facial anhidrosis. Disruption of any of the three neurons in the oculosympathetic pathway (first-order, second-order, or third-order) can cause Horner's syndrome.

SYNONYMS

Oculosympathetic paresis

Raeder's paratrigeminal syndrome: Horner's syndrome of the third-order neuron associated with pain in the trigeminal nerve distribution

ICD-9CM CODES
337.9 Horner's syndrome
ICD-10CM CODES
G90.2 Horner's Syndrome

EPIDEMIOLOGY & DEMOGRAPHICS

Congenital or acquired

PHYSICAL FINDINGS & CLINICAL PRESENTATION

- Ptosis is usually mild. It results from loss of sympathetic tone to Müller's muscle, which contributes approximately 2 mm of upper eyelid elevation. Weakness of the corresponding muscle in the lower eyelid causes it to elevate slightly. This combination causes narrowing of the palpebral fissure. Levator function of the eyelid is preserved.
- Miosis results from loss of sympathetic innervation to the iris dilator muscle (Fig. 1-480). The affected pupil reacts normally to bright light and accommodation. Anisocoria is greater in dim light.
  - Dilation lag: Horner's pupil dilates more slowly than the normal pupil when lights are dimmed (20 vs. 5 sec) because it dilates passively as a result of relaxation of the iris sphincter.
- Presence of facial anhidrosis is variable and depends on the site of injury. It occurs with lesions affecting first-order or second-order neurons.
- Congenital Horner's syndrome may result in heterochromia. The affected eye has a lighter-colored iris.
- Acute cases may also present with conjunctival injection from the loss of sympathetic vasoconstriction.

FIGURE 1-480 Horner's syndrome. The mild ptosis (1 to 2 mm) and the smaller pupil (in room light) can be seen on the affected right side. (From Palay D [ed]: *Ophthalmology for the primary care physician,* St Louis, 1997, Mosby.)

ETIOLOGY

Disruption of the ipsilateral sympathetic innervation to the eye and face. Lesions can damage any of the three neurons in the oculosympathetic pathway. (Fig. E1-481) First-order neuron lesions are least common but are usually caused by pathology in the hypothalamus, brainstem, or cervical spinal cord. Second-order neuron lesions are often caused by disease involving the cervicothoracic spinal cord, lung apex, or anterior neck. Third-order neuron lesions are usually seen with disease in the internal carotid artery, skull base, cavernous sinus, or orbital apex. Location is often suggested by the presence of associated findings. Vascular disease and neoplasm must be considered.

Mechanical:
- Syringomyelia
- Trauma
- Tumors: benign, malignant head and neck cancers (thyroid, apical lung, mediastinal)
- Lymphadenopathy
- Neurofibromatosis
- Cervical rib

Vascular (ischemia, hemorrhage or arteriovenous malformation):
- Brainstem lesion: commonly occlusion of the posterior inferior cerebellar artery but other arteries may be responsible (vertebral; superior, middle or inferior lateral medullary arteries; superior or anterior inferior cerebellar arteries)
- Carotid artery aneurysm or dissection. Can also be from injury to other major vessels (internal carotid artery, subclavian artery, ascending aorta)
- Cavernous sinus thrombosis
- Cluster headache, migraine

Miscellaneous:
- Idiopathic
- Congenital
- Demyelination (multiple sclerosis)
- Infection (apical tuberculosis, herpes zoster, Lyme disease)
- Myelitis
- Pneumothorax
- Iatrogenic (angiography, internal jugular/subclavian catheter, chest tube, neck or upper thoracic surgery, epidural spinal anesthesia)

DIAGNOSIS

DIFFERENTIAL DIAGNOSIS

Causes of anisocoria (unequal pupils):
- Normal variant
- Mydriatic use
- Prosthetic eye
- Prior eye surgery
- Unilateral cataract
- Iritis

Causes of ptosis are described in Section II.

PHARMACOLOGIC TESTING

- Topical cocaine test: confirms sympathetic denervation (drops dilate normal pupil but not Horner's pupil)
- Topical apraclonidine test: confirms diagnosis (drops reverse anisocoria by causing dilation of Horner's pupil and constriction of normal pupil)
- Topical hydroxyamphetamine test: distinguishes first- and second-order neuron lesions from third-order sympathetic lesions (drops dilate normal pupil and first- or second-order Horner's pupil, but not third-order Horner's pupil)

IMAGING STUDIES

Results of pharmacologic testing as well as accompanying signs and symptoms should guide imaging:
- MRI brain: brainstem (diplopia, vertigo, ataxia); cavernous sinus (eye movement abnormalities, sixth nerve palsy)
- MRI cervical and upper thoracic spinal cord: weakness of extremities, bowel/bladder dysfunction
- MR or CT angiography (ultrasound is less sensitive): carotid artery dissection (acute Horner's syndrome with face or neck pain)
- CT chest and neck: evaluate lung apex, perivertebral areas, mediastinum if symptoms do not localize to the central nervous system; brachial plexus lesion (arm/hand pain or weakness)

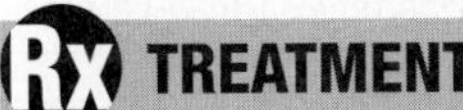

TREATMENT

- Treatment depends on underlying cause.
- Ptosis can be surgically corrected or treated with medication (phenylephrine drops).

REFERRAL

Ophthalmologist for pharmacologic testing to confirm diagnosis and localize lesion.

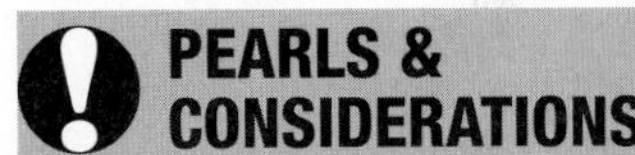

PEARLS & CONSIDERATIONS

- Normal variant anisocoria:
  - Occurs in 20% of people
  - Usually <1 mm difference between pupils
  - Pupils are round and display a normal, brisk constriction and dilation response to light

SUGGESTED READINGS
available at www.expertconsult.com

RELATED CONTENT

Lung Neoplasms, Primary (Related Key Topic)
Horner's Syndrome (Patient Information)

AUTHOR: **SUDEEP KAUR AULAKH, M.D.**

 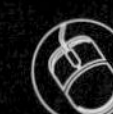

BASIC INFORMATION

DEFINITION

Hot flashes are sudden onset of intense warmth that begins in the neck or face, or in the chest and progresses to the neck and face; often associated with profuse sweating, anxiety, and palpitations.

ICD-9CM CODES
627.2 Hot flashes
ICD-10CM CODES
N95.1 Menopausal and female climacteric states
R23.2 Flushing

EPIDEMIOLOGY & DEMOGRAPHICS

- Hot flashes affect 75% of postmenopausal women.
- Most hot flashes begin 1 to 2 yr before menopause and resolve after 2 yr.
- 15% of women report duration of hot flashes >15 yr.

PHYSICAL FINDINGS & CLINICAL PRESENTATION

- Profuse sweating and red blotching of skin may be noted during the vasomotor event.
- Palpitations and hyperreflexia may be present during the hot flash.
- Hot flashes typically last 1 to 5 min.
- Each hot flash is associated with increase in temperature, increased pulse rate, and increased blood flow into the hands and face.
- Hot flashes during sleep are common and are referred to as *night sweats.*
- There is considerable variation in the frequency of hot flashes. One third of women report more than 10 flashes per day.

ETIOLOGY

- Dysfunction of central thermoregulatory centers caused by changes in estrogen level at the time of menopause
- Tamoxifen use
- Chemotherapy-induced ovarian failure
- Androgen ablation therapy for prostate carcinoma

DIAGNOSIS

DIFFERENTIAL DIAGNOSIS

- Carcinoid syndrome
- Anxiety disorder
- Idiopathic flushing
- Lymphoma (night sweats)
- Hyperthyroidism
- Hyperhidrosis

WORKUP

Evaluation of hot flashes is aimed at excluding the conditions listed in the differential diagnosis.

LABORATORY TESTS

- Follicle-stimulating hormone (FSH), luteinizing hormone, estradiol level. The serum FSH levels rather than estradiol levels are associated with greater severity of hot flashes in older postmenopausal women, suggesting that nonestrogen feedback systems may be important in modulating the severity of hot flashes. It is not necessary to obtain an FSH to make the diagnosis of menopausal status, however. An amenorrheic woman over age 50 with vasomotor symptoms is assumed to have made the menopausal transition and serum markers of menopause are not required to complete the diagnosis.
- Thyroid-stimulating hormone (TSH).

TREATMENT

NONPHARMACOLOGIC THERAPY

- Behavioral interventions such as relaxation training and paced respiration have been reported effective in reducing symptoms in some women.
- Avoidance of caffeine, alcohol, tobacco, and spicy foods may be beneficial.

GENERAL Rx

- Estrogen replacement therapy reduces hot flashes by 80% to 90%. Estrogen therapy, however, is contraindicated in many women, and others are fearful of its use. Potential risks and side effects should be considered before using estrogen in any patient. When using estrogen, it is best to use low-dose (e.g., Prempro [conjugated equine estrogen 0.45 mg or 0.3 mg plus medroxyprogesterone 1.5 mg]). Femring is an intravaginal ring that is changed every 3 mo and approved to treat vasomotor symptoms in women who have had a hysterectomy. It provides both local and systemic estrogen.
- Megestrol acetate, a progestational agent, is a safer alternative to estrogen in women with a history of receptor-positive breast or uterine cancer and in men receiving androgen ablation therapy for prostate cancer. Usual dose is 20 mg bid.
- The antidepressant venlafaxine has been reported to be 60% effective in reducing hot flashes and represents an alternative treatment modality in women unable or unwilling to use estrogens. Starting dose is 37.5 mg qd, increased as tolerated up to a maximum of 300 mg/day. Other antidepressants such as desvenlafaxine and escitalopram have also been shown to be effective in reducing the number and severity of menopausal hot flashes. A recent trial showed that paroxetine is also an effective agent for diminishing hot flashes in post-menopausal women and men receiving androgen ablation therapy.
- The anticonvulsant gabapentin (300 to 1200 mg/day) represents another nonhormonal alternative in the treatment of hot flashes and can be used alone or in combination with venlafaxine.
- The antihypertensive clonidine is also somewhat effective in reducing the frequency of hot flashes in mild cases. Adverse effects include dry mouth, sedation, and dizziness.
- Vitamin E (800 IU/day) may be effective in patients with mild symptoms that do not interfere with sleep or daily function.
- Soy protein (use of soy extracts that contain plant-derived estrogens [phytoestrogens]) is often used; however, clinical trials have not shown clear efficacy.
- Several classes of herbal remedies are available to patients and are commonly used, generally without significant benefit. Frequently used agents are *Cimicifuga racemosa* (black cohosh, snakeroot, bugbane), *Angelica sinensis,* and evening primrose (evening star). Recent trials using the isopropanolic extract of black cohosh rootstock (Remefemin) did show some improvement in controlling menopausal symptoms. Such alternative medications may be used to treat mild to moderate symptoms, but it is possible that symptomatic improvements may derive in part from a placebo effect.

SUGGESTED READINGS

available at www.expertconsult.com

RELATED CONTENT

Menopause (Related Key Topic)
Hot Flashes (Patient Information)

AUTHOR: **FRED F. FERRI, M.D.**

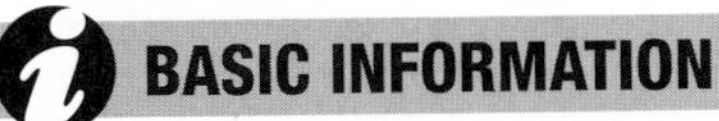

BASIC INFORMATION

DEFINITION

The human immunodeficiency virus, type 1 (HIV) is a retrovirus that is responsible for causing acquired immunodeficiency syndrome (AIDS). HIV infection does not necessarily mean a person has AIDS.

SYNONYMS

AIDS: The result of infection with HIV, which meets specific diagnostic criteria and leads to a weak immune system (See "Acquired Immunodeficiency Syndrome" in Section I.)

ICD-9CM CODES
042.9 HIV, unspecified
044.9 HIV, unspecified
ICD-10CM CODES
B20 Human immunodeficiency virus [HIV]

EPIDEMIOLOGY & DEMOGRAPHICS (U.S.)

- There are an estimated 1.1 million people infected with HIV in the United States, with approximately 1 out of 5 who do not know they are infected.
- In 2011 there were an estimated 49,273 new HIV infections according to the CDC.
- Greatest incidence is in men who have sex with men (MSM) and minority populations.

PREDOMINANT RISK GROUPS:

- Gay, bisexual, and other MSM are the groups most affected by HIV.
- In 2010, MSM accounted for 63% of all new infections according to the CDC.
- HIV disproportionately affects MSM of younger age and black/African American and Hispanic background.
- Heterosexual transmission and injection drug use accounted for 25% and 8% of new HIV infections in 2010, respectively.

RACIAL DATA:

- In 2010, blacks/African Americans accounted for 44% of new HIV infections despite being 12% of the U.S. population.
- In 2010, Hispanics/Latinos accounted for 21% of new HIV infections despite being 19% of the U.S. population.

GENETICS:

Familial Disposition:

Individuals with deletions in the *CCR5* gene are immune from infection with macrophage tropic virus (the predominant virus in sexual transmission). Other genetic variants may contribute to rapid progression or long-term control of the virus once infected. One in 300 individuals infected with HIV is an "elite controller" who is able to maintain a normal CD4 count and undetectable viral load through immune control.

Congenital Infection:

- 80% of childhood cases are caused by peripartum infection, which may occur in utero, during delivery, or after delivery via breastfeeding.
- No specific congenital abnormalities are associated with HIV infection, although risk of spontaneous abortion and low birth weight is greater.

Neonatal Infection:

- May occur during delivery or via breastfeeding
- Typically asymptomatic

PHYSICAL FINDINGS & CLINICAL PRESENTATION

- Signs and symptoms are variable with stage of disease.
- Acute HIV infection (0-3 mo, usually several wk):
  1. May cause a self-limited mononucleosis-like illness in 50% to 80% of individuals characterized by fever, sore throat, lymphadenopathy, headache, and a rash resembling roseola. Individuals may also be asymptomatic.
  2. In a minority of acute cases, aseptic meningitis, Bell's palsy, or peripheral neuropathy may occur.
  3. Rarely, opportunistic infections such as thrush or *Pneumocystis jiroveci* pneumonia (PJP) may occur.
- Chronic HIV infection is usually characterized by a prolonged asymptomatic phase followed by nonspecific symptoms of lymphadenopathy, fatigue, weight loss, diarrhea, and skin changes including seborrheic dermatitis, localized herpes zoster, and/or fungal infection.
- Advanced disease is characterized by the infections and malignancies associated with AIDS (see specific disorders).
- HIV infection in women may be associated with lower levels of viral load at comparable degrees of immunosuppression when compared with men. Furthermore, women may, on average, have higher CD4 lymphocyte counts at the time of AIDS diagnosis.
- Another special consideration in women infected with HIV is the high incidence of human papillomavirus (HPV) coinfection and the risk for cervical cancer that this presents. Even women with normal Pap smears should have this test repeated after 6 months and annually thereafter.
- Coinfection with HIV and hepatitis C is common because of similar transmission risk. Patients with HIV and hepatitis C progress faster to cirrhosis. Patients may already have signs of advanced liver disease at the time of diagnosis.

ETIOLOGY

- HIV-1 is a single-stranded RNA retrovirus (Fig. 1-482) that was derived from transmission of a simian immunodeficiency virus (SIV) from chimpanzees in Central Africa; a related virus, HIV-2 was derived from an SIV found in sooty mangabey monkeys from West Africa.

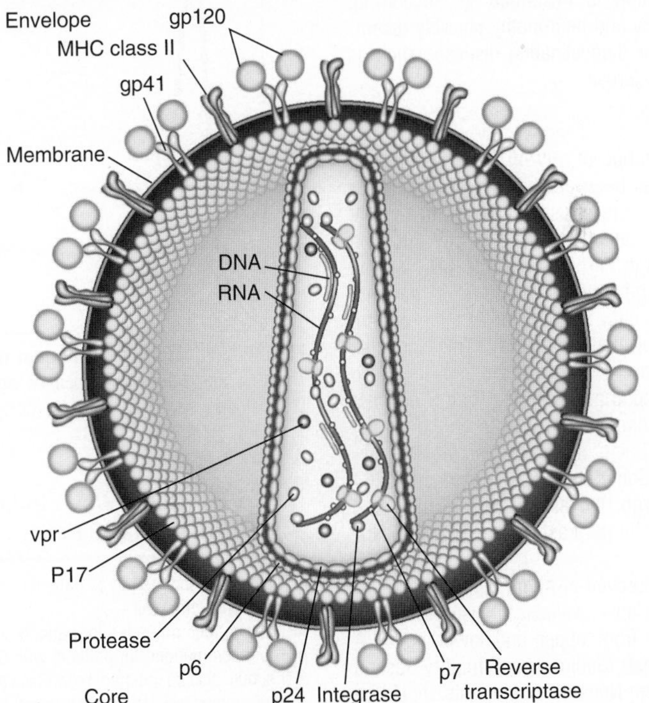

FIGURE 1-482 Structure of the HIV-1 virion. The viral envelope is formed from the host cell membrane, into which the HIV-1 envelope proteins gp41 and gp120 have been inserted and may include several host cell proteins, most significantly the major histocompatibility complex class II proteins. The matrix between the envelope and the core is formed predominantly from gag protein p17. The core contains the viral RNA, closely associated with gag protein p7, in addition to RT and integrase. It has also been proven that virions contain complementary DNA, as shown, synthesized by the RT. The major structural proteins of the core are gag proteins p24 and p6. Also present within the virion are the protease and two cleavage products from the gag precursor protein (p1 and p2, not shown) of undetermined position within the virion is also packaged in the virion and is thought to be localized within the core, as shown. (From Mandell GL et al: *Principles and practice of infectious diseases*, ed 7, Philadelphia, 2010, Saunders.)

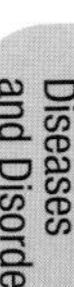

- HIV-1 is the predominant pathogenic retrovirus in human populations; HIV-2 has limited distribution (primarily in West Africa) and tends to progress less rapidly than HIV-1.
- HIV-1 is transmitted by sexual contact, shared needles, blood transfusion, or from mother to child during pregnancy, delivery, or breastfeeding.
- Primary target of infection: CD4 lymphocytes.
- Direct central nervous system (CNS) involvement: manifests as encephalopathy, myelopathy, or neuropathy in advanced cases.
- Renal failure, rheumatologic disorders, thrombocytopenia, or cardiac abnormalities may be seen in association with HIV-1.

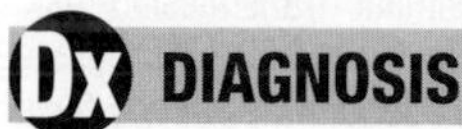

DIAGNOSIS

DIFFERENTIAL DIAGNOSIS

- Acute HIV infection: mononucleosis or other respiratory viral infections
- Late symptoms: similar to those produced by other wasting/chronic illnesses such as neoplasms, tuberculosis (TB), disseminated fungal infection (such as *Candida*), malabsorption, or depression
- HIV-related encephalopathy: confused with Alzheimer's disease or other causes of chronic dementia (cognitive impairment in HIV infection is described in Section II); myelopathy and neuropathy possibly resembling other demyelinating diseases such as multiple sclerosis

WORKUP

Since the debut of HIV/AIDS in the 1980s, diagnosis has been established by testing for antibodies to the virus. An algorithm for HIV detection in patients at risk for HIV infection is described in Fig. E1-483. The CDC is now recommending routine testing for patients in all health care settings unless the patient declines (opt-out screening). This includes routine testing of pregnant women. It is also recommended that separate written consent should no longer be required, although by law this is being addressed on a state-by-state basis. Generally, all persons aged 13-64 should undergo HIV testing at least once and more frequently (at least once a year) if sexually active.

- An FDA-approved at-home rapid HIV screening test is now available. It uses swabs of oral fluids from upper and lower gums. A positive test requires confirmatory testing in the office. Negative home tests should be repeated within 3 mo.

LABORATORY TESTS

HIV antibodies are detected by a two-step technique:

- ELISA (enzyme-linked immunosorbent assay), which is a sensitive screening test.
- Confirmation of positive ELISA tests with the more specific Western blot technique.
- ELISA antibody tests will measure HIV-1 and HIV-2 antibodies. The reflex Western blot will only look for HIV-1 proteins. If HIV-2 is suspected (i.e., the individual or sex partners are from Western Africa), a separate HIV-2 Western blot should be ordered.
- Baseline viral resistance testing is recommended for all newly diagnosed patients with HIV to guide choice of antiretroviral therapy (ART).
- The CD4 count and HIV RNA polymerase chain reaction (PCR) should be measured in all patients.
- The CD4 count is a marker of current immune status.
- The HIV RNA PCR (viral load) is predictive of disease progression.
- Rapid serologic tests have been increasingly used and are useful in specific settings: occupational exposures, pregnant women in labor without previous testing, and patients in high seroprevalence areas (for immediate results). Specimens are either blood or saliva and results are given within 1-20 min. Although sensitivity is high (99.1% to 99.7%), false-positive tests are more common in low seroprevalence populations. Thus, all positive results must be confirmed with standard serology, including Western blot.
- Early during infection (i.e., acute HIV infection), standard antibody tests may be negative ("window period"). The standard for diagnosing HIV during acute HIV infection is by testing for HIV RNA (viral load).
- In 2014, the Centers for Disease Control and Prevention released a revised surveillance case definition for HIV infection. This information has been added in the EBM section of this topic.

Fig. 1-484 describes the immunologic response to HIV infection.

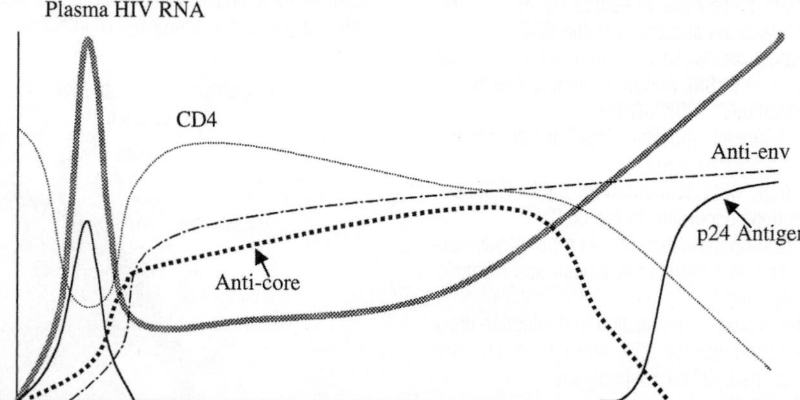

FIGURE 1-484 Course of human immunodeficiency virus infection. (From Mandell GL [ed]: *Mandell, Douglas, and Bennett's principles and practice of infectious diseases,* ed 6, New York, 2005, Churchill Livingstone.)

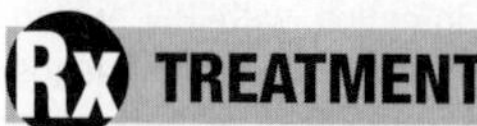

TREATMENT

NONPHARMACOLOGIC THERAPY

Maintenance of adequate nutrition

ACUTE GENERAL Rx

Acute management of opportunistic infections and malignancies (see AIDS-associated disorders, "*Pneumocystis jirovecii* Pneumonia," "Cryptococcosis," "Tuberculosis," "Toxoplasmosis" elsewhere in this text.)

CHRONIC Rx

All HIV-infected patients should be considered for ART regardless of CD4 cell count. The

TABLE 1-246 When to Initiate Antiretroviral Therapy (ART) in Treatment-Naïve Patients

ART should be initiated in all patients with a history of an AIDS-defining illness or with a CD4 count of <350 cells/mm^3 (AI).
ART is also recommended for patients with CD4 counts between 350 and 500 cells/mm^3 (AII).
ART is recommended for patients with CD4 counts greater than 500 cell/mm^3 (BIII).
ART should also be initiated, regardless of CD4 count, in patients with the following conditions: HIV-associated nephropathy (HIVAN) and HBV coinfection when treatment of HBV is indicated (AII).
A combination ARV drug regimen is also recommended for pregnant women who are not otherwise on treatment, with the goal to prevent perinatal transmission (AI).
Patients initiating ART should be willing and able to commit to lifelong treatment and should understand the benefits and risks of therapy and the importance of adherence.
Patients may choose to postpone therapy, and providers, on a case-by-case basis, may elect to defer therapy based on clinical and/or psychosocial factors.

Modified from Panel on Antiretroviral Guidelines for Adults and Adolescents. Guidelines for the use of antiretroviral agents in HIV-1–infected adults and adolescents. Department of Health and Human Services. March 27, 2012. http://www.aidsinfo.nih.gov/ContentFiles/AdultandAdolescentGL.pdf.

benefit of ART is well established in preventing progression to AIDS and associated comorbidities. Table 1-246 describes HIV treatment guidelines of the Department of Health and Human Services (DHHS) (www.aidsinfo.nih.gov/guidelines). Other considerations for initiation of antiretroviral therapy are described in Table 1-247. Prophylaxis to prevent first episode of HIV-related opportunistic disease is described in Table 1-248.

- Therapy is strongly recommended for all patients with symptomatic established HIV disease regardless of the CD4 count. Symptomatic HIV disease is defined as the presence of any of the following: thrush, vaginal candidiasis, herpes zoster, peripheral neuropathy, bacillary angiomatosis, cervical dysplasia in situ, constitutional symptoms such as fever or diarrhea for more than 1 month, ITP, PID, or listeriosis.
- In asymptomatic individuals, ART is now recommended regardless of CD4 cell counts. The updated recommendations are due to the safety and benefit of newer antivirals in preventing AIDS and decreasing both morbidity and mortality. Earlier treatment may also help reduce transmission of the virus to others due to reductions in viral loads.
- ART generally consists of using a 3-drug regimen to treat HIV-1 infection. Classes of antiretrovirals include:
    1. Nucleoside/nucleotide reverse transcriptase inhibitor (NRTI): zidovudine (AZT), lamivudine (3TC), emtricitabine (FTC), tenofovir (TDF), abacavir (ABC), stavudine (D4T), or didanosine (DDI).
    2. Protease inhibitors (PI): lopinavir/ritonavir, atazanavir, fosamprenavir, darunavir, saquinavir, amprenavir, tipranavir, nelfinavir, and indinavir. These PIs may be "boosted" by ritonavir to increase levels.
    3. Nonnucleoside reverse transcriptase inhibitors (NNRTI): Nevirapine, efavirenz, etravirine, delavirdine, or rilpivirine.
    4. Integrase Inhibitors (II): Raltegravir, elvitegravir, and dolutegravir. Raltegravir is a first-line agent according to the DHHS guidelines.
    5. Fusion Inhibitors: Enfuvirtide (T-20). This drug is administered through subcutaneous injections and is only used as part of a salvage regimen for individuals who have failed multiple other regimens.
    6. CCR5 Inhibitors: Maraviroc. Before using this drug, a viral trophism assay should be checked to determine if the virus uses the CCR5 co-receptor to infect cells. If the virus uses the CXCR4 co-receptor, this drug will not be effective. Adding a fourth drug to the three-drug regimen does not improve viral suppression or outcomes and is not recommended. Treatment interruptions based upon CD4 responses appear harmful in recent comparative studies versus standard continuous treatment protocols and should be avoided. Antiretroviral regimens for initial therapy are summarized in Table 1-249.
- Usual initial dosing regimen consists of two NRTIs and either a NNRTI, PI, or II. Data support inclusion of lamivudine or emtricitabine as one of the two NRTIs.

Standard NRTIs include:

- Truvada (tenofovir/emtricitabine) 1 tablet once daily.
    - Tenofovir: Individuals with underlying renal dysfunction or requiring other nephrotoxic agents may be at increased risk of renal toxicity.
    - Epzicom (abacavir/lamivudine) 1 tablet once daily
- Abacavir: may be associated with increased risk of myocardial infarction. Before using this drug, individuals should be checked for having HLA-B*5701. Individuals with this allele are at higher risk of serious hypersensitivity reactions and this drug should be avoided.
    - Combivir (Zidovudine/lamivudine) 1 tablet twice daily
    - Zidovudine: Associated with lipoatrophy and anemia. GI and CNS side effects.

Standard Backbone Regimens include:

- NNRTIs
    - Efavirenz 600 mg daily: not recommended for women in the first trimester or those who are contemplating pregnancy. This is considered the preferred agent within the class.
    - Nevirapine 200 mg two times a day: avoid with CD4 count >250 in men and >350 in women because of the risk of hepatitis. The newer agent rilpivirine had higher virologic failures and should be considered an alternative agent.
    - Etravirine 200 mg two times a day: This drug is generally used in patients that have failed other regimens. Etravirine retains activity in many patients that have developed resistance against efavirenz and nevirapine.
- PIs (ritonavir boosted)
    - Lopinavir/ritonavir (200 mg/50 mg) 2 tablets twice a day (or 4 tablets once a day): most likely to cause diarrhea and has the greatest negative effect on triglyceride levels.
    - Atazanavir and ritonavir (300 mg and 100 mg) 2 tablets a day: lower pill burden, but use with caution with acid reducing agents—can alter absorption. This is considered a preferred PI regimen within the DHHS guidelines.
    - Fosamprenavir and ritonavir (700 mg and 100 mg) 2 tablets twice a day (or 4 tablets once a day): cannot take fosamprenavir with sulfa allergy.
    - Darunavir and ritonavir: 800 mg and 100 mg a day. This is considered a preferred PI regimen within the DHHS guidelines.
    - Saquinavir and ritonavir.
- All these drugs have their own unique, as well as class-specific, side effects and require careful follow-up to achieve optimal antiviral effects. Compliance with the drug regimen and tolerance of common side effects are critically important to maintain drug efficacy. Antiviral response should be monitored by baseline HIV viral load and CD4 count and repeat measurement at 2 and 4 wk into treatment and then periodically (every 3 mo) to ensure viral suppression.
- All patients should have genotypic resistance testing upon entry into medical care and before initiation of ART.
- Later, an antiretroviral regimen should be constructed based on past antiretroviral experience and the results of genotypic or phenotypic testing.
- Patients with CD4 lymphocyte count <200/mm^3 should be given preventive therapy for PJP (see "*Pneumocystis jirovecii [P. carinii]* Pneumonia").
- Evaluation of chronic diarrhea in patients with HIV is described in the AIDS topic in Section I.
- Criteria for discontinuing and restarting opportunistic infection prophylaxis for adults and adolescents with HIV infection is described in Table 1-250.
- HIV infection in a pregnant woman poses special challenges and considerations. Appropriate and timely ART given to mother and newborn has been shown to dramatically reduce the risk of perinatal transmission of HIV. The goal of therapy is to achieve an undetectable viral load. For HIV-infected pregnant women who are already receiving ART: (1) Continue therapy if suppressing viral replication, but avoid use of efavirenz in the first trimester (substitution is recommended in the first trimester); (2) If viremia on therapy, genotypic testing is recommended; (3) Nevirapine should be continued, regardless of CD4 count, if there is viral suppression. For HIV-infected pregnant women who have never received ART: (1) Women who require ART for their own health should start on ART in the first trimester. Most antiretrovirals are safe in pregnancy, however, efavirenz should be avoided because of teratogenicity (Class D), DDI and D4T should be avoided (potential of lactic acidosis), and some protease inhibitors may be dose-altered in pregnancy. Nevirapine should not be initiated in an antiretroviral-naive pregnant patient with CD4 counts >250 because of the risk of hepatotoxicity. (2) Women who do not

TABLE 1-247 Conditions Favoring More Rapid Initiation of Antiretroviral Therapy

Pregnancy
AIDS-defining conditions
Acute opportunistic infections
Lower CD4 counts (e.g., <200 cells/mm^3)
Rapidly declining CD4 counts (e.g., >100 cells/mm^3 decrease per year)
Higher viral loads (e.g., >100,000 copies/ml)
HIV-associated nephropathy
Hepatitis B/C virus (HBV/HCV) coinfection

Modified from Panel on Antiretroviral Guidelines for Adults and Adolescents. Guidelines for the use of antiretroviral agents in HIV-1–infected adults and adolescents. Department of Health and Human Services. March 27, 2012. http://www.aidsinfo.nih.gov/ContentFiles/AdultandAdolescentGL.pdf.

TABLE 1-248 Prophylaxis to Prevent First Episode of HIV-related Opportunistic Disease

Pathogen	Indication	First Choice	Alternative
Pneumocystis jiroveci pneumonia (PJP, previously referred to as *Pneumocystis carinii,* PCP)	$CD4^+$ count <200 cells/mm^3 or oropharyngeal candidiasis $CD4^+$ <14% or history of AIDS-defining illness $CD4^+$ count >200 but <250 cells/mm^3 if monitoring $CD4^+$ count every 1-3 mo is not possible	Trimethoprim-sulfamethoxazole (TMP-SMX) 1 double-strength PO daily; *or* 1 single-strength daily	TMP-SMX 1 double-strength PO 3 times weekly; *or* Dapsone 100 mg PO daily or 50 mg PO bid; *or* Aerosolized pentamidine 300 mg via Respirgard II nebulizer every month; *or* Atovaquone 1500 mg PO daily
Toxoplasma gondii encephalitis	*Toxoplasma* IgG–positive patients with $CD4^+$ count <100 cells/mm^3 Seronegative patients receiving PCP prophylaxis not active against toxoplasmosis should have *Toxoplasma* serology retested if $CD4^+$ count declines to <100 cells/mm^3. Prophylaxis should be initiated if seroconversion occurred.	TMP-SMX, 1 double-strength PO daily	TMP-SMX 1 double-strength PO 3 times weekly; *or* TMP-SMX 1 single-strength PO daily; *or* Dapsone 50 mg PO daily + pyrimethamine 50 mg PO weekly + leucovorin 25 mg PO weekly; *or* Dapsone 200 mg PO weekly + pyrimethamine 75 mg PO weekly + leucovorin 25 mg PO weekly;
Mycobacterium tuberculosis infection (TB)(treatment of latent TB infection or LTBI)	(1) Diagnostic test for LTBI, no evidence of active TB, and no prior history of treatment for active or latent TB (2) Diagnostic test for LTBI, but close contact with a person with infectious pulmonary TB and no evidence of active TB (3) A history of untreated or inadequately treated healed TB (i.e., old fibrotic lesions) regardless of diagnostic tests for LTBI and no evidence of active TB	Isoniazid (INH) 300 mg PO daily or 900 mg PO twice weekly for 9 mo—both plus pyridoxine 50 mg PO daily; *or* For persons exposed to drug-resistant TB, selection of drugs after consultation with public health authorities	Rifampin (RIF) 600 mg PO daily × 3-4 mo; *or* Rifabutin (RFB) 300 mg once daily for 4 mo. Be careful of drug interactions with these medications (PIs and NNRTIs).
Disseminated *Mycobacterium avium* complex (MAC) disease	$CD4^+$ count <50 cells/mm^3—after ruling out active MAC infection	Azithromycin 1200 mg PO once weekly; *or* Clarithromycin 500 mg PO bid; *or* Azithromycin 600 mg PO twice weekly	RFB 300 mg PO daily (dosage adjustment based on drug-drug interactions with antiretroviral therapy); rule out active TB before starting RFB
Streptococcus pneumoniae infection	$CD4^+$ count >200 cells/mm^3 and no receipt of pneumococcal vaccine in the past 5 yr $CD4^+$ count <200 cells/mm^3—vaccination can be offered In patients who received polysaccharide pneumococcal vaccination (PPV) when $CD4^+$ count <200 cells/mm^3 but has increased to >200 cells/mm^3 in response to antiretroviral therapy	23-valent PPV 0.5 ml IM × 1 Revaccination every 5 yr may be considered	
Influenza A and B virus infection	All HIV-infected patients	Inactivated influenza vaccine 0.5 ml IM annually	
Histoplasma capsulatum infection	$CD4^+$ count ≤150 cells/mm^3 and at high risk because of occupational exposure or live in a community with a hyperendemic rate of histoplasmosis (>10 cases/100 patient-yr)	Itraconazole 200 mg PO daily	
Coccidioidomycosis	Positive IgM or IgG serologic test result in a patient from a disease-endemic area; and $CD4^+$ count <250 cells/mm^3	Fluconazole 400 mg PO daily Itraconazole 200 mg PO bid	
Varicella-zoster virus (VZV) infection	*Pre-exposure prevention:* Patients with $CD4^+$ count ≥200 cells/mm^3 who have not been vaccinated, have no history of varicella or herpes zoster, or who are seronegative for VZV Note: Routine VZV serologic testing in HIV-infected adults is not recommended. *Postexposure—close contact with a person who has active varicella or herpes zoster:* For susceptible patients (those who have no history of vaccination or of either condition, or are known to be VZV seronegative)	*Pre-exposure prevention:* Primary varicella vaccination (Varivax), 2 doses (0.5 ml SC) administered 3 mo apart If vaccination results in disease because of vaccine virus, treatment with acyclovir is recommended. *Postexposure therapy:* Varicella-zoster immune globulin (VariZIG) 125 IU per 10 kg (maximum of 625 IU) IM, administered within 96 hr after exposure to a person with active varicella or herpes zoster Note: As of June 2007, VariZIG can be obtained only under a treatment IND (1-800-843-7477, FFF Enterprises).	VZV-susceptible household contacts of susceptible HIV-infected persons should be vaccinated to prevent potential transmission of VZV to their HIV-infected contacts. *Alternative postexposure therapy:* Postexposure varicella vaccine (Varivax) 0.5 ml SC × 2 doses, 3 mo apart if $CD4^+$ count >200 cells/mm^3; *or* Preemptive acyclovir 800 mg PO 3×/day for 5 days These two alternatives have not been studied in the HIV population.
Human papillomavirus (HPV) infection	Women aged 11-26 yr. Men aged 11-21 yr	HPV quadrivalent vaccine 0.5 ml IM mo 0, 2, and 6	

Modified from Centers for Disease Control and Prevention. Guidelines for Prevention and treatment of opportunistic infections in HIV-infected adults and adolescents: Recommendations from CDC, the National Institutes of Health, and the HIV Medicine Association of the Infectious Disease Society of America, *MMWR Morb Mortal Wkly Rep* 58(RR-4), 2009.

Continued on following page

TABLE 1-248 Prophylaxis to Prevent First Episode of HIV-related Opportunistic Disease—*(Continued)*

Pathogen	Indication	First Choice	Alternative
Hepatitis A virus (HAV) infection	HAV-susceptible patients with chronic liver disease or who are injection-drug users, or men who have sex with men. Certain specialists might delay vaccination until CD4+ count >200 cells/mm³.	Hepatitis A vaccine 1 ml IM × 2 doses—at 0 and 6-12 mo IgG antibody response should be assessed 1 mo after vaccination; nonresponders should be revaccinated	
Hepatitis B virus (HBV) infection	All HIV patients without evidence of prior exposure to HBV should be vaccinated with HBV vaccine, including patients with CD4+ count <200 cells/mm³. *Patients with isolated anti-HBc:* consider screening for HBV DNA before vaccination to rule out occult chronic HBV infection	Hepatitis B vaccine IM (Engerix-B 20 μg/ml or Recombivax HB 10 μg/ml) at 0, 1, and 6 mo Anti-HBs should be obtained 1 mo after completion of the vaccine series.	Some experts recommend vaccinating with 40-μg doses of either vaccine.
	Vaccine nonresponders: Defined as anti-HBs <10 IU/ml 1 mo after a vaccination series For patients with low CD4+ count at the time of first vaccination series, certain specialists might delay revaccination until after a sustained increase in CD4+ count with antiretroviral therapy.	Revaccinate with a second vaccine series.	Some experts recommend revaccinating with 40-μg doses of either vaccine.

TABLE 1-249 What Antiretroviral Regimen to Choose for Initial Therapy

Preferred Regimens	Comments
NNRTI-based regimen EFV/TDF/FTC PI-based regimens (in alphabetical order) ATV/r + TDF/FTC DRV/r (once daily) + TDF/FTC Integrase inhibitor-based regimen RAL + TDF/FTC Preferred regimen for pregnant women LPV/r (twice daily) + ZDV/3TC	EFV should not be used during the first trimester of pregnancy or in women trying to conceive or not using effective and consistent contraception. ATV/r should not be used in patients who are on proton pump inhibitors or other antacids.
Alternative Regimens	***Comments***
NNRTI-based regimens (in alphabetical order) EFV + ABC/3TC RPV/TDF/FTC RPV + ABC/3TC PI-based regimens (in alphabetical order) ATV/r + ABC/3TC DRV + ABC/3TC FPV/r (once or twice daily) + either ABC/3TC or TDF/FTC LPV/r (once or twice daily) + either [(ABC or ZDV)/3TC] or TDF/FTC Integrase inhibitor-based regimens RAL + ABC/3TC	NVP should not be used in patients with moderate to severe hepatic impairment (Child-Pugh B or C) Should not be used in women with pre-treatment CD4 >250 cells/mm³ or men with CD4 >400 cells/mm³ ABC should not be used in patients who test positive for HLA-B*5701 Use with caution in patients with high risk of cardiovascular disease or with pretreatment HIV RNA >100,000 copies/mL Once-daily LPV/r is not recommended in pregnant women.
Acceptable Regimens	
EFV + AZT/3TC NVP + TDF/FTC or ABC/3TC or AZT/3TC RPV + AZT/3TC ATV + ABC/3TC or AZT/3TC ATV/r + AZT/3TC DRV/r + AZT/3TC FPV/r + AZT/3TC LPV/r + AZT/3TC RAL + AZT/3TC MVC + AZT/3TC or TDF/FTC or ABC/3TC	

3TC, Lamivudine; *ABC,* abacavir; *ATV,* atazanavir; *ddI,* didanosine; *DRV,* darunavir; *EFV,* efavirenz; *FPV,* fosamprenavir; *FTC,* emtricitabine; *INSTI,* integrase strand transfer inhibitor; *LPV,* lopinavir; *MRV,* maraviroc; *NNRTI,* nonnucleoside reverse transcriptase inhibitor; *NRTI,* nucleos(t)ide reverse transcriptase inhibitor; *NVP,* nevirapine; *PI,* protease inhibitor; *r,* low dose ritonavir; *RAL,* raltegravir; *RVP,* rilpivirine; *SQV,* saquinavir; *TDF,* tenofovir; *ZDV,* zidovudine.
The following combinations in the recommended list are available as fixed-dose combination formulations: ABC/3TC, EFV/TDF/FTC, LPV/r, TDF/FTC, RPV/TDF/FTC, and ZDV/3TC.
Modified from Panel on Antiretroviral Guidelines for Adults and Adolescents. Guidelines for the use of antiretroviral agents in HIV-1–infected adults and adolescents. Department of Health and Human Services 1-161, 2012. http://www.aidsinfo.nih.gov/ContentFiles/AdultandAdolescentGL.pdf.

TABLE 1-250 Criteria for Discontinuing and Restarting Opportunistic Infection Prophylaxis for Adults and Adolescents with Human Immunodeficiency Virus Infection

Opportunistic Infection	Criteria for Discontinuing Primary Prophylaxis	Criteria for Restarting Primary Prophylaxis	Criteria for Discontinuing Secondary Prophylaxis/Chronic Maintenance Therapy	Criteria for Restarting Secondary Prophylaxis/ Chronic Maintenance Therapy
Pneumocystis pneumonia (PJP)	$CD4^+$ count >200 cells/mm^3 for >3 mo in response to ART	$CD4^+$ count <200 cells/mm^3	$CD4^+$ count increased from <200 cells/mm^3 to >200 cells/mm^3 for ≥3 mo in response to ART If PJP is diagnosed when $CD4^+$ count >200 cells/mm^3, prophylaxis should probably be continued for life regardless of $CD4^+$ count rise in response to ART.	$CD4^+$ count <200 cells/mm^3, or if PCP recurred at a $CD4^+$ count >200 cells/ mm^3
Toxoplasma gondii encephalitis (TE)	$CD4^+$ count >200 cells/mm^3 for >3 mo in response to ART	$CD4^+$ count <100-200 cells/ mm^3	Successfully completed initial therapy, remain asymptomatic of signs and symptoms of TE, and $CD4^+$ count >200 cells/mm^3 for >6 mo in response to ART	$CD4^+$ count <200 cells/mm^3
Microsporidiosis	Not applicable	Not applicable	No signs and symptoms of non-ocular microsporidiosis and $CD4^+$ count >200 cells/mm^3 for >6 mo in response to ART Patients with ocular microsporidiosis should be on therapy indefinitely regardless of $CD4^+$ count.	No recommendation
Disseminated *Mycobacterium avium* complex (MAC) disease	$CD4^+$ count >100 cells/mm^3 for ≥3 mo in response to ART	$CD4^+$ count <50 cells/mm^3	If fulfill the following criteria Completed ≥12 mo therapy, and No signs and symptoms of MAC, and Have sustained (≥6 mo) $CD4^+$ count >100 cells/mm^3 in response to ART	$CD4^+$ count <100 cells/mm^3
Bartonellosis	Not applicable	Not applicable	If fulfill the following criteria Received 3-4 mo of treatment $CD4^+$ count >200 cells/mm^3 for ≥6 mo Certain specialists would discontinue therapy only if *Bartonella* titers have also decreased by fourfold.	No recommendation
Mucosal candidiasis	Not applicable	Not applicable	If used, reasonable to discontinue when $CD4^+$ count >200 cells/mm^3	No recommendation
Cryptococcal meningitis	Not applicable	Not applicable	If fulfill the following criteria Completed course of initial therapy Remain asymptomatic of cryptococcosis $CD4^+$ count ≥200 cells/mm^3 for >6 mo in response to ART Certain specialists would perform a lumbar puncture to determine if cerebrospinal fluid is culture and antigen negative before stopping therapy.	$CD4^+$ count <200 cells/mm^3
Histoplasma capsulatum infection	If used, $CD4^+$ count >150 cells/mm^3 for 6 mo on ART	For patients at high risk for acquiring histoplasmosis, restart at $CD4^+$ count ≤150 cells/mm^3.	If fulfill the following criteria Received itraconazole for ≥1 yr Negative blood cultures $CD4^+$ count >150 cells/mm^3 for ≥6 mo in response to ART Serum *Histoplasma* antigen <2 units	$CD4^+$ count ≤150 cells/mm^3
Coccidioidomycosis	If used, $CD4^+$ count ≥250 cells/mm^3 for ≥6 mo	If used, restart at $CD4^+$ count <250 cells/mm^3	**Only for patients with focal coccidioidal pneumonia:** Clinically responded to ≥12 mo of antifungal therapy $CD4^+$ count >250 cells/mm^3 Receiving ART Suppressive therapy should be continued indefinitely, even with increase in $CD4^+$ count on ART for patients with diffuse pulmonary, disseminated, or meningeal diseases.	No recommendation
Cytomegalovirus retinitis	Not applicable	Not applicable	$CD4^+$ count >100 cells/mm^3 for >3-6 mo in response to ART. Therapy should be discontinued only after consultation with an ophthalmologist, taking into account magnitude and duration of $CD4^+$ count increase, anatomic location of the lesions, vision in the contralateral eye, and the feasibility of regular ophthalmologic monitoring. Routine (every 3 mo) ophthalmologic follow-up is recommended for early detection of relapse or immune restoration uveitis.	$CD4^+$ count <100 cells/mm^3
Isospora belli infection	Not applicable	Not applicable	Sustained increase in $CD4^+$ count to >200 cells/ mm^3 for >6 mo in response to ART and without evidence of *I. belli* infection	No recommendation

Modified from Centers for Disease Control and Prevention. Guidelines for Prevention and treatment of opportunistic infections in HIV-infected adults and adolescents. Recommendations from CDC, the National Institutes of Health, and the HIV Medicine Association of the Infectious Disease Society of America. *MMWR Morb Mortal Wkly Rep* 58(RR-4), 2009.

need ART for their own health should also initiate three-drug therapy, but may do so at the end of the first trimester.

(3) Zidovudine (AZT) is recommended as a component of ART.

- Therapy should continue through the baby's birth. Zidovudine is given intravenously at the time of labor, regardless of whether it is an existing component of her three-drug regimen. In women with viral loads persistently >1000 copies/ml despite appropriate ART, cesarean section may further lower risk of transmission. Zidovudine (AZT) should also be given to the newborn for the first 6 weeks of life, and mothers should completely avoid nursing.

DISPOSITION

- Ongoing care consisting of frequent medical evaluations and T-lymphocyte subset analysis (CD4 counts) along with the plasma HIV loads.
- Long-term care focused on providing up-to-date ART and prophylaxis of PJP and other opportunistic infections, as well as early detection of complications (see Section III)
- Ongoing assessment for cardiovascular risk and other primary prevention interventions.
- Screening for hepatitis A, B, and C. Treatment where indicated. Drugs such as tenofovir and lamivudine have activity against both HIV and hepatitis B and may be used in patients with co-infection.
- Vaccinations including hepatitis A and B (when susceptible), Pneumovax, tetanus/diphtheria/pertussis, and influenza. Box 1-39 summarizes vaccinations in HIV-positive adults.
- Yearly screening for other sexually transmitted infections (*Chlamydia,* gonorrhea, syphilis).
- Consideration of AIDS (lymphomas, HPV) and non-AIDS related (screening for general population, age-specific cancers).

BOX 1-39 Vaccination in HIV-Positive Adults

Generally Avoid
- VZV
- BCG
- Oral polio
- Oral typhoid

Avoid if CD4+ Cells <200
- Yellow fever
- Measles

Give Routinely
- Tetanus/diphtheria (or Tdap)
- Hepatitis B
- *Streptococcus pneumoniae*
- Hib
- Influenza, yearly
- Hepatitis A

Give if Indicated for Travel
- Typhoid Vi
- Meningococcal
- Polio, IPV
- Rabies
- Japanese encephalitis
- Tick-borne encephalitis

From Auerbach P: *Wilderness medicine, expert consult* Premium Edition—Enhanced Online Features and Print, Philadelphia, 2012, Saunders.

REFERRAL

To a physician knowledgeable and experienced in the management of HIV infection and its complications

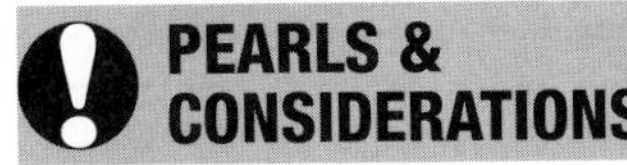

COMMENTS

- HIV chemoprophylaxis after occupational exposure is described in Section V.
- A recent analysis of the impact of ART indicates that ART has saved at least 3 million years of life since the introduction into medicine more than 10 years ago.
- In persons with HIV infection, screening for TB needs to include questions about combination of symptoms rather than only inquiring about chronic cough.
- Trials involving antiretroviral chemoprophylaxis before exposure for the prevention of HIV acquisition in MSM have shown that oral tenofovir disoproxil fumarate (FTC-TDF) provides protection against acquisition of HIV infection. Detected blood levels strongly correlated with the prophylactic effect.
- ART in combination with avoidance of breast-feeding and elective cesarean section in women with viremia reduces risk for mother-to-child transmission.

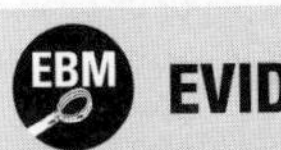

available at www.expertconsult.com

SUGGESTED READINGS

available at www.expertconsult.com

RELATED CONTENT

Human Immunodeficiency Virus (HIV) Infection (Patient Information)

Acquired Immunodeficiency Syndrome (Related Key Topic)

AUTHOR: **PHILIP A. CHAN, M.D., M.S.**

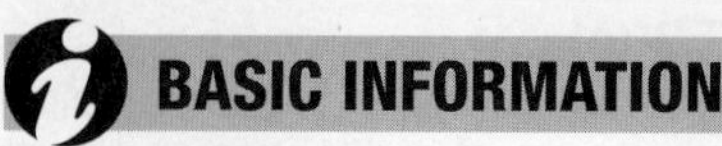

BASIC INFORMATION

DEFINITION

Huntington's disease is an autosomal dominant neurodegenerative disorder characterized by involuntary movements, psychiatric disturbance, and cognitive decline.

SYNONYMS

Huntington's chorea

ICD-9CM CODES
333.4 Huntington's chorea
ICD-10CM CODES
G10 Huntington's disease

EPIDEMIOLOGY & DEMOGRAPHICS

PEAK INCIDENCE: Late 30s and 40s, with onsets from ages 2 to 70 yr
PREVALENCE (IN U.S.): 4.1 to 8.4 cases/ 100,000 persons
PREDOMINANT SEX: Female = male
PREDOMINANT AGE: Adulthood
GENETICS: Autosomal dominant

PHYSICAL FINDINGS & CLINICAL PRESENTATION

- Chorea: irregular, rapid, flowing, nonstereotyped involuntary movements. When there is a writhing quality, it is referred to as choreoathetosis. Chorea is present early on and tends to decrease in end stages of disease.
- Dancelike, lurching gait, often caused by chorea.
- Westphal variant: cognitive dysfunction, bradykinesia, and rigidity. This variant is more commonly seen in juvenile-onset Huntington's.
- Oculomotor abnormalities are common early on and include increased latency of response and insuppressible eye blinking.
- Psychiatric disorders (can be present early on): depression is commonly seen as well as obsessive-compulsive behaviors and aggression associated with impaired impulse control.

ETIOLOGY

- Trinucleotide repeat disorder
- The responsible gene is the Huntington gene located on chromosome 4. Its function is not known.

Dx DIAGNOSIS

DIFFERENTIAL DIAGNOSIS

- Drug-induced chorea: dopamine, stimulants, anticonvulsants, antidepressants, and oral contraceptives have all been known to cause chorea.
- Sydenham's chorea: decreased incidence with decline of rheumatic fever.
- Benign hereditary chorea: autosomal dominant with onset in childhood; non-progressive and without associated dementia or behavioral problems.
- Senile chorea: possibly vascular in origin.
- Wilson's disease: autosomal recessive; tremor, dysarthria, and dystonia are more common presentations than chorea. A total of 95% of patients with neurologic manifestations will have Kayser-Fleischer rings.
- Postinfectious.
- Systemic lupus erythematosus: can be the presenting feature of lupus (rare).
- Chorea gravidarum: presents during first 4 to 5 mo of pregnancy and resolves after delivery.
- Paraneoplastic: seen most commonly in small-cell lung cancer and lymphoma.

WORKUP

Onset of symptoms in an individual with an established family history requires no additional investigation.

LABORATORY TESTS

- Genetic testing for CAG repeats
- If genetic tests are normal, obtain complete blood count with smear, erythrocyte sedimentation rate, electrolytes, serum ceruloplasmin, 24-hr urinary copper excretion, TFTs, antinuclear antibody, liver function tests, HIV, and ASO titer. Consider paraneoplastic markers.

IMAGING STUDIES

CT scan or MRI scan will show atrophy, most notably in the caudate and putamen. The cortex is involved to a lesser extent. A normal scan does not exclude the diagnosis.

Rx TREATMENT

NONPHARMACOLOGIC THERAPY

- Supportive counseling
- Physical and occupational therapy
- Home health care
- Genetic counseling

CHRONIC Rx

- Chorea does not need to be treated unless it is disabling.
- Tetrabenazine (TBZ) is approved by the FDA for the symptomatic treatment of chorea seen in Huntington's disease. It is a reversible inhibitor of the vesicle monoamine transporter type 2 (VMAT-2). It inhibits primarily dopamine and to a lesser degree serotonin and norepinephrine. Side effects include parkinsonism and severe depression.
- Neuroleptics, typical or atypical, can be used for symptomatic management of neuropsychiatric issues and chorea at low doses (e.g., haloperidol 1 to 10 mg/day).
- Amantadine (up to 300 to 400 mg divided tid).
- Depression with suicidal ideation is common; may improve with tricyclic antidepressants or SSRI

DISPOSITION

Relentless course of variable duration leading to progressive disability and death

REFERRAL

- Should refer to psychiatry and neurology for treatment of mood disorders and movement disorders
- Genetic counseling

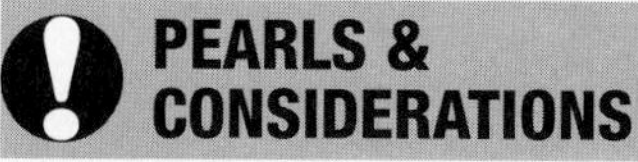

PEARLS & CONSIDERATIONS

- Suicide rate is fivefold that of the general population.
- The number of repeats does correlate with age of onset but does not clearly correlate with disease severity. Interpretation of number of repeats is still difficult at this time; therefore it is debatable whether to disclose this information to patients.

SUGGESTED READINGS

available at www.expertconsult.com

RELATED CONTENT

Huntington's Disease (Patient Information)

AUTHOR: **FARIHA ZAHEER, M.D.**

BASIC INFORMATION

DEFINITION

A hydrocele is a fluid collection in a serous scrotal space, usually between the layers of the tunica vaginalis (Fig. 1-485). A hydrocele that fills with fluid from the peritoneum is termed *communicating*. This is distinguished from a *noncommunicating* hydrocele by history of variation in size throughout the day and palpation of a thickened cord above the testicle on the affected side. A communicating hydrocele is a small inguinal hernia in which fluid, but not peritoneal structures, traverses the processus vaginalis. In noncommunicating hydrocele, the processus vaginalis was obliterated during development. An abdominoscrotal hydrocele is a rare variant of a hydrocele in which there is a large, tense hydrocele that extends into the lower abdominal cavity.

ICD-9CM CODES
603.9 Hydrocele
ICD-10CM CODES
N43.3 Hydrocele, unspecified
N43 Hydrocele and spermatocele
N43.0 Encysted hydrocele
N43.1 Infected hydrocele
N43.2 Other hydrocele

PHYSICAL FINDINGS & CLINICAL PRESENTATION

Symptoms:
- Scrotal enlargement
- Scrotal heaviness or discomfort radiating to the inguinal area
- Back pain

Physical findings:
- Most hydroceles are smooth and nontender. Scrotal distention may make it difficult to palpate the testis, but it is important to palpate the testis because some young men develop a hydrocele in association with a testis tumor
- Transillumination of the scrotum confirms the fluid-filled nature of the mass

ETIOLOGY

Hydroceles may occur as a congenital abnormality in which the processus vaginalis fails to close. In this case an inguinal hernia is virtually always associated with the malformation. Congenital hydroceles are most common in infants (1%-2% of neonates have hydroceles) and children. In adults, hydroceles are more frequently caused by infection, tumor, or trauma. Infection of the epididymis often results in the development of a secondary hydrocele. Tropical infections such as filariasis may produce hydroceles.

DIAGNOSIS

DIFFERENTIAL DIAGNOSIS

- Spermatocele
- Inguinoscrotal hernia
- Testicular tumor
- Varicocele
- Epididymitis

IMAGING STUDIES

Scrotal ultrasound is useful to rule out a testicular tumor as the cause of the hydrocele (Fig. 1-486). The acute development of a hydrocele might be associated with the onset of epididymitis, testicular tumor, trauma, and torsion of a testicular appendage. An ultrasound of the scrotum may provide important diagnostic information.

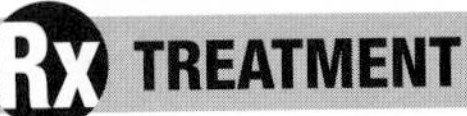

TREATMENT

- No treatment if asymptomatic and testis is believed to be normal. Most congenital hydroceles resolve by 12 months of age following reabsorption of the hydrocele fluid.
- Surgical repair should be considered if the hydrocele is tense and large. Communicating hydroceles should be repaired in the same manner as an indirect hernia. The indications for repair of a noncommunicating hydrocele include failure to resolve and increase in size to one that is large and tense.
- Surgical correction is similar to a herniorrhaphy: an inguinal incision is made, the spermatic cord is identified, the hydrocele fluid is drained, and a high ligation of the processus vaginalis is performed.

PEARLS & CONSIDERATIONS

- The long-term risk of a communicating hydrocele is the development of an inguinal hernia.
- An inguinal hernia/hydrocele is likely if compression of the fluid-filled mass completely reduces the hydrocele.

SUGGESTED READINGS

available at www.expertconsult.com

RELATED CONTENT

Hydrocele (Patient Information)

AUTHOR: **FRED F. FERRI, M.D.**

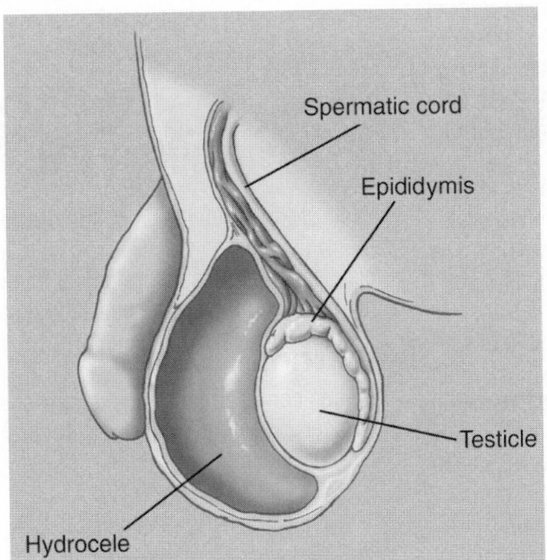

FIGURE 1-485 Schematic representation of the testicle, epididymis, spermatic cord, and a hydrocele. (From Lipshultz LI et al: *Urology and the primary care practitioner*, ed 3, Philadelphia, 2008, Elsevier.)

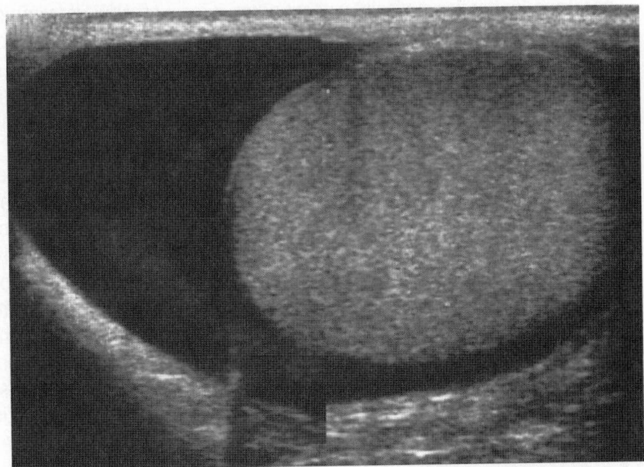

FIGURE 1-486 Longitudinal ultrasound view of normal testis and moderate hydrocele. (From Grainger RG et al [eds.]: *Grainger & Allison's diagnostic radiology*, ed 4, London, 2001, Harcourt.)

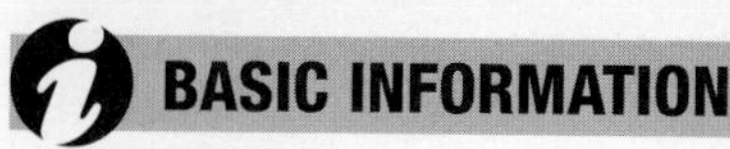

BASIC INFORMATION

DEFINITION

Normal pressure hydrocephalus (NPH) is a syndrome of symptomatic hydrocephalus in the setting of normal cerebrospinal fluid (CSF) pressure. The classic clinical triad of NPH includes gait disturbance, cognitive decline, and incontinence.

SYNONYMS

Occult hydrocephalus
Extraventricular obstructive hydrocephalus
Chronic hydrocephalus

ICD-9CM CODES
331.3 Communicating hydrocephalus
ICD-10CM CODES
G91.2 Normal pressure hydrocephalus
G91.8 Other hydrocephalus

EPIDEMIOLOGY & DEMOGRAPHICS

INCIDENCE: The exact incidence is not known. In one study the incidence was found to be 5.5 per 100,000, but it may account for up to 5% of dementia in the U.S. Hospital discharge data suggest approximately 11,500 new cases diagnosed annually (may be overestimated). The prevalence of NPH may be as high as 14% among extended care facility patients.
PREDOMINANT SEX: Males = females
PREDOMINANT AGE: NPH is more common with increasing age.

PHYSICAL FINDINGS & CLINICAL PRESENTATION

- Gait difficulty: patients often have difficulty initiating ambulation, and the gait may be broad based and shuffling, with the appearance that the feet are stuck to the floor ("magnetic gait" or "frontal gait disorder").
- Cognitive decline: mental slowing, forgetfulness and inattention typically without agnosia, aphasia, or other cortical disturbances.
- Incontinence: initially may have urinary urgency; incontinence later develops. Fecal incontinence also occasionally occurs.
- Gegenhalten (paratonia) or other frontal lobe signs may be seen.

ETIOLOGY

- Approximately 50% of cases are idiopathic; the remaining cases have a variety of causes, including prior subarachnoid hemorrhage, meningitis, head trauma, or intracranial surgery.
- Symptoms are presumed to result from stretching of sacral motor and limbic fibers that lie near the ventricles as dilation occurs.

Dx DIAGNOSIS

DIFFERENTIAL DIAGNOSIS

- Alzheimer's disease with extrapyramidal features
- Cognitive impairment in the setting of Parkinson's disease or parkinsonism-plus syndromes
- Diffuse Lewy body disease
- Frontotemporal dementia
- Cervical spondylosis with cord compromise in the setting of degenerative dementia
- Multiinfarct dementia
- HIV dementia

WORKUP

- Large-volume lumbar puncture:
  1. Mental status testing and time to walk a prespecified distance (usually 25 feet) are measured, followed by removal of 40 to 50 ml of CSF.
  2. Retest of mental status and timed walking are done later (sometimes at 1 and 4 hr). Patients who have significant improvement in gait or mental status may have a better surgical outcome; those with mild or negative response can have variable outcomes.
  3. Opening and closing pressure are measured; if pressure is elevated, alternative causes must be considered. Higher *normal* pressure may predict a good outcome from CSF shunting.
- Measurement of CSF outflow resistance by an infusion test or CSF pressure monitoring is sometimes used to help predict surgical outcome. External lumbar drainage (ELD) is being used more commonly.

LABORATORY TESTS

- CSF should be sent for routine fluid analysis to exclude other pathologies.
- CSF biomarkers may be useful in excluding Alzheimer's disease.
- The CSF protein lipocalin-type prostaglandin D synthase (L-PGDS) is being studied as a potential diagnostic biomarker in idiopathic NPH.

IMAGING STUDIES

- CT scan or MRI can be used to document ventriculomegaly. The distinguishing feature of NPH is ventricular enlargement out of proportion to sulcal atrophy (Fig. E1-487), and typically the frontal horn ratio exceeds 0.50. An algorithm for evaluation of patients with enlarged ventricles is described in Fig. E1-488.
- MRI has advantages over CT, including better ability to visualize structures in the posterior fossa, visualize transependymal CSF flow (seen as periventricular hyperintensity), and document extent of white matter lesions. On MRI a flow void in the aqueduct and third ventricle ("jet sign"), thinning and elevation of the corpus callosum on sagittal images, rounding of the frontal horns, and a narrow CSF space at the high convexity/midline areas relative to Sylvian fissure size may be seen.
- Isotope cisternography and dynamic MRI studies have not been shown to be superior in predicting shunt outcome.

Rx TREATMENT

There is no evidence that NPH can be effectively treated with medications.

NONPHARMACOLOGIC THERAPY

Response to ventriculoperitoneal shunting is variable. Some patients (variable depending on series reported) show significant improvement from shunting; however, effectiveness of shunting has never been demonstrated in a randomized-controlled trial. Gait is most likely to improve.

Factors that may predict positive outcome with surgery:

- NPH caused by prior trauma, subarachnoid hemorrhage, or meningitis
- History of mild impairment in cognition <2 yr duration
- Onset of gait abnormality before cognitive decline
- Imaging demonstrates hydrocephalus without sulcal enlargement, including normal-sized sylvian fissures and cortical sulci, and absent or mild white matter lesions.
- Transependymal CSF flow visualized on MRI
- Large-volume tap or ELD produces dramatic but temporary relief of symptoms
- High *normal* opening pressure

Factors that may predict negative outcome with surgery:

- Extensive white matter lesions or diffuse cerebral atrophy on MRI
- Moderate to severe cognitive impairment
- Onset of cognitive impairment before gait disorder
- History of alcohol abuse

ACUTE GENERAL Rx

Shunting in selected patients

DISPOSITION

Symptoms of NPH may progress over time. Prompt diagnosis may improve chances for treatment success.

REFERRAL

To neurologist for initial evaluation, including lumbar puncture, followed by neurosurgeon for shunting in appropriate patients

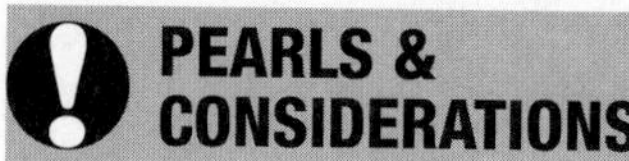

PEARLS & CONSIDERATIONS

Each of the cardinal symptoms of NPH is commonly seen in the elderly and occurs in multiple disease processes; therefore differential diagnoses should always be considered carefully.

CAUTION

Shunt complications, including subdural or intracerebral hematoma, may occur in 30% to 40% of patients.

SUGGESTED READINGS
available at www.expertconsult.com

RELATED CONTENT

Normal Pressure Hydrocephalus (Patient Information)

AUTHOR: **TAMARA G. FONG, M.D., PH.D.**

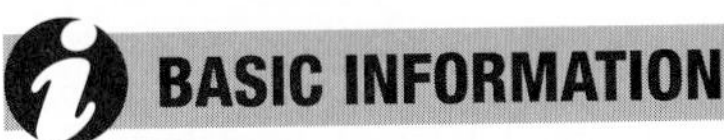

BASIC INFORMATION

DEFINITION

Hydronephrosis is dilation of the renal pyelocalyceal system, most often as a result of impairment of urinary flow.

SYNONYMS

Hydroureter (dilation of ureter, often seen with hydronephrosis when obstruction is in lower urinary tract)

Urinary tract obstruction

ICD-9CM CODES

591 Acquired hydronephrosis

753.2 Congenital hydronephrosis

ICD-10CM CODES

N13.30 Unspecified hydronephrosis

Q62.39 Other obstructive defects of renal pelvis and ureter

EPIDEMIOLOGY & DEMOGRAPHICS

Children usually have congenital malformations, whereas adults tend to have acquired defects as etiologies.

CLINICAL PRESENTATION

HISTORY:

- Pain is caused by distention of collecting system or renal capsule and is more related to the rate of onset than the degree of obstruction. It can vary in location from flank to the lower abdomen to the testes/labia. Pain in the flank occurring only on micturition is highly suggestive of vesicoureteral reflux.
- Anuria can occur with total obstruction of urinary flow (bilateral hydronephrosis, or unilateral if only one kidney is present).
- Polyuria or nocturia can occur with chronic (incomplete) obstruction because of deleterious effects on renal concentrating ability (nephrogenic diabetes insipidus).
- Urinary frequency, hesitancy, poor stream, and postvoid dribbling are all symptoms that can occur with obstruction at or below the bladder (e.g., prostatic hyperplasia).
- Chronic urinary infections can either result from chronic urinary obstruction (organisms favoring growth with stasis of urine) or lead to conditions (e.g., urine pH changes) that favor stone formation and subsequent obstruction.

PHYSICAL EXAMINATION:

- Hypertension can be caused by increased renin release in acute or subacute obstruction.
- Fever or costovertebral angle (CVA) tenderness can suggest urinary tract infection.
- Palpate bladder to detect if distention is present.
- Rectal examination to evaluate prostate for size and nodularity and also to check rectal sphincter tone.
- Pelvic examination to assess for vaginal anatomy, pelvic mass, or pelvic inflammatory disease.
- Penile examination to rule out meatal stenosis or phimosis.
- Bladder catheterization to assess postvoid residual volume if urinary tract obstruction is considered. Should rule out postrenal obstruction in unexplained acute renal failure.

ETIOLOGY

MECHANICAL IMPAIRMENTS:

Congenital:

- Ureteropelvic junction narrowing
- Ureterovesical junction narrowing
- Ureterocele
- Retrocaval ureter
- Bladder neck obstruction
- Urethral valve
- Urethral stricture
- Meatal stenosis

Acquired:

- Intrinsic to urinary tract:
  - Calculi
  - Inflammation
  - Trauma
  - Sloughed papillae
  - Ureteral tumor
  - Blood clots
  - Prostatic hypertrophy or cancer
  - Bladder cancer
  - Urethral stricture
  - Phimosis
- Extrinsic to urinary tract:
  - Gravid uterus
  - Retroperitoneal fibrosis or tumor (e.g., lymphoma)
  - Aortic aneurysm
  - Uterine fibroids
  - Trauma (surgical or nonsurgical)
  - Pelvic inflammatory disease
  - Pelvic malignancies (e.g., prostate, colorectal, cervical, uterine, bladder)

FUNCTIONAL IMPAIRMENTS:

- Neurogenic bladder (often with adynamic ureter) can occur with spinal cord disease or diabetic neuropathy.
- Pharmacologic agents such as alpha-adrenergic antagonists and anticholinergic drugs can inhibit bladder emptying.
- Vesicoureteral reflux may occur.
- Pregnancy can cause hydroureter and hydronephrosis (on the right more often than left) as early as the second month. Hormonal effects on ureteral tone combine with mechanical factors.

Dx DIAGNOSIS

DIFFERENTIAL DIAGNOSIS

- Urinary stones
- Neoplastic disease
- Prostatic hypertrophy
- Neurologic disease
- Urinary reflux
- Urinary tract infection
- Medication effects
- Trauma
- Congenital abnormality of urinary tract

LABORATORY TESTS

- Serum blood urea nitrogen and creatinine to assess for renal insufficiency (usually implies bilateral obstruction or unilateral obstruction of a solitary kidney).
- Electrolytes may reveal hypernatremia, hyperkalemia, or distal renal tubular acidosis.
- Urinalysis and examination of sediment may reveal white blood cells, red blood cells, or bacteria in the appropriate setting (e.g., infection, stones), but often the sediment is normal in obstructive renal disease.

IMAGING STUDIES

- Assess kidney and bladder size with ultrasound (Fig. 1-489) as well as contour of collecting system and ureters. Ultrasound is >90% sensitive and specific for hydronephrosis and is noninvasive.
- Abdominal CT scan without IV contrast provides excellent localization of the site of obstruction (Fig. 1-490).
- Magnetic Resonance (MR) Imaging is an alternative to CT. MR Urography has a similar diagnostic yield to CT but is not yet widely practiced. Poor renal function may preclude the use of gadolinium.
- Once diagnosed, antegrade or retrograde ureterograms can further delineate the point of obstruction.

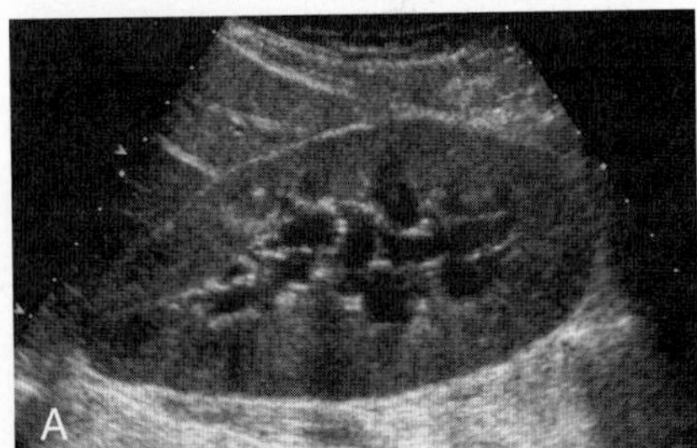

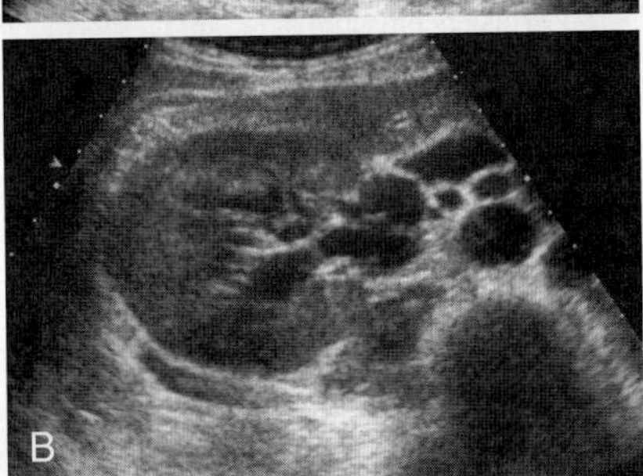

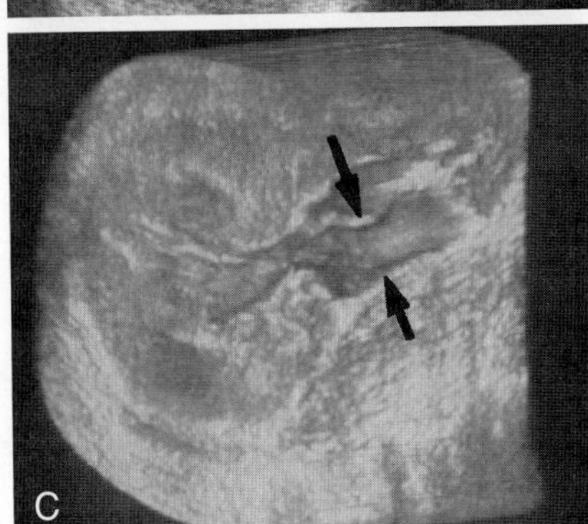

FIGURE 1-489 Renal ultrasound study demonstrating hydronephrosis. A, Sagittal image. **B,** Transverse image. **C,** Transverse three-dimensional surface-rendered image; *arrows* indicate the dilated proximal ureter. (From Floege J et al: *Comprehensive clinical nephrology,* ed 4, Philadelphia, 2010, Saunders.)

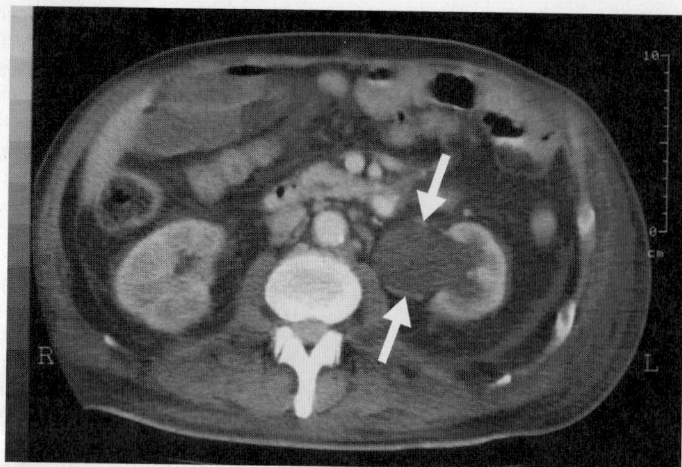

FIGURE 1-490 CT scan of the abdomen showing a grossly hydronephrotic kidney on the left. *Arrows* mark dilated renal pelvis. Dilated loops of small bowel are seen in the right hypochondrium. Sequential sections demonstrated that the ureter was dilated along its length and that there was a pelvic mass, which was responsible for both bowel and left ureteric obstruction. The mass was subsequently shown to be arising from a carcinoma of the colon. (From Johnson RJ, Feehally J: *Comprehensive clinical nephrology,* ed 2, St Louis, 2000, Mosby.)

- Voiding cystourethrogram is helpful in diagnosing vesicoureteral reflux and obstructions of the bladder neck or urethra.
- Diuretic renogram is sometimes used when there is hydronephrosis without apparent obstruction seen on any of the above studies. A loop diuretic is administered prior to a radionuclide scan. If obstruction is present, there will be slowed transit of the radioisotope during the scan, further dilation of the collecting system, and often reproduction of the patient's symptoms.
- A perfusion pressure flow study should be performed in a symptomatic patient with a negative or equivocal diuretic renogram.

Rx TREATMENT

NONPHARMACOLOGIC THERAPY

- Urgent treatment is required if urinary tract obstruction is associated with urinary tract infection, acute renal failure, or uncontrollable pain.
- Conservative management of calculi with IV fluids, IV antibiotics (if evidence of infection), and aggressive analgesia may be enough to treat acute unilateral urinary tract obstruction depending on the size (90% of stones <5 mm will pass spontaneously).
- Urethral catheter is adequate to relieve most obstructions at or distal to the bladder, but occasionally a suprapubic catheter will be required (e.g., impassable urethral stricture or urethral injury). Neurogenic bladder may require intermittent clean catheterization if frequent voiding and pharmacologic treatments are ineffective.
- Nephrostomy tube can be placed percutaneously to facilitate urinary drainage.
- Extracorporeal shock wave lithotripsy (ESWL) is used to fragment large stones to facilitate spontaneous passage or subsequent extraction. (Note: ESWL is contraindicated in pregnancy.)
- Nephroscopy is performed for extraction of proximal stones under direct visualization.
- Cystoscopy with ureteroscopy is used to remove distal ureteral stones with a loop or basket with or without fragmentation by ultrasonic or laser lithotripsy.
- Ureteral stents can be used for extrinsic and some intrinsic ureteral obstructions.
- Urethral dilation or internal urethrotomy can be used for urethral strictures.
- Nephrectomy or ureteral diversion may be required in severe cases (e.g., malignancy).
- Ureterovesical reimplantation can be used for reflux disease.
- Transurethral retrograde prostatectomy is used for severe obstruction from benign prostatic hypertrophy.
- IV fluid and electrolyte replacement are needed; the patient must be monitored closely during the postobstructive diuresis (usually lasting several days to a week).

ACUTE GENERAL Rx

Antibiotics if indicated

DISPOSITION

Aggressive treatment of infections and early relief of obstruction can usually prevent progressive loss of renal function; however, chronic bilateral obstruction (often from benign prostatic hypertrophy) can lead to chronic renal failure.

REFERRAL

- Urologist consultation early for diagnostic or therapeutic procedures
- Oncologist if a neoplasm is diagnosed
- Gynecologist if pregnancy or female pelvic anatomy is involved

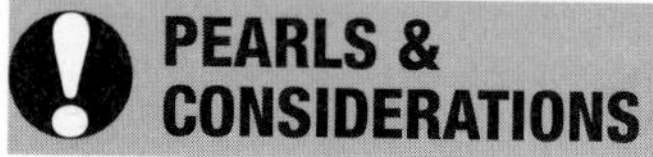

PEARLS & CONSIDERATIONS

COMMENTS

- Not a primary disorder: an underlying etiology should be sought.

PREVENTION

May be achieved through prevention of an underlying potential etiology (e.g., medical or surgical management of benign prostatic hypertrophy before obstruction occurring or medical treatment to avoid formation of renal stones).

SUGGESTED READINGS

available at www.expertconsult.com

RELATED CONTENT

Hydronephrosis (Patient Information)

AUTHORS: **SHEENAGH M. BODKIN, M.D.,** and **PAUL A. PIRRAGLIA, M.D., M.P.H.**

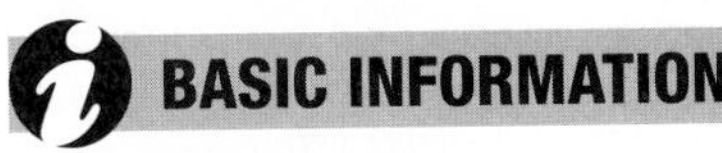

DEFINITION

Hypercholesterolemia refers to a blood cholesterol measurement ≥200 mg/dl.

SYNONYMS

Hypercholesteremia
Dyslipidemia
Type II familial hyperlipoproteinemia

ICD-9CM CODES
272.0 Pure hypercholesterolemia
ICD-10CM CODES
E78.0 Pure hypercholesterolemia

EPIDEMIOLOGY & DEMOGRAPHICS

- Over 105 million (37%) adults in the U.S. have total blood cholesterol levels higher than 200 mg/dl. Of this group, more than 36 million adults have extremely high-risk cholesterol levels over 240 mg/dl (~13%).
- For men over the age of 20 years, approximately 48% of white men, 45% of black men, and 50% of Hispanic men have high blood cholesterol.
- For women over the age of 20, approximately 50% of Hispanic women, 42% of black women, and 50% of white women have hypercholesterolemia.
- Prevalence of hypercholesterolemia increases with increasing age.
- According to NHANES data for 2009-2010, about 47% of adults had at least one of three risk factors for cardiovascular disease—uncontrolled high blood pressure, uncontrolled high levels of low-density lipoproteins (LDL) cholesterol, or current smoking.

PHYSICAL FINDINGS & CLINICAL PRESENTATION

- A detailed medication history should be performed because some medications may affect lipid levels (e.g., thiazides, corticosteroids, beta-blockers, and estrogens).
- The physical examination should include measurements of BMI and BP, thyroid and liver assessments, and examining peripheral pulses including carotids for bruits.
- Physical findings, particularly in the familial forms may include
  1. Tendon xanthomas
  2. Xanthelasma
  3. Arcus corneae
  4. Arterial bruits (young adulthood)

ETIOLOGY

Primary:
- Genetics
- Obesity
- Dietary intake

Secondary:
- Hypothyroidism
- Diabetes mellitus
- Nephrotic syndrome
- Obstructive liver disease: Hepatoma, extrahepatic biliary obstruction, primary biliary cirrhosis
- Alcohol or tobacco use
- Dysgammaglobulinemia (multiple myeloma, SLE)
- Drugs: Oral contraceptives, progesterone, corticosteroids, thiazide diuretics, β-blockers, androgenic steroids, retinoic acid derivatives, protease inhibitors

Dx DIAGNOSIS

DIFFERENTIAL DIAGNOSIS

- Always consider underlying secondary causes for the elevated cholesterol.
- Patients with very high LDL cholesterol usually have genetic forms of hypercholesterolemia (see *Hyperlipoproteinemia, Primary*). Early detection of these cases and family testing to identify similarly affected relatives is important.
- Metabolic syndrome:
  1. A constellation of lipid and nonlipid risk factors of a metabolic origin
  2. Diagnosed when three or more of the following are present: abdominal obesity (waist circumference >40 in in men and >35 in in women); fasting triglycerides >150 mg/dl; HDL <40 mg/dl in males and <50 mg/dl in females; systolic BP >130 mmHg and diastolic BP >85 mmHg; fasting glucose >110 mg/dl

WHO SHOULD BE SCREENED:

- AACE recommends screening of patients >20 yr of age for elevated cholesterol every 5 yr, males >45 yr and females >55 yr of age every 1-2 yr, and >65 yr of age every yr up to 75 yr of age regardless of CAD risk status. Patients above 75 yr of age with multiple CAD risk factors should still continue to get screened annually.
- The USPSTF supports routine screening for men aged >35 yr and women aged >45 yr by measurement of nonfasting total and HDL cholesterol alone.
- In 2010, the USPSTF recommended routine screening for overweight and obesity in persons aged <20 yr.
- In 2011, ACC/AHA recommended screening for hypertriglyceridemia by a nonfasting measurement. A nonfasting level of <200 mg/dl is commensurate with an optimal level of <100 mg/dl and no further testing is required. However, a nonfasting level of >200 mg/dl warrants further testing with a fasting lipid profile.

LABORATORY TESTS

- Obtain a fasting lipid profile.
- Risk assessment to modify LDL goals (Table 1-251)

TABLE 1-251 Risk Factors That Modify LDL Goals

1. Cigarette smoking
2. Hypertension (BP ≤140/90 mm Hg or on medications)
3. Low HDL cholesterol (<40 mg/dl)*
4. Family history of premature CHD (<55 yr in first-degree male relative or <65 yr in first-degree female relative)
5. Age (men ≥45 yr, women ≥55 yr)

*HDL cholesterol >60 mg/dl counts as a negative risk factor; its presence removes one risk factor from the total count.

TABLE 1-252 CHD Equivalents

1. Diabetes mellitus
2. Abdominal aortic aneurysm
3. Peripheral vascular disease (ABI <0.9)
4. Symptomatic carotid artery disease (stroke, transient ischemic attack)
5. 10-yr risk for coronary artery disease >20% using Framingham risk equation
6. Chronic kidney disease with plasma cr ≥1.5 mg/dl or estimated GFR <60 ml/min

Rx TREATMENT

NONPHARMACOLOGIC THERAPY

- First line of treatment: dietary therapy can result in 5% to 15% reduction in LDL cholesterol level.
- Composition of the TLC diet:
  1. Total fat 25% to 30% of total calories
  2. Polyunsaturated fat up to 10% of total calories
  3. Monounsaturated fat up to 20% of total calories
  4. Saturated fats <7% of total calories
  5. Carbohydrate 50% to 60% of total calories
  6. Protein 15% of total calories
  7. No more than 200 mg/day of cholesterol
  8. Fiber 20 to 30 g/day
- Increased physical activity: encourage 30 min of moderate intensity physical activity, four to six times a week (e.g., brisk walking, riding stationary bike, water aerobics)
- Weight reduction
- Smoking cessation
- Counseling on CAD risk factors
- Plant-based diets (including stanol-containing margarines, oat bran, and nuts) have shown effectiveness in controlling lipids.

ACUTE GENERAL Rx

No acute treatment needed

CHRONIC Rx

- The current guidelines represent a substantial departure from previous recommendations, which were based on LDL levels. The new guidelines identify four subgroups that benefit from statin therapy:
  1. Patients with clinically evident ASHD
  2. LDL ≥190 mg/dl
  3. DM and LDL ≥70 mg/dl
  4. Ten year risk for ASHD ≥7.5% and LDL ≥70 mg/dl

In these four patient groups, high-intensity statin therapy is recommended (Table 1-253)

- The 10-year risk of atherosclerotic CVD is calculated with the risk calculator available at http://my.americanheart.org/cvriskcalculator
- Non-statin LDL-cholesterol lowering agents, such as niacin or ezetimibe, are no longer recommended in statin-tolerant patients because they do not have a proven effect on reducing CVD risk.

- Routine assessment of LDL cholesterol levels in patients receiving statin therapy are no longer emphasized.
- Statin therapy is generally not recommended in patients older than 75 years unless they have atherosclerotic cardiovascular disease, NYHA class II, III, or IV heart failure, or those in need for hemodialysis.
- Bile acid sequestrants are the first-line drugs to lower cholesterol in children and in pregnant women.
- Bile acid sequestrants are the first-line drugs to lower cholesterol in children and in pregnant women.
- The management of metabolic syndrome includes weight reduction and increased physical activity and treatment of hypertension, elevated triglycerides, and low HDL cholesterol.
- In ten primary prevention clinical trials, statin use resulted in a 30% reduction in coronary events and a 12% reduction in total mortality.
- Statin use has been linked to an increased risk of diabetes (9% incidence). However, per JUPITER trial, in patients at risk for diabetes, statins prevented 134 vascular events vs. contributed to 54 new diabetes cases. There is no risk of new DM in statin-treated patients without DM risk factors.
- Fenofibrates have not been shown to reduce morbidity and mortality in patients.
- The AIM-HIGH trial found no cardiovascular benefit from taking extended-release niacin.

TABLE 1-253 High-Intensity and Moderate-Intensity Statin Therapy

- High-intensity statin therapy: Atorvastatin 40-80 mg/day; rosuvastatin 20-40 mg/day
  - LDL cholesterol level will decrease by ≥50% on average
- Moderate-intensity statin therapy: Atorvastatin 10-20 mg/day; rosuvastatin 5-10 mg/day, simvastatin 20-40 mg/day; pravastatin 40-80 mg/day
  - LDL cholesterol level will decrease by 30%-50% on average

DISPOSITION AND FOLLOW-UP

- LFT testing should be done prior to initiation of statin therapy and as clinically indicated thereafter. Routine monitoring is not necessary anymore.
- CK levels monitoring is not recommended unless a patient reports muscle weakness or myalgias.
- Counseling about behavioral lifestyle changes and risk factors for CHD should be provided at every follow-up visit.

REFERRAL

Patients with rare lipid disorders, hyperlipoproteinemias, patients resistant to treatment, on complex regimens, and with evidence of disease progression despite treatment should be referred to a lipid specialist.

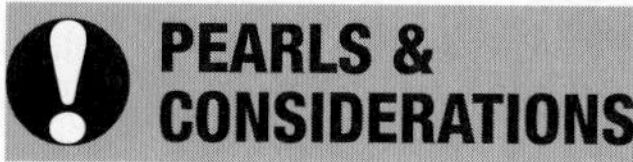

PEARLS & CONSIDERATIONS

COMMENTS

- The American Academy of Pediatrics (AAP) guideline (*Pediatrics* 122:198, 2008) recommends consideration toward pharmacologic treatment for children with LDL >190 mg/dl or >160 mg/dl if other risk factors are present.

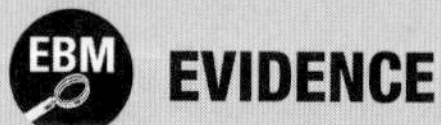

EVIDENCE

available at www.expertconsult.com

SUGGESTED READINGS

available at www.expertconsult.com

RELATED CONTENT

Hyperlipoproteinemia, Primary (Related Key Topic)
High Cholesterol (Patient Information)

AUTHORS: **PRIYA BANSAL, M.D., M.P.H.,** and **FRED F. FERRI, M.D.**

TABLE 1-254 Drugs Affecting Lipoprotein Metabolism

Drug Class	Agents and Daily Doses	Lipid/Lipoprotein Effects	Side Effects	Contraindications
HMG-CoA reductase inhibitors (statins)	Lovastatin (10-40 mg) Pravastatin (10-80 mg) Simvastatin† (5-80 mg) Fluvastatin (20-40 mg) Atorvastatin (10-80 mg) Rosuvastatin (5-40 mg) Pitavastatin (2-4 mg)	LDL ↓ 20%-60% HDL ↑ 5%-15% TG ↓ 7%-30%	Myalgias, myositis Increased liver enzymes New onset diabetes (with intensive therapy) Unproven concerns about memory loss	Active or chronic liver disease Pregnancy Concomitant use of certain drugs*
Bile acid sequestrants	Colestipol (5-20 g) Colesevelam‡ (2.6-3.8 g) Cholestyramine (4-16 g)	LDL ↓ 15%-30% HDL ↑ 3%-5% TG No change or increase	Gastrointestinal distress, constipation, drug interaction, hypertriglyceridemia Decreased absorption of fat-soluble vitamins	TG >300 mg/dl GI motility disorder
Omega-3 fatty acids	Fish oils (4-6 g)	TG ↓ 45% HDL ↑ 13%	Increased bleeding time Nausea	Caution with anticoagulant therapy
Nicotinic acid	Immediate release (niacin) (1.5-3 g) Extended-release (Niaspan) (1-2 g)	LDL ↓ 5%-25% HDL ↑ 15%-35% TG ↓ 20%-50%	Flushing Hyperglycemia Hyperuricemia (or gout) Upper GI distress Hepatotoxicity	Chronic liver disease Severe gout Diabetes Peptic ulcer disease Pregnancy/lactation
Fibric acids	Gemfibrozil (600 mg bid) Fenofibrate (45-145 mg)	LDL ↓ 5%-20% HDL ↑ 10%-20% TG ↓ 20%-50%	Dyspepsia Gallstones Myopathy	Severe renal disease Severe hepatic disease Caution with statins Can worsen LDL cholesterol
Ezetimibe (cholesterol absorption inhibitor)	Ezetimibe (10 mg)	LDL ↓ 18% HDL ↑ 1% TG ↓ 8%	Abdominal pain; myalgias	Liver disease Avoid with resins and fibrates

Modified from The National Cholesterol Education Program, *JAMA* 285:2486, 2001.
*Cyclosporine, macrolide antibiotics, various antifungal agents, and cytochrome P-450 inhibitors (fibrates and niacin should be used with appropriate caution).
†Dosages of 80 mg of simvastatin are no longer recommended. Potential interactions with amlodipine and ranolazine warrant doses ≤2 mg daily.
- Maintain patients on simvastatin 80 mg only if they have been taking this dose for 12 or more months without evidence of muscle toxicity.
- Do not start new patients on simvastatin 80 mg.
- Place patients who do not meet their LDL goal on simvastatin 40 mg on alternative LDL-C-lowering treatment(s) to reach goal.

‡Colesevelam reduces glucose and A1c ~0.5% and has been approved for treatment of diabetes with dyslipidemia.

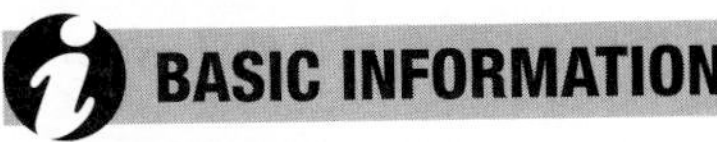

BASIC INFORMATION

DEFINITION

Hypercoagulable state is an inherited or acquired condition associated with an increased risk of thrombosis.

SYNONYMS

Thrombophilia

ICD-9CM CODES
289.8 Hypercoagulable state
ICD-10CM CODES
D68.5 Primary thrombophilia
D68.6 Other thrombophilia
D68.8 Other specified coagulation defects
D68.9 Coagulation defect, unspecified

EPIDEMIOLOGY & DEMOGRAPHICS

INCIDENCE: See Table 1-255.

PREVALENCE, PREDOMINANT SEX, AND AGE: Significant variations in the prevalence rates and thrombotic risks for thrombophilia are reported. This may reflect geographic variation in the prevalence of genetic defects, different populations, or the presence of other unidentified thrombophilic risk factors. When thrombosis occurs, it is often associated with an acquired risk factor (e.g., surgery, pregnancy, oral contraceptive [OC] use). Annual risk of thrombosis is <1%.

GENETICS:

- Most people with a genetic defect will not have thrombotic disease.
- Multiple genetic defects are not uncommon (1% to 2% prevalence in patients with idiopathic venous thromboembolism [VTE]); strong synergistic effect when multiple defects are present. Low risk of recurrent thrombosis in patients with a single genetic defect. Approximately half of patients with unprovoked thrombosis have an identifiable inherited thrombophilia.

RISK FACTORS: Family history of thrombosis, increasing age, tobacco use, immobility, surgery, prior history of DVT, pregnancy, hormone replacement therapy, trauma, connective tissue disease, underlying malignancy, medications (Megace, tamoxifen, birth control pills)

PHYSICAL FINDINGS & CLINICAL PRESENTATION

- Inherited thrombophilia is usually associated with VTE, most commonly deep vein thrombosis (DVT)
- Some acquired thrombophilias are associated with arterial thrombosis. Table E1-256 describes sites of thrombosis according to coagulation defect.
- Pregnancy complications
- Medical conditions associated with increased risk of thrombosis

ETIOLOGY

See Table 1-257A. The differential diagnosis of the patient presenting with thrombosis or thrombotic diathesis is described in Section II. Fig. E1-491 describes components of thrombus formation and actions of various antithrombotic and thrombolytic agents.

- Thrombosis is often a multifactorial process with genetic, environmental, and acquired factors. Table 1-257B describes causes of acquired deficiencies in antithrombin III, protein S, or protein C.
- Thrombotic risk increases with use of OCs or hormone replacement therapy (HRT) and during the pregnancy/postpartum period.
- Adverse pregnancy outcomes may be caused by thrombosis of the uteroplacental circulation.

Dx DIAGNOSIS

DIFFERENTIAL DIAGNOSIS

INHERITED:

Factor V Leiden (FVL) mutation:

- Autosomal-dominant mutation with low penetrance.
- Causes activated protein C resistance (APCR); 90% of APCR is caused by FVL mutation.
- Most common inherited thrombophilia; accounts for 40% to 50% of cases.
- OC use in heterozygous carriers is associated with an eightfold increased risk of VTE compared with noncarriers and a thirty-fivefold increased risk of VTE compared with noncarriers not using OCs.
- May be associated with cardiovascular disease in select high-risk subgroups.

Prothrombin G20210A mutation:

- Autosomal-dominant mutation with low penetrance.
- OC use in heterozygous carriers is associated with a sixteenfold increased risk of VTE compared with noncarriers not using OCs.

TABLE 1-257A Potential Prothrombotic States

Congenital
Deficiency of anticoagulants
AT-III, protein C or protein S, plasminogen
Resistance to cofactor proteolysis
Factor V Leiden
High levels of procoagulants
Prothrombin 20210 mutation
Elevated factor VIII levels
Damage to endothelium
Homocysteinemia
Acquired
Obstruction to flow
Indwelling lines
Pregnancy
Polycythemia/dehydration
Immobilization
Injury
Trauma, surgery, exercise
Inflammation
IBD, vasculitis, infection, Behçet syndrome
Hypercoagulability
Pregnancy
Malignancy
Antiphospholipid syndrome
Nephrotic syndrome
Oral contraceptives
L-Asparaginase
Elevated factor VIII levels
Rare Other Entities
Congenital
Dysfibrinogenemia
Acquired
Paroxysmal nocturnal hemoglobinuria
Thrombocythemia
Vascular grafts

AT-III, Antithrombin III; *IBD,* inflammatory bowel disease.
From Kliegman RM et al: *Nelson textbook of pediatrics,* ed 19, Philadelphia, 2011, Saunders.

TABLE 1-255 Hypercoagulable Conditions

	Prevalence in General Population (%)	Prevalence in Population with Thrombosis (%)	A/V Events	Relative Risk of Thrombosis
FVL mutation	5% of whites; rare in nonwhites	12%-40%	V	Heterozygous: 3-7; homozygous: 80
Prothrombin G20210A mutation	3% of whites; rare in nonwhites	6%-18%	V	3
AT deficiency	0.02%	1%-3%	V	20-50
PC deficiency	0.2%-0.4%	3%-5%	V	7-15
PS deficiency	0.03%-0.1%	1%-5%	V	5-11
Antiphospholipid antibody syndrome	1%-2%	5%-21%	V + A	2-11
Hyperhomocysteinemia	5%-7%	10%	V + A	3
Elevated factor VIII level	11%	25%	V + A	5

A, Arterial; *AT,* antithrombin; *FVL,* factor V Leiden; *PC,* protein C; *PS,* protein S; *V,* venous.

 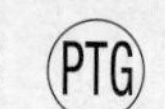

TABLE 1-257B Causes of Acquired Deficiencies in Antithrombin III, Protein C, or Protein S

Antithrombin III	Protein C	Protein S
Neonatal period	Neonatal period	Neonatal period
Pregnancy		Pregnancy
Liver disease	Liver disease	Liver disease
DIC	DIC	DIC
Nephrotic syndrome	Chemotherapy (CMF)	
Major surgery		Inflammatory states
Acute thrombosis	Acute thrombosis	Acute thrombosis
Treatment with:		
Heparin	Warfarin	Warfarin
L-Asparaginase	L-Asparaginase	L-Asparaginase
Estrogens		Estrogens

CMF, Cyclophosphamide, methotrexate, 5-fluorouracil; *DIC,* disseminated intravascular coagulation.
From Hoffman R et al: *Hematology, basic principles and practice,* ed 5, Philadelphia, 2009, Churchill Livingstone.

- May be associated with cardiovascular disease in select high-risk subgroups and young patients with ischemic stroke.

Protein C, protein S, antithrombin (AT) deficiency:
- Autosomal-dominant inheritance; many mutations identified for each of these conditions.
- Decreased level (type I deficiency) or abnormal function (type II deficiency).
- First episode of thrombosis is usually in young adults.

Protein C and protein S:
- Homozygous condition is very rare; usually associated with lethal thrombosis in infancy.
- Associated with warfarin-induced skin necrosis, which occurs secondary to depletion of vitamin K–dependent anticoagulant factors sooner than procoagulant factors in the first few days of therapy.

AT deficiency:
- Most thrombogenic of the inherited thrombophilias; 50% lifetime risk of thrombosis.
- Homozygous condition is very rare, probably not compatible with normal fetal development.
- Arterial thrombosis can occur rarely.
- Can cause heparin resistance.

Elevated factor VIII level:
- May be an important risk factor for thrombosis in African-American population.
- Increased risk of recurrent thrombosis.
- Genetic etiology is suspected but not yet identified.

Other possible causes: Non-O blood group, dysfibrinogenemia, elevated thrombin-activatable fibrinolysis inhibitor, elevated factor IX and factor XI levels

ACQUIRED:

Antiphospholipid antibody syndrome (APS):
- Most common cause of acquired thrombophilia.
- Can present as arterial or venous thrombosis, recurrent pregnancy loss, and adverse pregnancy outcomes.
- Thromboembolic events occur in up to 30% of population; high risk of recurrent thrombosis (up to 70% reported).
- See "Antiphospholipid Antibody Syndrome" for more information.

Hyperhomocysteinemia:
- Can be inherited (most commonly an autosomal recessive mutation in methylene tetrahydrofolate reductase gene) but more frequently acquired; folate, vitamin B_6, or vitamin B_{12} deficiency account for two thirds of cases. Other acquired causes include renal disease, hypothyroidism, malignancy, smoking, and certain medications.
- Acquired causes may be associated with VTE and atherosclerotic disease (cardiovascular, cerebrovascular, and peripheral vascular). Inherited causes may be associated with atherosclerotic disease and adverse pregnancy outcomes.

Conditions associated with increased risk of thrombosis:
- Prior thrombosis
- Trauma
- Medical illness: heart failure, respiratory failure, infection, diabetes mellitus, obesity, nephrotic syndrome, inflammatory bowel disease
- Chronic hemolysis–paroxysmal nocturnal hemoglobinuria, sickle cell anemia
- Pregnancy (sixfold increased risk of VTE), postpartum, OC use (fourfold increased risk, higher risk with third-generation OCs), transdermal contraceptive patch, HRT (twofold increased risk), tamoxifen, raloxifene
- Immobilization, travel
- Surgery (especially orthopedic), central venous catheters
- Hyperviscosity syndromes
- Myeloproliferative disorders
- Malignancy: disease or treatment related
- Heparin-induced thrombocytopenia and thrombosis
- Smoking

WORKUP

- History (presence of conditions or use of medications predisposing to thrombosis, family history of thrombosis), physical examination, laboratory tests, imaging studies.
- Age-appropriate cancer screening.
- No consensus exists regarding screening for thrombophilia; little cost-effectiveness or outcomes data are available. Screening laboratory evaluation for patients suspected of having a biologic defect predisposing to thrombosis is described in Box E1-40. Thrombophilia screening is probably overused, as results usually don't change management.
- Thrombophilia screening is not recommended for primary prevention of VTE; some advocate testing prior to OC use or pregnancy in women with a strong family history of thrombosis or thrombophilia.
- Screening not recommended if VTE was associated with an identified risk factor. A possible exception is thrombosis associated with pregnancy, the postpartum period or with OC use.
- Unprovoked VTE:
    - Screen individuals for APCR, prothrombin G20210A mutation, protein C, protein S, AT deficiency, and APS if any of the following are present: <50 yr of age at first episode of thrombosis, family history of thrombosis, recurrent thrombosis, thrombosis in unusual anatomic location, life-threatening thrombotic event, warfarin-induced skin necrosis, thrombosis in pregnancy/postpartum/with OC use, or characteristic pregnancy complications.
    - Screen all Caucasians <50 yr of age and all women on HRT for APCR, prothrombin G20210A mutation, and APS.
    - Screen all others for APS.
- Arterial thrombosis: Screen for APS.
- Note: Routine screening for factor VIII level or hyperhomocysteinemia is not recommended.

TIMING OF WORKUP:
- Ideally >3 wk after discontinuation of anticoagulation (except for APS, which requires prolonged anticoagulation).
- Note: Acute thrombosis, anticoagulation, pregnancy, and many medical conditions can affect the results and must be considered in the timing and interpretation of the workup.

LABORATORY TESTS

- CBC with peripheral smear, electrolytes, calcium, renal and liver function tests, prothrombin time/partial thromboplastin time, prostate-specific antigen (in men aged >50 yr), urinalysis
- Note: Genetic counseling and written informed consent should be obtained before genetic testing. Abnormal nongenetic tests should be repeated after 6 wk to decrease false-positive results.
- APCR: APC-resistance assay (using factor V–deficient plasma) and if positive confirm with genetic test for FVL mutation; use genetic test if lupus anticoagulant present.
- Prothrombin G20210A mutation test.
- AT, protein C, and protein S deficiency: functional assays; if decreased perform antigenic assay to determine type of deficiency. Antigenic assays for protein S should measure free and total levels. In protein C and protein S deficiency, the functional assay may be falsely low in the presence of APCR

or elevated factor VIII level and falsely high if lupus anticoagulant is present.

- APS: any of the following found on two occasions at least 12 wk apart: lupus anticoagulant or anticardiolipin antibodies or anti–B_2-glycoprotein-I antibodies.
- Hyperhomocysteinemia: fasting plasma homocysteine level (if normal but suspicion is high, can proceed with methionine loading test and genotyping for methylene tetrahydrofolate reductase).
- Factor VIII level functional assay.

IMAGING STUDIES

Chest radiograph and other tests as appropriate to diagnose thrombosis and rule out associated conditions

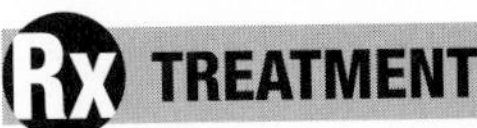

TREATMENT

NONPHARMACOLOGIC THERAPY

OC/HRT use and smoking should be avoided.

PROPHYLAXIS

- Prophylactic anticoagulation in high-risk situations.
- Patients with AT deficiency may benefit from antithrombin concentrates in high-risk situations.
- Although homocysteine levels can be lowered with folic acid, vitamin B_6, and vitamin B_{12} supplements, correcting hyperhomocysteinemia does not decrease risk of thrombosis and routine supplementation is not indicated.
- Vitamin E supplements may decrease risk of VTE in women.
- Pregnancy prophylaxis: timing and intensity of therapy is based on the patient's risk (genetic or acquired defect and clinical history). Women with thrombophilia and recurrent adverse pregnancy outcomes may benefit from prophylaxis with heparin and low-dose aspirin.

ACUTE GENERAL Rx

Initial therapy is the same as for individuals without thrombophilia (exceptions for protein C and AT deficiency).

Venous thrombosis:

- Begin low-molecular-weight heparin (LMWH) and warfarin simultaneously. Continue heparin for at least 5 days and until international normalized ratio (INR) is therapeutic for 2 consecutive days; continue warfarin for at least 3 mo. Aim for INR of 2 to 3. Unfractionated heparin (UH) or fondaparinux (factor Xa inhibitor) may be used as alternatives to LMWH. LMWH is preferred over UH (except in patients with massive pulmonary embolism, increased risk of bleeding or renal failure) because of equivalent or superior effectiveness and a better safety profile.
- Thrombophilia is not associated with a higher risk of recurrent VTE during warfarin therapy, with the exception of cancer patients in whom LMWH for 3 to 6 mo is associated with lower rates of recurrence than warfarin therapy.
- In pregnancy, anticoagulate with heparin throughout pregnancy and for at least 6 wk postpartum. Minimum duration of anticoagulation should be 6 mo. LMWH is preferred over UH. Warfarin may be used postpartum.
- Consider thrombolysis or thrombectomy in patients with massive pulmonary embolism or large proximal lower extremity DVT.

Protein C deficiency:

- Warfarin-induced skin necrosis: Discontinue warfarin, give vitamin K, and start heparin anticoagulation. Consider protein C replacement with protein C concentrate or fresh frozen plasma. Warfarin may be restarted at a low dose (2 mg daily for 3 days and increase by 2 to 3 mg daily until target INR is reached). Continue heparin for at least 5 days and until warfarin-induced anticoagulation is achieved.

AT deficiency:

- AT concentrates may be used if difficulty achieving anticoagulation (heparin resistance), severe thrombosis, or recurrent thrombosis despite adequate anticoagulation.

Arterial thrombosis:

- Anticoagulation and evaluation for thrombolysis or surgery.

CHRONIC Rx

- Optimal duration of anticoagulation remains unknown. Length of therapy may be individualized by assessing the risk of recurrence. Residual thrombosis (on ultrasonography) or elevated D-dimer levels after completion of anticoagulation are associated with an increased risk of recurrence. With these findings, consider prolonging anticoagulation.
- Must consider risk and benefit; risk of major bleeding 2% to 3% annually in general population on anticoagulation but higher in the elderly (7% to 9% per year). Long-term anticoagulation is usually not indicated given the low risk of recurrent thrombosis for most conditions and the bleeding risk associated with anticoagulation.
- Indefinite anticoagulation considered if ≥2 spontaneous thromboses or spontaneous thrombosis associated with any of the following:
  1. Life-threatening thrombosis or thrombosis at an unusual site
  2. More than a single genetic defect
  3. Presence of AT deficiency or APS
- Patients with active cancer may benefit from indefinite anticoagulation.

DISPOSITION

Depends on underlying condition

REFERRAL

Hematology, maternal-fetal medicine, obstetric medicine

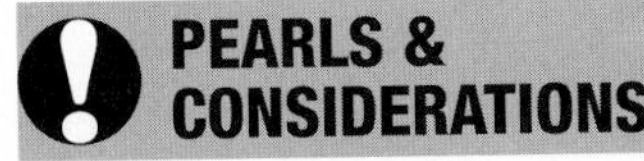

PEARLS & CONSIDERATIONS

COMMENTS

- Warfarin therapy effectively reduces the risk of recurrent VTE; when therapy is discontinued VTE risk increases.
- Previous episode of VTE is a major risk factor for recurrence regardless of the presence of thrombophilia. Risk is greatest in the first 2 yr after thrombosis. 20% of all patients with unprovoked VTE have recurrence within 5 yr.
- Genetic risk factors for thrombosis in nonwhites remain largely unknown.
- Interpreting workup: many medical conditions cause acquired abnormalities.
  - Acute thrombosis may be associated with lupus anticoagulant, increased anticardiolipin antibodies, and elevated factor VIII levels
  - Heparin therapy: antithrombin levels decrease by up to 30%; can affect lupus anticoagulant testing
  - Warfarin therapy: cannot measure protein C and protein S (levels and function decrease); antithrombin levels may increase; can affect lupus anticoagulant testing
  - Protein C, protein S, and antithrombin levels decrease with acute thrombosis (<2 wk), surgery, liver disease, disseminated intravascular coagulation, and chemotherapy. Protein C level also decreases with severe infection but levels increase with age and hyperlipidemia. Protein S and antithrombin levels also decrease with nephrotic syndrome, pregnancy, and estrogen therapy (HRT, OC)
  - APCR is increased with pregnancy, estrogen therapy (HRT, OCs), and certain cancers; elevated factor VIII level and antiphospholipid antibodies can cause APCR

PREVENTION

Risk of postthrombotic syndrome decreases if compression stockings are worn for at least 1 year, starting in the first month after the DVT.

PATIENT & FAMILY EDUCATION

National Blood Clot Alliance
120 White Plains Road, Suite 100
Tarrytown, NY 10591
http://www.stoptheclot.org/contact.htm

National Collaborative Outreach Project of the Blood Clot Outreach Program at the Hemophilia and Thrombosis Center University of North Carolina at Chapel Hill
http://www.clotconnect.org/about-clot-connect/about

Factor V Leiden Resources
http://www.fvleiden.org/resources/index.html

APS Foundation of America, Inc.
P. O. Box 801
LaCrosse, WI 54602-0801
http://www.apsfa.org/

SUGGESTED READINGS

available at www.expertconsult.com

RELATED CONTENT

Thrombophilia (Patient Information)

AUTHORS: **MATTHEW I. QUESENBERRY, M.D.**, and **SUDEEP KAUR AULAKH, M.D.**

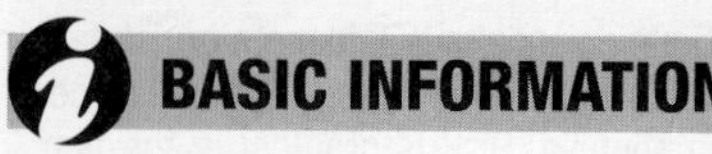

BASIC INFORMATION

DEFINITION

Hyperemesis gravidarum is a severe and persistent form of nausea and vomiting resulting in at least a 5% weight loss, dehydration, ketonuria, and electrolyte imbalance, with typical onset at 4 to 8 wk of pregnancy continuing through 14 to 16 wk of pregnancy.

ICD-9CM CODES
643.0 [0,1,3] Mild hyperemesis gravidarum
643.1 [0,1,3] Hyperemesis gravidarum with metabolic disturbance
ICD-10CM CODES
021.0 Mild hyperemesis gravidarum
021.1 Hyperemesis gravidarum with metabolic disturbance

EPIDEMIOLOGY & DEMOGRAPHICS

INCIDENCE: 0.5% to 2% of pregnancies
GENETICS: No genetic disposition
RISK FACTORS: Women with increased placental mass, including molar pregnancy or multiple gestation, family history or personal history of hyperemesis gravidarum, prior miscarriage, nulliparity, preexisting diabetes, hyperthyroid disorder, peptic ulceration or other gastrointestinal disorders, depression, and asthma. Female fetus increases the risk by 1.5-fold.

PHYSICAL FINDINGS & CLINICAL PRESENTATION

- Weight loss of more than 5% from pregravid weight
- Symptoms—nausea, vomiting, spitting, enhanced olfactory senses, food and/or fluid intolerance, lethargy
- Signs—dehydration, poor skin turgor, dry mucous membranes, ketonuria, anemia, tachycardia, hypotension
- Complications include inadequate caloric intake, nutritional deficiencies, dehydration, and electrolyte abnormalities including hyponatremia, hypocalcemia, hypokalemia, and in severe cases hypochloremic metabolic acidosis or Wernicke's encephalopathy from thiamine deficiency

ETIOLOGY

Unknown but likely multifactorial. Theories include gestational hyperestrogenemia, gastric dysrhythmias, and hyperthyroidism.

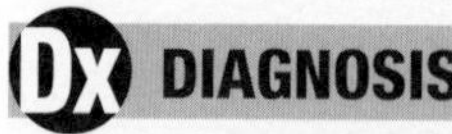

DIAGNOSIS

DIFFERENTIAL DIAGNOSIS

- Gastrointestinal conditions—gastroenteritis, gastroparesis, achalasia, biliary tract disease, hepatitis, intestinal obstruction, peptic ulcer disease, appendicitis
- Genitourinary tract conditions—pyelonephritis, uremia, ovarian torsion, kidney stones, degenerating uterine leiomyoma
- Metabolic disease—diabetic ketoacidosis, porphyria, Addison's disease, hyperthyroidism
- Neurologic conditions—pseudotumor cerebri, vestibular lesions, migraines, tumors of the central nervous system
- Miscellaneous—drug toxicity or intolerance, psychologic
- Pregnancy-related conditions—acute fatty liver of pregnancy, preeclampsia

WORKUP

Diagnosis is one of exclusion. History and physical examination along with laboratory tests to rule out other causes of vomiting should be performed.

LABORATORY TESTS

- Urinalysis may show elevated specific gravity, ketonuria, or proteinuria
- Liver enzymes (elevated but usually <300 U/L)
- Serum bilirubin (<4 mg/dl)
- Serum amylase or lipase (up to 5× greater than normal)
- BMP, may reveal hyponatremia, hypokalemia, low serum urea
- CBC
- Calcium
- TSH and free T4 (transient hyperthyroidism occurs in 2/3 of women with hyperemesis gravidarum; this is biochemical hyperthyroidism that usually resolves by 18 wk gestation; treatment should not be undertaken without evidence of intrinsic thyroid disease)

IMAGING STUDIES

- Ultrasound to evaluate for multiple gestation or molar pregnancy
- Right upper quadrant ultrasound to evaluate for biliary tract disease

Rx TREATMENT

NONPHARMACOLOGIC THERAPY

- Reassurance and support
- Avoidance of foods and smells that trigger nausea
- Oral ginger root
- Small frequent dry meals
- Eating prior to getting out of bed

ACUTE GENERAL Rx

- Nothing by mouth
- Intravenous fluid and electrolyte replacement with vitamin supplementation
- Thiamine administration prior to giving dextrose to avoid Wernicke's encephalopathy
- Pyridoxine (vitamin B_6)
- Doxylamine 25 mg qhs
- Antiemetics, including promethazine, phenothiazines, metoclopramide, and ondansetron, have been shown to be both safe and effective in improving pregnancy outcome
- Restart oral intake gradually no less than 48 hr after vomiting has stopped

CHRONIC Rx

- Nasogastric feedings are useful alternatives in severe cases
- Total parenteral nutrition may be necessary in life-threatening cases

COMPLEMENTARY AND ALTERNATIVE MEDICINE

- Supportive psychotherapy
- Acupuncture
- Acupressure with use of a wrist band

DISPOSITION

- Infants born to pregnancies complicated by hyperemesis are more likely to be premature and small for gestational age.
- Lower rates of miscarriage have also been documented when comparing pregnancies complicated by hyperemesis gravidarum vs. controls.

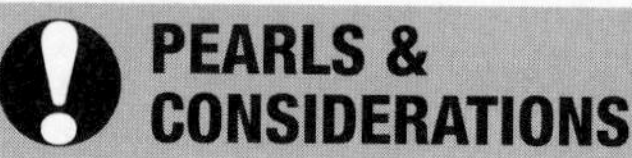

PEARLS & CONSIDERATIONS

COMMENTS

Nausea and vomiting in early pregnancy are associated with psychosocial morbidity.

PREVENTION

Taking a multivitamin at the time of conception

SUGGESTED READINGS

available at www.expertconsult.com

RELATED CONTENT

Hyperemesis Gravidarum (Patient Information)

AUTHOR: **ALISON PATTERSON, M.D.**

BASIC INFORMATION

DEFINITION

- Primary hyperlipoproteinemia is a group of genetic disorders of the lipid transport proteins in the blood that manifests as abnormally elevated levels of cholesterol, triglycerides, or both in the serum of affected patients.
- Usually defined as total cholesterol, LDL, triglycerides or lipoprotein A levels above 90th percentile or HDL or apo A-1 levels below the 10th percentile for the general population. Fig. E1-493 illustrates the structure of lipoproteins. Plasma lipoprotein composition is described in Table E1-258.

SYNONYMS

Hyperlipidemia

ICD-9CM CODES
272.4 Hyperlipoproteinemia
272.3 Fredrickson type I
272.0 Fredrickson type IIa
272.2 Fredrickson type IIb, III
272.1 Fredrickson type IV
272.3 Fredrickson type V
ICD-10CM CODES
E78.0 Pure hypercholesterolemia
E78.2 Mixed hyperlipidemia
E78.1 Pure hyperglyceridemia
E78.4 Other hyperlipidemia
E78.3 Hyperchylomicronemia

EPIDEMIOLOGY & DEMOGRAPHICS

INCIDENCE: The most common types are lipoprotein A excess, hypertriglyceridemia, and combined hyperlipidemia.

- Incidence of heterozygous familial hypercholesterolemia: –1:500.
- Incidence of homozygous familial hypercholesterolemia: –1:1 million.
- Familial hypercholesterolemia: autosomal-dominant disorder.
- Familial combined hyperlipidemia: possibly an autosomal-dominant disorder.
- Multifactorial predilection: apparent in majority of affected individuals.

GENETICS:

- Familial lipoprotein lipase deficiency: autosomal recessive, resulting in an elevation in the plasma chylomicrons and triglycerides
- Familial apoprotein CII deficiency: autosomal recessive, resulting in increased serum chylomicrons, very-low-density lipoprotein (VLDL), and hypertriglyceridemia
- Familial type 3 hyperlipoproteinemia: single-gene defect requiring contributory factors to manifest
- Familial hypercholesterolemia: autosomal-dominant defect of the LDL receptor, resulting in an elevated serum cholesterol level and normal triglycerides
- Familial hypertriglyceridemia: common, autosomal-dominant defect resulting in elevated VLDL and triglycerides
- Multiple lipoprotein–type hyperlipidemia: autosomal dominant, manifesting as isolated hypercholesterolemia, isolated hypertriglyceridemia, or hyperlipidemia
- Polygenic hypercholesterolemia: multifactorial
- Polygenic hyperalphalipoproteinemia: autosomal dominant or polygenic, causing an elevated high-density lipoprotein
- A classification of lipoprotein disorders is described in Table 1-259.

PHYSICAL FINDINGS & CLINICAL PRESENTATION

- Familial lipoprotein lipase deficiency: recurrent bouts of abdominal pain in infancy, eruptive xanthomas, hepatomegaly, splenomegaly, lipemia retinalis
- Familial apoprotein CII deficiency: occasional eruptive xanthomas
- Familial type 3 hyperlipoproteinemia: xanthoma striata palmaris or tuberoeruptive xanthomas, xanthelasmas, arterial bruits at a young age, gangrene of the lower extremities at a young age
- Familial hypercholesterolemia: tendon xanthomas, arcus corneae, xanthelasma
- Familial hypertriglyceridemia: associated obesity; eruptive xanthomas can develop with exacerbations

ETIOLOGY

- Genetic defects causing lipid abnormalities
- Environmental influences including diet, drugs, and alcohol intake

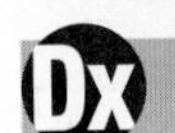

DIAGNOSIS

DIFFERENTIAL DIAGNOSIS

Secondary causes of hyperlipoproteinemias:

- Hypothyroidism
- Diabetes mellitus
- Pancreatitis
- Autoimmune hyperlipoproteinemia
- Nephrotic syndrome
- Biliary obstruction. Table E1-260 describes the differential diagnosis of hyperlipidemia and dyslipidemia.

WORKUP

- Family history for premature cardiac disease
- Personal history of recurrent pancreatitis
- Detailed physical examination

LABORATORY TESTS

- Standard lipid profile
- If normal, further testing with measurement of lipoprotein A, apo B, and apo A-1
- Lipoprotein electrophoresis and ultracentrifugation (for phenotypic classification)
- Workup for secondary causes: TSH, fasting glucose, liver function, renal function, urinary protein

TREATMENT

NONPHARMACOLOGIC THERAPY

- Cornerstone of treatment: dietary therapy
    - TLC diet (**t**herapeutic **l**ifestyle **c**hanges): see "Hypercholesterolemia" topic
- Risk factor reduction includes smoking cessation, treatment of hypertension, exercise
- Familial lipoprotein lipase deficiency and familial apoprotein CII deficiency: fat-free diet
- Remainder of cases, except those with polygenic hyperalphalipoproteinemia: fat- and cholesterol-restricted diets
- Interventions to improve adherence are described in Table 1-261

ACUTE GENERAL Rx

No acute treatment needed

CHRONIC Rx

- Familial lipoprotein lipase deficiency, polygenic hyperalphalipoproteinemia, or familial apoprotein CII deficiency: no chronic drug therapy
- Familial type 3 hyperlipoproteinemia: usually responds well to secondary causes being treated and diet therapy; if not, fibric acids may be tried
- Familial hypercholesterolemia: HMG-CoA reductase inhibitors, bile acid sequestrants, or niacin
- Familial hypertriglyceridemia: fibric acids (fenofibrate), niacin, omega-3 PUFA-containing fish oil capsules (lovaza, vascepa)
- Multiple lipoprotein–type hyperlipidemia: drug therapy aimed at the predominant lipid abnormality noted
- Recent data suggest in patients with lipoprotein abnormalities that treatment goals should be based on non-HDL cholesterol rather than LDL cholesterol
- The FDA has approved mipomersen and lomitapide in patients with homozygous familial hypercholesterolemia already taking maximum doses of other lipid-lowering drugs. Both medicines are hepatotoxic and very expensive.
- Table E1-262 describes the various drugs used to treat hyperlipidemia.

DISPOSITION

- Those with polygenic hyperalphalipoproteinemia: excellent prognosis for longevity
- Those with familial hypercholesterolemia, familial type 3 hypercholesterolemia, or multiple lipoprotein–type hyperlipidemia: even with aggressive treatment, at high risk for accelerated atherosclerosis and coronary artery disease

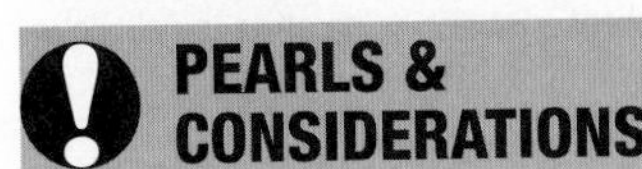

PEARLS & CONSIDERATIONS

COMMENTS

- Patient information is available through the American Heart Association.
- Lipid-lowering drug therapy is recommended for children ≥10 yr whose LDL-C levels remain extremely elevated after 6 mo to 1 yr of dietary modification. Drug therapy also can be considered for children with LDL-C levels of ≥190 mg/dl.

SUGGESTED READINGS

available at www.expertconsult.com

RELATED CONTENT

Hypercholesterolemia (Related Key Topic)

AUTHOR: **PRIYA BANSAL, M.D., M.P.H.**

TABLE 1-259 Classification of Lipoprotein Disorders by Phenotypes, Genotypes, and Corresponding Clinical Manifestations

Phenotype (Frederickson Type)	Genotype	Elevated Cholesterol Type	Genetic Defect	Xanthomas	Other Clinical Manifestations
I (rare)	Familial hyperchylomicronemia	Elevated chylomicrons	Familial lipoprotein lipase deficiency, Apo C-II deficiency	Eruptive skin xanthomas	Recurrent abdominal pain, hepatosplenomegaly
IIA	Familial hypercholesterolemia	Elevated LDL	FHC, LDL receptor deficiency	Tendon xanthomas, xanthelasma, tuberous; planar palmar (homozygous)	Premature CAD, arcus corneae, arthritic symptoms
IIB	Familial combined hypercholesterolemia	Elevated LDL and VLDL	Reduced LDL receptor and increased apo B		
III (rare)	Familial dysbetalipoproteinemia	Elevated IDL	Defective apo E2 synthesis	Tuberous, planar (palmar)	Premature CAD and peripheral vascular disease, male > female, obesity, abnormal glucose tolerance, hyperuricemia, aggravated by hypothyroiditis, good response to therapy
IV	Familial hyperlipemia	Elevated VLDL	Increased VLDL production	None	CAD and peripheral vascular disease, obesity, abnormal glucose tolerance, hyperuricemia, arthritic
V (rare)	Endogenous hypertriglyceridemia	Elevated VLDL, chylomicrons	Increased VLDL production and reduced LPL	Eruptive	

Apo, Apolipoprotein; *CAD,* coronary artery disease; *FHC,* familial hypercholesterolemia.
Modified from Graber MA: *The family practice handbook,* ed 4, St Louis, 2001, Mosby.

TABLE 1-261 Interventions to Improve Adherence

Focus on the Patient

Simplify medication regimens.
Provide explicit patient instruction and use good counseling techniques to teach the patient how to follow the prescribed treatment.
Encourage the use of prompts to help patients remember treatment regimens.
Use systems to reinforce adherence and maintain contact with the patient.
Encourage the support of family and friends.
Reinforce and reward adherence.
Increase visits for patients unable to achieve treatment goal.
Increase the convenience and access to care.
Involve patients in their care through self-monitoring.

Focus on the Physician and Medical Office

Teach physicians to implement lipid treatment guidelines.
Use reminders to prompt physicians to attend to lipid management.
Identify a patient advocate in the office to help deliver or prompt care.
Use patients to prompt preventive care.
Develop a standardized treatment plan to structure care.
Use feedback from past performance to foster change in future care.
Remind patients of appointments and follow up missed appointments.

Focus on the Health Delivery System

Provide lipid management through a lipid clinic.
Utilize case management by nurses.
Deploy telemedicine.
Utilize the collaborative care of pharmacists.
Execute critical care pathways in hospitals.

From Expert Panel on Detection, Evaluation, and Treatment of High Blood Cholesterol in Adults: Executive Summary of the Third Report of the National Cholesterol Education Program (NCEP) Expert Panel on Detection, Evaluation, and Treatment of High Blood Cholesterol in Adults (Adult Treatment Panel III), *JAMA* 285:2486-2497, 2001.

BASIC INFORMATION

DEFINITION

Hyperosmolar hyperglycemic syndrome (HHS) is characterized by severe hyperglycemia, hyperosmolarity, profound dehydration, and altered mental status in the absence of ketosis.

SYNONYMS

Hyperosmolar coma
Nonketotic hyperosmolar syndrome
Hyperosmolar nonketotic state
HHS

ICD-9CM CODES
250.2 Hyperosmolar coma
ICD-10CM CODES
E87.0 Hyperosmolality and hypernatremia

PHYSICAL FINDINGS & CLINICAL PRESENTATION

- Evidence of extreme dehydration (poor skin turgor, sunken eyeballs, dry mucous membranes)
- Neurologic defects (reversible hemiplegia, focal seizures)
- Orthostatic hypotension, tachycardia
- Evidence of precipitating factors (infection, myocardial ischemia, stroke)
- Suppressed mental status ranging from delirium to obtundation to coma (25% of patients)

ETIOLOGY

- Infections in up to 50% (e.g., pneumonia, urinary tract infection, sepsis)
- New or previously unrecognized diabetes (30%)
- Non-compliance, dose reduction, or recent discontinuation of diabetic medication
- Stress (myocardial infarction, cerebrovascular accident)
- Drugs: diuretics (dehydration), phenytoin, diazoxide (impairs insulin secretion), glucocorticoids, chemotherapeutic agents, calcium channel blockers, total parenteral nutrition, substance abuse (alcohol, cocaine)

DIAGNOSIS

DIFFERENTIAL DIAGNOSIS

- Diabetic ketoacidosis
- The differential diagnosis of coma is described in Section II

LABORATORY TESTS

- Hyperglycemia: serum glucose usually >600 mg/dl, serum/urine ketones absent or "small."
- Hyperosmolarity: serum osmolarity usually >320 mOsm/L.
- Serum sodium: may be low, normal, or high. Because glucose draws fluid from the intracellular space, decreasing the serum sodium, it is necessary to correct sodium for the serum glucose level. The corrected sodium can be obtained by increasing the serum sodium concentration by 1.6 mEq/dl for every 100 mg/dl increase in the serum glucose level over normal.
- Serum potassium: may be low, normal, or high; regardless of the initial serum level, the total body deficit is approximately 5 to 15 mEq/kg.
- Serum bicarbonate: usually >15 mEq/L (average 17 mEq/L).
- Arterial pH: usually >7.3; both serum bicarbonate and arterial pH may be lower if lactic acidosis is present.
- Blood urea nitrogen: generally ranges from 60 to 90 mg/dl due to severe dehydration and pro-renal azotemia.
- Phosphorus: hypophosphatemia (average deficit is 70 to 140 mmol).
- Calcium: hypocalcemia (average deficit is 50 to 100 mEq).
- Magnesium: hypomagnesemia (average deficit is 50 to 100 mEq).
- Complete blood count with differential, urinalysis, and blood and urine cultures should be performed to rule out infectious etiology.
- ECG to rule out a concomitant myocardial infarction.

IMAGING STUDIES

- Chest radiograph is useful to rule out infectious process. The initial radiograph may be negative if the patient has significant dehydration. Repeat chest x-ray after 24 hr of hydration if pulmonary infection is suspected.
- The need for additional imaging, such as CT scans, is determined by biochemical or physical exam findings.

TREATMENT

ACUTE GENERAL Rx

- Vigorous fluid replacement: the volume and rate of fluid replacement are determined by renal and cardiac function. Slower infusion rate may be used initially in patients with compromised cardiovascular or renal status. Frequent clinical monitoring of fluid status is essential.
  - During the first hour, infuse 1000 ml of 0.9% normal saline (NS) to expand the intravascular fluid volume.
  - Infuse a second liter of 0.9% NS in the next hour if the patient is persistently hypotensive.
  - Then begin replacing the free fluid deficit with 0.45% NS at 250 to 500 ml/hr. Taper the 0.45% NS to replace the estimated fluid deficit over 24 to 36 hours.
  - When serum glucose reaches 300 mg/dl, change to 5% dextrose with 0.45% NS.
- Correct hyperglycemia: the goal is to decrease plasma glucose by 50 to 100 mg/dl/hr.
  - Vigorous IV hydration will decrease the serum glucose level in most patients by 80 mg/dl/hr. Insulin should not be administered until serum potassium is >3.3 mEq/L to prevent life-threatening hypokalemia.
  - A regular insulin IV bolus (0.1 units/kg of body weight) is followed by an insulin fusion of 0.1 units/kg/hr, adjusted on an hourly basis as needed, until the serum glucose level approaches 300 mg/dl.
  - Before stopping the IV insulin infusion, administer an SC dose of insulin (dose varies with patient's demonstrated insulin sensitivity). Short (regular) or rapid-acting (aspart, lispro, glulisine) insulins should be administered SC 1 to 2 hr before stopping the IV insulin infusion. Intermediate (NPH) or long-acting (glargine, detemir) insulins should be administered SC 2 to 4 hr before stopping IV insulin infusion.
- Total daily insulin doses in insulin-naïve patients range from 0.5 to 0.8 units/kg/day. Approximately half of this dose should be given as intermediate or long-acting insulin, and half of this dose should be given as mealtime or prandial insulin if the patient is eating.
- Replace potassium: monitor potassium every 2 hours until the patient has stabilized. Confirm the patient is not anuric before starting potassium (K) replacement. Rate of K replacement can be based on presenting potassium level. If K is <3.3, give KCl 20 to 30 mEq/L of intravenous fluid (IVF) until K is >3.3. If K is 3.3 to 5.3, give KCl at 10 to 30 mEq/L IVF to maintain a K of >4. If K >5.3, hold potassium supplementation and check K every 2 hours. Continuous telemetry monitoring and hourly measurement of urinary output are recommended.
- Phosphate replacement: replacement can be considered if serum phosphate is <2 mEq/L or there is evidence of phosphate depletion syndrome rhabdomyolysis. In the absence of renal failure, phosphate can be administered at a rate of 0.1 mmol/kg/hr (5 to 10 mmol/hr) to a maximum of 80 to 120 mmol in 24 hr.
- Magnesium replacement, in the absence of renal failure, can be administered IM (0.05 to 0.10 ml/kg of 20% magnesium sulfate) or as IV infusion (4 to 8 ml of 20% magnesium sulfate [0.08 to 0.16 mEq/kg]).

PEARLS & CONSIDERATIONS

COMMENTS

- The typical patient is an elderly or bed-confined diabetic with impaired ability to communicate thirst who is evaluated after an interval of 1 to 2 wk of prolonged osmotic diuresis.

SUGGESTED READINGS

available at www.expertconsult.com

AUTHORS: **HILARY B. WHITLATCH, M.D., SAINATH GADDAM, M.D.,** and **FRED F. FERRI, M.D.**

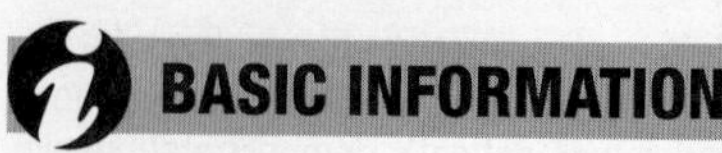

BASIC INFORMATION

DEFINITION

Hyperparathyroidism is an endocrine disorder caused by excessive secretion of parathyroid hormone (PTH) from the parathyroid glands. Autonomous production of PTH resulting in hypercalcemia defines primary hyperparathyroidism. Secondary hyperparathyroidism occurs when the parathyroid glands appropriately increase PTH production in response to low calcium or vitamin D states. Primary hyperparathyroidism is the focus of this section.

ICD-9CM CODES
252.00 Hyperparathyroidism, unspecified
252.01 Hyperparathyroidism, primary
252.02 Hyperparathyroidism, secondary
ICD-10CM CODES
E21.3 Hyperparathyroidism, unspecified
E21.0 Primary hyperparathyroidism

EPIDEMIOLOGY & DEMOGRAPHICS

INCIDENCE: 4 cases per 100,000 persons per year. Although malignancy is the most common cause of hypercalcemia in hospitalized patients, primary hyperparathyroidism is the most common cause of hypercalcemia in the outpatient setting.
PREVALENCE: 3 cases/1000 persons
PREDOMINANT SEX AND AGE: Higher prevalence in women (female:male ratio 2:1) and older age (peaks in the seventh decade of life).

PHYSICAL FINDINGS & CLINICAL PRESENTATION

The majority of patients with primary hyperparathyroidism are asymptomatic. Diagnosis is usually considered in patients after an incidental discovery of hypercalcemia or during the evaluation for decreased bone mass. The development of symptoms varies with severity and rapidity of disease progression and reflects both the hypercalcemic and hyperparathyroid components of the disease process.

- Cardiovascular: hypertension, shortened QT interval, bradycardia, arrhythmia, valvular calcification, left ventricular hypertrophy, increased mean carotid intima-media thickness.
- GI: anorexia, nausea, vomiting, constipation, abdominal pain, peptic ulcer disease, pancreatitis
- GU: nephrolithiasis, nephrocalcinosis, renal insufficiency, polyuria, nocturia, nephrogenic diabetes insipidus, renal tubular acidosis
- Musculoskeletal: weakness, myopathy, bone pain, osteopenia, osteoporosis, gout, pseudogout, chondrocalcinosis, osteitis fibrosa cystic, subperiosteal bone resorption (Fig. 1-494)
- CNS: confusion, anxiety, fatigue, lethargy, obtundation, depression, coma
- Other: pruritus, metastatic calcifications, band keratopathy

ETIOLOGY

- Most cases of primary hyperparathyroidism are sporadic but it can be associated with rare familial conditions such as multiple endocrine neoplasia (MEN-1 and MEN-2). Mutations in certain genes have been linked to tumor development in both sporadic and familial cases. Higher prevalence of hyperparathyroidism is noted with head and neck irradiation, chronic low calcium or vitamin D status, and lithium therapy.
- Pathologic characteristics include adenoma (80%-85%), hyperplasia (10%-15%), or carcinomas (<1%-2%).

Dx DIAGNOSIS

DIFFERENTIAL DIAGNOSIS

- Secondary hyperparathyroidism precipitated by conditions that result in hypocalcemia
  - Renal calcium loss (i.e., medication: loop diuretics and hypercalcuria)
  - Calcium deficiency
  - Vitamin D deficiency
  - Malabsorption
  - Chronic kidney disease (most common)
  - Pseudohypoparathyroidism (PTH resistance)
  - Inhibition of bone resorption (i.e., bisphosphonates)
- Other causes of hypercalcemia include:
  - Medications: thiazide diuretics, lithium therapy
  - Vitamin D intoxication, milk-alkali syndrome
  - Familial hypocalciuric hypercalcemia (FHH)
  - Renal failure (tertiary hyperparathyroidism)
  - Granulomatous disorders (e.g., sarcoidosis)
  - Malignancy (e.g., lung cancer, lymphoma, myeloma, bone metastasis)
  - Prolonged immobilization

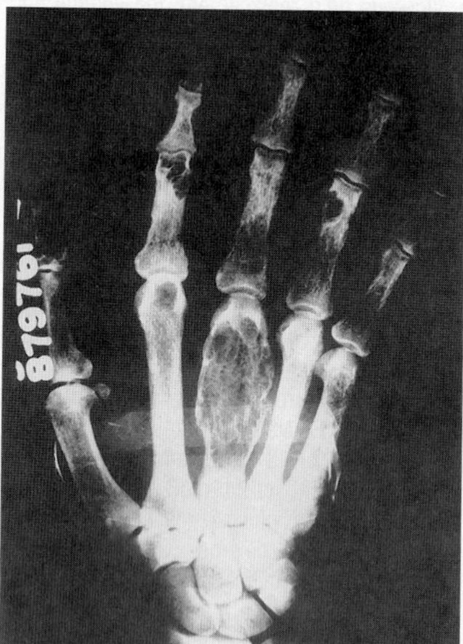

FIGURE 1-494 Radiograph of hand from a patient with severe primary hyperparathyroidism. Note the dramatic remodeling associated with the intense region of high bone turnover in the third metacarpal, in addition to widespread evidence of subperiosteal and trabecular resorption. (Courtesy Fuller Albright Collection, Massachusetts General Hospital. From Larsen PR et al [eds]: *Williams textbook of endocrinology,* ed 10, Philadelphia, 2003, Saunders.)

WORKUP

- Typically, primary hyperparathyroidism is confirmed with an elevated serum calcium and PTH level.
  - Two measurements of serum calcium are required for the confirmation of hypercalcemia. Total calcium should be corrected for low albumin utilizing the formula: Corrected Calcium = Serum Calcium + 0.8 × 4 − serum albumin). If a reliable laboratory is available, an ionized calcium should be considered especially in conditions associated with acid-base disturbances or low albumin states. Occasionally, patients with primary hyperparathyroidism can present with normal calcium levels. The most common reason for this finding is concomitant vitamin D deficiency and primary hyperparathyroidism.
  - The serum intact PTH (iPTH) level is the single best test to evaluate the etiology of hypercalcemia. PTH is elevated or in the high normal range (i.e., inappropriately normal for an elevated calcium state) in primary hyperparathyroidism. PTH is decreased in most other conditions associated with elevated calcium.
- Other causes of hypercalcemia should be ruled out. These are typically associated with low PTH levels. Exceptions include lithium use and FHH.
  - Review medication history to determine lithium, thiazide, vitamin D or calcium intake.
  - Check 24-hr urine calcium:creatinine to rule out FHH. Urine calcium is usually low in FHH. PTH can be low, normal, or high in FHH.
  - Consider PTH-related peptide (PTHrP) to evaluate hypercalcemia related to malignancies and vitamin D1,25 to assess hypercalcemia secondary to glaucomatous diseases or lymphomas.
  - Multiple myeloma and bone metastasis can also result in a high calcium state and therefore must be appropriately evaluated.
- Rule out other causes of elevated PTH (i.e., secondary hyperparathyroidism). Serum calcium is typically low or low-normal in secondary hyperparathyroidism.
  - Check calcium and 25 OH-vitamin D to rule out deficiency states.
  - Check creatinine to assess renal function and 24-hr urine calcium to evaluate renal loss

LABORATORY TESTS

- Serum calcium (ionized or corrected calcium): normal or elevated in primary hyperparathyroidism
- Serum phosphorus: low or low normal in primary hyperparathyroidism.

- PTH: elevated or high normal in primary hyperparathyroidism
- 24-hr urine calcium to evaluate risk for renal stones and to exclude FHH.
- Serum creatinine to assess GFR and renal status.
- PTHrP and 1,25 OH-vitamin D levels can be considered to rule out other causes of elevated calcium.
- Evaluation of 25 OH-vitamin D is recommended in all patients with hyperparathyroidism. Vitamin D deficiency can result in secondary hyperparathyroidism. Calcium levels are usually in the low-normal range in vitamin D deficiency.
- ECG may reveal shortening of the QT interval secondary to severe hypercalcemia (>12 mg/dl)

IMAGING STUDIES

- Neck imaging is not indicated for diagnosis but is useful for localization before planned parathyroidectomy.
- Parathyroid localization with technetium-99m sestamibi can identify potential adenomas.
- Bone mineral density of the spine, hip, and forearm (distal third) is recommended for all patients with hyperparathyroidism in order to assess the risk for osteoporosis and fragility fractures. Cortical bone loss (i.e., forearm or hip) is greater than trabecular bone loss (i.e., spine) in hyperparathyroidism.
- Renal ultrasound can be considered to assess asymptomatic renal stones.

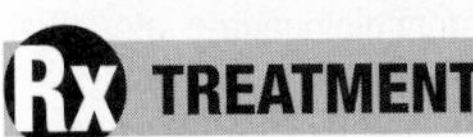

TREATMENT

Modality of treatment depends on disease progression and which patients are more likely to suffer end-organ effects of hyperparathyroidism or benefit the most from surgery.

NONPHARMACOLOGIC THERAPY

- Surgery is the only definitive treatment for symptomatic primary hyperparathyroidism. Surgery can normalize calcium levels, decrease the risk for kidney stones, improve bone mineral density and fracture risk, and enhance quality of life measures.
  - Indications for parathyroidectomy
    1. All patients younger than 50 yr
    2. Hypercalcemia (Ca >1 mg/dl above upper limit normal)
    3. Creatinine clearance <60 ml/min
    4. Osteoporosis (T-score < −2.5 or prior fragility fracture)
    5. Symptomatic hyperparathyroidism such as history of nephrolithiasis
  - Surgical approaches include:
    1. The conventional surgical approach is bilateral neck exploration under general anesthesia. An experienced endocrine surgeon cures >95% of patients undergoing bilateral neck exploration. Potential complications include transient and permanent hypocalcemia secondary to hypoparathyroidism and recurrent laryngeal nerve injury.
    2. Minimally invasive parathyroidectomy performed by experienced surgeons is an excellent alternative to conventional surgery. It can be performed under cervical block anesthesia as an outpatient procedure with intraoperative monitoring of PTH before and after removal to document the expected fall after abnormal glands are removed.
- Ablation therapy (e.g., ethanol, angiographic, radiofrequency) can be considered in patients who are not surgical candidates. Limited data is available on efficacy and side effects. Repeat ablations may be required if hypercalcemia persists.
- Medical monitoring is recommended for asymptomatic primary hyperparathyroidism. Majority of patients do not manifest disease progression during observation. However, approximately 25% of asymptomatic patients will require surgery over a 10-yr follow-up period.
  - Indications for medical monitoring
    1. Clinically asymptomatic and >50 yr old.
    2. Serum calcium level only mildly elevated (<1 mg/dl above upper limit normal)
    3. GFR > 60 ml/min and no nephrolithiasis or nephrocalcinosis
    4. No evidence of osteoporosis
    5. Medically unfit for surgery or refusing surgery
- Symptoms should be assessed regularly, serum calcium and creatinine should be checked yearly, and bone mineral density may be monitored every 2 yr.
- Medical management
  1. Avoid medications that precipitate hypercalcemia (e.g., thiazide or lithium)
  2. Since inadequate calcium and vitamin D status stimulates PTH, calcium and vitamin D intake should be the same as for patients without hyperparathyroidism (i.e., 1000 mg of elemental calcium and 600-800 IU of vitamin D daily).
  3. Encourage physical activity since immobilization increases bone resorption.
  4. Recommend adequate hydration (at least 2 L) to minimize the risk of nephrolithiasis.

PHARMACOLOGIC THERAPY

For patients who are not surgical candidates, pharmacologic options are available. Indications include symptomatic hyperparathyroidism or osteopenia associated with an increased fracture risk.

- Cinacalcet (Sensipar) is an oral calcimimetic agent that activates the calcium sensing receptor in the parathyroid gland. It decreases PTH production and subsequently serum calcium levels, without significant BMD changes. It is indicated for the treatment of secondary hyperparathyroidism associated with chronic kidney disease, for hypercalcemia associated with parathyroid carcinoma, and for the treatment of severe hypercalcemia in patients with primary hyperparathyroidism who are unable to undergo surgery.
- Agents that inhibit bone resorption such as bisphosphonates (e.g., alendronate, pamidronate, zoledronate), estrogens and selective estrogen receptor modulators (e.g., raloxifene) improve bone mineral density, and decrease calcium levels in patients with hyperparathyroidism. These agents should be considered when fracture reduction is the primary goal.

ACUTE GENERAL Rx

Severe and/or symptomatic hypercalcemia may require hospitalization especially if serum calcium >12 mg/dl. Acute management of hypercalcemia includes:

- Vigorous hydration with IV normal saline (2-4 L/day). Fluid status must be monitored in patients with cardiac dysfunction or renal insufficiency in order to avoid fluid overload.
- Bisphosphonates can effectively decrease calcium levels. Zoledronate (4 mg IV over 15 min) or pamidronate (60-90 mg IV over 4 hr) are both effective. Onset of action is 24 to 48 hr.
- Calcitonin (4 units/kg IM/SC every 12 hr) may be used with bisphosphonates to achieve a more rapid reduction of calcium levels. Onset of action is within hours.

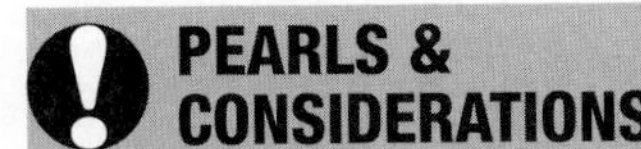

PEARLS & CONSIDERATIONS

COMMENTS

- Parathyroidectomy should be considered for all patients with symptomatic hyperparathyroidism. If surgery is contraindicated or not desired, cinacalcet can be considered.
- Asymptomatic patients can be monitored with serial creatinine, calcium, and bone mineral density measurements. Disease progression may result in surgery.
- Most patients can be managed medically by limiting factors that result in hypercalcemia (e.g., dehydration, immobilization, thiazide diuretics) and maintaining normal calcium and vitamin D intake.
- Patients with osteopenia and high fracture risk may require antiresorptive therapy such as bisphosphonates.

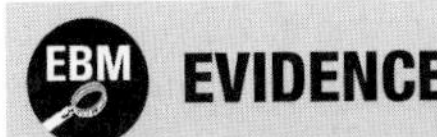

EVIDENCE

available at www.expertconsult.com

SUGGESTED READINGS

available at www.expertconsult.com

RELATED CONTENT

Hyperparathyroidism (Patient Information)

AUTHOR: **GEETHA GOPALAKRISHNAN, M.D.**

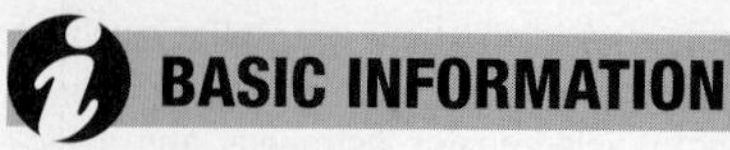

BASIC INFORMATION

DEFINITION

Hypersensitivity pneumonitis (HP) is a group of immunologically mediated pulmonary diseases, with or without systemic manifestations (e.g., fever, weight loss), caused by the inhalation of an antigen to which the patient is sensitized and hyperresponsive. Sensitization and exposure alone in the absence of symptoms do not define the disease.

SYNONYMS

Extrinsic allergic alveolitis (EAA)
Some specific examples:

- Bird fancier's lung
- Farmer's lung
- Chemical worker's lung
- Humidifier lung
- Hot tub lung
- Sauna taker's lung

ICD-9CM CODES
495.9 Pneumonitis, hypersensitivity
ICD-10CM CODES
J67.8 Hypersensitivity pneumonitis due to other organic dust
J67.9 Hypersensitivity pneumonitis due to unspecified organic dust

EPIDEMIOLOGY & DEMOGRAPHICS

- Prevalence and incidence of HP vary considerably.
- Depend on definition and methods to establish diagnosis, intensity of exposure, environmental conditions, and genetic risk factors that remain poorly understood.
- More than 300 causative agents have been identified, and the number continues to grow.
- Causative agents in residential and occupational exposures include birds, mold, humidifiers, fountains, steam irons, dry sausage molds, moldy cheese, contaminated wood, biofilm contained within wind instruments (e.g., trombone, saxophone), and organic and inorganic chemicals, including metalworking fluids. A large series of patients with HP associated with down pillows, feather duvets, and down-upholstered furniture has been published. Likely several genes are involved that cause an exaggerated lung response to an offending agent. The major histocompatibility complex is the most studied thus far.
- A viral connection has been implicated that may enhance clinical exposure to an offending agent.

PHYSICAL FINDINGS & CLINICAL PRESENTATION

Vary depending on frequency and intensity of antigen exposure.

- Acute: fever, cough, malaise, and dyspnea 4 to 6 hr after an intense exposure, lasting 18 to 24 hr
- Subacute: insidious onset of productive cough, dyspnea on exertion, anorexia, and weight loss, usually from a heavy, sustained exposure
- Chronic: gradually progressive cough, dyspnea, malaise, and weight loss, usually from low-grade or recurrent exposure
- Physical examination: cyanosis and crepitant rales, possible fever

ETIOLOGY

- Numerous environmental agents, often encountered in occupational settings
- Common sources of antigens: "moldy" hay, silage, grain, or vegetables; bird droppings or feathers (including those found commonly in down pillows, blankets, and upholstered furniture); low-molecular-weight chemicals (e.g., isocyanates); pharmaceutical products

Dx DIAGNOSIS

- Accurate diagnosis is important for differentiating HP from other interstitial disorders because the prognosis and treatment may differ.
- The clinical syndrome is indistinguishable from an acute respiratory infection without a history of illness occurring within hours of exposure to an antigen.
- Need high index of suspicion.
- Detailed occupational and home exposure history is required.
- Lung biopsy is often necessary for diagnosis.

DIFFERENTIAL DIAGNOSIS

Acute Stages	Chronic Stages
Acute bronchopulmonary aspergillosis	Idiopathic pulmonary fibrosis (IPF)
Pulmonary embolism	Bronchiectasis
Asthma	Chronic bronchitis
Aspiration pneumonia	Nonspecific interstitial pneumonia (NSIP)
Recurrent pneumonia	Connective tissue–related lung disease
Bronchiolitis obliterans–organizing pneumonia	
Sarcoidosis	
Churg-Strauss syndrome	
Wegener granulomatosis	

WORKUP

No single radiologic, physiologic, or immunologic test is specific for the diagnosis of HP. HP must be suspected in any patient presenting with cough, dyspnea, fever, and malaise. A thorough history focusing on potential exposures is essential. Table 1-263 describes examples of occupational causes of HP.

Environmental and occupational history questions should ask about grain dusts; animal handling; food processing; cooling towers; fountains; metalworking fluids; symptom improvement away from exposure; pets (particularly birds); hobbies involving chemicals, feathers, or fur; organic dusts; presence of humidifiers, dehumidifiers, or hot tubs/saunas; leaking or flooding indoors; visible fungal growth in living or working environment; feather pillows, bedding, or upholstered furniture.

Major criteria:

- History of symptoms compatible with HP that appear to worsen within hours after antigen exposure
- Confirmation of exposure to the offending agent by history, investigation of the environment, serum precipitin tests to potential agents (often referred to as a "hypersensitivity panel" by many labs), or bronchoalveolar lavage (BAL) antibody
- Compatible changes on chest radiograph or high-resolution CT (HRCT) of the chest
- BAL fluid lymphocytosis (if performed)
- Compatible histologic changes by lung biopsy (if performed): bronchiolocentric interstitial pneumonia, NSIP
- Positive natural challenge (reproduction of symptoms and laboratory abnormalities after exposure to the suspected environment) or controlled inhalation challenge

TABLE 1-263 Examples of Occupational Causes of Hypersensitivity Pneumonitis

Occupation	Cause
Farmer	Thermophilic actinomycetes in moldy hay
Metal worker	Contamination of metal-working fluids with microorganisms such as *Mycobacteria immunogens* or fungi
Worker exposed to humidifiers	Contamination with microorganisms such as protozoa or fungi
Sugarcane worker	Moldy sugarcane (bagassosis)
Maple bark stripper	Fungi
Chicken or turkey worker	Avian proteins
Pharmaceutical worker	Penicillin
Food handler	Soybeans
Office worker	Microorganisms contaminating air conditioners or humidifiers
Swimming pool attendant	Fungal contamination in sprays around pool area
Animal worker	Rat proteins
Mushroom worker	Fungi
Wheat farmer or handler	Weevil-infested flour
Greenhouse worker	Fungi
Workers spraying urethane paint or adhesives/sealants (or less often, other workers using diisocyanate)	Methylene diphenyl diisocyanate, hexamethylene diisocyanate, toluene diisocyanates
Chemical worker using plastics, resins, paints	Trimellitic anhydride

From Goldman L, Schafer AI: *Goldman's Cecil medicine,* ed 24, Philadelphia, 2012, Saunders.

Minor criteria:
- Basilar crackles
- Decreased diffusion capacity
- Arterial hypoxemia (either at rest or with exercise)

LABORATORY TESTS

- Routine laboratory tests do not make the diagnosis, but typically the erythrocyte sedimentation rate, C-reactive protein, lactate dehydrogenase, and leukocyte count are increased; elevated immunoglobulins IgG and IgM are nonspecific; rheumatoid factor (RF) and immune complexes are often positive; peripheral eosinophil count and serum IgE are generally normal.
- Lactate dehydrogenase (LDH) is increased and tends to decrease with improvement.
- Pulmonary function tests: restrictive ventilatory patterns are typically seen. Decreased FEV_1, decreased forced vital capacity, decreased total lung capacity, decreased diffusing capacity, and decreased static compliance.
- Arterial blood gases show mild hypoxemia (worsens with exercise).
- A-a gradient shows slight increase.
- Serum precipitin test for IgG antibodies against offending antigen detected in serum. It is sensitive but not specific for HP (asymptomatic patients may have IgG antibodies in serum). HP may also be present without a positive precipitin test.
- Skin testing: unclear if helpful. However, some believe it to be a safe, effective, and rapid procedure in the diagnosis and follow-up of patients with HP. Sensitivity is similar to that of the precipitin test but the specificity is higher.

IMAGING STUDIES

Chest x-ray: nonspecific; may be normal in early stage.
- Acute/subacute: bilateral interstitial and alveolar nodular infiltrates in a patchy or homogeneous distribution. Apices are often spared.
- Chronic: diffuse reticulonodular infiltrates and fibrosis.

High-resolution chest CT scan: no pathognomonic features but demonstrates airspace and interstitial patterns in the acute and subacute stage. The chronic stage reveals honeycombing and bronchiectasis.

Rx TREATMENT

NONPHARMACOLOGIC THERAPY

Early recognition and avoidance of the causative antigen

ACUTE GENERAL Rx

- Glucocorticoids accelerate initial lung recovery but may have no effect long term (from a controlled study in farmer's lung). No prospective, randomized, placebo-controlled trials for other types of HP or subacute and chronic stages.
- Prednisone 0.5 to 1 mg/kg usually over 1 to 2 wk then tapered over 4 wk. Some patients, particularly those with subacute or chronic presentation, may require a longer course of therapy.

DISPOSITION/PROGNOSIS

Prognosis is generally better in patients with acute or subacute HP, and with the finding of NSIP pathologically. Prognosis is worse in those with older age, desaturation during exercise, and findings of severe fibrosis by lung biopsy.

Acute: 4 to 48 hr
- Clinical: fever, chills, cough, hypoxia, malaise
- HRCT: ground-glass infiltrates
- Immunopathology: poorly formed, noncaseating granulomas or mononuclear cell infiltration in a peribronchial distribution, frequently with giant cells
- Prognosis: good

Subacute: weeks to 4 mo
- Clinical: dyspnea, cough, episodic flares
- HRCT: micronodules, air trapping
- Immunopathology: more well-formed, noncaseating granulomas, bronchiolitis, organizing pneumonia, and interstitial fibrosis
- Prognosis: good

Chronic: 4 mo to years
- Clinical: dyspnea, cough, fatigue, weight loss
- HRCT: fibrosis (possible), honeycombing, emphysema
- Immunopathology: granulomatous pneumonitides may be seen in addition to bronchiolitis obliterans (with or without organizing pneumonia) and honeycombing and fibrosis, lymphocytic infiltration, centrilobular and bridging fibrosis, neutrophil-mediated air space destruction, giant cells

REFERRAL

- Bronchoscopy: BAL provides useful supportive data in the diagnosis of HP. Usually reveals intense lymphocytosis (typically T cells >50%) of predominantly CD8+ suppressor cells. In the acute stage neutrophils predominate, but as the disease progresses to chronic form the ratio of CD4+ to CD8+ cells increases. When fibrosis is present the number of neutrophils increases.
- Lung biopsy: the histopathologic features of HP are distinctive but not pathognomonic. Bronchiolitis and interstitial pneumonitis with granuloma formation typically is seen. Variable degrees of interstitial fibrosis are seen in the chronic form. Chronic HP may be difficult to distinguish from IPF or NSIP pathologically.
- Laboratory inhalation challenge: testing to prove a direct relation between a suspected antigen and disease; extract of antigen is inhaled by nebulizer.

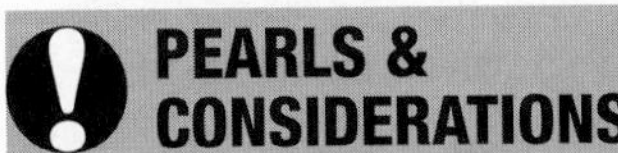

PEARLS & CONSIDERATIONS

A clinical prediction rule using six features has high specificity and sensitivity for the diagnosis of acute and subacute HP:
- Exposure to a known offending agent
- Positive specific precipitating antibody
- Recurrent episodes of symptoms
- Inspiratory crackles
- Symptoms occurring 4 to 8 hr after exposure
- Weight loss

HP occurs more frequently in smokers than nonsmokers (likely from an immunosuppressive effect).

SUGGESTED READINGS

available at www.expertconsult.com

RELATED CONTENT

Hypersensitivity Pneumonitis (Patient Information)

AUTHOR: **KRISTINA KRAMER, M.D.**

BASIC INFORMATION

DEFINITION

Hypersplenism is a syndrome characterized by splenomegaly, cytopenia (one or more of the following: anemia, thrombocytopenia, or leukopenia), and compensatory hyperplastic bone marrow. The cytopenias are correctable with splenectomy.

ICD-9CM CODES
289.4 Hypersplenism
ICD-10CM CODES
D73.1 Hypersplenism

EPIDEMIOLOGY & DEMOGRAPHICS

Most often seen in patients with liver disease, hematologic malignancy, and infection

PHYSICAL FINDINGS & CLINICAL PRESENTATION

- Symptoms depend on the size of the spleen, rate of growth, and underlying disease.
- History: early satiety, abdominal discomfort or fullness, left upper quadrant (LUQ) pleuritic pain (infarction), acute LUQ pain (sequestration crisis), referred pain to left shoulder
- Physical examination: splenomegaly (normal spleen usually not palpable), LUQ tenderness, presence of a rub in LUQ (suggestive of splenic infarct), stigmata of cytopenias

ETIOLOGY

The spleen is an important component of the hematologic and immune systems. It plays an important role in the synthesis, storage, and destruction of blood cells as well as antigen processing and antibody synthesis. The spleen has the unique function of filtering blood and removing defective blood cells and foreign particles. It removes microorganisms and other particulates (e.g., complement or antibody-coated cells) from the circulation. It is also responsible for the modification (removal of particles and parasites) and clearance of senescent or poorly deformable red blood cells (RBCs) from the circulation. The spleen is a platelet reservoir, storing 30% of platelet mass. It can become the site of hematopoiesis in certain disease states. The spleen's normal activities are augmented when enlarged.

- Splenomegaly increases the proportion of blood channeled through the red pulp, causing inappropriate splenic pooling of both normal and abnormal blood cells. The size of the spleen determines the amount of cell sequestration. Up to 90% of platelets may be pooled in an enlarged spleen.
- Prolonged sequestration leads to increased destruction of RBCs. Platelets and white blood cells (WBCs) have about normal survival time even when sequestered and may be available if needed.
- Splenomegaly exacerbates cytopenias by dilution, possibly due to plasma volume expansion.

DIAGNOSIS

DIFFERENTIAL DIAGNOSIS

Hypersplenism can be caused by splenomegaly of almost any cause.

- Splenic congestion: cirrhosis (portal hypertension); congestive heart failure; portal, splenic, or hepatic vein thrombosis
- Hematologic causes: hemolytic anemia, spherocytosis, elliptocytosis, sickle cell anemia, thalassemia, extramedullary hematopoiesis, chronic transfusions, following use of granulocyte colony-stimulating factor
- Infections: viral (hepatitis, infectious mononucleosis, cytomegalovirus, HIV/AIDS), bacterial (abscess, endocarditis, sepsis, tuberculosis, salmonella, brucella, Lyme's disease), parasitic (babesiosis, malaria, leishmaniasis, schistosomiasis, toxoplasmosis), fungal
- Malignancy: acute or chronic leukemia, lymphoma, histiocytosis, myeloproliferative diseases (polycythemia vera, essential thrombocythemia, myelofibrosis), metastatic tumors
- Inflammatory diseases: rheumatic fever, rheumatoid arthritis (Felty's syndrome), systemic lupus erythematosus, sarcoid, serum sickness
- Infiltrative diseases: amyloidosis, Gaucher's disease, Niemann-Pick disease, glycogen storage disease
- Anatomic abnormalities: cysts, hemangioma, hamartoma

LABORATORY TESTS

- CBC with differential: cytopenia, neutrophilia (infection)
- Peripheral smear: RBC and WBC morphology (abnormal cells may suggest infection, malignancy, bone marrow disease, rheumatologic disease), organisms (bacteria, malaria, babesiosis)
- Bone marrow aspiration/biopsy: hyperplasia of cytopenic cell lines; hematologic, infiltrative, or infectious disorders
- Tests to diagnose suspected cause of splenomegaly: liver function, hepatitis serology, HIV, rheumatoid factor, antinuclear antibody, tissue biopsy
- Note: red cell mass (^{51}Cr assay) may be used to assess severity of anemia. RBC mass measurement will differentiate true anemia (decrease in RBCs) from dilutional anemia (plasma volume expansion).

IMAGING STUDIES

- Ultrasound: splenic size, presence of cyst or abscess
- CT: estimate volume, obtain structural information: cyst, abscess, malignancy
- MRI: most useful for assessing vascular lesions and infections
- Nuclear medicine: liver-spleen scan: assess anatomy and function; may suggest presence of portal hypertension
- Consider other studies as suggested by history and examination: chest radiograph, echocardiogram, PET scan

TREATMENT

ACUTE GENERAL Rx

- Treat underlying disease
- Splenectomy is considered if:
  1. Indicated for the management of the underlying cause
  2. Persistent symptomatic disease (severe cytopenia) not responding to therapy
  3. Necessary for diagnosis

  Risks:
- Infections (especially encapsulated organisms): risk greatest in the first 2 yr after splenectomy. Mortality rate from sepsis is fiftyfold greater in asplenic patients. Attempts to decrease risk include:
  - Immunization with pneumococcal (PPSV23), meningococcal (2 doses), and *Haemophilus influenzae* vaccines at least 2 wk before splenectomy. Pneumococcal (PCV13) one-time vaccination >1 year after PPSV23. Revaccination for pneumococcal (PPSV23) in 5 yr and again after 65 yr. Revaccination for meningococcal every 5 yr. Annual influenza vaccination.
  - Prophylactic antibiotics after splenectomy in highest-risk patients.
  - Patient education regarding the importance of rapid initiation of antibiotics at the first sign of infection.
- Rapid increase in platelet count may cause thromboembolic complications.
- Possible increased risk of atherosclerotic heart disease.
- Splenectomy should not be performed if the spleen is the main site of hematopoiesis as a result of bone marrow failure (e.g., myelofibrosis).
- Other options include partial splenectomy, partial splenic embolization, radiofrequency ablation, portosystemic shunting (for congestive splenomegaly).

DISPOSITION

- Cytopenias usually correctable with splenectomy; normal cell counts in a few wk.
- Splenectomy may alleviate portal hypertension.
- Prognosis depends on the underlying disease.

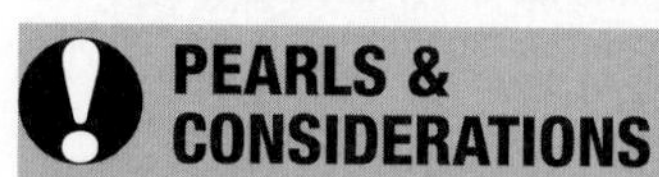

PEARLS & CONSIDERATIONS

- Thrombocytopenia in hypersplenism is usually moderately severe (>50 × 10^9/L) and asymptomatic; severe thrombocytopenia (<20 × 10^9/L) suggests another diagnosis.

SUGGESTED READINGS

available at www.expertconsult.com

RELATED CONTENT

Felty's Syndrome (Related Key Topic)
Fig. 3-179 Clinical approach to patient with splenomegaly (Algorithm)
Hypersplenism (Patient Information)

AUTHOR: **SUDEEP KAUR AULAKH, M.D.**

BASIC INFORMATION

DEFINITION

Normal blood pressure (BP) in adults can be defined as systolic BP <120 mm Hg and diastolic <80 mm Hg. *Prehypertension* is defined as systolic BP between 120 to 139 mm Hg or diastolic between 80 to 89 mm Hg. *Stage 1 hypertension* (HTN) is systolic BP from 140 to 159 mm Hg or diastolic BP from 90 to 99 mm Hg. *Stage 2 HTN* is systolic BP ≥160 mm Hg or diastolic BP ≥100 mm Hg.

SYNONYMS

Essential hypertension
Idiopathic hypertension
High BP

ICD-9CM CODES
401.1 Essential hypertension (HTN)
401.0-9 with 5th digit 1Renovascular hypertension
405 Secondary hypertension
642 Hypertension complicating pregnancy
437.2 Hypertensive encephalopathy

ICD-10CM CODES
I10 Essential (primary) hypertension
I15.0 Renovascular hypertension
O10.919 Unspecified pre-existing hypertension complicating pregnancy, unspecified trimester
I67.4 Hypertensive encephalopathy

EPIDEMIOLOGY & DEMOGRAPHICS

PREVALENCE: Based on NHANES data in 2005 to 2008, between 29% and 31% of U.S. adults have HTN (approximately 65 million) and only 31 million (46%) have it well controlled. There are around 1 billion individuals worldwide who meet the criteria for diagnosis of HTN.
PEAK PREVALENCE: Males and the elderly

PHYSICAL FINDINGS & CLINICAL PRESENTATION

Physical examination may be entirely within normal limits except for the presence of elevated BP. A proper initial physical examination on a hypertensive patient should include the following:

- The BP should be measured with an appropriately sized cuff (bladder of the cuff should cover at least two thirds of the circumference of the arm) and in both arms (the higher of the readings being used).
- The BP should be measured twice on each visit, and separated by at least 1 to 2 min to allow the return of trapped blood.
- Postural BP change should always be recorded in elderly to diagnose postural hypotension. This is assessed by taking BP in supine (after 5-minute rest) and standing (after 2 minutes) positions. A drop of ≥20 mm Hg in systolic, a drop of ≥10 mm Hg diastolic BP, or symptoms of cerebral hypoperfusion is suggestive of postural (orthostatic) hypotension.
- A diagnosis of HTN may be established if the BP is markedly elevated (>180/110 mm Hg) or has evidence of end organ damage; otherwise such a diagnosis should wait until BP is found elevated on at least 3-6 visits, spaced over a period of weeks to months.
- Measure heart rate, height, weight, body mass index, and waist circumference.
- Examine skin for the presence of café-au-lait spots (neurofibromatosis), uremic appearance (renal failure), and violaceous striae (Cushing's syndrome).
- Perform careful funduscopic examination; check for papilledema, retinal exudates, hemorrhages, arterial narrowing, arteriovenous compression.
- Examine neck for carotid bruits, distended neck veins, and enlarged thyroid gland.
- Perform extensive cardiopulmonary examination: check for loud aortic component of S_2, S_4, ventricular lift, murmurs, and arrhythmias.
- Palpate abdomen for renal masses (pheochromocytoma, polycystic kidneys), and auscultate for bruit over the aorta and renal arteries.
- Examine arterial pulses (dilated or absent femoral pulses and BP greater in upper extremities than lower extremities suggest aortic coarctation).
- Look for truncal obesity (Cushing's syndrome) and pedal edema (congestive heart failure [CHF]).
- The clinical evaluation should help to determine if the patient has primary or secondary (possibly reversible) HTN, if there is target organ disease present, and if there are additional cardiovascular risk factors. Table 1-264 provides a guide to evaluation of identifiable causes of HTN. Fig. E1-495 and Box E1-42 describe the investigation of suspected endocrine causes of HTN.

ETIOLOGY

- Essential (primary) HTN (85%)
- Drug induced or drug related (5%)
  1. NSAIDs
  2. Oral contraceptives
  3. Corticosteroids
- Renal HTN (5%)
  1. Renal parenchymal disease (3%)
  2. Renovascular HTN (RVH) (<2%)
- Endocrine (<2%)
  1. Primary aldosteronism (0.5%)
  2. Pheochromocytoma (0.2%)
  3. Cushing's syndrome and long-term steroid therapy (0.2%)
  4. Hyperparathyroidism or thyroid disease (0.2%)
- Coarctation of the aorta (0.2%)

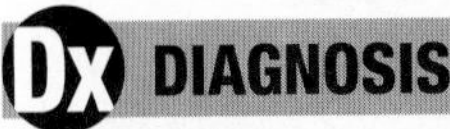

DIAGNOSIS

WORKUP

- The objective for the initial evaluation of HTN is to establish the diagnosis and stage of HTN.
- Gather office and nonoffice BP readings, assess presence of target organ damage (TOD), assess the level of global cardiovascular disease risk and produce a plan for individualized monitoring and therapy.
- ECG, CXR, renal imaging, and tests for plasma aldosterone/plasma renin activity are not routinely recommended at the initial evaluation stage of the patient with newly diagnosed HTN.
- Patient counseling and education should be prominent features of the initial evaluation.

TABLE 1-264 Guide to Evaluation of Identifiable Causes of Hypertension

Suspected Diagnosis	Clinical Clues	Diagnostic Testing
Chronic kidney disease	Estimated GFR <60 ml/min/1.73 m^2 Urine albumin-to-creatinine ratio ≥30 mg/g	Renal sonography
Renovascular disease	New elevation in serum creatinine, marked elevation in serum creatinine with ACEI or ARB, drug-resistant hypertension, flash pulmonary edema, abdominal, or flank bruit	Renal sonography (atrophic kidney), CT or MR angiography, invasive angiography
Coarctation of the aorta	Arm pulses > leg pulses, arm BP > leg BP, chest bruits, rib notching on chest radiography	MR angiography, TEE, invasive angiography
Primary aldosteronism	Hypokalemia, drug-resistant hypertension	Plasma renin and aldosterone, 24-hr urine aldosterone and potassium after oral salt loading, adrenal vein sampling
Cushing's syndrome	Truncal obesity, wide and blanching purple striae, muscle weakness	1 mg dexamethasone-suppression test, urinary cortisol after dexamethasone, adrenal CT
Pheochromocytoma	Paroxysms of hypertension, palpitations, perspiration, and pallor; diabetes	Plasma metanephrines, 24-hr urinary metanephrines and catecholamines, abdominal CT or MR imaging
Obstructive sleep apnea	Loud snoring, large neck, obesity, somnolence	Polysomography

ACEI, Angiotensin-converting enzyme inhibitor; *ARB,* angiotensin receptor blocker; *BP,* blood pressure; *CT,* computed tomography; *GFR,* glomerular filtration rate; *MR,* magnetic resonance; *TEE,* transesophageal echocardiography.
From Goldman L, Schafer AI: *Goldman's Cecil medicine,* ed 24, Philadelphia, 2012, Saunders.

- Pertinent history:
  - Age of onset of HTN, previous antihypertensive therapy
  - Family history of HTN, stroke, cardiovascular disease
- Diet, salt intake, alcohol, drugs (e.g., oral contraceptives, NSAIDs, decongestants, steroids)
- Occupation, lifestyle, socioeconomic status, psychologic factors
- Other cardiovascular risk factors: hyperlipidemia, obesity, diabetes mellitus
- Symptoms of secondary HTN:
  1. Headache, palpitations, excessive perspiration (possible pheochromocytoma)
  2. Weakness, polyuria (consider hyperaldosteronism)
  3. Claudication of lower extremities (seen with coarctation of aorta)

LABORATORY TESTS

- Urinalysis with microscopic evaluation, blood urea nitrogen and creatinine, and an albumin/creatinine ratio; for evidence of renal disease. High-serum creatinine is a predictor of cardiovascular risk in essential HTN.
- Nonoffice (home, workplace, 24-hr ambulatory) BP determination to establish the pattern of HTN (sustained, "white coat," or "masked" HTN).
- Serum electrolyte levels: low potassium is suggestive of primary aldosteronism or diuretic use.
- Screening for coexisting diseases that may adversely affect prognosis:
  1. Fasting serum glucose
  2. Serum lipid panel, uric acid, calcium
  3. If pheochromocytoma is suspected: 24-hr urine metanephrines

IMAGING STUDIES

- ECG: check for presence of left ventricular hypertrophy (LVH) with strain pattern.
- Magnetic resonance angiography of the renal arteries in suspected RVH (renal artery stenosis).

Rx TREATMENT

NONPHARMACOLOGIC THERAPY

Lifestyle modifications:

- Weight loss if overweight (target BMI <25).
- Limit alcohol intake to 1 oz of ethanol per day (<2 drinks/day) in men or 0.5 oz (<1 drink/day) in women.
- Regular aerobic exercise (at least 30 min/day on most days).
- Reduce sodium intake to <100 mmol/day (<1.5 g of sodium/day).
- Maintain adequate dietary potassium (>3500 mg/day) intake in patients with normal kidney function.
- Stop smoking.
- The BP reduction seen ranges from 2 to 20 mm Hg, most significant with substantial weight loss and the implementation of the Dietary Approaches to Stop Hypertension (DASH) eating plan, which relies on a diet high in fruits and vegetables, moderate in low-fat dairy products, and low in animal protein but with substantial amount of plant protein from legumes and nuts.

ACUTE GENERAL RX

According to the JNC 8[1]:

- In all patients, initiate pharmacologic treatment if diastolic BP is ≥90 mm Hg. In patients <60 years old, in diabetics, and in those with chronic kidney disease, pharmacologic treatment should be initiated for systolic BP ≥140 mm Hg, whereas in patients ≥60 years, the threshold for pharmacologic treatment for systolic BP has been raised to ≥150 mm Hg.
- In the general non-black population, preferred initial agents are thiazide-type diuretics, angiotensin-converting enzyme inhibitors (ACEi), calcium channel blockers (CCBs), or angiotensin receptor blockers (ARBs). ACEi or ARBs are preferred initial agents in diabetics and those with CKD in this population.
- Preferred initial agents in the black population (including diabetics) are thiazide-type diuretics or CCBs.
- When selecting drugs, try to give once per day dosages to improve compliance. Also consider the cost of the medication, metabolic and subjective side effects, and drug-drug interactions.
- The major advantages and limitations of each class of drugs are described as follows:
  1. Diuretics:
     a. Advantages: inexpensive, once-daily dosing. Useful in edematous states, CHF, chronic renal disease, elderly patients (decreased incidence of hip fractures in elderly patients)
     b. Disadvantages: significant adverse metabolic effects, increased risk of cardiac arrhythmias, sexual dysfunction, possible adverse effects on lipids and glucose levels
  2. Beta-blockers:
     a. Advantages: ideal in hypertensive patients with ischemic heart disease or status post MI. Favored in hyperkinetic, young patients (resting tachycardia, wide pulse pressure, hyperdynamic heart) and stable CHF patients.
     b. Disadvantages: adverse effect on quality of life (increased incidence of fatigue, depression, impotence), bronchospasm, hypoglycemia, peripheral vascular disease, adverse effects on lipids, masking of signs and symptoms of hypoglycemia in diabetics.
  3. Calcium antagonists:
     a. Advantages: helpful in hypertensive patients with ischemic heart disease. Generally favorable effect on quality of life; can be used in patients with bronchospastic disorders, renal disease, peripheral vascular disease, metabolic disorders, and salt sensitivity. CCBs BP-lowering effect is independent of Na^+ intake.
     b. Disadvantages: diltiazem and verapamil should be avoided in patients with CHF due to systolic dysfunction because of their negative inotropic effects; pedal edema may occur with nifedipine and amlodipine; constipation can be severe in elderly patients receiving verapamil. CCB-related edema is positional in nature, it improves with lying position; additional strategies include switching CCB classes, reducing dosage, giving the medication later in the day, and adding a venodilator (nitrates, an ACE, or an ARB); diuretics may improve edema, but at the expense of a reduction in plasma volume.
  4. ACE inhibitors:
     a. Advantages: well tolerated, favorable impact on quality of life; useful in HTN complicated by CHF; helpful in prevention of diabetic renal disease; effective in decreasing LVH.
     b. Disadvantages: cough is a frequent side effect (5% to 20% of patients); hyperkalemia may occur in patients with diabetes or severe renal insufficiency; hypotension may occur in volume-depleted patients; increased risk of renal failure in patients with renal artery stenosis; contraindicated in pregnancy.
  5. ARBs:
     a. Advantages: well tolerated, favorable impact on quality of life; useful in patients unable to tolerate ACE inhibitors because of persistent cough and in CHF and diabetic patients; single daily dose. An episode of renal insufficiency with ACE inhibitors does not rule out future therapy with an ARB unless high-grade bilateral renal artery stenosis exists.
     b. Disadvantages: excessive cost; hypotension may occur in volume-depleted patients; hyperkalemia; risk of renal failure in renal artery stenosis; contraindicated in pregnancy.
  6. Renin inhibitors: newest class of antihypertensives (Aliskiren):
     a. Advantages: generally well tolerated; once-daily dosing; can be used alone or in combination with other antihypertensive agents (avoid combining with ACEI or ARBs given increase of hyperkalemia)
     b. Disadvantages: contraindicated in pregnancy; should not be used in patients with impaired renal function; excessive cost; paucity of cardiovascular outcomes data showing benefit.
  7. Alpha-adrenergic blockers:
     a. Advantages: no adverse effect on blood lipids or insulin sensitivity; helpful in benign prostatic hypertrophy.

[1] James PA et al: 2014 Evidence-based guidelines for the management of high blood pressure in adults. Report from the panel members appointed to the eighth Joint National Committee (JNC8), *JAMA* 311(5):507-520, 2014.

b. Disadvantages: postural hypotension, sedation; syncope can be avoided by giving an initial low dose at bedtime.
8. Central alpha-antagonists:
   a. Oral clonidine mainstay of therapy for hypertensive urgencies because of the ease of administration and relative safety.
   b. Transdermal clonidine; useful in management of labile HTN, the hospitalized patient who cannot take medications by mouth, and patients subject to early morning BP surges. At equivalent doses, transdermal clonidine is more apt to precipitate salt and water retention than is the case with oral clonidine.
   c. Dose beyond 0.4 mg causes fatigue, sedation and dry mouth, salt and water retention, and rebound HTN upon abrupt termination of the medication.
9. Combined alpha- and beta-adrenergic receptor blockers:
   a. Labetalol, nebivolol, and carvedilol: Use is reserved to treat complicated hypertensive patient when an antihypertensive effect beyond beta-blockade is sought. IV labetalol is used for hypertensive emergencies. Carvedilol is shown to have less adverse effect on glycemic control than metoprolol and to reduce urinary protein excretion in hypertensive diabetic patients.

TREATMENT OF RENOVASCULAR HYPERTENSION: The therapeutic approach varies with the cause of the RVH (refer to "Renal Artery Stenosis" for additional information).

1. Young patients with fibromuscular dysplasia refractory to medical therapy can be treated with percutaneous transluminal renal angioplasty (PTRA).
2. Medical therapy is advisable in elderly patients with atheromatous RVH; useful agents are:
   a. Beta-blockers: highly effective in patients with elevated plasma renin
   b. ACE inhibitors: highly effective; however, should be avoided in patients with bilateral renal artery stenosis or with a solitary kidney and renal stenosis
   c. Diuretics: often used in combination with ACE inhibitors
3. Surgical revascularization: A recent trial revealed that renal-artery stenting does not confer a significant benefit with respect to the prevention of clinical events when added to comprehensive, multifactorial medical therapy in people with atherosclerotic renal-artery stenosis and hypertension or chronic kidney disease.[2]

HTN DURING PREGNANCY:

1. HTN complicates 5% to 12% of all pregnancies.
2. The American Obstetrical Committee defines BP of 130/80 mm Hg as the upper limit of normal at any time during pregnancy.
3. A rise of 30 mm Hg systolic or 15 mm Hg diastolic is also considered abnormal regardless of the absolute values obtained.
4. Chronic HTN (occurring before pregnancy) must be distinguished from preeclampsia because the risk to mother and fetus is much greater in the latter.
5. Treatment of chronic HTN during pregnancy is as follows:
   a. Initial treatment with conservative measures (proper nutrition, limited physical activity).
   b. When drug therapy is necessary, initiation of methyldopa, hydralazine, labetalol, or atenolol is preferred.
   c. ACE inhibitors can cause fetal and neonatal complications; their use should be avoided in pregnancy.
   d. The safety of CCBs remains unclear.
   e. Diuretics should be used only if there is a specific reason for initiating and maintaining their use (e.g., HTN associated with severe fluid overload or left ventricular dysfunction).

MALIGNANT HTN, HYPERTENSIVE EMERGENCIES, AND HYPERTENSIVE URGENCIES:

Definitions:

1. Malignant HTN is a potentially life-threatening situation caused by elevated BP.
   a. The rate of BP rise is a critical factor.
   b. The clinical manifestations are grade IV hypertensive retinopathy (exudates, hemorrhages, and papilledema); cardiovascular involvement (acute aortic dissection, acute left ventricular failure, acute myocardial infarction; cerebrovascular involvement), encephalopathy, intracerebral hemorrhage; or renal compromise.
   c. Requires immediate BP reduction (not necessarily into normal ranges) to prevent or limit target organ disease.
2. Hypertensive emergencies require rapid (within 1 hr) lowering of BP to prevent end-organ damage.
3. Hypertensive urgencies are significant BP elevations that should be corrected within 24 hr of presentation.

Therapy: The choice of therapeutic agents varies with the cause. IV medications are preferred in hypertensive emergencies.

1. Nitroprusside is the drug of choice in hypertensive encephalopathy, HTN and intracranial bleeding, malignant HTN, HTN and heart failure, dissecting aortic aneurysm (used in combination with propranolol); its onset of action is immediate.
2. Fenoldopam is a vasodilator agent useful for the short-term (up to 48 hr) management of severe HTN when rapid but quickly reversible reduction of BP is required. It should be avoided in patients with glaucoma.
3. Other commonly used agents are the IV CCBs nicardipine and clevidipine (useful for urgent treatment of HTN in the intensive care unit or operating room), the beta-blocker esmolol (useful in aortic dissection or postoperative HTN), labetalol (combined β-adrenergic and α-blocker useful in patients with coronary disease), phentolamine (useful for catecholamine-related emergencies), IV nitroglycerin (used in patients with cardiac ischemia and hypertensive crisis), and hydralazine (used for hypertensive emergencies in pregnancy).
4. Table 1-265 describes parenteral agents for management of hypertensive emergencies. *The following are important points to remember when treating hypertensive emergencies:*
   a. Introduce a plan for long-term therapy at the time of the initial emergency treatment.
   b. Agents that reduce arterial pressure can cause the kidney to retain sodium and water; therefore the judicious administration of diuretics should accompany their use.
   c. The initial goal of antihypertensive therapy is not to achieve a normal BP, but rather to gradually reduce the BP; cerebral hypoperfusion may occur if the mean BP is lowered >40% in the initial 24 hr.

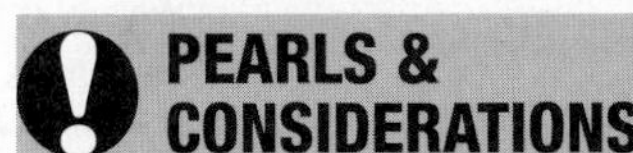

PEARLS & CONSIDERATIONS

COMMENTS

- For patients with prehypertension, every 20/10 mm Hg increase in BP doubles the risk of cardiovascular events.
- Most patients will require at least two medications for BP control.
- If BP is greater than 20/10 mm Hg above goal, therapy should be initiated with two drugs.
- A practical approach to multidrug therapy is use of fixed-dose antihypertensive combinations as an alternative to the sequenced addition of two or three drugs.
- Resistant HTN: HTN is considered resistant if the BP cannot be reduced below target levels in patients who are compliant with an optimal triple-drug regimen that includes a diuretic. Terms *refractory* and *resistant* are used interchangeably. Causes include pseudohypertension, measurement artifact, medication nonadherence, volume overload, and secondary HTN.
  - Pseudohypertension in elderly: hardened and sclerotic artery is not compressible hence falsely elevates BP measurement artifact
  - Measurement artifact: BP taken with a small cuff in people with large arm diameter. BP should be taken with the patient in the seated position and the arm supported at heart level, the bladder within the cuff should encircle at least 80% of the arm diameter.

Fig. E1-496 describes an approach to patients with resistant HTN.

- Renal sympathetic denervation: A recent blinded trial did not show a significant reduction of systolic blood pressure in patients with resistant hypertension 6 mo after renal artery denervation as compared with a sham control.[3]

[2] Cooper CJ et al: Stenting and medical therapy for atherosclerotic renal-artery stenosis, *N Engl J Med* 370:13-22, 2014.

[3] Bhatt DL et al: A controlled trial of renal denervation for resistant hypertension, *N Engl J Med* 370:1393-1401, 2014.

TABLE 1-265 Parenteral Agents for Management of Hypertensive Emergencies

Agent	Dose	Onset of Action	Precautions
Parenteral Vasodilators			
Sodium nitroprusside	0.25-10 mcg/kg/min IV infusion	Immediate	Thiocyanate toxicity with prolonged use
Nitroglycerin	5-100 mcg/min IV infusion	2-5 min	Headache, tachycardia, tolerance
Nicardipine	5-15 mg/hr IV infusion	1-5 min	Protracted hypotension after prolonged use
Fenoldopam mesylate	0.1-0.3 mcg/kg/min IV infusion	1-5 min	Headache, tachycardia, increased intraocular pressure
Hydralazine	5-10 mg as IV bolus or 10-40 mg IM; repeat every 4-6 hr	10 min IV 20 min IM	Unpredictable and excessive falls in blood pressure; tachycardia, angina exacerbation
Enalaprilat	0.625-1.25 mg every 6 hr IV bolus	15-60 min	Unpredictable and excessive falls in blood pressure; acute renal failure in patients with bilateral renal artery stenosis
Parenteral Adrenergic Inhibitors			
Labetalol	20-80 mg as slow IV injection every 10 min, or 0.5-2.0 mg/min IV as infusion	5-10 min	Bronchospasm, heart block, orthostatic hypotension
Metoprolol	5 mg IV every 10 min for three doses	5-10 min	Bronchospasm, heart block, heart failure, exacerbation of cocaine-induced myocardial ischemia
Esmolol	500 mcg/kg IV over 3 min; then 25-100 mg/kg/min as IV infusion	1-5 min	Bronchospasm, heart block, heart failure
Phentolamine	5-10 mg IV bolus every 5-15 min	1-2 min	Tachycardia, orthostatic hypotension

IM, Intramuscular; *IV*, intravenous.
From Andreoli TE et al: *Andreoli and Carpenter's Cecil essentials of medicine,* ed 8, Philadelphia, 2010, Saunders.

TABLE 1-266 Indications for Specialist Referral for Patients with Hypertension

Urgent Treatment Needed
Accelerated hypertension (severe hypertension with grade III-IV retinopathy)
Particularly severe hypertension (>220/120 mm Hg)
Impending complications (e.g., transient ischemic attack, left ventricular failure)
Possible Underlying Cause
Any clue in history or examination of a secondary cause (e.g., hypokalemia with increased or high–normal plasma sodium)
Elevated serum creatinine
Proteinuria or hematuria
Sudden onset or worsening of hypertension
Young age (any hypertension <20 years; needing treatment <30 years)
Therapeutic Problems
Multiple drug intolerances
Multiple drug contraindications
Persistent nonadherence or nonconcordance
Special Situations
Unusual blood pressure variability
Possible white coat hypertension
Hypertension in pregnancy

From Floege J et al: *Comprehensive clinical nephrology,* ed 4, Philadelphia, 2010, Saunders.

- Fig. E1-497 describes an algorithm for evaluation of secondary causes of HTN.
- Barriers to BP control: system issues, provider issues; patient issues, and behavior issues. The rate at which physicians adopt recommended changes based on evidence-based findings can be quite slow and has been properly described as "clinical inertia."
- ACE-ARB combination therapy has gained popularity in the primary care setting, but this practice should be discouraged. Recent studies assessing dual renin-angiotensin-aldosterone system blockade with ACE-ARB combination have not supported the use of this combination.
- Indications for specialist referral for patients with HTN are described in Table 1-266.

SUGGESTED READINGS

available at www.expertconsult.com

RELATED CONTENT

High Blood Pressure (Patient Information)
High Blood Pressure–Child (Patient Information)
Renal Artery Stenosis (Related Key Topic)

AUTHORS: **SAINATH GADDAM, M.D., FRED F. FERRI, M.D.,** and **HILARY B. WHITLATCH, M.D.**

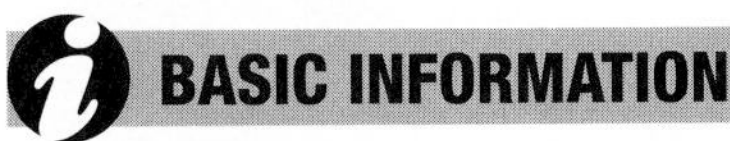

BASIC INFORMATION

DEFINITION

Hyperthyroidism is a hypermetabolic state resulting from excess thyroid hormone.

SYNONYMS

Thyrotoxicosis

ICD-9CM CODES
242.9 Hyperthyroidism
242.0 Hyperthyroidism with goiter
242.2 Hyperthyroidism, multinodular
242.3 Hyperthyroidism, uninodular
ICD-10CM CODES
E05.90 Thyrotoxicosis, unspecified without thyrotoxic crisis or storm
E05.00 Thyrotoxicosis with diffuse goiter without thyrotoxic crisis or storm
E05.20 Thyrotoxicosis with toxic multinodular goiter without thyrotoxic crisis or storm

EPIDEMIOLOGY & DEMOGRAPHICS

INCIDENCE/PREVALENCE:

- Hyperthyroidism affects 2% of women and 0.2% of men in their lifetimes.
- Toxic multinodular goiter usually occurs in women >55 yr and is more common than Graves' disease in the elderly.

PHYSICAL FINDINGS & CLINICAL PRESENTATION

- Patients with hyperthyroidism generally present with tachycardia, tremor, hyperreflexia, anxiety, irritability, emotional lability, panic attacks, heat intolerance, sweating, increased appetite, diarrhea, weight loss, menstrual dysfunction (oligomenorrhea, amenorrhea). Presentation may be different in elderly patients (see below).
- Patients with Graves' disease may present with exophthalmos, lid retraction, and lid lag (Graves' ophthalmopathy). The following signs and symptoms of ophthalmopathy may be present: blurring of vision, photophobia, increased lacrimation, double vision, and deep orbital pressure. Clubbing of fingers associated with periosteal new bone formation in other skeletal areas (Graves' acropachy) and pretibial myxedema may also be noted.
- Clinical signs of hyperthyroidism in the elderly may be masked by manifestations of coexisting disease (e.g., new-onset atrial fibrillation, exacerbation of congestive heart failure).

ETIOLOGY

- Graves' disease (diffuse toxic goiter): 80% to 90% of all cases of hyperthyroidism
- Toxic multinodular goiter (Plummer's disease)
- Toxic adenoma
- Iatrogenic and factitious
- Transient hyperthyroidism (subacute thyroiditis, Hashimoto's thyroiditis)
- Rare causes: hypersecretion of thyroid-stimulating hormone (TSH) (e.g., pituitary neoplasms), struma ovarii, ingestion of large amount of iodine in a patient with preexisting thyroid hyperplasia or adenoma (Jod-Basedow phenomenon), hydatidiform mole, carcinoma of thyroid, amiodarone therapy

DIAGNOSIS

DIFFERENTIAL DIAGNOSIS

- Anxiety disorder
- Pheochromocytoma
- Metastatic neoplasm
- Diabetes mellitus
- Premenopausal state

WORKUP

Suspected hyperthyroidism requires laboratory confirmation and identification of its etiology because treatment varies with cause. A detailed medical history will often provide clues to the diagnosis and etiology of the hyperthyroidism. Fig. E1-498 describes a diagnostic approach to suspected hyperthyroidism.

LABORATORY TESTS

- Elevated free thyroxine (T_4)
- Elevated free triiodothyronine (T_3): generally not necessary for diagnosis
- Low TSH (unless hyperthyroidism is a result of the rare hypersecretion of TSH from a pituitary adenoma)
- Thyroid autoantibodies useful in selected cases to differentiate Graves' disease from toxic multinodular goiter (absent thyroid antibodies)

IMAGING STUDIES

- 24-hr radioactive iodine uptake (RAIU) is useful to distinguish hyperthyroidism from iatrogenic thyroid hormone synthesis (thyrotoxicosis factitia) and from thyroiditis.
- An overactive thyroid shows increased uptake, whereas a normal underactive thyroid (iatrogenic thyroid ingestion, painless or subacute thyroiditis) shows normal or decreased uptake.
- The RAIU results also vary with the etiology of the hyperthyroidism:
  - Graves' disease: increased homogeneous uptake
  - Multinodular goiter: increased heterogeneous uptake
  - Hot nodule: single focus of increased uptake
- RAIU is also generally performed before the therapeutic administration of radioactive iodine to determine the appropriate dose.

TREATMENT

NONPHARMACOLOGIC THERAPY

Patient education regarding thyroid disease and discussion of the therapeutic options. Patients should be informed that radioiodine, antithyroid drugs, and surgery are all reasonable treatment options for hyperthyroidism. It is crucial for the physician to have a detailed discussion with the patient about the benefits and risks relative to lifestyle, patients' values, and coexisting conditions.

ACUTE GENERAL Rx

ANTITHYROID DRUGS (THIONAMIDES):

Propylthiouracil (PTU) and methimazole inhibit thyroid hormone synthesis by blocking production of thyroid peroxidase (PTU and methimazole) or inhibit peripheral conversion of T_4 to T_3 (PTU). Methimazole is favored by most endocrinologists because of the potential for hepatic failure with PTU. PTU is preferred in pregnant women because methimazole has been associated with aplasia cutis and with choanal and esophageal atresia. Complete blood count and differential should be obtained before their use.

1. Dosage: methimazole 15 to 30 mg/day given as a single dose; PTU 50 to 100 mg PO q8h.
2. Antithyroid drugs can be used as the primary form of treatment or as adjunctive therapy before radioactive therapy or surgery or afterward if the hyperthyroidism recurs.
3. Side effects: skin rash (3% to 5% of patients), arthralgias, myalgias, granulocytopenia (0.5%). Rare side effects are aplastic anemia, hepatic necrosis from PTU, cholestatic jaundice from methimazole.
4. When antithyroid drugs are used as primary therapy, they are usually given for 6 to 18 mo; prolonged therapy may cause hypothyroidism. Monitor thyroid function every 2 mo for 6 mo, then less frequently.
5. The use of antithyroid drugs before radioiodine therapy is best reserved for patients in whom exacerbation of hyperthyroidism after radioactive iodine therapy is hazardous (e.g., elderly patients with coronary artery disease or significant coexisting morbidity). In these patients the antithyroid drug can be stopped 2 days before radioactive iodine therapy, resumed 2 days later, and continued for 4 to 6 wk.

RADIOIODINE THERAPY (RADIOACTIVE IODINE [RAI; ^{131}I]):

1. RAI is the treatment of choice for patients aged >21 yr and younger patients who have not achieved remission after 1 yr of antithyroid drug therapy. RAI is also used in hyperthyroidism caused by toxic adenoma or toxic multinodular goiter.
2. Contraindicated during pregnancy (can cause fetal hypothyroidism) and lactation. Pregnancy should be excluded in women of childbearing age before RAI is administered.
3. A single dose of RAI is effective in inducing a euthyroid state in nearly 80% of patients.
4. There is a high incidence of post-RAI hypothyroidism (>50% within first year and 2%/yr thereafter); these patients should be frequently evaluated for the onset of hypothyroidism (see "Chronic Rx").

SURGICAL THERAPY (SUBTOTAL THYROIDECTOMY):

1. Indicated in obstructing goiters, in any patient who refuses RAI and cannot be adequately managed with antithyroid medications (e.g., patients with toxic adenoma or toxic multinodular goiter), and in pregnant

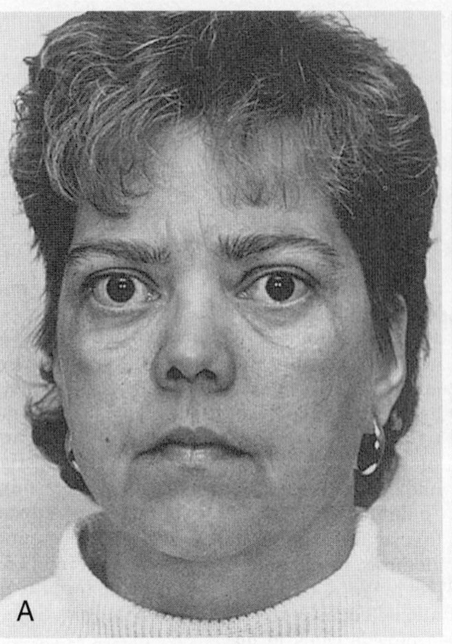

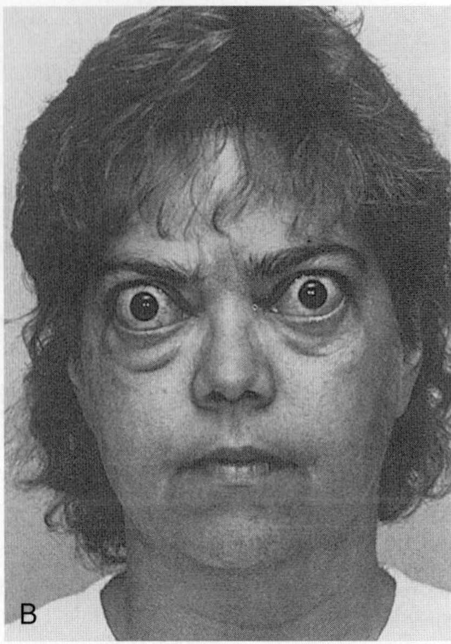

FIGURE 1-499 Characteristic signs of Graves' orbitopathy. A, Subsequently corrected by orbital decompression surgery. **B,** Note the thyroid stare, asymmetry, proptosis, and periorbital edema before correction. (Courtesy Dr. Jack Rootman, University of British Columbia, Vancouver, Canada. From Larsen PR et al [eds]: *Williams textbook of endocrinology,* ed 10, Philadelphia, 2003, Saunders.)

patients who cannot be adequately managed with antithyroid medication or develop side effects to them. Thyroidectomy can also be considered as primary therapy in refractory cases of amiodarone-induced hyperthyroidism. Thyroidectomy is not indicated for low RAIU hyperthyroidism.

2. Patients should be rendered euthyroid with antithyroid drugs before surgery.
3. Complications of surgery include hypothyroidism (28% to 43% after 10 yr), hypoparathyroidism, and vocal cord paralysis (1%).
4. Most patients should be started on replacement doses of levothyroxine (1.7 mcg/kg/day) before discharge from hospital.
5. Hyperthyroidism recurs after surgery in 10% to 15% of patients.

ADJUNCTIVE THERAPY: Propranolol alleviates the beta-adrenergic symptoms of hyperthyroidism; initial dose is 20 to 40 mg PO q6h; dosage is gradually increased until symptoms are controlled. Major contraindications to propranolol are congestive heart failure and bronchospasm. Diagnosis and treatment of thyrotoxic storm is also discussed in Section I.

CHRONIC Rx

- Patients undergoing treatment with antithyroid drugs should be seen every 1 to 3 mo until euthyroidism is achieved and every 3 to 4 mo while they remain on antithyroid therapy. After treatment is stopped, periodic monitoring of thyroid function tests with TSH is recommended every 3 mo for 1 yr, then every 6 mo for 1 yr, then annually.
- Orbital decompression surgery can be used to correct Graves' orbitopathy (Fig. 1-499). The administration of the antioxidant selenium (100 mcg PO bid) has been recently reported as effective in improving quality of life, reducing ocular involvement, and slowing progression of the disease in patients with mild Graves' orbitopathy. Its mechanism of action is believed to be an effect on the oxygen free radicals and cytokines that play a pathogenic role in Graves' orbitopathy.

DISPOSITION

Successful treatment of hyperthyroidism requires lifelong monitoring for the onset of hypothyroidism or the recurrence of thyrotoxicosis.

REFERRAL

- Endocrinology referral is recommended at the time of initial diagnosis and during treatment.
- Surgical referral in selected patients (see "Surgical Therapy").
- Hospitalization of all patients with thyroid storm.

PEARLS & CONSIDERATIONS

COMMENTS

- Elderly hyperthyroid patients may have only subtle signs (weight loss, tachycardia, fine skin, brittle nails). This form is known as ***apathetic hyperthyroidism*** and manifests with lethargy rather than hyperkinetic activity. An enlarged thyroid gland may be absent. Coexisting medical disorders (most commonly cardiac disease) may also mask the symptoms. These patients often have unexplained congestive heart failure, worsening of angina, or new-onset atrial fibrillation resistant to treatment. See the entry "Graves' Disease" for additional information on diagnosis and treatment.
- Subclinical hyperthyroidism is defined as a normal serum-free thyroxine and free triiodothyronine levels with a TSH level suppressed below the normal range and usually undetectable. These patients usually do not present with signs or symptoms of overt hyperthyroidism. Treatment options include observation or a therapeutic trial of low-dose antithyroid agents for 6 mo to attempt to induce remission.
- ***Thyrotoxic periodic paralysis (TPP)*** is a hyperthyroidism-related hypokalemia and muscle-weakening condition resulting from a sudden shift of potassium into cells. Many patients do not have other symptoms of hyperthyroidism. Typical presentation involves an Asian adult male with acute fatigue and muscle weakness initially presenting in the lower extremities. Physical examination reveals decreased deep tendon reflexes, hypertension, and tachycardia. ECG often reveals U waves, high QRS voltage, and first-degree atrioventricular block. Additional laboratory testing reveals normal acid-base state, hypokalemia with low urinary potassium excretion (spot urinary potassium concentration <20 mEq/L from potassium shift into cells), hypophosphatemia, hypophostaturia, and hypercalciuria. Electromyography during attacks shows low-amplitude compound muscle action potential of the tested muscle. Therapy consists of cautious potassium supplementation (increased risk of rebound hyperkalemia). Use of nonselective beta-blockers (e.g., propranolol) to counteract hyperadrenergic activity, which may be causing TPP, may also be useful.

SUGGESTED READINGS

available at www.expertconsult.com

RELATED CONTENT

Hyperthyroidism (Patient Information)
Graves Disease (Related Key Topic)
Thyrotoxic Storm (Related Key Topic)

AUTHOR: **FRED F. FERRI, M.D.**

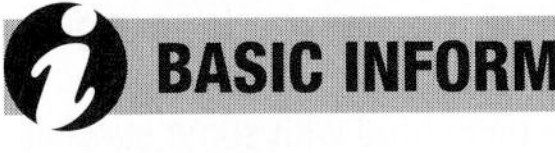

BASIC INFORMATION

DEFINITION

Hypertrophic osteoarthropathy (HOA) is a syndrome of clubbing of the digits, periostosis of long bones, abnormal proliferation of skin, and arthritis. Periostosis is usually involved with pain on palpation of the involved area. HOA may be primary or secondary to other underlying disease processes.

SYNONYMS

- Primary hypertrophic osteoarthropathy:
  1. Pachydermoperiostosis
  2. Idiopathic clubbing
  3. Touraine-Solente-Golé syndrome
- Secondary hypertrophic osteoarthropathy
- HOA

ICD-9CM CODES
731.2 Hypertrophic osteoarthropathy
ICD-10CM CODES
M89.3 Hypertrophy of bone
M89.40 Other hypertrophic osteoarthropathy, unspecified site

EPIDEMIOLOGY & DEMOGRAPHICS

- Fig. 1-500 provides a classification of HOA.
- Primary HOA is a familial autosomal-dominant disease affecting the age group between 1 and 20 yr and is rare. There is a male/female ratio of 9:1 in occurrence.
- Secondary HOA is more common, typically occurs in adults 55 to 75 years of age. 80% to 90% of secondary HOA is associated with non–small cell lung cancer, most frequently adenocarcinoma; other associated illnesses include:
  1. Pulmonary: mesothelioma, lung abscesses, empyema, bronchiectasis, cystic fibrosis, pulmonary fibrosis, sarcoidosis, arteriovenous malformations
  2. Gastrointestinal: Carcinoma of esophagus or colon, biliary atresia, inflammatory bowel disease (Crohn's disease, ulcerative colitis), hepatocellular carcinoma, liver cirrhosis, amebiasis
  3. Cardiac: infective endocarditis, right-to-left cardiac shunts, aortic aneurysms, infected aortic bypass graft
  4. Thymoma
  5. Hodgkin lymphoma
  6. Connective tissue diseases
  7. Thyroid acropachy
  8. HIV infection
  9. POEMS syndrome (polyneuropathy, organomegaly, endocrinopathy, M component, and skin changes)
  10. Thalassemia
  11. Osteosarcoma
  12. Nasopharyngeal sarcoma
  13. Osteosarcoma

PHYSICAL FINDINGS & CLINICAL PRESENTATION

- Primary HOA typically presents with the insidious onset of clubbing of the hands (Fig. 1-501) and feet, described as "spadelike." Finger clubbing is diagnosed by measurement of the digital index (Fig. 1-502). Other signs and symptoms of HOA include:
  1. Joint pain and swelling
  2. Decreased use of the fingers and hands
  3. Facial changes, coarse facial skin grooves, ptosis of the lids
  4. Thickening of the arms and legs
  5. Oily skin, diaphoresis, gynecomastia, and acne
  6. Thin and shiny appearance of the skin around the nail bed
  7. Nail convexity with nail "floating" sensation within the soft tissue is noticed on palpation of the base of the nail bed
  8. Edema, warmth, and tenderness of the extremities can be seen
- Secondary HOA patients may present with clinical symptoms before the underlying disorder can be detected. Signs and symptoms are similar to the above in addition to findings related to the underlying disease (e.g., bronchogenic carcinoma, infective endocarditis).
- Patients presenting with painful joints prior to developing clubbing can be misdiagnosed as inflammatory arthritis.

ETIOLOGY

The pathogenesis of HOA is not fully understood; current knowledge suggests that HOA results from the activation of one or more growth factors, such as vascular endothelial growth factor (VEGF) and platelet-derived growth factor, that are normally inactivated in the lungs and systemic circulation.

DIAGNOSIS

Diagnosis is primarily clinical; radiographs and bone scans can help confirm the diagnosis.

DIFFERENTIAL DIAGNOSIS

Paget's disease, Reiter's syndrome, psoriatic arthritis, syphilis, osteoarthritis, rheumatoid arthritis, osteomyelitis, scleromyxedema, and acromegaly.

WORKUP

HOA warrants an investigation into any associated illnesses.

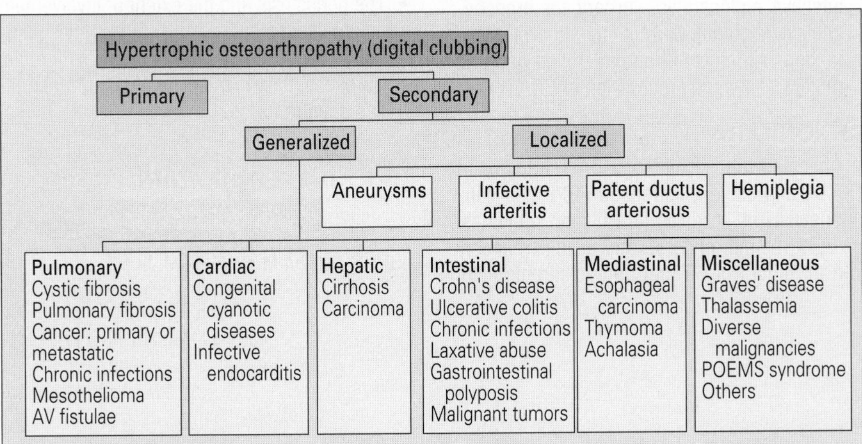

FIGURE 1-500 Classification of hypertrophic osteoarthropathy. *AV,* Arteriovenous; *POEMS,* polyneuropathy, organomegaly, endocrinopathy, monoclonal proteins, and skin changes. (From Hochberg MC et al: *Rheumatology,* ed 5, St Louis, 2011, Mosby.)

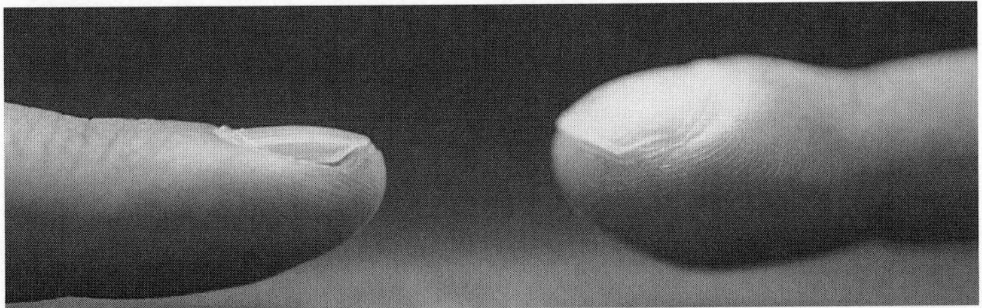

FIGURE 1-501 Clubbing deformity. The finger on the right is clubbed compared with the normal finger shape on the left. (From Hochberg MC et al: *Rheumatology,* ed 5, St Louis, 2011, Mosby.)

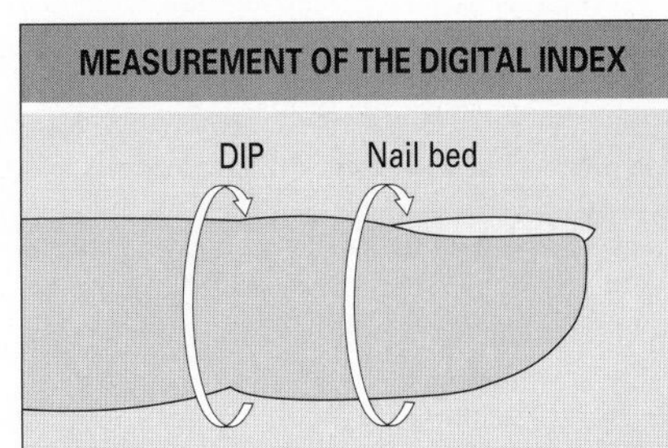

FIGURE 1-502 The digital index. The perimeter of each of the 10 fingers is measured at the nail bed (NB) and at the distal interphalangeal joint (DIP). If the sum of the 10 NB:DIP ratios is more than 10, clubbing is probably present. (From Hochberg MC et al: *Rheumatology,* ed 5, St Louis, 2011, Mosby.)

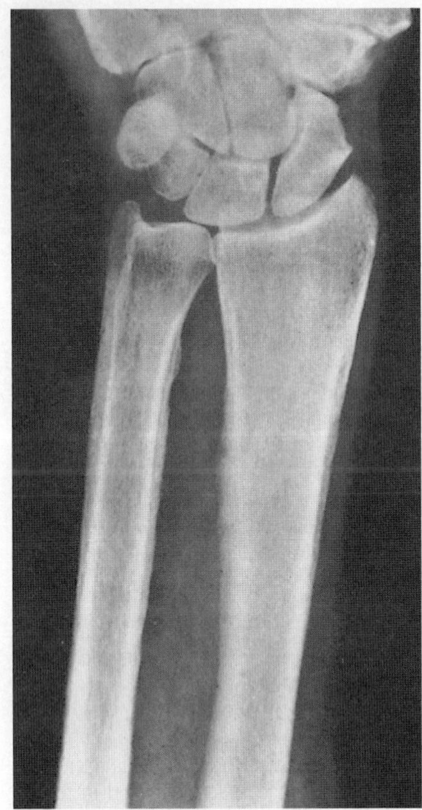

FIGURE 1-503 Hypertrophic osteoarthropathy. Wrist radiograph showing periostosis at the distal ends of the radius and ulna. The coarse, layered appearance is most evident along the diaphyses. The relative sparing of the radial epiphyses is characteristic. (From Hochberg MC et al: *Rheumatology*, ed 5, St Louis, 2011, Mosby.)

LABORATORY TESTS

- Routine laboratory studies such as blood count, electrolytes, and urine studies are typically normal in primary and secondary HOA.
- Erythrocyte sedimentation rate is elevated in secondary HOA.
- Liver function tests may be abnormal in patients with secondary HOA from gastrointestinal pathology.
- Alkaline phosphatase may be elevated as a result of periostosis of long bones.
- Analysis of the synovial fluid from joint effusions reveals a low white blood cell count with normal viscosity, color, and complement levels.

IMAGING STUDIES

- Radiographs of the long bones show periosteal new bone formation (Fig. 1-503).
- A chest radiograph should be obtained to rule out underlying lung cancer.
- Bone scan with technetium-99m reveals uptake along the long bones, phalanges, and periarticular joint spaces.
- Angiography findings may demonstrate hypervascularization of the finger pads.

Rx TREATMENT

ACUTE GENERAL Rx

- Treatment of primary HOA is symptomatic. Nonsteroidal anti-inflammatory medications such as aspirin, salicylate, ibuprofen, naproxen, indomethacin, corticosteroids, tamoxifen citrate, or retinoids can be used.
- Colchicine can be helpful for the pain due to subperiosteal new bone formation.
- Reconstructive surgery is indicated for correction of gross disfigurement.
- Treatment of secondary HOA is to eradicate the underlying disease (e.g., antibiotics for infective endocarditis, surgery for bronchogenic carcinoma). Correction of heart malformation or removal of an underlying tumor is rapidly followed by regression of HOA.

CHRONIC Rx

In patients with secondary HOA refractory to NSAIDs and aspirin, octreotide (100 mcg subcutaneously twice daily) and bisphosphonates, including pamidronate (1 mg/kg intravenously to a maximum of 60 mg) and zoledronic acid, which inhibit VEGF expression, have significantly reduced pain.

Vagotomy has been tried with some success. However, the definitive treatment is to treat the underlying disease.

DISPOSITION

- Patients with primary HOA typically have symptoms of joint pain and swelling for the early part of their life. However, the disease becomes quiescent thereafter.
- Prognosis and disease course in patients with secondary HOA will depend on the underlying cause. The insidious development of clubbing suggests an infectious process, whereas the rapid progression of clubbing may suggest underlying malignancy.

REFERRAL

Referral should be made to rheumatology when the diagnosis of HOA is suspected and the cause remains unclear.

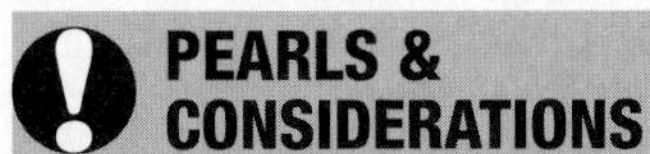

PEARLS & CONSIDERATIONS

Some cases of primary HOA may later be found to be associated with an underlying disease such as patent ductus arteriosus, Crohn's disease, or myelofibrosis, in which case they become secondary.

COMMENTS

- Infections and intrathoracic malignancies are the most common causes of secondary HOA.
- The periostosis and the extent of involvement do not depend on the form of the disease (primary or secondary), but rather on its duration.
- HOA secondary to infection of an arterial graft has been reported.

SUGGESTED READINGS

available at www.expertconsult.com

AUTHOR: **SYEDA M. SAYEED, M.D.**

BASIC INFORMATION

DEFINITION

Hyperuricemia may be defined as serum uric acid >7.0 mg/dl in males or >6.0 mg/dl in females. Some persons who are normouricemic by this definition will have levels of uric acid that exceed the limit of solubility of uric acid in tissue. Data from the Framingham study indicates that hyperuricemia increased from 4.8% of the population in the early 1970s to 9.3% in the mid-1980s. Age is an important risk factor in the increasing incidence of hyperuricemia and gout. Women become hyperuricemic at an older age than men due to the uricosuric effect of estrogen. Most people with hyperuricemia are asymptomatic and will remain so; however, 20% of those with serum uric acid >9 mg/dl will develop gout in 5 yr. Hyperuricemia is strongly associated with gout, obesity, diabetes, hypertension, and cardiovascular disease but has not been proven to cause any of these conditions.

ASYMPTOMATIC HYPERURICEMIA

Definition: laboratory evidence of elevated serum uric acid without clinical disease known to be caused by hyperuricemia

ETIOLOGY

Overproduction of uric acid accounts for a minority of cases of hyperuricemia. Most cases are due to decreased renal clearance of uric acid and high dietary purine consumption. Fig. 1-504 describes factors affecting urate balance. Table 1-267 describes a classification of hyperuricemia and gout.

ICD-10CM CODES
E79.0 Hyperuricemia without signs of inflammatory arthritis and tophaceous disease

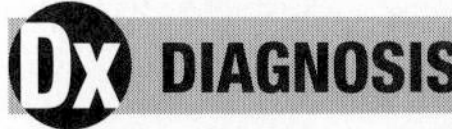

DIAGNOSIS

EVALUATION

The finding of hyperuricemia should prompt a thorough evaluation of potential causes and related diseases. Fig. E1-505 describes the evaluation of patients with hyperuricemia. If there is no clinical evidence of gout, nephrolithiasis, or acute kidney injury, the patient may be said to have asymptomatic hyperuricemia. Patients with hyperuricemia should be evaluated for potential causes of elevated uric acid including malignancy, renal insufficiency, toxins, lead toxicity, and dietary indiscretion. If a careful history and physical exam does not reveal an evident cause of persistent hyperuricemia, a 24-hr urine collection for uric acid and creatinine may be considered. Patients with urinary excretion of uric acid >800 mg/24 hr are likely to be overproducers of uric acid and should be investigated more thoroughly for the underlying cause of their hyperuricemia.

TABLE 1-267 Classification of Hyperuricemia and Gout

Impaired Uric Acid Excretion
Primary gout with decreased uric acid clearance
Secondary gout
Clinical conditions
Reduced glomerular filtration rate
Hypertension
Obesity
Systemic acidosis
Familial juvenile hyperuricemic nephropathy
Medullary cystic kidney disease
Lead nephropathy
Drugs
Diuretics
Ethanol
Low-dose salicylates (0.3-3.0 g/day)
Cyclosporine
Tacrolimus
Levodopa
Excessive Urate Production
Primary metabolic disorders
HPRT deficiency
PRPP synthetase overactivity
Glucose-6-phosphatase deficiency
Fructose-1-phosphate aldolase deficiency
Secondary causes
Clinical conditions
Myelo- and lymphoproliferative disorders
Obesity
Psoriasis
Glycogenoses III, V, VII
Drugs and dietary components
Nicotinic acid
Pancreatic extract
Cytotoxic drugs
Red meat, organ meat, shellfish
Alcoholic beverages (especially beer)
Fructose

HPRT, hypoxanthine-guanine phosphoribosyltransferase; *PRPP,* phosphoribosyl pyrophosphate.
From Goldman L, Schafer AI: *Goldman's Cecil medicine,* ed 24, Philadelphia, 2012, Saunders.

LABORATORY TESTS

- CBC with differential
- BUN/creatinine
- Urinalysis
- Lipid profile: Consider 24-hr urine collection

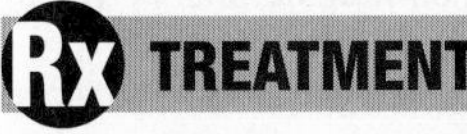

TREATMENT

No specific therapy is indicated for most patients with asymptomatic hyperuricemia. Lifestyle and dietary modification are often advisable.

NONPHARMACOLOGIC THERAPY

- Weight loss
- Reduce alcohol intake, especially beer
- Reduce consumption of foods known to be high in purines such as red meat, organ meat, and high-fructose soft drinks.

PEARLS & CONSIDERATIONS

- Research in progress suggests there may be a causal relationship between hyperuricemia and early hypertension.
- Very high levels of serum uric acid may warrant treatment even if asymptomatic.
- Patient with hyperuricemia and a family history of gout should be followed closely for the development of gouty arthritis.
- Hyperuricemia in patients with gout or presence of tophi (Fig. E1-506) should almost always be treated with urate-lowering medication (see "Gout").

SUGGESTED READINGS

available at www.expertconsult.com

RELATED CONTENT

Gout (Related Key Topic)

AUTHOR: **BERNARD ZIMMERMANN, M.D.**

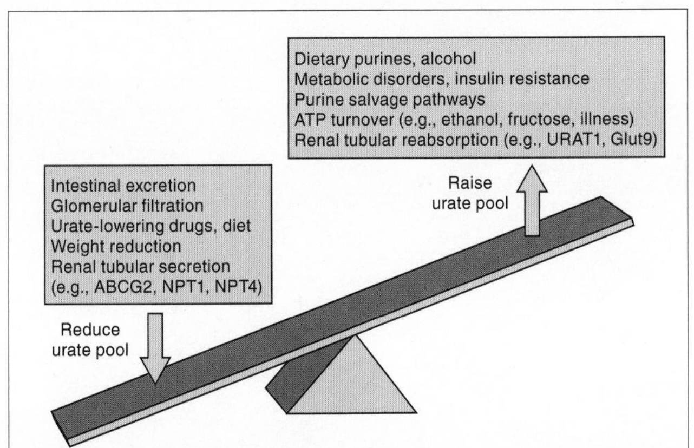

FIGURE 1-504 Factors affecting urate balance. The systemic urate pool and the likelihood of gout are determined by the dynamic balance among dietary purines, endogenous synthesis and recycling, and disposal by the kidney and gut. (From Hochberg MC et al: *Rheumatology,* ed 5, St Louis, 2011, Mosby.)

BASIC INFORMATION

DEFINITION

Hypoaldosteronism is defined as an aldosterone deficiency or impaired aldosterone function.

ICD-9CM CODES
255.4 Hypoadrenalism
ICD-10CM CODES
E27.40 Unspecified adrenocortical insufficiency
E27.3 Drug-induced adrenocortical insufficiency
E27.9 Disorder of adrenal gland, unspecified

EPIDEMIOLOGY & DEMOGRAPHICS

Selective hypoaldosteronism accounts for as many as 10% of cases of unexplained hyperkalemia.

PHYSICAL FINDINGS & CLINICAL PRESENTATION

- Physical examination may be entirely within normal limits.
- Hypertension may be present in some patients.
- Profound muscle weakness and cardiac arrhythmias may be present.

ETIOLOGY

- Hyporeninemic hypoaldosteronism (renin-angiotensin dependent): decreased aldosterone production as a result of decreased renin production; the typical patient has renal disease attributable to various factors (e.g., diabetes mellitus, interstitial nephritis, multiple myeloma).
- Hyperreninemic hypoaldosteronism (renin-angiotensin independent): renin production by the kidneys is intact; the defect is in aldosterone biosynthesis or in the action of angiotensin II. Common causes of this form of hypoaldosteronism are medications (ACE inhibitors, heparin), lead poisoning, aldosterone enzyme defects, and severe illness.

Dx DIAGNOSIS

DIFFERENTIAL DIAGNOSIS

Pseudohypoaldosteronism: renal unresponsiveness to aldosterone. In this condition both renin and aldosterone levels are elevated. Pseudohypoaldosteronism can be caused by medications (spironolactone), chronic interstitial nephritis, systemic disorders (systemic lupus erythematosus, amyloidosis), or primary mineralocorticoid resistance.

WORKUP

Measurement of plasma renin activity after 4 hr of upright posture can differentiate hyporeninemic from hyperreninemic causes. Renin levels in the normal or low range identify cases that are renin-angiotensin dependent, whereas high renin levels identify cases that are renin-angiotensin independent. The diagnosis and etiology of hypoaldosteronism can be confirmed with the renin-aldosterone stimulation test:

- Hyporeninemic hypoaldosteronism: low stimulated renin and aldosterone levels
- End-organ refractoriness to aldosterone action: high stimulated renin and aldosterone levels
- Adrenal gland abnormality: high stimulated renin and low aldosterone levels

LABORATORY TESTS

- Increased potassium, normal or decreased sodium
- Hyperchloremic metabolic acidosis (caused by the absence of hydrogen-secreting action of aldosterone)
- Increased BUN and creatinine (secondary to renal disease)
- Hyperglycemia (diabetes mellitus is common in these patients)

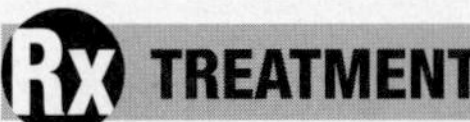

Rx TREATMENT

NONPHARMACOLOGIC THERAPY

- Low-potassium diet with liberal sodium intake (at least 4 g of sodium chloride per day)
- Avoidance of ACE inhibitors and potassium-sparing diuretics

ACUTE GENERAL Rx

- Judicious use of fludrocortisone (0.05 to 0.1 mg PO every morning) in patients with aldosterone deficiency associated with deficiency of adrenal glucocorticoid hormones
- Furosemide 20 to 40 mg qd to correct hyperkalemia of hyporeninemic hypoaldosteronism

DISPOSITION

Prognosis varies with the etiology of hypoaldosteronism and presence of associated disorders.

REFERRAL

Endocrinology referral for renin-aldosterone stimulation test

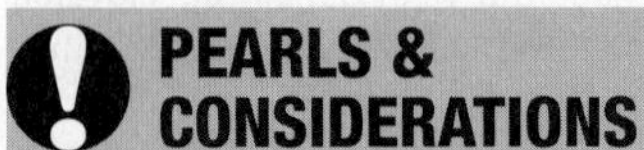

PEARLS & CONSIDERATIONS

COMMENTS

Treatment of pseudohypoaldosteronism is the same as for hypoaldosteronism; however, effect is limited because of impaired renal sensitivity.

AUTHOR: **FRED F. FERRI, M.D.**

BASIC INFORMATION

DEFINITION

Illness anxiety disorder (newly defined in DSM-5) is the preoccupation with the fear of having, or the idea that one has, a serious undiagnosed disease (previously defined as hypochondriasis), despite a lack of significant corresponding somatic symptoms or medical evidence. Whether or not another medical diagnosis is present, the severity of health-related anxiety is clearly disproportionate to the individual's health status. Existing medical literature (including that referenced here) explores the previously defined disorder hypochondriasis; it is unknown exactly how that evidence applies to illness anxiety disorder.

ICD-9CM and DSM-5 CODES
300.70
ICD-10CM CODES
F45.2 Hypochondriacal disorder

EPIDEMIOLOGY & DEMOGRAPHICS

PREVALENCE: 1% to 5% (based on estimates of DSM-III and DSM-IV disorder hypochondriasis), but may be higher (3-10%) in primary care outpatient settings.
PREDOMINANT SEX: Equal frequency in men and women.
PREDOMINANT AGE: Onset at any age, but most commonly between ages 20 and 30 yr
GENETICS/RISK: No known genetic component. May be more common in less-educated individuals. A comorbid major mental disorder (e.g., generalized anxiety, obsessive-compulsive disorder, and depression) is likely to affect over two-thirds of individuals with illness anxiety disorder; personality disorders and somatic symptom disorders may also be more common

PHYSICAL FINDINGS & CLINICAL PRESENTATION

- Somatic symptoms or signs are not present or are only mild; the focus of anxiety is the suspected medical diagnosis itself (i.e., concern for illness rather than symptoms per se).
- Mild somatic symptoms, if present, often include nonpathologic physical signs or sensations (e.g., belching, orthostatic lightheadedness).
- High health anxiety persists despite reassuring clinical evaluation (though without the intensity of a delusion).
- Illness anxiety symptoms often correlate with psychosocial stressors.
- Illness preoccupation lasts at least 6 mo (the specific illness feared may vary).
- Disruption in health-related quality of life and/or social, occupational, or other important areas of functioning.
- Two presentation types: care-seeking (medical attention frequently sought) and care-avoidant (maladaptive avoidance of health care).
- No specific physical examination findings.

ETIOLOGY

Unknown neurobiologic etiology. Serious childhood illness or trauma may be associated with illness anxiety disorder in adulthood.

DIAGNOSIS

DIFFERENTIAL DIAGNOSIS

- Underlying medical condition
- Adjustment disorder (health-related anxiety in response to illness)
- Somatic symptom disorder (excessive distress related to somatic symptom[s])
- Body dysmorphic disorder (restricted to a circumscribed concern about appearance)
- Factitious disorder
- Malingering
- Generalized anxiety disorder with health concerns as one worry among others
- Major depressive disorder with health concerns occurring only during depressive episodes
- Psychosis, as may occur with depression and schizophrenia

WORKUP

- History, physical examination, age-appropriate screenings, and laboratory and imaging tests, as appropriate, to exclude underlying medical condition.
- Symptom measures (e.g., Health Anxiety Inventory) may be used for detection and monitoring of severity over time.
- Evaluation for other psychiatric disorders associated with illness anxiety such as depression and generalized anxiety.

TREATMENT

NONPHARMACOLOGIC THERAPY

- Cognitive behavioral therapy (CBT) is the mainstay of treatment, with techniques to alter or restructure maladaptive thinking and behavior. Individual or group CBT, and mindfulness-based approaches, have demonstrated success.
- Regularly scheduled brief medical appointments.
- Avoidance of repeated or non-medically indicated diagnostic testing, referrals, or treatments.
- Limit on reading medical texts or websites.
- Benign interventions (e.g., exercise, massage).

CHRONIC Rx

- Antidepressants may be helpful even in individuals without features of depression: placebo-controlled trials of fluoxetine and paroxetine suggest benefit.
- Treatment of comorbid psychiatric conditions, if present.

DISPOSITION

Waxing and waning course over decades; recovery rates between 30% and 85%. Positive prognostic factors include shorter duration of illness and lack of comorbid psychiatric disorder.

REFERRAL

Referral for CBT is the mainstay of treatment; referral to a psychiatrist may be needed in the case of comorbid psychiatric condition.

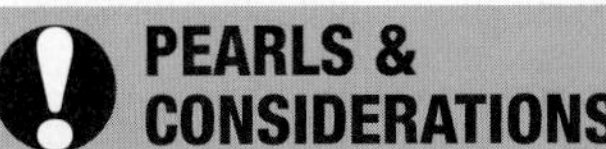

PEARLS & CONSIDERATIONS

- CBT and pharmacotherapy may be helpful treatment modalities for individuals open to treatment not directed at the perceived illness.
- In the updated DSM-5, hypochondriasis and related conditions were replaced by two new concepts: somatic symptom disorder (somatic symptoms present, with significant related distress) and illness anxiety disorder (somatic symptoms absent or minimal, concern focused on the idea of illness).

SUGGESTED READINGS

available at www.expertconsult.com

RELATED CONTENT

Somatization Disorder (Related Key Topic)
Somatization Disorder (Patient Information)

AUTHOR: **LUCY KALANITHI, M.D.**

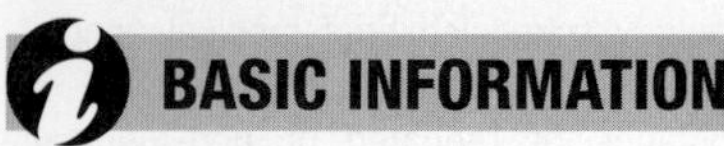

DEFINITION

Male hypogonadism is a clinical syndrome involving subnormal testosterone levels and/or impaired sperm production due to dysfunction at one or both levels of the hypothalamic-pituitary-testicular axis.

SYNONYMS

Testicular dysfunction

ICD-9CM CODES
257 Testicular dysfunction
ICD-10CM CODES
E29 Testicular dysfunction
E29.1 Testicular hypofunction
E29.8 Other testicular dysfunction
E29.9 Testicular dysfunction, unspecified

EPIDEMIOLOGY & DEMOGRAPHICS

INCIDENCE: Hypogonadism is the most common clinical disorder of the testis. Incidence is unclear due to the many possible underlying factors, nonspecificity of symptoms, and questions relating to the adequacy of a diagnostic serum total testosterone threshold.

PREVALENCE: Prevalence of hypogonadism increases with aging, obesity, diabetes mellitus, and other comorbidities. The average decrease in serum total testosterone levels in aging men is 1%-2% per year. Prevalence rises to 23% among men in their 70s. However, in population-based surveys of community-dwelling middle-aged and older males, prevalence of hypogonadism is approximately 6%.

GENETICS: Genetic abnormalities underlie a number of hypogonadal disorders including Klinefelter syndrome, Noonan syndrome, hemochromatosis, Kallmann syndrome, and Prader-Willi syndrome.

RISK FACTORS: These are many and include genetic abnormalities; the aging process; pituitary and testicular lesions and disorders; medications; drug abuse; HIV disease; acute illnesses; chronic cardiac, hepatic, renal, and pulmonary diseases; cancer; ionizing radiation; chemotherapy; obesity; and malnutrition.

PHYSICAL FINDINGS & CLINICAL PRESENTATION

Sexual (specific)
- Decrease in frequency of erections
- Erectile dysfunction
- Decrease in libido
- Decreased fertility
- Small or shrinking testes
- Gynecomastia
- Diminished sexual hair
- Hot flushes and sweats.

Neuro-psychological (less specific)
- Depression
- Inability to concentrate
- Diminished motivation and vitality
- Decrease in self-confidence
- Diminished energy and stamina
- Sleep disturbances.

Physical features and findings
- Diminished capacity for physical activity
- Decrease in physical endurance and performance
- Diminished muscle mass and strength
- Increase in body fat
- Decrease or loss of axillary and pubic hair and decrease in shaving frequency
- Fine wrinkling over the lateral aspects of the face
- Breast enlargement with or without tenderness
- Change in consistency and decrease in size of testes
- Fragility fractures
- Anemia

ETIOLOGY

- The importance of a careful history and examination cannot be overstated to determine the etiology of possible hypogonadism. Primary hypogonadism is a result of a decrease in testicular testosterone secretion and/or a decrease in spermatogenesis with an associated increase in gonadotropin levels as in Klinefelter syndrome, cryptorchidism, and following orchitis, testicular trauma, chemotherapy, and irradiation.
- Secondary hypogonadism is due to hypothalamic-pituitary dysfunction which results in a decrease in testosterone levels and/or spermatogenesis with gonadotropin levels that are subnormal or inappropriately within the normal range.
- Combined primary and secondary hypogonadism is a result of deficits at both the level of the hypothalamic-pituitary axis and testes with variable gonadotropin levels depending upon the predominance of the level of the defect.

Dx DIAGNOSIS (Fig. 1-507)

DIFFERENTIAL DIAGNOSIS

Hypogonadotropic or secondary hypogonadism
- Pituitary dysfunction—hypopituitarism, functioning or nonfunctioning pituitary tumor, lymphocytic hypophysitis, infiltrative disease as with sarcoidosis, hemochromatosis, and histiocytosis X
- Hyperprolactinemia—prolactinoma, medication-related, chronic kidney disease
- Genetic—Kallmann syndrome with anosmia, Prader-Willi syndrome with morbid obesity
- Acute and chronic illnesses, malnutrition, emotional disorders, HIV, sleep apnea, aging, malignancies, obesity, and renal, hepatic, pulmonary, and cardiac diseases
- Opioids, CNS—active medications, glucocorticoid excess, and GnRH analogs (androgen deprivation therapy)

Hypergonadotropic or primary hypogonadism
- Genetic—Klinefelter syndrome, Noonan syndrome, myotonic dystrophy
- Gonadal damage due to drugs, alcohol, radiation, chemotherapy, trauma
- Congenital anorchia (vanishing testis syndrome)
- Cryptorchidism
- Mumps orchitis, HIV orchitis
- Diabetes mellitus
- Hodgkin's disease
- Aging

Combined primary and secondary hypogonadism
- Hemochromatosis, sickle cell disease, thalassemia
- Alcoholism, glucocorticoid therapy, aging
- Chronic cardiac, hepatic, renal, pulmonary diseases, and HIV disease

WORKUP

- Determine the presence or absence of male hypogonadism on the basis of history, clinical manifestations and findings, and documentation of consistently low serum total testosterone levels and/or abnormal seminal fluid analysis.
- Morning serum total testosterone levels should be measured on at least 2 or 3 occasions for confirmation of diagnosis and when necessary followed by measurement of serum free or bioavailable testosterone.
- Serum FSH and LH levels are measured to determine whether hypogonadism is primary, secondary, or a result of combined defects of the hypothalamic-pituitary axis and testis.
- Hormonal assessment of gonadal status should not be done during an acute or subacute illness.

LABORATORY TESTS

- Serum total testosterone is tightly bound to sex hormone binding globulin (SHBG) and weakly bound to circulating albumin. 0.5-3% of serum total testosterone is unbound or free.
- Liquid chromatography tandem mass spectrometry assays for total serum testosterone are more accurate than immunoassays.
- Bioavailable testosterone refers to unbound testosterone plus the testosterone that is loosely bound to albumin.
- Free testosterone, if necessary, is best measured by equilibrium dialysis or centrifugal ultrafiltration.
- An SHBG measurement is helpful in determining the adequacy or normality of a serum total testosterone measurement. Conditions that lower SHBG include obesity, protein-losing states, androgens, hypothyroidism, and familial SHBG deficiency. Increases in SHBG occur in those with hyperthyroidism, hepatitis, cirrhosis, and HIV disease, aging, and by estrogens.
- The lower limit of normal for serum total testosterone in a healthy young male is approximately 240-280 ng/dl and a low-normal serum free testosterone in a young normal male is 9 pg/ml.
- Serum total testosterone levels can vary from day-to-day and there is a diurnal rhythm in young normal males with morning levels that are higher by approximately 20%-25% as compared with levels in the afternoon.
- In elderly males, the diurnal rhythm is diminished with levels approximately 10% lower in the afternoon as compared with morning levels.

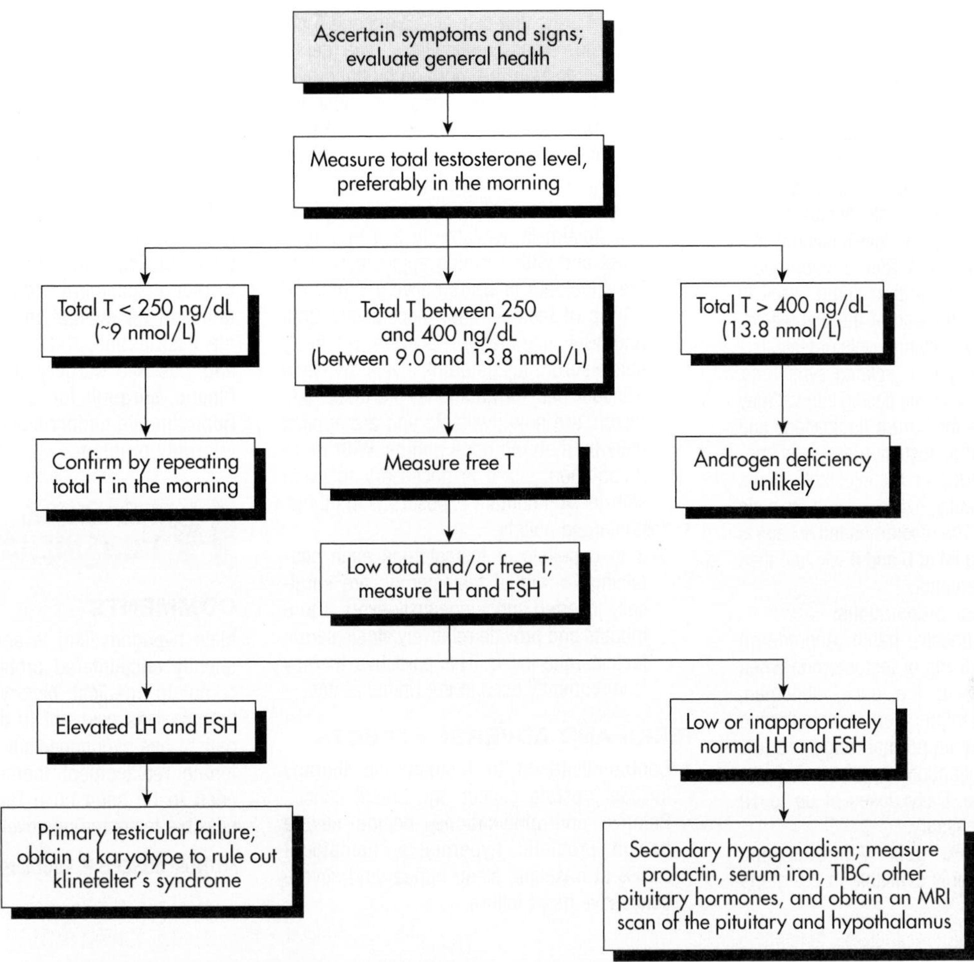

FIGURE 1-507 Algorithm showing an approach for the diagnostic evaluation of adult men suspected of having androgen deficiency. (From Shalender B, Shehzad B: Diagnosis and treatment of hypogonadism in men, *Best Pract Res Clin Endocrin* 25(2):251-270, 2011.)

- Serum FSH and LH measurements are important in delineating primary, secondary, and combined hypogonadism.
- Hypogonadal symptoms are more likely to be seen in those with total serum testosterone level below the lower limit of values for young normal males. Serum total testosterone levels of <150 ng/dl are unequivocally low.
- Transient suppression of total serum testosterone may occur during acute illness, in males that are being treated with glucocorticoid, in those taking opiates or CNS-active medications, in those with malnutrition or poor eating habits, and during excessive physical exercise.
- Quantity and quality of sperm counts and activity can vary in a significant way for a variety of reasons. Therefore, in assessing fertility, seminal fluid analysis should be done on two or more occasions each separated by two or more weeks and on semen collected within an hour of ejaculation after more than two days of abstinence.
- Depending on the clinical picture and examination, other studies may be necessary including a karyotype analysis, for example, for Klinefelter syndrome, or serum prolactin measurement for patients with possible hyperprolactinemia which may be drug-induced, related to a prolactinoma, or to chronic renal disease.

IMAGING STUDIES

- In males with severe androgen deficiency with low serum gonadotropin levels, increased serum prolactin levels, hypopituitarism, severe headaches, and visual defects, an MRI of the pituitary would be appropriate. In males with hypogonadism and a history of fractures, DXA measurements of spine and hip should be obtained to further delineate the status of the skeletal system.

Rx TREATMENT

- Testosterone replacement therapy is indicated when patients have symptoms and signs of hypogonadism and serum testosterone levels that are consistently subnormal with levels of <250 ng/dl. The goal of replacement therapy is to restore serum testosterone levels to within the normal range of values and to have a positive effect on the constellation of hypogonadal symptoms and signs. Subnormal spermatogenesis, if present in such patients, is not affected by testosterone therapy. In patients with hypogonadotropic or secondary hypogonadism, chorionic gonadotropin and/or GnRH therapy can optimize spermatogenesis, whereas, generally in patients with primary hypogonadism, subnormal spermatogenesis and infertility are irreversible.

NONPHARMACOLOGIC THERAPY

- Weight reduction, especially when it appears to be a major factor underlying male hypogonadism.
- Discontinuation of anabolic steroids, CNS-active medications, and narcotic abuse.
- Surgery or radiation therapy for patients with a pituitary functioning or nonfunctioning tumor with visual field abnormality and headaches who are not candidates for further medical therapy or have been unsuccessfully treated with medication.
- Surgery indicated for chronic gynecomastia and, occasionally, in cases with recent-onset gynecomastia that has not responded to testosterone replacement therapy.

CHRONIC THERAPY

Testosterone formulations:

- Parenteral testosterone preparations:
  - Testosterone enanthate (generic) and testosterone cypionate (Depotestosterone and generic) 150 to 200 mg are injected intramuscularly every 2 weeks. Following injections, there are appreciable fluctuations in serum testosterone, with levels rising within the first several days and a subsequent decrease to normal and in some cases to below normal at the end of the two weeks. As a result of the varying levels of testosterone, patients may have related symptoms. Adjustments in dose and dosing interval may help to alleviate the serum fluctuations and clinical symptoms. Testosterone undecanoate (AUEFD-ENDO) is an injectable depot formulation recently FDA-approved for male hypogonadism. The recommended dosage is 750 mg injected IM at 0 and 4 wk, and then every 10 wk thereafter.
- Topical testosterone preparations:
  - Testosterone adhesive patch (Androderm) delivers 2.5 or 5 mg of testosterone when applied nightly to the back, abdomen, upper arms, or thighs. Serum testosterone levels rise to within normal range in a few hours after application and, thereafter, are relatively stable. Daily doses of up to 10 mg may be necessary.
  - Testosterone 1% gels (AndroGel and Testim). Androgel is available in 2.5 g and 5 g gel units that deliver 2.5 mg and 5 mg of testosterone, respectively. The gel is applied daily in the morning by hand over the shoulder, upper arms, or abdomen. Adjustments in dose to 7.5 g or 10 g of gel may be necessary to optimize serum testosterone levels. AndroGel (1.62%) pump is also available for daily application. Testim is available in 5 g and 10 g tubes and with morning applications over the shoulders or arms delivers 5 mg and 10 mg of testosterone, respectively. Both AndroGel and Testim provide relatively stable serum testosterone levels. Two new transdermal formulations, Fortesta and Axiron, are now available and are applied daily by metered dose pumps. With these preparations, care is necessary to avoid skin-to-skin contact exposure with others.
- Testosterone pellets:
  - 3 to 6 pellets of testosterone each containing 75 mg of testosterone are surgically inserted subcutaneously every 3 to 6 months and provide relatively stable serum testosterone levels. This particular therapy is infrequently used in the United States.

RISKS AND ADVERSE EFFECTS

- Contraindications to testosterone therapy include prostate cancer and breast cancer. Relative contraindications include severe benign prostatic hyperplasia, hematocrit ≥50% at baseline, sleep apnea, and severe congestive heart failure.
- Patients on chronic testosterone therapy need to be followed carefully with prostate and PSA assessments and hematocrit measurements for possible excessive induction of erythrocytosis, initially at 3 to 6 months and at regular intervals thereafter.

REFERRAL

Endocrinology for full endocrine and metabolic assessment and therapy. Urology for further assessment and follow-up of the prostate and for evaluation and therapy of erectile dysfunction. Neurosurgery for evaluation and possible surgery for a pituitary lesion. Plastic surgery for chronic gynecomastia. Reproductive endocrinology for those with an infertility problem.

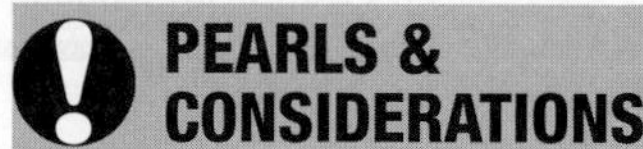

COMMENTS

Male hypogonadism is an important and frequently encountered problem that requires a complete medical history, examination, and hormonal assessment to determine whether a patient has hypogonadism and requires testosterone replacement therapy. Treated patients need to be seen on a regular basis to avoid possible testosterone adverse effects.

AUTHOR: **JOSEPH R. TUCCI, M.D., F.A.C.E., F.A.C.P.**

BASIC INFORMATION

DEFINITION

A decrease in parathyroid hormone (PTH) secretion or function results in hypoparathyroidism. In primary hypoparathyroidism, absence or dysfunction of the parathyroid gland results in inadequate PTH secretion and subsequent hypocalcemia and hyperphosphatemia. Surgical hypoparathyrodism is the most common etiology, followed by autoimmune disorders. Individuals with autoimmune polyglandular syndrome 1 typically present in childhood/adolescence with candidiasis, hypoparathyroidism, and adrenal insufficiency. Impaired function of PTH (i.e., PTH resistance) can also cause hypocalcemia and hyperphosphatemia but the measured PTH level is elevated in this circumstance. Maternally transmitted mutation in *GNAS1* gene results in PTH resistance (i.e., pseudohypoparathyroidism). It is associated with characteristic features that include developmental delay, short stature, round facies, and short 4th metacarpal known as Albright's Hereditary Osteodystrophy (AHO). Paternal transmission manifests with AHO without PTH resistance (i.e., pseudopseudohypoparathyroidism; Table 1-268). Secondary hypoparathyroidism, a condition in which PTH levels are low in response to hypercalcemic states, is discussed in Section IV (see hypercalcemia discussion in "Calcium" topic).

ICD-9CM CODES
252.1 Hypoparathyroidism
ICD-10CM CODES
E20.0 Idiopathic hypoparathyroidism
E20.1 Pseudohypoparathyroidism
E20.8 Other hypoparathyroidism
E20.9 Hypoparathyroidism, unspecified

EPIDEMIOLOGY & DEMOGRAPHICS

The incidence and prevalence of primary hypoparathyroidism depends on the etiology of the condition. Postoperative hypoparathyroidism is the most common etiology and occurs in the setting of thyroid or parathyroid surgery. Transient hypoparathyroidism can be as high as 20% postoperatively but permanent dysfunction is less common (3%). Autoimmune disorders are the subsequent most common cause of hypoparathyroidism in adults (female/male ratio of 1.4:1.0). Autoimmune polyglandular syndrome type I is reported to have an incidence worldwide of 1:1,000,000. Other etiologies of hypoparathyroidism are very rare.

PHYSICAL FINDINGS & CLINICAL PRESENTATION

The symptoms of hypoparathyroidism are primarily related to hypocalcemia. The presentation of symptoms varies with the severity and duration of illness.

- Cardiovascular: prolonged QT intervals, QRS and ST segment changes, ventricular arrhythmias
- Musculoskeletal: muscle cramps, laryngospasm, osteomalacia (adults), rickets (children), weakened tooth enamel, osteosclerosis
- CNS: tetany (Chvostek's sign and Trousseau's sign), seizures, paresthesias, visual impairment from cataract formation, altered mental status, papilledema, and basal ganglia calcifications with longstanding disease
- GI: abdominal pain
- Renal: hypercalciuria and nephrolithiasis
- Other: dry scaly skin, brittle nails, dry hair.

In addition to the hypocalcemia-related symptoms, syndromes associated with hypoparathyroidism can have distinct clinical findings. Conditions associated with hypoparathyroidism include:

- DiGeorge syndrome: dysmorphic facies, cleft palate
- Pseudohypoparathyroidism: developmental delay, short stature, round face, short 4th metacarpal (Albright's hereditary osteodystrophy)
- Hypoparathyroidism-retardation-dysmorphism syndrome: short stature, microcephaly, microphthalmia, small hands and feet, abnormal teeth
- Hypoparathyroidism-deafness-renal dysplasia syndrome: sensorineural deafness
- Autoimmune polyglandular syndrome type 1: mucocutaneous candidiasis and adrenal insufficiency

ETIOLOGY

There are several etiologies of hypoparathyroidism:

- Developmental defects of the parathyroids
  - Isolated hypoparathyroidism
  - Branchial dysembryogenesis (DiGeorge's syndrome)
  - Hypoparathyroidism-retardation-dysmorphism syndrome
  - Hypoparathyroidism-deafness-renal dysplasia syndrome
  - Mitochondrial dysfunction associated with hypoparathyroidism
- Destruction of the parathyroids
- Postoperative hypoparathyroidism
  - Autoimmune polyglandular syndrome type 1
  - Radiation to the neck
  - Infiltrative disease (e.g., metastatic carcinoma, Wilson's disease, hemochromatosis, thalassemia, granulomatous disease)
- Functional and secretory defects of the parathyroids
  - Activating mutation of the calcium-sensing receptor alters the set point of the receptor and decreases PTH secretion
  - Activating antibodies to calcium-sensing receptor alters the set point of the receptor and decreases PTH secretion
  - PTH resistance (i.e., target organs unresponsive to PTH action)
    - Pseudohypoparathyroidism (PHP): heterogeneous disorder presenting in childhood characterized by hypocalcemia, hyperphosphatemia, and elevated PTH levels. Table 1-269 summarizes the various types of PHP.
    - Hypermagnesemia and hypomagnesemia

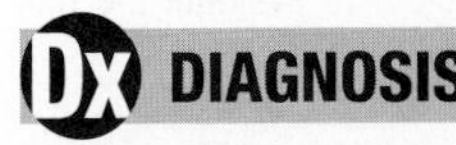

DIAGNOSIS

DIFFERENTIAL DIAGNOSIS

- Secondary hypoparathyroidism as a result of hypercalcemia (discussed in the "Hypercalcemia" section)
- Other conditions associated with hypocalcemia. These conditions are usually associated with an elevated PTH hormone level.

WORKUP

- Serum calcium is usually low and phosphorus is elevated
  - Two measurements of serum calcium are required for the confirmation of hypocalcemia. Total calcium should be corrected for low albumin utilizing the formula: Corrected Calcium = measured calcium + [(4 – albumin) × 0.8]. If a reliable laboratory is available, an ionized calcium should be considered especially in conditions associated with acid-base disturbances or low albumin states.
  - Serum phosphorus is usually high normal or elevated in primary hypoparathyroidism.
- The serum intact PTH (iPTH) level is the single best test to evaluate the etiology of hypocalcemia. Typically, PTH is decreased in hypoparathyroidism and elevated in most other conditions associated with low calcium levels. However, PTH is also elevated in disorders associated with impaired PTH function (i.e., pseudohypoparathyroidism). Genetic studies as indicated if medical or family history is suggestive.

LABORATORY TESTS

- Total and ionized calcium: low in hypoparathyroidism
- PTH: low in hypoparathyroidism and high in PTH resistance states like pseudohypoparathyroidism

TABLE 1-268 Types of Hypoparathyroidism

Type	Calcium	PO_4	PTH	Comments
Hypoparathyroidism	↓	↑	↓	Surgical removal (most common cause)
Pseudohypoparathyroidism	↓	↑	Ø↑	End-organ resistance to parathyroid hormone and Albright's hereditary osteodystrophy
Pseudo-pseudohypoparathyroidism	Normal	Normal	Normal	Only Albright hereditary osteodystrophy

Adapted from Weissleder R et al: *Primer of diagnostic imaging*, ed 5, St Louis, 2011, Mosby.

 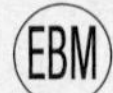

TABLE 1-269 Types of Pseudohypoparathyroidism (PHP)

Disorder	Urinary cAMP Response to PTH	Urinary PO_4 Response to PTH	Other Hormonal Resistance	AHO	Pathophysiology
PHP type 1A	Decreased	Decreased	Yes	Yes	$G_s\alpha$ mutation
Pseudo-PHP	Normal	Normal	No	Yes	$G_s\alpha$ mutation
PHP type 1B	Decreased	Decreased	No	No	*GNAS1* imprinting mutations
PHP type 1C	Decreased	Decreased	Yes	Yes	$G_s\alpha$ activity normal
PHP type 2	Normal	Decreased	No	No	Vitamin D deficiency or myotonic dystrophy in some cases

AHO, Albright's hereditary osteodystrophy; *cAMP*, cyclic adenosine monophosphate; *GNAS1*, portion of the *GNAS* complex locus encoding $G_s\alpha$; $G_s\alpha$, α-subunit of the stimulatory G protein; PO_4, phosphate; *PTH*, parathyroid hormone.
From Melmed: *Williams textbook of endocrinology*, ed 12, Philadelphia, 2011, Saunders.

- Phosphorus: high-normal or high in hypoparathyroidism
- Magnesium: both hypomagnesemia and hypermagnesemia can cause hypoparathyroidism
- ECG should be considered. Hypocalcemia associated with prolonged QT interval, rarely ST-segment elevations
- 24-hr urine for calcium to evaluate the risk for renal stones

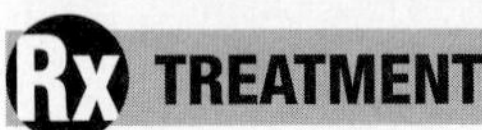

TREATMENT

NONPHARMACOLOGIC THERAPY

Parathyroid autotransplantation:
Hypoparathyroidism and subsequent hypocalcemia are common problems after neck exploration for total or near-total thyroidectomy or parathyroidectomy. In cases where there is concern for postoperative hypoparathyroidism, parathyroid autotransplantation of one or two parathyroid glands into the forearm or sternocleidomastoid muscle should be performed to prevent postoperative hypoparathyroidism.

PHARMACOLOGIC THERAPY

The mainstay of treatment for primary hypoparathyroidism is pharmacologic therapy with calcium and vitamin D supplementation. The goals of therapy are to control symptoms and minimize complications of therapy. The aim should be to achieve low-normal serum calcium (8.0-8.5 mg/dl), 24-hr urinary calcium <300 mg/day, and a calcium-phosphorus product <55.

- Vitamin D:
  - There are several vitamin D preparations available on the market but the treatment of choice for patients with primary hypoparathyroidism is calcitriol. It is an active metabolite that does not require hydroxylation in the liver or kidney and therefore bypasses the PTH-mediated 1-α hydroxylation defect that occurs with hypoparathyroidism.
  - Dose of 0.25 to 1 μg once or twice daily is usually required to correct hypocalcemia and improve symptoms. Its maximal effect is seen after 10 hr and it lasts for 2 to 3 days.
- Calcium:
  - Calcium carbonate or calcium citrates are common oral agents used for treatment of hypocalcemia associated with hypoparathyroidism. Calcium carbonate requires an acidic environment for effective absorption, and as a result, it must be taken with food. Its effectiveness is decreased with concomitant use of H_2 blockers or proton pump inhibitors. However, calcium carbonate is cheaper in cost than other calcium supplements and therefore it is first line in the management of hypocalcemia for some patients. The advantage of calcium citrate is that it does not require an acidic environment for effective absorption.
  - Start with a dose of 500 to 1000 mg of elemental calcium tid and adjust the dose for a desired calcium in the low-normal range.
- Magnesium:
  - Hypocalcemia is difficult to correct without normalizing magnesium levels.
  - Magnesium sulfate IV 2 g over 20 min followed by 1 g/hr infusion can be considered in severe deficiency states. Milder deficiencies can be managed with oral magnesium 100 mg tid.
- Thiazide diuretics:
  - Thiazide diuretics decrease urine calcium excretion and decrease kidney stones. They should be considered in individuals with urine calcium >250 mg/day.
- PTH replacement:
  - Preliminary studies involving injectable synthetic human PTH(1-34) and PTH (1-84) have been performed with results showing a decrease in urinary calcium excretion, maintenance of serum calcium in the normal range with reduced requirements for calcium and vitamin D supplementation, and increase in bone density at the spine. As expected, injectable PTH decreased forearm BMD.
  - It is not FDA approved for use in hypoparathyroidism.

ACUTE GENERAL Rx

Severe and/or symptomatic hypocalcemia requires hospitalization. Acute management of hypocalcemia includes:

- Telemetry monitoring for arrhythmias associated with severe hypocalcemia
- IV infusion of calcium gluconate 10 ml of 10% solution to receive a bolus of 90 mg of elemental calcium followed by an infusion of 0.5 to 2 mg/kg/hr until calcium levels are in the low–normal range.

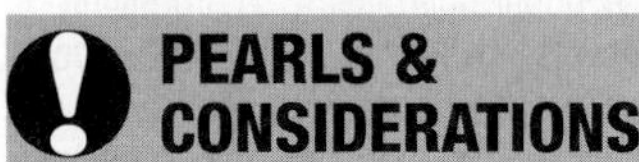

PEARLS & CONSIDERATIONS

COMMENTS

- The mainstay of treatment for primary hypoparathyroidism is calcitriol and calcium supplementation to maintain a goal serum calcium level in the low-normal range. IV calcium should be considered if calcium <7.0 mg/dl. Magnesium levels should be assessed and appropriately replaced in all patients with hypocalcemia. Clinical trials are under way to evaluate the role of recombinant PTH for the treatment of primary hypoparathyroidism.
- In patients undergoing neck exploration, consideration should be given to the parathyroid glands and autotransplantation of one or more parathyroid glands should be considered when appropriate to prevent postoperative hypoparathyroidism.

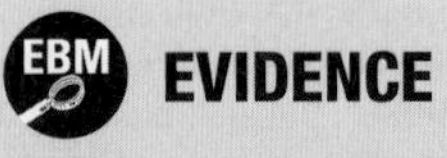

EVIDENCE

available at www.expertconsult.com

SUGGESTED READINGS

available at www.expertconsult.com

AUTHORS: **VICKY CHENG, M.D.**, and **GEETHA GOPALAKRISHNAN, M.D.**

BASIC INFORMATION

DEFINITION

Hypopituitarism (from the Latin *pituita,* meaning "phlegm") is the deficiency of one or more of the hormones of the anterior or posterior pituitary gland resulting from diseases of the hypothalamus or pituitary gland. Panhypopituitarism indicates the loss of all the pituitary hormones but is often used in clinical practice to describe patients deficient in growth hormone (GH), gonadotropins, corticotropin, or thyrotropin in whom posterior pituitary function remains intact.

SYNONYMS

Panhypopituitarism
Pituitary insufficiency

ICD-9CM CODES
253.2 Panhypopituitarism
ICD-10CM CODES
E23.0 Hypopituitarism

EPIDEMIOLOGY & DEMOGRAPHICS

Incidence of 4.2 cases per 100,000 persons

PHYSICAL FINDINGS & CLINICAL PRESENTATION

Symptoms depend on type of onset, number and severity of hormone deficiencies, their target organs, and age of onset.

- Mass effect of a pituitary tumor can cause headaches and visual disturbances (typically as bitemporal hemianopsia).
- Rhinorrhea.
- Corticotropin deficiency:
  - Fatigue and weakness, no appetite, abdominal pain, nausea, vomiting, failure to thrive in children, and hyponatremia. If the onset is abrupt, hypotension and shock
- Thyrotropin deficiency:
  - Fatigue and weakness, weight gain, cold intolerance, anemia, constipation
  - Bradycardia, hung-up reflexes, pretibial edema, change in voice, and hair loss
- Gonadotropin deficiency:
  - Loss of libido, erectile dysfunction, amenorrhea, hot flashes, dyspareunia, infertility, gynecomastia, decreased muscle mass, and anemia
- GH deficiency:
  - Growth retardation in children
  - Easy fatigue, hypoglycemia
  - Lean mass is reduced and fat mass is increased, leading to obesity
  - Decreased bone mineral density, increased low-density lipoprotein cholesterol, obesity, increased inflammatory cardiovascular markers (interleukin-6 and C-reactive protein)
- Hyperprolactinemia:
  - Galactorrhea, hypogonadism, inability to lactate after delivery
  - Posterior pituitary (vasopressin; antidiuretic hormone [ADH] deficiency): diabetes insipidus with polyuria, polydipsia, nocturia, hypotension, and dehydration

ETIOLOGY

It can be congenital or acquired:

- Congenital: mutations in transcription factors produce multiple hormonal deficiencies. Mutations in genes produce single hormonal deficiency.
- Acquired: the result of destruction of pituitary cells caused by:
  1. Pituitary apoplexy: hemorrhage or infarction of the pituitary gland. Predisposing factors include diabetes mellitus, anticoagulation therapy, head trauma, and radiation therapy. Sheehan's syndrome: postpartum necrosis, a rare complication after pregnancy.
  2. Infiltrative disease, including sarcoidosis, hemachromatosis, histiocytosis X, Wegener's granulomatosis, lymphocytic hypophysitis, and infection of the pituitary (tuberculosis, mycosis, syphilis).
  3. Primary empty sella syndrome: flattening of the pituitary gland caused by extension of the subarachnoid space and filling of cerebrospinal fluid into the sella turcica.
  4. Pituitary tumors: classified by size (microadenomas, <10 mm; macroadenomas, >10 mm) and function. Prolactin-secreting tumors and nonfunctioning tumors account for the majority of pituitary adenomas.
  5. Suprasellar tumors: craniopharyngiomas are the most common.

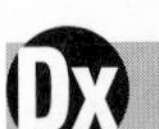

DIAGNOSIS

The diagnosis of hypopituitarism is suspected by clinical history and physical findings and is established by blood tests to confirm the presence of hormone deficiency.

DIFFERENTIAL DIAGNOSIS

The differential diagnosis is as outlined under "Etiology."

WORKUP

Includes baseline determination of each anterior pituitary hormone followed by dynamic provocative stimulation tests, radiograph imaging, and formal visual field testing. Table E1-270 summarizes testing for assessment of anterior pituitary function.

LABORATORY TESTS

- Corticotropin deficiency:
  1. The presence of a 9:00 am cortisol level >20 mcg/dl or <4 mcg/dl usually confirms sufficiency or deficiency, respectively.
  2. Corticotropin stimulation test using 250 mcg of corticotropin given IV and measuring serum cortisol before and 30 and 60 min after administration. A normal response is an increase in serum cortisol level >20 mcg/dl.
  3. With pituitary disease these test results may be indeterminate, and more dynamic testing such as an insulin-tolerance or metyrapone test may be necessary.
- Thyrotropin deficiency:
  1. Thyroid-stimulating hormone (TSH) and free T_4 measurements
  2. Primary hypothyroidism shows elevated TSH with low free T_4. Secondary hypothyroidism shows normal or low TSH with low free T_4 and low T_3 resin uptake.
- Gonadotropin deficiency:
  1. Follicle-stimulating hormone (FSH), luteinizing hormone (LH), estrogen, and testosterone measurements.
  2. In men, hypogonadotropic hypogonadism is seen with low testosterone levels and normal or low FSH and LH levels (ideally measured at 9:00 AM because of diurnal rhythm). Check free testosterone if patient is obese.
  3. In premenopausal women with amenorrhea, low estrogen with normal or low FSH and LH levels is typically seen.
- GH deficiency:
  1. Insulin-induced hypoglycemia stimulation test using 0.1 to 0.15 unit/kg regular insulin given IV and measuring GH 30, 60, and 120 min after administration. A normal response is a GH level >3 mcg/dl. This test is contraindicated in seizure disorder or ischemic heart disease.
  2. Combination of GH-releasing hormone plus arginine is an alternative test, with a diagnostic threshold of 9 mcg/L.
  3. Because the relation between serum insulinlike growth factor (IGF)-1 and GH levels blurs with age, a normal serum IGF-1 does not exclude the diagnosis in older adults.
- Hyperprolactinemia: prolactin levels may be elevated in prolactin-secreting pituitary adenomas.
- Vasopressin deficiency:
  1. Urinalysis shows low specific gravity.
  2. Urine osmolality is low.
  3. Serum osmolality is high.
  4. Fluid deprivation test over 18 hr with inability to concentrate the urine.
  5. Serum vasopressin level is low.
  6. Electrolytes may show hyponatremia and exclude hyperglycemia.

IMAGING STUDIES

- Imaging is the first step in identifying an underlying cause.
- MRI is more sensitive than CT in visualizing the pituitary fossa, sella turcica, optic chiasm, pituitary stalk, and cavernous sinuses. It is also more sensitive in detecting pituitary microadenomas. CT with contrast can be used if MRI is not available.
- Surveillance scan at baseline and 12 mo thereafter depending on protocol and clinical symptoms.

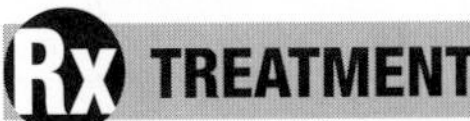

Threefold: removing underlying cause (surgery or radiation), treating hormonal deficiencies, and addressing any other repercussions from deficiency. Table E1-271 summarizes replacement therapy for adult hypopituitarism.

NONPHARMACOLOGIC THERAPY

- IV fluid resuscitation, correction of electrolyte and metabolic abnormalities with potassium bicarbonate, and oxygen therapy.
- Transsphenoidal surgery for tumors causing specific symptoms.
- Radiation or stereotactic radiosurgery ("gamma knife") for medically unresponsive, surgically unresectable tumors and tumors for which other modalities are contraindicated. It is both safe and effective for recurrent or residual pituitary adenomas.

ACUTE GENERAL Rx

Acute situations such as adrenal crisis or myxedema coma can occur in untreated hypopituitarism and should be treated accordingly with IV corticosteroids (e.g., hydrocortisone 100 to 250 mg bolus followed by hydrocortisone 100 mg IV q6h for 24 hr) and levothyroxine (e.g., 5 to 8 mcg/kg IV over 15 min, then 100 mcg IV q24h).

CHRONIC Rx

Treatment is lifelong:

- Adrenocorticotropic hormone (ACTH) deficiency: hydrocortisone 10 mg PO every morning and 5 mg PO every evening or prednisone 5 mg PO every morning and 2.5 mg PO every evening. Dexamethasone or prednisone is often preferred because of longer duration of action.
- LH and FSH deficiency:
  - In men, testosterone enanthate or propionate 200 to 300 mg IM every 2 to 3 wk, or transdermal testosterone scrotal patches can be tried.
  - In women who are not interested in fertility, conjugated estrogen 0.3 to 1.25 mg/day and held the last 5 to 7 days of each month with the addition of medroxyprogesterone 10 mg/day given during days 15 to 25 of the normal menstrual cycle. In those who have secondary hypogonadism and wish to become pregnant, pulsatile gonadotropic-releasing hormone may be of benefit.
- TSH deficiency: levothyroxine 0.05 to 0.15 mg/day.
- GH deficiency:
  - GH replacement in children is universally accepted.
  - GH replacement in adults is not generally recommended and requires careful consideration of each individual case. It may have effects on quality of life, body composition, bone density, and cardiovascular risk factors.
  - Side effects of replacement include peripheral edema, arthralgia, and headaches.
  - Usual GH dose is between 0.2 and 0.4 mg, determined by the age and gender of a patient and increments of 0.1 mg every 2 to 4 wk until serum IGF-1 is in the upper part of the normal range. Young adults and women taking estrogen require a higher dose.
- ADH deficiency:
  - Desmopressin (DDAVP) 10 to 20 mcg by intranasal spray or 0.05 to 0.1 mg PO bid is used in patients with diabetes insipidus.
  - Vasopressin: 5-10 U given IM or SC q6h.

DISPOSITION

- Hormone replacement therapy is adjusted according to serum hormone monitoring.
- If untreated can lead to adrenal crisis, severe hyponatremia and hypothyroidism, metabolic abnormalities, and death.
- Complications: visual deficit, adrenal crisis, susceptibility to infection and other stressors.
- Prognosis: stable patients have a favorable prognosis with replacement hormone therapy. Patients with acute decompensation are in critical condition with a high mortality rate.

REFERRAL

Consultation with an endocrinologist and neurosurgeon for surgical treatment

PEARLS & CONSIDERATIONS

- All patients sustaining moderate to severe head injury should undergo assessment of anterior pituitary function during the acute phase and at 6 mo.
- IGF-1 can be used as a marker of GH deficiency.
- All tests of GH secretion are more likely to give false-positive results in obese patients.
- The GH axis is the most vulnerable to the effects of radiotherapy; doses as low as 18 Gy in children have caused GH deficiency.
- Sequence of hormonal disruption: GH secretion then gonadotropin secretion. TSH and adrenocorticotropic hormone secretion are somewhat resistant.
- Thyroxine supplementation increases the rate of cortisol metabolism and can lead to adrenal crisis, so corticosteroids should be replaced first.
- All patients receiving glucocorticoid replacement therapy should wear proper identification stating the need for this therapy.
- Stress doses of corticosteroids are indicated before surgery or for any medical emergency (e.g., sepsis, acute myocardial infarction).
- Antidiuretic hormone deficiency may be masked if there is ACTH deficiency with symptoms only appearing when cortisol has been replaced.

COMMENTS

- Mineralocorticoid replacement is not necessary in secondary adrenal insufficiency because the renin-angiotensin-aldosterone system is unaffected by pituitary failure.
- Patients with adult-acquired GH deficiency must meet at least two criteria before replacement therapy: a poor GH response to at least two standard stimuli and hypopituitarism from pituitary or hypothalamic damage. The criteria are different in children in whom GH is required for normal growth.
- Prevention of acute decompensation can be accomplished by reminding patients to increase the dose of hydrocortisone in response to stress.
- Medical therapy should precede surgical therapy.

SUGGESTED READINGS

available at www.expertconsult.com

RELATED CONTENT

Hypopituitarism (Patient Information)

AUTHOR: **SHAHNAZ PUNJANI, M.D.**

BASIC INFORMATION

DEFINITION

Hypothermia is a rectal temperature <35° C (95.8° F). Accidental hypothermia is an unintentionally induced decrease in core temperature in the absence of preoptic anterior hypothalamic conditions.

ICD-9CM CODES
991.6 Accidental hypothermia
ICD-10CM CODES
T68 Hypothermia

EPIDEMIOLOGY & DEMOGRAPHICS

- Hypothermia occurs most frequently in the following groups: alcoholics; learning-impaired; patients with cardiovascular, cerebrovascular, or pituitary disorders; those using sedatives or tranquilizers; and elderly patients.
- >700 persons in the United States die from hypothermia annually.

PHYSICAL FINDINGS & CLINICAL PRESENTATION

The clinical presentation varies with the severity of hypothermia. Shivering may be absent if body temperature is <33.3° C (92° F) or in patients taking phenothiazines.

Hypothermia may masquerade as cerebrovascular accident, ataxia, or slurred speech, or the patient may appear comatose or clinically dead. Signs of hypothermia are summarized in Box E1-43.

Physiologic stages of hypothermia:

1. Mild hypothermia (32.2° to 35° C [90° to 95° F]): arrhythmias, ataxia
2. Moderate hypothermia (28° to 32.2° C [82.4° to 90° F]):
   a. Progressive decrease of level of consciousness, pulse, cardiac output, and respiration
   b. Fibrillation, dysrhythmias (increased susceptibility to ventricular tachycardia)
   c. Elimination of shivering mechanism for thermogenesis
3. Severe hypothermia (≤28° C [82.4° F]):
   a. Absence of reflexes or response to pain
   b. Decreased cerebral blood flow, decreased CO_2
   c. Increased risk of ventricular fibrillation or asystole

ETIOLOGY

Exposure to cold temperatures for a prolonged period. Contributing factors include:

1. Drugs: ethanol, phenothiazines, sedative-hypnotics
2. Skin disorders: extensive burns, severe psoriasis, exfoliative dermatitis
3. Metabolic disorders: hypopituitarism, hypothyroidism, hypoadrenalism
4. Neurologic abnormalities: stroke, head trauma, acute spinal cord transection, impaired shivering
5. Other: lack of acclimatization, aggressive fluid resuscitation, sepsis, heat stroke treatment
6. Box E1-44 summarizes factors predisposing to hypothermia

DIAGNOSIS

DIFFERENTIAL DIAGNOSIS

- It is crucial to determine an accurate core temperature measurement. Advantages and considerations of various methods to determine core temperature are summarized in Table 1-272.
- Cerebrovascular accident
- Myxedema coma
- Drug intoxication
- Hypoglycemia

LABORATORY TESTS

1. Metabolic and respiratory acidosis are usually present.
   a. When blood cools, the arterial pH increases, oxygen tension (Po_2) increases, and the Pco_2 falls:
      (1) pH increases 0.008 U/° F (or 0.015 U/° C), causing a decrease in temperature.
      (2) Pao_2 increases 3.3%/° F, causing a decrease in temperature. Oxygenation considerations during hypothermia are described in Box 1-45.
      (3) $Paco_2$ decreases 2.4%/° F, causing a decrease in temperature.
   b. Blood gas analyzers warm the blood to 37° C, increasing the partial pressure of dissolved gases, resulting in higher oxygen and carbon dioxide levels and a lower pH than the patient's actual values. Correction of arterial blood gases for temperature is unnecessary as a guide to therapy. The use of uncorrected values also permits reference to the standard acid–base nomograms.
2. A decrease in K^+ initially, then an increase in K^+ with increasing hypothermia; extreme hyperkalemia indicates a poor prognosis.
3. Hematocrit increases (caused by hemoconcentration), decreasing leukocytes and platelets (caused by splenic sequestration).
4. Blood viscosity, increased clotting time

IMAGING STUDIES

- Chest x-ray: generally not helpful; may reveal evidence of aspiration (e.g., intoxicated patient with aspiration pneumonia)
- ECG: prolonged PR, QT, and QRS segments, depressed ST segments, inverted T waves, atrioventricular block, and hypothermic J waves (Osborne waves) may appear at 25° to 30° C; characterized by notching of the junction of the QRS complex and ST segments (Fig. 1-509).

TABLE 1-272 Core Temperature Measurements

Type	Advantages	Considerations
Rectal	Convenient Continuous monitoring	Insert 15 cm (6 inches) Lags during transition from cooling to rewarming Falsely elevated with peritoneal lavage Falsely low if probe is in cold feces or when lower extremities are frozen
Esophageal	Convenient Continuous monitoring	Insert 24 cm (9.5 inches) below larynx Tracheal misplacement Aspiration Falsely elevated with heated inhalation
Tympanic	Approximates hypothalamic temperature via internal carotid artery	Probe: tympanic membrane perforation; canal hemorrhage Infrared: unreliable; cerumen effect
Bladder	Convenient Continuous monitoring	Unreliable Falsely elevated with peritoneal lavage Falsely low with cold diuresis

From Auerbach P: *Wilderness medicine, expert consult* Premium Edition—Enhanced Online Features and Print, Philadelphia, 2012, Saunders.

BOX 1-45 Oxygenation Considerations During Hypothermia

Detrimental Factors
Oxygen consumption increases with rise in temperature; caution if rapid rewarming; shivering also increases demand
Decreased temperature shifts oxyhemoglobin dissociation curve to the left
Ventilation-perfusion mismatch; atelectasis; decreased respiratory minute volume; bronchorrhea; decreased protective airway reflexes
Decreased tissue perfusion from vascoconstriction; increased viscocity
"Functional hemoglobin" concept: capability of hemoglobin to unload oxygen is lowered
Decreased thoracic elasticity and pulmonary compliance

Protective Factors
Reduction of oxygen consumption: 50% at 28° C (82.4° F); 75% at 22° C (71.6° F); 92% at 10° C (50° F)
Increased oxygen solubility in plasma
Decreased pH and increased $Paco_2$ shift oxyhemoglobin dissociation curve to right

From Auerbach P: *Wilderness medicine,* ed 4, St Louis, 2001, Mosby.

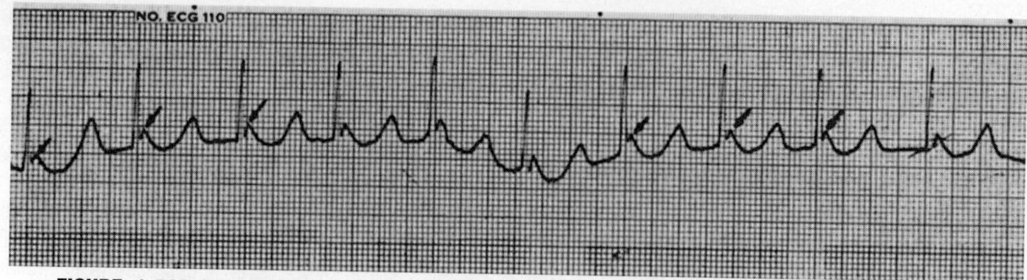

FIGURE 1-509 Hypothermic J waves (Osborne waves) ***(arrows)*** **in an 80-year-old man with core temperature of 86° F (30° C).** These waves disappeared with rewarming. (From Morse CD, Rial WY: Emergency medicine. In Rakel RE [ed]: *Textbook of family practice,* ed 4, Philadelphia, 1990, Saunders.)

Rx TREATMENT

NONPHARMACOLOGIC THERAPY

- Treatment of hypothermia varies with the following:
  1. Degree of hypothermia
  2. Existence of concomitant diseases (e.g., cardiovascular insufficiency)
  3. Patient's age and medical condition (e.g., elderly, debilitated patients vs. young, healthy patients)
- General measures:
  1. Secure an airway before warming all unconscious patients; precede endotracheal intubation with oxygenation (if possible) to minimize the risk of arrhythmias during the procedure.
  2. Peripheral vasoconstriction may impede placement of a peripheral intravenous catheter; consider femoral venous access as an alternative to the jugular or subclavian sites to avoid ventricular stimulation.
  3. A Foley catheter should be inserted, and urinary output should be monitored and maintained >0.5 to 1 ml/kg/hr with intravascular volume replacement.
  4. Box E1-46 summarizes measures for preparing hypothermic patients for transport.

ACUTE GENERAL Rx

- Continuous ECG monitoring of patients is recommended. Ventricular arrhythmias can be treated with bretylium; lidocaine is generally ineffective, and procainamide is associated with an increased incidence of ventricular fibrillation in hypothermic patients.
- Correct severe acidosis and electrolyte abnormalities.
- Hypothyroidism, if present, should be promptly treated (see "Myxedema Coma").
- If clinical evidence suggests adrenal insufficiency, administer IV methylprednisolone.

In patients unresponsive to verbal or noxious stimuli or with altered mental status, 100 mg of thiamine, 0.4 mg of naloxone, and 1 ampule of 50% dextrose may be given.

Warm (104° to 113° F [40° to 45° C]), humidified oxygen should also be given if available.

Specific treatment:

1. Mild hypothermia (rectal temperature <32.3° C [90° F]): passive external rewarming is indicated. Place the patient in a warm room (temperature >21° C [69.8° F]), and cover with insulating material after gently removing wet clothing; recommended rewarming rates vary between 0.5° and 20° C/hr but should not exceed 0.55° C/hr in elderly persons.
2. Moderate to severe hypothermia:
   a. Active core rewarming
      (1) Delivery of heat by way of fluids: warm gastrointestinal irrigation (with saline enemas and by nasogastric tube); IV fluids (usually D_5NS without potassium) warmed to 104° to 107.6° F (40° to 42° C), peritoneal dialysis with dialysate heated to 40.5° to 42.5° C.
      (2) Inhalation of heated, humidified oxygen (warmed to 40° C [104° F]) increases core temperature by 1° C (1.8° F) per hr and decreases evaporative heat loss from respiration.
   b. Active external rewarming: immersion in a bath of warm water (40° to 41° C); active external rewarming may produce shock because of excessive peripheral vasodilation. Ideal candidates are previously healthy, young patients with acute immersion hypothermia.
   c. Extracorporeal blood warming with cardiopulmonary bypass appears to be an efficacious rewarming technique in young, otherwise healthy persons.
   d. Patients with cardiac instability and those in cardiac arrest should be transported to a center capable of providing extracorporeal membrane oxygenation (ECMO) unless other conditions (e.g., trauma) require transport to a closer facility.

SUGGESTED READINGS

available at www.expertconsult.com

RELATED CONTENT

Hypothermia (Patient Information)

AUTHOR: **FRED F. FERRI, M.D.**

BASIC INFORMATION

DEFINITION

Hypothyroidism is a disorder caused by the inadequate secretion of thyroid hormone.

SYNONYMS

Myxedema

ICD-9CM CODES
244 Acquired hypothyroidism
243 Congenital hypothyroidism
244.1 Surgical hypothyroidism
244.3 Iatrogenic hypothyroidism
244.8 Pituitary hypothyroidism
246.1 Sporadic goitrous hypothyroidism

ICD-10CM CODES
E03.9 Hypothyroidism, unspecified
E00.9 Congenital iodine-deficiency syndrome, unspecified
E89.0 Postprocedural hypothyroidism
E03.2 Hypothyroidism due to medicaments and other exogenous substances
E01.8 Other iodine-deficiency related thyroid disorders and allied conditions
E07.1 Dyshormogenetic goiter

EPIDEMIOLOGY & DEMOGRAPHICS

INCIDENCE/PREVALENCE: 1.5% to 2% of women and 0.2% of men. Overall, about 1 in 300 persons in the United States has hypothyroidism.
PREDOMINANT AGE: Incidence of hypothyroidism increases with age; among persons older than 60 yr, 6% of women and 2.5% of men have laboratory evidence of hypothyroidism (thyroid-stimulating hormone [TSH] more than twice normal level).

PHYSICAL FINDINGS & CLINICAL PRESENTATION

- Hypothyroid patients generally present with the following signs and symptoms: fatigue, lethargy, weakness, constipation, weight gain, cold intolerance, muscle weakness, slow speech, slow cerebration with poor memory.
- Skin: dry, coarse, thick, cool, sallow (yellow color caused by carotenemia); nonpitting edema in skin of eyelids and hands (myxedema) secondary to infiltration of subcutaneous tissues by a hydrophilic mucopolysaccharide substance. (Fig. E1-510, A and B)
- Hair: brittle and coarse; loss of outer third of eyebrows.
- Facies: dulled expression, thickened tongue, thick and slow-moving lips.
- Thyroid gland: may or may not be palpable (depending on the cause of the hypothyroidism).
- Heart sounds: distant, possible pericardial effusion.
- Pulse: bradycardia.
- Neurologic: delayed relaxation phase of the deep tendon reflexes, cerebellar ataxia, hearing impairment, poor memory, peripheral neuropathies with paresthesia.
- Musculoskeletal: carpal tunnel syndrome, muscular stiffness, weakness.

ETIOLOGY

1. Primary hypothyroidism (thyroid gland dysfunction): the cause of >90% of the cases of hypothyroidism
   - Hashimoto's thyroiditis is the most common cause of hypothyroidism after age 8 yr
   - Idiopathic myxedema (nongoitrous form of Hashimoto's thyroiditis)
   - Previous treatment of hyperthyroidism (radioiodine therapy, subtotal thyroidectomy)
   - Subacute thyroiditis
   - Radiation therapy to the neck (usually for malignant disease)
   - Iodine deficiency or excess
   - Drugs (lithium, para-aminosalicylate, sulfonamides, phenylbutazone, amiodarone, thiourea)
   - Congenital (approximately one case per 4000 live births)
   - Prolonged treatment with iodides
2. Secondary hypothyroidism: pituitary dysfunction, postpartum necrosis, neoplasm, infiltrative disease causing deficiency of TSH
3. Tertiary hypothyroidism: hypothalamic disease (granuloma, neoplasm, or irradiation causing deficiency of thyrotropin-releasing hormone)
4. Tissue resistance to thyroid hormone: rare

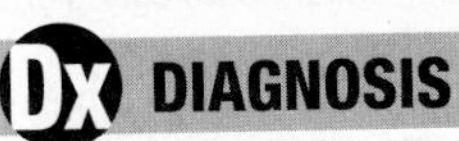

DIAGNOSIS

DIFFERENTIAL DIAGNOSIS

- Depression
- Dementia from other causes
- Systemic disorders (e.g., nephrotic syndrome, congestive heart failure, amyloidosis)

LABORATORY TESTS

- Increased TSH: TSH may be normal if patient has secondary or tertiary hypothyroidism, is receiving dopamine or corticosteroids, or the level is obtained after severe illness
- Decreased free T_4
- Other common laboratory abnormalities: hyperlipidemia, hyponatremia, and anemia
- Increased antimicrosomal and antithyroglobulin antibody titers: useful when autoimmune thyroiditis is suspected as the cause of the hypothyroidism
- Fig. E1-510, C describes a strategy for the laboratory evaluation of patients with suspected hypothyroidism

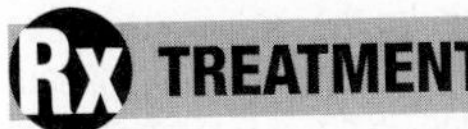

TREATMENT

NONPHARMACOLOGIC THERAPY

Patients should be educated regarding hypothyroidism and its possible complications. Patients should also be instructed about the need for lifelong treatment and monitoring of their thyroid abnormality.

ACUTE GENERAL Rx

Start replacement therapy with levothyroxine (L-thyroxine) 25 to 100 μg/day, depending on the patient's age and the severity of the disease. Physiologic combinations of L-thyroxine plus liothyronine do not offer any objective advantage over L-thyroxine alone. The levothyroxine dose may be increased every 6 to 8 wk, depending on the clinical response and serum TSH level. Elderly patients and patients with coronary artery disease should be started with 12.5 to 25 μg/day (higher doses may precipitate angina). The average maintenance dose of levothyroxine is 1.7 μg/kg/day (100 to 150 μg/day in adults). The elderly may require <1 μg/kg/day, whereas children generally require higher doses (up to 3 to 4 μg/kg/day). Pregnant patients also have increased requirements. Estrogen therapy may also increase the need for thyroxine. Women with hypothyroidism should increase their levothyroxine dose by approximately 30% as soon as pregnancy is confirmed. Close monitoring of serum thyrotropin levels and adjustment of levothyroxine dose is recommended throughout pregnancy. Table E1-273 summarizes conditions that alter levothyroxine requirements.

CHRONIC Rx

- Periodic monitoring of TSH level is an essential part of treatment. Patients should be evaluated initially with office visit and TSH levels every 6 to 8 wk until the patient is clinically euthyroid and the TSH level is normalized. The frequency of subsequent visits and TSH measurement can then be decreased to every 6 to 12 mo. Pregnant patients should be checked every trimester.
- For monitoring therapy in patients with central hypothyroidism, measurement of serum free thyroxine (free T_4 level) is appropriate and should be maintained in the upper half of the normal range.

REFERRAL

Admission to the hospital intensive care unit is recommended in all patients with myxedema coma. Additional information on the diagnosis and treatment of this life-threatening complication of hypothyroidism is available under "Myxedema Coma" in Section I.

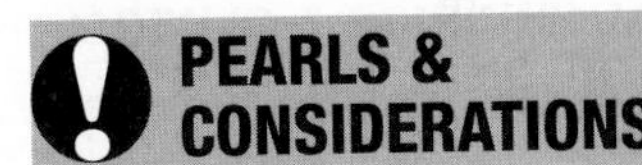

PEARLS & CONSIDERATIONS

COMMENTS

Subclinical hypothyroidism occurs in as many as 15% of elderly patients and is characterized by an elevated serum TSH and a normal free T_4 level. Subclinical hypothyroidism is associated with an increased risk of coronary heart disease events and mortality, particularly in those with a TSH concentration of 10 mU/L or greater. Treatment is individualized. In general, replacement therapy is recommended for all patients with serum TSH >10 mU/L and with presence of goiter or thyroid autoantibodies.

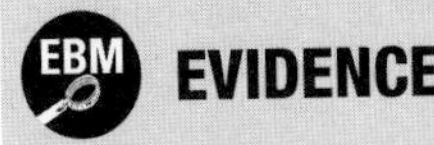

EVIDENCE

available at www.expertconsult.com

SUGGESTED READINGS

available at www.expertconsult.com

RELATED CONTENT

Hypothyroidism (Patient Information)

AUTHOR: **FRED F. FERRI, M.D.**

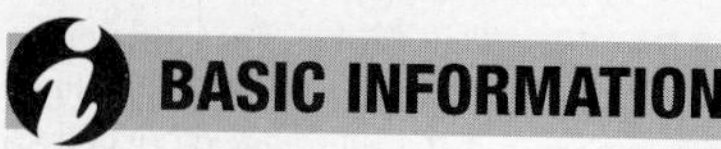

BASIC INFORMATION

DEFINITION

Idiopathic intracranial hypertension (IIH) is a syndrome of increased intracranial pressure (ICP) without underlying hydrocephalus or mass lesion and with normal cerebrospinal fluid analysis.

SYNONYMS

Pseudotumor cerebri
IIH
Benign intracranial hypertension

ICD-9CM CODES
348.2 Pseudotumor cerebri
ICD-10CM CODES
G93.2 Benign intracranial hypertension

EPIDEMIOLOGY & DEMOGRAPHICS

- Disease of obese women in childbearing age

INCIDENCE:

- General population: 1-2 per 100,000 (including children)
- Women (obese females in reproductive age group): 20 per 100,000
- Men: 0.3 to 1.5 cases per 100,000
- Female/male ratio 9:1
- More than 90% of IIH patients are obese
- Mean age at diagnosis is 30 yr

RISK FACTORS:

- Obesity
- Medications: vitamin A and retinoids (used in treatment of acne and leukemia), chronic oral medications used for acne (tetracycline, minocycline)
- Systemic conditions: chronic kidney disease, polycystic ovarian syndrome, obstructive sleep apnea

PHYSICAL FINDINGS & CLINICAL PRESENTATION

Symptoms:

- Headaches: generalized, throbbing, slowly progressive, worse with straining maneuvers, worse in the morning.
- Transient visual obscuration: a brief blurring of vision or scotomata lasting <30 sec; occurs with postural changes, Valsalva maneuver; may be monocular.
- Double vision: usually due to sixth nerve palsy.
- Pulsatile tinnitus: described as a "whooshing sound" that is synchronous with heartbeat; classic symptom that indicates raised ICP.
- Photopsia: lights, sparkles in the eyes.
- Pain: mainly retro-orbital. Pain may also be located in the shoulders or neck. Could be present without a headache. May be associated with Lhermitte's sign.

Signs:

- Papilledema: seen in virtually all cases; usually bilateral but may be asymmetric
- Sixth nerve palsy: seen in approximately 10% to 20% of patients
- Visual field defects: include enlarged physiologic blind spot, nasal field defects, and constricted visual fields. Ninety percent of patients exhibit some form of visual loss on perimetry.
- Loss of central vision: end result of long-standing and untreated IIH

ETIOLOGY

- The exact etiology remains unknown.
- Proposed pathophysiologic mechanisms underlying the raised ICP include increased brain water content, excess CSF production, reduced CSF absorption, and increased cerebral venous pressure either alone or in combination.
- Another proposed mechanism includes abnormal vitamin A metabolism leading to increased CSF retinol levels and decreased CSF absorption at the arachnoid granulations.

DIAGNOSIS

DIAGNOSTIC CRITERIA

MODIFIED DANDY CRITERIA FOR DIAGNOSIS OF IIH:

- Signs and symptoms of raised ICP (listed above)
- Absence of localizing focal neurologic signs (except 6th nerve palsy)
- CSF opening pressure of 25 cm H_2O or more with normal CSF composition
- Normal neuroimaging studies (MRI and MRV brain) including absence of cerebral venous thrombosis; stenosis of transverse sinuses may be seen in IIH without thrombosis.

DIFFERENTIAL DIAGNOSIS

- IIH is a diagnosis of exclusion and criteria listed above have to be satisfied.
- Causes of papilledema include intracranial space-occupying lesions such as tumors, abscesses, hematoma; venous sinus thrombosis; low CSF pressure; carcinomatous meningitis; chronic meningitides such as neurosarcoidosis, CNS lupus, neurosyphilis, cryptococcal meningitis, and tuberculous meningitis.

WORKUP

- Neuroimaging studies: MRI of brain with MR venogram; CT head and CT head venogram when MRI of brain cannot be obtained.
- Lumbar puncture: CSF opening pressure (OP) should be obtained in the lateral decubitus position with the legs stretched and patient relaxed. OP exceeding 25 cm H_2O is considered elevated. CSF composition should be normal.
- Ophthalmologic examination: all patients with IIH need an ophthalmologic examination including visual fields at baseline and follow-up visits.

LABORATORY TESTS

CSF analysis shows normal protein, glucose, and cell count.

IMAGING STUDIES

- MRI of the brain to rule out underlying structural lesions
  - Absence of specific causes of raised ICP listed above
  - Empty sella sign often associated with chronic raised ICP but not pathognomonic
- MR or CT venography to exclude cortical venous thrombosis
  - May show transverse sinus stenosis in IIH without thrombosis. Absence of specific causes of raised ICP listed above.
- CT head
  - May show slit-like ventricles

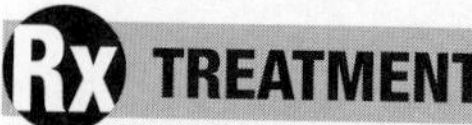

TREATMENT

NONPHARMACOLOGIC THERAPY

- Weight loss in obese patients
- Continuous positive airway pressure if obstructive sleep apnea is suspected

ACUTE GENERAL Rx

- Acetazolamide 250 mg to 4 g per day: reduces CSF production by inhibition of carbonic anhydrase, occasionally causing anorexia and resultant weight loss. Dose can be increased to a maximum of 4 g a day in resistant cases with visual loss.
- Furosemide 40 to 120 mg/day in divided doses: apparent mechanism of action is by reduced sodium transport, leading to decreased total CSF volume.
- Topiramate 100 to 400 mg/day: reported to be effective in treatment of IIH. It is a weak carbonic anhydrase inhibitor with weight loss as one of its primary side effects.
- Serial lumbar punctures: SHOULD NOT BE CONSIDERED AS STANDARD TREATMENT OF IIH. LP should be attempted in patients with severe headaches resistant to medical therapy. Goal is to reduce spinal fluid pressure to allow immediate reduction in headache severity. This treatment should be reserved for the most resistant cases and should be used as a conduit to future surgical intervention. Serial LP should not be used as treatment for IIH with progressive visual loss.

CHRONIC Rx

Surgical intervention is indicated in cases of treatment failure and progressive visual loss.

- Optic nerve fenestration: preferred for patients with visual loss and easily controlled headaches. Proposed mechanism is decompression of the optic nerve. Highly effective; however, has been associated with significant number of failure rates.
- CSF shunting: neurosurgical procedure; performed in patients with significant visual deterioration and difficult-to-control headaches. Provides rapid improvement in symptoms; however, reported to have significant rates of shunt revisions because of shunt malfunction.

DISPOSITION

- IIH is a potentially blinding condition, with severe vision loss in 5%-10% of patients; patients should be co-managed by neurologists and ophthalmologists (preferably by a neuro-ophthalmologist). Monthly follow-up is essential until visual fields stabilize.
- All patients with IIH should undergo MR or CT venography to rule out the possibility of venous sinus thrombosis.

REFERRAL

- Neuro-ophthalmologist for serial evaluation of visual fields and fundus photographs
- Nutritionist for weight loss
- General neurologist for the initial workup and eventual treatment of raised ICP

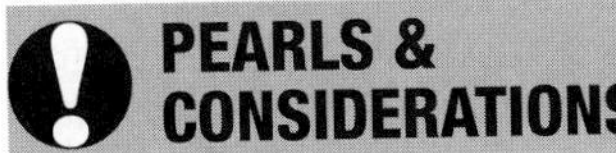

PEARLS & CONSIDERATIONS

COMMENTS

- IIH is a potentially blinding condition.
- IIH is a diagnosis of exclusion.
- IIH is a disease of young obese women.

PREVENTION

Maintenance of ideal body weight is one of the best preventive mechanisms for avoidance of IIH. However, it does occur in patients with normal body weight. In these cases there are no known preventable risk factors.

PATIENT & FAMILY EDUCATION

The combination of weight loss and medical therapy is highly effective in treatment of IIH. Given that most patients with IIH are young and otherwise healthy, high success rates can be accomplished.

SUGGESTED READINGS

available at www.expertconsult.com

RELATED CONTENT

Diplopia (Section II, Differential Diagnosis)
Optic Atrophy (Section II, Differential Diagnosis)
Papilledema (Section II, Differential Diagnosis)

AUTHOR: **SACHIN KEDAR, M.B.B.S, M.D.**

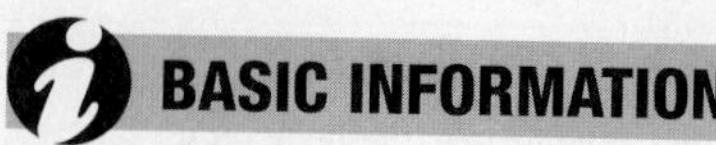

BASIC INFORMATION

DEFINITION

Idiopathic pulmonary fibrosis (IPF) is a specific form of chronic fibrosing interstitial pneumonia with histopathologic characteristics of usual interstitial pneumonia (UIP). Disease characterized by progressive parenchymal scarring and loss of pulmonary function.

SYNONYMS

Cryptogenic fibrosing alveolitis
IPF
Pulmonary fibrosis
Usual interstitial pneumonia

ICD-9CM CODES
516.3 Idiopathic pulmonary fibrosis
ICD-10CM CODES
J84.112 Idiopathic pulmonary fibrosis

EPIDEMIOLOGY & DEMOGRAPHICS

- Incidence: 7-16 cases/100,000 persons worldwide. Clinically IPF affects >50,000 people in the U.S.
- Most commonly presents in 5th and 6th decades
- More common in men than women
- More common in current and past smokers
- Familial forms account for 3% to 25% of cases. Genetic variants: include mutations in surfactant protein C and abnormal telomere shortening.
- No distinct geographic distribution; no clear racial predilection

PHYSICAL FINDINGS & CLINICAL PRESENTATION

- Most present with gradual onset (>6 mo) of exertional dyspnea and nonproductive cough. Progressive dyspnea is usually the most prominent symptom. Cough affects up to 80% of patients with IPF, is frequently disabling, and lacks effective therapy.
- Fine bibasilar inspiratory crackles in >80% of patients, with progression upward as the disease advances.
- Clubbing is found in 25% to 50% of patients.
- Cyanosis and right heart failure (cor pulmonale) may occur late in the disease course.
- Extrapulmonary involvement rarely occurs. Fever and wheezing are rare and suggest alternative diagnosis.

ETIOLOGY

- Unknown
- Cigarette smoking, environmental exposure, and microaspiration have been associated with IPF.
- Aberrant tissue repair and fibrosis are believed to play a greater role in the pathogenesis than generalized inflammation.

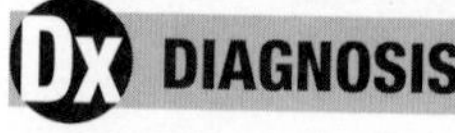

DIAGNOSIS

DIFFERENTIAL DIAGNOSIS

- Sarcoidosis
- Drug-induced interstitial lung disease
- Pulmonary manifestations of collagen vascular diseases (e.g., rheumatoid arthritis [RA], systemic sclerosis)
- Hypersensitivity pneumonitis (HP)
- Occupational exposures (e.g., asbestos, silica) may cause pneumoconiosis that mimics IPF
- Other idiopathic interstitial pneumonias:
  - Desquamative interstitial pneumonia (DIP)
  - Respiratory bronchitis–interstitial lung disease (RB-ILD)
  - Acute interstitial pneumonia (AIP)
  - Nonspecific interstitial pneumonia (NSIP)
  - Cryptogenic organizing pneumonia (COP)

WORKUP

- Almost all patients have abnormal chest radiograph at presentation, with bilateral reticular opacities most prominent in the periphery and lower lobes. Peripheral honeycombing may be seen.
- High-resolution CT scan shows patchy peripheral reticular abnormalities with intralobular linear opacities, irregular septal thickening, subpleural honeycombing, and may have ground-glass opacities.
- Pulmonary function testing shows restrictive pattern and reduced carbon monoxide diffusion into the lung.
- Six-minute walk test may show reduced exercise tolerance and/or exertional hypoxia.
- Laboratory abnormalities (nondiagnostic): mild anemia; increases in erythrocyte sedimentation rate, lactate dehydrogenase, C-reactive protein; low titer antinuclear antibody seen in up to 30% of patients.
- There is a limited role for bronchoalveolar lavage either in diagnosis or monitoring IPF.
- Gold standard for diagnosis is lung biopsy (open thoracotomy or video-assisted thoracoscopy). Hallmark features: heterogeneous distribution of parenchymal fibrosis against background of mild inflammation (UIP).
- Lung biopsy is critical to distinguish IPF from diseases with better prognosis and treatment options, especially in patients with any atypical features.

Rx TREATMENT

- No proven treatment for IPF and little evidence to support the routine use of any specific therapy. With the lack of evidence supporting specific therapies in IPF, evaluation for participation in clinical trials of new therapies may be warranted.
- In patients with advanced disease, treatment options include supportive care (pulmonary rehabilitation, supplemental oxygen, influenza and pneumococcal vaccination) and potential lung transplantation.
- Treatment of asymptomatic gastroesophageal reflux may be reasonable given association between pulmonary fibrosis and reflux or microaspiration.
- Lung transplantation is the only therapy shown to prolong survival in IPF. Posttransplant 5-yr survival for IPF patients is approximately 40%. Median survival time is longer after bilateral lung transplantation than single lung transplantation but is associated with more complications during the first year.
- The antifibrotic agent, pirfenidone, may have some effect with regards to slowing the progression of the disease; however, it is currently not available in the United States.
- Acute exacerbation of IPF, defined as worsening dyspnea (<1 mo), the presence of new opacities on radiograph, and the lack of evidence of infection, has an incidence of 10% to 57%. Progressive respiratory failure may require mechanical ventilation. Treatment often includes high-dose corticosteroids and broad-spectrum antibiotics.

DISPOSITION

- Spontaneous remissions do not occur.
- Natural history includes progressive loss of pulmonary function.
- There is an 8 to 14× increased risk of lung cancer.
- Mean survival after the diagnosis of biopsy-confirmed IPF is 2 to 5 yr.
- Respiratory failure is the most common cause of death.

REFERRAL

To pulmonologist for review of abnormal chest imaging and establishing diagnosis

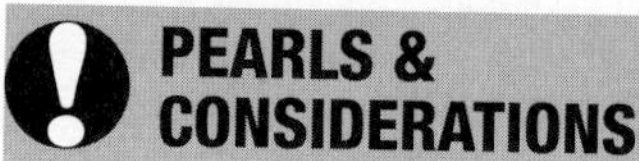

PEARLS & CONSIDERATIONS

- The course is progressive, with a high mortality rate.
- Among patients with IPF, a common risk polymorphism in MUC5B is associated with improved survival. Further research is necessary to refine the risk estimates and to determine the clinical implications of these findings.[1]
- Critical to differentiate IPF from other interstitial lung diseases because prognosis and response to treatment differ.
- There is no proven treatment for IPF. Recent studies have shown an increase in mortality, hospitalizations, and side effects with combination treatment (prednisone/azathioprine/NAC). Novel therapeutic agents targeting aberrant epithelial cell activation and repair may prove beneficial. The tyrosine kinase inhibitor BIBF 1120 at a dose of 150 mg bid has been reported to reduce the decline in lung function, with fewer exacerbations and preserved quality of life as compared to placebo. Trials involving thalidomide, a potent immunomodulary agent, have shown improvement in cough and respiratory quality of life.
- Consider early referral for lung transplant.

[1]Peljto AL et al: Association between the MUC5B promoter polymorphism and survival in patients with idiopathic pulmonary fibrosis, *JAMA* 309(21):2232-2239, 2013.

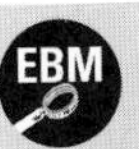

EVIDENCE

available at www.expertconsult.com

SUGGESTED READINGS

available at www.expertconsult.com

RELATED CONTENT

Idiopathic Pulmonary Fibrosis (Patient Information)

AUTHOR: **MICHAEL BLUNDIN, M.D.**

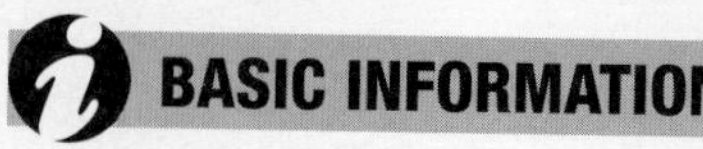

BASIC INFORMATION

DEFINITION

Immunoglobulin A (IgA) nephropathy is a proliferative glomerulonephritis associated with predominant deposition of IgA in the mesangium. The diagnostic hallmark of IgA nephropathy is the predominance of IgA deposits, either alone or with IgG, IgM, or both, in the glomerular mesangium.[1]

SYNONYMS

Berger's disease

ICD-9CM CODES
583.81 IgA Nephropathy
ICD-10CM CODES
N02.8 IgA nephropathy
N02.1 IgA nephropathy with glomerular lesion, focal and segmental hyalinosis or sclerosis
N02.3 IgA nephropathy with glomerular lesion, mesangial proliferative (diffuse)
N02.5 IgA nephropathy with glomerular lesion, membrane proliferative (diffuse)

EPIDEMIOLOGY & DEMOGRAPHICS

INCIDENCE: It is the most common type of glomerulonephropathy worldwide. The annual incidence of IgA nephropathy among children in the U.S. is about 0.5 cases per 100,000; however, in Japan, the incidence is 10 times as high.[1]

PREVALENCE: Prevalence rate is lower in the U.S. (10% to 15%) compared with Asian countries. Lower rates could be explained by a conservative approach by nephrologists in the U.S., who are reluctant to do renal biopsy in asymptomatic patients with minimal renal abnormalities. In most reports prevalence rates are expressed as a percentage of cases of primary glomerulonephritis or as a percentage of total series of renal biopsies.

PREDOMINANT SEX AND AGE: It is most prevalent in the second and third decades of life with a male/female ratio of 6:1 in the U.S.

GENETICS: Although it is considered a sporadic disease, genetic linkage to locus called *IgAN1* on 6q22 and 6q23 has been shown.

RISK FACTORS: It has a higher association with Asians, whites, and Native Americans and is rarely seen in African Americans.

PHYSICAL FINDINGS & CLINICAL PRESENTATION

- Two common presentations include (1) recurrent macroscopic hematuria often associated with upper respiratory infection and (2) persistent microscopic hematuria.
- Loin pain may be associated with macroscopic hematuria.
- Physical findings are usually unremarkable, except hypertension seen in 20% to 30% of patients with chronic disease and edema in 5% of patients with nephrotic-range proteinuria.
- Mild proteinuria is common.
- Rarely, IgA nephropathy presents as acute renal failure in 5% of patients and chronic renal failure in 10% to 20% of patients.

ETIOLOGY

- Most cases are idiopathic/primary.
- Secondary causes of IgA nephropathy include Henoch-Schönlein purpura; hepatitis B; alcoholic cirrhosis; celiac disease; inflammatory bowel disease; psoriasis; sarcoidosis; cystic fibrosis; cancer of the lungs, larynx, or pancreas; HIV infection; systemic lupus erythematosus; rheumatoid arthritis; diabetic nephropathy; Sjögren's syndrome; and Reiter's syndrome.
- Fig. 1-512 illustrates the pathogenesis of IgA nephropathy.

DIAGNOSIS

DIFFERENTIAL DIAGNOSIS

- Henoch-Schönlein purpura
- Hereditary nephritis
- Thin glomerular basement membrane disease
- Lupus nephritis
- Poststreptococcal nephritis
- Secondary causes associated with IgA nephropathy mentioned above

WORKUP

- The diagnosis is suspected on the basis of clinical history and laboratory data but is confirmed by renal biopsy showing IgA deposits in the mesangium.
- Renal biopsy is restricted to patients with sustained proteinuria >1 g/day or worsening renal function.

LABORATORY TESTS

- Urine analysis showing protein, red blood cells and casts, and white blood cells.
- Serum creatinine may be elevated.
- 24-hour urine assay for quantifying proteinuria and to check creatinine clearance.
- Serum IgA is elevated in only 50% of patients and has no clinical utility.

TREATMENT

Although initially considered a benign disease, IgA nephropathy is now recognized as a common cause of renal failure. Currently there is no cure. Table 1-274 summarizes treatment recommendations for IgA nephropathy.

NONPHARMACOLOGIC THERAPY

- Moderate dietary protein restriction
- Discourage smoking

ACUTE AND CHRONIC GENERAL Rx

- Aggressive therapy for hypertension, preferably with angiotensin-converting enzyme (ACE) inhibitors. Goal blood pressure is <125/75 mm Hg in the presence of proteinuria >1 g/day.
- Patients with recurrent gross hematuria or isolated microscopic hematuria, no or minimal proteinuria (<1 g/day), normal blood pressure, and normal kidney function should only be monitored every 6 to 12 mo to assess disease progression.

Pathogenesis of IgA nephropathy
Mucosal immune system
Polymeric IgA1 (pIgA1) production↓
IgA1 response to mucosal immunization↓
Bone marrow
pIgA1 production↑
pIgA1 response to systemic immunization↑
Circulation
Monomeric IgA1 (mIgA1)↑
pIgA1↑
IgA rheumatoid factors↑
Abnormal O-glycosylation of IgA↑
Kidney
pIgA1 deposition
± IgG/complement deposition
Liver
Impaired IgA1 clearance
Mesangial cell proliferation
Mesangial matrix↑
Sclerosis

FIGURE 1-512 Pathogenesis of IgA nephropathy. Abnormalities in IgA immunity leading to mesangial IgA deposition and injury. (Modified from Johnson RJ, Feehally J: *Comprehensive clinical nephrology,* ed 2, St Louis, 2000, Mosby.)

[1]Wyatt RJ, Julian BA: IgA nephropathy, *N Engl J Med* 368:2402-2414, 2013.

- If bouts of recurrent macroscopic hematuria are associated with tonsillitis, tonsillectomy may benefit these patients.
- Patients with persistent proteinuria >1 g/day with or without hypertension are treated with ACE inhibitors and/or angiotensin receptor blockers (ARBs). Steroids are reserved for patients with persistent proteinuria >1 g/day despite ACE and/or ARB administration.
- Patients with nephrotic syndrome, preserved kidney function, and minimal change in disease are treated with steroids for 6 mo.
- Patients with severe renal disease or crescentic, rapidly progressive glomerulonephritis in the absence of changes of chronic kidney disease in biopsy are treated with steroid and cyclophosphamide combination for the first 2 mo, followed by steroids and azathioprine for 2 yr for maintenance treatment.
- Patients with acute renal failure need renal biopsy to rule out acute tubular necrosis, which needs only supportive therapy, from crescentic IgA nephropathy, which needs aggressive medical management.
- Kidney transplantation is the treatment of choice for end-stage kidney disease. There is no difference in survival in living versus cadaver donors. At present, kidneys with IgA deposits are not used for transplantation.
- Statins are indicated for all IgA nephropathy patients with dyslipidemia, hypertension, and other cardiovascular risks.
- Role of mycophenolate and plasmapheresis is controversial.

TABLE 1-274 Treatment Recommendations for IgA Nephropathy

Treatment Recommendations for IgA Nephropathy
Recurrent Macroscopic Hematuria (Preserved Renal Function)
Aggressive hydration (no role for antibiotics or tonsillectomy)
Macroscopic Hematuria with Acute Kidney Injury
Renal biopsy mandatory if persistent acute kidney injury (see text) Acute tubular necrosis: supportive measures only Crescentic IgA nephropathy Induction: Prednisolone 0.5-1 mg/kg/day for up to 8 wk Cyclophosphamide 2 mg/kg/day for up to 8 wk (no evidence favoring oral or intravenous route—follow local practice) Maintenance: Prednisolone in reducing dosage Azathioprine 2.5 mg/kg/day
Proteinuria >1 g/24 h (±Microscopic Hematuria)
ACE inhibitor or ARB for urinary protein excretion of >18/day; increase dose depending on blood pressure
Nephrotic Syndrome with Minimal Change on Light Microscopy
Prednisolone 0.5-1 mg/kg/day (children 60 mg/m2/day) for up to 8 wk, then taper
Non-nephrotic Proteinuria <1 g/24 h (±Microscopic Hematuria)
ACE inhibitor and/or ARB (maximize dosage or combine to achieve target BP and proteinuria <0.5 g/day) If proteinuria still >1 g/24 h on maximal supportive therapy and GFR <70 ml/min, consider fish oil (12 g/daily for 6 mo). If further progression of renal failure, consider prednisolone (40 mg/day decreasing to 10 mg by 2 yr).
Hypertension
ACE inhibitors and ARB are agent of first choice—target BP: 130/80 mm Hg if proteinuria <1 g/24 h; 125/75 mm Hg if proteinuria >1 g/24 h
Transplantation
No special measures required

ACE, Angiotensin-converting enzyme; *ARB*, angiotensin receptor blocker; *BP*, blood pressure; *GFR*, glomerular filtration rate.
Modified from Floege J et al: *Comprehensive clinical nephrology*, ed 4, Philadelphia, 2010, Saunders.

BOX 1-47 Prognostic Markers at Presentation in IgA Nephropathy

Clinical

Poor Prognosis

Increasing age
Duration of preceding symptoms
Severity of proteinuria
Hyperuricemia
Hypertension
Renal impairment

Good Prognosis

Recurrent macroscopic hematuria

No Impact on Prognosis

Gender
Serum IgA level

Histopathologic

Poor Prognosis

Glomerular sclerosis
Tubular atrophy
Interstitial fibrosis
Vascular wall thickening
Capillary-loop IgA deposits

No Impact on Prognosis

Intensity of IgA deposits

None of the clinical or histopathologic adverse features, except capillary-loop IgA deposits, are specific to IgA nephropathy.
From Feehally J et al: *Comprehensive clinical nephrology*, ed 4, Philadelphia, 2010, Saunders.

COMPLEMENTARY & ALTERNATIVE MEDICINE

Role of fish oil is controversial.

DISPOSITION

- Complete remission occurs in <10% of patients.
- End-stage renal failure develops in 15% to 20% of patients within 10 yr of onset and in 30% to 35% of patients within 20 yr. Prognostic markers at presentation in IgA nephropathy are described in Box 1-47.
- Poor prognostic indicators include (1) male gender, (2) older age, (3) young age at the onset of the disease, (4) absence of episodes of recurrent macroscopic hematuria, (5) hypertension, (6) extent of renal insufficiency, (7) extent of proteinuria, (8) elevated serum uric acid, and (9) certain histologic changes seen in renal biopsy, such as crescents, glomerulosclerosis, and tubulointerstitial fibrosis or atrophy.
- The serum level of glycan-specific IgG antibodies is correlated with the level of urinary protein excretion and the risk of progression to end-stage renal disease (ESRD) or death.[1]

REFERRAL

Patients with IgA nephropathy are commonly referred to nephrologists.

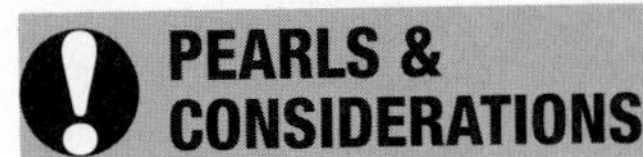

PEARLS & CONSIDERATIONS

COMMENTS

- IgA nephropathy seems to be a kidney-restricted form of Henoch-Schönlein purpura.
- IgA nephropathy is not an entirely benign condition, even when microhematuria is the only clinical presentation.

SUGGESTED READINGS

available at www.expertconsult.com

AUTHOR: **HEMANT K. SATPATHY, M.D.**

BASIC INFORMATION

DEFINITION

Immune thrombocytopenic purpura (ITP) is an autoimmune disorder in which antibody-coated or immune complex–coated platelets are destroyed prematurely by the reticuloendothelial system, resulting in peripheral thrombocytopenia. In primary ITP the thrombocytopenia is isolated, whereas in secondary ITP the condition is associated with other disorders (e.g., SLE, HIV).

ICD-9CM CODES
287.3 Idiopathic thrombocytopenic purpura (ITP)
ICD-10CM CODES
D69.3 Immune thrombocytopenic purpura

EPIDEMIOLOGY & DEMOGRAPHICS

INCIDENCE: Primary ITP incidence is 10 in 100,000 adults, 5 in 100,000 children

PREVALENCE: Five to 10 cases per 100,000 persons

PREDOMINANT SEX: 72% of patients > 10 yr are female; in children, males and females are affected equally

PREDOMINANT AGE: Children ages 2 to 4 yr and young women (70% are < 40 yr)

PHYSICAL FINDINGS & CLINICAL PRESENTATION

The presentation of ITP is different in children and adults:

- Children generally present with sudden onset of bruising and petechiae from severe thrombocytopenia.
- In adults the presentation is insidious; a history of prolonged purpura may be present; many patients are diagnosed incidentally on the basis of automated laboratory tests that now routinely include platelet counts.
- The physical examination may be entirely normal.
- Patients with severe thrombocytopenia may have petechiae, purpura, epistaxis, or heme-positive stool from gastrointestinal bleeding. Life-threatening bleeding is uncommon and generally confined to patients with platelets <10,000 per cubic mm.
- Splenomegaly is unusual; its presence should alert to the possibility of other etiologies of thrombocytopenia.
- The presence of dysmorphic features (skeletal anomalies, auditory abnormalities) may indicate a congenital disorder as the cause of the thrombocytopenia.

ETIOLOGY

Increased platelet destruction caused by autoantibodies to platelet-membrane antigens. Hundreds of medications can cause thrombocytopenia. Drugs commonly implicated are quinidine, heparin, antibiotics (linezolid, vancomycin, sulfonamides, rifampin), platelet inhibitors (tirofiban, abciximab, eptifibatide), cimetidine, NSAIDs, thiazide diuretics, antirheumatic agents (gold salts, penicillamine), acetaminophen, and chemotherapeutic agents (cyclosporine, fludarabine, oxaliplatin).

Dx DIAGNOSIS

DIFFERENTIAL DIAGNOSIS

- Falsely low platelet count (resulting from EDTA-dependent or cold-dependent agglutinins)
- Viral infections (e.g., HIV, hepatitis C, mononucleosis, rubella)
- Drug-induced (e.g., heparin, quinidine, sulfonamides)
- Hypersplenism resulting from liver disease
- Myelodysplastic and lymphoproliferative disorders
- Pregnancy, hypothyroidism
- SLE, TTP, hemolytic-uremic syndrome
- Congenital thrombocytopenia (e.g., Fanconi's syndrome, May-Hegglin anomaly, Bernard-Soulier syndrome)

LABORATORY TESTS

- Complete blood count, platelet count, and peripheral smear: platelets are decreased but are normal in size or may appear larger than normal (Fig. E1-513). Red blood cells and white blood cells have a normal morphology.
- Additional tests may be ordered to exclude other causes of the thrombocytopenia when clinically indicated (e.g., HIV, ANA, TSH, liver enzymes, bone marrow examination).
- The direct assay for the measurement of platelet-bound antibodies has an estimated positive predictive value of 80% to 83%. A negative test cannot be used to rule out the diagnosis.

IMAGING STUDIES

CT scan of abdomen/pelvis in patients with splenomegaly to exclude other disorders causing thrombocytopenia

Rx TREATMENT

NONPHARMACOLOGIC THERAPY

- Minimize activity to prevent injury or bruising (e.g., contact sports should be avoided).
- Stop any potentially offending drugs (see "Etiology"). Avoid medications that increase the risk of bleeding (e.g., aspirin and other NSAIDs).

ACUTE GENERAL Rx

- Treatment varies with the platelet count, patient's age, and bleeding status (Fig. 1-514).
- Observation and frequent monitoring of platelet count are needed in asymptomatic patients with platelet counts >30,000/mm^3.
- Oral prednisone 1 mg/kg/day in a tapering dose generally for 4 to 6 wk is the most common initial regimen. Methylprednisolone 30 mg/kg/day IV infused over a period of 20 to 30 min (maximum dose of 1 g/day for 2 or 3 days) plus IV immunoglobulin (1 g/kg/day for 2 or 3 days) and infusion of platelets should be given to patients with neurologic symptoms, internal bleeding, or those undergoing emergency surgery.
- Prednisone continued until the platelet count is normalized then slowly tapered off is indicated in adults with platelet counts <20,000/mm^3 and those who have counts <50,000/mm^3 and significant mucous membrane bleeding. Response rates range from 50% to 75%, and most responses occur within the first 3 wk. Oral dexamethasone at a dosage of 40 mg/day for 4 consecutive days has also been reported to induce a high response rate (85%). Continuation of corticosteriods is limited by long-term complications associated with its use (osteoporosis, weight gain, opportunistic infections, emotional lability)
- IV immunoglobulin (0.8-1.0 g/kg) is used in patients who have not responded to corticosteroids and often in pregnant patients. It rapidly increases platelet count in nearly 80% of patients, but its effect is transient. Anti-D immunoglobulin, a pooled IgG product derived from the plasma of Rh(D)-negative donors, is also effective. It can be given only to patients who are Rh(D) positive. Usual dose is 50-75 mcg/kg.
- Rituximab, a monoclonal antibody directed against the CD20 antigen, is used as a second-line agent. Usual dose is 375 mg/m^2 weekly x4 wk.
- Splenectomy is considered second-line treatment and should be considered in adults with platelet count <20,000/mm^3 after 6 wk of medical treatment or after 6 mo if more than 10 to 20 mg of prednisone per day is required to maintain a platelet count >30,000/mm^3. In children, splenectomy is generally reserved for persistent thrombocytopenia (>1 yr) and clinically significant bleeding. Appropriate immunizations (pneumococcal vaccine in adults and children, *Haemophilus influenzae* vaccine, meningococcal vaccine in children) should be administered before splenectomy.
- Additional second-line agents are thrombopoietin receptor agonists, azathioprine, cyclosporin A, cyclophosphamide, danazol, dapsone, mycophenolate mofetil, and *Vinca* alkaloids. Romiplostim, a recombinant fusion protein, and the oral thrombopoietin-receptor agonist eltrombopag are effective in increasing platelet count in adult patients with chronic ITP refractory to corticosteroids and/or splenectomy. The American Society of Hematology guidelines revised in 2011 recommend the use of thrombopoietin-receptor agonists for adult patients with ITP at risk for bleeding, who have a contraindication to splenectomy, or do not have a response to at least one other therapy.
- Platelet transfusion is needed only in case of life-threatening hemorrhage.
- Third-line therapy for ITP consists of combination chemotherapy and hematopoietic stem cell transplantation.

DISPOSITION

- More than 80% of children have a complete remission within 8 wk.
- In adults, the course of the disease is chronic; only 5% of adults have spontaneous remission.
- The principal cause of death from ITP is intracranial hemorrhage (1% of children, 5% of adults).

SUGGESTED READINGS

available at www.expertconsult.com

RELATED CONTENT

Immune Thrombocytopenic Purpura (Patient Information)

AUTHOR: **FRED F. FERRI, M.D.**

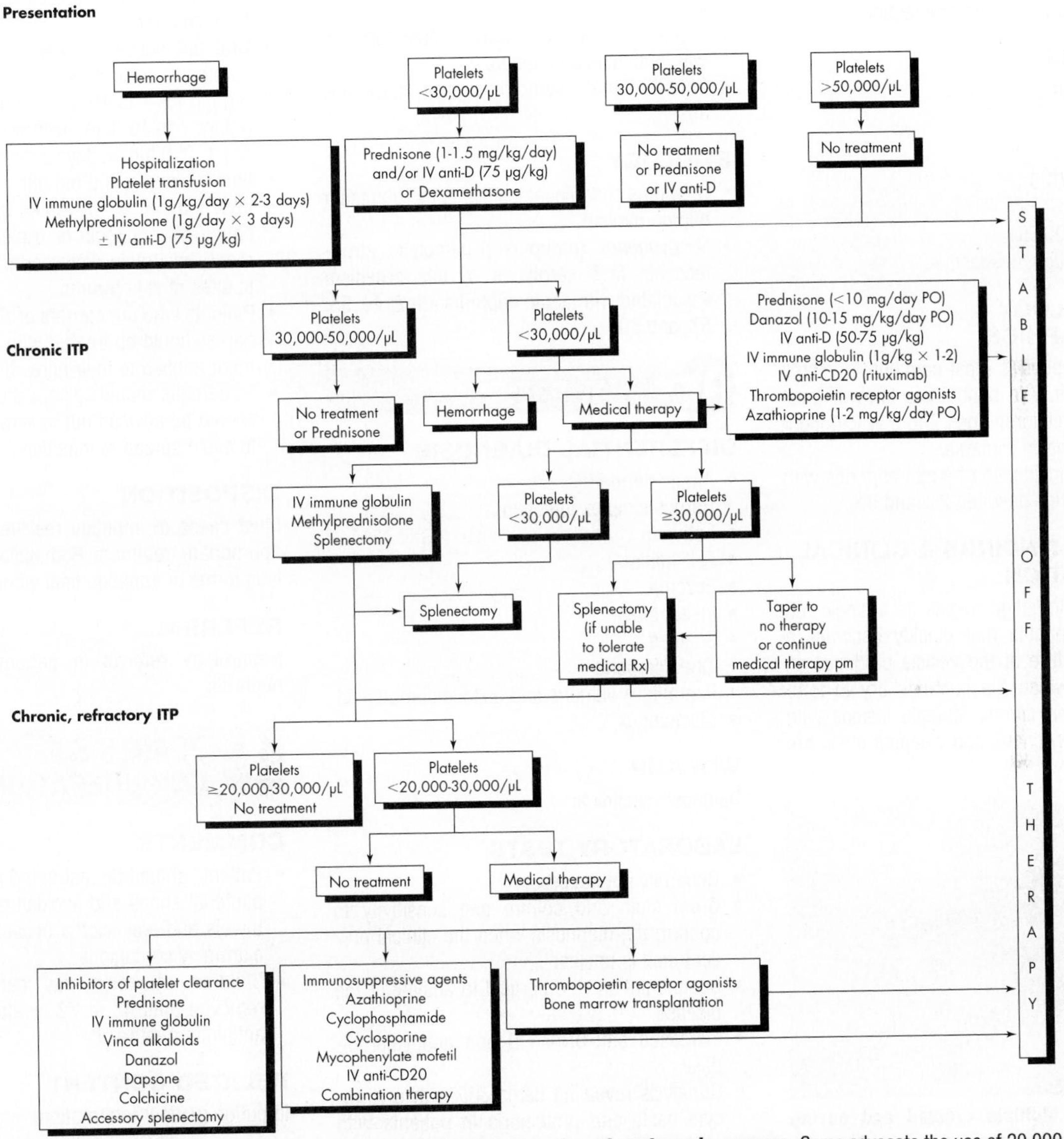

Presentation

Hemorrhage

Hospitalization
Platelet transfusion
IV immune globulin (1g/kg/day × 2-3 days)
Methylprednisolone (1g/day × 3 days)
± IV anti-D (75 μg/kg)

Platelets <30,000/μL

Prednisone (1-1.5 mg/kg/day) and/or IV anti-D (75 μg/kg) or Dexamethasone

Platelets 30,000-50,000/μL

No treatment or Prednisone or IV anti-D

Platelets >50,000/μL

No treatment

Chronic ITP

Platelets 30,000-50,000/μL

No treatment or Prednisone

Platelets <30,000/μL

Hemorrhage

Medical therapy

Prednisone (<10 mg/day PO)
Danazol (10-15 mg/kg/day PO)
IV anti-D (50-75 μg/kg)
IV immune globulin (1g/kg × 1-2)
IV anti-CD20 (rituximab)
Thrombopoietin receptor agonists
Azathioprine (1-2 mg/kg/day PO)

IV immune globulin
Methylprednisolone
Splenectomy

Platelets <30,000/μL

Platelets ≥30,000/μL

Splenectomy

Splenectomy (if unable to tolerate medical Rx)

Taper to no therapy or continue medical therapy prn

Chronic, refractory ITP

Platelets ≥20,000-30,000/μL
No treatment

Platelets <20,000-30,000/μL

No treatment

Medical therapy

Inhibitors of platelet clearance
Prednisone
IV immune globulin
Vinca alkaloids
Danazol
Dapsone
Colchicine
Accessory splenectomy

Immunosuppressive agents
Azathioprine
Cyclophosphamide
Cyclosporine
Mycophenylate mofetil
IV anti-CD20
Combination therapy

Thrombopoietin receptor agonists
Bone marrow transplantation

STABLE OFF THERAPY

FIGURE 1-514 Treatment algorithm for management of adult-onset immune thrombocytopenic purpura. Some advocate the use of 20,000/mcL as a guideline for therapy. The decision to treat patients with platelet counts lower than 50,000/mcL is based in part on evidence of bleeding, a history of bleeding, comorbid risk factors, lifestyle, and tolerance of therapy. There is no consensus as to duration of steroid therapy. The use of anti-D as initial therapy is appropriate only for Rh(D)-positive individuals who are not markedly anemic or hemolyzing. The goal of medical therapy is to attain a hemostatic platelet count, generally greater than 20,000 to 30,000/mcL. The threshold for treatment depends on comorbid risk factors for bleeding and risk of trauma. Higher platelet counts may be appropriate for surgery or after trauma. Medications can be used individually, but combinations of azathioprine and danazol (or corticosteroids) may provide added benefit and allow lower doses to be used. Intravenous immunoglobulin (IVIG) and anti-D are generally reserved for severe thrombocytopenia unresponsive to oral agents. The decision to proceed to splenectomy depends on intensity of therapy required, tolerance to side effects, risk of surgery, and patient preference. IVIG and/or methylprednisolone may help to increase the platelet count immediately prior to splenectomy. Laparoscopic and open splenectomy have comparable outcomes. The decision to treat patients who have platelet counts lower than 20,000 to 30,000/mcL after splenectomy involves an assessment of the risk of hemorrhage versus the side effects of each form of therapy. (Modified from Hoffman R et al: *Hematology, basic principles and practice,* ed 5, Philadelphia, 2009, Churchill Livingstone.)

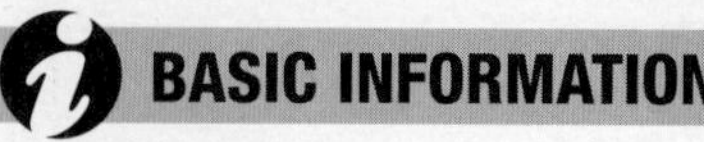

BASIC INFORMATION

DEFINITION

Impetigo is a superficial skin infection generally caused by *Staphylococcus aureus* and/or *Streptococcus* spp.

Common presentations are bullous impetigo (generally caused by staphylococcal disease) and nonbullous impetigo (from streptococcal infection and possible staphylococcal infection); the bullous form is caused by an epidermolytic toxin produced at the site of infection.

SYNONYMS

Impetigo vulgaris
Pyoderma

ICD-9CM CODES
684 Impetigo
ICD-10CM CODES
L01.00 Impetigo, unspecified

EPIDEMIOLOGY & DEMOGRAPHICS

- Bullous impetigo is most common in infants and children. The nonbullous form is most common in children ages 2 to 5 yr with poor hygiene in warm climates.
- The overall incidence of acute nephritis with impetigo varies between 2% and 5%.

PHYSICAL FINDINGS & CLINICAL PRESENTATION

- Nonbullous impetigo begins as a single red macule or papule that quickly becomes a vesicle. Rupture of the vesicle produces an erosion of which the contents dry to form honey-colored crusts. Multiple lesions with golden yellow crusts and weeping areas are often found on the skin around the nose, mouth (Fig. 1-515), and limbs.
- Bullous impetigo is manifested by the presence of vesicles that enlarge rapidly to form bullae with contents that vary from clear to cloudy. There is subsequent collapse of the center of the bullae; the peripheral areas may retain fluid, and a honey-colored crust may appear in the center. As the lesions enlarge and become contiguous with the others, a scaling border replaces the fluid-filled rim; there is minimal erythema surrounding the lesions.
- Regional lymphadenopathy is most common with nonbullous impetigo.
- Constitutional symptoms are generally absent.

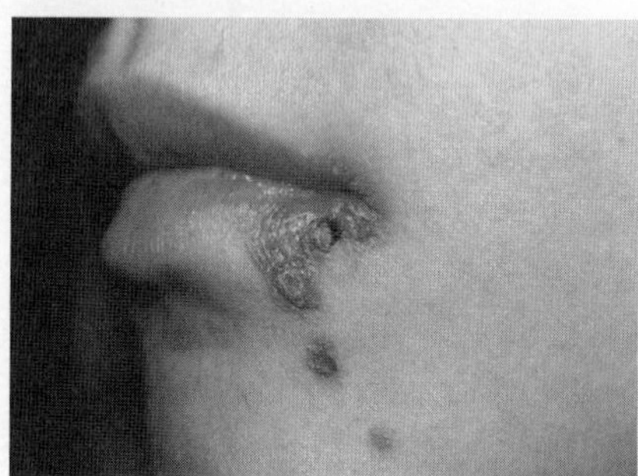

FIGURE 1-515 Multiple crusted and oozing lesions of impetigo. (From Kliegman RM et al: *Nelson textbook of pediatrics,* ed 19, Philadelphia, 2011, Saunders.)

ETIOLOGY

- *S. aureus* coagulase positive is the dominant microorganism.
- *S. pyogenes* (group A β-hemolytic streptococci): M-T serotypes of this organism associated with acute nephritis are 2, 49, 55, 57, and 60.

DIAGNOSIS

DIFFERENTIAL DIAGNOSIS

- Atopic dermatitis
- Herpes simplex infection
- Ecthyma
- Folliculitis
- Eczema
- Insect bites
- Scabies
- Tinea corporis
- Pemphigus vulgaris and bullous pemphigoid
- Chickenpox

WORKUP

Diagnosis is clinical.

LABORATORY TESTS

- Generally not necessary
- Gram stain and culture and sensitivity to confirm the diagnosis when the clinical presentation is unclear
- Sedimentation rate parallel to activity of the disease
- Increased anti-DNAse B and antihyaluronidase
- Urinalysis revealing hematuria with erythrocyte casts and proteinuria in patients with acute nephritis (most frequently occurring in children between ages 2 and 4 yr in the southern part of the U.S.)

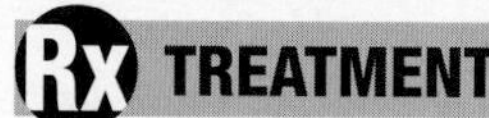

TREATMENT

NONPHARMACOLOGIC THERAPY

Remove crusts by soaking with wet cloth compresses (crusts block the penetration of antibacterial creams).

GENERAL Rx

- Application of 2% mupirocin ointment tid for 10 days or retapamulin 1% applied bid for 5 days to the affected area or until all lesions have cleared.
- Oral antibiotics are used in severe cases: commonly used agents are dicloxacillin 250 mg qid for 7 to 10 days, cephalexin 250 mg qid for 7 to 10 days, azithromycin 500 mg on day 1, 250 mg on days 2 through 5, amoxicillin/clavulanate 500 mg q8h.
- Impetigo can be prevented by prompt application of mupirocin or triple-antibiotic ointment (bacitracin, Polysporin, and neomycin) to sites of skin trauma.
- Patients who are carriers of *S. aureus* in their nares should be treated with mupirocin ointment applied to their nares bid for 5 days.
- Fingernails should be kept short, and patients should be advised not to scratch any lesions to avoid spread of infection.

DISPOSITION

Most cases of impetigo resolve promptly with appropriate treatment. Both bullous and nonbullous forms of impetigo heal without scarring.

REFERRAL

Nephrology referral in patients with acute nephritis

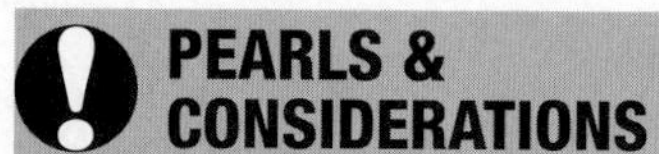

PEARLS & CONSIDERATIONS

COMMENTS

- Patients should be instructed on use of antibacterial soaps and avoidance of sharing of towels and washcloths because impetigo is extremely contagious.
- Children attending day care should be removed until 48 to 72 hr after initiation of antibiotic treatment.

RELATED CONTENT

Impetigo (Patient Information)

AUTHOR: **FRED F. FERRI, M.D.**

BASIC INFORMATION

DEFINITION

Inclusion body myositis (IBM) is the most common myopathy with onset after the age of 50 yr. Although classified among the inflammatory myopathies, its underlying pathophysiology has not yet been delineated.

SYNONYMS

None

ICD-9CM CODES
359.71 Inclusion body myositis
ICD-10CM CODES
G72.41 Inclusion body myositis [IBM]

EPIDEMIOLOGY & DEMOGRAPHICS

INCIDENCE: 0.22 to 0.79 cases/100,000 persons; uncommon in Asians and African Americans
PREVALENCE: 0.5 to 7.1 cases/100,000 persons
PREDOMINANT SEX: Male/female ratio 1.3:1
PREDOMINANT AGE: 87% older than 50 yr
PEAK INCIDENCE: Seventh decade
RISK FACTORS: None known
GENETICS: Less than 10% of cases familial

PHYSICAL FINDINGS & CLINICAL PRESENTATION

- Insidious onset of slowly progressive proximal leg and distal arm weakness.
- Time to diagnosis from symptom onset often lags by years to a decade.
- Functional loss of strength in the legs most often precedes arm weakness.
- The cardinal clinical features include early weakness and atrophy of quadriceps muscles (difficulty climbing stairs, arising from chairs, and getting out of cars) along with wrist and finger flexor muscles (difficulty grasping, opening jars, and turning doorknobs). Ankle dorsiflexion weakness may also be prominent leading to foot drop and tripping.
- When examining strength, side to side asymmetries are seen in one or more muscle groups in the majority of patients. This stands in contrast to the symmetrical, proximal involvement of polymyositis and most muscular dystrophies.
- Dysphagia and/or mild facial weakness are present in over half of cases. Dysphagia may be the presenting symptom.
- Although sensory symptoms are usually lacking, one third have evidence for peripheral neuropathy on physical examination and/or electrodiagnostic testing.
- 10% to 15% of patients have concomitant autoimmune disorders such as systemic lupus erythematosus, Sjögren's syndrome, scleroderma, sarcoidosis, or thrombocytopenia. However, different from polymyositis and dermatomyositis, IBM does not portend an increased risk of heart or lung disease nor cancer.

ETIOLOGY

The pathogenesis of IBM is not known. Inflammatory, degenerative, viral and prion etiologies have been postulated, but none substantiated.

Dx DIAGNOSIS

DIFFERENTIAL DIAGNOSIS

- Polymyositis (Table E1-275)
- Dermatomyositis
- Amyotrophic lateral sclerosis
- Late-onset muscular dystrophies
- Acid maltase deficiency

WORKUP

- Thorough neurologic examination with emphasis on the motor exam is important.
- Nerve conduction studies should be performed to exclude other causes and EMG to document a myopathy.
- The diagnosis of definite IBM requires the following features on muscle biopsy (Fig. E1-516): (1) inflammation, (2) inflammatory cells invading healthy muscle fibers, (3) vacuoles, and (4) amyloid deposits by Congo red staining, TDP-43 sarcoplasmic staining, or tubulofilaments on electron microscopy.

LABORATORY TESTS

Creatine kinase level (labs for collagen vascular diseases may be obtained after the diagnosis). A complete blood count and coagulation studies should be drawn in anticipation of the muscle biopsy.

IMAGING STUDIES

MRI may reveal atrophy and signal abnormalities in volar forearm muscle groups and quadriceps atrophy with relative preservation of the rectus femoris muscle.

Rx TREATMENT

NONPHARMACOLOGIC THERAPY

- Assistive devices for mobility such as canes, walkers, and wheelchairs are the mainstay of therapy.
- Occasionally knee orthoses or ankle-foot orthoses may improve and prolong ambulation.

ACUTE GENERAL Rx

None

CHRONIC Rx

- Experts have not found clinically significant improvement in functional strength with any pharmacologic therapy. Clinical trials of corticosteroids, methotrexate, intravenous immunoglobulin, anti-T lymphocyte globulin, etanercept, interferon β-1a, and oxandrolone have all failed to demonstrate functional improvements in limb strength.
- A short, small trial of a home exercise program demonstrated mild improvements in strength.
- IBM is generally refractory to therapy.

COMPLEMENTARY & ALTERNATIVE MEDICINE

Some patients choose to self-treat with creatine supplementation, coenzyme Q10, or lithium. There is no evidence supporting these treatments.

REFERRAL

- Patients with suspected IBM should be referred to a neurologist with subspecialty expertise in neuromuscular medicine.
- Physical therapy and occupational therapy consultations help the patient optimize ambulation and fine motor tasks, respectively.
- Speech therapy consultations can assist with symptomatic dysphagia.

PROGNOSIS

Life expectancy is not significantly altered in this late-onset, slowly progressive disorder. Some patients require wheelchair use 10 to 20 yr after disease onset.

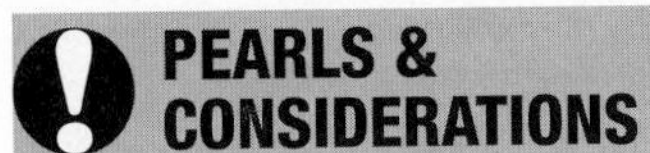

PEARLS & CONSIDERATIONS

COMMENTS

A key to diagnosis rests in finding weakness of wrist and/or finger flexors (especially the deep finger flexors at the DIP joints) on examination.

PREVENTION

None known

PATIENT/FAMILY EDUCATION

Patient information and support groups can be found at: www.ninds.nih.gov/disorders/inclusion_body_myositis and http://www.myositis.org.

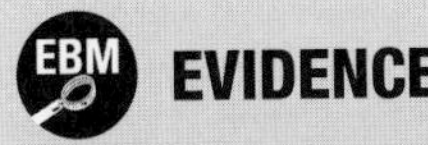

EVIDENCE

available at www.expertconsult.com

SUGGESTED READINGS

available at www.expertconsult.com

AUTHOR: **MATTHEW P. WICKLUND, M.D.**

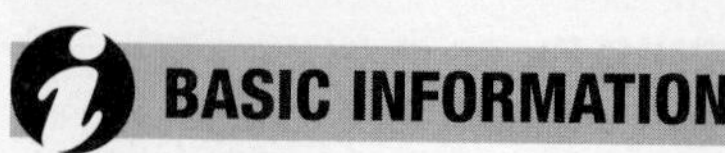

BASIC INFORMATION

DEFINITION

Fecal incontinence is defined as the involuntary loss of gas or liquid stool (minor incontinence) or the involuntary loss of solid stool (major incontinence).

SYNONYMS

Fecal Incontinence
Anal Incontinence

ICD-9CM CODES
787.6 Incontinence of feces
307.7 Encopresis of non-organic origin
ICD-10CM CODES
R15.9 Full incontinence of feces
F98.1 Encopresis not due to a substance or known physiological condition

EPIDEMIOLOGY & DEMOGRAPHICS

INCIDENCE: It affects 0.5% to 1.5% of the population younger than age 65 yr but >10% older than age 65. More commonly seen in institutionalized patients.

PREVALENCE: Varies widely; after age 65: 1%-10% of community dwellers, 14% of hospitalized, upto 54% of nursing-home residents. Prevalence increases greatly with age and body mass index (BMI) in women.

PREDOMINANT SEX AND AGE: More common in females as compared to males

RISK FACTORS:
- History of urinary incontinence
- Demented or cognitively impaired individuals
- Increasing age, especially >70 yr
- Presence of neurologic or psychiatric disease (depression in females)
- Poor mobility and poor general health
- Female sex
- Fecal impaction from chronic constipation or chronic diarrhea

PHYSICAL FINDINGS & CLINICAL PRESENTATION

- Should inspect perianal area and perform an internal digital rectal exam to evaluate for the presence of fecal material, prolapsing hemorrhoids, chemical dermatitis, scars, fistula or rectal prolapse.
- Assess for anocutaneous reflex. This is elicited by stroking skin in each perianal quadrant (normal response is a brisk anal wink).
- Assess resting and squeezing anal tone by asking the patient to bear down.
- Ask patient to strain and assess for rectal prolapse or excessive perianal descent.

ETIOLOGY

- Usually multifactorial
- Radiation-proctitis
- Inflammatory bowel disease (ulcerative colitis or Crohn's disease)
- Fecal impaction
- Idiopathic
- Neurologic disorders:
  - Status post stroke
  - Dementia
  - Multiple sclerosis
  - Spinal cord lesions
  - Diabetes mellitus
- Anal trauma
  - Anorectal surgery for hemorrhoids, fistula, and fissures
  - Vaginal delivery
- Number of births and episiotomies in females

Dx DIAGNOSIS

DIFFERENTIAL DIAGNOSIS

- Fecal encopresis

WORKUP

- Detailed history taking (Fig. E1-517 and Box E1-48) that includes the onset and precipitating events, duration and severity, stool consistency and urgency. Important to evaluate for history of urinary incontinence, anorectal surgery, neurologic disorders, or prior vaginal deliveries.
- Diagnostic workup includes anal manometry, endorectal ultrasound, proctosigmoidoscopy, defecography, pudendal nerve terminal latency, and anal electromyography (EMG).

IMAGING STUDIES

- Anal endosonography (simplest and least expensive)
- MRI

Rx TREATMENT

- Medications focus on decreasing stool frequency and improving consistency, and include loperamide, diphenoxylate/atropine sulfate, methylcellulose, anticholinergics (hyoscyamine).
- Solesta is a dextrananomer-hyaluronic gel that was FDA approved in 2011 for the treatment of fecal incontinence in adult patients who have failed conservative therapy (fiber therapy, diet, antimotility drugs). It consists of four 1ml injections into the deep submucosal layer of the anal canal, about 5 mm above the dentate line. It is hypothesized that Solesta may narrow the anal canal and allow for better sphincter control.

NONPHARMACOLOGIC THERAPY

- Supportive therapy:
  - Education, counseling, habit training
  - Diet (increase fiber)
- Biofeedback therapy:
  - Anal sphincter muscle training and strengthening
- Modified Kegel exercises
- Anal plugs (limited use)
- Surgery:
  - Overlapping sphincteroplasty (most common surgery)
  - Anterior overlap repair (usually after obstetric trauma)
  - Artificial anal sphincter
  - Sacral nerve stimulation
  - Anal electrical stimulation
  - Colostomy (if intractable symptoms and/or failed all other therapies)
  - Radiofrequency

REFERRAL

Colorectal surgery

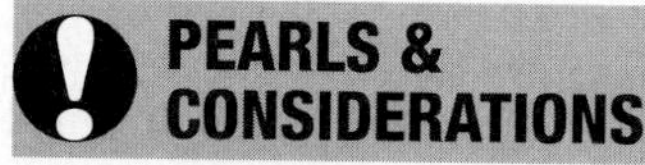

PEARLS & CONSIDERATIONS

COMMENTS

The shame, embarrassment, and stigma associated with fecal and urinary incontinence pose significant barriers to seeking professional treatment, which results in many people who suffer from these conditions without help. Therefore, during routine office visits, asking all patients >70 yr about incontinence may be helpful.

PREVENTION

- Endoanal ultrasound to detect and repair anal sphincter tears in women with second-degree perineal tears may reduce severe fecal incontinence (mid-level evidence).
- Routine episiotomy is the most easily preventable risk factor for fecal incontinence in females.

PATIENT/FAMILY EDUCATION

www.familydoctor.org/online/famdocen/home/seniors/common-older/067.html.digestive.niddk.nih.gov/ddiseases/pubs/fecalincontinencewww.nlm.nih.gov/medlineplus/ency/article/003135.htm

SUGGESTED READINGS

available at www.expertconsult.com

AUTHOR: **DAPHNE SCARMANGAS, M.D.**

BASIC INFORMATION

DEFINITION

Incontinence is the involuntary loss of urine.

ICD-9CM CODES

788.3	Incontinence
625.6	Stress incontinence
788.33	Mixed stress and urge incontinence
788.32	Male incontinence
788.39	Neurogenic incontinence
307.6	Nonorganic origin

ICD-10CM CODES

R32	Unspecified urinary incontinence
N39.3	Stress incontinence (female) (male)
N39.46	Mixed incontinence
N39.49	Disorder of urinary system, unspecified

EPIDEMIOLOGY & DEMOGRAPHICS

INCIDENCE/PREVALENCE: In the general population between the ages of 15 and 64 yr, 1.5% to 5% of men and 10% to 25% of women have incontinence. In the nursing home population, 50% of the population has some degree of incontinence. Nearly 20% of children through the mid-teenage years have episodes of urinary incontinence.

CLINICAL, PSYCHOLOGICAL, & SOCIAL IMPACT

Fewer than 50% of the individuals with incontinence living in the community consult health care providers, preferring to suffer silently, turning to home remedies, commercially available absorbent materials, and supportive aids. As their condition worsens, they become depressed, sacrifice their independence, suffer from recurrent urinary tract infection and its sequelae, limit social interaction, refrain from sexual intimacy, and become homebound. In terms of costs, for all ages living in the community, it is estimated that $7 billion is spent for incontinence annually.

MAJOR TYPES OF INCONTINENCE

- **Transient incontinence:** Incontinence occurring as a result or reaction to an acute medical problem affecting the lower urinary tract. Many of these problems can be reversed with treatment of the underlying problem.
- **Urge incontinence:** Involuntary loss of urine associated with an abrupt and strong desire to void. It is usually associated with involuntary detrusor contractions on urodynamic investigation. In neurologically impaired patients, the involuntary detrusor contraction is referred to as *detrusor hyperreflexia.* In neurologically normal patients the involuntary contraction is called *detrusor instability.*
- **Stress incontinence** (Fig. 1-518): The involuntary loss of urine with physical activities that increase abdominal pressure in the absence of a detrusor contraction or an overdistended bladder. Classification of stress incontinence:
  1. Type 0: Report of incontinence without demonstration of leakage.
  2. Type I: Incontinence in response to stress but with little descent of the bladder neck and urethra.
  3. Type II: Incontinence in response to stress with >2 cm descent of the bladder neck and urethra.
  4. Type III: Bladder neck and urethra wide open without bladder contraction; intrinsic sphincter deficiency; denervation of the urethra. The most common causes include urethral hypermobility and displacement of the bladder neck with exertion, intrinsic sphincter deficiency from failed antiincontinence surgery, prostatectomy, radiation, cord lesions, epispadias, and myelomeningocele.
- **Overflow incontinence:** Loss of urine resulting from overdistention of the bladder with resultant overflow or spilling of the urine. Causes include hypotonic-to-atonic bladder resulting from drug effect, fecal impaction, or neurologic conditions such as diabetes, spinal cord injury, surgery, or vitamin B_{12} deficiency. It is also caused by obstruction at the bladder neck and urethra. In this situation prostatism, prostatic cancer, urethral stenosis, antiincontinence surgery, pelvic prolapse, and detrusor-sphincter dyssynergia cause the incontinence.
- **Functional incontinence:** Involuntary loss of urine resulting from chronic impairments of physical and/or cognitive functioning. This is a diagnosis of exclusion. It consists of simply not getting to the toilet quickly enough due to significant mobility or cognitive impairment. The condition can sometimes be improved or cured by improving the patient's functional status, treating comorbidities, changing medications, and reducing environmental barriers.
- **Mixed stress and urge incontinence:** See Fig. 1-518.
- **Sensory urgency incontinence:** Involuntary loss of urine as a result of decreased bladder compliance and increased intravesical pressures accompanied by severe urgency and bladder hypersensitivity without detrusor overactivity. This is seen with radiation cystitis, interstitial cystitis, eosinophilic cystitis, myelomeningocele, and radical pelvic surgery. Nephropathy can occur as a complication of this vesicoureteral reflux.
- **Sphincteric incontinence:**
  1. *Urethral hypermobility:* The basic abnormality is a weakness of pelvic floor support. Because of this weakness, during increases in abdominal pressure there is rotational descent of the vesical neck and proximal urethra. If the urethra opens concomitantly, stress urinary incontinence ensues. Urethral hypermobility is often present in women who are not incontinent. Its mere presence is not sufficient evidence to make the diagnosis of sphincteric abnormality unless incontinence is shown.
  2. *Intrinsic sphincter deficiency:* There is an intrinsic malfunction of the sphincter itself. It is characterized by an open vesical neck at rest and a low leak point pressure (<65 cm water). Urethral hypermobility and intrinsic sphincter deficiency may coexist in the same patient. Causes of intrinsic sphincter deficiency are previous pelvic surgery, antiincontinence surgery, urethral diverticulectomy, radical hysterectomy, abdominoperineal resection of the rectum, urethrotomy, Y-V plasty of the vesical neck, myelodysplasia, anterior spinal artery syndrome, lumbosacral disease, aging, and hyperestrogenism.

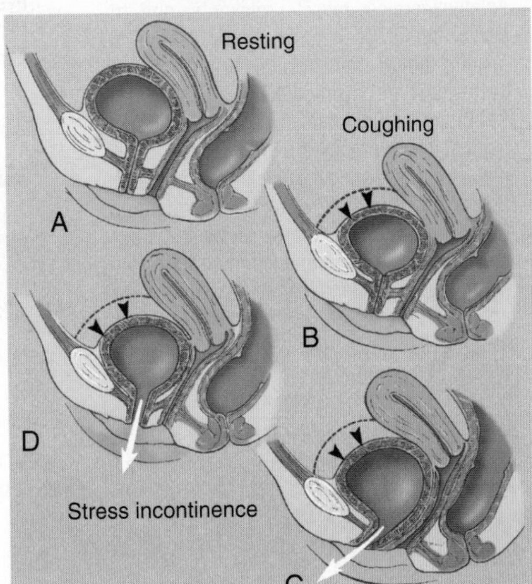

FIGURE 1-518 **A,** Bladder and urethra in normal position. **B,** Intra-abdominal pressure transmitted to the bladder. **C,** Bladder and urethra in abnormal position with loss of support (hypermobile). **D,** Loss of urethral closure. (From Lipshultz LI et al: *Urology and the primary care practitioner,* ed 3, Philadelphia, 2008, Elsevier.)

Dx DIAGNOSIS

HISTORY

- History of present illness, psychosocial factors, congenital disorders, access issues for the physically challenged, neurologic disorders, and disorders pertinent to the urologic tract

  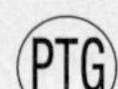

- Review of prescription and nonprescription medications
- Voiding diary to assess total voided volume, frequency of micturition, mean volume voided, largest single volume, diurnal distribution, nature and severity of incontinence

WORKUP

- Physical examination including general examination, gait of the patient (neuromuscular deficits), estrogen status, vaginal examination to include the periurethral region, evaluation for cystocele, rectocele, and enterocele
- Pelvic floor strength assessment
- Rectal examination to assess sphincter tone and bulbocavernosus reflex
- Neurologic examination
- Postvoid residual check with bladder scan or catheter

LABORATORY TESTS

Urinalysis, urine culture, urine cytology, blood urea nitrogen, creatinine

IMAGING STUDIES

- Radiography: a KUB (kidney, ureter, and bladder) to assess bony skeleton
- CT or intravenous pyelography (IVP) to rule out upper tract abnormalities, developmental anomalies, bladder configuration, and fistula
- Renal ultrasound if dye study is contraindicated

SPECIALIZED STUDIES

Simple cystometrogram, complex urodynamics for leak point pressures and uroflowmetry, endoscopic evaluation, cystogram

Rx TREATMENT

- Transient incontinence: treatment of underlying medical conditions and behavioral therapy to include habit training and timed voiding
- Urge incontinence: anticholinergic and antimuscarinic agents (tolterodine, oxybutynin, trospium chloride, fesoterodine, darifenacin, solifenacin). Anticholinergics bind to muscarinic receptors in the bladder and relax detrusor smooth muscle but can cause dry mouth, constipation, confusion, and cognition abnormalities in the elderly. Other treatment modalities include biofeedback, Kegel exercises, and surgical removal of obstructing or other pathologic lesions. A recent trial comparing oral anticholinergic therapy and onabotulinum toxin A by injection shows similar reductions in the frequency of daily episodes of urgency urinary incontinence. The group receiving onabotulinum toxin A was less likely to have dry mouth and more likely to have complete resolution of urgency urinary incontinence but higher rates of transient urinary retention and urinary tract infections. Mirabegron is a beta-3 adrenergic agonist recently FDA approved for overactive bladder. It is better tolerated than anticholinergic agents but has significant drug interactions and can cause urinary retention.
- Stress incontinence: pelvic floor muscle training (PFMT), Kegel exercises. Duloxetine improves incontinence rates and quality of life but does not cure incontinence. It can be tried if PFMT has been unsuccessful. PFMT is considered first-line therapy for stress incontinence and is also beneficial in mixed urge and stress incontinence. Midurethral-sling surgery is generally advocated when physiotherapy is unsuccessful. However, a recent trial[1] revealed that for women with stress incontinence, initial midurethral-sling surgery, as compared with initial physiotherapy, results in higher rates of subjective improvement and subjective and objective cure at 1 year.
  - Cystourethropexy (see Table E1-276): Burch procedure, Raz procedure, Stamey-Raz procedure, Gittes procedure, in situ transvaginal sling, pubovaginal sling with autologous or cadaver graft, laparoscopic Burch procedure, laparoscopic sling, tension-free vaginal tape
  - For intrinsic sphincter deficiency: bulking agents (e.g., collagen), sling, and artificial sphincter
- Overflow incontinence: surgical removal of any obstructing lesions, clean intermittent catheterization, indwelling catheter
- Functional incontinence: behavioral training to include habit training and timed voiding, incontinence undergarments and pads, external collecting devices, environmental manipulation
- Mixed urgency and stress incontinence: PFMT and use of measures recommended in the management of stress and urge incontinence
- Sensory urgency: bladder relaxants (e.g., anticholinergics, muscle relaxants, and tricyclic antidepressants), behavior therapy to include habit training and timed voiding, cystoscopy and hydrodilation
- Sphincteric deficiency: urethral bulking agents, sling procedure, artificial sphincter, mechanical clamp, external collection devices
- Botox (onabotulinum toxin A injection; Allergan) has been approved for the treatment of urinary incontinence in patients with neurologic conditions (e.g., spinal cord injury) and those with multiple sclerosis who have overactive bladder.

[1]Labrie J et al: Surgery versus physiotherapy for stress urinary incontinence, *N Engl J Med* 369:1124-1133, 2013.

TABLE 1-277 Transient Causes of Urinary Incontinence (DIAPPERS)

D	Delirium/confusional state
I	Infection—urinary (symptomatic)
A	Atrophic urethritis/vaginitis
P	Pharmaceuticals (diuretics, etc.)
P	Psychological, especially depression
E	Endocrine (hypercalcemia, hypokalemia, glycosuria)
R	Restricted mobility
S	Stool impaction

From Floege J et al: *Comprehensive clinical nephrology*, ed 4, Philadelphia, 2010, Saunders.

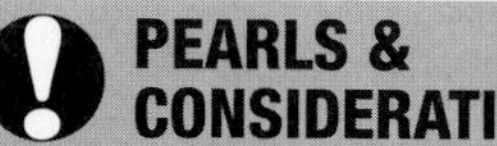

PEARLS & CONSIDERATIONS

COMMENTS

- Overweight and obese women with urinary incontinence have a high prevalence of monthly fecal incontinence (16% found to be associated with low dietary fiber intake after adjustment for other known risk factors for fecal incontinence). Transient causes of urinary incontinence in the elderly are described in Table 1-277.
- Other forms of incontinence:
  - Nocturnal enuresis (ICD-9CM code: 788.3): can be caused by sphincter abnormalities and detrusor overactivity; can occur as idiopathic, neurogenic, and with outlet obstruction
  - Postvoid dribble (ICD-9CM code: 599.2): a postsphincteric collection of urine seen with urethral diverticulum; can be idiopathic
  - Extraurethral incontinence: enterovesical (ICD-9CM codes: 596.1 and 596.2), urethral (ICD-9CM code: 599.1); also known as *fistula*
- Conditions that predispose to surgical failure: advanced age, postmenopausal state, hysterectomy, prior failed incontinence surgery, concurrent detrusor instability, abnormal perineal electromyography, pelvic radiation

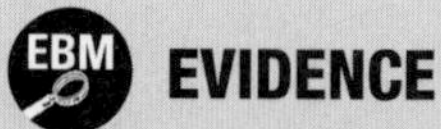

EVIDENCE

available at www.expertconsult.com

SUGGESTED READINGS

available at www.expertconsult.com

RELATED CONTENT

Pelvic Organ Prolapse (Related Key Topic)
Urinary Incontinence (Patient Information)

AUTHORS: **PHILIP J. ALIOTTA, M.D., M.S.H.A.,** and **RUBEN ALVERO, M.D.**

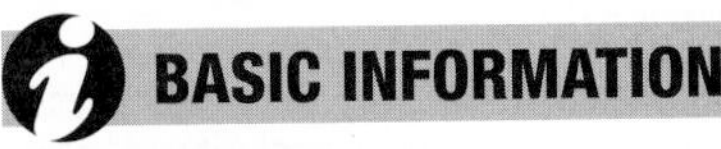

BASIC INFORMATION

DEFINITION

Infertility in a reproductive age couple is the inability to conceive after adequate coital attempts have been made for ≥1 yr. In couples where the female partner is >35 yr of age, an evaluation is justified after 6 mo without successful pregnancy.

SYNONYMS

Sterility

ICD-9CM CODES

628.0	Infertility, female, associated with anovulation
628.2	Infertility, female, of tubal origin
628.9	Infertility, of unspecified origin

ICD-10CM CODES

N97.0	Female infertility associated with anovulation
N97.1	Female infertility of tubal origin
N97.9	Female infertility, unspecified
N46	Male infertility

EPIDEMIOLOGY & DEMOGRAPHICS

PEAK INCIDENCE: The incidence of infertility increases with age. Subtle decreases in female fertility start as early as age 30. The rate of infertility increases dramatically after age 37 and spontaneous pregnancies become extremely uncommon as women reach the mid-40s. There is also a more subtle but still detectable decrease in male fertility that can also start as early as age 30.

PREVALENCE: One in eight reproductive age couples experience infertility. This prevalence is consistent in all developed countries and there is evidence that it is historically stable.

PREDOMINANT SEX AND AGE: By definition this is a diagnosis of reproductive age couples. Infertility increases with aging in both males and females but more dramatically in women. Male factor is responsible in ~40% of couples and the female factor is responsible in ~40% of couples. The remainder of the cases are either combined male and female or unexplained infertility, meaning a clear cause is not identified.

RISK FACTORS: Aging is among the most common of risk factors, predominantly among females. Women are increasingly deferring pregnancy as a result of careers, which is likely associated with the increasing prevalence in certain sectors of the population. Sexually transmitted disease with *Chlamydia* and gonorrhea is associated with pelvic inflammatory disease, which frequently results in tubal factor infertility. Extremes of weight, especially overweight, are associated with ovulatory dysfunction. Male factor infertility is most commonly idiopathic, although trauma, infection, varicocele, and exposure to environmental toxins may be associated with compromise of semen parameters. Smoking is the most common lifestyle choice that impairs fertility.

PHYSICAL FINDINGS & CLINICAL PRESENTATION

- Age (both partners)
- Previous fertility, particularly if no pregnancy has occurred in another relationship despite absence of contraception (both partners)
- Absence of secondary sexual characteristics (both partners)
- Irregular or absent menstruation (female)
- Hirsutism, acne and alopecia suggestive of hyperandrogenism (female)
- Pelvic exam suggestive of uterine abnormality such as fibroids (female)
- Trauma or torsion of the testes (male)
- Small, firm testes (male)

ETIOLOGY

- Advanced age, especially female
- Pelvic inflammatory disease (results in tubal factor infertility)
- Endometriosis (results in tubal factor infertility)
- Female anatomic (uterine fibroids, polyps, intrauterine adhesions)
- Oligoovulation, most frequently due to polycystic ovarian syndrome (PCOS)
- Idiopathic, both male and female

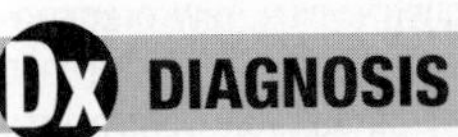

DIAGNOSIS

DIFFERENTIAL DIAGNOSIS

- Recurrent spontaneous abortion
- Ineffective attempts at natural conception
- Sterility due to previous permanent sterilization procedure

WORKUP

- The components of evaluation depend greatly on whether the female patient is reliably ovulating based on history (regular menses, premenstrual molimina such as breast tenderness) and laboratory testing (midluteal progesterone, basal body temperature testing, urinary LH predictor kits, mid-cycle ovulatory pain [Mittelschmerz], cervical mucus testing). Box E1-49 and Fig. E1-519 describe an approach to infertility diagnosis and management.
- Where the menstrual cycle is important in testing, the first day is defined as the first day of full menstrual flow
- If the female patient does not appear to be ovulating, testing should consist of:
  - TSH
  - Prolactin
  - Total testosterone/free testosterone (to assess for PCOS)
  - Transvaginal pelvic ultrasound to assess for polycystic-appearing ovaries
  - 17-Hydroxyprogesterone (to assess for cryptic congenital adrenal hyperplasia)
  - 2-hr glucose tolerance testing (if the patient has PCOS)
  - FSH/estradiol/anti-müllerian hormone on the second or third day of the menstrual cycle (if present)
  - Lipid panel (if the patient has PCOS, secondary to overlap with metabolic syndrome)
  - Liver function test (if the patient has PCOS, in case treatment with insulin-sensitizing agents indicated)
  - BUN/creatinine (if the patient has PCOS, in case treatment with insulin-sensitizing agents indicated)
  - Semen analysis in the male partner
  - Hysterosalpingogram (especially if the history suggests previous pelvic infection)
- If the female patient appears to be ovulating, testing should consist of:
  - Semen analysis in the male partner
  - Hysterosalpingogram (Fig. 1-520)
  - Mid-luteal progesterone, urinary LH predictor kits (to assess for ovulation)
  - FSH, estradiol, anti-müllerian hormone on day 2 to 3 of menstrual cycle (ovarian reserve testing)
  - Transvaginal pelvic ultrasound to assess for uterine anomalies and antral follicle count as a measure of ovarian reserve

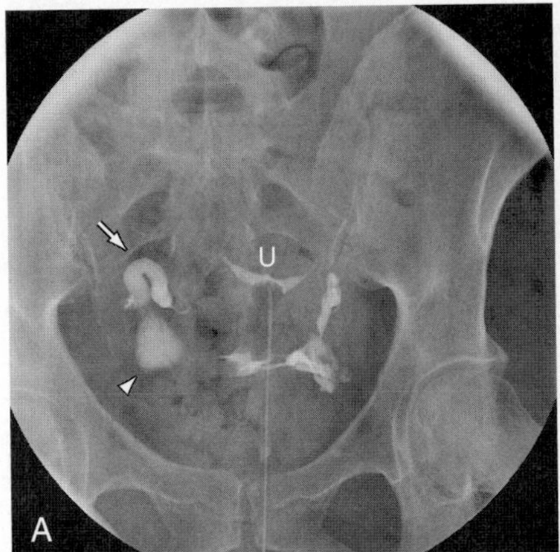

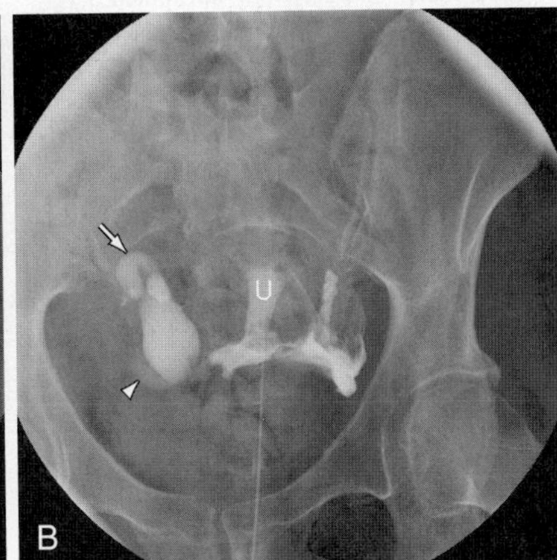

FIGURE 1-520 Hysterosalpingogram spot radiographs early **(A)** and late **(B)** demonstrate a rounded collection of contrast material *(arrowhead)* adjacent to the dilated ampullary portion of the right fallopian tube *(arrow)*, caused by peritubal pelvic adhesions related to previous pelvic inflammatory disease. Normal patient left fallopian tube. *U*, Uterus. (From Fielding JR et al: *Gynecologic imaging*, Philadelphia, 2011, Saunders.)

LABORATORY TESTS

- Semen analysis, using Kruger strict morphology after 2 to 3 days of abstinence (male)
- Day 2 or 3 FSH, estradiol, and anti-müllerian hormone as a measure of ovarian reserve (female)
- Mid-luteal progesterone (ideally 7 days after ovulatory surge). Given variability and absence of a reliable threshold, most practitioners use clinical criteria to diagnose ovulatory dysfunction.
- Urinary LH ovulatory kits
- See "Workup" for evaluation of couples where the female partner is oligo- or anovulatory

IMAGING STUDIES

- Hysterosalpingogram (between days 6 and 12 of the menstrual cycle)
- Day 2 or 3 transvaginal pelvic ultrasound to assess uterine abnormalities and to count the number of small antral follicles (2 to 9 mm) as a measure of ovarian reserve. If oligo- or anovulatory, to assess for polycystic-appearing ovary.
- Day 2 or 3 pelvic ultrasound assesses anatomic abnormalities and the number of antral ("resting") follicles; also a means of evaluating ovarian reserve.

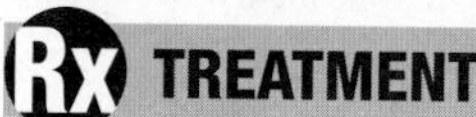

TREATMENT

Once the patient presents for evaluation, testing should be completed as quickly as possible, ideally within one menstrual cycle. The couple should follow up with the evaluating provider once all testing is completed and treatment initiated as abnormalities are found.

ACUTE GENERAL Rx

- Mild male factor infertility may be treated with intrauterine insemination but more severe forms will usually require assisted reproductive technologies (ART) with intracytoplasmic sperm injection (ICSI) in the laboratory, where sperm is injected directly into the oocyte.
- Tubal factor infertility may be treated surgically if mild and if the female patient is young and can afford the time to attempt pregnancy over multiple menstrual cycles. If the patient is older or if the tubal pathology is moderate to severe, the patient should use in vitro fertilization (IVF) to achieve pregnancy.
- Oligo- or anovulation should be treated with ovulation induction agents. Women with euestrogenic ovulatory dysfunction can be treated with clomiphene citrate as a first-line agent, using 50 mg in the first cycle attempt and increasing the dose by 50 mg up to a maximum dose of 200 mg if the patient fails to ovulate. Increasingly, aromatase inhibitors such as letrozole or anastrazole are being used both for ovulation induction in anovulatory patients and for superovulation in couples with unexplained infertility. A recent multicenter trial found that aromatase inhibitors achieved higher live birth rates than clomiphene citrate. Far less commonly, ovulatory dysfunction is the result of hypothalamic dysfunction. In these patients, once hypothalamic or pituitary abnormalities are excluded with MRI, ovulation can be achieved using injected gonadotropins.
- Uterine anatomic abnormalities such as submucous fibroids, polyps, or intrauterine adhesions should be corrected if they are identified. Fibroids that do not impact the uterine cavity probably do not interfere with fertility. Removal of intramural or subserosal fibroids is reserved for situations in which these cause excessive vaginal bleeding, pain, or pressure.
- Unexplained infertility can be treated empirically using superovulation with clomiphene citrate or gonadotropins combined with intrauterine insemination with partner's sperm. Most providers recommend using clomiphene citrate with insemination as a first-line superovulatory agent because it is inexpensive. After 3 to 4 such cycles, few pregnancies occur and the couple should be advised to become more aggressive. Controversy exists as to whether gonadotropins with insemination or IVF should be used after clomiphene citrate superovulation induction. There is evidence suggesting that moving to IVF in a *fast-track* fashion shortens the time interval to achieving pregnancy.

COMPLEMENTARY & ALTERNATIVE MEDICINE

Acupuncture is widely used by women being treated for infertility. Limited data suggest some benefit, with possible mechanisms of action including increasing blood flow to the uterus. Patients may additionally benefit from the stress relief that acupuncture provides.

DISPOSITION

- Most couples will achieve a pregnancy, provided that they are willing to use aggressive techniques, including ART such as IVF and gamete donation.
- Adoption is also a worthwhile and viable possibility for couples who cannot conceive. These couples should be ready to take on some challenges, such as limited availability of adoptable children, as well as related financial and bureaucratic hurdles.

REFERRAL

Couples should be referred to a reproductive endocrinologist once the complexity of treatment exceeds the comfort level of the provider, whether a family physician, internist or general gynecologist. Complex ovulation and superovulation induction and ART are usually managed by a board-certified reproductive endocrinologist.

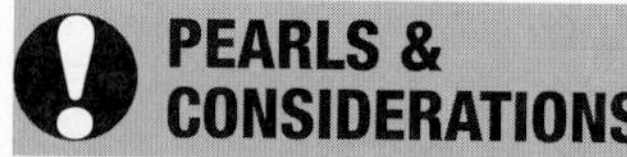

PEARLS & CONSIDERATIONS

COMMENTS

- >1% of all live births in the United States currently are the result of IVF.
- The incidence of heterotopic pregnancy in patients who have undergone IVF is relatively common; identification of a patient with ultrasound-proved intrauterine pregnancy who used ART to conceive should NOT necessarily exclude the possibility of an ectopic gestation.

PREVENTION

- Techniques that reduce the incidence of pelvic inflammatory disease, such as condom use, can reduce pelvic adhesions that are associated with tubal factor infertility.
- Women can be made aware of the fact that delaying pregnancy into the later reproductive years can reduce the chances for successful pregnancy.

PATIENT & FAMILY EDUCATION

Patient support groups such as *Resolve* (www.resolve.org) are available to help couples during evaluation and treatment of infertility, which can be extraordinarily stressful.

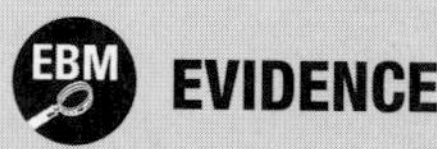

EVIDENCE

available at www.expertconsult.com

SUGGESTED READINGS

available at www.expertconsult.com

RELATED CONTENT

Amenorrhea (Related Key Topic)
Pelvic Inflammatory Disease (Related Key Topic)
Polycystic Ovary Syndrome (Related Key Topic)
Infertility (Patient Information)

AUTHOR: **RUBEN ALVERO, M.D.**

BASIC INFORMATION

DEFINITION

Influenza is an acute febrile illness caused by infection with influenza type A or B virus. Seasonal influenza can include the H1N1 virus. Severe acute respiratory syndrome (SARS) is a similar respiratory illness caused by a coronavirus called SARS-associated coronavirus (SARS-CoV). A new novel coronavirus was recognized in two patients in September 2012. This is a very different virus from the SARS agent; the two patients exhibited acute respiratory distress syndrome, renal failure, consumptive coagulopathy, and/or pericarditis. Now called the Middle East respiratory syndrome (MERS-CoV) virus, it has affected patients with connections to several Middle Eastern countries. Death rate has approached 50%. Dromedary camels are speculated to be a reservoir of MERS-CoV.

SYNONYMS

Flu

Influenza-like illness (ILI)

ICD-9CM CODES

487 Influenza

487.1 Influenza with other respiratory manifestations

ICD-10CM CODES

J10.1 Influenza due to other identified influenza virus with other respiratory manifestations

EPIDEMIOLOGY & DEMOGRAPHICS

PEAK INCIDENCE: Winter outbreaks lasting 5 to 6 wk

PREDOMINANT SEX: Male =female

PREDOMINANT AGE: Attack rates are higher among children than adults, although children are less prone to develop pulmonary complications.

INCIDENCE (IN U.S.): Annual incidence of influenza-related deaths is ~36,000 deaths/yr.

PANDEMICS

DEFINITION: Widespread human community-level outbreaks in ≥two countries in one World Health Organization (WHO) region.

HISTORICAL:

- In the twentieth century, pandemics occurred from H1N1 resulting in 40 to 100 million deaths worldwide in 1918, 70,000 deaths in the United States in 1957 from H2N2, and 36,000 deaths in the United States in 1968 from H3N2.
- H5N1 emerged in Hong Kong in 1997, quickly infecting poultry and birds. More than 400 humans were infected with avian flu (H5N1) by 2009, but transmission from human to human was not efficient.

Novel influenza A virus:

- WHO declared the H1N1 outbreaks a public health emergency in April 2009 and announced a global pandemic in June 2009. The U.S. emergency ended in June 2010, and the WHO declared an end to the global pandemic in August 2010.
- H1N1 is predicted to continue circulation as a seasonal virus for years to come.
- The 2009 H1N1 virus affected more young adults than the elderly.
- In 2009 in the United States, it is estimated that there were 43 million to 88 million cases, 192,000 to 398,000 hospitalizations, and as many as 18,000 deaths from H1N1.
- H3N2 variant virus (H3N2v) normally circulates in swine but sometimes infects humans. Infections occurred in 2012 and 2013, mostly associated with exposure to pigs at agricultural fairs. These are not sustained by efficient human-to-human community spread.
- The 2012 H3N2v viruses contain the matrix (M) gene from the 2009 pandemic influenza A (H1N1) virus.
- Influenza A H3N2v clinical presentation is similar to signs and symptoms of uncomplicated seasonal influenza, with vomiting and diarrhea in some pediatric cases. Symptoms can be milder, without fever, lasting 3-5 days.
- Avian influenza A (H7N9) virus caused severe human illness in China from February–May, 2013. Most symptomatic patients are older, male, with underlying conditions, and exposure to poultry. Recommended treatment is oral oseltamivir or inhaled zanamivir as early as possible.

PHYSICAL FINDINGS & CLINICAL PRESENTATION

- "Classic flu" is characterized by abrupt onset of fever, headache, myalgias, anorexia, and malaise after a 1- to 2-day incubation period.
- Clinical syndromes are similar to those produced by other respiratory viruses, including pharyngitis, common colds, tracheobronchitis, bronchiolitis, and croup.
- Respiratory symptoms such as cough, sore throat, and nasal discharge are usually present at the onset of illness, but systemic symptoms predominate.
- Elderly patients may experience fever, weakness, and confusion without any respiratory complaints.
- Acute deterioration to status asthmaticus may occur in patients with asthma.
- Influenza pneumonia: rapidly progressive cough, dyspnea, and cyanosis may occur after typical flu onset. This may be caused by primary influenza pneumonia or secondary bacterial pneumonia (often pneumococcal or staphylococcal co-infection).
- For influenza A (H3N2v), children younger than 10 years lack immunity. People 65 years and older and those with morbid obesity are at high risk.

ETIOLOGY

- Variation in the surface antigens of the influenza virus, hemagglutinin (HA) and neuraminidase (NA), leading to infection with variants to which immunity is inadequate in the population at risk
- Transmitted by small-particle aerosols and deposited on the respiratory tract epithelium

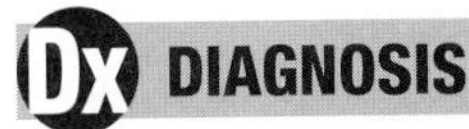

DIAGNOSIS

DIFFERENTIAL DIAGNOSIS

- Respiratory syncytial virus, adenovirus, parainfluenza virus infection
- Secondary bacterial pneumonia or mixed bacterial-viral pneumonia

WORKUP

- The accuracy of clinical diagnosis of influenza on the basis of symptoms alone is limited because symptoms from illness caused by other pathogens can overlap considerably with influenza. Diagnostic tests available for influenza include viral cultures, serology, rapid influenza diagnostic tests (RIDTs), reverse transcription-polymerase chain reaction (RT-PCR), and immunofluorescence assays.
- Virus isolation from nasal or throat swab or sputum specimens is the most rapid diagnostic method in the setting of acute illness.
- Specimens are placed into virus transport medium and processed by a reference laboratory.
- For serologic diagnosis:
  1. Paired serum specimens, acute and convalescent, the latter obtained 10 to 20 days later
  2. Fourfold rises or falls in the titer of antibodies (various techniques) considered diagnostic of recent infection
  3. Commercial rapid influenza diagnostic tests (RIDTs) are available. They can detect influenza virus antigens within 15 minutes of testing. Rapid flu test should be collected as early as possible, ideally within 4 days of onset. False-negative results are common during the flu season. A negative test result does NOT exclude diagnosis of influenza.
  4. Commercial RIDTs cannot determine if an H3N2 is a variant virus; when suspect H3N2v virus infection, send nasopharyngeal swab or aspirate in viral transport medium to state public health laboratory for rRT-PCR testing using CDC FLU rRT-PCR diagnostic panel assay.

LABORATORY TESTS

Septic syndrome presentation: CBC, ABG analysis, blood cultures

IMAGING STUDIES

- Chest x-ray examination when suspecting viral pneumonia: peribronchial and patchy interstitial infiltrates in multiple lobes with atelectasis. Table 1-279 describes x-ray pulmonary findings based on virus type.
- Possible progression to diffuse interstitial pneumonitis

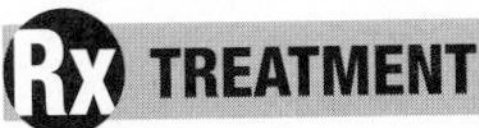

TREATMENT

NONPHARMACOLOGIC THERAPY

- Bed rest
- Hydration

ACUTE GENERAL Rx

- Supportive care: antipyretics; avoid use of aspirin in children because of the association with Reye's syndrome
- Antibiotics if bacterial pneumonia is proved or suspected
- Amantadine is NOT recommended due to resistant isolates.
- Neuraminidase inhibitors block release of virions from infected cells, resulting in shortened duration of symptoms and decrease in complications; effective against both influenza A and B, including A (H3N2v) for all hospitalized patients, those with severe and progressive illness, and high-risk patients with suspected or confirmed H3N2v.
    1. Zanamivir, administered via inhaler:
       For treatment, 10 mg (2 inhalations of 5 mg each) twice daily for 5 days
       For prevention in households, 10 mg (2 inhalations of 5 mg each) once daily for 17 days
    2. Oseltamivir, administered orally:
       For treatment, 75 mg PO twice daily for 5 days
       For prevention, 75 mg PO once daily for a minimum of 2 wk in an outbreak setting or 7 days after exposure for an adult
    3. Emergency use authorization by the Centers for Disease Control and Prevention (CDC) for intravenous peramivir during the H1N1 pandemic was terminated in June 2010. Intravenous peramivir is still available as an experimental drug.
- Placebo-controlled studies have suggested that antiviral therapy with any of the previously mentioned agents must ideally be initiated within 1 to 2 days of the onset of symptoms and reduces the duration of illness by ~1 day.
- Oseltamivir resistance developed on therapy in individuals with avian flu (H5N1) in Asia, and this is associated with poor outcome.
- Amantadine and rimantadine resistance are documented for novel (H1N1) influenza and H3N2 influenza virus.
- Systemic corticosteroids should not be routinely administered to patients with suspected or confirmed influenza, including H3N2v virus infection, except for patients on chronic corticosteroid therapy for COPD, asthma.

DISPOSITION

Patients are hospitalized if signs of pneumonia are present.

REFERRAL

Infectious disease and/or pulmonary consultation when influenza pneumonia is suspected

PEARLS & CONSIDERATIONS

COMMENTS

- Prevention of influenza in patients at high risk is an important goal of primary care.
- Vaccines reduce the risk of infection and the severity of illness.
    1. Antigenic composition of the vaccine is updated annually. The Northern Hemisphere's 2013 to 2014 season trivalent vaccine includes one influenza A (H3N2) (A/Victoria/361/2011), virus, one influenza A (H1N1)-like (A/California/7/2009(H1N1)pdm09-like) virus, and one influenza B-like virus (B/Massachusetts/2/2012-like). Quadrivalent vaccines contain these three antigens, plus an antigen from a second influenza B vaccine virus strain (B/Brisbane/60/2008-like).
    2. Revaccination is recommended annually even for those who received the vaccine in the previous season.
    3. Seasonal influenza vaccine does not provide protection against the influenza A (H3N2v) virus that is associated with agricultural fairs.
    4. Vaccination should be given at the start of the flu season (September-October) for all persons aged ≥6 mo. Vaccination is particularly important for persons who are at increased risk for severe complications from influenza. When vaccine supply is limited, vaccination efforts should focus on the following groups:
        a. All children aged 6 mo to 4 yr (59 mo).
        b. People 50 years and older
        c. Adults and children with chronic cardiac (except hypertension) or pulmonary (including asthma), renal, hepatic, neurologic, hematologic or metabolic disease (including diabetes mellitus)
        d. Immunocompromised patients (including HIV-infected persons or patients immunosuppressed due to medications)
        e. Women who are or will be pregnant during the influenza season
        f. Children aged 6 mo to 18 yr who are receiving long-term aspirin therapy
        g. Residents of nursing homes and other long-term care facilities
        h. American Indians/Alaska Natives
        i. Persons who are morbidly obese (BMI ≥40)
        j. Health care workers (HCWs)
        k. Household contacts and caregivers of persons in the previous groups
    5. Vaccination should be delayed for persons with moderate to severe acute febrile illness. Precautions include:
        a. Guillain-Barré syndrome within 6 wk following a previous dose of influenza vaccine
        b. Moderate or severe acute illness with or without fever (for trivalent inactivated influenza vaccine).
    6. Contraindication to receiving vaccine is a previous severe allergic reaction to influenza vaccine.
    7. Special efforts should be made to vaccinate high-risk patients <65 yr, only 10% to 15% of whom are vaccinated each year.
    8. HCW vaccination minimizes transmission to patients and coworkers. States are considering mandated vaccination of HCWs; some states and healthcare facilities promote the wearing of face masks for unvaccinated HCWs during the influenza season.
    9. Vaccine efficacy varies by age and by type of circulating virus.
- Alternate vaccine formulations
    1. Intradermal vaccine is available for injection into skin instead of muscle. This uses a smaller needle than the regular flu vaccine and might be preferred by adults aged 18 to 64 yr who do not like shots.

TABLE 1-279 Pulmonary Radiographic Findings Based on Virus Type

Virus	Centrilobular Nodules	Lobar Ground-Glass	Diffuse Ground-Glass	Thickened Interlobular Septa	Consolidation
Influenza	+++	+++	+		+
Epstein-Barr	+	+	+		+
Cytomegalovirus	++	++	++	+	+
Varicella-zoster	+++	+	+		
Herpes simplex	+	+++	+		+++
Measles	++	+	+		+
Hantavirus			+++	+	++
Adenovirus	++	+			+++

From Weissleder R et al: *Primer of diagnostic imaging*, ed 5, St Louis, 2011, Mosby.

2. Nasal spray, live-attenuated influenza vaccine (LAIV) is available for non-pregnant, healthy persons aged 2 to 49 yr. Note: give TIV if recipient has egg allergy or asthma or cares for immunosuppressed persons who require a protective environment.
3. High-dose inactivated vaccine (60 micrograms hemagglutinin each flu strain) is available for persons ≥65 yr.
4. Thimerosal-free vaccine is available.
5. Inactivated influenza vaccine (IIV) can be trivalent or quadrivalent, and egg-based or non-egg-based (cell culture or recombinant hemagglutinin).
6. There is no preference for live-attenuated influenza vaccine (LAIV) or IIV.
7. There is no preference for standard dose IIV, high dose IIV (age 65 or over) or intradermal IIV (age 18 - 64).
8. ACIP guidance is anticipated for egg allergies:
   - If a person with egg allergy experiences only hives, then administer trivalent recombinant hemagglutinin influenza vaccine (RIV3) if age 18-49, or IIV and observe for at least 30 minutes for reaction following vaccine.
   - If a person with egg allergy experiences other symptoms such as cardiovascular (e.g., hypotension), respiratory distress (e.g., wheezing), gastrointestinal (e.g., nausea/vomiting), reaction requiring epinephrine or emergency medical attention, administer RIV3 if age 18-49, or refer to a physician with expertise in management of allergic conditions.
   - If there is no known history of exposure to egg, but the person is suspected of having egg allergy, consult with a physician who has expertise in the management of allergies before vaccinating, or give RIV3 (if age 18-49).

- Chemoprophylaxis:
  1. Table 1-280 describes antiviral agents for influenza. Oseltamivir and zanamivir are recommended in the United States during the influenza season.
  2. Consider (after the current circulating strain of influenza has been shown to be sensitive):
     a. For high-risk patients in whom vaccination is contraindicated
     b. When the available vaccine is known not to include the circulating strain
     c. To provide added protection to immunosuppressed patients likely to have a diminished response to vaccination
     d. In the setting of an outbreak, when immediate protection of unvaccinated or recently vaccinated patients is desired
  3. Give for 2 wk in the case of late vaccination and for the duration of the flu season in all other patients
  4. Treatment should not wait for laboratory confirmation of influenza.
  5. Do not give aspirin or aspirin-containing products to children with influenza-like illness due to the risk of Reye's syndrome.
- Other prevention strategies:
  1. Hand hygiene, cough etiquette (cover your cough), respiratory hygiene (use of tissues, facemasks for the ill and proper disposal)
  2. Personal protective equipment (PPE)—wear gloves and gowns as for universal/standard precautions. Per Centers for Disease Control and Prevention, wear facemask, adhering to Droplet Precautions for 7 days after illness onset or until 24 hr after fever and respiratory symptoms are resolved, whichever is longer. Patient placement in a negative pressure room and N95 respirator for health care workers are recommended when procedures are conducted that generate respiratory aerosols.
  3. Management of ill health care workers—exclude from work until at least 24 hr after they no longer have a fever (without the use of fever-reducing medication). Extended exclusion time period when caring for severely immunocompromised patients.
  4. Standard cleaning and disinfection procedures.

SUGGESTED READINGS

available at www.expertconsult.com

RELATED CONTENT

Influenza (Flu) (Patient Information)

AUTHOR: **MARLENE FISHMAN WOLPERT, M.P.H., C.I.C.**

TABLE 1-280 Antiviral Agents for Influenza

	Amantadine	Rimantadine	Zanamivir	Oseltamivir
Protein target	M2	M2	Neuraminidase	Neuraminidase
Activity	A only (H1N1 and H3N2 are resistant)	A only (H1N1 and H3N2 are resistant)	A and B	A and B
Side effects	CNS (13%) GI (3%)	GI (6%)	? Bronchospasm	GI (9%)
Metabolism	None	Multiple (hepatic)	None	Hepatic
Excretion	Renal	Renal,+ others	Renal	Renal (tubular secretion)
Drug interactions	Antihistamines, anticholinergics	None	None	Probenecid (increased levels of oseltamivir)
Dose adjustments needed	≥65 yr old CrCl <50 ml/min	≥65 yr old CrCl <10 ml/min	None	CrCl <30 ml/min Severe liver dysfunction
Contraindications	Acute-angle glaucoma	Severe liver dysfunction	Underlying airway disease, asthma	
FDA-Approved Indications				
Therapy	Adults and children ≥1 yr old	Adults only	Adults and children ≥7 yr old	Adults and children ≥1 yr old*
Prophylaxis	Yes	Yes	Adults and children ≥5 yr old	Adults and children ≥13 yr old†

CrCl, Creatinine clearance; *FDA,* U.S. Food and Drug Administration; *GI,* gastrointestinal.
*FDA has authorized treatment of S-OIV (novel H1N1) virus with oseltamivir in children ≥3 mo of age.
†FDA has authorized prophylaxis for S-OIV (novel H1N1) virus with oseltamivir in children ≥1 yr of age.
From Mandell GL et al: *Principles and practice of infectious diseases,* ed 7, Philadelphia, 2010, Churchill Livingstone.

Diseases and Disorders I

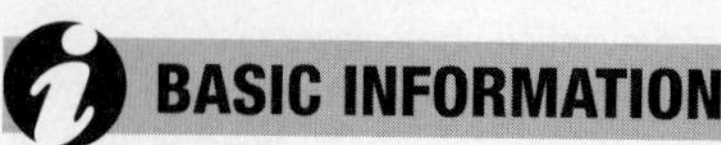

BASIC INFORMATION

DEFINITION

Insomnia is a disturbance of initiating or maintaining sleep. Restless, nonrestorative sleep may also be described as another specified insomnia. The disturbance occurs despite adequate circumstances and opportunity for sleep and is accompanied by significant distress or impairment in daytime functioning. It should be noted that in the new DSM-V the diagnosis of primary insomnia has been replaced with insomnia disorder in order to avoid the distinction between primary and secondary forms of the disorder. This paradigm shift relates to widely accepted research in the field suggesting that there is a bidirectional and interactive relationship between insomnia and any coexisting medical and/or mental disorders. As such it suggests that insomnia is deserving of direct clinical attention that may be expected to have beneficial impact on both the insomnia and comorbid disorder as well.

SYNONYMS

Sleeplessness

Sleep disorder, sleep disturbance, dyssomnia (NOTE: The terms *sleep disorder, sleep disturbance,* and *dyssomnia* are generic and can refer to disorders of wakefulness [hypersomnia] or sleep-related behavior disorders [parasomnias].)

ICD-9CM and DSM-5 CODES

780.52

ICD-10CM CODES

G47.0 Disorders of initiating and maintaining sleep (insomnias)

G47.9 Sleep disorder, unspecified

EPIDEMIOLOGY & DEMOGRAPHICS

INCIDENCE (IN U.S.): 30% to 45% of adults experience insomnia per year.

PREVALENCE (IN U.S.): 1% to 15% of all adults and 25% of older adults develop persistent insomnia.

PREDOMINANT SEX: More common in women.

PREDOMINANT AGE: Transient insomnia can occur at any age; persistent insomnia is more common after age 60 yr.

GENETICS: Can run in families and may be genetically influenced. Circadian rhythm disorders and narcolepsy have been traced to specific genes.

PHYSICAL FINDINGS & CLINICAL PRESENTATION

- Difficulty falling asleep, difficulty staying asleep, or early morning awakening.
- Significant distress or impairment in daytime functioning such as fatigue or low energy, sleepiness, cognitive impairments, mood disturbances, or behavioral problems.
- Difficulty occurs despite adequate opportunity for sleep.
- Symptoms may be acute and self-limited, chronic but intermittent, or chronic and frequent.

ETIOLOGY

- Transient insomnia:
  1. Stress
  2. Illness
  3. Travel (across time zones)
  4. Environmental disruptions (noise, heat, cold, poor bedding, bed partners, unfamiliar surroundings, etc.)
- Persistent insomnia:
  1. Mood and anxiety disorders (depression, hypomania/mania, PTSD)
  2. Psychophysiologic insomnia (conditioned arousal, extended sleep opportunity, sleep effort, poor sleep hygiene)
  3. Sleep-related breathing disorders (e.g., obstructive apnea and hypopnea, increased upper airway resistance)
  4. Chronobiologic (also known as circadian rhythm) disorder (delayed sleep phase, advanced sleep phase, shift work, free-running rhythm secondary to blindness)
  5. Drug and alcohol abuse
  6. Restless legs syndrome and periodic leg movements
  7. Neurodegenerative (Alzheimer's disease, Parkinson's disease, etc.)
  8. Medical (pain, GERD, nocturia, orthopnea, medications, etc.)

DIAGNOSIS

DIFFERENTIAL DIAGNOSIS

Insomnia disorder is only ruled out when the disorder is seen exclusively during other etiologies (see etiology). It can be precipitated by a "primary" medical mental health, or other sleep-wake disorder but continue as a comorbid condition even after the "primary disorder" has been treated.

WORKUP

- History (with bed partner interview, if possible)
- Sleep diary for 2 wk (sample sleep diary available at http://www.sleepfoundation.org)
- Wrist actigraphy (detects gross limb movements and can distinguish wake from sleep states) and as an adjunct to a diary—provides some objective verification of the diary data
- Validated sleep-quality rating scale (optional)
  1. Insomnia Severity Index
  2. Pittsburgh Sleep Quality Index
  3. Epworth Sleepiness Scale (see Daytime Sleepiness Test at http://www.sleepfoundation.org)

LABORATORY TESTS

- Evaluate for anemia, uremia (for restless legs), thyroid function (if other signs present).
- Polysomnography (in home or in sleep laboratory) is not standard for insomnia but should be reserved for patients whose history suggests specific sleep-related breathing or movement disorders. It is indicated for symptoms suggestive of daytime sleepiness (obstructive sleep apnea, narcolepsy), nonrestorative sleep (periodic leg movements, chronic pain conditions), or sleep behavior suggesting parasomnia (somnambulism, REM sleep behavior).

IMAGING STUDIES

- Not generally helpful for insomnia
- Brain CT or MRI for severe daytime sleepiness or acute onset

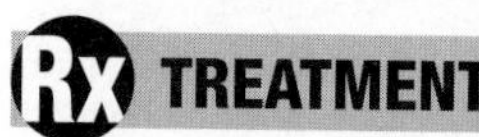

TREATMENT

NONPHARMACOLOGIC THERAPY

- Sleep hygiene measures (Box 1-50) as a monotherapy is not very effective. More useful combined with procedures described next.
- Cognitive-behavioral therapy for insomnia (CBT-I) has been shown to reduce time to fall asleep and time awake during the night, can reduce reliance on sleep medications, and has shown lasting effects after treatment has been discontinued.
- The standard components that comprise CBT-I are as follows:
  1. Stimulus Control, which addresses the conditioned cues that create arousal when attempting to sleep by restricting activity in bed to sleep and sex and not permitting sleep effort, worrying, watching TV, reading, etc., in bed (reconditioning of this type can take several days or weeks—patients should not come to expect positive changes on the first night)
  2. Sleep Restriction, which increases sleep drive by restricting sleep opportunity to the average amount of total sleep time the patient is getting as determined by baseline sleep diary data. Sleep time is

BOX 1-50 Sleep Habits (Sleep Hygiene Measures) That May Improve Sleep

1. Reduce caffeine, alcohol, or tobacco late in the day or especially evening.
2. Avoid heavy meals at night, but consider a light snack before bed such as toast or a handful of nuts.
3. Increase daytime activity, but avoid exercise within 3 hours of bedtime.
4. Increase daytime exposure to natural light.
5. Take warm bath as part of bedtime ritual.
6. Reduce liquids in the last 4 hours before bedtime.
7. Consider white noise as background sound for the sleep environment.
8. Maintain regular bed and wake times.
9. Go to bed with calm mind; resolve arguments or set a time earlier in the day to review problems and perhaps write down plans, solutions, or things to do.
10. Keep light exposure in the middle of the night to a minimum when awake and attenuate morning light in the bedroom.

increased incrementally based on improving sleep efficiency.

3. Cognitive Therapy, which involves education to address misconceptions and concerns about sleep that serve to increase anxiety
4. Sleep Hygiene, which is aimed at improving sleep habits (e.g., initiating or maintaining exercise, avoiding heavy meals at night, and avoiding or eliminating caffeine, nicotine, and alcohol intake). Environmental factors can also be addressed (e.g., using white noise and/or light attenuating bedroom). Although disruptive to sleep late in the day, caffeine sometimes can prove useful when used judiciously in the morning and early afternoon to combat the increased fatigue and somnolence that are produced early in therapy with sleep restriction and stimulus control.
5. Relaxation Exercises (e.g., progressive muscle relaxation, diaphragmatic breathing) may be considered good adjunctive therapy for insomnia treatment, especially in highly anxious patients, but are not thought to be essential in CBT-I. Mindfulness-based practices have also demonstrated some promise in the treatment of insomnia.

- Circadian Rhythm Disturbances, such as in shift workers, many blind individuals who lack light-dark cycle to synchronize body clock, adolescents and young adults with delayed sleep phase syndrome, and jet lag can be treated with chronobiologic therapies such as chronotherapy, bright light exposure, melatonin, or melatonin agonists. However, the timing of these interventions can be critical to outcome and constitutes therapies that are very different from standard medical and/or behavioral treatment for insomnia.

ACUTE GENERAL Rx

- Benzodiazepine receptor agonists zolpidem 5 mg and zaleplon 5 mg for sleep-onset insomnia, and zolpidem continuous-release formulation 6.25 to 12.5 mg and eszopiclone 1 to 3 mg for maintenance insomnia.
- Benzodiazepine sedative-hypnotics (e.g., temazepam 7.5 to 30 mg, triazolam 0.125 to 0.25 mg).
- A low-dose formulation (6 mg) of the tricyclic antidepressant doxepin, brand name Silenor, is also FDA approved for treatment of insomnia associated with sleep maintenance. This dose retains the hypnotic effect of doxepin without the typical tricyclic effects. A generic 10 mg/ml liquid formulation of doxepin is also available.
- In critical care: lorazepam 0.25 to 0.5 mg PO, SL, or IV as needed for sleep. In patients with acute delirium, haloperidol 0.25 to 0.5 mg IV as needed up to 2 mg/day may be less likely to worsen confusion.
- Melatonin agonist ramelteon 8 mg for sleep-onset insomnia when a mild agent without benzodiazepine side effects is desired.
- Avoid antihistamines except for occasional use.
- Optimize treatment of medical symptoms, especially pain.
- Most prescription and over-the-counter medications carry significant risk of adverse events and drug interactions, especially in the geriatric patient. Preferred pharmacotherapeutic agents in the elderly are zolpidem, zalepton, eszopiclone, and ramelteon.

CHRONIC Rx

- Considerable research supports the efficacy of CBT-I, with acute treatment outcomes equivalent to pharmacotherapy, with better long-term outcomes and maintenance of treatment gains. Three sedative-hypnotics—zolpidem continuous release, eszopiclone, and ramelteon—FDA approved for long-term use.
- Some evidence shows that benzodiazepines and benzodiazepine receptor agonists can be used for chronic insomnia on either intermittent or nightly use with moderate risk of tolerance and dependence but low risk of addiction.
- Sedating antidepressants (e.g., trazodone 25 to 150 mg, mirtazapine 7.5 to 30 mg, amitriptyline 25 to 50 mg, doxepin 10 mg) are in widespread use, with limited data on safety and efficacy. Amitriptyline should be avoided in older adults.
- Sedating antipsychotics (e.g., quetiapine 25 to 200 mg, olanzapine 2.5 to 10 mg at night) considered for severe mood or psychotic disorders associated with insomnia.

COMPLEMENTARY & ALTERNATIVE MEDICINE

Melatonin may shorten sleep-onset latency in some individuals. It may have more use in the treatment of circadian rhythm disorders. Timing of administration in these types of cases requires careful consideration and would not be often administered at bedtime.

DISPOSITION

- Transient insomnia: usually self-limited. May require follow-up if stress-related or illness-related because of risk of depression or persistence.
- Persistent insomnia: Studies have shown that patients who respond well to CBT-I often continue to maintain gains at 1- and 2-yr follow-ups. Insomnia patients may need periodic follow-up to reinforce good sleep hygiene and stimulus control and for reevaluation of pharmacologic therapies. There is now a compelling amount of evidence that insomnia is associated with significant negative mental and health effects over time, and if left untreated can interfere with treatment gains with other "primary disorders" and increase the chance for relapse.

REFERRAL

- A referral to a behavioral medicine specialist may be required for CBT-I or for circadian rhythmn disturbances
- Excessive daytime sleepiness not obviously caused by insomnia (e.g., narcolepsy, sleep-related breathing disorder)
- Nighttime behavior suggestive of a parasomnia (e.g., somnambulism, REM behavior disorder)
- Severe insomnia not responsive to basic interventions

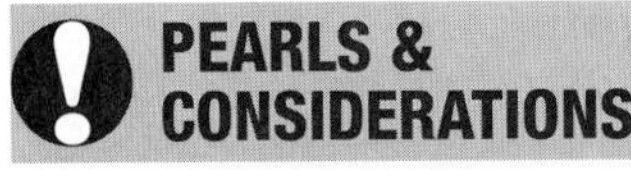

PEARLS & CONSIDERATIONS

COMMENTS

CBT-I often results in worse sleep and more fatigue in the short run. Patients often respond to initial worsening of symptoms as a sign of failure; however, they should be encouraged to see this as an important piece of the therapy and to stay the course as new conditioned patterns begin to emerge, sleep efficiency improves, and total sleep time gradually increases. Patients should avoid compensating for lost sleep by extending sleep opportunity in the form of sleeping in or napping. Therefore, early treatment should focus on helping patients to manage daytime fatigue and sleepiness by engaging in activities that help patients stay awake and maintain set bed and wake times.

MODE OF DELIVERY

Access to behavioral sleep medicine specialists can sometimes be limited especially in certain geographic regions. There is now some evidence that the use of Internet-based behavioral interventions for insomnia can have modest effect. Such interventions might be best thought of as part of a stepped care model in which this is one level of initial treatment. Patients who fail these attempts should still be encouraged to seek more tailored treatment with a specialist, especially when the insomnia is comorbid with other conditions.

PREVENTION

It is estimated that 50%-70% of individuals demonstrating the syndrome of insomnia (e.g., insomnia symptoms more than 3 days per week for a month along with deleterious daytime sequelae) are still syndromic 1-5 years later. Therefore early intervention with medication or education to prevent the development of maladaptive compensatory behaviors (e.g., napping, sleeping late, tossing and turning in bed, avoiding or decreasing daytime activity) may help to reduce the risk of developing persistent insomnia.

PATIENT & FAMILY EDUCATION

The National Sleep Foundation (http://www.sleepfoundation.org) is a comprehensive resource for health care providers and patients.

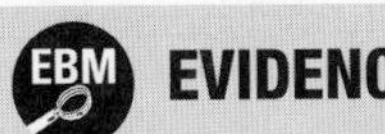

EVIDENCE

available at www.expertconsult.com

SUGGESTED READINGS

available at www.expertconsult.com

RELATED CONTENT

Fig. 3-177 Sleep disorders (Algorithm)
Insomnia (Patient Information)

AUTHOR: **DONN POSNER, PH.D., C.B.S.M.**

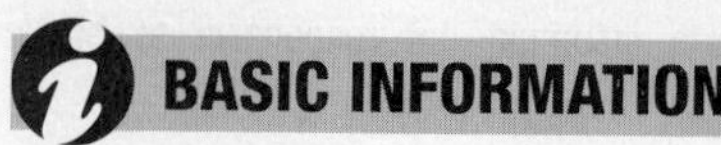

BASIC INFORMATION

DEFINITION

Insulinoma is a pancreatic insulin-secreting tumor that leads to inappropriately elevated plasma insulin or proinsulin levels with suppression of hepatic glucose output and subsequent hypoglycemia, especially during periods of fasting.

ICD-9CM CODES
M8151/0 Insulinoma
ICD-10CM CODES
C25.4 Malignant neoplasm of endocrine pancreas
D13.7 Benign neoplasm of endocrine pancreas
D37.7 Neoplasm of uncertain or unknown behavior of other digestive organs (pancreas)

EPIDEMIOLOGY & DEMOGRAPHICS

INCIDENCE: One case per 250,000 persons annually. 90% of insulinomas are benign.

PREDOMINANT SEX AND AGE: Insulinomas occur in both sexes (approximately 60% in women) and at all ages. In a Mayo Clinic series, the median age at diagnosis was 50 yr in sporadic cases but 23 yr in patients with multiple endocrine neoplasia, type 1 (MEN-1).

PHYSICAL FINDINGS & CLINICAL PRESENTATION

Symptoms typically occur in the morning before breakfast (i.e., fasting hypoglycemia as opposed to reactive hypoglycemia, which is not commonly associated with insulinoma).

Neuroglycopenic Symptoms	%
Various combinations of diplopia, blurred vision, sweating, palpitations, or weakness	85
Confusion or abnormal behavior	80
Unconsciousness or amnesia	53
Grand mal seizures	12
Adrenergic Symptoms	%
Sweating	43
Tremulousness	23
Hunger, nausea	12
Palpitations	10

ETIOLOGY, PATHOLOGY, PATHOPHYSIOLOGY

- Insulinomas are almost always solitary. Malignant insulinomas account for 5% of the total; they tend to be larger (6 cm). Metastases are usually to the liver (47%), regional lymph nodes (30%), or both.
- Insulinomas are evenly distributed in the head, body, and tail of the pancreas; ectopic insulinomas are rare (1% to 3%). Tumor size: 5% are ≤0.5 cm, 34% are 0.5 to 1 cm, 53% are 1 to 5 cm, and 8% are >5 cm.
- Histologic classification includes insulinoma in 86% of patients, adenomatosis in 5% to 15%, nesidioblastosis in 4%, and hyperplasia in 1%. Adenomatosis consists of multiple macroadenomas or microadenomas and occurs especially in patients with MEN-1. Nesidioblastosis is also a diffuse lesion in which islet cells form as buds on ductular structures.

Dx DIAGNOSIS

DIFFERENTIAL DIAGNOSIS (OF FASTING HYPOGLYCEMIA)

Hyperinsulinism:
- Insulinoma
- Nonpancreatic tumors
- Severe congestive heart failure
- Severe renal insufficiency in non-insulin-dependent diabetes

Hepatic enzyme deficiencies or decreased hepatic glucose output (primarily in infants and children):
- Glycogen storage diseases
- Endocrine hypofunction
- Hypopituitarism
- Addison's disease
- Liver failure
- Alcohol abuse
- Malnutrition

Exogenous agents:
- Sulfonylureas, biguanides
- Insulin
- Other drugs (aspirin, pentamidine)

Functional fasting hypoglycemia:
- Autoantibodies to insulin receptor or insulin

LABORATORY TESTS

- An overnight fasting blood sugar level combined with a simultaneous plasma insulin, proinsulin, and/or C peptide level will establish the existence of fasting organic hypoglycemia in 60% of patients. Table 1-281 describes biochemical patterns in patients with various causes of hyperinsulinemic hypoglycemia.
- If single overnight fasting glucose and insulin levels are nondiagnostic, a 72-hr fast is usually done with blood glucose and insulin levels determined at 2- to 4-hr intervals. A total of 75% of patients with insulinoma develop symptoms and a blood sugar level of <40 mg/dl by 24 hr, 92% to 98% develop these by 48 hr, and virtually all patients develop them by 72 hr. The test is considered positive for insulinoma if the plasma insulin/glucose ratio is more than 0.3. If at any point the patient becomes symptomatic, plasma insulin and glucose values should be obtained and IV glucose should be administered.
- The Endocrine Society guidelines for diagnosis of hypoglycemic disorders is based on glucose level <55 mg/dl (<3.1 mmol/L), elevated C-peptide level ≥0.61 ng/ml (≥0.2 nmol/L). Elevated insulin level ≥18 pmol/L, proinsulin level >5 pmol/L, and suppressed β-hydroxy-butyric acid level.
- An "amended" insulin-glucose ratio that accounts for the normal variation in insulin secretion according to prevailing glycemia has been shown to improve diagnostic accuracy of insulinomas. The "amended" insulin-glucose ratio is derived from the simple insulin-glucose ratio by subtracting 30 mg/dl (1.7 mmol/L) from the measured glucose concentrations.

IMAGING STUDIES

- Abdominal CT scan or MRI (Fig. E1-521) detects half to two thirds of insulinomas (abdominal ultrasound is not effective); should be done only after laboratory tests for insulinoma have confirmed the diagnosis
- Intraoperative ultrasound
- Arteriography
- Octreotide scan (Fig. E1-522)

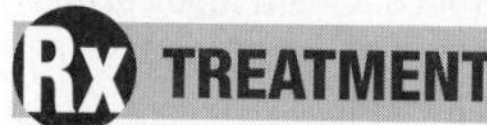

TREATMENT

NONPHARMACOLOGIC THERAPY

- Enucleation of single insulinoma
- Partial pancreatectomy for multiple adenomas

ACUTE GENERAL Rx

- Carbohydrate administration
- Diazoxide directly inhibits insulin release and has an extrapancreatic, hyperglycemic effect that enhances glycogenolysis
- Lanreotide and octreotide (somatostatin analogs)
- Streptozotocin

REFERRAL

To an endocrinologist and then to an endocrine surgeon.

SUGGESTED READINGS

available at www.expertconsult.com

RELATED CONTENT

Fig. E4-18 Diagnostic evaluation of patients with documented hypoglycemia and elevated insulin (Algorithm)

AUTHOR: **FRED F. FERRI, M.D.**

TABLE 1-281 Biochemical Patterns in Patients with Various Causes of Hyperinsulinemic Hypoglycemia

Insulin	C Peptide	Proinsulin	Sulfonylurea	Insulin Antibody	Diagnosis
↑	↓	↓	–	–	Exogenous insulin
↑	↑	↑*	–	–	Insulinoma, congenital hyperinsulinism
↑	↑	↑	+	–	Sulfonylurea
↑	↑†‡	↑†‡	–	+	Insulin autoimmune
±↑	↓	↓	–	–	Insulin receptor autoimmune‡

*> 20% of insulin value.
†Free C peptide and proinsulin ↓.
‡Insulin receptor antibody +.
From Larsen PR et al: *Williams textbook of endocrinology,* ed 10, Philadelphia, 2003, Saunders.

BASIC INFORMATION

DEFINITION

Multiple episodes of impulsive verbal or physical aggression out of proportion to perceived stressors or threats

ICD-9CM and DSM-5 CODES
312.34 Intermittent explosive disorder
ICD-10CM CODES
F63.8 Other habit and impulse disorders
F63.9 Habit and impulse disorder, unspecified

EPIDEMIOLOGY & DEMOGRAPHICS

INCIDENCE: Unknown
PEAK INCIDENCE: Occurs earlier in life
PREVALENCE: Lifetime prevalence of 6-7%
PREDOMINANT SEX AND AGE: Occurs more so in males and in people under the age of 50
GENETICS: Patients with intermittent explosive disorder (IED) are more likely to have first-degree relatives with the disorder. In addition, adoption and twin studies point to a greater than 50% of the variance in aggression related to genetic factors.
RISK FACTORS: Prior history of violence, exposure to trauma, comorbid depression, anxiety, substance abuse, or cluster B personality disorders

PHYSICAL FINDINGS & CLINICAL PRESENTATION

- Several episodes of verbal or physical aggression; the latter may include attacks on others or destruction of physical property.
- The aggression is out of proportion to any perceived stressors or threats.
- The aggression is impulsive.
- The aggression causes distress.
- The aggression is not accounted for by another disease process.
- The patient is at least 6 years of age.

ETIOLOGY

- Potentially an imbalance between aggression, originating from the amygdala and other limbic structures, and orbitofrontal and anterior cingulate cortices. This view is supported by multiple studies involving functional neuroimaging, specifically fMRI.
- From a neurochemical basis, a deficiency in the neurotransmitter serotonin appears involved. Serotonergic agents treat IED (see below) and PET imaging shows a decrease in serotonergic innervation in the anterior cingulate cortex.

Dx DIAGNOSIS

DIFFERENTIAL DIAGNOSIS

- Psychiatrically, patients may suffer from mood, anxiety, psychotic, and personality disorders (primarily antisocial and borderline). In addition, patients may be under the effects of substances, or in withdrawal from them.
- Neuropsychiatrically, dementia, delirium, temporal lobe epilepsy, cardiovascular disease, multiple sclerosis, and brain lesions can all cause similar behavior.
- If delirium is expected, a wider, more systemic differential diagnosis should be explored.

WORKUP

- A thorough mental status exam should be performed. In addition, there should be careful consideration for other neuropsychiatric conditions if the history points in that direction.

LABORATORY TESTS

- Urine toxicology screen, as substance abuse is highly comorbid
- Dementia workup when appropriate: CBC, head CT, Chem 7, B12, TSH, Folate, RPR
- Delirium workup when appropriate; associated signs and symptoms may be helpful for guidance, especially in clinical settings

IMAGING STUDIES

- Head CT or MRI, in cases where dementia, delirium, neurovascular disease, or brain lesions are expected. The appropriate test should be ordered depending on the particulars of the case (i.e., MRI to evaluate for MS).
- EEG is indicated to evaluate for seizure-related conditions.

Rx TREATMENT (Table 1-282)

- Selective serotonin reuptake inhibitors (SSRIs) are considered first-line therapy. Multiple studies have been performed on fluoxetine, up to 60 mg per day, though it is not unreasonable to try other SSRIs given similar mechanisms of action. Cost, side effects, drug half-life, and drug-drug interactions need to be considered. Starting at 20 mg per day, and increasing by 10 mg every other week, for a total of a 12-week trial, is recommended.
- Unless there is a contraindication to SSRIs, AEDs should be considered second line, given their potential side effects and toxicities.
- Multiple large trials and meta-analyses also point to the efficacy of phenytoin, lamotrigine, topiramate, and valproate.
- Lithium has also shown to be helpful.
- See Table 1-282 for details related to particular medications.

NONPHARMACOLOGIC THERAPY

- Cognitive-behavioral therapy has been shown to be helpful for patients with IED.
- Patients are taught to examine their thoughts in relation to stressful circumstances.
- Patients can be taught to examine their somatic sensations and change these through relaxation techniques.
- Relapse prevention is focused on helping patients avoid explosive behaviors in the future.

ACUTE GENERAL Rx

- See above

COMPLEMENTARY AND ALTERNATIVE MEDICINE

There is no evidence on the use of complementary or alternative medicine for this disorder.

REFERRAL

Referral to an outpatient mental health provider should be helpful.

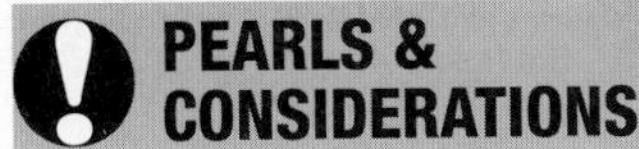

PEARLS & CONSIDERATIONS

PREVENTION

No prevention measures have been identified.

PATIENT/FAMILY EDUCATION

Psychoeducation to the patient and family may be helpful, especially in helping to identify triggers and supporting the use of coping skills

RELATED TOPICS

Bipolar disorder, personality disorders, substance abuse, conduct disorder, ADHD

AUTHOR: **ANTHONY GALLO, M.D.**

TABLE 1-282 Medications for Intermittent Explosive Disorder

Medication	Starting Dose	Blood Level	Adverse Outcomes	Cautionary Notes
Fluoxetine	10 mg PO qAM	N/A	Mania, sexual dysfunction, SIADH	Caution in patients with bipolar disorder
Phenytoin	100 mg PO tid	10-20 mcg/ml	Hepatotoxicity, gingival hyperplasia	Caution in patients with hepatic dysfunction
Topiramate	50 mg daily	N/A	Sedation	
Lamotrigine	25 mg daily	N/A	Rash, SJS	Slow titration schedule
Valproate	250 mg PO bid	75-125 mcg/ml	Hyperammonemia, pancreatitis, hepatic impairment	Caution in patients with hepatic impairment
Carbamazepine	200 mg PO bid	4-12 mcg/ml	Hepatic failure, SJS, blood dyscrasias, SIADH	Caution in patients with hepatic impairment
Lithium	300 mg PO bid	0.6-1.2 mEq/L	Hypothyroid, nephrotoxicity,	Caution in patients with renal impairment

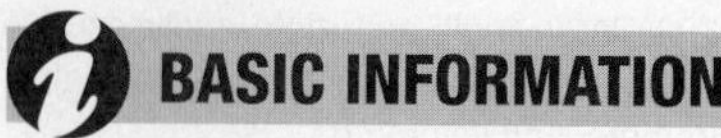

DEFINITION

The International Continence Society defines interstitial cystitis (IC), otherwise known as painful bladder syndrome, as a clinical syndrome consisting of suprapubic pain related to bladder filling and accompanied by other symptoms such as increased daytime and nighttime frequency in the absence of proven infection or other obvious pathology. The American Urological Association defines interstitial cystitis/bladder pain syndrome (IC/BPS) as an unpleasant sensation perceived to be related to the urinary bladder that is associated with lower urinary tract symptoms >6 weeks' duration, in the absence of infection or other unidentifiable causes.

SYNONYMS

Interstitial cystitis/bladder pain syndrome (IC/BPS)
Painful bladder syndrome
Tic douloureux of bladder

ICD-9CM CODES
595.1 Chronic interstitial cystitis
ICD-10CM CODES
N30.1 Interstitial cystitis (chronic)
N30.9 Cystitis, unspecified
N30.10 Interstitial cystitis (chronic) without hematuria

EPIDEMIOLOGY & DEMOGRAPHICS

INCIDENCE: 21 cases per 100,000 women and four cases per 100,000 men annually

PREVALENCE:

- 197 per 100,000 women and 41 per 100,000 men in the U.S.
- Because the disease is substantially underdiagnosed, it may actually affect one in five women and one in 20 men.
- More than 81% of women diagnosed with chronic pelvic pain and up to 84% of men initially diagnosed with chronic prostatitis actually have IC.
- More than 90% of patients diagnosed with overactive bladder who do not respond to anticholinergics are subsequently diagnosed with IC.

PREDOMINANT SEX AND AGE:

- White women constitute 95% of patients with IC.
- Female/male ratio of 5 to 10:1.
- Most prevalent in fourth and fifth decades of life.

PHYSICAL FINDINGS & CLINICAL PRESENTATION

- Urinary urgency, frequency (>8 in daytime), nocturia (>2 at night), and suprapubic pain are the most common symptoms.
- Suprapubic pain is worse with bladder filling or urinating and relieved after emptying.
- Dyspareunia.
- Symptoms lasting longer than 6 mo.
- Intensity of symptoms waxes and wanes.
- Insidious onset and worsens to the final stage within 5 to 15 yr.
- Exercise, stress, sexual activity, ejaculation, certain foods with high potassium and acids (beer, spices, bananas, tomatoes, chocolate, strawberries, artificial sweeteners, oranges, cranberries, caffeine), menstruation, prolonged sitting, and activation of allergies exacerbate the symptoms.
- Often associated with irritable bowel syndrome, migraine, endometriosis, skin sensitivities, multiple drug allergies, other allergies, vulvodynia, fibromyalgia, chronic fatigue syndrome, systemic lupus erythematosus, and mood disorders.
- Dysphoric mood.
- Lower abdominal tenderness.
- Tender prostate in digital rectal examination.
- Levator ani tenderness in female.
- Tenderness of anterior vaginal wall/bladder neck in female.

ETIOLOGY

Unknown

Dx DIAGNOSIS

DIFFERENTIAL DIAGNOSIS

- Chronic pelvic pain
- Overactive bladder
- Recurrent urinary tract infection
- Endometriosis
- Pelvic adhesions
- Vulvar vestibulitis
- Vulvodynia
- Urethral pain syndrome
- Chronic nonbacterial prostatitis
- Frequent vaginitis
- Benign prostatic hyperplasia

WORKUP

- IC can be considered a diagnosis of exclusion when no known cause of painful bladder can be identified.
- There is no definite diagnostic test.
- Validated questionnaires such as Pelvic Pain and Urgency/Frequency scale (PUF), O'Leary-Sant symptoms and problem index, and Wisconsin IC scale. PUF is the most commonly used.
- Voiding diary shows low-volume (<100 ml) and high-frequency voiding pattern.
- National Institute of Diabetes and Diseases of the Kidney diagnostic criteria misses 60% of IC patients and is not clinically used anymore.
- Anesthetic bladder challenge: with this test the symptoms dissipate on instillation of an anesthetic cocktail into the bladder.
- Cystoscopy and hydrodistention under general anesthesia may show terminal hematuria, glomerulation, Hunner's ulcers, and small bladder capacity of less than 350 ml. Cystoscopy and/or urodynamic testing should be considered when the diagnosis is in doubt, but the tests are not necessary to confirm an IC/BPS diagnosis in uncomplicated cases.
- Bladder biopsy is not essential for diagnosis of IC.
- Parson's potassium sensitivity test (PST).
- Urodynamics are unnecessary in diagnosis of IC.

LABORATORY TESTS

- Urine analysis and culture.
- Urine cytology should be performed if microscopic or gross hematuria is present, or with other risk factors such as smoking, age >40 yr, and other bladder cancer risk factors.
- Culture of sexually transmitted diseases if clinically indicated. Nonbacteriuric patients with pyuria should be screened for *Chlamydia*.
- Urine biomarkers (e.g., antiproliferative factor) are promising but not ready for clinical use.

IMAGING STUDIES

CT or ultrasound of abdomen and pelvis may be considered to rule out other pathology.

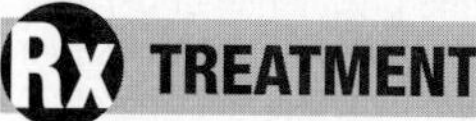

- There is no consensus for optimal management.
- There is no cure for this disease.

NONPHARMACOLOGIC THERAPY

- Avoidance of activities associated with flare-ups
- Avoidance of smoking
- Dietary restriction, avoiding common irritants (e.g., coffee, citrus fruits)
- Physical therapy
- Exercise
- Behavioral therapy
- Bladder retraining
- Biofeedback
- Warm sitz bath, ice, heating pad
- Thiele massage (transrectal and transvaginal manual therapy of pelvic floor muscle) in presence of pelvic floor muscle tenderness and spasm
- Hydrodistention only gives temporary relief, so it is not commonly used anymore

ACUTE AND CHRONIC Rx

- A course of empiric antibiotics if not tried yet. Long-term oral antibiotics are not recommended.
- Oral therapy is tried first.
- Pentosan polysulfate sodium (Elmiron) is the only FDA approved and most effective oral therapy.
- Most treatment takes 3 to 6 mo before maximum benefit is seen.
- Adjunct oral therapy includes tricyclic antidepressants (amitriptyline), cimetidine, antihistaminics (hydroxyzine, montelukast), neuroleptics (gabapentin, topiramate), analgesics (NSAIDs, opioid analgesics), and occasionally antimuscarinics.
- Oral therapies can be used in combination.
- Antihistaminics are preferred for patients with an allergy history or those who show mast cells in bladder biopsy.
- Oral prednisone is used in presence of Hunner's ulcers.
- Other drugs rarely used for IC are cyclosporin A, interleukin-10, imatinib, methotrexate, suplatast, misoprostol, and quercetin.

- Growth factor inhibitors, gene therapy, RDP 58, and vitamin B_3 analogue (BXL 628) may represent future therapies.
- Intravesical treatment is used when oral medications fail, for acute flare-ups, or before the oral medications take full effect.
- Dimethyl sulfoxide (DMSO), heparin, lidocaine, hyaluronic acid, capsaicin, botulinum toxin A, chondroitin sulfate, steroids, and Elmiron are drugs used for intravesical treatment.
- DMSO is the only FDA-approved intravesical treatment.
- DMSO is used less often now because of its side effects, specifically a garlic-like odor or taste on breath or skin that lasts 72 hr after treatment.
- Intravesical therapy typically involves mixture of heparin or Elmiron with lidocaine and sodium bicarbonate.
- Silver nitrate and Clorpactin have fallen out of favor.

SURGERY

- Major surgical intervention is not the mainstay of treatment.
- Patients whose condition is extreme and who are miserable may consider surgery if medications fail.
- Sacral neuromodulation (InterStim) is the current preferred surgical intervention.
- Laser ablation, fulguration, or resection is offered when Hunner's ulcers are seen in cystoscopy.
- Augmentation cystoplasty is not recommended.
- Cystourethrectomy with urinary diversion is rarely done.

COMPLEMENTARY & ALTERNATIVE MEDICINE

- Transcutaneous electric nerve stimulation
- Intravaginal electric nerve stimulation
- Acupuncture
- Urinary chelating agents such as Polycitra-K crystals, Urocit-K
- Prelief, an over-the-counter food additive
- Herbal remedies such as Algnot Plus, CystoProtek, Cysta-Q, aloe vera

DISPOSITION

- Close follow-up every month for 3 mo and every 3 mo thereafter.
- Voiding diary and symptom questionnaire are helpful to monitor response to treatment.

REFERRAL

- Urologist
- Pain specialist
- Physical therapist

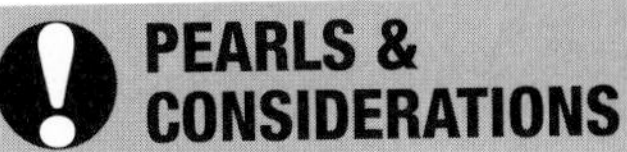

PEARLS & CONSIDERATIONS

COMMENTS

- On average these patients see five physicians and endure irritating voiding symptoms for 5 yr before the disease is identified.
- Besides symptom questionnaire and urine analysis, all other diagnostic tests are optional.
- PST is well tolerated.
- Negative cystoscopy does not rule out IC.

PREVENTION

Early identification and timely intervention improve patient outcome.

PATIENT & FAMILY EDUCATION

- IC support groups
- Interstitial Cystitis Association
- Interstitial Cystitis Network

SUGGESTED READINGS

available at www.expertconsult.com

AUTHOR: **HEMANT K. SATPATHY, M.D.**

BASIC INFORMATION

DEFINITION

The interstitial lung diseases (ILDs) include more than 150 nonmalignant disorders, characterized by varying degrees of damage to the lung parenchyma or interstitium via inflammation and fibrosis. The term "ILD" can be confusing as processes affecting the alveolar space (e.g., pulmonary alveolar proteinosis) are also lumped under the title.

SYNONYMS

Interstitial pulmonary disease
ILD
Diffuse parenchymal lung disease (DPLD)

ICD-9CM CODES

136.3	Acute interstitial lung disease
515	Chronic interstitial lung disease
516.30	Idiopathic interstitial pneumonia, NOS
516.31	Idiopathic pulmonary fibrosis

ICD-10CM CODES

J84	Other interstitial pulmonary disease
J84.1	Other interstitial pulmonary disease with fibrosis
J84.8	Other specified interstitial pulmonary diseases
J84.9	Interstitial pulmonary disease, unspecified

EPIDEMIOLOGY & DEMOGRAPHICS

PREVALENCE: Varies with type of ILD. The most common type of ILD is idiopathic interstitial fibrosis, with a prevalence of 20 cases/100,000 people in the general population, increasing with age to 175 cases/100,000 people aged 75 yr or older.

PREDOMINANT SEX & AGE: Some ILDs are more common in women, such as those resulting from connective tissue disorders. Lymphangiomyomatosis occurs exclusively in postmenopausal women. ILD caused by occupational exposures are more common in men. Generally, ILD occurs in people >50 yr.

RISK FACTORS: Although many ILDs are categorized as idiopathic, the most common identifiable risk factors include environmental exposures such as silicone, asbestos, or bird droppings; reactions to drugs such as chemotherapeutic agents, radiation therapy, cardiac medications, and some history of connective tissue disease such as rheumatoid arthritis or systemic lupus erythematosus.

PHYSICAL FINDINGS & CLINICAL PRESENTATION

- Shortness of breath (especially with exertion)
- Dyspnea
- Cough (dry)
- Tachypnea
- Bibasilar end-inspiratory dry crackles
- Pulmonary hypertension
- Cyanosis, clubbing

ETIOLOGY

- Hallmarks of ILD include a restrictive pattern and decreased diffusing capacity for carbon monoxide (DLCO) as demonstrated by pulmonary function testing. The restrictive process can be the result of a number of factors depending on the type of ILD. Different types of ILD are characterized by three distinct patterns:
  1. Acute inflammatory changes, which are potentially reversible
  2. Fibrotic changes
  3. Lung destruction
- Specific changes may be seen:
  - Granulomatous: accumulation of T lymphocytes, macrophages, and epithelioid cells into granulomas in lung parenchyma
  - Inflammation and fibrosis: injury to epithelium causes inflammation; if chronic, inflammation spreads to interstitium and vascular areas
- The MUC5B promoter polymorphism has been found to be associated with interstitial lung disease in the general population. Although this association was more apparent in older persons, it did not appear to be influenced by cigarette smoking.[1]

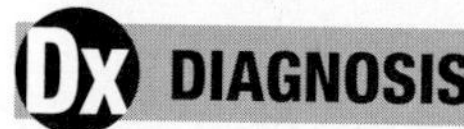

DIAGNOSIS

DIFFERENTIAL DIAGNOSIS

- Congestive heart failure
- Chronic renal failure
- Viral pneumonitis
- Pulmonary embolism
- Pulmonary hypertension

WORKUP

- Well-defined patterns in pulmonary function tests are usually consistent with restrictive defect (decreased FRC, RV, and TLC) owing to decreased lung compliance caused by alveolar wall thickening as a result of inflammation and fibrosis. Diffusion capacity is usually reduced also because of inflammation and thickening of alveolar walls, though nonspecific. FEV_1/FVC is usually normal or increased because lung stiffness keeps small airways open, although some conditions (e.g., sarcoidosis) may result in air trapping.
- Bronchoscopy and bronchoalveolar lavage (BAL) may help identify type of ILD. However, their role in defining stage of disease and response to therapy is controversial.
- If laboratory studies and imaging including HRCT fail in yielding a diagnosis, a surgical biopsy is required.
- Fig. 1-523 describes a diagnostic approach to occupational ILD.

Suspect occupational interstitial lung disease
Chest radiograph, pulmonary function testing
Normal radiograph Normal function
Abnormal radiograph
Normal radiograph Abnormal function
Follow-up
Nodular opacities
Linear opacities
High-resolution CT scan
Silicosis Coal workers' pneumoconiosis
Asbestosis Other ILD
Nodular pattern
Linear pattern
Silicosis Coal workers' pneumoconiosis
Asbestosis Other ILD

FIGURE 1-523 Diagnostic approach to occupational interstitial lung disease (ILD). *CT,* Computed tomography. (From Goldman L, Ausiello D [eds]: *Goldman's Cecil textbook of medicine,* ed 23, Philadelphia, 2008, Saunders.)

[1]Hunninghake GM et al: MUC5B promoter polymorphism and interstitial lung abnormalities, *N Engl J Med* 368:2192-2200, 2013.

LABORATORY TESTS

- ABGs may be normal or show respiratory alkalosis.
- Blood tests for connective tissue diseases, such as antinuclear antibodies, anti-immunoglobulin antibodies (rheumatoid factors), LDH.
- Serum precipitins confirm exposure if hypersensitivity pneumonitis is suspected.
- Antineutrophil cytoplasmic antibodies or anti-basement membrane antibodies if vasculitis is suspected.
- Elevation in angiotensin-converting enzyme level in sarcoidosis.

IMAGING STUDIES

- Chest x-ray may be normal but commonly shows a bibasilar reticular pattern.
- High-resolution CT (HRCT) (Fig. 1-524) is the gold standard for evaluating parenchymal opacities seen on chest x-ray; it is also useful for determining potential biopsy sights.
- Echocardiography may be useful to evaluate cardiac function/dilation or to evaluate for pulmonary hypertension.

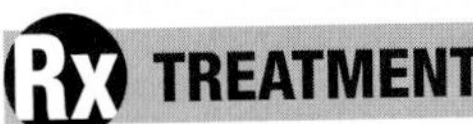

TREATMENT

NONPHARMACOLOGIC THERAPY

Avoidance of tobacco and occupational exposures

ACUTE GENERAL Rx

- Supplemental oxygen in patients with hypoxemia is helpful short and long term.
- Glucocorticoids are the mainstay of therapy, but success rate is low, and some guidelines recommend against use, especially long term. Patients should be reevaluated after this initial course of treatment. If they are stable, steroids may be tapered. If not, the same course may be maintained 4 additional wk. If patient's condition continues to decline, may consider adding second agent (cyclophosphamide, azathioprine).

CHRONIC GENERAL Rx

- Respiratory rehabilitation may be of value.
- Lung transplantation may be considered in appropriate patients in severe stages of the disease.

REFERRAL

- Surgical referral for biopsy
- Pulmonary referral for bronchoscopy and/or BAL

SUGGESTED READINGS

available at www.expertconsult.com

RELATED CONTENT

Interstitial Pulmonary Disease (Patient Information)

AUTHORS: **GRACE SHIH, M.D., CINDY GLEIT, M.D., JEFFREY BORKAN, M.D., PH.D.**, and **MICHAEL A. MARSH, M.D.**

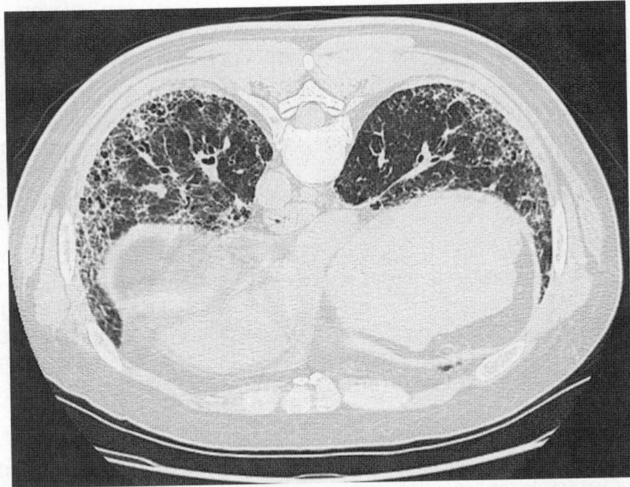

FIGURE 1-524 High-resolution computed tomography scan of the chest shows fibrotic changes in a subpleural distribution with honeycombing consistent with usual interstitial pneumonia. (From Hochberg MC et al: *Rheumatology*, ed 5, St Louis, 2011, Mosby.)

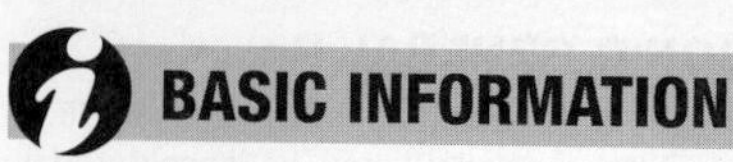

BASIC INFORMATION

DEFINITION

Can be classified into two broad categories:

Acute interstitial nephritis (AIN): Decrease in renal function resulting from immune-mediated injury characterized histopathologically with edema and inflammation of the renal interstitium, classically sparing the glomeruli and blood vessels. Most often drug-induced.

Chronic interstitial nephritis: Represents a large and diverse group of disorders characterized by interstitial fibrosis with mononuclear leukocyte infiltration and tubular atrophy. It is a final common pathway of many chronic kidney diseases including chronic bacterial infections, obstruction, and high-grade vesicoureteral reflux. Histopathologically seen as atrophy and fibrosis of the renal interstitium.

SYNONYMS

Acute tubulointerstitial nephritis
Contracted kidney
Cirrhosis of the kidney
Granular kidney
Gouty kidney
Renal sclerosis
Chronic productive nephritis without exudation

ICD-9CM CODES

583 Nephritis and nephropathy not specified as acute or chronic
583.7 Nephritis and nephropathy, not specific as acute or chronic, with lesion of renal medullary necrosis
583.8 Nephritis and nephropathy, not specific as acute or chronic, with other specified pathological lesion in kidney
583.9 With unspecified pathological lesions in the kidney

ICD-10CM CODES

N05.9 Unspecified nephritic syndrome with unspecified morphologic changes
N17.2 Acute kidney failure with medullary necrosis
N05.8 Unspecified nephritic syndrome with other morphologic changes

EPIDEMIOLOGY & DEMOGRAPHICS

PREVALENCE: The incidence in the US remains unknown. Best available estimates come from measuring the incidence of unexpected AIN at autopsy (<1%), in unselected renal biopsies (1% to 6%), and in renal biopsies selected for patients with acute renal failure (11% to 15%).

PREDOMINANT SEX AND AGE: Older patients generally at higher risk given reduced glomerular filtration rates.

PEAK INCIDENCE: Median age at presentation is 65 yr.

GENETICS: Risk of acute interstitial nephritis due to drugs (e.g., NSAIDs, penicillins, sulfa drugs, etc.) increases with volume depletion, underlying kidney disease, age >65 yr, congestive heart failure, and diabetes. Some autoimmune disorders are also risk factors.

PHYSICAL FINDINGS & CLINICAL PRESENTATION

Nonspecific but acutely can present with renal failure, oliguria, hematuria, malaise, mental status changes, rash, nausea, and vomiting. Classic triad of low-grade fever, rash, and arthralgias is present in only 5% of cases of AIN. Chronic interstitial nephritis can be asymptomatic with elevations in BUN or creatinine or the appearance of abnormal urinary sediment. Tubulointerstitial nephritis and uveitis (TINU) syndrome: Some patients present with interstitial nephritis and uveitis, and occasionally with systemic findings including fever, weight loss, malaise, fatigue, anorexia, asthenia, abdominal and flank pain, arthralgias, myalgias, headache, polyuria and/or nocturia.

ETIOLOGY

- Drug-induced (71%) usually hypersensitivity reaction occurring about 15 days after exposure to the drug: antibiotics (penicillins, cephalosporins, sulfonamides, rifampin, ciprofloxacin), NSAIDs, selective COX-2 inhibitors, diuretics, proton pump inhibitors (omeprazole, lansoprazole), anticonvulsants, indinavir, mesalamine
- Infection associated (15%) can be either primary renal infection (acute bacterial pyelonephritis, renal tuberculosis, and fungal nephritis) or complication of systemic infections
  - Bacterial: *Corynebacterium diphtheriae, Legionella,* staphylococci, streptococci, *Yersinia*
  - Viral: Cytomegalovirus, Epstein-Barr virus, hantaviruses, hepatitis C, herpes simplex virus, human immunodeficiency virus, mumps, polyomavirus
  - Other: *Mycobacterium, Mycoplasma, Rickettsia,* syphilis, toxoplasmosis
- Immune disorders: systemic lupus erythematosus, Sjögren's, and Wegener's
- Neoplastic disorders (multiple myeloma)
- Metabolic diseases (urate nephropathy, hypercalcemic nephropathy, hypokalemic nephropathy, oxalate nephropathy)
- Heavy metals (chronic form)
- Chronic urinary tract obstruction (chronic form)
- Sarcoidosis
- Other rare causes: IgG4 related tubulointerstitial nephritis, hypocomplementemic tubulointerstitial nephritis

Dx DIAGNOSIS

DIFFERENTIAL DIAGNOSIS

Any other causes of acute renal failure including acute tubular necrosis, glomerulonephritis, hypertensive nephrosclerosis, prerenal azotemia, obstructive nephropathy, renal vascular disease, and various electrolyte abnormalities

WORKUP

Medical history with focus on recent infection illness or new medication in the presence of acute to chronic onset of kidney failure; evaluation for underlying infection or insult

LABORATORY TESTS

- Urinalysis (white blood cells, red blood cells, white blood cell casts, eosinophils, proteinuria), urine microscopy (especially eosinophiluria although low sensitivity), serum chemistry profile (rise in plasma creatinine temporally related to administration of offending drug), complete blood count with differential (eosinophilia occurs in 50% of AIN patients), 24-hr urine specimen collection, consider serum IgE levels
- For patients who have AIN that is not believed to be related to a drug, following tests can be performed: chest x-ray to evaluate for sarcoidosis, tuberculosis, and other infections. Serum levels of angiotensin converting enzyme and serum calcium and urinary calcium excretion to evaluate for sarcoidosis. Serologic tests to exclude histoplasmosis, coccidiomycosis, toxoplasmosis, EBV. ANCA to exclude ANCA-associated vasculitides. ANA and dsDNA to exclude SLE. C3 and C4 to evaluate for SLE and IgG 4 related disease and hypocomplementemic AIN. Anti-Ro/SSA, anti-La/SSb antibodies, C-reactive protein and rheumatoid factor to exclude Sjogren's syndrome.
- Renal biopsy is the gold standard for diagnosis but is indicated only when diagnosis is unclear, removal of offending agent does not result in improvement, or steroid initiation is being considered. The major histologic changes are interstitial edema and a marked interstitial infiltrate consisting primarily of T lymphocytes and monocytes. Eosinophils, plasma cells, neutrophils also may be found.

IMAGING STUDIES

Neither ultrasound nor gallium 67 scan is diagnostic but may be useful for ruling out AIN

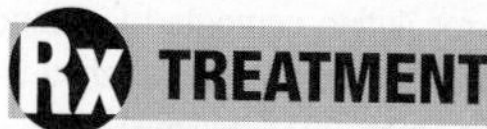

TREATMENT

NONPHARMACOLOGIC THERAPY

Largely supportive; removal of offending agent will resolve 60% of all cases.

ACUTE GENERAL Rx

- Correct fluid and electrolyte imbalances, maintain adequate hydration and urine output but avoid volume overload.
- Identify and treat infection as indicated.
- Remove offending drug, substitute as appropriate.
- Avoid medications that impair renal blood flow.
- Initiation of steroids is controversial, but retrospective studies have shown that early steroid treatment may reduce need for chronic dialysis in patients with drug-induced AIN. Reasonable to treat patients with corticosteroids if they do not have significant improvement in the serum creatinine within three to seven days after discontinuation of the offending agent.

CHRONIC Rx

- Limit exposure to known nephrotoxic agents.
- Renally adjust medications as indicated by glomerular filtration rate.
- Tight control of blood pressure, diabetes, and cholesterol to preserve kidney function as needed

DISPOSITION

With acute interstitial nephritis (AIN), 40% of patients will improve in time. Relapse is common with reexposure to offending agents.

REFERRAL

Refer to nephrology with questions in diagnosis, multiple comorbidities, with failure to respond to supportive care, or with decision to evaluate for biopsy.

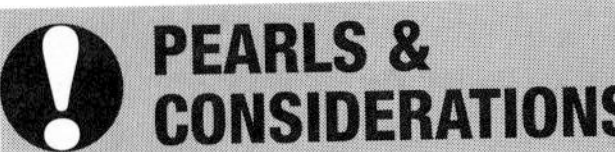

PEARLS & CONSIDERATIONS

COMMENTS

Once known mainly as a complication of streptococcal infection, today acute interstitial nephritis is most often due to drugs; 88% of the time, the drug was started in the past 30 days. Significant fibrosis of the tubules seen in biopsy is the best predictor of transition to chronic interstitial nephritis.

PREVENTION

Use known offending agents with care, especially in the elderly and those with known underlying kidney disease.

SUGGESTED READINGS

available at www.expertconsult.com

RELATED CONTENT

Interstitial Nephritis (Patient Information)

AUTHOR: **ELIZABETH J. BROWN, M.D.,** and **NADEEM MOHAMMED, M.D.**

BASIC INFORMATION

DEFINITION

Intraventricular conduction defect [IVCD] is a common clinical abnormality related to a conduction disturbance that occurs at the various levels of the branches in the His-Purkinje system. This defect does not meet criteria for right bundle branch, left bundle branch, or hemifascicular blocks. In adults, the QRS duration is >110 ms in adults, in children 4 to 16 yr of age is >100 ms, and in children less than 4 yr of age is >90 ms in the electrocardiogram (ECG). The conduction delay causing the prolonged QRS is considered to take place beyond the Purkinje's myocardial gates and arises from a slowing down in the cell-to-cell conduction.

SYNONYMS

IVCD
Nonspecific intraventricular conduction disturbance
Unspecified intraventricular conduction disturbance
Intraventricular conduction delay
Intraventicular block

ICD-9CM CODES
426.6 Intraventricular block, NOS
ICD-10CM CODES
145.4 Non-specific intraventricular block
145.8 Other specified conduction disorders
145.9 Conduction disorder, unspecified

EPIDEMIOLOGY

- Unknown in general population
- The reported prevalence in military aviators was similar to RBBB at 2:1000.

ETIOLOGY

- Any process that affects the intrinsic ventricular conduction system or slows down the intraventricular conduction can lead to the development of an intraventricular block or conduction delay.
- Nonspecific IVCDs are frequently found in patients with previous myocardial infarction and scar formation, on those who take Class I antiarrhythmic drugs, present left ventricular hypertrophy, and hyperkalemia. Etiology can also be unknown in many cases.
- Class IA antiarrhythmics (e.g., procainamide, disopyramide, quinidine) and class IC antiarrhythmics (e.g., flecainide, encainide, and propafenone), amantadine, carbamazepine, cocaine, diphenhydramine, mesoridazine, and thioridazine.
- In addition, propoxyphene and propranolol can also cause IVCD by sodium channel blockade

PHYSICAL FINDINGS & CLINICAL PRESENTATION

Nonspecific IVCD is asymptomatic and is recognizable only through an ECG.

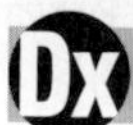

DIAGNOSIS

Usually IVCD is an ECG incidental finding. Lesions of the ventricular conduction system appear as blocks of the bundle branches or fascicles. Ventricular conduction system anomalies can be classified as unifascicular, bifascicular, or trifascicular blocks depending on the site of the lesion or lesions.

DIFFERENTIAL DIAGNOSIS

- Unifascicular block
- Bifascicular block
- Wolff-Parkinson-White (WPW) pattern and variants
- LBBB
- RBBB

WORKUP

Workup such as routine labs, cardiac biomarkers, and cardiac imaging should be targeted at the potential known etiologies and dictated by the clinical circumstances.

Clinical correlation is needed to identify associated cardiac problems. If there is history of heart failure or an abnormal cardiac exam, then an echocardiogram is indicated. If Q waves are present and there is history of myocardial infarction, then an echocardiogram and/or nuclear stress testing is indicated to determine if further therapy should be given to lessen the possibility of heart failure exacerbation, a future myocardial infarction, or other complications. If a Class I antiarrhythmic drug like quinidine or flecainide is being taken that relates temporally to the nonspecific IVCD, then increasing the dosage is not indicated. Blood chemistries can be helpful to assess for hyperkalemia.

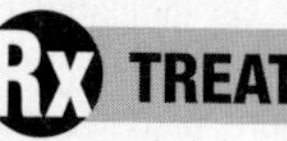

TREATMENT

Though cardiac resynchronization therapy has been effective in reducing clinical events in patients with LBBB (LBBB and RBBB are independent predictors of increased risk of cardiac death in patients with HF), patients with IVCDs do not correlate with worsened prognosis nor clinical improvement of heart failure. Therefore, no specific therapy is needed for IVCD. Patients are usually treated for their underlying heart diseases.

PROGNOSIS

In general population, nonspecific IVCD in the ECG is associated with increased all-cause mortality (RR2.01; 1.52-2.66; P <.001), increased cardiac mortality (RR 2.53; CI 1.64-3.90; P <.001) and a markedly elevated risk of sudden arrhythmic death (RR 3.11; CI 1.74-5.54; P = .001. Nevertheless, clinical correlation is needed because prognosis depends on underlying heart disease, if any.

REFERRAL

Refer to a cardiologist if there is history of heart failure, myocardial infarction, or an abnormal cardiac exam.

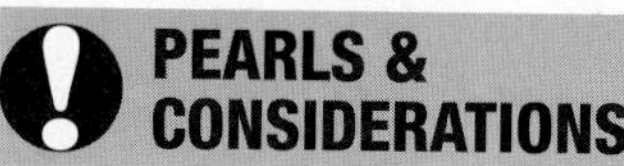

PEARLS & CONSIDERATIONS

Nonspecific IVCD can be due to drugs such as Class I antiarrhythmic drugs. Nonspecific IVCD can be a normal variant and is not always associated with cardiac pathology. Clinical correlation (history and physical exam) is needed to identify associated cardiac abnormalities. In patients with heart failure, cardiac resynchronization for IVCD does not influence prognosis or clinical improvement.

SUGGESTED READINGS

available at www.expertconsult.com

AUTHOR: **CLAUDIA SERRANO-GOMEZ, M.D.**

BASIC INFORMATION

DEFINITION

Irritable bowel syndrome (IBS) is a chronic functional disorder manifested by alteration in bowel habits and recurrent abdominal pain and bloating. IBS is a symptom complex influenced by a variety of physiologic determinants from gut to brain and back. The ROME III criteria for diagnosis of IBS are:

- Recurrent abdominal pain or discomfort at least 3 days per month in the past 3 mo associated with ≥ two of the following:
  - Pain is relieved or improved with defecation.
  - Its onset is associated with a change in the frequency of bowel movement.
  - Its onset is associated with a change in the form or appearance of the stool.
- The criteria must be fulfilled for at least the past 3 mo with symptom onset at least 6 mo before the diagnosis.

SYNONYMS

Irritable colon
Spastic colon
IBS

ICD-9CM CODES
564.1 Irritable bowel syndrome
ICD-10CM CODES
K58 Irritable bowel syndrome
K58.0 Irritable bowel syndrome
K58.9 Irritable bowel syndrome without diarrhea

EPIDEMIOLOGY & DEMOGRAPHICS

- IBS is the most common functional bowel disorder. An estimated 15 million people in the United States have IBS.
- IBS occurs in 20% of the population of industrialized countries and is responsible for >50% of gastrointestinal (GI) referrals. Worldwide adult prevalence is 12%. Incidence increases during adolescence and peaks in third and fourth decades of life.
- Female/male ratio is 2:1. Peak prevalence is from 20 to 39 years of age.
- Nearly 50% of patients have psychiatric abnormalities, with anxiety disorders being most common.

PHYSICAL FINDINGS & CLINICAL PRESENTATION

- The clinical presentation of IBS consists of abdominal pain and abnormalities of defecation, which may include loose stools, usually after meals and in the morning, alternating with episodes of constipation.
- Physical examination is generally normal.
- Nonspecific abdominal tenderness and distention may be present.

ETIOLOGY

- Unknown
- Associated pathophysiology includes altered GI motility, alteration in gut flora, and increased gut sensitivity
- Risk factors: anxiety, depression, personality disorders, history of childhood sexual abuse, and domestic abuse in women

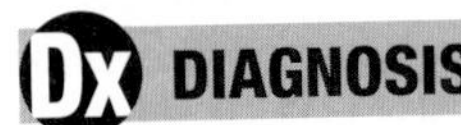

DIAGNOSIS

DIFFERENTIAL DIAGNOSIS

- Inflammatory bowel disease (IBD)
- Diverticulitis
- Colon malignancy
- Endometriosis
- Peptic ulcer disease
- Biliary liver disease
- Chronic pancreatitis
- Constipation caused by medications (opiates, calcium channel blockers, anticholinergics)
- Diarrhea caused by medications (metformin, colchicine, proton pump inhibitors, antacids, antibiotics)
- Small-bowel overgrowth
- Celiac disease
- Parasites
- Lymphoma of GI tract

WORKUP

Diagnostic workup (Fig. E1-525) is aimed primarily at excluding the conditions listed in the differential diagnoses. It is important to identify red flags of other diseases, such as weight loss, rectal bleeding, onset in patients >50 yr, fever, nocturnal pain, and family history of malignancy or IBD. Additional red flags include abnormal examination (e.g., mass, enlarged lymph nodes, stool positive for occult blood, muscle wasting) and abnormal laboratory values (anemia, leukocytosis, abnormal chemistry).

Common clinical criteria for diagnosis of IBS are >3 mo of symptoms, including abdominal pain that is relieved by a bowel movement, or pain accompanied by a change in bowel pattern, and abnormality in bowel movement 25% of the time, characterized by two of the following features:

- Abdominal distention
- Abnormal consistency
- Abnormal defecation (e.g., straining, sense of incomplete evacuation)
- Abnormal frequency
- Mucus with bowel movement

LABORATORY TESTS

- Blood work is generally normal. CBC is reasonable to evaluate for anemia. The presence of anemia should alert to the possibility of a colonic malignancy or IBD.
- Testing of stool for ova and parasites should be considered only in patients with chronic diarrhea. Evaluation of stool for *Clostridium difficile* may be helpful in patients with predominant diarrhea symptoms who have recently taken antibiotics.

IMAGING STUDIES

Imaging studies (e.g., flat and upright abdominal radiograph, small-bowel series, sonogram or CT of abdomen and pelvis) are normal and not necessary for diagnosis.

Lower endoscopy is generally normal except for the presence of some spasms. Colonoscopic imaging should be performed only in persons who have alarm features to rule out organic disease and in persons older than 50 yr to screen for colorectal cancer.

TREATMENT

NONPHARMACOLOGIC THERAPY

- The patient should be encouraged to maintain an adequate fiber intake and to eliminate foods that aggravate symptoms. Avoidance of caffeine, dairy products, fatty foods, and dietary excesses is also helpful.
- Cognitive-behavioral therapy is also recommended, particularly in younger patients because psychosocial stressors are important triggers of IBS. Reassurance and education about trigger avoidance and stress management are important.
- Importance of regular exercise and adequate fluid intake should be stressed.

GENERAL Rx

- The mainstay of treatment of IBS is a high-fiber diet. Fiber is helpful for relief of constipation but not for relief of pain. Because symptoms are chronic, the use of laxatives should generally be avoided.
- Soluble fiber (psyllium) is more effective in symptom relief than insoluble fiber (bran). Fiber supplementation with psyllium 1 tbsp bid or calcium polycarbophil (FiberCon) 2 tablets one to four times daily followed by 8 oz of water may be necessary in some patients.
- Patients should be instructed that there might be some increased bloating on initiation of fiber supplementation, which should resolve within 2 to 3 wk. It is important that patients take these fiber products on a regular basis and not only as needed. Fiber is not effective in patients with diarrhea-predominant IBS and may worsen symptoms in these patients.
- Patients who appear anxious can benefit from use of sedatives or selective serotonin reuptake inhibitors (SSRIs). Tricyclic antidepressants in low doses are also effective in some patients with diarrhea-predominant IBS.
- C-2 chloride channel activators: Lubiprostone (Amitiza) is a chloride channel activator that stimulates chloride-rich intestinal fluid secretion and accelerates small intestine and colonic transmit time. It may be effective in chronic constipation-predominant IBS unresponsive to conventional treatment. Usual dose is 8 to 24 mcg bid with food. Side effects include headache and nausea.
- Linaclotide (Linzess) is a guanylate cyclase-C (GC-C) agonist recently FDA approved for IBS with constipation. It stimulates secretion of chloride and bicarbonate into the intestinal lumen, mainly through activation of the CFTR ion channel, resulting in increased intestinal fluid and accelerated transit. Usual dose for IBS is 290 mcg 30 min before eating. The most common adverse effects are diarrhea, abdominal pain, flatulence, and abdominal distension.
- Loperamide is effective for diarrhea. Alosetron, a serotonin type-3 receptor antagonist

previously withdrawn because of severe constipation and ischemic colitis, has been reintroduced with limited availability. It is indicated only for women with severe chronic diarrhea-predominant IBS unresponsive to conventional therapy and not caused by anatomic or metabolic abnormality. Starting dose is 1 mg qd.

- Alterations in gut flora have been identified as potentially contributing to IBS (84% of IBS patients have an abnormal lactulose breath test, suggesting small-intestinal bacterial overgrowth). Rifaximin, a gut-selective antibiotic, has been used in recent trials to eradicate bacterial overgrowth (70% eradication rate). A dose of 400 mg tid for 10 days was reported effective in improving IBS symptoms up to 10 wk after discontinuation of therapy. Until additional evidence is available, use of rifaximin or other antibiotics in IBS should be reserved for patients with proven bacterial overgrowth.
- Antispasmodics-anticholinergics (e.g., dicyclomine, hyoscyamine) are often used, but efficacy data from clinical trials are inconclusive.
- Probiotics: Bifidobacteria and some combinations of probiotics have shown some limited efficacy. Lactobacilli do not appear to be effective for the treatment of IBS. Additional data showing efficacy is needed before probiotics can be endorsed for treatment of IBS.
- Antidepressants: SSRIs are more effective than placebo for relief of global IBS symptoms.

DISPOSITION

More than 60% of patients respond successfully to treatment over the initial 12 mo; however, IBS is a chronic, relapsing condition and requires prolonged therapy.

REFERRAL

GI referral is recommended in patients with rectal bleeding, fever, nocturnal diarrhea, anemia, weight loss, or onset of symptoms >40 yr. Consultation is also necessary if specialized diagnostic procedures such as endoscopy are necessary.

PEARLS & CONSIDERATIONS

COMMENTS

- Patients should be educated regarding maintenance of a high-fiber diet and elimination of stressors, which can precipitate attacks of IBS. They should be reassured that their condition does not lead to cancer.
- Recent drug efforts (alosetron, tegaserod) are aimed at serotonergic receptors in the gut because most of the serotonin in the body is found in the GI tract and is believed to be involved in the mediation of visceral sensation and motility.
- Cognitive-behavioral therapy is effective in the treatment of patients with IBS and should be considered as part of the armamentarium against this disorder.
- Some patients with IBS but without celiac disease show symptom improvement on a wheat-free diet. A 2- to 3-week trial of wheat avoidance may be reasonable in patients with treatment-resistant IBS.

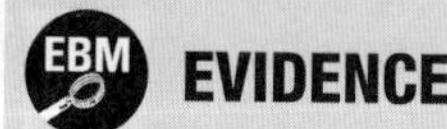

EVIDENCE

available at www.expertconsult.com

SUGGESTED READINGS

available at www.expertconsult.com

RELATED CONTENT

Irritable Bowel Syndrome (Patient Information)

AUTHOR: **FRED F. FERRI, M.D.**

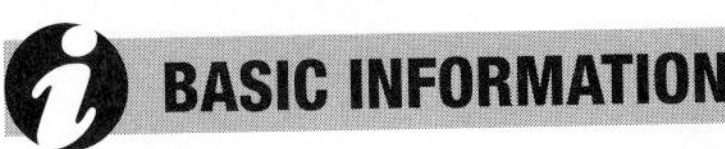

DEFINITION

Jaundice is a yellowish discoloration of the sclera (Fig. E1-526), skin, and mucous membranes caused by an excessive amount of bilirubin in the bloodstream. Clinically detectable jaundice in adults is a serum bilirubin of 2.5 to 3 mg/dl.

SYNONYMS

Icterus

ICD-9CM CODES
782.4 Jaundice
283.9 Hemolytic jaundice
576.8 Obstructive jaundice
ICD-10CM CODES
R17 Unspecified jaundice

EPIDEMIOLOGY & DEMOGRAPHICS

The major causes of jaundice by age and sex:
- Young adulthood (for either sex): viral hepatitis, Gilbert's disease
- Middle adulthood (for either sex): drug-induced hepatitis and cirrhosis
- Middle-aged and older men: alcoholic liver disease, pancreatic cancer, hepatoma, primary hemochromatosis
- Women: primary biliary cirrhosis, chronic active hepatitis, choledocholithiasis, carcinoma of the gallbladder

PHYSICAL FINDINGS & CLINICAL PRESENTATION

Presentation can vary from an incidental finding to acute and life threatening. History and physical examination give important clues to the underlying condition.
Key history of present illness findings:
- Duration of jaundice
- Associated symptoms: abdominal pain, fever, nausea, malaise, pruritus, chills, changes in urine and stool color, anorexia and/or weight loss

Key social history/exposure findings:
- Alcohol use, injection of illicit drugs, use of hepatotoxic medication or herbal products, blood transfusions, unprotected sex, ingestion of shellfish, travel, occupational exposure to toxins

Key past medical history findings:
- Prior abdominal/biliary surgery, prior episodes of jaundice, prior diagnosis of hepatitis B or C, inflammatory bowel disease

Key physical findings:
- Vital sign abnormalities: fever, hypotension, tachycardia
- Signs of acute disease: abdominal tenderness, splenomegaly, abdominal mass, encephalopathy, Murphy's sign
- Signs of chronic liver disease: palmar erythema, spider angiomas, bruising, gynecomastia, testicular atrophy, ascites, weight loss, Kayser-Fleischer rings (Wilson's), caput medusa, internal hemorrhoids, scleral icterus

ETIOLOGY

Disruption in any of the three phases of bilirubin metabolism can lead to jaundice:
- Prehepatic phase: an increase in heme degradation products from red blood cell catabolism, ineffective erythropoiesis, or breakdown of muscle myoglobin and cytochromes; leads to indirect (unconjugated) hyperbilirubinemia
- Intrahepatic phase: destruction of the hepatocytes or disruption of either of the two separate biochemical processes that conjugate bilirubin in the hepatocyte; may lead to indirect (unconjugated) or direct (conjugated) hyperbilirubinemia
- Posthepatic phase: blockage of the release of water-soluble bilirubin from the hepatobiliary system, preventing excretion into the stool or urine or recycling within the gut flora; leads to direct (conjugated) hyperbilirubinemia

Dx DIAGNOSIS

DIFFERENTIAL DIAGNOSIS

Prehepatic causes:
- Consider hemolysis (e.g., sickle cell disease, spherocytosis, thalassemia, G6PD, immune hemolysis, HUS), ineffective erythropoiesis (e.g., thalassemia, folate, severe iron deficiency), or large hematoma reabsorption.

Intrahepatic causes:
- If unconjugated hyperbilirubinemia: consider enzyme metabolism disorders, specifically Gilbert's disease, which is common and benign or Crigler-Najjar syndrome, which is rare and severe; drugs that alter the enzymatic pathways such as rifampin, isoniazid, and probenecid.
- If conjugated hyperbilirubinemia: consider intrahepatic cholestasis.
  1. Viruses: hepatitis A, B, and C; Epstein-Barr, hemorrhagic viruses (yellow fever, Ebola)
  2. Other infections: bacteria (leptospirosis, MAI), parasites (schistosomiasis, malaria, amebiasis), fungal (blastomyces, histoplasma)
  3. Alcohol: alcoholic hepatitis, alcoholic cirrhosis
  4. Autoimmune: primary biliary cirrhosis, primary sclerosing cholangitis, autoimmune hepatitis
  5. Hepatotoxic drug-induced: acetaminophen (most common), penicillins (specifically Augmentin), chlorpromazine, steroids (estrogenic or anabolic), NSAIDs, some herbals such as kava, ma huang, and off-market weight loss supplements
  6. Hereditary/metabolic: sickle cell disease and other RBC dyscrasias, hemochromatosis, Wilson's disease, Dubin-Johnson and Rotor's syndromes, α-antitrypsin deficiency, glycogen storage disease, NASH (non-alcoholic steatohepatitis), porphyria
  7. Systemic disease: invading liver: sarcoidosis, amyloidosis, hemochromatosis, tuberculosis, *Mycobacterium avium intracellulare*
  8. Other: cirrhosis, sepsis, total parenteral nutrition, pregnancy, graft-versus-host disease, environmental toxins, drugs related to intrahepatic cholestasis (PTU, Tylenol, erythromycin, anabolic steroids, contraceptive pills), benign postoperative state

Posthepatic causes:
- Intrinsic or extrinsic obstruction of the biliary system
  1. Blockage within hepatobiliary tree: strictures (congenital, traumatic, iatrogenic), cholangiocarcinoma, gallbladder cancer, carcinoma of ampulla of vater, infection (e.g., cytomegalovirus, *Cryptosporidium* in patients with AIDS, parasites), choledocholithiasis
  2. Blockage outside of hepatobiliary tree: pancreatitis, pancreatic carcinoma, pancreatic pseudocyst, lymphoma
- Pseudojaundice: not related to bilirubin but rather resulting from excessive ingestion of foods containing beta carotene (e.g., carrots, melons, squash)

WORKUP

History, physical examination, and first-line lab tests can often clarify diagnosis. Fig. 1-527 describes a clinical approach to jaundice.

LABORATORY TESTS

First-line tests:
- Serum total and direct bilirubin
- Urinalysis

If serum total bilirubin and direct bilirubin are elevated and urine is positive for bilirubin, consider intrahepatic or posthepatic process:
- Initial evaluation: liver function tests (AST, ALT, GGTP, alkaline phosphatase), CBC, liver synthetic function (albumin, PT, PTT), pancreatic function (amylase, lipase)
- Additional tests if diagnosis unclear:
  1. Screen for hepatitis A, B, and C; if still unclear then consider options 2 to 6 as follow
  2. Other viruses (Epstein-Barr virus, cytomegalovirus)
  3. Autoimmune disorders: antimitochondrial antibody, immunoglobulin (Ig) M (elevated in primary biliary cirrhosis); antismooth muscle antibody, antinuclear antibody, IgG (autoimmune chronic active hepatitis); antinuclear cytoplasmic antibody (primary sclerosing cholangitis)
  4. Ceruloplasmin (Wilson's disease)
  5. Alpha-1 antitrypsin deficiency (cirrhosis and emphysema)
  6. Ferritin, Fe saturation (elevated in hemochromatosis)

If serum total bilirubin is elevated but direct bilirubin is normal (unconjugated hyperbilirubinemia) and urine is negative for bilirubin, consider prehepatic or intrahepatic processes.
- Blood smear (abnormal RBC types)
- Diagnosis of exclusion: Gilbert's syndrome

Liver biopsy: essential in diagnosis of chronic hepatitis. Can be used for diagnosis of liver masses but carries a substantial risk.

Jaundice in the Adult Patient 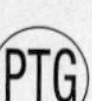 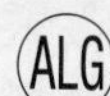

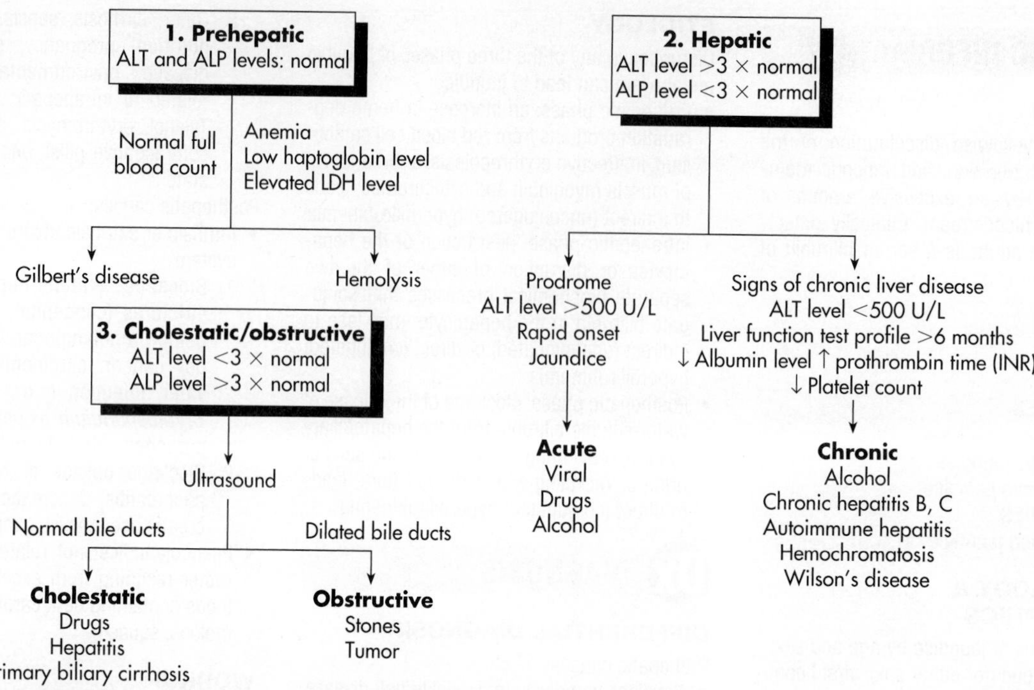

FIGURE E1-527 A clinical approach to jaundice. *ALP,* Alkaline phosphatase; *ALT,* alanine aminotransferase; *LDH,* lactate dehydrogenase. (Modified from Talley NJ, Martin CJ: *Clinical gastroenterology,* ed 2, Sydney, 2006, Churchill Livingstone.)

IMAGING STUDIES

- Abdominal ultrasound: first-line study (Figs. E1-528 and E1-529), may be completed bedside, most sensitive for proximal biliary tract disease; presence of dilated ducts hints at an extrahepatic process
- Abdominal CT: often necessary to elucidate more information on liver, pancreas, and distal biliary system
- Endoscopic retrograde cholangiopancreatography: rarely necessary for diagnostics. If needed, refer to GI consultant
- Percutaneous transhepatic cholangiography: rarely necessary for diagnostics. If needed, refer to GI consultant
- Magnetic resonance cholangiopancreatography: noninvasive visualization of bile and pancreatic ducts; becoming more available. If needed, refer to GI consultant.
- Endoscopic ultrasound: used for characterization and, if needed, biopsy of any focal lesions found within biliary tree and/or pancreas. If needed, refer to GI consultant

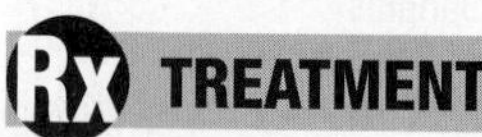

TREATMENT

NONPHARMACOLOGIC THERAPY

Depends on underlying cause of the jaundice and clinical stability of the patient. Generally, obstructive causes require surgical treatment, while nonobstructive causes require medical treatment.

ACUTE GENERAL Rx

Acute, life-threatening illness (e.g., cholecystitis or ascending cholangitis) requires prompt diagnosis with basic labs and bedside diagnostics, with early surgical and GI consultation in conjunction with medical management involving symptom relief with analgesia, IV fluids, correction of coagulopathy, and consideration for antibiotics. *N*-Acetylcysteine can be given for acetaminophen overdose.

CHRONIC Rx

Reversible causes must be ruled out first and suspicious medications or ETOH use must be stopped. For intrahepatic disease, consider GI consult for management of hepatitis B or C with interferon, Wilson's disease with penicillamine, hemochromatosis with phlebotomy, or for stent insertion with ERCP for post-hepatic obstruction related to strictures/cholangiocarcinoma to bypass unresectable lesion. Consider surgical consult for resection of pancreatic masses, cholecystecomy, etc.

Symptomatic pruritus may be treated with cholestyramine for bilirubin binding or with antihistamines to decrease the itch reflex. Ursodiol to treat primary biliary cirrhosis and for gallstone prevention/dissolution.

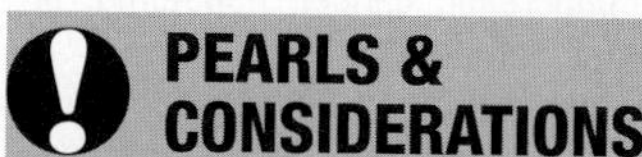

PEARLS & CONSIDERATIONS

COMMENTS

- Heed the warning signs of unstable vital signs to diagnose life-threatening illness; early collaboration with surgical and gastroenterology colleagues is helpful in complex patient care scenarios.
- Careful history and physical examination, basic labs, and prompt bedside imaging frequently lead to accurate diagnosis.
- Very high serum bilirubin (>15 mg/dl) is most likely to be seen in cirrhosis. Watch for hepatorenal syndrome in these patients.

SUGGESTED READINGS

available at www.expertconsult.com

RELATED CONTENT

Jaundice (Patient Information)

AUTHORS: **ALLA GOLDBURT, M.D.,** and **PAOLO G. PACE, M.A.SC., M.D.**

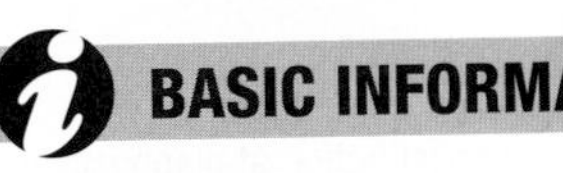

BASIC INFORMATION

DEFINITION

Juvenile idiopathic arthritis (JIA), previously referred to as juvenile rheumatoid arthritis (JRA), is a diverse spectrum of arthritides presenting before 16 yr of age. The arthritis symptoms must be persistent and objective in ≥one joints for at least 6 wk with the exclusion of any other known cause.

SYNONYMS

Still's disease
JIA
Juvenile rheumatoid arthritis

ICD-9CM CODES
714.3 Polyarticular juvenile rheumatoid arthritis, chronic or unspecified

ICD-10CM CODES
M08.00 Unspecified juvenile rheumatoid arthritis of unspecified site

EPIDEMIOLOGY & DEMOGRAPHICS

PREVALENCE (IN U.S.): 57 to 220 per 100,000 children

PHYSICAL FINDINGS & CLINICAL PRESENTATION

JIA is subdivided into seven categories based on the 2001 International League of Associations for Rheumatology (ILAR) classification criteria (subtype characteristics are summarized in Table 1-283).

Systemic onset JIA
- Arthritis in ≥one joints with or preceded by fever of at least 2 wk duration that is quotidian (once daily) for at least 3 days and associated with at least one of the following: (1) evanescent erythematous rash (Fig. E1-530), (2) generalized lymph node enlargement, (3) hepatomegaly, splenomegaly, or both, and (4) serositis such as pleuritis, pericarditis, or peritonitis.

Oligoarticular JIA (Fig. E1-531)
- Arthritis in one to four joints during a 6-mo period of time. There are two subtypes:
  - Persistent: ≤four joints throughout the disease course
  - Extended: ≤four joints during the first 6 mo extending to >four joints after 6 mo.

Polyarthritis, rheumatoid factor (RF) negative
- Arthritis involves >six joints during first 6 mo of the disease with negative RF.

Polyarthritis, RF positive
- Arthritis involves >six joints during first 6 mo of the disease with positive RF on at least two tests run 3 mo apart.
- Anti–cyclic citrullinated (CCP) antibodies may also be present
- Most likely to extend beyond childhood and most similar to adult rheumatoid arthritis

Psoriatic arthritis
- Psoriasis and arthritis or psoriasis and ≥two of the following:
  - Dactylitis, nail pitting, onycholysis, and psoriasis in a first-degree relative

Enthesitis-related arthritis
- Arthritis and enthesitis or arthritis or enthesitis and ≥two of the following:
  - Presence of or a history of SI joint pain, positive HLA-B27, boy aged >6 yr, acute anterior uveitis, or history of ankylosing spondylitis, reactive arthritis, sacroiliitis with inflammatory bowel disease or acute anterior uveitis in a first-degree relative

ETIOLOGY

Idiopathic: Both genetic and environmental triggers thought to play a role.

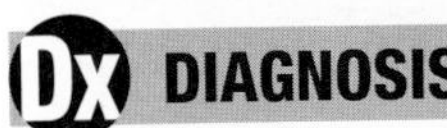

DIAGNOSIS

DIFFERENTIAL DIAGNOSIS

- Infection: viral or rheumatic fever
- Systemic lupus erythematosus (very rare under age 5)
- Malignancy
- Serum sickness
- Lyme arthritis

LABORATORY TESTS

- Increased erythrocyte sedimentation rate and CRP
- Low-grade anemia
- Leukocytosis
- Rheumatoid factor: rarely demonstrable in the serum of children
- Antinuclear antibodies: often found in children with ocular complications
- If macrophage activation syndrome suspected in patients with systemic JIA: decreased platelets, WBC, and fibrinogen with high ferritin and liver function tests. Bone marrow biopsy is needed to confirm diagnosis.

TABLE 1-283 Overview of the Main Features of the Subtypes of Juvenile Idiopathic Arthritis

ILAR Subtype	Peak Age of Onset (yr)	Female: Male; % of All JIA	Arthritis Pattern	Extraarticular Features	Investigations	Notes on Therapy
Systemic arthritis	2-4	1:1; ~10% of JIA cases	Polyarticular, often knees, wrists, and ankles; also fingers, neck, and hips	Daily fever; evanescent rash; pericarditis; pleuritis	Anemia; WBC↑↑; ESR↑↑; CRP↑↑; ferritin;↑ platelets↑↑ (normal or ↑ in MAS)	Less responsive to standard treatment with MTX and anti-TNF agents; consider IL-1Ra in resistant cases
Oligoarthritis	>6	4:1; 50%-60% of JIA (but ethnic variation)	Knees ++; ankles, fingers +	Uveitis in ~30%	ANA positive in 60%; other tests usually normal; may have mildly ↑ ESR/CRP	NSAIDs and intraarticular steroids; occasionally require MTX
Polyarthritis, RF negative	6-7	3:1; 30% of JIA cases	Symmetric or asymmetric; small and large joints; cervical spine; TMJ	Uveitis in ~10%	ANA positive in 40%; RF negative; ESR ↑ or; ↑↑ CRP↑/normal; mild anemia	Standard therapy with MTX and NSAIDs, then if nonresponsive, anti-TNF agents or other biologics
Polyarthritis, RF positive	9-12	9:1; >10% of JIA cases	Aggressive symmetric polyarthritis	Rheumatoid nodules in 10%; low-grade fever	RF positive; ESR ↑↑; CRP ↑/normal; mild anemia	Long-term remission unlikely; early aggressive therapy is warranted
Psoriatic arthritis	7-10	2:1; >10% of JIA cases	Asymmetric arthritis of small or medium sized joints	Uveitis in 10%; psoriasis in 50%	ANA positive in 50%; ESR ↑; CRP ↑/normal; mild anemia	NSAIDs and intraarticular steroids; second-line agents less commonly
Enthesitis-related arthritis	9-12	1:7; 10% of JIA cases	Predominantly lower limb joints affected; sometimes axial skeleton (but less than adult AS)	Acute anterior uveitis; association with reactive arthritis and IBD	80% HLA-B27$^+$	NSAIDs and intraarticular steroids; consider sulfasalazine as alternative to MTX

ANA, Antinuclear antibody; *AS*, ankylosing spondylitis; *CRP*, C-reactive protein; *ESR*, erythrocyte sedimentation rate; *IBD*, inflammatory bowel disease; *ILAR*, International League of Associations for Rheumatology; *IL-1Ra*, interleukin-1 receptor antagonist; *JIA*, juvenile idiopathic arthritis; *MAS*, macrophage activation syndrome; *MTX*, methotrexate; *NSAID*, nonsteroidal anti-inflammatory drug; *RF*, rheumatoid factor; *TMJ*, temporomandibular joint; *TNF*, tumor necrosis factor; *WBC*, white blood cell count.
From Firestein G et al: *Kelley's textbook of rheumatology*, ed 9, Philadelphia, 2013, Saunders.

IMAGING STUDIES

- Roentgenographic findings (Fig. E1-532) are similar to those in adult, with soft tissue swelling and periarticular osteopenia early in the disease.
- Joint destruction (Fig. E1-533) is less frequent.
- Bony erosion and cyst formation may be present as a result of synovial hypertrophy.

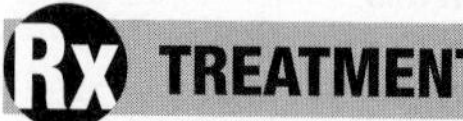

TREATMENT

NONPHARMACOLOGIC THERAPY

Proper management requires close cooperation among primary physician, physical and occupational therapists, pediatric rheumatologist, social workers, and orthopedist.

- Rest
- Physical and occupational therapy
- Patient and family education
- Proper diet and weight maintenance (Fig. 1-534)

ACUTE GENERAL Rx

- NSAIDs
- DMARDs: methotrexate, leflunomide, sulfasalazine
- Patients with polyarticular disease are less likely to respond to methotrexate if they have longer disease duration, positive ANA, higher level of disability, and bilateral wrist arthritis. It may be reasonable to start with anti-TNF therapy first in these cases.
- Axial involvement is also less likely to respond to methotrexate
- Biologics:
  - Tumor necrosis factor blockers such as etanercept and adalimumab
  - T-cell modulator CTLA-4 fusion protein, abatacept, is FDA approved for patients with polyarticular JIA who have not responded to anti-TNF therapy
  - IL-6 (tocilizumab) and IL-1 inhibitors (anakinra, canakinumab) for systemic JIA
- Intraarticular steroids can prevent leg length discrepancies in oligoarticular JIA
- Systemic corticosteroids

DISPOSITION

- Complete remission occurs in the majority of patients and may occur at any age.
- 70% to 85% of children regain normal function.
- Mortality is three- to fourteenfold greater than in the general population of the same age. Macrophage activation syndrome is a life-threatening complication in systemic JIA.
- Oligoarticular JIA patients with positive ANA are at the highest risk for blindness due to chronic iridocyclitis and require frequent ophthalmologic monitoring.
- Systemic and localized growth disturbance can lead to generalized growth failure and leg length discrepancies.
- Arthritis of the temporomandibular joint can lead to jaw malformation.

REFERRAL

- Early rheumatology consultation
- Ophthalmology consultation at diagnosis and regularly thereafter particularly in ANA+, oligoarticular JIA
- Orthopedic consultation for corrective surgery

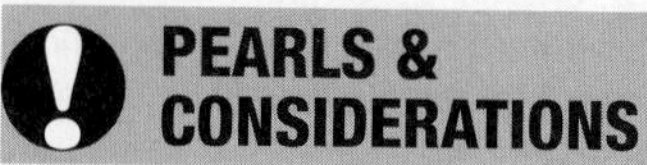

PEARLS & CONSIDERATIONS

COMMENTS

The spontaneous adverse event reports (SERS) in the FDA surveillance system has recently reported a warning for risk of malignancy related to anti-TNF agents in the pediatric population. However, baseline risk of malignancy in children with JIA is unknown and the SERS reporting system has limitations, including incomplete adverse event reporting. Initiation of anti-TNF therapy should be a decision made between families and pediatric rheumatologists.

SUGGESTED READINGS

available at www.expertconsult.com

RELATED CONTENT

Juvenile Rheumatoid Arthritis (Patient Information)

AUTHOR: **ELISABETH B. MATSON, D.O.**

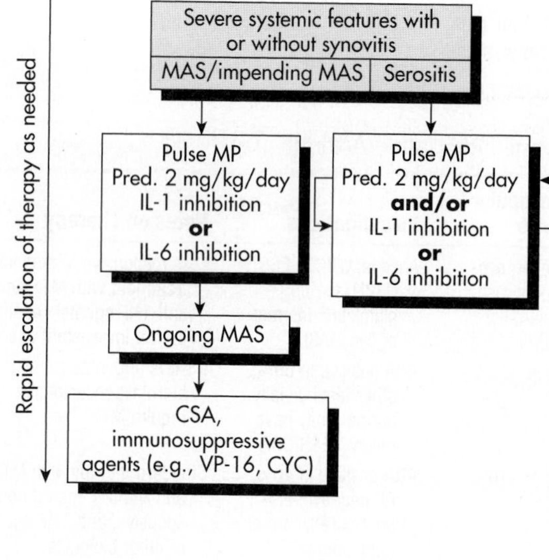

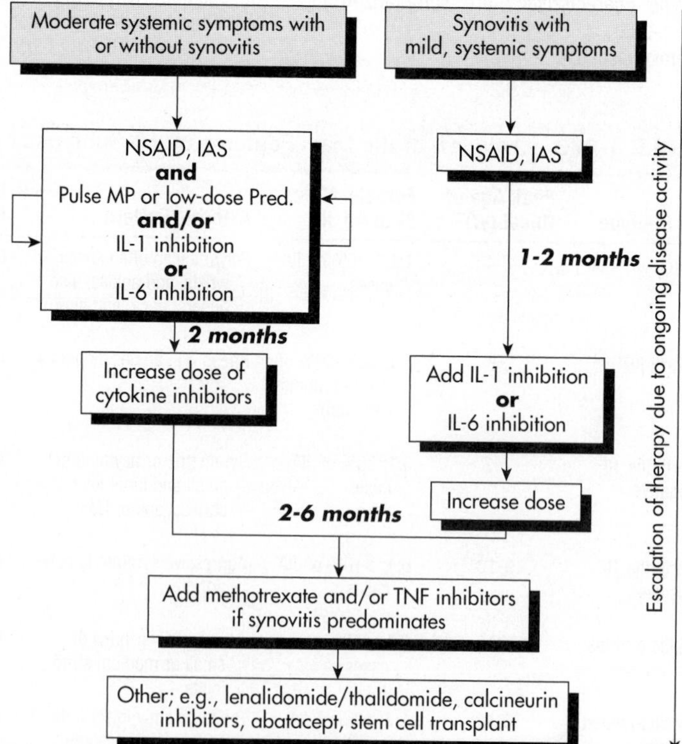

FIGURE 1-534 Systemic juvenile idiopathic arthritis treatment algorithm. The treatment goal is remission of disease activity, both systemic and articular, and is stratified by severity of disease. Algorithm is divided into severe systemic disease manifestations (macrophage activation syndrome [MAS], serositis) or synovitis with milder systemic disease. Currently there is significant variability in practice regarding using corticosteroid as initial systemic therapy or moving directly to inflammatory cytokine inhibitors. At the time of this writing, interleukin (IL)-1 inhibition and IL-6 inhibition are currently in trials, and more information is likely to be available in the future. *CSA*, cyclosporine A; *CYC*, cyclophosphamide; *IAS*, intraarticular steroid; *MP*, methylprednisolone; *NSAID*, nonsteroidal anti-inflammatory drug; *Pred.*, prednisone; *TNF*, tumor necrosis factor. (From Firestein GS et al: *Kelly's textbook of rheumatology*, ed 9, Philadelphia, 2013, Saunders.)

BASIC INFORMATION

DEFINITION

Kaposi's sarcoma (KS) is a vascular neoplasm most frequently occurring in AIDS patients. It can be divided into the following four subsets:

1. Classic KS: most frequently found in elderly Eastern European and Mediterranean males. It consists initially of violaceous macules and papules with subsequent development of plaques and red-purple nodules. Growth is slow, and most of the patients die of unrelated causes.
2. Epidemic or AIDS-related KS: most frequently occurs in homosexual men. Lesions are generally multifocal and widespread. Lymphadenopathy may be associated.
3. Endemic KS: usually affects African children and adults. An aggressive lymphadenopathic form affects African children in particular.
4. Immunosuppression-associated, or transplantation-associated, KS: usually associated with chemotherapy.

SYNONYMS

KS

ICD-9CM CODES
173.9 Malignant neoplasm of the skin
ICD-10CM CODES
C46.9 Kaposi's sarcoma, unspecified

EPIDEMIOLOGY & DEMOGRAPHICS

- AIDS-related KS affects >35% of AIDS cases.
- Highest incidence is in homosexual men.

PHYSICAL FINDINGS & CLINICAL PRESENTATION

- AIDS-related KS: multifocal and widespread red-purple (Fig. E1-535) or dark plaques (Fig. E1-536) and/or nodules on cutaneous or mucosal surfaces (Fig. 1-537).
- Generalized lymphadenopathy at the time of diagnosis is present in >50% of patients with AIDS-related KS; the initial lesions have a rust-colored appearance; subsequent progression to red or purple nodules or plaques occurs.
- Most frequently affected areas are the face, trunk, oral cavity, and upper and lower extremities.

ETIOLOGY

A herpesvirus (HHV-8, KS-associated herpesvirus KSHV) has been isolated from patients with most forms of KS and is believed to be the causative agent. It can be transmitted sexually (homosexual or heterosexual activities) and by other forms of nonsexual contact such as maternal-infant transmission (common in African countries).

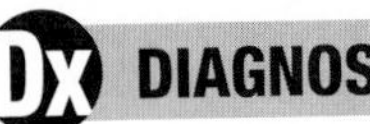

DIAGNOSIS

DIFFERENTIAL DIAGNOSIS

- Stasis dermatitis
- Pyogenic granuloma
- Capillary hemangiomas
- Granulation tissue
- Postinflammatory hyperpigmentation
- Cutaneous lymphoma
- Melanoma
- Dermatofibroma
- Hematoma
- Prurigo nodularis

The differential diagnosis of cutaneous lesions in patients with HIV infection is described in Section II.

WORKUP

Diagnosis can generally be made on clinical appearance; tissue biopsy will confirm diagnosis.

LABORATORY TESTS

HIV in patients suspected of AIDS

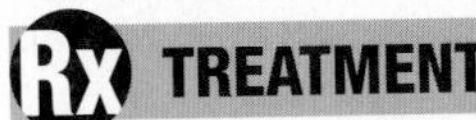

TREATMENT

NONPHARMACOLOGIC THERAPY

Observation is a reasonable option in patients with slowly progressive disease.

GENERAL Rx

- Excisional biopsy often provides adequate treatment for single lesions and resected recurrences in classic KS.
- Liquid nitrogen cryotherapy can result in complete response in 80% of lesions.
- Interlesional chemotherapy with vinblastine is useful for nodular lesions >1 cm in diameter. Intralesional injection of interferon alfa-2b has also been reported as effective and well tolerated.
- Radiation therapy is effective in non-AIDS KS and for large tumor masses that interfere with normal function.
- Systemic therapy with interferon is also effective in AIDS-related KS and is often used in combination with zidovudine.
- Systemic chemotherapy (vinblastine, bleomycin, doxorubicin, and dacarbazine) can be used for rapidly progressive disease and for classic and African endemic KS.
- Sirolimus (rapamycin), an immunosuppressive drug, is effective in inhibiting the progression of dermal KS in kidney transplant recipients.
- Oral etoposide is also effective and has less myelosuppression than vinblastine.
- Paclitaxel is also effective in patients with advanced KS and represents an excellent second-line therapy.
- Thalidomide, retinoids.

DISPOSITION

- Prognosis is poor in AIDS-related KS. Death is often a result of other AIDS-defining illnesses.
- Prognosis is better in African cutaneous KS and classic sarcoma (patients usually die of unrelated causes).

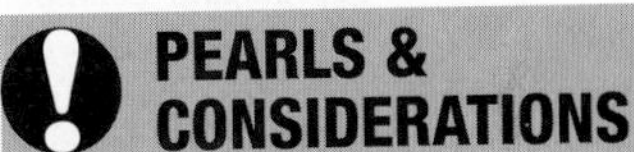

PEARLS & CONSIDERATIONS

COMMENTS

Immunosuppression-associated KS usually regresses with the cessation, reduction, or modification of immunosuppression therapy in most patients. Similarly, in HIV patients KS responds concurrently with the decrease in serum HIV RNA and increase in the CD4 count.

SUGGESTED READINGS

available at www.expertconsult.com

RELATED CONTENT

Kaposi's Sarcoma (Patient Information)

AUTHOR: **FRED F. FERRI, M.D.**

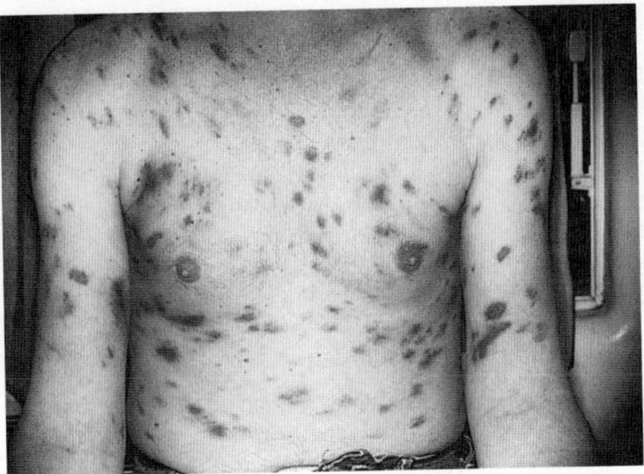

FIGURE 1-537 Kaposi's sarcoma. More advanced lesions. Note widespread hemorrhagic plaques and nodules. (From Noble J [ed]: *Textbook of primary care medicine,* ed 2, St Louis, 1995, Mosby.)

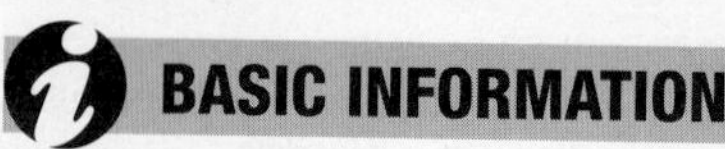

DEFINITION

Kawasaki disease (KD) is an acute, febrile vasculitis of small and medium-size blood vessels that predominantly affects children. It is usually a self-limiting condition lasting for an average of 12 days if not treated.

SYNONYMS

Kawasaki syndrome
Mucocutaneous lymph node syndrome
Infantile polyarteritis

ICD-9CM CODES
446.1 Kawasaki disease
ICD-10CM CODES
M30.3 Mucocutaneous lymph node syndrome [Kawasaki]

EPIDEMIOLOGY & DEMOGRAPHICS

- KD is the leading cause of acquired heart disease in children in developing countries and in the U.S. and Japan.
- Commonly occurs in children <5 yr (80%); peak incidence is in infants aged 9 to 11 mo to 24 mo. Occurrence is rare after late childhood.
- More prevalent in boys than girls (1.5:1).
- The highest incidence is found in Japan (~174 cases/100,000 children).
- Temporal clustering and winter to spring predominance have been observed in KD cases in Japan.
- Incidence of KD in the U.S. is 17 to 18 cases/100,000 children <5 yr.
- Children of Asian descent have the highest incidence of KD compared with those of European or African descent.
- ~4200 new cases are diagnosed each year in the U.S.
- 1% of patients with KD in Japan have a positive family history of KD.
- In the U.S., KD has now surpassed acute rheumatic fever as the leading cause of acquired heart disease in children.

PHYSICAL FINDINGS & CLINICAL PRESENTATION

- The clinical presentations reflect inflammation of small and medium-sized blood vessels. Diagnosis of KD is based on characteristic clinical signs and symptoms and includes fever persisting for >5 days and the presence of at least four of the following five principal features:
  1. Bilateral, painless bulbar conjunctival injection without exudate
  2. Oral mucosal changes: erythema and fissured lips, strawberry tongue (Fig. E1-538, *B*), diffuse injection of the oropharyngeal mucosae
  3. Polymorphous exanthema (usually in truncal region) (Fig. E1-539, *A* and *B*)
  4. Extremity changes: (a) acute: erythema and edema of hands and feet (Fig. E1-538, *A*); (b) convalescent: membranous desquamation of fingertips
  5. Cervical lymph node enlargement (at least one lymph node >1.5 cm in diameter).
- The fever of KD is mildly responsive to antipyretics and is usually higher than 102.2° F (39° C) and often >104.0° F (40° C). If untreated, it lasts for an average of 12 days.
- The rash of KD can be maculopapular or can take various forms; however, vesicles, bullae, purpura, and petechia are never observed.
- Coronary artery aneurysms can develop in as many as 25% to 60% of untreated children between 1 to 4 weeks of illness. This subset of patients can develop ischemic heart disease, myocardial infarction, and congestive heart failure over time, and, occasionally, death. New aneurysms seldom form after 6 weeks. Half of the aneurysms show angiographic regression in 1-2 years
- Morbidity and mortality rates are highest if aneurysm diameter is >8 mm.
- Children with KD who are <1 yr or >6 yr are more likely to develop the cardiac sequelae and are least likely to respond to treatment.
- Patients with fever and fewer than four principal symptoms but evidence of coronary artery disease are diagnosed as having atypical or incomplete KD (10%).
- Cervical lymphadenopathy is the most common physical manifestation absent in atypical KD, followed by exanthema and then extremity changes.
- Oral mucosal changes are the most common manifestations of KD affecting approximately 90% of cases (either typical or atypical).
- Patients may also develop sensitivity to light and uveitis along with conjunctival injection.
- Redness and induration can be seen at the site of bacille Calmette-Guérin (BCG) inoculation.
- Beau's lines (transverse grooves of the nails), diarrhea, acute myocarditis, cough, rhinorrhea, dyspnea, arthralgia, and myalgia may also be seen.
- Aseptic meningitis can develop in 40% of cases.
- Interstitial nephritis, acute renal failure in rare cases, KD shock syndrome, and macrophage activation syndrome can also occur.
- Self-limiting arthritis involving large joints including knees, ankles and hips were reported in 7.5% to 25% of patients.

ETIOLOGY

The cause of KD is not known, although evidence suggests an infectious etiology precipitating an immune-mediated reaction in genetically susceptible individuals.

Dx DIAGNOSIS

Diagnosis of KD is made on the basis of clinical features (see "Physical Findings & Clinical Presentation"). The hallmark of KD is fever lasting >5 days. Typically, the clinical signs appear over the course of several days. Laboratory evaluation may be helpful in making the diagnosis in atypical KD. The timely diagnosis and treatment of KD are important in preventing complications.

DIFFERENTIAL DIAGNOSIS

- Scarlet fever
- Stevens-Johnson syndrome
- Drug eruption
- Henoch-Schönlein purpura
- Toxic shock syndrome
- Measles
- Rocky Mountain spotted fever
- Epstein-Barr virus, adenovirus, echovirus, and enterovirus
- Juvenile rheumatoid arthritis
- Mercury hypersensitivity (acrodynia)
- Leptospirosis

WORKUP

Clinical findings in addition to laboratory and imaging studies are useful in searching for multiorgan system involvement and complications (e.g., cardiac, lung, liver).

LABORATORY TESTS

Inflammatory markers will be increased in KD.

Clinical and laboratory findings observed in patients with this disease are frequently helpful in diagnosis:

- Complete blood count commonly shows a normochromic normocytic anemia, elevated white blood cell count with neutrophil predominance and elevated platelet count, which usually rises by the second week.
- Abnormal liver function tests are found: elevated transaminases (hepatic congestion), elevated bilirubin (gallbladder hydrops), low albumin.
- Elevated erythrocyte sedimentation rate is found (often >40 mm/hr and not uncommonly elevated to levels of >100 mm/hr).
- Hyponatremia is associated with increased risk of coronary aneurysms.
- Elevated C-reactive protein.
- Urinalysis may show sterile pyuria.
- Impaired serum lipid profiles with decreased high-density lipoproteins (HDL) and elevated triglycerides and low-density lipoproteins (LDL) can occur.
- Cerebrospinal fluid (CSF) with increased white cell count without elevated CSF protein is found.
- Arthrocentesis of joints usually demonstrates pleocytosis with 125,000 to 300,000 white cells/mm^3.

IMAGING STUDIES

- Chest radiograph may reveal pulmonary infiltrates; cardiomegaly may also be present.
- Echocardiogram is recommended at the time of illness, and repeat in 6 wk and 6 mo. Echocardiogram should include careful assessment of the coronary arteries for size and aneurysms, mural or intraluminal thrombi, effusions, valve function, and myocardial function.
- Coronary angiogram, computed tomography angiography, and magnetic resonance angiography can be used to visualize the arterial system and the presence of coronary artery aneurysms. Echocardiography may be able to visualize these aneurysms in infants.
- Intravascular ultrasound can assess for luminal irregularities of the coronary arteries.

- Exercise testing with myocardial perfusion studies can be done to assess for coronary blood flow and the presence of myocardial ischemia.
- ECG changes (arrhythmias, abnormal Q waves, prolonged PR and/or QT intervals, occasionally low voltage, or ST-T wave changes) can be seen.

Rx TREATMENT

The goal of treatment of KD in the acute phase is directed at reducing clinical symptoms and reducing inflammation in the systemic and coronary arteries and preventing arterial thrombosis.Long-term therapy in individuals who develop coronary aneurysms is aimed at preventing myocardial ischemia or infarction.

NONPHARMACOLOGIC THERAPY

- Oxygen in selected patients
- Salt restriction in patients with congestive heart failure
- Emollient creams for peeling skin and balms for fissured lips

ACUTE GENERAL Rx

- IV immunoglobulin (IVIG) 2 g/kg over 8 to 12 hr as a single infusion is the treatment of choice in children diagnosed with KD, and ideally should be given within the first 7 to 10 days of the illness.
- Aspirin 80 to 100 mg/kg/day (anti-inflammatory dosing) given in four divided doses until the patient is no longer febrile for 48 hr. Thereafter, aspirin 3 to 5 mg/kg/day (antiplatelet dosing) is continued until laboratory studies (e.g., platelet count, sedimentation rate) return to normal, generally within 6 to 8 wk after disease onset if there are no coronary artery abnormalities or indefinitely if abnormalities are present.
- In patients who do not defervesce within 48 hr or have recrudescent fever after initial IVIG treatment, a second dose of IVIG 2 g/kg IV over 8 to 12 hr should be considered.
- NSAIDs are not effective in the treatment of KD.
- Efficacy of treatment with IVIG along with aspirin is higher than aspirin alone in decreasing risk of coronary artery aneurysms.
- The effect of corticosteroids on coronary artery aneurysms is unclear. Therefore most experts recommend withholding steroids unless fever persists after at least two courses of IVIG. Pulse methyprednisolone at 30 mg/kg daily is given to such patients for 1 to 3 days.
- Other therapies, including urinary trypsin inhibitor (Ulinastatin), pentoxifylline, etanercept, infliximab (monoclonal antibody against tumor necrosis factor-α), plasma exchange, abciximab (platelet glycoprotein IIb/IIIa receptor inhibitor), and immunosuppressive agents have been used, but data are limited on their success.
- Acute coronary thrombosis should be managed with thrombolytic agents under cardiology supervision.
- Most patients with large or giant coronary artery aneurysms (diameter >8 mm) are maintained on aspirin (or clopidogrel) and warfarin to prevent thrombosis within the aneurysm and myocardial infarction.

CHRONIC Rx

Interventional and surgical procedures can be tried in children who have developed cardiac complications of KD:

- Percutaneous transluminal coronary angioplasty with or without stenting may be performed, but the data is limited.
- Coronary bypass graft surgery using the internal mammary artery or the gastroepiploic artery has met with greater patency success than saphenous vein grafts and is done in those with severe obstructive lesions such as involving the left main coronary artery or multivessel disease.
- Cardiac transplantation is an option and is indicated in patients with:
  - Severe left ventricular failure
  - Malignant arrhythmias
  - Multivessel coronary artery disease
- For patients with persistent giant (≥8 mm) aneurysms, anticoagulation with warfarin for a goal international normalized ratio of 2.0 to 2.5 should be considered.

DISPOSITION

- Mortality rate of children with KD is 0.5% to 2.8%, usually from coronary aneurysm thrombosis and myocardial infarction.
- Death usually occurs in the third to fourth week of the illness.
- Before the use of IVIG, ~20% of all patients with KD developed coronary artery aneurysms.
- ~>50% of coronary artery aneurysms return to normal lumen diameter by 1 to 2 yr after onset of illness.
- Treatment with IVIG has reduced the incidence of coronary aneurysms by 80%.
- Aspirin in high dose decreases the coronary artery involvement to <5% from 25%.
- IVIG has also been shown to improve left ventricular function during the acute stages of the disease.
- Risk factors for the development of coronary aneurysms or giant coronary aneurysms 8 mm or greater are:
  - Fever lasting >10 days
  - Age <1 yr or >6 yr
  - Male
  - Recurrence of fever
- Recurrence is in about 1% to 3% of cases most commonly within 1 yr of the initial occurrence.
- Aspirin should be discontinued upon exposure to varicella or influenza to decrease the risk of developing Reye's syndrome.

REFERRAL

Multiple specialists may be consulted to assist in the diagnosis of KD, including dermatology, rheumatology, and infectious disease. Cardiology consultation is recommended in any patient with cardiac involvement and in the long-term follow-up of patients with KD.

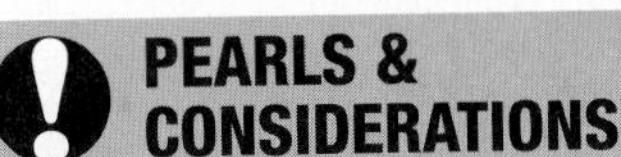

PEARLS & CONSIDERATIONS

COMMENTS

- The mechanism of action of IVIG therapy for KD remains unknown.
- Failure of corticosteroids suggests that the inflammatory response is different compared with other vasculitic conditions.
- Increased risk of atherosclerotic heart disease in adulthood is unclear in patients with history of KD during childhood with normal echocardiographic findings.
- Live vaccine (varicella, measles) administration is suggested to be postponed for 11 mo in children treated with IVIG, since it interferes with vaccine immunogenicity.

PREVENTION

- Without a known etiologic agent for KD, primary prevention is not possible.
- Thrombosis leading to myocardial infarction in a stenotic or aneurysmal coronary artery is the leading cause of death in these children and occurs most often in the first year after illness onset. Therefore serial imaging and stress tests are necessary in patients with significant coronary artery abnormalities (by coronary angiography).

SUGGESTED READINGS

available at www.expertconsult.com

RELATED CONTENT

Kawasaki Disease (Patient Information)

AUTHOR: **SYEDA M. SAYEED, M.D.**

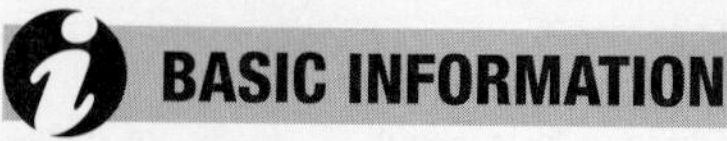

BASIC INFORMATION

DESCRIPTION

Keloid may be defined as a benign growth of dense fibrous tissue developing from an abnormal healing response to cutaneous injury, extending beyond the original borders of the wound or inflammatory response (Fig. 1-540).

In 1806, Alibert used the term *cheloide,* derived from the Greek *chele,* or crab's claw, to describe lateral growth of tissue into unaffected skin.

ICD-9CM CODES
701.4 Keloid scar
ICD-10CM CODES
L91.0 Hypertrophic scar

EPIDEMIOLOGY

- Keloid is seen 5 to 15 times more often in pigmented ethnic groups than in whites.
- Its prevalence is 16% in blacks and Hispanics.
- The highest incidence is seen in the second decade.
- It affects both sexes equally.
- Combined incidence of keloid and hypertrophic scar ranges from 40% to 70% following surgery to up to 91% following burns.

ETIOLOGY

- Wounds from trauma, surgery, or body piercing (Fig. 1-541)
- Burn
- Other injuries such as insect bites, vaccination, folliculitis, or acne
- Rarely can be spontaneous without obvious injury
- Familial predisposition seen in some patients

RISK FACTORS

- Family history of keloids
- Personal history of keloids
- Blacks, Hispanics, and Asians
- Pregnancy
- Puberty
- Patients with blood group A
- Injury over bones

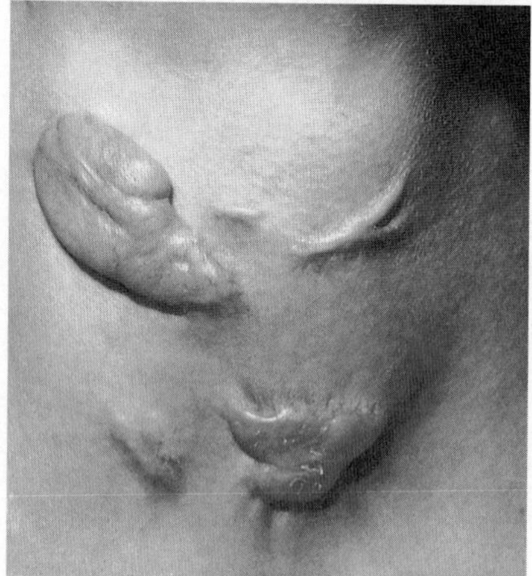

FIGURE 1-540 Keloids. An abnormal reparative reaction to skin injury, keloids are characterized by proliferation of fibroblasts and collagen that extends beyond the margins of the original wound. (From Zitelli BJ, Davis HW: *Atlas of pediatric physical diagnosis,* ed 5, Philadelphia, 2007, Mosby.)

PATHOGENESIS

- Pathophysiology of keloid is not completely understood
- Caused by benign dermal fibroproliferation because of disorder in the regulation of cellularity during the wound healing process

CLINICAL FEATURES

- Keloids usually appear within a few months of the injury, in contrast to the hypertrophic scars, which develop within a few weeks. At times it could take up to a year to appear because the growth is slow.
- Keloids are often symptomatic in the early stages. Common complaints are pruritus, burning, pain, and tenderness.
- Keloids are commonly seen on the shoulders, sternum, upper back, nape of neck, ear lobes, mandibular border, and cheek. Hands and feet are often spared.
- Skin lesions vary from papules to nodules to large tuberous lesions. They have the normal skin color most of the time with well-defined borders. Early on they can appear erythematous, whereas older lesions may be hypo- or hyperpigmented. They can be firm to hard in consistency with smooth surface and are tender to touch. Hair follicles are absent in these keloids.
- Unlike with hypertrophic scar, in keloids the scar extends beyond the margin of the initial wound.

DIAGNOSIS

- Workup is usually not necessary because it is a clinical diagnosis.
- Biopsy is usually avoided because it may increase the keloid size. When biopsy is done, the histology shows randomly organized large collagen fibers in a dense connective tissue matrix. In fact, both major components of extracellular matrix, collagen and glycosaminoglycans, are increased.

DIFFERENTIAL DIAGNOSIS

- Hypertrophic scar
- Dermatofibroma
- Dermatofibrosarcoma protuberance
- Desmoid tumor
- Foreign body granuloma
- Scar with sarcoidosis
- Lobomycosis

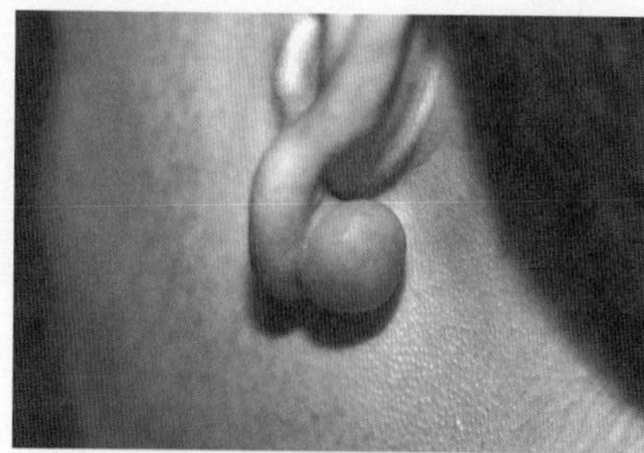

FIGURE 1-541 Keloid of ear lobe after piercing. (From Kliegman RM et al: *Nelson textbook of pediatrics,* Philadelphia, 2011, Saunders.)

TREATMENT

- There is no universally accepted treatment protocol. Prevention is the best strategy.
- Combination treatment is most effective.
- Surgical excision using cold knife followed by intralesional steroids is the preferred method.
- Treatment outcome is the best when it is initiated shortly after the keloid formation.
- Different treatment options include:
  1. Unlike with hypertrophic scars, **surgery** alone is associated with a 55% to 100% recurrence rate in patients with keloids. Results are significantly better when it is followed by intralesional steroids, radiotherapy, pressure therapy, or silicone application. Both complete and near total excision has been advocated. Few recommend core extirpation. Use of Z-plasties or any wound lengthening techniques is strongly discouraged.
  2. **Intralesional steroid** every 2 to 4 wk is administered either alone or following surgery. Duration of treatment depends on the treatment response. Triamcinolone is the most studied steroid and is used at a concentration of 10 to 40 mg/ml. Higher concentration is used for denser, more calcitrant lesions, and those located in trunks or extremities. It could be used in combination with lidocaine to reduce the discomfort. A 27- to 30-gauge needle is used for its administration. To distribute the suspension evenly, it should be injected while continuously advancing the needle. No more than 20 to 30 mg of the drug is used during each treatment. Liquid nitrogen is applied to the injection briefly for 2 to 4 seconds about 10 to 15 min prior to steroid injection for better dispersal of the steroid and to minimize deposition into surrounding normal tissue. Hypopigmentation, skin atrophy, ulceration, and telangiectasia are the side effects associated with this treatment.
  3. **Cryotherapy** has been used for smaller lesions. When this treatment is chosen, the entire lesion is treated with 2 to 3 freeze-thaw cycles of 30 seconds' duration each. Most lesions need 2 to 10 treatment sessions at 4-wk intervals. Pain and hypopigmentation are the main adverse events.
  4. **Silicone gel sheeting or cushioning** can prevent keloids from recurring after surgery. These are applied as soon as re-epithelialization is achieved and are worn for at least 12 hr/day for 2 to 4 mo.
  5. **Application of pressure** by compression devices has been advocated in the treatment of keloids. These compression treatments include button compression,

pressure earrings, pressure gradient garments, ACE bandages, elastic adhesive bandages, compression wraps, Spandex or Elastane bandages, and support bandages. About 24 to 40 mm Hg pressure must be maintained. It must be instituted for long periods (>23 hr/day for 6 to 12 mo) before significant effect can be achieved. Unfortunately, many parts of the body are not amenable to this pressure. Patient discomfort frequently reduces compliance.

6. **Radiation** following surgery can also reduce the recurrence rate. X-rays of 700 to 1500 cGy in fractions over 5 to 6 treatments are the most frequently used treatment. Radiation is usually initiated within 10 days, preferably within 24 hr of surgery. It is avoided in pediatric and pregnant patients. At times brachytherapy with interstitial iridium 192 is used. Most physicians use radiation only for keloids over the extremities. The reported risk of radiation-induced malignancy is theoretical.
7. **5-Fluorouracil** can be used as an individual agent, following surgery, or in combination with intralesional steroids. Weekly injection of 0.5 to 2 ml at a 50 mg/ml concentration of 5-fluorouracil for 12 wk is the recommended dose.
8. Superiority of **laser** use to simple excision currently has not been demonstrated.
9. Topical 5% **imiquimod** cream has some role when used following surgery locally every night for a minimum of 2 mo.
10. Other treatments include Cordran tape, bleomycin, interferon, vitamin A, nitrogen mustard, antihistamines, zinc, tacrolimus, sirolimus, allantoin, botulinum toxin, colchicine, salicylic acid, calcipotriol, NSAIDs, d-penicillamine, relaxin, quercetin, dinoprostone, doxorubicin, ACE inhibitors, hyaluronidase, pentoxifylline, tranilast, mitomycin-C, tamoxifen, silver sulfadiazine, onion extract, vitamin E, intralesional verapamil.

FOLLOW-UP

Because of the high risk of recurrence, a follow-up of at least 12 mo is necessary to fully evaluate the effectiveness of therapy.

PREVENTION

- Avoid nonessential surgery such as body piercing, which carries a high risk for keloid formation.
- LASIK eye surgery and CO_2 laser resurfacing should be avoided in patients with a tendency for keloids.
- Use a laparoscopic approach when surgery is needed.
- Avoid making incisions over joint spaces or over midchest, and ensure that they follow skin creases.
- Handle tissue gently during surgery.
- Ensure good hemostasis intraoperatively.
- Use tension-free primary wound closure.
- Use monofilament, synthetic permanent sutures.
- Use adhesives instead of sutures when possible for closure of wounds.
- Compressive pressure dressing is preferred in high-risk patients following surgery.
- Avoid wound infection.
- Avoid tattoos.
- Aggressively treat inflammatory acnes.

COMPLICATIONS

- Psychological effects secondary to disfigurement.
- Contracture from keloids may result in loss of function if overlying a joint.

PROGNOSIS

- Unlike hypertrophic scars, keloids do not regress with time. However, they may continue to expand in size for decades.
- Regardless of the type of treatment there is a high recurrence rate.
- Keloids never become malignant.

SUGGESTED READINGS

available at www.expertconsult.com

RELATED CONTENT

Keloids (Patient Information)

AUTHOR: **HEMANT K. SAPATHY, M.D.**

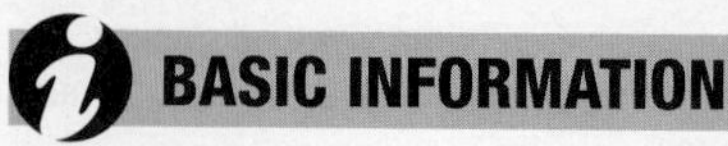

BASIC INFORMATION

DEFINITION

Labyrinthitis is a peripheral vestibulopathy characterized by acute onset of vertigo usually associated with nausea and vomiting. It may be associated with hearing loss. It may be either serous or purulent.

SYNONYMS

Acute labyrinthitis
Acute vestibular neuronopathy
Vestibular neuronitis
Viral neurolabyrinthitis

ICD-9CM CODES

386.12 Vestibular neuronitis (active and recurrent)
386.3 Labyrinthitis

ICD-10CM CODES

H81.23 Vestibular neuronitis, bilateral
H83.09 Labyrinthitis, unspecified ear

EPIDEMIOLOGY & DEMOGRAPHICS

INCIDENCE (IN U.S.): Most common cause of prolonged spontaneous vertigo associated with nausea at any age

PREDOMINANT AGE: Any

CLINICAL PRESENTATION

- Vertigo, nausea, and vomiting with onset over several hours.
- Symptoms usually peak within 24 hr, then resolve gradually over several weeks.
- During the first day, the patient usually has difficulty focusing the eyes because of spontaneous nystagmus.
- Usually has benign course, with complete recovery within 1 to 3 mo, although older patients may have intractable dizziness that persists for many months.

PHYSICAL FINDINGS

- Nystagmus
- Nausea
- Vomiting
- Vertigo worsening with head movement
- Abnormal caloric ENG tests
- May have hearing loss in the affected ear
- Normal otoscopic exam typically
- Normal neurologic exam; may have signs of vestibular loss, such as a positive head thrust test

ETIOLOGY

Symptoms often preceded for 1 to 2 wk by a viral-like illness. It may be either bacterial or viral, and be either tympanogenic (i.e., resulting from spread of infection into the inner ear from the middle ear, antrum, or petrous apex), meningogenic, or hematogenic from encephalitis or brain abscess. The round window membrane is considered the most likely pathway of inflammatory mediators from the middle to the inner ear that subsequently give rise to labyrinthitis.

Dx DIAGNOSIS

DIFFERENTIAL DIAGNOSIS

- Acute labyrinthine ischemia (vascular insufficiency)
- Other forms of labyrinthitis (bacterial and syphilitic)
- Labyrinthine fistula
- Benign positional vertigo
- Meniere's syndrome
- Cholesteatoma
- Drug induced
- Eighth nerve tumor
- Head trauma
- Vertebrobasilar stroke

WORKUP

- Otoscopic examination
- Neurologic examination, with close attention to cranial nerves
- Bedside test of vestibular function, that is, head thrust or head heave test
- Audiogram if symptoms accompanied by hearing loss
- Caloric test if presentation is atypical

LABORATORY TESTS

- Routine laboratory tests are generally not helpful.
- If there is a history of significant emesis, check electrolytes, BUN, and creatinine.

IMAGING STUDIES

- Imaging studies are usually not necessary.
- Contrasted MRI may show enhancement of bony labyrinth. MRI of the brain with and without contrast with fine cuts through the internal auditory canal is indicated if there is an abnormal cranial nerve exam or suspicion of eighth nerve tumor.
- Head CT with fine cuts through temporal bones is indicated if there is a history of trauma or suspicion of cholesteatoma.

Rx TREATMENT

NONPHARMACOLOGIC THERAPY

- Reassurance.
- Initial bed rest, then encourage increase in activity as tolerated.

ACUTE GENERAL Rx

- Phenergan or other antiemetics are typically effective.
- Vestibular suppressant: meclizine 12.5 to 25 mg qid is often used. Scopolamine patch is also effective.
- Methylprednisolone 100 mg per day for 3 days, with slow taper over 3 wk.
- Valacyclovir has not been shown to be helpful.

CHRONIC Rx

No specific chronic therapy

DISPOSITION

Usually does not require hospital admission unless the patient is unable to tolerate oral intake of liquids.

REFERRAL

- Refer if symptoms persist or neurologic abnormalities are present.
- Consider vestibular rehabilitation, particularly in the elderly.

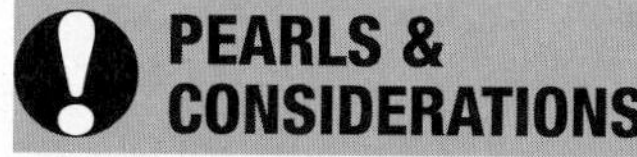

PEARLS & CONSIDERATIONS

COMMENTS

Labyrinthitis is a term that usually implies peripheral vestibulopathy associated with hearing loss. The term vestibular neuronitis is typically used when hearing is not affected. Despite this technical distinction, many physicians use these terms interchangeably.

SUGGESTED READINGS

available at www.expertconsult.com

RELATED CONTENT

Labyrinthitis (Patient Information)

AUTHOR: **SHARON S. HARTMAN POLENSEK, M.D., PH.D.**

BASIC INFORMATION

DEFINITION

Lactose intolerance is the insufficient concentration of lactase enzyme, leading to fermentation of malabsorbed lactose by intestinal bacteria with subsequent production of intestinal gas and various organic acids, manifesting clinically with diarrhea, abdominal pain, flatulence, or bloating after lactose intake. *Lactose malabsorption* occurs when a substantial amount of lactose is not absorbed in the intestine. *Lactase deficiency* is defined as brush-border lactase activity that is markedly reduced relative to the activity observed in infants.

SYNONYMS

Lactase deficiency
Milk intolerance

ICD-9CM CODES
271.3 Lactose intolerance
ICD-10CM CODES
E73.9 Lactose intolerance, unspecified

EPIDEMIOLOGY & DEMOGRAPHICS

Nearly 50 million people in the United States have partial or complete lactose intolerance. There are racial differences, with <25% of white adults being lactose intolerant but >85% of Asian Americans and >60% of African Americans having some form of lactose intolerance.

PHYSICAL FINDINGS & CLINICAL PRESENTATION

- Abdominal tenderness and cramping, bloating, flatulence
- Diarrhea
- Symptoms are directly related to the osmotic pressure of substrate in the colon and occur approximately 2 hr after ingestion of lactose
- Physical examination: may be entirely within normal limits

ETIOLOGY

- Congenital lactase deficiency: common in premature infants; rare in term infants and generally inherited as a chromosomal recessive trait
- Secondary lactose intolerance: usually a result of injury of the intestinal mucosa (Crohn's disease, viral gastroenteritis, AIDS enteropathy, cryptosporidiosis, Whipple's disease, sprue)

DIAGNOSIS

DIFFERENTIAL DIAGNOSIS

- Inflammatory bowel disease
- Irritable bowel syndrome
- Pancreatic insufficiency
- Nontropical and tropical sprue
- Cystic fibrosis
- Diverticular disease
- Bowel neoplasm
- Laxative abuse
- Celiac disease
- Parasitic disease (e.g., giardiasis)
- Viral or bacterial infections

WORKUP

- The diagnosis can usually be made on the basis of the history and improvement with dietary manipulation.
- Diagnostic workup may include confirming the diagnosis with hydrogen breath test and excluding other conditions listed in the differential diagnosis that may also coexist with lactase deficiency.

LABORATORY TESTS

- Lactose breath hydrogen test: a rise in breath hydrogen >20 ppm within 90 min of ingestion of 50 g of lactose is positive for lactase deficiency. This test is positive in 90% of patients with lactose malabsorption. Common causes of false-negative results are recent use of oral antibiotics or recent high colonic enema.
- The lactose tolerance test is an older and less accurate testing modality (20% rate of false-positive and false-negative results). The patient is administered an oral dose of 1 to 1.5 g of lactose/kg body weight. Serial measurement of blood glucose level on an hourly basis for 3 hr is then performed. The test is considered positive if the patient develops intestinal symptoms and the blood glucose level rises <20 mg/dl above the fasting baseline level.
- Diarrhea associated with lactase deficiency is osmotic in nature with an osmotic gap and a pH <6.5.

IMAGING STUDIES

Imaging studies are generally not indicated. A small bowel series may be useful in patients with significant malabsorption.

TREATMENT

NONPHARMACOLOGIC THERAPY

Management consists of reducing lactose exposure by avoiding milk and milk-containing products or using milk in which the lactose has been prehydrolized with lactase. A lactose-free diet generally results in prompt resolution of symptoms. Lactose is primarily found in dairy products but may be present as an ingredient or component of common foods and beverages. Possible sources of lactose include breads, candies, cold cuts, dessert mixes, cream soups, bologna, commercial sauces and gravies, chocolate, drink mixes, salad dressings, and medications. Labels should be read carefully to identify sources of lactose.

ACUTE GENERAL Rx

- Addition of lactase enzyme supplement (Lactaid tablets, Dairy Ease) before the ingestion of milk products may prevent symptoms in some patients. However, it is not effective for all lactose-intolerant patients.
- Lactose-intolerant patients must ensure adequate calcium intake. Calcium supplementation is recommended to prevent osteoporosis.

CHRONIC Rx

Patient education regarding foods high in lactose, such as milk, cottage cheese, or ice cream, is recommended.

DISPOSITION

Clinical improvement with restriction or elimination of milk products

REFERRAL

GI referral for endoscopic procedures if concomitant GI disorders are suspected

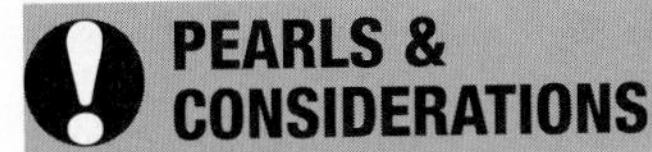

PEARLS & CONSIDERATIONS

COMMENTS

- There is great variability in signs and symptoms in patients with lactose intolerance depending on the degree of lactase deficiency. Most individuals with presumed lactose malabsorption can tolerate 12 to 15 g of lactose or up to 12 oz of milk daily without symptoms.
- Nondairy synthetic drinks (e.g., Coffee-Mate) and use of rice milk are well tolerated.

SUGGESTED READINGS

available at www.expertconsult.com

RELATED CONTENT

Lactose Intolerance (Patient Information)

AUTHOR: **FRED F. FERRI, M.D.**

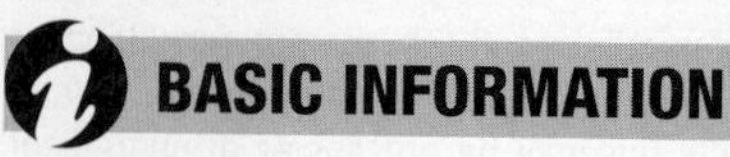

BASIC INFORMATION

DEFINITION

Lambert-Eaton myasthenic syndrome (LEMS) is a disorder of neuromuscular transmission caused by antibodies directed against presynaptic voltage-gated P/Q calcium channels on motor and autonomic nerve terminals. There are two forms: paraneoplastic (most common) and nonparaneoplastic (autoimmune).

SYNONYMS

Eaton-Lambert syndrome

ICD-9CM CODES
199.1 Malignant neoplasm without specification of site, other
ICD-10CM CODES
G73.1 Lambert-Eaton syndrom (C00-D48+)
G70.8 Other specified myoneural disorders

EPIDEMIOLOGY & DEMOGRAPHICS

INCIDENCE: Uncertain; estimated at five cases per 1 million persons annually (in U.S.)
PEAK INCIDENCE: Sixth decade
PREVALENCE: Uncertain; estimated at one per 100,000 (in U.S.). Up to 3% of small cell lung cancer (SCLC) patients are estimated to develop LEMS.
PREDOMINANT SEX: Male:female ratio of 2:1.

PHYSICAL FINDINGS & CLINICAL PRESENTATION

- Weakness with diminished or absent muscle stretch reflexes
- Proximal lower-extremity muscles affected most
- Ocular and bulbar muscles less commonly affected
- Transient strength improvement with brief exercise
- Reflexes may be facilitated by repeatedly tapping the tendon or after brief exercise
- Autonomic dysfunction common (dry mouth [75%], sexual dysfunction, blurred vision, constipation, orthostasis, etc.)

ETIOLOGY

- Antibodies directed against presynaptic voltage-gated P/Q calcium channels are present in most patients. The reduction in calcium influx causes a reduction in presynaptic acetylcholine release at motor and autonomic nerve terminals.
- Paraneoplastic forms, usually associated with SCLC, account for 50% to 70% of patients.
- Autoimmune forms, usually in patients with other autoimmune diseases, occur in 10% to 30% of patients.

Dx DIAGNOSIS

DIFFERENTIAL DIAGNOSIS

- Myasthenia gravis
- Polymyositis
- Primary myopathies
- Carcinomatous myopathies
- Polymyalgia rheumatica
- Botulism
- Guillain-Barré syndrome

WORKUP

Diagnosis is confirmed on basis of characteristic electrodiagnostic (EMG/NCS) findings: reduced motor amplitudes with normal sensory studies; >10% decrement in motor amplitudes on slow repetitive nerve stimulation (RNS) at 2 to 5 Hz, with >100% increment on fast RNS (20 to 50 Hz) or immediately after 10 sec of maximum exercise (postexercise facilitation).

LABORATORY TESTS

Check P/Q calcium channel antibody titers (commercially available).

IMAGING STUDIES

Screen for an underlying malignancy. Presentation with LEMS may precede diagnosis of SCLC by up to 5 yr; hence chest radiograph or CT of the chest may be required every 6 to 12 mo for SCLC.

Rx TREATMENT

NONPHARMACOLOGIC THERAPY

Symptomatic treatment for autonomic dysfunction.

ACUTE GENERAL Rx

- Anticholinesterase agents (pyridostigmine 30 to 60 mg q4-6h) may yield some improvement.
- Guanidine hydrochloride: start 5 to 10 mg/kg/day up to 30 mg/kg/day in 3-day intervals.
- Plasma exchange (200 to 250 ml/kg over 10 to 14 days) or IV immunoglobulins (2 g/kg divided over 2 to 5 days) often produce significant, temporary improvement.
- Prednisone 1.0 to 1.5 mg/kg/day can be gradually tapered over months to minimal effective dose.
- Azathioprine can be given alone or in combination with prednisone. Give up to 2.5 mg/kg/day. If patient is intolerant, can administer cyclosporine up to 3 mg/kg/day instead.
- 3,4-Diaminopyridine (3,4-DAP) 10 to 20 mg PO qid (maximum of 100 mg/day) may improve muscle strength and reduce autonomic symptoms in up to 85% of patients in uncontrolled series. It is available in Europe and may be available in the U.S. on a compassionate use basis.

CHRONIC Rx

Treat underlying malignancy if present.

DISPOSITION

- Gradually progressive weakness leading to impaired mobility if untreated
- Clinical remission may occur with chronic immunosuppressive therapy in 43% of cases
- Possible substantial improvement with successful treatment of underlying malignancy

REFERRAL

1. Referral to a neurologist is highly recommended because this is a rare disease requiring highly specialized treatment in the context of weighing risk vs. benefit of the different therapeutic options.
2. Referral to specialist centers for 3,4-DAP therapy may be warranted in the U.S.
3. Surgical referral for tumor debulking in paraneoplastic forms necessary.

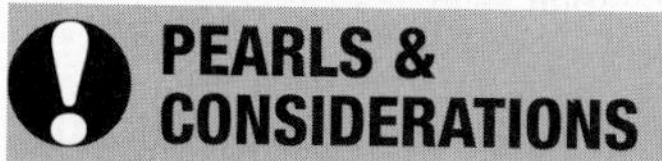

PEARLS & CONSIDERATIONS

COMMENTS

- Prominent autonomic symptoms (dry eyes, dry mouth, impotence, orthostasis) are often clues to the diagnosis in the appropriate clinical context.
- Many drugs may worsen weakness and should be used only if absolutely necessary. Included are succinylcholine, d-tubocurarine, quinine, quinidine, procainamide, aminoglycoside antibiotics, β-blockers, and calcium channel blockers.

PATIENT INFORMATION

Available through the website http://www.lems.com/resources.

SUGGESTED READINGS

available at www.expertconsult.com

AUTHOR: **DIVYA SINGHAL, M.D.**

BASIC INFORMATION

DEFINITION

Laryngeal carcinoma is cancer of the larynx, including the vocal cords (glottis), supraglottis, and subglottis.

SYNONYMS

Laryngeal cancer

Head and neck cancer (subsite); other sites include oral cavity, pharynx, paranasal sinus, and salivary glands

ICD-9CM CODES

231.0 Carcinoma of larynx

ICD-10CM CODES

D02.0 Carcinoma in situ of larynx

EPIDEMIOLOGY & DEMOGRAPHICS

INCIDENCE: 12,000 new cases per year in the U.S.

PEAK INCIDENCE: Sixth decade

PREDOMINANT SEX: 80% male predominance (current, with past and projected increase in female rates as a result of changing smoking habits)

PHYSICAL FINDINGS & CLINICAL PRESENTATION

- Glottis: Early diagnosis possible because of voice change (hoarseness). Any voice change of more than 2-wk duration should prompt a laryngeal examination.
- Supraglottis:
  1. No early symptom
  2. Cervical lymphadenopathy
  3. Neck pain or ear pain
  4. Discomfort during swallowing
  5. Odynophagia
  6. Later: hoarseness, dysphagia, airway obstruction
- Subglottis: Even more subtle than supraglottic lesion; the same signs occur, only later in the course.

ETIOLOGY

- Smoking (cigarette, cigar, or pipe)
- Alcohol intake/abuse
- Diet and nutritional deficiencies
- Gastroesophageal reflux
- Voice abuse
- Chronic laryngitis
- Exposure to wood dust
- Asbestosis
- Exposure to radiation
- Possible role of human papillomavirus

DIAGNOSIS

DIFFERENTIAL DIAGNOSIS

- Laryngitis
- Allergic and nonallergic rhinosinusitis
- Gastroesophageal reflux
- Voice abuse leading to hoarseness
- Laryngeal papilloma
- Vocal cord paralysis attributable to a neurologic condition or entrapment of the recurrent laryngeal nerve caused by mediastinal compression
- Tracheomalacia

STAGING:

Supraglottic:

T_1: Tumor limited to one subsite with normal cord mobility

T_2: Tumor invades mucosa of more than one subsite (e.g., base of tongue, vallecula, pyriform sinus) without fixation of larynx

T_3: Tumor limited to larynx with vocal cord fixation or invasion of postcricoid area or preepiglottis

T_4: Tumor invades thyroid cartilage or extends into soft tissue of the neck, thyroid, or esophagus

Glottic:

T_1: Tumor limited to vocal cord with normal mobility

T_{1a}: Tumor limited to one vocal cord

T_{1b}: Tumor involves both vocal cords

T_2: Tumor extends to supra- or subglottis or impairs cord mobility

T_3: Tumor limited to larynx with cord fixation

T_4: Tumor invades through cartilage or other tissues beyond larynx

Stage grouping:

Stage I (one anatomic site within the larynx): T_1, N0, M0

Stage II (one anatomic region within the larynx): T_2, N0, M0

Stage III (extending beyond one anatomic region but confined to the larynx): T_3, N0, M0

T_1, T_2, T_3, N1, M0

Stage IV (distant metastasis): T_4, N0, N1, M0

Any T, N2, N3, M0

Any T, any N or M >0

WORKUP

- Laboratory: none
- Endoscopic laryngeal inspection
- After (and only after) diagnosis of the malignancy, imaging with CT or MRI should be undertaken to stage the disease

HISTOLOGIC CLASSIFICATION

Epithelial cancers:

- Squamous cell carcinoma in situ
- Superficially invasive cancer
- Verrucous carcinoma
- Pseudosarcoma
- Anaplastic cancer
- Transitional cell carcinoma
- Lymphoepithelial cancer
- Adenocarcinoma
- Neuroendocrine tumors, including small cell and carcinoid

Sarcomas:

- Metastatic malignancies

TREATMENT

ACUTE GENERAL Rx

- Early stage (T or T_2) has two options:
  1. Conservative surgery (partial laryngectomy) with neck dissection
  2. Primary radiation
- Intermediate stage has four options:
  1. Primary radiation alone
  2. Supraglottic laryngectomy with neck dissection
  3. Supraglottic laryngectomy with postoperative radiation
  4. Chemotherapy with radiation
- Advanced stage:
  1. Chemotherapy and radiation with total laryngectomy reserved for treatment failure

Glottis:

- Carcinoma in situ
  1. Microexcision
  2. Laser vaporization
  3. Radiation
- Early stage (T or T_2) has two options:
  1. Voice conservation surgery
  2. Radiation
- Intermediate stage (T_3)
  1. Combined radiation and chemotherapy (cisplatin and 5-fluoruracil)
  2. Total laryngectomy for treatment failure
- Advanced stage (T_4)
  1. Combined radiation and chemotherapy
  2. Total laryngectomy and neck dissection followed by postoperative radiation in unfavorable lesion or treatment failure

Subglottis:

- Total laryngectomy and approximate neck surgery to excise the tumor, followed by radiation

Unresected cancers:

- Induction chemotherapy and radiation followed by neck dissection in chemosensitive tumors, or by laryngectomy and neck dissection in chemoresistant tumors
- If hypopharyngeal involvement exists: laryngopharyngectomy, neck dissection, and postoperative radiation

DISPOSITION

Supraglottis 5-yr control:

- T_1: 95% to 100%
- T_2: 80% to 90%
- T_3: 65% to 85%
- T_4: 40% to 55%

Glottis 5-yr control:

- T_1: 95% to 100%
- T_2: 50% to 85%
- T_3: 35% to 85%
- T_4: 20% to 65%

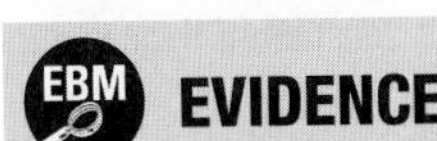

EVIDENCE

available at www.expertconsult.com

RELATED CONTENT

Laryngeal Cancer (Patient Information)

AUTHOR: **FRED F. FERRI, M.D.**

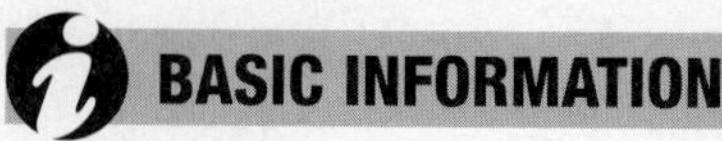

BASIC INFORMATION

DEFINITION

Laryngitis is an acute or chronic inflammation of the laryngeal mucous membranes.

SYNONYMS

Lower respiratory tract infection

ICD-9CM CODES
464.0 Acute laryngitis
476.0 Chronic laryngitis
ICD-10CM CODES
J04.0 Acute laryngitis
J37.0 Chronic laryngitis

EPIDEMIOLOGY & DEMOGRAPHICS

It is a common illness worldwide in both genders and all age groups, but the diagnosis is imprecise and, therefore, statistics are not readily available with respect to incidence and prevalence.

PHYSICAL FINDINGS & CLINICAL PRESENTATION

ACUTE LARYNGITIS:

- Clinical syndrome characterized by the onset of hoarseness, voice breaks, or episodes of aphonia; may also have accompanying sore throat, cough, nasal congestion, and rhinorrhea
- Usually associated with viral upper respiratory infection
- Larynx with diffuse erythema, edema, and vascular engorgement of the vocal folds, and occasionally mucosal ulceration
- In young children subglottis is often affected, resulting in airway narrowing with marked hoarseness, inspiratory stridor, dyspnea, and restlessness
- Respiratory compromise rare in adults

CHRONIC LARYNGITIS: Characterized by hoarseness or dysphonia persisting for longer than 2 wk

ETIOLOGY

ACUTE LARYNGITIS:

- Most often caused by viruses so treatment consists of supportive measures as outlined in "Nonpharmacologic Therapy" section.
- Studies evaluating the use of antibiotics (erythromycin, penicillin) in acute laryngitis failed to show objective clinical benefit over placebo so they are not routinely recommended. Antibiotics and other antimicrobials may be indicated in cases in which specific treatable pathogens are identified.
- Avoid decongestants because of their drying effect.
- Guaifenesin may be a useful adjunct as a mucolytic agent.
- In gastroesophageal reflux disease (GERD)-associated laryngitis use acid-suppressive therapy (H_2 blockers, proton pump inhibitors) and nocturnal antireflux precautions.

CHRONIC LARYNGITIS:

- Results from any of the following: tuberculosis, usually through bronchogenic spread; leprosy, from nasopharyngeal or oropharyngeal spread; syphilis, in secondary and tertiary stages; rhinoscleroma, extending from the nose and nasopharynx; actinomycosis; cryptococcosis; histoplasmosis; blastomycosis; paracoccidiomycosis; coccidiosis; candidiasis; aspergillosis; sporotrichosis; rhinosporidiosis; parasitic infections including leishmaniasis and *Clinostomum* infection following raw fresh-water fish ingestion.
- Noninfectious causes of both acute and chronic laryngitis include malignancy, voice abuse (singers), GERD, and chemical or environmental irritants such as cigarettes and allergens. Other causes of inflammatory or granulomatous lesions of the larynx include relapsing polychondritis, Wegener's granulomatosis, and sarcoidosis.

Dx DIAGNOSIS

DIFFERENTIAL DIAGNOSIS

- Young children with signs of airway obstruction:
  - Supraglottitis (epiglottitis)
  - Laryngotracheobronchitis
  - Tracheitis
  - Foreign body aspiration
- Adults with persistent hoarseness, consider noninfectious causes of laryngitis as listed previously

WORKUP

- History and physical examination: diagnosis is usually apparent.
- Laryngoscopy for severe or persistent cases.
- Laryngeal cultures should be performed if a cause other than acute viral infection is suspected.
- Imaging not indicated unless there is evidence of airway compromise. Obtain plain radiographs of neck, anteroposterior and lateral views, to differentiate laryngitis from acute laryngotracheobronchitis or supraglottitis.

Rx TREATMENT

NONPHARMACOLOGIC THERAPY

- Rest the voice.
- Use an air humidifier.
- Ensure adequate hydration. Avoid alcohol and caffeine because of diuretic effect.

ACUTE GENERAL Rx

- Antibiotics and other antimicrobials should generally not be used. They are indicated only when a specific pathogen is isolated; commonly employed antibacterial agents are macrolides; clarithromycin 500 mg by mouth bid for 5 to 7 days or azithromycin 500 mg followed by 250 mg once daily for 4 to 5 days if the cause of laryngitis is found to be *Mycoplasma pneumoniae* or *Chlamydophila pneumoniae* (the new name for what was formerly known as *Chlamydia pneumoniae*).
- Avoid decongestants because of their drying effect.
- Guaifenesin may be a useful adjunct as a mucolytic agent.
- In GERD-associated laryngitis use acid-suppressive therapy (H_2 blockers, proton pump inhibitors) and nocturnal antireflux precautions.

DISPOSITION

Uncomplicated laryngitis is usually benign, with gradual resolution of symptoms.

REFERRAL

- If symptoms persist for >2 wk, refer to otolaryngologist for laryngoscopy.
- Consider referral to gastroenterologist if GERD is suspected.

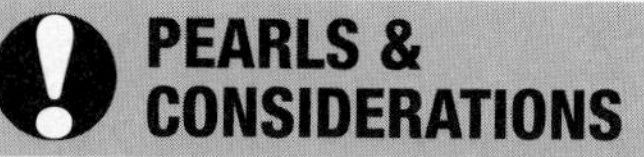

PEARLS & CONSIDERATIONS

- Most cases of uncomplicated acute laryngitis are viral in origin, and antibacterial agents should not be routinely administered.
- A recent Cochrane analysis in 2013 found no evidence for the use of empiric antibiotics in adults with laryngitis.
- The most difficult clinical challenge is often convincing patients with acute laryngitis that they do not need and will not benefit from antibacterial agents.

SUGGESTED READINGS

available at www.expertconsult.com

RELATED CONTENT

Laryngitis (Patient Information)

AUTHOR: **GLENN G. FORT, M.D., M.P.H.**

BASIC INFORMATION

DEFINITION

Acute laryngotracheobronchitis is a viral infection of the upper and lower respiratory tract leading to erythema and edema of the tracheal walls and narrowing of the subglottic region. Laryngotracheitis, which is limited to larynx and trachea, is also known as croup.

SYNONYMS

Croup

ICD-9CM CODES
464.4 Croup
ICD-10CM CODES
J05.0 Acute obstructive laryngitis [croup]

EPIDEMIOLOGY & DEMOGRAPHICS

- Croup is primarily a disease of children occurring between the ages of 1 and 6 yr.
- The peak incidence of croup is between 6 and 36 mo.
- Most cases occur in the fall and represent parainfluenza type 1 viral infection.
- Winter outbreaks usually represent infection by influenza A and B viruses.
- Croup accounts for 10% to 15% of lower respiratory tract infections in young children.
- Boys are affected more often than girls in a ratio of 1.4:1.

PHYSICAL FINDINGS & CLINICAL PRESENTATION

Most children with croup present with symptoms of an upper respiratory infection for several days.

- Rhinorrhea
- Cough
- Low-grade fever
- Barking cough that usually occurs at night and awakens the child
- Sore throat
- Stridor
- Apprehension
- Use of accessory muscles of respiration
- Tachypnea
- Tachycardia
- Wheezing

ETIOLOGY

- Parainfluenza viruses (types 1, 2, and 3) are the most common causes of croup in the U.S. Type 1 is the most common cause of fall and winter outbreaks, with type 2 causing milder disease outbreaks. Parainfluenza type 3, while sporadic, can be more severe than other types.
- Respiratory syncytial virus (RSV) and adenovirus are common causes of croup as well.
- Human coronavirus NL63, rhinoviruses, enteroviruses such as Coxsackie and echovirus.
- Influenza A and B, although not common causes of croup, do lead to more severe cases of the disease.
- *Mycoplasma pneumoniae* (rare).

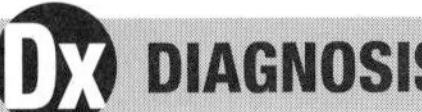

DIAGNOSIS

The diagnosis of croup is usually based on the characteristic clinical presentation of a young child between the ages of 1 and 6 yr waking up with a barking cough ("seal's bark") and stridor.

DIFFERENTIAL DIAGNOSIS

- Spasmodic croup
- Epiglottitis
- Bacterial tracheitis
- Angioneurotic edema
- Diphtheria
- Peritonsillar abscess
- Retropharyngeal abscess
- Smoke inhalation
- Foreign body

WORKUP

- The workup of a child with croup is to differentiate viral laryngotracheobronchitis from noninfectious causes of stridor, bacterial tracheitis, and epiglottitis caused by *H. influenzae* (Table E1-285).
- The clinical presentation and plain films of the soft tissues of the neck assist in differentiating viral from nonviral and noninfectious causes.

LABORATORY TESTS

- Laboratory tests are not often used to make the diagnosis of viral tracheobronchitis.
- CBC, viral serology, and tissue cultures can be ordered and may detect the infecting agent in up to 65% of cases.
- Pulse oximetry and ABG determination for patients with tachypnea and respiratory distress.

IMAGING STUDIES

- Plain (AP and lateral) films of the soft tissues of the neck (Fig. E1-542) may show the classic radiographic finding of subglottic stenosis or "steeple" sign.
- CT scan of the soft tissues of the neck may be performed in cases in which the differentiation between croup, epiglottitis, and noninfectious causes is more difficult.
- Direct visualization via laryngoscopy may be useful in some situations under a controlled setting.

Rx TREATMENT

Treatment of croup focuses on airway management.

NONPHARMACOLOGIC THERAPY

- Humidified oxygen or humidified air
- Cool mist
- Hot steam

ACUTE GENERAL Rx

- 0.25 to 0.75 ml of 2.25% racemic epinephrine every 20 min is used in children with severe respiratory symptoms, rest stridor, and impending intubation.
- Corticosteroids (e.g., dexamethasone 0.6 mg/kg IV or PO, prednisone 2 mg/kg/day) have been shown to be effective.
- Budesonide, a nebulized corticosteroid given at 4 mg, has been shown to improve symptoms in patients with moderate to severe croup.

DISPOSITION

- Croup is usually benign and self-limited, resolving within 3 to 4 days.
- Complications include:
  1. Airway obstruction
  2. Otitis media
  3. Pneumonia
  4. Dehydration

REFERRAL

If intubation is needed (rarely), an emergency consultation with ENT and/or anesthesiology is recommended.

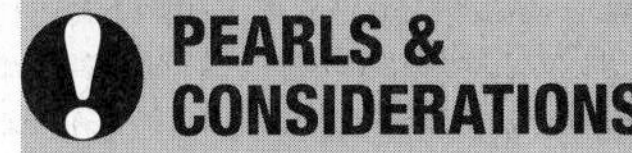

PEARLS & CONSIDERATIONS

COMMENTS

- Most patients with croup can be managed at home (e.g., patients without stridor and in no respiratory distress).
- Hospitalization and observation are required for children with moderate to severe croup (e.g., rest stridor, respiratory distress refractory to the previously mentioned acute treatments). A family history of croup is a risk factor for croup and recurrent croup.

SUGGESTED READINGS

available at www.expertconsult.com

RELATED CONTENT

Croup (Patient Information)

AUTHOR: **GLENN G. FORT, M.D., M.P.H.**

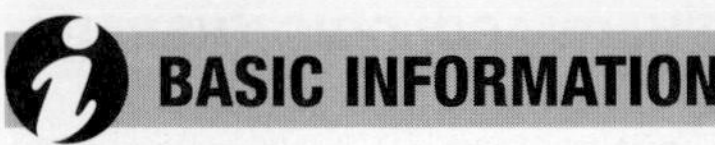

BASIC INFORMATION

DEFINITION

Lead is a potent, pervasive neurotoxicant. Lead poisoning refers to multisystem abnormalities resulting from excessive lead exposure.

SYNONYMS

Plumbism

ICD-9CM CODES
984.0 Lead poisoning
ICD-10CM CODES
T56.0X1A Toxic effect of lead and its compounds, accidental (unintentional), initial encounter

EPIDEMIOLOGY & DEMOGRAPHICS

- Lead poisoning is most common in children ages 1 to 5 yr (17,000 cases/100,000 persons). The highest rates are among blacks, those with low income, and urban children.
- In 1991 the Centers for Disease Control and Prevention (CDC) lowered the definition of a safe blood lead level to <10 mcg/dl of whole blood (a blood lead level of 25 mcg/dl was considered acceptable before 1991).
- It is estimated that >15% of preschoolers in the U.S. have a blood lead level >15 mcg/dl.

PHYSICAL FINDINGS & CLINICAL PRESENTATION

- Findings vary with the degree of toxicity. Examination may be normal in patients with mild toxicity.
- Myalgias, irritability, headache, and general fatigue may be present initially.
- Abdominal cramping, constipation, weight loss, tremor, paresthesias and peripheral neuritis, seizures, and coma may occur with severe toxicity.
- Motor neuropathy is common in children with lead poisoning; learning disorders are also frequent.

ETIOLOGY

Chronic, repeated exposure to paint containing lead, plumbing, storage of batteries, pottery, or lead soldering. Concentration of lead is generally highest in lead-based paint on exterior surfaces. Among interior surfaces, windows are most likely to have the highest lead content.

Dx DIAGNOSIS

DIFFERENTIAL DIAGNOSIS

- Polyneuropathies from other sources
- Anxiety disorder, attention deficit disorder
- Malabsorption, acute abdomen
- Iron-deficiency anemia

WORKUP

Laboratory screening: all U.S. children should be considered to be at risk for lead poisoning and should be screened routinely starting at age 1 yr for low-risk children and age 6 mo for high-risk children.

LABORATORY TESTS

- Venous blood lead level: normal level, <5 mcg/dl; levels of 50 to 70 mcg/dl, indicative of moderate toxicity; levels >70 mcg/dl, associated with severe poisoning
- Mild anemia with basophilic stippling on peripheral smear
- Elevated zinc protoporphyrin levels or free erythrocyte protoporphyrin level
- An increased body burden of lead with previous high-level exposure in patients with occupational lead poisoning can be demonstrated by measuring the excretion of lead in urine after premedication with calcium ethylenediamine tetraacetic acid (EDTA) or another chelating agent

IMAGING STUDIES

- Imaging studies are generally not necessary.
- A plain abdominal film can visualize lead particles in the gut.
- "Lead lines" may be noted on x-ray films of long bones.

Rx TREATMENT

NONPHARMACOLOGIC THERAPY

- Provide adequate amounts of calcium, iron, zinc, and protein in patient's diet
- Family education on sources of lead exposure and potential adverse health effects

ACUTE GENERAL Rx

- For children with blood levels of 10 to 19 mcg/dl, the CDC recommends nonpharmacologic interventions (see "Nonpharmacologic Therapy").
- For children with blood levels between 20 and 44 mcg/dl, the CDC recommendations include case management by a qualified social worker, clinical management, environmental assessment, and lead hazard control. Chelation therapy should be considered in children with refractory blood lead levels.

Chelation therapy (Table E1-286) is indicated in children with blood lead levels >45 mcg/dl:

- Succimer (DMSA) 10 mg/kg PO q8h for 5 days then q12h for 2 wk can be used in patients with levels between 45 and 70 mcg/dl.
- Edetate calcium disodium (EDTA) and dimercaprol (BAL) are effective in patients with severe toxicity.
- Use of both EDTA and DMSA is indicated in children with blood levels >70 mcg/dl.
- d-Penicillamine (Cuprimine) can also be used for lead poisoning, but it is not FDA approved for this condition.

CHRONIC Rx

- Reduce exposure, remove any potential lead sources.
- Correct iron deficiency and any other nutritional deficiencies.
- Recheck blood lead level 7 to 21 days after chelation therapy.

DISPOSITION

Patients with mild to moderate toxicity generally improve without any residual deficits. The presence of encephalopathy at diagnosis is a poor prognostic sign. Residual neurologic deficits may persist in these patients. Chelation therapy seems to slow the progression of renal insufficiency in patients with mildly elevated body lead burden.

REFERRAL

If exposure to lead is work related, it should be reported to the Office of the United States Occupational Safety and Health Administration (OSHA). Follow-up testing is mandatory in all patients after an abnormal screening blood lead level.

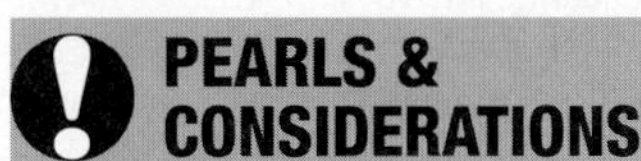

PEARLS & CONSIDERATIONS

COMMENTS

- Even blood lead concentrations as low as 5-10 mcg/dl are inversely associated with children's IQ scores at age 3 and 5 yr.
- Screening of household members of affected individuals is recommended.
- In children with blood lead levels of >45 mg/dl, treatment with succimer does not improve scores on tests of cognition, behavior, or neuropsychological function.
- Lead toxicity may delay growth and pubertal development in girls.
- Low-level environmental lead exposure may accelerate progressive renal insufficiency in patients without diabetes who have chronic renal disease. Repeated chelation therapy may improve renal function and slow the progression of renal failure.

SUGGESTED READINGS

available at www.expertconsult.com

RELATED CONTENT

Lead Poisoning (Patient Information)

AUTHOR: **FRED F. FERRI, M.D.**

BASIC INFORMATION

DEFINITION

Legg-Calvé-Perthes disease (LCPD) is characterized by circulatory compromise of the immature proximal femoral head leading to avascular necrosis. The classification of LCPD is outlined in Fig. 1-543.

SYNONYMS

Perthes disease
Coxa plana
Capital femoral osteochondrosis
Osteonecrosis of the proximal femoral epiphysis
LCPD

ICD-9CM CODES
732.1 Perthes' disease
ICD-10CM CODES
M91.10 Juvenile osteochondrosis of head of femur [Legg-Calvé-Perthes], unspecified leg

EPIDEMIOLOGY & DEMOGRAPHICS

PREVALENCE: One case in 1300 children. More common in Caucasians
INCIDENCE: One in 1200 children, younger than 15 years of age
PREDOMINANT SEX: Male/female ratio of 4:1
PREDOMINANT AGE: 4 to 10 yr

PHYSICAL FINDINGS & CLINICAL PRESENTATION

- Initial symptom: usually a mildly painful limp
- Pain referred down the inner aspect of the thigh to the knee
- Positive roll test: with the patient in the supine position, rolling of the affected extremity into internal and external rotation elicits guarding, with limited range of motion
- Pain at the extremes of movement and tenderness over anterior hip joint
- No history of trauma
- Condition is bilateral in 10% to 20% of patients

ETIOLOGY

Unknown

DIAGNOSIS

DIFFERENTIAL DIAGNOSIS UNILATERAL DISEASE

- Transient synovitis
- Sickle cell disease
- Septic arthritis
- Neoplasm
- Spondyloepiphyseal dysplasia tarda

BILATERAL DISEASE

- Multiple epiphyseal dysplasia (MED)
- Sickle cell disease
- Juvenile idiopathic arthritis

WORKUP

Diagnosis is usually based on the physical findings and eventual radiographic findings.

IMAGING STUDIES

- Plain roentgenography to establish the diagnosis
- Anteroposterior and frog-leg lateral radiographs (Fig. 1-544)
- Technetium bone scanning to help confirm the diagnosis in early cases

TREATMENT

ACUTE GENERAL Rx

- A brief period of bed rest (1 to 3 days) followed by bracing (except in mild cases)
- Bracing may be required for 2 to 3 yr in a small percent of patients
- NSAIDs and non-weight-bearing for pain control
- Range-of-motion physical therapy exercises (physiotherapy)
- Surgical therapy in refractory cases: tenotomy, various osteotomies

DISPOSITION

- Prognosis depends on age of patient and degree of involvement of the femoral head at onset.
- In patients younger than 6 yr, outcome is generally positive regardless of treatment
- Patients over the age of 8 yr at onset often have poorer outcomes. Females tend to do worse than males in this age group.
- A few patients eventually develop degenerative arthritis.

REFERRAL

Referral to orthopedics or rheumatology for consultation when diagnosis is suspected

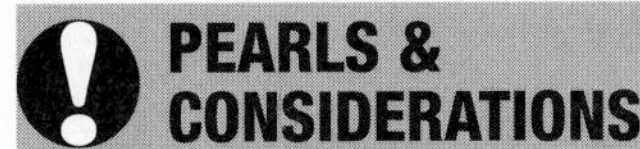

PEARLS & CONSIDERATIONS

Both the etiology and the treatment of LCPD remain controversial. Treatment recommendations vary widely and continue to evolve. Children greater than 6-8 yr at age of onset may benefit from early surgical intervention.

COMMENTS

There is great uncertainty regarding treatment and its effect on outcome. Bracing may have limited efficacy in augmenting the natural course of the disease.

SUGGESTED READINGS
available at www.expertconsult.com

RELATED CONTENT

Legg-Calvé-Perthes Disease (Patient Information)

AUTHOR: **MATTHEW J. STANISHEWSKI, D.O.**

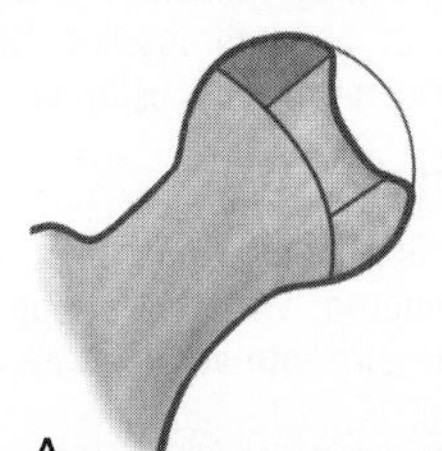

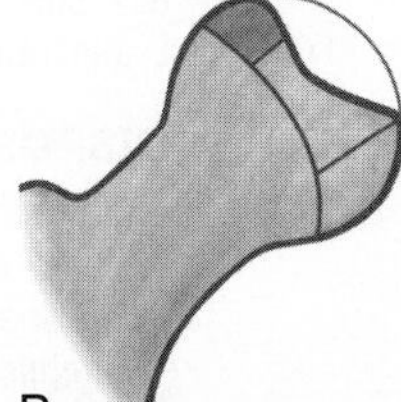

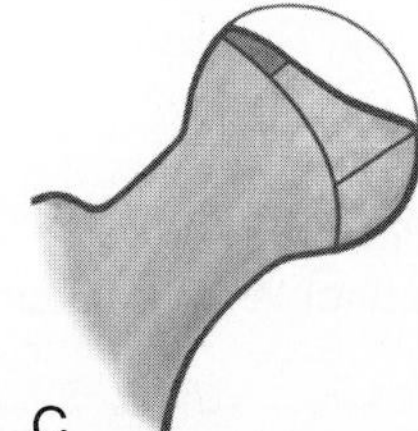

FIGURE 1-543 Lateral pillar classification for Legg-Calvé-Perthes disease. A, There is no involvement of the lateral pillar. **B,** More than 50% of the lateral pillar height is maintained. **C,** Less than 50% of the lateral pillar height is maintained. (From Kliegman RM et al: *Nelson textbook of pediatrics,* ed 19, Philadelphia, 2011, Saunders.)

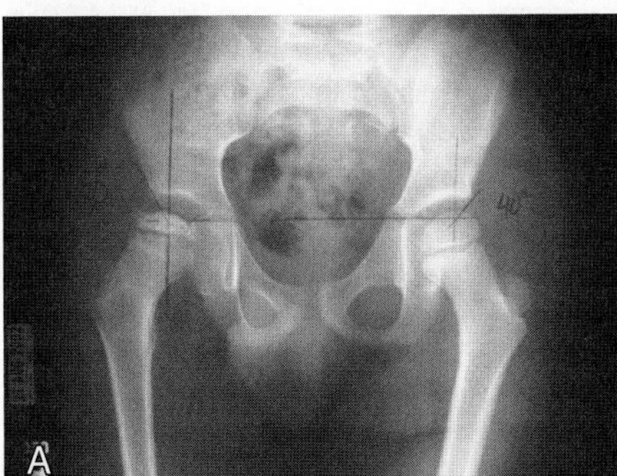

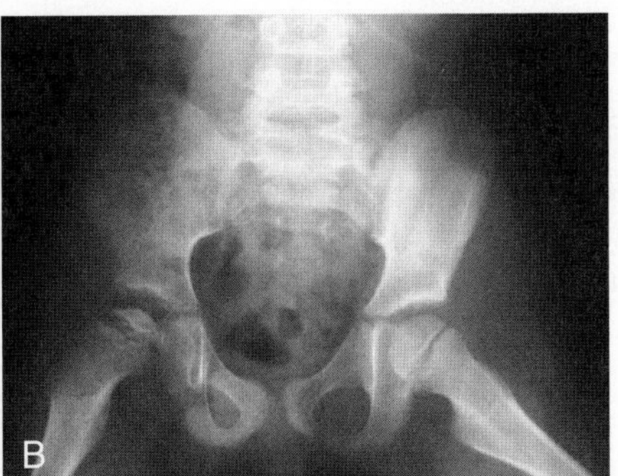

FIGURE 1-544 A, Anteroposterior radiograph of the pelvis shows epiphyseal fragmentation in the right hip, characteristic of the fragmentation phase of Legg-Calvé-Perthes disease. **B,** The frog-leg lateral view demonstrates subchondral fracture, increased density of the femoral head, and some collapse. (From Kliegman RM et al: *Nelson textbook of pediatrics,* ed 19, Philadelphia, 2011, Saunders.)

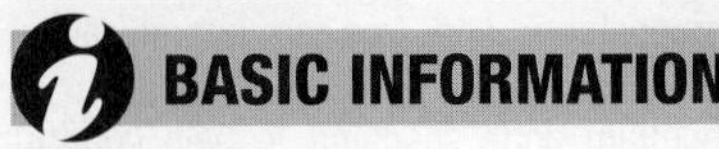

BASIC INFORMATION

DEFINITION

Acute lymphoblastic leukemia (ALL) is a malignancy of B or T lymphoblasts characterized by uncontrolled proliferation of abnormal, immature lymphocytes and their progenitors, ultimately replacing normal bone marrow elements.

SYNONYMS

Lymphoid leukemia
ALL

ICD-9CM CODES
204.0 Acute lymphoblastic leukemia
ICD-10CM CODES
C91.00 Acute lymphoblastic leukemia not having achieved remission

EPIDEMIOLOGY & DEMOGRAPHICS

- ALL is primarily a disease of children (peak incidence from ages 2 to 10 yr).
- It is diagnosed in 3000 to 4000 persons in the U.S. each year; two thirds are children. It is the most common malignancy of childhood.

PHYSICAL FINDINGS & CLINICAL PRESENTATION

- Skin pallor, purpura, or easy bruising
- Lymphadenopathy or hepatosplenomegaly
- Fever, bone pain, oliguria, weakness, weight loss, mental status changes

ETIOLOGY

- Unknown; increased risk in patients with a previous use of antineoplastic agents (e.g., chemotherapy of non-Hodgkin's lymphoma, Hodgkin's disease, ovarian cancer, myeloma)
- Environmental factors (e.g., ionizing radiation), toxins (e.g., benzene)

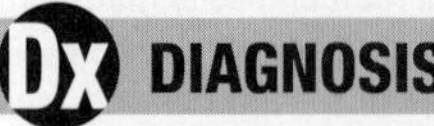

DIAGNOSIS

DIFFERENTIAL DIAGNOSIS

- Acute myeloid leukemia (AML): the distinction between ALL and AML (see Table 1-288) and the classification of the various subtypes are based on the following factors:
  1. Cell morphology
     - Lymphoblasts: a high nucleus/cytoplasmic ratio; cytoplasmic granules are usually not present.
     - Myeloblasts: abundant cytoplasm; cytoplasmic granules (Auer rods) are often present.
  2. Histochemical stains
     - Peroxidase and Sudan black stains: negative in ALL; useful to distinguish nonlymphoid from lymphoid cells.
     - Chloroacetate esterase: a pink cytoplasmic reaction identifies granulocytes; useful to distinguish granulocytes from monocytes in patients with AML.
  3. Cytogenic/molecular markers (Table 1-289)
- Lymphoblastic lymphoma
- Aplastic anemia
- Infectious mononucleosis
- Leukemoid reaction to infection
- Multiple myeloma

WORKUP

- Laboratory evaluation
- Bone marrow examination (with biopsy, cytochemistry, immunophenotyping, and cytogenetics) (Fig. E1-548)
- Lumbar puncture and imaging studies

LABORATORY TESTS

- Complete blood count reveals normochromic, normocytic anemia, thrombocytopenia.
- Peripheral smear will reveal lymphoblasts.
- Initial blood work should also include blood urea nitrogen, creatinine, serum electrolytes, uric acid, and lactate dehydrogenase.
- Special diagnostic tests include immunophenotyping, cytogenetics, and cytochemistry.
- The French, American, British (FAB) Cooperative Study Group has classified ALL into three groups (L1 to L3) on the basis of cell size, cytoplasmic appearance, nucleus shape, and chromatin pattern. The most common form is the L2 type.
- Immunologic classification is made on the basis of expression of surface antigens by blast cells: T lineage and B lineage.

IMAGING STUDIES

- Chest x-ray to evaluate for the presence of mediastinal mass
- CT scan or ultrasound of abdomen/pelvis to assess splenomegaly or leukemic infiltration of abdominal organs

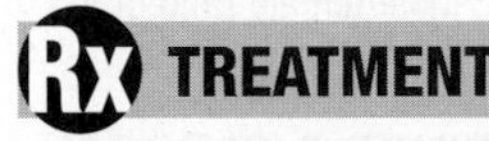

TREATMENT

ACUTE GENERAL Rx

Table 1-290 summarizes the preferred approach to the treatment of adult ALL patients. For younger adults, induction therapy usually consists of an anthracycline, vincristine, L-asparaginase, and a corticosteroid.

DISPOSITION

- Prognosis is generally poorer in adult disease compared with childhood disease (40% adult cure rate versus 80% cure rate in children).
- Five-year leukemia-free survival is <40%.
- The different clinical outcomes associated with the various subtypes of ALL can be attributed primarily to drug sensitivity or resistance of leukemic blasts harboring specific genetic abnormalities. For example, cases of ALL expressing the TEL-AML1 fusion protein are very responsive to intensive chemotherapy with asparaginase, whereas the presence of Philadelphia chromosome (Ph{∑Y}+{/∑Y}), monosomy 5 and 7, and abnormalities of 11q23 are bad prognostic signs in ALL.
- Genetic alteration (deletion) of IKZF1 is associated with a very poor outcome in B-cell-progenitor ALL.
- Outcome of adult ALL patients according to subgroups is summarized in Table 1-291.

REFERRAL

Referral to a hematologist is indicated in all cases of ALL.

TABLE 1-288 Morphologic, Cytochemical, and Biochemical Characteristics Helpful in Distinguishing Acute Lymphoblastic Leukemia from Acute Myelocytic Leukemia

Morphologic Features	ALL	AML
Nuclear/cytoplasmic ratio	High	Low
Nuclear chromatin	Clumped	Spongy
Nucleoli	0-2	2-5
Granules	–	+
Auer rods	–	+/–
Cytoplasm	Blue	Blue-gray
Cytochemical Reaction		
Peroxidase	–	+
Sudan black B	–	+
Periodic acid–Schiff	+/–	–
Naphthyl AS-D chloroacetate esterase	–	+/–
α-Naphthyl acetate esterase	–	+/–
α-Naphthyl butyrate esterase	–	–
Terminal deoxynucleotidyl transferase	+*	–

Table provides information on characteristics that may be useful in differentiating acute lymphoblastic leukemia (ALL) from acute myelocytic leukemia (AML) (see text for details). Wide variation in morphology is encountered in both disease categories. Diagnostic evaluation should include more refined classification of disease according to FAB subtype.
*Terminal deoxynucleotidyl transferase is usually negative in FAB L3 ALL.
From Hoffman R et al: *Hematology, basic principles and practice,* ed 5, Philadelphia, 2009, Churchill Livingstone.

TABLE 1-289 Preferred Approach to the Treatment of Adult Acute Lymphocytic Leukemia Patients

	Low-Risk ALL	High-Risk ALL	Very High-Risk ALL	Mature B-ALL
Definition	*B-lineage* WBC <30,000/mL Time to CR <4 wk No Pro-B/ t(4;11) *T-lineage* Thy ALL Molecular CR	*B-lineage* WBC >30,000/mL Time to CR >4 wk Pro-B/ t(4;11) *T-lineage* Early T, mature T No molecular CR	Ph/BCR-ABL positive	
Multidrug-induction	Yes	Yes	Yes + imatinib	Short intensive cycles including HDM, fractionated C, HDAC, and other drugs Rituximab
CNS prophylaxis*	Yes	Yes	Yes	Yes
Consolidation (also other combinations)	Alternating cycles, e.g., HDM, HDAC, asparaginase reinduction	One cycle	One cycle + imatinib	6 cycles
SCT in CR1	None	Allogeneic SCT (if matched related or unrelated donor) Autologous SCT After additional (if no donor and negative MRD, consolidation)		None
Maintenance	6-MP/M + intensification for 2-2½ yr		Imatinib	None

AC, Cytosine arabinoside; *ALL,* acute lymphocytic leukemia; *CR,* complete remission; *HDM,* high-dose methotrexate; *MRD,* minimal residual disease; *SCT,* stem cell transplantation; *Thy ALL,* thymic ALL.
*Intrathecal therapy with M or triple combination (M, AC, steroid) continued during maintenance therapy; additional CNS irradiation and/or high-dose chemotherapy according to subgroup.
From Hoffman R et al: *Hematology, basic principles and practice,* ed 5, Philadelphia, 2009, Churchill Livingstone.

TABLE 1-290 Outcome of Adult Lymphocytic Leukemia Patients According to Subgroup*

Subgroup	No. of Patients	CR Rate	No. of Patients	LFS
Age				
<30	669	88%	510	42%-60%‡
30-59	610	79%	412	33%
≥60	215	58%	141	15%
Subtype				
T-ALL†	976	88%	850	40%-60%‡
B-Precursor ALL	2366	82%	2036	40%-60%
Pro-B-ALL	987	75%	107	37%-60%§
Cytogenetics				
Ph/bcr-abl + (without imatinib)	633	72%	633	21%
Ph/bcr-abl + (with imatinib + chemo)		90%		50%
WBC				
<30,000/mL	698	81%	746	40%
>30,000/mL	387	75%	409	28%
Time to CR				
<4 wk			1433	44%
>4 wk			253	36%

CR, Complete remission; *LFS,* leukemia-free survival; *MRD,* median remission duration.
*Pooled data from published studies.
†Depends on T-ALL subtype.
‡Depending on protocol and subtype.
§Including allogeneic SCT.
From Hoffman R et al: *Hematology: basic principles and practice,* ed 5, Philadelphia, 2009, Churchill Livingstone.

SUGGESTED READINGS

available at www.expertconsult.com

RELATED CONTENT

Acute Lymphocytic Leukemia (ALL) (Patient Information)

AUTHOR: **FRED F. FERRI, M.D.**

TABLE 1-291 Immunologic Subtypes of Acute Lymphocytic Leukemia and Corresponding Cytogenetic/Molecular Markers

Subgroups	Most Important Markers	Incidence in Children (*n* = 1756)	Incidence in Adults (*n* = 946)	Cytogenetic/Molecular Marker
B-Lineage	HLA-DR+, TdT+, CD19+ and/or CD79a+ and/or CD22+	85%	72%	
Pro-B (B-I)	CD10−, no other differentiation markers	5%	11%	6% t(4;11)/ALL1-AF4 (70% in pro-B) (20% Flt3 in MLL+)
Common ALL (B-II)	CD10+	65%	51%	33% t(9;22)/BCR-ABL (30%-50% in c/pre-B)
Pre-B (B-III)	cy IgM+	15%	10%	4% t(1;19)/PBX-E2A
Mature B	cy or s kappa or lambda	3%	4%	5% t(8;14)/c-myc-IgH
T-Lineage	cy or s CD3+, CD7+		26%	
Early T	cy CD3+, CD7+, CD5±, CD2−, sCD3−, CD1a−	1%	7%	5% t(10;14)/HOX11-TCR <5% t(11;14)LMO/TCR 2% SIL-TAL1
Cortical (thymic) T	CD2+, CD5+, CD1a+, sCD3±		13%	4% NUP213-ABL1 (in T-ALL), 33% HOX11
Mature T (T-IV)	CD2+, CD5+, sCD3+, CD1a−		7%	5% HOX11L2 (in T-ALL) 50% Notch1 (in T-ALL)

a, And; *cy*, intracytoplasmic; *o*, or; *s*, surface.
From Hoffman R et al: *Hematology, basic principles and practice*, ed 5, Philadelphia, 2009, Churchill Livingstone.

BASIC INFORMATION

DEFINITION

Acute myelogenous leukemia (AML) is a malignancy of myeloid progenitor cells. It is characterized by uncontrolled proliferation of primitive myeloid cells (blasts), ultimately replacing normal bone marrow elements and frequently resulting in hematopoietic insufficiency (granulocytopenia, thrombocytopenia, or anemia) with or without leukocytosis.

SYNONYMS

Acute nonlymphoblastic leukemia (ANLL)
Acute nonlymphocytic leukemia
Acute myeloid leukemia (AML)

ICD-9CM CODES
205.0 Acute myelogenous leukemia
ICD-10CM CODES
C92.00 Acute myeloblastic leukemia, not having achieved remission

EPIDEMIOLOGY & DEMOGRAPHICS

- AML usually affects adults (most patients are 30 to 60 yr; median age at presentation is 50 yr).
- Annual incidence is 2 to 4 cases/100,000 persons.

PHYSICAL FINDINGS & CLINICAL PRESENTATION

Patients generally come to medical attention because of the effects of the cytopenias:

- Anemia manifests with weakness or fatigue.
- Thrombocytopenia can manifest with bleeding, petechiae, and ecchymosis.
- Neutropenia can result in infections and fever.
- Physical examination may reveal skin pallor, bruises, petechiae; abdominal examination may reveal hepatosplenomegaly; peripheral lymphadenopathy may also be present.
- Hyperleukocytosis can lead to symptoms of leukostasis, such as ocular and cerebrovascular dysfunction or bleeding.

ETIOLOGY

Risk factors are previous use of antineoplastic agents, chromosomal abnormalities, ionizing radiation, toxins, immunodeficiency states, and chronic myeloproliferative disorders. Congenital disorders or acquired factors predisposing to AML are described in Table 1-292.

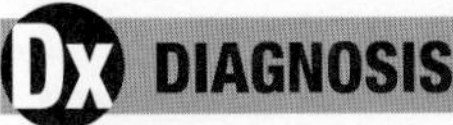

DIAGNOSIS

DIFFERENTIAL DIAGNOSIS

- Acute lymphocytic leukemia
- Leukemoid reaction
- Myelodysplastic syndrome
- Infiltrative diseases of the bone marrow
- Epstein-Barr virus, other viral infection

LABORATORY TESTS

- Complete blood count reveals anemia and thrombocytopenia. Peripheral white blood cell count varies from $<5000/mm^3$ to $>100,000/mm^3$.
- Additional laboratory findings may include elevated lactate dehydrogenase and uric acid levels, decreased fibrinogen, and increased fibrin degradation product as a result of disseminated intravascular coagulation (DIC).
- Cytogenetic abnormalities are common (chromosome 8 is most frequently involved in AML). Table 1-293 describes gene mutations in patients with AML. DNMT3A mutations are highly recurrent in patients with de novo AML with an intermediate-risk cytogenetic profile and are independently associated with a poor outcome.
- The distinction between acute lymphoblastic leukemia (ALL) and AML and the classification of the various subtypes are based on the following factors:
  1. Cell morphology: myeloblasts reveal abundant cytoplasm; cytoplasmic granules are often present (Auer rods).
  2. Histochemical stains:
     - Peroxidase and Sudan black stains are negative in ALL.
     - Chloroacetate esterase: a pink cytoplasmic reaction identifies granulocytes; useful to distinguish granulocytes from monocytes in patients with AML.

TABLE 1-292 Congenital Disorders or Acquired Factors Predisposing to Acute Myeloid Leukemia

Genetic Factors
Down syndrome
Fanconi anemia
Bloom syndrome
Neurofibromatosis type I
Klinefelter syndrome
Turner syndrome
Congenital Bone Marrow Failure Syndromes
Kostmann syndrome
Diamond-Blackfan anemia
Drugs
Benzene
Alkylating agents
Epipodophyllotoxins
Ionizing radiation
Myelodysplastic syndromes

From Hoffman R et al: *Hematology: basic principles and practice*, ed 6, Philadelphia, 2013, Elsevier.

TABLE 1-293 Gene Mutations in Patients with Acute Myelogenous Leukemia, and Normal Karyotype

Gene Mutation	Frequency (%)	Prognosis
NPM	45-63	Favorable
FLT3	23-33	Adverse
MLL	5-30	Adverse
C/EBP	8-19	Favorable

From Hoffman R et al: *Hematology: basic principles and practice*, ed 6, Philadelphia, 2013, Elsevier.

- AML is diagnosed by the presence of at least 30% blast cells and positive peroxidase or Sudan black histochemical stain in the bone marrow aspirate.
- The French, American, British (FAB) Cooperative Study Group has classified AML into seven categories (M1 to M7) based on the type and percentage of immature cells. The World Health Organization classification of AML is described in Table 1-294. A summary of diagnostic features of AML in the FAB classification is outline in Table 1-295.
- A stepwise algorithm for diagnosis and classification of AML using cytomorphology, cytochemistry, immunophenotyping, cytogenetics, and molecular genetics is described in Box 1-51 and in Fig. E1-549. Cytogenetic risk categories in AML are described in Table 1-296. Bone marrow findings are described in Fig. E1-550.

IMAGING STUDIES

- Chest x-ray is useful to evaluate for the presence of mediastinal masses.
- CT scan of the abdomen may reveal hepatosplenomegaly or leukemic involvement of other organs.

Rx TREATMENT

ACUTE GENERAL Rx

- Emergency treatment consisting of one or more of the following is indicated in patients with intracerebral leukostasis:
  1. Cranial irradiation
  2. Leukapheresis
  3. Oral hydroxyurea
- Urate nephropathy can be prevented by vigorous hydration and lowering uric acid level with allopurinol and urine alkalinization with acetazolamide.
- Infections must be aggressively treated with broad-spectrum antibiotics.
- Correct significant thrombocytopenia with platelet transfusions.
- Bleeding from DIC is treated with heparin and replacement of clotting factors.
- Intensive induction chemotherapy to destroy a significant number of leukemic cells and achieve remission usually consists of cytarabine and daunorubicin. It is a 7 + 3 regimen consisting of 7 days of continuous IV infusion of cytarabine and 3 days of daunorubicin. With this regimen, the chance of obtaining a complete remission is 65% to 70% with significantly lower rates in older patients (.56 yr old). All-trans retinoic acid is effective for the induction of remission of AML M3 subtype (acute promyelocytic leukemia).
- High-dose cytarabine (ARA-C) (HiDAC) can be used in patients with refractory or relapsed AML. It usually takes 28 to 32 days from the start of therapy to achieve remission. The duration of remission is variable; the median duration of remission in an adult with AML is 1 yr.
- Postremission therapy following complete remission with induction chemotherapy may include either allogeneic bone marrow

transplant (younger patients with donor match) or consolidation chemotherapy.

- Consolidation therapy consists of an aggressive course of chemotherapy with or without radiation shortly after complete remission has been obtained; its purpose is to prolong the remission period or cure. Complications of consolidation therapy are usually attributable to severe bone marrow suppression (anemia, thrombocytopenia, granulocytopenia).
- Goal of therapy is to maintain a state of remission. A postinduction course of high-dose cytarabine can provide equivalent disease-free survival and somewhat better overall survival than autologous marrow transplantation in adults.
- Autologous bone marrow transplantation is indicated in patients <55 yr without a sibling donor. Allogeneic bone marrow transplantation is generally available to <20% of patients; it is usually performed only in patients <40 yr because of higher incidence of graft-versus-host disease with advancing age.

DISPOSITION

- Remission can be achieved in nearly 80% of patients <55 yr. Remission rates are highest in children. Patient characteristics relating to duration of remission are described in Table 1-297.
- Allogeneic stem cell transplantation (SCT) after myoablative conditioning is a curative option in younger patients with AML in first complete remission (CR1). However, concerns related to toxicity limit its use. Cure for allogeneic bone marrow transplantation approaches 60%; cure rates with autologous transplantation are lower. Compared with nonallogeneic SCT therapies, allogeneic SCT has significant relapse-free survival (RFS) and overall survival benefit for intermediate- and poor-risk AML but not for good-risk AML in first complete remission.
- Favorable cytogenics are inv (16) (p13;q22) and t(8;21), t(15;17).
- High expression of an LSC (leukemic stem cell) gene signature is independently associated with adverse outcomes with AML.

PEARLS & CONSIDERATIONS

- The major complication of chemotherapy is profound marrow depression with pancytopenia lasting 3 to 4 wk. Treatment is aimed at red blood cell and platelet replacement and aggressive monitoring and treatment of suspected infections.
- Low doses of arsenic trioxide can induce complete remission in patients with acute promyelocytic leukemia.

SUGGESTED READINGS

available at www.expertconsult.com

RELATED CONTENT

Acute Myelogenous Leukemia (Patient Information)

AUTHOR: **FRED F. FERRI, M.D.**

TABLE 1-294 World Health Organization Classification of Acute Myeloid Leukemia

Acute myeloid leukemia with recurrent genetic abnormalities
Acute myeloid leukemia with t(8;21)(q22;q22), (AML1/ETO)
Acute myeloid leukemia with abnormal bone marrow eosinophils and inv(16)(p13;q22) or t(16;16)(p13;q22), (CBFb/MYH11)
Acute promyelocytic leukemia with t(15;17)(q22;q12), (PML/RARα) and variants
Acute myeloid leukemia with 11q23 (MLL) abnormalities
Acute myeloid leukemia with multilineage dysplasia
Following MDS or MDS/MPD
Without antecedent MDS or MDS/MPD, but with dysplasia in at least 50% of cells in two or more myeloid lineages
Acute myeloid leukemia and myelodysplastic syndromes, therapy related
Alkylating agent/radiation-related type
Topoisomerase II inhibitor-related type (some may be lymphoid)
Others
Acute myeloid leukemia, not otherwise categorized
Classify as:
Acute myeloid leukemia, minimally differentiated
Acute myeloid leukemia without maturation
Acute myeloid leukemia with maturation
Acute myelomonocytic leukemia
Acute monoblastic/acute monocytic leukemia
Acute erythroid leukemia (erythroid/myeloid and pure erythroleukemia)
Acute megakaryoblastic leukemia
Acute basophilic leukemia
Acute panmyelosis with myelofibrosis
Myeloid sarcoma

From Hoffman R et al: *Hematology: basic principles and practice*, ed 5, Philadelphia, 2009, Churchill Livingstone.

TABLE 1-295 Summary of Diagnostic Features of Acute Myeloid Leukemia in the FAB Classification

FAB Subtype (%)	Diagnostic Features
AML-M0 (3%-5%)	≥30% blasts; >3% blasts reactive to MPO, SBB, or NSE; immunophenotyping $CD33^+$, $CD13^+$, may be $CD34^+$, TdT^+
AML-M1 (15%-20%)	≥30% blasts; ≥3% blasts reactive to MPO or SBB; <10% of marrow nucleated cells are promyelocytes or more mature neutrophils
AML-M2 (25%-30%)	≥30% blasts; ≥3% blasts reactive for MPO or SBB; ≥10% of marrow nucleated cells are promyelocytes or more mature neutrophils; t(8:21) chromosome abnormality
AML-M3 (10%-15%)	≥30% blasts and abnormal promyelocytes; intense MPO and SBB reactivity; promyelocytes and blasts with multiple Auer rods (faggot cells); t(15:17) cytogenetic abnormality
AML-M4 (20%-30%)	≥30% myeloblasts, monoblasts, and promonocytes; ≥20% monocytic cells in marrow; ≤5 × 10^9/L monocytic cells in blood: ≥20% neutrophils and precursors in marrow; monocytic cells reactive for NSE; abnormal eosinophils in M4 with associated inv(16) chromosome abnormality
AML-M5a (2%-7%)	≥80% monocytic cells; monoblasts ≥80% of monocytic cells; monoblasts and promonocytes NSE positive; monoblasts usually MPO and SBB negative
AML-M5b (2%-5%)	≥80% monocytic cells; monoblasts ≥80% of monocytic cells; promonocytes predominate; monoblasts and promonocytes NSE positive; promonocytes may have scattered MPO- and SBB-positive granules
AML-M6 (3%-5%)	≥50% erythroid precursors: ≥30% of nonerythroid precursors are myeloblasts; Auer rods may be present in myeloblasts; dysplastic erythroid precursors frequently are PAS positive
AML-M7 (3%-5%)	≥30% blasts; ≥50% cells megakaryoblasts by morphology or electron microscopy; immunophenotyping $CD41^+$, $CD61^+$

AML, Acute myeloid leukemia; *CD,* cluster designation; *FAB,* French-American-British; *MPO,* myeloperoxidase; *NSE,* nonspecific esterase; *PAS,* periodic acid–Schiff; *SBB,* Sudan black B; *TdT,* terminal deoxynucleotidyl transferase.
Percent of all AML.
From Hoffman R et al: *Hematology: basic principles and practice,* ed 5, Philadelphia, 2009, Churchill Livingstone.

BOX 1-51 Stepwise Algorithm for Diagnosis and Classification of Acute Myelogenous Leukemia Using Cytomorphology, Cytochemistry, Immunophenotyping, Cytogenetics, and Molecular Cytogenetics

The criteria are based on Wright-Giemsa–stained blood and marrow smears and biopsy. The percentage of blast cells separates acute myeloid leukemia (AML) from myelodysplastic syndrome (MDS). The World Health Organization (WHO) classification defines AML as greater than 20% blasts in the marrow or blood. The next step is to define the blast population by immunophenotyping and/or immunohistochemistry. The initial evaluation separates AML from ALL. A history of exposure to prior cytoxic chemotherapy or agents associated with AML defines the leukemia as *therapy-related acute myeloid leukemia* (t-AML). The WHO recognizes the unique clinical and biologic features of the therapy-related leukemias (t-AML). This subtype results from prior exposure to cytotoxic chemotherapy and/or radiation therapy. A majority of patients will have clonal cytogenetic abnormalities and now account for more than 40% of all patients with AML. The WHO recognizes two types of t-AML based on the type of prior exposure or treatment: alkylating agent–related AML and topoisomerase II inhibitor–related AML. The WHO classification defines major subgroups of AML that manifest recurring cytogenetic abnormalities. As a group, these AMLs have chromosomal translocations that result in the production of chimeric proteins, which are pivotal in the leukemogenic process. The genetic abnormalities define a specific biology, clinical course, and prognosis and therefore it is important to classify them separately. In this group of patients, the diagnosis is defined by the cytogenetic abnormality independent of the percentage of blasts. There are four recurrent translocations in this group. The diagnosis is defined by the cytogenetic abnormalities and is not dependent on the number of blasts: (a) AML with t(8;21)(q22;q22), (AML1/ETO) (RUNX/CBFA2T1); (b) AML with abnormal bone marrow eosinophils and inv[16](p13;q22) or t(16;16)(p13;q22), (CBFB/MYH11); (c) acute promyelocytic leukemia: AML with t(15;17)(q22;q21) (PML/RARA) or t(11;17)(q23;q12) (PLZF/RARA) or t(5;17)(q23;q12)(NPM/RARA), or t(11;17)(q13;q12) (NuMA/RARA); and (d) AML with 11q23 (MLL) abnormalities. If multilineage dysplasia is present, then the leukemia is classified as *acute leukemia with multilineage dysplasia.*

AML with multilineage dysplasia is characterized by the presence of 20% or more blasts in the marrow and dysplasia in at least 50% of the cells of at least two of the three main hemopoietic lines. The leukemia may occur de novo or after a preceding myelodysplastic, myeloproliferative, or overlap myelodysplastic/myeloproliferative syndrome unrelated to prior exposure to chemotherapy. If such a syndrome preceded the development of acute leukemia, the AML is best designated as AML "evolving from a myelodysplastic syndrome." When a leukemia fails to satisfy the cytogenetic, morphologic, or clinical criteria for the newly defined subgroups, it is classified as AML not otherwise categorized. The *not otherwise categorized* designation essentially applies the original FAB classification with some modifications, namely, acute promyelocytic leukemia (M3) is no longer included; a pure erythroleukemia has been distinguished from erythroleukemia, acute erythroid/myeloid type; and acute basophilic leukemia (very rare) has been added, as is a rare entity termed acute panmyelosis with myelofibrosis and the solid tumor myeloid sarcoma.

CD, Cluster designation; *MPO,* myeloperoxidase; *NEC,* nonerythroid cells; *NSE,* nonspecific esterase; *PAS,* periodic acid–Schiff; *SBB,* Sudan black B; *TdT,* terminal deoxynucleotidyl transferase; *TNC,* total nucleated cells.

From Hoffman R et al: *Hematology, basic principles and practice*, ed 5, Philadelphia, 2009, Churchill Livingstone.

TABLE 1-296 Cytogenetic Risk Categories in Acute Myelogenous Leukemia

Category	Abnormality
Favorable	t(8;21),* t(15;17), inv(16) with or without other abnormalities
Intermediate	Normal, +6, +8, +21, +22 −Y, del(9q)
Unfavorable	−5/del(5q), −7/del(7q), abn(3q) t(9;22),t(6;9), abn(11q), 20q or 21q, abn(17p), complex karyotype

*Without deletion 9q or complex karyotype.

From Hoffman R et al: *Hematology: basic principles and practice*, ed 5, Philadelphia, 2009, Churchill Livingstone.

TABLE 1-297 Patient Characteristics Relating to Duration of Remission

Characteristics	Favorable Value
Cytogenetics	t(15;17), t(8;21), inv(16)
Leukocyte count	$<100{,}000/\mu L^{-1}$
Secondary acute myeloid leukemia	Not present
FAB subtype	M1 or M2 with Auer rods, M3 and M4eo
FLT3	Wild-type
Courses to complete remission	1

From Hoffman R et al: *Hematology: basic principles and practice*, ed 5, Philadelphia, 2009, Churchill Livingstone.

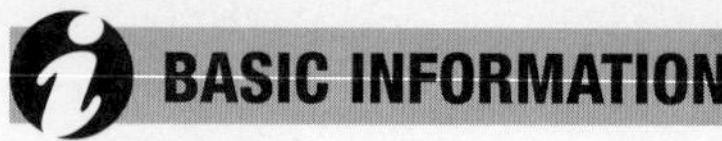

DEFINITION

Chronic lymphocytic leukemia (CLL) is a lymphoproliferative disorder characterized by proliferation and accumulation of mature-appearing neoplastic lymphocytes.

SYNONYMS

CLL

ICD-9CM CODES
204.1 Leukemia, chronic lymphocytic
ICD-10CM CODES
C91.10 Chronic lymphocytic leukemia of B-cell type not having achieved remission

EPIDEMIOLOGY & DEMOGRAPHICS

- Most frequent form of leukemia in Western countries (10,000 new cases annually in the United States). Incidence rate is 2-6 cases per 100,000 per year, and increases to 13 cases per 100,000 at age 65. It is more common in Caucasians and in those with a family history of CLL or other lymphoid malignancy.
- Generally occurs in elderly patients (70% of diagnoses are made in patients >65 yr of age). Mean age at diagnosis is 65 yr.
- Male/female ratio of 2:1
- CLL accounts for 11% of all hematologic neoplasms.

PHYSICAL FINDINGS & CLINICAL PRESENTATION

- At presentation most patients are asymptomatic. Many cases are diagnosed on the basis of laboratory results obtained after routine physical examination
- Lymphadenopathy, splenomegaly, and hepatomegaly in the majority of patients
- Variable clinical presentation according to stage of the disease
- Some patients come to medical attention because of weakness and fatigue (as a result of anemia) or lymphadenopathy

ETIOLOGY

CLL is a disease derived from antigen-experienced B lymphocytes that differ in the level of immunoglobulin V-gene mutations.

Dx DIAGNOSIS

- Identification of cells bearing the phenotype of CLL in peripheral blood (CD5-positive/CD19-positive)
- Absolute B lymphocyte count in the peripheral blood ≥5000/μL for >3 mo with a preponderant population of morphologically mature-appearing small lymphocytes (Fig. E1-551)
- Demonstration of clonality of circulating B lymphocytes by flow cytometry of peripheral blood
- Table 1-298 describes the evaluation of CLL patients at diagnosis

TABLE 1-298 Evaluation of Chronic Lymphocytic Leukemia (CLL) Patients at Diagnosis

History
B-symptom and fatigue assessment
Infectious history assessment
Occupational assessment for chemical exposure
Familial history of CLL and lymphoproliferative disorders
Preventive interventions for infections and secondary cancers
Physical Exam
Laboratory Assessment
Complete blood count with differential
Morphology assessment of lymphocytes
Chemistry, LFT enzymes, LDH
Flow cytometry assessment to confirm immunophenotype of CLL
Serum immunoglobulins
Serum b_2M levels
Interphase cytogenetics for del(17p13.1), del(11q22.3), del(13q14), del(6q21), and trisomy 12
IgV_H mutational analysis
Stimulated metaphase karyotype (if available)
Selected Tests Under Certain Circumstances
Direct antiglobulin test (DAT), haptoglobin, reticulocyte count if anemia present
CT scan if unexplained abdominal pain or enlargement present
PET scan and/or biopsy if large nodal mass present
Bone marrow aspirate and biopsy if cytopenias present
Familial counseling if first-degree relative with CLL
Teaching
Varicella zoster identification instruction
Skin cancer identification
Disease education (Leukemia and Lymphoma Society, CLL Topics, ACOR)

From Hoffmann R et al: *Hematology: basic principles and practice*, ed 6, Philadelphia, 2013, Elsevier.

DIFFERENTIAL DIAGNOSIS

- Hairy cell leukemia
- Adult T-cell lymphoma. Table 1-299 describes major diagnostic features of CLL and small lymphocytic lymphoma (SLL)
- Prolymphocytic leukemia
- Viral infections
- Waldenström's macroglobulinemia

LABORATORY TESTS

- Proliferative lymphocytosis (≥15,000/dl) of well-differentiated lymphocytes is the hallmark of CLL. B-cell clones are early markers for CLL and can be detected in peripheral blood >6 yr before a CLL diagnosis.
- There is monotonous replacement of the bone marrow by small lymphocytes (marrow contains ≥30% of well-differentiated lymphocytes). With the use of cell surface markers for clonality determination, the use of bone marrow aspirate and biopsy has become unnecessary for diagnosis or prognosis.
- Hypogammaglobulinemia and elevated lactate dehydrogenase may be present at the time of diagnosis.
- Anemia or thrombocytopenia, if present, indicates poor prognosis.
- Trisomy-12 is the most common chromosomal abnormality, followed by 14 q+, 13 q, and 11 q; these all indicate a poor prognosis.
- New laboratory techniques (CD 38, fluorescence in situ hybridization) can identify patients with early-stage CLL at higher risk of rapid disease progression. Staining of mononuclear cells by a two-color (fluorescein isothiocyanate/phycoerythrin) flow cytometric assay using antibodies to the chemokine receptors (CXCR1, CXCR2, etc.) can help in the staging and prognosis of patients. Increase in expression of chemokine receptors CXCR4 and CCR7 correlates with advanced Rai stage (stage IV). The presence of V-gene mutations, CD38+, or ZAP-70+ cells also has prognostic relevance.

TABLE 1-299 Major Diagnostic Features of Chronic Lymphocytic Leukemia (CLL) and Small Lymphocytic Lymphoma (SLL)

CLL
- Absolute mature lymphocytosis of ≥5×10^9/L sustained for at least 3 months
- Monoclonal B cell with mature phenotype, CD5 coexpression, weak CD20, weak surface immunoglobulin, CD23, weak CD22, weak CD11c
- Antigens typically *not* expressed include CD10, FMC7, and CD79b

SLL
- Extramedullary sites of disease predominate
- Diffuse infiltrate of small lymphocytes, proliferation foci
- Monoclonal B cell with mature phenotype similar to CLL

From Jaffe ES et al: *Hematopathology*, Philadelphia, 2011, Saunders.

BASIC INFORMATION

DEFINITION

Hairy cell leukemia is a lymphoid neoplasm characterized by the proliferation of mature B cells with prominent cytoplasmic projections (hairs).

SYNONYMS

HCL
Leukemic reticuloendotheliosis

ICD-9CM CODES
202.4 Hairy cell leukemia
ICD-10CM CODES
C91.40 Hairy cell leukemia not having achieved remission

EPIDEMIOLOGY & DEMOGRAPHICS

PREVALENCE: Occurs predominantly in men between ages 40 and 60 yr. Approximately 2% of leukemia cases are of the hairy cell type.
PREDOMINANT SEX: Male/female ratio of 4:1

PHYSICAL FINDINGS & CLINICAL PRESENTATION

- Usually, splenomegaly (present in >90% of cases) caused by tumor cell infiltration (Fig. E1-555)
- Pallor, ecchymosis, and evidence of infection if the pancytopenia is severe
- Weakness, lethargy, and fatigue
- Infections (resulting from impaired resistance caused by neutropenia) and easy bruising (caused by thrombocytopenia) also common

ETIOLOGY

Neoplastic disease of the lymphoreticular system of unknown etiology. A heterozygous mutation in BRAF that results in a BRAF V6000E variant protein has been identified in all patients with hairy cell leukemia

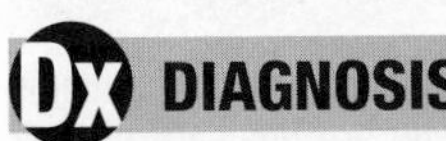

DIAGNOSIS

DIFFERENTIAL DIAGNOSIS

- Other forms of leukemia
- Lymphoma
- Viral syndrome

WORKUP

Comprehensive history, physical examination, and laboratory evaluation to confirm the diagnosis. Table 1-300 describes major diagnostic features of hairy cell leukemia.

LABORATORY TESTS

- Pancytopenia involving erythrocytes, neutrophils, and platelets is common; anemia is usually present and varies from minimal to severe.
- Hairy cells (Fig. 1-556) can account for 5% to 80% of cells in the peripheral blood. The cytoplasmic projections on the cells are redundant plasma membranes.
- Leukemic cells stain positively for tartrate-resistant acid phosphatase stain.
- A bone marrow biopsy (Fig. E1-557) is essential for confirmation and to quantify the degree of hairy cell infiltration. Bone marrow may result in a "dry tap" (because of increased marrow reticulin).

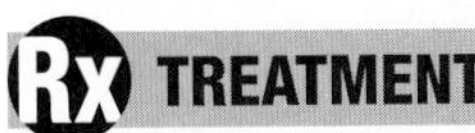

TREATMENT

NONPHARMACOLOGIC THERAPY

Approximately 8% to 10% of patients are asymptomatic and have minimal splenomegaly and minor cytopenia. They are usually detected on routine laboratory evaluation and do not require initial therapy. They should, however, be frequently monitored for progression of disease. Patients require treatment when they have significant cytopenias or occasionally recurrent infections from immunocompromise.

ACUTE GENERAL Rx

- Drugs of choice are the purine analogues 2-chloro-2 deoxyadenosine (cladribine) or 2-deoxycoformycin (DCF, pentostatin). They induce complete remissions in up to 85% of patients and partial responses in 5% to 25%.

TABLE 1-300 Major Diagnostic Features of Hairy Cell Leukemia

Study	Findings
Morphology of hairy cells	Oval or indented nuclei and abundant pale blue cytoplasm Absent or inconspicuous nucleoli Circumferential cell surface "ruffled" projections
Bone marrow biopsy morphology	Diffuse or interstitial bone marrow infiltration, without discrete nodular aggregates Clear cells with "fried egg" or spindled appearance Reticulin fibrosis
Flow cytometry	Clonal B cells expressing *CD103, CD25,* and *CD11c* and lacking *CD5* expression
Immunohistochemistry	Positive for DBA.44, TRAP, and ANXA1

From Jaffe ES et al: *Hematopathology,* Philadelphia, 2011, Saunders.

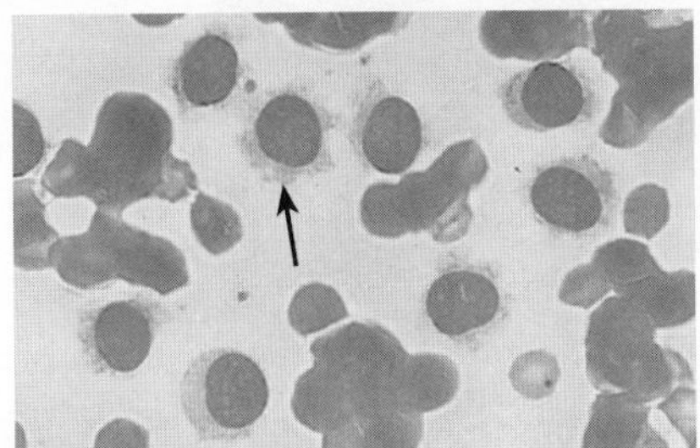

FIGURE 1-556 Hairy cell leukemia. Note the lymphocytes with hairlike cytoplasmic projections surrounding the nucleus. (From Rodak BF: *Diagnostic hematology,* Philadelphia, 1995, Saunders.)

- Cladribine may be preferred because it is easy to administer (0.14 mg/kg qd for 7 days), has minimal toxicity, and is able to induce complete durable responses with a single course of therapy.
- The anti-CD 22 recombinant immunotoxin BL 22 can induce complete remission in patients with hairy cell leukemia resistant to treatment with purine analogues.

CHRONIC Rx

- Patients should be monitored with periodic examination and laboratory tests for progression of disease.
- Approximately 40% of patients with HCL eventually relapse. Relapsed patients can be re-treated with purine analogs or the monoclonal CD20 antibody rituximab. If the prior response was <18 months in duration, rituximab may be preferred over retreatment with cladribine.

DISPOSITION

Prognosis has become increasingly favorable with the newer agents. Approximately 90% of patients who are treated have a complete or partial response.

REFERRAL

Hematology consultation is recommended in all patients.

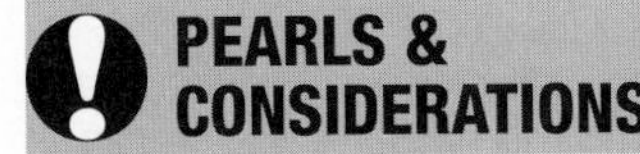

PEARLS & CONSIDERATIONS

COMMENTS

The diagnosis of hairy cell leukemia is occasionally missed and subsequently made by the histopathologist after removal of the spleen for diagnostic purposes.

SUGGESTED READINGS

available at www.expertconsult.com

RELATED CONTENT

Hairy Cell Leukemia (Patient Information)

AUTHOR: **FRED F. FERRI, M.D.**

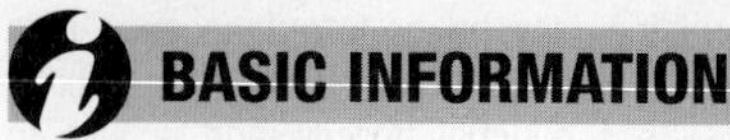

BASIC INFORMATION

DEFINITION

Oral hairy leukoplakia (OHL) is a painless, white, nonremovable, plaquelike lesion typically located on the lateral aspect of the tongue.

ICD-9CM CODES
528.6 Oral hairy leukoplakia
ICD-10CM CODES
K13.3 Hairy leukoplakia

EPIDEMIOLOGY & DEMOGRAPHICS

INCIDENCE AND PREVALENCE: Incidence of Epstein-Barr virus (EBV) seroprevalence is high in individuals who are HIV seropositive. However, OHL occurs in only 25% of these cases.

RISK FACTORS: OHL is usually found in HIV-seropositive individuals (median CD4 count is 468/μL) but may also be identified in smokers and other immunocompromised patients such as transplant recipients (particularly renal) and patients taking steroids. Diagnosing OHL is an indication to institute a workup to evaluate and manage HIV disease.

PHYSICAL FINDINGS & CLINICAL PRESENTATION

- Varying morphology and appearance, which may change daily.
- May be unilateral or bilateral.
- White plaques can be small with fine, vertical corrugations on the lateral margin of the tongue (Fig. 1-558). The plaques from OHL are adherent to the tongue surface (in contrast to candidal plaques, which may be easily scraped off).
- Irregular surface; may have prominent folds or projection, occasionally markedly resembling hairs.
- May spread to cover the entire dorsal surface or spread onto the ventral surface of the tongue where the lesions usually appear flat.
- Rarely, lesions can manifest on the soft palate, buccal mucosa, or posterior oropharynx.
- Usually asymptomatic, but some patients have mouth pain, soreness, or a burning sensation; impaired taste; or difficulty eating; others complain of its unsightly appearance.
- OHL may rarely progress to oral squamous cell carcinoma particularly in smokers, which has a poor prognosis.

ETIOLOGY

EBV is implicated in its etiology, and OHL is a result of replication EBV in the epithelium of keratinized cells. OHL differs from most EBV-related diseases in that infection is predominantly lytic rather than latent.

DIAGNOSIS

DIFFERENTIAL DIAGNOSIS

- *Candida albicans*
- Lichen planus
- Idiopathic leukoplakia
- White sponge nevus
- Dysplasia
- Squamous cell carcinoma

WORKUP

Requires physical examination and evaluation of HIV disease

LABORATORY TESTS

The *provisional* diagnosis is clinical and based on:

- Visual inspection
- Inability to scrape the lesion off the tongue with a blade
- Failure to respond to antifungal therapy

The *presumptive* diagnosis requires biopsy and histologic demonstration of:

- Epithelial hyperplasia with hairs
- Absence of inflammatory cell infiltrate

The *definitive* diagnosis requires:

- In situ hybridization of histologic or cytologic specimens revealing EBV DNA *or*
- Electron microscopy of specimens revealing herpes-like particles
- Measurement of the DNA content in cells of oral leukoplakia may be used to predict the risk of oral carcinoma

NOTE: Specimens obtained from lesions may demonstrate hyphae of *Candida albicans,* which may coexist and potentiate EBV-induced OHL.

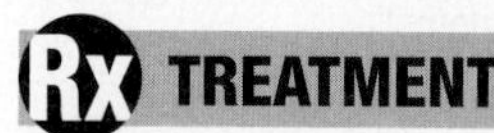

TREATMENT

NONPHARMACOLOGIC THERAPY

OHL is usually asymptomatic and requires no specific therapy. It may resolve spontaneously and is generally benign in HIV-seropositive patients.

ACUTE GENERAL Rx

- Antiretroviral therapy (ART) has considerably changed the frequency of oral lesions caused by opportunistic infections in HIV-seropositive individuals.
- Topical retinoids (0.1% vitamin A) may improve the appearance of OHL-affected oral surfaces through their dekeratinizing and immunomodulation effects; however, they are expensive and prolonged use may result in a burning sensation over the treated area.
- Topical podophyllin resin 25% solution has been reported to induce resolution.
- Surgical excision and cryotherapy may help, but the lesions may recur.
- High-dose acyclovir 800 mg five times per day, valacyclovir 1000 mg tid, famciclovir 500 mg tid, ganciclovir 1000 mg tid, or foscarnet 40 mg/kg IV tid will cause lesions to resolve but only temporarily.

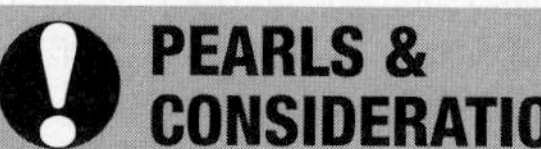

PEARLS & CONSIDERATIONS

- OHL may be the presenting sign of patients infected with HIV who are unaware of their status.
- The incidence has decreased significantly in the era of ART.

SUGGESTED READINGS
available at www.expertconsult.com

RELATED CONTENT

Epstein-Barr Virus Infection (Related Key Topic)
Human Immunodeficiency Virus (Related Key Topic)
Leukoplakia (Patient Information)

AUTHOR: **SAJEEV HANDA, M.D., S.F.H.M.**

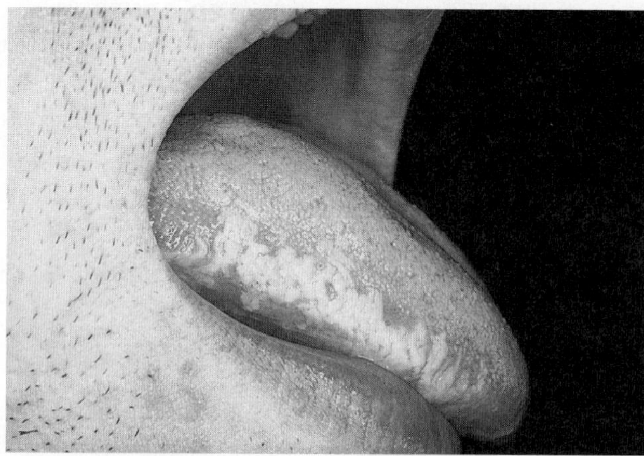

FIGURE 1-558 Oral hairy leukoplakia. Note white verrucoid plaques on the lateral border of the tongue. (From Noble J: *Primary care medicine,* ed 3, St Louis, 2001, Mosby.)

Patients with clones having few or no V-gene mutations or many CD38+ or ZAP-70+ B cells are associated with an aggressive, usually fatal course.

- The percentage of smudge cells (CLL cells ruptured during smear preparation) is associated with mutated IgVH gene status, a favorable prognostic factor. A high percentage of smudge cells on peripheral smear indicates a longer time to treatment from initial diagnosis and better overall survival in patients with early stage CLL.

STAGING:

Rai et al divided CLL into five clinical stages:

- Stage 0: Characterized by lymphocytosis only (>15,000/mm^3 on peripheral smear, bone marrow aspirate ≥40% lymphocytes). The coexistence of lymphocytosis and other factors increases the clinical stage.
- Stage 1: Lymphadenopathy
- Stage 2: Lymphadenopathy/hepatomegaly
- Stage 3: Anemia (hemoglobin [Hgb] <11 g/mm^3)
- Stage 4: Thrombocytopenia (platelets <100,000/mm^3)

Another well-known staging system developed by Binet divides CLL into three stages:

- Stage A: Hgb >10 g/dl, platelets >100,000/mm^3, and fewer than three areas involved (the cervical, axillary, and inguinal lymph nodes [whether unilaterally or bilaterally]; the spleen; and the liver)
- Stage B: Hgb >10 g/dl, platelets >100,000/mm^3, and three or more areas involved
- Stage C: Hgb <10 g/dl, low platelets (<100,000/mm^3), or both (independent of the areas involved)

IMAGING STUDIES

CT scans at diagnosis for assessment of end-organ involvement are not recommended in diagnostic guidelines. However, CT scan of abdomen may be done to evaluate for hepatomegaly and splenomegaly in patients with poor prognostic features.

Rx TREATMENT

NONPHARMACOLOGIC THERAPY

- Treatment goals are relief of symptoms and prolongation of life.
- Observation is appropriate for patients in Rai stage 0 or Binet stage A.
- There are no survival benefits and a slight trend toward worse survival for patients who have early intervention versus deferred chemotherapy.

ACUTE GENERAL Rx

- Symptomatic patients in Rai stage I or II or Binet stage B: fludarabine-based combination chemotherapy: local irradiation for isolated symptomatic lymphadenopathy and lymph nodes that interfere with vital organs.
- Best response rates are seen when combination chemotherapy and retuximab are used (>70% complete response, median time to disease progression >4 years).
- Rai stages III or IV, Binet stage C: chlorambucil chemotherapy with or without prednisone:
  1. Fludarabine, CAP (***c***yclophosphamide, ***A***driamycin, ***p***rednisone), or cyclophosphamide, doxorubicin, vincristine, and prednisone (mini-CHOP) can be used in patients who respond poorly to chlorambucil.
  2. Monoclonal antibodies: rituximab, ofatumumab, or alemtuzumab is useful for treatment of patients with CLL refractory to fludarabine.
  3. Splenic irradiation can be used in selected patients with advanced disease.
  4. Bendamustine, an alkylator in the nitrogen mustard family, is well tolerated and can also be used in some patients with CLL.
  5. Combination therapy with fludarabine (F), cyclophosphamide (C), rituximab (R) [FCR] provides additional benefits beyond single-agent therapy. It has shown to improve progression-free and overall survival in patients with CLL who do not have deletion of chromosome 17p and who are considered fit enough for fludarabine-based chemotherapy.
  6. Recent trials[1] have shown that ibrutinib, an oral covalent inhibitor of Bruton's tyrosine kinase (BKT), an essential component of B-cell receptor signaling, is associated with a high frequency of durable remissions in patients with relapsed or refractory CLL.
- An algorithm to treatment approach to first relapsed CLL is described in Fig. 1-552.

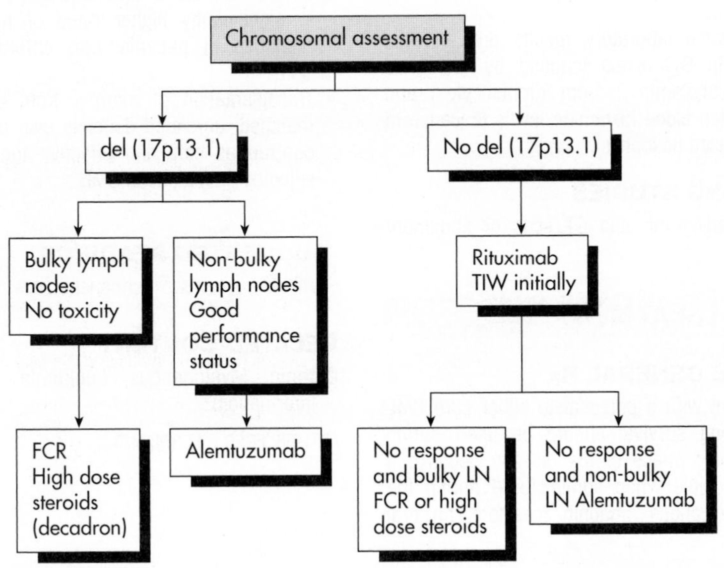

FIGURE 1-552 Algorithm to treatment approach to first relapsed chronic lymphocytic leukemia. (Modified from Hoffman R et al: *Hematology: basic principles and practice*, ed 5, Philadelphia, 2009, Churchill Livingstone.)

CHRONIC Rx

Treatment of systemic complications:

- Hypogammaglobulinemia is frequent in CLL and is the chief cause of infections. Immune globulin (250 mg/kg IV every 4 wk) may prevent infections but has no effect on survival rate. Infections should be treated with broad-spectrum antibiotics. Patients should be monitored for opportunistic infections.
- Recombinant hematopoietic cofactors (e.g., granulocyte-macrophage colony stimulating factor and granulocyte colony stimulating factor) may be useful to overcome neutropenia related to treatment.
- Erythropoietin may be useful to treat anemia that is unresponsive to other measures.

DISPOSITION

The patient's prognosis is generally directly related to the clinical stage (e.g., the average survival in patients in Rai stage 0 or Binet stage A is >120 mo, whereas for Rai stage 4 or Binet stage C it is approximately 30 mo). Overall 5-yr survival is 60%. Measurement of ZAP-70 intracellular protein (where available) is also a useful indicator of prognosis.

SUGGESTED READINGS

available at www.expertconsult.com

RELATED CONTENT

Chronic Lymphocytic Leukemia (Patient Information)

AUTHOR: **FRED F. FERRI, M.D.**

[1]Byrd JC et al: Targeting BTK with ibrutinib in relapsed chronic lymphocytic leukemia, *N Engl J Med* 369:32-42, 2013.

BASIC INFORMATION

DEFINITION

Chronic myelogenous leukemia (CML) is a malignant clonal stem disease caused by an acquired somatic mutation that fuses, through chromosomal translocation, the *ABL* and *BCR* genes on chromosomes 9 and 22 and is characterized by abnormal proliferation and accumulation of immature granulocytes. CML manifests with a chronic phase (CP-CML) lasting months to years, followed by an advanced phase (AP-CML) characterized by poor response to therapy, worsening anemia, or decreased platelet count; the second phase then evolves into a terminal phase (acute transformation) that degenerates into acute leukemia (mostly myeloid and approximately 20% lymphoid subtype), characterized by elevated number of blast cells and numerous complications (e.g., sepsis, bleeding).

SYNONYMS

CML
Chronic granulocytic leukemia
Chronic myeloid leukemia

ICD-9CM CODES
201.1 Chronic myelogenous leukemia
ICD-10CM CODES
C92.10 Chronic myeloid leukemia, BCR/ABL-positive, not having achieved remission

EPIDEMIOLOGY & DEMOGRAPHICS

- CML usually affects elderly patients (median age at presentation is 65 yr) and accounts for 15% of adult cases of leukemia
- Incidence is one to two cases per 100,000 people annually

PHYSICAL FINDINGS & CLINICAL PRESENTATION

- The chronic phase usually reveals splenomegaly; hepatomegaly is not infrequent, but lymphadenopathy is highly unusual and generally indicates the accelerated proliferative phase of the disease.
- Common symptoms at the time of diagnosis are weakness or discomfort from an enlarged spleen (abdominal discomfort or pain). Splenomegaly is present in up to 40% of patients at time of diagnosis.
- 40% of patients are asymptomatic, and diagnosis is based solely on an abnormal blood count.

ETIOLOGY

Current evidence strongly implicates the chromosome translocation t(9;22) (q34;q11.2) as the cause of chronic granulocytic leukemia. This translocation is present in >95% of patients. The remaining patients have a complex or variant translocation involving additional chromosomes that have the same end result (fusion of the *BCR* [break point cluster region] gene on chromosome 22 to *ABL* [Ableson leukemia virus] gene on chromosome 9).

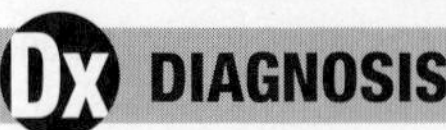

DIAGNOSIS

DIFFERENTIAL DIAGNOSIS

- Splenic lymphoma
- Chronic lymphocytic leukemia
- Myelodysplastic syndrome

LABORATORY TESTS

- Elevated white blood cell count (generally >100,000/mm^3) with broad spectrum of granulocytic forms.
- Bone marrow demonstrates hypercellularity with granulocytic hyperplasia, increased ratio of myeloid cells to erythroid cells, and increased number of megakaryocytes (Fig. E1-553). Blasts and promyelocytes constitute <10% of all cells.
- The Philadelphia chromosome results from the reciprocal translocation between the long arms of chromosomes 9 and 22 [Fig. E1-554] and is present in >95% of patients with CML; its presence (Ph^1) is a major prognostic factor because survival rate of patients with Philadelphia chromosome is approximately eight times better than that of those without it. Some believe that Ph^1(+) defines CML and that those who are Ph^1(–) have another disease.
- Leukocyte alkaline phosphatase is markedly decreased (used to distinguish CML from other myeloproliferative disorders).
- Anemia and thrombocytosis are often present.
- Additional laboratory results are elevated vitamin B_{12} levels (caused by increased transcobalamin 1 from granulocytes) and elevated blood histamine levels (because of increased basophils).

IMAGING STUDIES

Chest radiograph and CT scan of abdomen/pelvis

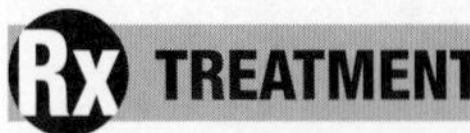

TREATMENT

ACUTE GENERAL Rx

Treatment with a potential to either cure CML or prolong survival should be used during the chronic phase of the disease because it is often futile when administered during the advanced phase. Imatinib mesylate, an oral tyrosine kinase inhibitor, is effective and indicated as first-line treatment for CML myeloid blast crisis, accelerated phase, or CML in its chronic phase. More than 75% of patients have major cytogenetic response (<35% Philadelphia chromosome-positive cells in the marrow), and more than 80% have progression-free survival after 24 mo. Complete hematologic response usually occurs in <1 mo. Nilotinib and dasatinib are newer, more effective agents that also inhibit the activity of the BCR-ABL fusion protein by binding to a particular site and can be used after failure of imatinib and eventually may become first-line agents. Ponatinib is a newer oral tyrosine kinase inhibitor that blocks native and mutated BCR-ABL and has been shown to be highly active in pretreated patients with Ph-positive leukemias with resistance to other tyrosine kinase inhibitors.

- Symptomatic hyperleukocytosis (e.g., central nervous system symptoms) can be treated with leukapheresis and hydroxyurea; allopurinol should be started to prevent urate nephropathy after the rapid lysis of the leukemia cells.
- Allogeneic stem-cell transplantation (SCT) is the only curative treatment for CML in the chronic phase unresponsive to imatinib. In general only 20% of patients are candidates for SCT given the limitations of age or lack of HLA-matched related donors.
    1. It should be considered in "young" patients (increased survival in patients <55 yr) with compatible siblings.
    2. Early transplantation is also important for patient's survival.
- Interferon-alfa is an acceptable alternative in the early chronic phase for patients who do not tolerate tyrosine kinase inhibitors.
- Recent trials have shown that as compared with other treatments, the addition of peginterferon alfa-2a to imatinib therapy resulted in significantly higher rates of molecular response in patients with chronic-phase CML.
- Transplantation of marrow from an HLA-matched, unrelated donor is also now recognized as safe and effective therapy for selected patients with CML.

SUGGESTED READINGS

available at www.expertconsult.com

RELATED CONTENT

Chronic Myelogenous Leukemia (Patient Information)

AUTHOR: **FRED F. FERRI, M.D.**

BASIC INFORMATION

DEFINITION

Lichen planus (LP) refers to an idiopathic inflammatory disease manifesting with a papular skin eruption characteristically found over the flexor surfaces of the extremities, genitalia, and mucous membranes.

SYNONYMS

Lichen
Lichen planus et atrophicus
LP

ICD-9CM CODES
697.0 Lichen planus
ICD-10CM CODES
L43 Lichen planus
L43.0 Hypertrophic lichen planus
L43.1 Bullous lichen planus
L43.9 Lichen planus, unspecified
L43.8 Other lichen planus

EPIDEMIOLOGY & DEMOGRAPHICS

INCIDENCE: One in every 100 new patients seen in dermatology clinics in the U.S. is diagnosed with LP
PREVALENCE: 440 cases/100,000 persons
PREDOMINANT SEX: Found equally between males and females (1:1)
PREDOMINANT AGE: Usually found in people between the ages of 30 and 60 yr
PREDISPOSING FACTORS:
1. Associated with other autoimmune disorders (e.g., primary biliary cirrhosis, myasthenia gravis, ulcerative colitis, diabetes)
2. Associated with hepatitis C infection
3. Drug-induced form affects any area of the body surface (e.g., beta-blocker, methyldopa, penicillamine, quinidine, nonsteroidal antiinflammatory drugs, angiotensin-converting enzyme inhibitors, sulfonylurea agents)

PHYSICAL FINDINGS & CLINICAL PRESENTATION

The clinical presentation varies depending on the area involved.
History:
- Usually starts on an extremity and may remain localized or spread to involve other areas over a 1- to 4-mo period
- Pruritic

Physical findings:
- Anatomic distribution:
  1. Flexor surface of wrists, forearms, shins, and upper thighs
  2. Neck and back area
  3. Nails (5%-10% of patients)
  4. Scalp (lichen planopilaris)
  5. Oral mucosa, buccal mucosa, tongue, gingiva, and lips; oral lichen planus can cause extensive dequamative gingivitis
  6. Vulva, penis

Genital mucosa:
- Lesion configuration:
  1. Linear
  2. Annular (more common)
  3. Reticular pattern noted on oral mucosa and genital area
- Lesion morphology:
  1. Papules most common presentation (flat, smooth, shiny) (Fig. 1-559)
  2. Hypertrophic
  3. Follicular
  4. Vesicular
- Color:
  1. Dark red, bluish red, purplish-violaceous color is noted in cutaneous LP.
  2. Individual lesions characteristically have white lines visible (Wickham's striae).
  3. Oral and genital LP has a reticular network of white lines that may be raised or annular in appearance.
- Scalp lesions may result in alopecia.

ETIOLOGY

The cause of LP is unknown. It is believed that LP represents a T-cell–mediated inflammatory disorder.

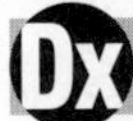

DIAGNOSIS

- Clinical history and physical findings usually establish the diagnosis of LP.
- Skin biopsy (deep shave or punch biopsy of the most developed lesion) can be performed to confirm the diagnosis.

DIFFERENTIAL DIAGNOSIS

Drug eruption, psoriasis, Bowen's disease, leukoplakia, candidiasis, lupus rash, secondary syphilis, seborrheic dermatitis, chronic graft vs. host disease

WORKUP

If the diagnosis is questionable, a skin biopsy is performed.

LABORATORY TESTS

Laboratory tests are not specific for the diagnosis of LP. Lipid panels screening is useful since increases in serum triglycerides and decreases in HDL cholesterol are common in patients with LP.

IMAGING STUDIES

Imaging studies are not helpful in diagnosing LP.

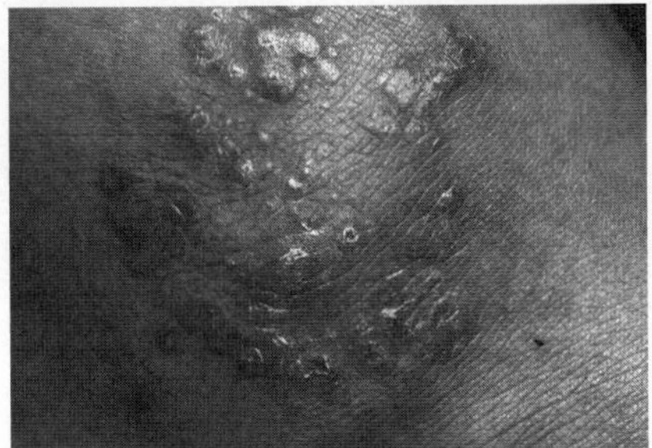

FIGURE 1-559 Flat-topped, purple polygonal papules of the lichen planus. (From Morelli JG: Diseases of the epidermis. In Kliegman RM et al [eds]: *Nelson textbook of pediatrics,* ed 19, Philadelphia, 2011, Saunders.)

TREATMENT

NONPHARMACOLOGIC THERAPY

- Avoid scratching.
- Use mild soaps and emollients after bathing to prevent dryness.

ACUTE GENERAL Rx

For cutaneous LP:
- Topical steroids (e.g., triamcinolone acetonide 0.1%, fluocinonide 0.05%, clobetasol propionate 0.05% cream or ointment) with occlusion used twice daily.
- Acitretin 30 mg/day PO for 8 wk.
- Systemic prednisone 30 to 60 mg/day as a starting dose and tapered to 15 to 20 mg/day maintenance for 6 wk.
- Intradermal steroid triamcinolone acetonide 5 mg/ml can be tried for thick hyperkeratotic lesions.
- Hydroxyzine 25 mg PO q6h can be used for pruritus.
- Phototherapy: PUVA or narrow-band ultraviolet B therapy: 2 or 3 times per week, for a total of 12 sessions (i.e., one cycle).

For oral LP:
- Topical steroid fluocinonide in an adhesive base used six times/day for 9 wk.
- Topical calcineurin in steroid-unresponsive cases.
- Topical or systemic retinoids 0.1% retinoic acid in an adhesive base or gel.
- Etretinate 75 mg/day for 2 mo.

CHRONIC Rx

Refer to "Acute General Rx."

DISPOSITION

- Spontaneous remissions of cutaneous LP occur in more than 65% of cases within the first year.
- Spontaneous remission of oral LP usually occurs by 5 yr.
- Approximately 10% to 20% of patients will have recurrence.

REFERRAL

To dermatologist if diagnosis is unclear

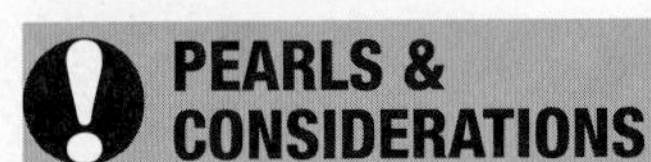

PEARLS & CONSIDERATIONS

COMMENTS

- LP can be remembered as purple, planar, pruritic, polygonal, papules, and plaques (six P's).
- Lesions can develop at the site of prior skin injury (Koebner's phenomenon).
- Although there is an increased risk of squamous cell carcinoma in chronic lesions of mucosal LP, transformation to skin cancer is uncommon.

SUGGESTED READINGS

available at www.expertconsult.com

RELATED CONTENT

Lichen Planus (Patient Information)

AUTHOR: **TANYA ALI, M.D.**

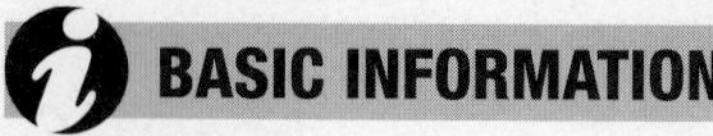

BASIC INFORMATION

DEFINITION

Lichen sclerosus is a chronic inflammatory condition of the skin usually affecting the vulva, perianal area, and groin.

ICD-9CM CODES
701.0 Lichen sclerosus
ICD-10CM CODES
L90.0 Lichen sclerosus et atrophicus

EPIDEMIOLOGY & DEMOGRAPHICS

- Most common in postmenopausal women and men between ages 40 and 60 yr
- More common in females (female/male ratio of 5:1)
- Can occur in children (usually prepubertal girls with involvement of the vulva and perineum)

PHYSICAL FINDINGS & CLINICAL PRESENTATION

- Erythema may be the only initial sign. A characteristic finding is the presence of ivory-white atrophic lesions on the involved area.
- Close inspection of the affected area will reveal the presence of white-to-brown follicular plugs on the surface (dells).
- When the genitals are involved, the white, parchment-like skin assumes an hourglass configuration around the introital and perianal area ("keyhole" distribution; Fig. 1-560). Inflammation, subepithelial hemorrhages, and chronic ulceration may develop.
- Dyspareunia, genital bleeding, and anal bleeding are common.

ETIOLOGY

Unknown. There may be an autoimmune association and a genetic familial component.

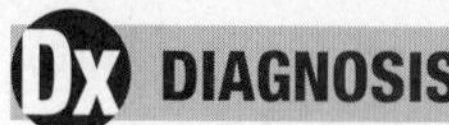

DIAGNOSIS

DIFFERENTIAL DIAGNOSIS

- Localized scleroderma (morphea)
- Cutaneous discoid lupus erythematosus
- Atrophic lichen planus
- Psoriasis

WORKUP

Diagnosis is based on close examination of the lesions for the presence of ivory-white atrophic lesions and typical location.

LABORATORY TESTS

Punch or deep shave biopsy can be used to confirm the diagnosis.

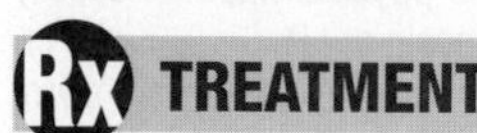

TREATMENT

NONPHARMACOLOGIC THERAPY

Attention to hygiene and elimination of irritants or excessive bathing with harsh soaps

GENERAL Rx

- Application of clobetasol propionate 0.05% topically bid for up to 4 wk is usually effective. Repeat courses of corticosteroids may be necessary because of the chronic nature of this disorder. Continual application of topical steroids may lead to atrophy of the vulva.
- There is no substantial evidence that use of topical sex hormones (e.g., topical testosterone [2%]) is effective in genital lichen sclerosus.
- Lubricants (e.g., Nutraplus cream) are useful to soothe dry tissues.
- Hydroxyzine 25 mg at bedtime is effective in decreasing nocturnal itching.
- Use of intralesional steroids, etretinate, and surgical management is usually reserved for refractory cases.

DISPOSITION

- The disease persists in approximately one third of patients.
- Most prepubertal girls improve spontaneously at menarche.
- Squamous cell carcinoma can develop within the lesions in 3% to 10% of older patients; therefore periodic examination and biopsy of suspicious areas are indicated.

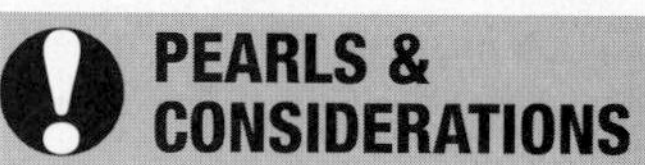

PEARLS & CONSIDERATIONS

COMMENTS

- Prepubertal lichen sclerosus may be confused with sexual abuse in prepubertal girls and may lead to false accusations and investigations.
- Lichen sclerosus of the vulva (kraurosis vulvae) usually occurs after menopause and is generally chronic. It can be painful and interfere with sexual activity.
- Lichen sclerosus of the penis (balanitis xerotica obliterans) is seen more commonly in uncircumcised males. It affects the glans and prepuce and may lead to stricture if it encroaches into the urinary meatus.

SUGGESTED READINGS

available at www.expertconsult.com

RELATED CONTENT

Lichen Sclerosus (Patient Information)

AUTHOR: **FRED F. FERRI, M.D.**

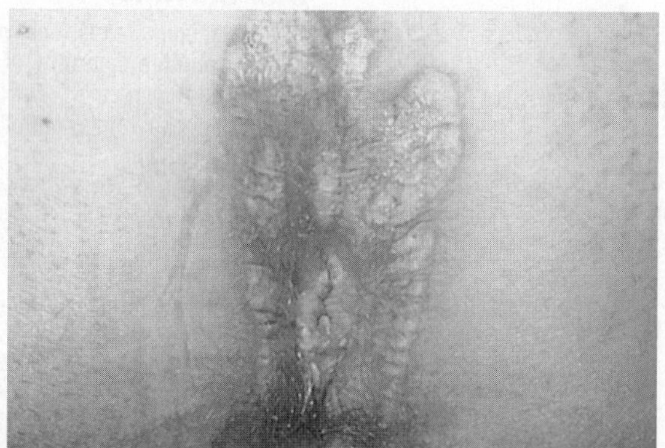

FIGURE 1-560 Lichen sclerosus. Perianal area is thinned and chalk white (keyhole distribution). (Courtesy Department of Dermatology, University of North Carolina at Chapel Hill. From Goldstein BG, Goldstein AO: *Practical dermatology,* ed 2, St Louis, 1997, Mosby.)

BASIC INFORMATION

DEFINITION

Lichen simplex chronicus is neurodermatitis manifesting with localized areas of thickened, hyperplastic scaly skin due to prolonged and severe scratching in patients with no underlying dermatologic condition.

SYNONYMS

Neurodermatitis from rubbing

ICD-9CM CODES
698.3 Lichenification and lichen simplex chronicus
ICD-10CM CODES
L28.0 Lichen simplex chronicus

EPIDEMIOLOGY & DEMOGRAPHICS

PEAK INCIDENCE: Between 35 and 50 yr old
PREVALENCE: Increased in patients with underlying anxiety disorders
PREDOMINANT SEX AND AGE:

- Sex: Females > males (2:1)
- Age: Adults over 60

RISK FACTORS: Anxiety disorders, dry skin, insect bites

PHYSICAL FINDINGS & CLINICAL PRESENTATION

- Patients present with profound pruritus and localized scaly plaques with accentuated skin markings said to resemble tree bark (Fig. 1-561).
- Lichenified circumscribed plaques. Trauma from rubbing and scratching accounts for persistence of the plaque.
- Commonly involved areas include hands and wrists (Fig. 1-562), back and sides of neck, anterior tibias, anogenital areas, and ankles.

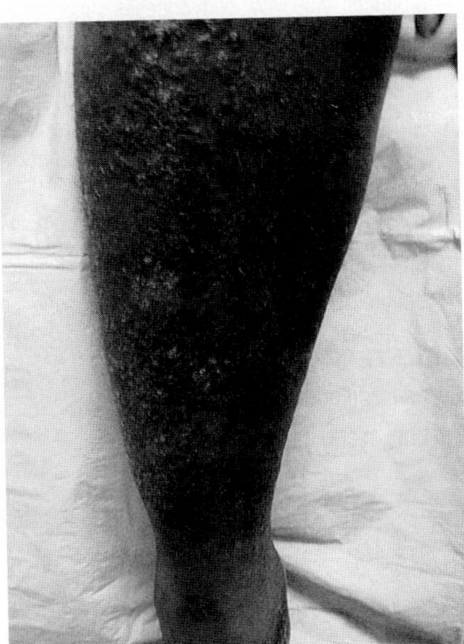

FIGURE 1-561 Lichenified skin of the lower extremity caused by habitual rubbing. The confluence of multiple scaling papules has formed a large plaque of palpably thickened skin. (From Ferri FF et al: *Ferri's fast facts in dermatology,* Philadelphia, 2010, Saunders.)

ETIOLOGY

- Neurodermatitis
- Common triggers are excess dryness of skin, heat, sweat, and psychological stress. It can also accompany other conditions such as the fungal infections candidiasis or tinea cruris, or psoriasis, lichen sclerosus, and neoplasia, leading to squamous cell hyperplasia.
- Other causes include atrophic dermatitis and insect bites. Rare cases have shown links to lithium use, hair dye containing PPD, and long-term exposure to vehicle pollution.

Dx DIAGNOSIS

DIFFERENTIAL DIAGNOSIS

- Lichen planus
- Psoriasis
- Atopic dermatitis
- Insect bite
- Nummular eczema
- Contact dermatitis
- Stasis dermatitis

WORKUP

Patient history and skin examination. Skin biopsy when diagnosis is unclear or persistent symptoms.

LABORATORY TESTS

- Not generally necessary
- Biopsy reveals hyperkeratosis, acanthosis, and mild to moderate lymphohistocytic inflammatory infiltrate with prominent lichenification.

Rx TREATMENT

NONPHARMACOLOGIC THERAPY

- Patient education is essential to break the itch-scratch cycle and facilitate treatment of any underlying dermatitis.
- Psychotherapy

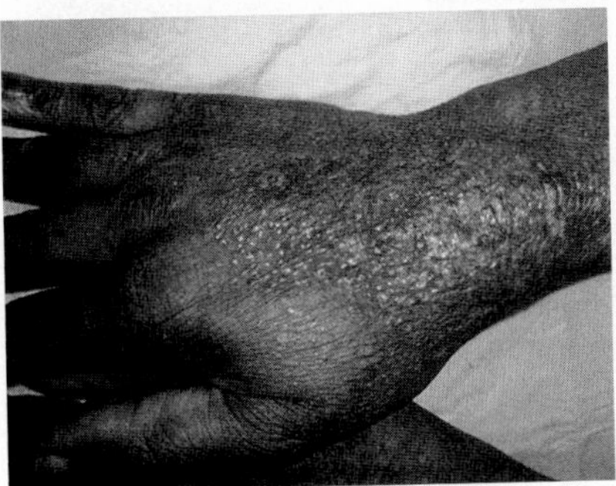

FIGURE 1-562 Longstanding pruritus and scratching resulted in this thickened, hyperpigmented skin on the wrist consisting of numerous 1- to 2-mm papules. This "follicular" pattern is more common in African Americans. (From Ferri FF et al: *Ferri's fast facts in dermatology,* Philadelphia, 2010, Saunders.)

ACUTE GENERAL Rx

- Antihistamine hydroxyzine 25 mg at bedtime is effective in decreasing nocturnal itching.
- Topical corticosteroids
- Intralesional corticosteroids
- Anxiolytics, SSRIs
- Oral doxepin (an antidepressant and anxiolytic)
- Mirtazapine
- Tropical calcineurin inhibitor for vulvar lichenification

Cyclosporin A

Topical tacrolimus, 0.1% ointment, can be used for sensitive skin—face.

Botulinum intradermal injections

Alitretinoin, 30 mg daily for 3 mo, has shown some clinical improvement in case studies but needs further investigation as a potential rx.

CHRONIC Rx

Constant irritation of the skin must be avoided. Keeping skin moisturized, a covering to prevent scratching, or nail filing may be necessary.

DISPOSITION

Psychological intervention improves recovery. Regular follow-up visits facilitate long-term management.

REFERRAL

Refer to a psychologist for psychological evaluation and consultation, and a dermatologist in resistant cases.

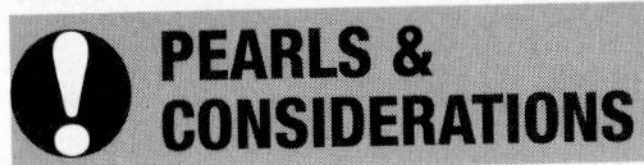

PEARLS & CONSIDERATIONS

- Significant scratching may occur during nocturnal hours.
- The involved area is always at a site that is easily reached for scratching.
- Chronic scratching can also cause keratinocyte necrosis and the development of amyloid in the papillary dermis, called lichen amyloidosis.

COMMENTS

Patients may be at increased risk for scarring of the skin, changes in skin pigmentation, and bacterial and fungal infections of the involved skin.

PREVENTION

Prevent future incidences by continued therapy, stress management, and avoidance of common triggers and accompanying conditions.

SUGGESTED READINGS
available at www.expertconsult.com

AUTHORS: **FRED F. FERRI, M.D.,** and **HEATHER FERRI, D.O.**

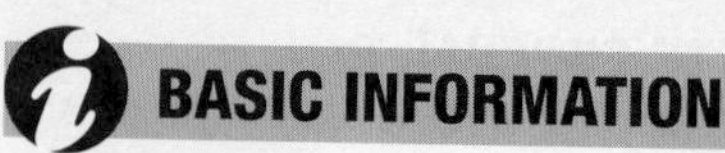

BASIC INFORMATION

DEFINITION

Listeriosis is a systemic infection caused by the gram-positive aerobic bacterium *Listeria monocytogenes.*

SYNONYMS

Listerial infection
Granulomatosis infantisepticum

ICD-9CM CODES

027.0	Listeriosis
771.2	Congenital listeriosis
771.2	Fetal listeriosis
665.4	Suspected fetal damage affecting management of pregnancy

ICD-10CM CODES

A32	Listeriosis
A32.0	Cutaneous listeriosis
A32.7	Listerial sepsis
A32.8	Other forms of listeriosis
A32.9	Listeriosis, unspecified
A32.11	Listerial meningitis

EPIDEMIOLOGY & DEMOGRAPHICS

INCIDENCE (IN U.S.):

- *Listeria* meningitis: about 0.7 cases/100,000 persons (fourth most common cause of community-acquired bacterial meningitis in adults)
- Perinatal listeriosis: 8.6 cases/100,000 persons
- Nonperinatal listeriosis: 3 cases/1 million persons

PREDOMINANT SEX: Pregnant women are more susceptible to *Listeria* bacteremia, accounting for up to one third of reported cases.

PREDOMINANT AGE:

- Pregnant women
- Immunocompromised patients of any age
- Elderly patients are susceptible even in the absence of recognized immunocompromised states

GENETICS:

Congenital infection:

- With transplacental transmission, syndrome termed *granulomatosis infantisepticum* in neonate
- Characterized by disseminated abscesses in multiple organs, skin lesions, and conjunctivitis
- Mortality: 33% to 100%

Neonatal infection:

- Infant becoming ill after 3 days of age; mother invariably asymptomatic
- Clinical picture of sepsis of unknown origin

PHYSICAL FINDINGS & CLINICAL PRESENTATION

Infections in pregnancy

1. More common in third trimester
2. Usually present with fever and chills without localizing symptoms or signs of infection

Meningoencephalitis

1. More common in neonates and immunocompromised patients, but up to 30% of adults have no underlying condition
2. In neonates: poor appetite with or without fever possibly the only presenting signs
3. In adults: presentation often subacute, with low-grade fever and personality change as only signs
4. Focal neurologic signs seen without demonstrable brain abscess on CT scan

Cerebritis/rhombencephalitis

1. Headache and fever may be only presenting complaints
2. Progressive cranial nerve palsies, hemiparesis, seizures, depressed level of consciousness, cerebellar signs, respiratory insufficiency may also be seen

Focal infections

1. Ocular infections (purulent conjunctivitis) and skin lesions (granulomatosis infantisepticum) as a result of inadvertent inoculation by laboratory and veterinary personnel
2. Others: arthritis, prosthetic joint infections, peritonitis, osteomyelitis, organ abscesses, cholecystitis

ETIOLOGY

- Direct invasion of skin and eye has been documented, but mechanism of GI entry is unclear.
- Organism's intracellular life cycle explanatory of:
  1. Importance of cell-mediated immunity in host defense
  2. Increased infection in neonates, pregnant women, and immunocompromised hosts

DIAGNOSIS

DIFFERENTIAL DIAGNOSIS

- Meningitis caused by other bacteria, mycobacteria, or fungi
- CNS sarcoidosis
- Brain neoplasm or abscess
- Tuberculous and fungal (especially cryptococcal) meningitis
- Cerebral toxoplasmosis
- Lyme disease
- Sarcoidosis

WORKUP

Dictated by age, end-organ involvement, and immune status

LABORATORY TESTS

- Cultures of blood and other appropriate body fluids
- Variable CSF findings, but neutrophils usually predominate
- Organisms uncommonly seen on Gram stain and may be difficult to identify morphologically
- Monoclonal antibodies, polymerase chain reaction, and DNA probe techniques to detect *Listeria* in foods

IMAGING STUDIES

- If focal cerebral involvement suspected: CT scan or MRI
- MRI most sensitive for evaluation of brainstem and cerebellum

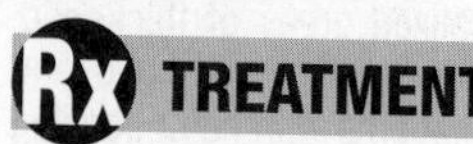

TREATMENT

Empiric therapy should be administered when diagnosis is suspected because overall mortality is 23%.

ACUTE GENERAL Rx

- Drugs of choice:
  1. IV ampicillin 8 to 12 g/day in divided doses
  2. IV penicillin 12 to 24 million U/day in divided doses
- Continuation of therapy for 2 wk
- Alternative (if penicillin allergic): trimethoprim/sulfamethoxazole or vancomycin
- Gentamicin added to provide synergy in meningitis or endocarditis

CHRONIC Rx

Relapses reported, especially in immunocompromised hosts, after 2 wk of therapy.

DISPOSITION

Long-term follow-up of immunodeficiency state

REFERRAL

Infectious disease consultation for all patients

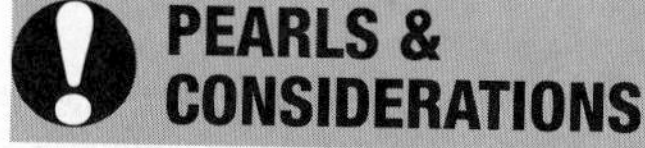

PEARLS & CONSIDERATIONS

COMMENTS

- Foodborne cases have been linked to various products: coleslaw, soft cheeses, unpasteurized milk and milk products, vegetables, undercooked chicken, hot dogs, luncheon meats, refrigerated smoked seafood, and so on.
- Complete decontamination of food products is difficult because *Listeria* is resistant to pasteurization and refrigeration.

SUGGESTED READINGS

available at www.expertconsult.com

RELATED CONTENT

Listeriosis (Patient Information)

AUTHOR: **GLENN G. FORT, M.D., M.P.H.**

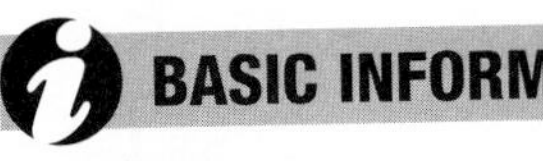

BASIC INFORMATION

DEFINITION

Long QT syndrome (LQTS) is a disorder of myocardial repolarization characterized by a prolongation of the QT interval on the ECG associated with an increased risk of developing life-threatening ventricular arrhythmias, most commonly torsades de pointes (a specific type of polymorphic ventricular tachycardia), which may lead to ventricular fibrillation and sudden cardiac death (SCD). This syndrome may be either genetic or acquired.

SYNONYMS

LQTS
Congenital forms:
- Jervell and Lange-Nielsen syndrome (associated with deafness)
- Romano-Ward syndrome (associated with normal hearing)

ICD-9CM CODES
427.9 Unspecified cardiac dysrhythmia
ICD-10CM CODES
I45.81 Long QT syndrome

EPIDEMIOLOGY & DEMOGRAPHICS

- Congenital LQTS is thought to account for more than 3000 deaths in childhood per year in the United States.
- Incidence of LQTS is thought to be between 1:2500 and 1:10,000 in the general population, although it has been difficult to estimate due to incomplete penetrance.
- Congenital form associated with deafness is autosomal recessive (Jervell and Lange Nielsen syndrome) and is less common than the autosomal dominant form as well as more severe.
- Congenital form associated with normal hearing (Romano-Ward syndrome) is autosomal dominant. Although inheritance of LQTS is autosomal dominant, female predominance has often been observed and has been attributed to an increased susceptibility to cardiac arrhythmias in women.
- At least 13 different LQTS genes have been identified to date.
- LQTS is more common in women than in men.
- Mortality rate is estimated to be about 1% per year.
- Genetic mutations in the congenital LQTS are described in Table 1-301. Common types of LQTS are described in Table 1-302.

PHYSICAL FINDINGS & CLINICAL PRESENTATION

- Many episodes are stress mediated.
- Palpitations, presyncope
- Syncope caused by ventricular tachycardia
- SCD
- Seizure
- Family history of LQTS, but a family history of SCD has not been proved to be a risk factor for SCD in patients with LQTS
- Abnormal ECG (prolonged QT) in asymptomatic relatives of known case
- Prolonged QTc interval on ECG (QTc should be >460 ms in women and >440 ms in men)
- In case of congenital LQTS, the presentation of syncope or SCD is typically triggered by exercise and swimming in LQT1 patients, in LQT2 patients by emotion, pregnancy, or noise, and patients with LQT3 are at highest risk of events when at rest or asleep

ETIOLOGY

- Cardiac repolarization abnormality
- Congenital cause (hundreds of mutations on more than 10 genes have been identified)
- Most of the gene mutations affect function of ion channels leading to prolonged repolarization (i.e., sodium and potassium channels resulting in either increased Na^+ influx or decreased K^+ efflux). These mutations prolong depolarization and predispose the patient to torsades de pointes.
- Acquired causes:
  - Drugs: dofetilide, ibutilide, bepridil, quinidine, procainamide, sotalol, amiodarone, ranolazine, disopyramide, phenothiazines and antiemetic agents (droperidol, domperidone), tricyclic antidepressants, antipsychotics (quetiapine, ziprasidone, iloperidone), citalopram, antihistamines, quinolones, azithromycin, astemizole or cisapride given with ketoconazole or erythromycin,

TABLE 1-301 Genetic Mutations in Congenital Long QT Syndrome

		Location	Gene	Current	Effect
Romano-Ward syndrome (autosomal-dominant inheritance)	*LQT1*	11p15.5	*KCNQ1* (K^+ channel)	I_{Ks}	↓ Function ↓ Repolarization
	LQT2	7q35-36	*KCNH2* (K^+ channel)	I_{Kr}	↓ Function ↓ Repolarization
	LQT3	3q21-24	*SCN5A* (Na^+ channel)	I_{Na}	↑ Function ↑ Depolarization
	LQT4	4q25-27	*ANK2*	Unknown	Unknown
	LQT5	21q22	*KCNE1* (K^+ channel, subunit minK)	I_{Ks}	↓ Function ↓ Repolarization
Jervell and Lange-Nielsen syndrome (autosomal-recessive inheritance)		11p15.5	*KvLQT1* (K^+ channel)	I_{Ks}	↓ Function ↓ Repolarization
		21q22	*KCNE* 1 (K^+ channel, subunit minK)	I_{Ks}	↓ Function ↓ Repolarization

From Crawford MH et al (eds): *Cardiology*, ed 2, St Louis, 2004, Mosby.

TABLE 1-302 Common Types of Long QT (LQT) Syndrome

	LQT1	LQT2	LQT3
Pathophysiology			
Gene	*KCNQ1 (KvLQT1)*	*KCNH2 (HERG)*	*SCN5A*
Protein	$K_v7.1$	$K_v11.1$	$Na_v1.5$
Ionic current	Decreased I_{Ks}	Decreased I_{Kr}	Increased late I_{Na}
Clinical Presentation			
Incidence of cardiac events	63%	46%	18%
Incidence of SCD	4%	4%	4%
Arrhythmia triggers	Emotional/physical stress (swimming, diving)	Emotional stress, arousal (alarm clock, telephone), rest	Sleep/rest
ECG	Broad-based T wave	Low-amplitude, bifid T wave	Long isoelectric ST segment
QT response to exercise	Attenuated QTc shortening and an exaggerated QTc prolongation during early and peak exercise	Normal QT during exercise but with exaggerated QT hysteresis	Supernormal QT shortening
Management			
Exercise restriction	+++	++	?
Response to beta blockers	+++	+++	?
Potassium supplement	+	++	+
Left cervicothoracic sympathectomy	++	++	++
Response to mexiletine	+	+	++

From Issa Z et al: *Clinical arrhythmology and electrophysiology*, ed 2, Philadelphia, 2012, Saunders.

clarithromycin, and antimalarials, particularly among patients with asthma or those using potassium-lowering medications; also common in patients receiving methadone
- Hypokalemia, hypomagnesemia, hypocalcemia (especially in patients with malabsorption syndrome)
- Liquid protein diet
- Central nervous system lesions
- Ischemia
- Hypothyroidism

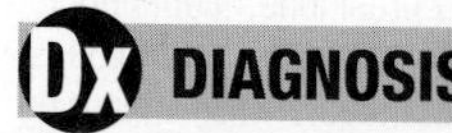

DIAGNOSIS

DIFFERENTIAL DIAGNOSIS

See "Syncope." Brugada's syndrome, arrhythmogenic right ventricular dysplasia, and LQTS are major causes of genetic sudden death syndromes (Fig. 1-563).

Diagnostic criteria for the congenital LQTS:

ECG Criteria	
QTc >480 ms	3 points
QTc 460-480 ms	2 points
QTc 450-460 ms (males)	1 point
Torsades de pointes	2 points
T-wave alternans	1 point
Notched T wave in 3 leads	1 point
Bradycardia	0.5 point
History	
Syncope with stress	2 points
Syncope without stress	1 point
Congenital deafness	0.5 point
Definite family history of long QT	1 point
Unexplained cardiac death in first-degree relative <30 yr	0.5 point

Total score = 4: definite LQTS; total score = 2 to 3: intermediate probability; total score = 1: low probability.

WORKUP

Cardiology referral is recommended for all cases.

Genetic analysis is an essential step for risk stratification of patients with congenital prolonged QT and is important for identification of potential mutation carriers within the proband family. There is evidence for gene-specific triggers of events and therapeutic efficacy. Molecular screening should become part of the routine clinical management of LQTS.

In relatives of known patients with LQTS or in young patients with syncope:
- Stress test may prolong the QT interval or cause T-wave alternans
- Valsalva maneuver: may prolong the QT interval or cause T-wave alternans
- Prolonged ECG monitoring with various stimulations aimed at increasing catecholamines and assess for QT prolongation (perform in a setting that can provide resuscitation with α- and β-antagonists readily available).
- Epinephrine-induced prolongation of the QT interval (epinephrine infusion QT stress test)
- Genetic analysis
  - *LQT1* locus of *KCNQ1* potassium channel gene
  - *LQT2* locus of *KCNH2* potassium channel gene
  - *LQT3* locus of *SCN5A* sodium channel gene
  - These three variants account for >90% of all genotyped LQTS patients, whereas the remaining genes are responsible for a minority of cases
- Risk stratification for each genetic variant on the basis of gender and QTc: groups are defined on the basis of the probability of the first cardiac event (syncope, cardiac arrest, or sudden death) before the age of 40 years or before therapy. QT interval duration was the strongest predictor of risk for cardiac events; a QTc exceeding 500 ms identifies patients with the highest risk.
  - High risk (>50% of cardiac event): QTc ≥ 500 ms and *LQT1* or *LQT2*, or male with *LQT3*
  - Moderate risk (30% to 50%): QTc <500 ms in male with *LQT3* or in female with *LQT2 or LQT3*, and female with *LQT3 with QTc ≥ 500 ms*
  - Low risk (<30%): QTc <500 ms and *LQT1* or male *LQT2 with QTc <500 ms*
  - Prophylactic treatment should be considered in all patients with moderate or high risk for cardiac events based on the above risk stratification scheme (Table 1-303)

Rx TREATMENT

NONPHARMACOLOGIC

- Focuses on exclusion of triggers of life-threatening arrhythmia—there are gene-specific triggers for symptoms:
  - *LQT1* patients experience 90% of lethal events under physical and emotional stress. Swimming and diving should be avoided or performed under supervision.
  - *LQT2* patients are at highest risk during arousal or emotions, also during sleep and at rest but not at all during exercise; avoid sudden or excessive acoustic stimuli, especially during sleep (e.g., avoid telephone and/or alarm clock in the proximity)—as opposed to *LQT3* patients, in whom 80% of the events occur at rest or while asleep.
- Avoid competitive sports.
- Implantation of an implantable cardioverter-defibrillator (ICD) is recommended according to the ACC/AHA guidelines for patients with a good functional status for more than 1 yr and the following conditions (Table 1-304):
  - Survivors of cardiac arrest (class 1)
  - Patients with syncope or ventricular tachycardia while receiving β-blockers (class IIa)
  - Prophylaxis of SCD with use of β-blocker in patients with characteristics that suggest high risk (such as *LQT2* and *LQT3, QTc >500 ms*) (class IIb)

PHARMACOLOGIC

- With few exceptions (mostly borderline QTc and *LQT1* males older than age 25 to 30 yr), all mutation carriers should be treated because of the risk of SCD during first cardiac event. All symptomatic patients should be treated as well.

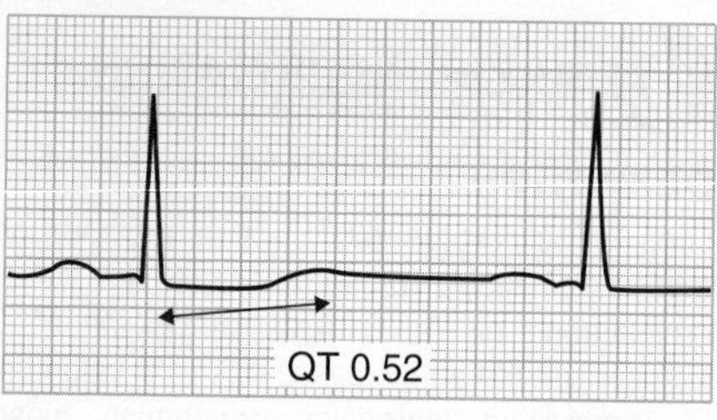

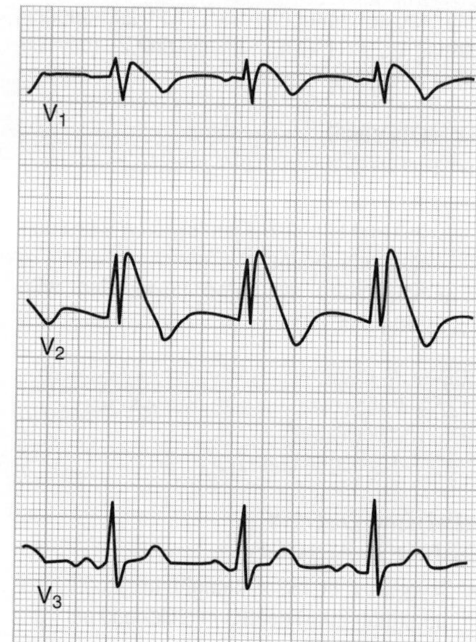

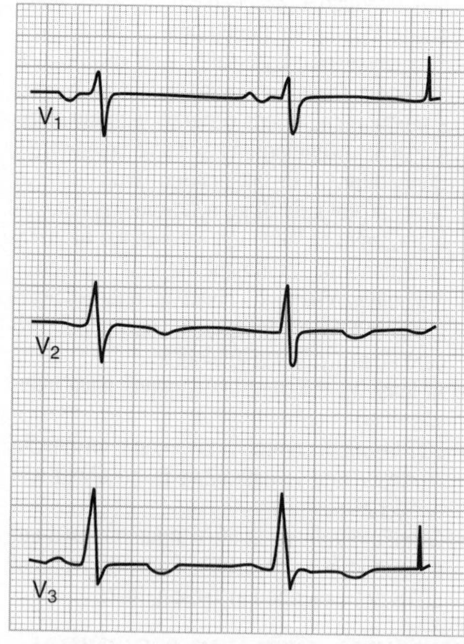

FIGURE 1-563 Sinus rhythm electrocardiogram findings in three genetic sudden death syndromes. A, QT prolongation during sinus rhythm in a patient with long QT syndrome. **B,** ST elevation in V_1 and V_2 in a patient with Brugada's syndrome. **C,** T wave inversion in V_1-V_3 in a patient with arrhythmogenic right ventricular dysplasia. (From Goldman L, Schafer AI: *Goldman's Cecil medicine*, ed 24, Philadelphia, 2012, Saunders.)

TABLE 1-303 Cardiac Event Risk Stratification Scheme Based on Genes, Gender, and QTc

Genetic Subtype	QTc <500 ms		QTc ≥5500 ms	
	Male	**Female**	**Male**	**Female**
LQT1	Low	Low	High	High
LQT2	Low	Intermediate	High	High
LQT3	Intermediate	Intermediate	High	Intermediate

Probability of the first cardiac event (syncope, cardiac arrest, or sudden death) before the age of 40 years or before therapy. High = >50%, Intermediate = 30%-50%, Low = <30%.

TABLE 1-304 Management of Patients with Long QT Syndrome

Type of Syndrome	Management	Indication
Congenital	Beta-blockers	Asymptomatic patients, symptomatic patients (who do not have bronchospasm)
	Cervicothoracic sympathectomy	Refractory symptoms, especially in pediatric patients
	Cardiac pacing	Refractory symptoms associated with bradycardia, pauses
	Implantable cardioverter-defibrillator	Cardiac arrest, refractory syncope, prophylaxis for moderate- to high-risk patients for cardiac events
Acquired	Elimination of causative drug or condition	All patients
	Magnesium sulfate	Nonsustained ventricular tachycardia, torsades de pointes (even with a normal serum magnesium concentration)
	Administration of potassium (to keep serum K^+ >4.5 mEq/L)	Serum K^+ <4.5 mEq/L
	Maneuvers to increase heart rate (cardiac pacing, isoproterenol)	Bradycardia, arrhythmias refractory to magnesium sulfate

K^+, Potassium.
Adapted from Crawford MH et al (eds): *Cardiology*, ed 2, St Louis, 2004, Mosby.

- Beta-blockers an initial therapy of choice—there are differential responses to β-blocker therapy among different genetic variants; especially effective among *LQT1* patients. Studies showed the efficacy of β-blockers with an overall mortality <2% over a mean follow-up exceeding 5 yr.
- In patients with LQT3, mexiletine shortens the QTc and can be given with a β-blocker.
- From 20% to 30% of patients who continue to have symptoms on a β-blocker, the main options are either left cardiac sympathetic denervation (LCSD) or the prophylactic implantation of an ICD.
- In patients with frequent ICD shocks or in those with high risk for SCD where ICD placement cannot be performed, cardiac pacing and/or LCSD may be indicated.
- In patients with recurrent syncope and/or aborted cardiac arrest despite combined ICD and β-blocker, LCSD as adjunctive therapy can be performed.
- Correctable factors including electrolyte disorder—hypokalemia and hypomagnesemia—and avoidance of precipating drugs that may further prolong the QT interval is mandatory.
- For patients with acquired form and torsades de pointes, IV magnesium and atrial or ventricular pacing are initial choices.
- Table 1-304 summarizes management of patients with LQTS.

PROGNOSIS

In carefully treated patients, mortality is around 0.5% to 1% over 20 years.

The timing and frequency of syncope, QTc prolongation, and gender are predictive of risk for aborted cardiac arrest and SCD during adolescence. Higher risk is present in those with one or two or more episodes of syncope in the last 10 yr compared with those with no syncopal episodes, those with QTc >530 ms, and males aged 10 to 12 yr.

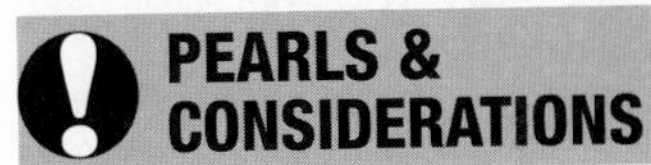

PEARLS & CONSIDERATIONS

COMMENTS

Family history should be assessed for a history of sudden death and other deaths that may have occurred as manifestations of LQTS (e.g., sudden infant death, drowning, and loss of consciousness while driving).

SUGGESTED READINGS

available at www.expertconsult.com

RELATED CONTENT

Long QT Syndrome (Patient Information)
Torsades de Pointes (Related Key Topic)

AUTHOR: **BARRY FINE, M.D., Ph.D.**

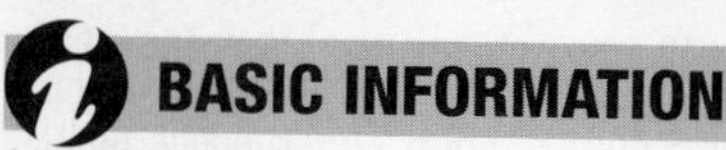

BASIC INFORMATION

DEFINITION

Lumbar disc syndrome includes diseases resulting from disk disorder, either herniation or degenerative change (spondylosis). Massive disk protrusion may rarely lead to paralysis in the lower extremity, a condition termed *cauda equina syndrome*. Gradual narrowing of the spinal canal (lumbar stenosis), usually from spondylosis, may also cause lower extremity symptoms.

SYNONYMS

Lumbago
Sciatica

ICD-9CM CODES
722.10 Lumbar disc displacement
724.02 Lumbar stenosis
344.60 Cauda equina syndrome
721.3 Lumbar spondylosis
ICD-10CM CODES
M51.26 Other intervertebral disc displacement, lumbar region
M48.06 Spinal stenosis, lumbar region
G83.4 Cauda equina syndrome
M47.817 Spondylosis without myelopathy or radiculopathy, lumbosacral region

EPIDEMIOLOGY & DEMOGRAPHICS

PREVALENCE:
- Variable
- At least one episode in 80% of adults

PREDOMINANT SEX: Approximately equal
PREDOMINANT AGE:
- Herniation: 20 to 40 yr
- Stenosis: >40 to 50 yr
- Disc symptoms: rare <20 yr

PHYSICAL FINDINGS & CLINICAL PRESENTATION

- Overlapping clinical syndromes that may result:
  1. Mild herniation without nerve root compression
  2. Herniation with nerve root compression
  3. Cauda equina syndrome
  4. Chronic degenerative disease with or without leg symptoms
  5. Spinal stenosis
- Low back pain, often worsened by activity or coughing and sneezing
- Local lumbar or lumbosacral tenderness
- Paresthesias, usually unilateral (Fig. 1-564)
- Restricted low back motion
- Increased pain on bending toward affected side
- Weakness and reflex changes (L4—knee jerk and quadriceps, L5—extensor hallucis longus, S1—ankle jerk and toe walking) (Table 1-305)
- Sensory examination usually not helpful
- Lumbar stenosis that possibly produces symptoms (pseudoclaudication), which are often misinterpreted as being vascular. Pseudoclaudication usually recovers quickly with sitting or spine flexion. Vascular disease is unaffected by spine position and is typically associated with atrophic skin changes and diminished pulses.)
- Positive straight leg raising test if nerve root compression is present

ETIOLOGY

Multifactorial

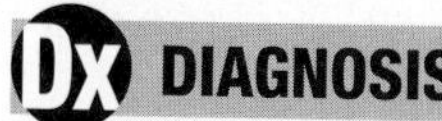

DIAGNOSIS

DIFFERENTIAL DIAGNOSIS

- Soft tissue strain or sprain
- Tumor
- Degenerative arthritis of hip
- Insufficiency fracture of hip or pelvis

Section II describes the differential diagnosis of common low back pain syndromes. Table 1-306 differentiates the various causes of mechanical low back pain. Red flags for potentially serious underlying causes of low back pain are described in Table E1-307.

WORKUP

In most cases the diagnosis can be established on a clinical basis alone.

IMAGING STUDIES

- Imaging is not warranted for most patients with acute low back pain.
- Plain roentgenograms may be indicated within the first few weeks for persistent pain; they are usually normal in soft disc herniation, but with chronic degenerative disc disease loss of height of the disk space and osteophyte formation can occur.
- MRI (Fig. E1-565) may be indicated in patients whose symptoms do not resolve or when other spinal pathology may be suspected.
- Electrodiagnostic studies may confirm the diagnosis or rule out peripheral nerve disorders.

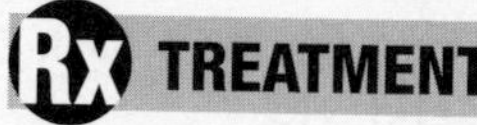

TREATMENT

NONPHARMACOLOGIC THERAPY

- Short course (3 to 5 days) of limited physical activity for acute disc herniation with leg pain
- Physical therapy for modalities plus a careful gradual exercise program. Physical therapists generally use the McKenzie method (see http://www.mckenziemdt.org/approach.cfm or http://www.youtube.com/watch?v=bPz9A4TWMCQ) for the treatment of low back pain.
- Lumbosacral corset brace during rehabilitation process in conjunction with exercise program is beneficial only in some cases.
- Percutaneous electrical nerve stimulation may be beneficial in selected patients with chronic back pain.

ACUTE GENERAL Rx

- NSAIDs
- Muscle relaxants for sedative effect
- Analgesics
- Injection therapy for low back pain and sciatica has limited clinical benefit and is generally not recommended. Epidural steroid injection for leg symptoms only in selected patients

DISPOSITION

- Almost all lumbar disc syndromes improve with time.
- Recurrent episodes usually respond to medical management.
- Recovery from the rare paralytic event is often incomplete.

REFERRAL

- For orthopedic or neurosurgical consultation for intractable pain or significant neurologic deficit
- Emergency referral for cauda equina syndrome
- Table 1-308 summarizes indications for surgical referral

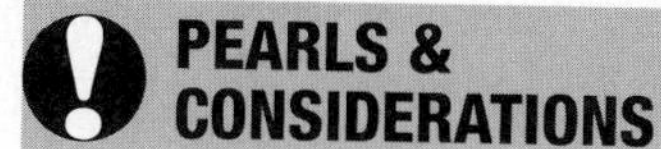

PEARLS & CONSIDERATIONS

Red flags suggesting a more serious condition as a cause of the back pain include:
1. Fever
2. History of malignancy
3. Pain at rest

TABLE 1-305 Symptoms and Signs of Common Root Compression Syndromes Produced by Lumbar Disc Prolapse

Root Lesion	Pain	Sensory Loss	Motor Weakness	Reflex Lost	Other Signs
S1	From buttock down back of thigh and leg to ankle and foot	Sole of foot and posterior calf	Plantar flexion of ankle and toes	Ankle jerk	Diminished straight leg raising
L5	From buttock to lateral aspect of leg and dorsum of foot	Dorsum of foot and antero-lateral aspect of lower leg	Dorsiflexion of foot and toes	None	As above
L4	Lateral aspect of thigh to medial side of calf	Medial aspect of calf and shin	Dorsiflexion and inversion of ankle; extension of knee	Knee jerk	Positive femoral stretch test

From Ballinger A: *Kumar & Clark's essentials of clinical medicine*, ed 6, Edinburgh, 2012, Saunders.

TABLE 1-306 Mechanical Low Back Pain

	Muscle Strain	Herniated Nucleus Pulposus	Osteoarthritis	Spinal Stenosis	Spondylolisthesis	Scoliosis
Age (yr)	20-40	30-50	>50	>60	20	30
Pain pattern location	Back (unilateral)	Back (unilateral)	Back (unilateral)	Leg (bilateral)	Back	Back
Onset	Acute	Acute (prior episodes)	Insidious	Insidious	Insidious	Insidious
Standing	↑	↓	↑	↑	↑	↑
Sitting	↓	↑	↓	↓	↓	↓
Bending	↑	↑	↓	↓	↑	↑
Straight leg	−	+	−	+ (stress)	−	−
Plain radiography	−	−	+	+	+	+

From Borenstein DG et al: *Low back pain: medical diagnosis and comprehensive management,* ed 2, Philadelphia, 1995, Saunders.

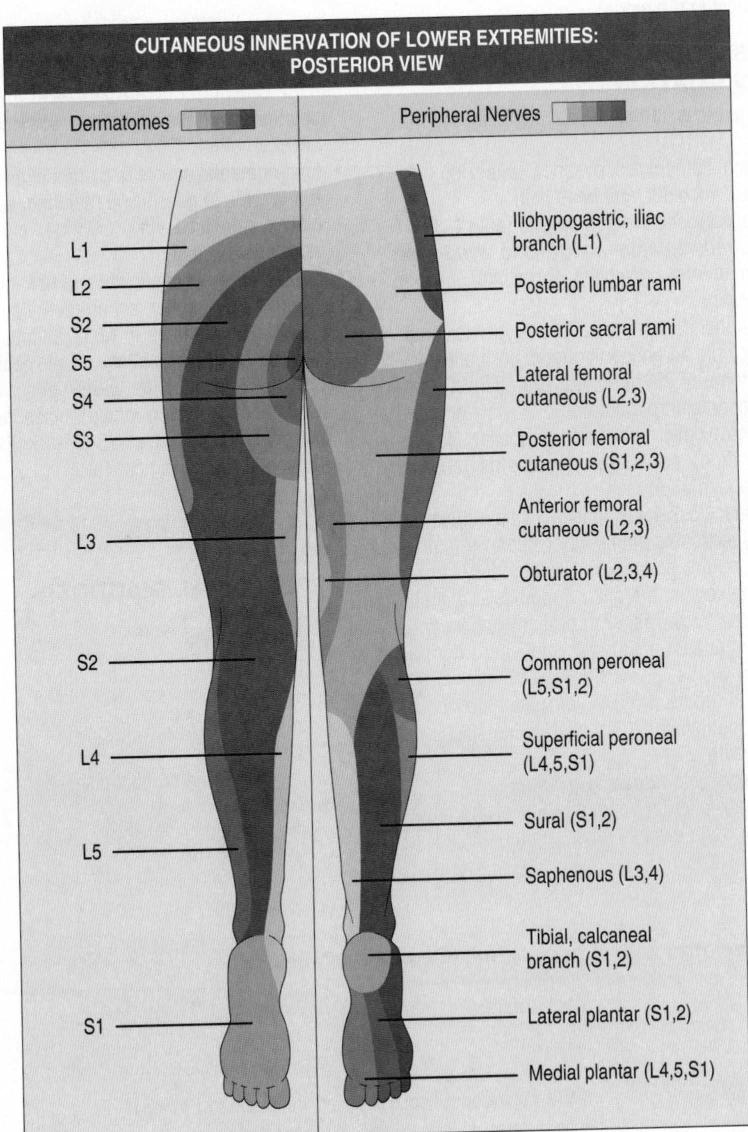

FIGURE 1-564 Lumbar disk syndrome. Cutaneous sensory innervation. Posterior view of lower extremities illustrating skin areas supplied by nerve roots *(left)* and peripheral nerves *(right)*. (From Hochberg MC et al: *Rheumatology,* ed 5, St Louis, 2011, Mosby.)

TABLE 1-308 Indications for Surgical Referral

Disk Herniation

- Cauda equina syndrome (emergency)
- Serious neurologic deficit
- Progressive neurologic deficit
- Greater than 6 weeks of disabling radiculopathy (elective)

Spinal Stenosis

- Serious neurologic deficit
- Progressive neurologic deficit
- Persistent and disabling pseudoclaudication (elective)

Spondylolisthesis

- Serious or progressive neurologic deficit

From Firestein GS et al: *Kelly's textbook of rheumatology,* ed 9, Philadelphia, 2013, Saunders.

4. Incontinence
5. Sudden worsening in level of pain
6. Weight loss
7. Significant motor loss, especially if associated with saddle anesthesia

COMMENTS

- Surgery is most consistently helpful when leg pain (not back pain) predominates.
- No substantial benefit has been shown with oral steroids, traction, epidural corticosteroid injections, or lumbar support.

SUGGESTED READINGS

available at www.expertconsult.com

RELATED CONTENT

Lumbar Disc Syndrome (Patient Information)

AUTHOR: **FRED F. FERRI, M.D.**

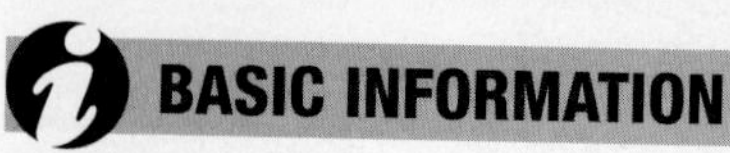

DEFINITION

A primary lung neoplasm is a malignancy arising from lung tissue. The World Health Organization distinguishes 12 types of pulmonary neoplasms. The major types are squamous cell carcinoma, adenocarcinoma, small cell carcinoma, and large cell carcinoma. However, the crucial difference in the diagnosis of lung cancer is between small cell lung cancer (SCLC) and non–small cell lung cancer (NSCLC) because the prognosis and therapeutic approach are different.

ADENOCARCINOMA: Represents 35% to 40% of lung carcinomas; frequently located in mid-lung and periphery; initial metastases are to lymphatics; frequently associated with peripheral scars; adenocarcinoma is described as preinvasive, minimally invasive, or invasive

SQUAMOUS CELL (EPIDERMOID): 20% to 30% of lung cancers; central location; metastasis by local invasion; frequent cavitation and obstructive phenomena

SMALL CELL (OAT CELL): 20% of lung carcinomas; central location; metastasis through lymphatics; associated with lesion of the short arm of chromosome 3; high cavitation rate

LARGE CELL: 10% to 15% of lung carcinomas; frequently located in the periphery; metastasis to central nervous system and mediastinum; rapid growth rate with early metastasis

LEPIDIC-PREDOMINANT PATTERN (BRONCHOALVEOLAR): 5% of lung carcinomas; frequently located in the periphery; may be bilateral; initial metastasis through lymphatic, hematogenous, and local invasion; no correlation with cigarette smoking; cavitation rare

SYNONYMS

Lung cancer

ICD-9CM CODES
162.9 Malignant neoplasm of bronchus and lung, unspecified

ICD-10CM CODES
C34.90 Malignant neoplasm of unspecified part of unspecified bronchus or lung

EPIDEMIOLOGY & DEMOGRAPHICS

- Lung cancer is responsible for >30% of cancer deaths in males and >25% of cancer deaths in females. It has been the most common cancer in the world since 1985 and is the leading cause of cancer-related death.
- Tobacco smoking is implicated in 90% of cases; second-hand smoke is responsible for approximately 20% of cases.
- There are >200,000 new cases of lung cancer yearly in the U.S., most occurring at age >50 yr (<4% in patients <40 yr).
- Among women there has been a 600% increase in incidence of lung cancer during the past 80 years. The rates of death among women with lung cancer in the U.S. are the highest in the world.

PHYSICAL FINDINGS & CLINICAL PRESENTATION

- Weight loss, fatigue, fever, anorexia, dysphagia
- Cough, hemoptysis, dyspnea, wheezing
- Chest, shoulder, and bone pain
- Paraneoplastic syndromes (see Table 1-309):
  - ***Lambert-Eaton myasthenic syndrome:*** myopathy involving proximal muscle groups
  - Endocrine manifestations: hypercalcemia, ectopic adrenocorticotropic hormone, syndrome of inappropriate excretion of adrenocorticotropic hormone
  - Neurologic: subacute cerebellar degeneration, peripheral neuropathy, cortical degeneration
  - Musculoskeletal: polymyositis, clubbing, hypertrophic pulmonary osteoarthropathy
  - Hematologic or vascular: migratory thrombophlebitis, marantic thrombosis, anemia, thrombocytosis, or thrombocytopenia
  - Cutaneous: acanthosis nigricans, dermatomyositis
- Pleural effusion (10% of patients), recurrent pneumonias (from obstruction), localized wheezing
- ***Superior vena cava syndrome:***
  - Obstruction of venous return of the superior vena cava is most commonly caused by bronchogenic carcinoma or metastasis to paratracheal nodes.
  - The patient usually reports headache, nausea, dizziness, visual changes, syncope, and respiratory distress.
  - Physical examination reveals distention of thoracic and neck veins, edema of face and upper extremities, facial plethora, and cyanosis.
- ***Horner's syndrome:*** constricted pupil, ptosis, facial anhidrosis caused by spinal cord damage between C8 and T1 as a result of a superior sulcus tumor (bronchogenic carcinoma of the extreme lung apex)
- ***Pancoast tumor:*** a superior sulcus tumor associated with ipsilateral Horner's syndrome and shoulder pain

ETIOLOGY

- Tobacco abuse; the chance of developing lung cancer for a 40-pack-year persistent smoker is 20 times that of someone who never smoked
- Environmental agents (e.g., radon) and industrial agents (e.g., ionizing radiation, asbestos, nickel, uranium, vinyl chloride, chromium, arsenic, coal dust)
- Lung cancer susceptibility and risk increased in inherited cancer syndromes caused by germ-line mutations in p53, retinoblastoma, and germ-line mutation in the epidermal growth factor receptor *(EGFR)* gene; also an association between single-nucleotide polymorphism variation at 15q24-15q25.1 and susceptibility to lung cancer

Dx DIAGNOSIS

DIFFERENTIAL DIAGNOSIS

- Pneumonia
- Tuberculosis (TB)
- Metastatic carcinoma to the lung
- Lung abscess
- Granulomatous disease
- Carcinoid tumor
- Mycobacterial and fungal diseases
- Sarcoidosis
- Viral pneumonitis

TABLE 1-309 Paraneoplastic Syndromes Associated with Bronchogenic Carcinoma

Syndrome	Cell Type	Mechanism
Hypertrophic pulmonary osteoarthropathy and clubbing	All except small cell	Unknown
Hyponatremia	Small cell most common; may be any type	SIADH, ectopic antidiuretic hormone production by tumor
Hypercalcemia	Usually squamous cell	Bone metastases, osteoclast-activating factor, parathyroid hormone–like hormone, prostaglandins
Cushing's syndrome	Usually small cell	Ectopic ACTH production
Lambert-Eaton myasthenic syndrome	Usually small cell	Voltage-sensitive calcium channel antibodies in >75%; affects presynaptic neuronal calcium channel activity
Other neuromyopathic disorders	Small cell most common; may be any type	Antineuronal nuclear antibodies, also known as anti-Hu; others unknown
Thrombophlebitis	All types	Unknown

ACTH, Adrenocorticotropic hormone; *SIADH,* syndrome of inappropriate secretion of antidiuretic hormone.
From Andreoli TE et al: *Andreoli and Carpenter's Cecil essentials of medicine,* ed 8, Philadelphia, 2010, Saunders.

- Benign lesions that simulate thoracic malignancy:
  - Lobar atelectasis: pneumonia, TB, chronic inflammatory disease, allergic bronchopulmonary aspergillosis
  - Multiple pulmonary nodules: septic emboli, Wegener's granulomatosis, sarcoidosis, rheumatoid nodules, fungal disease, multiple pulmonary atrioventricular fistulas
  - Mediastinal adenopathy: sarcoidosis, lymphoma, primary TB, fungal disease, silicosis, pneumoconiosis, drug-induced (e.g., phenytoin, trimethadione)
  - Pleural effusion: congestive heart failure, pneumonia with parapneumonic effusion, TB, viral pneumonitis, ascites, pancreatitis, collagen-vascular disease

WORKUP

Workup generally includes chest radiograph, CT scan of chest, positron-emission tomographic (PET) scan, and tissue biopsy. Lab tests should include CBC, serum calcium, and liver chemistry studies. Diagnosis and staging of lung cancer should be performed simultaneously to minimize invasive testing.

LABORATORY TESTS

Obtain tissue diagnosis. Various modalities are available:

- Biopsy of any suspicious lymph nodes (e.g., supraclavicular node)
- Flexible fiberoptic bronchoscopy: brush and biopsy specimens are obtained from any visualized endobronchial lesions
- Transbronchial needle aspiration: done with a special needle passed through the bronchoscope; this technique is useful to sample mediastinal masses or paratracheal lymph nodes
- Transthoracic fine-needle aspiration biopsy with fluoroscopic or CT scan guidance to evaluate peripheral pulmonary nodules
- Mediastinoscopy and anteromedial sternotomy in suspected tumor involvement of the mediastinum
- Pleural biopsy in patients with pleural effusion
- Thoracentesis of pleural effusion and cytologic evaluation of the obtained fluid: may confirm diagnosis

IMAGING STUDIES

- Chest radiograph (Fig. 1-566): The radiographic presentation often varies with the cell type. Pleural effusion, lobar atelectasis, and mediastinal adenopathy can accompany any cell types.
- CT scan of chest (Fig. 1-567) is performed to evaluate mediastinal and pleural extension of suspected lung neoplasms. The chest CT should include liver and adrenal glands (common sites of metastases). CT or MRI of brain should be considered in a patient presenting with neurologic symptoms (e.g., headaches, vision disturbances).
- PET with ^{18}F-fluorodeoxyglucose (^{18}FDG-PET), a metabolic marker of malignant tissue, is superior to CT scan in detecting mediastinal and distant metastases in NSCLC. It is useful for preoperative staging of NSCLC.
- The use of PET-CT for preoperative staging of NSCLC reduces both the total number of thoracotomies and the number of futile thoracotomies but does not affect overall mortality.
- The combination of endoluminal ultrasound (EUS) and endobronchial ultrasound (EBUS) with fine-needle aspiration has been reported to have a 93% sensitivity and 97% specificity for establishing the presence of mediastinal disease in lung cancer patients.

STAGING

After confirmation of diagnosis, patients should undergo staging:

1. The international staging system is the most widely accepted staging system for NSCLC. In this system, stage I (N0 [no lymph node involvement]) and stage II (N1 [spread to ipsilateral bronchopulmonary or hilar lymph nodes]) include localized tumors for which surgical resection is the preferred treatment. Stage III is subdivided into IIIA (potentially resectable) and IIIB. The surgical management of stage IIIA disease (N2 [involvement of ipsilateral mediastinal nodes]) is controversial. Only 20% of N2 disease is considered minimal disease

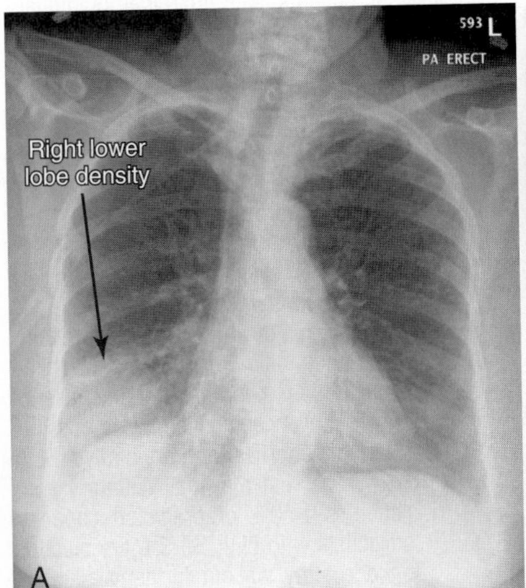

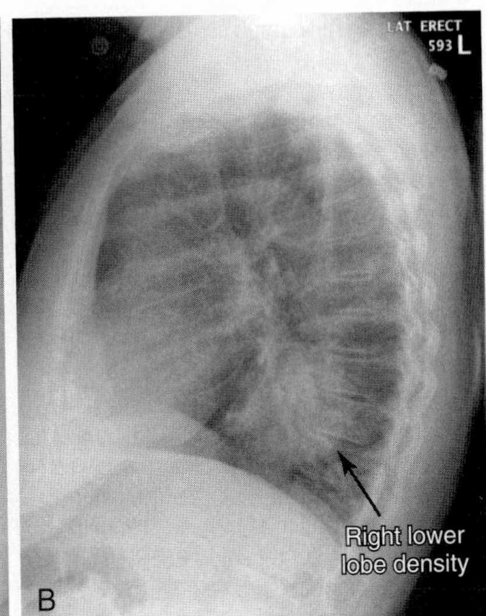

FIGURE 1-566 Lung neoplasm, primary. Lung mass presenting with hemoptysis. **A,** Posterior-anterior (PA) chest x-ray. **B,** Lateral chest x-ray. This 83-year-old female presented with hemoptysis of a quarter-sized clot. Her posterior-anterior chest x-ray shows a rounded right lower lobe density. On the lateral view, this is visible in the retrocardiac space. This density measures 7.6 cm in diameter. Pneumonia, neoplasm, or abscess could have this appearance on chest x-ray. Computed tomography was performed to further delineate the pathology (see Fig. 1-567). (From Broder JS: *Diagnostic imaging for the emergency physician,* Philadelphia, 2011, Saunders.)

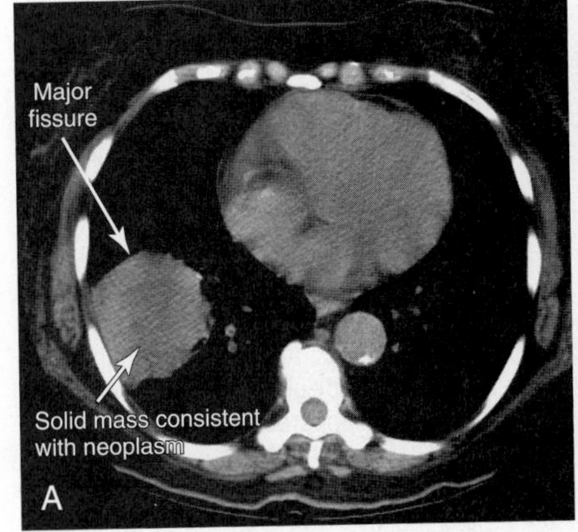

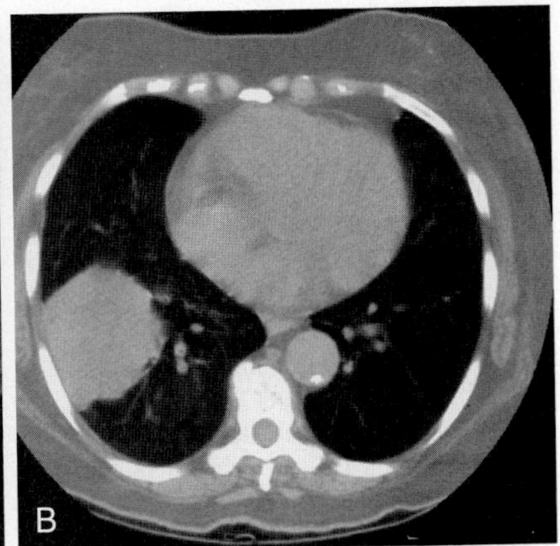

FIGURE 1-567 Lung neoplasm, primary. Lung mass presenting with hemoptysis. Same patient as in Fig. 1-566. Noncontrast computed tomography was performed (contrast was withheld as a consequence of the patient's renal dysfunction) and shows a 6 by 6 cm round lesion abutting the oblique fissure (also called the major fissure) and lateral chest wall. **A,** Soft tissue windows. **B,** Lung windows. On soft tissue windows, the center appears slightly darker, indicating lower density that may represent central necrosis. If IV contrast had been given, an area of necrosis would have failed to enhance. Infection or infarction is technically possible, but a pulmonary neoplasm is the most likely explanation for this lesion. Biopsy showed this to be a moderately differentiated squamous cell carcinoma. (From Broder JS: *Diagnostic imaging for the emergency physician,* Philadelphia, 2011, Saunders.)

(involvement of only one node) and technically resectable. Stage IV indicates metastatic disease. The pathologic staging system uses a tumor/nodal involvement/metastasis system.
2. In patients with SCLC, a more practical accepted staging system is the one developed by the Veterans Administration Lung Cancer Study Group. This system contains two stages:
   a. Limited-stage disease: confined to the regional lymph nodes and to one hemithorax (excluding pleural surfaces)
   b. Extensive-stage disease: spread beyond the confines of limited-stage disease
3. Pretreatment staging procedures for lung cancer patients, in addition to complete history and physical examination, generally include the following tests:
   a. Chest radiograph (posteroanterior and lateral), ECG
   b. Laboratory evaluation: complete blood count, complete metabolic panel, arterial blood gases, pulse oximetry. The identification of molecular signatures of lung cancer to predict prognosis with data from microarray and/or reverse-transcription polymerase chain reaction analysis has been validated in recent trials. A five-gene signature (*DUSP6, MMD, STAT1, ERBB3,* and *LCK*) is closely associated with relapse-free and overall survival among patients with NSCLC. Anaplastic lymphoma kinase (ALK) translocation is found in about 4% to 5% of lung cancers. Detection of mutations in epidermal growth factor receptor (EGFR) in circulating tumor cells from the blood of patients with lung cancer offers the possibility of monitoring changes in epithelial tumor genotypes during the course of treatment
   c. Pulmonary function studies
   d. CT scan of chest and PET scan: a recent Dutch trial revealed a 51% relative reduction in futile thoracotomies for patients with suspected NSCLC who underwent preoperative assessment with PET with the tracer ^{18}FDG-PET in addition to conventional workup
   e. Mediastinoscopy or anterior mediastinotomy in patients being considered for possible curative lung resection
   f. Biopsy of any accessible suspect lesions
   g. CT scan of liver and brain; radionuclide scans of bone in all patients with small cell carcinoma of the lung and patients with NSCLC neoplasms suspected of involving these organs
   h. Bone marrow aspiration and biopsy only in selected patients with small cell carcinoma of the lung. In the absence of an increased lactate dehydrogenase or cytopenia, routine bone marrow examination not recommended
   i. Newer technologies in preoperative staging include endoscopic bronchial ultrasonography and esophageal ultrasonography to guide biopsies; however, cervical mediastinoscopy is standard criterion in preoperative nodal staging (sensitivity >93%, specificity >95%)

Rx TREATMENT

NONPHARMACOLOGIC THERAPY

- Nutritional support
- Avoidance of tobacco and other substances toxic to the lungs
- Supplemental O_2 prn

ACUTE GENERAL Rx

NON–SMALL CELL CARCINOMA:

- Surgical resection is the best hope for cure in patients with operable NSCLC (stage I or II when the patient is a surgical candidate). Lobectomy is the best standard surgical approach. Lesser resections may be necessary in patients with marginal pulmonary reserve. Video-assisted thoracic surgery (VATS) is helpful in decreasing morbidity and shortening hospital stay.
  1. Surgical resection is indicated in patients with limited disease (not involving mediastinal nodes, ribs, pleura, or distant sites). This represents approximately 15% to 30% of diagnosed cases.
  2. Preoperative evaluation includes review of cardiac status (e.g., recent myocardial infarction, major arrhythmias) and evaluation of pulmonary function (to determine if the patient can tolerate any loss of lung tissue). Pneumonectomy is possible if the patient has a preoperative FEV_1 = 2 L or if the maximal voluntary ventilation is >50% of predicted capacity. Individuals with FEV_1 >1.5 L are suitable for lobectomy without further evaluation unless there is evidence of interstitial lung disease or undue dyspnea on exertion. In that case, carbon dioxide diffusion in the lung (DLCO) should be measured. If the DLCO is <80% predicted normal, the individual is not clearly operable.
  3. Preoperative chemotherapy should be considered in patients with more advanced disease (stage IIIA) who are being considered for surgery because it increases the median survival time in patients with NSCLC compared with the use of surgery alone. Gene expression profiles that predict the risk of recurrence in patients with early stage (IA) NSCLC have been identified. These patients are at high risk of recurrence and may also benefit from adjuvant chemotherapy.
  4. Postoperative adjuvant chemotherapy (chemotherapy given after surgical resection of an apparently localized tumor to eradicate occult metastases) with vinorelbine plus cisplatin significantly increases 5-yr survival (69% vs. 54%) in patients with completely resected stage IB or stage II NSCLC and good performance status. Adjuvant chemotherapy is generally indicated for patients with resected stages IIA through IIIA.
- Treatment of unresectable NSCLC:
  1. Radiotherapy can be used alone or in combination with chemotherapy; it is used primarily for treatment of central nervous system and skeletal metastases, superior vena cava syndrome, and obstructive atelectasis. Although thoracic radiotherapy is generally considered standard therapy for stage 3 disease, it has limited effect on survival. Palliative radiotherapy should be delayed until symptoms occur because immediate therapy offers no advantage over delayed therapy and results in more adverse events from the radiotherapy. Conventional radiotherapy fails to durably control the primary lung tumor in nearly 70% of patients and 2-yr survival is less than 40%. Stereotactic body radiation (SBRT) uses several highly focused radiation beams to deliver high doses in 15 treatments and appears to be more effective than conventional radiotherapy, with a survival rate of 55.8% at 3 yr for inoperable early stage lung cancer.
  2. Chemotherapy remains the mainstay of treatment for advanced stage IIIB and stage IV NSCLC. (stage I or II when the patient is a surgical candidate). Lobectomy is the best standard surgical approach. Lesser resections may be necessary in patients with marginal pulmonary reserve. Video-assisted thoracic surgery (VATS) is helpful in decreasing morbidity and shortening hospital stay.. A platinum-based treatment is recommended for fit patients, and single agents can be offered in elderly patients and in those with poor performance status. Various combination regimens are available. Current drugs of choice are paclitaxel plus either carboplatin or cisplatin, cisplatin plus vinorelbine, gemcitabine plus cisplatin, and carboplatin or cisplatin plus docetaxel. The overall results are disappointing, and none of the standard regimens for NSCLC is clearly superior to the others. The addition of bevacizumab to paclitaxel plus carboplatin results in significant survival benefit but carries an increased risk of treatment-related death. Gefitinib and erlotinib are oral inhibitors of *EGFR* tyrosine kinase. Activating mutations in the *EGFR* gene confer hypersensitivity to these medications. Sensitivity of lung neoplasms to these agents is seen primarily in tumors with somatic mutations in the tyrosine kinase domain (more common in adenocarcinomas found in patients who never smoked and in Asian patients). Recent trials revealed that gefitinib is superior to carboplatin-paclitaxel as an initial treatment for pulmonary adenocarcinoma among nonsmokers or former smokers in East Asia. In these patients the presence in the tumor of a mutation of the *EGFR* gene was a strong predictor of a better outcome with gefitinib. The National Comprehensive Cancer Network (NCCN) recognizes erlotinib as an option for second- or third-line therapy in patients with advanced NSCLC who have a performance status

of 0 to 3. It also recommends erlotinib monotherapy as first line for patients with an EGFR mutation. Erlotinib can also be used as a salvage treatment in this subgroup and as a maintenance agent for patients with stable or responsive disease after first-line platinum-based chemotherapy.Oncogenic fusion genes consisting of EML4 and anaplastic lymphoma kinase (ALK) are present in a subgroup of NSCLCs, representing 4% to 5% of such tumors. The inhibition of ALK in lung tumors with crizotinib, an orally available small-molecule inhibitor of the ALK tyrosine kinase, has resulted in tumor shrinkage and significant prolonged progression-free survival. Crizotinib was recently approved by the FDA for locally advanced or metastatic NSCLC with ALK translocation, which is found in about 5% of lung cancers. Recent trials[1] have shown that crizotinib is superior to standard chemotherapy in patients with previously treated advanced non–small-cell cancer with ALK rearrangement.

3. The addition of chemotherapy to radiotherapy improves survival in patients with locally advanced, unresectable NSCLC. The absolute benefit is relatively small, however, and should be balanced against the increased toxicity associated with the addition of chemotherapy.
4. Early initiation of palliative care focusing on management of symptoms, psychosocial support, and assistance with decision making in patients with metastatic NSCLC leads to improved quality of life, longer survival, and less use of aggressive end-of-life care.

[1]Shaw AT et al: Crizotinib versus chemotherapy in advanced ALK-positive lung cancer, *N Engl J Med* 368:2385-2394, 2013.

SMALL CELL LUNG CANCER:

- Limited-stage disease: standard treatments include thoracic radiotherapy and chemotherapy (cisplatin and etoposide).
- Extensive-stage disease: standard treatments include combination chemotherapy (cisplatin or carboplatin plus etoposide or combination of irinotecan and cisplatin).
- Prophylactic cranial irradiation for patients in complete remission to decrease the risk of central nervous system metastasis.
- Despite high initial response rates, most patients eventually relapse. Topotecan may be an option for these patients.

DISPOSITION

- The 5-yr survival of patients with NSCLC when the disease is resectable is approximately 30%.
- Median survival time in patients with limited-stage disease and SCLC is 15 mo; in patients with extensive stage disease, it is 9 mo. Among patients with metastatic NSCLC, early palliative care results in longer survival and significant improvements in both quality of life and mood.
- Methylation of the promoter region of certain genes (*P16, CDH13, APC,* and *RASSF1A*) in a resected NSCLC specimen is associated with recurrence of the tumor.

PEARLS & CONSIDERATIONS

COMMENTS

- CT screening with use of low-dose computed tomography (LDCT) for detection of lung cancer among persons with a heavy history of smoking increases the percentage of lung cancer cases that are diagnosed in stage 1 and reduces mortality from lung cancer. The National Lung Screening Trial (NLST) showed that lung cancer screening with LDCT resulted in a 20% reduction in mortality from lung cancer. New guidelines from the American College of Chest Physicians, the American Society of Clinical Oncology, and the National Comprehensive Cancer Network recommend annual LDCT for those who are current or former smokers aged 55-74. The U.S. Preventive Services Task Force (USPSTF) recommends annual screening for lung cancer with LDCT in adults aged 55 to 80 years who have a 30 pack-year smoking history and currently smoke or have quit within the past 15 years. Screening should be discontinued once a person has not smoked for 15 years or develops a health problem that substantially limits life expectancy or the ability or willingness to have curative lung surgery.[2]
- Quitting smoking is the most effective method to reduce risk for lung cancer. Following smoking cessation, the risk of lung cancer remains higher than normal based on duration and quantity of smoking but does not increase further as in a continuing smoker.

SUGGESTED READINGS

available at www.expertconsult.com

RELATED CONTENT

Lung Cancer Diagnosis
Lung Cancer Screening (Patient Information)

AUTHOR: **FRED F. FERRI, M.D.**

[2]Moyer VA on behalf of U.S. Preventive Services Task Force: Screening for lung cancer: U.S. Preventive Services Task Force recommendation statement, *Ann Intern Med* 160:330-338, 2014.

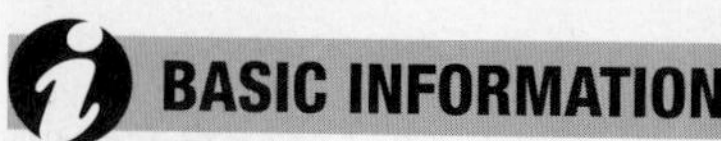

BASIC INFORMATION

DEFINITION

Lyme disease is a multisystem inflammatory disorder caused by the transmission of a spirochete, *Borrelia burgdorferi*. Lyme disease is spread by the bite of infected *Ixodes* ticks, taking 36 to 48 hr for a tick to feed and transmit the infecting organism *B. burgdorferi* to the host.

SYNONYMS

Bannworth's syndrome (Europe)
Acrodermatitis chronica atrophicans

ICD-9CM CODES
088.8 Lyme disease
ICD-10CM CODES
A69.20 Lyme disease, unspecified

EPIDEMIOLOGY & DEMOGRAPHICS

INCIDENCE (IN U.S.): 4.4 cases/100,000 persons; 90% of cases in the U.S. are found in: Massachusetts, Connecticut, Rhode Island, New York, New Jersey, Pennsylvania, Minnesota, Wisconsin, and California.
PEAK INCIDENCE: May to November
PREDOMINANT SEX: Male = female
PREDOMINANT AGE: Median age of 28 yr

PHYSICAL FINDINGS & CLINICAL PRESENTATION

Lyme disease may present in the following stages:

- *Early localized stage (incubation period 3-30 days):* early Lyme disease, erythema migrans (EM); skin rash, often at site of tick bite (the CDC has defined EM rash as an expanding red macule or papule that must reach at least 5 cm in size, with or without central clearing); possible fever, myalgias 3 to 32 days after tick bite
- *Early disseminated stage (incubation period 3-6 weeks):* days to weeks later; multiorgan system involvement, including CNS with aseptic meningitis–type picture or Bell's palsy, joints (arthritis or arthralgias), cardiac including varying degrees of heart block; related to dissemination of spirochete
- *Late stage (incubation period months to years):* mo to yr after tick exposure; affects central and peripheral nervous system, cardiac, joints

Common presenting signs and symptoms include:

- EM (Fig. E1-568)
- Lymphadenopathy, neck pains, pharyngeal erythema, myalgias, hepatosplenomegaly.
- Patients will complain of malaise, fatigue, lethargy, headache, fever/chills, neck pain, myalgias, back pain.

ETIOLOGY

B. burgdorferi transmitted from bite of an *Ixodes* tick (mostly in the nymph stage, but can also be from adult ticks)

Dx DIAGNOSIS

Clinical presentation, exposure to ticks in endemic area, and diagnostic testing for antibody response to *B. burgdorferi*

DIFFERENTIAL DIAGNOSIS

- Chronic fatigue/fibromyalgia
- Acute viral illnesses
- Babesiosis
- Ehrlichiosis

WORKUP

- ELISA testing and if positive or equivocal then followed by a Western blot IgM and IgG (Table 1-310). A Western blot IgM assay is positive if 2 of 3 bands present. The Western blot IgG is positive if 5 of 10 bands present.
- Early disease often difficult to diagnose serologically secondary to slow immune response
- Culturing of skin lesions (EM) and polymerase chain reaction (PCR) of skin biopsy and blood to give definitive diagnosis (available only in reference laboratories)

IMAGING STUDIES

- Echocardiogram if conduction abnormalities are present with cardiac involvement
- CT scan, MRI of head for CNS involvement

TREATMENT

Early localized Lyme disease:

- Doxycycline 100 mg bid or amoxicillin 500 mg tid for 14 days (doxycycline should be avoided in children >8 yr and pregnant females).
- Alternative treatments: cefuroxime axetil 500 mg bid for 14 to 21 days, azithromycin 500 mg PO for 7 to 10 days but should not be used as a first-line agent.
- A single dose of 200 mg doxycycline given within 72 hr of *Ixodes* tick bite can prevent development of Lyme disease.

Early disseminated and late persistent infection:

- 28 days of treatment necessary; doxycycline and ceftriaxone appear equally effective for acute disseminated Lyme disease.
- Arthritis: 28 days of doxycycline or amoxicillin plus probenecid.
- Neurologic involvement requires parenteral antibiotics. Those who fail to respond should be treated with IV ceftriaxone or cefotaxime.
- Ceftriaxone 2 g/day IV for 21 to 28 days; alternative: cefotaxime 2 g q8h IV; alternative: penicillin G 5 million U qid.
- Cardiac involvement: IV ceftriaxone or penicillin plus cardiac monitoring.
- Prolonged treatment with IV or PO antibiotic therapy for up to 90 days did not improve symptoms more than placebo.

Post–Lyme disease syndrome:

- Antibiotics are not indicated. Antibiotic treatment of patients with persistent unexplained symptoms despite previous antibiotic treatment of Lyme disease provides little, if any, benefit and carries significant risk.
- Supportive care

DISPOSITION

- The patient often needs careful follow-up and supportive care for the arthralgia-neuritis symptoms.
- Repeat episodes of EM in appropriately treated patients are due to reinfection and not to relapse.

REFERRAL

- To a neurologist if significant neurologic complications (meningitis, myelitis, ophthalmoplegia, Bell's palsy)
- To a cardiologist if the patient develops evidence of cardiac conduction disturbances or pericarditis

PEARLS & CONSIDERATIONS

- A physician diagnosis of classic EM in an endemic region of Lyme disease is sufficient to make a definitive diagnosis.
- In some patients with Lyme disease, nonspecific complaints such as headache, fatigue, and arthralgia may persist for months after appropriate (and ultimately successful) antibiotic treatment.
- There is no evidence of current or previous *Borrelia burgdorferi* infection in most patients evaluated at university-based Lyme disease referral centers. Psychiatric comorbidity and other psychological factors are prominent in the presentation and outcome of some patients who inaccurately ascribe longstanding symptoms to "chronic Lyme disease."

SUGGESTED READINGS

available at www.expertconsult.com

RELATED CONTENT

Lyme Disease (Patient Information)

AUTHOR: **GLENN G. FORT, M.D., M.P.H.**

TABLE 1-310 Criteria for Western Blot Interpretation in the Serologic Confirmation of Lyme Disease

Duration of Disease	Isotype Tested	Criteria for Positive Test
First month of infection	IgM	2 of the following 3 bands are present: 23 kD (OspC), 39 kD (BmpA), and 41 kD (Fla)
After first month of infection	IgG	5 of 10 bands are present: 18 kD, 21 kD, 28 kD, 30 kD, 39 kD, 41 kD, 45 kD, 58 kD (not GroEL), 66 kD, and 93 kD

Modified from Centers for Disease Control and Prevention: Recommendations for test performance and interpretation from the Second National Conference on Serologic Diagnosis of Lyme Disease, *MMWR Morb Mortal Wkly Rep* 44:590–591, 1995.

BASIC INFORMATION

DEFINITION

Lymphangitis refers to the inflammation of lymphatic vessels due to infectious or noninfectious causes. Infectious causes include bacteria, mycobacteria, viruses, fungi, and parasites.

SYNONYMS

Nodular lymphangitis
Sporotrichoid lymphangitis

ICD-9CM CODES
457.2 Lymphangitis
ICD-10CM CODES
I89.1 Lymphangitis

EPIDEMIOLOGY & DEMOGRAPHICS

INCIDENCE (IN U.S.): Several hundred cases/yr of sporotrichoid lymphangitis

PHYSICAL FINDINGS & CLINICAL PRESENTATION

ACUTE LYMPHANGITIS:

- Commonly associated with a bacterial cellulitis
- Usually develops after cutaneous inoculation of microorganisms into the lymphatic vessels through a skin wound or as a result of spread from a distal infection
- May or may not recognize site of skin trauma (i.e., laceration, puncture, ulcer)
- In hours to days, distal appearance of erythema, edema, and tenderness, with linear erythematous streaks extending proximally to regional lymph nodes
- Possible lymphadenitis and fever
- Predisposition to group A streptococcal infection of the skin in those with chronic lymphedema and superficial fungal infections (e.g., tinea pedis)

SPOROTRICHOID OR NODULAR LYMPHANGITIS:

- Includes subcutaneous nodules that develop along the path of involved lymphatics
- Most commonly results from inoculation of the skin of the hand
- Usually preceded by well-defined episode of cutaneous inoculation or trauma
- Lesions apparent from one to several wk after inoculation
- Initially, nodular or papular lesion; may ulcerate
- May have frank pus or a serosanguineous discharge
- Systemic complaints uncommon, but infection with certain microorganisms associated with fever, chills, myalgias, and headache

ETIOLOGY

- Acute lymphangitis: usually associated with *Streptococcus pyogenes* (group A streptococcus), but staphylococcal organisms are increasingly recognized as a cause of severe soft tissue infections such as lymphangitis, including community-acquired methicillin-resistant *S. aureus* (CA-MRSA)
- Nodular lymphangitis caused by one of several organisms
  1. *Sporothrix schenckii*
     a. Most common recognized cause in the U.S., usually in the Midwest
     b. Found in soil and plant debris
  2. *Nocardia brasiliensis:* found in soil
  3. *Mycobacterium marinum:* associated with trauma related to water (e.g., aquariums, swimming pools, fish)
  4. *Leishmania brasiliensis*
     a. Protozoal parasite transmitted to humans by sandflies, mostly to travelers in endemic areas
     b. Small endemic focus in Texas
  5. *Francisella tularensis*
     a. Most often in Midwestern states
     b. Associated with contact with infected mammals (e.g., rabbits) or tick bites

DIAGNOSIS

DIFFERENTIAL DIAGNOSIS

- Nodular lymphangitis
- Insect or snake bites
- Filariasis

WORKUP

- Acute lymphangitis: blood cultures
- Nodular lymphangitis: various stains and cultures of drainage or biopsy specimens of inoculation sites to make definitive diagnosis

LABORATORY TESTS

- WBCs possibly elevated with cellulitis
- Eosinophilia common with helminthic infections

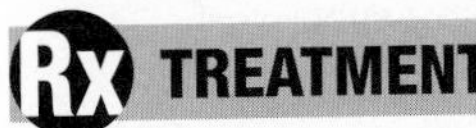

NONPHARMACOLOGIC THERAPY

Limb elevation

ACUTE GENERAL Rx

- Penicillin possibly sufficient, but 1 wk of dicloxacillin or cephalexin 500 mg PO qid commonly used to ensure antistaphylococcal coverage; if CA-MRSA suspected, then use oral Bactrim DS: one PO bid is the best oral agent and with vancomycin 1 g IV every 12 hr being reserved for patients requiring IV therapy.
- If allergic to penicillin:
  1. Clindamycin 300 mg PO qid for 7 days *or*
  2. Erythromycin 500 mg PO qid for 7 days
  3. Levaquin 500 mg PO daily or moxifloxacin 400 mg PO daily for 7 days
- Nodular lymphangitis: specific therapy directed at etiologic agent.
- For superficial fungal infections: treatment may prevent recurrence of acute lymphangitis.

DISPOSITION

- Acute lymphangitis: usually resolves with therapy
- Recurrent attacks: may lead to chronic lymphedema of limb, rarely resulting in elephantiasis nostras (nonfilarial elephantiasis)
- Nodular lymphangitis: usually responds to appropriate therapy

REFERRAL

- If acute lymphangitis is more than a mild disease or involves the face
- If nodular lymphangitis or filariasis is suspected

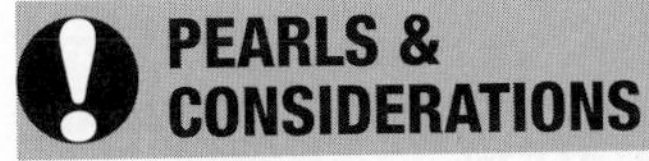

COMMENTS

- Outside of the U.S., initial episodes of filariasis caused by *Brugia malayi* resemble acute lymphangitis.
- Chronic lymphedema or elephantiasis results from recurrent episodes.

SUGGESTED READINGS
available at www.expertconsult.com

RELATED CONTENT

Lymphangitis (Patient Information)

AUTHOR: **GLENN G. FORT, M.D., M.P.H.**

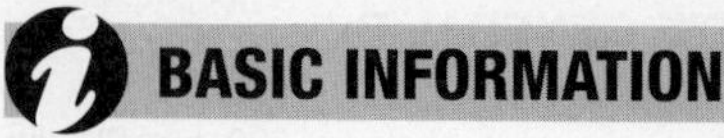

BASIC INFORMATION

DEFINITION

A primary role of the lymphatic system is to transport proteins from the interstitium to the heart. When the transport capacity of the lymphatic system is reduced, proteins accumulate in the interstitium. Accumulated proteins attract water which creates a high protein swelling in the subcutaneous tissues called lymphedema.

SYNONYMS

Elephantiasis

ICD-9CM CODES

457.0 Lymphedema: secondary to breast cancer
457.1 Lymphedema: secondary to all other causes
757 Lymphedema: primary

ICD-10CM CODES

I97.2 Postmastectomy lymphedema syndrome
I89.0 Lymphedema, not elsewhere classified

EPIDEMIOLOGY & DEMOGRAPHICS

PRIMARY LYMPHEDEMA:

- Found in 1.1/100,000 people aged <20 yr
- Females outnumber males 3.5:1.
- Incidence peaks between ages 12 and 16 (puberty)

SECONDARY LYMPHEDEMA: See specific etiology below.

PHYSICAL FINDINGS & CLINICAL PRESENTATION

Lymphedema is a slow onset, progressive disease characterized by an asymmetrical, inflammatory swelling, traveling distal to proximal, that can affect any body part including limbs, trunk, head/neck and genitals (Fig. 1-569). Box 1-52 summarizes lymphedema staging from the International Society of Lymphology.

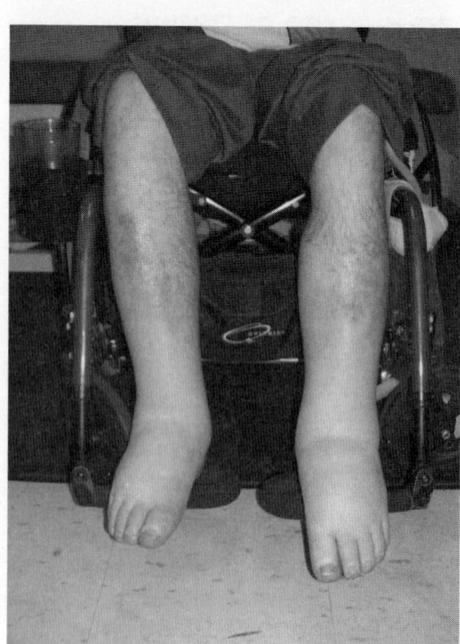

FIGURE 1-569 Lymphedema before treatment.

STAGE 0: LATENCY

- Decreased lymphatic system transport capacity due to primary or secondary etiology
- Subjective complaints of affected body part feeling heavy or achy
- No objective findings, no apparent swelling

STAGE I: REVERSIBLE

- Edema is observable, soft, pitting and reversible with elevation
- No secondary skin changes are present

STAGE II: SPONTANEOUSLY IRREVERSIBLE

- Skin becomes more firm/fibrotic, therefore less pitting
- Edema does not reverse to normal with elevation
- Possibility of infections (cellulitis), wounds or weeping (lymphorrhea)

STAGE III: ELEPHANTIASIS

- Skin becomes very firm/fibrotic, therefore non-pitting
- Evidence of substantial skin changes (e.g., papillomas, lobules, *"peau d' orange"*)

ETIOLOGY

Lymphedema is caused by a reduction in lymphatic system transport and is classified into primary and secondary forms.

PRIMARY LYMPHEDEMA:

- Occurs when the lymphatic system does not maturate properly during fetal development
  1. Aplasia
  2. Hypoplasia
  3. Hyperplasia
- Can be familial, genetic or hereditary
- Lymphedema congenital: symptoms present at birth
- Lymphedema praecox: symptoms onset prior to age of 35 (commonly during puberty)
- Lymphedema tardum: symptoms onset at the age of 35 or after

SECONDARY LYMPHEDEMA:

- Occurs secondary to a disruption or obstruction of the lymphatic system caused by
  1. Filariasis (#1 cause worldwide)
  2. Lymph node surgery/radiation due to cancer (#1 cause in the United States)
  3. Other: chronic venous insufficiency (CVI), deep vein thrombosis (DVT), infection, surgery/trauma, lipedema and obesity

BOX 1-52 Lymphedema Staging

Stage 0: Latent

- Impaired lymphatic function
- No evident edema; subclinical
- May last months or years before progression

Stage I: Spontaneously Reversible

- Early accumulation of protein-rich fluid
- Pitting edema
- Subsides with elevation

Stage II: Spontaneously Irreversible

- Accumulation of protein-rich fluid
- Pitting edema progresses to fibrosis
- Does not resolve with elevation alone

Stage III: Lymphostatic Elephantiasis

- Nonpitting
- Significant fibrosis
- Trophic skin changes

From International Society of Lymphology: The diagnosis and treatment of peripheral edema: 2009 consensus document of the International Society of Lymphology, *Lymphology* 42(2):51-60, 2009.

DIAGNOSIS

- Lymphedema is primarily a clinical diagnosis made on the basis of past medical history and objective findings that distinguish it from other causes of chronic edema
- A Stemmer's sign is often used to identify lymphedema (inability to pick up or pinch a fold of skin at the base of the second toe or finger)
- When physical examination is inconclusive, other available imaging tests can help make the diagnosis (see imaging studies below)

DIFFERENTIAL DIAGNOSIS

Other causes of edema that should be ruled out prior to treatment for lymphedema include cardiac, renal, hepatic, and thyroid dysfunction.

WORKUP

A detailed history and physical examination should help exclude most of the differential diagnoses.

LABORATORY TESTS

- Blood urea nitrogen, creatinine, liver function tests, albumin, urine analysis, and thyroid function tests are obtained to exclude possible systemic causes of edema
- Genetic testing may be practical in defining a specific hereditary syndrome with a discrete gene mutation such as lymphedema distichiasis (*FOXC2*), Milroy's disease (*VEGFR-3*), Meige's disease or Klippel-Trenaunay-Weber syndrome

IMAGING STUDIES

- Lymphoscintigraphy: diagnostic image of choice for lymphedema (if needed)
- Indocyanine green (ICG) fluorescent lymphography: can now be used to identify sentinel nodes, to demonstrate superficial lymph channels and functional lymphatics, to indicate treatment pathways, and to confirm the effectiveness of therapeutic techniques.
- Magnetic resonance imaging (MRI): primarily used in tumor diagnosis
- Duplex ultrasound: determines venous involvement in the edema
- Computed axial tomography (CAT): distinguishes between fatty tissue and accumulations of protein-rich fluids
- Lymphography: phased out in favor of less invasive techniques

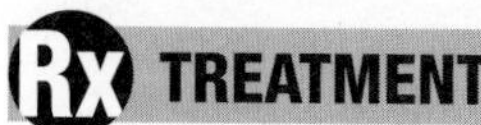

TREATMENT

NONPHARMACOLOGIC THERAPY

- Complete decongestive therapy (CDT) is backed by longstanding research and experience as the primary treatment of choice for lymphedema in both children and adults (Fig. 1-570). It should be delivered by a certified lymphedema therapist (CLT). CDT involves a two-phase treatment program:

- Phase 1—Reduce tissue congestion of affected body part with daily treatments:
  1. Manual lymph drainage
  2. Skin care
  3. Compression wrapping of limb
  4. Decongestive exercises
- Phase 2—Maintain decongestion with Home Maintenance Program:
  1. Daily use of elastic and inelastic compression garments that are properly fitted according to circumference and length to prevent lymphedema from returning
  2. Compression is graduated; most of the compression is distal with decreasing compression in the stocking proximally
  3. Different knits and compression classes are available for different stages of lymphedema
  4. Choices of garments include below the knee stockings, thigh-high stockings, pantyhose, sleeves, bras, and truncal garments

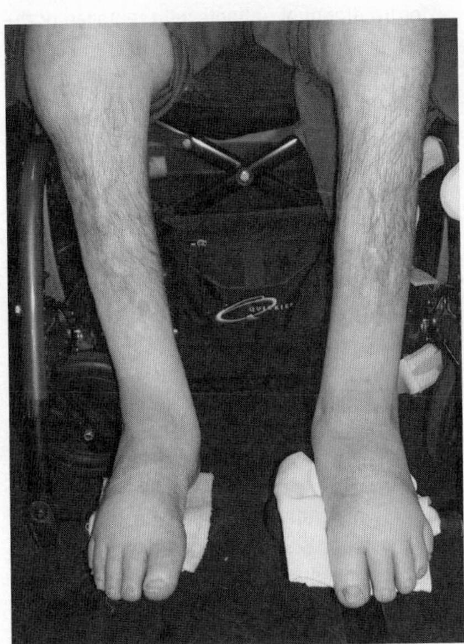

FIGURE 1-570 Lymphedema after treatment.

- Massage (or any modality that increases blood flow) can have negative effects on lymphedema by increasing vasodilation. Therefore it is contraindicated on the lymphedematous quadrants
- Compression pumps have not been found to be effective in removing proteins from lymphedematous quadrants
- Nutritional therapy (reducing the amount of proteins ingested) is ineffective in the treatment of lymphedema

PHARMACOLOGIC THERAPY

No drugs have been shown to be beneficial in the treatment of lymphedema. Diuretics, in particular, have not been found to be effective in removing proteins from lymphedematous quadrants and may promote the development of volume depletion.

SURGERY

Surgery for lymphedema has been proven largely unsuccessful and should not be considered prior to CDT. Surgical procedures are divided into two types:

- Physiologic procedures: those performed to improve lymph node drainage (e.g., anastomoses of the lymph system with the venous system, lymph node transplant)
- Excisional or debulking procedures: those performed to excise the subcutaneous tissue (e.g., Charles' procedure, Thompson's procedure, the modified Homans' procedure, and liposuction). Liposuction-circumferential suction-assisted lipectomy represents a newly proposed method to reduce morbidity involved in the traditional excisional techniques

PEARLS & CONSIDERATIONS

- Lymphedema is a chronic, generally incurable but very manageable condition that requires lifelong care and attention along with psychosocial support
- Children and adolescents (along with parents and adults) should be encouraged to pursue a normal life, participating in school activities and sports (preferably noncontact, such as swimming)
- Infections such as cellulitis should be treated promptly
- If the etiology is filariasis caused by the parasites *Wuchereria bancrofti* or *Brugia malayi*, treatment is diethylcarbamazine citrate 5 mg/kg in divided doses for 3 wk.
- Patients with lymphedema commonly manifest psychiatric comorbidities as a result of their disease, such as anxiety, depression, adjustment problems, and difficulty in vocational, domestic, or social domains
- Lymphedema can be complicated in rare cases by development of lymphangiosarcomata or other cutaneous malignancies
- Gene therapy to develop new lymphangioles in the affected body parts is a potential clinical remedy in the future

SUGGESTED READINGS

available at www.expertconsult.com

RELATED CONTENT

Lymphedema (Patient Information)

AUTHORS: **FRANK G. FORT, M.D., F.A.C.S.,** and **KATHRYN TAYLOR ANILOWSKI, M.S., P.T., C.L.T.-L.A.N.A.**

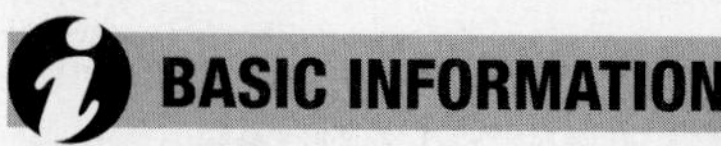

DEFINITION

Non-Hodgkin lymphoma (NHL) is a heterogeneous group of malignancies of the lymphoreticular system.

SYNONYMS

NHL

ICD-9CM CODES
201.9 Lymphoma, non-Hodgkin
ICD-10CM CODES
C85.90 Non-Hodgkin lymphoma, unspecified, unspecified site

EPIDEMIOLOGY & DEMOGRAPHICS

INCIDENCE (IN U.S.): Sixth most common neoplasm (56,000 new cases annually). Incidence increases with age; majority of patients are above 60 years of age.

- In patients with HIV, NHL is the second most common tumor (after Kaposi's sarcoma).
- Diffuse large B-cell lymphoma (DLBCL) is the most common type of HIV-associated lymphoma, accounting for 80% to 90% of cases.
- Primary CNS lymphoma (PCNSL) accounts for 2% of the cases of lymphoma in patients with HIV infection, but it accounts for 10% of the cases in patients with a diagnosis of AIDS.
- More common in men than women.
- Higher rates seen in Europe, Australia, and the U.S.

PREDOMINANT AGE: Median age at time of diagnosis is 50 yr.

PHYSICAL FINDINGS & CLINICAL PRESENTATION

- Patients often present with asymptomatic lymphadenopathy.
- Approximately one third of NHLs originate extranodally. Involvement of extranodal sites can result in unusual presentations (e.g., gastrointestinal tract involvement can simulate peptic ulcer disease).
- Presence of B symptoms like unexplained weight loss, fever, fatigue, and night sweats.
- NHL cases associated with HIV occur predominantly in the brain.
- Pruritus
- Hepatomegaly and splenomegaly may be present.
- Cough, dyspnea in pulmonary involvement.

Dx DIAGNOSIS

DIFFERENTIAL DIAGNOSIS

- Hodgkin's disease
- Viral infections
- Metastatic carcinoma
- Autoimmune conditions

A clinical algorithm for evaluation of lymphadenopathy is described in Section III. The differential diagnosis of lymphadenopathy is described in Section II.

WORKUP

Initial laboratory evaluation may reveal only mild anemia and elevated lactate dehydrogenase (LDH) and erythrocyte sedimentation rate (ESR). Proper staging of NHL requires the following:

- A thorough history, physical examination, and excisional or surgical biopsy. Laparoscopic lymph node biopsy can be used on an outpatient basis for most patients with intraabdominal lymphoma.
- Routine laboratory evaluation (complete blood count, flow cytometry, ESR, urinalysis, LDH, blood urea nitrogen, creatinine, serum calcium, uric acid, liver function tests, serum protein electrophoresis).
- Chest x-ray (posteroanterior and lateral).
- Bone marrow evaluation (aspirate and full bone core biopsy) (Fig. E1-571).
- CT scan of abdomen and pelvis; CT scan of chest if chest x-ray films abnormal.
- Fluorine-18 fluorodeoxyglucose (FDG) positron emission tomography (PET) integrated with CT has emerged as a powerful tool for staging, response evaluation, and posttreatment surveillance in patients with NHL.
- Bone scan (particularly in patients with histiocytic lymphoma).
- Depending on the histopathology (Table E1-311), the results of the above studies and the planned therapy, some other tests may be performed.
- β-2 microglobulin levels should be obtained initially (prognostic value) and serially in patients with low-grade lymphomas (useful to monitor therapeutic response of the tumor).
- Serum interleukin levels have prognostic value in diffuse large cell lymphoma.
- HIV testing.

CLASSIFICATION: The working formulation of NHL for clinical use subdivides lymphomas into low grade, intermediate grade, high grade, and miscellaneous (Table 1-312).

STAGING: The Ann Arbor staging system with Cotswold modification is described in Table 1-313. Histopathology has greater therapeutic implications in NHL than in Hodgkin's disease. The frequency of indolent lymphomas among all lymphomas is described in Table 1-314. The classification of aggressive lymphomas is described in Table 1-315.

Rx TREATMENT

ACUTE GENERAL Rx

The therapeutic regimen varies with the histologic type and pathologic stage. Following are the commonly used therapeutic modalities:

LOW-GRADE NHL (e.g., NODULAR, POORLY DIFFERENTIATED)

1. Local radiotherapy for symptomatic obstructive adenopathy.
2. Deferment of therapy and careful observation in asymptomatic patients with indolent lymphomas.
3. Single-agent chemotherapy with cyclophosphamide or chlorambucil and glucocorticoids is infrequently used.
4. Combination chemotherapy alone or with radiotherapy: generally indicated only when the lymphoma becomes more invasive, with poor response to less aggressive treatment. Radiation therapy without chemotherapy is not recommended due to increased relapse rate.
5. Monoclonal antibodies directed against B-cell surface antigens can also be used to treat follicular lymphomas resistant to conventional therapy. The anti-CD20 monoclonal antibody rituximab is effective against low-grade NHL in patients who have not received previous treatment. The addition of rituximab to cyclophosphamide, doxorubicin, vincristine, and prednisone (CHOP-R) is generally well tolerated.
6. Ibritumomab tiuxetan, an immunoconjugate that combines the linker-chelator tiuxetan with the monoclonal antibody ibritumomab, can be used as part of a two-step regimen for treatment of patients with relapsed or refractory low-grade, follicular, or transformed B-cell NHL refractory to rituximab.
7. New purine analogs (FLAMP, 2CDA) can be used in salvage treatment of refractory lymphomas. They all have activity in follicular lymphomas.
8. Table 1-316 summarizes treatment strategies for indolent lymphomas.

INTERMEDIATE- AND HIGH-GRADE LYMPHOMAS (e.g., DIFFUSE HISTIOCYTIC LYMPHOMA)

Combination chemotherapy regimens (e.g., CHOP, PRO-MACE-CYTABOM, MACOP-B, M-BACOD). An anthracycline-containing regimen (such as CHOP) given in standard doses and schedule is generally best for treatment of older patients with advanced stage, aggressive-histology lymphoma who do not have significant comorbid illness.

1. High-dose sequential therapy is superior to standard-dose MACOP-B for patients with diffuse large-cell lymphoma of the B-cell type.
2. Dose-modified chemotherapy should be considered for most HIV-infected patients with lymphoma.
   - Three cycles of CHOP followed by involved-field radiotherapy may be superior to eight cycles of CHOP alone in patients with localized intermediate- and high-grade NHL.
   - High-dose chemotherapy with autologous stem-cell support has been reported to be superior to CHOP in adults with disseminated aggressive lymphoma.
   - The addition of rituximab against CD20 B-cell lymphoma to the CHOP regimen (CHOP-R) increases the complete response rate and prolongs event-free and overall survival in elderly patients with diffuse large B-cell lymphoma without a clinically significant increase in toxicity. Bexxar, a combination of the mononuclear antibody tositumomab and radiolabeled iodine-131, can be used for a single treatment of relapsed follicular NHL in patients who are refractory to rituximab.

TABLE 1-312 Classification Systems for Grading Lymphomas

Kiel Classification	Working Formulation	Revised European-American Classification
Low-grade malignancy	Low grade	B-cell lymphomas
Lymphocytic, CLL	A. Malignant lymphoma, small lymphocytic	
Lymphocytic, other	Consistent with CLL	B-CLL/SLL
Lymphoplasmacytoid		Lymphoplasmacytoid lymphoma
Centrocytic	B. Malignant lymphoma, follicular, predominantly small cleaved cell	Follicle center lymphomas
Centroblastic/centrocytic		Marginal zone lymphomas (MALT)
Follicular without sclerosis	Diffuse areas	Mantle cell lymphoma
Follicular with sclerosis	Sclerosis	
Follicular and diffuse, without sclerosis	C. Malignant lymphoma, follicular mixed, small cleaved and large cell	
Follicular and diffuse, with sclerosis	Diffuse areas	Diffuse large B-cell lymphoma
Diffuse	Sclerosis	Primary mediastinal large B-cell lymphoma
Low-grade malignant lymphoma, unclassified	Intermediate grade	Burkitt's lymphoma
High-grade malignancy	D. Malignant lymphoma, follicular	T-cell lymphomas
Centroblastic	Diffuse areas	
Lymphoblastic, Burkitt's type	E. Malignant lymphoma, diffuse small cleaved cell	
Lymphoblastic, convoluted cell type		T-CLL
Lymphoblastic, other (unclassified) immunoblastic		Mycosis fungoides/Sézary syndrome
High-grade malignant lymphoma, unclassified	F. Malignant lymphoma, diffuse mixed, small and large cell sclerosis	
Malignant lymphoma unclassified (unable to specify high grade or low grade)	G. Malignant lymphoma diffuse	Peripheral T-cell lymphoma, unspecified
Composite lymphoma	Large cell	Angioimmunoblastic T-cell lymphoma
	Cleaved cell	Angiocentric lymphoma
	Noncleaved cell	Intestinal T-cell lymphoma
	Sclerosis	Adult T-cell lymphoma/leukemia
	High grade	Anaplastic large cell lymphoma
	H. Malignant lymphoma large cell, immunoblastic	Precursor T-lymphoid lymphoma/leukemia
	Plasmacytoid	
	Clear cell	
	Polymorphous	
	Epithelioid cell component	
	I. Malignant lymphoma lymphoblastic	
	Convoluted cell	
	Nonconvoluted cell	
	J. Malignant lymphoma small noncleaved cell	
	Burkitt's	
	Follicular areas	

B-CLL, B-cell chronic lymphoid leukemia; *CLL,* chronic lymphocytic leukemia; *MALT,* mucosa-associated lymphoid tumor; *SLL,* lymphoid leukemia; *T-CLL,* T-cell CLL.
From Abeloff MD: *Clinical oncology,* ed 3, New York, 2004, Churchill Livingstone.

TABLE 1-313 Ann Arbor Staging System for Lymphomas

Stage*	Cotswold Modification of Ann Arbor Classification
I	Involvement of a single lymph node region or lymphoid structure
II	Involvement of two or more lymph node regions on the same side of the diaphragm (the mediastinum is considered a single site, whereas the hilar lymph nodes are considered bilaterally); the number of anatomic sites should be indicated by a subscript (e.g., II_3)
III	Involvement of lymph node regions on both sides of the diaphragm: III_1 (with or without involvement of splenic hilar, celiac, or portal nodes) and III_2 (with involvement of para-aortic, iliac, and mesenteric nodes)
IV	Involvement of one or more extranodal sites in addition to a site for which the designation E has been used

*All cases are subclassified to indicate the absence (A) or presence (B) of the systemic symptoms of significant fever (>38.0° C [100.4° F]), night sweats, and unexplained weight loss exceeding 10% of normal body weight within the previous 6 months. The clinical stage (CS) denotes the stage as determined by all diagnostic examinations and a single diagnostic biopsy only. In the Ann Arbor classification, the term pathologic stage (PS) is used if a second biopsy of any kind has been obtained, whether negative or positive. In the Cotswold modification, the PS is determined by laparotomy; X designates bulky disease (widening of the mediastinum by more than one third or the presence of a nodal mass >10 cm), and E designates involvement of a single extranodal site that is contiguous or proximal to the known nodal site.
From Hoffmann R et al: *Hematology: basic principles and practice,* ed 5, Philadelphia, 2009, Churchill Livingstone.

TABLE 1-314 Frequency of Indolent Lymphomas Among All Lymphomas in the World Health Organization Classification

Follicular lymphoma	22.1%
Extranodal marginal zone lymphoma of mucosa-associated lymphoid tissue type	7.6%
Small lymphocytic lymphoma/chronic lymphocytic leukemia	6.7%
Mantle cell	6.0%
Splenic marginal zone lymphoma	1.8%
Lymphoplasmacytic lymphoma	1.2%
Nodal marginal zone B-cell lymphoma (±monocytoid B cells)	1.0%

From Hoffman R et al: *Hematology: basic principles and practice,* ed 5, Philadelphia, 2009, Churchill Livingstone.

TABLE 1-315 Classification of Aggressive Lymphomas

B-cell Neoplasms
Precursor B-cell lymphoma
Precursor B lymphoblastic leukemia/lymphoma
Mature B-cell lymphoma
Mantle cell lymphoma
Diffuse large B-cell lymphoma
Mediastinal (thymic) large B-cell lymphoma
Intravascular large B-cell lymphoma
Primary effusion lymphoma
Burkitt lymphoma/leukemia
B-cell proliferations of uncertain malignant potential
Lymphomatoid granulomatosis
Posttransplant lymphoproliferative disorder, polymorphic
T-cell and NK-cell Neoplasms
Precursor T-cell
Precursor T lymphoblastic leukemia/lymphoma
Blastic NK cell lymphoma
Mature T-cell and NK-cell lymphoma
Adult T-cell leukemia/lymphoma
Extranodal NK/T cell lymphoma, nasal type
Hepatosplenic T-cell lymphoma
Peripheral T-cell lymphoma, unspecified
Angioimmunoblastic T-cell lymphoma
Anaplastic large cell lymphoma

NK, Natural killer.
From Hoffman R et al: *Hematology: basic principles and practice*, ed 5, Philadelphia, 2009, Churchill Livingstone.

TABLE 1-316 Treatment Strategies for Indolent Lymphomas

Advanced Stage Disease
"Watchful waiting"
Alkylating agents
Purine analogs
Combination chemotherapy
Monoclonal antibodies Unconjugated Conjugated – radioimmunoconjugates and immunotoxins
Chemotherapy + monoclonal antibodies (chemoimmunotherapy)
High dose chemotherapy plus autologous/allogeneic hematopoietic cell transplantation
Reduced intensity conditioning allogeneic transplantation
Palliative radiotherapy
Localized Disease
Radiotherapy
"Watchful waiting"

From Hoffman R et al: *Hematology: basic principles and practice*, ed 5, Philadelphia, 2009, Churchill Livingstone.

- In patients <61 yr, chemotherapy with three cycles of ACVBP (doxorubicin, cyclophosphamide, vindesine, bleomycin, and prednisone) followed by sequential consolidation has been reported to be superior to three cycles of CHOP plus radiotherapy for treatment of newly diagnosed aggressive lymphoma (diffuse mixed, diffuse large cell, or immunoblastic according to the working formulation).
- Granulocyte-colony stimulating factor: may be effective in reducing the risk of infection in patients with aggressive lymphoma undergoing chemotherapy.
- Radioimmunotherapy with (^{131}I) anti-B1 antibody therapy for NHL either by itself or in combination with other treatments represents a new modality in the armamentarium against lymphomas.
- Treatment with high-dose chemotherapy and autologous bone marrow transplant: compared with conventional chemotherapy, increases event-free and overall survival in patients with chemotherapy-sensitive NHL in relapse.
- An algorithm for the management of NHL in pediatric patients is described in Fig. E1-572. Combination chemotherapy regimens for NHL are described in Table 1-317.

DISPOSITION

- Patients with low-grade lymphoma, despite their long-term survival (6 to 10 yr average), are rarely cured, and the great majority (if not all) eventually die of the lymphoma, whereas patients with a high-grade lymphoma may achieve a cure with aggressive chemotherapy.
- Complete remission occurs in 35% to 50% of patients with intermediate- and high-grade lymphoma. Prognostic factors include the histiologic subtype, age of patient, and bulk of disease. Table E1-318 describes the International Prognostic Index for aggressive lymphomas.
- Patients who present with AIDS-related NHL and a low CD4 cell count have a poor prognosis (median duration of survival is 15 to 34 mo). Despite therapeutic advances, the management of HIV-associated lymphomas is challenging due to potential pharmacologic interactions and increased risk of infectious complications. It is important to optimize the CD4 cell count during treatment. Referral to an HIV oncologist is recommended.

TABLE 1-317 Combination Chemotherapy Regimens for Non-Hodgkin Lymphoma

Regimen	Dose	Days of Administration	Frequency
CHOP-R			Every 21 days
Cyclophosphamide	750 mg/m² IV	1	
Doxorubicin	50 mg/m² IV	1	
Vincristine	1.4 mg/m² IV*	1	
Prednisone, fixed dose	100 mg PO	1-5	
Rituximab	375 mg/m² IV	1	
CVP-R			Every 21 days
Cyclophosphamide	1000 mg/m² IV	1	
Vincristine	1.4 mg/m² IV*	1	
Prednisone, fixed dose	100 mg PO	1-5	
Rituximab	375 mg/m² IV	1	
FCR			Every 28 days
Fludarabine	25 mg/m² IV	1-3	
Cyclophosphamide	250 mg/m² IV	1-3	
Rituximab	375 mg/m²	1	

*Vincristine dose often capped at 2 mg total.
From Goldman L, Schafer AI: *Goldman's Cecil medicine*, ed 24, Philadelphia, 2012, Saunders.

SUGGESTED READINGS
available at www.expertconsult.com

RELATED CONTENT
Non-Hodgkin's Lymphoma (Patient Information)

AUTHORS: **SYEDA M. SAYEED, M.D.,** and **FRED F. FERRI, M.D.**

BASIC INFORMATION

DEFINITION

Lynch syndrome is a hereditary predisposition to malignancy of the colon that is explained by a germline mutation in a DNA mismatch repair gene.

SYNONYMS

Hereditary nonpolyposis colorectal cancer
Hereditary site-specific colon cancer

ICD-9CM CODES
1539 Lynch syndrome
ICD-10CM CODES
C18.9 Malignant neoplasm of colon, unspecified

EPIDEMIOLOGY & DEMOGRAPHICS

The lifetime risk for developing colon cancer in the U.S. is approximately 6%. Of these cases, 2% to 3% may be attributable to Lynch syndrome. The incidence of Lynch syndrome is estimated to be between 1:660 and 1:2000. Lynch syndrome is the most common form of hereditary colon cancer. The average age of diagnosis for Lynch syndrome is 48 years, although diagnosis can occur as early as the 20s or as late as the 70s.

RISK FACTORS: Family history of colon cancer or other hereditary nonpolyposis colorectal cancer (HNPCC)-related cancers such as endometrial (up to 40% of women with Lynch syndrome may develop endometrial cancer), biliary tract, ovarian, stomach, upper urinary tract, or brain.

GENETICS: Autosomal-dominant inheritance pattern

ETIOLOGY

Lynch syndrome is thought to be secondary to germline mutations in DNA mismatch repair genes. The predominant genes involved are *MSH2* and *MLH1,* which are tumor suppressor genes, although other genes have documented involvement *(PMS1, PMS2, MSH6, MLH3).* Mutations in these genes prevent repair of DNA mismatches during DNA replication. This is most prevalent in regions of DNA called microsatellites causing DNA microsatellite instability and leading to an increased risk for malignancy, especially colon cancer. *MSH6* mutations are associated with a markedly lower cancer risk than *MLH1* or *MSH2* mutations.

PHYSICAL FINDINGS & CLINICAL PRESENTATION

- Changes in bowel habits (prolonged constipation)
- Melena
- Hematochezia
- Abdominal pain
- Unexplained weight loss
- Decreased appetite

Dx DIAGNOSIS

DIFFERENTIAL DIAGNOSIS

- Familial adenomatosis polyposis
- Peutz-Jeghers syndrome
- Juvenile polyposis
- Nonhereditary colorectal cancer
- Gardner syndrome

WORKUP

If an individual presents with numerous adenomatous polyps or has multiple relatives with cancer at a young age, a family history complete with pedigree must be obtained. Clinical diagnosis of the Lynch syndrome can be made with the Amsterdam or Bethesda criteria.

- Revised Amsterdam (II) criteria (must meet all criteria):
  1. HNPCC associated carrier diagnosis in at least three individuals in the family
  2. One of the patients is a first-degree family member of two other patients
  3. Involved patients occur in at least two successive generations with diagnosis of HNPCC
  4. At least one diagnosis in family of HNPCC was made before age 50
  5. The diagnoses are histologically confirmed
  6. Familial adenomatous polyposis is excluded
- Bethesda criteria (must meet all criteria):
  1. Colorectal cancer before age 50
  2. Multiple colorectal cancers or other HNPCC-related cancers such as biliary tract, endometrial, stomach, or ovary
  3. Colorectal cancer with microsatellite instability histology <60 yr of age
  4. Colorectal cancer or HNPCC-related cancer in first-degree relative <50 yr of age
  5. Colorectal cancer or HNPCC-related cancer in at least two first- or second-degree relatives, any age
- If criteria for the Lynch syndrome are not met, no further analysis is necessary (although a genetic syndrome cannot be definitively excluded and genetic referral may be warranted).

LABORATORY TESTS

- If a patient meets criteria for Lynch syndrome, immunohistochemistry can be performed for the presence or absence of mismatch repair genes *MLH1, MSH2, MSH6,* and *PMS2.* Rarely, *MLH3* is identified.
- Microsatellite instability analysis should also be performed if criteria for Lynch syndrome are met.

Rx TREATMENT

- If the mutation has been identified in a family member, screening for this mutation can be performed via genetic testing. Informed consent must be obtained after a thorough explanation has been provided to each individual.
- Surveillance using colonoscopy can be performed in individuals who screen positive, while those who screen negative can be discharged. The mismatch repair gene that is mutated guides screening.
- According to the Netherlands Surveillance Protocol, for example, individuals with mutations in *MLH1, MSH2,* or *MSH6* should have colonoscopies every 1 to 2 yr starting at age 20 to 25 yr; urine cytology every 1 to 2 yr starting at age 30 to 35 yr; gastroscopy every 1 to 2 yr starting at age 30 to 35 yr; and, in females, ultrasound of endometrium and CA-125 every 1 to 2 yr starting at age 30 to 35 yr.

REFERRALS

- To gastroenterology for surveillance colonoscopies
- To genetic counselor if patient satisfies Bethesda criteria
- To psychologist as necessary for psychologic support

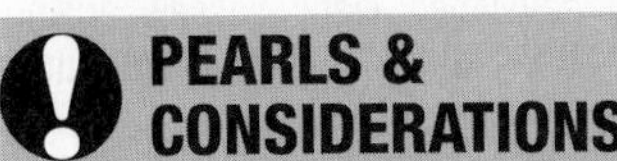

PEARLS & CONSIDERATIONS

- Prior to genetic testing being instituted, informed consent must be obtained because consequences of this testing include the necessity of lifelong screenings such as colonoscopies.
- The risk of pancreatic cancer is increased in families with Lynch syndrome compared with the U.S. population.

PATIENT & FAMILY EDUCATION

- For information on local genetic counselors, visit the National Society of Genetic Counselors Web site at www.nsgc.org.
- For information on Lynch syndrome, visit www.mayoclinic.com/health/lynch-syndrome/DS00669.

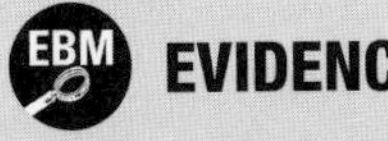

EVIDENCE

available at www.expertconsult.com

SUGGESTED READINGS

available at www.expertconsult.com

RELATED CONTENT

Colorectal Cancer (Related Key Topic)

AUTHORS: **PAUL F. GEORGE, M.D.,** and **JOANNE M. SILVIA, M.D.**

BASIC INFORMATION

DEFINITION

Macular degeneration refers to a group of diseases associated with loss of central vision and damage to the macula. Degenerative changes occur in the pigment, neural, and vascular layers of the macula. Dry macular degeneration is usually ischemic in etiology, and wet macular degeneration is associated with leakage of fluid from blood vessels, usually referred to as *age-related macular degeneration* (AMD).

ICD-9CM CODES
362.5 Degeneration of macula and posterior pole
ICD-10CM CODES
H35.30 Unspecified macular degeneration

EPIDEMIOLOGY & DEMOGRAPHICS

INCIDENCE (IN U.S.):
- Leading cause of irreversible blindness in people ≥50 yr in the developed world.
- Increases with age.
- More than 8 million Americans have AMD. The overall prevalence is projected to increase by >50% by 2020.
- About 10% of patients with AMD have the neovascular form manifested by an often rapid decrease in central visual acuity caused by newly developed leaky vessels arising from the choroid towards the subretinal space.

PEAK INCIDENCE:
- Ages 75 to 80 yr
- Dramatically increases in incidence and prevalence with age until ~80% of people ≥75 yr have senile macular degeneration

PREVALENCE (IN U.S.): Varies, but ~5% of people >50 yr have some signs of macular degeneration

PREDOMINANT SEX: Males and females are affected equally (15% of white women >80 yr have severe AMD)

PREDOMINANT AGE: >50 yr

RISK FACTORS:
- Advancing age
- Genetic factors
- Complement factor H, Tyr402His variant
- *LOC387715/ARMS2*, Ala69Ser variant
- History of smoking within past 20 yr
- Dietary factors (low intake of antioxidants and zinc, high fat intake)
- Obesity
- White race

PHYSICAL FINDINGS & CLINICAL PRESENTATION

- Decreased central vision
- Macular hemorrhage, pigmentation, edema, atrophy
- The most common abnormality seen in AMD is the presence of drusen, or yellowish deposits deep to the retina; this may be early in the course of disease
- Choroidal neovascular membrane (CNVM) develops with rapid change in vision

ETIOLOGY

- Subretinal neovascular membrane early
- Pigmentary and vascular changes with exudate, edema, and scar tissue development
- Dry-type atrophy of macular pigment epithelium
- The main mediator of neovascularization in wet AMD is the vascular endothelial growth factor (VEGF). It induces angiogenesis and increases inflammation and vascular permeability

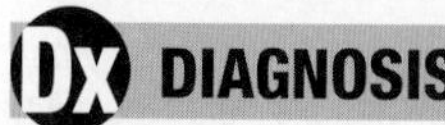

DIAGNOSIS

DIFFERENTIAL DIAGNOSIS

- Diabetic retinopathy (with neovascularization, can mimic CNVM)
- Hypertension
- Histoplasmosis (less common cause of CNVM)
- Trauma with scar

WORKUP

- Complete eye examination, including visual field and fluorescein angiography
- Optical coherence tomography (OCT)

LABORATORY TESTS

Evaluate for diabetes and other metabolic problems as well as vascular diseases

IMAGING STUDIES

- OCT
- Fluorescein angiography

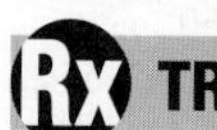

TREATMENT

NONPHARMACOLOGIC THERAPY

- There is no proven treatment for dry AMD.
- Laser treatment to stop progression of disease; photodynamic treatment with verteporfin IV
- Laser (argon) for certain classic membranes (CNVM)
- A high dietary intake of antioxidants, vitamins C and E, and zinc has been reported to substantially reduce the risk of AMD in elderly persons

ACUTE GENERAL Rx

- The introduction of therapies blocking VEGF dramatically changed the management of AMD and it is now standard practice for clinicians to offer intravitreal injections of anti-VEGF agents (ranibizumab, bevacizumab) as first-line treatment for neovascular AMD. Intravitreal administration of ranibizumab, a monoclonal antibody Fab that neutralizes all active forms of VEGF A, has shown to be effective in preventing vision loss and improving mean visual acuity in patients with AMD. It has also been reported to be superior to photodynamic therapy with verteporfin in the treatment of predominantly classic neovascular AMD. Bevacizumab, a monoclonal antibody to VEGF, is also often used off-label as intravitreal therapy. Its cost per intravitreal dose is significantly lower than that of ranibizumab. A major concern regarding anti-VEGF treatment is the potential increased risk of stroke and cardiovascular disease.
- Intravitreous injections of pegaptanib, a more selective anti-VEGF, appear to be less effective therapy in slowing vision loss in neovascular AMD than bevacizumab or ranibizumab. Pegaptanib is administered once every 6 wk by intravitreous injection into one eye.
- Afibercept, a fusion protein that competes for binding of VEGF, has recently been FDA approved for the treatment of wet (neovascular) AMD. It is injected intravitreally every 8 weeks. It appears to be as effective as ranibizumab and bevacizumab but is more expensive.
- Laser photocoagulation therapy may be useful in patients with extrafoveal lesions but is no longer routinely recommended for wet AMD.

CHRONIC Rx

- Laser phototherapy is not recommended for dry AMD.
- Antioxidants and zinc may slow progression of AMD

DISPOSITION

- Follow closely by ophthalmologist, retinal specialist.
- Most bevacizumab or ranibizumab treatment failures are due to missed follow-up visits. Patients should be reminded repeatedly to call if their vision worsens. There should also be a system in place for calling patients who have been lost to follow-up due to the high risk of recurrent neovascularization and vision loss in these patients.

REFERRAL

- To ophthalmologist early in the course of the disease if vision is to be saved
- Immediate referral if any change in vision

PEARLS & CONSIDERATIONS

COMMENTS

- Sildenafil has no significant effect on macular degeneration.
- Statistically, the vision of only 1 of 10 affected persons can be saved, but the disease is so devastating that vigorous therapy should be considered in all patients.
- Statins plus aspirin may slow progression.
- Vitamins with zinc and antioxidants may slow progression of AMD.
- Quitting smoking significantly reduces the risk of developing AMD.

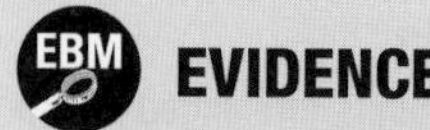

EVIDENCE

available at www.expertconsult.com

SUGGESTED READINGS

available at www.expertconsult.com

RELATED CONTENT

Macular Degeneration (Patient Information)

AUTHORS: **MELVYN KOBY, M.D.**, and **R. SCOTT HOFFMAN, M.D.**

BASIC INFORMATION

DEFINITION

Malaria is a protozoan disease caused by the genus *Plasmodium* and transmitted by female *Anopheles* spp. mosquitoes. It is endemic throughout most of the tropics and is characterized by hectic fever and often presents with classic malarial paroxysm. Five species of genus *Plasmodium* usually infect humans (Table 1-319):

- *P. falciparum*
- *P. vivax*
- *P. malariae*
- *P. ovale*
- *P. knowlesi*

SYNONYMS

Periodic fever
Tertian malaria
Quartan malaria
Tropical splenomegaly

ICD-9CM CODES
084.6 Malaria
ICD-10CM CODES
B54 Unspecified malaria
B50.9 *Plasmodium faluparum* malaria, unspecified
B51.9 *Plasmodium vivax* malaria without complications
B52.9 *Plasmodium malariae* malaria without complications
53.0 *Plasmodium ovale* malaria
B53.8 Other parasitologically confirmed malaria, not elsewhere classified

EPIDEMIOLOGY & DEMOGRAPHICS

Global:

- ~300 million cases a year in more than 100 countries
- Around 900,000 deaths per year, with more than 80% of the deaths ocurring in children of sub-Saharan Africa
- 3 billion people live in malaria-endemic areas

U.S.:

- ~1500 cases reported to the CDC in the United States each year. In the majority of reported cases, U.S. civilians who acquired infection abroad had not adhered to a chemoprophylaxis regimen that was appropriate for the country in which they acquired malaria.
- More than 50% of the reported cases in the U.S. are *P. falciparum.* On average, there are six deaths per year in the United States.
- Most infections limited to:
  1. Immigrant population
  2. Returned travelers or troops from endemic area
- Occasionally, transmission through exposure to infected blood product or shared intravenous needles by users of injection drugs.
- Congenital transmission is possible.
- Local mosquito-borne transmission has been reported.
- Competent mosquito vectors are present.
  1. *A. albimanus* in eastern United States
  2. *A. freeborni* in western United States

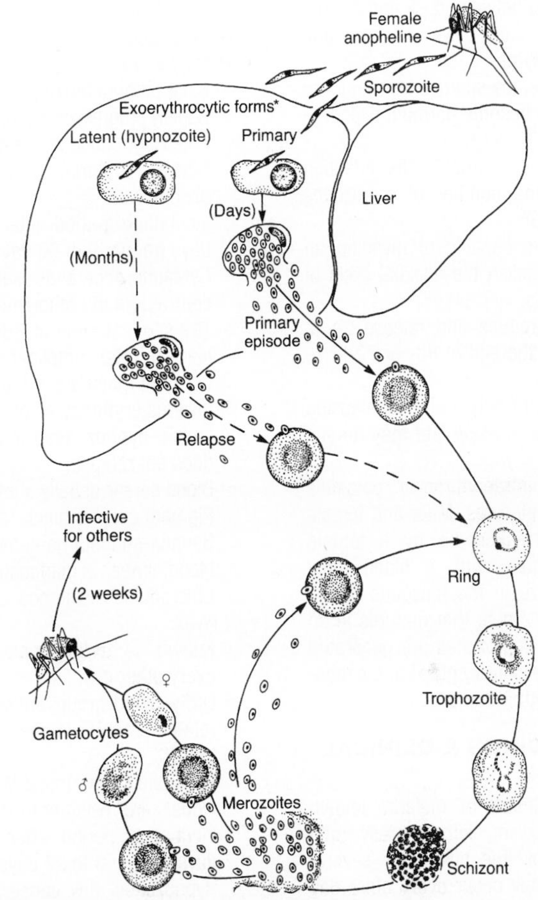

FIGURE 1-573 Life cycle of plasmodia in humans. Exoerythrocytic forms are also called schizonts. (From Gorbach SL: *Infectious diseases,* ed 2, Philadelphia, 1998, Saunders.)

TABLE 1-319 Features of the Five Species of Malaria Known to Cause Disease in Humans

	Plasmodium falciparum	*Plasmodium vivax*	*Plasmodium ovale*	*Plasmodium malariae*	*Plasmodium knowlesi*
Incubation period (days)	6-25	8-27	8-27	16-40	12
Asexual cycle (hours)	48 (tertian)	48 (tertian)	48 (tertian)	72 (quartan)	24 (tertian)
Relapse	No	Yes*	Yes*	No†	No
Chloroquine resistance	Yes‡	Rare§	No	No‖	No
Characteristic on thin blood film	Rings predominate, multiply infected RBCs, high parasitemia, rings with thread-like cytoplasm, double nuclei, banana-shaped gametocytes	Enlarged RBCs, Schüffner's dots, trophozoite cytoplasm ameboid, 12-24 merozoites in mature schizont	Oval RBCs with fringed edges, Schüffner's dots, trophozoite cytoplasm compact, 6-16 merozoites in mature schizont	Trophozoite cytoplasm compact (band forms), 6-12 merozoites in mature schizont, RBC unchanged	Similar to *P. malariae*, 8-10 merozoites in mature schizont, often in rosette pattern with central clump of pigment

*Relapses may appear months to years after initial infection due to dormant hypnozoites in the liver.
†Although relapse does not occur, *P. malariae* can produce persistent infections that remain below detectable limits in the blood for 20 to 30 years or more.
‡*P. falciparum* resistance to sulfadoxine/pyrimethamine, mefloquine, halofantrine, and artemisinin have also been reported in some areas, along with partial resistance to quinine and quinidine.
§*P. vivax* resistance to chloroquine now reported in some areas of Southeast Asia, Oceania, and South America.
‖Chloroquine-resistant *P. malariae* has also been reported in south Sumatra, Indonesia.
From Vincent JL et al: *Textbook of critical care,* ed 6, Philadelphia, 2011, Saunders.

Geographic distribution:

- *P. falciparum:* Sub-Saharan Africa, Papua New Guinea, Solomon Islands, Haiti, Indian subcontinent
- *P. vivax:* Central America, South America, North Africa, Middle East, Indian subcontinent
- *P. ovale:* West Africa
- *P. malariae:* worldwide

Parasite life cycle (Fig. 1-573):

- Human infection begins when a female anopheline mosquito bites (only female anopheline mosquito takes blood meal) and inoculates plasmodial sporozoites into bloodstream. The bite usually occurs between dusk and dawn.
- The sporozoites then travel to liver and invade to hepatocytes.
- In the hepatocytes, the sporozoites mature to tissue schizont or become dormant hypnozoites.
- The tissue schizonts amplify the infection by producing large number of merozoites (10,000 to 30,000).
- Each merozoite is capable of invading an RBC and can establish the asexual cycle of replication in RBCs.
- Asexual cycles produce and release 24 to 32 merozoites at the end of 48- or 72-hr *(P. malariae)* cycles.
- The hypnozoites are only found in relapsing malaria *P. vivax* or *P. ovale* and may remain dormant for up to 5 yr.
- Eventually some intraerythrocytic parasites develop into gametocytes. Male and female gametocytes are taken up by a female anopheline mosquito with a blood meal where they fertilize in the mosquito gut to produce a diploid zygote that matures to an ookinete; haploid sporozoites are generated that migrate to the salivary gland of the mosquito to infect another human.

PHYSICAL FINDINGS & CLINICAL PRESENTATION

- Fever is the hallmark of malaria, known as malarial paroxysm, initially daily until synchronization of infection after several wk, when fever may occur every other day (tertian) in *P. vivax, P. ovale,* or *P. falciparum* malaria or every third day (quartan) in *P. malariae* malaria. Table 1-320 describes the WHO criteria for severe malaria.
- Classic malarial paroxysm characterized by
  1. Cold stage: abrupt onset of cold feeling associated with rigors, shakes
  2. Hot stage: high fever (~40° C) associated with restlessness
  3. Sweating stage: patient defervesces
- Nonspecific symptoms are
  1. Headache
  2. Cough
  3. Myalgia
  4. Vomiting
  5. Diarrhea
  6. Jaundice
- *P. falciparum:*
  - Most pathogenic of the four species.
  - Rapidly progresses to high-level parasitemia.
  - Important cause of the fatal malaria.
  - Classic malarial paroxysm is usually absent.
  - Incubation period after exposure is 12 days (range: 9 to 60 days).
  - Cytoadherence and resetting of RBCs play central role in pathogenesis.
  - The sequestration of RBCs in vital organs leads to fatal complications.
  - Cerebral malaria is a feared complication.
  - Invades erythrocytes of all ages.
  - Lacks hypnozoites (intrahepatic stage), does not relapse.
  - Blood smear usually shows ring form only.
  - Pigment color is black.
  - Banana-shaped gametocytes; if seen in blood, smear is diagnostic.
  - Chloroquine resistance is widely present.
- *P. vivax:*
  - Known as tertian malaria: fever occurs every other day.
  - Duffy blood-group antigen FYA- or FYB-related receptor is needed for attachment to RBC.
  - FyFy phenotype (most West African) individuals are resistant to *P. vivax* malaria.
  - Incubation period after exposure is 14 days (range: 8 to 27 days).
  - Hypnozoites may cause relapse of infection after years.
  - Infects mainly reticulocytes.
  - Irregularly shaped large rings and trophozoites, enlarged RBCs, and Schüffner's dots are seen in peripheral blood smear (Fig. 1-574).
  - Pigment color is yellow-brown.
  - *P. vivax* from Papua New Guinea have reduced sensitivity to chloroquine.
  - Primaquine is needed to eradicate the hypnozoites.
- *P. ovale:*
  - Also known as tertian malaria; fever occurs every other day.
  - Occurs mainly in tropical Africa.
  - Incubation period after exposure is 14 days (range: 8 to 27 days).
  - Hypnozoites may cause relapse of infection.
  - Infects mainly reticulocytes.
  - Infected RBC is seen as enlarged, oval shape containing large ring or trophozoites with Schüffner's dots.
  - Pigment color is dark brown.
  - Primaquine needed to eradicate the hypnozoites.
  - No chloroquine resistance has been encountered.
- *P. malariae:*
  - Known as quartan malaria; fever occurs every third day.
  - Common cause of chronic malarial infection.
  - May persist for 20 to 30 yr after leaving the endemic area.
  - Worldwide distribution.
  - Incubation period after exposure is 30 days (range: 16 to 60 days).
  - Lacks hypnozoites (intrahepatic stage).
  - May persist in blood for many years if treated inadequately.
  - Chronic infection may cause soluble immune-complex, resulting in nephritic syndrome.
  - Infects mainly mature RBCs.
  - Band or rectangular forms of trophozoites are commonly seen in peripheral blood smear.
  - Pigment color is brown-black.
- Cerebral malaria:
  - Feared complication of *P. falciparum* infection.
  - Mortality is ~20%.

TABLE 1-320 World Health Organization Criteria for Severe Malaria, 2000

Impaired consciousness
Prostration
Respiratory distress
Multiple seizures
Jaundice
Hemoglobinuria
Abnormal bleeding
Severe anemia
Circulatory collapse
Pulmonary edema

From Kliegman RM et al: *Nelson textbook of pediatrics,* ed 19, Philadelphia, 2011, Saunders.

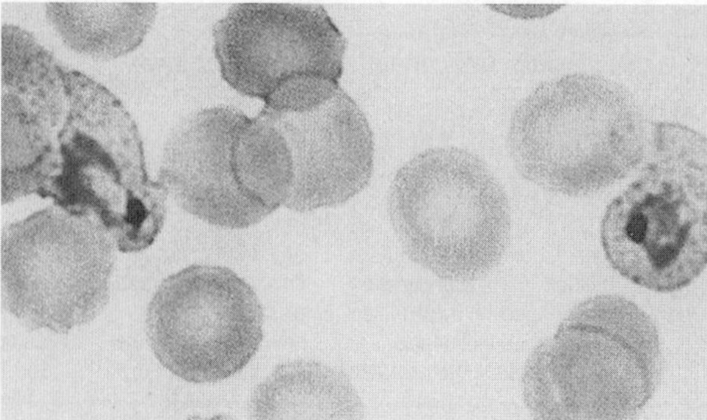

FIGURE 1-574 Giemsa-stained blood smear in *Plasmodium vivax* malaria. Asexual parasites. Note that the parasites are large and ameboid; the infected erythrocytes are the largest cells in the field (because they are reticulocytes), and the erythrocytes contain numerous pink dots (Schüffner's dots) (×2000). (From Klippel JH et al [eds]: *Internal medicine,* ed 5, St Louis, 1998, Mosby.)

- Pathogenesis is poorly understood.
- Ischemia as a result of sequestration of parasites or cytokines induced by parasite toxin(s) is the key debate.
- Seizure and altered mental status leading to coma are cardinal manifestation.
- Hypoglycemia, lactic acidosis, and elevated circulating TNF-α may be present.
- CSF studies: no increase of WBC count or protein, raised lactate concentrate, and increased opening pressure, especially in children, may be present.

Dx DIAGNOSIS

DIFFERENTIAL DIAGNOSIS

- Typhoid fever
- Dengue fever
- Yellow fever
- Viral hepatitis
- Influenza
- Brucellosis
- UTI
- Leishmaniasis
- Trypanosomiasis
- Rickettsial diseases
- Leptospirosis

WORKUP

- Clinical diagnosis is notoriously inaccurate.
- Demonstration of malarial parasites in blood smear is essential.
- Newer molecular diagnostic techniques (polymerase chain reaction, rapid diagnostic tests) are promising.

LABORATORY TESTS

- The thick and thin blood film is required to identify malarial parasites. A Giemsa-stained film of the patient's peripheral blood should be examined for parasites as soon as possible.
- The thick smears are more sensitive and primarily used to detect the presence of parasites.
- The thin smears are used for species differentiation and parasite density estimation.
- A patient who is suspected of having malaria but who has no parasite seen in blood smears should have blood smears repeated every 12 to 24 hr for 3 consecutive days.

PREPARATION OF BLOOD SMEAR:

- Must be prepared from fresh blood obtained by pricking the fingers.
- The thin smear is fixed in methanol before staining.
- The thick smear is stained unfixed.
- The smear should be stained with a 3% Giemsa solution (pH of 7.2) for 30 to 45 min.
- The parasite density should be estimated by counting the percentage of RBCs infected, not the number of parasites, under an oil immersion lens on thin film.

COMMON ERRORS IN READING MALARIAL SMEARS:

- Platelets overlying an RBC
- Misreading artifacts as parasites
- Concern about missing a positive slide

MOLECULAR DIAGNOSIS OF MALARIA:

- Rapid diagnostic tests (RDT)
  1. Employ immunochromatographic lateral flow technology for antigen detection.
  2. Thus far only one RDT has been FDA approved: BinaxNOW Malaria test kit.
  3. This kit is based on antigens HRP-2 and aldolase.
  4. For *P. falciparum:* sensitivity 95% and specificity 94%.
  5. For *P. vivax:* sensitivity 69% and specificity 100%.
- Limitations of the BinaxNOW Malaria test:
  1. Not approved for mixed infections
  2. Should not be used for *P. malariae* and *P. ovale* as data are limited
  3. Positive test must be confirmed by microscopy
  4. Negative results require confirmation by thick and thin smears
  5. This test cannot be used to monitor therapy as antigen persists after the elimination of the parasite, causing false positives
- Other diagnostic tests available include:
  1. Tagged monoclonal antibodies for malaria antigen detection
  2. Nucleic acid amplification and detection: PCR can detect parasites down to a level of 1 to 5 parasites per microliter of blood. PCR can detect mixed species infection
  3. Fluorescence microscopy with acridine orange or other staining
  4. Dark field microscopy

Rx TREATMENT

NONPHARMACOLOGIC THERAPY

ANTIMOSQUITO MEASURES:

1. Eradication of mosquito breeding places by chemical spray
2. Use of mosquito nets properly in the endemic areas
3. Use of protective clothing
4. Use of insect spray (permethrin), mosquito coils, or repellents such as diethyltoluamide (DEET). For adults, DEET (30% to 50%) is generally protective for at least 4 hr. For smaller children, use DEET at ≤20% concentration.

ACUTE GENERAL Rx

A definitive diagnosis of malaria is essential for specific antimalarial chemotherapy.

NON-FALCIPARUM MALARIA:

- Chloroquine 600 mg base (1000 mg chloroquine phosphate) PO loading dose, 6 hr later 300 mg base (500 mg salt), then 300 mg base (500 mg salt) daily for 2 days.
- In the case of *P. vivax* and *P. ovale,* treatment with primaquine 15 mg daily for 14 days is needed to eradicate the exoerythrocytic forms, especially the hypnozoites responsible for relapses.
- G6PD should be measured before primaquine is given. Primaquine is not recommended for those who are glucose-6-phosphate dehydrogenase deficient, because primaquine can cause hemolysis and even death in G6PD-deficient persons. Normal G6PD levels must be documented before using primaquine for either chemoprophylaxis or treatment.
- Chloroquine-resistant *P. vivax* has been documented; in that case, quinine is given.

FALCIPARUM MALARIA:

- Chloroquine can be used cautiously for *falciparum* malaria acquired in chloroquine-sensitive areas (chloroquine is more rapidly effective than quinine)
- Mainstay of treatment is oral quinine sulfate 10 mg (salt)/kg (usually 650 mg) q8h for 3 to 7 days + doxycycline 100 mg PO bid both for 7 days for adults. Pediatrics: quinine sulfate: 10 mg/kg PO tid plus clindamycin: 20 mg/kg per day divided in tid dose both for 7 days.
- Atovaquone-proguanil (Malarone): 250 mg atovaquone/100 mg proguanil): 4 adult tabs PO once a day for 3 days with food in adults or for pediatrics: pediatric tablets (62.5 mg atovaquone/25 mg proguanil) are used based on weight:
  - 5 to 8 kg: 2 pediatric tabs PO once daily for 3 days
  - 9 to 10 kg: 3 pediatric tabs PO once daily for 3 days
  - 11 to 20 kg: 1 adult tab PO once daily for 3 days
  - 21 to 30 kg: 2 adult tabs PO once daily for 3 days
  - 31 to 40 kg: 3 adult tabs PO once daily for 3 days
- >40 kg: 4 adult tabs PO once daily for 3 days artemether-lumefantrine (Coartem) tablets: 4 tabs PO (at time zero and 8 hr later) then bid × 2 days for a total of six doses. For pediatrics:
  - 5 to <15 kg: 1 tablet per dose
  - 15 to <25 kg: 2 tablets per dose
  - 25 to <35 kg: 3 tablets per dose
  - >35 kg: 4 tablets per dose. The child should receive initial dose based on weight, then followed by second dose 8 hr later, then 1 dose PO bid for following 2 days

ALTERNATIVES:

- Quinine sulfate plus clindamycin 900 mg tid for 7 days in adults, or
- Mefloquine 750 mg PO then 500 mg PO 6 to 12 hr later in adults

NOTE: Parasitemia may paradoxically rise in the first 24 to 36 hr and is not an indication of treatment failure.

SEVERE *FALCIPARUM* MALARIA:

- It is a medical emergency; intensive care is preferred.
- Measurement of blood glucose, lactate, ABG is important.
- IV quinidine gluconate 10 mg salt/kg loading dose (maximum 600 mg) in NS; infuse slowly over 1 to 2 hr, followed by continuous infusion of 0.02 mg/kg/min until patient can swallow.
- Need to monitor ECG for observation of QT interval as can prolong. Also need to monitor blood pressure and glucose to avoid hypoglycemia.
- Alternatively, IV artesunate: 2.4 mg/kg IV first dose then at 12 and 24 hr followed by 2.4 mg/kg once daily. One recent study showed the superiority of parenteral artesunate over

parenteral quinine in adults and children who could not take an oral medication.
- Plasmapheresis is an option for parasitemia >30% or in pregnant women and in elderly with severe malaria.

NOTE: WHO recommends IV artesunate as the treatment of choice for severe malaria in adults and children in area of low transmission. Data on children in high-transmission regions are limited, and WHO recommends treatment with artesunate, artemether, or quinine.

MULTIDRUG-RESISTANT MALARIA:
- Mefloquine 1250 mg as a single dose, or
- Halofantrine 500 mg every 6 hr for 3 doses, repeat same course after 1 wk
- Combination therapy usually preferred

DISPOSITION

RISK FACTORS FOR FATAL MALARIA:
- Failure to take chemoprophylaxis
- Delay in seeking medical care
- Misdiagnosis

COMPLICATIONS OF MALARIA:
- Anemia
- Acidosis
- Hypoglycemia
- Respiratory distress
- DIC
- Blackwater fever
- Renal failure
- Shock

REFERRAL

- To an infectious disease specialist or travel medicine expert for severe malaria complications
- To an intensive care specialist if severe cerebral malaria or other major organ failure develops
- All malaria cases are mandated to be reported to local and state health departments by health care providers or laboratory staff

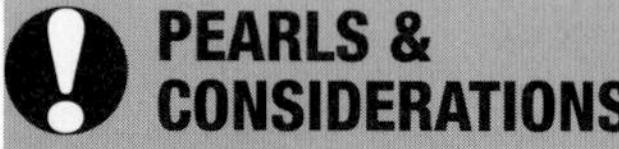

PEARLS & CONSIDERATIONS

HOST RESPONSE:
- The specific immune response to malaria confers protection from high-level parasitemia and disease, but not from infection.
- Asymptomatic parasitemia without illness (premunition) is common among adults in endemic areas.
- Immunity is specific for both the species and the strain of infecting malarial parasites.
- Immunity to all strains is never achieved.
- Normal spleen function is an important host factor because of immunologic as well as filtering functions of the spleen.
- Both humoral and cellular immunity is necessary for protection.
- Polyclonal increase in serum level of IgG, IgM, and IgA occurs in immune individuals.
- Antibody to antigenically variant protein PfEMP1 is important for protection in case of *P. falciparum* malaria.
- Passively transferred IgG from immune individuals has been shown to be protective.
- Maternal antibody confers relative protection of infants from severe disease.
- Genetic disorders (sickle cell disease, thalassemia, and G6PD deficiency) confer protection from death because parasites are unable to grow efficiently in low-oxygen tensions, thus preventing high-level parasitemias.
- Individuals deficient of Duffy factor in RBCs are resistant to infection by *P. vivax.*
- Nonspecific defense mechanisms, such as cytokines (TNF-α, IL-1, -6, -8), also play an important role in protection, causing fever (temperatures of 40° C damage mature parasites) and other pathologic effects.

PREVENTION OF MALARIA:

Medications are available for the prophylaxis of malaria and will vary depending on level of chloroquine resistance in a given area.

Areas free of chloroquine-resistant Falciparum malaria: Chloroquine 300 mg base (500 mg chloroquine phosphate) PO/wk. Start 1 wk prior to arrival in malaria area, then weekly while there and for 4 wk on leaving malaria area. Pediatric dose: 8.3 mg/kg (5 mg/kg base). Alternatives for adults include atovaquone-proguanil (Malarone): 1 adult tablet per day starting 1 to 2 days prior to arriving in malaria area, then daily while there and then for 7 days daily on leaving malaria area. For children, atovaquone-proguanil pediatric tablets based on weight:

11 to 20 kg 1 pediatric tablet
21 to 30 kg 2 pediatric tablets
31 to 40 kg 3 pediatric tablets
>40 kg 1 adult tablet

Areas with chloroquine-resistant Falciparum malaria:
- Atovaquone-proguanil (Malarone): dosing as above
- Mefloquine 250 mg (228 mg base) PO/wk, starting 1 wk before arriving in malaria area, weekly while there and then weekly for 4 wk on return. In children, mefloquine dose is based on weight:
  <15 kg 5 mg/kg
  15 to 19 kg ¼ adult dose
  20 to 30 kg ½ adult dose
  31 to 45 kg ¾ adult dose
  >45 kg adult dose
- Doxycycline 100 mg PO/day for adults and children aged >8. Start 1 to 2 days before travel, daily while in malaria area, and then daily for 4 wk on return.

SPECIAL CONSIDERATIONS:
- Long-term visitors or travelers
- Children aged <12 yr
- Immunocompromised host
- Pregnant women: chloroquine and mefloquine are safe in pregnancy but not atovaquone-proguanil. Avoid doxycycline and primaquine.

VACCINATION:
- No effective and safe vaccine available yet
- A live, attenuated, whole sporozoite vaccine shown to work
- A synthetic peptide (SPf66) vaccine proved ineffective
- New DNA-based vaccines are in development

MALARIA INFORMATION:
- CDC Travelers' Health Hotline (877) 394–8747; CDC Travelers' Health Fax (888) 232–3299
- CDC Malaria Epidemiology (770) 488–7788; internet: www.cdc.gov

SUGGESTED READINGS

available at www.expertconsult.com

RELATED CONTENT

Malaria (Patient Information)

AUTHOR: **GLENN G. FORT, M.D., M.P.H.**

BASIC INFORMATION

DEFINITION

Malignant hyperthermia is a rare yet life-threatening subclinical myopathy that occurs in susceptible individuals after exposure to triggering agents, most commonly inhaled anesthetics (such as halothane, isoflurane, sevoflurane, and desflurane) or depolarizing agents (such as succinylcholine). Recently, there have been case reports of malignant hyperthermia with ondansetron and endosulfan poisoning. Initial signs include rising end-tidal carbon dioxide, tachypnea, tachycardia, hyperpyrexia, as well as skeletal muscle and masseter rigidity.

SYNONYMS

Malignant hyperthermia of anesthesia
Malignant hyperpyrexia
MH

ICD-9CM CODES
995.86 Malignant hyperthermia of anesthesia
ICD-10CM CODES
T88.3 Malignant hyperthermia due to anesthesia, initial encounter

EPIDEMIOLOGY & DEMOGRAPHICS

INCIDENCE: Incidence in the general population is 1:100,000; however, the incidence in a clinical population largely depends on the prevalence of susceptibility and the use of triggering anesthetics.
PEAK INCIDENCE: Children account for 42% to 52% of cases, however, any age may be affected.
PREVALENCE: Prevalence of MH in the general population is estimated at 1:2000. In susceptible cohorts, the prevalence ranges from 1:200 to 1:5000.
PREDOMINANT AGE AND SEX: Males are affected more frequently than females. Pediatric patients are the most frequently affected age group.
GENETICS: MH susceptibility is a heritable disorder of skeletal muscle calcium homeostasis most commonly inherited in an autosomal dominant fashion in 50% of cases. There is significant clinical variability due to incomplete penetrance and variable expressivity. The mutation most commonly involves the genes coding for the ryanodine receptor and the dihydropyridine receptor of skeletal muscle sarcoplasmic reticulum.
RISK FACTORS: Family history of malignant hyperthermia or significant problems with general anesthesia may indicate risk. Additionally, patients with dystrophinopathies such as Duchenne and Becker muscular dystrophy, enzymopathies of skeletal muscle such as McArdle's disease, and other genetic syndromes such as osteogenesis imperfecta, myotonia, and neuroleptic malignant syndrome may all contribute to risk elevation for developing MH crisis.

PHYSICAL FINDINGS & CLINICAL PRESENTATION

- Within minutes to hours after the triggering anesthetic is administered, the patient develops muscle rigidity (especially masseter spasm), hyperthermia (up to 45° C), tachycardia that may progress to other dysrhythmias, and hypotension. Skin initially reddens but then becomes cyanotic and mottled. There is also increased carbon dioxide production.
- Rhabdomyolysis, acute renal failure, and disseminated intravascular coagulation may soon follow.
- Box 1-53 summarizes positive findings consistent with malignant hyperthermia.

ETIOLOGY

- In contrast to fever, in which elevated core temperature is related to hypothalamus set point adjustment by cytokines, malignant hyperthermia results from overproduction of heat via skeletal muscle metabolism in the context of a normal hypothalamic set point.
- In genetically susceptible individuals, administration of anesthetic agents results in release of calcium from the sarcoplasmic reticulum of skeletal muscles, causing muscle rigidity and cellular hypermetabolism. This results in significant heat production that overwhelms the body's normal ability to dissipate heat.

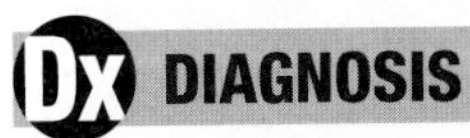

DIFFERENTIAL DIAGNOSIS

- Neuroleptic malignant syndrome
- Fever
- Heat stroke
- Thyrotoxicosis
- Pheochromocytoma
- Central nervous system infection or space-occupying lesion
- MDMA (Ecstasy), cocaine, alcohol withdrawal, or amphetamine use
- Serotonin syndrome
- Adverse reaction to monoamine oxidase inhibitor or anticholinergic drug
- Strychnine poisoning
- Delirium tremens
- Sepsis associated with renal and respiratory failure
- Drug withdrawal
- Rhabdomyolysis
- Blood transfusion reaction

WORKUP

Based on history, malignant hyperthermia can be distinguished from other causes of hyperthermia; however, the most dependable method for confirming MH susceptibility is a muscle biopsy test. The biopsy involves excising a sample of skeletal muscle and placing it in a small bath mixture of caffeine and halothane. A positive test is indicated by significant muscle contracture. This test provides a reliability of 95% for MH susceptibility.

LABORATORY TESTS

- If the cause of hyperthermia is uncertain, a complete blood count, thyroid function studies, toxicology screen, and urine vanillylmandelic acid (VMA) may be useful.
- Once diagnosis is established, it is important to follow electrolytes (especially potassium, calcium, and phosphorus), creatinine, blood urea nitrogen, liver transaminases, and creatinine kinase.
- Prothrombin time and partial thromboplastin time should be followed to evaluate for disseminated intravascular coagulation.
- Testing for susceptibility to MH can involve genetic testing or an in vitro muscle contracture test, as discussed previously.

IMAGING STUDIES

CT scan to assess for space-occupying lesion if diagnosis is uncertain

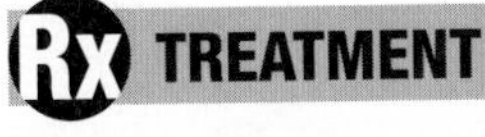

The most important measures for treatment include immediate discontinuation of the triggering agent, hyperventilation on 100% oxygen, dantrolene administration, physical cooling with ice packs and ice lavage, sodium bicarbonate

BOX 1-53 Positive Findings Consistent with Malignant Hyperthermia (MH)

History of recent exposure to trigger agent, including volatile anesthetic agents or succinylcholine
Family or personal history of MH susceptibility
Total body rigidity
Masseter spasm
Inappropriately elevated (38.8° C) or rapidly increasing temperature (>1.5° C over 5 min)
Inappropriate tachypnea
Profuse sweating
Mottled, cyanotic skin
Dark urine, urine dipstick testing shows a positive result from blood without red cells in the sediment and no hemolysis
Unexplained, excessive bleeding
Unexplained ventricular tachycardia or fibrillation
Inappropriate hypercarbia (venous $Paco_2$ >65 mm Hg, arterial $Paco_2$ >55 mm Hg) if the patient is receiving positive-pressure ventilation or is spontaneously breathing with greater than normal minute ventilation
Arterial base excess more negative than −8 mEq/L
Arterial pH <7.25
Potassium concentration >6 mEq/L
Creatine kinase >10,000 IU/L

From Fuhrman BP et al: *Pediatric critical care*, ed 4, Philadelphia, 2011, Saunders.

to combat metabolic acidosis, and dextrose and insulin to treat hyperkalemia while monitoring critical indicators such as arterial blood gas, serum electrolytes, clotting studies, urine output, central venous pressure, and capnograph.

NONPHARMACOLOGIC THERAPY

- Cooling by ice bath, ice packs in the groin and axillae, cool spray with fans, or cooling blankets. In severe instances extracorporeal partial bypass or iced peritoneal lavage may be used. Stop cooling when core temperature reaches 38° C to prevent overcooling.
- Careful monitoring of cardiovascular and respiratory status with constant core temperature measurements. Hyperventilation may be helpful.

ACUTE GENERAL Rx

(see Box 1-54)

- Dantrolene is the mainstay of treatment and is to be administered at 2.5 mg/kg IV given every five minutes until symptoms subside.
- Beta-blockers or lidocaine may be useful for dysrhythmias, but verapamil should be avoided as its use with dantrolene has been shown to depress cardiac function.
- Sodium bicarbonate may be necessary to reverse acidosis.
- Aggressive hydration with forced diuresis and urine alkalinization should be instituted as treatment for rhabdomyolysis.

CHRONIC Rx

This is an acute illness.

BOX 1-54 Management of an Acute Malignant Hyperthermia Episode in the Intensive Care Unit

1. Administer high-flow 100% oxygen via a nonrebreathing mask, and consider endotracheal intubation.
2. For ventilated patients, administer an Fio2 of 1.0 and increase minute ventilation to control $Paco_2$.
3. Administer dantrolene (2.5 mg/kg intravenously) over 10 min, and repeat until acidosis and muscle rigidity have resolved. Repeat dantrolene (1 mg/kg) every 6 hr.
4. Initiate cooling with ice packs in the axillae and groin; decrease room temperature; use hypothermia blankets, iced intravenous saline solution (10 mL/kg over 10 min, repeated as needed), and lavage body cavities with cold saline solution if temperature is greater than 39° C. Stop cooling when core temperature falls to 38° C.
5. Correct metabolic acidosis with sodium bicarbonate (1-2 mEq/kg initially), and give subsequent doses based on base excess and body weight.
6. Administer calcium chloride (10 mg/kg) or calcium gluconate (100-200 mg/kg) to cardiotoxicity associated with hyperkalemia.
7. Give regular insulin (0.1 U/kg) and glucose (0.3-0.5 g/kg) to correct hyperkalemia.
8. Administer lidocaine (1 mg/kg) to treat ventricular arrhythmias. Consider amiodarone (5 mg/kg IV) for refractory, stable ventricular tachycardia. Do not delay defibrillation or cardiopulmonary resuscitation if indicated by cardiovascular instability.
9. Maintain urine output of 2 ml/kg/hr with aggressive cold fluid administration, furosemide (0.5-1 mg/kg), and additional mannitol (0.25-0.3 g/kg) if needed.
10. Consider quantitative end-tidal CO_2 monitoring.
11. Monitor core temperature (pulmonary artery, esophageal temperature probe, rectal probe).
12. Place arterial catheter for invasive blood pressure monitoring and frequent blood sampling. Consider central venous catheter and/or pulmonary artery catheter if indicated by cardiovascular instability.
13. Repeat venous blood gas and electrolytes analysis until these normalize. Repeat CK at least every 6 hr while the patient is in ICU and then daily until CK returns to normal. Assess glucose, clotting function, and hepatic and renal functions, and treat symptomatically. Repeat lactic acid measurement after each dantrolene administration.
14. Consider hemodialysis if indicated.
15. Consider intensive care monitoring for at least 24 hr after MH episode or after recrudescence of MH.
16. Refer the patient for muscle caffeine-halothane contracture testing and consider exam of RYR1. Pursue a pathologic diagnosis for other occult myopathies.

CK, Creatine kinase; *ICU,* intensive care unit; *MH,* malignant hyperthermia.
From Fuhrman BP et al: *Pediatric critical care,* ed 4, Philadelphia, 2011, Saunders.

COMPLEMENTARY & ALTERNATIVE MEDICINE

None

DISPOSITION

Patient will likely need intensive monitoring for at least 24 hours, necessitating an intensive care unit bed.

REFERRAL

Anesthesia consultants will likely already be involved. Consider cardiac, renal, or hematologic consult if sequelae are significant.

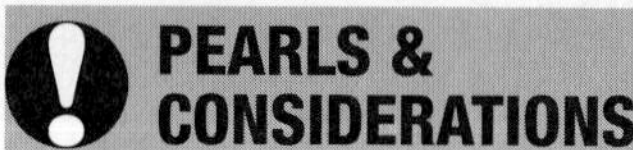

PEARLS & CONSIDERATIONS

COMMENTS

Malignant hyperthermia is a life-threatening condition that requires prompt recognition of the signs and symptoms to minimize illness and end-organ damage.

PREVENTION

- Careful family or personal history of significant adverse effects with general anesthesia is an important tip-off.
- Prophylactic dantrolene therapy is no longer recommended in susceptible individuals.

PATIENT & FAMILY EDUCATION

The importance of awareness of family history for patients and families with malignant hyperthermia susceptibility is to be emphasized.

SUGGESTED READINGS

available at www.expertconsult.com

AUTHORS: **STEPHANIE A. CURRY, M.D.,** and **MARINA GARAS, B.S., OMS-III**

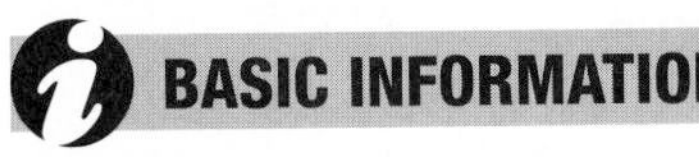

BASIC INFORMATION

DEFINITION

A Mallory-Weiss tear (MWT) is a longitudinal mucosal laceration in the region of the gastroesophageal junction.

SYNONYMS

Mallory-Weiss syndrome

ICD-9CM CODES
530.7 Gastroesophageal laceration-hemorrhage syndrome
530.82 Esophageal hemorrhage
ICD-10CM CODES
K22.6 Mallory-Weiss syndrome

EPIDEMIOLOGY & DEMOGRAPHICS

- Accounts for 5% to 15% of cases of upper gastrointestinal (GI) bleeding
- Reported from early childhood to old age; the majority of patients are age 40 to 60 yr
- More common in males
- Alcohol use is present in 30% to 60%

PHYSICAL FINDINGS & CLINICAL PRESENTATION

- Vomiting, retching, or vigorous coughing will often, but not always, precede hematemesis.
- Patients may be clinically stable or present with tachycardia, hypotension, melena, or hematochezia.
- Bleeding may be self-limited or severe.
- Tears may be seen in association with other upper GI tract lesions, including hiatus hernia (present in as many as 90% of patients), ulcers, and esophageal varices, particularly in alcoholics.

ETIOLOGY

- An acute increase in intraabdominal pressure is transmitted to the esophagus, resulting in mucosal laceration.
- Vomiting may be associated with alcohol use, ketoacidosis, ulcer disease, uremia, pancreatitis, cholecystitis, pregnancy (in particular associated with hyperemesis gravidarum), myocardial infarction, or the postoperative period.
- Tears may be iatrogenic, related to routine endoscopy (especially in struggling or retching patients), enteroscopy with or without overtubes, esophageal dilation, lower esophageal pneumatic disruption therapy for achalasia, endoscopic submucosal dissection, transesophageal echocardiography, or in association with polyethylene glycol electrolyte colonic lavage preparation.

Dx DIAGNOSIS

DIFFERENTIAL DIAGNOSIS

- Esophageal or gastric varices
- Esophagitis or esophageal ulcers (peptic or pill-induced)
- Gastric erosions
- Gastric or duodenal ulcer
- Dieulafoy lesion
- Arteriovenous malformations
- Neoplasms (usually gastric)
- Boerhaave's syndrome

WORKUP

Endoscopy is the diagnostic method of choice.

LABORATORY TESTS

- Complete blood count, prothrombin time, partial thromboplastin time
- Electrolytes, blood urea nitrogen, creatinine, liver function tests, pregnancy test, tests to evaluate for predisposing conditions

IMAGING STUDIES

Upper GI series is usually not sensitive. Patients with concurrent chest pain, dyspnea, shock, or physical examination findings of crepitus or pleural effusion should have a chest radiograph or CT to exclude Boerhaave's syndrome.

Rx TREATMENT

NONPHARMACOLOGIC THERAPY

- Supportive care
- Avoidance of aspirin, nonsteroidal anti-inflammatory drugs, and anticoagulants

ACUTE GENERAL Rx

- Patients with active bleeding or hemodynamic instability require large-bore IVs, fluid resuscitation, and transfusion of blood products (red blood cells, fresh frozen plasma, and platelets) as appropriate.
- Nasogastric decompression and antiemetics may be considered.
- Endoscopic therapy for patients with active or ongoing hemorrhage (Fig. 1-575). Therapeutic modalities include electrocoagulation, injection (e.g., 1:10,000 epinephrine, polidocanol), sclerotherapy (for bleeding associated with esophageal varices), band ligation, or endoscopic hemoclips (therapies may be used alone or in combination) (Fig. E1-576).
- Arterial embolization in patients with active bleeding who are poor surgical candidates.
- Laparotomy, with gastrotomy and oversewing of the tear, is required in a small percentage of patients with uncontrolled bleeding.

CHRONIC Rx

- Healing will usually occur without specific therapy.
- H_2 blockers or proton pump inhibitors may be given to help facilitate healing but should not be used long term unless appropriate indications are present.

DISPOSITION

- Prognosis is good, with spontaneous cessation of bleeding in upwards of 90% of patients. Endoscopic features can guide treatment. Blatchford score <6 suggests no need for transfusion or endoscopic intervention.
- Delayed rebleeding is described in patients with high-risk stigmata (shock at initial presentation, spurting or oozing at initial endoscopy).
- Death has been reported in 3% to 12%, often in association with severe bleeding and underlying comorbid conditions such as advanced age, coagulopathy, elevated transaminases, thrombocytopenia, alcohol use, presentation with a very low hemoglobin level or melena, and multisystem organ failure.

REFERRAL

- Gastrointestinal referral for endoscopy
- Surgical referral for bleeding unresponsive to endoscopic treatment or in the setting of coexistent perforation

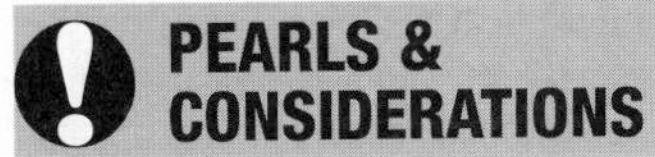

PEARLS & CONSIDERATIONS

Conditions predisposing to retching or vomiting should be identified and treated at presentation.

SUGGESTED READINGS

available at www.expertconsult.com

RELATED CONTENT

Mallory-Weiss Tear (Patient Information)

AUTHOR: **HARLAN G. RICH, M.D., F.A.C.P., A.G.A.F.**

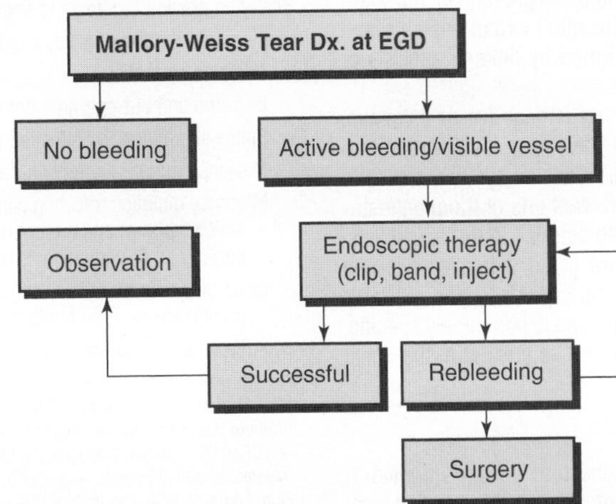

FIGURE 1-575 Treatment algorithm for Mallory-Weiss tear. *EGD,* Esophagogastroduodenoscopy. (From Cameron JL, Cameron AM: *Current surgical therapy,* ed 10, Philadelphia, 2011, Saunders.)

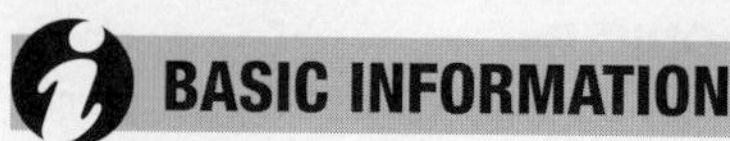

BASIC INFORMATION

DEFINITION

Marfan's syndrome is an inherited disorder of connective tissue involving the skeleton, cardiovascular system, eyes, lungs, and central nervous system.

ICD-9CM CODES
759.82 Marfan's syndrome
ICD-10CM CODES
Q87.40 Marfan's syndrome, unspecified

EPIDEMIOLOGY & DEMOGRAPHICS

PREVALENCE:

- One case per 10,000 persons.
- Both sexes are affected equally by this autosomal-dominant syndrome.
- Approximately 30% of cases are a new mutation.

PHYSICAL FINDINGS & CLINICAL PRESENTATION

Diagnostic criteria for Marfan's syndrome (Table 1-321):

- Skeleton: joint hypermobility (Fig. 1-577), tall stature (Fig. 1-578, *A*), pectus excavatum, reduced thoracic kyphosis, scoliosis, arachnodactyly (Fig. 1-578, *B*), dolichostenomelia, pectus carinatum, and erosion of the lumbosacral vertebrae from dural ectasia*
- Eye: myopia, retinal detachment, elongated globe, ectopia lentis*
- Cardiovascular: mitral valve prolapse, endocarditis, arrhythmia, dilated mitral annulus, mitral regurgitation, tricuspid valve prolapse, aortic regurgitation, aortic dissection,* dilation of the aortic root*
- Pulmonary: apical blebs, spontaneous pneumothorax
- Skin and integument: inguinal hernias, incisional hernias, striae atrophicae
- Central nervous system: attention deficit disorder, hyperactivity, verbal-performance discrepancy, dural ectasia, anterior pelvic meningocele*

If the family history is positive for a close relative clearly affected by Marfan's syndrome, manifestations should be present in the skeleton and one of the other organ systems and the diagnosis confirmed by linkage analysis or mutation detection.

If the family history is negative or unknown, the patient should have manifestations in the skeleton, the cardiovascular system, and one other system and at least one of the manifestations indicated by an asterisk in the above lists.

Manifestations are listed within each organ system in increasing specificity for Marfan's syndrome; although none is completely specific, those indicated by an asterisk are the most specific.

ETIOLOGY

Mutations in the gene that encodes fibrillin-1, the major constituent of microfibrils, which form the frame for elastic fibers. All the manifestations of Marfan's syndrome can be explained by the defective microfibrils.

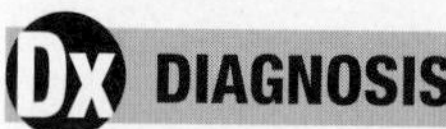

DIAGNOSIS

DIFFERENTIAL DIAGNOSIS

Each of the clinical manifestations of the syndrome may have other causes; however, if the diagnostic criteria are met, the diagnosis is made.

WORKUP

- Echocardiography to establish:
  1. Mitral valve prolapse
  2. Mitral regurgitation
  3. Tricuspid valve prolapse
  4. Aortic regurgitation
  5. Dilation of the aortic root
- Chest radiograph
- Transesophageal echocardiography, chest CT scan, chest MRI, or aortography for suspected aortic dissection

TABLE 1-321 Diagnostic Criteria for Marfan's Syndrome

In the absence of a family history of MFS, a diagnosis can be reached in 1 of 4 scenarios:
1. Aortic diameter at Sinuses of Valsalva Z-score ≥2 AND Ectopia Lentis = MFS*
2. Aortic diameter at Sinuses of Valsalva Z-score ≥2 AND *FBN1* mutation = MFS
3. Aortic diameter at Sinuses of Valsalva Z-score ≥2 AND Systemic Score ≥7 = MFS*
4. Ectopia Lentis AND *FBN1* mutation known to associate with aortic aneurysm = MFS

In the absence of a family history of MFS, alternative diagnoses to MFS include:
1. Ectopia Lentis ± Systemic Score AND *FBN1* mutation not known to associate with aortic aneurysm or no *FBN1* mutation = Ectopia Lentis syndrome
2. Aortic diameter at Sinuses of Valsalva Z-score >2 AND Systemic Score 2:5 (with at least one skeletal feature) without Ectopia Lentis = MASS phenotype
3. Mitral Valve Prolapse AND Aortic diameter at Sinuses of Valsalva Z-score <2 AND Systemic Score <5 without Ectopia Lentis = Mitral Valve Prolapse syndrome

In the presence of a family history of MFS, a diagnosis can be reached in 1 of 3 scenarios:
1. Ectopia Lentis AND Family History of MFS = MFS
2. Systemic Score ≥7 AND Family History of MFS = MFS*
3. Aortic diameter at Sinuses of Valsalva Z-score ≥2 if older than 20 yr or ≥3 if younger than 20 yr AND Family History of MFS = MFS*

Scoring of Systemic Features (in points)†

Wrist AND thumb sign = 3 (wrist OR thumb sign = 1)
Pectus carinatum deformity = 2 (pectus excavatum or chest asymmetry = 1)
Hindfoot deformity = 2 (plain pes planus = 1)
Pneumothorax = 2
Dural ectasia = 2
Protrusio acetabuli = 2
Reduced US/LS AND increased arm/height AND no severe scoliosis = 1
Scoliosis or thoracolumbar kyphosis = 1
Reduced elbow extension = 1
Facial features (3/5) = 1 (dolichocephaly, enophthalmos, downslanting palpebral fissures, malar hypoplasia, retrognathia)
Skin striae = 1
Myopia >3 diopters = 1
Mitral valve prolapse (all types) = 1

Criteria for Causal *FBN1* Mutation

Mutation previously shown to segregate in a Marfan family
Any one of the following *de novo* mutations (with proven paternity and absence of disease in parents):
- Nonsense mutation
- In-frame and out-of-frame deletion/insertion
- Splice site mutations affecting canonical splice sequence or shown to alter splicing on mRNA/cDNA level
- Missense mutation affecting/creating cysteine residues
- Missense mutation affecting conserved residues of the EGF consensus sequence [(D/N)X(D/N)(E/Q)Xm(D/N)Xn(Y/F), with m and n representing variable number of residues; D, aspartic acid; N, asparagine; E, glutamic acid; Q, glutamine; Y, tyrosine; F, phenylalanine]
- Other missense mutations: segregation in family, if possible, + absence in 400 ethnically matched control chromosomes; if no family history, absence in 400 ethnically matched control chromosomes

Linkage of haplotype for n≥6 meioses to the *FBN1* locus

MFS, Marfan's syndrome; *US/LS*, upper segment/lower segment ratio.
*Without discriminating features of Shprintzen-Goldberg syndrome, Loeys-Dietz syndrome, or Ehlers-Danlos syndrome *and* after TGFBR1/2, collagen biochemistry, COL3A1 testing if indicated. Other conditions/genes will emerge with time.
†Maximum total: 20 points; score ≥7 indicates systemic involvement.
From Loeys BL et al: The revised Ghent nosology for the Marfan syndrome, *J Med Genet* 47:476-485, 2010.

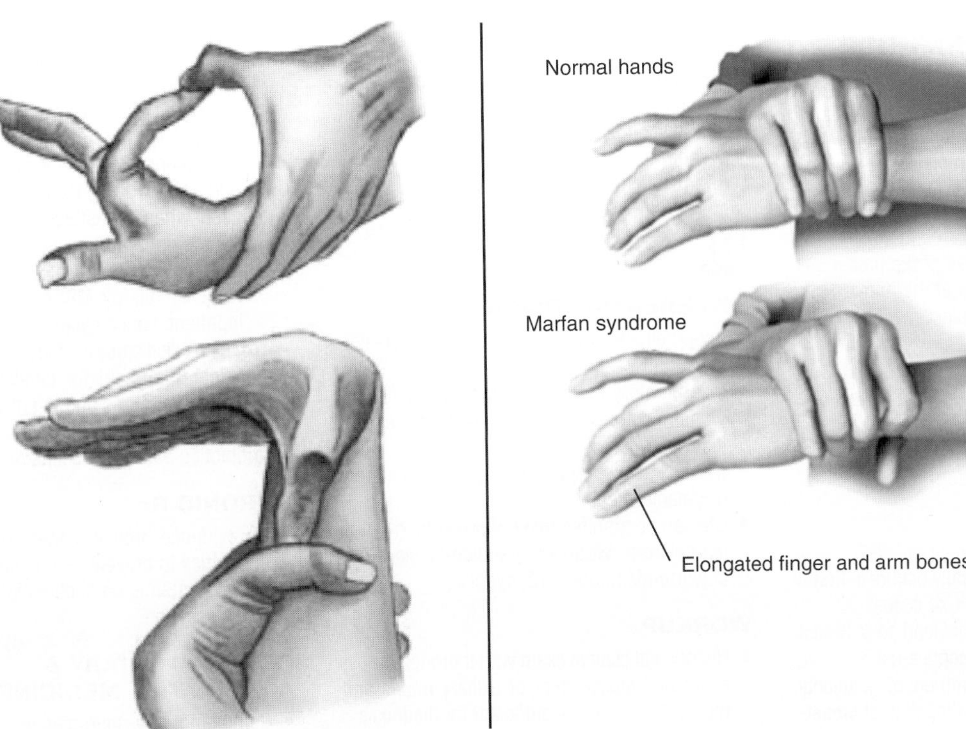

FIGURE 1-577 Marfan syndrome. The Steinberg test (thumb) and the Walker-Murdoch test (wrist) show arachnodactyly. (From Firestein GS et al: *Kelley's textbook of rheumatology,* ed 9, Philadelphia, 2013, Saunders, Elsevier.)

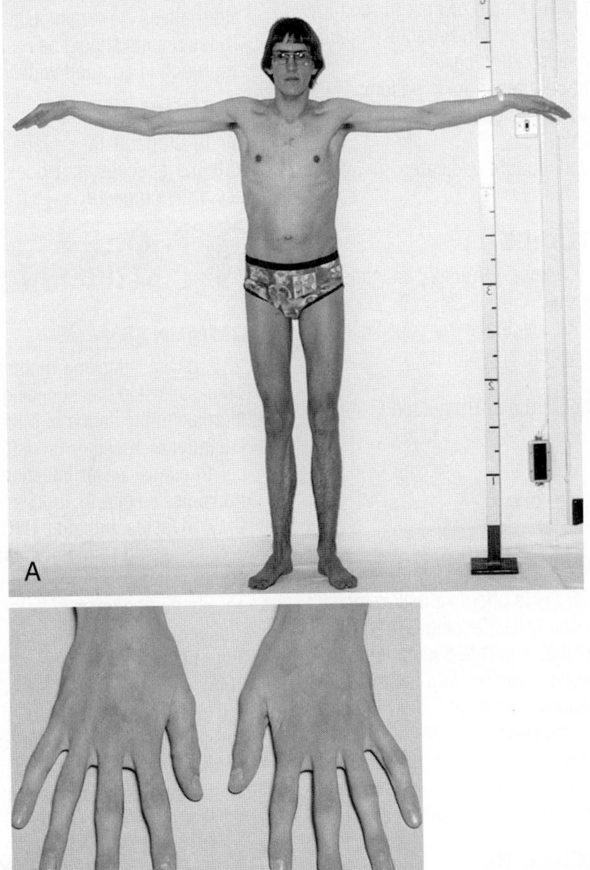

FIGURE 1-578 A, Long limbs compared with the trunk. **B,** Arachnodactyly. (From Kanski JJ, Bowling B: *Clinical ophthalmology, a system approach,* ed 7, Philadelphia, 2010, Saunders.)

- Chest radiograph for pulmonary apical bullae
- Ophthalmologic examination by ophthalmologist

Rx TREATMENT

- Regular cardiac and aorta monitoring by physical examination and echocardiography.
- Endocarditis prophylaxis.
- Restriction of contact sports, weight lifting, and overexertion.
- Beta-blockers are commonly prescribed to slow the rate of aortic root dilation. Patients with Marfan's syndrome and associated aneurysm should be receiving beta-blockers unless there is a contraindication to their use. Recent reports indicate that use of angiotensin receptor blockers significantly also slowed the rate of progressive aortic root dilation independent of hemodynamic effects.
- Early use of angiotensin-converting enzyme inhibitors in young patients with Marfan's syndrome and valvular regurgitation should be considered.
- Genetic counseling.
- Monitor aorta during pregnancy because of the increased risk of dissection.

SUGGESTED READINGS

available at www.expertconsult.com

RELATED CONTENT

Marfan's Syndrome (Patient Information)

AUTHOR: **FRED F. FERRI, M.D.**

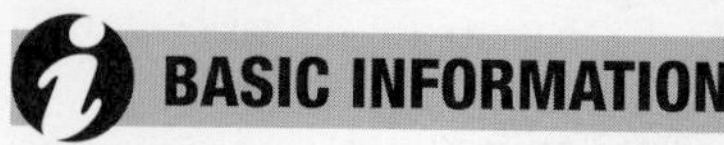

BASIC INFORMATION

DEFINITION

Mastitis is local painful inflammation of the breast that may or may not be accompanied by infection, flulike symptoms, and abscess formation.

ICD-9CM CODES

611.0 Inflammatory disease of the breast
675.1 Postpartum abscess of the breast
675.2 Postpartum nonpurulent mastitis

ICD-10CM CODES

N61 Inflammatory disorders of breast
O91.12 Abscess of breast associated with the puerperium
O91.22 Nonpurulent mastitis associated with the puerperium

EPIDEMIOLOGY & DEMOGRAPHICS

- In lactating mothers, typically occurs in first 3 mo postpartum (74%-95% of cases)
- When severe, mastitis can lead to a breast abscess (5% to 11%) or septicemia
- Delayed diagnosis and treatment of lactational mastitis can lead to discontinuation of breastfeeding, breast tissue damage, recurrence
- In nonlactating women of childbearing age, often presents as granulomatous mastitis (GM)
- In older nonlactating women it is called periductal mastitis (PM) and is caused by inflamed milk ducts near the nipple
- Mastitis can occur in infancy, when breast hypertrophy from maternal hormone leads to infection

PREVALENCE: Lactational mastitis occurs in up to 33% of mothers

PREDOMINANT SEX: Females

RISK FACTORS:

- Previous mastitis
- Milk stasis and missed feedings
- Cracked, fissured, or sore nipples
- Primiparity and infant attachment difficulties
- Cleft lip or palate or short frenulum in infant
- Poor maternal nutrition
- Use of manual breast pump
- Diabetes
- Breast implants
- Nipple piercings

PHYSICAL FINDINGS & CLINICAL PRESENTATION

- Warmth, redness, tenderness in breast
- Unilateral or bilateral
- Malaise, myalgias, fevers, chills
- Decreased milk output
- Breast is hard, wedge shaped, and swollen
- In PM, breast mass near nipple with retraction or discharge
- In GM, enlarged axillary lymph nodes or sinus tract formation

ETIOLOGY

- Milk stasis and irritation of the milk ducts due to local immune response to milk proteins.
- Bacterial infection of subcutaneous tissue due to breaks in skin.
- Most commonly, *S. aureus;* less common, group A beta-hemolytic streptococci, *S. pneumoniae, E. coli, Candida albicans, M. tuberculosis.*
- GM from inflammation with epithelioid histiocytes and multinucleated giant cells can be caused by etiologies like tuberculosis, sarcoidosis, foreign body reaction, parasitic and mycotic infections, or idiopathic (IGM).
- Neonatal mastitis caused by *S. aureus* or gram-negative enteric bacteria.

Dx DIAGNOSIS

DIFFERENTIAL DIAGNOSIS

- Engorgement, plugged duct (see Table E1-322)
- Breast abscess
- Inflammatory or other breast cancer (3% of women diagnosed with breast cancer are lactating)
- Mastitis as a symptom of hyperprolactinemia or galactorrhea
- GM can be manifestation of systemic disease (sarcoidosis, Wegener granulomatosis, GCA, polyarteritis nodosa, TB, syphilis)

WORKUP

- History and clinical exam with thorough breast exam and assessment of axillary nodes and nipple discharge are sufficient for diagnosis
- Recurrent mastitis should include workup for underlying breast disease

LABORATORY TESTS

- Simple mastitis requires no milk culture or laboratory studies
- Obtain midstream sample of milk for culture for antibiotic sensitivities in refractory mastitis or in MRSA-suspected cases
- CBC and blood cultures in toxic patients
- In abscess formation, culture of drainage or aspirate fluid
- Gram stain and culture indicated in infant mastitis

IMAGING STUDIES

- Not necessary unless refractory mastitis or abscess suspected
- Consider US to evaluate for abscess or mammogram when appropriate to exclude carcinoma
- In GM, mammogram and US guided FNA are standard

Rx TREATMENT

NONPHARMACOLOGIC THERAPY

- Mainstay of therapy is effective milk removal through continued breastfeeding or pumping
- Consider referral to a certified lactation consultant to improve breastfeeding technique
- Warm compresses, increased fluid intake, good nutrition, and rest
- In abscess formation, surgical drainage or needle aspiration is necessary, followed by antibiotic therapy based on sensitivities of culture

ACUTE GENERAL Rx

- NSAIDs and analgesics (e.g., acetaminophen, ibuprofen). There is insufficient evidence to support or refute the effectiveness of antibiotic therapy. Common regimens include:
- No history of MRSA:
  - Dicloxacillin 500 mg 4x/d for 10-14 d
  - Cephalexin 500 mg 4x/d for 10-14 d
  - Inpatient nafcillin or oxacillin 2 g IV q4h
- Suspected MRSA:
  - Trimethoprim/sulfamethoxazole 160 mg/800 mg 2x/d for 10-14 d; should not be used when breastfeeding healthy infants <2 mo or compromised infants
  - Clindamycin 300 mg 4x/d for 10-14 d (for penicillin allergy, MRSA coverage)
  - Inpatient: vancomycin 1 g IV q12h
- Oxytocin nasal spray if letdown reflex disturbed
- Consider treatment for candidal infection if bilateral symptoms and infant with thrush
- Mastitis in infant treated with parenteral antibiotics based on results of Gram stain

CHRONIC Rx

- No evidence proving benefit of prophylactic antibiotics to prevent lactational mastitis
- In GM, systemic corticosteroids or wide surgical resection.

COMPLEMENTARY & ALTERNATIVE MEDICINE

- Complementary therapies not assessed in prospective studies: *Belladonna, Phytolacca, Chamomilla,* sulfur, *Bellis perennis*
- Several strains of lactobacilli have shown promise as probiotic agents that might be useful in treating mastitis. *L. fermentum* and *L. salivarius* have been found effective alternatives to antibiotics in recent trials. These results should be replicated before this approach is adopted widely.

REFERRAL

Refer to surgeon for severe PM or significant lactational abscess that does not resolve with conservative measures

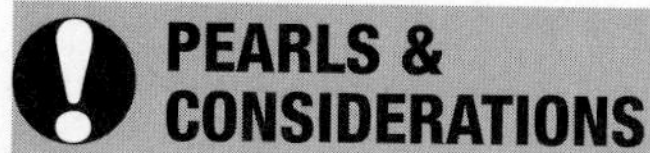

PEARLS & CONSIDERATIONS

COMMENTS

- 25% of breastfeeding mothers with 1 episode of mastitis stop breastfeeding.
- Increasing incidence of MRSA mastitis.
- Lactational mastitis is risk factor for vertical transmission of infections (i.e., increased transmission of retroviruses [especially HIV-1], CMV, measles, hepatitis B, C.
- In reassessing refractory nonlactational mastitis, the most important consideration is the possibility of cancer.
- Nonlactational mastitis can be a manifestation of systemic disease.
- GM mimics breast cancer both clinically and radiologically (>50% of reported cases are initially mistaken for carcinoma). This includes fine needle aspiration, which is sometimes interpreted as malignant.

SUGGESTED READINGS

available at www.expertconsult.com

AUTHORS: **MARY BETH SUTTER, M.D.,** and **ANDREI LEVCHENKO, Ph.D.**

BASIC INFORMATION

DEFINITION

- Pain in the breast
- Usually cyclic condition but may be noncyclic or extramammary

SYNONYMS

Mastalgia

ICD-9CM CODES
611.71 Mastodynia
ICD-10CM CODES
N64.4 Mastodynia

EPIDEMIOLOGY & DEMOGRAPHICS

- Mastodynia affects up to 70% of women at some time in their reproductive lives.
- Severe cyclic mastodynia lasting more than 5 days/mo and of sufficient intensity to interfere with sexual, physical, social, and work-related activities is reported among 30% of premenopausal women.
- Underlying fear of breast cancer is the reason most of these women seek medical consultation.
- One tenth of women with mastodynia require pain-relieving therapy.

PHYSICAL FINDINGS & CLINICAL PRESENTATION

- Usually the breasts are normal bilaterally
- Full, tender breasts
- Generalized breast nodularity without discrete lumps
- Chest wall tenderness: extramammary breast pain
- Distinguishing mammary from extramammary pain can be difficult
- With the patient lying on her side so that the breast tissue falls away from the chest wall, tenderness can then be reproduced by direct pressure over the offending site
- Cyclic mastodynia presents in the luteal phase of the menstrual cycle
- Women with cyclic mastodynia tend to have abdominal bloating, leg swelling, and other symptoms of premenstrual syndrome
- Noncyclic mastodynia, on the other hand, is unrelated to the menstrual cycle
- Extramammary breast pain simulates noncyclic mastodynia

ETIOLOGY

- Hormonal imbalance
- Abnormal lipid metabolism
- Premenstrual syndrome (20%)
- Fibrocystic breast disease
- Emotional abuse and anxiety
- Excessive caffeine intake
- Breast cancer (10%)
- Tietze syndrome (idiopathic costochondritis)

DIAGNOSIS

DIFFERENTIAL DIAGNOSIS

- See "Etiology."
- The majority of women with mastodynia have no underlying abnormality.
- Breast fullness and tenderness associated with hormonal changes fluctuate with the menstrual cycle.
- Similarly, breast nodularity, which may or may not be the result of fibrocystic breast disease, also fluctuates with the menstrual cycle.
- Discrete breast lumps need full evaluation to rule out malignancy.
- Tietze syndrome is usually unilateral and may be associated with chest wall swelling.

LABORATORY TESTS

Although hormonal imbalance and abnormal lipid metabolism have been implicated in the etiopathogenesis of mastodynia, there is no good evidence to support any consistent pattern of serum hormonal or lipid profile in women with mastodynia. These tests are therefore not recommended.

IMAGING STUDIES

- Mammography should be part of the baseline investigation if the woman is >35 yr.
- Ultrasound can be performed as needed; it is particularly helpful in the assessment of cystic breast lesions.
- In women <35 yr, imaging investigations are not helpful unless a lump has been palpated clinically. Consideration of family history for breast disease is important.
- There are no radiologic features associated with mastodynia: rather, radiologic investigations are performed to exclude the rare presence of a subclinical carcinoma.

TREATMENT

NONPHARMACOLOGIC THERAPY

- 85% of the women with mastodynia can be reassured after full clinical evaluation.
- The remaining 15% require some form of therapy in addition to reassurance.
- A firm, supportive brassiere designed for postpartum use is particularly helpful if mastodynia is associated with breast swelling.
- Follow a low-fat, high-carbohydrate diet.
- Reduce caffeine intake.

ACUTE GENERAL Rx

- Evening primrose oil, which contains gamma-linolenic acid, has been shown to have some effectiveness and is an acceptable treatment for mastodynia.
- Topical NSAID preparations may confer some benefit and can be prescribed for these women.
- Hormonal therapy is the mainstay of treatment.
- Danazol is the only drug approved by the FDA for the treatment of mastodynia. Danazol has some androgenic and peripheral antiestrogenic effects. Its efficacy is well established, with significant relief of mastodynia in 70% to 93% of cases.
  - Widespread use of danazol is limited because of its adverse side effects. These include menstrual irregularities, depression, acne, hirsutism, and, in severe cases, voice deepening. Women taking danazol should be advised to use effective nonhormonal contraception because of the drug's potential adverse effects on the fetus.
- The side effects of danazol can be significantly reduced by using a low dose (100 mg daily) and confining treatment to 2 wk preceding menstruation. However, alternatives should be explored.
- Tamoxifen, a synthetic antiestrogen, has also been shown to be effective in the treatment of mastodynia. Although effective in relieving symptoms, its use is extremely limited because of side effects. When used, it should be at a low dosage of 10 mg/day and duration should be limited to 6 mo at a time. In the U.S. this agent is not approved for use in women with mastodynia.
- Bromocriptine is a dopamine-receptor agonist whose primary action is inhibition of prolactin release. It has been used extensively in the treatment of severe cyclic mastodynia and is effective. Again, side effects such as headache and lightheadedness have limited its use.
- Lisuride maleate was recently found to be effective by one study.
- Other hormonal agents that have been reported to be effective in small studies cannot be recommended. Either they have unacceptable side effect profiles or their efficacy is not established. These agents include gestrinone, gonadotropin-releasing hormone analogues, progesterone, and hormone replacement therapy.

CHRONIC Rx

- Longstanding cases of mastodynia can be managed with intermittent low-dose danazol therapy to limit side effects. In between these courses of hormone, nonpharmacologic and nonhormonal therapy can be used.
- Severe, unremitting mastodynia that does not respond to medical treatment may require mastectomy; this is rare.

DISPOSITION

- Cyclic mastodynia resolves spontaneously in 20% to 30% of women.
- Up to 60% of women may develop recurrent symptoms 2 yr after treatment.
- Noncyclic mastodynia responds poorly to treatment but may resolve spontaneously in up to 50% of women.

SUGGESTED READINGS

available at www.expertconsult.com

RELATED CONTENT

Abscess, Breast (Related Key Topic)
Fibrocystic Breast Disease (Related Key Topic)
Breast Pain (Patient Information)

AUTHORS: **ALEXANDER B. OLAWAIYE, M.D.,** and **RUBEN ALVERO, M.D.**

BASIC INFORMATION

DEFINITION

Mastoiditis is inflammation of the mastoid process and air cells, a complication of otitis media.

SYNONYMS

Mastoid abscess

ICD-9CM CODES
383.00 Mastoiditis, acute or subacute
383.1 Mastoiditis, chronic
ICD-10CM CODES
H70.0 Acute mastoiditis
H40.1 Chronic mastoiditis
H70.8 Other mastoiditis and related conditions
H70.9 Mastoiditis, unspecified

EPIDEMIOLOGY & DEMOGRAPHICS

INCIDENCE (IN U.S.): Since the introduction of antibiotic therapy and use of broad-spectrum antibiotics, there has been a marked decline in the incidence of acute mastoiditis.
PREDOMINANT SEX: More common in males
PREDOMINANT AGE: 2 mo to 18 yr
PEAK INCIDENCE: Early childhood

PHYSICAL FINDINGS & CLINICAL PRESENTATION

- Acute mastoiditis is usually a complication of acute otitis media.
- Most common presenting symptom is pain and tenderness in the postauricular region.
- Other signs or symptoms include:
  1. Fever
  2. Postauricular erythema and edema
  3. Protrusion of the pinna inferiorly and anteriorly
  4. Tympanic membrane usually intact with signs of acute otitis media
- Complications of acute mastoiditis include:
  1. Subperiosteal abscess (most common complication)
  2. Hearing loss
  3. Facial nerve palsy
  4. Labyrinthitis
  5. Intracranial complications such as hydrocephalus, meningitis, encephalitis, intracranial abscess, and lateral sinus thrombosis
- Chronic mastoiditis is characterized by chronic otorrhea and chronic tympanic membrane perforation.

ETIOLOGY

- Continuity exists between the middle air space and the mastoid cavity.
- Initial hyperemia and edema of the mucosal lining of the air cells results in accumulation of purulent exudate.
- Dissolution of calcium from bony septa and osteoclastic activity in the inflamed periosteum lead to bone necrosis and coalescence of air cells.
- Most common bacterial isolates are:
  1. *Streptococcus pneumoniae*
  2. *Streptococcus pyogenes*
  3. *Haemophilus influenzae*
  4. *Moraxella catarrhalis*
  5. *Staphylococcus aureus*
- Often, there are multiple organisms in chronic mastoiditis, with predominance of anaerobes and gram-negative bacteria.
- *Mycobacterium tuberculosis,* nontuberculous mycobacteria, *Aspergillus,* and *Rhodococcus equi* have been reported in cases of mastoiditis in severely immunocompromised individuals.

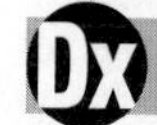

DIAGNOSIS

DIFFERENTIAL DIAGNOSIS

- Children
  1. Rhabdomyosarcoma
  2. Histiocytosis X
  3. Leukemia
  4. Kawasaki syndrome
- Adults
  1. Fulminant otitis externa
  2. Histiocytosis X
  3. Metastatic disease

WORKUP

A thorough history and physical examination are important in establishing diagnosis.

LABORATORY TESTS

- Fluid for Gram stain and culture may be obtained by myringotomy.
- If there is a perforation in the tympanic membrane with drainage, cultures of this may be taken after carefully cleaning the external canal.

IMAGING STUDIES

- Plain x-rays of the mastoid region may demonstrate clouding or opacification in areas of pneumatization.
- CT scan can demonstrate early involvement of bone (mastoiditis with bone destruction).
- MRI is more sensitive than CT scan in evaluating soft-tissue involvement and is useful in conjunction with CT scan to investigate other complications of mastoiditis.

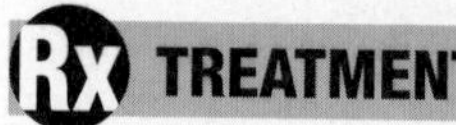

TREATMENT

NONPHARMACOLOGIC THERAPY

Myringotomy, if the ear is not already draining

ACUTE GENERAL Rx

- Initiated with IV antibiotics directed against the common organisms *S. pneumoniae* and *H. influenzae.* Useful agents are amoxicillin/clavulanate, ceftriaxone, and cefotaxime. If the disease in the mastoid has had a prolonged course, coverage for *S. aureus* with gram-negative enteric bacilli may be considered for initial therapy until results of cultures become available. Add vancomycin if MRSA suspected or nafcillin/oxacillin if culture is positive for *S. aureus*, methicillin susceptible.
- Antibiotics continued until all signs of mastoiditis have resolved
- Directed against enteric gram-negative organisms and anaerobes in chronic mastoiditis
- Indications for mastoidectomy:
  1. Failure to improve after 72 hr of therapy
  2. Persistent fever
  3. Imminent or overt signs of intracranial complications
  4. Evidence of a subperiosteal abscess in the mastoid bone

DISPOSITION

Proceed with mastoidectomy when medical therapy fails.

REFERRAL

- To otorhinolaryngologist:
  1. If diagnosis is in doubt
  2. If aural complications present
  3. To evaluate for surgical intervention
- To neurosurgeon if intratemporal or intracranial extension of infection suspected
  1. Aural complications: bone destruction, subperiosteal abscess, petrositis, facial paralysis, labyrinthitis
  2. Intracranial complications: extradural abscess, lateral sinus thrombophlebitis or thrombosis, subdural abscess, meningitis, brain abscess, otitic hydrocephalus

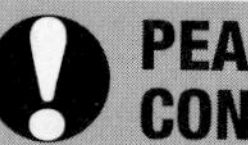

PEARLS & CONSIDERATIONS

Mastoiditis is particularly difficult to eradicate because the mastoid air cells are poorly vascularized and difficult to drain.

SUGGESTED READINGS

available at www.expertconsult.com

RELATED CONTENT

Mastoiditis (Patient Information)

AUTHOR: **GLENN G. FORT, M.D., M.P.H.**

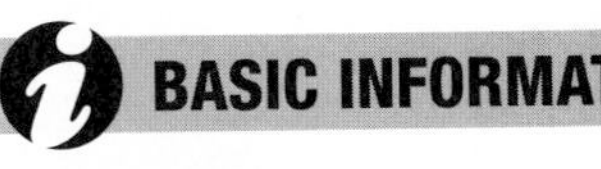

BASIC INFORMATION

DEFINITION

Meckel diverticulum is an ileal diverticulum located 100 cm proximal to the cecum. It results from failure of the omphalomesenteric duct to obliterate completely (as it should by the eighth week of gestation).

SYNONYMS

MD

ICD-9CM CODES
751.0 Meckel diverticulum
ICD-10CM CODES
Q43.0 Meckel's diverticulum (displaced) (hypertrophic)

EPIDEMIOLOGY & DEMOGRAPHICS

- Meckel diverticulum, based on autopsy studies and intraoperative evidence, occurs in 0.3% to 4% of the population and is the most prevalent congenital anomaly of the gastrointestinal (GI) tract. Complications occur more frequently in males.
- Most patients who develop symptoms are <10 yr.
- The lifetime risk of complications developing in a case of Meckel diverticulum is 4%.
- In adults, complications (small bowel obstruction [25% to 40%], diverticulitis [20%]) are usually attributable to factors other than heterotopic mucosa.
- Tumors have rarely been reported in symptomatic Meckel diverticulum, with carcinoid being the most common type.

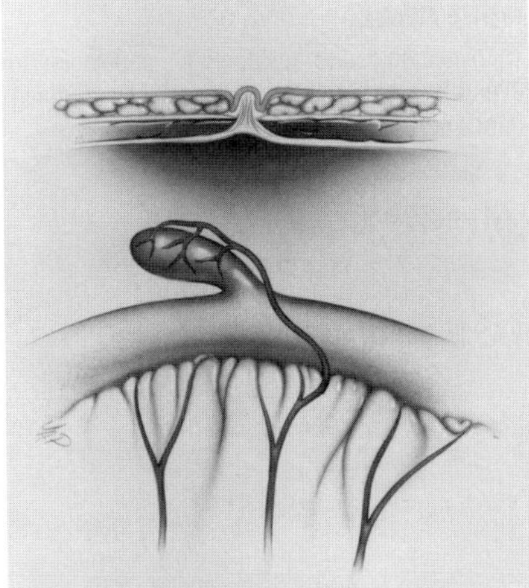

FIGURE 1-582 Typical Meckel diverticulum located on the antimesenteric border. (From Kliegman RM et al: *Nelson textbook of pediatrics,* ed 19, Philadelphia, 2011, Saunders.)

PHYSICAL FINDINGS & CLINICAL PRESENTATION

- Painless lower GI bleeding (4%)
- Intestinal obstruction caused by intussusception, volvulus, herniation, or entrapment of a loop of bowel through a defect in the diverticular mesentery (6%)
- Meckel's diverticulitis mimics acute appendicitis (5%)
- Rare primary tumor arising from diverticulum (carcinoid, sarcoma, leiomyoma, adenocarcinoma)
- Asymptomatic (80% to 95%)

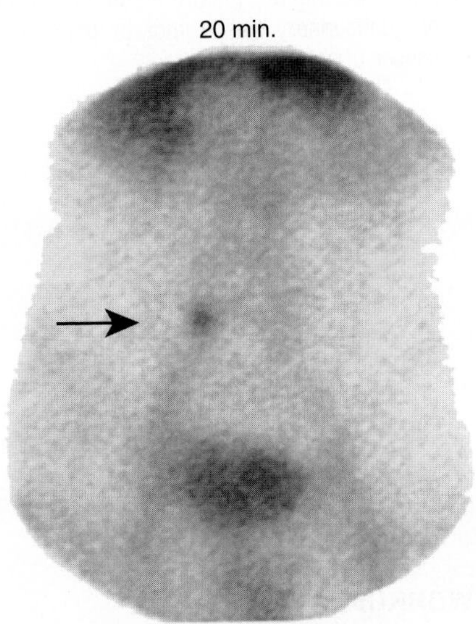

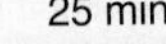

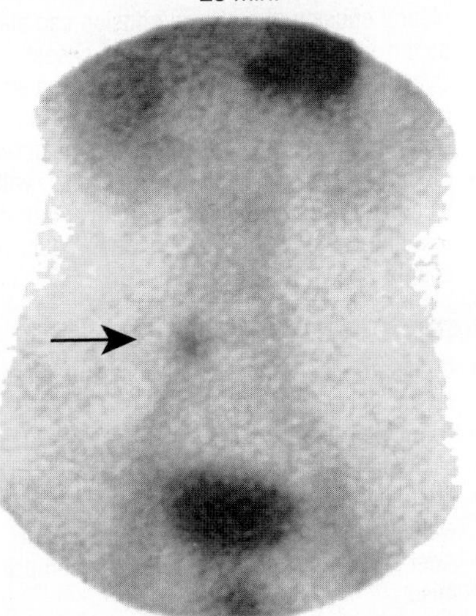

FIGURE 1-583 Meckel scan demonstrating accumulation in the stomach superior bladder (inferior) and in the acid-secreting mucosa of a Meckel diverticulum. (From Kliegman RM et al: *Nelson textbook of pediatrics,* ed 19, Philadelphia, 2011, Saunders.)

ETIOLOGY & PATHOGENESIS

- As a remnant of the omphalomesenteric duct, Meckel diverticulum contains all layers of the intestinal wall and has its own mesentery and blood supply (branch of the superior mesenteric artery) (Fig. 1-582).
- The majority of complicated cases of Meckel diverticulum contain ectopic mucosa (75% gastric, 15% pancreatic). It causes ulceration and bleeding of ileal mucosa adjacent to the acidic ectopic gastric secretions. Alkaline secretions of ectopic pancreatic tissue can also cause ulcerations.

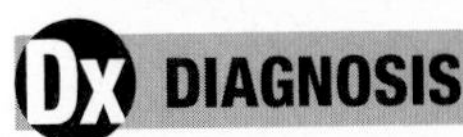

DIAGNOSIS

DIFFERENTIAL DIAGNOSIS

- Appendicitis
- Crohn's disease
- All causes of lower GI bleeding (polyp, colon cancer, arteriovenous malformation, diverticulosis, hemorrhoids)

WORKUP

- Diagnosis is often made intraoperatively when the preoperative diagnosis is appendicitis.
- Preoperative detection of symptomatic Meckel diverticulum requires a high index of suspicion.
- Meckel scan: In the case of GI bleeding of unknown source, a technetium scan will identify Meckel diverticulum (sensitivity: 85% in children, 62% in adults; specificity: 95% in children, 9% in adults) (Fig. 1-583).
- In patients with suspected small-bowel obstruction, intussusception, or diverticulitis, a CT scan of the abdomen and pelvis is helpful.

TREATMENT

- Surgical resection in symptomatic patients.
- There is controversy regarding the need to remove an incidentally found diverticulum, with most surgeons arguing in favor of resection.

SUGGESTED READINGS
available at www.expertconsult.com

RELATED CONTENT

Meckel Diverticulum (Patient Information)

AUTHOR: **FRED F. FERRI, M.D.**

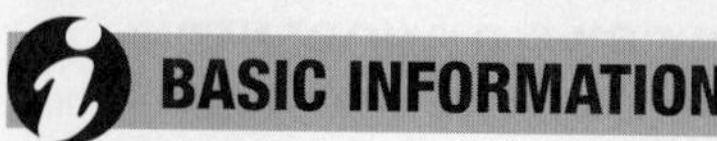

BASIC INFORMATION

DEFINITION

Meigs' syndrome is characterized by the presence of a benign solid ovarian tumor associated with ascites and predominantly right hydrothorax that disappear after tumor removal.

ICD-9CM CODES

620.2 Ovarian mass (unspecified)
789.5 Ascites
511.9 Pleural effusion

ICD-10CM CODES

D27.9 Benign neoplasm of ovary
R18 Ascites
J91.8 Pleural effusion in other conditions classified elsewhere

EPIDEMIOLOGY & DEMOGRAPHICS

- Occurs in <1% of ovarian fibromas (associated with approximately 0.004% of ovarian tumors)
- Most frequently encountered during middle age (average age, approximately 48 yr)

PHYSICAL FINDINGS & CLINICAL PRESENTATION

- Asymptomatic pelvic mass on bimanual examination
- Intermittent pelvic pain (intermittent torsion)
- Acute pelvic tenderness
- Acute abdominal tenderness
- Abdominal pelvic mass
- Abdominal bloating
- Fluid wave
- Shifting dullness
- "Puddle sign"
- Hyperresonance or flatness to chest percussion, absence of tactile and vocal fremitus
- Absent or loud bronchial breath sounds, rales, mediastinal displacement, tracheal shift
- Weight loss and emaciation

ETIOLOGY

- Not specifically known
- Usually associated with "edematous" fibromas (or other benign ovarian solid tumor) in excess of 10 cm
- Plausible that large fibroma with narrow stalk has inadequate lymphatic drainage; when coupled with intermittent torsion, results in backflow transudation into the peritoneal cavity; accumulated peritoneal ascites then pass to the right pleural cavity by the lymphatics (overloaded thoracic duct) or abdominal pleural commutation (i.e., foramen of Bochdalek)

Dx DIAGNOSIS

DIFFERENTIAL DIAGNOSIS

- Abdominal ovarian malignancy
- Various gynecologic disorders:
  1. Uterus; endometrial tumor, sarcoma, leiomyoma ("pseudo-Meigs' syndrome")
  2. Fallopian tube: hydrosalpinx, granulomatous salpingitis, fallopian tube malignancy
  3. Ovary: benign, serous, mucinous, endometrioid, clear cell, Brenner tumor, granulosa, stromal, dysgerminoma, fibroma, metastatic tumor
- Nongynecologic (gastrointestinal tract or genitourinary tract tumor or pathology) causes of pelvic mass
  1. Ascites
  2. Portal vein obstruction
  3. Inferior vena cava obstruction
  4. Hypoproteinemia
  5. Thoracic duct obstruction
  6. Tuberculosis
  7. Amyloidosis
  8. Pancreatitis
  9. Neoplasm
  10. Ovarian hyperstimulation
  11. Pleural effusion
  12. Congestive heart failure
  13. Malignancy
  14. Collagen-vascular disease
  15. Pancreatitis
  16. Cirrhosis

WORKUP

- Clinical condition characterized by ovarian mass, ascites, and predominantly right-sided pleural effusion (the pleural effusion can also be left-sided in a small number of cases)
- Ovarian malignancy and the other causes (see "Differential Diagnosis") of pelvic mass, ascites, and pleural effusion to be considered
- History of early satiety, weight loss with increased abdominal girth, bloating, intermittent abdominal pain, dyspnea, nonproductive cough

LABORATORY TESTS

- Complete blood count to rule out inflammatory process
- Tumor markers (CA-125, hCG, AFP, CEA) to evaluate malignancy
- Chemical and liver function testing profile to evaluate metabolic or hepatic involvement
- Arterial blood gases if respiratory compromise

IMAGING STUDIES

- Pelvic sonography (color-flow Doppler evaluation of adnexal mass) initially to evaluate pelvic pathology (CT scan or MRI to further delineate neoplastic lesions [Fig. E1-584])
- Chest x-ray

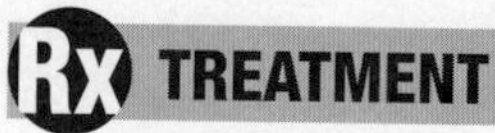

TREATMENT

NONPHARMACOLOGIC THERAPY

- Informed consent and proper preparation of patient for possible staging laparotomy (total abdominal hysterectomy and bilateral salpingo-oophorectomy, omentectomy, possible bowel resection, pelvic/periaortic lymphadenectomy)
- Bowel prep if considering pelvic malignancy

ACUTE GENERAL Rx

Depending on clinical presentation, size of pelvic mass, amount of ascites, and pleural effusion:

- If pelvic mass <10 cm with minimal ascites/pleural effusion: consider diagnostic laparoscopy (possible exploratory laparotomy) and salpingo-oophorectomy with removal of ovarian fibroma (tumor).
- If pelvic mass >10 cm with moderate/large amount ascites/pleural effusion: consider pleurocentesis if respiratory compromise (cytology: AFB) and exploratory laparotomy with salpingo-oophorectomy and removal of ovarian fibroma (tumor).
- Treat pelvic malignancy, gastrointestinal or genitourinary tumor as indicated.

CHRONIC Rx

- Resolution of ascites and right-sided pleural effusion after removal of ovarian fibroma
- No long-term follow-up for benign ovarian fibroma

DISPOSITION

Excellent progress and complete survival are expected.

REFERRAL

To gynecologist or gynecologic oncologist for evaluation and treatment, especially if malignancy considered or encountered

SUGGESTED READINGS

available at www.expertconsult.com

AUTHOR: **RUBEN ALVERO, M.D.**

BASIC INFORMATION

DEFINITION

Melanoma is a skin neoplasm arising from the malignant degeneration of melanocytes. It is classically subdivided in four types:

1. Superficial spreading melanoma (70%) (Fig. 1-585, *A*)
2. Nodular melanoma (15% to 20%) (Fig. 1-585, *B*)
3. Lentigo maligna melanoma (5% to 10%)
4. Acral lentiginous melanoma (7% to 10%)

SYNONYMS

Malignant melanoma
Cutaneous malignant melanoma
CMM

ICD-9CM CODES
172.9 Melanoma of the skin, site unspecified
ICD-10CM CODES
C43.9 Malignant melanoma of skin, unspecified

EPIDEMIOLOGY & DEMOGRAPHICS

- Annual incidence of melanoma is 13 cases per 100,000 persons. By 2015 the estimated lifetime risk of the development of cutaneous melanoma will be 1 in 50.
- Melanoma has doubled to tripled in incidence over the past 25 yr.
- Melanoma is the most common cancer among women ages 20 to 29 yr.
- Melanoma is much more common in whites (17.2/100,000 white men) than in African Americans (1 in 100,000 African American men). Increased risk of developing melanomas is found in patients with fair skin, red hair, light eyes, abundance of freckles, atypical moles or large amount of moles (>50). A personal history of non-melanoma skin cancer or a family history of melanoma also increases the risk.
- Lifetime risk of cutaneous melanoma for white Americans is 1 in 90. White men >50 yr old are the most likely to have rapidly growing melanomas.
- Melanoma is the leading cause of death from skin disease. Although melanoma represents less than 10% of all skin-cancer diagnoses, at least 70% of deaths that are related to skin cancer are attributed to melanoma.
- Median age at diagnosis is 53 yr.
- Superficial spreading melanoma occurs most often in young adults on sun-exposed areas.
- Acral lentiginous melanoma is most often found in Asian Americans and African Americans and is not related to sun exposure.
- Death rate for white men with melanoma is 3 per 100,000.
- 8% to 10% of melanomas arise in people with a family history of the disease.

PHYSICAL FINDINGS & CLINICAL PRESENTATION

Variable depending on the subtype of melanoma:

- Superficial spreading melanoma is most often found on the lower legs, arms, and upper back. It may have a combination of many colors or may be uniformly brown or black.
- Nodular melanoma can be found anywhere on the body, but it most frequently occurs on the trunk on sun-exposed areas. It has a dark-brown or red-brown appearance and can be dome shaped or pedunculated. Lesions are frequently misdiagnosed because they may resemble a blood blister or hemangioma and may also be amelanotic.
- Lentigo maligna melanoma is generally found in older adults in areas continually exposed to the sun and frequently arising from lentigo maligna (Hutchinson's freckle) or melanoma in situ. It might have a complex pattern and variable shape; color is more uniform than in superficial spreading melanoma.
- Acral lentiginous melanoma frequently occurs on soles, subungual mucous membranes, and palms (sole of the foot is the most prevalent site). Unlike other types of melanoma, it has a similar incidence in all ethnic groups.
- The warning signs that the lesion may be a melanoma can be summarized with the ABCDE mnemonic:
  - **A:** Asymmetry (e.g., lesion is bisected and halves are not identical)
  - **B:** Border irregularity (uneven, ragged border)
  - **C:** Color variegation (presence of various shades of pigmentation)
  - **D:** Diameter enlargement (>6 mm)
  - **E:** Evolving (mole changing in size, shape, or color, or mole that differs visibly from surrounding moles ["ugly duckling" sign]) (Fig. 1-586)

ETIOLOGY

- Ultraviolet light is the most important cause of malignant melanoma.
- There is a modest increase in melanoma risk in patients with small nondysplastic nevi and a much greater risk in those with dysplastic lesions.
- The *CDKN2A* gene, residing at the *9p21* locus, is often deleted in people with familial melanoma.
- A mutated signal transduction molecule v-raf murine sarcoma viral oncogene homolog B_1 (BRAF) has been identified in about 50% of patients with metastatic melanoma.

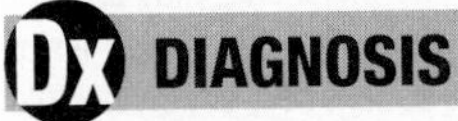

DIAGNOSIS

DIFFERENTIAL DIAGNOSIS

- Dysplastic nevi
- Solar lentigo
- Vascular lesions
- Blue nevus
- Basal cell carcinoma
- Seborrheic keratosis

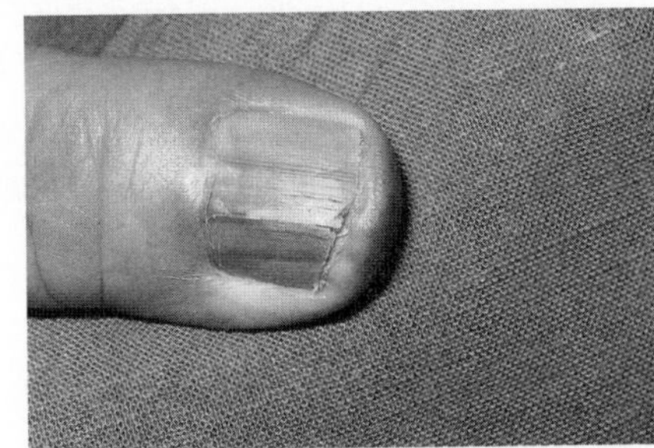

FIGURE 1-586 Subungual melanoma with Hutchinson sign (pigment spreading from under the nail to involve the adjacent skin, usually of the proximal or lateral nail fold). These lesions are thought to emanate from the nail matrix. (From White GM, Cox NH [eds]: *Diseases of the skin, a color atlas and text,* ed 2, St Louis, 2006, Mosby.)

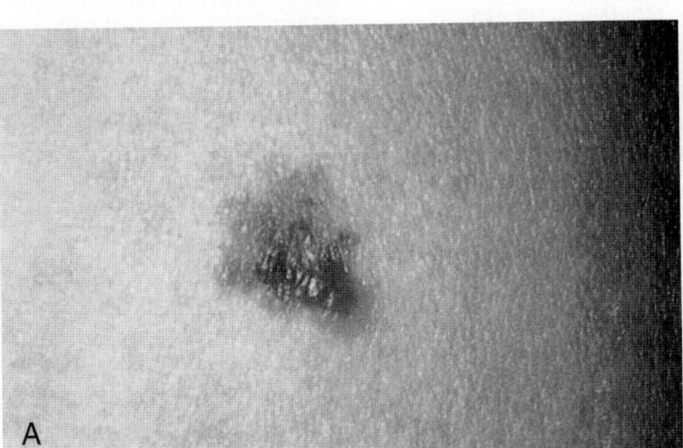

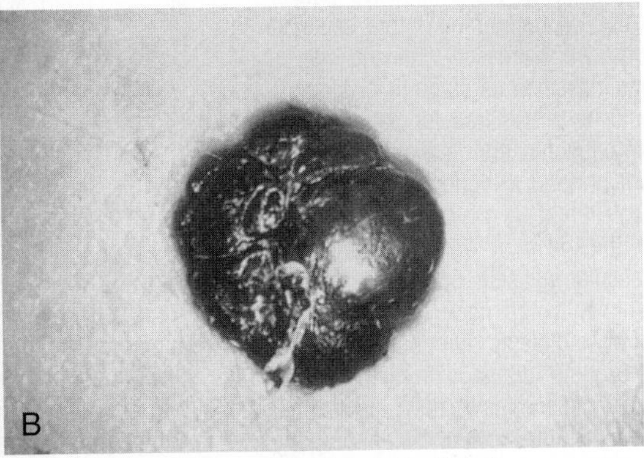

FIGURE 1-585 A, Superficial spreading melanoma. **B,** Nodular melanoma. (From Abeloff MD [ed]: *Clinical oncology,* ed 3, New York, 2004, Churchill Livingstone.)

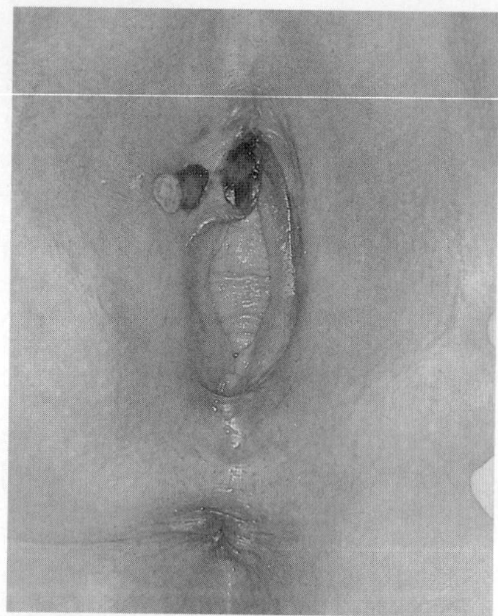

FIGURE 1-587 Melanoma of the vulva. Benign nevi, vulva melanosis, and melanoma may occur in the vulvar region. Any suspicious pigmented lesion should be biopsied. The patient here is 75 years old. (Courtesy Paul Koonings, M.D. From White GM, Cox NH [eds]: *Diseases of the skin, a color atlas and text,* ed 2, St Louis, 2006, Mosby.)

WORKUP

- Dermoscopy (use of an instrument that shines polarized light on skin surfaces and magnifies skin lesions) can increase the accuracy in diagnosing melanoma by 10% to 27%.
- Any suspicious lesion (Fig. 1-587) should be biopsied. Perform excisional biopsy with elliptical excision that includes 1 to 2 mm of normal skin surrounding the lesion and extends to the subcutaneous tissue; incisional punch biopsy is sometimes necessary in surgically sensitive areas (e.g., digits, nose). It is essential that the size of the specimen be adequate to determine the histologic depth of penetration, which is known as the Breslow depth.
- Sentinel lymph node excision (SLNE) is probably the most important diagnostic and potentially therapeutic procedure for patients with melanoma. It should be considered in patients with intermediate (1 to 4 mm) melanomas or high-risk skin tumors to obtain information regarding a patient's subclinical lymph node status with minimal morbidity. The National Comprehensive Cancer Network (NCCN) recommends that sentinel-node biopsy be discussed with and offered to patients classified as stage IB or stage II, and should be considered for patients with stage IA melanoma and "adverse" features that might portend a higher risk of sentinel node involvement (e.g., Clark level IV or V, tumor thickness of 0.75 mm or more, lymphovascular invasion, positive deep margins). Sentinel lymph node biopsy involves the use of radiologic lymphoscintigraphy to map lymphatic drainage from the site of the primary melanoma to the first sentinel lymph node in the region. When properly performed, if the sentinel node is negative the remaining lymph nodes in the region will not have metastases in more than 98% of cases. If the sentinel nodes are negative, no additional regional surgery is recommended. The staging of intermediate thickness (1.2 to 3.5 mm) primary melanomas, according to the results of sentinel node biopsy, provides important prognostic information and identifies patients with nodal metastases whose survival can be prolonged by immediate lymphadenectomy. SPECT/CT is helpful in detecting micrometastatic melanoma. Among patients with clinically lymph node-negative melanoma, the use of SPECT/CT-aided SLNE compared with SNLE alone is associated with a higher frequency of metastatic involvement and a higher rate of disease-free survival.
- The staging system for melanoma adapted by the American Joint Committee on Cancer (AJCC) is as follows:

T*	Thickness of primary tumor
Tis	In situ
T1	≤1.0 mm
T2	1.01-2.0 mm
T3	2.01-4.0 mm
T4	>4.0 mm
N†	Number of positive lymph nodes
N0	0
N1	1
N2	2 or 3
N3	≥4 (or combination of in-transit metastases, satellite lesions, or an ulcerated primary lesion with any number of nodes)
M	Metastases
M0	0
M1	Distant subcutaneous or lymph node metastases
M2	Lung metastases
M3	All other visceral or any distant metastases or an elevated lactate dehydrogenase level not attributable to another cause
Clinical Stage	
0	(T0N0M0)
IA	(T1aN0M0)
IB	(T1bN0M0) (T2aN0M0)
IIA	(T2bN0M0) (T3aN0M0)
IIB	(T3bN0M0) (T4aN0M0)
IIC	(T4bN0M0)
IIIA	(T1-T4aN1bM0)
IIIB	(T1-T4aN2bM0)
IIIC	(AnyT, N2c, M0) (Any T, N3, M0)
IV	(Any T, Any N, >M1)

**a,* Without ulceration; *b,* with ulceration.
†*a,* Micrometastasis; *b,* macrometastases; *c,* in-transit metastases with metastatic lymph nodes.

LABORATORY TESTS

The pathology report should indicate the following:

- Tumor thickness (Breslow microstage).
- Tumor depth: the depth of invasion is the most important histologic prognostic parameter in evaluating the primary tumor.
- Mitotic rate: tabulated as mitoses per square millimeter in the dermal part of the tumor in which most mitoses are identified.
- Radial growth rates versus vertical growth rate: radial growth phase describes the growth of melanoma within the epidermis and along the dermal-epidermal junction.
- Tumor infiltrating lymphocytes have a strong predictive value in vertical growth phase melanomas and are defined as brisk, nonbrisk, or absent.
- Histologic regression: characterized by the absence of melanoma in the epidermis and dermis flanked on one or both sides by melanoma.
- Reverse-transcription polymerase chain reaction assay for tyrosine messenger RNA is a useful marker for the presence of melanoma cells. It is performed on sentinel lymph node biopsy and is useful for detection of submicroscopic metastases.
- Identification of somatic mutations in the gene encoding the serine-threonine protein kinase B-RAF (*BRAF*). This mutation is found in approximately 50% of melanomas.

Rx TREATMENT

- Initial excision of the melanoma
- Reexcision of the involved area after histologic diagnosis:
  1. The margins of reexcision depend on the Breslow depth. For melanoma in situ with Breslow depth ≤2.0 mm, recommended surgical margin is 1 cm. If Breslow depth is ≤2.0 mm, margin should be 2 cm. For melanoma in situ, margin should be 5 mm.
  2. Low-risk or intermediate-risk tumors require excision of 1 to 3 cm.
  3. Melanomas of moderate thickness (0.9 to 2.0 mm) can be excised safely with 2-cm margins.
  4. A 1-cm margin of excision for melanoma with a poor prognosis (as defined by a tumor thickness ≥2 mm) is associated with a significantly greater risk of regional recurrence than is a 3-cm margin, but with a similar overall survival rate. Randomized clinical trials have also shown that radical surgery with 2 cm excision margins did not differ from that with 4 cm margins for survival in patients with cutaneous melanoma >2 mm thick.
- Lymph node dissection: recommended in all patients with enlarged lymph nodes. Lymph node evaluation is important in patients with melanoma 1 mm in depth because it determines the overall prognosis and need for therapeutic lymph node dissection or adjuvant treatment.
  1. Elective lymph node dissection remains controversial.
  2. It is indicated with positive sentinel node. It may be considered in those with a primary melanoma between 1 and 4 mm thick (especially in patients >60 yr).
- Adjuvant therapy with interferon alfa-2b (intron A) in patients with metastatic melanoma is approved by the FDA for AJCC stages IIb and III melanoma; however, its statisti-

cal benefit remains unclear. Peginterferon alfa-2b (which has a longer duration of action and can be given once a week compared to 3-5 times/week for standard interferon) has now also been FDA approved for adjuvant treatment of node-positive melanoma after surgical resection.

- Dacarbazine and interleukin-2 can be used in metastatic melanoma. Results are generally poor, with median survival time in patients with distant metastatic melanoma approximately 6 mo.
- Recent attention has focused on combinations of dacarbazine and cisplatin with interleukin-2 and interferon-alfa (biochemotherapy). Novel therapeutics involve cancer vaccines and use of granulocyte-macrophage colony-stimulating factor and angiogenesis inhibitors. Preliminary trials involving the stimulation of immune response with vaccines using high-dose interleukin-2 plus the gp100:209-217 (210 M) peptide vaccine in patients with advanced melanoma have shown increased survival. Trials with ipilimumab, an agent that blocks cytotoxic T-lymphocyte–associated antigen 4 to potentiate an antitumor T-cell response, have shown improved overall survival in patients with previously treated metastatic melanoma. Ipilimumab when used with dacarbazine also showed improved overall survival in patients with previously untreated metastatic melanoma.
- In patients that carry the V600E *BRAF* mutation, trials involving treatment with vemurafenib (PLX4032), an oral inhibitor of mutated *BRAF*, have shown complete or partial tumor regression in the majority of patients with metastatic melanoma and improved rates of overall and progression-free survival in patients with previously untreated melanoma. The oral selective MEK inhibitor trametinib has also shown improved rates of progression-free and overall survival among patients who had metastatic melanoma with a BRAF V600E or V600K mutation.
- Some melanomas harbor activating mutations and amplification of the type III transmembrane receptor tyrosine kinase KIT. In these patients with advanced melanomas harboring KIT alterations, treatment with imatinib mesylate results in significant clinical responses in a subset of patients.
- Patients with a history of melanoma should be followed up with skin examinations every 6 mo or sooner if patient detects any new lesions; the assessments usually consist of medical history, physical examination, laboratory values, and chest radiograph.

DISPOSITION

- Prognosis varies with the stage of the melanoma. The 5-yr survival related to thickness is as follows: <0.76 mm, 99% survival; 0.6 to 1.49 mm, 85%; 1.5 to 2.49 mm, 84%; 2.5 to 3.9 mm, 70%; >4 mm, 44%.
- The 5-yr survival in patients with distant metastasis is <10%.
- Treatment of advanced disease consists (in addition to surgical excision and lymph node dissection) of chemotherapy, immunotherapy, and radiation therapy.

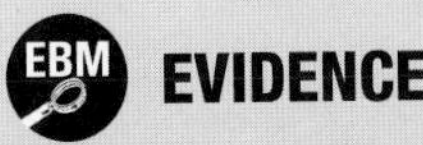

EVIDENCE

available at www.expertconsult.com

SUGGESTED READINGS

available at www.expertconsult.com

RELATED CONTENT

Melanoma (Patient Information)

AUTHOR: **FRED F. FERRI, M.D.**

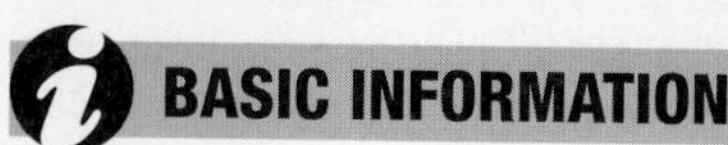

BASIC INFORMATION

DEFINITION

Ménière's disease is a syndrome characterized by recurrent vertigo with fluctuating hearing loss, tinnitus, and fullness in the ear.

SYNONYMS

Endolymphatic hydrops
Lermoyez's syndrome
Idiopathic endolymphatic hydrops

ICD-9CM CODES
386.01 Ménière's disease
ICD-10CM CODES
H81.09 Ménière's disease, unspecified ear

EPIDEMIOLOGY & DEMOGRAPHICS

INCIDENCE (IN U.S.): Varies between 4.3 and 15.3/100,000 persons
PREDOMINANT SEX: Female to male ratio of 1.3:1
PEAK INCIDENCE: Fourth to sixth decade of life

PHYSICAL FINDINGS & CLINICAL PRESENTATION

- Hearing may be unilaterally decreased.
- Pallor, sweating, and nausea may occur during a severe attack.
- Usually the patient develops a sensation of fullness and pressure along with decreased hearing and tinnitus in a single ear.
- The patient typically experiences severe vertigo, which peaks within minutes, then slowly subsides over hours.
- May see spontaneous nystagmus on examination.
- Persistent sense of disequilibrium for days is typical after an acute episode
- May have vestibulopathy demonstrable with a positive head thrust test.

ETIOLOGY

- Unknown; viral, autoimmune, and genetic causes have been suggested.
- Endolymphatic hydrops is the postmortem histologic hallmark. Recent research suggests that endolymphatic hydrops may create cytochemical changes which disturb endolymphatic fluid homeostasis leading to spiral ganglion cell death.

Dx DIAGNOSIS

Proposed guidelines by the American Academy of Otolaryngology-Head and Neck Surgery (AAO-HNS) for diagnosis of Ménière's disease:

DIFFERENTIAL DIAGNOSIS

- Acoustic neuroma
- Migrainous vertigo
- Multiple sclerosis
- Autoimmune inner ear syndrome
- Otitis media
- Vertebrobasilar disease
- Labyrinthitis

WORKUP

- Diagnosis is primarily made by history, although further diagnostic tests may help support the diagnosis. Guidelines to define Ménière's disease are described in Table 1-323.
- Audiogram may show sensorineural hearing loss, with lower frequencies primarily affected. Hearing loss may recover either partially or completely after an attack. Recurrent attacks may lead to a persistent and progressive sensorineural hearing loss.
- Electronystagmography may show peripheral vestibular deficit.
- Electrocochleography (ECoG) records the summating potential and action potential of the eighth cranial nerve in response to auditory stimuli and may indicate significant endolymphatic hydrops if the ratio of summating potential to action potential (SP:AP) is greater than 0.35. Unfortunately, sensitivity and specificity of ECoG to diagnosis of Ménière's disease are low, due to their variability related to severity and chronicity of disease.
- More recently, the vestibular-evoked myogenic potential (VEMP), a short latency inhibitory potential of sternocleidomastoid muscle evoked by brief and loud monaural clicks or tone bursts, has been shown to be elevated or absent in some patients with Ménière's disease, reflecting impaired function of the saccule. However, this test also lacks significant sensitivity and specificity to Ménière's disease and has not yet been widely used in the clinical setting.

LABORATORY TESTS

No laboratory serologic test is specific for Ménière's disease. A thyroid panel, glucose, hemoglobin A1C, antinuclear antibodies, urinalysis, chemistry panel, Venereal Disease Research Laboratory (VDRL) Test, fluorescent treponemal antibody (FTA-ABS), Lyme disease antibodies, and allergy testing can be ordered to screen for other disorders such as thyroid or autoimmune diseases, diabetes, otorenal syndrome, syphilis, Lyme disease, and allergy-mediated Ménière's disease.

IMAGING STUDIES

- MRI to rule out acoustic neuroma, or other retrocochlear lesion, especially if cerebellar or CNS dysfunction is present
- Recent efforts have shown a role for MRI with intratympanic gadolinium.

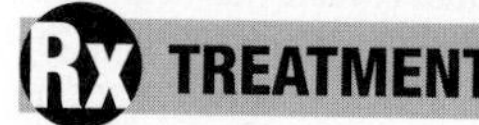

TREATMENT

NONPHARMACOLOGIC THERAPY

Limit activity during attacks

ACUTE GENERAL Rx

- Prochlorperazine 5 to 10 mg PO q6h or 25 mg PO bid
- Promethazine 12.5 to 25 mg PO q4 to 6h
- Diazepam 5 to 10 mg IV/PO for acute attack
- Meclizine 25 mg q6h
- Scopolamine patch

CHRONIC Rx

- Diuretics such as hydrochlorothiazide or acetazolamide, salt restriction, and avoidance of caffeine are traditional.
- For refractory cases, intratympanic gentamicin injections to the affected ear, endolymphatic sac surgery

DISPOSITION

- Patients are usually followed by an otoneurologist or ENT specialist.
- Usual course of disease consists of alternating attacks and remissions.
- Majority of patients can be managed medically. Of patients, 10% to 30% will undergo surgical intervention for persistent incapacitating vertigo.

REFERRAL

To an otolaryngologist for surgical intervention if attacks persist despite medical therapy

SUGGESTED READINGS
available at www.expertconsult.com

RELATED CONTENT

Ménière's Disease (Patient Information)

AUTHOR: **SHARON S. HARTMAN POLENSEK, M.D., PH.D.**

TABLE 1-323 Guidelines to define Ménière's disease

Definition	Symptoms
Certain Ménière's disease	Definite Ménière's disease + histopathologic confirmation
Definite Ménière's disease	≥2 definitive spontaneous episodes of vertigo 20 min or longer Audiometrically documented hearing loss on at least one occasion Tinnitus or aural fullness in the treated ear Other causes excluded
Probable Ménière's disease	One definite episode of vertigo Audiometrically documented hearing loss on at least one occasion Tinnitus or aural fullness in the treated ear Other causes excluded
Possible Ménière's disease	Episodic vertigo without documented hearing loss, or sensorineural hearing loss (SNHL) fluctuating or fixed, with disequilibrium but nonepisodic Other causes excluded

BASIC INFORMATION

DEFINITION

Meningiomas are generally slow-growing tumors arising from arachnoid cells of the arachnoid villi; 90% are benign.

ICD-9CM CODES
225.2 Cerebral meninges
ICD-10CM CODES
D32.0 Benign neoplasm of cerebral meninges

EPIDEMIOLOGY & DEMOGRAPHICS

INCIDENCE: 6/100,000 persons/yr; account for about one third of primary brain tumors and are the second most common brain tumor in adults; often underreported.

PREDOMINANT SEX AND AGE: Female/male ratio of almost 3:1 in the brain and up to 6:1 in the spinal cord; male = female in childhood

PEAK INCIDENCE: Males: sixth decade, females: seventh decade, incidence increases with age; rare in childhood

RISK FACTORS: Ionizing radiation results in increased incidence and a shorter latency period. Neurofibromatosis type 2 (NF2) is an autosomal dominant genetic disorder that predisposes to multiple intracranial tumors. Approximately half of all individuals with NF2 have meningiomas, most of which are intracranial. Studies have suggested a link between hormonal factors and development of meningioma. At present, there is no conclusive evidence to support a causal relationship with cell phone usage and subsequent development of meningioma.

GENETICS: Meningiomas may be isolated or found in association with other genetic diseases, such as neurofibromatosis type 2 and familial meningioma. Approximately half of meningiomas have allelic losses involving of the *NF2* and *DAL-1* genes. Allelic losses of chromosomes 1p, 2p, 6q, 9q, 10q, 14q, 17p, and 18q may be associated with histologic progression.

TABLE 1-324 Locations and Presentations of Meningiomas

Location	Presenting Manifestation
Parasagittal	Urinary incontinence, dementia, gradual paraparesis, seizures
Lateral convexity	Variable depending on structures compressed, including slow hemiparesis, speech abnormalities
Olfactory groove	Anosmia, visual disturbance, dementia, Foster-Kennedy syndrome
Suprasellar	Hormonal failure, bitemporal hemianopia, optic atrophy
Sphenoid ridge	Extraocular nerve paresis, exostoses, proptosis, seizures

From Goetz CG, Pappert EJ: *Textbook of clinical neurology,* Philadelphia, 1999, Saunders.

PHYSICAL FINDINGS & CLINICAL PRESENTATION

- Neurologic symptoms vary with location and size (see Table 1-324); meningiomas can arise from the dura at any site, although most commonly occur within the skull and at sites of dural reflection, such as the cerebral convexities and the falx. Other less common locations include the sphenoid wing, olfactory groove, and optic nerve sheath. Focal symptoms such as vision loss, hearing loss, or mental status change depend on the site of origin and the time course of growth.
- Most common presentation is with a focal or generalized seizure or gradually worsening neurologic deficit. Seizures are present preoperatively in 30% to 40%.
- Typically are slow growing and asymptomatic; many meningiomas are asymptomatic and/or discovered incidentally on a neuroimaging study or at autopsy.

ETIOLOGY

- Meningiomas are thought to arise from a multistep progression of genetic changes.
- Mutations of the *NF2* gene on chromosome 22 are found in patients with neurofibromatosis type 2 and >50% of sporadic meningiomas. This gene is thought to act as a tumor suppressor gene; the protein product, merlin, is also involved in cytoskeletal organization.
- *DAL-1* is another tumor suppressor gene, located on chromosome 18p, that has been identified in a subset of the approximately 40% of sporadic meningiomas with neither the *NF2* gene mutations nor allelic loss of chromosome 22q.
- Cranial radiation may be responsible for some cases following an appropriate latency period from 10 to 20 yr. Meningiomas that result from radiation are generally more aggressive.
- The link with steroid hormones and their receptors is suggested by the increase in growth rate and/or development of meningiomas during pregnancy and increased incidence in women who use postmenopausal hormones or in association with breast carcinomas.

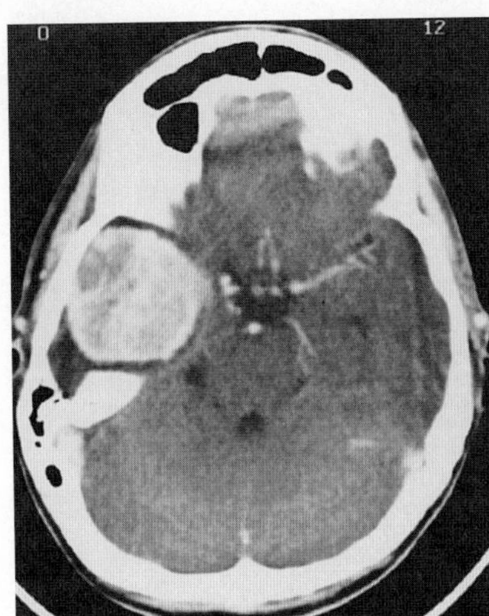

FIGURE 1-588 Contrast-enhanced CT scan demonstrates a large contrast-enhancing right sphenoid wing meningioma. (From Specht N [ed]: *Practical guide to diagnostic imaging,* St Louis, 1998, Mosby.)

DIAGNOSIS

DIFFERENTIAL DIAGNOSIS

Other well-circumscribed intracranial tumors that involve the dura or subdural space.

- Acoustic schwannoma (typically at the pontocerebellar junction)
- Ependymoma, lipoma, and metastases within spinal cord
- Metastatic disease from lymphoma/adenocarcinoma, inflammatory disease such as sarcoidosis and Wegener's granulomatosis, or infections such as tuberculosis

WORKUP

Imaging studies with CT or MRI, followed by surgical removal with histologic confirmation

LABORATORY TESTS

According to the World Health Organization (WHO) classification, there are nine benign histologic variants (account for 90% of all meningiomas) and four variants associated with increased recurrence and rates of metastasis. Ninety percent of meningiomas are classified as benign meningiomas or WHO grade I.

IMAGING STUDIES

- Cranial CT scanning or MRI can detect and determine the extent of meningiomas (Fig. 1-588). CT can show hyperostosis and/or intratumoral calcifications. MRI (Fig. 1-589) is the imaging modality of choice to

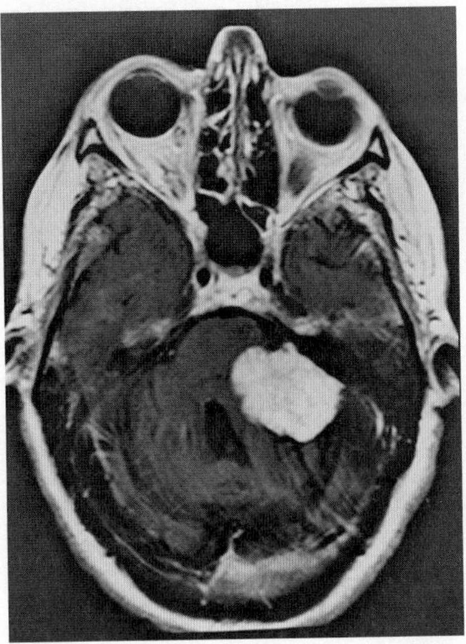

FIGURE 1-589 MRI picture of a posterior fossa meningioma, demonstrated an extra-axial homogeneously contrast-enhanced mass arising from the tentorium and compressing the cerebellar hemisphere. (From Goetz CG, Pappert EJ: *Textbook of clinical neurology,* Philadelphia, 1999, Saunders.)

demonstrate the dural origin of the tumor in most cases, with the characteristic "tail" sign.
- On nonenhanced scans, meningiomas typically are isodense or slightly hyperdense to brain and are homogeneous in appearance. They show homogeneous contrast enhancement; gadolinium can facilitate imaging of smaller additional lesions that are missed on unenhanced images.
- Indistinct margins, marked edema, mushroomlike projections from tumor, brain parenchymal infiltration, and heterogeneous enhancement are suggestive of more aggressive behavior.
- PET scan may help in predicting the aggressiveness of the tumor and the potential for recurrence, but it is not used routinely.

Rx TREATMENT

Primary management depends on signs or symptoms, age of patient, and location and size of tumor. Observation may be appropriate if tumors are discovered incidentally and/or if growth is indolent and unlikely to cause symptoms.

PHARMACOLOGIC THERAPY

- Although a variety of chemotherapeutic agents have been studied, such as hydroxyurea, there is no established effective systemic therapy.
- Inhibition of hormone receptors, such as progesterone, estrogen, and androgen, has failed to demonstrate clinical benefit.
- Treatment with molecularly targeted approaches, such as angiogenesis inhibition, is currently under way.

NONPHARMACOLOGIC THERAPY

- The mainstay of treatment for meningiomas remains surgical removal. Complete resection is usually attempted, when feasible. After total excision, recurrence rates of 0% to 20% have been observed, while 20% to 50% of patients recur within 5 yr of a subtotal resection.
- Active surveillance to monitor for tumor recurrence is important.
- Radiation therapy is the only validated form of adjuvant therapy and may be beneficial in patients with incomplete resections or inoperable tumors. Stereotactic radiosurgery can provide local control with more limited toxicity.

ACUTE GENERAL Rx

- For lesions that cause significant mass effect, steroids are sometimes used to decrease brain edema.
- Anticonvulsants are used if the patient presents with seizures.

CHRONIC Rx

- Prophylactic use of anticonvulsants is not recommended in patients without a history of seizures.
- There is limited data on the efficacy of traditional chemotherapy, and the evidence is largely anecdotal. The most extensively evaluated agents are hydroxyurea, mifepristone (RU486), and interferon alfa-2b. Recently, somatostatin analogs have been evaluated in multicenter clinical trials.

DISPOSITION

- Estimated surgical mortality is 7%. Significant morbidity and mortality can be observed in meningiomas with otherwise favorable pathology secondary to unfavorable location (e.g., skull base).
- Long-term outcome varies, based on pathology, tumor grade, location, and completeness of resection.
- Most incidentally discovered meningiomas remain asymptomatic and have a slow rate of growth. Calcified tumors may be less likely to progress than noncalcified ones.
- Meningiomas may recur after surgical resection. In addition, some tumors show histologic progression to a higher grade. Features suggesting increased rate of recurrence include multiple allelic chromosomal losses,local brain invasion, high rate of mitosis, and highly anaplastic features.

REFERRAL

- Neurosurgical consultation for all cases
- Neurology, radiation oncology, and oncology depending on presence of other sequelae and in setting of recurrence

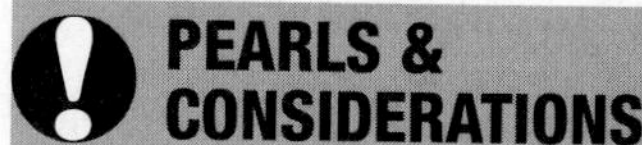

PEARLS & CONSIDERATIONS

COMMENTS

- Many meningiomas are discovered incidentally; most are benign and remain asymptomatic.
- "Dural tail" is classic finding on neuroimaging studies.
- Individuals with neurofibromatosis type 2 are at high risk to develop meningiomas.

PATIENT & FAMILY EDUCATION

Meningioma mommas: www.meningiomamommas.org
Meningioma Support and Patient Information Group
National Brain Tumor Society
Meningioma Online Support Group: http://www.brainstrust.org/meningioma.htm

SUGGESTED READINGS

available at www.expertconsult.com

RELATED CONTENT

Meningioma (Patient Information)

AUTHOR: **NICOLE J. ULLRICH, M.D., PH.D.**

BASIC INFORMATION

DEFINITION

Bacterial meningitis is an inflammation of meninges with increased intracranial pressure, and pleocytosis or increased WBCs in cerebrospinal fluid (CSF) secondary to bacteria in the pia-subarachnoid space and ventricles, leading to neurologic sequelae and abnormalities.

SYNONYMS

Spinal meningitis

ICD-9CM CODES
320 Bacterial meningitis
ICD-10CM CODES
G00.9 Bacterial meningitis, unspecified

EPIDEMIOLOGY & DEMOGRAPHICS

INCIDENCE (IN U.S.): 1.3 to 2.0 cases/100,000 persons; 1.2 million cases per year in the world; 135,000 deaths annually worldwide. The rate of bacterial meningitis declined dramatically in the U.S. starting in the early 1990s with the introduction of the *Haemophilus influenzae* type b (Hib) vaccine and in 2000 with the introduction of the conjugate pneumococcal vaccine.

PREDOMINANT SEX: Male = female

PREDOMINANT AGE: All ages, neonate to geriatric

PHYSICAL FINDINGS & CLINICAL PRESENTATION

- Fever
- Headache
- Neck stiffness, nuchal rigidity, meningismus
- Altered mental state, lethargy
- Vomiting, nausea
- Photophobia
- Seizures
- Coma; lethargy, stupor
- Rash: petechial associated with meningococcal infection (Fig. 1-590), purpura fulminans (Fig. 1-591)
- Myalgia
- Cranial nerve abnormality (unilateral)
- Papilledema
- Dilated, nonreactive pupil(s)
- Posturing: decorticate/decerebrate
- Physical examination findings of Kernig's sign and Brudzinski's sign in adults with meningitis are often not helpful in determining meningeal inflammation

ETIOLOGY

The bacterial etiology of meningitis depends on the age of the patient. *Neisseria meningitidis* is now more common than *Haemophilus influenzae* as a cause of bacterial meningitis in children as well as adults, and streptococci are still common causes of bacterial meningitis. *H. influenzae* is the cause of >30% of cases of meningitis (usually in infants and children <6 yr of age). It is associated with sinusitis, otitis media.

- Neonates: group B streptococcus, gram-negative rods such as *E. coli, Listeria monocytogenes*
- Infants ≥1 mo and <3 mo: group B streptococci (40%), gram-negative rods (30%), *Streptococcus pneumoniae* (14%), and *Neisseria meningitidis* (12%)
- Infants ≥3 mo and <3 yr:
  1. *S. pneumoniae* (45%)
  2. *N. meningitidis* (34%)
  3. *S. agalactiae* (group B streptococci) (11%)
  4. *H. influenzae*
  5. *E. coli*
- Ages ≥3 yr and <10 yr:
  1. *S. pneumoniae* (47%)
  2. *N. meningitidis* (32%)
- Ages ≥10 yr and <19 yr
  1. *N. meningitidis* (55%)
  2. *S. pneumoniae*
- Adults: *S. pneumoniae, N. meningitidis,* and *L. monocytogenes* (especially over age 50-60 or with cell-mediated immune deficiencies)
- People with HIV/AIDS are at increased risk for invasive meningococcal disease (IMD).

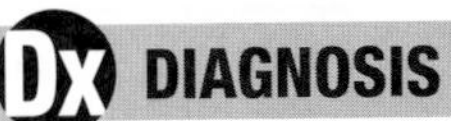

DIAGNOSIS

Diagnostic approach is based on patient presentation and physical examination (Fig. 1-592). Lumbar puncture should be performed as soon as possible. Key elements to diagnosis are CSF evaluation and CT scan or MRI if the patient is in a coma or has focal neurologic deficits, pupillary abnormalities, or papilledema.

DIFFERENTIAL DIAGNOSIS

- Endocarditis, bacteremia
- Intracranial tumor
- Lyme disease
- Brain abscess
- Partially treated bacterial meningitis
- Medications
- SLE
- Seizures
- Acute mononucleosis
- Other infectious meningitides

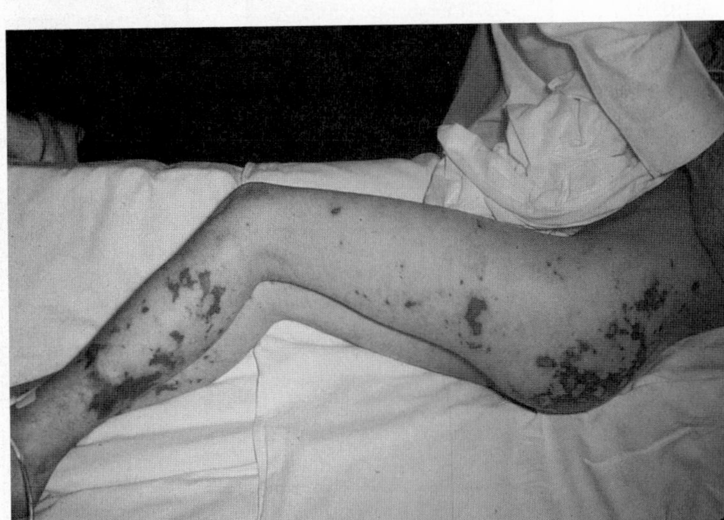

FIGURE 1-590 Fully developed, almost pathognomonic hemorrhagic rash of meningococcal sepsis. (From Cohen J, Powderly WG: *Infectious diseases,* ed 2, St Louis, 2004, Mosby.)

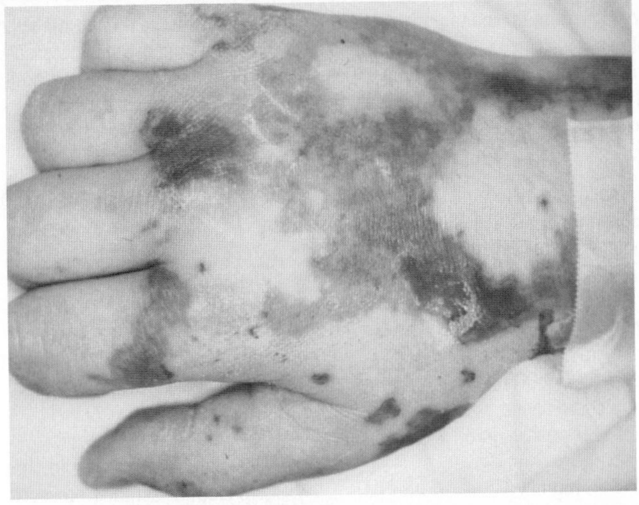

FIGURE 1-591 Meningococcal purpura fulminans in overwhelming meningococcal meningitis. (From Adams JG et al: *Emergency medicine, clinical essentials,* ed 2, Philadelphia, 2013, Elsevier.)

 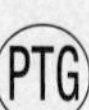 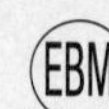 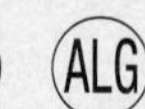

Management of Adults with Acute Meningitis Syndrome
(Fulminant course (<48 h) with fever, headache, usually with impaired sensorium and stiff neck. This protocol is not applicable if the dominant clinical impression is subarachnoid hemorrhage or acute psychosis.)

H&P STAT Labs Including 2 Sets of Blood Cultures

1. *Comatose*
2. *Inadequate History* (patient unable to provide history and no family available)
3. *Risk of Mass Lesion* (papilledema, focal neurologic defects, recent head trauma, malignant neoplasm, or history of CNS mass lesion)
4. *Immunosuppressed* (HIV, transplant, neoplasm, steroids)

No → STAT lumbar puncture

Yes → STAT CT or MRI scan‡ → Focal defect? Yes → Subacute CNS infection syndrome; No → STAT lumbar puncture. (Treatment Protocol given before STAT CT or MRI scan)

Treatment Protocol (in order)
1. Dexamethasone 10 mg IV q6h for 4 days
2. Ceftriaxone 2 g IV q12h*
3. Vancomycin 1 g IV q12h
4. Ampicillin 2 g IV q4h†

STAT lumbar puncture → CSF cloudy or high clinical suspicion of bacterial meningitis? Yes → Treatment Protocol; No →

Bacteria on Gram stain?
or
CSF WBC >1000/mm³
or
CSF PMN >100/mm³
or
CSF/Serum glucose <0.5 mg/dL
or
CSF/Blood glucose <0.42 mg/dL

Yes → Treatment Protocol; No → Prior antibiotics and abnormal CSF? Yes → Treatment Protocol; No → Subacute CNS infection syndrome

FIGURE 1-592 Algorithm for management of adult patients with acute meningitis syndrome. *For severe cephalosporin allergy, consider meropenem or moxifloxacin. †Ampicillin is indicated if there is a history of alcoholism, organ transplant, malignancy, pregnancy, or age older than 50 years. For penicillin-allergic patients, an alternative is trimethoprim-sulfamethoxazole. ‡Consider magnetic resonance imaging *(MRI)* if the patient is known or suspected to have human immunodeficiency virus *(HIV)*, if it can be obtained rapidly. *CNS*, Central nervous system; *CSF*, cerebrospinal fluid; *CT*, computed tomography; *H&P*, history and physical examination; *PMN*, polymorphonuclear leukocyte; *WBC*, white blood cell. (From Vincent JL et al: *Textbook of critical care*, ed 6, Philadelphia, 2011, Saunders.)

- Neuroleptic malignant syndrome
- Subdural empyema
- Rocky Mountain spotted fever

WORKUP

CSF examination:
- Opening pressure >100 to 200 mm Hg
- WBC usually >1000 WBC/mm³
- Neutrophilic predominance: >80%
- Gram stain of CSF: positive in 60% to 90% of patients
- CSF protein: >50 mg/dl
- CSF glucose: <40 mg/dl
- Culture: positive in 65% to 90% of cases
- CSF bacterial antigen: 50% to 100% sensitivity
- E-test for susceptibility of pneumococcal isolates

LABORATORY TESTS

Blood culturing, WBC with differential, and CSF examination (see "Workup")

IMAGING STUDIES

- CT scan or MRI of head: necessary with increased intracranial pressure, coma, neurologic deficits
- Sinus CT: if sinusitis suspected

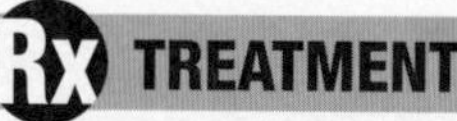

TREATMENT

Empiric therapy is necessary with IV antibiotic treatment if patient has purulent CSF fluid at time of lumbar puncture, is asplenic, or has signs of DIC/sepsis pending Gram stain and culture results. Try to obtain blood and CSF cultures before starting antimicrobial therapy, but do not delay therapy if obtaining them is not possible. Therapy after Gram stain pending cultures is recommended for the following:

1. Neonates: ampicillin: 200-400 mg/kg per day divided q6 to 8 hr plus gentamicin: 7.5 mg/kg

IV in 3 divided doses plus a third-generation cephalosporin: cefotaxime or ceftriaxone

2. 1-23 months: vancomycin: 60 mg/kg per day IV (maximum up to 4 g/day) divided in 4 doses plus third-generation cephalosporin: ceftriaxone: 100 mg/kg (maximum dose 4 g/day) in 1 or 2 divided doses or cefotaxime: 300 mg/kg per day IV (maximum dose of 12 g/day) in 3 or 4 divided doses
3. Children: vancomycin: 60 mg/kg per day IV (maximum dose 4 g/day) in 4 divided doses plus third-generation cephalosporin: ceftriaxone 100 mg/kg per day IV (maximum 4 g/day) or cefotaxime: 300 mg/kg IV (maximum dose of 12 g/day) in 3 or 4 divided doses
4. Adults: vancomycin: 15-20 mg/kg IV every 8 to 12 hours plus third-generation cephalosporin: ceftriaxone: 2 g IV q12 hours or cefotaxime: 2 g IV q4 to 6 hr. For adults over 50 yr of age also add ampicillin 2 g IV every 4 hr to cover *Listeria*
5. Immunocompromised patients: vancomycin *plus* ampicillin *plus* either cefepime 2 g IV every 8 hr to cover *Pseudomonas* or meropenem 2 g IV q8 hr for adults, which also covers *Pseudomonas*
   - Use of corticosteroids in adults: dexamethasone 0.15 mg/kg q6h for first 4 days of therapy should be used for adults in developed countries with known or suspected bacterial meningitis. Decreased mortality and neurologic sequelae are seen with adjunct therapy. The benefit of dexamethasone is less clear in developing countries with high HIV prevalence and malnutrition or with delayed clinical presentations.
   - Dexamethasone also benefits children with Hib meningitis if given at the same time or before the first dose of the antibiotic: 0.15 mg/kg per dose q6 hr for 2 to 4 d. The use and benefit of corticosteroids in suspected or pneumococcal or meningococcal meningitis to prevent neurologic sequelae is not as clear and should be individualized after analysis of risk and benefits.

DISPOSITION

Bacterial meningitis is a reportable disease that needs to be reported to local health authorities. Droplet precautions should be used for first 24 hr of therapy for suspected or confirmed *N. meningitidis* infection.

REFERRAL

- To a neurologist if persistent neurologic sequelae develop after bacterial meningitis
- To an infectious disease consultant if a patient has recurrent bacterial meningitis; such patients deserve a workup for an anatomic (CSF dural leak) or immunologic defect (complement defect, hyposplenism, immunoglobulin deficiency)

PEARLS & CONSIDERATIONS

COMMENTS

- Nosocomial bacterial meningitis may result from invasive procedures (e.g., placement of ventricular catheters, lumbar puncture, craniotomy, spinal anesthesia). Treatment of this different spectrum of microorganisms requires empirical antimicrobial therapy with vancomycin plus either cefepime, ceftazidime, or meropenem. In cases of basilar skull fracture, effective empirical antimicrobial therapy consists of vancomycin plus a third-generation cephalosporin.
- Prevention of meningitis can be achieved through chemoprophylaxis of close contacts (household members and anyone exposed to oral secretions).
- Effective medications are rifampin 10 mg/kg PO bid for 2 days or ceftriaxone 250 mg IM single dose in patients older than age 12; 125 mg IM if age 12 or younger.
- Ciprofloxacin 500 mg for prevention of *Neisseria* meningitis can be given to patients older than 18 yr who cannot tolerate rifampin to eradicate pharyngeal colonization.
- Menactra: a protein-conjugate vaccine against serogroup A, C, Y, W-135 capsular polysaccharides is available for adults (up to 55 yr) and children older than 2 yr.

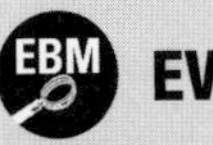

EVIDENCE

available at www.expertconsult.com

SUGGESTED READINGS

available at www.expertconsult.com

RELATED CONTENT

Meningitis (Patient Information)
Meningitis, Viral (Related Key Topic)

AUTHOR: **GLENN G. FORT, M.D., M.P.H.**

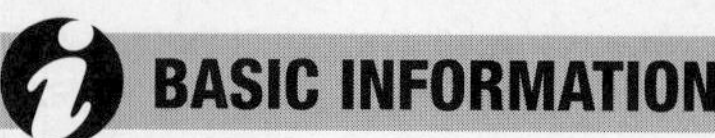

BASIC INFORMATION

DEFINITION

Fungal meningitis is an infection of the meninges and/or central nervous system that is usually more subacute than acute and caused by a variety of different fungi or molds. The most common causes in the U.S. are *Cryptococcus neoformans* and *Coccidioides immitis* meningitis but there has been a recent multi-state outbreak in the U.S. of fungal central nervous system infections and septic arthritis mostly caused by *Exserohilum rostartum* transmitted via epidural or paraspinal injections of methylprednisolone produced at a single compounding pharmacy. See Table 1-325. This chapter will cover this outbreak. See chapters on Crytococcosis and Coccidioidomycosis.

SYNONYMS

Fungal central nervous system infections

ICD-9CM Codes

321.1 Meningitis in other fungal diseases

ICD-10CM CODES

B37.5+	Candidal meningitis
B38.4+	Coccidiodomycosis meningitis
B40.7	Disseminated blastomycosis
B39.3	Disseminated histoplasmosis capsulati
B47.7	Disseminated sporotrichiosis
B45.1	Cerebral cyptococcosis
B46.1	Rhinocerebral mucormycosis
B49	Unspecified mycosis

EPIDEMIOLOGY & DEMOGRAPHICS

- Outbreak started in September 2012
- As of August 2013 there have been 750 cases, including 64 deaths
- Cases have been reported in 20 states but Michigan, Tennessee, and Indiana have had the most cases
- Some 14,000 patients may have been injected with vials of the methylprednisolone that were potentially contaminated with the mold

INCIDENCE:

Overall attack rate is calculated at 4.4 cases per 100 persons potentially exposed.

PEAK INCIDENCE:

Occurs within 6 wk of receiving an epidural or paraspinal injection of methylprednisolone contaminated with the mold, but cases have been detected after 3 mo.

PREDOMINANT SEX AND AGE:

- Median age of affected patient is 64 yr (range 16 to 92).
- Females represent 60% of the cases.

RISK FACTORS:

The source of this outbreak has been traced to a single compounding pharmacy (New England Compounding Center). *E. rostratum* has been detected in two of three implicated lots of unopened vials of preservative-free methylprednisolone.

TABLE 1-325 Mycoses as a Cause of Fungal Meningitis

Crytococcus neoformans and Crytococcus gatti
Cocciodioides immitis
Histoplasma capsulatum
Candida albicans and other *Candida* species
Sprorthrix schenckii
Blastomyces dermatitidis
Molds: *Scedosporium, Aspergillus*
Molds with dark cell walls containing melanin: many species including
Cladophialophora
Exophiala species
Exserohilum rostratum

- 17,000 vials were potentially contaminated.
- 75 health care facilities (hospital and outpatient treatment centers) in 23 states received vials with lots that were subsequently recalled.
- Infection is only acquired via injection of the steroid and *not* transmitted person to person.
- Eventually all products manufactured at that facility were recalled and the facility closed.
- Contamination was felt to have occurred due to lack of sterility controls in manufacturing.
- Green-black material was visibly seen in 83 of 321 vials from one of the recalled lots.

PHYSICAL FINDINGS & CLINICAL PRESENTATION

Most patients present 1 to 4 wk after injection.

- Meningitis, stroke, and injection site infections
  - Meningitis: new or worsening headache, neck stiffness, photophobia
  - Stroke: neurologic deficit with weakness, slurred speech, vertigo, ataxia, or diplopia. Stroke usually involves posterior circulation causing a basilar stroke.
  - Injection site infections: epidural abscess, arachnoiditis, discitis, vertebral osteomyelitis, or persistent back pain
  - Peripheral joint infections: 35 patients have developed only a peripheral joint infection due to an injection into that joint with a steroid from a contaminated lot
- Pathogenesis: the steroid itself may impair local host defenses and facilitate the fungal infection into the central nervous system. The fungus accesses the CSF and spreads upward to the basal cisterns and then invades the basilar arteries.
- Fever has not been a consistent symptom.
- Some patients were found to have injection site infections on screening MRI but had no clinical symptoms yet.

ETIOLOGY

- Only about a third of the clinical cases have a proven culture result.
- *Exserohilum rostratum* is the documented cause in about 30% of clinical cases.
  - Part of the Dematiaceae fungi group (darkly pigmented due to melanin)
  - Found in soil and part of living or dead plant material
  - Sensitive to voriconazole and amphotericin B but resistant to fluconazole
- Thirteen other mold species have been isolated in patients including *Aspergillus* species, *Alternaria* species, *Cladosporium* species, *Penicillium* species, and other species.
- Four different types of molds were isolated from the contaminated vials.

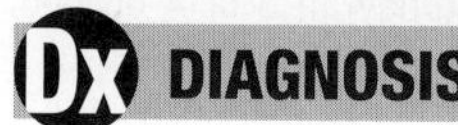

DIAGNOSIS

DIFFERENTIAL DIAGNOSIS

- Meningitis: bacterial, viral, or mycobacterial pathogens
- Stroke: cardioembolic stroke, hemorrhagic stroke
- Tumors of the central nervous system
- Epidural abscess by bacterial pathogens
- Osteomyelitis of bacterial etiology

WORKUP

Should be considered in any patient who has received an injection from a steroid manufactured at New England Compounding Center. Information is available on website: http://www.cdc.gov/hai/outbreaks/meningitis-facilities-map.html

- A negative culture from a clinical specimen does not rule out the infection.
- Local health department should be contacted if case suspected.

LABORATORY TESTS

- CSF: if meningitis suspected perform LP. Obtain at least 10 to 20 ml of CSF.
  - Obtain routine tests: Gram stain, culture, cell count, protein, glucose
  - At least 10 cc for fungal culture and hold for a minimum of 2 wk
  - Send unspun CSF to CDC for a PCR for *E. rostratum*
- Other tests: routine CBC with differential, Bun/Cr, liver function tests

IMAGING STUDIES

Neuroimaging via MRI or MRI/MRA or CT can detect:

- Infarcts/strokes
- Large vessel involvement of the posterior circulation
- Dural and leptomeningeal enhancement
- Arachnoiditis
- Osteomyelitis/discitis of the spine
- Epidural abscess

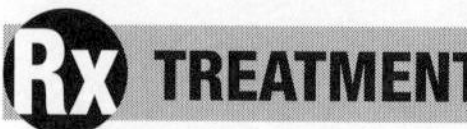

TREATMENT

ACUTE GENERAL Rx

Will depend on site of infection and severity:

- Meningitis: Voriconazole with or without liposomal amphotericin B

- Voriconazole: 6 mg/kg q12h IV for severe cases or oral for mild cases has good penetration into CSF; side effects include changes in color vision or hallucinations
- Liposomal amphotericin B (AmBisome): 7.5 mg/kg IV q24h can be added to voriconazole for the most severe cases or for patients who are not responding to voriconazole alone or relapse. Can cause nephrotoxicity that can be ameliorated by giving 1 L of IV normal saline prior to dose.

• Injection site infections: epidural abscess, discitis, vertebral osteomyelitis, etc.
  - Voriconazole: 6 mg/kg q12h IV or oral depending on presentation and can consider adding liposomal amphotericin B at 5-6 mg/kg IV q24h.

CHRONIC Rx

- Meningitis: meningitis therapy should last at least 3 mo, but stroke or severe CNS disease may require 6 mo to one yr. Monitor liver function tests, and obtain a voriconazole trough concentration on day 5 of treatment that should be between >2 mcg/ml and <5 mcg/ml. Monitor for neurologic side effects of voriconazole. For patients on liposomal amphotericin B, kidney function and electrolytes (K+) need to be monitored frequently.
- Injection site infections: therapy should last at least 3 to 6 mo.

DISPOSITION

Mortality has been about 8.8%, and highest risk factor is development of a stroke.

REFERRAL

Infectious diseases physician for guidance on initial and long-term antifungal therapy

Neurologist for evaluation and diagnosis

Neuroradiologist for MRI/MRA interpretation

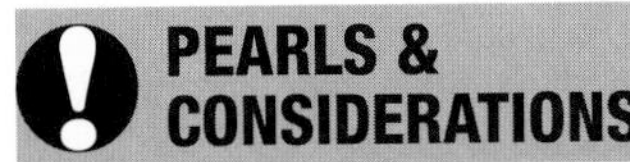

PEARLS & CONSIDERATIONS

PATIENT & FAMILY EDUCATION

This fungal disease is transmitted by the contaminated steroid injection and is not transmitted person to person and thus not contagious.

RELATED CONTENT

Meningitis, Bacterial (Related Key Topic)

Meningitis, Viral (Related Key Topic)

AUTHOR: **GLENN G. FORT, M.D., M.P.H.**

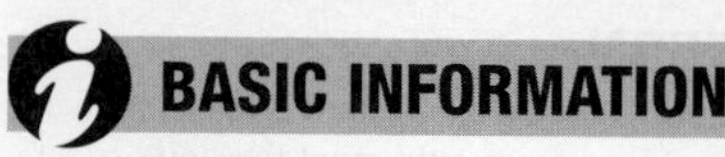

BASIC INFORMATION

DEFINITION

Viral meningitis is an acute febrile illness with signs and symptoms of meningeal irritation, usually with a lymphocytic pleocytosis of the cerebrospinal fluid (CSF) and negative CSF bacterial stains and cultures.

SYNONYMS

Aseptic meningitis

ICD-9CM CODES
047.8 Meningitis, aseptic
ICD-10CM CODES
A87.8 Other viral meningitis
A87.9 Viral meningitis, unspecified
A87.2 Lymphocytic choriomeningitis

EPIDEMIOLOGY & DEMOGRAPHICS (Table 1-326)

INCIDENCE (IN U.S.): 11 cases/100,000 persons. Leads to 26,000 to 42,000 hospitalizations a year.
PREDOMINANT SEX: Male = female
GENETICS: Those with abnormal humoral immunity and agammaglobulinemia have associated difficulty with viral clearance.

PHYSICAL FINDINGS & CLINICAL PRESENTATION

- Fever
- Headache
- Nuchal rigidity
- Photophobia
- Myalgias
- Vomiting
- Rash

ETIOLOGY

- Enterovirus: 85% to 95% of all cases. Most common are coxsackie viruses and echoviruses
- Parechoviruses
- Mumps virus
- Measles
- Arboviruses from mosquitoes: EEE, West Nile, St Louis
- Herpes: HSV-1, HSV-2, VZV, HHV-6, and HHV-7
- Acute HIV
- Lymphocytic choriomeningitis virus
- Adenovirus
- CMV and EBV
- Other arthropod-borne viruses: Powassan virus
- Influenza A and B virus

Dx DIAGNOSIS

The diagnostic approach is similar to that for bacterial meningitis (see "Meningitis, Bacterial"); the foremost need is to rule out bacterial meningitis with CSF evaluation. Presentation may be similar to that of meningitis with bacterial involvement.

DIFFERENTIAL DIAGNOSIS

- Bacterial meningitis
- Meningitis secondary to Lyme disease, TB, syphilis, amebiasis, leptospirosis
- Rickettsial illnesses: Rocky Mountain spotted fever
- Migraine headache
- Medications
- SLE
- Acute mononucleosis/Epstein-Barr virus
- Seizures
- Carcinomatous meningitis

WORKUP

CSF examination:

- Usually shows pleocytosis
- Lymphocytic predominance (neutrophils in early stages)
- Opening pressure: 200 to 250 mm Hg
- WBC: 100 to 1000 mm^3
- Increased CSF protein
- Decreased or normal CSF glucose
- Negative Gram stain, cultures, CIE, latex agglutination
- Viral cultures or serologic testing may be diagnostic
- Polymerase chain reaction for HSV, West Nile, or enterovirus (which could shorten duration of antibiotic treatment and hospitalization if bacterial meningitis was suspected)

LABORATORY TESTS

CBC with differential, blood culturing, and CSF examination (see "Workup")

IMAGING STUDIES

CT scan or MRI: if cerebral edema, focal neurologic findings develop

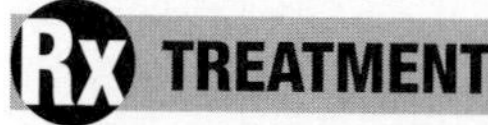

TREATMENT

No specific antiviral therapy for most viruses. Treatment is supportive unless HSV is detected, which would be treated with IV acyclovir: 10 mg/kg q8h in adults for 14-21 days. Up to 20 mg/kg q8h in children >12 yr.

DISPOSITION

Viral meningitis is almost always an uncomplicated illness that will resolve; however, relapsing headache, myalgia, and weakness may occur for 2 to 3 wk after onset of symptoms.

PEARLS & CONSIDERATIONS

- Enteroviruses are the most common cause of viral meningitis and are transmitted by fecal-oral route and less commonly by the respiratory route. They are more common in summer and fall months. From 2000 to 2005, the most common serotypes were coxsackie viruses A9, B5, and B1 and echoviruses 6, 9, 13, 18, and 30.
- Herpes simplex type 2 (HSV-2) can be a cause of a primary episode of meningitis and also be a cause of and recurrent episodes of lymphocytic meningitis. HSV-2 meningitis presents most often without a history of genital herpes or genital symptoms. Recurrent aseptic meningitis also known as Mollaret's disease is predominantly caused by HSV-2 infection.

SUGGESTED READINGS
available at www.expertconsult.com

RELATED CONTENT

Meningitis (Patient Information)

AUTHOR: **GLENN G. FORT, M.D., M.P.H.**

TABLE 1-326 Epidemiology of Acute Viral Meningitis

EPIDEMIOLOGIC FACTORS*				
Season	**Patient's Age (yr)**	**Patient's Sex**	**Risk Factor**	**Suggested Viral Agent**
Summer-fall	Infant	—	Infected mother	Coxsackievirus B
	1-15	—	Swimming pools, closed communities	Enteroviruses
			Geographic area: California, southeastern United States	California serogroup virus
Winter	1-15	—	School exposure	Varicella virus, measles virus
		Male/female 3:1		Mumps virus
	16-21	—	College exposure	Measles virus
		Male/female 3:1		Mumps virus
		—		Epstein-Barr virus (mononucleosis)
	Any	—	Mice, rats, hamsters	Lymphocytic choriomeningitis virus
	Adults	—	Varicella-zoster	Varicella-zoster virus
Any	Any	—	Immunocompromise	Adenovirus
		—	Acquired immunodeficiency syndrome	Human immunodeficiency virus

*Epidemiologic factors are suggestive but should not be used to exclude diagnoses in individual cases.
From Gorbach SI: *Infectious diseases*, ed 2, Philadelphia, 1998, Saunders.

BASIC INFORMATION

DEFINITION

Menopause is the permanent cessation of menstrual periods for 1 yr after age 40 yr or permanent cessation of ovulation after lost ovarian activity. It is the reproductive stage of life marked by waxing and waning estrogen levels followed by decreasing ovarian function. Premature ovarian failure (recently also referred to as Premature Ovarian Insufficiency) and no menstrual periods may also occur because of depletion of ovarian follicles before the age of 40 yr.

SYNONYMS

Change of life
Climacteric ovarian failure

ICD-9CM CODES

627 Premenopausal menorrhagia
627.2 Menopausal or female climacteric states
627.4 States associated with artificial menopause

ICD-10CM CODES

Z78.0 Asymptomatic menopausal state
N95.1 Menopausal and female climacteric states
N95.8 Other specified menopausal and perimenopausal disorders

EPIDEMIOLOGY & DEMOGRAPHICS

- Average age of menopause in the United States is 51 yr.
- Age at which menopause occurs is primarily genetically determined.
- Smokers experience menopause an average of 1.5 yr earlier than nonsmokers.
- More than one third of a woman's life will be spent after menopause.
- Onset of perimenopause is usually in a woman's mid- to late-40s.
- Approximately 4000 women each day begin menopause.

PHYSICAL FINDINGS & CLINICAL PRESENTATION

- Atrophic vaginitis, which can cause burning, itching, bleeding, dyspareunia
- Either complete cessation of menses or a period of irregular cycles and diminished or heavier bleeding
- Osteoporosis
- Psychological dysfunction:
  1. Anxiety
  2. Depression
  3. Insomnia
  4. Nervousness
  5. Irritability
  6. Inability to concentrate
- Sexual changes, decreased libido, dyspareunia
- Urinary incontinence
- Vasomotor symptoms (hot flashes, flushes), night sweats, cardiovascular disease, coronary artery disease, atherosclerosis, headaches, tiredness, and lethargy. A recent study from the University of Pennsylvania noted that the median duration of moderate-to-severe hot flashes is 10.2 yr but that the length of hot flashes was largely dictated by how early these began in the perimenopause.

ETIOLOGY

- The most common etiology: physiologic, caused by depleted granulosa and theca cells that fail to react to endogenous gonadotropins, producing less estrogen; decreased negative feedback in the hypothalamic pituitary access, increased follicle-stimulating hormone (FSH), and increased luteinizing hormone (LH), which leads to stromal cells that continue to produce androgens as a result of the LH stimulation
- Surgical castration
- Family history of early menopause, cigarette smoking, blindness, abnormal chromosomal karyotype (Turner's syndrome, gonadal dysgenesis), precocious puberty, and left-handedness

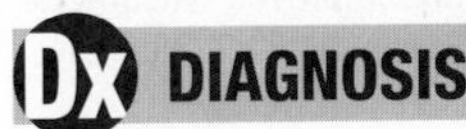

DIAGNOSIS

DIFFERENTIAL DIAGNOSIS

- Asherman's syndrome
- Hypothalamic dysfunction
- Hypothyroidism
- Pituitary tumors
- Adrenal abnormalities
- Ovarian abnormalities
- Polycystic ovarian syndrome
- Pregnancy
- Ovarian neoplasm
- Tuberculosis of the endometrium

WORKUP

- If the clinical picture is highly suggestive of menopause, estrogen can be prescribed. If all symptoms resolve, then diagnosis has essentially been made. Before estrogen is prescribed, a complete history and physical examination are needed. If a patient has estrogen-dependent malignancy, unexplained abnormal uterine bleeding, history of thrombophlebitis, or acute liver disease, estrogen therapy is contraindicated.
- Progesterone challenge test: medroxyprogesterone 10 to 20 mg PO or progesterone 100 mg IM to induce withdrawal bleeding. If no withdrawal bleeding is obtained, a hypoestrogenic state is assumed to be present. This test is increasingly controversial even if very commonly performed.
- Physical examination, height, weight, blood pressure, breast examination, and pelvic examination are needed.
- Assess risk for coronary artery disease, osteoporosis, cigarette smoking, personal history, history of breast cancer, liver disease, active coagulation disorder, or any unexplained vaginal bleeding.

LABORATORY TESTS

- FSH, LH, and estrogen levels: markedly elevated FSH and markedly depressed estrogen level constitute laboratory diagnosis of ovarian failure; LH only if polycystic ovarian disease is to be ruled out in a younger patient. It is not necessary to obtain an FSH if the patient fulfills the clinical criteria for menopause. Similarly, since estradiol levels vary during the menstrual cycle, estradiol levels are rarely necessary or informative
- TSH to rule out thyroid dysfunction and prolactin level if patient has symptoms of galactorrhea and if suspicion of pituitary adenoma exists
- A general chemistry profile to check for any systemic diseases
- Pap smear, endometrial biopsy, or dilation and curettage in patients who have had irregular periods or intermenstrual or postmenopausal bleeding
- Mammogram

IMAGING STUDIES

- CT scan or MRI of sella if pituitary tumor is suspected
- Bone density studies if high-risk condition for osteoporosis exists
- Pelvic ultrasound to check endometrial stripe

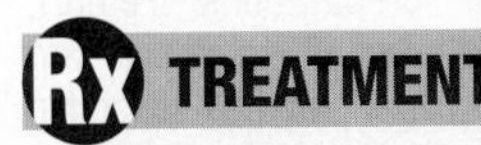

TREATMENT

NONPHARMACOLOGIC THERAPY

- A balanced diet: low in fat, with total fat intake being <30% of calories; total calories sufficient to maintain body weight or produce weight loss if that is needed
- Avoidance of smoking and excessive alcohol or caffeine intake
- Exercise: weight-bearing exercise for osteoporosis prevention
- Kegel exercises for strengthening the pelvic floor
- Adequate calcium intake: 1500 mg qd is necessary to maintain zero calcium balance in postmenopausal women
- Change in the ambient temperature (may ameliorate hot flashes and reduce night sweats)
- Vitamin E
- Avoidance of caffeine, alcohol, and spicy foods if they trigger hot flashes
- Vaginal lubricants to help with the dyspareunia attributable to vaginal dryness (e.g., Replens, K-Y Jelly, or Gyne-Moistrin cream)

ACUTE GENERAL Rx

Estrogen replacement in symptomatic patients can be done in a variety of forms, including oral estrogen and transdermal estrogen patch. The lowest effective dose should be prescribed.

- Examples of oral estrogen include:
  1. Conjugated estrogens: start with 0.3 mg qd and increase to 1.25 mg qd depending on symptoms.
  2. Estradiol: start with 0.5 mg qd and increase to 2 mg qd.

3. Esterified estrogens: start with 0.3 to 1.25 mg qd.
4. Estropipate: start with 0.625 to 2.5 mg qd.
5. Esterified estrogen/testosterone combination: give 1.25 mg and methyltestosterone 2.5 mg (Estratest) and esterified estrogen 0.625 mg and methyltestosterone 1.25 mg (Estratest HS [half-strength]). May improve sexual enjoyment and libido.

- If the patient has had a hysterectomy for benign disease, estrogen alone is sufficient. However, if she still has her uterus, progestin is necessary to prevent endometrial hyperplasia associated with unopposed estrogen which is protective against endometrial cancer. Progestins can be prescribed as continual daily dose or cyclic fashion. Most commonly prescribed progestins include medroxyprogesterone acetate 2.5 mg, 5 mg, and 10 mg; Prometrium 100 mg, 200 mg, and 400 mg; and Aygestin 5 mg. Continuous hormone replacement therapy is preferred because after time the patient should be amenorrheic. Patients should be counseled that they may experience some irregular spotting for the first 6 to 9 mo after starting the hormone replacement therapy. Cyclic therapy will cause withdrawal bleeding.
- Combination oral preparations Femhrt, Prefest, Prempro, Activella, Premphase are commonly used. However, the U.S. Preventive Services Task Force recommends against the use of combined estrogen and progestin for the prevention of chronic conditions in postmenopausal women.
- Transdermal patches can be either estradiol (Estraderm, Vivelle, FemPatch) 0.025 to 0.1 mg applied twice weekly or Climara 0.025 to 0.1 mg used once a week. With these preparations, progesterone should be used in a similar fashion. Apply CombiPatch twice weekly (combination estrogen and progesterone) or Climara Pro once per week (one patch).
- Vaginal creams can be used; these should be reserved for local therapy of atrophic vaginitis. Systemic absorption does occur; however, blood levels are unpredictable. Usual dose 0.5 to 2 g intravaginally daily, cyclically 3 wk on 1 wk off. When symptoms improve, once to twice weekly is adequate maintenance.
- Vagifem estradiol vaginal tablets. Initial dosage: one Vagifem tablet, inserted vaginally, qd for 2 wk. Maintenance dose: one Vagifem tablet, inserted vaginally, twice weekly.
- Femring vaginal ring delivering the equivalent of 0.5 mg/day inserted every 3 mo or Estring 0.0075 mg/day.
- EstroGel 0.06% (estradiol gel) One Pump (1.25 g/day) applied to one arm from wrist to shoulder.
- The FDA contraindications to menopause hormone therapy include the following diseases and disorders: active liver disease; current, past, or suspected breast cancer; active or recent anterior thrombembolic disease (angina, myocardial infarction); known or suspected estrogen-sensitive malignant conditions; known hypersensitivity to the active substance of the therapy or to any of the excipients; porphyria cutanea tarda; previous idiopathic or current venous thromboembolism; undiagnosed genital bleeding; untreated hypertension; untreated endometrial hyperplasia.
- For women in whom estrogen is contraindicated or for those who do not wish to take estrogen, the following regimens can be used:
  1. Serotonin reuptake inhibitors
  2. Depo-Provera 150 mg IM every month (may be helpful in alleviating hot flashes)
  3. Clonidine 0.05 to 0.15 mg PO qd (questionable efficacy) or transdermal clonidine patch
  4. Bellergal-S (questionable efficacy)
- Tibolone significantly improves vasomotor symptoms, libido, and vaginal lubrication. Not available in the U.S.

CHRONIC Rx

Hormone replacement therapy should be used only for the short term unless benefits outweigh the risks of long-term use. As a result of the results of the Women's Health Initiative (WHI), the FDA has instituted a "black box" warning on postmenopausal hormone replacement products suggesting that the lowest dose should be used for the shortest period of time. This necessitates a considered and nuanced counseling session with patients contemplating hormone replacement prior to the initiation of therapy and then on a periodic basis after that, usually at least a yearly basis.

DISPOSITION

If treated, the patient should have resolution of her symptoms and reduced incidence of osteoporosis. Lifelong medical supervision is necessary to monitor adequacy of treatment and prevention of complications. This should include annual Pap smears, pelvic examinations, breast examinations, mammography, and endometrial sampling of any type of abnormal bleeding. If untreated, the vasomotor symptoms will eventually disappear; however, this may take several years in a small percentage of women. Some women who are in their 80s have experienced hot flashes. Urogenital atrophy will continue to worsen. Osteoporosis and coronary artery disease risks will increase with every passing year.

REFERRAL

Most menopausal women are managed by their gynecologists. However, this condition can be managed adequately by the patient's primary care physician who has an interest in treating menopausal women.

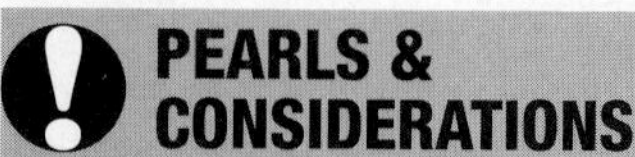

PEARLS & CONSIDERATIONS

COMMENTS

- Short-term risks of hormone replacement therapy (HRT) include an eighteenfold increased rise for cholecystitis, three-and-a-half-fold risk of a thrombocardiac event in the first year, and possible increased risk of stroke and myocardial infarction.
- Results of the WHI study found that for every 10,000 women taking HRT (combination of both estrogen and progesterone) for 1 yr (10,000 person-yr), seven more would have coronary events, eight would have more strokes, eight would have more pulmonary emboli, and eight would have earlier breast cancer than would 10,000 women taking placebo. Benefits of HRT were six fewer cases of colorectal cancer and five fewer hip fractures per 10,000 women.
- HRT should not be initiated or continued for the primary or secondary prevention of coronary heart disease.
- Estrogen-replacement therapy or HRT should only be prescribed for patients with sufficient menopausal symptoms that impact the patient's quality of life.
- Interestingly, women who start hormone therapy early in menopause may have cardiac and other benefits. The Women's Health Initiative had an average age at the start of therapy of 61, and this may have skewed the results of the study.

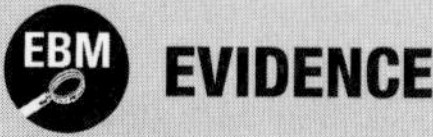

EVIDENCE

available at www.expertconsult.com

SUGGESTED READINGS

available at www.expertconsult.com

RELATED CONTENT

Osteoporosis (Related Key Topic)
Hot Flashes (Related Key Topic)
Menopause (Patient Information)

AUTHOR: **RUBEN ALVERO, M.D.**

BASIC INFORMATION

DEFINITION

Menorrhagia is menstrual blood loss greater than 80 mL.

Metrorrhagia is bleeding between menses.

Polymenorrhea is bleeding that occurs more often than every 21 days.

Oligomenorrhea is bleeding less than every 35 days.

The new FIGO classification of abnormal uterine bleeding further defines abnormal bleeding by etiology. The acronym PALM-COEIN (polyp, adenomyosis, leiomyoma, malignancy or hyperplasia, coagulopathy, ovulatory dysfunction, endometrial, iatrogenic, or not yet classified) is now used to define abnormal uterine bleeding.

SYNONYMS

Abnormal uterine bleeding
Menometrorrhagia
Dysfunctional uterine bleeding

ICD-9CM CODES
626.2 Menorrhagia
ICD-10CM CODES
N92.0 Excessive and frequent menstruation with regular cycle
N92.1 Excessive and frequent menstruation with irregular cycle
N92.4 Excessive bleeding in the premenopausal period
N92.2 Excessive menstruation at puberty
N92.6 Irregular menstruation, unspecified

EPIDEMIOLOGY & DEMOGRAPHICS

PREVALENCE: 30% of women in their lifetime; 5% of medical visits for women

PREDOMINANT SEX AND AGE: Female; peak in adolescence and perimenopausal periods

GENETICS: Von Willebrand disease; hereditary platelet dysfunction disorders; 20% of women at any age have underlying bleeding disorder

RISK FACTORS: genetic predisposition, anticoagulation treatment, obesity

PHYSICAL FINDINGS & CLINICAL PRESENTATION

- History: age, age of menarche or menopause, menstrual bleeding patterns, severity of bleeding, pain, underlying medical conditions, surgical history, use of medications, signs and symptoms of hemostatic disorder including history of heavy bleeding since menarche, postpartum hemorrhage, surgery-related bleeding, bleeding from dental work, easy bruising, epistaxis, and frequent gum bleeding, family history of bleeding disorder
- Physical exam: general findings including excessive weight, signs of polycystic ovarian syndrome (PCOS) (hirsutism and acne), signs of thyroid disease (nodule), signs of insulin resistance (acanthosis nigricans), signs of bleeding disorder including petechiae, ecchymoses, pallor, swollen joints, pelvic examination including external, speculum, and bimanual exam

ETIOLOGY

- Pregnancy/miscarriage
- Endometrial polyps
- Adenomyosis
- Uterine leiomyoma
- Endometrial hyperplasia or carcinoma
- Coagulopathy, inherited or acquired
- Ovulatory dysfunction, most likely PCOS
- Endometrial
- Iatrogenic

DIAGNOSIS

DIFFERENTIAL DIAGNOSIS

Pregnancy, STD, PCOS, thyroid dysfunction, anovulation due to immature hypothalamic-pituitary-ovarian axis, perimenopausal transition, uterine pathology including endometrial hyperplasia or carcinoma, leiomyoma, adenomyosis, or endometrial polyp, von Willebrand's disease, platelet dysfunction disorder, iatrogenic due to medications including oral contraceptives or anticoagulants (warfarin)

WORKUP

- History
- Physical exam to evaluate for uterine pathology
- Laboratory, pathology, and imaging studies to determine etiology

LABORATORY TESTS

- Pregnancy test
- CBC with platelets to assess for anemia or platelet dysfunction
- TSH to assess for hypothyroidism or hyperthyroidism
- Chlamydia trachomatis testing if high risk for evaluation of pelvic infection
- Evaluation for cyclic menses
- Prothrombin time and partial thromboplastin time
- Testing for von Willebrand disease if clinically suspected (von Willebrand–ristocetin cofactor activity, von Willebrand factor antigen, and factor VIII)
- Endometrial sampling by endometrial biopsy or hysteroscopic sampling for women >45 yr or <45 yr with history of unopposed estrogen (PCOS, obesity), failed medical management, or persistent abnormal bleeding

IMAGING STUDIES

- Transvaginal ultrasound if abnormal exam or persistent symptoms
- Sonohysterography or hysteroscopy if ultrasound not adequate or suspicion for endometrial polyp or submucosal leiomyoma
- Transabdominal ultrasound in adolescents may be considered
- MRI not indicated initially

TREATMENT

NONPHARMACOLOGIC THERAPY

- Dilation and curettage
- Uterine artery embolization
- Hysteroscopic resection of uterine pathology including endometrial polyps and submucosal leiomyoma
- Endometrial ablation
- Hysterectomy

ACUTE GENERAL Rx

- Progestin
- Oral contraceptive pills
- Conjugated estrogens
- Surgical management if indicated including dilation and curettage, uterine artery embolization, or hysterectomy
- Hospitalization to maintain hemostasis and administer blood transfusion if severe menorrhagia

CHRONIC Rx

- Oral contraceptive pills. Can be used cyclically or continuously.
- Levonorgestrel intrauterine device: high degree of efficacy
- Gonadotropin-releasing hormone agonist (goserelin)
- Nonsteroidal anti-inflammatory drugs
- Tranexamic acid, aminocaproic acid
- Danazol (significant side-effect profile requires justification for use; this is rare)
- Surgery for anatomic causes including resection of leiomyoma and hysterectomy
- Endometrial ablation if completed childbearing

REFERRAL

- If concern for uterine pathology as etiology for menorrhagia, referral to a gynecologist for surgical management indicated
- If endometrial sampling reveals endometrial hyperplasia or malignancy, referral to a gynecologist is indicated. Cyclic progestogen therapy is necessary with resampling. If endometrial hyperplasia associated with complex glands or atypia, consultation with gynecologic oncologist is important because of high degree of progression to malignancy.

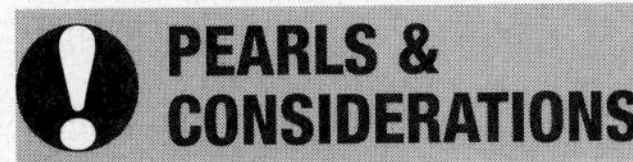

PEARLS & CONSIDERATIONS

PREVENTION

Weight reduction

Intervention in women with chronic oligoovulation due to chronic exposure to unopposed estrogen.

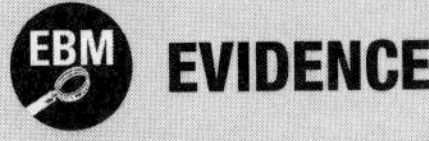

EVIDENCE

available at www.expertconsult.com

SUGGESTED READINGS

available at www.expertconsult.com

RELATED CONTENT

Dysfunctional Uterine Bleeding (Related Topic)

AUTHOR: **ERIN MEDLIN, M.D.**

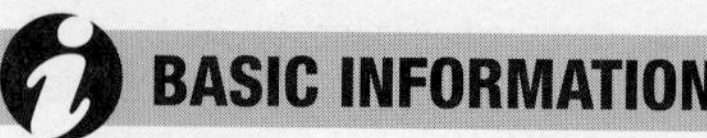

BASIC INFORMATION

DEFINITION

Acute mesenteric lymphadenitis is a syndrome of acute right lower quadrant abdominal pain associated with mesenteric lymph node enlargement and a normal appendix.

ICD-9CM CODES
289.2 Mesenteric adenitis
ICD-10CM CODES
I88.0 Nonspecific mesenteric lymphadenitis

EPIDEMIOLOGY & DEMOGRAPHICS

- Incidence unknown
- Affects mostly children (<18 yr) with no sex preference
- When *Yersinia* enterocolitis is the cause, boys are more frequently involved

PHYSICAL FINDINGS & CLINICAL PRESENTATION

- Abdominal pain of variable severity (mild ache to severe colic) beginning in upper abdomen or right lower quadrant; eventually localizes in the right side but not in a precise location (unlike appendicitis)
- In *Yersinia* infection outbreaks (see Table E1-327), symptoms include abdominal pain (84%), diarrhea (78%), fever (43%), anorexia (22%), nausea (13%), and vomiting (8%)
- Physical findings:
  - Other lymphadenopathy (20% of cases)
  - Right lower quadrant tenderness (site of maximal tenderness may vary from one examination to the next)
  - Guarding (rare)
  - Mild fever

ETIOLOGY & PATHOGENESIS

- Reactive hyperplasia of lymph nodes that drain the ileocecal region, similar to that seen in inflammatory or allergic conditions. One study reported that approximately two thirds of cases are secondary (reactive) and one third are primary (no demonstrable associated inflammatory process).
- *Yersinia enterocolitica, Y. pseudotuberculosis, Salmonella* species, *Escherichia coli,* and streptococci have been implicated in mesenteric adenitis. Clinical manifestations of yersiniosis are described in Table E1-328.

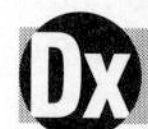

DIAGNOSIS

In general, the diagnosis is made on exploration of the abdomen of a patient suspected of having acute appendicitis. On examination the appendix appears normal, and enlarged mesenteric lymph nodes are noted. Excision of an enlarged lymph node with culture and nodal histology may provide information regarding the etiology but is not routinely used.

DIFFERENTIAL DIAGNOSIS

- Acute appendicitis (5% to 10% of patients admitted to hospitals with a diagnosis of appendicitis are discharged with a diagnosis of mesenteric adenitis)
- Crohn's disease

Section II describes the differential diagnosis of right lower quadrant abdominal pain.

LABORATORY TESTS

- Complete blood count may show leukocytosis
- Abdominal sonography and CT scan with IV and oral contrast (Fig. 1-594) may be useful
- Laparotomy if appendicitis is suspected

PROGNOSIS

Recurrent bouts are common; therefore if laparotomy is performed and a normal appendix is found, it should be removed.

SUGGESTED READINGS

available at www.expertconsult.com

AUTHOR: **FRED F. FERRI, M.D.**

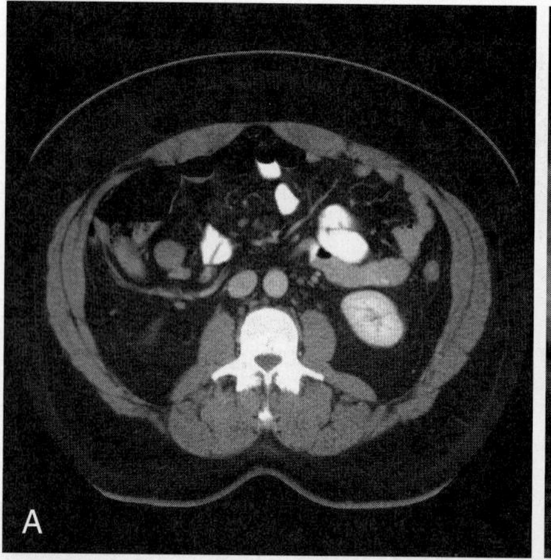

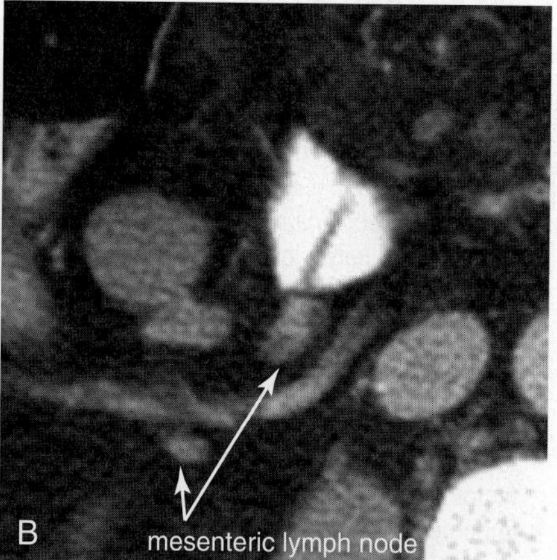

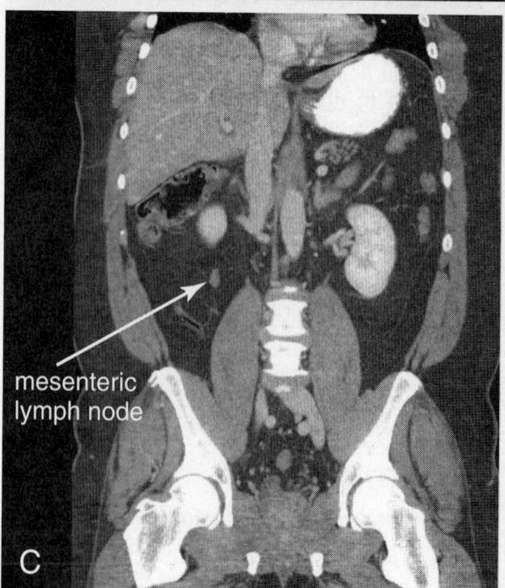

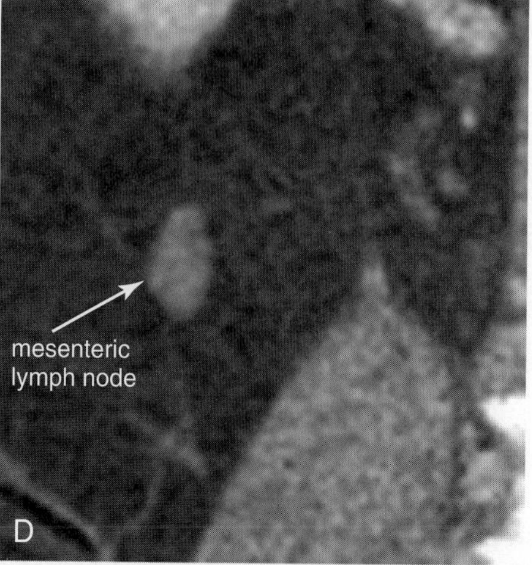

FIGURE 1-594 Mesenteric adenitis, CT with IV and oral contrast, soft-tissue window. Mesenteric adenitis can mimic appendicitis in its clinical presentation. Enlarged lymph nodes are visible on CT. Lymph nodes have soft-tissue density and appear as discrete, rounded structures. On a single image they may appear similar to blood vessels or to the appendix, but on inspection of adjacent images it becomes clear that lymph nodes are rounded, not tubular like a blood vessel or the appendix. **A,** Axial image. **B,** Close-up from **A. C,** Coronal reconstruction. **D,** Close-up from **C.** (From Broder JS: *Diagnostic imaging for the emergency physician,* Philadelphia, 2011, Saunders.)

BASIC INFORMATION

DEFINITION

Acute mesenteric ischemia (AMI) is the sudden onset of intestinal hypoperfusion to all or part of the small bowel caused by emboli, arterial or venous thrombosis (Fig. 1-595), or vasoconstriction from low-flow states.

ICD-9CM CODES
ICD-557.1 Mesenteric vascular insufficiency
ICD-10CM CODES
K55.0 Acute vascular disorders of intestine

EPIDEMIOLOGY & DEMOGRAPHICS

INCIDENCE:
- AMI accounts for 0.1% of hospital admissions.
- The incidence appears to be increasing, likely due to increased awareness among clinicians and aging of the population. The mortality rate is 60% to 85%.
- Improved intensive care, and longer survival of sicker patients, has allowed mesenteric ischemia to occur more frequently as a complication of the initial illnesses.

PREDOMINANT SEX AND AGE:
- AMI caused by arterial embolism or thrombosis occurs more frequently in the elderly.
- AMI from mesenteric venous thrombosis often presents in younger age groups.

GENETICS: No specific genetic predisposition but may be related to underlying factors such as cardiac disease, atherosclerosis, and hypercoagulable states.

RISK FACTORS:
- Advanced age, atherosclerosis, low cardiac output (especially atrial fibrillation), severe cardiac valvular disease, intraabdominal malignancy.
- In the subgroup of cases caused by venous thrombosis, risk factors include hypercoagulable states, portal hypertension, abdominal infection, blunt trauma, pancreatitis, and portal malignancy.
- Additional risk factors for AMI caused by nonocclusive mesenteric ischemia include recent cardiac surgery, dialysis, and cocaine use.
- Table E1-329 summarizes risk factors for ischemic bowel disease.
- AMI may occur rarely in patients with no identifiable risk factors.

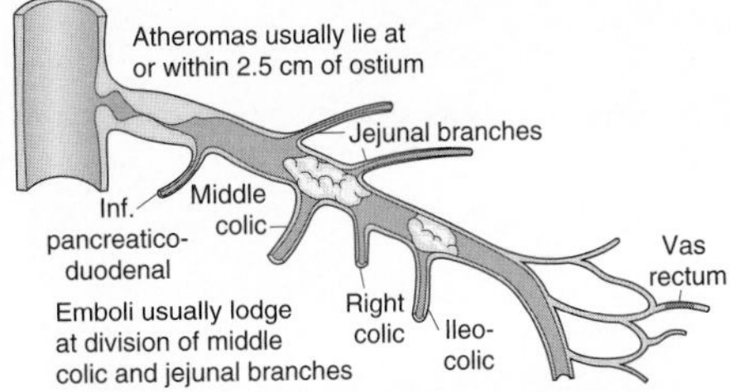

FIGURE 1-595 Typical location of superior mesenteric artery obstruction in patients with embolic and thrombotic occlusion. (From Donaldson MC: Mesenteric vascular disease. In Braunwald S, Creager MA [eds]: *Atlas of heart diseases*, St Louis, 1996, Mosby.)

PHYSICAL FINDINGS & CLINICAL PRESENTATION

- The classic presentation is rapid onset of severe periumbilical pain out of proportion to physical examination findings.
- Nausea and vomiting are commonly associated.
- Initial abdominal examination may be normal, with no rebound or guarding, or may include minimal distention or stool positive for occult blood.
- Later in the course the patient may present with gross distention, absence of bowel sounds, and peritoneal signs. In the elderly, mental status changes may occur.

ETIOLOGY

The pathophysiologic mechanisms that cause AMI include:
- Mesenteric arterial embolism: typically from the left atrium, left ventricle, or cardiac valves. The superior mesenteric artery is most commonly affected.
- Mesenteric arterial thrombosis: often in patients with prior progressive atherosclerotic stenoses, with superimposed abdominal trauma or infection.
- Mesenteric venous thrombosis may occur in the setting of hypercoagulable states (acquired or inherited), blunt trauma, abdominal infection, portal hypertension, pancreatitis, and portal malignancy.
- Nonocclusive mesenteric ischemia is caused by reduced intestinal perfusion, such as may be seen in a patient with an acute cardiovascular disease process being treated with drugs that reduce intestinal perfusion, or with use of ergot, cocaine, or amphetamines.

DIAGNOSIS

DIFFERENTIAL DIAGNOSIS

Initially include other causes of abdominal pain of acute onset, including perforated peptic ulcer and early appendicitis. Ultimately, the varied causes of peritonitis.

WORKUP

- Early diagnosis is key. Treatment success is related to the duration of symptoms before diagnosis.
- Consider early laparotomy for diagnosis in cases with a high index of suspicion when angiography is not available.

LABORATORY TESTS

- Laboratory test results are nonspecific, especially early in the course. Elevated lactic acid, leukocytosis, acidosis, and elevated hematocrit from hemoconcentration can occur later in the course, often after progression to bowel necrosis has occurred, hence are not useful for early diagnosis.
- When a hypercoagulable state is suspected, workup may include proteins C and S, antithrombin III, and factor V Leiden. This will likely not affect the diagnosis of AMI but may help guide long-term therapy.
- D-dimer testing has been reported to be useful for the early diagnosis of AMI but is very nonspecific.

IMAGING STUDIES

- Biphasic contrast-enhanced CT is the preferred diagnostic mode. It is more easily available and has similar sensitivity to angiography.
- With strong clinical suspicion, workup should proceed directly to angiography without delay for CT scan (Fig. 1-596) or other testing. If angiography cannot be done emergently, diagnositic laparotomy should not be delayed.
- Plain films are normal 25% of the time in the early stages. Suggestive findings may include ileus, bowel wall thickening, or intramural gas. Intraluminal barium should not be used as it is rarely helpful in making a positive diagnosis and will interfere with angiographic studies.
- Doppler ultrasound evaluation of intestinal blood flow is often limited by the presence of air-filled loops of bowel and is not an appropriate part of the diagnostic workup if AMI is the leading working diagnosis.
- Plain CT findings also are commonly nonspecific and more often found late in the course. Portal venous gas or intramural gas may be seen after the development of gangrene; in many cases, even at that advanced stage CT findings remain nonspecific. The use of IV contrast material may affect interpretation of subsequent angiography.
- CT scanning is more useful in cases of mesenteric vein thrombosis causing AMI, with sensitivity approaching 90%. It has also been found useful in monitoring the progress of patients with superior mesenteric venous thrombosis who are treated nonsurgically.

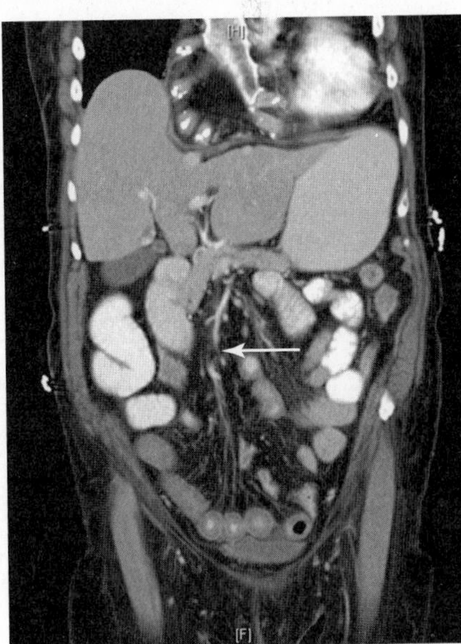

FIGURE 1-596 Mesenteric ischemia, acute. CT after administration of oral and intravenous contrast in patient with embolism to superior mesenteric artery and ischemia of small bowel and right colon. *Arrow* points to embolus in superior mesenteric artery. (From Vincent JL et al: *Textbook of critical care*, ed 6, Philadelphia, 2011, Saunders.)

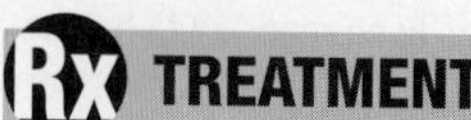

TREATMENT

- The goal of treatment is to restore blood flow as rapidly as possible to ischemic bowel before the occurrence of infarction.
- Treatment varies depending on etiology.

ACUTE GENERAL Rx

- Initial management should include hemodynamic monitoring and support, correction of acidosis, administration of broad-spectrum antibiotics, and gastric decompression by nasogastric tube.
- Vasoconstricting agents should be avoided.
- Systemic anticoagulation may be started. Optimal timing of initiation is unclear.

NONPHARMACOLOGIC THERAPY

- Signs of peritonitis mandate early laparotomy and resection of infarcted bowel.
- When workup is positive for major superior mesenteric artery (SMA) embolus, embolectomy is considered standard treatment in the absence of peritoneal signs. Depending on the location and degree of occlusion of the embolus, surgical revascularization, intraarterial infusion of thrombolytics or vasodilators, or systemic anticoagulation may be considered.
- In cases of SMA thrombosis, emergency surgical revascularization is the treatment of choice; stent placement may be a viable alternative.
- Angiography is needed to diagnose nonocclusive mesenteric ischemia before infarct and should be followed up by intraarterial vasodilator infusion. This approach has been shown to significantly reduce mortality rate in this situation.
- In patients with mesenteric vein thrombosis, treatment depends on the presence or absence of peritoneal signs. Laparotomy and resection of infarcted bowel is indicated in more advanced cases. If there are no peritoneal signs, immediate anticoagulant therapy with heparin, and ultimately warfarin, may be adequate treatment.
- Percutaneous treatment with lytic therapy, balloon angioplasty, or stenting may be limited by the frequent presence of nonviable bowel, which would require laparotomy despite success with the percutaneous treatment.

CHRONIC Rx

In the subgroup of patients with mesenteric venous thrombosis, prevention of further thrombosis is indicated. The optimal duration of anticoagulation is unclear.

DISPOSITION

- Prognosis is best in AMI due to mesenteric venous thrombosis and after surgical treatment for acute arterial embolism. It remains poor in cases of arterial thrombosis and nonocclusive ischemia.
- With delayed diagnosis, intestinal infarction—resulting in perforation or gangrenous bowel, sepsis, shock, and death—is typical.

REFERRAL

- Early surgical consultation should be considered. There should be no delay with peritoneal signs.
- If diagnostic angiography is unavailable, surgery may be warranted for diagnostic purposes.

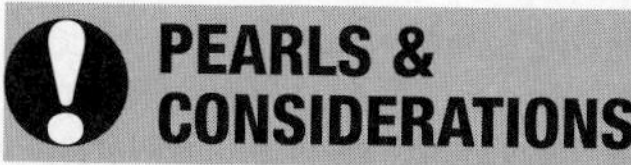

PEARLS & CONSIDERATIONS

COMMENTS

- The diagnosis of AMI should be considered in any patient with acute onset of abdominal pain out of proportion to physical findings, particularly in at-risk patients.
- Early diagnosis, before intestinal infarction occurs, is critical and correlates with improved survival rates.
- In a recent case series, the primary location of the ischemic colitis was in the right, transverse, left, and distal colon in 25%, 10%, 33%, and 25% of cases, respectively; 7% were pancolonic.

PREVENTION

Prevention of the underlying factors, most notably atherosclerotic disease

SUGGESTED READINGS

available at www.expertconsult.com

RELATED CONTENT

Mesenteric Venous Thrombosis (Related Key Topic)

AUTHOR: **MARGARET TRYFOROS, M.D.**

BASIC INFORMATION

DEFINITION

Mesenteric venous thrombosis (MVT) is a thrombotic occlusion of the mesenteric venous system involving major trunks or smaller branches and leading to intestinal infarction in its acute form.

ICD-9CM CODES
557.0 Mesenteric venous thrombosis

ICD-10CM CODES
K55.0 Acute vascular disorders of intestine
K55.1 Chronic vascular disorders of intestine

EPIDEMIOLOGY & DEMOGRAPHICS

Between 5% and 15% of patients with acute mesenteric infarction have MVT. MVT is slightly more common in men than women. The typical age of occurrence is 50 to 60 yr. Table 1-330 summarizes the incidence of ischemic bowel disease.

PHYSICAL FINDINGS & CLINICAL PRESENTATION

Acute MVT:
- Symptoms: abdominal pain in 90% of patients, typically out of proportion to the physical findings. Nausea and vomiting occur in 50% and gastrointestinal (GI) bleeding occurs in 50% (occult) and 15% (gross).
- Physical findings:
  - Early: abdominal tenderness, decreased bowel sounds, abdominal distention
  - Later: guarding and rebound tenderness, fever, septic shock

Subacute MVT:
- Symptoms: nonspecific abdominal pain for weeks or months
- Physical findings: none

Chronic MVT:
- Symptoms: upper GI hemorrhage from bleeding varices
- Physical findings: none other than signs of blood loss if significant

ETIOLOGY & PATHOGENESIS

Hypercoagulable states:
- Peripheral deep venous thrombosis
- Neoplasms
- Antithrombin III, protein C, protein S deficiencies
- Lupus anticoagulant (antiphospholipid antibody)
- Oral contraceptive use, pregnancy
- Polycythemia vera
- Thrombocytosis
- Paroxysmal nocturnal hemoglobinuria

Portal hypertension:
- Cirrhosis

Inflammation:
- Pancreatitis
- Peritonitis (e.g., appendicitis, diverticulitis, perforated viscus)
- Inflammatory bowel disease
- Pelvic or intraabdominal abscess
- Intraabdominal cancer

Postoperative state or trauma:
- Blunt abdominal trauma
- Postoperative states (abdominal surgery)

Thrombosis may begin in small mesenteric branches (e.g., in hypercoagulable states) and propagate to the major venous mesenteric trunks or begin in large veins (e.g., in cirrhosis, intraabdominal cancer, surgery) and extend distally. If collateral drainage is inadequate, the intestine becomes congested, edematous, cyanotic, and hemorrhagic and eventually may infarct.

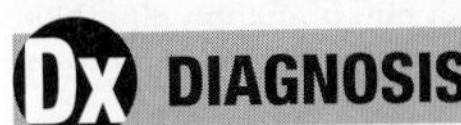

DIAGNOSIS

DIFFERENTIAL DIAGNOSIS

All other causes of abdominal pain (e.g., peritonitis, intestinal obstruction, pancreatitis, peptic ulcer disease, gastritis, inflammatory bowel disease, perforated viscus). Also to be considered in the differential diagnosis of GI hemorrhage.

WORKUP

Laboratory tests and imaging studies

LABORATORY TESTS

- Complete blood count: leukocytosis
- Electrolytes: metabolic acidosis (lactic) indicates bowel infarction
- Elevated amylase
- Tests for hypercoagulable status

IMAGING STUDIES

- Abdominal plain radiograph: ileus, ascites, bowel dilation, bowel wall thickening, loop separation, thumbprinting
- Abdominal CT scan (diagnostic in 90%): bowel wall thickening, venous dilation, venous thrombus
- Arteriography if CT scan is not diagnostic
- Diagnosis occasionally made by laparotomy

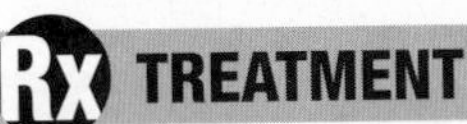

TREATMENT

- Anticoagulation or thrombolytic therapy
- Laparotomy if intestinal infarction is suspected
- Short ischemic segment: resection
- Long ischemic segment:
  1. Nonviable: resection or close
  2. Viable: intraarterial papaverine and/or thrombectomy followed by "second look" intervention
- Treatment of chronic MVT is the same as for portal hypertension

PROGNOSIS

- Mortality rate of acute MVT: 20% to 50%
- Recurrence rate: 15% to 25%

SUGGESTED READINGS

available at www.expertconsult.com

AUTHOR: **FRED F. FERRI, M.D.**

TABLE 1-330 Incidence of Ischemic Bowel Diseases

Disease	Incidence (%)*
Superior mesenteric artery (SMA) embolism: • The SMA is susceptible to embolism because of large vessel caliber and a narrow angle of departure from the aorta. • The proximal SMA is most commonly obstructed within 6-8 cm of the aorta.	50
Nonocclusive ischemia	25
SMA thrombosis	20
Mesenteric venous thrombosis	5

*Percentage of all cases of acute mesenteric ischemia.
From Adams JG et al: *Emergency medicine, clinical essentials,* ed 2, Philadelphia, 2013, Elsevier.

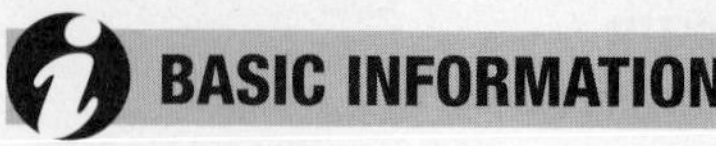

BASIC INFORMATION

DEFINITION

Malignant mesothelioma is a neoplasm that originates from the mesothelial surfaces of the pleural cavities (80%) or peritoneal cavities (20%).There are three major histologic subtypes: epithelial (most common), sarcomatous, and mixed (epithelial/sarcomatous).

ICD-9CM CODES
199.1 Malignant mesothelioma, site NOS
ICD-10CM CODES
C45.0 Mesothelioma of pleura
C45.1 Mesothelioma of peritoneum
C45.2 Mesothelioma of pericardium
C45.7 Mesothelioma of other sites
C45.9 Mesothelioma, unspecified

EPIDEMIOLOGY & DEMOGRAPHICS

- Associated with asbestos exposure (all fiber types)
- More than 3000 new cases diagnosed in the United States annually
- More common in men as a result of asbestos exposure in the workplace
- Right-sided involvement is more common
- Incidence of mesothelioma increases with age; median age at presentation is >60 yr
- More than 8 million persons in the United States are currently at risk for mesothelioma because of prior asbestos exposure

PHYSICAL FINDINGS & CLINICAL PRESENTATION

- Dyspnea
- Nonpleuritic chest pain
- Fever, weight loss, sweats, fatigue, loss of appetite
- Dysphagia, superior vena cava syndrome, Horner's syndrome in advanced stages
- Auscultation may reveal unilateral loss of breath sounds
- Dullness on percussion may be present

ETIOLOGY

- Asbestos exposure (>70% of patients)
- Other reported potentially causal factors include prior radiation therapy and extravasated Thorotrast, zeolite, and erionite fibers

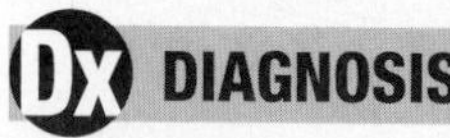

DIAGNOSIS

DIFFERENTIAL DIAGNOSIS

Metastatic adenocarcinomas (from lung, breast, ovary, kidney, stomach, prostate)

WORKUP

- Staging evaluation (Fig. E1-597) includes complete history (including occupational history), physical examination, and testing to determine potential operability (CT, bone scan, pulmonary function tests [PFTs])
- Thoracoscopy, pleuroscopy, and open-lung biopsy are useful in obtaining adequate tissue samples for diagnosis
- Pulmonary function tests
- Staging: the International Union Against Cancer (UICC) staging uses the TNM categories to organize mesothelioma in stages I to IV in a manner similar to that used for non–small cell lung cancer

LABORATORY TESTS

- Diagnostic thoracentesis is generally insufficient for diagnosis because pleural effusions may only reveal atypical mesothelial cells.
- Immunohistochemistry is useful to distinguish adenocarcinoma from epithelial malignant mesothelioma (mesotheliomas are generally carcinoembryonic antigen negative and cytokeratin positive).
- Thrombocytosis and anemia may be found on initial laboratory evaluation.
- Fibulin-3 may be useful as a blood and effusion biomarker for pleural mesothelioma. Recent data reveal that plasma fibulin-3 levels can distinguish healthy persons with exposure to asbestos from patients with mesothelioma. In conjunction with effusion fibulin-3 levels, plasma fibulin-3 levels can further differentiate mesothelioma effusions from other malignant and benign effusions.
- Serum osteopontin levels (when available) can also be used to distinguish persons with exposure to asbestos who do not have cancer from those with exposure to asbestos who have pleural mesothelioma.

IMAGING STUDIES

- Chest radiographs may reveal pleural plaques (Fig. 1-598) or calcifications in the diaphragm.
- CT scans of the chest and abdomen and bone scan are used to assess the extent of disease.

TREATMENT

GENERAL Rx

- Operable patient (epithelial type, no positive nodes, confined to pleura, adequate PFTs): the two surgical techniques for therapeutic intervention are decortication (pleurectomy) and extrapleural pneumonectomy. Postoperative chemotherapy with cisplatin, doxorubicin, and cyclophosphamide and subsequent external-beam radiation are used in some centers with limited success.
- Inoperable patient (disease too extensive, sarcomatous or mixed histology type, poor PFTs): supportive care with or without radiation therapy for symptoms or supportive care plus chemotherapy. Combined modality therapies (surgery, radiation therapy, chemotherapy, and biologics) have also been used to reduce both local and distant recurrences. The combination of pemetrexed (an antimetabolite that inhibits enzymes involved in folate metabolism) and cisplatin is used for chemotherapy of unresectable malignant pleural mesothelioma.
- Intrapleural instillation of cisplatin or biologics (e.g., interferons, interleukin-2) is generally limited to very early disease because it can only penetrate a very limited depth of the tumor and there is a propensity of the pleural space to become progressively obliterated with advancing disease.
- The role of radiation therapy in the treatment of mesotheliomas remains uncertain. It is often used for palliation of local pain despite lack of trials to prove its utility.
- Obliteration of the pleural space (pleurodesis) with instillation of tetracycline, bleomycin, or biologic substances such as *Cryptosporidium parvum* into the pleural cavity is often attempted in the treatment of recurrent symptomatic pleural effusions.

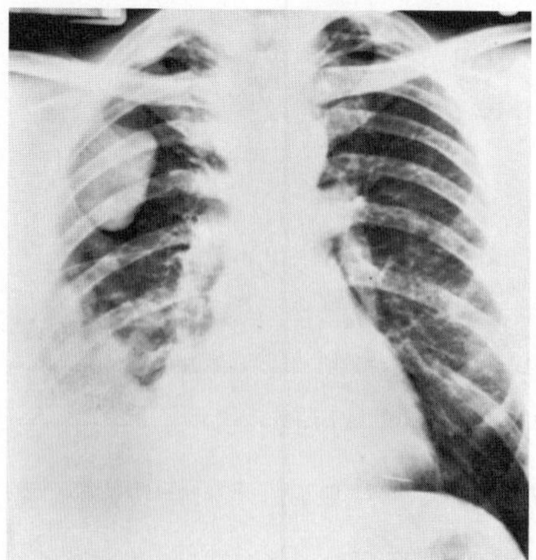

FIGURE 1-598 Chest radiograph of patient with mesothelioma. Note several lobulated, pleural-based masses in right hemithorax accompanied by right pleural effusion. (From Weinberg SE et al: *Principles of pulmonary medicine,* ed 5, Philadelphia, 2008, Saunders.)

DISPOSITION

Median survival is from 6.7 to 21 mo for patients undergoing pleurectomy and ranges from 4 to 21 mo for extrapleural pneumonectomy. Survival is better for patients with the epithelial form.

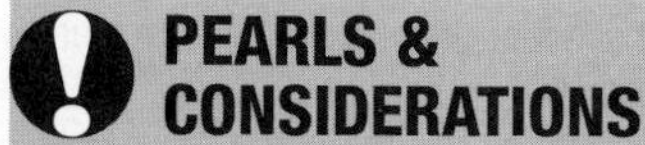

PEARLS & CONSIDERATIONS

COMMENTS

Patients with early disease should be referred to treatment centers specializing in mesothelioma treatment before attempts are made to obliterate the pleural space with pleurodesis.

SUGGESTED READINGS

available at www.expertconsult.com

RELATED CONTENT

Mesothelioma (Patient Information)

AUTHOR: **FRED F. FERRI, M.D.**

BASIC INFORMATION

DEFINITION

Hyperglycemia, dyslipidemia, abdominal obesity, and hypertension are critical components of metabolic syndrome. Over the years, many definitions of the syndrome have been proposed and debated (see Table 1-331). In 2009, a consensus statement from several organizations including the International Diabetes Federation (IDF) and American Heart Association defined "metabolic syndrome" as the presence of any three of the following criteria:

- Abdominal waist circumference >94 cm (37 in) in men and >80 cm (31 in) in women (the use of population- and country-specific definitions is suggested; however, until better data are available, IDF recommends using these cutoffs)
- Serum hypertriglyceridemia ≥150 mg/dl (1.7 mmol/L) or drug treatment for elevated triglycerides
- Serum high-density lipoprotein (HDL) cholesterol <40 mg/dl (1 mmol/L) in men and <50 mg/dl (1.3 mmol/L) in women or drug treatment for low HDL-C
- Blood pressure ≥130/85 mm Hg or drug treatment for elevated blood pressure
- Fasting glucose ≥100 mg/dl (5.6 mmol/L) or drug treatment for elevated blood glucose

SYNONYMS

Syndrome X
Insulin resistance syndrome
Obesity dyslipidemia syndrome

ICD-9CM CODES
277.7 Metabolic syndrome
ICD-10CM CODES
E88.81 Metabolic syndrome

EPIDEMIOLOGY & DEMOGRAPHICS

- Affects 22% of U.S. adults.
- Prevalence increases with age, affecting more than 40% of individuals >60 yr.
- Increasing prevalence among women, especially in the African American and Mexican American populations.
- Prevalence increases with weight. Metabolic syndrome is noted in 5% of normal weight, 22% of overweight, and 60% of obese individuals.
- Other risk factors include low socioeconomic status, lack of physical activity, high-carbohydrate diet, no alcohol intake, smoking, genetic predisposition, use of atypical antipsychotics, and postmenopausal status.

TABLE 1-331 Common Definitions for Metabolic Syndrome

Criterion	NCEP ATP III (3 or more criteria)
Abdominal obesity	Waist circumferance
Men	>40 inches (>102 cm)
Women	>35 inches (>88 cm)
Hypertriglyceridemia	>150 mg/dl (≥1.7 mmol/l)
Low HDL	
Men	<40 mg/dl (<1.03 mmol/l)
Women	<50 mg/dl (<1.30 mmol/l)
Hypertension	≥130/85 mm Hg or on antihypertensive medication
Impaired fasting glucose or diabetes	>100 mg/dl (5.6 mmol/l) or taking insulin or hypoglycemic medication

From Floege J et al: *Comprehensive clinical nephrology*, ed 4, Philadelphia, 2010, Saunders.

CLINICAL PRESENTATION

- Obesity, hypertension, dyslipidemia, and hyperglycemia as defined.
  - Blood pressure: ≥130/85 mm Hg
  - Abdominal obesity with waist circumference: >94 cm (37 in) in men and >80 cm (31 in) in women
  - Triglycerides: ≥150 mg/dl (1.7 mmol/L)
  - HDL: <40 mg/dl (1 mmol/L) in men and >50 mg/dl (1.3 mmol/L) in women
  - High fasting glucose: ≥100 mg/dl (5.6 mmol/L)
- Patients with the metabolic syndrome are at twice the risk of developing cardiovascular disease and have a sevenfold increase in risk for type 2 diabetes and a 1.5-fold increase in all-cause mortality compared to patients without the syndrome. Other complications include cognitive decline in the elderly, fatty liver disease, polycystic ovary syndrome, obstructive sleep apnea, gout, and chronic kidney disease.
- Focus history on symptoms of diabetes and its complications, obesity and its complications, coronary artery disease (angina), and polycystic ovary syndrome.
- Complete physical examination, including height, weight, waist circumference, and blood pressure.

ETIOLOGY

- Genetic and environmental factors associated with obesity increase the risk of developing metabolic syndrome.
- Abdominal obesity is associated with insulin resistance and hyperinsulinemia.
- Insulin resistance results in ineffective glucose and fatty acid utilization leading to type 2 diabetes mellitus (Fig. 1-599).
- Hyperinsulinemia and inflammatory markers/cytokines play an important role in development of abnormal lipid profile, hypertension, and vascular endothelial dysfunction, which can lead to the development of atherosclerotic cardiovascular disease.

DIAGNOSIS

DIFFERENTIAL DIAGNOSIS

- Other causes of weight gain or obesity (Cushing's syndrome, hypothyroidism)
- Other causes of hyperlipidemia (familial hyperlipidemia, hypothyroidism)
- Other causes of hypertension (Cushing's syndrome, hyperaldosteronism)
- Other forms of diabetes (type 1)

LABORATORY TESTS

- Fasting lipid profile (total cholesterol, low-density lipoprotein [LDL] cholesterol, HDL cholesterol, and triglycerides)
- Fasting glucose

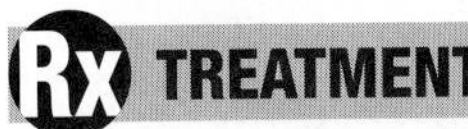

TREATMENT

NONPHARMACOLOGIC THERAPY

- Lifestyle modification:
  - Dietary modifications aimed at weight loss
  - Physical activity of moderate intensity (i.e., brisk walking): 30 min daily
  - Smoking cessation
- Consider bariatric surgery in the management of obesity:
  - Body mass index (BMI) ≥40 kg/m^2 in patients who have not responded to diet and exercise (with or without drug therapy).
  - Individuals with BMI >35 kg/m^2 and comorbidities (hypertension, impaired glucose tolerance, diabetes mellitus, dyslipidemia, sleep apnea) are also potential surgical candidates.

ACUTE GENERAL Rx

- Treat obesity (see "Obesity"): Pharmacologic treatment: consider orlistat and other approved agents in patients who have not responded to diet and exercise if BMI >30 kg/m^2 or a BMI of 27 to 30 kg/m^2 with comorbid conditions. Drug therapy still needs to be in conjunction with diet and exercise.
- Treat hypertension (see "Hypertension"): Systolic blood pressures >130/80 mm Hg: consider angiotensin-converting enzyme inhibitors or angiotensin II receptor blocker as first-line therapy.
- Treat hyperlipidemia: In the 2013 guidelines from the American College of Cardiology and American Heart Association (ACC/AHA), treatment goals for LDL-C and non-HDL-C are no longer recommended and there are no guidelines for treating high triglyceride levels. The new guidelines specify four groups that merit intensive or moderately intensive statin therapy[1]:
  - People with clinical atherosclerotic cardiovascular disease (ASCVD)
  - People with LDL-C levels of ≥190 mg/dL
  - People with diabetes, age 40 to 75
  - People without diabetes, age 40 to 75 with LDL-C levels 70-190 mg/dL, and a 10-year ASCVD risk of 7.5% or higher as determined by the new risk calculator.[2]
- Treat diabetes:
  - Goal HgAIC <7.0%
  - Metformin as first-line therapy to improve insulin sensitivity

[1]Raymond C et al: New cholesterol guidelines: worth the wait? *Clev Clin J Med* 81:11-19, 2014.

[2]American Heart Association: *2013 Prevention Guideline Tools. CV risk calculator.* Available at http://my.americanheart.org/professional/statementsguidelines/preventionguidelines/preventionguidelines_VCM_subhomepage.jsp

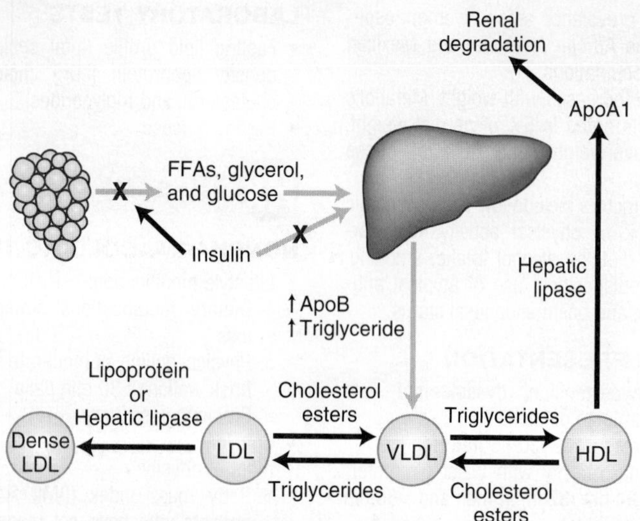

FIGURE 1-599 Insulin resistance and dyslipidemia. The suppression of lipoprotein lipase and very-low-density lipoprotein (VLDL) production by insulin is defective in insulin resistance, leading to increased flux of free fatty acids (FFAs) to the liver and increased VLDL production, which results in increased circulating triglyceride concentrations. The triglycerides are transferred to low-density lipoprotein (LDL) and high-density lipoprotein (HDL), and the VLDL particles gain cholesterol esters by the action of the cholesterol ester transfer protein (CETP). This leads to increased catabolism of HDL particles by the liver and loss of apolipoprotein (Apo) A, resulting in low HDL concentrations. The triglyceride-rich LDL particle is stripped of its triglycerides, resulting in the accumulation of atherogenic small, dense LDL particles. (From Melmed S: *Williams textbook of endocrinology,* ed 12, Philadelphia, 2011, Saunders.)

- Treat cardiovascular risk factors:
  - Consider aspirin. Aspirin should be started in patients with metabolic syndrome and an intermediate or elevated Framingham cardiovascular risk, if there are no contraindications.
  - Risk can be lowered with weight loss, exercise, smoking cessation, blood pressure control, diabetes management, and treatment of hyperlipidemia.

CHRONIC RX

- Encourage lifestyle modification as above.
- Pharmacologic and surgical management to maintain therapeutic goals described above.

DISPOSITION

Weight loss can prevent disease progression. Appropriate treatment of obesity, hypertension, hyperlipidemia, and diabetes can improve morbidity and mortality rates.

REFERRAL

- To nutritionist for dietary counseling
- To weight loss and exercise programs
- To endocrinologist if difficulty reaching therapeutic goals
- To bariatric surgeon if patient meets surgical criteria (as noted previously)

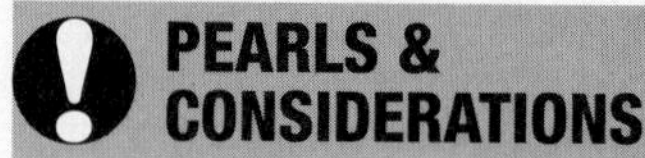

PEARLS & CONSIDERATIONS

PREVENTION

- Weight loss is essential for the prevention and treatment of metabolic syndrome.
- Recommend dietary modifications and moderate physical activity.
- Consider pharmacologic and surgical options in select individuals (as above).

PATIENT & FAMILY EDUCATION

- Weight reduction programs, including Weight Watchers, Curves, etc.
- American Diabetes Association: http://www.diabetes.org
- Polycystic Ovarian Syndrome Association: http://www.pcosupport.org
- The Hormone Foundation: http://www.hormone.org

SUGGESTED READINGS

available at www.expertconsult.com

RELATED CONTENT

Obesity (Related Key Topic)
Metabolic Syndrome (Patient Information)

AUTHOR: **GEETHA GOPALAKRISHNAN, M.D.**

BASIC INFORMATION

DEFINITION

The diagnosis of metatarsalgia includes multiple etiologies of pain involving the plantar aspect of the lesser metatarsal heads or metatarsophalangeal joints (Fig. 1-600).

ICD-9CM CODES
726.7 Metatarsalgia
ICD-10CM CODES
M77.40 Metatarsalgia, unspecified foot

PHYSICAL FINDINGS & CLINICAL PRESENTATION

- Pain beneath any or all of metatarsal heads 2, 3, 4, and 5
- Pain on metatarsophalangeal joint range of motion
- Often associated with hammertoe deformity and gastrocnemius/soleus equinus
- May include predislocation syndrome
- Common with bunion deformity
- Often obesity, recent weight gain, or increased/change in type of activity

ETIOLOGY

- Primary structural/functional factors, all yielding increased submetatarsal pressure:
  - Structural: sagittal plane (cavus foot, ankle equinus, pseudoequinus, elongated lesser metatarsal[s] relative to the optimal metatarsal parabola) or frontal plane (relative fixed dorsiflexion or plantarflexion of adjacent metatarsals)
  - Functional causes yielding transferred pressure (from hypermobile first or fifth rays) or friction (secondary to compensation for transverse plane deformities or lack of sufficient rearfoot mobility).
- Local factors: decreased shock absorption due to hammertoe deformity, predislocation syndrome, translocation of the plantar fat pad, plantar fat pad atrophy.
- Trauma: rupture of plantar plate, metatarsophalangeal joint capsule, or any associated tendon
- Degenerative joint diseases (osteoarthritis, rheumatoid arthritis, psoriatic arthritis, etc.)

DIAGNOSIS

DIFFERENTIAL DIAGNOSIS

- Interdigital neuroma, most commonly third interspace (Morton's)
- Metatarsal traumatic fracture or stress fracture
- Foreign body, infection/abscess
- Freiberg's infraction, usually of second metatarsal head, frequently in teenage females
- Secondary systemic findings: rheumatoid nodules, gout
- Neoplasms: ganglion cyst, bone tumor
- Skin: verrucous plantaris, intractable plantar keratoma, tinea pedis, etc.
- Neuropathy or peripheral vascular disease

LABORATORY TESTS

As necessary if suspicion of a systemic cause of joint arthritis/destruction

IMAGING STUDIES

- X-rays: rule out fracture, tumor, avascular necrosis, arthritic process/joint disease.
- MRI: evaluate for any plantar plate injury, capsular injury, tendon rupture, or neuroma.
- Bone scan: if stress fracture suspected (may take 2 wk to show up on x-ray).

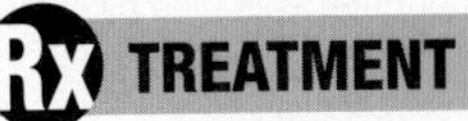

TREATMENT

- Silicone padding provides symptomatic relief, works well for fat pad atrophy.
- Moleskin or padding will reduce frictional forces without adding bulk for long-term use.
- Custom orthotics with proximal metatarsal pad or submetatarsal cutout to offload.
- Heel lift or shoes with short heel or wedge are effective when equinus is etiology.
- Rocker-bottom to prevent motion in severe or high-risk diabetic patients
- Nonsteroidal anti-inflammatory drugs
- Intraarticular injection if indicated, based on underlying etiology
- **Caution with injection:** risk of plantar plate ruptures; use only if absolutely indicated!

DISPOSITION

Varies depending on etiology

REFERRAL

To podiatric or foot/ankle orthopedic surgeon for biomechanical exam/orthotic management or surgical consultation

SUGGESTED READINGS
available at www.expertconsult.com

RELATED CONTENT

Metatarsalgia (Patient Information)

AUTHOR: **BROOKE E. KEELEY, D.P.M.**

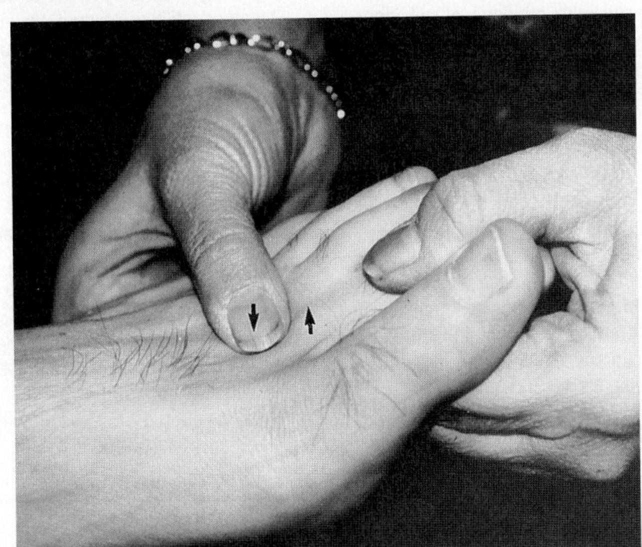

FIGURE 1-600 Vertical stress test for metatarsophalangeal stability. One of the examiner's hands stabilizes the metatarsal head while the other grasps the proximal phalanx. Examiner attempts to displace the proximal phalanx dorsally. A positive test result is the ability to displace dorsally while reproducing symptoms. (From Scuderi G [ed]: *Sports medicine: principles of primary care,* St Louis, 1997, Mosby.)

BASIC INFORMATION

DEFINITION

An accidental or intentional ingestion of 1 g/kg of methanol or ethylene glycol is considered lethal, although even small amounts can be toxic. Inhalation and dermal exposures rarely cause toxicity.

SYNONYMS

Antifreeze and moonshine overdose

ICD-9CM CODES
980.1 Toxic effect of methyl alcohol
980.8 Toxic effect of other specified alcohols
ICD-10CM CODES
T51.8 Toxic effect of other alcohols (ethylene glycol)
T51.1 Toxic effect of methanol

EPIDEMIOLOGY & DEMOGRAPHICS

INCIDENCE: In 2011, the American Association of Poison Control Centers reported 7014 and 1300 single-exposure cases of ethylene glycol and methanol poisoning, respectively. Most cases reported are in adults older than 19 yr and predominantly males. Accidental exposure is common in children, while alcoholism, polysubstance abuse, depression, and suicide are seen in adults.

PHYSICAL FINDINGS & CLINICAL PRESENTATION

- Clinical manifestations of both substances depends on the quantity of ingestion, duration of time since the ingestion, and whether co-ingestion of ethanol or other substances occurs.
- Early ingestions of both substances can mimic ethanol ingestion with nausea, vomiting, inebriation, and CNS depression. Late effects include progressive CNS depression including seizure and coma, as well as both respiratory and cardiopulmonary failure.
- Visual symptoms ranging from blurry or snowy vision to complete visual loss and findings of papillary edema, afferent pupillary defect, retinal hyperemia, and parkinsonian-like syndrome are indicative of methanol poisoning
- Abdominal pain, oliguria, hematuria, calcium oxalate crystalluria, tetany, and acute kidney injury suggest ethylene glycol toxicity

ETIOLOGY

- Toxicity of these alcohols is related to its metabolites rather than the parent compound
- Sequential metabolism by alcohol and aldehyde dehydrogenase converts methanol to formic acid and ethylene glycol to glycolic acid and oxalate, resulting in toxicity
- While methanol metabolites primarily cause retinal injury, ethylene glycol metabolites cause renal tubular injury and calcium oxalate stones
  - Formic acid prevents oxygen utilization by mitochondria, resulting in an array of organ dysfunction, including within the central nervous system, specifically affecting the retinal and optic neurons and the basal ganglia.
  - Oxalate forms calcium oxalate renal stones, which are responsible for direct renal injury.

DIAGNOSIS

DIFFERENTIAL DIAGNOSIS

- Other causes of anion gap metabolic acidosis include lactic acidosis, diabetic/alcoholic ketoacidosis, renal failure, toluene, and salicylate intoxication
- Elevated plasma osmolal gap can also be seen in ethyl alcohol or isopropyl alcohol ingestion and other serious illnesses like septic shock

WORKUP

- Diagnosis depends on history, clinical presentation, and laboratory abnormalities
- Anion gap metabolic acidosis (AG >12 mEq/L) with elevated plasma osmolal gap (>10 mOsm/L) in an appropriate clinical setting should raise the suspicion for methanol or ethylene glycol ingestion. In both intoxications, an osmolar gap will initially be positive, but as the parent compound is converted to its metabolites, the osmolar gap will normalize and the serum anion gap will then be positive.
- Serum methanol and ethylene glycol levels are elevated in respective ingestions.
  - While those with ethylene glycol ingestion may have fewer toxicities and may present without acidosis, anion gap, or symptoms, the osmolar gap will remain elevated.
- Acute kidney injury, hypocalcemia with prolonged QT interval, and calcium oxalate crystalluria can been seen due to ethylene glycol toxicity
- Wood's lamp fluorescence uses ultraviolet light to detect fluorescein contained in ethylene glycol preparations but lacks sensitivity as not all preparations contain fluorescein and also lacks specificity due to high rate of false positivity

LABORATORY TESTS

- Calculation of the anion gap and serum osmolar gap
  - Anion gap determination: electrolytes, albumin
  - Osmolal gap determination: measured and calculated serum osmolality (sodium, BUN, glucose, ± ethanol)
- Arterial blood gas analysis, lactate, calcium, and creatinine kinase
- Creatinine, urine analysis to assess kidney function, tubular injury, and calcium oxalate crystals
- ECG to assess QT interval
- Toxicology screen and quantification: acetaminophen, salicylate, ethanol, methanol, ethylene glycol, and isopropyl alcohol

TREATMENT

High index of suspicion and immediate recognition with early treatment remain crucial to reduce mortality. Box 1-55 describes common commercial products that may contain ethylene glycol.

NONPHARMACOLOGIC THERAPY

- Securing patient's airway, breathing, and circulation and advanced cardiac life support measures instituted as indicated.
- While data are limitied, gastric decontamination (charcoal and/or gastric lavage) is of limited use unless done within 1 hr of ingestion as alcohols are rapidly absorbed. Induction of vomiting is contraindicated even in conscious patients given the risks of development of central nervous system depression in these patients.

ACUTE GENERAL Rx

- The principles of therapy include prevention of formation of toxic metabolites, correction of acidosis, and toxin removal.
- Ethanol, as a competitive substrate, and fomepizole, a competitive inhibitor of alcohol dehydrogenase, prevent the formation of toxic metabolites of ethylene glycol and methanol. Fomepizole is preferred over ethanol given the increased incidence of adverse events with ethanol administration, which are likely secondary to the erratic pharmacokinetic profile of ethanol. Volume expansion with isotonic fluids facilitates urinary excretion of the toxins.
- When acidosis is present (pH <7.3), isotonic bicarbonate should be preferentially utilized for volume expansion as reversal of acidosis helps prevent end-organ damage from toxic metabolites. The goal pH range is 7.35-7.45.
- Treatment with medications and/or hemodialysis is continued until the methanol or ethylene glycol concentration is <20 mg/dl.
- Ethanol:
  - Target ethanol concentration is 100-200 mg/dl requiring close monitoring
  - Loading dose: 800 mg/kg in a 10% vol/vol solution of D5W which will raise serum ethanol by 100 mg/dl

BOX 1-55 Common Commercial Products That May Contain Ethylene Glycol

Paints and lacquers
Polishes and detergents
Inks
Cosmetics
Hydraulic brake fluids
Solar collector fluids
Car wash fluids

Data from Kruse JA: Methanol, ethylene glycol, and related intoxications. In Carlson RW, Geheb MA (eds): *Principles and practice of medical intensive care,* Philadelphia, 1993, Saunders.

- Maintenance dose: infusion of 80-160 mg/kg/hr based on the levels
- Fomepizole: preferred antidote
- Indications for fomepizole use:
  - Plasma concentration of methanol or ethylene glycol >20 mg/dl OR
  - Documented ingestion with an osmolal gap >10 mOsm/L OR
  - Suspected ingestion with at least two of the following criteria:
  - Arterial pH <7.3
  - Serum bicarbonate <20 mEq/L
  - Osmolal gap >10 mOsm/L
  - Urinary oxalate crystals in the case of ethylene glycol toxicity
- Fomepizole (4-methylpyrazole) dosing:
  - Loading dose: 15 mg/kg body weight
  - Maintenance dose: 10 mg/kg body weight every 12 hr for 4 doses then 15 mg/kg body weight every 12 hr (if blood levels do not reach goal by 48 hr).
  - During hemodialysis: Add 1 to 1.5 mg/kg body weight per hr
- Ethanol:
  - Target ethanol concentration is 100-200 mg/dl requiring close monitoring
  - Loading dose: 800 mg/kg in a 10% vol/vol solution of D5W which will raise serum ethanol by 100 mg/dl
  - Maintenance dose: infusion of 80-160 mg/kg/hr based on the levels
- Hemodialysis should be considered in patients with significant metabolic acidosis (pH <7.25-7.30), renal failure, visual abnormalities, electrolyte imbalances refractory to pharmacologic treatments, hemodynamic instability, and serum concentrations >50 mg/dl.
- Duration of hemodialysis can be estimated using the formula: Time (hr) equals $-V \ln(5/A)/0.06\ k$, where V is the Watson estimate of total body water (in liters); A is the initial alcohol concentration (in mmol/L); and k is 80% of the manufacturer's specified urea clearance (in ml/min). Average duration of dialysis in studies was 8.4 ± 3.2 hr.

ADJUNCTIVE Rx

- In cases of ethylene glycol poisoning, thiamine and pyridoxine may decrease oxalic acid formation and shift metabolism to less toxic metabolites.
- Folinic acid at doses of 1 mg/kg given intravenously every 4 to 6 hr may be used to increase the metabolism of formic acid in methanol overdose.
  - Correct electrolyte abnormalities (hypocalcemia, etc.).
  - Treat seizures.

DISPOSITION

Transfer to a hospital with intensive care and hemodialysis capability should be considered early in the patient's course.

REFERRAL

- Regional poison center (toxicologist) and nephrology recommended to avoid treatment delays
- Ophthalmology for patients with visual symptoms
- Psychiatry if depression and suicidal ideation
- Detoxification centers for patients with substance abuse

PROGNOSIS

- Coma or seizures at presentation and prolonged severe acidosis correlated with increased mortality

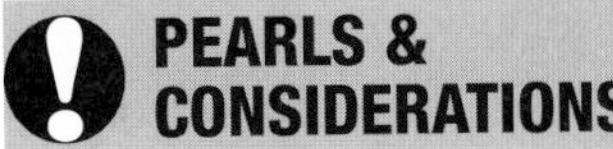

- Profound plasma osmolar gap or anion gap metabolic acidosis should raise suspicion for ethylene glycol and/or methanol ingestion. A high index of suspicion and early treatment remain crucial to reduce mortality. The metabolites of methanol and ethylene glycol cause clinical toxicity rather than the agents themselves.
- Complaints of visual blurring, central scotomata, and blindness suggest methanol poisoning.
- Calcium oxalate crystalluria, oliguria, and hematuria suggest ethylene glycol poisoning.
- Fomepizole is favored over ethanol due to complications associated with ethanol use.
- Emergent hemodialysis is indicated in the setting of end organ damage and severe metabolic acidosis.

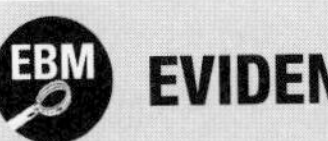

available at www.expertconsult.com

SUGGESTED READINGS

available at www.expertconsult.com

RELATED CONTENT

Fig. 3-153 Algorithm for the management of acute poisoning (Algorithm)

AUTHORS: **CLAIRE KASSAKIAN, M.D.,** and **SUSIE L. HU, M.D.**

BASIC INFORMATION

DEFINITION

Methicillin-resistant *Staphylococcus aureus* (MRSA) is a common bacterial pathogen with resistance to many antibiotics. It is defined as a *S. aureus* that shows a minimum inhibitory concentration (MIC) of greater than or equal to 4 mcg/ml to oxacillin. There are now two types of MRSA:

- HA-MRSA: hospital-acquired MRSA, usually multidrug resistant
- CA-MRSA: community-acquired MRSA; an emerging pathogen, usually acquired outside of the hospital setting; resistance may differ from HA-MRSA and is generally susceptible to more antibiotics than HA-MRSA

SYNONYMS

Multidrug-resistant *Staphylococcus aureus*
Oxacillin-resistant *Staphylococcus aureus*

ICD-9CM CODES
041.12 Methicillin-resistant *Staphylococcus aureus* in conditions classified elsewhere and of unspecified site
ICD-10CM CODES
B95.62 Methicillin-resistant *Staphylococcus aureus* infection as the cause of diseases classified elsewhere

EPIDEMIOLOGY & DEMOGRAPHICS

INCIDENCE: 1:3000
PEAK INCIDENCE: Occurs year round; may peak during summer and fall months for CA-MRSA
PREVALENCE: The national rate of MRSA colonization or infection is 46.3 per 10,000 inpatients. Hospital prevalence rate of MRSA is as high as 60% in hospitals, which means that 60% of *S. aureus* strains in that hospital will be MRSA.
PREDOMINANT SEX AND AGE: All ages and both sexes
GENETICS: NA
RISK FACTORS:

- HA-MRSA: hospitalization; invasive medical device; residing in long-term nursing facility
- CA-MRSA: initially seen in young men engaged in athletic activities and in gyms, prisons, military barracks, etc., but has now spread to the entire age spectrum including neonates and the elderly.

PHYSICAL FINDINGS & CLINICAL PRESENTATION

- CA-MRSA: can present with skin infection, associated with opening in the skin; red bump, pustule, or boil; erythema, swelling; edema, often fluctuant and very painful
- HA-MRSA: bacteremia; infection associated with intravenous device
  - Catheters: pneumonia
  - Skin: cellulitis
  - Bone: osteomyelitis
  - Endocarditis
  - Abscesses: skin or organ
  - Pneumonia: nosocomial

ETIOLOGY

- CA-MRSA: the most prevalent strain in the US on pulse field electrophoresis (PFGE) is called USA 300
  - CA-MRSA: common cause of skin and soft tissue infections in the emergency room. It can, however, also cause necrotizing pneumonia, sepsis, osteomyelitis, etc.
  - Virulence factors particular to CA-MRSA: Panton-Valentine leukocidin (PVL) toxin, alpha-hemolysin toxin, phenol soluble modulins, etc., that enhance ability to cause infection
- HA-MRSA: most strains on PFGE are USA 100 or USA 200 and tend to have multidrug resistance. Patients with HA-MRSA infection have higher mortality and morbidity than patients with a methicillin-sensitive *S. aureus* (MSSA) infection.

Dx DIAGNOSIS

DIFFERENTIAL DIAGNOSIS

- Skin: spider bite (many patients with CA-MRSA feel as if they were bitten by a spider)
- Cellulitis: other organism(s) such as streptococci and methicillin-sensitive *S. aureus* (MSSA)
- Pneumonia: not due to MRSA
- Bacteria: not due to MRSA

WORKUP

- Culture of wound, abscess, blood, sputum; rule out colonization; culture of nares or axillae

LABORATORY TESTS

- See above.
- PFGE: usually done only for epidemiologic or outbreak purposes.

IMAGING STUDIES

- Radiographs or computed tomography scan of suspected organ
- Echocardiogram if endocarditis suspected

Rx TREATMENT

- CA-MRSA: oral antibiotics that may be effective include trimethoprim-sulfamethoxazole, doxycycline, minocycline, or clindamycin; linezolid is another option but very expensive.
- HA-MRSA: intravenous antibiotics, vancomycin, linezolid, daptomycin, tigecycline

NONPHARMACOLOGIC THERAPY

Abscess surgically drained

ACUTE GENERAL Rx

- Trimethoprim-sulfamethoxazole, one double-strength tablet PO bid, is useful in cases of CA-MRSA since 95% of community-acquired MRSA strains are susceptible to it in vitro. Other agents that can be used for CA-MRSA include:
  1. Clindamycin: 300 to 450 mg q6-8h also inhibits toxin production. If strain tests sensitive to clindamycin but resistant to erythromycin, then a D test must be done to ensure there will not be inducible resistance while on therapy with the clindamycin.
  2. Doxycycline: 100 mg PO q12h and minocycline also have some activity against MRSA.
  3. Rifampin: never used alone but can be used with one of the other oral agents
- Vancomycin 15-20 mg/kg IV q8 to 12h is the mainstay of parenteral therapy for MRSA infections. There is an increasing concern of MRSA strains developing tolerance to vancomycin, requiring higher doses to achieve eradication. True vancomycin resistant strains (MIC ≥32 mg/L) remain rare. Vancomycin trough levels of at least 15 to 20 mcg/ml are recommended to treat MRSA infections.
- Linezolid 600 mg PO or IV bid is a synthetic oxazolidinone FDA-approved for MRSA skin and soft tissue infections and pneumonia. It has been shown to be more effective than vancomycin for MRSA pneumonia. However, its cost is more than 10 times as much as vancomycin.
- Daptomycin: 4 mg/kg/day to 6 mg/kg/day IV is approved for skin and soft tissue infections, bacteremia and right-sided endocarditis but should not be used for pneumonia as it is inactivated by pulmonary surfactant.
- Tigecycline: 100 mg IV load, then 50 mg IV q12h, is approved for MRSA skin and soft tissue infections and intraabdominal abscess.
- Ceftaroline is a fifth-generation cephalosporin, also effective against MRSA but only skin and soft tissue infections, not pneumonia: 600 mg IV q12h.

CHRONIC Rx

- Patients with MRSA colonization may have reexposure or may be unable to eradicate colonized state.
- Oral agents used to attempt eradication of colonization are rifampin, tetracycline, and minocycline.

COMPLEMENTARY & ALTERNATIVE MEDICINE

- Mupirocin ointment may be administered to the nares to attempt to decolonize; it can also be applied to infected skin sites.
- Chlorhexidine 2% or 4% wash may be used to lower skin burden of colonization.

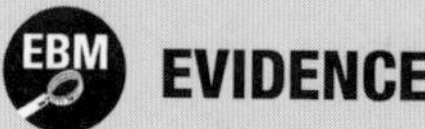

EVIDENCE

available at www.expertconsult.com

SUGGESTED READINGS

available at www.expertconsult.com

AUTHOR: **GLENN G. FORT, M.D., M.P.H.**

BASIC INFORMATION

DEFINITION

Microscopic polyangiitis (MPA) is an ANCA (antineutrophil cytoplasmic autoantibody)-associated small to medium vessel systemic vasculitis. It is characterized by necrotizing, pauci-immune, small vessel vasculitis in the absence of granulomatous inflammation. It commonly affects the kidney and can also affect the lower respiratory tract, skin, nervous system, and gastrointestinal (GI) tract. Renal involvement can lead to glomerulonephritis and renal failure. MPA belongs to a category of vasculitides that also includes granulomatosis with polyangiitis (GPA) and Churg-Strauss syndrome (Table 1-332).

TABLE 1-332 Classification Scheme of Vasculitides According to Size of Predominant Blood Vessels Involved

PREDOMINANTLY LARGE-VESSEL VASCULITIDES
Takayasu's arteritis
Giant cell arteritis
Cogan's syndrome
Behçet's syndrome*
PREDOMINANTLY MEDIUM-VESSEL VASCULITIDES
Classic polyarteritis nodosa
Cutaneous polyarteritis nodosa
Rheumatoid vasculitis†
Buerger's disease
Kawasaki disease
Primary angiitis of the central nervous system
PREDOMINANTLY SMALL-VESSEL VASCULITIDES
Immune complex mediated
• Cutaneous leukocytoclastic angiitis ("hypersensitivity" vasculitis)
• Henoch-Schönlein purpura
• Urticarial vasculitis
• Cryoglobulinemia†
"ANCA-associated" disorders
• Wegener's granulomatosis†
• Microscopic polyangiitis†
• Churg-Strauss syndrome†
Miscellaneous small-vessel vasculitides
• Connective tissue disorders†
• Paraneoplastic diseases
• Infection
• Inflammatory bowel disease

ANCA, Antineutrophil cytoplasmic antibody.
*May involve small, medium, and large blood vessels.
†Frequent overlap of involvement of small- and medium-sized blood vessels.
From Goldman L, Schafer AI: *Goldman's Cecil medicine*, ed 24, Philadelphia, 2012, Saunders.

ICD-9CM CODES
446 Polyarteritis nodosa and allied conditions
ICD-10CM CODES
M31.7 Microscopic polyangiitis

SYNONYMS

Microscopic polyarteritis
MPA

ICD-10CM Codes
M31.7 Microscopic polyangiitis

EPIDEMIOLOGY & DEMOGRAPHICS

- Incidence is 3.6 per 1,000,000 annually in U.S.
- Prevalence is 1 to 2 cases in 100,000.
- More common in Caucasians as compared to African Americans.
- Equally present in both males and females.
- Average age is approximately 50 years depending on the population studied.

PHYSICAL FINDINGS & CLINICAL PRESENTATION

- Constitutional symptoms like fatigue, fever, "flu-like" symptoms, weight loss, anorexia
- Macroscopic hematuria, proteinuria, edema, decreased urinary output
- Pulmonary symptoms like hemoptysis, cough, dyspnea, pulmonary hemorrhage, pleuritic pain
- Palpable purpura 41% and livedo reticularis 12%
- Inflammation of visceral blood and gut vessels causes pain, bloody stools, and perforation
- Kidney involvement 90%
- Weight loss >70%
- Peripheral neuropathy 60%
- Myalgias 50%
- Chest pain, heart failure symptoms

ETIOLOGY

- Autoimmune process of unknown etiology. ANCA, most specifically those directed at cytoplasmic myeloperoxidase, are felt to contribute to the inflammatory process. Once bound to their cellular epitope, anti-myeloperoxidase (MPO) antibodies likely contribute to degranulation of the neutrophil, which presumably contributes to endothelial injury. Most recently, investigators have demonstrated that anti- MPO antibodies alone can cause necrotizing and crescentic glomerulonephritis.

DIAGNOSIS

DIFFERENTIAL DIAGNOSIS

- Polyarteritis nodosa
- Kawasaki's disease
- Infective endocarditis
- Lymphoma
- Amyloidosis
- Hypercoagulable states
- Systemic lupus erythematosus
- Paraproteinemias

MPA is distinguished from GPA and Churg-Strauss syndrome by the absence of granuloma formation (Table 1-333) and the absence of asthma and eosinophilia characteristic of Churg-Strauss syndrome.

WORKUP

- Medical history to look for the presence of MPA symptoms
- Physical examination to detect sites of organ involvement and to exclude other illnesses that may have a similar appearance

LABORATORY TESTS

- Laboratory testing may reveal elevated sedimentation rate (ESR), C-reactive protein, leukocytosis, anemia
- Elevated serum blood urea nitrogen (BUN) and creatinine suggestive of renal impairment
- Urinalysis to detect proteinuria, hematuria, erythrocyte casts, abnormal urine sediment
- ANCA positive 82% to 94%
- Perinuclear ANCA directed at myeloperoxidase 60%
- Cytoplasmic ANCA directed at proteinase –3 40%
- Serum complement levels
- Increased aspartate aminotransferase, alanine aminotransferase, and creatine phosphokinase may indicate liver or muscle (skeletal or cardiac) involvement
- Blood cultures to rule out bacterial endocarditis
- Intestinal angina is often a result of mesenteric ischemia and can be assessed using mesenteric angiography when renal function permits
- Tissue for pathology diagnosis is usually required to confirm the diagnosis
- Biopsy of the skin reveals nonspecific leukocytoclastic vasculitis with little or no complement and immunoglobulin on immunofluorescence.
- Kidney biopsy usually reveals necrotizing crescentic glomerulonephritis, that is usually pauci-immune on immunofluorescence and necrotizing vasculitis of microscopic vessels (small arteries, arterioles, capillaries,venules) (Figure 1-601).

IMAGING STUDIES

- Chest radiograph would show diffuse parenchymal infiltrates secondary to pulmonary alveolar hemorrhages.
- Computed tomographic (CT) scanning may disclose previously undetected nodules, unsuspected cavitation in nodules, alveolar opacities, large-airway inflammation or stenotic lesions, and pleural-based lesions.
- An EMG may reveal a sensorimotor peripheral neuropathy in patients with neuropathy.
- Electrocardiography is indicated in myocardial infection, pericarditis, and congestive heart failure.
- Gastrointestinal endoscopy and mesenteric angiography in cases of gastrointestinal involvement.

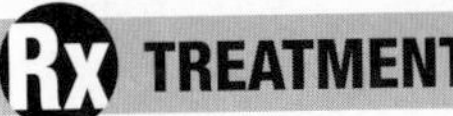

TREATMENT

ACUTE GENERAL Rx

Induction

- Corticosteroids combined with immunomodulatory drugs, such as cyclophosphamide or azathioprine and methotrexate.
- Rituximab is an effective alternative to cyclophosphamide initial treatment as well as for relapse.

TABLE 1-333 Names and Definitions of Vasculitis Adopted by the Chapel Hill Consensus Conference on the Nomenclature of Systemic Vasculitis

Name	Large-Vessel Vasculitis*
Giant cell (temporal arteritis)	Granulomatous arteritis of the aorta and its major branches, with a predilection for the extracranial branches of the carotid artery. Often involves the temporal artery. Usually occurs in patients older than 50 yr and often is associated with polymyalgia rheumatica
Takayasu's arteritis	Granulomatous inflammation of the aorta and its major branches. Usually occurs in patients younger than 50 yr
	Medium-Sized Vessel Vasculitis*
Polyarteritis nodosa (classic polyarteritis nodosa)	Necrotizing inflammation of medium-sized or small arteries without glomerulonephritis or vasculitis in arterioles, capillaries, or venules. Kawasaki's disease arteritis involving large, medium-sized, and small arteries and associated with mucocutaneous lymph node syndrome. Coronary arteries are often involved. Aorta and veins may be involved. Usually occurs in children
	Small-Vessel Vasculitis*
Wegener's granulomatosis†,‡	Granulomatous inflammation involving the respiratory tract and necrotizing vasculitis affecting small- to medium-sized vessels, e.g., capillaries, venules, arterioles, and arteries. Necrotizing glomerulonephritis is common
Churg-Strauss syndrome†,‡	Eosinophil-rich and granulomatous inflammation involving the respiratory tract and necrotizing vasculitis affecting small- to medium-sized vessels and associated with asthma and blood eosinophilia
Microscopic polyangiitis (microscopic polyarteritis)†,‡	Necrotizing vasculitis with few or no immune deposits affecting small vessels, e.g., capillaries, venules, or arterioles. Necrotizing arteritis involving small- and medium-sized arteries may be present. Necrotizing glomerulonephritis is very common. Pulmonary capillaritis often occurs
Henoch-Schönlein purpura‡	Vasculitis with immunoglobulin A–dominant immune deposits affecting small vessels, e.g., capillaries, venules, or arterioles. Typically involves the skin, gut, and glomeruli and is associated with arthralgias or arthritis
Essential cryoglobulinemic vasculitis‡	Vasculitis with cryoglobulin immune deposits affecting small vessels, e.g., capillaries, venules, or arterioles, and associated with cryoglobulins in serum. Skin and glomeruli are often involved
Cutaneous leukocytoclastic angiitis	Isolated cutaneous leukocytoclastic angiitis without systemic vasculitis or glomerulonephritis

Large artery refers to the aorta and the largest branches directed toward major body regions (e.g., to the extremities and the head and neck); *medium-sized artery* refers to the main visceral arteries (e.g., renal, hepatic, coronary, and mesenteric arteries); and *small artery* refers to the distal arterial radicals that connect with arterioles (e.g., renal arcuate and interlobular arteries). Note that some small- and large-vessel vasculitides may involve medium-sized arteries; but large- and medium-sized vessel vasculitides do not involve vessels smaller than arteries.

†Strongly associated with antineutrophil cytoplasmic autoantibodies (ANCA).

‡May be accompanied by glomerulonephritis and can manifest as nephritis or pulmonary renal vasculitic syndrome.

From Runge MS, Greganti MA. *Netter's Internal Medicine,* ed 2 (Netter Clinical Science); Philadelphia, 2008, Saunders, p. 1053; Originally adapted from Jennette JC et al: Nomenclature of systemic vasculitides. Proposal of an international consensus conference. *Arthritis Rheum* 37(2):187-192, 1994.

- Plasmapheresis is an option for patients with bleeding in the lungs or kidney failure leading to dialysis to remove ANCA.

CHRONIC Rx

Maintenance therapy

- Low-dose steroids, azathioprine, methotrexate, and rituximab have been demonstrated to be non-inferior to cyclophosphamide and can be used for maintenance therapy as well although dosing intervals and duration of therapy are still being determined.
- Prophylaxis for opportunistic infections like *Pneumocystis carinii (jiroveci)* pneumonia (PCP) is with low-dose sulfamethoxazole/trimethoprim given as one double-strength tablet three times weekly.

Relapse therapy

- Mild or non-life-threatening relapses while on maintenance therapy can be treated by increasing glucocorticoid dose or azathioprine or methotrexate most commonly.
- In severe cases, treatment is the same as in remission induction; however, rituximab is often preferred over cyclophosphamide.

DISPOSITION

- Poor prognosis if untreated.
- Prompt diagnosis is important to permit initiation of therapy that may be life-saving and organ sparing.
- Renal failure and pulmonary involvement are the major causes of morbidity and mortality.
- With treatment, 2-5-yr survival rates are 74%.

REFERRAL

Nephrology consultation is needed with the diagnosis and management of renal involvement and possible need for dialysis.

Multiple specialists may be consulted depending on system involvement.

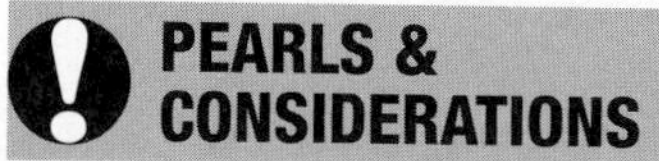

PEARLS & CONSIDERATIONS

Relapse occurs in one third of the cases.

PCP occurs in 6% of the patients as a complication of immunosuppressive therapy.

AUTHOR: **SYEDA M. SAYEED, M.D.**

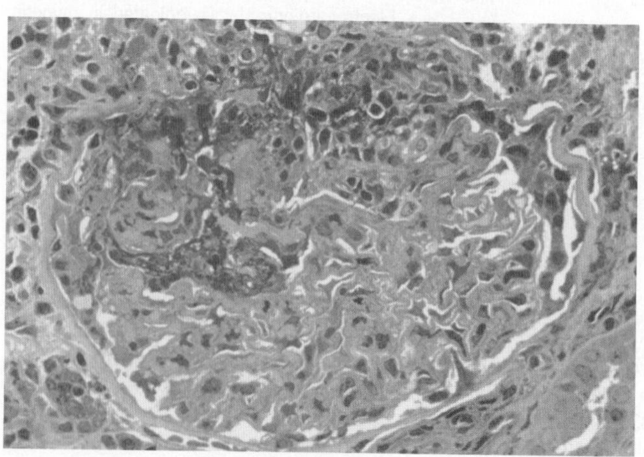

FIGURE 1-601 ANCA-associated crescentic glomerulonephritis. This toluidine blue–stained plastic section demonstrates a glomerulus with a cellular crescent. There is partial obliteration of Bowman's space by a proliferation of epithelial cells and macrophages. All types of crescentic glomerulonephritis appear similar by light microscopy, and immunofluorescence is needed to distinguish among pauci-immune, immune complex, and anti–glomerular basement membrane subtypes. (Courtesy of Dr. J. Myles.) (From Firestein GS et al: *Kelley's textbook of rheumatology,* ed 9, Philadelphia, 2013, Saunders, p. 1439.)

BASIC INFORMATION

DEFINITION

Significant cognitive impairment in the absence of dementia with preserved activities of daily living (ADLs). Mild cognitive impairment (MCI) is an intermediate state between normal cognitive function and dementia.

SYNONYMS

Isolated short-term memory loss
Cognitive impairment not dementia (CIND)
Pre-dementia
Dementia prodrome
Mild neurocognitive disorder
MCI

ICD-9CM CODES
331.83 Mild cognitive impairment, so stated
ICD-10CM CODES
G31.84 Mild cognitive impairment, so stated

EPIDEMIOLOGY & DEMOGRAPHICS

INCIDENCE:
- 12 to 15 cases per 1000 person-yr age ≥65
- 51 to 77 cases per 1000 person-yr age ≥75

PEAK INCIDENCE: In the elderly
PREVALENCE: 15% to 25% in those older than age 70.
PREDOMINANT SEX AND AGE: Male, age ≥75
GENETICS: *APOE4* genotype
- Various pathways result in amyloid accumulation and deposition in pre-Alzheimer's presenting as MCI.

RISK FACTORS: Male sex, age, lower socioeconomic status, lower educational level

CLINICAL PRESENTATION

- Subjective memory problems, preferably corroborated by another person.
- Preserved functional status (ADLs).
- Normal general thinking and reasoning skills.
- Subtypes of MCI include amnestic (mainly involves memory loss) vs. nonamnestic with involvement of other cognitive domains (single domain vs. multiple domains).
- Domains affected in MCI include memory, visuospatial skills, language, attention, and executive function.

ETIOLOGY

Neurodegenerative, vascular, traumatic, depression, or due to underlying medical condition

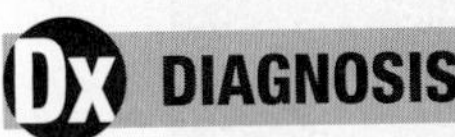

DIAGNOSIS

DIFFERENTIAL DIAGNOSIS:

- Delirium
- Dementia
- Depression
- "Reversible" cognitive impairment:
  - Medication related (anticholinergics)
  - Hypothyroidism
  - Vitamin B_{12} deficiency
- Reversible CNS conditions
  - Subdural hematoma
  - Normal pressure hydrocephalus
  - Metastatic disease

WORKUP

History
- Focus on cognitive deficits and impairment.
- Review all medications that may impact cognition (i.e., anticholinergics).
- Rule out depression and delirium.
- Perform functional assessment.

Physical exam
- Check blood pressure
- Neurologic exam to rule out reversible CNS causes of cognitive impairment

Cognitive function testing:
Brief mental status testing using MOCA (Montreal Cognitive Assessment) or SLUMS (Saint Louis University Mental Status) for office screening followed by neuropsychological testing if appropriate for specific deficits in cognitive domains.

LABORATORY TESTS

- Complete blood count
- Comprehensive metabolic profile
- TSH
- Vitamin B_{12}
- Lipids
- Vitamin D level

IMAGING STUDIES

- CT imaging can detect most reversible CNS conditions leading to cognitive impairment.
- MRI further evaluates vascular, infectious, neoplastic, and inflammatory conditions.

Rx TREATMENT

- There is insufficient evidence to recommend use of cholinesterase inhibitors (Table E1-334) for MCI. They are not approved for treating MCI, have shown little efficacy in altering progression to dementia, and can have significant side effects.
- Consider treatment with these medications only if memory complaints appear to be affecting day-to-day quality of life in individual patients or in amnestic subtypes of MCI.

NONPHARMACOLOGIC THERAPY

- Role of cognitive rehabilitation to target specific deficits
- Caregiver education and counseling
- Physical and mental exercises to maintain cognition should be recommended

COMPLEMENTARY & ALTERNATIVE MEDICINE

No clear indications for antioxidants, and studies in humans are inconclusive.

DISPOSITION

- Progression to Alzheimer's at the rate of 5% to 15% per year
  - Risk factors for progression to dementia include presence of vascular risk factors, significant cognitive impairment, depression, and presence of extrapyramidal signs.
- Mortality of those with MCI is twice that of those without MCI.
- Two- to threefold increase in risk of nursing home placement in those with MCI.

REFERRAL

Consider referral to a memory specialist if more than just memory is involved or for further evaluation of specific deficits.

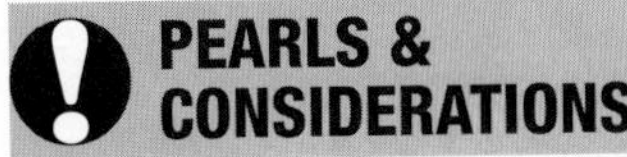

PEARLS & CONSIDERATIONS

COMMENTS

Patients with MCI usually report short-term memory concerns such as misplacing things, not remembering names of people, word-finding difficulties, forgetting day-to-day tasks, not being able to read a book, or not being able to follow a conversation.

MCI becomes clinically relevant when quality of life is affected such as problems making financial decisions and problems with personal day-to-day interactions.

Depression should be ruled out prior to making a diagnosis of MCI since it is highly prevalent in the elderly.

Anticholinergic medication use should be evaluated carefully prior to making a diagnosis of MCI.

PREVENTION

Patients with MCI should be counseled on strategies to prevent progression to dementia. They should remain physically and mentally active, have a well-balanced diet, continue activities that are socially engaging, reduce stress in their lives, and aggressively pursue treatment of vascular risk factors.

PATIENT & FAMILY EDUCATION

- Patients with MCI typically have poor retention and rapid loss of newly learned information.
- For additional information for patients, families, and clinicians: Alzheimer's Association (www.alzheimers.org)

SUGGESTED READINGS
available at www.expertconsult.com

AUTHORS: **BIRJU B. PATEL, M.D., F.A.C.P.,** and **N. WILSON HOLLAND, M.D., F.A.C.P.**

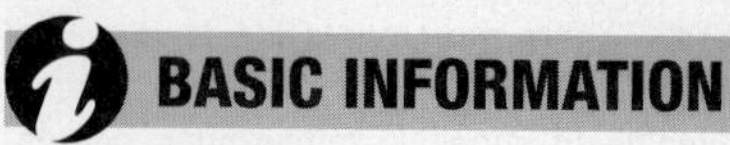

BASIC INFORMATION

DEFINITION

Mitral regurgitation (MR) is retrograde blood flow into the left atrium resulting from an incompetent mitral valve. This condition can lead to left ventricular (LV) failure as well as increased left atrial and pulmonary pressures, with consequent pulmonary hypertension and right heart failure.

SYNONYMS

Mitral insufficiency

ICD-9CM CODES
424.0 Mitral regurgitation
ICD-10CM CODES
I34.0 Nonrheumatic mitral (valve) insufficiency
I05.1 Rheumatic mitral insufficiency
I05.9 Mitral valve disease, unspecified

EPIDEMIOLOGY & DEMOGRAPHICS

The incidence of MR has increased over the past 30 yr; however, this may be due to increasing availability of echocardiography and MR diagnosis rather than any real increase in the prevalence of this condition.

PHYSICAL FINDINGS & CLINICAL PRESENTATION

- Holosystolic, high-pitched, "blowing" murmur at apex with radiation to base, left axilla, or back; there is a poor correlation between the intensity of the systolic murmur and the degree of regurgitation. However, an early diastolic to mid-diastolic rumble (pseudomitral stenosis) suggests severe MR.
- The murmur of acute MR (e.g., from papillary muscle rupture) can be very soft or inaudible due to a large regurgitant volume entering a noncompliant left atrium, leading to an acute rise in left atrial pressure and thus lack of significant gradient for an audible murmur.
- Hyperdynamic apex, sometimes with palpable LV lift and apical thrill.
- Many patients with mild to moderate MR will remain asymptomatic and without evidence of hemodynamic compromise for years.
- Diminished S1, reflecting failure of valve leaflets to coapt completely, widely split S2 (decreased LV ejection time results in early A2)
- Symptomatic patients with MR generally present with the following:
  - Symptoms suggestive of heart failure (fatigue, dyspnea, orthopnea, paroxysmal nocturnal dyspnea, edema)
  - Hemoptysis (caused by pulmonary hypertension)
  - Atrial fibrillation

ETIOLOGY

Primary MR
- Idiopathic myxomatous degeneration of the mitral valve, mitral valve prolapse (most common cause of MR in industrialized countries)
- Papillary muscle dysfunction or rupture (typically as a result of an inferior wall myocardial infarction)
- Ruptured chordae tendineae
- Infective endocarditis
- Calcified mitral valve annulus
- Rheumatic valvulitis (may be combined with mitral stenosis; common in developing countries)
- Systemic lupus erythematosus (Libman-Sacks endocarditis)
- Drugs: fenfluramine, dexfenfluramine, pergolide, cabergoline
- Congenital cleft valve
- Ischemic mitral regurgitation due to papillary muscle dysfunction from multivessel CAD

Secondary MR
- Hypertrophic cardiomyopathy
- LV dilation (e.g., secondary to dilated cardiomyopathy)

Dx DIAGNOSIS

DIFFERENTIAL DIAGNOSIS

- Hypertrophic cardiomyopathy
- Tricuspid regurgitation
- Aortic stenosis
- Aortic sclerosis
- Ventricular septal defect
- Atrial septal defect

WORKUP

- Diagnostic workup consists of echocardiography, ECG, and chest radiograph; cardiac catheterization sometimes needed to confirm severity of the disease.
- Recent studies suggest that in patients with severe asymptomatic MR and normal LV function, elevations of brain natriuretic peptide (BNP) >105 pg/ml have an independent and additive prognostic value that may identify patients at high risk and aid in the selection of patients for early surgery.

IMAGING STUDIES

- Echocardiography (Fig. 1-602): dilated left atrium, hyperdynamic left ventricle (erratic motion of the leaflet is seen in patients with ruptured chordae tendineae); color flow Doppler will show evidence of MR. The most important aspect of the echocardiographic examination is the quantification of the severity of MR (Table 1-336), LV systolic performance, and estimated right ventricular (RV) systolic pressure vena contracta width >0.6 cm, regurgitant volume >60 ml, regurgitant orifice area >0.40 cm^2 by PISA (proximal isovelocity surface area), and systolic pulmonary vein flow reversal are all echocardiographic criteria of severe MR.
- Chest x-ray:
  - Left atrial enlargement, LV enlargement
  - Possible pulmonary congestion, although most often normal

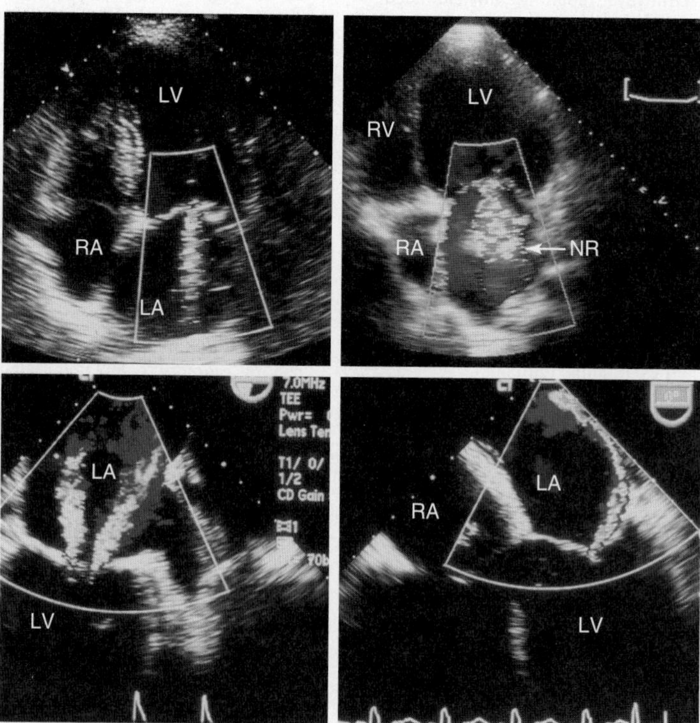

FIGURE 1-602 Mitral regurgitation. Four panels depicting varying degrees of mitral regurgitation; the two *top panels* are apical four-chamber transthoracic views showing, on the *left,* mild mitral regurgitation and, on the *right,* moderate to severe mitral regurgitation. On the *left,* note the relatively narrow jet directed from the tips of the mitral valve toward the posterior left atrial wall. On the right, note the larger jet, filling approximately 40 percent of the left atrial cavity. The two *bottom panels* are transesophageal echocardiograms. On the *left,* note the mitral regurgitation occurring in two discrete jets and, on the *right,* the highly eccentric jet, which courses along the extreme lateral wall of the left atrium. *LA,* Left atrium; *LV,* left ventricle; *RA,* right atrium; *RV,* right ventricle. (From Zipes DP et al [eds]: *Braunwald's heart disease,* ed 7, Philadelphia, 2005, Saunders.)

TABLE 1-336 Mitral Regurgitation Severity*

	(Mild)	II	III	IV (Severe)
MR = jet (%LA)	<15	15-30	35-50	>50
Spectral Doppler	Faint	—	—	Dense
Vena contracta	<3 mm	—	—	>6 mm
Pulmonary vein flow	S > D	—	—	Systolic reversed
RV (ml)	<30	30-44	45-59	≥60
ERO (cm^2)	<0.2	0.2-0.29	0.3-0.39	≥0.40
PISA	Small	—	—	Large

D, Antegrade flow in diastole; *ERO,* effective regurgitant orifice; *%LA,* percentage of left atrial area encompassed by the *MR* jet with color flow Doppler; *MR,* mitral regurgitation; *PISA,* proximal isovelocity surface area; *RV,* regurgitant volume; *S,* antegrade flow in systole.

*For some parameters, the observation is valid at the extremes of MR severity and there may be marked overlap in intermediate (grades II, III) MR. In these instances, no value is presented.

From Zipes DP et al (eds): *Braunwald's heart disease,* ed 7, Philadelphia, 2005, Saunders and the 2003 American Society of Echocardiography Guidelines.

- ECG:
  - Left atrial enlargement
  - LV hypertrophy
  - Atrial fibrillation
- Cardiac catheterization: to confirm severity of MR, or to rule out presence of coronary artery disease in patients being evaluated for surgical replacement
- Can consider cardiac MRI in cases where echocardiography is limited or LV function/dimensions are borderline, or when clinical condition and echocardiographic findings are discordant.

Rx TREATMENT

NONPHARMACOLOGIC THERAPY

Salt restriction

ACUTE GENERAL Rx

- Medical: medical therapy is primarily directed toward treatment of the source or its complications (e.g., atrial fibrillation, ischemic heart disease, infective endocarditis, hypertension, and heart failure).
  - The utility of afterload reduction (to decrease the regurgitant fraction and to increase cardiac output) depends upon the etiology of MR and the administration of afterload reducers. In acute MR, intravenous nitroprusside has shown some utility. Long-term use of oral afterload reducers (e.g., ACE inhibitors or angiotensin receptor blockers [ARBs]) do not slow the progression of mitral regurgitation, and their use should be only for other indications such as hypertension and LV dysfunction.
  - Control ventricular response only if atrial fibrillation with rapid ventricular response is present.
  - Anticoagulants if atrial fibrillation occurs.
- Surgery: surgery is the only definitive treatment for MR. Although no randomized trial of mitral valve repair vs. replacement exists, repair is favored over replacement in degenerative mitral valve disease due to its lower perioperative risk, improved event-free survival, freedom from complications of prosthetic valves, and better postoperative LV function. It is a class I indication in patients with:
  - Acute severe MR
  - Symptomatic patients with severe MR despite optimal medical therapy and LVEF >30%, LV end-systolic dimension <55 mm.
  - Asymptomatic patients with severe MR but with evidence of declining LV function (EF <60%) or progressive dilation (LV at end-systole >40 mm)
- Surgery is a class IIa (reasonable) recommendation in:
  - Severe MR with new-onset atrial fibrillation, even if asymptomatic
  - Asymptomatic severe MR with pulmonary hypertension (≥50 mm Hg at rest or ≥60 mm Hg during exercise)
  - Asymptomatic severe MR secondary to flail leaflet
  - A recent study of early surgical intervention for severe MR secondary to a flail leaflet in patients with asymptomatic disease shows greater long-term survival and reduced rates of heart failure when compared to medical therapy alone.
  - Symptomatic severe MR with severe LV dysfunction or dilatation (LVEF <30% or LV at end-systole >55 mm, respectively) in whom LV dysfunction is not the primary cause for the MR (as opposed to the other way around)
  - Asymptomatic severe MR with preserved LVEF (>60%) and size (<40 mm in end-systole) in whom the likelihood of successful repair without residual MR is >95% and operative mortality is <1%
- Quantitative grading of MR is a powerful predictor of the clinical outcome of asymptomatic MR. In general, patients with regurgitant orifice areas of ≥40 mm^2 should be considered for prompt surgery, whereas those with orifices between 20 and 39 mm^2 can be followed closely
- Percutaneous mitral valve repair methods are currently being investigated, and the MitraClip device is now FDA approved for use in patients with significant symptomatic degenerative MR (>3+) who have too high a risk for surgery. Early data have not demonstrated a significant efficacy in MR reduction compared to surgical replacement; however, it has been shown to improve NYHA functional class and quality of life measures.

DISPOSITION

Prognosis is generally good unless there is significant impairment of left ventricular function or significantly elevated pulmonary artery pressures. Most patients remain asymptomatic for many years (average interval from diagnosis to onset of symptoms is 16 yr). In patients with chronic severe MR, MR is commonly progressive, with onset of other symptoms or left ventricular dysfunction within 6-10 yr. However surgery should be advised well before the onset of symptoms in case of worsening LVEF and LV systolic dimensions and presence of pulmonary hypertension or atrial fibrillation, all of which are poor prognostic signs.

REFERRAL

- Surgical referral in selected patients (see "Acute General Rx"). Emergency surgery is usually necessary in patients with acute MR caused by ruptured papillary muscle or chordae tendineae after myocardial infarction.
- Mitral valve repair can also be accomplished with an investigational procedure that involves the percutaneous implantation of a clip that grasps and approximates the edges of the mitral leaflets at the origin of the regurgitant jet. Preliminary data reveals that although percutaneous repair is less effective at reducing MR than conventional surgery, the procedure is associated with superior safety and similar improvements in clinical outcomes.

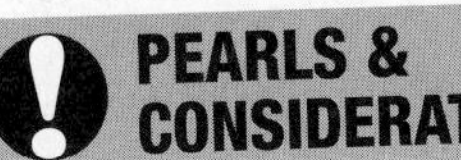

PEARLS & CONSIDERATIONS

COMMENTS

- Although vasodilators and other agents should be used to treat hypertension in patients with severe mitral regurgitation, there is no evidence that they will delay the need for eventual valve surgery, which is the definitive treatment for severe MR.
- In 2007, the AHA guidelines for prevention of infectious endocarditis were revised and routine antibiotic prophylaxis to undergo dental or other invasive procedures is no longer recommended, unless the patient has prior endocarditis.

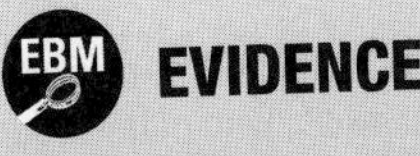

EVIDENCE

available at www.expertconsult.com

SUGGESTED READINGS

available at www.expertconsult.com

RELATED CONTENT

Mitral Regurgitation (Patient Information)

AUTHORS: **SHALINE D. RAO, M.D.,** and **VEERANNA MERLA, M.D.**

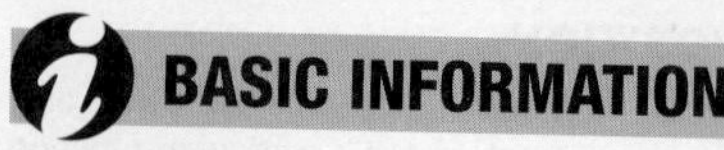

BASIC INFORMATION

DEFINITION

Mitral stenosis is a narrowing of the mitral valve orifice that prevents proper opening during diastole and obstruction of blood flow from the left atrium to the left ventricle. Due to thickening of the leaflets there is restricted movement. The cross section of a normal orifice measures 4 to 6 cm^2. Symptoms usually develop with exercise when the orifice measures <2.5 cm^2, and symptoms may develop at rest when the orifice is <1.5 cm^2.

SYNONYMS

MS

ICD-9CM CODES
394.0 Mitral stenosis
ICD-10CM CODES
I05.0 Mitral stenosis
I05.2 Mitral stenosis with insufficiency

EPIDEMIOLOGY & DEMOGRAPHICS

- The predominant cause of mitral stenosis is rheumatic heart disease; however, the occurrence of mitral valve stenosis has decreased worldwide over the past 30 yr (particularly in developed countries) as a result of declining incidence of rheumatic fever due to appropriate antibiotic use.
- Rheumatic heart disease has a predilection for the mitral valve, aortic valve, and to some extent the tricuspid valve.
- The incidence of MS is higher in women (2:1 female-to-male ratio).
- Of note, the majority of the world's population live in developing countries with high prevalence of rheumatic heart disease.
- Outbreaks of rheumatic fever in the U.S. are due to increased virulence of a streptococcal strain or enhanced immigration from where rheumatic heart disease is prevalent.

PHYSICAL FINDINGS & CLINICAL PRESENTATION

- Dyspnea is the most common symptom along with fatigue and decreased exercise capacity. These occur secondary to an inability to increase cardiac output, especially with exercise, and elevated pulmonary capillary wedge pressures, with resultant increase in pulmonary artery pressures.
- The left ventricle is unaffected in pure MS; however, MS often coexists with mitral regurgitation and occasionally with aortic valve dysfunction, both of which can cause left ventricular dysfunction.
- "Mitral facies" which are pinkish-purple patches on the cheek due to low cardiac output and vasoconstriction, usually indicate severe MS.
- Paroxysmal nocturnal dyspnea (PND) and orthopnea secondary to elevated left atrial pressure may occur.
- Acute pulmonary edema may occur after an increase in flow across the mitral valve secondary to an increase in cardiac output or heart rate (exertion, tachyarrhythmias, fever, anemia, etc.).
- Pulmonary hypertension that results from chronically elevated pulmonary capillary wedge pressures can lead to right ventricular (RV) dysfunction and signs and symptoms of right heart failure (hepatomegaly, pulsatile liver, peripheral edema, ascites).
- The left ventricle is typically "protected" in mitral stenosis and exists in a low pressure state.
- Hemoptysis can be present secondary to rupture of thin-walled dilated bronchial veins due to an abrupt increase in left atrial pressure.
- Systemic embolic events are caused by left atrial thrombi. These are associated with atrial fibrillation 80% of the time, since mitral stenosis leads to left atrial enlargement, which is a predisposing factor to atrial arrhythmias.
- Atrial fibrillation is more prevalent in patients with more severe MS, increasing age, and other valvular abnormalities.
- Chest pain can be caused by RV pressure overload and/or concomitant coronary artery disease in up to 15% of patients.
- Irregularly irregular pulse caused by atrial fibrillation.
- Loud first heart sound (S_1) caused by delayed valve closure preceded by an opening snap and rapid rising left ventricular (LV) pressure.
- A low-pitched rumbling diastolic murmur heard best at the apex. The intensity of the murmur is not related to the severity of the stenosis, but the duration is holodiastolic in severe MS.
- An opening snap (OS) caused by tensing of the valve leaflets after the cusps have opened completely. The OS follows S_2 by 0.03 to 0.14 sec, and the shorter the S_2-OS interval, the more severe the MS, due to higher left atrial pressures.
- Prominent A wave on the pulmonary capillary wedge pressure tracing. This is homologous to the prominent A wave seen in systemic venous pressure tracings with tricuspid stenosis.
- A diastolic thrill may be palpable at the apex, especially with the patient in the left lateral recumbent position.
- An RV lift may be palpable at the left sternal border secondary to RV hypertrophy and pulmonary hypertension.
- An accentuated P_2 and/or a soft, early diastolic decrescendo murmur *(Graham Steell murmur)* caused by pulmonary regurgitation may be present in patients with pulmonary hypertension (not specific for mitral stenosis).
- Hoarseness due to the enlargement of the left atrium compressing the recurrent laryngeal nerve.
- Straightening of the left heart border seen on chest radiography indicative of left atrial enlargement.

ETIOLOGY

- Rheumatic fever (RF) is the predominant cause of MS. RF causes thickening of the leaflet tips, commissure fusion, and chordal shortening and fusion. This leads to the classic doming of the leaflets in diastole due to fusion of the leaflet tips at the commisures. Rheumatic fever involves the leaflet tips first with progression towards the annulus. This is opposite of mitral annular calcification, which typically starts in the annulus and proceeds out to the leaflet tips, leading to mitral stenosis in severe cases.
- Congenital defect (parachute valve) has the usual two mitral leaflets, but the chordae, instead of diverging to insert into two papillary muscles, converge into one major papillary muscle, which allows little mobility of the leaflets, cor triatriatum in which there is a thin membrane which obstructs the pulmonary vein flow and simulates mitral stenosis.
- Rare causes are severe mitral annular calcification usually seen in end stage renal disease patients, endomyocardial fibroelastosis, malignant carcinoid syndrome, systemic lupus erythematosus, Whipple disease, Fabry disease, and rheumatoid arthritis.

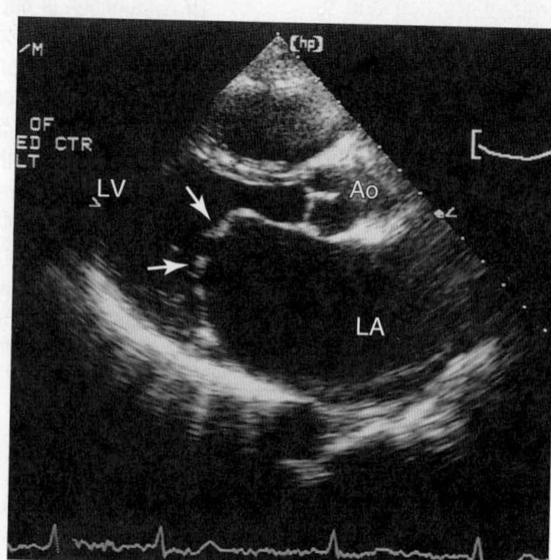

FIGURE 1-603 Mitral stenosis. Parasternal long-axis view of a patient with mitral stenosis and a pliable noncalcified mitral valve leaflet. Note the "doming" motion of the mitral valve leaflets *(arrows)*. Valves with these morphologic features are excellent candidates for percutaneous balloon valvotomy. *Ao,* Aorta; *LA,* left atrium; *LV,* left ventricle. (From Zipes DP et al [eds]: *Braunwald's heart disease,* ed 7, Philadelphia, 2005, Saunders.)

- Atrial septal defect in association with rheumatic mitral stenosis is termed Lutembacher syndrome.
- Medications: methysergide

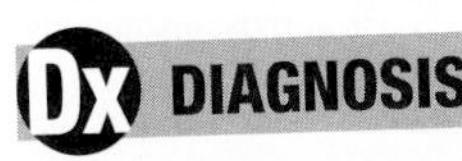

DIAGNOSIS

DIFFERENTIAL DIAGNOSIS

- Left atrial myxoma
- Ball valve thrombus
- Other valvular abnormalities (e.g., tricuspid stenosis, mitral regurgitation)
- Atrial septal defect

WORKUP

Physical examination and echocardiography

IMAGING STUDIES

- Echocardiography (Fig. 1-603):
  - Two-dimensional echocardiogram can measure valve area by direct planimetry or calculate it by the Doppler pressure half-time method (this may be inaccurate in patients with concomitant diastolic dysfunction or aortic insufficiency and in patients who have recently undergone mitral valvuloplasty) or the continuity equation can be used to calculate the valve area. A valve area less than 1 cm^2 is consistent with severe MS. The transmitral gradient can also be calculated. A mean gradient of >10 mm Hg indicates severe MS. 5-10 mm Hg is consistent with moderate MS, and 0-5 mm Hg is consistent with mild MS or no MS.
  - Echocardiography will also show a markedly diminished E-to-F slope of the anterior mitral valve leaflet during diastole; there is also fusion of the commissures, resulting in "doming" of the leaflets during diastole.
  - Grading of leaflet thickness, mobility, calcification, and subvalvular thickening (mitral valvuloplasty score); with a score of 0 to 4 for each characteristic can predict hemodynamic results and outcome of balloon mitral valvuloplasty (a low score of less than 8 is favorable for balloon valvuloplasty and a high score is unfavorable). A score above 8 would favor a surgical approach. In addition, mitral regurgitation that is greater than mild would preclude a balloon mitral valvuloplasty procedure.
  - Doppler echocardiography can be used to assess for pulmonary hypertension and to give an estimate of the pulmonary artery systolic pressure at rest and with exercise.
- Chest radiograph:
  - Straightening of the left cardiac border caused by enlarged left atrium
  - Left atrial enlargement on lateral chest radiograph
  - Prominence of pulmonary arteries that indicates pulmonary hypertension
  - Possible pulmonary congestion and edema (Kerley B lines)
- ECG:
  - RV hypertrophy; right axis deviation caused by pulmonary hypertension
  - Left atrial enlargement (broad, biphasic P waves in lead V1 and duration of P-waves >0.11 sec in lead II). This is termed "P-mitrale."
  - Atrial fibrillation
- Cardiac catheterization:
  - Allows the measurement of pulmonary artery pressure and transmitral pressure gradients at rest or with exercise (supine biking or raising weights with arms while lying supine).
  - Allows the measurement of transmitral flow and calculation of the valve area.
  - Is not routinely recommended for the evaluation of MS but is useful when the echocardiographic findings are nondiagnostic or discrepant with the clinical scenario.
  - Cardiac catheterization in addition to echocardiography can be used to monitor the hemodynamics during a balloon mitral valvuloplasty procedure.

Rx TREATMENT

NONPHARMACOLOGIC THERAPY

Decrease level of activity in symptomatic patients and salt restriction if pulmonary congestion is present.

ACUTE GENERAL Rx

- Medical:
  - Anticoagulation for the prevention of systemic embolic events in patients with MS and:
    1. Atrial fibrillation
    2. Prior embolic event
    3. Documented left atrial thrombus or left atrial appendage thrombus
    4. Severe mitral stenosis if associated with severe left atrial enlargement and spontaneous echo contrast indicating stagnant blood flow (class 2b indication)
  - Ventricular rate control (to increase diastolic filling period) with beta-blockers, non-dihydropyridine calcium channel blockers, or digitalis and aggressive treatment of tachyarrhythmias.
  - Treat congestive heart failure with loop diuretics and sodium restriction.
  - Antibiotic prophylaxis to prevent recurrent rheumatic fever is usually not indicated unless presence of high-risk features such as prior endocarditis, prosthetic heart valves, valvulopathy of the transplanted heart, and certain cases of cyanotic congenital heart disease. Pregnancy in females with advanced MS may be poorly tolerated due to the hemodynamic changes such as increased cardiac output. Whereas pregnant females with mild to moderate MS may tolerate pregnancy very well with medical therapy alone.
  - Pregnancy in females with advanced MS may be poorly tolerated due to the hemodynamic changes such as increased cardiac output. Whereas pregnant females with mild to moderate MS may tolerate pregnancy very well with medical therapy alone.
- Table 1-337 summarizes approaches to mechanical relief of mitral stenosis.
- Percutaneous balloon mitral valvotomy (BMV) is the therapy of choice for symptomatic patients with moderate to severe MS (valve area ≤1.5 cm^2) with a favorable valvuloplasty score, minimal or no mitral regurgitation and no left atrial thrombus. Balloon valvotomy is

TABLE 1-337 Approaches to Mechanical Relief of Mitral Stenosis

Approach	Advantages	Disadvantages
Closed surgical valvotomy	Inexpensive Relatively simple Good hemodynamic results in selected patients Good long-term outcome	No direct visualization of valve Only feasible with flexible, noncalcified valves Contraindicated if MR >2+ Surgical procedure with general anesthesia
Open surgical valvotomy	Visualization of valve allows directed valvotomy Concurrent annuloplasty for MR is feasible	Best results with flexible, noncalcified valves Surgical procedure with general anesthesia
Valve replacement	Feasible in all patients regardless of extent of valve calcification or severity of MR	Surgical procedure with general anesthesia Effect of loss of annular-papillary muscle continuity on LV function Prosthetic valve Chronic anticoagulation
Balloon mitral valvotomy	Percutaneous approach Local anesthesia Good hemodynamic results in selected patients Good long-term outcome	No direct visualization of valve Only feasible with flexible, noncalcified valves Contraindicated if MR >2+

LV, Left ventricular; *MR,* mitral regurgitation.
From Otto CM: *Valvular heart disease*, ed 2, Philadelphia, 2004, Saunders.

M

Diseases and Disorders I

also indicated in asymptomatic patients with moderate to severe MS that has resulted in pulmonary artery pressures of 50 mm Hg at rest or 60 mm Hg with exercise. Percutaneous BMV is also considered the procedure of choice in pregnant women with rheumatic MS and in NYHA class 3 to 4 heart failure and/or unresponsive to adequate medical treatment. In addition, it is a reasonable option for patients who are at high risk for surgery even when their valve morphology is not ideal (class 2a indication).

- Surgical intervention is indicated for patients with moderate to severe symptomatic MS when BMV is not available or is contraindicated (valvuloplasty score greater than or equal to 8) or the valve is calcified, MR that is more than mild, there is presence of left atrial thrombus and when the surgical risk is acceptable. The surgical approaches include closed mitral valvotomy, open valvotomy and repair (preferred) and mitral valve replacement when repair is not possible.

DISPOSITION

- Prognosis is generally good except in patients with chronic pulmonary hypertension.
- Operative mortality rates for mitral valve replacement are 1% to 5% at most institutions.

RELATED CONTENT

Mitral Stenosis (Patient Information)

AUTHORS: **PHILLIP RUISI, D.O.,** and **ARAVIND RAO KOKKIRALA, M.D.**

BASIC INFORMATION

DEFINITION

Mitral valve prolapse (MVP) is the bulging of one or both of the mitral valve leaflets into the left atrium during systole. MVP syndrome refers to a constellation of MVP and associated symptoms (e.g., autonomic dysfunction, palpitations) or other physical abnormalities (e.g., pectus excavatum). Table 1-338 describes a classification of mitral valve prolapse.

SYNONYMS

MVP
Mitral click murmur syndrome
Barlow's syndrome

ICD-9CM CODES
424.0 Mitral valve disorders
394.9 Other and unspecified mitral valve diseases
ICD-10CM CODES
I34.1 Mitral valve prolapse
I34.0 Nonrheumatic mitral (valve) insufficiency

EPIDEMIOLOGY & DEMOGRAPHICS

- MVP can be found by echocardiogram in 1% to 4% of the general population, with some studies suggesting that it is more common in women than in men.
- Increased incidence is seen with autoimmune thyroid disorders, Ehlers-Danlos syndrome, Marfan's syndrome, osteogenesis imperfecta, pseudoxanthoma elasticum, pectus excavatum, anorexia nervosa, and bulimia.
- Compared to men, women with MVP have less posterior prolapse (22% vs. 31%), less flail (2% vs. 8%), more leaflet thickening (32% vs. 28%), and less frequent severe mitral regurgitation (MR) (10% vs. 23%).
- Although MVP is more common in women than men, men more often develop severe regurgitation requiring surgical intervention.

TABLE 1-338 Classification of Mitral Valve Prolapse

Mitral Valve Prolapse Syndrome

- Younger age (20-50 yr)
- Predominantly female
- Click or click-murmur on physical examination
- Thin leaflets with systolic displacement on echocardiography
- Associated with low blood pressure, orthostatic hypotension, palpitations
- Benign long-term course

Myxomatous Mitral Valve Disease

- Older age (40-70 yr)
- Predominantly male
- Thickened, redundant valve leaflets
- Mitral regurgitation on physical exam and echocardiography
- High likelihood of progressive disease requiring mitral valve surgery

Secondary Mitral Valve Prolapse

- Marfan syndrome
- Hypertrophic cardiomyopathy
- Ehlers-Danlos syndrome
- Other connective tissue diseases

Modified from Otto CM: *Valvular Heart Disease,* ed 2, Philadelphia, 2004, WB Saunders, p. 369.

PHYSICAL FINDINGS & CLINICAL PRESENTATION

- Mid to late systolic click, heard best at the apex
- If regurgitation is present, a crescendo mid to late systolic murmur, may be heard that worsens with standing and Valsalva's maneuver
- Timing of click within the cardiac cycle varies with loading conditions within the left ventricle (i.e., may occur earlier with standing or Valsalva and later with squatting or expiration)
- May be associated with small anteroposterior chest diameter, scoliosis, pectus excavatum, or low BMI.
- Most patients with MVP are asymptomatic; symptoms (if present) consist primarily of chest pain, palpitations, fatigue, dyspnea, or and anxiety
- Neurologic abnormalities (e.g., transient ischemic attack [TIA] or stroke) are rare
- A spectrum of arrhythmias, mainly paroxysmal supraventricular tachycardia and atrial and ventricular premature beats, etc., is also observed with mitral valve prolapse. There is also an increased association with Wolff-Parkinson-White syndrome and QT prolongation

ETIOLOGY

- Myxomatous degeneration of connective tissue within mitral valve, usually involving multiple leaflet segments. In contrast, fibroelastic deficiency of single leaflet segment develops in elderly patients.
- Congenital deformity of mitral valve and supportive structures
- Secondary to other disorders of connective tissue such as Ehlers-Danlos, Marfan, or pseudoxanthoma elasticum; association with other connective tissue disorders suggests MVP result of defective embryogenesis in cells of mesenchymal origin

DIAGNOSIS

DIFFERENTIAL DIAGNOSIS

- Other valvular abnormalities (especially mitral regurgitation [MR])
- Anxiety/panic disorders
- Pulmonary embolism
- Atypical chest pain

WORKUP

- Medical history and physical examination, with increased suspicion in patients with other findings of connective tissue disorder.
- Two or three-dimensional echocardiography in patients with a systolic click or murmur on careful auscultation.
- Cardiac MRI is an emerging tool for the evaluation and diagnosis of MVP but has not yet been independently validated.
- ECG is most often normal but may show nonspecific ST-T wave changes, prolonged QT interval, or prominent Q waves.

IMAGING STUDIES

Echocardiography (Fig. 1-604) shows one or more leaflets prolapsing >2 mm into the left atrium during systole in a long axis view. Mitral leaflets may be thickened (>5 mm). MR is typically present, though sometimes only during exertion. If moderate or severe MR is present, findings of dilated left atrium, LV dilation and/or dysfunction, and elevated estimated RV systolic pressures may also be present. There is an increased incidence of secundum-type atrial septal defects (ASDs) in patients with MVP, which may also be identified with echocardiography.

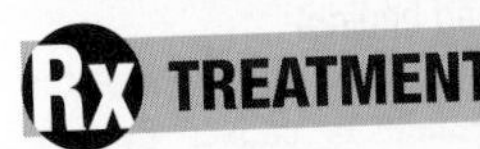

TREATMENT

NONPHARMACOLOGIC THERAPY

Avoidance of stimulants (e.g., caffeine, nicotine) in patients with palpitations. Sometimes, reassurance is sufficient to reduce the severity of symptoms in many patients.

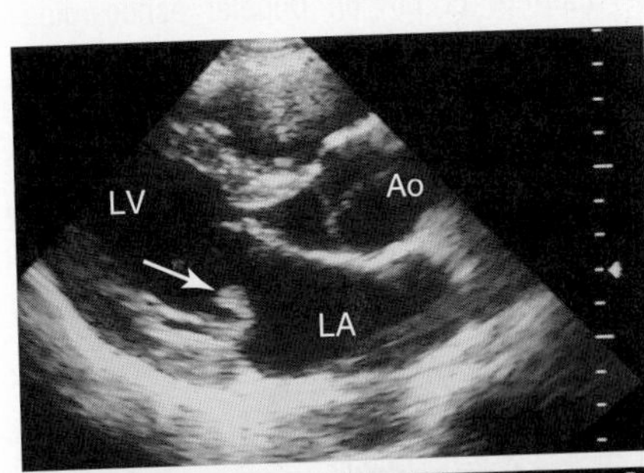

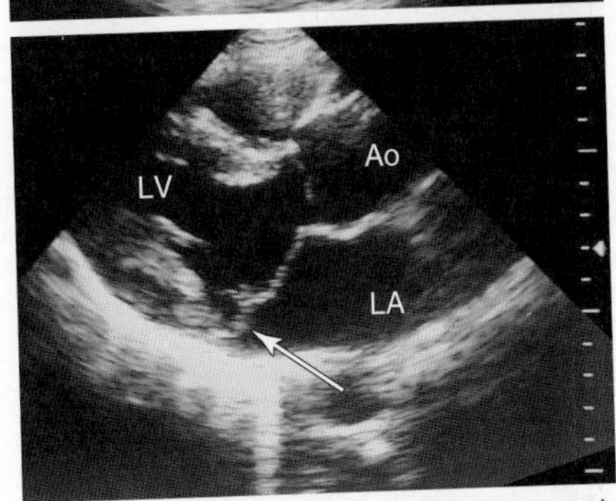

FIGURE 1-604 Mitral valve prolapse. Parasternal long-axis view in diastole *(top)* and systole *(bottom)* in a patient with mitral valve prolapse and myxomatous changes. In the *upper panel,* note the open mitral valve and the diffuse thickening of the posterior mitral valve leaflet *(arrow).* The *lower panel* was recorded in systole. Note that both leaflets prolapse behind the plane of the mitral valve annulus. The prolapse of the posterior leaflet is somewhat more prominent *(arrow). Ao,* Aorta; *LA,* left atrium; *LV,* left ventricle. (From Zipes DP et al [eds]: *Braunwald's heart disease,* ed 7, Philadelphia, 2005, Saunders.)

ACUTE GENERAL Rx

β-blockers may be tried in symptomatic patients (e.g., palpitations, chest pain); they decrease the heart rate and contractility, thus potentially decreasing the stretch on the prolapsing valve leaflets.

CHRONIC Rx

Monitoring for complications:

- Mitral regurgitation (most common complication); on rare occasion may occur acutely due to rupture of chordae tendineae.
- Bacterial endocarditis (risk is three to eight times that of the general population); higher risk in patients with regurgitation than without
- TIA or stroke caused by embolic phenomena (from fibrin and platelet thrombi) in patients with thickened leaflets; risk in young patients is <0.05% per year; if present aspirin (75-325 mg) is indicated for secondary prevention
- Cardiac arrhythmias (the vast majority are supraventricular and benign)
- Sudden death (rare); most often associated with acute flail leaflets or caused by ventricular arrhythmias associated with other structural heart disease
- The incidence of complications of MVP is very low (<1% per year) if mitral leaflet thickness (≤0.5 mm); young patients (age <45 yr) with absence of mitral systolic murmur or MR on Doppler echocardiography, all of which are at low risk for any complications. Table 1-339 describes predictors of clinical outcome in mitral valve prolapse.
- Risk factors that predict higher risk of complications are presence of moderate to severe MR, LV ejection fraction <50%, LA dimension >40 mm, age >50 years

TABLE 1-339 Predictors of Clinical Outcome in Mitral Valve Prolapse

Predictor	Survival	Valve Surgery	Arrhythmias or Sudden Death	Endocarditis
Age	+++	+++	–	–
Gender	++	++	–	–
Leaflet thickness or redundancy	+++	+++	++++	++++
Severity of mitral regurgitation	++++	++++	++++	++++
Systolic click	+	–	–	–
Left ventricular dilation	+	++++	++	–
Left atrial dilation	–	++	+	–

Symbols indicate the relative predictive value of each variable for the listed clinical outcomes on a scale of no predictive value (–) to strongly predictive (++++).

From Bonow RO et al: *Braunwald's heart disease: a textbook of cardiovascular medicine,* Philadelphia, 2012, Saunders.

SURGICAL REFERRAL

Surgical referral may be necessary in patients who develop progressive MR with surgical indications as per guidelines for valvular heart disease (see topic on mitral regurgitation).

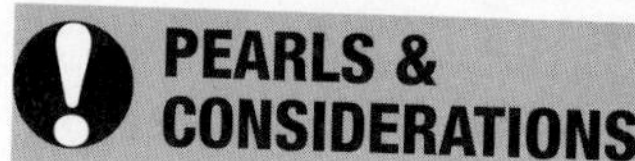

PEARLS & CONSIDERATIONS

COMMENTS

- Recent studies suggest that the prevalence of MVP and its propensity to cause symptoms and serious complications have been overestimated in the past.
- The relationship between MVP syndrome and sudden cardiac death is unclear, and the best evidence suggests that there is only a slight risk in subsets of patients with MVP who have severe MR, severe valvular deformity, complex ventricular arrhythmias, QT prolongation, and a history of syncope.
- Asymptomatic patients with MVP and mild or no MR can be evaluated clinically every 3 to 5 yr. High-risk patients (those with symptoms, arrhythmias, or significant regurgitation) should undergo a follow-up examination once a year.
- In 2007, the AHA guidelines for prevention of infectious endocarditis were revised and prophylactic antibiotics are no longer recommended for patients with MVP without previous endocarditis.

PATIENT & FAMILY EDUCATION

www.themitralvalve.org

SUGGESTED READINGS

available at www.expertconsult.com

RELATED CONTENT

Mitral Valve Prolapse (Patient Information)

AUTHOR: **AMANDA C. DORAN, M.D., Ph.D.**

BASIC INFORMATION

DEFINITION

An overlap syndrome with clinical features seen in systemic lupus erythematosus (SLE), polymyositis (PM), and systemic sclerosis (Scl) in association with high titer of anti U1-RNP antibodies, especially to the 68-70 kD epitope. Not all clinical features are present initially, and it usually takes several years before enough overlapping features are present to be confident that mixed connective tissue disease (MCTD) is the most likely diagnosis. Because of the nonspecific signs and symptoms at presentation, most of the patients may be initially classified as having undifferentiated connective tissue disease.

SYNONYMS

MCTD

ICD-9CM CODES
710.9 Diffuse connective tissue disease NOS
ICD-10CM CODES
M35.1 Other overlap syndrome
M35.9 Systemic involvement of connective tissue, unspecified

EPIDEMIOLOGY & DEMOGRAPHICS

PREVALENCE: Variable by population.
PREDOMINANT SEX: Female/male ratio of 10:1
PREDOMINANT AGE: Age at onset generally in the second or third decade

PHYSICAL FINDINGS & CLINICAL PRESENTATION

- General: exertional dyspnea, malaise, fatigue, fever
- Joints: arthalgias are an early symptom that can evolve to arthritis resembling RA but without severe erosions. Sausage-shaped fingers (Fig. 1-605)
- Skin and mucosas: Raynaud's phenomenon is an early finding. Malar rash, discoid plaques, oral or genital ulcers, sicca symptoms, subcutaneous nodules, abnormal nail fold capillaries can be seen
- Muscle: myalgias, inflammatory myopathy
- Lung: interstitial lung disease leading to pulmonary fibrosis
- Heart: pulmonary hypertension, pericardial effusion (most frequent cardiac manifestation), pericarditis
- Hematopoietic: anemia of chronic disease, lymphopenia, thrombocytopenia
- Gastrointestinal tract: altered motility, mesenteric vasculitis, pancreatitis, hepatitis
- Kidney: membranous glomerulonephritis, diffuse proliferative glomerulonephritis; kidney involvement is uncommon
- Nervous system: trigeminal neuropathy, headache, aseptic meningitis

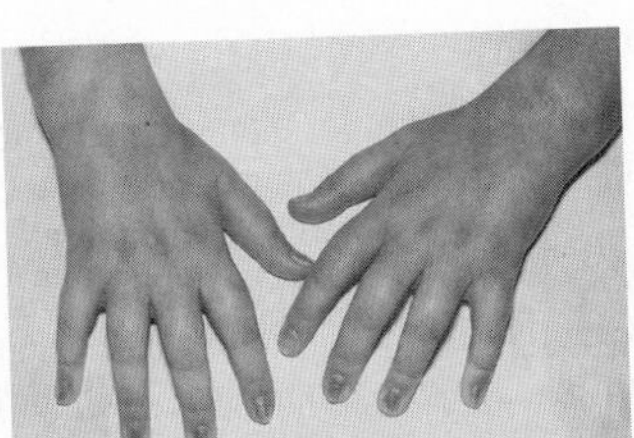

FIGURE 1-605 Sausage-shaped fingers in a patient with mixed connective tissue disease. An identical appearance may be found in patients with early scleroderma and eosinophilic fasciitis. (From Hochberg MC et al: *Rheumatology,* ed 5, St Louis, 2011, Mosby.)

ETIOLOGY

Autoimmune disorder

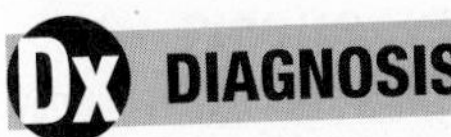

DIAGNOSIS

DIFFERENTIAL DIAGNOSIS

Other connective tissue disorders (SLE, progressive Scl, PM, infection, malignancy)

WORKUP

Table 1-340 summarizes diagnostic criteria.

Alarcon-Segovia: Serologic criterion accompanied by three or more clinical criteria, one of which must be synovitis or myositis (sensitivity 81.3%, specificity 86.2%).

Kahn: Serologic criterion accompanied by Raynaud's phenomenon and at least two of the three remaining clinical criteria.

LABORATORY TESTS

- Positive antinuclear antibody (ANA) speckled pattern often >1:1280 titer
- U1-RNP antibodies especially to the 68-70 kD antigen (high titers)
- SLE-specific autoantibodies are generally absent.
- Rheumatoid factor and anti-CCP positive (50% to 70%)

TABLE 1-340 Diagnostic Criteria by Alarcon-Segovia and Kahn

	Alarcon-Segovia Criteria	Kahn Criteria
Serology	Anti-RNP at hemagglutination titer of ≥1:1600	High-titer anti-RNP corresponding to a speckled ANA of ≥1:1200
Clinical	Swollen hands Synovitis Myositis Raynaud's phenomenon Acrosclerosis	Swollen fingers Synovitis Myositis Raynaud's phenomenon

TREATMENT

- Considered to be a steroid-responsive disease, especially features seen in SLE and myositis
- Aimed at the specific features of the overlap syndrome
- Arthralgias, arthritis, fatigue, myalgias usually respond to NSAIDs, antimalarials, and/or steroids. Immunosuppressive medications such as methotrexate and azathioprine can also be used
- Keeping warm, avoiding beta-blockers, smoking cessation, and dihydropiridine calcium channel blockers can be used for Raynaud's phenomenon
- Pulmonary hypertension and lung disease: Therapies include steroids, cyclophosphamide, low-dose aspirin, anticoagulation, ACE inhibitors, endothelin receptor antagonist, IV prostacyclin, cyclic GMP phosphodiesterase type 5 inhibitors like sildenafil, tadalafil, and mycophenolate mofetil.
- Calcium, vitamin D, and bisphosphonates are used for bone health

DISPOSITION

- Patients with high titers of U1-RNP antibodies have low prevalence of serious renal disease and life-threatening neurologic disorders.
- Disease-related mortality is usually related to pulmonary hypertension and its cardiac sequelae.

REFERRAL

Rheumatology consultation for clarification and assistance in treatment

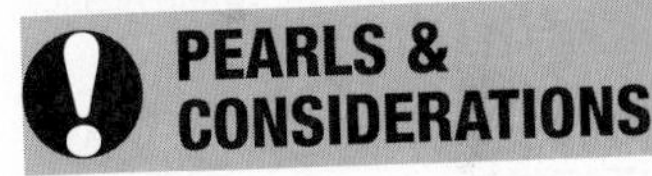

PEARLS & CONSIDERATIONS

COMMENTS

Pulmonary arterial hypertension (PAH) is diagnosed by cardiac catheterization. It is the main disease-related cause of death. Early detection of PAH and aggressive treatment may improve prognosis.

SUGGESTED READINGS

available at www.expertconsult.com

RELATED CONTENT

Scleroderma (Systemic Sclerosis) (Related Key Topic)

AUTHOR: **DANIEL E. MENDEZ-ALLWOOD, M.D.**

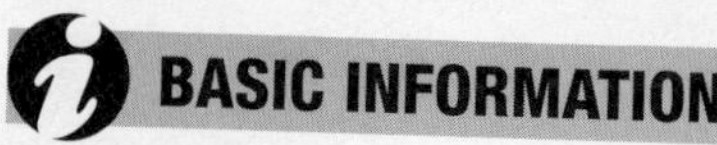

BASIC INFORMATION

DEFINITION

Molar pregnancy is a premalignant gestational disorder. Molar pregnancies are classified as complete or partial based on morphologic and pathologic examination. Both complete and partial molar pregnancies have an abnormal placenta with enlargement and swelling of the chorionic villi and hyperplasia of the villous trophoblastic cells. Most molar pregnancies are complete and are characterized by generalized hydropic villous changes with no fetal tissue. Partial moles are characterized by a mixture of large hydropic villi and normal placental tissue and often have fetal tissue present. The risk of malignant sequelae (gestational trophoblastic neoplasia) for a complete mole is 18% to 29% and for a partial mole is 0% to 11%.

SYNONYMS

Hydatidiform mole
Gestational trophoblastic disease

ICD-9CM CODES
630 Hydatidiform mole
ICD-10CM CODES
001.9 Hydatidiform mole, unspecified

EPIDEMIOLOGY & DEMOGRAPHICS

INCIDENCE: 0.57 to 2/1000 pregnancies with wide regional variation

PREDOMINANT SEX AND AGE: Females of reproductive age, highest rates at extremes of reproductive ages

RISK FACTORS: Extremes of reproductive age (<21 and >40 yr), previous molar pregnancy, history of spontaneous abortion

PHYSICAL FINDINGS & CLINICAL PRESENTATION

Complete molar pregnancy:
- 80% to 90% present with vaginal bleeding at 6 to 16 wk gestational age
- 28% with uterine enlargement greater than expected for gestational age
- 8% with hyperemesis gravidarum
- 1% with gestational hypertension in the first or second trimester
- 15% with bilateral theca lutein cysts
- 15% will have a beta hCG >100,000 mIU/ml

Partial molar pregnancy
- 90% present with an incomplete or missed abortion
- 75% present with vaginal bleeding
- <10% will have a beta hCG of >100,000 mIU/ml

ETIOLOGY

Complete molar pregnancy
- Fertilization of an oocyte with absent or inactive maternal chromosomes and duplication of paternal chromosomes (90% are 46, XX) or fertilization of an empty oocyte with 2 sperm (46, XY or XX)
- Uniform villous enlargement and no development of a fetus

Partial molar pregnancy
- Fertilization of a normal oocyte with 2 sperm (usually 69, XXY)
- Focal villous edema with identifiable fetus

Dx DIAGNOSIS

DIFFERENTIAL DIAGNOSIS

Complete mole, partial mole, ectopic pregnancy, abortion (incomplete or spontaneous), normal intrauterine pregnancy

WORKUP

- Pelvic exam to evaluate for uterine size and bleeding
- Blood pressure to assess for gestational hypertension or preeclampsia (systolic blood pressure >140 or diastolic blood pressure >90)

LABORATORY TESTS

- Quantitative beta human chorionic growth hormone (beta hCG); significantly elevated levels >100,000 will raise suspicion for molar pregnancy
- Complete blood count (CBC) to assess for acute anemia from vaginal bleeding
- Comprehensive metabolic panel to evaluate for renal or liver disease
- TSH to evaluate for hyperthyroidism
- Urinalysis for proteinuria to evaluate for pre-eclampsia
- Type and screen to evaluate Rh and to prepare for surgery

IMAGING STUDIES

- Pelvic ultrasound (Fig. 1-606)
  - Complete molar pregnancy will show diffuse vesicular changes with no evidence of fetal tissue and may show theca lutein cysts
  - Partial molar pregnancy will show focal cystic changes in the placenta and fetal tissue may be present
- Baseline chest x-ray to use for comparison if malignant trophoblastic disease develops

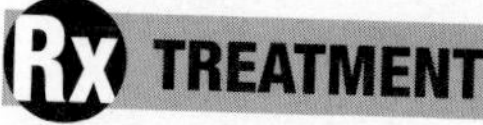

TREATMENT

NONPHARMACOLOGIC THERAPY

Surgical uterine evacuation with dilatation and curettage (D&C)

ACUTE GENERAL Rx

D&C, Rh immune globulin if Rh negative

CHRONIC Rx & DISPOSITION

If pathology results are consistent with complete or partial mole, patients must be followed to evaluate for trophoblastic neoplasia. 15% to 20% of complete moles and 1% to 5% of partial moles will develop into trophoblastic neoplasia. Quantitative beta hCG should be followed weekly until three consecutive results show normal levels. After that, check quantitative beta hCG every 3 mo for a total of 6 mo. Patients should remain on reliable contraception during this time to prevent confusion from a rising beta hCG in the case of a new pregnancy.

REFERRAL

- If there is concern for a molar pregnancy, the patient should be managed by a gynecologist for uterine evacuation and follow-up.
- If there is a plateau or rise of the beta hCG during follow-up, the patient should be referred to a gynecologic oncologist for treatment with chemotherapy.

SUGGESTED READINGS

available at www.expertconsult.com

RELATED CONTENT

Spontaneous Miscarriage (Related Key Topic)
Vaginal Bleeding During Pregnancy (Related Key Topic)

AUTHOR: **LAUREN ROTH, M.D.**

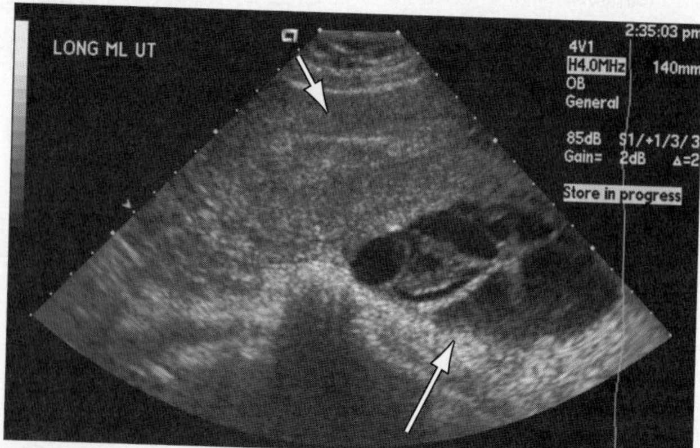

FIGURE 1-606 Endovaginal ultrasound of the theca lutein cyst with early molar pregnancy. Note enlarged anechoic cystic spaces within the ovary *(arrows)*. (From Fielding JR et al: *Gynecology imaging,* Philadelphia, 2011, Saunders.)

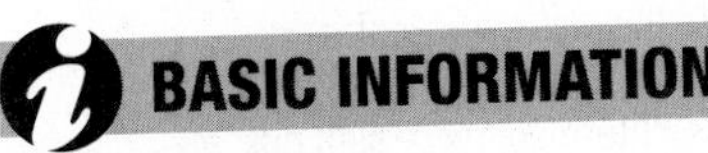

BASIC INFORMATION

DEFINITION

Molluscum contagiosum is a viral infection characterized by discrete skin lesions with central umbilication.

SYNONYMS

MC

ICD-9CM CODES
078.0 Molluscum contagiosum
ICD-10CM CODES
B08.1 Molluscum contagiosum

EPIDEMIOLOGY & DEMOGRAPHICS

- Molluscum contagiosum spreads by autoinoculation, scratching, or touching a lesion.
- It usually occurs in young children. It is also common in sexually active adults and patients with HIV infection.
- Incubation period varies between 4 and 8 wk.
- Spontaneous resolution in immunocompetent patients can occur after several months.

PHYSICAL FINDINGS & CLINICAL PRESENTATION

- The individual lesion appears initially as a small (2-3 mm), flesh-colored, firm, smooth-surfaced papule with subsequent central umbilication. Lesions are frequently grouped (Fig. 1-607). The size of each lesion generally varies from 2 to 6 mm in diameter.
- Typical distribution in children involves the face, extremities, and trunk. Mucous membranes are spared.

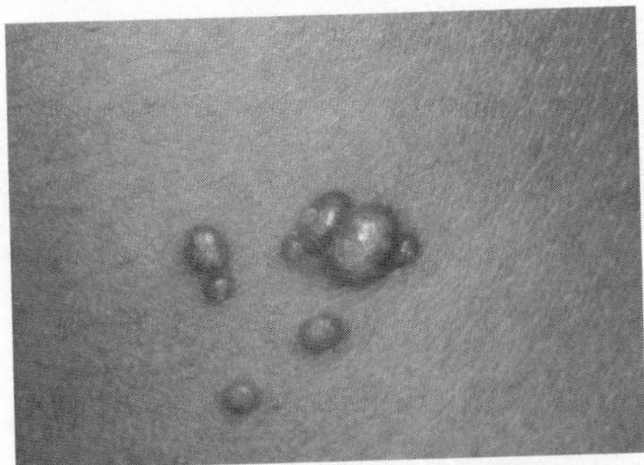

FIGURE 1-607 Grouped molluscum. (From Kliegman RM et al: *Nelson textbook of pediatrics*, ed 19, Philadelphia, 2011, Saunders.)

- Distribution in adults generally involves pubic and genital areas.
- Erythema and scaling at the periphery of the lesions may be present as a result of scratching or hypersensitivity reaction.
- Lesions are not present on the palms and soles.

ETIOLOGY

Viral infection of epithelial cells caused by a poxvirus, molluscum contagiosum

Dx DIAGNOSIS

Diagnosis is usually established by the clinical appearance of the lesions (distribution and central umbilication). A magnifying lens can be used to observe the central umbilication. If necessary, the diagnosis can be confirmed by removing a typical lesion with a curette and examining the content on a slide after adding potassium hydroxide and gentle heating. Staining with toluidine blue will identify viral inclusions.

DIFFERENTIAL DIAGNOSIS

- Verruca plana (flat warts): no central umbilication, not dome shaped, irregular surface, can involve palms and soles
- Herpes simplex: lesions become rapidly umbilicated
- Varicella: blisters and vesicles are present
- Folliculitis: no central umbilication, presence of hair piercing the pustule or papule
- Cutaneous cryptococcosis in AIDS patients: budding yeasts will be present on cytologic examination of the lesions
- Basal cell carcinoma: multiple lesions are absent
- Cellulitis

WORKUP

Careful examination of the papules

LABORATORY TESTS

Generally not indicated in children. Screening for other sexually transmitted diseases is recommended in all cases of genital molluscum contagiosum.

Rx TREATMENT

GENERAL THERAPY

- Therapy is individualized depending on number of lesions, immune status, and patient's age and preference.
- Observation for spontaneous resolution is reasonable in patients with few, small, nonirritated, and nonspreading lesions. Genital lesions should be treated in all sexually active patients.
- Liquid nitrogen cryotherapy
- Carbon dioxide laser
- Curettage after pretreatment of the area with combination prilocaine 2.5% with lidocaine 2.5% cream (EMLA) for anesthesia is useful for treatment of a few lesions. Curettage should be avoided in cosmetically sensitive areas because scarring may develop.
- Treatments with liquid nitrogen therapy in combination with curettage are effective in older patients who do not object to some discomfort.
- Application of cantharidin 0.7% to individual lesions covered with clear tape will result in blistering over 24 hr and possible clearing without scarring. This medication should be avoided on facial lesions.
- Other treatment measures include use of imiquimod cream or tretinoin 0.025% gel or 0.1% cream at bedtime, daily use of salicylic acid (Occlusal) at bedtime, and use of laser therapy.
- Trichloroacetic acid peel generally repeated every 2 wk for several weeks is useful in immunocompromised patients with extensive lesions.

DISPOSITION

Most patients respond well to the therapeutic modalities listed previously. Spontaneous resolution can occur after 6 to 9 mo in some immunocompetent patients.

REFERRAL

To dermatology when diagnosis is in doubt or in patients with extensive lesions

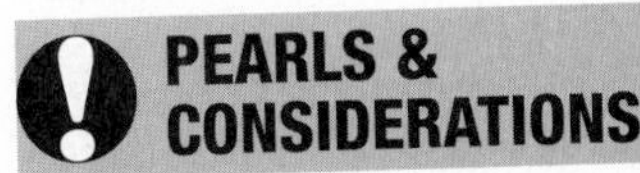

PEARLS & CONSIDERATIONS

COMMENTS

Genital molluscum contagiosum in children may be indicative of sexual abuse.

RELATED CONTENT

Molluscum Contagiosum (Patient Information)

AUTHOR: **FRED F. FERRI, M.D.**

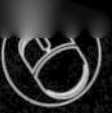

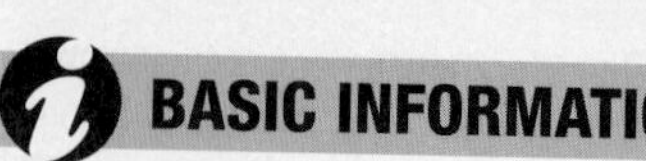

BASIC INFORMATION

DEFINITION

Monoclonal gammopathy of undetermined significance (MGUS) is defined by the presence of a monoclonal protein in persons with no features of multiple myeloma or other malignant gammopathies (Table 1-341). Patients with MGUS have a serum monoclonal protein concentration <3 g/dl, <10% plasma cells on the bone marrow, and no clinical manifestations related to the monoclonal gammopathy.

SYNONYMS

Non-IgM MGUS
IgM MGUS
Light chain MGUS

ICD-9CM CODES
273.1 Monoclonal gammopathy
ICD-10CM CODES
D47.2 Monoclonal gammopathy of undetermined significance (MGUS)

EPIDEMIOLOGY & DEMOGRAPHICS

INCIDENCE: The annual incidence of MGUS in men is 120 per 100,000 population at age 50 yr and increases to 530 per 100,000 at age 80 yr. The rates for women are 60 per 100,000 at 50 yr and 370 per 100,000 at 80 yr.
PREVALENCE: Prevalence is higher in blacks than in whites
PREDOMINANT SEX AND AGE: Median age of diagnosis is about 70 yr. Prevalence is higher in men than in women.
RISK FACTORS: Race (African American), older age, male sex, exposure to pesticides and family history of MGUS or multiple myeloma

PHYSICAL FINDINGS & CLINICAL PRESENTATION

- MGUS typically detected after a routine blood test reveals an elevated total protein concentration
- Asymptomatic
- Physical exam is normal

ETIOLOGY

- Unknown mechanism
- Characterized by a rearrangement of immunoglobulin genes that results in the production of a monoclonal protein

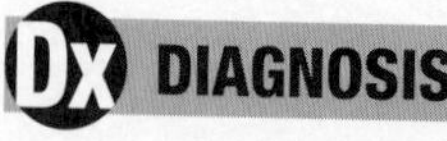

DIAGNOSIS

DIFFERENTIAL DIAGNOSIS

Smoldering myeloma (Table E1-342)
Multiple myeloma
Waldenström's gammaglobulinemia
Secondary monoclonal gammopathies
- Chronic liver disease
- Rheumatologic diseases
- Chronic myelomonocytic leukemia
- Chronic neutrophilic leukemia
- Lichen myxedematosus

Pyoderma gangrenosum

LABORATORY TESTS

Protein studies:
- Serum protein electrophoresis (Fig. 1-608)
  - IgG most common, followed by IgM and IgA
- 24-hour urine protein excretion and urine electrophoresis
- Serum and urine immunofixation
- Determination of serum free light chain ratio (kappa and lambda free light chains)

Hemoglobin
Serum calcium and creatinine
Examination of the bone marrow aspirate

IMAGING STUDIES

- Skeletal survey
- Bone mineral density resting at baseline (MGUS is associated with increased risk of osteoporosis)

Rx TREATMENT

International Myeloma Working Group Recommendation
1. Risk stratification
   - Abnormal free light chain ratio
   - Bone marrow plasma cells >10%
   - Serum M protein >3 g/dl

   1, 2, or 3 risk factors had 5-yr progression rates of 25%, 51%, and 76%, respectively; time to progression 10, 5.1, and 1.9 yr, respectively
2. Follow up by risk category
   - Low risk: every 2-3 yr
   - Intermediate or high risk: after diagnosis, reevaluation at 2-3 mo. If results are stable, re-evaluation every 4-6 mo for 1 yr. If results remain stable, reevaluation every 6-12 mo.

Reevaluation consists of:
- Total serum protein–serum electrophoresis
- 24-hour urine protein excretion
- Hemoglobin
- Serum creatinine and calcium

DISPOSITION

- Risk of myeloma at 25 yr is 30%.
- Annual risk of transformation to myeloma is 1% per year after diagnosis.

REFERRAL

To hematologist/oncologist for evaluation

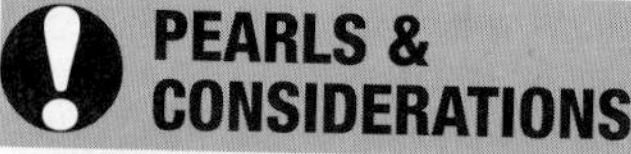

PEARLS & CONSIDERATIONS

- Approximately 55% of 70-yr-old patients diagnosed as having MGUS have had the condition for more than 10 yr.
- Most patients with MGUS should be monitored every 6 to 12 mo for signs and symptoms of progression.
- There is no indicated treatment.

SUGGESTED READINGS

available at www.expertconsult.com

AUTHOR: **KIMBERLY PEREZ, M.D.**

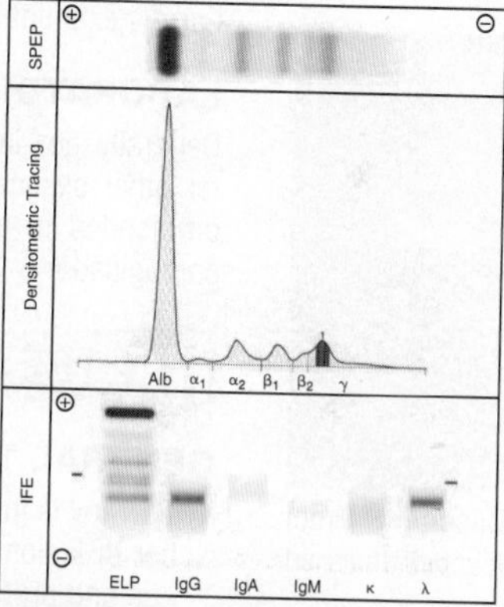

FIGURE 1-608 Serum electrophoresis from a 73-year-old man with monoclonal gammopathy of undetermined significance. The patient has no clinical, hematologic, or imaging evidence of a plasma cell dyscrasia, except for a persistent, modest (0.4 g/dl), single M protein peak on the densitometric tracing *(shaded area, middle panel)* of the serum protein electrophoresis pattern *(SPEP)*. The M protein was identified by immunofixation electrophoresis *(IFE)* as IgGλ, located in the β_2 region of the electrophoresis *(ELP)* pattern. (Courtesy Drs. Frank H. Wians Jr. and Dennis C. Wooten, Department of Pathology, University of Texas Southwestern Medical Center, Dallas. From Jaffe ES et al: *Hematopathology,* Philadelphia, 2011, Saunders.)

M

TABLE 1-341 Disease Definitions for the Monoclonal Gammopathies: MGUS and Related Disorders

Type of Monoclonal Gammopathy	Premalignancy with a Low Risk of Progression (1%-2% per year)	Premalignancy with a High Risk of Progression (10% per year)	Malignancy
IgG and IgA (non-IgM) monoclonal gammopathies*	**Non-IgM MGUS** All 3 criteria must be met: • Serum monoclonal protein <3 g/dl • Clonal bone marrow plasma cells <10%, and • Absence of end-organ damage such as hypercalcemia, renal insufficiency, anemia, and bone lesions (CRAB) that can be attributed to the plasma cell proliferative disorder	**Smoldering multiple myeloma** Both criteria must be met: • Serum monoclonal protein (IgG or IgA) ≥3 g/dl and/or clonal bone marrow plasma cells ≥10%, and • Absence of end-organ damage such as lytic bone lesions, anemia, hypercalcemia, or renal failure that can be attributed to a plasma cell proliferative disorder	**Multiple myeloma** All 3 criteria must be met except as noted: • Clonal bone marrow plasma cells ≥10% • Presence of serum and/or urinary monoclonal protein (except in patients with true nonsecretory multiple myeloma), and • Evidence of end-organ damage that can be attributed to the underlying plasma cell proliferative disorder, specifically ○ Hypercalcemia: serum calcium >11.5 mg/dL or ○ Renal insufficiency: serum creatinine >2 mg/dL or estimated creatinine clearance <40 mL/min ○ Anemia: normochromic, normocytic with a hemoglobin value of >2 g/dL below the lower limit of normal or a hemoglobin value <10 g/dL ○ Bone lesions: lytic lesions or severe osteopenia attributed to a plasma cell proliferative disorder or pathologic fractures
IgM monoclonal gammopathies	**IgM MGUS†** All 3 criteria must be met: • Serum monoclonal protein <3 g/dl • Clonal bone marrow lymphoplasmacytic cells <10%, and • Absence of end-organ damage such as anemia, constitutional symptoms, hyperviscosity, lymphadenopathy, or hepatosplenomegaly that can be attributed to the underlying lymphoproliferative disorder	**Smoldering Waldenström macroglobulinemia** Both criteria must be met: • Serum IgM monoclonal protein ≥3 g/dl and/or bone marrow lymphoplasmacytic infiltration ≥10%, and • No evidence of anemia, constitutional symptoms, hyperviscosity, lymphadenopathy, or hepatosplenomegaly that can be attributed to the underlying lymphoproliferative disorder	**Waldenström macroglobulinemia** All criteria must be met: • IgM monoclonal gammopathy (regardless of the size of the M-protein), and • ≥10% bone marrow lymphoplasmacytic infiltration (usually intertrabecular) by small lymphocytes that exhibit plasmacytoid or plasma cell differentiation and a typical immunophenotype (eg, surface IgM^+, $CD5^{+/-}$, $CD10^-$, $CD19^+$, $CD20^+$, $CD23^-$) that satisfactorily excludes other lymphoproliferative disorders including chronic lymphocytic leukemia and mantle cell lymphoma • Evidence of anemia, constitutional symptoms, hyperviscosity, lymphadenopathy, or hepatosplenomegaly that can be attributed to the underlying lymphoproliferative disorder. **IgM myeloma** All criteria must be met: • Symptomatic monoclonal plasma cell proliferative disorder characterized by a serum IgM monoclonal protein regardless of size • Presence of 10% plasma cells on bone marrow biopsy • Presence of lytic bone lesions related to the underlying plasma cell disorder and/or translocation t(11;14) on fluorescence in situ hybridization.
Light-chain monoclonal gammopathies	**Light-chain MGUS** All criteria must be met: • Abnormal FLC ratio (<0.26 or >1.65) • Increased level of the appropriate involved light-chain (increased kappa FLC in patients with ratio >1.65 and increased lambda FLC in patients with ratio <0.26) • No immunoglobulin heavy-chain expression on immunofixation • Clonal bone marrow plasma cells <10%, and • Absence of end-organ damage such as hypercalcemia, renal insufficiency, anemia, and bone lesions (CRAB) that can be attributed to the plasma cell proliferative disorder	**Idiopathic Bence Jones proteinuria** All criteria must be met: • Urinary monoclonal protein on urine protein electrophoresis ≥500 mg/24 h and/or clonal bone marrow plasma cells ≥10% • No immunoglobulin heavy-chain expression on immunofixation • Absence of end-organ damage such as hypercalcemia, renal insufficiency, anemia, and bone lesions (CRAB) that can be attributed to the plasma cell proliferative disorder	**Light-chain multiple myeloma†** • Same as multiple myeloma except no evidence of immunoglobulin heavy-chain expression

FLC, Free light chain; *MGUS*, monoclonal gammopathy of undetermined significance.
*Occasionally patients with IgD and IgE monoclonal gammopathies have been described and will be considered to be part of this category as well.
†Note that conventionally IgM MGUS is considered a subtype of MGUS, and similarly light-chain multiple myeloma is considered as a subtype of multiple myeloma. Unless specifically distinguished, when the terms MGUS and multiple myeloma are used in general, they include IgM MGUS and light-chain multiple myeloma, respectively.
From Rajkumar SV et al: Advances in the diagnosis, classification, risk stratification, and management of monoclonal gammopathy of undetermined significance: implications for recategorizing disease entities in the presence of evolving scientific evidence, *Mayo Clin Proc* 85(10):945-948, 2010.

BASIC INFORMATION

DEFINITION

Mononucleosis is a symptomatic infection caused by Epstein-Barr virus (EBV) and characterized by fever, tonsillar pharyngitis, and lymphadenopathy.

SYNONYMS

Infectious mononucleosis (IM)

ICD-9CM CODES
075 Infectious mononucleosis
ICD-10CM CODES
B27 Infections mononucleosis
B27.0 Gamma herpesviral mononucleosis
B27.1 Cytomegaloviral mononucleosis
B27.8 Other infectious mononucleosis
B27.9 Infectious mononucleosis

EPIDEMIOLOGY & DEMOGRAPHICS

INCIDENCE (IN U.S.): 500 cases/100,000 persons/yr

PREDOMINANT SEX: Incidence is the same, but occurs earlier in females.

PREDOMINANT AGE: Most common between the ages of 15 and 24 yr.

PHYSICAL FINDINGS & CLINICAL PRESENTATION

- Following an incubation period of 1 to 2 mo, a prodrome may occur, with fever, chills, malaise, and anorexia for several days. This is followed by the classic triad, which includes pharyngitis, fever, and adenopathy. Although fatigue and malaise may be prominent, pharyngitis is usually the most severe symptom. Exudates are common.
- Lymphadenopathy is most prominent in the cervical region but may be diffuse.
- Splenomegaly may occur, most commonly during the second wk of illness.
- Rash is uncommon but will occur in nearly all patients who receive ampicillin.
- At times, IM can present as fever and adenopathy without pharyngitis. Although complications may be severe, they are uncommon and tend to resolve completely. Involvement of the hematologic, pulmonary, cardiac, or nervous system may occur; splenic rupture is rare. IM is usually a self-limited illness, but symptoms of malaise and fatigue may last months before resolving.

ETIOLOGY

The cause of IM is primary infection with EBV. Primary infection during childhood causes few or no symptoms. Infection during childhood is more common in lower socioeconomic groups. The frequency of IM in late adolescence is attributed to the onset of social contact between the sexes. Close personal contact is usually necessary for transmission. Transfer via saliva while kissing may be responsible for many cases. Virus can persist in oropharynx of patients with IM for up to 18 mo. Transmission may also occur sexually as EBV can be isolated in cervical epithelial cells and male seminal fluid and can also be transmitted by blood transfusion.

DIAGNOSIS

DIFFERENTIAL DIAGNOSIS

- Heterophile-negative IM caused by cytomegalovirus (CMV); although clinical presentation may be similar, CMV more frequently follows transfusion
- Bacterial and viral causes of pharyngitis
- Toxoplasmosis
- Acute retroviral syndrome of HIV, lymphoma

WORKUP

Initial testing consists of heterophile antibody (monospot) and CBC with differential. Fig. E1-609 illustrates a diagnostic algorithm for EBV infection and IM.

LABORATORY TESTS

- Increased WBC is common, with a relative lymphocytosis and neutropenia. Atypical lymphocytes (Fig. E1-610) are the hallmark of IM, but are not pathognomonic. Mild thrombocytopenia is common. A falling hematocrit may signal splenic rupture or severe immune-mediated hemolytic anemia. Elevated hepatocellular enzymes and cryoglobulins occur in most cases. Heterophile antibody, as measured by the monospot test, may be positive at presentation, or may appear later in the course of illness. A negative test should be repeated if clinical suspicion is high. If this test remains negative for 8 wk, other causes of IM are likely. The monospot usually remains positive for 3 to 6 mo, but can last for 1 yr.
- A positive test has been reported with primary HIV infection.
- In addition to the heterophile antibody, virus-specific antibodies may result in response to IM. Determination of these EBV-specific antibodies is rarely necessary to diagnose IM, although early diagnosis in monospot negative cases may be made by isolating IgM to the viral capsid antigen, which is usually positive during the acute illness.

IMAGING STUDIES

Chest x-ray may rarely show infiltrates. An elevated left hemidiaphragm may occur in cases of splenic rupture.

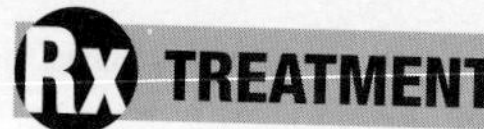

TREATMENT

NONPHARMACOLOGIC THERAPY

- Supportive rest is advocated by some, but effect on outcome is not clear.
- Splenectomy if rupture occurs; transfusions for severe anemia or thrombocytopenia

ACUTE GENERAL Rx

- Pharmacologic therapy is not indicated in uncomplicated illness.
- The use of steroids (Fig. E1-611) is suggested in patients who have severe thrombocytopenia or hemolytic anemia, or impending airway obstruction as a result of enlarged tonsils. Prednisone, 60 to 80 mg PO qid for 3 days, then tapered over 1 to 2 wk. There is no role for antiviral agents such as acyclovir in the management of IM.

CHRONIC Rx

A rare, chronic form of IM with persistent organ infection and inflammation has been described. This should not be confused with chronic fatigue syndrome, which is unrelated to EBV.

DISPOSITION

Eventual resolution of all symptoms is the rule.

REFERRAL

More than mild illness

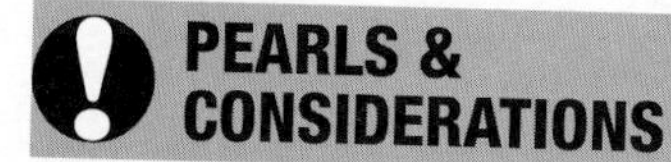

PEARLS & CONSIDERATIONS

COMMENTS

- Contact sports should be avoided during the first month of illness, because splenic rupture can occur, even in the absence of clinically detectable splenomegaly.
- Between 30% and 75% of college freshmen are seronegative for EBV. Each year nearly 20% of susceptible persons become infected and up to 50% of these persons develop IM.

SUGGESTED READINGS

available at www.expertconsult.com

RELATED CONTENT

Mononucleosis (Patient Information)

AUTHOR: **GLENN G. FORT, M.D., M.P.H.**

BASIC INFORMATION

DEFINITION

Morton neuroma is an entrapment neuropathy involving one of the common plantar digital nerves of the foot. This condition manifests as pain in the plantar aspect of the forefoot, often localized between the metatarsal heads.

SYNONYMS

Morton metatarsalgia
Morton toe
Interdigital neuroma
Plantar neuroma
Metatarsal neuralgia

ICD-9CM CODES
355.6 Morton's neuroma
ICD-10CM CODES
G57.6 Lesion of plantar nerve
G57.8 Other mononeuropathies of lower limb
G57.9 Mononeuropathy of lower limb, unspecified

EPIDEMIOLOGY & DEMOGRAPHICS

- Morton neuroma affects one of the common plantar digital nerves located at any of the four interspaces of the foot.
  - It most commonly affects the third common plantar digital proper nerve, located in the third interspace.
  - It occurs most frequently in patients who wear tight-fitting, high-heeled shoes.
- Morton neuroma is usually unilateral.
- The condition occurs most frequently in women.
- It usually presents between the fourth and sixth decade of life.

PHYSICAL FINDINGS & CLINICAL PRESENTATION

- Patients with Morton neuroma will present complaining of pain to the plantar aspect of the foot, typically localized between the metatarsal heads of the affected interspace.
- The pain may be described as stabbing, burning, tingling, or "electric" and may radiate to the digits.
- The pain is exacerbated by the use of tight-fitting shoes. The typical indication of a Morton neuroma is the patient's desire to remove shoes and rub the forefoot.
- The pain can often be recreated by applying pressure at the plantar aspect of the inter space, starting just proximal to the metatarsal heads and proceeding distally.
- Mulder's sign: Compression of the forefoot at the level of the metatarsophalangeal joints, combined with plantar pressure at the affected interspace, elicits a palpable "click."

ETIOLOGY

- Morton neuroma is considered to be an entrapment neuropathy of the affected common digital plantar nerve. The etiology remains obscure.
- The common plantar digital nerves are branches of the medial plantar nerve, coursing distally to supply the digits of the foot, passing just beneath the deep transverse intermetatarsal ligament. The third common plantar nerve is often supplied by a communicating branch of the lateral plantar nerve. This anatomic variation results in a thicker nerve that is more prone to trauma, a reason often cited to explain the prevalence of Morton neuroma in the third common plantar digital nerve.
- The deep transverse intermetatarsal ligament may also be implicated in the cause of a neuroma. If it is thickened or has aberrant bands, it may cause compression of the affected nerve.
- Soft tissue masses, such as a plantar lipoma, may also cause compression of the nerve against the ligament, leading to the formation of a neuroma.
- Histologic examination of resected Morton neuroma exhibits increased neural width, demyelination, intraneural fibrosis, and thickened endoneural capillaries.

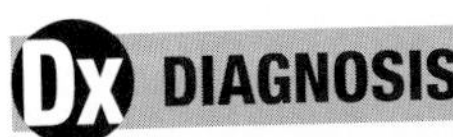

DIAGNOSIS

The diagnosis of Morton neuroma is primarily a clinical diagnosis. Laboratory tests and imaging modalities are generally not necessary for diagnosis.

DIFFERENTIAL DIAGNOSIS

- Peripheral neuropathy
- Tarsal tunnel syndrome
- Metatarsal stress fracture
- Freiberg's infraction
- Metatarsophalangeal joint capsulitis
- Osteoarthritis
- Rheumatoid arthritis

WORKUP

Exclude other causes mentioned in "Differential Diagnosis".

LABORATORY TESTS

There is no specific laboratory study that can be used to diagnose Morton neuroma.

IMAGING STUDIES

- Weight-bearing radiographs may be performed to exclude other pathologic conditions.
- MRI may be used to detect and localize a neuroma. The mass is best visualized on a T1-weighted image.
  - MRI is best for patients with recurrent neuromas and atypical symptoms.
  - Ultrasound imaging can be used to visualize a neuroma. It will typically present as a hypoechoic mass.

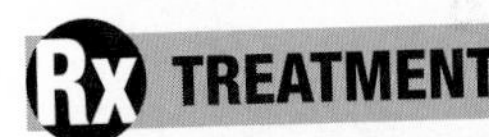

TREATMENT

NONPHARMACOLOGIC THERAPY

- Altering footwear is the first line of treatment.
- Wide shoes with a low heel are recommended.
- A metatarsal pad may also provide relief, as it splays the metatarsal heads, thereby decreasing the pressure on the neuroma.
- If adequate relief is noted with the above, then orthotics may also be considered.

ACUTE GENERAL Rx

- If conservative measures are unsuccessful, other treatment options include serial injections (Fig. 1-612) with corticosteroids or a sclerosing agent. The sclerosing solution is commonly composed of bupivacaine and ethyl alcohol. Recent trials[1] showed that corticosteroid injection is a reasonable temporizing intervention for some patients with Morton neuroma. Pain relief was, however,

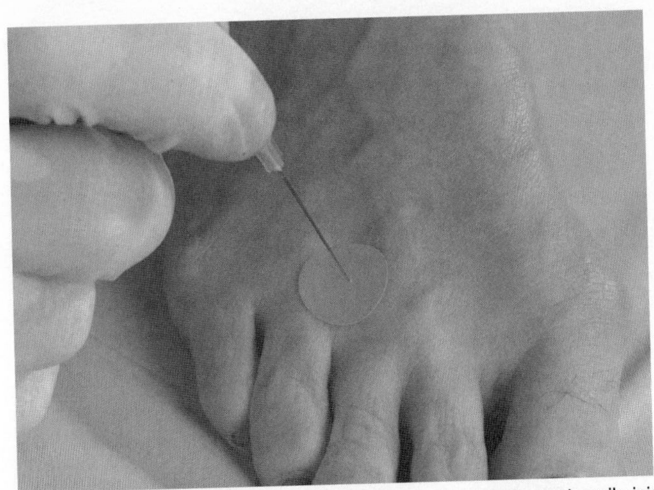

FIGURE 1-612 Injection for interdigital (Morton) neuroma. The area is most easily injected from the dorsal aspect, usually between the metatarsal heads of the third and fourth toes. The area of tenderness is marked, the needle is inserted to 1 inch, and steroid with anesthetic is injected. (From Firestein GS et al: *Kelly's textbook of rheumatology*, ed 9, Philadelphia, 2013, Saunders.)

[1]Thomson CE et al: Methylprednisolone injections for the treatment of Morton neuroma: a patient-blinded randomized trial, *J Bone Joint Surg Am* P5:790, 2013.

limited, and one third of steroid recipients underwent surgery at some point after 3 mo.
- Nonsteroidal anti-inflammatory agents may also provide relief.

CHRONIC Rx

- If conservative treatment fails to provide a resolution to symptoms, then surgical intervention should be considered.
- Surgical excision of the neuroma is performed in an operating room under monitored anesthesia care.
- Possible complications of surgery include hematoma formation, numbness, infection, and recurrent neuroma.

DISPOSITION

- Following surgery, patients are often placed on a partial weight-bearing status to the affected foot. Sutures are removed 2 to 3 weeks following the initial surgery. Patients generally return to their previous activity level in 4 to 6 weeks.
- Should a neuroma recur, a second surgical procedure may be performed.

REFERRAL

If surgery is being considered, a consultation with either a podiatrist or a foot and ankle specialized orthopedic surgeon is indicated.

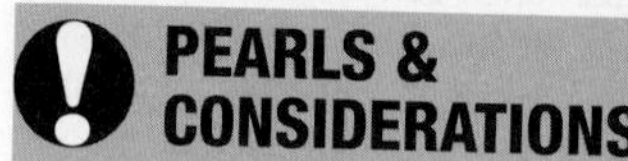

PEARLS & CONSIDERATIONS

COMMENTS

- Dr. Thomas G. Morton is given credit for describing this disorder in 1876.
- Morton neuroma may occur in any of the four interspaces of the foot but most commonly affects the third interspace.
- If conservative treatment and serial injections fail, surgery should be considered for the excision of the neuroma.

SUGGESTED READINGS

available at www.expertconsult.com

RELATED CONTENT

Morton's Neuroma (Patient Information)

AUTHOR: **NATHALIA DOOBAY, D.P.M.**

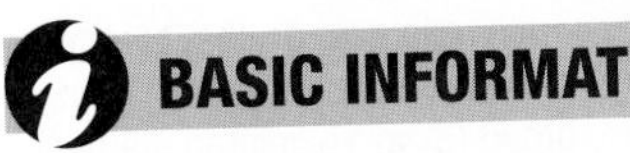

BASIC INFORMATION

DEFINITION

Motion sickness is a clinical syndrome associated with motion or perception of motion. Patients with motion sickness suffer perspiration, nausea, vomiting, increased salivation, and generalized malaise in response to movement.

SYNONYMS

Physiologic vertigo

ICD-9CM CODES
994.6 Motion sickness
ICD-10CM CODES
T75.3 Motion sickness

EPIDEMIOLOGY & DEMOGRAPHICS

INCIDENCE (IN U.S.): Common
PEAK INCIDENCE: Any age
PREVALENCE (IN U.S.): Common
PREDOMINANT SEX: Male = female
PREDOMINANT AGE: Any age
GENETICS: Not known to be genetic

PHYSICAL FINDINGS & CLINICAL PRESENTATION

- Vomiting
- Sweating
- Pallor

ETIOLOGY

- Motion (e.g., amusement rides, rides in automobiles or planes)
- Exacerbated by anxiety, fumes (e.g., industrial pollutants), visual stimuli

Dx DIAGNOSIS

DIFFERENTIAL DIAGNOSIS

- Acute labyrinthitis
- Gastroenteritis
- Metabolic disorders
- Viral syndrome

WORKUP

None necessary in routine case

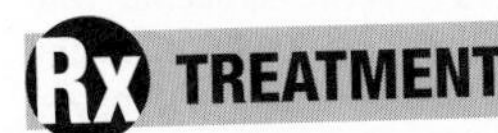

TREATMENT

NONPHARMACOLOGIC THERAPY

- Fixate on far object
- Cease motion
- Avoid reading
- Avoid alcohol

ACUTE GENERAL Rx

- Scopolamine patch is most effective. It should be applied to a hairless area behind the ear every 3 days prn. It should be applied >4 hr before antiemetic effect is required.
- Over-the-counter oral preparations (e.g., Dramamine) are less effective.
- Meclizine 12.5 to 25 mg q6h may be effective.

CHRONIC Rx

- Rarely chronic
- Symptoms generally resolve completely with cessation of motion exposure.

DISPOSITION

Follow-up is not needed.

REFERRAL

If another diagnosis is suspected (e.g., purulent ear, fever, cranial nerve abnormalities)

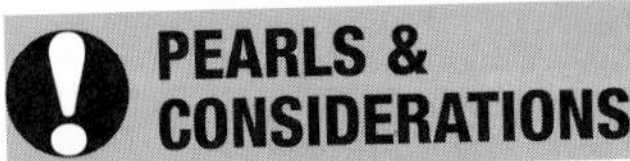

PEARLS & CONSIDERATIONS

COMMENTS

- Many patients with migraine report having had severe motion sickness as a child.
- Improved ventilation, avoidance of large meals before travel, semirecumbent sitting, and avoidance of reading while in motion will minimize the risk of motion sickness.

SUGGESTED READINGS

available at www.expertconsult.com

RELATED CONTENT

Motion Sickness (Patient Information)

AUTHOR: **FRED F. FERRI, M.D.**

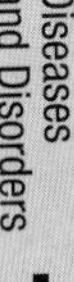

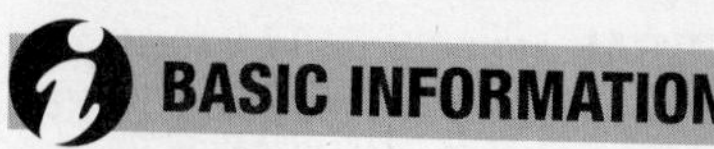

BASIC INFORMATION

DEFINITION

Mucormycosis is a fungal infection by Zygomycetes fungi and includes species in the order Mucorales (*Rhizopus* sp., *Rhizomucor, Cunninghamella, Apophysomyces, Saksenaea, Absidia, Syncephalastrum, Cokeromyces, Mortierella*) and in the order Entomophthorales (*Conidiobolus* and *Basidiobolus*).

ICD-9CM CODES
117.7 Mucormycosis
ICD-10CM CODES
B46.5 Mucormycosis, unspecified
B46.1 Rhinocerebral mucormycosis
B46.0 Pulmonary mucormycosis
B46.3 Cutaneous mucormycosis
B46.4 Disseminated mucormycosis

EPIDEMIOLOGY & DEMOGRAPHICS

- These fungi are ubiquitous in nature and can be found in soil and decaying vegetation. Infection is seen in association with underlying conditions, including diabetes mellitus especially with ketoacidosis, hematologic malignancies, stem cell or solid organ transplants, severe burns or trauma, treatment with deferoxamine or iron overload states, steroid treatment, immunodeficiency states (e.g., AIDS), injection drug use, and malnutrition. Immunocompetent hosts may become infected in tropical climates.
- The fungus gains entry to the body most commonly through the respiratory tract. The spores are deposited in the nasal turbinates and may be inhaled into the pulmonary alveoli. In cases of cutaneous mucormycosis, the spores are introduced directly into the skin lesion.
- After a tornado with winds >200 mph struck Joplin, Missouri, in May 2011, there were 13 confirmed cases of mucormycosis *(Apophysomyces trapeziformis),* including five deaths. While two patients had diabetes, none were immunocompromised. It was felt that the fungus entered through wounds sustained during the tornado. Wooden splinters were found in four patients.

PHYSICAL FINDINGS & CLINICAL PRESENTATION

- Rhinocerebral-rhinoorbital-paranasal syndrome may present with fever, facial and orbital pain, headache, diplopia, loss of vision, facial or orbital cellulitis, facial anesthesia, cranial nerve dysfunction, black nasal discharge, epistaxis, and seizure. Physical findings in this situation include proptosis; chemosis; nasal, palatal, or pharyngeal necrotic ulcerations; and retinal infarction. Thrombosis of the cavernous sinus or internal carotid artery may occur. This form of mucormycosis is found most commonly in diabetics, primarily in the presence of acidosis, and in patients with leukemia and neutropenia.
- Pulmonary mucormycosis can present with pneumonia, lung abscess, pulmonary infarction, pleurisy, pleural effusion, hemoptysis, chills, and fever. This form of mucormycosis is found most commonly in immunocompromised neutropenic hosts after chemotherapy for hematologic malignancies.
- Gastrointestinal zygomycosis presents with abdominal pain, diarrhea, gastrointestinal hemorrhage, ulcers, peritonitis, and bowel infarction. This form of mucormycosis is found most commonly in patients with extreme malnutrition and is believed to arise from ingestion of spores of the fungi.
- Cutaneous zygomycosis presents as nodular lesions (hematogenous seeding) or a wound infection. It primarily involves the epidermis and dermis after use of occlusive dressings that have not been properly sterilized.
- Cardiac mucormycosis is a form of endocarditis.
- Septic arthritis and osteomyelitis
- Brain abscess occurs most often from extension of the fungus from the nose or paranasal sinuses through adjacent bones in severely debilitated patients.
- Disseminated zygomycosis (rare but uniformly fatal)
- Physical findings depend on the location of the infection.

ETIOLOGY & PATHOGENESIS

The cause of mucormycosis is infection by a fungus of the Zygomycetes class (see "Definition"). Normal host defenses include leukocytes and pulmonary macrophages. Quantitative (e.g., neutropenia) or qualitative (e.g., diabetes mellitus or steroid treatment) disruption in the host defenses predisposes the patient to infection.

Dx DIAGNOSIS

The hallmark of mucormycosis is infarction and necrosis of host tissues that result from invasion of the vasculature by the fungal elements. Black eschars and discharges should be closely evaluated. Diagnosis depends on the demonstration of the organism in the tissue of a biopsy specimen.

DIFFERENTIAL DIAGNOSIS

- Infection of the sites described previously by other organisms (bacterial [including tuberculosis and leprosy], viral, fungal, or protozoan)
- Noninfectious tissue necrosis (e.g., neoplasia, vasculitis, degenerative) of the sites described previously

WORKUP

- Biopsy of infected tissue with direct-light microscopy examination establishes the diagnosis within minutes of the biopsy in the case of nasopharyngeal infection. Fungal hyphae are broad (5- to 15-micron diameter) and irregularly branched and have rare septations, in contrast to molds such as *Aspergillus,* which are narrower, have regular branching, and have many septations.
- Bronchoalveolar lavage or bronchoscopy with biopsy for smear, culture, and histologic examination
- Radiographs and other imaging studies such as CT of symptomatic sites may be required before infection is suspected and tissue specimens are obtained.

Rx TREATMENT

Aggressive correction of underlying disease (e.g., hyperglycemia, high steroid doses, use of immunosuppressive drugs) should be undertaken.

Standard therapy consists of aggressive surgical debridement of involved tissues and antifungal therapy. For invasive mucormycosis recommended treatment is with a lipid formulation of amphotericin B that allows higher doses with less nephrotoxicity. The start dose is 5 mg/kg of liposomal amphotericin B or amphotericin B lipid complex. Doses as high as 10 mg/kg have also been used.

Traditional amphotericin B given IV at a daily dose of 1.0 to 1.5 mg/kg infused over 2 to 4 hr daily for a total of 1 to 4 g can also still be used, but are associated with significant nephrotoxicity and adverse reactions such as fever, chills, myalgias, vomiting, and electrolyte disturbances.

- Other antifungals do not appear to be effective except possibly posaconazole, which may serve as an oral step-down therapy after amphotericin B at a dose of 400 mg bid with a fatty meal.
- Some studies suggest that caspofungin with amphotericin B may be synergistic for *Rhizopus oryzae* infections only.
- The role of colony-stimulating factors remains unclear, beyond that of increasing the neutrophil count in patients with neutropenia.
- Hyperbaric oxygen has been used in some patients but its utility in therapy is still not clear.

PROGNOSIS

- Sinus infection with no underlying disease: 75% survival
- Sinus infection with diabetes: 60% survival
- Sinus infection with renal disease: 25% survival

SUGGESTED READINGS
available at www.expertconsult.com

AUTHOR: **GLENN G. FORT, M.D., M.P.H.**

BASIC INFORMATION

DEFINITION

These are gram-negative bacteria that are resistant to at least one antimicrobial in three or more antimicrobial classes (antipseudomonal penicillins, third-generation cephalosporins, fluoroquinolones, carbapenems, and aminoglycosides).

SYNONYMS

CRE: carbapenam-resistant Enterobacteriaceae
ESBL: extended-spectrum beta-lactamases
MDR-GNB: multidrug-resistant gram-negative bacilli
MDRO: multidrug-resistant organisms
NDM-1: New Delhi metallo-beta-lactamase-1

ICD-9CM CODES
V09.9 Infection with drug-resistant microorganisms, unspecified
V09.1 Infection with microorganisms resistant to cephalosporins and other beta-lactam antibiotics
ICD-10CM CODES
Z16.30 Resistance to unspecified antimicrobial drugs
Z16.10 Resistance to unspecified beta lactam antibiotics

EPIDEMIOLOGY & DEMOGRAPHICS

INCIDENCE: There is an increasing incidence of these bacteria in hospitals and long-term care facilities in the U.S. and around the world. ESBL bacteria were first discovered in Europe in 1984 and in the U.S. in 1988. CRE bacteria were first described in the late 1990s in the U.S. The NDM-1 bacteria were first noted in 2009 in Sweden in a patient from India.

PREDOMINANT SEX AND AGE: These bacteria can be seen in any age group. They may be more frequent in women due to increased risk of urinary tract sepsis.

RISK FACTORS: In general, these bacteria are more common in hospitals and long-term care facilities, but they are spread nosocomially through patient care and thus are now entering the community, where the incidence is also increasing. Specific risk factors include:
- Length of stay in the hospital
- Length of ICU stay
- Use of central line catheters
- Abdominal surgery
- Presence of gastrostomy or jejunostomy tube
- Prior administration of any antibiotic
- Prior residence in a long-term care facility
- Presence of indwelling urinary catheter

ETIOLOGY

- Several different classes of MDR-GNRs exist based on their resistance mechanism.
  1. ESBL: These bacteria contain enzymes that break open the beta-lactam ring of penicillins, cephalosporins, and aztreonam and thus inactivate antibiotics from those classes. Enzymes conferring resistance include:
     - TEM beta-lactamases
     - SHV beta-lactamases
     - CTX-M beta lactamases
     - OXA beta-lactamases

     These enzymes are plasmid-mediated and thus can spread from one gram-negative bacteria to another, causing outbreaks in a single institution.
  2. CRE: Enzymes conferring resistance include:
     - Class A beta-lactamases: encoded on chromosomes or plasmids (e.g., *Klebsiella pneumoniae* carbapenamase [KPC], which has caused outbreaks in hospitals around the world)
     - Class B: metallo-beta-lactamases (e.g., New Delhi metallo-beta-lactamase-1). Encoded on a mobile plasmid that can spread to other gram-negative bacteria.
     - Class C and Class D beta-lactamases
- *Stenotrophomonas maltophilia*: MDR-GNR that acts as an opportunistic pathogen among mostly hospitalized patients with high morbidity and mortality. It has intrinsic or acquired resistance mechanisms to multiple antibiotic classes and has the ability to adhere to foreign materials and form a biofilm, which escapes host defenses.
- *Acinetobacter* sp. (e.g., *Acinetobacter baumannii*): strains have emerged that are resistant to all commercially available antibiotics. These bacteria have the capability to acquire diverse mechanisms of resistance including:
  - AmpC beta-lactamases
  - Beta-lactamases: serine and metallo-beta-lactamases

CLINICAL PRESENTATION

All these resistant bacteria have the capability of causing diverse infections, including
- Pneumonia
- Bacteremia
- Urinary tract sepsis
- Central line–associated infections
- Ventilator-associated pneumonia (VAP)
- Surgical site infections

VAP from *A. baumannii* now accounts for 8.4% of GNR pneumonias in the ICU.

DIAGNOSIS

DIFFERENTIAL DIAGNOSIS

Other gram-negative rods such as:
- *Pseudomonas aeruginosa*
- *Klebsiella pneumoniae* that are not ESBL or CRE by resistance pattern
- *Morganella morgani*
- *Providencia, Proteus* sp., *Serratia*

WORKUP

Detection of ESBL and CRE bacteria can pose problems for the clinical microbiology laboratory:
1. To detect ESBL bacteria: automated systems such as Vitek use disk diffusion or broth dilution techniques, or double disk test or E-test strip with clavulanate
2. To detect CRE: modified Hodge test to detect carbapenamase-producing bacteria
3. In 2010, testing guidelines with respect to susceptibility involving several beta-lactam antibiotics were changed to better identify these bacteria via automated systems.

LABORATORY TESTS

Clinical testing is the same in infections from these resistant organisms as with nonresistant organisms:
- Cultures of any wounds, blood, sputum, urine, catheter tips
- CBC, liver function tests, urinalysis

IMAGING STUDIES

Studies depend on the clinical presentation but are similar to those for nonresistant bacteria causing infections.

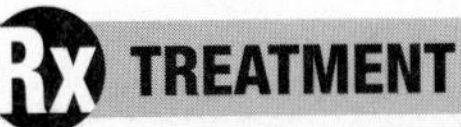

TREATMENT

Because of multidrug resistance, only a few reliable antibiotics are available to treat these infections.
1. ESBL bacteria: carbapenem antibiotics such as imipenem, meropenem, ertapenem, or the cephalosporin cefoxitin or tigecycline.
2. CRE bacteria: selection of antibiotic will depend on testing but tigecycline may be used clinically. Other alternatives include:
   - IV colistin
   - *Stenotrophomonas maltophilia:* only available agents are Bactrim (drug of choice), levaquin, and minocycline
   - *A. baumannii:* will depend on susceptibility testing, but ampicillin-sulbactam, imipenem or meropenem, or tigecycline can be used for MDR strains. For pan-resistant strains, IV colistin ± rifampin can be used. Inhaled colistin can be used for pneumonia patients.

DISPOSITION

Morbidity and mortality can be quite high with infections from these MDR bacteria.
1. Nosocomial *Acinetobacter* pneumonia carries a mortality rate of 35% to 70%.
2. *Stenotrophomonas* infections carry a mortality rate of 21% to 69%.
3. ESBL infections carry a mortality rate of 3.7% despite therapy with carbapenem antibiotics.

REFERRAL

- Infectious diseases specialist for selection of best antibiotic choice and follow-up
- Microbiologist for specialized testing and interpretation of results
- Pulmonary specialist for severe forms of pneumonia
- Infection control officer to help prevent spread of these bacteria in an institution

SUGGESTED READINGS

available at www.expertconsult.com

AUTHOR: **GLENN G. FORT, M.D., M.P.H.**

Multifocal Atrial Tachycardia 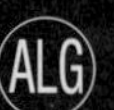 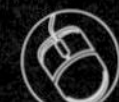

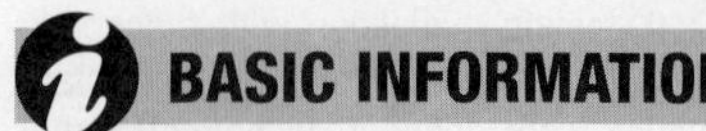

BASIC INFORMATION

DEFINITION

Multifocal atrial tachycardia (MAT) is a supraventricular, tachyarrhythmia (rate greater than 100 beats/min) with P waves having at least three or more different morphologies and irregular P-P intervals. An isoelectric baseline further differentiates MAT from atrial fibrillation or atrial flutter. Each P wave is thought to originate from a different atrial focus.

SYNONYMS

Chaotic atrial rhythm

Chronic atrial tachycardia

Repetitive multifocal paroxysmal atrial tachycardia

The term *wandering pacemaker* is used for a similar arrhythmia associated with a normal or slow heart rate (<100 beats/min).

ICD-9CM CODES
427.89 Multifocal atrial tachycardia
ICD-10CM CODES
I47.1 Supraventricular tachycardia

EPIDEMIOLOGY & DEMOGRAPHICS

Estimated prevalence in hospitalized patients of 0.05% to 0.32%. Average age is 70s. Usually associated with underlying pulmonary disease with right atrial electromechanical delay. Chronic obstructive pulmonary disease (COPD) is present in approximately 55% of patients with MAT.

PHYSICAL FINDINGS & CLINICAL PRESENTATION

Symptoms:
- Palpitation
- Lightheadedness
- Syncope
- Symptoms of the underlying pulmonary disease
- Physical findings associated with the underlying pulmonary disease

ETIOLOGY

- Exact mechanism unknown
- Exacerbated by underlying pulmonary disease (COPD, hypoxia, pulmonary embolism, pneumonia), cardiac disease, hypercarbia, acidosis, electrolyte disturbances, digitalis toxicity

DIAGNOSIS

DIFFERENTIAL DIAGNOSIS

- Atrial fibrillation
- Atrial flutter with variable AV conduction
- Sinus tachycardia
- Paroxysmal atrial tachycardia
- Extrasystole

WORKUP

- ECG (Fig. 1-613)
- Chest x-ray
- Pulmonary function tests
- Electrolytes
- Arterial blood gases
- Digoxin level (if patient on digoxin)

TREATMENT

- Correction and/or improvement in the underlying pulmonary or metabolic dysfunction if possible and avoiding drugs such as digoxin, theophylline, etc.
- Electrolyte repletion, especially magnesium and potassium
- Calcium channel blockers
- β-blockers are typically contraindicated by obstructive lung disease or acute heart failure
- If the arrhythmia is asymptomatic, it can be left untreated
- Direct current cardioversion is ineffective
- No significant role for antiarrhythmics
- In extreme cases of refractory MAT in symptomatic patients who cannot tolerate medical therapy or in MAT resistant to medical therapy, AV nodal ablation with pacemaker implantation has been performed.

SUGGESTED READINGS
available at www.expertconsult.com

RELATED CONTENT

Fig. 3-138 Algorithm for evaluating patients with symptoms of palpitation, dizziness, or syncope (Algorithm)

Fig. 3-185 Stepwise approach to the diagnosis of type of tachycardia based on 12-lead electrocardiogram during the episode (Algorithm)

Fig. 3-186 Evaluation and management of narrow complex tachycardia (Algorithm)

AUTHOR: **BARRY FINE, M.D., PH.D**

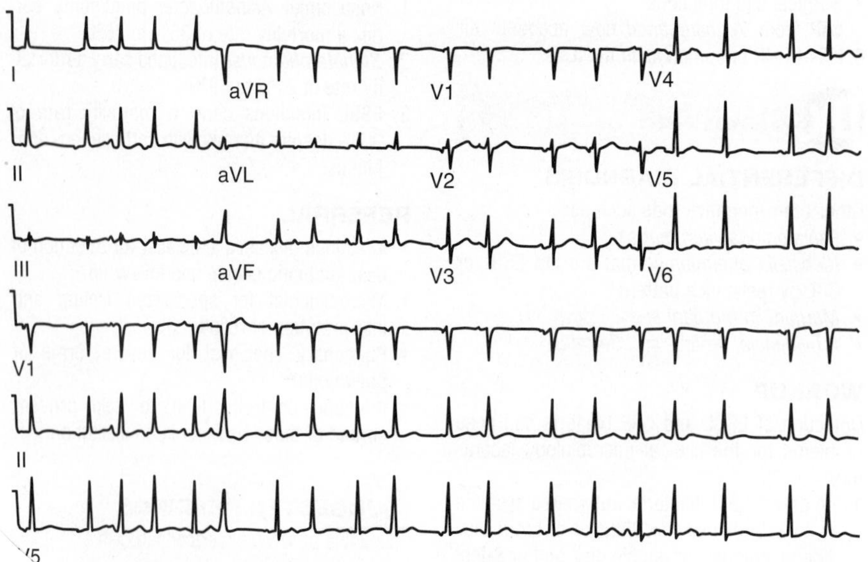

E 1-613 Surface ECG of multifocal atrial tachycardia. Note the varying morphology of the P waves [illegible] intervals. (From Issa Z et al: *Clinical arrhythmology and electrophysiology*, ed 2, Philadelphia, 2012,

BASIC INFORMATION

DEFINITION

Multiple myeloma is a malignancy of plasma cells characterized by clonal proliferation of malignant plasma cells in the bone marrow, monoclonal protein in the blood or urine, and associated organ dysfunction. Diagnostic criteria require the following:

1. Presence of ≥10% plasma cells on examination of the bone marrow (or biopsy of a tissue with monoclonal plasma cells).
2. Monoclonal protein in the serum or urine. Occasional patients without detectable monoclonal protein are considered to have nonsecretory myeloma.
3. Evidence of end-organ damage (***c***alcium elevation, ***r***enal insufficiency, ***a***nemia, or ***b***one lesions [CRAB]).

ICD-9CM CODES
203.0 Multiple myeloma
ICD-10CM CODES
C90.0 Multiple myeloma

EPIDEMIOLOGY & DEMOGRAPHICS

ANNUAL INCIDENCE: Five cases/100,000 persons (blacks affected twice as frequently as whites, males more than females); multiple myeloma accounts for 10% of all hematologic cancers. It is the most common primary bone malignancy. More than 20,000 new cases are diagnosed annually in the United States.

PREDOMINANT AGE: Peak incidence is in the seventh decade at a median age of 70 yr.

PHYSICAL FINDINGS & CLINICAL PRESENTATION

The patient usually comes to medical attention because of one or more of the following:

- Bone pain (58%) (back, thorax) or pathologic fractures (30%) caused by osteolytic lesions
- Fatigue (32%) or weakness because of anemia from bone marrow infiltration with plasma cells
- Recurrent infections as a result of impaired neutrophil function and deficiency of normal immunoglobulins
- Nausea and vomiting caused by constipation and uremia
- Delirium resulting from hypercalcemia
- Neurologic complications, such as spinal cord or nerve root compression, blurred vision from hyperviscosity
- Pallor and generalized weakness from anemia
- Purpura, epistaxis from thrombocytopenia
- Evidence of infections from impaired immune system
- Paresthesias (5%), weight loss (24%)
- Swelling on ribs, vertebrae, and other bones

DIAGNOSIS

DIFFERENTIAL DIAGNOSIS

- Metastatic carcinoma
- Lymphoma (B-cell non-Hodgkin lymphoma)
- Bone neoplasms (e.g., sarcoma)
- Monoclonal gammopathy of undetermined significance
- Primary amyloidosis
- Chronic lymphocytic leukemia
- Waldenström's macroglobulinemia
- Figure E1-614 describes a diagnostic approach to multiple myeloma

LABORATORY TESTS

- Normochromic, normocytic anemia; rouleaux formation on peripheral smear (Fig. 1-615)
- Hypercalcemia is present in 15% of patients at diagnosis.
- Elevated blood urea nitrogen, creatinine, uric acid, and total protein
- Urine protein immunoelectrophoresis: proteinuria from overproduction and secretion of free monoclonal kappa or lambda chains (Bence Jones protein)
- Serum protein immunoelectrophoresis: tall homogeneous monoclonal spike (M spike) on protein immunoelectrophoresis in approximately 75% of patients (Fig. 1-616); decreased levels of normal immunoglobulins (Ig)
    1. The increased immunoglobulins are generally IgG (75%) and IgA (15%).
    2. Approximately 17% of patients have a flat level of immunoglobulins but increased light chains in the urine by electrophoresis.
    3. A small percentage (<2%) of patients have nonsecreting myeloma (no increase in immunoglobulins and no light chains in the urine) but have other evidence of the disease (e.g., positive bone marrow examination).
- Reduced ion gap from the positive charge of the M proteins and the frequent presence of hyponatremia in myeloma patients
- Hyponatremia, serum hyperviscosity (more common with production of IgA)
- Bone marrow examination: usually demonstrates nests or sheets of plasma cells, which comprise >30% of the bone marrow; ≥10% are immature
- Serum beta-2 microglobulin has little diagnostic value; it is useful for prognosis because levels >8 mg/L indicate high tumor mass and aggressive disease.
- Elevated serum levels of lactate dehydrogenase at the time of diagnosis define a subgroup of myeloma patients with very poor prognosis.
- Increased interleukin-6 in serum during active stage of myeloma
- The production of DKK1, an inhibitor of osteoblast differentiation, by myeloma cells is associated with the presence of lytic bone lesions in patients with multiple myeloma.
- Nearly all patients with myeloma present with abnormal chromosomes identified by fluorescence in situ hybridization (FISH). The Mayo Clinic Stratification of Myeloma, for purposes of therapy, identifies high-risk patients (<25% of patients at diagnosis) as those who have any of the following: FISH deletion 17p, FISH translocation 4;14, FISH translocation 14;16, cytogenetic deletion 13q, cytogenetic hypodiploidy, or plasma cell labeling index ≥3%.

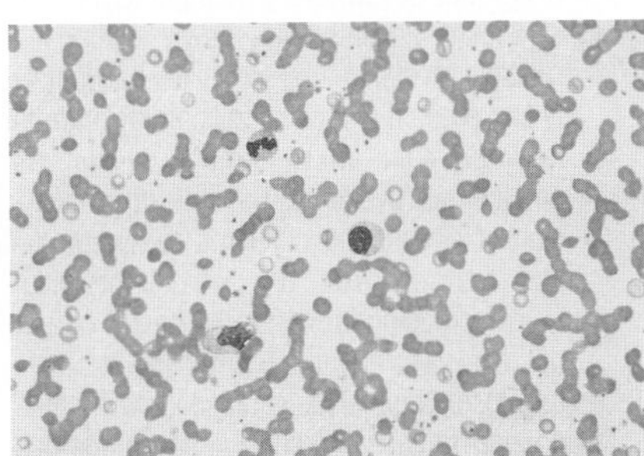

FIGURE 1-615 Increased rouleaux formation is seen in this blood smear from a patient with a large M protein. Marked rouleaux formation is often a clue to the diagnosis of a plasma cell neoplasm, but may also be observed in other conditions (Wright-Giemsa stain). (From Jaffe ES et al: *Hematopathology,* Philadelphia, 2011, Saunders.)

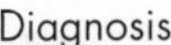
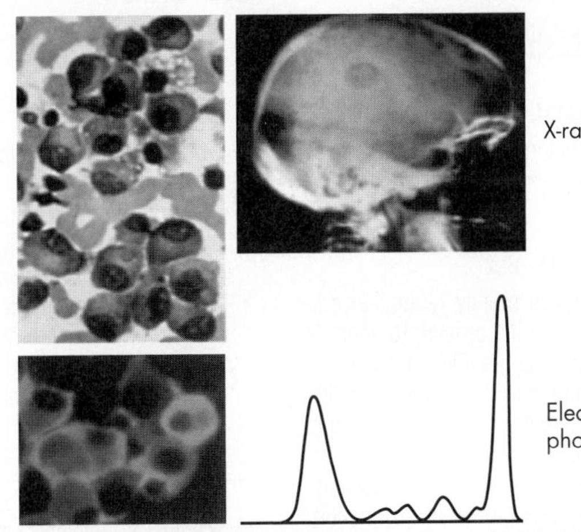

FIGURE 1-616 Common diagnostic features in multiple myeloma. Light chain-restricted plasma cells in a bone marrow aspirate; multiple lytic lesions in a skull radiograph; large monoclonal spike in the γ-globulin area in serum electrophoresis. (From Hoffman R et al: *Hematology, basic principles and practice,* ed 5, Philadelphia, 2009, Churchill Livingstone.)

TABLE 1-343 Myeloma Staging System

Stage	Criteria
I	All of the following: 1. Hemoglobin >10 g/dl 2. Serum calcium <12 mg/dl 3. Normal bone radiograph or solitary lesion 4. Low M-component production a. IgG level <5 g/dl b. IgA level <3 g/dl c. Urine light chain <4 g/24 hr
II	Fitting neither I nor III
III	One or more of the following: 1. Hemoglobin <8.5 g/dl 2. Serum calcium >12 mg/dl 3. Advanced lytic bone lesions 4. High M-component production a. IgG level >7 g/dl b. IgA level >5 g/dl c. Urine light chains >12 g/24 hr

Subclassification:
A Serum creatinine <2 mg/dl
B Serum creatinine <2 mg/dl

IMAGING STUDIES

Radiograph films of painful areas may demonstrate punched-out lytic lesions or osteoporosis (Fig. 1-616). MRI is the preferred technique for suspected spinal compression or soft tissue plasmacytomas. Bone scans are not useful because lesions are not blastic. PET and MRI scans are emerging as useful tools to detect early bone involvement or extramedullary disease.

STAGING

Table 1-343 describes a historical multiple myeloma staging system. With use of newer tumor biology factors (see "Disposition") that can affect prognosis, along with tumor burden described in Table 1-343 and patient-related factors, it is possible to classify patients in three risk groups (high, intermediate, and standard).

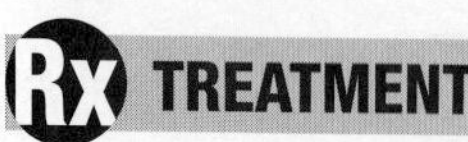

TREATMENT

NONPHARMACOLOGIC THERAPY

Prevention of renal failure with adequate hydration and avoidance of nephrotoxic agents and dye contrast studies

ACUTE GENERAL Rx

- Treatment strategy is mainly related to age and comorbidities. It is crucial to identify transplant-eligible patients (Fig. E1-617).
  1. Initiation of induction therapy with thalidomide, lenalidomide, or bortezomib plus autologous stem cell transplant (ASCT) for patients <70 yr who do not have substantial heart, lung, renal, or liver dysfunction. [illegible]SCT with a reduced-intensity condition-[illegible]imen should be considered in older [illegible], or those with coexisting condi-
  3. Conventional therapy combined with thalidomide, lenalidomide, or bortezomib should be administered in patients >70 yr.
- Induction therapy in patients ineligible for transplantation (old age, coexisting conditions, poor physical conditions) includes the following chemotherapeutic agents:
  1. Thalidomide in combination with melphalan and prednisone.
  2. Melphalan, bortezomib, and prednisone
  3. Bortezomib-thalidomide-prednisone
  4. Melphalan-prednisone-lenalidomide (MPR-R)
  5. Lenalidomide and low-dose dexamethasone
- Therapy for relapsed and refractory myeloma:
  1. If the relapse occurs more than 6 mo after conventional therapy is stopped, the initial chemotherapy regimen can be reinstituted.
  2. Consider autologous stem cell transplantation as salvage therapy in patients who had stem cells cryopreserved early in the course of the disease.
  3. The proteasome inhibitors bortezomib and carfilzomib are FDA-approved for treatment of refractory multiple myeloma.
- ~15% of patients with newly diagnosed multiple myeloma are recognized incidentally and present without significant symptoms (asymptomatic MM, formerly known as smoldering myeloma). The rate of progression of smoldering myeloma to symptomatic disease is 10% per year for the initial 5 yr, decreasing to 5% for the next 5 yr, and decreasing further to 1.5% per year thereafter. Observation alone is reasonable in these patients because no survival advantage has been demonstrated by treating them.
- An exception to this may be in high-risk smoldering myeloma patients.[1] A recent trial[2] has shown that early treatment with lenalidomine plus doxamethasone of patients with high-risk smoldering myeloma delays progression to active disease and increases overall survival.

CHRONIC Rx

- Promptly diagnose and treat infections. Common bacterial agents are *Streptococcus pneumoniae* and *Haemophilus influenzae.* Prophylactic therapy against *Pneumocystis jirovecii* with trimethoprim-sulfamethoxazole must be considered in patients receiving chemotherapy and high-dose corticosteroid regimens. Vaccinate against *S. pneumoniae,* influenza, and *H. influenzae.*
- Control hypercalcemia with IV fluids and corticosteroids. Monthly infusions of the bisphosphonate pamidronate provide significant protection against skeletal complications and improve the quality of life of patients with advanced multiple myeloma. Zoledronic acid at doses of 2 mg and 4 mg in patients with osteolytic lesions has been shown to be as effective as pamidronate in terms of reducing the need for radiation to bone, increasing bone mineral density, and decreasing bone resorption. It can be infused over 15 min for treatment of hypercalcemia of malignancy. Bisphosphonates (pamidronate, zoledronate, and ibandronate) also appear to have an antitumor effect.
- Control pain with analgesics; radiation therapy to treat painful bone lesions or cord compression. Perform surgical stabilization of pathologic fractures. Consider vertebroplasty or kyphoplasty for selected vertebral lesions.
- Treat anemia with erythropoietin.
- Aggressive treatment of reversible causes of renal failure such as dehydration, hypercalcemia, and hyperuricemia.

DISPOSITION

- In patients presenting at an age <60 yr, the 10-year survival is approximately 30%. The median length of survival after diagnosis is now 8 yr. Prognosis is better in asymptomatic patients with indolent or smoldering myeloma. Median survival time is approximately 10 yr in persons with no lytic bone lesions and a serum myeloma protein concentration <3 g/dl. Adverse outcome is associated with increased levels of beta-2 microglobulin, low levels of serum albumin, circulating plasma cells, plasmablastic features in bone marrow, increased plasma cell labeling index, complete deletion of chromosome 13 or its long arm, t (4;14) or t (14;16) translocation, and increased density of bone marrow microvessels. In general any chromosomal abnormality that is detected on standard cytogenetic analysis is associated with a worse outcome than that associated with a normal karyotype.
- Compared with a single autologous stem cell transplantation, double transplantation (two successive autologous stem cell transplantations) improves survival among patients with myeloma, especially those who do not have a very good partial response after undergoing one transplantation.
- Recent trials reveal that among patients with newly diagnosed myeloma, survival in recipients of a hematopoietic stem cell autograft followed by a stem cell allograft from an HLA-identical sibling is superior to that in recipients of tandem stem cell autografts.

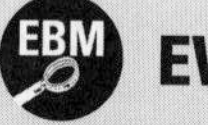

EVIDENCE

available at www.expertconsult.com

SUGGESTED READINGS

available at www.expertconsult.com

RELATED CONTENT

Multiple Myeloma (Patient Information)

AUTHOR: **FRED F. FERRI, M.D.**

[1]Kyle RA et al: Clinical course and prognosis of smoldering (asymptomatic) multiple myeloma, *N Engl J Med* 356:2582-2590, 2007.

[2]Mateos MV et al: Lenalidomide plus dexamethasone for high-risk smoldering multiple myeloma, *N Engl J Med* 369:438-447, 2013.

BASIC INFORMATION

DEFINITION

Multiple sclerosis (MS) is a chronic autoimmune demyelinating disease of the central nervous system (CNS) characterized by subacute neurologic impairment correlated with CNS lesions separated in time and space that cannot be explained by other disease. Most forms involve relapses, which are defined as a subacute onset of neurologic dysfunction that lasts for at least 24 hr.

Subtypes include:

- Relapsing-remitting MS (RRMS) (82%): relapses followed by complete or near-complete recovery, 50% to 85% of which later transition to secondary progressive MS
- Secondary progressive MS (SPMS): progression of disability with few or no relapses
- Primary progressive MS (PPMS) (18%): progression from the onset, typically without relapses
- Progressive relapsing or relapsing progressive courses can be incorporated into SPMS or PPMS, respectively.

Rare MS variants include:

- Marburg's disease (malignant MS): MRI reveals a tumorlike lesion with notable edema in one cerebral hemisphere. Pathology shows severe inflammation with necrosis: typically acute onset with a fulminant course, leading to coma or death.
- Balo's concentric sclerosis: Neuroimaging and pathology show alternating rings of myelination and demyelination—typically more fulminant progression than classic MS.
- Schilder's diffuse sclerosis: childhood onset with one to two large symmetric lesions
- Relapsing optic neuritis

SYNONYMS

MS
Disseminated sclerosis

ICD-9CM CODES
340 Multiple sclerosis
ICD-10CM CODES
G35 Multiple sclerosis

EPIDEMIOLOGY & DEMOGRAPHICS

PEAK INCIDENCE: 20 to 40 yr in two thirds of patients; mean age of onset is 37.5 yr, range is infancy to 70.

PREVALENCE: More common in people raised in northern latitudes and in certain genetic clusters. Prevalence per 10,000 varies from 20 in southern Europe to 150-180 in Canada, northern United States, and northern Europe; and less than 10 in Asia, Central America, and most of Africa. Estimated 400,000 people in the U.S. and 2.5 million people worldwide with MS.

PREDOMINANT SEX & AGE: Female/male ratio is 2 to 3:1.

GENETICS: Frequency of MS in dizygotic twins and siblings is 3% to 5% and 20% to 40% in monozygotic twins. Most common associations include human leukocyte antigen classes I and II *(DRB1*1501, DQA1*0102, DQB1*0602)*, *(DRB1*0405-DQA1*0301-DQB1*0302* in Mediterranean population).

PHYSICAL FINDINGS & CLINICAL PRESENTATION

- Common: nonspecific complaints such as fatigue, blurred vision, diplopia, vertigo, falls, hemiparesis, paraparesis, monoparesis, numbness, paresthesias, ataxia, cognitive deficits, depression, sexual dysfunction, and urinary dysfunction
- Visual abnormalities: horizontal nystagmus, visual field defects, ***Marcus Gunn pupil*** (i.e., relative afferent papillary defect—normal direct and consensual light reflexes; however, when swinging flashlight from one eye to the other, direct light causes dilatation of pupil of affected eye), ***internuclear ophthalmoplegia*** (paresis of the adducting eye on conjugate lateral gaze with horizontal nystagmus of the abducting eye [Fig. 1-618])
- Corticospinal tract(s) involvement: leads to upper motor neuron signs such as spasticity, hyperreflexia, clonus, extensor plantar responses, and UMN pattern of weakness (shoulder abduction, elbow, hand and finger extension, hip and knee flexion, foot dorsiflexion)
- Sensory loss: numbness and tingling may or may not follow anatomic distribution, dermatomal loss of pain and temperature, loss of vibration (common) and position sense, and a thoracic band of sensory loss
- Ataxia: intention tremor, heel-to-shin ataxia, inability to tandem gait
- Bladder dysfunction: detrusor hyperreflexia (urge incontinence), flaccidity (neurogenic bladder), and dyssynergia (bladder contracts against a closed sphincter)
- ***Lhermitte's sign:*** flexion of the neck elicits an electrical sensation extending down the spine and occasionally into the extremities
- ***Uhthoff's phenomenon:*** transient worsening of preexisting symptoms with small increases in body temperature (during exercise or exposure to warm environments)

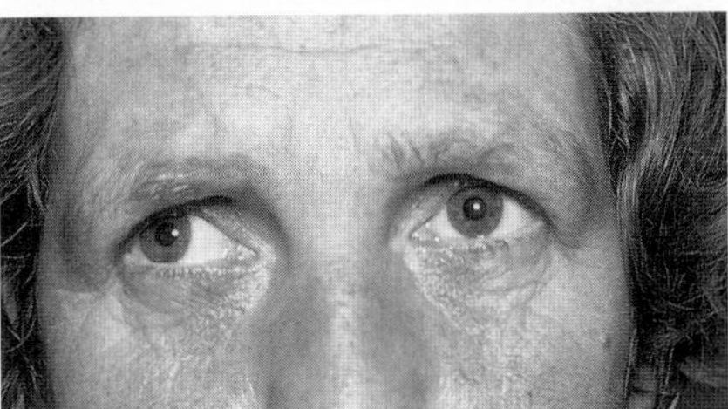

FIGURE 1-618 Internuclear ophthalmoplegia may be an initial feature of brain stem involvement in multiple sclerosis. On lateral gaze to the right, adduction of the left eye is incomplete. On convergence, eye movement was normal. The lesion is in the left medial longitudinal bundle, between the nucleus in the pons and the third nerve nucleus on the opposite side. (From Forbes CD, Jackson WF. *Color atlas and text of clinical medicine,* ed 3, London, 2003, Mosby.)

ETIOLOGY

Remains unknown but likely multifactorial with evidence for autoimmunity (autoreactive T and B cells) and genetics. It is believed that an interaction between multiple genes influencing the immune system and environmental factors (such as certain viruses [e.g., Epstein-Barr virus and human herpes virus 6], low vitamin D level, smoking, and sun exposure) are important factors.

DIAGNOSIS

- MS: based on revised 2010 McDonald criteria (Table 1-344)
- RRMS: at least two relapses—two clinical lesions distinctly separated in space and time *or* one clinical lesion plus paraclinical testing (Table 1-344)
- PPMS: insidious progression of disability with a positive CSF and either dissemination in both space and time *or* ongoing progression for at least 1 yr

TABLE 1-344 Summary of Revised 2005-2010 McDonald Criteria for Diagnosis of Multiple Sclerosis

RRMS/Clinical Attacks	Clinical Lesions	Paraclinical Testing Needed
2	2	None
2	1	MRI dissemination in space *or* two lesions on MRI consistent with multiple sclerosis plus positive CSF
1	2	MRI dissemination in time
1	1	MRI dissemination in space *or* two MRI lesions consistent with multiple sclerosis and positive CSF, *and* MRI dissemination in time
		PPMS/No attacks
		Consistent MRI
		At least 2 out of 3 needed 1 yr of progression
		Dissemination in space, >2 lesions in the spinal cord, or positive CSF

Evidence of clinical lesions by physical examination or evoked potentials.
CSF, Cerebrospinal fluid; *MRI,* magnetic resonance imaging; *MRI dissemination in space;* ≥1 T2 lesions in 2 of the 4 typical areas for MS lesions – periventricular, juxtacortical, infratentorial or spinal cord; *MRI dissemination in time,* a new lesion at follow-up MRI at any time, or presence of both an enhancing and nonenhancing lesion at any time.

DIFFERENTIAL DIAGNOSIS

- Autoimmune: acute disseminated encephalomyelitis (ADEM), postvaccination encephalomyelitis
- Degenerative: subacute combined degeneration of the cord (vitamin B_{12} deficiency), amyotrophic lateral sclerosis
- Infections: Lyme disease, neurosyphilis, HIV, tropical spastic paraparesis, progressive multifocal leukoencephalopathy, Whipple's disease
- Inflammatory: systemic lupus erythematosus, vasculitis, sarcoidosis, Sjögren's disease, Behçet's disease, celiac disease
- Inherited metabolic disorders: leukodystrophies
- Mitochondrial: Leber's hereditary optic neuropathy, mitochondrial encephalopathy, lactic acidosis, and strokelike episodes (MELAS)
- Neoplasms: CNS lymphoma, metastases
- Vascular: subcortical infarcts, Binswanger's disease

WORKUP

- Lumbar puncture may be considered for cases that are atypical or do not satisfy the diagnostic criteria for MS. Typical CSF abnormalities include increased protein (less than 100 mg/dl), mild elevation of mononuclear white blood cells, and increased IgG synthesis rate. An elevated CSF immunoglobulin (Ig) G index and positive oligoclonal bands are seen in 70% and 90%, respectively, of clinically definite MS. (Serum MS profile needs to be sent to lab simultaneously with CSF MS profile.) False-positive results with IgG index and rarely with positive OCBs (at least two CSF OCBs with polyclonal or negative serum) can be seen in CNS infections (SSPE, neurosyphilis), inflammation (vasculitis), and CNS lymphoma.
- Serum: complete blood count (CBC), erythrocyte sedimentation rate, chemistry panel, liver function tests (LFTs), antinuclear antibody, vitamin B_{12}, vitamin D.
- Consider: collagen vascular serum tests, neuromyelitis optica IgG antibody, Lyme titer, angiotensin-converting enzyme, TSH, free T_4, anti–thyroglobulin antibody, very-long-chain fatty acids, arylsulfatase A.
- Consider optical coherence tomography or evoked potentials (visual, somatosensory and brain stem auditory evoked response). Demyelination causes slow conduction velocities. Visual evoked potentials reveal prolongation of P100.

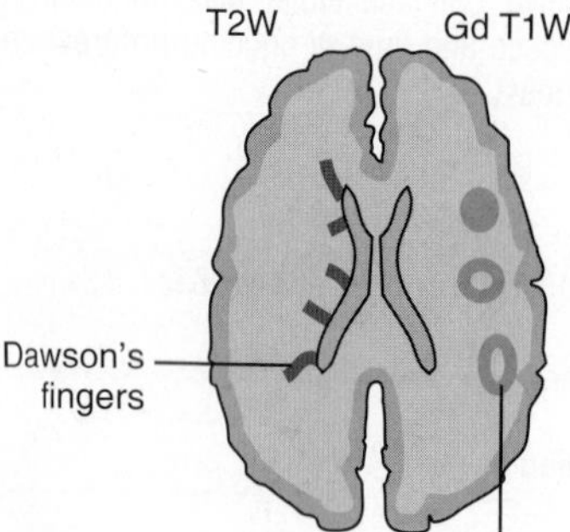

FIGURE 1-619 Imaging features. MRI appearance of plaques.

- Plaques are most commonly multiple. To support the diagnosis of multiple sclerosis, at least three plaques of >5 mm should be present.
- Average size range: 0.5 to 3 cm
- Contrast enhancement may be homogeneous, ...glike, or patchy.
- ... plaques do not enhance.
- ... intensity on T2W and PDW images

(...erer R et al: *Primer of diagnostic* ..., St Louis, 2011, Mosby.)

IMAGING STUDIES

Head imaging (MRI) ± gadolinium is recommended in all cases. Figs. 1-619 and 1-620 illustrate imaging features of MS. MRI of the head with gadolinium is the modality of choice. MRI of the cervical spine can be helpful. MRI assesses disease load, acute lesions, and atrophy. A normal MRI of the brain does not conclusively exclude MS.

Rx TREATMENT

NONPHARMACOLOGIC THERAPY

Patient education regarding disease characteristics, treatment options, and prognosis. Often patients need intermittent rest periods on a daily basis and avoid exposure to heat, which typically worsens symptoms. Provide encouragement regarding improved quality of life with new disease-modifying drug options.

Recommend physical therapy for new weakness, incoordination, or for spasticity.

ACUTE GENERAL Rx

Relapses: high-dose IV methylprednisolone (3 to 5 days of 1 g/day; alternative dose is 15 mg/kg/day), often followed by a 7- to 10-day prednisone taper. High-dose corticosteroids typically do not alter the long-term course of disease.

CHRONIC Rx

- Disease-modifying injection therapy for RRMS is typically, but not exclusively, first-line therapy: includes interferon beta-1a (IM Avonex, SC Rebif), interferon beta-1b (SC Betaseron), and glatiramer acetate (SC Copaxone). Common side effects for Copaxone include injection site reactions and chest tightness, but no serum studies are needed. Common side effects for interferons include flulike symptoms, liver toxicity, and leukopenia; CBC and LFTs (initially q1mo, then q3mo).
- Disease-modifying oral therapy:

  Typically monthly CBC and liver function tests for 6 mo then q3mo.

  1. Fingolimod (Gilenya), a sphingosine-1-phosphate receptor modulator and immunosuppressant, was approved for RRMS. Common side effects: liver toxicity, bradycardia with first dose only (requiring cardiac monitoring and ECG for at least 8 hr after administration of first dose), pancytopenia.
  2. Teriflunomide (Aubagio), reversible inhibitor of pyrimidine synthesis and immunosuppressant, was approved for relapsing MS. Common side effects: diarrhea, abnormal liver function tests, nausea, and hair loss; pregnancy category X.
  3. Dimethyl fumarate (Tecfidera), mechanism includes inhibition of transcription of NF-KB and immunosuppressant, is approved for relapsing MS. Common side effects include nausea, abdominal discomfort, and flushing—especially during the first month—and leukopenia.
- Disease modifying IV therapy:
  1. Natalizumab (Tysabri) is monoclonal humanized Ab which binds integrin-α4, and is approved for treatment of RRMS. It has been associated with a higher risk of developing progressive multifocal leukoencephalopathy (JC virus), but other

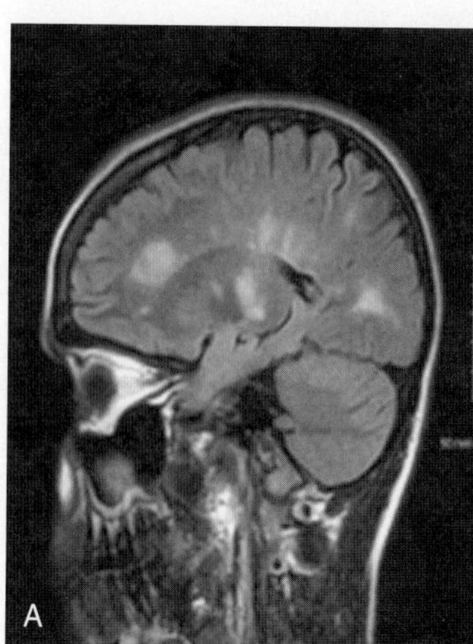

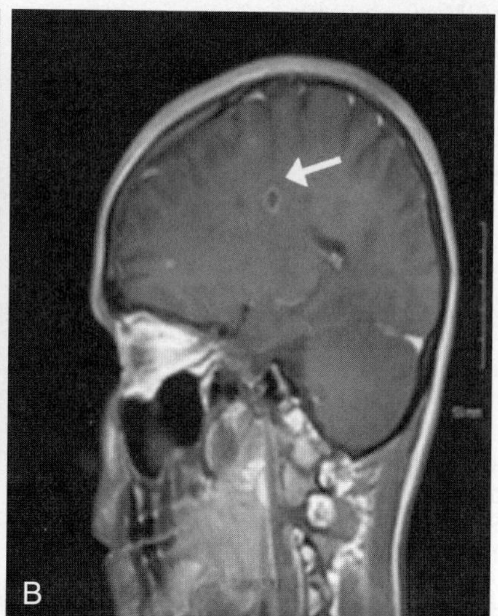

FIGURE 1-620 Multiple sclerosis. A, Sagittal FLAIR image magnetic resonance scan shows multiple lesions in corpus callosum (periventricular and perpendicular to corpus callosum, known as "Dawson's fingers") along with lesions in right frontal, occipital lobes. **B,** Gadolinium-enhanced scan shows one enhancing lesion *(arrow).*

immunosuppressants also carry risk. Test for JC virus Ab at least annually, and when detected, PML is still rare but is more likely with increased length of therapy, history of chemotherapy, concomitant immunosuppressants, or interferons.

2. Cytotoxic cyclophosphamide or mitoxantrone for rapidly progressive or frequent relapses on other maximum therapy.

Strong immunosuppressant with long-term effects, increases risk of infections, and especially mitoxantrone; risk of hematopoietic malignancy and dose-dependent cardiotoxicity.

- Symptomatic therapy:
- Dalfampridine (Ampyra) is a potassium channel blocker recently approved to improve walking speed in patients with MS.

Treat spasticity with baclofen or tizanidine. In acute worsenings, rule out infection. Onabotulinum toxin type A injection is an alternative for focal intractable spasticity.

Treat urge incontinence with anticholinergic/muscarinic therapy such as oxybutynin or tolterodine. Treat urinary retention with tamsulosin. In both cases, always rule out a bladder infection.

Treat dysesthesias with gabapentin or oxycarbazepine.

Fatigue: consider amantadine 100 mg bid, modafinil, stimulant, or fluoxetine.

Tremor: clonazepam, carbamazepine, propranolol, or gabapentin. Wrist splints may be helpful.

Depression: selective serotonin receptor inhibitors or tricyclic antidepressants.

DISPOSITION

Most patients have complete or near-complete recovery weeks to months after a relapse. Typically, two flares occur in RRMS patient per year (75% will have at least one flare). Although the rate of disease progression is highly variable, higher risk of greater long-term disability with frequent relapse rate during the first 2-5 yr, poor recovery, older age of onset, involvement of multiple systems, male sex, and primary progressive disease.

REFERRAL

- Referral to neurologist is highly recommended.
- Consider referrals for physical therapy and occupational therapy to prevent/minimize disability. Consider referral to urology if post-void residual by bladder scan is more than 100 ml.
- Referral to MS specialist should be strongly considered in case of poor response to therapy, possibility of cytotoxic treatment, and/or concern for complications of disease-modifying therapies.

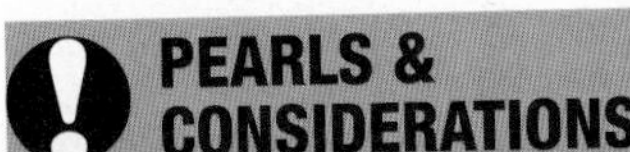

PEARLS & CONSIDERATIONS

- Clinically isolated syndrome (CIS): patient with an isolated demyelinating event such as optic neuritis with no prior history of neurologic symptoms. If brain MRI is completely normal, there is 20% to 25% chance of subsequent MS. If there are two or more T2 hyperintensities on neuroimaging, there is a 70% to 90% chance of subsequent MS.
- Pseudorelapses may occur with heat, fever, or infections (urinary tract infections common in patients with MS).
- In an African American patient with clinical suspicion for MS, strongly consider possibility of neurosarcoidosis and order CXR, CSF angiotensin-converting enzyme level, and perhaps noncontrast chest CT.

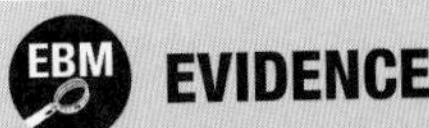

EVIDENCE

available at www.expertconsult.com

SUGGESTED READINGS

available at www.expertconsult.com

RELATED CONTENT

Multiple Sclerosis (Patient Information)

AUTHOR: **DIVYA SINGHAL, M.D.**

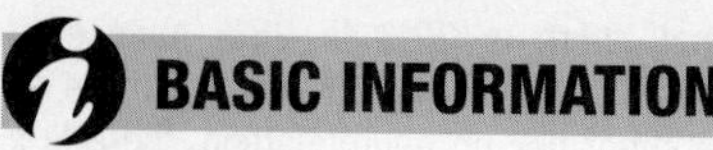

BASIC INFORMATION

DEFINITION

Mumps is an acute generalized viral infection that is usually characterized by nonsuppurative swelling and tenderness of one or both parotid glands. It is caused by mumps virus, a single-stranded RNA paramyxovirus, of which humans are the only natural host.

SYNONYMS

Viral parotitis
Parotitis

ICD-9CM CODES
072.9 Mumps
ICD-10CM CODES
B26.9 Mumps without complication
B26.0+ Mumps orchitis
B26.1+ Mumps meningitis
B26.2+ Mumps encepalitis
B26.3+ Mumps pancreatitis

EPIDEMIOLOGY & DEMOGRAPHICS

INCIDENCE (IN U.S.):

- About 300 infections/yr. Sporadic outbreaks still occur in schools, colleges, military posts, or summer camps started by an unvaccinated person.
- More than 150,000 cases/yr before licensure of mumps vaccine in 1967

PREDOMINANT SEX: Males = females
PREDOMINANT AGE: 75% of disease in teenage years
PEAK INCIDENCE:
Late winter and early spring months
GENETICS:
Congenital infection:

- First-trimester infection is associated with excessive fetal deaths.
- Second- and third-trimester infection is not associated with increased fetal mortality.

Neonatal infection:

- Uncommon
- Uncommon in infants <1 yr because of passive immunity conferred by placental transfer of maternal antibody

PHYSICAL FINDINGS & CLINICAL PRESENTATION

- Prodromal period: includes low-grade fever, malaise, anorexia, and headache
- Parotid swelling (Fig. 1-621) and tenderness; often the first signs of infection:
  1. Progresses over 2 to 3 days, then opposite side may become involved
  2. Unilateral parotitis in 25% of cases
  3. Considerable pain with parotid swelling, causing trismus and difficulty with mastication and pronunciation
  4. Pain exacerbated by eating or drinking citrus and other acidic foods
  5. Possible fever with parotid swelling, ranging up to 40° C
  6. Parotid swelling, usually resolving within 1 wk
- CNS involvement:
  1. May occur from 1 wk before to 2 wk after the onset of parotitis or even in its absence
  2. Meningitis:
     a. Occurs in 1% to 10% of patients with mumps parotitis
     b. Occurs three times more often in males than females
     c. Symptoms: headache, fever, nuchal rigidity, and vomiting
     d. Full recovery with no sequelae
  3. Encephalitis:
     a. May develop early, as a result of direct viral invasion of neurons, or late, around the second wk after onset of parotitis, and is a postinfectious demyelinating process.
     b. Mumps accounted for only 0.5% of viral meningitis.
     c. Symptoms: fever, alterations in the level of consciousness, possible seizures, paresis or paralysis, and aphasia. Fever can be quite high (40° to 41° C).
     d. Cerebellitis and hydrocephalus are serious complications of mumps encephalitis.
     e. May result in permanent sequelae or death.
  4. Other rare neurologic complications: include cerebellar ataxia, transverse myeli tis, Guillain-Barré syndrome, and facial palsy.
- Epididymoorchitis:
  1. Most common extrasalivary gland complication of mumps in adult men
  2. Occurs in 38% of postpubertal males who have mumps
  3. Most often unilateral but is bilateral in 30% of males who develop this complication
  4. May precede development of parotitis and may be only manifestation of mumps
  5. Two thirds of cases develop during first week of parotitis
  6. Symptoms:
     a. Severe pain, swelling, and tenderness of the testes and scrotal erythema
     b. Fever and chills
  7. Some degree of testicular atrophy in 50% of cases, mo to yr later
  8. Sterility from bilateral orchitis is rare
- Involvement of pancreas and ovaries:
  1. Pancreas: abdominal pain, fever, and vomiting
  2. Ovaries: oophoritis
     a. Occurs in 5% of postpubertal women with mumps
     b. Symptoms include fever, nausea, vomiting, and lower abdominal pain
     c. May rarely result in decreased fertility and premature menopause
- Transient renal impairment: common and manifested by hematura and polyuria
- Joint involvement:
  1. Migratory polyarthritis is most frequent
  2. Infrequently affects adults with mumps
  3. Occurs rarely in children
  4. Self-limited, with complete resolution
- Deafness:
  1. Most often unilateral, involving high frequencies; may rarely cause bilateral involvement
  2. Most patients recover
  3. Permanent unilateral deafness reported in 1 in 20,000 cases
  4. Labyrinthitis and end lymphatic hydrops also reported
- Myocardial involvement:
  1. Uncommon
  2. Rarely causes progressive and fulminant fatal myocarditis with dilated cardiomyopathy
  3. Refractory arrhythmia and congestive heart failure
  4. Coronary artery involvement
- Eye involvement:
  1. Corneal endothelitis following mumps parotitis

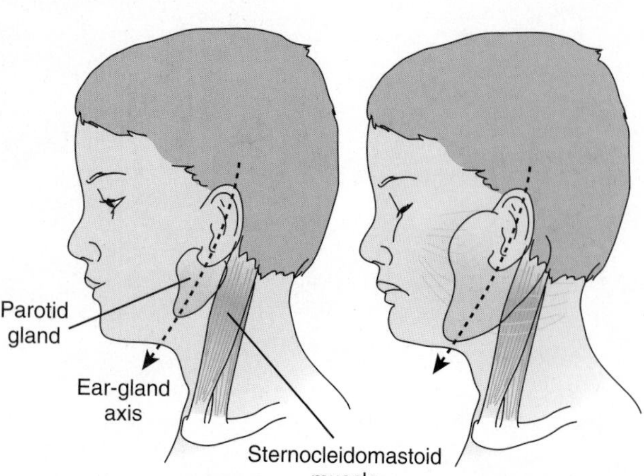

FIGURE 1-621 Schematic drawing of a parotid gland infected with mumps *(right)* compared with a normal gland *(left)*. An imaginary line bisecting the long axis of the ear divides the parotid gland into two equal parts. These anatomic relationships are not altered in the enlarged gland. An enlarged cervical lymph node is usually posterior to the imaginary line. (From Mumps [epidemic parotitis]. In Krugman S et al [eds]: *Infectious diseases in children,* ed 6, St Louis, 1977, Mosby.)

ETIOLOGY

- Virus is spread via direct contact, droplet nuclei, fomites, or oral or nasal secretions.
- Patients are contagious from 48 hr before to 9 days after parotid swelling.

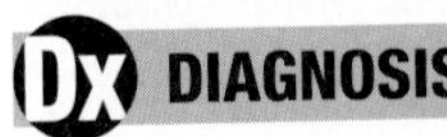

DIFFERENTIAL DIAGNOSIS

- Other viruses that may cause acute parotitis:
  1. Parainfluenza types 1 and 3
  2. Coxsackie viruses
  3. Influenza A
  4. Cytomegalovirus
- Suppurative parotitis:
  1. Most often caused by *Staphylococcus aureus*
  2. May be differentiated from mumps
     a. Extreme indurations, tenderness and erythema overlying the gland
     b. Ability to express pus from Stensen's duct or massage of parotid
- Other conditions that may occur with parotid enlargement or swelling:
  1. Sjögren's syndrome
  2. Leukemia
  3. Diabetes mellitus
  4. Uremia
  5. Malnutrition
  6. Cirrhosis
- Drugs that cause parotid swelling:
  1. Phenothiazines
  2. Phenylbutazone
  3. Thiouracil
  4. Iodides
- Conditions that cause unilateral swelling:
  1. Tumors
  2. Cysts
  3. Stones causing obstruction
  4. Strictures causing obstruction

WORKUP

- Diagnosis based on history of exposure and physical finding of parotid tenderness with mild to moderate constitutional symptoms.
- Diagnosis is confirmed by a variety of serologic tests or isolation of the virus.

LABORATORY TESTS

- Diagnosis is confirmed by a positive IgM mumps antibody or by fourfold rise between acute and convalescent sera by CF, ELISA, or neutralization tests. However, serologic mumps testing is particularly unhelpful in some vaccinated individuals who can have mumps without having the usual immunoglobin M (IgM) spike. A polymerase chain reaction (PCR) assay is also available.
- Virus can be isolated from the saliva, usually from 2 to 3 days before to 4 to 5 days after the onset of parotitis. Researchers have shown that many cases labeled as "parotitis" are actually caused by other viruses (EB virus, human herpesvirus 6B, human parainfluenza virus).[1]
- Virus can be cultured from CSF in patients with meningitis during the first 3 days of meningeal findings. More rapid confirmation of mumps in the CSF is IgM antibody capture immunoassay and nested PCR assay.
- Virus can be detected in urine during the first 2 wk of infection.
- WBC:
  1. May be normal or possible mild leukopenia with a relative lymphocytosis
  2. Leukocytosis with left shift with extra–salivary gland involvement, such as meningitis, orchitis, or pancreatitis
- Serum amylase:
  1. Elevated in the presence of parotitis
  2. May remain elevated for 2 to 3 wk
  3. May be differentiated from mumps and parotids by isoenzyme analysis or serum pancreatic lipase
- Mumps meningitis:
  1. CSF WBCs from 10 to 2000 WBC/mm^3 with a predominance of lymphocytes
  2. In 20% to 25% of patients, predominance of polymorphonuclear cells
  3. CSF protein normal or mildly elevated
  4. CSF glucose low, <40 mg/dl, in 6% to 30% of patients

Rx TREATMENT

NONPHARMACOLOGIC THERAPY

- Supportive treatment
- Adequate hydration and nutrition

ACUTE GENERAL Rx

- Analgesics and antipyretics to relieve pain and fever
- Narcotic analgesics, along with bed rest, ice packs, and a testicular bridge, to relieve pain associated with mumps orchitis
- IV fluids for patients with frequent vomiting associated with mumps pancreatitis or meningitis

[1]Barshey AE et al: Viruses detected among sporadic cases of parotitis, United States 2009-2011, *J Infect Dis* 208:1979, 2013.

DISPOSITION

Most patients recover without incident.

REFERRAL

- To a neurologist if significant neurologic complications develop during or following mumps (myelitis, encephalitis, cranial nerve involvement, cerebellar ataxia, etc.)
- To a cardiologist if viral perimyocarditis develops
- To a urologist if orchitis develops

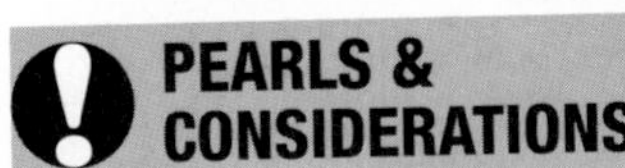

COMMENTS

Prevention:

- Attenuated live mumps virus vaccine has been available since 1967.
  1. Usually given in combination with measles and rubella vaccines (MMR)
  2. Should be given at 12-15 mo of age, and again at 5 to 12 yr
  3. Seroconversion in about 100% of infants given the vaccine
  4. Contraindicated in pregnant women and immunocompromised patients
  5. Patients with asymptomatic HIV infection and patients with symptomatic HIV infection, in the absence of severe immunosuppression, can safely receive mumps, measles, and rubella (MMR) vaccine
  6. Adverse events of vaccination include local pain, indurations, thrombocytopenic purpura, Guillain-Barré syndrome, and cerebellar ataxia
- The CDC and American Academy of Pediatrics (AAP) recommend that patients with mumps stay home from work or school for 5 days after onset of clinical symptoms.
- Because virus may be shed before the onset of parotid swelling, isolation possibly not of great value in limiting spread of infection. Use droplet precautions as per CDC and AAP.
- Mumps is an notifiable disease in all U.S. states.

SUGGESTED READINGS

available at www.expertconsult.com

RELATED CONTENT

Mumps (Patient Information)

AUTHOR: **GLENN G. FORT, M.D., M.P.H.**

BASIC INFORMATION

DEFINITION

Muscular dystrophy (MD) refers to a heterogeneous group of inherited disorders resulting in characteristic patterns of muscle weakness, some with cardiac involvement. Only disorders with childhood or adult onset are considered here (i.e., excluding congenital myopathies).

ICD-9CM CODES
359 Muscular dystrophies and other myopathies
359.1 Hereditary progressive muscular dystrophy
ICD-10CM CODES
G71.0 Muscular dystrophy

EPIDEMIOLOGY & DEMOGRAPHICS

INCIDENCE:

- Most common childhood MD is Duchenne's muscular dystrophy (DMD) with an incidence of 1/3500 male births.
- Most common adult MD is myotonic dystrophy with an incidence as high as 1/8000.

GENETICS:

- **Dystrophinopathies:** X-linked recessive defect in dystrophin gene resulting in either absence (DMD) or reduced/defective (Becker's MD [BMD]) dystrophin (Fig. 1-622)
- **Myotonic Dystrophy:** Autosomal dominant (AD) CTG trinucleotide repeat (see "Myotonia")
- **Limb-Girdle Muscular Dystrophy:** The majority are autosomal recessive, also autosomal dominant forms. Associated with deficiencies identified in multiple proteins (sarcoglycan, calpain, dystroglycan, and dysferlin may be most common; also may involve telethonin, lamin A/C, myotilin, and caveolin-3)
- **Emery-Dreifuss Muscular Dystrophy:** X-linked recessive defect in nuclear protein emerin or AR/AD defect in inner nuclear lamina proteins lamin A/C
- **Facioscapulohumeral Muscular Dystrophy:** AD; genetic mutation causes deletion of 3.3 kb repeat
- **Oculopharyngeal Muscular Dystrophy:** AD GCG trinucleotide repeat resulting in deficient mRNA transfer from nucleus

PHYSICAL FINDINGS & CLINICAL PRESENTATION

- **Dystrophinopathies:** Proximal arm and leg weakness with hypertrophic calf muscles (Fig. 1-623), delayed motor milestones, cognitive impairment, cardiac involvement, progressive course resulting in respiratory complications and respiratory failure
  - DMD (Fig. 1-624) onset at 2 to 3 yr old, typically wheelchair-bound by 12 yr
  - BMD onset at 5 to 15 yr old, ambulatory beyond age 15
- **Myotonic Dystrophy:** Variable age of onset and severity manifesting as predominantly distal weakness with long face, percussion and grip myotonia, temporalis and masseter wasting, ptosis, hypersomnolence, cognitive impairment, and cardiac conduction defects. May be associated with frontal balding, cataracts, impaired glucose tolerance, and male infertility.
- **Limb-Girdle MD:** Phenotypically and genetically heterogenous characterized by proximal hip and shoulder girdle weakness, some genotypes featuring cardiac involvement
- **Emery-Dreifuss MD:** Early adulthood onset with predominantly humeroperoneal weakness, early contractures, and cardiac dysfunction
- **Facioscapulohumeral MD:** Onset typically in late childhood or adolescence with weakness mostly in face and shoulder girdle musculature and possible later, mild involvement of lower extremities
- **Oculopharyngeal MD:** Symptom onset typically in mid-adult life with ptosis, dysphagia, dysarthria, and proximal muscle weakness

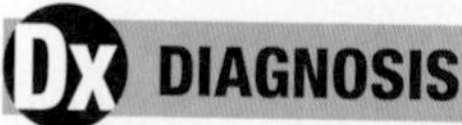

DIAGNOSIS

DIFFERENTIAL DIAGNOSIS

Myasthenia gravis, inflammatory myopathy, metabolic myopathy, endocrine myopathy, toxic myopathy, mitochondrial myopathy

WORKUP

- CK
- ECG, Holter monitor, echocardiography

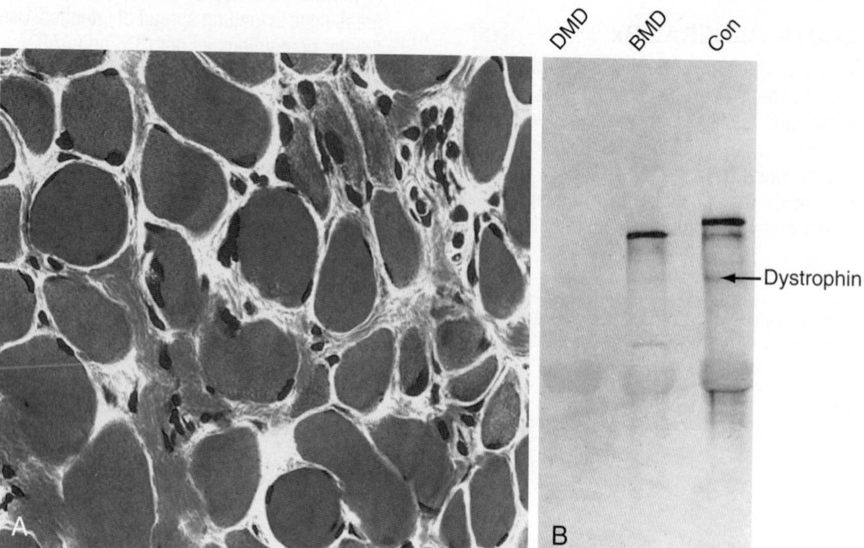

FIGURE 1-622 A, Duchenne muscular dystrophy showing variation in muscle fiber size, increased endomysial connective tissue, and regenerating fibers. **B,** Western blot showing absence of dystrophin in DMD and altered dystrophin size in Becker muscular dystrophy (BMD) compared with control (Con). (Courtesy Dr. L. Kunkel, Children's Hospital, Boston. From Kumar V et al: *Robbins and Cotran pathologic basis of disease,* ed 7, Philadelphia, 2005, Saunders.)

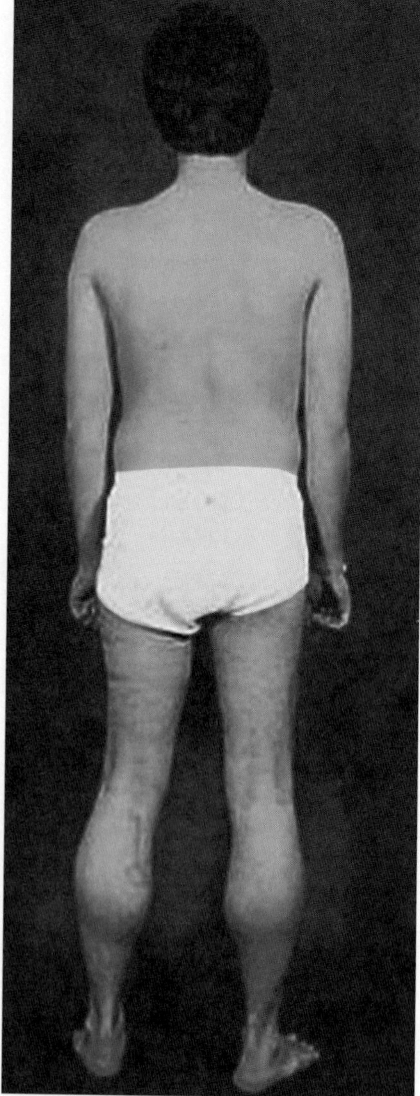

FIGURE 1-623 Becker muscular dystrophy in a 24-year-old male. There is dystrophy of the shoulder girdle and calf pseudohypertrophy. (Courtesy Dr. R. Pascuzzi. From Libby PL et al: *Braunwald's heart disease: a textbook of cardiovascular medicine,* ed 8, Philadelphia, 2007, Saunders.)

- EMG
- Muscle biopsy with immunohistochemistry useful for diagnosis of dystrophinopathies and limb-girdle MD
- DNA analysis helpful if clinical suspicion is for myotonic, Emery-Dreifuss, facioscapulohumeral, and oculopharyngeal MDs
- Assessment of respiratory parameters, including forced vital capacity (FVC)

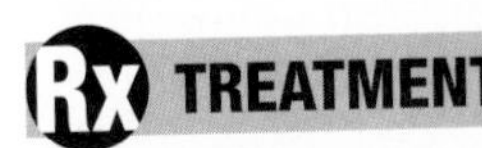

TREATMENT

NONPHARMACOLOGIC THERAPY

- Genetic counseling
- Physical, occupational, respiratory, speech therapy as symptoms dictate
- Screening for sleep-disordered breathing with overnight polysomnogram (PSG) if clinically indicated
- Pacemaker placement may be necessary if cardiac conduction defect present

ACUTE GENERAL Rx

Prednisone may modestly prolong ambulation in DMD. A dose of 0.75 mg/kg/day may improve muscle strength and function over 6 months to 2 years. These short-term benefits must be weighed against the side effects of long-term steroid therapy.

CHRONIC Rx

Vigilance to avoid cardiac and respiratory complications, joint contractures

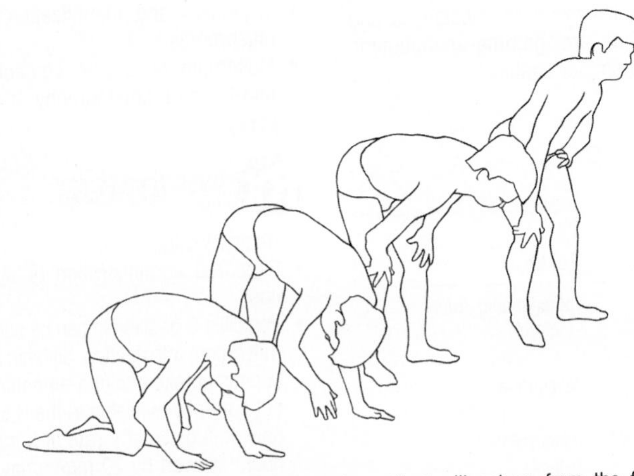

FIGURE 1-624 In Duchenne's muscular dystrophy, the patient will get up from the floor with Gower's maneuver. The boy will "walk up" his body with his hands as he arises. (From Remmel KS et al: *Handbook of symptom-oriented neurology,* ed 3, St Louis, 2002, Mosby.)

DISPOSITION

Variable course, because severity of phenotype is contingent upon both diagnosis and genotype

REFERRAL

- Surgical referral for correction of scoliosis or contractures may be necessary
- Assessment and follow-up in an MD specialty clinic

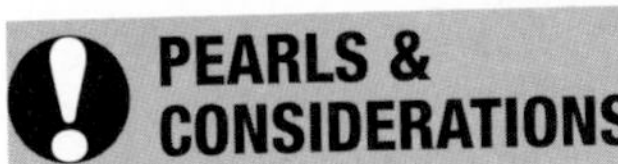

PEARLS & CONSIDERATIONS

Formal evaluation by anesthetist is recommended before any operation with general anesthesia in patients with dystrophinopathy.

SUGGESTED READINGS

available at www.expertconsult.com

RELATED CONTENT

Muscular Dystrophy (Patient Information)

AUTHOR: **TAYLOR HARRISON, M.D.**

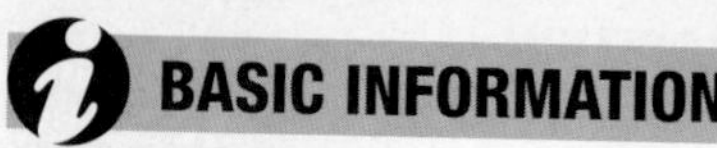

BASIC INFORMATION

DEFINITION

Mushroom poisoning is intoxication resulting from ingestion of poisonous mushrooms.

ICD-9CM CODES
988.1 Mushroom poisoning
ICD-10CM CODES
T62.0X1A Toxic effect of ingested mushrooms, accidental (unintentional), initial encounter

EPIDEMIOLOGY & DEMOGRAPHICS

- 5% of all mushrooms are poisonous. Distinction between poisonous and edible mushrooms may be difficult even by experienced persons.
- Common poisonous species include *Amanita, Russula, Gyromitra,* and *Omphalotus.*

PHYSICAL FINDINGS & CLINICAL PRESENTATION (Table 1-345)

- *Russula* causes confusion, delirium, visual disturbance, tachycardia, and diarrhea within a few hours of ingestion. Prognosis: spontaneous recovery (mortality rate >1%).
- *Amanita* and *Gyromitra* intoxication begins with symptoms of gastroenteritis (nausea, vomiting, diarrhea, abdominal cramps) approximately 10 hr after ingestion. *Amanita* then causes cardiomyopathy and hepatic and renal failure. *Gyromitra* produces jaundice and seizures. Both mushrooms are associated with a 50% mortality rate.
- *Omphalotus* causes symptoms of gastroenteritis that subside spontaneously within 24 hr.

ETIOLOGY

- *Amanita* contains cytotoxic substances and isoxazoles that are gamma-aminobutyric acid neurotransmitter analogs.
- *Gyromitra* contains a pyridoxine antagonist that disrupts the gastrointestinal mucosa and causes hemolysis.
- *Russula* contains a cholinergic substance.

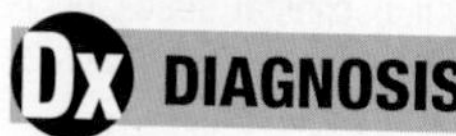

DIAGNOSIS

DIFFERENTIAL DIAGNOSIS

- Food poisoning
- Overdose of prescription or illegal drug
- Other intoxications
- See topic on specific organ failure (e.g., renal or hepatic failure) for differential diagnosis of those conditions

WORKUP

- History
- Inspection and identification of suspected mushrooms
- Mushroom or gastric content analysis (by thin-layer chromatography or radioimmunoassay)

TREATMENT

- Gastric lavage
- Repeated administration of activated charcoal
- Penicillin G or silibinin can be used for *Amanita* mushroom intoxication. Silibinin interferes with hepatic uptake of alpha-amanitin. IV silibinin is not currently available in the U.S. Where available, it is given at a rate of 5 mg/kg IV over 1 hour, followed by 20 mg/kg/day. An oral form of silibinin is available in health food stores as an extract from milk thistle called silymarin. Dose is 1 g PO qid. IV benzyl penicillin reduces hepatocyte uptake of amatoxin.
- Supportive care as needed (may require respiratory assistance, hemodialysis, or emergency liver transplantation)

RELATED CONTENT

Mushroom Poisoning (Patient Information)

AUTHOR: **FRED F. FERRI, M.D.**

TABLE 1-345 Mushroom Poisoning Syndromes

Syndrome	Incubation Period (hr)	Species	Toxin
Confusion, restlessness, visual disturbances, lethargy	2	*Amanita muscaria* *Amanita pantherina*	Ibotenic acid, muscimol
Parasympathetic activity	2	*Inocybe* spp. *Clitocybe* spp.	Muscarine
Hallucinations	2	*Psilocybe* spp. *Panacolus* spp.	Psilocybin Psilocin
Disulfiram	2	*Coprinus atramentarius*	Disulfiram-like substances
Gastroenteritis	2	Many	Unknown
Hepatorenal failure	6-24	*Amanita phalloides* *Amanita virosa* *Amanita verna* *Galerina autumnalis* *Galerina marginata* *Galerina venenata*	Amatoxins Phallotoxins
Hepatic failure	6-24	*Gyromitra* spp.	Gyromitrin

From Gorbach SL: *Infectious diseases,* ed 2, Philadelphia, 1998, Saunders.

BASIC INFORMATION

DEFINITION

Myasthenia gravis (MG) is an autoimmune disorder that affects postsynaptic neuromuscular transmission classically mediated by antibodies directed against the nicotinic acetylcholine receptor (AChR) of the neuromuscular junction, resulting in a decrease in functional postsynaptic ACh receptors and consequent weakness. More recently, antibodies against muscle-specific tyrosine kinase (MuSK) have been described, which impact both pre- and postsynaptic function of the neuromuscular junction.

ICD-9CM CODES
358.0 Myasthenia gravis
ICD-10CM CODES
G70.00 Myasthenia gravis without (acute) exacerbation

EPIDEMIOLOGY & DEMOGRAPHICS

INCIDENCE (IN U.S.): 10 to 20 cases annually per 1 million persons. It is the most common disorder of neuromuscular junction transmission.
PEAK INCIDENCE: Female, second to third decades; male, sixth to eighth decades
PREVALENCE (IN U.S.): One per 20,000 persons
PREDOMINANT SEX: Females are affected more often than males (3:2) in adults; they are equally affected in the elderly
GENETICS: Increased frequency of HLA-B8, DR3

PHYSICAL FINDINGS & CLINICAL PRESENTATION

- The hallmark of MG is fluctuating weakness worsened with exercise and improved with rest.
- Generalized weakness involving proximal muscles, diaphragm, and neck extensors is common.
- Weakness is confined to eyelids and extraocular muscles in approximately 15% of patients.
- Bulbar symptoms of ptosis, diplopia, dysarthria, and dysphagia are common.
- Reflexes, sensation, and coordination are normal.

ETIOLOGY

Antibody-mediated decrease in nicotinic AChR in the postsynaptic neuromuscular junction resulting in defective neuromuscular transmission and subsequent muscle weakness and fatigue. MuSK antibodies have been recognized since 2001 and present with a similar syndrome to AchR MG although they may have more bulbar weakness, proximal muscle atrophy, and either lack of or paradoxical response to pyridostigmine.

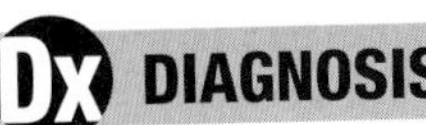

DIAGNOSIS

DIFFERENTIAL DIAGNOSIS

Lambert-Eaton myasthenic syndrome, botulism, medication-induced myasthenia, chronic progressive external ophthalmoplegia, congenital myasthenic syndromes, thyroid disease, basilarmeningitis, intracranial mass lesion with cranial neuropathy, Miller-Fisher variant of Guillain-Barré syndrome

WORKUP

- Edrophonium (Tensilon) test (Fig. E1-625): useful in MG patients with ocular symptoms. Cardiac monitoring and atropine ready at the bedside are essential. Patients with MG may also have a positive ice test (Fig. E1-626).
- Repetitive nerve stimulation: successive stimulation shows decrement of muscle action potential in clinically weak muscle; may be negative in up to 50%.
- Single-fiber electromyography: highly sensitive; abnormal in up to 95% of patients.
- Serum AChR antibodies found in up to 80% of patients.
- A subset of patients (an estimated 40%-60%) with seronegative MG may have MuSK antibodies.

ADDITIONAL TESTS

- Spirometry to document pulmonary function
- CT scan or MRI with contrast of anterior chest to look for thymoma or residual thymic tissue
- Thyroid-stimulating hormone, free T_4 to rule out thyroid disease

TREATMENT

NONPHARMACOLOGIC THERAPY

- Patient education to facilitate recognition of worsening symptoms and impress need for medical evaluation at onset of clinical deterioration
- Avoidance of selected drugs known to provoke exacerbations of MG (beta-blockers, aminoglycoside and quinolone antibiotics, penicillamine, interferons, class I antiarrhythmics [procainamide, quinidine, etc.])
- Prompt treatment of infections, diet modification, and speech evaluation with dysphagia

ACUTE GENERAL Rx

- Symptomatic treatment with acetylcholinesterase inhibitors:
  1. Pyridostigmine 30 to 60 mg PO q4 to 6h initially; onset of effects is 30 min, duration 4 hr. May be titrated up to 120 mg every 4 hr. GI upset is not uncommon with higher doses and may respond to hyoscyamine.
- Immunosuppressive treatment with corticosteroids, azathioprine, cyclosporine for long-term disease-modifying therapy
  1. Prednisone initiated at 15 to 20 mg qd titrate by 5-mg increments to effect or dose of 1 mg/kg/day with improvement in 2 to 4 wk and maximal response by 3 to 6 mo
  2. Azathioprine initiated at 50 mg qd titrated to 2 to 3 mg/kg/day with clinical effect in 6 to 12 mo
  3. Cyclosporine initiated at 5 mg/kg/day with clinical effect within 1 to 2 mo
- Plasmapheresis and IV immunoglobulin are short-term options for immunotherapy during an exacerbation.
- Mechanical ventilation is lifesaving in setting of a myasthenic crisis. Consider elective intubation if forced vital capacity <15 ml/kg, maximal expiratory pressure <40 cm H_2O, or negative inspiratory pressure <25 cm H_2O.

SURGICAL Rx

- In thymomatous MG, thymectomy is indicated in all patients. If the tumor cannot be surgically resected, chemotherapy can be considered for prevention of local invasion and symptom relief.
- For nonthymomatous autoimmune MG, thymectomy is an option in select patients, typically <40 yr.

DISPOSITION

Course of disease is highly variable. Mortality rate has decreased from 75% to 4.5% over past 4 decades.

REFERRAL

Surgical referral for thymectomy in selected cases (see "Surgical Rx")

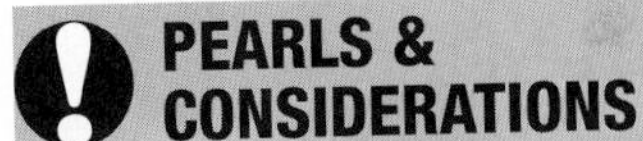

PEARLS & CONSIDERATIONS

- Sustained upward or lateral gaze and arm abduction for 120 sec may be necessary to elicit subtle signs on examination.
- Myasthenic patients can worsen rapidly and warrant close, careful observation during an exacerbation.

SUGGESTED READINGS

available at www.expertconsult.com

RELATED CONTENT

Myasthenia Gravis (Patient Information)

AUTHOR: **TAYLOR HARRISON, M.D.**

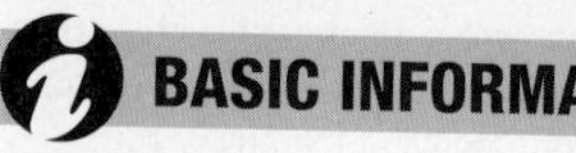

BASIC INFORMATION

DEFINITION

Mycosis fungoides refers to a T-cell lymphoproliferative disorder with characteristic cutaneous skin lesions and the potential to disseminate into lymph nodes and viscera.

SYNONYMS

Cutaneous T-cell lymphoma

ICD-9CM CODES
202.1 Mycosis fungoides
ICD-10CM CODES
C84.00 Mycosis fungoides, unspecified site

EPIDEMIOLOGY & DEMOGRAPHICS

- Incidence of mycosis fungoides is four cases per 1 million persons.
- ~1000 new cases are diagnosed annually in the United States.
- More commonly affects males than females (2:1).
- Affects blacks more often than whites (2:1).
- Usually found in males ages 40 to 60.

PHYSICAL FINDINGS & CLINICAL PRESENTATION

Mycosis fungoides characteristically progresses through three phases:

- A *premycotic phase* featuring scaly, erythematous patches that can last from months to years. During this stage the diagnosis can only be suspected because the histopathologic features are not definitive for mycosis fungoides. Lesions are pruritic and can appear anywhere but are usually found in sun-shielded areas. Parapsoriasis in plaques, poikilodermatous parapsoriasis, parapsoriasis lichenoides, and variegata are skin lesions suspicious of representing premycotic cutaneous T-cell lymphoma.
- The *infiltrative plaque phase* features raised, indurated erythematous palpable plaques that are pruritic and may be associated with alopecia.
  - Stage IA disease is defined as a patch or plaque skin disease involving <10% of the skin surface area and with absence of blood involvement or with low blood tumor burden (<5% of atypical T cells [Sézary cells] in the peripheral blood).
  - Stage IB disease (Fig. 1-627) is defined as a patch or plaque skin disease involving ≥10% of the skin surface area (Fig. E1-628) with absence of blood involvement or low blood tumor burden (<5% Sézary cells).
- The *tumor phase* is characterized by large, lumpy nodules arising from a premycotic patch, plaque, or unaffected skin and represents systemic infiltration and spreading. The tumors can be pruritic and large (>10 cm) and ulceration can occur.
  - Stage IIA and stage IIB diseases are defined by the presence of tumors with or without clinically abnormal peripheral lymph nodes with absence of blood involvement or low blood tumor burden. In approximately 5% of cases of mycosis fungoides, the presentation may be a diffuse, painful, pruritic erythroderma with Sézary cells (Fig. E1-629) in the peripheral blood (known as Sézary syndrome) (Fig. E1-630).
  - Stage III disease is defined by the presence of generalized erythroderma from the spread of cancer cells through the skin but not yet to the lymph nodes.
- Lymphadenopathy can occur during the plaque or tumor stages and may be regional or diffuse.
  - Stage IVA disease is defined by a lymph node biopsy showing large clusters of atypical cells, more than six cells, or total effacement by atypical cells.
- Infiltration of the liver, spleen, lungs, bone marrow, kidney, stomach, and brain can occur.
  - Stage IVB disease is defined by the presence of visceral involvement.

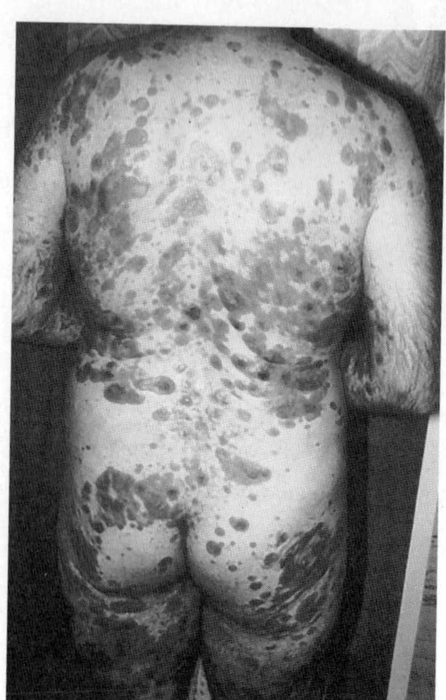

FIGURE 1-627 Cutaneous T-cell lymphoma (mycosis fungoides). Note patch, plaque, and tumor stages. (From Noble J [ed]: *Textbook of primary care medicine,* ed 2, St Louis, 1996, Mosby.)

ETIOLOGY

The specific cause of mycosis fungoides is not known. Infection with the retrovirus HTLV-1 has been suspected, given the association of individuals infected with HTLV-1 and those with T-cell leukemia. Other considerations listed but unsubstantiated include environmental toxins (e.g., tobacco, pesticides, herbicides, and solvents) and genetic predisposition.

Dx DIAGNOSIS

The diagnosis of mycosis fungoides is established by skin biopsy. This may be difficult to differentiate from other skin lesions in the early phases of the disease (e.g., premycotic patch or early plaque lesions); therefore the diagnosis can only be suspected.

DIFFERENTIAL DIAGNOSIS

- Contact dermatitis
- Atopic dermatitis
- Nummular dermatitis
- Parapsoriases
- Superficial fungal infections
- Drug eruptions
- Psoriasis
- Photodermatitis
- Alopecia mucinosa
- Lymphomatoid papulosis

WORKUP

Any patient who is suspected of having mycosis fungoides should have a staging workup. Prognosis in patients with mycosis fungoides depends on the type of skin lesions and the extent of disease. The workup should focus on:

1. Complete physical examination:
   - The type of skin lesion and the extent of skin involvement of the body (e.g., skin involvement is >10% or <10% of the skin surface)
   - Identification of palpable lymph node (especially those >1.5 cm in largest diameter)
   - Identification of organomegaly (e.g., lungs, liver)
2. Skin biopsy:
   - Biopsy of the most indurated area
   - Immunophenotyping
   - Evaluation for clonality
3. Blood test:
   - Complete blood count with differential, liver function tests, lactate dehydrogenase, chemistry
   - T-cell receptor gene rearrangement
   - Determination of Sézary cell count and/or flow cytometry
4. Radiologic tests
   - Depending on the stage of the disease, chest radiograph; ultrasound; and CT scan of the chest, abdomen, and pelvis alone, with or without fluorodeoxyglucose positron emission tomography scan
5. Lymph node biopsy
   - Excisional biopsy
   - Biopsy of the largest lymph node
   - If multiple nodes enlarged, order of preference is cervical, axillary, and inguinal areas
   - Histopathology, flow cytometry, T-cell receptor gene rearrangement

Rx TREATMENT

Treatment is guided according to the stage of disease. A treatment algorithm is described in Fig. E1-631.

NONPHARMACOLOGIC THERAPY

- For dry, cracking skin, emollients (e.g., lanolin and petrolatum) are applied bid.
- Moisturizing lotion (e.g., ammonium lactate) applied bid.

- Topical antibiotics (e.g., bacitracin) are used on ulcerative tumors.

ACUTE GENERAL Rx

- Treatment of patients with stage IA limited patch or plaque phase includes:
  - Topical agents such as corticosteroids and retinoids are used when cutaneous symptoms develop.
  - Psoralen ultraviolet A (PUVA) light therapy where 0.6 mg/kg of 8-methoxypsoralen is ingested 1 to 2 hr before exposure of the skin to UVA light (320 to 400 nm). This is done three times per wk and tapered to twice per wk until all the lesions have cleared. This is typically continued for 6 mo with a 90% complete remission rate.
- Treatment of patients with stage IB and IIA disease is similar to stage IA, with topical corticosteroids and retinoids or PUVA.
  - Total skin electron beam therapy is considered in patients with thick plaques.
  - Interferon-alpha 5 million units SQ three times weekly can be considered in patients with stage IB or IIA disease.
  - Retinoids in combination with PUVA are used in refractory cases. Isotretinoin 1 mg/kg per day or acitretin 25 to 50 mg per day is the standard dosing.
- Treatment of patients with stage IIB disease with generalized tumor and plaque disease:
  - Total skin electron beam therapy in doses of 3000 to 3600 cGy given over 8 to 10 wk followed by adjuvant therapy with topical mustard can be used.
- Patients with advanced disease may receive combination chemotherapy (CHOP). Allogeneic HSCT should also be considered and may be curative in patients. Alemtuzumab has been reported effective in patients with organ involvement.

CHRONIC Rx

- In patients developing diffuse erythroderma, stage III disease (e.g., Sézary syndrome, extracorporeal photophoresis), 8-methoxypsoralen is ingested and peripheral blood is exposed to UVA through a membrane filter.
- In stage IV disease, interferon and other systemic chemotherapeutic agents (e.g., methotrexate, cyclophosphamide, doxorubicin, vincristine, prednisone) and alemtuzumab are considered.

DISPOSITION

- The patients with limited patch or plaque disease have excellent prognosis with long-term life expectancy that is similar to an age-, sex-, and race-matched control population.
- The patients with generalized patch or plaque without evidence of extracutaneous involvement have a median survival of greater than 11 yr.
- The patients with cutaneous tumor and generalized erythroderma without extracutaneous involvement have a median survival of 3 to 4.6 yr.
- The patients with extracutaneous disease at presentation involving either lymph node or viscera have median survival of 13 mo.

REFERRAL

Any patient with suspected mycosis fungoides should be referred to a dermatologist for definitive diagnosis and initial therapy. Oncology consultation is also indicated in patients with more advanced disease.

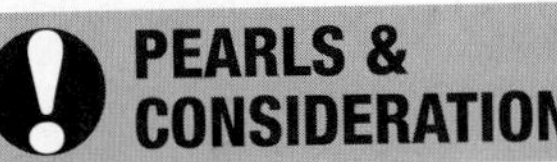

PEARLS & CONSIDERATIONS

A TNM staging classification of mycosis fungoides has been in use for guiding therapy since 1979. The International Society for Cutaneous Lymphomas (ISCL) and the Cutaneous Lymphoma Task Force of the European Organization of Research and Treatment of Cancer (EORTC) recommended revisions to the TNM classification and staging system of cutaneous T-cell lymphoma in 2007. Table 1-346 compares EORTC and WHO classifications of primary cutaneous lymphoma.

COMMENTS

Mycosis fungoides is thought to represent one class of the spectrum of cutaneous T-cell lymphomas.

TABLE 1-346 Comparison of EORTC and WHO Classifications of Primary Cutaneous Lymphoma

EORTC Classification	WHO Classification
Cutaneous T-Cell Lymphoma	
Indolent clinical behavior	Mycosis fungoides
Mycosis fungoides variants	Mycosis fungoides variants
Follicular mycosis fungoides	Follicular mycosis fungoides
Pagetoid reticulosis	Pagetoid reticulosis
CTCL, large cell, $CD30^+$	Primary cutaneous $CD30^+$ ALCA ($CD30^+$ lymphoproliferative disease, including lymphomatoid papulosis)
Lymphomatoid papulosis	
Aggressive clinical behavior	Sézary syndrome
Sézary syndrome	Peripheral T-cell lymphoma, unspecified (most); extranodal NK/T-cell lymphoma, nasal type
CTCL, large cell, $CD30^-$	
Provisional entities	
CTCL, pleomorphic, small/medium sized	
Subcutaneous panniculitis-like T-cell lymphoma	Subcutaneous panniculitis-like T-cell lymphoma
Cutaneous B-Cell Lymphoma	
Indolent clinical behavior	Extranodal marginal zone B-cell lymphoma
Primary cutaneous immunocytoma (marginal zone B-cell lymphoma)	
Follicle center cell lymphoma (any grade)	
Intermediate clinical behavior	
Primary cutaneous large B-cell	
Lymphoma of the leg	
Provisional Entities	
Primary cutaneous plasmacytoma	Plasmacytoma
Intravascular large B-cell lymphoma	Diffuse large B-cell lymphoma (intravascular)

ALCL, Anaplastic large cell lymphoma; *CTCL,* cutaneous T-cell lymphoma; *EORTC,* European Organization for the Research and Treatment of Cancer; *NK,* natural killer; *WHO,* World Health Organization.
From Hoffman R et al: *Hematology: basic principles and practice,* ed 5, Philadelphia, 2009, Churchill Livingstone.

SUGGESTED READINGS

available at www.expertconsult.com

AUTHOR: **TANYA ALI, M.D.**

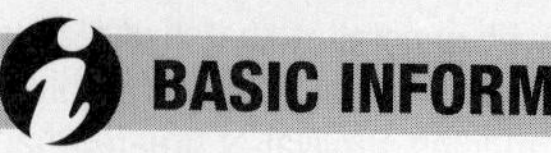

BASIC INFORMATION

DEFINITION

Myelodysplastic syndrome (MDS) is a group of acquired clonal disorders affecting the hemopoietic stem cells and characterized by cytopenias with hypercellular bone marrow and various morphologic abnormalities in the hemopoietic cell lines. MDS shows abnormal (dysplastic) hemopoietic maturation. Marrow cellularity is increased, reflecting an effective hematopoiesis, but inadequate maturation results in peripheral cytopenias.

CLASSIFICATION

- Myelodysplasia encompasses several heterogenous syndromes. The French-American-British (FAB) classification of MDSs is based on the proportion of immature blast cells in the blood and marrow and on the presence or absence of ringed sideroblasts or peripheral monocytosis (Table 1-347). It includes refractory anemia, refractory anemia with ringed sideroblasts, refractory anemia with excess blasts, chronic myelomonocytic leukemia, and refractory anemia with excess blasts in transformation.
- In 1999 the World Health Organization modified the FAB by incorporating newer morphologic insights and cytogenetic findings. It includes the disease subtypes refractory anemia, refractory anemia with ringed sideroblasts, refractory cytopenia with multilineage dysplasia, refractory cytopenia with multilineage dysplasia and ringed sideroblasts, refractory anemia with excessive blasts (1, 2), unclassified MDS, and MDS associated with isolated del(5q).

SYNONYMS

MDS
Preleukemia
Dysmyelopoietic syndrome

ICD-9CM CODES
238.7 Myelodysplastic syndrome
ICD-10CM CODES
D46.9 Myelodysplastic syndrome, unspecified

EPIDEMIOLOGY & DEMOGRAPHICS

INCIDENCE (IN U.S.): Approximately 82 cases/100,000 persons per yr. An estimated 7000 to 12,000 new cases are diagnosed annually in the U.S.

PREDOMINANT AGE: More common in elderly patients; median age, >65 yr

PHYSICAL FINDINGS & CLINICAL PRESENTATION

- Splenomegaly, skin pallor, mucosal bleeding, and ecchymosis may be present.
- Patients often present with fatigue.
- Fever, infection, and dyspnea are common.

ETIOLOGY

Unknown. However, exposure to radiation, chemotherapeutic agents, benzene, or other organic compounds is associated with myelodysplasia. Table 1-348 describes predisposing factors and epidemiologic associations of patients with MDS. Recently targeted resequencing of the gene encoding RNA splicing factor 3B, subunit 1 (SF3B1) has shown that mutations in SF3B1 implicate abnormalities of messenger RNA splicing in the pathogenesis of MDS.

DIAGNOSIS

DIFFERENTIAL DIAGNOSIS

- Hereditary dysplasias (e.g., Fanconi's anemia, Diamond-Blackfan syndrome)
- Vitamin B_{12}/folate deficiency
- Exposure to toxins (drugs, alcohol, chemotherapy)
- Renal failure
- Irradiation
- Autoimmune disease
- Infections (tuberculosis, viral infections)
- Paroxysmal nocturnal hemoglobinuria

WORKUP

Diagnostic workup (Fig. E1-632) includes laboratory evaluation (Table E1-349) and bone marrow examination (Fig. E1-633). Cytogenetic analysis (Box E1-56) by conventional metaphase karyotyping should be performed in patients with MDS. Physical examination, medical history, and laboratory tests aiding in diagnosis of MDS are described in Table 1-350.

TABLE 1-347 French-American-British Classification Criteria

Subtype	Abbreviation	Peripheral Blood	Bone Marrow
Refractory anemia	RA	Blasts <1%	Blasts <5%
Refractory anemia with ringed sideroblasts	RARS	Blasts <1%	Blasts >5%, and >15% ringed sideroblasts
Refractory anemia with excess blasts	RAEB	Blasts <5%	Blasts 5%-20%
Refractory anemia with excess blasts in transformation	RAEB-T	Blasts >5%	Blasts 20%-30% or Auer rods
Chronic myelomonocytic leukemia	CMML	Monocytes $>1 \times 10^9$/L	Any of the above
Acute myelogenous leukemia	AML	Blasts >30%	

From Hoffmann R et al: *Hematology, basic principles and practice*, ed 5, Philadelphia, 2009, Churchill Livingstone.

TABLE 1-348 Predisposing Factors and Epidemiologic Associations of Patients with Myelodysplastic Syndrome

Heritable
Constitutional Genetic Disorders
Trisomy 8 mosaicism Familial monosomy 7 Down syndrome (trisomy 21) Neurofibromatosis 1 Germ cell tumors [embryonal dysgenesis del(12p)]
Congenital Neutropenia
Kostmann syndrome Shwachman-Diamond syndrome
DNA Repair Deficiencies
Fanconi anemia Ataxia-telangiectasia Bloom syndrome Xeroderma pigmentosum Pharmacogenomic polymorphisms (GSTq1-null)
Acquired
Senescence
Mutagen Exposure
Alkylator therapy (chlorambucil, cyclophosphamide, melphalan, N-mustards) Topoisomerase II inhibitors (anthracyclines)β Emitters (32p) Autologous stem cell transplantation Environmental/occupational (benzene) Tobacco Aplastic anemia Paroxysmal nocturnal hemoglobinuria

From Hoffman R et al: *Hematology, basic principles and practice*, ed 5, Philadelphia, 2009, Churchill Livingstone.

Rx TREATMENT

NONPHARMACOLOGIC THERAPY

Red blood cell transfusions in patients with severe symptomatic anemia

ACUTE GENERAL Rx

- Erythropoietin (10,000 to 40,000 U/wk) in patient with symptomatic anemia.
- DNA methyltransferase inhibitors: Azacitidine (Vidaza), a pyrimidine nucleoside analog of cytidine, has been shown to improve the quality of life for patients with MDS and probably prolong survival. Decitabine (Dacogen), another nucleoside analog, has also been FDA approved for patients with MDS. These agents may also be useful in preventing the transition of MDS to AML.
- Immunomodulators: Lenalidomide (Revlimid), a novel analogue of thalidomide, has demonstrated hematologic activity in patients with low-rise MDS who have no response to erythropoietin or who are unlikely to benefit from conventional therapy. Lenalidomide can also reduce transfusion requirements and reverse cytologic and cytogenetic abnormalities in patients who have MDS with the 5q31 deletion.
- Allogeneic stem cell transplantation should be considered in patients ≤60 yr because this is the established procedure with cure potential (Fig. E1-634).
- Results of chemotherapy are generally disappointing. Combination chemotherapy regimens (e.g., cytarabine plus doxorubicin) generally induce a complete response in only a minority of patients, and the average duration of response is <1 yr.
- The role of myeloid growth factors (granulocyte colony-stimulating factor [G-CSF], granulocyte-macrophage CSF) and immunotherapy is undefined. In a recent trial, 34% of patients treated with antithymocyte globulin (40 mg/kg for 4 days) became transfusion independent. Response was also associated with a statistically significantly longer survival.

TABLE 1-350 Physical Examination, Medical History, and Laboratory Tests Aiding in Diagnosis of Myelodysplastic Syndrome

Medical History
Duration of symptoms
History of blood disease
History of exposure to occupational toxins or cytotoxic agents
Medication history
Alcohol intake
Comorbid conditions
Physical Examination
Pallor
Petechiae
Purpura
Bruising
Tachypnea
Signs of infection
Splenomegaly
Laboratory Testing
Complete blood count with a manual differential
Reticulocyte count
Vitamin B_{12} and folate levels
Consider methylmalonic acid and red blood cell folate levels
Iron, total iron-binding capacity, and ferritin level
Thyroid-stimulating hormone level
Lactate dehydrogenase
Antinuclear antibody
Coombs test and haptoglobin
Serum erythropoietin level
Human leukocyte antigen (histocompatibility antigens) typing in appropriate patients
Paroxysmal nocturnal hemoglobinuria screen
Bone Marrow Testing
Hematopathology
Percentage of blasts on 200 cell aspirate differential
Presence or absence of Auer rods
Percentage of cellularity of bone marrow biopsy
Iron stain on aspirate (ringed sideroblasts)
Iron stain on biopsy (storage)
Dysplastic features (% and number of dysplastic lineages)
Cytogenetics (karyotype of 20 metaphase cells)
Fluorescent in situ hybridization
Flow cytometry (not useful for quantitation)

From Hoffman R et al: *Hematology, basic principles and practice*, ed 5, Philadelphia, 2009, Churchill Livingstone.

CHRONIC Rx

Monitor for infections, bleeding, and complications of anemia. Supportive measures include blood transfusions and erythropoietin for anemia and antibiotics to treat opportunistic infections. Iron overload from frequent transfusions may require iron chelation therapy.

DISPOSITION

- Cure rates in young patients with allogeneic bone marrow transplantation approach 30% to 50%.
- The risk of transformation to acute myelogenous leukemia varies with the percentage of blasts in the bone marrow.
- Advanced age, male sex, and deletion of chromosomes 5 and 7 are associated with a poor prognosis.
- The 1997 International Prognostic Scoring System uses the following three elements for staging: (1) the proportion of myeloblasts in the patient's marrow, (2) the number of blood cell lineage deficits, and (3) the type of chromosomal abnormality present (e.g., poor risk includes abnormalities of chromosome 7; good risk includes clonal loss of the Y chromosome). According to the International Myelodysplastic Syndrome Risk Analysis Workshop, the most important variables in disease outcome are the specific cytogenetic abnormalities, the percentage of blasts in the bone marrow, and the number of hematopoietic lineages involved in the cytopenias.

REFERRAL

Hematology referral in all patients with MDS

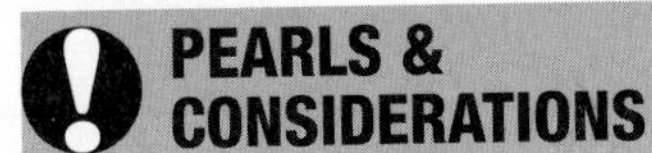

PEARLS & CONSIDERATIONS

COMMENTS

- Somatic point mutations in TP53, EZH2, ETV6, RUNX1, and ASXL1 are predictors of poor overall survival in patients with MDS independent of established risk factors. Patients with cytogenetic abnormalities associated with poor prognosis should be considered for aggressive treatment with high-dose chemotherapy and stem cell transplantation.
- Many younger patients who respond to immunosuppressive therapy with drugs such as antithymocyte globulin and cyclosporine have clonal expansions of cytotoxic $CD8^+$ T cells that suppress normal hematopoiesis, as well as expansion of $CD4^+$ helper T-cell subsets that promote and sustain autoimmunity.
- Nearly 50% of the deaths that result from MDS are the result of cytopenia associated with bone marrow failure.

SUGGESTED READINGS

available at www.expertconsult.com

RELATED CONTENT

Myelodysplastic Syndrome (Patient Information)

AUTHOR: **FRED F. FERRI, M.D.**

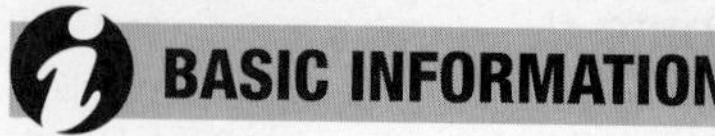

BASIC INFORMATION

DEFINITION

Primary myelofibrosis (PMF) is a clonal stem cell disorder characterized by chronic myeloproliferation, atypical megakaryocytic hyperplasia, bone marrow fibrosis (Fig. 1-635A) and extramedullary hematopoiesis in the spleen. PMF is a myeloproliferative neoplasm; however, it does not include patients who present with myelofibrosis with an associated antecedent diagnosis.

ICD-9CM CODES
238.76 Primary myelofibrosis
ICD-10CM CODES
C94.4 Acute panmyelosis with myelofibrosis
D47.1 Chronic myeloproliferative disease

EPIDEMIOLOGY & DEMOGRAPHICS

INCIDENCE (IN U.S.): ~0.21 per 100,000
PREDOMINANT SEX AND AGE:
- No sex association
- Median age of diagnosis is ~67 years of age

PHYSICAL FINDINGS & CLINICAL PRESENTATION

- Fatigue
- Symptoms related to splenomegaly: abdominal fullness, early satiety
- Acute left upper quadrant pain with the development of spontaneous splenic infarction
- Due to extramedullary hematopoiesis: hepatomegaly and portal hypertension, lymphadenopathy, ascites, or pleural effusions
- Infection
- Skeletal changes
- Leukemic transformation
  - Incidence 3.9% to 20%
  - Within the first 10 yr of diagnosis
  - >20% blasts in the bone marrow or extramedullary leukemic deposits
- Thrombohemorrhagic events

ETIOLOGY

- Clonal disorder of multipotent hematopoietic progenitors arising from the hematopoietic stem cell compartment
- Single mutation in Janus family of cytoplasmic nonreceptor tyrosine kinase (JAK)–2, which is a guanine-to-thymine mutation resulting in a substitution of valine to phenylalanine codon 617 within the pseudokinase domain (JH2) of JAK2 (JAK2V617F)
- JAK2 mutation results in autoinhibition and constitutive JAK2 activity
- Present in 40% to 50% of PMF patients
- Alternative alleles: somatic mutations at codon 515 of the thrombopoietin receptor gene MPL (three different substitutions—W515L (leucine), W515K (lysine), or W515A (alanine)—present in 10% of JAK2V617F-negative patients

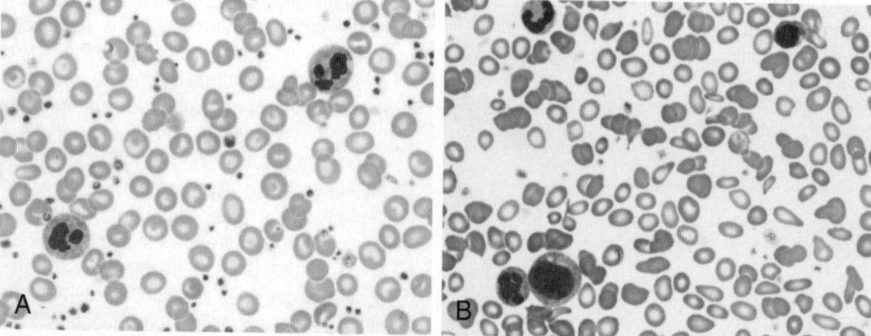

FIGURE 1-635A Blood smears from prefibrotic and fibrotic stages of primary myelofibrosis. A, This smear from the prefibrotic stage shows neutrophilia and thrombocytosis but minimal red cell changes. **B,** This smear from the fibrotic stage shows leukoerythroblastosis with marked red cell abnormalities, including many teardrop forms. (From Jaffe ES et al: *Hematopathology,* Philadelphia, 2011, Saunders.)

BOX 1-57 World Health Organization Classification of Myeloid Malignancies and Operational Subcategorization of Myeloproliferative Neoplasms

1. Acute myeloid leukemia and related precursor neoplasms
2. Myelodysplastic syndromes (MDS)
3. Myeloproliferative neoplasms (MPN)
   a. Classic MPN
      i. Chronic myelogenous leukemia (CML), BCR-ABL1 positive
      ii. Polycythemia vera (PV)
         (1) Chronic phase PV
         (2) Post-PV MF
         (3) Blast phase PV
      iii. Essential thrombocythemia (ET)
         (1) Chronic phase ET
         (2) Post-ET MF
         (3) Blast phase ET
      iv. Primary myelofibrosis (PMF)
         (1) Chronic phase PMF
         (2) Blast phase PMF
   b. Nonclassic MPN
      i. Chronic neutrophilic leukemia
      ii. Chronic eosinophilic leukemia, not otherwise specified
      iii. Mastocytosis
      iv. Myeloproliferative neoplasm, unclassifiable (MPN-U)
4. MDS/MPN
5. Myeloid and lymphoid neoplasms with eosinophilia and abnormalities of PDGFRA,*PDGFRB, *FGFR1*

*Genetic rearrangements involving platelet-derived growth factor receptor α/β (PDGFRA/PDGFRB) or fibroblast growth factor receptor 1 (FGFR1).
From Tefferi A: How I treat myelofibrosis, ***Blood*** 117:3494-3504, 2011.

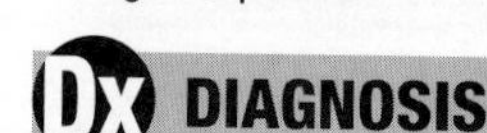

DIAGNOSIS

DIFFERENTIAL DIAGNOSIS

- Myelofibrosis in the setting of preexisting PV or ET (MPN)
- Chronic myelogenous leukemia
- Myelodysplastic syndrome with marrow fibrosis
- Acute myelofibrosis of acute megakaryocytic leukemia
- Marrow fibrosis associated with hairy cell leukemia, lymphoma, and multiple myeloma
- Nonhematologic disorders with bone marrow fibrosis: solid tumor metastases to the bone marrow, autoimmune disorders, and secondary hyperparathyroidism with vitamin D deficiency

WORKUP

- WHO criteria for PMF (3 major, 2 minor; Boxes 1-57 and 1-58)
- Major criteria:
  - Presence of megakaryocytic proliferation and atypia, usually accompanied by reticulin and/or collagen fibrosis, or, in the absence of significant reticulin fibrosis, the megakaryocyte changes must be accompanied by an increased bone marrow cellularity characterized by granulocytic proliferation and often decreased erythropoiesis
  - *Not* polycythemia vera, chronic myelogenous leukemia, myelodysplastic syndrome or other myeloid neoplasm
  - Demonstration of JAK2V617F or other clonal marker (MPLW515K/L), or, in the absence of a clonal marker, no evidence of bone marrow fibrosis due to underlying inflammatory or other neoplastic diseases

- Minor criteria:
  - Leukoerythroblastosis: nucleated red blood cells, granulocyte precursors, and teardrop-shaped erythrocytes
  - Increase in serum lactate dehydrogenase level
  - Anemia
  - Palpable splenomegaly

LABORATORY TESTS

- Anemia (hemoglobin <10g/dl)
- Platelet count and white blood cell count vary widely
- Peripheral blood smear: nucleated red blood cells, granulocyte precursors, and teardrop-shaped erythrocytes (leukoerythroblastosis)
- Bone marrow is fibrotic, megakaryocytic dysplasia
- Presence of JAK2V617F mutation

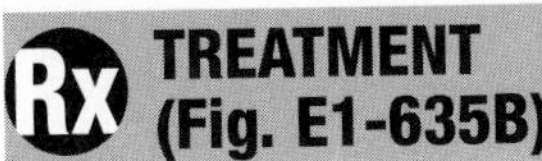

TREATMENT (Fig. E1-635B)

Risk factors are based on Dynamic International Prognostic Scoring System plus (DIPSS-plus).

- Age >65 years
- Hemoglobin <10 g/dl
- Leukocyte count $>25 \times 10^9$/L
- Circulating blasts >1%
- Presence of constitutional symptoms
- Red cell transfusion need
- Platelet $<100 \times 10^9$/L
- Unfavorable karyotype (complex or presence of +8, −7/7q−, i(17q), inv(3), −5/5q−, 12p−, or 11q23 rearrangement)

Scoring: low (0 risk factors); intermediate 1 (1 risk factor); intermediate 2 (2 or 3 risk factors), and high (>4 risk factors)

LOW AND INTERMEDIATE 1 RISK

- Asymptomatic - observation
- Conventional drug therapy if symptomatic (response rates to each of the following agents is ~15%-25%):
  - Anemia – thalidomide and prednisone
  - Patients who are not transplant candidates–an androgen preparation or danazol or erythropoiesis-stimulating agent
  - Patients with a 5q deletion–lenalidomide
  - Treatment failure with thalidomide, danazol, or androgens–lenalidomide
  - Symptomatic splenomegaly–hydroxyurea

INTERMEDIATE 2 AND HIGH RISK

- Palliative options:
  - Conventional drug therapy (see above) Splenectomy – hydroxyurea refractory splenomegaly
  - Radiotherapy - hydroxyurea refractory splenomegaly
  - Experimental drug therapy
  - JAK2 inhibitor ATP mimetics
  - mTOR inhibitors
- Curative options:
  - Allogeneic stem cell transplant (5-year disease-free survival 33% and treatment-related mortality 35%-50%)

DISPOSITION:

Median survival between 3.5 and 5 years based on above DIPSS-plus scoring system

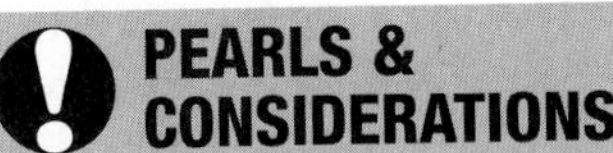

PEARLS & CONSIDERATIONS

- PMF is a clonal stem cell disorder.
- Significant proportion of PMF patients have JAK2V617F or MPL mutations.
- The only curative treatment is autologous stem cell transplant.

SUGGESTED READINGS

available at www.expertconsult.com

AUTHOR: **KIMBERLY PEREZ, M.D.**

BOX 1-58 Diagnostic Criteria for Primary Myelofibrosis

WHO Diagnostic Criteria for PMF Requires Meeting All 3 Major Criteria and ≥2 Minor Criteria Outlined

Major Criteria

1. Megakaryocyte proliferation, including small-to-large megakaryocytes, with aberrant nuclear/cytoplasmic ratio and hyperchromatic and irregularly folded nuclei and dense clustering accompanied by either reticulin and/or collagen fibrosis, or in the absence of reticulin fibrosis (i.e., prefibrotic PMF), the megakaryocyte changes must be accompanied by increased marrow cellularity, granulocytic proliferation, and often decreased erythropoiesis
2. Not meeting WHO criteria for chronic myelogenous leukemia, polycythemia vera, myelodysplastic syndromes, or other myeloid neoplasm
3. Demonstration of JAK2V617F or other clonal marker or no evidence of reactive marrow fibrosis

Minor Criteria

1. Leukoerythroblastosis
2. Increased serum lactate dehydrogenase
3. Anemia
4. Palpable splenomegaly

International Working Group for Myeloproliferative Neoplasms Research and Treatment Criteria for Post–Polycythemia Vera/Essential Thrombocythemia (post-PV/ET) Myelofibrosis Requires Meeting Both Major Criteria and ≥2 Minor Criteria

Major Criteria

1. Documentation of a previous diagnosis of PV or ET as defined by the WHO criteria
2. Bone marrow fibrosis grade 2-3 (on 0-3 scale) or grade 3-4 (on 0-4 scale)*

Minor Criteria

1. A leukoerythroblastic peripheral blood picture (for both PV and ET)
2. Increasing splenomegaly defined as either an increase in palpable splenomegaly of ≥5 cm (distance of the tip of the spleen from the left costal margin) or the appearance of a newly palpable splenomegaly (for both PV and ET)
3. Development of ≥1 of 3 constitutional symptoms: >10% weight loss in 6 months, night sweats, unexplained fever (>37.5° C) (for both PV and ET)
4. Anemia or sustained loss of requirement for phlebotomy in the absence of cytoreductive therapy (for PV)
5. Anemia and a decrease of hemoglobin level ≥2 g/dl from baseline (for ET)
6. Increased serum lactate dehydrogenase (for ET)

*Grade 2-3 according to the European classification: diffuse, often coarse fiber network with no evidence of collagenization (negative trichrome stain) or diffuse, coarse fiber network with areas of collagenization (positive trichrome stain). Grade 3-4 according to the standard classification: diffuse and dense increase in reticulin with extensive intersections, occasionally with only focal bundles of collagen and/or focal osteosclerosis or diffuse and dense increase in reticulin with extensive intersections with coarse bundles of collagen, often associated with significant osteosclerosis.

From Tefferi A: How I treat myelofibrosis, *Blood* 117:3494-3504, 2011.

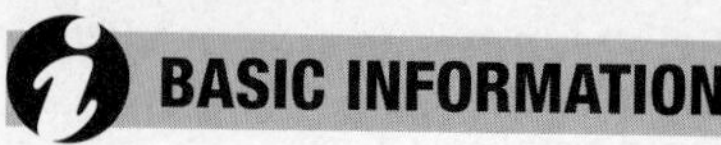

BASIC INFORMATION

DEFINITION

Myocardial infarction (MI) is a clinical syndrome characterized by symptoms of myocardial ischemia, persistent electrocardiographic (ECG) changes, and release of biomarkers of myocardial necrosis resulting from an insufficient supply of oxygenated blood to an area of the heart. According to the European Society of Cardiology/American College of Cardiology, either one of the following criteria for acute evolving or recent MI satisfies the diagnosis:

1. Detection of the rise and/or fall of cardiac biomarkers (preferably cTn) with at least 1 value above the 99th percentile and with at least 1 of the following:
2. Symptoms if ischemia
3. New, or presumed new, significant ST-T changes or new LBBB. New ST elevation at the J point in at least 2 contiguous leads of ≥2 mm (0.2 mV) in men or ≥1.5 mm (0.15 mV) in women in leads V2–V3 and/or of ≥1 mm (0.1 mV) in other contiguous chest leads or the limb leads
4. Development of pathologic Q waves on the ECG
5. Imaging evidence of new loss of viable myocardium or a new regional wall motion abnormality
6. Identification of an intracoronary thrombus by angiography or autopsy

- Pathologic findings of acute MI

MI may be classified as ST-segment elevation MI (STEMI) and non–ST-segment elevation MI [NSTEMI]) depending on the ECG findings on MI presentation. This entry discusses STEMI. For a discussion of NSTEMI, see "Acute Coronary Syndromes."

The *European Heart Journal* and the *Journal of the American College of Cardiology* published a new definition of acute MI that includes 5 subtypes of acute MI, imaging tests supporting the diagnosis, and biomarker thresholds after percutaneous coronary intervention (PCI) or coronary artery bypass grafting (CABG).

- Type 1: Spontaneous MI related to ischemia due to a primary coronary event such as plaque erosion and/or rupture, fissuring, or dissection
- Type 2: MI secondary to ischemia due to either increased oxygen demand or decreased supply (e.g., coronary artery spasm, coronary embolism, anemia, arrhythmias, hypertension, or hypotension)
- Type 3: Sudden unexpected cardiac death, including cardiac arrest, often with symptoms suggestive of myocardial ischemia, accompanied by presumably new ST elevation, new left bundle branch block, or evidence of fresh thrombus in a coronary artery by angiography and/or at autopsy, but death occurring before blood samples could be obtained or at a time before the appearance of cardiac biomarkers in the blood
- Type 4a: MI associated with percutaneous coronary intervention
- Type 4b: MI associated with stent thrombosis as documented by angiography or at autopsy
- Type 5: MI associated with coronary artery bypass grafting

SYNONYMS

MI
Myocardial infarction
ST-elevation MI
Heart attack
Acute myocardial infarction
AMI
Coronary thrombosis
Coronary occlusion

ICD-9CM CODES
410.9 Acute myocardial infarction, unspecified site

ICD-10CM CODES
I21 Acute myocardial infarction
I21.0 Acute transmural myocardial infarction of anterior wall
I21.1 Acute transmural myocardial infarction of inferior wall
I21.2 Acute transmural myocardial infarction of other sites
I21.3 Acute transmural myocardial infarction of unspecified site
I21.9 Acute myocardial infarction, unspecified

EPIDEMIOLOGY & DEMOGRAPHICS

INCIDENCE/PREVALENCE (IN U.S.):

- In 2009, around 683,000 patients were discharged from U.S. hospitals with a diagnosis of acute coronary syndrome (ACS). Community incidence rates as well as mortality rates from STEMI have declined over the past decade, whereas those for NSTEMI have increased. At present, STEMI comprises approximately 25% to 40% of MI presentations. In-hospital (approximately 5% to 6%) and 1-year (approximately 7% to 18%)
- It is more prominent in males between the ages of 40 and 65 yr; no predominant sex after the age of 65 yr
- Women comprised 30% of STEMI patients. They experience more lethal and severe first acute MIs than men regardless of comorbidity, previous angina, or age. Being a woman constituted a strong independent predictor of failure to receive reperfusion therapy, have longer reperfusion times, be less often given the standard of care treatment within 24 hours of presentation, and have higher risk for bleeding with antithrombotic therapy.
- At least one fourth of all MIs are clinically unrecognized. Approximately 23% of patients with STEMI in the U.S. have diabetes mellitus, and three quarters of all deaths among patients with diabetes mellitus are related to coronary artery disease. Diabetes mellitus is associated with higher short- and long-term mortality after STEMI. In CRUSADE trial, 7% of eligible patients did not receive reperfusion therapy. The most important factor for not providing reperfusion therapy in eligible patients was increasing age.

PHYSICAL FINDINGS & CLINICAL PRESENTATION

Clinical presentation: Myocardial infarction is usually based on a history of chest pain lasting for 20 min or more that does not respond to nitroglycerin. Important clues are history of CAD and radiation of the pain to the neck, lower jaw, or left arm. The pain may not be severe. Some patients may present less-typical symptoms such as nausea/vomiting, shortness of breath, fatigue, palpitations, or syncope. These patients, who tend to present typical symptoms later, are more likely to be women, diabetic patients, or elderly patients and less frequently receive reperfusion therapy and other evidence-based therapies than patients with a typical chest pain presentation. Records show that up to 30% of patients with STEMI present with atypical symptoms.

Physical findings:

- Skin may be diaphoretic and exhibit pallor (because of decreased oxygen).
- Rales may be present at the bases of lungs (indicative of heart failure [HF]).
- Cardiac auscultation may reveal an apical systolic murmur caused by mitral regurgitation from papillary muscle dysfunction; S_3 or S_4 may also be present.
- Physical examination may be completely normal.

ETIOLOGY

- Coronary atherosclerosis and plaque rupture
- Coronary artery spasm
- Coronary embolism (caused by infective endocarditis, rheumatic heart disease, intracavitary thrombus)
- Periarteritis and other coronary artery inflammatory diseases
- Dissection into coronary arteries (aneurysmal or iatrogenic)
- Calcium supplementation may promote vascular calcification. Studies have shown that calcium supplementation (but not dietary calcium intake) is associated with elevated risk for MI.
- MI with normal coronaries: more frequent in younger patients and cocaine addicts. The risk of acute MI is increased by a factor of 24 during the 60 min after the use of cocaine in persons who are otherwise at relatively low risk. Most patients with cocaine-related MI are young, nonwhite, male cigarette smokers without other risk factors for coronary heart disease who have a history of repeated cocaine use. Blood and urine toxicology screen for cocaine is recommended in all young patients who present with acute MI.
- Hypercoagulable states, increased blood viscosity (polycythemia vera)

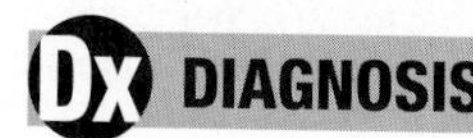

DIAGNOSIS

DIFFERENTIAL DIAGNOSIS

The various causes of myocardial ischemia are described along with the differential diagnosis of chest pain.

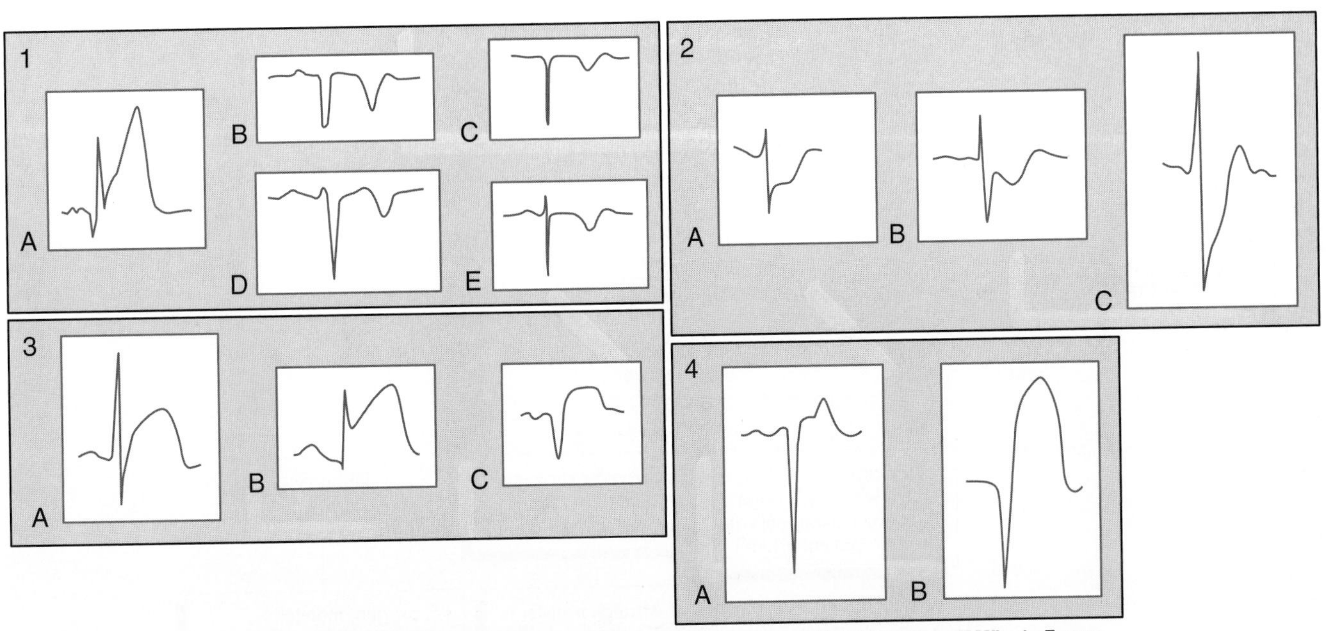

FIGURE 1-636 Electrocardiographic findings of acute myocardial infarction (AMI). 1, T-wave abnormalities of AMI. *A,* Prominent "hyperacute" T wave. *B-E,* T-wave inversions of non-ST-segment elevation MI (NSTEMI). **2,** ST-segment depression. *A,* Flat. *B,* Downsloping. *C,* Upsloping. **3,** ST-segment elevation. *A,* Convex ST-segment elevation. *B,* Obliquely straight ST-segment elevation. *C,* Convex ST-segment elevation. **4,** Pathologic Q waves. *A,* Pathologic Q wave of completed myocardial infarction. *B,* Simultaneous ST-segment elevation with pathologic Q wave 2 hours into the course of ST-segment elevation MI (STEMI). (From Vincent JL et al: *Textbook of critical care,* ed 6, Philadelphia, 2011, Saunders.)

LABORATORY TESTS

- Electrocardiogram (Fig. 1-636): a 12-lead ECG should be performed and shown to an experienced emergency physician within 10 min of ED arrival for all patients with chest discomfort (or anginal equivalent) or other symptoms suggestive of STEMI. If the initial ECG is not diagnostic for STEMI but the patient remains symptomatic and there is a high clinical suspicion for STEMI, serial ECGs at 5- to 10-minute intervals or continuous 12-lead ST-segment monitoring should be performed to detect the potential development of ST elevation. In patients with inferior STEMI, right-sided ECG leads should be obtained to look for ST elevation suggestive of right ventricular (RV) infarction. The joint ESC/ACCF/AHA committee for the definition of MI established the definition for the diagnosis of ST-elevation MI, which is considered to be present when there is an ST-segment elevation in two contiguous leads, ≥0.20 mm for men and ≥1.5 mm for women, or ≥1 mm in other leads. ST-segment elevation is measured at 0.08 sec after the J point (the junction between the end of the QRS and the beginning of the ST segment). ECG findings alone, without laboratory results, are sufficient to diagnose STEMI; therefore, treatment should not be delayed until biomarkers are available.
- Cardiac troponin levels: Cardiac-specific troponin T (cTnT) and cardiac-specific troponin I (cTnI) are generally indicative of myocardial injury with increases in serum levels of >99th percentile of a normal reference population. Detection of a rise and fall pattern of the measurements is essential to the diagnosis of AMI. The rise may occur relatively early after muscle damage (3-12 hr), peak at 24-48 hr, and may be present for several days after MI (up to 7 days for cTnI and up to 10 to 14 days for cTnT). cTnT or cTnI tests can be falsely positive in patients with renal failure. Recently, highly sensitive troponin assays (hs-cTnI, hs-cTnT) have also been developed to facilitate an early diagnosis of AMI. Most patients can be diagnosed with AMI within the first 2-3 hours of presentation. However, an initial negative high-sensitivity troponin at the time of presentation is not sensitive enough to completely rule out AMI. MI can be excluded in most patients by 6 hours of presentation, but guidelines suggest serial samples be obtained if there is a high degree of suspicion to definitively rule out MI.
- CK-MB isoenzyme is also a useful marker for MI if troponin levels are not available. It is released in the circulation in amounts that correlate with the size of the infarct. An increased CK-MB value for the diagnosis of MI is defined as a measurement above the 99th percentile of the upper reference limit. Troponin, however, is the preferred marker for the diagnosis of myocardial necrosis because of its increased sensitivity and specificity as compared to CK-MB. This preference was recommended by the 2007 Joint ESC/ACCF/AHA Task Force for the Definition of Myocardial Infarction. Because troponins need 7-14 days to be cleared by the kidneys, they are not sensitive enough to detect a recurrent MI within days from the initial MI. Therefore CK-MB isoenzyme can be useful in such circumstances.

IMAGING STUDIES

- Imaging studies such as a high-quality portable chest x-ray, echocardiography, and a contrast chest CT scan, or an MRI scan should be used to differentiate STEMI from aortic dissection in patients for whom this distinction is initially unclear.

RISK ASSESSMENT

Several risk assessment models are available. Some of the independent predictors of early death from STEMI include age (≥65), Killip class (≥2), time to reperfusion, cardiac arrest, tachycardia (>100 beats/min), hypotension (<100 mm Hg), anterior infarct location, prior infarction, diabetes mellitus, smoking status, renal function, and biomarker findings. Also weight >67 kg, anterior ST elevation or left bundle branch block, and time to treatment >4 hr. The higher the score, the higher the 30-day mortality rate. Risk assessment is a continuous process that should be repeated throughout hospitalization and at time of discharge.

Rx TREATMENT

NONPHARMACOLOGIC THERAPY

- Limit patient's activity: bed rest for the initial 12 to 24 hr; if the patient remains stable, gradually increase activity.
- Diet: nothing by mouth until stable, then a low-salt and a low-cholesterol diet.
- Patient education to decrease the risk of subsequent cardiac events (proper diet, smoking cessation, regular exercise) should be initiated when the patient is medically stable.

ACUTE GENERAL Rx

- Fig. 1-637 shows a treatment algorithm for STEMI. Assessment and treatment algorithm

 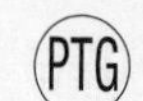

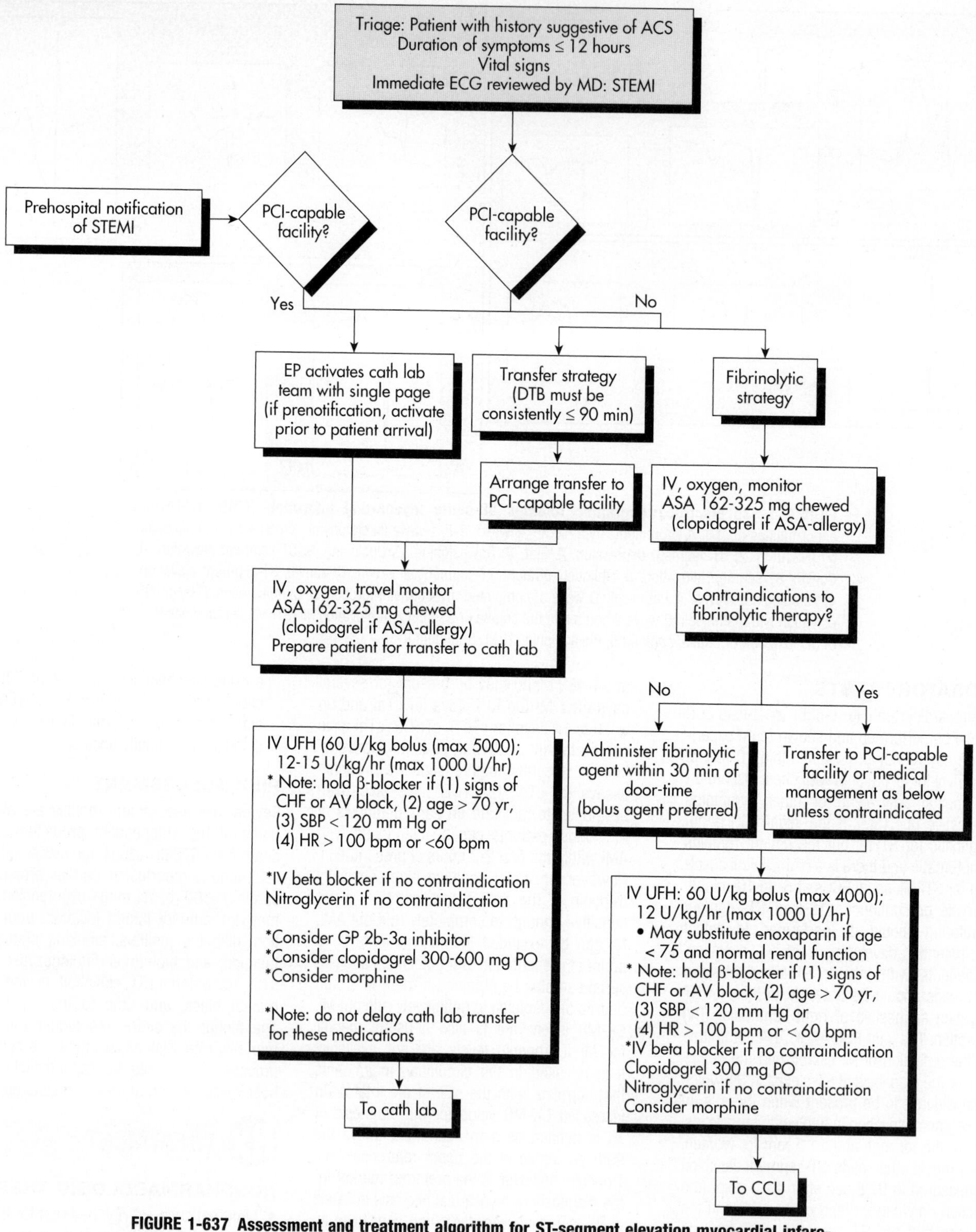

Triage: Patient with history suggestive of ACS
Duration of symptoms ≤ 12 hours
Vital signs
Immediate ECG reviewed by MD: STEMI

Prehospital notification of STEMI → PCI-capable facility?

PCI-capable facility?

Yes:

EP activates cath lab team with single page (if prenotification, activate prior to patient arrival)

No:

Transfer strategy (DTB must be consistently ≤ 90 min) → Arrange transfer to PCI-capable facility

Fibrinolytic strategy → IV, oxygen, monitor ASA 162-325 mg chewed (clopidogrel if ASA-allergy) → Contraindications to fibrinolytic therapy?

- No: Administer fibrinolytic agent within 30 min of door-time (bolus agent preferred)
- Yes: Transfer to PCI-capable facility or medical management as below unless contraindicated

IV, oxygen, travel monitor
ASA 162-325 mg chewed
(clopidogrel if ASA-allergy)
Prepare patient for transfer to cath lab

IV UFH (60 U/kg bolus (max 5000);
12-15 U/kg/hr (max 1000 U/hr)
* Note: hold β-blocker if (1) signs of CHF or AV block, (2) age > 70 yr, (3) SBP < 120 mm Hg or (4) HR > 100 bpm or <60 bpm

*IV beta blocker if no contraindication
Nitroglycerin if no contraindication

*Consider GP 2b-3a inhibitor
*Consider clopidogrel 300-600 mg PO
*Consider morphine

*Note: do not delay cath lab transfer for these medications

To cath lab

IV UFH: 60 U/kg bolus (max 4000);
12 U/kg/hr (max 1000 U/hr)
• May substitute enoxaparin if age < 75 and normal renal function
* Note: hold β-blocker if (1) signs of CHF or AV block, (2) age > 70 yr, (3) SBP < 120 mm Hg or (4) HR > 100 bpm or < 60 bpm
*IV beta blocker if no contraindication
Clopidogrel 300 mg PO
Nitroglycerin if no contraindication
Consider morphine

To CCU

FIGURE 1-637 Assessment and treatment algorithm for ST-segment elevation myocardial infarction (STEMI). *ACS*, Acute coronary syndrome; *ASA*, acetylsalicylic acid; *AV*, atrioventricular; *bpm*, beats per minute; *cath lab*, catheterization laboratory; *CCU*, cardiac care unit; *CHF*, congestive heart failure; *DTB*, door-to-balloon time; *ECG*, electrocardiogram; *EP*, emergency physician; *GP*, glycoprotein; *HR*, heart rate; *IV*, intravenous/intravenous line; *PCI*, percutaneous coronary intervention; *PO*, orally; *SBP*, systolic blood pressure; *UFH*, unfractionated heparin. (From Adams JG et al: *Emergency medicine, clinical essentials*, ed 2, Philadelphia, 2013, Elsevier.)

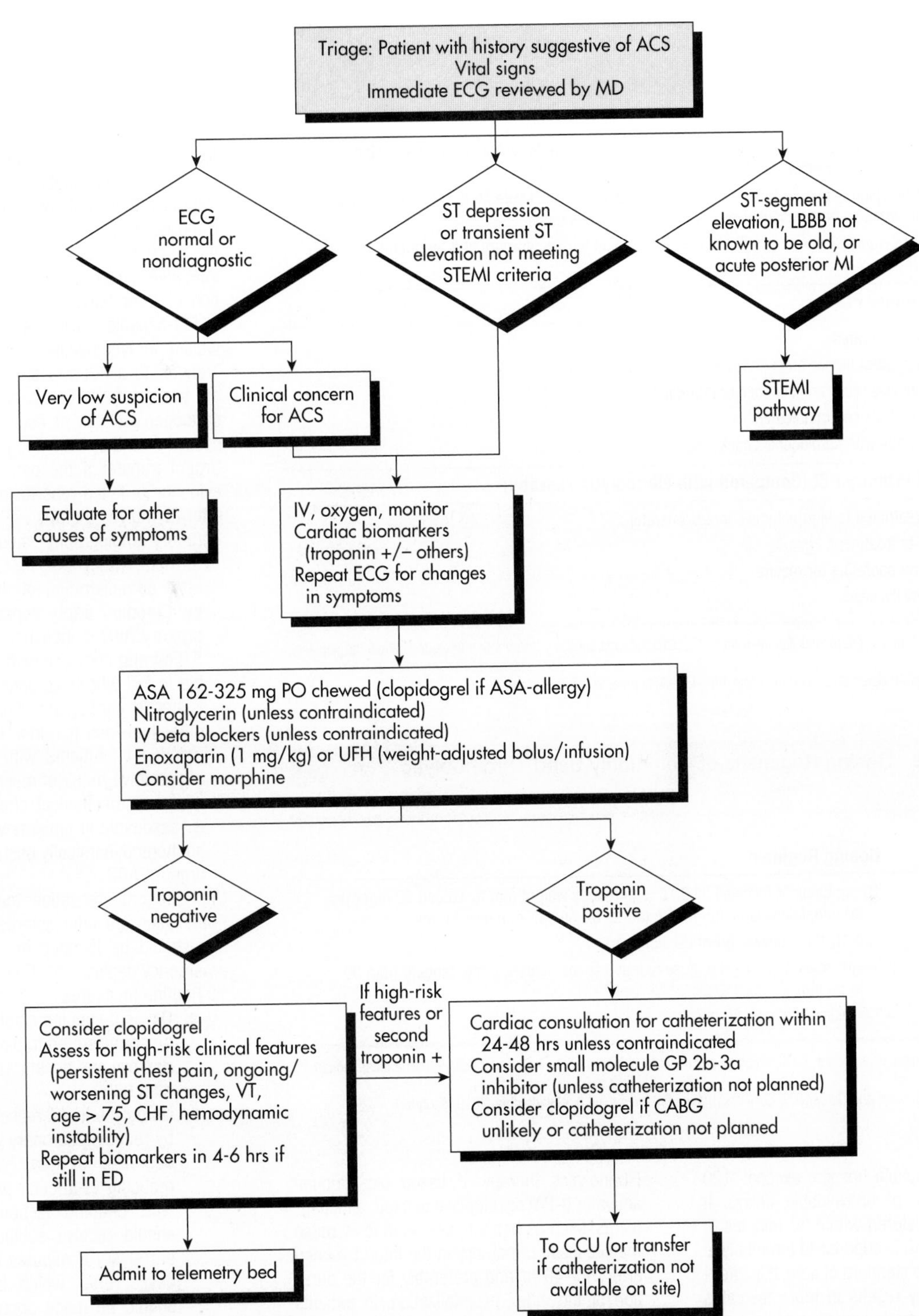

FIGURE 1-638 Assessment and treatment algorithm for non–ST-segment elevation myocardial infarction. *ACS,* Acute coronary syndrome; *ASA,* acetylsalicylic acid; *CABG,* coronary artery bypass grafting; *CCU,* cardiac care unit; *CHF,* congestive heart failure; *ED,* emergency department; *ECG,* electrocardiogram; *GP,* glycoprotein; *IV,* intravenous/intravenous line; *LBBB,* left bundle branch block; *MI,* myocardial infarction; *STEMI,* ST-segment elevation myocardial infarction; *UFH,* unfractionated heparin; *VT,* ventricular tachycardia. (From Adams JG et al: *Emergency medicine, clinical essentials,* ed 2, Philadelphia, 2013, Elsevier.)

for non-ST-segment MI is described in Fig. 1-638. Rationale of the treatment of a patient with STEMI is based on "time is muscle." Therefore, all communities should create and maintain a regional system of STEMI care that includes assessment and continuous quality improvement of EMS and hospital-based activities. A 12-lead ECG must be done by EMS personnel at the site of first medical contact (FMC).

- Reperfusion therapy should be administered to all eligible patients with STEMI with symptom onset within 12 hours. Indications for primary angioplasty and comparison with fibrinolytic therapy are described in Table 1-351. Primary PCI (Fig. E1-369) is the recommended method of reperfusion when it can be performed in a timely fashion by experienced operators with an ideal FMC-to-device time system goal of 90 minutes or less. In the absence of contraindications, fibrinolytic therapy (Table 1-352) should be administered to patients with STEMI at non-PCI-capable hospitals when the anticipated FMC-to-device

TABLE 1-351 Indications for Primary Angioplasty and Comparison with Fibrinolytic Therapy

Indications
Alternative recanalization strategy for ST segment elevation or LBBB acute MI within 12 hr of symptom onset (or >12 hr if symptoms persist)
Cardiogenic shock developing within 36 hr of ST segment elevation/Q wave acute MI or LBBB acute MI in patients >75 yr old who can be revascularized within 18 hr of shock onset
Recommended only at centers performing >200 PCI/yr with backup cardiac surgery and for operators performing <75 PCI/yr
Advantages of Primary PCI
Higher initial recanalization rates
Reduced risk of intracerebral hemorrhage
Less residual stenosis; less recurrent ischemia or infarction
Usefulness when fibrinolysis contraindicated
Improvement in outcomes with cardiogenic shock
Disadvantages of Primary PCI (Compared with Fibrinolytic Therapy)
Access, advantages restricted to high-volume centers, operators
Longer average time to treatment
Greater dependence on operators for results
Higher system complexity, costs

LBBB, Left bundle branch block; *MI,* myocardial infarction; *PCI,* percutaneous coronary intervention (includes balloon angioplasty, stenting).
From Goldman L, Schafer AI: *Goldman's Cecil medicine,* ed 24, Philadelphia, 2012, Saunders.

TABLE 1-352 Dosing Regimens of Commonly Used Thrombolytic Agents

Thrombolytic Agents	Dosing Regimen
t-PA (alteplase)	15 mg bolus IV, followed by 0.75 mg/kg body weight (not to exceed 50 mg) over 30 min, followed by 0.5 mg/kg (not to exceed 35 mg) over 60 min
r-PA (reteplase)	Two 10-U IV boluses, given 30 min apart
TNK–t-PA (tenecteplase)	Single bolus IV 0.5 mg/kg (dose rounded to the nearest 5 mg, ranging from 30 to 50 mg)
Streptokinase	1.5 million U IV over 60 min

IV, Intravenous; *PA,* plasminogen activator; *r-PA,* reteplase plasminogen activator; *TNK–t-PA,* tenecteplase tissue plasminogen activator; *U,* units.
From Andreoli TE et al: *Andreoli and Carpenter's Cecil essentials of medicine,* ed 8, Philadelphia, 2010, Saunders.

time at a PCI-capable hospital exceeds 120 minutes because of unavoidable delays. It should be administered within 30 minutes of hospital arrival. PCI is superior to thrombolytic therapy and is the standard of care. It is effective and generally results in more favorable outcomes than thrombolytic therapy.

- Primary PCI should be performed in patients with STEMI and persistent ischemic symptoms and who have contraindications to fibrinolytic therapy, irrespective of the time delay from FMC, or with cardiogenic shock or acute severe HF irrespective of time delay from myocardial infarction (MI) onset. Coronary stents (drug-eluting or bare-metal) are useful in patients with STEMI.
- Because the effectiveness of thrombolytics is time dependent, these agents should ideally be administered either in the field or within 30 min of the patient's arrival to the emergency department (door-to-needle time).

Fibrinolytics therapy: if tissue plasminogen activator (t-PA) or reteplase is used, anticoagulants, such as heparin, are given to increase the likelihood of patency in the infarct-related artery for 48 hr and preferably for the duration of the index hospitalization. In patients receiving fibrinolysis for STEMI, treatment with enoxaparin is superior to treatment with unfractionated heparin for 48 hr but is associated with an increase in major bleeding episodes. In patients receiving streptokinase or APSAC, heparin after thrombolysis is not indicated because it does not offer any additional benefit and can result in increased bleeding complications. Tenecteplase and reteplase are comparable with accelerated infusion recombinant t-PA in terms of efficacy and safety but are more convenient because they are administered by bolus injection. Lanoplase and heparin bolus plus infusion are as effective as tPA with regard to mortality rate, but the rate of intracranial hemorrhage is significantly higher. Absolute contraindications to thrombolytic therapy (Table 1-353) include aortic dissection, active internal bleeding, intracranial neoplasm or arteriovenous malformation, intracranial surgery in the last 6 mo, ischemic stroke in the last yr, head trauma with loss of consciousness in the last 6 mo, surgery in noncompressible location in the last 6 wk, alteration in mental status, and infectious endocarditis. After the administration of thrombolytics, immediate transfer to a PCI-capable facility is advisable without waiting for lytic results.

- Transfer to a PCI-capable hospital: immediate transfer for STEMI patients who develop cardiogenic shock or acute severe HF, irrespective of the time delay from MI onset. Urgent transfer if the patient demonstrates evidence of failed reperfusion or reocclusion after fibrinolytic therapy.

  Coronary angiography should not be performed within the first 2 to 3 hours after administration of fibrinolytic therapy. Coronary artery bypass graft (CABG): urgent CABG is indicated in patients with STEMI and coronary anatomy not amenable to PCI who have ongoing or recurrent ischemia, cardiogenic shock, severe HF, or other high-risk features. CABG is recommended in patients with STEMI at time of operative repair of mechanical defects.

  The use of mechanical circulatory support is reasonable in patients with STEMI who are hemodynamically unstable and require urgent CABG.
- Until the catheterization team is ready or fibrinolytics are administered, medical therapy should be initiated immediately in the emergency department. This includes:
  1. Routine measures
     a. Oxygen: supplemental oxygen should be administered to patients with arterial oxygen desaturation (SaO_2 less than 90%).
     b. Nitroglycerin: increase oxygen supply by reducing coronary vasospasm and decrease oxygen consumption by reducing ventricular preload. Patients with ongoing ischemic discomfort should receive sublingual nitroglycerin every 5 minutes for a total of 3 doses, after which an assessment should be made about the need for intravenous nitroglycerin. Intravenous nitroglycerin is indicated for relief of ongoing ischemic discomfort, control of hypertension, or management of pulmonary congestion. Nitrates should not be administered to patients whose systolic blood pressure is <90 mm Hg or ≥30 mm Hg below baseline or severe bradycardia (<50 beats/min), tachycardia (>100 beats/min), or suspected RV infarction. Nitrates should not be administered to patients who have received a phosphodiesterase inhibitor for erectile dysfunction within the last 24 hr (48 hr for tadalafil).

TABLE 1-353 Contraindications to Thrombolytic Therapy in Acute Myocardial Infarction

Absolute
Suspected aortic dissection
Active bleeding*
Any prior cerebral hemorrhage
Intracranial neoplasm
Cerebral aneurysm or arteriovenous malformation
Ischemic cerebrovascular accident within 3 mo
Relative
Bleeding diathesis, coagulopathy, or anticoagulant use
Major surgery within 3 wk
Puncture of a noncompressible vessel, internal bleeding, or head or major body trauma within previous 2 wk
Nonhemorrhagic stroke or gastrointestinal hemorrhage within 6 mo
Proliferative retinopathy
Active peptic ulcer disease
History of chronic, severe, poorly controlled hypertension
Severe uncontrolled hypertension on presentation (systolic blood pressure >180 mm Hg or diastolic blood pressure >110 mm Hg)
Traumatic or prolonged (>10 min) cardiopulmonary resuscitation
Pregnancy

*Does not include menstrual bleeding.
From Andreoli TE et al: *Andreoli and Carpenter's Cecil essentials of medicine*, ed 8, Philadelphia, 2010, Saunders.

c. Adequate analgesia: morphine sulfate 2-4 mg IV initially with increments of 2-8 mg IV at 5- to 10-min intervals can be given for severe pain unrelieved by nitroglycerin. Morphine can reduce the catecholamine surge caused by anxiety and pain, which in turn can reduce the increased cardiac workload and oxygen demand, leading to decreased ischemia. Hypotension from morphine can be treated with careful IV hydration with saline solution. If sinus bradycardia accompanies hypotension, use atropine (0.5 to 1.0 mg IV q5min prn to a total dose of 2.5 mg). Respiratory depression caused by morphine can be reversed with naloxone 0.8 mg.

d. Aspirin 162-325 mg PO should be crushed and chewed to enhance drug absorption and delivery. It should be given as soon as possible and continued indefinitely, at 81 mg daily. Depending on the clinical and ECG findings, if the patient is suspected to have a coronary anatomy that needs CABG rather than PCI, thienopyridine (clopidogrel) should be avoided because it increases the perioperative bleeding risk; otherwise, surgery is deferred for 5-7 days. However, if the coronary artery disease is likely to benefit from PCI alone, then a loading dose of clopidogrel 600 mg or ticagrelor 180 mg PO should be given as early as possible or prasugrel 60 mg as early as possible and no later than 1 hour after PCI. Thienopyridines should be continued for at least 1 yr after STEMI.

- In patients receiving fibrinolytics only or balloon angioplasty without stent, thienopyridines can be given for as little as 14 d.
- Beta-adrenergic blocking agents should generally be given to all patients. Beta-blockers are useful to reduce myocardial oxygen consumption and prevent tachyarrhythmias. Early IV beta blockage (in the initial 24 hr) followed by institution of an oral maintenance regimen is also effective in reducing recurrent infarction and ischemia. Oral beta-blockers should be initiated in the first 24 hr in patients with STEMI who do not have any of the following: signs of HF, evidence of a low-output state, increased risk for cardiogenic shock, or other contraindications for its use (PR interval more than 0.24 seconds, second- or third-degree heart block, active asthma, or reactive airways disease).

  They should be continued during and after hospitalization for all patients with STEMI and with no contraindications to their use for at least 2 yr. Patients with initial contraindications to the use of beta-blockers in the first 24 hr after STEMI should be reevaluated to determine their subsequent eligibility.

  It is reasonable to administer intravenous beta-blockers at the time of presentation to patients with STEMI and no contraindications to their use who are hypertensive or have ongoing ischemia.
- Anticoagulation therapy: STEMI is due to plaque rupture exposing the underlying collagen platelets that are activated and the coagulation cascade is initiated. IV unfractionated heparin or bivalirudin, or subcutaneous enoxaparin or fondaparinux can be used. In patients at high risk of bleeding, use of bivalirudin is reasonable. Anticoagulation therapy is usually continued for 48 hours after administration of lytic therapy unless streptokinase or APSAC is used.
- Neither facilitation of PCI with reteplase plus abciximab nor facilitation with abciximab alone significantly improves the clinical outcomes compared with abciximab given at the time of PCI in patients with STEMI. In patients with acute MI, treatment with drug-eluting stents is associated with decreased 2-yr mortality rates and a reduction in the need for repeated revascularization procedures compared with treatment including bare-metal stents.

CHRONIC Rx

- Discharge medications in all patients with MI (unless contraindicated) should include antiischemic medications (e.g., nitroglycerin, beta-blocker), lipid-lowering agents, and antiplatelet therapy (aspirin and/or clopidogrel).
- Aspirin, 81 mg (baby dose) PO daily, but should be continued indefinitely unless not tolerated (e.g., GI bleed). Clopidogrel 75 mg PO daily; ticagrelor, 90 mg bid, or prasugrel, 10 mg PO daily, can be combined with aspirin and should be continued without interruption for 30 days after bare-metal stent placement or for 12 months after drug-eluting stent placement, but preferably, if no contraindications, should be given for at least 1 yr and can be discontinued after completion of duration; however, aspirin should be continued indefinitely. Combining thienopyridines with aspirin reduces risk for in-stent restenosis. If there is an elective surgical intervention pending, it is recommended to defer the surgery until completion of the full course of the thienopyridine treatment.
- Angiotensin-converting enzyme inhibitors (ACEIs) should be started within the first 24 hours of STEMI to all patients having STEMI with anterior infarction, pulmonary congestion, or LV EF <40%, in the absence of hypotension. They reduce LV dysfunction and dilation and slow the progression to HF during and after acute MI. Angiotensin receptor blockers should be given to patients who have indication but are intolerant of ACEIs. IV formulations of ACEIs should not be given within the first 24 hours of STEMI due to risk of hypotension. Angiotensin receptor blockers (ARBs) offer no advantage over ACEIs and should be considered only in patients who are intolerant to ACEIs.
  - Commonly used ACEIs are ramipril 2.5 mg PO qd, captopril 12.5 mg PO bid, enalapril 2.5 mg PO bid, and lisinopril 2.5-5 mg PO qd initially, with subsequent titration as needed. Ramipril is associated with a lower mortality rate than most ACEIs.
  - ACEIs may be stopped in patients without complications and no evidence of LV dysfunction after 6 to 8 weeks.
  - ACEIs should be continued indefinitely in patients with impaired LV function (EF <40%) or clinical HF.
- Long-term aldosterone antagonist therapy should be prescribed for post-STEMI patients without significant renal dysfunction (creatinine ≤2.5 mg/dl in men and ≤2.0 mg/dl in women) or hyperkalemia who are already taking an ACEI, a beta-blocker, and have LV EF <40% with symptomatic HF or diabetes.

- Statins should be started as early as possible in all patients with STEMI regardless of lipid panel, not only for their lipid-lowering effects, but also their anti-inflammatory properties (JUPITER trial), which can stabilize the ruptured plaque. Atorvastatin 80 mg can be used (PROVE IT-TIMI 22 and MIRACL trials). Lipid panel should be checked during the first 24 hr of hospital course and the intensive therapy can be stepped down if appropriate. Goal LDL cholesterol is <70 mg/dl. Consider addition of fenofibrate or niacin if triglycerides are significantly elevated. Recent data showed no improvement in outcome with increasing HDL cholesterol therapy using niacin; therefore its use to decrease HDL cholesterol is questionable.

COMPLICATIONS OF STEMI

Cardiogenic shock: emergent revascularization with either PCI or CABG is the recommended treatment.

Sustained ventricular tachycardia: cardioverter-defibrillator therapy is indicated before discharge in patients who develop sustained ventricular tachycardia/ventricular fibrillation more than 48 hr after STEMI, provided the arrhythmia is not due to transient or reversible ischemia, reinfarction, or metabolic abnormalities.

Pacing in STEMI: temporary pacing is indicated for symptomatic bradyarrhythmias unresponsive to medical treatment and after revascularization. A lot of AV blocks and bradyarrhythmias may be transient and resolve within 2 wk of an MI.

Pericarditis after STEMI: aspirin is recommended for treatment of pericarditis after STEMI. Glucocorticoids and nonsteroidal anti-inflammatory drugs are potentially harmful for treatment of pericarditis after STEMI.

EVALUATION OF POST-MI PATIENTS:

- Noninvasive testing for ischemia should be performed before discharge to assess the presence and extent of inducible ischemia in patients with STEMI who have not had coronary angiography and do not have high-risk clinical features for which coronary angiography would be warranted. It might be considered before discharge to evaluate the functional significance of a noninfarct artery stenosis previously identified at angiography and/or before discharge to guide the postdischarge exercise prescription.
- Assessment of LV function: LV ejection fraction should be measured in all patients with STEMI.

Echocardiography to rule out presence of mural thrombi in patients suspected of having an extensive infarction (more common with anterior wall MI); contrast echocardiography is added if mural thrombosis is suspected

  - Assessment of risk for sudden cardiac death: patients with an initially reduced LV ejection fraction who are possible candidates for implantable cardioverter-defibrillator therapy should undergo reevaluation of LV ejection fraction <35% and NYHA class II or III heart failure and should then be considered for implanted defibrillator if the life expectancy is >1 yr.
- Cardiac rehabilitation/secondary prevention programs are recommended for patients with STEMI
- Lifestyle risk factors modification

DISPOSITION

The prognosis after MI depends on multiple factors:

- New bundle branch block, Mobitz II second-degree block, and third-degree heart block adversely affect outcome.
- Size of infarct: the larger it is, the higher the post-MI mortality rate. Significant myocardial stunning with subsequent improvement of ventricular function occurs in most patients after anterior MI. A lower level of creatine kinase, an estimate of the extent of necrosis, is independently predictive of recovery of function.
- Site of infarct: inferior wall MI carries a better prognosis than anterior wall MI; however, patients with inferior wall MI and right ventricular involvement have a high risk for arrhythmic complications and cardiogenic shock.
- Ejection fraction after MI: the lower the LV ejection fraction, the higher the mortality rate after MI. The risk of death is higher in the first 30 days after MI among patients with LV dysfunction, HF, or both.
- Presence of post-MI angina indicates a high mortality rate.
- Performance on low-level exercise test: the presence of ST-segment changes during the test is a predictor of high mortality rate during the first year.
- Presence of pericarditis during the acute phase of MI increases mortality rate at 1 yr.
- Type A behavior (competitive drive, ambitiousness, hostility) is associated with a lower mortality rate after symptomatic MI.
- The Killip classification is an independent predictor of all-cause 30-day mortality:
  - Killip class I includes individuals with no clinical signs of HF. Mortality rate is 6%.
  - Killip class II includes individuals with rales or crackles in the lungs, S_3 gallop, and elevated jugular venous pressure. Mortality rate is 17%.
  - Killip class III describes individuals with frank acute pulmonary edema. Mortality rate is 38%.
  - Killip class IV describes individuals in cardiogenic shock or hypotension (measured as systolic blood pressure <90 mm Hg) and evidence of peripheral vasoconstriction (oliguria, cyanosis, or sweating). Mortality rate is 67%.
- Self-reported moderate alcohol consumption in the year before acute MI is associated with reduced 1-yr mortality rate.
- Discharge medication in patients with MI should include lipid-lowering agents. Statins may also lower vascular inflammation and damage by mechanisms other than reduction of low-density lipoprotein cholesterol. Early initiation of statin treatment in patients with acute MI is associated with reduced 1-yr mortality rate.
- Additional poor prognostic factors include cigarette smoking, history of hypertension or prior MI, presence of ST-segment depression in acute MI, older age, diabetes mellitus, and female sex (especially women >50 yr).
- Renal disease, even mild, as assessed by the estimated glomerular filtration rate, is a major risk factor for cardiovascular complications after MI.
- Although black patients with MI have worse outcomes than white patients, these differences did not persist after adjustment for patient factors and site of care.

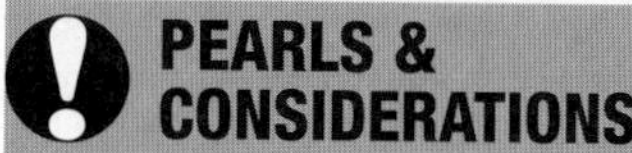

PEARLS & CONSIDERATIONS

COMMENTS

- Approximately 1.5 million patients undergo PCI in the United States each year. Depending on local practices and the diagnostic criteria used, 5% to 30% of these patients have evidence of a periprocedural MI.
- The 12-lead ECG has low sensitivity for the detection of MI if the culprit lesion is in the left circumflex artery (LCX). If the initial 12-lead ECG is not diagnostic and high clinical suspicion for acute coronary syndrome exists it is reasonable to obtain additional posterior chest leads (V_7 to V_9) to detect LCX occlusion.

SUGGESTED READINGS

available at www.expertconsult.com

RELATED CONTENT

Acute Coronary Syndrome (Related Key Topic)
Angina Pectoris (Related Key Topic)
Heart Attack (Patient Information)

AUTHOR: **CLAUDIA SERRANO-GOMEZ, M.D.**

BASIC INFORMATION

DEFINITION

Myocarditis broadly refers to inflammation of the heart muscle. This may result from exposure to discrete external antigens such as viruses, bacteria, parasites, and drugs or from internal triggers such as autoimmune conditions.

ICD-9CM CODES
429.0 Myocarditis, nonspecific
391.2 Myocarditis, rheumatic
422.91 Myocarditis, viral (except Coxsackie)
074.23 Myocarditis, Coxsackie
422.92 Myocarditis, bacterial
ICD-10CM CODES
I40 Acute myocarditis
I40.0 Infective myocarditis
I40.1 Isolated myocarditis
I40.8 Other acute myocarditis
I40.4 Acute myocarditis, unspecified

EPIDEMIOLOGY & DEMOGRAPHICS

- The incidence of focal myocarditis reported at autopsy is 1% to 9% in asymptomatic patients and 50% in patients infected with HIV.
- Myocarditis is a major cause of sudden unexpected death (as high as 8% to 9%) in young adults <40 years of age, especially in cases of idiopathic dilated cardiomyopathy, where myocarditis may account for 10% to 40% of the cases overall.

PHYSICAL FINDINGS & CLINICAL PRESENTATION

- Persistent tachycardia out of proportion to fever
- Faint S_1, S_3, and S_4 gallops on auscultation
- Murmur of functional mitral regurgitation and functional tricuspid regurgitation caused by severe left ventricular dilatation
- Pericardial friction rub if associated with pericarditis as in myopericarditis
- Chest pain especially pleuritic and positional when the pericardium is involved.
- Presyncope or syncope
- Viral prodrome and fatigue
- Congestive heart failure (CHF) symptoms that usually manifest with fatigue and decreased exercise capacity
- If myocarditis is severe and diffuse and rapid in evolution, it can present with acute CHF symptoms leading to cardiogenic shock and death.
- Signs of biventricular failure (hypotension, hepatomegaly, peripheral edema, distention of neck veins, S_3 sounds)
- Patients may present with a history of recent flulike syndrome (fever, arthralgias, malaise); children often have a more fulminant presentation. Difficulty breathing is the most common presentation of pediatric myocarditis.
- The most common presentations are dyspnea (72% of patients), chest pain (32%), and arrhythmias (sinus tachycardia, atrial and ventricular premature contractions) (18%).
- Acute coronary syndrome, which can occur because of local coronary spasm and inflammation and can present on ECG as infarction or ischemic changes
- Sudden cardiac death from ventricular tachycardia/ventricular fibrillation mediated by inflammation and/or scar

ETIOLOGY

- Infection
  1. Viral (adenovirus, parvovirus B19, hepatitis C virus (HCV), Coxsackie B virus, cytomegalovirus, echovirus, poliovirus, mumps, HIV, Epstein-Barr virus). Viruses are the most common cause of myocarditis in developed countries. In the 1980s and 1990s, enteroviruses were frequently associated with myocarditis and dilated cardiomyopathy. In the past 10 years, however, other viruses such as adenovirus, HCV, parvovirus B19, and herpesvirus 6 (HH6) have emerged as the significant pathogens.
  2. Bacterial (*Staphylococcus aureus, Clostridium perfringens,* diphtheria, and any severe bacterial infection)
  3. *Mycoplasma*
  4. Mycotic *(Candida, Mucor, Aspergillus)*
  5. Parasitic (*Trypanosoma cruzi*—most common worldwide, *Trichinella, Echinococcus, Amoeba, Toxoplasma*)
  6. *Rickettsia rickettsii*
  7. Spirochetal *(Borrelia burgdorferi*–Lyme carditis)
- Rheumatic fever
- Systemic lupus erythematosus
- Wegener's granulomatosis
- Giant cell arteritis and Takayasu's arteritis
- Drugs (e.g., cocaine, emetine, doxorubicin, sulfonamides, isoniazid, methyldopa, amphotericin B, tetracycline, phenylbutazone, lithium, 5-fluorouracil, phenothiazines, interferon-alfa, tricyclic antidepressants, cyclophosphamides, smallpox vaccination)
- Toxins (carbon monoxide, ethanol, diphtheria toxin, lead, arsenicals)
- Systemic and collagen-vascular disease (scleroderma, sarcoidosis, celiac disease, Sjögren's syndrome, Kawasaki syndrome, etc.)
- Radiation
- Postpartum status

Dx DIAGNOSIS

DIFFERENTIAL DIAGNOSIS

- Ischemic cardiomyopathies and other, nonischemic cardiomyopathies
- Acute coronary syndromes
- Valvulopathies
- Infiltrative diseases of the myocardium, such as sarcoidosis, amyloidosis, hemochromatosis, and Chagas' disease.

The differential diagnosis of chest pain is described in Section II.

WORKUP

- Medical history: the clinical presentation of myocarditis is nonspecific and can consist of fatigue, palpitations, dyspnea, precordial discomfort, and myalgias.
- Diagnostic workup includes chest x-ray examination, ECG, laboratory evaluation, echocardiogram, cardiac catheterization, and endomyocardial biopsy (in selected patients on the basis of the likelihood of finding specific treatable disorders such as giant cell myocarditis). Of note, endomyocardial biopsy has a sensitivity of only 10% to 35% using standard histologic criteria. This is due to variability in interpretation and sampling error.

LABORATORY TESTS

- Elevated cardiac troponin T is suggestive of myocarditis in patients with clinically suspected myocarditis. Troponin I specificity is 89%; sensitivity is 34% to 53%. A normal level does not rule out the diagnosis.
- Increased creatine kinase (CK) (with elevated MB fraction, lactate dehydrogenase), and aspartate aminotransferase from myocardial necrosis.
- Elevation of cardiac troponin I or T is more common than CK-MB elevation in patients with biopsy-proven myocarditis.
- The elevations of cardiac troponin I were correlated with a short duration (typically less than 1 mo) of CHF symptoms, indicating that the majority of myocardial necrosis occurs early in the disease course.
- Persistent elevations of cardiac biomarkers are indicative of ongoing myocardial necrosis.
- Increased erythrocyte sedimentation rate (nonspecific but may be of value in following the progress of the disease and the response to therapy).
- Increased white blood cell count (increased eosinophils if parasitic infection).
- Viral titers (acute and convalescent).
- Cold agglutinin titer, antistreptolysin O titer, blood cultures.
- Lyme disease antibody titer.
- RPR, VDRL.

IMAGING STUDIES

- Chest radiograph: enlargement of cardiac silhouette
- ECG: sinus tachycardia with nonspecific ST-T wave changes unless there is concomitant pericarditis in which the ECG changes are more specific; interventricular conduction defects and bundle branch block are uncommon in typical viral myocarditis but are common manifestations in cardiac sarcoid and idiopathic giant cell myocarditis.
  1. Lyme disease and diphtheria cause all degrees of heart block.
  2. Changes mimicking acute myocardial infarction can occur with focal necrosis.
- Echocardiogram:
  1. The most useful test in detecting decreased ventricular function in suspected myocarditis even when subclinical.

 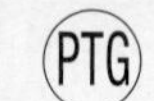

2. The spheroid dysfunctional ventricle in acute myocarditis tends to remodel to the more normal elliptical shape over several months.
3. Dilated and hypokinetic chambers
4. The dysfunction is generally global but may be regional or segmental.
5. Abnormal tissue Doppler signal can provide additional evidence for the presence of myocarditis.
6. The echocardiogram can also be helpful with diagnosing coexisting pericardial involvement.

- Cardiac catheterization and angiography:
  1. To rule out coronary artery disease and valvular disease. Coronary angiography is most commonly normal with no evidence of coronary artery disease.
  2. A right ventricular endomyocardial biopsy can confirm the diagnosis, although a negative biopsy result does not exclude myocarditis owing to the low sensitivity of this test. Recent studies have shown that myocardial biopsy may be unnecessary because immunosuppression therapy based on biopsy results is generally ineffective. However, if idiopathic giant cell myocarditis is suspected, biopsy can confirm this diagnosis, and immunosuppression therapy is often helpful in this patient cohort.
- Cardiac MRI (Fig. 1-640):
  1. Can be used to detect myocardial edema and myocyte injury in myocarditis.
  2. Increased focal or global signal intensity can be used to calculate an edema ratio.
  3. Late gadolinium enhancement (LGE) and the presence of increased focal and global myocardial contrast enhancement relative to skeletal muscle.
  4. Any combination of two of the above has a sensitivity and specificity of 86% and 95%, respectively, and is probably the gold standard for diagnosis of myocarditis today.
  5. Cardiac MRI has demonstrated that myocarditis tends to start as a focal process and becomes a more global process over time, with the extent of myocardial enhancement correlating with clinical status and left ventricular function.
  6. Some viral pathogens have focal involvement of the myocardium. Parvovirus B19 involves the subepicardial lateral wall of the left ventricle. HHV6 and especially the combination of HHV6/parvovirus B19 tend to involve the septum and present with more acute and chronic heart failure symptoms.
  7. The pattern of LGE is different from that in ischemic cardiomyopathy. LGE in myocarditis tends to involve the epicardium with variable extension into the midmyocardium and sparing of the endocardium.
- Indium-111-labeled antimyosin antibody scintigraphy is positive in myocarditis with a sensitivity of up to 65%.

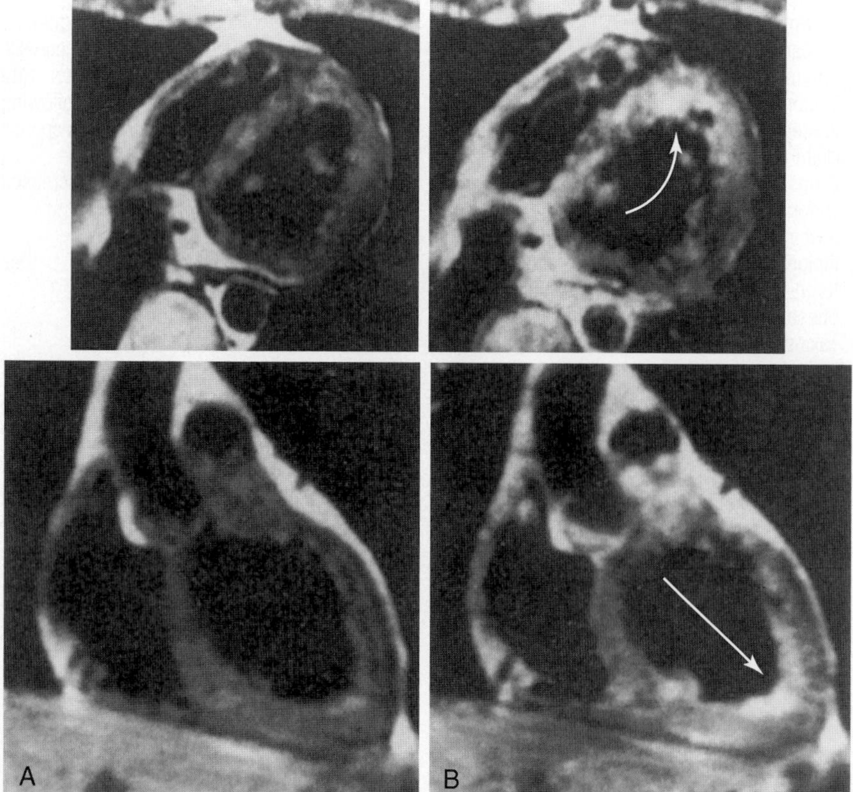

FIGURE 1-640 A, Precontrast T1-weighted transaxial *(upper)* and coronal *(lower)* magnetic resonance images through the left ventricle in a patient with myocarditis. **B,** Postcontrast magnetic resonance images at the same levels after contrast injection. Note enhancement of the myocardial signal in the septum and apical region *(arrows)*. (From Zipes DP et al [eds]: *Braunwald's heart disease*, ed 7, Philadelphia, 2005, Saunders.)

Rx TREATMENT

NONPHARMACOLOGIC THERAPY

- Supportive care is the first line of therapy for patients with myocarditis.
- Restrict physical activity (to decrease cardiac work). Bed rest is advisable during viremia.

ACUTE GENERAL RX

- Treat underlying cause (e.g., use specific antibiotics for bacterial infection).
- Treat congestive heart failure (CHF) with diuretics, angiotensin-converting enzyme inhibitors (ACE inhibitors), and salt restriction. A beta-blocker may be added once clinical stability has been achieved. Digoxin should be used with caution and only at low doses.
- Patients who are left with an LVEF ≤35% despite optimal medical therapy, who have a good functional status, and who have a prognosis >1 yr will benefit from primary prevention with implantable cardioverter-defibrillator (ICD) implantation as in patients with ischemic cardiomyopathy and other nonischemic cardiomyopathies.
- Antiarrhythmics if needed for ventricular arrhythmias. ICD implantation for secondary prevention in patients with life-threatening ventricular arrhythmias who have good functional status and a prognosis >1 yr.
- In patients with chronic CHF from myocarditis, only ACE inhibitors, beta-blockers, and possibly aldosterone receptor antagonists will decrease their mortality in the long run.
- Provide anticoagulation to prevent thromboembolism in atrial fibrillation, in severe left ventricular dysfunction with an EF >20%, and in patients with severe segmental wall motion abnormality of the apex.
- Inotropes or mechanical assist devices such as intra-aortic balloon pumps, Impella device, and left ventricular assist device (LVAD) if severe heart failure or if cardiogenic shock persists despite medical therapy.
- Cardiac transplantation in patients with chronic myocarditis with intractable cardiomyopathy and persistent CHF.
- Corticosteroid use is contraindicated in early infectious myocarditis; it may be justified in only selected patients with intractable CHF, severe systemic toxicity, and severe life-threatening arrhythmias.
- Immunosuppressive drugs (prednisone with cyclosporine or azathioprine) do not have any significant effect on the prognosis of myocarditis and should not be used in the routine treatment of patients with myocarditis. Immunosuppression may have a role in the treatment of myocarditis from systemic autoimmune disease (e.g., lupus, scleroderma), in patients with idiopathic giant cell myocarditis, myocarditis caused by hypersensitivity reactions, or severe hemodynamic compromise.
- In patients with ongoing viral genomic expression, treatment with interferons may improve both symptoms and left ventricular function when compared with standard heart

failure therapy and is currently showing promising data in Phase III clinical trials.

- IV immunoglobulins have been studied, but because of lack of efficacy data, at present there is no indication for their use except in some pediatric cases or those refractory to immunosuppressive therapy.
- A treatment algorithm for patients with myocarditis is described in Fig. 1-641.

DISPOSITION

- Most patients with acute myocarditis and mild cardiac involvement have a partial or a full clinical recovery. In some cases, however, the process may continue subclinically with eventual progression to a cardiomyopathy. Therefore all patients with myocarditis should be followed up at least initially at intervals of 1 to 3 mo. Of those with advanced cardiac dysfunction, one third will have residual cardiac dysfunction and 25% may progress to cardiac transplantation or death.
- Prognosis is best for patients with fulminant lymphocytic myocarditis (severe hemodynamic compromise, rapid onset of symptoms, or high fever). These patients tend to have complete recovery with total resolution of myocarditis on repeat biopsy.
- In contrast, patients with giant cell myocarditis have an extremely poor prognosis with a median survival of <6 mo, and most require cardiac transplantation.

REFERRAL

Consider heart transplant if intractable CHF develops.

SUGGESTED READINGS

available at www.expertconsult.com

RELATED CONTENT

Myocarditis (Patient Information)

AUTHORS: **PHILLIP RUISI, D.O.**, and **ARAVIND RAO KOKKIRALA, M.D.**

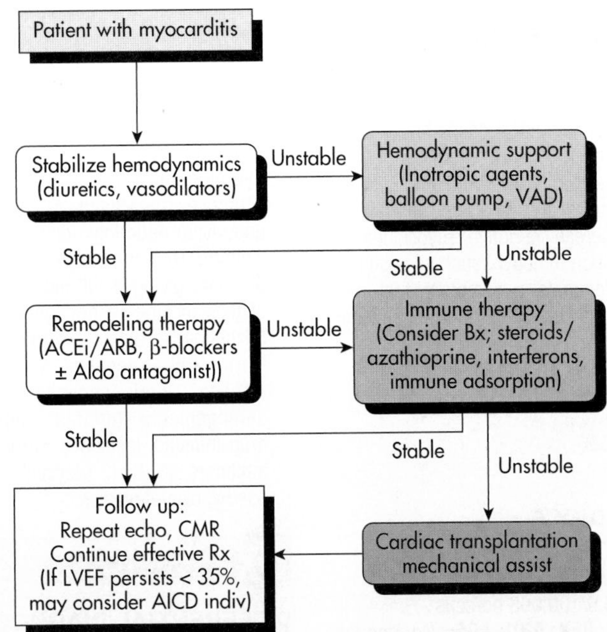

FIGURE 1-641 Treatment algorithms for patients with myocarditis, depending on hemodynamic stability and response to general supportive and remodeling treatment regimen at each step. All patients should have aggressive support and appropriate follow-up. Immune therapy at present is still mainly to support those who have failed to improve spontaneously. *ACEi*, Angiotensin-converting enzyme inhibitors; *AICD*, automatic implantable cardioverter-defibrillator; *Aldo*, aldosterone; *ARB*, angiotensin receptor blockers; *Bx*, biopsy; *CMR*, cardiac magnetic resonance; *indiv*, based on individual assessment of risk versus benefit; *LVEF*, left ventricular ejection fraction; *VAD*, ventricular assist device. (From Bonow RO et al: *Heart disease*, ed 9, Philadelphia, 2012 ,Saunders.)

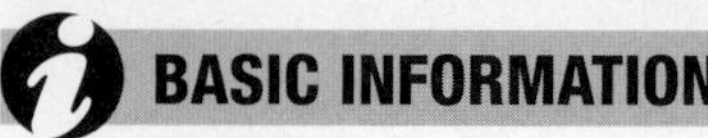

BASIC INFORMATION

DEFINITION

Myoclonus is defined as sudden, brief, jerky, "shocklike" involuntary movements that can involve the muscles of the extremities, face, or trunk. Positive myoclonus is caused by muscle contraction, whereas negative myoclonus is caused by inhibition of active (such as postural) muscles. Myoclonus is a symptom that can be seen in a number of different neurologic disorders.

ICD-9CM CODES
333.2 Myoclonus
ICD-10CM CODES
G25.3 Myoclonus

EPIDEMIOLOGY & DEMOGRAPHICS

INCIDENCE: 1.3/100,000 persons
PREVALENCE: 8.6/100,000 persons
PREDOMINANT SEX AND AGE: No gender preference; age at onset varies by the etiology of the myoclonus.
GENETICS: Varies by etiology, can be hereditary or sporadic

PHYSICAL FINDINGS & CLINICAL PRESENTATION

- Clinically, myoclonus can be classified by its distribution: focal (only one body part involved), multifocal, segmental (spread to adjacent body parts), axial (muscles innervated by one or several spinal levels), or generalized. It can be stimulus-induced or occur at rest.
- Myoclonus can be seen with involvement or lesions of the cerebral cortex, brain stem, spinal cord, or peripheral nerve. The location of the lesion may not always influence the characteristics of the myoclonus.
- Negative myoclonus is typically seen in postural muscles of the legs, causing a "bobbing" while walking. Asterixis is another form of negative myoclonus.

ETIOLOGY

- The causes of myoclonus are numerous and can be grouped into the categories of physiologic, essential, epileptic, and symptomatic.
- Physiologic myoclonus ranges from sleep (hypnic) jerks to exercise-induced myoclonus and can be seen in normal subjects.
- Essential myoclonus occurs in the absence of other neurologic symptoms and is usually autosomal dominant. When dystonia is present, it is called myoclonus-dystonia. The myoclonus is often responsive to alcohol in this condition.
- In epileptic myoclonus, seizures dominate the clinical picture. Syndromes include infantile spasms and juvenile myoclonic epilepsy among others.
- Symptomatic or secondary myoclonus comprises myoclonus in the setting of an underlying neurologic disorder or other precipitant. The number of secondary causes prevents giving a full list, but common etiologies include neurodegenerative diseases (Alzheimer's, atypical forms of parkinsonism), CNS infections (Creutzfeldt-Jakob disease, viral encephalitis), metabolic derangements (uremia, hepatic failure), drug-induced (selective serotonin reuptake inhibitors [SSRIs], tricyclics, lithium), and posthypoxic etiologies.

Dx DIAGNOSIS

DIFFERENTIAL DIAGNOSIS

- Tremor: a rhythmic oscillation around a point; slower than myoclonus
- Tic: complex patterned movements that can be suppressed voluntarily for a short time unlike myoclonus, which is simple jerks that are persistent
- Dystonia: patterned contractions of agonist/antagonist muscles causing twisting or pulling; slower than myoclonus
- Chorea: typically slower, writhing, patterned movements
- Psychogenic myoclonus: variable in duration and location, distractible, or entrainable

LABORATORY TESTS

- Evaluate for metabolic precipitants (renal and hepatic function, Mg, Ca, thyroid studies)
- Toxicology screen
- Lumbar puncture if encephalitis is suspected
- Electroencephalography (EEG) to evaluate for epileptic myoclonus

IMAGING STUDIES

MRI of the brain can evaluate for a seizure focus if the myoclonus is epileptic. Creutzfeldt-Jakob disease can show diffusion weighted abnormalities in the striatum and cortex.

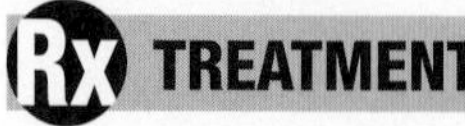

Rx TREATMENT

NONPHARMACOLOGIC THERAPY

- Treatment should be directed toward correcting the underlying cause if it is reversible (e.g., hepatic or renal failure).
- Carefully remove or decrease potentially causative medications.

ACUTE GENERAL Rx

For acute treatment of epileptic myoclonus, antiepileptic drugs such as valproic acid, levetiracetam, or clonazepam are helpful.

CHRONIC Rx

- Clonazepam, valproic acid, levetiracetam are typically used for all forms of myoclonus, and often combinations of several medications seem to be more effective.
- If dystonia is present (myoclonus-dystonia), a trial of levodopa is worthwhile although only rarely responsive. Anticholinergics may also help dystonia. Botulinum toxin injections are used for focal dystonias.
- Peripheral focal myoclonus can also be helped by botulinum toxin injections.

DISPOSITION

The ultimate prognosis depends on the etiology of the myoclonus.

REFERRAL

Referral to a general neurologist or movement disorders center is appropriate.

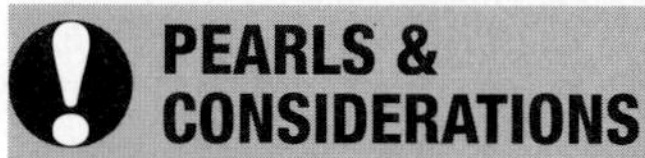

PEARLS & CONSIDERATIONS

COMMENTS

- When myoclonus is seen with parkinsonism, atypical forms of parkinsonism should be high on the differential such as dementia with Lewy bodies, corticobasal degeneration, and multiple system atrophy. Myoclonus is only rarely seen in idiopathic Parkinson's disease.
- Symptomatic palatal myoclonus is a specific syndrome that is often associated with a focal brain-stem lesion. In essential palatal myoclonus (no lesion), ear "clicking" is an additional symptom, which is not seen in the symptomatic form.

SUGGESTED READINGS
available at www.expertconsult.com

AUTHOR: **ANDREW DUKER, M.D.**

BASIC INFORMATION

DEFINITION

Inflammatory myopathies are idiopathic diseases of muscle characterized clinically by muscle weakness and pathologically by inflammation and muscle fiber breakdown. The three most common are dermatomyositis (DM), polymyositis (PM), and inclusion body myositis (IBM). See separate topic on "Inclusion Body Myositis" for details regarding the latter.

SYNONYMS

Idiopathic inflammatory myopathies
Myositis syndromes
Polymyositis
Dermatomyositis

ICD-9CM CODES
710.3 Dermatomyositis
710.4 Polymyositis
ICD-10CM CODES
M33.90 Dermatopolymyositis, unspecified, organ involvement unspecified
M33.20 Polymyositis, organ involvement unspecified

EPIDEMIOLOGY & DEMOGRAPHICS

DM:

- Occurs in children and in adults (bimodal age peak)
- Average age at diagnosis is 40 yr in adults. Age range in children: 5 to 14 yr
- More common in females than in males (2:1)
- Incidence 1:100,000
- Prevalence 1 to 10 cases/million in adults and 1 to 3.2 cases/million in children
- Up to one third of patients older than 50 with DM have an associated malignancy

PM:

- Occurs mostly in adults, very rare in children
- Average age at diagnosis >20 yr
- More common in females
- Least common inflammatory myopathy
- Exact incidence unknown

PHYSICAL FINDINGS & CLINICAL PRESENTATION

DM and PM:

- Most patients have a subacute onset over weeks to months.
- Pattern is typically symmetric proximal muscle weakness involving the proximal limbs (shoulder and pelvic girdles).
- Weakness of neck flexion and extension is common.
- Difficulty getting up from a chair, climbing stairs, reaching for objects above head, or combing hair.
- Distal muscle and ocular involvement is uncommon.
- Sensation is preserved.
- Reflexes may be preserved or diminished.
- Dysphagia and dysphonia result from involvement of striated muscle of the pharynx and proximal esophagus.
- Esophageal dysmotility is common in DM.
- Respiratory failure from associated pulmonary fibrosis.
- Cardiac conduction abnormalities can be seen with DM.
- Systemic autoimmune disease occurs frequently in PM, and rarely in DM.
- Skin findings in DM:
  - Heliotrope rash on the upper eyelids (Fig. 1-642)
  - Erythematous rash on the face (see Fig. 1-642)
  - May also involve the back and shoulders (shawl sign), neck and chest (V-shape), knees (Fig. 1-643), and elbows
  - Photosensitivity
  - Gottron's papules (violaceous papules overlying dorsal interphalangeal or metacarpophalangeal areas, elbow or knee joints—Fig. 1-644)
  - Nail cracking, thickening, and irregularity (Fig. 1-645) with periungual telangiectasia (see Fig. 1-644)
  - Mechanic's hand: fissured, hyperpigmented, scaly, and hyperkeratotic; also associated with increased risk of interstitial lung disease

ETIOLOGY

DM: complex, immune-mediated microangiopathy. Adaptive immune response via humorally mediated complement attack

PM: unknown:

- Cell-mediated immune major histocompatibility-I (MHC-1) process directed against muscle fibers is likely, given biopsy features.
- A viral etiology has been proposed secondary to the presence of autoantibodies to histidyl transferase, anti-Jo-1, and signal recognition particle.

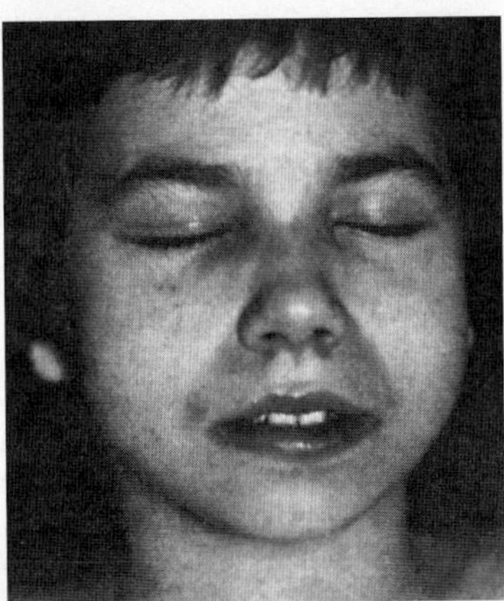

FIGURE 1-642 The facial rash of juvenile dermatomyositis. There is erythema over the bridge of the nose and malar areas, with violaceous (heliotropic) discoloration of the upper eyelids. (From Behrman RE: *Nelson textbook of pediatrics,* ed 17, Philadelphia, 2004, Saunders.)

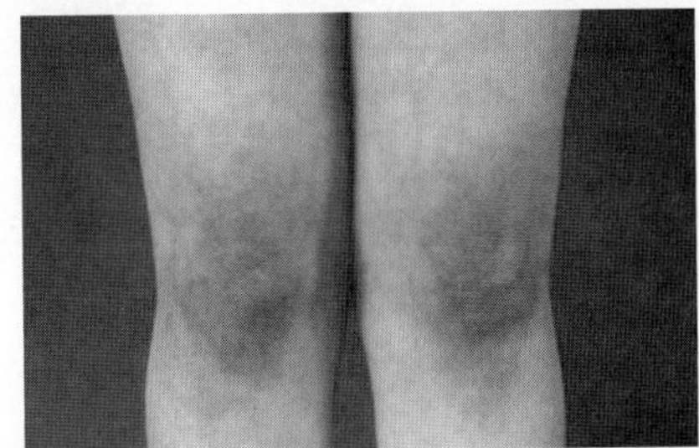

FIGURE 1-643 Violaceous plaques on the knees in a patient with dermatomyositis (Gottron sign). (From Hochberg MC et al: *Rheumatology,* ed 5, St Louis, 2011, Mosby.)

DIAGNOSIS

- Myopathic pattern of muscle weakness
- Characteristic rash in DM
- EMG shows myopathic (small-amplitude, short-duration, polyphasic) motor potentials with early recruitment
- Majority of patients have "irritable" features (fibrillations and positive sharp waves) on EMG
- See "Laboratory Tests."
- Biopsy is required for diagnosis and should confirm inflammation before treatment is started. Table E1-354 describes histologic features of idiopathic inflammatory myopathies. In idiopathic inflammatory myopathies, myopathic features (variation in fiber size, fiber splitting, fatty replacement of muscle tissue, and increased endomysial connective tissue) should be seen in addition to the following:
  - DM: perifascicular atrophy, MAC deposition along capillaries

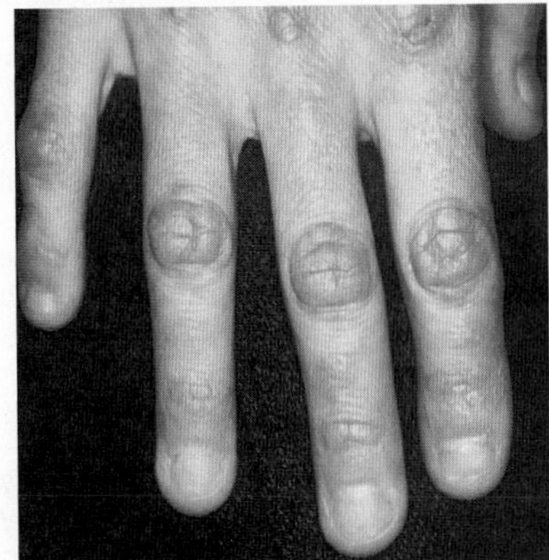

FIGURE 1-644 Dermatomyositis (Gottron's papules). Note erythematous papules over joints and periungual telangiectasias. (From Noble J [ed]: *Textbook of primary care medicine,* ed 2, St Louis, 1996, Mosby.)

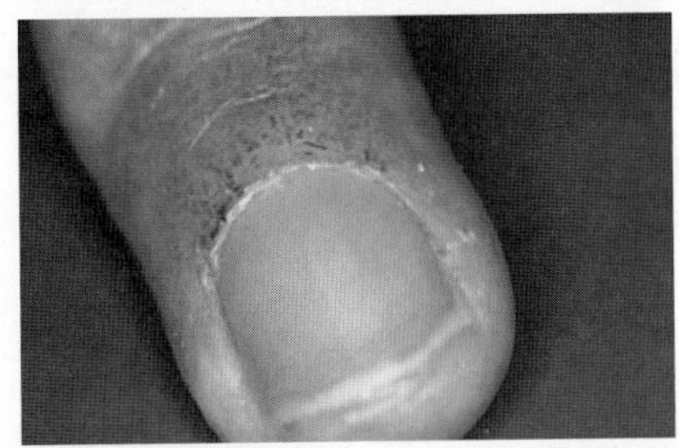

FIGURE 1-645 Enlarged nailfold capillaries in a patient with dermatomyositis. (From Hochberg MC et al: *Rheumatology,* ed 5, St Louis, 2011, Mosby.)

- PM: endomysial infiltrates composed of CD8+ T cells and macrophages invading nonnecrotic muscle fibers that express MHC-I antigen

DIFFERENTIAL DIAGNOSIS

- IBM
- Muscular dystrophies
- Amyloid myoneuropathy
- Amyotrophic lateral sclerosis
- Myasthenia gravis
- Eaton-Lambert syndrome
- Drug-induced myopathies (e.g., quinidine, NSAIDs, penicillamine, HMG CoA-reductase inhibitors)
- Diabetic amyotrophy
- Guillain-Barré syndrome
- Hyperthyroidism or hypothyroidism
- Lichen planus
- Amyopathic DM (rash without weakness)
- DM sine rash (weakness with characteristic biopsy, but no rash)
- Systemic lupus erythematosus (SLE)
- Contact atopic or seborrheic dermatitis
- Psoriasis

LABORATORY TESTS

- Creatine kinase (CK) is the most sensitive muscle enzyme test for muscle breakdown. It should be checked at onset, and serially monitored several times during treatment.
- CK is typically elevated (5-50x normal) in active PM.
- CK may be normal or only slightly elevated in DM.
- Aldolase, AST, ALT, alkaline phosphatase, and LDH may be elevated.
- Anti-Jo-1 antibodies are seen in myositis with associated interstitial lung disease but are not specific for either DM or PM.
- Electrolytes, thyroid-stimulating hormone (TSH), Ca, and Mg should be evaluated to exclude other causes of weakness.
- Check ECG for cardiac involvement.

IMAGING STUDIES

- Chest x-ray is used to rule out pulmonary involvement. If suspicious for pulmonary interstitial disease, a high-resolution CT scan of the chest may be helpful.
- Video fluoroscopy or barium swallow study to look for upper esophageal dysfunction in patients with dysphagia and DM.

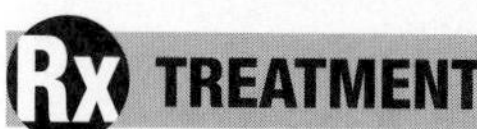

TREATMENT

Goal: maintain function, minimize disease/iatrogenic sequelae

NONPHARMACOLOGIC THERAPY

- Sun-blocking agents with SPF 15 or greater for skin protection in patients with DM
- Physical therapy beneficial for gait training and increasing muscle tone and strength
- Occupational therapy assists with activities of daily living
- Speech therapy to monitor patients with swallowing dysfunction

ACUTE GENERAL Rx

- Corticosteroids are the mainstay of therapy. Start prednisone 1 to 2 mg/kg per day, up to a maximum dose of 100 mg/day. Continue until muscle strength improves or muscle enzymes have normalized for at least 4 wk. Begin tapering by 10 mg/mo until 60 mg/day, then slowly taper by 5 mg/mo. Consider every-other-day prednisone treatment at same dose (may decrease side effects).
- Consider IV immunoglobulin (IVIG) if patient fails to improve on prednisone, or muscle enzymes begin rising when tapering off prednisone. See "Chronic Rx" for specific dosage.
- Hydroxychloroquine can be used to treat the cutaneous lesions of DM.
- A treatment algorithm for adult patients with PM and DM is described in Fig. E1-646.

CHRONIC RX

- Chronic prednisone therapy may be needed for years, but other immunosuppressive ("steroid-sparing") agents may be added early to decrease long-term steroid side effects.
- Azathioprine 2 to 3 mg/kg per day tapered to 1 mg/kg per day once steroid is tapered to 15 mg/day. Reduce dosage monthly by 25-mg intervals. Maintenance dosage is 50 mg/day.
- Methotrexate 7.5 to 10 mg PO/wk, increased by 2.5 mg/wk to total of 25 mg/wk; consider IM dosing if PO is ineffective.
- IV immunoglobulin 2 g/kg total dose over 2 to 5 days.
- IV cyclophosphamide 1 g/M^2 monthly for 6 mo is preferred to oral dosing for refractory cases. However, oral dosing of cyclophosphamide is 1 to 3 mg/kg per day PO or 2 to 4 mg/kg per day in conjunction with prednisone.
- Cyclosporin A: initial dose 2.0 to 2.5 mg/kg bid; long-term maintenance is lowest effective dose.
- Mycophenolate mofetil 500 mg PO bid, titrate to 1500 mg PO bid over 1 to 2 mo.
- Hydroxychloroquine 200 mg PO daily; monitor for visual changes.

DISPOSITION

- 30% to 40% of patients achieve clinical remission with treatment.
- In patients with residual weakness, deficits typically remain stable over long-term follow-up.
- 10% experience recurrent disease.
- Serum CK often returns to normal before symptoms improve.
- During exacerbations, enzymes may rise before clinical symptoms appear.
- Poor prognostic indicators include delay in diagnosis, older age, recalcitrant disease, malignancy, interstitial pulmonary fibrosis, dysphagia, leukocytosis, fever, and anorexia.
- Infection, malignancy, and cardiac and pulmonary dysfunction are the most common causes of death.
- With early treatment, 5- and 8-yr survival rates of 80% and 73%, respectively, have been reported.

REFERRAL

Neurology or rheumatology referral should be made to help establish the diagnosis and implement treatment.

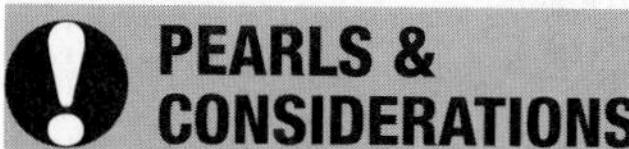

PEARLS & CONSIDERATIONS

- Do not implement treatment before muscle biopsy.
- When assessing response to treatment, clinical muscle strength is more important than muscle enzyme tests.
- The concern for malignancies (ovary, lung, breast, GI) associated with DM is legitimate and merits screening in patients older than age 40 at time of diagnosis and every 2 to 3 yr thereafter.
- There does not appear to be any association between juvenile DM and malignancy.
- Overlap syndrome refers to patients with DM who also meet criteria for a connective tissue disorder (e.g., rheumatoid arthritis, scleroderma, SLE).
- In any patient taking steroids, closely monitor for:
  - Diabetes or glucose intolerance (2-hour oral glucose tolerance test)
  - Osteopenia/osteoporosis (DEXA scan q6mo)
  - Cataracts (yearly ophthalmologic appointment)
  - Hypertension
  - Psychiatric side effects including depression or psychosis
  - Poor sleep
  - Peptic ulcer disease (prescribe H_2 antagonist or proton pump inhibitor)
- Clinical and immune response features can be used for categorizing heterogeneous myositis syndromes and mutually exclusive and stable phenotypes and are useful for predicting clinical signs and symptoms, associated environmental and genetic risk factors, and responses to therapy and prognosis.

RELATED CONTENT

Dermatomyositis and Polymyositis (Patient Information)

AUTHOR: **GAVIN BROWN, M.D.**

BASIC INFORMATION

DEFINITION

Myotonia is a type of muscular dystrophy in which relaxation of a muscle after contraction is delayed or prolonged. The most common type of muscular dystrophy with myotonia is myotonic dystrophy. The nondystrophic myotonias (NDMs) are rare disorders (prevalence 1:100,000) caused by mutations in skeletal muscle chloride and sodium channels with the common clinical feature of myotonia without muscle wasting.[1]

SYNONYMS

Myotonic dystrophy

ICD-9CM CODES

359.2 Myotonic disorders
728.85 Muscle spasm

ICD-10CM CODES

G71.1 Myotonic disorders
M62.89 Other specified disorders of muscle
M62.40 Contracture of muscle, unspecified site

EPIDEMIOLOGY & DEMOGRAPHICS

- Three to five cases/100,000 persons
- Genetic disorder inherited as an autosomal-dominant illness
- Symptoms usually manifest during adolescence or early adulthood. Cases of infantile myotonic dystrophy have been described.

PHYSICAL FINDINGS & CLINICAL PRESENTATION

- Usual first symptom is distal extremity weakness sometimes associated with muscle stiffness, cramps, or difficulty relaxing grasp.
- Weakness spreads to eventually involve all muscle groups. Flexor neck muscle weakness and masseter and temporal wasting are often prominent features, as is dysarthria.
- Percussion of a muscle produces a slow contraction followed by prolonged relaxation. The myotonic reflex is best tested by percussing the thenar muscles and observing a slow flexion followed by slow relaxation of the thumb.
- As the disease progresses, generalized weakness becomes more pronounced and myotonia becomes less evident.
- Extramuscular involvement:
  - Mental retardation of variable severity (may be absent)
  - Frontal baldness (Fig. 1-647)
  - Cataracts
  - Diabetes mellitus
  - Hypogonadism
  - Adrenal failure
  - Cardiomyopathy
- Infantile myotonic dystrophy presents as neonatal extreme hypotonia with "shark mouth" deformity (upper lip forming an inverted V).

ETIOLOGY & PATHOGENESIS

Genetic disorder encoded on chromosome 19 leading to sustained firing of the muscle membrane, causing prolonged muscle contraction. Myotonic dystrophy 1 (the more common form) is caused by an expanded CTG repeat within the noncoding 3′ untranslated region of the myotonic dystrophy protein kinase *(DMPK)* gene. The less common form (myotonic dystrophy 2) is caused by an expanded CCTG repeat in the first intron of the zinc finger protein 9 *(ZNF9)* gene.

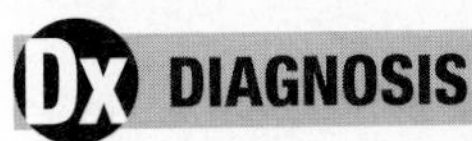

DIAGNOSIS

DIFFERENTIAL DIAGNOSIS

The disease is limited to muscles and causes hypertrophy and stiffness after rest. Muscle function normalizes with exercise. There is no weakness. Symptoms are exacerbated by exposure to cold.

- Myotonia congenita (Thomsen's disease)
- May be autosomal dominant or recessive (two distinct varieties)
- Paramyotonia congenita (autosomal-dominant disease): weakness and stiffness of facial muscles and distal upper extremities, especially or exclusively on cold exposure
- Muscular dystrophies
- Inflammatory myopathies (polymyositis)
- Metabolic muscle diseases
- Myasthenic syndromes
- Motor neuron disease

WORKUP

- History and physical examination usually sufficient
- Muscle enzymes usually abnormal (creatine phosphokinase, aldolase, aspartate aminotransferase)
- Electromyography: typical myotonic "dive bomber" bursts
- Muscle biopsy: type I fiber atrophy, ring fibers, increased central nucleation

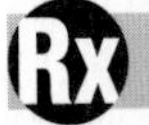

TREATMENT

- Phenytoin
- Quinine
- Quinidine
- Procainamide
- Acetazolamide
- Genetic counseling
- Assistive devices, orthotics
- In recent trials,[1] the use of mexiletine resulted in improvement of patient-reported stiffness in patients with nondystrophic myotonias.

DISPOSITION

- In myotonic dystrophy, death is usually caused by the wasting of skeletal muscle and defects in cardiac function.
- Among patients with myotonic dystrophy type 1, an invasive strategy based on systemic electrophysiological studies and prophylactic permanent pacing is associated with longer survival than a non-invasive strategy.[2]

REFERRAL

To neurologist

SUGGESTED READINGS

available at www.expertconsult.com

AUTHOR: **FRED F. FERRI, M.D.**

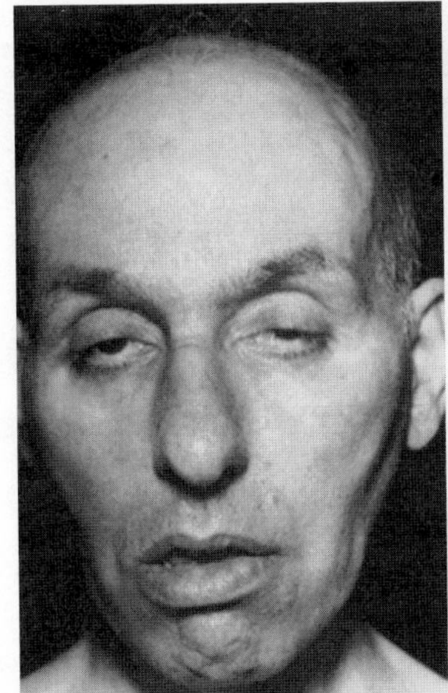
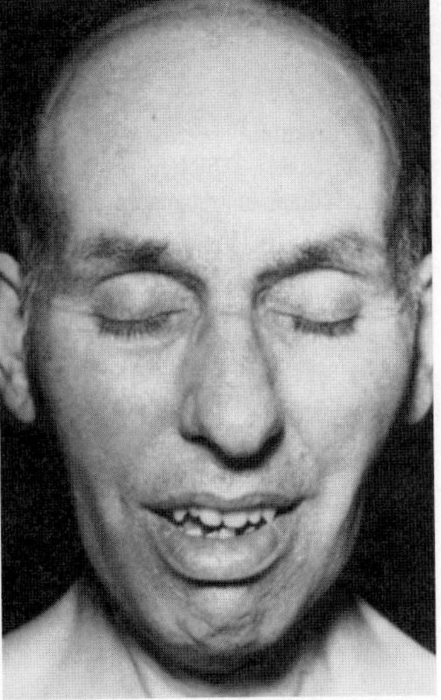

FIGURE 1-647 Myotonic dystrophy with typical myopathic facies, frontal balding, and sunken cheeks. (From Dubowitz V: *Muscle disorders in childhood,* London, 1995, Saunders.)

[1]Statland JM et al: Mexiletine for symptoms and signs of myotonia in nondystrophic myotonia, *JAMA* 308(13): 1357-1365, 2012.

[2]Wahbi K et al: Electrophysiological study with prophylactic pacing and survival in adults with myotonic dystrophy and conduction system disease, *JAMA* 307(12):1292-1301, 2012.

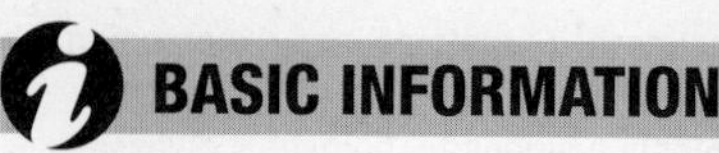

BASIC INFORMATION

DEFINITION

Myxedema coma is a life-threatening complication of hypothyroidism characterized by profound lethargy or coma and usually accompanied by hypothermia.

ICD-9CM CODES
244.8 Myxedema, pituitary
244.1 Myxedema, primary
ICD-10CM CODES
E03.5 Myxedema coma
E03.8 Other specified hypothyroidism
E03.9 Hypothyroidism, unspecified

PHYSICAL FINDINGS & CLINICAL PRESENTATION

- Mental obtuntation, profound lethargy or coma
- Hypothermia (rectal temperature <35° C [95° F]); often missed by using ordinary thermometers graduated only to 34.5° C or because the mercury is not shaken below 36° C
- Bradycardia, hypotension (attributable to circulatory collapse)
- Delayed relaxation phase of deep tendon reflexes, areflexia
- Myxedema facies (Fig. 1-648)
- Alopecia, macroglossia, ptosis, periorbital edema, nonpitting edema, doughy skin
- Bladder dystonia and distention
- Pleural, pericardial, and peritoneal effusions

ETIOLOGY

Decompensation of hypothyroidism from:

- Sepsis
- Exposure to cold weather
- Central nervous system depressants (sedatives, narcotics, antidepressants)
- Trauma, surgery
- Stroke, congestive heart failure, burns
- Intravascular volume contraction (GI blood loss, diuretic use)

Dx DIAGNOSIS

DIFFERENTIAL DIAGNOSIS

- Severe depression, primary psychosis
- Drug overdose
- Cerebrovascular accident, liver failure, renal failure
- Hypoglycemia, CO_2 narcosis, encephalitis

WORKUP

Diagnosis of hypothyroidism and exclusion of contributing factors (e.g., sepsis, cerebrovascular accident) with laboratory and radiographic studies (see "Laboratory Tests")

LABORATORY TESTS

- Markedly increased thyroid-stimulating hormone (if primary hypothyroidism), decreased serum free T_4
- Complete blood count with differential, urine and blood cultures to rule out infectious process
- Electrolytes, blood urea nitrogen, creatinine, liver function tests, calcium, glucose
- Arterial blood gases to rule out hypoxemia and carbon dioxide retention
- Cortisol level to rule out adrenal insufficiency
- Elevated CPK
- Hyperlipidemia

IMAGING STUDIES

- CT scan of head in suspected cerebrovascular accident
- Chest x-ray to rule out infectious process

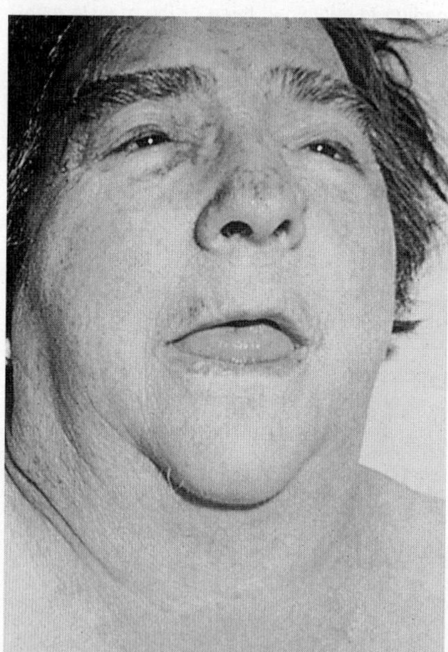

FIGURE 1-648 Myxedema facies. Note dull, puffy, yellowed skin; coarse, sparse hair; temporal loss of eyebrows; periorbital edema; prominent tongue. (Courtesy Paul W. Ladenson, M.D., The Johns Hopkins University and Hospital, Baltimore. In Seidel HM [ed]: *Mosby's guide to physical examination,* ed 5, St Louis, 2004, Mosby.)

Rx TREATMENT

NONPHARMACOLOGIC THERAPY

- Prevent further heat loss; cover the patient but avoid external rewarming because it may produce vascular collapse.
- Support respiratory function; intubation and mechanical ventilation may be required.
- Monitor patient in the intensive care unit.

ACUTE GENERAL Rx

- Give levothyroxine 5 to 8 mcg/kg (300 to 500 mcg) IV infused over 15 min, then 100 mcg IV q24h.
- Glucocorticoids should also be administered until coexistent adrenal insufficiency can be ruled out. Hydrocortisone hemisuccinate 100 mg IV bolus is initially given, followed by 100 mg IV q8h until initial plasma cortisol level is confirmed normal.
- IV hydration with D_5NS is used to correct hypotension and hypoglycemia (if present); avoid overhydration and possible water intoxication because clearance of free water is impaired in these patients.
- Rule out and treat precipitating factors (e.g., antibiotics in suspected sepsis).

CHRONIC Rx

Refer to "Hypothyroidism" in Section I.

DISPOSITION

Mortality rate in myxedema coma is 20% to 50%.

REFERRAL

Endocrinology consultation

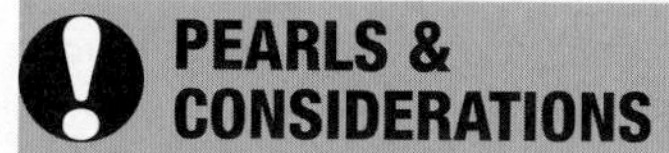

PEARLS & CONSIDERATIONS

COMMENTS

If the diagnosis is suspected, initiate treatment immediately without waiting for confirming laboratory results.

RELATED CONTENT

Hypothyroidism (Related Key Topic)
Hypothyroidism (Patient Information)

AUTHOR: **FRED F. FERRI, M.D.**

BASIC INFORMATION

DEFINITION

Narcissistic personality disorder (NPD) is characterized by a pattern of grandiosity, need for admiration, and lack of empathy that begins by early adulthood and causes significant distress or impairment in multiple domains of functioning. The individual must meet five or more of the following criteria:

1. Grandiose sense of self-importance. For example, the person may exaggerate achievements and talents or expect recognition as superior without commensurate achievements.
2. Preoccupied with fantasies of unlimited success, power, brilliance, beauty, or ideal love.
3. Views self as "special" and unique and should only associate with other special or highly regarded people and institutions.
4. Requires excessive admiration.
5. Sense of entitlement. For example, unreasonable expectations of especially favorable treatment or automatic compliance with his or her expectations.
6. Interpersonally exploitative.
7. Lacks empathy—unwilling to recognize or identify with the feelings or needs of others.
8. Often envious of others or believes others envious of him or her.
9. Shows arrogant or haughty behaviors.

SYNONYMS

None

ICD-9CM and DSM-5 CODES
301.81
ICD-10CM CODES
F60.8 Other specific personality disorder

EPIDEMIOLOGY & DEMOGRAPHICS

PREVALENCE: Less than 1% of the general population; estimates range from 2% to 16% in the clinical population

PREDOMINANT SEX: More commonly diagnosed in males (up to 3:1)

PREDOMINANT AGE: 20s and 30s

CLINICAL PRESENTATION

- Patients have an underlying sense of inferiority and inadequacy.
- May be related to the failure of parents or parental surrogates to impart a sense of self-worth.
- To avoid these beliefs and their associated painful effects, patients seek to convince self and others that they are special, the best, or unusually talented.
- Astutely aware of status, pecking order.
- Vulnerability in self-esteem makes these patients exquisitely sensitive to criticism, defeat, or perceived weakness, which in turn can lead to feeling humiliated, degraded, and empty.
- These patients react to perceived slights with either more intense grandiosity and admiration seeking or with disdain and rage. Either approach seeks to bolster their sense of self often by devaluing or criticizing the other person.
- Experiences of self-deflation lead to social withdrawal or depressed mood or to feigned humility that protects grandiosity.
- Interpersonal relationships are typically shallow and limited.
- Although ambition and confidence may lead to high achievement, vocational functioning may be disrupted by intolerance for criticism.

ETIOLOGY

- Limited knowledge about role of genetic loading and neurobiologic vulnerability.
- Prevailing hypotheses focus on impaired development of self as "worthy" because of insufficient affirmation and warmth from parents.

Dx DIAGNOSIS

DIFFERENTIAL DIAGNOSIS

- Mania and hypomania
- Dysthymia and major depressive episode
- Substance-induced euphoria, especially cocaine abuse
- Histrionic, borderline, antisocial, and paranoid personality disorders share common features and are often comorbid
- Personality changes from a general medical condition, including central nervous system processes in the frontal-temporal regions of the brain

WORKUP

- History: collateral information essential to establishing presence of longstanding interpersonal pattern in multiple domains of the patient's life
- Physical examination
- Mental status examination

LABORATORY TESTS

Tests necessary to rule out medical causes of personality changes

IMAGING STUDIES

Those necessary to rule out medical causes of personality changes

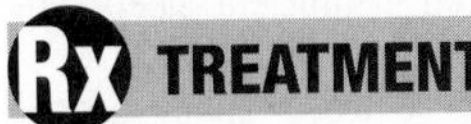

TREATMENT

NONPHARMACOLOGIC THERAPY

- Cognitive-behavioral therapy to help patients control rage, manage perceived criticism, and develop social skills
- Psychodynamic psychotherapy to help develop improved self-concept, affect tolerance, and interpersonal functioning

ACUTE GENERAL Rx

Benzodiazepines or low-dose antipsychotics to control rage

CHRONIC Rx

- Selective serotonin reuptake inhibitors for impulsivity or comorbid depression
- Mood stabilizers if comorbid bipolar or to improve impulse control

DISPOSITION

- Severity is variable and course is chronic. The majority of patients obtain greater functioning in fifth decade and beyond when pessimism replaces grandiosity. Often lifelong difficulty maintaining intimate relationships.
- At increased risk for major depressive disorder and substance abuse or dependence (especially cocaine).

REFERRAL

If pharmacotherapy is contemplated

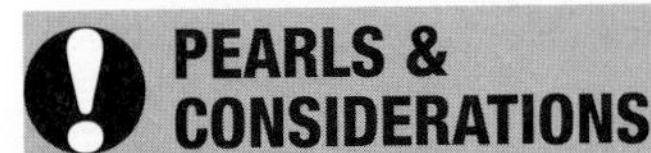

PEARLS & CONSIDERATIONS

COMMENTS

- Illness threatens these patients' image of superiority.
- To defend against this threat, patients may minimize symptoms or deny presence of illness.
- Patients will commonly demand special treatment from senior and well-known physicians.
- Patients may devalue, criticize, or question the behavior or credentials of the treating physician.
- Management guidelines:
  1. Be respectful and nonconfrontational.
  2. Help patient use self-perceived talents in service of treatment.
  3. Do not personalize patient's devaluation, but understand their criticalness as an attempt to manage their own intense insecurity.
  4. Appeal to the patient's narcissism. In other words, agree with the patient that he or she is "entitled" to appropriate care.

SUGGESTED READINGS

available at www.expertconsult.com

RELATED CONTENT

Narcissistic Personality Disorder (Patient Information)

AUTHOR: **JOHN Q. YOUNG, M.D., M.P.P.**

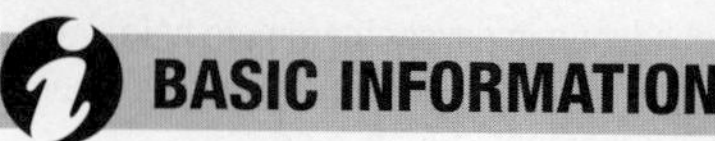

BASIC INFORMATION

DEFINITION

Narcolepsy is a chronic neurologic sleep disorder characterized by excessive daytime sleepiness and dysregulation of rapid eye movement (REM) sleep. It is the second most common cause of disabling daytime sleepiness after obstructive sleep apnea. Symptoms of REM sleep dysregulation include cataplexy, sleep paralysis, and hallucinations during transition between wake and sleep. Difficulty sleeping with either frequent awakenings or disrupted sleep may also occur.

SYNONYMS

Hypersomnia of central origin
Narcolepsy with cataplexy
Narcolepsy-cataplexy syndrome
Narcolepsy with hypocretin deficiency
Gelineau syndrome

ICD-9CM CODES
347.00 Narcolepsy without cataplexy
347.01 Narcolepsy with cataplexy
ICD-10CM CODES
G47.419 Narcolepsy without cataplexy
G47.411 Narcolepsy with cataplexy

EPIDEMIOLOGY & DEMOGRAPHICS

INCIDENCE: 0.74/100,000 persons/yr
PREVALENCE: 5 to 50/100,000 people
PREDOMINANT SEX: Males and females are equally affected.
AGE OF ONSET: Peak 15 to 30 yr (range, 10-55 yr)
GENETICS:
- Associated with human leukocyte antigen (HLA) subtypes, specifically, *DQB1*0602,* which is present in 95% of patients with cataplexy and 96% of patients with hypocretin deficiency.
- Risk of narcolepsy increases 20 to 40 times if a family member is affected.
- Monozygotic twin concordance rate is 17% to 36%, thus indicating an incomplete penetrance and suggesting an environmental factor in the disease process.

RISK FACTORS: Anesthesia, head injury, history of meningitis or encephalitis, family history of narcolepsy, tumor, vascular malformations, stroke, and obesity.

PHYSICAL FINDINGS & CLINICAL PRESENTATION

- Overwhelming urge to sleep with chronic hypersomnia may occur during the day.
- Cataplexy occurs in 60% to 100% of patients with narcolepsy and is reported as a partial or complete loss of voluntary muscle control with preserved consciousness that is precipitated by a strong emotion, more commonly with laughter. This is the most specific symptom and is considered pathognomonic for narcolepsy.
- Hypnagogic (wake to sleep) or hypnopompic (sleep to wake) hallucinations have been reported in 60% to 80% of patients with narcolepsy.
- Sleep paralysis, defined as loss of muscle tone during the transition between sleep and wakefulness, occurs in 60% to 80% of patients with narcolepsy. It may occur with hallucinations and can be interrupted by sensory stimuli.
- Only about one third of patients will have all four symptoms: chronic daytime sleepiness, cataplexy, hypnagogic hallucinations, and sleep paralysis.
- Fragmented sleep is seen in 60% to 80% of narcolepsy patients and can often be mistaken for insomnia or other intrinsic sleep disorder.
- Other symptoms that have been reported in narcolepsy include automatic behavior or semipurposeful movements in 40% of patients and memory disturbance in 50% of patients.

ETIOLOGY

The loss of hypocretin/orexin signaling, genetic factors, and brain lesions are presently identified factors in the development of narcolepsy.
HYPOCRETIN/OREXIN:
- Loss of hypocretin-1 and hypocretin-2 (also known as orexin-A and orexin-B) producing neurons in the lateral hypothalamus.
- Human cerebrospinal fluid (CSF) levels of hypocretin-1 are low to undetectable in narcoleptics with cataplexy.
- Narcolepsy without cataplexy may have a different cause because CSF hypocretin levels are usually normal in these patients, so there may be a completely separate mechanism in these patients, or it may result from less extensive loss of hypocretin neurons or impaired signaling.

SECONDARY ETIOLOGIES:
- Tumors, vascular malformations, and strokes have all been reported to cause secondary narcolepsy.
- Direct injury to the hypocretin neurons or their projections is the most likely cause of secondary narcolepsy due to central nervous system lesions.
- Narcolepsy has been reported in genetic syndromes, including Prader-Willi syndrome and Niemann-Pick disease type C, as well as paraneoplastic syndromes.

Dx DIAGNOSIS

DIFFERENTIAL DIAGNOSIS

Excessive daytime somnolence:
- Autism
- Autosomal dominant cerebellar ataxia, deafness, and narcolepsy
- Behaviorally induced insufficient sleep syndrome
- Central or obstructive sleep apnea (sleep-disordered breathing)
- Circadian rhythm disorder
- Depression
- Diencephalic lesions
- Drug or alcohol abuse
- Hypothyroidism
- Idiopathic hypersomnia with long or short sleep time
- Inadequate sleep hygiene
- Insufficient sleep
- Increased intracranial pressure
- Insomnia
- Kleine-Levin syndrome
- Medication effect
- Menstrual-related hypersomnia
- Posttraumatic narcolepsy
- Seizures
- Sleep fragmentation (multiple causes)

Cataplexy:
- Seizures
- Periodic paralysis
- Cardiovascular insufficiency
- Psychogenic (multiple causes)
- Lesions of the hypothalamus or brain stem

WORKUP

- Narcolepsy is often diagnosed by clinical history. The Epworth Sleepiness Scale is very useful in determining the degree of excessive daytime sleepiness (Table 1-355).
- The diagnosis of narcolepsy can be made if there is a clear history of cataplexy in the setting of excessive daytime somnolence, without need for further diagnostic testing. Sleep laboratory testing or possibly laboratory testing is required if these symptoms do not exist.
- The medical history should include questions regarding severity of daytime hypersomnia while also evaluating for sleep-disordered breathing, transient muscle weakness triggered by emotion, hallucinations while falling asleep or upon awakening, and inability to move after awakening. The clinical evaluation should also address symptoms of seizures and paraneoplastic disorders while also asking about previous stroke or genetic disorders. A detailed family history is imperative. Hypothalamic dysfunction such as unexplained weight gain, endocrine abnormalities, circadian dysrhythmias, and autonomic nervous system problems may provide useful insight.
- A thorough examination including a detailed neurologic examination should be performed.
- Nocturnal polysomnography followed by a multiple sleep latency test (MSLT) remains the gold standard for the diagnosis of narcolepsy. A drug screen should also be performed to rule out pharmacologic modulations of sleep.

LABORATORY TESTS

HLA subtyping and CSF hypocretin/orexin levels may be attempted in suspected cases of narcolepsy. CSF hypocretin/orexin analysis is primarily a research tool. CSF hypocretin levels below 110 pg/ml are indicative of narcolepsy, but normal or high CSF hypocretin levels do not exclude the diagnosis.

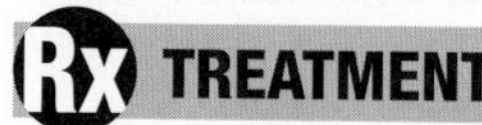

TREATMENT

NONPHARMACOLOGIC THERAPY

Avoidance of over-the-counter drugs and illicit drugs, optimal sleep hygiene and scheduled daily naps, and psychosocial support can be used for symptoms of excessive daytime somnolence. However, nonpharmacologic therapy is typically not sufficient for treatment of narcolepsy alone but is often used as adjunct therapy with medications.

PHARMACOLOGIC THERAPY

For excessive daytime somnolence:

- Sodium oxybate: a central nervous system depressant that can be used for the treatment of cataplexy and REM-related symptoms
- Modafinil 200 to 600 mg PO every morning or divided bid
- Armodafinil 150 or 250 mg PO as a single dose in the morning
- Methylphenidate 5 to 15 mg PO bid to tid
- Methylphenidate SR 18 to 54 mg PO every morning or divided bid
- Dextroamphetamine 10 to 60 mg PO qd
- Eldepryl 5 mg PO bid

For cataplexy:

- Sodium oxybate: a central nervous system depressant that can be used for the treatment of cataplexy and REM-related symptoms
- Fluoxetine 20 mg PO qd initially
- Sertraline 25 mg PO qd initially
- Venlafaxine 25 mg PO qd initially
- Clomipramine 25 mg/day initially
- Protriptyline 5 mg tid initially
- Imipramine 25 to 50 mg/day initially
- Desipramine 10 mg bid initially

DISPOSITION

This is a chronic sleep disorder that may worsen for the first few years and then persist for life.

REFERRAL

Because of the complexity of this disorder and its ever-changing management and treatment, patients should be referred to centers or programs with highly trained sleep specialists with expertise caring for these patients, especially if sodium oxybate (Xyrem) therapy is needed.

PEARLS & CONSIDERATIONS

Many narcoleptics report the onset of symptoms beginning in childhood to early adulthood with a long delay of actual diagnosis on the order of 10 to 15 yr. Typically, excessive daytime sleepiness is the initial symptom followed by REM dysregulation (e.g., cataplexy, sleep paralysis, hypnagogic hallucinations). Patients with narcolepsy also have higher than expected incidence of other sleep disorders, including obstructive sleep apnea, periodic limb movements of sleep, and REM sleep behavior disorder.

COMMENTS

Narcolepsy is a rare disorder that is underdiagnosed. Cataplexy is specific for narcolepsy, but other symptoms of REM dysregulation, including sleep paralysis and hypnagogic or hypnopompic hallucinations, can occur even in normal patients. Sleep-onset REM or REM periods on an MSLT may occur as a result of sleep deprivation or withdrawal from REM-suppressing drugs.

SUGGESTED READINGS

available at www.expertconsult.com

RELATED CONTENT

Narcolepsy (Patient Information)

AUTHOR: **DON HAYES, JR., M.D., M.S.**

TABLE 1-355 Epworth Sleepiness Scale

How likely are you to doze off or fall asleep in the following situations, in contrast to just feeling tired? This refers to your usual way of life in recent time. Even if you have not done some of these things recently, try to work out how they would have affected you. Use the following scale to choose the most appropriate number for each situation.

0 = would never doze

1 = slight chance of dozing

2 = moderate chance of dozing

3 = high chance of dozing

Situation	Chance of Dozing
Sitting and reading	
Watching TV	
Sitting and inactive in a public place (theater or meeting)	
As a passenger in a car for an hour without a break	
Lying down to rest in the afternoon when circumstances permit	
Sitting and talking to someone	
Sitting quietly after lunch (without alcohol)	
In a car, while stopped for a few minutes in traffic	
TOTAL	

From Johns MW: A new method for measuring daytime sleepiness: the Epworth Sleepiness Scale, *Sleep* 14:540-545, 1991.

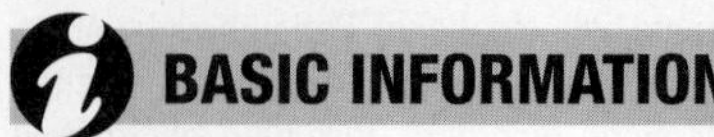

BASIC INFORMATION

DEFINITION

Necrotizing fasciitis is a rapidly spreading bacterial infection of the deep fascia, with associated inflammation, leading to necrosis of subcutaneous tissue planes. This infection can occur in wounds from trauma or surgical wounds or can be spontaneous or idiopathic. There are two clinical types, both of which carry a high rate of morbidity and mortality.

SYNONYMS

Soft tissue gangrene
Flesh eating bacteria
Fournier's gangrene
Hemolytic streptococcal gangrene

ICD-9CM CODES
728.86 Necrotizing fasciitis
ICD-10CM CODES
M72.6 Necrotizing fasciitis

EPIDEMIOLOGY & DEMOGRAPHICS

PREDOMINANT SEX: Male > female
PREDOMINANT AGE: 6-50 yr; rare in children
EPIDEMIOLOGY: Invasive group A *Streptococcus* infection occurs at a rate of 3.5 cases per 100,000 persons, with a case fatality rate of around 24%.

PHYSICAL FINDINGS & CLINICAL PRESENTATION

CLINICAL TYPES OF NECROTIZING FASCIITIS

- Type I necrotizing fasciitis: at least one anaerobic species is isolated in conjunction with one or more facultative anaerobic species, such as streptococci (not group A), *and* members of the Enterobacteriaceae:
  - Anaerobic bacteria, most commonly *Bacteroides* or *Peptostreptococcus* spp.
  - Enterobacteriaceae: *Escherichia coli*, *Klebsiella* spp., *Proteus* spp., *Enterobacter* spp.
  - Usually associated with diabetes or peripheral vascular disease
  - Example of type I: Fournier's gangrene of the perineum
- Type II necrotizing fasciitis: Group A *Streptococcus* is isolated alone or in combination with other bacteria, most likely *Staphylococcus aureus.* Also known as hemolytic streptococcal gangrene
  - Example of type II: Invasive group A *Streptococcus*, associated with virulence factors type 1 and type 3 M protein

EXAMPLES OF NECROTIZING FASCIITIS

- Fournier's gangrene: Aggressive type I infection of the perineum usually caused by penetration of the gastrointestinal or urethral mucosa by enteric organisms. Can rapidly spread to involve the scrotum, penis, and abdominal wall or gluteal muscles, causing gangrene.
- Clostridial cellulitis: Caused by *Clostridium perfringens* associated by local trauma or surgery and crepitus caused by gas production; generally noted in the skin, with deeper tissues generally spared.

PHYSICAL FINDINGS

Minor skin trauma, toxic-appearing patient:

- Open skin wound
- Severe pain at injury or surgical site
- Fever, confusion, weakness, diarrhea
- Early skin erythema, quickly spreading in hours to days
- Skin redness changes to purple discoloration
- Gangrenous skin changes may develop
- Loosening of skin and subcutaneous skin in association with deep fascial necrosis (Fig. 1-649)
- Muscle involvement, thrombosis of blood vessels, and myonecrosis may develop
- Bullae and gas formation at site

ETIOLOGY

- Polymicrobial: mixture of anaerobes and aerobic enteric gram-negative rods
- Group A streptococci *(S. pyogenes)*
- *S. aureus*
- *C. perfringens*
- *Bacteroides fragilis*
- *Vibrio vulnificus*
- Methicillin-resistant *S. aureus* (MRSA), especially community-acquired MRSA

DIAGNOSIS

DIFFERENTIAL DIAGNOSIS

- Cellulitis
- Pyomyositis
- Gas gangrene
- A classification of necrotizing skin, soft-tissue, and muscle infections is described in Table 1-356.

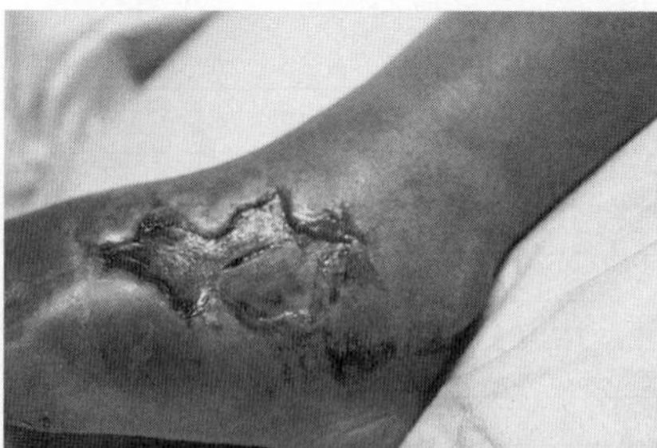

FIGURE 1-649 Necrotizing fasciitis. The so-called flesh-eating bacteria, group A β-hemolytic *Streptococcus,* can cause significant tissue destruction rapidly. This 32-year-old woman had pain, erythema, and swelling of the foot followed by necrotic ulceration over a week. There was no history of trauma. (Courtesy Roger Bitar, MD. From White GM, Cox NH [eds]: *Diseases of the skin, a color atlas and text,* ed 2, St Louis, 2006, Mosby.)

WORKUP

- Diagnosis of necrotizing fasciitis generally requires incision and probing. In patients with necrotizing fasciitis, there is no resistance to probing subcut and there is fascial plane involvement.
- Laboratory tests:
  - Complete blood cell count (CBC) with differential
  - Cultures of skin, soft tissue, or debrided tissue, aerobically and anaerobically. Blood cultures are positive in 60% of patients with type II infections and 20% with type I infections.
- Imaging:
  - Radiographs show subcutaneous gas in fascial planes (Fig. 1-650).
  - Computed tomography (CT)/magnetic resonance imaging (MRI) may be helpful because they can detect gas in the tissues.

TREATMENT

- Aggressive surgical debridement of involved necrotic tissues is essential as soon as possible to reduce mortality.
- Fasciotomies of extremities may be necessary.
- Empiric antibiotic treatment:
  - Type I: Piperacillin/tazobactam; carbapenems such as imipenem, meropenem, or doripenem; and third-generation cephalosporin + metronidazole or aminoglycoside + clindamycin are reasonable choices pending cultures. It is important to always have anaerobic coverage.
  - Type II: For group A *Streptococcus,* give intravenous (IV) penicillin G, 4 million U q4h in patients who weigh more than 60 kg with clindamycin, 600-900 mg IV q8h.
  - Clindamycin has the added effect of suppressing toxin production. If community associated-MRSA is suspected, add vancomycin.
- Intravenous gammaglobulin, 2 g/kg, neutralizes circulating streptococcal toxins and has been shown beneficial in severe forms of invasive group A streptococcal infections.
- Hyperbaric oxygen evaluation as an adjunct to surgery and IV antibiotics.

SUGGESTED READINGS

available at www.expertconsult.com

AUTHOR: **GLENN G. FORT, M.D., M.P.H.**

TABLE 1-356 Classification of Necrotizing Skin, Soft-Tissue, and Muscle Infections

Disease	Bacteriology	Comments
Necrotizing Cellulitis		
Clostridial cellulitis	*Clostridium perfringens*	Local trauma, recent surgery; fascial/deep muscle spared
Nonclostridial cellulitis	Mixed: *Escherichia coli, Enterobacter, Peptostreptococcus* spp., *Bacteroides fragilis*	Diabetes mellitus predisposes; produces foul odor
Meleney's synergistic gangrene	*Staphylococcus aureus,* microaerophilic streptococci	Rare infection; postoperative; slowly expanding, indolent, ulceration in superficial fascia
Synergistic necrotizing cellulitis	Mixed aerobic and anaerobic, including *B. fragilis, Peptostreptococcus* spp.	Diabetes mellitus predisposes; variant of necrotizing fasciitis type I; involves skin, muscle, fat, and fascia
Necrotizing Fasciitis		
Type I	Mixed aerobic and anaerobic; staphylococci, *B. fragilis, E. coli,* group A streptococci, *Peptostreptococcus* spp., *Prevotella, Porphyromonas* spp., *Clostridium* spp.	Usually requires a breach in the mucous membrane layer either through surgery or penetrating injuries or from chronic medical conditions such as diabetes, peripheral vascular disease, malignancy, and anal fissures
Type II	Group A streptococci	Increasing in frequency and severity since 1985; very high mortality; often begins at site of nonpenetrating minor trauma such as a bruise or muscle strain but often no identified precursor Predisposing factors: blunt/penetrating trauma, varicella (chickenpox), intravenous drug abuse, surgical procedures, childbirth, nonsteroidal anti-inflammatory drug use
Myonecrosis		
Clostridial myonecrosis	*Clostridium* spp.	Predisposing factors: deep/penetrating injury, bowel and biliary tract surgery, improperly performed abortion and retained placenta, prolonged rupture of the membranes, and intrauterine fetal demise or missed abortion in postpartum patients. Recurrent gas gangrene occurs at sites of previous gas gangrene.
Streptococcal myonecrosis	Streptococci	
Special Type of Necrotizing Soft-Tissue Infection		
Fournier's gangrene	Polymicrobial, with *E. coli* the predominant aerobe and *Bacteroides* the predominant anaerobe. Other microflora: *Proteus, Staphylococcus, Enterococcus,* aerobic and anaerobic *Streptococcus, Pseudomonas, Klebsiella,* and *Clostridium*	Necrosis of the scrotum or perineum that starts with scrotal pain and erythema and rapidly spreads onto anterior abdominal wall and gluteal muscle. It is more often seen in diabetics and can be associated with trauma.

From Vincent JL et al: *Textbook of critical care,* ed 6, Philadelphia, 2011, Saunders.

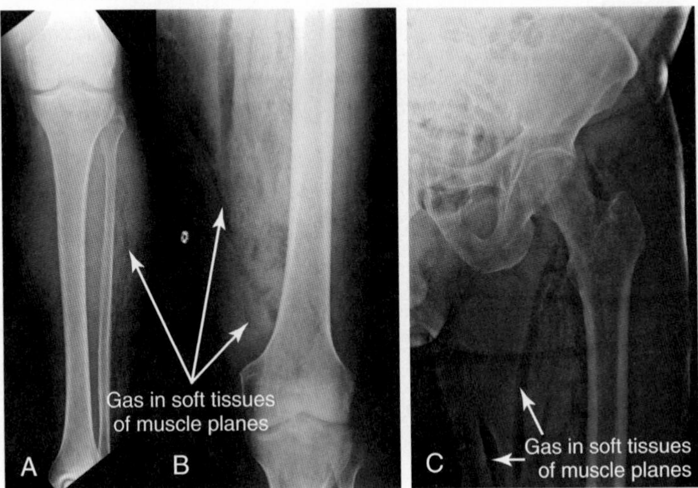

FIGURE 1-650 Necrotizing fasciitis. This 71-year-old man with aplastic anemia presented with fevers to 38.9° C, leg weakness, and extreme leg pain. Initially, the patient was thought to have neuropathic pain and weakness, possibly indicating spinal disease such as epidural abscess. He rapidly developed crepitus of his legs. Radiographs of the patient's legs were obtained, followed by noncontrast CT. **A,** Anterior-posterior (AP) tibia and fibula. **B,** AP femur. **C,** AP hip. Air is seen dissecting in muscle planes of the legs. On radiograph, air appears black. Given the wide distribution of air, a focal abscess is unlikely, and necrotizing fasciitis with gas-producing organisms should be suspected. (From Broder JS: *Diagnostic imaging for the emergency physician,* Philadelphia, 2011, Saunders.)

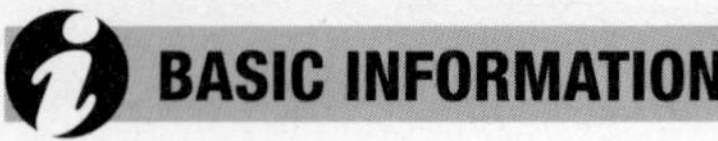

BASIC INFORMATION

DEFINITION

Nephroblastoma is a malignant renal tumor derived from primitive metanephric blastoma. Most tumors are unicentric, but some are multifocal in one or both kidneys. Associated anomalies may be present.

SYNONYMS

Wilms' tumor

ICD-9CM CODES
189.0 Nephroblastoma
ICD-10CM CODES
C64 Malignant neoplasm of kidney

EPIDEMIOLOGY & DEMOGRAPHICS

- Pediatric malignancy mean presentation is at 41.5 mo in boys and 46.9 mo in girls.
- Slightly more frequent in girls
- Incidence rate is 7.9 cases per year per 1 million white children <15 yr (a little over 500 new cases annually in the U.S.); the incidence is double in black children.
- Associated syndromes (Table 1-357):
  1. Cryptorchidism
  2. Hypospadias
  3. Hemihypertrophy with or without the Beckwith-Wiedemann syndrome, aniridia
  4. Denys-Drash syndrome (nephroblastoma, pseudohermaphroditism, glomerulonephritis)
  5. WAGR syndrome (***W***ilms' tumor, ***a***niridia, ***g***enitourinary malformations, and mental ***r***etardation)
- Familial nephroblastoma occurs in 1.5% (with younger age at diagnosis and more frequent multifocal tumors).

PHYSICAL FINDINGS & CLINICAL PRESENTATION

- Nephroblastoma often is discovered when a parent notices a mass while bathing or dressing a child, most commonly a child who is approximately age 3 yr, or during a routine physical examination. The mass is unilateral, firm, and nontender and below the costal margin.
- Abdominal swelling and/or pain
- Nausea
- Vomiting
- Constipation
- Loss of appetite
- Fever of unknown origin
- Night sweats
- Hematuria (less common than in adult renal malignancies)
- Malaise
- High blood pressure that is triggered when the tumor obstructs the renal artery
- Varicocele
- Signs of associated syndromes

ETIOLOGY & PATHOGENESIS

- Three cell types: blastomal, stromal, and epithelial may be present. Structural diversity is characteristic.
- Anaplasia is evidenced by the presence of gigantic polyploid nuclei. The term *focal anaplasia* is used to describe such findings when it is confined within the primary tumor in the kidney.
- Staging:
  Stage I: Tumor limited to the kidney whose capsule is intact. The tumor is completely excised.
  Stage II: Tumor extends beyond the kidney but is completely excised. No peritoneal involvement.
  Stage III: Residual tumor confined to the abdomen after surgery. No hematogenous metastases.
  Stage IV: Hematogenous metastases present.
  Stage V: Bilateral renal involvement at time of initial diagnosis.

DIAGNOSIS

DIFFERENTIAL DIAGNOSIS

- Other renal malignancies
  1. Hypernephroma
  2. Transitional cell carcinoma
  3. Lymphoma
  4. Clear cell sarcoma
  5. Rhabdoid tumor of the kidney
- Renal cyst
- Other intraabdominal or retroperitoneal tumors

LABORATORY TESTS

- Complete blood count
- Transaminases (alanine aminotransferase, aspartate aminotransferase)
- Alkaline phosphatase
- Blood urea nitrogen and creatinine
- Serum calcium
- Urinalysis

IMAGING STUDIES

- Renal ultrasound to confirm existence of a solid mass in a kidney
- Abdominal CT scan with contrast
- Chest radiograph or CT scan

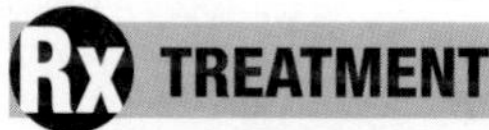

TREATMENT

- Surgical resection and surgical staging:
  1. Stages I and II: surgery followed by chemotherapy
  2. Stages III and IV: surgery followed by radiation and chemotherapy
- Chemotherapeutic agents used in the treatment of nephroblastoma include vincristine, dactinomycin, and doxorubicin

PROGNOSIS

- Stage I: 95% survival
- Stage II: 91% survival
- Stage III: 91% survival
- Stage IV: 81% survival
- Prognosis is better for patients <2 yr

AUTHOR: **FRED F. FERRI, M.D.**

TABLE 1-357 Syndromes associated with Wilms' Tumor

Syndrome	Clinical Characteristics	Genetic Anomalies
Wilms' tumor, aniridia, genitourinary abnormalities, and mental retardation (WAGR syndrome)	Aniridia, genitourinary abnormalities, mental retardation	Del 11p13 (*WT1* and *PAX6*)
Denys-Drash syndrome	Early-onset renal failure with renal mesangial sclerosis, male pseudohermaphroditism	*WT1* missense mutation
Beckwith-Wiedemann syndrome (BWS)	Organomegaly (liver, kidney, adrenal, pancreas) macroglossia, omphalocele, hemihypertrophy	Unilateral paternal disomy, duplication of 11p15.5 loss of imprinting, mutation of *p57KIP57* Del 11p15.5 *IGF2* and *H19* imprinting control region

From Kliegman RM et al: *Nelson textbook of pediatrics,* ed 19, Philadelphia, 2011, Saunders.

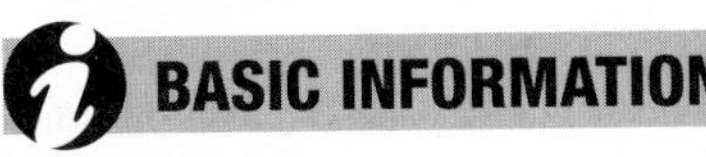

BASIC INFORMATION

DEFINITION

Multiorgan systemic fibrosis related to gadolinium-based contrast exposure

SYNONYMS

Nephrogenic fibrosing dermopathy
Gadolinium-associated nephrogenic systemic fibrosis

ICD-9CM CODES
710.8 Other specified diffuse diseases of connective tissue
ICD-10CM CODES
M35.5 Multifocal fibrosclerosis

EPIDEMIOLOGY & DEMOGRAPHICS

INCIDENCE: 4%
PREDOMINANT SEX AND AGE: No predilection for sex or age
RISK FACTORS: Linear, ionically charged gadolinium-based contrast agents including gadodiamide (Omniscan), gadopentetate (Magnevist), and gadoversetamide (OptiMARK) exposure among patients with severe renal dysfunction (Stage 4/GFR <30 ml/min per 1.73 m^2 or worse), including dialysis patients, with the highest risk in patients on peritoneal dialysis or acute kidney injury (AKI), particularly hepatorenal in origin. Proinflammatory states including major surgery, thrombotic events, infection, and malignancy as well as high-dose erythropoietin use in this population are associated with higher risk of nephrogenic systemic fibrosis.

PHYSICAL FINDINGS & CLINICAL PRESENTATION

- History of gadolinium-based contrast media in a patient with renal dysfunction (GFR <30 ml/min) or AKI, particularly in those patients with proinflammatory states
- Presentation time varies from day of exposure to several months later, with a median of 11.5 days.
- Primary presentation with pruritic, erythematous plaques with induration and edema. Skin presentations typically are symmetric and involve the extremities and trunk, generally sparing the face. Fibrosis can be extradermal, leading to multiorgan dysfunction. For example, fibrosis can lead to respiratory failure from muscular involvement of the diaphragm. It can also affect the eyes and blood vessels.

ETIOLOGY

- Pathophysiology remains unclear, but current postulation is that free gadolinium ions deposit in the tissues after being displaced from its chelating agent. Displacement of gadolinium from its chelating agent is postulated to occur more readily in proinflammatory states. In renal failure, when the duration of gadolinium exposure is highest due to a decreased clearance of gadolinium, tissue deposition is higher. Deposition leads to fibrocyte recruitment and further contribution to the proinflammatory states, leading to further tissue injury and fibrocyte recruitment and ultimately tissue fibrosis.

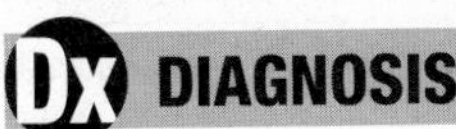

DIAGNOSIS

DIFFERENTIAL DIAGNOSIS

- Scleroderma

WORKUP

- Skin biopsy

LABORATORY TESTS

- None

IMAGING STUDIES

- None

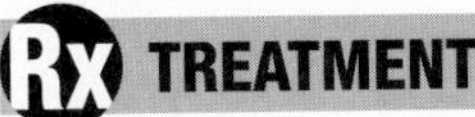

TREATMENT

No current effective treatment. There are no randomized clinical trials available. Case reports implementing corticosteroids, plasmapheresis, thalidomide, and methotrexate suggest little to no benefit, whereas case reports implementing photopheresis and sodium thiosulfate have shown modest benefit. Hemodialysis can effectively remove gadolinium contrast media, but no current evidence demonstrates that immediate hemodialysis is protective against development of nephrogenic systemic fibrosis. It is reasonable to perform dialysis following gadolinium contrast exposure in patients currently on dialysis.

REFERRAL

- Dermatology for biopsy

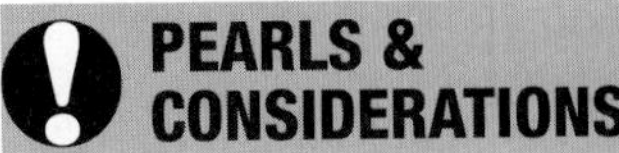

PEARLS & CONSIDERATIONS

COMMENTS

Given the lack of treatment modalities, prevention of this disease by avoidance of gadolinium-based contrast administration is best among patients with advanced CKD. All patients intended to receive gadolinium-based contrast for renal dysfunction should be screened.

PREVENTION

Unless essential diagnostic information is needed from a gadolinium-based contrast medium, these studies should be avoided in patients with a GFR less than 30 ml per minute per 1.73m^2 or with AKI. Caution should also be used in children under one year and pregnant women.

RELATED TOPICS

Information on gadolinium-based contrast agents:
http://www.fda.gov/Drugs/DrugSafety/PostmarketDrugSafetyInformationforPatientsandProviders/ucm142882.htm

AUTHOR: **SUSIE L. HU, M.D.**

BASIC INFORMATION

DEFINITION

Nephrotic syndrome is characterized by high urine protein excretion (>3.5 g/1.73 m^3/24 hr), peripheral edema, and metabolic abnormalities (hypoalbuminemia, hypercholesterolemia). Table 1-358 describes definitions of terms used in idiopathic nephrotic syndrome in adults and children. Fig. 1-651 illustrates the mechanism of nephrotic edema.

ICD-9CM CODES
581.9 Nephrotic syndrome
ICD-10CM CODES
N04.9 Nephrotic syndrome with unspecified morphologic changes

EPIDEMIOLOGY & DEMOGRAPHICS

- Nephrotic syndrome occurs predominantly in children ages 2 to 6 yr (2 new cases/100,000 persons/yr) and in adults of all ages (3 to 4 new cases/100,000 persons/yr).
- Membranous glomerulonephritis is the most common cause of nephrotic syndrome.

PHYSICAL FINDINGS & CLINICAL PRESENTATION

- Peripheral edema, eyelid edema (Fig. 1-652)
- Ascites, anasarca
- Hypertension
- Pleural effusion
- Typically patients present with severe peripheral edema, exertional dyspnea, and abdominal fullness secondary to ascites. There is a significant amount of weight gain in most patients.

ETIOLOGY

- Idiopathic (may be secondary to the following glomerular diseases: minimal change disease [nil disease, lipoid nephrosis], focal segmental glomerular sclerosis (20% of cases of nephrotic syndrome), membranous nephropathy, membranoproliferative glomerular nephropathy). PLA 2 R is a major antigen in the majority of patients with idiopathic membranous nephropathy. An HLA-DQA_1 allele on chromosome 6p21 is most closely associated with idiopathic membranous nephropathy in persons of white ancestry. This allele may facilitate an autoimmune response against targets such as variants of PLA 2 R1.
- Associated with systemic diseases (diabetes mellitus, systemic lupus erythematosus [SLE], amyloidosis). Amyloidosis and dysproteinemias should be considered in patients >40 yr.

TABLE 1-358 Nephrotic Syndrome (NS): Definitions

Term	NS DEFINITIONS: Adult	NS DEFINITIONS: Pediatric
Relapse	Proteinuria ≥3.5 g/day occurring after complete remission has been obtained for >1 mo	Albu-stix 3+ or proteinuria >40 mg/m/h occurring on 3 days within 1 wk
Frequently relapsing	2+ relapses within 6 mo	2+ relapses within 6 mo
Complete remission	Reduction of proteinuria to ≤0.20 g/day and serum albumin >35 g/L	<4 mg/m/h on at least 3 occasions within 7 days serum albumin >35 g/L
Partial remission	Reduction of proteinuria to between 0.21 g/day and 3.4 g/day ± decrease in proteinuria of ≥50% from baseline	Disappearance of edema. Increase in serum albumin >35 g/L and persisting proteinuria >4 mg/m/h or >100 mg/m/day
Steroid-resistant	Persistence of proteinuria despite prednisone therapy 1 mg/kg/day × 4 mo	Persistence of proteinuria despite prednisone therapy 60 mg/m × 4 wk*
Steroid-dependent—NS recurs when stop or decrease treatment	Two consecutive relapses occurring during therapy or within 14 days of completing steroid therapy	Two relapses of proteinuria within 14 days after stopping or during alternate day steroid therapy

Definition of terms used in idiopathic nephrotic syndrome in adults and children. The definitions were generated by a consensus of the International Society for Kidney Diseases in and the German Pediatric Nephrology Society.
*Or persistence of proteinuria despite prednisone therapy 60 mg m^{-2} × 4 weeks and three methylprednisolone pulses.
From Floege J et al: *Comprehensive clinical nephrology,* ed 4, Philadelphia, 2010, Saunders.

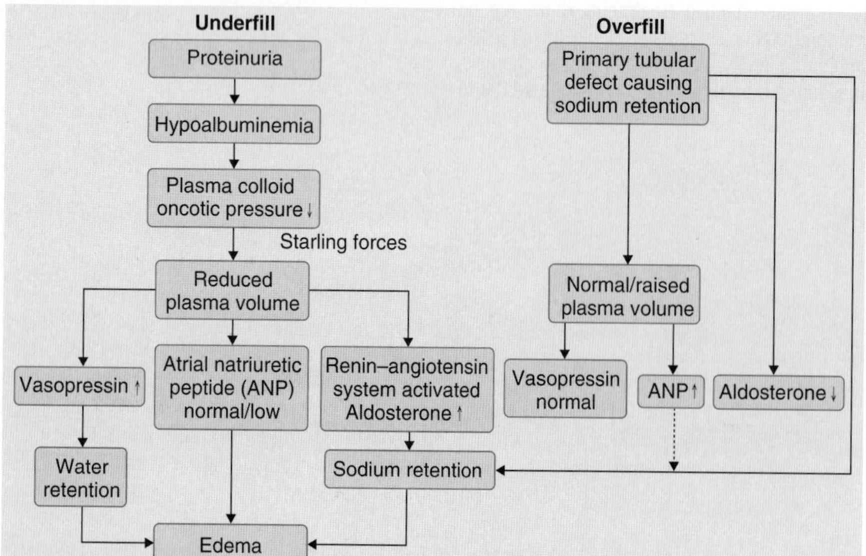

FIGURE 1-651 Mechanisms of nephrotic edema. The kidney is relatively resistant to ANP in this setting, so ANP has little effect in countering sodium retention. (From Floege J et al: *Comprehensive clinical nephrology,* ed 4, Philadelphia, 2010, Saunders.

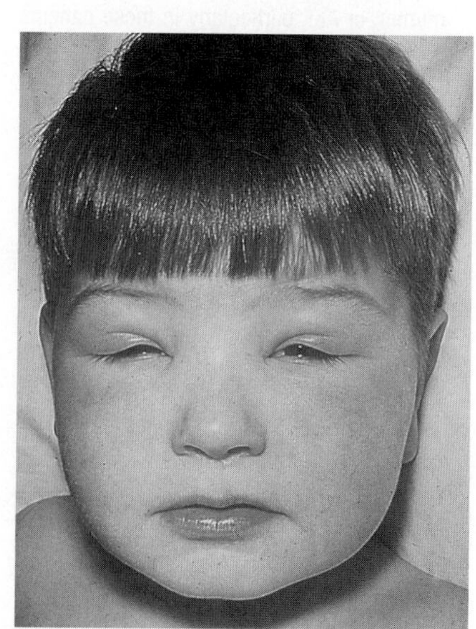

FIGURE 1-652 Nephrotic edema. Periorbital edema in the early morning in a nephrotic child. The edema resolves during the day under the influence of gravity. (From Floege J et al: *Comprehensive clinical nephrology,* ed 4, Philadelphia, 2010, Saunders.)

- Majority of children with nephrotic syndrome have minimal change disease (this form also associated with allergy, nonsteroidals, and Hodgkin's disease).
- Focal glomerular disease: can be associated with HIV infection, heroin abuse. A more severe form of nephrotic syndrome associated with rapid progression to end-stage renal failure within months can also occur in HIV seropositive patients and is known as "collapsing glomerulopathy."
- Membranous nephropathy: can occur with Hodgkin's lymphoma, carcinomas, SLE, gold therapy
- Membranoproliferative glomerulonephropathy: often associated with upper respiratory infections

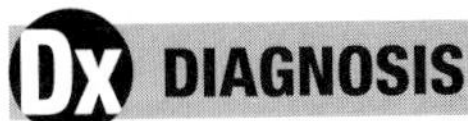

DIAGNOSIS

DIFFERENTIAL DIAGNOSIS

- Other edema states (CHF, cirrhosis)
- Primary renal disease (e.g., focal glomerulonephritis, membranoproliferative glomerulonephritis [MPGN]). The differentiation between nephrotic syndrome and nephritic syndrome is described in Table 1-359.

TABLE 1-359 Differentiation between Nephrotic Syndrome and Nephritic Syndrome

Typical Features	Nephrotic	Nephritic
Onset	Insidious	Abrupt
Edema	++++	++
Blood pressure	Normal	Raised
Jugular venous pressure	Normal/low	Raised
Proteinuria	++++	++
Hematuria	May/may not occur	+++
Red-cell casts	Absent	Present
Serum albumin	Low	Normal/slightly reduced

From Johnson RJ, Feehally J: *Comprehensive clinical nephrology,* ed 2, St Louis, 2000, Mosby.

Table 1-360 summarizes primary renal diseases that present as idiopathic nephrotic syndrome.

- Carcinoma, infections
- Malignant hypertension
- Polyarteritis nodosa
- Serum sickness
- Toxemia of pregnancy

WORKUP

Diagnostic workup consists of family history and history of drug use or toxin exposure and laboratory evaluation. Renal biopsy is generally performed in individuals with persistent proteinuria in whom the etiology of the proteinuria is unclear.

LABORATORY TESTS

- Urinalysis reveals proteinuria. The presence of hematuria, cellular casts, and pyuria is suggestive of nephritic syndrome. Oval fat bodies (tubular epithelial cells with cholesterol esters) are also found in the urine in patients with nephrotic syndrome.
- 24-hr urine protein excretion is >3.5 g/1.73 m^3/24 hr.
- Abnormalities of blood chemistries include serum albumin <3 g/dl, decreased total protein, elevated serum cholesterol, glucose, azotemia.

TABLE 1-360 Summary of Primary Renal Diseases That Present as Idiopathic Nephrotic Syndrome

	Minimal-Change Nephropathy Syndrome	Focal Segmental Sclerosis	Membranous Nephrotic	MEMBRANOPROLIFERATIVE GLOMERULONEPHRITIS Type I	MEMBRANOPROLIFERATIVE GLOMERULONEPHRITIS Type II
Frequency*					
Children	75%	10%	<5%	10%	10%
Adults	15%	15%	50%	10%	10%
Clinical Manifestations					
Age (yr)	2-6	2-10	40-50	5-15	5-15
Sex	2:1 female	1.3:1 female	2:1 male	Male-female	Male-female
Nephrotic syndrome	100%	90%	80%	60%	60%
Asymptomatic proteinuria	0	10%	20%	40%	40%
Hematuria	10%-20%	60%-80%	60%	80%	80%
Hypertension	10%	20% early	Infrequent	35%	35%
Rate of progression to renal failure	Does not progress	10 years	50% in 10-20 yr	10-20 yr	5-15 yr
Associated conditions	Allergy? Hodgkin's disease, usually none	None	Renal vein thrombosis, cancer, SLE, hepatitis B	None	Partial lipodystrophy
Laboratory Findings	Manifestations of nephrotic syndrome ↑ BUN in 15%-30%	Manifestations of nephrotic syndrome ↑ BUN in 20%-40%	Manifestations of nephrotic syndrome	Low C1, C4, C3-C9	Normal C1, C4, low C3-C9
Immunogenetics	HLA-B8, B12 (3.5)†	Not established	HLA-DRW3 (12–32)†	Not established	C3 nephritic factor Not established
Renal Pathology					
Light microscopy	Normal	Focal	Thickened	Thickened	Lobulation
Immunofluorescence	Negative	IgM	Fine	Granular	C3 only
Electron microscopy	Foot process fusion	Foot	Subepithelial	Mesangial	Dense deposits
Response of Steroids	90%	15%-20%	May slow progression	Not established	Not established

*Approximate frequency as a cause of idiopathic nephrotic syndrome. About 10% of adult nephrotic syndrome is due to various diseases that usually present with acute glomerulonephritis.
†Relative risk.
↑, Elevated; *BUN,* blood urea nitrogen; *C,* complement; *GBM,* glomerular basement membrane; *hepatitis B,* hepatitis B virus; *HLA,* human leukocyte antigen; *Ig,* immunoglobulin; *SLE,* systemic lupus erythematosus.
Modified from Goldman L, Ausiello D (eds): *Cecil textbook of medicine,* ed 22, Philadelphia, 2004, Saunders.

 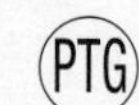

- Additional tests in patients with nephrotic syndromes depending on the history and physical examination are ANA, serum and urine immunoelectrophoresis, C3, C4, CH-50, LDH, liver enzymes, alkaline phosphatase, hepatitis B and C screening, and HIV.

IMAGING STUDIES

- Ultrasound of kidneys
- Chest x-ray

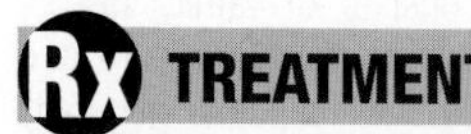

TREATMENT

NONPHARMACOLOGIC THERAPY

- Bed rest as tolerated, avoidance of nephrotoxic drugs, low-fat diet, fluid restriction in hyponatremic patients; normal protein intake unless urinary protein loss exceeds 10 g/24 hr (some patients may require additional dietary protein to prevent negative nitrogen balance and significant protein malnutrition)
- Improved urinary protein excretion and serum lipid changes have been observed with a low-fat soy protein diet providing 0.7 g of protein/kg/day. However, because of increased risk of malnutrition, many nephrologists recommend normal protein intake.
- Strict sodium restriction to help manage peripheral edema
- Close monitoring of patients for development of peripheral venous thrombosis and renal vein thrombosis because of hypercoagulable state secondary to loss of antithrombin III and other proteins involved in the clotting mechanism

ACUTE GENERAL Rx

- Furosemide is useful for severe edema (Fig. 1-653).
- Use of ACE inhibitors to reduce proteinuria is generally indicated even in normotensive patients.
- Anticoagulant therapy should be administered as long as patients have nephrotic proteinuria, an albumin level <20 g/L, or both.

The mainstay of therapy is treatment of the underlying disorder:

- Minimal change disease generally responds to prednisone 1 mg/kg/day. Relapses can occur when steroids are discontinued. In these individuals, cyclophosphamide and chlorambucil may be useful.
- Focal segmental glomerulosclerosis: children—empiric therapy with prednisone (60 mg/square meter of BSA) for 4-6 wk because 80% will have glucocorticoid-responsive minimal change disease. Adults receive RAS blockade (ACE inhibitors, ARBs) and dietary sodium restriction. Some genetic forms may respond to empiric therapy with calcineurin inhibitors.
- Membranous glomerulonephritis: prednisone 2 mg/kg/day may be useful in inducing remission. Cytotoxic agents can be added if there is poor response to prednisone.
- MPGN: most patients are treated with steroid therapy and antiplatelet drugs. Despite treatment, the majority of patients will progress to end-stage renal disease within 5 yr.

CHRONIC Rx

- Patients should be monitored for azotemia and should be aggressively treated for hypertension and hyperlipidemia. Furosemide is useful for severe edema. Anticoagulants may be necessary for thromboembolic events. Prophylactic anticoagulation should be considered in patients with membranous glomerulonephritis.
- Oral vitamin D is useful in the treatment of hypocalcemia (because of vitamin D loss).

REFERRAL

Nephrology consultation is recommended in all cases of nephrotic syndrome.

SUGGESTED READINGS

available at www.expertconsult.com

RELATED CONTENT

Nephrotic Syndrome (Patient Information)

AUTHOR: **FRED F. FERRI, M.D.**

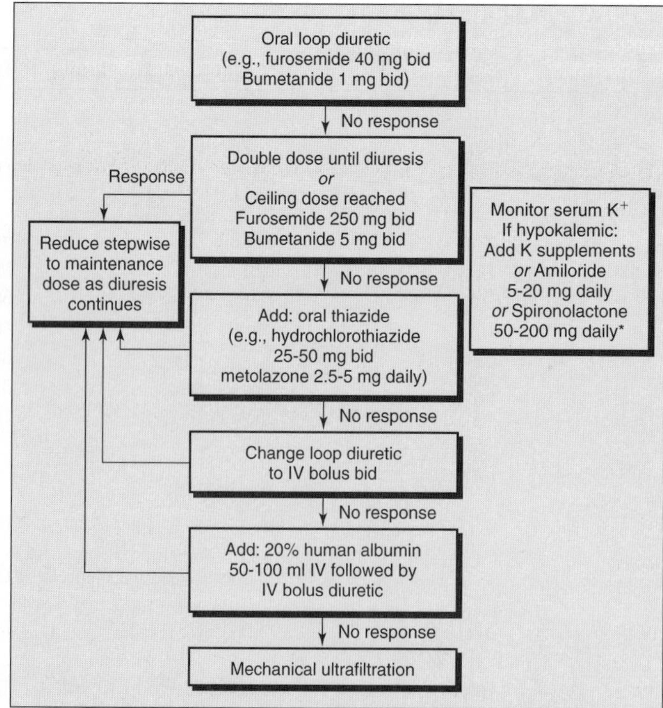

FIGURE 1-653 Management of edema in nephrotic syndrome. Edema is often diuretic resistant, but the response is not predictable. Therefore, stepwise escalation of therapy is appropriate until diuresis occurs. Even when there is anasarca, diuresis should not proceed faster than 2 kg/day in adults to minimize the risk of clinically significant hypovolemia. Mechanical ultrafiltration is rarely required for nephrotic edema unless there is associated renal insufficiency. *Spironolactone is less effective in nephrotic syndrome than in cirrhosis and is often poorly tolerated because of gastrointestinal side effects. Spironolactone should be used with great caution if the glomerular filtration rate is very low. (From Floege J et al: *Comprehensive clinical nephrology,* ed 4, Philadelphia, 2010, Saunders.)

BASIC INFORMATION

DEFINITION

Neuroblastomas are tumors of postganglionic sympathetic neurons that typically originate in the adrenal medulla or the sympathetic chain/ganglion. Often present at birth, but not diagnosed until later, when the child shows symptoms of the disease. They are almost exclusively a disease of childhood.

ICD-9CM CODES
194.0 Neuroblastoma, unspecified site
ICD-10CM CODES
C74.90 Malignant neoplasm of unspecified part of unspecified adrenal gland

EPIDEMIOLOGY & DEMOGRAPHICS

INCIDENCE (IN U.S.): 8%-10% of all solid tumors of childhood (third most common childhood cancer, after leukemia and brain tumors); 1/10,000 children <15 yr.
PREDOMINANT SEX: Male/female ratio of 1:1.3
PEAK AGE: Early childhood. Mean age of onset is 18 mo; 33% onset by 1 year; 75% onset by 5 year; 97% by 10 year. In rare cases, neuroblastoma can be discovered by fetal ultrasound.
GENETICS: Chromosomal deletions (loss of heterozygosity) found in nearly half of tumors, most commonly localized to chromosomes 1p, 11q, and 14q. Deletion of 1p36 (leading to amplification and overexpression of *N-MYC* protooncogene) associated with poor prognosis. There is a small subset with an autosomal dominant pattern of inheritance. Somatic recurrent mutations (ATRX gene) in tumors from patients with stage 4 neuroblastoma correlate with age at diagnosis and telomere length in children and young adults.

PHYSICAL FINDINGS & CLINICAL PRESENTATION

- Neuroblastomas can arise anywhere along the sympathetic nervous system. The most common primary site is the adrenal gland (40%), followed by a mass in the abdomen (25%), thorax (15%), neck (5%), and pelvis (5%). In approximately 1% of cases a primary site cannot be identified. 70% to 80% of children have regional lymph node involvement or distant metastases to bone marrow, cortical bone, orbits, liver, and skin at time of presentation.
- Spinal cord/paraspinal: can present with localized back pain, signs of compression—paraplegia, stool/urine retention, scoliosis
- Abdominal mass, pain, or constipation
- Horner's syndrome (ptosis, miosis, anhidrosis)
- Thoracic: difficulty breathing, dysphagia, infections, chronic cough
- Secondary symptoms referable to metastatic disease: fatigue, chronic pain (typically bony pain), pancytopenia, periorbital ecchymosis, proptosis, anorexia, weight loss, unexplained fever, multiple subcutaneous bluish nodules, irritability
- Paraneoplastic syndromes: opsoclonus-myoclonus syndrome (OMS) is described as "dancing eyes, dancing feet," which manifest as myoclonic jerks and chaotic eye movements in all directions. This may be initial presentation before tumor diagnosis; present in 1% to 3% of patients with neuroblastoma; of all patients with opsoclonus-myoclonus, approximately 50% have an underlying neuroblastoma. Patients who present with this syndrome must be evaluated for neuroblastoma; when present, the neuroblastoma often has more favorable biologic features.
- Progressive cerebellar ataxia.
- Abnormal secretion of vasoactive intestinal peptide by the tumor, leading to distention of the abdomen and secretory diarrhea.

DIAGNOSIS

WORKUP

- Careful general physical examination to look for mass
- Biopsy and resection of tumor when possible

LABORATORY TESTS

- Complete blood count, coagulation studies, erythrocyte sedimentation rate.
- 24-hour urine for catecholamines: homovanillic acid (HVA) and vanillylmandelic acid (VMA) are secreted by up to 90% of tumors.
- Nonspecific serum markers such as neuron-specific enolase, lactate dehydrogenase, and ferritin.
- Bone marrow biopsy and aspirate: karyotype, DNA index, *N-MYC* copy number.
- Minimum criteria for diagnosis is based on one of the following: (1) unequivocal pathologic diagnosis made from tumor tissue or (2) combination of bone marrow aspirate with unequivocal tumor cells and increased levels of serum or urinary catecholamine metabolites, as described above.
- Genetic/biologic variables have been studied in children with neuroblastoma, in particular the histology, aneuploidy of tumor DNA, and amplification of the *N-MYC* oncogene within tumor tissue, because treatment decisions may be based on these factors.
    - Hyperdiploid DNA is associated with favorable prognosis, especially in infants.
    - *N-MYC* amplification is associated with poor prognosis, regardless of patient age, likely due to association with deletion of chromosome 1p and gain of chromosome 17q.
    - Other biologic factors studied include profile of GABAergic receptors, expression of neurotrophin receptors, level of telomerase RNA and serum ferritin and lactate dehydrogenase.

IMAGING STUDIES

- Chest x-ray, abdominal plain film, skeletal survey, abdominal and renal/bladder ultrasound
- CT scan or MRI of the chest and abdomen to provide information about regional lymph nodes, vessel invasion, and distant metastases (Fig. 1-654)
- Body scan with ^{131}I-MIBG (meta-iodobenzylguanidine), which is taken up by neuroblasts and is sensitive to metastases in the bone and soft tissue
- Bone scan with Tc-99 MDP to visualize lytic bone lesions and metastases
- Urine catecholamines: elevated in 90% to 95% of patients with neuroblastomas
- STAGING (staged according to the International Neuroblastoma Staging System [INSS])

I.	Confined to single organ
IIA.	Localized tumor with incomplete gross resection; lymph nodes negative
IIB.	Localized tumor with incomplete gross resection; ipsilateral lymph nodes positive
III.	Extension across midline, with or without lymph node involvement
IV.	Distant metastases to lymph nodes, bone, bone marrow, liver, skin
IVs.	Localized primary tumor with dissemination limited to skin, liver, or bone marrow; limited to infants

DIFFERENTIAL DIAGNOSIS

- Other small, round, blue-cell childhood tumors, such as lymphoma, rhabdomyosarcoma, soft tissue sarcoma, and primitive neuroectodermal tumors (PNETs)
- Wilms' tumor. Table 1-361 describes features distinguishing between Wilms' tumor and neuroblastoma.
- Hepatoblastoma. Opsoclonus myoclonus may occur with other tumors such as hepatoblastoma, infections (e.g., Coxsackie virus, Lyme disease, rickettsia, HIV), ingestions (phenytoin,

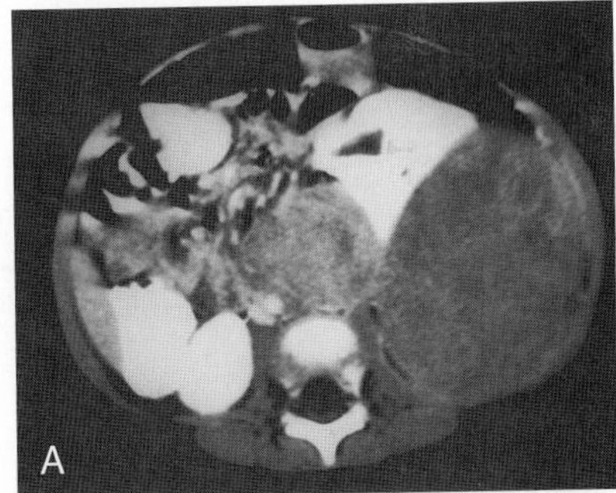

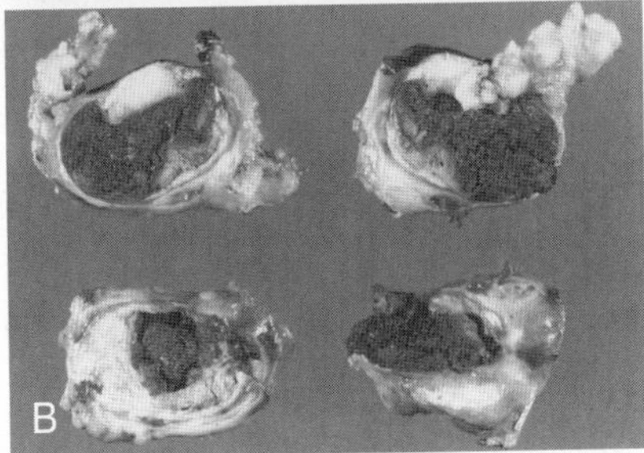

FIGURE 1-654 Computed tomographic scan **(A)** shows adrenal neuroblastoma at diagnosis. Serial sections through adrenal neuroblastoma **(B)** show tumor with large areas of diffuse hemorrhage and calcification. (From Abeloff MD [ed]: *Clinical oncology,* ed 3, Philadelphia, 2004, Saunders.)

 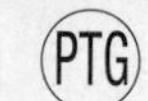

amitriptyline, diazepam), toxic exposures, and metabolic derangements (biotin-responsive multiple carboxylase deficiency).

Rx TREATMENT

- Assure patient and family that there is hope for recovery with aggressive treatment.
- Overall, treatment will be determined by several factors, including age at diagnosis, stage of disease, site of primary tumor and metastases, tumor histology, and quantitative DNA content of the tumor.
- Surgery: particularly for low-risk tumors.
- Radiation therapy may be tried for unresectable tumors or tumors that are not responsive to chemotherapy.
- Multiagent chemotherapy is mainstay of treatment (e.g., cisplatinum, etoposide, Adriamycin, cyclophosphamide, carboplatin).
- Autologous bone marrow transplantation following aggressive chemotherapy for stage IV disease or patients who are at highest risk based on presence of disseminated disease or unfavorable markers such as *N-MYC* amplification.
- Novel therapies include immunotherapy using monoclonal antibodies and vaccines that attempt to initiate an immune reaction against the disease and targeting of tumor cells with drugs that induce apoptosis or have antiangiogenic effect. Immunotherapy with ch14.18, a monoclonal antibody against the tumor-associated disialoganglioside GD2, has activity against neuroblastoma. Recent trials have shown that immunotherapy with ch14.18, GM-CSF, and interleukin-2 is associated with a significantly improved outcome as compared with standard therapy in patients with high-risk neuroblastoma. Treatment with MIBG in conjunction with autologous peripheral blood stem cell rescue.
- Adrenocorticotropic hormone (ACTH) treatment is thought to be effective for patients with opsoclonus/myoclonus syndrome.

DISPOSITION

- Overall survival is >40%. Children under the age of 1 yr have a cure rate as high as 90%.
- Approximately 70% of patients with neuroblastoma have metastases at diagnoses.
- Prognosis is related to age at time of diagnosis, clinical stage, and regional lymph node involvement. Children with localized disease and infants <1 year at diagnosis and favorable disease characteristics have better prognosis whereas poorer prognosis is noted in older children with stage IV disease (20% survival compared with >95% in stage I), age >1 year at diagnosis, increased number of *N-MYC* copies, adrenal tumor, and chronic 1p deletion.
- Children treated for neuroblastoma may be at risk for second malignancies, including renal cell carcinoma.

REFERRAL

Multidisciplinary oncology team with experience in treating cancers of childhood and adolescence.

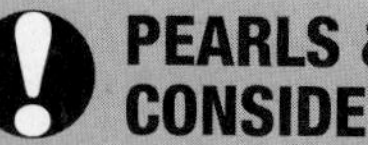

PEARLS & CONSIDERATIONS

- Neuroblastoma is predominantly a tumor of early childhood that originates in the sites where the sympathetic nervous system tissue is present.
- Symptoms occur due to tumor mass or bone pain from metastases.
- Children can present with classic paraneoplastic neurologic symptoms, including cerebellar ataxia and opsoclonus myoclonus.
- Recent trials have shown a very high rate of survival among patients with intermediate-risk neuroblastoma with biologically based treatment assignment involving a substantially reduced duration of chemotherapy and reduced doses of chemotherapeutic agents as compared with regimens used in earlier trials. These data provide support for further reduction in chemotherapy with more refined risk stratifications.
- Despite recent advances, 50% to 60% of patients with high-risk neuroblastoma have a relapse and currently there are no salvage treatment regimens known to be curative.

SUGGESTED READINGS

available at www.expertconsult.com

RELATED CONTENT

Neuroblastoma (Patient Information)

AUTHOR: **NICOLE J. ULLRICH, M.D., PH.D.**

TABLE 1-361 Features Distinguishing Between Wilms' Tumor and Neuroblastoma

Feature	Wilms' Tumor	Neuroblastoma
Age	2-3 years	<2 years
Origin	Kidney	Retroperitoneal neural crest
Renal mass effect	Intrinsic mass effect	External compression
Laterality	10% bilateral	Almost always
Calcification	<15%	85%-95%
Vessel involvement	Renal vein invasion in 5%-10%	Frequent encasement

From Weissleder R et al: *Primer of diagnostic imaging,* ed 5, St Louis, 2011, Mosby.

BASIC INFORMATION

DEFINITION

Neurofibromatosis (NF) is an autosomal-dominant disorder affecting bone, the nervous system, soft tissue, and skin. There are three major subtypes of NF disorders: NF type 1 (NF1), NF type 2 (NF2), and schwannomatosis. Schwannomatosis has only recently been recognized as a distinct disorder; currently very little is known about it.

SYNONYMS

NF1: von Recklinghausen disease, peripheral NF
NF2: bilateral acoustic neurofibromatosis, central NF

ICD-9CM CODES
237.70 Neurofibromatosis, unspecified
237.71 Type 1, von Recklinghausen's
237.72 Type 2, acoustic
ICD-10CM CODES
Q85.00 Neurofibromatosis, unspecified
Q85.01 Neurofibromatosis, type 1
Q85.02 Neurofibromatosis, type 2

EPIDEMIOLOGY & DEMOGRAPHICS

- Incidence of NF1 (one case/3000 live births), NF2 (one case/25,000 live births).
- Prevalence of NF1 (one case/5000 persons), NF2 (one case/210,000 persons).
- NF1 and NF2 are autosomal dominant; approximately 50% of cases have no family history.
- The two disorders affect approximately 100,000 people in the U.S.
- Affects males and females equally.
- NF1 may be associated with optic gliomas, astrocytomas, spinal neurofibromas, pheochromocytomas, and chronic myeloid leukemia.
- NF2 may be associated with meningiomas, spinal schwannomas, and cataracts.
- For schwannomatosis, the incidence is one per 30,000 persons, and the disease is mostly sporadic in nature.

PHYSICAL FINDINGS & CLINICAL PRESENTATION

- Common features of NF1 include:
  1. Café-au-lait macules (100% of children by age 2 yr)
     a. Hyperpigmented skin lesions (Fig. 1-655) occurring anywhere on the body except the face, palms, and soles
     b. Appear early in life and increase in size and number during puberty
     c. Are focal or diffuse
  2. Axillary and inguinal freckling (70%)
  3. Multiple neurofibromas (Figs. 1-656 and 1-657) can be soft or firm; three subtypes:
     a. Cutaneous: circumscribed, not specific for NF1
     b. Subcutaneous: circumscribed, not specific for NF1
     c. Plexiform: noncircumscribed, thick and irregular; can cause disfigurement of supportive structures and specific for NF1
  4. Lisch nodule (small hamartoma of the iris) found in >90% of adult cases.
  5. Visual defects possibly related to optic gliomas (2% to 5%).
  6. Neurodevelopment problems such as learning disability and mental retardation (30% to 40%).
  7. Skeletal disorders, including long bone dysplasia, pseudoarthrosis, scoliosis, short stature, and decreased bone mineral density.
- Common features of NF2 include:
  1. Hearing loss and tinnitus related to bilateral acoustic neuromas (>90% of adults)
  2. Cataracts (81%)
  3. Headache
  4. Unsteady gait
  5. Cutaneous and subcutaneous neurofibromas but fewer than in NF1
  6. Café-au-lait macules (1%)
- Common features of schwannomatosis include painful multiple schwannomas of the spinal, peripheral, or cranial nerves *except* the vestibular nerve.

ETIOLOGY

- NF1 is caused by DNA mutations located on the long arm of chromosome 17 responsible for encoding the protein neurofibromin.
- NF2 is caused by DNA mutations located in the middle of the long arm of chromosome 22 responsible for encoding the protein merlin, which is a potent inhibitor of glioma growth.
- Both proteins are speculated to act as tumor suppressors.
- The etiology of schwannomatosis remains unclear; however, biallelic NF2 mutations are found in the schwannomas but nowhere else, suggesting that they are secondary mutations.

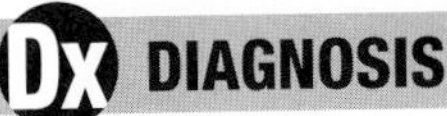

DIAGNOSIS

- NF1 is diagnosed if the person has two or more of the following features:
  1. Six or more café-au-lait macules >5 mm in prepubertal patients and >15 mm in postpubertal patients
  2. Two or more neurofibromas of any type or one plexiform neurofibroma
  3. Axillary or inguinal freckling
  4. Optic glioma
  5. Two or more Lisch nodules (iris hamartomas)
  6. Sphenoid wing dysplasia or cortical thinning of long bones, with or without pseudoarthrosis
  7. A first-degree relative (parent, sibling, or child) with NF1 based on the previous criteria
- NF2 is diagnosed if the person has either of the following two criteria:
  1. Bilateral eighth nerve masses seen by appropriate imaging studies (e.g., CT, MRI)
  2. A first-degree relative with NF2 and either a unilateral eighth nerve mass or two of the following: neurofibroma, meningioma, glioma, schwannoma, or juvenile posterior subcapsular lenticular opacity
- Schwannomatosis is diagnosed in an individual >30 yr having either of the following two criteria:
  1. Two nonintradermal schwannomas, no vestibular tumor found on MRI scan, no NF2 mutation
  2. One nonvestibular schwannoma and a first-degree relative fitting the above criteria

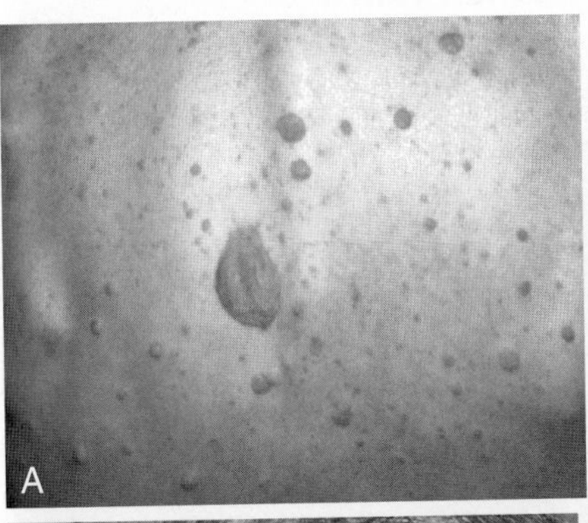

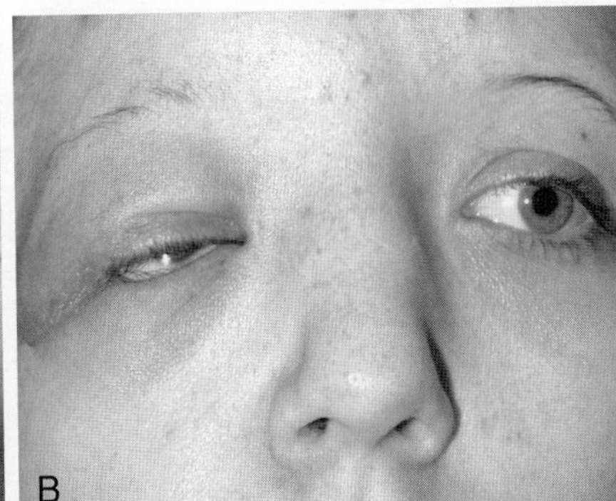

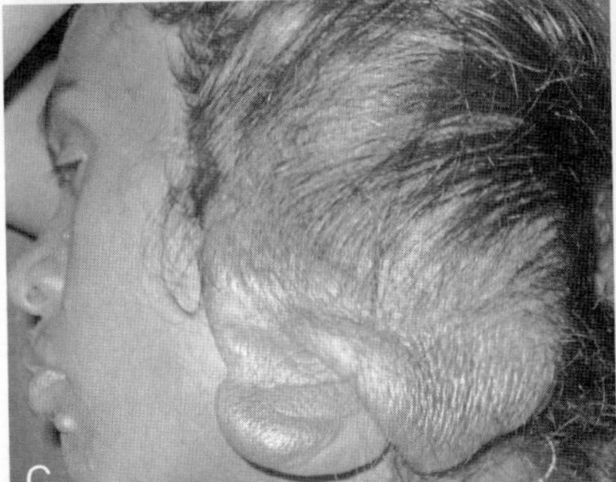

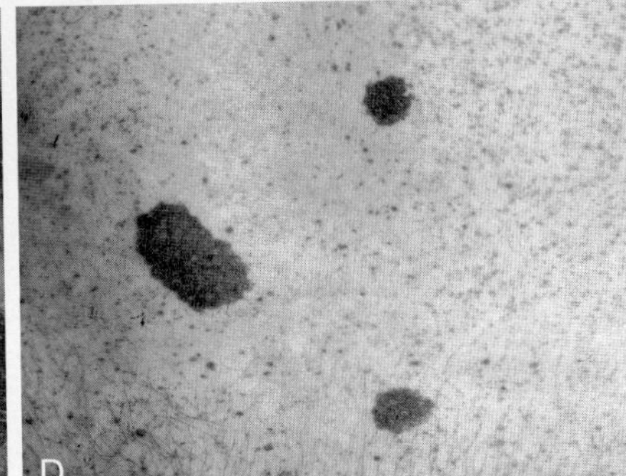

FIGURE 1-655 Systemic features of NF1. A, Discrete neurofibromas. **B,** Nodular plexiform neurofibroma of the eyelid. **C,** Elephantiasis nervosa. **D,** Cafe-au-lait spots. (**C** courtesy S. Kumar Puri. From Kanski JJ, Bowling B: *Clinical ophthalmology, a systematic approach,* ed 7, Philadelphia, 2010, Saunders.)

 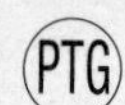

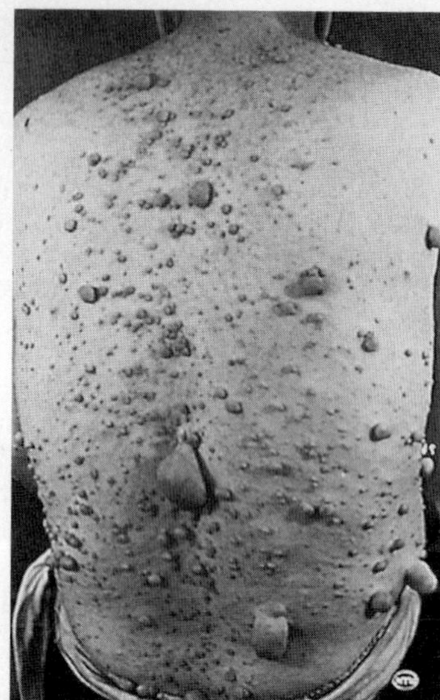

FIGURE 1-656 Nodules. Solid, large (>1 cm), deep-seated mass in dermal or subcutaneous tissues. These nodules are neurofibromas in a patient with neurofibromatosis. (From Goldman L, Ausiello D [eds]: *Cecil textbook of medicine,* ed 22, Philadelphia, 2004, Saunders.)

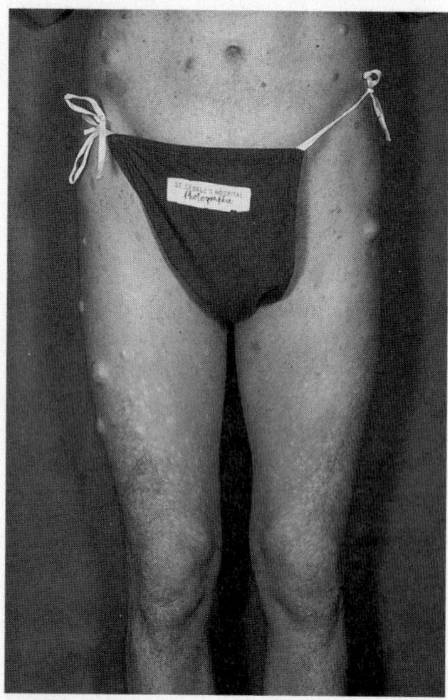

FIGURE 1-657 Type 1 neurofibromatosis: widespread cutaneous neurofibromata are a prominent feature of the classical variant. (Courtesy of R.A. Marsden, M.D., St George's Hospital, London. From McKee PH, Calonje E, Granter SR [eds]: *Pathology of the skin with clinical correlations,* ed 3, St Louis, 2005, Mosby.)

DIFFERENTIAL DIAGNOSIS

- Abdominal NF
- Myxoid lipoma
- Nodular fasciitis
- Fibrous histiocytoma
- Segmental NF

WORKUP

The diagnosis of NF is usually self-evident. Workup is dictated by clinical symptoms in NF1 and usually includes MRI evaluation of the head and spine in NF2 and schwannomatosis. In fact, if NF2 is suspected but no vestibular nerve schwannomas are found, the diagnosis points to schwannomatosis.

LABORATORY TESTS

- Genetic testing is possible in individuals who desire prenatal diagnosis for NF1. There is no single standard test and multiple tests are required. Results can only tell if an individual is affected but cannot predict the severity of the disease due to variable expression.
- In NF2, linkage analysis testing provides a >99% certainty the individual has NF2.

IMAGING STUDIES

- MRI with gadolinium is the imaging study of choice in both NF1 and NF2 patients. MRI increases detection of optic gliomas, tumors of the spine, acoustic neuromas, and "bright spots" believed to represent hamartomas.
- MRI of the spine is recommended in all patients diagnosed with NF2 to exclude intramedullary tumors.

OTHER TESTS

- Wood lamp examination may be useful in patients with very pale skin for visualizing café-au-lait spots.
- Slit-lamp examination is recommended for children >6 yr to confirm the presence of Lisch nodules and subcapsular opacity.

Rx TREATMENT

Treatment is directed primarily at symptoms and complications of NF1 and NF2. As for schwannomatosis, resection should be reserved for tumors that are symptomatic or threaten to cause spinal cord compression.

NONPHARMACOLOGIC THERAPY

- Counseling addressing prognosis and genetic, psychological, and social issues
- Hearing testing and speech pathology evaluation

ACUTE GENERAL Rx

- Surgery is usually not done on skin tumors unless cosmetically requested or if suspicion of malignant transformation exists.
- Surgery may be indicated for spinal or cranial neurofibromas, gliomas, or meningiomas.
- Acoustic neuromas can be treated by surgical excision.

CHRONIC Rx

- Radiation may be indicated in optic nerve gliomas and patients whose central nervous system tumors show radiographic progression.
- Stereotactic radiosurgery with a gamma knife may be an alternative approach to surgery for acoustic neuromas.

DISPOSITION

- Prognosis varies according to the severity of involvement.
- There is no cure for NF.

REFERRAL

A multidisciplinary team of consultants is needed in patients with NF, including neurosurgeon, otolaryngologist, dermatologist, neurologist, audiologist, speech pathologist, geneticist, and neuropsychologist.

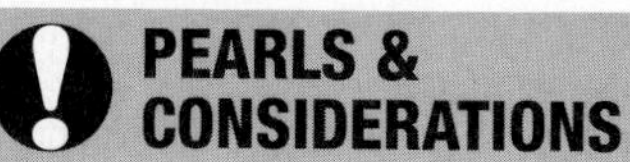

PEARLS & CONSIDERATIONS

- Friedrich Daniel von Recklinghausen first reported his cases in 1882, although there had been similar accounts dating back to the 1600s.
- A high SPRED1 mutation detection rate has been identified in NF1 mutation-negative families with an autosomal dominant phenotype of CALMs with or without freckling and no other NF1 features.

COMMENTS

For additional information and patient resources, refer to the National Neurofibromatosis Foundation (www.nf.org) or Neurofibromatosis Inc. (www.nfinc.org).

SUGGESTED READINGS

available at www.expertconsult.com

RELATED CONTENT

Neurofibromatosis Type 1 (Patient Information)

AUTHORS: **MARK F. BRADY, M.D., M.P.H., M.M.S.,** and **WEN Y. WU-CHEN, M.D.**

BASIC INFORMATION

DEFINITION

Neuroleptic malignant syndrome (NMS) is a disorder characterized by hyperthermia, muscular rigidity, autonomic dysfunction, and depressed/fluctuating levels of arousal that evolve over 24 to 72 hr. This occurs as an idiosyncratic adverse reaction to medications that affect the central dopaminergic system, usually D2 receptors blockade.

SYNONYMS

NMS

ICD-9CM CODES
333.92 Neuroleptic malignant syndrome
ICD-10CM CODES
G21.0 Malignant neuroleptic syndrome

EPIDEMIOLOGY & DEMOGRAPHICS

INCIDENCE (IN U.S.): 0.07% to 0.15% annual incidence in psychiatric population.
PREDOMINANT SEX: More than two thirds of patients are male.
PREDOMINANT AGE: Young and middle-aged adults
PREDISPOSING FACTORS:
- History of intake of dopamine antagonists e.g., antipsychotics

PHYSICAL FINDINGS & CLINICAL PRESENTATION

- Syndrome typically begins abruptly while the patient is taking therapeutic (not toxic) dosages of neuroleptics and reaches maximum severity within 72 hr.
- Severe muscle rigidity (hypertonia, cogwheeling, or "lead pipe" rigidity)
- Hyperthermia (38.6° to 42.3° C, usually <40° C)
- Autonomic symptoms: diaphoresis, dysphagia, sialorrhea, skin pallor, urinary incontinence
- Tachycardia, tachypnea
- Labile blood pressure (hypertension or postural hypotension)
- Agitation, catatonia, fluctuating consciousness, obtundation

ETIOLOGY

- Exact etiology is unknown, but it has been suggested that sudden and marked dopamine receptor blockade in nigrostriatal, hypothalamic, mesolimbic, and mesocortical pathways leads to clinical manifestations seen in NMS.
- Neuroleptic drugs have different potencies for inducing NMS:
  1. Typical neuroleptics: high potency, haloperidol; medium potency, chlorpromazine, fluphenazine; low potency, levomepromazine, loxapine
  2. Atypical neuroleptics: low potency, risperidone, olanzapine, clozapine, quetiapine

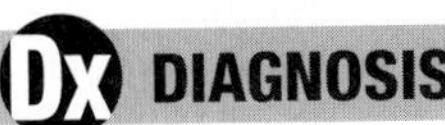

DIAGNOSIS

DIFFERENTIAL DIAGNOSIS

- Heatstroke, drug-induced states and overdose (Ecstasy abuse, phencyclidine), thyrotoxicosis, pheochromocytoma, serotonin syndrome
- Malignant hyperthermia, catatonia, acute psychosis with agitation
- CNS or systemic infections, including sepsis

WORKUP

Careful drug history

LABORATORY TESTS

- Elevated creatine phosphokinase (CPK) (sensitivity 0.71)
- Urinary myoglobin
- Leukocytosis, usually 10,000 to 40,000/mm^3
- Electrolytes and renal function
- Blood gases
- Drug levels

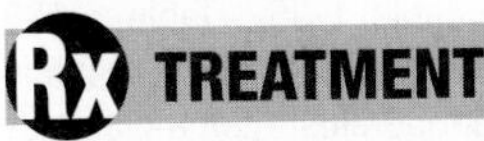

TREATMENT

NONPHARMACOLOGIC THERAPY

- Stop all neuroleptic drugs and reinstitute any recently discontinued dopaminergic agonists.
- Respiratory support; nutritional support in cases with dysphagia or comatose.
- Careful fluid balance monitoring with adequate hydration (intravenous in severe cases).
- Active cooling (cooling blanket and antipyretics).
- Skilled nursing care is necessary to prevent decubitus ulcers in bed-confined patients.

ACUTE GENERAL Rx

- Bromocriptine, a dopamine receptor agonist, is the mainstay of therapy for patients with NMS. Initial doses of 2.5 to 10 mg are given IV q8h and are increased by 5 mg/day until clinical improvement is seen. The drug should be continued for at least 10 days after the syndrome has been controlled and then tapered slowly.
- Dantrolene therapy can inhibit the excessive muscle contractions that generate myoglobinemia. Initially, patients can be given 0.25 mg/kg IV q6-12h, followed by a maintenance dose up to 3 mg/kg/day. After 2 to 3 days, patients may be given the drug orally (25 to 600 mg/day in divided doses). Oral dantrolene therapy (50 to 600 mg/day) may be continued for several days afterward.
- Amantadine, an NMDA receptor antagonist with possible dopaminergic properties, administered orally at doses of 100 to 200 mg PO bid, has also been shown to reduce mortality in comparison to supportive therapy alone.
- IV benzodiazepines (e.g., diazepam 2 to 10 mg, with total daily dose of 10 to 60 mg) to relax muscles and control agitation.
- Electroconvulsive therapy with neuromuscular blockage in pharmacologically refractory cases. Succinylcholine should not be used because it may cause hyperkalemia and cardiac arrhythmias in patients with rhabdomyolysis or dysautonomia.

CHRONIC Rx

- Respiratory care, nutritional support, and physical therapy may be required in more severe cases.
- Appropriate therapy would be required in patients with persistent neuropsychiatric sequelae of NMS (e.g., antidepressants for depression, cognitive behavioral therapy for cognitive deficits, rehabilitation for contractures).

DISPOSITION

- Mortality rate is currently 5% to 10% despite therapeutic measures. Serious sequelae may occur in a further 20%. Complete recovery occurs in >70% of patients. Causes of death include cardiac arrhythmias, myocardial infarction, renal failure secondary to rhabdomyolysis, seizures, pulmonary edema, and bronchopneumonia.
- Factors adversely affecting mortality are development of renal failure and core temperature >104° F (40° C).
- Late neuropsychiatric sequelae.
- Monitor closely for future complications of pharmacologic therapy.

REFERRAL

If the patient's condition is critical, it is preferable to treat the patient in a medical/neurologic ICU.

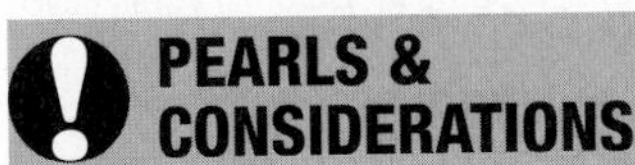

PEARLS & CONSIDERATIONS

COMMENTS

- Early detection and diagnosis lead to a more favorable outcome. Refer to recent consensus diagnostic criteria as a guide. Treatment is a medical emergency.
- Sudden withdrawal from dopaminergic agents (such as those used in Parkinson's disease) may lead to "levodopa withdrawal syndrome" that presents with similar clinical manifestations.

SUGGESTED READINGS

available at www.expertconsult.com

AUTHOR: **FARIHA ZAHEER, M.D.**

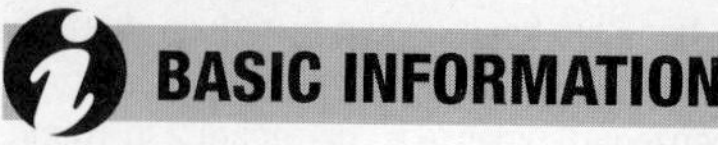

BASIC INFORMATION

DEFINITION

Neuropathic pain is not itself a disease, but rather a symptom that is associated with multiple different diseases. Thus it is not enough to define its presence without searching for a cause. It is defined as the sensation derived from the abnormal discharges of impaired or injured neural structures in either the peripheral or central nervous system. Descriptors include:

- Hyperesthesia: heightened sensitivity to nonpainful stimuli (e.g., light touch)
- Hyperalgesia: heightened sensitivity to painful stimuli (e.g., pinprick), or reduced threshold to feel pain
- Allodynia: pain provoked by a stimulus that is not normally painful

SYNONYMS

Neuralgia

ICD-9CM CODES
782.0 Numbness, paresthesias
729.1 Myositis/myalgia, not otherwise specified
729.2 Neuralgia, neuritis, or radiculitis, not otherwise specified
ICD-10CM CODES
G58.0 Intercostal neuropathy
G58.7 Mononeuritis multiplex
G58.8 Other specified mononeuropathies
G58.9 Mononeuropathy, unspecified
G60.0 Hereditary sensory and motor neuropathy
G61.9 Inflammatory polyneuropathy, unspecified
G62.0 Drug-induced polyneuropathy
G62.1 Alcoholic polyneuropathy
G62.9 Polyneuropathy, unspecified
G63.2 Diabetic polyneuropathy
G63.5 Polyneuropathy in systemic connective tissue disease
G63.8 Polyneuropathy in other diseases classified elsewhere

EPIDEMIOLOGY & DEMOGRAPHICS

- Estimates of the prevalence of neuropathic pain in the general population range from 1.6% to 8.2%.
- Demographics vary widely depending on etiology, for example:
  - Postherpetic neuralgia: affects elderly, pain seen in almost 100% of cases
  - AIDS: 30% of patients affected
  - Diabetes mellitus: 20% to 24% affected (prevalence rates vary, increasing with longer disease duration)
  - Fabry disease: affects mostly children, pain in 81% to 90% of patients

PHYSICAL FINDINGS & CLINICAL PRESENATION

- History: localize the disease with questions
  - Quality (description) of neuropathic pain: burning, hot or cold, "icy hot," "pins and needles," stinging, lancinating, sharp, shooting
  - Distribution of symptoms may aid in localization (i.e., "stocking-glove" symptoms in generalized neuropathy, numbness in a peripheral nerve territory in focal neuropathy)
  - Generalized small fiber neuropathy: dysesthesias without numbness common, but many etiologies (e.g., diabetes) cause both small and large fiber dysfunction
  - Large fiber neuropathy (LFPN): coexisting numbness, hyporeflexia, or weakness may be seen, usually worse distally
  - Nerve root: coexisting neck or low back pain that radiates along a specific dermatome; most common cause is structural compression
  - Spinal cord symptoms: coexisting spasticity, bowel or bladder involvement, sensory level
  - Prior history of thalamic stroke in central thalamic pain syndrome (Dejerine-Roussy syndrome)
  - Family history may suggest a genetic cause
- Examination: see Table 1-362. Table 1-363 describes joint involvement in neuropathic arthropathy. Fig. 1-659 illustrates a diagnostic approach to neuropathic pain. Fig. 1-658 shows a neuropathic ankle.

ETIOLOGY & LABORATORY EVALUATION (Table 1-364)

- Metabolic: diabetes mellitus; malnutrition and alcoholism; vitamin B_{12} deficiency; thiamine deficiency; porphyria; Fabry's disease
- Inflammatory: immune vasculitides (lupus, Sjögren's syndrome, polyarteritis nodosa, etc.), acute inflammatory demyelinating polyneuropathy (classically presents with ascend-

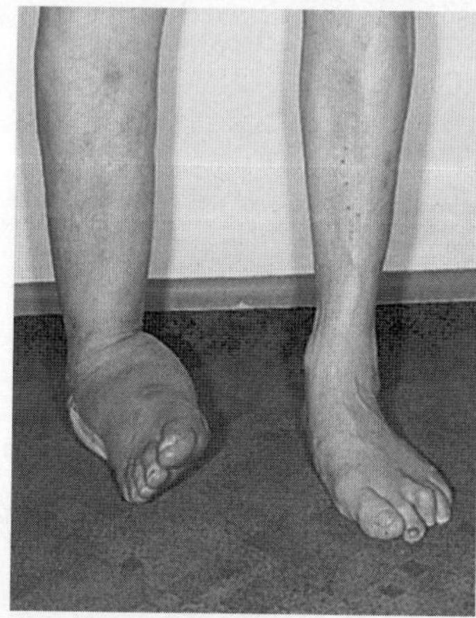

FIGURE 1-658 Neuropathic ankle. Marked instability of the subtalar and midtarsal joints is seen with collapse on weight bearing. (From Hochberg MC et al: *Rheumatology,* ed 5, St Louis, 2011, Mosby.)

TABLE 1-362 Examination

Exam Finding	Localization
Pinprick/temperature loss alone	Small fibers only
Pinprick/temperature loss + vibratory/proprioceptive loss	Small and large fibers
Sensory loss and motor dysfunction worse distally than proximal	Large fiber neuropathy
Sensory loss and motor dysfunction along single nerve distribution	Single nerve
Sensory loss and motor dysfunction along multiple single nerves	Multiple mononeuropathies (i.e., mononeuropathy multiplex)
Motor and sensory loss involving multiple nerves belonging to specific region of brachial or lumbar plexus	Plexopathy
Sensory loss along dermatome with multiple myotomal muscles affected	Nerve root lesion
Asymmetric sensory loss without weakness and pseudoathetosis	Dorsal root ganglion
Vibratory/proprioceptive loss without pinprick/temperature loss	Dorsal column dysfunction (from compressive lesion, B_{12} deficiency, or tabes dorsalis from neurosyphilis)
Sensory level with weakness below the level of lesion and long tract signs (spasticity/Babinski's sign)	Spinal cord lesion
Hemisensory hyperalgesia	Contralateral thalamus

TABLE 1-363 Joint Involvement in Neuropathic Arthropathy

Disease	Site of Involvement
Diabetes mellitus	Midtarsal, metatarsophalangeal, tarsometatarsal
Syringomyelia	Shoulder, elbow, wrist
Amyloidosis	Knee, ankle
Congenital sensory neuropathy	Knee, ankle, intertarsal, metatarsophalangeal
Tabes dorsalis	Knee, hip, ankle
Leprosy	Tarsal, tarsometatarsal

From Hochberg MC et al: *Rheumatology,* ed 5, St Louis, 2011, Mosby.

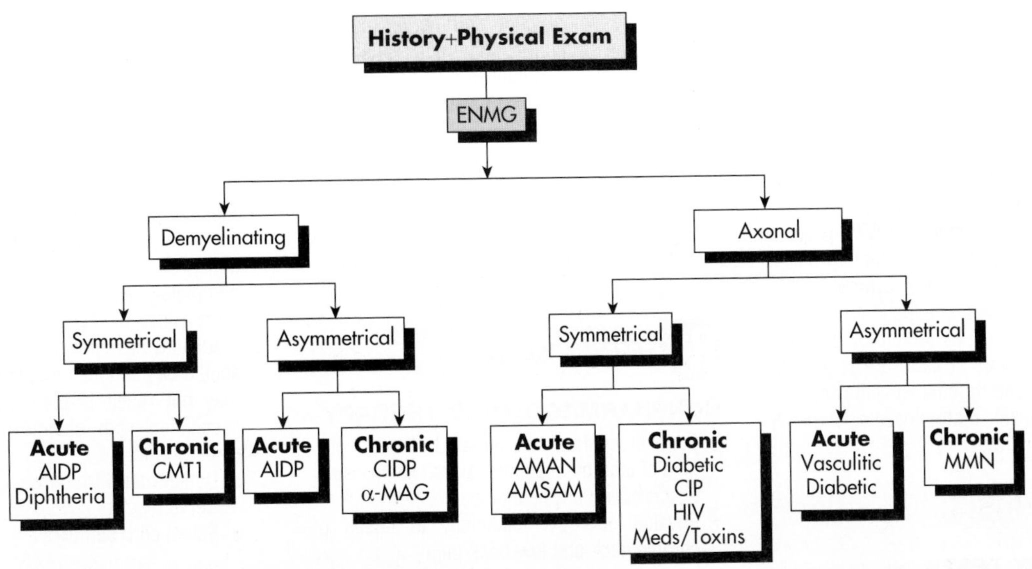

FIGURE 1-659 A systematic approach to evaluate neuropathy. The diseases listed are examples of neuropathies associated with specific neurophysiologic and clinical findings. Diabetic distal, predominantly sensory neuropathies are manifested as chronic axonal neuropathies; acute asymmetric neuropathies can also occur with diabetes. Most neuropathies caused by toxins or by side effects of medication are chronic, symmetric axonal neuropathies. AIDP, AMAN, and AMSAN are subtypes of Guillain-Barré syndrome. These and other examples are discussed in more detail in the text. *AIDP,* Acute inflammatory demyelinating polyradiculoneuropathy; *AMAN,* acute motor axonal neuropathy; *AMSAN,* acute motor and sensory axonal neuropathy; *CIDP,* chronic inflammatory polyradiculoneuropathy; *CIP,* chronic illness polyneuropathy; *CMT1,* Charcot-Marie-Tooth disease type 1, a genetic disorder; *ENMG,* electroneuromyography; *HIV,* human immunodeficiency virus–related neuropathy; *α-MAG,* anti-myelin-associated glycoprotein; *MMN,* multifocal motor neuropathy. (From Goldman L, Schafer AI: *Goldman's Cecil medicine,* ed 24, Philadelphia, 2012, Saunders.)

TABLE 1-364 Clinical Presentation and Laboratory Findings

Neuropathy Type	Predisposition	Examination Findings	EMG/NCS	Laboratory Analysis
Idiopathic small fiber PN	Age >50	Strength: normal Reflexes: normal Pos/Vib: normal Pain/Temp: decreased distally	Normal	Serum studies: normal Skin biopsy: abnormal Sudomotor studies: abnormal
Diabetic PN	Longstanding disease Family history	Strength normal to reduced, sensation reduced distally	Abnormal	Abnormal glucose tolerance High fasting glucose
Inherited PN	Family history	Pes cavus, hammer toes, reduced reflexes, sensation reduced distally	Abnormal	Genetic studies may be abnormal, other studies normal
Familial amyloid PN	Family history	Pain/temp loss Reduced reflexes Orthostasis	Abnormal if large fibers affected; also carpal tunnel syndrome	Transthyretin genetic study
Acquired amyloid PN	Monoclonal gammopathy	Pain/temp loss Reduced reflexes Orthostasis	Abnormal if large fibers affected; also carpal tunnel syndrome	SPEP, UPEP, immunofixation abnormal
Fabry's disease	Age Renal failure Strokes	Normal; possible reduced pain/temp sensation	Normal	α-Galactosidase levels in cultured fibroblasts
PN + mixed connective tissue disease	History of lupus, rheumatoid arthritis, Sjögren's syndrome	Reduced reflexes and distal sensation	Abnormal	ANA, RF, SS-A/SS-B may be abnormal
Peripheral nerve vasculitis	Asymmetric disease	Multiple peripheral nerves involved	Abnormal	ANA, RF, SS-A/SS-B, ANCA, cryoglobulins may be abnormal
Paraneoplastic neuropathy	Lung cancer risk factors, chemical exposures	Asymmetric sensory loss, pseudoathetosis, relatively preserved strength	Abnormal	Anti-Hu
Sarcoidosis	Pulmonary sarcoid	Multiple mononeuropathies	Abnormal	Abnormal biopsy, elevated serum ACE, CXR abnormal
Arsenic	Pesticides, copper smelting	Reduced reflexes and distal sensation	Abnormal	Elevated arsenic in plasma, urine, and hair
HIV	Promiscuity, unprotected sex, IV drug abuse, blood transfusion	Variable, but most often reduced reflexes and distal sensation	Abnormal if large fibers involved	HIV antibody

ACE, Angiotensin-converting enzyme; *ANA,* antibody to nuclear antigens; *ANCA,* antineutrophil cytoplasmic antibodies; *CXR,* chest x-ray; *EMG,* electromyography; *HbA1C,* glycosylated hemoglobin; *HIV,* human immunodeficiency virus; *IV,* intravenous; *NCS,* nerve conduction studies; *PN,* polyneuropathy; *Pos,* position sensation; *RF,* rheumatoid factor; *SPEP,* serum protein electrophoresis; *SS-A,* Sjögren syndrome A; *SS-B,* Sjögren syndrome B; *Temp,* temperature sensation; *UPEP,* urine protein electrophoresis; *Vib,* vibration sensation.
Adapted from Mendell JR, Sahenk Z: Painful sensory neuropathy, *N Engl J Med* 348(13):1243, 2003.

ing weakness and numbness, although pain is also a common feature), chronic inflammatory demyelinating polyneuropathy, sarcoid, multiple sclerosis
- Infiltrative: amyloidosis, paraproteinemias (e.g., monoclonal gammopathy of uncertain significance [MGUS])
- Infectious: postviral (brachial neuritis), HIV/AIDS, HSV, varicella-zoster virus (VZV; postherpetic neuralgia), Lyme disease, leprosy (thickened nerves and skin lesions), syphilis
- Neoplastic and paraneoplastic-carcinomatous infiltration of nerve/nerve root, anti-Hu
- Drugs/toxins: history of exposure to alcohol, chemotherapeutic agents (paclitaxel, vincristine), isoniazid, metronidazole, or heavy metals (thallium, arsenic)

Dx DIAGNOSIS

LABORATORY TESTS

- Fasting blood glucose (FBG)
- 2-hour oral glucose tolerance test (OGTT)
- Vitamin B_1 level
- If B_{12} level normal: serum methylmalonic acid and homocysteine levels
- Serum erythrocyte sedimentation rate (ESR), ANA, SS-A and SS-B, c-ANCA, p-ANCA
- RPR or FTA-ABS
- Serum ACE level (sarcoid)
- HIV antibody
- SPEP, UPEP, immunofixation
- Urine and stool protoporphyrins, if porphyria is suspected clinically
- Hu antibody: can be seen in both small cell and non–small cell lung cancers, may be positive without evidence of lung cancer
- Lumbar puncture: protein elevation, oligoclonal bands, CSF/serum IgG index, herpes simplex virus (HSV), VZV, Lyme polymerase chain reaction (PCR), VDRL

ELECTROPHYSIOLOGY STUDIES

- Electrophysiologic testing (electromyography with nerve conduction studies): may be normal in small fiber neuropathies or CNS lesion, but is often abnormal in large fiber neuropathies
- Quantitative sensory testing: abnormal in small and large fiber neuropathy
- Evoked potentials (only if suspicion for spinal cord lesion)

PATHOLOGY STUDIES

- Nerve biopsy is occasionally useful in selected cases, particularly when vasculitis, sarcoid, or amyloid neuropathy are in the differential.
- Skin biopsy for intraepidermal nerve fiber (IENF) density may be useful for small fiber neuropathy when other studies are normal.
- Rectal or abdominal fat pad biopsy may show amyloid deposition in systemic amyloidosis.

IMAGING STUDIES

- MRI (with and without contrast):
  - Of the brain to exclude thalamic pathology if symptoms and signs are consistent with thalamic lesion
  - Of the spinal cord and nerve roots to exclude structural, inflammatory, neoplastic, or infectious causes
  - Of the lumbar spine to evaluate for arachnoiditis
- If MRI cannot be performed, consider:
  - CT of the brain for thalamic pathology
  - CT myelography of the spinal cord to evaluate for structural/neoplastic disease, but only if clinical signs of spinal or nerve root compromise are present

Rx TREATMENT

NONPHARMACOLOGIC THERAPY

- Counseling should be initiated at the beginning of therapy to address psychologic issues exacerbating physiologic pain
- Physical therapy: especially in cases of chronic neck and low back pain

ACUTE GENERAL Rx

- Antidepressants:
  - Tricyclic antidepressants (TCAs): nortriptyline preferred over amitriptyline (fewer anticholinergic side effects with nortriptyline). Begin 25 mg PO qd in adults, or 10 mg qd in elderly. Increase dose by 25 mg every week as tolerated until usual maximal effective dose of 150 mg/day.
  - Paroxetine: begin 10 mg PO qd, increase by 10 mg/wk to a max dose of 60 mg qd.
  - Duloxetine: begin 30 mg daily, increase to 60 to 120 mg daily. Duloxetine is effective in diabetic neuropathy, post-herpetic neuropathy, and chemotherapy-induced painful peripheral neuropathy.
- Antiepileptics:
  - Gabapentin: begin 300 mg PO qd, advance to 300 mg PO tid by the end of the first week. Effective dose: higher than 1600 mg/day. Max dose: 1500 mg PO tid.
  - Carbamazepine: for trigeminal neuralgia. Begin 400 mg PO bid, increase to tid if necessary. Side effects and drug levels help to determine optimal dosing. Risk of aplastic anemia and hyponatremia (monitor CBC and chemistries).
  - Oxcarbazepine: better tolerated than carbamazepine. Start 150 mg PO bid and gradually increase to a maximal dose of 600 mg bid.
  - Lamotrigine: begin 25 mg PO bid, increase slowly (by 100 mg biweekly) until maximum effective dose of 200 to 300 mg PO bid. Risk: Stevens-Johnson syndrome.
  - Pregabalin: begin 50 mg PO tid, increase slowly to 100 to 200 mg PO tid.
- Analgesics:
  - Tramadol: 150 mg/day (50 mg tid), increase by 50 mg/wk, max 200 to 400 mg/day.
  - Morphine (oral): 15 to 30 mg q8h, max 90 to 360 mg/day.
  - Oxycodone: 20 mg q12h, increase by 10 mg/wk, max 40 to 160 mg/day.
  - Fentanyl patch: 25 to 100 mcg transdermally q3 days.
- Topical anesthetics:
  - 5% lidocaine patch, apply to area of pain, max three patches every 12 hr.
  - Capsaicin is inconsistent in its ability to relieve pain and may exacerbate it. Use not recommended.
- Procedural/surgical: this option is considered mostly when the patient suffers from pain secondary to spinal cord or cauda equina injury. Studies are limited and benefit is not completely established. Procedures should be considered only when all other therapeutic modalities have failed. In addition, the patient should be cautioned that surgical procedures may not result in pain relief and may be associated with significant morbidity and even mortality.
  - Dorsal root rhizotomy
  - Nerve blocks
  - Spinal cord stimulator

DISPOSITION

Prognosis depends on multiple factors, including:
- Etiology of pain
- Treatment of any underlying condition
- Initiation of appropriate (often multiple) therapeutic modalities
- Patient compliance with prescribed regimen

Most care is accomplished in the outpatient setting, except when surgery is required.

REFERRAL

- Pain clinic
- Neurology
- Psychiatry
- Psychology
- Physiatry
- Anesthesiology (nerve blocks)
- Neurosurgery if considering surgical management

PEARLS & CONSIDERATIONS

- Factitious disorder and malingering frequently manifest with pain complaints. These are diagnoses of exclusion, and require negative evaluation for organic etiologies before diagnosis is made.
- Peripheral neuropathy in diabetics increases the risk of foot ulceration by sevenfold. Abnormal results in monofilament testing and vibratory perception (alone or in combination with the appearance of the feet, ulceration, and ankle reflexes) are the most helpful sign for the detection of LFPN.

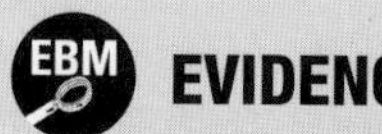

EVIDENCE

available at www.expertconsult.com

SUGGESTED READINGS

available at www.expertconsult.com

AUTHOR: **GAVIN BROWN, M.D.**

N

Diseases and Disorders

BASIC INFORMATION

DEFINITION

Any disorder affecting the peripheral nervous system, including nerve roots, plexuses, and individual peripheral nerves, that has a genetic basis of inheritance and has been or is capable of being transmitted along generations.

There are many different types of hereditary peripheral neuropathies, including Dejerine-Sottas disease, inherited metabolic neuropathies, hereditary sensory and autonomic neuropathies (HSANs), and hereditary motor neuropathies. Most disorders are diagnosed in infancy or childhood; as such, adult clinicians rarely see these patients. For this reason, this chapter discusses only the hereditary motor and sensory neuropathies that an adult clinician might encounter.

SYNONYMS

Charcot-Marie-Tooth (CMT) disease, a.k.a. hereditary motor-sensory neuropathy (HMSN)

Hereditary neuropathy with liability to pressure-sensitive palsies (HNPP)

ICD-9CM CODES

CMT: 356.1

HNPP: 689

ICD-10CM CODES

G60.0 Hereditary motor and sensory neuropathy

G60.8 Other hereditary and idiopathic neuropathies

G60.9 Hereditary and idiopathic neuropathy, unspecified

EPIDEMIOLOGY & DEMOGRAPHICS

All CMT: approximately 30 per 100,000

- CMT type 1 (demyelinating pathophysiology): 1 in 2500
- CMT type 2 (axonal pathophysiology): 7 in 1000
- CMT type 4 and CMT-X: rare (either axonal or demyelinating pathophysiology)

HNPP: 2 to 5 per 100,000

PHYSICAL FINDINGS & CLINICAL PRESENTATION

CMT: Highly variable

- Age at onset earlier for CMT-1 than CMT-2, but both may present from childhood to old age.
- Severely affected patients have severe distal weakness and muscle atrophy with hand (prominently affecting interossei) and foot deformities (pes cavus, high arched feet, hammer toes).
- Mildly affected patients may have only foot deformity (pes cavus) with little or no weakness/sensory loss.
- Legs can be affected greater than arms, and patients will complain of gait abnormalities (steppage), which cause them to trip and fall.
- Sensory complaints (paresthesias, numbness, dysesthesia) are uncommon despite physical findings of impaired sensation.
- Decreased or absent reflexes.
- Some patients may have postural tremor of the upper limbs.

HNPP (a.k.a. tomaculous neuropathy):

- Age at onset is commonly adolescence.
- Disorder is characterized by recurrent entrapment of peripheral nerves with accompanying signs and symptoms (paresthesias and/or weakness in anatomic distributions). Most common are:
  1. Median nerve at the wrist (carpal tunnel syndrome)
  2. Ulnar nerve at the elbow (cubital tunnel syndrome)
  3. Painless brachial plexopathies
  4. Lateral femoral cutaneous nerve (meralgia paresthetica)
  5. Peroneal nerve at the fibular head
- May be associated with a generalized polyneuropathy.

ETIOLOGY

CMT: more than 30 subgroups have been identified and have various chromosomal abnormalities.

- Most common mutation is PMP-22 duplication, giving rise to CMT 1A demyelinating phenotype.
- Other mutations include P0 (demyelinating) and neurofilament light chain mutations (demyelinating or axonal phenotype)—see the following.
- Updated information may be available at http://www.neuro.wustl.edu/neuromuscular.

HNPP: deletion of chromosome 17p11.2–12.

DIAGNOSIS

DIFFERENTIAL DIAGNOSIS

CMT: other genetic, metabolic, and multisystem disorders including:

- Spinocerebellar ataxias
- Friedreich's ataxia
- Leukodystrophies
- Refsum's disease (elevated serum phytanic acid)
- Distal spinal muscular atrophies and distal myopathies, which can present with pes cavus and other foot deformities
- Chronic inflammatory demyelinating polyneuropathy (CIDP)

HNPP:

- Hereditary neuralgic amyotrophy (HNA), which typically is painful rather than painless. In addition, in HNA, there is no evidence of generalized polyneuropathy.
- Multifocal motor neuropathy with conduction block (MMNCB)—autoimmune-mediated pure motor neuropathy
- Neuropathy associated with renal failure
- Lead neuropathy
- Neuropathy relating to paraproteinemia (demyelinating pathophysiology)

EVALUATION

CMT

- History of gradual onset symptoms is important to distinguish CMT from other forms of neuropathy.
- Detailed family history with *pedigree* is essential. Consider examination of multiple family members.
- History should evaluate for potential heavy metal exposure.
- History of dysesthesias is uncommon and should prompt search for acquired neuropathy or other inherited neuropathies (e.g., Fabry's disease).

HNPP: genetic testing after identification of multiple entrapment neuropathies on EMG and nerve conduction studies

LABORATORY TESTS

- Neurophysiology: electromyography (EMG) and nerve conduction studies (NCSs) must be done first to determine type of pathophysiology: demyelinating or axonal. This will guide genetic testing.
- NCSs in CMT-1 will reveal demyelinating physiology characterized by very slow conduction velocities (around 15 to 30 m/s) with prolonged distal latencies. Inherited demyelinating disorders can be distinguished from acquired demyelinating disorders (e.g., chronic inflammatory demyelinating polyneuropathy or CIDP) by the presence of conduction block in the latter.
- In HNPP, diffusely prolonged distal latencies with superimposed entrapment neuropathies at common sites will be seen on NCSs.
- EMG will reveal reinnervation characterized by long-duration, large-amplitude, polyphasic motor unit potentials (MUPs) with decreased MUP recruitment.
- Genetic tests are available for some CMT subtypes:
  1. CMT-1A: chromosome 17p11-PMP-22 duplication
  2. CMT-1B: chromosome 1q22-P0 mutation
  3. CMT-2E: chromosome 8p21-neurofilament light chain (NF-L) point mutation
  4. CMT-X: connexin 32 mutations
  5. HNPP: chromosome 17p11 deletion, which includes the PMP-22 gene
- Serum and 24-hour urine levels of heavy metals (arsenic, lead, etc.)
- SPEP, UPEP, immunofixation (for paraprotein).
- Anti-GM1 antibody (positive in ~50% of patients with MMNCB).
- Lumbar puncture may reveal elevated CSF protein in CIDP.
- Peripheral nerve biopsy:
  1. Demyelination with "onion bulb formation." Tomaculae, or focal thickening of myelin sheaths, seen in HNPP
  2. Generally not indicated unless diagnosis is uncertain

IMAGING STUDIES

- Spine plain films: for evaluation of scoliosis.
- MRI: indicated if dissociative sensory loss (dorsal column dysfunction with intact spinothalamic tract function) or if upper motor neuron findings (spasticity, Babinski's sign, clonus, increased tendon reflexes) are present.
- Exclusion of involvement of brain or spinal cord compressive lesions causing arm or leg weakness.

- Some inherited peripheral demyelinating disorders (i.e., CMT-X) are associated with intracerebral white matter abnormalities on MRI.
- Exclusion of structural, infectious, or inflammatory nerve root pathology.

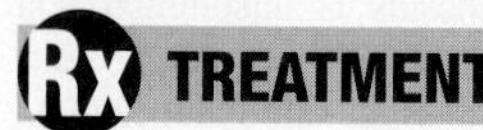

TREATMENT

There is no known cure for any of these disorders. Management is supportive.

NONPHARMACOLOGIC THERAPY

- Physical therapy (PT) and occupational therapy (OT) to provide assistance with gait and coordination.
- PT and OT might provide walking aid such as ankle foot orthosis (AFO), cane, walker, or wheelchair depending on the severity of the neuropathy.
- Wrist splints for superimposed carpal tunnel syndrome.
- Elbow pads (Heelbo Pads) to cushion the ulnar nerve at the elbow.
- Heel-cord strengthening.
- Stretching exercises.
- Analgesics for pain associated with foot deformity.
- Surgical correction of foot deformities by orthopedic surgeons if indicated.

Vincristine may worsen existing neuropathy (important for oncologist to know if patient develops cancer requiring chemotherapy).

SURGICAL TREATMENT

- Patients with HNPP should probably not undergo surgical decompression of the median nerve at the wrist or the ulnar nerve at the elbow; these nerves are sensitive to manipulation. Poor results have been reported with ulnar nerve transposition.
- Anesthesiologists should be aware of HNPP diagnosis in patients undergoing surgery to prevent compression neuropathies from occurring during surgical procedures.

GENETIC COUNSELING

Must be routinely done for patient and family when diagnosis is established. Many aspects of the patient and family's life are affected, including:

- Future progeny of patient and/or patient's parents or children
- Psychosocial aspects including social functioning, marriage, employment
- Financial needs
- Medical and life insurability

PROGNOSIS

- CMT: slowly progressive, and patients often remain ambulatory until late in life. Life expectancy is normal. Patients with respiratory involvement (i.e., phrenic nerve involvement with diaphragm paresis) may have shorter life expectancy.
- HNPP: benign prognosis.

DISPOSITION

Outpatient care. Routine follow-up appointments should be done initially every 6 mo, and then every 1 to 2 yr.

REFERRAL

- Neurology and/or neuromuscular disease specialist
- Podiatry for recurrent foot problems, including appropriate arches

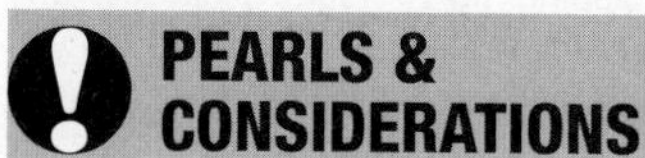

PEARLS & CONSIDERATIONS

PATIENT & FAMILY EDUCATION

Patients can benefit from use of Muscular Dystrophy Association (MDA) resources.

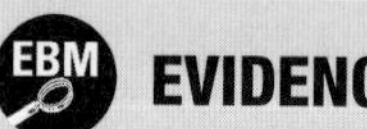

EVIDENCE

available at www.expertconsult.com

SUGGESTED READINGS

available at www.expertconsult.com

RELATED CONTENT

Fig. E1-590 Neuropathic pain, diagnostic approach (Algorithm)

Charcot-Marie-Tooth Disease (Related Key Topic)

AUTHOR: **GAVIN BROWN, M.D.**

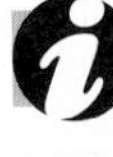

BASIC INFORMATION

DEFINITION

Nocardiosis is an infection caused by aerobic actinomycetes found in soil and characterized by lung, soft tissue, or central nervous system (CNS) involvement.

SYNONYMS

Mycetoma
Nocardia

ICD-9CM CODES
039 Actinomycotic infections
039.9 Nocardiosis NOS, of unspecified site
ICD-10CM CODES
A43.0 Pulmonary nocardiosis
A43.1 Cutaneous nocardiosis
A43.8 Other forms of nocardiosis
A43.9 Nocardiosis, unspecified
A42.9 Actinomycosis, unspecified

EPIDEMIOLOGY & DEMOGRAPHICS

- *Nocardia* species are found worldwide in the soil.
- Nocardiosis is found most commonly in patients who are immunocompromised (e.g., those receiving steroids or immunosuppressive therapy; those with lymphoma, leukemia, or lung cancer; transplant recipients; and those with pulmonary infections).
- Other underlying conditions associated with nocardiosis are pemphigus vulgaris, Whipple's disease, Goodpasture's syndrome, Cushing's disease, cirrhosis, ulcerative colitis, and rheumatoid arthritis.
- Use of steroids is an independent risk factor for developing nocardiosis.
- Between 500 and 1000 new cases are diagnosed each year in the U.S.
- Approximately 2% of patients with AIDS develop nocardiosis.
- Occurs more commonly in men than in women (2:1).
- Adults are affected more often than children.

PHYSICAL FINDINGS & CLINICAL PRESENTATION

- Inhalation of *Nocardia* organisms is the most common mode of entry, and pneumonia is the most common presentation, with 75% manifesting with fever, chills, dyspnea, and a productive cough (Fig. 1-660).
  1. Presentation can be acute, subacute, or chronic.
  2. Nocardiosis should be suspected if soft tissue abscesses or CNS tumors or abscesses form in conjunction with the pulmonary infection.
  3. Pulmonary infection may spread into the pericardium, mediastinum, and superior vena cava.
- Cutaneous disease usually occurs by direct inoculation of the organism as a result of skin puncture by a thorn or splinter, surgery, IV catheter use, or animal scratches or bites manifesting in:
  1. Cellulitis
  2. Lymphocutaneous nodules appearing along lymphatic sites draining the infected puncture wound
  3. Mycetoma (Madura foot), a chronic deep nodular infection usually involving the hands or feet that can cause skin breakdown or fistula formation and that spreads along the fascial planes to infect surrounding skin, subcutaneous tissue, and bone
- The CNS is infected in approximately one third of all cases. Brain abscess is the most common pathologic finding.
- Dissemination of nocardiosis may infect other tissues and organs, including the kidney, heart, skin, and bone.

ETIOLOGY

- The most common *Nocardia* species leading to infection in human beings are:
  1. *N. asteroides* (causing more than 80% of the cases of pulmonary nocardiosis)
  2. *N. brasiliensis* (most common cause of mycetoma)
  3. *N. otitidiscaviarum*
- *N. asteroides* has two subgroups:
  1. *N. farcinica*
  2. *N. nova*

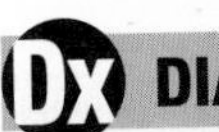

DIAGNOSIS

The diagnosis of nocardiosis requires a high index of suspicion in the proper clinical setting and is confirmed by bacteriologic staining and growth of the organism in culture.

DIFFERENTIAL DIAGNOSIS

There are no pathognomonic findings separating nocardiosis pneumonia from other infectious etiologies of the lung. Diagnoses presenting in a similar manner and often confused for nocardiosis include:

1. Tuberculosis
2. Lung abscess
3. Lung tumor
4. Other causes of pneumonia
5. Actinomycosis
6. Mycosis
7. Cellulitis
8. Coccidioidomycosis
9. Histoplasmosis
10. Aspergillosis
11. Kaposi's sarcoma

WORKUP

All patients with suspected nocardiosis need laboratory identification of the microorganism by obtaining sputum in the case of pneumonia, cultures of the infected skin lesions in mycetoma or lymphocutaneous disease, or the sampling of any purulent material (e.g., brain abscess, lung abscess, or pleural effusion).

LABORATORY TESTS

- Blood tests are not very sensitive in the diagnosis of nocardiosis.
- Gram stain shows gram-positive beaded filaments with multiple branches (Fig. 1-661).
- Gomori methenamine silver staining may detect the organism.
- *Nocardia* species are acid-fast on a modified Ziehl-Neelsen stain.
- *Nocardia* are slow-growing organisms; colony growth in cultures may take up to 2 to 3 wk.

IMAGING STUDIES

- Chest radiograph may demonstrate infiltrates, densities, nodules, cavitary masses, or multiple abscesses.

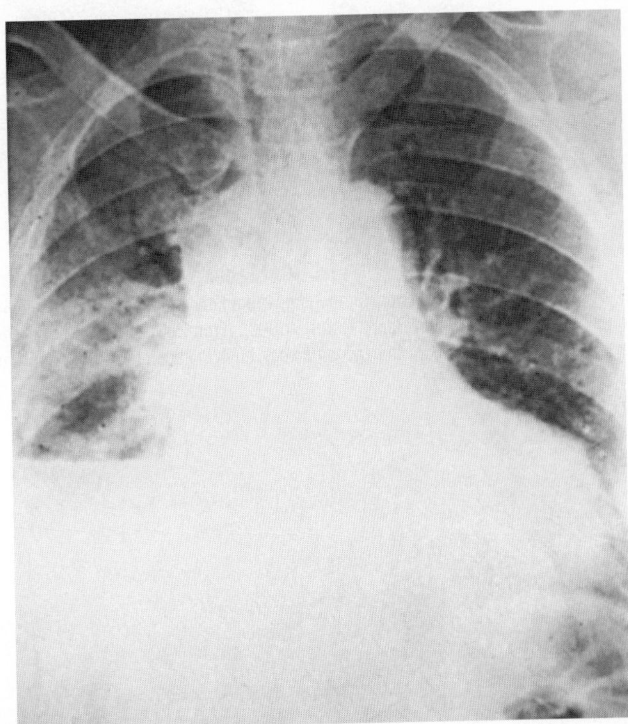

FIGURE 1-660 Right lower lobe *Nocardia* pneumonia in a kidney transplant recipient. (From Gorbach SL: *Infectious diseases,* ed 2, Philadelphia, 1998, Saunders.

- CT scan of the brain is indicated in the appropriate clinical setting to exclude CNS brain abscesses.

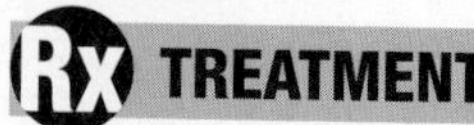

TREATMENT

NONPHARMACOLOGIC THERAPY

- Supportive therapy with oxygen in patients with pneumonia
- Chest physiotherapy
- For any abscess formation, surgical drainage is indicated (e.g., skin, lung, or brain)

ACUTE GENERAL Rx

- There are no prospective, randomized trials to date highlighting the most effective treatment of nocardiosis. Culture and sensitivity should always be done on the specimen.
- For cutaneous infection, trimethoprim-sulfamethoxazole (TMX-SMX) 5 mg/kg of the trimethoprim component divided in 2 doses
- *Nocardia* infection that does not involve CNS: TMX-SMX (15 mg/kg/day of TMP component IV in 2-4 divided doses) *plus* (amikacin 7.5 mg/kg q12h). An alternate regimen consists of imipenem 500 mg IV q6h *plus* amikacin 7.5 mg/kg IV q12h.
- In patients with CNS disease, (TMX-SMX 15 mg/kg/day of TMP component IV divided in 2-4 doses) *plus* imipenem 500 mg q6h IV. If multiorgan involvement, add amikacin 7.5 mg/kg q12h. Measure peak sulfonamide levels; target is 100-150 mcg/ml 2 hours post dose. An alterative regimen consists of linezolid 600 mg IV or PO q12h *plus* meropenem 2 g q8h.For infections without involvement of the CNS the patient can be switched to oral therapy after the initial IV therapy for 3-6 weeks or until clinical improvement. For infections involving CNS the initial IV therapy should be continued for minimum of 6 weeks and clear evidence of clinical improvement before switching to combination oral therapy.The combination oral antibiotics that can be used following initial IV therapy include:
- Sulfonamide-resistant disease: following two-drug regimens is recommended: imipenem (500 mg IV q6h), and amikacin (7.5 mg/kg IV q12h).
- Alternative drug treatment includes:
  1. Third-generation cephalosporin
  2. Minocycline 100 to 200 mg bid
  3. Extended-spectrum fluoroquinolones (moxifloxacin)
  4. Linezolid (use of linezolid >4 wk is associated with hematologic toxicity)
  5. Tigecycline
  6. Dapsone

CHRONIC Rx

- Although the optimal duration of therapy has not been determined, long-term therapy is generally recommended for all infections caused by *Nocardia.*
- Patients with cellulitis and lymphocutaneous syndrome are treated for 2 to 4 mo depending on whether there is bone involvement.
- Mycetomas are best treated with antibiotics for 6 to 12 mo but may require surgical drainage.
- Pulmonary and systemic nocardiosis excluding the CNS is treated for at least 6 mo in immunocompromised hosts.
- CNS involvement is treated with drainage and antibiotics for 12 mo.
- All immunosuppressed patients should receive 12 mo of antibiotic therapy.

DISPOSITION

- Patients with pulmonary nocardiosis have a mortality rate of 15% to 30%.
- CNS involvement carries a >40% mortality rate.
- Isolated skin lesions have a low mortality rate.

REFERRAL

Whenever the diagnosis of nocardiosis is suspected, consultation with infectious disease is indicated. Pulmonary evaluation and assistance may be needed in pulmonary nocardiosis. Neurosurgery consultation is indicated in patients with single or multiple brain abscesses.

PEARLS & CONSIDERATIONS

- Nocardiosis does not spread from animal to animal.
- Nocardiosis is not transmitted from person to person.
- Nocardiosis is distinguished by its ability to disseminate to any organ and its tendency to relapse despite appropriate antibiotic therapy.

COMMENTS

Tuberculosis and nocardiosis may coexist in the same patient.

SUGGESTED READINGS

available at www.expertconsult.com

RELATED CONTENT

Nocardiosis (Patient Information)

AUTHOR: **TANYA ALI, M.D.**

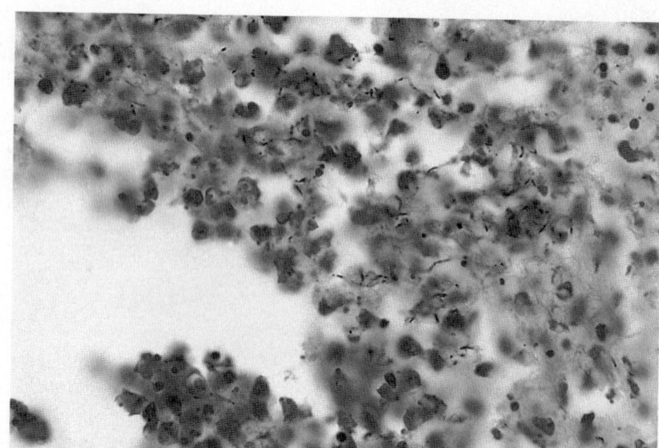

FIGURE 1-661 ***Nocardia* pneumonia.** Thin, branching, irregularly staining gram-positive bacilli course through necrotic pulmonary tissue (Brown-Hopps Gram, ×1000). (From Silverberg SG et al [eds]: *Silverberg's principles and practice of surgical pathology and cytopathology,* ed 4, Philadelphia, 2006, Churchill Livingstone.)

BASIC INFORMATION

DEFINITION

Nonalcoholic fatty liver disease (NAFLD) is a spectrum of diseases based on histiopathologic findings and representing a morphologic rather than a clinical diagnosis. It is liver disease occurring in patients who do not abuse alcohol and manifesting histologically by mononuclear cells and/or polymorphonuclear cells, hepatocyte ballooning, and spotty necrosis. Nonalcoholic steatohepatitis (NASH) is a subset of NAFLD. A diagnosis of NAFLD is contingent on the following factors:

1. Alcohol consumption in amounts less than those considered hepatotoxic
2. Absence of serologic evidence of other hepatic diseases or disorders
3. Liver biopsy showing predominant macrovesicular steatosis or steatohepatitis

SYNONYMS

Nonalcoholic steatohepatitis (NASH)
NAFLD
Fatty liver hepatitis
Diabetes hepatitis
Alcohol-like liver disease
Laënnec's disease

ICD-9CM CODES
571.8 Fatty liver
ICD-10CM CODES
K76.0 Fatty (change of) liver, not elsewhere classified

EPIDEMIOLOGY & DEMOGRAPHICS

- NAFLD affects 10% to 24% of the general population.
- Increased prevalence in obese persons (57% to 74%), type 2 diabetes mellitus, and hyperlipidemia (primarily hypertriglyceridemia)
- Most common cause of abnormal liver test results in adults in the United States (accounts for up to 90% of cases of asymptomatic ALT elevations)
- 30 million obese adults have steatosis; 8.6 million may have steatohepatitis.
- There is a 3:1 female-to-male predominance.

PHYSICAL FINDINGS & CLINICAL PRESENTATION

- Most patients are asymptomatic.
- Patients may report a sensation of fullness or discomfort on the right side of the upper abdomen.
- Nonspecific complaints of fatigue or malaise may be reported.
- Hepatomegaly is generally the only positive finding on physical examination.
- Acanthosis nigricans may be found in children.

ETIOLOGY

- Insulin resistance is the most reproducible factor in the development of NAFLD. High baseline and continuously increasing fasting insulin levels are independent determinants for future development of NFLD.
- Risk factors are obesity (especially truncal obesity), diabetes mellitus, hyperlipidemia.

DIAGNOSIS

DIFFERENTIAL DIAGNOSIS

- Alcohol-induced liver disease (a daily alcohol intake of 20 g in females and 30 g in males [three 12-oz beers or 12 oz of wine] may be enough to cause alcohol-induced liver disease)
- Viral hepatitis
- Autoimmune hepatitis
- Toxin- or drug-induced liver disease

WORKUP

Diagnosis is usually suspected on the basis of hepatomegaly, asymptomatic elevations of transaminases, or "fatty liver" on sonogram of abdomen in obese patients with little or no alcohol use. Liver biopsy will confirm diagnosis and provide prognostic information. It should be considered in patients with suspected advanced liver fibrosis (presence of obesity or type 2 diabetes, AST/ALT ratio 1, age 45 yr).

LABORATORY TESTS

- Elevated ALT, AST: AST/ALT ratio is usually <1, but can increase as fibrosis advances
- Negative serology for infectious hepatitis; generally normal GGTP and serum alkaline phosphatase
- Hyperlipidemia (primarily hypertriglyceridemia) may be present.
- Elevated glucose levels may be present.
- Prolonged prothrombin time, hypoalbuminuria, and elevated bilirubin may be present in advanced stages.
- Elevated serum ferritin and increased transferrin saturation may be found in up to 10% of patients; however, hepatic iron index and hepatic iron level are normal.
- Liver biopsy may show a wide spectrum of liver damage, ranging from simple steatosis to advanced fibrosis and cirrhosis.

IMAGING STUDIES

- Ultrasound generally reveals diffuse increase in echogenicity as compared with that of the kidneys; CT scan reveals diffuse low-density hepatic parenchyma.
- Occasionally patients may have focal rather than diffuse steatosis, which may be misinterpreted as a liver mass on ultrasound or CT; use of MRI in these cases will identify focal fatty infiltration.

TREATMENT

NONPHARMACOLOGIC THERAPY

- Weight reduction in all obese patients. The American Gastroenterological Association recommends that the initial target weight loss be 10% of baseline weight at a rate of 1 to 2 lb (0.45 to 0.90 kg) per week.
- Increase physical activity.
- Alcohol has a deleterious effect on NAFLD and should be avoided.

GENERAL Rx

- No medications have been proved to directly improve liver damage from NAFLD.
- Medications to control hyperlipidemia (e.g., fenofibrates for elevated triglycerides) and hyperglycemia (e.g., metformin) can lead to improvement in abnormal liver test results.
- Pioglitazone therapy (30 mg/day) and vitamin E (800 IU/day) provide modest benefits in NASH.

DISPOSITION

- Patients with pure steatosis on liver biopsy generally have a relatively benign course.
- The presence of steatohepatitis or advanced fibrosis on liver biopsy is associated with a worse prognosis.

REFERRAL

- Liver transplantation should be considered in patients with decompensated, end-stage disease; however, in these patients there may be a recurrence of NAFLD post transplantation.

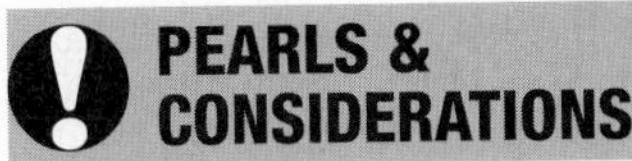

COMMENTS

- NAFLD is closely associated with metabolic disorders, even in nonobese, nondiabetic subjects. It can be considered an early predictor of metabolic disorders, particularly in the normal-weight population. The presence of metabolic syndrome is a strong predictor of NAFLD.
- NAFLD is associated with an increased risk of incident cardiovascular disease that is independent of the risk conferred by traditional risk factors and components of the metabolic syndrome.

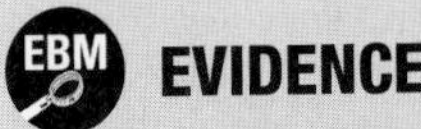

available at www.expertconsult.com

SUGGESTED READINGS

available at www.expertconsult.com

RELATED CONTENT

Fatty Liver (Patient Information)

AUTHOR: **FRED F. FERRI, M.D.**

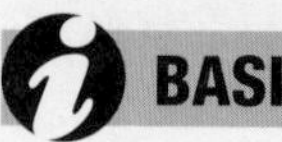

BASIC INFORMATION

DEFINITION

Obesity refers to having an excess amount of body fat in relation to lean body mass, or a body mass index (BMI) of ≥30 kg/m^2. Overweight is defined as BMI of 25 to 29.9 kg/m^2 and morbid obesity refers to adults with a BMI ≥40 kg/m^2. BMI is used as a surrogate measure of obesity. These conditions result from an imbalance between energy intake and expenditure.

ICD-9CM CODES
278.0 Obesity
ICD-10CM CODES
E66.9 Obesity, unspecified

EPIDEMIOLOGY & DEMOGRAPHICS

- The World Health Organization first recognized obesity as a worldwide epidemic in 1997. As of 2005, 1.6 billion adults worldwide were classified as overweight, 400 million of whom were obese. It is predicted that the combination of overweight and obesity will soon eclipse public health issues such as malnutrition and infectious diseases as the most significant cause of poor health.
- Based on U.S. National Health and Nutrition Examination (NHANES) data from 2009-2010, the prevalence of obesity in the U.S. was 35.7%. By 2015, it is estimated that two in every five adults and one in every four children in the U.S. will be obese.
- The present cost of obesity in the U.S. population is estimated at $100 billion annually.
- For persons with a BMI ≥30 kg/m^2, all-cause mortality is increased by 50% to 100% above that of persons with BMI in the range of 20 to 25 kg/m^2.
- Obesity is an independent risk factor for cardiovascular disease (CVD) and CVD risks associated with obesity have also been documented in children.
- Obese individuals are at increased risk of morbidity and death from type 2 diabetes, hypertension, coronary heart disease (CHD), cancer (particularly colon, prostate, and breast cancer), sleep apnea, degenerative joint disease, thromboembolic disorders, digestive tract diseases (gallstones), and dermatologic disorders.
- Significant morbidity and risk of death are projected to begin in young adulthood, resulting in more than 100,000 excess cases of CHD by 2035, even with the most modest projection of future obesity.
- When children enter kindergarten, 12.4% are obese, and another 14.9% are overweight. Data show that incident obesity between the ages of 5 and 14 years is more likely to have occurred at younger ages.[1]
- Obesity in adolescence is significantly associated with increased risk of incident severe obesity in adulthood, with variations by sex and race/ethnicity. Overweight or obese adults who were obese as children have increased risk of type 2 DM, dyslipidemia, hypertension, and carotid artery atherosclerosis.
- Obesity is a major preventable cause of death and disability in the United States (the other is tobacco).
- Extensive data indicate that weight loss can reverse or arrest the harmful effects of obesity.

PHYSICAL FINDINGS & CLINICAL PRESENTATION

- Physical examination should assess the degree and distribution of body fat and signs of secondary causes of obesity.
- Increased waist circumference is apparent. Excess abdominal fat is clinically defined as a waist circumference >40 inches (>102 cm) in men and >35 inches (>88 cm) in women (in Asian men and women, >36 inches and >33 inches, respectively).
- Symptoms associated with hypertension, coronary artery disease (CAD), and diabetes (e.g., polyuria, polydipsia, acanthosis nigricans, retinopathy, and neuropathy) may be present.
- Obesity is associated with cardiac hypertrophy, diastolic dysfunction, and decreased aortic compliance, which are independent predictors of cardiovascular risk.
- Joint pain and swelling are associated with degenerative joint disease secondary to obesity.
- The physical exam and ECG often underestimate the presence and extent of cardiac dysfunction in obese patients. Jugular venous distention and hepatojugular reflux may not be seen and heart sounds are frequently distant. Obesity is associated with changes in the ECG, including a reduction in voltage and nonspecific ST-T changes that may interfere with diagnosis of left ventricular hypertrophy (LVH) or CAD.
- A large quantity of fluid is present in the interstitial space of adipose tissue, as the interstitial space is ~10% of the tissue wet weight. This excess fluid in this compartment if redistributed into the circulation, can have negative repercussions in obese individuals with heart failure. Obese individuals have higher cardiac output and a lower total peripheral resistance than do lean individuals, and obesity is associated with persistence of elevated cardiac filling pressure during exercise.
- Obesity predisposes to heart failure through several different mechanisms: increased total blood volume, increased cardiac output, LVH, left ventricular diastolic dysfunction, and adipositas cordis (excessive epicardial fat and fatty infiltration of the myocardium).

ETIOLOGY

- The pathophysiology of obesity is complex and poorly understood, but includes social, nutritional, physiologic, psychological, and genetic factors.
- Environmental factors such as a sedentary lifestyle and chronic ingestion of excess calories can cause obesity.
- Obesity may be related to genetic factors, which are thought to be polygenic. Genetic studies with adopted children have demonstrated that they have similar BMIs to their biologic parents but not their adoptive parents. Twin studies also demonstrate a genetic influence on BMI.

Dx DIAGNOSIS

- BMI will establish the diagnosis of obesity. BMI is a measure of an adult's weight in relation to his or her height—more specifically, the adult's weight in kilograms divided by the square of his or her height—and is closely correlated with total body fat content.
- BMI values can categorize patients into three classes of obesity:
  - Class I (mild): BMI of 30.0 to 34.9 kg/m^2
  - Class II (moderate): BMI of 35.0 to 39.9 kg/m^2
  - Class III (severe): BMI of ≥40 kg/m^2
- Although BMI is commonly used to define obesity, it is not a highly accurate indicator of body fat composition in children, who are undergoing rapid changes in height, or in bodybuilders or athletes who have large amounts of muscle tissue.
- Waist circumference or waist-hip ratio is indicative of visceral adipose tissue/intraabdominal fat, which may be more deleterious than overall overweight or obesity.

DIFFERENTIAL DIAGNOSIS

It is important to evaluate obese patients for secondary medical causes of obesity. Hypothalamic disorders, hypothyroidism, Cushing's syndrome, insulinoma, depression, and drugs (corticosteroids, antidepressants, second-generation antipsychotics, and HIV protease inhibitors) can cause obesity. In children, certain genetic conditions, such as Prader-Willi syndrome, are associated with obesity.

WORKUP

History should be obtained regarding weight change, family history of obesity, and eating and exercise behavior. Assessment for eating disorders and depression should be made. Attention should be directed to the use of nutritional supplements, over-the-counter medications, hormones, diuretics, and laxatives. The workup of an obese patient typically requires laboratory work to assess for risks and complications as well as to rule out underlying causative medical conditions. Fig. E1-662 describes the evaluation of patients with suspected endocrine cause of obesity.

LABORATORY TESTS

- Obese patients should be assessed for medical consequences of their obesity by screening for metabolic syndrome. This includes measurement of fasting lipid profile, blood pressure, and waist circumference, and screening for diabetes or prediabetes (oral glucose tolerance test, fasting glucose, or hemoglobin A1C).

---

[1]Cunningham SA et al: Incidence of childhood obesity in the United States, *N Engl J Med,* 370:403-411, 2014.

- In the proper clinical setting, thyroid function studies and dexamethasone suppression testing will exclude hypothyroidism and Cushing's syndrome as underlying causes of obesity. If insulinoma is suspected, the patient will need to undergo a 72-hour fast to confirm hypoglycemia with inappropriate insulin secretion.

IMAGING STUDIES

- Several methods are available for determining or calculating total body fat but offer no significant advantage over the BMI. These include measurement of total body water, total body potassium, bioelectrical impedance, and dual-energy x-ray absorptiometry.
- Buoyancy testing is an accurate method for determining total body fat composition.

OTHER STUDIES

Obesity increases the risk of obstructive sleep apnea, which, in turn, increases the risks of hypertension, cardiac arrhythmias, CVD, stroke, and heart failure. Therefore one should have a low threshold to screen obese patients for obstructive sleep apnea via sleep study/polysomnography.

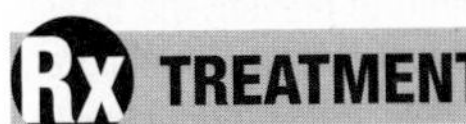

TREATMENT

The National Heart, Lung, and Blood Institute (NHLBI) developed guidelines for selecting treatment strategies for overweight and obese patients based on BMI and comorbidities. They recommend a combination of dietary management, physical activity management, and behavior therapy for anyone with a BMI ≥25 or with a high-risk waist circumference and two or more obesity-associated comorbidities. Pharmacotherapy should be considered for patients with a BMI ≥30 or ≥27 with comorbidities.

Surgery is indicated for patients with a BMI ≥35 with comorbidities and for any patient with a BMI ≥40 (Table 1-365).

NONPHARMACOLOGIC THERAPY

- The cornerstones for weight management and reduction are calorie restriction, exercise, and behavioral modification.
- The NHLBI guidelines recommend an initial diet to produce a calorie deficit of 500 to 1000 kcal/day. This has been shown to reduce total body weight by an average of 8% over 3 to 12 mo.
- These guidelines recommend the use of a food diary to focus on dietary substitutes.
- Thirty minutes of moderate-intensity activity on 5 or more days of the week results in health benefits for obese individuals. Moreover, several studies indicate that 60 to 80 min of moderate to vigorous physical activity may provide additional benefit.
- Increased physical activity without caloric restriction (minimal or no weight loss) can reduce abdominal (visceral) adipose tissue and improve insulin resistance.
- The key features of the standard behavioral modification program include goal setting, self-monitoring, stimulus control (modification of one's environment to enhance behaviors that will support weight management), cognitive restructuring (increased awareness of perceptions of oneself and one's weight), and prevention of relapse (weight regain).
- Mammalian sleep is closely integrated with the regulation of energy balance. Trials have shown that the amount of human sleep contributes to the maintenance of fat-free body mass at times of decreased energy intake. Lack of sufficient sleep may compromise the efficacy of typical dietary interventions for weight loss and related metabolic risk reduction.

TABLE 1-365 Weight-Loss Treatment Guidelines from the National Heart, Lung, and Blood Institute*

	BMI				
Treatment	**25.0-26.9**	**27.0-29.9**	**30.0-34.9**	**35.0-39.9**	**>40.0**
Diet, physical activity, behavioral therapy, or all three	Yes	Yes	Yes	Yes	Yes
Pharmacotherapy†		In patients with obesity-related diseases	Yes	Yes	Yes
Surgery‡				In patients with obesity-related diseases	Yes

*Data are from www.nhlbi.nih.gov/guidelines/obesity/ob_home.htm. These guidelines are generally consistent with those from the American Heart Association, the American Medical Association, the American Diabetic Association, the Obesity Society (Practical Guide), the American Diabetes Association, the American Academy of Family Physicians, the American College of Sports Medicine, and the American Cancer Society. *BMI* denotes body mass index, calculated as the weight in kilograms divided by the square of the height in meters.

†Pharmacotherapy should be considered only in patients who are not able to achieve adequate weight loss with available conventional lifestyle modifications and who have no absolute contraindications for drug therapy.

‡Bariatric surgery should be considered only in patients who are unable to lose weight with available conventional therapy and who have no absolute contraindications for surgery.

ACUTE GENERAL Rx

- According to the NHLBI *Guidelines on the Identification, Evaluation, and Treatment of Overweight and Obesity in Adults* and the U.S. Food and Drug Administration (FDA), pharmacotherapy is indicated for:
  - Obese patients with a BMI ≥30
  - Overweight patients with a BMI of ≥27 and concomitant obesity-related risk factors or diseases, such as hypertension, diabetes, or dyslipidemia
- Pharmacologic treatment options include:
  - Gastrointestinal lipase inhibitors: Orlistat is the only drug available for long-term treatment of obesity. It blocks the digestion and absorption of ingested dietary fat. It is a reversible inhibitor of pancreatic, gastric, and carboxyl ester lipases and phospholipase A2, which are required for the hydrolysis of dietary fat in the gastrointestinal tract. Side effects include flatulence, fecal incontinence, cramps, and oily spotting. There can also be impairment of absorption of vitamin A, E, and beta-carotene. Oxalate-associated acute kidney injury and rare severe liver injury have also been reported.
  - C Serotonin agonists: Lorcaserin is a selective serotonin agonist that acts centrally to reduce appetite, aiding weight loss. Adverse effects include headache, upper respiratory infections, dizziness, and nausea. While there is little evidence of serotonin-associated cardiac valvular disease (as seen with nonselective serotonergic agonists fenfluramine and dexfenfluramine), long-term data is currently limited.
  - Sympathomimetic medications: Phentermine and diethylpropion are currently approved for short-term treatment of obesity. They reduce food intake by causing early satiety. Side effects include increased blood pressure and increased pulse. They are Schedule IV drugs with a potential for abuse. Other sympathomimetic drugs that have been removed from the market due to concerns about cardiovascular safety are sibutramine, phenylpropanolamine, and ephedrine.
  - Antidepressants: While not FDA-approved for treatment of obesity alone, bupropion and fluoxetine are antidepressants that have been associated with modest weight loss.
  - Antiepileptic drugs: Zonisamide and topiramate (also used in migraine therapy) have been associated with weight loss in clinical trials but are not currently FDA-approved for treatment of obesity alone.
  - Diabetes drugs: While not FDA-approved for treatment of obesity alone, metformin, pramlintide (synthetic human amylin), and glucagon-like polypeptide-1 agonists (exenatide, liraglutide) have been associated with weight loss in the treatment of individuals with diabetes. Weight loss was also reported in a trial of liraglutide in patients without diabetes.

CHRONIC Rx

- According to the NHLBI guidelines, surgical intervention is an option for selected patients with clinically severe obesity (a BMI ≥40 or a BMI ≥35 with comorbid conditions), when patients are at high risk for obesity-associated morbidity or death, and when less invasive methods of weight loss have failed.
- Bariatric surgery for weight loss falls into one of three general categories:
  - Restrictive surgeries limit the amount of food the stomach can hold and slow the rate of gastric emptying. These include vertical banded gastroplasty and laparoscopic adjustable silicone gastric banding LAGB [Fig. E1-663]). Band slippage is the most common LAGB complication. Gastric necrosis of the stomach wall is a rarer late complication that results from ischemia caused by a combination of gastric prolapse—the part of the stomach below the band herniates up through the device (Fig. E1-664)—pressure from the band.
  - Malabsorptive surgeries reduce nutrient absorption by shortening length of small intestine. These include jejunoileal bypass and the duodenal switch operation (DS).
  - Restrictive malabsorptive bypass procedures combine the elements of gastric restriction and selective malabsorption. These include Roux-en-Y gastric bypass (considered the gold standard because of its high level of effectiveness and durability) and biliopancreatic diversion.
- Compared with usual care, bariatric surgery is associated with reduced number of cardiovascular deaths and lower incidence of cardiovascular events in obese adults. A study on bariatric surgery patients demonstrated a significant reduction in long-term cardiovascular events. Ten-year follow-up estimated relative risk reductions ranging from 18% to 79% according to the Framingham risk score and 8% to 62% with the PROCAM risk score.
- Liposuction is removal of fat by aspiration after injection of physiologic saline. This technique reduces the subcutaneous fat but has failed to improve insulin sensitivity or risk factors for CHD.

DISPOSITION

- The incidence of venous thromboembolism in the upper tertile of BMI was 2.42 times that of the lowest BMI tertile. Obese patients have a higher incidence of postoperative thromboembolic events when undergoing noncardiac surgery.
- Perioperative obesity (>140% ideal body weight) may increase morbidity and mortality rates after heart transplantation.
- Weight stable obese subjects have an increased risk of arrhythmias and sudden death even in the absence of cardiac dysfunction.
- Obesity and the cardiac autonomic nervous system are intrinsically related. A 10% increase in body weight is associated with a decline in parasympathetic tone accompanied by a rise in mean heart rate. Conversely, a 10% weight loss in severely obese patients is associated with significant improvement in autonomic nervous system cardiac modulation, including decreased heart rate and increased heart rate variability.
- Postmortem Determinants of Atherosclerosis in Youth (PDAY) study data provided convincing evidence that obesity in adolescents and young adults accelerates the progression of atherosclerosis decades before the appearance of clinical manifestations.
- Obesity accelerates the progression of native coronary atherosclerosis and after coronary artery bypass grafting.
- In older adults, obesity is associated with protection against hip fracture, but this protective effect on bone status does not offset the extensive array of potential adverse effects on conditions common in the older population.

REFERRAL

- Obesity is commonly seen in the primary care setting. If pharmacologic therapy is considered, consultation with physicians specializing in obesity and experienced with the use of the drug is recommended. In addition, consultation with nutritionists and behavioral therapists is helpful. A consultation with general surgery is indicated in patients being considered for surgical intervention.
- Recent trials have shown that among adolescents, use of gastric banding compared with lifestyle intervention results in a greater percentage achieving a loss of 50% of excess weight corrected for age. There were associated benefits to health and quality of life.

PEARLS & CONSIDERATIONS

COMMENTS

- Enhanced weight-loss counseling helps about one third of obese patients achieve long-term, clinically meaningful weight loss.
- The NHLBI launched the Obesity Education Initiative in January 1991. The overall purpose of the initiative is to help reduce the prevalence of overweight along with the prevalence of physical inactivity to reduce the risk of CHD and overall morbidity and mortality rates from CHD.
- The American Medical Association, in association with the Robert Wood Johnson Foundation and the U.S. Department of Health and Human Services, produced a primer for the assessment and management of adult obesity. The primer consists of 10 booklets that offer practical recommendations for addressing adult obesity in the primary care setting and is available for free at: http://www.ama-assn.org/ama/pub/physician-resources.
- Recent research indicates that brown adipose tissue represents a natural target for the modulation of energy expenditure. The presence of brown adipose tissue in humans may be quantified with the use of ^{18}F-FDG PET-CT. The amount of brown adipose tissue is inversely correlated with BMI, suggesting a potential role of brown adipose tissue in adult human metabolism.
- Obesity, glucose intolerance, and hypertension in childhood are strongly associated with increased rates of premature death from endogenous causes in this population.
- Recent trials have shown that among persons living in a controlled setting, calories alone account for the increase in fat. Protein affected energy expenditure and storage of lean body mass, but not body fat storage.

PREVENTION

- Prevention of overweight and obesity involves both increasing physical activity and dietary modification to reduce caloric intake.
- There is compelling evidence that prevention of weight regain in formerly obese individuals requires 60 to 90 min of moderate intensity activity or lesser amounts of vigorous intensity activity.
- Moderate intensity activity of approximately 45 to 60 min per day, or 1.7 physical activity level (PAL), is required to prevent the transition to overweight or obesity. For children, even more activity time is recommended.
- Clinicians can help guide patients to develop personalized eating plans and help them recognize the contributions of fat, concentrated carbohydrates, and large portion sizes.
- Clinicians must work with patients to modify other risk factors such as tobacco use, high glycemic intake, and elevated blood pressure to prevent the long-term chronic disease sequelae of obesity.
- Regular screening of body weight and BMI measurements at routine office visits can help identify early weight gain.

PATIENT & FAMILY EDUCATION

Information can be obtained on the American Obesity Association website (http://www.obesity.org) and the American Medical Association website (http://www.ama-assn.org).

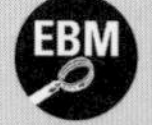

EVIDENCE

available at www.expertconsult.com

SUGGESTED READINGS

available at www.expertconsult.com

RELATED CONTENT

Fig. 3-203 Weight gain (Algorithm)
Obesity, Female (Patient Information)
Obesity, Male (Patient Information)

AUTHORS: **HILARY B. WHITLACH, M.D., SAINATH GADDAM, M.D.,** and **FRED F. FERRI, M.D.**

BASIC INFORMATION

DEFINITION

Obsessive-compulsive disorder (OCD) is characterized by obsessions (recurrent and persistent thoughts, urges, or images experienced as intrusive and unwanted) and/or compulsions (repetitive behaviors or mental acts performed in response to obsessions, or according to rules that must be applied rigidly) that are time-consuming (e.g., >1 hr/day) or cause marked impairment or distress. The symptoms are usually perceived as excessive and unreasonable.

SYNONYMS

OCD

ICD-9CM and DSM-5 CODES
300.3
ICD-10CM CODES
F42 Obsessive-compulsive disorder

EPIDEMIOLOGY & DEMOGRAPHICS

PEAK INCIDENCE: Mean age at onset is 19.6 yr.
12-MONTH PREVALENCE: 1.2% of adults in U.S., international prevalence estimates are similar (1.1%-1.8%)
PREDOMINANT SEX: Approximately equal distribution between sexes
PREDOMINANT AGE:

- Modal age of onset for females is between 20 and 29 yr.
- Modal age of onset for males is between 6 and 15 yr.

DISEASE COURSE:

- Condition is chronic with waxing and waning pattern.
- Symptoms typically worsen with stress.
- 15% show progressive deterioration, whereas 5% show an episodic course with little impairment between episodes.

GENETICS:

- There is no clear genetic pattern.
- Rate of concordance is higher in monozygotic (57%) compared with dizygotic (27%) twins.
- Rate of disorder is also much higher in first-degree relatives of individuals with OCD and Tourette's disorder than in the general population.

PHYSICAL FINDINGS & CLINICAL PRESENTATION

- Persistent and recurrent intrusive and egodystonic obsessive ideas, thoughts, urges, or images that are perceived as alien and beyond one's control.
- Frequent experiencing of obsessions related to contamination (e.g., when using the telephone), excessive doubt (e.g., was the door locked?), organization (the need for a particular order), violent impulses (e.g., to yell obscenities in church), or intrusive sexual imagery.
- Compulsive behaviors (e.g., repeated hand washing, checking, rearranging) or mental rituals (e.g., counting, repeating phrases) meant to temporarily ameliorate anxiety caused by obsessions.
- Obsessions and compulsions almost always accompanied by high anxiety and subjective distress. Both are usually seen as excessive and unreasonable.

ETIOLOGY

- Strong evidence of neurobiologic etiology.
- OCD onset may be temporally associated with infectious illness of CNS (e.g., Von Economo's encephalitis, Sydenham's chorea).
- OCD may follow head trauma or other premorbid neurologic condition, including birth hypoxia and Tourette's syndrome.
- Serotonergic pathways believed important in some ritualistic instinctual behaviors, with dysfunction of these pathways possibly giving rise to OCD.

DIAGNOSIS

DIFFERENTIAL DIAGNOSIS

- Obsessive-compulsive personality disorder (OCPD) is a maladaptive personality style defined by excessive rigidity, need for order and control, preoccupation with details, and excessive perfectionism. Unlike OCD, OCPD is ego-syntonic.
- Other psychiatric disorders in which obsessive or intrusive thoughts occur (e.g., body dysmorphic disorder, eating disorders, hypochondriasis, phobias, posttraumatic stress disorder).
- Impulse control disorders (e.g., trichotillomania [hair-pulling disorder], excoriation (skin-picking) disorder, pathologic gambling disorder, compulsive shopping, kleptomania, paraphilias/sexual compulsions).
- Neurologic disorders with repetitive behaviors (e.g., Tourette's syndrome, Sydenham's chorea, torticollis, autism).
- Delusions or psychosis, which may be mistaken for obsessive thoughts; unlike OCD, these individuals do not believe their obsessions are unreal and may likely meet criteria for another psychotic spectrum disorder that fully accounts for the obsessions (e.g., schizophrenia).

WORKUP

- Careful history leading to diagnosis
- Neurologic examination to rule out concomitant Tourette's or other tic disorder
- In adolescents and children: psychological testing to reveal learning disabilities

TREATMENT

NONPHARMACOLOGIC THERAPY

- Treatment will help ~50% of patients achieve partial remission within the first 6 mo.
- Cognitive-behavioral therapy (CBT), especially exposure/response prevention, is successful in up to 70% of patients, but nearly 25% drop out of treatment because of the initial anxiety the exposures create. Best results are found for contamination obsessions and washing compulsions.

GENERAL Rx

- Antidepressants with serotonin reuptake blockade, including clomipramine, fluvoxamine, fluoxetine, paroxetine, sertraline, citalopram and escitalopram, venlafaxine, and duloxetine; optimal dosages are typically at the high end of the prescription range. Risk/benefit/alternatives discussion is crucial (e.g., dose-related risk of QT interval prolongation with clomipramine and citalopram).
- Clonazepam may be helpful in patients with extreme anxiety.
- Most improve with treatment, but few become symptom-free. No response in 15% of patients.
- Likely indefinite treatment. Relapse is common if medications are discontinued.
- Recent studies suggest that combination CBT and pharmacotherapy yields superior outcomes. More severe symptoms warrant combination therapy.
- Patients who do not respond to first-line treatments and those with comorbid psychosis and/or tic disorders may benefit from augmentation with a first- or second-generation antipsychotic medication (e.g., haloperidol, olanzapine, risperidone).
- Surgical intervention (e.g., cingulotomy, deep brain stimulation) is an option for the most extreme, refractory cases.

DISPOSITION

- Most mild to moderate cases can be managed on a regular outpatient basis. Treatment should typically start with SSRI monotherapy with regular follow-up to assess treatment response and side-effect management. Dose should be increased to maximum tolerated.
- Patient and family education may help improve medical adherence and support.

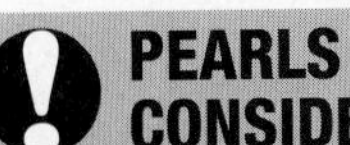

PEARLS & CONSIDERATIONS

Patients with OCD typically have insight regarding the irrationality of their obsessions and compulsions but lack the ability to control them. This may cause intense shame and avoidance of medical care unless patient education and support are provided. Screen for OCD, especially among patients who present with "depression" or "anxiety."

SUGGESTED READINGS

available at www.expertconsult.com

RELATED CONTENT

Obsessive-Compulsive Disorder (OCD) (Patient Information)

AUTHORS: **AGUSTIN G. YIP, M.D., PH.D.,** and **JASON M. SATTERFIELD, PH.D.**

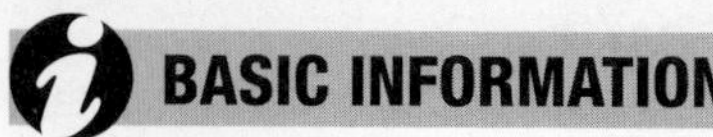

BASIC INFORMATION

DEFINITION

The term *ocular foreign body* refers to a foreign body on the surface of the corneal epithelium.

ICD-9CM CODES
930 Foreign body in external eye
ICD-10CM CODES
T15 Foreign body on external eye
T15.0 Foreign body in cornea
T15.1 Foreign body in conjunctival sac
T15.8 Foreign body in other and multiple parts of external eye
T15.9 Foreign body on external eye, part unspecified

EPIDEMIOLOGY & DEMOGRAPHICS

INCIDENCE (IN U.S.): Universal, with a predominance in active people

PEAK INCIDENCE: Childhood through active adult years

PREDOMINANT SEX: Perhaps slightly more common in men

PREDOMINANT AGE: Childhood through active adult years

PHYSICAL FINDINGS & CLINICAL PRESENTATION

- Pain is most common symptom.
- Causes of most common foreign bodies:
  - Grinding (Fig. 1-665)
  - Drilling
  - Auto repair
  - Working beneath cars
  - Airborne particles, such as blown by fans

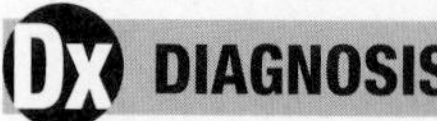

DIAGNOSIS

DIFFERENTIAL DIAGNOSIS

- History of corneal foreign body seen
- Hemorrhage, loss of vision
- Distorted anterior chamber, soft eye
- Corneal abrasion
- Corneal ulceration or laceration
- Glaucoma
- Herpes ulcers
- Infection
- Other keratitis
- Intraocular foreign body

WORKUP

- Fluorescein stain, slit-lamp examination if no foreign body is found
- Ultrasound examination
- Plain radiographs

LABORATORY TESTS

Intraocular pressure to make certain that eye has not been penetrated

IMAGING STUDIES

Occasionally, MRI of the orbits to identify foreign bodies not found by other means. Do not perform MRI if suspect metallic foreign body. Plain radiographs and ultrasound are sufficient.

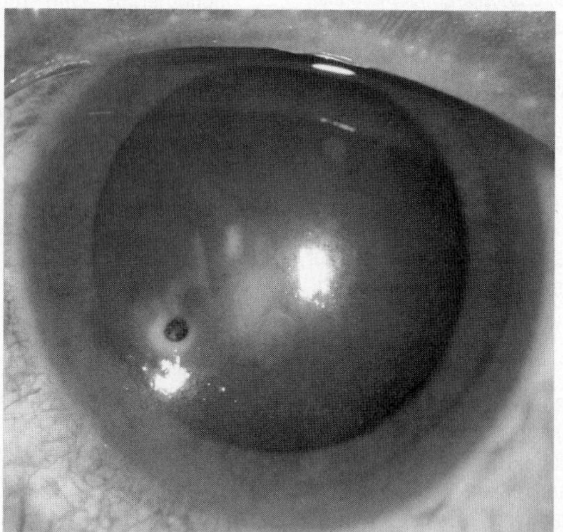

FIGURE 1-665 A small iron foreign body may be seen on external examination. (Courtesy Department of Dermatology, University of North Carolina at Chapel Hill. In Goldstein GB, Goldstein AO: *Practical dermatology,* ed 2, St Louis, 1997, Mosby.)

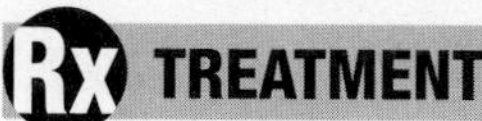

TREATMENT

NONPHARMACOLOGIC THERAPY

- Remove foreign body
- Treat infection
- Repair eye if ruptured
- Treat corneal abrasion or injury

ACUTE GENERAL Rx

- Saline irrigation
- Removal of foreign body with moist cotton-tipped applicator after instillation of topical anesthetic drops
- Use burr or more aggressive treatment if needed
- Cycloplegics, antibiotics, and pressure dressing after removal of foreign body
- Repair corneal laceration or damaged eye

DISPOSITION

If symptoms persist 24 hr after examination, refer to an ophthalmologist.

REFERRAL

To ophthalmology within 24 hr if patient not completely comfortable

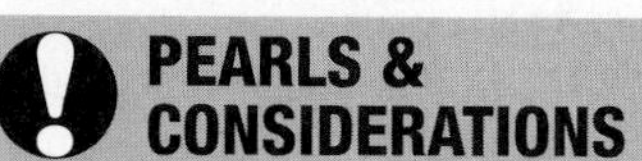

PEARLS & CONSIDERATIONS

COMMENTS

- Make sure foreign body is not intraocular (inside eye).
- Alkaline or acidic chemical foreign bodies can be dangerous; pH test must be performed if either of these is suspected (for all chemical foreign bodies).

SUGGESTED READINGS

available at www.expertconsult.com

RELATED CONTENT

Corneal Foreign Body (Patient Information)

AUTHORS: **MELVYN KOBY, M.D.**, and
R. SCOTT HOFFMAN, M.D.

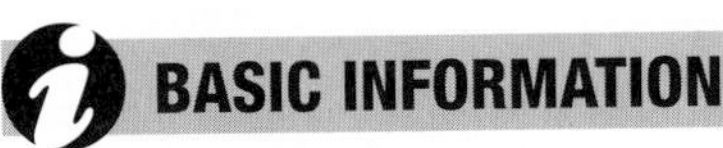

BASIC INFORMATION

DEFINITION

Onychomycosis is defined as a persistent fungal infection affecting the toenails and fingernails.

SYNONYMS

Tinea unguium
Ringworm of the nails

ICD-9CM CODES
110.1 Onychomycosis
ICD-10CM CODES
B35.1 Tinea unguium

EPIDEMIOLOGY & DEMOGRAPHICS

- Onychomycosis is most commonly found in people between the ages of 40 and 60 yr.
- Onychomycosis rarely occurs before puberty.
- Incidence: 20 to 100 cases/1000 population.
- Toenail infection is 4 to 6 times more common than fingernail infection.

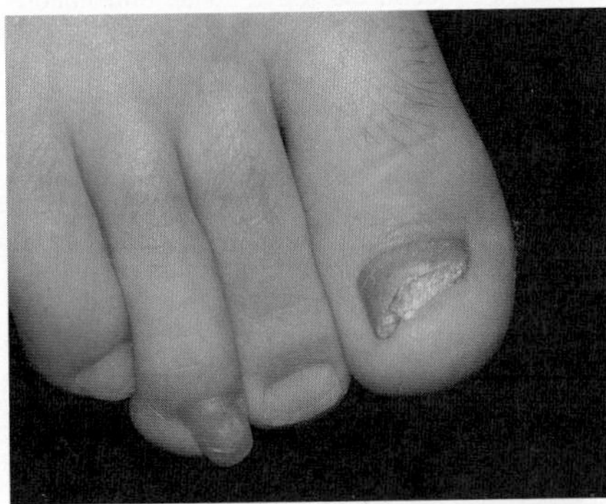

FIGURE 1-666 Distal subungual onychomycosis in a 5-year-old. Note how heavily infected nails occur adjacent to totally normal nails. Cutting back the big toe's nail plate has revealed the friable subungual debris. This material is the most desirable for culture. (From White GM, Cox NH [eds]: *Diseases of the skin, a color atlas and text,* ed 2, St Louis, 2006, Mosby.)

- Onychomycosis affects men more often than women.
- Occurs more frequently in patients with diabetes, peripheral vascular disease, and any conditions resulting in the suppression of the immune system.
- Occlusive footwear, physical exercise followed by communal showering, and incompletely drying the feet predispose the individual to developing onychomycosis.

PHYSICAL FINDINGS & CLINICAL PRESENTATION

- Onychomycosis causes nails to become thick, brittle, hard, distorted, and discolored (yellow to brown color) (Fig. 1-666). Eventually, the nail may loosen, separate from the nail bed, and fall off (Fig. 1-667).
- Onychomycosis is frequently associated with tinea pedis (athlete's foot).

ETIOLOGY

- The most common causes of onychomycosis are dermatophyte, yeast, and nondermatophyte molds.
- The dermatophyte *Trichophyton rubrum* accounts for 80% of all nail infections caused by fungus.
- *Trichophyton interdigitale* and *Trichophyton mentagrophytes* are other fungi causing onychomycosis.
- The yeast *Candida albicans* is responsible for 5% of the cases of onychomycosis and tends to involve fingernails more than toenails.
- Nondermatophyte molds *Scopulariopsis brevicaulis* and *Aspergillus niger,* although rare, can also cause onychomycosis.
- Onychomycosis is classified according to the clinical pattern of nail bed involvement. The main types are:
  1. Distal and lateral subungual onychomycosis (DLSO)
  2. Superficial onychomycosis
  3. Proximal subungual onychomycosis
  4. Endonyx onychomycosis
  5. Total dystrophic onychomycosis

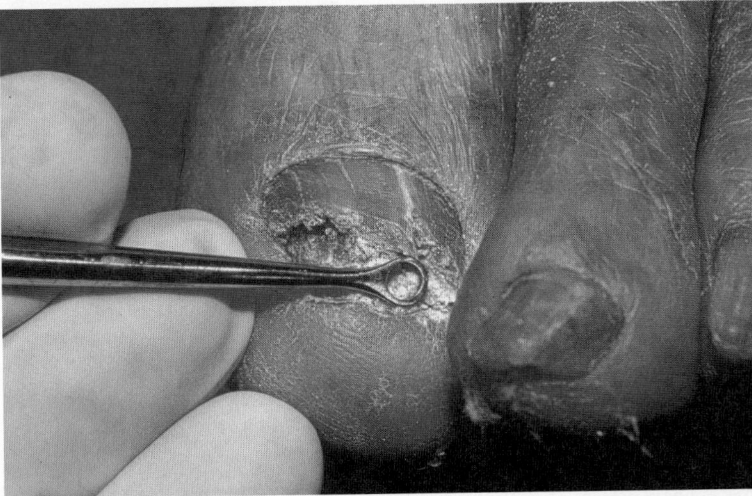

FIGURE 1-667 Collection of nail for culture. The subungual debris is the most valuable material for culture. After the nail is cut back, a curette may be used. Clippings of the nail may be added to the culture. (From White GM, Cox NH [eds]: *Diseases of the skin, a color atlas and text,* ed 2, St Louis, 2006, Mosby.)

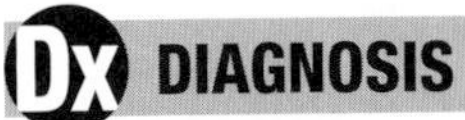

DIAGNOSIS

The diagnosis of onychomycosis is based on the clinical nail findings and confirmed by direct microscopy and culture.

DIFFERENTIAL DIAGNOSIS

- Psoriasis
- Contact dermatitis
- Lichen planus
- Subungual keratosis
- Paronychia
- Infection (e.g., *Pseudomonas*)
- Trauma
- Peripheral vascular disease
- Yellow nail syndrome

WORKUP

The workup of suspected onychomycosis is directed at confirming the diagnosis of onychomycosis by visualizing hyphae under the microscope by KOH prep or by culturing the organism. Although the standard for the diagnosis of fungal nail disease is a positive result on microscopic examination and culture of nail clippings with subungal debris or from surface debris in superficial white onychomycosis, treatment is often prescribed in absence of confirmatory findings.

LABORATORY TESTS

- KOH prep: specificity is high but sensitivity is variable
- Fungal cultures on Sabouraud medium: culture may take 4 to 6 wk
- Dermatophyte test medium (DTM): an alternative to Sabouraud's that takes only 3 to 7 days and can be done in office setting. A color change indicates dermatophyte growth.
- Nail plate biopsy with periodic acid–Schiff (PAS) stain
- Blood tests are not specific in the diagnosis of onychomycosis and therefore not useful

IMAGING STUDIES

- Imaging studies are not very specific in making the diagnosis of onychomycosis and not useful.
- If an infection is present and osteomyelitis is a consideration, an x-ray of the specific area and a bone scan may help establish the diagnosis.

CLASSIFICATION

- The Onychomycosis Severity Index (OSI) is a new classification system for grading the severity of onychomycosis.
- The OSI score is obtained by multiplying the score for the area of involvement (range, 0-5) by the score for the proximity of the disease to the matrix (range, 1-5). Ten points are added for the presence of a longitudinal streak or a patch (dermatophytoma) or for >2 mm of subungual hyperkeratosis.
- Mild onychomycosis corresponds to a score of 1-5; moderate to a score of 6-15; severe to a score of 16-35.

TREATMENT

NONPHARMACOLOGIC THERAPY

- Surgical removal of the nail plate is a treatment option; however, the relapse rate is high.
- Prevention of reinfection by wearing properly fitted shoes, avoiding public showers, and keeping feet and nails clean and dry.
- Short-pulse laser therapy is fungicidal and is a newer treatment modality for onychomycosis. Most patients will require 2-4 treatments, each lasting 15-30 minutes. Laser therapy is useful in patients with contraindications to oral agents. It is, however, expensive ($250-$1,000 per treatment) and not covered by most insurance plans.

ACUTE GENERAL Rx

- Topical antifungal creams are used for early superficial nail infections.
  1. Miconazole 2% cream applied over the nail plate bid
  2. Clotrimazole 1% cream bid
  3. Ciclopirox: topical antifungal nail lacquer can be used for moderate onychomycosis that spares the lunula. Success rate <10%
  4. Amorolfine: nail lacquer for infection that spares lunula but is not available in the U.S.
- Oral agents.
  1. Terbinafine
     a. For toenails: 250 mg/day for 3 mo
     b. For fingernails: 250 mg/day for 6 wk
  2. Itraconazole
     a. For toenails: 200 mg PO daily for 3 mo
     b. For fingernails: 200 mg PO daily for 6 wk
  3. Fluconazole: not as effective as terbinafine or itraconazole
     a. For toenails: 150 to 300 mg once weekly for 18 to 26 wk
     b. For fingernails: 150 to 300 mg once weekly for 12 to 16 wk
- All oral agents used for onychomycosis require periodic monitoring of liver function blood tests. Patients should be advised to watch for symptoms of drug-induced hepatitis (anorexia, fatigue, nausea, right upper quadrant pain) while taking these oral antifungal agents. They should stop their medication and contact their physician immediately if symptoms occur.
- Itraconazole is contraindicated in patients taking cisapride, astemizole, triazolam, midazolam, and terfenadine. Statins should be discontinued during itraconazole therapy. Itraconazole requires gastric acidity for absorption; patients should be advised not to take oral antacids, H_2 blockers, or proton pump inhibitors while taking itraconazole.
- Fluconazole is contraindicated in patients taking cisapride and terfenadine.
- Oral antifungal agents should not be initiated during pregnancy.

DISPOSITION

- Spontaneous remission of onychomycosis is rare.
- A disease-free toenail is reported to occur in approximately 25% to 50% of patients treated with the oral antifungal agents mentioned previously.

REFERRAL

- Podiatry consultation is indicated in diabetic patients for proper instruction in foot care, footwear, and nail debridement or surgical removal of the toenail.
- Dermatology consultation is indicated in patients refractory to treatment or if another diagnosis is considered (e.g., psoriasis).

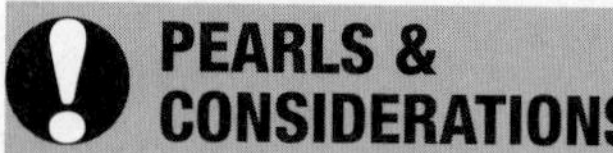

PEARLS & CONSIDERATIONS

COMMENTS

- The growth of fungus on an infected nail typically begins at the end of the nail and spreads under the nail plate to infect the nail bed as well.
- Carefully consider the informational insert regarding drug-drug interactions and contraindications before initiating oral antifungal agents.
- Meta-analysis showed cure rates with the oral agents as follows: terbinafine (about 75%), itraconazole (60%-65%), and fluconazole (about 50%).

SUGGESTED READINGS

available at www.expertconsult.com

RELATED CONTENT

Ringworm (Patient Information)

AUTHOR: **GLENN G. FORT, M.D., M.P.H.**

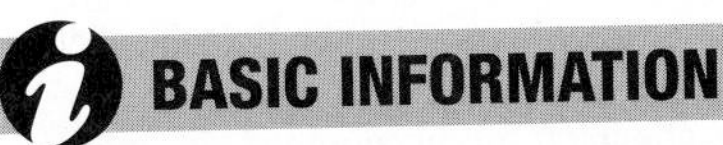

BASIC INFORMATION

DEFINITION

- Opioid addiction/dependence is defined as a cluster of cognitive, behavioral, and physiologic symptoms in which the individual continues use of opiates despite significant opiate-induced problems. Opiate dependence is a chronic, relapsing disorder characterized by repeated self-administration that usually results in opiate tolerance, withdrawal, and compulsive drug use. Tolerance is the need to increase dose to achieve the same effect. Dependence may occur with or without the physiologic symptoms of tolerance and withdrawal.
- There are four stages of addiction:
  1. Stage I, acute drug effects: rewarding effects of drug result from neurobiologic changes in response to the acute drug use. Duration varies from hours to days.
  2. Stage II, transformation to addiction: associated with changes in neuronal function that accumulate with repeated administration and diminish over days or weeks after discontinuation of drug use.
  3. Stage III, relapse after extended periods of abstinence: precipitated by an incubation of cue-induced craving (people, places, and things as triggers) and priming (relapse precipitated by drug exposure).
  4. Stage IV, end-stage addiction: vulnerability to relapse endures for years and results from prolonged changes at the cellular level.
- Pseudoaddiction: undertreatment of pain resulting in "opiate-seeking" behaviors such as "doctor shopping" and multiple emergency department visits. These behaviors disappear with adequate treatment of pain.

SYNONYMS

Opiate addiction
Opiate abuse
Narcotic addiction
Narcotic abuse

ICD-9CM CODES
304.7X/304.8X Opioid dependence
ICD-10CM CODES

F11.0	Mental and behavioral disorders due to use of opioids, acute intoxication
F11.2	Mental and behavioral disorders due to use of opioids, dependence syndrome
F11.3	Mental and behavioral disorders due to use of opioids, withdrawal stage
F19.20	Other psychoactive substance dependence, uncomplicated

EPIDEMIOLOGY & DEMOGRAPHICS

INCIDENCE: There are 980,000 opiate addicts in the U.S.; less than one third are in treatment.
PREVALENCE:

- Approximately 6 million persons age ≥12 yr used psychotherapeutic drugs for nonmedical purposes in 2004, which represents 2.5% of the population. Most of them reported abusing opiate pain relievers.
- In 2004, 2.4 million persons age ≥12 yr initiated nonmedical use of prescription pain relievers, surpassing for the first time those who initiated abuse of marijuana (2.1 million).
- Opiate addiction is becoming an adolescent disease. Among twelfth-graders, in 2005, 9.5% reported past-year nonmedical use of oxycodone (Vicodin) and 5.5% reported past-year nonmedical use of oxycodone slow-release tablets (OxyContin).
- The percentage of eighth-, tenth-, and twelfth-graders who have used heroin has more than doubled since the late 1990s. This increase has largely been attributed to decreased price and increased purity in the last decade.

PREDOMINANT SEX: Males abuse opiates more commonly than females, with a male/female ratio of 3:1 for heroin and 1.5:1 for prescription opiates.
PEAK INCIDENCE: The majority of new abusers of opiates are <26 yr.
RISK FACTORS:

- Family history
- Prior history of addiction
- Psychiatric disorders

GENETICS:

- Genetic epidemiologic studies suggest a high degree of heritable vulnerability for opiate dependence.
- Gene polymorphism for dopamine receptor/transporters, opioid receptors, serotonin receptors/transporters, proenkephalin, and catechol-*O*-methyltransferase all appear to be associated with vulnerability to opiate dependence. Future interventions for opiate dependence may include medications identified through genetic research.

PHYSICAL FINDINGS & CLINICAL PRESENTATION

- Physical examination is often noncontributory.
- Small-sized pupils may be the only observable sign of use because only mild tolerance develops for miosis.
- Scars or tracks from chronic IV use may be visible over the veins of the arms, hands, ankles, neck, and breasts.
- Inflamed nasal mucosa or respiratory wheezing may be apparent in patients who are snorting heroin or OxyContin.
- Patients in withdrawal may have more dramatic findings such as tachycardia, hypertension, fever, piloerection (goose flesh), mydriasis, lacrimation, central nervous system (CNS) arousal, irritability, and repeated yawning. In patients with sympathetic overactivity and panic attacks, use of CNS stimulants, such as amphetamines or cocaine, should also be ruled out.
- Although gastrointestinal symptoms of nausea, vomiting, and abdominal pain are common in opiate withdrawal, other causes such as gastroenteritis, pancreatitis, peptic ulcer disease, and intestinal obstruction need to be ruled out.
- The history may provide relevant information in making the diagnosis. Significant findings may include:
  1. A long history of opiate self-administration, typically by the IV or intranasal route but sometimes through smoking as well.
  2. Polysubstance use. Intoxication by drugs other than narcotics (e.g., benzodiazepines, barbiturates) should be ruled out in unconscious patients.
  3. A high incidence of non-opiate-related psychiatric disorders (>80%).
  4. History of problems at work, school, or relationships associated with drug use.
  5. History of legal problems associated with drug use, such as arrest for possession, robbery, or prostitution.
  6. History of interpersonal violence (as perpetrator or victim).
  7. History of physical problems such as skin infections, phlebitis, endocarditis, or liver diseases attributable to acetaminophen toxicity (Vicodin/Percocet) or viral hepatitis. Hepatitis C is the most prevalent blood-borne pathogen. It is present in approximately 90% of opiate-dependent people and is often spread by sharing IV drug paraphernalia or snorting devices. There is also a higher incidence of HIV infection.

ETIOLOGY

Opioid dependence is a biopsychosocial disorder. Pharmacologic, social, genetic, and psychodynamic factors interact to influence abusive behaviors. Pharmacologic factors are especially prominent in opiate addiction because these drugs are strong reinforcing agents because of their euphoric effects and their ability to reduce anxiety and increase self-esteem and the patient's subjective feelings of improved ability to cope with daily challenges.

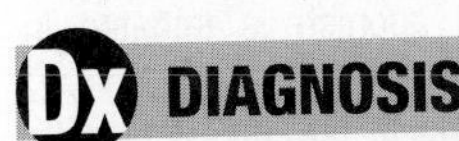

DIAGNOSIS

DIFFERENTIAL DIAGNOSIS

- Psychiatric disorders (e.g., anxiety, depression, bipolar disorder).
- Acute medical illness (e.g., hypoglycemia, seizure disorder, sepsis, renal or hepatic insufficiency) may mimic opiate withdrawal symptoms.

WORKUP

- The history is the most important part of the workup.
- Observation of opiate withdrawal is indicative of opiate addiction.
- Observation of purposeful behaviors such as complaints and manipulations directed at getting more drugs and anxiety during withdrawal is suggestive of opiate addiction.
- Screen blood and urine for opiate metabolites.
- Screen for communicable diseases: HIV, hepatitis B and hepatitis C, tuberculosis.

- Screen for endocarditis in patients with newly diagnosed murmurs.

LABORATORY TESTS

- Urine and serum toxicology screen
- Complete blood count
- Chemistries (alanine aminotransferase, aspartate aminotransferase, serum creatinine): elevated liver function test (LFT) results may be from viral hepatitis or acetaminophen toxicity
- Hepatitis screen: if hepatitis C antibody positive, follow up with hepatitis C polymerase chain reaction (viral load) even in patients with normal LFTs
- HIV
- PPD

IMAGING STUDIES

Generally not helpful in routine diagnosis and treatment. Consider echocardiography in patients with heart murmurs and liver sonography or CT scan in patients with elevated LFTs or who are positive for hepatitis C or B (increased risk of hepatocellular carcinoma).

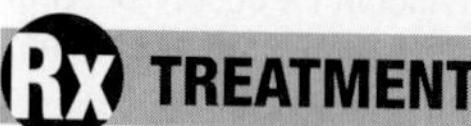

TREATMENT

NONPHARMACOLOGIC THERAPY

- Brief counseling interventions during a visit with their primary care physician or OB/GYN have proved efficacious in motivating patients for treatment.
- Therapeutic communities (residential).
- 12-step or other self-help groups (e.g., Alcoholics Anonymous, Narcotics Anonymous).
- Relapse prevention (counseling).

ACUTE Rx

- Medical withdrawal (not overdosed).
- Short- (30 days) or long-term (30 to 180 days) protocols.
- Buprenorphine (opioid partial agonist) or methadone (opioid agonist) is initiated in tapering doses.
- Clonidine 0.1 mg bid to tid can be used to minimize autonomic symptoms (sweating) and craving.
- Nonsteroidal anti-inflammatory drugs for body and muscle aches.
- The anticholinergic dicyclomine can be used to minimize gastrointestinal hyperactivity.
- Nonbenzodiazepine hypnotics, low-dose atypical antipsychotics (e.g., quetiapine), or low-dose tricyclic antidepressants are effective for promoting adequate sleep.

CHRONIC Rx

Opioid antagonist treatment:

- Naltrexone: does not stabilize neuronal circuitry like partial or full opioid agonists and generally results in poor outcomes, much like Antabuse for alcohol.
- Opioid partial agonist therapy: buprenorphine.
- Opioid agonist therapy: methadone.

NOTE: Buprenorphine and methadone are both metabolized by the cytochrome P450 3a4 and 2d6 I isoenzyme pathways. Prescribers should be aware of multiple possible drug interactions.

PATIENT SELECTION FOR BUPRENORPHINE OR METHADONE

- Appropriate patients for buprenorphine office-based treatment:
  - Patients interested (highly motivated) in treatment
  - Have no major contraindications (see following)
  - Can be expected to be reasonably compliant with treatment
  - Understand the benefits and risks of buprenorphine treatment
  - Willing to follow safety precautions
- Less likely to be appropriate for office-based treatment:
  - Have comorbid dependence on benzodiazepines or other CNS depressants (including ethylene alcohol)
  - Have significant untreated psychiatric comorbidities
  - Have active or chronic suicidal or homicidal ideation or attempts
  - Have multiple previous treatments with frequent relapses
  - Have poor response to previous treatment with buprenorphine
  - Have significant medical complications (e.g., hepatic insufficiency, bacterial endocarditis, active tuberculosis)
- Methadone maintenance: narcotic treatment program (clinic setting) indications
- Evidence of opiate addiction >1 yr
- Two failed previous treatment attempts
- Patients not appropriate for office-based treatment
- Eligible without active "use" if prior methadone maintenance patient within previous 2 mo
- Pregnancy

DISPOSITION

- Opioid addiction is a chronic, relapsing disease.
- High rate of relapse after "detox."
- Relapse potential after medically supervised withdrawal from methadone:
  - 90% after 1 yr stable in treatment
  - 80% after 3 yr stable in treatment
  - 70% after 5 yr stable in treatment

REFERRAL

Refer to addiction medicine specialist or narcotic treatment program when the neurobiologic disease of opioid addiction is identified.

PEARLS & CONSIDERATIONS

COMMENTS

- Methadone maintenance is the gold standard for the pregnant opiate-addicted patient regardless of the duration of the addiction or prior treatment attempts. Detoxification is contraindicated during pregnancy.
- Breastfeeding is encouraged in mothers on methadone maintenance. The American Academy of Pediatrics statement regarding "Transfer of Drugs and Other Chemicals into Human Milk" has placed methadone into the "usually compatible with breastfeeding" group based on the assumption that maternal urine is monitored to detect use of illicit drugs. The U.S. Department of Health and Human Services also recommends that mothers on methadone be encouraged to breastfeed.
- When a physician identifies a patient as a "drug seeker," it is imperative that the physician avoid abruptly stopping the opiate prescription because this will often result in the patient's buying the drugs illegally. These patients should be counseled and referred for treatment.
- Patients on methadone or buprenorphine who have pain resulting from an acute injury will need pain medication in addition to their daily dose of methadone or buprenorphine. They will require higher than usual doses of pain medications because of opiate receptor blockade attributable to their methadone or buprenorphine use.
- Opiate-dependent patients have a lower pain threshold resulting from hyperalgesia caused by the long-term use of opiates.

PREVENTION

Education is the hallmark of prevention.

- School drug prevention education programs.
- Educate children about their family medical history, including diseases of addiction.
- Address childhood psychiatric disorders to prevent self-medicating.

PATIENT & FAMILY EDUCATION

- Stigma of addictions and treatment often interferes with good treatment.
- Family needs to be educated so they can support the patient's efforts.
- Encourage family meeting with addiction specialist, counselor.
- Recommend support groups for family members.

SUGGESTED READINGS

available at www.expertconsult.com

RELATED CONTENT

Drug Abuse (Patient Information)

AUTHOR: **STEVEN PELIGIAN, D.O.**

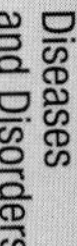

BASIC INFORMATION

DEFINITION

- *Optic atrophy* refers to the degeneration of axons of the optic nerve.
- It is a sign indicative of optic nerve insult rather than a distinct disease entity.

SYNONYMS

Unilateral/bilateral optic atrophy

ICD-9CM CODES
377.10 Optic atrophy NOS
377.11 Optic atrophy, primary
377.12 Optic atrophy, post-inflammatory
377.13 Optic atrophy, retinal dystrophy
377.15 Optic atrophy, partial
377.16 Optic atrophy, hereditary
ICD-10 CM CODES
H47.2 Optic atrophy

EPIDEMIOLOGY & DEMOGRAPHICS

PREDOMINANT SEX: Depends on etiology; <50 yr demyelinating diseases more likely and >50 yr, ischemic optic neuropathy more likely
PREDOMINANT AGE: Variable
PEAK INCIDENCE: Varies depending on cause

PHYSICAL FINDINGS & CLINICAL PRESENTATION

- Optic atrophy is identified weeks to months after an initial insult such as optic neuritis, trauma, or ischemia. Frequently, it is noted by the physician during a routine eye exam.
- Asymmetry of disc color is often first subtle finding.
- Temporal part of optic disc is pale initially (Fig. 1-668); later the entire disc becomes pale/white.
- Optic disc pallor occurs 4 to 6 wk after optic nerve insult.
- Unilateral lesion produces a relative afferent pupillary defect (RAPD): swing flashlight eye to eye; abnormal pupil dilates to direct light.
- Decreased visual acuity, blurred vision, visual field deficits (e.g., central scotoma), abnormal color vision (e.g., red desaturation).

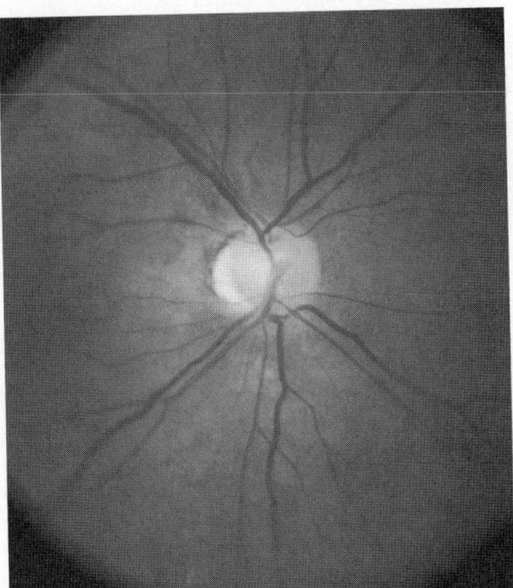

FIGURE 1-668 Optic atrophy. Patient's right eye shows atrophy. (Courtesy John W. Payne, M.D., The Wilmer Ophthalmological Institute, The Johns Hopkins University and Hospital, Baltimore. From Seidel HM [ed]: *Mosby's guide to physical examination,* ed 4, St Louis, 1999, Mosby.)

ETIOLOGY

- Optic neuritis—MS, sarcoidosis, infections (syphilis, CMV, HIV, Lyme disease)
- Vascular—ischemic optic neuropathy, central retinal artery occlusion, temporal arteritis
- Compression—glaucoma, pituitary tumor, meningioma, thyroid eye disease
- Hereditary—Leber's hereditary optic neuropathy
- Nutritional, toxic, and metabolic—amiodarone, isoniazid, B_{12} deficiency, tobacco, alcohol
- Trauma

DIAGNOSIS

DIFFERENTIAL DIAGNOSIS

- Optic disc anomalies such as myelinated nerve fibers, "blonde" fundus

WORKUP

- A detailed history to identify onset and course, exposure to risk factors such as toxic/nutritional factors, detailed family history, and associated findings such as headache, eye pain, proptosis, or neurologic deficits
- Ophthalmic examination to document deficits of visual acuity, color vision, contrast sensitivity, and visual fields must be performed. Relative afferent pupillary defect (RAPD) on swinging flashlight examination is sine qua non for unilateral optic nerve disease and must be documented. Absence indicates retinal disease or bilateral lesions.
- General examination and neurologic examination can provide clues to an underlying cause.
- Pertinent laboratory testing as noted below; genetic studies with a consultation can be obtained in cases with a suggestive history. Lumbar puncture should be obtained in patients with unexplained optic atrophy especially with neurologic deficits.
- In the absence of an obvious cause, contrasted MRI of brain and orbits should be obtained to evaluate for demyelinating lesions and compressive lesions of the anterior visual pathways.

LABORATORY TESTS

- Depends on suspected cause: none for trauma, tumor, or MS
- Serum B_{12}
- Autoimmune diseases: ESR, ANA, ACE

IMAGING STUDIES

- MRI of the brain with contrast, fat suppression, and special (thin) cuts through orbits is necessary to identify compressive lesions in all patients with unexplained optic atrophy; especially important in patients with positive-predictive factors for abnormal imaging (e.g., young age, progression, bilateral findings).
- If sarcoid is suspected, order chest x-ray.

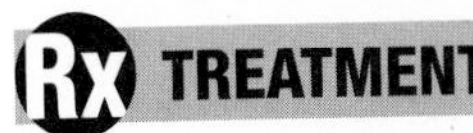

TREATMENT

ACUTE GENERAL Rx

Treat the underlying cause—discontinue identifiable toxins, use B_{12} replacement, neurosurgical intervention is necessary if tumor is found; consider IV steroids if there is evidence for active demyelinating disease.

CHRONIC Rx

The optic nerve does not regenerate, although symptoms often improve.

DISPOSITION

- Visual loss usually occurs over weeks to months.
- Appointment with neurologist or ophthalmologist

REFERRAL

Depends on the underlying disease process

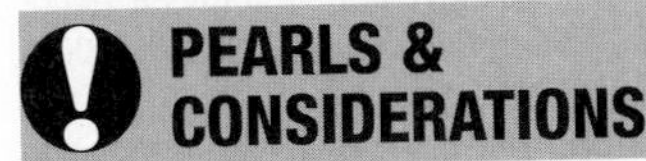

PEARLS & CONSIDERATIONS

COMMENTS

- An experienced clinician should be able to identify pale optic discs and an RAPD.
- Pupillary dilation with mydriatic agents (e.g., pilocarpine) may be necessary to optimize funduscopic examination.
- Patient education material can be obtained from the National Eye Institute, Department of Health and Human Services, 9000 Rockville Pike, Bethesda, MD 20892.

SUGGESTED READINGS

available at www.expertconsult.com

AUTHOR: **SACHIN KEDAR, M.B.B.S., M.D.**

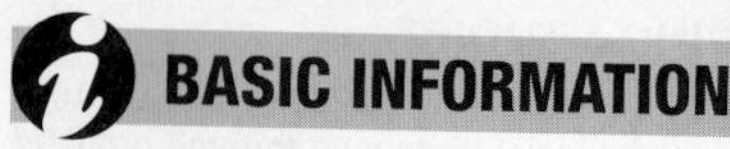

BASIC INFORMATION

DEFINITION

Optic neuritis is an inflammation of the optic nerve resulting in impaired visual function.

SYNONYMS

Optic papillitis
Retrobulbar neuritis

ICD-9CM CODES
377.3 Optic neuritis
ICD-10CM CODES
H46.9 Unspecified optic neuritis

EPIDEMIOLOGY & DEMOGRAPHICS

INCIDENCE (IN U.S.): 1 to 5/100,000 person(s) per year; rates vary according to incidence of multiple sclerosis (MS)
PREVALENCE (IN U.S.): Common in patients with MS
PREDOMINANT SEX: Female/male ratio: 1.8:1
PEAK INCIDENCE: 20 to 49 yr, mean 30
GENETICS: Unknown. If due to MS, it is more common in patients with certain HLA blood types and in monozygotic twins of affected siblings. See topic "Multiple Sclerosis."

PHYSICAL FINDINGS & CLINICAL PRESENTATION

- Presents with acute or subacute (days) visual loss, often accompanied by periocular pain that worsens with eye movements.
- **Marcus Gunn pupil** (relative afferent pupillary defect [RAPD]): direct and consensual response is normal; however, when flashlight is swung from eye to eye, the affected eye's pupil dilates to direct light.
- Decreased visual acuity
- Unilateral visual field abnormalities—often a central scotoma (Fig. E1-669)
- Color desaturation; red is most often affected
- Normal orbit and fundus; occasionally there is disc edema acutely (Fig. 1-670), uveitis, or periphlebitis.
- May have movement or light-induced phosphenes (flashes of light lasting 1 to 2 sec).

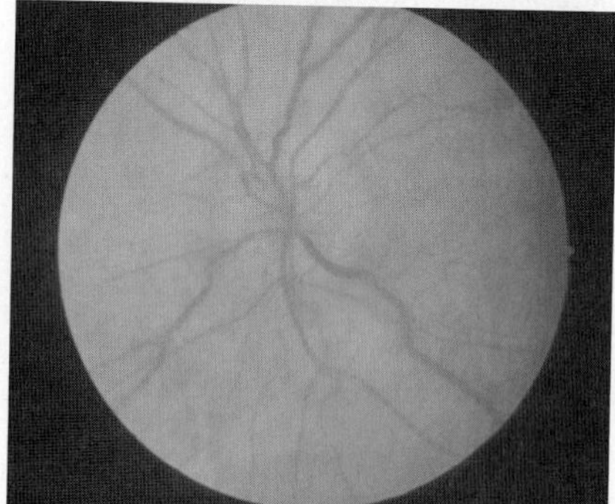

FIGURE 1-670 A case of optic neuritis. The optic disc edema seen here is often not present. Note the otherwise normal fundus. (Courtesy of J. Barton, M.D., Beth Israel Deaconess Medical Center, Boston.)

- Uhthoff's phenomenon (benign exercise–or heat-induced deterioration of vision) is seen in some. Vision may also worsen in bright sunlight.
- Over time the optic disc may atrophy and become pale.

ETIOLOGY

An inflammatory response associated with an infection, autoimmune disease (such as collagen vascular disease, granulomatous disease, MS, or neuromyelitis optica), or, rarely, a mitochondrial disorder

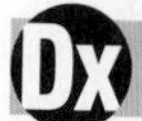

DIAGNOSIS

Consistent clinical presentation and exclusion of alternate ocular pathology, infection, and CNS mass lesions. Classic triad includes loss of vision, retroorbital pain, and dyschromatopsia. 70% of cases are unilateral and 30% bilateral.

DIFFERENTIAL DIAGNOSIS

For optic neuritis (usually with retroorbital tenderness)

- Inflammatory: MS, neuromyelitis optica (NMO), sarcoidosis, lupus, Sjögren's, Behçet's, postinfectious, postvaccination, neuroretinitis, acute disseminated encephalomyelitis, paraneoplastic, autoimmune optic neuropathy (with retinopathy is ARRONS)
- Infectious: syphilis, TB, Lyme disease, *Bartonella,* HIV, CMV, herpes, helminths, chickenpox. Q fever, periorbital infections, *Toxocara* sp. For optic neuropathy typically without ocular pain
- Ischemic: anterior and posterior ischemic optic neuropathies, diabetic papillopathy, branch or central retinal artery or vein occlusion
- Mitochondrial: Leber's hereditary optic neuropathy

For loss of vision typically without ocular pain

- Mass lesion: pituitary tumor, aneurysm, meningioma, glioma, metastases, and sinus mucocele
- Ocular: optic drusen, retinal detachment, vitreous hemorrhage, uveitis, posterior scleritis, neuroretinitis, maculopathies, and retinopathies
- Drugs, toxins, and nutritional: toxins (arsenic, tobacco, etc.), medications (amiodarone, cyclosporine, etc.), and vitamin deficiencies (B_{12}, B_1, B_6, niacin)
- Other: acute papilledema, retinal migraine, factitious visual loss

WORKUP

A thorough neurologic examination; recommend dilated ophthalmoscopy

LABORATORY TESTS

- Recommend CBC, ANA, ACE, ESR.
- Consider HIV Ab, Lyme titer, RPR, other autoimmune or infectious causes.
- Bilateral or recurrent ON:NMO IgG; paraneoplastic CRMP-5-IgG
- Visual field tests

IMAGING STUDIES

- MRI of the brain and orbits (thin section fat-suppressed T_2-weighted) ± gadolinium to look for compressive and infiltrative causes and the risk to develop MS can be assessed. Often enhancement of the optic nerve is seen.
- Consider using optical coherence tomography to follow optic nerve atrophy objectively longitudinally.

Rx TREATMENT

NONPHARMACOLOGIC THERAPY

Assure patient that in most cases there is near complete recovery of vision.

ACUTE Rx

Treat if the visual loss is severe or if there is an abnormal MRI (higher risk of MS). Treatment is with methylprednisolone (MP) 250 mg IV every 6 hr (or 1 g IV daily) for 3 days followed by an oral prednisone taper of 11 days.

CHRONIC Rx

None, unless at significant risk to develop MS. See topic "Multiple Sclerosis."

DISPOSITION

Most often vision is worst at the end of week 1, followed by recovery over months. In the Optic Neuritis Treatment Trial (ONTT), 90% had 20/40 or better vision at 1 yr and 3% had 20/200 or worse. Of initial 20/200 or worse cases, only 5% remained in that group at 6 mo.

REFERRAL

- To neurologist for other neurologic signs and to assess risk of developing MS; urgently needed if proptosis or ophthalmoplegia present
- To ophthalmologist when atypical features or slowly progressive; urgently when other ocular pathology is present or if vision worsens or does not improve after several wk, pain is severe or persistent, or vision deteriorates as steroids are tapered

PEARLS & CONSIDERATIONS

- Bilateral optic neuritis suggests a systemic inflammatory disorder, infection, NMO, or paraneoplastic but can also occur in MS.
- Acute bilateral loss of vision with a severe headache or diplopia should raise concern for pituitary apoplexy and/or giant cell arteritis in the elderly.

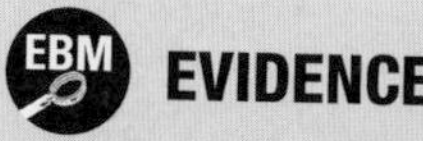

EVIDENCE

available at www.expertconsult.com

SUGGESTED READINGS

available at www.expertconsult.com

RELATED CONTENT

Multiple Sclerosis (Related Key Topic)

AUTHOR: **ALEXANDRA DEGENHARDT, M.D., M.M.S.**

BASIC INFORMATION

DEFINITION

Oral cancer is malignant cell formation in the oral cavity and may occur as a primary lesion initiating in any of the oral tissues, by metastasis from a distant site of origin, or by extension from a neighboring anatomic structure such as the nasal cavity or the maxillary sinus.

SYNONYMS

Oral cancer
Oropharyngeal cancer
Oral malignant neoplasm

ICD-9CM CODES

Code	Description
140.0-149.0	Code varies with specific anatomic structure

ICD-10CM CODES

Code	Description
C01	Malignant neoplasm of base of tongue
C03	Malignant neoplasm of gum
C04	Malignant neoplasm of floor of mouth
C05	Malignant neoplasm of palate
C06	Malignant neoplasm of other and unspecified parts of mouth
C09	Malignant neoplasm of tonsil
C10	Malignant neoplasm of oropharynx
C11	Malignant neoplasm of nasopharynx
C12	Malignant neoplasm of piriform sinus
C13	Malignant neoplasm of hypopharynx
C14	Malignant neoplasm of other and ill-defined sites of lip, oral cavity and larynx
C14.0	Malignant neoplasm of pharynx, unspecified
C14.2	Malignant neoplasm of Waldeyer's ring
C14.8	Malignant neoplasm of overlapping sites of lip, oral cavity and pharynx

EPIDEMIOLOGY & DEMOGRAPHICS

INCIDENCE & PREVALENCE: Oral and pharyngeal cancer is the sixth most common cancer in the world. An estimated half a million cases are diagnosed annually around the globe and the rates have been rising, particularly in young people and among minorities. In 2011, oropharyngeal squamous cell carcinoma (OP-SCCA) affected >12,000 new patients, with the most common sites being the tonsillar fossa and base of the tongue. In the U.S., the incidence of OP-SCCA linked to alcohol and tobacco use has been declining, whereas those linked to human papillomavirus (HPV), primarily HPV type 16, is on the rise. In Asian countries where chewing betel nut is customary, oral cancer accounts for up to 40% of cancers in some regions (Ayaz, 2011). Squamous cell carcinoma is the most common malignancy that occurs in the oral cavity. Minor salivary gland cancers, lymphomas, and sarcomas are less common. For more detailed data please see the Surveillance, Epidemiology, and End Results (SEER) Program of the National Cancer Institute.

PREDOMINANT SEX & AGE:

- Predominantly male, middle aged
- Black males have a higher early incidence in the 50- to 60-yr age group, but with increasing age, white men predominate.

GENETICS: There is no specific genetic factor or translocation, but the human papillomavirus (HPV)–induced oral squamous cell cancer typically seen in younger populations is associated with loss of p53 tumor suppressor due to inactivation by E6 protein from the virus.

RISK FACTORS:

- Tobacco use of any kind
- HPV infection (primarily types 16 and 18)
- Alcohol
- Immune deficiency
- Syphilis
- Radiation
- Vitamin A, C, E deficiency
- Betel nut consumption
- Solar radiation

PHYSICAL FINDINGS & CLINICAL PRESENTATION

- Often starts as a tiny, unnoticed white or red spot or sore anywhere in the oropharyngeal cavity or lip.
- Most lesions begin on the tongue or buccal mucosa.
- Clinically, oral cancer can present as:
  - Erythroplakia (flat red patch) Can mimic inflammatory or traumatic lesions.
  - Leukoplakia (white patch; Fig. 1-671)
  - Raised lesion
  - Ulcerated lesion
  - White warty lesion or growth
- The borders of the oral cavity can be defined as from the skin-vermilion junction of the lips to the junction of the hard and soft palate above and to the line of the circumvallate papilla of the tongue below. The lateral boundary between the oral cavity and oropharynx consists of the anterior tonsillar pillars and glossotonsillar folds.
- Oral cavity cancer can present on the lip, floor of the mouth, oral tongue (anterior two thirds of the tongue), lower alveolar ridge, upper alveolar ridge, retromolar trigone (retromolar gingiva), hard palate, salivary glands, and buccal mucosa.
- Oral cavity tumors often present with local invasion, tissue destruction, and lymph node metastases.
- Oral cancers rarely have distant metastases at the time of presentation, although this may vary depending on the length of time until presentation.

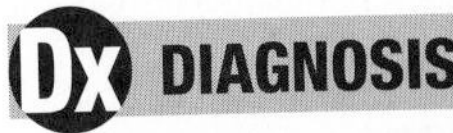

DIAGNOSIS

DIFFERENTIAL DIAGNOSIS

- Oral leukoplakia
- Traumatic ulcerative granuloma with stromal eosinophilia, especially on the tongue
- Deep fungal infections
- Chancre of early syphilis and gumma of tertiary syphilis
- Chronic ulcer

WORKUP

- Primary workup includes incisional biopsy with vital staining of the presenting lesion for histopathologic analysis.
- Pretreatment evaluation: Tumor size, the extent of invasion, and the presence or absence of regional lymph node metastases are critical for planning treatment.
- Workup includes staging the cancer: The tumor-node-metastasis (TNM) staging system of the American Joint Committee on Cancer (AJCC) and the International Union for Cancer Control (UICC) is used to classify lip and oral cavity carcinoma.
- By definition, patients with early (stage I and II) disease have tumors <4 cm in greatest

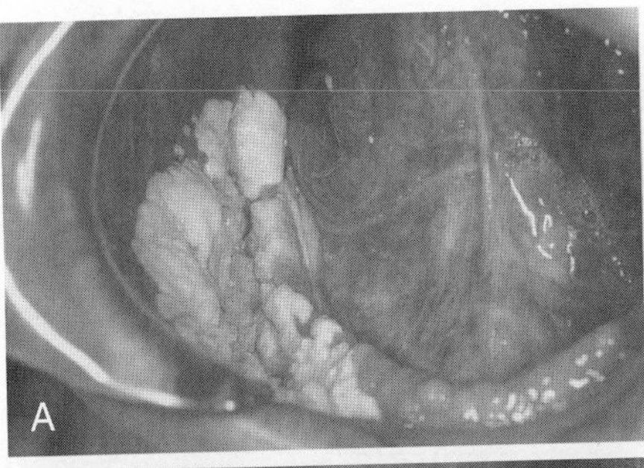

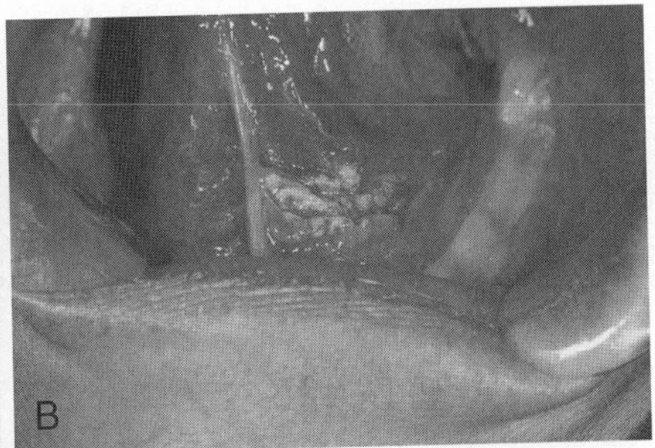

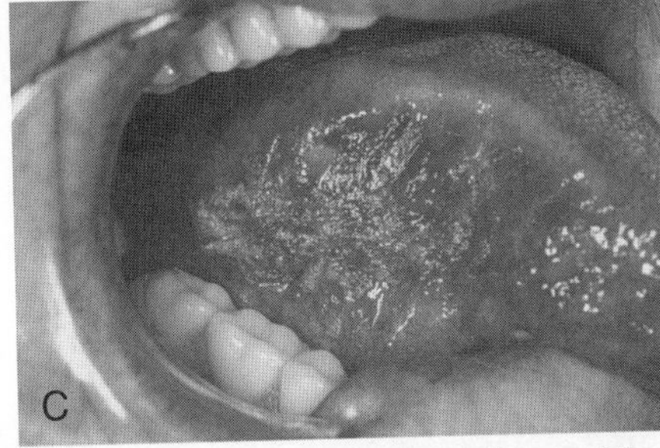

FIGURE 1-671 Squamous cell carcinoma of the oral mucosa. A, Leukoplakia. **B,** Invasive carcinoma of the floor of the mouth. **C,** Invasive carcinoma of the tongue. (Courtesy G. Putnam. In White GM, Cox NH [eds]: *Diseases of the skin: a color atlas and text,* ed 2, St Louis, 2006, Mosby.)

dimension without deep invasion into surrounding structures and have no evidence of lymph node involvement.

- Oral cavity cancers tend to invade bone and soft tissue early in their natural history. Therefore, pretreatment imaging studies, such as magnetic resonance imaging (MRI) and computed tomography (CT), are required in addition to a thorough inspection and deep palpation of the oral cavity.

LABORATORY TESTS

Send biopsy specimen to oral and maxillofacial pathology, head and neck pathology, or general pathology.

IMAGING STUDIES

Consider MRI or CT based on the extent of clinical presentation.

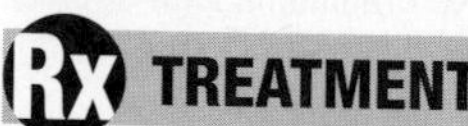

TREATMENT

- Surgery vs. radiation therapy:
  - Both primary surgery and definitive radiation therapy are options for patients with oral cavity cancer.
  - Outcomes with primary surgery and definitive radiation therapy appear to be similar based on retrospective studies, but the two modes of treatment have not been compared in randomized controlled trials.
- Surgery is generally favored because it is typically associated with less morbidity than radiation therapy. Surgical therapy traditionally involved wide-exposure approaches (mandibulotomy, transpharyngeal access). Newer surgical techniques allow tumor resection through the mouth. Recently, transoral robotic surgery (TORS) has been developed to improve access to oropharyngeal squamous cell carcinomas with excellent oncologic outcomes.
  - Acute surgical complications can include infection, bleeding, aspiration, wound breakdown, fistula, and flap loss.
  - Surgical procedures can cause functional deficits in speech and swallowing, but these adverse effects can be minimized by appropriate reconstruction and prostheses.
- Definitive radiation therapy is reserved for patients who cannot tolerate surgery or for whom surgical resection would result in particularly severe functional impairment.
  - Radiation therapy can include external beam radiation and brachytherapy.
  - Radiation therapy side effects include mucositis, skin reaction, loss of taste, dysphagia, and xerostomia.
  - Late complications can include skin and soft tissue atrophy and fibrosis, osteoradionecrosis, and trismus.
- Close margins, typically defined as <5 mm, are associated with a worse prognosis.
- Adjuvant chemotherapy may also be an option in treatment regimen.

DISPOSITION

- Prognosis depends on the cancer cell type and staging.
- Tumor HPV status is a strong and independent prognostic factor for survival among patients with oropharyngeal cancer.

REFERRAL

Refer to oral and maxillofacial or ear, nose, and throat surgeon.

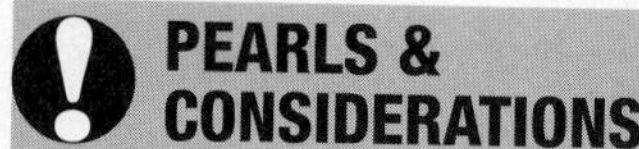

PEARLS & CONSIDERATIONS

COMMENTS

- Oral and pharyngeal cancer is the sixth most common cancer globally.
- Biopsy is the key for diagnosis.
- Posttreatment surveillance is important.

PREVENTION

- Encourage patients to stop using any type of tobacco and drinking alcohol.
- Examine oral cavities at annual checkups and work up suspicious lesions.

PATIENT & FAMILY EDUCATION

http://globocan.iarc.fr/factsheets/populations/factsheet.asp?uno=900.

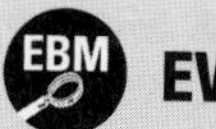

EVIDENCE

available at www.expertconsult.com

SUGGESTED READINGS

available at www.expertconsult.com

RELATED CONTENT

Mouth Cancer (Patient Information)

AUTHORS: **PRIYA SARIN GUPTA, M.D., M.P.H.,** and **KEVIN PLUMLEY, M.D.**

BASIC INFORMATION

DEFINITION

Orchitis is an inflammatory process (usually infectious) involving the testicles. Infection may be viral or bacterial and can be associated with infection of other male sex organs (prostate, epididymis, or bladder) or lower urogenital tract or sexually transmitted diseases often via hematogenous spread. Common causes are:

- Viral: mumps—20% postpubertal; coxsackie B virus
- Bacterial: pyogenic via spread from involving epididymis; bacteria include *Escherichia coli, Klebsiella pneumoniae, P. aeruginosa, Staphylococcus, Streptococcus* or *Rickettsia, Brucella* spp.
- Other:
  - Viral—HIV-associated, CMV
  - Fungi
    1. Cryptococcosis
    2. Histoplasmosis
    3. *Candida*
    4. Blastomycosis
    5. Syphilis
  - *Mycobacterium tuberculosis* and *M. leprae*
  - Parasitic causes: toxoplasmosis, filiariasis, schistosomiasis
- Table 1-366 describes a classification of epididymitis and orchitis based on etiology.

SYNONYMS

Epididymoorchitis
Testicular infection
Testicular inflammation

ICD-9CM CODES
0.72 Mumps
098.13 Acute gonococcal orchitis
095.8 Syphilitic orchitis
016.50 Tuberculous orchitis, unspecified
ICD-10CM CODES
N45.9 Orchitis, epididymitis, and epididymo-orchitis without abscess
A54.1 Gonococcal orchitis
A56.1 Chlamydial orchitis
N51.1 Mumps orchitis

EPIDEMIOLOGY & DEMOGRAPHICS

PREDOMINANT SEX: Male
PREDOMINANT ORGANISM: The leading cause of viral orchitis is mumps. The mumps virus rarely causes orchitis in prepubertal males but involves one or both testicles in nearly 30% of postpubertal males.

PHYSICAL FINDINGS & CLINICAL PRESENTATION

- Testicular pain, unilateral or bilateral swelling
- May have associated epididymitis, prostatitis, fever, scrotal edema, erythema, cellulitis
- Inguinal lymphadenopathy
- Acute hydrocele (bacterial)
- Rare development: abscess formation, pyocele of scrotum, testicular infarction
- Spermatic cord tenderness may be present
- Granulomatous

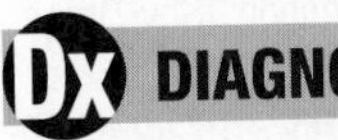

DIAGNOSIS

Clinical presentation as described previously with possible history of acute viral illness or concomitant epididymitis.

DIFFERENTIAL DIAGNOSIS

- Epididymoorchitis-gonococcal
- Autoimmune disease
- Vasculitis
- Epididymyosis
- Mumps, with or without parotitis
- Neoplasm
- Hematoma
- Spermatic cord torsion

LABORATORY TESTS

- CBC with differential
- Urinalysis
- Viral titer—mumps
- Urine culture
- Ultrasound of testicle to rule out abscess

IMAGING STUDIES

Ultrasound if abscess suspected

TREATMENT

- Dependent on cause
- Viral (mumps): observation; bed rest, ice packs, analgesics, and a scrotal sling for support may provide some relief of discomfort that accompanies mumps orchitis
- Bacterial: empiric antibiotic treatment with parenteral antibiotic treatment until pathogen identified: ceftriaxone (250 mg IM once) plus doxycycline (100 mg PO bid for 10 days), in men <35 yr old to cover *Neisseria gonorrhoeae* and Chlamydia trachomatis. In homosexual men or men >35 yr old: levofloxacin 500-750 mg IV/PO qd for 10-14 days *or* ampicillin-sulbactam *or* third-generation cephalosporin or ticarcillin-clavulanate.
- Surgery for abscess, pyogenic process

DISPOSITION

Follow-up for evidence of recurrence, hypogonadism, and infertility may be needed with bilateral orchitis.

REFERRAL

- To a urologist if surgical drainage is needed
- To an endocrinologist if hypogonadism develops
- To a fertility specialist if infertility develops

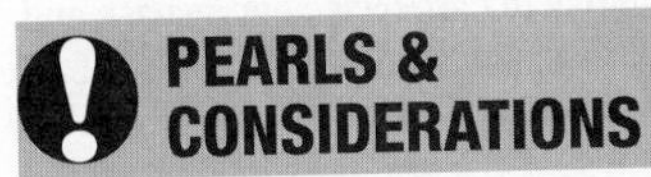

PEARLS & CONSIDERATIONS

Consider tuberculous orchitis if symptoms fail to respond to standard antibacterial therapy, even in the absence of chest radiographic evidence of pulmonary tuberculosis.

SUGGESTED READINGS

available at www.expertconsult.com

RELATED CONTENT

Orchitis (Patient Information)
Epididymitis (Related Key Topic)
Mumps (Related Key Topic)

AUTHOR: **GLENN G. FORT, M.D., M.P.H.**

TABLE 1-366 Classification of Epididymitis and Orchitis

Acute Epididymitis or Epididymoorchitis	Granulomatous Epididymitis or Orchitis	Viral Orchitis
Neisseria gonorrhoeae	*Mycobacterium tuberculosis*	Mumps
Chlamydia trachomatis	*Treponema pallidum*	Enteroviruses
Escherichia coli		
Streptococcus pneumoniae	*Brucella* spp.	
Klebsiella spp.	Sarcoid	
Salmonella spp.	Fungal	
Other urinary tract pathogens	Parasitic	
Idiopathic	Idiopathic	

From Cohen J, Powderly WG: *Infectious diseases*, ed 2, St Louis, 2004, Mosby.

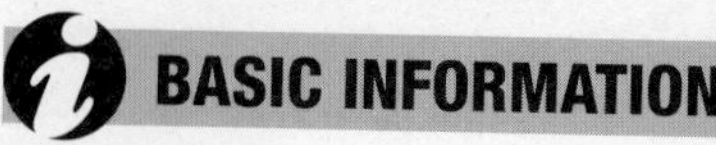

BASIC INFORMATION

DEFINITION

Orthostatic hypotension (OH) is defined as the presence of at least one of the following: a decrease in systolic blood pressure by ≥20 mm Hg or a decrease in diastolic blood pressure by ≥10 mm Hg within 3 min of standing. It is a physical sign that requires further investigation to discern its underlying etiology.

SYNONYMS

Postural hypotension

ICD-9CM CODES
458.0 Orthostatic hypotension
ICD-10CM CODES
I95.1 Orthostatic hypotension

EPIDEMIOLOGY & DEMOGRAPHICS

- The incidence of OH is increased in older people and in those with diseases associated with autonomic dysfunction (e.g., Parkinson disease, diabetes mellitus).
- OH may cause up to 30% of all syncopal events in the elderly, and OH is associated with an increased risk of heart failure among those aged 45 to 55 yr and an increased risk of cardiovascular disease and all-cause mortality among those aged 55 yr and older.

PHYSICAL FINDINGS & CLINICAL PRESENTATION

- Symptoms may include dizziness, lightheadedness, syncope, visual and auditory disturbances, weakness, diaphoresis, pallor, and nausea. OH may also be asymptomatic, especially in older hypertensive patients.
- Associated with increased autonomic activity during meals (from increased splanchnic blood flow), exercise, and hot weather.
- Supine and nocturnal hypertension in patients with OH may indicate an underlying autonomic dysfunction.

ETIOLOGY

- The assumption of an upright posture results in the pooling of approximately 500 ml of blood in the lower extremities due to gravity and decreased venous return, decreased cardiac output, and decreased arterial pressure. The consequent increase in sympathetic tone due to increased carotid baroreceptor activity causes arterial and venous constriction as well as positive inotropic and chronotropic effects, thereby limiting the fall in upright blood pressure. Peripheral vasoconstriction is also mediated by increased activity of the renin-angiotensin system and decreased activity of atrial natriuretic factor.
- Impairment of the baroreceptor reflex, as in central or peripheral autonomic dysfunction and aging, may cause OH because decreased blood pressure cannot be counteracted by the aforementioned regulatory mechanisms.

Dx DIAGNOSIS

DIFFERENTIAL DIAGNOSIS

Common:

- Medications: antihypertensives, antidepressants (tricyclics), antipsychotics (phenothiazines), alcohol, narcotics, barbiturates, insulin, nitrates, PDE-5 inhibitors, alpha-adrenergic antagonists
- Reduced intravascular volume (hemorrhage, dehydration, hyperglycemia, hypoalbuminemia)
- Postprandial effect (especially in the elderly)
- Vasovagal syncope
- Deconditioning
- Central autonomic dysfunction (Parkinson's disease)
- Peripheral autonomic dysfunction (diabetes mellitus, Guillain-Barré syndrome)

Uncommon:

- Central autonomic dysfunction (Shy-Drager syndrome)
- Postganglionic autonomic dysfunction: impaired norepinephrine release
- Autoimmune autonomic dysfunction: nicotinic acetylcholine receptor autoantibodies
- Paraneoplastic autonomic dysfunction: anti-Hu antibodies (in small-cell lung cancer)
- Postural tachycardia syndrome (POTS): usually occurs in young women; an abnormally large increase in heart rate is observed in the upright position caused by increased venous pooling from autonomic dysfunction of the lower extremities, but blood pressure is not affected because of an excess of plasma norepinephrine
- Impaired cardiac output (myocardial infarction, aortic stenosis, arrhythmias)
- Cerebrovascular accident
- Adrenal insufficiency
- Deconditioning
- Carotid sinus hypersensitivity
- Anxiety, panic attacks
- Seizures
- Sepsis
- Idiopathic

WORKUP

- Measure supine blood pressure after the patient has been resting comfortably, stand for 3 min, then measure upright blood pressure. The blood pressure cuff must be held at the level of the right atrium; holding the cuff below this level will result in a 5 to 10 mm Hg underestimation of blood pressure.
- Thorough neurologic examination should be performed.
- Rule out treatable causes (e.g., medications, volume depletion).

LABORATORY TESTS

- Hemoglobin and hematocrit
- Consider when treatable causes of OH have been ruled out:
  - Blood pressure and heart rate monitoring with a tilt table test
  - Plasma norepinephrine measurements (to distinguish postganglionic from preganglionic autonomic dysfunction)
  - Other methods, which use the Valsalva maneuver or measure sweating as indirect means of evaluating the autonomic nervous system

IMAGING STUDIES

None

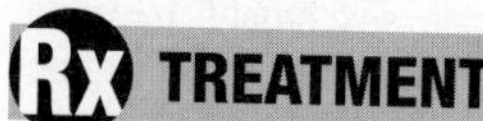

TREATMENT

NONPHARMACOLOGIC THERAPY

- Patient education (leg crossing, prolonged sitting before first standing in the morning, avoid excessive straining and hot baths)
- High-salt diet (e.g., bouillon cubes); caution if history of heart failure
- Liberal fluid intake
- Take needed antihypertensive medications at different times of the day
- Raise the head of the bed at night
- Compression stockings (to include splanchnic circulation)
- Multiple low-carbohydrate meals to avoid postprandial OH
- Avoid large carbohydrate loads and excess alcohol consumption

ACUTE GENERAL Rx

- Correction of volume status
- Review medication list and attempt to eliminate those potentially contributing to OH

CHRONIC Rx

- Fludrocortisone: 0.1 mg/day (may combine with an alpha-1 agonist to lower the dose of each); monitor for electrolyte disturbances and supine hypertension
- Midodrine (alpha-1 agonist): 10 mg three times a day; monitor for supine hypertension
- Erythropoietin (consider if anemic)
- Caffeine (for postprandial hypotension)

OTHER TREATMENTS

- Pyridostigmine (enhances renal sodium reabsorption): 0.2 to 0.6 mg/day (not FDA approved for this indication)
- Octreotide: 300 to 600 mg/day (not FDA-approved for this indication)
- Indomethacin (prostaglandin inhibitor)
- DDAVP (experimental)

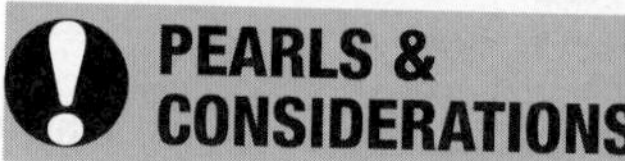

PEARLS & CONSIDERATIONS

COMMENTS

- The presence of OH should always trigger a search for an underlying etiology.
- OH is diagnosed by observing changes in blood pressure, not heart rate.
- Volume depletion should cause an increased heart rate on standing; a lack of heart rate response in this setting suggests autonomic dysfunction.
- Pharmacotherapy with mineralocorticoids may require concomitant potassium replenishment and monitoring for hypertension.

- Evidence to support the efficacy of pharmacologic interventions to treat OH, including midodrine, is limited.
- The etiology of OH is often multifactorial in older patients, but increased susceptibility to volume depletion due to decreased baroreceptor reflexes frequently contributes.
- Evidence suggests that nursing home residents with more stringent SBP control (<140 mm Hg) have a lower risk of OH than nursing home residents with less stringent SBP control.
- The physical examination of patients with dizziness, gait disturbance, and/or falls should include an assessment for OH.
- Because OH may be asymptomatic, physical examination of those at risk must include assessment of blood pressure in both the supine and upright positions.

SUGGESTED READINGS

available at www.expertconsult.com

AUTHOR: **TIMOTHY W. FARRELL, M.D.**

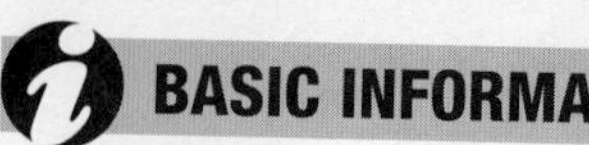

BASIC INFORMATION

DEFINITION

Osgood-Schlatter disease is painful swelling of the growing tibial tuberosity in adolescents.

SYNONYMS

Juvenile osteochondrosis

ICD-9CM CODES
732.4 Osgood-Schlatter disease
ICD-10CM CODES
M92.40 Juvenile osteochondrosis of patella, unspecified knee

EPIDEMIOLOGY & DEMOGRAPHICS

PREVALENCE: 4 cases/100 adolescents
PREDOMINANT SEX: Male/female ratio of 3:1
PREDOMINANT AGE: Males: age 12-15 yr, females: age 8-12 yr

PHYSICAL FINDINGS & CLINICAL PRESENTATION

- Gradual onset of pain and swelling of the tibial tubercle
- Worsening of pain after athletic activity
- Reproduction of pain with resisted knee extension

ETIOLOGY

- Repetitive microtrauma and avulsion of the developing ossification center of the tibial tuberosity
- Anatomic variants such as patella alta

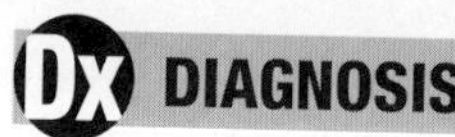

DIAGNOSIS

DIFFERENTIAL DIAGNOSIS

- Stress fracture of the proximal tibia
- Hoffa disease
- Sinding-Larsen-Johansson syndrome
- Patellar tendinitis

WORKUP

- The diagnosis of Osgood-Schlatter disease is generally made on clinical grounds.
- Imaging to exclude fracture or bony tumors.

IMAGING STUDIES

- Lateral x-rays may show separation and fragmentation of the upper tibial epiphysis (Fig. 1-672).
- Musculoskeletal ultrasound can also be used and may be helpful in evaluating soft tissue, tendons, and noncalcified cartilage.

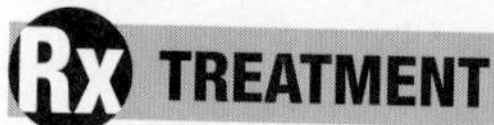

TREATMENT

NONPHARMACOLOGIC THERAPY

- Activity modification with increased periods of rest
- Physical therapy

ACUTE GENERAL Rx

- Ice, especially after exercise
- Nonsteroidal anti-inflammatory drugs
- Quadriceps stretching exercises

DISPOSITION

- Condition usually heals when the epiphysis closes.
- 90% of patients respond to conservative treatment.
- Recent studies have shown promising results with the use of hyperosmolar dextrose injections in recalcitrant disease
- Surgery is rarely needed in the treatment of Osgood-Schlatter disease but can be used for relief of persistent symptoms in which patients have separated ossicles or an abnormally ossified tibial tuberosity.

REFERRAL

Orthopedic consultation is recommended when symptoms persist more than 6 to 8 weeks with conservative treatment.

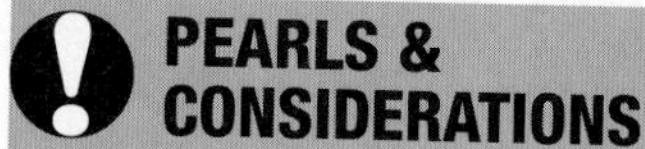

PEARLS & CONSIDERATIONS

COMMENTS

Larsen-Johansson disease is a similar disorder. While the diagnosis of Osgood-Schlatter disease is clinical, imaging should be performed to rule out infection, fracture, and malignancy as causes of unilateral anterior knee pain in adolescents.

SUGGESTED READINGS

available at www.expertconsult.com

RELATED CONTENT

Osgood-Schlatter Disease (Patient Information)

AUTHOR: **AMY L. LUNDHOLM, D.O.**

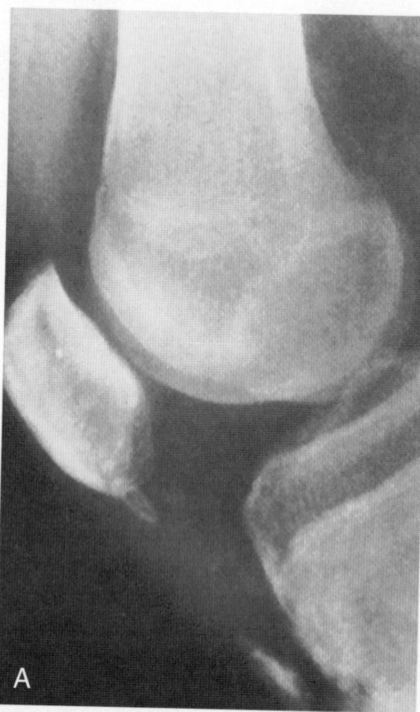

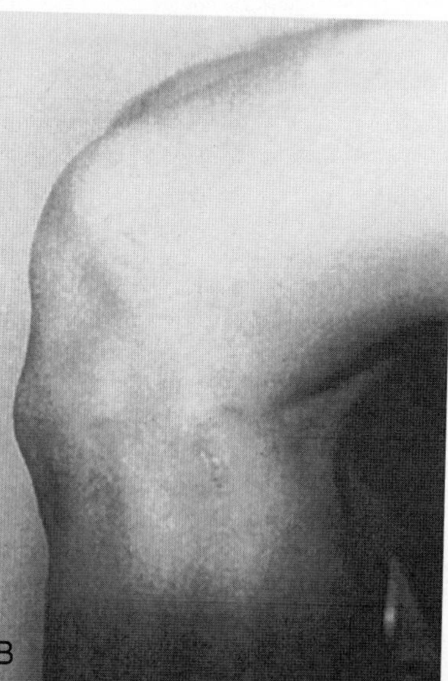

FIGURE 1-672 **A,** Radiograph of Osgood-Schlatter disease demonstrating thickening of patella tendon, fragmentation of the tibial tubercle, and soft tissue swelling. **B,** Clinical picture of bony prominence anteriorly at the tibial tubercle. (From Scuderi G [ed]: *Sports medicine: principles of primary care,* St Louis, 1997, Mosby.)

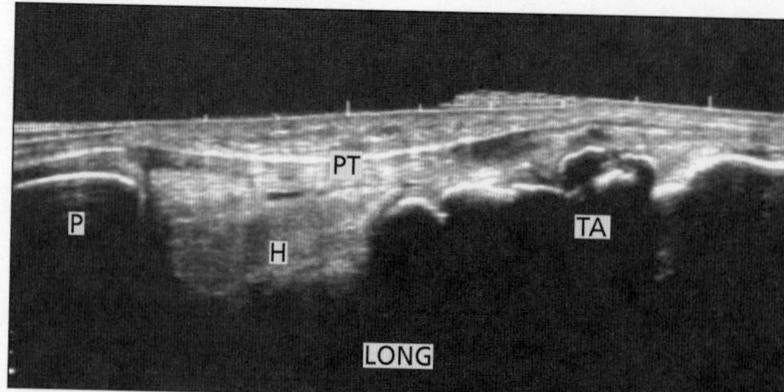

FIGURE 1-673 EFOV of a patient with Osgood-Schlatter disease in the long axis with a knee in extension showing irregularity and fragmentation of the distal tibial apophysis. *P,* Patella; TA, tibial apophysis, PT, patella tendon, H, Hoffa's fat. (From McNally E: *Practical musculoskeletal ultrasound,* ed 1, New York, 2005, Churchill Livingstone, p. 146.)

BASIC INFORMATION

DEFINITION

Osteoarthritis (OA) is a progressive disease of the joint representing failed repair of joint damage that results from intraarticular stresses that may be initiated by abnormalities in articular cartilage, subchondral bone, ligaments, menisci (when present), periarticular muscles, peripheral nerves, or synovium. This ultimately results in the breakdown of cartilage and bone, leading to symptoms of pain, stiffness, and functional disability. As a disease, it is aptly defined as structural abnormalities visualized on plain radiographs and MRI (magnetic resonance imaging), while as an illness, it encompasses a symptom complex of pain, aching, discomfort, stiffness, fatigue, and sleep disturbance that results in functional limitation, physical disability, and reduced health-related quality of life.

SYNONYMS

Degenerative joint disease
Osteoarthrosis
Arthrosis

ICD-9CM CODES
715.0 Osteoarthrosis and allied disorders
ICD-10CM CODES
M15.9 Polyarthrosis, unspecified
M17 Gonarthrosis (arthrosis of knee)
M18 Arthrosis of first metacarpal joint
M19 Other arthrosis
M19.8 Other specified arthrosis
M19.9 Arthrosis, unspecified

EPIDEMIOLOGY & DEMOGRAPHICS

PREVALENCE: 2% to 6% of general population
PREDOMINANT SEX: Females slightly more than males in a 2:1 ratio
PREDOMINANT AGE: >50 yr
GENETICS: 39% to 65% heritability rate in twin studies of women who have generalized OA, concordance rate of 0.64 in monozygotic twins.
RISK FACTORS: Nonmodifiable are age, female gender, hormonal status, geographic, genetic, and presence of congenital or developmental conditions. Modifiable risk factors such as obesity, smoking, high bone density, nutritional deficiencies such as vitamin D deficiency, and presence of crystal arthropathies such as gout. Local factors are trauma during physical activities, type of occupation, muscle strength, anatomic malalignment of the lower extremities, as well as biomechanical factors such as knee laxity, leg length discrepancy, and proprioceptive deficits.

PHYSICAL FINDINGS & CLINICAL PRESENTATION

- Similar symptoms in most forms: stiffness, pain, crepitus
- Joint tenderness, swelling
- Decreased range of motion
- Crepitus with motion
- Bouchard's nodes: bony enlargement on the proximal interphalangeal (PIP) joints of the hand
- Heberden's nodes: bony enlargement of the distal interphalangeal (DIP) joints of the hand (Fig. 1-675)
- Pain with range of motion

ETIOLOGY

- Primary or idiopathic OA can be mono-, oligo-, or polyarticular.
- Secondary OA is due to an identifiable condition such as trauma, type of occupation, developmental, mechanical, metabolic, and inflammatory conditions.

DIAGNOSIS

DIFFERENTIAL DIAGNOSIS

- Bursitis, tendinitis
- Inflammatory arthritides
- Infectious arthritis
- Crystal arthropathies such as gout and pseudogout
- Rheumatoid arthritis (Fig. 1-676)

WORKUP

- No diagnostic test exists for degenerative joint disease.
- Laboratory evaluation is normal.
- Rheumatoid factor, erythrocyte sedimentation rate, complete blood count, and antinuclear antibody tests may be required if inflammatory component is suggested by history.
- Arthrocentesis of swollen joints: synovial fluid examination is generally normal or noninflammatory in character.

IMAGING STUDIES

- Plain x-ray of the involved joints is the first step and usually of high diagnostic value.
- Roentgenographic evaluation (Fig. 1-677) reveals:
  1. Joint space narrowing
  2. Subchondral sclerosis
  3. New bone formation in the form of osteophytes

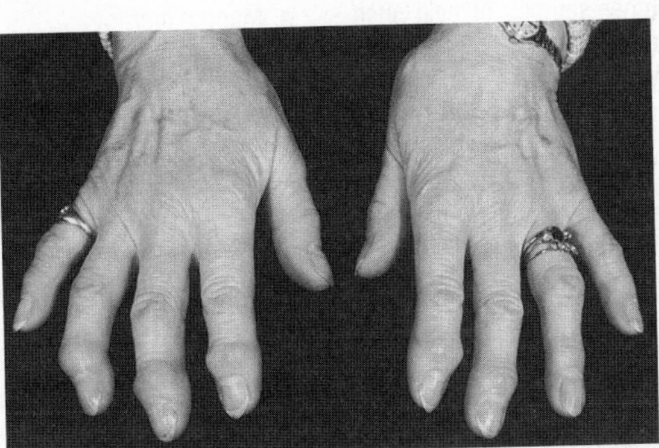

FIGURE 1-675 Osteoarthritis of the distal interphalangeal (DIP) joints. This patient has the typical clinical findings of advanced osteoarthritis of the DIP joints, including large, firm swellings (Heberden's nodes), some of which are tender and red because of associated inflammation of the periarticular tissues and the joint. (From Klippel J et al [eds]: *Primary care rheumatology,* London, 1999, Mosby.)

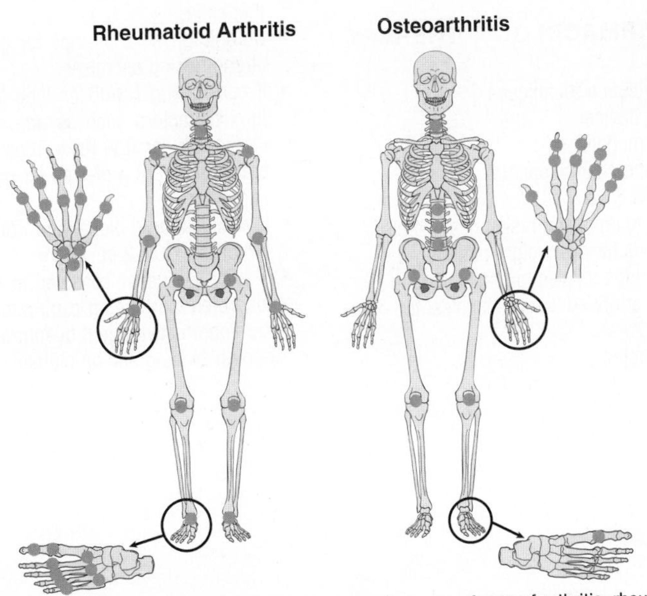

FIGURE 1-676 Distribution of involved joints in the two most common forms of arthritis: rheumatoid arthritis and osteoarthritis. *Shaded circles* are shown over the involved joint areas. (From Goldman L, Schafer AI: *Goldman's Cecil medicine,* ed 24, Philadelphia, 2012, Saunders.)

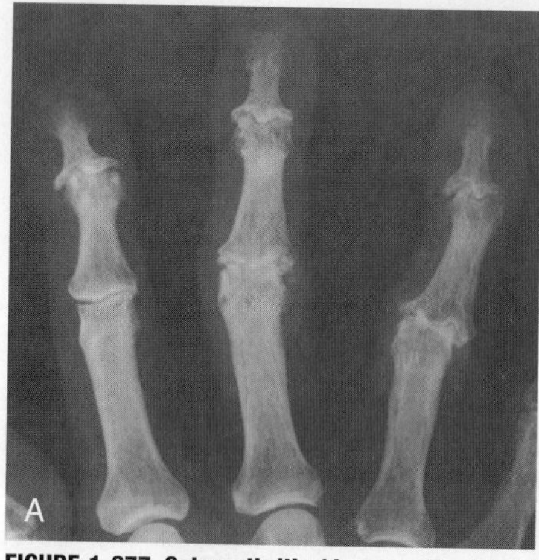

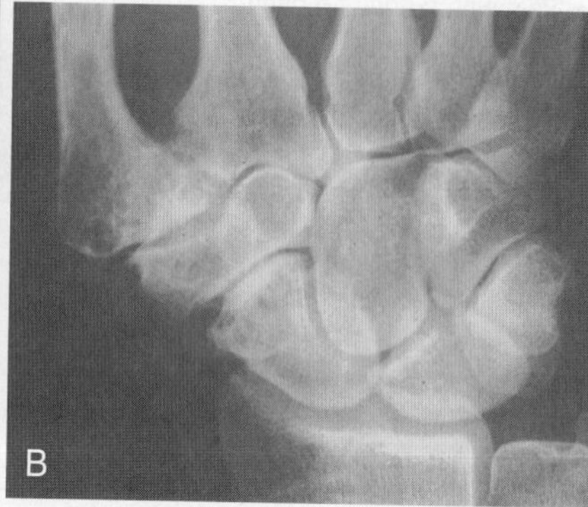

FIGURE 1-677 Osteoarthritis (degenerative joint disease). A, Primary osteoarthritis of the fingers with characteristic cartilage loss, deviations, and spurs of the proximal (Bouchard's nodes) and distal (Heberden's nodes) interphalangeal joints. **B,** Primary osteoarthritis of the carpus showing characteristic involvement of the radial side with cartilage loss, subchondral sclerosis, and small spur formation from the base of the first metacarpal to the distal articular surface of the scaphoid. (From Grainger RG, Allison D: *Grainger & Allison's diagnostic radiology, a textbook of medical imaging,* ed 4, London, 2001, Churchill Livingstone.)

- MRI can detect other sources of pain such as synovial thickening, effusions, bone marrow edema, bony attrition, and periarticular lesions.
- Musculoskeletal ultrasound (MSKUS) is emerging as an alternative, fast, and inexpensive modality to identify joint damage, presence of osteophytes, effusions, and noninflammatory synovial proliferation identified using Doppler studies. This is otherwise operator-dependent.

Rx TREATMENT

- Optimal use of both pharmacologic and nonpharmacologic measures. Fig. E1-678 describes an algorithm for the management of OA.
- Education and reassurance

NONPHARMACOLOGIC THERAPY

HAND OA

- Joint protection techniques
- Assistive devices
- Thermal modalities
- Trapeziometacarpal splints

HIP AND KNEE OA

- Aerobic, aquatic, and resistance exercises
- Weight loss for overweight patients
- Medial wedge insoles for valgus knee
- Subtalar strapped lateral insoles for varus knees
- Patellar taping
- Manual therapy
- Assistive devices such as canes or walkers
- Thermal agents
- Tai chi

ACUTE GENERAL Rx/ PHARMACOLOGIC Rx

- Rest and ice
- Acetaminophen recommended for mild to moderate pain
- May add weak opioids such as tramadol
- Oral and topical NSAIDs. Capsaicin may be used.
- Arthrocentesis of the acutely swollen joint followed by intraarticular steroid injection
- Duloxetine, tramadol if above initial treatment fails
- Opioid analgesics recommended only for severe pain unresponsive to other treatment modalities
- Chronic physical therapy for gentle assisted strengthening exercises
- If considering NSAID as long term, evaluate for risk factors such as age, GI bleed, and cardiovascular (CV) risks. Topical rather than oral NSAIDs are preferred for patients age 75 and older.
- If with risk for GI bleed (age <60 yr), may add PPI or use COX-2 inhibitors
- If with CV risks, consider using naproxen. Ibuprofen may render aspirin ineffective as a cardioprotective agent by interfering with the aspirin-binding site on platelets.
- Nutritional supplements (glucosamine and chondroitin) are unproven. Trials have shown that neither glucosamine sulfate or glucosamine hydrochloride reduces pain compared with placebo in knee or hip osteoarthritis.
- Use of intraarticular hyaluronan injection is controversial. A recent trial in patients with knee OA found viscosupplementation associated with a small and clinically irrelevant benefit and an increased risk for serious adverse events.

DISPOSITION

Progression is not always inevitable, and the prognosis is variable depending on the site and extent of the disease.

REFERRAL

Surgical consultation for patients not responding to nonpharmacologic and pharmacologic management

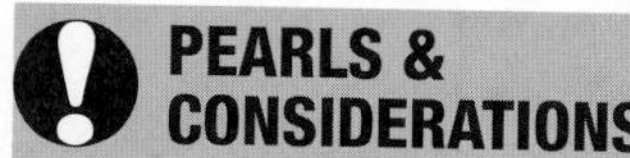

PEARLS & CONSIDERATIONS

COMMENTS

Surgical intervention is generally helpful in degenerative joint disease. Arthroplasty, arthrodesis, and realignment osteotomy are the most common procedures performed. Arthroscopic debridement (of the knee) appears to be of questionable value. In patients needing hip arthroplasty, resurfacing hip arthroplasty (in which the femoral head is resurfaced with a cap and the neck is preserved) is increasingly popular among younger patients because it results in more hip movement and allows total hip arthroplasty later in the patient's life if necessary.

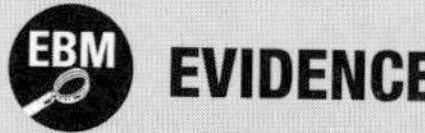

EVIDENCE

available at www.expertconsult.com

SUGGESTED READINGS

available at www.expertconsult.com

RELATED CONTENT

Osteoarthritis (Patient Information)

AUTHOR: **CRISOSTOMO R. BALIOG, JR, M.D.**

BASIC INFORMATION

DEFINITION

Osteochondritis dissecans (OCD) refers to a localized necrosis of the bone with detachment of the overlying subchondral bone and cartilage. The suffix "-itis" is a misnomer, as the disease does not involve inflammation.

SYNONYMS

Osteochondrosis

Avascular necrosis (AVN), aseptic necrosis, ischemic necrosis—AVN and OCD have the same pathophysiology; AVN is a more generic term, whereas OCD is used specifically when a detached fragment of bone and/or cartilage is seen on imaging.

ICD-9CM CODE

732.7 Osteochondritis dissecans

ICD-10CM CODES

M93.20 Osteochondritis dissecans of unspecified site

ETIOLOGY & PATHOPHYSIOLOGY

- While the cause remains unknown, predisposing factors have been identified, including genetic predisposition, repetitive microtrauma, and single trauma followed by bone ischemia. The sequence of events likely entails bone injury, hypovascularization with defective repair, bone necrosis with structural collapse, and detachment of the overlying subchondral bone and cartilage.
- OCD is seen more often in children and adolescents and is more commonly associated with repetitive trauma and sports.

EPIDEMIOLOGY & DEMOGRAPHICS

PREVALENCE: 2 cases/10,000 persons

PREDOMINANT SEX: Male/female ratio of 3:1

PREDOMINANT AGE: Typically between 10 and 20 years of age

CLINICAL PRESENTATION & PHYSICAL FINDINGS

- OCD most commonly affects the knee (75%) followed by the elbow (6%) and the ankle (4%); the other joints are affected in 15% of cases.
- Early lesions cause nonspecific pain with activity.
- As the disease progresses, stiffness and intermittent swelling occurs.
- Range of motion is usually intact in the knees.
- If a loose fragment becomes detached, it can cause locking or catching.
- Physical exam reveals tenderness at the site of the lesion; crepitus may also be present.
- When the knee is involved, a positive Wilson sign can sometimes be found (pain with knee extension and internal rotation); antalgic gait and limp can occur in chronic cases.
- Rare asymptomatic cases have been reported.

DIAGNOSIS

DIFFERENTIAL DIAGNOSIS

- Knee: torn meniscus, patellofemoral syndrome, medial plica syndrome, stress fracture
- Elbow: Panner's disease, Little League elbow, epicondyle fracture, epicondilitis
- Talus: ankle sprain, os trigonum tarsal coalition

IMAGING STUDIES

- X-rays including "tunnel views" are the initial test of choice.
- Early, small lesions can look normal or show only increased subchondral bone density.
- The defining lesion of OCD is seen on x-ray as a subchondral bone fragment surrounded by a radiolucent, crescent-shaped line (Fig. 1-679).
- MRI (Fig. 1-680) is the most sensitive test (91%) and is useful to identify OCD in symptomatic patients with normal x-rays.
- Contrast is used to evaluate blood supply to the affected fragment, evaluating stability.

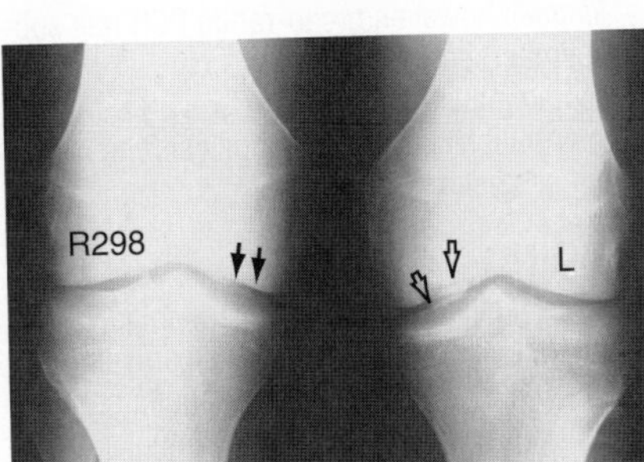

FIGURE 1-679 Bilateral, asymmetrical osteochondritis dissecans with a healed right lesion *(black arrows)* and an unhealed, unstable left lesion *(open arrows)* in a 17-year-old tennis player. (From DeLee D, Drez D [eds]: *DeLee and Drez's orthopaedic sports medicine,* ed 2, Philadelphia, 2003, Saunders.)

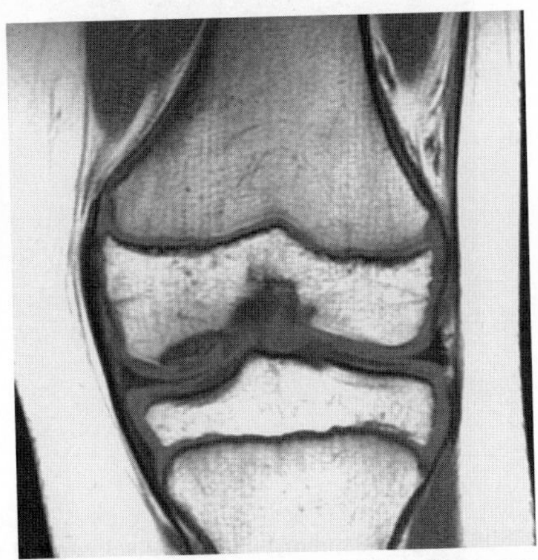

FIGURE 1-680 Osteochondritis dissecans (OCD). A coronal MRI of an OCD lesion of the medial femoral condyle. (From Frontera WR: *Clinical sports medicine: medical management and rehabilitation,* Philadelphia, 2006, Saunders.)

TREATMENT

ACUTE GENERAL Rx

- Conservative management: usually indicated in juvenile OCD without an intraarticular foreign body and for adult patients who have a small, stable fragment
- Non–weight bearing and immobilization for 4-6 wk; physical therapy once healing starts
- Surgery: indicated for juvenile OCD with a loose body and in cases that fail to improve after 4-6 mo of conservative management; also indicated in adults with OCD

DISPOSITION & PROGNOSIS

- Office follow-ups are initially frequent, every 2 wk.
- X-ray changes should be monitored every 6 wk while immobilized.
- Once bone healing has been seen on x-rays, follow-ups can be spaced every 3 mo.
- Return to activity can be attempted once the patient is pain free and has an intact active full range of motion; it usually takes from 3 to 6 mo.
- Once complete healing occurs, joint function usually returns to normal.
- Complete healing is frequent in skeletally immature children with small lesions (95%), but in adults with larger lesions complete healing is less common (50%).

REFERRAL

- Orthopedic consultation is helpful in most symptomatic children and adults with OCD for staging and management options.
- Surgical options include arthroscopic drilling, fixation with Kirschner wires, special screws, and chondrocyte transplantation.

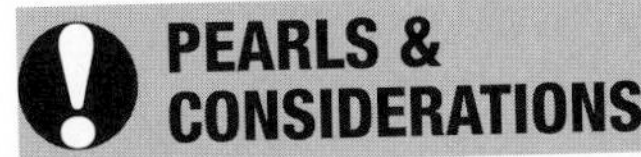

PEARLS & CONSIDERATIONS

COMMENTS

- Although inflammation is suggested by the name, it has not been shown to be of significance in this disorder. *Osteochondral lesion* or *osteochondrosis dissecans* may be more appropriate terms to describe these disorders.
- Repetitive trauma with ischemic necrosis is the most likely cause.
- The condition is often bilateral, especially in the knee, which could suggest the possibility of an endocrine or genetic basis.
- This condition should always be considered in the patient whose "sprained ankle" does not improve over the usual course of treatment.

SUGGESTED READINGS

available at www.expertconsult.com

RELATED CONTENT

Osteochondritis Dissecans (Patient Information)

AUTHOR: **DAN A. CRISTESCU, M.D.**

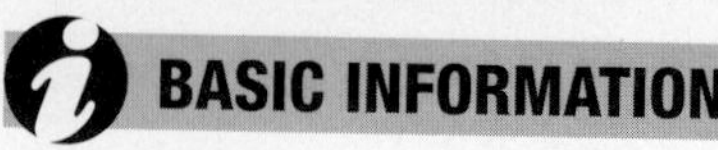

BASIC INFORMATION

DEFINITION

Osteomyelitis is an acute or chronic infection of the bone secondary to the hematogenous or contiguous source of infection or direct traumatic inoculation, which is usually bacterial.

SYNONYMS

Bone infection

ICD-9CM CODES
730.1 Chronic osteomyelitis
730.2 Acute or subacute osteomyelitis
ICD-10CM CODES
M86 Osteomyelitis
M86.0 Acute hematogenous osteomyelitis
M86.1 Other acute osteomyelitis
M86.2 Subacute osteomyelitis
M86.3 Chronic multifocal osteomyelitis
M86.6 Other chronic osteomyelitis
M86.9 Osteomyelitis, unspecified

EPIDEMIOLOGY & DEMOGRAPHICS

PREDOMINANT SEX: Male > female
PREDOMINANT AGE: All ages

PHYSICAL FINDINGS & CLINICAL PRESENTATION

HEMATOGENOUS OSTEOMYELITIS:
- Usually occurs in tibia/fibula (children)
- Localized inflammation: often secondary to trauma with accompanying hematoma or cellulitis
- Abrupt fever
- Lethargy
- Irritability
- Pain in involved bone

VERTEBRAL OSTEOMYELITIS:
- Usually hematogenous
- Fever: 50%
- Localized pain/tenderness. Back pain is the most common initial symptom (86% of cases)
- Neurologic defects: motor/sensory (sensory loss, weakness, radiculopathy)

CONTIGUOUS OSTEOMYELITIS:
- Direct inoculation
- Associated with trauma, fractures, surgical fixation
- Chronic infection of skin/soft tissue
- Fever, drainage from surgical site

CHRONIC OSTEOMYELITIS:
- Bone pain
- Sinus tract drainage, nonhealing ulcer
- Chronic low-grade fever
- Chronic localized pain

ETIOLOGY

- *Staphylococcus aureus*
- *S. aureus* (methicillin-resistant)
- *Pseudomonas aeruginosa*
- Enterobacteriaceae
- *Streptococcus pyogenes*
- *Enterococcus*
- Mycobacteria
- Fungi
- Coagulase-negative staphylococci
- *Salmonella* (in sickle cell disease)

Dx DIAGNOSIS

DIFFERENTIAL DIAGNOSIS

- Gaucher's disease
- Bone infarction
- Charcot's joint
- Fracture

WORKUP

- ESR, C-reactive protein
- Blood culturing
- Bone culture. A culture of a biopsy specimen has a significantly higher overall diagnostic yield than does a blood culture. Bone samples should be cultured for aerobic and anaerobic bacteria and for fungi
- Pathologic evaluation of bone biopsy for acute/chronic changes consistent with necrosis or acute inflammation
- PCR analysis of specimens obtained by means of biopsy or puncture may be useful for organisms that are difficult to identify (anaerobic bacteria, *Bartonella* sp., *Kingella kingae*); however, broad-range PCR has suboptimal sensitivity and specificity due to contamination and may not provide sufficient information on the susceptibility of the microorganisms to antibiotics

IMAGING STUDIES

- Bone radiograph examination: initial study but not sensitive in early osteomyelitis as may not show changes for as much as 2 wk
- MRI (Fig. 1-681): most accurate imaging study. CT only if patient has contraindication to MRI
- Triple-phase technetium-99m bone scan (Fig. 1-682). Typically positive within a few days after onset of symptoms but accuracy is lower than that of MRI
- Gallium scan (Ga-67) scintigraphy with single-photon emission CT (SPECT) has higher accuracy than bone scan but is less sensitive for detection of epidural abscess in vertebral osteomyelitis
- Indium-111–labeled leukocyte scintigraphy scan; low sensitivity (<20%) for vertebral osteomyelitis
- Positron-emission tomography (PET) scanning with ^{18}F-fluorodeoxyglucose has high accuracy (similar to MRI) and is useful in patients with metallic implants

Rx TREATMENT

- Surgical debridement in biopsy-positive cases will guide direction for antibiotic therapy. This will vary with type of osteomyelitis. Duration of therapy is usually 6 wk for acute osteomyelitis; chronic osteomyelitis may need a longer course of medication
- *S. aureus:* cefazolin IV, nafcillin IV, vancomycin IV (in patient allergic to penicillin)
- *S. aureus* (methicillin resistant): vancomycin IV, linezolid, daptomycin, or tigecycline
- *Streptococcus* spp.: ceftriaxone, IV penicillin G in sensitive species
- *P. aeruginosa:* cefepime plus ciprofloxacin, piperacillin/tazobactam plus ciprofloxacin, or imipenem/cilastatin plus aminoglycoside
- Enterobacteriaceae quinolone-susceptible: fluoroquinolone or ceftriaxone
- Enterobacteriaceae quinolone-resistant: carbapenem (such as imipenem, meropenem, or doripenem)

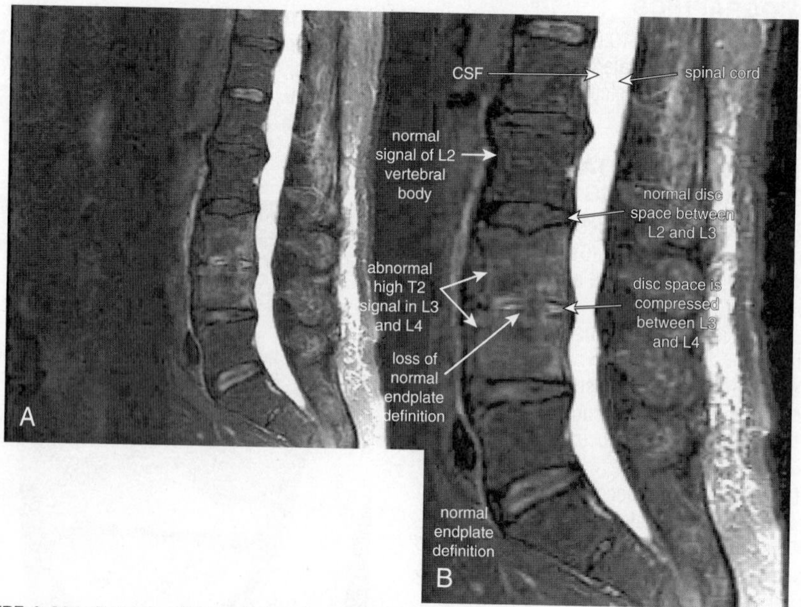

FIGURE 1-681 Osteomyelitis and discitis of L3 and L4. A, T2-weighted fast spin–echo magnetic resonance imaging without contrast demonstrates typical findings of vertebral osteomyelitis and discitis. **B,** Close-up. The inferior endplate of L3 and the superior endplate of L4 are abnormal and ill-defined. The L3 and L4 vertebral bodies show a high T2 signal, indicating an abnormally high fluid content. In comparison, L2 shows a normal marrow signal and appears dark gray due to a normal fat signal. *CSF,* Cerebrospinal fluid. (From Broder JS: *Diagnostic imaging for the emergency physician,* Philadelphia, 2011, Saunders.)

- Anaerobes: clindamycin, ticarcillin clavulanate, cefotetan, or metronidazole
- Table 1-367 summarizes antimicrobial therapy for selected microorganisms in osteomyelitis
- Hyperbaric oxygen therapy: may be useful in chronic osteomyelitis
- Surgical debridement of all devitalized bone and tissue
- Immobilization of affected bone (plaster, traction) if bone is unstable

DISPOSITION

Acute hematogenous osteomyelitis usually resolves without recurrence or long-term complications, but contiguous focus osteomyelitis, bone infections from open fractures, or osteomyelitis frequently recurs.

REFERRAL

- To an orthopedic surgeon if chronic osteomyelitis with need for bone debridement, bone grafting, or stabilization of infected tissue adjacent to a bone fracture
- To an infectious disease specialist for appropriate treatment for difficult-to-treat or recalcitrant infections
- To a hyperbaric oxygen chamber service for nonhealing, chronic osteomyelitis

PEARLS & CONSIDERATIONS

Chronic osteomyelitis is one of the most challenging infections to treat; the high failure rate is a consequence of poor vascular supply, nondistensible bone tissue, and limited penetration of bone tissue.

SUGGESTED READINGS

available at www.expertconsult.com

RELATED CONTENT

Osteomyelitis (Patient Information)

AUTHOR: **GLENN G. FORT, M.D., M.P.H.**

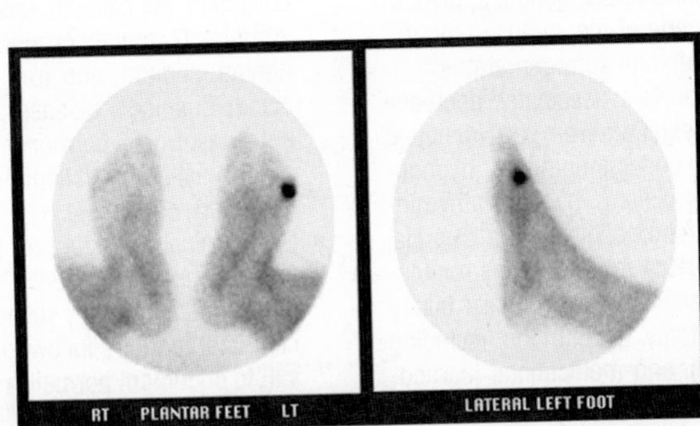

FIGURE 1-682 Osteomyelitis. Intense accumulation of Tc-99m WBCs in proximal phalanx of fifth digit of left foot at 4 hr after injection. (From Specht N [ed]: *Practical guide to diagnostic imaging,* St Louis, 1998, Mosby.)

TABLE 1-367 Antimicrobial Therapy for Selected Microorganisms in Osteomyelitis or Septic Arthritis in Adults

Microorganism	First Choice*	Alternative Choice
Methicillin/oxacillin/nafcillin-sensitive staphylococci	Nafcillin sodium or oxacillin sodium 1.5-2 g IV q4-6h for 4-6 wk *or* cefazolin 1-2 g IV q8h	Vancomycin 15 mg/kg IV q12h for 4-6 wk
Methicillin/oxacillin/nafcillin-resistant staphylococci (MRSA)	Vancomycin† 15 mg/kg IV q12h *or* daptomycin 6 mg/kg IV q24h	Linezolid 600 mg PO/IV q12h *or* levofloxacin† 500-750 mg PO/IV daily
Penicillin-sensitive streptococci	Aqueous penicillin G 20 × 10^6 U/24 hr IV either continuously or in six equally divided daily doses *or* ceftriaxone 1-2 g IV q24h *or* cefazolin 1-2 g IV q8h	Vancomycin 15 mg/kg IV q12h
Enterococci	Aqueous crystalline penicillin G 20 × 10^6 U/24 hr IV either continuously or in six equally divided daily doses *or* ampicillin sodium 12 g/24 hr IV either continuously or in six equally divided daily doses; the addition of gentamicin sulfate 1 mg/kg IV or IM q8h for 1-2 wk is *optional*	Vancomycin† 15 mg/kg IV q12h; the addition of gentamicin sulfate 1 mg/kg IV or IM q8h for 1-2 wk is *optional*
Enterobacteriaceae, quinolone resistant	Ticarcillin clavulanate, 3.1 g IV q4h or piperacillin/tazobactam, 3.375 g IV q6h	Ceftriaxone 1-2 g IV q24h
Pseudomonas aeruginosa	Cefepime 2 g IV q12h plus ciprofloxacin 400 mg IV q8-12h	Imipenem/cilastatin 1 g IV q8h, plus aminoglycoside

*Antimicrobial selection should be based on in vitro sensitivity data, as well as allergies, intolerances, and drug interactions in individual patients.
†Doses shown are based on normal renal and hepatic function and may need to be adjusted or serum levels monitored (vancomycin).
MRSA, Methicillin-resistant *Staphylococcus aureus.*
Adapted from Berbari EF et al: Osteomyelitis. In Mandell GL et al (eds): *Mandell, Douglas, and Bennett's principles and practice of infectious diseases,* ed 7, Philadelphia, 2010, Churchill Livingstone.

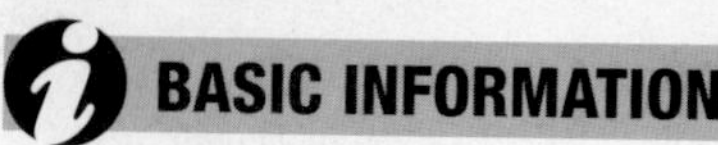

DEFINITION

Osteoporosis is characterized by a progressive decrease in bone mass that results in increased bone fragility and a higher fracture risk. The various types are as follows:

PRIMARY OSTEOPOROSIS: Affects 80% of women and 60% of men with osteoporosis.

- Idiopathic osteoporosis: unknown pathogenesis; may occur in children and young adults
- Type I osteoporosis: may occur in postmenopausal women (ages 51 to 75); characterized by accelerated and disproportionate trabecular bone loss and associated with vertebral body and distal forearm fractures (estrogen withdrawal effect)
- Type II osteoporosis (involutional): occurs in both men and women aged >70 yr; characterized by both trabecular and cortical bone loss and associated with fractures of the proximal humerus and tibia, femoral neck, and pelvis

SECONDARY OSTEOPOROSIS: Affects 20% of women and 40% of men with osteoporosis; osteoporosis that exists as a common feature of another disease process, heritable disorder of connective tissue, or drug side effect (see "Differential Diagnosis")

ICD-9CM CODES
733.0 Osteoporosis
ICD-10CM CODES
M81.0 Age-related osteoporosis without current pathological fracture
M81.4 Drug-induced osteoporosis
M81.5 Idiopathic osteoporosis
M81.6 Localized osteoporosis

EPIDEMIOLOGY & DEMOGRAPHICS

PREVALENCE (IN U.S.):

- <25 million men and women
- Twice as common in women
- Results in 1.5 million fractures annually (70% women)
- Osteoporosis-related fractures in 50% of women and 20% of men aged >65 yr
- Results: institutionalization, death, and costs in excess of $10 billion annually

RISK FACTORS:

- Age: each decade after 40 yr associated with a fivefold increased risk
- Genetics:
  1. Ethnicity (white/Asian are affected more often than blacks, with Polynesians affected the least)
  2. Gender (females affected more often than males)
  3. Family history (hip fracture in first-degree relative)
- Environmental factors: poor nutrition, calcium deficiency, physical inactivity, medication (chronic corticosteroid use [>3 mo], PPIs, aromatase inhibitors, anticonvulsants, anticoagulants, SSRIs), tobacco use, alcohol use (>3 drinks/day), traumatic injury, high caffeine intake
- Chronic disease states: estrogen deficiency, androgen deficiency, hyperthyroidism, inflammatory bowel disease, diabetes mellitus, hypercortisolism, cirrhosis, malabsorption, gastrectomy, multiple myeloma

PHYSICAL FINDINGS & CLINICAL PRESENTATION

- Most commonly silent with no signs and symptoms
- Insidious and progressive development of dorsal kyphosis ***(dowager's hump),*** loss of height, and skeletal pain typically associated with fracture; other physical findings related to other conditions with associated increased risk for osteoporosis (see "Risk Factors")

ETIOLOGY

- Primary osteoporosis: multifactorial, resulting from a combination of factors including nutrition, peak bone mass, genetics, level of physical activity, age of menopause (spontaneous vs. surgical), and estrogen status
- Secondary osteoporosis: associated decrease in bone mass resulting from an identified cause, including endocrinopathies, hypogonadism, hyperthyroidism, hyperparathyroidism, Cushing's syndrome, hyperprolactinemia, acromegaly, diabetes mellitus, gastrointestinal disease, malabsorption, primary biliary cirrhosis, gastrectomy, malnutrition (including anorexia nervosa), and medications (corticosteroids, PPIs, rosiglitazone, pioglitazone)

Dx DIAGNOSIS

DIFFERENTIAL DIAGNOSIS

- Malignancy (multiple myeloma, lymphoma, leukemia, metastatic carcinoma)
- Primary hyperparathyroidism
- Osteomalacia
- Paget's disease
- Osteogenesis imperfecta: types I, III, and IV (see also "Epidemiology & Demographics" and "Etiology")

WORKUP

- History and physical examination (20% of women with type I osteoporosis have associated secondary cause), with appropriate evaluation for identified risk factors and secondary causes
- Diagnosis of osteoporosis made by bone mineral density (BMD) determination (BMD should ideally evaluate the hip, spine, and wrist)
  - Dual-energy x-ray absorptiometry (DEXA) is the gold standard for screening and monitoring changes in BMD due to excellent precision, widespread availability, low cost, and minimal radiation exposure. DEXA is indicated in all women 65 years and older and in postmenopausal women younger than 65 years of age who are at risk for fracture (e.g., weight <127 lbs, parental history of hip fracture, use of medications that cause bone loss, smoking, alcoholism, rheumatoid arthritis, or presence of diseases that cause bone loss).
- Recommendations as to when to repeat bone density testing should be based on initial T scores. Data from the Study of Osteoporotic Fractures indicates that in women with normal bone density or mild osteopenia, repeat testing might not be necessary for another 10-15 yr. For women with moderate osteopenia, a screening interval of 3-5 yr may be appropriate. Annual testing may be indicated for women with advanced osteopenia.

LABORATORY TESTS

- Biochemical profile to evaluate renal and hepatic function, primary hyperparathyroidism, and malnutrition
- CBC: for nutritional status and myeloma
- TSH to rule out the presence of hyperthyroidism
- Vitamin D level. Consideration of 24-hr urine collection for calcium (excess skeletal loss, vitamin D malabsorption/deficiency), creatinine, sodium, and free cortisol (to detect occult Cushing's disease); no need to measure calcitropic hormones (parathyroid hormone, calcitriol, calcitonin) unless specifically indicated
- Biochemical markers of bone remodeling; may be useful to predict rate of bone loss and/or follow therapy response; specific biochemical markers followed (e.g., 3-mo interval) to document normalization as a response to therapy
  1. High-turnover osteoporosis: high levels of resorption markers (lysyl pyridinoline, deoxy lysyl pyridinoline, n-telopeptide of collagen cross-links, C-telopeptide of collagen cross-links) and formation markers (osteocalcin, bone-specific alkaline phosphatase, carboxy-terminal extension peptide of type I procollagen); accelerated bone loss responding best to antiresorptive therapy
  2. Low-normal-turnover osteoporosis: normal or low levels of the markers of resorption and formation (see "high turnover osteoporosis" listed previously); no accelerated bone loss; responds best to drugs that enhance bone formation

IMAGING STUDIES

- BMD determination (see "Workup") should be performed on all women with determined risk factors and/or associated secondary causes; criteria for diagnosis of osteoporosis based on measurement of bone density and T score equivalent cut points are summarized in Table 1-368 and Fig. E1-683.
  1. Normal: BMD <1 SD of the young adult reference mean
  2. Osteopenia: BMD 1 to 2.5 SD below the young adult reference mean
  3. Osteoporosis: BMD >2.5 SD below the young adult reference mean
- For patient undergoing treatment: annual BMD to follow response to therapy
- X-ray exam of appropriate part of skeleton to evaluate clinical osteoporotic fracture only

TABLE 1-368 1994 WHO Criteria for the Diagnosis of Osteoporosis Based on the Measurement of Bone Density and T Score Equivalent Cut Points

Diagnostic Category	Standard Deviations Below the Young-Adult Mean	T Score
Normal	≤1 SD	Equal to or better than −1
Osteopenia (low bone mass)	Between 1 and 2.5 SD	Between −1 and −2.5
Osteoporosis	≥2.5 SD	Equal to or poorer than −2.5
Severe (established) osteoporosis	≥2.5 SD + a fragility fracture	Equal to or poorer than −2.5 + a fragility fracture

From Hochberg MC et al: *Rheumatology,* ed 5, St Louis, 2011, Mosby.

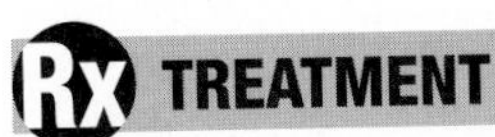

TREATMENT

NONPHARMACOLOGIC THERAPY

Prevention:

- Identification and minimization of risk factors
- Appropriate diagnosis and treatment of secondary causes
- Behavioral modification: proper nutrition, physical activity, fracture prevention strategies

ACUTE GENERAL Rx

- Vitamin D supplement: 600 IU/day for persons 19 to 70 years of age and 800 IU/day for persons 71 years and older
- Calcium supplement: The recommended dietary intake of calcium for women 19 to 50 years of age and men 19 to 70 years of age is 1000 mg/day; women older than age 50 and men older than age 70 require 1200 mg/day. Calcium intake above 25000 mg/day (2000 mg/day in persons >50 years of age) should be avoided. Consumption of calcium-rich foods and beverages is the preferred approach to ensuring adequate calcium intake.[1]
- Oral bisphosphonates (ibandronate, alendronate, risendronate): they decrease bone resorption by attenuating osteoclast activity. They are first-line therapy for the treatment of most patients with osteoporosis, with proven efficacy to reduce fracture risk. Ibandronate is given 150 mg once monthly, swallowed whole with 8 oz water on empty stomach, with no oral intake for at least 60 min. Do not lie down for 60 min after dose. Alendronate is given 70 mg once weekly on awakening, with 8 oz water on empty stomach, with no oral intake for at least 30 min. Use 70-mg dose for treatment of postmenopausal osteoporosis and a 35-mg tablet for the prevention of osteoporosis in postmenopausal women. Risedronate is given 35 mg once weekly or 75 mg taken on 2 consecutive days per month on awakening, with 8 oz water on empty stomach, with no oral intake for at least 30 min.
- Raloxifene: 60 mg qd. Selective estrogen-receptor moderator, it has suppressive effects on osteoclast and bone resorption.
- Zoledronic acid: a bisphosphonate given by IV infusion over at least 15 min, 5 mg once/year
- Teriparatide is a recombinant human parathyroid hormone used for postmenopausal women with osteoporosis who are at high risk for fracture. It is also used in men with primary or hypogonadal osteoporosis who are at high risk of fracture. It is administered by injection 20 mcg qd SQ into the thigh or abdominal wall. Use for >2 yr not recommended. It stimulates bone formation and reduces the risk of fracture but may increase the risk of stroke in older women with osteoporosis.
- Denosumab is a human monoclonal antibody that decreases bone resorption by inhibiting the formation and activity of osteoclasts. It was recently approved for treatment of postmenopausal osteoporosis. Dosage is 60 mg subcutaneously every 6 months. Cost of 1 yr of therapy is approximately $2000. Recent trials[2] have also shown that the monoclonal antibody romosozumab can also increase bone mineral density and bone formation and decrease bone resorption.
- Other FDA-approved drugs (without osteoporosis indication) used to treat osteoporosis:
  1. Calcitriol
  2. Etidronate
  3. Thiazide
- Estrogen (conjugated equine estrogen or equivalent): 0.3 to 0.625 mg/day
- Progestin: continuous (e.g., 2.5 mg medroxyprogesterone acetate/day or equivalent) or cyclic (e.g., 10 mg medroxyprogesterone acetate days for 10 days each mo or equivalent) coadministered in women with a uterus in place.
- Combination estrogen/alendronate or estrogen-progestin/alendronate may be considered in individualized patients on hormone replacement therapy with identified osteoporosis. BMD baseline obtained before onset of therapy and at 1 yr; decrease of 2% or greater results in dosage adjustment or medication change.
- A recent trial on the effects of lasofoxifene on the risk of fractures showed that in postmenopausal women with osteoporosis, lasofoxifene (0.5 mg/day) decreased risk of vertebral and nonvertebral fractures. It also lowered the risk of ER-positive breast cancer, coronary heart disease, and stroke but it increased the risk of venous thromboembolic events.
- Baseline biochemical markers of remodeling baseline considered; identified high-turnover osteoporosis patients rescreened at 3 mo to document marker return to normal

[1]Bauer DC: Calcium supplements and fracture prevention, *N Engl J Med* 369:1537-1543, 2013.

[2]McClung MR et al: Romosozumab in postmenopausal women with low bone mineral density, *N Engl J Med* 370:412-420, 2014.

CHRONIC Rx

- Lifelong disorder requiring lifelong attention to behavior modification issues (nutrition, physical activity, fracture prevention strategies) and compliance with pharmacologic intervention. There is little evidence to guide physicians about long-term bisphosphonate therapy. Evidence is accumulating that the risk of atypical fracture of the femur increases after 5 years of bisphosphonate use. It is reasonable to stop bisphosphonates at 3 to 5 yr in women at the lowest risk (T score better than −2.5 and no fractures) and then monitor patients with markers of bone turnover. Continued treatment may be advisable in those at highest risk.
- Continuing need to eliminate high-risk factors when possible and to diagnose and optimally manage secondary causes of osteoporosis

DISPOSITION

Goal for diagnosis and treatment: identification of women at risk; initiation of preventive measures for all women lifelong; institution of treatment modalities that will result in a decrease in fracture risk; and reduction of morbidity, mortality, and unnecessary institutionalization, thereby improving quality of independent life and productivity.

REFERRAL

- To reproductive endocrinologist, medical endocrinologist, gynecologist, or rheumatologist if unfamiliar with diagnosis and management of osteoporosis
- If multidisciplinary management is required, to other specialties depending on presence of acute fracture and/or secondary associated disorders

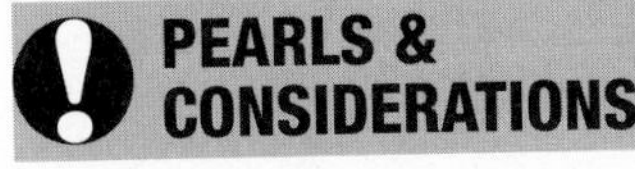

PEARLS & CONSIDERATIONS

COMMENTS

- Osteonecrosis of the jaw is a known complication of high-dose IV bisphosphonate therapy for cancer; however, there is considerable debate on whether low-dose bisphosphonates used for osteoporosis can also cause this disorder. Evidence for this is inconclusive.
- Long-term use (>10 yr) of bisphosphonates has been reported to increase risk of atypical subtrochanteric or femoral shaft fractures in several uncontrolled case series. A prodrome of thigh pain, lack of trauma prior to the procedure, and specific radiologic

characteristics have been reported. The evidence remains inconclusive. Patients can be reassured that short or intermediate use of bisphosphonates does not increase the risk of atypical femoral fractures. Current strategies should include considering a 12-mo interruption in therapy after 5 yr in patients who are clinically stable and considering teriparatide treatment in individuals who experience an atypical fracture while receiving bisphosphonate therapy.

- Increased risk of esophageal cancer and atrial fibrillation have been reported as possible adverse effects of bisphosphonate therapy.

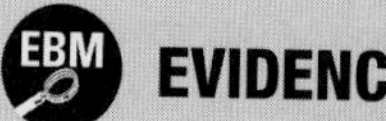

EVIDENCE

available at www.expertconsult.com

SUGGESTED READINGS

available at www.expertconsult.com

RELATED CONTENT

Osteoporosis (Patient Information)
Biphosphonate-Related Osteonecrosis of Jaw (Related Key Topic)

AUTHORS: **DENNIS M. WEPPNER, M.D.**, and **RUBEN ALVERO, M.D.**

BASIC INFORMATION

DEFINITION

Otitis externa is a term encompassing a variety of conditions causing inflammation and/or infection of the external auditory canal (and/or auricle and tympanic membrane). There are six subgroups of otitis externa:

1. Acute localized otitis externa (furunculosis)
2. Acute diffuse bacterial otitis externa (swimmer's ear)
3. Chronic otitis externa
4. Eczematous otitis externa
5. Fungal otitis externa (otomycosis)
6. Invasive or necrotizing (malignant) otitis externa (Fig. 1-684)

SYNONYMS

See "Definition."

ICD-9CM CODES
38.10 Otitis externa
ICD-10CM CODES

H60.90	Unspecified otitis externa, unspecified ear
H60.2	Malignant otitis externa
H60.3	Other infective otitis externa
H60.5	Acute otitis externa, non-infective
H60.8	Other otitis externa

EPIDEMIOLOGY & DEMOGRAPHICS

INCIDENCE (IN U.S.):

- Among the most common disorders
- Affects 3% to 10% of patients seeking otologic care

PREVALENCE (IN U.S.):

- Diffuse otitis externa (swimmer's ear) is most often seen in swimmers and in hot, humid climates, conditions that lead to water retention in the ear canal.
- Necrotizing otitis externa is more common in elderly, diabetics, and immunocompromised patients.

PREDOMINANT SEX: None
PREDOMINANT AGE:

- Occurs at all ages
- Necrotizing otitis externa: typically occurs in elderly: mean age >65 yr

PHYSICAL FINDINGS & CLINICAL PRESENTATION

The two most common symptoms are otalgia, ranging from pruritus to severe pain exacerbated by motion (e.g., chewing), and otorrhea. Patients may also experience aural fullness and hearing loss as a result of swelling with occlusion of the canal. More intense symptoms may occur with bacterial otitis externa, with or without fever, and lymphadenopathy (anterior to tragus). There are also findings unique to the various forms of the infection:

- Acute localized otitis externa (furunculosis):
  1. Occurs from infected hair follicles, usually in the outer third of the ear canal, forming pustules and furuncles
  2. Furuncles are superficial and pointing or deep and diffuse
- Impetigo:
  1. In contrast to furunculosis, this is a superficial spreading infection of the ear canal that may also involve the concha and the auricle
  2. Begins as a small blister that ruptures, releasing straw-colored fluid that dries as a golden crust
- Erysipelas:
  1. Caused by group A *Streptococcus*
  2. May involve the concha and canal
  3. May involve the dermis and deeper tissues
  4. Area of cellulitis, often with severe pain
  5. Fever, chills, malaise
  6. Regional adenopathy
- Eczematous otitis externa:
  1. Stems from a variety of dermatologic problems that can involve the external auditory canal
  2. Severe itching, erythema, scaling, crusting, and fissuring possible

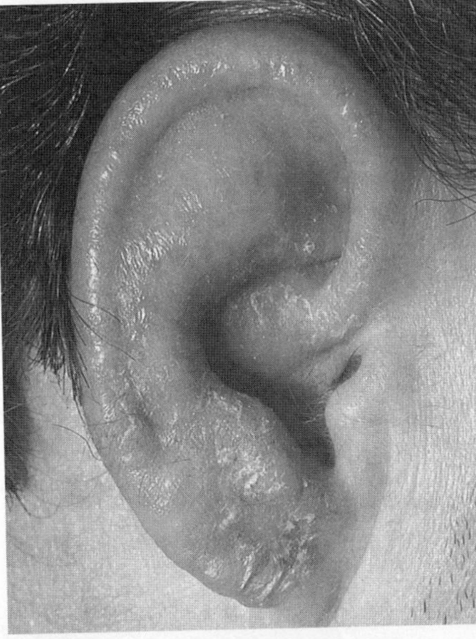

FIGURE 1-684 Malignant external otitis. Severe infection of the ear has occurred after months of chronic inflammation of the pinna. (From Habif TP: *Clinical dermatology: a color guide to diagnosis and therapy,* ed 3, St Louis, 1996, Mosby.)

- Acute diffuse otitis externa (swimmer's ear):
  1. Begins with itching and a feeling of pressure and fullness in the ear that becomes increasingly tender and painful
  2. Mild erythema and edema of the external auditory canal, which may cause narrowing and occlusion of the canal, leading to hearing loss
  3. Minimal serous secretions, which may become profuse and purulent
  4. Tympanic membrane may appear dull and infected
  5. Usually absence of systemic symptoms such as fever, chills
- Otomycosis:
  1. Chronic superficial infection of the ear canal and tympanic membrane
  2. In primary fungal infection, major symptom is intense itching
  3. In secondary infection (fungal infection superimposed on bacterial infection), major symptom is pain
  4. Fungal growth of variety of colors
- Chronic otitis externa:
  1. Dry and atrophic canal
  2. Typically lack of cerumen
  3. Itching, often severe, and mild discomfort rather than pain
  4. Occasionally mucopurulent discharge
  5. With time, thickening of the walls of the canal, causing narrowing of the lumen
- Necrotizing otitis externa (also known as malignant otitis externa). Typically seen in older patients with diabetes or in patients who are immunocompromised.
  1. Redness, swelling, and tenderness of the ear canal
  2. Classic finding of granulation tissue on the floor of the canal and the bone–cartilage junction
  3. Small ulceration of necrotic soft tissue at bone–cartilage junction
  4. Most common symptoms: pain (often severe) and otorrhea
  5. Lessening of purulent drainage as infection advances
  6. Facial nerve palsy often the first and only cranial nerve defect
  7. Possible involvement of other cranial nerves

ETIOLOGY

- Acute localized otitis externa: *Staphylococcus aureus*
- Impetigo:
  1. *S. aureus* including MRSA
  2. *Streptococcus pyogenes*
- Erysipelas: *S. pyogenes*
- Eczematous otitis externa:
  1. Seborrheic dermatitis
  2. Atopic dermatitis
  3. Psoriasis
  4. Neurodermatitis
  5. Lupus erythematosus
- Acute diffuse otitis externa:
  1. Swimming
  2. Hot, humid climates
  3. Tightly fitting hearing aids
  4. Use of ear plugs
  5. *Pseudomonas aeruginosa*
  6. *S. aureus* including MRSA

- Otomycosis:
  1. Prolonged use of topical antibiotics and steroid preparations
  2. *Aspergillus* (80% to 90%)
  3. *Candida*
- Chronic otitis externa: persistent low-grade infection and inflammation
- Necrotizing otitis externa (NOE):
  1. Complication of persistent otitis externa
  2. Extends through Santorini's fissures, small apertures at the bone-cartilage junction of the canal, into the mastoid and along the base of the skull
  3. *P. aeruginosa*

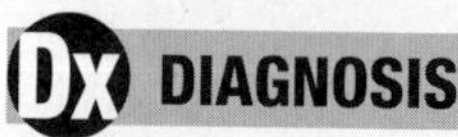

DIAGNOSIS

DIFFERENTIAL DIAGNOSIS

- Acute otitis media
- Bullous myringitis
- Mastoiditis
- Foreign bodies
- Neoplasms
- Contact dermatitis
- Eczema
- Ramsey-Hunt syndrome
- Seborrhea
- Otomycosis
- Referred pain

WORKUP

Thorough history and physical examination

LABORATORY TESTS

- Cultures from the canal are usually not necessary unless the condition does not respond to treatment.
- Leukocyte count normal or mildly elevated.
- Erythrocyte sedimentation rate is often quite elevated in malignant otitis externa.

IMAGING STUDIES

- CT scan is the best technique for defining bone involvement and extent of disease in malignant otitis externa.
- MRI is slightly more sensitive in evaluation of soft tissue changes.
- Gallium scans are more specific than bone scans in diagnosing NOE.
- Follow-up scans are helpful in determining efficacy of treatment.

NOTE: Expert opinion supports history and physical examination as the best means of diagnosis. Persistent pain that is constant and severe should raise the question of NOE (particularly in the elderly, diabetics, and immunocompromised patients).

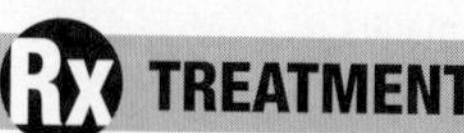

TREATMENT

NONPHARMACOLOGIC THERAPY

- Cleansing and debridement of the ear canal with cotton swabs and hydrogen peroxide or other antiseptic solution allows a more thorough examination of the ear.
- If the canal lumen is edematous and too narrow to allow adequate cleansing, a cotton wick or gauze strip inserted into the canal serves as a conduit for topical medications to be drawn into the canal. Usually remove wick after 2 days.
- Local heat is useful in treating deep furunculosis.
- Incision and drainage is indicated in treatment of superficial pointing furunculosis.

ACUTE GENERAL Rx

Topical medications:

- An acidifying agent such as 2% acetic acid (Vosol) inhibits growth of bacteria and fungi
- Topical antibiotics (in the form of otic or ophthalmic solutions) or antifungals, often in combination with an acidifying agent and a steroid preparation
- The following are some of the available preparations:
  1. Neomycin otic solutions and suspensions:
     a. With polymyxin-B-hydrocortisone (Corticosporin)
     b. With hydrocortisone-thonzonium (Coly-Mycin S)
  2. Polymyxin-B-hydrocortisone (Otobiotic)
  3. Quinolone otic solutions:
     a. Ofloxacin 0.3% solution (Floxin Otic)
     b. Ciprofloxacin 0.3% with hydrocortisone (Cipro HC)
  4. Quinolone ophthalmic solutions:
     a. Ofloxacin 0.3% (Ocuflox)
     b. Ciprofloxacin 0.3% (Ciloxan)
  5. Aminoglycoside ophthalmic solutions:
     a. Gentamicin sulfate 0.3% (Garamycin)
     b. Tobramycin sulfate 0.3% (Tobrex)
     c. Tobramycin 0.3% and dexamethasone 0.1% (TobraDex)
  6. Chloramphenicol 0.5% otic solution or 0.25% ophthalmic solution (Chloromycetin)
  7. Gentian violet (methylrosaniline chloride 1%, 2%)
  8. Antifungals:
     a. Amphotericin B 3% (Fungizone lotion)
     b. Clotrimazole 1% solution (Lotrimin)
     c. Tolnaftate 1% (Tinactin)
- Topical preparations should be applied qid (bid for quinolones, antifungals), generally for 3 days after cessation of symptoms (average 10 to 14 days total)

Systemic antibiotics:

- Reserved for when the infection has spread beyond the ear canal
- Treatment usually for 10 days with ciprofloxacin 750 mg q12h or ofloxacin 400 mg q12h, or with antistaphylococcal agent (e.g., dicloxacillin or cephalexin 500 mg q6h). Use Bactrim when MRSA suspected or cultured at one DS twice a day instead of cephalexin or dicloxacillin. For malignant otitis externa (due to *Pseudomonas aeruginosa* in >90% of cases), effective agents are imipenem-cilastatin 0.5 g IV q6h or ciprofloxacin 400 mg IV q12h or 750 mg PO q12h or cefepime 2 g q12h.

Treatment for NOE:

- Requires prolonged therapy up to 3 mo; whether to use oral parenteral therapy based on clinical judgment
- Oral quinolones, ciprofloxacin 750 mg q12h or ofloxacin 400 mg q12h may be appropriate initial therapy or used to shorten the course of IV therapy
- Intravenous antipseudomonals with or without aminoglycosides are also appropriate
- Local debridement

Pain control:

- May require NSAIDs or opioids
- Topical corticosteroids to reduce swelling and inflammation

CHRONIC Rx

- Patients prone to recurrent infections should try to identify and avoid precipitants to infection.
- Swimmers should try tight-fitting ear plugs or tight-fitting bathing caps and remove all excess water from the ears after swimming.
- Treat underlying systemic diseases and dermatologic conditions that predispose to infection.

DISPOSITION

Inadequate treatment of otitis externa may lead to NOE and mastoiditis.

REFERRAL

To an otolaryngologist:

- NOE
- Treatment failure
- Severe pain

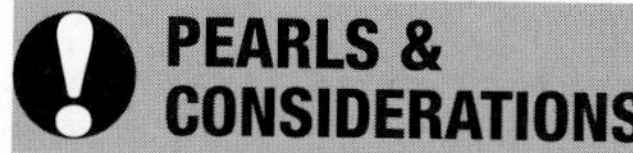

PEARLS & CONSIDERATIONS

Otitis externa varies in severity from a mild irritation of the external acoustic canal (swimmer's ear) that resolves spontaneously by simply removing the offending agent (stay out of fresh water or wear ear plugs) to a life-threatening infection with the risk of intracranial extension, gram-negative bacterial meningitis, and severe neurologic impairment with multiple cranial neuropathy. Do not miss severe malignant otitis externa in patients who are diabetic or immunocompromised.

SUGGESTED READINGS

available at www.expertconsult.com

RELATED CONTENT

Otitis Externa (Patient Information)

AUTHOR: **GLENN G. FORT, M.D., M.P.H.**

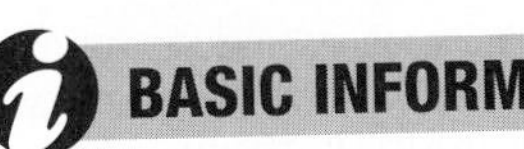

BASIC INFORMATION

DEFINITION

Otitis media is the rapid onset of signs and symptoms of inflammation in the middle ear.

SYNONYMS

Acute suppurative otitis media
Purulent otitis media
Acute otitis media
AOM

ICD-9CM CODES
382.9 Acute or chronic otitis media
381.00 Acute non-suppurative otitis media
ICD-10CM CODES
H65.0 Acute serous otitis media
H65.1 Other acute nonsuppurative otitis media
H65.9 Nonsuppurative otitis media, unspecified
H65.2 Chronic serous otitis media
H65.3 Chronic mucoid otitis media
H65.6 Other chronic nonsuppurative otitis media
H66.0 Acute suppurative otitis media
H66.4 Suppurative otitis media, unspecified
H66.9 Otitis media, unspecified
H66.1 Chronic tubotympanic suppurative otitis media
H66.2 Chronic atticoantral suppurative otitis media

EPIDEMIOLOGY & DEMOGRAPHICS

INCIDENCE (IN U.S.):

- Affects patients of all ages but is largely a disease of infants and young children.
- Affects approximately 80% of all children by age 5 yr.
- Occurs three or more times in one third of all children by age 3 yr.
- In 2000, costs associated with otitis media were approximately $5 billion, with 40% of the costs occurring from patients ages 1-3
- From 1995 to 2006, 80% of children diagnosed with otitis media received an antibiotic at initial visit.

PEAK INCIDENCE:

- Between 9 and 15 mo
- Second peak between ages 4 and 6 yr
- Fall, winter, early spring (coincident with peak respiratory virus prevalence in the community)

PREDOMINANT SEX: Males

PREDOMINANT AGE:

- 47% to 60% of all children have their first episode of otitis media during their first year of life and 80% by their fifth birthday.
- Incidence of infection declines with age; seen infrequently in adults.

GENETICS:

Familial disposition:

- Native Americans
- Eskimos
- Australian aborigines
- Those with a strong family history
- Immune globulin G (IgG) or subclass deficiencies

Congenital infection: high incidence in children born with cleft palates and other craniofacial abnormalities

PHYSICAL FINDINGS & CLINICAL PRESENTATION

- Moderate to severe bulging of the tympanic membrane
- Fluid in the middle ear along with signs and symptoms of local inflammation (Figs. 1-685 and 1-686).
  1. Erythema with diminished light reflex
- As infection progresses, middle ear exudation occurs (exudative phase); the exudate rapidly changes from serous to purulent (suppurative phase).
  1. Retraction and poor motility of the tympanic membrane, which then becomes bulging and convex
- At any time during the suppurative phase the tympanic membrane may rupture, releasing the middle ear contents.
- Erythema of the tympanic membrane without other abnormalities is not a diagnostic criterion for acute otitis media (AOM) because it may occur with any inflammation of the upper respiratory tract, crying, or nose blowing.
- Symptoms:
  1. Rapid- or recent-onset otalgia, ranging from slight discomfort to severe, spreading to the temporal region
  2. Ear stuffiness and hearing loss may precede or follow otalgia
  3. Otorrhea if tympanic membrane has ruptured
  4. Vertigo, nystagmus, tinnitus, fever, lethargy, irritability, nausea, vomiting, anorexia
- After an episode of AOM:
  1. Persistence of effusion for weeks or months (called secretory, serous, or nonsuppurative otitis media)
  2. Fever and otalgia usually absent
  3. Hearing loss possible (10 to 50 dB, with predominant involvement of the low frequencies)

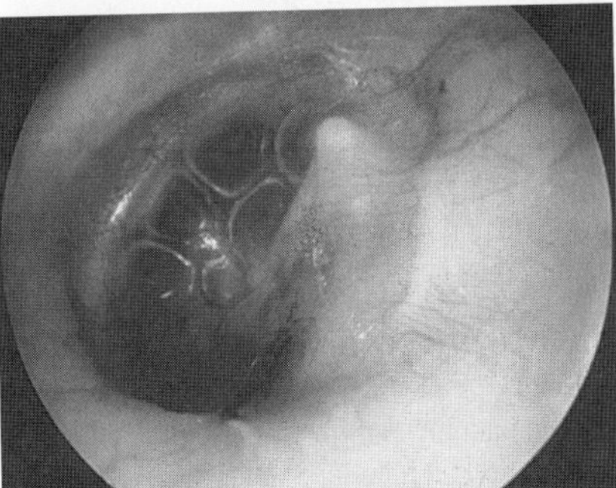

FIGURE 1-685 Otitis media with effusion of left ear. Retracted eardrum, prominent short process of malleus, and air bubbles seen anteriorly through the tympanic membrane. (From Behrman RE: *Nelson textbook of pediatrics,* ed 16, Philadelphia, 1996, Saunders.)

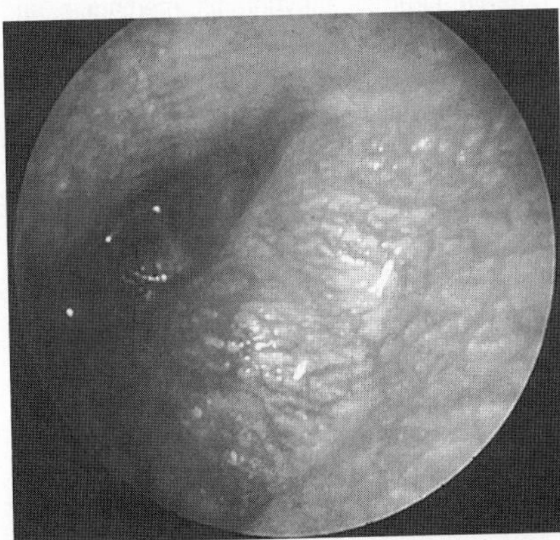

FIGURE 1-686 Acute left otitis media. (From Behrman RE: *Nelson textbook of pediatrics,* ed 16, Philadelphia, 1996, Saunders.)

ETIOLOGY

- Most common etiologic factor is a viral upper respiratory tract infection, which causes inflammation and dysfunction of the eustachian tube and transient aspiration of nasopharyngeal secretions into the middle ear. Bacterial colonization from the nasopharynx in conjunction with eustachian tube dysfunction leads to infection.
- May occasionally develop as a result of hematogenous spread or by direct invasion from the nasopharynx.
- Conjugated pneumococcal vaccination of children has resulted in decreases in *Streptococcus pneumoniae* causing AOM.
- Most common bacterial pathogens:
  1. *S. pneumoniae* causes 30% to 40% of cases and is the least likely of the major pathogens to resolve without treatment
  2. *Haemophilus influenzae* causes up to 50% of cases
  3. *Moraxella catarrhalis* causes 10% to 20% of cases
  4. Of increasing importance, infection caused by penicillin-nonsusceptible *S. pneumoniae* (MIC >0.1 μg/ml), ranging from 8% to 34%. About 50% of PNSSP isolates are penicillin-intermediate (MIC 0.1 to 2.0 μg/ml)
- Viral pathogens:
  1. Respiratory syncytial virus
  2. Rhinovirus
  3. Adenovirus
  4. Influenza
- Others:
  1. *Mycoplasma pneumoniae*
  2. *Chlamydia trachomatis*

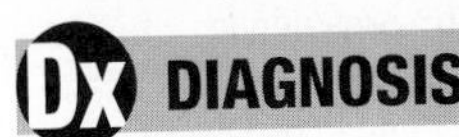

DIAGNOSIS

DIFFERENTIAL DIAGNOSIS

- Otitis externa
- Referred pain
  1. Mouth
  2. Nasopharynx
  3. Tonsils
  4. Other parts of the upper respiratory tract
- Section II describes the differential diagnosis of earache

 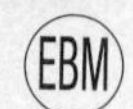

WORKUP

Thorough otoscopic examination. Adequate visualization of the tympanic membrane may require removal of cerumen and debris.

- Tympanometry
  1. Measures compliance of the tympanic membrane and middle ear pressure
  2. Detects the presence of fluid
- Acoustic reflectometry
  1. Measures sound waves reflected from the middle ear
  2. Useful in infants >3 mo
  3. Increased reflected sound correlated with the presence of effusion

LABORATORY TESTS

- Tympanocentesis
  1. Not necessary in most cases because the microbiology of middle ear effusions has been shown to be quite consistent
  2. May be indicated in:
     a. Highly toxic patients
     b. Patients who do not respond to treatment in 48 to 72 hr
     c. Immunocompromised patients
- Cultures of the nasopharynx: sensitive but not specific
- Blood counts (generally not necessary): usually show a leukocytosis with polymorphonuclear elevation
- Plain mastoid radiographs: generally not indicated; will reveal haziness in the periantral cells that may extend to entire mastoid
- CT or MRI may be indicated if serious complications suspected (meningitis, brain abscess, severe mastoiditis)

Rx TREATMENT

ACUTE GENERAL Rx

Hydration, avoidance of irritants (e.g., tobacco smoke), nasal systemic decongestants, cool mist humidifier

Antimicrobials:

NOTE: Most uncomplicated cases of AOM resolve spontaneously, without complications. Studies have demonstrated limited therapeutic benefit from antibiotic therapy. Watchful waiting is appropriate for children who look well, can be comforted with supportive care, and are old enough to easily evaluate. However, when opting to use antibiotic therapy:

- Amoxicillin remains the drug of choice for first-line treatment of uncomplicated AOM despite increasing prevalence of drug-resistant *S. pneumoniae.*
- Treatment failure is defined by lack of clinical improvement of signs or symptoms after 3 days of therapy.
- With treatment failure, in the absence of an identified etiologic pathogen, therapy should be redirected to cover:
  1. Drug-resistant *S. pneumoniae*
  2. β-lactamase–producing strains of *H. influenzae* and *M. catarrhalis*
- Agents fulfilling these criteria include amoxicillin/clavulanate, second-generation (e.g., cefuroxime axetil, cefaclor) or third-generation cephalosporins (e.g., oral cefdinir or cefpodxime or IM ceftriaxone). Do not use cefaclor, cefixime, loracarbef, and ceftibuten given limited activity against pneumococci.
- TMP/SMX and macrolides have been used as first- and second-line agents, but pneumococcal resistance to these agents is rising (up to 25% resistance to TMP/SMX and up to 10% resistance to erythromycin).
- Cross-resistance between these drugs and the β-lactams exists; therefore patients who do not respond to amoxicillin are more likely to have infections resistant to TMP/SMX and macrolides.
- Fluoroquinolones are not indicated as first- or second-line therapy for AOM and should be avoided in young children due to risks of musculoskeletal effects and lack of dosing guidance.
- Treatment should be modified according to cultures and sensitivities when available.
- Generally treatment course is 10 days for children <2 yr and those with severe symptoms, 7 days for children age 2-5 yr, and 5-7 days for children ≥6 yr.
- Follow up should be tailored to clinical improvement and concern for neurocognitive development delays in at-risk children. Standard follow-up of all cases is no longer required.

NOTE: Effusions may persist for 8 wk or longer in many cases of adequately treated otitis media.

SURGICAL Rx

- No evidence to support the routine use of myringotomy, but in severe cases it provides prompt pain relief and accelerates resolution of infection.
- Purulent secretions retained in the middle ear can lead to increased pressure that may lead to spread of infection to contiguous areas. Myringotomy to decompress the middle ear is sometimes necessary to avoid complications.
- Complications include mastoiditis, facial nerve paralysis, labyrinthitis, meningitis, and brain abscess.
- Other procedures used for drainage of the middle ear include insertion of a ventilation tube and/or simple mastoidectomy.

CHRONIC Rx

- Myringotomy and tympanostomy tube placement for persistent or recurrent middle ear effusion unresponsive to medical therapy for ≥3 mo if bilateral or ≥6 mo if unilateral.
- Adenoidectomy, with or without tonsillectomy, often advocated for treatment of recurrent otitis media, although indications for this procedure are controversial.
- Long-term complications include tympanic membrane perforations, cholesteatoma, tympanosclerosis, ossicular necrosis, toxic or suppurative labyrinthitis, hearing loss, and intracranial suppuration.

DISPOSITION

Patients can be treated at home as outpatients with the rare exception of patients with evidence of local suppurative complications (e.g., meningitis, acute mastoiditis, brain abscess, cavernous sinus, or lateral vein thrombosis).

REFERRAL

- To otorhinolaryngologist if:
  1. Medical treatment failure
  2. Diagnosis uncertain: adults with one or more episodes of otitis media should be referred for ear-nose-throat evaluation to rule out underlying process (e.g., malignancy)
  3. Any of the above-mentioned acute and chronic complications

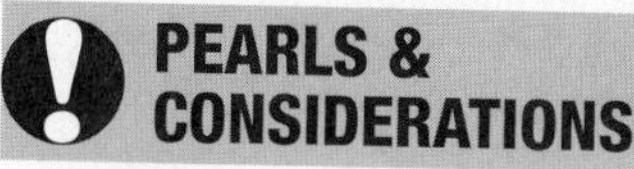

PEARLS & CONSIDERATIONS

COMMENTS

- Otoscopic findings are critical for accurate AOM diagnosis. AOM microbiology has changed with use of pneumococcal conjugate vaccine (PCV13). Antibiotics are modestly more effective than no treatment but cause adverse effects in 4% to 10% of children. Most antibiotics have comparable clinical success.

Prevention:

- Multiple component conjugate vaccines have helped decrease recurrent episodes of AOM
- Breastfeed and bottle-feed infants in an upright position
- Avoidance of irritants (e.g., tobacco smoke)

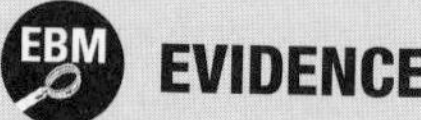

EVIDENCE

available at www.expertconsult.com

SUGGESTED READINGS

available at www.expertconsult.com

AUTHORS: **GLENN G. FORT, M.D., M.P.H.** and **RUSSELL J. MCCULLOH, M.D., M.P.H.**

BASIC INFORMATION

DEFINITION

Ovarian tumors can be benign, requiring operative intervention but not recurring or metastasizing; malignant, recurring, metastasizing, and having decreased survival; or borderline, having a small risk of recurrence or metastases and generally having a good prognosis. An emerging concept is the possibility that many ovarian cancers have origins on nonovarian tissues such as distal fallopian tube and endometriotic implants.

SYNONYMS

Epithelial ovarian cancer
Germ cell tumor
Sex cord stromal tumor
Ovarian tumor of low malignant potential

ICD-9CM CODES
183.0 Malignant neoplasm of ovary
ICD-10CM CODES
C56.9 Malignant neoplasm of unspecified ovary

EPIDEMIOLOGY & DEMOGRAPHICS

INCIDENCE: 12.9 to 15.1 cases/100,000 persons; ~25,000 new cases annually
PREVALENCE: Median age of 61 yr; peaks at age 75 to 79 yr (54/100,000)
RISK FACTORS: Low parity, delayed childbearing, use of talc on the perineum (unlikely), high-fat diet, fertility drugs (unlikely), Lynch II syndrome (nonpolyposis colon cancer, endometrial cancer, breast cancer, and ovarian cancer clusters in first- and second-degree relatives), breast-ovarian familial cancer syndrome, site-specific familial ovarian cancer.
GENETICS: The greatest risk factors of ovarian cancer are a family history and associated genetic syndromes. Familial susceptibility has been shown with the *BRCA1* gene located on 17q12 to 21. This correlates with breast-ovarian cancer syndrome.

PHYSICAL FINDINGS & CLINICAL PRESENTATION

- 60% present with advanced disease
- Abdominal fullness, early satiety, dyspepsia
- Pelvic pain, back pain, constipation
- Pelvic or abdominal mass
- Lymphadenopathy (inguinal)
- Sister Mary Joseph nodule (umbilical mass)

ETIOLOGY

- Can be inherited as site-specific familial ovarian cancer (two or more first-degree relatives have ovarian cancer)
- Breast-ovarian cancer syndrome (clusters of breast and ovarian cancer among first- and second-degree relatives)
- Lynch syndrome
- No family history and unknown etiology in the majority of ovarian cancer cases

Dx DIAGNOSIS

DIFFERENTIAL DIAGNOSIS

- Primary peritoneal cancer mesothelioma
- Benign ovarian tumor
- Functional ovarian cyst
- Endometriosis
- Ovarian torsion
- Pelvic kidney
- Pedunculated uterine fibroid
- Primary cancer from breast, gastrointestinal tract, or other pelvic organ metastasized to the ovary

WORKUP

- Definitive diagnosis made at laparotomy; epithelial ovarian cancer most common type of ovarian cancer
- Careful physical and history, including family history
- Exclusion of nongynecologic etiologies
- Observation of small cystic masses in premenopausal women for regression for 2 mo
- FIGO classification of ovarian carcinoma is described in Table 1-370.

LABORATORY TESTS

- Complete blood count
- Chemistry profile
- CA-125 or lysophosphatidic acid level. Use of these tests for annual screening is controversial. Only about 50% of early-stage ovarian cancers will be associated with elevated CA-125. Additionally, false elevations may occur with uterine leiomyoma, endometriosis, pregnancy, and intraabdominal infections. The PLCO cancer screening trial revealed that annual screening based on CA-125 and vaginal ultrasound is ineffective and diagnostic follow-up of false positives resulted in 15% serious complication rate.
- Consider: human chorionic gonadotropin, inhibin, alpha-fetoprotein, neuron-specific enolase, and lactate dehydrogenase in patients at risk for germ cell tumors.
- A panel of 3 serum biomarkers (apolipoprotein A-1 [ApoA-1], transthyretin [TTR], and transferrin [TF]) has been reported useful in distinguishing normal samples from early-stage ovarian cancer with a sensitivity of 84% and normal samples from late-stage ovarian cancer with a sensitivity of 97%.

IMAGING STUDIES

- Ultrasound
- Chest x-ray
- Mammogram
- CT scan to help evaluate extent of disease (Fig. 1-688)
- Other studies (MRI, intravenous pyelogram, etc.) as clinically indicated

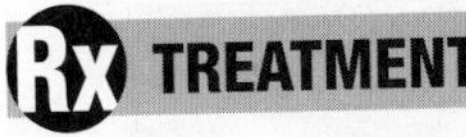

Rx TREATMENT

NONPHARMACOLOGIC THERAPY

Virtually all cases of ovarian cancer involve surgical exploration. This includes:

- Abdominal cytology
- Total abdominal hysterectomy and bilateral salpingo-oophorectomy (except in early stages in which fertility preservation is an issue)
- Omentectomy

TABLE 1-370 FIGO Classification of Ovarian Carcinoma

Stage I	Growth limited to the ovaries:
	Stage IA: Growth limited to one ovary, no ascites and no tumor present on the external surface; capsule intact
	Stage IB: Growth limited to both ovaries, no ascites and no tumor present on the external surface; capsule intact
	Stage IC: Stage 1A or 1B where there is tumor on the surface of either ovary; or with ruptured capsules or with ascites containing malignant cells or positive peritoneal washings. Surgical spillage of a malignant cyst upgrades the patient to IC although it is unlikely that this event affects prognosis.
Stage II	Growth involving one or both ovaries with pelvic extension:
	Stage IIA: Extension and/or metastases to the uterus and tubes
	Stage IIB: Extension to other pelvic tissues
	Stage IIC: Stage IIA or IIB with tumor on the surface of either ovary or positive peritoneal washings or malignant ascites
Stage III	Growth involving one or both ovaries with peritoneal implants outside the pelvis or positive retroperitoneal or inguinal lymph nodes:
	Stage IIIA: Microscopic seeding of abdominal peritoneal surfaces
	Stage IIIB: Macroscopic disease outside the pelvis less than 2 cm in diameter
	Stage IIIC: Abdominal implants greater than 2 cm and/or positive nodes
Stage IV	Growth involving one or both ovaries with distant metastases including parenchymal (but not superficial) liver metastases and pleural effusions containing malignant cells

From Symonds EM, Symonds IM: *Essential obstetrics and gynaecology*, ed 4, London, 2004, Churchill Livingstone.

- Diaphragm sampling
- Selective lymphadenectomy (pelvic and paraaortic nodes)
- Primary cytoreduction with a goal of residual tumor diameter <2 cm
- Bowel surgery, splenectomy if needed to obtain optimal (<2 cm) cytoreduction
- Conventional treatment includes surgical debulking (cytoreduction) followed by chemotherapy. However, patients with low-grade, well-differentiated stage I ovarian cancer do not benefit from adjuvant chemotherapy.

ACUTE GENERAL Rx

- Optimal cytoreduction is generally followed by chemotherapy (except in some early-stage disease).
- Cisplatin-based combination chemotherapy is used for stage II or greater, 6-mo treatment. Compared with IV paclitaxel plus cisplatin, IV paclitaxel plus intraperitoneal cisplatin and paclitaxel improves survival rates in patients with optimally debulked stage III ovarian cancer.
- Chemotherapy regimens continue to change as research continues. Bevacizumab, a humanized antivascular endothelial growth factor monoclonal antibody, has been shown to be effective in improving progression-free survival in women with ovarian cancer. Trials using bevacizumab during and up to 10 months after carboplatin and paclitaxel chemotherapy have shown prolongation of the median progression-free survival by about 4 months in patients with advanced epithelial ovarian cancer. Olaparib, an oral polymerase inhibitor, has shown antitumor activity in patients with high-grade serous ovarian cancer with or without BRCA1 and BRCA2 germline mutations. Trials have shown that olaparib as maintenance treatment significantly improved progression-free survival among patients with platinum-sensitive, relapsed high-grade serous ovarian cancer.
- Second-look surgery when chemotherapy is complete generally is no longer recommended because this procedure has not been shown to improve survival.
- Recent trials have shown that neoadjuvant chemotherapy followed by interval debulking surgery is not inferior to debulking surgery followed by chemotherapy as a treatment option for patients with bulky stage IIIC or IV ovarian carcinoma. Complete resection of all macroscopic disease, whether performed as primary treatment or after neoadjuvant chemotherapy, remains the objective whenever cytoreductive surgery is performed.

CHRONIC Rx

- If CA-125 elevated, may have recurrent disease
- Physical and pelvic examinations every 3 mo for 2 yr, every 4 mo during third year, then every 6 mo
- CA-125 every visit
- Yearly Pap smear

DISPOSITION

- Overall 5-yr survival rates remain low because of the preponderance of late-stage disease:
  - Stage I and II: 80% to 100%
  - Stage III: 15% to 20%
  - Stage IV: 5%
- Younger patients (<50 yr) in all stages have a considerably better 5-yr survival than older patients (40% vs. 15%).
- Among women with high-grade serous ovarian cancer, *BRCA2* mutation, but not *BRCA1* deficiency, is associated with improved survival, improved chemotherapy response, and genome instability compared with *BRCA* wild-type.
- Among patients with invasive epithelial ovarian cancer (EOC), having a germline mutation in *BRCA1* or *BRCA2* is associated with improved 5-yr overall survival. *BRCA2* carriers have the best prognosis.

COMMENTS

- The U.S. Preventive Services Task Force has concluded that current evidence does not show any mortality benefit to routine screening for ovarian cancer with transvaginal ultrasonography or single-threshold serum CA-125 testing and that the harms of such screening are at least moderate.
- Patients at high risk for developing ovarian cancer (BRCA1/BRCA2 gene mutation, hereditary nonpolyposis colorectal cancer syndrome) should consider prophylactic salpingo-oophorectomy after childbearing is complete. If surgery is declined, the National Comprehensive Cancer Network guidelines recommend intensive surveillance with pelvic and abdominal sonogram and serum CA-125 every 6 mo starting at age 35 or 10 yr earlier than cancer diagnosis in family member.

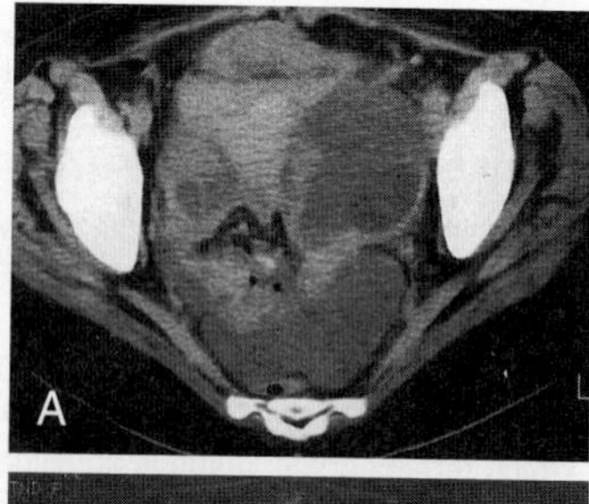

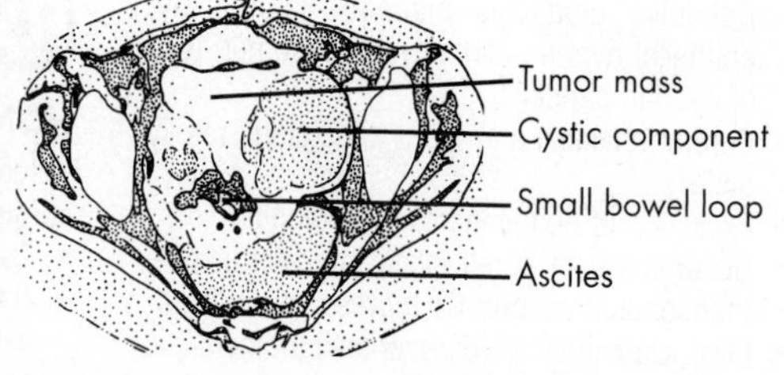

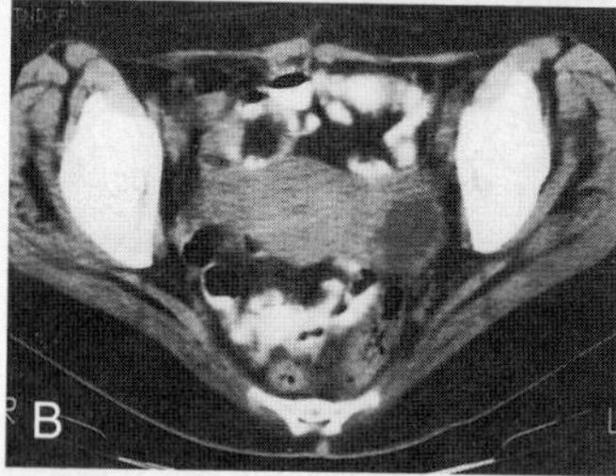

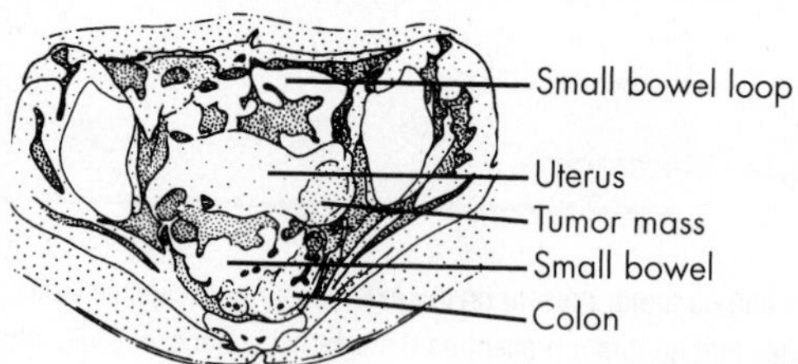

FIGURE 1-688 Response to chemotherapy. A 51-year-old woman presented with a rapid increase in abdominal girth. **A,** On CT scan, she was found to have a 12 x 8 cm ovarian mass with a cystic component; peritoneal involvement was extensive and 6 L of ascites was removed. Pathologic examination showed a poorly differentiated tumor. The tumor was not resectable, and she was treated with combination chemotherapy. After one cycle of therapy, her abdomen returned to normal size. **B,** A CT scan reveals only a small residual ovarian mass. Surgery after four cycles of chemotherapy showed no gross or microscopic tumor. She received four more cycles of chemotherapy but relapsed 1 year later with abdominal metastases. (From Skarin AT: *Atlas of diagnostic oncology,* ed 3, St Louis, 2003, Mosby.)

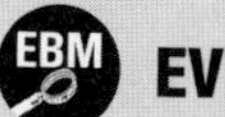

EVIDENCE

available at www.expertconsult.com

SUGGESTED READINGS

available at www.expertconsult.com

RELATED CONTENT

Ovarian Neoplasm, Benign (Related Key Topic)
Ovarian Cancer (Patient Information)

AUTHOR: **RUBEN ALVERO, M.D.**

BASIC INFORMATION

DEFINITION

Benign ovarian neoplasms are often clinically indistinguishable from their malignant counterparts. Therefore all persistent adnexal masses must be considered malignant until proven otherwise. Nonneoplastic tumors include:

- Germinal inclusion cyst
- Follicle cyst
- Corpus luteum cyst
- Pregnancy luteoma
- Theca lutein cysts
- Sclerocystic ovaries
- Endometrioma

Neoplastic tumors derived from coelomic epithelium include:

- Cystic tumors: serous cystadenoma, mucinous cystadenoma, mixed forms
- Tumors with stromal overgrowth: fibroma, adenofibroma, Brenner tumor

Tumors derived from germ cells are dermoids (benign cystic teratomas).

ICD-9CM CODES
220 Benign neoplasm of ovary
ICD-10CM CODES
D27.9 Benign neoplasm of unspecified ovary

EPIDEMIOLOGY & DEMOGRAPHICS

- Reproductive years:
  1. Most common benign ovarian neoplasms: serous cystadenoma and benign cystic teratoma
  2. Most common adnexal mass: functional cyst
- Risk of malignancy increases after age 40 yr.
- Infants: adnexal masses are usually follicular cysts attributable to maternal hormone stimulation that regress during first few months of life.
- Childhood:
  1. Adnexal masses are rare
  2. 8% malignant
  3. Almost always dysgerminomas or teratomas (germ cell origin)
  4. Frequency of malignancy inversely correlated with age
- Adolescence:
  1. Most common adnexal mass is a functional cyst.
  2. Most common neoplastic ovarian tumor is a benign cystic teratoma.
  3. Solid/cystic adnexal tumors are rare and almost always dysgerminomas or malignant teratomas.

PHYSICAL FINDINGS & CLINICAL PRESENTATION

- Usually asymptomatic
- Pelvic pain or pressure
- Dyspareunia
- Abdominal pain ranging from mild to severe peritoneal irritation
- Increasing abdominal girth or distention
- Adnexal mass of pelvic examination
- Children: abdominal or rectal mass

ETIOLOGY

- Physiologic
- Endometriosis
- Unknown

Dx DIAGNOSIS

DIFFERENTIAL DIAGNOSIS

- Ovarian torsion
- Malignancy: ovary, fallopian tube, colon
- Uterine fibroid
- Diverticular abscess, diverticulitis
- Appendiceal abscess, appendicitis (especially in children)
- Tubo-ovarian abscess
- Paraovarian cyst
- Distended bladder
- Pelvic kidney
- Ectopic pregnancy
- Retroperitoneal cyst or neoplasm

WORKUP

- Complete history and physical examination
- Pelvic or rectovaginal examination to reveal firm, irregular, mobile mass
- Laparoscopy or laparotomy to establish diagnosis

LABORATORY TESTS

- Pregnancy test
- Serum tumor markers:
  1. Cancer antigen 125 (CA-125)
  2. Alpha-fetoprotein (endodermal sinus tumor, immature teratoma)
  3. Beta-human chorionic gonadotropin
  4. Lactate dehydrogenase (dysgerminoma)

IMAGING STUDIES

Ultrasound (Fig. 1-689):

- May differentiate adnexal mass from other pelvic masses
- Features that increase risk of malignancy include solid component, papillae, multiple septations or solitary thick septa, ascites, matted bowel, bilaterality, irregular borders
- CT scan with contrast
- Colonoscopy or barium enema, if symptomatic

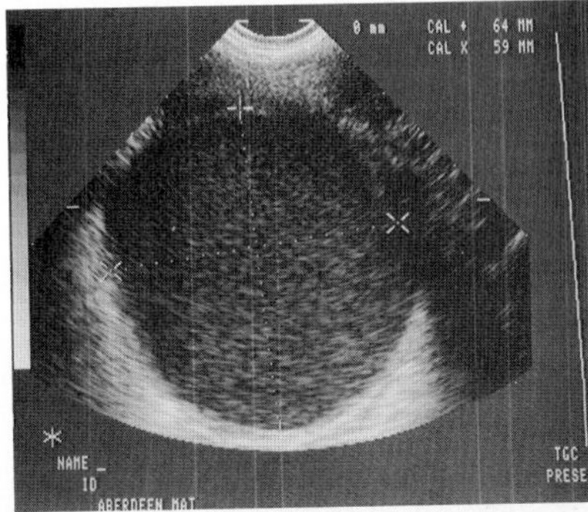

FIGURE 1-689 Ultrasonogram, which reveals a cyst 6.5 cm across, which was found at laparotomy to be an endometrioma, full of altered blood: the so-called chocolate cyst. This may cause cyclical or chronic pelvic pain. (From Greer IA et al: *Mosby's color atlas and text of obstetrics and gynecology,* London, 2000, Harcourt.)

Rx TREATMENT

NONPHARMACOLOGIC THERAPY

Repeat pelvic examination for premenopausal women in 4 to 6 wk

ACUTE GENERAL Rx

Indications for surgery:

- Postmenopausal or premenarcheal palpable adnexal mass
- Adnexal mass with suspicious ultrasound features
- Premenopausal woman with persistent cyst >5 cm
- Any adnexal mass >10 cm
- Suspected torsion or rupture

CHRONIC Rx

- Depends on diagnosis
- Possible suppression of formation of new cysts by oral contraceptives

DISPOSITION

Depends on diagnosis

REFERRAL

- If malignancy suspected
- If surgery required

SUGGESTED READINGS

available at www.expertconsult.com

RELATED CONTENT

Ovarian Cysts (Patient Information)

AUTHOR: **RUBEN ALVERO, M.D.**

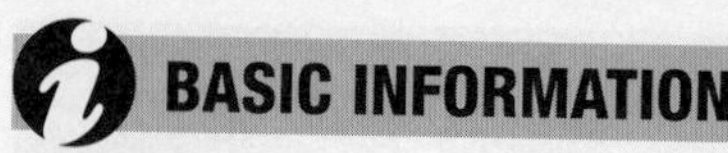

BASIC INFORMATION

DEFINITION

Paget's disease of bone is a focal disorder of chaotic bone remodeling with increased osteoblastic and osteoclastic activity that results in disorganized woven and lamellar bone in one or more skeletal sites. The end result is bone of poor quality that is enlarged, hypervascular, and susceptible to deformation and fracture.

SYNONYMS

Osteitis deformans

ICD-9CM CODES
731.0 Paget's disease (osteitis deformans)
ICD-10CM CODES
M88.9 Osteitis deformans of unspecified bone

EPIDEMIOLOGY & DEMOGRAPHICS

Epidemiologic data suggest an origin of Paget's disease in Great Britain spreading to other areas by English colonists beginning in the seventeenth century. Highest prevalence occurs in Eastern and Western Europe and in those who have emigrated to New Zealand, Australia, South Africa, and North America. Rarely seen in Japanese, Chinese, Asian Indians, sub-Saharan Africans, and Middle Eastern Arabs.

Most commonly diagnosed in those aged >50 yr and rare before 40 yr.

Prevalence estimates of up to 3% of population aged >50 yr and up to 10% in those aged >90 yr.

PREDOMINANT SEX: Variable preponderance of males.

PREDOMINANT AGE: Middle or advanced years.

FAMILIAL INCIDENCE: Common, family history positive in up to 40% of cases.

PHYSICAL FINDINGS & CLINICAL PRESENTATION

- Most common sites of involvement: pelvis, spine, sacrum, femur, skull, tibia (Fig. E1-690), humerus, scapula.
- Uncommon: hand, foot, fibula.
- Lesions in one (monostotic) or more bones (polyostotic).
- Gradual progression of disease in affected bone(s) with rare appearance at new site(s).
- Many patients are asymptomatic, but up to 40% of patients who come to medical attention present with bone pain.
- Symptoms and signs include bone and articular pain often related to secondary arthritis, bone deformities and enlargement, increased warmth over pagetic bone, skull enlargement, nerve entrapment or compression syndromes, cranial nerve deficits especially deafness, spinal cord compression and vascular steal syndromes, fissure fractures, fractures, and neoplastic degeneration.

ETIOLOGY

Etiology remains unknown.

Extensive epidemiologic and laboratory data are in keeping with potential role of paramyxoviral infection of osteoclasts in a genetically susceptible individual with or without documented genetic mutations.

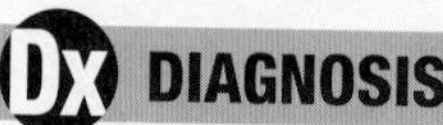

DIAGNOSIS

DIFFERENTIAL DIAGNOSIS

- Osteosclerosis
- Hyperphosphatasia
- Familial expansile osteolysis
- Fibrous dysplasia
- Skeletal neoplasm (primary or metastatic)
- Osteomalacia with secondary hyperparathyroidism

LABORATORY TESTS

- Increase in serum alkaline phosphatase or bone-specific alkaline phosphatase
- Increase in urine NTx/creatinine ratio or plasma CTx
- Bone biopsy may be necessary to rule out sarcomatous degeneration or metastasic disease

IMAGING STUDIES (Fig. E1-691)

Bone scintigraphy is the most sensitive test for delineating the extent and site of pagetic lesions but nonspecific in that areas of uptake may be related to arthritis or metastatic lesions. Radiographs (Fig. 1-692) will further delineate characteristic pagetic changes.

Rx TREATMENT

Indications for therapy include extensive or symptomatic disease; neurologic complications; involvement of weight-bearing bones, skull, vertebrae, and other areas of critical involvement, for example, in proximity to joints; and prevention of excess bleeding from an orthopedic procedure on pagetic bone.

NONPHARMACOLOGIC THERAPY

Optimization of calcium and vitamin D intake and appropriate guidance regarding ambulatory needs.

SPECIFIC THERAPY

Bisphosphonates are the mainstay of therapy and include oral alendronate or risedronate and intravenous pamidronate or zoledronic acid.

- SC salmon calcitonin when bisphosphonates are not tolerated or are contraindicated as in those with GFR of <35 ml/min
- Acetaminophen, aspirin, and nonsteroidal drugs for relief of pain

DISPOSITION

- Without treatment, progression of disease is common
- With treatment, remissions of varying duration in most patients. Bisphosphonates can normalize bone turnover in a high proportion of patients, but evidence that long-term suppression of bone turnover prevents complications or improves the clinical outcome is currently inconclusive.
- Careful and regular clinical and biochemical followup at 3- to 6-mo intervals with necessity of retreatment in patients with continued pagetic activity or reactivation
- With first ever intravenous dose of pamidronate or zoledronic acid, patients may experience a flu-like syndrome for several days that may be prevented with acetaminophen

SUGGESTED READINGS

available at www.expertconsult.com

RELATED CONTENT

Paget's Disease of Bone (Patient Information)

AUTHOR: **JOSEPH R. TUCCI, M.D., F.A.C.P., F.A.C.E.**

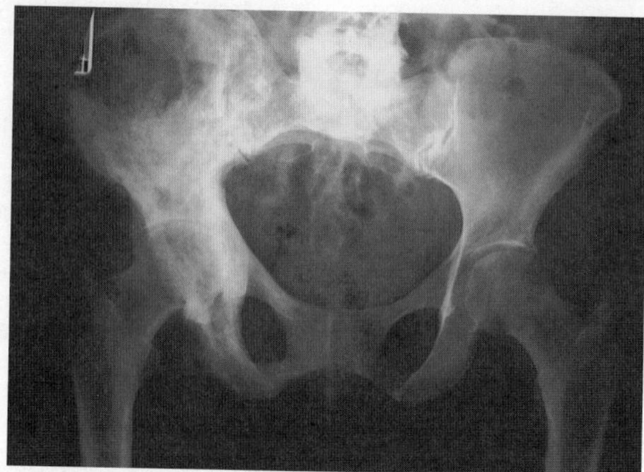

FIGURE 1-692 Paget's disease of the bone. Frontal radiograph of the pelvis shows marked prominence of the trabeculae in the right ilium, ischium, and pubic bones, with small lytic areas identified as compatible with the later stages of Paget's disease. (From Specht N [ed]: *Practical guide to diagnostic imaging,* St Louis, 1998, Mosby.)

BASIC INFORMATION

DEFINITION

Paget's disease of the breast is a malignant disease that presents itself as a scaly, sore, eroding, bleeding ulcer of the nipple. It represents an extension of a ductal adenocarcinoma of the breast. Microscopically, typical large clear cells (Paget's cells) with pale and abundant cytoplasm and hyperchromatic nuclei with prominent nucleoli are found in the epidermal layer. Paget's disease is more often associated with primary invasive or in situ carcinoma of the breast.

ICD-9CM CODES
174.0 Malignant neoplasm of female breast, nipple, and areola
ICD-10CM CODES
C50.0 Malignant neoplasm of nipple and areola
C50.019 Malignant neoplasm of nipple and areola, unspecified female breast

EPIDEMIOLOGY & DEMOGRAPHICS

- Not common
- Found in one in 100 to 200 breast cancer patients

PHYSICAL FINDINGS & CLINICAL PRESENTATION

- Variable; most often reveals an erythematous, irregularly bordered plaque on the nipple.
- Itching or burning nipple and/or reported lump
- Very minimal scaly lesion that may bleed when scales are lifted
- Typical ulcer located on nipple with serous fluid weeping or small amount of bleeding coming from it (Fig. 1-693)
- Palpable carcinoma in the breast of some patients

ETIOLOGY

- Exact origin unknown
- Possibly migration of either in situ or invasive carcinoma cells in breast to nipple skin to produce Paget's disease

Dx DIAGNOSIS

DIFFERENTIAL DIAGNOSIS

- Chronic dermatitis
- Florid papillomatosis of the nipple or nipple adenoma
- Eczema

WORKUP

- Clinically apparent
- Careful breast examination with diagnosis in mind
- Palpable mass or mammographic lesions in 60% to 70% of patients

A clinical algorithm for the evaluation of nipple discharge is described in Section III, "Breast, Nipple Discharge Evaluation."

LABORATORY TESTS

Biopsy of nipple lesion

IMAGING STUDIES

Mammograms to search for possible primary carcinoma

Rx TREATMENT

NONPHARMACOLOGIC THERAPY

- Fewer patients:
  1. Paget's disease of nipple only finding when mammographically negative breast
  2. Consideration of wide excision of nipple with or without radiation
- Other patients: additional invasive or in situ carcinoma recognized
- Either modified mastectomy or breast conservation treatment
- Presence of underlying in situ or invasive carcinoma in mastectomy specimen of majority of patients

ACUTE GENERAL Rx

Systemic adjuvant therapy depending on extent of invasive carcinoma found

DISPOSITION

- Parallel prognosis to that of breast cancer patient without Paget's disease
- Regular follow-up as in other invasive or in situ carcinoma patients

REFERRAL

At outset, all suspicious nipple lesions should be referred for evaluation and treatment.

SUGGESTED READINGS

available at www.expertconsult.com

RELATED CONTENT

Breast Cancer (Related Key Topic)
Paget's Disease of the Breast (Patient Information)

AUTHOR: **RUBEN ALVERO, M.D.**

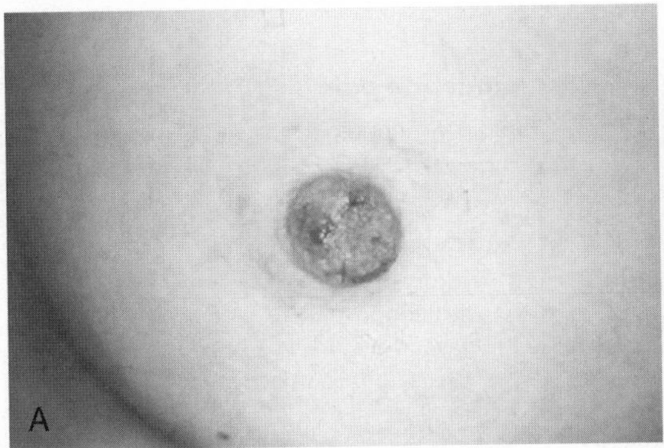

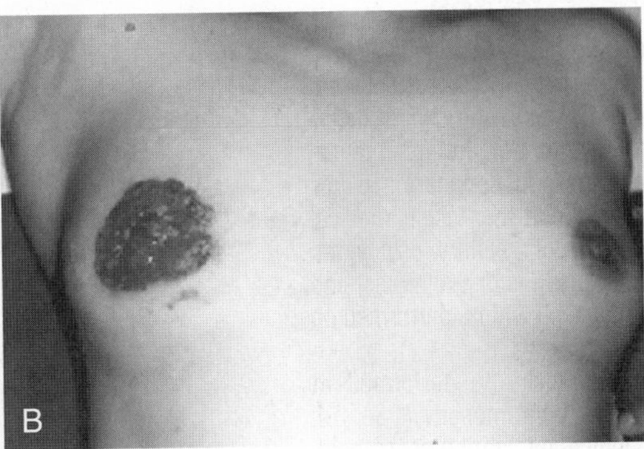

FIGURE 1-693 A and B: Paget disease of the nipple. (Courtesy Sehwan Han, MD.)

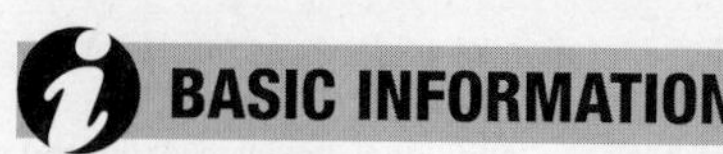

BASIC INFORMATION

DEFINITION

Chronic pain is pain that persists for longer than the expected time frame or that is associated with progressive, nonmalignant disease. Pain is an unpleasant sensory and emotional experience associated with actual or potential tissue damage or described in terms of such damage. The perception of pain is influenced by physiologic, psychological, and social factors.

SYNONYMS

Nonmalignant chronic pain

ICD-9CM CODES

338.29	Chronic Pain
338.4	Chronic Pain Syndrome
780.96	Generalized Pain

ICD-10CM CODES

G89.4	Chronic pain syndrome
R52	Pain, unspecified
G89.29	Other chronic pain

EPIDEMIOLOGY & DEMOGRAPHICS

Estimates of the prevalence of chronic pain in the United States vary widely. Data from one national survey (1999-2002 National Health and Nutrition Examination Survey [NHANES]) reported a prevalence of chronic regional and widespread pain of 11% and 3.6%, respectively, while the National Center for Health Statistics estimates that 32.8% of the U.S. population suffers from some form of chronic pain. Chronic pain is the third leading cause of physical impairment in the U.S., and related costs are estimated to be tens of billions annually. Patients with chronic pain may also experience changes in mood, depression, sleep disturbances, and fatigue, and decreased overall physical functioning.

CLINICAL PRESENTATION

- History: Comprehensive patient assessment, including history of present illness (cause of pain, location timing, characteristics, exacerbating/relieving factors, triggers), past therapies (pharmacologic and nonpharmacologic and outcomes of these therapies), medical history, family and social history, psychiatric history, substance use history, allergies, and current medications, should be performed on initial evaluation.
- Pain assessment should be performed at each visit; includes pain intensity (1 to 10), response to medication, attributes of pain, and assessment of function (cognitive, emotional, employment, sleep, mobility, and self-care). Standardized templates for both initial and follow-up pain assessment have been developed by various organizations. The website Pain Treatment Topics contains many of these assessment tools (http://pain-topics.org/clinical_concepts/assess.php).
- Physical examination: Directed at systems affected by pain and neurologic examination.

ETIOLOGY

Chronic pain can generally be categorized as originating from one of five etiologies: musculoskeletal, neuropathic, inflammatory, mechanical, or mixed. Chronic pain may include such diagnoses as headache, low back pain, previous trauma, arthritis, neurogenic (e.g., trigeminal neuralgia), psychogenic (related to depression or anxiety), fibromyalgia, reflex sympathetic dystrophy, myofascial pain syndrome, phantom limb pain, idiopathic, or unknown.

Dx DIAGNOSIS

DIFFERENTIAL DIAGNOSIS

- Depends on etiology.
- Depression and anxiety disorders can be both a cause and a result of chronic pain, so temporal association of these disorders is important.

WORKUP

- Laboratory testing, imaging studies, and/or electromyographic studies should be used when etiology of chronic pain is unknown or unclear, when comorbidities are suspected, and as the history and physical examination direct.
- Consider use of random urine drug screens or other tests to screen for presence of illegal drugs, unreported prescribed medications, or alcohol use.

Rx TREATMENT

- Studies increasingly support the application of a multidisciplinary approach that addresses the multiple facets of pain (e.g., physical, psychological, social aspects).
- Therapeutic goal is the reduction of pain (elimination of chronic pain is generally unlikely and providers need to discuss these limitations with patients at outset).
- Fig. E1-694 describes an algorithm for the treatment of pain.

NONPHARMACOLOGIC THERAPY

- Exercise
- Modalities: heat therapy, cold therapy, transcutaneous electrical nerve stimulation (TENS) units, cognitive behavioral therapy, psychological counseling, and physical therapy
- Electrostimulation therapy: TENS units
- Behavioral therapies: cognitive behavioral therapy, hypnosis, biofeedback, relaxation therapy
- Music therapy (in conjunction with other types of therapy)
- Surgery

ACUTE GENERAL Rx

- Short-acting anti-inflammatory and analgesic medications (e.g., acetaminophen/NSAIDs/opioids)
- Trigger point or joint injections (immediate anesthetic plus long-acting corticosteroids)
- Epidural steroid injections
- Nerve blocks

CHRONIC Rx

- Pain management with long-acting pharmacologic agents is considered a key aspect of therapy but is often underused. Fig. 1-695 illustrates a strategy for pharmacologic management of pain using the World Health Organization (WHO) analgesic ladder.
- Long-acting NSAIDs. Table 1-371 describes adjuvant analgesic drugs for chronic pain.

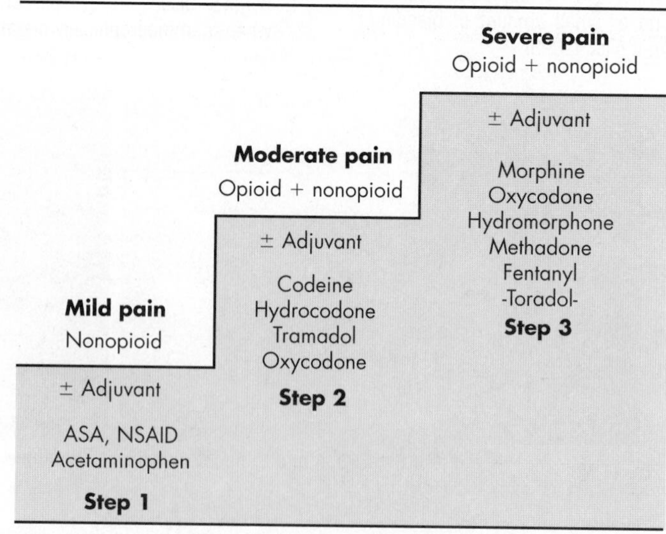

FIGURE 1-695 Strategy for pharmacologic management of pain using the World Health Organization (*WHO*) analgesic ladder. Multiagent therapy is usually required for optimal pain management. Patients with mild pain should be started on a nonopioid analgesic, and those with moderate pain on a step 2 opioid. Many patients can benefit from the addition of a nonopioid to the opioid (e.g., for bone pain) or an adjuvant agent to the opioid (e.g., for neuropathic pain). If this combination does not produce adequate relief or the patient has severe pain, step 3 opioids should be started initially. Toradol (ketorolac) is a nonsteroidal anti-inflammatory drug *(NSAID)* with the pain-relieving potency of a step 3 opioid. Many patients can benefit from the addition of nonopioid analgesics or adjuvants, if indicated. *ASA*, Aspirin. (From Hoffman R et al: *Hematology, basic principles and practice,* ed 5, Philadelphia, 2009, Churchill Livingstone.)

TABLE 1-371 Adjuvant Analgesic Drugs for Chronic Pain

Drug	Dosage	Indications	Adverse Effects	Comments
Tricyclic Antidepressants				
Amitriptyline, imipramine, desipramine, nortriptyline	10-150 mg/day	Peripheral neuropathy, postherpetic neuralgia, other types of peripheral neuropathic pain, central pain, facial pain, fibromyalgia, headache prophylaxis, irritable bowel syndrome, and chronic low back pain with or without radiculopathy	Sedation, dry mouth, confusion, weight gain, constipation, urinary retention, ataxia, cardiac conduction delay (QTc prolongation)	First-line agents for neuropathic pain and headache prophylaxis Secondary amine drugs (e.g., nortriptyline) have fewer side effects than tertiary amines (e.g., amitriptyline) Contraindicated in glaucoma
Serotonin-Norepinephrine Reuptake Inhibitors				
Venlafaxine	75-225 mg/day	Peripheral neuropathy, headache prophylaxis	Sedation, dry mouth, constipation, ataxia, hypertension, hyperhidrosis	Dose adjustment in patients with renal dysfunction
Duloxetine	60-120 mg/day	Peripheral neuropathy, fibromyalgia, chronic back pain	Sedation, dry mouth, constipation, hyperhidrosis	U.S. Food and Drug Administration (FDA)-approved for fibromyalgia and diabetic neuropathy Contraindicated in glaucoma
Anticonvulsants				
Gabapentin	600-3600 mg/day	Peripheral neuropathy, postherpetic neuralgia, other types of peripheral neuropathic pain, central pain, pelvic pain, headache prophylaxis, radiculopathy, chronic postsurgical pain	Sedation, weight gain, dry mouth, ataxia, edema	First-line agent for neuropathic pain FDA-approved for postherpetic neuralgia Effective preemptively for postoperative pain
Pregabalin	150-600 mg/day	Peripheral neuropathy, postherpetic neuralgia, central pain, fibromyalgia	Sedation, weight gain, dry mouth, ataxia, edema	First-line agent for neuropathic pain FDA-approved for diabetic neuropathy, postherpetic neuralgia, fibromyalgia Effective preemptively for postoperative pain Same mechanism of action as gabapentin
Carbamazepine	200-1600 mg/day	Facial neuralgias, diabetic neuropathy	Sedation, ataxia, diplopia, hyponatremia, agranulocytosis, diarrhea, aplastic anemia, hepatotoxicity, Stevens-Johnson syndrome	First-line agent and FDA-approved for trigeminal and glossopharyngeal neuralgia Contraindicated in patients with porphyria and atrioventricular conduction block
Topiramate	50-400 mg/day	Headache prophylaxis, chronic low back pain with or without radiculopathy	Sedation, ataxia, diplopia, weight loss, diarrhea, metabolic acidosis, kidney stones	First-line agent and FDA-approved for migraine prophylaxis Often used as appetite suppressant
Corticosteroids (Systemic)				
Prednisone	5-60 mg/day	Inflammatory arthritis, other inflammatory pain conditions (e.g., inflammatory bowel disease), traumatic nerve injury, complex regional pain syndrome	Myriad psychiatric, gastrointestinal, neurologic, and cardiac side effects; immunosuppression, weakness, edema, weight gain, elevated glucose, poor wound healing, others	Stronger evidence supports local (i.e., injection) administration More effective for acute pain Strong anti-inflammatory effects
Miscellaneous				
Muscle relaxants	Variable depending on drug	Skeletal muscle spasm, acute spinal pain, temporomandibular disorder Baclofen effective for spasticity, dystonia, and trigeminal neuralgia	Sedation, ataxia, blurred vision, confusion, asthenia, xerostomia and other gastrointestinal effects, palpitations	First-line agents for acute back pain and skeletal muscle spasm
Lidocaine patch	1-3 patches every 12 hr	Postherpetic neuralgia, peripheral neuropathy, other types of neuropathic and possibly myofascial pain associated with allodynia	Minimal systemic side effects when applied appropriately	Second-line agent and FDA-approved for postherpetic neuralgia
Capsaicin cream	0.025% applied three or four times per day	Postherpetic neuralgia, peripheral neuropathy and other types of neuropathic pain, chronic postsurgical pain, arthritis, and other musculoskeletal conditions	Burning on application Minimal systemic side effects when applied appropriately	FDA-approved for arthritis Second-line agent for postherpetic neuralgia and third-line agent for peripheral neuropathy Single application 8% patch providing up to 3 mo of pain relief was recently approved for postherpetic neuralgia
Cannabinoids	Variable depending on drug and delivery route	Strongest evidence is for multiple sclerosis May be effective for peripheral neuropathy and other types of neuropathic pain spasticity	Myriad psychiatric, neurologic, and cardiac effects; xerostomia, abdominal pain, and other gastrointestinal effects	Fourth-line agent with narrow therapeutic index Modest analgesic effect comparable to codeine

From Goldman L, Schafer AI: *Goldman's Cecil medicine*, ed 24, Philadelphia, 2012, Saunders.

- Sustained-release opioids (used for moderate to severe pain that has failed other therapeutic interventions): oxycodone, morphine SR, methadone (use with caution), or Duragesic patch; short-acting opioids can be used in conjunction with these agents for management of breakthrough pain. Conversion to a long-acting opioid should be based on an equianalgesic conversion (http://www.acpinternist.org/archives/2008/01/extra/pain_charts.pdf). Table E1-372 provides guidelines for opioid dose selection, conservative initial starting doses for opioid-naïve individuals, and conversion ratios for opioid rotation in patients on chronic opioids.
- Antidepressants (tricyclic and selective serotonin reuptake inhibitor)
- Anticonvulsant medications particularly helpful for neuropathic conditions (e.g., carbamazepine, valproic acid, gabapentin, pregabalin)
- Implantable methods, epidural and intrathecal drug delivery systems, dorsal column stimulators

COMPLEMENTARY & ALTERNATIVE MEDICINE

Acupuncture and massage (evidence based for some indications). Acupuncture is most likely to benefit patients with low back pain, neck pain, chronic idiopathic or tension headache, migraine, and knee osteoarthritis.

REFERRAL

- Pain medicine specialist or multidisciplinary pain clinic: useful when primary therapies fail, in patients with complex pain conditions, or for invasive therapies
- Consider referral to an addiction specialist if patient has a history of substance abuse or addiction
- Psychiatry/psychological services for counseling, if needed

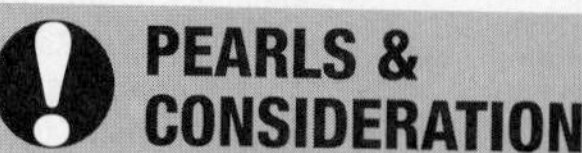

PEARLS & CONSIDERATIONS

- Patient consent should be obtained in the form of a written treatment agreement before initiating treatment. This agreement should outline the goals of therapy, use of a single provider or treatment team and a single pharmacy, limitations on dose and number of prescribed medications, prohibition on use with alcohol or sedating medications, keeping medication safe and secure, prohibition on selling or sharing medication, limitations on refills, compliance with all components of the treatment plan, the role of drug screening, and consequences of nonadherence.
- Follow-up assessment should occur every 1 to 6 mo and include a complete pain assessment (see earlier), review of the type of long-acting analgesic used and dosage, use of breakthrough analgesics, side effects and their management, use of nonpharmacologic therapies, and adjunct medication use.

COMMENTS

- Medication dependence and addiction should not be confused. Most patients receiving chronic opioid therapy can become dependent on these medications for pain relief but opioid addiction does not occur. Patients exhibiting signs of addiction often will seek escalating doses of medication, request refills of prescriptions earlier than planned, and engage in drug-seeking activities (e.g., emergency department visits between prescriptions, seeking multiple prescriptions).
- Side effects need not preclude use of opioid medications and should be anticipated. Antiemetics can aid in controlling nausea. Constipation can be managed with stool softeners and laxatives.
- The emphasis of comprehensive pain management for non–cancer-related chronic pain has led to a fourfold increase in prescribing of opioid medications in the United States. This increase in opiate use has also led to a rise in the misuse and abuse of these medications. Providers should proceed with caution before initiating pain management with opiate medications and should familiarize themselves with processes and tools for pain assessment and medication management. Forty-two states have developed prescription drug monitoring programs (PDMPs) to assist providers in identifying issues of abuse, polypharmacy, and misuse of controlled substances.

PATIENT & FAMILY EDUCATION

National Pain Foundation
(http://www.painconnection.org)
American Pain Foundation
(http://www.painfoundation.org)
National Institutes of Health
(http://www.nih.gov)

SUGGESTED READINGS

available at www.expertconsult.com

AUTHOR: **ANNGENE G. ANTHONY, M.D., M.P.H., F.A.A.F.P.**

BASIC INFORMATION

DEFINITION

Pancreatic cancer is an adenocarcinoma derived from the epithelium of the pancreatic duct.

ICD-9CM CODES
157.9 Pancreatic cancer
157.0 (head)
157.1 (body)
157.2 (tail)
157.3 (duct)
230.9 (in situ)

ICD-10CM CODES
C25.9 Malignant neoplasm of pancreas, unspecified
C25.0 Malignant neoplasm of head of pancreas
C25.1 Malignant neoplasm of body of pancreas
C25.2 Malignant neoplasm of tail of pancreas
C25.3 Malignant neoplasm of pancreatic duct

EPIDEMIOLOGY & DEMOGRAPHICS

INCIDENCE: One case in 10,000 persons annually. In the U.S. there are >35,000 patients diagnosed with pancreatic cancer and >35,000 deaths yearly. It is the fourth leading cause of cancer-related death in the U.S. Less than 20% of patients present with localized, potentially respectable tumors.

PREDOMINANT SEX: Male/female ratio of 2:1

PREDOMINANT AGE: Seventh and eighth decades of life

PHYSICAL FINDINGS & CLINICAL PRESENTATION

Presenting symptoms:
- Jaundice
- Abdominal pain: generally dull upper abdominal pain or vague abdominal discomfort
- Weight loss
- Anorexia/change in taste, asthenia
- Nausea
- Uncommonly: depression, gastrointestinal bleeding, acute pancreatitis (from obstruction of the pancreatic duct), back pain
- Trousseau syndrome (hypercoagulability in the setting of malignancy) may be initial presentation in some patients.

Physical findings:
- Icterus
- Cachexia, temporal wasting
- Ascites, peripheral lymphadenopathy, hepatomegaly
- Excoriations from scratching pruritic skin

ETIOLOGY

Unknown, but several conditions have been associated with pancreatic cancer:
- Smoking
- Alcoholism
- Genetics: 5% to 10% of patients have a family history of the disease
- Gallstones
- Diabetes mellitus
- Chronic pancreatitis
- Diet rich in animal fat
- Occupational exposures: oil refining, paper manufacturing, chemical industry
- Overweight or obesity during early adulthood is associated with a greater risk of pancreatic cancer and a younger age of disease onset. Obesity at an older age is associated with a lower overall survival in patients with pancreatic cancer.
- Possible increased risk for certain type-2 diabetes medications (GLP-1 receptor agonists and DPP-4 inhibitors

Dx DIAGNOSIS

DIFFERENTIAL DIAGNOSIS

- Common duct cholelithiasis
- Cholangiocarcinoma
- Common duct stricture
- Sclerosing cholangitis
- Primary biliary cirrhosis
- Autoimmune pancreatitis
- Drug-induced cholestasis (e.g., phenothiazines)
- Chronic hepatitis
- Sarcoidosis
- Other pancreatic tumors (islet cell tumor, cystadenocarcinoma, epidermoid carcinoma, sarcomas, lymphomas)

WORKUP

Routine Laboratory Tests	*% Abnormal*
Alkaline phosphatase	80
Bilirubin	55
Total protein	15
Amylase	15
Hematocrit	60

Ca 19-9: Not useful as a screening tool because it may be elevated in other conditions, such as cholestasis, but is useful for therapeutic monitoring and early detection of recurrent disease after treatment

IMAGING STUDIES

Multidetector helical CT with IV administration of contrast is the imaging procedure of choice for initial evaluation. Endoscopic ultrasonography is useful when there is no identifiable mass on CT and diagnosis is strongly suspected and in obtaining tissue for diagnostic purposes. Fine-needle aspiration biopsy combined with endoscopic ultrasonography is the preferred modality for evaluation of cystic or mass lesions to determine malignancy. Endoscopic retrograde cholangiopancreatography (ERCP) is useful in patients with jaundice needing an endoscopic stent to relieve obstruction.

Noninvasive Imaging	*% Abnormal*
Abdominal ultrasonography	60
Abdominal CT scan (with contrast) (Fig. 1-696)	90
Abdominal MRI scan	90
Invasive Imaging	
ERCP	90
CT scan or ultrasonography-guided needle aspiration cytology	90-95

STAGING FOR PANCREATIC CANCER

PRIMARY TUMOR (T):

TX	Primary tumor cannot be assessed
T0	No evidence of primary tumor
T1	Tumor <2 cm
T2	Tumor >2 cm, confined to the pancreas
T3	Tumor extends locally beyond the pancreas
T4	Tumor involves celiac or superior mesenteric arteries

LYMPH NODES (N):

NX	Regional lymph nodes cannot be assessed
N0	No regional lymph node metastasis
N1	Regional lymph node metastasis

DISTANT METASTASES (M):

MX	Presence of distant metastasis cannot be assessed
M0	No distant metastasis
M1	Distant metastasis

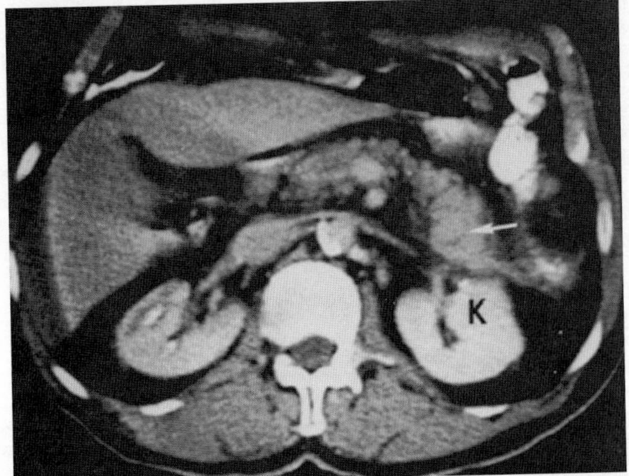

FIGURE 1-696 CT scan of a patient with adenocarcinoma of the body and tail of the pancreas. The tumor *(arrow)* is seen anterior and adjacent to the left kidney *(K)*. At operation, the tumor was invading Gerota's fascia. (From Sabiston D: *Textbook of surgery,* ed 17, Philadelphia, 2005, Saunders.)

STAGING GROUP:

IA	T1, N0, M0
IB	T2, N0, M0
IIA	T3, N0, M0
IIB	T1-3, N1, M0
III	T4, N0-1, M0
IV	T1-4, N0-1, M1

A clinical/radiographic staging system for adenocarcinoma of the pancreatic head and uncinate process is described in Table 1-373.

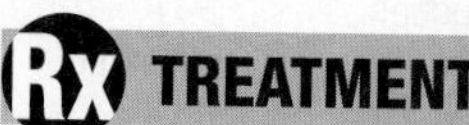

TREATMENT

SURGERY

Curative cephalic pancreatoduodenectomy (Whipple's procedure) is appropriate for only 10% to 20% of patients whose lesion is <5 cm, solitary, and without metastases. Surgical mortality rate is 5%. Adjuvant chemotherapy may improve postoperative survival. The addition of gemcitabine to adjuvant fluorouracil and leucovorin chemotherapy has been reported to have a survival benefit for patients with resected pancreatic cancer. An emerging strategy is the use of neoadjuvant preoperative treatment in patients with resectable pancreatic cancer

PALLIATIVE SURGERY (FOR BILIARY DECOMPRESSION/DIVERSION)

Palliative therapeutic ERCP with stents

CHEMOTHERAPY

In patients with advanced disease an accepted approach is the administration of gemcitabine given alone or combined with a platinum agent, the oral EGFR inhibitor erlotinib, or fluoropyrimidine. Combination therapy consisting of oxaliplatin, irinotecan, fluorouracil, and leucovorin (FOLFIRINOX) offers increased median survival in metastatic pancreatic cancer when compared to gemcitabine (11.1 mo versus 6.8 mo) but increased toxicity.

- A recent trial revealed that in patients with metastatic pancreatic adenocarcinoma, NAB-paclitaxel plus gemcitabine significantly improved overall survival, progression-free survival, and response rate, but rates of peripheral neuropathy and myelosuppression were increased.[1]

RADIATION

- External-beam radiation for palliation of pain.
- Combined chemotherapy and radiation provides a median survival of 11 mo.
- Celiac plexus block by an experienced anesthesiologist provides pain relief in 80% to 90% of cases.

DISPOSITION

- Adjunct chemotherapy has a significant survival benefit in patients with resected pancreatic cancer.
- Recent trials have shown that adjuvant postoperative chemotherapy with gemcitabine significantly delays the development of recurrent disease after complete resection of pancreatic cancer. Among patients with macroscopic complete removal of pancreatic cancer, the use of adjuvant gemcitabine for 6 mo compared with observation alone resulted in increased overall survival as well as disease-free survival. These findings provide strong support for use of gemcitabine in this setting.[2]
- Median survival for locally unresectable disease is about 1 yr. Median survival for metastatic cancer is 4-6 mo.

[1]Von Hoff DD et al: Increased survival in pancreatic cancer with NAB-paclitaxel plus gemcitabine, *N Engl J Med* 369:1691-1703, 2013.

[2]Dettel H et al: Adjuvant chemotherapy with gemcitabine and long-term outcomes among patients with resected pancreatic cancer, the CONKO-001 randomized trial, *JAMA* 310(14):1473-1481, 2013.

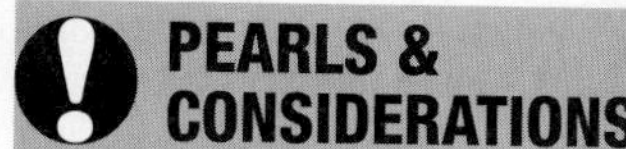

PEARLS & CONSIDERATIONS

COMMENTS

- The U.S. Preventive Services Task Force (USPSTF) recommends against routine screening for pancreatic cancer in asymptomatic adults by abdominal palpation, ultrasonography, or serologic markers. The USPSTF found no evidence that screening for pancreatic cancer is effective in reducing mortality rates. There is potential for significant harm because of the low prevalence of pancreatic cancer, limited accuracy of available screening tests, invasive nature of diagnostic tests, and poor outcome of treatment. As a result, the USPSTF concluded that the harms of screening for pancreatic cancer exceed any potential benefits.
- Recent trials indicate that pancreatic cancer may have a distinct microRNA (miRNA) expression pattern that may differentiate it from normal pancreas and chronic pancreatitis. Current research is aimed at using miRNA expression patterns to distinguish between long- and short-term survivors.
- Alcohol consumption, specifically liquor consumption of three or more drinks per day, increases pancreatic cancer mortality independent of smoking.

SUGGESTED READINGS

available at www.expertconsult.com

RELATED CONTENT

Pancreatic Cancer (Patient Information)

AUTHOR: **FRED F. FERRI, M.D.**

TABLE 1-373 Clinical/Radiographic Staging System for Adenocarcinoma of the Pancreatic Head and Uncinate Process

Clinical Stage	AJCC Stage	TUMOR-VESSEL RELATIONSHIP ON COMPUTED TOMOGRAPHY			
		SMA	Celiac Axis	CHA*	SMV-PV
Resectable (all four are required to be resectable)†	I/II	Normal tissue plane between tumor and vessel	Normal tissue plane between tumor and vessel	Normal tissue plane between tumor and vessel	Patent (may include tumor abutment or encasement)
Borderline resectable (only one of the four required)	III	Abutment	Abutment	Abutment or short segment encasement	May have short segment occlusion if reconstruction possible
Locally advanced (only one of the four required)	III	Encasement	Encasement	Extensive encasement with no technical option for reconstruction	Occluded with no technical option for reconstruction

AJCC, American Joint Commission for Cancer; *CHA,* common hepatic artery; *SMV–PV,* superior mesenteric vein–portal vein confluence.
Abutment refers to ≤180 degrees or ≤50% of the vessel circumference; encasement is <180 degrees or <50% of the vessel circumference.
*Assumes normal vascular anatomy; for example, encasement of the CHA is not a limitation in performing PD when there is an uninvolved replaced right hepatic artery arising from the superior mesenteric artery.
†Assumes the technical ability to resect and reconstruct the SMV, PV, or SMV-PV confluence when necessary. Others would consider tumor-vein abutment/encasement, which results in deformity of the vein as borderline resectable.
From Cameron JL, Cameron AM: *Current surgical therapy,* ed 10, Philadelphia, 2011, Saunders.

BASIC INFORMATION

DEFINITION

- Acute pancreatitis is an inflammatory process of the pancreas with intrapancreatic activation of enzymes that may also involve peripancreatic tissue and/or remote organ systems.
- Commonly used scoring systems for acute pancreatitis are described in Table 1-374. Severe acute pancreatitis (SAP) is diagnosed by the presence of any of the following four criteria:
  1. Organ failure with one or more of the following: shock (systolic blood pressure <90 mm Hg), pulmonary insufficiency (Pa_{O_2} ≤60 mm Hg), renal failure (serum creatinine >2 mg/dl after rehydration), and gastrointestinal bleeding (>500 ml/24 hr)
  2. Local complications such as necrosis, pseudocyst, or abscess
  3. At least three of Ranson's criteria (see below) *or*
  4. At least eight of the Acute Physiology and Chronic Health Evaluation II (APACHE II) criteria

ICD-9CM CODES
577.0 Acute pancreatitis
ICD-10CM CODES
K85.9 Acute pancreatitis, unspecified
K85.0 Idiopathic acute pancreatitis
K85.1 Biliary acute pancreatitis
K85.2 Alcohol-induced pancreatitis
K85.3 Drug-induced pancreatitis
K8.5 Other acute pancreatitis

EPIDEMIOLOGY & DEMOGRAPHICS

- There are >240,000 cases of acute pancreatitis reported annually in the U.S., with nearly 50% due to gallstone disease.
- Acute pancreatitis is most often secondary to biliary tract disease and alcohol. The rate of pancreatitis continues to rise and ranges from 10-45 cases/100,000 in Western countries.
- Incidence in urban areas is twice that of rural areas (20/100,000 persons in urban areas).
- 20% of patients have necrotizing pancreatitis; the remainder have interstitial, or edematous, pancreatitis.
- Acute pancreatitis accounts for >220,000 hospital admissions in the U.S. each year.

PHYSICAL FINDINGS & CLINICAL PRESENTATION

- Epigastric tenderness and guarding, often radiating to the back; pain usually developing suddenly, reaching peak intensity within 10 to 30 min, severe and lasting several hours without relief
- Hypoactive bowel sounds (from ileus)
- Tachycardia, shock (from decreased intravascular volume)
- Confusion (from metabolic disturbances)
- Fever
- Tachycardia, decreased breath sounds (atelectasis, pleural effusions, acute respiratory distress syndrome [ARDS])
- Jaundice (from obstruction or compression of biliary tract)
- Ascites (from tear in pancreatic duct, leaking pseudocyst)
- Palpable abdominal mass (pseudocyst, phlegmon, abscess, carcinoma)
- Evidence of hypocalcemia (Chvostek's sign, Trousseau's sign)
- Evidence of intraabdominal bleeding (hemorrhagic pancreatitis):
  1. Gray-blue discoloration around the umbilicus ***(Cullen's sign)***
  2. Bluish discoloration involving the flanks ***(Grey Turner's sign)***
- Tender subcutaneous nodules (caused by subcutaneous fat necrosis)

ETIOLOGY

- In >90% of cases: biliary tract disease (calculi or sludge) or alcohol, most common after 5-10 yr of heavy drinking
- Drugs (e.g., thiazides, furosemide, corticosteroids, tetracycline, estrogens, valproic acid, metronidazole, azathioprine, methyldopa, pentamidine, ethacrynic acid, procainamide, sulindac, nitrofurantoin, angiotensin-converting enzyme inhibitors, danazol, cimetidine, piroxicam, gold, ranitidine, sulfasalazine, isoniazid, acetaminophen, cisplatin, opiates, erythromycin, metformin, GLP-1 receptor antagonists, incretin mimetics)
- Abdominal trauma
- Surgery
- Endoscopic retrograde cholangiopancreatography (ERCP)
- Infections (predominantly viral infections)
- Peptic ulcer (penetrating duodenal ulcer)
- Pancreas divisum (congenital failure to fuse of dorsal or ventral pancreas)
- Idiopathic
- Pregnancy
- Vascular (vasculitis, ischemic)
- Hypolipoproteinemia (types I, IV, and V)
- Hypercalcemia
- Pancreatic carcinoma (primary or metastatic)
- Renal failure
- Hereditary pancreatitis
- Occupational exposure to chemicals: methanol, cobalt, zinc, mercuric chloride, creosol, lead, organophosphates, chlorinated naphthalenes
- Others: scorpion bite, obstruction at ampulla region (neoplasm, duodenal diverticula, Crohn's disease), hypotensive shock, autoimmune pancreatitis

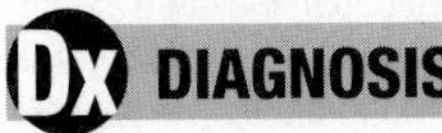

DIAGNOSIS

DIFFERENTIAL DIAGNOSIS

- PUD
- Acute cholangitis, biliary colic
- High intestinal obstruction
- Early acute appendicitis

TABLE 1-374 Commonly Used Scoring Systems: Advantages and Disadvantages

System	Scoring	Advantages	Disadvantages
Ranson's criteria on admission: 1. Age >55 yr 2. WBC >16 × 10^9/L 3. LDH >350 U/L 4. AST >250 U/L 5. Glucose >200 mg/dl During initial 48 hr: 1. Hgb falls below 10 mg/dl 2. BUN rises by >5 mg/dl 3. Ca <8 mg/dl 4. Pa_{O_2} <60 mm Hg 5. Base deficit >4 mEq/L 6. Fluid sequestration >6 L	1 point for each factor listed; score >3 indicates SAP	Well known, relatively easy to calculate	Requires 48 hr to complete evaluation
APACHE II*	Score >8 predicts SAP	Can be calculated within 24 hr of admission	Requires large dataset for processing
BISAP 1. BUN >25 mg/dl 2. Altered mental status 3. Presence of SIRS 4. Age >60 yr 5. Pleural effusions	1 point for each factor listed; score >3 indicates SAP	Ease of use, available within 24 hr of admission	Significantly lower sensitivity than either Ranson's or APACHE II; results in greater likelihood of missing severe AP
CTSI	Based on radiographic data	Excellent predictor of local complications; can show infected pancreatic necrosis	Requires 72 to 96 hr, making it a poor test for guiding decisions at admission

**Based on diverse variables, including age, physiology, and long-term health; equation available at www.sfar.org/scores2/apache22.html#calcul. Adding body mass index (BMI) to APACHE II (the APACHE O score) increases discrimination (1 point added for BMI 26-30; 2 points for BMI >30).*

APACHE, Acute Physiology and Chronic Health Evaluation; *AST,* Aspartate aminotransferase; *BISAP,* Bedside Index for Severity in Acute Pancreatitis; *BUN,* blood urea nitrogen; *Ca,* serum calcium; *CTSI,* Computed Tomography Severity Index; *Hgb,* hemoglobin; *LDH,* lactate dehydrogenase; *SAP,* severe acute pancreatitis; *SIRS,* systemic inflammatory response syndrome; *WBC,* white blood cell count.

Modified from Cameron JL, Cameron AM: *Current surgical therapy,* ed 10, Philadelphia, 2011, Saunders.

- Mesenteric vascular obstruction
- DKA
- Pneumonia (basilar)
- Myocardial infarction (inferior wall)
- Renal colic
- Ruptured or dissecting aortic aneurysm
- Mesenteric ischemia

LABORATORY TESTS

Pancreatic enzymes:

- Amylase is increased, usually elevated in the initial 3 to 5 days of acute pancreatitis. Isoamylase determinations (separation of pancreatic cell isoenzyme components of amylase) are useful in excluding occasional cases of salivary hyperamylasemia. The use of isoamylase rather than total serum amylase reduces the risk of erroneously diagnosing pancreatitis and is preferred by some as initial biochemical test in patients suspected of having acute pancreatitis.
- Urinary amylase determinations are useful to diagnose acute pancreatitis in patients with lipemic serum, to rule out elevated serum amylase caused by macroamylasemia, and to diagnose acute pancreatitis in patients whose serum amylase is normal.
- Serum lipase levels are elevated in acute pancreatitis; the elevation is less transient than serum amylase; concomitant evaluation of serum amylase and lipase increases diagnostic accuracy of acute pancreatitis. An elevated lipase/amylase ratio is suggestive of alcoholic pancreatitis.
- Elevated serum trypsin levels are diagnostic of pancreatitis (in absence of renal failure).
- Serum C-reactive protein at 48 hr is an excellent laboratory marker of severity.
- Rapid measurement of urinary trypsinogen-2 (if available) is useful in the emergency department as a screening test for acute pancreatitis in patients with abdominal pain; a negative dipstick test for urinary trypsinogen-2 rules out acute pancreatitis with a high degree of probability, whereas a positive test indicates need for further evaluation.

Additional tests:

- Complete blood count: reveals leukocytosis; hematocrit (Hct) may be initially increased as a result of hemoconcentration; decreased Hct may indicate hemorrhage or hemolysis.
- Blood urea nitrogen (BUN) is increased because of dehydration. Serial BUN measurements are the most valuable lab test for predicting mortality during the initial 48 hr.
- Elevation of serum glucose in a previously normal patient correlates with the degree of pancreatic malfunction and may be related to increased release of glycogen, catecholamines, and glucocorticoid release and decreased insulin release.
- Liver profile: aspartate aminotransferase (AST) and lactate dehydrogenase (LDH) are increased as a result of tissue necrosis; bilirubin and alkaline phosphatase may be increased from common bile duct obstruction. A threefold or greater rise in serum alanine aminotransferase concentrations is an excellent indicator (95% probability) of biliary pancreatitis.
- Serum calcium is decreased as a result of saponification, precipitation, and decreased parathyroid hormone response.
- Arterial blood gases: Pa_{O_2} may be decreased as a result of ARDS, pleural effusion(s); pH may be decreased as a result of lactic acidosis, respiratory acidosis, and renal insufficiency.
- Serum electrolytes: potassium may be increased from acidosis or renal insufficiency; sodium may be increased from dehydration.

IMAGING STUDIES

- Abdominal plain films are useful initially to distinguish other conditions that may mimic pancreatitis (perforated viscus). They may reveal localized ileus (sentinel loop), pancreatic calcifications (chronic pancreatitis), blurring of left psoas shadow, dilation of transverse colon, calcified gallstones.
- Chest x-ray may reveal elevation of one or both diaphragms, pleural effusions, basilar infiltrates, or platelike atelectasis.
- Abdominal ultrasonography is useful in detecting gallstones (sensitivity of 60% to 70% for detecting stones associated with pancreatitis). It is also useful for detecting pancreatic pseudocysts. Its availability and noninvasive nature make it the initial imaging study of choice; its major limitation is the presence of distended bowel loops overlying the pancreas.
- CT scan (Fig. 1-697) is superior to ultrasonography in identifying pancreatitis and defining its extent, and it also plays a role in diagnosing pseudocysts (they appear as a well-defined area surrounded by a high-density capsule); gastrointestinal fistulation or infection of a pseudocyst can also be identified by the presence of gas within the pseudocyst. Sequential contrast-enhanced CT is useful for detection of pancreatic necrosis. The severity of pancreatitis can also be graded by CT scan (Table E1-375). (A = normal pancreas, B = enlarged pancreas [1 point], C = pancreatic and/or peripancreatic inflammation [2 points], D = single peripancreatic collection [3 points], E = at least two peripancreatic collections and/or retroperitoneal air [4 points]. Percentage of pancreatic necrosis <30% [2 points], 30% to 50% [4 points], >50% [6 points]. The CT severity index is calculated by adding grade points to points assigned for percentage of necrosis.)
- Magnetic resonance cholangiopancreatography (MRCP) has >90% sensitivity for choledocholithiasis and can identify other anatomic abnormalities.
- Endoscopic ultrasonography (EUS) is a minimally invasive test that provides high-resolution imaging of the pancreas. It is useful to identify anatomic abnormalities of the pancreas and has good sensitivity and specificity for small gallstones (≤5 mm).
- ERCP indications: useful to perform biliary sphincterotomy and stone removal in the presence of a retained bile duct stone seen on imaging. The role and timing of ERCP in patients with acute biliary pancreatitis has been controversial. Guidelines from the American College of Gastroenterology suggest that urgent ERCP (within 24 hr of admission) is indicated in patients with biliary pancreatitis who have concurrent acute cholangitis, but it is not needed in most patients who do not have evidence of ongoing biliary obstruction.[1,2]

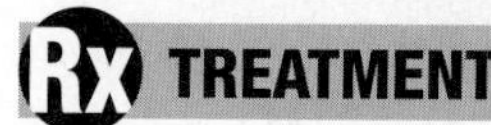

NONPHARMACOLOGIC THERAPY

- Bowel rest with avoidance of liquids or solids during the acute illness
- Avoidance of alcohol and any drugs associated with pancreatitis

[1]Fogel EL, Sherman S: ERCP for gallstone pancreatitis, *N Engl J Med* 370:150-157, 2014.

[2]Tenner S et al: American College of Gastroenterology guidelines: management of acute pancreatitis, *Am J Gastroenterol* 108:1400-1415, 2013.

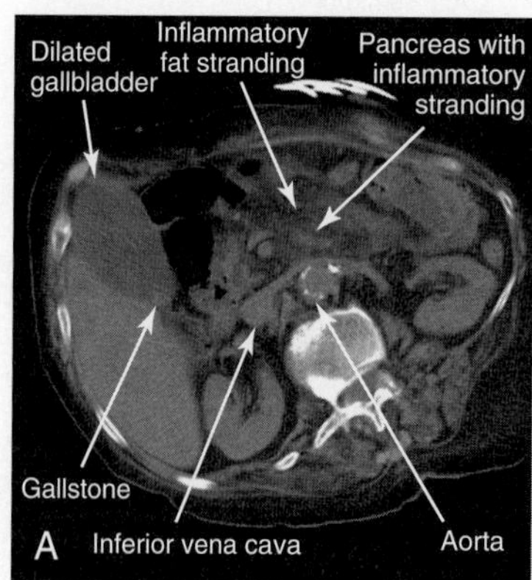

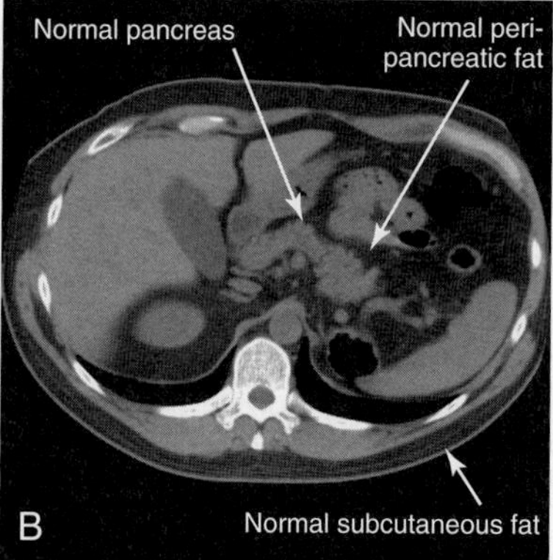

FIGURE 1-697 Gallstone pancreatitis and normal pancreas for comparison, axial CT without contrast. A, Gallstone pancreatitis CT. A dilated gallbladder is visible with a hyperdense dependent lesion consistent with a gallstone. The region of the pancreas shows significant inflammatory stranding. In this patient, the pancreas lies just anterior to the left renal vein, which can be seen crossing anterior to the aorta and entering the inferior vena cava. **B,** A normal pancreas is visible. This pancreas is surrounded by uninflamed fat, which is dark (nearly black). Compare this normal fat with normal subcutaneous fat. (From Broder JS: *Diagnostic imaging for the emergency physician,* Philadelphia, 2011, Saunders.)

ACUTE GENERAL Rx

General measures:

- Assess severity of pancreatitis (see Table 1-374).
- Maintain adequate intravascular volume with vigorous IV hydration. Aggressive fluid resuscitation is critical in managing acute pancreatitis.
- Patient should remain NPO until clinically improved, stable, and hungry. Enteral feedings are preferred over total parenteral nutrition. Enteral nutrition reduces mortality, multiple organ failure, systemic infections, and operative interventions more than total parenteral nutrition does in patients with acute pancreatitis. Parenteral nutrition may be necessary in patients who do not tolerate enteral feeding or in whom an adequate infusion rate cannot be reached within 2 to 4 days.
- Nasogastric suction is useful only in severe pancreatitis to decompress the abdomen in patients with ileus.
- Control pain: IV morphine or fentanyl. Meperidine and hydromorphone are also commonly used narcotics for pain control.
- Correct metabolic abnormalities (e.g., replace calcium and magnesium as necessary).

Specific measures:

- Pancreatic or peripancreatic infection develops in 40% to 70% of patients with pancreatic necrosis. However, IV antibiotics should not be used prophylactically for all cases of pancreatitis; their use is justified if the patient has evidence of septicemia, pancreatic abscess, or pancreatitis caused by biliary calculi. Their use should generally be limited to 5 to 7 days to prevent development of fungal superinfection. Appropriate empiric antibiotic therapy should cover:
  - *Bacteroides fragilis* and other anaerobes (cefotetan, cefoxitin, metronidazole, or clindamycin plus aminoglycoside)
  - *Enterococcus* (ampicillin)
- Surgical therapy has a limited role in acute pancreatitis; it is indicated in the following:
  - Gallstone-induced pancreatitis: cholecystectomy when acute pancreatitis subsides. However, randomized trials have shown that patients with mild gallstone pancreatitis can undergo cholecystectomy safely during the first 48 hr of hospitalization.
  - Perforated peptic ulcer.
  - Necrotizing pancreatitis with infected necrotic tissue is associated with an elevated rate of complications and increased risk of death. Traditional treatment has been open necrosectomy; surgical necrosectomy induces a proinflammatory response and is associated with a high complication rate. Recent trials have shown that a step-up approach consisting of percutaneous drainage followed, if necessary, by minimally invasive retroperitoneal necrosectomy may have a lower rate of complications and death. Endoscopic transgastric necrosectomy, a form of natural orifice transluminal endoscopic surgery, has been shown in recent trials to be effective in reducing the proinflammatory response as well as reducing complications.
- Identification and treatment of complications:
  - **Pseudocyst:** round or spheroid collection of fluid, tissue, pancreatic enzymes, and blood.
    - Diagnosed by CT scan or sonography
    - Treatment: Pancreatic pseudocysts can be drained surgically or endoscopically. The endoscopic approach is preferable when the patient's anatomy is suitable and an experienced endoscopist is available. CT scan or ultrasound-guided percutaneous drainage (with a pigtail catheter left in place for continuous drainage) can be used, but the recurrence rate is high; the conservative approach is to reevaluate the pseudocyst (with CT scan or sonography) after 6 to 7 wk and surgically drain it if the pseudocyst has not decreased in size.

      Generally, pseudocysts <5 cm in diameter are reabsorbed without intervention, whereas those >5 cm require surgical intervention after the wall has matured.
  - **Phlegmon:** represents pancreatic edema. It can be diagnosed by CT scan or sonography. Treatment is supportive because it usually resolves spontaneously.
  - **Pancreatic abscess:** diagnosed by CT scan (presence of bubbles in the retroperitoneum); Gram staining and cultures of fluid obtained from guided percutaneous aspiration usually identify bacterial organism. Therapy is surgical (or catheter) drainage and IV antibiotics (imipenem-cilastatin is the drug of choice).
  - **Pancreatic ascites:** usually caused by leaking of pseudocyst or tear in pancreatic duct. Paracentesis reveals very high amylase and lipase levels in the pancreatic fluid; ERCP may demonstrate the lesion. Treatment is surgical correction if exudative ascites from severe pancreatitis does not resolve spontaneously.
  - Gastrointestinal bleeding: caused by alcoholic gastritis, bleeding varices, stress ulceration, or disseminated intravascular coagulation (DIC).
  - Renal failure: caused by hypovolemia, resulting in oliguria or anuria, cortical or tubular necrosis (shock, DIC), or thrombosis of renal artery or vein.
  - Hypoxia: caused by ARDS, pleural effusion, or atelectasis.

THERAPY OF UNCOMMON FORMS OF PANCREATITIS

1. **Autoimmune pancreatitis (AIP):** Fibroinflammatory disease characterized by an IgG4 lymphoplasmacytic infiltrate. It has been associated with other autoimmune disorders (e.g., primary sclerosing cholangitis, Sjögren syndrome). The inflammatory process is generally responsive to corticosteroid therapy. Type II autoimmune hepatitis (idiopathic duct-centric chronic pancreatitis) is associated with inflammatory bowel disease and not related to IgG4 cell deposition.
2. **Hypertriglyceridemic pancreatitis (HTGP):** Beneficial results have been reported with early (within 48 hr) initiation of apheresis with IV heparin and insulin in addition to conventional treatment modalities for acute pancreatitis when there is concomitant hyperglycemia with severe acute pancreatitis.

DISPOSITION

Prognosis varies with the severity of pancreatitis; overall mortality rate in acute pancreatitis is 5% to 10%. Prognostic criteria for acute pancreatitis are described in Table E1-376.

REFERRAL

- Hospitalization is indicated in moderate to severe cases of pancreatitis.
- Surgical consultation is needed in suspected gallstone pancreatitis, perforated peptic ulcer, or presence of necrotic or infected foci. Acute pancreatitis can generally be attributed to gallstones when patients have both abnormal liver enzymes and gallstones (or sludge) on imaging. Such patients should consider cholecystectomy to prevent recurrent pancreatitis.
- Gastroenterology consultation in severe or recurrent pancreatitis, when ERCP is needed for gallstone pancreatitis, or when the cause of pancreatitis is unclear.

PEARLS & CONSIDERATIONS

- Acute pancreatitis is the most common major complication of ERCP. NSAIDs are potent inhibitors of phospholipase A_2, cyclooxygenase, and neutrophil-endothelial interactions, which play an important role in the pathogenesis of acute pancreatitis. Preliminary trials show that among patients at high risk for post-ERCP pancreatitis, rectal indomethacin (given as two 50 mg indomethacin suppositories administered immediately after ERCP) significantly reduced the incidence of post-ERCP pancreatitis.
- Pancreatic stent placement decreases the risk of post-ERCP pancreatitis.
- Statins reduce risk for pancreatitis in adults. Fibrates do not affect risk for pancreatitis.

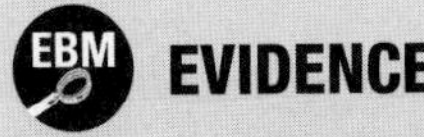

EVIDENCE

available at www.expertconsult.com

SUGGESTED READINGS

available at www.expertconsult.com

RELATED CONTENT

Acute Pancreatitis (Patient Information)

AUTHOR: **FRED F. FERRI, M.D.**

BASIC INFORMATION

DEFINITION

Chronic pancreatitis is a recurrent or persistent inflammatory process of the pancreas characterized by chronic pain and by pancreatic exocrine and/or endocrine insufficiency.

ICD-9CM CODES
577.1 Chronic pancreatitis
ICD-10CM CODES
K86.1 Other chronic pancreatitis
K86.0 Alcohol-induced chronic pancreatitis

EPIDEMIOLOGY & DEMOGRAPHICS

- Chronic pancreatitis occurs in approximately five to 10 per 100,000 persons in industrialized countries.
- Average age at diagnosis is 35 to 55 yr; male/female ratio is 5:1.

PHYSICAL FINDINGS & CLINICAL PRESENTATION

- Persistent or recurrent epigastric and left upper quadrant pain that may radiate to the back
- Tenderness over the pancreas, muscle guarding
- Significant weight loss
- Bulky, foul-smelling stools, greasy in appearance
- Epigastric mass (10% of patients)
- Jaundice (5% to 10% of patients)

ETIOLOGY

- Chronic alcoholism
- Obstruction (ampullary stenosis, tumor, trauma, pancreas divisum, annular pancreas)
- Hereditary pancreatitis
- Severe malnutrition
- Idiopathic
- Untreated hyperparathyroidism (hypercalcemia)
- Mutations of the cystic fibrosis transmembrane conductance regulator *(CFTR)* gene and the TF genotype
- ***Autoimmune pancreatitis (AIP):*** (5% of chronic pancreatitis cases): presents clinically with jaundice (63% of patients) and abdominal pain (35%). CT may reveal diffusely enlarged pancreas, enhanced peripheral rim of hypoattenuation "halo," and low-attenuation mass in head of pancreas. Laboratory values reveal elevated serum immunoglobulin (Ig) G4, elevated serum Ig or gamma-globulin level, presence of antilactoferrin antibody (ALA), anticarbonic anhydrase (ACA) II level, anti-smooth-muscle antibody (ASMA), or antinuclear antibody (ANA).
- ***Sclerosing pancreatitis:*** a form of chronic pancreatitis characterized by infrequent attacks of abdominal pain, irregular narrowing of the pancreatic duct, and swelling of the pancreatic parenchyma; patients have high levels of serum immunoglobulins (IgG4). Chronic sclerosing pancreatitis is also known as *autoimmune pancreatitis.*

DIAGNOSIS

DIFFERENTIAL DIAGNOSIS

- Pancreatic cancer
- Peptic ulcer disease
- Cholelithiasis with biliary obstruction
- Malabsorption from other etiologies
- Recurrent acute pancreatitis
- Renal insufficiency
- Intestinal ischemia or infarction
- Other: Crohn's disease, gastroparesis, inflammatory bowel disease

WORKUP

Medical history with focus on alcohol use, laboratory tests, diagnostic imaging

LABORATORY TESTS

- Serum amylase and lipase may be elevated (normal amylase levels, however, do not exclude the diagnosis).
- Hyperglycemia, glycosuria, hyperbilirubinemia, and elevated serum alkaline phosphatase may also be present.
- 72-hr fecal fat determination (rarely performed) reveals excess fecal fat. Fecal elastase test requires only 20 g of stool.
- Secretin stimulation test is the best test for diagnosing pancreatic exocrine insufficiency.
- Lipid panel: significantly elevated triglycerides can cause pancreatitis.
- Serum calcium: hyperparathyroidism is a rare cause of chronic pancreatitis.
- Elevated levels of serum IgG4 are found in sclerosing pancreatitis and AIP.
- Elevated serum Ig or gamma-globulin level, presence of ALA, ACA II level, ASMA, or ANA in AIP.

IMAGING STUDIES

- Plain abdominal radiographs (Fig. E1-698) may reveal pancreatic calcifications (95% specific for chronic pancreatitis).
- Ultrasound of abdomen may reveal duct dilation, pseudocyst, calcification, and presence of ascites.
- Contrast-enhanced CT scan of abdomen is the initial modality of choice. It is useful to detect calcifications, evaluate for ductal dilation, and rule out pancreatic cancer.
- Endoscopic retrograde cholangiopancreatography (ERCP) had been traditionally used to evaluate for the presence of dilated ducts, strictures, pseudocysts, and intraductal stones. However, for the evaluation of pancreatic parenchyma and duct system newer, less invasive modalities such as magnetic resonance cholangiopancreatography and endoscopic ultrasonography (EUS) are preferred. EUS (Fig. E1-699) has a sensitivity of 97% and a specificity of 60% for chronic pancreatitis and a very low complication rate. Fine-needle aspiration biopsy combined with EUS is the preferred modality for evaluation of cystic or mass lesions to determine malignancy.

TREATMENT

NONPHARMACOLOGIC THERAPY

- Avoidance of alcohol and tobacco
- Frequent, small-volume, low-fat meals

ACUTE GENERAL Rx

- Avoidance of narcotics if possible (simple analgesics or NSAIDs can be used). Fig. E1-700 describes an approach to the patient with painful chronic pancreatitis.
- Treatment of steatorrhea with pancreatic supplements (e.g., Pancrease, Creon, Pancrelipase titrated prn based on the amount of steatorrhea and patient's weight loss). All non–enteric-coated enzymes should be used with acid-suppressing medications. Proton pump inhibitors and H_2 blockers reduce inactivation of the enzymes from gastric acid.
- Antioxidants (vitamin A, selenium, vitamin E) may be helpful for pain control in chronic pancreatitis.
- Percutaneous or via EUS celiac plexus blockade with corticosteroids or neurolysis with ethanol may provide temporary pain relief.
- Treatment of complications (e.g., type 1 diabetes mellitus).
- Glucocorticoid therapy in patients with AIP and sclerosing pancreatitis can induce clinical remission and significantly decrease serum concentrations of IgG4, immune complexes, and the IgG4 subclass of immune complexes.

CHRONIC Rx

- Surgical intervention may be necessary to eliminate biliary tract disease and improve flow of bile into the duodenum by eliminating obstruction of pancreatic duct.
- ERCP with endoscopic sphincterectomy and stone extraction is useful in selected patients.
- Transduodenal sphincteroplasty or pancreaticojejunostomy in selected patients. Surgery should also be considered in patients with intractable pain.

DISPOSITION

- Long-term survival is poor (50% of patients die within 10 yr from chronic pancreatitis or malignancy).
- Prognosis is best in patients with recurrent acute pancreatitis resulting from cholelithiasis, hyperparathyroidism, or stenosis of the sphincter of Oddi.

REFERRAL

Gastrointestinal referral for ERCP, surgical referral in selected patients (see "Chronic Rx")

SUGGESTED READINGS
available at www.expertconsult.com

RELATED CONTENT

Chronic Pancreatitis (Patient Information)

AUTHOR: **FRED F. FERRI, M.D.**

BASIC INFORMATION

DEFINITION

- A **panic attack** is a relatively brief, sudden episode of intense fear or apprehension, often associated with a sense of impending doom and various uncomfortable and disquieting physical symptoms. Panic attacks may be uncued ("out of the blue") or cued (i.e., triggered by a particular object or situation). Panic attacks may be present in a variety of different anxiety-related disorders (e.g., phobias, social anxiety, obsessive-compulsive disorder). Table 1-377 describes criteria for diagnosis of panic attack.
- **Panic disorder** is diagnosed at least after two uncued panic attacks have occurred followed by at least 1 mo (or more) of significant concern about future attacks, worry about their implications, or a major change in behavior related to these attacks. The criteria for diagnosis of panic disorder is summarized in Table 1-378. **Agoraphobia** is anxiety about, and avoidance of, places or situations in which the ability to escape is perceived to be limited or embarrassing or in which help might not be available in the event of having a panic attack.

SYNONYMS

Anxiety attacks
Fear attacks
Ataque de nervios

ICD-9CM and DSM-5 CODES
300.01
ICD-10CM CODES
F41.0 Panic disorder
F40.0 Agoraphobia

EPIDEMIOLOGY & DEMOGRAPHiCS

INCIDENCE (IN U.S.): 1% 1-mo incidence of panic attacks

TABLE 1-377 Criteria for Diagnosis of a Panic Attack

A discrete period of intense fear or discomfort, in which ≥4 of the following symptoms developed abruptly and reached a peak within 10 min

- Palpitations, pounding heart, or accelerated heart rate
- Sweating
- Trembling or shaking
- Sensations of shortness of breath or being smothered
- Feeling of choking
- Chest pain or discomfort
- Nausea or abdominal distress
- Feeling dizzy, unsteady, light-headed, or faint
- Derealization (feelings of unreality) or depersonalization (being detached from oneself)
- Fear of losing control or going crazy
- Paresthesias (numbness or tingling sensations)
- Chills or hot flashes

From Kliegman RM et al: *Nelson essentials of pediatrics*, ed 5, Philadelphia, 2006, Saunders.

PREVALENCE (IN U.S.):
- 15% to 20% lifetime prevalence of one or more panic attacks.
- Panic disorder is much more uncommon, with a lifetime prevalence of 1.5% to 3.5%; chronicity of condition reflected by a similar 1-yr prevalence rate of 1% to 2%.
- Agoraphobia is relatively rare; 0.3% to 1% lifetime prevalence; 30% to 50% of patients diagnosed with panic disorder also have agoraphobia.

PEAK INCIDENCE:
- Chronic condition with a waxing and waning course.
- Bimodal incidence peaks noted, with the first peak between ages 15 and 24 yr and second peak between ages 35 and 44 yr.

PREDOMINANT SEX:
- Women more commonly affected (>85% of clinical population).
- Panic disorder twice as common in women.
- Panic disorder with agoraphobia three times as common in women.

PREDOMINANT AGE:
- Age of onset is typically late adolescence to mid-30s. Onset earlier in males (24 yr) than females (28 yr).
- Onset after age 45 yr is rare and should raise suspicion of different etiology.

GENETICS:
- Risk of developing panic disorder in first-degree relatives of individuals with panic disorder is four to seven times that of general population.
- Findings in twin studies: approximately 60% of contributing factors to panic are genetic.

PHYSICAL FINDINGS & CLINICAL PRESENTATION

Panic disorder:
- Present either with a panic attack or with fear and anxiety related to anticipation of a future panic attack or its implications.
- Typical presentation: unexpected, untriggered periods of intense anxiety and fear with associated physiologic changes (e.g., palpitations, sweating, tremulousness, shortness of breath, chest pain, gastrointestinal distress, faintness, derealization, paresthesia). This is accompanied by associated fears of dying, heart attack, stroke, passing out, losing control, or losing one's mind. Panic attacks are often described as "the most terrifying" episode an individual has experienced.
- Emergency or physician visits often occasioned by physical symptoms such as chest pain, dizziness, or difficulty breathing. Thirty percent of patients presenting with chest pain have panic disorder.

TABLE 1-378 Criteria for Diagnosis of Panic Disorder

1. Recurrent unexpected panic attacks with associated worry or behavior change
2. Not due to effects of a drug, medication, or medical condition

Agoraphobia:
- Rare complaints to physician. May manifest in missed office visits or tardiness. Patients may request home visits or telephone care.
- Activities usually self-limited by avoiding public situations where the patient believes he or she might experience a panic attack and would be unable to exit readily, such as the following:
  1. Crowded public areas (stores, public transportation, flying, church)
  2. Individual interactions (hairdresser, dentist, neighborhood meetings)
  3. Driving (especially if alone, far from home over bridges, through tunnels, on highways or on isolated roads)
- On exposure to or anticipation of exposure to feared situations, significant anxiety occurs. Anxiety may generate somatic symptoms that trigger a full-blown panic attack. Patients believe that escape from these situations reduces the alarming symptoms, thus reinforcing future avoidance. In actuality, symptom relief stems from adrenaline breaking down in the body after approximately 20 minutes.

ETIOLOGY

Hypotheses (NOTE: There are sufficient data to support each model. Models are not mutually exclusive.)
1. Central dyscontrol of autonomic arousal (typically localized to the locus ceruleus); similar symptoms may be chemically induced with yohimbine, caffeine, or cholecystokinin.
2. Cognitive overreaction (i.e., "catastrophic misinterpretation") to relatively mild or benign physiologic cues that then triggers a genuine autonomic cascade and further misinterpretations.
3. Dysfunction of a central suffocation alarm mechanism; some signs of compensated respiratory alkalosis. Can be experimentally induced with sodium lactate or carbon dioxide.

Dx DIAGNOSIS

DIFFERENTIAL DIAGNOSIS

Medical conditions:
- Endocrinopathies:
  1. Hyperthyroidism
  2. Hyperparathyroidism
  3. Pheochromocytoma
  4. Carcinoid tumor
- Cardiac and respiratory diseases:
  1. Arrhythmias
  2. Myocardial infarction
  3. Chronic obstructive pulmonary disease
  4. Asthma
  5. Mitral valve prolapse
- Metabolic:
  1. Hypoglycemia
  2. Electrolyte imbalances
  3. Porphyria
- Seizure disorders
- Psychiatric disorders (NOTE: Panic attacks are common in a variety of psychiatric

 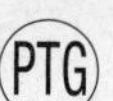

disorders. Panic disorder could be conceptualized as a phobia of the somatic sensations or situations that have become paired with panic attacks.)

1. Phobias (e.g., specific phobia or social phobia). Note that fear of going on a plane because of crashing would be a specific phobia, whereas fear of going on a plane because one is then trapped and worries about panic is more suggestive of panic disorder with agoraphobia.
2. Obsessive-compulsive disorder (cued by exposure to the object of the obsession)
3. Posttraumatic stress disorder (cued by recall of a stressor)
4. Generalized anxiety disorder (cued by excessive worry)

- Therapeutic (theophylline, steroids) and recreational (cocaine, amphetamine, caffeine, diet pills) drugs and drug withdrawal (alcohol, cannabis, barbiturates, benzodiazepines)

WORKUP

- Emergency presentation: cardiac, respiratory, or neurologic symptoms
- History and physical examination to rule out a concomitant medical or substance-related condition

NOTE: Panic disorder and agoraphobia are not diagnoses of exclusion, but exclusion of other conditions is usually required.

LABORATORY TESTS

- Thyroid profile
- Electrolyte measures, including calcium
- Toxicology screen
- ECG
- Acute cases: possible monitoring and cardiac enzymes to rule out arrhythmia or ischemia

IMAGING STUDIES

- For temporal lobe dysfunction (e.g., temporal lesions or as ictal or interictal manifestation of temporal lobe seizures): brain CT scan or MRI or an electroencephalogram in some patients
- Holter monitor to rule out occult or episodic arrhythmias
- Chest x-ray, arterial blood gases, or pulmonary function tests if respiratory compromise suspected

Rx TREATMENT

NONPHARMACOLOGIC THERAPY

Cognitive-behavioral therapy (CBT), in particular Panic Controlled Treatment developed by David Barlow, PhD, and Michelle Craske, PhD, is generally very effective, with strongest results for cognitive restructuring (i.e., challenging catastrophic misinterpretations of somatic symptoms), in vivo or imaginal exposures (i.e., exposure to panic triggers in a controlled graded hierarchical fashion from least to most difficult with the goal of habituation and extinction of the fear response), and interoceptive exposures (i.e., repeated recreation and management of feared somatic sensations via activities such as chair spinning, straw breathing, and hyperventilation). CBT effect sizes are equal to or larger than for pharmacotherapy, attrition rates are lower, and relapse rates are lower. Treatment may take several sessions spread over weeks and may require referral to a behavioral specialist.

ACUTE GENERAL Rx

- Benzodiazepines, particularly alprazolam: highly effective in the acute setting although long-term use is contraindicated for effective outcome.
- Low-dose alprazolam for patients with rare panic attacks and asymptomatic periods (0.25 to 0.5 mg PO or sublingually prn).
- Start patient on selective serotonin reuptake inhibitor (SSRI) or similar agent and taper patient off of benzodiazepine by wk 2 to 3.

CHRONIC Rx

- Preferred pharmacologic agents: antidepressants with a significant serotonin reuptake inhibitory action. Generally start at low dose and titrate upward. Minimum treatment duration is 6 to 8 mo, but many patients need to take medications indefinitely.
  1. SSRIs: paroxetine (10 to 60 mg/day), sertraline (50 to 200 mg/day), citalopram (20 to 60 mg/day), escitalopram (5 to 30 mg/day), and fluoxetine (5 to 60 mg/day)
  2. Imipramine (100 to 300 mg/day)
  3. Venlafaxine (75 to 225 mg/day)
- Combination CBT plus SSRI has shown good long-term effects and is somewhat better than antidepressants or CBT alone. Combination CBT plus benzodiazepine does not provide any added benefit and may undermine CBT (interoceptive and in-vivo exposures may be less effective if the benzodiazepine is completely controlling the anxiety).

DISPOSITION

- Typical course is chronic but with significant waxing and waning (common to have long periods of remission).
- Presence of agoraphobia associated with a more chronic course.
- Findings with long-term follow-up studies: 6 to 10 yr after treatment some 30% are in remission, 40% to 50% have improved with residual symptoms, and the remainder are either unchanged or worse.

REFERRAL

- If patients do not respond to an SSRI
- Cognitive-behavioral therapy is the preferred treatment.

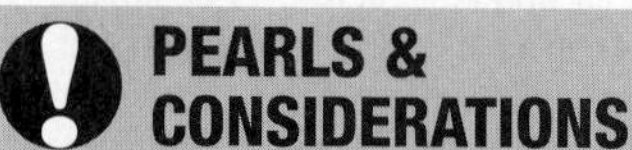

PEARLS & CONSIDERATIONS

- Patient and family education is an important first step in the management of panic disorder. Education provides more adaptive explanations for the benign somatic sensations paired with panic. Presentation of genetic information and explanation of the benign nature of the physiology of each of the symptoms the patient experiences serve as a good start to allay fears and reduce stigma.
- Resumption of avoided activities or situations is a positive prognostic sign and may promote further therapeutic gains.

SUGGESTED READINGS

available at www.expertconsult.com

RELATED CONTENT

Panic Disorder (Patient Information)

AUTHORS: **JEFFREY P. WINCZE, PH.D**, and **JASON M. SATTERFIELD, PH.D.**

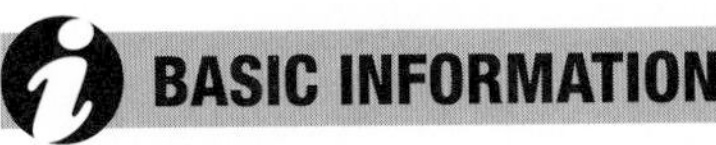

BASIC INFORMATION

DEFINITION

Panniculitis refers to inflammation of subcutaneous fat. Panniculitis can be separated into groups based on histopathologic findings from a skin biopsy, depending on where the cellular infiltrates are more predominantly located. Panniculitis can be classified into lobular or septal panniculitis, based on if the inflammation is seen in the fat lobules or septae, respectively (Box 1-59). It can be further classified based on whether the inflammation is associated with or without vasculitis (Table 1-379). Lastly, the inflammatory infiltrate is examined to determine the types of cells involved, that is, lymphocytes, neutrophils, etc.

SYNONYMS

None

ICD-9CM CODES

729.3 Panniculitis, unspecified

ICD-10CM CODES

M79.3 Unspecified panniculitis
M5400 Panniculitis affecting regions of neck and back, site unspecified
M5401 Panniculitis affecting regions of neck and back, occipito-atlanto-axial region
M5402 Panniculitis affecting regions of neck and back, cervical region

EPIDEMIOLOGY & DEMOGRAPHICS

The epidemiology of the various panniculitides varies with each disease process. The most common panniculitis is erythema nodosum (refer to chapter on erythema nodosum). Another common panniculitis seen in the clinical setting is lipodermatosclerosis (LDS), which is usually seen in young, overweight females with associated venous insufficiency.

PHYSICAL FINDINGS & CLINICAL PRESENTATION

- Skin lesions can appear as nonspecific areas of erythema or erythematous nodules and/or plaques. The nodules can be palpated beneath the dermis. Ulceration, atrophy, and sclerosis can be associated clinical features of these lesions.
- The lesions are frequently painful and tender to palpation.
- Associated constitutional symptoms such as low-grade fevers, malaise, fatigue, myalgias, and arthralgias may be present.
- These skin findings usually are found on the lower limbs; however, the location of these lesions can vary with each specific panniculitis, that is, erythema nodosum is found on the pretibial areas of the lower extremities, erythema induratum occurs on the calf, and lupus panniculitis occurs on the upper arms, shoulders, and face.
- Skin findings tend to evolve as the types of inflammatory cells change over the course of a few days.

ETIOLOGY

Panniculitis can be either primary/idiopathic or secondary. Common secondary etiologies can be classified into the following broad categories:

- Infections: bacterial (streptococci), mycobacterial, fungal, parasitic, and viral
- Inflammatory/connective tissue disease: erythema nodosum, erythema induratum, lipodermatosclerosis, lupus panniculitis, cutaneous polyarteritis nodosa, dermatomyositis-associated panniculitis
- Malignancy: subcutaneous panniculitis-like type T cell lymphoma
- Pancreatic disease: pancreatic panniculitis, which is associated with pancreatitis or pancreatic carcinoma
- Immunodeficiency states: alpha-1 antitrypsin deficiency panniculitis, which is associated with pulmonary and hepatic disease
- Trauma: cold panniculitis, traumatic panniculitis, and factitial panniculitis, which is due to injection of medication or foreign substances into the subcutaneous fat
- Deposition: calciphylaxis, gout

Panniculitis can be a sign of an underlying systemic disease. Lupus panniculitis can occur alone or may present before or after the onset of either discoid lupus erythematosus or systemic lupus erythematosus.

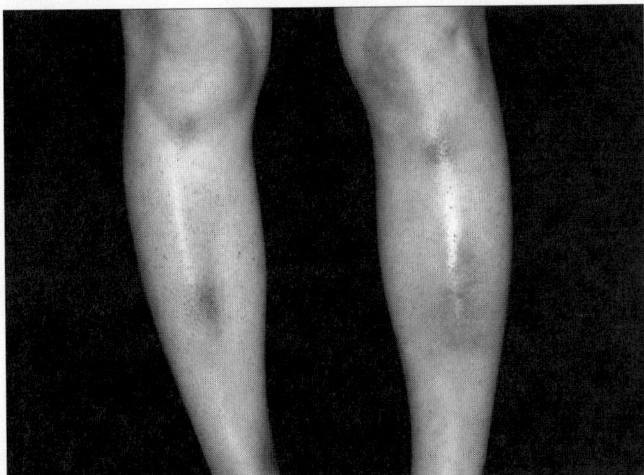

FIGURE 1-701 Erythema nodosum secondary to acute sarcoidosis. (From Hochberg MC et al: *Rheumatology*, ed 5, St Louis, 2011, Mosby.)

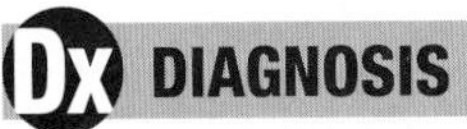

DIAGNOSIS

DIFFERENTIAL DIAGNOSIS

- The skin lesions of panniculitis need to be distinguished from other skin lesions that may manifest similarly, such as insect bites, thrombophlebitis, and cellulitis.
- Disorders affecting the deep dermis or fascia (i.e., plaque morphea, eosinophilic fasciitis), benign or malignant tumors manifesting as subcutaneous nodules, and nodules with deep bruising may have similar clinical findings and be difficult to distinguish from panniculitis.

WORKUP

- Diagnosis of panniculitis depends on a thorough history and physical exam, evaluation of patient's risk factors, skin lesion appearance and distribution, as well as any associated clinical findings.
- If the diagnosis is unclear or needs to be confirmed, a skin biopsy should be performed.
- The preferred biopsy is an excisional biopsy. Alternatively, a large 6-8 mm punch biopsy may be performed.
- The sample can be classified based on the histopathologic findings characteristic of the sample, such as the location of the inflammation, infiltrate composition, and presence or absence of vasculitis.

Although the previous often establishes a diagnosis, there are times when it is difficult to accurately diagnose a specific panniculitis. Different forms of panniculitides have similar clinical findings while others are rare, complicating the presentation. Biopsy specimens may be too superifical to assess for the involvement of the subcutaneous fat or to assess for the presence of a vasculitis. Inflammation of the subcutaneous fat is a changing process, with varying histologic findings as well as physical characteristics of skin lesions based on the stage of evolution. Cellular infiltrates may not be confined to one location in the subcutaneous fat, and may overlap between septa and lobules.

LABORATORY TESTS

Depending on the suspected underlying disorder, the following workup may be considered:

- Throat swab for rapid streptococcal screen, ASO titer, CBC, PPD, chest radiograph, tissue cultures, and histologic stains for organisms
- Amylase, lipase
- Serum alpha-1 antitrypsin level
- ESR, workup for possible connective tissue disease
- Further special studies of biopsy sample to determine cell type if malignancy is suspected

IMAGING STUDIES

- CXR
- Assessment for peripheral vascular disease with ankle-brachial index (LDS)
- Further imaging based on clinical suspicion of disease (i.e., CT scan of abdomen for pancreatitis)

TABLE 1-379 Classification of Panniculitis

I. Without prominent vasculitis
  A. Septal inflammation
    1. Lymphocytic and mixed: erythema nodosum and variants
    2. Granulomatous: palisaded granulomatous diseases, sarcoidosis, subcutaneous infection: tuberculosis, syphilis
    3. Sclerotic: scleroderma, eosinophilic fasciitis, lipodermatosclerosis, toxins
  B. Lobular inflammation
    1. Neutrophilic: infection, ruptured folliculitis and cysts, pancreatic fat necrosis
    2. Lymphocytic: lupus panniculitis, poststeroid panniculitis, lymphoma/leukemia
    3. Macrophagic: histiocytic cytophagic panniculitis
    4. Granulomatous: erythema induratum/nodular vasculitis, palisaded granulomatous diseases, sarcoidosis, Crohn's disease
    5. Mixed inflammation with many foam cells: $\alpha 1$-antitrypsin deficiency, traumatic fat necrosis
    6. Eosinophilic: eosinophilic panniculitis, arthropod bites, parasites
    7. Enzymatic fat necrosis: pancreatic enzyme panniculitis
    8. Crystal deposits: sclerema neonatorum, subcutaneous fat necrosis of the newborn, gout, oxalosis
    9. Embryonic fat pattern: lipoatrophy, lipodystrophy

II. With prominent vasculitis (septal or lobular)
  A. Neutrophilic: leukocytoclastic vasculitis, subcutaneous polyarteritis nodosa, thrombophlebitis, ENL
  B. Lymphocytic: nodular vasculitis, perniosis, angiocentric lymphomas
  C. Granulomatous: nodular vasculitis/erythema induratum, ENL, granulomatosis with polyangiitis, Churg-Strauss allergic granulomatosis

III. Mixed patterns

ENL, Erythema nodosum leprosum.
From Lee L, Werth V: The skin and rheumatic diseases: panniculitis. In Firestein G et al (eds): *Kelley's textbook of rheumatology*, ed 9, Philadelphia, 2013, Elsevier Saunders, p, 611.)

BOX 1-59 Classification of the Panniculitides

Mostly septal panniculitis without vasculitis
- Erythema nodosum
- Vilanova's disease: subacute nodular migratory panniculitis

Mostly lobular panniculitis without vasculitis
- Idiopathic neutrophilic panniculitis
- Subcutaneous fat necrosis of the newborn
- Postcorticosteroid panniculitis
- Calcifying panniculitis
- Pancreatic panniculitis
- α_1-Antitrypsin deficiency
- Physical or factitial panniculitis
- Histiocytic cytophagic panniculitis
- Lipodystrophy syndromes
- Connective tissue panniculitis
- Subcutaneous panniculitis–like T-cell lymphoma
- Sclerosing panniculitis: lipodermatosclerosis

Mixed panniculitis
- Lupus profundus: lupus erythematosus panniculitis
- Erythema nodosum–like lesions of Behçet's syndrome

Panniculitis with vasculitis
- Small vessel vasculitis (postcapillary venule), also known as leukocytoclastic vasculitis
- Medium-sized vessel vasculitis (arterioles or small arteries): polyarteritis nodosa
- Erythema induratum, also known as nodular vasculitis

From Hochberg MC et al: *Rheumatology*, ed 5, St Louis, 2011, Mosby.

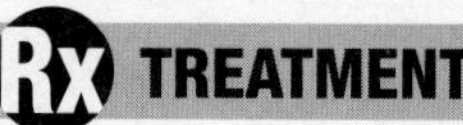

TREATMENT

Treatment of panniculitis is toward treatment of the underlying etiology. Any suspected medications should be discontinued. Appropriate antibiotics to treat underlying infections should be prescribed.

NONPHARMACOLOGIC THERAPY

Certain skin lesions can be treated with potassium iodide, support hosiery, leg elevation, or bed rest.

ACUTE GENERAL Rx

- Anti-inflammatory medications, such as NSAIDs

CHRONIC Rx

- Chronic treatment is based on the underlying disorder.

REFERRAL

- Dermatology for biopsy of skin lesions
- Specific specialists based on underlying etiology

RELATED TOPICS

Erythema nodosum

AUTHOR: **JOANNE SZCZGIEL CUNHA, M.D.**

BASIC INFORMATION

DEFINITION

Paraneoplastic syndromes are a large group of syndromes caused by hormonal, immunologic, or other soluble factors due to the presence of a malignancy. Findings and symptoms are specific to each syndrome. Paraneoplastic syndromes affect most organ systems, predominantly the central and peripheral nervous systems, endocrine system, kidneys, and skin.

ICD-9CM CODES

275.42 Hypercalcemia of malignancy
253.6 Syndrome of inappropriate antidiuretic hormone (SIADH)
255.0 Cushing's syndrome
323 Limbic encephalitis (LE)
334.9 Paraneoplastic cerebellar degeneration (PCD)
358.1 Lambert-Eaton myasthenia syndrome (LEMS)
358.0 Myasthenia gravis (MG)

ICD-10CM CODES

G13.0 Paraneoplastic neuromyopathy and neuropathy
G13.1 Other systemic atrophy primarily affecting central nervous system in neoplastic disease
E83.5 Disorders of calcium metabolism
E73.1 Lambert-Eaton syndrome
E73.2 Other myasthenic syndromes in neoplastic disease

EPIDEMIOLOGY & DEMOGRAPHICS

- Paraneoplastic syndromes may affect as many as 8% of cancer patients.
- See Table 1-380 for epidemiology of each syndrome.

TABLE 1-380 Epidemiology of Each Paraneoplastic Syndrome

Condition	Prevalence	Risk Factors
Hypercalcemia of malignancy	Up to 10%-20% of all cancer patients	Squamous cell cancers (lung, head, and neck), breast, kidney, bladder, and ovarian cancers, lymphoma
Syndrome of inappropriate antidiuretic hormone (SIADH)	Up to 1%-2% of all cancer patients Found in 10%-45% of SCLC patients	SCLC
Cushing's syndrome	Approximately 2% in all cancer patients (50% of these are SCLC)	SCLC Pituitary adenoma, benign and malignant adrenal tumors, carcinoid tumors
Limbic encephalitis (LE)	Less than 1%	SCLC Testicular germ cell tumor Breast cancer
Paraneoplastic cerebellar degeneration	Less than 1%	SCLC Hodgkin's lymphoma Breast cancer
Lambert-Eaton myasthenia syndrome (LEMS)	3% of SCLC patients	SCLC, prostate cancer lymphoma
Myasthenia gravis (MG)	15% of thymoma patients	Thymoma

SCLC, Small cell lung cancer.

PHYSICAL FINDINGS & CLINICAL PRESENTATION

Hypercalcemia of malignancy

- Nausea/vomiting
- Constipation
- Abdominal pain
- Anorexia
- Fatigue
- Altered mental status (from confusion to coma)
- Depression/anxiety
- Renal failure

SIADH

- Headache
- Weakness
- Anorexia
- Nausea
- Vomiting
- Memory impairment, irritability, restlessness
- Mental status changes may progress to obtundation or coma if hyponatremia is >125 mEq/L.

Cushing's syndrome

- Rapid weight gain
- Muscle weakness
- Generalized edema
- Centripetal fat distribution, which often progressed to obesity; limbs are often spared or wasted
- Hypertension
- Characteristic "moon face" due to accumulation of fat deposition in the cheeks
- Skin atrophy, easy bruising, and purple abdominal striae due to skin fragility
- Hyperpigmentation, notably in sun-exposed areas
- Menstrual irregularity, mild hirsutism in women

Limbic encephalitis (LE)

- Slow progression of mood changes
- Hallucinations
- Short-term memory loss
- If hypothalamus is involved, may develop hyperthermia or somnolence.
- Two thirds develop multifocal nervous system involvement.

Paraneoplastic cerebellar degeneration (PCD)

- May develop prodrome of dizziness, nausea, vomiting.
- Ataxia
- Diplopia
- Dysphagia
- Dysarthria

Lambert-Eaton myasthenia syndrome (LEMS)

- Gradual onset of pelvic girdle and lower extremity weakness, progressing in caudocranial direction
- Hyporeflexia
- Fatigue
- Mild bulbar dysfunction
- Dysautonomia, especially erectile dysfunction

Myasthenia gravis (MG)

- Ocular symptoms: ptosis and diplopia
- Weakness of facial muscles, notably with fatigable chewing
- Lower extremity weakness that starts distally and progresses proximally
- May progress to involve muscles of respiration and respiratory crisis

Paraneoplastic dermatologic and rheumatologic syndromes

- Acanthosis nigricans
- Dermatomyositis (DM)
- Erythroderma
- Hypertrophic osteoarthropathy
- Leukocytoclastic vasculitis
- Paraneoplastic pemphigus (PNP)
- Polymyalgia rheumatica (PMR)
- Sweet syndrome (acute febrile neutrophilic dermatosis)

ETIOLOGY

Paraneoplastic endocrine syndromes (PES) are due to tumor production of hormones or peptides that lead to metabolic derangements:

Hypercalcemia of malignancy:

Humoral hypercalcemia of malignancy (HHM): 80% of hypercalcemia of malignancy cases. Most commonly due to production of parathyroid hormone–related peptide (PTHrP) in lung and breast cancer (also seen in renal, bladder, and ovarian cancer). More rarely, can see 1,25-dihydroxyvitamin D production from increased 1α-hydroxylase activity in Hodgkin and non-Hodgkin lymphomas or ectopic production of parathyroid hormone (PTH) by the tumor.

Osteolytic activity: 20% of hypercalcemia of malignancy cases. Tumor cells metastasize, infiltrate bone, and produce local factors that stimulate osteoclast activation.

SIADH: production of antidiuretic hormone (arginine vasopressin, atrial natriuretic peptide) by tumor cells

Cushing's syndrome: ectopic ACTH promotes excess production of cortisol and other glucocorticoids from the adrenal glands, which do not respond to normal HPA feedback

Paraneoplastic neurologic syndromes (PNS) are due to immune cross-reactivity between tumor cells and components of the nervous system. Tumor-directed antibodies (onconeural antibodies) are produced by the patient in response to a developing cancer. These onconeural antibodies and associated onconeural antigen-specific T lymphocytes inadvertently attack components of the nervous system because of antigenic similarity:

LE, PCD, LEMS, MG: cross-reactive autoantibodies against various components of the central and peripheral nervous system

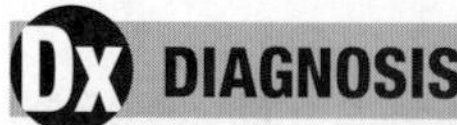

DIAGNOSIS

DIFFERENTIAL DIAGNOSIS

Hypercalcemia of malignancy: primary hyperparathyroidism, familial hypocalciuric hypercalcemia, excess calcium intake, vitamin D toxicity, thiazide diuretics. It is important to differentiate between HHM and osteolytic causes of malignancy-associated hypercalcemia because prognosis and response to treatment differ.

SIADH: hypovolemic hyponatremia, reset osmostat, psychogenic polydipsia

Cushing's syndrome: excess glucocorticoid administration, pituitary adenoma, benign or malignant adrenal tumors

LE, PCD, LEMS, MG: multiple sclerosis, stroke, meningitis, encephalitis

WORKUP

- History and physical examination. Box E1-60 summarizes the evaluation and diagnosis of paraneoplastic syndromes.
- Age-appropriate cancer screening
- EEG, EMG

LABORATORY TESTS

Hypercalcemia of malignancy

- Serum calcium and albumin levels to measure corrected calcium (HHM more common when serum Ca^{2+} >13 mg/dl)
- Ionized serum calcium
- PTH (low to normal)
- PTHrP (elevated)
- 1,25$(OH)_2$D levels (if the above values are inconclusive)

SIADH

- Serum and urine sodium (serum sodium <135 mEq/L or urine sodium >40 mEq/L)
- Serum and urine osmolality (serum osm <280 mOsm/kg of water and/or urine osm >100 mOsm/kg of water)

Cushing's syndrome

- High-dose dexamethasone suppression: 2 mg dexamethasone by mouth every 6 hr for 72 hr, with measurement of urinary 17-hydroxycorticosteroid at 9 A.M. and midnight days 2 and 3
- Low-dose dexamethasone suppression: 1 mg dexamethasone given with measurement of morning serum cortisol
- Dexamethasone suppression test distinguishes pituitary vs. ectopic source of ACTH
- Potassium and glucose should be monitored closely due to increased risk of hypokalemia and hyperglycemia

LE: Anti-Hu, Anti-Ma2, Anti-CRMP5, anti-amphiphysin, CSF analysis

PCD: Anti-Yo, Anti-Hu, Anti-Ma, Anti-Ri, Anti-VGCC, Anti-mGluR1, CSF analysis

LEMS: Anti-VGCC (P/Q), CSF analysis

MG: Anti-AchR, Anti-MuSk, CSF analysis

IMAGING STUDIES

Hypercalcemia of malignancy: CT imaging to evaluate for breast lesion, lung mass, or lymphadenopathy

SIADH: CT imaging to evaluate for brain or lung mass

Cushing's syndrome: CT scan, MRI, or octreotide scan

LE, PCD, LEMS, MG: CT chest, FDG-PET scan, MRI

Rx TREATMENT

NONPHARMACOLOGIC THERAPY

Hypercalcemia of malignancy

- Treatment of underlying malignancy, either surgical resection or chemotherapy/radiation of identified tumors
- Fluid resuscitation, typically 1 L bolus followed by 200-300 ml/hr to achieve euvolemia; followed by maintenance hydration

SIADH

- Surgical resection of identified tumors
- Fluid restriction

Cushing's syndrome

- Surgical resection of identified tumors

LE, PCD, LEMS, MG

- IVIG
- Plasma exchange

ACUTE GENERAL Rx

Hypercalcemia of malignancy

- Furosemide intravenously once euvolemia has been reached, although clinical efficacy is debatable
- Bisphosphonates, either pamidronate or zoledronic acid intravenous infusions (treatment side effects are renal dysfunction and osteonecrosis of the jaw)
- Calcitonin weight-based dosing, although tachyphylaxis occurs after 48 hours of administration
- Corticosteroids in cases of myeloma and lymphoma
- Hemodialysis in severe cases

SIADH

- If urine sodium is >308 mOsm/kg and patient develops seizure or obtundation, then sodium replacement with hypertonic saline (3%) is indicated
- Sodium should not be corrected at a rate faster than 1-2 mEq/L/hr to decrease chances of osmotic demyelination syndrome

Cushing's syndrome

- Management of volume status and blood pressure with diuretics and antihypertensive agents

CHRONIC Rx

- Chronic treatment of all is centered on treatment of the underlying malignancy.

Hypercalcemia of malignancy

- Bisphosphonate therapy every 4 weeks in cases of bone metastasis
- Chronic calcitonin use can be considered

SIADH

- Demeclocycline and vasopressin receptor antagonists (vaptans; conivaptan and tolvaptan, although both are approved for initial administration in hospitalized patients only)
- Cessation of any possible causative medications
- Maintain adequate dietary protein and salt intake

Cushing's syndrome: inhibition of steroid production with ketoconazole, mitotane, metyrapone, aminoglutethimide

LE/PCD: Glucocorticoids, cyclophosphamide, rituximab

LEMS: 3,4-diaminopyridine, pyridostigmine, azathioprine

MG: Pyridostigmine, azathioprine, cyclosporin A, tacrolimus, mycophenolate, rituximab

DISPOSITION

Specific to each condition; however, humoral hypercalcemia of malignancy carries a poor overall prognosis with 30-day mortality of 50%.

REFERRAL

Oncology, endocrinology, neurology, nephrology

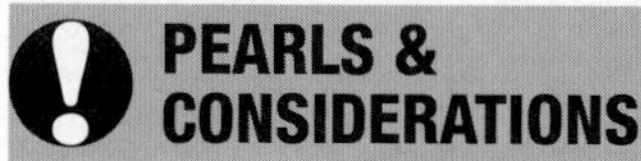

PEARLS & CONSIDERATIONS

COMMENTS

- Signs or symptoms of a paraneoplastic syndrome may manifest prior to the identification of a malignancy.
- If paraneoplastic syndrome is suspected, a thorough workup for a tumor is indicated.
- With treatment of the primary tumor, the clinical effects of hypercalcemia of malignancy, SIADH, and Cushing's syndrome may improve or resolve.
- The effects of the neurologic paraneoplastic syndromes can be long-term, due to permanent CNS or PNS damage. In neurologic paraneoplastic syndromes, tumor detection can be difficult, since the immune system, which is causing the syndrome, i.e., the immune system, is also keeping the tumor in check.

PREVENTION

- Smoking cessation
- Age-appropriate cancer screening

PATIENT & FAMILY EDUCATION

Conditions with autoimmune etiology (LE, PCD, LEMS, MG) symptoms may not improve even if tumor is identified and treated, as damage to the nervous system may be sustained or permanent

SUGGESTED READINGS

available at www.expertconsult.com

AUTHORS: **KENNETH D. BISHOP, M.D., Ph.D., JOHN L. REAGAN, M.D.,** and **ANGELA M. TABER (PLETTE), M.D.**

BASIC INFORMATION

DEFINITION

Paranoid personality disorder (PPD) is characterized by a pattern of pervasive distrust and suspiciousness of others that leads the person to assign malevolence to the motives of others. PPD begins by early adulthood and causes significant distress or impairment in multiple domains of functioning. Individuals must meet four or more of the following criteria:

1. Suspect, without justification, that others are exploiting, harming, or deceiving them.
2. Preoccupied with unwarranted doubts about the loyalty or trustworthiness of friends or associates.
3. Reluctant to confide in others because of unjustified fear that the information will be used against them in a malicious fashion.
4. Infer demeaning or threatening statements from benign remarks or events.
5. Bear grudges for extended periods. For example, PPD patients are unforgiving of perceived or real insults and slights.
6. Perceive attacks on their character that are not apparent to others. Quick to react angrily or to counterattack.
7. Recurrent suspicions, without justification, regarding fidelity of spouse or partner.

SYNONYMS

PPD

ICD-9CM and DSM-5 CODES
301.0
ICD-10CM CODES
F60.0 Paranoid personality disorder

EPIDEMIOLOGY & DEMOGRAPHICS

PREVALENCE: From 0.5% to 4.4% in the general population, 10% to 30% in inpatient psychiatric settings, and 2% to 10% in outpatient mental health clinics.

PREDOMINANT SEX: More commonly diagnosed in males in clinical samples.

GENETICS: Increased prevalence of PPD in relatives of probands with schizophrenia and delusional disorder, paranoid type.

CLINICAL PRESENTATION

- Signs of PPD in childhood include solitariness, poor peer relationships, social anxiety, underachievement in school, hypersensitivity, peculiar thoughts and language, and idiosyncratic fantasies.
- As children, these patients may have appeared "odd" or "eccentric" and attracted teasing.
- Their excessive suspiciousness often leads to either overt argumentativeness and recurrent complaining or quiet, hostile aloofness.
- These patients maintain interpersonal distance and may refuse to answer personal questions, saying the information is "nobody's business."
- Misinterpret benign actions by others as malicious assaults. PPD patients may, for example, interpret an honest mistake as a deliberate attempt to harm, a casual humorous remark as a serious character attack, a compliment as a veiled criticism, and an offer of help as a judgment of failure.
- Close relationships are impaired by hypervigilance for threats and associated guardedness. May appear as "cold." Suspiciousness can lead to pathologic jealousy where they gather circumstantial evidence to support contention of betrayal.
- To protect themselves from the perceived malice of others, these patients often maintain a high degree of control of relationships and interactions, constantly questioning the whereabouts, intentions, or actions of the other.
- Often rigid and critical of others but have great difficulty accepting criticism themselves.
- Given their lack of trust of others, PPD patients have an excessive need for self-sufficiency and autonomy.
- Quick to counterattack and may be litigious.
- May join "cults" or groups that share their paranoid belief system.
- In response to stress, may experience very brief psychotic episodes (minutes to hours).

ETIOLOGY

- At this point, limited knowledge about role of genetic loading and neurobiologic vulnerability.
- However, increased prevalence in families of probands with schizophrenia and delusional disorder, paranoid type, suggests possible genetic role.

Dx DIAGNOSIS

DIFFERENTIAL DIAGNOSIS

- Schizophrenia, paranoid type, delusional disorder, paranoid type, and mood disorder with psychotic symptoms: require presence of persistent positive psychotic symptoms such as delusions and hallucinations. To give an additional diagnosis of PPD, the personality disorder must be present before the onset of psychotic symptoms and must persist when the psychotic symptoms are in remission.
- Substance-induced paranoia, especially in the context of cocaine, PCP, or methamphetamine abuse or dependence.
- Personality changes caused by a general medical condition that affects the central nervous system.
- Paranoid traits associated with a sensory disability; for example, hearing impairment.
- Increased risk for major depressive disorder, obsessive-compulsive disorder, agoraphobia, and substance abuse or dependence.
- The most common co-occurring personality disorders are schizotypal, schizoid, narcissistic, avoidant, and borderline:
  1. Schizotypal personality disorder includes magical thinking and unusual perceptual experiences.
  2. Schizoid and borderline personality disorders do not have prominent paranoid ideation.
  3. Avoidant personality disorder includes fear of embarrassment.
  4. Narcissistic personality disorder includes the fear that hidden "flaws" or "inferiority" may be revealed.

WORKUP

- History: collateral information is essential to establishing the presence of longstanding interpersonal pattern in multiple domains of the patient's life.
- Physical examination
- Mental status examination

LABORATORY TESTS

Those necessary to rule out medical causes of personality changes

IMAGING STUDIES

Those necessary to rule out medical causes of personality changes

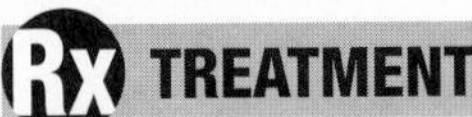

Rx TREATMENT

NONPHARMACOLOGIC THERAPY

- Cognitive-behavioral therapy to help patients control rage, manage perceived criticism, and develop social skills
- Psychodynamic psychotherapy to help patient develop capacity to trust and improve interpersonal functioning.

ACUTE GENERAL Rx

Benzodiazepines or low-dose antipsychotics to control hostility and paranoia

CHRONIC Rx

- Low-dose antipsychotic medication. Increase dose in small increments to minimize risk of side effects.
- Selective serotonin reuptake inhibitors if comorbid depression, obsessive-compulsive disorder, or agoraphobia
- Substance abuse treatment if comorbid dependence

COMPLEMENTARY & ALTERNATIVE MEDICINE

No evidence of efficacy in PPD

DISPOSITION

- Severity is variable and course is chronic. Often lifelong difficulty maintaining intimate relationships.
- At increased risk for major depressive disorder, obsessive-compulsive disorder, agoraphobia, and substance abuse or dependence.
- In some cases, PPD is a prepsychotic antecedent of delusional disorder, paranoid type.

REFERRAL

- If pharmacotherapy or psychotherapy is contemplated
- If patient's social or occupational functioning is impaired

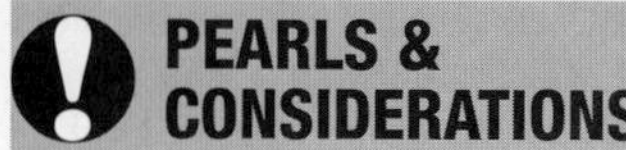

PEARLS & CONSIDERATIONS

COMMENTS

- Illness exacerbates these patients' sense of vulnerability.
- Communicating personal information to the physician challenges the guarded, self-protective approach to others and will often heighten PPD patients' fear that the physician will harm them.
- The encounter with the physician intensifies hypervigilance. As a result, innocuous or even overtly helpful behaviors by the physician may be perceived as manipulating or threatening.
- With the perceived threat, these patients will often confront and challenge the physician on their motives and their rationale for diagnosis and treatment. Conflict and argument are not uncommon.
- Thus establishing an alliance with the patient can be challenging.
- Faced with such a patient, physicians may understandably react defensively to unfounded suspicion or distance and not respond to the patient's concerns. Both responses increase the patient's anxiety and paranoia.
- Management guidelines:
  1. Convey intent "to do no harm."
  2. Address the patient's fears and concerns, no matter how irrational, in a clear, direct, and detailed manner.
  3. Remember that behind the patient's hostility lie fears that are real to him or her.
  4. Maintain a professional and neutral stance.
  5. Responding with too much warmth and friendliness will intensify paranoia.
  6. Give patient detailed and factual information about treatment plan.
  7. Give patient as much control as possible, including maximum participation at each decision node.
  8. Do not personalize patient's hostility and suspicion, but understand his or her distrust as an attempt to manage intense fear.
  9. Validate patient's concerns about the diagnosis or treatment plan.

SUGGESTED READINGS

available at www.expertconsult.com

RELATED CONTENT

Paranoid Personality Disorder (Patient Information)

AUTHOR: **JOHN Q. YOUNG, M.D., M.P.P.**

BASIC INFORMATION

DEFINITION

Idiopathic Parkinson's disease (PD) is a progressive neurodegenerative disorder characterized clinically by rigidity, tremor, postural instability, and slowness of movement (bradykinesia).

SYNONYMS

Paralysis agitans

ICD-9CM CODES

332.0 Idiopathic Parkinson's disease, primary
332.1 Parkinson's disease, secondary

ICD-10CM CODES

G20 Parkinson's disease
G21.11 Neuroleptic induced parkinsonism
G21.1 Other drug-induced secondary parkinsonism
G21.2 Secondary parkinsonism due to other external agents
G21.3 Postencephalitic parkinsonism
G21.4 Vascular parkinsonism
G21.8 Other secondary parkinsonism
G21.9 Secondary parkinsonism, unspecified

EPIDEMIOLOGY & DEMOGRAPHICS

PREVALENCE:

- Affects more than 1 million people in North America.
- In age group <40 yr, <5/100,000 are affected.
- In those aged >70 yr, 700/100,000 are affected.
- Highest incidence in whites, lowest incidence in Asians and African Americans

PHYSICAL FINDINGS & CLINICAL PRESENTATION

- Tremor (Fig. 1-702)—typically a resting tremor with a frequency of 4 to 6 Hz that is often first noted in the hand as a pill-rolling tremor (thumb and forefinger). Can also involve the leg and lip. Tremor improves with purposeful movement. Usually starts asymmetrically.
- Rigidity—increased muscle tone that persists throughout the range of passive movement of a joint. This, too, is usually asymmetric at onset.
- Akinesia/bradykinesia—slowness in initiating movement
- Postural instability—tested by "pull test." Ask patient to stand in place with back to examiner. Examiner pulls patient back by the shoulders, and proper response would be to take no steps back or very few steps back without falling. Retropulsion is a positive test as is falling straight back. This is not usually severe early on. If falls and postural reflexes are greatly impaired early on, then consider other disorders.
- Masked facies (hypomimia)—face seems expressionless, giving the appearance of depression. Decreased blink; often there is excess drooling.
- Gait disturbance
- Stooped posture, decreased arm swing
- Difficulty initiating the first step; small shuffling steps that increase in speed (festinating gait). Steps become progressively faster and shorter while the trunk inclines further forward.
- Other complaints and findings early on include handwriting becoming smaller (micrographia), and voice becoming softer and often "gruffer" (hypophonia).

ETIOLOGY

- Unknown
- Most cases are sporadic, with age being the most common risk factor, although there is probably a combination of both environmental and genetic factors contributing to disease expression. There are rare familial forms with at least seven different genes identified; these include the parkin gene, which is a significant cause of early-onset autosomal recessive PD and LRRK2, which is the most common cause of familial and sporadic parkinsonism.

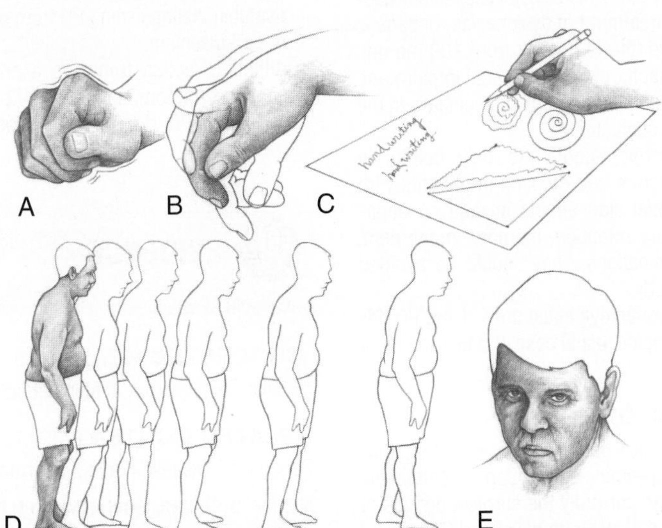

FIGURE 1-702 The parkinsonian syndrome. A, The "pill-rolling" tremor. **B,** Tremor that can worsen with emotional stress. **C,** Handwriting abnormalities, which include micrographia. **D,** Typical posture and gait, which becomes faster (festination). **E,** Lack of facial expression as well as "stare" from decreased blinking. (From Remmel KS et al: *Handbook of symptom oriented neurology,* ed 3, St Louis, 2002, Mosby.)

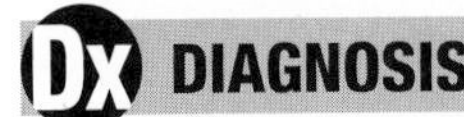

DIAGNOSIS

A clinical diagnosis can be made based on a comprehensive history and physical examination. The four cardinal signs used to diagnose PD are (mnemonic = TRAP):

1. **T**remor (resting, typically 4-6 Hz)
2. **R**igidity, of the cogwheel type
3. **A**kinesia/bradykinesia—slowness of movement
4. **P**ostural instability—failure of postural "righting" reflexes leading to poor balance and falls

One need not demonstrate all four cardinal signs to make a presumptive diagnosis of PD and begin treatment.

DIFFERENTIAL DIAGNOSIS

- Multiple system atrophy—distinguishing features include autonomic dysfunction (including urinary incontinence, orthostatic hypotension, and erectile dysfunction), parkinsonism, cerebellar signs, and normal cognition.
- Diffuse Lewy body disease—parkinsonism with concomitant dementia: patients often have early hallucinations and fluctuations in level of alertness and mental status.
- Corticobasal degeneration—often begins asymmetrically with apraxia, cortical sensory loss in one limb, and sometimes alien limb phenomenon.
- Progressive supranuclear palsy—tends to have axial rigidity greater than appendicular (limb) rigidity. These patients have early and severe postural instability. Hallmark is supranuclear gaze palsy that usually involves vertical gaze (especially downward) before horizontal.
- Essential tremor—bilateral postural and action tremor
- Secondary (acquired) parkinsonism
    1. Iatrogenic—any of the neuroleptics and antipsychotics. The high-potency D_2-blocker neuroleptics are most likely to cause parkinsonism. Quetiapine is an atypical antipsychotic with lower risk of causing parkinsonism. Metoclopramide can also cause parkinsonism. Abuse of methamphetamine has been recently linked to risk of PD.
    2. Postinfectious parkinsonism—von Economo's encephalitis
    3. Parkinson's pugilistica—after repeated head trauma
    4. Toxins (e.g., MPTP, manganese, carbon monoxide)
    5. Cerebrovascular disease "vascular parkinsonism" (basal ganglia infarcts); often lower limbs (especially gait) affected more than upper extremities

 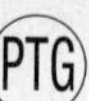

WORKUP

- Identification of clinical signs and symptoms associated with PD (see "Physical Findings") and elimination of conditions that may mimic it with a comprehensive history and physical examination
- Routine genetic testing is not recommended.

IMAGING STUDIES

Computed tomographic (CT) scan has almost no role in investigations. Magnetic resonance imaging (MRI) of the head may sometimes distinguish between idiopathic PD and other conditions that present with signs of parkinsonism (see "Differential Diagnosis").

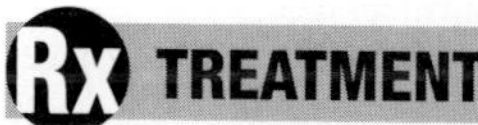

TREATMENT

NONPHARMACOLOGIC THERAPY

- Physical therapy, patient education and reassurance, treatment of associated conditions (e.g., depression) are important. A safe, practical, and reasonable exercise regimen must be encouraged, individualized to the patient's access to resources and motivation. Recent trials reveal that t'ai chi training is effective in reducing balance impairment and falls and improving functional capacity.
- Avoidance of drugs that can induce or worsen parkinsonism: neuroleptics (especially high potency), certain antiemetics (prochlorperazine, trimethobenzamide), metoclopramide, nonselective MAO inhibitors (may induce hypertensive crisis), reserpine, methyldopa

ACUTE GENERAL Rx

- There continues to be controversy whether levodopa or dopamine agonists should be the initial treatment. In younger patients, agonists are usually the drug of choice; in patients >70 yr, levodopa is typically the preferred initial therapy.
- It is appropriate to initiate pharmacotherapy when required by symptoms; prior practice of waiting for limitation of ADLs is now outdated. Fig. E1-703 describes an approach to patients with parkinsonism.
- Motor complications do develop during the course of the disease and likely reflect the combination of disease progression together with the side effects of dopaminergic medications.

CHRONIC RX

- Levodopa therapy
  1. Cornerstone of symptomatic therapy—should be used with a peripheral dopa decarboxylase inhibitor (carbidopa) to minimize side effects (nausea, lightheadedness, postural hypotension). The combination of the two drugs is marketed under the trade name Sinemet. Levodopa therapy has been found to reduce morbidity and mortality in PD patients.
  2. Usual starting dose is 25/100 mg (carbidopa/levodopa) tid 1 hr before (or after) meals.
  3. Controlled-release preparations (e.g., Sinemet CR) are available, but their use should be deferred to a neurologist.
  4. Stalevo (combination Sinemet and entacapone, a COMT inhibitor). Useful for patients with motor fluctuations (wearing off); has no role in treating early patients with PD.
- Dopamine receptor agonists (ropinirole and pramipexole) are not as potent as levodopa, but they are often used as initial treatment in younger patients to attempt to delay the onset of complications (dyskinesias, motor fluctuations) associated with levodopa therapy. These medications are more expensive than levodopa. In general, they cause more side effects than levodopa, including nausea, vomiting, light-headedness, peripheral edema, confusion, and somnolence. They can also cause impulse control behaviors such as hypersexuality, binge eating, and compulsive shopping and gambling. Presence of these must be assessed at each visit.
  1. Ropinirole: initial dose is 0.25 mg tid
  2. Pramipexole: initial dose is 0.125 mg tid
- MAO-B inhibitors can be used as monotherapy early in the disease or as adjunctive therapy in later stages; they have been shown to have milder symptomatic benefit than dopamine agonists or levodopa. Well tolerated and easy to titrate. Concurrent use of stimulants and sympathomimetics should be avoided. Certain food restrictions may apply.
  1. Rasagiline: initial dose is 0.5 mg qd, then 1 mg daily. A recent study, ADAGIO, suggests that 1 mg rasagiline may have disease-modifying benefits, but results must be interpreted with caution.
  2. Selegiline: Usual dose, 5 mg bid with breakfast and lunch. Has amphetamine byproduct so has mild stimulant-like effects, which can be beneficial in some patients.
- Amantadine (unclear mechanism of action, but reported to modulate the dopamine and glutamate systems in the CNS) can be used alone early in the disease. It is especially useful in the treatment of dyskinesias. Dosage is 100 mg tid (titrate q week from 100 mg qd). Must adjust for elderly and renal impairment. The most notable side effect, especially in the elderly, is confusion.
- Anticholinergic agents are only helpful in treating tremor and drooling in patients with PD. Potential side effects include constipation, urinary retention, memory impairment, and hallucinations. They should be avoided in the elderly.
  1. Trihexyphenidyl: initial dose, 1 mg PO tid
  2. Benztropine: usual dose, 0.5 to 1 mg qd or bid

SURGICAL OPTIONS

- Pallidal (globus pallidus interna) and subthalamic deep-brain stimulation (subthalamic nucleus) are currently the surgical options of choice for patients with advanced PD; similar improvement in motor function and adverse effects has been reported after either procedure. Compared with ablative procedures, DBS has the advantage of being reversible and adjustable. Thalamic DBS may be useful for refractory tremor. It improves the cardinal motor symptoms, extends medication "on" time, and reduces motor fluctuations during the day. In general, patients are likely to benefit from this therapy if they show a clear response to levodopa. Therefore, when considering DBS, patients should be evaluated for motor response to levodopa by stopping levodopa overnight and evaluating motor response before and after a dose of levodopa.
- Surgery is often limited to patients with disabling, medically refractory problems, and patients must still have a good response to L-dopa to undergo surgery. Yet for many patients, earlier stimulation might provide an improved motor benefit before disability from other symptoms has occurred and should be considered at an earlier stage of PD. DBS results in decreased dyskinesias, fluctuations, rigidity, and tremor.

DISPOSITION

PD usually follows a slowly progressive course leading to disability over the course of several years. However, every patient will progress individually, and patients should be reassured that this diagnosis does not, by definition, result in being either wheelchair- or bed-bound.

REFERRAL

- Neurology consultation is recommended at initial diagnosis of PD.
- Exercise is important for all patients with PD.
- Participation in outpatient physical therapy program is recommended for patients with moderate to advanced disease.

PEARLS & CONSIDERATIONS

- Asymmetry of symptoms at onset is very useful in distinguishing PD from other causes of parkinsonism.
- Although resting tremor is a common presenting symptom, up to 25% of patients with idiopathic PD do not have classic resting tremor.

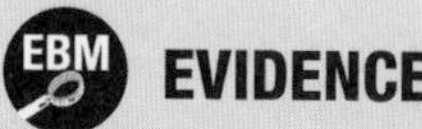

EVIDENCE

available at www.expertconsult.com

SUGGESTED READINGS

available at www.expertconsult.com

RELATED CONTENT

Parkinson's Disease (Patient Information)

AUTHOR: **U. SHIVRAJ SOHUR, M.D., PH.D.**

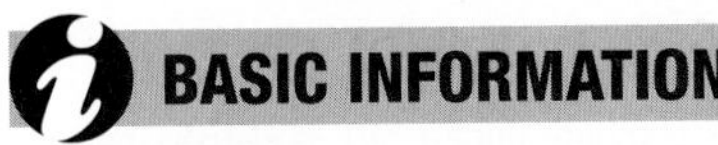

BASIC INFORMATION

DEFINITION

Paronychia is a localized superficial infection or abscess of the lateral and proximal nail fold. Paronychia may be acute or chronic.

SYNONYMS

Nail bed infection
Nail bed abscess

ICD-9CM CODES
681.9 Paronychia
ICD-10CM CODES
L03.019 Cellulitis of unspecified finger

EPIDEMIOLOGY & DEMOGRAPHICS

- Acute paronychia affects males and females equally.
- Chronic paronychia is more common in females than males (9:1).
- Acute paronychia most often occurs in children.
- Chronic paronychia usually presents in the fifth or sixth decade of life.
- Paronychia is the most common infection of the hand.

PHYSICAL FINDINGS & CLINICAL PRESENTATION

- Acute paronychia usually presents with the sudden onset of redness, swelling, and pain with abscess or cellulitis formation in the nail fold. Fluid with purulence is often present.
- Chronic paronychia is insidious, presenting with mild swelling and erythema of the nail folds.
- Acute paronychia usually involves only one finger.
- Chronic paronychia may involve more than one finger.
- Acute paronychia usually involves the thumb.
- Chronic paronychia commonly involves the middle finger.

ETIOLOGY

- Any disruption of the seal between the proximal nail fold and the nail plate can cause paronychial infections.
- Acute paronychia is almost always bacterial in origin (e.g., methicillin-sensitive *Staphylococcus aureus* [most common, but also consider MRSA], *Streptococcus pyogenes, Enterococcus faecalis, Proteus* and *Pseudomonas* species, and anaerobes).
- Chronic paronychia is commonly caused by *Candida albicans* (70%), with bacterial organisms accounting for the remaining 30%.
- Trauma, nail biting, hangnails, diabetes, and long-term exposure to water are common predisposing features of paronychia.

Dx DIAGNOSIS

The diagnosis of paronychia is self-evident on physical examination.

DIFFERENTIAL DIAGNOSIS

- Herpetic whitlow caused by herpes simplex
- Pyogenic granuloma
- Viral warts
- Ganglions
- Squamous cell carcinoma

WORKUP

A workup is usually not pursued unless there is treatment failure.

LABORATORY TESTS

- Gram stain and culture any purulent drainage.
- Potassium hydroxide mount may show pseudohyphae.

IMAGING STUDIES

Radiographs of the digit if concerned about osteomyelitis.

Rx TREATMENT

NONPHARMACOLOGIC THERAPY

- For acute paronychia without purulent drainage, warm soaks tid or qid are helpful. If pus is present, surgical drainage is required (Fig. 1-704).
- For chronic paronychia, avoid frequent immersion in water or exposure to moisture.

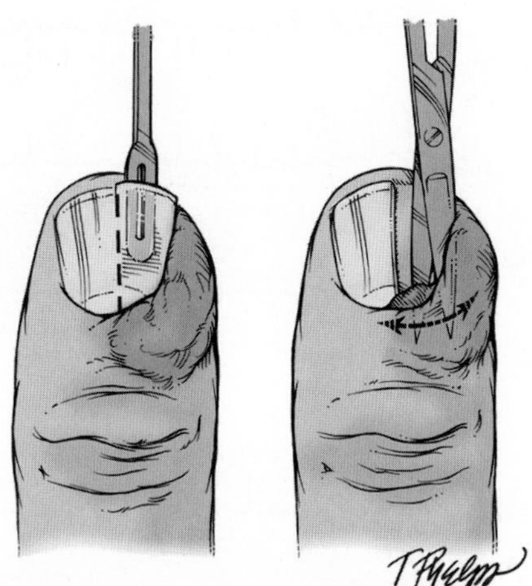

FIGURE 1-704 Surgical drainage of acute paronychia. The lateral nail on the affected side is gently elevated from the nail bed, and a longitudinal strip of nail is removed. If this does not decompress the infection adequately, the margins of the nail fold are opened gently to drain the adjacent soft tissues. (From Cameron JL, Cameron AM: *Current surgical therapy,* ed 10, Philadelphia, 2011, Saunders.)

ACUTE GENERAL Rx

- Trimethoprim-sulfamethoxazole DS ī PO bid for 7 days is usually the antibiotic of choice for acute paronychia.
- Alternative antibiotic choices include dicloxacillin 500 mg qid, cephalexin 500 mg qid, clindamycin, and amoxicillin-clavulanate potassium.
- Surgical drainage is indicated if purulent discharge is noted.
- A No. 11 blade scalpel is used to lift the lateral perionychium and proximal eponychium off the nail, facilitating drainage.
- If the pus is located beneath the nail, the lateral edge of the nail can be lifted off the nail bed and excised.

CHRONIC Rx

- If no fungal organism is found, tincture of iodine (2 drops bid) helps keep the nail and skin dry.
- Chronic paronychia caused by *Candida albicans* is treated with topical antifungal agents (e.g., miconazole or ketoconazole applied tid).
- Unresponsive cases may be treated with itraconazole or fluconazole, but this should be done in consultation with dermatology and/or infectious disease.
- Surgery may be needed in refractory cases.

DISPOSITION

- Most acute paronychias with appropriate treatment resolve within 7 to 10 days.
- Osteomyelitis is a potential complication of paronychia.
- Untreated chronic paronychia leads to thickening and discoloration with eventual nail loss.

REFERRAL

Chronic paronychia refractory to topical medical therapy is best referred to dermatology and/or infectious disease. A hand surgeon is consulted if abscess drainage or surgery is being considered.

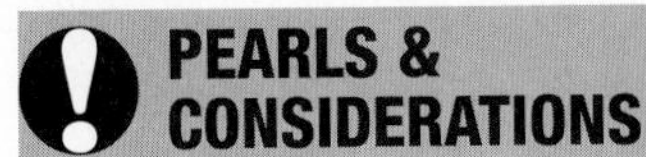

PEARLS & CONSIDERATIONS

COMMENTS

The gastrointestinal tract, including the mouth and bowel, and the genitourinary tract in women are the usual sources of *C. albicans* in chronic paronychia.

SUGGESTED READINGS

available at www.expertconsult.com

RELATED CONTENT

Paronychia (Patient Information)

AUTHOR: **GLENN G. FORT, M.D., M.P.H.**

BASIC INFORMATION

DEFINITION

Paroxysmal supraventricular tachycardia (SVT) is a group of tachyarrhythmias that originate from within or above the atrioventricular (AV) node and are characterized by sudden onset and abrupt termination. They include AV nodal reentrant tachycardia (AVNRT), AV reentrant tachycardia (AVRT), atrial fibrillation, atrial flutter, sinus tachycardia, and atrial tachycardia.

SYNONYMS

PSVT
Supraventricular tachycardia (SVT)

ICD-9CM CODES
427.0 Paroxysmal atrial tachycardia
ICD-10CM CODES
I47.1 Supraventricular tachycardia

PHYSICAL FINDINGS & CLINICAL PRESENTATION

- Patients may be either symptomatic or asymptomatic.
- Patient may be aware of "fast" heartbeat (palpitations) or have presyncope, syncope, or chest pain.
- Hemodynamic status during arrhythmia may vary and can depend on the patient's comorbidities and presence of underlying structural heart disease.

ETIOLOGY

- AVNRT—Dual electrical pathways within or near the AV node
- AVRT (Wolff-Parkinson-White syndrome)—accessory pathway mediated, either orthodromic (antegrade through the AV node and retrograde through the accessory pathway) or antidromic (antegrade through the accessory pathway and retrograde through the AV node)
- Atrial fibrillation and atrial flutter are covered in separate topics.
- Paroxysmal atrial tachycardia and multifocal atrial tachycardia—abnormal automaticity of atrial tissue or triggered activity

Dx DIAGNOSIS

DIFFERENTIAL DIAGNOSIS

Other arrhythmias that present with narrow complex tachycardia like PSVT are:
1. Fascicular VT
2. Junctional tachycardias
3. Artifact such as with Parkinson's

PSVT can be broad complex as well, and the features to distinguish it from ventricular tachycardia are outlined in Table 1-382.

WORKUP

- Electrocardiography
- Shows a rhythm <100 beats/min.
- P waves may or may not be seen (the presence of P waves depends on the relation of atrial to ventricular depolarization). P wave morphology can be useful in discriminating rhythms. P waves with a similar axis to the sinus node can be atrial tachycardias and sinus tachycardias. P waves with retrograde depolarization of the atria (seen as inverted in the inferior leads) can be seen in AVNRT, AVRT, and atrial tachycardia. Sawtooth P waves are indicative of classical counterclockwise type I flutter, and an absence of P waves with irregular R-R intervals points to atrial fibrillation. Variable (>3) morphologies of P wave are suggestive of multifocal atrial tachycardia.
- Wide QRS complex (>0.12 sec) with initial slurring (delta wave) during sinus rhythm and short PR (<0.12 sec) is characteristic of WPW syndrome.
- QRS complex during SVT is usually narrow; however, may be widened because of intrinsic conduction disease, myocardial disease, or rate-related bundle branch block. It may also be widened if the patient has antidromic AVRT.
- Pseudo r and pseudo S waves may be seen in atrioventricular nodal tachycardia (Fig. 1-706).
- Fig. 1-707 illustrates the differential diagnosis of different types of SVT based on timing of atrial activity (RP and PR intervals).
- Holter or event monitor to document the arrhythmias if they are paroxysmal

TABLE 1-382 Features That May Differentiate Ventricular Tachycardia from Supraventricular Tachycardia with Aberrancy

Helpful Features	Implications
Positive QRS concordance	Diagnostic of VT
Presence of AV dissociation, capture beats, or fusion beats	Diagnostic of VT
Atypical RBBB (monophasic R, QR, RS, or triphasic QRS in V_1; R:S ratio < 1, QS or QR, monophasic R in V_6)	Suggests VT
Atypical LBBB (R >30 min or R to S [nadir or notch] >60 min in V_1 or V_2; R:S ratio < 1, QS or QR in V_6)	Suggests VT
Shift of axis from baseline	Suggests VT
History of CAD	Suggests VT
QRS during tachycardia identical to QRS during sinus rhythm	Suggests SVT
Termination with adenosine	Suggests SVT

AV, Atrioventricular; *CAD,* coronary artery disease; *LBBB,* left bundle branch block; *RBBB,* right bundle branch block; *SVT,* supraventricular tachycardia; *VT,* ventricular tachycardia.
From Andreoli TG et al (eds): *Andreoli and Carpenter's Cecil essentials of medicine,* ed 8, Philadelphia, 2010, Saunders.

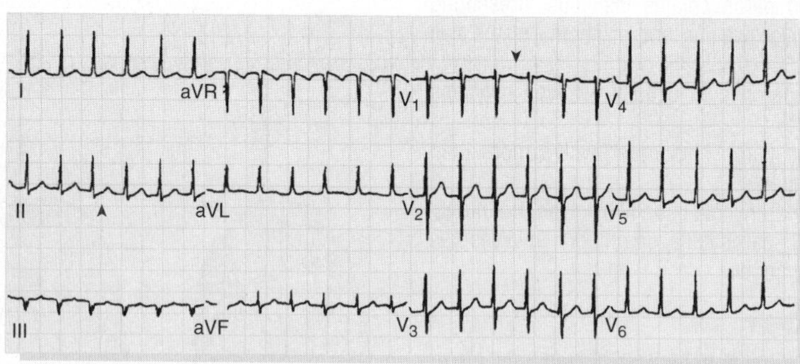

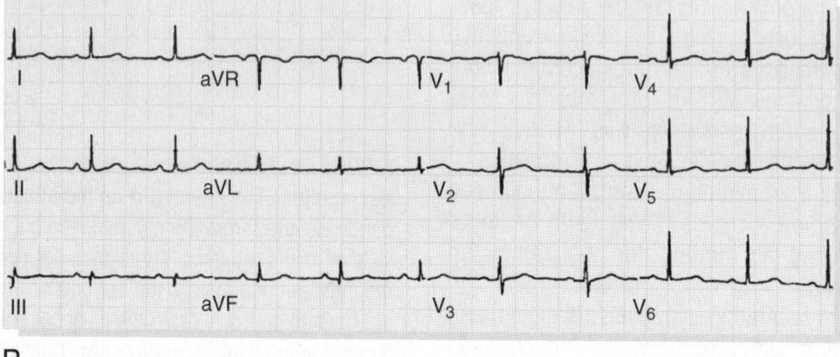

FIGURE 1-706 Twelve-lead electrocardiogram of atrioventricular nodal reentrant tachycardia. A, During tachycardia a pseudo-r wave is seen in lead V_1 *(arrowhead),* and pseudo-S waves *(arrowhead)* are seen in leads II, III, and aVF. **B,** These waves become more obvious when compared with the QRS complexes during sinus rhythm. (From Jaffe ES et al: *Hematopathology,* Philadelphia, 2011, Saunders.)

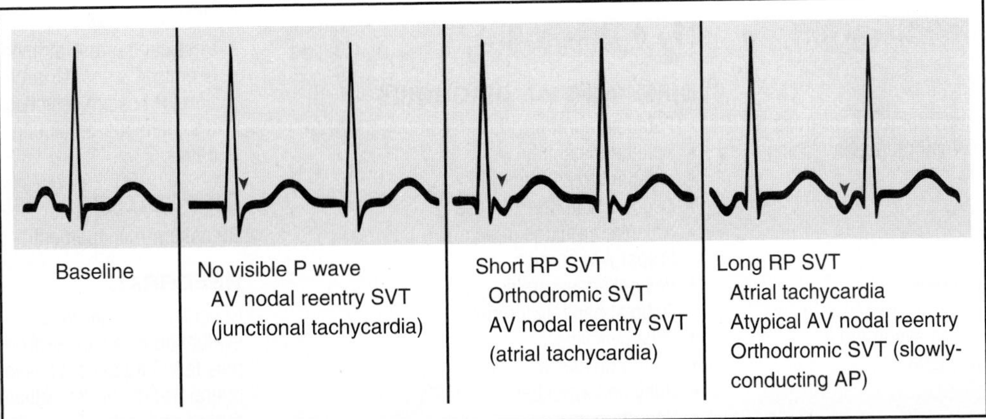

FIGURE 1-707 Differential diagnosis of different types of supraventricular tachycardia (SVT) based on timing of atrial activity (RP and PR intervals). Left, normal beat. Different types of tachycardia are listed below the representative electrocardiographic patterns that they can produce, categorized by P wave position relative to the QRS complex. *Red arrowhead* shows the location of the P wave in each example. *AV*, Atrioventricular; *AP*, accessory pathway. (From Bonow RO et al: *Braunwald's heart disease: a textbook of cardiovascular medicine,* Philadelphia, 2012, Saunders.)

- Echocardiography is appropriate to assess for the presence of underlying structural heart disease.
- Laboratory workup including thyroid function tests, electrolytes, etc.
- Evaluation for obstructive sleep apnea, lung disease, drugs such as theophylline, etc., which may be triggers

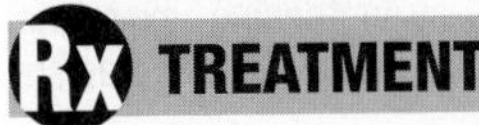

TREATMENT

NONPHARMACOLOGIC THERAPY

- Valsalva maneuver in the supine position is the most effective way to terminate most types of SVT; carotid sinus massage (after excluding occlusive carotid disease) is also commonly used to elicit vagal efferent impulses. These are effective in terminating AVRT, AVNRT, and some types of atrial tachycardia but only transiently slow down AV conduction in case of sinus tachycardia, atrial flutter, and atrial fibrillation without terminating the actual tachycardia.
- Synchronized DC shock is used if patient shows signs of hemodynamic instability.
- Table 1-382 describes useful features to differentiate ventricular tachycardia from SVT with aberrancy.

ACUTE GENERAL Rx

- Adenosine is useful for treatment of orthodromic AVRT and AVNRT and can uncover the underlying rhythm in paroxysmal atrial tachycardia; it is the first choice of therapy for treatment of almost all episodes of SVT unresponsive to vagal maneuvers (see Fig 3-186). The dose is 12 mg given as a rapid IV bolus; tachycardia is usually terminated within a few seconds. If necessary, may repeat with 12-mg IV bolus. Contraindications are second- or third-degree atrioventricular block, sick sinus syndrome, and chronic use of drugs such as dipyridamole, theophylline, or aminophylline. Adenosine may cause bronchospasm in asthmatics.
- Verapamil 5 to 10 mg IV is given over 5 min; if no effect, may repeat in 30 min.
  1. Verapamil should be used cautiously in patients with SVT associated with hypotension.
  2. Slow injection of calcium chloride (10 ml of a 10% solution given over 5 to 8 min before verapamil administration) decreases the hypotensive effect without compromising its antiarrhythmic effect.
- Repeat carotid massage after IV verapamil if SVT persists.
- Metoprolol (IV 5 mg/2 min up to 15 mg) or esmolol (500 μg/kg IV bolus, then 50 μg/kg/min) may be effective in the treatment of SVT.
- IV digoxin (0.75 to 1 mg slow IV loading in increments of 0.25 mg over several hours) if other agents are not effective.
  1. Repeat carotid massage 30 min later; if not successful, give additional 0.25 mg IV digoxin and repeat carotid sinus massage 1 hr later.
  2. Digoxin, beta-blockers, and calcium-channel blockers should be avoided in patients with pre-excitation syndrome to avoid increased conduction through the accessory pathway.

DISPOSITION

Most patients respond well with resolution of the paroxysmal atrial tachycardia upon treatment (see "Acute General Rx"). Some patients may need chronic AV blocking agents for recurrence.

REFERRAL

Radiofrequency ablation (RFA) is the procedure of choice in symptomatic patients who are refractory to medical therapy especially in AVRT, AVNRT, and atrial flutter. RFA has high efficacy rates (single procedure success is 93.2%), low all-cause mortality (0.1%), and low adverse events (2.9%). Despite high reported success rates, RFA appears to be underused in clinical practice.

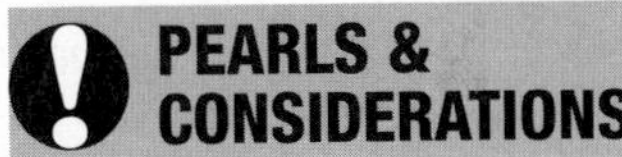

PEARLS & CONSIDERATIONS

COMMENTS

Accessory pathways occur in 0.1% to 0.3% of the general population.

SUGGESTED READINGS

available at www.expertconsult.com

RELATED CONTENT

Fig. 3-186 Evaluation and management of narrow complex tachycardia (Algorithm)

AUTHOR: **BARRY FINE, M.D., PH.D.**

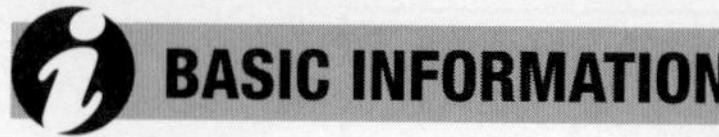

BASIC INFORMATION

DEFINITION

Patellofemoral pain syndrome is overuse or overload of the patellofemoral region leading to anterior knee pain.

SYNONYMS

PFPS
Retropatellar pain syndrome
Runner's knee
Lateral facet compression syndrome
Idiopathic anterior knee pain

ICD-9CM CODES
719.46 Patellofemoral pain syndrome
ICD-10CM CODES
M22.2 Patellofemoral disorders
M25.569 Pain in unspecified knee

EPIDEMIOLOGY & DEMOGRAPHICS

PREVALENCE: Estimated >20% of adolescents. PFPS is the most common diagnosis in outpatients presenting with knee pain. PFPS also constitutes 16% to 25% of all injuries to runners.

PREDOMINANT SEX AND AGE: Nearly 2:1 female predominance; disproportionately affects active adolescents and adults in the second and third decades of life

RISK FACTORS: Increase in physical activity intensity or duration, overuse, joint overload, trauma, anatomic abnormalities, malalignment, patellar hypermobility, quadriceps weakness

PHYSICAL FINDINGS & CLINICAL PRESENTATION

- Gradual or acute onset of anterior knee pain
- Sometimes localized under or around the patella
- Also described as a catching sensation under the patella
- Worsened pain with squatting, running, prolonged sitting, or ascending or descending steps
- Effusion implies intraarticular pathology not explained by PFPS
- Pain may be elicited by compression of the patella into the trochlear groove while the leg is extended

ETIOLOGY

No clear consensus; likely multifactorial, including muscle overuse or joint overload with malalignment and/or trauma potentially contributing resulting in imbalances in the forces controlling patellar tracking during knee flexion and extension

Dx DIAGNOSIS

DIFFERENTIAL DIAGNOSIS

- Patellofemoral arthritis
- Patellar instability
- Patellar stress fracture
- Osgood-Schlatter disease
- Articular cartilage injury
- Prepatellar bursitis
- Pes anserine bursitis
- Iliotibial band syndrome
- Plica synovitis
- Chondromalacia
- Bony abnormalities
- Bone tumors
- Patellar tendinopathy
- Other: Referred pain from lumbar spine or hip joint pathology, loose bodies, osteochondritis dissecans, Sinding-Larsen-Johansson syndrome, symptomatic bipartite patella

WORKUP

- PFPS is a clinical diagnosis of exclusion; evaluate and rule out other possibilities on the differential. Dynamic patellar tracking can be assessed by having the patient perform a single leg squat and stand. Physical exam should also include patellar mobility testing (displacement >3 quadrants is considered hypermobile), patellar grind (or inhibition) test (positive test if pain is produced), and patellar tilt test to assess for tightness of the lateral structures.
- Physical exam findings consistent with PFPS include eliciting pain by compression of the patella into the trochlear groove while the leg is extended.

IMAGING STUDIES

- No imaging is necessary in the initial workup.
- Consider plain films if symptoms do not improve after 1 to 2 mo of therapy.

Rx TREATMENT

There is a general lack of consensus. Management should focus on the implementation of a comprehensive rehabilitation program.

NONPHARMACOLOGIC THERAPY

Physical therapy; quadriceps, hamstring, iliotibial band, and calf-stretching exercises; quadriceps and hip abductor strengthening

ACUTE GENERAL Rx

Short-term (2 to 3 wk) nonsteroidal anti-inflammatory drugs or acetaminophen for pain relief; activity modification; ice for 10 to 20 min after activity

CHRONIC Rx

- Physical therapy; strengthening and flexibility exercises; consider arch supports or evaluation for custom orthotics.
- Spontaneous resolution may occur in some cases.

DISPOSITION

Outpatient management

REFERRAL

Consider referral to orthopedics for surgical evaluation as a last resort if conservative therapies fail. Surgical options include release of the lateral retinaculum; articular cartilage procedures; and proximal realignment, usually with anteromedialization of the tibial tubercle.

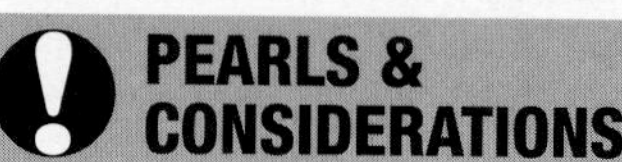

PEARLS & CONSIDERATIONS

COMMENTS

Treatment is most successful when the patient has a disciplined approach.

PATIENT & FAMILY EDUCATION

The American Academy of Family Practice website www.familydoctor.org contains frequently asked questions, patient information, and example stretching and strengthening exercises. Information is available in English and Spanish.

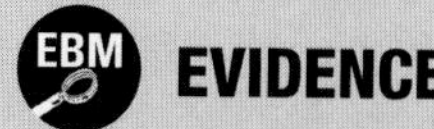

EVIDENCE

available at www.expertconsult.com

SUGGESTED READINGS

available at www.expertconsult.com

RELATED CONTENT

Knee Pain (Patient Information)
Patellofemoral Pain Syndrome (Patient Information)

AUTHOR: **KATE MAVRICH, M.D.**

BASIC INFORMATION

DEFINITION

- Patent foramen ovale (PFO) is a vestige of the fetal circulation, and results from failure of the primum and secundum septa to fuse postnatally. Persistence of the one-way flap valve overlying this foramen ovale allows right to left blood flow when right atrial pressure exceeds that of the left.
- Foramen ovale remains open during intrauterine life, in a valve-like manner, to allow highly oxygenated blood to reach the left atrium from the inferior vena cava. High right atrial pressure in the fetus keeps it open.
- Soon after birth, as the pulmonary circulation fills, the left atrial pressure rises higher than that of the right atrium. This pushes the septum primum against septum secondum, closing the right-to-left pathway through the foramen ovale.

ICD-9CM CODES
745.5 Patent foramen ovale
ICD-10CM CODES
Q21.1 Atrial septal defect

EPIDEMIOLOGY & DEMOGRAPHICS

- PFO fails to close in as much as a fourth of the population.
- PFO has similar frequency among males and females.

PHYSICAL FINDINGS & CLINICAL PRESENTATION

- Most patients with isolated PFO are asymptomatic.
- It cannot be detected on clinical examination.

COMPLICATIONS

- Cryptogenic stroke (particularly <55 yr).
- The proposed mechanism of stroke with PFO includes paradoxical embolization, in situ thrombosis within the canal of the PFO, associated atrial arrhythmia, and concomitant hypercoagulable state.
- Migraine with aura.
- Decompression sickness and air embolism.
- Increases risk of hypoxemia during sleep in patients with obstructive sleep apnea.
- Platypnea-orthodeoxia syndrome (characterized by both dyspnea and arterial desaturation in the upright position with improvement in supine position).
- Increased risk of postoperative atrial fibrillation and hypoxemia, in off-pump coronary artery bypass surgery.

ETIOLOGY

Unknown

DIAGNOSIS

- Testing for PFO is primarily performed in patients with a cerebral ischemic event of uncertain origin.
- A variety of echocardiography modalities have been used to diagnose PFO. These include:
  1. Transthoracic echocardiography (TTE)
  2. Transesophageal echocardiogram (TEE) (Fig. 1-708)
  3. Transmitral Doppler (TMD)
  4. Transcranial Doppler (TCD) of middle cerebral artery after injection of agitated saline peripherally
- TEE, especially when performed with contrast injected during a cough or Valsalva, is the most sensitive and preferred test for diagnosing PFO.
- Essentially, a PFO is suggested by the presence of echo dropout in the atrial septum visualized in more than one plane during echocardiography. The appearance of microbubbles in the left atrium within three to five cardiac cycles after injection of agitated saline peripherally is considered diagnostic of PFO with associated right-to-left shunt (RLS).
- The diagnosis of PFO is enhanced with multiple intravenous contrast injections with maneuvers that cause transient elevations of right atrial pressure (cough or Valsalva) to enhance RLS.
- TCD has the advantage of being noninvasive and easy to perform at bedside. But it can only detect a right-to-left shunt, not the location of the shunt or other cardiac structural anomalies.

TREATMENT

- Management guidelines from professional societies are shown in Table 1-383.
- Most patients with a PFO as an isolated finding receive no special treatment. This is because the yearly risk of cryptogenic stroke in healthy persons with PFO may be as low as 0.1%.
- As it is not associated with increased risk for endocarditis, antibiotic prophylaxis is not indicated.

PHARMACOLOGIC TREATMENT

When PFO is associated with an otherwise unexplained neurologic event, traditional treatment has been antiplatelet treatment (e.g., aspirin) therapy alone in low-risk patients and combined with therapeutic anticoagulants (e.g., warfarin) in high-risk patients.

Risk factors associated with a higher risk of complications, particularly stroke, include:

- Coexisting atrial septal aneurysm
- Large PFO
- Spontaneous right-to-left shunting
- Major shunt (>50 bubbles)
- Valsalva-provoking activity preceding the onset of stroke
- Presence of Chiari network (a congenital remnant of the right valve of the sinus venosus)
- Eustachian valves
- Younger age (<55 yr)
- Multiple clinical events or infarcts
- Pulmonary hypertension
- Failure or contraindications to anticoagulants
- High risk for recurrent deep venous thrombosis
- Pulmonary embolism at time of initial event
- Hypercoagulable state

PERCUTANEOUS TRANSCATHETER CLOSURE OF PFO

Percutaneous method of closure is usually preferred over open surgical closure because of invasiveness, procedure time, and patient convenience.

- Indications:
  1. Recurrent cryptogenic stroke due to presumed paradoxical embolism through PFO while on adequate medical treatment with antiplatelets or anticoagulants. The

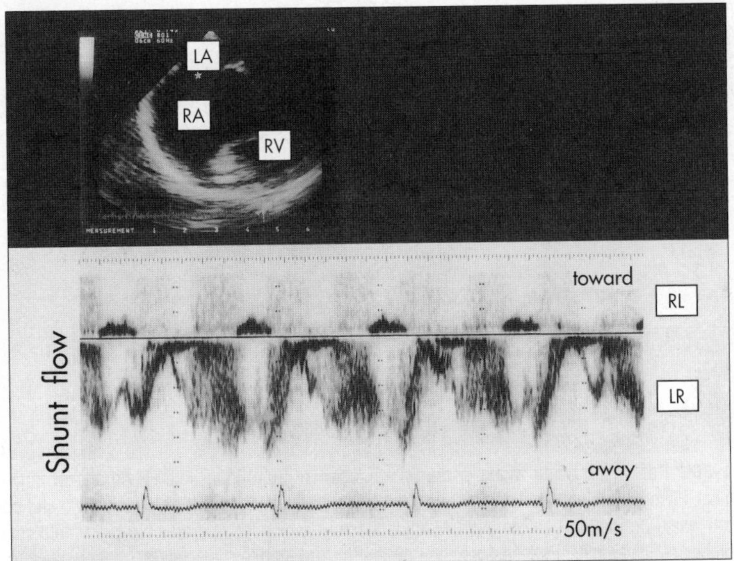

FIGURE 1-708 Transesophageal echocardiography of an internal defect and pulsed Doppler flow signal. Pulsed Doppler echocardiographic signal is consistent with left-to-right level. *LA,* Left atrium; *RA,* right atrium; *RV,* right ventricle; *LR,* left-to-right shunt signal; *RL,* right-to-left shunt signal. (From Crawford MH et al [eds]: *Cardiology,* ed 2, St Louis, 2004, Mosby.)

American Heart Association and American College of Cardiology have discouraged the use of devices to close a PFO as a means of preventing recurrent stroke. A recent trial (CLOSURE I) revealed that in patients with cryptogenic stroke or TIA who had a PFO, closure with a device did not offer a greater benefit than medical therapy alone for the prevention of recurrent stroke or TIA.

2. In presence of contraindications to anticoagulants

- Contraindications:
  1. Presence of thrombus on the implant site or in the venous system used for access
  2. Active endocarditis or bacteremia
  3. Inadequate size of femoral vein for access
  4. Atrial septal anatomy without an adequate rim to hold the device
  5. Atrial septal anatomy that may result in the occluder obstructing an intracardiac structure
  6. Known hypercoagulable state
  7. Presence of an intracardiac mass or vegetation
- The Food and Drug Administration (FDA) has approved CardioSEAL Septal Occlusion System and Amplatzer PFO Occluder devices for percutaneous PFO closure (Fig. 1-709).
- Requires SBE prophylaxis and antiplatelets (aspirin and clopidogrel for first 3 mo, followed by aspirin for another 3 mo) for 6 mo postprocedure. During this period of endothelialization, the risk of recurrent stroke is highest.
- The 1-yr rate of recurrent neurologic events ranged from 0% to 5% with percutaneous closure group vs. 4% to 12% with medical therapy group.
- MRI or metal detectors do not affect these implants, as they are not metallic in nature.

TABLE 1-383 Management Guidelines from Professional Societies

	American Academy of Neurology	American College of Chest Physicians
PFO	1. Evidence is insufficient to determine whether warfarin or aspirin is superior in preventing recurrent strokes or death, but minor bleeding is more frequent with warfarin. 2. There is insufficient evidence to evaluate the efficacy of surgical or endovascular closure.	
PFO alone		1. Antiplatelet therapy recommended over no therapy 2. Antiplatelet therapy suggested over warfarin
PFO with other risk factors		Inadequate data available to allow recommendation of optimal medical therapy vs. endovascular or surgical closure
PFO with concomitant deep vein thrombosis or pulmonary embolism	At least 3 mo of anticoagulation	Anticoagulation recommended

SURGICAL CLOSURE (OPEN THORACOTOMY)

Indications:
1. PFO >25 mm in size
2. Inadequate rim of tissue around the defect
3. Percutaneous device failure
4. In presence of other indication for open heart surgery

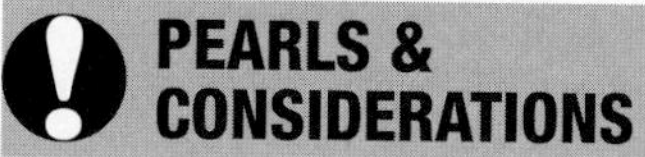

PEARLS & CONSIDERATIONS

COMMENTS

PFO is found on transesophageal echocardiography in about 50% of young survivors of stroke without clear cause for their stroke. In these patients, it is unclear whether the PFO was the cause of the stroke or whether it was an incidental finding. Trials have shown that closure of a PFO for secondary prevention of cryptogenic embolism did not result in a significant reduction in the risk of recurrent embolic events or death as compared with medical therapy.

SUGGESTED READINGS

available at www.expertconsult.com

AUTHOR: **HEMANT K. SATPATHY, M.D.**

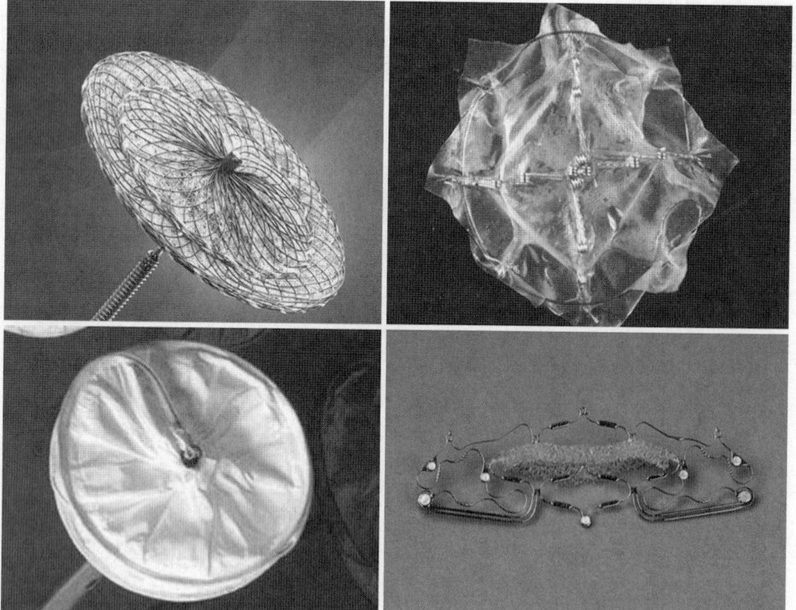

FIGURE 1-709 Patent foramen ovale occluders. Clockwise from upper left: (1) Amplatzer PFO occluder (AGA Medical, Plymouth, Minn) fashioned of two nitinol alloy disks, each with embedded fabric and connected by a central waist; (2) BioSTAR device (NMT Medical, Boston), which incorporates biodegradable collagenous disks fashioned similarly to its predecessors, the CardioSEAL and StarFlex devices; (3) Coherex device (Coherex Medical, Salt Lake City), which stretches the defect in one dimension while approximating the edges of the defect; and (4) Helex device (WL Gore & Associates, Newark, Del) with a single spiral coil of nitinol wire covered in fabric. (From Bonow RO et al: *Braunwald's heart disease: a textbook of cardiovascular medicine,* Philadelphia, 2012, Saunders.)

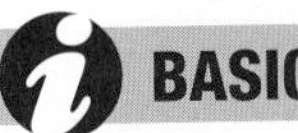

BASIC INFORMATION

DEFINITION

Pediculosis is lice infestation. Human beings can be infested with three kinds of lice: *Pediculus capitis* (head louse), *Pediculus corporis* (body louse), and *Phthirus pubis* (pubic, or crab, louse). Lice feed on human blood and deposit their eggs (nits) on the hair shafts (head lice and pubic lice) and along the seams of clothing (body lice). Nits generally hatch within 7 to 10 days. Lice are obligate human parasites and cannot survive away from their hosts for longer than 7 to 10 days.

SYNONYMS

Lice

ICD-9CM CODES
132.9 Pediculosis
ICD-10CM CODES
B85.2 Pediculosis, unspecified

EPIDEMIOLOGY & DEMOGRAPHICS

- There are 6 to 12 million cases of head lice in the U.S. yearly. The estimated annual direct and indirect cost of head louse infestation in the U.S. is $1 billion.
- Lice infestation of the scalp is most common in children (girls affected more often than boys).
- Infestation of the eyelashes is most frequently seen in children and may indicate sexual abuse.
- The chance of acquiring pubic lice from one sexual exposure with an infested partner is >90% (most contagious STD known).
- Body lice is most common in conditions of poor hygiene.

PHYSICAL FINDINGS & CLINICAL PRESENTATION

- Pruritus with excoriation may be caused by hypersensitivity reaction, inflammation from saliva, and fecal material from the lice.
- Nits can be identified by examining hair shafts.
- The presence of nits on clothes is indicative of body lice.
- Lymphadenopathy may be present (cervical adenopathy with head lice, inguinal lymphadenopathy with pubic lice).
- Head lice is most frequently found in the back of the head and neck, behind the ears.
- Scratching can result in pustules and crusting.
- Pubic lice may affect the hair around the anus.

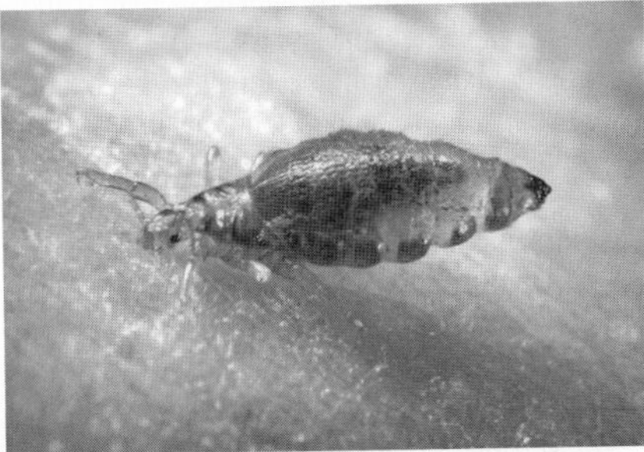

FIGURE 1-710 Body louse, *Pediculus humanus var. corporis*, as it was obtaining a blood meal from human host. (Courtesy Public Health Image Library, Centers for Disease Control and Prevention. From Vincent JL et al: *Textbook of critical care,* ed 6, Philadelphia, 2011, Saunders.)

ETIOLOGY

Lice are transmitted by close personal contact or use of contaminated objects (e.g., combs, clothing, bed linen, hats).

Dx DIAGNOSIS

DIFFERENTIAL DIAGNOSIS

- Seborrheic dermatitis
- Scabies
- Eczema
- Other: pilar casts, trichonodosis (knotted hair), monilethrix

WORKUP

Diagnosis is made by seeing the lice (Fig. 1-710) or their nits. Combing hair with a fine-toothed comb is recommended because visual inspection of the hair and scalp may miss more than 50% of infestations.

LABORATORY TESTS

Wood's light examination is useful to screen a large number of children: live nits fluoresce, empty nits have a gray fluorescence, nits with unborn louse reveal white fluorescence.

Rx TREATMENT

NONPHARMACOLOGIC THERAPY

- Patients with body lice should discard infested clothes and improve their hygiene.
- Combing out nits is a widely recommended but unproven adjunctive therapy.
- Personal items such as combs and brushes should be soaked in hot water for 15 to 30 min.
- Close contacts and household members should also be examined for the presence of lice.

ACUTE GENERAL Rx

The following products are available for treatment of lice:

- Permethrin: available over the counter (1% permethrin [Nix]) or by prescription (5% permethrin [Elimite]); should be applied to the hair and scalp and rinsed out after 10 min. A repeat application 7 days later is generally not necessary in patients with head lice. It can be applied to clean, dry hair and left on overnight (8 to 14 hours) under a shower cap. Resistance to permethrin is now widespread.
- Malathion, an organophosphate, is effective in head lice. It is available by prescription. Use should be avoided in children ≤2 yr. It is not commonly used because of its objectionable odor, fear of flammability, and prolonged application time (8 to 12 hr).
- Spinosad (Natroba) is a newer FDA-approved product for head lice. It is a topical suspension applied to dry hair for 10 min, then rinsed. It may be repeated 7 days later if necessary. It is more effective than permethrin but also much more expensive. It is safe in pregnancy (category B—no evidence of risk in humans).
- Benzyl alcohol lotion, 5% (Ulesfia) can be used for treatment of head lice in patients >6 mo old. The lotion is applied to dry hair and left on for 10 min. Treatment must be repeated after 7 days because the drug is not ovicidal.
- Eyelash infestation can be treated with the application of petroleum jelly rubbed into the eyelashes three times a day for 5 to 7 days. The application of baby shampoo to the eyelashes and brows three or four times a day for 5 days is also effective. The use of fluorescein drops applied to the lids and eyelashes is also toxic to lice.
- In patients who have previously not responded to treatment or in whom resistance with 1% permethrin cream rinse occurs, a 10-day course of trimethoprim-sulfamethoxazole (TMP-SMX) 8 mg/kg/day in divided doses is an effective treatment for head lice infestation, especially for eyelash infestations with *Phthirus pubis*.
- Ivermectin, an antiparasitic drug, given as an oral dose of 400 mcg/kg of body weight on days 1 and 8, is effective for head lice resistant to other treatments (currently not FDA approved for pediculosis). Ivermectin 0.5% lotion is FDA approved as a single-use topical treatment for head lice in patients 6 mo or older. Cost is more than $200 for 4 oz.

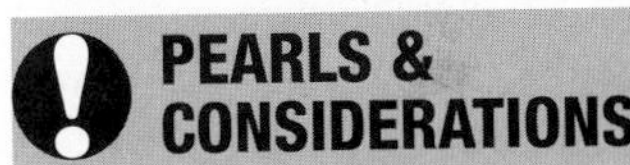

PEARLS & CONSIDERATIONS

COMMENTS

- Patients with pubic lice should notify their sexual contacts. Sex partners within the last month should be treated.
- Parents of patients should also be educated that head lice infestation (unlike body lice) does not indicate poor hygiene.

SUGGESTED READINGS

available at www.expertconsult.com

RELATED CONTENT

Lice (Patient Information)

AUTHOR: **FRED F. FERRI, M.D.**

BASIC INFORMATION

DEFINITION

According to the DSM-5, pedophilic disorder (PD) is one of eight identified paraphiliac disorders. A paraphilic disorder is described as a paraphilia or "any intense and persistent sexual interest other than sexual interest in genital stimulation or preparatory fondling with phenotypically normal, physically mature, consenting human partners," that either causes distress or functional impairment to the individual or entails personal harm or risk of harm to others. The diagnostic criteria for PD include the presence of recurrent, intense sexually arousing fantasies, sexual urges, or behaviors involving sexual activity with a prepubescent child or children (generally age 13 years or younger) that occur over a period of at least six months. The individual has acted on these urges or the urges have caused significant distress or interpersonal difficulty. The individual must be at least 16 yr and at least 5 yr older than the object of the sexual interest. DSM-5 subtypes pedophilic disorder into categories based on his/her victim gender preference (males, females, or both), on the exclusivity of the sexual urges (attracted only to children or not), and on his/her relationship with the victim ("limited to incest"). Individuals in late adolescence involved in ongoing sexual relationships with 12- or 13-year-old children are not included for this disorder in DSM-5.

ICD-9CM and DSM-5 CODES
302.2 Pedophilia
ICD-10CM CODES
F65.4 Pedophilia

EPIDEMIOLOGY & DEMOGRAPHICS

PREVALENCE: Unknown, with likely maximum of 5% in the male population and much smaller in the female population.
ONSET: Around the time of puberty, as adolescents begin to develop sexual interest.
PREDOMINANT SEX: The significant majority of pedophiles are men (females commit roughly 1% to 6% of child sexual assault).

PHYSICAL FINDINGS & CLINICAL PRESENTATION

- Diagnosis is made by clinical interview and is often complicated by reluctance to disclose symptoms unless the behaviors have already been identified.
- Legal involvement is common and may be the reason for presentation for care.
- Sex offenders have higher rates of *general* crime recidivism than *sexual* crime recidivism. When known child molesters are rearrested, ~40% of their rearrests are for sexual offenses.

DIAGNOSIS

DIFFERENTIAL DIAGNOSIS

- Antisocial personality disorder
- Conduct disorder
- Substance use disorder or intoxication
- Obsessive compulsive disorder

WORKUP

Requires comprehensive data from multiple sources, including self-report, past sexual offense convictions, past and present partner report, psychophysiologic assessments, forensic computer analysis, and/or assessment tools. Deviant sexual preferences and lifestyle instability/criminality are strongly associated with general sexual recidivism. Therefore, clinical interview should explore sexual preferences (sex drive, paraphilic interests, victim characteristics), past sexual behaviors (including inquiry into the use of child pornography), and a history of rule violation, substance abuse, and risk taking. It is also important to explore opportunities that the individual has to be around children as well as exploring an individual's strengths and protective factors.

SCALES AND LABORATORY TESTS

- Penile plethysmography: The penile volume or circumference is measured in response to a variety of sexual materials. The result may be a predictor of sexual recidivism for individuals who have committed sexual offenses. However, ~20% to 30% of individuals tested are considered low or nonresponders. Further, in the U.S., possession of the viewing material (child pornography) presents a legal dilemma for researchers. Other limitations include its lack of applicability to females, lack of applicability to males with impotence, and ability of individuals to try to suppress sexual feelings via distraction. This form of testing is not currently admissible in court for the purpose of determining guilt.
- Viewing Time: Viewing time is correlated with self-reported sexual interest and phallometric sexual arousal to children. No studies report that this measure predicts recidivism.
- Both of the above tests require the provider to show visual stimuli that may violate U.S. laws around possession of child pornography.
- Scales: For the prediction of general sexual recidivism, the most accurate approach appears to be the use of certain actuarial and mechanical measures. Some of the measures include the Static 99, MNSOST-3, Risk Matrix-2000, and the SVR 20 for adults, or the J-SOAP-II, ERASOR, and J-SORRAT-II for juveniles+. An individual's likelihood to recidivate is estimated based on the average risk of a group of individuals with similar characteristics.

TREATMENT

NONPHARMACOLOGIC THERAPY

- Treatment for sexually aggressive behaviors in general typically incorporates multiple modalities, including individual, group, family, social skills, behavioral, and educational therapies.
- Key elements of treatment include taking responsibility for behaviors, developing empathy for victims, developing skills to prevent re-offending
- General goals of treatment include improved control of deviant behaviors, impulse control, and coping; enhanced conflict resolution, anger management, and social skills; enhanced sense of empathy; understanding of cycle of thoughts, feelings, and events leading to inappropriate behaviors; respect within male-female relationships; and sexual education promoting healthy sexual behaviors (especially when working with juveniles).
- Community interventions might include the education of parents (re: high-risk situations, neighborhood sex offenders) and the education of children (re: assertiveness training, etc.).

PHARMACOLOGIC THERAPY

All used off-label in adults, adolescents, and children

Goals of treatment include suppression and elimination of deviant sexual fantasies, elimination of deviant sexual urges and behaviors, and reduction of risk for recidivism.

Selective serotonin reuptake inhibitors (SSRIs)

- Primary choice in adolescents, since few side effects (especially on adolescent physiological development)
- Case reports and small studies supporting use of fluoxetine, sertraline

Antiandrogens and hormonal agents

- Medroxyprogesterone acetate (MPA)
  - Most common hormonal agent in U.S.
  - Evidence mostly based on open trials
  - Reduces sex drive, sexual fantasy, sexual activity
  - Reduces sex drive, sexual fantasy, sexual activity
  - Side effects include nausea, vomiting, feminization, weight gain, decreased sperm production, diabetes mellitus, headaches, deep vein thrombosis, hot flashes
  - Induces testosterone-reductase in the liver, increasing metabolic clearance of testosterone and decreasing plasma testosterone
  - Also has progestinic effect, leading to reduction of gonadotropin secretion
- Cyproterone acetate (CPA)
  - Most common in Canada
  - Antiandrogenic, antigonadotropic, progesteinic effects
  - Principal effect at androgen receptors—blocks intracellular testosterone uptake and metabolism of androgen

- Similar effects to MPA
- Effects dose dependent
- Research indicates decrease in posttreatment recidivism rates for paraphilias
- Side effects include decreased erections, masturbation, and sexual intercourse; liver dysfunction; adrenal suppression; osteoporosis; osteopenia

- Only should be used rarely by psychiatrists with experience in conjunction with pediatric endocrinologist for severe behaviors (short-term use)

Luteinizing hormone-releasing hormone (LHRH) agonists

- Leuprolide acetate most common in U.S.
- Goserelin acetate available, triptorelin acetate likely available soon
- Specifically target paraphilias
- Pharmacologic castration effect
- Not recommended in children <18 yr, only indicated for severe symptoms in adults
- Overstimulation of hypothalamic-pituitary axis leading to inhibition of gonadotropin secretion
- Reduction or elimination of testosterone makes them useful in treating prostate cancer

REFERRAL

Refer to specialty mental health.

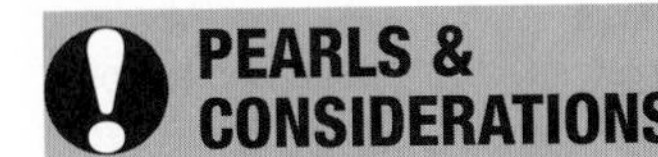

PEARLS & CONSIDERATIONS

- Individuals with pedophilia who have had no known risk of prior sexual contacts with children are at unknown risk to offend.
- Physicians must be aware of reporting requirements in their jurisdiction.

SUGGESTED READINGS

available at www.expertconsult.com

RELATED CONTENT

Pedophilia (Patient Information)

AUTHORS: **ELIZABETH A. LOWENHAUPT, M.D.,** and **SARAH L. XAVIER, D.O.**

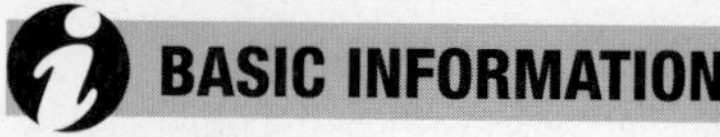

DEFINITION

Pelvic inflammatory disease (PID) is a polymicrobial infection of the upper genital tract, including a combination of any of the following:

- Endometritis, salpingitis, tubo-ovarian abscess, or pelvic peritonitis
- Resulting from an ascending lower genital tract infection
- Not related to obstetric or surgical intervention

SYNONYMS

PID
Adnexitis
Pyosalpinx
Salpingitis
Tubo-ovarian abscess

ICD-9CM CODES
614.9 Unspecified inflammatory disease of female pelvic organs and tissue
ICD-10CM CODES
A54.2 Gonococcal pelviperitonitis and other gonococcal genitourinary infections
A56.1 Chlamydial infection of pelviperitoneum and other genitourinary organs
N73.9 Female pelvic inflammatory disease, unspecified

EPIDEMIOLOGY & DEMOGRAPHICS

INCIDENCE/PREVALENCE:

- Estimated 600,000 to 1 million cases annually (U.S.), affecting primarily young sexually active women
- Diagnosed in 2% to 5% of women seen in sexually transmitted disease clinics
- Very common cause of female infertility and ectopic pregnancy

RISK FACTORS:

- Adolescent sexually active females <20 yr
- Previous episode of gonococcal PID
- Multiple sexual partners

PHYSICAL FINDINGS & CLINICAL PRESENTATION

- Lower abdominal pain
- Abnormal vaginal discharge
- Abnormal uterine bleeding
- Dysuria
- Dyspareunia
- Nausea and vomiting (suggestive of peritonitis)
- Fever
- Right upper quadrant tenderness (perihepatitis): 5% of PID cases
- Cervical motion tenderness and adnexal tenderness
- Adnexal mass

ETIOLOGY

- *Chlamydia trachomatis*
- *Neisseria gonorrhoeae*
- Polymicrobial infection: *Bacteroides fragilis, Escherichia coli, Gardnerella vaginalis, Haemophilus influenzae, Mycoplasma hominis, Ureaplasma urealyticum*
- *Mycobacterium tuberculosis* (an important cause in developing countries)
- Cytomegalovirus (CMV)

Dx DIAGNOSIS

DIFFERENTIAL DIAGNOSIS

- Ectopic pregnancy
- Appendicitis
- Ruptured ovarian cyst
- Endometriosis
- Urinary tract infection (cystitis or pyelonephritis)
- Renal calculus
- Adnexal torsion
- Proctocolitis

WORKUP

Diagnostic considerations:

- Clinical diagnosis is difficult and imprecise. The spectrum of disease ranges from asymptomatic to life-threatening tubo-ovarian abscess. PID should be suspected in at-risk patients who present with pelvic or lower abdominal pain.
- Clinical diagnosis of symptomatic PID has a positive predictive value of 65% to 90% compared with laparoscopy as the standard.
- No single historical, physical, or laboratory finding is both sensitive and specific for the diagnosis of PID.
- Empiric treatment for PID should be initiated in sexually active young women and other women at risk for STDs if they are experiencing pelvic or lower abdominal pain, if no cause for the illness other than PID can be identified, and if one or more of the following minimum criteria are present on pelvic examination:
    - Uterine tenderness
    - Adnexal tenderness
    - Cervical motion tenderness
- The requirement that all three minimum criteria be present before the initiation of empiric treatment could result in insufficient sensitivity for the diagnosis of PID. The presence of signs of lower genital tract inflammation (predominance of leukocytes in vaginal secretions), in addition to one of the three minimum criteria, increases the specificity of the diagnosis.
- Additional criteria to increase the specificity of the diagnosis of PID in women with severe clinical signs:
    - Oral temperature >38.3° C (101° F)
    - Abnormal cervical or vaginal discharge
    - Elevated erythrocyte sedimentation rate (ESR)
    - Elevated C-reactive protein
    - Laboratory documentation of cervical infection with *N. gonorrhoeae* or *C. trachomatis*
- Presence of abundant numbers of WBCs on saline microscopy of vaginal fluid.
- Definitive criteria for diagnosing PID warranted in selected cases:
    - Laparoscopic abnormalities consistent with PID
    - Histopathologic evidence of endometritis on biopsy. Endometrial biopsy is warranted in women undergoing laparoscopy who do not have visual evidence of salpingitis because endometritis is the only sign of PID in some women
    - Transvaginal sonography or other imaging techniques showing thickened fluid-filled tubes with or without free pelvic fluid or tubo-ovarian complex

LABORATORY TESTS

- Leukocytosis
- Elevated acute phase reactants: ESR >15 mm/hr, C-reactive protein
- Gram stain of endocervical exudate: >30 polymorphonuclear cells per high-power field correlates with chlamydial or gonococcal infection
- Endocervical cultures for *N. gonorrhoeae* and *C. trachomatis*
- Fallopian tube aspirate or peritoneal exudate culture if laparoscopy performed
- Human chorionic gonadotropin to rule out ectopic pregnancy

IMAGING STUDIES

- Transvaginal ultrasound to look for adnexal mass has sensitivity for PID of 81%, specificity of 78%, and accuracy of 80%.
- MRI has sensitivity for PID of 95%, specificity of 89%, and accuracy of 93%. It is useful for establishing the diagnosis of PID and detecting other processes responsible for the symptoms. Disadvantages are its higher cost and limited availability.
- CT scan (Fig. 1-711).

Rx TREATMENT

NONPHARMACOLOGIC THERAPY

- Most patients are treated as outpatients.
- Criteria for hospitalization (CDC, 2006) as follows:
    - Surgical emergencies such as appendicitis cannot be excluded
    - Tubo-ovarian abscess
    - Pregnant patient
    - Patient is immunodeficient
    - Severe illness, nausea, or vomiting precluding outpatient management
    - Patient unable to follow or tolerate outpatient regimens
    - No clinical response to outpatient therapy

ACUTE GENERAL Rx

Regimens for treatment of PID should also be effective against *N. gonorrhoeae* and *C. trachomatis* because endocervical screening for these organisms does not rule out upper reproductive tract infections.

INPATIENT REGIMENS:

Recommended parenteral regimen A

- Cefotetan 2 g IV q12h OR
- Cefoxitin 2 g IV q6h PLUS
- Doxycycline 100 mg PO or IV q12h

Recommended parenteral regimen B

- Clindamycin 900 mg IV q8h PLUS

- Gentamicin loading dose IV or IM (2 mg/kg of body weight), followed by a maintenance dose (1.5 mg/kg) q8h. Single daily dosing (3 to 5 mg/kg) can be substituted.

Alternative parenteral regimens

- Ampicillin/sulbactam 3 g IV q6h
  PLUS
- Doxycycline 100 mg PO or IV q12h

OUTPATIENT REGIMENS:

Recommended regimen

- Ceftriaxone 250 mg IM in a single dose
  PLUS
- Doxycycline 100 mg PO bid for 14 days
  WITH or WITHOUT
- Metronidazole 500 mg PO bid for 14 days
  OR
- Cefoxitin 2 g IM in a single dose and probenecid, 1 g PO administered concurrently in a single dose
  PLUS
- Doxycycline 100 mg PO bid for 14 days
  WITH or WITHOUT
- Metronidazole 500 mg PO bid for 14 days
  OR
- Other parenteral third-generation cephalosporin (e.g., ceftizoxime or cefotaxime)
  PLUS
- Doxycycline 100 mg PO bid for 14 days
  WITH or WITHOUT
- Metronidazole 500 mg PO bid for 14 days

CHRONIC Rx

Hospitalized patients receiving IV therapy:

1. Significant clinical improvement is characterized by defervescence, decreased abdominal tenderness, and decreased uterine, adnexal, and cervical motion tenderness within 3 to 5 days.
2. If no clinical improvement occurs, further diagnostic workup is necessary, including possible surgical intervention.

DISPOSITION

- Long-term sequelae of PID: recurrent PID, chronic pelvic pain, ectopic pregnancy, infertility, Fitz-Hugh-Curtis syndrome (Fig. 1-712)
- Risk of tubal infertility related to episodes of PID: first episode, 8%; second episode, 20%; third episode, 40%
- Essential to evaluate and treat male sex partners

REFERRAL

If there is no clinical improvement with outpatient therapy observed within 72 hr, patient should be hospitalized and gynecology consult requested.

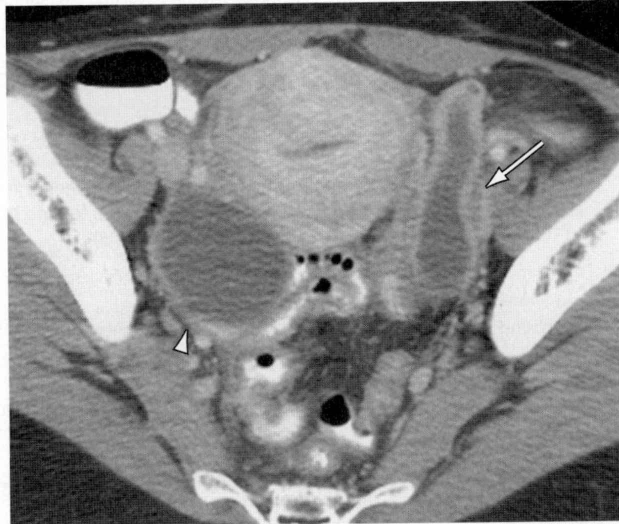

FIGURE 1-711 Pelvic inflammatory disease with pyosalpinx in a 26-yr-old patient. Computed tomographic image through pelvis shows cystic tubular structure with thick enhancing walls *(arrow)* lateral to the uterus, which, in absence of oral contrast, could be mistaken for a loop of small bowel. (From Fielding JR et al: *Gynecologic imaging,* Philadelphia, 2011, Saunders.)

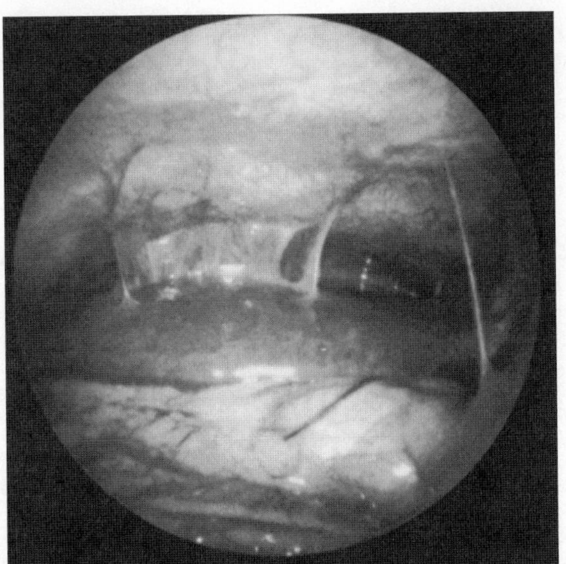

FIGURE 1-712 "Violin string" adhesions are visualized in this patient with Fitz-Hugh-Curtis syndrome. (From Copeland LJ: *Textbook of gynecology,* ed 2, Philadelphia, 2000, Saunders.)

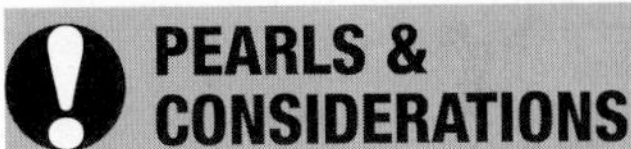

PEARLS & CONSIDERATIONS

COMMENTS

- Maintain a low threshold for the diagnosis of PID.
- Women with documented chlamydial or gonococcal infections have a high rate of reinfection within 6 mo of treatment. Repeat testing of all women who have been diagnosed with chlamydia or gonorrhea is recommended 3 to 6 mo after treatment, regardless of whether their sex partners were treated.
- All women diagnosed with acute PID should be offered HIV testing.
- Male sex partners of women with PID should be examined and treated if they had sexual contact with the patient during 60 days preceding the patient's onset of symptoms. If a patient's last sexual intercourse was >60 days before onset of symptoms or diagnosis, the patient's most recent sex partner should be treated.
- Patients should be instructed to abstain from sexual intercourse until therapy is completed and until they and their sex partners no longer have symptoms.

SUGGESTED READINGS

available at www.expertconsult.com

RELATED CONTENT

Abscess, Pelvic (Related Key Topic)
Chlamydia Genital Infections (Related Key Topic)
Gonorrhea (Related Key Topic)
Pelvic Inflammatory Disease (Patient Information)

AUTHOR: **RUBEN ALVERO, M.D.**

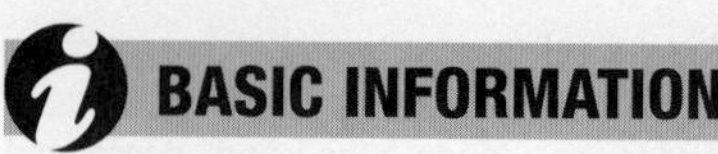

BASIC INFORMATION

DEFINITION

Pelvic organ prolapse (POP) or *uterine prolapse* refers to the protrusion of the uterus into or out of the vaginal canal. In a first-degree uterine prolapse, the cervix is visible when the perineum is depressed. In a second-degree uterine prolapse, the uterine cervix has prolapsed through the vaginal introitus, with the fundus remaining within the pelvis proper. In a third-degree uterine prolapse (i.e., complete uterine prolapse, uterine procidentia), the entire uterus is outside the introitus. Table 1-384 compares the various types of prolapse.

SYNONYMS

Genital prolapse
Uterine descensus
Uterine prolapse
POP

ICD-9CM CODES
618.8 Genital prolapse
618.1 Uterine descensus
618.8 Pelvic organ prolapse
ICD-10CM CODES
N81.4 Uterovaginal prolapse, unspecified
N81.5 Vaginal enterocele
N81.6 Rectocele
N81.I8 Other female genital prolapse
N81.89 Other female genital prolapse
N81.2 Incomplete uterovaginal prolapse
N81.82 Incompetence or weakening of pubocervical tissue

EPIDEMIOLOGY & DEMOGRAPHICS

PREVALENCE: Most prevalent in postmenopausal multiparous women.

RISK FACTORS:
- Pregnancy, especially POP symptoms during pregnancy
- Labor
- Vaginal childbirth
- Obesity
- Chronic coughing
- Constipation
- Pelvic tumors
- Ascites
- Strenuous physical exertion, especially during pregnancy
- Maternal history of prolapse
- Caucasian race

GENETICS: Increased incidence in women with spina bifida occulta.

PHYSICAL FINDINGS & CLINICAL PRESENTATION

- Pelvic pressure
- Bearing-down sensation
- Bilateral groin pain
- Sacral backache
- Coital difficulty
- Protrusion from vagina
- Spotting
- Ulceration
- Bleeding
- Examination of patient in lithotomy, sitting, and standing positions and before, during, and after a maximum Valsalva effort
- Erosion or ulceration of the cervix possible in the most dependent area of the protrusion

ETIOLOGY

- Vaginal childbirth and chronic increases in intraabdominal pressure leading to detachments, lacerations, and denervations of the vaginal support system
- Further weakening of pelvic support system by hypoestrogenic atrophy
- Direct injury to the levator ani, neurologic injury from stretching of the pudendal nerves
- Some cases from congenital or inherited weaknesses within the pelvic support system
- Neonatal uterine prolapse mostly coexistent with congenital spinal defects

DIAGNOSIS

DIFFERENTIAL DIAGNOSIS

- Occasionally, elongated cervix; body of the uterus remains undescended.
- Diagnosis is based on history and physical examination. Currently there is only one genital tract prolapse classification system that has attained international acceptance and recognition: the patient pelvic organ prolapse quantification (POP-Q) (Boxes 1-61 and 1-62).

WORKUP

- If erosion or ulceration of the cervix is present, a Pap smear followed by a cervical biopsy should be performed if indicated.
- If urinary symptoms are significant, further urodynamic workup is indicated, looking for concurrent cystourethrocele, cystocele, enterocele, or rectocele.

TABLE 1-384 Types of Genital Prolapse

Original Position of Organs	Prolapse	Symptoms (in addition to the general symptoms of discomfort, dragging, the feeling of a "lump" and, rarely, coital problems)
Anterior	Urethrocele Cystocele	Urinary symptoms (stress incontinence, urinary frequency)
Central	Cervix/uterus: 1st, 2nd, and 3rd degree Procidentia	Bleeding and/or discharge from ulceration in association with procidentia
Posterior	Rectocele Enterocele	Bowel symptoms, particularly the feeling of incomplete evacuation and sometimes having to press the posterior wall backwards to pass stool

From Drife J, Magowan B: *Clinical obstetrics and gynaecology,* Philadelphia, 2004, Saunders.

BOX 1-61 Staging of Pelvic Organ Prolapse Based on POP-Q Examination

Stage 0	No prolapse.
Stage I	Most distal prolapse >1 cm above hymenal ring.
Stage II	Most distal point is ≤1 cm above hymenal ring.
Stage III	Most distal point is >1 cm below the hymenal ring but not farther than 2 cm less than the total vaginal length (TVL) (i.e., ≥1 cm but ≤ [TVL – 2] cm).
Stage IV	Complete vaginal eversion.

From Pemberton J (ed): *The pelvic floor,* Philadelphia, 2002, Saunders.

BOX 1-62 Points of Reference for POP-Q

Point A: 3 cm above the hymen on anterior vaginal wall (Aa) or posterior vaginal wall (Ap). Point Aa roughly corresponds with the urethrovesical junction.
Point B: The lowest extent of the segment of vagina between point A and the apex of the vagina. Unlike point A, it is not fixed but will be the same as A if point A is the most protruding point. In maximal prolapse it will be the same as point C.
Point C: The most distal part of the cervix or vaginal vault.
Point D: The posterior fornix, which is omitted in women with prior hysterectomy.
Genital hiatus: From midline external urethral meatus to inferior hymenal ring.
Perineal body: From inferior hymenal ring to middle of anal orifice.
Vaginal length: This should be measured without undue stretching of the vagina.

From Pemberton J (ed): *The pelvic floor,* Philadelphia, 2002, Saunders.

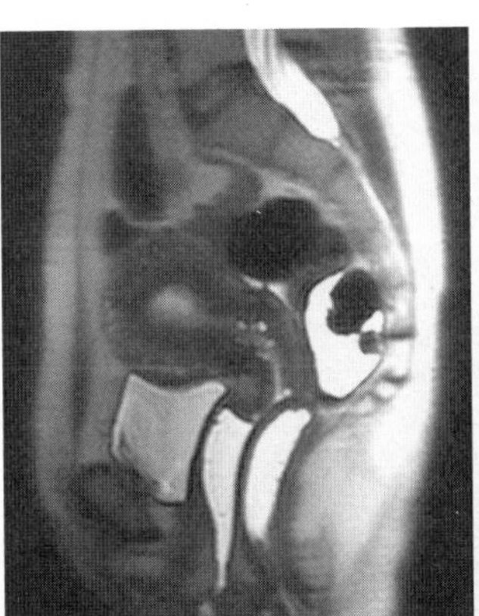

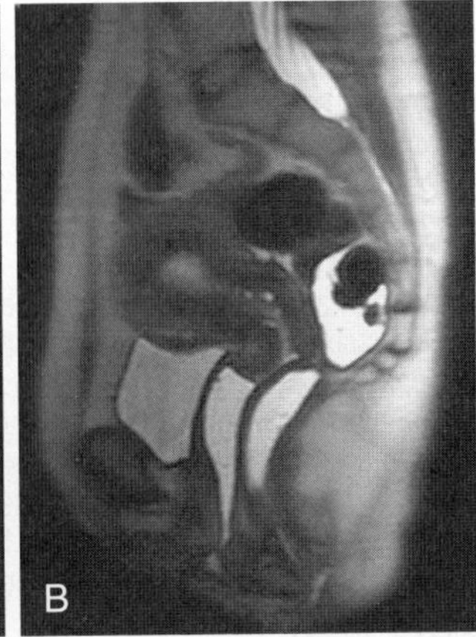

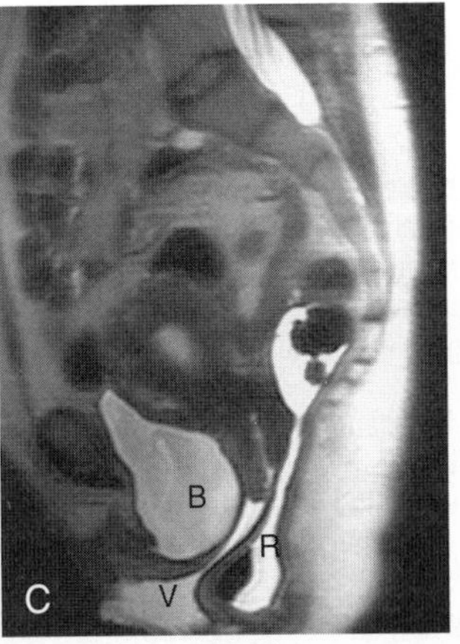

FIGURE 1-713 **A**, Moderate global pelvic prolapse in a woman with stress urinary incontinence, pelvic heaviness, and constipation after three vaginal deliveries. At rest, all viscera are normally situated in the pelvis. **B**, With Kegel contraction, note that all viscera remain normally situated in the pelvis. **C**, With maximal strain, bladder *(B)*, vagina *(V)*, and rectum *(R)* are well below the pelvic floor. (From Fielding JR et al: *Gynecologic imaging,* Philadelphia, 2011, Saunders.)

LABORATORY TESTS

Urine culture

IMAGING STUDIES

Ultrasound if concurrent fibroids need further evaluation, CT or MRI (Fig. 1-713) in symptomatic patients with unclear diagnosis

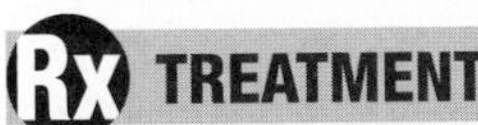

TREATMENT

NONPHARMACOLOGIC THERAPY

- Prophylactic measures
  1. Diagnosis and treatment of chronic respiratory and metabolic disorders
  2. Correction of constipation
  3. Weight control, nutrition, and smoking cessation counseling
  4. Pelvic muscle exercises
- Supportive pessary therapy
  1. Ring-type pessary useful for first- or second-degree prolapse
  2. Gellhorn pessary preferred for more advanced prolapse
  3. Use of pessaries in conjunction with continuous hormone replacement therapy, unless contraindicated
  4. Perineorrhaphy under local anesthesia possibly needed to support the pessary if the vaginal outlet is very relaxed

ACUTE GENERAL Rx

- Patients who are only infrequently symptomatic: insertion of a tampon or diaphragm for temporary relief when prolonged standing is anticipated
- Neonatal uterine prolapse: simple digital reduction or the use of a small pessary

CHRONIC Rx

- Hormone replacement therapy at the time of menopause helps preserve tissue strength, maintain elasticity of the vagina, and promote the durability of surgical repairs.
- Gold standard for therapy is vaginal hysterectomy.
- Vaginal apex should be well suspended, but a prophylactic sacrospinous ligament fixation is not routinely required.
- If occult enterocele present, McCall culdoplasty is performed.
- If vaginal approach to hysterectomy is contraindicated, abdominal hysterectomy is performed; vaginal apex likewise well supported. Use of laparoscopically assisted approaches, including robotically assisted approaches are increasingly being used. Questions do exist as to whether the robotic approach is cost-effective for this indication.
- Colpocleisis is considered for the elderly patient who is sexually inactive and is a high-risk patient from a surgical point of view; can be done rapidly under local anesthesia with mild sedation if necessary.
- For symptomatic women who desire childbearing: management with pessaries or pelvic muscle exercises is recommended; if surgical correction is required, transvaginal sacrospinous fixation is the preferred method.
- Other surgical options are sling operations and sacral cervicopexy.
- Trials have shown that as compared with anterior colporrhaphy, use of a standardized, trocar-guided mesh kit for cystocele repair results in higher short-term rates of successful treatment but also in higher rates of surgical complications and postoperative adverse events.
- Women without stress incontinence undergoing vaginal surgery for POP are at risk for postoperative urinary incontinence. Use of a prophylactic midurethral sling inserted during vaginal prolapse surgery has been shown to result in a lower rate of urinary incontinence at 3 and 12 months but a higher rate of adverse events (UTIs, major bleeding complications, incomplete bladder emptying).

DISPOSITION

If untreated, uterine prolapse progressively worsens.

REFERRAL

To a gynecologist/urologist if pessary fitting or surgical intervention is needed

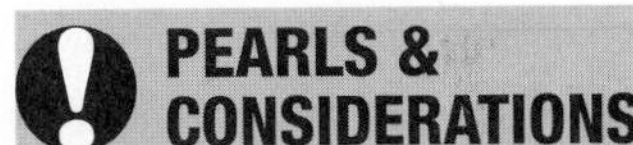

PEARLS & CONSIDERATIONS

COMMENTS

- More than 300,000 surgeries are performed annually in the U.S. for pelvic organ prolapse
- Surgery contraindicated in mild or asymptomatic uterine prolapse because the patient will seldom benefit from the operation although exposed to its risks.
- The Optimal Randomized Trial compared the sacrospinous ligament fixation (SSLF) and uterosacral ligament suspension (ULS) surgical approaches to correct apical prolapse and also whether perioperative behavioral therapy with pelvic floor muscle training (BPMT) improved outcomes of prolapse surgery. The trial showed that two years after vaginal surgery for prolapse and stress urinary incontinence, neither ULS or SSLF was significantly superior to the other for anatomic, functional, or adverse event outcomes. Perioperative BPMT did not improve urinary symptoms at 6 mo or prolapse outcomes at 2 yr.[1]

SUGGESTED READINGS

available at www.expertconsult.com

RELATED CONTENT

Incontinence, Urinary (Related Key Topic)
Fig. E3-197 Management of vaginal prolapse (Algorithm)
Uterine Prolapse (Patient Information)

AUTHORS: **ARUNDATHI G. PRASAD, M.D.,** and **RUBEN ALVERO, M.D.**

[1]Barber MD et al: Comparison of 2 transvaginal surgical approaches and perioperative behavioral therapy for apical vaginal prolapse, the Optimal Randomized Trial, *JAMA* 311(10):1023-1034, 2014

BASIC INFORMATION

DEFINITION

- *Pemphigus* refers to a group of rare, potentially fatal, chronic, autoimmune blistering diseases of the skin and mucous membranes
- Pemphigus has four main subtypes:
  1. Pemphigus vulgaris (PV) (most common) (Fig. 1-714)
     - Pemphigus vegetans, a rare clinical variant of PV
  2. Pemphigus foliaceus (PF)
     - Pemphigus erythematosus, a variant of PF
  3. Paraneoplastic pemphigus
  4. Immunoglobulin (Ig) A pemphigus

SYNONYMS

Pemphigus
Fogo selvagem: endemic pemphigus foliaceus
Senear-Usher syndrome: pemphigus erythematosus

ICD-9CM CODES
694.4 Pemphigus
ICD-10CM CODES
L10.0 Pemphigus vulgaris

EPIDEMIOLOGY & DEMOGRAPHICS

- Incidence is approximately one case per 100,000 persons and varies substantially by geographic region.
- More common in Ashkenazi Jews and people of Middle Eastern descent.
- Typically occurs in the fourth and fifth decades of life, although range of ages affected is broad and it may occur in the very young or elderly.
- No gender predilection

PHYSICAL FINDINGS & CLINICAL PRESENTATION

- History:
  1. Multiple oropharyngeal ulcerations and erosions typically occur first, which can then be followed by a more generalized bullous eruption involving the skin within several weeks or months
  2. Blisters are fragile and rupture easily, leaving painful erosions and ulcerations that may be the predominant clinical finding
  3. Pain associated with oral mucosal blistering often results in dysphagia and hoarseness
  4. Not commonly pruritic
- Physical findings:
  1. Anatomic distribution
     a. Oral mucosa
     b. Can also involve the pharynx, larynx, vagina, penis, anus, and conjunctival mucosa
     c. Generalized cutaneous involvement (Figs. 1-715 and 1-716)
  2. Lesion configuration
     a. Any stratified squamous epithelial surfaces can become involved
  3. Lesion morphology
     a. Flaccid bullae and vesicles
     b. Erosion with crusting commonly occurs
  4. Positive Nikolsky sign: when the clinician applies lateral pressure to normal-appearing skin at the periphery of active lesions, separation of the superficial epidermis occurs

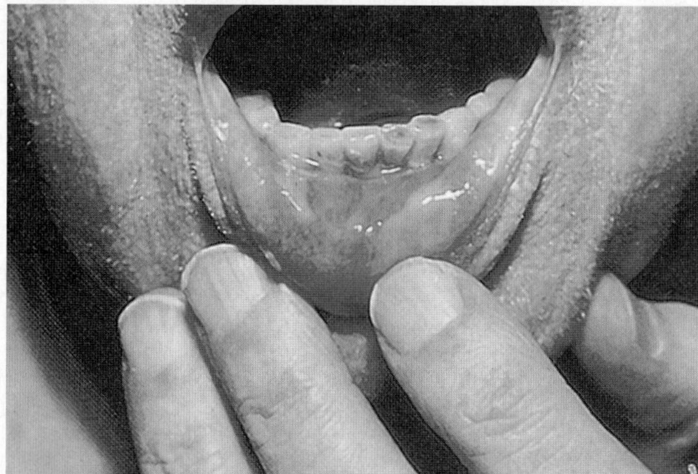

FIGURE 1-714 Pemphigus vulgaris with oral lesions and no intact bullae. (Courtesy Department of Dermatology, University of North Carolina at Chapel Hill. From Goldstein BG, Goldstein AO: *Practical dermatology,* ed 2, St Louis, 1997, Mosby.)

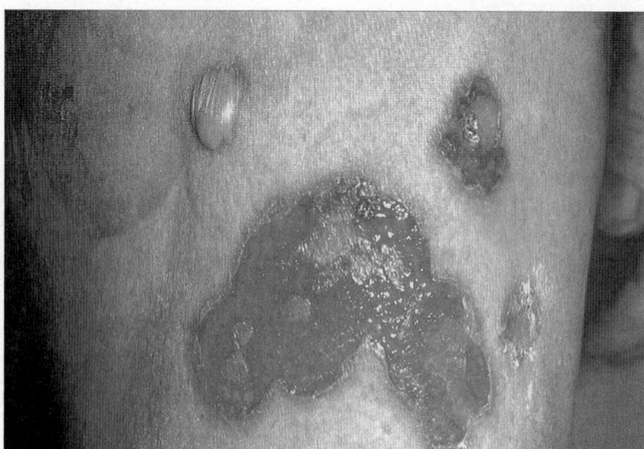

FIGURE 1-715 Pemphigus vulgaris; extensive erosions and blisters are present on the shin. (Courtesy R. A. Marsden, M.D., St. George's Hospital, London. From McKee PH et al [eds]: *Pathology of the skin with clinical correlations,* ed 3, St Louis, 2005, Mosby.)

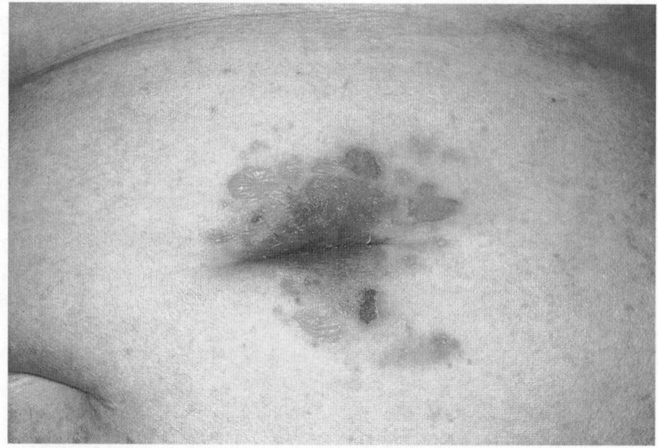

FIGURE 1-716 Pemphigus vulgaris: umbilical lesions showing intact blisters as well as raw erosions. (Courtesy R. A. Marsden, M.D., St. George's Hospital, London. From McKee PH et al [eds]: *Pathology of the skin with clinical correlations,* ed 3, St Louis, 2005, Mosby.)

ETIOLOGY

Autoimmune disease caused by autoantibodies against the cell surface of keratinocytes. The predominant antibody in PV is directed against desmoglein 3; in PF it is directed against desmoglein 1.

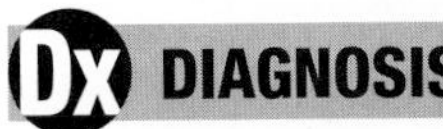

DIAGNOSIS

The diagnosis of pemphigus vulgaris should be suspected in patients with painful oral erosions and flaccid bullae or erosions on the skin.

DIFFERENTIAL DIAGNOSIS

- Bullous pemphigoid (Table 1-385)
- Cicatricial pemphigoid
- Behçet's syndrome
- Erythema multiforme
- Hailey-Hailey disease
- Aphthous stomatitis
- Bullous lupus erythematosus
- Drug eruptions
- Dermatitis herpetiformis
- Epidermolysis bullosa acquisita
- IgA pemphigus
- Paraneoplastic pemphigus
- Pemphigus foliaceus

WORKUP

Skin biopsy is diagnostic; specimens should be sent for routine histochemical staining and direct immunofluorescence. Certain laboratory values may also be useful in establishing the diagnosis of pemphigus.

LABORATORY TESTS

- Skin biopsy reveals intraepidermal vesicles, also called *acantholysis* (loss of cell adhesion between the epidermal cells).
- Indirect immunofluorescence may detect circulating autoantibodies.
- Direct immunofluorescence studies of perilesional skin demonstrate IgG directed against keratinocyte surfaces in the epidermis.

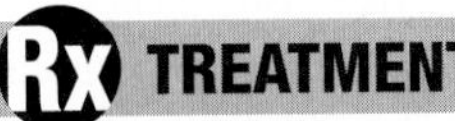

TREATMENT

NONPHARMACOLOGIC THERAPY

- Mild soaps and emollients to skin
- Burow's solution may be useful for weeping erosions.
- Soft diet and viscous lidocaine can be used in patients with oral lesions.

ACUTE GENERAL Rx

- For localized disease, topical steroids may be effective.
- For generalized disease, systemic corticosteroids (prednisone) are the mainstay of therapy and often work rapidly to halt blistering.
  - Initial dose of prednisone is usually 1 mg/kg/day, then tapered over weeks as blistering decreases.
  - Steroid-sparing immunosuppressive therapies are often initiated simultaneously with prednisone to minimize the side effects of prolonged corticosteroid therapy.

CHRONIC Rx

- Adjuvant therapy such as immunosuppressants, anti-inflammatories, chemotherapeutic agents, and biologics are useful for disease control and to shorten the length of treatment with oral steroids; treatment duration and dosing are determined by clinical response:
  1. Azathioprine 50 to 100 mg/day
  2. Cyclophosphamide 1 to 3 mg/kg/day
  3. Mycophenolate mofetil 500 mg to 2 g daily
- Refractory disease:
  1. IV Ig
  2. Rituximab (anti-CD20 monoclonal antibody)
  3. Plasmapheresis

DISPOSITION

- Before the use of oral corticosteroids, pemphigus was usually a fatal disease with most patients dying within 5 yr of diagnosis.
- Combined corticosteroids and adjuvant therapy have decreased mortality rates to <10%.
- Death generally occurs from sepsis or complications related to medical therapy.

REFERRAL

Dermatology
Otolaryngology

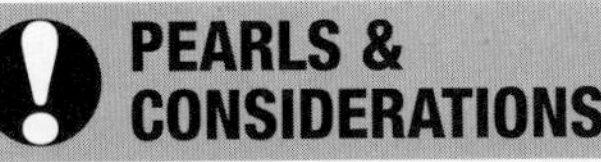

PEARLS & CONSIDERATIONS

COMMENTS

- PV, unlike bullous pemphigoid, is a disease of middle-aged persons.
- Early diagnosis of pemphigus is important to initiate prompt treatment.
- Oral corticosteroids have many substantial side effects, and patients should be monitored for osteoporosis, hypertension, and diabetes.

SUGGESTED READINGS

available at www.expertconsult.com

RELATED CONTENT

Pemphigus Vulgaris (Patient Information)

AUTHORS: **JESSICA CORWIN, M.D., M.P.H.,** and **KACHIU LEE, B.A.**

TABLE 1-385 Differentiation of Pemphigus Vulgaris and Bullous Pemphigoid

Characteristics	Pemphigus Vulgaris	Bullous Pemphigoid
Age	Usually occurs in middle-aged persons	>60 yr
Site	Oral mucosa, face, chest, groin	Flexural areas, groin, axilla; less often involving mucosal surfaces
Findings	Flaccid bullae and erosions, intraepidermal blisters, IgG autoantibodies against keratinocyte surfaces	Intact bullae, subepidermal blisters, IgG autoantibodies against hemidesmosomal antigens
Treatment	Prednisone 1 mg/kg/day with adjuvant immunosuppressant agents; refractory disease may require intravenous immunoglobulin, plasmapheresis, or rituximab	Prednisone 1 mg/kg/day with adjuvant immunosuppressant therapy; localized disease may be controlled with topical steroids
Prognosis	>90% respond; steroid side effects significant	>90% respond; remissions and recurrences common

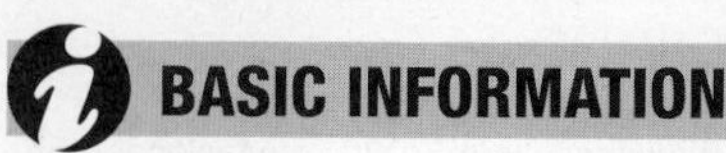

BASIC INFORMATION

DEFINITION

Peptic ulcer disease (PUD) is an ulceration in the stomach or duodenum resulting from an imbalance between mucosal protective factors and various mucosal damaging mechanisms (see "Etiology").

SYNONYMS

PUD
Duodenal ulcer (DU)
Gastric ulcer (GU)

ICD-9CM CODES
536.8 Peptic ulcer disease
531.3 Peptic ulcer, stomach, acute
531.7 Peptic ulcer, stomach, chronic
532.3 Peptic ulcer, duodenum, acute
532.7 Peptic ulcer, duodenum, chronic

ICD-10CM CODES
K25.3 Acute gastric ulcer without hemorrhage or perforation
K25.7 Chronic gastric ulcer without hemorrhage or perforation
K26.3 Acute duodenal ulcer without hemorrhage or perforation
K26.7 Chronic duodenal ulcer without hemorrhage or perforation

EPIDEMIOLOGY & DEMOGRAPHICS

- Incidence: 250,000 to 500,000 (200,000 to 400,000 duodenal; 50,000 to 100,000 gastric) annually; duodenal ulcer/gastric ulcer ratio is 4:1.
- Anatomic location: <90% of duodenal ulcers occur in the first portion of the duodenum; gastric ulcers occur most frequently in the lesser curvature near the incisura angularis.

PHYSICAL FINDINGS & CLINICAL PRESENTATION

- Physical examination is often unremarkable.
- Patient may have epigastric tenderness, tachycardia, pallor, hypotension (from acute or chronic blood loss), nausea and vomiting (if pyloric channel is obstructed), boardlike abdomen and rebound tenderness (if perforated), and hematemesis or melena (with a bleeding ulcer). Box 1-63 describes key symptoms and signs of peptic ulcer.

ETIOLOGY

Often multifactorial. The following are common mucosal damaging factors:

- *Helicobacter pylori* infection. *H. pylori* is the major cause of PUD. It is found in more than 70% of patients with duodenal ulcers and gastric ulcers in the U.S. Rates are much higher (>90%) in other parts of the world. Eradication of *H. pylori* markedly reduces peptic ulcer recurrence.
- Medications (NSAIDs, glucocorticoids). Risk factors for development of NSAID-related ulcers are described in Table 1-386.
- Incompetent pylorus or lower esophageal sphincter
- Bile acids
- Impaired proximal duodenal bicarbonate secretion
- Decreased blood flow to gastric mucosa
- Acid secreted by parietal cells and pepsin secreted as pepsinogen by chief cells
- Cigarette smoking
- Alcohol

TABLE 1-386 Risk Factors for Development of NSAID-Related Ulcers

Definite
Advanced age
History of ulcer
Concomitant corticosteroid therapy
Concomitant anticoagulation therapy
High doses of NSAIDs
Serious systemic disorders
Possible
Concomitant infection with *Helicobacter pylori*
Cigarette smoking
Consumption of alcohol

NSAIDs, Nonsteroidal anti-inflammatory drugs.
From Andreoli TE et al: *Andreoli and Carpenter's Cecil essentials of medicine,* ed 8, Philadelphia, 2010, Saunders.

BOX 1-63 Key Symptoms and Signs of Peptic Ulcer

Uncomplicated Ulcer
No symptoms ("silent ulcer" in up to 40% of cases)
Epigastric pain
Pain may radiate to the back, thorax, other parts of abdomen (cephalad most likely, caudad least likely)
Pain may be nocturnal (most specific), "painful hunger" relieved by food, or continuous (least specific)
Nausea
Vomiting
Heartburn (mimics or associated with gastroesophageal reflux)

Complicated Ulcer
Acute perforation
Severe abdominal pain
Shock
Abdominal boardlike rigidity (and rebound and other signs of peritoneal irritation)
Free intraperitoneal air
Hemorrhage
Hematemesis and/or melena
Hemodynamic changes, anemia
Previous history of ulcer symptoms (80%)
Gastric outlet obstruction
Satiation, inability to ingest food, eructation
Nausea, vomiting (and related disturbances)
Weight loss

From Goldman L, Schafer AI: *Goldman's Cecil medicine,* ed 24, Philadelphia, 2012, Saunders.

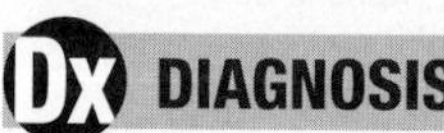

DIAGNOSIS

DIFFERENTIAL DIAGNOSIS

- Gastroesophageal reflux disease
- Cholelithiasis syndrome
- Pancreatitis
- Gastritis
- Nonulcer dyspepsia
- Neoplasm (gastric carcinoma, lymphoma, pancreatic carcinoma)
- Angina pectoris, myocardial infarction, pericarditis
- Dissecting aneurysm
- Other: high small-bowel obstruction, pneumonia, subphrenic abscess, early appendicitis

WORKUP

Comprehensive history and physical exam to exclude other diagnoses. Diagnostic modalities include endoscopy or upper GI series. Endoscopy is preferred.

LABORATORY TESTS

- Routine laboratory evaluation is usually unremarkable.
- Anemia may be present in patients with significant GI bleeding.
- *H. pylori* testing by endoscopic biopsy, urea breath test, stool antigen test (*H. pylori* stool antigen), or specific antibody test is recommended:
  1. Serologic testing for antibodies to *H. pylori* is easy and inexpensive; however, the presence of antibodies demonstrates previous but not necessarily current infection. Antibodies to *H. pylori* can remain elevated for months to years after infection has cleared; therefore antibody levels must be interpreted in light of the patient's symptoms and other test results (e.g., PUD seen on upper GI series).
  2. The urea breath test documents active infection (sensitivity and specificity >90%). The patient ingests a small amount of urea labeled with carbon 13 or carbon 14. If urease is present (produced by the organism), the urea is hydrolyzed and the patient exhales labeled carbon dioxide that is then collected and measured. This test is more expensive and not as readily available. Use of proton pump inhibitors (PPI) within 2 wk of the urea breath test may interfere with test results. Recently

a new card test for ^{14}C urea has been developed, providing a testing option in primary care settings. It uses a flat breath card that is read by a small analyzer.
3. Histologic evaluation of endoscopic biopsy samples is considered by many the gold standard for accurate diagnosis of *H. pylori* infection. However, detection of *H. pylori* depends on the site and number of biopsy samples, the method of staining, and experience of the pathologist.
4. Stool antigen test is an ELISA that identifies *H. pylori* antigen in a stool specimen through a polyclonal anti–*H. pylori* antibody. It is as accurate as the urea breath test for diagnosis of active infection and follow-up evaluation of patients treated for *H. pylori.* A negative result on the stool antigen test 6 wk after completion of therapy identifies patients in whom eradication of *H. pylori* was successful.

- Additional laboratory evaluation is indicated only in specific cases (e.g., amylase level in suspected pancreatitis, serum gastrin level in suspected Zollinger-Ellison [ZE] syndrome).

IMAGING STUDIES

Conventional upper GI barium studies identify approximately 70% to 80% of PUD; accuracy can be increased to approximately 90% by using double contrast.

Rx TREATMENT

NONPHARMACOLOGIC THERAPY

- Stop smoking; smoking increases the risk of PUD, decreases the healing rate, and increases the frequency of recurrence.
- Avoid NSAIDs and alcohol.
- Special diets have been proved unrelated to ulcer development and healing; however, avoid foods that cause symptoms.

ACUTE GENERAL Rx

Eradication of *H. pylori,* when present, can be accomplished with various regimens:

1. PPI (e.g., omeprazole 20 mg bid or lansoprazole 30 mg bid, esomeprazole 40 mg qd) *plus* clarithromycin 500 mg bid *and* amoxicillin 1000 mg bid for 10 days. This regimen achieves an eradication rate of 80% to 90% and can be used as first-line therapy for patients not allergic to penicillin.
2. PPI bid *plus* amoxicillin 500 mg bid *plus* metronidazole 500 mg bid for 10 days.
3. PPI bid *plus* clarithromycin 500 mg bid *and* metronidazole 500 mg bid for 10 days. This regimen is useful in those with penicillin allergy.
4. A 1-day quadruple therapy may be as effective as a 7-day triple-therapy regimen. The 1-day quadruple-therapy regimen consists of 2 tablets of 262-mg bismuth subsalicylate qid, 1 500-mg metronidazole tablet qid, 2 g of amoxicillin suspension qid, and 2 capsules of 30 mg of lansoprazole.
5. Bismuth compound qid *plus* tetracycline 500 mg qid *and* metronidazole 500 mg qid for 14 days.
6. A combination of levofloxacin 250 mg bid, amoxicillin 1000 mg bid, and a PPI bid for 10 to 14 days can be used as salvage therapy after unsuccessful attempts to eradicate *H. pylori* using other regimens.

A 10-day sequential therapy has been reported to be superior to standard triple therapy for eradication of *H. pylori.* It consists of 5 days of treatment with a PPI and one antibiotic (usually amoxicillin) followed by 5-day treatment with the PPI and two other antibiotics (usually clarithromycin and metronidazole).

PUD patients testing negative for *H. pylori* should be treated with antisecretory agents:

- H_2 receptor antagonists (H_2RAs): cimetidine, ranitidine, famotidine, and nizatidine are all effective; they are usually given in split dose or at nighttime.
- PPIs: can also induce rapid healing; they are usually given 30 min before meals.

Antacids and sucralfate are also effective agents for the treatment and prevention of PUD.

CHRONIC Rx

Maintenance therapy in duodenal ulcer patients is indicated in the following situations:

- Persistent smokers
- Recurrent ulcerations
- Long-term treatment with NSAIDs, glucocorticoids
- Elderly or debilitated patients
- Aggressive or complicated ulcer disease (e.g., perforation, hemorrhage)
- Asymptomatic bleeders

Misoprostol therapy (100 μg qid with food, increased to 200 μg qid if well tolerated) is useful for the prevention of NSAID-induced gastric ulcers in all patients on long-term NSAID therapy; it is contraindicated in women of childbearing age because of its abortifacient properties. PPIs are at least as effective as misoprostol and more effective than H_2 receptor antagonists at healing ulcers and maintaining remission in patients on long-term NSAIDs.

DISPOSITION

- The recurrence rate for untreated PUD is ~60% (>70% in smokers). Treatment decreases the recurrence rate by nearly 30%.
- Patients with recurrent ulcers should be re-treated for an additional 8 wk and then placed on maintenance therapy with H_2RAs, PPIs, sucralfate, or antacids.
- An ulcer is considered refractory to treatment if healing is not evident after 8 wk for duodenal ulcers and 12 wk for gastric ulcers. In these patients maximum acid inhibition (e.g., esomeprazole 40 mg bid) is preferred over continued therapy with standard antiulcer therapy.
- Eradication of *H. pylori* (when present) is indicated in all patients. A negative stool antigen test for *H. pylori* 6 wk after treatment accurately confirms cure of *H. pylori* infection with reasonable sensitivity in initially seropositive healthy subjects.
- Screening for ZE syndrome should also be considered in patients with multiple recurrent ulcers; in patients with ZE, the serum gastrin level is >1000 pg/ml and the basal acid output is usually >15 mEq/hr.
- Surgery for refractory ulcers is now only rarely performed; it consists of highly selective vagotomy for duodenal ulcers or ulcer removal with antrectomy or hemigastrectomy without vagotomy for gastric ulcers.

REFERRAL

- GI referral for patients requiring endoscopy
- Surgical referral for patients with nonhealing ulcers despite appropriate medical therapy

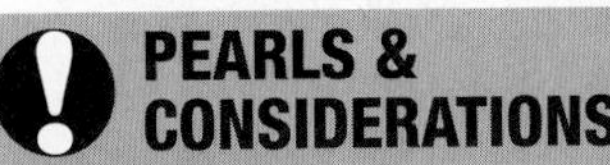

PEARLS & CONSIDERATIONS

COMMENTS

- Patients with gastric ulcers should have repeat endoscopy after 4 to 6 wk of therapy to document healing and test exfoliative cytology for gastric carcinoma.
- After endoscopic treatment of bleeding peptic ulcers, bleeding recurs in up to 20% of patients. PPI administration intravenously by continuous infusion substantially reduces the risk of recurrent bleeding. High-dose IV esomeprazole (80 mg IV bolus followed by 8 mg/hr infusion over 72 hr) given after successful endoscopic therapy to patients with high-risk peptic ulcer bleeding has been reported to reduce recurrent bleeding at 72 hr and to maintain sustained clinical benefits for up to 30 days.
- Among low-dose aspirin recipients who had peptic ulcer bleeding, continuous aspirin therapy may increase the risk for recurrent bleeding; however, mortality was reported higher among those who stopped aspirin therapy and were at risk for cardiovascular events.

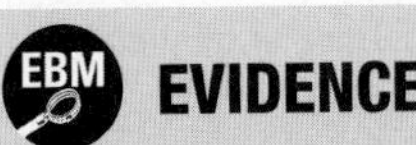

EVIDENCE

available at www.expertconsult.com

SUGGESTED READINGS

available at www.expertconsult.com

RELATED CONTENT

Peptic Ulcer (Patient Information)

AUTHOR: **FRED F. FERRI, M.D.**

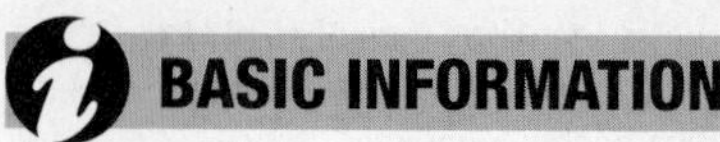

BASIC INFORMATION

DEFINITION

Pericarditis is the inflammation (or infiltration) of the pericardium. Acute pericarditis is a syndrome characterized by typical chest pain, a pathognomonic pericardial friction rub on auscultation, and specific electrocardiogram (ECG) changes.

ICD-9CM CODES
420.91 Pericarditis
ICD-10CM CODES

I30.0	Acute nonspecific idiopathic pericarditis
I30.1	Infectious pericarditis
I30.8	Other forms of acute pericarditis
I30.9	Acute pericarditis, unspecified
I301.0	Chronic adhesive pericarditis
I31.1	Chronic constrictive pericarditis
I31.3	Pericardial effusion (non-inflammatory)
I31.9	Diabetes of pericardium, unspecified (tamponade)
I31.2	Hemopericardium

EPIDEMIOLOGY & DEMOGRAPHICS

- The exact incidence of acute pericarditis is not known. However, it is approximately 0.1% of hospitalized patients, and 5% of patients seen in the emergency room for nonacute myocardial infarction chest pain.
- Increased incidence found in males and in adults compared with children.
- The use of thrombolytic agents and early revascularization has greatly reduced the incidence of both early postinfarction pericarditis and Dressler's syndrome.

PHYSICAL FINDINGS & CLINICAL PRESENTATION

- Severe, constant pain that localizes over the anterior chest and may radiate to the arms and back. As opposed to ischemic pain, the pain is pleuritic and is improved by sitting up and leaning forward. While present in the majority of cases, chest pain may be absent, particularly when uremia or rheumatologic causes are the underlying etiology.
- A pericardial friction rub is virtually pathognomonic of acute pericarditis, although is not present in all patients. When present, it is virtually pathognomonic of acute pericarditis. It is best heard with the patient sitting up and leaning forward and by pressing the diaphragm of the stethoscope firmly against the chest at the lower left sternal border during inspiration. It consists of three short, scratchy sounds, corresponding to a systolic, diastolic, and late diastolic component. In many patients, the rub is not clearly triphasic.
- The physical exam is important in assessing the presence of cardiac tamponade which may occur as a complication of large or rapidly accumulating effusions. Classic tamponade findings include hypotension, jugular venous distention, and muffled heart sounds (Beck's triad). In addition, tachycardia and pulsus paradoxus are usually present.

ETIOLOGY

- Most common causes of pericarditis are idiopathic or viral: 80%-90% of cases
- Other infectious agents (bacterial [1%-2%], tuberculous [4%-9%], HIV fungal, amebic, toxoplasmosis)
- Collagen-vascular disease (systemic lupus erythematosus, rheumatoid arthritis, scleroderma, vasculitis, dermatomyositis): 3% to 4% of cases
- Neoplasm (primary or metastatic [breast, lung, leukemia, lymphoma]): 7%-13% of cases
- Drug-induced: procainamide, hydralazine, phenytoin, isoniazid, rifampin, doxorubicin, mesalamine, adalimumab
- Acute myocardial infarction and post-MI (Dressler's syndrome, usually 2 weeks post MI)
- Trauma, including iatrogenic causes (post-pericardiotomy, postpacemaker lead placement, postcatheter ablation, post-CPR)
- Postmediastinal radiation (e.g., patients with Hodgkin's disease)
- Metabolic (hypothyroidism, uremia)
- Leakage of aortic aneurysm into pericardial sac

Dx DIAGNOSIS

DIFFERENTIAL DIAGNOSIS

- Angina pectoris
- Dissecting aortic aneurysm
- Pulmonary causes: embolism, infarction, pneumothorax, pneumonia with pleurisy
- Dissecting aneurysm
- Gastrointestinal causes: hepatitis, cholecystitis, GERD, hiatal hernia, esophageal rupture
- Musculoskeletal strain

WORKUP

Diagnosis is clinical, based on history and physical examination. ECG may help confirm the diagnosis if typical changes are found. Echocardiogram may diagnose an associated pericardial effusion if present; however, it may be present only in up to 50% to 60% cases of acute pericarditis, and its presence should not be used as a cornerstone of diagnosing pericarditis. Laboratory tests may help elucidate the underlying cause.

LABORATORY TESTS

Laboratory tests will not confirm the diagnosis, but can help determine a specific etiology. Initial blood work should be limited to the following tests:

- Complete blood count with differential
- Erythrocyte sedimentation rate, C-reactive protein (not specific but may be of value in following the course of the disease and the response to therapy)
- Blood urea nitrogen, creatinine
- Troponin I (plasma troponins are elevated in 35% to 50% of patients with pericarditis, and indicate involvement of the myocardium, i.e., myopericarditis)

The following tests may be useful when specific etiologies of pericarditis are suspected:

- HIV
- PPD
- Antinuclear antibody, rheumatoid factor

PERICARDIAL SAMPLING

- Pericardiocentesis is indicated in patients with tamponade physiology, in those with purulent pericarditis, when a neoplastic origin is suspected, and in patients with a significant idiopathic pericardial effusion that has not resolved by 3 mo. The fluid should be analyzed for red and white blood cell counts, cytology, glucose, lactate dehydrogenase, protein, pH, triglyceride level, and culture. Polymerase chain reaction assays or elevated levels of adenosine deaminase activity are useful when suspecting tuberculous pericarditis.
- Pericardial biopsy may be helpful in recurrent pericardial effusion if the diagnosis remains elusive. It should also be considered whenever malignancy or tuberculosis is suspected.

IMAGING STUDIES

- Echocardiogram to detect and determine amount of pericardial effusion (present in 50%-60% of patients) (Fig. 1-717); absence of effusion. Moreover, an echocardiogram will help to rule out cardiac tamponade, suggest a possible etiology of the pericarditis, and also help to assess for any associated acute myocarditis.
- ECG: the changes vary with the evolutionary stage of pericarditis. If there is myocardial involvement, there may be focal EKG changes that mimic territorial ischemia. Patients with acute STEMI, but not those with acute pericarditis, show prolongation of QRS complex and shortening of QT interval in ECG leads with ST-segment elevation.[1] ECG changes in pericarditis are as follows:
    1. Acute phase: PR-segment depression and diffuse ST-segment elevations (particularly evident in the precordial leads), which can be distinguished from acute MI by the lack of reciprocal changes and the absence of Q waves
    2. Intermediate phase: return of PR and ST segments to baseline, and T-wave inversion in leads previously showing ST-segment elevation (Fig. 1-718)
    3. Late phase: resolution of the T-wave changes
- Chest x-ray: done primarily to rule out abnormalities of the mediastinum or lung fields that may cause chest pain

  Cardiac silhouette may appear enlarged in patients with pericardial effusion if ≥200 ml of fluid has accumulated (Fig. 1-719).

  Calcifications around the heart may be seen with constrictive pericarditis.

---

[1]Rossello X et al: New electrocardiographic criteria to differentiate acute pericarditis and mycardial infarction, *Am J Med* 127:223-239, 2014.

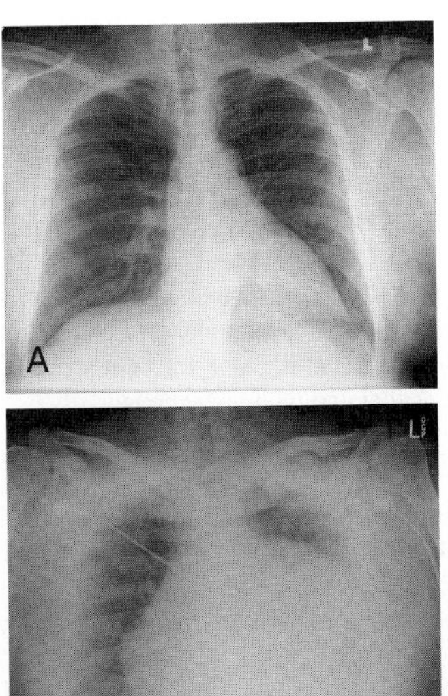

FIGURE 1-717 Bedside ultrasound image showing large pericardial effusion. A, Patient's chest radiograph 1 year before presentation with cardiac tamponade. **B,** Same patient's chest radiograph on presentation to the emergency department with cardiac tamponade.(From Adams JG et al: *Emergency medicine, clinical essentials,* ed 2, Philadelphia, 2013, Elsevier.)

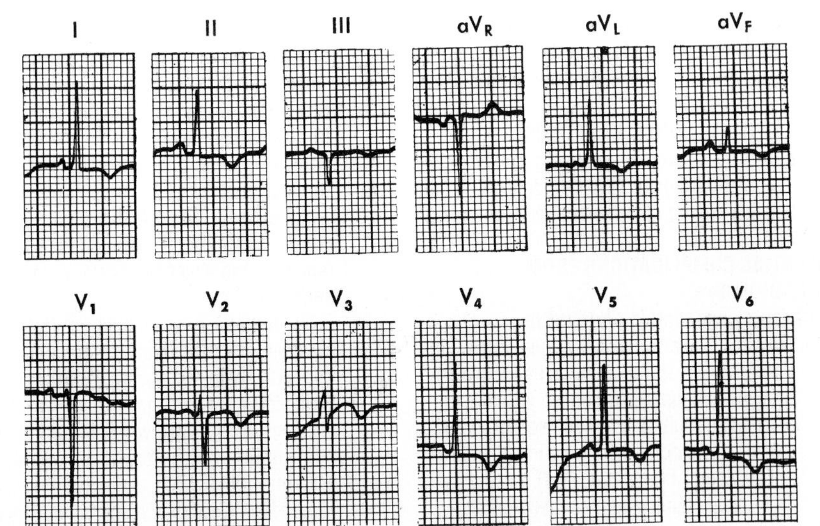

FIGURE 1-718 Pericarditis, evolving pattern. Note the diffuse T-wave inversions in leads I, II, III, aVL, aVF, and V2 to V6. (From Goldberg AL [ed]: *Clinical electrocardiography,* ed 5, St Louis, 1994, Mosby.)

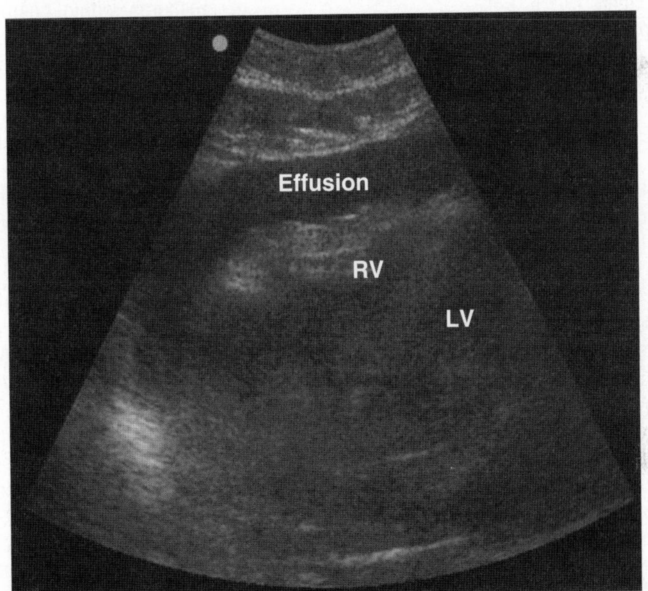

FIGURE 1-719 The patient subsequently had 2 L drained from this effusion. *LV,* Left ventricle; *RV,* right ventricle. (From Adams JG et al: *Emergency medicine, clinical essentials,* ed 2, Philadelphia, 2013, Elsevier.)

- MRI (Fig. 1-720) may be useful in patients with constrictive pericarditis and when malignancy is suspected.

Rx TREATMENT

NONPHARMACOLOGIC THERAPY

- Limitation of activity until the pain abates
- Patient education regarding potential complications (e.g., cardiac tamponade, constrictive pericarditis)

ACUTE GENERAL Rx

- Aspirin 650-1000 mg tid. NSAIDs can be used in place of aspirin (e.g., ibuprofen 600-800 mg tid, indomethacin 50 mg tid). NSAIDs are contraindicated in patients with recent MI and CHF.
- Colchicine 0.5-0.6 mg bid should be used in combination with aspirin/NSAIDs. Several randomized trials (ICAP, COPE, COPPS) have demonstrated that colchicine is effective in both reducing symptoms and the rates of recurrent pericarditis. Its use is recommended for first episodes but is not currently approved for recurrent disease.
- Use of corticosteroids is controversial. There is evidence of their use being associated with increased recurrence, side effects, and hospitalizations. Current guidelines recommend that systemic steroid therapy be restricted to patients with underlying connective tissue disease, autoimmune disease or uremia pericarditis. One study found that using a lower dose (0.25 to 0.5 mg/kg per day) maintained for 4 weeks and followed by a slow taper had same efficacy and fewer adverse effects than with higher conventional doses (1 mg/kg/day for 2-4 weeks).

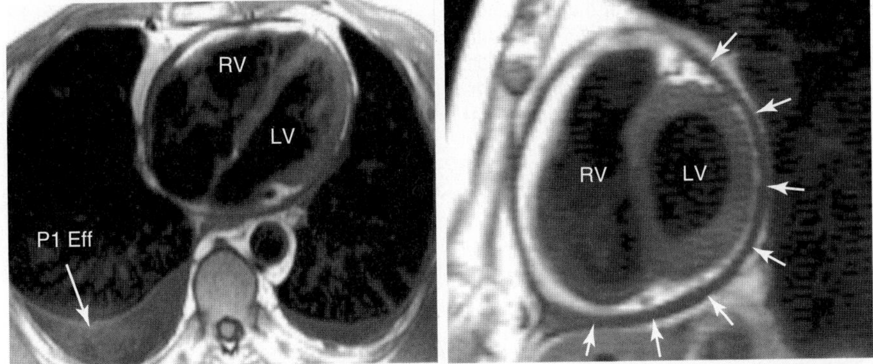

FIGURE 1-720 Cardiovascular magnetic resonance in a patient with constrictive pericarditis. On the *right* is a basal short-axis view of the ventricles showing a thickened pericardium encasing the heart *(arrows).* On the *left* is a transaxial view, again showing the thickened pericardium, particularly over the right heart, but also a pleural effusion *(P1 Eff). LV,* Left ventricle; *RV,* right ventricle. (From Zipes DP et al [eds]: *Braunwald's heart disease,* ed 7, Philadelphia, 2005, Saunders.)

- Close observation of patients when there is suspicion for cardiac tamponade.
- Avoidance of anticoagulants (increased risk of hemopericardium).

TREATMENT OF UNDERLYING CAUSE:

- Bacterial pericarditis: systemic antibiotics and surgical drainage of pericardium
- Collagen vascular disease: prednisone
- Uremic: dialysis

POTENTIAL COMPLICATIONS FROM PERICARDITIS:

1. **Chronic constrictive pericarditis:**
   a. Physical examination: jugular venous distention, Kussmaul's sign (increase in jugular venous distention during inspiration as a result of increased venous pressure), pericardial knock (early diastolic filling sound heard 0.06 to 0.1 sec after S_2), clear lungs, tender hepatomegaly, pedal edema, ascites, scrotal edema, and possible anasarca.
   b. Chest radiograph: clear lung fields, normal or slightly enlarged heart, pericardial calcification.
   c. ECG: low-voltage QRS complex.
   d. Echocardiography: may show respiratory inflow variation over the mitral and tricuspid valves (due to variations in the diastolic ventricular pressure gradients with respiration), pericardial thickening or may be normal.
   e. Cardiac catheterization: elevation of right-sided filling pressures: shows a prominent y descent in the right atrial tracing, a "dip and plateau" tracing of the right ventricular pressure and discordance of right ventricular and left ventricular systolic pressures during respiration.
   f. Therapy: surgical stripping or removal of both layers of the constricting pericardium.
2. **Cardiac tamponade:** occurs in 5% to 15% of patients with idiopathic pericarditis but in up to 60% of those with neoplastic, tuberculous, or purulent pericarditis.
   a. Signs and symptoms: dyspnea, orthopnea, interscapular pain.
   b. Physical examination: distended neck veins, distant heart sounds, decreased apical impulse, diaphoresis, tachypnea, tachycardia, Ewart's sign (an area of dullness at the angle of the left scapula caused by compression of the lungs by the pericardial effusion), hypotension, narrowed pulse pressure, or pulsus paradoxus (decrease in systolic blood pressure ≥10 mm Hg during inspiration; most specific sign). Of all the clinical signs, a pulsus paradoxus >10 mm Hg in patients with pericardial effusion is the most specific for tamponade.
   c. Chest x-ray: cardiomegaly ("water-bottle" configuration of the cardiac silhouette may be seen) with clear lungs; may be normal when acute tamponade occurs rapidly in the absence of prior pericardial effusion.
   d. ECG: decreased amplitude of the QRS complex, electrical alternans (occurs more frequently with neoplastic effusions).
   e. Echocardiography: may show diastolic collapse of the right ventricle and/or the right atrium, respiratory inflow variation over the mitral valve and tricuspid valve (due to transmission of respiratory changes in intrathoracic pressure to the ventricles), or paradoxical wall motion may also be seen.
   f. Cardiac catheterization: equalization of pressures within chambers of the heart, elevation of right atrial pressure with a prominent x but no significant y descent.
   g. Therapy: immediate pericardiocentesis, preferably by needle paracentesis with the use of echocardiography, fluoroscopy, or CT In patients with recurrent effusions (e.g., neoplasms), placement of a percutaneous drainage catheter or pericardial window may be necessary.
3. **Effusive-constrictive pericarditis:** Uncommon syndrome characterized by concomitant tamponade caused by tense pericardial effusion and constriction caused by the visceral pericardium.
   a. Signs and symptoms: in addition to features of tamponade and/or constriction, may demonstrate decreased breath sounds (pleural effusions), peripheral edema, ascites, pulsatile hepatomegaly, and cachexia. Kussmaul's sign is typically not present.
   b. Echocardiography: typically not sensitive enough to distinguish effusive-constrictive pericarditis from other types.
   c. Cardiac catheterization: mixed picture with features of constriction and tamponade. Prior to drainage, Y descent is usually less prominent than expected and right atrial v wave persists. After drainage, may continue to have elevated right atrial and pulmonary wedge pressures.
   d. Therapy: extensive epicardiectomy (with disruption of the visceral layer of pericardium) is the procedure of choice in symptomatic patients.
4. **Myopericarditis**: myocardial injury unrelated to MI. It occurs in up to 15% of patients with pericarditis. ECG reveals concave downward ST-segment elevation and/or deep T wave inversions; cardiac enzymes are positive. May be associated with arrhythmias.

DISPOSITION

- Complete resolution of pain and other signs and symptoms during the initial 3 wk of therapy.
- Recurrence in 10% to 15% of patients within the initial 12 mo. The recurrence rate increases up to 50% after a first recurrence.
- Recurrence of large effusion after pericardiocentesis is common in patients with idiopathic chronic pericardial effusion. Pericardiectomy should be considered in these patients.
- Most cases of pericarditis can be treated in the outpatient setting. Indications for hospitalization are fever >38° C, immunosuppressed state, history of trauma, subacute onset, oral anticoagulant therapy, presence of myocarditis (myopericarditis), large pericardial effusion or tamponade, and failure to respond to 1 week of outpatient treatment.
- In patients with pericardial effusion after cardiac surgery, use of NSAIDs is not recommended because they have not been shown to reduce the size of the effusions or prevent late cardiac tamponade. One randomized trial (COPPS) suggested that prophylactic colchicine may reduce the risk of developing a postpericardiotomy syndrome.

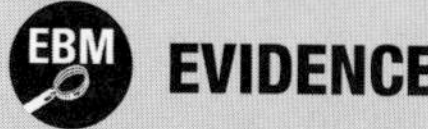

EVIDENCE

available at www.expertconsult.com

SUGGESTED READINGS

available at www.expertconsult.com

RELATED CONTENT

Pericarditis (Patient Information)

AUTHORS: **AMANDA C. DORAN, M.D., Ph.D.,** and **VEERANNA MERLA, M.D**

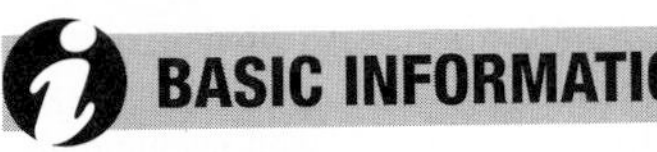

BASIC INFORMATION

DEFINITION

Peripheral arterial disease (PAD) refers to atherosclerotic, inflammatory, occlusive, and aneurysmal diseases involving the abdominal aorta and its branch arteries. (We will focus on lower extremity PAD.)

SYNONYMS

PAD
Peripheral vascular disease (PVD)
Arteriosclerosis obliterans
Atherosclerotic occlusive disease
Atherosclerosis of the extremities
Peripheral arterial stenosis
Vaso-occlusive disease of the legs
Chronic critical limb ischemia

ICD-9CM CODES
443.9 Peripheral vascular disease
ICD-10CM CODES
I73.9 Peripheral vascular disease, unspecified
I79 Disorders of arteries, arterioles and capillaries in diseases classified elsewhere

EPIDEMIOLOGY & DEMOGRAPHICS

- Approximately 4.3% to 5.28% of the adult population over the age of 40 has PAD, and the prevalence is nearly equal in men and women. It increases with age, from 5.28% in those aged 40 to 49 yr to 18.83% in those aged 70 to 79 yr. However symptoms of claudication are more likely to be present in males with PAD (50%) vs. women with PAD (25%).
- As per the PARTNERS study, the prevalence of PAD in patients >70 yr or 50-69 yr with history of smoking or diabetes was 29%.
- Risk factors that increase risk of PAD according to a 2013 meta-analysis of 112,027 studied patients include:
- Smoking (odds ratio 2.72)
- Diabetes (odds ratio 1.88)
- Hypertension (odds ratio 1.55)
- Hypercholesterolemia (odds ratio 1.19)
- Black race/ethnicity has greater prevalence according to NHANES data (odds ratio 2.83)
- Patients with newly diagnosed PAD are six times more likely to die within the next 10 yr when compared with patients without PAD.

PHYSICAL FINDINGS & CLINICAL PRESENTATION

- Peripheral arterial disease may present in a variety of ways:
- 20% to 50% of patients are asymptomatic.
- 10% to 35% of patients present with intermittent claudication (aching pain, cramping, or numbness of the calf induced by exercise, relieved by rest).
- 40% to 50% of patients present with atypical symptoms of claudication involving the calf, thigh, or buttock.
- 1% to 2% of patients may present with critical limb ischemia manifested as tissue loss or rest pain in a limb with nonhealing ulcers, necrotic tissue, or gangrene (Fig. 1-721).
- Diminished pulses and/or cool skin temperature of lower extremities.
- Bruits heard over the distal aorta, iliac, or femoral arteries.
- Changes in skin color, especially on feet (rubor with prolonged capillary refill on dependency or delayed pallor), livedo reticularis.
- Trophic changes of hair loss, brittle nails, and muscle atrophy.
- Weakness, numbness, or a feeling of heaviness in legs.
- Aching or burning in toes and feet during rest and especially while lying flat, which may be a sign of ischemia and more serious PAD.

ETIOLOGY

PAD is primarily the result of atherosclerotic disease and the formation of plaques that consist of a lipid core of cholesterol and inflammatory mediators with a fibrous intravascular covering. Symptoms of claudication are a product of physiologically significant luminal stenoses of the peripheral vessels, limiting blood flow to limb muscles.

Dx DIAGNOSIS

DIFFERENTIAL DIAGNOSIS

- Spinal stenosis
- Musculoskeletal disorder
- Lumbar spinal stenosis or nerve root compression (neurogenic or pseudoclaudication)
- Peripheral neuropathy
- Reflex sympathetic dystrophy
- Raynaud's disease
- Compartment syndrome

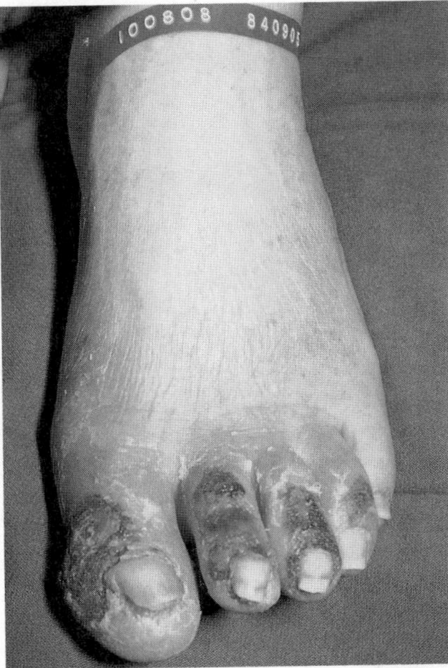

FIGURE 1-721 Ischemic skin ulcer induced by trauma from shoes. This patient with peripheral arterial occlusive disease suffered severe superficial skin necrosis of several toes because of shoes that were too tight. (From Crawford MH et al [eds]: *Cardiology,* ed 2, St Louis, 2004, Mosby.)

- Deep venous thrombosis
- Popliteal entrapment syndrome
- Direct vascular injury

WORKUP

- Thorough history, including symptoms regarding walking impairment, claudication, ischemic rest pain, or nonhealing wounds in patients ≥70 yr or those ≥50 yr with a history of smoking and/or diabetes:
- Measurement of blood pressure in both arms and notation of asymmetry.
- Palpation and recording of carotid pulses, upstroke, amplitude, and presence of bruits.
- Auscultation and palpation of abdomen for bruits, aortic pulsation, and diameter.
- Palpation of brachial, radial, ulnar, femoral, popliteal, dorsalis pedis, and posterior tibial pulses. Pulse intensity should be recorded as follows: 0, absent; 1+, diminished; 2+, normal; 3+, bounding.
- Auscultation of femoral arteries for the presence of bruits.
- Extremities should be inspected for color, temperature, integrity of the skin, hair loss, and hypertrophic nails.

The most widely used classification schemes are Fontaine's stages and Rutherford's categories.

- Fontaine's staging system is as follows:
  - I: Asymptomatic
  - IIa: Mild claudication
  - IIb: Moderate-severe claudication
  - III: Ischemic rest pain
  - IV: Ulceration or gangrene
- Rutherford's categories are as follows:
  - Grade 0, Category 0: Asymptomatic
  - Grade I, Category 1: Mild claudication
  - Grade I, Category 2: Moderate claudication
  - Grade I, Category 3: Severe claudication
  - Grade II, Category 4: Ischemic rest pain
  - Grade III, Category 5: Minor tissue loss
  - Category IV, Category 6: Major tissue loss
- Measurement of resting ankle-brachial index (ABI) should be performed to establish diagnosis of lower extremity PAD in patients with suspected lower extremity PAD (individuals with one or more of the following exertional leg symptoms: nonhealing wounds, age >65, or age >50 with smoking or diabetes history). ABI should be measured in both legs in all new patients (Fig. 1-722).
- Toe-brachial index should be used in patients suspected of PAD with unreliable ABI due to noncompressible vessels.
- The severity of PAD is based on the ABI at rest and during treadmill exercise (1 to 2 mph, 5 min, or symptom limited).
  - Noncompressible: >1.3
  - Normal: 1.00 to 1.29 at rest
  - Borderline: 0.91 to 0.99 at rest
  - Mild: ABI at rest 0.71 to 0.90 or ABI during exercise 0.50 to 0.90
  - Moderate: ABI at rest 0.41 to 0.70 or ABI during exercise 0.20 to 0.50
  - Severe: ABI at rest <0.40 or ABI during exercise <0.20
- Table 1-387 describes the Fontaine classification of peripheral arterial disease.

 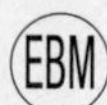 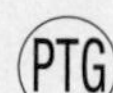

LABORATORY TESTS

Laboratory tests can help identify risk factors and allow for their modification. These include lipid profile, hemoglobin A_{1C}, homocysteine levels, fibrinogen, D-dimer, and CRP.

PHYSIOLOGIC TESTING AND IMAGING STUDIES

- The diagnosis of PAD can be confirmed by measuring the ABI or toe-brachial index.
- Rest or exercise pulse volume recordings (PVRs) and segmental limb pressures are also useful. PVRs measure volume of limb flow per pulse in different segments of the limb (e.g., thigh, calf, ankle, metatarsal, and toes). They help to assess the location and severity of the lesion with alterations in the pulse volume contour and amplitude indicating proximal arterial obstruction.
- Conventional angiography remains the gold standard, but ultrasonography, computed tomography angiography (CTA), and magnetic resonance angiography (MRA) have largely replaced catheter-based angiography in the initial diagnostic evaluation. CT is 92% sensitive and 91% specific. MRA is 93% to 100% sensitive and 96% to 100% specific for PAD.
- Contrast angiography (Fig. 1-723) is now reserved for patients with PAD who are being considered for endovascular revascularization and can provide physiologic information such as pressure gradients prior to percutaneous intervention.

Rx TREATMENT

The treatment goal in patients with PAD is to focus on cardiovascular risk-factor reduction to decrease morbidity and mortality as well as to improve limb-related symptoms. There are also medical and surgical approaches to management of limb-related symptoms.

CHRONIC MEDICAL Rx

LOWERING CARDIOVASCULAR MORBIDITY AND MORTALITY:

- Medical therapy for PAD is mainly aimed at decreasing cardiovascular risk; however, smoking may decrease progression of PAD.
- Smoking cessation should be emphasized in patients with PAD at each visit with assistance of behavioral and pharmacologic treatment (Class I).
- Proper foot care, including use of appropriate footwear, chiropody/podiatric medicine, daily foot inspection, skin cleansing, and use of topical moisturizing creams, should be encouraged, and skin lesions and ulcerations should be addressed urgently in all patients with diabetes and lower extremity PAD (Class I).

TABLE 1-387 Fontaine Classification of Peripheral Artery Disease

Stage	Symptoms
I	Asymptomatic
II	Intermittent claudication
IIa	Pain free, claudication walking >200 m
IIb	Pain free, claudication walking <200 m
III	Rest and nocturnal pain
IV	Necrosis, gangrene

From Bonow RO et al: *Braunwald's heart disease: a textbook of cardiovascular medicine,* ed 9, Philadelphia, 2012, Saunders.

- Antiplatelet therapy is indicated to reduce risk of myocardial infarction, stroke, and vascular death in individuals with symptomatic PAD with either aspirin (75 to 325 mg) or clopidogrel (75 mg) (Class I) and in asymptomatic patients (Class IIa).
- Warfarin is not indicated.
- Goal LDL cholesterol is <100 mg/dl and possibly <70 mg/dl in high-risk patients.
- If triglycerides are >200 mg/dl, non-HDL cholesterol should be lowered to <130 mg/dl.
- Management of hypertension with a goal of <140/90 mm Hg or <130/80 mm Hg if the patient has diabetes or chronic renal disease. Ramipril use has been reported to improve walking ability and quality of life in PAD patients with intermittent claudication.
- No clear benefit has been observed with combination aspirin and clopidogrel therapy.

TREATMENT OF CLAUDICATION:

- Exercise therapy: Supervised training should be performed for a minimum of 30 to 45 min, in sessions performed at least three times per week for a minimum of 12 wk. Studies have shown that a rigorous exercise-training program may be as beneficial as lower-extremity bypass surgery in symptomatic improvement. Supervised treadmill training and resistance training improve functional performance measured by treadmill walking and quality of life evaluation.
- Pharmacologic therapy with cilostazol (Pletal) 100 mg bid has been shown to increase pain-free and maximal walking distance by 40% to 60% in symptomatic patients with infrainguinal PAD after 12 to 24 wk of therapy, and has been demonstrated to improve ABI.
- Cilostazol has also been shown to be superior to pentoxifylline but is contraindicated in patients with systolic heart failure.

REVASCULARIZATION

There is no difference in percutaneous vs. surgical revascularization in iliac and femoropopliteal disease except for the higher morbidity with surgery and greater re-interventions in the percutaneous approach.

- The 2011 ACC/AHA guidelines on PAD have suggested that the following factors be considered prior to revascularization with either percutaneous/endovascular or surgical methods:
  - Considerations in percutaneous/endovascular treatment:
    1. Should be considered in those who have a vocational or lifestyle-limiting disability due to intermittent claudication when clinical features suggest a reasonable likelihood of symptomatic improvement with endovascular intervention and (a) there has been an inadequate response to exercise or pharmacologic therapy and/or (b) there is a very favorable risk-benefit ratio (e.g., focal aortoiliac occlusive disease).
    2. In TASC (TransAtlantic Inter-Society Consensus) type A iliac and femoropopliteal arterial lesions.

How to Perform and Calculate the ABI

Partners Program ABI Interpretation
Above 0.90—Normal
0.71–0.90—Mild Obstruction
0.41–0.70—Moderate Obstruction
0.00–0.40—Severe Obstruction

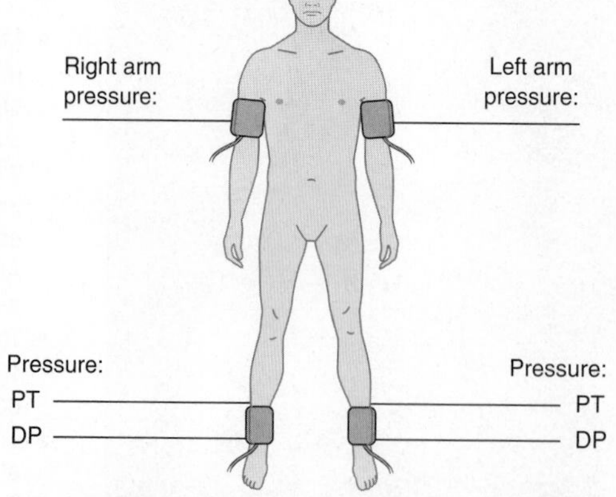

RIGHT ABI

Higher right ankle pressure / Higher arm pressure = mm Hg / mm Hg = ______

LEFT ABI

Higher left ankle pressure / Higher arm pressure = mm Hg / mm Hg = ______

EXAMPLE

Higher ankle pressure / Higher arm pressure = 92 mm Hg / 164 mm Hg = 0.56 See ABI Chart

FIGURE 1-722 Performing pressure measurements and calculating the ankle-brachial index (ABI). To calculate the ABI, systolic pressures are determined in both arms and both ankles with the use of a handheld Doppler instrument. The highest readings for the dorsalis pedis (DP) and posterior tibial (PT) arteries are used to calculate the index. (From Goldman L, Schafer AI: *Goldman's Cecil medicine,* ed 24, Philadelphia, 2012, Saunders.)

3. Endovascular therapy is preferred in patients aged 50 yr or younger, because they have a higher risk of graft failure after surgical therapy than older patients.
4. Endovascular intervention is not indicated as prophylactic therapy in an asymptomatic patient with lower-extremity PAD, or if there is no significant pressure gradient across a stenosis even after augmentation of flow with vasodilators.
5. Stenting is effective as primary therapy for common iliac artery stenosis and occlusions, and in external iliac artery stenoses and occlusions but not for infra-inguinal disease in the femoral, popliteal, and tibial arteries where it should be reserved for those who fail balloon dilatation.

- Considerations in surgical revascularization:
    1. Individuals with claudication symptoms who have a significant functional disability that is vocational or lifestyle limiting. These patients need to also be unresponsive to exercise or pharmacotherapy and should have a reasonable likelihood of symptomatic improvement with an acceptable surgical risk.
    2. Iliac or femoropopliteal disease with long segments; multifocal segments; long segment occlusions; and eccentric, calcified stenosis, which are less amenable to percutaneous interventions.
    3. Surgical intervention is not indicated to prevent progression to limb-threatening ischemia in patients with intermittent claudication as generally claudication does not progress to severe ischemia.
    4. Prior to any surgical therapy, patients should have a preoperative cardiovascular risk evaluation as it is a high risk surgery and is associated with a higher morbidity compared to percutaneous revascularization.

DISPOSITION

Risk factors for atherosclerosis should be assessed, and appropriate modification instituted. Focus should be placed on smoking cessation, dietary adjustment, and pharmacotherapy for dyslipidemia, hyperglycemia, and hypertension. All patients with PAD should receive aspirin therapy unless contraindicated. Revascularization is performed if the symptoms of PAD do not improve with conservative therapy as discussed previously.

REFERRAL

Consultation with vascular medicine, vascular surgery, or other physicians with expertise in PAD is recommended in patients with rest pain, functional disability from pain, ABI <0.50 at rest, or any physical signs of limb ischemia or gangrene.

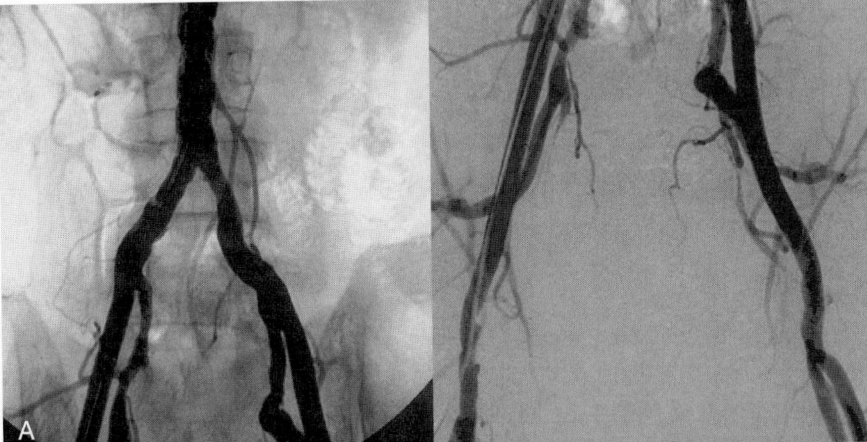

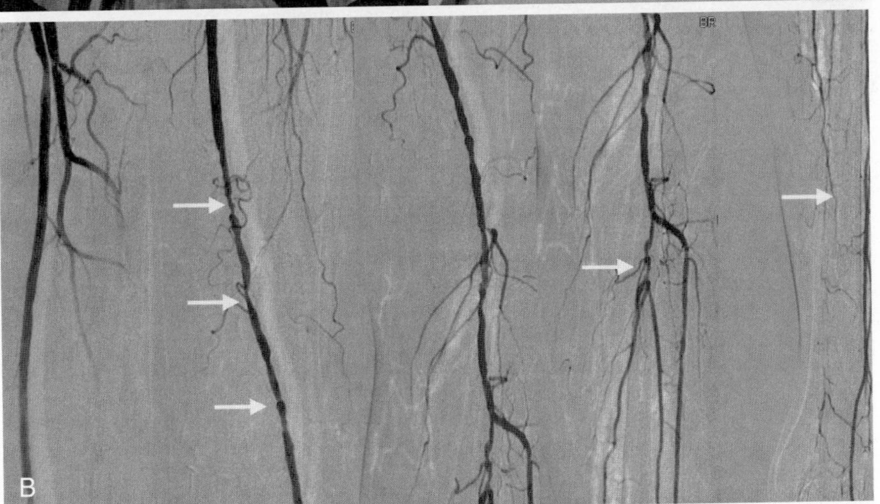

FIGURE 1-723 Angiogram of a patient with disabling left calf claudication. A, The aorta and bilateral common iliac arteries are patent. **B,** The left superficial femoral artery has multiple stenotic lesions *(arrows)*. There is a significant stenosis of the left tibioperoneal trunk and left posterior tibial artery *(arrows)*. (From Zipes DP et al [eds]: *Braunwauld's heart disease,* ed 7, Philadelphia, 2005, Saunders.)

PEARLS & CONSIDERATIONS

COMMENTS

- PAD remains underdiagnosed and undertreated.
- Medical treatment is aimed mainly at cardiovascular risk factor modification, except for cilostazol.
- Studies of the natural history of claudication show the relative safety of initial conservative treatment of PAD in the absence of critical limb ischemia.
- When PAD limits a patient's ability to walk and exercise, percutaneous revascularization can be considered.
- Exercise training is an important and often neglected treatment strategy that has proven beneficial.
- Surgical intervention should be considered in patients who meet the criteria for intervention but have lesions that are not amenable to PTA/stenting or in older patients with a low surgical risk. In younger patients, due to the high risk of graft failure and recurrence, surgery should be a last resort.

PREVENTION

Cardiovascular disease is the major cause of death in patients with intermittent claudication. Therefore, the treatment of claudication is directed not only at improving walking distance but also at reducing cardiovascular risk.

PATIENT & FAMILY EDUCATION

The following organizations offer more information about PAD:

- American College of Cardiology (http://www.acc.org)
- Vascular Disease Foundation (http://www.vdf.org)

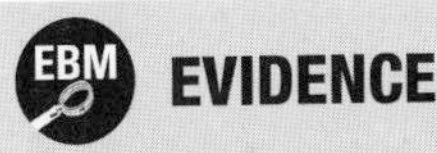

available at www.expertconsult.com

SUGGESTED READINGS

available at www.expertconsult.com

RELATED CONTENT

Peripheral Arterial Disease (Patient Information)

AUTHORS: **PRANAV M. PATEL, M.D., F.A.C.C., F.S.C.A.I.,** and **RAHUL BHARDWAJ, M.D.**

BASIC INFORMATION

DEFINITION

Peritonitis refers to the acute onset of severe abdominal pain caused by peritoneal inflammation.

Secondary peritonitis is a localized (abscess) or diffuse peritonitis originating from a defect in abdominal viscus.

SYNONYMS

Acute abdomen
Surgical abdomen

ICD-9CM CODES
567.2 Peritonitis
ICD-10CM CODES
K65.0 Generalized (acute) peritonitis
K65.8 Other peritonitis
K65.9 Peritonitis, unspecified

EPIDEMIOLOGY & DEMOGRAPHICS

Common presentation as a result of diverse etiologies; for example, 5% to 10% of the population has acute appendicitis at some point in their lives.

PHYSICAL FINDINGS & CLINICAL PRESENTATION

- Acute abdominal pain
- Abdominal distention and ascites
- Abdominal rigidity, rebound, and guarding
- Fever, chills
- Exacerbation with movement
- Anorexia, nausea, and vomiting
- Constipation
- Decreased bowel sounds
- Hypotension and tachycardia
- Tachypnea, dyspnea

ETIOLOGY

- Microbiology: most common is gram-negative bacteria (*Escherichia coli, Enterobacter, Klebsiella, Proteus*), gram-positive bacteria (enterococci, streptococci, staphylococci), anaerobic bacteria (*Bacteroides, Clostridium*), and fungi
- Acute perforation peritonitis: gastrointestinal perforation, intestinal ischemia, pelvic peritonitis, and other forms
- Postoperative peritonitis: anastomotic leak, accidental perforation, and devascularization
- Posttraumatic peritonitis: after blunt or penetrating abdominal trauma

Dx DIAGNOSIS

DIFFERENTIAL DIAGNOSIS

- Postoperative: abscess, sepsis, bowel obstruction, injury to internal organs
- Gastrointestinal: perforated viscus, appendicitis, inflammatory bowel disease, infectious colitis, diverticulitis, acute cholecystitis, peptic ulcer perforation, pancreatitis, bowel obstruction
- Gynecologic: ruptured ectopic pregnancy, pelvic inflammatory disease, ruptured hemorrhagic ovarian cyst, ovarian torsion, degenerating leiomyoma
- Urologic: nephrolithiasis, interstitial cystitis
- Miscellaneous: abdominal trauma, penetrating wounds, infections caused by intraperitoneal dialysis

WORKUP

- Acute peritonitis is mainly a clinical diagnosis based on patient history and physical examination.
- Laboratory and imaging studies (see "Laboratory Tests") assist in determining the need for and type of intervention.
- If patient is hemodynamically unstable, immediate diagnostic laparotomy should be performed in lieu of adjuvant diagnostic studies.

LABORATORY TESTS

- Complete blood count: leukocytosis, left shift, anemia
- SMA7: electrolyte imbalances, kidney dysfunction
- Liver function tests: ascites from liver disease, cholelithiasis
- Amylase: pancreatitis
- Blood cultures: bacteremia, sepsis
- Peritoneal cultures: infectious etiology
- Blood gas: respiratory versus metabolic acidosis
- Ascitic fluid analysis: exudate versus transudate
- Urinalysis and culture: urinary tract infection
- Cervical cultures for gonorrhea and *Chlamydia*
- Urine/serum human chorionic gonadotropin

IMAGING STUDIES

- Abdominal series: free air from perforation, small or large bowel dilation from obstruction, identification of fecalith
- Chest x-ray examination: elevated diaphragm, pneumonia
- Pelvic/abdominal ultrasound: abscess formation, abdominal mass, intrauterine versus ectopic pregnancy, identify free fluid suggestive of hemorrhage or ascites
- CT: mass, ascites

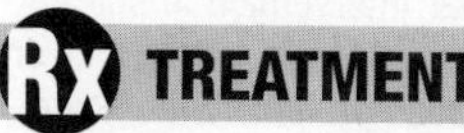

Rx TREATMENT

NONPHARMACOLOGIC THERAPY

- IV hydration to correct dehydration, hypovolemia
- Blood transfusion to correct anemia from hemorrhage
- Nasogastric decompression, especially if obstruction is present
- Oxygen: intubation if necessary
- Bed rest

ACUTE GENERAL Rx

- Surgery to correct underlying pathology, such as controlling hemorrhage, correcting perforation, draining abscess
- Broad-spectrum antibiotics to cover both gram-negative aerobic and gram-negative anaerobic bacteria:
  1. Mild-moderate disease: piperacillin-tazobactam 3.375 g IV q6h or 4.5 g IV q8h *or* ticarcillin-clavulanate 3.1 g IV q6h. Alternative agents are ciprofloxacin 400 mg IV q12h or levofloxacin 750 mg IV q24h *plus* metronidazole 1 g IV q12h.
  2. Severe life-threatening disease: imipenem 500 mg IV q6h or meropenem 1 g IV q8h. Alternative agents are ampicillin *plus* metronidazole *plus* ciprofloxacin.
- Pain control: morphine or meperidine as needed (hold until diagnosis confirmed)

DISPOSITION

Depends on etiology of peritonitis, age of patient, coexisting medical disease, and duration of process before presentation

REFERRAL

Surgical consultation is required in all cases of acute peritonitis.

SUGGESTED READINGS
available at www.expertconsult.com

AUTHORS: **ARUNDATHI G. PRASAD, M.D.**, and **RUBEN ALVERO, M.D.**

BASIC INFORMATION

DEFINITION

Spontaneous bacterial peritonitis (SBP) is an inflammatory reaction of the peritoneum secondary to the presence of bacteria or other microorganisms. More specifically, SBP is defined as an ascitic fluid infection without an evident intra-abdominal surgically treatable source occurring primarily in patients with advanced cirrhosis of the liver.

SYNONYMS

Primary peritonitis
SBP

ICD-9CM CODES
567.2 Peritonitis
ICD-10CM CODES
K65.2 Spontaneous bacterial peritonitis

EPIDEMIOLOGY & DEMOGRAPHICS

PREVALENCE: The prevalence of SBP in cirrhotic patients admitted to the hospital has been estimated at 10% to 30%.

PREDOMINANT SEX: Males affected more often than females

PHYSICAL FINDINGS & CLINICAL PRESENTATION

- Acute fever with accompanying abdominal pain/ascites, nausea, vomiting, diarrhea
- In cirrhotic patients, presentation may be subtle with a low-grade temperature (100° F) with or without abdominal abnormalities
- In patients with ascites, a heightened degree of awareness is necessary for detection
- Jaundice and encephalopathy
- Deterioration of mental status and/or renal function

ETIOLOGY

- *Escherichia coli*
- *Klebsiella pneumoniae*
- *Streptococcus pneumoniae*
- *Streptococcus* and *Enterococcus* spp.
- *Staphylococcus aureus*
- Anaerobic pathogens: *Bacteroides, Clostridium* organisms
- Other: fungal, mycobacterial, viral

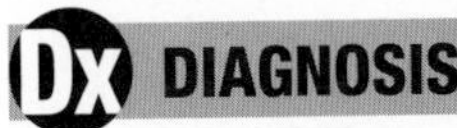

DIAGNOSIS

The diagnosis of SBP is established by a positive ascitic fluid bacterial culture and an elevated ascitic fluid absolute polymorphonuclear leukocyte count (≥250 cells/mm^3).

DIFFERENTIAL DIAGNOSIS

- Appendicitis (in children)
- Perforated peptic ulcer
- Secondary bacterial peritonitis
- Peritoneal abscess
- Splenic, hepatic, or pancreatic abscess
- Cholecystitis
- Cholangitis

WORKUP

Paracentesis and ascitic fluid analysis will confirm diagnosis (see "Laboratory Tests").

LABORATORY TESTS

Ascitic fluid analysis reveals the following:

- Cell count with an absolute polymorphonuclear cell count >250/mm^3
- Presence of bacteria on Gram stain
- pH <7.31
- Lactic acid >32 mg/dl
- Protein <1 g/dl
- Glucose >50 mg/dl
- Lactate dehydrogenase <225 mU/ml
- Positive culture of peritoneal fluid
- Measurement of the serum/ascites/albumin gradient: The serum/ascites/albumin gradient indirectly measures portal pressure. The albumin concentration of ascitic fluid and serum must be obtained on the same day. The ascitic fluid value is subtracted from the serum value to obtain the gradient. If the difference (not a ratio) is >1.1 g/dl, the patient has portal hypertension, with 97% accuracy. If the difference is <1.1 g/dl, portal hypertension is not present. The majority of patients with SBP have portal hypertension as a result of cirrhosis.

IMAGING STUDIES

- Abdominal ultrasound: if there is clinical difficulty in performing paracentesis
- CT scan: to rule out secondary peritonitis (if indicated) and to exclude abscess, mass

Rx TREATMENT

ACUTE GENERAL Rx

- Cefotaxime (2 g IV q12h) or ceftriaxone (2 g IV q24h) or ticarcillin-clavulanate or piperacillin-tazobactam. Continue therapy for 7 days. Repeat diagnostic paracentesis at day 2. Repeat paracentesis at 48 hours will demonstrate a significant decrease in polymorphonuclear count in patients with SBP. If ascites PMN count decreases by at least 25% at day 2, IV therapy can be switched to PO (levofloxacin 250 mg PO bid) to complete 7 days of therapy.
- IV albumin (1 g/kg of body weight) if BUN >30 mg/dL, bilirubin >4 mg/dL; repeat at day 3 if renal dysfunction persists

PROPHYLAXIS

- Oral norfloxacin 400 mg PO qd or ciprofloxacin 500 mg PO qd or levofloxacin 250 mg PO qd
- Alternative therapy: TMP-SMX one double-strength tablet PO qd
- Prophylaxis should be continued until disappearance of ascites or until liver transplantation

DISPOSITION

- The overall mortality rate from an episode of SBP is 20%, and following an episode, the 1-year mortality rate approaches 70%.

REFERRAL

- To a gastroenterologist for management of ascites and prevention of recurrent SBP
- To an infectious disease specialist for management of difficult-to-treat infections, antibiotic-resistant bacterial infections, or antibiotic drug intolerance

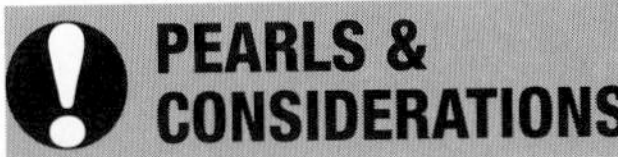

PEARLS & CONSIDERATIONS

COMMENTS

- Renal failure is a major cause of morbidity in cirrhotic patients with SBP. The use of IV albumin (1.5 g/kg at the time of diagnosis and 1 g/kg on day 3) may lower the rate of renal failure and mortality in patients with SBP.
- The criteria for the diagnosis of SBP require that abdominal paracentesis be performed and ascitic fluid be analyzed before a diagnosis of SBP can be made.
- Culturing ascitic fluid as if it were blood (with bedside inoculation of at least 10 ml of ascitic fluid directly into blood culture bottles at the bedside) has been shown to significantly increase the culture positivity of the ascitic fluid in the 80% to 100% range.
- Avoid therapeutic paracenteses during active infection
- Positive blood cultures in an individual with ascites require exclusion of a peritoneal source by paracentesis.

SUGGESTED READINGS
available at www.expertconsult.com

AUTHOR: **GLENN G. FORT, M.D., M.P.H.**

BASIC INFORMATION

DEFINITION

Pertussis is a prolonged bacterial infection of the upper respiratory tract characterized by paroxysms of an intense cough.

SYNONYMS

Whooping cough

ICD-9CM CODES
033.9 Pertussis
ICD-10CM CODES
A37.90 Whooping cough, unspecified species without pneumonia

EPIDEMIOLOGY

INCIDENCE (IN U.S.): Provisional case counts for 2012 have surpassed the last peak year, 2010, with 41,880 pertussis cases and 14 deaths in infants aged <12 months.

PEAK INCIDENCE:
- Childhood
- Usually affects children aged <1 yr

PREDOMINANT AGE:
- 50% in children aged <1 yr
- 20% in children aged >15 yr
- Classically an infection of infants and young children, pertussis is often overlooked as a cause of chronic cough in adults. However, a resurgence of pertussis has been observed in recent years, with nearly 50% of all cases identified in adolescents and adults, likely due to waning immunity and decreased effectiveness of acellular vaccines in early childhood compared to older, whole-cell-derived vaccines.

PHYSICAL FINDINGS & CLINICAL PRESENTATION

- Infection is characterized by 3 phases: catarrhal, paroxysmal, and convalescent
- Catarrhal phase: Usually begins with a 1- to 2-wk prodrome that resembles a common cold. This phase may be mild or absent in adolescents and adults given partial immunity from prior immunization
- After this initial phase, increased production of mucus occurs. Excessive lacrimation and conjunctival infection should heighten the suspicion for pertussis
- Paroxysmal phase: Increased mucus production is followed by an intense, paroxysmal cough, ending with gasps and an inspiratory whoop
- In some children, apnea, cyanosis and anoxia are noted; posttussive gagging and vomiting are characteristic of pertussis
- Cases can be severe and life-threatening in young infants, particularly children <6 months old
- When prolonged, frank exhaustion and even apnea occur. The paroxysmal phase lasts from 2 wk to 2 mo
- Convalescent phase: Lasts over 2 months and is characterized by cough of decreasing severity

ETIOLOGY

Bordetella pertussis, a gram-negative rod which adheres to human cilia and respiratory epithelia

Dx DIAGNOSIS

DIFFERENTIAL DIAGNOSIS

- Croup
- Epiglottitis
- Foreign body aspiration
- Bacterial pneumonia
- Viral pneumonia

WORKUP

Pertussis is often overlooked as a cause of chronic cough, especially in adolescents and adults. The presence of posttussive emesis and/or inspiratory whoop increases the likelihood of pertussis but only modestly. Therefore, clinicians must use their overall impression in pursuing the diagnosis.

- Enzyme-linked immunosorbent assay for detection of antibody to pertussis. Polymerase chain reaction (PCR) is the most sensitive method for rapid detection of pertussis. PCR testing should be used only to confirm a diagnosis in persons with signs and symptoms consistent with pertussis. PCR testing sensitivity declines and is unlikely to be positive after 1 month of infection. PCR testing after 5 days of treatment with antibiotics can cause false-negative results and is generally not recommended
- Blood cultures in hospitalized patients
- Chest x-ray
- Culture of bacteria, usually from nasopharynx by aspiration or by swabbing the posterior nasopharynx with a polyester-tipped, rayon-tipped, or nylon-flocked swab
- Immunofluorescent staining of nasopharyngeal secretions
- Serologic tests for immunoglobulin G (IgG) or A (IgA) are available. A twofold increase between acute and convalescent sera is considered proof of seroconversion. A single elevated IgG or IgA titer is considered diagnostic when no acute serum is available. Can be useful for diagnosis later in illness.

LABORATORY TESTS

Complete blood count, which usually demonstrates marked lymphocytosis:
- Up to 18,000 white blood cells
- 70% to 80% lymphocytes

IMAGING STUDIES

Chest x-ray examination is of value if secondary bacterial pneumonia is suspected.

Rx TREATMENT

ACUTE GENERAL Rx

- Intensive supportive care:
  1. Adequate hydration
  2. Control of secretions
  3. Maintenance of airway
- Antibiotics (Table E1-388) are indicated even though their ability to alter the course of the disease is controversial.
  1. Azithromycin 500 mg on day 1, followed by 250 mg for days 2 to 5. Erythromycin 50 mg/kg/day for 14 days. Recent literature reports indicate that a 7-day treatment regimen may be as effective as a 14-day course of erythromycin. TMP/SMX 320/1600 mg per day in divided doses can be used in patients with allergy or intolerance to macrolides.
  2. Although unproved, dexamethasone 1 mg/kg/day in four doses for severe, life-threatening paroxysms.
  3. Ceftriaxone 75 mg/kg/day in two doses for broad coverage of secondary bacterial pneumonias.
  4. Close observation of infants <6 months old as risk for apnea is high in this age group.
- Vaccination is successful in preventing the disease: universal vaccination is advised for all children and adults. The Advisory Committee on Immunization Practices (ACIP) updated Tdap recommendations to include a single dose of Tdap vaccine in place of routine Td for adults age 19-64 yr and a single-dose Tdap for adults 65 yr and older who have or will have close contact with an infant (>12 mo). The ACIP also recommends that all pregnant women receive a dose of Tdap with every pregnancy, preferably during weeks 27-36 of gestation.
- Erythromycin is recommended for all close contacts in the household: TMP/SMX in two oral doses per day for those intolerant to erythromycin.

DISPOSITION

Close attention to accepted vaccination schedules is the best prevention.

REFERRAL

To intensive care setting for life-threatening infections:
- Pulmonologist
- Infectious disease specialist

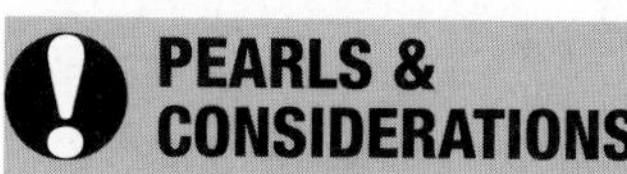

PEARLS & CONSIDERATIONS

- The diagnosis of pertussis in a young child is easily recognized, but in adults pertussis can be a subtle diagnosis and is often missed. The tip-off is often a persistent, hacking, and productive cough with minor or no fever in a previously healthy person that lasts < 2 wk.
- Approximately 11% of pertussis cases in the pediatric population are attributable to vaccine refusal, dispelling the myth that herd immunity protects children whose parents refuse pertussis vaccine.

SUGGESTED READINGS

available at www.expertconsult.com

RELATED CONTENT

Pertussis (Patient Information)

AUTHOR: **RUSSELL J. MCCULLOH, M.D.**

BASIC INFORMATION

DEFINITION

- A hamartomatous polyp is a benign intestinal growth that may contain all components of the intestinal mucosa. In gastrointestinal polyposis, multiple such polyps coexist within the intestinal tract, and associated manifestations are usually also present.
- Juvenile polyps are benign polyps composed of cystic dilatations of glandular structures within the fibroblastic stroma of the lamina propria. They may cause bleeding or intussusception.
- Commonly recognized syndromes are Peutz-Jeghers syndrome, juvenile polyposis syndrome, Cowden's disease, Bannagan-Ruvalcaba-Riley syndrome, and Cronkhite-Canada syndrome. Other, lesser known inherited hamartomatous polyposis syndromes are hereditary mixed polyposis syndrome, intestinal ganglioneuromatosis and neurofibromatosis (variant of von Recklinghausen's syndrome), Devon family syndrome, basal cell nevus syndrome, and tuberous sclerosis (may involve gastrointestinal tract). Table 1-389 describes general features of some inherited colorectal cancer syndromes.

ICD-9CM CODES
759.6 (Peutz-Jeghers syndrome)
211.3 (Cronkhite-Canada syndrome)
ICD-10CM CODES
D12.6 Colon, unspecified (adenomatosis of colon, hereditary polyposis)

EPIDEMIOLOGY

- Colonic adenomas, the precursors of nearly all colorectal cancers, are found in nearly 40% of patients by age 60 yr.
- 25% of men and 15% of women who undergo colonoscopy are found to have one or more adenomas.
- Detection of any adenoma in patients <60 yr confers an increased risk of colorectal cancer (by a factor of 2.6) in their first-degree relatives.

PHYSICAL FINDINGS & CLINICAL PRESENTATION

PEUTZ-JEGHERS SYNDROME:

- Transmission: autosomal dominant with incomplete penetrance
- Disease expression:
  - Stomach, small and large intestinal hamartomas with bands of smooth muscle in the lamina propria
  - Pigmented lesions around mouth (lips and buccal mucosa), nose, hands, feet, genitals, and perineal areas
  - Ovarian tumors
  - Sertoli cell testicular tumors
  - Airway polyps
  - Pancreatic cancer
  - Breast cancer
  - Urinary tract polyps
- Cumulative lifetime cancer risk
  - Colon cancer: 39%
  - Stomach cancer: 29%
  - Small intestine cancer: 13%
  - Pancreatic cancer: 36%
  - Breast cancer: 54%
  - Ovarian cancer: 10%
  - Sertoli cell tumor: 9%
  - Overall cancer risk: 93%
- Clinical manifestation:
  - Gastrointestinal, small-bowel obstruction, intussusception, gastrointestinal bleeding
  - See chapters on relevant malignancies for their signs and symptoms

JUVENILE POLYPOSIS SYNDROME:

- Transmission: autosomal dominant
- Disease expression
  - Solitary juvenile polyps numbering 10 or more in the rectum or throughout the gastrointestinal tract; the polyps are smooth and covered with normal epithelium
  - Various congenital abnormalities coexist in 20%
- Cumulative cancer risk is increased (may be as high as 50%)
- Clinical manifestation
  - Intestinal obstruction
  - Intussusception
  - Gastrointestinal bleeding

COWDEN'S DISEASE:

- Transmission: autosomal dominant, rare
- Disease expression
  - Juvenile intestinal polyposis
  - Orocutaneous hamartomas
  - Fibrocystic breast disease and breast cancer
  - Goiter and thyroid cancer
  - Facial tricholemmomas (papules) in 83%
- Cumulative cancer risk
  - Gastrointestinal: same as general population
  - Thyroid: 3% to 10%
  - Breast: 25% to 50%

BANNAGAN-RUVALCABA-RILEY SYNDROME:

- Transmission: autosomal dominant, rare
- Disease expression
  - Juvenile intestinal polyposis
  - Macrocephaly
  - Developmental delay
  - Penile pigmented spots
  - Cumulative cancer risk unknown

CRONKHITE-CANADA SYNDROME:

- Transmission: acquired
- Age of onset: midlife
- Disease expression
  - Diffuse gastrointestinal juvenile polyposis (50% to 95% of cases)
  - Chronic diarrhea and protein-losing enteropathy (the entire intestinal mucosa may be inflamed), which leads to abdominal pain, weight loss, and various complications of malnutrition
  - Dystrophic nails
  - Alopecia
  - Hyperpigmentation
- Cumulative cancer risk: same as the average population

TABLE 1-389 General Features of the Inherited Colorectal Cancer Syndromes

Syndrome	Polyp Histology	Polyp Distribution	Age of Onset	Risk of Colon Cancer	Genetic Lesion	Clinical Manifestations	Associated Lesions
Familial adenomatous polyposis	Adenoma	Large intestine, duodenum	16 yr (range, 8-34 yr)	100%	5q (*APC* gene)	Rectal bleeding, abdominal pain, bowel obstruction	Desmoids, CHRPE
Peutz-Jeghers syndrome	Hamartoma	Large and small intestine	First decade	Slightly above average	19p (*STK11* gene)	Possible rectal bleeding, abdominal pain, intussusception	Orocutaneous melanin pigment spots, other tumors
MUTYH-associated polyposis	Adenoma	Large intestine, duodenum	45-50 yr (range, 13-60 yr)	75% (range, 50%-100%)	1p (*MYH* gene)	Rectal bleeding, abdominal pain, bowel obstruction	CHRPE, osteomas
Juvenile polyposis	Hamartoma (rarely adenoma)	Large and small intestine	First decade	≈9%	*PTEN, SMAD4, BMPR1*	Possible rectal bleeding, abdominal pain, intussusception	Pulmonary AVMs
Hereditary nonpolyposis colon cancer	Adenoma	Large intestine	40 yr (range, 18-65 yr)	30%	Mismatch repair genes*	Rectal bleeding, abdominal pain, bowel obstruction	Other tumors (e.g., ovary, uterus, pancreas, stomach)

AVM, Arteriovenous malformation; *CHRPE,* congenital hypertrophy of the retinal pigment epithelium; *MUTYH,* mutY homolog *(Escherichia coli).*
*Including *hMSH2, hMSH3, hMSH6, hMLH1, hPMS1,* and *hPMS2.*
From Goldman L, Schafer AI: *Goldman's Cecil medicine,* ed 24, Philadelphia, 2012, Saunders.

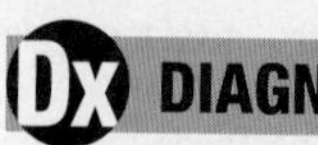

DIAGNOSIS

Diagnosis is suggested in many cases by family history and confirmed by colonoscopy and physical findings described previously.

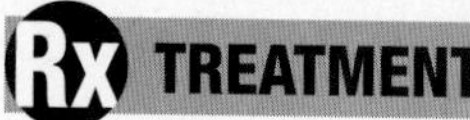

TREATMENT

GENERAL Rx

Peutz-Jeghers syndrome:
- Colonoscopies with polypectomies
- Screening for breast cancer, testicular cancer, possibly ovarian cancer

Juvenile polyposis syndrome:
- Colonoscopies with polypectomies if few colon polyps
- Total colectomy if numerous polyps
- Esophagogastroscopies and polypectomies

Cowden's disease:
- Rigorous breast cancer screening or prophylactic simple bilateral mastectomy with reconstruction.

Cronkhite-Canada syndrome:
- Progressive malabsorption syndrome is the hallmark of this syndrome, and no specific treatment exists. Enteral or parenteral feeding is the cornerstone of management and can result in remission.

DISPOSITION

- The screening of first-degree relatives of patients with colonic adenomas detected before 60 yr of age is controversial. Some recommend beginning colonoscopic screening at age 40 yr or 10 yr younger than the age at diagnosis of the youngest person in the family with an adenoma.
- Recommended interval between colonoscopies from the U.S. Consensus Guidelines for Colonoscopic Surveillance after Polypectomy are as follows:
  - 10 yr for small, rectal hyperplastic polyps
  - 5 to 10 yr for one to two low-risk adenomas (tubular adenomas <1 cm)
  - 3 yr for low-risk adenomas or any high-risk adenoma (large [≥1 cm] or histologically advanced adenomas [tubulovillous or villous adenomas or villous adenomas and those with high-grade dysplasia])
  - <3 yr for presence of >10 adenomas
  - 2 to 6 mo for inadequately removed adenomas

SUGGESTED READINGS

available at www.expertconsult.com

RELATED CONTENT

Peutz-Jeghers Syndrome (Patient Information)

AUTHOR: **FRED F. FERRI, M.D.**

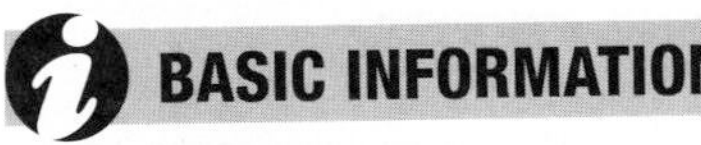

BASIC INFORMATION

DEFINITION

Peyronie's disease is an abnormal curvature and shortening of the penis during an erection. This is caused by scarring of the tunica albuginea of the corpora cavernosa.

SYNONYMS

Plastic induration of the penis
Penile fibromatosis

ICD-9CM CODES
607.89 Peyronie's disease
ICD-10CM CODES
N48.6 Induratio penis plastica

EPIDEMIOLOGY & DEMOGRAPHICS

- Peyronie's disease occurs in approximately 1% of men.
- It is commonly seen between the ages of 45 and 60 yr.
- A genetic predisposition has been suggested.
- There are no incidence and prevalence data available in the literature.

PHYSICAL FINDINGS & CLINICAL PRESENTATION

- Painful erections
- Tenderness over the scar tissue area
- Erectile dysfunction
- Curvature of the erected penis interfering with penetration
- Dupuytren's contracture is a commonly associated finding in patients with Peyronie's disease

ETIOLOGY

- Specific cause is unknown. It is believed that scar tissue forms on either the dorsal or ventral midline surface of the penile shaft. The scar restricts expansion at the involved site, causing the penis to bend or curve in one direction.
- The precipitating factor appears to be trauma from repetitive microvascular injury caused by vigorous sexual intercourse, accidents, or prior surgeries (e.g., transurethral or radical prostatectomy, cystoscopy).

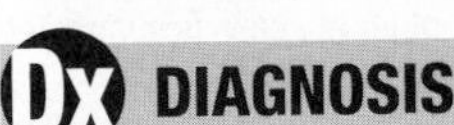

DIAGNOSIS

Diagnosis is based on the clinical findings.

DIFFERENTIAL DIAGNOSIS

- The history differentiates congenital from acquired curvatures of the penis.
- Other causes of erectile dysfunction must be excluded, including metabolic, diabetic, thyroid, and renal causes, in addition to hypogonadism and hyperprolactinemia.

WORKUP

History and physical examination alone will usually establish the diagnosis of Peyronie's disease.

LABORATORY TESTS

There are no specific blood tests to diagnose Peyronie's disease. Electrolytes, blood urea nitrogen, creatinine, glucose, thyroid function tests (thyroid-stimulating hormone, T_3U, T_4), testosterone, and prolactin levels are blood tests to exclude other medical causes of erectile dysfunction.

IMAGING STUDIES

Imaging studies are not specific.

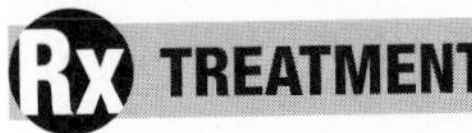

TREATMENT

NONPHARMACOLOGIC THERAPY

A conservative approach of reassurance and observation is taken at first because the disease process may be self-limiting.

ACUTE GENERAL Rx

Although not substantiated by direct randomized, controlled clinical trials, the following treatment modalities have been tried:

- Vitamin E 400 mg bid.
- Paraaminobenzoic acid 12 g/day.
- Colchicine 0.6 mg bid for 2 to 3 wk.
- Fexofenadine 60 mg bid for 3 mo.
- Steroid injection into the scar tissue.
- Collagenase injection into the scar tissue.
- Radiation to the scar tissue area.
- Extracorporeal shockwave therapy (ESWT): Current evidence on the safety, but not the efficacy, of ESWT appears adequate. From comparative studies, the main benefits of ESWT were the alleviation of pain and reduction of angulation of the penis. In one comparative study, 10 of 20 patients receiving ESWT had a decrease in the curvature of at least 30%. Case series evidence also suggested some improvement of sexual performance.
- Other medications that can be helpful include verapamil, tamoxifen, and interferon.

CHRONIC Rx

In patients who have progressed to intractable pain with erection or erectile dysfunction, surgical treatment with excision of the plaque and skin grafting may be indicated.

DISPOSITION

Peyronie's disease evolves slowly and in some cases can resolve on its own. Waiting for 1 yr before proceeding with surgical attempts is recommended.

REFERRAL

A urologic consultation is recommended in patients with progressive symptoms and erectile dysfunction.

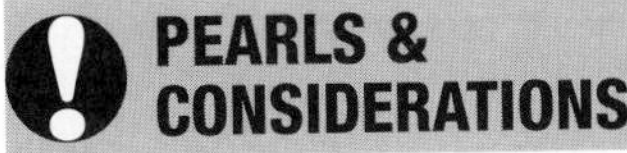

PEARLS & CONSIDERATIONS

COMMENTS

- Peyronie's disease is not commonly seen in younger patients because they are able to sustain intracorporeal pressures high enough to stretch the scar tissue, preventing it from deforming the penis during erection.
- Trauma from buckling of the erected penis is thought to be the precipitant cause of scar formation and Peyronie's disease. It is found more often in men who are sexually very active and vigorous, having sexual intercourse daily or almost daily.
- Sexual positions with the woman being on top or thrusting the penis into the anterior vaginal wall are thought to increase the chances of developing Peyronie's disease.

SUGGESTED READINGS

available at www.expertconsult.com

RELATED CONTENT

Peyronie's Disease (Patient Information)

AUTHOR: **TANYA ALI, M.D.**

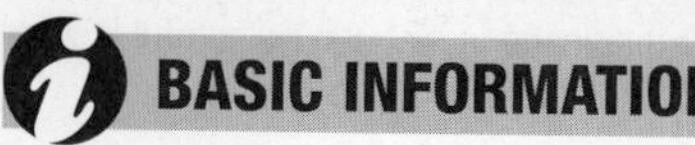

BASIC INFORMATION

DEFINITION

Inflammation of the pharynx or tonsils

SYNONYMS

Sore throat
Group A streptococci (GAS)

ICD-9CM CODES
462 Pharyngitis
ICD-10CM CODES
J02.9 Acute pharyngitis, unspecified
J03.0 Acute tonsillitis
J03.9 Acute tonsillitis, unspecified
J04.0 Acute laryngitis

EPIDEMIOLOGY & DEMOGRAPHICS

Acute pharyngitis accounts for 1.3% of outpatient visits to health care providers in the U.S.
PEAK INCIDENCE: Late winter/early spring (GAS infections)
PREDOMINANT SEX: Females = males
PREDOMINANT AGE:
- All ages affected
- Streptococcal pharyngitis most common among school-age children (5-15 yr of age). GAS are responsible for 5%-15% of cases of pharyngitis in adults and 20%-30% of cases in children (5-15 yr of age).

PHYSICAL FINDINGS & CLINICAL PRESENTATION

- Pharynx:
  1. May appear normal to severely erythematous
  2. Tonsillar hypertrophy and exudates commonly seen but do not indicate etiology
- Viral infection:
  1. Rhinorrhea
  2. Conjunctivitis
  3. Cough
- Bacterial infection, especially GAS:
  1. High fever
  2. Systemic signs of infection
- Herpes simplex or enterovirus infection: vesicles
- Streptococcal infection:
  1. Rare complications:
     a. Scarlet fever
     b. Rheumatic fever
     c. Acute glomerulonephritis
  2. Extension of infection: tonsillar, parapharyngeal, or retropharyngeal abscess presenting with severe pain, high fever, trismus
- Streptococcal tonsillitis is manifested as acute onset of fever, headache, neck pain, odynophagia, sore throat, otalgia, red tongue with enlargement of papillae, sore throat, red swollen uvula, and tender anterior cervical adenitis.
- Peritonsillar abscess (accumulation of pus between the tonsil and its capsule) is the most common complication of acute tonsillitis. Clinical signs include deformed posterior pharynx, medial displacement of the uvula, trismus, and muffled voice (hot-potato voice).
- Table 1-390 describes seven danger signs in patients with sore throat.

ETIOLOGY

- Viruses:
  1. Respiratory syncytial virus
  2. Influenza A and B
  3. Epstein-Barr virus
  4. Adenovirus
  5. Herpes simplex
- Bacteria:
  1. GAS: *Streptococcus pyogenes.* β-Hemolytic GAS are the most common cause of acute tonsillitis.
  2. *Neisseria gonorrhoeae*
  3. *Arcanobacterium haemolyticum*
- Other organisms:
  1. *Mycoplasma pneumoniae*
  2. *Chlamydophila pneumoniae*

DIAGNOSIS

DIFFERENTIAL DIAGNOSIS

- Sore throat associated with granulocytopenia, thyroiditis
- Tonsillar hypertrophy associated with lymphoma
- Section II describes the differential diagnosis of sore throat.

WORKUP

The Centor criteria to identify patients at risk for GAS consists of (1) fever subjective or measured >38.1° C (100.5° F), (2) absence of cough, (3) tonsilar exudates, (4) tender anterior cervical lymphadenopathy. Patients with ≤1 criteria are at low risk and do not need additional testing. The McIsaac criteria adds 1 point for age 3-14 and subtracts a point for age ≥45 yr.
- Rapid streptococcal antigen test (culture should be performed if rapid test negative)
- Throat swab for culture to exclude *S. pyogenes, N. gonorrhoeae* (requires specific transport medium) in selected cases

LABORATORY TESTS

- Bloodwork is only rarely necessary
- Complete blood count with differential
  1. May help support diagnosis of bacterial infection when diagnosis is unclear
  2. Streptococcal infection suggested by leukocytosis >15,000/mm^3
- Viral cultures, serologic studies rarely needed
- Monospot if diagnosis is unclear

TABLE 1-390 Seven Danger Signs in Patients with Sore Throat

1. Persistence of symptoms longer than 1 wk without improvement
2. Respiratory difficulty, particularly stridor
3. Difficulty in handling secretions
4. Difficulty in swallowing
5. Severe pain in the absence of erythema
6. A palpable mass
7. Blood, even in small amounts, in the pharynx or ear

From Andreoli TE et al: *Andreoli and Carpenter's Cecil essentials of medicine*, ed 8, Philadelphia, 2010, Saunders.

IMAGING STUDIES

Seldom indicated. If necessary to distinguish between tonsillitis and peritonsillar abscess, CT or MRI of the neck can be done.

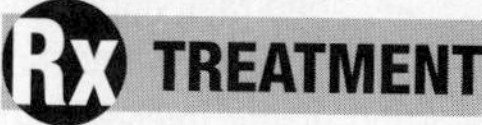

TREATMENT

NONPHARMACOLOGIC THERAPY

- Fluids
- Salt water gargles

ACUTE GENERAL Rx

- Analgesics: aspirin (adults) or acetaminophen or ibuprofen (adults and children)
- If streptococcal infection proven or suspected:
  1. Penicillin V 500 mg PO bid for 10 days or benzathine penicillin 1.2 million U IM once (adults). Children: penicillin V 250 mg bid or tid
  2. Erythromycin 500 mg PO bid or 250 mg qid for 10 days or azithromycin if penicillin allergic
- If gonococcal infection proven or suspected: ceftriaxone 125 mg IM once
- Amoxicillin 500 mg tid for 10 days is the primary antibiotic treatment of streptococcal tonsillitis. Macrolides or clindamycin can be used in penicillin-allergic patients.
- Treatment of peritonsillar abscess is drainage through needle or incision.

CHRONIC Rx

- Recurrent streptococcal infections are common and may represent reinfection from other household members, including pets.
- There is no conclusive evidence from randomized clinical trials that tonsillectomy is superior to antibiotic therapy for recurrent tonsillitis in adults.
- Tonsillopharyngitis is generally managed in an outpatient setting with follow-up arranged in 1 to 2 wk. Admission to the hospital is indicated for local suppurative complications (peritonsillar abscess; lateral pharyngeal or posterior pharyngeal abscess; impending airway closure; or inability to swallow food, medications, or water).

REFERRAL

- To otolaryngologist:
  1. If peritonsillar or other abscess is suspected
  2. If tonsillar hypertrophy persists

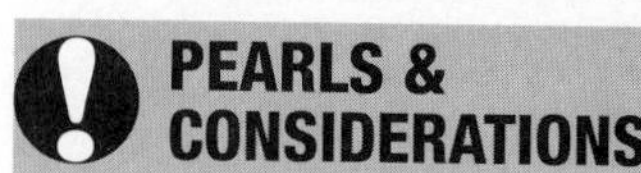

PEARLS & CONSIDERATIONS

COMMENTS

- Antibiotic therapy should be avoided unless bacterial etiology is suspected or proven, especially in adults.

SUGGESTED READINGS

available at www.expertconsult.com

RELATED CONTENT

Tonsillitis (Patient Information)
Sore Throat (Patient Information)

AUTHOR: **GLENN G. FORT, M.D., M.P.H.**

 BASIC INFORMATION

DEFINITION

Pheochromocytomas are catecholamine-producing tumors that originate from chromaffin cells of the adrenergic system. They generally secrete both norepinephrine and epinephrine, but norepinephrine is usually the predominant amine.

SYNONYMS

Paraganglioma

ICD-9CM CODES
194.0 Pheochromocytoma
255.6 Medulloadrenal hyperfunction
ICD-10CM CODES
C74.9 Malignant neoplasm of adrenal gland, unspecified
C75.9 Malignant neoplasm of endocrine gland, unspecified
E27.5 Adrenomedullary hyperfunction

EPIDEMIOLOGY & DEMOGRAPHICS

- Incidence: 0.05% of population; peak incidence in 30s and 40s.
- Approximately 25% of patients with apparently sporadic pheochromocytoma may be carriers of mutations.
- Approximately 25% of pheochromocytomas are familial and associated with genetic disorders (Table E1-391). Pheochromocytoma is a feature of two disorders with an autosomal-dominant pattern of inheritance:
  1. Multiple endocrine neoplasia (MEN) type 2
  2. Von Hippel-Lindau disease: angioma of the retina, hemangioblastoma of the central nervous system, renal cell carcinoma, pancreatic cysts, and epididymal cystoadenoma
- Pheochromocytomas occur in 5% of patients with neurofibromatosis type 1.

PHYSICAL FINDINGS & CLINICAL PRESENTATION

- Hypertension: can be sustained (55%) or paroxysmal (45%).
- Headache (80%): usually paroxysmal in nature and described as "pounding" and severe.
- Palpitations (70%): can be present with or without tachycardia.
- Hyperhidrosis (60%): most evident during paroxysmal attacks of hypertension.
- Physical examination may be entirely normal if done in a symptom-free interval; during a paroxysm the patient may demonstrate marked increase in both systolic and diastolic pressure, profuse sweating, visual disturbances (caused by hypertensive retinopathy), dilated pupils (from catecholamine excess), paresthesias in the lower extremities (caused by severe vasoconstriction), tremor, tachycardia.
- Orthostatic hypotension is common among patients with pheochromocytoma due to reduction of blood volume and desensitization of adrenergic receptors by the chronic excess of catecholamines.

ETIOLOGY

- Catecholamine-producing tumors that are usually located in the adrenal medulla.
- Specific mutations of the RET protooncogene cause familial predisposition to pheochromocytoma in MEN 2.
- Mutations in the von Hippel-Lindau tumor suppressor gene (*VHL* gene) cause familial disposition to pheochromocytoma in von Hippel-Lindau disease.
- Recently identified genes for succinate dehydrogenase subunit D *(SDHD)* and succinate dehydrogenase subunit B *(SDHB)* predispose carriers to pheochromocytoma and globus tumors.

Dx DIAGNOSIS

DIFFERENTIAL DIAGNOSIS

- Anxiety disorder
- Thyrotoxicosis
- Amphetamine or cocaine abuse
- Carcinoid
- Essential hypertension

WORKUP

Laboratory evaluation and imaging studies to locate the neoplasm (Fig. E1-724). Misdiagnosis of pheochromocytoma is not uncommon. Correct interpretation of biochemical tests and imaging is crucial to a correct diagnosis.

LABORATORY TESTS

- Although there is no consensus on the best test, plasma-free metanephrines have been suggested as the test of first choice for excluding the tumor. Elevated plasma concentrations of normetanephrines or metanephrine have a sensitivity of up to 100%, but the specificity is markedly lower.
- 24-hr urine collection for metanephrines (up to 100% sensitive) will also show increased metanephrines; the accuracy of the 24-hr urinary levels for metanephrines can be improved by indexing urinary metanephrine levels by urine creatinine levels.

IMAGING STUDIES

- Abdominal CT scan (Fig. E1-725) with and without contrast (88% sensitivity) is useful in locating pheochromocytomas >0.5 inch in diameter (90% to 95% accurate).
- MRI with contrast: pheochromocytomas demonstrate a distinctive MRI appearance (up to 100% sensitivity); MRI may become the diagnostic imaging modality of choice.
- Scintigraphy with 131 or 1-123 I-MIBG (up to 100% sensitivity) (Fig. E1-725): this norepinephrine analog localizes in adrenergic tissue; it is particularly useful in locating extraadrenal pheochromocytomas.
- 6-[^{18}F]Fluorodopamine positron emission tomography is reserved for cases in which clinical symptoms and signs suggest pheochromocytoma and results of biochemical tests are positive but conventional imaging studies cannot locate the tumor. An alternative approach is to use vena caval sampling for plasma catecholamines and metanephrines.

Rx TREATMENT

GENERAL Rx

Laparoscopic adrenalectomy (surgical resection for both benign and malignant disease):

1. Preoperative stabilization with combination of alpha-adrenergic blocking agents (prazosin, doxazosin, terazosin, or phenoxybenzamine), beta-blocker, and liberal fluid and salt intake starting 10 to 14 days before surgery. Beta-blockers should be avoided until patients receive adequate alpha-adrenergic blockade for several days to avoid hypertensive crisis due to unopposed alpha stimulation. Amlodipine or verapamil can be added to beta-blockers if blood pressure control is still inadequate. Table E1-392 describes orally administered drugs to treat pheochromocytoma.
2. Hypertensive crisis preoperatively and intraoperatively can be controlled with nitroprusside. Table E1-393 summarizes intravenously administered drugs used to treat pheochromocytoma.

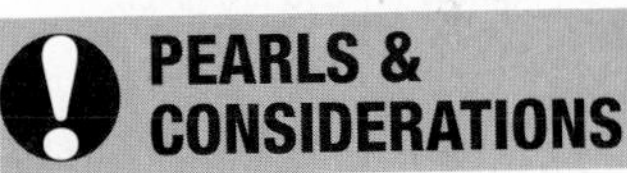

PEARLS & CONSIDERATIONS

COMMENTS

- Obtaining a detailed family history is important because 25% of pheochromocytomas are familial.
- Screening for pheochromocytoma should be considered in patients with any of the following:
  1. Malignant hypertension
  2. Poor response to antihypertensive therapy
  3. Paradoxical hypertensive response
  4. Hypertension during induction of anesthesia, parturition, surgery, or thyrotropin-releasing hormone testing
  5. Hypertension associated with imipramine or desipramine
  6. Neurofibromatosis (increased incidence of pheochromocytoma)
- All patients with pheochromocytoma should be screened for MEN-2 and von Hippel-Lindau disease with the pentagastrin test, serum parathyroid hormone, ophthalmoscopy, MRI of the brain, CT scan of the kidneys and pancreas, and ultrasonography of the testes.
- In patients with pheochromocytoma, routine analysis for mutations of *RET, VHL, SDHD,* and *SDHB* is indicated to identify pheochromocytoma-associated syndromes.

SUGGESTED READINGS

available at www.expertconsult.com

RELATED CONTENT

Pheochromocytoma (Patient Information)

AUTHORS: **MARK F. BRADY, M.D., M.P.H.,** and **FRED F. FERRI, M.D.**

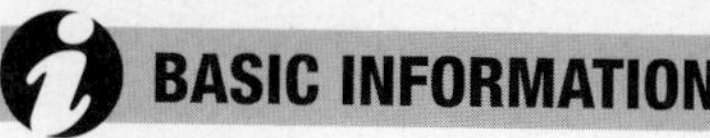

DEFINITION

Specific phobias are anxiety disorders characterized by an excessive, persistent fear elicited by a specific object or situation that is then avoided or tolerated with intense distress. The provoking stimulus may be a specific object, such as an animal or insect; natural environments, such as heights or water; or a specific situation, such as the sight of blood, the receipt of an injection, or being in a tunnel or on a bridge. Social anxiety disorder (formerly named social phobia) is a specific, separately diagnosed disorder characterized by a fear of being in social or performance situations. Agoraphobia also is a separately diagnosed disorder, characterized by an intense anxiety about being in a place or situation from which they would not be able to escape in the event of a panic attack or panic-like symptoms. Such situations include being in enclosed/crowded spaces or being more than a certain distance from home alone. If agoraphobia is present in individuals with panic disorder, both diagnoses are given.

SYNONYMS

Simple phobia (obsolete name for specific phobia)

Phobias named for the provoking stimulus, such as arachnophobia (fear of spiders) and acrophobia (fear of heights)

Specific phobias are codes:
ICD-9CM and DSM-5
300.29
ICD-10CM
F40.2xx
Social Phobia:
ICD-9CM and DSM-5
300.23
ICD-10CM
F40.10
Agoraphobia:
ICD-9CM and DSM-5
300.22
ICD-10CM
F40.00

EPIDEMIOLOGY & DEMOGRAPHICS

PEAK INCIDENCE: The majority of cases of specific phobia tend to onset prior to age 10; median onset is from ages 7-10.

PREVALENCE (IN U.S.):

- Specific phobias are prevalent in 7% to 9% of the general population (12-month prevalence rate).
- Social anxiety disorder is prevalent in approximately 7% to 13% of the general population.
- Agoraphobia is prevalent in approximately 1.7% of the general population per year.

PREDOMINANT SEX AND AGE:

- Females with specific phobias outnumber males 2:1, though rates vary by phobia.
- More women than men are affected with social anxiety disorder (odds ratios ranging from 1.5-2.2).
- Agoraphobia is more prevalent in women than men (2:1).
- Most specific phobias have childhood onset, although it is possible for them to develop at any age.
- Situational phobias tend to have a later age of onset compared to natural environment, animal, or blood-injection phobias.
- Onset of social anxiety disorder usually occurs in the mid-teens, with onset after age 25 being unusual; this disorder is generally lifelong.
- Onset of agoraphobia typically occurs in late adolescence or early adulthood; two thirds of cases onset prior to age 35.

GENETICS: Specific phobia and social anxiety disorder are more common in first-degree relatives.

PHYSICAL FINDINGS & CLINICAL PRESENTATION

- When approaching the phobic stimulus, the experience of extreme anxiety is often accompanied by autonomic symptoms such as tachycardia, tremor, and diaphoresis; depersonalization may occur. In blood or injection phobias, symptoms are often followed by a parasympathetic response that can cause vasovagal syncope.
- Specific phobias frequently occur with other anxiety disorders.

ETIOLOGY

There is no clear etiology and likely is a combination of factors including temperamental (e.g., behavioral inhibition, neuroticism), environmental (e.g., negative encounters with the feared stimulus, parental overprotection), and genetic.

Dx DIAGNOSIS

DIFFERENTIAL DIAGNOSIS

- Social anxiety disorder is distinguished from specific phobias in that what is feared is humiliation or embarrassment in social interaction or performance situations, rather than fear of a specific object or environment.
- Panic attacks (with or without agoraphobia): anxiety symptoms seen in specific phobia may resemble symptoms of panic attacks, but the stimulus in the specific or social situation is clear, whereas panic attacks do not have a clearly associated provoking stimulus (i.e., they occur unexpectedly in the absence of a trigger).
- Posttraumatic stress disorder (PTSD): anxiety and physiologic arousal associated with specific cues from the traumatic event defining the PTSD may resemble the symptoms induced by a phobia.
- Generalized anxiety disorder (GAD): may be difficult to distinguish from social anxiety disorder, but in social anxiety disorder the focus is fear of embarrassment or humiliation in the presence of other people, whereas GAD has no specific focus for the worry.
- Avoidant personality disorder is often comorbid with social anxiety disorder.
- Psychotic disorders can present with a fear of being in public that arises from delusions.

WORKUP

- History: usually diagnostic. This should include information about other medical disorders, medications, any history of past trauma, and substance abuse.
- Physical examination: to confirm absence of cardiovascular abnormalities such as arrhythmias or evidence of endocrinologic reasons for hyperarousal such as an enlarged or tender thyroid gland.

LABORATORY TESTS

No specific laboratory tests are indicated.

IMAGING STUDIES

No specific imaging studies are recommended.

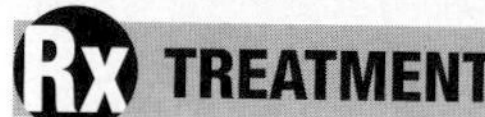

NONPHARMACOLOGIC THERAPY

- Cognitive-behavioral therapy (CBT) and exposure-based treatments have been effective for treating specific phobia and social anxiety disorder in controlled trials and are considered an appropriate first-line treatment.
- Behavioral treatments sometimes involve relaxation training, often paired with visualization and progressive desensitization.
- Success rates in treating specific phobias are higher when the phobia is not complicated by other anxiety disorders.

ACUTE GENERAL Rx

- Although benzodiazepines provide rapid relief of anxiety associated with exposure to provoking stimuli, they are associated with adverse effects including somnolence, accidents, abuse, and dependence, and thus are not recommended as a first-line treatment.
- Beta-blockers (e.g., propranolol) have been used to decrease autonomic hyperarousal and tremor associated with performance situations (e.g., before public speaking), but are not recommended for more generalized forms of social anxiety disorder.

CHRONIC Rx

- If the phobic stimulus is rarely encountered, benzodiazepines used on an as-needed basis can be an appropriate long-term treatment; however, there is a risk of abuse and dependence that makes them a less desirable choice for long-term treatment.
- Selective serotonin reuptake inhibitors are the most effective pharmacologic treatment in reducing symptoms and improving function for people with social anxiety disorder.
- Monoamine oxidase inhibitors are also effective for treatment of social anxiety disorder, but are rarely used due to dietary restrictions and adverse effects.

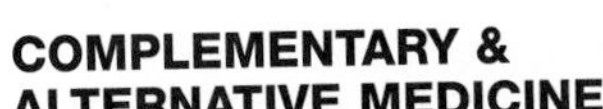

COMPLEMENTARY & ALTERNATIVE MEDICINE

No definitive evidence supports complementary or alternative medicines in the treatment of phobic disorders.

DISPOSITION

Phobic disorders are generally present for life, although outpatient-based treatment may effectively reduce symptoms.

REFERRAL

Recommended for confirmation of diagnosis and for evaluation for psychotherapy and other treatment modalities.

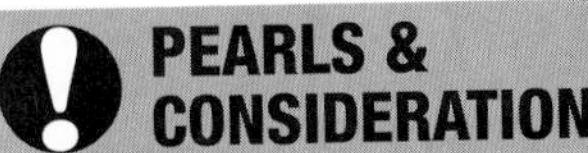

PEARLS & CONSIDERATIONS

People with social anxiety disorder often have low self-esteem and fear being scrutinized by others such that they avoid or are fearful of any situation in which others may assess or evaluate them directly or indirectly. More than half are concurrently affected by another anxiety disorder, and alcohol and other substance dependence is common because these patients often use substances to mask their anxiety.

SUGGESTED READINGS

available at www.expertconsult.com

RELATED CONTENT

Social Anxiety Disorder (Related Key Topic)
Posttraumatic Stress Disorder (Related Key Topic)
Phobias (Patient Information)

AUTHOR: **KRISTY L. DALRYMPLE, PH.D.**

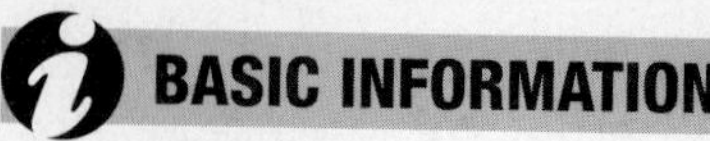

BASIC INFORMATION

DEFINITION

From the Latin words *pilus,* meaning "hair," and *nidus,* meaning "nest."

A *pilonidal sinus* is a short tract that extends from the skin surface and most likely represents a distended hair follicle. It is most commonly found in the intergluteal fold sacrococcygeal region, but it can also occur in the interdigital area, umbilicus, chest wall, and scalp. An *acute pilonidal abscess,* which consists of pus and a wall of edematous fat, results from rupture of an infected follicle into fat. A *chronic pilonidal abscess* results when an infected follicle ruptures directly into surrounding tissues; the wall of a chronic pilonidal abscess consists of fibrous tissue. A *pilonidal cyst* develops from a chronic abscess of long duration as a thin and flat lining of epithelium grows into the cavity from the skin surface.

SYNONYMS

Jeep disease

ICD-9CM CODES
685.1 Pilonidal cyst
ICD-10CM CODES
L05 Pilonidal cyst
L05.0 Pilonidal cyst with abscess
L05.9 Pilonidal cysts without abscess

EPIDEMIOLOGY & DEMOGRAPHICS

INCIDENCE: 26 cases per 100,000 persons
PREDOMINANT SEX: Males are more commonly affected than females (2.2:1).
AVERAGE AGE OF PRESENTATION: 21 yr
RISK FACTORS:
- Male sex
- Caucasian race
- Family predisposition
- Obesity
- Sedentary lifestyle
- Occupation requiring prolonged sitting
- Local hirsutism
- Poor hygiene
- Increased sweat activity

PHYSICAL FINDINGS & CLINICAL PRESENTATION

- May manifest as asymptomatic pits or pores in the natal cleft (Fig. E1-726)
- Tenderness after physical activity or prolonged sitting
- Acute pilonidal abscess in 20% of patients with pilonidal disease
- Presents as a hot, tender, fluctuant swelling just lateral to the midline over the sacrum that may exude pus through the midline pit
- Chronic pilonidal abscess in 80% of patients with pilonidal disease
- Acute suppuration, tenderness, swelling, and heat
- Infrequently, systemic reaction: occasionally fever, leukocytosis, and malaise

ETIOLOGY

- Currently believed to be acquired rather than congenital.
- Drilling of hair shed from the perineum or the head into sebaceous or hair follicles in the natal cleft.
- Drilling is facilitated by the friction of the natal cleft.
- Subsequent infection by skin organisms leads to pilonidal abscess.

Dx DIAGNOSIS

DIFFERENTIAL DIAGNOSIS

- Perianal abscess arising from the posterior midline crypt
- Hidradenitis suppurativa
- Carbuncle
- Furuncle
- Osteomyelitis
- Anal fistula
- Coccygeal sinus

WORKUP

- Diagnosis is based on history and physical examination.
- Midline pits present behind the anus overlying the sacrum and coccyx.
- Broken hairs are often seen extruding from the midline pits.
- Insert probe in pilonidal sinus in path away from the anus.
- Complicated anal fistula may be angulating posteriorly before passing into a retrorectal abscess, but thorough examination of the anal cavity usually discloses point of origin.

LABORATORY TESTS

Complete blood count

IMAGING STUDIES

CT scan in advanced, recurrent cases

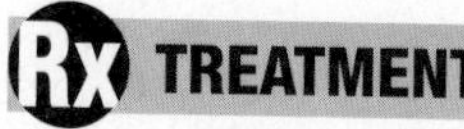

Rx TREATMENT

NONPHARMACOLOGIC THERAPY

Prevention of exacerbations:
1. Local hygiene
2. Avoidance of prolonged sitting position
3. Weight reduction

ACUTE GENERAL Rx

- Procedure of choice for first-episode acute abscess: simple incision and drainage in an outpatient setting. Box E1-64 describes surgical options for the treatment of pilonidal sinus.
- Cure rate of 76% after 18 mo
- Antibiotics: generally not indicated unless the patient has a medical condition such as rheumatic heart disease or is immunosuppressed

CHRONIC Rx

Elective treatment of pilonidal disease:
1. Minimal surgery:
   a. Remove hair from midline pits and shave buttocks.
   b. May use a fine wire brush with local anesthesia to clear the pits and any lateral openings of granulation tissue and hair.
   c. Keep area clean.
2. Fistulotomy and curettage:
   a. Used when minimal surgery does not control episodes of suppuration
   b. Pass probe to outline the pilonidal sinus and open tract surgically
   c. Curette granulation tissue at the base of the sinus and excise edges of the skin
   d. Keep open granulating wound meticulously clean and allow to heal
   e. If complete healing does not take place, use a skin graft or advancement flap to close the defect
3. Marsupialization:
   a. This is the treatment of choice for chronic pilonidal disease.
   b. Wide excision of the pilonidal area is performed, including all affected skin and subcutaneous tissues down to the presacral fascia.
   c. Wound is left open, allowed to marsupialize, or closed as a primary procedure.
   d. Give antibiotics for 24 hr (particularly those directed against *Staphylococcus* and *Bacteroides* species).
4. Other procedures:
   a. Excision and closure
   b. Excision and skin grafting
   c. Bascom procedure (follicle removal and lateral drainage)
   d. Flaps: *Z*-plasty, V-Y advancement flap, rhomboid flap, gluteus maximus myocutaneous flap

DISPOSITION

- Recurrence rate for excision (most definitive procedure): 1% to 6%
- Incidence of squamous cell carcinoma in a chronic, recurrent pilonidal sinus is rare <1%

REFERRAL

- Emergency department for incision and drainage for an acute abscess
- To a surgeon for elective treatment or management of chronic or recurrent disease

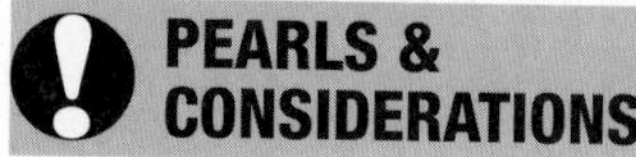

PEARLS & CONSIDERATIONS

COMMENTS

Because of significant associated morbidity, the elective surgical procedures outlined are performed only after the potential risks versus benefits are carefully weighed.

SUGGESTED READINGS

available at www.expertconsult.com

RELATED CONTENT

Pilonidal Cyst (Patient Information)

AUTHORS: **ARUNDATHI G. PRASAD, M.D.,** and **RUBEN ALVERO, M.D.**

BASIC INFORMATION

DEFINITION

Pinworms are a noninvasive infestation of the intestinal tract by *Enterobius vermicularis,* a helminth of the nematode family. It is a small (1 cm in length), white, thread-like roundworm that typically inhabits the cecum, appendix, and adjacent areas of the ileum and ascending colon.

SYNONYMS

Enterobiasis

ICD-9CM CODES
127.4 Enterobiasis
ICD-10CM CODES
B80 Enterobiasis

EPIDEMIOLOGY & DEMOGRAPHICS

- Most common intestinal nematode; approximately 30,000 cases annually in the U.S.
- Worldwide distribution, but most common in temperate climates.
- The prevalence of pinworm infection is lowest in infants and reaches highest infection rate in school-age children (ages 5 to 14 yr).
- Eggs are infective within 6 hr of oviposition and may remain so for 20 days.
- Clusters are found in families, institutionalized persons, and homosexual men.

PHYSICAL FINDINGS & CLINICAL PRESENTATION

- Most infested persons are asymptomatic.
- Perianal itching is the most common reported symptom, with scratching leading to excoriation and sometimes secondary infection.
- Rarely insomnia, irritability, anorexia, and weight loss are described.
- Granulomas have been described in various organs resulting from worms wandering outside the intestines and dying there.

ETIOLOGY & PATHOGENESIS

- *E. vermicularis* is highly prevalent throughout the world, particularly in countries of the temperate zone. Human beings are the only host for this worm. Infestation is by fecal-oral route; ingested eggs hatch in the stomach and the larvae migrate to the colon, where they mature. Gravid female worms containing an average of 10,000 ova migrate to the perianal skin at night, lay their eggs there, and die. The eggs embryonate within 6 hr and cause itching; scratching causes egg deposition under fingernails, from which they can contaminate food or lead to autoreinfection.
- *E. vermicularis* may be transmitted between sexual partners, especially those engaging in oral-anal sex.

DIAGNOSIS

DIFFERENTIAL DIAGNOSIS

- Perianal itching related to poor hygiene
- Hemorrhoidal disease and anal fissures
- Perineal yeast/fungal infections

Section II describes the causes of pruritus ani.

WORKUP

Identification of adult worms or eggs. *E. vermicularis* ova are ovoid but flattened on one side and measure approximately 56 × 27 micrometers (Fig. 1-727). The eggs can be identified on transparent tape placed on the perianal skin on awakening. (NOTE: Five consecutive negative tests rule out the diagnosis.) A single examination detects 50% of infections, three examinations detect 90%, and five examinations detect 99%.

TREATMENT

- Single dose of mebendazole (100 mg) with a repeat dose given after 2 wk results in cure rates of 90% to 100%.
- Single dose of albendazole (400 mg) with a second dose given 2 wk later is also highly effective.
- Pyrantel pamoate (11 mg/kg up to 1 g) can prevent against *E. vermicularis.* It is available as a suspension and has minimal toxicity (mild transient gastrointestinal symptoms, headache, drowsiness). A repeat dose after 2 wk is recommended because of the frequency of reinfection and autoinfection.
- Other infected family members, classmates, or residents of long-term care facilities should be treated at the same time as the index case.

PEARLS & CONSIDERATIONS

- Eosinophilia is not observed in most cases because tissue invasion does not occur.
- Good hand hygiene is the most effective method of prevention.
- Frequent changing of underclothes, bed clothes, and bed sheets is helpful to decrease risk of autoinfection.

SUGGESTED READINGS

available at www.expertconsult.com

RELATED CONTENT

Pinworms (Patient Information)

AUTHOR: **FRED F. FERRI, M.D.**

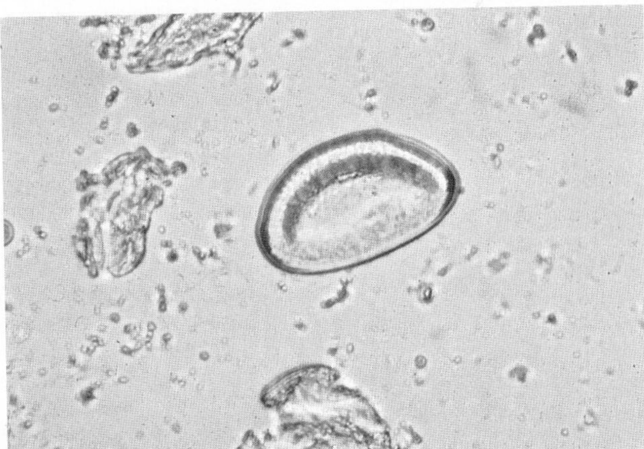

FIGURE 1-727 Enterobius vermicularis embryonated egg. Note larva inside (40 × 10 μm). (From Gorbach SL et al [eds]: *Infectious diseases,* ed 2, Philadelphia, 1998, Saunders.)

BASIC INFORMATION

DEFINITION

Piriformis syndrome is a form of low back pain characterized by pain and instability. The pain is usually present in the hip, groin, buttock, coccyx, and distal part of the lower extremity.

ICD-9CM CODES
956.0 Injury to sciatic nerve
ICD-10-CM CODES
S74.00 Injury of sciatic nerve at hip and thigh level

EPIDEMIOLOGY & DEMOGRAPHICS

- Women are affected more than men.
- Female-to-male incidence ratio is 6:1.
- About 6% of patients with sciatica have piriformis syndrome.

PHYSICAL FINDING & CLINICAL PRESENTATION

CLINICAL PRESENTATION

Patients with piriformis syndrome may present the following symptoms:

- Pain in the buttocks
  - This may be chronic,
  - Which may radiate to the distal part of the lower extremities,
  - Which worsens with squatting or walking.
- Pain on defecation
- Hip movements (especially adduction and internal rotation) cause pain.
- Labia majora or scrotal pain
- Dyspareunia in women
- Pain and discomfort on sitting

PHYSICAL FINDINGS

- Piriformis syndrome is a diagnosis of exclusion.
- There are no neurologic deficits in patients with piriformis syndrome.
- There is tenderness over the gluteal area.
- Other signs used in diagnosing piriformis syndrome include:
  - *Lasègue sign*—Extension of the knee with the hip flexed to 90 degrees produces pain in the vicinity of the greater sciatic notch.
  - *Pace sign*—Resisted abduction-external rotation of the thigh causes pain and weakness on the affected side.
  - *Freiberg sign*—With the patient in the supine position, passive internal rotation of the extended thigh causes pain.
  - Pain in the back when the patients lies with the painful side up and involved leg flexed

ETIOLOGY

1. Trauma to the buttocks/gluteal region
2. Spinal stenosis
3. Anatomic variations of the division of the sciatic nerve
4. As the sciatic nerve passes through the greater sciatic foramen, it is in close proximity to the piriformis muscle (Fig. 1-728). Pain results from compression of the sciatic nerve by the piriformis muscle.

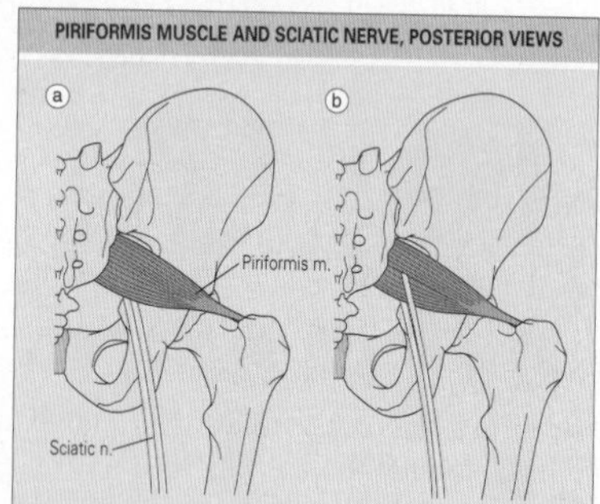

FIGURE 1-728 Piriformis muscle and sciatic nerve, posterior views. The piriformis muscle arises from the anterior surface of the sacrum and the gluteal surface of the ilium and crosses the greater sciatic foramen to insert onto the superior border of the greater trochanter. **A,** In most instances, the sciatic nerve passes along the anterior surface of the piriformis muscle and exits the pelvis below the piriformis muscle, passing posteriorly along its inferior border. **B,** In some individuals, a portion of the sciatic nerve passes through the piriformis muscle. Other anatomic variants have been described. (From Hochberg MC et al: *Rheumatology,* ed 5, St Louis, 2011, Mosby.)

Dx DIAGNOSIS

DIFFERENTIAL DIAGNOSIS

1. Lumbosacral disc or spine injury
2. Sacroiliac joint injury
3. Hamstring injury
4. Sciatic nerve entrapment
5. Paraspinal muscle spasm

WORKUP

Usually involves imaging studies

- Computed tomography scan:
  - Used to identify spinal stenosis
  - May show a large mass anterior to the piriformis muscle
- Magnetic resonance imaging:
  - May show an enlarged piriformis muscle on a T_1- or T_2-weighted images
- Electromyogram (EMG):
  - Normal EMG findings in the gluteus minimus, gluteus medius, and tensor fasciae latae muscles
  - Abnormal EMG findings in the gluteus maximus and piriformis muscles

Rx TREATMENT

TREATMENT DURING ACUTE PHASE

- Stop offending activities
- Start physical therapy (PT) treatment
  a) PT
    - The basic PT treatment is **stretching** and **manual therapy.**
    - PT modalities are most beneficial when used in conjunction with stretching exercise.
    - Ultrasound and/or moist heat is recommended before stretching.
    - Massage of the lumbosacral and gluteal areas reduces muscle tightness and sciatic nerve irritation.
    - Cold pack and/or electrical stimulation may be applied after exercise.

  b) Occupational therapy. Advise patients to:
    - Avoid sitting for prolonged periods.
    - Make frequent stops when driving to get up and stretch.

  c) Surgical intervention. Promising results include:
    - Piriformis tendon release
    - Sciatic neurolysis

  d) Other treatment modalities
    - Local injection of anesthetics into trigger points
    - Nonsteroidal anti-inflammatory drugs and opiates
    - Transrectal message

TREATMENT DURING RECOVERY PHASE

- Start gradual strengthening activities for the piriformis and gluteal muscles.
- Continue therapeutic modalities.
- Start light sport-specific activities and functional training if patient is asymptomatic.
- Some athletes may consider changing their footwear to avoid additional stress on the piriformis muscle.

TREATMENT DURING MAINTENANCE PHASE

- Continue performing a home exercise program for increasing flexibility and strength.
- Athletes may increase their training volume as tolerated.
- Compliance to a daily stretching program is crucial to avoid recurrence of this syndrome.

REFERRAL

- Physical therapist: to instruct patients about stretching and pain-relieving maneuvers
- Orthopedic: when diagnosis is in doubt, the patient failed conservative treatment, and surgical evaluation is needed
- Neurologist: for EMG studies

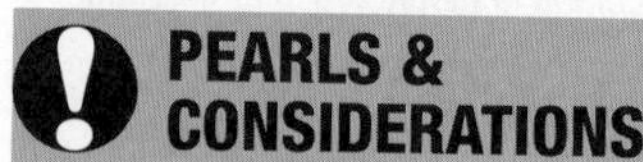

PEARLS & CONSIDERATIONS

COMMENTS

Athletes may return to play when:

- They are pain free with full range of motion.
- They have full strength in the affected side.

PREVENTION

To prevent the recurrence of pain:

- Avoid risk factors.
- Continue stretching exercises.

SUGGESTED READING

available at www.expertconsult.com

AUTHOR: **DANIEL K. ASIEDU, M.D., PH.D., F.A.C.P.**

BASIC INFORMATION

DEFINITION

Pituitary adenoma is a benign neoplasm of the anterior lobe of the pituitary that causes symptoms, either by excess secretion of hormones or by a local mass effect as the tumor impinges on other, nearby structures (e.g., optic chiasm, hypothalamus, pituitary stalk). Pituitary adenomas are classified by their size, function, and features that characterize their appearance. Microadenomas are <10 mm in size, and macroadenomas are ≥10 mm in size.

- *Acromegaly* is the disease state characterized by a pituitary adenoma that secretes growth hormone (GH).
- A *prolactinoma* secretes prolactin (PRL).
- *Cushing's disease* is a disease state of hypersecretion of adrenocorticotropic hormone (ACTH).
- *Thyrotropin-secreting pituitary adenomas* secrete primarily thyroid-stimulating hormone (TSH).
- *Nonsecretory pituitary adenomas* are those in which the neoplasm is a space-occupying lesion whose secretory products do not cause a specific disease state.

ICD-9CM CODES
253 Pituitary adenoma
ICD-10CM CODES
D35.2 Benign neoplasm of pituitary gland

EPIDEMIOLOGY & DEMOGRAPHICS

CLASSIFICATION (BY HORMONE SECRETED):

- PRL only: 35%
- No hormone: 30%
- GH only: 20%
- PRL and GH: 7%
- ACTH: 7%
- Luteinizing hormone (LH), follicle-stimulating hormone (FSH), TSH: 1%

PREVALENCE/INCIDENCE:

- Pituitary adenomas: up to 10% to 15% of all intracranial neoplasms; 3% to 27% at autopsy series
- Prolactinomas: up to 20% in women with unexplained primary or secondary amenorrhea
- GH-secreting pituitary adenoma: 50 to 60 cases per 1 million persons
- Thyrotropin-secreting pituitary adenoma: 2.8% of pituitary adenomas with a slight female/male predominance of 1.7:1
- Corticotropin-secreting pituitary adenomas: female/male predominance of 8:1 but overall rare diagnosis

PHYSICAL FINDINGS & CLINICAL PRESENTATION

PROLACTINOMAS:

- Females:
    1. Galactorrhea
    2. Amenorrhea
    3. Oligomenorrhea with anovulation
    4. Infertility
    5. Estrogen deficiency leading to hirsutism
    6. Decreased vaginal lubrication
    7. Osteopenia
- Males:
    1. Large tumors more common as a result of delayed diagnosis
    2. Possible impotence, decreased libido, or hypogonadism
    3. Galactorrhea rare because males lack the estrogen-dependent breast growth and differentiation

GH-SECRETING PITUITARY ADENOMA: ACROMEGALY:

- Coarse facial features
- Oily skin
- Prognathism
- Carpal tunnel syndrome
- Osteoarthritis
- History of increased hat, glove, or shoe size
- Decreased exercise capacity
- Visual field deficits
- Diabetes mellitus

CORTICOTROPIN-SECRETING PITUITARY ADENOMA: CUSHING'S DISEASE:

- Usually present when the tumor is small (1 to 2 mm)
- 50% of the tumors <5 mm
- Other symptoms:
    1. Truncal obesity
    2. Round facies (moon face)
    3. Dorsocervical fat accumulation (buffalo hump)
    4. Hirsutism
    5. Acne
    6. Menstrual disorders
    7. Hypertension
    8. Striae
    9. Bruising
    10. Thin skin
    11. Hyperglycemia

THYROTROPIN-SECRETING PITUITARY ADENOMA:

- In males, larger, more invasive, and more rapidly growing tumors that present later in life
- Other symptoms: thyrotoxicosis, goiter, visual impairment

NONSECRETORY PITUITARY ADENOMAS (ENDOCRINE INACTIVE PITUITARY ADENOMA):

- Usually large at the time of diagnosis
- Symptoms:
    1. Bitemporal hemianopsia as a result of compression of the optic chiasm
    2. Hypopituitarism from compression of the pituitary gland
    3. Hypogonadism in men and in premenopausal women
    4. Cranial nerve deficits caused by extension into the cavernous sinus
    5. Hydrocephalus from extension into the third ventricle, compressing the foramen of Monro
    6. Diabetes insipidus resulting from compression of the hypothalamus or pituitary stalk (a rare complication)

ETIOLOGY

Benign neoplasms of epithelial origin

Dx DIAGNOSIS

DIFFERENTIAL DIAGNOSIS

PROLACTINOMA:

- Pregnancy
- Postpartum puerperium
- Primary hypothyroidism
- Breast disease
- Breast stimulation
- Drug ingestion (especially phenothiazines, antidepressants, haloperidol, methyldopa, reserpine, opiates, amphetamines, and cimetidine)
- Chronic renal failure
- Liver disease
- Polycystic ovarian disease
- Chest wall disorders
- Spinal cord lesions
- Previous cranial irradiation

ACROMEGALY: Ectopic production of GH-releasing hormone from a carcinoid or other neuroendocrine tumor

CUSHING'S DISEASE:

- Diseases that cause ectopic sources of ACTH overproduction (including small-cell carcinoma of the lung, bronchial carcinoid, intestinal carcinoid, pancreatic islet cell tumor, medullary thyroid carcinoma, or pheochromocytoma)
- Adrenal adenomas, adrenal carcinoma
- Nelson's syndrome

THYROTROPIN-SECRETING PITUITARY ADENOMAS: Primary hypothyroidism

NONSECRETORY PITUITARY ADENOMA: Nonneoplastic mass lesions of various etiologies (e.g., infectious, granulomatous)

WORKUP

Screening tests for functional pituitary adenomas are described in Table 1-394.

PROLACTINOMA:

First step: measurement of basal PRL levels (practitioners should be aware of discriminatory values in their own institutions)

- Elevated PRL levels are correlated with tumor size.
- Level >200 ng/ml indicates likely prolactinoma, with levels of 100 to 200 ng/ml being equivocal and possibly associated with medications or other sources.
- Basal PRL levels between 20 and 100 suggest a microadenoma as well as other conditions such as psychotropic drug ingestion, recent breast examination, and even a recent meal.
- Basal level <20 ng/ml is usually considered normal. Each laboratory should develop its own normative values, however, and practitioner should refer to these values.
- Threshold level for obtaining imaging such as MRI should be developed by individual providers depending on the level of specificity and sensitivity desired.

ACROMEGALY:

- First screening tests are the measurement of the serum insulin-like growth factor I level, postprandial serum GH, and TRH stimulation test.

 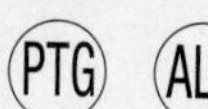

TABLE 1-394 Screening Tests for Functional Pituitary Adenomas

Disorder	Test	Comments
Acromegaly	IGF1 OGTT with GH obtained at 0, 30, and 60 min	Interpret IGF1 relative to age- and gender-matched controls. Normal subjects should suppress GH to <1 μg/L.
Prolactinoma	Serum PRL level	A level >500 μg/L is pathognomonic for macroprolactinoma. If >200 μg/L, prolactinoma is likely.*
Cushing's disease	24-hr UFC Nighttime salivary cortisol Dexamethasone (1 mg) at 11 P.M and fasting plasma cortisol measured at 8 A.M ACTH assay	Ensure that urine collection is total and accurate by measuring urinary creatinine. Free salivary cortisol reflects circadian rhythm and elevated levels may indicate Cushing's disease. Normal subjects suppress to <1.8 μg/dL. Distinguishes adrenal adenoma from ectopic ACTH or Cushing's disease.
TSH-secreting tumor	TSH measurement Free T_4 by dialysis Total T_3	If T_4 or T_3 is elevated and TSH is measurable or elevated, a TSH-secreting tumor may be present.

ACTH, Adrenocorticotropic hormone; GH, growth hormone; IGF1, insulin-like growth factor type 1; OGTT, oral glucose tolerance test; PRL, prolactin; T3, triiodothyronine; T4, thyroxine; TSH, thyroid-stimulating hormone; UFC, urinary free cortisol.
*Risperidol may result in prolactin levels >200 μg/L.
From Melmed S et al: *Williams textbook of endocrinology*, ed 12, Philadelphia, 2011, Saunders.

- Follow with an oral glucose tolerance test.
- Failure to suppress serum GH to <2 ng/ml with an oral load of 100 g glucose is considered conclusive.
- A GH-releasing hormone level >300 ng/ml is indicative of an ectopic source of GH.

CUSHING'S DISEASE:
- Normal or slightly elevated corticotropin levels ranging from 20 to 200 pg/ml; normal is 10 to 50 pg/ml (normative data should be developed by each institution for its population).
- Level <10 pg/ml usually indicates an autonomously secreting adrenal tumor.
- Level >200 pg/ml suggests an ectopic corticotropin-secreting neoplasm.
- Cushing's disease can be assessed by absence of cortisol suppression with the low-dose dexamethasone test but with the presence of cortisol suppression after the high-dose test. As a method to distinguish Cushing's disease from an ectopic source of ACTH, this test is robust.
- 24-hr urine collection should demonstrate an increased level of cortisol excretion.

THYROTROPIN-SECRETING PITUITARY ADENOMA:
- Highly sensitive thyrotropin assays, which evaluate the presence of thyrotoxicosis, are one way to detect a thyrotropin-secreting tumor.
- Free alpha subunit is secreted by >80% of tumors, with the ratio of the alpha subunit to thyrotropin <1.
- With central resistance to thyroid hormone, ratio is <1 and the sella is normal.
- Laboratory tests show elevated serum levels of both T_3 and T_4.

NONSECRETORY PITUITARY ADENOMA:
- Visual field testing
- Assessment of the pituitary and organ function to determine if there is hypopituitarism or hypersecretion of hormones (even if the effects of hypersecretion are subclinical)
- TRH to provoke secretion of FSH, LH, and LH-beta-subunit; will not elicit response in normal persons
- Exclusion of Klinefelter's syndrome in patient with longstanding primary hypogonadism, elevated gonadotropin levels, and enlargement of the sella

IMAGING STUDIES

Study of choice: MRI of the pituitary (Fig. E1-729) and hypothalamus
- When evaluating Cushing's disease, small size at the onset of symptoms noted
- MRI, in this case, only 60% sensitive at best and may yield false-positive results
- CT scan only when MRI is unavailable or is otherwise contraindicated

Rx TREATMENT

NONPHARMACOLOGIC THERAPY

SURGERY:
- Selective transsphenoidal resection of the adenoma (Table E1-395) is the treatment of choice for acromegaly, Cushing's disease, and thyrotropin-secreting pituitary adenomas, all of which tend to be microadenomas at the time of onset of symptoms.
- Macroadenomas, such as the nonsecretory pituitary adenoma, may also be surgically removed, but risk of recurrence is greater with these tumors and adjunctive therapy such as irradiation may also be necessary.
- Bilateral adrenalectomy has been performed in patients with Cushing's disease after failure of other therapies; complications requiring lifelong hormone replacement or Nelson's syndrome (rapid enlargement of pituitary tumor due to adrenal resection) may occur.

RADIOTHERAPY
- Radiotherapy is used primarily as adjuvant treatment. It is reserved for patients who have not responded to surgical treatment and who still have symptoms of the adenoma.
- Used with varying degrees of success in all the different pituitary adenomas
- Radiotherapy complications include long-term hypopituitarism (40% of patients) and secondary neoplasms (1.5% of patients).

ACUTE GENERAL Rx

PROLACTINOMA:
- Bromocriptine, a dopamine analogue, is generally given orally in divided doses of 1.5 to 10 mg. Cabergoline is given once or twice weekly. It is better tolerated and more effective than bromocriptine for tumor shrinkage but more expensive.
- Side effects include orthostatic hypotension, nausea, and dizziness; avoided by beginning with low-dose therapy.
- Other compounds include pergolide mesylate, a long-acting ergot derivative with dopaminergic properties, as well as other nonergot derivatives.

ACROMEGALY:
- Somatostatin analogues: octreotide, lanreotide administered as monthly injections
- Cabergoline or bromocriptine can also be used. They have modest activity but can be administered orally and are less expensive than somatostatin analogues.
- Pegvisomant can also be used to normalize IGF-1 levels.

CUSHING'S DISEASE:
- Ketoconazole, which inhibits the cytochrome P-450 enzymes involved in steroid biosynthesis, is effective in managing mild to moderate disease in daily oral doses of 600 to 1200 mg.
- Metyrapone and aminoglutethimide can be used to control hypersecretion of cortisol but are generally used when preparing a patient for surgery or while waiting for a response to radiotherapy.

THYROTROPIN-SECRETING PITUITARY ADENOMA:
- Ablative therapy with either radioactive iodide or surgery is indicated.
- Treatment directed to the thyroid alone may accelerate growth of the pituitary adenoma.
- Octreotide has been shown to be effective in doses similar to those used for acromegaly.

NONSECRETORY PITUITARY ADENOMA:
- There is no role for medical therapy at this time.
- Surgery and radiotherapy may be indicated. An algorithm for the management of nonfunctioning pituitary adenomas is described in Fig. 1-730.

CHRONIC Rx

For all pituitary adenomas:
- Careful follow-up is important. Patients undergoing transsphenoidal microsurgical resection should be seen in 4 to 6 wk to ensure that the adenoma has been completely removed and that the endocrine hypersecretion is resolved.

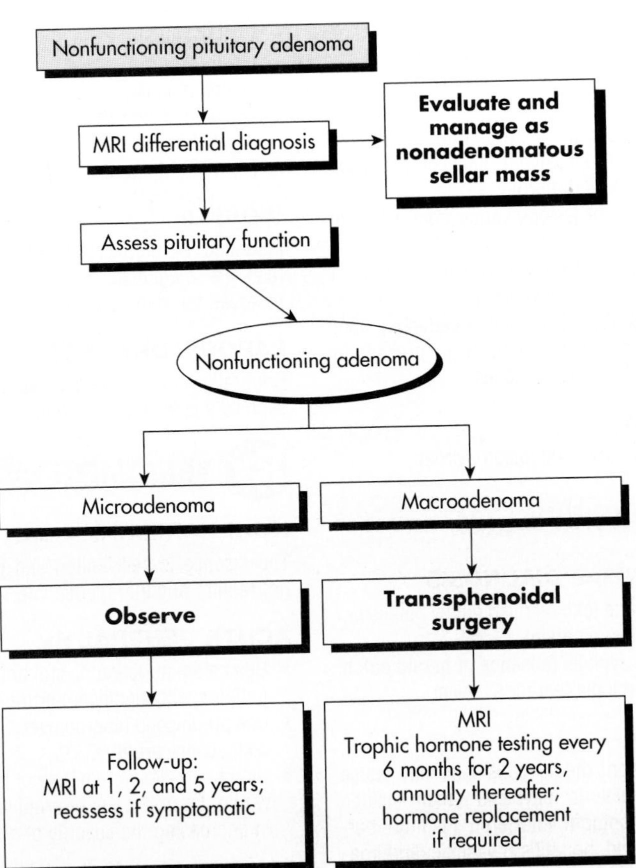

FIGURE 1-730 Management of nonfunctioning pituitary adenomas. Skilled interpretation of magnetic resonance images is crucial to diagnose a nonadenomatous mass such as a meningioma, aneurysm, or other sellar lesion. (From Melmed S et al: *Williams textbook of endocrinology*, ed 12, Philadelphia, 2011, Saunders.)

- If there is good clinical response, patient should be monitored yearly for recurrence and to follow the level of the hypersecreted hormone.
- Patients who have undergone irradiation should have close follow-up with backup medical therapy because response to radiotherapy may be delayed; incidence of hypopituitarism also increases with time.

SUGGESTED READINGS

available at www.expertconsult.com

RELATED CONTENT

Acromegaly (Related Key Topic)
Amenorrhea (Related Key Topic)
Cushing's Disease and Syndrome (Related Key Topic)
Galactorrhea (Related Key Topic)
Prolactinoma (Related Key Topic)
Evaluation of suspected pituitary tumor (Algorithm in Section II)
Pituitary Adenoma (Patient Information)

AUTHORS: **BETH J. WUTZ, M.D.,** and **RUBEN ALVERO, M.D.**

BASIC INFORMATION

DEFINITION

Pityriasis is a common self-limiting skin eruption of unknown etiology.

ICD-9CM CODES
696.3 Pityriasis rosea
ICD-10CM CODES
L42 Pityriasis rosea

EPIDEMIOLOGY & DEMOGRAPHICS

- Most cases of pityriasis rosea occur between ages 10 and 35 yr; mean age is 23 yr.
- The incidence of disease is highest in the fall and spring.
- Female/male ratio is 1.5:1.

PHYSICAL FINDINGS & CLINICAL PRESENTATION

- Initial lesion (herald patch), an annular pink patch with trailing scale, precedes the eruption by approximately 1 to 2 wk; typically measures 3 to 6 cm; it is round to oval in appearance and most frequently located on the trunk (Fig. 1-731).
- Eruptive phase follows within 2 wk and peaks after 7 to 14 days.
- Lesions are most frequently located in the lower abdominal area. They have a salmon-pink appearance in whites and a hyperpigmented appearance in blacks.
- Most lesions are 4 to 5 mm in diameter; center has a "cigarette paper" appearance; border has a characteristic ring of scale (collarette).
- Lesions occur in a symmetric distribution and follow the cleavage lines of the trunk (Christmas tree pattern).
- The number of lesions varies from a few to hundreds.
- Most patients are asymptomatic; pruritus is the most common symptom.
- History of recent fatigue, headache, sore throat, and low-grade fever is present in approximately 25% of cases.

ETIOLOGY

Unknown, possibly viral (picornavirus)

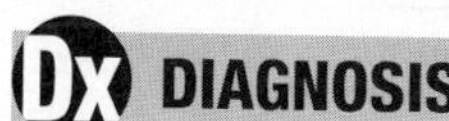

DIAGNOSIS

DIFFERENTIAL DIAGNOSIS

- Tinea corporis (can be ruled out by potassium hydroxide examination)
- Secondary syphilis (absence of herald patch, positive serologic test for syphilis)
- Psoriasis
- Nummular eczema
- Drug eruption: medications that may cause rashes similar to pityriasis rosea include clonidine, captopril, interferon, bismuth, barbiturates, gold, hepatitis B vaccine, and imatinib mesylate
- Viral exanthem
- Eczema
- Lichen planus
- Tinea versicolor (the lesions are more brown and the borders are not as ovoid)
- Erythema migrans

WORKUP

Presence of herald lesion and characteristic rash are diagnostic. Skin biopsy is generally reserved for atypical cases.

LABORATORY TESTS

Generally not necessary; serologic test for syphilis if clinically indicated

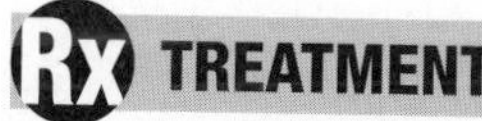

TREATMENT

NONPHARMACOLOGIC THERAPY

The disease is self-limited and generally does not require any therapeutic intervention.

ACUTE GENERAL Rx

- Use calamine lotion or oral antihistamines in patients with significant pruritus.
- Use prednisone tapered over 2 wk in patients with severe pruritus.
- Direct sun exposure or use of ultraviolet light within the first week of eruption is beneficial in decreasing the severity of disease.

DISPOSITION

- Spontaneous complete resolution of the rash within 4 to 8 wk
- Recurrence rare (<2% of cases)

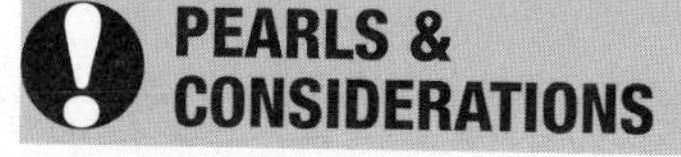

PEARLS & CONSIDERATIONS

COMMENTS

Reassure patient that the disease is not contagious and its course is benign.

SUGGESTED READINGS
available at www.expertconsult.com

RELATED CONTENT

Pityriasis Rosea (Patient Information)

AUTHOR: **FRED F. FERRI, M.D.**

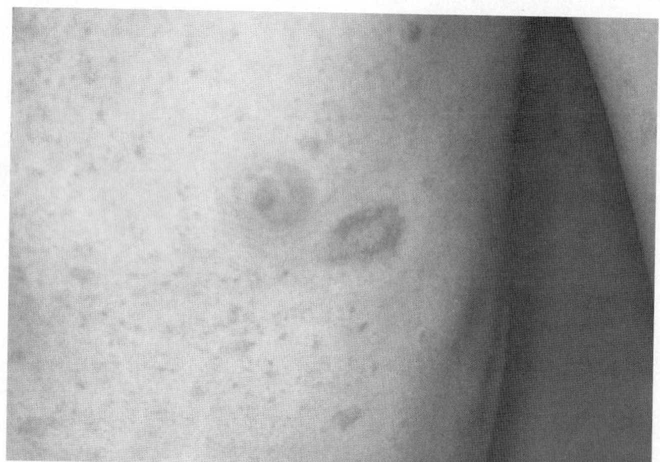

FIGURE 1-731 Herald patch and surrounding pityriasis rosea. (From Kliegman RM et al: *Nelson textbook of pediatrics,* ed 19, Philadelphia, 2011, Saunders.)

BASIC INFORMATION

DEFINITION

Placenta previa is the implantation of the placenta over the internal os. Four degrees of this abnormality (Fig. 1-732) have been traditionally defined; however, the accurate localization of the placental edge in relation to the discrete point of the internal os with transvaginal sonography makes the following terms outmoded:

1. Total placenta previa: the internal os is covered completely.
2. Partial placenta previa: the internal os is partially covered.
3. Marginal placenta previa: the edge of the placenta is at the margin of the internal os.
4. Low-lying placenta: the placenta is implanted in the lower uterine segment and, although its edge does not reach the internal os, is in close proximity to it.

ICD-9CM CODES
641.1 Placenta previa
ICD-10CM CODES
044 Placenta previa
044.0 Placenta previa specified as without hemorrhage
044.1 Placenta previa specified as with hemorrhage

EPIDEMIOLOGY & DEMOGRAPHICS

INCIDENCE: 0.26% to 0.7% of pregnancies

RISK FACTORS:
- Previous cesarean delivery (after one cesarean delivery, the risk is 1% to 4%; after four or more, the risk approaches 10%).
- Multiparity has also been associated with placenta previa.

PHYSICAL FINDINGS & CLINICAL PRESENTATION

The classic presentation of placenta previa is painless vaginal bleeding, usually in the second or third trimester. Uterine contractions may or may not be present. On physical examination, the uterus is soft and pain free. The fetus is often in breech, transverse lie, or high. Fetal distress is usually not present.

DIAGNOSIS

DIFFERENTIAL DIAGNOSIS

- Placenta accreta
- Placenta percreta
- Placenta increta
- Vasa previa
- Abruptio placentae
- Vaginal or cervical trauma
- Labor
- Local malignancy

WORKUP

- Do *not* perform a digital vaginal examination.
- The diagnosis of placenta previa can seldom be firmly established by physical examination alone. A speculum examination in a hospital setting to exclude any local bleeding may be performed.
- This diagnosis should not be dismissed until thorough evaluation, including sonography, has completely excluded its presence.

LABORATORY TESTS

- A complete blood count can be used to monitor hemoglobin and hematocrit.
- A Kleihauer-Betke preparation of maternal blood in all Rh-negative women and Rh-immune globulin when indicated

IMAGING STUDIES

- The simplest and safest method of placental localization is transabdominal sonography with confirmatory imaging by transvaginal ultrasonography (TVS). Transabdominal ultrasound alone is inaccurate in the diagnosis of placenta previa and should be used only as a screening tool. TVS has become the gold standard for the diagnosis of placenta previa. It is safe even in the presence of active bleeding. A distance of ≤20 mm from placental edge to interior cervical os is becoming a new criterion for performing term cesarean delivery in women with placenta previa.
- MRI has also been effective in detecting placenta previa, although sonography remains the preferred method.

TREATMENT

NONPHARMACOLOGIC THERAPY

- In preterm pregnancies with no active bleeding, close observation and expectant management are indicated. In those with active bleeding, conservative management, including blood transfusions for severe bleeds, is appropriate. The woman should stay in the hospital for at least 48 hr after the bleeding has stopped.
- Bed rest, preferably in a hospital setting, should be prescribed.

ACUTE GENERAL Rx

- Initial assessment for signs of maternal hemodynamic compromise or hemorrhagic shock; large-bore IV access with crystalloid fluid resuscitation
- Assess fetal status and gestational age by sonogram and continuous fetal heart rate monitoring
- Cross-matched blood should be made available during bleeding episodes; if the hemorrhage is severe, cesarean delivery is indicated despite fetal immaturity
- Tocolytic therapy may be considered in those women in preterm labor, as well as the administration of corticosteroids to enhance fetal lung maturity

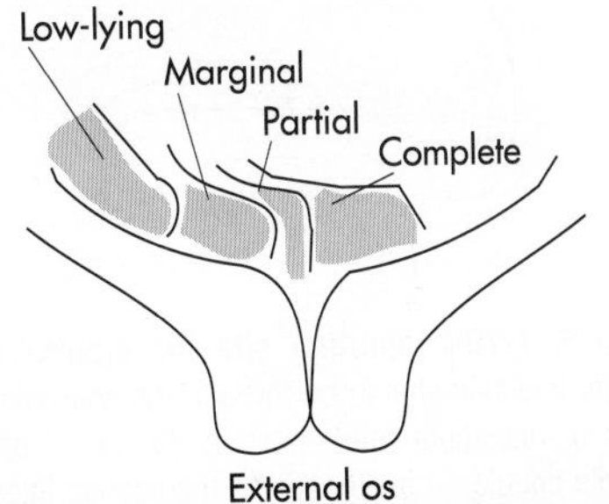

FIGURE 1-732 Depiction of degrees of placenta previa. (From Weissleder R et al: *Primer of diagnostic imaging,* St Louis, 2007, Mosby.)

CHRONIC Rx

- Cesarean delivery is necessary in nearly all cases of placenta previa.
- Uncontrollable hemorrhage after placental removal should be anticipated as a result of the poorly contractile nature of the lower uterine segment. The need for hysterectomy to control bleeding should be discussed with the patient before delivery, if possible.

DISPOSITION

Because of the unpredictable nature of placenta previa, not all women with placenta previa can be treated expectantly.

REFERRAL

Affected women and their families should be aware of all signs and symptoms that would necessitate immediate transport to the hospital. The possibility of hysterectomy should also be discussed early during pregnancy.

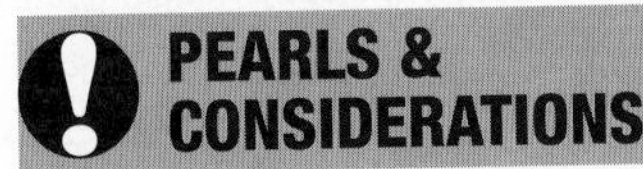

PEARLS & CONSIDERATIONS

COMMENTS

Third-trimester measurement of the distance from the placental edge to the internal cervical os by TVS commonly is used to gauge the likelihood of need for cesarean section. The decision to offer women with a placenta that is situated 11 to 20 mm away a trial of labor remains controversial. Recent reports by Vergani et al indicate that more than two thirds of women with a placental edge to cervical os distance of >10 mm fewer than 28 days before delivery can deliver vaginally without increased risk of hemorrhage

SUGGESTED READINGS

available at www.expertconsult.com

RELATED CONTENT

Vaginal Bleeding During Pregnancy (Related Key Topic)
Placenta Previa (Patient Information)

AUTHORS: **SONYA S. ABDEL-RAZEQ, M.D.,** and **RUBEN ALVERO, M.D.**

BASIC INFORMATION

DEFINITION

The plantar fascia arises from the calcaneal tuberosity and has various attachments as it travels longitudinally, ending at the digital level (Fig. 1-733). It acts as a tension band supporting the medial longitudinal arch of the foot. Plantar fasciitis describes the local inflammation and subsequent pain occurring at the insertion at the medial calcaneal tuberosity or along the course of the fascial band.

SYNONYMS

Heel pain syndrome

ICD-9CM CODES
728.71 Plantar fasciitis
726.73 Calcaneal spur
ICD-10CM CODES
M72.2 Plantar fascial fibromatosis
M77.30 Calcaneal spur, unspecified foot

EPIDEMIOLOGY & DEMOGRAPHICS

INCIDENCE: Plantar fasciitis affects >1 million persons/yr in the U.S. and two thirds of patients will seek care from their primary care physician for this condition. It is one of the more common causes of heel pain in adults.
PREDOMINANT SEX: Females slightly greater than males, studies vary
PREDOMINANT AGE: Commonly middle aged; any age group possible
RISK FACTORS: Weight gain, obesity (present in 90% of patients), increased activity, change in activity type, prolonged standing, hard surfaces, trauma, certain activities (see "Etiology").

PHYSICAL FINDINGS & CLINICAL PRESENTATION

- Pain is localized to the heel or along the course of the plantar fascia.
- Pain is greatest upon first steps in the morning and upon standing after rest (poststatic dyskinesia).
- Symptoms may improve throughout the day or with ambulation, but may persist or increase with prolonged standing.
- Pain may be elicited with ankle dorsiflexion and simultaneous subtalar eversion.
- Often exquisitely tender upon palpation of the medial calcaneal tuberosity
- May have localized or medial heel edema.

ETIOLOGY

- Any factor that increases the tension at the insertion of the fascia on the medial calcaneal tuberosity, creating local inflammation. Evidence suggests that plantar spurs are secondary rather than an etiology; these are an incidental finding in about 30% of asymptomatic patients.
- Achilles/ankle equinus or pseudoequinus
- Active STJ/rearfoot pronation, such as with calcaneal or forefoot varus
- A strain of the fascia or dorsiflexory force of the forefoot on the midfoot or vice versa. Example: jumping from a height, sprinting from starting blocks, reaching on a ladder.

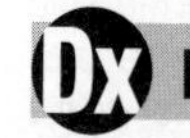

DIAGNOSIS

DIFFERENTIAL DIAGNOSIS

- Calcaneal fracture, including traumatic or stress fracture, or bone bruise
- Tarsal tunnel syndrome
- Calcaneal osteomyelitis
- Bone cyst or bone tumor
- Posterior tibial tendon dysfunction (often misdiagnosed as plantar fasciitis)
- Plantar fascial fibromatosis (thickening/soft tissue mass along the plantar fascial band)
- Systemic cause: gout, Paget's disease of the bone, psoriasis, Reiter's syndrome, etc.
- Plantar fascia rupture

STUDIES

- Weight-bearing x-rays: rule out tumor or trauma (lateral, oblique, calcaneal axial views)
- MRI/bone scan to rule out stress fracture (takes 2 wk to show on x-ray)
- MRI or ultrasound if suspected plantar fascial fibromatosis
- May need to rule out tarsal tunnel syndrome with nerve studies

TREATMENT

- Supportive lace-up sneakers with firm, cushioned sole. Weight loss for obese patients
- Ice, stretching exercises, NSAIDs, limit activity
- Low-dye strapping/taping
- Steroid/local anesthetic injections (Fig. 1-734) via several techniques. Although corticosteroid injection is often used to alleviate pain from plantar fasciitis, evidence supporting this treatment is limited. Trials have shown that pain improvement after steroid injection is slightly faster than placebo and benefits are likely to be short lived.
- Custom orthotics will limit subtalar joint overpronation and other faulty biomechanics.
- Add heel cushion to orthotics if acute pain/inflammation.
- Heel lifts if the etiology is Achilles equinus or pseudoequinus
- Night splints maintain ankle dorsiflexion overnight.
- Severe cases may require a cast or cast walker for 4 to 6 wk.
- Recalcitrant cases may require surgical endoscopic or open fasciotomy.

DISPOSITION

Cases that are treated sooner and acute cases with sudden onset have a higher likelihood of resolving completely. Chronic, recalcitrant cases may require surgery.

REFERRAL

- For biomechanical exam or surgical consult (podiatric/orthopedic foot/ankle surgeon)
- Physical therapy is often beneficial when first-line therapy fails.

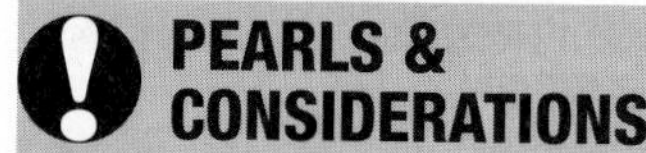

PEARLS & CONSIDERATIONS

COMMENTS

Caution: common, seemingly simple diagnosis. Do not overlook differential diagnosis.

PREVENTION

- Avoid shoes with bendable/flexible soles and shoes without laces/straps.
- Maintain foot/ankle flexibility with stretching exercises.
- Seek treatment at first signs of pain. Faster recovery rate with early diagnosis and treatment.

SUGGESTED READINGS

available at www.expertconsult.com

RELATED CONTENT

Plantar Fasciitis (Patient Information)

AUTHOR: **BROOKE E. KEELEY, D.P.M.**

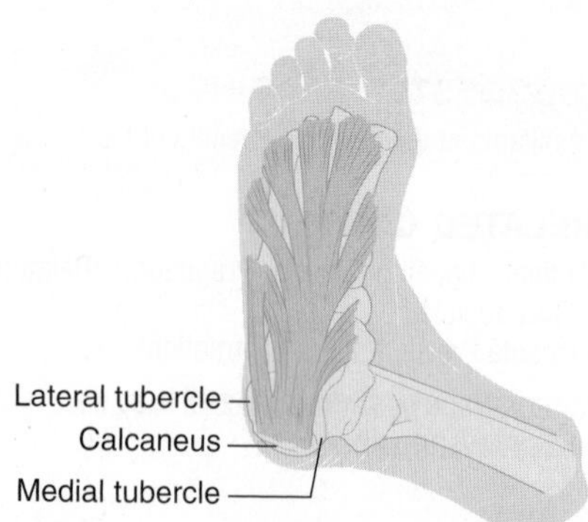

FIGURE 1-733 Plantar view of origin and insertion of plantar fascia. (From Frontera WR: *Essentials of physical medicine and rehabilitation*, ed 2, Philadelphia, 2008, Saunders.)

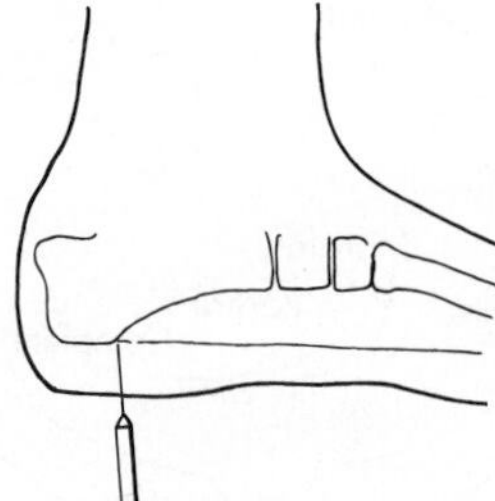

FIGURE 1-734 Injection site for plantar fasciitis. Injection should be through the sole into the area of maximum tenderness. A 25- or 27-gauge needle should be used and the medication injected slowly because some pain may occur. The total volume should be no greater than 1.5 ml. (From Mercier L: *Practical orthopedics*, ed 5, St Louis, 2002, Mosby.)

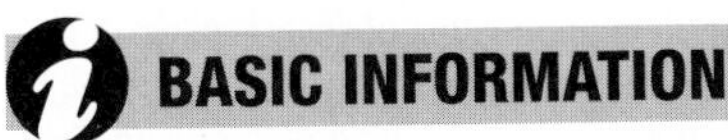

BASIC INFORMATION

DEFINITION

Pleurisy refers to the inflammation of the parietal pleura. This inflammation results in pleuritic chest pain that is characteristically worsened with respiration or movement.

SYNONYMS

Pleuritis

ICD-9CM CODES
511.0 Pleurisy
ICD-10CM CODES
R09.1 Pleurisy

EPIDEMIOLOGY & DEMOGRAPHICS

INCIDENCE: One of the most common causes of pleuritic chest pain is viral pleurisy. However, there are a variety of disorders that may result in pleurisy. Infectious diseases, rheumatologic disorders, thromboembolic events, and trauma may all lead to pleural inflammation. Therefore, the incidence of pleurisy varies in accordance with the underlying etiology.

PHYSICAL FINDINGS & CLINICAL PRESENTATION

- The defining characteristic of pleurisy is chest pain that worsens with respiration, coughing, or sneezing.
- Pleuritic chest pain is typically described as sharp or stabbing. However, pleuritic chest pain may also be described as dull pain, burning pain, or a "catch" while breathing.
- Movements of the trunk or chest wall may exacerbate pain. Patients with pleurisy may locate the position of minimal discomfort and remain still in that position.
- Dyspnea may be associated with pleurisy.
- Physical exam may be remarkable for a pleural friction rub.
- Decreased breath sounds, rales, or egophony may be appreciated if pneumonia is the underlying etiology of the patient's pleurisy.

ETIOLOGY

- Pleurisy is caused by inflammation of the parietal pleura. The visceral pleura is not innervated by nociceptors. However, injury or inflammation at the periphery of the lung parenchyma often results in inflammation of the overlying parietal pleura. The parietal pleura, which lines the rib cage and the lateral portion of each hemidiaphragm, is innervated by intercostal nerves; therefore pain is localized to the cutaneous distribution of those nerves (over the chest wall). The parietal pleura of the central diaphragm is innervated by fibers that travel with the phrenic nerve; therefore pain associated with inflammation in this area is referred to the ipsilateral shoulder or neck.
- Various underlying etiologies may result in pleurisy, including:
  1. Thromboembolism (pulmonary embolism)
  2. Viral infection (coxsackieviruses, respiratory syncytial virus [RSV], cytomegalovirus [CMV], adenovirus, Epstein-Barr virus [EBV], parainfluenza, influenza)
  3. Bacterial infection (pneumonia or tuberculous pleuritis)
  4. Fungal infection (coccidioidomycosis, histoplasmosis)
  5. Rheumatologic disease (rheumatoid arthritis, systemic lupus erythematosus [SLE])
  6. Medications
  7. Malignancy of the lung or pleura
  8. Trauma (rib fracture)
  9. Hereditary (familial Mediterranean fever, sickle cell disease)

Dx DIAGNOSIS

DIFFERENTIAL DIAGNOSIS

- Cardiac: myocardial infarction, ischemia, pericarditis
- Intraabdominal process: pancreatitis, cholecystitis
- Thromboembolic: pulmonary embolism, infarction of lung parenchyma
- Traumatic/mechanical: rib fracture or pneumothorax
- Viral infection: viral infections may lead to epidemic pleurodynia (also known as Bornholm's disease). Implicated viruses include coxsackieviruses, RSV, CMV, adenovirus, EBV, parainfluenza, influenza. Of note, viral pleurisy is a diagnosis of exclusion.
- Bacterial infection: pneumonia or tuberculous pleurisy
- Fungal infection: coccidioidomycosis, histoplasmosis
- Rheumatologic disease: rheumatoid arthritis, SLE
- Medications: drug-induced lupus
- Hereditary causes: familial Mediterranean fever, sickle cell disease
- Malignancy: malignancy affecting the lung or pleura
- Uremia

WORKUP

- A thorough history and physical exam of all patients presenting with pleuritic chest pain should be taken. The time course of the patient's symptoms can provide valuable diagnostic clues. Acute onset of symptoms is suggestive of traumatic injuries, spontaneous pneumothorax, pulmonary embolism, or myocardial infarction. Subacute onset of symptoms suggests a potential infectious, rheumatologic, or medication-induced cause. Viral pleurisy is often associated with prodromal symptoms of upper respiratory infection. Chronic or recurrent symptoms suggest a potential malignant, tuberculous, or hereditary cause.
- Chest x-ray to evaluate for pneumonia, pneumothorax, or pleural effusion
- ECG to evaluate for infarction, ischemia, or pericarditis
- Evaluation for pulmonary embolism should be undertaken if clinical suspicion exists.

LABORATORY TESTS

- Laboratory testing varies based on suspected underlying etiology.
- If a pleural effusion is present, diagnostic thoracentesis may provide valuable diagnostic clues to the underlying etiology.

IMAGING STUDIES

- Chest x-ray
- ECG

Rx TREATMENT

- Treatment of pleurisy consists of pain control as well as treating the underlying condition.
- NSAIDs are the preferred first-line agent to control pain associated with pleurisy. Human studies have been limited to trials using indomethacin for pain control, although an NSAID class effect is presumed.
- Indomethacin 50 mg orally up to three times a day has been found to be effective in relieving pain and is associated with an improvement in mechanical lung function.

SUGGESTED READINGS

available at www.expertconsult.com

AUTHOR: **MARISA E. VAN POZNAK, M.D.**

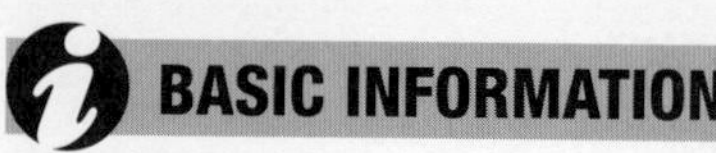

BASIC INFORMATION

DEFINITION

Aspiration pneumonia is a vague term that refers to pulmonary abnormalities following abnormal entry of endogenous or exogenous substances in the lower airways. It is generally classified as:

- Aspiration (chemical pneumonitis)
- Primary bacterial aspiration pneumonia
- Secondary bacterial infection of chemical pneumonitis

ICD-9CM CODES
507.0 Aspiration pneumonia
ICD-10CM CODES
J69.0 Pneumonitis due to inhalation of food and vomit

EPIDEMIOLOGY & DEMOGRAPHICS

INCIDENCE (IN U.S.):

- Few reliable data
- 20% to 35% of all pneumonias
- 5% to 15% of all community-acquired pneumonias

PEAK INCIDENCE: Elderly patients in hospitals or nursing homes

PREVALENCE (IN U.S.): Unknown (unreliable data)

PREDOMINANT SEX: Males and females affected equally

PREDOMINANT AGE: Elderly

PHYSICAL FINDINGS & CLINICAL PRESENTATION

- Shortness of breath, tachypnea, cough, sputum, fever after vomiting, or difficulty swallowing
- Rales, rhonchi, often diffusely throughout lung

ETIOLOGY

Complex interaction of etiologies, ranging from chemical (often acid) pneumonitis after aspiration of sterile gastric contents (generally not requiring antibiotic treatment) to bacterial aspiration

COMMUNITY-ACQUIRED ASPIRATION PNEUMONIA:

- Generally results from predominantly anaerobic mouth bacteria (anaerobic and microaerophilic streptococci, fusobacteria, gram-positive anaerobic non–spore-forming rods), *Bacteroides* species *(melaninogenicus, intermedius, oralis, ureolyticus), Haemophilus influenzae,* and *Streptococcus pneumoniae*
- Rarely caused by *Bacteroides fragilis* (of uncertain validity in published studies) or *Eikenella corrodens*
- High-risk groups: the elderly; alcoholics; IV drug users; patients who are obtunded; stroke victims; and those with esophageal disorders, seizures, poor dentition, or recent dental manipulations.

HOSPITAL-ACQUIRED ASPIRATION PNEUMONIA:

- Often occurs among elderly patients and others with diminished gag reflex; those with nasogastric tubes, intestinal obstruction, or ventilator support; and especially those exposed to contaminated nebulizers or unsterile suctioning.
- High-risk groups: seriously ill hospitalized patients (especially patients with coma, acidosis, alcoholism, uremia, diabetes mellitus, nasogastric intubation, or recent antimicrobial therapy, who are frequently colonized with aerobic gram-negative rods); patients undergoing anesthesia; those with strokes, dementia, or swallowing disorders; the elderly; and those receiving antacids or H_2 blockers (but not sucralfate).
- Hypoxic patients receiving concentrated O_2 have diminished ciliary activity, encouraging aspiration.
- Causative organisms:
  1. Anaerobes listed above, although in many studies gram-negative aerobes (60%) and gram-positive aerobes (20%) predominate.
  2. *E. coli, P. aeruginosa, S. aureus* including MRSA, *Klebsiella, Enterobacter, Serratia, Proteus* spp., *H. influenzae, S. pneumoniae, Legionella,* and *Acinetobacter* spp. (sporadic pneumonias) in two thirds of cases.
  3. Fungi, including *Candida albicans,* in fewer than 1%.

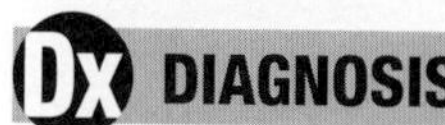

DIAGNOSIS

DIFFERENTIAL DIAGNOSIS

- Other necrotizing or cavitary pneumonias (especially tuberculosis, gram-negative pneumonias)
- See "Pulmonary Tuberculosis."

WORKUP

- Chest x-ray examination
- Complete blood count (CBC), blood cultures
- Sputum Gram stain and culture
- Consideration of tracheal aspirate

LABORATORY TESTS

- CBC: leukocytosis often present
- Sputum Gram stain
  1. Often useful when carefully prepared immediately after obtaining suctioned or expectorated specimen, examined by experienced observer.
  2. Only specimens with multiple white blood cells and rare or absent epithelial cells should be examined.
  3. Unlike nonaspiration pneumonias (e.g., pneumococcal), multiple organisms may be present.
  4. Long, slender rods suggest anaerobes.
  5. Sputum from pneumonia caused by acid aspiration may be devoid of organisms.
  6. Cultures should be interpreted in light of morphology of visualized organisms.

IMAGING STUDIES

- Chest x-ray often reveals bilateral, diffuse, patchy infiltrates and posterior segment upper lobes. Chemical pneumonitis typically affects the most dependent regions of the lungs.
- Aspiration pneumonia of several days' or longer duration may reveal necrosis (especially community-acquired anaerobic pneumonias) and even cavitation with air-fluid levels, indicating lung abscess.

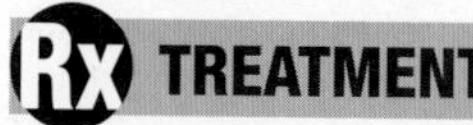

TREATMENT

NONPHARMACOLOGIC THERAPY

- Airway management to prevent repeated aspiration
- Ventilatory support if necessary

ACUTE GENERAL Rx

Acute aspiration of acidic gastric contents without bacteria may not require antibiotic therapy; consult infectious disease or pulmonary expert.

- Community-acquired anaerobic aspiration pneumonia: clindamycin (600 mg IV twice daily followed by 300 mg q6h orally). Intravenous penicillin G (1 to 2 million U q4 to 6h) can also still be used. Alternative oral agents include: amoxicillin-clavulanate (875 mg orally twice daily), amoxicillin plus metronidazole or oral moxifloxacin (400 mg orally once daily). Do not use metronidazole alone, as this is associated with high failure rates.
- Nursing home aspirations: levofloxacin 500-750 mg qd or piperacillin-tazobactam 3.375 g q6h or ceftazidime 2 g q8h +/− vancomycin if MRSA suspected or known
- Hospital-acquired aspiration pneumonia:
  - Piperacillin-tazobactam 3.375 g IV q6h, or cefoxitin 2 g IV q8h +/− vancomycin IV to cover MRSA. Alternative agents are ceftriaxone 1 g IV q24h *plus* metronidazole 500 mg IV q6h or 1 g IV q12h.
  - Knowledge of resident flora in the microenvironment of the aspiration within the hospital is crucial to intelligent antibiotic selection; consult infection control nurses or hospital epidemiologist.
  - Confirmed *Pseudomonas* pneumonia should be treated with antipseudomonal beta-lactam agent plus an aminoglycoside until antimicrobial sensitivities confirm that less toxic agents may replace the aminoglycoside.
  - Do not use metronidazole alone for anaerobes.

DISPOSITION

Repeat chest x-ray examination in 6 to 8 wk.

REFERRAL

For consultation with infectious disease and/or pulmonary experts for patients with respiratory distress, hypoxia, ventilatory support, pneumonia in more than one lobe, or necrosis or cavitation on x-ray examination or for those not responding to antibiotic therapy within 2 to 3 days.

SUGGESTED READINGS

available at www.expertconsult.com

RELATED CONTENT

Aspiration Pneumonia (Patient Information)

AUTHOR: **GLENN G. FORT, M.D., M.P.H.**

BASIC INFORMATION

DEFINITION

Bacterial pneumonia is an infection involving the lung parenchyma.

ICD-9CM CODES
486.0 Pneumonia, acute
507.0 Pneumonia, aspiration
482.9 Pneumonia, bacterial
481 Pneumonia, pneumococcal
482.1 Pneumonia, *Pseudomonas*
482.4 Pneumonia, staphylococcal
482.0 Pneumonia, *Klebsiella*
482.2 Pneumonia, *Haemophilus influenzae*
ICD-10CM CODES
J15.9 Unspecified bacterial pneumonia
J69.0 Pneumonitis due to inhalation of food and vomit
J15.9 Unspecified bacterial pneumonia
J13 Pneumonia due to *Streptococcus pneumoniae*
J15.1 Pneumonia due to *Pseudomonas*
J15.20 Pneumonia due to staphylococcus, unspecified
J15.0 Pneumonia due to *Klebsiella pneumoniae*
J14 Pneumonia due to *Haemophilus influenzae*

EPIDEMIOLOGY & DEMOGRAPHICS

- The incidence of community-acquired pneumonia (CAP) is 1 in 100 persons. CAP is the most common infectious cause of death in the U.S.
- The incidence of health care facility–acquired pneumonia (HCAP) is 8 cases per 1000 persons annually.
- Primary care physicians see an average of 10 cases of pneumonia annually.
- Hospitalization rate for pneumonia is 15% to 20%.
- Most cases of pneumonia occur in the winter and in elderly patients.

PHYSICAL FINDINGS & CLINICAL PRESENTATION

- Fever, tachypnea, chills, tachycardia, cough
- Presentation varies with the cause of pneumonia, the patient's age, and the clinical situation:
  - Patients with streptococcal pneumonia usually present with high fever, shaking chills, pleuritic chest pain, cough, and copious production of rusty-appearing purulent sputum. Pleurisy and parapneumonic effusions are also common. Potential complications include bacteremia, empyema, and distant infections (e.g., meningitis).
  - *Mycoplasma pneumoniae:* insidious onset; headache; dry, paroxysmal cough that is worse at night; myalgias; malaise; sore throat; extrapulmonary manifestations (e.g., erythema multiforme, aseptic meningitis, urticaria, erythema nodosum) may be present.
  - *Chlamydia pneumoniae:* persistent, nonproductive cough, low-grade fever, headache, sore throat.
  - *Legionella pneumophila:* high fever, mild cough, mental status change, myalgias, diarrhea, respiratory failure.
  - MRSA pneumonia: often preceded by influenza, may present with shock and respiratory failure.
  - Elderly or immunocompromised hosts with pneumonia may initially present with only minimal symptoms (e.g., low-grade fever, confusion); respiratory and nonrespiratory symptoms are less commonly reported by older patients with pneumonia.
  - In general, auscultation of patients with pneumonia reveals crackles and diminished breath sounds.
  - Percussion dullness is present if the patient has pleural effusion.
  - The clinical impression of pneumonia has an overall sensitivity of 70% to 90%; specificity ranges from 40% to 70%.

ETIOLOGY

- *Streptococcus pneumoniae* (20% to 60% of CAP cases)
- *Haemophilus influenzae* (3% to 10% of CAP cases)
- *L. pneumophila* (1% to 5% of adult pneumonias) (2% to 8% of CAP cases)
- *Klebsiella, Pseudomonas, Escherichia coli*
- *Staphylococcus aureus* (3% to 5% of CAP cases)
- Atypical organisms such as *M. pneumoniae, C. pneumoniae,* and *L. pneumophila* implicated in up to 40% of cases of CAP
- Pneumococcal infection responsible for 50% to 75% of CAPs. Influenza infection is one of the important predisposing factors to *S. pneumoniae* and *S. aureus* pneumonia; gram-negative organisms cause >80% of nosocomial pneumonias
- Predisposing factors:
  1. Chronic obstructive pulmonary disease: *H. influenzae, S. pneumoniae, Legionella*
  2. Seizures: aspiration pneumonia
  3. Compromised hosts: *Legionella,* gram-negative organisms
  4. Alcoholism: *Klebsiella, S. pneumoniae, H. influenzae*
  5. HIV: *S. pneumoniae*
  6. IV drug addicts with right-sided bacterial endocarditis: *S. aureus*
  7. Older patient with comorbid diseases: *C. pneumoniae*

DIAGNOSIS

DIFFERENTIAL DIAGNOSIS

- Exacerbation of chronic bronchitis
- Pulmonary embolism or infarction
- Lung neoplasm
- Bronchiolitis
- Sarcoidosis
- Hypersensitivity pneumonitis
- Pulmonary edema
- Drug-induced lung injury
- Viral pneumonias
- Fungal pneumonias
- Parasitic pneumonias
- Atypical pneumonia
- Tuberculosis

WORKUP

Laboratory evaluation and chest x-ray. Table E1-396 summarizes diagnostic testing for CAP. Useful tools for assessing severity of illness are the *CURB-65* (see following) and *Pneumonia Severity Index.* Poor prognostic indicators are hypotension (SBP <90 or DBP <60), respiratory rate >30/min, hyperpyrexia (>40° C), or hypothermia (<35° C). None of these indices is as valuable as clinical judgment of the physician.

LABORATORY TESTS

- Complete blood count with differential; white blood cell count is elevated, usually with left shift
- Blood cultures (hospitalized patients only): positive in approximately 20% of cases of pneumococcal pneumonia
- Pneumococcal urinary antigen test can be used to detect the C-polysaccharide antigen of *S. pneumoniae.* It is a useful tool in the treatment of hospitalized adult patients with CAP.
- Direct immunofluorescent examination of sputum when suspecting *Legionella* (e.g., direct fluorescent antibody stain is a highly specific and rapid test for detecting legionellae in clinical specimen) or urine *Legionella* antigen test
- Serologic testing for HIV in selected patients
- Serum electrolytes (hyponatremia in suspected *Legionella* pneumonia), BUN, creatinine
- Pulse oximetry or arterial blood gases: hypoxemia with partial pressure of oxygen <60 mm Hg while the patient is breathing room air, a standard criterion for hospital admission

IMAGING STUDIES

Chest x-ray (Fig. 1-735): findings vary with the stage and type of pneumonia and the hydration of the patient:

- Classically, pneumococcal pneumonia presents with a segmental lobe infiltrate.
- Diffuse infiltrates on chest x-ray can be seen with *L. pneumophila, M. pneumoniae,* viral pneumonias, *P. jirovecii (carinii),* miliary tuberculosis, aspiration, aspergillosis.
- An initial chest x-ray is also useful to rule out the presence of any complications (pneumothorax, empyema, abscesses).

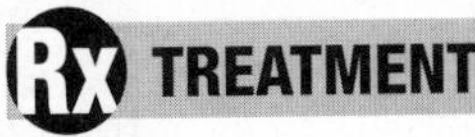

TREATMENT

NONPHARMACOLOGIC THERAPY

- Avoidance of tobacco use
- Oxygen to maintain partial oxygen pressure in arterial blood >60 mm Hg
- IV hydration, correction of dehydration
- Assisted ventilation in patients with significant respiratory failure

ACUTE GENERAL Rx

- Initial antibiotic therapy should be based on clinical, radiographic, and laboratory evaluation.
- Macrolides (azithromycin or clarithromycin) or levofloxacin is recommended for empiric outpatient treatment of CAP. Box E1-65 summarizes empirical therapy regimens for severe CAP. Cefotaxime or a beta-lactam/beta-lactamase inhibitor can be added in patients with more severe presentation who insist on outpatient therapy. Duration of treatment ranges from 7 to 14 days. The treatment of choice in suspected *Legionella* pneumonia is either a quinolone (e.g., moxifloxacin) or a macrolide (e.g., azithromycin) antibiotic.
- In the hospital setting, patients admitted to the general ward can be treated empirically with a second- or third-generation cephalosporin (ceftriaxone, ceftizoxime, cefotaxime, or cefuroxime) plus a macrolide (azithromycin or clarithromycin) or doxycycline. An antipseudomonal quinolone (levofloxacin or moxifloxacin) can be substituted in place of the macrolide or doxycycline.
- Empiric therapy in ICU patients: IV beta-lactam (ceftriaxone, cefotaxime, ampicillin-sulbactam) plus an IV quinolone (levofloxacin, moxifloxacin) or IV azithromycin.
- In hospitalized patients at risk for *P. aeruginosa* infection, empiric treatment should consist of an antipseudomonal beta-lactam (meropenem, doripenem, imipenem, or piperacillin-tazobactam) plus an aminoglycoside plus an antipseudomonal quinolone.
- In patients with suspected methicillin-resistant *S. aureus,* vancomycin or linezolid is effective.

CHRONIC Rx

Parapneumonic effusion empyema can be managed with chest tube placement for drainage. Instillation of fibrinolytic agents (streptokinase, urokinase) by chest tube may be necessary in resistant cases.

DISPOSITION

- Most patients respond well to antibiotic therapy. Risk factors for a poor outcome from CAP are summarized in Box E1-66.
- Indications for hospital admission are:
  1. Hypoxemia (oxygen saturation <90% while patient is breathing room air)
  2. Hemodynamic instability
  3. Inability to tolerate medications
  4. Active coexisting condition requiring hospitalization.

  A criterion often used to determine hospital admission is known as the "CURB-65": **C**onfusion, B**U**N >19.6 mg/dl, **R**espiratory rate >30 breaths/min, systolic **B**P <90 mg Hg, and diastolic BP ≤60 mm Hg, age ≥**65**. Patients are generally admitted to the hospital if they fulfill 2 or more criteria and to the ICU if they have 3 or more criteria

PEARLS & CONSIDERATIONS

COMMENTS

- Use of gastric acid suppressive therapy (H_2 receptor antagonists, proton pump inhibitors [PPIs]) has been associated with an increased risk of CAP. It appears that PPI therapy started within the previous 30 days is associated with an increased risk for CAP, whereas longer-term current use is not.
- Causes of slowly resolving or nonresolving pneumonia:
  1. Difficult to treat infections: viral pneumonia, *Legionella,* pneumococci or staphylococci with impaired host response, tuberculosis, fungi
  2. Neoplasm: lung, lymphoma, metastasis
  3. Congestive heart failure
  4. Pulmonary embolism
  5. Immunologic or idiopathic: Wegener granulomatosis, pulmonary eosinophilic syndromes, systemic lupus erythematosus
  6. Drug toxicity (e.g., amiodarone)
- If patients with pneumonia are not doing well, repeat films should be taken promptly. In those with complete clinical recovery, it is reasonable to wait 6 to 8 wk before repeating the radiograph to document clearing of the infiltrate. The benefit of routine radiography after pneumonia has been questioned due to the low 1 yr incidence of lung cancer. Opponents propose a selective approach limiting follow-up chest x-ray to middle-aged and older adults.

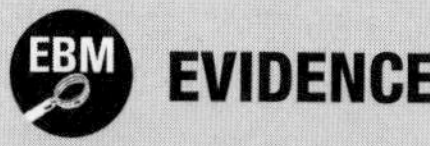

EVIDENCE

available at www.expertconsult.com

SUGGESTED READINGS

available at www.expertconsult.com

RELATED CONTENT

Bacterial Pneumonia (Patient Information)

AUTHOR: **FRED F. FERRI, M.D.**

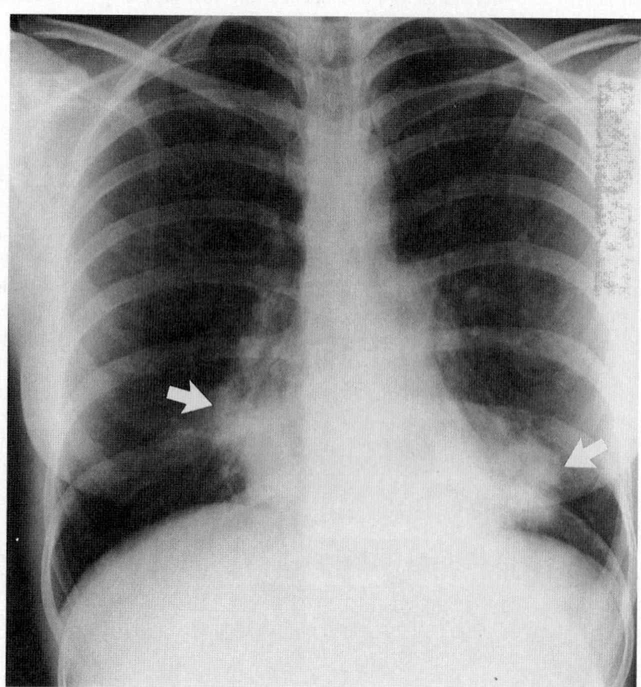

FIGURE 1-735 *Streptococcus pneumoniae* pneumonia, bilateral lower zone consolidation *(arrows).* Although penumococcal pneumonia is typically unifocal, multifocal involvement is not uncommon. (From Grainger RG et al: *Grainger and Allison's diagnostic radiology,* ed 4, London, 2001, Harcourt.)

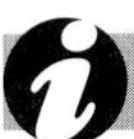

BASIC INFORMATION

DEFINITION

Mycoplasma pneumonia is an infection of the lung parenchyma caused by a small bacterium, *Mycoplasma pneumoniae.*

SYNONYMS

Primary atypical pneumonia
Eaton's pneumonia
Walking pneumonia

ICD-9CM CODES
483 *Mycoplasma* pneumonia
ICD-10CM CODES
J15.7 Pneumonia due to *Mycoplasma pneumoniae*

EPIDEMIOLOGY & DEMOGRAPHICS

INCIDENCE (IN U.S.):
- It is a frequent cause of community-acquired pneumonia. CDC estimates 2 million cases a yr with 100,000 pneumonia-related hospitalizations.
- Many cases probably resolve without coming to medical attention.
- Incidence is estimated at one case per 1000 persons annually.
- Incidence is estimated to at least triple every (approximately) 5 yr during epidemics.

PEAK INCIDENCE:
- Some increased incidence in fall to early winter
- Seems more prevalent in temperate climates

PREVALENCE (IN U.S.):
- Estimated to be present in one in every five patients hospitalized for pneumonia (generally a self-limited disease, so its true prevalence is unknown)
- Estimated to cause 7% of all cases of pneumonia and approximately half the cases in those aged 5 to 20 yr

PREDOMINANT SEX: Equal distribution
PREDOMINANT AGE:
- Most commonly affected: school-age children and young adults (ages 5 to 20 yr)
- Occurs in older adults as well, especially with household exposure to a young child
- More severe infections in affected elderly patients

GENETICS: Familial disposition:
- None known
- May be more severe in patients with sickle cell anemia

Neonatal infection: severe respiratory distress, sometimes requiring intubation, attributed to this disease in infants.

PHYSICAL FINDINGS & CLINICAL PRESENTATION

- Nonexudative pharyngitis (common)
- Headache, otalgia common
- Fever may be mild or not present
- Rhonchi or rales without evidence of consolidation (common) in lower lung zones
- Associated with bullous myringitis (nonspecific finding; perhaps no more frequently than in other pneumonias)
- Skin rashes in up to one fourth of patients
  1. Morbilliform
  2. Urticaria
  3. Erythema nodosum (unusual)
  4. Erythema multiforme (unusual)
  5. Stevens-Johnson syndrome (rare)
- Muscle tenderness (<50% of the patients)
- On examination (and confirmed with testing):
  1. Mononeuritis or polyneuritis
  2. Transverse myelitis
  3. Cranial nerve palsies
  4. Meningoencephalitis
- Lymphadenopathy and splenomegaly
- Conjunctivitis
- Table 1-397 summarizes the clinical manifestations of *Mycoplasma pneumoniae.*

ETIOLOGY

Infection is spread person-to-person via respiratory droplets or secretions with an incubation period of 1 to 4 wk.

Dx DIAGNOSIS

DIFFERENTIAL DIAGNOSIS

- *Chlamydia* (now known as *Chlamydophila*) *pneumoniae*
- *Chlamydophila psittaci*
- *Legionella* spp.
- *Coxiella burnetii*
- Several viral agents
- Q fever
- *Streptococcus pneumoniae*
- Pulmonary embolism or infarction

WORKUP

- Chest x-ray
- Thorough history and physical examination
- Laboratory tests
- Evaluation guided by symptoms and findings

TABLE 1-397 Clinical Manifestations of *Mycoplasma Pneumoniae* Infection

Respiratory tract	Pharyngitis, laryngitis, acute bronchitis, bronchopneumonia
Skin and mucosa	Maculopapular and vesicular exanthema, urticaria, purpura, erythema nodosum, erythema multiforme, Stevens-Johnson syndrome
Central nervous system	Meningitis, meningoencephalitis, acute psychosis, cerebellitis, Guillain-Barré syndrome?
Parenchymatous organs	Pancreatitis, diabetes mellitus, nonspecific reactive hepatitis, subacute thyroiditis?
Miscellaneous	Hemorrhagic bullous myringitis, hemolytic anemia, pericarditis, thromboembolism?

Some association remains uncertain.
From Cohen J, Powderly WG: *Infectious diseases,* ed 2, St Louis, 2004, Mosby.

LABORATORY TESTS

- White blood cells (WBCs):
  1. WBC count $>10,000/mm^3$ in approximately one fourth of patients
  2. Differential count nonspecific
  3. Leukopenia rare
- Cold agglutinins:
  1. Detected in approximately half of the patients
  2. Also may be found in:
     a. Lymphoproliferative diseases
     b. Influenza
     c. Mononucleosis
     d. Adenovirus infections
     e. Occasionally, Legionnaires' disease
  3. Titers typically >1:64
     a. May be detectable with bedside testing
     b. Appear between days 5 and 10 of the illness (so may be demonstrable when patient is first examined) and disappear within 1 mo
- Complement fixation testing assay specific for mycoplasm antigens of paired sera (fourfold rise) or a single titer ≥1:32 in patients with pneumonia and a compatible history:
  1. Considered diagnostic in the appropriate clinical setting
  2. Other assays include ELISA, antigen capture-enzyme immunoassay, and PCR
- Culture of the organism from specimens
  1. Only truly specific test for infection
  2. Technically difficult and done reliably by few laboratories
  3. May require weeks to get results
- Sputum
  1. Often no sputum produced for laboratory testing
  2. When present, Gram-stained specimens show polymorphonuclear cells without organisms
- Infection occasionally complicated by pancreatitis or glomerulitis
- Disseminated intravascular coagulation is a rare complication
- Electrocardiographic evidence of pericarditis or myocarditis may be present

IMAGING STUDIES

- Predilection for lower lobe involvement (upper lobes involved in less than a fourth), with radiographic abnormalities frequently out of proportion to those on physical examination (Fig. 1-736)
- Small pleural effusions in approximately 30% of patients
- Large effusions: rare
- Infiltrates: patchy, unilateral, and with a segmental distribution, although multilobar involvement may be seen
- Evidence of hilar adenopathy on chest radiographs in 20% to 25%
- Rare cases reported:
  1. Associated lung abscess
  2. Residual pneumatoceles
  3. Lobar collapse
  4. Hyperlucent lung syndrome

 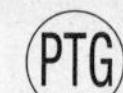

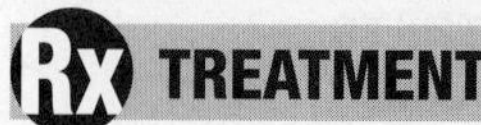

TREATMENT

ACUTE GENERAL Rx

- Therapy: azithromycin 500 mg qd × 3 or 500 mg initially, then 250 mg daily for 4 days for adults. For children: 10 mg/kg in one dose on first day, then 5 mg/kg in one dose for 4 days or clarithromycin: 500 mg bid for 10 days in adults, 15 mg/kg per day in two divided doses for 10 days in children. Alternatives include erythromycin (500 mg qid) for adults or 30 to 40 mg/kg per day in four divided doses in children or doxycycline: 2 to 4 mg/kg per day in one or two divided doses for 10 days, maximum daily dose: 100 to 200 mg, but this agent cannot be used in young children or women of childbearing age. Respiratory fluoroquinolones such as Levaquin or moxifloxacin are alternative agents for treatment in adults but should not be used in young children.
- Therapy shortens the duration and severity of symptoms and may hasten radiographic clearing, but the disease is self-limiting.

CHRONIC Rx

- Effective antimicrobial therapy does not eliminate the organism from the respiratory secretions, which may be positive for weeks.
- Serum antibody response does not necessarily provide lifelong immunity.
- Chronic symptoms do not occur, although clinical relapses may occur 7 to 10 days after the initial response and may be associated with new areas of infiltration.

DISPOSITION

- Clinical improvement is almost universal within 10 days.
- Infiltrates generally clear within 5 to 8 wk.
- Rare deaths are likely attributable to underlying medical diseases.
- Person-to-person spread can be minimized by avoiding open coughing, especially in enclosed areas.

REFERRAL

- Not responding to treatment
- Severe infection
- Severe extrapulmonary manifestations
- Multilobe involvement accompanied by respiratory embarrassment (very rare)

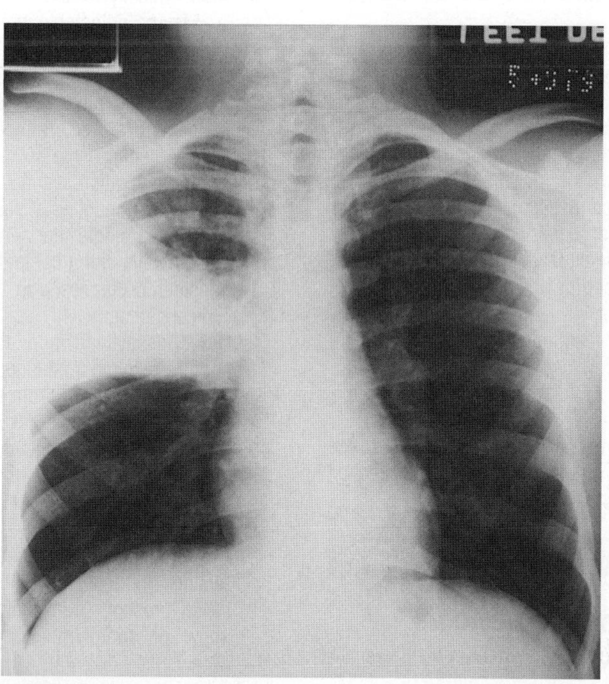

FIGURE 1-736 Localized airspace opacification resulting from *Mycoplasma pneumoniae.* (From Specht N [ed]: *Practical guide to diagnostic imaging,* St Louis, 1998, Mosby.)

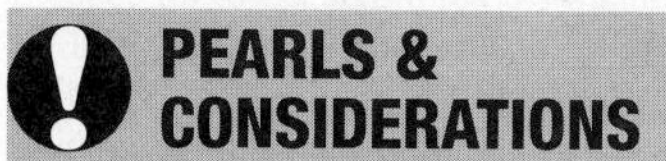

PEARLS & CONSIDERATIONS

COMMENTS

X-ray resolution complete by 8 wk in approximately 90% of patients.

SUGGESTED READINGS

available at www.expertconsult.com

RELATED CONTENT

Mycoplasma Pneumonia (Patient Information)

AUTHOR: **GLENN G. FORT, M.D., M.P.H.**

BASIC INFORMATION

DEFINITION

Pneumocystis jirovecii pneumonia (PJP) is a serious respiratory infection caused by the fungal or protozoal organism *P. jirovecii* (formerly known as *P. carinii*).

SYNONYMS

PCP
PJP

ICD-9CM CODES
136.3 *Pneumocystis jirovecii (P. carinii)* pneumonia
ICD-10CM CODES
B59 Pneumocystosis

EPIDEMIOLOGY & DEMOGRAPHICS

INCIDENCE (IN U.S.):
- Seen primarily in the setting of AIDS.
- Approximately 11 cases per 100 patient-years among HIV-infected patients with CD4 lymphocyte counts <100/mm^3.
- Also seen in other immunocompromised patients with severe cell-mediated immune deficiency (congenital T-cell deficiency, acute leukemia, lymphoma, bone marrow or organ transplant deficiency).
- Rituximab use has been associated with PJP in HIV-negative patients, most of whom had hematologic cancers.

PEAK INCIDENCE: Age 20 to 40 yr (parallel to AIDS epidemic).
PREDOMINANT SEX: Equal incidence when corrected for HIV status.
PREDOMINANT AGE:
- 20 to 40 yr

GENETICS: Neonatal infection:
- Most frequent opportunistic infection among HIV-infected children, occurring in approximately 30%.
- Neonatal occurrence unusual.

PHYSICAL FINDINGS & CLINICAL PRESENTATION

- Fever, cough, shortness of breath present in almost all cases. May be subacute or insidious.
- Lungs frequently clear to auscultation, although rales occasionally present.
- Cyanosis and pronounced tachypnea in severe cases.
- Hemoptysis unusual.
- Spontaneous pneumothorax.

ETIOLOGY

- *P. jirovecii* (formerly *P. carinii*) recently reclassified as a fungal organism.
- Reactivation of dormant infection.
- Extrapulmonary involvement rare.

Dx DIAGNOSIS

DIFFERENTIAL DIAGNOSIS

- Other opportunistic respiratory infections:
  1. Tuberculosis
  2. Histoplasmosis
  3. Cryptococcosis
- Nonopportunistic infections:
  1. Bacterial pneumonia
  2. Viral pneumonia
  3. Mycoplasmal pneumonia
  4. Legionellosis
- Occurs virtually exclusively in the setting of profound depression of cellular immunity.

WORKUP

- Chest x-ray (Fig. E1-737) or chest CT.
- Arterial blood gases.
- Because *Pneumocystis* cannot be cultured, diagnosis relies on detection of the organism by colorimetric or immunofluorescent stains or PCR.
- Cannot be cultured. Sputum examination for cysts of PJP and to exclude other pathogens.
- Bronchoscopy with bronchoalveolar lavage or lung biopsy for diagnosis if sputum examination is negative or equivocal. Stains such as Gomori methenamine silver stain or toluidine blue O are used to identify the organism.

LABORATORY TESTS

- Arterial blood gas monitoring.
- Elevated lactate dehydrogenase in majority of cases.
- HIV antibody test and CD4 cell count if cause of underlying immune deficiency state is unclear.

IMAGING STUDIES

- CT scan of the chest in selected patients (Fig. E1-738).
- PJP may appear as diffuse, unilateral, bilateral, or interstitial infiltrates on chest x-ray or CT. Imaging may be normal in up to one quarter of individuals. Pneumothoraces may also occur.

Rx TREATMENT

NONPHARMACOLOGIC THERAPY

- Supplemental oxygen.
- Ventilatory support if needed.
- Prompt thoracotomy if pneumothorax develops.

ACUTE GENERAL Rx

For confirmed or suspected PJP:
- Trimethoprim-sulfamethoxazole (15 to 20 mg/kg trimethoprim and 75 to 100 mg/kg sulfamethoxazole qd) PO or IV per day divided and given q6 to 8h.
- Pentamidine (4 mg/kg IV qd) (severe cases with a contraindication to trimethoprim/sulfamethoxazole).
- Either regimen with prednisone (40 mg PO bid):
  1. If arterial oxygen pressure <70 mm Hg.
  2. If arterial-alveolar oxygen pressure difference >35 mm Hg.
  3. Dose tapered to 20 mg bid after 5 days and 20 mg qd after 10 days.
- Therapy continued for 3 wk.
- Alternative therapies available for patients unable to tolerate conventional therapy:
  1. Dapsone/trimethoprim
  2. Clindamycin/primaquine
  3. Atovaquone

CHRONIC Rx

- After completion of therapy, prophylaxis should be maintained with trimethoprim-sulfamethoxazole (one single-strength tablet PO qd or double-strength three times weekly) until the CD4 cell count is >200 for 3 mo.
- Patients intolerant of this therapy should be treated with dapsone (100 mg PO qd) or atovaquone (1500 mg PO qd).
- Inhaled pentamidine (300 mg monthly by standardized nebulizer) is less effective and is reserved for patients intolerant to other forms of prophylaxis.

DISPOSITION

After completion of therapy, long-term ambulatory follow-up is mandatory to provide secondary prevention of PJP (see "Chronic Rx" above) and management of the underlying immunodeficiency syndrome.

REFERRAL

- To pulmonologist for bronchoscopy if diagnosis cannot be confirmed by sputum examination.
- To an infectious disease specialist if case is severe or difficult to manage.

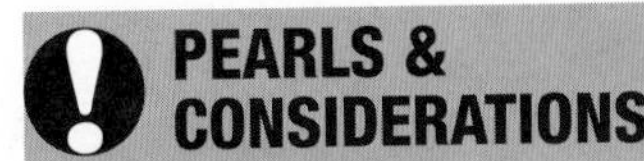

COMMENTS

- All patients, especially those with severe infection or intolerant of conventional therapy, should be followed by a physician experienced in the management of PJP and, if appropriate, in the long-term management of HIV infection or other underlying disease.
- Severe and life-threatening hypoglycemia may occur after 1 or 2 wk after start of IV pentamidine. Monitor closely and advise the patient of symptoms of hypoglycemia.

SUGGESTED READINGS
available at www.expertconsult.com

RELATED CONTENT

Pneumocystis Pneumonia (Patient Information)

AUTHOR: **PHILIP A. CHAN, M.D., M.S.**

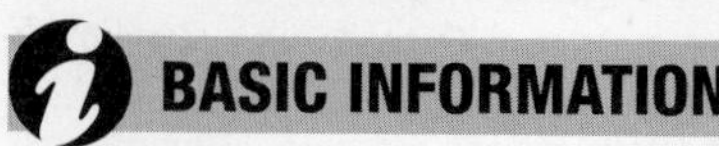

BASIC INFORMATION

DEFINITION

Viral pneumonia is infection of the pulmonary parenchyma caused by any of a large number of viral agents. The most important viruses are discussed.

SYNONYMS

Nonbacterial pneumonia
Atypical pneumonia

ICD-9CM CODES
480.8 Viral pneumonia
487.0 Viral pneumonia due to influenza
ICD-10CM COES
J12.9 Viral pneumonia, unspecified

EPIDEMIOLOGY & DEMOGRAPHICS

INCIDENCE (IN U.S.):

- Influenza virus:
  1. 10% to 20% of population in temperate zones infected during 1-2 mo epidemics occurring yearly during winter months.
  2. Up to 50% infected during pandemics.
  3. Pneumonia develops in small percentage of infected persons.
- Incidence of other important viral pneumonias is not known precisely.

PEAK INCIDENCE:

- Influenza:
  1. Winter months for influenza A
  2. Year round for influenza B
  3. Peak of pneumonia seen weeks into the outbreak of infection
- Respiratory syncytial virus (RSV) and parainfluenza virus:
  1. Winter and spring
- Adenovirus:
  1. Endemic (miliary)
- Varicella:
  1. Spring in temperate zones
- Measles:
  1. Year round
- Cytomegalovirus (CMV):
  1. Year round

PREVALENCE (IN U.S.):

- Often related to immune status of the population or presence of an epidemic
- Normal hosts (estimates):
  1. 86% of cases of pneumonia resulting in hospitalization in American adults
  2. 16% of pediatric pneumonias managed as outpatients
  3. 49% of hospitalized infants with pneumonia
- Important problem in hosts with impaired immunity

PREDOMINANT SEX:

- None generally
- Male sex may predispose to more severe respiratory disease in RSV infection

PREDOMINANT AGE:

- Influenza:
  1. Overall incidence greatest at age 5 yr
  2. Lower with increasing age
  3. The most serious sequelae in those with chronic medical illnesses, especially cardiopulmonary disease
  4. Hospitalizations greatest in infants and adults aged >64 yr
- RSV and parainfluenza virus:
  1. Young children (as the major cause of pneumonia)
  2. Occurs throughout life
- Adenoviruses:
  1. Young children
  2. Adults, primarily military recruits
- Varicella:
  1. Approximately 16% of adults (not infected in childhood) who contract chickenpox
  2. Acute varicella during pregnancy more likely to be complicated by severe pneumonia
  3. 90% of reported varicella pneumonia cases are in adults (highest incidence ages 20 to 60 yr)
- Measles:
  1. Young adults and older children who received a single vaccination (5% failure rate)
  2. Measles during pregnancy more likely to be complicated by pneumonia
  3. Underlying cardiopulmonary diseases and immunosuppression predispose to serious pneumonia complicating measles
  4. Before availability of measles vaccine, 90% of pneumonias in those <10 yr
  5. Currently more than one third of U.S. patients >14 yr
  6. 3% to 50% of measles cases are complicated by pneumonia
- CMV:
  1. Neonatal through adult
  2. Immunosuppression is key predisposing factor

GENETICS:

Familial disposition:

- Close contact, not genetics, is important in acquisition
- Congenital anomalies and immunosuppression worsen course of RSV pneumonia

Congenital infection:

- CMV is the most common intrauterine infection in the U.S.
- Pneumonia occurs occasionally in infants with symptomatic congenital infection.

Neonatal infection:

- Severe RSV pneumonia
- Adenovirus pneumonia
  1. 5% to 20% mortality rate
  2. Can lead to residual restrictive or obstructive functional abnormalities
- "Varicella neonatorum"
  1. Disseminated visceral disease including pneumonia
  2. May develop in neonates whose mothers develop peripartum chickenpox
- CMV pneumonia
  1. Generally fatal
  2. Associated with severe cerebral damage in this population

PHYSICAL FINDINGS & CLINICAL PRESENTATION

1. Influenza:
   - Fever, cough, or sore throat (referred to as influenza-like illness [ILI])
   - Uncomfortable or lethargic appearance
   - Prominent dry cough (rarely hemoptysis)
   - Flushed integument and erythematous mucous membranes
   - Rales or rhonchi
2. RSV and parainfluenza:
   - Fever
   - Tachypnea
   - Prolonged expiration
   - Wheezes and rales
3. Adenoviruses:
   - Hoarseness
   - Pharyngitis
   - Tachypnea
   - Cervical adenitis
4. Measles:
   - Conjunctivitis
   - Rhinorrhea
   - Koplik's spots (white lesions on the buccal mucosa)
   - Exanthem (maculopapular rash that starts on the head, then moves down to rest of body)
   - Pneumonitis
     a. May occur as a complication in 3% to 4% of adolescents and young adults
     b. Coincident with rash
     c. May also develop after apparent recovery from measles
   - Fever
   - Dry cough
5. Varicella:
   - Fever
   - Maculopapular or vesicular rash (all lesions at the same stage)
     a. Becomes encrusted
     b. Pneumonia typical 1 to 6 days after rash appears
     c. Pneumonia accompanied by cough and occasionally hemoptysis
   - Few auscultatory abnormalities noted on examination of the lungs
6. CMV:
   - Fever
   - Paroxysmal cough
   - Occasional hemoptysis
   - Diffuse adenopathy when pneumonia occurs after transfusion

ETIOLOGY

Viral infection can lead to pneumonia in both immunocompetent and immunocompromised hosts.

Dx DIAGNOSIS

DIFFERENTIAL DIAGNOSIS

- Bacterial pneumonia, which frequently complicates (i.e., can follow or be simultaneous with) viral pneumonia
- Other causes of atypical pneumonia:
  1. *Mycoplasma* spp.
  2. *Chlamydia* spp.
  3. *Coxiella* spp.
  4. Legionnaires' disease
- Acute respiratory distress syndrome (ARDS)
- Physical findings and associated hypoxemia confused with pulmonary emboli

WORKUP

- Information about the current prevalent strain of influenza virus can be obtained from local health departments or from the Centers for Disease Control and Prevention.

- Influenza and other viruses may be cultured from respiratory secretions during the initial few days of the illness (special media and techniques necessary).
- Respiratory viral panels that use PCR-based assays to test for a variety of viruses are extremely sensitive and are becoming the test of choice.
- Rapid flu tests have a 50% sensitivity in diagnosing influenza (a negative test does not mean the patient does not have influenza).
- Measles and adenovirus pneumonia are usually diagnosed clinically and can be confirmed with serology.
- CMV may be grown in culture or PCR amplified from bronchoalveolar lavage samples. An algorithm for the workup and management of suspected severe influenza pneumonia in the critical care unit is described in Fig. E1-739. Open lung biopsy is required for a definite diagnosis of CMV pneumonia.

LABORATORY TESTS

- Sputum Gram stain (usually produced in scanty amounts) typically shows few polymorphonuclear leukocytes and few bacteria.
- White blood cell count may vary from leukopenic to modest elevation, usually without a leftward shift.
- Disseminated intravascular coagulation occasionally complicates adenovirus type 7 pneumonia.
- Multinucleated giant cells on Tzanck preparation of an unroofed vesicular lesion are useful in diagnosing varicella in a patient with an infiltrate (also found in herpes simplex).
- Severe immunosuppression is associated with symptomatic CMV pneumonia (usually reactivation of latent infection or in previously seronegative recipients from the donor).
- Hypoxemia may be profound.
- Cultures may be helpful in identifying superinfecting bacterial pathogens.
- When they occur, parapneumonic pleural effusions are exudative.

IMAGING STUDIES

- Chest radiographs may demonstrate a spectrum of findings from ill-defined, patchy, or generalized interstitial infiltrates, which can be associated with ARDS.
- A localized dense alveolar infiltrate suggests a superimposed bacterial pneumonia.
- Small calcified nodules may develop as a radiographic residual of varicella pneumonia.

Rx TREATMENT

NONPHARMACOLOGIC THERAPY

General:

- Measures to diminish person-to-person transmission
- Modified bed rest
- Maintenance of adequate hydration
- Possible ventilatory support for severe pneumonia or ARDS

Influenza:

- Yearly prophylactic strain-specific influenza vaccination (only subvirion vaccine should be used in children <13 yr) can be given to prevent infection.
- Live, attenuated influenza vaccines administered by nose drops as effective as injected inactivated viral vaccines.

RSV:

- Isolation techniques are important in limiting spread of RSV infections.
- Immunoglobulins with a high RSV-neutralizing antibody titer are beneficial in treatment.

Adenoviruses:

- Intestinal inoculation of respiratory adenoviruses has been used to successfully immunize military recruits.
- Although they produce no disease in recipients, the viruses may be shed chronically and may infect others at a later date.
- These vaccines are not available for civilian populations.

Varicella:

- Live, attenuated varicella vaccine has been successfully used in clinical trials.
- Varicella-zoster immune globulin should be administered within 4 days of exposure to prevent or modify the disease in susceptible persons.
- Nonimmunized persons exposed to varicella are potentially infectious between 10 and 21 days after exposure.

Measles:

- Effective measles vaccine is available:
  - The vaccine should be administered at age 15 mo.
  - A second dose should be administered at the time of school entry.
- Live, attenuated vaccine or gamma-globulin can prevent measles in unvaccinated persons if administered early after exposure.
- Vitamin A given PO for 2 days reduces morbidity and mortality rates from measles in exposed children.

Severe acute respiratory syndrome (SARS)-associated coronaviruses:

- No vaccine currently available.
- Supportive care: ribavirin ineffective, use of steroids or interferon-alpha of unclear value.

ACUTE GENERAL Rx

- **General:** Administer appropriate antibiotics for bacterial superinfections.
- **Influenza:**
  - Amantadine and rimantadine for influenza A (not active against influenza B). Early use can speed recovery from small airways dysfunction, but whether it influences the development or course of pneumonia is uncertain.
  - The neuraminidase inhibitors oseltamivir and zanamivir are effective if given in the first 48 hours of symptoms of influenza; their efficacy in established influenza pneumonia is unclear.
  - Aerosolized ribavirin or amantadine may have a role in severe influenza pneumonia but have not been approved for this indication.
- **RSV and parainfluenza:**
  - Ribavirin aerosol is effective for severe RSV pneumonia.
  - There is no approved antiviral therapy for parainfluenza virus pneumonia.
- **Adenoviruses:** no effective agent; some case reports of cidofovir use but unproved.
- **Varicella:**
  - Varicella pneumonia can be treated with IV acyclovir.
  - Adults who develop chickenpox should be considered for acyclovir treatment, which may prevent the development of pneumonia.
- **Measles:** no effective antimeasles agent.
- **CMV:**
  - Acyclovir can prevent CMV infection in renal transplant recipients.
  - Ganciclovir and foscarnet, with or without CMV hyperimmune globulin, show promise in the treatment of serious CMV infection, including pneumonia, in compromised hosts.

DISPOSITION

- Supportive therapy is useful.
- Death is possible during acute illness.
- Residual functional abnormalities may be persistent or develop into or predispose to chronic respiratory diseases in later life.
- Morbidity and mortality rates after most viral pneumonias are increased by bacterial superinfection.

REFERRAL

- Uncertainty about the diagnosis in a compromised host.
- Symptoms or findings are progressive.
- Severe respiratory compromise, diffuse infiltrates, or the development of ARDS.

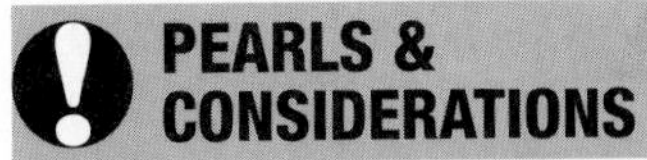

PEARLS & CONSIDERATIONS

COMMENTS

- Influenza spreads by close contact and by small droplets transmitted by cough.
- RSV is effectively transmitted by fomites and by direct contact (little by aerosol).
- Varicella is transmitted by direct contact or by aerosol.
- Of the three major forms of parainfluenza viruses (types 1 to 3), type 3 is the most common cause of viral pneumonia; types 1 and 2 primarily cause laryngotracheitis.
- Recent evidence indicates that a newly discovered virus known as metapneumovirus is a common cause of upper respiratory infections worldwide; this virus can cause pneumonia.

SUGGESTED READINGS

available at www.expertconsult.com

RELATED CONTENT

Viral Pneumonia (Patient Information)

AUTHORS: **PHILIP A. CHAN, M.D.,** and **GLENN G. FORT, M.D., M.P.H.**

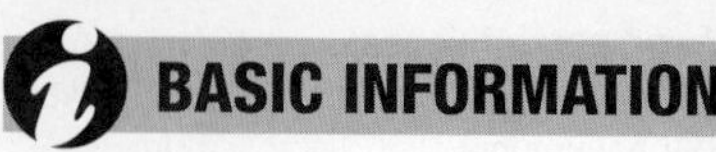

BASIC INFORMATION

DEFINITION

A spontaneous pneumothorax (SP) is defined as the accumulation of air into the pleural space, collapsing the lung without a precipitating event. This can be primary SP (without any obvious underlying lung disease) or secondary SP (with underlying lung disease).

SYNONYMS

Primary spontaneous pneumothorax
Secondary spontaneous pneumothorax

ICD-9CM CODES
512.0S Spontaneous tension pneumothorax
512.8 Other spontaneous pneumothorax
ICD-10CM CODES
J93.83 Other pneumothorax
J93.9 Pneumothorax, unspecified

EPIDEMIOLOGY & DEMOGRAPHICS

- Approximately 20,000 new cases of SP occur each year in the U.S.
- SP is more common in men than women (6:1).
- Incidence of primary SP is 7.4 per 100,000 in men and 1.2 per 100,000 in women.
- Incidence of secondary SP is 6.3 per 100,000 in men and 2.0 per 100,000 in women.
- SP is commonly seen in tall, thin young men aged 20 to 40 yr.
- Risk factors include smoking, family history, Marfan's syndrome, homocystinuria, and thoracic endometriosis.

PHYSICAL FINDINGS & CLINICAL PRESENTATION

- Sudden onset of pleuritic chest pain (90%), usually at rest, which often becomes dull after a few hours
- Pain is usually unilateral and can be sharp and agonizing and associated with considerable apprehension.
- Dyspnea (80%), which often resolves within 24 hr, despite persistence of pneumothorax
- Cough (10%)
- Asymptomatic (5%); may take up to 7 days to come to medical attention
- Tachycardia
- Hypoxemia
- Decreased chest excursion on the affected side
- Diminished breath sounds
- Subcutaneous emphysema may be present.
- Hyperresonance on percussion

ETIOLOGY

- In primary SP, rupture of small blebs, usually located near the apex of the upper lobes, is a common cause. The check-valve mechanism is uncommon in this case; therefore, tension pneumothorax rarely occurs.
- In secondary SP, chronic obstructive pulmonary disease is the most common cause, but it can also be associated with pneumonia, bronchogenic carcinoma, mesothelioma, sarcoidosis, tuberculosis, cystic fibrosis, and many other lung diseases (Fig. 1-740).

Dx DIAGNOSIS

Established by the chest x-ray (Fig. 1-741)

DIFFERENTIAL DIAGNOSIS

- Pleurisy
- Pulmonary embolism
- Myocardial infarction
- Pericarditis
- Asthma
- Pneumonia

WORKUP

Includes CXR and, in some inconclusive cases, CT scan of the chest

LABORATORY TESTS

Arterial blood gases may show hypoxemia and hypocapnia as a result of hyperventilation.

IMAGING STUDIES

- SP is usually confirmed by upright CXR:
  1. A white visceral pleural line. The absence of vessel markings peripheral to this line helps differentiate from mimicking conditions such as an overlying skin fold.

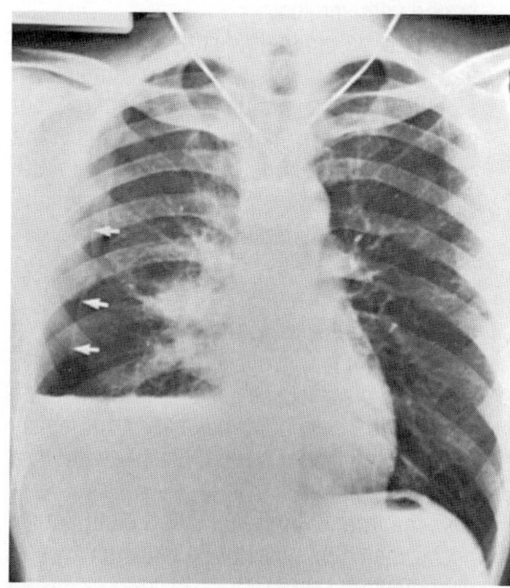

FIGURE 1-741 Chest radiograph shows right hydropneumothorax. Horizontal line in lower right hemithorax is interface between air and liquid in pleural space. *Arrows* point to visceral pleura above level of effusion. There is air in pleural space between visceral pleura and chest wall. (From Weinberg SE et al: *Principles of pulmonary medicine,* ed 5, Philadelphia, 2008, Saunders.)

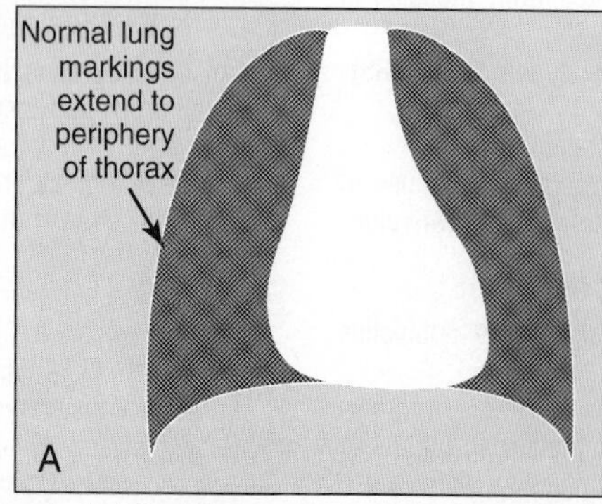

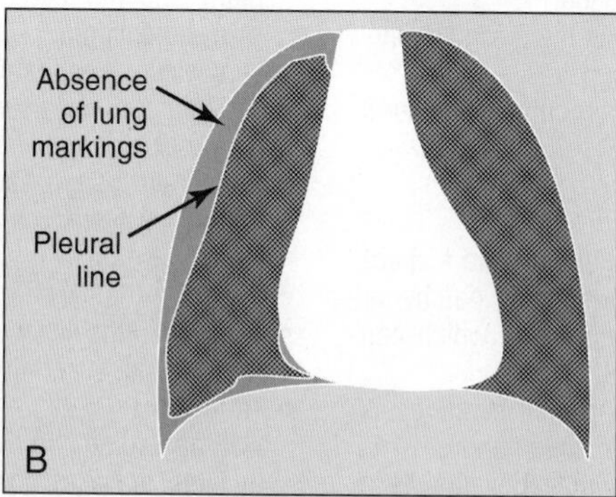

FIGURE 1-740 Pneumothorax. A, Schematic of normal lung. **B,** Schematic of pneumothorax. Pneumothoraces can range in size from tiny to massive. Because of the variability in their size and location, pneumothoraces can be difficult to detect on chest x-ray. For example, a pneumothorax that is anterior or posterior rather than lateral may be hidden on frontal chest x-ray, particularly one taken in the supine position. An upright chest x-ray should be obtained if possible. An expiratory film is thought to be more sensitive, because the lung and thorax decrease in size during expiration, but air trapped in the pleural space remains the same size and thus appears relatively larger. Subtle pneumothoraces may not be visible on chest x-ray. In some cases, subcutaneous air may be the only visible clue to underlying lung injury. CT is extremely sensitive for pneumothorax, although controversy remains over the proper management of pneumothoraces seen only on CT. Ultrasound is also thought to be more sensitive than chest x-ray for detection of pneumothorax, although, again, the management of pneumothorax seen only on ultrasound is uncertain because this is a relatively newly described method of detection. The chest x-ray findings of pneumothorax include a lack of the normal lung markings, which should be visible to the periphery of the chest wall. Sometimes a line marking the boundary of the lung and visceral pleura is visible, although this can be confused with ribs and with the medial margin of the scapula. Depending on the degree of pneumothorax and lung collapse, the lung parenchyma may appear denser than the opposite side. In extreme cases of tension pneumothorax, the pressure exerted by the air in the pleural space may begin to displace other structures, including the diaphragm and mediastinum. In tension pneumothorax, the hyperinflated hemithorax may also have abnormally positioned ribs, with a position more horizontal than usual. (From Broder JS: *Diagnostic imaging for the emergency physician,* Philadelphia, 2011, Saunders.)

A lateral width of 1 cm corresponds to 10% pneumothorax.
2. The left lateral decubitus position is the most sensitive and the supine position the least sensitive. Inspiratory and expiratory films have equal sensitivities.
3. As little as 50 ml of air can be detected on upright film.

- Tension pneumothorax (Fig. E1-742) is a medical emergency and should be suspected when the patient is hemodynamically unstable or with contralateral tracheal and mediastinal deviation and ipsilateral flattening or inversion of the diaphragm on the CXR (Fig. E1-743).
- CT scan can be done in suspected but difficult-to-visualize pneumothoraces, to differentiate from large subpleural bullae or to evaluate for underlying lung pathology, especially in patients with secondary pneumothorax.

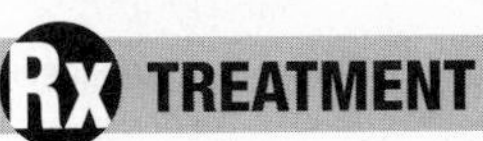

TREATMENT

INITIAL MANAGEMENT

- 100% oxygen administration reduces the partial pressure of nitrogen in pleural capillaries, consequently quadrupling the rate of pneumothorax absorption, and should be administered to all patients with pneumothorax.
- Further treatment is based on the size of the pneumothorax.
  - If the pneumothorax is small (<3 cm between lung and chest wall on CXR), the patient can be treated with observation alone. Repeat imaging should be performed to ensure stability/resorption of the pneumothorax.
  - If the pneumothorax is >3 cm, or if the patient is symptomatic with chest pain and dyspnea, initial management should focus on removing air from the pleural space. Needle aspiration is the treatment of choice in the clinically stable patient.
- Needle aspiration can be done at the bedside using a large-bore angiocatheter needle or commercially available needle thoracotomy kit. The needle is introduced in the second intercostal space midclavicular line. The catheter is left in place and attached to a three-way stopcock and a large syringe. Air is aspirated until resistance is met or the patient experiences significant coughing. Repeat CXR is done immediately after aspiration and again in 4 to 24 hr to document reexpansion of the lung. If the pneumothorax fails to resolve with aspiration, a chest tube should be placed.
- If there is improvement but not complete resolution of pneumothorax after the aspiration, the catheter can be attached to a Heimlich (one-way) valve to allow further lung expansion. Some stable patients can be discharged home with this device in place if close follow-up monitoring can be obtained. An alternative approach is to perform an autologous blood patch. This involves withdrawal of peripheral blood and infusion into the pleural space through a chest tube.
- Chest tube insertion has been recommended for patients with primary SP who do not respond to simple aspiration and for all patients with secondary SP, recurrent pneumothorax, or tension pneumothorax. Most patients can be managed with small chest tubes (<22 Fr). The chest tube can be connected to a water seal device, with or without suction, and left in position until the pneumothorax has resolved.
- An algorithmic approach to the treatment of primary spontaneous pneumothorax is outlined in Fig. E1-744.

PREVENTION

- Approximately 25% to 50% of patients with primary SP with have a recurrence within 1 yr.
- Multiple techniques have been used to prevent recurrence, including intrapleural instillation of sclerosing agents, pleurectomy, laser abrasion of parietal pleura, and pleural abrasion with dry gauze.
- The current recommended approach is the use of video-assisted thoracoscopy (VATS) with an aim to excise the associated bullae or perform guided pleurodesis or treatment. Most pulmonologists recommend definitive management after the first recurrence. However, high-risk occupations such as divers or pilots should be considered for surgery after their first pneumothorax. Similarly, complex conditions such as patients with persistent bronchopleural fistula suggested by a persistent air leak from the chest tube should also be considered for VATS and early surgical intervention. The overall recurrence rate is estimated at <5% after VATS.
- The recurrence rates for the instillation of sclerosing agents (minocycline 5 mg/kg in 50 ml of normal saline or doxycycline 500 mg in 50 ml of normal saline) are higher than for VATS-guided therapy (<25%). Therefore this mode of therapy should be reserved for patients who are poor surgical candidates.
- Talc has also been used as a sclerosing agent with favorable results; however, concerns persist due to case reports describing acute respiratory distress syndrome and pleural calcification occurring after use.
- Open thoracotomy is performed in patients who do not respond to VATS or when VATS is not available.

DISPOSITION

- Smoking cessation should be advised.
- Death from primary SP is uncommon. In patients with secondary SP and chronic obstructive pulmonary disease, mortality rates range from 1% to 16%.

REFERRAL

A pulmonary specialist and surgical consultation are recommended.

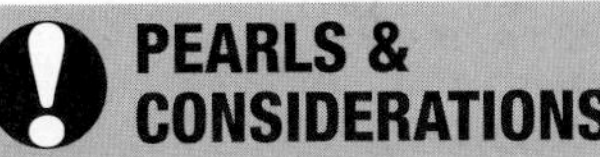

PEARLS & CONSIDERATIONS

- The rate of pleural air absorption is approximately 1.25% of the volume of the hemithorax per day. Therefore the interval for complete resolution of pneumothorax with observation can be estimated.
- Catamenial pneumothorax is a rare condition characterized by recurrent SP coinciding with the onset of menses. It usually affects the right lung and is believed to be caused by endometriosis with involvement of the diaphragm and/or pleura. It is believed to be hormonally related, and treatment is aimed at endometrial suppression.

COMMENTS

- Patients with AIDS and *Pneumocystis carinii* infection have a high incidence of SP. Treatment typically requires chest tube placement and either thoracoscopy or open thoracotomy.

SUGGESTED READINGS

available at www.expertconsult.com

RELATED CONTENT

Pneumothorax (Patient Information)

AUTHORS: **JOHANNES STEINER, M.D.**, and **RICHARD REGNANTE, M.D.**

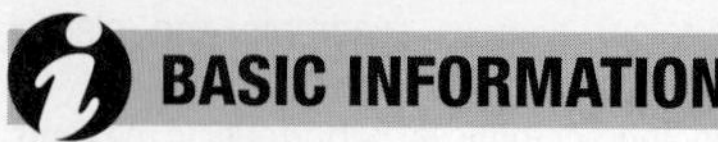

BASIC INFORMATION

DEFINITION

Poison ivy dermatitis is a contact dermatitis caused by exposure to urushiol, the oil of plants of the genus *Toxicodendron,* which includes poison ivy, poison oak, and poison sumac.

SYNONYMS

Rhus dermatitis
Toxicodendron dermatitis

ICD-9CM CODES
692.6 Dermatitis due to plant
ICD-10CM CODES
L23.7 Allergic contact dermatitis due to plants, except food

EPIDEMIOLOGY & DEMOGRAPHICS

INCIDENCE: Affects 10 million to 40 million Americans annually.
PEAK INCIDENCE: More frequent in months when outdoor activity is more common.
PREVALENCE: From 50% to 75% of the adult population is clinically sensitive to these plants. Sensitivity rates are lower in urban areas. (Tolerance is found in 10% to 15% of the population.)
PREDOMINANT SEX AND AGE: Sensitization occurs most commonly between ages 8 and 14 yr. Sensitivity wanes with age, especially with limited exposure and prior mild reactions.
GENETICS: There is believed to be a genetic susceptibility to sensitivity; however, the rash occurs in all ethnicities and skin types.
RISK FACTORS: Firefighters, forestry workers, farmers, and outdoor workers in general as well as those who participate in outdoor recreation. These plants are indigenous to the United States, Canada, and Mexico, and cases are most common in these areas.

PHYSICAL FINDINGS & CLINICAL PRESENTATION

- Patients typically present with intense pruritus and rash. The patient may not be aware of exposure to the plant.
- Symptoms typically peak from 1 to 14 days after exposure depending on the degree of exposure and thickness of affected skin.
- Dermatitis may initially present as erythema and may develop into papules, vesicles, and bullae.
- Lesions may be found in the classic linear configuration, typically in exposed areas likely to have been in contact with plants (Fig. E1-745). Atypical appearance or location of dermatitis is more common with secondary exposure, such as through pets or infected tools or clothing.
- Face and genital involvement may present with significant edema.
- Inhalation of urushiol aerosolized by fire can cause significant respiratory tract inflammation. This can be a particular occupational hazard of forest firefighters.
- Postinflammatory hyperpigmentation may occur, more commonly in dark skin types. This usually resolves with treatment.

ETIOLOGY

- Initial contact with oil of plants in this genus, which is released with damage to plant parts, causes a classic T-lymphocyte–mediated delayed-type allergic reaction.
- Subsequent exposures cause a cell-mediated cytotoxic immune response.

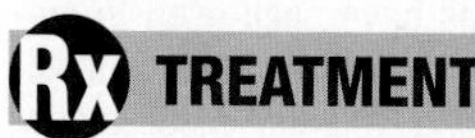

DIAGNOSIS

DIFFERENTIAL DIAGNOSIS

- Allergic contact dermatitis from other plants or nonplant substances
- Irritant contact dermatitis
- Nummular dermatitis
- Arthropod reactions, including scabies and bedbug bites

WORKUP

Typically not needed. Diagnosis is based on characteristic rash and possibly history of exposure.

TREATMENT

Prevention is the most effective treatment.

NONPHARMACOLOGIC THERAPY

- After known exposure, patients should remove contaminated clothing and wash the skin gently with soap and water. Washing after appearance of dermatitis does not prevent further lesions.
- Calamine lotion, cool compresses, baking soda, or colloidal oatmeal baths may provide symptomatic relief.
- Keep nails short and clean to help prevent secondary bacterial infection.
- Exposed clothing, as well as tools, pets, and equipment, should be washed with soap and water to prevent secondary exposure.

ACUTE GENERAL Rx

- Topical steroids generally should be avoided. They may be effective in mild, early cases with erythema and pruritus but no vesiculation.
- Topical antibiotics should be avoided.
- Use of antihistamines for associated pruritus may be effective, but this has not been extensively studied.
- Systemic corticosteroids offer significant relief in moderate to severe *Rhus* dermatitis, including generalized rash or severe facial or genital involvement.
- Effective dosing of oral prednisone is 1 mg/kg/day over 7 to 10 days (maximum 60 mg initial dose), with tapering over an additional 7 to 10 days.
- Inadequate doses or too-rapid tapering of systemic steroids may cause symptom rebound.
- IM treatment with long-acting triamcinolone suspension may be considered for patients intolerant of oral therapy.

CHRONIC Rx

- Recurrence may be caused by repeated exposure to fomites, including contaminated clothing, equipment, or pets.
- Secondary bacterial infection of the skin is the most common complication of *Rhus* dermatitis. Staph and strep are the most common pathogens, but MRSA must be considered.

DISPOSITION

Untreated *Rhus* dermatitis will resolve in 1 to 3 weeks.

REFERRAL

Refer to dermatology if there is diagnostic confusion.

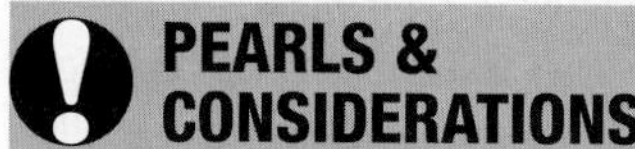

PEARLS & CONSIDERATIONS

PREVENTION

- Patients should be educated regarding identification and avoidance as well as washing to remove the oil after known exposure.
- Total avoidance of the plants may not be practical.
- The use of barrier creams applied before exposure to prevent dermatitis may be of some benefit, particularly in potential occupational (therefore predictable) exposure.
- Products available for postexposure prophylaxis are effective; however, equal efficacy may be obtained from less expensive liquid dishwashing soap.
- Desensitization has not been found to be effective.

PATIENT & FAMILY EDUCATION

- "Leaves of three, let it be," is a helpful reminder for patients.
- Patient education material, including access to photographs of the leaves of these plants in a variety of seasons and conditions, may be useful.

SUGGESTED READINGS
available at www.expertconsult.com

RELATED CONTENT

Poison Ivy (Patient Information)

AUTHOR: **MARGARET TRYFOROS, M.D.**

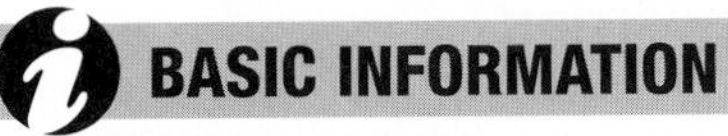

BASIC INFORMATION

DEFINITION

Polyarteritis nodosa (PAN) is a systemic vasculitic syndrome involving medium-sized to small arteries, characterized histologically by necrotizing inflammation of the arterial media and inflammatory cell infiltration.

SYNONYMS

Periarteritis nodosa
PAN
Necrotizing arteritis

ICD-9CM CODES
446.0 Polyarteritis nodosa
ICD-10CM CODES
M30.0 Polyarteritis nodosa

EPIDEMIOLOGY & DEMOGRAPHICS

- Incidence is 1/100,000 persons annually. Increased incidence in patients with hepatitis B surface antigen or hepatitis C virus.
- Male/female ratio of 2:1
- Can occur in any age group, more commonly between 40 yr and 60 yr.
- No racial predilection is observed.
- Prevalence is 2 to 33/1,000,000.
- Is also associated with hairy cell leukemia.

PHYSICAL FINDINGS & CLINICAL PRESENTATION

- Typical presentation is subacute, with the onset of constitutional symptoms over weeks to months in more than 90% of cases
- Nausea, vomiting, headache
- Testicular pain or tenderness
- Myalgias, weakness, or leg tenderness in 24% to 80% of cases
- Neuropathy (mononeuritis multiplex), foot drop
- Skin lesions are observed in one third of patients with tender nodules, livedo reticularis, palpable purpura, ulceration of digits
- Abdominal pain after meals, hematemesis, hematochezia, occasionally with diarrhea and gastrointestinal bleeding in severe cases
- Asymmetric polyarthritis (tending to involve large joints of lower extremities); true synovitis occurs only in a minority of patients
- Presence of lung vasculitis suggests other causes
- Fever (PAN is often a cause of fever of unknown origin) can range from intermittent, low-grade fevers to high fevers with chills
- Chest pain secondary to ischemic infarcts in the coronary arteries, pericarditis, congestive heart failure, and arrhythmias are seen with cardiac involvement
- Tachycardia is common and often striking
- Hypertension can occur due to renal artery involvement

ETIOLOGY

- Unknown
- Hepatitis B virus–associated PAN appears to be an immune complex–mediated disease.
- Hepatitis C and hairy cell leukemia are also associated in some cases.

Dx DIAGNOSIS

DIFFERENTIAL DIAGNOSIS

- Cryoglobulinemia
- Systemic lupus erythematosus
- Infections (e.g., subacute bacterial endocarditis, trichinosis, *Rickettsia*)
- Lymphoma
- Henoch-Schönlein purpura
- Wegener granulomatosis
- Microscopic polyangiitis
- Kawasaki disease
- Churg-Strauss syndrome
- Giant cell arteritis
- Human immunodeficiency virus

WORKUP

- Laboratory evaluation, arteriography, and biopsy of small or medium-sized arteries can confirm diagnosis. Clinical manifestations are variable and depend on the arteries involved and the organs affected (e.g., kidney involvement occurs in >80% of cases).

Table 1-398 summarizes investigations for patients with suspected PAN.

- The presence of any three of the following 10 items allows the diagnosis of PAN with a sensitivity of 82% and a specificity of 86%:
  1. Weight loss >4 kg
  2. Livedo reticularis
  3. Testicular pain or tenderness
  4. Myalgias, weakness, or leg tenderness
  5. Neuropathy
  6. Diastolic blood pressure <90 mm Hg
  7. Elevated blood urea nitrogen (BUN) or creatinine
  8. Positive test for hepatitis B virus
  9. Arteriography revealing small or large aneurysms and focal constrictions between dilated segments
  10. Biopsy of small or medium-sized artery containing necrotizing inflammatory infiltrate.

LABORATORY TESTS

- Elevated BUN or creatinine, positive test for hepatitis B virus or hepatitis C.
- Elevated erythrocyte sedimentation rate and C-reactive protein, anemia, elevated platelets, eosinophilia, proteinuria, hematuria.

TABLE 1-398 Investigations for Patients with Suspected Polyarteritis Nodosa (PAN)

Test	Supports Diagnosis of PAN	Supports an Alternative Diagnosis	Comment
Elevated C-reactive protein	+		Supports the presence of systemic inflammation
Elevated sedimentation rate	+		Supports the presence of systemic inflammation
Elevated serum creatinine	+/−	+/−	Raised serum creatinine, typically without hematuria or proteinuria on urinalysis, may indicate renal ischemia or infarction. Significant proteinuria or hematuria (especially red cell casts) would suggest glomerular disease, which is *not* a feature of PAN
Abnormal liver function tests	+		May suggest hepatitis, either from HBV or as a result of ischemic hepatitis from PAN affecting the hepatic arteries
Positive HBV serology	+		Seen in HBV PAN
Anemia	+		Due to chronic inflammation or from gastrointestinal blood loss
Positive ANCA		+	A positive ANCA would suggest an alternative type of vasculitis such as granulomatosis with polyangiitis or MPA
Elevated creatine kinase	+/−	+/−	Normal or mildly elevated, despite any muscle involvement
Blood cultures		+	To exclude endocarditis or other infective mimic of vasculitis
Positive HCV serology and cryoglobulins		+	HCV associated with a skin limited manifestation of PAN, but typically it is associated with a small vessel vasculitis related to cryoglobulinemia
Positive rheumatoid factor and ACPA		+	To rule out rheumatoid arthritis, especially in the context of a patient presenting predominantly with arthritis
Positive ANA and anti-dsDNA		+	In patients with clinical features consistent with SLE or other connective tissue disease
HIV positive		+	

ACPA, Anticitrullinated protein antibody; *ANA,* antinuclear antibody; *ANCA,* antineutrophil cytoplasm antibody; *dsDNA,* double-stranded deoxyribonucleic acid; *ESR,* erythrocyte sedimentation rate; *HBV,* hepatitis B virus; *HCV,* hepatitis C virus; *HIV,* human immunodeficiency virus; *MPA,* microscopic polyangiitis; *SLE,* systemic lupus erythematosus.
From Firestein GS et al: *Kelly's textbook of rheumatology,* ed 9, Philadelphia, 2013, Saunders.

- Biopsy of small or medium-sized artery of symptomatic sites (muscle, nerve) is >90% specific. Biopsy of the gastrocnemius muscle and sural nerve is commonly performed.
- Circumferential or segmental vessel wall involvement with necrotizing mixed cell inflammation with fibrinoid necrosis is characteristic lesion of active PAN.
- Assays for antinuclear antibody and rheumatoid factor are negative; however, low, nonspecific titers may be detected.
- Serum and urine immunofixation electrophoresis for monoclonal gammopathy and human immunodeficiency virus should also be tested for alternative diagnoses

IMAGING STUDIES

Arteriography can be done in patients with negative biopsies or if there are no symptomatic sites. Mesenteric angiography will reveal aneurysmal dilation of the renal, mesenteric (Fig. 1-746), or hepatic arteries. Less invasive techniques, such as computed tomography (CT) and MRI angiography, also help evaluate the extent and resolution of the disease.

Nerve conduction studies are useful in patients with neuropathy suggesting PAN, helping to evaluate nerves or muscles to biopsy.

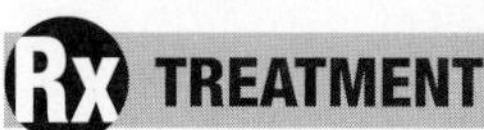

TREATMENT

NONPHARMACOLOGIC THERAPY

Low-sodium diet in hypertensive patients

ACUTE GENERAL Rx

- Prednisone 1 to 2 mg/kg/day with higher doses initially, then tapering the doses slowly with overall course of average 9 mo or longer.
- Patients with isolated cutaneous involvement may be treated with steroids alone or in combination with methotrexate.

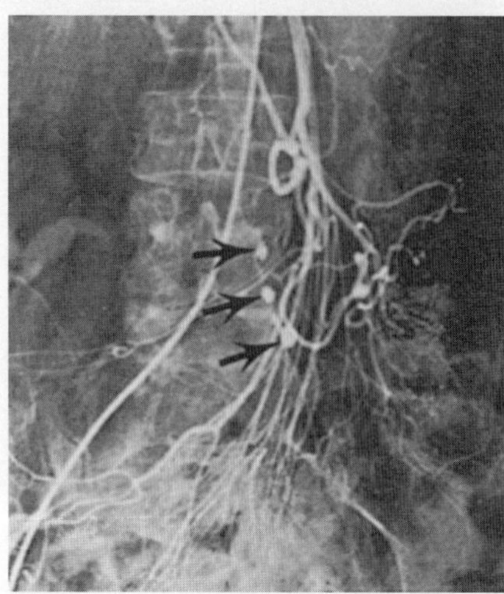

FIGURE 1-746 Superior mesenteric arteriogram in patients with polyarteritis. Several small aneurysms *(arrows)* are present in branches of superior mesenteric artery. (Courtesy Dr. A.W. Stanson. From Harris ED et al: *Kelley's textbook of rheumatology*, ed 7, 2005, Saunders.)

- Severe PAN with multiorgan involvement treated with a combination of cyclophosphamide 1.5 to 2 mg/kg per day and glucocorticoids has shown good disease outcomes. Once patient achieves stable remission, transition to a less toxic immunomodulatory therapy such as methotrexate or azathioprine, along with tapering doses of oral prednisone, is indicated for chronic therapy.
- If hepatitis B is identified, then appropriate antiviral treatment (interferon alfa-2b or lamivudine with or without plasma exchange) is initiated.

CHRONIC Rx

Monitoring for infections and potential complications such as thrombosis, infarction, or organ necrosis. Hypertension in patients with renal involvement in PAN is treated with angiotensin-converting enzyme inhibitor.

DISPOSITION

The 5-yr survival is <20% in untreated patients. Treatment with corticosteroids increases survival to approximately 50%. Use of both corticosteroids and immunosuppressive drugs may increase 5-yr survival to >80%. Poor prognostic signs are severe renal or gastrointestinal involvement. Patients on cyclophosphamide should have regular white cell count monitoring for leukopenia. Cyclophosphamide can cause increased risk of infertility, myelodysplsia, lymphoma, bladder malignancy, and when given in combination of high-dose corticosteroids can predispose patients to infection with *Pneumocystis jirovecii (carinii)* pneumonia. Therefore, close follow-up and PCP prophylaxis are recommended.

REFERRAL

Patients with suspected diagnosis of PAN should be immediately referred to a rheumatologist.

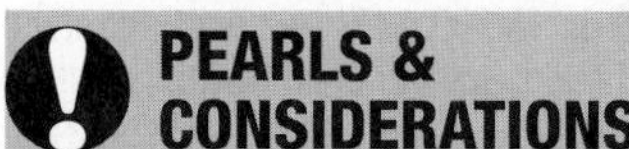

PEARLS & CONSIDERATIONS

- After treatment, patients should be followed up closely for relapse throughout their lifetime.
- Smoking cessation, exercise, and lifestyle modifications should be discussed to decrease vascular complications.

SUGGESTED READINGS

available at www.expertconsult.com

AUTHORS: **SYEDA M. SAYEED, M.D.,** and **HARALD A. HALL, M.D.**

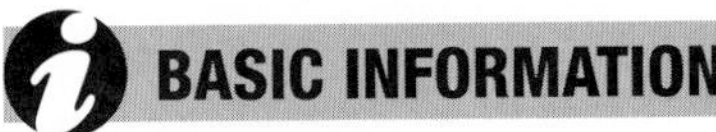

BASIC INFORMATION

DEFINITION

Polycystic kidney disease (PKD) refers to a systemic hereditary disorder characterized by the formation of cysts in the cortex and medulla of both kidneys (Figs. 1-747 and 1-748).

SYNONYMS

Autosomal-dominant polycystic kidney disease (ADPKD)

ICD-9CM CODES
753.1 Polycystic kidney, unspecified type
753.13 Polycystic kidney, autosomal dominant

ICD-10CM CODES
Q61.3 Polycystic kidney, unspecified
Q61.2 Polycystic kidney, adult type

EPIDEMIOLOGY & DEMOGRAPHICS

- The most common mendelian disorder of the kidneys
- Affects all racial groups worldwide
- Results in kidney failure in the majority of individuals by the fifth to sixth decade
- PKD occurs in one in 1000 persons
- Usually presents in the third to fourth decades of life and generally leads to end-stage renal disease (ESRD) in the sixth or seventh decade of life
- ADPKD comprises 5% of the ESRD population in the U.S.

PHYSICAL FINDINGS & CLINICAL PRESENTATION

- Characterized by focal development of renal and extrarenal cysts in an age-dependent manner, resulting in a slow, gradual, and massive kidney enlargement.

Symptoms:
- Pain (60%): acute pain can be associated with renal hemorrhage, passage of stones (20% of patients; usually uric acid or calcium oxalate), and urinary tract infections
- Palpable flank mass
- Hypertension: >60% of patients; usually develops before the loss of renal function
- Headache
- Nocturia, hematuria

Renal manifestations:
- Kidney and cyst volumes and renal blood flow (or vascular resistance) are the strongest predictors of renal function decline. Kidney function does not decline in individuals with PKD until kidney size is at least five times greater than normal.
- Morphometric analysis of sequential CT was shown to be sufficiently accurate to monitor rates of renal enlargement in PKD, and MRI-based methods have been developed. Two general groups of kidney volume increase: those with rapid rates (>5% increase in total kidney volume per year) and those with rates of progression <5% per year. Intervals between measurements as short as 6 mo may be adequate to determine an effect of treatment that reduces the rates of volume progression >50% in those with rapidly progressive disease.
- All cysts develop from preexisting renal tubule segments, and only a small portion of the nephrons (1%) undergoes cystic formation.
- Renal failure: in most patients renal function is maintained within normal range, despite relentless growth of cysts, until the fourth to sixth decades of life.
- Nephrolithiasis (20%)
- Urinary tract infection

Extrarenal manifestations:
- Associated with liver cysts (50% to 70%), pancreatic cysts (10%), splenic cysts (5%), central nervous system arachnoid cysts (5%), and cerebral aneurysms (20%)
- Polycystic liver disease: most common extrarenal manifestation—associated with both *PKD1* and non-*PKD1* genotypes
- Vascular manifestations: intracranial aneurysms (occur in approximately 6% of patients with a negative family history of aneurysms and 16% of those with a positive history), thoracic aortic and cervicocephalic artery dissection, and coronary artery aneurysms
- Increased incidence of diverticular disease and mitral valve prolapse

ETIOLOGY

- Dominantly inherited heterogenic systemic disease: mutations in *PKD1* (chromosome region 16p13.3; 85% of cases) or *PKD2* (4q21; approximately 15% of cases).
- Polycystin 1 and polycystin 2 are the protein products of PKD1 and PKD2, which interact and coassemble and seem to function together to regulate the morphologic configuration of epithelial cells. Although individuals with PKD1 are clinically indistinguishable from individuals with PKD2, patients with PKD2 have a less severe course of disease with a later mean age of diagnosis, hypertension, and end-stage renal disease (ESRD).
- Disease penetrance is 100%.

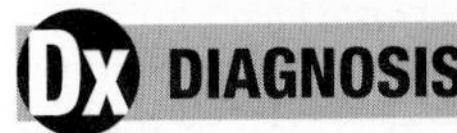

DIAGNOSIS

Sonographic imaging or CT scan:
1. In an individual with a family history for the disease, including:
   - Age <30 yr: at least two unilateral or bilateral cysts
   - 30 to 59 yr: two cysts in each kidney
   - ≥60 yr: four cysts in each kidney
2. In the absence of a family history: bilateral renal enlargement or cysts or the presence of multiple bilateral cysts with hepatic cysts together and in the absence of other manifestations suggesting a different renal cyst disease
   - Genetic testing can be used when the imaging results are equivocal and when a definitive diagnosis is required in a younger individual, such as a potential living related kidney donor.

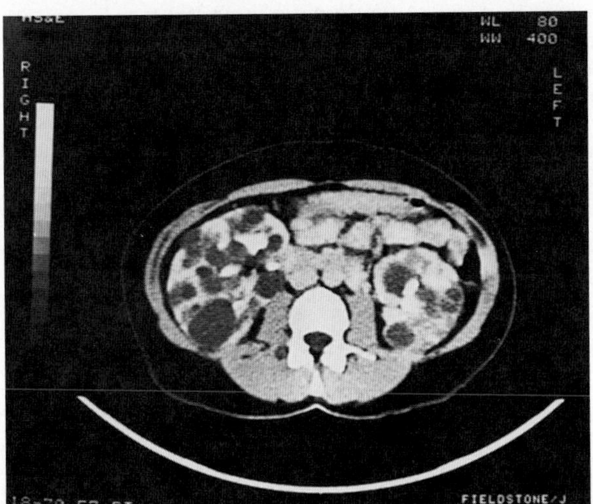

FIGURE 1-747 Tomogram of autosomal-dominant polycystic kidney disease. Kidney cysts. (From Stein JH [ed]: *Internal medicine,* ed 5, St Louis, 1998, Mosby.)

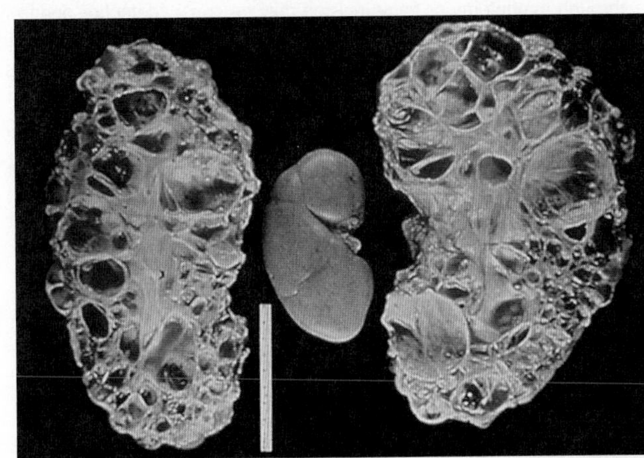

FIGURE 1-748 Markedly enlarged polycystic kidneys from a patient with autosomal-dominant polycystic kidney disease compared with a normal kidney *(middle).* (From Johnson RJ, Feehally J: *Comprehensive clinical nephrology,* ed 2, St Louis, 2000, Mosby.)

 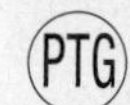

DIFFERENTIAL DIAGNOSIS

- Simple cysts
- Autosomal-recessive PKD in children
- Tuberous sclerosis
- von Hippel-Lindau syndrome
- Acquired cystic kidney disease

LABORATORY TESTS

- Hemoglobin and hematocrit are elevated because of increased secretion of erythropoietin from functioning renal cysts.
- Electrolyte abnormalities commonly seen in any patients with renal insufficiency.
- Blood urea nitrogen and creatinine can be elevated.
- Urinalysis can show microscopic hematuria and proteinuria (seldom >1 g/24 hr). Proteinuria >2 g/day is unusual and suggests the presence of another kidney disease.

IMAGING STUDIES

- A cyst is considered to be present if it measures >2 mm in diameter.
- Abdominal renal ultrasound is the easiest and most cost-efficient test for renal cysts. Renal ultrasound can detect cysts from 1 to 1.5 cm.
- Abdominal CT scan is more sensitive than ultrasound and can detect cysts as small as 0.5 cm.
- Both studies can detect associated hepatic, splenic, and pancreatic cysts.
- MRI is more sensitive than ultrasound and may help distinguish renal cell carcinomas from simple cysts.

Rx TREATMENT

NONPHARMACOLOGIC THERAPY

- Treatment consists of the standard therapies for chronic renal disease, including good blood pressure control and control of hyperlipidemia.
- When conservative measures fail to control the pain, infection, or bleeding, surgical interventions such as cystic decompression by aspiration under ultrasound or CT guidance or laparoscopic or surgical cyst fenestration through lumbotomy or flank incision may be of benefit.
- When above measures fail, nephrectomy should be undertaken in ESRD.
- Combined percutaneous cyst drainage and antibiotic treatment provide the best treatment results for hepatic cyst infection.

ACUTE GENERAL Rx

- Kidney infections should be treated with antibiotics known to penetrate the cyst (e.g., trimethoprim-sulfamethoxazole 1 tablet PO bid or ciprofloxacin 250 mg PO bid).
- Early detection and treatment of hypertension are important because cardiovascular disease is the main cause of death.

CHRONIC Rx

- Dialysis for end-stage renal failure.
- Pretransplant nephrectomy is reserved for patients with a history of infected cyst or frequent bleeding.
- Renal transplantation is the treatment of choice for ESRD.
- Cyst infections are often difficult to treat. Lipophilic agents penetrate the cysts consistently. If fever persists after 1 to 2 wk of appropriate antimicrobial treatment, percutaneous or surgical drainage of the cysts may be needed. Several months of antibiotic treatment may be needed to eradicate the infection.
- Most cases of polycystic liver disease do not need treatment; patients should avoid estrogens and compounds that promote cyclic adenosine monophosphate accumulation (e.g., caffeine).

DISPOSITION

- Most patients with PKD will progress to renal failure.
- Gross hematuria is usually self-limited.

REFERRAL

- Nephrology consultation
- Urology can also be consulted in patients with nephrolithiasis, for recurrent episodes of gross hematuria, or for consideration for nephrectomy before transplantation.
- Counseling should be done before PKD genetic testing. Benefits include certainty of diagnosis that could affect family planning, early detection and treatment of disease complications, and selection of genetically unaffected family members for living related donor transplantation. Potential discrimination in terms of insurability and employment associated with a positive diagnosis should be discussed.

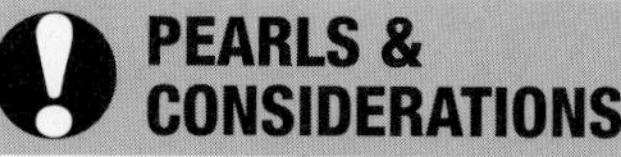

PEARLS & CONSIDERATIONS

- ESRD patients with PKD do better on dialysis than do patients with other causes of ESRD.
- There is no difference in patient survival after transplantation between patients with PKD and other ESRD populations.
- Widespread screening is not indicated. Indications for screening include family history of aneurysm, subarachnoid hemorrhage, previous aneurysm rupture, preparation for major elective surgery, high-risk occupations (airplane pilots), and patient anxiety despite adequate information.
- Kidney and cyst volumes are the strongest predictors of renal function decline.

COMMENTS

- Conservative management is recommended for patients with a small (<7 mm) cerebral aneurysm, particularly in the anterior circulation. Rescreening of patients with a family history of intracranial aneurysm after 5 to 10 yr seems reasonable.
- Trials with treatment protocols involving vasopressin antagonists (tolvaptan) are under way to slow the progression of PKD. The TEMPO (Tolvaptan Efficacy and Safety in Management of Autosomal Dominant Polycystic Kidney Disease and Its Outcome) showed that tolvaptan prolonged the median age at ESRD onset by 6.5 yr and increased life expectancy by 2.6 yr. At $5,760 per mo, tolvaptan cost $744,100 per quality-adjusted life-year compared with standard care.[1]

SUGGESTED READINGS

available at www.expertconsult.com

RELATED CONTENT

Polycystic Kidney Disease (Patient Information)

AUTHOR: **SHAHNAZ PUNJANI, M.D.**

[1]Erickson KR et al: Cost-effectiveness of tolvaptan in autosomal dominant polycystic kidney disease, *Ann Int Med* 159:382-389, 2013.

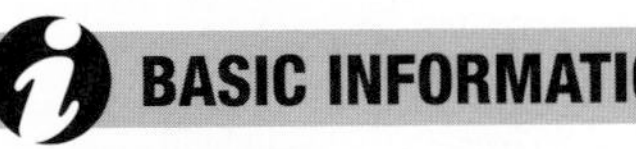

BASIC INFORMATION

DEFINITION

Polycystic ovary syndrome (PCOS) is characterized by an accumulation of incompletely developed follicles in the ovaries due to anovulation and associated with ovarian androgen production. In its complete form, it is associated with polycystic ovaries, amenorrhea, hirsutism, and obesity. Criteria for PCOS according to published definitions are described in Table 1-399.

SYNONYMS

Stein-Leventhal syndrome
PCOS

ICD-9CM CODES
256.4 Polycystic ovary syndrome
ICD-10CM CODES
E28.2 Polycystic ovarian syndrome

EPIDEMIOLOGY & DEMOGRAPHICS

- 5% to 15% of reproductive-age women (most common endocrine disorder in this population).
- Symptoms usually begin around the time of menarche, and the diagnosis is often made during adolescence or young adulthood.
- Increased risk of endometrial and ovarian cancers.
- PCOS is the most common cause of anovulatory infertility

PHYSICAL FINDINGS & CLINICAL PRESENTATION

- Oligomenorrhea or amenorrhea
- Dysfunctional uterine bleeding
- Infertility
- Hirsutism
- Acne, alopecia, acanthosis nigricans (Fig. 1-749)
- Obesity (40% only), predominantly abdominal obesity
- Insulin resistance (type 2 diabetes mellitus)
- Hypertension

ETIOLOGY & PATHOGENESIS

Elevated serum luteinizing hormone (LH) concentrations and an increased serum LH/follicle-stimulating hormone (FSH) ratio result either from an increased gonadotropin-releasing hormone hypothalamic secretion or less likely from a primary pituitary abnormality. This results in dysregulation of androgen secretion and increased intraovarian androgen, the effect of which in the ovary is follicular atresia, maturation arrest, polycystic ovaries, and anovulation. Hyperinsulinemia is a contributing factor to ovarian hyperandrogenism, independent of LH excess. A role for insulin growth factor (IGF) receptors has been postulated for the association of PCOS and diabetes. Fig. E1-750 illustrates the pathologic mechanisms in PCOS.

Dx DIAGNOSIS

The diagnosis of PCOS excludes secondary causes (androgen-producing neoplasm, hyperprolactinemia, adult-onset congenital adrenal hyperplasia).
Clinical:

- The symptoms, signs, and biochemical features of PCOS vary greatly among women and may change over time.
- PCOS is the most common cause of chronic anovulation with estrogen present. A positive progesterone withdrawal test establishes the presence of estrogen. Medroxyprogesterone (Provera) 10 mg qd is administered for 5 days and bleeding occurs if estrogen is present.
- The presence of oligomenorrhea, hirsutism, obesity, and documented polycystic ovaries establishes the diagnosis.

DIFFERENTIAL DIAGNOSIS

Causes of amenorrhea:

- Primary (unusual in PCOS)
  1. Genetic disorder (Turner's syndrome)
  2. Anatomic abnormality (e.g., imperforate hymen)
- Secondary
  1. Pregnancy
  2. Functional (cause unknown, anorexia nervosa, stress, excessive exercise, hyperthyroidism, less commonly hypothyroidism, adrenal dysfunction, pituitary dysfunction, severe systemic illness, drugs such as oral contraceptives, estrogens, or dopamine agonists)
  3. Abnormalities of the genital tract (uterine tumor, endometrial scarring, ovarian tumor)

LABORATORY TESTS

- Glucose tolerance test at the initial presentation and every 2 yr thereafter (rule out diabetes mellitus). Impaired glucose tolerance is very common, occurring in approximately 30% of women with PCOS
- Fasting lipid panel (rule out dyslipidemia), alanine aminotransferase, aspartate aminotransferase (rule out hepatic steatosis)
- Elevated LH/FSH ratio >2.5
- Prolactin level elevation in 25%
- Elevated androgens (testosterone [free and total levels], DHEA-S) (rule out androgen-secreting tumor)
- Other: thyroid-stimulating hormone (rule out hypothyroidism), 17-hydroxyprogesterone (rule out congenital adrenal hyperplasia), 24-hr urine for cortisol and creatinine (rule out Cushing's syndrome)

IMAGING STUDIES

Pelvic ultrasound (Fig. 1-751) (or CT scan) reveals the presence of twofold to fivefold ovarian enlargement with a thickened tunica albuginea, thecal hyperplasia, and 20 or more subcapsular follicles from 1 to 15 mm in diameter (Fig. 1-752). It is important to note that having polycystic ovaries alone does not make the diagnosis of PCOS because 20% of women with polycystic ovaries have no symptoms.

Rx TREATMENT

The goal is to interrupt the self-perpetuating abnormal hormone cycle:

- Reduction of ovarian androgen secretion by laparoscopic ovarian wedge resection. Laparoscopic ovarian surgery (laparoscopic ovarian drilling [LOD]) is a useful alternative that does not trigger ovarian hyperstimulation

TABLE 1-399 Criteria for Polycystic Ovary Syndrome according to Published Definitions

	NICHD/NIH/1990	Rotterdam 2003	AE-PCOS/2009
Diagnostic criteria	Requires simultaneous presence of: • Clinical and/or biochemical hyperandrogenism • Menstrual dysfunction	Requires the presence of at least two criteria: • Clinical and/or biochemical hyperandrogenism • Ovulatory dysfunction • PCOM	Requires the presence of: • Hyperandrogenism and/or hyperandrogenemia • Ovarian dysfunction: oligoovulation or anovulation and/or polycystic ovaries
Exclusion criteria	Congenital adrenal hyperplasia, androgen-secreting tumors, Cushing's syndrome, and hyperprolactinemia	Congenital adrenal hyperplasia, androgen-secreting tumors, and Cushing's syndrome	21-hydroxylase-deficient nonclassic adrenal hyperplasia, androgen-secreting neoplasms, androgenic–anabolic drug use or abuse, the hyperandrogenic-insulin resistance-acanthosis nigricans syndrome, thyroid dysfunction, and hyperprolactinemia
Clinical traits	Hirsutism, acne, and alopecia	Hirsutism, acne, and androgenic alopecia	Hirsutism
PCOM	Not included	At least one ovary showing either: • Twelve or more follicles of 2-9 mm in diameter • Ovarian volume, 10 ml	At least one ovary showing either: • Twelve or more follicles of 2-9 mm in diameter • Ovarian volume, 10 ml

AE-PCOS, Androgen Excess and PCOS Society; *NICHD/NIH,* National Institute for Child Health and Human Development/National Institutes of Health; *PCOM,* polycystic ovarian morphology.
From Fielding JR et al: *Gynecologic imaging,* Philadelphia, 2011, Saunders.

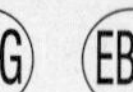

- Reduction of ovarian androgen secretion by using oral contraceptives or LH-releasing hormone (LHRH) analogs
- Weight reduction for all obese women with PCOS. Loss of abdominal fat seems to be crucial to restore ovulation
- FSH stimulation with clomiphene HMG or pulsatile LHRH
- Urofollitropin (pure FSH) administration
- Metformin improves ovulation, insulin sensitivity, and possibly hyperandrogenemia

Choice of treatment:

- The management of hirsutism without risking pregnancy includes oral contraceptives, glucocorticoids, LHRH analogs, or spironolactone (an antiandrogen). Finasteride and flutamide may be similarly effective in reducing hirsutism as spironolactone.
- Pregnancy can be achieved with clomiphene (alone or with glucocorticoids, human chorionic gonadotropin, or bromocriptine), HMG, urofollitropin, pulsatile LHRH, or ovarian wedge resection. (Metformin may induce ovulation.)
- Psychological screening for depression is recommended. Women with PCOS are fourfold more likely to have abnormal depression scores.

SUGGESTED READINGS

available at www.expertconsult.com

RELATED CONTENT

Polycystic Ovarian Syndrome (Patient Information)

AUTHOR: **FRED F. FERRI, M.D.**

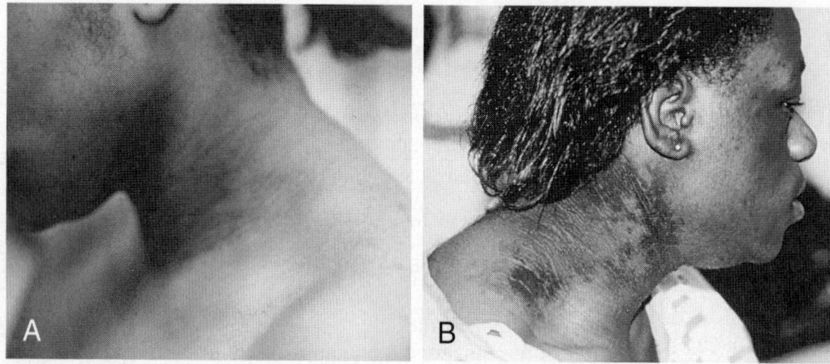

FIGURE 1-749 Acanthosis nigricans. A, Moderate acanthosis nigricans (i.e., darkening and thickening of skin) at the lateral lower fold of the neck. Notice facial hirsutism (sideburns) in the same patient. **B,** Severe acanthosis nigricans in another patient with severe insulin resistance. (**B,** Courtesy of Dr. R. Ann Word, Dallas, Texas. From Melmed S et al: *Williams textbook of endocrinology*, ed 12, Philadelphia, 2011, Saunders.)

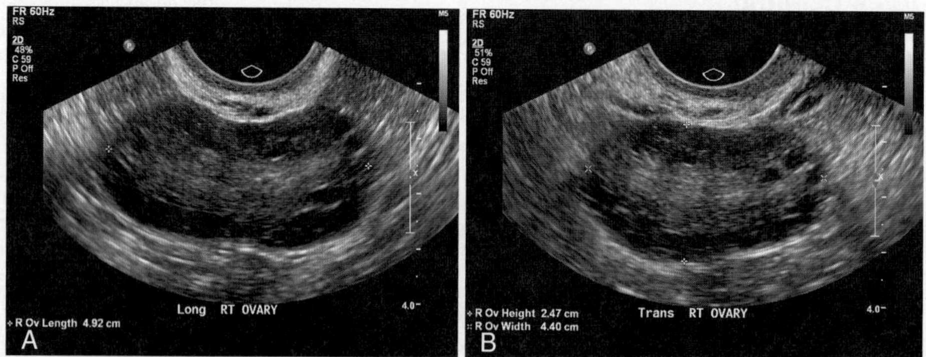

FIGURE 1-751 A, Transvaginal ultrasound in the longitudinal plane showing polycystic ovary morphology. Numerous small follicles surround an echogenic central stroma. **B,** Transvaginal ultrasound in the transverse plane in the same patient. (From Fielding JR et al: *Gynecologic imaging,* Philadelphia, 2011, Saunders.)

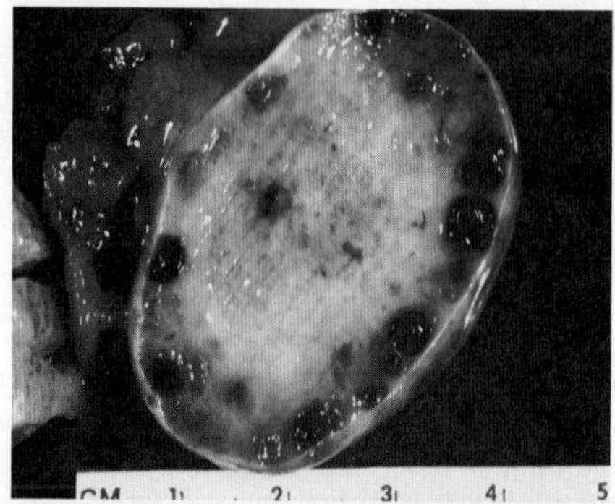

FIGURE 1-752 Sagittal section of a polycystic ovary illustrating large number of follicular cysts and thickened stroma. (From Mishell DR: *Comprehensive gynecology,* ed 3, St Louis, 1997, Mosby.)

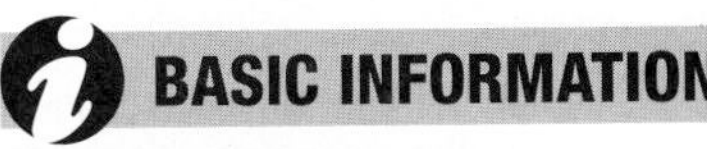

BASIC INFORMATION

DEFINITION

Polycythemia vera is a chronic myeloproliferative disorder that originates from a pluripotent hematopoietic stem cell and is characterized mainly by erythrocytosis (increase in red blood cell [RBC] mass).

SYNONYMS

Primary polycythemia
Vaquez disease

ICD-9CM CODES
238.4 Polycythemia vera
ICD-10CM CODES
D45 Polycythemia vera

EPIDEMIOLOGY & DEMOGRAPHICS

INCIDENCE: 1 case per 100,000 persons. Occurs most commonly in patients aged 50 to 75 years. Mean age at onset is 60 yr; men are affected more often than are women.

PHYSICAL FINDINGS & CLINICAL PRESENTATION

Polycythemia vera has a latent, proliferative, and spent phase. The patient generally comes to medical attention because of symptoms associated with increased blood volume and viscosity or impaired platelet function:

- Impaired cerebral circulation resulting in headache, vertigo, blurred vision, dizziness, transient ischemic attack, cerebrovascular accident
- Fatigue, poor exercise tolerance
- Pruritus, particularly after bathing (caused by overproduction of histamine)
- Bleeding: epistaxis, upper gastrointestinal bleeding (increased incidence of peptic ulcer disease)
- Abdominal discomfort from splenomegaly; hepatomegaly may be present
- Hyperuricemia may result in nephrolithiasis and gouty arthritis
- Nearly 20% of patients experience arterial or venous thrombosis as their initial symptom.

The physical examination may reveal:

- Facial plethora, congestion of oral mucosa, ruddy complexion
- Enlargement and tortuosity of retinal veins
- Splenomegaly (found in >75% of patients)

Dx DIAGNOSIS

DIFFERENTIAL DIAGNOSIS

Smoking:

- Polycythemia is caused by increased carboxyhemoglobin, resulting in left shift in the hemoglobin (Hgb) dissociation curve.
- Laboratory evaluation shows increased hematocrit (Hct), RBC mass, erythropoietin level, and carboxyhemoglobin.
- Splenomegaly is not present on physical examination.

Hypoxemia (secondary polycythemia):

- Living for prolonged periods at high altitudes, pulmonary fibrosis, congenital cardiac lesions with right-to-left shunts.
- Laboratory evaluation shows decreased arterial oxygen saturation and elevated erythropoietin level.
- Splenomegaly is not present on physical examination.

Erythropoietin-producing states:

- Renal cell carcinoma, hepatoma, cerebral hemangioma, uterine fibroids, polycystic kidneys.
- The erythropoietin level is elevated in these patients, and the arterial oxygen saturation is normal.
- Splenomegaly may be present with metastatic neoplasms.

Stress polycythemia (Gaisböck's syndrome, relative polycythemia):

- Laboratory evaluation demonstrates normal RBC mass, arterial oxygen saturation, and erythropoietin level; plasma volume is decreased.
- Splenomegaly is not present on physical examination.

Hemoglobinopathies associated with high oxygen affinity:

- An abnormal oxyhemoglobin-dissociation curve (P50) is present.

WORKUP

Recent developments in molecular biology have identified a single, acquired point mutation in the Janus kinase 2 *(JAK2)* gene in the majority of patients with polycythemia vera and other pH-negative myeloproliferative disorders. The *JAK2* mutation is found in >95% of patients with polycythemia vera and can be used for diagnostic purposes. Testing for the *JAK2 V617F* mutation with polymerase chain reaction assay is now available. In patients with high hematocrit (>52% in men or >48% in women) and in the absence of coexisting secondary erythrocytosis, the presence of the *JAK2* mutation is sufficient for the diagnosis of polycythemia vera.

The World Health Organization diagnostic criteria for polycythemia vera are described in Table 1-400.

LABORATORY TESTS

- Elevated RBC count (>6 million/mm^3), elevated Hgb (>18 g/dl in men, >16 g/dl in women), elevated Hct (<54% in men, <49% in women)
- Increased white blood cell count (often with basophilia); thrombocytosis in the majority of patients
- Elevated leukocyte alkaline phosphatase, serum vitamin B_{12}, and uric acid levels
- Low serum erythropoietin level
- Bone marrow aspiration revealing RBC hyperplasia (Fig. E1-753) and absent iron stores

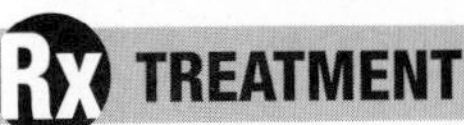

TREATMENT

NONPHARMACOLOGIC THERAPY

Phlebotomy to keep Hct >45% in men and >42% in women is the mainstay of therapy. Phlebotomy, however, has no effect on the development of myelofibrosis.

ACUTE GENERAL Rx

- Hydroxyurea can be used in conjunction with phlebotomy to decrease the incidence of thrombotic events.
- Interferon-alpha-2b is also effective in controlling RBC values without significant side effects.
- Myelosuppressive therapy with chlorambucil is effective but should not be routinely used because of its leukemogenic potential.
- Box 1-67 describes an algorithm for management of patients with polycythemia vera.

CHRONIC Rx

- Patient education regarding need for lifelong monitoring and treatment.
- Adjunctive therapy: treatment of pruritus with antihistamines, control of significant hyperuricemia with allopurinol, reduction of gastric hyperacidity with antacids of H_2 blockers, low-dose aspirin to treat vasomotor symptoms in patients without bleeding diathesis. Low-dose aspirin can safely prevent thrombotic complications in patients with polycythemia vera and should be given to all patients in absence of contraindications.

TABLE 1-400 World Health Organization 2008 Diagnostic Criteria for Polycythemia Vera

Major Criteria

1. Hemoglobin (Hgb) >18.5 g/dl (men), >16.5 (women); *or* Hgb or hematocrit (Hct) >99% reference range for age, sex, or altitude of residence; *or* Hgb >17 g/dl (men), >15 g/dl (women) if associated with a sustained increase of ≥2 g/dl from baseline that cannot be attributed to correction of iron deficiency; *or* elevated red cell mass (>25% above mean normal predicted value)
2. Presence of *JAK2 V617F* or similar mutation

Minor Criteria

1. Bone marrow trilineage myeloproliferation
2. Subnormal serum erythropoietin level
3. Endogenous erythroid colony formation in vitro

Either both major criteria and one minor criterion *or* the first major criterion and two minor criteria must be met for diagnosis of polycythemia vera.

From Andreoli TE et al: *Andreoli and Carpenter's Cecil essentials of medicine,* ed 8, Philadelphia, 2010, Saunders.

 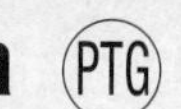

BOX 1-67 Management of Patients with Polycythemia Vera

Low-risk young patients (<60 yr) and no prior history of thrombosis, platelet count $<1.5 \times 10^6$ mm^{-3}

Phlebotomy + low-dose aspirin (81 mg/d) to maintain Hct <45% in males and <42% in females. Aspirin should not be used in patients with histories of hemorrhagic episode or with extreme thrombocytosis ($>1.5 \times 10^6$ mm^{-3}) or acquired von Willebrand syndrome.

↓

Thrombosis or hemorrhage
Systemic symptoms
Severe pruritus refractory to histamine antagonists
Painful splenomegaly

↓

Pegylated interferon 90 to 180 μg/wk or interferon α (3×10^6 units three times/wk; alter dose depending on response and toxicity). Consider the use of pegylated interferon, which can be administered once/wk.

↓

If platelet control is inadequate or patient cannot tolerate interferon, one option could be the use of anagrelide. However, the use of this drug is controversial. In this case, supplemental phlebotomy is required to maintain Hct <45% in males and <42% in females, and the use of hydroxyurea should be considered, especially if patient continues to have thrombotic episodes.

↓

If the patient has increasing splenomegaly, systemic symptoms, or repeated thromboses in spite of adequate dose of hydroxyurea (2 to 3 g/d) start busulphan 4 to 6 mg/d PO for 4 to 8 wk. It should be mentioned that the sequential use of hydroxyurea and busulphan may be associated with an increased risk of leukemia. Supplemental phlebotomy may be required.

↓

Painful splenomegaly
Splenectomy + continued systemic therapy

High-risk patients (>60 yr), previous thrombosis, platelet count $>1.5 \times 10^6$ mm^{-3}
Phlebotomy to Hct <42% in females and <45% in males
Aspirin (81 mg/d) to be given only in patients with platelet counts $<1.5 \times 10^6$ mm^{-2}
Myelosuppressive therapy with hydroxyurea 30 mg/kg PO for 1 wk

↓

Then 15 to 20 mg/kg

If patient continues to have thrombotic episodes and has extreme thrombocytosis or cannot tolerate hydroxyurea, consider pegylated interferon 90 to 180 μg/wk or add busulphan 4 to 6 mg/d PO for 4 to 8 wk.

Stop when blood counts are normalized or platelet count is <300,000 mm^{-3}.

Occasional supplemental phlebotomy if Hct is >42% in females and >45% in males; when patient relapses (patient is symptomatic), initiate busulphan therapy again at same dose.

↓

If patient is poorly compliant, consider ^{32}P: 2.3 mCi/m^2 IV every 12 wk as needed (limit 5 mCi per dose).

Increase dose by 25% if no response

Patient age >70 yr
Phlebotomy + low-dose aspirin + hydroxyurea

↓

No response or poor compliance

Busulphan 4 to 6 mg/d PO for 4 to 8 wk. Stop when blood counts are normalized or platelet count is >300,000 mm^{-3}.

↓

No response to ^{32}P

From Hoffmann R et al: *Hematology: basic principles and practice,* ed 5, Philadelphia, 2009, Churchill Livingstone.

DISPOSITION

- The median survival time without treatment is 6 to 18 mo after diagnosis; phlebotomy extends the average survival time to 12 yr.
- Patients with polycythemia vera with a hematocrit <45% have a significantly lower rate of cardiovascular death and major thrombosis than those with hematocrit of 45% to 50%.
- Prognosis is worse in patients >60 yr and those with a history of thrombosis.

SUGGESTED READINGS

available at www.expertconsult.com

RELATED CONTENT

Polycythemia Vera (Patient Information)

AUTHOR: **FRED F. FERRI, M.D.**

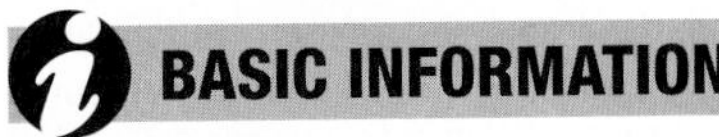

BASIC INFORMATION

DEFINITION

Polymyalgia rheumatica (PMR) is an inflammatory condition characterized by shoulder and pelvic girdle muscle pain and stiffness.

SYNONYMS

Anarthritic rheumatoid syndrome
PMR

ICD-9CM CODES
725.0 Polymyalgia rheumatica
ICD-10CM CODES
M35.3 Polymyalgia rheumatica

EPIDEMIOLOGY & DEMOGRAPHICS

PREVALENCE: Some geographic variation with rates of 59 per 100,000 in Minnesota; 84 per 100,000 in UK; rare in African Americans
PREDOMINANT SEX: Female/male ratio of 2:1
PREDOMINANT AGE: Age >50 years with greater incidence as age increases

PHYSICAL FINDINGS & CLINICAL PRESENTATION

- In majority of patients, sudden onset of muscle pain and stiffness
- Neck, shoulders, and arms are most often affected. Pelvic girdle and thigh muscles also involved.
- Patients often note severe pain and stiffness.
- Constitutional symptoms of fatigue, malaise, and loss of appetite may accompany pain and stiffness.
- Physical exam is fairly benign; passive range of motion is typically preserved; may find minimal joint swelling, and strength testing is normal.
- Presence of fever, chills, night sweats, visual disturbances, headaches, or jaw claudication suggests concomitant giant cell arteritis and warrants further evaluation.

ETIOLOGY

Appears to be related to the presence of HLA-D4 haplotypes, which confer susceptibility to activation of the innate immune system leading to inflammation.

DIAGNOSIS

DIFFERENTIAL DIAGNOSIS

See Box E1-68.

WORKUP

- Elderly patients with PMR symptoms should have initial laboratory evaluation with ESR, CBC, CPK.
- ESR >40 is seen in majority of patients.
- May have a normocytic, normochromic anemia and thrombocytosis.
- An algorithm for diagnosing polymyalgia rheumatica without giant cell arteritis is described in Fig. 1-754.
- Table 1-401 describes diagnostic criteria for PMR.

TREATMENT

ACUTE GENERAL Rx

- Prednisone 10 to 20 mg/day with dramatic improvement in symptoms typically noted in 24 to 48 hr.
- Initial dose of prednisone maintained for 2 to 4 wk with steroid dose reduced by 10% every 4 wk as long as patient remains symptom free.
- It is prudent to start a proton-pump inhibitor at initiation of therapy given the need for gastric protection in an elderly age group at high risk for GI toxicity.
- Attention should be paid to bone health given most patients are on steroids for 1 to 2 yr. Calcium and vitamin D supplementation should be started early on with possible bisphosphonate use if indicated by bone density measurement.

PEARLS & CONSIDERATIONS

Patients with PMR should be monitored carefully for the development of giant cell arteritis. Patients who have incomplete response to treatment with prednisone or have an evolving pattern of pain and swelling should be reevaluated for the possibility of a different diagnosis.

SUGGESTED READINGS

available at www.expertconsult.com

RELATED CONTENT

Giant Cell Arteritis (Related Key Topic)
Vasculitis, Systemic (Related Key Topic)
Polymyalgia Rheumatica (PMR) (Patient Information)

AUTHOR: **NUHA R. SAID, M.D.**

Polymyalgia rheumatica without giant cell arteritis suspected
Prednisone up to 20 mg/day for 7 days
No or poor response after ~7 days
Increase prednisone to 30 mg/day for ~7 days
Excellent response
No response to prednisone 30 mg/day
Diagnosis supported
Continue to monitor for emergence of giant cell arteritis
Reject diagnosis of polymyalgia rheumatica; search for alternative diagnosis

FIGURE 1-754 Algorithm for diagnosing polymyalgia rheumatica without giant cell arteritis. (From Firestein GS et al: *Kelly's textbook of rheumatology*, ed 9, Philadelphia, 2013, Saunders.)

TABLE 1-401 Polymyalgia Rheumatica: Diagnostic Criteria

Chuang et al 1982	Healey 1984
• Age of onset = 50 yr or older • Erythrocyte sedimentation rate >40 mm/h • Bilateral aching and stiffness for =1 mo and involving two of the following areas: neck or torso, shoulders or proximal regions of the arms, and hips or proximal aspects of the thighs • Exclusion of all other diagnoses causing PMR-like symptoms	• Age of onset = 50 yr or older • Erythrocyte sedimentation rate >40 mm/h • Pain persisting for =1 mo and involving two of the following areas: neck, shoulders, and pelvic girdle • Absence of other diseases capable of causing the musculoskeletal symptoms • Morning stiffness lasting more than 1 hr • Rapid response to prednisone (=20 mg/day)

From Hochberg M: *Rheumatology*, ed 4, Philadelphia, 2007, Mosby.

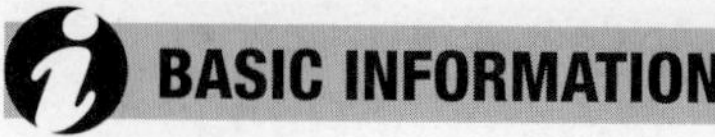

BASIC INFORMATION

DEFINITION

Clinically significant portal hypertension is defined as a portal vein pressure >10 mm Hg, most commonly attributable to liver disease.

SYNONYMS

None

ICD-9CM CODES
572.3 Portal hypertension
ICD-10CM CODES
K76.6 Portal hypertension

EPIDEMIOLOGY & DEMOGRAPHICS

- Incidence of portal hypertension is not known.
- Cirrhosis is the most common cause of portal hypertension in the U.S.
- More than 90% of patients with cirrhosis develop portal hypertension.
- Alcoholic and viral liver diseases are the most common causes of cirrhosis and portal hypertension in the U.S.
- Schistosomiasis is the main cause of portal hypertension outside the U.S.
- Esophageal varices may appear when portal vein pressure rises to >10 mm Hg.
- Variceal hemorrhage is the most serious complication of portal hypertension and may occur when portal pressures rise >12 mm Hg.

PHYSICAL FINDINGS & CLINICAL PRESENTATION

- Jaundice
- Ascites (Fig. 1-755)
- Spider angiomata
- Testicular atrophy
- Gynecomastia
- Palmar erythema
- Dupuytren's contracture
- Asterixis (with advanced liver failure)
- Irritability, encephalopathy
- Splenomegaly
- Dilated veins in the anterior abdominal wall
- Venous pattern on the flanks
- Caput medusae (tortuous collateral veins around the umbilicus)
- Hemorrhoids
- Hematemesis
- Melena
- Pruritus

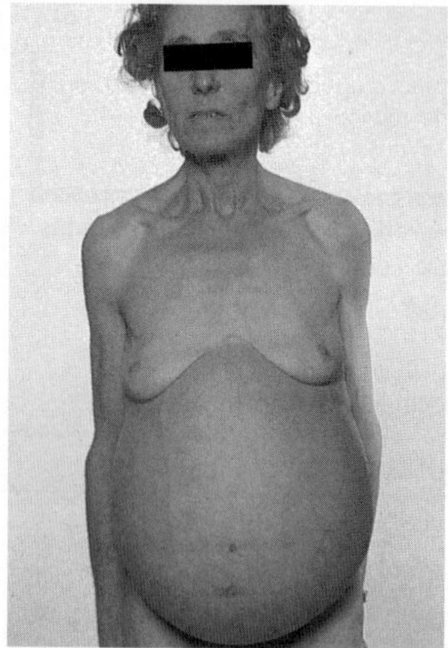

FIGURE 1-755 Ascites secondary to portal hypertension. Note the dilated collateral vein running up the right side of the abdomen. (From Forbes A et al [eds]: *Atlas of clinical gastroenterology,* ed 3, Oxford, 2005, Mosby.)

ETIOLOGY

Pathophysiologically caused by:

1. Conditions resulting in an increased resistance to flow
   - Prehepatic (e.g., portal vein thrombosis, splenic vein thrombosis, congenital stenosis)
   - Hepatic (e.g., cirrhosis, alcoholic liver disease, primary biliary cirrhosis, schistosomiasis)
   - Posthepatic (e.g., Budd-Chiari syndrome, constrictive pericarditis, inferior vena cava obstruction, cor pulmonale, tricuspid regurgitation)
2. Conditions leading to increase in portal blood flow
   - Splanchnic arterial vasodilation accompanying portal hypertension, mediated by local release of nitric oxide
   - Arterial-portal venous fistulae

Table 1-402 summarizes the etiology of portal hypertension.

DIAGNOSIS

- The diagnosis of portal hypertension is made on clinical grounds after a comprehensive history and physical examination.
- Noninvasive and invasive procedures confirm diagnosis and determine the severity of portal hypertension.

DIFFERENTIAL DIAGNOSIS

- Ascites from infection, neoplasm, or other inflammatory processes
- Obesity
- Abdominal organomegaly

WORKUP

The workup of portal hypertension includes blood tests and noninvasive imaging studies to determine if the cause of portal hypertension is prehepatic, hepatic, or posthepatic. Ascitic fluid analysis is a key part of the diagnosis.

LABORATORY TESTS

- Complete blood count with platelets
- Liver function tests with serum albumin
- Prothrombin and partial thromboplastin times
- Hepatitis B surface antigen and antibody
- Hepatitis C antibody
- In selected cases: iron, total iron-binding capacity, and ferritin; antinuclear antibody, anti–smooth muscle antibodies, antimitochondrial antibody, ceruloplasmin, alpha-1 antitrypsin.
- Ascitic fluid analysis: a serum-ascites albumin gradient ≥1.1 mg/dl suggests portal hypertension. Polymorphonuclear cells ≥250 cells/ml or positive Gram stain or culture suggest complicating spontaneous bacterial peritonitis (SBP).

IMAGING STUDIES

- Duplex-Doppler ultrasound is effective in screening for portal hypertension.
- Less commonly, CT/MRI/MRA scanning (Fig. 1-756) or liver-spleen nuclear medicine scanning can be used if the results from ultrasound are equivocal.
- Upper endoscopy is the most reliable test documenting the presence of esophageal varices.

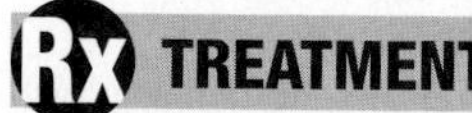

TREATMENT

The treatment of portal hypertension is complex and involves measures to reduce the hypertension directly, minimize volume overload, correct underlying disorders, and prevent complications (most notably SBP and variceal bleeding).

NONPHARMACOLOGIC THERAPY

Dietary sodium restriction to generally 2000 mg/day forms the basis of therapy to limit fluid overload.

ACUTE GENERAL Rx

- For tense ascites, serial large-volume paracentesis (LVP) is generally recommended. The use of albumin infusion (8 to 10 g/L of ascites fluid removed) during LVP >5 L has been shown to reduce the incidence of postparacentesis circulatory dysfunction, although its use remains somewhat controversial.
- IV diuretics, typically furosemide and spironolactone, are used to achieve natriuresis and net negative salt and water balance. Renal function and serum electrolytes are monitored frequently, with transition to an oral regimen for long-term therapy.
- SBP is treated with IV antibiotics directed against enteric bacteria.
- Acute variceal hemorrhage is treated with crystalloid and blood product resuscitation, IV octreotide, terlipressin/vasopressin or somatostatin, and urgent upper endoscopy, often with sclerotherapy or band ligation. Patients with acute variceal hemorrhage should receive antibiotic prophylaxis against SBP.
- Traditionally, a transjugular intrahepatic portosystemic shunt (TIPS) or surgical shunt placement may be considered in patients not responding to above measures. However, recent data show early TIPS placement improved outcomes in acute variceal hemorrhage.

CHRONIC Rx

- Dietary sodium restriction in combination with diuretics: the typical ratio of furosemide 40 mg to spironolactone 100 mg retains normal serum potassium levels in most patients.

TABLE 1-402 Etiology of Portal Hypertension

Condition	Site of Increased Resistance	FHVP	WHVP	HVPG	SPP	Liver Disease
Cirrhosis	Intrahepatic sinusoidal	Normal	Increased	Increased	Increased	Yes
Alcoholic hepatitis	Intrahepatic sinusoidal	Normal	Increased	Increased	Increased	Yes
Extrahepatic portal, splenic, or mesenteric vein thrombosis	Extrahepatic presinusoidal	Normal	Normal	Normal	Increased	No
Early primary biliary cirrhosis, PSC, sarcoid, schistosomiasis, congestive heart failure, noncirrhotic portal fibrosis, NRH	Intrahepatic presinusoidal	Normal	Normal/?raised	Normal/?raised	Increased	No
Hemochromatosis, peliosis, infiltrative disease, acute fatty liver of pregnancy	Intrahepatic sinusoidal hypertension	Normal	Increased	Increased	Increased	Yes
Veno-occlusive disease, posttransplant rejection	Intrahepatic postsinusoidal hypertension	Normal	?Increased	?Decreased	Increased	Yes
Budd-Chiari syndrome (noncirrhotic)	Extrahepatic postsinusoidal hypertension	Increased	Increased	Normal	Increased	Depends on severity
Constrictive pericarditis, inferior vena cava obstruction, congenital inferior vena cava web, right heart failure	Extrahepatic postsinusoidal hypertension	Increased	Increased	Normal	Increased	Depends on severity

FHVP, Free hepatic venous pressure; *HVPG,* hepatic venous pressure gradient; *SPP,* systolic pulse pressure; *WHVP,* wedged hepatic venous pressure.
From Vincent JL et al: *Textbook of critical care,* ed 6, Philadelphia, 2011, Saunders.

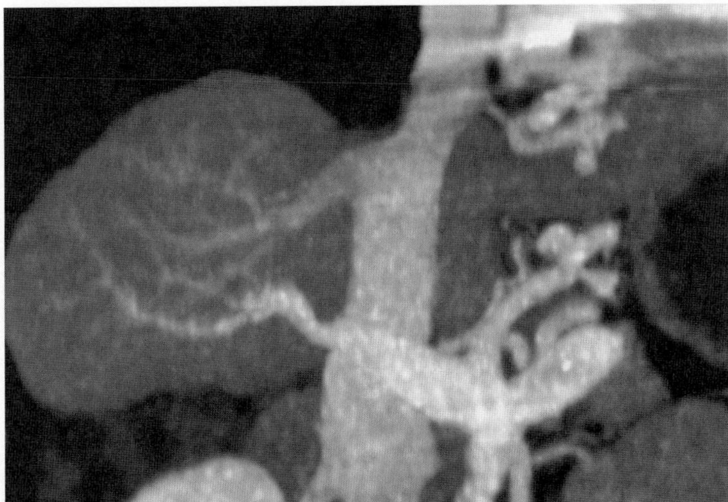

FIGURE 1-756 MR angiography showing portal hypertension with collaterals. The shrunken liver and collateral are obvious. (From Forbes A et al [eds]: *Atlas of clinical gastroenterology,* ed 3, St Louis, 2005, Mosby.)

- Nonselective beta-blockers (propranolol and nadolol) in dosages sufficient to reduce the resting heart rate by 25% have been shown to be effective in primary prophylaxis for first-time variceal bleeding and for preventing recurrent variceal bleeding. Dosages are usually given bid and decreased if heart rate falls to <55 beats/min or systolic blood pressure drops to <90 mm Hg. The addition of a long-acting nitrate (e.g., isosorbide-5-mononitrate) has been shown to improve portal hemodynamics. Findings of a prospective trial of beta-blockers to prevent the formation of varices were negative. The combination of beta-blockade plus endoscopic esophageal variceal banding is superior to either intervention alone.
- Intermittent LVP may be needed in "diuretic resistant" patients.
- Patients with prior SBP merit lifelong antibiotics for secondary prevention.
- Abstinence from alcohol or treatment for hepatitis B or hepatitis C. Vaccination for hepatitis A and B as appropriate.
- Hepatic transplantation is an option in selected patients.

DISPOSITION

- The most common complication associated with portal hypertension is variceal bleeding. The risk of bleeding from varices is approximately 15% at 1 yr.
- Development of the hepatorenal syndrome (HRS) is associated with high near-term mortality. In particular, HRS may complicate SBP, which emphasizes the importance of making the diagnosis of SBP and instituting appropriate prophylaxis.

REFERRAL

Consultation with a gastroenterologist is recommended in all patients with portal hypertension to screen for esophageal varices.

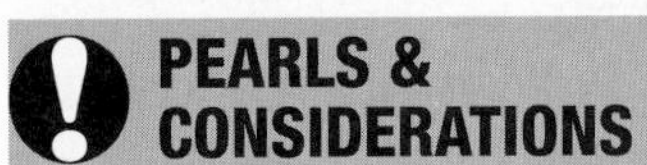

PEARLS & CONSIDERATIONS

Splanchnic arterial vasodilation is increasingly recognized as an important component of the pathophysiology of portal hypertension and ascites. There may be vasodilation in other capillary beds as well; of note, pulmonary arteriolar vasodilation can create a significant shunt fraction and resultant hypoxemia in the absence of chest radiograph or CT chest evidence of parenchymal disease. The diagnosis is suspected when otherwise unexplained hypoxia arises in a patient with cirrhosis, along with platypnea (dyspnea worse when sitting upright) and orthodeoxia (desaturation with upright posture). The diagnosis is confirmed by echocardiography with agitated saline, in which there is delayed appearance of bubbles in the left heart after injection into a peripheral vein.

COMMENTS

Portal hypertension and its complications carry significant morbidity and mortality rates. Emphasize ethanol abstinence, provide vaccinations and prophylactic therapy where indicated, and consider early referral to a specialist for assistance with management and consideration for hepatic transplantation.

SUGGESTED READINGS

available at www.expertconsult.com

AUTHOR: **MEL L. ANDERSON, M.D.**

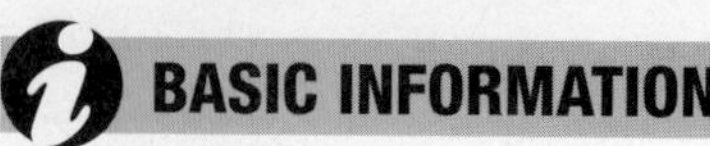

BASIC INFORMATION

DEFINITION

Portal vein thrombosis (PVT) is thrombotic occlusion of the portal vein. The thrombus can also involve segments of the mesenteric veins and/or the splenic vein.

SYNONYMS

Pylethrombosis
PVT

ICD-9CM CODES
452 Portal vein thrombosis
ICD-10CM CODES
I81 Portal vein thrombosis

EPIDEMIOLOGY & DEMOGRAPHICS

Occurs with equal frequency in children (peak age: 6 yr) and adults (peak age: 40 yr)

PHYSICAL FINDINGS & CLINICAL PRESENTATION

- Acute PVT may present with sudden onset of fever and abdominal pain (when there is mesenteric extension).
- Upper gastrointestinal hemorrhage (hematemesis and/or melena) caused by esophageal varices

ETIOLOGY & PATHOPHYSIOLOGY

In children: umbilical sepsis (pathophysiology unknown). In adults:

1. Hypercoagulable states
   - Antiphospholipid syndrome
   - Neoplasm (common cause)
   - Paroxysmal nocturnal hemoglobinuria
   - Myeloproliferative diseases
   - Oral contraceptives
   - Polycythemia vera
   - Pregnancy
   - Protein S or C deficiency
   - Sickle cell disease
   - Thrombocytosis
2. Inflammatory diseases
   - Crohn's disease
   - Pancreatitis
   - Ulcerative colitis
3. Complications of medical intervention
   - Ambulatory dialysis
   - Chemoembolization
   - Liver transplantation
   - Partial hepatectomy
   - Sclerotherapy
   - Splenectomy
   - Transjugular intrahepatic portosystemic shunt
4. Infections
   - Appendicitis
   - Diverticulitis
   - Cholecystitis
5. Miscellaneous
   - Cirrhosis (common cause)
   - Bladder cancer

Pathophysiology: PVT results in portal hypertension, leading to esophageal and gastrointestinal varices. The liver sustained by the hepatic artery maintains normal function.

Dx DIAGNOSIS

DIFFERENTIAL DIAGNOSIS

Causes of upper gastrointestinal hemorrhage are covered in Section II.

WORKUP

- Abdominal ultrasound (Fig. 1-757) or MRI may show the PVT. Abdominal ultrasound color Doppler imaging has a 98% negative predictive value and is considered the imaging modality of choice in diagnosing PVT.
- Determination of underlying cirrhosis of the liver should be the foremost step.
- Esophagogastroscopy shows esophageal varices.

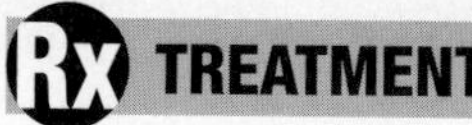

TREATMENT

- Anticoagulation data on thrombolytic therapy are inconclusive. In patients with chronic PVT and concomitant cirrhosis, long-term anticoagulation is generally not recommended.
- Variceal sclerotherapy or banding
- Surgical mesocaval or splenorenal shunt
- The roles of thrombolysis and transjugular intrahepatic portosystemic shunt continue to evolve

REFERRAL

- To surgeon to rule out intestinal infarction
- To gastroenterologist

SUGGESTED READINGS
available at www.expertconsult.com

AUTHOR: **FRED F. FERRI, M.D.**

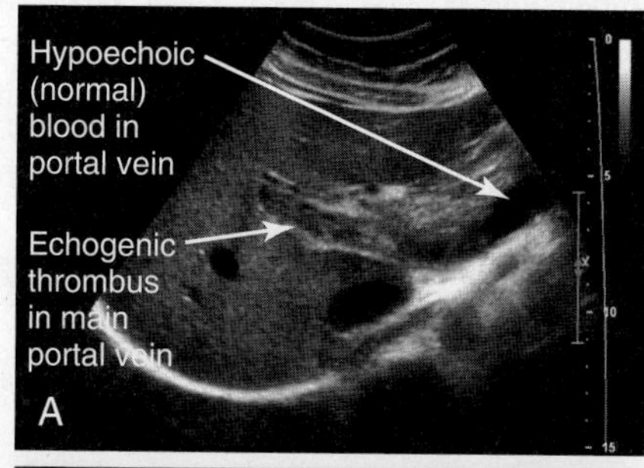

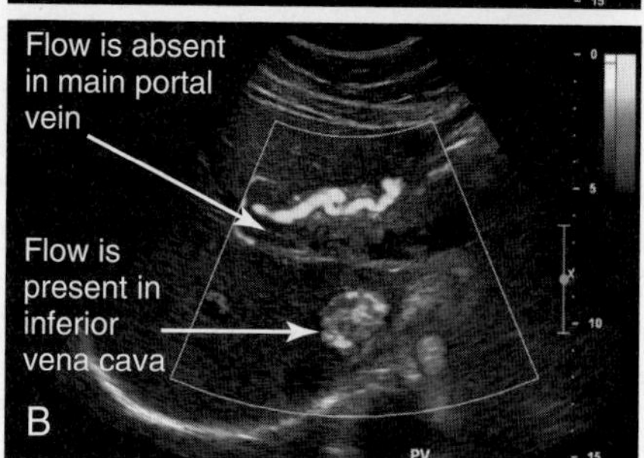

FIGURE 1-757 Portal vein thrombosis: ultrasound. This 22-year-old female, 2 months postpartum, presented with 1 week of right upper quadrant pain. Ultrasound was performed to evaluate for suspected cholecystitis or symptomatic cholelithiasis. Instead, portal vein thrombosis was discovered. The postpartum state is a risk factor for this condition. Hypercoagulable states and inflammatory or neoplastic abdominal conditions, including pancreatitis and abdominal malignancies, also can result in portal vein thrombosis. **A,** Ultrasound gray scale image showing thrombus in the main portal vein. **B,** Doppler ultrasound showing no flow within the portal vein. (From Broder JS: *Diagnostic imaging for the emergency physician,* Philadelphia, 2011, Saunders.)

BASIC INFORMATION

DEFINITION

Postconcussive syndrome (PCS) refers to persistent neurologic cognitive, and psychological symptoms that result from traumatic brain injury (TBI), usually beyond 3 months. PCS can also follow moderate and severe brain injury, although it is more commonly associated with mild brain injury or concussion. Concussion is an acute trauma-induced alteration of mental function lasting <24 hr, with or without preceding loss of consciousness.

SYNONYMS

PCS
Postconcussion syndrome
Posttraumatic nervous instability or brain injury
Postcontusion syndrome or encephalopathy
Status post commotio cerebri

ICD-9CM CODES
310.2 Postconcussion syndrome
ICD-10CM CODES
F07.81 Postconcussional syndrome

EPIDEMIOLOGY & DEMOGRAPHICS

- Incidence is approximately 27 cases per 100,000 persons/year.
- From 30% to 80% of patients with mild to moderate brain injury will experience some symptoms of PCS.
- Female gender and increasing age are risk factors for PCS.
- Usually seen in the young, ages 20 to 30 yr.

PHYSICAL FINDINGS & CLINICAL PRESENTATION

- Usually present without focal neurologic deficits on examination.
- Symptoms start within a few days after the head injury and usually persist after 3 mo.
- Can be divided into early and late or persistent (>6 mo).
- 15% of patients will have persistent symptoms 1 yr later.
- Symptoms include (at least three of the following after TBI to meet ICD-10 criteria):
  1. Headache (usually of fronto-occipital location and showing characteristics of tension or migraine headache). The International Headache Society suggests that coding and attribution of headaches with characteristics of primary headaches but in the setting of an inciting event should be attributed to the event, unless there was a known history of the headache and the inciting event was seen as aggravating/initiating the preexisting migraine/tension headache.
  2. Fatigue
  3. Dizziness and/or vertigo
  4. Impaired memory
  5. Difficulty in concentrating
  6. Insomnia
  7. Irritability
  8. Lowered tolerance of stress, emotion, or alcohol
- Other associated symptoms: noise sensitivity, neck pain, nondermatomal paresthesias, interference with social role functioning.

ETIOLOGY

- Caused by TBI from events such as falls, motor vehicle accidents, and contact sports.
- Postmortem findings reveal diffuse axonal injury as the primary pathologic finding along with small petechial hemorrhages and local edema.
- The primary injury triggers a slew of pathophysiological changes at the cellular level secondary to the axonal stretching and injury, leading to alterations in membrane and intracellular physiology. These changes are believed to be a factor in determining whether the outcome will be an apparent normal recovery or persistent postconcussion symptoms.
- Diffuse axon injury is believed to lead to altered neurotransmission and possibly to clinical manifestations.
- A psychogenic origin has been suggested by a number of empiric and clinical observations; however, limitations in methodology and differing definitions preclude firm conclusions. Prior history of anxiety is a strong risk factor for occurrence of PCS.

DIAGNOSIS

A careful history, a nonfocal neurologic examination, and normal neurologic testing will usually establish the diagnosis.

DIFFERENTIAL DIAGNOSIS

- Headache (dissection of the vertebral artery, occipital neuralgia)
- Epidural hematoma
- Subdural hematoma
- Skull fracture
- Cervical spine disk disease
- Whiplash
- Cerebrovascular accident
- Depression
- Anxiety

WORKUP

To exclude other causes of neurologic symptoms after TBI:
- Normal results of electroencephalography
- Normal evoked potentials
- Neuropsychological testing, which often reveals difficulties in concentration, memory, language, and executive function

LABORATORY TESTS

Various biomarkers in blood and cerebrospinal fluid and genetic testing have been proposed and studied in patients with TBI, but these tests are not specific and are not routinely used.

IMAGING STUDIES

- 10% of CT scans of the head following mild TBI are abnormal, showing mild subarachnoid hemorrhage, subdural hemorrhage, or contusions.
- MRI of the head is abnormal in 30% of patients with normal CT scans and may show irregular brain contours or old cerebral contusions.
- Recent improvements in imaging modalities, including diffuse tensor imaging (DTI) and susceptibility weighted imaging (SWI) in MRI, functional MRI (fMRI), and metabolic imaging such as magnetic resonance spectroscopy (MRS), positron emission tomography (PET), and single-photon emission computed tomography (SPECT) imaging, appear to be promising in elucidating the underlying pathophysiology of TBI and PCS, although they have not found a major role in clinical practice yet.

TREATMENT

Must be recognized as a physiologic and psychological problem and treated accordingly.

GENERAL Rx

- Must be individualized to the patient's particular symptoms.
- Simple reassurance is often the major treatment.
- Supportive care may include the use of nonnarcotic analgesics and antiemetics.
- Pain management.
- Amitriptyline has been widely used for posttraumatic tension-type headaches as well as for nonspecific symptoms such as irritability, dizziness, insomnia, and depression.
- Posttraumatic migraine-type headaches can be treated with a trial of propranolol or amitriptyline alone or in combination.
- Depression can be treated with selective serotonin reuptake inhibitors but may not respond as well when compared with patients without PCS who have depression.
- Some patients may be admitted for severe symptoms; most can be managed as outpatients.
- There may be a role for cognitive behavioral therapy in treating symptoms.

NONPHARMACOLOGIC THERAPY

- Early psychological intervention and cognitive rehabilitation are key for full recovery.
- Physical and occupational therapy.
- Avoidance of alcohol, narcotics, and sleep deprivation.
- Explanation of symptoms and expectations, combined with early follow-up with reassurance, may hasten resolution of symptoms.

DISPOSITION

- Most patients improve after mild TBI without any residual deficits within 3 months.
- Although good improvement is typically seen within the first 6 mo, patients can continue to show improvement for up to 12-18 mo.
- Patients with very severe brain injuries (low Glasgow Coma Scale [GCS] score) and prolonged anterograde amnesia are at increased risk of development of some degree of permanent cognitive and personality disturbance.

 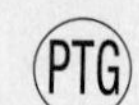

- Predictors for the development of persistent PCS include:
  - Female sex
  - Ongoing litigation (conflicting studies)
  - Low socioeconomic status
  - Prior headaches
  - Prior TBI
  - Prior psychiatric illnesses such as anxiety

REFERRAL

Early consultations with psychologists, psychiatrists, neurologists, and rehabilitation specialists in an outpatient setting may be beneficial.

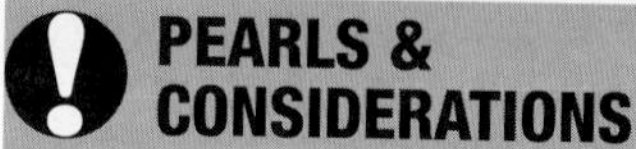

PEARLS & CONSIDERATIONS

- PCS starts within a few days after the injury.
- Recognizing depression and treating pain symptoms early in the course may help prevent the development of persistent PCS (>1 yr).
- The severity of the trauma does not clearly predict the risk of PCS.
- The severity of brain injury is usually documented by initial GCS score, duration of loss of consciousness, and duration of amnesia; however, there is a move toward tests of function, such as neuropsychological testing or fMRI.

COMMENTS

- Attempts to determine how much of a role psychological and/or neurologic factors play in the PCS are important but very difficult.
- No medication at hospital discharge has been proved to change the natural course of the disease.

SUGGESTED READINGS

available at www.expertconsult.com

RELATED CONTENT

Post-concussion Syndrome (Patient Information)

AUTHOR: **PRASHANTH KRISHNAMOHAN, M.B.B.S, M.D**

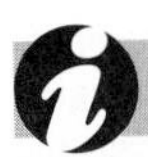

BASIC INFORMATION

DEFINITION

Postpartum hemorrhage (PPH) is classically defined as estimated blood loss >500 ml after a vaginal birth or >1000 ml after a cesarean section. Primary PPH is hemorrhage within the first 24 hr after delivery. Secondary PPH is hemorrhage after 24 hr and within 6-12 wk.

SYNONYMS

Obstetric hemorrhage

ICD-9CM CODES
666 Postpartum hemorrhage
ICD-10CM CODES
O72.1 Other immediate postpartum hemorrhage

EPIDEMIOLOGY & DEMOGRAPHICS

INCIDENCE: 4%-6%
PREDOMINANT SEX AND AGE: Female of reproductive age
RISK FACTORS: Prolonged labor, augmented labor, rapid labor, history of PPH, episiotomy, preeclampsia, multiple gestation, macrosomic infant, operative delivery, chorioamniotis, bleeding dyscrasia, Asian or Hispanic ethnicity

PHYSICAL FINDINGS & CLINICAL PRESENTATION (Table 1-403)

- Bleeding is generally brisk at time of delivery.
- Examination findings include boggy uterus with continued passage of clot or blood with fundal pressure.
- Objective findings can also include hypotension, tachycardia, and oliguria with substantial blood loss.

ETIOLOGY

- Primary: uterine atony (>80%), retained placenta, coagulopathies, lacerations
- Secondary: subinvolution of placental site, retained products, infection, coagulopathies

DIAGNOSIS

WORKUP

- Bladder should be emptied
- Bimanual examination to evaluate for atony; massage if it is present
- Examination to verify that no lacerations are present, including cervical examination with necessary lighting and retractors
- Ultrasonography at bedside to evaluate for retained tissue or clot
- Examination to verify that placenta is intact

LABORATORY TESTS

Significant hemorrhage can lead to disseminated intravascular coagulation (DIC). If DIC is suspected, complete blood count and coagulation panels should be ordered. Similarly, if coagulopathy is suspected, evaluation of clotting factors should be ordered.

IMAGING STUDIES

Ultrasonography can be used to scan for retained products, including clot or placenta. It can be performed to assess the need for more invasive measures, such as instrumentation or a manual sweep.

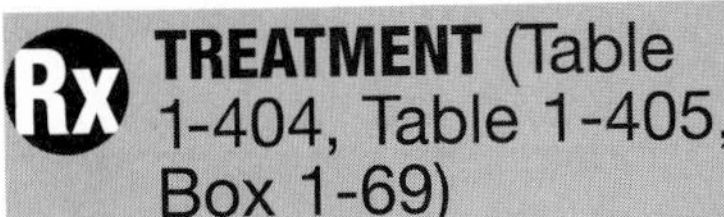

TREATMENT (Table 1-404, Table 1-405, Box 1-69)

Medical management with uterotonics is generally the first line of treatment:

- Oxytocin (IV, 10-40 units diluted into IV solution, or 10 units IM); often given prophylactically immediately after delivery
- Methergine (IM, 0.2 mg)
- Hemabate (IM, 0.25 mg)
- Misoprostol (800-1000 mcg rectally)

NONPHARMACOLOGIC THERAPY

Secondary management includes the following:

- Packing with gauze, Foley catheter, or tamponade balloon
- Uterine curettage for suspected retained products
- Uterine artery embolization
- Surgical management with laparotomy
  - Hypogastric artery ligation
  - Bilateral uterine artery ligation (O'Leary sutures)
  - B-lynch sutures
  - Hysterectomy

ACUTE GENERAL Rx

Uterotonics, surgical management, embolization, blood transfusion

CHRONIC Rx

For anemia: ferrous sulfate supplementation to support new red blood cell production

TABLE 1-403 Presentation of Symptoms in Postpartum Hemorrhage

% Blood loss (ml)	Systolic blood pressure (mm Hg)	Signs and symptoms
10-15 (500-1000)	Normal	Tachycardia, palpitations, dizziness
15-25 (1000-1500)	Low-normal	Tachycardia, weakness, diaphoresis
25-35 (1500-2000)	70-80	Restlessness, pallor, oliguria
35-45 (2000-3000)	50-70	Collapse, air hunger, anuria

From Vincent JL et al: *Textbook of critical care,* ed 6, Philadelphia, 2011, Saunders.

TABLE 1-404 Therapeutic Response to Initial Fluid Resuscitation

Response	Description	Follow-up treatment
Rapid response	<20% of blood volume lost	No additional fluids or blood are needed.
Transient response	20%-40% of blood volume lost; responds to initial fluid bolus but later has worsening vital signs	Continue fluids and consider blood transfusions.
Minimal or no response	Ongoing severe hemorrhage with >40% blood volume lost	Continue aggressive fluid and blood product replacements.

From Vincent JL et al: *Textbook of critical care,* ed 6, Philadelphia, 2011, Saunders.

TABLE 1-405 Dosing Regimens for Oxytocic Drugs

Drug	Regimens
Oxytocin (Pitocin)	5-unit IV bolus
	Add 20-40 units oxytocin to 1 L of fluids
	10 units intramyometrially
Methylergonovine (Methergine)	0.2 mg IM every 2-4 hr
Ergonovine (Ergotrate Maleate)	100-125 mcg IM or intramyometrially every 2-4 hr
	200-250 mcg IM
	Total dose 1.25 mg
Carboprost (Hemabate)	250 mcg IM or intramyometrially every 15-90 min
	Total dose 2 mg
Misoprostol	800 mcg PR or 800 mcg of sublingual misoprostol

IM, Intramuscular; *IV,* intravenous; *PR,* per rectum.
From Vincent JL et al: *Textbook of critical care,* ed 6, Philadelphia, 2011, Saunders.

DISPOSITION

- The patient should be closely watched for at least 24 hr after a postpartum hemorrhage. Laboratory findings should be monitored to follow trends on the Hunt and Hess scale. Vital signs should be monitored for evidence of hemodynamic stability and appropriate response to anemia.
- Morbidity can include shock, acute respiratory distress syndrome, Sheehan's syndrome, and loss of fertility.

REFERRAL

During the course of a postpartum hemorrhage, the anesthesiology department should be notified and adequate nursing should be available. Early considerations should be made to notify obstetricians. If bleeding is brisk or estimated blood loss is considerable, preparation should be made for transfusion of blood products, including drawing blood for typing and notifying the blood bank.

AUTHOR: **LEO HAN, M.D.**

BOX 1-69 Blood Product Replacement

Cross-matched blood
Type-specific or "saline cross-matched" blood
Compatible ABO and Rh blood types
Rh-negative blood is preferable.
Warm the blood, if possible, especially if the rate of infusion is >100 ml/min or if the total volume transfused is high; cold blood is associated with an increased incidence of arrhythmias and paradoxical hypotension.
Administer calcium if blood is transfused rapidly at >100 ml/min because of binding of calcium by anticoagulants in banked blood.
Give 6-10 units fresh frozen plasma (FFP) for every 10 units of packed red blood cell transfusions.
Give 10-12 units of platelets if the platelet count decreases to <50 × 109/L.
Cryoprecipitate can be given to replace fibrinogen in addition to the FFP.
Consider 60-120 mcg/kg intravenous bolus injection of recombinant activated factor VII (rFVIIa).

From Vincent JL et al: *Textbook of critical care*, ed 6, Philadelphia, 2011, Saunders.

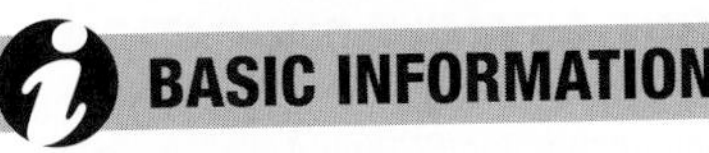

BASIC INFORMATION

DEFINITION

Postpoliomyelitis syndrome (PPS) is a disorder typically characterized by the gradual onset and slow progression of new weakness, fatigue, and pain in survivors of paralytic poliomyelitis after a period of partial or complete recovery and many years of neurologic stability. The symptoms are persistent and cannot be explained by the presence of other neurologic, medical, or orthopedic conditions.

SYNONYMS

Post-polio syndrome
Progressive postpoliomyelitis muscular atrophy

ICD-9CM CODE
138 Late effects of acute poliomyelitis
ICD-10 CM CODE
G14 Post-polio myelitic syndrome
B91 Sequelae of poliomyelitis
Excludes 1: sequelae of poliomyelitis (B91)

EPIDEMIOLOGY & DEMOGRAPHICS

INCIDENCE: Estimates vary from 22% to 85% of individuals who survive acute poliomyelitis
PEAK INCIDENCE: About 30 to 36 years following acute poliomyelitis, although cases have been reported between 8 and 71 years.
RISK FACTORS:
- Increasing age and greater length of time since the episode of acute poliomyelitis
- Acute poliomyelitis at an older age
- Greater severity of the acute poliomyelitis or chronic deficits after recovery

PHYSICAL FINDINGS & CLINICAL PRESENTATION

- The most common clinical features are new weakness (20% to 60%), fatigue (59% to 89%), and pain (38% to 86%).
- The symptoms typically have an insidious onset with gradual progression.
- The new weakness is typically, but not exclusively, in muscles that were previously affected by the acute poliomyelitis.
- Fatigue may be described as general or muscular in nature and is often the most disabling symptom.
- Pain is usually described as severe aching, cramping, or burning localized to the muscles or joints, particularly in areas previously affected by acute poliomyelitis
- Respiratory weakness and sleep-disordered breathing with nocturnal hypoventilation occur less frequently
- Other less common features include fasciculations, dysphagia, dysarthria, and cold intolerance
- Neurologic examination reveals evidence of asymmetric, lower motor neuron weakness with or without musculoskeletal deformities secondary to longstanding polio such as asymmetric limb size, kyphoscoliosis, degenerative joint disease, and joint instability.

ETIOLOGY

The pathophysiologic basis of PPS remains unclear, although there are several proposed mechanisms. The most popular hypothesis is that the reduced population of enlarged motor units after acute poliomyelitis is subject to increased stress and overuse over the course of years. This leads to distal degeneration of the motor units and worsening denervation, causing clinical symptoms.

Dx DIAGNOSIS

DIFFERENTIAL DIAGNOSIS

PPS is a diagnosis of exclusion. A particular individual's symptoms will determine the differential, but some commonly considered entities:
- Amyotrophic lateral sclerosis (ALS)
- Cervical or lumbosacral radiculopathy
- Acquired demyelinating polyneuropathies
- Myasthenia gravis
- Fibromyalgia
- Chronic fatigue syndrome
- Anemia
- Hypothyroidism
- Arthritis
- Depression
- Normal aging

WORKUP

- A detailed history should confirm a past history of acute poliomyelitis followed by a period of stability prior to emergence of the new symptoms
- A neurologic exam confirms weakness of the lower motor neuron pattern
- Nerve conduction studies and electromyography confirm the presence of denervation and help exclude other potential causes of weakness.
- A sleep study should be strongly considered to evaluate for the presence of sleep-disordered breathing.
- Pulmonary function tests should be strongly considered to evaluate for evidence of respiratory weakness.
- A swallow study should be performed in patients with difficulty swallowing.

LABORATORY TESTS

Complete blood count, electrolytes, and thyroid function tests are conducted to exclude other causes of fatigue. Erythrocyte sedimentation rate is typically normal, and increase in creatinine kinase levels (if any) is nonspecific.

IMAGING STUDIES

Magnetic resonance imaging of the brain and spine can be helpful in excluding other potential causes of weakness.

CRITERIA FOR DIAGNOSING POSTPOLIOMYELITIS SYNDROME

1. Prior episode of poliomyelitis with evidence of residual lower motor neuron loss
2. Duration of acute onset of polio and neurologic and functional stability of 15 or more years
3. Gradual onset of persistent new weakness and abnormal muscle fatigability (lasting 1 year or longer)
4. Exclusion of other conditions mentioned in the previous differential diagnosis section

Rx TREATMENT

There is no specific therapy for PPS. However, a multidisciplinary management program tailored to the patient's presentation can be very helpful in the management of symptoms, resulting in improved functionality and quality of life.
- Most individuals will benefit from physical activity regimens (i.e., nonfatiguing exercise programs) designed by a physical therapist to focus on energy conservation and pacing.
- Orthoses and assistive devices may facilitate ambulation and other activities of daily living as well as reduce the risk of falls.
- Pain can often be controlled with conservative measures such as activity and lifestyle modifications, but analgesic medications may be necessary in some cases. Amitriptyline has been found to help with relief of pain and fatigue in anecdotal cases.
- Trials indicate that drugs such as IVIG and lamotrigine as well as application of static magnetic fields over identified trigger points may be beneficial in treating muscle weakness and pain; however, these treatments warrant further investigation.
- Several studies evaluating the use of pyridostigmine for the treatment of weakness and fatigue in PPS have had conflicting results.
- Studies evaluating amantadine, modafinil, prednisone, and human growth hormone have failed to show any definitive benefit.
- There have been promising initial results with limited studies of lamotrigine and intravenous immunoglobulin, but further trials are needed.

DISPOSITION

- The symptoms of PPS tend to be slowly progressive and may stabilize over the course of years.
- The weakness, fatigue, and pain may result in disability.
- Rarely fatal, but individuals with respiratory weakness and dysphagia are at increased risk and may benefit from early use of noninvasive respiratory support.

REFERRAL

- Neuromuscular specialist can assist in diagnosis and management.
- Physiatry, physical therapy, and occupational therapy for rehabilitation and assistive devices.
- Speech therapy referral is useful in patients with dysarthria or dysphagia.
- Pulmonary consult should be obtained for patients with symptoms or signs of respiratory weakness.
- Orthopedic consult may be necessary for patients requiring surgical correction of joint deformities.

- A mental health professional can assist with management of depression and other psychosocial issues.

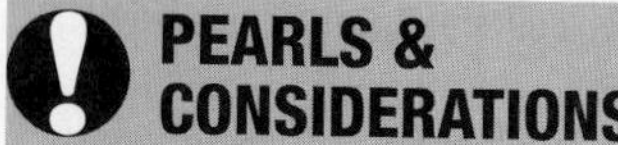

PEARLS & CONSIDERATIONS

COMMENTS

- A diagnosis of PPS should only be made after a thorough evaluation for other potential causes of the patient's symptoms has been completed.
- Due to the high incidence of PPS among the large number of poliomyelitis survivors, PPS is the most common motor neuron disease worldwide.
- For patients with PPS who need to undergo surgical procedures, shorter-acting anesthetic agents should be used due to these patients' impaired baseline respiratory status and their potentially increased sensitivity to anesthetic and nondepolarizing neuromuscular blocking agents.

PATIENT & FAMILY EDUCATION

Website: http://www.mayoclinic.com/health/post-polio-syndrome/DS00494

SUGGESTED READINGS

available at www.expertconsult.com

AUTHOR: **DIVYA SINGHAL, M.D.**

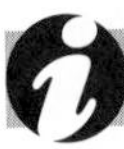

BASIC INFORMATION

DEFINITION

Posttraumatic stress disorder (PTSD) is an anxiety disorder that may arise when an individual has witnessed or experienced a potentially fatal or serious injury during which he or she felt helpless or horrified. The individual continues to experience the event in the form of flashbacks (reliving the trauma), intrusive recollections, dreams, or physiologic reactivity. These responses are associated with persistent hyperarousal (e.g., hypervigilance, exaggerated startle response, sleep disturbance, irritability, and difficulty concentrating) and avoidance (both physically and cognitively) of stimuli associated with the traumatic event. In children, the horror may be expressed by disorganized or agitated behavior.

SYNONYMS (Historical)

Soldier's heart
Effort syndrome
Shell shock
Irritable heart
Traumatic necrosis
Survivor syndrome
Concentration camp syndrome

ICD-9CM and DSM-5 CODES
309.81
ICD-10CM CODES
F43.1 Post-traumatic stress disorder

EPIDEMIOLOGY & DEMOGRAPHICS

INCIDENCE: Fewer than 10% of individuals who have experienced a traumatic event will develop PTSD.

PREVALENCE (IN U.S.):
- One of the most common psychiatric disorders; estimated lifetime prevalence 7.8% to 12.3%
- Prevalence among high-risk populations (e.g., combat veterans or victims of violent crimes) up to 58%
- ~80% psychiatric comorbidity (depression, anxiety disorder, or substance use)
- Factors most associated with development are subsequent life stress and perceived lack of social support

PREDOMINANT SEX: Twice as many women as men are affected (prevalence 10% to 14% for women and 5% to 6% for men). More than 50% of cases in women are related to sexual assault.

PREDOMINANT AGE: No predisposing age factors

GENETICS: Twin studies have demonstrated genetic vulnerability related to combat.

PHYSICAL FINDINGS & CLINICAL PRESENTATION

Core symptom clusters include intrusion, avoidance, negative mood and cognition, hyperarousal, and sometimes dissociative symptoms. Individuals present with different variations of these symptoms. Symptoms must occur for more than one month and result in significant distress and functional impairment.

Key PTSD symptoms:
1. Distressing memories or dreams of the event. Note: Children older than 6 may express this symptom in repetitive play.
2. Flashbacks
3. Intense distress after reminders of the event.
4. Avoidance due to trauma-related thoughts or feelings.
5. Persistent negative trauma-related emotions.
6. Feeling detached
7. Aggressive or reckless behavior
8. Hypervigilance
9. Problems with concentration or sleep
10. Depersonalization

ETIOLOGY

- Interpersonal violence is more likely to give rise to PTSD than events such as motor vehicle accidents or natural disasters.
- Severity of physical injury is a weaker predictor of PTSD than the psychological distress; stress duration is the most important factor.
- Proposed mechanisms include activation of the amygdala, disruption of prefrontal cortex modulation of the amygdala, and excessive stress-induced HPA and alpha-1 receptor activation.

Dx DIAGNOSIS

Diagnosis is made when the stressor is consistent with DSM-5 definition (follows), and the individual experiences symptoms of re-experiencing, avoidance, negative mood and cognition, and arousal and reactivity as defined under "Clinical Presentation." The symptoms must be present for more than one month, must cause impairment in functioning, and must not be attributable to substance use or other medical conditions. Subtypes meet specified criteria and in addition have dissociative symptoms or delayed onset (meeting full criteria at least six months after the event.)

Definition of Stressor
Exposure to death, threatened death, actual or threatened serious injury, or actual or threatened sexual violence, as follows: (1 required)
1. Directly experiencing the event.
2. Witnessing the event occur to others.
3. Indirectly, by learning that a close relative or close friend was exposed to trauma. If the event involved actual or threatened death, it must have been violent or accidental.
4. Repeated or extreme indirect exposure to aversive details of the event(s), usually in the course of professional duties (e.g., first responders collecting body parts; professionals repeatedly exposed to details of child abuse). This does not include indirect nonprofessional exposure through electronic media, television, movies, or pictures, unless the exposure is work related.

DIFFERENTIAL DIAGNOSIS

- Adjustment disorders: precipitating stress is less catastrophic and psychological reaction is less specific.
- Acute stress disorder: duration of symptoms from 48 hr to 4 wk after trauma.

Anxiety disorder and obsessive-compulsive disorder
- Major depressive disorder
- Personality disorders
- Dissociative disorders
- Conversion disorder (functional neurological symptom disorder)
- Psychotic disorder
- Traumatic brain injury

WORKUP

- Among self-report questionnaires and structured diagnostic instruments, the best validated is the Posttraumatic Diagnostic Scale.
- Laboratory and imaging are not clinically useful.
- Primary care PTSD (PC-PTSD) screen recommended by the Veterans Administration. "Yes" answers to three of four of the questions is a positive screen:
  In your life, have you ever had any experience that was so frightening, horrible, or upsetting that, in the past month, you:
  1. Have had nightmares about it or thought about it when you did not want to?
  2. Tried hard not to think about it or went out of your way to avoid situations that reminded you of it?
  3. Were constantly on guard, watchful, or easily startled?
  4. Felt numb or detached from others, activities, or your surroundings?

Rx TREATMENT

MEDICATIONS

There is no definitive cure for PTSD, and individuals have varying responses to different medications. Sertraline and paroxotine, both SSRIs, are the only FDA-approved medications for PTSD. Other medication use is off-label with differing levels of evidence to support use. Medications are used to target symptoms and the physiologic changes associated with PTSD.
- SSRIs, SNRIs: sertraline, paroxotine, fluoxetine, venlafaxine.
- Other antidepressants: mirtazapine, nefazadone
- Mood stabilizers: topiramate has been shown to be effective in some studies. Other mood stabilizers are sometimes used off-label to target individual patient symptoms, such as severe irritability, anxiety, aggression, or depression.
- Guanfacine may be helpful in treating arousal symptoms.
- Prazosin may decrease distressing dreams and improve sleep quality.
- Atypical antipsychotics: risperidone been shown to be effective in some studies. Other antipsychotics are sometimes used off-label to target individual patient symptoms such as paranoia, extreme anxiety, or angry outbursts.

NONPHARMACOLOGIC THERAPY

- Talk therapy, either psychodynamic or CBT with sensitivity to pacing, readiness, containment, and dissociation, can decrease symptom intensity and frequency. Prolonged exposure (PE), a type of CBT that includes education on stress response, breathing training, and prolonged recounting of the event including sensory details, was found to be more effective than standard CBT in female veterans. There is some controversy regarding appropriateness of exposure therapy for all patients, particularly those with "complex PTSD" from multiple lifetime traumatic events, and the potential for "retraumatization."
- Group therapy is helpful, particularly for combat veterans.
- Eye movement desensitization reprocessing (EMDR) has shown efficacy in controlled trials.

ACUTE GENERAL Rx

- Immediate postincident debriefing may worsen outcome.
- A brief course of benzodiazepines may be helpful acutely but has not been shown to decrease development of core symptoms.
- Beta-adrenergic blockers may be helpful if given within hours after the trauma to disrupt the physiologic stress response.
- Sedating antidepressants or sleep aids may be helpful for initial insomnia.

COMPLEMENTARY & ALTERNATIVE APPROACHES

Acupuncture has been shown to be effective in decreasing symptoms of PTSD.

DISPOSITION

- Recovery rates are highest in the first 12 mo after onset.
- Average duration of symptoms is 36 mo for those who undergo treatment and 64 mo for those never treated.
- 50% chance of remission at 2 yr; 50% have chronic symptoms.
- Predictors of chronic course include previous trauma, premorbid psychiatric function, panic reaction at time of event, prolonged terror, or dissociation at time of event.

REFERRAL

Because early intervention improves outcome, refer to psychiatry as soon as diagnosis made.

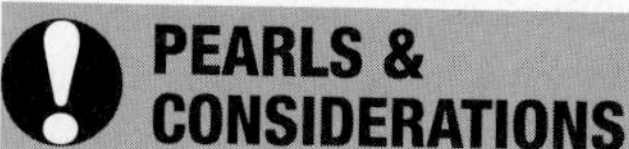

PEARLS & CONSIDERATIONS

- PTSD can be associated with suicidal ideation and attempts
- PTSD can be associated with aggressive and violent behavior
- Individuals with PTSD are 80% more likely to have a comorbid psychiatric disorder, including substance abuse
- Among combat veterans of recent wars, there is a 41% co-occurrence with mild TBI
- PTSD may vary culturally and present as culturally specific syndromes and idioms of distress
- Treatment can be effective even if it begins years after the traumatic event occurred.
- PTSD is increasingly being conceived of as a stress-induced fear-circuitry disorder of the limbic system.
- Evidence-based treatments for PTSD have not been established for adolescents despite high prevalence of PTSD in this population. A recent trial that examined the effects of counselor-delivered prolonged exposure therapy compared with supportive counseling for adolescents with PTSD revealed that adolescent girls with sexual abuse-related PTSD experienced greater benefit from prolonged exposure therapy than from supportive counseling even when delivered by counselors who typically provide supportive counseling.[1]

SUGGESTED READINGS

available at www.expertconsult.com

RELATED CONTENT

Posttraumatic Stress Disorder (PTSD) (Patient Information)

AUTHORS: **KAILA COMPTON, M.D., Ph.D.,** and **ALISON C. MAY, M.D.**

[1]Foa EB et al: Prolonged exposure vs supportive counseling for sexual abuse-related PTSD in adolescent girls, a randomized clinical trial, *JAMA* 310(24):2650-2657, 2013.

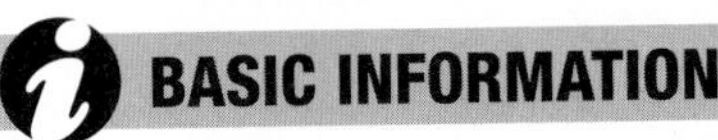

BASIC INFORMATION

DEFINITION

Precocious puberty is defined as sexual development occurring before age 8 yr in females and 9 yr in males.

SYNONYMS

Pubertas praecox

ICD-9CM CODES
259.1 Precocious puberty
ICD-10CM CODES
E30.1 Precocious puberty

EPIDEMIOLOGY & DEMOGRAPHICS

INCIDENCE: Estimated to be between one in 5000 to 10,000.
PREDOMINANT SEX: Females are affected more often than males for the idiopathic variant; for other causes, dependent on the underlying etiology.
GENETICS: The genetics for some of the etiologies of precocious puberty is known. Deficiency of *MKRN3* causes central precocious puberty in humans.

PHYSICAL FINDINGS & CLINICAL PRESENTATION

- In females: breast development, pubic hair development, accelerated growth, menarche
- In males: increase in testicular volume and penile length, pubic hair development, accelerated growth, muscular development, acne, change in voice, penile erections

ETIOLOGY

- Idiopathic or true: diagnosis of exclusion
- Central nervous system (CNS) pathology: tumors, hydrocephalus, ventricular cysts, benign lesions
- Severe hypothyroidism
- Posttraumatic head injury
- Genetic disorders: neurofibromatosis, tuberous sclerosis, McCune-Albright syndrome, congenital adrenal hyperplasia
- Gonadal tumors
- Nongonadal tumors: hepatoblastoma
- Exposure to exogenous sex steroids

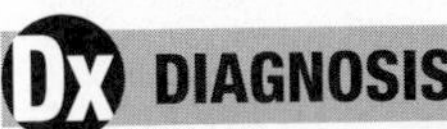

DIAGNOSIS

DIFFERENTIAL DIAGNOSIS

- Most common diagnoses to consider: premature thelarche and premature adrenarche
- Gonadotropin hormone-releasing hormone (GnRH)-dependent precocious puberty: idiopathic, CNS tumors, hypothalamic hamartomas, neurofibromatosis, tuberous sclerosis, hydrocephalus, status after acute head injury, ventricular cysts, status after CNS infection
- GnRH-independent precocious puberty: congenital adrenal hyperplasia, adrenocortical tumors (males), McCune-Albright syndrome (females), gonadal tumors, ectopic human chorionic gonadotropin (hCG)-secreting tumors (chorioblastoma, hepatoblastoma), exposure to exogenous sex steroids, severe hypothyroidism
- Table E1-406 summarizes the differential diagnosis of sexual precocity

WORKUP

Thorough history and physical examination are essential to determine if the patient has true precocious puberty. Particular attention should be paid to growth, development, order of appearance of the secondary sexual characteristics, pubertal development in family members, medications, neurologic symptoms, Tanner staging, abdominal and neurologic examination. Flowcharts for diagnosing sexual precocity in females and males are shown in Figs. E1-758 and E1-759.

LABORATORY TESTS

- GnRH testing will help determine if dependent or independent cause
- Sex hormone studies: luteinizing hormone, follicle-stimulating hormone, hCG, testosterone (males), estrogen (females). Levels of sex steroids should be determined in the morning, with use of assays that have detection limits adapted to pediatric values. In girls, serum estradiol levels are highly variable and have a rather low sensitivity for the diagnosis of precocious puberty.
- T_4, thyroid-stimulating hormone

IMAGING STUDIES

- CT scan or MRI of the brain to evaluate for CNS pathology
- Consideration of pelvic ultrasound in female patients to evaluate for ovarian cysts or tumors
- Abdominal imaging with CT scan if intraabdominal pathology suspected

Rx TREATMENT

NONPHARMACOLOGIC THERAPY

- Good communication with the parents is essential to care.
- Psychological support for the child may be needed with regard to self-image and problems with peer acceptance.

ACUTE GENERAL Rx

There is no acute therapy for precocious puberty.

CHRONIC Rx

Therapy depends on the etiology of precocious puberty. For the treatment of central or gonadotropin-dependent precocious puberty depot GnRH agonists (leuprorelin, leuprolide, triptorelin, goserelin, histrelin, buserelin) are effective.

- Leuprolide is given 0.25 to 0.3 mg/kg with a 7.5 mg minimum IM every 4 wk. Local side effects include pain, erythema, and inflammatory reactions. Other side effects include headaches and menopausal-like symptoms (asthenia, hot flashes).
- For other CNS lesions and extragonadal tumors, therapy is dependent on the type of lesion, location of the lesion, and the overall prognosis of the underlying problem.
- For severe hypothyroidism, treatment with thyroid hormone will result in regression of the sexual development. The child will subsequently undergo appropriate pubertal development later in life.
- For familial male gonadotropin-independent precocious puberty, the androgen-synthesis inhibitor ketoconazole can be used at doses of 600 mg/day divided tid, or a combination of the aromatase inhibitor testolactone and spironolactone can be used.

DISPOSITION

- For true precocious puberty and some CNS lesions, long-term outcome is usually very good. When drug therapy is instituted, it is continued until a time when further pubertal development is appropriate. It is then discontinued, allowing the child to progress through puberty.
- For other cases, long-term outcomes depend on the prognosis of the underlying cause.

REFERRAL

- Initial workup can be instituted by the primary care provider.
- Referral to an endocrinologist is indicated for most children because they will need long-term management, monitoring, and treatment.
- Attention to the emotional needs of the child is important.

SUGGESTED READINGS

available at www.expertconsult.com

RELATED CONTENT

Precocious Puberty (Patient Information)

AUTHORS: **BETH J. WUTZ, M.D.,** and **RUBEN ALVERO, M.D.**

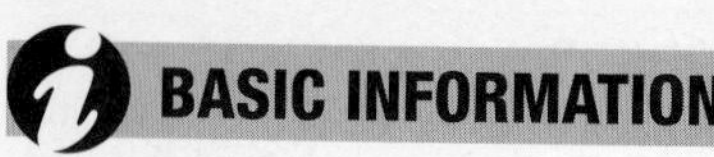

BASIC INFORMATION

DEFINITION

Preeclampsia involves the triad of hypertension, proteinuria, and edema that develops after the twentieth week of gestation. Mild preeclampsia is defined as a blood pressure of >140/90 mm Hg. Severe preeclampsia (Table 1-407) is associated with a blood pressure <160/110 mm Hg, proteinuria <5 g in a 24-hr urine collection, oliguria (>400 ml/24 hr), cerebral or visual disturbances, epigastric pain, pulmonary edema, thrombocytopenia, hepatic dysfunction, or severe intrauterine growth restriction. Table 1-408 differentiates preeclampsia from chronic hypertension.

SYNONYMS

Pregnancy-induced hypertension
Toxemia of pregnancy

ICD-9CM CODES
642.6 Preeclampsia
ICD-10CM CODES
014.0 Moderate pre-eclampsia
014.1 Severe pre-eclampsia
014.9 Pre-eclampsia, unspecified

EPIDEMIOLOGY & DEMOGRAPHICS

INCIDENCE: 0% to 14% in primigravidas, 5.7% to 7.3% in multigravidas
RISK FACTORS: Increased incidence and severity with multiple gestations or renal or collagen-vascular diseases. Extremes of reproductive age, <20 or >35 yr, obesity, African American race, thrombophilia, previous preeclampsia.
GENETICS: Positive correlation with maternal and paternal family history

PHYSICAL FINDINGS & CLINICAL PRESENTATION

- Preeclampsia typically presents with hypertension, peripheral edema, and proteinuria, most commonly in the third semester of pregnancy.
- Generalized swelling or nondependent edema, possibly manifested by rapid weight gain (>4 lb/wk) even in the absence of edema
- Auscultation of pulmonary rales
- Right upper quadrant pain (HELLP syndrome [hemolysis, elevated liver enzymes, and low platelet count] or subcapsular liver hematoma)
- Hyperreflexia or clonus
- Vaginal bleeding (placental abruption)
- Acute or chronic fetal compromise manifested by intrauterine growth restriction or fetal tachycardia with late decelerations, respectively
- Wide range of symptoms attributable to multiorgan system dysfunction, involving hepatic, hematologic, renal, pulmonary, and central nervous systems
- Possibility of severe disease despite "normal" blood pressure readings, so a high index of suspicion must be maintained in high-risk situations

ETIOLOGY

- Exact etiology or toxic substance is unknown
- Theories:
  - Imbalance between thromboxane A_2 (vasoconstrictor and platelet aggregator) and prostacyclin (vasodilator)
  - Abnormal trophoblastic invasion of spiral arteries
  - Increased sensitivity to angiotensin II by the muscular walls of the arteries
  - Excess circulating soluble fms-like tyrosine kinase 1 (*sFlt1*), which binds placental growth factor (PIGF) and vascular endothelial growth factor (VEGF), may have a pathogenic role
- Potential secondary effects of the metabolic, inflammatory endothelial alternatives in preeclampsia are described in Table 1-409.

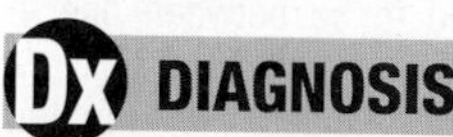

DIAGNOSIS

DIFFERENTIAL DIAGNOSIS

- Acute fatty liver of pregnancy
- Appendicitis
- Diabetic ketoacidosis
- Gallbladder disease

TABLE 1-407 Criteria for the Diagnosis of Severe Preeclampsia

In patients with preeclampsia, **severe preeclampsia** can be diagnosed if any one of the following criteria is present:

Blood pressure
≥160 mm Hg systolic or ≥110 mm Hg diastolic on two separate occasions at least 6 hours apart
Proteinuria
Random urine protein-creatinine ratio ≥5 mg/ml (500 mg/mmol) *or* proteinuria ≥5 g/24 h
Oliguria <500 ml in 24 hours
Cerebral or visual disturbances such as cerebrovascular accident, seizures, or visual loss
Pulmonary edema
Epigastric or right upper quadrant pain
Hepatocellular injury (serum transaminases at least twice normal)
Serum lactate dehydrogenase: >600 IU/L
Thrombocytopenia <100,000
Fetal growth restriction (birth weight less than 10th percentile for the gestational age)

From Floege J et al: *Comprehensive clinical nephrology,* ed 4, Philadelphia, 2010, Saunders.

TABLE 1-408 Differences between Preeclampsia and Chronic Hypertension

Feature	Preeclampsia	Chronic Hypertension
Age (yr)	Young (<20)	Older (>30)
Parity	Primigravida	Multigravida
Onset	After 20 wk of pregnancy	Before 20 wk of pregnancy
Weight gain and edema	Sudden	Gradual
Systolic blood pressure	<160 mm Hg	>160 mm Hg
Funduscopic findings	Spasm, edema	Arteriovenous nicking, exudates
Left ventricular hypertrophy	Rare	More common
Proteinuria	Present	Absent
Plasma uric acid	Increased	Normal
Blood pressure after delivery	Normal	Elevated

From Zipes DP et al (eds): *Braunwald's heart disease,* ed 7, Philadelphia, 2005, Saunders.

TABLE 1-409 Potential Secondary Effects of the Metabolic, Inflammatory Endothelial Alternatives in Preeclampsia

CVS	Increased peripheral resistance leading to hypertension Increased vascular permeability and reduced maternal plasma volume
Lungs	Laryngeal and pulmonary edema
Renal	Glomerular damage leading to proteinuria, hypoproteinemia, and reduced oncotic pressure, which further exacerbates the hypovolemia. May develop acute renal failure ± cortical necrosis
Clotting	Hypercoagulability, with increased fibrin formation and increased fibrinolysis, i.e., disseminated intravascular coagulation
Liver	HELLP syndrome Hepatic rupture
CNS	Thrombosis and fibrinoid necrosis of the cerebral arterioles Eclampsia (convulsions), cerebral hemorrhage, and cerebral edema
Fetus	Impaired uteroplacental circulation, potentially leading to FGR, hypoxemia, and intrauterine death

CVS, Cardiovascular system; *CNS,* central nervous system; *FGR,* fetal growth restriction; *HELLP,* hemolysis, elevated liver enzymes, low platelets.
From Drife J, Magowan B: *Clinical obstetrics and gynecology,* Philadelphia, 2004, Saunders.

- Gastroenteritis
- Glomerulonephritis
- Hemolytic-uremic syndrome
- Hepatic encephalopathy
- Hyperemesis gravidarum
- Idiopathic thrombocytopenia
- Thrombotic thrombocytopenic purpura
- Nephrolithiasis
- Pyelonephritis
- Peptic ulcer disease
- Systemic lupus erythematosus
- Viral hepatitis

WORKUP

- Two blood pressure measurements with the patient in lateral recumbent position 6 hr apart, with an absolute pressure >140/90 mm Hg or an increase of 30 mm Hg systolic or 15 mm Hg diastolic from baseline, an increase in the mean arterial pressure (MAP) of 20 mm Hg, or an absolute MAP >105 mm Hg
- Evaluation for proteinuria as defined by >0.1 g/L on urine dipstick or >300 mg protein on a 24-hr urine collection
- Evaluation of fetal status for evidence of intrauterine growth restriction, oligohydramnios, alteration in umbilical or uterine artery Doppler flow, or acute compromise, such as abruption
- Because of the insidious nature of the disease with potential for multiple organ involvement, complete evaluation for preeclampsia in any pregnant patient presenting with central nervous system derangement or gastrointestinal symptoms after 20 wk of gestation
- Evaluation for associated conditions such as disseminated intravascular coagulation, hepatic dysfunction, or subcapsular hematoma

LABORATORY TESTS

- High-risk patients: baseline assessment of renal function (24-hr urine collection for protein and creatinine clearance), platelets, blood urea nitrogen, creatinine, liver function tests (LFTs), and uric acid should be obtained at the first prenatal visit.
- Complete blood count (hemoglobin, hematocrit, platelets) may show signs of volume contraction or HELLP syndrome.
- LFTs (aspartate aminotransferase, alanine aminotransferase, lactate dehydrogenase) are useful in evaluation for HELLP syndrome or to exclude important differentials.
- Hyperuricemia or increased creatinine may indicate decreasing renal function.
- Prothrombin time, partial thromboplastin time, and fibrinogen should be checked to rule out disseminated intravascular coagulation.
- Peripheral smear may demonstrate microangiopathic hemolytic anemia.
- Complement levels can be used to differentiate from an acute exacerbation of a collagen-vascular disease.
- Increased levels of *sFlt1* and reduced levels of PIGF predict subsequent development of preeclampsia.

IMAGING STUDIES

- CT scan of head if atypical presentation of eclampsia, possibility of intracerebral bleed, or prolonged postictal state
- Sonogram of fetus to evaluate for intrauterine growth restriction (Fig. 1-760), amniotic fluid, placenta
- Sonogram of maternal liver if suspect subcapsular hematoma

TREATMENT

NONPHARMACOLOGIC THERAPY

Bed rest in left lateral decubitus position

ACUTE GENERAL Rx

Delivery is the treatment of choice and the only cure for the disease. This must be taken in the context of the gestational age of the fetus, severity of the preeclampsia, and the likelihood of a successful induction and reliability of patient.

- Administer magnesium sulfate 6 g IV loading dose, with 2 to 3 g maintenance or phenytoin at 10 to 15 mg/kg loading dose, then 200 mg IV q8h starting 12 hr after loading dose.
- Hydralazine 10 mg IV, labetalol hydrochloride 20 to 40 mg IV, nifedipine 20 mg SL can be used for acute blood pressure control.
- Continuous fetal monitoring is needed.
- Epidural is anesthesia of choice for pain management in labor or cesarean section.
- All patients undergoing induction of labor should receive antiseizure medications regardless of severity of disease.

CHRONIC Rx

- Mild preeclampsia <37 wk: close observation for worsening maternal or fetal condition, with delivery at >37 wk with favorable cervix or at 40 wk regardless of cervical status.
- Severe preeclampsia: delivery in the presence of maternal or fetal compromise, labor, or >34 wk; at 28 to 34 wk consider steroids with close monitoring, and at <24 wk consider termination of pregnancy.
- Methyldopa is drug of choice for long-term blood pressure control during pregnancy.

DISPOSITION

Preeclampsia is a progressive and unpredictable disease process; a course of expectancy should be managed with caution. Up to 20% of patients who have seizures are normotensive.

REFERRAL

Obstetric management is indicated because of the insidious nature of the disease, with transfer of all cases <34 wk to a facility with a level three nursery.

PEARLS & CONSIDERATIONS

COMMENTS

- Low-dose aspirin 81 mg qd and calcium supplementation 1500 mg qd can be considered in high-risk patients to decrease the risk of recurrence.
- Begin after first trimester.
- Although the absolute risk of ESRD in women who have had preeclampsia is low, preeclampsia is a marker for an increased risk of subsequent ESRD.
- The development of preeclampsia may be one of the earliest identifiable risk markers for potential future cardiovascular disease in women. It has been shown that women who develop preeclampsia have a higher incidence of cardiovascular risk factors including components of the metabolic syndrome within 1 yr of delivery.

SUGGESTED READINGS

available at www.expertconsult.com

RELATED CONTENT

Eclampsia (Related Key Topic)
Preeclampsia (Patient Information)

AUTHOR: **RUBEN ALVERO, M.D.**

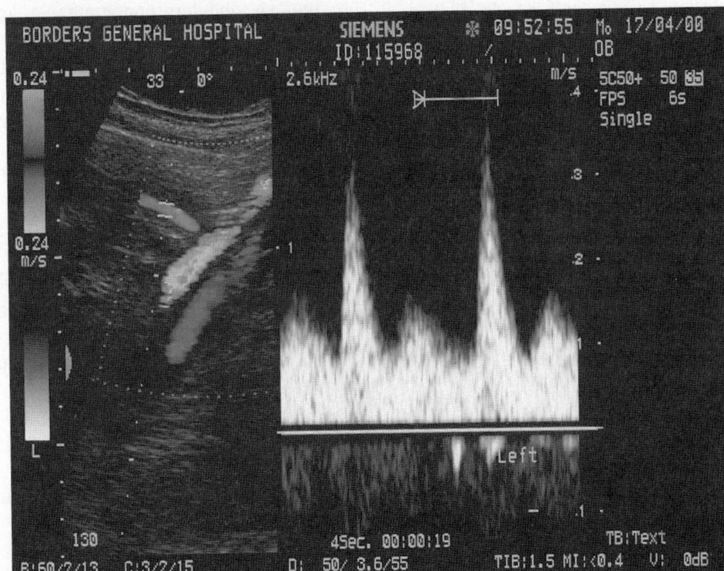

FIGURE 1-760 Uterine artery Doppler notching at 24 wk is predictive of preeclampsia and intrauterine growth restriction in high-risk mothers. (From Drife J, Magowan B: *Clinical obstetrics and gynecology*, Philadelphia, 2004, Saunders.)

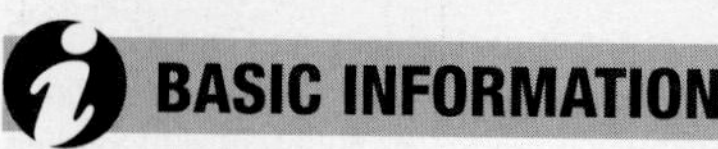

BASIC INFORMATION

DEFINITION

Premature labor is defined as regular contractions that result in cervical dilation or effacement prior to 37 wk gestation.

SYNONYMS

Preterm labor

ICD-9CM CODES
644.0
ICD-10CM CODES
O60.0 Preterm labor without delivery
O60.1 Preterm spontaneous labor with preterm delivery
O60.2 Preterm spontaneous labor with term delivery

EPIDEMIOLOGY & DEMOGRAPHICS

INCIDENCE: The incidence of preterm births in the U.S. has increased over the past two decades from 9.5% in 1981 to 12.7% in 2006. Between 40% and 45% of these births follow spontaneous preterm labor; either the remaining preterm births result from preterm premature rupture of membranes (PPROM), or they occur secondary to maternal or fetal indications.

PREDOMINANT SEX AND AGE: Pregnant women at the extremes of reproductive age (<17 yr and >35 yr) are at greatest risk.

GENETICS: A genetic component has been suggested. Women with sisters who have had preterm births and women with grandparents who were born preterm may be at increased risk for having preterm deliveries themselves. Single-nucleotide polymorphisms have also been associated with preterm labor.

RISK FACTORS: Risk factors for premature labor include a prior preterm delivery, intrauterine infection, systemic or genital tract infections, interpregnancy interval (<6 mo), short cervical length (<25 to 30 mm), low pre-pregnancy BMI (<19.8 kg/m^2), age <17 yr or >35 yr, a history of elective pregnancy termination, history of prior stillbirth, African-American ethnicity, vaginal bleeding, polyhydramnios or oligohydramnios, multiple gestation, structural abnormalities of the uterus, history of cervical cone biopsy or loop electrocautery excision, in vitro fertilization or ovulation induction, tobacco use, heavy alcohol consumption, cocaine use, heroin use, and psychological or social stress.

PHYSICAL FINDINGS & CLINICAL PRESENTATION

Presenting symptoms include increased pelvic pressure, abdominal cramping or contractions, increased vaginal discharge, vaginal spotting, or leakage of fluid.

ETIOLOGY

Causes of premature labor are varied and often difficult to determine. Premature labor may be secondary to infection, systemic illness, trauma, anatomic abnormalities (i.e., uterine anomaly such as lateral fusion defects like unicornuate or bicornuate uterus), or a combination of factors. It is thought that cervical ripening is the most common first step to premature labor or delivery. Subsequently, decidual-membrane activation occurs, as do contractions.

Dx DIAGNOSIS

DIFFERENTIAL DIAGNOSIS

The differential should include premature labor, preterm rupture of membranes, preterm contractions (contractions prior to 37 wk gestation that do not result in cervical change), and abdominal pain or cramping secondary to other medical conditions. There are many conditions that may cause preterm contractions or premature labor. These include:

- Infection
    - Chorioamnionitis
    - Genital tract infections, including bacterial vaginosis, gonorrhea, chlamydia
    - Urinary tract infections, including pyelonephritis, cystitis, or asymptomatic bacteruria
    - Gastroenteritis
- Trauma
- Placental abruption
- Illicit drug use
- Preterm premature rupture of membranes
- Appendicitis
- Nephrolithiasis
- Pancreatitis
- Cholelithiasis

WORKUP

- History and physical exam to rule out trauma, abuse, other causes of abdominal pain, and infection
- Fetal heart rate monitoring and tocometry to determine fetal status and contraction frequency
- Speculum exam to visually assess the cervix and assess for rupture of membranes, bleeding, infection, or advanced cervical dilation
    - If the patient is <35 wk gestation, a Fetal Fibronectin (FFN) test should be collected prior to performing a digital exam or transvaginal ultrasound. A FFN test can help predict preterm delivery if the patient has a cervical length on transvaginal ultrasound of <30 mm
- Digital exam to determine cervical dilation and effacement, and fetal station

LABORATORY TESTS

- CBC
- Urine analysis and culture
- Urine toxicology screen
- Collect tests for GBS, gonorrhea, and *Chlamydia*
- Perform a wet prep for yeast, bacterial vaginosis, and *Trichomonas*
- Fetal fibronectin
- Consider PT, PTT, INR, CMP, amylase, and lipase
- Amniocentesis may be performed if an intraamniotic infection is suspected

IMAGING STUDIES

A formal ultrasound is indicated to determine estimated fetal weight, fetal presentation, amniotic fluid volume, placental location and appearance, and cervical length.

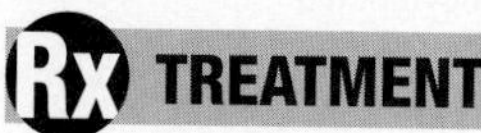

TREATMENT

Patients with premature labor should be delivered promptly when an intraamniotic infection is suspected or when they have cervical dilation >5 cm, a persistently nonreassuring fetal heart rate tracing, intrauterine growth restriction, or vaginal bleeding concerning for placental abruption.

NONPHARMACOLOGIC THERAPY

- Smoking cessation
- Bedrest, activity restriction, and pelvic rest are often recommended, but there are insufficient data to support this practice.

ACUTE GENERAL Rx

- Antenatal administration of corticosteroids between 24 wk and 33 6/7 wk gestation is recommended for women at risk of preterm delivery to prevent neonatal respiratory distress syndrome and decrease the incidence of intraventricular hemorrhage and necrotizing enterocolitis.
- Numerous tocolytic agents have been used in an attempt to inhibit contractions. Although efficacy is unclear, they can be utilized during an observation period in an effort to prolong gestation for administration of steroids or to transfer the mother to a facility capable of caring for preterm infants. This, of course, assumes there are no maternal or fetal medical contraindications to use of tocolytic drugs and no indications for rapid delivery. The most commonly used tocolytics are beta-mimetics (terbutaline), magnesium sulfate, calcium channel blockers (nifedipine), or prostaglandin synthetase inhibitors (indomethacin, ketorolac, sulindac).
- Routine antibiotic use has failed to show benefit in the absence of a known infection. But all mothers in preterm labor (without a documented negative group B strep culture) should be given antibiotics to prevent neonatal infection.

CHRONIC Rx

- Patients with a history of prior spontaneous preterm birth may be candidates for prophylactic use of 17 alpha-hydroxyprogesterone caproate between 16 wk and 36 wk gestation.
- Patients with a history of preterm birth and short cervix may also be candidates for prophylactic or rescue cerclage.
- There is no evidence supporting the use of maintenance tocolytic therapy

REFERRAL

- Women who present in preterm labor should be referred to an obstetrician and transferred to a facility with a neonatal intensive care unit.
- For women who present for prenatal care with a history of preterm delivery, early referral to an obstetrician is also recommended

SUGGESTED READINGS

available at www.expertconsult.com

RELATED CONTENT

Abruptio Placentae (Related Key Topic)
Breech Birth (Related Key Topic)

AUTHOR: **LAUREN MAY, M.D.**

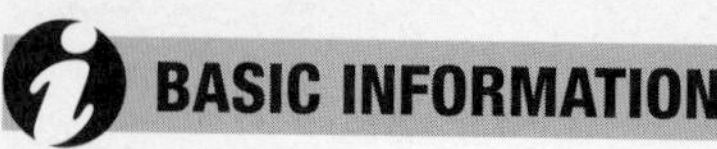

BASIC INFORMATION

DEFINITION

Premenstrual syndrome (PMS) is a cyclic recurrence during the luteal phase of the menstrual cycle of somatic, affective, and behavioral disturbances that are of sufficient severity to affect interpersonal relationships adversely or interfere with normal activities.

SYNONYMS

PMS
PMDD

ICD-9CM CODES
625.4 Premenstrual tension syndromes
ICD-10CM CODES
N94.3 Premenstrual tension syndrome

EPIDEMIOLOGY & DEMOGRAPHICS

- PMS is believed to be extremely prevalent, intermittently affecting approximately one third of all premenopausal women.
- Severe cases occur in approximately 2% to 10% of women with PMS.
- Those seeking treatment for PMS are usually in their 30s or 40s.
- The natural history of PMS has not been clearly elucidated.

PHYSICAL FINDINGS & CLINICAL PRESENTATION

- Diverse and potentially disabling symptoms. Table 1-410 summarizes common symptoms of cyclic PMS.
- Associated with >150 psychological, physical, and behavioral symptoms
- Most frequent reason for seeking treatment: emotional symptoms
- Most common emotional symptoms: depression, irritability, anxiety, labile moods, anger, crying easily, sadness, extreme sensitivity, nervous tension
- Most common physical symptoms: headache, bloating, cramps, breast tenderness, migraines, fatigue, weight gain, aches and pains, palpitations
- Most common behavior symptom: food cravings
- Other behavioral symptoms: increased appetite, increased alcohol intake, decreased motivation, decreased efficiency, avoidance of activities, staying home, sleep changes, libido changes, forgetfulness, decreased concentration

ETIOLOGY

- Etiology remains obscure.
- Because of the multifactorial, multiorgan nature of PMS, a single etiologic cause is unlikely.

DIAGNOSIS

DIFFERENTIAL DIAGNOSIS

- A diagnosis of exclusion, so other medical or psychological disorders should be ruled out.
- Most common disorders: depression or anxiety, thyroid disease.

WORKUP

- History
- Physical examination
- Laboratory studies to rule out alternative diagnosis
- If no alternative diagnosis confirms diagnosis of PMS, basal body temperature charting is used to determine if the patient is ovulating:
  1. If she is not ovulating, it is not PMS.
  2. If she is ovulating, symptoms should be charted for at least two cycles to determine if the symptoms occur in the luteal phase.
  3. If symptoms are not occurring in the luteal phase, it is not PMS and further investigation is needed.
     a. If symptoms occur in the follicular phase, patient has premenstrual exacerbation of another condition.
     b. If symptoms do not occur in the follicular phase, diagnosis of PMS is confirmed.

LABORATORY TESTS

- None available to specifically confirm the diagnosis of PMS
- Thyroid function tests to rule out thyroid disease

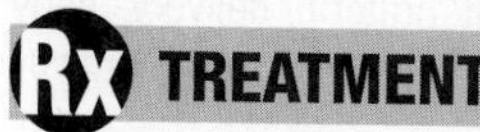

TREATMENT

NONPHARMACOLOGIC THERAPY

- Individualization of the treatment plan to maximize therapeutic response
- Psychosocial intervention:
  - Education
  - Stress management
  - Environmental changes
  - Adequate rest and sleep
  - Regular exercise
- Nutritional recommendations:
  - Regularly eaten, well-balanced meals
  - Adequate amounts of protein, fiber, and complex carbohydrates; low fat
  - Avoidance of foods that are high in salt and simple sugars; may promote water retention, weight gain, and physical discomfort
  - Avoidance of caffeine-containing beverages; stimulant effects of caffeine may worsen tension, irritability, and insomnia
  - Avoidance of alcohol and illicit drugs; may worsen emotional lability
  - Calcium supplementation (1000 mg/day for women 19 to 50 yr, 1300 mg/day for girls 14 to 18 yr) to reduce the physical and emotional symptoms
  - Magnesium (360 mg/day) to reduce water retention and the negative effect associated with PMS
  - Pyridoxine (vitamin B_6) 50 mg bid to improve depression, fatigue, irritability, and natural diuretic ability; neurotoxicity observed at higher dosages

ACUTE GENERAL Rx

Suppression of ovulation:

- Oral contraceptives: one pill per day
- Progestin-only oral contraceptive: one pill per day
- Oral micronized progesterone: 100 mg every morning and 200 mg every evening on days 17 through 28 of menstrual cycle
- Progestin suppository: 200 to 400 mg bid on days 17 through 28 of menstrual cycle
- Oral contraceptive containing drosperinone/ethinyl estradiol: very effective in decreasing physical symptoms
- Medroxyprogesterone: 150 mg IM q3mo
- Levonorgestrel implants: surgical insertion every 5 yr
- Transdermal estradiol: one or two 100-μg patches every 3 days
- Danazol: 100 to 200 mg/day (ovulation not suppressed at this dose); has significant side-effect profile
- Gonadotropin-releasing hormone (GnRH) agonists: daily by intranasal spray or monthly by depot injection; profound hypoestrogenism, concerns for osteoporosis and vasomotor symptoms

TABLE 1-410 Common Symptoms of Cyclic Premenstrual Syndrome

Somatic Symptoms	
Abdominal bloating	Constipation or diarrhea
Acne	Headache
Alcohol intolerance	Peripheral edema
Breast engorgement and tenderness	Weight gain
Clumsiness	
Emotional and Mental Symptoms	
Anxiety	Insomnia
Change in libido	Irritability
Depression	Lethargy
Fatigue	Mood swings
Food cravings (especially salt and sugar)	Panic attacks
Hostility	Paranoia
Inability to concentrate	Violence toward self and others
Increased appetite	Withdrawal from others

From Goldman L, Schafer AI: *Goldman's Cecil medicine*, ed 24, Philadelphia, 2012, Saunders.

Suppression of physical symptoms:

- Spironolactone: 25 to 50 mg bid on days 14 through 28 of menstrual cycle
- Mefenamic acid
  - For fluid retention: 250 mg tid on days 24 through 28 of cycle
  - For pain: 500 mg tid on days 19 through 28 of cycle
- Bromocriptine: 5 mg/day on days 10 through 26 of cycle
- Danazol: 200 mg/day on days 19 through 28 of cycle
- Naproxen: 550 mg bid on days 17 through 28 of cycle, Naprosyn-500 mg bid on days 17 through 28 of cycle

Suppression of psychological symptoms:

- Nortriptyline: 50 to 125 mg/day
- Fluoxetine: 20 mg/day or 90 mg weekly (this medication has indications for premenstrual dysphoric disorder)
- Buspirone: 10 mg bid or tid on days 16 through 28 of cycle, then taper drug
- Alprazolam: 25 mg tid on days 16 through 28 of cycle, then taper drug
- Clonidine: 0.1 mg bid
- Naltrexone: 0.25 mg/day on days 9 through 18 of cycle
- Atenolol: 50 mg/day
- Paroxetine: 20 mg/day
- Sertraline: 50 to 100 mg/day
- Nefazodone: initial dosage 100 mg bid; after 1 wk increase to 150 mg bid
- Propranolol: 20 to 40 mg bid
- Verapamil: 100 to 320 mg qd

CHRONIC Rx

- Therapy is largely trial and error, with the goal of providing effective treatment with the safest and most simple therapy.
- For severe intractable PMS: bilateral oophorectomy; give trial of GnRH therapy or danazol before surgery (bilateral oophorectomy should be exceedingly rare).
- Estrogen replacement therapy recommended postoperatively to reduce the risk of osteoporosis, heart disease, and genitourinary atrophy.

DISPOSITION

Improved symptoms in 90% of women over time

REFERRAL

- For counseling with a psychologist or psychiatrist if underlying psychiatric disorder is discovered (cognitive-behavioral therapy)
- To a gynecologist if surgical therapy is contemplated

SUGGESTED READINGS

available at www.expertconsult.com

RELATED CONTENT

Dysmenorrhea (Related Key Topic)
Premenstrual Syndrome (Patient Information)
Premenstrual Dysphoric Disorder (Related Key Topic)

AUTHOR: **RUBEN ALVERO, M.D.**

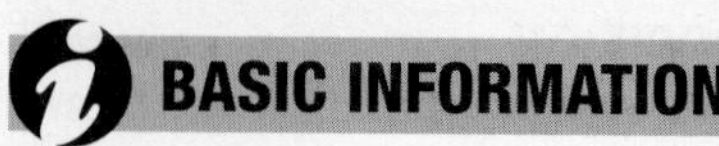

BASIC INFORMATION

DEFINITION

Preoperative evaluation is the clinical risk evaluation for patients undergoing surgery. It is an overall assessment of patient's health and surgery's risk. The goal of the assessment is not to "clear" the patient for the surgery, because there is always some level of risk, but to provide accurate preoperative risk stratification and implement possible risk reduction strategies. Preoperative evaluation should also include functional assessment and determine social support. It also provides the opportunity for discussion and helps to alleviate patient's anxiety before surgery.

SYNONYMS

Preoperative evaluation and risk reduction
Risk reduction in patients undergoing invasive procedures
Preoperative clearance

ICD-9CM CODES
ICD-V72.81–ICD-V72.84
ICD-10CM CODES
Z01.810 Encounter for preprocedural cardiovascular examination
Z01.811 Encounter for preprocedural respiratory examination
Z01.818 Encounter for other preprocedural examination
Z01.812 Encounter for preprocedural laboratory examination

EPIDEMIOLOGY & DEMOGRAPHICS

The number of outpatient surgical procedures performed in the United States has been gradually expanding over the years. By the end of 2010, outpatient procedures accounted for more than 50% of all surgeries compared with less than 33% in 2000. (U.S. Surgical Procedure Volumes Report #A626, February 2012).

Some studies have shown the benefits of preoperative testing while others have shown no added benefit. Lack of added benefit has been particularly true for otherwise healthy individuals: the prevalence of significant unrecognized disease and the predictive value of tests are both low for this population–leading to an excess of false positive tests.

In a trial of 1061 ambulatory surgical patients randomly assigned to preoperative testing or no testing, there was no difference in perioperative adverse events or events within 30 days of the surgery (Chung F et al., 2009).

Certain risk factors do exist that may be helpful: The nature and extent of surgery appear to play a role, as do increasing age, exercise capacity, and certain medications. Box 1-70 describes stratification of risk of common noncardiac surgical procedures.

Preoperative evaluation may be a good opportunity to reach out to patients about other preventive, screening, and routine health care issues as well. The primary care physician is uniquely poised to provide an accurate assessment and risk stratification of patients and to develop care plans for follow-up. This information can then be used to help surgeons counsel patients and guide patients' decision making.

PEAK INCIDENCE: When there are adverse consequences from surgery, cardiovascular complications account for a majority of the morbidity and mortality in patients. Perioperative MIs (PMI) is one of the most important predictors of short- and long-term morbidity and mortality associated surgery. The highest incidence of PMI is in the first 3 to 5 days after surgery.

PHYSICAL FINDINGS & CLINICAL PRESENTATION

The history, physical, and other studies need to assess the risks for myocardial infarction, arrhythmias, heart failure, endocarditis, stroke, venous thrombosis and pulmonary embolism, prolonged mechanical ventilation and respiratory failure, hemorrhage, diabetic acidosis, renal or hepatic failure, and infection.

WORKUP (Fig. 1-761)

HISTORY

A thorough medical history is the most valuable tool. Assess the urgency of the surgical procedure. A conversation with the surgical team is helpful for urgent and emergent procedures.

Some standard screening questionnaires have been adapted to help identify patients who would benefit from formal preoperative evaluation.

- Age is important to consider because age is often associated with an increasing number of comorbidities, which are in turn associated with an increase in perioperative risk.
- All patients should be asked about their exercise capacity before surgery. One way to assess functional capacity is in metabolic equivalents (METS) (*Circulation,* 2009) (Table 1-411). Studies have shown that those who have a low exercise capacity have twice as much risk for postoperative complications compared to those who have high exercise capacity.
- Evaluate for evidence of active cardiac conditions: unstable angina, recent MI (<30 days), significant arrhythmia, decompensated CHF, and severe valvular disease.
- Other medical conditions and risk factors:
    - Stable CAD, compensated CHF, HTN
    - Chronic lung diseases, obstructive sleep apnea
    - Other medical comorbidities: CVA, diabetes mellitus (DM), CKD, liver diseases
    - Personal or family history of anesthetic complications
    - Personal or family history of hypercoagulable states or bleeding disorders
    - Medications such as anticoagulants, antiplatelets, NSAIDs, and oral hypoglycemic agents
    - Smoking
    - Alcohol
        - Obesity
        - Pregnancy
- Consider further testing based on above risk factors. The decision to order preoperative tests should be guided by the patient's clinical history, comorbidities, and physical examination findings. Cardiac evaluation algorithm for noncardiac surgery is described later (Fleisher et al, 2007).

PHYSICAL EXAMINATION

- Vital signs: blood pressure, heart rate and rhythm, rate and ease of respirations, and temperature.
- Cardiovascular exam. Auscultate heart to check for heart murmurs, pathologic heart sounds, and ventricular systolic or diastolic dysfunction.
- Respiratory exam. Auscultate lungs for crackles, wheezes, decreased breath sounds.
- Vascular exam. Examine for carotid, abdominal, and femoral bruits.
- Integumentary exam. Check for evidence of venous stasis in lower extremities, petechiae, and unusual bruises.
- Mental status. Conduct a mini-mental exam.

LABORATORY TESTS & IMAGING STUDIES

- Determine the patient's age, height, weight.
- Routine laboratory studies are not necessary unless there is a specific medical indication. (*Anesthesiology,* 2002). Testing need not be repeated if results are recently available, unless there has been a change in clinical status.

BOX 1-70 Stratification of Risk of Common Noncardiac Surgical Procedures

High risk (>5%)	Emergent and urgent major operations, especially in the elderly Aortic and noncarotid major vascular surgery Surgery associated with large fluid status change or blood loss
Intermediate risk (1%-5%)	Head and neck surgery Carotid endarterectomy surgery Major thoracic surgery Major abdominal surgery Orthopedic surgery Prostate surgery
Low risk (<1%)	Eye and skin surgery Endoscopy Breast Ambulatory procedure

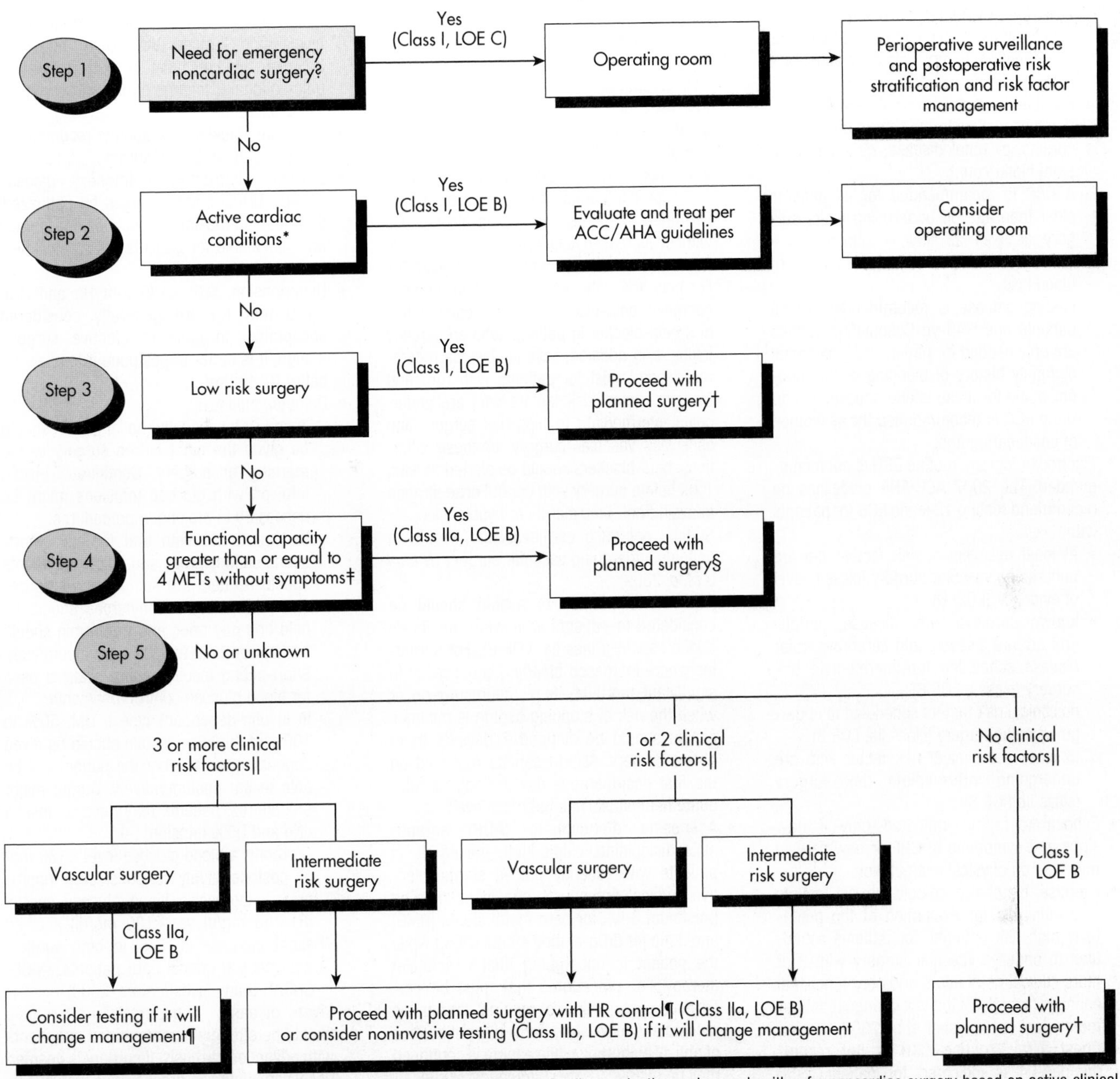

- **Step 1**: Need for emergency noncardiac surgery?
  - Yes (Class I, LOE C) → Operating room → Perioperative surveillance and postoperative risk stratification and risk factor management
  - No ↓
- **Step 2**: Active cardiac conditions*
  - Yes (Class I, LOE B) → Evaluate and treat per ACC/AHA guidelines → Consider operating room
  - No ↓
- **Step 3**: Low risk surgery
  - Yes (Class I, LOE B) → Proceed with planned surgery†
  - No ↓
- **Step 4**: Functional capacity greater than or equal to 4 METs without symptoms‡
  - Yes (Class IIa, LOE B) → Proceed with planned surgery§
- **Step 5**: No or unknown
  - 3 or more clinical risk factors||
    - Vascular surgery → Class IIa, LOE B → Consider testing if it will change management¶
    - Intermediate risk surgery → Proceed with planned surgery with HR control¶ (Class IIa, LOE B) or consider noninvasive testing (Class IIb, LOE B) if it will change management
  - 1 or 2 clinical risk factors||
    - Vascular surgery → Proceed with planned surgery with HR control¶ (Class IIa, LOE B) or consider noninvasive testing (Class IIb, LOE B) if it will change management
    - Intermediate risk surgery → Proceed with planned surgery with HR control¶ (Class IIa, LOE B) or consider noninvasive testing (Class IIb, LOE B) if it will change management
  - No clinical risk factors|| → Class I, LOE B → Proceed with planned surgery†

FIGURE 1-761 Stepwise approach to preoperative cardiac assessment. Cardiac evaluation and care algorithm for noncardiac surgery based on active clinical conditions, known cardiovascular disease, or cardiac risk factors for patients 50 years of age or older. (Adapted from Fleisher LA et al: ACC/AHA 2007 Guidelines on Perioperative Cardiovascular Evaluation and Care for Noncardiac Surgery, *Circulation* 116: e418-e500, 2007.)

Table 1-411 Functional Capacity (Metabolic Equivalents)

<4 METS	4-10 METS	>10 METS
Daily living activities	Heavy housework	Strenuous exercise
Walking (2 mph)	Walking up a hill	Skiing
Walk 1-2 blocks	Walking (4 mph)	Tennis (single)
	Cycling	
	Golf	
	Tennis (double)	

(1 MET: energy expenditure of 70-kg man sitting quietly)

Adapted from Fleisher LA et al: ACC/AHA 2007 Guidelines on perioperative cardiovascular evaluation and care for noncardiac surgery, *Circulation* 116:e418-e500, 2007.

- Low-risk procedures do not require routine basic metabolic panel, blood glucose, liver function, hemostasis evaluation, or a urine analysis.
- For intermediate- and high-risk procedures as well as in the setting of diabetes, cardiac, or renal disease, obtain a complete blood count.
- A CBC is recommended for all patients older than age 65 undergoing major surgery as well as anyone undergoing a surgery with expected large amounts of blood loss.
- Fasting glucose is recommended for all patients age >45 yr. Coagulation studies are only needed for patients with personal or family history of bleeding or thrombophilia and for those taking anticoagulants.
- Urine hCG is recommended for all women of childbearing age.

- Electrocardiogram: routine ECG is not recommended. The 2007 ACC/AHA guidelines do recommend resting 12 leads ECG for patients with:
  - at least one clinical risk factor who are undergoing vascular surgery (class I, level of evidence (LOE) B)
  - known cardiovascular disease, peripheral arterial disease, and cerebrovascular disease scheduled for intermediate risk surgery (class I, LOE C)
  - no clinical risk factors scheduled to undergo vascular surgery (class IIa, LOE B)
  - at least one clinical risk factor who are undergoing intermediate risk surgery (class IIb LOE B)
- Echocardiography: indicated only if new signs and symptoms of CHF or new cardiac murmurs on physical examination.
- Exercise or pharmacologic stress testing: only indicated for evaluation of the potentially high-risk patients: for patients scheduled to undergo vascular surgery with 3 or more clinical risk factors and poor functional capacity (<4 METS) if it will change management (class IIa) (Fleisher et al, 2007).
- Chest x-ray: routine CXR is not recommended. It is indicated for patients >50 years of age undergoing high-risk procedures (American College of Physicians [ACP] recommendations) and patients with new respiratory symptoms, suspected congestive heart failure, or valvular heart disease.
- Pulmonary function tests: It is only recommended for patients undergoing lung resection surgery but can be considered in:
  - Patients with COPD or asthma, only if clinical evaluation cannot determine if they are at their best baseline.
  - Patients with dyspnea or exercise intolerance that remains unexplained after clinical evaluation.
- Arterial blood gas: should be obtained only when clinically significant (to determine if lung disease is compensated).

TREATMENT

- Beta blockers: While routine administration of perioperative beta-blockers was advocated for many years, conflicting evidence currently exists regarding their efficacy. While confirming a decrease in cardiac events with aggressive preoperative beta-blockade, the POISE trial (extended-release metoprolol beginning on day of surgery) showed an increase in mortality and stroke risk (*Lancet*, 2008). On the other hand, DECREASE IV (fluvastatin + bisoprolol) demonstrated a cardioprotective effect of perioperative beta-blocker use without increased incidence in perioperative stroke or mortality (Dunkelgrun M et al, 2009). For now, the only class I indication for perioperative beta-blockers is the continuation of a beta-blocker in patients who are already taking it. In addition, several class IIa recommendations exist for patients with CAD and multiple clinical risk factors who are undergoing intermediate to high-risk surgery and especially vascular surgery. In these situations, beta-blockers should be started at least 1 wk before surgery with careful dose titration to avoid frank bradycardia or hypotension.
- Statins: decrease cardiovascular events in patients undergoing vascular surgery (*N Engl J Med,* 2009).
- Aspirin: continuation of aspirin should be considered in patients who were previously taking aspirin (Class IIa, LOE B). For surgeries where increased bleeding could result in significant morbidity (e.g., neurosurgery) or when the risk of stopping aspirin is minimal, aspirin should be stopped 7 days or more before surgery. Aspirin can be restarted on the first postoperative day as long as adequate hemostasis has been achieved.
- Adenosine diphosphate (ADP) antagonists (ticlopidine, clopidogrel, prasugrel): in patients with recently placed stents, elective surgical procedures should be delayed (minimum 3 wk for bare metal stents [BMS] and 3 mo for drug-eluting stents [DES]) while the patient is undergoing dual antiplatelet therapy. For procedures that must be performed, continuation of aspirin therapy is recommended. A short-term discontinuation of anti-ADP therapy while aspirin is continued may be relatively safe (*Circulation,* 2009).
- Anticoagulation therapy: patients taking warfarin who have a high risk of thromboembolism should be bridged with low-molecular-weight heparin (LMWH) (with last dose 24 h before surgery) or unfractionated heparin (UFH) (with drip stopped 4 hr before surgery). Resumption of bridging therapy within 24 hr is safe for minor procedures but is associated with unacceptable, high bleeding rates in patients undergoing major surgery (Dunn et al, 2007). Therefore, it is recommended to wait 48 to 72 hr postoperatively to resume bridging therapy in patients who had major surgery. Another alternative regimen is to resume warfarin 12 to 24 hr postoperatively without any bridging therapy (Douketis et al, 2008).
- NSAIDs: NSAID therapy is almost never necessary, and it should be stopped before surgery (5-10 days prior).
- Pacemakers and defibrillators: consultation with an electrophysiologist is recommended. Pacemaker should be reprogrammed to an asynchronous mode (VOO, DOO), and defibrillation function must be set off to avoid unintentional discharge during surgery (electrocauterization).
- Smoking: smoking cessation is recommended at least 8 wk before surgery.
- Chronic obstructive pulmonary disease (COPD): COPD therapy should be optimized. Steroids and maximal bronchodilator therapy are reasonable for patients not at their best baseline.
- Hypertension: SBP <180 mm Hg and DBP <110 mm Hg are generally considered acceptable. In case of elective surgery, though, it is better to postpone it to allow for better BP control.
- Diabetes mellitus:
  - Type I DM: scheduled basal insulin should be given the night before surgery or the morning of surgery. Continuous insulin infusion with glucose infusions might be necessary in prolonged procedures.
  - In type II DM with oral therapy: short-acting sulfonylureas and other oral agents should be held the same day. Metformin and long-acting sulfonylureas should be held one day prior, and metformin should be kept on hold for 48 hr postoperatively. Short-acting insulin sliding scale is used for blood glucose control meanwhile.
  - In insulin-dependent type II DM: 50% to 100% of the basal insulin should be given depending on whether the patient will be able to eat postoperatively. During major procedures, patients may need an insulin drip and D5% infusion.
  - Currently, a blood glucose level <180 mg/dl postoperatively is considered appropriate. Aggressive blood glucose control (81-108 mg/dl vs. <180 mg/dl) showed slight increase in risks in both surgical and medical critical care patients. (NICE-SUGAR Study Investigators, 2009).
- Liver disease: nonoperative alternative should be strongly recommended in patients with advanced cirrhosis. If surgery is deemed necessary, optimize preoperative status: correct coagulopathy, thrombocytopenia, volume status, electrolytes, ascites, and encephalopathy.
- End-stage renal disease: achieve euvolemia and correct electrolytes. Patients receiving hemodialysis should undergo dialysis the day before surgery. In patients with a prior history of uremic bleeding, desmopressin administration should be considered.
- Corticosteroid management and adrenal insufficiency: in patients taking exogenous steroids, continuation of the same steroid regimen is reasonable. In those with chronic adrenal insufficiency, steroid supplementation is generally recommended with the dose titrated to the level of stress of the surgical procedure.

PEARLS & CONSIDERATIONS

COMMENTS

Although most individuals will not require any significant preoperative testing, certain conditions will require further workup.

- Ischemic heart disease
  - If patient has angina, determine frequency, precipitating factors, response to rest and nitroglycerin
  - If patient has had prior cardiac catheterizations or coronary revascularizations, obtain previous records
- Dysrhythmias and pacemakers
  - Examine current and prior ECGs for high-grade atrioventricular block, symptomatic ventricular arrhythmias, and supraventricular tachycardias at uncontrolled rates.
  - If patient has a pacemaker, establish the type and mode, date of implantation, and when it was last interrogated.
- Valvular and congenital heart disease
  - Look for signs of severe valvular heart disease on last echocardiographic evaluations.
- Cerebrovascular disease
  - Inquire about prior carotid artery ultrasounds
- Venous thromboembolism
  - Determine results of studies for thrombophilia (factor V Leiden mutation, lupus anticoagulant, antithrombin III, protein C or S).
- Tools for cardiac risk assessment:
  - http://www.statcoder.com
  - http://www.infopoems.com

PATIENT & FAMILY EDUCATION

Advise patients that their preoperative evaluation visit with their PCP is another opportunity for them to bring up concerns or get questions answered about their upcoming procedure.

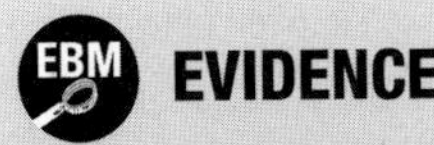

EVIDENCE

available at www.expertconsult.com

SUGGESTED READINGS

available at www.expertconsult.com

AUTHORS: **PRIYA SARIN GUPTA , M.D.** and **TONY ABDO, M.D.**

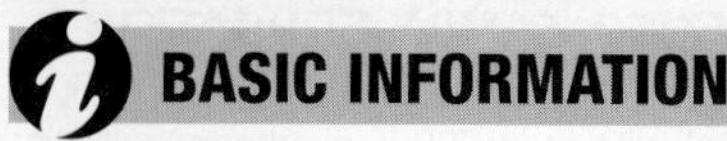

BASIC INFORMATION

DEFINITION

Pressure ulcers are ischemic soft tissue injuries that result from pressure, shearing forces, and moisture that usually occur over bony prominences over a long period.

SYNONYMS

Decubitus ulcers
Pressure sores
Bedsores
Decubiti

ICD-9CM CODES
707.0
ICD-10CM CODES
L89 Pressure ulcers
Subcategories of codes determined by stage and location of ulcer
L89.153 Example: Stage 3 ulcer of sacral area

EPIDEMIOLOGY & DEMOGRAPHICS

- Occurs in all health care settings from hospitals to nursing homes and even at home. Incidence approaches as many as 40% of affected individuals. Prevalence has declined among all nursing home residents over the past decade. It is highest in institutions with lower staffing levels of certified nurses and nursing assistants, reflecting emphasis on health care resources more than medical decision-making.
- Associated with decreased quality of life and significant morbidity and mortality. One-year mortality rate approaches 40%.
- Pain occurs in two thirds of patients with stage II or greater pressure ulcers.
- Complicated by cellulitis, osteomyelitis, abscesses, and sepsis.

CLINICAL PRESENTATION

The National Pressure Ulcer Advisory Panel in 2007 has outlined the staging system of pressure ulcers as follows:

Stage I: Nonblanchable erythema of intact skin usually over a bony prominence or boggy, mushy feeling of skin

Stage II: Partial-thickness skin loss involving the epidermis, dermis, or both. May also present as an intact or ruptured serum-filled blister.

Stage III: Full-thickness skin loss involving damage or necrosis of subcutaneous tissue that may extend down to, but not through, underlying fascia or muscle. There may be undermining and tunneling.

Stage IV: Full-thickness skin loss with exposed muscle, bone, or supporting structures (e.g., tendons, joint capsule). Sloughing or eschar may be present. These ulcers often include undermining and tunneling (Fig. 1-762).

Deep tissue injury: Purple or maroon localized area of discolored, intact skin or blood-filled blister due to damage of underlying tissue from pressure and/or shear.

Unstageable: Full-thicknesss tissue loss with the base of the ulcer covered by slough or eschar in the wound bed.

Only pressure ulcers are classified by stage.

ETIOLOGY

Pressure ulcers are ischemic soft tissue injuries caused by constant, unrelieved pressure in tissues over bony prominences. The four main external factors include pressure, shearing forces, friction, and moisture. Host factors include immobility, incontinence, malnutrition, and compromised skin perfusion. A number of neurologic and nonneurologic diseases may contribute, lead, or exacerbate the development of pressure ulcers. However, further studies need to be performed to identify whether these are independent predictors.

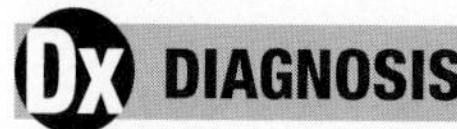

DIAGNOSIS

DIFFERENTIAL DIAGNOSIS

- Venous stasis ulcers
- Arterial ulcers
- Diabetic ulcers
- Skin cancer
- Cellulitis
- Kennedy ulcers (rapidly progressing ulcers that occur at the end of life)

WORKUP

Evaluate ulcer characteristics, including its stage, appearance, location, and size (documented on a clock face, with the patient's head at 12 o'clock and feet at 6 o'clock). For stages III and IV, describe the wound bed (epithelialization, granulation tissue, necrotic tissue, eschar); presence of exudates, including type and amount; depth and wound edges (undermining, sinus tracts, tunneling, or fistulas); signs of infection (purulent drainage, odor, surrounding cellulitis); and pain. In addition, pressure ulcer risk factors and causes should be reassessed.

LABORATORY TESTS

- Directed at identifying cause of risk factors or any complications arising from the pressure ulcer (e.g., abscess or osteomyelitis).
- Cultures of wound bed are not believed to be helpful and should be avoided. Deep tissue biopsy is the gold standard if a culture is indicated.
- Markers for malnutrition include prealbumin, albumin, transferrin, lymphocyte count, and total cholesterol level.
- Complete blood count if systemic infection is suspected.

IMAGING STUDIES

- Ultrasound not proven to be effective.
- Plain radiographs, MRI, and bone scan may help identify osteomyelitis when clinically suspected.
- A comparison study of 44 patients scheduled for open biopsy did not show MRI to have superior diagnostic benefit over plain radiography.

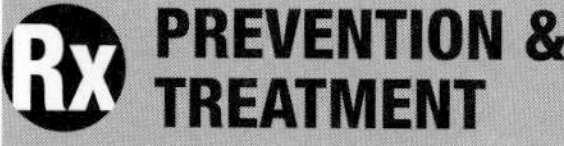

PREVENTION & TREATMENT

- Identify high-risk patients using standardized risk assessment scales (e.g., Braden, Norton, and Waterlow scales)
- Routine skin inspection and good skin care for high-risk patients.
- Minimize prolonged skin exposure to moisture, urine, or stool.
- Treat dry, cracking skin.
- Use repositioning and pressure-reducing devices (e.g., foam mattresses, low–air loss beds, pillows, or foam wedges when in bed or in a chair).
  - Patient repositioning:
    A recent multicenter trial demonstrated no difference in pressure ulcer formation in high-risk nursing home patients turned at 2-, 3-, and 4-hour intervals when on a high-density foam mattress.
  - Bed surface
    Air-fluidized beds
    a. Two RCTs found that use of air-fluidized beds contributed to the healing of a greater number of ulcers after 15 days compared with standard care.
    b. Systematic review revealed no differences in rate of pressure ulcer healing with use of either alternating-pressure mattresses or low–air loss beds compared with standard care.

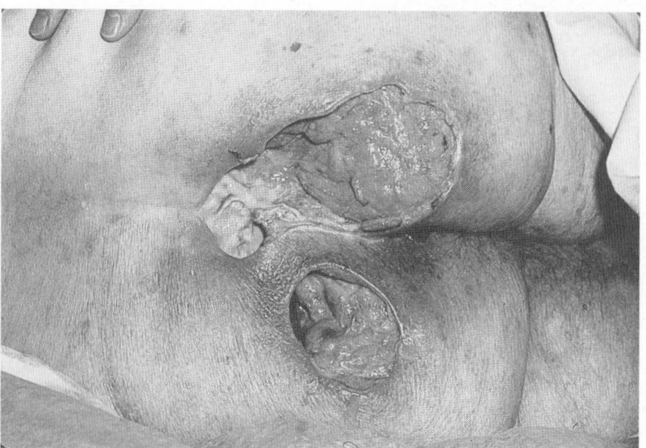

FIGURE 1-762 Natural debridement of pressure injury at 2 weeks. (From Tallis R, Fillit H: *Brockelhurst's textbook of geriatric medicine and gerontology*, ed 6, London, 2003, Churchill Livingstone.)

Pressure-relieving overlays

a. One RCT demonstrated that a viscoelastic pad on the operating table significantly reduced incidence of postoperative pressure ulcers compared with a standard operating table.

Foam alternatives

a. Forty-one RCTs demonstrated that patients lying on standard hospital mattresses are more likely to develop pressure ulcers than those patients lying on higher specification foam mattresses.

- Use adequate support surfaces while in bed or in a chair to prevent "bottoming out" (defined as less than 1 inch between patient and support surface; measured by putting hand under support surface and feeling thickness to patient).
- Recent systematic review of pressure ulcer prevention strategies showed poor methodology in most studies. Use of support surfaces, repositioning, optimized nutrition, and sacral skin moisturizing was most appropriate.
  - The 2010 consensus statement from the National Pressure Ulcer Advisory Panel said that not all pressure ulcers are avoidable because there are patient situations where pressure cannot be relieved and perfusion cannot be improved.

NONPHARMACOLOGIC THERAPY

- Should be cleaned at each dressing change; necrotic tissue should be debrided quickly because it delays wound healing (except for heel ulcers).
- Wound irrigation should not exceed 15 psi and is best done with an 18-gauge angiocatheter.
- No single dressing or product is superior; should be used to keep ulcer bed moist and protect it from urine/stool. Silver dressings (which are felt to be antimicrobial), topical phenytoin, and growth factors should be limited to difficult-to-heal wounds, chronic ulcers, and extensive burns given their extra cost and limited scientific validation.
- Avoid agents that are cytotoxic to epithelial cells (e.g., iodine, iodophor, sodium hypochlorite, hydrogen peroxide, acetic acid, alcohol).
- Reduce pressure by using foam mattress, dynamic support surface (e.g., low–air loss bed), and frequent repositioning (e.g., q2h or, in cases of poor perfusion, more frequently).
- Hyperbaric oxygen, ultrasound, ultraviolet, electromagnetic therapy, and low-energy radiation either are ineffective or have not been extensively evaluated for efficacy.
- Negative pressure devices (Vac devices) may help in wounds that have significant drainage. They also may improve healing by promoting angiogenesis, improving tissue perfusion, and decreasing bacterial count. Calcium alginate and foam dressings may also be beneficial for such wounds.
- Although correcting poor nutrition has been shown to be beneficial, a recent large investigation demonstrated that feeding tube insertion did not prevent or heal pressure ulcers, but increased the risk for developing a pressure ulcer.
- Minimize or promptly remove urinary and/or fecal contamination.
- Use a standardized assessment tool to monitor wound healing on weekly basis. Examples of monitoring scales include the Pressure Sore Status Tool (PSST) and Pressure Ulcer Scale for Healing (PUSH) in addition to the NPUAP staging system.
- No RCTs have compared debridement versus without debridement in the treatment of pressure ulcers.
- Thirty-two RCTs have compared different debridement agents, but there is insufficient evidence to promote the use of one particular agent.
- One RCT demonstrated ulcers treated with collagenase healed significantly more quickly than those treated with hydrocolloid.
- One RCT comparing honey-treated dressing with dressing soaked with saline showed faster healing times with the honey-treated group.
- A meta-analysis and one RCT found significant benefit in rates of healing with use of hydrocolloid dressings versus traditional saline gauze dressings but not over other forms such as hydrogels, foam dressings, or collagenase.
- No benefit was found with nutritional and vitamin supplements, artificial nutrition, or ultrasound therapy.

ACUTE GENERAL Rx

- Management of pressure ulcers is contingent on the stage of the ulcer.
- The cornerstone of therapy involves use of appropriate wound dressings, pressure-relieving devices, treatment of infection, debridement, and surgical consultation when appropriate.
- Adjunctive therapies such as electrical stimulation, negative pressure wound therapy, therapeutic ultrasound, hyperbaric oxygen, topical oxygen, and application of growth factors to the wound are being investigated.
- Pain medications are necessary because pressure ulcers are often painful. One study found that excruciating pain was more prevalent in nursing home residents with pressure ulcers.

CHRONIC Rx

- Continue vigilance with pressure reduction because pressure ulcers can recur with minimal trauma.
- Consider radiologic evaluation for infected ulcer bed, occult osteomyelitis, or abscess.

COMPLEMENTARY & ALTERNATIVE MEDICINE

Vitamin C, zinc, and multivitamin supplements may be of benefit to optimize nutrition.

DISPOSITION

- When systematic risk assessments are done and preventive measures are followed, most pressure ulcers can be prevented. Most ulcers heal when appropriate management strategies are followed.
- Stage IV ulcers in high-risk patients (e.g., paraplegics) can take months or years to heal.

REFERRAL

- Physical and occupational therapists to improve bed and chair mobility.
- Wounds with necrotic tissue need referral to persons trained in sharp debridement.
- To plastic surgeons for operative repair for large stage III or IV ulcers that do not respond to optimal care.
- To a specialty wound center for nonhealing ulcers.

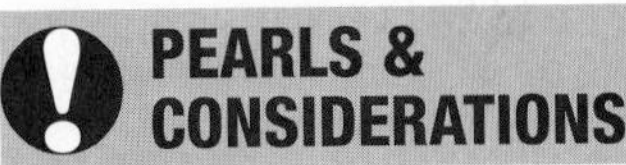

PEARLS & CONSIDERATIONS

COMMENTS

- Up to 10% of older persons will have a pressure ulcer.
- Because 70% of pressure ulcers occur in older persons, the approach should be similar to other multifactorial geriatric syndromes with a multidisciplinary team approach. Identify and reduce all modifiable risk factors for pressure ulcers.
- Treat the pain associated with pressure ulcers.
- Proper skin care, use of support surfaces, mobilization, and attention to nutrition are key for prevention and treatment.
- Clinical studies have not revealed if any one dressing product is superior.
- Nonhealing ulcers require assessment for debridement, infection, abscess, and/or referral to a wound center.

PATIENT & FAMILY EDUCATION

- Educate patient and family members on the risk factors for pressure ulcers.
- Encourage mobility and adequate nutritional intake and avoid bed rest.

SUGGESTED READINGS

available at www.expertconsult.com

RELATED CONTENT

Bed Sores (Patient Information)

AUTHORS: **RACHEL ROACH, A.P.R.N.-B.C.,** and **NOEL S. C. JAVIER, M.D.**

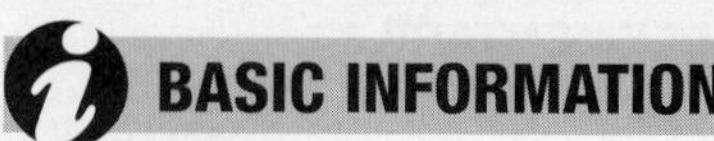

BASIC INFORMATION

DEFINITION

Priapism is the persistent, usually painful erection associated or unassociated with sexual stimulation. There are two major forms: low-flow (veno-occlusive) priapism and high-flow priapism (associated with increased arterial inflow without increased venous outflow resistance).

ICD-9CM CODES
607.3 Priapism
ICD-10CM CODES
N48.30 Priapism, unspecified

EPIDEMIOLOGY & DEMOGRAPHICS

- Peak incidence is seen from ages 5 to 10 yr and 20 to 50 yr.
- In the younger group, priapism is often associated with sickle cell disease or neoplasm. In the older group it is often caused by pharmacologic agents.
- Low-flow (venoocclusive priapism [type I]) is much more common than high-flow (type II).

PHYSICAL FINDINGS & CLINICAL PRESENTATION

- In idiopathic priapism the initial erection is associated with prolonged sexual excitement. Previous transient episodes are frequently reported. The erection involves the corpora cavernosa alone. Detumescence does not occur spontaneously.
- In secondary priapism, sexual excitement need not be involved. Otherwise the clinical picture is the same as in idiopathic priapism.
- Table 1-412 compares normal erection and priapism.

ETIOLOGY

Idiopathic: prolonged sexual arousal
Secondary or associated causes:
- Sickle cell disease
- Diabetes
- Leukemia (especially chronic myelogenous leukemia)
- Solid tumor (malignant) penile infiltration
- Spinal cord injury
- Perineal or penile trauma
- Iatrogenic
- Total parenteral nutrition, which includes a fat emulsion
- Hyperosmolar IV contrast
- Spinal or general anesthesia
- Anticoagulant therapy
- Phenothiazines
- Trazodone
- Intracorporeal injection therapy for impotence
- Phosphodiesterase type 5 inhibitors (e.g., sildenafil [Viagra], tadalafil [Cialis], vardenafil [Levitra])

PATHOPHYSIOLOGY

- Low-flow priapism: prolonged erection leads to edema of the cavernosal trabeculae, resulting in a sequence of stasis, thrombosis, venous occlusion, fibrosis, scarring, and possibly impotence.
- High-flow priapism: cavernosal artery rupture leading to an arteriocavernous fistula.

Dx DIAGNOSIS

WORKUP

None if the associated underlying causes are known to be present. Otherwise they should be ruled out. Low-flow priapism can be distinguished from high-flow priapism by obtaining a corporeal blood gas value. A Po_2 <30 mm Hg, Pco_2 >60 mm Hg, and a pH <7.25 are consistent with low-flow priapism. High-flow priapism can be confirmed by a perineal Doppler ultrasound or arteriography (useful to identify arterial-lacunar fistula).

Rx TREATMENT

Goal: achieve detumescence with preservation of potency.

1. Medical therapies:
   - Ice packs
   - Ice water enemas
   - Hot water enemas
   - Pressure dressing
   - Sedatives
   - Analgesics
   - Antispasmodic/anticholinergic drugs
   - Estrogens
   - Anticoagulants
   - Procaine
   - Amyl nitrite
   - Local or general anesthesia
   - Ketamine (1 mg/lb)
2. In the patient with sickle cell disease: intravenous hydration, alkalinization, transfusion or exchange transfusion, oxygen.
3. Corporeal irrigation with normal saline may be used for low-flow priapism. The midshaft of the penis can be injected with a small-gauge butterfly needle and irrigated with 10 to 20 ml of normal saline, followed by an intracorporeal injection of an alpha-adrenergic agonist every 5 min until detumescence. Commonly used intracavernous vasoconstrictor agents are epinephrine (10 to 20 mcg), phenylephrine (250 to 500 mcg), and ephedrine (50 to 100 mg). It is mandatory to monitor the patient's blood pressure and pulse when using alpha-adrenergic agonists.
4. Surgery:
   - Cavernospongiosum shunt
   - Glans-cavernosum shunt
   - Cavernosaphenous shunt
   - In the less common situation of high-flow priapism (diagnosed by the finding of bright red arterial blood on aspiration), arterial embolization or surgical ligation is recommended.

PROGNOSIS

Impotence is associated with the duration of priapism, with 36 hr being an important threshold.

REFERRAL

To urologist

RELATED CONTENT

Priapism (Patient Information)

AUTHOR: **FRED F. FERRI, M.D.**

TABLE 1-412 Comparison of Normal Erection and Priapism

Factor	Normal Erection	Priapism
Portion of penis involved	Corpora cavernosa and corpus spongiosum and glans	Corpora cavernosa
Cause	Vasodilatation of penile arteries	Obstruction of venous outflow Disturbance of neuroarterial mechanism (imbalance between it and adrenergic activity) Increased viscosity
Sexual desire	Present	Absent
Pain	Absent	Present
Duration	Minutes to hours	Hours to days

From Nseyo UO (ed): *Urology for primary care physicians,* Philadelphia, 1999, Saunders.

BASIC INFORMATION

DEFINITION

Primary biliary cirrhosis (PBC) is a chronic, variably progressive cholestatic liver disease most often affecting women and characterized by destruction of the small intrahepatic bile ducts leading to portal inflammation, fibrosis, cirrhosis, and ultimately, liver failure.

SYNONYMS

Biliary cirrhosis
Nonsuppurative destructive cholangitis
Autoimmune cholangiopathy

ICD-9CM CODES
571.6 Biliary cirrhosis
ICD-10CM CODES
K74.3 Primary biliary cirrhosis

EPIDEMIOLOGY & DEMOGRAPHICS

INCIDENCE:

- PBC affects all races and accounts for 0.6% to 2% of deaths from cirrhosis worldwide.
- Annual incidence rates range from 0.7 to 49 cases per million.

PREVALENCE: Prevalence is greatest in the U.K., Scandinavia, Canada, and the U.S., and varies tremendously by geographic areas, ranging from 6.7 to 402 cases per million. Disease burden seems to be increasing, which may be a result of better detection rather than true rise in disease incidence.

PREDOMINANT SEX: Female to male ratio of up to 10:1.

PREDOMINANT AGE: Onset typically occurs between the ages of 30 and 65 yr, and it is uncommon before age 25 yr.

PREDOMINANT RACE: Predominantly Caucasian but can be seen in other races.

GENETICS:

- Although there are no clearly identified genetic factors associated with PBC, there is a clear familial occurrence. Prevalence among first-degree relatives is 5% to 6%, and 1% to 6% of all patients have at least one affected family member. The concordance rate among monozygotic twins is 63%.
- Up to 84% of patients with PBC have at least one other autoimmune disorder, such as thyroiditis, Sjögren's syndrome, rheumatoid arthritis, Raynaud's phenomenon, or scleroderma. A variant form of PBC exists as an overlap syndrome with autoimmune hepatitis (AIH).
- PBC is closely associated with a greater risk of hepatocellular carcinoma as well as an overall greater risk of cancer.

ETIOLOGY

- Although the cause of PBC remains unknown, it is believed to require both a genetic susceptibility as well as an environmental trigger, ultimately leading to the modification of mitochondrial proteins triggering a persistent T lymphocyte–mediated attack on intralobular bile duct epithelial cells.
- PBC is associated with the DRB1*08 family of alleles, but there is a great deal of variation among ethnicities.
- Possible environmental triggers include cigarette smoking, urinary tract infections, reproductive hormone replacement, nail polish, and toxic waste sites (particularly exposure to halogenated hydrocarbons), as well as xenobiotics in animal models of PBC.
- Recent studies have identified a group of autoantigens collectively known as the "M2 subtype" of autoantigens that play a major role in the early pathogenesis of PBC. These are peptides within the mitochondrial membrane that share structural homology. The enzyme complex subunit (PDC-E2) is one of the key autoantigens in this group. Patients with PBC have a tenfold increased concentration of cytotoxic $CD8^+$ lymphocytes recognizing this peptide in their livers compared with their blood, and most antimitochondrial antibodies (AMAs), which are the serologic hallmark of this disease, react to the PDC-E2 subunit. In addition, bile duct epithelial cells handle PDC-E2 in a unique way that exposes them to immune-mediated attack by PDC-E2–oriented cytotoxic T cells. Future therapies may be specific immunomodulation directed at these peptides.
- In addition to the T lymphocyte–mediated direct destruction of small bile ducts, secondary damage to hepatocytes results from the chronic accumulation of bile acids.

PHYSICAL FINDINGS & CLINICAL PRESENTATION

Clinical stages:

- Asymptomatic
- Symptomatic
- Cirrhotic
- Hepatic failure

Symptoms:

- 50% to 60% of patients may be asymptomatic; 40% to 100% of these patients will develop symptoms, and nearly 25% of symptomatic patients at diagnosis will progress to liver failure within 10 yr without treatment.
- Fatigue (78% of patients) and pruritus (20% to 70% of patients) are the usual presenting symptoms.
- Pruritus is worse at night, under constricting, coarse garments; in association with dry skin; and in hot, humid weather. The cause is unknown; it is no longer believed to be a result of the retention of bile acids in skin. Pruritus may first occur during pregnancy but is distinguished from pruritus of pregnancy because it persists into the postpartum period and beyond.
- Other common symptoms include jaundice, unexplained right upper quadrant pain (10%), manifestations of portal hypertension, sicca symptoms, and scleroderma-like lesions.
- Musculoskeletal complaints caused by inflammatory arthropathy in 40% to 70% of patients: 5% to 10% experience development of chronic rheumatoid arthritis and 10% experience development of "arthritis of PBC."
- Steatorrhea may be seen in advanced disease.

Physical:

- Variable: Results depend on stage of disease at time of presentation; patients at the early stage may be completely unaffected.
- Excoriations may be present.
- Hepatomegaly (70%) and splenomegaly (initially 35%) may be present in more advanced disease.
- Xanthomas and jaundice appear in advanced disease. Kayser-Fleischer rings are rare and result from copper retention. Hyperpigmentation of the skin due to melanin deposition may be present.
- Late physical findings mirror those of cirrhosis: spider nevi, temporal and proximal limb wasting, ascites, and edema.

Dx DIAGNOSIS

The diagnosis of PBC can be established when two of the following three criteria are met.

- Positive serum AMA, titer >1:40
- Biochemical evidence of cholestasis (mainly alkaline phosphatase elevation)
- Characteristic liver histology: nonsuppurative destructive cholangitis and destruction of interlobular bile ducts

DIFFERENTIAL DIAGNOSIS

- Drug-induced cholestasis
- PBC-AIH overlap syndrome: reported in almost 10% of adults with AIH or PBC; transition from stable PBC to AIH and vice versa also seen
- Other etiologies of chronic liver disease and cirrhosis, such as alcoholic cirrhosis, chronic viral hepatitis, primary sclerosing cholangitis, AIH, sarcoidosis, chemical/toxin-induced cirrhosis, other hereditary or familial disorders (e.g., cystic fibrosis, α-1-antitrypsin deficiency)
- Biliary obstruction

WORKUP

History, physical examination, laboratory evaluation, liver biopsy

LABORATORY TESTS

- AMAs found in 95% of patients with PBC and are 98% specific.
- Antinuclear antibodies (ANAs) and AMAs found in approximately 50% of patients. In approximately 5% of patients, AMAs are absent or present only in low titer (AMA-negative PBC). Nearly all of these patients have ANA or AMAs, or both.
- Cholestatic pattern of liver biochemical markers, that is, markedly increased alkaline phosphatase (of hepatic origin).
- γ-Glutamyl transpeptidase is increased.
- Serum IgM levels are increased (lower in AMA-negative PBC).
- Bilirubin level is normal early; increases with disease progression (direct and indirect) in 60% of patients. Increased serum bilirubin level is a poor prognostic sign.
- Aminotransferase level may be normal and, if increased, is rarely more than five times the upper limit of normal.

- Markedly increased serum lipids in more than 50% of patients. Total cholesterol may exceed 1000 mg/dl. No increased risk for death from atherosclerosis seen, possibly because of high levels of LP-X, an anti-atherogenic low-density lipoprotein particle, very-high-density lipoprotein levels, and low serum levels of lipoprotein(a).
- Percutaneous liver biopsy confirms or rules out the diagnosis, allows staging, but is not essential in order to initiate medical therapy in patients with typical liver chemistry and positive AMA test.
- Histology is not uniform, so histologic stage is based on the most advanced lesion present.
    - Stage I: Lymphocytic infiltration of the epithelial cells of the small bile ducts with granuloma-like lesions, limited to portal triads (bridging fibrosis)
    - Stage II: Extension of inflammatory cells to periportal parenchyma, invasion by foamy macrophages, and development of biliary piecemeal necrosis
    - Stage III: Fibrous septa link portal triads
    - Stage IV: Frank cirrhosis; hyaline deposits and accumulation of stainable copper are also seen

IMAGING STUDIES

If history, physical examination, blood tests, and liver biopsy are all consistent with PBC, neither imaging nor cholangiography is necessary (Fig. E1-763).

PROGNOSIS

- Median survival was 10 yr but may be getting longer with earlier diagnosis and initiation of treatment.
- Mean time of progression from stage I or II disease to cirrhosis with no medical treatment is 4 to 6 yr.
- Neither presence nor total titer level of AMAs predicts survival, disease progression, or response to therapy.
- Prognostic laboratory measures: Serum bilirubin is most important.
- Response to ursodiol therapy can be prognostic: Patients with a decrease in alkaline phosphatase level of at least 40% or to the reference range after 1 yr of treatment with ursodeoxycholic acid (UDCA) may have a prognosis similar to an age-matched healthy population. Similarly, the Mayo Risk score, a predictor of short-term survival probability (http://www.mayoclinic.org/gi-rst/mayomodel1.html), can also reliably predict life expectancy when calculated after 6 mo of ursodiol therapy.
- Poorer prognosis exists with jaundice, advanced histologic stage, advanced age, edema, coagulopathy, and ascites.

Rx TREATMENT

- Treatment is according to the clinical stage of the disease.
- Asymptomatic stage: Follow bilirubin every 3 mo. Once liver function test results become abnormal, begin UDCA at 13 to 15 mg/kg/day in a twice-daily divided dose regardless of histologic stage. Side effects may include weight gain of approximately 5 lbs during the first 1 to 2 yr and, less commonly, thinning of hair and loose stools. Watch for interactions with cholestyramine and other bile-acid sequestrants, as well as antacids, which may interfere with UDCA absorption. Efficacy is best if started during stage I or II disease but should be started at any stage of disease. Lifelong therapy is currently recommended, but benefits are still observed if therapy is interrupted and restarted.
- Treatment also includes treatment of associated conditions such as pruritus, osteoporosis, increased low-density lipoprotein level, and any eventual complications of cirrhosis.
- 20% of patients will not respond to medical therapy and will proceed to liver transplantation, which is the only definitive treatment for this disease.

ACUTE GENERAL Rx

- Symptomatic stage: Goals of treatment are resolution of pruritus, decrease of alkaline phosphatase levels, and delay of progression to liver failure.
- Ursodiol can significantly improve bilirubin and alkaline phosphatase levels, prolong survival without liver transplantation, and delay progression of liver fibrosis and development of portal hypertension.
- The addition of colchicine, methotrexate, or benzafibrate has not been found to be of benefit to mortality or time to liver transplantation in controlled trials.
- Prednisone, azathioprine, penicillamine, and cyclosporine are no longer used because of limited efficacy and significant toxicity.
- For the pruritus of PBC, cholestyramine resin (4 g/dose; maximum, 16 g/day) reduces pruritus in most patients but must be given at least 2 to 4 hr apart from ursodiol to avoid reducing the efficacy of that drug. Antihistamines at bedtime help nighttime symptoms. Rifampin (150 to 300 mg bid) or oral opiate antagonists such as naltrexone (50 mg daily) can be used for pruritus refractory to bile acid sequestrants. Intractable pruritus can be an indication for liver transplantation.

CHRONIC Rx

- Liver function tests should be checked every 3 to 6 mo.
- Management of sicca syndrome: Artificial tears can be used initially for dry eyes. Saliva substitutes can be used for xerostomia and dysphagia; pilocarpine or cevimeline for refractory cases. Moisturizers can be given for vaginal dryness.
- Treatment/Prevention of osteopenia/osteoporosis: Patients with PBC should be provided 1000 to 1500 mg calcium and 1000 IU of vitamin D daily in the diet and as supplements if needed. Bone densitometry should be done every 2 to 4 yr. Alendronate (70 mg weekly) should be considered if patients are osteopenic in the absence of acid reflux or known varices.
- Hyperlipidemia is common in patients with cholestatic liver disease. Statins are safe in patients who may need treatment even if liver chemistry is abnormal.
- Vitamin A, K, and E deficiencies can be clinically important in advanced cases and respond to oral replacement.
- Upper endoscopy to assess for varices should be done every 2 to 3 yr in patients with cirrhosis or Mayo risk score >4.1. Nonselective beta-blockers or endoscopic banding can be considered for prevention of variceal hemorrhage.
- Regular screening for hepatocellular carcinoma with ultrasound and α-fetoprotein every 6 to 12 mo is recommended for patients with cirrhosis.
- Liver transplantation is the only effective treatment for patients with liver failure. Indications for transplantation include hepatic decompensation (ascites, encephalopathy, jaundice), hepatocellular carcinoma fulfilling Milan criteria (see "Hepatocellular Carcinoma"), and intractable pruritus.
- The outcome of liver transplantation for patients with PBC is more favorable than that of nearly all other liver disease categories. The survival rates are 85% to 90% and 80% to 85% at 1 and 5 yr, respectively. Although recurrent disease may develop in 20% to 25% of patients after liver transplantation over 10 yr, patient and graft survival is usually not affected.

DISPOSITION

Definitive treatment requires liver transplantation; survival is 7 to 16 yr depending on symptoms at time of diagnosis.

REFERRAL

Gastroenterology and/or hepatology for treatment, evaluation for liver transplantation, and management of portal hypertension

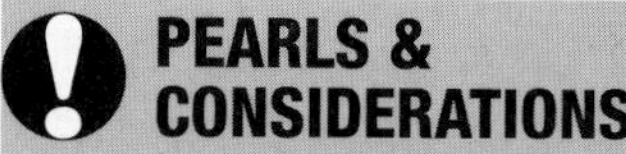

PEARLS & CONSIDERATIONS

- AMA is the serologic hallmark of PBC.
- The prototypical patient with PBC is a middle-aged, Caucasian woman reporting fatigue and pruritus.
- Ursodiol should be started as soon as liver biochemical markers begin to increase and is most effective when started early in the course of the disease.
- Associated illnesses must be detected and treated.
- Liver transplantation is the only effective treatment for PBC with end-stage liver failure.

SUGGESTED READINGS

available at www.expertconsult.com

RELATED CONTENT

Primary Biliary Cirrhosis (PBC) (Patient Information)

AUTHORS: **MICHAEL ENGELS, M.D.**, and **JEANETTE G. SMITH, M.D.**, and **KITTICHAI PROMRAT, M.D.**

BASIC INFORMATION

DEFINITION

- Woman younger than 40 yr of age with amenorrhea, oligomenorrhea, or dysfunctional uterine bleeding for 4 mo or more along with follicle stimulating hormone (FSH) levels in the menopausal range meet diagnostic criteria for primary ovarian insufficiency.
- Menopause younger than the age of 40 yr.

SYNONYMS

Hypergonadotropic hypogonadism
Premature ovarian failure
Premature menopause
Gonadal dysgenesis

ICD-9CM CODES
256.31 Premature menopause
ICD-10CM CODES
E28.3 Primary ovarian failure
E28.9 Ovarian dysfunction, unspecified
E28.310 Symptomatic premature menopause

EPIDEMIOLOGY & DEMOGRAPHICS

INCIDENCE: Affects 1% to 4% of the female population in the U.S.
PREDOMINANT AGE: 1:250 incident cases by age 35 and 1:100 by age 40

PHYSICAL FINDINGS & CLINICAL PRESENTATION

- The most common presentation is disturbance in menstrual pattern due to intermittent ovarian function.
- Between 5% and 30% of affected women have another affected female relative.
- Between 10% and 30% of affected women already have a concurrent autoimmune condition, the most common of which is hypothyroidism.
- Symptoms of estrogen deficiency include hot flashes, night sweat, poor concentration, drying of the vagina, and infertility.
- Physical exam may reveal stigmata of an autoimmune condition such as vitiligo, thyroid enlargement, or Turner's syndrome (webbed neck, short stature, and high-arched palate).

ETIOLOGY (see Table 1-413)

Idiopathic in 95% of cases

DIAGNOSIS

DIFFERENTIAL DIAGNOSIS

- Pregnancy
- Causes of secondary amenorrhea include eating disorder, exercise, drugs, sarcoidosis, polycystic ovarian disease, hypothalamic amenorrhea, hyperprolactinemia/prolactinoma, and Cushing's disease.

WORKUP

- After pregnancy is ruled out, the initial evaluation should include the measurement of serum prolactin, FSH, and thyrotropin (TSH) levels.
- If the FSH level is in the menopausal range (>40 uIU/ml by radioimmunoassay), the test should be repeated in 1 month along with a serum estradiol measurement to confirm the diagnosis of primary ovarian insufficiency.

LABORATORY TESTS

Once a diagnosis of premature ovarian failure is made, other evaluations include:

- Autoimmune disorders, adrenal insufficiency (seen in 3% of cases): serum anti-adrenal and anti-21 hydroxylase antibodies should be measured.
- Hypothyroidism: serum TSH, T_4, and anti-TPO antibodies
- All cases should be screened for osteoporosis by DXA for bone mineral density.
- A karyotype analysis should be performed for all patients to look for chromosomal defects including Turner's variant or deletions of the X chromosome.
- Permutations for the fragile X syndrome (FMR1 gene) should be checked for as well.

IMAGING STUDIES

Pelvic ultrasound has no proven benefit in the management of these patients.

TREATMENT

NONPHARMACOLOGIC THERAPY

Counseling or patient support group should be offered to all women with low self-esteem and depression due to the psychological scar left by the diagnosis.

ACUTE GENERAL Rx

- Physiologic estrogen and progestin replacement is reasonable in the cases of young women until they reach the age of natural menopause.
- A dose of 100 mcg of estradiol per day, administered by transdermal patch, achieves average estradiol level observed in normal menstruating women and effectively treats symptoms.
- Cyclic medroxyprogesterone at a dose of 10 mg per day for 12 days each month is the preferred progestin to provide protection against endometrial cancer.
- Pregnancy may occur while a woman is taking estrogen and progesterone therapy and the therapy should be stopped immediately if the pregnancy test is found to be positive.

TABLE 1-413 Mechanisms and Causes of Primary Ovarian Insufficiency

Accelerated Follicular Depletion
Genetic: Turner's syndrome, fragile X premutations, galactosemia
Toxic: Chemotherapy, radiation, infections such as mumps or cytomegalovirus
Automimmune: Polyglandular failure, hypothyroidism, Addison's disease, vitiligo, myasthenia gravis
Abnormal Follicular Stimulation
Gonadotropin receptor function: follicle stimulating hormone/luteinizing hormone receptor mutation
Enzyme defects: Aromatase deficiency
Luteinized follicles

CHRONIC Rx

- Intake of 1200 mg of elemental calcium and 800 units of vitamin D_3 per day should be encouraged to prevent bone loss. A serum 25-hydroxyvitamin D level of 30 ng per ml or higher should be maintained.
- Patients with positive tests for adrenal antibodies should be evaluated annually for adrenal insufficiency by corticotropin stimulation test.
- Patients who wish to avoid pregnancy should use a barrier method or an IUD.
- Options for parenthood include adoption, foster parenthood, egg donation, and embryo donation.

DISPOSITION

Women with the known diagnosis should be encouraged to maintain a lifestyle that optimizes bone and cardiovascular health, including regular weight-bearing exercises, adequate intake of calcium (1200 mg daily) and vitamin D (800 IU daily), healthy diet to prevent obesity, and screening for cardiovascular risk factors.

REFERRAL

Referral to gynecologist and reproductive endocrinologist may be helpful in patients who decide to pursue parenthood.

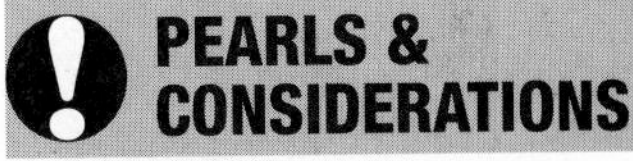

PEARLS & CONSIDERATIONS

COMMENTS

- Common etiologies should be ruled out, including chromosomal abnormalities, fragile X premutations, and autoimmune causes.
- Management directed at symptom resolution and bone protection primarily, but should include psychosocial support for women facing this devastating diagnosis.

PREVENTION

Early diagnosis of primary ovarian insufficiency important for osteoporosis prevention and possibly prevention of coronary artery disease.

PATIENT & FAMILY EDUCATION

www.pofsupport.org
poi.nichd.nih.gov

SUGGESTED READINGS
available at www.expertconsult.com

AUTHOR: **PRIYA BANSAL, M.D., M.P.H.**

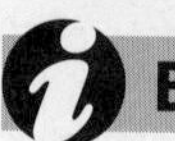

BASIC INFORMATION

DEFINITION

Primary sclerosing cholangitis (PSC) is a chronic progressive cholestatic liver disease characterized by segmental fibrosing and inflammation of intrahepatic and extrahepatic bile ducts complicated by recurrent cholangitis, cholangiocarcinoma, cirrhosis, and portal hypertension.

SYNONYMS

Chronic obliterative cholangitis
Fibrosing cholangitis
Stenosing cholangitis
PSC

ICD-9CM CODES
567.1 Cholangitis
ICD-10CM CODES
K83.0 Cholangitis
K83.0 Disease of biliary tract, unspecified

EPIDEMIOLOGY & DEMOGRAPHICS

- The incidence and prevalence of PSC are 0.9 to 1.3 cases and 8.5 to 16.2 cases per 100,000 population, respectively.
- About 65% of patients with PSC are men
- Mean age of presentation is 30 to 40 yr.
- 60% to 80% of patients with PSC also have inflammatory bowel disease (IBD). 4% of patients with ulcerative colitis (UC) will develop PSC. PSC is an independent risk factor for developing colon cancer in patients with IBD.
- PSC can coexist with other autoimmune liver disease. Autoimmune hepatitis (AIH) and PSC overlap syndrome can be seen in young adults and children.
- Cholangiocarcinoma is present in 1% to 2% of PSC patients at diagnosis. The lifetime risk is 5% to 10%.
- The median survival from time of diagnosis is 10 to 15 yr without liver transplantation.

PHYSICAL FINDINGS & CLINICAL PRESENTATION

- Most patients are asymptomatic (15% to 40%) at the time of diagnosis with normal physical findings.
- More than 75% of asymptomatic patients develop symptoms, the most common of which are pruritus (70%) and fatigue (70%). Physicial findings of symptomatic patients may reveal jaundice, skin excoriation and hyperpigmentation from scratching, hepatosplenomegaly, and xanthelasma. Other symptoms include abdominal discomfort, steatorrhea, jaundice, and weight loss, which are concerning for advanced PSC, sepsis or mechanical obstruction (i.e., cholangitis), and malignancy (i.e., cholangiocarcinoma).
- Patients can also present with advanced liver disease and decompensated cirrhosis (i.e., ascites, spontaneous bacterial peritonitis, hepatic encephalopathy, and variceal hemorrhage) or hepatic failure. Physical findings in these patients may reveal a shrunken nodular liver and evidence of portal hypertension.
- Physical findings of symptomatic patients may reveal jaundice, skin excoriation and hyperpigmentation from scratching due to pruritus, hepatosplenomegaly, and xanthelasma. In patients with cirrhosis, physical findings may reveal a shrunken nodular liver and evidence of portal hypertension.

ETIOLOGY

- The cause of PSC is unknown, but mechanisms include genetic factors, bile acid toxicity, environmental gut microbiota translocation, and gut liver lymphocyte homing mechanisms.
- Genetic and immunologic factors are supported by reports of familial occurrence of this disorder and increased frequency of HLA B8 and DR3. Genome-wide association studies have discovered novel loci associated with PSC, but the functional aspects of these genes are still unknown.
- Portosystemic inflammation caused by translocation of the gut microbiota is an increasing area of research. The close association with UC and PSC may be secondary to gut-activated T lymphocytes in IBD causing portal inflammation because of overlapping adhesion molecules in the gut and liver.

Dx DIAGNOSIS

Diagnosis is based on characteristic cholangiographic findings in combination with clinical, biochemical, and in some cases histologic features. Table 1-414 describes staging of PSC.

DIFFERENTIAL DIAGNOSIS

- Choledocholithiasis
- Surgical biliary trauma
- Recurrent pyogenic cholangitis
- Ischemic cholangitis
- Cholangiocarcinoma
- IgG4-associated cholangitis (IAC)
- Intraarterial chemotherapy
- Diffuse intrahepatic metastasis
- Histiocytosis X

TABLE 1-414 Staging of Primary Sclerosing Cholangitis

Stage	Description
I—Portal	Portal edema, inflammation, ductal proliferation; abnormalities do not extend beyond the limiting plate
II—Periportal	Periportal fibrosis with or without inflammation extending beyond the limiting plate
III—Septal	Septal fibrosis, bridging necrosis, or both
IV—Cirrhotic	Biliary cirrhosis

From Cameron JL, Cameron AM: *Current surgical therapy,* ed 10, Philadelphia, 2011, Saunders.

WORKUP

History, physical examination, laboratory evaluation, imaging studies, and possible liver biopsy

LABORATORY TESTS

- Serum biochemical tests usually indicate cholestasis with predominant elevation in the serum alkaline phosphatase (three to ten times the upper limit of normal); however, this value can vary and be normal during the disease course. Serum aminotransferase levels are elevated in the majority of patients (two to three times the upper limits of normal). Serum bilirubin is usually normal at the time of diagnosis unless patient has advanced stricturing disease.
- A wide range of autoantibodies can be detected in patients with PSC; however, they are nonspecific for PSC, including the perinuclear antineutrophil cytoplasmic antibody (pANCA). However, autoantibodies such as antinuclear antibody (ANA), anti-smooth muscle antibody (ASMA), and serum IgG levels are useful in the diagnosis of PSC-AIH overlap syndrome and IAC with autoimmune pancreatitis.

IMAGING STUDIES

- Cholangiography is considered to be the gold standard for the diagnosis of PSC. Characteristic findings reveal segmental fibrosis of bile ducts with saccular dilatation of normal intervening areas resulting in a "beads-on-a-string" appearance (Fig. 1-764).
- Magnetic resonance cholangiopancreatography (MRCP) has an overall diagnostic accuracy rate of 90%. It is the imaging modality of choice when PSC is suspected because endoscopic retrograde cholangiopancreatography (ERCP) can be associated with serious complications (i.e., pancreatitis and cholangitis).

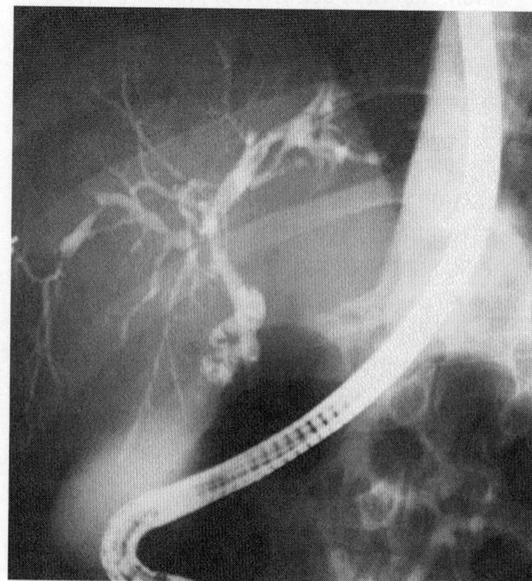

FIGURE 1-764 A 29-year-old male patient who was diagnosed with PSC 5 years previously. Both the intra- and extrahepatic bile ducts are involved at cholangiography. (From Parlak E et al: An endoscopic finding in patients with primary sclerosing cholangitis: retraction of the main duodenal papilla into the duodenum wall, *Gastrointest Endosc* 65[3]:535, 2007.)

- Liver biopsy is not necessary for the diagnosis of PSC in patients with typical cholangiographic findings. Biopsies are subject to sample variation, and the typical onion skin–type periductal fibrosis finding is rare. Liver biopsy may help in the diagnosis of PSC-AIH overlap syndrome, small-duct PSC (normal cholangiogram), or IAC.

Rx TREATMENT

- No medical therapy has been proved to be effective in halting the disease progression of PSC.
- Management of PSC patients is aimed at symptom relief and management of complications from PSC (i.e., obstruction/strictures, early detection of carcinomas, and timely referral for liver transplantation).
- Ursodeoxycholic acid (UDCA) has not shown benefit in randomized controlled trials. It is unclear if UDCA slows the progression of PSC-related liver disease, and in high doses it has been shown to be harmful. Therefore UDCA is not recommended as medical therapy in patients with PSC.
- The use of corticosteroids and other immunosuppressive agents is not recommended in patients with PSC alone; however, it is recommended in patients with PSC-AIH overlap syndrome.
- Use of tumor necrosis factor inhibitors has been ineffective in PSC. Other monoclonal antibody therapies targeting lymphocyte trafficking, tyrosine kinase signaling, and liver fibrosis are being studied.

ACUTE GENERAL Rx

- Bile acid sequestrants (i.e., cholestyramine 16 g/day) are the preferred choice for the initial management of pruritus. Alternative agents for pruritus refractory to bile acid sequestrants include rifampicin 150 to 300 mg twice daily, naltrexone 50 mg daily, and sertraline 75 to 100 mg daily.
- Patients who present with increasing serum bilirubin and/or worsening pruritus, progressive bile duct dilatation on imaging studies, or cholangitis need to be evaluated for dominant strictures. with imaging. A dominant stricture is a stenosis $\leq$1.5 mm in the common bile duct or $\geq$1 mm in the hepatic duct
- ERCP with brushings, cytology, and fluorescent in situ hybridization (FISH) is recommended to evaluate dominant strictures for cholangiocarcinoma. Once malignancy is excluded, balloon dilatation with or without stenting is recommended to treat symptoms. If ERCP is unsuccessful, percutaneous cholangiopancreatography with stenting should be considered.
- In noncirrhotic patients with dominant strictures refractory to endoscopic or percutaneous management, surgery should be considered, although this may complicate future liver transplantation surgery.
- Antibiotic usage is recommended in patients with dominant strictures/obstructions both acutely and for long-term prophylaxis in patients with recurrent cholangitis.

CHRONIC Rx

- Avoidance of alcohol and vaccination against hepatitis A and B are advised.
- Patients with PSC are at risk for osteoporosis and osteopenia. At time of diagnosis a DEXA scan is recommended and should be repeated in 2 to 3 yr. Calcium (1000 to 1500 mg) and vitamin D 600-800 IU daily are recommended for patients with osteopenia and the addition of bisphosphonate is recommended in patients with osteoporosis.
- Patients with newly diagnosed PSC should have a full colonoscopy with biopsies to exclude concurrent IBD and for surveillance of colorectal cancer. In patients with IBD, continued surveillance colonoscopy with biopsies at 1- to 2-yr intervals is recommended. In patients without IBD, a suggested 5-yr surveillance interval has been recommended due to an increased risk of colorectal cancer.
- Annual transabdominal ultrasound is recommended due to the increased risk of gallbladder malignancy. If masses are detected, cholecystectomy should be performed.
- Patients with cirrhosis are recommended to have gastroesophageal variceal and hepatocellular carcinoma (HCC) surveillance at regular intervals.
- Annual surveillance for cholangiocarcinoma with MRCP or ultrasound and CA 19-9 testing can be considered.
- All patients with deterioration in clinical performance status or liver biochemical parameters should be evaluated for development of cholangiocarcinoma and in patients with cirrhosis the development of hepatocellular carcinoma.

DISPOSITION

Liver transplantation is the only effective treatment for patients with end-stage liver disease, portal hypertension, liver failure, and recurrent or intractable bacterial cholangitis. Survival is excellent, with 90% and 80% survival rates at 1 and 5 yr, respectively. The recurrence of PSC after transplant is reportedly 5% to 20%.

REFERRAL

Gastroenterology and/or hepatology for treatment of PSC, management of its complications, surveillance of associated malignancy, and evaluation for liver transplantation.

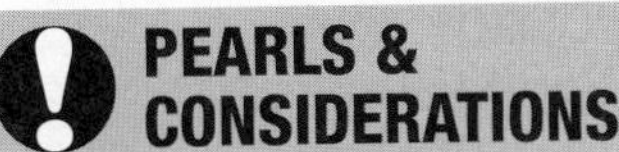

PEARLS & CONSIDERATIONS

- Management of PSC targets symptom relief, complications of PSC, cirrhosis, early carcinoma detection, and timely referral for liver transplantation.
- Patients are at increased risk for the development of colorectal cancer, gallbladder cancer, and cholangiocarcinoma and need surveillance.
- In patients with cirrhosis, surveillance for gastroesophageal varices and HCC is recommended.
- Liver transplant remains the only definitive therapy for complications of PSC.

SUGGESTED READINGS

available at www.expertconsult.com

RELATED CONTENT

Ulcerative Colitis (Related Key Topic)

AUTHORS: **CHARLES WANG, M.D.,** and **AMANDA PRESSMAN, M.D.**

BASIC INFORMATION

DEFINITION

Progressive multifocal leukoencephalopathy (PML) is an uncommon and often fatal subacute demyelinating disease of the white matter, caused by reactivation of the JC virus (JCV) infection in an immunocompromised individual. JCV was isolated in 1971 and is named for the initials of the first patient from whose brain it was isolated.

ICD-9CM CODES
046.3 Progressive multifocal leukoencephalopathy
ICD-10CM CODES
A81.2 Progressive multifocal leukoencephalopathy

EPIDEMIOLOGY & DEMOGRAPHICS

RISK FACTORS: Typically seen in patients with profound immunosuppression and impaired cell-mediated immunity. These include patients with AIDS, lymphoproliferative disorders, chronic infections such as tuberculosis, and, more recently, patients on immunosuppressive or immunomodulating medications such as natalizumab, rituximab, efalizumab, brentuximab-vedotin, and mycophenolate mofetil.

INCIDENCE & PREVALANCE:

- Two population groups—HIV and natalizumab-treated patients—have seen a significant increase in PML.
- HIV: a 50-fold increase in PML cases was reported with HIV epidemic. 3%-5% patients with HIV will develop PML. PML is an AIDS-defining illness. Highly active retroviral therapy (HAART) has led to some decline in PML cases.
- Incidence of PML in natalizumab-treated patients 3 to 4/1000 patients and depends on treatment duration.
- Seroepidemiologic studies have shown that asymptomatic primary infection with JCV occurs at an early age, and by adult life 30% to 90% of the population is seropositive.

PREDOMINANT SEX & AGE: Males and females are equally affected. There is no specific age distribution.

GENETICS: Unknown

PHYSICAL FINDINGS & CLINICAL PRESENTATION

- Subacute neurologic deficits are common; can also present acutely as a stroke mimic.
- The clinical course spans weeks to months leading to severe disability and death.
- PML lesions usually involve cerebral hemispheres; cerebellum and brainstem involvement may be seen in AIDS. Multifocal asymmetric white matter involvement is common; rarely there can be gray matter involvement including cerebellar granular cells.
- Non–AIDS-associated PML: early lesions involve occipital subcortical white matter and cause visual-field deficits (homonymous hemianopia) or cortical blindness. Motor weakness and altered mentation may be seen, while headache, seizures, and extrapyramidal syndromes are rare.
- AIDS-related PML: motor weakness is more common. Abnormalities of speech, cognition, gait, sensation, and visual impairment may also be seen.
- Natalizumab-associated PML: frontal lobe is commonly involved, leading to cognitive impairment, neurobehavioral changes, motor disorders, language disorders, and visual defects.
- Immune reconstitution inflammatory syndrome (IRIS): a paradoxical clinical deterioration that occurs during immunologic recovery in previously immunocompromised patients, such as antiretroviral therapy–treated HIV-seropositive patients, or cessation of immunomodulating treatment, such as natalizumab. An increase in the number or size of lesions on neuroimaging with contrast enhancement of brain lesions and brain edema may be seen.

ETIOLOGY & PATHOGENESIS

- JCV infection may be acquired through respiratory tissue or oropharyngeal route; seroconversion usually occurs in childhood.
- A cytotoxic-specific response against JCV acts as a containing mechanism for PML. Immunosuppression leads to development of PML either as primary infection of the CNS following immunosuppression or reactivation of a dormant infection. The virus produces lytic infection of the oligodendrocytes and causes demyelination. Neuronal infection does not usually occur except in granule cell neurons of the cerebellum.

DIAGNOSIS

DIFFERENTIAL DIAGNOSIS

- Multiple sclerosis
- Acute disseminated encephalomyelitis
- Vasculitis
- HIV encephalitis
- Mitochondrial encephalopathies (e.g., MELAS)
- Posterior reversible encephalopathy syndrome

WORKUP

- Diagnosis is based on compatible clinical presentation, MRI brain features, and detection of JCV in CSF.
- Brain biopsy is the gold standard and demonstrates a triad of histopathologic findings—demyelination, bizarre astrocytes, and enlarged oligodendrocytic nuclei.

LABORATORY TESTS

- CSF examination: usually normal; may show mild lymphocytic pleocytosis (20-25 leukocytes/ml) and elevated protein (usually <65 mg/dl).
- CSF PCR for JCV has a sensitivity of 95% and specificity of 99% using ultrasensitive PCR techniques, but may be lower depending on the techniques used.

IMAGING STUDIES

- MRI brain is the neuroimaging of choice and shows demyelinating lesions that are hyperintense on T2 and FLAIR sequences, hypointense on T1, and may enhance with gadolinium.
- CT head may show subcortical hypodensities with faint contrast enhancement.
- MR spectroscopy will demonstrate features of demyelination—decreased N-acetyl acetate, increased choline, and increased lactate.

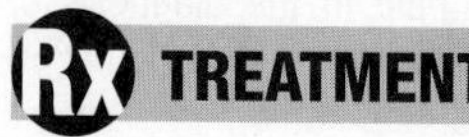

TREATMENT

There is no specific treatment for PML. Treatment is aimed at reversal of the underlying causes of immunosuppression.

NONPHARMACOLOGIC THERAPY

Plasma exchange and immunoadsorption for natalizumab-treated patients to rapidly reduce blood levels of natalizumab and hasten restoration of immune function

ACUTE GENERAL Rx

- HIV-positive patients: antiretroviral therapy should be optimized.
- HIV-negative patients: immunosuppressive medication should be discontinued; plasma exchange may be considered for natalizumab-treated patients.
- IRIS: treatment with steroids should be considered.

CHRONIC Rx

No specific pharmacologic therapy exists for chronic treatment.

DISPOSITION

Of all HIV-related cerebral disorders, PML probably has the worst prognosis. Pre-AIDS era survival was 6 months. With HAART, incidence and prognosis of PML has improved. A lower CSF JCV load and better CD4 counts have better prognoses. Natalizumab-treated patients have worse prognoses seen with longer time to diagnosis, presence of widespread disease, and brainstem involvement.

REFERRAL

Refer to neurology if patients have neurologic deficits of uncertain etiology, especially in the setting of AIDS or immunosuppression.

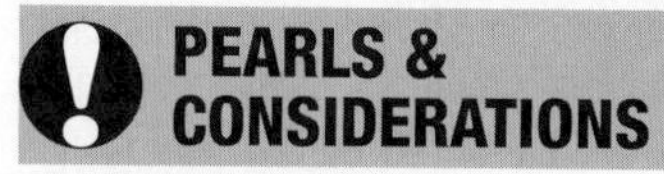

PEARLS & CONSIDERATIONS

COMMENTS

PML is a fatal opportunistic cerebral infection that should be considered in all immunosuppressed individuals presenting with neurologic deficits and demyelinating cerebral lesions. Early referral to a center with neurologic expertise, especially neuroimmunology or neuroinfectious diseases, should be considered.

SUGGESTED READINGS
available at www.expertconsult.com

AUTHORS: **PADMAJA SUDHAKAR, M.B.B.S.,** and **SACHIN KEDAR, M.B.B.S., M.D.**

BASIC INFORMATION

DEFINITION

Progressive supranuclear palsy (PSP) is an atypical parkinsonian syndrome characterized by supranuclear gaze impairment, prominent and early postural instability with falls, axial greater than appendicular rigidity, and poor or absent response to levodopa.

SYNONYMS

Steele-Richardson-Olszewski syndrome
Progressive supranuclear ophthalmoplegia

ICD-9CM CODES
333.0 Other degenerative diseases of the basal ganglia
ICD-10CM CODES
G23.1 Progressive supranuclear ophthalmoplegia
G23.9 Degenerative disease of basal ganglia, unspecified

EPIDEMIOLOGY & DEMOGRAPHICS

INCIDENCE: 1.1 per 100,000 (5.3 per 100,000 over age 50)
PREVALENCE: 4.9 per 100,000 (6.4 per 100,000 age-adjusted)
PREDOMINANT SEX AND AGE: Slight male predominance; mean age onset 63 yr, very uncommon for onset <50 yr
GENETICS: Familial cases have been reported only rarely. The vast majority of cases are sporadic.

PHYSICAL FINDINGS & CLINICAL PRESENTATION

Tremorless parkinsonism is the general clinical presentation, and differentiation from idiopathic Parkinson's disease can be challenging early in the disease course. However, there are certain symptoms that can serve as "red flags" to consider PSP:

- Early postural instability and retropulsion leads to frequent falls; falls within the first year of onset of symptoms is typically the rule.
- Supranuclear gaze palsy is often preceded by slowing of vertical saccades; square wave jerks can be present; blepharospasm is common.
- Dystonia of the frontalis and procerus muscles gives the PSP patient a "surprised" or "frightened" expression as opposed to the hypomimia of Parkinson's disease (Fig. 1-765).
- Speech is typically strained, spastic, hypernasal, with a low-pitched dysarthria.
- Pseudobulbar affect and "emotional incontinence" can be seen, with easy crying or laughter.
- Early cognitive impairment, most commonly with apathy, disinhibition, and anxiety.

ETIOLOGY

PSP is caused by neuronal degeneration of nuclei in the midbrain and basal ganglia, as a result of abnormal tau protein accumulation, most commonly in astrocyte inclusions and neurofibrillary tangles.

DIAGNOSIS

DIFFERENTIAL DIAGNOSIS

- Parkinson's disease: responds more robustly to levodopa, progression much slower, and lacks "red flag" symptoms above
- Corticobasal degeneration: also a tauopathy like PSP, but characterized by parkinsonism with prominent asymmetric dystonia, cortical sensory signs such as astereognosis, typically progressing to apraxia and sometimes an "alien hand" syndrome
- Multiple system atrophy: distinguished by autonomic involvement such as orthostatic hypotension, cerebellar ataxia, and inspiratory stridor
- Dementia with Lewy bodies: dementia coincident with parkinsonism, fluctuating mental status, visual hallucinations often preceding onset of dopaminergic treatment

WORKUP

- PSP is a clinical diagnosis, best made by a neurologist familiar with the disorder such as a movement disorders specialist.
- A robust response to a trial of levodopa may help to lead consideration away from PSP.
- MRI scan (see below) can be helpful.

LABORATORY TESTS

There are no diagnostic laboratory tests.

IMAGING STUDIES

- Dorsal midbrain atrophy is commonly seen on MRI.
- MRI regional apparent diffusion coefficients (rADC) in specific nuclei on diffusion-weighted imaging can reliably differentiate PSP from Parkinson's disease, although not from multiple system atrophy.

TREATMENT

NONPHARMACOLOGIC THERAPY

- Physical therapy, in particular focusing on fall prevention, is essential for avoiding the morbidity associated with frequent falls. Assistive devices such as a walker or wheelchair should be encouraged.
- Dysphagia is a common finding and should be monitored for closely in conjunction with a speech therapist.
- Prisms may be helpful in some patients for the eye movement abnormalities that can result in misalignment and diplopia; however, benefits, if noted, tend to be short-lived as the disease progresses.

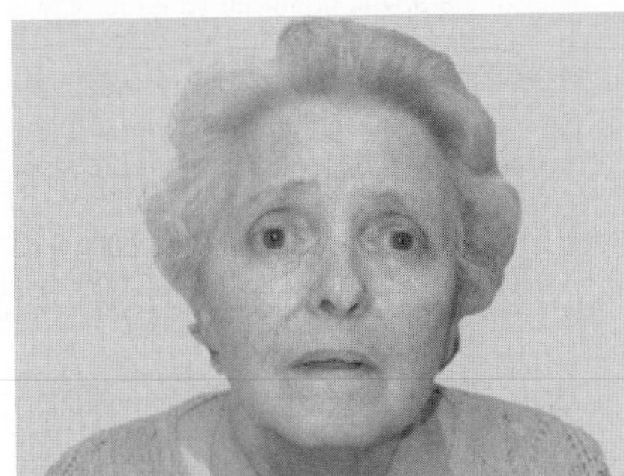

FIGURE 1-765 A patient with progressive supranuclear palsy with staring expression, frontalis overactivity, and retrocolitis. She is wearing a neck sling for a fractured wrist sustained in a fall. (From Burn D, Lees A: Progressive supranuclear palsy: where are we now? *Lancet Neurol* 1:359, 2002.)

CHRONIC Rx

- Although classically felt to be unresponsive to levodopa, there is often a transient response to this medication and it can be useful. The poor response to levodopa is most likely due to the loss of postsynaptic dopamine receptors.
- Anticholinergic medications should be avoided.
- Blepharospasm can be effectively treated with botulinum toxin injections.

DISPOSITION

Median latency from symptom onset to wheelchair-bound state is 5 yr and to death is 7 yr.

REFERRAL

Referral to a general neurologist or movement disorders center is appropriate.

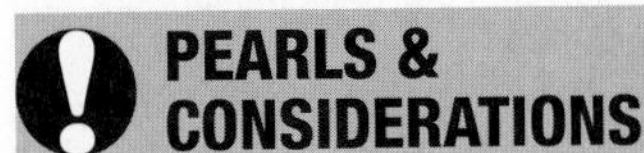

PEARLS & CONSIDERATIONS

COMMENTS

Consider PSP in a parkinsonian patient with the onset of falls within 1 yr of diagnosis, vertical eye movement abnormalities, early cognitive impairment, pseudobulbar affect, frontonasal dystonia, or poor response to levodopa.

PATIENT & FAMILY EDUCATION

Patient and caregiver information and resources can be found at www.wemove.org (a comprehensive movement disorders website) as well as the Society for Progressive Supranuclear Palsy at www.curepsp.org.

SUGGESTED READINGS

available at www.expertconsult.com

AUTHOR: **ANDREW DUKER, M.D.**

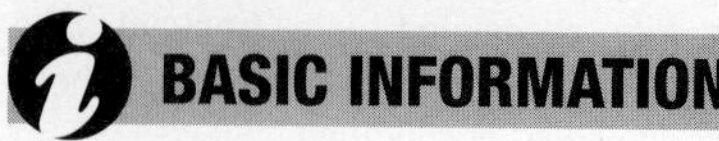

BASIC INFORMATION

DEFINITION

Prolactinomas are monoclonal tumors that secrete prolactin.

ICD-9CM CODES
253.1 Forbes-Albright syndrome
ICD-10CM CODES
D35.2 Benign neoplasm of pituitary gland
E22.8 Other hyperfunction of pituitary gland

EPIDEMIOLOGY & DEMOGRAPHICS

INCIDENCE: Most common pituitary tumor; nearly 30% of all pituitary adenomas secrete enough prolactin to cause hyperprolactinemia.
PREDOMINANT SEX: Microadenomas are more common in women; macroadenomas are found more frequently in men.

PHYSICAL FINDINGS & CLINICAL PRESENTATION

- Men: decreased facial and body hair, infertility, small testicles; may also have decreased libido, erectile dysfunction, and delayed puberty (caused by decreased testosterone as a result of inhibition of gonadotropin secretion).
- Women: physical examination may be normal; history may reveal amenorrhea, galactorrhea (Fig. E1-766), oligomenorrhea, and anovulation.
- Both sexes: visual field defects and headache may occur depending on size of tumor and its expansion.

ETIOLOGY

Prolactin-secreting pituitary adenomas: microadenomas (<10 mm diameter) or macroadenomas (>10 mm diameter). No risk factors have been identified for sporadic prolactinomas. Rarely prolactinomas can be part of multiple endocrine neoplasia (MEN) type 1 syndrome.

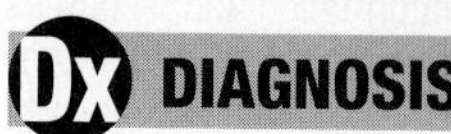

DIAGNOSIS

DIFFERENTIAL DIAGNOSIS

Secretion of prolactin is under tonic inhibitory control by hypothalamic dopamine. Hyperprolactinemia may be caused by the following:

- Drugs: risperidone, phenothiazines, methyldopa, reserpine, monoamine oxidase inhibitors, androgens, progesterone, cimetidine, tricyclic antidepressants, haloperidol, meprobamate, chlordiazepoxide, estrogens, narcotics, metoclopramide, verapamil, amoxapine, cocaine, oral contraceptives
- Hepatic cirrhosis, renal failure, primary hypothyroidism
- Ectopic prolactin-secreting tumors (hypernephroma, bronchogenic carcinoma)
- Infiltrating diseases of the pituitary (sarcoidosis, histiocytosis)
- Head trauma, chest wall injury, spinal cord injury
- Polycystic ovary disease, pregnancy, nipple stimulation
- Idiopathic hyperprolactinemia, stress, exercise

WORKUP

- The diagnosis of prolactinoma is established by demonstration of an elevated serum prolactin level (after exclusion of other causes of hyperprolactinemia) and radiographic evidence of a pituitary adenoma.
  1. Normal mean prolactin levels are 8 ng/ml in women and 5 ng/ml in men.
  2. Levels >300 ng/ml are virtually diagnostic of prolactinomas.
  3. Prolactin levels can vary with time of day, stress, sleep cycle, and meals. More accurate measurements can be obtained 2 to 3 hr after awakening, preprandially, and when patient is not distressed.
  4. Serial measurements are recommended in patients with mild prolactin elevations.
- TSH, free T_4, BUN, Creat, ALT, AST are useful tests. Pregnancy test in all women of childbearing age.
- All patients with prolactinomas should undergo visual field testing. Serial evaluation is recommended, particularly during pregnancy in patients with macroadenomas.

IMAGING STUDIES

- MRI with gadolinium enhancement is the procedure of choice in the radiographic evaluation of pituitary disease.
- In absence of MRI, a radiographic diagnosis is best accomplished with a high-resolution CT scanner and special coronal cuts through the pituitary region.

TREATMENT

NONPHARMACOLOGIC THERAPY

Pregnancy and breastfeeding should be avoided because they can encourage tumor growth.

ACUTE GENERAL Rx

- Management of prolactinomas depends on their size and encroachment on the optic chiasm and other vital structures, the presence or absence of gonadal dysfunction, and the patient's desires regarding fertility. Fig. E1-767 describes a management algorithm for prolactinomas.
- Medical therapy is preferred when fertility is an important consideration.
  1. Bromocriptine: initial dose is 0.625 mg at bedtime for the first week. After 1 wk, add morning dose of 1.25 mg. Gradually increase dose by 1.25 mg/wk until dose of 5 to 10 mg/day is achieved. Bromocriptine decreases size of the tumor and generally lowers the prolactin level into the normal range when the initial serum prolactin is <500 ng/ml. Side effects of bromocriptine are nausea, constipation, dizziness, and nasal stuffiness. Bromocriptine appears to be safe during pregnancy.
  2. Cabergoline is a longer-acting dopamine agonist that is more expensive but may be more effective and better tolerated than bromocriptine; initial dose is 0.25 mg twice weekly.
- Transsphenoidal resection: option in an infertile patient who cannot tolerate bromocriptine or cabergoline or when medical therapy is ineffective. The success rate depends on the location of the tumor (entirely intrasellar), experience of the neurosurgeon, and size of the tumor (<10 mm in diameter); the recurrence rate may reach 80% within 5 yr. Possible complications of transsphenoidal surgery vary with experience and skill of the neurosurgeon and tumor anatomy and include transient diabetes insipidus, hypopituitarism, cerebrospinal fluid rhinorrhea, and infections (meningitis, wound infection).
- Pituitary irradiation is useful as adjunctive therapy of macroadenomas (>10 mm in diameter) and in patients with persistent hypersecretion after surgery. Potential complications include cranial nerve damage, radionecrosis, and cognitive abnormalities.
- Stereotactic radiosurgery (gamma knife) has become popular as a modality in the treatment of prolactinomas. A high dose of ionizing radiation is delivered to the tumor through multiple ports. Its advantage is minimal irradiation to surrounding tissues. Proximity of the tumor to the optic chiasm limits this therapeutic modality.

CHRONIC Rx

- Patients on medical therapy require periodic measurement of prolactin levels. An attempt to reduce the dose of bromocriptine or cabergoline can be made after the prolactin level has been normal for 2 yr. An MRI scan of the pituitary should be obtained to rule out tumor enlargement within 6 mo of initiation of tapering regimen.
- Evaluation and monitoring of pituitary function are recommended after transsphenoidal surgery.

DISPOSITION

- Transsphenoidal surgery will result in a cure in nearly 50% to 75% of patients with microadenomas and 10% to 20% of patients with macroadenomas.
- Nearly 20% of microprolactinomas resolve during long-term dopamine agonist treatment.

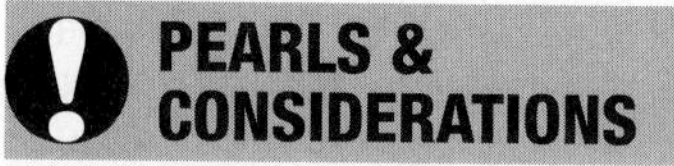

PEARLS & CONSIDERATIONS

COMMENTS

- Patients must be monitored for several years after surgery because up to 50% of microadenomas and nearly 90% of macroadenomas can recur.
- Pituitary microadenomas are found in 10.9% of autopsies, and 44% of these microadenomas are prolactinomas.

SUGGESTED READINGS

available at www.expertconsult.com

RELATED CONTENT

Prolactinoma (Patient Information)

AUTHOR: **FRED F. FERRI, M.D.**

BASIC INFORMATION

DEFINITION

Pronator syndrome is a form of compression neuropathy of the median nerve in the proximal forearm caused primarily by the pronator teres muscle (Fig. 1-768). Occasionally, only the anterior interosseus motor branch is affected, sometimes causing a specific separate clinical presentation.

SYNONYMS

Kiloh-Nevin syndrome (anterior interosseus syndrome)

ICD-9CM CODES

354.1 Median nerve entrapment
354.9 Mononeuritis of upper limb

ICD-10CM CODES

G56.10 Other lesions of median nerve, unspecified upper limb
G56.90 Unspecified mononeuropathy of unspecified upper limb

EPIDEMIOLOGY & DEMOGRAPHICS

PREDOMINANT SEX: Males are affected more often than females.

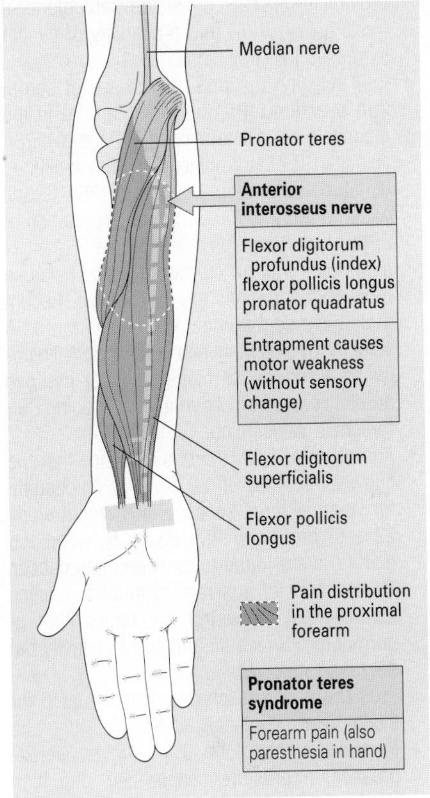

FIGURE 1-768 Forearm entrapment regions. The median nerve may be compressed at several locations in the forearm, most commonly as it traverses the pronator teres muscle. The anterior interosseus branch of the median nerve is solely motor, thus entrapment produces no sensory deficit. (From Hochberg MC et al [eds]: *Rheumatology,* ed 3, St Louis, 2003, Mosby.)

INCIDENCE: Rare (comprises <1% of median nerve entrapment disorders); most common in dominant arm.

PHYSICAL FINDINGS & CLINICAL PRESENTATION

- Forearm discomfort and fatigue, often resulting from repetitive pronation
- Insidious onset
- Nocturnal paresthesias are not typical.
- Vague numbness in hand, primarily in thumb and index finger, may be present.
- Tenderness and enlargement of the pronator teres may be present.
- Tinel's sign may be positive at the site of compression.
- Although there are no reliable provocative tests, painful paresthesias may occasionally be elicited with forced pronation of the forearm against resistance.
- Motor impairment is rare.

Anterior interosseus nerve syndrome:

- Forearm pain and weakness
- Patient may be unable to form a circle when trying to pinch the index finger and thumb because of the inability to flex distal phalanges of thumb and index finger.
- Sensation to the hand is not affected.

ETIOLOGY

- Localized anatomic compression
- Trauma
- Traumatic cutdown or phlebotomy

DIAGNOSIS

DIFFERENTIAL DIAGNOSIS

- Carpal tunnel syndrome
- Cervical disc syndrome with radiculopathy
- Tendon rupture
- Tendinitis

WORKUP

- Electrodiagnostic studies may be helpful; they are indicated if symptoms persist >4 to 6 wk or if motor weakness is suspected
- Plain radiography to rule out bony abnormalities causing compression

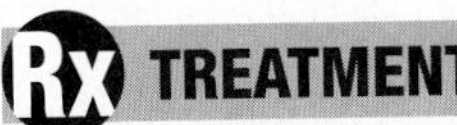

TREATMENT

- Rest, bracing of forearm, sling
- Stretching exercises, physical therapy
- Nonsteroidal anti-inflammatory drugs

DISPOSITION

Patients whose symptoms are mainly subjective often respond to nonsurgical management. Motor deficits may not be reversible despite surgery.

REFERRAL

Surgical referral in cases of failed medical management or when motor weakness is present

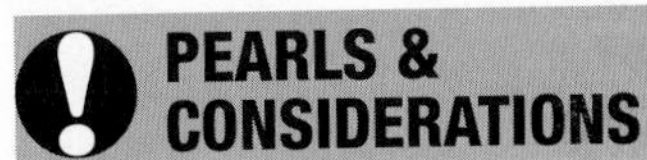

PEARLS & CONSIDERATIONS

COMMENTS

Prognosis for recovery is good. When indicated, surgical intervention is most effective if the diagnosis can be firmly established by objective testing.

SUGGESTED READINGS

available at www.expertconsult.com

AUTHORS: **LONNIE R. MERCIER, M.D.**, and **FRED F. FERRI, M.D.**

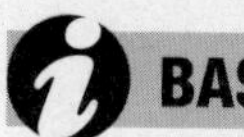

BASIC INFORMATION

DEFINITION & CLASSIFICATION

Prostate cancer is a neoplasm involving the prostate. Various classifications have been developed to evaluate malignancy potential and prognosis.

- The degree of malignancy varies with the stage:
  1. Stage A: Confined to the prostate, no nodule palpable
  2. Stage B: Palpable nodule confined to the gland
  3. Stage C: Local extension
  4. Stage D: Regional lymph nodes or distant metastases
- In the Gleason classification, two histologic patterns are independently assigned numbers 1 to 5 (best to least differentiated). These numbers are added to give a total tumor score between 2 and 10. Prognosis is best for highly differentiated tumors (e.g., Gleason score 2 to 4) compared with most poorly differentiated tumors (Gleason score 7 to 10).
- Another commonly used classification is the Tumor-Node-Metastasis (TNM) classification of prostate cancer.

ICD-9CM CODES
185 Malignant neoplasm of prostate
ICD-10CM CODES
C61 Malignant neoplasm of prostate

EPIDEMIOLOGY & DEMOGRAPHICS

- Prostate cancer has surpassed lung cancer as the most common nonskin cancer in men.
- In the U.S. nearly 200,000 cases are diagnosed yearly, and nearly 30,000 males die from prostate cancer each year (second leading cause of death from cancer in U.S. men).
- Incidence of prostate cancer increases with age: uncommon <50 yr; 80% of new cases are diagnosed in patients aged ≥65 yr. Widespread PSA testing has doubled the incidence of prostate cancer and the lifetime risk for prostate cancer to approximately 16%. Prostate cancer is also diagnosed earlier, and the incidence of clinically "silent" T1 tumors has increased from 17% in 1989 to 48% in 2001 since the advent of PSA screening.
- Average age at time of diagnosis is 72 yr.
- Blacks in the U.S. have the highest incidence of prostate cancer in the world (one in every nine males).
- Incidence is low in Asians.
- Approximately 9% of all prostate cancers may be familial. Obesity is a risk factor for prostate cancer. High-fat, low-fiber diet increases risk. High insulin levels may also increase the risk of prostate cancer. Dietary supplementation with vitamin E has been reported to significantly increase the risk of prostate cancer among healthy men. Linkage studies have implicated chromosome 17p21-22 as a possible location of a prostate-cancer susceptibility gene. Germline mutations in *HOXB13* are associated with a significantly increased risk of hereditary prostate cancer.
- Mortality rates of prostate cancer have declined substantially in the past 15 yr from 34% in 1990 to <20% currently.

PHYSICAL FINDINGS & CLINICAL PRESENTATION

- Generally silent disease until it reaches advanced stages.
- Bone pain and pathologic fractures may be initial symptoms of prostate cancer.
- Local growth can cause symptoms of outflow obstruction.
- Digital rectal examination (DRE) may reveal an area of increased firmness; 10% of patients will have a negative DRE.
- Prostate may be hard, fixed, with extension of tumor to the seminal vesicles in advanced stages.

Dx DIAGNOSIS

DIFFERENTIAL DIAGNOSIS

- Benign prostatic hypertrophy
- Prostatitis
- Prostate stones

LABORATORY TESTS

- Fig. E1-769 describes the assessment and treatment of patients with prostate cancer suspected on the grounds of a DRE and PSA. Measurement of prostate-specific antigen (PSA) is controversial in early diagnosis of prostate cancer. PSA screening is associated with psychological harm, and its potential benefits remain uncertain. In asymptomatic men with no history of prostate cancer, screening using PSA does not reduce all-cause mortality or death from prostate cancer. Normal PSA is found in >20% of patients with prostate cancer, whereas only 20% of men with PSA levels between 4 ng/ml and 10 ng/ml have prostate cancer. Most guidelines encourage a shared decision-making approach between patient and physician regarding PSA testing. Available evidence favors clinician discussion of the pros and cons of PSA screening with average-risk men aged 65-69 yr. Only men who express a definite preference for screening should have PSA testing.[1] The American Cancer Society recommends offering the PSA test and DRE yearly to men aged ≥50 yr who have a life expectancy of at least 10 yr. Earlier testing, starting at age 40-45 yr, is recommended for men at high risk (e.g., blacks, men with family history of prostate cancer). An isolated elevation in PSA level should be confirmed several weeks later before proceeding with further testing, including prostate biopsy. Screening for prostate cancer in men aged ≥75 yr is controversial and generally not recommended. The American College of Physicians (ACP) recommends that clinicians should not screen for prostate cancer using the PSA in average-risk men under age 50, men over age 69, or men with a life expectancy of less than 10 to 15 yr.[2] The U.S. Preventive Services Task Force (USPSTF) recommends against PSA-based screening for prostate cancer in all age groups. According to the USPSTF:
  - The magnitude of harms from screening (e.g., falsely high PSA levels, psychological effects, unnecessary biopsies, overdiagnosis of indolent tumors) is "at least small."
  - The magnitude of treatment-associated harms (i.e., adverse effects of surgery, radiation, and hormonal therapy) is "at least moderate."
  - The 10-yr mortality benefit of PSA-based prostate cancer screening is "small to none."
  - The overall balance of benefits and harms results in "moderate certainty that PSA-based screening has no net benefit."
- Free PSA: the use of serum free PSA for prostate screening has been proposed by some urologists as a means to decrease unwarranted biopsies without missing a significant number of prostate cancers. This approach is based on the higher free PSA in men with benign prostatic hyperplasia and the higher protein-bound PSA levels in men with prostate cancer. For example, in men with total PSA levels of 4 to 10 ng/ml, the cancer probability is 0.25, but if the percentage of free PSA is ≤17%, the probability of cancer increases to 0.45.
- PSA velocity: the rate of increase of serum PSA over time (PSA velocity) can aid in the diagnosis of prostate cancer. A yearly PSA velocity >0.75 ng/ml increases the likelihood of later malignancy when total PSA is still within normal range. Proper interpretation of PSA velocity requires at least three PSA measurements over an 18-month period because most PSA variations are physiologic. Recent trials have cast a doubt on the value of PSA velocity by showing that adding PSA velocity as a trigger for biopsy did not improve predictive accuracy beyond that of using PSA threshold values alone.
- Age-adjusted PSA: there is evidence that the current threshold of 4.0 ng/ml is inadequate for younger men, because in a recent study 22% of men with PSA levels between 2.6 and 4.0 were found to have prostate cancer. The concept of age-related cutoffs remains controversial. Lowering the upper limit of normal for PSA would improve sensitivity but decrease specificity.
- Prostatic acid phosphatase can be used for evaluation of nonlocalized disease.
- Prostate cancer gene 3 *(PCA3)* is overexpressed in prostate cancer cell, and high levels are suggestive of prostate cancer. Measurement of *PCA3* in urine specimens collected after digital exams is helpful to

---

[1]Hayes JH, Barry MJ: Screening for prostate cancer with the prostate-specific antigen test, a review of current evidence, *JAMA* 311(11):1143-1149, 2014.

[2]Qaseem A et al: Screening for prostate cancer: a guidance statement from the clinical guidelines committee of the American College of Physicians, *Ann Int Med* 158:761-768, 2013.

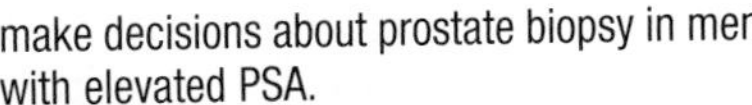

make decisions about prostate biopsy in men with elevated PSA.

- Transrectal biopsy and fine-needle aspiration of prostate can confirm the diagnosis. Indications for biopsy include an abnormal PSA level, an abnormal DRE, or a previous biopsy specimen that showed prostatic intraepithelial neoplasia or prostatic atypia. The number of cores taken is patient specific, typically including a minimum of 10 cores. Prostate volume negatively affects cancer detection rate (23% in glands >50 cm^3, 38% in glands <50 cm^3).

IMAGING STUDIES

- Bone scan is useful to evaluate bone metastasis (present or eventually develops in almost 80% of patients). However, according to the American Urological Association (AUA), the routine use of bone scanning is not required for staging of prostate cancer in asymptomatic men with clinically localized cancer if the PSA level is ≤20 ng/ml.
- CT scan, MRI, and transrectal ultrasonography may be useful in selected patients to assess extent of prostate cancer. High-resolution MRI with magnetic nanoparticles has been used for the detection of small and otherwise undetectable lymph node metastases in patients with prostate cancer. However, according to the AUA, transrectal ultrasonography adds little to the combination of PSA and DRE. Similarly, CT and MRI imaging are generally not indicated for cancer staging in men with clinically localized cancer and PSA <25 ng/ml. With regard to pelvic lymph node dissection in staging, the AUA states that it may not be required in patients with PSA levels <10 ng/ml and when PSA level is <20 ng/ml and the Gleason score is <6.

Rx TREATMENT

NONPHARMACOLOGIC THERAPY

Watchful waiting is reasonable in selected patients with early-stage (T-IA) and projected life expectancy <10 yr or in patients with focal and moderately differentiated carcinoma.

ACUTE GENERAL Rx

- Therapeutic approach varies with the following:
  1. Stage of the tumor
  2. Patient's life expectancy
  3. General medical condition
  4. Patient's treatment preference (e.g., patient may be opposed to orchiectomy)
- The optimal treatment of clinically localized prostate cancer is unclear. It's important to remember that all forms of treatment have potential adverse effects. Management requires careful consideration of the potential benefits and harms of intervention, the patient's age, health status, and individual preferences.
  1. Radical prostatectomy is generally performed in patients with localized prostate cancer and life expectancy >10 yr. Radical prostatectomy reduces disease-specific mortality, overall mortality, and the risks of metastasis and local progression. The absolute reduction in the risk of death after 10 yr is small, but the reductions in the risks of metastasis and local tumor progression are substantial. Postoperative complications of radical prostatectomy include urinary incontinence (10% to 20% depending on degree of neurovascular bundle and urethral preservation, patient age, and correct mucosal apposition) and erectile dysfunction (percentage exceeds 50% and varies with patient age, preoperative erectile dysfunction, stage of tumor at time of surgery, and preservation of neurovascular bundle). Lower complication rates occur in hospitals that perform a large number of prostatectomies. Fewer men will have postsurgical erectile dysfunction after unilateral or bilateral nerve-sparing surgery. In men undergoing prostatectomy, robotic-assisted laparoscopic surgery represents an alternative to open retropubic radical prostatectomy. Despite advertisements that suggest that there are fewer complications after robotic surgery, recent data show that sexual dysfunction occurs postoperatively in about 88% of patients who have undergone robotic-assisted or conventional prostatectomy and that incontinence problems are more prevalent (33%) with robotic surgery than with open retropubic radical prostatectomy (RPP) (27%). Recent trials have shown that prostatectomy is preferred over "watchful waiting" in patients with localized prostate cancer detected by PSA if the PSA level is >10 ng/ml. In this subgroup, the 10-year mortality is 48.4% with prostatectomy versus 61.6% with watchful waiting. In men who have low-risk disease (PSA level <10 mcg/L, stage <T2a, Gleason score ≤3 + 3), and less than 6% risk for prostate cancer–specific death at 15 yr, watchful waiting (WW) and active surveillance (AS) are reasonable and underutilized options.[3]
  2. Radiation therapy (external-beam irradiation or brachytherapy with implantation of radioactive pellets [iodine-125 or palladium-103 seeds] into the prostate gland) represents an alternative in patients with localized prostate cancer, especially poor surgical candidates or patients with a high-grade malignancy. The efficacy of brachytherapy is comparable to external radiation. In patients receiving external-beam radiation, a total dose of 79.2 Gy (high dose) compared with a total dose of 70.2 Gy (conventional dose) has been reported to lower the risk of recurrence without increased risk of morbidity and mortality. Newer radiation treatments such as intensity-modulated radiation therapy (IMRT) and proton therapy are becoming increasingly popular and replacing the older technique of conformal radiation therapy over the past 10 years. Trials have shown that among patients with nonmetastatic prostate cancer, the use of IMRT compared with conformal therapy is associated with less gastrointestinal morbidity and fewer hip fractures but more erectile dysfunction; IMRT compared with proton therapy is associated with less GI morbidity. Patients with localized prostate cancer and high risk for extraprostatic disease and disease recurrence (e.g., Gleason score ≤7 with multiple positive biopsy cores and clinical stage T1b-T2b) may benefit (increased overall survival) with the addition of 6 mo of androgen suppression therapy to radiation therapy.
  3. Watchful waiting is reasonable in patients who are too old or too ill to survive longer than 10 yr. If the cancer progresses to the point where it becomes symptomatic, palliation can be attempted with several methods. Conservative management is also reasonable for patients with Gleason score of 2 to 4 because these patients do not have a shortened life expectancy and treatment is associated with long-term side effects. Watchful waiting also appears to be safe in older men with less-aggressive disease. Individual preferences play a central role in the decision whether to treat or to pursue active surveillance.
- Patients with advanced disease and projected life expectancy <10 yr are candidates for radiation therapy and hormonal therapy (diethylstilbestrol, luteinizing hormone–releasing hormone analogs, antiandrogens, bilateral orchiectomy).
- Recommended treatment of patients with regional metastatic prostate cancer with projected life expectancy ≥10 yr includes radiation therapy and hormonal therapy.
- Prostate cancer is an androgen-receptor-dependent disease, and the blocking of androgen-receptor signaling is an effective treatment modality. Androgen deprivation therapy (ADT) is the mainstay of treatment for metastatic prostate cancer. Adverse effects of ADT include decreased libido, impotence, hot flashes, osteopenia with increased fracture risk, metabolic alterations, and changes in mood and cognition. Adjuvant treatment with luteinizing hormone-releasing hormone (LHRH) agonists (goserelin, leuprolide, or triptorelin) plus antiandrogens (flutamide, bicalutamide, or nilutamide), when started simultaneously with external-beam radiation, improves local control and survival in patients with locally advanced prostate cancer. Pamidronate inhibits osteoclast-mediated bone resorption and prevents bone loss in the hip and lumbar spine in men receiving treatment for prostate cancer. Gonadotropin-releasing hormone (GnRH) receptor antagonists can be used for rapid medical castration of men with advanced prostate cancer. Degarelix is an injectable GnRH agonist useful to suppress

[3]Hayes JH et al: Observation versus initial treatment for men with localized, low-risk prostate cancer, *Ann Int Med* 158:853-860, 2013.

testosterone in patients with prostate cancer who are not good candidates for LHRH agonists and refuse surgical castration. Assessment of bone density and treatment with once-weekly oral alendronate can prevent and improve the bone loss that occurs in men receiving ADT for prostate cancer.

- Docetaxel plus prednisone or docetaxel plus estramustine can be used in metastatic hormone–refractory prostate cancer. Newer treatments for hormone-refractory prostate cancer (castration-resistant cancer) include immunotherapy with sipuleucel and cabazitaxel, a microtubule inhibitor that interferes with cell mitosis and replication. Both agents can prolong survival but adverse effects can be severe and both agents are very expensive. Abiraterone is an oral agent that blocks biosynthesis of androgens by inhibiting CYP17, an enzyme required for androgen biosynthesis. It has been FDA approved for oral treatment, in combination with prednisone, of metastatic castration-resistant prostate cancer in patients previously treated with docetaxel.
- Enzalutamide is a newer nonsteroidal antiandrogen. Trials have shown it to be highly effective in extending survival in patients with metastatic castration-resistant prostate cancer. It can be used sequentially with other agents such as docetaxel, abiraterone, cabazitaxel, and immunotherapy. Radium-223, an alpha emitter, selectively targets bone metastases and has been found effective in improving survival in men with castration-resistant prostate cancer and bone metastases.[4]

CHRONIC Rx

- Patients should be monitored at 3- to 6-mo intervals with clinical examination and PSA for the first year, then every 6 mo for the second year, then yearly if stable. For patients who have undergone radical prostatectomy, a rising PSA level suggests evidence of residual or recurrent prostate cancer. Salvage radiotherapy may potentially cure patients with disease recurrence after radical prostatectomy.
- Chest radiography and bone scan should be performed yearly or sooner if patient develops symptoms.

DISPOSITION

- Prognosis varies with the stage of the disease and the Gleason classification (see "Definition"). For patients between ages 65 and 69 yr at diagnosis and a Gleason score of 2 to 4, the probability of dying from prostate cancer 15 yr after diagnosis is 0.06 and that of dying from other causes is 0.56. If the Gleason score is 7 to 10, the probability of dying from prostate cancer increases to 0.72 and from other causes varies from 0.25 to 0.36.
- The ploidy of the tumor also has prognostic value; prognosis is better with diploid tumor cells and worse with aneuploid tumor cells.
- For grade 1 tumors, the extended 10-yr, disease-specific survival is similar for patients with prostatectomy (94%), radiotherapy (90%), and conservative management (93%); survival rate is better with surgery than with radiotherapy or conservative management in patients with grade 2 or 3 localized prostate cancer.
- Expression of the gene *EZH2* has been identified as an important factor in the determination of the aggressiveness of prostate cancer. A recent study revealed that expression of the *EZH2* gene may be a better predictor of clinical failure than Gleason score, tumor stage, or surgical margin status. Testing for *EZH2* protein in prostate cancer tissue may be useful to determine prognosis and direct treatment.
- Preoperative PSA level and PSA velocity have prognostic significance. Men whose PSA level increases by >2.0 mcg/ml during the year before the diagnosis of cancer may have a relatively high risk of death from prostate cancer despite undergoing radical prostatectomy.
- Extraprostatic disease is detected at radical prostatectomy in 38% to 52% of patients and is associated with a risk of disease recurrence, progression, and death. In these patients, adjuvant radiotherapy results in significantly reduced risk of PSA relapse and disease recurrence; however, the improvements in metastases-free survival and overall survival are not statistically significant.
- The Prostate Cancer Prevention trial revealed that the use of 5-alpha-reductase inhibitors lowers the incidence of prostate cancer but also increases the incidence of high-grade tumors (Gleason score >7). It is possible that these agents delay diagnosis of prostate cancer by lowering PSA levels and decreasing prostate size. The trade-off inherent in using 5-alpha-reductase inhibitors for prostate cancer prevention is risk of one additional high-grade cancer in order to avert three or four lower-grade cancers. Based on these results, the FDA's Oncologic Drugs Advisory Committee concluded that finasteride and dutasteride do not have a favorable risk-benefit profile for chemoprevention of prostate cancer in healthy men.
- Patients undergoing prostatectomy are more likely to have urinary incontinence than those undergoing radiotherapy at 2 years and 5 years. However, at 15 years there are no significant relative differences in disease-specific functional outcomes among men undergoing prostatectomy or radiotherapy.

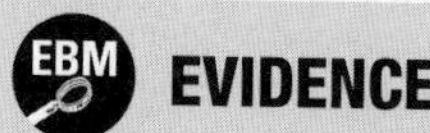

available at www.expertconsult.com

SUGGESTED READINGS

available at www.expertconsult.com

RELATED CONTENT

Prostate Cancer (Patient Information)

AUTHOR: **FRED F. FERRI, M.D.**

[4]Nilsson CP et al: Alpha emitter radium-223 and survival in metastatic prostate cancer, *N Engl J Med* 369:213-223, 2013.

BASIC INFORMATION

DEFINITION

Benign prostatic hyperplasia (BPH) is the benign growth of the prostate, generally originating in the periureteral and transition zones, with subsequent obstructive and irritative voiding symptoms.

SYNONYMS

BPH
Prostatic hypertrophy

ICD-9CM CODES
600 Benign prostatic hyperplasia
ICD-10CM CODES
N40 Hyperplasia of prostate
N40.0 Enlarged prostate without lower urinary tract symptoms

EPIDEMIOLOGY & DEMOGRAPHICS

- 80% of men have evidence of BPH by age 80 yr.
- Medical and surgical intervention for problems caused by BPH is required in <20% of males by age 75 yr.
- Transurethral resection of the prostate (TURP) is the tenth most common operative procedure (<400,000/yr in U.S.).
- 10% to 30% of men with BPH have occult prostate cancer.

PHYSICAL FINDINGS & CLINICAL PRESENTATION

- Digital rectal examination (DRE) reveals enlargement of the prostate.
- Focal enlargement may be indicative of malignancy.
- There is poor correlation between size of prostate and symptoms (BPH may be asymptomatic if it does not encroach on the urethral lumen).
- Most patients with BPH report difficulty in initiating urination (hesitancy), decrease in caliber and force of stream, incomplete emptying of bladder often resulting in double voiding (need to urinate again a few minutes after voiding), postvoid "dribbling," and nocturia.

ETIOLOGY

Multifactorial; a functioning testicle is necessary for development of BPH (as evidenced by the absence in males who were castrated before puberty).

DIAGNOSIS

DIFFERENTIAL DIAGNOSIS

- Prostatitis
- Prostate cancer
- Strictures (urethral)
- Medications interfering with the muscle fibers in the prostate and also with bladder function
  - Opiates: impaired autonomic function
  - Decongestants: increased sphincter tone
  - Antihistamines: decreased parasympathetic tone
  - Tricyclic antidepressants: anticholinergic effects
- Neurogenic bladder
- Bladder cancer

WORKUP

Symptom assessment (use of American Urological Association [AUA] Symptom Index for BPH [Table 1-415]), laboratory tests, and imaging studies Fig. E1-770 describes a diagnostic approach to patients with BPH.

LABORATORY TESTS

- Prostate-specific antigen (PSA): protease secreted by epithelial cells of the prostate; elevated in 30% to 50% of patients with BPH. Testing for PSA increases detection rate for prostate cancer and tends to detect cancer at an earlier stage. However, the PSA test does not discriminate well between patients with symptomatic BPH and those with prostate cancer, particularly if the cancer is pathologically localized and curable. The test may also trigger additional evaluation, including ultrasound biopsy of the prostate. Asymptomatic men with PSA levels >2 ng/ml do not need annual testing. According to the AUA, PSA testing and DRE should be offered to any asymptomatic man <50 yr with a life expectancy of 10 yr. PSA testing can also be offered at an earlier age in men at higher risk of prostatic cancer (e.g., first-degree relatives with prostate cancer; African American race).
- Measurement of "free" PSA is useful to assess the probability of prostate cancer in patients with normal DRE and total PSA between 4 and 10 ng/ml. In these patients the global risk of prostate cancer is 25%. However, if the free PSA is >25%, the risk of prostate cancer decreases to 8%, whereas if the free PSA is <10%, the risk of cancer

TABLE 1-415 International Prostate Symptom Score (I-PSS)

	SCORE						
Symptom	**Not at All**	**Less than 1 Time in 5**	**Less than Half the Time**	**About Half the Time**	**More than Half the Time**	**Almost Always**	**Total Score**
Incomplete emptying: Over the past month, how often have you had a sensation of not emptying your bladder completely after you finished urinating?	0	1	2	3	4	5	
Frequency: Over the past month, how often have you had to urinate again <2 hr after you finished urinating?	0	1	2	3	4	5	
Intermittency: Over the past month, how often have you found you stopped and started again several times when you urinated?	0	1	2	3	4	5	
Urgency: Over the past month, how often have you found it difficult to postpone urination?	0	1	2	3	4	5	
Weak stream: Over the past month, how often have you had a weak urinary stream?	0	1	2	3	4	5	
Straining: Over the past month, how often have you had to push or strain to begin urination?	0	1	2	3	4	5	
	None	**1 Time**	**2 Times**	**3 Times**	**4 Times**	**5 or More Times**	
Nocturia: Over the past month, how many times did you most typically get up to urinate from the time you went to bed at night until the time you got up in the morning?	0	1	2	3	4	5	
Total I-PSS score =							

increases to 56%. Free PSA is also useful to evaluate the aggressiveness of prostate cancer. A low free PSA percentage generally indicates a high-grade cancer, whereas a high free PSA percentage is generally associated with a slower growing tumor.
- Elevated measurement of prostate cancer gene 3 *(PCA3)* in urine specimens collected after digital exam is helpful in deciding about prostate biopsy in men with elevated PSA (increased *PCA3* = increased likelihood of prostate cancer).
- Urinalysis, urine culture, and sensitivity to rule out infection (if suspected).
- Blood urea nitrogen and creatinine to rule out postrenal insufficiency.

IMAGING STUDIES

- Transrectal ultrasound may be indicated in patients with palpable nodules or significant elevation of PSA. It is also useful to estimate prostate size. BPH may also be evident in suprapubic ultrasound and MRI.
- Uroflowmetry may be used to determine relative impact of obstruction on urine flow. Urethral pressure profile is useful to predict prostatic hypertrophy within the urethral lumen.
- Pressure flow studies, although invasive, are particularly helpful in patients whose history and/or examination suggest primary bladder dysfunction as a cause of symptoms of prostatism. They are also useful in patients for whom a distinction between prostatic obstruction and impaired detrusor contractility may affect the choice of therapy. However, pressure flow studies may not be useful in the workup of the usual patient with symptoms of prostatism.
- Postvoid residual urine measurement has not been proved useful in predicting the need for or response to treatment; it may be useful in monitoring the course of the disease in patients who elect nonsurgical treatment.
- Urethral cystoscopy is an option during later evaluation if invasive treatment is being planned.

Rx TREATMENT

NONPHARMACOLOGIC THERAPY

- Avoidance of caffeine or any other foods that may exacerbate symptoms
- Avoidance of medications that may exacerbate symptoms (e.g., most cold and allergy remedies)

GENERAL Rx

- Asymptomatic patients with prostate enlargement caused by BPH generally do not require treatment. Patients with mild to moderate symptoms are candidates for pharmacologic treatment (see below). For patients who have specific complications from BPH, prostate surgery is usually the most appropriate form of treatment. However, surgery may result in significant complications (e.g., incontinence, infection).
- Alpha-blockers (e.g., tamsulosin, alfuzosin, doxazosin, prazosin, terazosin) relax smooth muscle of the bladder neck and prostate and can increase peak urinary flow rate. They have no effect on the size of the prostate. Alpha-1 blockers are useful in symptomatic patients to relieve symptoms of obstruction by causing relaxation of smooth muscle tone in the prostatic capsule, urethra, and bladder neck.
- Hormonal manipulation with finasteride, a 5-alpha-reductase inhibitor that blocks conversion of testosterone to dihydrotestosterone, can reduce the size of the prostate. Usual dose is 5 mg qd. Treatment requires ≥6 mo for maximal effect.
- Dutasteride is also a 5-alpha-reductase inhibitor useful to decrease prostate size and improve urinary flow. In addition to inhibiting the isoform of 5-alpha-reductase located in the prostate, the medication inhibits a second isoform and reduces dihydrotestosterone formation in the skin and liver. Usual dose is 0.5 mg qd.
- Tadalafil 5 mg qd has been FDA-approved to treat patients with signs and symptoms of BPH and patients with both ED and signs and symptoms of BPH. Tadalafil can potentiate the hypotensive effect of alpha-blockers and should not be used in combination with alpha-blockers.
- The dietary supplement saw palmetto is commonly used for relief of symptoms of BPH. Recent trials using 160 mg of saw palmetto bid did not improve symptoms of BPH. This contrasts with the positive findings of many previous studies. Trials with higher dose-ranging protocols are currently in progress.
- TURP is the most commonly used surgical procedure for BPH. Transurethral incision of the prostate (TUIP), a procedure almost equivalent in efficacy, is limited to patients whose estimated resection tissue weight would be 30 g or less. TUIP can be performed in an ambulatory setting or during a 1-day hospitalization. Open prostatectomy is typically performed on patients with very large prostates.
- Laser therapy for BPH is a less invasive alternative to TURP; YAG laser enucleation has minimal effect on potency, libido, or patient satisfaction with his sex life and is associated with retrograde ejaculation. However, recent studies indicate that at least in the initial 7 mo after surgery, TURP is moderately more effective than laser therapy in relieving symptoms of BPH.
- Transurethral needle ablation with radiofrequency to remove periurethral prostate tissue is being increasingly used in patients with prostate volume >60 ml and moderate symptoms. It has a low morbidity rate, but treatment failure is approximately 25% at 5 yr and <80% at 10 yr.
- Balloon dilation of the prostatic urethra is less effective than surgery for relieving symptoms but is associated with fewer complications. It is a reasonable treatment option for patients with smaller prostates and no middle lobe enlargement.
- Surgery need not be the treatment of last resort for most patients; that is, patients need not undergo other treatments for BPH before they can have surgery. However, recommending surgery on the grounds that a patient's surgical risk will "only increase with age" is generally inappropriate.

DISPOSITION

With appropriate therapy, symptoms improve or stabilize in <70% of patients with BPH.

REFERRAL

Urology referral for patients with severe or intolerable symptoms and for any patient suspected of having prostate cancer (10% to 30% of men with BPH)

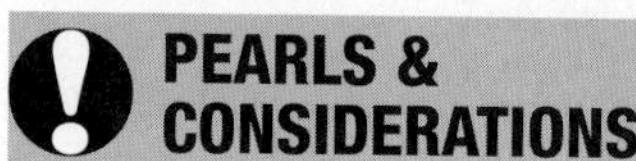

PEARLS & CONSIDERATIONS

COMMENTS

- Emerging technologies for treating BPH, including transurethral holmium laser enucleation, transurethral electrovaporization, and transurethral microwave thermotherapy of the prostate, appear promising; however, long-term effectiveness has not yet been demonstrated.
- The increase in the use of pharmacologic management has resulted in <30% reduction in the total number of TURP procedures.
- Combined drug therapy for BPH with an alpha-blocker and a 5-alpha-reductase inhibitor is superior to monotherapy with either agent.
- Saw palmetto extract is ineffective for BPH symptoms. Trials have shown that even at three times the standard dosing, saw palmetto extract had no greater effect than placebo on improving lower urinary symptoms associated with BPH.

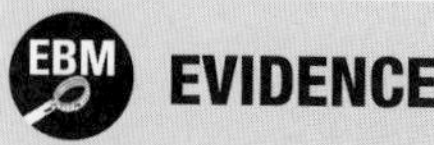

EVIDENCE

available at www.expertconsult.com

SUGGESTED READINGS

available at www.expertconsult.com

RELATED CONTENT

Enlarged Prostate (Patient Information)

AUTHOR: **FRED F. FERRI, M.D.**

BASIC INFORMATION

DEFINITION

Prostatitis refers to inflammation of the prostate gland. There are four major categories:

1. Acute bacterial prostatitis (type I)
2. Chronic bacterial prostatitis (type II)
3. Chronic prostatitis/pelvic pain syndrome (CP/CPPS) (type III): subdivided into type IIIA (inflammatory) and IIIB (noninflammatory)
4. Asymptomatic inflammatory prostatitis (type IV)

ICD-9CM CODES
601.0 Prostatitis (acute)
601.1 Prostatitis (chronic)
ICD-10CM CODES
N41.0 Acute prostatitis
N41.1 Chronic prostatitis

EPIDEMIOLOGY & DEMOGRAPHICS

- 50% of men will have symptoms of prostatitis in their lifetime.
- Prostatitis accounts for >8% of visits to urologists and 1% of visits to primary care physicians.
- The prevalence of chronic bacterial prostatitis is 5% to 10%.
- CP/CPPS is the most common of the clinically defined prostatitis syndromes, with prevalence ranging from 9%-12% of men.

PHYSICAL FINDINGS & CLINICAL PRESENTATION

1. Acute bacterial prostatitis:
   - Sudden or rapidly progressive onset of:
     - Dysuria
     - Frequency
     - Urgency
     - Nocturia
     - Perineal pain that may radiate to the back, rectum, or penis
   - Hematuria or a purulent urethral discharge may occur.
   - Occasionally urinary retention complicates the course.
   - Fever, chills, and signs of sepsis can also be part of the clinical picture.
   - On rectal examination the prostate is typically tender.
2. Chronic bacterial prostatitis:
   - Characterized by positive culture of expressed prostatic secretions. May cause symptoms such as suprapubic, low back, or perineal pain; mild urgency, frequency, and dysuria with urination; and possibly recurrent urinary tract infections.
   - May be asymptomatic when the infection is confined to the prostate.
   - May present as an increase in severity of baseline symptoms of benign prostatic hypertrophy (BPH).
   - When cystitis is also present, urinary frequency, urgency, and burning may be reported.
   - Hematuria may be a presenting complaint.
   - In elderly men, new onset of urinary incontinence may be noted.
3. CP/CPPS:
   - Presents similarly with pain in the pelvic region lasting >3 mo. Symptoms also can include pain in the suprapubic region, low back, penis, testes, or scrotum.
   - The symptoms can be of variable severity and may include lower urinary tract symptoms, sexual dysfunction, and reduced quality of life.

ETIOLOGY

1. Acute bacterial prostatitis:
   - Acute, usually gram-negative infection of the prostate gland. *E. coli* is the most commonly isolated organism.
     - Generally associated with cystitis
     - Results from the ascent of bacteria into the urethra
   - Occasionally the route of infection is hematogenous or a lymphatogenous spread of rectal bacteria.
   - Consider *Neisseria gonorrhoeae* or *Chlamydia trachomatis* in young patients (age <35 yr) with risk of sexually transmitted disease (STD).
2. Chronic bacterial prostatitis:
   - Often asymptomatic. *E. coli* is the most commonly isolated organism.
   - Exacerbation of symptoms of BPH caused by the same mechanism as in acute bacterial prostatitis.
3. CP/CPPS:
   - Type IIIA: refers to symptoms of prostatic inflammation associated with the presence of white blood cells in prostatic secretions with no identifiable bacterial organism.
   - *Chlamydia* infection may be etiologically implicated in some cases.
   - Type IIIB: refers to symptoms of prostatic inflammation with no or few white blood cells in the prostatic secretion.
   - Its cause is unknown. Spasm in the bladder neck or urethra may be responsible for the symptoms.

DIAGNOSIS

DIFFERENTIAL DIAGNOSIS

- BPH with lower urinary tract symptoms
- Prostate cancer

WORKUP

- Rectal examination:
  1. Tender prostate most suggestive of acute bacterial prostatitis
  2. Enlarged prostate common in chronic bacterial prostatitis
  3. Normal prostate is consistent with chronic bacterial prostatitis and CP/CPPS.
- Expression of prostatic secretions by prostate massage is contraindicated in acute bacterial prostatitis but is appropriate in the other three situations.

LABORATORY TESTS

- Urinalysis
- Urine culture and sensitivity
- Bacterial localization studies can be performed but are cumbersome and impractical in most clinical settings.
- Cell count and culture of expressed prostatic secretions
- Prostate-specific antigen (PSA) is not used to diagnose prostatitis and is not recommended unless a nodule is present on digital examination. A rapid rise over baseline should raise the possibility of prostatitis even in the absence of symptoms. In such cases, a follow-up PSA after treatment of prostatitis is appropriate.
- Complete blood count and blood cultures if fever, chills, or signs of sepsis exist.

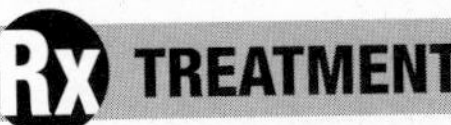

TREATMENT

1. Acute bacterial prostatitis:
   - Uncomplicated (with risk of STD, age <35 yr): ceftriaxone 250 mg IM × 1 dose *or* cefixime 400 mg PO × 1 *then* doxycycline 100 mg bid × 10 days
   - Uncomplicated with low risk of STD: levofloxacin 500 mg qd or ciprofloxacin 500 mg bid × 10-14 days
2. Chronic bacterial prostatitis:
   - First-line choice is a quinolone (ciprofloxacin or levofloxacin) for 4 wk.
   - Trimethoprim-sulfamethoxazole (TMP-SMX) is second-line choice for 1-3 mo if the organism is sensitive. Tissue penetration for TMP-SMX is not as good as quinolones, and there is evidence of increasing uropathogenic resistance.
3. CP/CPPS:
   - No specific treatment. A brief course of NSAIDs may be tried until urine localization cultures are completed. Alfuzosin may reduce symptoms in men who have not received prior therapy with an alpha-blocker.
   - Recent trials have shown modest improvement with quinolones (possibly secondary to their anti-inflammatory and analgesic effects), but antibiotics are not generally effective and should be avoided in patients who are afebrile and have normal urinalysis results.

SUGGESTED READINGS

available at www.expertconsult.com

RELATED CONTENT

Prostatitis (Patient Information)

AUTHOR: **FRED F. FERRI, M.D.**

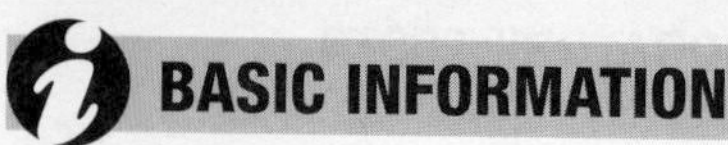

BASIC INFORMATION

DEFINITION

Pruritus ani refers to an intense chronic itching of the anus and perianal skin.

ICD-9CM CODES
698.0 Pruritus ani
ICD-10CM CODES
L29.0 Pruritus ani

EPIDEMIOLOGY & DEMOGRAPHICS

- Any age can be affected.
- Occurs in 1% to 5% of the population.
- Male/female predominance of 4:1

PHYSICAL FINDINGS & CLINICAL PRESENTATION

- Anal itching
- Anal fissures
- Hemorrhoids
- Excoriations
- Pinworms
- Fecal incontinence

ETIOLOGY

Anorectal diseases and fecal contamination:
- Diarrhea
- Anal incontinence
- Hemorrhoids
- Fissures
- Fistulae
- Rectal prolapse
- Malignancy: Bowen's disease, epidermoid cancer, perianal Paget's disease

Infections:
- Fungal: candidiasis, dermatophytes
- Parasitic: pinworms, scabies
- Bacterial: *Staphylococcus aureus,* erythrasma
- Lymphogranuloma venereum
- Granuloma inguinale
- Chancroid
- Molluscum contagiosum
- Trichomoniasis
- Venereal: herpes, gonococcal syphilis, human papillomavirus

Local irritants:
- Moisture, obesity, excessive perspiration
- Soaps, hygiene products
- Toilet paper: perfumed, dyed
- Underwear: irritating fabrics, detergents
- Anal creams, suppositories
- Dietary: coffee, beer, acidic foods
- Drugs: mineral oil, ascorbic acid, hydrocortisone sodium succinate, quinine, colchicine

Dermatologic diseases:
- Psoriasis
- Atopic dermatitis
- Seborrheic dermatitis

Section II also describes the various causes of pruritus ani.

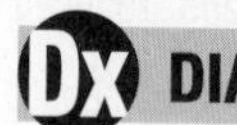

DIAGNOSIS

DIFFERENTIAL DIAGNOSIS

- Allergies
- Anxiety
- Dermatologic conditions
- Infections
- Parasites
- Diabetes mellitus
- Chronic liver disease
- Neoplasia
- Proctalgia fugax

WORKUP

- Detailed history regarding bowel habits, hygiene, use of perfumed products, and medical history
- Inspection of perianal area
- Possible biopsy to exclude neoplasia
- Microscopic inspection of scrapings
- Colposcopy of perineum

LABORATORY TESTS

- Chemistry profile
- Urinalysis
- Cultures
- Stool for ova and parasites
- Tape test
- Glucose tolerance test, if necessary

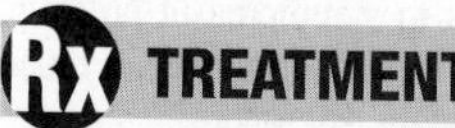

TREATMENT

NONPHARMACOLOGIC THERAPY

- Avoidance of tight, nonbreathable clothing and underclothing
- Discontinuation or curtailment of coffee, beer, citrus fruits, tomatoes, chocolate, and tea. Dietary modification is frequently recommended, although its effectiveness has not been established.
- Cleansing of anal area after bowel movements with a premoistened pad or tissue and avoidance of perfumes and dyes present in toilet paper and soaps
- Avoidance of excessive perspiration
- Aggressive management of fecal leakage or incontinence to avoid soiling of perianal skin

ACUTE GENERAL Rx

- Minimization of frequent loose stools with antidiarrheals and fiber agents if appropriate
- Use of a 1% hydrocortisone cream sparingly bid during the acute phase of pruritus ani but not for >2 wk to avoid atrophy
- Protective ointments such as zinc oxide may be helpful.
- Treatment of predisposing factors, such as parasites, diabetes, liver disease, hemorrhoids, and other infections

CHRONIC Rx

- Possible complications: excoriation and secondary bacterial infection; must be treated aggressively
- Longstanding, intractable pruritus ani: good response to intracutaneous injections of methylene blue and other agents, steroid injection

DISPOSITION

- Usually good results with total resolution of symptoms
- In some, persistent and recurrent symptoms

REFERRAL

To colorectal specialist if conservative measures fail or if patient experiences rectal bleeding or change in bowel movements

SUGGESTED READINGS

available at www.expertconsult.com

RELATED CONTENT

Hemorrhoids (Related Key Topic)
Anal Itching (Patient Information)

AUTHOR: **RUBEN ALVERO, M.D.**

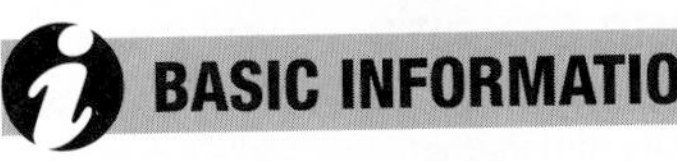

BASIC INFORMATION

DEFINITION

Pruritus vulvae refers to intense itching of the female external genitalia.

SYNONYMS

Vulvodynia

ICD-9CM CODES
698.1 Pruritus of genital organs
ICD-10CM CODES
L29.2 Pruritus vulvae
L29.3 Anogenital pruritus, unspecified

EPIDEMIOLOGY & DEMOGRAPHICS

- A female disorder that can affect women at any age
- Young girls: infection is usually causative
- Postmenopausal women: frequently affected because of hypoestrogenic state

PHYSICAL FINDINGS & CLINICAL PRESENTATION

Constant, intense itching or burning of the vulva

ETIOLOGY

- Approximately 50% are caused by monilial infection or trichomoniasis.
- Other infectious causes are herpes simplex, condylomata acuminata, and molluscum contagiosum.
- Other causes:
  1. Infestations with scabies, pediculosis pubis, and pinworms
  2. Dermatoses such as hypertrophic dystrophy, lichen sclerosus, lichen planus, and psoriasis
  3. Neoplasms such as Bowen's disease, Paget's disease, and squamous cell carcinoma
  4. Allergic or chemical dermatitis caused by dyes in clothing or toilet paper, detergents, contraceptive gels, vaginal medications, douches, or soaps
  5. Vulvar or vaginal atrophy
- Severe pruritus is probably caused by degeneration and inflammation of terminal nerve fibers.
- Most intense itching occurs with hyperplastic lesions.
- Children typically (75%) have nonspecific pruritus, lichen sclerosus, bacterial infections, yeast infection, or pinworm infestation.

Dx DIAGNOSIS

DIFFERENTIAL DIAGNOSIS

- Vulvitis
- Vaginitis
- Lichen sclerosus
- Squamous cell hyperplasia
- Pinworms
- Vulvar cancer
- Syringoma of the vulva

WORKUP

- Inspection of vulva, vagina, and perianal area for infection, fissures, ulcerations, induration, or thick plaques
- Must rule out trichomoniasis, candidiasis, bacterial vaginosis, allergy, vitamin deficiencies, diabetes. Fig. E1-771 describes a diagnostic approach to the diagnosis of vulvar pruritus.

LABORATORY TESTS

- Wet prep of saline and potassium hydroxide of vaginal discharge
- Tape test to look for pinworms
- Vaginal cultures
- Biopsy when needed (punch biopsy commonly used)

Rx TREATMENT

NONPHARMACOLOGIC THERAPY

- Keep vulva clean and dry.
- Wear white cotton panties.
- Avoid perfumes and body creams over vulvar area because they can cause irritation.
- Reduce stress.
- Apply wet dressings with aluminum acetate (Burow's) solution frequently.
- Avoid coffee and caffeine-containing beverages, chocolate, and tomatoes.
- Sitz baths may be helpful.

ACUTE GENERAL Rx

Need to treat underlying problem:

- Yeast infection: any of the vaginal creams or difluconazole 150-mg one-time dose
- Trichomoniasis or *Gardnerella vaginalis:* metronidazole 500 mg or 375 mg PO bid for 7 days
- Urinary tract infection: treatment of specific organism
- Estrogen replacement therapy if atrophy is the cause of pruritus
- Pinworms: mebendazole 100 mg 1 tablet at diagnosis and repeated in 1 to 2 wk; also treat other members in family aged >2 yr
- Squamous cell hyperplasia: local application of corticosteroids
  1. One of the high- or medium-potency corticosteroids (0.025% or 0.01% fluocinolone acetonide or 0.01% triamcinolone acetonide) can be used to relieve itching.
  2. Rub into vulva bid or tid for 4 to 6 wk.
  3. Once itching is controlled, fluorinated steroid can be discontinued and patient can be switched to hydrocortisone preparation.
- Lichen sclerosus: topical 2% testosterone in petrolatum massaged into the vulvar tissue bid or tid; clobetasol propionate gel 0.05% tid for 5 days is effective
- Treatment with immune response modifiers

CHRONIC Rx

- If not relieved by topical measures: intradermal injection of triamcinolone (10 mg/ml diluted 2:1 saline); 0.1 ml of the suspension injected at 1-cm intervals and tissue gently massaged
- If symptoms still uncontrollable: SC injection of absolute alcohol 0.1 ml at 1-cm intervals

DISPOSITION

Usually controlled with conservative measures and topical steroids

REFERRAL

To a gynecologist for further workup if conservative measures do not give relief

SUGGESTED READINGS
available at www.expertconsult.com

RELATED CONTENT

Vaginitis, Estrogen-Deficient (Related Key Topic)
Vaginitis, Fungal (Related Key Topic)
Vaginitis, Prepubescent (Related Key Topic)
Vaginitis, Trichomonas (Related Key Topic)

AUTHOR: **RUBEN ALVERO, M.D.**

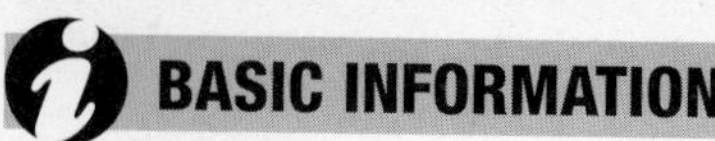

BASIC INFORMATION

DEFINITION

Psittacosis is a systemic infection caused by the bacterium *Chlamydophila psittaci* (formerly known as *Chlamydia psittaci*) and is predominantly transmitted by birds.

SYNONYMS

Ornithosis
Parrot pneumonia

ICD-9CM CODES
073.9 Psittacosis
ICD-10CM
A70 Chlamydia psittaci infections

EPIDEMIOLOGY & DEMOGRAPHICS

INCIDENCE (IN U.S.):
- Between 2000 and 2009 there were between 8 and 25 cases a year but only 4 cases in 2010.
- True incidence possibly higher because infections may be subclinical
- Highest incidence among pet owners and people working with birds

PEAK INCIDENCE: Age 30 to 60 yr
PREVALENCE (IN U.S.):
- Low among human beings
- More than 130 avian species serve as hosts of the bacterium and between 5% to 8% of birds carry the organism, including poultry, seagulls, and geese.
- Most human infections are from birds of the order Psittaformes, which includes cockatiels, parrots, cockatoos, and budgerigars

PREDOMINANT SEX: Equal sex distribution
PREDOMINANT AGE: More common in adults

PHYSICAL FINDINGS & CLINICAL PRESENTATION

- Incubation period of 5 to 15 days
- Subclinical infection
- Onset abrupt or insidious
- Most common symptoms:
  1. Fever
  2. Myalgias
  3. Chills
  4. Cough
- Most common clinical syndrome: atypical pneumonia with fever, headache, dry cough, and a chest radiograph more dramatically abnormal than the physical examination
- Ranges from mild disease to respiratory failure and death, although this is extremely unusual
- Other clinical presentations:
  1. Mononucleosis-like syndrome
  2. Typhoidal form
- Most frequent physical findings:
  1. Fever
  2. Pharyngeal erythema
  3. Rales
  4. Hepatomegaly
- Less common findings:
  1. Somnolence
  2. Confusion
  3. Relative bradycardia
  4. Pleural rub
  5. Adenopathy
  6. Splenomegaly
  7. Horder's spots (pink blanching maculopapular rash)
- Besides the lungs, other specific end-organ involvement:
  1. Pericarditis
  2. Myocarditis
  3. Endocarditis
  4. Hepatitis
  5. Joints
  6. Kidneys (glomerulonephritis)
  7. Central nervous system

ETIOLOGY

- *C. psittaci* is an obligate intracellular bacterium.
- Infection is usually spread by the respiratory route from infected birds, by direct contact or aerosolization of dried feces or bird feather dust, and rarely from a bite.
- There is a history of exposure to birds in 85% of patients, mostly with birds as pets.
- Strains from turkeys and psittacine birds are most virulent for human beings.
- Cows, goats, and sheep are occasionally implicated.

DIAGNOSIS

DIFFERENTIAL DIAGNOSIS

- *Legionella*
- *Mycoplasma*
- *Chlamydophila pneumoniae*
- Viral respiratory infections
- Typhoid fever
- Viral hepatitis
- Aseptic meningitis
- Mononucleosis

WORKUP

- Complete blood count, renal and liver function tests
- *Chlamydophila* serology
- Chest x-ray examination
- Special immunostaining of respiratory secretions

LABORATORY TESTS

- White blood count is normal or slightly elevated.
- ESR and C-reactive protein are generally elevated.
- Mild liver function abnormalities are common (50%).
- Blood cultures are almost always negative.
- Studies on respiratory secretions:
  1. Direct immunofluorescent antibody of respiratory secretions with monoclonal antibodies to chlamydial antigens
  2. *Chlamydophila* lipopolysaccharide antigen by enzyme immunoassay
  3. Polymerase chain reaction
- Serologic studies:
  1. Complement-fixing antibodies
  2. Microimmunofluorescence
  3. Possible false-negative results and cross-reaction with other chlamydial species with both techniques

IMAGING STUDIES

- Chest x-ray is abnormal in 50% to 90% with a variety of patterns.
- Pleural effusions are common.

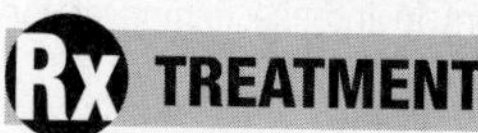

TREATMENT

NONPHARMACOLOGIC THERAPY

Oxygen supplementation as needed

ACUTE GENERAL Rx

- Doxycycline (100 mg PO bid) for 10 to 14 days after fever declines *or*
- Tetracycline (500 mg PO qid)
- Macrolides such as erythromycin or azithromycin are considered second-line agents in adults but first-line agents in children.
- Quinolones such as ciprofloxacin and moxifloxacin are effective in vitro, but more studies are needed for clinical use.

CHRONIC Rx

In the rare cases of endocarditis, combination of heart valve replacement and prolonged antibiotic course may be the treatment of choice.

DISPOSITION

- Mortality rate is low (0.7%)
- Poor prognostic factors:
  1. Advanced age
  2. Leukopenia
  3. Severe hypoxemia
  4. Renal failure
  5. Confusion
  6. Multilobe pulmonary involvement
- Possible reinfection

REFERRAL

- To infectious disease expert:
  1. Complicated atypical pneumonia or other end-organ involvement
  2. Suspicion of an outbreak
- To pulmonologist for diagnostic bronchoscopy

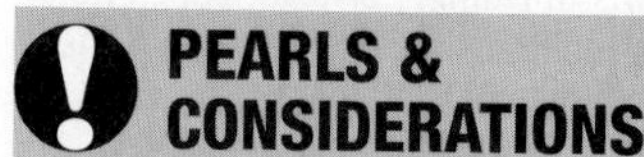

PEARLS & CONSIDERATIONS

COMMENTS

- Hospitalized patients do not require specific isolation precautions.
- Any confirmed or suspected case of psittacosis should be reported to public health authorities.
- Recent evidence indicates that *C. psittaci* may be associated with induction of a rare form of lymphoma found in the ocular adnexa; case reports have described regression of ocular lymphoma with antibiotic treatment for *C. psittaci*.

SUGGESTED READINGS

available at www.expertconsult.com

AUTHOR: **GLENN G. FORT, M.D., M.P.H.**

BASIC INFORMATION

DEFINITION

Psoriasis is a chronic skin disorder characterized by excessive proliferation of keratinocytes, resulting in the formation of thickened scaly plaques, itching, and inflammatory changes of the epidermis and dermis. The various forms of psoriasis include guttate, pustular, and arthritis variants.

ICD-9CM CODES

696.0 Psoriasis, arthritis, arthropathic
696.1 Psoriasis, any type except arthropathic

ICD-10CM CODES

L40	Psoriasis
L40.4	Guttate psoriasis
L40.1	Generalized pustular psoriasis
L40.8	Other psoriasis
L40.9	Psoriasis unspecified
L40.54	Psoriatic juvenile arthropathy
L40.0	Psoriasis vulgaris

EPIDEMIOLOGY & DEMOGRAPHICS

- Psoriasis affects 1% to 3% of the world's population. Most patients have limited psoriasis involving <5% of their body surface.
- There is a strong association between psoriasis and human leukocyte antigens (HLAs) B13, B17, and B27 (pustular psoriasis).
- Peak age of onset is bimodal (adolescents and at age 60 yr).
- Men and women are affected equally.

PHYSICAL FINDINGS & CLINICAL PRESENTATION

- Approximately 85% of patients with psoriasis have mild-to-moderate disease.
- The primary psoriatic lesion is an erythematous papule topped by a loosely adherent scale. Scraping the scale results in several bleeding points ***(Auspitz sign)***.
- Chronic plaque psoriasis generally manifests with symmetric, sharply demarcated, erythematous, silver-scaled patches affecting primarily the intergluteal folds, elbows, scalp, fingernails, toenails, and knees (Fig. 1-772). This form accounts for 80% of psoriasis cases.
- Psoriasis can also develop at the site of any physical trauma (sunburn, scratching). This is known as ***Koebner's phenomenon***.
- Nail involvement is common (pitting of the nail plate), resulting in hyperkeratosis, onychodystrophy with onycholysis.
- Pruritus is variable; soreness and bleeding may occur.
- Joint involvement can result in sacroiliitis and spondylitis.
- Guttate psoriasis is generally preceded by streptococcal pharyngitis and manifests with multiple droplike lesions on the extremities and the trunk.
- Adverse effect on psychological and social functioning, with affected persons often feeling stigmatized.

ETIOLOGY

- Unknown, but there is a strong genetic component and high heritability. There are at least nine chromosomal loci with linkage to psoriasis. These loci are called psoriasis susceptibility 1 through 9 (PSORS1-PSORS9). PSORS1 locus in the major histocompatibility complex (MHC) region on chromosome 6 is considered the most important susceptibility locus and is believed to account for 35% to 50% of the heritability of the disease.
- Familial clustering (genetic transmission with a dominant mode with variable penetrants).
- One third of persons affected have a positive family history.

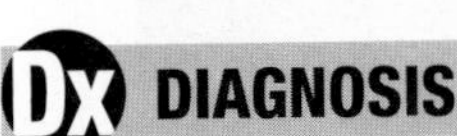

DIAGNOSIS

DIFFERENTIAL DIAGNOSIS

- Contact dermatitis
- Atopic dermatitis
- Stasis dermatitis
- Tinea
- Nummular dermatitis
- Candidiasis
- Mycosis fungoides
- Cutaneous systemic lupus erythematosus
- Secondary and tertiary syphilis
- Drug eruption

WORKUP

- Diagnosis is clinical. Blood work is rarely needed.
- Skin biopsy is rarely necessary.

LABORATORY TESTS

Generally not necessary for diagnosis

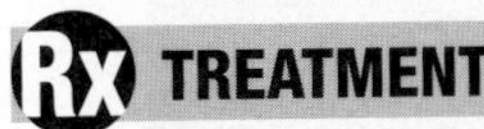

TREATMENT

NONPHARMACOLOGIC THERAPY

- Sunbathing generally leads to improvement.
- Eliminate triggering factors (e.g., stress, certain medications [e.g., lithium, beta-blockers, antimalarials]).
- Patients with psoriasis benefit from a daily bath in warm water followed by application of a cream or ointment moisturizer. Regular use of an emollient moisturizer limits evaporation of water from the skin and allows the stratum corneum to rehydrate itself.

GENERAL Rx

Therapeutic options vary according to the extent of disease. Approximately 70% to 80% of all patients can be treated adequately with topical therapy.

- Patients with limited disease (<20% of the body) can be treated with the following:
  1. Topical steroids: disadvantages are brief remissions, expense, and decreased effect with continued use. Salicylic acid can be compounded by pharmacist in concentrations of 2% to 10% and used in combination with a corticosteroid to decrease the amount of scale.
  2. Calcipotriene: a vitamin D analogue effective for moderate plaque psoriasis. Adults should comb the hair, apply solution to the lesions, and rub it in, avoiding uninvolved skin. Disadvantages include its cost and potential burning and skin irritation. It should not be used concurrently with salicylic acid because calcipotriene is inactivated by the acidic nature of salicylic acid. Taclonex ointment is a combination of calcipotriene and the high-potency corticosteroid betamethasone dipropionate. It is well tolerated and more effective than either agent used alone but also much more expensive.
  3. Tar products (Estar, LCD, Psorigel) can be used overnight and are most effective when combined with ultraviolet B (UVB) light (Goeckerman regimen).
  4. Anthralin: useful for chronic plaques; can result in purple-brown staining; best used with UVB light.
  5. Retinoids such as tazarotene 0.05%, 0.1% cream or gel, are effective in thinning plaques but are expensive and can cause irritation.
  6. Other useful measures include tape or occlusive dressing, UVB and lubricating agents, and interlesional steroids.
- Therapeutic options for persons with generalized disease (affecting >20% of the body) and for those with inadequate response to topical agents:
  1. UVB light exposure three times a week: this therapy does not require administration of a systemic drug (unlike psoralen plus ultraviolet A [PUVA]), but to be effective, it requires removal of scale with keratolytic agents and emollients.
  2. Oral PUVA administered two to three times weekly is effective for generalized disease. It is often considered in patients for whom narrow-band UVB therapy is ineffective. However, many PUVA treatments are required, necessitating frequent office visits, and it may be associated with phototoxicity, such as erythema and blistering, and increased risk of skin cancer.
- Systemic treatments include methotrexate 25 mg/wk for severe psoriasis. Etretinate (a synthetic retinoid) is most effective for palmar-plantar pustular psoriasis. Dose is 0.5 to 1 mg/kg/day. It can cause liver enzyme and lipid abnormalities and is teratogenic.
- Cyclosporine is also effective in severe psoriasis; however, relapses are common.
- Chronic plaque psoriasis may be treated with alefacept, a recombinant protein that selectively targets T lymphocytes. Treatment with alefacept for 12 wk (0.025, 0.075, or 0.150 mg/kg of body weight IV weekly) may result in significant improvement. Some patients also demonstrate a sustained clinical response after the cessation of treatment. This medication is very expensive (a 12-wk course costs >$8000).
- TNF inhibitors: Treatment with etanercept, a tumor necrosis factor (TNF) antagonist,

for 24 wk can also lead to a reduction in severity of plaque psoriasis. Efalizumab, a humanized monoclonal antibody that inhibits the activation of T cells, has also been reported to produce significant improvement in plaque psoriasis treatment period. Adalimumab—a fully human, anti-TNF-alpha monoclonal antibody—has been reported to be effective for joint and skin manifestations of psoriasis.

- Newer biologic agents in patients with moderate to severe plaque psoriasis are ustekinumab (an interleukin-12 and interleukin-23 blocker), brodalumab, an anti–interleukin-17 receptor antibody, and briakinumab, a monoclonal antibody against the p40 molecule shared by interleukin-12 and interleukin-23, which is overexpressed in psoriatic skin lesions. Trials have shown efficacy in the treatment of moderate-to-severe psoriasis.

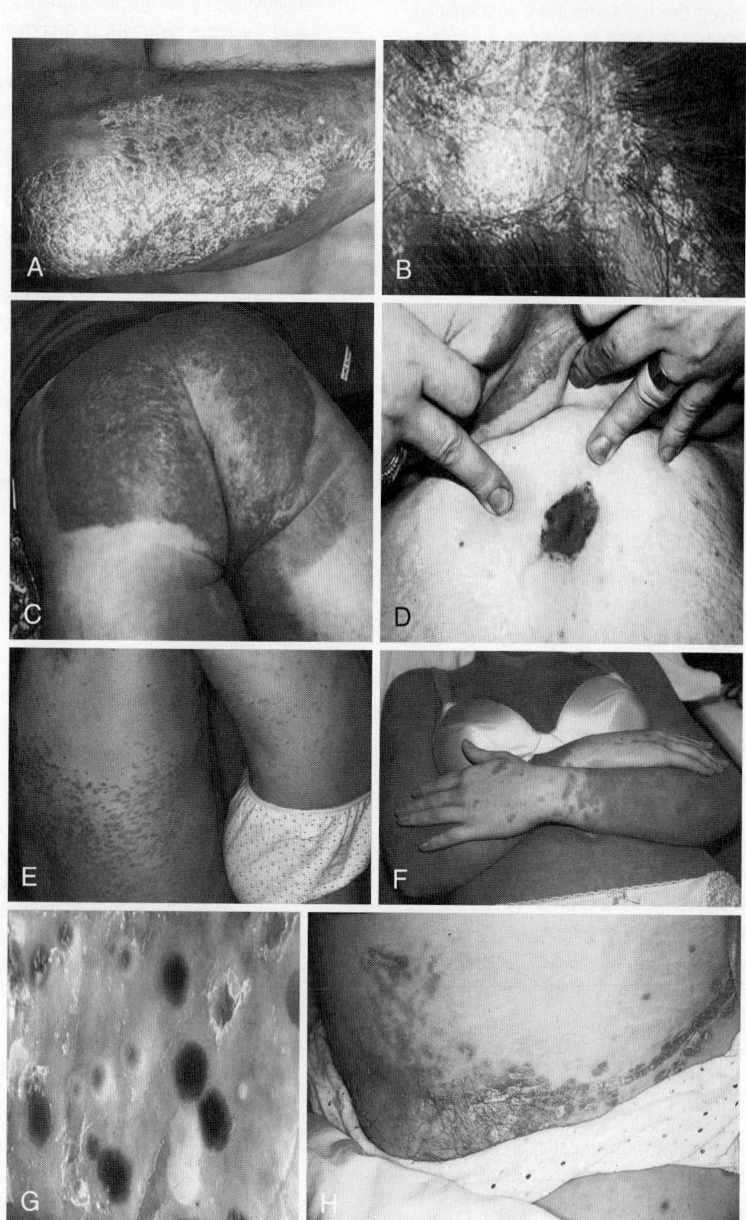

FIGURE 1-772 Clinical phenotypes in psoriasis: plaque psoriasis (psoriasis vulgaris). **A,** At extensor surface of elbow and on scalp (**B**). **C,** Genital psoriasis. **D,** Inframammary and umbilical flexural psoriasis. **E,** Guttate psoriasis in a father and child. **F,** Erythrodermic psoriasis on the trunk and upper limbs. **G,** Pustular psoriasis on the foot. **H,** The Koebner phenomenon on a surgical abdominal wound. (From Firestein GS et al: *Kelly's textbook of rheumatology,* ed 9, Philadelphia, 2013, Saunders.)

DISPOSITION

The course of psoriasis is chronic, and the disease may be refractory to treatment.

REFERRAL

- Dermatology referral is recommended in all patients with generalized disease.
- Hospital admission may be necessary for severe diffuse or poorly responsive psoriasis. The Goeckerman regimen combines daily application of tar with UVB exposure and can result in prolonged remissions.

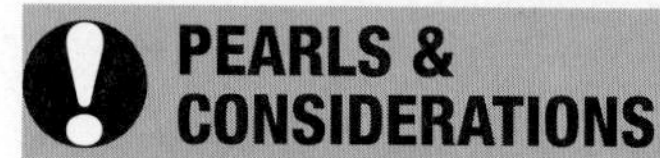

PEARLS & CONSIDERATIONS

COMMENTS

Psoriasis is more emotionally than physically disabling for most patients. Counseling may be indicated, particularly when it affects younger patients.

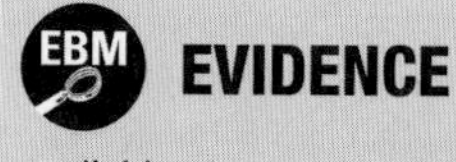

EVIDENCE

available at www.expertconsult.com

SUGGESTED READINGS

available at www.expertconsult.com

RELATED CONTENT

Psoriasis (Patient Information)

AUTHOR: **FRED F. FERRI, M.D.**

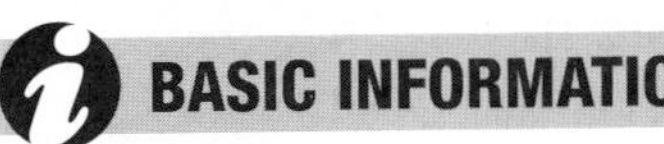

BASIC INFORMATION

DEFINITION

Psoriatic arthritis is an inflammatory arthropathy occurring in association with skin psoriasis and generally in the absence of rheumatoid factor (RF). It is often included in a class of disorders called the *seronegative spondyloarthropathies,* a family of diseases characterized by inflammation of the spine, peripheral joints, and enthesial sites (sites of insertion of tendon into bone). Classifications of psoriatic arthritis are described in Table 1-416.

ICD-9CM CODES
696.0 Psoriatic arthritis
ICD-10CM CODES
L40.5+ Arthropathic psoriasis
L40.54 Psoriatic juvenile arthropathy

EPIDEMIOLOGY & DEMOGRAPHICS

PREVALENCE: 0.1% to 0.2% overall, variable estimates of 7% to 30% of patients with psoriasis (psoriasis incidence varies by population but overall estimated prevalence of 1% to 2% of general population)

PREDOMINANT SEX: Equal male/female distribution of 1:1

PREDOMINANT AGE: Symptom onset generally age 30 to 55 yr

PHYSICAL FINDINGS & CLINICAL PRESENTATION

- Variably arthritis, dactylitis, spondylitis, and enthesitis occur in the setting of known psoriasis although joint symptoms may predate skin psoriasis in ~15% of patients.
    - Arthritis is inflammatory in nature, commonly characterized by prolonged morning stiffness, joint erythema, warmth, or swelling including joint effusions.
- Distribution of joint involvement follows five classically described patterns (Box 1-71).
- Often more than one classical pattern will occur simultaneously and patterns can evolve over time in an individual patient. Subtypes of psoriatic arthritis are described in Box 1-71.
- Dactylitis refers to diffuse swelling of a digit, either finger or toe, which is typically the result of inflammation in both small joints of the digit as well as associated tenosynovitis of digital tendons. Dactylitis is common in psoriatic arthritis and occurs in approximately 30% to 40% of patients during the course of disease.
- Enthesitis commonly occurs at the Achilles tendon insertion into the calcaneus as well as the insertion of the plantar fascia. Findings on physical exam may include swelling and tenderness.
- Dystrophic changes of the nails (pitting, onycholysis) may occur in association with joint inflammation in involved digits.
- Spondyloarthritis may include sacroiliitis as well as inflammation of the axial spine, but is generally less likely to cause contiguous fusion to the extent seen in ankylosing spondylitis.

ETIOLOGY

Unknown

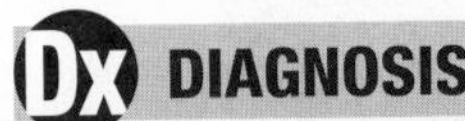

DIAGNOSIS

DIFFERENTIAL DIAGNOSIS

- Rheumatoid arthritis
- Erosive osteoarthritis
- Crystal arthritis including gout and pseudogout
- Other seronegative spondyloarthropathies, including reactive arthritis, enteropathic arthritis, and ankylosing spondylitis
- The differential diagnosis of spondyloarthropathies is described in Section III

WORKUP

- Diagnosis generally made on clinical grounds based on history, exam, and radiographic findings given lack of specific lab findings. An algorithm for the diagnosis of psoriatic arthritis is described in Fig. 1-773.
- Early diagnosis may be difficult to establish when the arthritis develops before skin lesions appear.

LABORATORY TESTS

- No specific/diagnostic lab tests
- Acute phase reactants such as ESR and CRP may be elevated although less commonly than in patients with rheumatoid arthritis.
- Anemia of chronic disease may be seen.
- RF, while generally negative, can be present in >10% of patients.
- *HLA B27* is significantly more common in patients with axial inflammation (note that *HLA B27* positivity is present in up to 8% of general population).
- Arthrocentesis of active joint generally demonstrates inflammatory synovial fluid and absence of crystals.

IMAGING STUDIES

- Radiographic findings (Fig. 1-774) of involved joints may include soft tissue swelling, joint space narrowing, subluxation, erosive changes, and new bone formation such as periostitis and fusion.
- Severe digital erosive change with adjacent heterotopic bone formation may give rise

BOX 1-71 Subtypes of Psoriatic Arthritis

Distal interphalangeal joint–predominant arthritis (10%) (Fig. 1-775)
Symmetric polyarthritis–predominant arthritis (5%-20%)
Asymmetric oligoarthritis or monoarthritis (70%-80%)
Axial disease–predominant (spondylitis and/or sacroiliitis) (5%-20%)
Arthritis mutilans (rare)

From Hochberg MC et al: *Rheumatology,* ed 5, St Louis, 2011, Mosby.

TABLE 1-416 Classifications of Psoriatic Arthritis

Moll and Wright	CLASSIFICATION CRITERIA FOR PSORIATIC ARTHRITIS (CASPAR)* Points	Category	Description
Presence of psoriasis and: 1) An inflammatory arthritis (peripheral arthritis and/or sacroiliitis or spondylitis) 2) The (usual) absence of serologic tests for rheumatoid factor	2	Current psoriasis or personal or family history of psoriasis	Psoriatic skin or scalp disease confirmed by dermatologist or rheumatologist; history of psoriasis from patient, family physician, dermatologist, rheumatologist, or other qualified practitioner; patient-reported history of psoriasis in first- or second-degree relative
	1	Psoriatic nail dystrophy on current physical examination	Includes onycholysis, pitting, and hyperkeratosis
	1	Negative for rheumatoid factor	Enzyme-linked immunosorbent assay or nephelometry preferred (no latex) using local laboratory reference range
	1	Current dactylitis or history of dactylitis documented by a rheumatologist	Swelling of entire digit
	1	Radiographic evidence of juxta-articular new bone formation	Ill-defined ossification near joint margins excluding osteophyte formation on plain radiographs of hand or foot

*Psoriatic arthritis is diagnosed when ≥3 points are assigned in the presence of inflammatory articular disease (joint, spine, or entheseal).
From Hochberg MC et al: Rheumatology, ed 5, St Louis, 2011, Mosby.

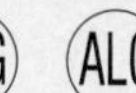

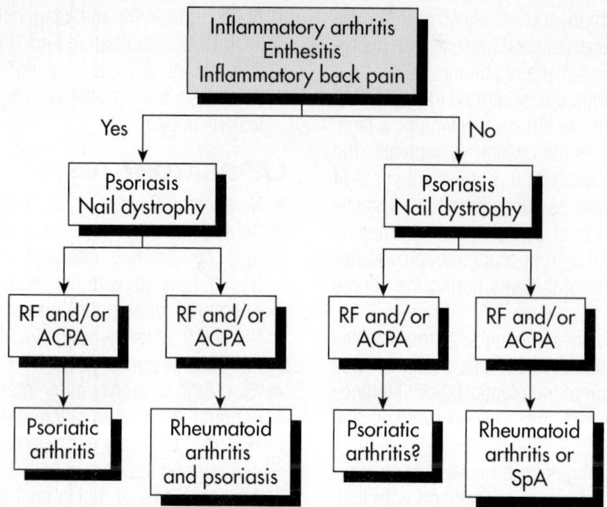

FIGURE 1-773 Algorithm to be used in the diagnosis of individual patients presenting with possible psoriatic arthritis. Some patients may present with typical articular manifestations of psoriatic arthritis, but in the absence of skin or nail disease. They can be diagnosed as having definite psoriatic arthritis only when psoriasis subsequently develops. *ACPA,* Anticitrullinated protein antibody; *RF,* rheumatoid factor; *SpA,* spondyloarthropathy. (Firestein GS et al: *Kelly's textbook of rheumatology,* ed 9, Philadelphia, 2013, Saunders.)

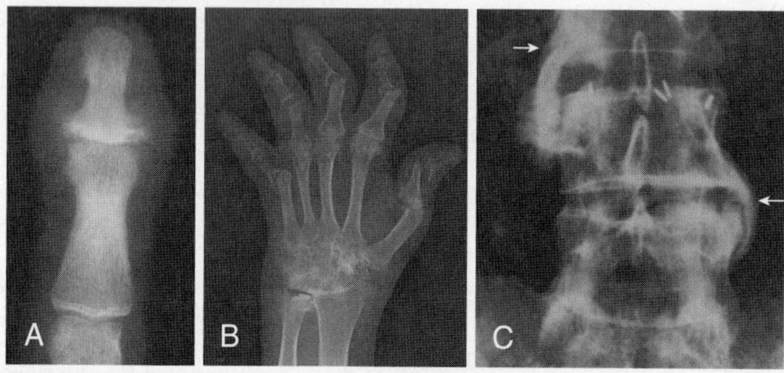

FIGURE 1-774 Psoriatic arthritis (x-ray). **A,** Distal interphalangeal joint with classic radiographic findings, including soft tissue swelling, bone erosions with accompanying bone proliferation, and lack of osteoporosis. **B,** Arthritis mutilans resulting from psoriatic arthritis with destructive changes and joint deformity of the hand and pancompartmental ankylosis of the wrist. **C,** Psoriatic spondylitis. Thick asymmetric paravertebral ossifications (*arrows*), which are characteristic of psoriatic spondylitis and reactive arthritis. (From Resnick D, Niwayama G: *Diagnosis of bone and joint disorders,* Philadelphia, 1988, WB Saunders.)

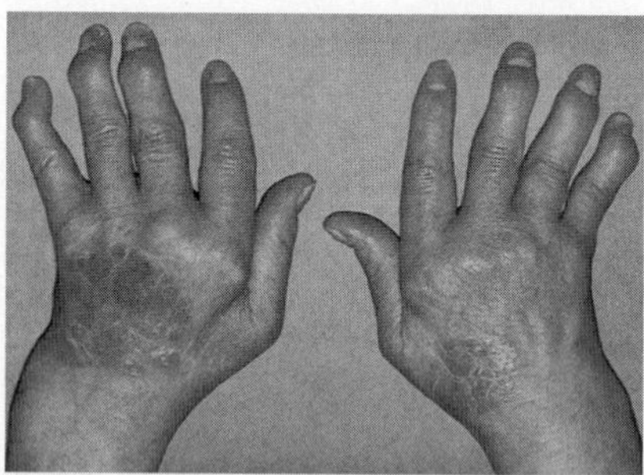

FIGURE 1-775 The hands of a woman with symmetric polyarthritis. Initially, this was indistinguishable from rheumatoid disease, but note the distal interphalangeal joint involvement, which is uncommon in rheumatoid arthritis, as well as the skin psoriasis. (From Klippel J et al [eds]: *Primary care rheumatology,* London, 1999, Mosby.)

to "pencil in cup" deformity seen in arthritis mutilans.

- Findings in patients with spondylitis may include sacroiliitis and development of vertebral syndesmophytes that often bridge adjacent vertebral bodies.
- Musculoskeletal ultrasound may be helpful in the evaluation of an inflamed enthesis or joint.
- MRI may be helpful in the evaluation of sacroiliitis or spinal involvement.

Rx TREATMENT

ACUTE GENERAL Rx

- NSAIDs may be used for mild symptoms or limited involvement.
- Intraarticular corticosteroid injections can be used as adjunctive therapy in involved joints.

CHRONIC Rx

- NSAIDs for mild or limited disease
- In patients with several sites of active peripheral disease, elevated acute phase reactants, or with evidence of erosive changes on imaging, traditional DMARDs such as methotrexate, sulfasalazine, and leflunamide should be considered early in disease.
- In patients with peripheral arthritis who fail to respond to traditional DMARD therapy, additional therapy with a tumor necrosis factor (TNF) inhibitor should be considered.
- In patients with predominant axial disease not responsive to NSAIDs, anti-TNF therapy should be considered for initial disease-modifying therapy.
- Enthesitis and dactylitis are poorly responsive to oral DMARD therapy but like spondylitis will often respond to anti-TNF therapy.

REFERRAL

Rheumatology for confirmation of diagnosis and management

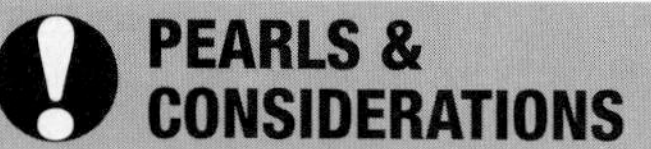

PEARLS & CONSIDERATIONS

- Patients frequently have a positive family history of psoriasis or psoriatic arthritis.
- Severity of skin psoriasis and activity of inflammatory arthritis are frequently discordant.

SUGGESTED READINGS

available at www.expertconsult.com

RELATED CONTENT

Psoriatic Arthritis (Patient Information)

AUTHOR: **HARALD A. HALL, M.D.**

BASIC INFORMATION

DEFINITION

Psychosis is a state in which external reality is distorted by delusions and/or hallucinations (a delusion is a fixed false idiosyncratic belief; a hallucination is a false auditory, visual, olfactory, tactile, or taste perception).

SYNONYMS

Psychosis is a key finding in many mental illnesses, such as brief psychotic disorder, delusional disorder, schizoaffective disorder, schizophrenia, schizophreniform disorder, or shared psychotic disorder. Psychosis can also present as part of the evolution of a mood disorder (depression and bipolar disorder), a sign of an underlying medical condition, or a manifestation of a toxic state, i.e., abuse of substances or withdrawal state.

ICD-10CM CODES

F09	Unspecified organic or symptomatic mental disorder
F10.5	Psychotic disorder due to psychoactive substance use
F05	Delirium not induced by alcohol and other psychoactive substances
F06.0	Organic hallucinosis
F32.3	Major depressive disorder, single episode, severe with psychotic features

EPIDEMIOLOGY & DEMOGRAPHICS

One-year prevalence: 4.5 per 1000. The demographics of psychosis depends on the underlying disorder.

PHYSICAL FINDINGS & CLINICAL PRESENTATION

History:

- Past and current medical history important to identify potential medical etiologies
- Medication use
- Use of illicit substances or alcohol
- Identification of functional and social impairment
- Behavior that is odd or unpredictable; patient may be acting based on misinterpretation of their reality or false perceptions (delusions or hallucinations)

Examination:

- Examine for symptoms of:
  - Mood disorder: delusions or hallucinations are usually congruent with the mood (e.g., auditory hallucinations in a depressed patient may tell the patient what a terrible person he is)
  - Altered or disorganized thought pattern: usually reflected in disorganized speech (including word salad, thought blocking, rhyming, clang associations)
  - Lack of insight into problems
  - Signs of Parkinson's disease, dementia

ETIOLOGY

- Involves an interaction among:
  1. Dopaminergic overactivity (particularly in the mesolimbic, nigrostriatal, and mesocortical systems)
  2. Environmental, social, or childhood factors
  3. Genetic predisposition

Dx DIAGNOSIS

WORKUP

- Evaluate for potential confounding factors. Fig. E1-776 describes an algorithmic approach to evaluation of the psychotic patient.
- Underlying mental disorder: schizophrenia, major depression, brief psychotic disorder, delusional disorder, schizoaffective disorder, schizophreniform disorder
- Underlying personality disorder: borderline, paranoid, schizoid, schizotypal
- Underlying medical conditions: infections ranging from UTIs to HIV/AIDS, Parkinson's disease, Huntington's disease, leprosy, malaria, sarcoidosis, systemic lupus erythematosus, prion disease, hypoglycemia, postpartum state, cerebrovascular event, temporal lobe epilepsy, brain neoplasm
- Medications: systemic steroids, anticonvulsants, antiparkinsonian medications, some chemotherapy, scopolamine
- Underlying dementia: Alzheimer's disease, Lewy body dementia, vascular dementia
- Illicit drugs (usually with chronic use; can be caused by intoxication or withdrawal): LSD, PCP, cocaine, gamma-hydroxybutyrate (GHB; withdrawal), alcohol, amphetamines, marijuana. New substances of abuse (e.g., "bath salts", synthetic cannabinoids) may not be detected by current toxicology panels.
- Traumatic brain injury
- Intensive care unit stay: hypoxia, decreased cardiac output, infection, medications, sleep deprivation, alteration of diurnal cycle, sensory deprivation or overload, pain
- Emotional stress

LABORATORY TESTS

Consider checking chemistry panel (calcium), complete blood count, UA, liver function tests, cortisol, HIV, rapid plasma reagin, thyroid-stimulating hormone, toxicology screen, lumbar puncture (LP).

IMAGING STUDIES

Consider chest x-ray (rule out sarcoid), electroencephalography, head CT or MRI.

Rx TREATMENT

NONPHARMACOLOGIC THERAPY

- Cognitive-behavioral therapy
- Social and behavioral skills training
- Training for self-management of disease
- Aforementioned strategies favored over psychoanalytic techniques given the relative inability for abstract thought and lack of insight in psychotic patients
- Family intervention, including education and strategies to reduce emotional expression
- Counseling for substance abuse

ACUTE GENERAL Rx

- Antipsychotics, such as haloperidol combined with anticholinergics like benztropine to reduce side effects; low doses should control first episode. Use with caution in elderly patients because adverse effects limit effectiveness. Second-generation antipsychotics are also useful starting with low doses. Newer formulations are available in rapid injectable form or oral disintegrating tablets.
- Benzodiazepines if agitation is severe
- Discontinue offending medication if present.

CHRONIC Rx

Second-generation antipsychotics may reduce the incidence of tardive dyskinesia but may increase incidence of metabolic disorders compared with first-generation antipsychotics. Multicenter trials showed similar efficacy between first and second generation. Consider economic, including insurance formulary, factors when selecting a maintenance regimen.

DISPOSITION

Prognosis varies according to etiology of psychosis. In general, the more severe and longer the psychotic episode, the worse the prognosis.

REFERRAL

Patient should be admitted for acute stabilization if actively psychotic to prevent harm to self and others as well as ensure administration of medications.

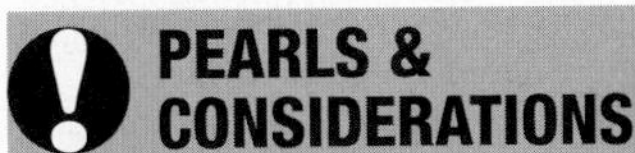

PEARLS & CONSIDERATIONS

- Delusions and/or hallucinations are hallmarks of psychosis.
- Rule out medical or drug causes of psychosis.
- Antipsychotics are the mainstay of acute and chronic treatment.
- Consider alternatives to antipsychotics in elderly or intellectually disabled patients (see "Nonpharmacologic Therapy").

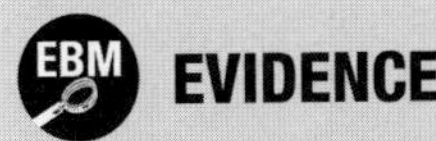

EVIDENCE

available at www.expertconsult.com

SUGGESTED READINGS

available at www.expertconsult.com

RELATED CONTENT

Psychosis (Patient Information)
Delirium (Related Key Topic)

AUTHORS: **ARNOLDO A. BERGES, M.D., RICHARD J. GOLDBERG, M.D., M.S.,** and **MICHAEL K. ONG, M.D., PH.D.**

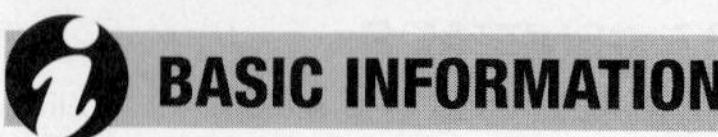

BASIC INFORMATION

DEFINITION

Acute cardiogenic pulmonary edema (ACPE) is a life-threatening condition that may occur when there is elevated left ventricular (LV) filling pressure related to systolic or diastolic LV dysfunction.

SYNONYMS

Cardiogenic pulmonary edema
Acute cardiogenic pulmonary edema
ACPE Acute heart failure [AHF] with pulmonary edema

ICD-9CM CODES
428.1 Acute pulmonary edema with heart disease
ICD-10CM CODES
I50.1 Left ventricular failure

EPIDEMIOLOGY & DEMOGRAPHICS

- Leading cause of hospitalization (6.5 million hospital days in the U.S. each year)
- In-hospital mortality rate is 10% to 20%, particularly when associated with acute MI.

PHYSICAL FINDINGS & CLINICAL PRESENTATION

- Dyspnea (exertional, paroxysmal nocturnal dyspnea, orthopnea, or at rest)
- Cough and wheezing
- Diaphoresis, perioral and peripheral cyanosis
- Pink, frothy sputum
- Moist, bilateral pulmonary rales are the most common findings and noted in up to 87% of the patients
- Increased pulmonary second sound, S_3 gallop. S3 gallop is present in up to one-third of the patients and correlates well with the degree of LV systolic dysfunction and BNP levels.
- Hypertension (unless in cardiogenic shock and hypotensive)
- Tachycardia
- Bulging neck veins with elevated jugular venous pressure and positive hepatojugular reflex
- Altered mental status or drowsiness due to hypoperfusion
- Peripheral edema

ETIOLOGY

Increased pulmonary capillary pressure attributable to:
- Acute myocardial infarction
- Exacerbation of chronic congestive heart failure due to poor dietary or medical compliance, use of concomitant nonsteroidal anti-inflammatory drugs, calcium antagonists such as verapamil and diltiazem, excessive alcohol consumption, anemia or inadequately treated hypertension
- Valvular regurgitation (e.g., mitral regurgitation)
- Ventricular septal defect
- Severe myocardial ischemia
- Mitral stenosis
- Other: cardiac tamponade, endocarditis, myocarditis, arrhythmias, cardiomyopathy, hypertensive crisis, endocrine abnormalities such as thyrotoxicosis

Dx DIAGNOSIS

DIFFERENTIAL DIAGNOSIS

- Noncardiogenic pulmonary edema (see Fig. 1-777)
- Pulmonary embolism
- Exacerbation of asthma
- Exacerbation of chronic obstructive pulmonary disease
- Sarcoidosis
- Pulmonary fibrosis
- Lymphangitic carcinomatosis
- Pulmonary fibrosis
- Viral pneumonitis and other pulmonary infections

LABORATORY TESTS

- Arterial blood gases (ABGs): respiratory and metabolic acidosis, decreased Pa_{O_2}, increased Pa_{CO_2}, low pH. (NOTE: The patient may initially show respiratory alkalosis as a result of hyperventilation in attempts to maintain Pa_{O_2}.)
- Measurement of plasma brain natriuretic peptide (elevated). The Breathing Not Properly [BNP] Multinational Study demonstrated that elevated BNP levels are able to distinguish dyspnea caused by heart failure from those caused by pulmonary disease. The BASEL study with nt-pro-BNP demonstrated similar results in patients presenting with acute dyspnea.
- Cardiac biomarkers: troponin I levels to evaluate for possible acute myocardial infarction.
- Basic chemistries: hyponatremia is common in chronic heart failure; evaluate renal function.

IMAGING STUDIES

- ECG:
  1. May have evidence of ischemia, arrhythmias, or LV hypertrophy (often seen in diastolic dysfunction)
- Chest x-ray (Fig. 1-778):
  1. Pulmonary congestion with Kerley B lines; fluffy perihilar infiltrates in the early stages; bilateral interstitial alveolar infiltrates
  2. Pleural effusions
  3. Enlarged cardiac silhouette
- Echocardiogram:
  1. Useful to evaluate valvular abnormalities, diastolic versus systolic dysfunction
  2. Can help differentiate cardiogenic versus noncardiogenic pulmonary edema
  3. Can also estimate pulmonary capillary wedge pressure using E/E' ratio, where E = early diastolic transmitral blood flow velocity and E' = early diastolic mitral annular tissue velocity.
- Right heart catheterization (RHC): May be used in selected patients such as those in shock or unclear hemodynamics. RHC in pulmonary edema will show increased pulmonary artery diastolic pressure and pulmonary capillary wedge pressure (PCWP) generally ≥25 mm Hg; low mixed venous oxyhemoglobin saturation. In the ESCAPE trial, use of RHC did not significantly affect in-hospital or 6 mo mortality or days of hospitalization compared to clinical assessment alone and was related to more adverse events.

Signs	Cardiac	Renal	Lung Injury
Heart size	Enlarged	Normal	Normal
Blood flow	Inverted	Balanced	Normal
Kerley lines	Common	Common	Absent
Edema	Basilar	Central: butterfly	Diffuse
Air bronchograms	Not common	Not common	Very common
Pleural effusions	Very common	Common	Not common

FIGURE 1-777 Types of pulmonary edema. (From Weissleder R et al: *Primer of diagnostic imaging,* St Louis, 2007, Mosby.)

P

Diseases and Disorders

I

TREATMENT

ACUTE GENERAL Rx

All the following steps can be performed concomitantly:

- 100% oxygen by face mask. Noninvasive ventilation (continuous positive airway pressure [CPAP]) or bilevel noninvasive positive-pressure ventilation [NPPV]) reduces dyspnea and corrects metabolic abnormalities more rapidly than does standard oxygen therapy, and may reduce the need for endotracheal intubation. Both CPAP and bilevel NPPV systems can improve oxygenation and lower carbon dioxide tensions. Monitor ABGs; if marked hypoxemia or severe respiratory acidosis, intubate the patient and place on a mechanical ventilator. Positive pressure ventilation (invasive or noninvasive) decreases preload and afterload and reduces the work of breathing, while positive end expiratory pressure improves oxygenation.
- Pharmacologic preload reducers:
  1. Furosemide: 1 mg/kg IV bolus (typically 40 to 100 mg) to rapidly establish diuresis and decrease venous return through its venodilator action; may double the dose in 30 min if no effect. As per the DOSE trial (NEJM March 3, 2011), among patients with acute decompensated heart failure, there were no significant differences in patients' global assessment of symptoms or in the change in renal function when diuretic therapy was administered by bolus as compared with continuous infusion or at a high dose as compared with a low dose
  2. Nitrates: particularly useful if the patient has concomitant chest pain or is hypertensive.
     a. Nitroglycerin: 150 to 600 mcg SL or nitroglycerin spray may be given immediately on arrival and repeated multiple times if the patient remains symptomatic and blood pressure remains stable.
     b. 2% nitroglycerin ointment: 1 to 3 inches out of the tube applied continuously; absorption may be erratic.
     c. IV nitroglycerin: 100 mg in 500 ml of D_5W solution; start at 6 mcg/min (2 ml/hr).
  3. Morphine: 2 to 4 mg IV, SC, or IM; may repeat q15min prn. It decreases venous return, anxiety, and systemic vascular resistance (naloxone should be available at bedside to reverse the effects of morphine if respiratory depression occurs). However, potential adverse effects of morphine administration may outweigh these physiologic benefits, and the role of morphine in treatment of ACPE has recently been questioned.
- Vasodilator therapy:
  1. Angiotensin-converting enzyme (ACE) inhibitors: captopril 25 mg PO tablet can be used for SL administration (placing a drop or two of water on the tablet and placing it under the tongue helps dissolve it); onset of action is <10 min, peak effect can be reached in 30 min. ACE inhibitors can also be given IV (e.g., enalapril at 1 mg IV given q2h prn).
  2. Nitroprusside: useful for afterload reduction in hypertensive patients with decreased cardiac index (CI).
     a. Increases the CI and decreases LV filling pressure.
     b. Nitroprusside use in patients with acute myocardial infarction is controversial because it may increase ischemia by decreasing blood flow to the myocardium.
  3. Nesiritide (recombinant human BNP) causes potent vasodilation in the venous and arterial vessels, including coronary vasculature, produces significant reduction in venous and ventricular filling pressures, and mildly increases cardiac output. However, its high cost and potential safety concerns, including increased mortality, have limited its use.
- Inotropes:
  1. Dobutamine: parenteral inotropic agent of choice in severe cases of cardiogenic pulmonary edema. It can be administered at a dosage of 2.5 to 10 mcg/kg/min IV.
  2. IV phosphodiesterase inhibitors (amrinone, milrinone, and enoximone [available only in Europe]) may be useful in refractory cases. Milrinone may be associated with increased hypotension and new atrial arrhythmias with increased mortality in patients with ischemia HF and should be used with caution.
- Levosimendan is a novel agent that increases myocardial contractility and produces peripheral vasodilation through calcium sensitization. In clinical trials such as REVIVE-II and SURVIVE, levosimendan has been shown to significantly increase cardiac output, reduce PCWP and afterload, and improve dyspnea compared to standard care. It has however been associated with increased atrial fibrillation and hypotension.
- Potential future therapies: Istaroxime, natriuretic peptides, adenosine antagonists, vasopressin antagonists, endothelin antagonists.
- Mechanical support:
  1. Intra-arterial Balloon Pump (IABP): decreases afterload
  2. Ultrafiltration/Aquapheresis

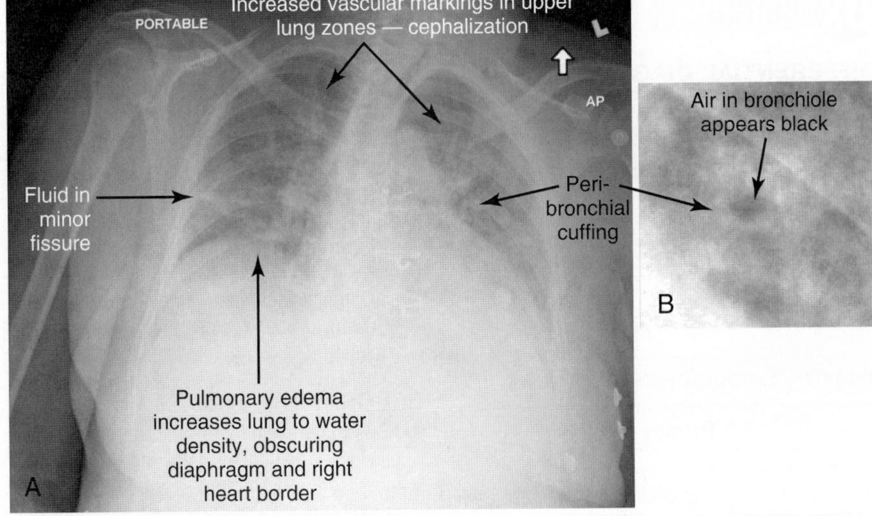

FIGURE 1-778 Pulmonary edema. A, Anterior-posterior chest x-ray. **B,** Close-up from **A.** This 53-year-old female with end-stage renal disease missed dialysis and presented to the emergency department. Her examination demonstrated bilateral rales. Her x-ray shows mild cardiomegaly, bilateral interstitial opacities, and cephalization of the pulmonary vascular markings. The minor fissure appears thickened. These findings are consistent with pulmonary edema. In addition, peribronchial cuffing is present. As discussed elsewhere, this is a nonspecific thickening of the bronchial wall that can occur from edema in the setting of heart failure, asthma, viral illness, or even infections such as pertussis. The thickened wall appears white, whereas the air-filled bronchiole appears black and has a circular short-axis cross section. (From Broder JS: *Diagnostic imaging for the emergency physician,* Philadelphia, 2011, Saunders.)

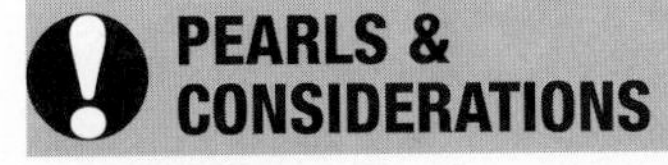

PEARLS & CONSIDERATIONS

COMMENTS

Accumulated evidence still favors the use of noninvasive ventilation, especially CPAP, in patients with ACPE, especially as this therapy reduces dyspnea and helps correct metabolic abnormalities more rapidly than standard oxygen therapy. The role of morphine in the treatment of ACPE has come into question. Also refer to section on Heart Failure.

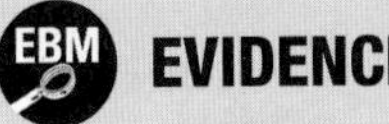

EVIDENCE

available at www.expertconsult.com

SUGGESTED READINGS

available at www.expertconsult.com

AUTHORS: **MARC PAUL WAASE, M.D., Ph.D.,** and **VEERANNA MERLA, M.D.**

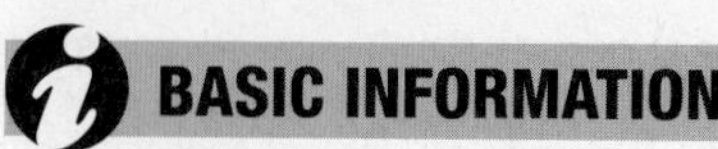

BASIC INFORMATION

DEFINITION

Pulmonary embolism (PE) refers to the lodging of a thrombus or other embolic material from a distant site in the pulmonary circulation. A classification of acute pulmonary embolism is described in Table 1-417.

SYNONYMS

Pulmonary thromboembolism
PE

ICD-9CM CODES
415.1 Pulmonary embolism and infarction
ICD-10CM CODES
I26 Pulmonary embolism
I26.0 Pulmonary embolism with acute cor pulmonale

EPIDEMIOLOGY & DEMOGRAPHICS

- 650,000 cases of PE occur in the U.S. each year (increased incidence in women and with advanced age); annually, as many as 300,000 people in the U.S. die from acute PE, and the diagnosis is often not made until after autopsy. The incidence of PE is increasing with the increasing use of spiral CT scans, with a lower severity of illness and lower mortality, suggesting the increase is caused by earlier diagnosis.
- More than 90% of pulmonary emboli originate in the deep venous system of the lower extremities.
- Pulmonary thromboembolism is associated with >200,000 hospitalizations each yr in the U.S.
- 8% to 10% of victims of PE die within the first hr.

PHYSICAL FINDINGS & CLINICAL PRESENTATION

- Most common symptom: dyspnea (82% to 85%)
- Tachypnea (30% to 60%)
- Chest pain: may be nonpleuritic or pleuritic (infarction) (40% to 49%)
- Syncope (massive PE) (10% to 14%)
- Fever, diaphoresis, apprehension
- Hemoptysis (2%)
- Evidence of DVT may be present (e.g., swelling and tenderness of extremities)
- Cardiac examination may reveal: tachycardia (23%), increased pulmonic component of S2, murmur of tricuspid insufficiency, right ventricular heave, right-sided S3
- Pulmonary examination: may demonstrate rales, localized wheezing, friction rub

ETIOLOGY

- Thrombus, fat, or other foreign material
- Risk factors for PE:
  1. Prolonged immobilization, reduced mobility
  2. Postoperative state, major surgery
  3. Trauma to lower extremities, immobilizer, or cast
  4. Estrogen-containing birth control pills, hormone replacement therapy
  5. Prior history of DVT or PE
  6. CHF
  7. Pregnancy and early puerperium
  8. Visceral cancer (lung, pancreas, alimentary and genitourinary tracts)
  9. Spinal cord injury
  10. Advanced age
  11. Obesity
  12. Hematologic disease (e.g., factor V Leiden mutation, antithrombin III deficiency, protein C deficiency, protein S deficiency, lupus anticoagulant, polycythemia vera, dysfibrinogenemia, paroxysmal nocturnal hemoglobinuria, acquired protein C resistance without factor V Leiden, G20210A prothrombin mutation)
  13. COPD, diabetes mellitus, acute medical illness
  14. Prolonged air travel
  15. Central venous catheterization
  16. Autoimmune diseases (SLE, IBD, RA)

Dx DIAGNOSIS

DIFFERENTIAL DIAGNOSIS

- Myocardial infarction
- Pericarditis
- Pneumonia
- Pneumothorax
- Chest wall pain
- GI abnormalities (e.g., peptic ulcer, esophageal rupture, gastritis)
- CHF
- Pleuritis
- Anxiety disorder with hyperventilation
- Pericardial tamponade
- Dissection of aorta
- Asthma

WORKUP

- Clinical assessment alone is insufficient to diagnose or rule out PE. It is also important to remember that no single noninvasive test has both high sensitivity and high specificity for PE. Consequently, in addition to clinical assessment, most patients require an imaging test to diagnose PE. Figs. 1-779 and E1-780 are diagnostic algorithms for suspected PE. The Wells prediction rules can be used to estimate the probability of PE. Each of the following findings is assigned a score:
  1. Clinical signs/symptoms of deep vein thrombosis (score = 3.0)
  2. No alternate diagnosis as likely or more likely than PE (score = 3.0)
  3. Heart rate >100/min (score = 1.5)
  4. Immobilization or surgery in last 4 weeks (score = 1.5)
  5. Previous history of DVT or PE (score = 1.5)
  6. Hemoptysis (score = 1.0)
  7. Cancer actively treated within last 6 months (score = 1.0)
- The probability of PE is high if total score is >6, moderate if 2-6; and low if <2.
- The modified Wells score divides PE as likely (>4 points) or unlikely (<4 points)
- A low clinical probability of PE in association with a normal plasma D-dimer measurement essentially rules out PE, and further imaging is not needed. If clinical probability is intermediate or high, and/or the D-dimer measurement is abnormal, further workup with imaging is needed.
- Spiral chest CT with contrast (see Fig. 1-781) is an excellent diagnostic modality (83% sensitivity and 96% specificity).
- V/Q scan is reserved for patients with clinically significant contrast allergies or renal insufficiency.
- Pulmonary angiogram (gold standard) can confirm the diagnosis, but is rarely used.
- Serial compressive duplex ultrasonography of lower extremities can be used in patients with "low-probability" lung scan and high clinical suspicion (see "Imaging Studies"). It is useful if positive; negative results do not exclude PE.

LABORATORY TESTS

- ABGs may reveal hypoxemia and respiratory alkalosis (decreased Pa_{O_2} and Pa_{CO_2} and increased pH); normal results do not rule out PE.
- Alveolar-arteriolar (A-a) oxygen gradient, a measure of the difference in oxygen concentration between alveoli and arterial blood, may be elevated. However, a normal A-a gradient does not rule out PE.
- Plasma D-dimer measurement: D-dimer assays by ELISA detect the presence of plasmin-mediated degradation products of

TABLE 1-417 Classification of Acute Pulmonary Embolism

Classification	Presentation	Therapy
Massive PE	Systolic blood pressure <90 mm Hg or poor tissue perfusion or multisystem organ failure plus right or left main pulmonary artery thrombus or "high clot burden"	Thrombolysis or embolectomy or inferior vena caval filter plus anticoagulation
Submassive PE	Hemodynamically stable but moderate or severe right ventricular dysfunction or enlargement	Addition of thrombolysis, embolectomy, or filter remains controversial
Small to moderate PE	Normal hemodynamics and normal right ventricular size and function	Anticoagulation

From Bonow RO et al: *Heart disease*, ed 9, Philadelphia, 2012 ,Saunders.

fibrin that contain cross-linked D fragments in the whole blood or plasma. A normal plasma D-dimer level is useful to exclude PE in patients with a low pretest probability of PE. However, it cannot be used to "rule in" the diagnosis because it increases with many other disorders (e.g., metastatic cancer, trauma, sepsis, postoperative state). Plasma D-dimer can also be used in conjunction with lower-extremity compression ultrasonography in patients with indeterminate V/Q and spiral CT scans. Absence of DVT and presence of a normal D-dimer level in these settings generally rules out clinically significant PE.

- Elevated cardiac troponin levels also occur in patients with PE because of right ventricular dilation and myocardial injury; therefore, PE should be considered in the differential diagnosis of all patients presenting with chest pain or dyspnea and elevated cardiac troponin levels.
- Elevated serum BNP levels in patients with acute PE may reflect RV overload.
- ECG is abnormal in 85% of patients with acute PE. Frequent abnormalities are sinus tachycardia; nonspecific ST-segment or T-wave changes; S-1, Q-3, T-3 pattern (10% of patients); S-1, S-2, S-3 pattern; T-wave inversion in V_1 to V_6; acute RBBB; new-onset atrial fibrillation; ST segment depression in lead II; right ventricular strain. A right ventricular strain pattern on ECG in patients with PE and normal blood pressure is associated with adverse short-term outcome and adds incremental prognostic value to echocardiographic evidence of right ventricular function.

IMAGING STUDIES

- Chest x-ray may be normal; suggestive findings include elevated diaphragm, pleural effusion, dilation of pulmonary artery, infiltrate or consolidation, abrupt vessel cut-off, oligemia distal to the PE (**Westermark sign**), or atelectasis. A wedge-shaped consolidation in the middle and lower lobes is suggestive of a pulmonary infarction and is known as "**Hampton's hump**."
- CT angiography is an accurate, noninvasive tool in the diagnosis of PE at the main, lobar, and segmental pulmonary artery levels. A major advantage of CT angiography over standard pulmonary angiography is its ability to diagnose intrathoracic disease other than PE that may account for the patient's clinical picture. It is also less invasive, less costly, and more widely available. Its major shortcoming is its poor sensitivity for subsegmental emboli.
- Lung scan (in patient with normal chest x-ray examination):
  1. A normal lung scan rules out PE.
  2. A ventilation-perfusion mismatch is suggestive of PE, and a lung scan interpretation of high probability is confirmatory (Fig. 1-782).
  3. If the clinical suspicion of PE is high and the lung scan is interpreted as low probability, moderate probability, or indeterminate, a pulmonary arteriogram is diagnostic; a positive arteriogram confirms diagnosis; a positive compressive duplex ultrasonography for DVT obviates the need for an arteriogram, because treatment with IV anticoagulants is indicated in these patients; the overall sensitivity of compressive ultrasonography for DVT in patients with PE is 29%, specificity 97%; adding ultrasonography in patients with

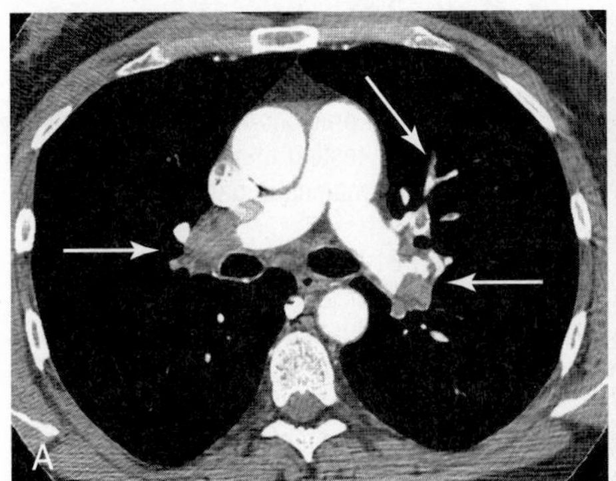

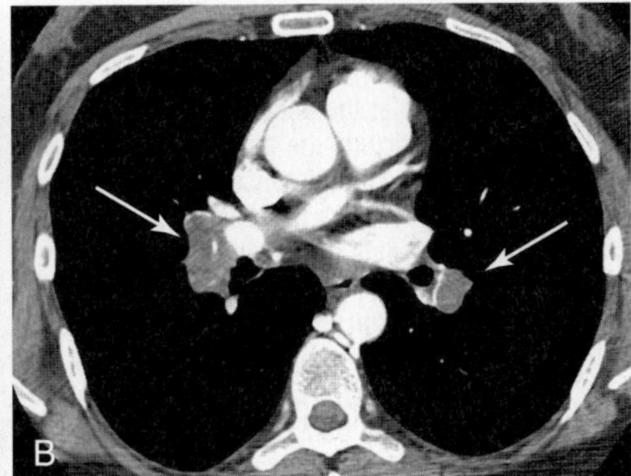

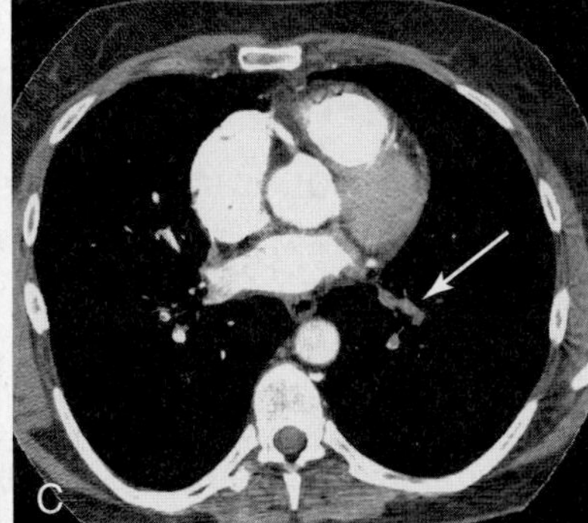

FIGURE 1-781 A 46-year-old woman presented with acute shortness of breath and hypoxia. Chest radiograph was normal. **A,** Chest computed tomography shows a low-attenuation filling defect in left and right main pulmonary arteries *(arrows)* and left upper lobe segmental artery *(arrow)*, representing massive pulmonary embolism. Emboli extend to left and right interlobar arteries (*arrows*), as well as a left lower lobe segmental artery *(arrow)*, seen in **B** and **C,** respectively. (From Vincent JL et al: *Textbook of critical care,* ed 6, Philadelphia, 2011, Saunders.)

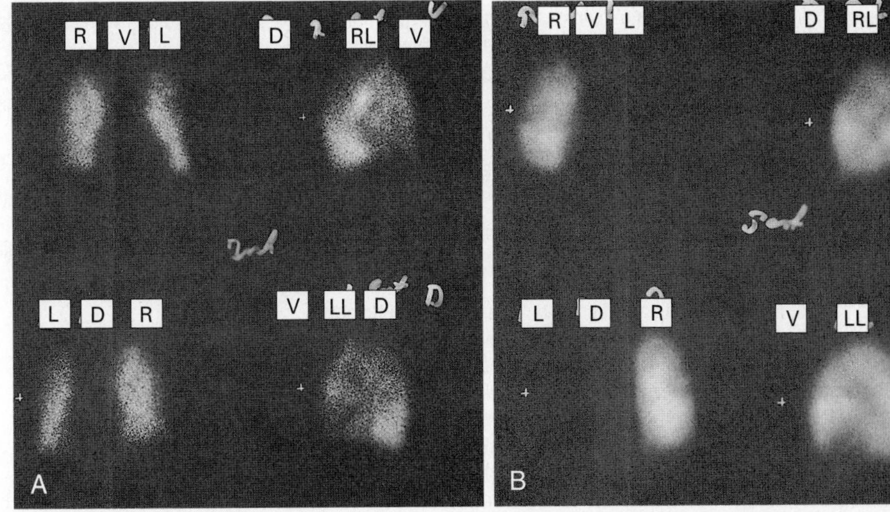

FIGURE 1-782 Ventilation-perfusion lung scan in massive pulmonary embolism. A, A normal pattern on the ventilation scan. **B,** The complete disappearance of the entire left lung from the perfusion scan indicates proximal occlusion of the left pulmonary artery. *D,* Dorsal; *L,* left; *LL,* left lobe; *R,* right; *RL,* right lobe; *V,* ventral. (From Crawford MH et al [eds]: *Cardiology*, ed 2, St Louis, 2004, Mosby.)

a nondiagnostic lung scan prevents 9% of angiographies; however, this improvement in efficacy is achieved at the cost of unnecessary anticoagulant therapy in 26% of patients who have false-positive ultrasonography results.

- Angiography: pulmonary angiography is the historic gold standard; however, it is invasive, expensive, and not readily available in some clinical settings. False-positive pulmonary angiograms may result from mediastinal disorders such as radiation fibrosis and tumors.
- Gadolinium-enhanced magnetic resonance angiography (MRA) of the pulmonary arteries has a moderate sensitivity and high specificity for the diagnosis of PE at experienced centers, but obtaining acceptable images is technically challenging and should only be performed if other imaging tests are contraindicated.
- Echocardiography: useful for identifying patients with PE who may have poor prognosis. Moderate or severe hypokinesis, persistent pulmonary hypertension, patent foramen ovale, and free-floating right heart thrombus are markers for increased risk of death or recurrent thrombosis. Such patients should be considered for thrombolysis or embolectomy.

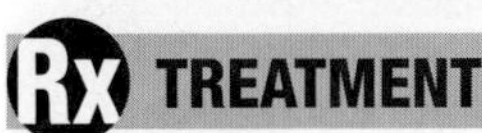

TREATMENT

NONPHARMACOLOGIC THERAPY

Correction of risk factors (see "Etiology") to prevent future PE

ACUTE GENERAL Rx

- Anticoagulant drugs for initial treatment of PE are described in Table E1-418. Unfractionated heparin (UFH) (IV or subcutaneous), subcutaneous low-molecular-weight heparin (LMWH), or subcutaneous fondaparinux is recommended for the initial treatment for at least 5 days. If IV unfractionated heparin is used, a bolus dose (80 U/kg) followed by a weight-based (18 U/kg/hr) continuous infusion to achieve therapeutic anti-factor Xa (or aPTT) levels should be used. LMWH and fondaparinux should be avoided in patients with severe renal failure.
- Oral rivaroxaban, a factor Xa inhibitor (15 mg bid for 3 wk, then 20 mg/d), has been studied as a treatment for DVT and for PE, without prior parenteral therapy. For both DVT and PE, treatment with rivaroxaban alone was noninferior to treatment with LMWH followed by a vitamin K antagonist with regard to the endpoint of recurrent venous thromboembolism. Use of rivaroxaban should be avoided in patients with severe renal failure.
- Thrombolytic agents (urokinase, tPA, streptokinase): provide rapid resolution of clots with increased risk of major bleeding (up to 3% incidence of intracranial hemorrhage); thrombolytic agent are the treatment of choice in patients with massive PE who are hemodynamically unstable and with no contraindication to their use. The use of thrombolytic agent in the treatment of hemodynamically stable patients with acute submassive PE remains controversial, although there is some evidence that half dose tPA has some efficacy. Use of the thrombolytic agents alteplase (100 mg IV over 2-hr period) in normotensive patients with moderate or severe right ventricular dysfunction identified by ECG has been advocated by some physicians. Use of alteplase in conjunction with heparin has been shown to improve the clinical course of stable patients who have acute submassive PE without internal bleeding, mainly by reducing need for subsequent thrombolytic use. Additional studies are needed to confirm these findings before recommending routine use of this therapeutic approach.
- Long-term treatment for PE not associated with malignancy can be carried out with warfarin therapy or rivaroxaban.
- For PE associated with malignancy, LMWH is recommended for long-term therapy.
- For PE occurring in the setting of a reversible risk factor, anticoagulation should be continued for 3 mo. For patients with an unprovoked PE, longer-term anticoagulation should be considered, and indefinite long-term anticoagulation should be used in patients with recurrent unprovoked PE. Important factors to consider in the decision to extend anticoagulation include the patient's risk of bleeding and patient preferences after an informed discussion of risks and benefits.
- If thrombolytics and anticoagulants are contraindicated (e.g., GI bleeding, recent CNS surgery, recent trauma) or if the patient continues to have recurrent PE despite anticoagulation therapy, vena caval interruption is indicated by transvenous placement of an inferior vena caval filter.
- IVC filters are also strongly associated with reduced in-hospital fatality rate in stable patients who received thrombolytic therapy. It seems prudent to consider a vena cava filter in patients with PE who are receiving thrombolytic therapy.
- Acute pulmonary artery surgical embolectomy or catheter-based thrombectomy may be indicated in a patient with massive PE who cannot receive thrombolytic therapy. Pulmonary embolectomy is also recommended for those whose critical status does not allow sufficient time for thrombolytic therapy to be effective and for those who remain unstable after receiving fibrinolysis.

CHRONIC Rx

- Elimination of risk factors (see "Etiology")
- Patients with unprovoked DVT/PE have a high rate of recurrent VTE. Longer durations of chronic anticoagulation after unprovoked DVT/PE result in lower rates of recurrent DVT/PE while on anticoagulation, but benefits are lost once anticoagulation is halted. The use of indefinite anticoagulation in selected individuals with apparently unprovoked DVT/PE must be weighed against ongoing bleeding risk and other factors.
- A recent study demonstrated that aspirin (100 mg daily) is superior to placebo in preventing recurrence of venous thromboembolism in patients with a first-ever unprovoked venous thromboembolism (VTE) who had already completed 6 to 18 months of oral anticoagulation. This suggests that aspirin could be offered as an alternative to oral anticoagulants for prevention of recurrent VTE in patients who refuse to or cannot continue oral anticoagulant therapy but who have a high risk of recurrent VTE.

DISPOSITION

- Mortality can be reduced to <10% by rapid and effective treatment. Stratification of risk of death associated with PE and severity-adjusted treatment is described in Table E1-419.
- Mortality from recurrent pulmonary emboli is 8% with effective treatment and >30% in patients with untreated pulmonary emboli.

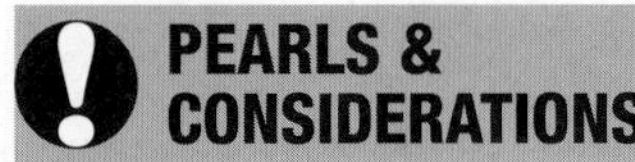

PEARLS & CONSIDERATIONS

COMMENTS

- Use of clinical prediction rules in association with D-dimer testing may reduce the use of unnecessary imaging in patients in whom PE is unlikely.
- Massive PE (PE associated with hypotension, shock, or circulatory arrest) remains the clearest situation in which thrombolytics should be employed. Submassive PE (PE associated with right ventricular dysfunction or injury but without hypotension) remains an area of controversy with regards to thrombolytic use.

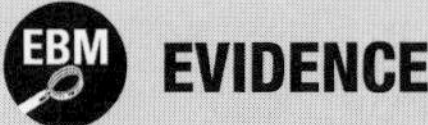

EVIDENCE

available at www.expertconsult.com

SUGGESTED READINGS

available at www.expertconsult.com

RELATED CONTENT

Pulmonary Embolism (PE) (Patient Information)
Deep Vein Thrombosis (Related Key Topic)
Hypercoagulable State (Related Key Topic)

AUTHOR: **BARRY FINE, M.D., PH.D**

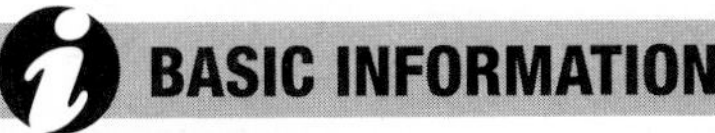

DEFINITION

Pulmonary hypertension (PH) is defined as the presence of an abnormally elevated pulmonary arterial pressure. A mean pulmonary artery pressure (PAP) >25 mm Hg at rest or pulmonary artery systolic pressure >35 mm Hg is considered abnormal. Pulmonary arterial hypertension (PAH) is a syndrome with various causes and is defined as pulmonary hypertension with a normal pulmonary capillary wedge pressure, left atrial pressure, or left ventricular end diastolic pressure ≤5 mm Hg, and a pulmonary vascular resistance greater than 3 Wood units on right heart catheterization. Idiopathic pulmonary arterial hypertension (IPAH) is diagnosed when PAH is present without any apparent cause. Pulmonary hypertension from lung disease is covered under the separate topic Cor Pulmonale

SYNONYMS

Idiopathic pulmonary arterial hypertension (IPAH)
Secondary pulmonary arterial hypertension (PAH)
Group I Pulmonary Hypertension

ICD-9CM CODES
416.0 Primary pulmonary hypertension
416.8 Secondary pulmonary hypertension
ICD-10CM CODES
I27.0 Primary pulmonary hypertension
I27.2 Other secondary pulmonary hypertension

EPIDEMIOLOGY & DEMOGRAPHICS

- IPAH is rare, occurring in one to two cases per 1 million people per year, with an overall prevalence estimated at 1300 per 1 million.
- IPAH is more common in women than men (3:1), usually presenting in the third to fourth decades of life.
- In adults the most common cause of pulmonary hypertension is lung disease
- IPAH incidence ranges from 1-2 per million per year, and prevalence is 0.1-0.2% of all post mortem examinations
- Prevalence of secondary PAH could range from 8-12% in cases of scleroderma, 0.5% of HIV, 23-53% of mixed connective tissue disorders, and 1-4% cases of systemic lupus erythromatosus

PHYSICAL FINDINGS & CLINICAL PRESENTATION

- Insidious, may go undetected for years
- Exertional dyspnea most common presenting symptom (60%)
- Fatigue and weakness
- Syncope, classically exertion-related or after a warm shower with peripheral vasodilation
- Chest pain
- Hoarse voice from compression of recurrent laryngeal nerve by an enlarged pulmonary artery (Ortner's syndrome)
- Loud P2 component of the second heart sound and paradoxical splitting of second heart sound
- Right-sided S4
- Jugular venous distention
- Abdominal distention and ascites
- Prominent parasternal (right ventricular [RV]) impulse
- Holosystolic tricuspid regurgitation murmur heard best along the left fourth parasternal line that increases in intensity with inspiration
- Peripheral edema

ETIOLOGY

- The etiology of IPAH is unknown. Most cases are sporadic, but there is a 6% to 12% familial incidence.
- PH is associated with several known risk factors: connective tissue disorders, portal hypertension and liver cirrhosis, appetite-suppressant drugs (fenfluramine), hemoglobinopathies, and infections including schistosomiasis and HIV disease. It is estimated that 10% of patients with hemoglobinopathies and 0.5% of patients with HIV infection develop moderate to severe PH. Schistosomiasis, sickle cell disease, and HIV disease may be the most common causes of PH worldwide, although pulmonary venous hypertension from left ventricular failure and PH related to COPD are more common causes of PH in developed nations.
- Several genetic abnormalities have been associated with the familial form of IPAH, many of which are mutations in the genes that code for members of the tumor growth factor-beta family of receptors (BMPR-II, ALK-1, endoglin) on chromosome 2q33. A recent study[1] has identified the association of a novel gene, *KCNK3,* with familial and idiopathic pulmonary arterial hypertension.
- Familial PAH is an autosomal-dominant disease with variable penetrance, affecting only about 10% to 20% of carriers.
- Several factors play a role in the pathogenesis of PAH, including a genetic predisposition, endothelial cell dysfunction, abnormalities in vasomotor control, thrombotic obliteration of the vascular lumen, and vascular remodeling through cell proliferation and matrix production.
- SSRI use in late pregnancy is associated with increased persistent PH in newborns.
- The updated clinical classification of PAH is described in Table 1-420.

Dx DIAGNOSIS

- PAH is a hemodynamic diagnosis involving the detection of elevated pressure in the pulmonary arteries and elevated pulmonary vascular resistance in the pulmonary vascular bed, occurring in the absence of significant pulmonary venous hypertension; characterization of this abnormality determines its etiology.
- Right-sided heart catheterization must be performed in all patients suspected of having PAH to establish the diagnosis and to assess pulmonary hemodynamics and acute vasoreactivity response testing.

[1]Ma L et al: A novel channelopathy in pulmonary arterial hypertension, *N Engl J Med* 369:351-361, 2013.

TABLE 1-420 Updated Clinical Classification of Pulmonary Hypertension

Group 1
Pulmonary arterial hypertension
Idiopathic pulmonary arterial hypertension
Heritable
BMPR2
ALK1, endoglin (with or without hereditary hemorrhagic telangiectasia)
Unknown
Drug- and toxin-induced
Associated with:
Connective tissue diseases
HIV infection
Portal hypertension
Congenital heart diseases
Schistosomiasis
Chronic hemolytic anemia
Persistent pulmonary hypertension of the newborn
Pulmonary veno-occlusive disease with left to right shunts and/or pulmonary capillary hemangiomatosis
Group 2
Pulmonary hypertension owing to left heart disease
Systolic dysfunction
Diastolic dysfunction
Valvular disease
Group 3
Pulmonary hypertension owing to lung diseases and/or hypoxia
Chronic obstructive pulmonary disease
Interstitial lung disease
Other pulmonary diseases with mixed restrictive and obstructive pattern
Sleep-disordered breathing
Alveolar hypoventilation disorders
Chronic exposure to high altitude
Developmental abnormalities
Group 4
Chronic thromboembolic pulmonary hypertension
Group 5
Pulmonary hypertension with unclear multifactorial mechanisms
Hematologic disorders: myeloproliferative disorders, splenectomy
Systemic disorders: sarcoidosis, pulmonary Langerhans cell histiocytosis: lymphangioleiomyomatosis, neurofibromatosis, vasculitis
Metabolic disorders: glycogen storage disease, Gaucher's disease, thyroid disorders
Others: tumoral obstruction, fibrosing mediastinitis, chronic renal failure on dialysis

ALK1, Activin receptor-like kinase type 1; *BMPR2,* bone morphogenetic protein receptor type 2; *HIV,* human immunodeficiency virus.
From Simonneau G et al: Updated clinical classification of pulmonary hypertension, *J Am Coll Cardiol* 54:S43-S54, 2009.

- IPAH is a diagnosis that rests on the detection of PH with exclusion of known causes of high pulmonary arterial pressure.

DIFFERENTIAL DIAGNOSIS

The differential diagnosis is as listed under "Etiology."

EVALUATION

- Consists of establishing the diagnosis and etiology.
- Echocardiography with Doppler technique can provide a noninvasive but limited estimation of systolic PAP. Common findings include tricuspid regurgitation, right heart enlargement, abnormal movement of septum and, rarely, pericardial effusion. However, the diagnosis of PH cannot be established by echocardiography alone, as echocardiography can overestimate or underestimate PAP.
- ECG shows RV enlargement, strain pattern, and right axis deviation.
- Chest radiograph (Fig. 1-783) shows enlarged central pulmonary arteries and right heart enlargement. Chest radiography is abnormal in 90% of patients at diagnosis.
- A normal chest radiograph does not rule out the diagnosis. High-resolution computed tomography (CT) (Fig. 1-784) can assist in the evaluation for emphysema or interstitial lung disease. Ventilation-perfusion lung scan has high sensitivity for chronic thromboembolic disease. The diagnosis should be confirmed by pulmonary angiography, which has high specificity.
- Pulmonary function tests may show obstructive (airway disease) and/or restrictive disease (parenchymal disease) depending on etiology. Diffusion capacity of carbon monoxide in the lung is reduced due to pulmonary vascular destruction in PAH.
- Right heart catheterization is required to assess pulmonary hemodynamics, exclude shunts and left heart disease, and perform acute vasoreactivity response testing.
- Screening for the presence of PAH with Doppler echocardiography is warranted in individuals with a known predisposing genetic mutation or first-degree relative with IPAH, connective tissue diseases (especially scleroderma), congenital heart disease with left-to-right shunt, or portal hypertension undergoing evaluation for orthotopic liver transplantation.
- Determining the degree of functional impairment, as assessed by the WHO functional classification system (Classes I-IV) and the 6-min walk test (6MWT), is a useful way to monitor disease progression and assess response to treatment.

LABORATORY TESTS

- Complete blood count is usually normal in PAH but may show secondary polycythemia.
- Arterial blood gases show low PO_2 and oxygen saturation.
- Overnight oximetry and/or sleep study to rule out sleep apnea or hypopnea.
- Other blood tests: antinuclear antibody (ANA), antineutrophil cytoplasmic antibodies (ANCA), anti-Scl-70, anticentromere, ribonucleoprotein antibody levels, and rheumatoid factor (RF) to screen for underlying connective tissue disease, HIV serology, liver function tests, and antiphospholipid antibodies.
- Brain natriuretic peptide (BNP) level can provide prognostic information, with elevation in BNP level being associated with increased mortality.
- Ventilation-perfusion lung scan has high sensitivity for chronic thromboembolic PAH. The diagnosis should be confirmed by pulmonary angiography, which has high specificity.

Rx TREATMENT

- Most of the evidence in management of PAH is limited to IPAH. There is some evidence in treatment of PAH associated with connective tissue disease, especially scleroderma, and congenital heart disease. The recommendations for treating PAH associated with other causes are limited to case studies and expert opinions.
- There is some evidence for the use of advanced therapies for sarcoidosis-associated PH. The heterogeneity of sarcoid-associated PH complicates the interpretation.

NONPHARMACOLOGIC THERAPY

- Oxygen therapy to improve alveolar oxygen flow in both idiopathic and secondary PH. Goal oxygen saturation >90%
- Avoidance of vigorous exercise and pregnancy

GENERAL TREATMENT:

1. Diuretics (e.g., furosemide 40 to 80 mg qd) improve dyspnea by reducing preload and peripheral edema. Avoid excessive diuresis in patients who are preload dependent.
2. Digoxin 0.25 mg qd has been used in patients with IPAH with inconclusive benefits.
3. Oral anticoagulation with warfarin is recommended especially for IPAH, as per a 1984 retrospective study by Fuster et al that showed improved long term survival. This practice is supported by the high incidence of antemortem clots found in autopsy in the small pulmonary arteries and arterioles of patients with IPAH. Recommended goal for INR is lower at 1.5 to 2.5.

CHRONIC Rx

- Acute vasoreactivity response testing should be done in all patients at the time of right heart catheterization. Epoprostenol, adenosine, or nitric oxide is generally used to assess the response. A positive response is a fall in mean PAP of >10 mm Hg to a value of <40 mm Hg, with increased or unchanged cardiac output. Fewer than 10% of patients are responders in IPAH.
- The positive responders may benefit from treatment with calcium channel blockers (diltiazem, amlodipine, or nifedipine). Verapamil is not recommended because of its negative inotropic effects. All patients should be reassessed in 6 to 8 wk to demonstrate sustained benefit from the calcium channel blocker.

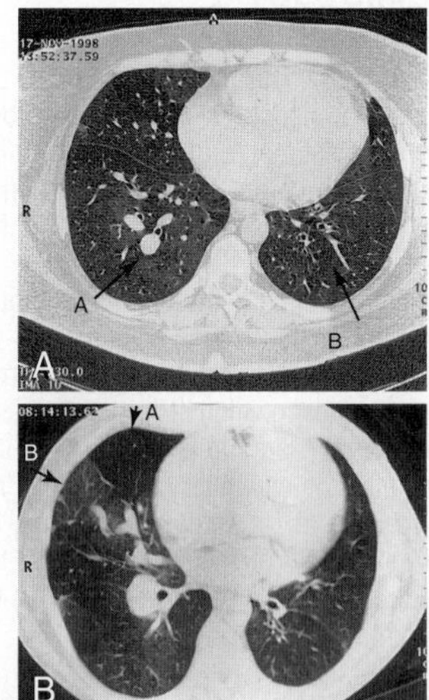

FIGURE 1-784 Chest computed tomographic scans in a patient with chronic thromboembolic pulmonary hypertension. A, Helical scan with contrast medium enhancement of the pulmonary vasculature shows a marked disparity in vessel size between the involved vessels *(A),* which are enlarged from thrombus, and the uninvolved vessels *(B).* **B,** Non-contrast-enhanced high-resolution scan illustrates a marked mosaic pattern manifest by differences in density of regions of the lung parenchyma reflecting the perfused areas *(B)* and the nonperfused areas *(A),* also consistent with underlying thromboembolic disease. (From Zipes DP et al [eds]: *Braunwauld's heart disease,* ed 7, Philadelphia, 2005, Saunders.)

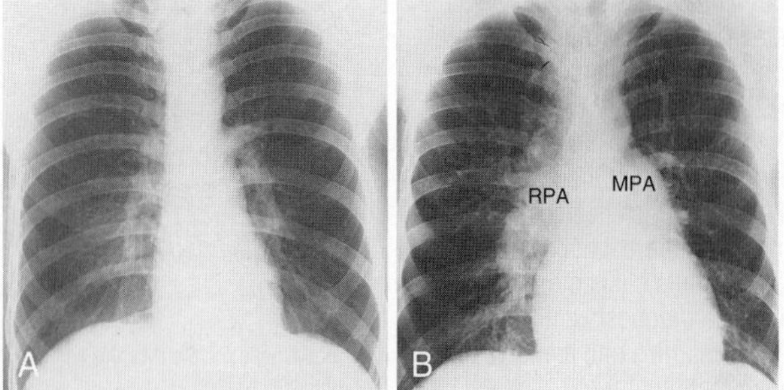

FIGURE 1-783 Progressive pulmonary arterial hypertension. This patient initially presented with a relatively normal chest radiograph **(A).** However, several years later **(B)** there is increasing heart size and marked dilation of the main pulmonary artery *(MPA)* and right pulmonary artery *(RPA).* Rapid tapering of the arteries as they proceed peripherally is suggestive of pulmonary hypertension and is sometimes referred to as pruning. (From Mettler FA [ed]: *Primary care radiology,* Philadelphia, 2000, Saunders.)

- Nonresponders or nonsustained responders are eligible for selective pulmonary vasodilators.
- Prostanoids (epoprostenol, treprostinil, iloprost, and beraprost) act as potent vasodilators of pulmonary arteries and inhibitors of platelet aggregation. Ideal for class IV patients.
  1. Epoprostenol: IV formulation with very short half-life. Requires long-term IV access with associated risks of infection and thrombosis. Rapid tachyphylaxis, and therefore dose escalation, is seen. Common side effects include jaw pain, abdominal cramping, and diarrhea. Limited evidence exists for use in secondary PAH patients.
  2. Treprostinil: IV and SQ formulation with longer half-life. Main disadvantage is pain at SQ pump site (no long-term evidence for IV formulation). Treprostinil is also available as a nebulized inhaled solution.
  3. Iloprost: aerosolized formulation with short half-life requiring 6 to 8 treatments/day.
  4. Beraprost: PO formulation. Not approved in U.S.
- Endothelin receptor antagonists (ERAs):
  1. Bosentan (nonselective endothelin A and B receptor blocker): oral pulmonary vasodilator, requires monthly liver function tests, often response delay by weeks. Thus, it is not an ideal starting therapy for WHO class IV patients. They are effective in class II and III patients.
  2. Sitaxsentan and ambrisentan (selective endothelin A receptor blockers).
  3. Macitentan
- Phosphodiesterase (PDE-5) inhibitors (sildenafil and tadalafil): act by increasing concentration of nitric oxide. Sildenafil is administered as 20 mg PO tid up to 80 mg PO tid. Tadalafil dose is 40 mg once daily. Highly effective in WHO class II patients, both in IPAH and scleroderma-associated PAH.
- Low risk, functional class I-III patients may be treated with PDE-5 inhibitors, oral ERAs or inhaled prostacyclins
- High risk, functional class III-IV patients should be treated with intravenous or subcutaneous prostacyclins. They should then be revaluated and considered for combination therapy
- Combination therapies: considered when there is no improvement or deterioration on monotherapy.
- Bosentan + inhaled iloprost (STEP trial) showed some benefit over monotherapy.
- IV epoprostenol + oral bosentan (BREATH-2 trial) did not show much difference.
- IV epoprostenol + oral sildenafil (PACES trial) showed benefit over monotherapy.
- Lung transplantation and heart-lung transplantation are other options in patients with end-stage class IV disease. Atrial septostomy may be performed as a bridge to transplant. The defect can be closed at the time of transplantation.
- Atrial septostomy is recommended for individuals with a room air SaO_2 >90% who have severe right-sided heart failure (with refractory ascites) despite maximal diuretic therapy, or who have signs of impaired systemic blood flow (such as syncope) from reduced left heart filling.
- Lung transplant recipients with IPAH had survival rates of 73% at 1 yr, 55% at 3 yr, and 45% at 5 yr.

TREATMENT OF SECONDARY PAH:

- Directed toward cause. Some situations merit mention.
- PAH with uncorrected congenital heart disease: Eisenmenger's syndrome. Medical treatment generally ineffective. Heart-lung transplantation required in most patients. PH may persist after surgical correction of congenital heart disease, and pulmonary vasodilators can be effective therapies in this patient population.
- PAH with scleroderma: selective pulmonary vasodilators are effective.
- PAH with lung disease or hypoxia: oxygen therapy, for hypoxemia, CPAP (for OSA), control of primary disease process.
- PAH with chronic thromboembolic disease: may consider pulmonary vasodilators after anticoagulation and pulmonary thromboendarterectomy (or if thromboendarterectomy is not an option) if continued symptoms and elevation in PVR and transpulmonary gradient.
- PAH with HIV: control of viral load by antiretroviral therapy.

FOLLOW-UP

Regular follow-up at 3-mo intervals with clinical assessment: WHO class and 6MWT, 6- to 12-mo objective assessment of RV function by ECG and cardiac catheterization studies.

DISPOSITION

- The 6MWT is predictive of survival in patients with idiopathic PAH. A baseline 6MWT less than 250 m is associated with a 50% risk of death at 2 yr. Drop in O_2 saturation >10% during the test increases mortality risk 2.9 times over a median follow-up of 26 mo.
- A BNP level ≥350 pg/ml at baseline evaluation is associated with a 25% risk of death at 2 yr.
- WHO class II and III patients with PAH have a mean survival of 3.5 yr.
- WHO class IV patients have a mean survival of 6 mo.
- As per the REVEAL (Registry to Evaluate Early and Long-term Pulmonary Arterial Hypertension Disease Management) risk score, poor prognostic signs include:
  1. Signs of RV failure
  2. WHO functional class III or IV
  3. Salk distance of <165 meters in 6-min walk test
  4. Peak VO2 <15 ml/min/kg in cardiopulmonary testing
  5. Elevated BNP levels >180 pg/ml
  6. Presence of pericardial effusion
  7. TAPSE [tricuspid annular plane systolic excursion] <2 cm on echo of right ventricle
  8. Right atrial pressure >20 mm Hg or pulmonary vascular resistance of >32 Wood units on right heart catheterization
  9. Increased heart rate >92 or BP <109 mm Hg
  10. Male gender >60 years of age
  11. Concomitant renal dysfunction with estimated glomerular filtration rate ≤30/mL/min/m
  12. Diffusion capacity of lung for carbon monoxide (DLCO) <33%

REFERRAL

If the diagnosis of IPAH is suspected, a consultation with a pulmonary specialist is recommended. Secondary causes of PH may require disease-specific consultations.

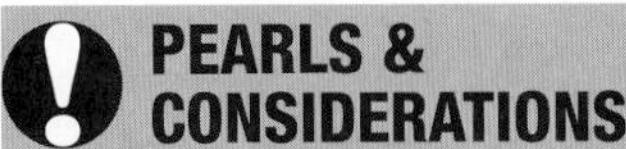

PEARLS & CONSIDERATIONS

- The exertional dyspnea of PAH is typically described by patients as being relentlessly progressive over several months to a year, often out of proportion to, or in the absence of, underlying heart or lung disease.
- Over 20% of patients in the Registry to Evaluate Early and Long-term PAH Disease Management had symptoms for more than 2 years before PAH was recognized. Consideration of the diagnosis of PAH in the differential diagnosis of unexplained dyspnea, especially in younger individuals, is essential.
- Chest x-ray may reveal evidence of interstitial fluid or fibrosis within the lungs in cases of secondary PH. IPAH is not associated with infiltrates on chest radiograph.

COMMENTS

- RV systolic pressure (RVSP) as estimated by echocardiography is not a good indicator of the presence of PAH because RVSP increases with age and body mass index. Athletically conditioned men also have a higher resting RVSP. Thus, these measurements can be misleading.
- Abrupt development of pulmonary edema during acute vasodilator testing suggests pulmonary veno-occlusive disease or pulmonary capillary hemangiomatosis and is a contraindication to long-term vasodilator treatment.
- In advanced PAH, heart rate increase is the main compensatory mechanism and reflects increased sympathetic tone. A higher heart rate at rest is an important marker of prognosis and should be assessed at frequent intervals after initiation of treatment for PAH.

FUTURE DIRECTIONS

- Serotonin receptor modulators, platelet-derived growth factor and Rho kinase inhibitors
- Gene analysis to identify genes that determine individual disease susceptibility and help identify targeted therapy

SUGGESTED READINGS

available at www.expertconsult.com

RELATED CONTENT

Pulmonary Hypertension (Patient Information)

AUTHOR: **RABIA ARSHAD, M.D.**

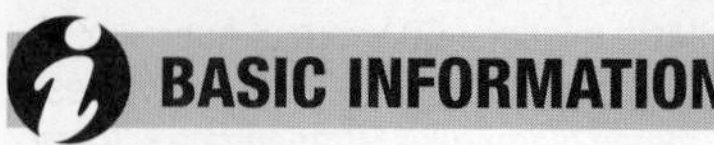

BASIC INFORMATION

DEFINITION

Pulseless electrical activity (PEA) is defined as the presence of organized electrical activity without sufficient mechanical contraction of the heart to produce a palpable pulse or measurable blood pressure.

SYNONYMS

Electromechanical dissociation (EMD)

ICD-9CM CODES
427.5 Cardiac arrest
ICD-10CM CODES
I46.9 Cardiac arrest, cause unspecified
I49.9 Cardiac arrythmia, unspecified

EPIDEMIOLOGY & DEMOGRAPHICS

- Accounts for about 35% of cardiac arrest cases
- Increasingly recognized as the cause of sudden cardiac death in patients with implantable cardioverter-defibrillators

PHYSICAL FINDINGS & CLINICAL PRESENTATION

PRIMARY PEA:
- Organized electrical activity (not VT/VF)
- No detectable pulse

SECONDARY PEA: As in primary PEA and may also have:
- Bradycardia: drug overdose
- Tachycardia: hypovolemia, massive PE
- Decreased jugular venous pressure (JVP): hypovolemia
- Elevated JVP and no pulse with CPR: cardiac tamponade, massive PE, tension pneumothorax
- Absent unilateral breath sounds and tracheal deviation: tension pneumothorax
- Cyanosis: hypoxia

ETIOLOGY

PRIMARY PEA: Myocardial electromechanical uncoupling secondary to advanced heart muscle disease

SECONDARY PEA: Because of changes in the loading conditions of the heart, ischemia, myocardial depressants
- Massive MI
- Massive PE
- Hypovolemia
- Cardiac tamponade
- Tension pneumothorax
- Hypoxia
- Hypothermia
- Acidosis
- Hyperkalemia/hypokalemia
- Drug overdose: β-blockers, calcium channel blockers, digoxin, tricyclic antidepressants, benzodiazepines, opioids

DIAGNOSIS

WORKUP

- Stabilizing patient and workup to establish etiology should proceed simultaneously
- History, physical examination, laboratory tests, imaging studies

LABORATORY TESTS

- CBC, potassium, magnesium, CK-MB, troponin, toxicology screen
- Arterial blood gas
- ECG (Fig. 1-785):
  Low voltage: tamponade
  Right heart strain: PE, pneumothorax
  Arrhythmias: MI, metabolic abnormalities, drug effects
  ST changes, Q waves: MI

IMAGING STUDIES

- Chest radiograph: rule out pneumothorax, aortic dissection
- Chest CT/pulmonary arteriogram: rule out PE
- Echocardiogram: rule out tamponade, ischemia (LV contractility, wall motion), valve dysfunction, tumors, and clots. May help diagnose aortic dissection and PE and assess intravascular volume status
- Abdominal radiograph: rule out ruptured abdominal aortic aneurysm

TREATMENT

Identifying and treating a reversible cause is critical.

Physiologic parameters can help monitor quality of CPR and detect the return of spontaneous circulation (ROSC). Suggested methods include quantitative waveform capnography (if intubated), arterial relaxation "diastolic" pressure (if arterial catheter in place), or central venous oxygen saturation (if central venous catheter in superior vena cava).

NONPHARMACOLOGIC THERAPY

- Activate emergency response service
- Begin CPR; ensure high quality, minimize interruptions. Perform CPR for 2 min between pauses to assess rhythm and circulation
- Attach cardiac monitor/defibrillator
- Obtain IV/intraosseous (IO) access
- Consider advanced airway placement
- Confirm absence of blood flow with Doppler ultrasound, arterial line, or bedside echocardiogram

FIGURE 1-785 Sinus rhythm with pulseless electrical activity (PEA). Although the ECG showed sinus rhythm, the patient had no pulse or blood pressure. In this case the PEA was a result of depressed myocardial function after a cardiac arrest. (From Goldberg AL: *Clinical electrocardiography*, ed 5, St Louis, 1994, Mosby.)

ACUTE GENERAL Rx

- Treat specific cause if known
- Give 100% oxygen
- Epinephrine 1 mg IV push/IO, q3 to 5min; vasopressin 40 U IV/IO may be used to replace the first or second dose of epinephrine
- Give normal saline (20 ml) bolus after peripheral IV administration of medication to improve its distribution
- Medication can be given via endotracheal tube if IV/IO access cannot be obtained; IV/IO routes preferred because they provide more predictable drug delivery and pharmacologic effects. Give 2 to 2.5× the IV dose in 10 ml of sterile water.
- If rhythm changes to VF or pulseless VT
  - Defibrillate
  - For refractory VF or pulseless VT consider amiodarone
- If achieve ROSC, initiate post–cardiac arrest care

DISPOSITION

Of hospitalized patients who develop PEA, <15% survive to discharge. Survival rates much lower in patients with prehospital PEA. Survivors often have poor neurologic outcomes.

REFERRAL

As needed for underlying condition

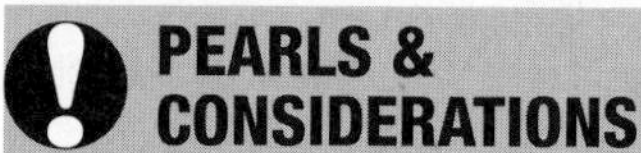

PEARLS & CONSIDERATIONS

- 2010 American Heart Association guidelines for cardiopulmonary resuscitation and emergency cardiovascular care recommend the use of epinephrine in PEA resuscitation. New data suggest that epinephrine use may be associated with worse neurologic outcomes and increased long-term mortality. Recent study suggests that the use of steroids in resuscitation and for post-resuscitation shock improved neurologic outcomes and survival to hospital discharge.
- Termination of resuscitation guidelines exist for out-of-hospital cardiac arrest. Similar guidelines for in-hospital cardiac arrest are not available; termination of resuscitation is based on multiple patient factors.
- Therapeutic hypothermia (32° to 34° C for 12 to 24 hr) may improve neurologic outcomes and reduce mortality in comatose cardiac arrest survivors.
- Prognosis may be guided by testing, but no single exam finding or test is definitive. Delay testing for at least 24 hr after ROSC. Available tests include median nerve somatosensory-evoked potentials, EEG, or corneal and pupillary reflexes. Prognostication is more difficult in patients treated with hypothermia; wait >72 hr before attempting to predict outcome.

SUGGESTED READINGS

available at www.expertconsult.com

AUTHOR: **SUDEEP KAUR AULAKH, M.D.**

BASIC INFORMATION

DEFINITION

Pyelonephritis is an infection, usually bacterial in origin, of the upper urinary tract.

SYNONYMS

Acute pyelonephritis
Pyonephrosis
Renal carbuncle
Lobar nephronia
Acute bacterial nephritis

ICD-9CM CODES
590.81 Pyelonephritis
599.0 Urinary tract infection
595.9 Cystitis

ICD-10CM CODES
N10 Acute tubulo-interstitial nephritis
N11 Chronic tubulo-interstitial nephritis
N11.0 Nonobstructive reflux-associated chronic pyelonephritis
N11.1 Chronic obstructive pyelonephritis
N11.8 Other chronic tubulo-interstitial nephritis
N11.9 Chronic tubulo-interstitial nephritis, unspecified
N12 Tubulo-instertitial nephritis, not specified as acute or chronic

EPIDEMIOLOGY & DEMOGRAPHICS

INCIDENCE (IN U.S.): Extremely common
PREDOMINANT SEX: Female
PREDOMINANT AGE:

- Sexually active years in women
- Usually age >50 yr in men

GENETICS: Congenital urologic structural disorders may predispose to infections at an early age.

PHYSICAL FINDINGS & CLINICAL PRESENTATION

- Fever, rigors, chills
- Flank pain
- Dysuria
- Polyuria
- Hematuria
- Toxic feeling and appearance
- Nausea and vomiting
- Headache
- Diarrhea
- Physical examination notable
  1. Costovertebral angle tenderness
  2. Exquisite flank pain

ETIOLOGY

- Gram-negative bacilli such as *Escherichia coli* and *Klebsiella* spp. in more than 95% of cases
- Other, more unusual gram-negative organisms, especially if instrumentation of the urinary system has occurred
- Resistant gram-negative organisms or even fungi in hospitalized patients with indwelling catheters
- Gram-positive organisms such as enterococci
- *Staphylococcus aureus:* presence in urine indicates hematogenous origin
- Viruses: rarely, but these are usually limited to the lower tract

DIAGNOSIS

DIFFERENTIAL DIAGNOSIS

- Nephrolithiasis
- Appendicitis
- Ovarian cyst torsion or rupture
- Acute glomerulonephritis
- Pelvic inflammatory disease
- Endometritis
- Other causes of acute abdomen
- Perinephric abscess
- Hydronephrosis

WORKUP

- No workup usually indicated in sexually active women
- Poorly responding infections, especially with azotemia and frank bacteremia
- Renal sonogram or CT scan (Fig. 1-787) to assess for underlying urologic pathology such as hydronephrosis
- Urologic imaging studies in all young men and boys
- Prostate assessment in older men

LABORATORY TESTS

- Complete blood count with differential
- Renal panel
- Blood cultures
- Gram stain of urine, urinalysis, and urine cultures

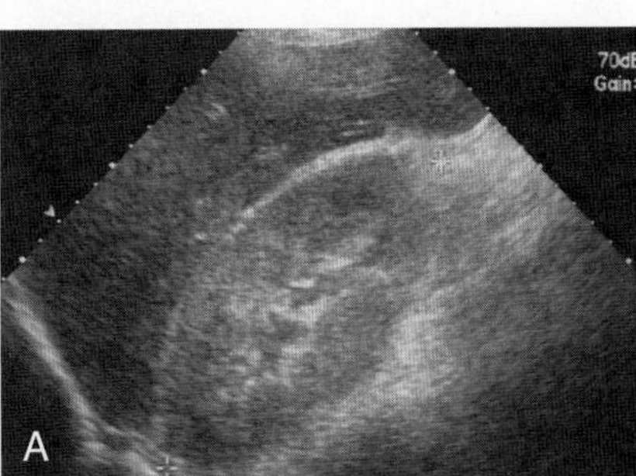

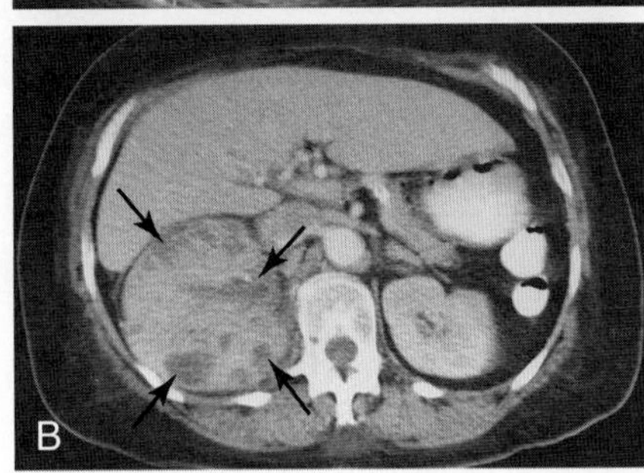

FIGURE 1-787 Acute pyelonephritis. A, Ultrasound image demonstrates an enlarged echogenic kidney. Bipolar length of kidney is 12.9 cm. **B,** CT scan with contrast enhancement obtained 24 hours later demonstrates multiple nonenhancing abscesses *(arrows)*. (From Floege J et al: *Comprehensive clinical nephrology,* ed 4, Philadelphia, 2010, Saunders.)

- Urgent renal sonography if obstruction or closed space infection suspected
- CT scans may better define the extent of collections of pus and can identify emphysematous pyelonephritis
- Helical CT scans excellent to detect calculi

TREATMENT

ACUTE GENERAL Rx

- Hospitalization for:
  1. Toxic patients
  2. Complicated infections
  3. Diabetes
  4. Suspected bacteremia
- Keep patients well hydrated.
- IV fluids are indicated for those unable to take adequate amounts of liquids.
- Give antipyretics such as acetaminophen when necessary.
- Antibiotic therapy should be initiated after cultures are obtained and guided by the results of culture and sensitivity testing.
  1. Oral quinolones such as ciprofloxacin (500 mg PO bid usually for 10 to 14 days) or Levaquin (500 or 750 mg for 10 to 14 days) are typically used for stable patients who can tolerate oral medications with sensitive pathogens. The optimum duration of therapy for acute pyelonephritis is unclear. Recent trials have shown that a short course (7 days) is not inferior to a 14-day course in women with uncomplicated pyelonephritis.
  2. IV antibiotic options for more toxic patients pending cultures include ceftriaxone (1 to 2 g q day), IV cipro (400 mg q12h) or IV Levaquin (500 to 750 mg IV q day), piperacillin/tazobactam (3.375 g IV q6h) or carbapenems such as meropenem or imipenem (500 mg IV q6-8h)
  3. Ceftazidime 1 to 2 g IV 8h, piperacillin/tazobactam, and carbapenems are best choices for *Pseudomonas.* There is increasing resistance of *Pseudomonas* to ciprofloxacin
  4. Aminoglycosides such as gentamicin (2 mg/kg IV load followed by 1 mg/kg IV q8h adjusted for renal function) added, but nephrotoxicity possible, especially in diabetics with azotemia
  5. Vancomycin 1 g IV q12h or linezolid to cover gram-positive cocci such as enterococci or staphylococci
  6. Ampicillin 1 to 2 g IV q4 to 6h to cover enterococci with an aminoglycoside for synergy
- Prompt drainage with nephrostomy tube placement for obstruction.
- Surgical drainage of large collections of pus to control infection.
- Diabetic patients, as well as those with indwelling catheters, are especially prone to complicated infections and abscess formation.

CHRONIC Rx

- Repair underlying structural problems, especially when renal function is compromised.

1. Reflux
2. Obstruction
3. Nephrolithiasis should be considered

- Patients with diabetes mellitus and indwelling urinary catheters are at particular risk of severe and complicated infections.
- When possible, remove catheters.

DISPOSITION

Most patients with uncomplicated pyelonephritis are now treated as outpatients or in short hospitalizations. Indications to admit a patient with pyelonephritis include pregnancy, suspected urinary obstruction, suspected renal abscess or perinephric abscess, bacterial sepsis, diabetes or other immunocompromised states, recurrent or refractory pyelonephritis, or infection with an unusual or antibiotic-resistant microorganism.

REFERRAL

- To a surgeon for correction of underlying urologic problems (e.g., reflux and hydronephrosis)
- To a pediatrician for detection of reflux to avoid recurrent urinary tract infection and loss of renal function
- To an internist for aggressive metabolic and urologic evaluation for patients with nephrolithiasis

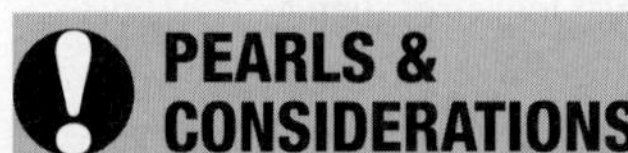

PEARLS & CONSIDERATIONS

Pyelonephritis is a systemic illness and may be a source of bacteremia and sepsis, especially if accompanied by urinary obstruction. Workup for abscess, obstruction, papillary necrosis, and other local complications of pyelonephritis should be initiated if the patient is septic, if patient does not respond to antibiotic therapy after 72 hr of treatment, or if infection is accompanied by worsening renal function.

SUGGESTED READINGS

available at www.expertconsult.com

RELATED CONTENT

Pyelonephritis (Patient Information)

AUTHOR: **GLENN G. FORT, M.D., M.P.H.**

BASIC INFORMATION

DEFINITION

Pyogenic granuloma is a benign vascular lesion of the skin and mucous membranes. The lesions are caused by capillary proliferation, generally the result of trauma.

SYNONYMS

Granuloma pyogenicum
Tumor of pregnancy
Eruptive hemangioma
Lobular capillary hemangioma
Granulation tissue–type hemangioma

ICD-9CM CODES
686.1 Pyogenic granuloma
ICD-10CM CODES
L98.0 Pyogenic granuloma

EPIDEMIOLOGY & DEMOGRAPHICS

- Common in children and young adults. Also found more frequently in pregnant women.
- Equally prevalent in males and females, with no racial or familial predisposition.
- Caused by trauma or surgery.
- Gingival lesions occur more frequently during pregnancy.

PHYSICAL FINDINGS & CLINICAL PRESENTATION

- Small (<1 cm), yellow to red, dome-shaped lesions
- May have surrounding scale at base (Fig. 1-789)
- Most commonly found on the head, neck, and extremities
- Often found on the gingiva during pregnancy (called *epulis*)
- Extremely friable, can easily ulcerate, and may bleed profusely with minor trauma

ETIOLOGY

Trauma causing focal capillary growth. These lesions are neither infectious in etiology nor granulomatous in histology.

DIAGNOSIS

DIFFERENTIAL DIAGNOSIS

- Amelanotic melanoma
- Bacillary angiomatosis
- Glomus tumor
- Hemangioma
- Irritated nevus
- Wart
- Kaposi's sarcoma

WORKUP

Diagnosis is based on clinical history and appearance. Generally begins with trauma followed by the development of an erythematous papule. The lesion tends to bleed easily and develops over several days to weeks.

LABORATORY TESTS

Pathologic examination should be performed after excision to rule out melanoma.

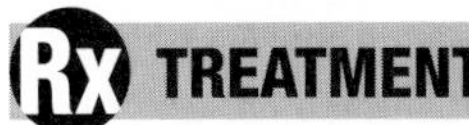

TREATMENT

ACUTE GENERAL Rx

- Excision: using 1% lidocaine for anesthesia, shave or curette at base and border. Follow with electrocauterization or cryotherapy.
- Pulsed-dye laser is also a safe and effective treatment modality.
- Pregnancy epulis generally resolves spontaneously after childbirth.

REFERRAL

Dermatology referral recommended if lesion recurs or multiple satellite lesions occur after excision

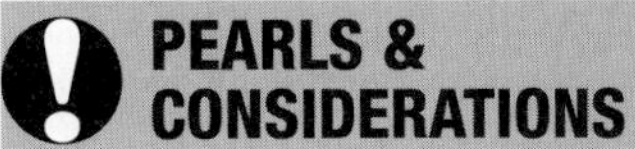

PEARLS & CONSIDERATIONS

COMMENTS

- Removal of entire lesion is essential because lesions may recur at the site of residual tissue.
- Patients and parents should be alerted to the possibility of recurrence after removal.
- Multiple satellite lesions occasionally develop near a primary pyogenic granuloma, usually after destruction of that lesion.

AUTHOR: **FRED F. FERRI, M.D.**

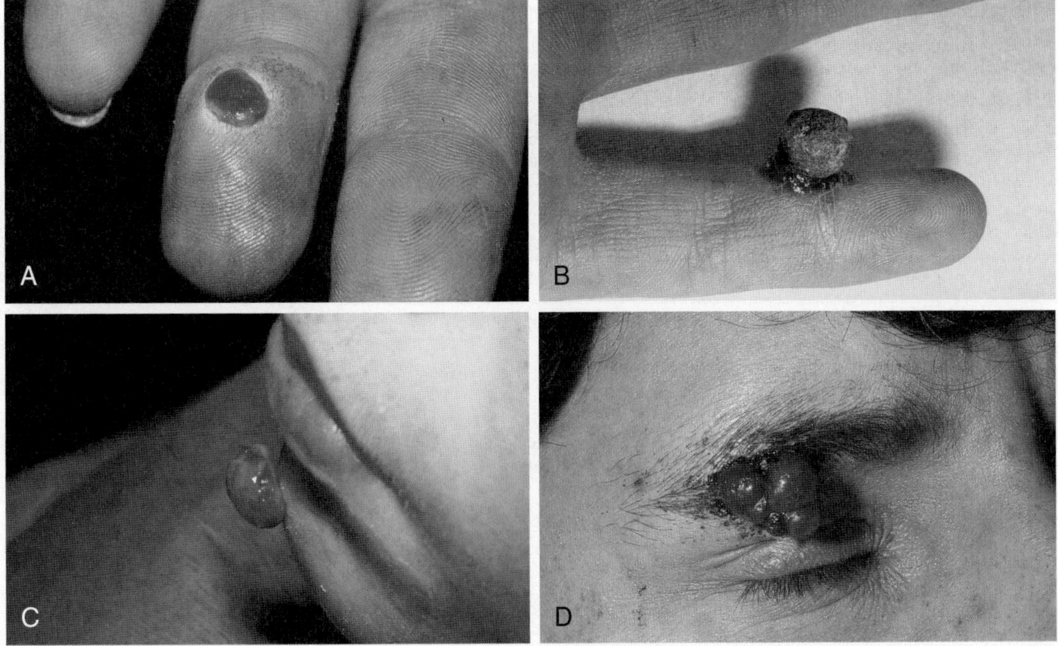

FIGURE 1-789 Pyogenic granuloma. A, This is the classic appearance of a red, friable nodule growing rapidly on the finger. There is often a portion that extends under the skin laterally. **B,** Pyogenic granuloma on the finger. This lesion is more dry and crusted. **C,** Pyogenic granuloma on the chin of an adult. The fingers, lip, palms, soles, and face are typical sites. **D,** Pyogenic granuloma of the eyebrow. (From White GM, Cox NH [eds]: *Diseases of the skin, a color atlas and text,* ed 2, St Louis, 2006, Mosby.)

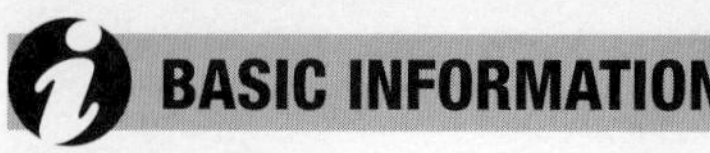

BASIC INFORMATION

DEFINITION

Radiation is the emission of energy as electromagnetic waves or moving subatomic particles. It can be natural or man-made. Natural radiation can come from a cosmic source, such as the sun, or a terrestrial source, such as naturally occurring radionuclides. Man-made radiation can come from nuclear reactors and x-ray machines. Radiation with the potential for human tissue injury is called ionizing radiation. Examples of ionizing radiation include x-rays, gamma rays, and photons.

UNITS OF RADIATION

- Roentgen (R): unit of exposure in air
- Radiation absorbed dose (rad): amount of radiation absorbed in a material; 100 rad =1 gray (Gy)
- Roentgen equivalent man (rem): amount of radiation biologic damage; 100 rem = 1 Sievert (Sv). It takes into account differential sensitivity among tissues (quality factor) (Table 1-426).

SYNONYMS

For large exposures (deterministic, or nonstochastic, effects of radiation):
Acute radiation syndrome
Radiation sickness
Chronic low-dose exposures produce stochastic effects. This has no common synonyms.

ICD-9CM CODES
990 Radiation exposure
ICD-10CM CODES
W88 Exposure to ionizing radiation
T66 Unspecified effects of radiation

EPIDEMIOLOGY & DEMOGRAPHICS

- High-dose radiation doses are limited to nuclear disasters.
- Epidemiology of cumulative low-level radiation is not well understood and is based on the following two theories:
  - Stochastic effects of radiation exposure: there is a probability of damage-increased effect with dose, but there is no dose threshold and severity is not dose related.
  - Deterministic effects: severity of damage is dose related but with a threshold below which there is no negative outcome.

PHYSICAL FINDINGS & CLINICAL PRESENTATION

- Low-level radiation: Low-level radiation over time may present clinically with various malignancies that may be at increased incidence compared with background rates of malignancies, but there remains much controversy.
- Exposure to radiation from medical imaging tests has been implicated in secondary cancer; the rate of cancer has been found to be dose dependent and exposure increases incremental risk.
- Occupational radiation exposure has been associated with cancer risk, both non-CLL leukemia and other cancers. Occupational exposure has been implicated to cause cataracts in medical professionals who get exposure in a dose-dependent relationship.
- The clinical course of acute radiation syndrome depends on absorbed radiation dose and distribution. The hematopoietic system and skin are particularly important in acute radiation exposure syndromes.
- Acute radiation syndrome: Effects of acute radiation exposure are better studied based on previous nuclear disasters and are summarized in Table 1-427. Rapidly dividing cells such as hematopoietic cells are most prone to radiation. Radiation sickness symptoms are most apparent with doses >1 Gy.
  1. Stage 1 (prodromal phase): flulike syndrome with anorexia, apathy, nausea, vomiting, diarrhea, fever, tachycardia, and/or headache, usually occurring in the first 48 hours.
  2. Stage 2 (latent phase): a short period characterized by improvement in symptoms, lasting for several days to a month.

TABLE 1-427 Dose Estimates for Common Life and Medical Activities

Activity	Dose Estimate
Natural background and man-made radiation (annual average dose equivalent, including radon)	360 mrem
Diagnostic chest x-ray	6-10 mrem
Flight from Los Angeles to Paris	800 mrem
Barium enema	5 mrem
Smoking 1.5 packs per day for 1 year	16,000 mrem = 16 rem
Heart catheterization	45,000 mrad = 45 rad = 0.45 Gy
Mild acute radiation syndrome	200 rad = 2 Gy
LD_{50} for acute whole body irradiation	450 rad = 4.5 Gy
Occupational limit for a radiation worker	5 rem = 0.05 Sv
Limit of a member of the public	0.1 rem = 0.001 Sv = 1 mSv

Gy, Gray; *LD50,* median lethal dose; *mrad,* millirad; *mrem,* millirem; *mSv,* millisievert; *rad,* radiation absorbed dose; *rem,* roentgen equivalent man; *Sv,* sievert.
Modified from Goans RE: Medical management of radiation incidents. In Shannon MW et al (eds): *Haddad and Winchester's clinical management of poisoning and drug overdose,* ed 4, Philadelphia, 2007, Saunders.

TABLE 1-426 Symptoms, Therapy, and Prognosis of Whole Body Ionizing Radiation Injury

	0-1 SV	1-2 SV	2-6 SV	6-10 SV	10-20 SV	>50 SV
Therapeutic needs	None	Observation	Specific treatment	Possible treatment	Palliative	Palliative
Vomiting	None	5%-50%	>3 Gy, 100%	100%	100%	100%
Time to nausea, vomiting	—	3 hr	2 hr	1 hr	30 min	<30 min
Main locus of injury	None	Lymphocytes	Bone marrow	Bone marrow	Small bowel	Brain
Symptoms and signs	—	Moderate leukopenia, epilation	Leukopenia, hemorrhage, epilation	Leukopenia, hemorrhage, epilation	Diarrhea, fever, electrolyte imbalance	Ataxia, coma, convulsions
Critical period	—	—	4-6 wk	4-6 wk	5-14 days	1-4 hr
Therapy	Reassurance	Observation	Transfusion of granulocytes, platelets	Transfusion, antibiotics, bone marrow transplantation	Fluids and salts, possible bone marrow transplantation	Palliative
Prognosis	Excellent	Excellent	Guarded	Guarded	Poor	Hopeless
Lethality	0	0	0%-80%	80%-100%	100%	100%
Time of death	—	—	2 mo	1-2 mo	2 wk	1-2 days
Cause of death	—	—	Infection, hemorrhage	Hemorrhage, infection, pneumonitis	Enteritis, infection	Cerebral edema

Modified from Phillips TL: Radiation injury. In Wyngaarden JB et al (eds): *Cecil textbook of medicine,* ed 24, Philadelphia, 2012, Saunders.

3. Stage 3 (manifest illness phase): if the person survives this stage, recovery is likely.
   - Hematopoietic syndrome: effects can occur with exposure >1 Gy and include pancytopenia, increased infection risk, and bleeding disorders.
   - GI syndrome: radiation induces loss of intestinal crypts, resulting in abdominal pain, nausea, vomiting, anorexia, and diarrhea.
   - Central nervous system: symptoms occur with a very high level of acute radiation (>5 Gy) and include ataxia, confusion, and coma.
4. Stage 4: recovery, lasting weeks to months. If patients survive, they will need lifelong follow-up because of the potential for unusual infections, organ dysfunction, and carcinogenesis.
   - Radiation "burn": Prolonged exposure from fluoroscopy can lead to acute radiodermatitis presenting as red patches but over a few weeks can lead to tissue necrosis.

PROGNOSIS

ACUTE RADIATION SYNDROME

- Exposure <1 Gy: almost certain survival
- Exposure 1 to 2 Gy: 90% survival with medical care
- Exposure 2 to 3.5 Gy: probable survival with medical care
- Exposure 3.5 to 5.5 Gy: 50% survival with medical care
- Exposure 5.5 to 10 Gy: probable death
- Exposure >10 Gy: certain death

CHRONIC LOW-DOSE EXPOSURE: excess cancer not detected below 100 mSv

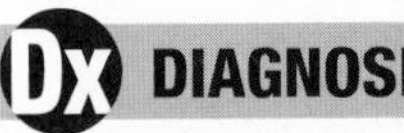

DIAGNOSIS

ACUTE RADIATION SYNDROME

- Diagnosis usually accompanies a nuclear disaster and therefore suspicion is already very high.
- Workup can include measuring radiation levels at site. Estimation of exposure may be accomplished using tools such as the METREPOL (Medical Treatment Protocols for Radiation Accident) clinical grading system, which is useful for prognosis.
- Laboratory studies: in the acute setting, CBC, brain imaging

CHRONIC LOW-DOSE EXPOSURE

Currently impossible to determine whether a subsequently diagnosed malignancy is radiation induced. Workup is for underlying malignancy evaluation.

ETIOLOGY

ACUTE RADIATION SYNDROME: usually nuclear disaster

CHRONIC LOW-DOSE EXPOSURE: The average annual dose to residents of the U.S. is approximately 3.6 mSv.

- Cosmic: positive-charged ions that interact with atmosphere to create secondary radiation
- Terrestrial: radon, potassium-40, thorium, and uranium
- Man-made: medical radiation including x-rays, CT scans, PET scans, nuclear stress tests, nuclear weapon fallout, fluoroscopy, and smoking

Rx TREATMENT

- For all accidental radiation contamination, such as nuclear medicine materials, the following decontamination steps are considered mandatory:
  1. Perform at site of exposure unless there is continued radiation exposure.
  2. Remove all clothing (and treat as radioactive waste). Providers should use strict isolation precautions, including donning of gown, mask, cap, double gloves, and shoe covers, when evaluating and treating contaminated patients.
  3. Wash patient with mild soap (neutral pH) and tepid water. Dispose of contaminated water as radioactive waste.
  4. Scrub any open wound.
  5. Depending on the situation, the regional emergency response system should be called for additional measures such as evacuation.
- Management of acute radiation syndrome:
  1. Establish IV access.
  2. Monitor physiologic signs.
  3. Manage the airway.
  4. Manage burns.
  5. Identify and treat other injuries.
  6. Provide analgesia.
  7. Give antiemetics (e.g., ondansetron).
  8. Manage bleeding and transfuse if necessary.
  9. Diagnose and treat sepsis. Administration of antibiotics reduces the mortality rate. In nonneutropenic patients, use of antibiotics should be reserved for obvious foci of infection secondary to extensive burns, penetrating wounds, and/or abdominal/visceral trauma.
  10. Confirm initial dose estimate using chromosome aberration cytogenetic bioassay when possible.
  11. Consider colony-stimulating factors (CSFs). In any adult with whole-body or significant partial body exposure >3 Gy, treatment with CSFs should be rapidly initiated (e.g., G-CSF or filgrastim, 5 mcg/kg of body weight per day). CSFs may be withdrawn when the absolute neutrophil count reaches a level greater than 1.0×10^9 after recovery from the nadir.
  12. Consider stem cell transplantation in people with exposure dose of 7 to 10 Gy who do not have significant burns or other major organ toxicity and who have an appropriate donor.
  13. Provide counseling; 75% of individuals exposed to nuclear weapon detonations exhibit some form of psychological symptoms, ranging from insomnia to difficulty concentrating and social withdrawal.
- Chronic low-dose exposures: Treatment of radiation-induced organ damage would not differ significantly from non–radiation-induced cancers, cataracts, or skin lesions.

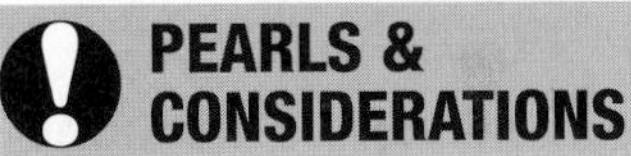

PEARLS & CONSIDERATIONS

COMMENTS

- It is difficult to make a link between exposure to chronic low-level radiation and a specific malignancy in an individual.
- Positioning patients for fluoroscopy procedures and monitoring amount of x-ray radiation are very important to prevent radiation burns.
- Humans are consistently exposed to background/naturally occurring radiation.
- Ionizing radiation from medical imaging procedures is not negligible. Since the early 1980s, the per capita dose of radiation from medical imaging has increased by a factor of nearly 6. Radiation exposure from imaging at current rates is predicted to be responsible for 2% of future cancers.

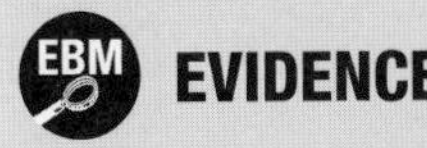

EVIDENCE

available at www.expertconsult.com

SUGGESTED READINGS

available at www.expertconsult.com

AUTHORS: **RAHUL BHARDWAJ, M.D.** and **PRANAV M. PATEL, M.D., F.A.C.C., F.S.C.A.I.**

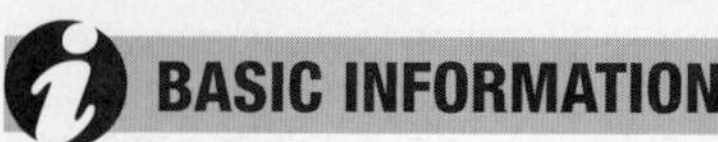

BASIC INFORMATION

DEFINITION

Ramsay Hunt syndrome is a localized herpes zoster infection involving the seventh nerve and geniculate ganglia, resulting in hearing loss, vertigo, and facial nerve palsy.

SYNONYMS

Herpes zoster oticus
Geniculate herpes
Herpetic geniculate ganglionitis

ICD-9CM CODES
053.11 Ramsay Hunt syndrome
ICD-10CM CODES
B02.21 Postherpetic geniculate ganglionitis

EPIDEMIOLOGY & DEMOGRAPHICS

PREDOMINANT SEX: Equal sex distribution
PREDOMINANT AGE:
- Increasingly common with advancing age
- Rare in childhood

PHYSICAL FINDINGS & CLINICAL PRESENTATION

- Characteristic vesicles:
  1. On pinna
  2. In external auditory canal (Fig. 1-792)
  3. In distribution of the facial nerve and, occasionally, adjacent cranial nerves
- Facial paralysis on the involved side

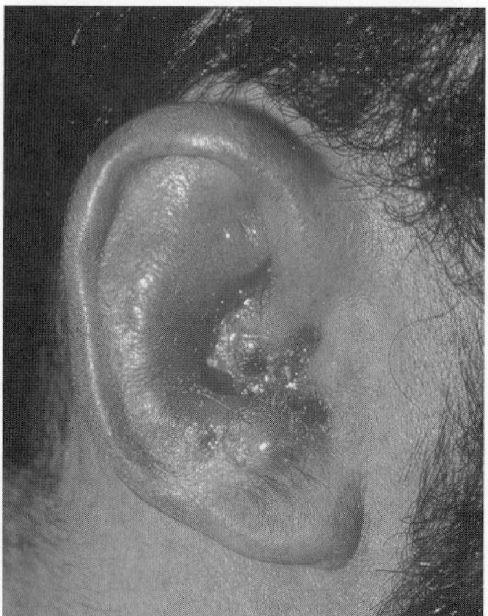

FIGURE 1-792 Herpes zoster of the geniculate ganglion resulting in vesicles on the ear (as shown here) and tympanic membrane occurs in Ramsay Hunt syndrome. Both seventh and eighth cranial nerve functions may be affected. (From White GM, Cox NH [eds]: *Diseases of the skin: color atlas and text,* ed 2, St Louis, 2006, Mosby.)

ETIOLOGY

Reactivation of dormant infection with varicella-zoster virus after primary varicella

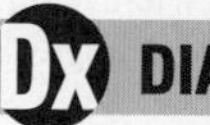

DIAGNOSIS

- Usually made by recognition of the clinical features detailed previously
- Viral culture and/or microscopic examination of specimens taken from active vesicles

DIFFERENTIAL DIAGNOSIS

- Herpes simplex
- External otitis
- Impetigo
- Enteroviral infection
- Bell's palsy of other etiologies
- Acoustic neuroma (before appearance of skin lesions)

The differential diagnosis of headache and facial pain is described in Section II.

WORKUP

If the diagnosis is in doubt, confirm varicella-zoster virus infection.

LABORATORY TESTS

- Generally not necessary
- Viral culture of specimens of vesicular fluid and scrapings of the vesicle base
- Tzanck preparation, which may reveal multinucleated giant cells
- Direct immunofluorescent staining of scrapings

IMAGING STUDIES

MRI may demonstrate enhancement of the facial and vestibulocochlear nerves before appearance of vesicles.

TREATMENT

ACUTE GENERAL Rx

- Use of corticosteroids is controversial.
- Acyclovir (800 mg PO five times qd for 10 days), famciclovir (500 mg tid for 7 days), or valacyclovir (1 g q8h for 7 days) may hasten healing.
- Prednisone (40 mg PO for 2 days, 30 mg for 7 days, followed by tapering course) is recommended by some authors.
- Analgesics should be used as indicated.

CHRONIC Rx

- Duloxetine and amitriptyline are effective in postherpetic pain.
- Other agents for postherpetic pain include gabapentin and pregabalin.
- Narcotic analgesics may occasionally be necessary.

DISPOSITION

Recurrences are unusual.

REFERRAL

To otolaryngologist: patients with persistent facial paralysis for potential surgical decompression of the facial nerve

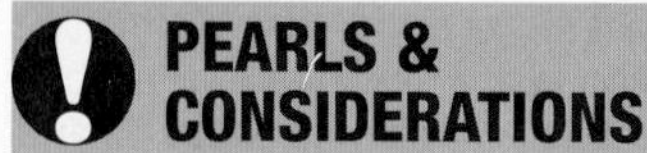

PEARLS & CONSIDERATIONS

COMMENTS

Immunodeficiency states, particularly HIV infection, should be considered in:
- Younger patients
- Severe cases
- Patients with a history of specific risk behavior

SUGGESTED READINGS

available at www.expertconsult.com

RELATED CONTENT

Ramsay Hunt Syndrome (Patient Information)

AUTHOR: **GLENN G. FORT, M.D., M.P.H.**

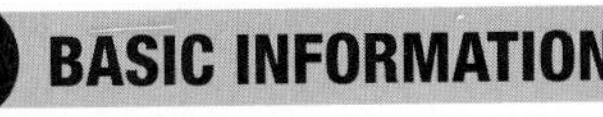

BASIC INFORMATION

DEFINITION

Raynaud's phenomenon (RP) is a vasospastic disorder that causes an exaggerated response to cold temperatures and/or emotional stress, resulting in episodic digital ischemia. It presents as a cold-induced, symmetric, sharply demarcated white or blue discoloration of the distal fingers or toes, followed by erythema at a variable time after rewarming.

SYNONYMS

Primary Raynaud's phenomenon or Raynaud's disease
Secondary Raynaud's phenomenon

ICD-9CM CODES
443.0 Raynaud's syndrome, Raynaud's disease, Raynaud's phenomenon (secondary)
ICD-10CM CODES
I73.0 Raynaud's syndrome

EPIDEMIOLOGY & DEMOGRAPHICS

- RP is classified clinically into primary or secondary forms and affects approximately 3% to 5% of the general population, 15% of children younger than 12 yr, and less than 1% of adults older than 60 yr.
- Primary RP usually occurs between the ages of 12 and 25 yr.
- It is more likely to affect women than men (4:1) and appears to be more common in colder climates.
- 5% to 15% of patients with primary Raynaud's phenomenon develop a secondary cause later in the course of the disease (mostly a connective tissue disorder).
- Secondary RP tends to begin after age 35 to 40 yr.
- Secondary RP occurs in more than 90% of patients with scleroderma and in approximately 30% of patients with systemic lupus erythematosus or Sjögren's syndrome.

PHYSICAL FINDINGS & CLINICAL PRESENTATION

- The typical manifestation of RP is the biphasic color response of the digits to cold exposure and rewarming, which may or may not be accompanied by pain. RP most often affects the hand (Fig. 1-793).
  1. White (pallor) or blue (cyanotic) discoloration of the digit(s) resulting from vasospasm on cold or vibration exposure.
  2. Red (rubor) with or without pain and paresthesia when vasospasm resolves and blood returns to the digit.
- Color changes can sometimes be induced by placing the hand in an ice bath, although this is not recommended as a diagnostic maneuver because responses may be inconsistent even in patients with definite RP.
- Color changes are well delineated, symmetric, and usually bilateral, involving the fingers and toes. The index, middle, and ring fingers are commonly involved and the thumb infrequently; however, if the thumb is involved, that suggests secondary causes of RP.
- Fingertips are most often involved, but feet, ears, nose, tongue, and nipples can also be affected.
- Patients with RP may exhibit a violaceous or reticular pattern of skin of arms and legs, sometimes with regular, unbroken circles (livedo reticularis).
- Duration of attacks can range from seconds to hours and averages 15 to 20 min.
- Chronic skin changes resulting from repeated attacks may include skin thickening and brittle nails. Ulcerations and, rarely, gangrene may occur.
- Physical examination should also include examination for symptoms associated with autoimmune disease, such as fever, rash, arthritis, dry eyes, dry mouth, myalgias, or cardiopulmonary abnormalities.

ETIOLOGY

- Primary RP can also be called idiopathic Raynaud's phenomenon, primary Raynaud's syndrome, or Raynaud's disease. It occurs in the absence of any associated disease.
- With primary RP, the possibility that another first-degree family member is affected is reported as approximately 25%.
- Secondary RP is associated with an underlying pathologic condition or disorder, use of certain drugs, or related occupation. Secondary RP is associated with:
  1. CREST syndrome (calcinosis, RP, esophageal involvement, sclerodactyly, and telangiectasia)
  2. Scleroderma, Sjögren's syndrome, mixed connective tissue disease, polymyositis, and dermatomyositis
  3. Primary pulmonary hypertension
  4. Systemic lupus erythematosus, arteritis
  5. Rheumatoid arthritis
  6. Thromboangiitis obliterans (Buerger's disease)
  7. Drugs (beta-blockers, ergotamine, methysergide, vinblastine, bleomycin, oral contraceptives, nicotine, clonidine, cocaine, caffeine, vinyl chloride, tegafur, interferon alfa, interferon beta)
  8. Hematologic disorders (polycythemia, cryoglobulinemia, cold agglutinins, paraproteinemia, cryofibrinogenemia)
  9. Carpal tunnel syndrome
  10. Use of tools that vibrate
  11. Endocrine disorders (hypothyroidism, carcinoid syndrome, pheochromocytoma, metabolic syndrome)
  12. Estrogen replacement therapy without progesterone
  13. Hypercoagulable states, protein C, protein S, antithrombin III deficiency, factor V Leiden deficiency, and antiphospholipid syndrome
  14. Poliomyelitis is a rare cause
  15. Primary biliary cirrhosis
  16. Vasospastic disorders (migraines, Prinzmetal angina)
  17. Malignancies (angiocentric lymphoma, ovarian cancer)

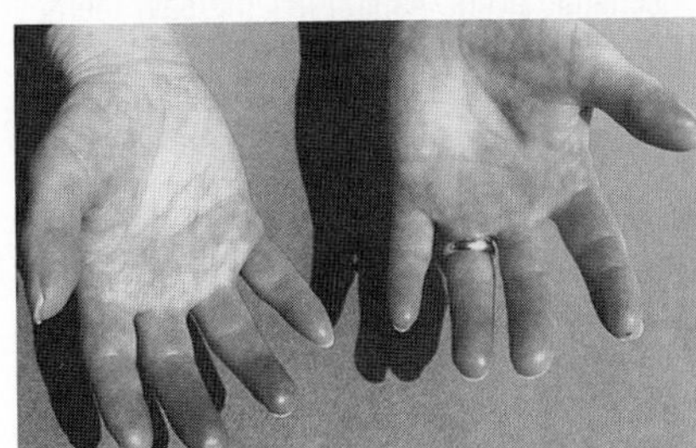

FIGURE 1-793 Raynaud's phenomenon. Sharply demarcated cyanosis of the fingers with proximal venular congestion (livedo reticularis) is seen. (From Klippel J et al [eds]: *Primary care rheumatology,* London, 1999, Mosby.)

Dx DIAGNOSIS

Clinical criteria:
- Definite RP: repeated episodes of biphasic color change on cold exposure
- Possible RP: Uniphasic color changes plus numbness or paresthesia on cold exposure
- No RP: No color change on cold exposure

The suggested criteria for primary RP are:
- Symmetric attacks
- Absence of tissue necrosis, ulceration, gangrene, or peripheral vascular disease
- Absence of a secondary cause on the basis of a patient's history and general physical examination
- Negative nail-fold capillary examination
- Negative test for antinuclear antibody (ANA)
- Normal erythrocyte sedimentation rate (ESR)

Secondary RP is suggested by the following findings:
- Onset of symptoms after age 30 yr
- Male gender
- Episodes that are painful, asymmetric, or associated with ischemic skin lesions
- Clinical features suggestive of a connective-tissue disease
- Elevated specific autoantibody tests and ESR
- Evidence of microvascular disease on microscopy of nail-fold capillaries

DIFFERENTIAL DIAGNOSIS

- Neurogenic thoracic outlet syndrome or carpal tunnel syndrome
- Frostbite or cold weather injury
- Medication reaction (ergotamine, chemotherapeutic agents)
- Atherosclerosis, thromboembolic disease
- Buerger's disease, embolic disease
- Acrocyanosis
- Livedo reticularis
- Injury from repetitive motion

WORKUP

- Fig. E1-794 describes an approach to diagnosis of Raynaud's phenomenon. Once the diagnosis of RP is established, differentiating primary from secondary is helpful in treatment and prognosis.
- Patients who are younger when their symptoms occur, have a normal history and physical examination and normal nail-fold

capillaries, and have no history of digital ischemic lesions can be considered as having primary RP. These patients can be monitored clinically without any further testing.
- If a secondary cause of RP is suspected, appropriate laboratory testing is recommended (see "Laboratory Tests"). Secondary RP has associated abnormal nail-fold microscopy.

LABORATORY TESTS

- CBC, serum electrolytes, blood urea nitrogen, creatinine, ESR, ANAs, VDRL antibody test, rheumatoid factor, and urinalysis should be included in the initial evaluation.
- If the history, physical examination, and initial laboratory tests suggest a possible secondary cause, specific serologic testing (e.g., anticentromere antibodies, anti-Scl 70, cryoglobulins, complement testing, and serum protein electrophoresis) may be indicated.
- Noninvasive vascular testing includes finger systolic blood pressures, segmental blood pressure measurements, cold recovery time (measure vasoconstrictor and vasodilator responses of finger to cold), fingertip thermography, and laser Doppler with thermal challenge (measures relative change in skin blood flow with ambient warming).

IMAGING STUDIES

- The diagnosis of RP should not be made on the basis of laboratory tests, and imaging studies should not replace a good history and physical examination.
- Duplex ultrasound can image the palmar arch and digital arteries for patency.
- Magnetic resonance angiography is useful for imaging larger arteries.
- Contrast angiography is the gold standard for arterial imaging.
- Nail-fold capillary microscopy can differentiate primary from secondary RP.
- Videomicroscopy and thermography are also useful for diagnosis of RP.

Rx TREATMENT

NONPHARMACOLOGIC THERAPY

- Avoid drugs that may precipitate RP (see "Etiology").
- Avoid cold exposure and sudden temperature shifts. Use warm gloves, hats, and garments during the winter months or before going into cold environments (e.g., air-conditioned rooms).
- Avoid stressful situations, and use relaxation techniques in preventing RP attacks.

ACUTE GENERAL Rx

- Acute measures to terminate an attack include rotating the arms in a windmill pattern, placing the hands under warm water or in a warm body fold such as the axilla, and the swing-arm maneuver.
- Medications are indicated in the treatment of RP if there are signs of critical ischemia or if the quality of life of the patient is affected to the degree that activities of normal living are no longer possible and preventive techniques do not work.

CHRONIC Rx

- Dihydropyridine calcium channel blockers (e.g., nifedipine, amlodipine, felodipine, nisoldipine, isradipine) are the most effective pharmacologic treatment for RP and are the drugs of choice. Verapamil is ineffective for patients with severe RP.
- Nifedipine is most often prescribed at a dose of 10 to 20 mg 30 min before cold exposure. If symptoms occur with long duration, nifedipine XL 30 to 180 mg PO qd is often effective.
- Patients who do not tolerate or do not respond to calcium channel blocker therapy can sometimes benefit from other drugs that directly or indirectly cause vasodilation, either alone or in combination, although data for these therapies are less robust. Some potential therapeutic options include direct vasodilators such as nitroprusside, hydralazine, papaverine, minoxidil, niacin, and griseofulvin. Topical 1% nitroglycerin or topical l-arginine, ethyl nicotinate, hexyl nicotinate, thurfyl salicylate may also be useful, particularly if low blood pressure is a concern.
- Phosphodiesterase inhibitors (cilostazol, pentoxifylline, and sildenafil), angiotensin 2 receptor antagonists (losartan), and selective serotonin reuptake inhibitors (fluoxetine) have been used with some limited success.
- Alpha receptor antagonists such as prazosin and phenoxybenzamine have shown some effectiveness in treating RP.
- The prostaglandins, including inhaled iloprost, IV epoprostenol, alprostadil, and tadalafil, may be promising in severe RP. However, additional experience and controlled studies are needed.
- Antioxidants like zinc gluconate have been used to decrease tissue damage.
- *N*-Acetylcysteine and probucol have been shown to lead to improvement in RP.
- Anticoagulation with IV unfractionated heparin or subcutaneous low-molecular-weight heparin and addition of aspirin can be considered during the acute phase of a severe ischemic event. Aspirin (81 mg/day) therapy can be considered in all patients with secondary RP with a history of ischemic ulcers or thrombotic events; however, caution should be exercised because aspirin can theoretically worsen vasospasm by the inhibition of prostacyclin. Long-term anticoagulation with heparin or warfarin is not recommended unless there is evidence of a hypercoagulable state.
- Bypass surgery can be performed for severe RP associated with reconstructible arterial occlusive disease.
- Sympathectomy is available for unreconstructible occlusive disease or pure vasospastic disease refractory to medical treatment.
- Microsurgical revascularization of the hand and digital reconstruction may improve digital vascular perfusion and heal digital ulcers when proximal arterial occlusion is associated with digital vasospasm.
- Ischemic digital lesions should be treated with topical antibiotics and daily cleansing with soap and water. Digits that progress to dry gangrene should be permitted to undergo autoamputation. Surgical amputation is limited for intractable pain or deep tissue infection.

DISPOSITION

The prognosis of patients with RP depends on the etiology.

- Primary RP is fairly benign, usually remaining stable and controlled with nonpharmacologic medical treatment.
- Remission of primary RP can occur spontaneously.
- Patients with secondary RP, specifically those with scleroderma, CREST syndrome, or thromboangiitis obliterans, may develop severe ischemic digits with ulceration, gangrene, and autoamputation.

REFERRAL

- Rheumatology consult is indicated if secondary collagen vascular disease is diagnosed.
- Vascular surgery consult is indicated if ulcers, gangrene, or threatened digit loss is noted.

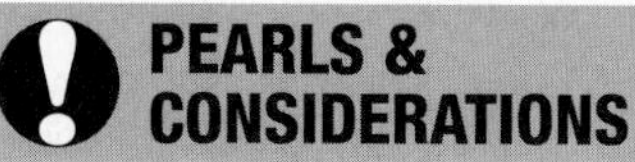

PEARLS & CONSIDERATIONS

- Most patients with RP can be managed by a primary care provider.
- It is important to differentiate primary from secondary forms. Secondary forms may become manifest as far out as 10 yr from the diagnosis of RP. It is important to take immediate action during an attack, and patients are encouraged to:
  1. Keep warm
  2. Not use tobacco products
  3. Avoid aggravating medications
  4. Control stress
  5. Exercise
  6. Follow up with a physician

SUGGESTED READINGS

available at www.expertconsult.com

RELATED CONTENT

Raynaud's Phenomenon (Patient Information)

AUTHORS: **SYEDA M. SAYEED, M.D.**, and **FRED F. FERRI, M.D.**

BASIC INFORMATION

DEFINITION

Reiter's syndrome is one of the seronegative spondyloarthropathies, so called because serum rheumatoid factor is not present in these forms of inflammatory arthritis. There is an international consensus that the term *reactive arthritis* (ReA) should replace the name "Reiter's syndrome" to describe this constellation of signs and symptoms. Unfortunately, the original name is still associated with the syndrome. Reiter's syndrome is an asymmetric polyarthritis that affects mainly the lower extremities and is associated with one or more of the following:

- Urethritis
- Cervicitis
- Dysentery
- Inflammatory eye disease
- Mucocutaneous lesions

SYNONYMS

Reiter's disease
Reactive arthritis
Seronegative spondyloarthropathy

ICD-9CM CODES
099.3 Reiter's syndrome
ICD-10CM CODES
M02.30 Reiter's disease, unspecified site

EPIDEMIOLOGY & DEMOGRAPHICS

INCIDENCE (IN U.S.): 0.0035% annually of men ≤50 yr
PEAK INCIDENCE: Most common in the third decade
PREDOMINANT SEX: Male
PREDOMINANT AGE: 20 to 40 yr
GENETICS: Familial disposition: strongly associated with HLA-B27 (63% to 96%)

PHYSICAL FINDINGS & CLINICAL PRESENTATION

- Polyarthritis
  1. Affecting the knee and ankle
  2. Commonly asymmetric
- Heel pain and Achilles tendinitis, especially at the insertion of the Achilles tendon
- Plantar fasciitis
- Large effusions
- Dactylitis, or "sausage toe"
- Urethritis
- Uveitis or conjunctivitis; uveitis can progress to blindness without treatment
- Keratoderma blennorrhagicum, circinate balanitis
  1. Hyperkeratotic lesions on soles of the feet (Fig. E1-795), toes, penis (Fig. E1-796), hands
  2. Closely resembles psoriasis
- Aortic regurgitation similar to that seen in ankylosing spondylitis

ETIOLOGY

- Epidemic Reiter's syndrome after outbreaks of dysentery has been well described.
- Genetically susceptible HLA-B27 individuals are at risk for developing Reiter's syndrome after infection with certain pathogens:
  - *Salmonella*
  - *Shigella*
  - *Yersinia enterocolitica*
  - *Chlamydia trachomatis*
- Symptom complex indistinguishable from Reiter's syndrome has been described in association with HIV infection.

DIAGNOSIS

DIFFERENTIAL DIAGNOSIS

- Ankylosing spondylitis
- Psoriatic arthritis
- Rheumatoid arthritis
- Gonococcal arthritis-tenosynovitis
- Rheumatic fever

WORKUP

- X-ray examination of affected joints
- Synovial fluid examination and culture
- Careful examination of eyes and skin
- Cultures for gonococcus (urethral, cervical, stool)

LABORATORY TESTS

- Elevated but nonspecific erythrocyte sedimentation rate
- No specific laboratory tests to diagnose Reiter's syndrome
- Do not use HLA-B27 testing as a diagnostic tool

IMAGING STUDIES

Plain radiographs:

- Juxtaarticular osteopenia of affected joints
- Erosions and joint space narrowing in more advanced disease
- Periostitis and reactive new bone formation at the insertions of the Achilles tendon and the plantar fascia
- Sacroiliitis:
  1. Unilateral or bilateral
  2. Indistinguishable from ankylosing spondylitis
- Vertebral bridging osteophytes

TREATMENT

NONPHARMACOLOGIC THERAPY

Physical therapy to maintain range of motion of the spine and other joints

ACUTE GENERAL Rx

- Flares treated with nonsteroidal anti-inflammatory drugs such as indomethacin (25 to 50 mg PO tid).
- Enteric or urethral infection should be treated with appropriate antibiotic coverage.
- Uveitis should be treated with steroid eye drops in consultation with an ophthalmologist.
- Achilles tendinitis and plantar fasciitis should be treated with injections of methylprednisolone (40 to 80 mg).
- Sulfasalazine (2 to 3 g PO tid) may be effective.
- Careful monitoring for the following is essential:
  - Gastrointestinal toxicity
  - Hypersensitivity
  - Bone marrow suppression
- Persistent and uncontrolled disease should be managed with cytotoxic drugs (methotrexate, azathioprine) in consultation with a rheumatologist.

CHRONIC Rx

Chronic disease is best managed by a team approach with the collaboration of a rheumatologist or other experienced physician and physical therapist.

DISPOSITION

- Recurrences are frequent, even with treatment.
- Long-term sequelae:
  - Persistent polyarthritis
  - Chronic back pain
  - Heel pain
  - Progressive iridocyclitis
  - Aortic regurgitation

REFERRAL

- To ophthalmologist if uveitis is suspected
- To rheumatologist if arthritis and tendinitis fail to improve rapidly after a course of nonsteroidal anti-inflammatory drugs

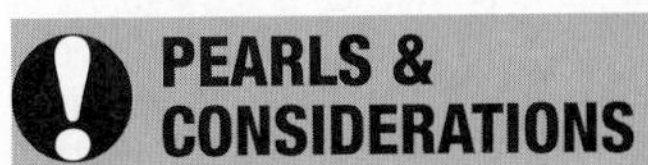

PEARLS & CONSIDERATIONS

COMMENTS

- Infection with HIV is associated with particularly severe cases of Reiter's syndrome.
- HIV testing is recommended, especially if risk factors such as unprotected sexual activity or IV drug use are identified.

SUGGESTED READINGS

available at www.expertconsult.com

RELATED CONTENT

Reiter's Syndrome (Patient Information)

AUTHOR: **GLENN G. FORT, M.D., M.P.H.**

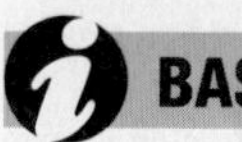

BASIC INFORMATION

DEFINITION

Renal artery stenosis (RAS) is the progressive narrowing of the renal artery, which is most commonly due to atherosclerosis or fibromuscular dysplasia. RAS is an important, potentially reversible cause of hypertension and ischemic nephropathy. RAS increases the risk of acute renal artery occlusion, which usually results from cardioemboli, vascular emboli, or in situ thrombosis.

SYNONYMS

Acute:
- Renal artery thrombosis
- Renal artery embolism

Chronic:
- Renovascular hypertension

ICD-9CM CODES

440.1 Renal artery stenosis
405.01 Renovascular hypertension, secondary
447.9 Renal artery hyperplasia

ICD-10CM CODES

I70.1 Atherosclerosis of renal artery
I15.0 Renovascular hypertension
I77.9 Disorder of arteries and arterioles, unspecified

EPIDEMIOLOGY & DEMOGRAPHICS

- Chronic RAS:
  1. Atherosclerotic RAS (ARAS) accounts for about 90% of chronic RAS. True prevalence is unknown.
     a. General population autopsy studies show prevalence of 4% and 2% to 5% in hypertensive patients.
     b. In the general population >65 yr of age, the prevalence is 6.8% (5.5% of women, 9.1% of men, 6.7% of African Americans, and 6.9% of Caucasians). Of those with ARAS, 12% had bilateral disease.
     c. In patients with malignant hypertension, the prevalence is 43% in Caucasians and 7% in African Americans. In patients with mild hypertension, the prevalence is <1%.
     d. In patients with peripheral artery disease, the prevalence is 22% to 59%.
  2. Fibromuscular dysplasia accounts for approximately 10% of chronic RAS. It is typically seen in women (81%) aged <50 yr. 26% have bilateral disease.
     - Acute renal artery occlusion: epidemiology depends on the underlying cause. The incidence on autopsy study was 1.4%.

PHYSICAL FINDINGS & CLINICAL PRESENTATION

Progressive RAS:
- Majority of patients with RAS are asymptomatic.
- Fibromuscular dysplasia: new-onset hypertension at age <50 yr or hypertension in any patient without family history or risk factors
- Atherosclerotic renal artery disease: new-onset hypertension at age >55 yr, with risk factors for or evidence of atherosclerotic disease
- Uncontrolled hypertension refractory to three or more medications including a diuretic
- Abdominal bruit (40% of cases)
- Chronic kidney disease
- Hypertensive retinopathy
- Pulmonary edema in a hypertensive patient
- Hypokalemia
- Acute kidney injury (AKI) after the administration of an ACE inhibitor (ACEI) has previously been considered a marker for bilateral RAS but is neither sensitive nor specific.

Acute renal artery occlusion:
- Flank or abdominal pain
- Fever
- Nausea and/or vomiting
- Leukocytosis
- Hematuria (microscopic or gross)
- Elevated aspartate aminotransferase, lactate dehydrogenase, and alkaline phosphatase
- Oliguric renal failure if occlusion is bilateral; normal or near-normal renal function in unilateral occlusion
- Cholesterol or septic emboli: depending on distribution of emboli, patients may have multisystem manifestations such as visual disturbance, painful distal extremities, abdominal pain, signs of organ or limb ischemia; laboratory findings include eosinophiluria, proteinuria, AKI, elevated erythrocyte sedimentation rate

ETIOLOGY

RAS and thrombosis:
- Atherosclerosis: risk factors for atherosclerosis include family history, smoking, diabetes, hypertension, and hyperlipidemia. Typically involves the ostium and proximal third of the main renal artery.
- Fibromuscular dysplasia (Fig. 1-797): etiology unknown. Classified into three categories based on the layer of arterial wall affected: medial (>90%), intimal (<10%), adventitial (<1%). Typically involves the distal main renal artery and intrarenal branches.
- Extrinsic compression (e.g., neoplasm)
- Neurofibromatosis and fibrous bands
- Vasculitides, including autoimmune (Takayasu's, antiphospholipid syndrome), infectious (syphilis)
- Renal artery aneurysm
- Hypercoagulable state
- Complication of renal transplantation (role of cyclosporine)

Renal artery embolism (cardiac conditions contribute 90%):
- Left ventricular thrombus (may be the result of myocardial infarction or other cardiomyopathy)
- Atrial fibrillation
- Endocarditis
- Paradoxical emboli from deep vein thrombosis in patient with atrioventricular or ventricular septal defect
- Atheromatous plaques (cholesterol emboli)

PATHOGENESIS

- Pathogenesis of fibromuscular dysplasia is unknown.
- The pathogenesis of hypertension is related to the neurohormonal cascade resulting from

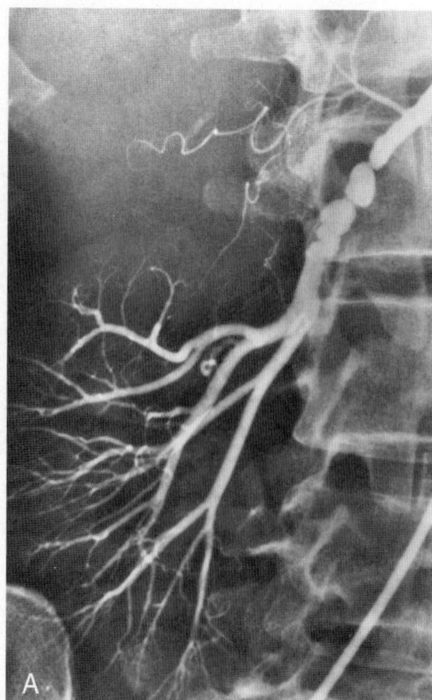

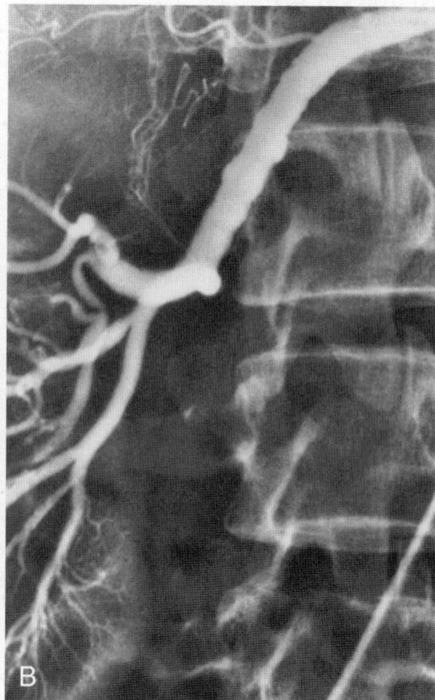

FIGURE 1-797 Fibromuscular dysplasia. A, Selective renal arteriogram illustrating the beaded appearance of fibromuscular dysplasia with multiple webs characteristic of medial fibroplasia in a 39-yr-old woman. **B,** Selective injection of the same renal artery after technically successful percutaneous transluminal renal angioplasty. (Courtesy Michael McKusick, M.D., Mayo Clinic, Rochester, Minnesota. From Floege J et al: *Comprehensive clinical nephrology,* ed 4, Philadelphia, 2010, Saunders.)

R

Diseases and Disorders

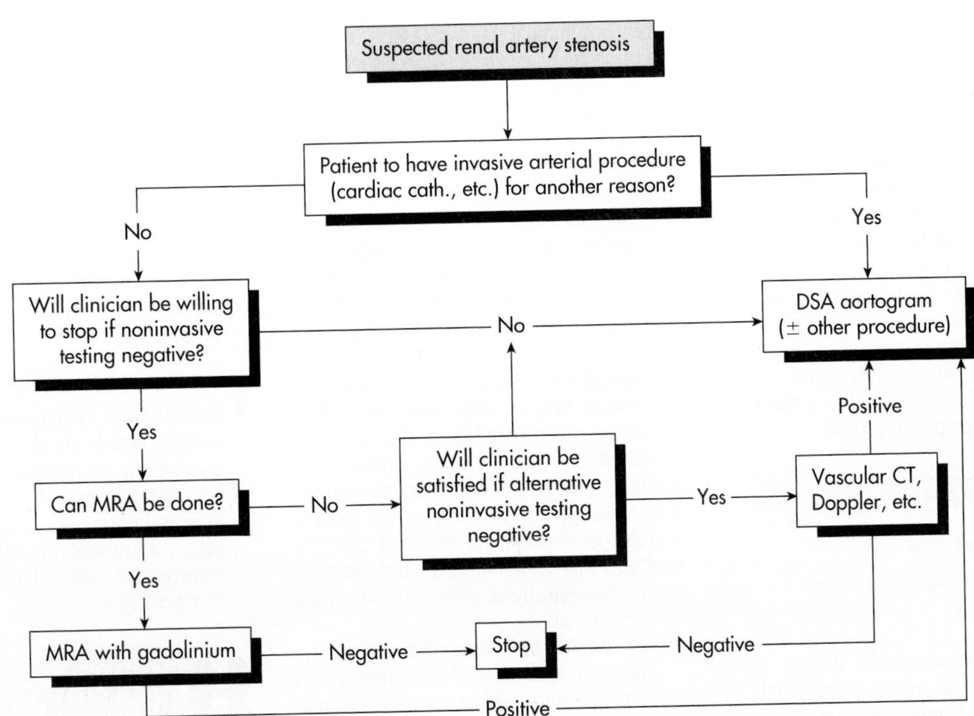

FIGURE 1-798 Approach to the anatomic evaluation of renal artery stenosis. Once stenosis is suspected, if the patient is to have another invasive arterial procedure, noninvasive imaging is deferred and a low-volume digital subtraction aortogram *(DSA)* is done at the time of that procedure. In other cases, the clinician should assess whether a negative noninvasive test would be sufficient evidence to acquit the renal arteries. If so, noninvasive testing should be performed. If not, consideration should be given to DSA and selective angiography. *Cath,* Catherization; *CT,* computed tomography; *MRA,* magnetic resonance angiography. (From Zipes DP et al [eds]: *Braunwald's heart disease,* ed 7, Philadelphia, 2005, Saunders.)

renal ischemia. The macula densa of the kidney senses a decreased systemic blood pressure caused by the reduced blood flow through the stenotic artery leading to a decrease in the glomerular filtration rate. Renal hypoperfusion or ischemia produces an increase in plasma renin that stimulates the conversion of angiotensin I to angiotensin II, causing vasoconstriction and aldosterone secretion, sodium retention, and potassium wasting. Hypertension results and can be self-sustaining, even in the case of unilateral RAS, because of hypertensive damage to the contralateral kidney.

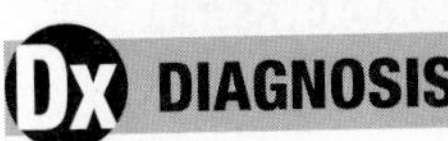

Dx DIAGNOSIS

SCREENING

American College of Cardiology and American Heart Association (ACC/AHA) guidelines for identifying patients who should be screened for RAS:

- Onset of hypertension at age <30 yr or severe hypertension at age >55 yr
- Clinical findings that suggest secondary hypertension as opposed to essential hypertension in the absence of another more likely cause of secondary hypertension such as pheochromocytoma
- Malignant hypertension: hypertension with coexistent evidence of acute end-organ damage (acute renal failure, acute decompensated heart failure, new visual or neurologic disturbance, and/or advanced retinopathy)
- Accelerated hypertension: sudden and persistent worsening of previously controlled hypertension
- Resistant hypertension: full doses of a three-drug regimen that includes a diuretic
- Sudden unexplained pulmonary edema
- New azotemia or acute renal failure after ACEI or angiotensin receptor blockers (ARBs)
- Unexplained atrophic kidney or variation in size of both kidneys by >1.5 cm, smaller kidney likely affected by RAS

LABORATORY TESTS

- Basic chemistry, including sodium, potassium, blood urea nitrogen, and creatinine
- Glomerular filtration rate
- Urinalysis and urine cultures
- Electrocardiogram to evaluate for atrial fibrillation and signs of coronary artery disease/myocardial infarction
- Hypercoaguable workup in setting of thrombosis or embolic disease

IMAGING STUDIES

- Duplex Doppler ultrasonography, CT angiography, and magnetic resonance angiography (MRA) are effective diagnostic screening methods. The choice of imaging modality will depend on the availability of the diagnostic tool, the experience and local accuracy of each modality, and patient characteristics, including body size, renal function, contrast allergy, and presence of prior stents. Fig. 1-798 describes an approach to the anatomic evaluation of RAS. An approach to the angiographic evaluation and treatment of RAS is described in Fig. E1-799.
- Duplex Doppler ultrasonography is safe and inexpensive. When compared with angiography, duplex ultrasound has a sensitivity of 84% to 98% and a specificity of 62% to 99% for detecting RAS. An end-diastolic velocity of >150 cm/sec predicts severe RAS (>80% stenosis). Peak systolic velocity >285 cm/sec, renal/aorta ratio >3.5, and/or renal resistive index >0.15 correlated with RAS >60%. Duplex Doppler ultrasonography may also be used to measure the renal dimensions. US is a good surveillance test to monitor stent patency after intervention. Limitations include operator-dependent imaging, patient body habitus, and poor visualization of accessory renal arteries.
- MRA (Fig. 1-800) provides good visualization of both main and accessory renal arteries. The test has high sensitivity (90%-100%) and a specificity of 76% to 94%. Limitations include the associated risk of nephrogenic systemic fibrosis with gadolinium infusion, high cost, inability to image within a previously placed metallic stent, and lack of widespread availability.
- CT angiography is fast and effective. When compared with angiography, CT has a sensitivity of 59% to 96% and a specificity of 82% to 99%. CT has good spatial resolution and can detect restenosis through metal stents

but requires radiation exposure and infusion of potentially nephrotoxic iodinated contrast.

- IV digital subtraction catheter angiography (88% sensitivity, 90% specificity) is the gold standard for anatomic diagnosis of RAS. It is not a first-line screening tool but is recommended, if noninvasive tests are inconclusive but clinical suspicion is high. Renal fractional flow reserve (FFR) at the time of catheter angiography can be used to assess severity of RAS using maximal vasodilatation. A hyperemeic systolic gradient of at least 21 mm Hg or renal fractional flow reserve of <0.90 can be considered hemodynamically significant. This modality should be reserved for patients with a high likelihood of intervention.

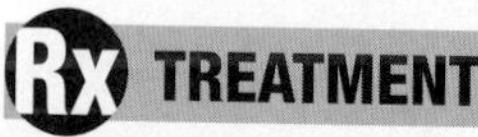

TREATMENT

ACUTE GENERAL Rx

Acute renal artery thrombosis:

- Thrombolytic therapy
- Anticoagulation
- Revascularization (endovascular therapy or surgery). Endovascular renal artery stenting is favored over surgery, and has shown better clinical results when compared with balloon angioplasty (without stenting) in ARAS. Balloon angioplasty with bailout stent placement if necessary is recommended for FMD. Primary open revascularization with vascular reconstruction can be considered selectively for patients with complex disease that extends into segmental arteries, small renal arteries, or early primary branching of the main renal artery.
- Acute blood pressure control with IV antihypertensives

CHRONIC Rx

Renal artery thrombosis/emboli: anticoagulation based upon underlying condition. If the patient has atrial fibrillation with therapeutic INR, consider INR 2.5 to 3.5.

Cholesterol emboli:

- Supportive care

RAS:

- Because of the activation of the renin-angiotensin-aldosterone system in RAS, ACEI/ARBs are recommended and well tolerated (92%) for the treatment of renovascular hypertension. Renal function should be monitored carefully when initiating or titrating these medications, particularly in patients with bilateral RAS (78% tolerability) or unilateral stenosis with solitary kidney, so as to avoid precipitating AKI.
- Beta-blockers and calcium channel blockers are recommended for the treatment of hypertension in patients with RAS of all types.
- Antiplatelet therapy and statin therapy in patients with atherosclerotic RAS.
- Percutaneous intervention or surgical revascularization should be reserved for patients whose blood pressure control with medication is difficult and for patients with progressive disease. The ACC/AHA guidelines for clinical indications of renal artery revascularization in the presence of significant stenosis include:
  1. Accelerated, resistant, or malignant hypertension (class IIa)
  2. Hypertension with unilateral small kidney (class IIa)
  3. Hypertension with intolerance to medication (class IIa)
  4. Treatment of cardiac destabilization syndromes such as unexplained heart failure exacerbations or episodes of flash pulmonary edema (class I), and refractory or unstable angina (class IIa)
  5. Progressive chronic kidney disease with bilateral RAS or RAS associated with a solitary functioning kidney (class IIa)
- Randomized control trials (e.g., DRASTIC and ASTRAL) have shown no benefit to percutaneous therapy when compared with medical therapy, with endpoints of blood pressure control, renal function, and cardiovascular events. However, these trials did have several inherent limitations.
  1. The DRASTIC trial was a small angioplasty-only trial that showed no difference in blood pressure but did show decrease in daily doses of antihypertensive drugs and number of drugs in the intervention group.
  2. The ASTRAL trial was a moderate-sized trial of stenting versus medication in moderate RAS that showed no difference in blood pressure control or the number of antihypertensives but had increased risks associated with intervention.
  3. CORAL is a large prospective multicenter trial comparing stenting versus medication in severe RAS (>60% stenosis); this study confirms that in patients with atherosclerotic renal-artery stenosis and hypertension, clinical outcomes are not improved by stenting, and renal artery stenting is futile in those patients.

NATURAL HISTORY

- RAS caused by fibromuscular dysplasia generally does not progress. Fibromuscular dysplasia RAS responds well to angioplasty with long-term patency of the lesion typically observed.
- RAS associated with atherosclerosis is progressive. Of patients with >60% stenosis, 5% progress to total occlusion in 1 yr and 11% progress in 2 yr.
- An increased pulse pressure (PP), defined as systolic minus diastolic blood pressure, has been implicated in the development and progression of small-vessel disease and has been shown to reflect more advanced renal disease. It can help identify patients who are less likely to benefit from percutaneous interventions.

DISPOSITION & REFERRAL

- Patients with uncontrolled hypertension on multiple agents should be referred for management by a specialist.
- Decision for percutaneous intervention for atherosclerotic RAS requires weighing the risks and benefits in detail and should be reserved for selected patients until further data are available.

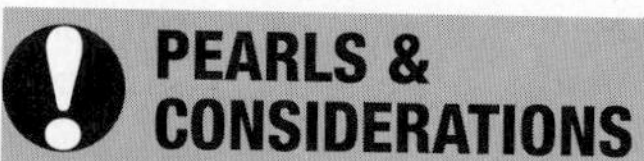

PEARLS & CONSIDERATIONS

- Symptoms for acute renal artery occlusion are nonspecific and can be confused with nephrolithiasis and pyelonephritis among other causes. Evaluation with LDH and liver enzymes can be very helpful. LDH four times the normal range without significant transaminitis is consistent with renal infarction.
- Renal artery stenting currently requires more data to address its utility in both unilateral and bilateral RAS.
- The modality for the type of imaging should depend on the expertise of the institution.

SUGGESTED READINGS

available at www.expertconsult.com

RELATED CONTENT

Renal Artery Stenosis (Patient Information)
Hypertension (Related Key Topic)

AUTHORS: **MEGHA AGARWAL, M.D.** and **PRANAV M. PATEL, M.D., F.A.C.C., F.S.C.A.I.**

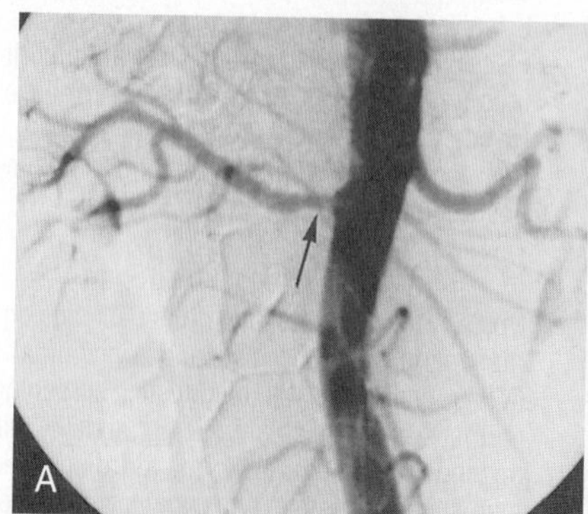

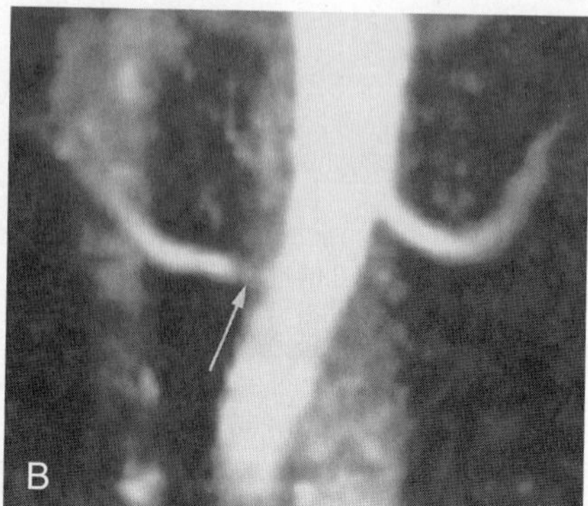

FIGURE 1-800 Renal arteriograms. A, Conventional renal digital subtraction (DSA) showing mild renal stenosis *(arrows)* on the right. **B,** Magnetic resonance angiogram (MRA) of the same patient. The stenosed segment *(arrows)* is clearly seen in this coronal projection. (Courtesy Dr. W. Gedroyc. From Souhami RL, Moxham J: *Textbook of medicine,* ed 4, London, 2002, Churchill Livingstone.)

BASIC INFORMATION

DEFINITION

Renal cell adenocarcinoma (RCA) is a primary adenocarcinoma originating in the renal parenchyma from the malignant transformation of proximal renal tubular epithelial cells. Most renal cell cancers are of clear cell type. Papillary tumors comprise 15% of renal cancers, and chromophobe tumors make up 10%.

SYNONYMS

Hypernephroma
Clear cell carcinoma of the kidney
Grawitz tumor

ICD-9CM CODES
189.0 Adenocarcinoma of kidney
189.1 (Renal pelvis)
ICD-10CM CODES
C64.9 Malignant neoplasm of kidney, except renal pelvis
C65.9 Malignant neoplasm of renal pelvis

EPIDEMIOLOGY & DEMOGRAPHICS

INCIDENCE: Approximately one in 10,000 persons annually (3% of all adult malignancies). In the U.S., renal cancer is the seventh leading malignant condition among men and twelfth among women. Two percent of cases of renal cancer are associated with inherited syndromes.
PREDOMINANT SEX: Male/female ratio of 2:1
PREDOMINANT AGE: Peaks at age 50 to 70 yr

PHYSICAL FINDINGS & CLINICAL PRESENTATION

The classic presentation of RCA includes the triad of flank pain, hematuria, and a palpable abdominal mass. This now represents an unusual presentation. Current presenting findings in RCA patients now include:

Hematuria	50% to 60%
Elevated erythrocyte sedimentation rate	50% to 60%
Abdominal mass	25% to 45%
Anemia	20% to 40%
Flank pain	35% to 40%
Hypertension	20% to 40%
Weight loss	30% to 35%
Fever	5% to 15%
Hepatic dysfunction	10% to 15%
Classic triad (hematuria, abdominal mass, flank pain)	5% to 10%
Hypercalcemia	3% to 6%
Erythrocytosis	3% to 4%
Varicocele	2% to 3%

ETIOLOGY

Hereditary forms:
- Familial renal carcinoma
- Renal carcinoma associated with von Hippel-Lindau disease
- Hereditary papillary renal cell carcinoma

Risk factors:
- Cigarette smoking
- Obesity
- Use of diuretics
- Phenacetin-containing analgesics
- Asbestos exposure
- Gasoline and other petroleum products
- Lead
- Cadmium
- Thorotrast
- Role of the *VHL* gene on chromosome 3

DIAGNOSIS

DIFFERENTIAL DIAGNOSIS

- Transitional cell carcinomas of the renal pelvis (8% of all renal cancers)
- Wilms' tumor
- Other rare primary renal carcinomas and sarcomas
- Renal cysts
- All causes of hematuria (see Section II)
- Retroperitoneal tumors

WORKUP

Laboratory tests and imaging studies

LABORATORY TESTS

- Urinalysis: hematuria
- Complete blood count: anemia or erythrocytosis
- Nonmetastatic hepatic dysfunction with elevated alkaline phosphatase, prolonged prothrombin time, and hypoalbuminemia
- Hypercalcemia (caused by parathyroid-related protein)
- Other: elevated ferritin, elevated insulin and glucagon levels, elevated alpha-fetoprotein, and elevated beta–human chorionic gonadotropin
- Recent reports indicate that urine AQP1 and ADFP concentrations quantified by Western blot appear to be sensitive and specific biomarkers of kidney cancers of proximal tubule origin and may be useful to diagnose an imaged renal mass and screen for kidney cancer at an early stage. Additional investigations are under way to determine if these tests should become standard tumor markers in the investigation of renal masses.

IMAGING STUDIES

Nearly 50% of renal cancers are now detected because a renal mass is incidentally detected on radiographic evaluation.
- Renal ultrasound
- Abdominal CT scan with contrast (Fig. 1-801); CT-guided biopsy is generally not necessary for diagnosis of solid masses >4 cm (high likelihood of cancer)
- MRI
- Renal arteriogram
- Intravenous pyelography

STAGING

See Table 1-428.

COMMON SITES OF METASTASES

Lung	50% to 60%
Bone	30% to 40%
Regional nodes	15% to 30%
Main renal vein	15% to 20%
Perirenal fat	10% to 20%
Adrenal (ipsilateral)	10% to 15%
Vena cava	10% to 15%
Brain	10% to 15%
Adjacent organs (colon, pancreas)	10%
Kidney (contralateral)	2%

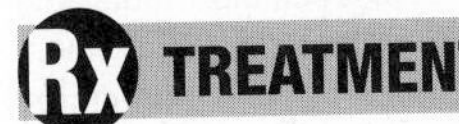

TREATMENT

- Surgery
  - Surgical nephrectomy (open procedure or laparoscopic approach) is the only effective management for stages I, II, and

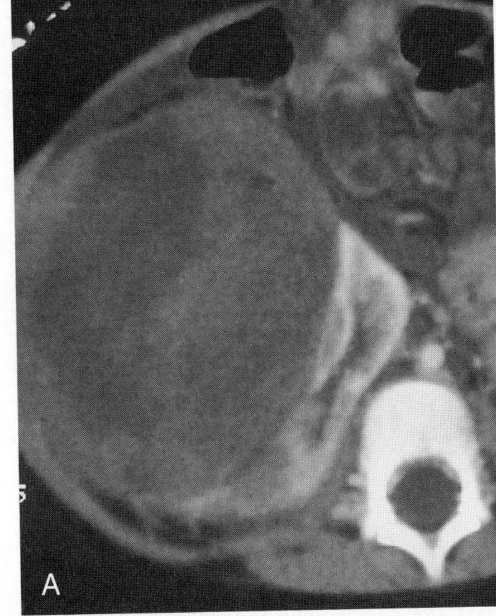

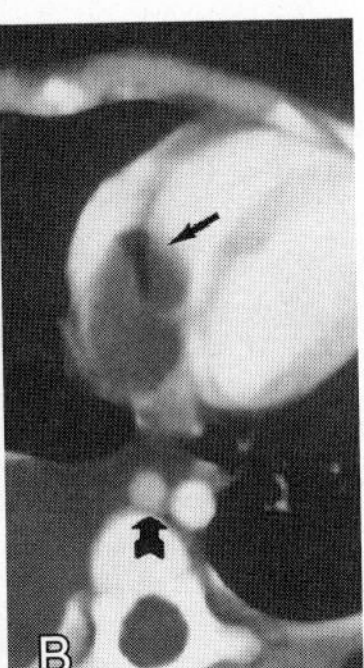

FIGURE 1-801 Renal cell carcinoma. Ultrasound demonstrates a 17-mm hyperreflective mass in the left kidney with posterior shadowing. (From Grainger RG et al [eds]: *Grainger & Allison's diagnostic radiology,* ed 4, London, 2001, Harcourt.)

TABLE 1-428 Comparison of Conventional and TNM Staging Classification of Renal Cell Carcinomas

Robson Stage	T	N	M
I: Tumor confined by capsule	T_1 (tumor ≤2.5 cm) T_2 (tumor >2.5 cm, limited to kidney)		
II: Tumor extension to perirenal fat or ipsilateral adrenal but confined by Gerota's fascia	T_3a (tumor invades adrenal gland or perinephric fat but not beyond Gerota's fascia)		
IIIa: Renal vein or inferior vena caval involvement	T_3b (renal vein or caval involvement below diaphragm)	N_0 (nodes negative)	M_0 (no distant metastases)
IIIb: Lymphatic involvement	T_{1-4}	N_1 (single lymph node ≤2 cm) N_2 (single node 2 to 5 cm, or multiple) N_3 (single or multiple nodes >5 cm)	T_3c (caval involvement above nodes <5 cm)
IIIc: Combination of IIIa and IIIb	$T_{3,4}$		
IVa: Spread to contiguous	T_4 (tumor extends beyond organs except ipsilateral adrenal Gerota's fascia)		
IVb: Distant metastases	T_{1-4}		M_1 (distant metastases)

some stage III tumors. Although radical nephrectomy had long been the standard treatment, retrospective studies have shown that partial rather than radical nephrectomy is associated with improved survival and is appropriate for patients with renal cell neoplasms <4 cm that are not adjacent to renal pelvis.

- Various forms of partial nephrectomy may be available for patients with bilateral cancers or with a solitary kidney.
- The role of nephrectomy in patients with metastatic renal cell carcinoma is controversial and should probably be reserved for patients who have a solitary metastasis amenable to surgical resection. However, there are data showing that nephrectomy before immunotherapy improves survival in patients with metastatic renal cell cancer compared with immunotherapy alone.

- Angioinfarction (for palliation)
- Radiotherapy (for palliation)
- Chemotherapy: In patients with unresectable disease, inhibitors of vascular endothelial growth factor (VEGF) such as the antivascular endothelial growth factor antibody bevacizumab, mTOR kinase inhibitors such as everolimus and temsirolimus, and the tyrosine kinase inhibitors axitinib, sunitinib, pazopanib, and sorafenib can be used as first-line therapy.
- Hormonal therapy (high-dose progesterone may achieve a 15% to 20% response rate)
- Immunotherapy: interleukin-2 may achieve a 15% to 30% response rate; alpha-, beta-, and gamma-interferons are somewhat less effective and now used less frequently

PROGNOSIS

Prognosis of surgically treated patients:

TNM Stage	*5-yr Survival (%)*
I	95
II	88
III (renal vein or vena cava)	50 to 60
III (nodal involvement)	15 to 25
IV	5 to 20

REFERRAL

To urologist

SUGGESTED READINGS

available at www.expertconsult.com

RELATED CONTENT

Kidney Cancer (Patient Information)

AUTHOR: **FRED F. FERRI, M.D.**

BASIC INFORMATION

DEFINITION

Renal tubular acidosis (RTA) is a disorder characterized by inability to excrete H^+ or inadequate generation of new HCO_3^-. RTA syndromes are summarized in Table E1-429. Factors differentiating types of RTA are described in Table 1-430. Four main types of RTA are described in the medical literature:

- Type I (classic, distal RTA): abnormality in distal hydrogen secretion, resulting in hypokalemic hyperchloremic metabolic acidosis.
- Type II (proximal RTA): decreased proximal bicarbonate reabsorption, resulting in hypokalemic hyperchloremic metabolic acidosis.
- Type III (RTA of glomerular insufficiency): normokalemic hyperchloremic metabolic acidosis as a result of impaired ability to generate sufficient NH_3 in the setting of decreased glomerular filtration rate (<30 ml/min). This type of RTA is described in older textbooks and is considered by many not to be a distinct entity.
- Type IV (hyporeninemic hypoaldosteronemic RTA): aldosterone deficiency or antagonism, resulting in decreased distal acidification and decreased distal sodium reabsorption with subsequent hyperkalemic hyperchloremic acidosis.

SYNONYMS

RTA

ICD-9CM CODES
588.8 Renal tubular acidosis
ICD-10CM CODES
N25.89 Other disorders resulting from impaired renal tubular function

EPIDEMIOLOGY & DEMOGRAPHICS

RTA type IV affects mostly adults, whereas RTA types I and II are more frequent in children.

PHYSICAL FINDINGS & CLINICAL PRESENTATION

- Examination may be normal.
- Poor skin turgor may be present from dehydration.
- Muscle weakness and muscle aches from hypokalemia may occur.
- Low back pain and bone pain may be present in patients with abnormalities of calcium metabolism (RTA II).
- There is failure to thrive in children (RTA II).

ETIOLOGY

- Type I RTA: autoimmune disorders, primary biliary cirrhosis and other liver diseases, medications (amphotericin, nonsteroidals), systemic lupus erythematosus, Sjögren's syndrome, genetic disorders (Ehlers-Danlos syndrome, Marfan syndrome, hereditary elliptocytosis), toxins (toluene), disorders with nephrocalcinosis (hyperparathyroidism, vitamin D intoxication, idiopathic hypercalciuria), tubulointerstitial disease (obstructive uropathy, renal transplantation)
- Type II RTA: Fanconi's syndrome, primary hyperparathyroidism, multiple myeloma, medications (acetazolamide)
- Type IV RTA: diabetes mellitus, sickle cell disease, Addison's disease, urinary obstruction

DIAGNOSIS

DIFFERENTIAL DIAGNOSIS

- Diarrhea with significant bicarbonate loss
- Other causes of metabolic acidosis
- Respiratory acidosis

WORKUP

Detection of hyperchloremic metabolic acidosis with arterial blood gases (ABGs) and serum electrolytes and evaluation of potential causes (see "Etiology"). Fig. E1-802 describes an approach to the patient with RTA.

LABORATORY TESTS

- ABGs reveal metabolic acidosis; serum potassium is low in RTA types I and II, normal in type III, and high in type IV.
- Minimal urine pH is >5.5 in RTA type I and <5.5 in types II, III, and IV.
- Urinary anion gap is 0 or positive in all types of RTA.
- Additional useful studies include serum calcium level and urine calcium.
- Anion gap is normal.
- Parathyroid hormone measurement is useful in patients suspected of primary hyperparathyroidism (may be associated with type II RTA).

IMAGING STUDIES

- Plain abdominal radiography is useful to evaluate for nephrocalcinosis.
- Renal sonogram can be used to evaluate renal size or presence of stones.
- Intravenous pyelogram in patients with nephrocalcinosis or nephrolithiasis.

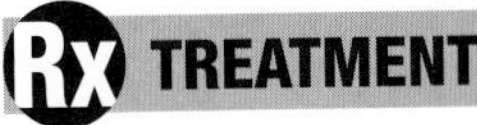

TREATMENT

ACUTE GENERAL Rx

- Types I and II are treated with oral sodium bicarbonate (1 to 2 mEq/kg/day in RTA I, 2 to 4 mEq/kg/day in RTA type II) titrated to correct acidosis.
- Potassium supplementation is needed in hypokalemic patients.
- Type IV RTA can be treated with furosemide to lower elevated potassium levels and sodium bicarbonate to correct significant acidosis. Fludrocortisone 100 to 300 mg/day can be used to correct mineralocorticoid deficiency.

CHRONIC Rx

- Frequent monitoring of potassium levels in RTA type IV
- Monitoring for bone disease in RTA type II
- Monitoring for nephrocalcinosis and nephrolithiasis in RTA type I

DISPOSITION

- Prognosis varies with the presence of associated conditions (see "Etiology").
- Untreated distal RTA may result in hypercalcemia, hyperphosphaturia, nephrolithiasis, and nephrocalcinosis.

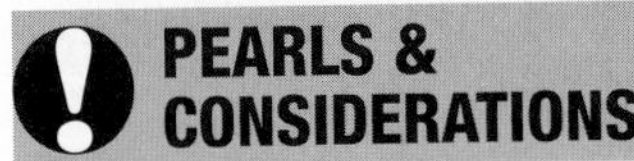

PEARLS & CONSIDERATIONS

COMMENTS

Patient education material can be obtained from the National Kidney and Urologic Diseases Information Clearinghouse, Box NKUDIC, Bethesda, MD 20893.

AUTHOR: **FRED F. FERRI, M.D.**

TABLE 1-430 Factors Differentiating Type 1, Type 2, and Type 4 Renal Tubular Acidosis (RTA)

	Type 1 RTA	Type 2 RTA	Type 4 RTA
Serum K^+	Low	Low	High
Renal function	Normal or near normal	Normal or near normal	Stage 3, 4, or 5 chronic kidney disease
Urine pH during acidosis	High	Low	Low or high
Serum HCO_3^- (mmol/L)	10-20	16-18	16-22
Urine pCO_2 (mm Hg)	<40	<40	>70
Urine citrate	Low	High	Low
Fanconi syndrome	No	May be present	No

From Floege J et al: *Comprehensive clinical nephrology,* ed 4, Philadelphia, 2010, Saunders.

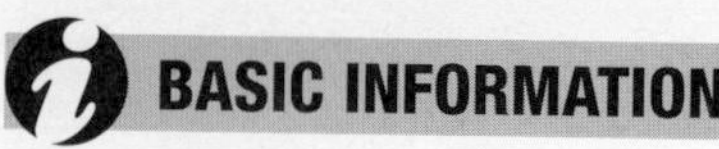

BASIC INFORMATION

DEFINITION

Renal vein thrombosis is the thrombotic occlusion of one or both renal veins.

ICD-9CM CODES
453.3 Renal vein thrombosis
ICD-10CM CODES
I82.3 Embolism and thrombosis of renal vein

EPIDEMIOLOGY & DEMOGRAPHICS

- Incidence unknown; probably an underdiagnosed condition
- May occur at any age with no gender preference
- Epidemiology tied to the underlying cause

PHYSICAL FINDINGS & CLINICAL PRESENTATION

Acute bilateral renal vein thrombosis:
- Back and bilateral flank pain
- Acute renal failure

Acute unilateral renal vein thrombosis:
- Flank pain
- Decline in renal function
- Hematuria
- Increase in the amount of proteinuria if associated with nephrotic syndrome

Chronic unilateral renal vein thrombosis:
- May be silent
- Pulmonary emboli and hemolysis
- Back pain
- Deep vein thrombosis in lower extremities
- Edema
- Glycosuria
- Hyperchloremic acidosis
- Left varicocele (if the left renal vein is thrombosed)
- Dilated abdominal veins

ETIOLOGY & PATHOGENESIS

- Extrinsic compression by a tumor or retroperitoneal mass
- Invasion of the renal vein or inferior vena cava by tumor (almost always renal cell cancer)
- Trauma
- Hypercoagulable states
- Dehydration
- Glomerulopathies (membranous glomerulonephritis, crescentic glomerulonephritis, systemic lupus erythematosus, amyloidosis) especially in the presence of nephrotic syndrome when the serum albumin is <2 g/dl
- NOTE: For unknown reasons, diabetic nephropathy is not commonly associated with renal vein thrombosis even if the nephrotic syndrome is present

A controversy has existed regarding whether the renal vein thrombosis association with nephrotic syndrome is a complication of nephrotic syndrome or whether renal vein thrombosis occurring in the setting of increased renal vein pressure (e.g., with congestive heart failure, constrictive pericarditis, or extrinsic compression) can independently cause proteinuria. Current evidence is that renal vein thrombosis does not cause nephrotic syndrome.

Dx DIAGNOSIS

DIFFERENTIAL DIAGNOSIS

The diagnosis of renal vein thrombosis does not include any differential consideration. The differential diagnosis is that of proteinuria. Renal vein thrombosis should be considered if proteinuria worsens or if renal function worsens in a patient with glomerulonephritis. Renal vein thrombosis should also be considered in patients with pulmonary emboli and no lower-extremity deep vein thrombosis.

WORKUP

Clinical suspicion (see "Differential Diagnosis") and imaging studies

IMAGING STUDIES

- Abdominal ultrasound
- Abdominal MRI or CT with contrast (Fig. 1-803)
- Renal arteriography (delayed films during venous phase)
- Selective renal vein venography (inferior venacavogram images should be obtained before advancing the catheter in the vena cava because clots, if present, could be dislodged)
- Renal biopsy may be indicated if evidence of nephritis is present (e.g., active urinary sediment)

Rx TREATMENT

- Anticoagulation in acute renal vein thrombosis to prevent pulmonary emboli and in attempt to improve renal function and decrease proteinuria
- Thrombolytic therapy or surgical thrombectomy has also been reported to be effective
- The value of anticoagulation in chronic renal vein thrombosis is dubious except in nephrotic patients with membranous glomerulonephritis with profound hypoalbuminemia where prolonged prophylactic anticoagulation may be of benefit even if renal vein thrombosis has not been documented

PROGNOSIS

Probable worsening of the underlying glomerulonephritis by acute renal vein thrombosis; the effect of chronic renal vein thrombosis is unclear.

AUTHOR: **FRED F. FERRI, M.D.**

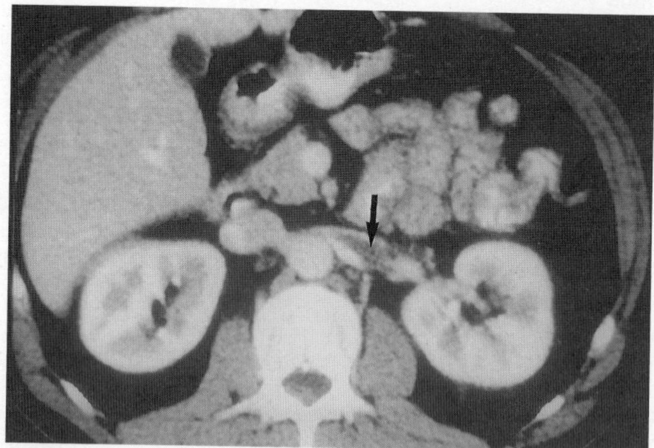

FIGURE 1-803 Renal vein thrombus in a patient with nephritic syndrome. Contrast medium–enhanced CT at the level of the renal vein shows thrombus in the left renal vein *(arrow)*. (From Grainger RG et al [eds]: *Grainger & Allison's diagnostic radiology,* ed 4, Philadelphia, 2001, Churchill Livingstone.)

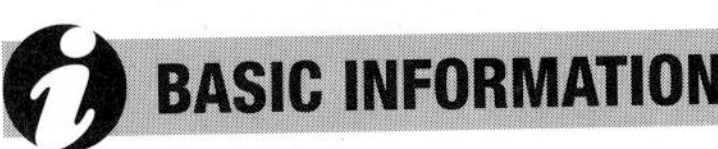

BASIC INFORMATION

DEFINITION

Restless legs syndrome (RLS) is an awake phenomenon consisting of an urge to move legs, usually associated with feeling of discomfort in legs.

SYNONYMS

RLS
Wittmaack-Ekbom syndrome

ICD-9CM CODES
333.94 Restless leg syndrome
ICD-10CM CODES
G25.81 Restless legs syndrome

EPIDEMIOLOGY & DEMOGRAPHICS

PREVALENCE: Average prevalence rate is 1% to 29%. Prevalence estimates in Europe are around 10%, and 0.1% to 12% in East Asian population.
PEAK PREVALENCE: 10% in persons aged 30 to 79 and 19% in persons aged 80 or above.
PREDOMINANT SEX: Early-onset RLS is more common in females, with 2:1 female/male ratio.
PREDOMINANT AGE: Prevalence of RLS increases with age, and it is more commonly seen in elderly population.
GENETICS: Genetic basis of RLS has been reported, particularly in early-onset RLS.

- Autosomal dominant disorder
- Common among first-degree relatives
- RLS associated with certain sequences in chromosome 6p,12q, 14q, 9p, 20p, 2p, 16p

RISK FACTORS: Diabetes mellitus (most consistent risk factor for RLS), iron deficiency anemia (IDA), end-stage renal disease (ESRD) requiring hemodialysis, pregnancy, rheumatoid arthritis, Parkinson's disease, neuropathy, and myelopathy

CLASSIFICATION

- Primary RLS is without any obvious cause, with no associated disorder.
- Secondary RLS results from other medical conditions; the most frequently found associations are pregnancy, IDA, ESRD, and Parkinson disease.

PHYSICAL FINDINGS & CLINICAL PRESENTATION

- Wide spectrum of severity of clinical manifestations has been reported in RLS.
- Most common symptom is unpleasant sensations in legs ("dysesthesias"), reported as discomfort or "creepy-crawling" sensations, mostly bilateral. Arms are occasionally involved.
- There is an extreme urge to move legs and relief is sustained as long as the movement continues.
- Symptoms are worse at night or evening. Best sleep is usually early in the morning.

ETIOLOGY

The exact etiology remains unknown. Pharmacologic, pathologic, physiologic, and imaging studies have implicated dopaminergic pathways, brain iron metabolism, and endogenous opioid pathways.

DIAGNOSIS

DIFFERENTIAL DIAGNOSIS

- Periodic limb movement disorder (PLMD)
- Nocturnal leg cramps
- Painful peripheral neuropathy
- Akathisia
- Positional discomfort
- Volitional movements, foot tapping, leg rocking

WORKUP

- Diagnosis of RLS is based on established clinical criteria (Table 1-431) and normal neurologic examination.
- Testing is done to determine possible cause of secondary RLS.
- Polysomnography to document periodic limb movements during sleep
- Leg activity monitors to determine limb movements during sleep but they are unable to distinguish periodic limb movements from periodic movements associated with sleep apnea.
- Nerve conduction studies and electromyography for associated peripheral neuropathy

LABORATORY TESTS

- Iron status: serum ferritin, total iron binding capacity, percent saturation
- CBC for anemia in case of iron deficiency
- Metabolic panel: blood urea nitrogen and serum creatinine for renal insufficiency

IMAGING STUDIES

No imaging studies are required for diagnosis for RLS.

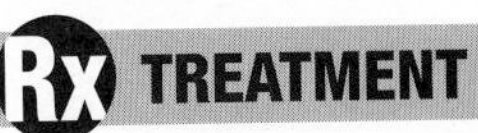

TREATMENT

Treatment options for RLS include:

- Dopaminergic agents, levodopa, and dopamine agonists help to ameliorate RLS symptoms, decrease periodic limb movements, and improve sleep. Dopamine agonists, pramipexole and ropinirole, are first-line agents in the treatment of RLS.
- Anticonvulsants, such as gabapentin, have been shown to be effective in multiple studies. A recent trial has shown that pregabalin is also effective and well tolerated for RLS.[1] Limited case reports reveal use of lamotrigine, Gabatril, and topiramate in patients who are intolerant to other agents.
- Opiates, mostly methadone, are generally reserved as last line of treatment.
- Iron replacement should be started in case of iron deficiency.

NONPHARMACOLOGIC THERAPY

- Avoidance of caffeine, alcohol, nicotine, and medications that exacerbate RLS
- Physical and mental activity
- Good sleep hygiene

ACUTE GENERAL Rx

Once the diagnosis of RLS is considered based on clinical criteria as mentioned in Table 1-431 and causes impairment of quality of life, a dopamine agonist (bromocriptine, pramipexole, or ropinirole) should be started at low dose and then gradually tapered depending on tolerance. Dopaminergic medications have the potential to cause iatrogenic worsening (augmentation) of RLS with long-term treatment.

REFERRAL

Refer to neurologist if diagnosis is uncertain or an underlying disorder is suspected.

SUGGESTED READINGS

available at www.expertconsult.com

RELATED CONTENT

Restless Legs Syndrome (Patient Information)

AUTHOR: **FARIHA ZAHEER, M.D.**

TABLE 1-431 Diagnostic Criteria for Restless Legs Syndrome

Minimal Criteria
1. Desire to move the legs usually associated with paresthesias.
2. Motor restlessness, as characterized by floor pacing, leg rubbing, stretching, and flexing.
3. Worse at rest, with relief by activity.
4. Worse at night.
Additional Criteria
1. Sleep disturbances, as difficulty in sleep onset and maintaining sleep, daytime fatigue, or somnolence.
2. Involuntary movements, as periodic limb or leg movements in sleep and periodic or aperiodic limb movements while awake.
3. Neurologic examination is normal in idiopathic restless legs syndrome.
4. Clinical course may begin at any age but most severe in middle and older age.
5. Family history suggests autosomal dominant mode of inheritance in 1/3 of the cases.

From Stiansy K et al: Clinical symptomatology and treatment of restless leg syndrome and periodic limb movement disorder, *Sleep Med Rev* 6(4):253-265, 2002.

[1]Allen RP et al: Comparison of pregabalin with pramipexole for restless legs syndrome, *N Engl J Med* 370:621-631, 2014.

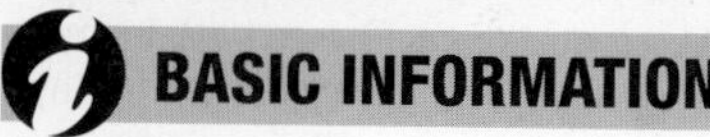

BASIC INFORMATION

DEFINITION

Retinal detachment is the separation of the neurosensory retina (NSR) from the retinal pigment epithelium (RPE). This results in the accumulation of subretinal fluid (SRF) in the potential space between the NSR and the RPE. The main types of retinal detachment are rhegmatogenous, tractional, exudating, and combined tractional-rhegmatogenous.

SYNONYMS

Inflammatory lesions of choroid
Uveitis
Tumor
Vascular lesions
Congenital disorders

ICD-9CM CODES
361 Retinal detachment and defects
ICD-10CM CODES
H33 Retinal detachment and breaks
H33.2 Serous retinal detachment
H33.5 Other retinal detachments
H33.0 Retinal detachment with retinal break

EPIDEMIOLOGY & DEMOGRAPHICS

INCIDENCE (IN U.S.):
- 0.02% of the population
- Particularly common in patients with high myopia of 5 diopters or more

PEAK INCIDENCE: Incidence increases with increasing age or increasing myopia.

PREVALENCE (IN U.S.): Busy ophthalmologists may see one or two acute retinal detachments per month.

PREDOMINANT AGE:
- Congenital in younger patients
- Usually trauma in patients aged 30 to 40 yr and older
- High myopia a predisposition

PHYSICAL FINDINGS & CLINICAL PRESENTATION

- Elevation of retina and vessels associated with tears in the retina (Fig. 1-804 and Fig. 1-805), fluid, and/or hemorrhage beneath the retina and changes in the vitreous.
- Reports of flashing lights and floaters.
- After a variable period of time, the patient notices a relative peripheral visual field defect that may progress to involve central vision.

ETIOLOGY

- Trauma
- Tears in the retina
- Uveitis
- Fluid accumulation beneath the retina
- Tumors
- Scleritis
- Inflammatory disease
- Diabetes
- Collagen-vascular disease
- Vascular abnormalities
- Oral fluoroquinolones (higher risk of retinal detachment compared with nonusers, although the absolute risk is small)

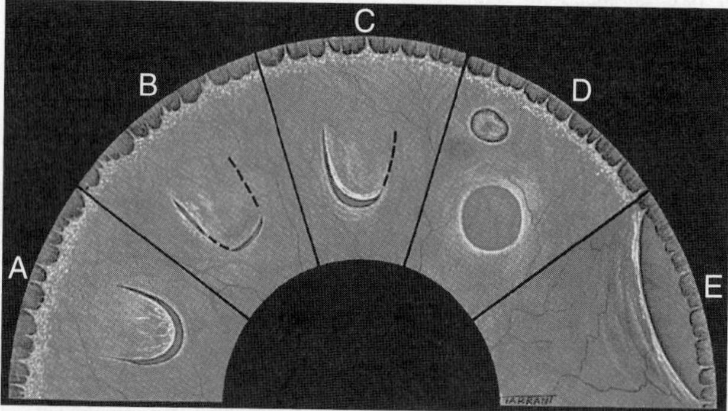

FIGURE 1-804 Retinal tears. A, Complete U-shaped; **B,** linear; **C,** L-shaped; **D,** operculated; **E,** dialysis. (From Kanski JJ, Bowling B: *Clinical ophthalmology: a systematic approach,* ed 7, Philadelphia, 2010, Saunders.)

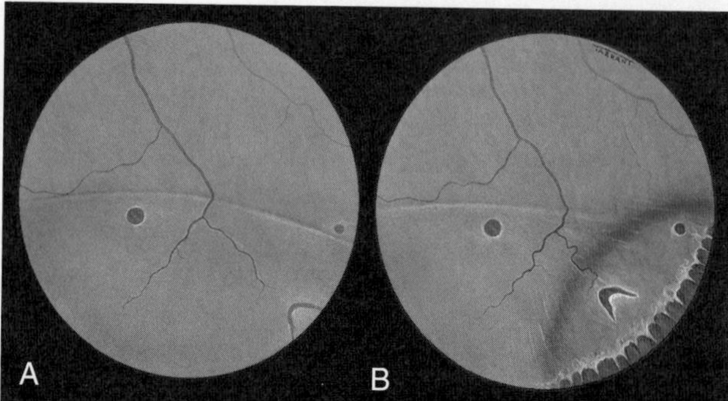

FIGURE 1-805 Appearance of retinal breaks in detached retina. A, Without scleral indentation; **B,** with indentation. (From Kanski JJ, Bowling B: *Clinical ophthalmology, a systematic approach,* ed 7, Philadelphia, 2010, Saunders.)

DIAGNOSIS

DIFFERENTIAL DIAGNOSIS

- Degenerative retinoschisis
- Uveal effusion syndrome
- Choroidal detachment
- Hemorrhage
- Tumors

WORKUP

- Full eye examination
- Fluorescein angiography
- Visual fields
- Ultrasonography to show the retinal detachment or tumors beneath it
- Medical workup only when inflammation or systemic disease considered

LABORATORY TESTS

Usually not necessary

IMAGING STUDIES

B scan ultrasonography (US) of the eye

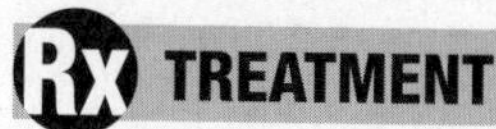

TREATMENT

NONPHARMACOLOGIC THERAPY

Immediate surgery. The three principal methods for reattachment of the retina in patients with primary retinal detachment are scleral buckling, vitrectomy, and pneumatic retinopexy. There is a paucity of randomized trials comparing these procedures and the choice remains subjective. Some data suggest that vitrectomy may be preferable for detachment in pseudophakic eyes, whereas primary detachment in phakic eyes with complexity exceeding the original indications for rheumatic retinopexy may be treated with scleral buckling or vitrectomy.

ACUTE GENERAL Rx

- Early surgery to repair the detachment
- Treatment of the underlying disorder

CHRONIC Rx

Occasionally, steroids or other treatment of underlying disease is indicated.

DISPOSITION

- Immediately refer to an ophthalmologist.
- Early intervention improves outcomes.

REFERRAL

Immediately

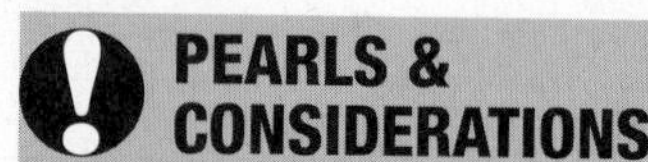

PEARLS & CONSIDERATIONS

COMMENTS

If treated early, most patients will recover a substantial portion of their vision.

SUGGESTED READINGS

available at www.expertconsult.com

AUTHORS: **MELVYN KOBY, M.D.,** and **R. SCOTT HOFFMAN, M.D.**

BASIC INFORMATION

DEFINITION

In a retinal hemorrhage, blood accumulates in or on the surface of the retina, in the subretinal space, or in the vitreous cavity. Generally, these hemorrhages are abnormal and causes should be sought (see "Etiology").

SYNONYMS

Retinal hemorrhage, vitreous hemorrhage
Subretinal or preretinal hemorrhages
Splinter hemorrhage, dot and blot hemorrhages
Roth spots (small white centered blood, traditionally associated with endocarditis)

ICD-9CM CODES
362.81 Retinal hemorrhage
ICD-10CM CODES
H35.60 Retinal hemorrhage, unspecified eye

EPIDEMIOLOGY & DEMOGRAPHICS

INCIDENCE (IN U.S.): Busy ophthalmologists see one or two cases a month.

PEAK INCIDENCE:
- In children: associated primarily with trauma and hematologic disorders (must consider shaken baby syndrome), rare retinal vascular diseases of children (Coat's, Eale's disease)
- Associated with trauma, diabetes, vascular disease (hypertensive retinopathy, retinal vascular occlusions, sickle cell disease, anemia), macular degeneration, altitude changes (mountain climbing)

PREDOMINANT AGE: Usually vascular disease in older patients

PHYSICAL FINDINGS & CLINICAL PRESENTATION

- Hemorrhage within the retina or subretinal area (Fig. 1-806)
- Evidence of retinal tears, tumors, and inflammation; macular degeneration, drugs, diabetes

ETIOLOGY

- Diabetes
- Hypertension
- Trauma
- Inflammation
- Tumors
- Subretinal neovascularization
- Associated with diabetes and aging
- Rapid changes in altitude (mountain climbing or scuba diving)

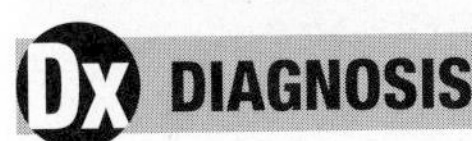

DIAGNOSIS

DIFFERENTIAL DIAGNOSIS

- Evaluate patients for local and systemic diseases.
- Trauma in children or adults
- Venous or arterial occlusion associated with atherosclerotic or heart disease may cause retinal hemorrhage.
- Rule out malignant melanoma, trauma, hypertensive cardiovascular disease.

Section II describes the differential diagnosis of acute painless loss of vision.

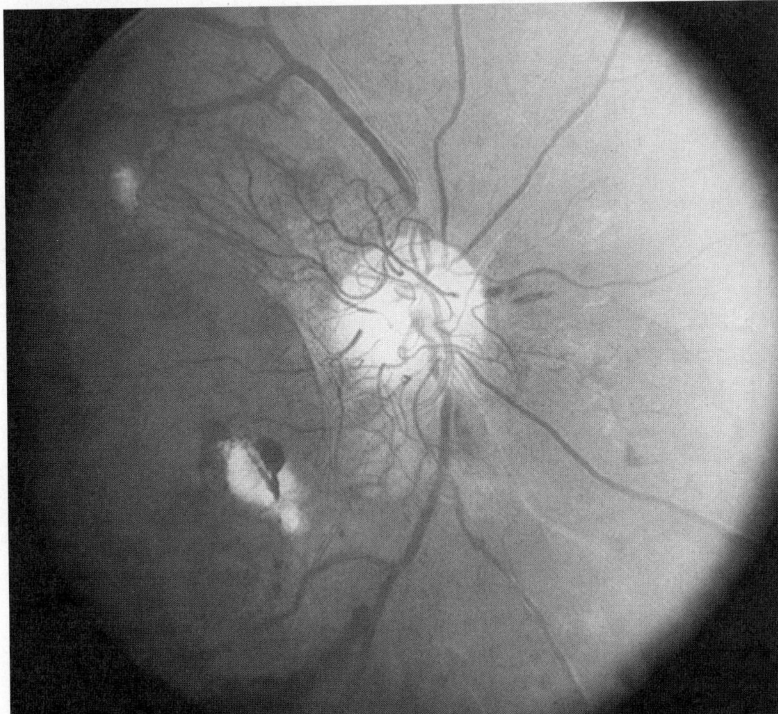

FIGURE 1-806 Fronds of neovascularization on the disc are present in this right eye. Temporally, two cotton-wool spots have adjacent intraretinal hemorrhage and preretinal hemorrhage. Native retinal arteries are narrowed and show evidence of sclerosis. (From Palay D [ed]: *Ophthalmology for the primary care physician*, St Louis, 1997, Mosby.)

WORKUP

Complete general physical examination, evaluate for trauma; look for systemic diseases and medication etiologies.

LABORATORY TESTS

- Minimum: complete blood count, erythrocyte sedimentation rate, complete blood chemistries
- Visual field testing

IMAGING STUDIES

- Usually not necessary
- Trauma: skull radiographs or head CT (evaluate for fractures)
- Ultrasound
- Fluorescein angiography (evaluate retinal vascular diseases and macular degeneration)

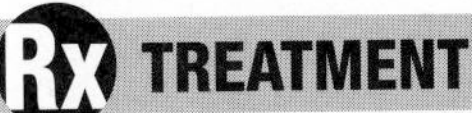

TREATMENT

NONPHARMACOLOGIC THERAPY

- Laser or treatment of underlying disorder
- Treat medical problems (age-related macular degeneration, etc.)

ACUTE GENERAL Rx

- Laser treatment may be indicated for certain retinal diseases.
- Treatment may be indicated with wet macular degeneration (intravitreal injection).
- Treat underlying disease.
- Repair any damage from trauma.

CHRONIC Rx

- Vitamin therapy: high in zinc and antioxidants for macular degeneration
- Treatment will differ depending on various causes of bleeding.
- Encourage adequate control of underlying medical disorders.

DISPOSITION

If present, hemorrhage in the retina is generally considered abnormal; refer to ophthalmologist for evaluation.

REFERRAL

Immediate referral to an ophthalmologist, especially if there is a significant change in vision; early treatment significantly affects outcome

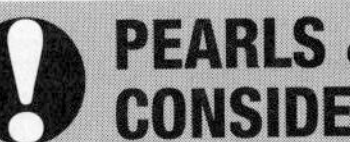

PEARLS & CONSIDERATIONS

COMMENTS

- Vision may return substantially.
- Complete recovery of vision depends on cause.
- Chronic situations have poor prognosis.

SUGGESTED READINGS

available at www.expertconsult.com

RELATED CONTENT

Diabetic Retinopathy (Patient Information)

AUTHORS: **MELVYN KOBY, M.D.,** and
R. SCOTT HOFFMAN, M.D.

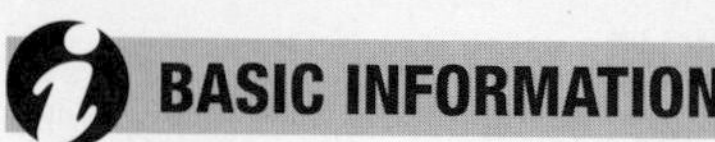

BASIC INFORMATION

DEFINITION

Retinitis pigmentosa (RP) refers to a clinically and genetically diverse group of diffuse retinal dystrophies initially predominantly affecting the rod photoreceptor cells with subsequent degeneration of cones (rod-cone dystrophy).

ICD-9CM CODES
362.74 Retinitis pigmentosa, pigmentary retinal dystrophy
ICD-10CM CODES
H35.5 Hereditary retinal dystrophy

EPIDEMIOLOGY & DEMOGRAPHICS

PEAK INCIDENCE:
- Recessive incidence: in the 20s
- Dominant form: in the 40s

PREVALENCE (IN U.S.): One in 5000 persons. It is the most commonly encountered hereditary fundus dystrophy.

PREDOMINANT SEX: Depends on inheritance

PREDOMINANT AGE: The age of onset, rate of progression, eventual vision loss, and associated ocular features are frequently related to the mode of inheritance.

GENETICS:
- 19% dominant
- 19% recessive
- 8% X-linked
- 46% not known to be genetically related (mutations)
- 8% undetermined cause

PHYSICAL FINDINGS & CLINICAL PRESENTATION

- Deposition of retinal pigment in midperiphery and centrally in the retina (Fig. E1-807) with a pale optic nerve and narrowing of blood vessels (Fig. 1-808)
- Possible cataracts and macular edema
- Decrease in night vision and peripheral vision. Patients typically lose night vision to a greater extent than they lose day vision, and they lose peripheral vision before losing central vision.

ETIOLOGY

RP may occur as an isolated sporadic disorder, or may be inherited as AD, AR, or XL. Many cases are due to mutation of the rhodopsin gene. XL is the least common but most severe form, and may result in complete blindness by the third or fourth decade.

Dx DIAGNOSIS

DIFFERENTIAL DIAGNOSIS

- Syphilis
- Old inflammatory scars
- Old hemorrhage
- Diabetes
- Toxic retinopathies (phenothiazines, chloroquine)

WORKUP

- Electrophysiologic studies
- Dark adaptation studies
- Visual fields

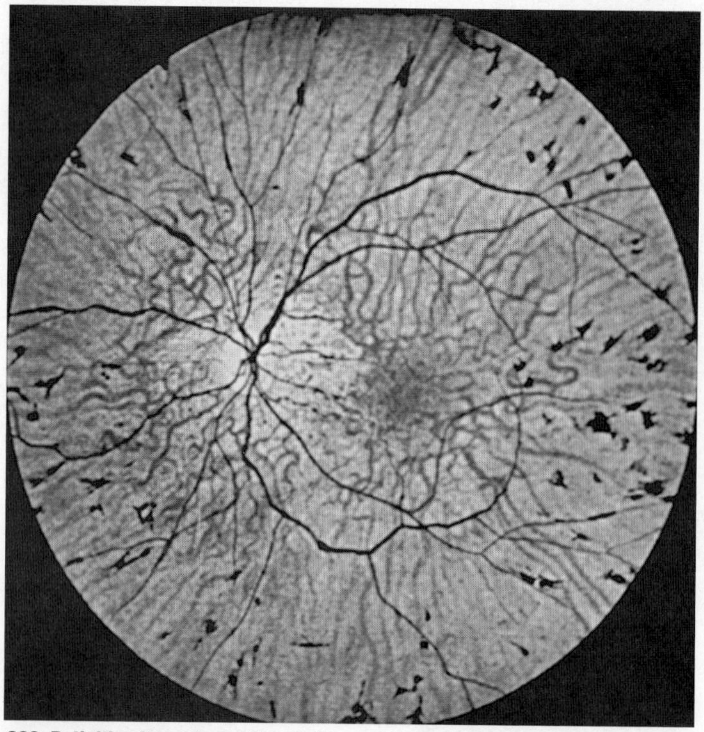

LABORATORY TESTS

- Usually not necessary
- VDRL (syphilis), glucose (selected patients)

IMAGING STUDIES

- Usually not necessary
- Rate of decline of vision for different groups cannot be accurately determined; decline rates are fastest with patients with mutations

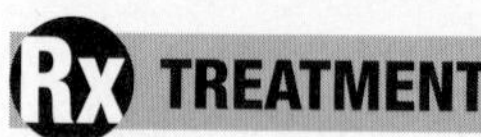

TREATMENT

CHRONIC Rx

- No proven effective therapy
- Correction of biochemical abnormalities. Some success has been reported with subretinal gene therapy in which patients with mutations in the gene encoding RPE65 were treated with delivery under the retina of a normal RPE65 gene by intraocular injection
- Nutritional supplements: sometimes vitamin E or vitamin A may be helpful
- In patients with advanced disease, treatment options may include attempts to regenerate photoreceptors by transplantation or genetic manipulation of nonphotoreceptor retinal cell types

DISPOSITION

Disease may be either mild or severe, but if the patient is expected to progress to total blindness, counseling and early education are important.

REFERRAL

To ophthalmologist to confirm diagnosis

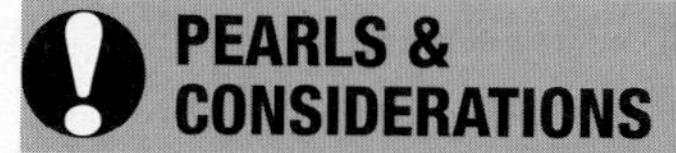

PEARLS & CONSIDERATIONS

COMMENTS

- The spider web–like appearance of macular degeneration should not be confused with the extra pigments sometimes seen in dark-skinned individuals.
- Patient education material can be obtained from the Retinitis Pigmentosa Foundation Fighting Blindness, 1401 Mt. Royal Avenue, 4th Floor, Baltimore, MD 21217.
- Research in fetal retinal pigment transplantation and computer chip implantation is ongoing.

FIGURE 1-808 Retinitis pigmentosa. (From Behrman RE [ed]: *Nelson textbook of pediatrics,* Philadelphia, 2005, Saunders.)

SUGGESTED READINGS

available at www.expertconsult.com

RELATED CONTENT

Retinitis Pigmentosa (Patient Information)

AUTHORS: **MELVYN KOBY, M.D.,** and **R. SCOTT HOFFMAN, M.D.**

BASIC INFORMATION

DEFINITION

Retinoblastoma is an inherited, highly malignant congenital neoplasm arising from the neural layers of the retina.

ICD-9CM CODES
190.5 Retinoblastoma, malignant neoplasm of eyes, retina
ICD-10CM CODES
C69.20 Malignant neoplasm of unspecified retina

EPIDEMIOLOGY & DEMOGRAPHICS

INCIDENCE (IN U.S.): Retinoblastoma affects 1 in 15,000 children, with ~300 children newly diagnosed each year in the United States. It is the most common primary intraocular malignancy of childhood.

PEAK INCIDENCE:
- 6 to 13 mo. Mean age at diagnosis is 12 mo for bilateral tumors and 24 mo for unilateral tumors.
- 72% diagnosed by age 3 yr
- 90% diagnosed by age 4 yr

PREDOMINANT AGE: 8 mo

GENETICS:
- Gene mutation or an autosomal-dominant gene with 80% to 95% penetration
- 5% mutations

PHYSICAL FINDINGS & CLINICAL PRESENTATION

- Leukocoria (white reflex or white pupil) (Fig. 1-809)
- White elevated retinal masses
- Strabismus
- Glaucoma
- Uveitis
- Vitreous masses and opacity

ETIOLOGY

The retinoblastoma gene is a tumor suppressor gene located on the long arm of chromosome 13 at region 14 that codes for the RB protein. ~60% of retinoblastomas are attributable to somatic, nonhereditary mutations.

DIAGNOSIS

DIFFERENTIAL DIAGNOSIS

Examination of eye
- Strabismus
- Retinal detachment
- Uveitis
- Other tumors
- Glaucoma
- Coats' disease (pathologic telangiectatic retinal vessels that leak and lead to accumulation of subretinal fluid and lipid)
- Endophthalmitis
- Cataract
- Infectious

WORKUP

Diagnosis is by ophthalmologic examination. An awake examination to determine if the patient can fixate and extent of eye mobility should be done. Examination should also include visual acuity, papillary examination, extraocular movements, slit-lamp examination for evidence of iris neovascularization, hyphema or hypopyon, indirect ophthalmoscopy with 360 degrees of scleral depression, and fundus photographs documenting all lesions. Ophthalmologic examination is followed by ultrasonography of the eye and MRI of the orbits and brain to exclude extraocular extension and trilateral retinoblastoma.

CLASSIFICATION

Retinoblastoma is separated into intraocular and extraocular disease. The Reese-Ellsworth classification system became outdated as chemoreduction strategies became widely used for salvage therapy and a new international classification system for intraocular retinoblastoma was formulated in 2003, which more accurately reflects response to standardized chemotherapy regimen used in conjunction with focal consolidative therapy. The international classification system is subdivided into group A (small), group B (medium), group C (confined, medium), group D (diffuse, large), and group E (enucleation, advanced)

IMAGING STUDIES

- MRI: may show calcifications in retina
- Ultrasonography: good delineation of mass

TREATMENT

Usually treated by a multidisciplinary team consisting of a pediatrician, an ophthalmologist, a pediatric oncologist, and pediatric radiation oncologist. Treatment depends on location and stage of tumor when diagnosed:
- Chemotherapy for larger tumors usually with carboplatin, etoposide, and vincristine. The goal of chemotherapy is to reduce the tumor volume for focal therapy with cryotherapy, laser, thermotherapy, or plaque brachytherapy.
- Radioactive plaque brachytherapy with iodine 125 or ruthenium 106 plaques and cryotherapy
- Surgical enucleation of the eye
- Radiation and chemotherapy

DISPOSITION

Overall there is a high cure rate (93% 5-yr survival in the United States) for retinoblastoma. Group A tumors generally have good visual and survival prognosis with focal consolidative therapy alone, groups B and C are treated with chemotherapy and focal therapy with good results (vision salvage rates up to 93%), group D patients often eventually require enucleation despite treatment.

REFERRAL

- To ophthalmologist, pediatric oncologist, and pediatric radiation oncologist
- Prospective parents with a family history of retinoblastoma should be referred for genetic counseling. Genetic testing should be carried out for most retinoblastoma patients unless it is declined.

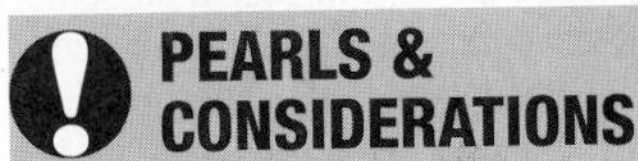

PEARLS & CONSIDERATIONS

COMMENTS

- High incidence of second tumor in survivors compared with general population
- High incidence of lung cancer, bladder cancer, and other epithelial cancers

SUGGESTED READINGS

available at www.expertconsult.com

RELATED CONTENT

Retinoblastoma (Patient Information)

AUTHORS: **MELVYN KOBY, M.D.,** and **R. SCOTT HOFFMAN, M.D.**

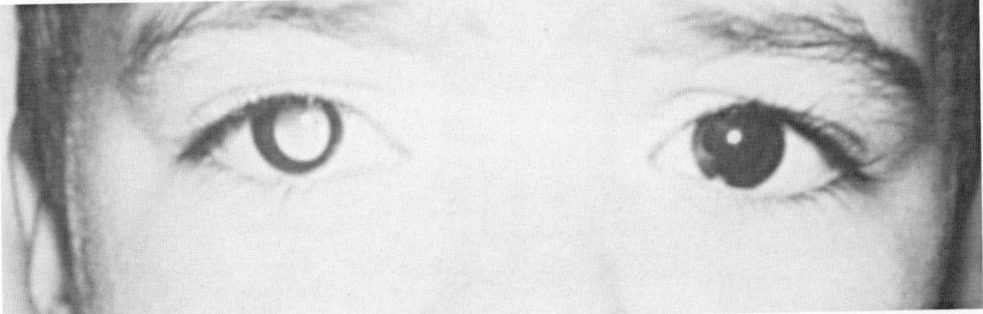

FIGURE 1-809 Leukocoria. White papillary reflex in a child with retinoblastoma. (From Behrman RE [ed]: *Nelson textbook of pediatrics,* Philadelphia, 2005, Saunders.)

BASIC INFORMATION

DEFINITION

Rh incompatibility occurs when an absence of the D antigen on maternal red blood cells (RBCs) and its presence on fetal RBCs cause risk of isoimmunization.

ICD-9CM CODES
656.1 Rh incompatibility
ICD-10CM CODES
O36.0910 Maternal care for other rhesus isoimmunization, first trimester, not applicable or unspecified
T80.4 Rh incompatibility reaction
T80.4 Unspecified complication following infusion, transfusion, and therapeutic injection

EPIDEMIOLOGY & DEMOGRAPHICS

INCIDENCE:

- The absence of the D antigen (Rh− blood type) occurs in 15% of whites, 8% of blacks, and virtually no Asians or Native Americans. If the father's blood type is not known, the chance that an Rh− pregnant woman is bearing an Rh+ fetus is approximately 60%.
- Of those pregnancies complicated by Rh incompatibility, the risk of maternal isoimmunization to the D antigen is approximately 8% for each ABO-compatible pregnancy if no prophylaxis is given.
- Maternal-fetal ABO incompatibility is somewhat protective against Rh isoimmunization.

GENETICS: Five major loci determine Rh status: C, D, E, c, e. The presence of the D antigen results in an Rh+ individual. Its absence results in an Rh− individual. Of Rh+ fathers, 45% are homozygotes, and 55% are heterozygotes. For homozygous Rh+ fathers, the probability of an Rh+ offspring is 100%. The probability for heterozygotes is approximately 50%.

RISK FACTORS:

- Antepartum: fetal-to-maternal transfusion
- Intrapartum: fetal-to-maternal transfusion, spontaneous abortion, ectopic pregnancy, abruptio placentae, abdominal trauma, chorionic villus sampling, amniocentesis, percutaneous umbilical blood sampling (PUBS), external cephalic version, manual removal of the placenta, therapeutic abortion, autologous blood product administration

ETIOLOGY

The initial response to D antigen exposure is production of immunoglobulin (Ig) M (molecular weight 900,000) that does not cross the placenta. With a repeated exposure, IgG (MW 160,000) is produced. IgG can cross the placenta and enter the fetal circulation, producing hemolysis in the fetus. This may produce erythroblastosis fetalis or hemolytic disease in the newborn, resulting in antepartum or neonatal death or neurologic damage to the fetus because of hyperbilirubinemia and kernicterus.

DIAGNOSIS

LABORATORY TESTS

ABO and Rh blood type and an antibody screen as part of the initial prenatal profile

- If antibody screen negative:
    1. Repeat antibody screen at 28 wk gestation.
    2. Obtain neonatal blood type after delivery.
    3. If Rh incompatibility is confirmed by the neonatal blood type, a Kleihauer-Betke or rosette test should be performed to determine the amount of fetomaternal transfusion in the following high-risk circumstances: abruptio placentae, placenta previa, cesarean delivery, intrauterine manipulation, manual removal of the placenta.
- If anti-D antibody screen is positive:
    1. Maternal indirect Coombs test is needed to determine antibody titer.
    2. Determine paternal Rh status and zygosity.
    3. If father is heterozygous, PUBS or amniotic fluid is needed to determine fetal Rh status.

IMAGING STUDIES

Ultrasound evaluation can diagnose hydrops fetalis, but it cannot predict it.

TREATMENT

PREVENTION OF D ISOIMMUNIZATION

- 50 mcg of D immunoglobulin: after spontaneous or induced abortion or ectopic pregnancy <13 wk gestation.
- 300 mcg of D immunoglobulin (protects against 30 ml of fetal blood):
    1. After spontaneous or induced abortion >13 wk gestation, amniocentesis, chorionic villous sampling, PUBS, external cephalic version, or other intrauterine manipulation.
    2. As antepartum prophylaxis at 28 wk gestation. Maternal anti-D prophylaxis does not cause hemolysis in the fetus or newborn.
    3. At delivery if the neonate is D- or Du-positive.
    4. If Kleihauer-Betke or rosette test confirms >30 ml of fetal red blood in maternal circulation, additional D immunoglobulin is indicated. Confirm adequacy of therapy by a maternal indirect Coombs test 48 to 72 hr after Rh immune globulin is given.

MANAGEMENT OF D ISOIMMUNIZED PREGNANCIES

- Serial amniocentesis for assessment of OD_{450} after 25 wk gestation with interpretation of the Delta OD_{450} according to criteria established by Liley
- PUBS if ultrasonographic evidence of hydrops, rising zone II Delta OD_{450} values on amniocentesis, or maternal history of a severely affected child
- Intrauterine exchange transfusion if severe anemia is documented remote from term
- Initiation of steroids for lung maturation at 28 wk in severely affected pregnancies with delivery at lung maturity
- Delivery as soon as lung maturation is achieved in mild to moderately affected pregnancies

DISPOSITION

Survival of nonhydropic infants is 90%. Of infants with hydrops, 82% survive.

REFERRAL

Refer all Rh isoimmunized pregnancies to a tertiary care center before 18 to 20 wk gestation.

SUGGESTED READING

available at www.expertconsult.com

AUTHOR: **LAUREL M. WHITE, M.D.**

BASIC INFORMATION

DEFINITION

Rhabdomyolysis is the dissolution or disintegration of muscle, which causes membrane lysis and leakage of muscle constituents, resulting in the excretion of myoglobin in the urine. In general CK levels in excess of 5× normal and the presence of myoglobinuria with the appropriate clinical presentation (see below) are sufficient criteria for the diagnosis of rhabdomyolysis. Renal damage can occur as a result of tubular obstruction by myoglobin as well as hypovolemia.

ICD-9CM CODES
728.89 Rhabdomyolysis
ICD-10CM CODES
M62.9 Disorder of muscle, unspecified
T79.6 Traumatic ischemia of muscle
M62.89 Other specified disorders of muscle

EPIDEMIOLOGY & DEMOGRAPHICS

PREDOMINANT AGE: Rare in children. Increased risk in advanced age (>80 yr).
MORTALITY RATE: 8%
ONSET: The average length of time on statin therapy before rhabdomyolysis is 1 yr. Average time for onset of rhabdomyolysis after addition of fibrate to statin therapy is 32 days.

PHYSICAL FINDINGS & CLINICAL PRESENTATION

- Variable muscle tenderness. Rhabdomyolysis apart from statin use presents with muscle symptoms only 50% of the time.
- Weakness
- Muscular rigidity
- Fever
- Altered consciousness
- Muscle swelling
- Malaise, fatigue. In statin-induced rhabdomyolysis, fatigue (74%) is nearly as common as muscle pain (88%).
- Dark urine: myoglobinuria may cause the urine to be reddish-brown

ETIOLOGY

- Exertion (exercise-induced). Genetic mutations associated with exertional rhabdomyolysis are described in Table 1-434.
- Electrical injury
- Drug-induced (statins, combination of statins with fibrates, or erythromycin, simvastatin and amiodarone, amphetamines, haloperidol)
- Compartment syndrome
- Multiple trauma
- Malignant hyperthermia
- Limb ischemia
- Reperfusion after revascularization procedures for ischemia
- Extensive surgical (spinal) dissection, bariatric surgery
- Tourniquet ischemia
- Prolonged static positioning during surgery
- Infectious and inflammatory myositis
- Metabolic myopathies
- Hypovolemia and urinary acidification are important precipitating causes in the development of acute renal failure
- Sickle cell trait is a predisposing condition
- Hypothyroidism
- Alcoholism
- Seizures
- Table 1-435 summarizes the various causes of rhabdomyolysis.

DIAGNOSIS

DIFFERENTIAL DIAGNOSIS

"Creatine Kinase Elevation" in Section IV describes a clinical algorithm for the evaluation of creatine phosphokinase (CPK) elevation.

LABORATORY TESTS

- Screening for myoglobinuria with a simple urine dipstick test using orthotoluidine or benzidine. Myoglobinuria does not occur in the absence of rhabdomyolysis; therefore, when present, it is the best marker and diagnostic cornerstone of rhabdomyolysis
- Blood urea nitrogen, creatinine

TABLE 1-434 Genetic Mutations Associated with Exertional Rhabdomyolysis

Gene	
Ryanodine receptor 1	*RyR1*
Myoadenylate deaminase	*AMPDA1*
Carnitine palmitoyltransferase II	*CPT2*
Myophosphorylase	*PYGM*
Phosphofructokinase	*PFKM*
Phosphorylase *b* kinase	*PHKA1*
Very long chain acyl coenzyme-A dehydrogenase	*ACAD9*
Phosphoglycerate mutase	*PGAMM*
Phosphoglycerate kinase	*PGK1*
Lactate dehydrogenase	*LDHA*
Cytochrome *c* oxidase	*COX I, II,* and *III*
Cytochrome *b* (complex III)	*CYTB*
Mitochondrial tRNA	*Mt-tRNA*
β-Sarcoglycan	*SGCB*

From Goldman L, Schafer AI: *Goldman's Cecil medicine,* ed 24, Philadelphia, 2012, Saunders.

- Increased CK: CK levels typically peak 2 to 5 days after the initial insult (Fig. 1-811). Levels above 15,000 U/L are more likely to be associated with renal injury
- Hyperkalemia
- Hypocalcemia: due to influx and deposition of of Ca^{2+} in damaged muscle tissue. Hypercalcemia may follow resolution of rhabdomyolysis with subsequent release of calcium back into the circulation
- Hyperphosphatemia
- Elevations in serum myoglobin precede the rise in CK, but it is rapidly eliminated, making this test a less reliable marker of muscle injury
- Pigmented granular casts
- Hyperuricemia
- Anion gap metabolic acidosis may be present due to the release of organic acids from damaged muscle
- Box 1-72 summarizes laboratory abnormalities observed with rhabdomyolysis

TREATMENT

ACUTE GENERAL Rx

- Early, aggressive, high-volume IV fluid replacement. Fluid repletion reduces the accumulation of toxic intracellular contents caused by the rapid breakdown of muscle and subsequent renal damage. Fig. 1-812 describes a treatment algorithm for rhabdomyolysis.

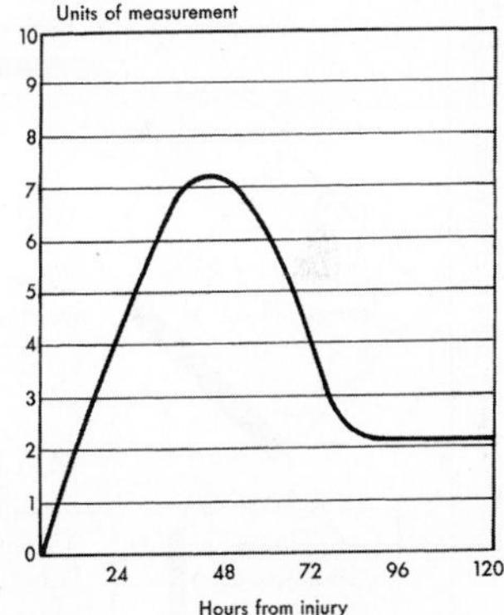

FIGURE 1-811 Typical creatine kinase elimination curve. (From Rosen P [ed]: *Emergency medicine,* ed 4, St Louis, 1998, Mosby.)

TABLE 1-435 Causes of Rhabdomyolysis

Muscle injury/ischemia	Trauma, pressure necrosis, electric shock, burns, acute vascular disease
Myofiber exhaustion	Seizures, excessive exercise, heat exhaustion
Toxins	Alcohol, cocaine, heroin, amphetamines, Ecstasy, phencyclidine, snakebite
Drugs	Statins, fibrates, zidovudine, neuroleptic malignant syndrome, azathioprine, theophylline, lithium, diuretics
Electrolyte disorders	Hypophosphatemia, hypokalemia, excess water shifts (hyperosmolality)
Infections	Viral (influenza, HIV, Coxsackievirus, Epstein-Barr virus), bacterial *(Legionella, Francisella, Streptococcus pneumoniae, Salmonella, Staphylococcus aureus)*
Familial	McArdle's disease, carnitine palmitoyl transferase deficiency, malignant hyperthermia
Other	Hypothyroidism, polymyositis, dermatomyositis

From Floege J et al: *Comprehensive clinical nephrology,* ed 4, Philadelphia, 2010, Saunders

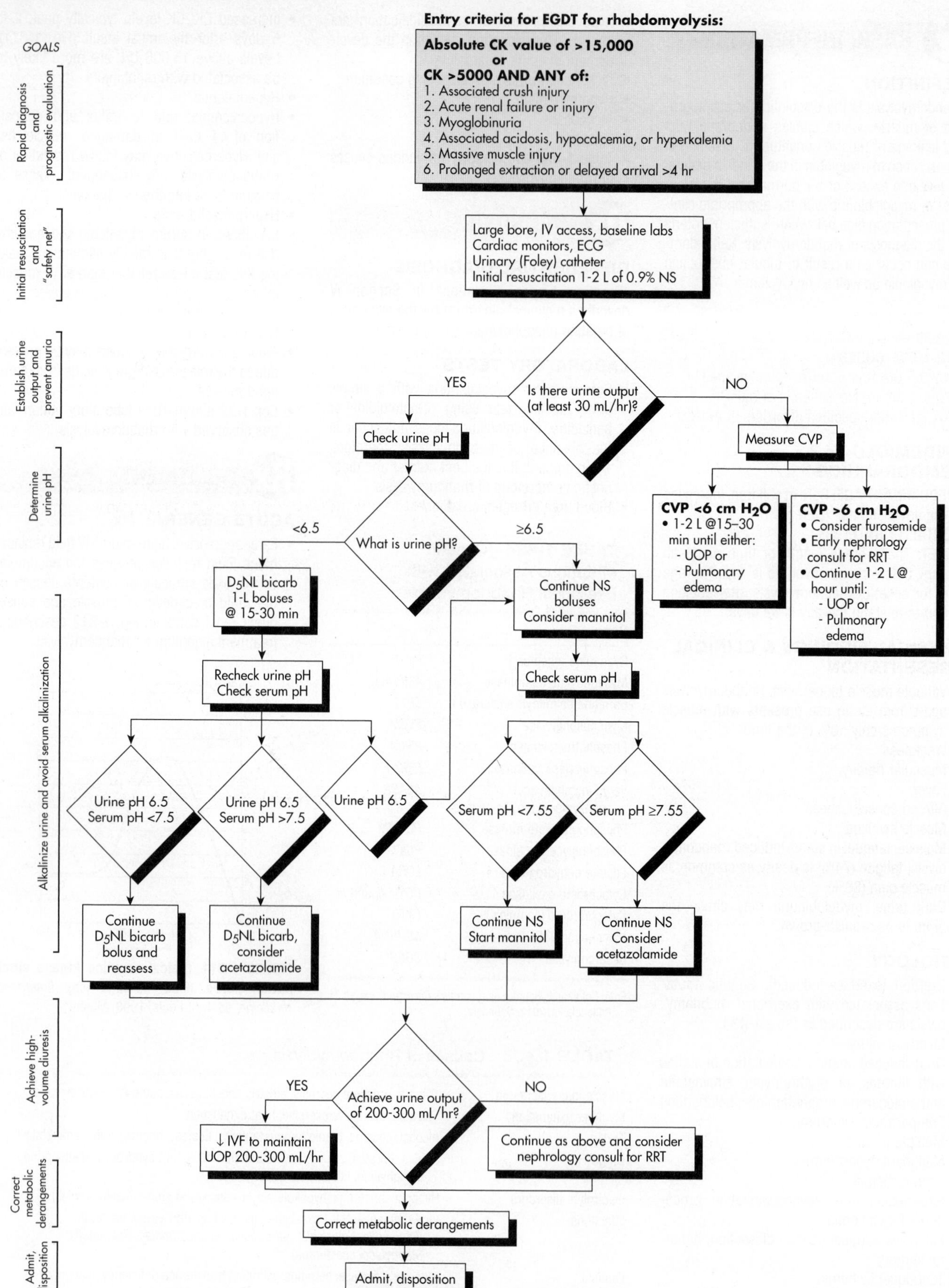

FIGURE 1-812 Early goal-directed therapy for rhabdomyolysis. *CK*, Creatine kinase; *CVP*, central venous pressure; *D5NL bicarb*, 5% dextrose in normal sodium bicarbonate solution; *EGDT*, early goal-directed therapy; *IV*, intravenous; *IVF*, intravenous fluid; *NS*, normal saline; *RRT*, renal replacement therapy; *UOP*, urinary output. (From Adams JG et al: Emergency Medicine, Clinical Essentials, 2nd ed, Philadelphia, Elsevier 2013.)

BOX 1-72 Laboratory Abnormalities Observed with Rhabdomyolysis

Potassium
Elevated
Risk for acute kidney injury

Bicarbonate
Decreased (20 mEq/L)
Metabolic acidosis

Uric Acid
Elevated (>7 mg/dL)
Marker of acute renal failure

Sodium
Usually normal
Can decrease with mannitol therapy
Use serum osmolarity values as a guide

Phosphate
Elevated
Risk for precipitation of calcium phosphate
May need phosphate binders if phosphate >7 mg/dL

Creatine Kinase
Elevated
Associated with creatine kinase level of 15 to 75,000

Blood Urea Nitrogen
Elevated (>20 mg/dL)

Creatinine
Elevated

Calcium
Initially low, sometimes markedly so
Rebound phase may demonstrate hypercalcemia

Liver Function Tests
Sometimes elevated
Serum aspartate transaminase, lactate dehydrogenase, aldolase, muscle enzyme levels elevated

Troponin
Normal
Suspect myocardial damage as a cause (or effect) if elevated
Seven percent false-positive rate for troponin I

Anion Gap
Sometimes elevated
May be predictive of acute renal failure

Prothrombin Time, Partial Thromboplastin Time, D-Dimer
Disseminated intravascular coagulation in up to 30% of severe cases
Associated with higher mortality

(From Adams JG et al: Emergency Medicine, Clinical Essentials, 2nd ed, Philadelphia, Elsevier 2013.)

- Initiate volume repletion with normal saline at a rate of 200 to 1000 ml/hour depending on the setting and severity. Consider treatment with mannitol (up to 200 g/day and cumulative dose up to 800 g) to induce diuresis to prevent acute renal failure. Typically a 20% mannitol infusion at a dose of 0.5 g/kg is given over a 15-min period followed by an infusion at 0.1 g/kg/hr. Fluids should be administered at a rate that results in a urine output of 200 ml/hr until CK levels begin to decrease. Check for plasma osmolality and plasma osmolal gap. Discontinue mannitol if diuresis (>20 ml/hr) is not established. Maintain volume repletion until myoglobinuria is cleared (negative urine dipstick for blood).
- Monitor serum potassium frequently. Correct electrolyte imbalances. Correct hypocalcemia only if symptomatic or if severe hyperkalemia occurs.
- Treatment of electrolyte imbalances
- Alkalinization of urine (to maintain urine pH between 6 and 7 and keep serum pH at 7.50) is controversial but appears helpful in research models when administered early in the course of rhabdomyolysis. Urine alkalinization may trap myoglobin, thereby preventing toxic myoglobin precipitation, and lowers lipid peroxidation, reactive oxygen species formation, and myoglobin-induced vasoconstriction.
- Fasciotomy is indicated in compartment syndrome for preservation of muscle and nerve function. Fasciotomy can lead to rapid decompression of compartment syndrome.

DISPOSITION

Early diagnosis and management are necessary to avoid renal failure, which occurs in 30% of cases. Rhabdomyolysis accounts for 7% to 10% of all cases of acute kidney injury.

REFERRAL

Renal consultation

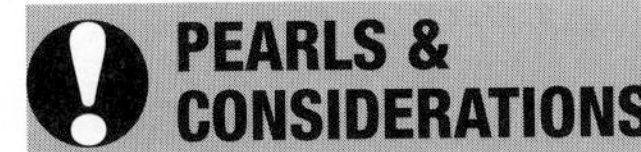

PEARLS & CONSIDERATIONS

COMMENTS

- A clinical algorithm for the evaluation of muscle cramps and aches is described in Section III.
- Statin-induced rhabdomyolysis is 12× more frequent when statins are combined with fibrates compared with statin monotherapy.
- Short-term high-dose corticosteroids (500 to 1000 mg of methylprednisolone) have been successfully used in the treatment of alcohol-induced rhabdomyolysis unresponsive to fluid repletion and may be reasonable in cases of severe rhabdomyolysis refractory to conventional treatment. Corticosteroids block the response of neutrophils to damage tissues and inhibit the chemotaxis of monocytes and neutrophils to sites of inflammation. It has been hypothesized that corticosteroid administration may help diminish the inflammatory exacerbation of muscle damage.

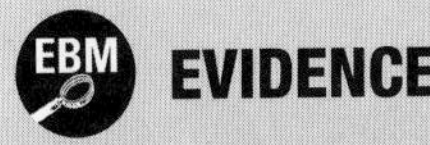

EVIDENCE

available at www.expertconsult.com

SUGGESTED READINGS

available at www.expertconsult.com

RELATED CONTENT

Statin-Induced Muscle Syndromes (Related Key Topic)
Rhabdomyolysis (Patient Information)

AUTHOR: **FRED F. FERRI, M.D.**

R

Diseases and Disorders I

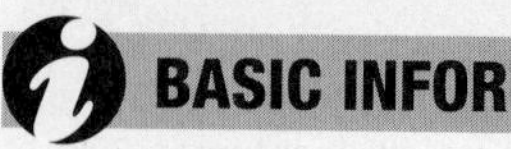

BASIC INFORMATION

DEFINITION

Rheumatoid arthritis (RA) is a systemic autoimmune disease characterized by inflammatory polyarthritis, which affects peripheral joints, especially the small joints of the hands and feet. Chronic untreated inflammation may lead to joint erosions and joint destruction.

ICD-9CM CODES
714.0 Rheumatoid arthritis
ICD-10CM CODES
M06.9 Rheumatoid arthritis, unspecified

EPIDEMIOLOGY & DEMOGRAPHICS

INCIDENCE: Annual incidence in northern Europe and U.S. 0.15 to 0.60 per 1000

PEAK INCIDENCE: Steadily increases with age until the mid-70s

PREVALENCE: 0.5% to 1.0% of the worldwide population

PREDOMINANT SEX AND AGE: Male/female ratio of 1:2; prevalence increases with age

GENETICS: Genetic factors account for more than 50% of risk of disease. RA is polygenic; identified genetic associations include *HLA-DRB1, PTPN22,* and *PADI4.*

RISK FACTORS: Female sex, age, tobacco use, silica exposure, obesity

PHYSICAL FINDINGS & CLINICAL PRESENTATION

Initial presentation:

>6 wk of pain, swelling, warmth in one or more peripheral joints, frequently with symmetric joint involvement involving wrists, hands, and/or feet, and often associated with >1 hr of morning stiffness.

Most common joints involved include metacarpophalangeal (MCP), proximal interphalangeal (PIP), wrists, metatarsophalangeal (MTP), and ankles.

Also elbows, shoulders, hips, and knees.

Distal interphalangeal (DIP) joints are spared.

Sacroiliac and vertebral joints are spared except for C1 to C2.

Chronic longstanding disease:

"Swan-neck" (DIP flexion and PIP hyperextension) and "boutonniere" PIP flexion and DIP hyperextension) deformities (Fig. 1-813), as well as MCP subluxation resulting in ulnar drift (Fig. 1-814).

C1-C2 (atlantoaxial) inflammation can lead to odontoid erosion and transverse ligament laxity, resulting in atlantoaxial subluxation and cord compression.

Joint damage of wrists, elbows, shoulders, hips, and knees can lead to severe osteoarthritis, necessitating joint surgery and/or replacement.

Extraarticular manifestations:

Secondary Sjögren's syndrome (~35%): immune-mediated inflammation of lacrimal and salivary glands resulting in dry mouth and eyes (sicca syndrome).

Rheumatoid nodules (25%): on extensor surfaces and pressure points, in rheumatoid factor positive (RF+) disease. Histopathology demonstrates palisading histiocytes surrounding fibrinoid necrosis.

Normocytic normochromic anemia

Felty's syndrome: RA with splenomegaly and leukopenia

Pulmonary disease

- Pleural disease (effusions, pleuritis)
- Interstitial lung disease (up to 10% clinically significant)

Vasculitis

Cardiac disease

- Pericarditis
- ↑ Risk cardiovascular disease

Ocular disease

- Keratoconjunctivitis sicca (dry eye, without dry mouth/secondary Sjögren's) (10%)
- Episcleritis, scleritis

Amyloidosis: longstanding RA. Can affect heart, kidney, liver, spleen, intestines, and skin.

ETIOLOGY

Unknown. It is likely that a combination of genetic and environmental factors leads to aberrant immune activation and inflammatory response in the joint. Stages of disease development presumably include:

- Initiation of immune response (trigger unknown, but environmental exposures such as tobacco and silica have been implicated.)
- Perpetuation of inflammatory response, with migration of inflammatory cells into joint space, activation of macrophage-like and fibroblast-like synoviocytes, and development of "synovial pannus," a thickened synovial membrane
- The pannus releases proinflammatory cytokines (TNF-α, IL-1, IL-6, IL-8), as well as proteases, which erode cartilage and bone
- Many of the new "biologic" disease-modifying antirheumatic drugs (DMARDs) are engineered to target these cytokines

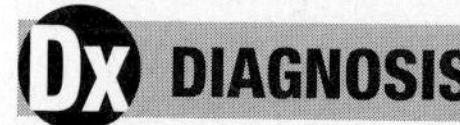

DIAGNOSIS

The American College of Rheumatology and the European League Against Rheumatism have developed new classification criteria for RA. Four variables constitute the new criteria:

1. The number and size of involved joints (score 0 to 5, with higher scores for a larger number of small joints affected)
2. Results of rheumatoid factor (RF) and anti-citrullinated protein antibody testing (score 0 to 3, with more points for a high positive RF or anti-CCP)
3. Abnormal sedimentation rate or elevated C-reactive protein (1 point)
4. Symptom duration >6 wk (1 point)

Scores ≥6 points are considered to have "definite RA." Maximum score is 10 points.

DIFFERENTIAL DIAGNOSIS

- Infections: parvovirus B19, hepatitis B, hepatitis C, poststreptococcal reactive arthritis, acute rheumatic fever
- Systemic lupus erythematosus
- Seronegative spondyloarthropathies
- Calcium pyrophosphate deposition (CPPD or "pseudo-RA")
- Polymyalgia rheumatica
- Hemochromatosis
- Scleroderma
- Osteoarthritis (see Table 1-436)

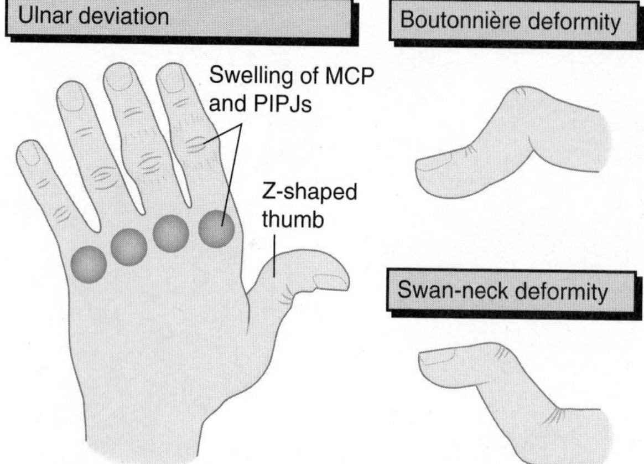

FIGURE 1-813 Characteristic hand deformities in rheumatoid arthritis. *MCP,* Metacarpophalanges; *PIPJs,* proximal interphalangeal joints. (From Ballinger A: *Kumar & Clark's essentials of clinical medicine,* ed 6, Edinburgh, 2012, Saunders.)

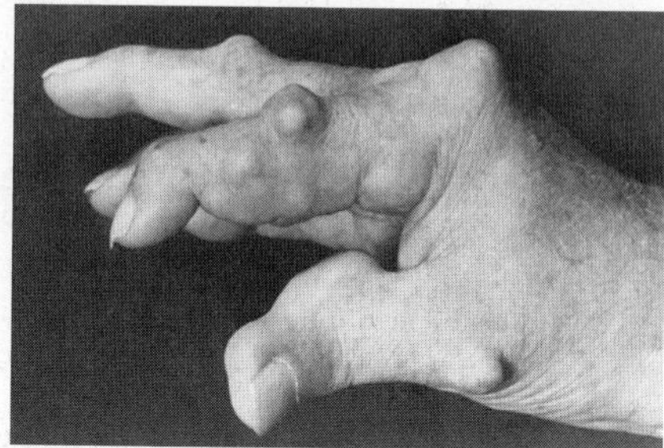

FIGURE 1-814 Rheumatoid arthritis. Hand of a 60-year-old man with seropositive rheumatoid arthritis. There are fixed deformities and gross rheumatoid nodules. (From Canoso JJ: *Rheumatology in primary care,* Philadelphia, 1997, Saunders.)

TABLE 1-436 Factors Useful for Differentiating Early Rheumatoid Arthritis from Osteoarthritis

	Rheumatoid Arthritis	Osteoarthritis
Age at onset	Childhood and adults, peak incidence in 50s	Increases with age
Predisposing factors	Susceptibility epitopes (HLA-DR4, HLA-DR1) *PTPN22, PADI4* polymorphisms, and others Smoking	Trauma Congenital abnormalities (e.g., shallow acetabulum)
Early symptoms	Morning stiffness	Pain increases through the day and with use
Joints involved	Metacarpophalangeal joints, wrists, proximal interphalangeal joints most often; distal interphalangeal joints almost never	Distal interphalangeal joints (Heberden's nodes), weight-bearing joints (hips, knees)
Physical findings	Soft tissue swelling, warmth	Bony osteophytes, minimal soft tissue swelling early
Radiologic findings	Periarticular osteopenia, marginal erosions	Subchondral sclerosis, osteophytes
Laboratory findings	Increased C-reactive protein, rheumatoid factor, anticitrullinated protein antibody, anemia, leukocytosis	Normal

From Firestein GS et al (eds): *Kelly's textbook of rheumatology*, ed 9, Philadelphia, 2013, Saunders.

LABORATORY TESTS

- RF. An immunoglobulin directed against the Fc region of the IgG
  - Sensitivity ~60%
  - Specificity ~80%. False positives are seen with hepatitis C, subacute bacterial endocarditis, sarcoidosis, malignancy, Sjögren's, SLE, increasing age
- Anti-cyclic citrullinated peptide (anti-CCP) antibodies. More specific than RF for RA (up to 95% to 98%). Sensitivity similar to RF. The presence of either RF or anti-CCP ("seropositive RA") is associated with more severe RA.
- ↑ Erythrocyte sedimentation rate (ESR), C-reactive protein (CRP)
- ↑ CBC with differential: possible mild anemia and leukocytosis
- Synovial fluid: inflammatory, with >2000 PMNs.

IMAGING STUDIES

Plain radiography:

- Earlier changes include soft tissue swelling, joint space narrowing, and periarticular osteopenia.
- Later changes include periarticular erosions, especially in MCPs, PIPs, MTPs, and wrist. This reflects cartilage and bone destruction secondary to pannus (Fig. 1-815).
- MRI and musculoskeletal ultrasound are more sensitive for detecting erosive disease and joint effusion/synovitis.

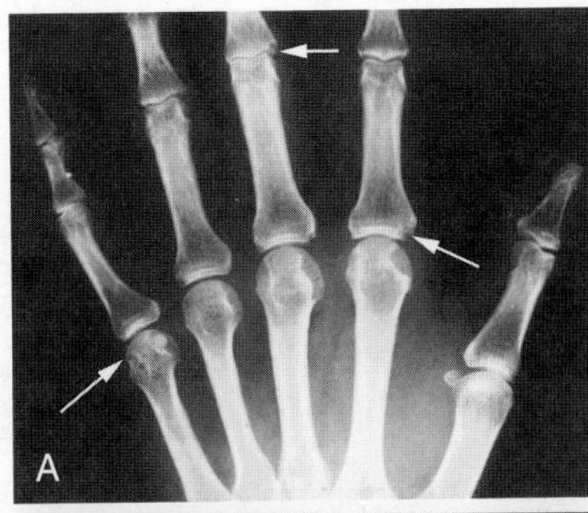

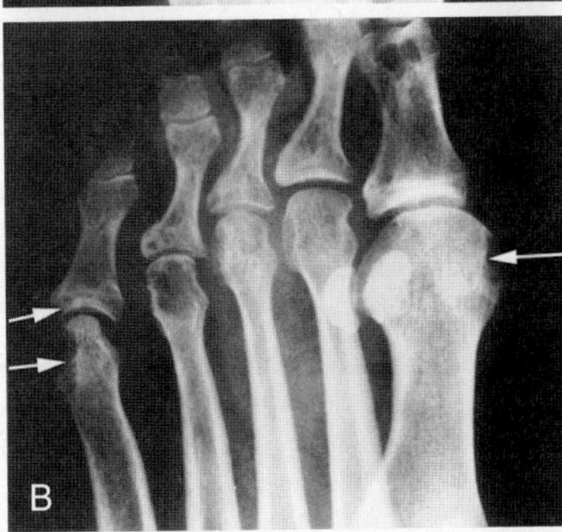

FIGURE 1-815 Rheumatoid arthritis. A, Periarticular osteopenia and marginal erosions in metacarpophalangeal joints and a proximal interphalangeal *(arrows)*. **B,** In the same patient, marginal erosions at metatarsal heads. (From Canoso JJ [ed]: *Rheumatology in primary care,* Philadelphia, 1997, Saunders.)

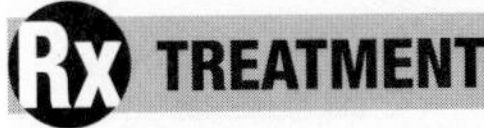

TREATMENT

Early identification and treatment of RA with DMARDs are crucial. More than half of patients have radiographic joint damage within 2 yr of disease onset, but early aggressive treatment (with DMARDs) is associated with less damage. Fig. 1-816 describes the American College of Rheumatology recommendations for treatment of rheumatoid arthritis.

ACUTE GENERAL Rx

- NSAIDs: Sometimes used initially to relieve pain and mild inflammation, or used later in the disease course for additional control of mild pain. NSAIDs are NOT disease modifying.
- Corticosteroids: oral or intraarticular, frequently used initially to reduce inflammation rapidly until oral DMARD treatments take effect. They may also be used during acute flares or in low doses for additional control of inflammation. They have many side effects, including but not limited to weight gain, increased risk of diabetes, osteoporosis, and avascular necrosis.

CHRONIC Rx

DMARDs: Can be classified into "nonbiologic" and "biologic" treatments.

Nonbiologic DMARDs: commonly used agents are methotrexate (MTX), hydroxychloroquine (HCQ), sulfasalazine (SSZ), and leflunomide. Most of these are associated with potential toxicity and require close monitoring. They are also slow-acting drugs that require >8 wk to become fully effective.

MTX is the most commonly used DMARD worldwide for the treatment of RA.

"Triple therapy"—MTX, HCQ, and SSZ are superior to MTX alone.

Biologic DMARDs: newer biologically engineered therapies, which target cytokines and cells involved in the RA inflammatory response. Major side effects include an increased risk of severe infection, most notably reactivation of tuberculosis with anti-TNF agents. A negative PPD is a prerequisite to initiate therapy. Biologic DMARDs are most effective when used in combination with a nonbiologic DMARD, usually MTX.

Tumor necrosis factor α inhibitors (TNFI). Includes infliximab, etanercept, adalimumab, certolizumab pegol, and golimumab.

Abatacept (CTLA-4Ig). A recombinant protein that prevents costimulatory binding of antigen presenting cell to T cell, preventing T cell activation.

Tocilizumab (anti–IL-6). A monoclonal antibody against the IL-6 receptor.

Tofacitinib (JAK3 inhibitor). Inhibits the JAK-STAT intracellular signaling pathway, thus preventing the production of inflammatory mediators. The first oral biologic DMARD.

Rituximab (anti-CD20). A monoclonal antibody against CD20 antigen on B lymphocytes.

DISPOSITION

- Remissions and exacerbations are common, but condition is chronically progressive in the majority of cases.
- Joint degeneration and deformity often lead to disability. Joint replacement is indicated for patients with severe joint damage whose symptoms are poorly controlled by medical management.
- Early and aggressive diagnosis and treatment are crucial in preventing or slowing joint destruction.

REFERRAL

- Early referral to rheumatologist
- Orthopedic consultation for corrective surgery

PEARLS & CONSIDERATIONS

RA sometimes develops acutely in the postpartum patient; conversely, many patients with RA will experience remission during pregnancy.

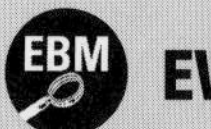

EVIDENCE

available at www.expertconsult.com

SUGGESTED READINGS

available at www.expertconsult.com

RELATED CONTENT

Rheumatoid Arthritis (Patient Information)

AUTHOR: **KERRI BATRA, M.D.**

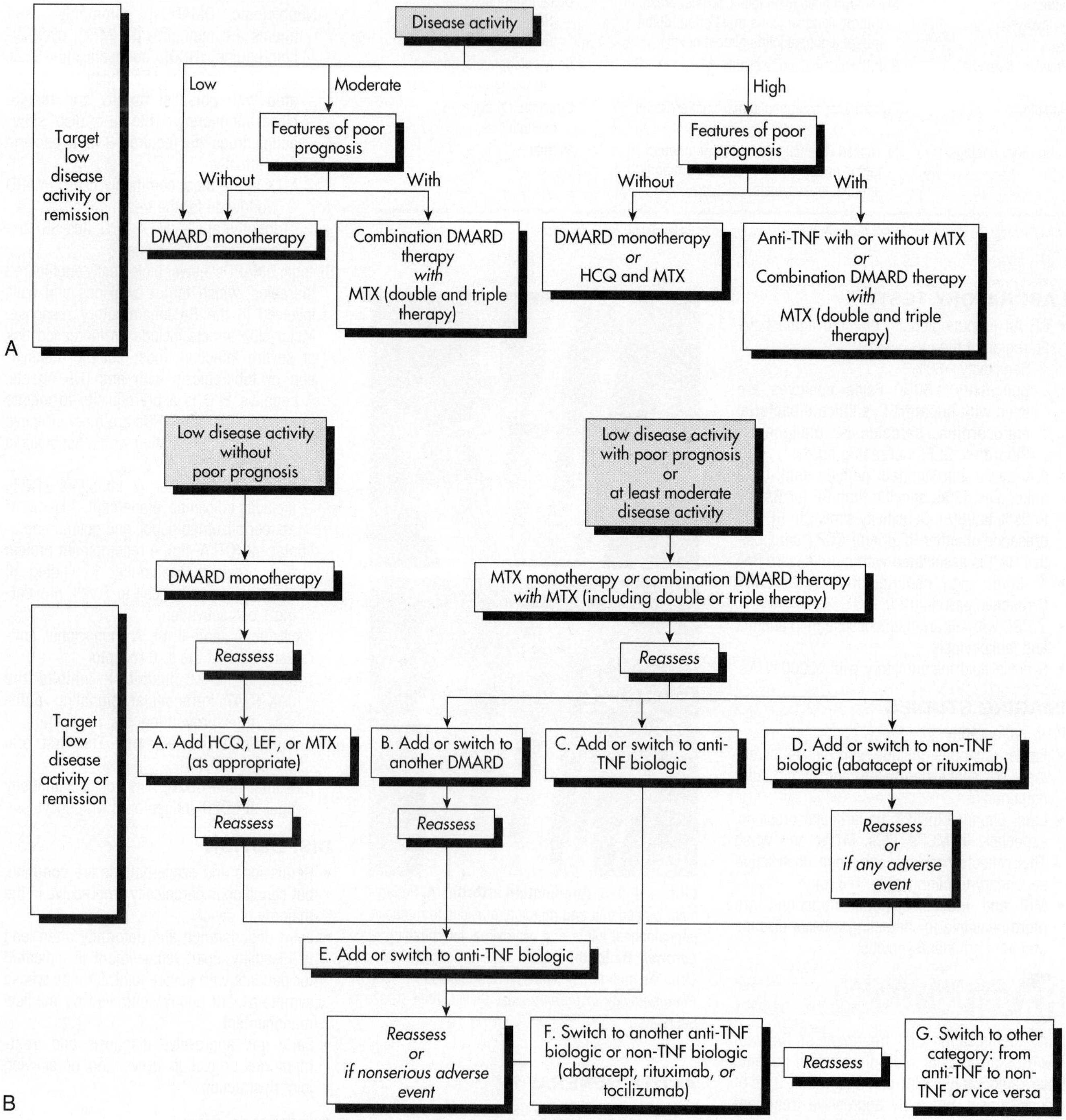

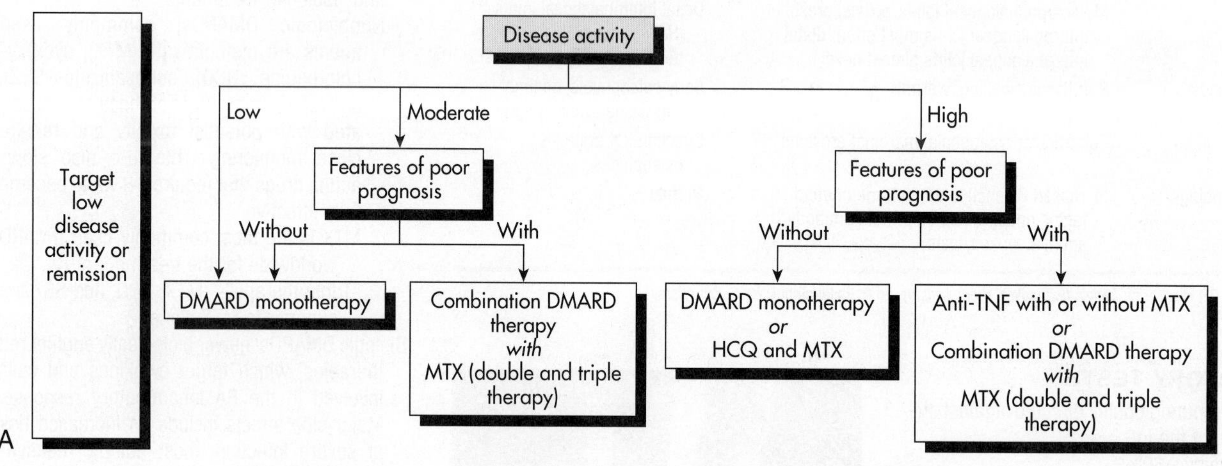

FIGURE 1-816 American College of Rheumatology recommendations for treatment of rheumatoid arthritis. A, Early disease. **B**, Established disease. *DMARD*, Disease-modifying antirheumatic drug; *HCQ*, hydroxychloroquine; *LEF*, leflunomide; *MTX*, methotrexate; *TNF*, tumor necrosis factor. (From Firestein GS et al [eds]: *Kelly's textbook of rheumatology*, ed 9, Philadelphia, 2013, Saunders.)

BASIC INFORMATION

DEFINITION

Rickets is a result of deficient mineralization causing softening and weakening of bones in infants and children. The mineralization impairment may be secondary to abnormal calcium, phosphorus, or vitamin D metabolism leading to accumulation of osteoid before epiphyseal closure, compromising bone stability. When this occurs in adulthood after epiphyseal closure, it is referred to as osteomalacia. Renal osteodystrophy is a term used to describe a similar condition in patients with chronic kidney disease. Certain forms of the disorder may respond only to high doses of vitamin D and are referred to as vitamin D–resistant rickets (VDRR).

ICD-9CM CODES

268.0 Active rickets
268.1 Late effect rickets
275.3 Vitamin D–resistant rickets, familial hypophosphatemia
588.0 Renal rickets (renal osteodystrophy)
268.2 Osteomalacia

ICD-10CM CODES

E55.0 Rickets, active
E83.30 Disorder of phosphorus metabolism, unspecified
N25.0 Renal osteodystrophy
M83.9 Adult osteomalacia, unspecified

RISK FACTORS

- Children ages 6 to 24 months
- Premature infants
- Residents of northern latitudes with inadequate sunlight exposure
- Solely breastfed infants
- Darker skin pigmentation
- Use of anticonvulsants

PHYSICAL FINDINGS & CLINICAL PRESENTATION

The classic clinical presentation of children with rickets includes the following:

- Apathy, muscle weakness, delayed growth
- Skeletal pain and swollen joints
- Protuberant abdomen due to muscle hypotonia
- Widened sutures, delayed closure of fontanelles, and frontal bossing of head
- Craniotabes (softening of skull bones)
- Delayed eruption and poorly mineralized teeth
- Bowing deformity of lower extremities, specifically femur and tibia (Fig. 1-817)
- Rachitic rosary (enlargement and cupping of the costochondral junctions)
- Harrison's groove (indentation of the lower ribs)
- Pathologic fractures

The less pronounced clinical presentation of adults with osteomalacia includes the following:

- Skeletal pain and bone tenderness
- Muscle hypotonia and proximal muscle weakness
- Pathologic fractures
- Gait disturbances

ETIOLOGY

The most common cause of rickets and osteomalacia is vitamin D deficiency. This may arise from various conditions, including inadequate dietary intake, malabsorption, and the additional risk factors listed previously. Malabsorption that causes inefficient mineralization is observed in such diseases as cystic fibrosis and celiac disease. Vitamin D is required for adequate calcium absorption in the GI tract. If a deficiency of vitamin D is present, dietary calcium is not absorbed properly, and this leads to hypocalcemia.

Other causes specifically include vitamin D–dependent rickets, VDRR, and hereditary hypophosphatemic rickets.

- VDRR type I results from abnormalities in the gene coding for 25 (OH)D3-1-alpha-hydroxylase, and type II results from defective vitamin D receptors.
- Chronic renal failure can produce renal osteodystrophy (renal rickets). This results in decreased excretion of phosphate, therefore elevating serum phosphorus, along with elevated parathyroid hormone (PTH) and low levels of 1,25-OH vitamin D.

DIAGNOSIS

DIFFERENTIAL DIAGNOSIS

- Osteoporosis
- Hyperparathyroidism
- Hyperthyroidism
- Hypophosphatasia
- Metaphyseal dysostoses

WORKUP

Diagnosis is clinically based, and it is often challenging to determine the exact cause. A dietary and medication history for children is important. Bone biopsy is generally not performed; however, it is the diagnostic gold standard.

LABORATORY TESTS

- Requires a high degree of interest because many of the conditions are so similar that only a complicated laboratory evaluation may establish the diagnosis.
- Blood testing would include serum calcium, inorganic phosphorus (Pi), alkaline phosphate, PTH, 25-OH vitamin D, creatinine, and liver enzymes.

IMAGING STUDIES

- In rickets, characteristic radiologic findings include irregular epiphyseal-metaphyseal junctions with widening and flaring of the epiphyses of long bones, causing bowing.
- Pseudofractures (Looser zones) and narrow radiolucent lines may be seen as a result of microfractures at high stress points or at the location of entry of blood vessels into the bone and are observed in severe rickets and osteomalacia.

TREATMENT

- Treatment is dependent on the underlying cause.
- VDRR type I is treated with vitamin D. The earliest biochemical change after initiation of treatment is an increase in the level of phosphorus followed by a rise in calcium level. Serum calcium, phosphorus, alkaline phosphatase, and calcidiol levels and urine calcium and phosphorus levels should be obtained within 2 wk of initiation of therapy and periodically. The treatment of type II is more complex and requires the expertise of an endocrinologist and/or nephrologists.
- Familial hypophosphatemic rickets is treated with calcitriol and oral phosphorus.
- Oral phosphorus alone is the treatment of choice for hereditary hypophosphatemic rickets with hypercalciuria.

REFERRAL

- Because of the complex nature of many of these disorders, a qualified endocrinologist and nephrologist should be consulted for treatment.
- Orthopedic consultation may be required for some cases of bowlegs or spinal deformities, which may require specific bracing for long-term growth of the bones. If the deformity is very severe, it may require surgery.
- Surgical care is indicated for slipped capital femoral epiphysis, which is fairly common in renal rickets.

SUGGESTED READINGS

available at www.expertconsult.com

RELATED CONTENT

Vitamin D Deficiency (Patient Information)

AUTHOR: **STEPHANIE A. CURRY, M.D.**

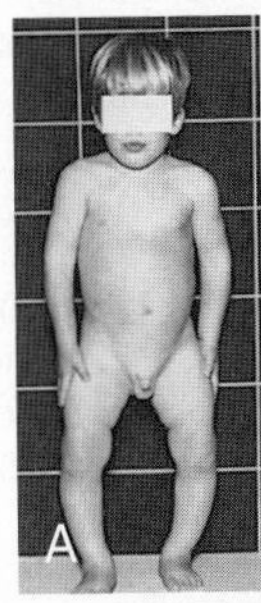

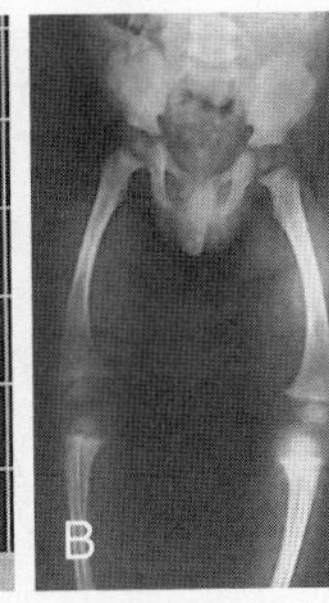

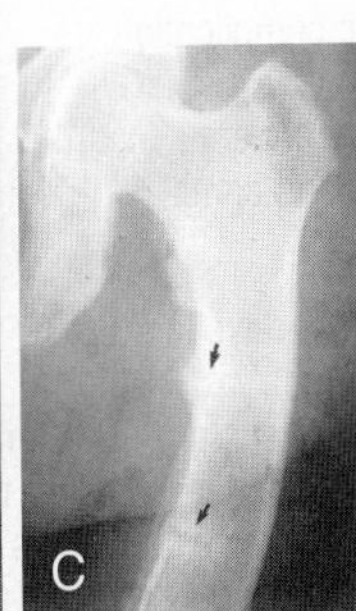

FIGURE 1-817 A, A typical example of rickets. Note the bowing of the femurs and tibiae, which may result from vitamin D deficiency, phosphate deficiency, or other causes. **B,** A skeletal radiograph of a child with rickets. Note that the weight-bearing bones of the lower extremities are bowed and that the epiphyses are open, mottled, and overgrown. **C,** Looser zones or pseudofractures that are characteristic of osteomalacia or rickets. Because the epiphyses are closed, the patient is an adult. This radiograph is diagnostic of osteomalacia. (From Stewart A: Metabolic bone diseases. In Andreoli TE et al [eds]: *Cecil essentials of medicine,* ed 8, Philadelphia, 2010, Saunders.)

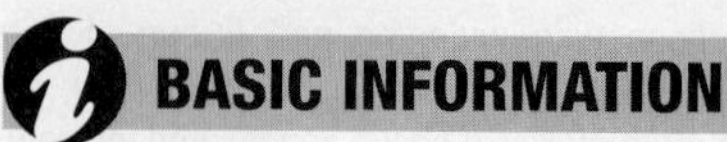

BASIC INFORMATION

DEFINITION

Rocky Mountain spotted fever (RMSF) is a life-threatening, tick-borne febrile illness caused by infection with *Rickettsia rickettsii*. The infection occurs when *R. rickettsii* in the salivary glands of a vector tick is transmitted into the dermis, spreading and replicating in the cytoplasm of endothelial cells and eliciting widespread vasculitis and end-organ damage.

ICD-9CM CODES
082.0 Rocky Mountain spotted fever
ICD-10CM CODES
A77.0 Spotted fever due to Rickettsia rickettsii

EPIDEMIOLOGY & DEMOGRAPHICS

INCIDENCE: 0.18 to 0.32 cases per 100,000 person-years
PREVALENCE: Most prevalent in the Southeast, followed by the South Central states, but seen anywhere (Fig. E1-818). It has recently been reported in eastern Arizona, with common brown dog ticks *(Rhipicephalus sanguineus)* implicated as a vector of *R. rickettsii*.
PREDOMINANT SEX: Affects both genders equally
PREDOMINANT AGE: Occurs at any age, but more likely in children ages 5 to 14 yr

PHYSICAL FINDINGS & CLINICAL PRESENTATION

- Incubation: 2 to 14 days
- First symptoms: fever, headache, malaise, myalgias

Common History, Signs, or Symptoms	*%*
Tick bite	65
Fever	100
Rash	90
Rash on palms and soles (Fig. E1-819)	80
Headache	90
Myalgia	75
Nausea or vomiting	60
Abdominal pain	40
Conjunctivitis	30
Edema	20
Pneumonitis	15
Any severe neurologic complication (including stupor, delirium, seizures, ataxia, papilledema, focal neurologic deficits, and coma)	30

- Rash:
  - Appears during first 3 days in 50%; by day 5, 80% have it. No rash in 10%.
  - Initial appearance: blanching erythematous macules on wrists and ankles that then spread to trunk, palms, and soles.
  - Lesions may evolve into papules and eventually become nonblanching (petechiae or palpable purpura).
- Gastrointestinal symptoms:
  - Nausea, vomiting, and abdominal pain are common
  - Occasionally may mimic an "acute abdomen" (e.g., appendicitis, cholecystitis)
  - Mild hepatitis
- Cardiopulmonary involvement:
  - Interstitial pneumonitis
  - Myocarditis
- Renal problems:
  - Prerenal azotemia
  - Interstitial nephritis
  - Glomerulonephritis
- Neurologic involvement:
  - Encephalitis (confusion, lethargy, delirium)
  - Ataxia
  - Convulsion
  - Cranial nerve palsy
  - Speech impediment
  - Hemiparesis or paraparesis
  - Spasticity
- Fulminant RMSF:
  - Early, widespread vascular necrosis leading to multisystem illness and death

ETIOLOGY & PATHOGENESIS

- Infectious agent: *R. rickettsii* (an intracellular bacterium)
- Vector: dog tick and wood tick (vertical transmission exists in ticks, but horizontal transmission involving rodents represents an important reservoir for the agent). In the United States *R. rickettsii* is transmitted mainly by the American dog tick *(Dermacentor variabilis)* and the Rocky Mountain wood tick *(D. andersoni)*.
- Pathogenesis: the spread of *R. rickettsii* is hematogenous with attachment to the vascular endothelium, causing a vasculitis. The manifestations of this illness are caused by increased vascular permeability.

Dx DIAGNOSIS

DIFFERENTIAL DIAGNOSIS

Influenza A, enteroviral infection, typhoid fever, leptospirosis, infectious mononucleosis, viral hepatitis, sepsis, ehrlichiosis, gastroenteritis, acute abdomen, bronchitis, pneumonia, meningococcemia, disseminated gonococcal infection, secondary syphilis, bacterial endocarditis, toxic shock syndrome, scarlet fever, rheumatic fever, measles, rubella, typhus, rickettsialpox, Lyme disease, drug hypersensitivity reactions, idiopathic thrombocytopenic purpura, thrombotic thrombocytopenic purpura, Kawasaki disease, immune complex vasculitis, connective tissue disorders.

WORKUP

Consider RMSF in any patient with an acute febrile illness with headache and myalgia, especially with an associated history of tick exposure. Absence of rash does not rule out the diagnosis.

LABORATORY TESTS

Routine Tests	*%*
White cell count	
$<10{,}000/mm^3$	72
>10% bands	69
Platelet count	
$<150{,}000/mm^3$	52
$<99{,}000/mm^3$	32
Serum sodium value <132 mEq/L	56
Aspartate aminotransferase ≥2× normal	62
Alanine aminotransferase ≥2× normal	39
Bilirubin value >1.4 mg/dl	30
Cerebrospinal fluid	
Opening pressure ≥250 mm H_2O	14
Glucose value ≤50 mg/dl	8
Protein value ≥50 mg/dl	35
White cell count $\geq 5/mm^3$	38
Mononuclear cell predominance	46
Polymorphonuclear cell predominance	50

- Etiologic tests:
  - Antibody titers to *R. rickettsii* (by indirect fluorescent antibody test). The diagnosis of RMSF requires a fourfold increase 2 wk apart and thus is not helpful in the care of the patients despite a sensitivity and specificity of near 100%.
  - The only test that can provide a timely diagnosis is the immunohistologic demonstration of *R. rickettsii* in skin biopsy specimens.

Rx TREATMENT

- Oral or IV doxycycline, 200 mg/day in 2 divided doses for 7 days or for 2 days after defervescence
- Chloramphenicol, 50 mg/kg/day in 4 divided doses; chloramphenicol may be preferred during pregnancy because of the effects of doxycycline on fetal bones and teeth; therapy continued for at least 2 days after defervescence

PROGNOSIS

Fatality rate: 1% to 4% (five times greater if treatment is initiated after day 5 of illness, which is more likely in the absence of rash and during seasonal nonpeak tick activity). Long-term sequelae seen in patients who recover from severe RMSF: paraparesis, hearing loss; peripheral neuropathy; bladder and bowel incontinence; cerebellar, vestibular, and motor dysfunction; language disorders; limb amputation; and scrotal pain after cutaneous necrosis.

SUGGESTED READINGS

available at www.expertconsult.com

RELATED CONTENT

Rocky Mountain Spotted Fever (Patient Information)

AUTHOR: **FRED F. FERRI, M.D.**

BASIC INFORMATION

DEFINITION

Rosacea is a chronic skin disorder characterized by papules and pustules affecting the face and often associated with flushing and erythema.

SYNONYMS

Acne rosacea

ICD-9CM CODES
695.3 Rosacea
ICD-10CM CODES
L71 Rosacea
L71.9 Rosacea unspecified
L71.1 Rhinophyma
L71.8 Other rosacea
L71.0 Perioral dermatitis

EPIDEMIOLOGY & DEMOGRAPHICS

- Rosacea occurs in one in 20 Americans
- Onset often between ages 30 and 50 yr
- More common in people of Celtic origin; however, this disease may be overlooked in nonwhites because skin pigmentation results in atypical presentation
- Female/male ratio of 3:1

PHYSICAL FINDINGS & CLINICAL PRESENTATION

- Facial erythema, presence of papules, pustules, and telangiectasia.
- Excessive facial warmth and redness are the predominant presenting symptoms.
- Itching is generally absent.
- Comedones are absent (unlike acne).
- Women are more likely to show symptoms on the chin and cheeks, whereas in men the nose is commonly involved.
- Ocular findings (mild dryness and irritation with blepharitis, conjunctival injection, burning, stinging, tearing, eyelid inflammation, swelling, and redness) are present in 50% of patients.

Rosacea can be classified into four major subtypes:

1. Erythematotelangiectatic (vascular): erythema in central part of face, telangiectasia, flushing
2. Papulopustular (inflammatory): presence of dome-shaped erythematous papules and small pustules, in addition to facial erythema, flushing, and telangiectasia
3. Phymatosis (Fig. E1-820): presence of thickened skin with prominent pores that may affect the nose (rhinophyma), chin (gnathophyma), forehead (metophyma), eyelids (blepharophyma), and ears (otophyma)
4. Ocular: conjunctival injection, sensation of foreign body in the eye, telangiectasia and erythema of lid margins, scaling.

ETIOLOGY

- Unknown but believed to involve the vasculature
- Hot drinks, alcohol, and sun exposure may accentuate the erythema by causing vasodilation of the skin.
- Flare-ups may also result from reactions to medications (e.g., simvastatin, angiotensin-converting enzyme inhibitors, vasodilators, fluorinated corticosteroids), stress, extreme heat or cold, wind, humidity, strenuous exercise, spicy drinks, menstruation.

Dx DIAGNOSIS

DIFFERENTIAL DIAGNOSIS

- Drug eruption
- Acne vulgaris
- Contact dermatitis
- Systemic lupus erythematosus
- Carcinoid flush
- Idiopathic facial flushing
- Seborrheic dermatitis
- Facial sarcoidosis
- Photodermatitis
- Mastocytosis
- Perioral dermatitis
- Granulomas of the skin

WORKUP

Diagnosis is based on clinical findings. Distinguishing features between acne and rosacea are the presence of telangiectasia and deep diffuse erythema and absence of comedones in rosacea.

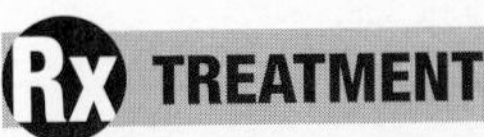

TREATMENT

NONPHARMACOLOGIC THERAPY

- Avoid alcohol, excessive sun exposure, and hot drinks of any type.
- Use of mild, nondrying soap is recommended; local skin irritants should be avoided.
- Reassure patient that rosacea is completely unrelated to poor hygiene.
- Vascular laser surgery is effective for telangiectasia.
- Surgical options are available for rhinophyma.

GENERAL Rx

- Several classes of drugs are used in treatment of rosacea, including the metronidazole family, the tetracycline family, and azelaic acid.
- Vascular rosacea: topical therapy with metronidazole aqueous gel (MetroGel) applied bid is effective as initial therapy for mild cases. A new 1% formulation of metronidazole (Noritate) applied daily may improve patient compliance. Clindamycin lotion (Cleocin), sulfacetamide, or erythromycin 2% solution may also be effective. Brimonidine (mirvaso) is a selective alpha$_2$-adrenergic receptor agonist recently FDA-approved as a gel preparation for topical treatment of adults with persistent facial erythema of rosacea.
- Pustular and ocular rosacea: systemic antibiotics (doxycycline 100 mg qd or tetracycline 250 mg qid until symptoms diminish, then taper off). Minocycline 50 to 100 mg qd should be used only in resistant cases because this medication is expensive. Oral metronidazole (200 mg qd to bid) for 4 to 6 wk is also effective.
- Isotretinoin (Accutane) 0.5 to 1 mg/kg/day in two divided doses for 15 to 20 wk can be used for refractory papular and pustular rosacea; use of retinoids may, however, worsen erythema and telangiectasis.
- Laser treatment is an option for progressive telangiectasias or rhinophyma.
- Erythema and flushing may respond to low-dose clonidine (0.05 mg bid).
- Treatment of phymatous rosacea: oral tetracyclines, oral isotretinoin, ablative/pulsed dye laser therapy, electrosurgery.
- Treatment of ocular rosacea: topical or oral tetracyclines, artificial tears, and/or lid cleansing for eyelid hygiene.

DISPOSITION

- Rosacea is often resistant to initial treatment and recurrent. Periods of remission and relapse are common.
- The progression of rosacea is variable. Typical stages include:
  1. Facial flushing
  2. Erythema and/or edema and ocular symptoms
  3. Papules and pustules
  4. Rhinophyma

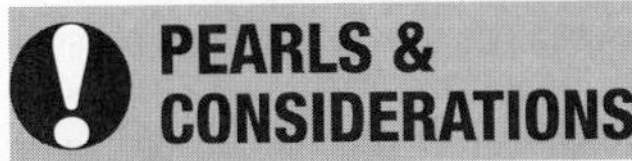

PEARLS & CONSIDERATIONS

COMMENTS

- The course of the disease is typically chronic, with remissions and relapses.
- Patients with resistant cases may have *Demodex folliculorum* mite infestation or tinea infection (diagnosis can be confirmed with potassium hydroxide examination); the role of *D. folliculorum* in rosacea is unclear. These mites can sometimes be found in large numbers in the lesions; however, their numbers do not generally decline with treatment.
- Rosacea can result in emotional and social stigmas, especially because many people associate rosacea and rhinophyma with alcohol abuse.
- Early consultation with an ophthalmologist is recommended in patients with suspected ocular involvement.

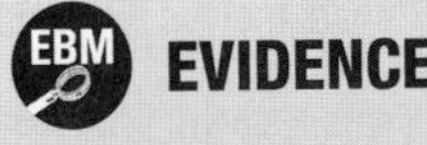

EVIDENCE

available at www.expertconsult.com

SUGGESTED READINGS

available at www.expertconsult.com

RELATED CONTENT

Rosacea (Patient Information)

AUTHOR: **FRED F. FERRI, M.D.**

BASIC INFORMATION

DEFINITION

Roseola is a benign viral illness found in infants and characterized by high fevers that last 3 or 4 days, followed by defervescence and development of a macular or maculopapular rash.

SYNONYMS

Exanthem subitum
Sixth disease
Roseola infantum
Pseudorubella
Human herpesvirus 6 (HHV-6), human herpesvirus 7 (HHV-7)

ICD-9CM CODES
057.8 Roseola
ICD-10CM CODES
B08.2 Exanthema subitum (sixth disease)

EPIDEMIOLOGY & DEMOGRAPHICS

- Nearly one third of all infants develop roseola before the age of 2 yr.
- Peak prevalence is between 7 and 13 mo.
- More than 90% of children older than 2 yr of age are seropositive for the virus causing roseola.
- Roseola is spread from person to person. It is not known how it is spread, but it must be very efficiently spread and presumably via the respiratory tract.
- There is no predilection for gender or time of year.

PHYSICAL FINDINGS & CLINICAL PRESENTATION

- Typically the child develops a high fever, usually up to 104° F (40° C), that lasts for 3 to 5 days
- Fever may be associated with a runny nose, irritability, and fatigue
- A rash appears within 48 hr of defervescence, begins on the neck or trunk and then spreads to extremities, and persists for a few hours to 2 days.
- Faint pink maculopapular rash that blanches when palpated (Fig. E1-821) and generally nonpruritic
- Other common findings: cervical and/or occipital adenopathy, erythematous tympanic membranes, anorexia
- Nagayama spots: red papules on the soft palate or base of the uvula
- Seizures
- Less common: febrile seizures (≤6% of cases), cough, diarrhea, aseptic meningitis

ETIOLOGY

- Roseola is usually caused by human herpesvirus-6 (HHV-6) in the great majority of cases but other causes include human herpesvirus-7, enteroviruses, adenoviruses, and parainfluenza virus type 1. A small percentage of children may have primary infection with HHV-7.
- The incubation period is between 5 and 15 days.

DIAGNOSIS

The diagnosis of roseola is usually made by the clinical presentation as stated previously. It can be confirmed serologically by indirect immunofluorescence assays, ELISA, neutralization assays, and immunoblot. Viral culture is the gold standard to document active viral replication but is expensive, time consuming, and available only in research laboratories.

DIFFERENTIAL DIAGNOSIS

- Rubeola (measles)
- Rubella
- Fifth disease (erythema infectiosum) caused by parvovirus B19
- Enteroviral infections
- Drug eruption
- Mononucleosis
- All causes of fever (e.g., otitis media, pneumonia, and urinary tract infection)
- Meningitis

WORKUP

- If unsure of the diagnosis of roseola in a febrile infant, a fever workup is done to rule out other infectious causes.
- The decision to proceed with a fever workup is a clinical judgment call.

LABORATORY TESTS

- CBC with differential usually shows relative neutropenia and mild atypical lymphocytosis.
- Erythrocyte sedimentation rate (ESR), blood cultures as indicated
- Urinalysis and urine cultures
- Stool cultures if diarrhea is present
- Lumbar puncture if needed to rule out meningitis in patients with mental status changes
- Commercial assays can be used to detect HHV-6-specific IgG antibody responses but IgM assays are not always reliable for acute infection

IMAGING STUDIES

Chest x-ray to rule out pneumonia

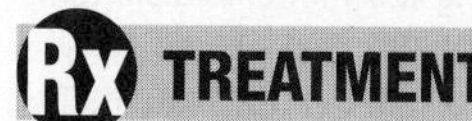

TREATMENT

NONPHARMACOLOGIC THERAPY

- Supportive care
- Maintain hydration by drinking clear fluids: water, fruit juice, lemonade, and so forth
- Sponge bathe with lukewarm water if febrile

ACUTE GENERAL Rx

- Acetaminophen 10 to 15 mg/kg per dose at 4-hr intervals for fever
- Ibuprofen 5 to 10 mg/kg per dose at 6-hr intervals (maximal dose 600 mg)

CHRONIC Rx

Roseola is a viral disease that is short lasting; chronic treatment is usually not an issue.

DISPOSITION

- Roseola is generally a benign, self-limited disease that usually lasts approximately 1 wk.
- Complications, although rare, can occur and include:
  1. Febrile seizures
  2. Meningitis
  3. Encephalitis
  4. Pneumonitis
  5. Hepatitis

REFERRAL

Subspecialty consultation is made with the appropriate discipline if any of the previously mentioned complications occur (e.g., neurology for seizures).

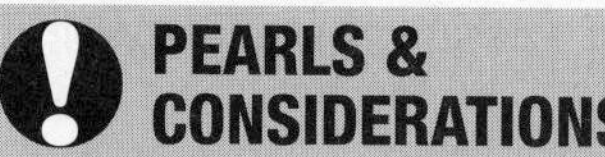

PEARLS & CONSIDERATIONS

COMMENTS

- A child with fever and rash should be excluded from day care.
- HHV-6 is named accordingly because it is the sixth herpesvirus discovered after herpes simplex 1 (HSV-1), HSV-2, cytomegalovirus (CMV), Epstein-Barr virus (EBV), and varicella-zoster virus (VZV).
- Roseola is called sixth disease because it represents the sixth childhood "exanthem"; the other five are measles, scarlet fever, rubella, Dukes disease, and erythema infectiosum.

SUGGESTED READINGS

available at www.expertconsult.com

RELATED CONTENT

Roseola (Patient Information)

AUTHOR: **GLENN G. FORT, M.D., M.P.H.**

BASIC INFORMATION

DEFINITION

- The rotator cuff syndrome is a spectrum of afflictions involving the four rotator cuff muscles of the shoulder: supraspinatus, infraspinatus, teres minor, and subscapularis.
- It consists of subacromial bursitis, rotator cuff tendinopathy, and partial- or full-thickness muscle or tendon tear.

SYNONYMS

Shoulder impingement syndrome
Painful arc syndrome
Supraspinatus syndrome

ICD-9CM CODES
726.10 Rotator cuff syndrome
727.61 Rotator cuff rupture
ICD-10CM CODES
M75.1 Rotator cuff syndrome
M75.100 Unspecified rotator cuff tear or rupture of unspecified shoulder, not specified as traumatic

EPIDEMIOLOGY & DEMOGRAPHICS

PREVALENCE: 5% to 10% of the population
PREDOMINANT SEX: Males more than females
PREDOMINANT AGE: >40 yr
RISK FACTORS: Repetitive overhead activity, advanced age, obesity, smoking, trauma

PHYSICAL FINDINGS & CLINICAL PRESENTATION

- Lateral shoulder pain with overhead activity
- Pain at night when lying on the shoulder
- Muscle weakness indicates a tear
- Atrophy and sunken appearance of the scapular muscles with longstanding disease
- Tenderness over the affected muscle or under the acromion (Fig. E1-822)
- Useful clinical tests:
  - ***Hawkins-Kennedy sign:*** shoulder and elbow are flexed at 90 degrees; shoulder pain is elicited with passive internal rotation (Fig. 1-823, *A*)
  - ***Painful arc sign:*** pain with active abduction of the shoulder between 70% to 120%
  - ***Drop arc sign:*** failure to smoothly control shoulder adduction
  - Painful resisted external rotation and forced passive full-forward flexion (Fig. 1-823, *B, C*)
- The combination of Hawkins-Kennedy sign, the painful arc sign, and weakness in external rotation yields the best probability (95%) for any degree of impingement
- The combination of drop arm sign, painful arc sign, and weakness in external rotation accurately predicts full-thickness tears (91%)
- A subacromial lidocaine injection can be used to distinguish weakness from rotator cuff tendinopathy and true tears—normal strength after injection indicates tendinopathy

ETIOLOGY

A combination of tendon overload, microvascular compromise, and compression by surrounding structures

Dx DIAGNOSIS

DIFFERENTIAL DIAGNOSIS

- Bicipital tendinitis, labrum tears, adhesive capsulitis, glenohumeral osteoarthritis, acromioclavicular injury, subscapular bursitis, avascular necrosis. Table E1-437 describes the differential diagnosis of shoulder pain.
- Neurologic and visceral etiologies need to be ruled out.

IMAGING STUDIES

- Plain radiography: not routinely needed; can reveal tendon calcifications and migration of humeral head, indicating a large tear
- Ultrasonography: accurate tool for initial evaluation but has limitations; partial tears are difficult to identify; highly operator-dependent
- MRI is the test of choice for shoulder soft tissue lesions

Rx TREATMENT

ACUTE GENERAL Rx

- Ice and rest without overhead activity
- Physical therapy
- NSAIDs for 7 to 10 days, then as needed
- Subacromial glucocorticoid injections can be used in patients with severe pain and without suspected tears
- Surgery is reserved for healthy patients with acute full-thickness tears or with chronic partial tears who fail conservative management

DISPOSITION

Return to work or sport should be gradual and is based upon the ability to exhibit full ROM and appropriate strength without discomfort.

REFERRAL

Orthopedic consultation should be obtained in patients with a clinically significant rotator cuff tear and in patients who fail to improve with medical management.

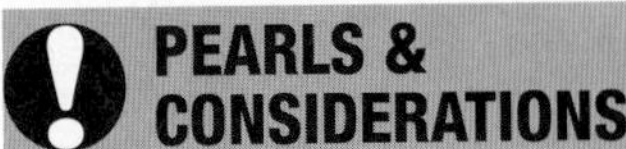

COMMENTS

- Supraspinatus is the most commonly injured muscle.
- Rotator cuff tears can be asymptomatic.
- Identification of partial tears remains a clinical challenge and imaging is often needed.
- It is important to differentiate tears from tendinopathy because they require different management.
- Most patients respond to conservative management.
- Untreated, longstanding rotator cuff tendinopathy can cause significant loss in range of motion and adhesive capsulitis.

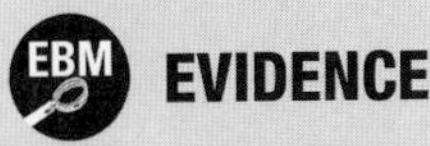

available at www.expertconsult.com

SUGGESTED READINGS

available at www.expertconsult.com

RELATED CONTENT

Bursitis (Related Key Topic)
Rotator Cuff Tendinitis (Patient Information)
Rotator Cuff Pain (Patient Information)
Rotator Cuff Tear (Patient Information)
Rotator Cuff Tendinosis (Patient Information)

AUTHOR: **DAN A. CRISTESCU, M.D.**

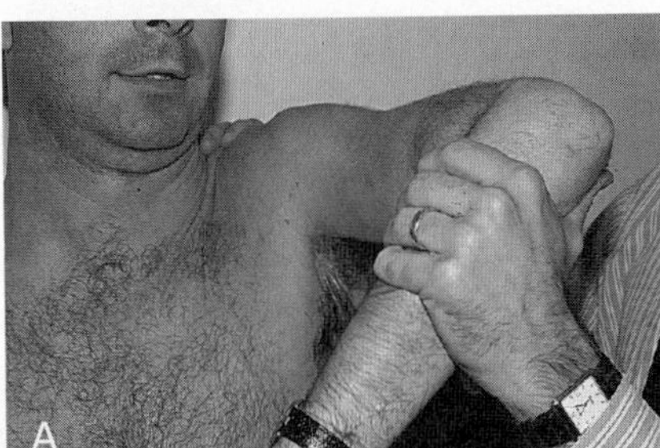

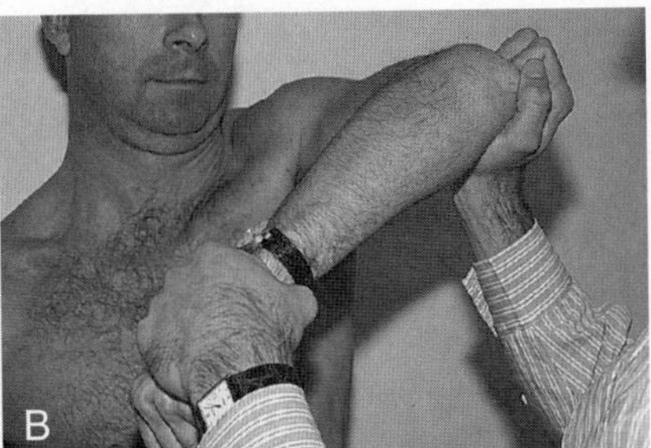

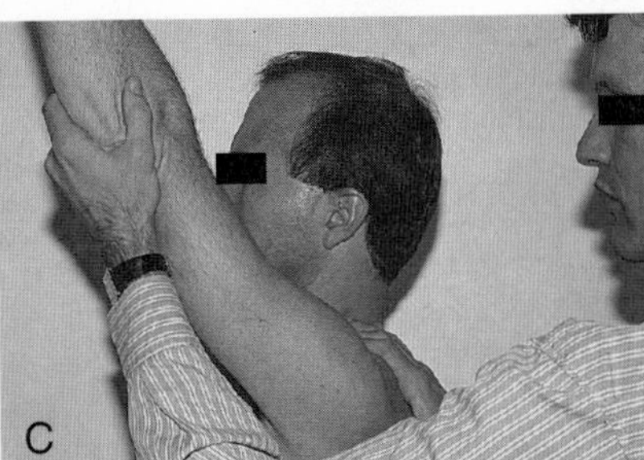

FIGURE 1-823 Impingement tests. A, Forced passive internal rotation. **B,** Resisted external rotation. **C,** Forced passive full forward flexion. (From Hochberg MC et al: *Rheumatology*, ed 5, St Louis, 2011, Mosby.)

BASIC INFORMATION

DEFINITION

Salivary gland neoplasms are benign or malignant tumors of a salivary gland (parotid, submandibular, or sublingual).

SYNONYMS

These tumors are often named according to their histologic type (see "Diagnosis").

ICD-9CM CODES
142.9 Salivary gland neoplasm
142.0 (Parotid)
142.1 (Submandibular)
142.2 (Sublingual)

ICD-10CM CODES
C08.9 Malignant neoplasm of major salivary gland, unspecified
C07 Malignant neoplasm of parotid gland
C08.0 Malignant neoplasm of submandibular gland
C08.1 Malignant neoplasm of sublingual gland

EPIDEMIOLOGY & DEMOGRAPHICS

INCIDENCE: One to two cases per 100,000 person-years (1% of all head and neck tumors)

DISTRIBUTION:
- Parotid gland, 85% (80% are benign)
- Submandibular gland, 10% (55% are benign)
- Sublingual and minor glands, 5% (35% are benign)

PHYSICAL FINDINGS & CLINICAL PRESENTATION

- Parotid gland:
  1. Painless swelling overlying the masseter muscle (under the temporomandibular joint)
  2. Pain
  3. Facial nerve palsy
  4. Cervical lymph nodes
  5. Mass in oral cavity
- Submandibular gland: swelling under anterior portion of the mandible
- Sublingual gland: intraoral swelling under the tongue, medial to the mandible

DIAGNOSIS

PATHOLOGY

HISTORY:

Benign Tumors:
- Mixed tumor (usually parotid)
- Adenolymphoma (Warthin's tumor)
- Pleomorphic adenoma
- Capillary hemangioma, lymphangioma (in children)
- Intraductal papilloma
- Other (e.g., myoepithelioma, canalicular adenoma, basal cell adenoma)

MALIGNANT TUMORS:
- Mucoepidermoid carcinoma (most common malignant tumor of the parotid gland)
- Adenoid cystic carcinoma
- Adenocarcinoma
- Malignant mixed tumor
- Squamous cell carcinoma
- Other

STAGE (TNM):

T_0 No evidence of primary tumor
T_1 Tumor <2 cm
T_2 Tumor 2 to 4 cm
T_3 Tumor 4 to 6 cm
T_4 Tumor >6 cm

All subdivided into
- Without local extension
- With local extension

N_0 No lymph node metastasis
N_1 Single ipsilateral node <3 cm
N_2 Ipsilateral, contralateral, or bilateral node <6 cm
N_3 Any node >6 cm
M_0 No distant metastasis
M_1 Distant metastasis

Stage I T_{1a} or $_{2a}N_0M_0$
Stage II $T_{1b,2b,3a}$ N_0M_0
Stage III $T_{3b,4a}$ N_0M_0 or any T except $_{4b}N_1M_0$
Stage IV T_{4b} any N any M or any T $N_{2,3}M_0$ or any T, any N_1M_1

WORKUP

- Fine-needle aspiration. The sensitivity, specificity, and accuracy of parotid gland aspirates are approximately 92%, 100%, and 98%, respectively
- Imaging by CT scan or MRI
- Open biopsy (rarely indicated)

TREATMENT

Malignant tumors:
- Surgery is the mainstay of treatment; gland resection and neck dissection if lymph nodes are involved.
- A lateral lobectomy with preservation of facial nerve should be considered for tumors confined to the superficial lobe of the parotid gland. Gross tumor should not be left in situ, but if the facial nerve is able to be preserved by "peeling" tumor off the nerve, it should be attempted, followed by radiation therapy for microscopic disease.
- Postoperative radiation is indicated for high-grade malignancies demonstrating extraglandular disease, perineural invasion, direct invasion of surrounding tissues, or regional metastases.
- Chemotherapy.

Benign tumors: surgery for tumor resection

PROGNOSIS OF MALIGNANT TUMORS

Five-year survival rates:
- Mucoepidermoid carcinoma: 75% to 95%
- Adenoid cystic carcinoma: 40% to 80%
- Adenocarcinoma: 20% to 75%
- Malignant mixed tumor: 35% to 75%
- Squamous cell carcinoma: 25% to 60%

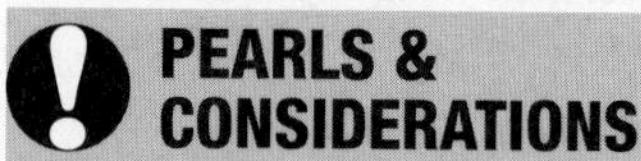

PEARLS & CONSIDERATIONS

COMMENTS

Salivary gland neoplasms most often present as slow-growing, well-circumscribed masses. Pain, rapid growth, nerve weakness, fixation to skin or underlying muscle, and paresthesias usually are indicative of malignancy.

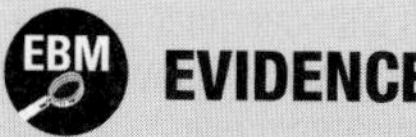

EVIDENCE

available at www.expertconsult.com

SUGGESTED READING

available at www.expertconsult.com

RELATED CONTENT

Salivary Gland Tumors (Patient Information)

AUTHOR: **FRED F. FERRI, M.D.**

BASIC INFORMATION

DEFINITION

Salmonellosis is an infection caused by one of several serotypes of a gram-negative bacillus of the genus *Salmonella.* Current *Salmonella* nomenclature is described in Table 1-439.

SYNONYMS

Typhoid fever
Paratyphoid fever
Enteric fever

ICD-9CM CODES
003.0 Salmonellosis
ICD-10CM CODES
A02.0 Salmonella enteritis
A02.1 Salmonella sepsis
A02.2 Localized salmonella infections
A02.8 Other specified salmonella infections
A0.9 Salmonella infection, unspecified

EPIDEMIOLOGY & DEMOGRAPHICS

INCIDENCE (IN U.S.):

- Epidemiologically, the clinical syndromes are divided into those that cause a typhoidal type of infection (systemic illness with fever and abdominal pain) such as *Salmonella typhi* and those that do not: nontyphoidal *Salmonella* infections (gastroenteritis) such as *S. enteritidis, S. newport,* and *S. typhimurium.*
- Estimated 1 million cases/yr of nontyphoidal salmonellosis in the U.S.
- Approximately 500 cases of *Salmonella typhi* infection reported each yr. In 2009 contaminated peanut butter and peanut products caused a nationwide *Salmonella typhimurium* outbreak in 46 states, affecting more than 700 individuals.
- Largest outbreak: 200,000 people who ingested contaminated milk

PEAK INCIDENCE: Summer and fall

PREDOMINANT AGE:

- <20 yr old
- >70 yr old
- Highest rates of infection in infants, especially neonates

GENETICS

Neonatal infection:

- Highly susceptible to infection with nontyphoidal *Salmonella*

PHYSICAL FINDINGS & CLINICAL PRESENTATION

- Infections
  1. Localized to GI tract (gastroenteritis)
  2. Systemic (typhoid fever)
  3. Localized outside of GI tract
- Gastroenteritis
  1. Incubation period: 12 to 48 hr
  2. Nausea, vomiting
  3. Diarrhea, abdominal cramps
  4. Fever
  5. Bacteremia: occurs mostly in the immunocompromised host or those with underlying conditions, including HIV infection
  6. Self-limited illness lasting 3 or 4 days
  7. Colonization of GI tract persistent for months, especially in those treated with antibiotics
- Typhoid fever
  1. Incubation period of few days to several wk
  2. Prolonged fever, often with a stepwise-increasing temperature pattern
  3. Myalgias
  4. Headache, cough, sore throat
  5. Malaise, anorexia
  6. Abdominal pain
  7. Hepatosplenomegaly
  8. Diarrhea or constipation early in the course of illness
  9. Rose spots (faint, maculopapular, blanching lesions) sometimes seen on chest or abdomen
- Untreated disease
  1. Fever lasting 1 to 2 mo
  2. Main complication: GI bleeding caused by perforation from ulceration of Peyer's patches in the ileum
  3. Rare complications:
     a. Mental status changes
     b. Shock
  4. Relapse rate of approximately 10%
- Infections outside GI tract
  1. Can occur in virtually any location
  2. Usually occur in patients with underlying diseases
  3. Endocarditis, endovascular infections are caused by seeding of atherosclerotic plaques or aneurysms
  4. Hepatic or splenic abscesses in patients with underlying disease in these organs
  5. Urinary tract infections in patients with renal TB or schistosomiasis
  6. Salmonellae are a frequent cause of gram-negative meningitis in neonates
  7. Osteomyelitis in children with hemoglobinopathies (particularly sickle cell disease)

ETIOLOGY

- More than 2000 serotypes of *Salmonella* exist, but only a few cause disease in humans. Host factors and conditions predisposing to the development of systemic disease with nontyphoidal *Salmonella* strains are described in Table 1-440.
- Raw produce is an increasingly recognized vehicle for salmonellosis. In 2008 there was a large outbreak of *Salmonella* Saintpaul involving 1500 persons, of whom 21% were hospitalized and 2 died. It was due to contaminated jalapeno and serrano peppers. More recently outbreaks of human *Salmonella* infections have been increasingly associated with contact with live poultry.
- Some found only in humans are the cause of enteric fever.
  1. *S. typhi*
  2. *S. paratyphi*
- Some responsible for gastroenteritis and frequently isolated from raw meat and poultry and uncooked or undercooked eggs.
  1. *S. typhimurium*
  2. *S. enteritidis*
- *S. choleraesuis* is a prototype organism that causes extraintestinal nontyphoidal disease.
- Transmission generally via ingestion of contaminated food or drink.
- Outbreaks of gastroenteritis related to contaminated poultry, meat, and dairy products are common.
- Typhoid fever is a systemic illness caused by serotypes exclusive to humans.
  1. Acquisition by ingestion of food or water contaminated by other humans
  2. Most cases in the U.S. are:
     a. Acquired during foreign travel
     b. Acquired by ingestion of food prepared by chronic carriers, many of whom have acquired the organism outside of the U.S.

TABLE 1-440 Host Factors and Conditions Predisposing to the Development of Systemic Disease with Nontyphoidal *Salmonella* Strains

Neonates and young infants (≤3 mo of age)
HIV/AIDS
Other immunodeficiencies and chronic granulomatous disease
Immunosuppressive and corticosteroid therapies
Malignancies, especially leukemia and lymphoma
Hemolytic anemia, including sickle cell disease, malaria, and bartonellosis
Collagen vascular disease
Inflammatory bowel disease
Achlorhydria or use of antacid medications
Impaired intestinal motility
Schistosomiasis, malaria
Malnutrition

From Kliegman RM et al: *Nelson textbook of pediatrics,* ed 19, Philadelphia, 2011, Saunders.

TABLE 1-439 *Salmonella* Nomenclature

Traditional Usage	Formal Name	CDC Designation
S. typhi	*S. enterica** subsp. enterica ser. Typhi	*S.* ser. Typhi
S. dublin	*S. enterica* subsp. enterica ser. Dublin	*S.* ser. Dublin
S. typhimurium	*S. enterica* subsp. enterica ser. Typhimurium	*S.* ser. Typhimurium
S. choleraesuis	*S. enterica* subsp. enterica ser. Choleraesuis	*S.* ser. Choleraesuis
S. marina	*S. enterica* subsp. houtenae ser. Marina	*S.* ser. Marina

CDC, Centers for Disease Control and Prevention; *ser.,* serovar; *subsp.,* subspecies.
*Some authorities prefer *S. choleraesuis* or *S. enteritidis* rather than *S. enterica* to describe the species.
From Kliegman RM et al: *Nelson textbook of pediatrics,* ed 19, Philadelphia, 2011, Saunders.

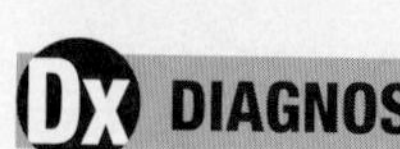

DIAGNOSIS

DIFFERENTIAL DIAGNOSIS

- Other causes of prolonged fever:
  1. Malaria
  2. TB
  3. Brucellosis
  4. Amebic liver abscess
- Other causes of gastroenteritis:
  1. Bacterial: *Shigella, Yersinia, Campylobacter* spp.
  2. Viral: Norwalk virus, rotavirus
  3. Parasitic: *Entamoeba histolytica, Giardia lamblia*
  4. Toxic: enterotoxigenic *E. coli, Clostridium difficile*

WORKUP

- Typhoid fever
  1. Cultures of blood, stool, urine; repeat if initially negative.
  2. Blood cultures are more likely to be positive early in the course of illness.
  3. Stool and urine cultures are more commonly positive in the second and third wk of illness.
  4. Highest yield with bone marrow biopsy cultures: 90% positive.
  5. Serology using Widal's test is helpful in retrospect, showing a fourfold increase in convalescent titers.
- Gastroenteritis: stool cultures
- Extraintestinal localized infection:
  1. Blood cultures
  2. Cultures from the site of infection

LABORATORY TESTS

- Neutropenia is common
- Transaminitis is possible
- Culture to grow organism: blood, body fluids, biopsy specimens

IMAGING STUDIES

- Not routinely indicated
- Radiographs of bone may be suggestive of osteomyelitis (particularly in patients with sickle cell disease and bone infarctions).
- CT scan or sonogram of abdomen:
  1. May reveal hepatic or splenic abscesses or pleural involvement
  2. May reveal aortic aneurysm

TREATMENT

NONPHARMACOLOGIC THERAPY

Adequate hydration and electrolyte replacement in people with diarrhea

ACUTE GENERAL Rx

- Typhoid fever:
  1. Ciprofloxacin 500 mg PO bid or 400 mg IV bid *or* levofloxacin 750 mg PO/IV q24h for 7-10 days. Should not be used as first line in patients from South Asia due to resistance unless known to be susceptible.
  2. Ceftriaxone 2 g IV qd for 7-14 days or cefixime (20-30 mg/kg/day orally divided into q12h dosing for 7-14 days)
  3. Another alternative agent: azithromycin (1 g orally then 500 mg daily for 5-7 days)
  4. Children: see Table 1-441. In general, quinolones are avoided in children unless a multidrug-resistant strain is involved due to concerns of possible cartilage damage. Another alternative for children: azithromycin (10-20 mg/kg to 1 g maximum once daily for 5-7 days)
  5. If tests show susceptibility, can also use amoxicillin or Bactrim in adults and children
  6. Dexamethasone 3 mg IV initially, followed by 1 mg IV q6h for eight doses for patients with shock or mental status changes
- Gastroenteritis:
  1. Usually not indicated for gastroenteritis alone because this illness usually self-limited
  2. Treatment may prolong the carrier state and is discouraged for healthy patients <50 yr of age who have relatively mild disease.
  3. Prophylactic treatment for patients who are at high risk of developing complications from bacteremia (see Table 1-441)
     a. Neonates
     b. Patients with hemoglobinopathies
     c. Patients with atherosclerosis
     d. Patients with aneurysms
     e. Patients with prosthetic devices
     f. Immunocompromised patients

TABLE 1-441 Treatment of *Salmonella* Gastroenteritis

Organism and Indication	Dose and Duration of Treatment
Salmonella infections in infants <3 mo of age or immunocompromised persons (in addition to appropriate treatment for underlying disorder)	Cefotaxime 100-200 mg/kg/day every 6 hr for 5-14 days *or* Ceftriaxone 75 mg/kg/day once daily for 7 days *or* Ampicillin 100 mg/kg/day every 6 hr for 7 days *or* Cefixime 15 mg/kg/day for 7-10 days

From Kliegman RM et al: *Nelson textbook of pediatrics,* ed 19, Philadelphia, 2011, Saunders.

CHRONIC Rx

- Carrier states are possible in those with typhoid fever.
- More common in people >60 yr of age and in people with gallstones.
- Usual site of colonization is the gallbladder.
- Treatment should be considered for those with persistently positive stool cultures and for food handlers.
- Suggested regimens for eradication of carrier state:
  1. Ciprofloxacin 500 mg PO bid for 4 wk
  2. SMX/TMP 1 to 2 DS tabs PO bid for 6 wk (if susceptible)
  3. Amoxicillin 2 g PO q8h for 6 wk (if susceptible)
- Cholecystectomy may be required in carriers with gallstones who fail medical therapy, but this is rarely indicated for nontyphoidal salmonellosis currently.
- Prolonged course of oral therapy or lifetime suppression for patients with AIDS who have chronic infection.

DISPOSITION

- Typhoid fever
  1. Treated patients usually respond to therapy; small percentage of chronic carriers.
  2. Untreated patients may have serious complications.
- Gastroenteritis
  1. Usually self-limited
  2. May be recurrent or persistent in AIDS patients

REFERRAL

- If gastroenteritis is persistent or recurrent
- If there is evidence of extraintestinal infection, typhoid fever, or chronic carriers

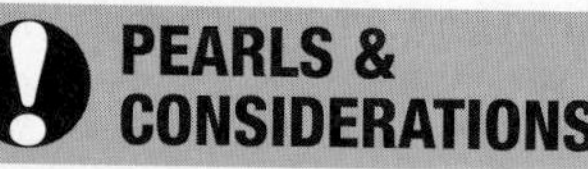

PEARLS & CONSIDERATIONS

COMMENTS

- Quinolones should not be used in children or pregnant women.
- Infections should be reported to local health departments.
- Recent outbreaks in the U.S. have been traced back to raw tomatoes, peanut butter, pet turtles, and frozen pot pies.

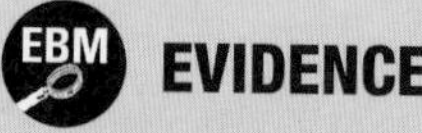

EVIDENCE

available at www.expertconsult.com

SUGGESTED READINGS

available at www.expertconsult.com

RELATED CONTENT

Salmonellosis (Patient Information)

AUTHOR: **GLENN G. FORT, M.D., M.P.H.**

BASIC INFORMATION

DEFINITION

Sarcoidosis is a chronic multisystem granulomatous disease characterized histologically by the presence of nonspecific, noncaseating granulomas.

SYNONYMS Boeck's sarcoid

ICD-9CM CODES
135.0 Sarcoidosis
ICD-10CM CODES
D86 Sarcoidosis
D86.0 Sarcoidosis of lung
D86.1 Sarcoidosis of lymph nodes
D86.2 Sarcoidosis of lung with sarcoidosis of lymph nodes
D86.3 Sarcoidosis of skin
D86.8 Sarcoidosis of other and combined sites
D86.9 Sarcoidosis, unspecified

EPIDEMIOLOGY & DEMOGRAPHICS

INCIDENCE (IN U.S.): 11 in 100,000 whites and 35 in 100,000 blacks; presents most commonly in the winter and early spring

PREDOMINANT SEX: Increased incidence in females

PREDOMINANT AGE: 20 to 40 yr

GENETICS: Familial clustering has been described. Having a first-degree relative with sarcoidosis increases the risk for disease fivefold.

PHYSICAL FINDINGS & CLINICAL PRESENTATION

- Clinical manifestations often vary with the stage of the disease and degree of organ involvement. Patients may be asymptomatic, but a chest radiograph may demonstrate findings consistent with sarcoidosis (see "Imaging Studies"). Nearly 50% of patients with sarcoidosis are diagnosed by incidental findings on chest radiograph. Thoracic involvement occurs in >90% of patients with sarcoidosis.
- Frequent manifestations:
  1. Pulmonary manifestations: dry, nonproductive cough; dyspnea; chest discomfort
  2. Constitutional symptoms: fatigue, weight loss, anorexia, malaise
  3. Visual disturbances: blurred vision, ocular discomfort, conjunctivitis, iritis, uveitis (65% of patients)
  4. Dermatologic manifestations (30% of patients): erythema nodosum (10% of patients), macules, papules, subcutaneous nodules, hyperpigmentation, lupus pernio (indurated violaceous lesions on the nose, lips, ears, and cheeks that can erode into underlying cartilage and bone) (Fig. E1-826)
  5. Myocardial disturbances, arrhythmias, cardiomyopathy. Cardiac sarcoidosis is much more common than clinically appreciated and is found in up to 25% of patients in the United States
  6. Splenomegaly, hepatomegaly
  7. Rheumatologic manifestations: arthralgias have been reported in up to 40% of patients
  8. Neurologic and other manifestations: cranial nerve palsies, diabetes insipidus, meningeal involvement, parotid enlargement, hypothalamic and pituitary lesions, peripheral adenopathy. Neurosarcoidosis is detected in up to 25% of patients and can occur in the absence of apparent disease elsewhere

ETIOLOGY Unknown. A cardinal feature of sarcoidosis is the presence of CD4+ T cells that interact with antigen-presenting cells to initiate the formation and maintenance of granulomas. Multiple lines of evidence suggest that sarcoidosis may result from the interaction of multiple genes with environmental exposures or infection.

Dx DIAGNOSIS

DIFFERENTIAL DIAGNOSIS

- Tuberculosis
- Lymphoma
- Hodgkin's disease
- Metastases
- Pneumoconioses
- Enlarged pulmonary arteries
- Infectious mononucleosis
- Lymphangitic carcinomatosis
- Idiopathic hemosiderosis
- Alveolar cell carcinoma
- Pulmonary eosinophilia
- Hypersensitivity pneumonitis
- Fibrosing alveolitis
- Collagen disorders
- Parasitic infection

Section II describes the differential diagnosis of granulomatous lung disease and a classification of granulomatous disorders.

WORKUP

- No pathognomonic diagnostic test exists for sarcoidosis, so the diagnosis remains one of exclusion. Workup is aimed at excluding critical organ involvement, determining extent and severity of disease, and excluding other disease. The presence of noncaseating granulomas does not establish the diagnosis, because conditions such as tuberculosis and malignancies, among others, can cause granulomas. A complete neurologic and ophthalmologic examination is mandatory. A complete occupational and environmental exposure history is recommended.
- Initial laboratory evaluation should include complete blood count, serum chemistries (alanine aminotransferase, aspartate aminotransferase, alkaline phosphatase, electrolytes, blood urea nitrogen, creatinine, serum calcium), urinalysis, 24-hour urinary excretion of calcium, CRP, ESR, and tuberculin skin test.
- Chest radiograph and ECG should also be obtained in all patients with sarcoidosis.
- Pulmonary function testing: spirometry, diffusion capacity of carbon monoxide–single breath.
- Biopsy should be done on accessible tissues suspected of sarcoid involvement (conjunctiva, skin, lymph nodes); bronchoscopy with transbronchial biopsy (85% diagnostic yield) is often performed in patients without any readily accessible site. Endobronchial ultrasound-guided fine-needle aspiration of intrathoracic lymph nodes also has high diagnostic yield and makes use of mediastinoscopy mostly unnecessary. Among patients with suspected Stage I/II pulmonary sarcoidosis undergoing tissue confirmation, the use of endosonographic nodal aspiration compared with bronchoscopic biopsy resulted in greater diagnostic yield.[1]

LABORATORY TESTS

Laboratory abnormalities:

- Hypergammaglobulinemia, anemia, leukopenia may be present
- Liver function test abnormalities are common
- Hypercalcemia (11% of patients), hypercalciuria (40% of patients; attributable to increased gastrointestinal absorption, abnormal vitamin D metabolism, and increased calcitriol production by sarcoid granuloma)
- Angiotensin-converting enzyme: elevated in approximately 60% of patients with sarcoidosis; nonspecific and generally not useful as a diagnostic tool and in following the course of the disease

IMAGING STUDIES

- Chest radiograph (Fig. 1-827): adenopathy of the hilar and paratracheal nodes is a frequent finding. Parenchymal changes may also be present, depending on the stage of the disease (stage 0, normal radiograph; stage I, bilateral hilar adenopathy; stage II, stage I plus pulmonary infiltrate; stage III, pulmonary infiltrate without adenopathy; stage IV, advanced fibrosis with evidence of "honeycombing," hilar retraction, bullae, cysts, and emphysema).
- Pulmonary function tests (spirometry and diffusing capacity of the lung for carbon dioxide): may be normal or may reveal a restrictive ventilatory defect with reduced forced vital capacity, reduced DLCO, or both.
- For patients without apparent lung involvement, ^{18}F-fluorodeoxyglucose positron emission tomography (FDG-PET) is useful in identifying sites for diagnostic biopsy.
- CT imaging is generally unnecessary for most patients with sarcoidosis. It is indicated when the chest radiograph is atypical for sarcoidosis or if the patient has hemoptysis.
- FDG-PET and MRI with gadolinium are useful in patients with suspected cardiac and neurologic involvement.
- Gallium-67 scan: represents an older testing modality. It will localize in areas of granulomatous infiltrates; however, it is not specific and not necessary. The "panda" sign (localization in the lacrimal and salivary glands, giving a "panda" appearance to the face) is suggestive of sarcoidosis.

---

[1]Von Bartheld MB et al: Endoscopy vs conventional bronchoscopy for the diagnosis of sarcoidosis, *JAMA* 309(23):2457-2464, 2013.

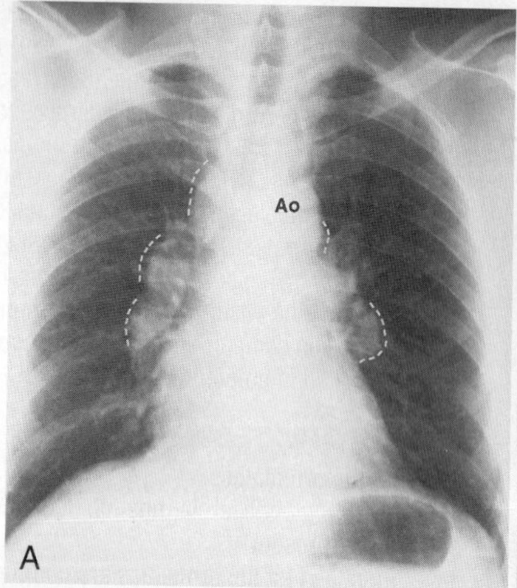

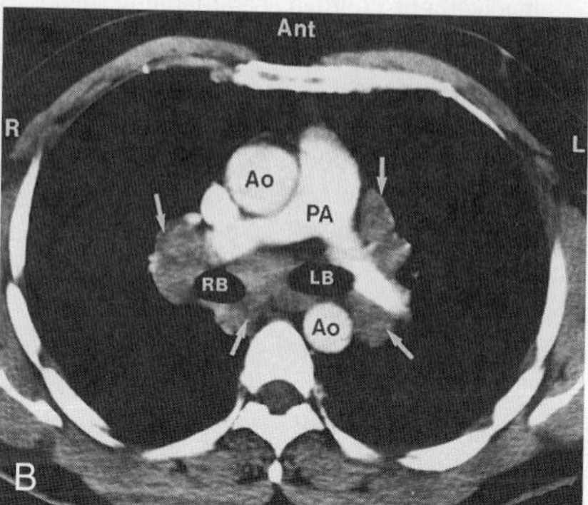

FIGURE 1-827 Sarcoid. Marked lymphadenopathy *(dotted lines)* is seen in the region of both hila in the right paratracheal region **(A)**. The transverse contrast-enhanced CT scan of the upper chest **(B)** clearly shows the ascending and descending aorta *(Ao)* as well as the pulmonary artery *(PA)* and superior vena cava. The right and left mainstem bronchus area is also seen. The arrows indicate the extensive lymphadenopathy. *LB,* Left bronchus; *RB,* right bronchus. (From Mettler FA [ed]: *Primary care radiology,* Philadelphia, 2000, Saunders.)

TABLE 1-442 Indications for Use of Corticosteroids in Sarcoidosis

Disorder	Treatment
Iridocyclitis	Corticosteroid eye drops; local subconjunctival deposit of cortisone
Posterior uveitis	Oral prednisone
Pulmonary involvement	Steroids rarely recommended for stage I; typically used if infiltrate remains static or worsens over 3-mo period or the patient is symptomatic
Upper airway obstruction	Rare indication for intravenous steroids
Lupus pernio	Oral prednisone shrinks the disfiguring lesions
Hypercalcemia	Responds well to corticosteroids
Cardiac involvement	Corticosteroids usually recommended if patient has arrhythmias or conduction disturbances
Central nervous system involvement	Response is best in patients with acute symptoms
Lacrimal/salivary gland involvement	Corticosteroids recommended for disordered function, not gland swelling
Bone cysts	Corticosteroids recommended if symptomatic

From Andreoli TE (ed): *Cecil essentials of medicine,* ed 8, Philadelphia, 2010, Saunders.

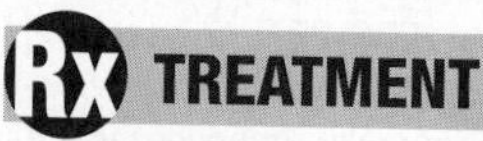

TREATMENT

GENERAL Rx

- Many patients with sarcoidosis will not require any treatment. In general, treatment should be instituted when organ function is threatened. Corticosteroids (Table 1-442) are the mainstay of therapy when treatment is required (e.g., prednisone 40 mg qd for 8 to 12 wk with gradual tapering of the dose to 10 mg qod over 8 to 12 mo); corticosteroids should be considered in patients with severe symptoms (e.g., dyspnea, chest pain); hypercalcemia; ocular, central nervous system, or cardiac involvement; or progressive pulmonary disease. Patients with interstitial lung disease benefit from oral steroid therapy for 6 to 24 mo.
- A lack of benefit from steroid therapy may be due to the presence of irreversible fibrotic disease. Patients with progressive disease refractory to corticosteroids may be treated with methotrexate 7.5 to 15 mg once per week or another immunosuppressant such as azathioprine or mycophenolate mofetil.
- Hydroxychloroquine is effective for chronic disfiguring skin lesions, hypercalcemia, and neurologic involvement.
- Nonsteroidal anti-inflammatory drugs are useful for musculoskeletal symptoms and erythema nodosum.
- Pulmonary rehabilitation in patients with significant respiratory insufficiency. Consider liver and lung transplantation in patients unresponsive to conventional treatment.

DISPOSITION

- The majority of patients with sarcoidosis have spontaneous remission within 2 yr and do not require treatment. Their course can be followed by periodic clinical evaluation, chest radiographs, and pulmonary function tests.
- Blacks have increased rates of pulmonary involvement, a worse long-term prognosis, and more frequent relapses.
- Up to one third of patients have unrelenting disease, leading to clinically significant organ impairment. Adverse prognostic factors in sarcoidosis include age of onset >40 yr, cardiac involvement, neurosarcoidosis, progressive pulmonary fibrosis, chronic hypercalcemia, chronic uveitis, involvement of nasal mucosa, nephrocalcinosis, and presence of cystic bone lesions and lupus pernio.

REFERRAL Ophthalmologic examination is indicated in all patients with suspected sarcoidosis because ocular findings (iridocyclitis, uveitis, conjunctivitis, and keratopathy) are found in ≥25% of documented cases.

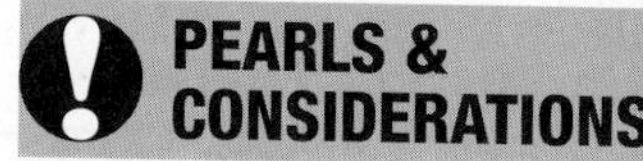

PEARLS & CONSIDERATIONS

COMMENTS

- Serial spirometry and measurement of DLCO can be useful in following response to therapy and disease progression.
- Approximately 15% to 20% of patients with lung involvement advance to irreversible lung impairment (bronchiectasis, cavitation, progressive fibrosis, pneumothorax, and respiratory failure). Death from pulmonary failure occurs in 5% to 7% of patients with sarcoidosis.
- Newer treatment approaches are aimed at targeting mechanisms involving CD4 type 1 helper T cells.
- The diagnosis of sarcoidosis should be reconsidered in the presence of atypical manifestations or persistent/progressive disease despite appropriate therapy.

SUGGESTED READINGS

available at www.expertconsult.com

RELATED CONTENT

Sarcoidosis (Patient Information)

AUTHOR: **FRED F. FERRI, M.D.**

BASIC INFORMATION

DEFINITION

Sarcomas are heterogenous groups of malignant tumors of connective tissue. They show a wide range of differentiation—blood vessels (angiosarcoma), fat tissue (liposarcoma), bone (osteosarcoma). Sarcomas occur in soft tissues and bones, but are more common in soft tissues. They affect virtually all tissues, but 75% occur in the limbs. Sarcomas of bone are extremely rare. There are three histiogenic types: osteosarcoma, Ewing's sarcoma, and chondrosarcoma.

ICD-9CM CODES

171.0 Malignant neoplasm of connective and other soft tissue of head, face, and neck (depends on type)

ICD-10CM CODES

C40 Malignant neoplasm of bone and articular cartilage of limbs

C41 Malignant neoplasm of bone and articular cartilage of other unspecified sites

C22.3 Angiosarcoma of liver

C49.9 Malignant neoplasm of connective and soft tissue, unspecified

C49.0 Malignant neoplasm of connective and soft tissue of head, face, and neck

EPIDEMIOLOGY & DEMOGRAPHICS

INCIDENCE:

Soft tissue sarcoma: 30 cases per million per annum.

Sarcoma of bone: 8 cases per million per annum.

Soft tissue sarcoma can occur at any age.
- In the United States there are 7800 new cases per year.
- Incidence increases with age.
- Average age of diagnosis is 57 yr.
- Men and women are affected equally.
- Soft tissue sarcomas represent <1% of all newly diagnosed malignancies.

Sarcomas of bone represent 0.2% of all new cancers.
- About 2600 new cases in the United States each year.
- Osteosarcoma and Ewing's sarcoma (the two most common bone tumors) occur predominantly during childhood and adolescence.

GENETICS: See "Etiology."

PHYSICAL FINDINGS & CLINICAL PRESENTATION

- Bone sarcomas. Clinical presentation usually includes:
  - Pain—at rest or at night
  - Swelling or mass at the site
  - Pathologic fractures
- Soft tissue sarcomas:
  Present with painless mass (usually >5 cm). Mass grows slowly for months or years.

ETIOLOGY

- Most sarcomas arise sporadically.
- Genetic predispositions:
  1. Familial retinoblastoma (mutation of the *RBI* gene at 13q14) predisposes to osteosarcoma.
  2. Neurofibromatosis type 1 (mutation of *NF1* gene at 17q11) predisposes to malignant peripheral nerve sheath tumor.
  3. Diaphyseal aclasis (an autosomal inherited condition) is associated with increased risk of peripheral chondrosarcoma.
- Environmental causes:
  1. Previous radiotherapy (e.g., for cervical or breast cancer): predisposes to sarcoma 4 yr or so later.
  2. Chronic lymphedema: associated with the development of angiosarcoma.
  3. Exposure to chemicals (e.g., dioxins, phenoxyacetic herbicides, vinyl choride).
  4. Viruses (e.g., human herpesvirus 8 causes Kaposi's sarcoma).
  5. Foreign body (shrapnel, medical implants)

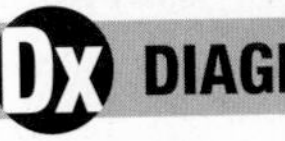

DIAGNOSIS

WORKUP

- Soft tissue sarcoma: any unexplained superficial soft tissue mass >5 cm or deep-seated, soft tissue mass should be regarded as malignant until proven otherwise.
- Bone sarcoma: patients with unexplained bone pain, persistent bone tenderness, or nonmechanical bone pain (especially when it disturbs sleep or rest) have bone cancer until proven otherwise.
- Patients with suspected spontaneous fracture or recurrence of the fracture with minor trauma should be considered as having bone cancer.
- Referral to a sarcoma treatment center of all patients with a suspected sarcoma is recommended.

IMAGING STUDIES

- A chest spiral CT scan is compulsory for staging purposes. Chest spiral CT helps detect lung metastasis, since metastasis through blood to the lungs is the principal form of spread.
- Staging aids in estimating prognosis, survival, and plan management.
- The American Joint Committee on Cancer (AJCC) and International Union Against Cancer (IUCC) are widely used for staging classification.

Soft tissue sarcoma
- Magnetic resonance imaging (MRI) is the initial imaging modality of choice, especially for soft tissue sarcoma of the extremities, trunk, and head and neck. CT with IV contrast is also useful for diagnosis.
- Ultrasound is used to help differentiate between benign and suspicious lesions.

Bone sarcoma
- Radiograph (Fig. 1-828) is the initial imaging of choice. It helps to rule out bone tumor, shows calcification, and reveals bone erosions.
- A multidisciplinary approach is essential. The team should include radiologist, surgeons, pathologist, medical oncologist, and radiation therapists.

BIOPSY

- In nearly all cases a biopsy is needed to establish a tissue diagnosis.
- Multiple core needle biopsies are usually done.
- An excisional biopsy may be used for superficial lesions <5 cm.
- In carefully selected cases an open biopsy may be done (rarely used because of its high complication rate).
- For difficult to palpate or necrotic soft sarcomas, ultrasound or computed tomography (CT)–guided biopsies are performed.
- Biopsy results are interpreted collaboratively by the specialist sarcoma pathologist, surgeon, and radiologist together.

HISTOLOGIC DIAGNOSIS

- Treatment planning is guided by a histologic diagnosis.
- Histologic diagnosis is made according to the World Health Organization (WHO) classification.
- WHO has defined more than 50 histologic subtypes of soft tissue sarcoma.
- Newer methods such as immunocytochemistry and cytogenetics can aid diagnosis. They identify tumor lineage.

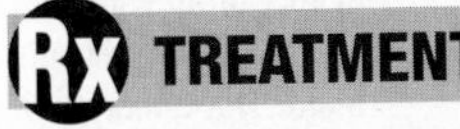

TREATMENT

Treatment depends on the extent of the disease and falls into several groups.

ACUTE GENERAL Rx

- Tumors treated by surgery: for example, in most adults soft tissue sarcoma and sarcoma of bone are not sensitive to chemotherapy.
  1. Surgery must be done by surgeon trained to treat this disease.
  2. Wide excision with negative margins is the standard surgical procedure.
  3. For bone sarcomas amputation has been the standard procedure. Recent advances permit the avoidance of amputation with limb-sparing surgery followed by reconstruction by endoprosthetic replacement.
- Chemotherapy followed by local therapy: for example, osteosarcoma.
  1. Early chemotherapy to reduce disseminated micrometastasis and tumor size.
- Follow-up of bone sarcoma after treatment includes:
  - Periodic monitoring with radiographs and other imaging modalities
  - CT scan of the chest
  - Bone scan
- Follow-up of soft tissue sarcoma (extremities):
  - Physical exam detects 97% of recurrence.
  - Physical exam is done every 3-6 mo for 3 yr, then every 6 mo for the next 2 yr for stage II and III cancers, then annually.

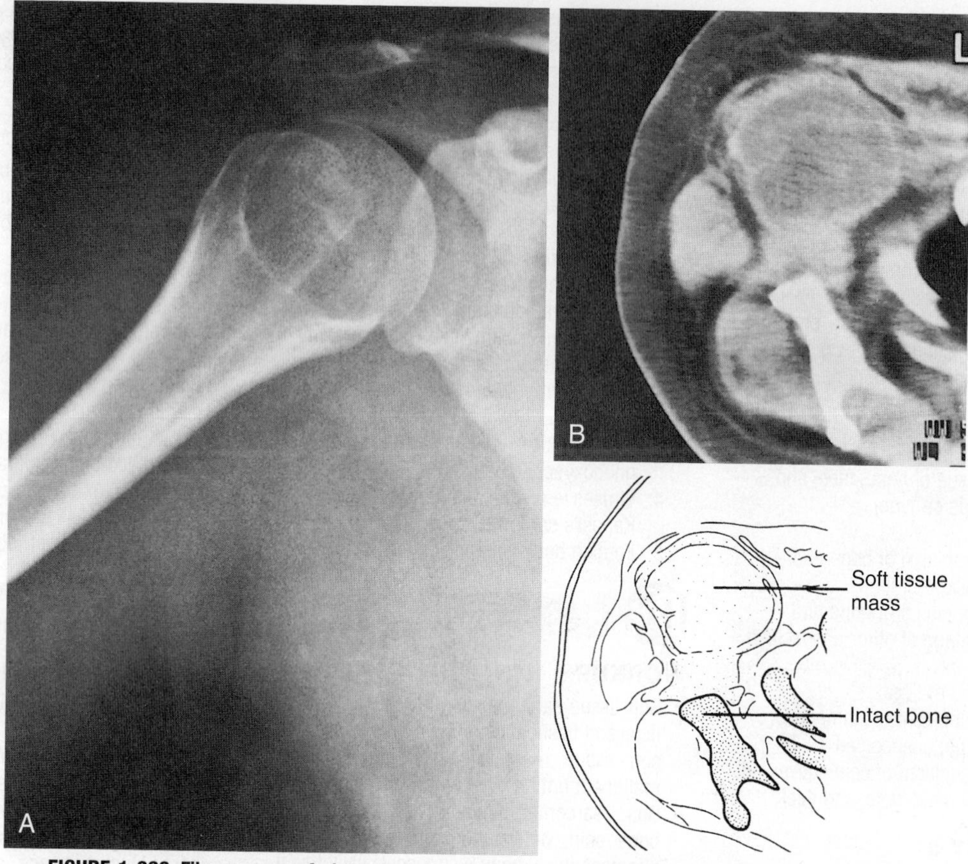

FIGURE 1-828 Fibrosarcoma. A, Anteroposterior plain film of the shoulder of a 40-year-old woman with a history of an enlarging mass in the right axilla shows an ill-defined mass adjacent to the lateral border of the scapula. **B,** CT section with contrast enhancement shows the extent of the mass and the lack of bone involvement. The tumor proved to be a fibrosarcoma. (From Skarin AT: *Atlas of diagnostic oncology,* ed 3, St Louis, 2003, Mosby.)

- Imaging
  - Stage I: CXR every 6-12 mo
  - Stages II and III: image the primary site with MRI or CT
  - Chest x-ray or chest CT every 3-6 mo for 5 yr, then annually

REFERRAL

- Because sarcomas are relatively uncommon yet comprise a wide variety of different entities, evaluation by oncology teams who have expertise in the field is recommended.
- Treatment and follow-up guidelines have been published by the National Comprehensive Cancer Network (www.nccn.org).

SUGGESTED READINGS

available at www.expertconsult.com

AUTHOR: **DANIEL K. ASIEDU, M.D., PH.D., F.A.C.P.**

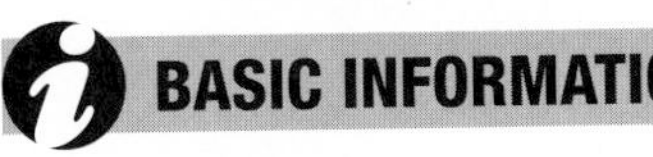

BASIC INFORMATION

DEFINITION

Scabies is a contagious disease caused by the mite *Sarcoptes scabiei.*

ICD-9CM CODES
133.0 Scabies
ICD-10CM CODES
B86 Scabies

EPIDEMIOLOGY & DEMOGRAPHICS

- Scabies is generally acquired by sleeping with or in the bedding of infested individuals.
- It is generally associated with poor living conditions and is also common in hospitals and nursing homes.

PHYSICAL FINDINGS & CLINICAL PRESENTATION

- Primary lesions are caused when the female mite burrows within the stratum corneum, laying eggs within the tract she leaves behind; burrows (linear or serpiginous tracts, see Fig. 1-829) end with a minute papule or vesicle.
- Primary lesions are most commonly found in the web spaces of the hands, wrists, buttocks, scrotum, penis, breasts, axillae, and knees. They are often confused with eczema (Fig. 1-830).
- Secondary lesions result from scratching or infection.
- Intense pruritus, especially nocturnal, is common; it is caused by an acquired sensitivity to the mite or fecal pellets and is usually noted 1 to 4 wk after the primary infestation.
- Examination of the skin may reveal burrows, tiny vesicles, excoriations, inflammatory papules.
- Widespread and crusted lesions (Norwegian or crusted scabies) may be seen in elderly and immunocompromised patients.

ETIOLOGY

Human scabies is caused by the mite *S. scabiei,* var. *hominis* (Fig. 1-831). After impregnation on the skin surface, the gravid female burrows in the stratum corneum within 30 min and gradually extends the tract along the boundary with the stratum granulosum depositing 10 to 25 oval eggs in a 4- to 5-wk period. The eggs hatch in 3 to 5 days, and larvae move to the skin surface and mature in 2 to 3 wk, resuming the cycle.

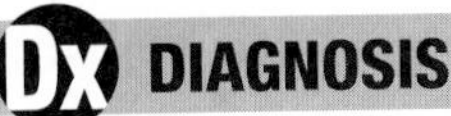

DIAGNOSIS

DIFFERENTIAL DIAGNOSIS

- Pediculosis
- Atopic dermatitis
- Flea bites
- Seborrheic dermatitis
- Dermatitis herpetiformis
- Contact dermatitis
- Nummular eczema
- Syphilis
- Other insect infestation

WORKUP

Diagnosis is made on the clinical presentation and on the demonstration of mites, eggs, or mite feces.

LABORATORY TESTS

- Microscopic demonstration of the organism, feces, or eggs: a drop of mineral oil may be placed over the suspected lesion before removal; the scrapings are transferred directly to a glass slide; a drop of potassium hydroxide is added and a cover slip is applied.
- Skin biopsy is rarely necessary to make the diagnosis.

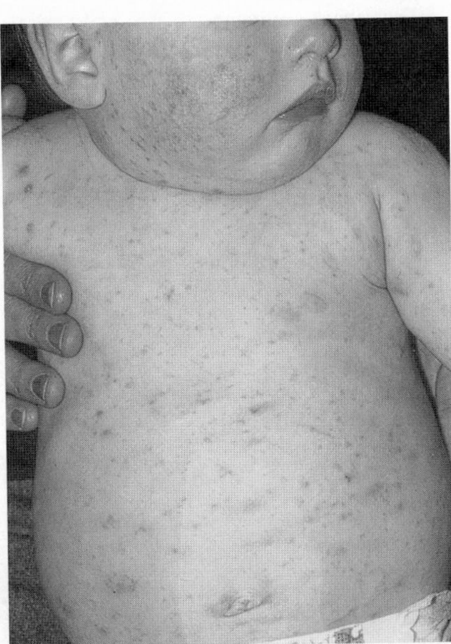

FIGURE 1-830 Scabies in an infant. Diffuse pruritic, eczematous lesions on an infant are often confused with eczema. (From White GM, Cox NH [eds]: *Diseases of the skin: a color atlas and text,* ed 2, St Louis, 2006, Mosby.)

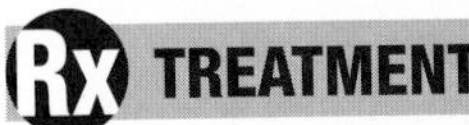

TREATMENT

NONPHARMACOLOGIC THERAPY

Clothing, underwear, and towels used in the 48 hr before treatment must be laundered.

ACUTE GENERAL Rx

- Permethrin 5% cream (Elimite) is usually effective with one treatment; it should be massaged into the skin from head to soles of feet and applied under fingernails and toenails; remove 8 to 14 hr later by washing. Repeat in 1 to 2 wk. Permethrin is safe for children >2 mo old.
- A single dose (150 to 200 micrograms/kg in 6-mg tablets) of ivermectin, an antihelmintic agent, is also effective for the treatment of scabies. It is the best treatment for generalized crusted scabies.
- Pruritus generally abates 24 to 48 hr after treatment but can last up to 2 wk; oral antihistamines are effective in decreasing postscabietic pruritus.
- Topical corticosteroid creams may hasten the resolution of secondary eczematous dermatitis.
- If the patient is a resident of an extended care facility, it is important to educate the patients, staff, family, and frequent visitors about scabies and the need to have full cooperation in treatment. Scabicide should be applied to all patients, staff, and frequent visitors, whether symptomatic or not; symptomatic family members of staff and visitors should also receive treatment.

DISPOSITION

Refractory cases usually are seen with immunocompromised hosts or patients with underlying skin diseases. ***Norwegian scabies*** refers to a highly contagious variant often found in institutions caring for physically and mentally disabled individuals.

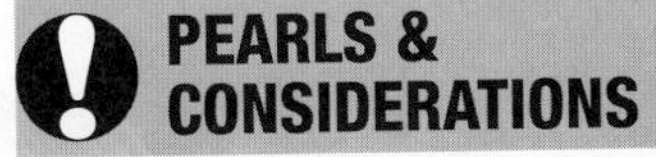

PEARLS & CONSIDERATIONS

COMMENTS

- Lindane is potentially neurotoxic and should not be used on infants or pregnant women (permethrin is safe and effective in these situations).
- Sexual partners should be notified and treated.

SUGGESTED READINGS

available at www.expertconsult.com

RELATED CONTENT

Scabies (Patient Information)

AUTHOR: **FRED F. FERRI, M.D.**

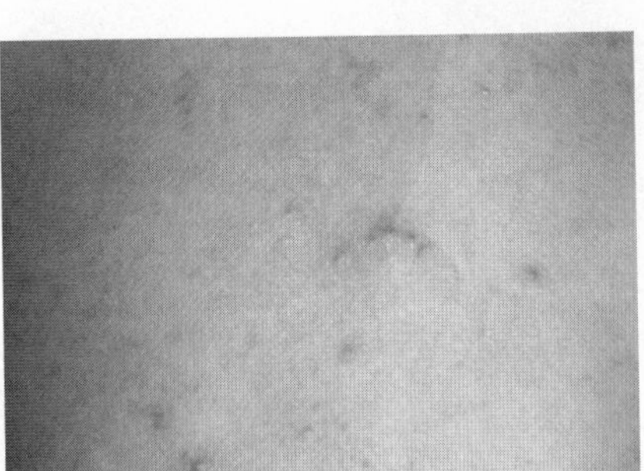

FIGURE 1-829 Classic scabies burrow. (From Kliegman RM et al: *Nelson textbook of pediatrics,* ed 19, Philadelphia, 2011, Saunders.)

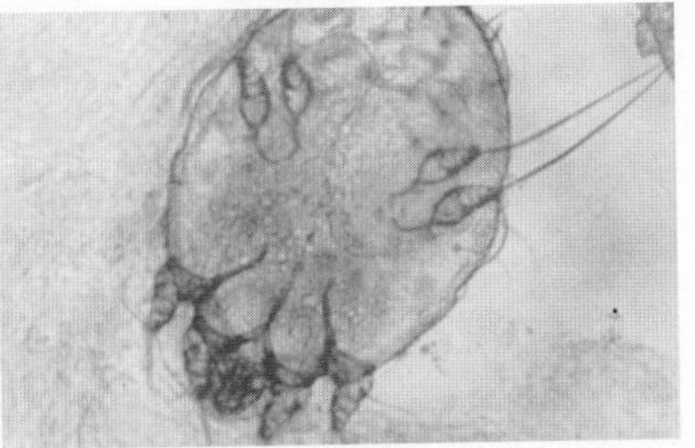

FIGURE 1-831 Scabies organism in a wet mount preparation. (From Mandell GL: *Mandell, Douglas, and Bennett's principles and practice of infectious diseases,* ed 5, New York, 2000, Churchill Livingstone.)

BASIC INFORMATION

DEFINITION

Scarlet fever is a rash involving the skin and tongue and complicating streptococcal group A pharyngitis.

SYNONYMS

Scarlatina
SF

ICD-9CM CODES
034.1 Scarlet fever
ICD-10CM CODES
A38 Scarlet fever
A38.9 Scarlet fever, uncomplicated

EPIDEMIOLOGY & DEMOGRAPHICS

- Same as streptococcal pharyngitis; namely, children ages 5 to 15 yr. May also complicate impetigo.
- Most common in cooler climates during the late fall, winter, and early spring.
- Most cases follow tonsillitis or pharyngitis; however, it has also been reported after wounds ("surgical scarlet fever"), burns, and pelvic or puerperal infections.

PHYSICAL FINDINGS & CLINICAL PRESENTATION

- Diffuse erythema, beginning on face and spreading to neck, back, chest, rest of trunk, and extremities (Fig. 1-832, *A*). Most intense on inner aspects of arms and thighs.
- Erythema blanches, but nonblanching petechiae may be present or produced by a tourniquet.
- Strawberry or raspberry tongue (Fig. 1-832 *B, C*).
- Rash lasts approximately 1 wk and then desquamates.
- Febrile illness with headache, malaise, anorexia, and pharyngitis begins after a 2- to 4-day incubation period.
- Scarlatinal rash begins 1 or 2 days after the onset of pharyngitis.

ETIOLOGY

Caused by group A beta-hemolytic *Streptococcus* infection, which produces one of three erythrogenic toxins (NOTE: *Some streptococcal species have the ability to cause both scarlet fever and rheumatic fever*).

Dx DIAGNOSIS

DIFFERENTIAL DIAGNOSIS

- Viral exanthems (covered in Section II)
- Kawasaki disease
- Toxic shock syndrome
- Drug rashes

See differential diagnosis of "Pharyngitis" in Section I.

WORKUP

- Identification of group A *Streptococcus* by throat culture
- Streptolysin O antibody titers

Rx TREATMENT

- Penicillin 250 mg PO qid for 10 days or erythromycin 250 mg PO qid for 10 days in penicillin-allergic patients. A clinical response can be expected in 24 to 48 hr.
- Benzathine penicillin 1 to 2 million U IM once; may be used for a patient who cannot swallow pills.

COMPLICATIONS (RARE)

- Peritonsillar abscess
- Mastoiditis
- Otitis media
- Pneumonia
- Sepsis and distant foci of infection
- Acute rheumatic fever
- Inability to swallow liquids or upper airway obstruction requiring hospitalization

NOTE: Failure to respond to penicillin should raise doubt about the diagnosis because *Streptococcus* may be carried in the pharynx without causing infection.

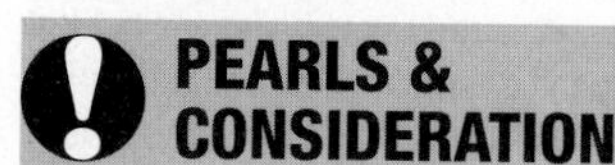

PEARLS & CONSIDERATIONS

COMMENTS

Patients with antibodies against the toxin are spared the rash but still develop other symptoms of the infection (e.g., sore throat).

RELATED CONTENT

Scarlet Fever (Patient Information)

AUTHOR: **FRED F. FERRI, M.D.**

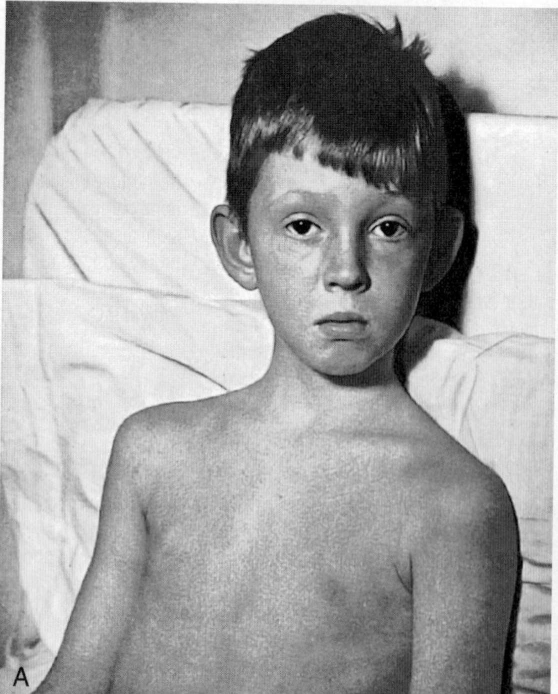

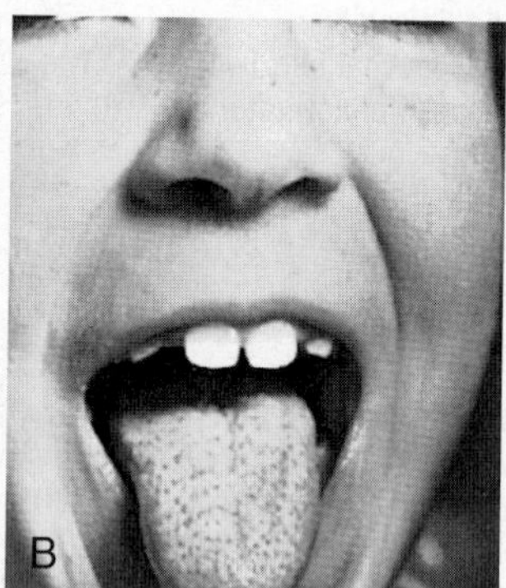

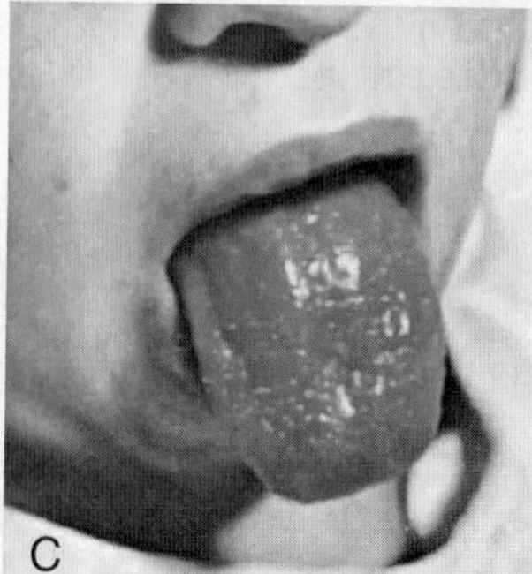

FIGURE 1-832 Scarlet fever. A, Punctate, erythematous rash (2nd day). **B,** White strawberry tongue (1st day). **C,** Red, strawberry tongue (3rd day). (Courtesy Dr. Franklin H. Top, Professor and Head of the Department of Hygiene and Preventive Medicine, State University of Iowa, College of Medicine, Iowa City, IA; and Parke, Davis & Company's Therapeutic Notes. From Gershon AA et al: *Krugman's infectious diseases of children*, ed 11, Philadelphia, 2004, Mosby.)

BASIC INFORMATION

DEFINITION

Schizophrenia is a disorder that causes significant distortions in thinking, perception, speech, and behavior. Characteristics include psychosis, apathy, social withdrawal, and cognitive impairment, which result in significant social impairment.

SYNONYMS

Dementia praecox

ICD-9CM and DSM-5 CODES
295.90
ICD-10CM CODES
F20 Schizophrenia
F20.0 Paranoid schizophrenia
F20.1 Hebephrenic schizophrenia
F20.2 Catatonic schizophrenia
F20.3 Undifferentiated schizophrenia
F20.5 Residual schizophrenia
F20.6 Simple schizophrenia
F20.8 Other schizophrenia
F20.9 Schizophrenia, unspecified

EPIDEMIOLOGY & DEMOGRAPHICS

INCIDENCE: 0.2 per 1000
PREVALENCE: 0.5%; lifetime prevalence risk, 0.4%
PREDOMINANT SEX: Males have a more severe illness with earlier onset. Prevalence in males approximately 1.4 times higher.
PREDOMINANT AGE:
- Age of onset of psychotic symptoms is the early 20s for males and the late 20s for females.
- Age of onset of negative symptoms is usually earlier (i.e., the mid-teenage years).

PEAK INCIDENCE: Between ages of 16 and 30 yr
GENETICS:
- Genetics accounts for 70% of risk; the remaining 30% associated with other factors such as urban environments, migration, or cannabis use.
- First-degree relatives have a 10 times greater chance of becoming schizophrenic.
- Discordant rates among identical twins are higher than expected with the simple inheritance pattern.
- Associations with several chromosomes have been described, but none has been replicated.
- Evidence exists that triplet nucleotide repeat expansion (e.g., such as that seen with Huntington's disease) may play a role in the inheritance of the disease.

PHYSICAL FINDINGS & CLINICAL PRESENTATION

- Schizophrenia is best defined as a dementing illness that begins early in life and that progresses slowly throughout the lifetime.
- Frequent structural brain imaging findings include the enlargement of the ventricular system, a loss of brain volume and cortical gray matter, and an alteration of the white matter tracts.
- The initial "negative" symptoms of adolescence (prodromal phase)—cognitive decline, social withdrawal and awkwardness, loss of motivation and pleasure, and loss of emotional expressiveness—begin after a period of normal development.
- During early adulthood, positive symptoms of psychosis and thought disturbance occur; psychotic symptoms then wax and wane throughout life. Treatment ameliorates positive symptoms but generally does little for negative ones.
- The condition is also accompanied by cognitive impairment, including problems with attention and concentration, psychomotor speed, learning, memory, and executive functions (e.g., abstract thinking, problem solving, planning).
- Social and occupational dysfunction can be profound.

ETIOLOGY

- The basic determination of whether this is a degenerative or developmental condition has not been made.
- The major hypothesis is that abnormality of the mesocortical pathways produces the hypofrontality and the negative symptoms. This occurs along with a compensatory hyperactivation of the mesolimbic pathways, which produces the positive symptoms of psychosis.

Dx DIAGNOSIS

DIFFERENTIAL DIAGNOSIS

- Schizophrenia is diagnosed when an individual has experienced at least 6 mo (1 mo if using ICD-10 criteria) of hallucinations, delusions, thought disorders, catatonia, or negative symptoms (e.g., avolition, anhedonia, social isolation, affective flattening).
- Any medical condition, medicine, or substance that can affect brain homeostasis can cause psychosis; this is distinguished from schizophrenia by a relatively brief course and an alteration in mental status that suggests an underlying delirium.
- Other neurologic conditions that have psychosis as the initial presentation (e.g., Huntington's disease) need to be ruled out.
- Mood disorders with psychosis: these are indistinguishable from schizophrenia cross-sectionally but have a longitudinal course that includes full recovery.
- Delusional disorder involves nonbizarre delusions and lacks the thought disturbance, hallucinations, and negative symptoms of schizophrenia.
- Autism in the adult has an early age of onset and lacks significant hallucinations or delusions.

WORKUP

- History and physical examination to help determine whether the psychosis is primary or secondary
- Neurologic examination to uncover the soft neurologic signs (e.g., clumsiness, cortical thumb, loss of fine motor movements) that are common with schizophrenia

LABORATORY TESTS

- No laboratory tests are specific.
- Laboratory examinations (e.g., chemistry profile, blood count, sedimentation rate, toxicology screen, urinalysis) are geared toward excluding a primary medical condition or toxic state. Note that new common drugs of abuse may not be detectable with regular screening tests.

IMAGING STUDIES

- CT or MRI of the brain during the initial workup; repeated if the course of the illness varies from what is expected
- EEG may reveal slowing when psychosis is the result of an encephalopathy. Findings can be similar as a result of common medication use for treatment of psychosis

Rx TREATMENT

NONPHARMACOLOGIC THERAPY

- Significant social support is required by most schizophrenic patients, but available support services are grossly inadequate. Schizophrenic patients constitute nearly one third of all homeless individuals. They usually require help with basic social, occupational, and interaction skills.
- Family stress can precipitate relapse and rehospitalization. Family interventions can reduce morbidity.
- Cognitive behavioral therapy can reduce the severity of both psychotic and negative symptoms.
- Illness management training for patients can increase medication adherence and reduce symptom distress.
- Integrated treatment that includes assertive community treatment, family involvement programs, and social skills training reduces the severity of both psychotic and negative symptoms, reduces comorbid substance misuse, reduces hospital days, increases adherence to treatment, and increases satisfaction with treatment.

ACUTE GENERAL RX

- Acute psychosis is usually adequately controlled with antipsychotic agents.
- Few differences in effectiveness exist between first-generation antipsychotics (e.g., haloperidol, perphenazine, fluphenazine, chlorpromazine) and second-generation antipsychotics (e.g., risperidone, olanzapine, quetiapine, ziprasidone, aripiprazole, clozapine, lurasidone) for nonrefractory patients. First-generation antipsychotics are slightly more likely than second-generation antipsychotics to cause a parkinsonian state and eventual tardive dyskinesia (rate of tardive dyskinesia, 15% to 30%). Antiparkinsonian drugs (e.g., benztropine, amantadine) are used to ameliorate the parkinsonism. Risperidone has been shown to be superior to haloperidol for the prevention of acute psychotic relapse.
- Sedatives (i.e., benzodiazepines and, to a lesser degree, barbiturates) can be used transiently if a patient is in an agitated state.

CHRONIC RX

- Relapse prevention is a major goal of treatment. Noncompliance is common and leads to high relapse rates. Antipsychotic agents usually must be continued at the same doses that controlled psychosis. For noncompliant patients, long-acting injectable preparations given biweekly or monthly can be used.
- Most patients frequently switch among antipsychotics; there is considerable individual variability with regard to antipsychotic response and vulnerability to specific adverse effects.
- Clozapine is more effective than other agents for treatment-refractory patients. However, it requires monitoring to prevent life-threatening adverse effects. Olanzapine may also be more effective than less expensive first-generation drugs but has substantial adverse metabolic effects. Lurasidone is a newer second-generation antipsychotic that appears to be better tolerated, but longer-term studies are needed.
- Neurocognitive improvement associated with antipsychotic treatment among patients with schizophrenia is small and does not differ between first-generation and second-generation antipsychotics.
- Antiparkinsonian agents may also need to be continued for the long term.
- Tardive dyskinesia (i.e., choreoathetoid movements of the muscles of tongue and face and occasionally of other muscle groups) can occur in as many as 30% of patients with the long-term use of neuroleptics.
- The negative symptoms of schizophrenia can resemble depression. In addition, depressive disorders may occur in schizophrenic patients. Antidepressant treatment of the negative symptoms is usually not effective. However, antidepressants can improve the symptoms of a comorbid depressive episode.
- Mood stabilizers (e.g., lithium, valproate, carbamazepine) are of little use unless the patient has a comorbid impulse control disorder.
- Substance abuse is a major problem for more than a third of schizophrenic patients. More than half of these patients smoke cigarettes. Unfortunately, these individuals do poorly in traditional substance abuse treatment programs. Specialized "dual-diagnosis" programs with highly structured aftercare are required.
- Specific antipsychotic medications have been associated with weight gain (i.e., olanzapine and clozapine) and QT prolongation. Hyperlipidemia and diabetes mellitus are associated with second-generation antipsychotics, and hyperprolactinemia is associated with first-generation antipsychotics. (Risperidone, a second-generation antipsychotic, can also produce hyperprolactinemia). Clozapine is associated with agranulocytosis. Metabolic status and weight should be screened before the start of treatment and at regular intervals.
- Patients with schizophrenia have a higher lifetime incidence of suicide, with 20% attempting on one of more occasions and 5% to 6% completing suicide. Comorbid use of substances and hopelessness are associated risk factors.

DISPOSITION

- The positive symptoms of as many as 20% to 30% of schizophrenic patients do not respond to available treatments. A much higher fraction of patients experience relapse as a result of poor compliance.
- Negative symptoms are responsible for the 50% to 70% of patients in whom deterioration in occupational and social function continues.
- Approximately 10% of schizophrenic patients will complete suicide.
- The course of the illness is most strongly predicted by level of social development attained at the onset of psychosis.
- Schizophrenic patients die 12 to 15 yr sooner than the average population, mostly as a result of physical causes related to a lack of access to health care or as a result of health risk factors (e.g., smoking, obesity).

REFERRAL

- If hospitalization is required
- If patient is noncompliant
- If patient is resistant to treatment

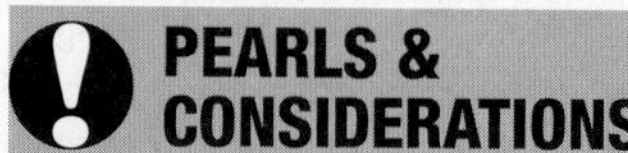

PEARLS & CONSIDERATIONS

- Rule out delirium caused by medical conditions, medications, or substance abuse before diagnosing an individual's psychotic behavior as schizophrenia.
- All antipsychotic medications have high discontinuation rates in chronic schizophrenia treatment. Olanzapine and clozapine may be more effective than other antipsychotics for chronic treatment, but they have significant side effects.
- Significant social support is required for most patients with schizophrenia. Nonpharmacologic therapy should be used in conjunction with pharmacotherapy.

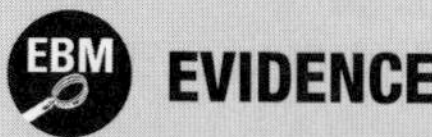

EVIDENCE

available at www.expertconsult.com

SUGGESTED READINGS

available at www.expertconsult.com

RELATED CONTENT

Schizophrenia (Patient Information)

AUTHORS: **ARNALDO A. BERGES, M.D., RICHARD J. GOLDBERG, M.D.,** and **MICHAEL K. ONG, M.D., PH.D.**

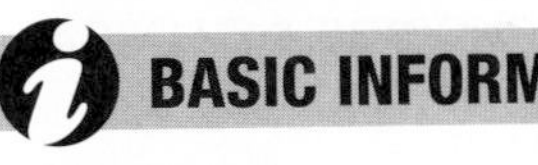

BASIC INFORMATION

DEFINITION

Scleritis is inflammation of the sclera (the fibrous layer of the eye underlying the conjunctiva and episclera). It is characterized by edema and cellular infiltration of the entire thickness of the sclera.

Classification of immune:

1. Anterior nonnecrotizing scleritis: can be subdivided into diffuse or nodular
2. Anterior necrotizing scleritis with inflammation: subdivided into vasoocclusive, granulomatous, surgically induced. Aggressive form of scleritis. Average age of onset is 60 yr. Bilateral in 60% of patients
3. Scleromalacia perforans: typically affects elderly women with longstanding rheumatoid arthritis
4. Posterior scleritis: involves the deeper tissues of the eye and is potentially blinding. Age of onset is often under 40 yr. Bilateral in 35% of cases

SYNONYMS

Anterior scleritis
Diffuse nodular, necrotizing scleritis
Scleromalacia perforans
Scleral melt syndrome

ICD-9CM CODES
379.0 Scleritis and episcleritis
ICD-10CM CODES
H15.0 Scleritis
H15.1 Episcleritis

EPIDEMIOLOGY & DEMOGRAPHICS

PEAK INCIDENCE: Increases with increasing age
INCIDENCE (IN U.S.): Busy ophthalmologists may see one or two cases a year
PREVALENCE (IN U.S.): Relatively rare
PREDOMINANT SEX: 61% women
PREDOMINANT AGE: 52 yr

PHYSICAL FINDINGS & CLINICAL PRESENTATION

- Deep, boring (dull) eye pain that may awaken patient from sleep
- Photophobia
- Tearing
- Painful eye movements
- Globe is tender to touch
- Conjunctival injection (Fig. 1-835)
- Thinning of the sclera
- More than 50% of patients have an underlying systemic autoimmune disease. Most common rheumatic problem is rheumatoid arthritis. Most patients with systemic disease are diagnosed before development of scleritis.

ETIOLOGY

- Inflammatory (seen with rheumatoid arthritis, granulomatosis with polyangiitis [Wegener granulomatosis], relapsing polychondritis, polyarteritis nodosa), lupus, sarcoidosis
- Allergic
- Bisphosponates: risk of scleritis is 50% higher among new bisphosphonate users than among nonusers.
- Infectious scleritis (herpes zoster, tuberculosis, Lyme disease, syphilis, *Pseudomonas aeruginosa, Nocardia,* leprosy) is uncommon, accounting for 4% to 18% of cases
- Approximately 50% of patients with scleritis have an underlying systemic disease (vasculitis, infectious disease).

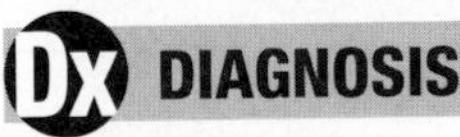

DIAGNOSIS

DIFFERENTIAL DIAGNOSIS

- Most common causes are rheumatoid arthritis and other collagen-vascular diseases.
- Occasionally there are allergic, infectious, or traumatic causes.
- Conjunctivitis, iritis, and episcleritis should be considered in the differential diagnosis. Patients with episcleritis generally have less pain and vision is unaffected.

WORKUP

- Eye examination
- Visual field examination
- Workup for autoimmune disease (e.g., vasculitis, collagen vascular diseases)

LABORATORY TESTS

Rheumatoid factor, antinuclear antibody, erythrocyte sedimentation rate, ANCA (c-ANCA, p-ANCA), antiphospholipid antibodies, may be useful for underlying etiology

IMAGING STUDIES

Usually not necessary; CT scan of orbit may be useful in selected patients for collagen vascular disease or vasculitis

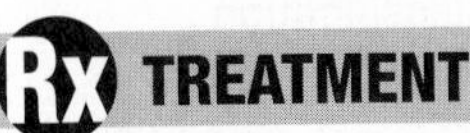

TREATMENT

NONPHARMACOLOGIC THERAPY

- Bandage lenses
- Surgery if thinning of the sclera is severe to prevent eye rupture

ACUTE GENERAL Rx

Immunotherapy:

- Steroids (topical, periocular, and systemic)
- Cycloplegic drops
- Nonsteroidal anti-inflammatory drugs (topical and systemic); systemic more effective than topical
- Cytotoxic agents (cyclophosphamide, azathioprine, mycophenolate mofetil, methotrexate)
- Immune modulators (cyclosporin, tacrolimus)
- Specific antibodies (infliximab, rituximab)

CHRONIC RX

- Systemic steroids can be given for the underlying disease.
- Local steroids may be helpful.
- Control underlying disease.

DISPOSITION

Urgent referral to ophthalmologist because this disorder can be a sight-threatening condition

REFERRAL

If not referred to an ophthalmologist early, patients may develop uveitis and other complications.

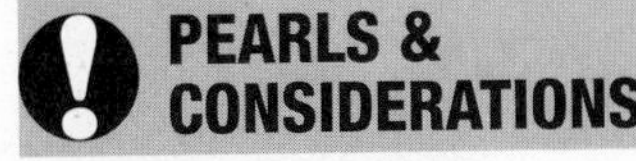

PEARLS & CONSIDERATIONS

COMMENTS

An ominous diagnosis because these patients often have other severe underlying debilitating disease processes.

SUGGESTED READINGS
available at www.expertconsult.com

AUTHORS: **MELVYN KOBY, M.D.,** and **R. SCOTT HOFFMAN, M.D.**

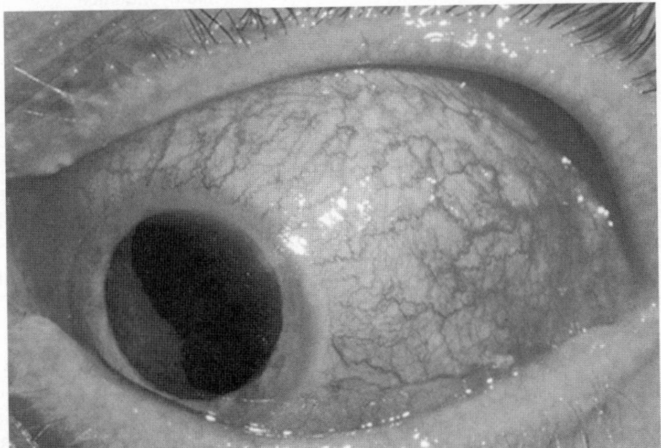

FIGURE 1-835 In diffuse anterior scleritis, widespread injection of the conjunctival and deep episcleral vessels occurs. (From Palay D [ed]: *Ophthalmology for the primary care physician,* St Louis, 1997, Mosby.)

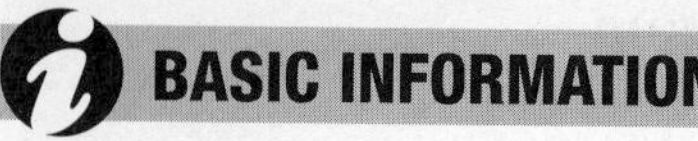

BASIC INFORMATION

DEFINITION

Scleroderma (systemic sclerosis [SSc]) is a connective tissue disorder that is characterized by thickening and fibrosis of the skin and variably severe involvement of diverse internal organs. It can be subdivided into two major subgroups: (1) limited cutaneous SSc (lcSSc), which involves mainly the face, neck, arms, and hands; and (2) diffuse cutaneous SSc (dcSSc), which affects the skin in a more generalized distribution including the entire extremities, face, neck, and trunk. Both subgroups typically have characteristic internal organ involvement. Table 1-443 compares localized scleroderma and SSc. A classification of scleroderma is described in Box 1-73.

BOX 1-73 Classification of Scleroderma

I. Localized scleroderma
   A. Morphea
   B. Linear scleroderma
   C. Scleroderma en coup de sabre
II. Systemic sclerosis
   A. Limited cutaneous systemic sclerosis
   B. Diffuse cutaneous systemic sclerosis

From Hochberg MC et al: *Rheumatology,* ed 5, St Louis, 2011, Mosby.

SYNONYMS

Systemic sclerosis

Morphea applies to localized scleroderma that affects only the skin

Scleredema is a disease of the skin that is distinct from scleroderma.

ICD-9CM CODES
710.1 Scleroderma
701.0 Morphea
ICD-10CM CODES
M34.0 Progressive systemic sclerosis
L94.0 Localized scleroderma (morphea)
L94.1 Linear scleroderma

EPIDEMIOLOGY & DEMOGRAPHICS

INCIDENCE: There are 2.3 to 22.8 cases per 1 million persons per yr, but many mild cases go unrecognized.

PREVALENCE: 50 to 300 cases per 1 million persons

PREDOMINANT SEX: Female/male ratio of 4:1

PREDOMINANT AGE: 30 to 50 yr

DISTRIBUTION: Worldwide

TABLE 1-443 Comparison of Localized Scleroderma and Systemic Sclerosis

Feature	Localized Scleroderma/Morphea	Systemic Sclerosis
Skin findings	Patches or linear distribution of thickened skin	Sclerodactyly ± proximal skin thickening
Raynaud's phenomenon	Absent	Present
Digital ischemic changes	Absent	Usually present (digital pitting scars or ulcers, loss of fingerpad substance)
Internal organ disease	Absent	Present
Antinuclear antibody	Positive in ≥50% of cases	Positive in ≥85% of cases
Scleroderma-specific autoantibodies*	Negative	Positive in 60% of cases
Biopsy—histologic findings	Dermal fibrosis	Dermal fibrosis

*Scleroderma-specific antibodies include antibodies to centromere, topoisomerase-1 (Scl 70), and RNA polymerase III.
From Hochberg MC et al: *Rheumatology,* ed 5, St Louis, 2011, Mosby.

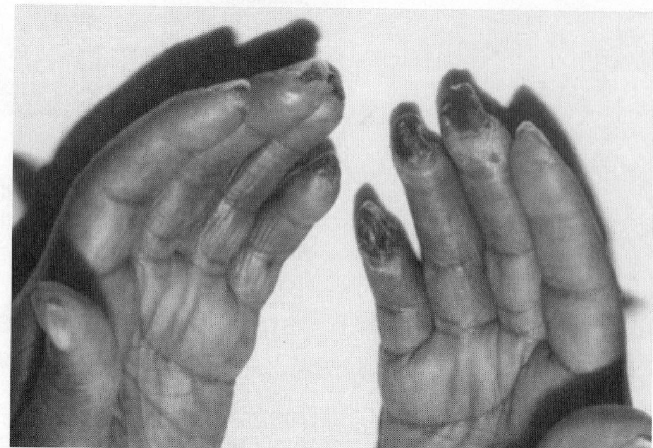

FIGURE 1-839 Digital gangrene on the fingertips of a patient with scleroderma. (From Hochberg MC et al: *Rheumatology,* ed 5, St Louis, 2011, Mosby.)

PHYSICAL FINDINGS & CLINICAL PRESENTATION

PHYSICAL FINDINGS:

1. Skin
   - Tightening of the skin begins on the hands and then progresses to the forearms, face, and neck; the skin is shiny, taut, and sometimes red, with a loss of creases and hair. Skin involvement in scleroderma is subdivided into "limited" and "diffuse" cutaneous forms (Fig. E1-836). Fig E1-837 illustrates the method used to semi-quantify skin thickness in scleroderma.
   - Later, skin tightening may limit movement by causing flexion contractures of the fingers, wrists, and elbows. Perioral skin tightening (Fig. E1-838) results in decreased oral aperture, furrowing around the lips, and dry membranes.
   - Pigmentary changes may occur.
   - Skin atrophy and digital gangrene of fingertips (Fig. 1-839) occurs during later stages.
2. Musculoskeletal
   - Joint pain and swelling
   - Symmetric inflammatory arthritis
   - Myopathy
3. Gastrointestinal involvement
   - Esophageal dysmotility with heartburn, dysphagia, and odynophagia
   - Delayed gastric emptying
   - Small-bowel dysmotility with abdominal cramps and diarrhea
   - Colon dysmotility with constipation
   - Primary biliary cirrhosis (see "Cirrhosis, Primary Biliary" in Section I)
4. Pulmonary manifestations
   - Pulmonary fibrosis with symptoms of dyspnea and nonproductive cough as well as fine inspiratory crackles on examination
   - Pulmonary hypertension
5. Cardiac involvement
   - Myocardial fibrosis that leads to congestive heart failure
6. Renal involvement
   - Malignant hypertension
   - Rapidly progressive renal failure
7. Other organ involvement
   - Hypothyroidism
   - Erectile dysfunction
   - Sjögren's syndrome
   - Entrapment neuropathies
8. CREST syndrome (term now replaced by lcSSc)
   - Calcinosis, Raynaud's syndrome, Esophageal dysmotility, Sclerodactyly (Fig. 1-840), Telangiectasias—with CREST syndrome, scleroderma is limited to the distal extremities. This acronym is now considered obsolete by many because it does not accurately reflect the burden of internal organ involvement.

CLINICAL PRESENTATION:

- Raynaud's phenomenon: initial complaint in 70% of patients (NOTE: The prevalence of Raynaud's phenomenon is 5% to 10% in the general population; most cases do not progress to scleroderma.)
- Finger or hand swelling that is sometimes associated with carpal tunnel syndrome

- Arthralgias/arthritis
- Internal organ involvement

ETIOLOGY

The etiology of this condition is unknown. Genetic profiles show clustering of different alleles according to the subtype of SSc. There is abnormal selection of fibroblasts and aberrant control of connective tissue synthesis by fibroblasts and other cells. Although there are characteristic autoantibodies detected, it is not clear that they directly participate in the pathogenesis of the disease.

- Extracellular connective tissue activation
- Frequent immunologic abnormalities including autoantibodies
- Inflammation in the early stages of disease
- Vasoconstriction

Dx DIAGNOSIS

DIFFERENTIAL DIAGNOSIS

DERMATOLOGIC:

- Scleredema
- Amyloidosis
- Porphyria cutanea tarda
- Eosinophilic fasciitis
- Reflex sympathetic dystrophy
- Nephrogenic systemic fibrosis

SYSTEMIC:

- Idiopathic pulmonary fibrosis
- Primary pulmonary hypertension
- Primary biliary cirrhosis
- Cardiomyopathies
- Gastrointestinal dysmotility problems
- Systemic lupus erythematosus and overlap syndromes

WORKUP

Laboratory tests and imaging studies

LABORATORY TESTS

- Antinuclear antibodies (homogeneous, speckled, or nucleolar patterns)
- Negative antibody to native DNA
- Negative anti–smooth muscle antibody
- Autoantibodies against ribonucleoprotein positive in 20% of patients

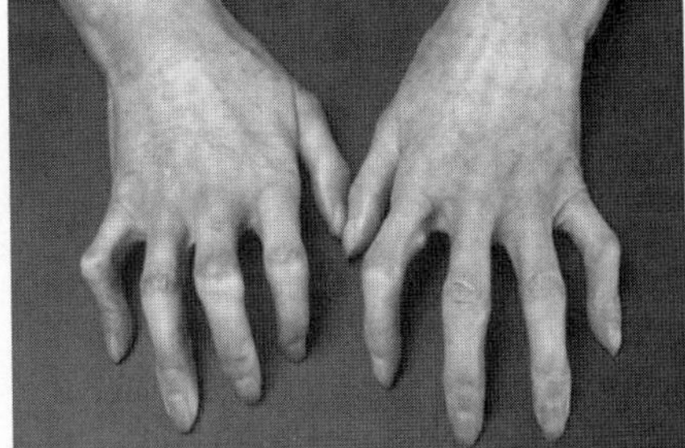

FIGURE 1-840 Sclerodactyly in a patient with systemic sclerosis. (From Hochberg MC et al: *Rheumatology,* ed 5, St Louis, 2011, Mosby.)

- Rheumatoid factor positive in 20% of patients
- Anticentromere antibodies in one third of patients with lcSSc
- Positive extractable nuclear antibody to Scl-70 in 40% of patients with dcSSc
- Routine biochemistry tests may indicate specific organ involvement (e.g., liver, kidney, muscle)

IMAGING AND OTHER STUDIES

1. Arthritis: joint radiographs
2. Gastrointestinal
   - Endoscopy (diagnostic procedure of choice; may be therapeutic)
   - Cine-esophagography (in rare circumstances)
   - Barium swallow (occasionally indicated)
   - Esophageal manometry (almost never necessary)
3. Pulmonary
   - Chest x-ray
   - Pulmonary function tests (especially single-breath diffusion capacity for CO)
   - Chest computed tomography (CT) scan
   - Bronchoscopy with biopsy
   - Gallium lung scan
   - Bronchoalveolar lavage
4. Heart
   - ECG
   - Ambulatory (Holter) ECG monitoring
   - Echocardiography
   - Cardiac catheterization
5. Kidney: renal biopsy
6. Skin: skin biopsy

Rx TREATMENT

1. Fig. E1-841 illustrates management strategies in SSc. No disease-modifying therapy available. Immunosuppressive agents used in individual patients. Prednisone should be used with extreme caution, especially in doses >20 mg/day. Table E1-444 summarizes current recommendations for treatment of scleroderma.
2. Raynaud's syndrome:
   - Calcium channel blockers (i.e., long-acting dihydropyridines)
   - Peripheral α_1-adrenergic blockers
   - Angiotensin II receptor blockers
   - Pentoxifylline
   - Phosphodiesterase inhibitors
   - Stellate ganglionic blockades
   - Digital sympathectomy
3. Arthralgias: nonsteroidal anti-inflammatory drugs
4. Skin: for extensive skin fibrosis, immunomodulatory drugs have been used such as methotrexate, mycophenalate mofetil, and cyclophosphamide but have not been proved to be beneficial
5. Esophageal reflux
   - H_2-receptor blockers
   - Proton pump inhibitors
6. Pulmonary hypertension and fibrosis
   - Oxygen
   - Diuretics (with caution)
   - Endothelin-1 receptor inhibitors (bosentan, ambrisentan)
   - Sildenafil, tadalafil
   - Prostacyclin analogues (epoprostenol, iloprost, treprostinil)
   - Lung transplantation
   - Cyclophosphamide chemotherapy for symptomatic scleroderma-related interstitial lung disease
7. Renal involvement
   - Angiotensin-converting enzyme inhibitors
   - Dialysis
   - Renal transplantation

REFERRAL

Rheumatology consultation

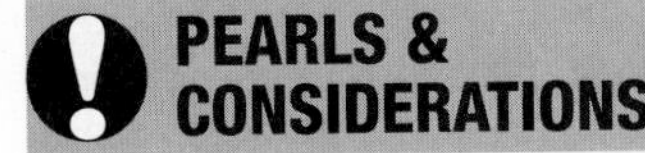

PEARLS & CONSIDERATIONS

COMMENTS

- Plasmacytoid dendritic cells have been implicated in the pathogenesis of systemic sclerosis. CXCL4 is the predominant protein secreted by plasmacytoid dendritic cells in systemic sclerosis and could be used as a biomarker in systemic sclerosis. Plasma levels of CXCL4 are elevated in patients with systemic sclerosis and correlated with the presence and progression of complications, such as long fibrosis and pulmonary arterial hypertension.[1]

RELATED CONTENT

Scleroderma (Patient Information)

AUTHORS: **EDWARD V. LALLY, M.D.,** and **FRED F. FERRI, M.D.**

[1]Van Bon L et al: Proteome-wide analysis and CXCL4 as a biomarker in systemic sclerosis, *N Engl J Med* 370:433-443, 2014.

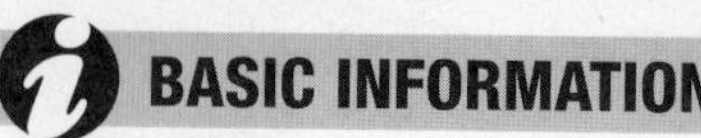

BASIC INFORMATION

DEFINITION

Scoliosis is a lateral curvature of the spine in the upright position, usually 10 degrees or greater. Scoliosis may be classified as either structural (fixed, nonflexible) or nonstructural (flexible, correctable).

ICD-9CM CODES

737.30 Idiopathic scoliosis
737.39 Paralytic scoliosis
754.2 Congenital scoliosis
737.43 Associated with neurofibromatosis

ICD-10CM CODES

M41 Scoliosis
M41.0 Infantile idiopathic scoliosis
M41.1 Juvenile idiopathic scoliosis
M41.3 Thoracogenic scoliosis
M41.20 Other idiopathic scoliosis, site unspecified
M41.80 Other forms of scoliosis, site unspecified
Q67.5 Congenital deformity of spin
M41.40 Neuromuscular scoliosis, site unspecified

EPIDEMIOLOGY & DEMOGRAPHICS (IDIOPATHIC FORM)

PREDOMINANT SEX: The incidence of scoliosis is the same in males and females; however, females have up to a 10-fold greater risk of curve progression.

PREVALENCE: Four cases per 1000 persons. Idiopathic scoliosis is present in 2%-4% of adolescents.

PREDOMINANT AGE:

- Onset variable
- Most curves found in adolescents (age ≥11 yr)

PHYSICAL FINDINGS & CLINICAL PRESENTATION

- Record patient age (in years plus months) and height.
- Perform neurologic examination to rule out neuromuscular disease.
- Inspect the shoulders and iliac crests to determine if they are level.
- Palpate the spinous processes to determine their alignment.
- Have the patient bend forward symmetrically at the waist with the arms hanging free (Adams' position); observe from the back or front to detect abnormal spine rotation (Fig. 1-842).

ETIOLOGY

- 90% unknown, usually referred to as *idiopathic* (genetic)
- Congenital spine deformity
- Neuromuscular disease
- Leg-length inequality
- Local inflammation or infection
- Acute pain (disk disease)
- Chronic degenerative disk disease with asymmetric disk narrowing

Curves of an idiopathic nature or those accompanying congenital deformity or neuromuscular disease are associated with structural changes. The nonstructural types (leg-length discrepancy, inflammation, or acute pain) disappear when the offending disorder is corrected.

DIAGNOSIS

WORKUP

- Curvatures associated with congenital spine abnormalities, neuromuscular disease, and other less common forms of scoliosis can usually be identified by history or associated radiographic or physical findings.
- The diagnosis of scoliosis is suspected on the basis of physical examination and confirmed by radiography performed while the patient is in a standing position. Physical examination with the Adams' forward bend test and scoliometer measurement can identify scoliosis and the radiologic testing for Cobb angle measurement can confirm the diagnosis. The Risser grade measures ossification. It consists of 5 grades ranging from 25% ossification in grade 1 to fusion of ossified epiphysis to the iliac wing in grade 5. Scoliosis screening is described in Fig. E1-843.

IMAGING STUDIES

- Diagnosis of idiopathic scoliosis is confirmed by a standing roentgenogram of the spine.
- Severity of the curve is measured in degrees, usually by the Cobb method (Fig. E1-844).
- MRI is usually not indicated unless there is pain, a neurologic deficit, or a left thoracic curve (which is often associated with an underlying spinal disorder).

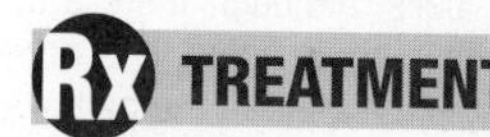

TREATMENT

ACUTE GENERAL Rx

- Treatment or correction of cause if curve is nonstructural
- Early detection is key in treating genetic curve
- Regular observation for curves <20 degrees
- Bracing for idiopathic curves of 25 to 45 degrees in patients with an immature skeleton to prevent progression
- Surgery for idiopathic curves >45 degrees in patients with an immature skeleton

DISPOSITION

- The larger the curve at detection, the greater the chance of progression.
- Progression is more common in young children who are beginning their growth spurt.
- Curves in females are more likely to progress.
- Curves <20 degrees will improve spontaneously >50% of the time.
- Failure to diagnose and treat these curves may allow progressive deformity, pain, and cardiopulmonary compromise to develop.
- Spinal deformities >50 degrees in adults may progress and eventually become painful.
- There is no difference in the rate of back pain in the general population and patients with adolescent idiopathic scoliosis.

REFERRAL

For orthopedic consultation if structural curve is present

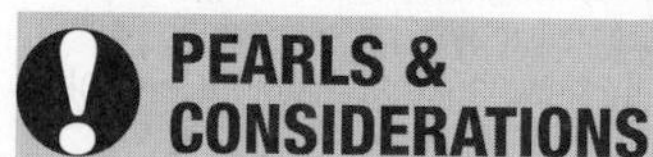

PEARLS & CONSIDERATIONS

COMMENTS

- Congenital scoliosis has a high incidence of cardiac and urinary tract abnormalities.
- Bracing is not intended to completely straighten the idiopathic curve. It may improve the curvature but is mainly used to stabilize and prevent progression.
- The initial Cobb angle magnitude (≥25 degrees) is the most important predictor of long-term curve progression.

SUGGESTED READINGS

available at www.expertconsult.com

RELATED CONTENT

Scoliosis (Patient Information)

AUTHORS: **LONNIE R. MERCIER, M.D.,** AND **FRED FERRI, M.D.**

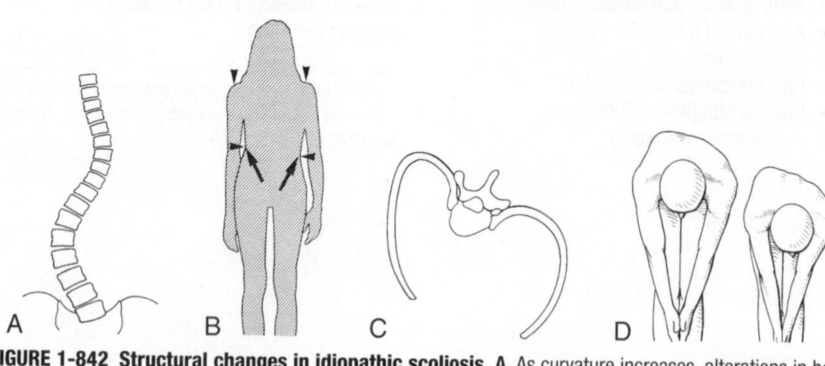

FIGURE 1-842 Structural changes in idiopathic scoliosis. A, As curvature increases, alterations in body configuration develop in both the primary and compensatory curve regions. **B,** Asymmetries of shoulder height, waistline, and the elbow-to-flank distance are common findings. **C,** Vertebral rotation and associated posterior displacement of the ribs on the convex side of the curve are responsible for the characteristic deformity of the chest wall in scoliosis patients. **D,** In the school screening examination for scoliosis, the patient bends forward at the waist. Rib asymmetry of even a small degree is obvious. (From Scoles PV: Spinal deformity in childhood and adolescence. In Behrman RE, Vaughn VC III [eds]: *Nelson textbook of pediatrics*, ed 5, Philadelphia, 1989, Saunders.)

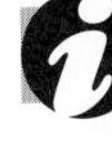

BASIC INFORMATION

DEFINITION

Recurrent depressive episodes during autumn and winter alternating with nondepressive episodes during spring and summer. Patients with seasonal affective disorder (SAD) have experienced two episodes of major depression in the past 2 yr that demonstrate the temporal seasonal relations and have had no nonseasonal episodes over this period.

SYNONYMS

SAD
Seasonal depression
Winter depression
Wintertime blues

ICD-9CM and DSM-5 CODES
296.30

ICD-10CM CODES

F33	Recurrent depressive disorder
F33.0	Recurrent depressive disorder, current episode, mild
F33.1	Recurrent depressive disorder, moderate
F33.2	Recurrent depressive disorder, severe without psychotic symptoms
F33.3	Recurrent depressive disorder, severe with psychotic symptoms
F33.4	Recurrent depressive disorder, currently in remission
F33.9	Recurrent depressive disorder, unspecified

EPIDEMIOLOGY & DEMOGRAPHICS

- Climate, genetic vulnerability, and sociocultural factors all play a role. The risk of seasonal mood swings is clearly associated with northern latitudes. The prevalence of SAD is estimated to be 0.5% to 1.5% in northern European populations, but up to 10% to 20% of these populations report milder, recurrent episodes consistent with subsyndromal SAD. In the U.S. it is estimated that about 5% of the population experiences SAD.
- As with other depressive disorders, women are affected disproportionately.
- Younger age, as well as greater familiarity with SAD, is associated with increased prevalence.

PHYSICAL FINDINGS & CLINICAL PRESENTATION

- The symptoms of SAD can be identical to those of other depressive episodes but tend to include features associated with atypical major depression, including low energy, irritability, weight gain, and overeating.
- Average duration is 5 mo, generally beginning in November.

ETIOLOGY

- Explanations focus on diathesis-stress models. An interaction between biologic and cognitive-affective factors appears to contribute to SAD. Retinal sensitivity anomalies and emotional reactivity to light stimuli, circadian rhythm disturbance, and irregularities in melatonin and melatonin-serotonin interaction have been identified as potential risk factors. Shorter photoperiod and decrease in sunlight are hypothesized to be the triggers.
- Several neurotransmitters implicated, including dopamine, serotonin, and norepinephrine.
- Cognitive risk factors include elevated rumination and negative cognitions related to the winter season and its impact on one's mood.
- Low activity and exercise levels, which are also implicated in nonseasonal depression, have been shown in some studies to characterize SAD.

Dx DIAGNOSIS

Diagnostic workup similar to that for major depression

DIFFERENTIAL DIAGNOSIS

- Major depressive disorder
- Minor depression or adjustment disorder
- Bipolar affective disorder
- Evaluate for substance use (especially alcohol)
- Medical illness or medications that may contribute to depression (e.g., endocrine disorders, neurologic disease)

WORKUP

- As with major depression, consider medical etiologies and rule out as indicated by the presenting signs and symptoms. Consider endocrine evaluation, especially thyroid function; sleep studies and a toxicology screen might be considered.
- Structured Interview Guide for the Hamilton Depression Rating Scale–Seasonal Affective Disorders Version (SIGH-SAD) used in research settings.
- In patients with major depressive disorder treated longitudinally, the routine use of depression scales to monitor outcome can help identify seasonal fluctuations of symptoms.

LABORATORY TESTS

As directed by presenting symptoms

IMAGING STUDIES

Generally not indicated

Rx TREATMENT

NONPHARMACOLOGIC THERAPY

- Phototherapy presupposes that artificial light at a similar strength to natural sunlight will prevent the biologic changes that mediate SAD.
- Many studies have demonstrated efficacy of light therapy in individuals with SAD. Recent studies indicate that light therapy may also be efficacious, with various subtypes of depression, including both melancholic and atypical, and for individuals with nonseasonal depression
- Light therapy may be used as a first-line treatment; choice of light therapy vs. medication or psychotherapy depends on various factors, however, including severity of symptoms and suicidality, prior response to medication or light therapy, feasibility, and patient preference.
- Some studies showing retinal sensitivity anomalies in SAD normalize following phototherapy.
- Phototherapy tends to use 2500 to 10,000 lux delivered by a commercial light box or a portable head-mounted unit. Phototherapy is recommended to begin within 2 wk of the start of symptoms and continue through the winter months. Patients are instructed to sit ~18 in from the light box for 30 min up to several hours once or twice per day for a minimum of 1 wk.
- A recent meta-analysis demonstrated efficacy of high-density negative ions in reducing depressive severity, although further research is needed to determine whether efficacy is comparable to light therapy.
- Small trials have demonstrated the efficacy of cognitive-behavioral therapy tailored specifically for SAD, either alone or with possible additive effects to light therapy. CBT for SAD appears to operate through distinct mechanisms than light therapy (e.g., reducing rumination and negative SAD-related cognitions).

PHARMACOLOGIC THERAPY

Bupropion effective in preventing recurrence

ACUTE GENERAL Rx

Necessary if patient is suicidal

CHRONIC Rx

- Growing support for use of SSRIs for SAD (e.g., fluoxetine, sertraline), although more research is needed.
- Preliminary studies demonstrated efficacy of novel antidepressants that act on melatonin (i.e., agomelatine), but further research is needed.

DISPOSITION

Psychiatric referral may be helpful to confirm diagnosis. Recommended for high-risk and suicidal patients.

REFERRAL

For active suicidal ideation, psychosis, symptoms suggestive of bipolar disorder

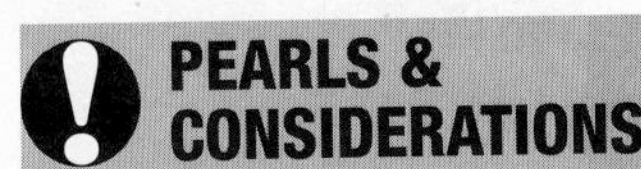

PEARLS & CONSIDERATIONS

Patients with SAD may present with a complaint of overeating, particularly food high in carbohydrates.

SUGGESTED READINGS

available at www.expertconsult.com

RELATED CONTENT

Seasonal Affective Disorder (SAD) (Patient Information)

AUTHORS: **MARK ZIMMERMAN, M.D.,** and **CATHERINE D'AVANZATO, PH.D.**

BASIC INFORMATION

DEFINITION

Seborrheic dermatitis (SD) is a common, inflammatory skin condition characterized by a mild to severe rash with scaling and erythema that occurs in areas of the skin rich in sebaceous glands.

SYNONYMS

SD
Dandruff
Cradle cap (Fig. 1-845)
Sebopsoriasis
Seborrheic eczema
Pityriasis capitis
Seborrhea

ICD-9CM CODES
690.10 Seborrheic dermatitis
ICD-10CM CODES
L21.9 Seborrheic dermatitis, unspecified

EPIDEMIOLOGY & DEMOGRAPHICS

PREVALENCE: Affects between 3% and 5% of otherwise healthy adults.

PREDOMINANT SEX AND AGE: Can occur from infancy through old age, with peak incidence in adolescents and young adults and increasing again after age 50 yr. More common in men than women.

RISK FACTORS: More common in patients with HIV/AIDS, Parkinson's disease, other neurologic disorders, mood disorders, chronic alcoholic pancreatitis, hepatitis, cancer, and genetic disorders (e.g., Down syndrome). Occurs more often during winter season.

PHYSICAL FINDINGS & CLINICAL PRESENTATION

Mild, greasy scaling of the scalp and nasolabial folds, postauricular skin, beard area, eyebrows, trunk, and sometimes the central face. Blepharitis, otitis externa, and coexisting acne vulgaris or pityriasis may also be present. Itching and stinging of lesions can occur. Increased occurrence during times of stress or sleep deprivation.

ETIOLOGY

Actual etiology is unknown but has been linked to hormone levels, fungal infections, altered immune function, nutritional deficits, and neurogenic factors. Fungal infections of the *Malassezia* species have been associated with SD.

Dx DIAGNOSIS

DIFFERENTIAL DIAGNOSIS

- Atopic dermatitis
- Candidiasis
- Dermatophytosis
- Langerhans cell histiocytosis
- Psoriasis
- Rosacea
- Systemic lupus erythematosus
- Tinea infection

WORKUP

- Diagnosis usually based on clinical identification of lesions
- Skin biopsies can be performed, if warranted, to distinguish SD from similar disorders

LABORATORY TESTS

Microscopic examination with special stains can be used to determine if yeast cells are present in keratinocytes

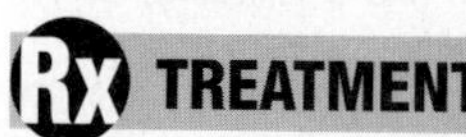

Rx TREATMENT

NONPHARMACOLOGIC THERAPY

- Patient education that SD is a chronic condition and treatment is aimed at resolving lesions but does not prevent recurrence.
- General recommendations: wash skin regularly, soften and remove scales, and apply moisturizing emollients after washing.
- Scale removal can be accomplished through the application of mineral or olive oil and removed with a comb or brush after 1 hr.

ACUTE GENERAL Rx

- Topical steroids: can be in the form of shampoos, creams, or ointments. Can be used alone or in more severe SD with antifungals.
- Antifungals (e.g., Nizoral, selenium sulfide, ketoconazole [the most evidence for effectiveness among antifungals], ciclopirox, fluconazole). Reserve oral antifungal therapy for patients with widespread SD or SD that is refractory to topical therapy. Itraconazole 200 mg/day for 7 days is a sample oral regimen.
- Calcineurin inhibitors (e.g., tacrolimus ointment, pimecrolimus cream): good when face and ears are affected
- Keratolytics (e.g., tar, salicylic acid, zinc pyrithione)
- Treatment of any secondary bacterial infection with oral antibiotics

CHRONIC Rx

Recalcitrant SD: topical azole combined with desonide regimen (limit use to 2 wk)

COMPLEMENTARY & ALTERNATIVE MEDICINE

Tea tree oil (melaleuca oil)

REFERRAL

Consider referral to dermatology for recalcitrant cases or uncertain diagnosis

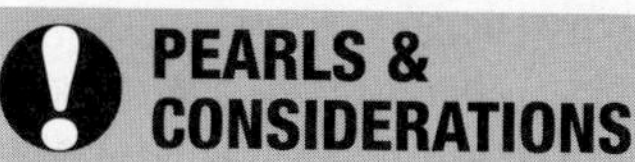

PEARLS & CONSIDERATIONS

- Use a combination of topical steroids and antifungal cream for severe SD
- Limit use of steroids to 2-wk course of treatment due to risk of cutaneous atrophy and telangiectasias
- SD of the scalp can be treated with an antifungal (e.g., 2% ketoconazole) or keratolytic shampoo. Limit use of antifungal shampoos to twice a week to prevent drying of the scalp. Alternate the use of antifungal shampoos with a moisturizing shampoo.
- In patients with widespread SD, consider testing for HIV infection

SUGGESTED READINGS

available at www.expertconsult.com

AUTHOR: **ANNGENE G. ANTHONY, M.D., M.P.H., F.A.A.F.P.**

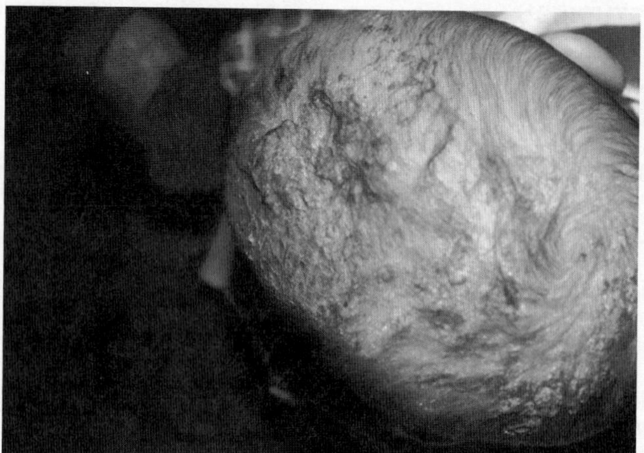

FIGURE 1-845 Cradle cap in an infant. (From Kliegman RM et al: *Nelson textbook of pediatrics*, ed 19, Philadelphia, 2011, Saunders.)

BASIC INFORMATION

DEFINITION

Absence seizures are a type of generalized seizures, characterized by brief episodes of staring with impairment of consciousness (absence). They usually last a few seconds, up to 20 to 30 sec. The onset and the end of the seizures are sudden. Usually the patients are not aware of them and resume the activity they were doing prior to the seizure. The electroencephalogram signature of absence seizures consists of generalized 3-Hz spike and slow wave discharges.

SYNONYMS

Childhood absence epilepsy
Petit mal epilepsy

ICD-9CM CODES
345.0 Generalized nonconvulsive epilepsy
ICD-10CM CODES
G40.309 Generalized idiopathic epilepsy and epileptic syndromes, not intractable, without status epilepticus

EPIDEMIOLOGY & DEMOGRAPHICS

INCIDENCE: 1 to 10 cases per 100,000 population
PEAK INCIDENCE: 6 to 7 yr
PREVALENCE: Represent up to 18% of all pediatric epilepsy syndromes
PREDOMINANT SEX AND AGE: More common in girls than in boys, absences typically begin between 4 and 8 yr

PHYSICAL FINDINGS & CLINICAL PRESENTATION

- Patients with absence seizures usually have normal physical and neurologic examinations.
- During the seizures, the patients are unresponsive and can have motor phenomena (automatisms, eye blinks, mouth and hand movements).
- Tonic clonic seizures are not usually a feature of this syndrome. If this is the case, other etiologies should be investigated, such as juvenile absence epilepsy, juvenile myoclonic epilepsy, complex partial seizures, etc.

ETIOLOGY

Genetic

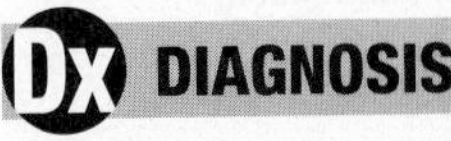

DIAGNOSIS

DIFFERENTIAL DIAGNOSIS

- Juvenile absence epilepsy
- Juvenile myoclonic epilepsy
- Complex partial seizures

WORKUP

- EEG with hyperventilation and photic stimulation is crucial in the diagnosis.
- Ambulatory EEG and video EEG are recommended for patients with diagnostic uncertainty.

LABORATORY TESTS

No specific studies needed

IMAGING STUDIES

- MRI of the brain should be performed in all epilepsy patients, especially if the EEG does not show the typical characteristic of absence seizures (3-Hz spike and slow wave discharges).
- CT scans of the head should be avoided in children due to unnecessary exposure to radiation and low yield of the test except when MRI cannot be obtained.

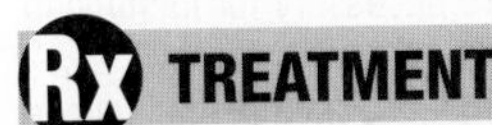

TREATMENT

The medication of choice based on the best current data available is ethosuximide, followed by valproic acid and lamotrigine.

NONPHARMACOLOGIC THERAPY

Not applicable

GENERAL Rx

- Ethosuximide: initial dose: 10 mg/kg/day; then after 7 days, 20 mg/kg
- Valproic acid (Depakote): initial dose: 5-10 mg/kg/day (divided bid), maximum dose 60 mg/kg/day
- Lamotrigine: dose for patients on no other antiepileptic drugs. Wk 1 and 2: 0.3 mg/kg/day. Wk 3 and 4: 0.6 mg/kg/day. Wk 5 onward: increase every 1 to 2 wk by 0.6 mg/kg/day. Maintenance: 4.5 to 7.5 mg/kg/day. Warning: should be used with caution due to the potential for toxicity and Stevens-Johnson syndrome. Patients on other antiepileptic drugs can also have severe adverse reactions.

CHRONIC Rx

- Children with recurrent seizures require chronic treatment.
- If children are seizure free for a period of 1 to 2 yr, a trial on no medications should be considered; children, unlike adults, can "outgrow" seizures.

COMPLEMENTARY & ALTERNATIVE MEDICINE

Not applicable

DISPOSITION

- Response to treatment is excellent.
- Absence seizures tend to remit in teenage years.

REFERRAL

Patients with epilepsy and seizures should be referred for a consultation by a neurologist, preferably one specializing in epilepsy.

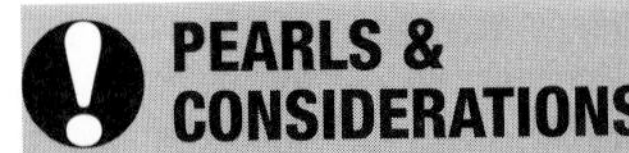

PEARLS & CONSIDERATIONS

COMMENTS

- Absence seizures can be present in other epilepsy syndromes.
- Valproic acid should be avoided in girls and women with childbearing potential due to the risk of teratogenicity.
- Carbamazepine and phenytoin should be avoided in the treatment of absence seizures, since these medications may worsen seizures and could provoke absence status epilepticus.
- All women of childbearing age taking antiepileptic drugs should take folic acid supplementation (1 to 4 mg/day) for the prevention of neural tube defects.

PREVENTION

Sleep deprivation and alcohol consumption should be avoided.

PATIENT & FAMILY EDUCATION

- Patients with epilepsy have normal lives.
- The goal of treatment is no seizures and no side effects to medications.
- Patient education and information can be obtained from the Epilepsy Foundation: www.epilepsyfoundation.org
- Pregnant women with epilepsy should visit the Antiepileptic Drug Pregnancy Registry website for information and assistance: www2.massgeneral.org/aed
- Patients with ongoing seizures are forbidden from driving; check state regulations and laws regarding driving and epilepsy.

SUGGESTED READINGS

available at www.expertconsult.com

RELATED CONTENT

Absence Seizures (Patient Information)

AUTHOR: **PATRICIO SEBASTIAN ESPINOSA, M.D., M.P.H.**

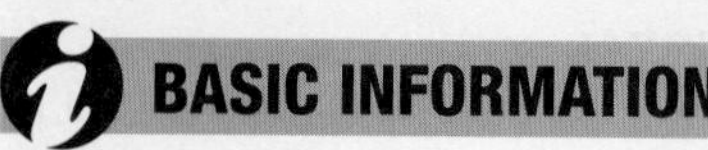

BASIC INFORMATION

DEFINITION

Febrile seizures are seizures that occur in febrile children (fever of at least 100.4° F [38° C]) between the ages of 6 and 60 mo in the absence of infection of the central nervous system (CNS), metabolic disturbance, or history of neonatal seizures or a previous unprovoked seizures. Febrile seizures are subdivided into 2 categories: simple and complex. Simple febrile seizures last <15 min, are generalized (without a focal component), and occur once in a 24-hr period, whereas complex febrile seizures are prolonged (>15 min), show focal neurologic signs, or occur more than once in 24 hr.

SYNONYMS

Febrile convulsions

ICD-9CM CODES
780.6 Febrile seizures
ICD-10CM CODES
R56.0 Febrile convulsions

EPIDEMIOLOGY & DEMOGRAPHICS

INCIDENCE: Febrile seizures are the most common seizures of childhood. 2% to 5% of children will have a febrile seizure by age 60 mo. Simple febrile seizures represent 65% to 90% of febrile seizures.
PREDOMINANT SEX AND AGE: Slightly more common in boys than girls.
PEAK INCIDENCE: 6 to 60 mo
PREVALENCE: Represent up to 18% of all pediatric epilepsy syndromes

PHYSICAL FINDINGS & CLINICAL PRESENTATION

- Children with febrile seizures have normal physical and neurologic examinations.
- Viral illnesses are the predominant cause of febrile seizures.

ETIOLOGY

- Viral infections are a common cause of fever that triggers febrile seizures.
- Febrile seizures tend to occur in families. Although clear evidence exists for a genetic basis of febrile seizures, the mode of inheritance is unknown.
- Febrile seizures are likely multifactorial with genetic and environmental factors.

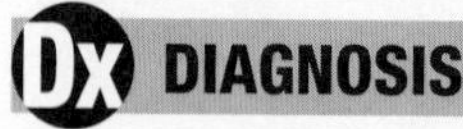

DIAGNOSIS

DIFFERENTIAL DIAGNOSIS

- CNS infection (i.e., meningitis)
- Epilepsy

WORKUP

- It is important to first investigate whether an underlying infection exists. Fig. E1-846 describes guidelines for febrile seizure evaluation.
- In patients with simple self-limited febrile seizures with rapid return to consciousness and a normal neurologic examination, further workup is not routinely recommended.
- In patients with complex febrile seizures, laboratory workup and brain imaging are recommended.
- EEG is not routinely recommended in the evaluation of a neurologically healthy child with simple partial seizures.

LABORATORY TESTS

- Routine blood workup (CBC with differential, CMP, electrolytes), blood and urine cultures are often performed but there is no evidence that these tests are necessary for identifying the cause of a simple febrile seizure.
- CSF analysis: lumbar puncture guidelines (American Academy of Pediatrics)
  - Lumbar puncture should be performed in children with febrile seizures and signs and symptoms of meningitis (e.g., neck stiffness, Kernig sign, Brudzinski sign), or if the patient history or examination suggests the presence of meningitis or intracranial infection.
  - In infants 6 to 12 months of age with febrile seizures, lumbar puncture is an option if they have not received the recommended *Haemophilus influenza* type b (Hib) or pneumococcal vaccinations, or if their immunization status is unknown.
  - Lumbar puncture is also considered an option in children with febrile seizures pretreated with antibiotics.

IMAGING STUDIES

- MRI of the brain is not required in the routine evaluation of patients with simple febrile seizures.
- Imaging of the brain should be considered in children with complex febrile seizures and in children with focal neurologic deficits.
- CT scans of the head should be avoided in children, if possible, due to exposure to radiation and the relative low yield of the test compared to MRI. CT scans of the head are reserved for neurologic emergencies and are adjusted for weight in children.

Rx TREATMENT

Febrile seizures do not usually require antiepileptic drug treatment.

NONPHARMACOLOGIC THERAPY

Not applicable

GENERAL Rx

Symptomatic treatment of fever

CHRONIC Rx

No chronic treatment for febrile seizures is recommended.

COMPLEMENTARY & ALTERNATIVE MEDICINE

Not applicable

DISPOSITION

- Treatment is not recommended.
- Febrile seizures should stop by age 60 mo.
- Risk of recurrence in the first 2 years after initial febrile seizure is 15% to 70%.

REFERRAL

Patients with recurrent febrile seizures need to be referred for a consultation by a pediatric neurologist.

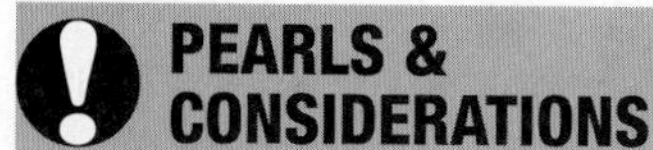

PEARLS & CONSIDERATIONS

COMMENTS

- It is crucial to find out the etiology of the fever and to treat it appropriately.
- Patient with seizures and fever after age 60 mo are not classified as febrile seizures.

PREVENTION

Antipyretics do not reduce the recurrence risk of febrile seizures. However, fever should be treated and worked up independently of the diagnosis of febrile seizures.

PATIENT & FAMILY EDUCATION

- Children with febrile seizures do not need antiepileptic drug treatment.
- Patient education and information can be obtained at the Epilepsy Foundation: www.epilepsyfoundation.org. Parents should be reassured that children without underlying developmental problems will usually not have lasting neurologic effects from febrile seizures.

SUGGESTED READINGS

available at www.expertconsult.com

RELATED CONTENT

Fever Seizures (Patient Information)

AUTHOR: **PATRICIO SEBASTIAN ESPINOSA, M.D., M.P.H.**

BASIC INFORMATION

DEFINITION

Tonic clonic seizures are characterized by sudden loss of consciousness, muscle contraction (tonic phase) followed by rhythmic jerking activity (clonic phase).

SYNONYMS

Convulsive seizures
Grand mal seizures

ICD-9CM CODES
345.1 Generalized convulsive epilepsy
ICD-10CM CODES
G40.6 Grand mal seizures, unspecified
G41.0 Grand mal status epilepticus

EPIDEMIOLOGY & DEMOGRAPHICS

INCIDENCE: 30 to 50 cases per 100,000 person-yr (epilepsy incidence)
PEAK INCIDENCE: Not applicable
PREVALENCE: 5 to 8 cases per 1000 persons (epilepsy incidence)
PREDOMINANT SEX AND AGE: No gender preference

PHYSICAL FINDINGS & CLINICAL PRESENTATION

- Patients with tonic clonic seizures usually have normal physical and neurologic examinations.
- During the seizures, the patients are unresponsive and can have violent postures with severe repetitive muscle contractions.
- After the seizure, the patients are usually lethargic and confused.
- Tonic clonic seizures are associated with injuries, bladder incontinence, and tongue biting.
- Focal postictal weakness may point toward a focal neurologic lesion (Todd's paralysis).

ETIOLOGY

- Seizures are a cardinal sign of cortical neurologic injury.
- The etiology of seizures can be idiopathic (likely genetic), cryptogenic (possibly genetic), and symptomatic (due to a neurologic injury/infection).

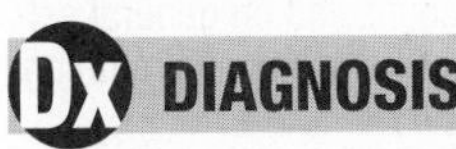

DIAGNOSIS

DIFFERENTIAL DIAGNOSIS

- Convulsive syncope
- Nonepileptic spells

WORKUP

- EEG
- Ambulatory EEG and/or video EEG recommended for patients with diagnostic uncertainty
- MRI of the brain

LABORATORY TESTS

- Routine blood workup (CBC, CMP, glucose, electrolytes)
- Urine drug screen
- Lumbar puncture is recommended in patients with suspicion of meningitis

IMAGING STUDIES

- Neurodiagnostic imaging studies such as CT of the head or, preferably, MRI of the brain should be performed in all patients with first unprovoked seizure.
- CT scans of the head should be avoided in children due to unnecessary exposure to radiation and the low yield of the test. CT scans of the head are reserved for neurologic emergencies and are adjusted for weight in children.

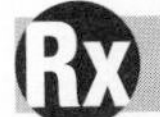

TREATMENT

- Treatment is based on the type and etiology of seizures (i.e., metabolic disturbance, infectious, etc.).
- Levetiracetam is an effective and well-tolerated antiepileptic drug for treating generalized tonic clonic seizures.
- Valproic acid is better tolerated than topiramate and more efficacious than lamotrigine in patients with generalized and unclassified epilepsy types.
- Valproic acid should be avoided in girls and women with childbearing potential due to the risk of teratogenicity.

NONPHARMACOLOGIC THERAPY

Not applicable

GENERAL Rx

- First unprovoked seizure with normal imaging, EEG, and laboratory workup requires no treatment.
- Recurrent seizures and seizures with abnormal studies require treatment depending on the etiology.
- Levetiracetam (Keppra): Initial dose 250 to 500 bid, maximum dose 1500 mg bid.
- Valproic acid (Depakote): Initial dose: 10 to 15 mg/kg/day (divided bid), maximum dose 60 mg/kg/day.

CHRONIC Rx

Chronic treatment with antiepileptic drugs is indicated for ≥2 unprovoked seizures or in patients with one seizure with abnormal workup.

COMPLEMENTARY & ALTERNATIVE MEDICINE

Not applicable

DISPOSITION

- Patients should avoid situations that may cause injuries or accidents in the event of a seizure.
- No driving until seizure freedom in accordance with local laws and regulations.

REFERRAL

Patients with epilepsy and seizures should be referred for a consultation by a neurologist, preferably one with epilepsy training.

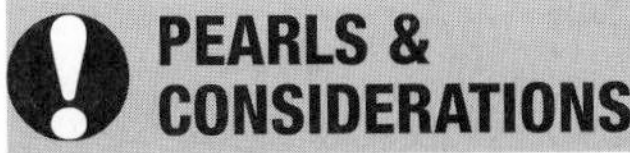

PEARLS & CONSIDERATIONS

COMMENTS

- It is crucial to understand that tonic clonic seizures can occur in variety of acute neurologic diseases.
- Successful treatment depends on the correct choice of antiepileptic drugs based on the type (partial vs. generalized in onset) and etiology of the seizures.
- Valproic acid should be avoided in girls and women with childbearing potential due to the risk of teratogenicity.
- All women of childbearing age taking antiepileptic drugs should take folic acid supplementation (1-4 mg/day) for the prevention of neural tube defects.

PREVENTION

Sleep deprivation and alcohol consumption should be avoided.

PATIENT & FAMILY EDUCATION

- Patients with epilepsy have normal lives.
- The goal of treatment is no seizures and no side effects to medications.
- Patient education and information can be obtained at the Epilepsy Foundation: www.epilepsyfoundation.org
- Pregnant women with epilepsy should visit the Antiepileptic Drug Pregnancy Registry website for information and assistance: www2.massgeneral.org/aed
- Patients with ongoing seizures are forbidden from driving; check your state regulations and laws regarding driving and epilepsy.

SUGGESTED READINGS

available at www.expertconsult.com

RELATED CONTENT

Generalized Tonic-Clonic Seizures (Patient Information)
Status Epilepticus (Related Key Topic)

AUTHOR: **PATRICIO SEBASTIAN ESPINOSA, M.D., M.P.H.**

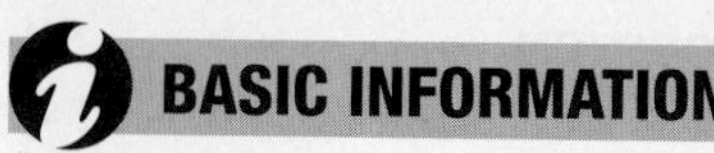

BASIC INFORMATION

DEFINITION

Partial seizures are characterized by focal cortical discharges that provoke seizure symptoms related to the area of the brain involved. Simple partial seizures do not cause impairment of consciousness. However, partial seizures can evolve into complex partial and/or tonic clonic seizures.

SYNONYMS

Simple partial seizures
Focal seizures

ICD-9CM CODES
345.5 Localization-related (focal) (partial) epilepsy and epileptic syndromes with simple partial seizures
ICD-10CM CODES
G40.0 Localization-related (focal) (partial) idiopathic epilepsy and epileptic syndromes with seizures of localized onset
G40.109 Localization-related (focal) (partial) symptomatic epilepsy and epileptic syndromes with simple partial seizures, not intractable, without status epilepticus

EPIDEMIOLOGY & DEMOGRAPHICS

INCIDENCE: 30 to 50 cases per 100,000 person-yr
PREVALENCE: 5 to 8 cases per 1000 persons
PREDOMINANT SEX AND AGE: No gender preference

PHYSICAL FINDINGS & CLINICAL PRESENTATION

- Patients with partial seizures usually have normal physical and neurologic examinations unless the focal seizures are due to a structural abnormality such as a stroke, wherein the patient will have a neurologic exam consistent with the area of CNS structural damage.
- During partial seizures the patients are conscious, unless there is spread of the epileptic focus causing secondary generalization and unresponsiveness. A focal seizure can evolve to a generalized tonic clonic seizure.
- Patients with partial seizures can experience postictal weakness/paralysis that usually resolves within 24 hr (Todd's paralysis). However, focal neurologic deficits may also be indicative of a structural brain lesion.

ETIOLOGY

- Seizures in general are a cardinal sign of cortical neurologic injury.
- The etiology of partial seizures can be idiopathic (likely genetic), cryptogenic (unknown, possibly genetic), and symptomatic (due to a neurologic injury).
- Frequent causes of partial seizures are tumor, stroke, CNS infections (cysticercosis, abscesses), arteriovenous malformations (AVMs), traumatic brain injury, cortical malformations, and others.

Dx DIAGNOSIS

DIFFERENTIAL DIAGNOSIS

- Transient ischemic attack
- Movement disorders
- Nonepileptic spells

WORKUP

- EEG
- Ambulatory EEG and/or video EEG recommended for patients with diagnostic uncertainty

LABORATORY TESTS

Routine blood workup (CBC, CMP, glucose, electrolytes) may be considered in appropriate clinical situations.

IMAGING STUDIES

- In the acute setting, a CT scan of the head is high yield to rule out space-occupying lesions.
- MRI of the brain with a defined epilepsy protocol should be performed in all patients with recurrent seizures.
- CT scans of the head should be avoided in children if possible, unless in an emergency setting.

Rx TREATMENT

- Carbamazepine traditionally has been the standard initial drug treatment for partial seizures.
- Lamotrigine and levetiracetam are effective and well-tolerated antiepileptic drugs for treating partial seizures.
- Other antiepileptic drugs (e.g., lacosamide, oxcarbazepine, ezogabine) may be used by an epilepsy specialist in specific cases.
- Surgical treatments (e.g., temporal lobectomy in mesial temporal sclerosis) may be indicated in refractory cases of partial seizures.

GENERAL Rx

- After a first unprovoked seizure with normal examination, imaging, and EEG, no treatment is required.
- Recurrent seizures and seizures with abnormal studies require treatment.

DISPOSITION

- Response to treatment often depends on the etiology of the partial seizures.
- 47% of patients become seizure free with monotherapy and 67% with polytherapy.
- No driving until seizure freedom in accordance with local laws and regulations.

REFERRAL

Patients with epilepsy and seizures should be referred for a consultation by a neurologist, preferably one with a special interest in epilepsy.

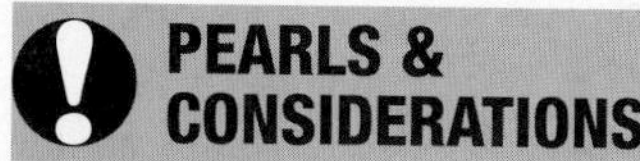

PEARLS & CONSIDERATIONS

COMMENTS

- It is crucial to understand that partial seizures can be due to a variety of neurologic diseases.
- Successful treatment depends on the correct choice of antiepileptic drugs based on patient's gender and comorbidities.
- Valproic acid should be avoided in girls and women with childbearing potential due to the risk of teratogenicity.
- All women in childbearing age taking antiepileptic drugs should take folic acid supplementation (1 to 4 mg/day) for the prevention of neural tube defects.

PREVENTION

- Sleep deprivation and alcohol consumption should be avoided.
- Drug compliance is compulsory to prevent seizure recurrence.

PATIENT & FAMILY EDUCATION

- People with epilepsy can lead normal lives.
- The goal of treatment is no seizures and no side effects to medications.
- Patient education and information can be obtained at the Epilepsy Foundation: www.epilepsyfoundation.org
- Pregnant women with epilepsy should visit the Antiepileptic Drug Pregnancy Registry website for information and assistance: www2.massgeneral.org/aed
- Patients with ongoing seizures are forbidden from driving; check your state regulations and laws regarding driving and epilepsy.
- Patients should be counseled on general seizure precautions such as swimming, bathing, and heights.

SUGGESTED READINGS

available at www.expertconsult.com

RELATED CONTENT

Partial Motor Seizures (Patient Information)

AUTHOR: **PATRICIO SEBASTIAN ESPINOSA, M.D., M.P.H.**

BASIC INFORMATION

DEFINITION

Sepsis is an exaggerated inflammatory response to an infectious stimulus. It is generally caused by generalized bacterial or fungal infection and characterized by evidence of infection, fever or hypothermia, hypotension, and evidence of end-organ compromise.

SYNONYMS

Septicemia
Sepsis syndrome
Severe sepsis
Systemic inflammatory response syndrome
Septic shock

ICD-9CM CODES
038.9 Sepsis
038.40 Sepsis, gram-negative bacteremia
038.1 Sepsis, *Staphylococcus*
ICD-10CM CODES
A41.9 Sepsis, unspecified organism
A41.50 Gram-negative sepsis, unspecified
A41.2 Sepsis due to unspecified *Staphylococcus*

EPIDEMIOLOGY & DEMOGRAPHICS

INCIDENCE (IN U.S.):
- Exact incidence is unknown
- Approximately 750,000 cases of severe sepsis occur among hospitalized patients each year in the U.S.
- Complicates a minority of bacteremia cases and may occur in the absence of documented bacteremia

PREDOMINANT SEX: Males slightly more commonly affected than females

PREDOMINANT AGE:
- Neonatal period
- Patients >65 yr of age account for 60% of all cases of severe sepsis

GENETICS:
- Familial disposition: a great variety of congenital immunodeficiency states and other inherited disorders may predispose to septicemia.
- Neonatal infection: incidence is high in neonatal period.

PHYSICAL FINDINGS & CLINICAL PRESENTATION

- Fever or hypothermia
- Hypotension
- Tachycardia
- Tachypnea
- Altered mental status
- Bleeding diathesis
- Skin rashes
- Symptoms that reflect primary site of infection: urinary tract, GI tract, CNS, respiratory tract
- Table 1-445 describes some clinical signs and symptoms of sepsis.

ETIOLOGY

- Disseminated infection with a great variety of bacteria:
  A. Gram-negative bacteria
    1. *Escherichia coli*
    2. *Klebsiella* spp.
    3. *Pseudomonas aeruginosa*
    4. *Proteus* spp.
    5. *Neisseria meningitidis*
  B. Gram-positive bacteria
    1. *Staphylococcus aureus* (including MRSA)
    2. *Streptococcus* spp.
    3. *Enterococcus* spp.
- Less common infections:
  1. Fungal
  2. Viral
  3. Rickettsial
  4. Parasitic
- Sepsis is a complex dysregulation of both inflammation and coagulation. There is activation of coagulation, inflammatory cytokines, complement, and kinin cascades with release of a variety of vasoactive endogenous mediators
- Predisposing host factors:
  1. General medical condition
  2. Extremes of age
  3. Immunosuppressive therapy
  4. Recent surgery
  5. Granulocytopenia
  6. Hyposplenism
  7. Diabetes
  8. Instrumentation

DIAGNOSIS

DIFFERENTIAL DIAGNOSIS

- Cardiogenic shock
- Acute pancreatitis
- Pulmonary embolism
- Systemic vasculitis
- Toxic ingestion
- Exposure-induced hypothermia
- Fulminant hepatic failure
- Collagen-vascular diseases

WORKUP

- Evaluation should focus on identifying a specific pathogen and localizing the site of primary infection. Fig. E1-847 illustrates workup following results of blood cultures.
- Hemodynamic, metabolic, coagulation disorders should be carefully characterized.
- Intensive monitoring, including the use of central venous catheters.

LABORATORY TESTS

- Cultures of blood and examination and culture of sputum, urine, wound drainage, stool, and CSF
- CBC with differential, coagulation profile
- Routine chemistries, LFTs
- ABGs, lactic acid level; procalcitonin might be useful as a general marker of infection/sepsis
- Urinalysis

IMAGING STUDIES

- Chest x-ray examination
- Other radiographic and radioisotope procedures according to suspected site of primary infection

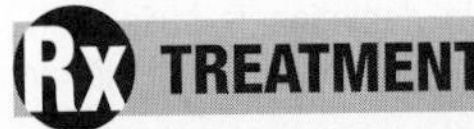

TREATMENT

NONPHARMACOLOGIC THERAPY

- Tissue oxygenation: mixed venous oxygen saturation maintained >70% if possible; early mechanical ventilation with low title volume (6 ml/kg predicted body weight) to protect lung parenchyma from overstretching and "volutrauma"
- Focal infection should be drained if possible, and potentially infected catheters should be removed

ACUTE GENERAL Rx

- Blood pressure support, rapid IV fluid resuscitation and vasopressors, if needed, with the goal of reestablishing a mean arterial blood pressure >65 mm Hg; reduction in blood lactate and mixed venous oxygen saturation >70% within 6 hr of recognition of septic shock is associated with improved survival. Measure vena cava oxygen saturation ($ScvO_2$) to assess adequacy of resuscitation. If the $ScvO_2$ is <70%, consider packed red

TABLE 1-445 Clinical Signs and Symptoms of Sepsis

Infection	General	Inflammatory	Hemodynamic	Tissue Perfusion
Documented or suspected	Temperature >38°C or <36°C Heart rate >90 beats/min Respiratory rate ≥20 breaths/min Altered mental status Hyperglycemia Third spacing of fluid	WBC count <4000 or >12,000 cells/mcL or ≥10% bands	Hypotension: systolic blood pressure <90 mm Hg MAP <70 mm Hg SVo_2 >70 CI >3.5 L/min/m^2	Hypoxemia: (Pao_2/Fio_2 <300) Acute oliguria (urine output <0.5 ml/kg/hr) Coagulopathy Abnormal liver function tests Platelet count <100,000 cells/μL Lactic acidosis Skin mottling

CI, Cardiac index; *MAP,* mean arterial pressure; *SVo_2,* mixed venous oxygen saturation; *WBC,* white blood cell.
From Cameron, JL, Cameron AM: *Current surgical therapy*, ed 10, Philadelphia, 2011, Saunders.

TABLE 1-446 Initial Antibiotic Recommendations for Septic Patients*

Empiric coverage	Vancomycin 15 mg/kg q12h plus either piperacillin-tazobactam† 3.375 g IV q6h or imipenem 0.5 g IV q6h or meropenem 1.0 g IV q8h with or without an aminoglycoside (e.g., tobramycin 5 mg/kg IV q24).‡
Community-acquired pneumonia	Ceftriaxone 1 g IV q24h plus azithromycin 500 mg IV q24h or a fluoroquinolone (e.g., moxifloxacin 400 mg IV q24h or levofloxacin 750 mg IV q24h).§
Community-acquired urosepsis	Ciprofloxacin 400 mg IV q24h or ampicillin 2 g IV q6h plus gentamicin 5 mg/kg IV q24h.
Meningitis	Vancomycin 500-750 mg IV q6h plus ceftriaxone 2 g IV q12h plus dexamethasone 0.15 mg/kg IV q6h × 2-4 days preferably before antibiotics; add ampicillin 2 g IV q4h if *Listeria* is suspected.
Nosocomial pneumonia	Vancomycin 15 mg/kg q12h plus either piperacillin-tazobactam 4.5 g IV q6h or imipenem 0.5 g IV q6h or meropenem 1 g IV q8h or cefepime 2 g IV q12h plus either an aminoglycoside (e.g., amikacin 15 mg/kg IV q24h or tobramycin 7 mg/kg IV q24h) or levofloxacin 750 mg IV q24h. Some authorities would substitute linezolid 600 mg IV q12h for vancomycin if methicillin-resistant *Staphylococcus aureus* is of significant concern or known to be the cause.
Neutropenia	Cefepime 2 g IV q8h; add vancomycin 15 mg/kg IV q12h if a central line is present and infection is a concern. Add antifungal coverage with liposomal amphotericin B 3-5 mg/kg q24h or caspofungin 70 mg IV × 1 then 50 mg IV q24h if fever persists ≥5 days. If invasive aspergillosis is highly suspected or proven, voriconazole 6 mg/kg IV q12h × 2 then 4 mg/kg IV q12h should be used.
Cellulitis and skin infections	Vancomycin 15 mg/kg IV q12h. Add piperacillin-tazobactam 4.5 g IV q6h in diabetics or immunocompromised patients. If necrotizing fasciitis is suspected, add clindamycin 900 mg IV; surgical debridement is crucial.

*Assumes normal renal function; dose adjustments required with impaired creatinine clearance.
†Substitute aztreonam 2 g IV q8h if penicillin allergic.
‡Monitor drug levels of aminoglycosides (i.e., peak and trough).
§Use ceftriaxone and azithromycin if the patient is admitted to the intensive care unit.
From Andreoli TE et al: *Andreoli and Carpenter's Cecil essentials of medicine,* ed 8, Philadelphia, 2010, Saunders.

blood cell transfusion to achieve Hct >30%. Start inotropic agents (dobutamine) if $ScvO_2$ is <70% despite transfusion.
1. IV hydration; crystalloids are as effective as colloids as resuscitation fluids, give 30 ml/kg IV if fluid depletion is suspected. Most patients need 4 to 6 L of fluid in the first 6 hours.
2. Therapy with vasopressors (e.g., norepinephrine, epinephrine, vasopressin) if mean arterial blood pressure of >65 mm Hg cannot be maintained by hydration alone. A recent trial comparing low-dose vasopressin with norepinephrine revealed that low-dose vasopressin did not reduce mortality rates as compared with norepinephrine among patients with septic shock who were treated with catecholamine vasopressors.

- Correction of acidosis by improving the tissue perfusion, not by giving bicarbonate
  1. Mechanical ventilation
- Antibiotics
  1. Directed at the most likely sources of infection. Table 1-446 describes initial antibiotic recommendations for septic patients.
  2. Should generally provide broad coverage of gram-positive and gram-negative bacteria (or fungi if clinically indicated).
  3. Antibiotics should be administered within 1 hr of the diagnosis of septic shock—this is a medical emergency.
  4. The role of corticosteroids in the acute management of septicemia has long been debated. Previous trials had shown that corticosteroid therapy improved hemodynamic outcomes in patients with severe septic shock. Patients with relative adrenal insufficiency may benefit from low-dose therapy with hydrocortisone (200 mg IV by continuous infusion for 7 days). Recent trials, however, revealed that hydrocortisone did not improve survival or reversal of shock, either overall or in patients who did not have a response to corticotropin, although hydrocortisone hastened reversal of shock in patients in whom shock was reversed. Until definitive data are available, the decision to administer corticosteroids for septic shock should be based on the individual patient's severity of illness versus risk of corticosteroid administration. The corticotropin (ACTH) stimulation test is not helpful and should not be used to determine the need for corticosteroid in these patients.

CHRONIC Rx

- Adjust antibiotic therapy on the basis of culture results.
- In general, continue therapy for a minimum of 7 to 10 days.
- If hyperglycemia develops during treatment start continuous insulin IV infusion, maintain blood glucose in the 110-180 mg/dl level, and avoid insulin-induced hypoglycemia.

DISPOSITION

All patients with suspected septicemia should be hospitalized and given access to intensive monitoring and nursing care.

REFERRAL

- To infectious diseases expert
- To physician experienced in critical care

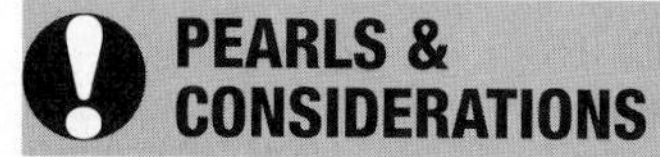

PEARLS & CONSIDERATIONS

COMMENTS

- Mortality rises quickly if antibiotic therapy is not instituted promptly (preferably within 1 hr of onset of shock) and metabolic derangements are not treated aggressively.
- Human recombinant activated protein C (drotrecogin alfa activated) was taken off the market as a treatment for sepsis after followup studies showed no added benefit to standard sepsis care.

SUGGESTED READINGS

available at www.expertconsult.com

AUTHOR: **STEVEN M. OPAL, M.D.**

BASIC INFORMATION

DEFINITION

Septic arthritis is a highly destructive form of joint disease most often caused by hematogenous spread of organisms from a distant site of infection. Direct penetration of the joint as a result of trauma or surgery and spread from adjacent osteomyelitis may also cause bacterial arthritis. Any joint in the body may be affected.

SYNONYMS

Infectious arthritis
Bacterial arthritis
Pyogenic arthritis

ICD-9CM CODES
711 Pyogenic arthritis, site unspecified
ICD-10CM CODES
M00.9 Pyogenic arthritis, unspecified

EPIDEMIOLOGY & DEMOGRAPHICS

INCIDENCE (IN U.S.): Unknown
PREVALENCE (IN U.S.): Unknown
PREDOMINANT SEX: Gonococcal arthritis in females
PREDOMINANT AGE: Gonococcal arthritis in sexually active adults
PEAK INCIDENCE:
- Gonococcal arthritis: young adults
- Other bacterial causes: all ages

PHYSICAL FINDINGS & CLINICAL PRESENTATION

- Hallmark: acute onset of monoarticular joint pain, erythema, heat, and immobility
- Limited range of motion of the joint
- Effusion, with varying degrees of erythema and increased warmth around the joint
- Single joint affected in 80% to 90% of cases of nongonococcal arthritis
- Gonococcal dermatitis-arthritis syndrome
  - Typical pattern is a migratory polyarthritis or tenosynovitis
  - Small pustules on the trunk or extremities
- Febrile patient at presentation
- Most commonly affected joints in adult: knee and hip, but any joint may be involved; in children: hip

ETIOLOGY

- Bacteria spread from another locus of infection
  - Highly vascular synovium is invaded by hematogenously spread bacteria.
  - WBC enzymes cause necrosis of synovium, cartilage, and bone.
  - Extensive joint destruction is rapid if infection is not treated with appropriate IV antibiotics and drainage of necrotic material.
- Predisposing factors: rheumatoid arthritis, prosthetic joints, advanced age, immunodeficiency (HIV, DM, immunosuppressive drugs), sexual activity (gonococcal arthritis), skin infections, cutaneous ulcers (contiguous spread), recent joint surgery, recent intraarticular infection. Fig. E1-848 illustrates routes by which bacteria can reach the joint.
- The most common nongonococcal organisms are staphylococci (40%), streptococci (28%), and gram-negative bacilli (19%). Less common are mycobacteria (8%), gram-negative cocci (3%), anaerobes (1%), and gram-positive bacilli (1%).
- Staphylococci (*S. aureus* and coagulase-negative staphylococcal species) account for >50% of prosthetic-hip and prosthetic-knee infections. *S. aureus* is very common in patients with rheumatoid arthritis.

Dx DIAGNOSIS

DIFFERENTIAL DIAGNOSIS

- Gout
- Pseudogout
- Trauma
- Hemarthrosis
- Rheumatic fever
- Adult or juvenile rheumatoid arthritis
- Spondyloarthropathies such as reactive arthritis (Reiter's syndrome)
- Osteomyelitis
- Viral arthritides
- Septic bursitis
- Lyme disease caused by *Borrelia burgdorferi*

WORKUP

- Joint aspiration, Gram stain, and culture of the synovial fluid. Fig. E1-849 describes an algorithm for synovial fluid analysis in septic arthritis.
- Immediate arthrocentesis before other studies are undertaken or antibiotics instituted. Synovial fluid should be evaluated at bedside and then sent for lab evaluation

LABORATORY TESTS

- Joint fluid analysis
  - Synovial fluid leukocyte count is usually elevated >50,000 cells/mm^3 with > 80% polymorphonuclear cells.
  - Counts are highly variable, with similar findings in gout, pseudogout, or rheumatoid arthritis. Lower WBC counts can occur in joint replacement, disseminated gonococcal disease, and peripheral leukopenia.
  - Synovial fluid glucose or protein is not helpful because results are not specific for septic arthritis. The differential diagnosis of synovial fluid abnormalities is described in Section III.
  - PCR testing: useful for detection of uncommon organisms (e.g., Lyme disease)
  - Crystal analysis: septic arthritis can coexist with crystal arthropathy; therefore, the presence of crystals does not preclude a diagnosis of septic arthritis.
- Blood cultures: positive in 25% to 50% of patients with septic arthritis
- Culture of possible extraarticular sources of infection
- Elevated peripheral WBC count, ESR (nonspecific), C-reactive protein (CRP) (nonspecific). When elevated, ESR and CRP may be useful to monitor therapeutic response.
- If gonococcus is suspected, perform nucleic acid amplification tests (NAATs) on synovial fluid.

IMAGING STUDIES

- Radiograph of the affected joint (Fig. E1-850): useful to rule out osteomyelitis, fractures, chondrocalcinosis, or inflammatory arthritis
- MRI: findings that suggest an acute intraarticular infection include the combination of bony erosions with marrow edema
- CT scan: useful for early diagnosis of infections of the spine, hips, and sternoclavicular and sacroiliac joints
- Ultrasound: can be useful for detecting effusions in joints that are more difficult to examine (e.g., hip)

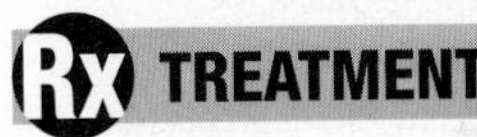

TREATMENT

NONPHARMACOLOGIC THERAPY

- Affected joints aspirated daily to remove necrotic material and to follow serial WBC counts and cultures
- If no resolution with IV antibiotics and closed drainage: open debridement and lavage, particularly in nongonococcal infections
- Prevention of contractures:
  - After acute stage of inflammation, range-of-motion exercises of the affected joint
  - Physical therapy helpful

ACUTE GENERAL Rx

- IV antibiotics immediately after joint aspiration and Gram stain of the synovial fluid. Empiric antibiotic therapy is based on organism found on Gram stain of synovial fluid:
  - Gram-positive cocci: vancomycin
  - Gram-negative cocci: ceftriaxone
  - Gram-negative rods: ceftazidime, cefepime, piperacillin-tazobactam. Aztreonam or fluoroquinolones can be used in patients with allergy to penicillin or cephalosporins
  - Negative Gram stain: vancomycin plus either ceftazidime or a carbapenem such as meropenem or ertapenem.

SUGGESTED READINGS

available at www.expertconsult.com

RELATED CONTENT

Septic Arthritis (Patient Information)

AUTHOR: **GLENN G. FORT, M.D., M.P.H.**

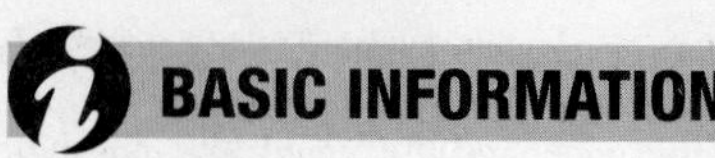

BASIC INFORMATION

DEFINITION

Serotonin syndrome (SS) refers to a group of symptoms resulting from increased activity of serotonin (5-hydroxytryptamine) in the CNS. SS is a drug-induced disorder that is classically characterized by a change in mental status and alteration in neuromuscular activity and autonomic function.

SYNONYMS

SS
Hyperserotonemia
Serotonergic syndrome
Serotonin toxicity

ICD-9CM CODES
333.99 Syndrome serotonin
ICD-10CM CODES

Y49	Adverse effects due to psychotropic drugs
Y49.0	Adverse effects due to tricyclic and tetracyclic antidepressants
Y49.1	Adverse effects due to monoamino-oxidase-inhibitor antidepressants
Y49.2	Adverse effects due to other and unspecified antidepressants
Y49.3	Adverse effects due to phenothiazine antipsychotics and neuroleptics
G25.89	Other specified extrapyramidal and movement disorders

EPIDEMIOLOGY & DEMOGRAPHICS

- The incidence of SS is not known.
- SS is seen in all age groups, from neonates to elderly.
- SS classically occurs in patients receiving two or more serotonergic drugs, but it can also occur with monotherapy—selective serotonin reuptake inhibitor (SSRI) monotherapy has an incidence of 0.5 to 0.9 cases of SS per 1000 patient-mo. Although there is an FDA alert, it has been argued that there is a lack of sufficient evidence showing that SSRIs and triptans cause serious SS.
- Concomitant use of an SSRI with a monoamine oxidase inhibitor (MAOI) poses the greatest risk of developing SS.
- Combination of SSRIs with other serotonergic drugs (e.g., tryptophan, illicit drugs like cocaine and MDMA, "Ecstasy") or drugs with serotonergic properties (e.g., lithium, meperidine, triptans, linezolid) may also lead to SS.

PHYSICAL FINDINGS & CLINICAL PRESENTATION

- Findings of clonus with hyperreflexia in the setting of recent (<5 wk) use of serotonergic agents strongly suggest the diagnosis of SS.
- Symptoms can manifest within minutes to hours after starting a new psychopharmacologic treatment, increasing the dose of a serotonergic drug, or administering a second serotonergic drug.
- Clonus (inducible, spontaneous, and ocular) is the key finding in establishing a diagnosis of SS.
- Other pertinent findings include:
  - Confusion, agitation, hypomania
  - Fever >38° C (100° F), tachycardia, and tachypnea
  - Nausea, vomiting, abdominal pain, and diaphoresis
  - Diarrhea, tremors, shivering, and seizures
  - Hyperreflexia and muscle rigidity

ETIOLOGY

- Hyperstimulation of the brain stem and spinal cord serotonin receptors leading to the neuromuscular and autonomic symptoms.
- Psychopharmacologic drugs—in particular, fluoxetine and sertraline co-administered with MAOI (e.g., tranylcypromine and phenelzine)—have been cited in the literature as a common cause of SS. Triptans (serotonin-receptor agonists used in the treatment of migraines) may also precipitate the SS when used in combination with SSRIs and serotonin-norepinephrine reuptake inhibitors (SNRIs). Box 1-74 describes classes of medications that produce SS in psychiatric patients.

BOX 1-74 Classes of Medications That Produce Serotonin Syndrome in Psychiatric Patients

Selective serotonin reuptake inhibitors
Monoamine oxidase inhibitors
Atypical antipsychotics
Heterocyclic antidepressants
Trazodone
Dual-uptake inhibitors
Psychostimulants
Buspirone
Mood stabilizers
Analgesics
Antiemetics
Cough suppressants
Dietary supplements

From Goldman L, Schafer AI: *Goldman's Cecil medicine,* ed 24, Philadelphia, 2012, Saunders.

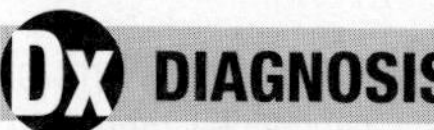

DIAGNOSIS

- The diagnosis of SS is made on clinical grounds. There are no specific laboratory tests for SS. A high index of suspicion along with a detailed medication history is the mainstay of diagnosis.
- Diagnostic criteria: most accurate is Hunter Serotonin Toxicity Criteria (sensitivity 84%, specificity 97%, confirmation by toxicologist). Sternbach's diagnostic criteria (Table 1-447) is also commonly used.
- To fulfill Hunter criteria a patient must have consumed a serotonergic drug and have one of the following:
  1. Spontaneous clonus
  2. Inducible clonus plus agitation or diaphoresis
  3. Ocular clonus plus agitation or diaphoresis
  4. Tremor and hyperreflexia
  5. Temperature greater than 38° C (100° F) plus hypertonia plus ocular clonus or inducible clonus

DIFFERENTIAL DIAGNOSIS

- Neuroleptic malignant syndrome (NMS), substance abuse (e.g., cocaine, amphetamines), anticholinergic toxicity, thyroid storm, infection (e.g., meningitis, encephalitis), alcohol and opioid withdrawal.
- Classic features in differentiation of NMS from SS are that SS develops over 24 hr, involves neuromuscular hyperactivity, and begins to resolve within 24 hr with appropriate therapy, whereas NMS develops gradually over days to weeks, involves sluggish neuromuscular response, and resolves over an average period of 1 wk to 10 days.

TABLE 1-447 Criteria to Determine Serotonin Syndrome and Toxicity

Sternbach's diagnostic criteria for serotonin syndrome	1. Recent addition or increase of proserotonergic medication 2. At least three of the following: • Agitation • Ataxia • Diaphoresis • Diarrhea • Hyperreflexia • Hyperthermia • Mental status changes • Myoclonus • Shivering • Tremor 3. Neuroleptic agent not added or dose increased before the onset of symptoms 4. Diagnosis of infections, withdrawal, and other poisoning or metabolic disruptions excluded
Hunter's criteria for serotonin toxicity (context of serotonergic medications)	1. If patient has spontaneous clonus, serotonin toxicity present 2. If no spontaneous clonus, one of the following needed for a diagnosis of serotonin toxicity: • Inducible clonus *and* agitation *or* diaphoresis • Ocular clonus *and* agitation *or* diaphoresis • Tremor *and* hyperreflexia • Temperature >38° C *and* ocular clonus *or* inducible clonus

From Adams JG et al: *Emergency medicine, clinical essentials,* ed 2, Philadelphia, 2013, Elsevier.

WORKUP

- Because SS is a clinical diagnosis, there is no laboratory test that confirms the diagnosis, and serum serotonin concentration does not correlate with clinical picture. Other causes are described in "Differential Diagnosis." Thus, all patients should have blood tests and diagnostic imaging studies to rule out infectious, toxic, and metabolic causes.
- Additional laboratory tests are performed to exclude complicating features of SS (e.g., renal failure secondary to rhabdomyolysis).

LABORATORY TESTS

- CBC with differential to rule out sepsis
- Electrolytes, BUN, and creatinine to rule out acidosis and renal failure
- Blood and urine toxicology screen
- Thyroid function tests
- Creatine-phosphokinase (CPK) with isoenzymes
- Urine and blood cultures
- ECG because ventricular rhythm disturbance is a potentially fatal complication

IMAGING STUDIES

Imaging studies are not specific in the diagnosis of SS and are only ordered to exclude other causes with similar clinical presentations as SS.

Rx TREATMENT

- Once a diagnosis of SS is established, appropriate consultation with a medical toxicologist, clinical pharmacologist, and/or poison control center should be sought.
- Management includes:
    - Discontinue use of all potential precipitating drugs
    - Provide supportive management
    - Control agitation
    - Administer serotonin antagonists
    - Control autonomic instability
    - Control hyperthermia
    - Reassess the need to resume the use of the serotonergic agent once the symptoms have resolved

NONPHARMACOLOGIC THERAPY

- Discontinuation of the drug is the mainstay of therapy.
- Treatment is supportive: maintaining oxygenation and blood pressure and monitoring respiratory status. Hypotensive patients may require both IV fluids and vasopressor therapy.
- Patients who are severely hyperthermic with temperatures greater than 41° C (106° F) should be given IV sedation, paralyzed, and intubated. Cooling blankets can be used for patients with mild to moderate hyperthermia. There is no role for acetaminophen here.
- Intubation is recommended for patients unable to protect their airways as a result of mental status changes or seizures.

ACUTE GENERAL Rx

- Benzodiazepines for control of agitation are preferred to physical restraints.
    1. Lorazepam 1 to 2 mg IV every 30 min has been used effectively in treating agitation, muscle rigidity, myoclonus, and seizure complications.
    2. Diazepam is an alternative choice.
- Blood pressure management with short-acting agents such as esmolol and nitroprusside.
- Serotonin antagonists should be titrated to clinical effectiveness in patients for whom nonpharmacologic therapy and benzodiazepines are not achieving adequate response, although substantial and rigorous data are lacking.
    1. Cyproheptadine 4-mg tablet or 2 mg/5 ml syrup is given 12 mg initially followed by 2 mg every 2 hr until therapeutic response is achieved in adults (up to 32 mg/day); children ages 7 to 14 should receive 4 mg every 6 hr (up to 16 mg/day), children ages 2 to 6 should receive 2 mg every 6 hr (up to 12 mg/day), and children younger than 2 yr should receive a maximum of 0.25 mg/kg/day as 0.06 mg/kg every 6 hr.
    2. Atypical antipsychotic agents with serotonin antagonist properties (e.g., olanzapine 10 mg SL) have been tried with some success.
    3. Chlorpromazine 50 to 100 mg IM may be considered in severe cases.

CHRONIC Rx

For patients not requiring hospital admission, cyproheptadine and lorazepam can be given in an oral dose on a prn basis with close follow-up.

DISPOSITION

- SS is a potentially life-threatening condition if not recognized early, although it does exist on a spectrum.
- Prompt diagnosis and withdrawal of the medication result in improvement of symptoms within 24 hr.
- Seizures, rhabdomyolysis, hyperthermia, ventricular arrhythmia, respiratory arrest, and coma are all complicating features of SS.

REFERRAL

All cases of SS secondary to psychotropic medications should be referred to a psychiatrist.

PREVENTION

Modify prescription practices by avoiding multidrug regimens.

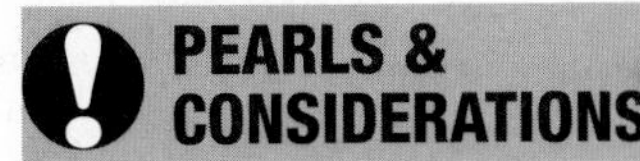

PEARLS & CONSIDERATIONS

The combined use of SSRIs and MAOIs is contraindicated.

COMMENTS

- The use of SSRIs and other serotonergic agents is not an absolute contraindication; however, prompt withdrawal of the medication is recommended if any symptoms suggesting SS occur.
- SS is usually found in patients being treated for depression, bipolar disorders, obsessive-compulsive disorder, attention-deficit disorder, and Parkinson's disease.

SUGGESTED READINGS

available at www.expertconsult.com

AUTHOR: **MARK F. BRADY, M.D., M.P.H., M.M.S.**

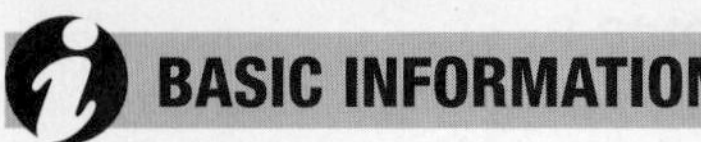

BASIC INFORMATION

DEFINITION

Sexual assault is any sexual act performed by one person on another without consent, resulting from the use of force, the threat of force or from the victim's inability to give consent.

SYNONYMS

Rape

ICD-9CM CODES
E960.1 Rape
ICD-10CM CODES
Y05 Sexual assault by bodily force

EPIDEMIOLOGY & DEMOGRAPHICS

INCIDENCE: 17.6% of women, 3% of men
PEAK INCIDENCE: As high as 25%
PREVALENCE (IN U.S.): 17.7 million women, 2.8 million men
PREDOMINANT SEX AND AGE: Female, age 16-24
RISK FACTORS: Alcohol/drug consumption, prior history of being sexually/physically abused, multiple sexual partners, involvement in sex work, poverty, incarceration/institutionalization, mental retardation

PHYSICAL FINDINGS & CLINICAL PRESENTATION

- Extragenital trauma: 70%: bruises, abrasions, erythema on thigh, arms, face, neck
- Anogenital trauma: 27%: injury to breasts, external genitalia, vagina, anus, rectum
- Physical findings more likely if examined within 72 hr of event, if event occurred outdoors, and if perpetrator was unknown

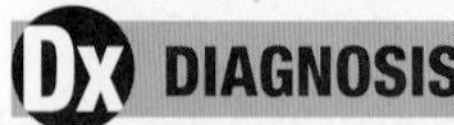

DIAGNOSIS

WORKUP

- History
  - Circumstances of assault: date, time, location
  - Physical description of perpetrator
  - Areas of trauma, specifically details of oral, vaginal, anorectal contact, or penetration
  - Condom use
  - Ejaculation: presence or absence
  - Presence of bleeding in victim or perpetrator
  - Recent consensual sexual activity
  - Showering, bathing, changing of clothes since event
- Physical examination
  - Ideally performed by individual trained to perform sexual assault examinations, i.e., SANE (Sexual Assault Nurse Evaluation) providers: www.sane-sart.com
  - Physical exam can take 3-6 hr to complete
  - Components
    - Physical examination of entire body
    - Forensic evidence collection
    - STD evaluation and treatment
    - Pregnancy risk evaluation
    - Care of injuries
  - General physical exam components
    - Documentation of any physical trauma, including photographs
    - Colposcopy: may reveal areas of minor genital trauma
    - Wood's light: to reveal foreign debris or semen
  - Forensic evaluation: not required, but should be offered; written informed consent needed
    - Commercially made specimen collection kits available: once completed, kits need to be sealed and handled according to kit instructions
    - U.S.: States required to provide free specimen collection
    - Samples of blood, saliva, mucosal swabs: buccal/vaginal/rectal, fingernail scrapings/clippings, hair specimens
    - Clothing: if unchanged since event
- Box E1-75 summarizes potential specimens to be gathered for forensic evidence collection.
- Fig. E1-851 describes an algorithm for emergency department management of patients after sexual assault.

LABORATORY TESTS

- Pregnancy test (if applicable)
- STD testing
  - GC/CT: recommended for all, may be excluded if individual elects for prophylactic treatment
  - Wet mount or vaginal swab for *Trichomonas*
  - Baseline HIV/hepatitis/syphilis testing: individual basis
    - Retest for HIV/syphilis at 6 wk, 3 mo, and 6 mo from incident

IMAGING STUDIES

Use of imaging studies as dictated by other injuries sustained for diagnosis/treatment of fractures, soft tissue, and other traumatic injuries

TREATMENT

NONPHARMACOLOGIC THERAPY

Acute crisis counseling: to support mental health needs of victim in immediate post-assault period

ACUTE GENERAL Rx

- Sexually transmitted infections
  - Empiric treatment recommended secondary to poor follow-up rates
  - Gonorrhea: ceftriaxone 250 mg IM *or* cefixime 400 mg PO
  - *Chlamydia:* azithromycin 1 g (single dose) *or* doxycycline 100 mg bid × 7 days
  - Trichomoniasis: metronidazole 2 g PO (single dose)
- Hepatitis B
  - If perpetrator known to be infected: HBIG + Hep B vaccination
  - If perpetrator disease status unknown: Hep B vaccination alone
  - If victim has already been vaccinated with documented immunity: no treatment necessary
- HIV
  - Use of antiretrovirals after sexual assault is controversial.
  - Overall risk of acquiring HIV is unknown but higher in certain situations.
    - Male-on-male rapists
    - Assault occurring in area with high local prevalence
    - Multiple assailants
    - Anal sexual assault
    - Presence of trauma, bleeding, or genital lesions in either victim/assailant
  - Antiretroviral drugs should be offered in all situations.
  - Ideally, antiretrovirals are initiated within 4 hr; should not start if >72 hr.
- Pregnancy
  - Pregnancy risk is estimated to be 5% per rape in women age 12-45.
  - Emergency contraception should be offered in all cases.
    - Levonorgestrel: 0.75 mg q12h for two doses or 1.5 mg single dose
    - Yuzpe regimen: 100 mcg ethinyl estradiol + 0.5 mg levonorgestrel, repeated in 12 hr
    - Ulipristal (selective progesterone receptor modulator): preferred method when >72 hr from assault
  - Antiemetics: EC + antibiotics for STD prophylaxis commonly causes nausea.

CHRONIC Rx

- No chronic prescriptions
- Long-term psychiatric counseling may be needed.

REFERRAL

Mental health professional

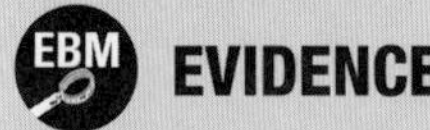

EVIDENCE

available at www.expertconsult.com

SUGGESTED READINGS

available at www.expertconsult.com

RELATED CONTENT

Chlamydia Genital Infections (Related Key Topic)
Contraception (Related Key Topic)
Gonorrhea (Related Key Topic)
Syphilis (Related Key Topic)

AUTHOR: **SARAH L. CHISHOLM, M.D.**

S

Diseases and Disorders

BASIC INFORMATION

DEFINITION

A sexual dysfunction in a woman is any disorder that interferes with female sexuality and that causes marked distress to that person. These disorders are generally categorized into four types:

1. Disorders of desire (most common)
2. Disorders of arousal
3. Orgasmic disorders
4. Sexual pain disorders (including dyspareunia, vaginismus, and vulvodynia)

Female sexual dysfunction is also further categorized as lifelong (primary) or acquired (secondary), situational (e.g., current partner) or generalized (all partners and settings).

SYNONYMS

Female sexual dysfunction

ICD-9CM CODES
302.70 Decreased libido
302.72 Disorders of arousal
302.73 Orgasmic disorders
ICD-10CM CODES
R37 Sexual dysfunction, unspecified
F52.31 Female orgasmic disorder

EPIDEMIOLOGY & DEMOGRAPHICS

INCIDENCE: According to the National Health and Social Life Survey, in 1999, ~20% to 50% of women reported some form of sexual dysfunction during their lifetimes. One third of women reported a decrease in sexual interest, and one fourth reported an inability to achieve orgasm.

PREVALENCE: A more recent survey of women 18 yr of age and older found an age-adjusted prevalence of any sexual problem to be ~43%.

PREDOMINANT AGE: Sexually related personal distress was more common in middle-aged women (aged 45 to 64) than in younger or older women.

RISK FACTORS:

- Correlates of distressing sexual problems include poor self-assessed health, low education level, depression, anxiety, thyroid conditions, and urinary incontinence.
- Obesity and overweight body status have been associated with lower sexual satisfaction and desire.

PHYSICAL FINDINGS & CLINICAL PRESENTATION

- History:
  - Important to obtain the patient's definition of the dysfunction, including its onset and duration; to determine whether the dysfunction is situational or global; and to determine whether more than one dysfunction exists and the interrelationship among the dysfunctions
  - Related medical and gynecologic conditions (including prior gynecologic surgery)
  - Psychosocial factors, including sexual abuse, sexual orientation, depression and anxiety, status of current relationships and sexual activity, personal and family beliefs about sexuality
  - Current medications including OTC and herbal preparations, alcohol, tobacco and drug use, and birth control method
- Physical examination:
  - The gynecologic examination can aid in identifying signs of decreased estrogen and androgen levels, infection, endometriosis, pelvic floor dysfunction, and systemic disease
  - Other body systems as indicated (e.g., cardiovascular, thyroid)

ETIOLOGY

- Chronic medical conditions (e.g., diabetes, coronary vascular disease, arthritis, urinary incontinence)
- Medication induced (e.g., antihypertensives, selective serotonin reuptake inhibitors [SSRIs])
- Gynecologic conditions (e.g., cystitis, posthysterectomy, gynecologic cancers, breast cancer [femininity/self-image issues; chemotherapy effects], postpregnancy, postmenopausal)
- Psychosocial (e.g., religion, taboos, identity conflicts, guilt, relationship problems, abuse, rape, life stressors)
- Fig. E1-852 illustrates the four phases of the human sexual response as postulated by Masters and Johnson.

Dx DIAGNOSIS

DIFFERENTIAL DIAGNOSIS

- Depression
- Psychosocial stressors
- Medical disease (e.g., thyroid dysfunction)

LABORATORY TESTS

- Cervical cultures and vaginal swabs for infectious disease
- Pap smear
- Appropriate laboratory tests if comorbid or chronic disease is suspected

IMAGING STUDIES

Appropriate imaging studies if comorbid or chronic disease is suspected

Rx TREATMENT

NONPHARMACOLOGIC THERAPY

- Education including a discussion of normal sexual behavior
- Stress management
- Activities to enhance stimulation and eliminate routine
- Distraction techniques
- Noncoital behavior
- Position changes (e.g., female astride)
- Lubricants (e.g., nonpetroleum based). There are several over-the-counter lubricants and massage oils, some of which are hypoallergenic, that can be safely applied to female genitalia

ACUTE GENERAL Rx

NSAIDs before intercourse for sexual pain disorders

CHRONIC Rx

- Treat underlying medical, gynecologic, or psychological conditions.
- Reduce comorbidities, including weight loss.
- Increase physical activity (associated with increased satisfaction and sexual engagement).
- For medication-induced conditions, decrease dose or change medication.
- For postmenopausal women or those with hypoestrogenism, try estrogen replacement therapy with or without progesterone.
- Testosterone therapy (still in Phase III clinical trials): results show increase in satisfying sexual activity and sexual desire.
- Sildenafil (evidence from RCTs for use in patients with neurodegenerative disease and antidepressant-induced FSD after traditional therapy has failed). Data are conflicting. Phosphodiesterase inhibitors may increase blood flow to the genitalia but generally appear to have little benefit in treating arousal disorders.
- Bupropion 300 to 400 mg/day was shown to increase sexual arousal and orgasm completion in a recent trial. In addition, adjunctive treatment with bupropion significantly improved key aspects of sexual function in women with SSRI-induced sexual dysfunction.
- Behavioral therapy (e.g., cognitive-behavioral therapy to reduce anxiety).
- Table E1-448 summarizes investigational pharmacotherapy for women's sexual dysfunctions.

REFERRAL

- Gynecologic referral for conditions that may be amenable to surgical therapy
- Psychological referral for conditions (e.g., depression, abuse) that may benefit from counseling or psychotherapy
- Social services referrals for active abuse issues

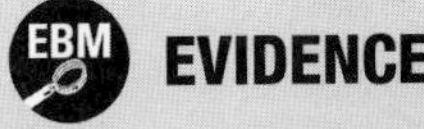

EVIDENCE

available at www.expertconsult.com

SUGGESTED READINGS

available at www.expertconsult.com

RELATED CONTENT

Female Sexual Dysfunction (Patient Information)

AUTHOR: **ANNGENE G. ANTHONY, M.D., M.P.H., F.A.A.F.P.**

BASIC INFORMATION

DEFINITION

Shaken baby syndrome is a potentially life-threatening and severe form of abuse in which an infant or child is violently shaken. Intracranial injury is caused by rapid acceleration and rotation of the cranium (sometimes associated with impact on a solid object which leads to rapid angular deceleration). The classic injury pattern associated with shaking includes diffuse subdural hemorrhage, retinal hemorrhages, and diffuse brain injury (Fig. 1-853). The diagnosis is often difficult to make because the clinical manifestations are nonspecific, perpetrators are unlikely to report a history of trauma, and there may be little to no external signs of injury.

SYNONYMS

Shaken infant syndrome
Abusive head trauma
Nonaccidental head injury

ICD-9CM CODES
995.55 Shaken infant syndrome
ICD-10CM CODES
T74.1 Physical abuse
T74.4 Shaken infant syndrome, initial encounter

EPIDEMIOLOGY & DEMOGRAPHICS

INCIDENCE: Most common cause of death or serious neurologic injury resulting from child abuse. It is specific to infancy, when children have unique anatomic features. A population-based study conducted in the U.S. showed an incidence of abusive head trauma in children <2 yr of 17 per 100,000 persons with a higher incidence in the first year of life compared to the second. Population-based studies in Europe show similar incidence in the first yr.
PEAK INCIDENCE: Shaken babies are typically younger than 1 yr; with median age of 4 mo.

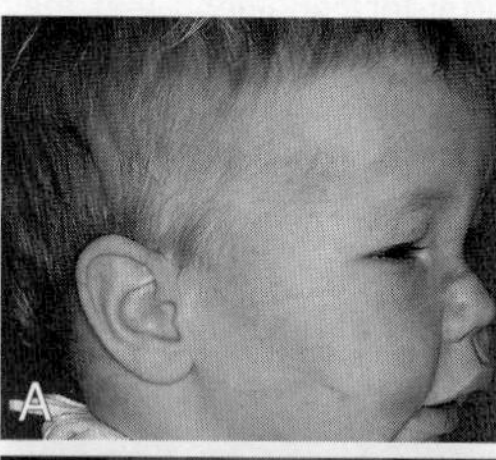

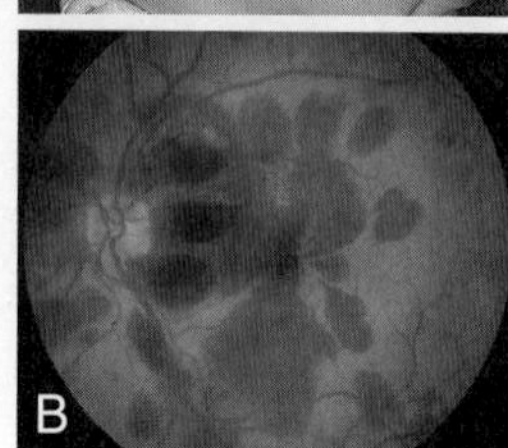

FIGURE 1-853 Shaken baby syndrome. A, Facial bruising. **B,** Fundus hemorrhages involving different levels. (Courtesy R. Bates. From Kanski JJ, Bowling B: *Clinical ophthalmology, a systematic approach,* ed 7, Philadelphia, 2010, Saunders.)

PREVALENCE: ~25% of clinically diagnosed babies with shaken baby syndrome die, and ~80% of the remaining suffer lifelong neurologic damage.
PREDOMINANT SEX: About 60% of identified victims of shaking injury are male. Children of families who live at or below the poverty level are at an increased risk for these injuries as well as any type of child abuse.
RISK FACTORS: History of abuse, history of domestic violence, low socioeconomic status, perinatal illness, incessant crying, and family dysfunction. The perpetrators in 65%-90% of cases are males and are most commonly the father.

PHYSICAL FINDINGS & CLINICAL PRESENTATION

In several retrospective series, no history of a traumatic event was offered in 64%-97% of cases. One study of 364 children with shaken baby syndrome found that 40% had no signs of external injury on initial evaluation. Majority will have an abnormal neurologic examination. Generally present with nonspecific symptoms (i.e., seizures, failure to thrive, vomiting associated with lethargy or drowsiness, decreased feeding, hypothermia, bradycardia, hypertension or hypotension, respiratory irregularities, apnea, coma or death). Retinal and cranial hemorrhages and brain injury are hallmarks of the syndrome. Other signs of abuse such as skull fractures, occult fractures (particularly of ribs and long bone diaphysis) and abdominal injury may be present.

ETIOLOGY

Angular deceleration forces cause primary parenchymal injury including traumatic axonal injury. Neuropathology and imaging techniques have established the cause of brain injury as hypoxic ischemic encephalopathy.

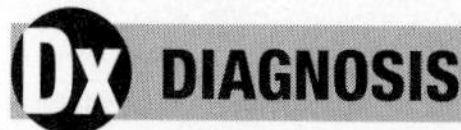

DIAGNOSIS

DIFFERENTIAL DIAGNOSIS

Head trauma from other etiology vs. infection vs. bleeding disorder vs. other etiology

WORKUP

Imaging of the brain, skeletal survey

LABORATORY TESTS

CBC, chemistry, coagulation study, lumbar puncture if meningitis is considered

IMAGING STUDIES

Initial study of unenhanced CT scan and skeletal survey. MRI should be done as follow up in patients with abnormal CT findings and is indicated for infants who are asymptomatic but require neuroimaging after finding noncranial injuries.

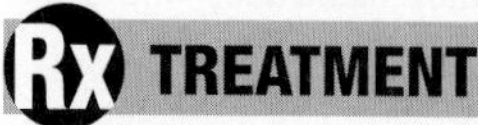

TREATMENT

Treatment focused on targeting specific injuries and also on prevention of future injuries.

NONPHARMACOLOGIC THERAPY

Admission to a hospital for observation.

ACUTE GENERAL Rx

Supportive care and interventions as dictated by the clinical, laboratory, and imaging findings

CHRONIC Rx

Counseling, working with the child's school to optimize academic development

REFERRAL

Neurologist and neurosurgery (if needed)

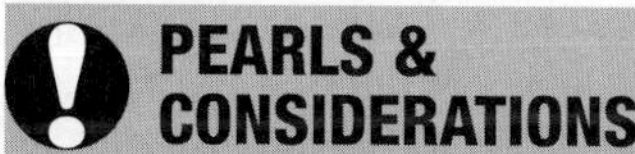

PEARLS & CONSIDERATIONS

PREVENTION

The National Center on Shaken Baby Syndrome offers a prevention program. Additionally, researchers like Harvey Karp have suggested ideas.

PATIENT & FAMILY EDUCATION

Shaken baby syndrome can result in lifelong, irreversible injuries. Prevention is a key component. Infants crying most commonly leads to shaking. Therefore the National Center on Shaken Baby Syndrome offers a prevention program, the **Period of Purple Crying,** which seeks to help parents and other caregivers understand crying in normal infants. By defining and describing the sometimes inconsolable infant crying that can sometimes cause stress, anger, and frustration in parents and caregivers, the program hopes to educate and empower people to prevent abusive head trauma.

Another method that may help is one suggested by author Dr. Harvey Karp's "five S's":

1. Shushing: use "white noise" or rhythmic sounds that mimic the constant whir of noise in the womb.
2. Side/stomach positioning: place the baby on the left side to help digestion.
3. Sucking: let the baby breast-feed or bottle-feed, or give the baby a pacifier or finger to suck on.
4. Swaddling: wrap the baby up snugly in a blanket to help him or her feel more secure.
5. Swinging gently: rock in a chair, use an infant swing, or take a car ride to help duplicate the constant motion the baby felt in the womb.

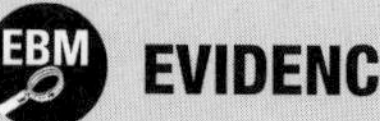

EVIDENCE

available at www.expertconsult.com

SUGGESTED READINGS

available at www.expertconsult.com

AUTHORS: **PRIYA SARIN GUPTA, M.D, M.P.H., LEANNA R. GARBUS, OMS III,** and **POOJA VERMA, M.D.**

BASIC INFORMATION

DEFINITION

Shigellosis is an inflammatory disease of the bowel caused by one of several species of *Shigella.* It is the third most common cause of diarrhea in the U.S. after *Salmonella* and *Campylobacter* and the most common cause of bacillary dysentery in the U.S.

SYNONYMS

Bacillary dysentery

ICD-9CM CODES
004.9 Shigellosis
ICD-10CM CODES
A03.9 Shigellosis, unspecified

EPIDEMIOLOGY & DEMOGRAPHICS

INCIDENCE (IN U.S.): 6.59 cases per 100,000 population with approximately 450,000 cases/yr
PREDOMINANT SEX: Male homosexuals at increased risk
PREDOMINANT AGE: Shigellosis predominantly affects children with 28 cases per 100,000 population in children less than 4 yr old and 25.67 cases per 100,000 population in children aged 4 to 11.
PEAK INCIDENCE: Summer
GENETICS: Neonatal infection: rare but severe

PHYSICAL FINDINGS & CLINICAL PRESENTATION

- Possibly asymptomatic, but incubation period can range from 1 to 7 days with an average of 3 days
- Mild illness that is usually self-limited, resolving in a few days
- High fever
- Watery diarrhea
- Bloody diarrhea
- Dysentery (abdominal cramps, tenesmus, and numerous, small-volume stools with blood, mucus, and pus)
- Descending intestinal tract illness, reflecting infection of small bowel first and then the colon
- Severe disease is more common in children and elderly and outside of U.S.
- Complications of severe illness:
  1. Seizures
  2. Megacolon
  3. Intestinal perforation
  4. Death
- Extraintestinal manifestations are rare
- Bacteremia is more common in children; in adults it has been described in patients with AIDS, the elderly, and diabetics
- Hemolytic-uremic syndrome (HUS): can be caused by *S. dysenteriae* 1.
- Reactive arthritis, sometimes as part of Reiter's syndrome following *S. flexneri* infection

ETIOLOGY

- *Shigella:* gram-negative rod bacteria that are less susceptible to stomach acid and thus as few as 10 to 100 bacteria can cause disease. The bacteria invade colonic tissue and cause inflammation.
  1. *S. flexneri*
  2. *S. dysenteriae*
  3. *S. sonnei*
  4. *S. boydii*
- *S. sonnei* is the most commonly isolated species in the U.S. (over 75% of cases), and it usually causes a mild watery diarrhea.
- Direct person-to-person transmission is thought to be the most common route. Outbreaks among men who have sex with men have occurred because of direct or indirect oral-anal contact.
- Contaminated food or water may transmit disease.
- Outbreaks have occurred in day care centers, a community wading pool frequented by toddlers, and residential institutions.

DIAGNOSIS

DIFFERENTIAL DIAGNOSIS

- May mimic other bacterial gastroenteritis, such as *Clostridium difficile, Salmonella, Campylobacter,* and *Yersinia.*
- Dysentery can also be caused by *Entamoeba histolytica.*
- Bloody diarrhea may resemble disease caused by invasive *E. coli* (IEC).
- Hemolytic-uremic syndrome caused by enterohemorrhagic *E. coli* (O157:H7).

LABORATORY TESTS

- The diagnosis is established by bacterial stool culture.
- Stool should be cultured from fresh samples, because the yield is increased by processing the specimen soon after passage. The best yield is from the mucoid part of the stool.
- Serology is available but rarely useful.
- Polymerase chain reaction (PCR) is available but due to cost used mainly for outbreak investigations.
- Fecal leukocyte preparation may show WBCs.
- Total WBCs may be low, normal, or high. Leukemoid reactions can occur in children.

IMAGING STUDIES

Abdominal radiographs may suggest megacolon or perforation in rare, severe cases.

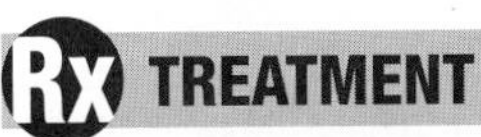

TREATMENT

NONPHARMACOLOGIC THERAPY

- Adequate hydration
- Electrolyte replacement

ACUTE GENERAL Rx

Antibiotics:

- To shorten course of illness
- To limit transmission of illness
- For adults: Pending susceptibilities, ciprofloxacin 750 mg PO bid for 3 days or levofloxacin 500-750 mg q day for 3 days should be used. An alternative is azithromycin 500 mg q day for 3 days.
- For children: IV ceftriaxone (50 mg/kg/day) for 5 days in cases of severe disease. For oral therapy, can use cefixime: 8 mg/kg/day as single daily dose or divided q12h for 5 days *or* azithromycin: 10 mg/kg/day in a single daily dose for 3 days. A short course of an oral quinolone can also be used safely although they are not approved for children.

DISPOSITION

- Most disease is self-limited.
- Severe illness may be fatal.

REFERRAL

For severe illness or complications

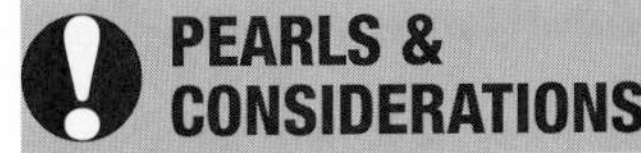

PEARLS & CONSIDERATIONS

COMMENTS

- *Shigella* is one cause of "gay bowel syndrome."
- Illness is worsened by agents that decrease intestinal motility.
- Food handlers, child care providers, and health care workers should have a negative stool culture documented following treatment.

SUGGESTED READINGS

available at www.expertconsult.com

RELATED CONTENT

Shigellosis (Patient Information)

AUTHOR: **GLENN G. FORT, M.D., M.P.H.**

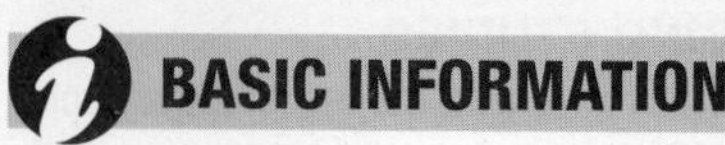

BASIC INFORMATION

DEFINITION

Short bowel syndrome (SBS) is a malabsorption syndrome that results from extensive small intestinal resection or congenital causes (Table 1-449).

SYNONYMS

Short bowel
SBS

ICD-9CM CODES
579.3 (Postsurgical malabsorption)
ICD-10CM CODES
K91.2 Postsurgical malabsorption, not elsewhere classified

EPIDEMIOLOGY & DEMOGRAPHICS

- Parallels Crohn's disease (see "Crohn's Disease" in Section I), which is the most common cause of the syndrome in adults.
- In children, two thirds of short bowels are related to congenital abnormalities (intestinal atresia, gastroschisis, volvulus, aganglionosis) and one third are related to necrotizing enterocolitis.
- Prevalence: 10,000 to 20,000 cases are estimated to exist in the U.S.

PHYSICAL FINDINGS & CLINICAL PRESENTATION

- Diarrhea and steatorrhea
- Weight loss
- Anemia related to iron or vitamin B_{12} absorption
- Bleeding diathesis related to vitamin K malabsorption
- Osteoporosis/osteomalacia related to vitamin D and calcium malabsorption
- Hyponatremia, hypokalemia
- Hypovolemia
- Other macronutrient or micronutrient deficiency states

TABLE 1-449 Causes of Short Bowel Syndrome

Congenital
Congenital short bowel syndrome
Multiple atresias
Gastroschisis
Bowel Resection
Necrotizing enterocolitis
Volvulus with or without malrotation
Long-segment Hirschsprung disease
Meconium peritonitis
Crohn's disease
Trauma

From Kliegman RM et al: *Nelson textbook of pediatrics,* ed 19, Philadelphia, 2011, Saunders.

ETIOLOGY

- Extensive bowel resection for treatment of the conditions mentioned previously (see "Epidemiology").
- Congenital (Table 1-449).

The human intestine is 3 to 8 m in length. Removal of up to half of the small intestine produces no disruption in nutrient absorption, and most patients can maintain nutritional balance on oral feeding if they have more than 100 cm (3 ft) of jejunum. Similarly, 100 cm of intact jejunum can maintain a normal water, sodium, and potassium balance under normal circumstances. The presence of an intact colon can compensate for some small intestine loss.

Site-specific functions:

- Calcium, magnesium, phosphorus, iron, and vitamins are absorbed in the duodenum and proximal jejunum.
- Vitamin B_{12} and bile acids are absorbed in the ileum. The resection of more than 60 cm of ileum results in vitamin B_{12} malabsorption. The loss of more than 100 cm results in fat malabsorption (from the loss of bile acids).
- The loss of gastrointestinal endocrine hormones can affect intestinal motility.
- Intestinal bacterial overgrowth may also occur, especially if the ileocecal valve is lost.

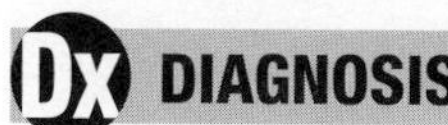

DIAGNOSIS

Presence of macronutrient and/or micronutrient loss in a patient with a known history of bowel resection

DIFFERENTIAL DIAGNOSIS

Because the history of significant bowel resection is typically known, there is no differential diagnosis. If that history is not known, all causes of weight loss, malabsorption, and diarrhea must be considered.

TABLE 1-450 Management Strategies for Short Bowel Syndrome

1. Acute phase
   a. Treat postoperative complications
   b. Maintain full support via the parenteral route
   c. Initiate low-rate trophic enteral feeds
   d. Document amount and site of remaining bowel and underlying disease
2. Early adaptation (up to 1 yr postsurgery)
   a. Increase enteral nutrition to tolerance; supplement with glutamine
   b. Achieve permanent parenteral access, if indicated
   c. Maximize antiperistaltic agents
   d. Octreotide for high-output ostomy or fistula
   e. Dietary counseling
   f. Clinical trials of trophic growth factors
3. Long-term adaptation (>1 yr postsurgery)
   a. Recruit bypassed bowel
   b. Bowel-lengthening procedure (Bianchi or STEP)
   c. Monitor for development of TPN-associated complications, and refer for transplant prior to recurrent sepsis, thrombosis, or end-stage liver disease

From Cameron JL, Cameron AM: *Current surgical therapy,* ed 10, Philadelphia, 2011, Saunders.

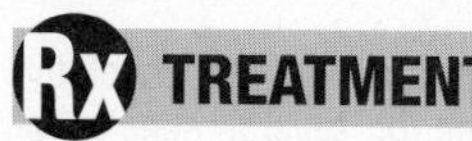

TREATMENT

Extensive small bowel resection with colectomy (<100 cm of jejunum)

- Rx: long-term total parenteral nutrition (TPN). Some patients can switch to oral intake after 1 to 2 yr of TPN. In jejunostomy patients, excessive fluid loss can be reduced with H_2 blockers, proton pump inhibitors, or octreotide. Micronutrients are supplemented.

Extensive small bowel resection with partial colectomy (usually patients with Crohn's disease)

- Rx: oral intake alone is possible in all patients with >100 cm of jejunum. In addition to vitamin B_{12} deficiency, these patients often have diarrhea. Consider lactose malabsorption and bacterial overgrowth treated, respectively, with lactose restriction and antibiotics (tetracycline 250 mg tid or metronidazole 500 mg tid for 2 wk). Nonspecific antidiarrheal agents may also be indicated (e.g., Imodium or codeine). The patient must be monitored for micronutrient losses.
- Table 1-450 summarizes management strategies for SBS. Intestinal transplantation is performed mostly in children at selective centers.
- FDA-approved medications for SBS in patients receiving nutritional support are:
  - Recombinant growth hormone somatropin (Zorbtive): effective in increasing weight and reducing parenteral nutrition volume. These effects do not persist when the drug is stopped.
  - Teduglutide (Gattex), a recombinant DNA analog of glucagon-like peptide-2. It promotes mucosal growth in the small bowel through stimulation of crypt cell proliferation and inhibition of enterocyte apoptosis. This drug may have to be continued indefinitely for effects to persist.

COMPLICATIONS

- Oxalate kidney stones
- Cholesterol gallstones
- D-Lactic acidosis

PROGNOSIS

- Directly dependent on the extent of the bowel resection and in the case of Crohn's disease by the underlying illness
- Whether the colon remains in continuity with the small bowel is an important factor in the patient's ability to adapt after significant small bowel resection.

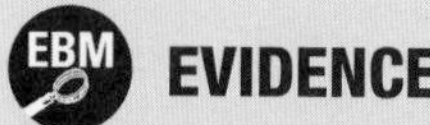

EVIDENCE

available at www.expertconsult.com

RELATED CONTENT

Short Bowel Syndrome (Patient Information)

AUTHOR: **FRED F. FERRI, M.D.**

S

Diseases and Disorders

DEFINITION

Short QT syndrome (SQTS) is a genetically inherited disorder of cardiac repolarization characterized by a severely shortened QT interval on the ECG, leading to atrial and ventricular arrhythmias and sudden cardiac death in affected individuals. This is a primary electrical disorder and patients have structurally normal hearts.

SYNONYMS

SQTS

ICD 9CM CODES
426.89 Other specified conduction disorders
ICD 10CM CODES
I45.89 Other specified conduction disorders

EPIDEMIOLOGY AND DEMOGRAPHICS

- Unknown; disease described for the first time only in 2000 (Gussak et al., 2000)
- This is primarily because, while there is near-unanimity on what constitutes the upper limit of a normal QT interval, no such consensus exists about the lower limit. In most (but not all) cases of the SQTS, the QT or QTc (corrected QT interval) has been <360 msec; however, there are many individuals with that QT interval who are clinically unaffected. Consequently, the incidence and prevalence is unknown, especially given the extremely small number of individuals diagnosed with the syndrome.
- Genetics: the disease is genetically heterogeneous and transmitted in an autosomal dominant fashion. So far, six variants have been identified. Three represent gain of function mutations, and three represent loss of function mutations. SQT1 is the most common variant described, due to a mutation in the cardiac ion channel KCNH2(HERG).

PHYSICAL FINDINGS AND CLINICAL PRESENTATION

- Seen across all age groups, though most patients are children or young adults.
- Syncope and cardiac arrest are the most common presenting features. Syncope is likely due to ventricular arrhythmias. Sudden death can happen with exercise as well as at rest.
- Atrial fibrillation and flutter are well described as being part of the syndrome.
- A significant percentage of patients are asymptomatic

ETIOLOGY

- Cardiac repolarization abnormality
- Genetic channelopathy transmitted via autosomal dominant mode, caused by missense mutations on genes (six identified so far)
- Mutations cause an increase in net outward current from either a reduction in inward depolarizing currents INa or ICa or augmentation of outward repolarizing currents I to, I K1, I K-ATP, I ACh, I Kr or I Ks. The resultant shortening of the action potential causes a shortening of the effective refractory period, with subsequent increased susceptibility of both atrial and ventricular muscle to premature depolarizations that lead to AF and VF.
- Acquired causes—see "Differential Diagnosis"

Dx DIAGNOSIS

- The differential diagnosis of a short QT includes various conditions such as hyperkalemia, hypercalcemia, acidosis, digitalis toxicity, effect of acetylcholine or epinephrine, sinus tachycardia, or hyperthermia. All these are possible causes of an acquired short QT interval that must be ruled out before a diagnosis of SQTS can be entertained.
- It must be remembered that merely having a short QT on the surface ECG does not confer a diagnosis of SQTS. The clinical history, including family history and genetic testing, are included in the criterion necessary to establish a diagnosis of SQTS, and are invaluable in making the diagnosis (Table 1-451).

WORK-UP

- Evaluation of any survivor of sudden death starts with a detailed history and physical examination, with particular emphasis on family history. Many patients with SQTS have unexplained syncope or palpitations prior to resuscitated sudden death. Atrial fibrillation is common in SQTS patients and a family history of lone AF should also be sought, in addition to resuscitated VF arrest.
- Physical examination is mostly normal in patients with SQTS.
- ECG findings in SQTS include not only an abnormally short QT interval (usually <360 msec), but usually also a short or even absent ST interval, with the T-wave appearing to emanate directly from the S-wave. T-waves are usually any combination of tall, narrow, and symmetric, with a prolonged Tpeak-Tend ratio (Fig. 1-854). Another feature to look for is the lack of adaptation of the QT interval to the heart rate (diminished rate dependence) as a result of which the corrected QT interval can be misleading; therefore, QT measurement on resting ECG in SQTS is more accurate with heart rate as close to 60 as possible.
- Echocardiogram and cardiac MRI should be performed to confirm a lack of structural heart disease.
- Holter recordings and stress tests can document a lack of variation of the QT interval in relation to the RR cycle; this is an important aspect of establishing the diagnosis. The QT interval shortens only slightly with increasing heart rates, so the QT and QTc values approach normal levels during faster heart rates. The QT fails to lengthen at slower heart rates.
- At electrophysiology study, the atrial and ventricular refractory periods are usually very short (140-200 msec at a CL of 400-600 msec). Sustained atrial fibrillation or flutter with rapid ventricular rates are often induced with programmed stimulation in the atrium. The inducibility of VF in SQTS patients at EPS is about 60%. EPS has a role in adding to the diagnosis by demonstrating short A and V refractory periods (also seen in other channelopathies such as Brugada Syndrome), but given its low sensitivity it cannot be used for risk stratification.

TABLE 1-451 SQTS Diagnostic Criteria

	Points
QT_c, msec	
<370	1
<350	2
<330	3
Jpoint-Tpeak interval <120 msec	1
Clinical history	
History of sudden cardiac arrest	2
Documented polymorphic VT or VF	2
Unexplained syncope	1
Atrial fibrillation	1
Family history	
First- or second-degree relative with high-probability SQTS	2
First- or second-degree relative with autopsy-negative sudden cardiac death	1
Sudden infant death syndrome	1
Genotype	
Genotype positive	2
Mutation of undetermined significance in a culprit gene	1

A minimum of 1 point must be obtained in the electrocardiographic section in order to obtain additional points.
High-probability SQTS: ≥4 points; intermediate-probability SQTS; 3 points, low-probability SQTS: ≤2 points. Electrocardiogram: must be recorded in the absence of modifiers known to shorten the QT. Jpoint-Tpeak interval must be measured in the precordial lead with the greatest amplitude T-wave. Clinical history: events must occur in the absence of an identifiable etiology, including structural heart disease. Points can only be received for 1 of cardiac arrest, documented polymorphic VT, or unexplained syncope. Family history: points can only be received once in this section.
VF, ventricular fibrillation; *VT*, ventricular tachycardia;
Adapted from Gollob MH, Redpath CJ, Roberts JD: The short QT syndrome: proposed diagnostic criteria, *J Am Coll Cardiol* 57(7):802-812, 2011. http://dx.doi.org/10.1016/j.jacc.2010.09.048)

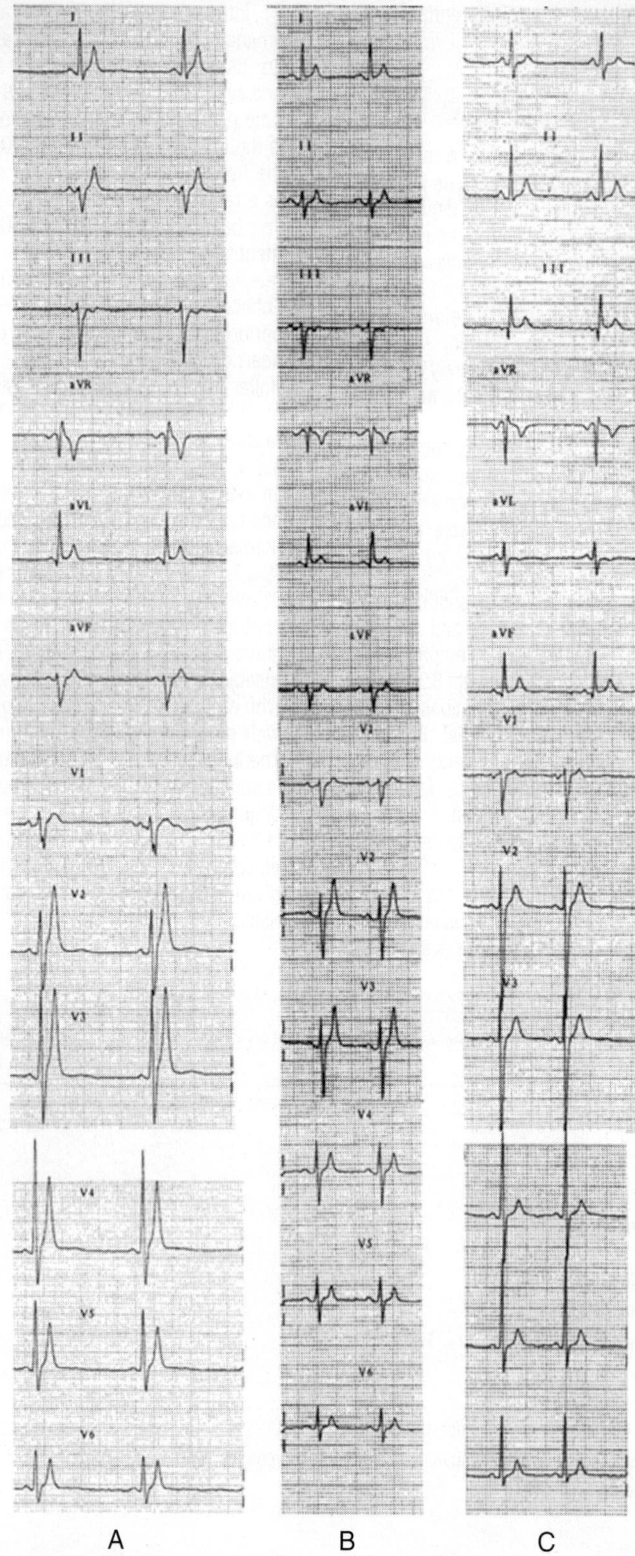

A B C

FIGURE 1-854 Twelve-lead ECG (25 mm/s paper speed) of family 1 patients. A, Patient 1 (IV, 3): sinus rhythm, heart rate 52 beats per minute (bpm); left-axis deviation, QT 280 msec. **B,** Patient 2 (IV, 2): sinus rhythm, heart rate 96 bpm; left-axis deviation, QT 220 msec. **C,** Patient 3 (V, 1): sinus rhythm with mean heart rate 92 bpm, QT 260 msec. (Adapted with permission from Gaita F et al: Short QT syndrome: a familial cause of death, *Circulation* 108:965-970, 2003.)

LABORATORY TESTS

Genetic testing is recommended for all patients in whom a diagnosis of SQTS is suspected. This is especially true if they have a clinical or family history of syncope or sudden death.

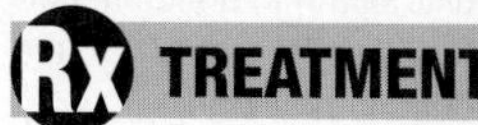

TREATMENT

- There is no significant clinical data on how to approach patients with an isolated short QT interval but no family or clinical history or genotype criterion (low and intermediate probability of SQTS). Risk stratification of these patients is not possible at this time; however, they should be referred to an electrophysiologist with expertise on this topic for comprehensive testing, including genetic testing.
- Patients with QT <330 msec and one criterion from clinical/family history or genetic testing fall in the high probability category of SQTS and hence a higher risk subgroup for sudden cardiac death. An ICD implant is recommended in this group for secondary and possibly also primary prevention against sudden cardiac death.
- A peculiar issue in patients with SQTS implanted with an ICD is double counting of peaked T-waves that are closely coupled to the QRS complex. This often leads to inappropriate ICD shocks. Most ICDs have programming modifications that can be turned on to get around this problem.
- Pharmacologic therapy is usually only advised in patients with multiple and frequent appropriate ICD shocks.
- However, they may be the mainstay of therapy in patients in whom an ICD cannot be implanted for various reasons, including in children in whom technical challenges are significant.
- While many drugs, such as flecainide, sotalol, ibutilide, hydroquinone, and amiodarone, have been used in an attempt to increase the QT interval, most of the available data favor hydroquinidine as the drug of choice across all forms of the SQTS.

REFERRAL

Consultation with an electrophysiologist is strongly recommended if SQTS is suspected.

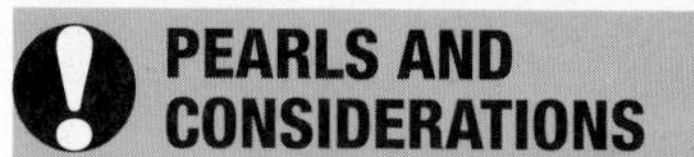

PEARLS AND CONSIDERATIONS

- SQTS is a rare genetic syndrome causing arrhythmias and sudden death.
- Should be suspected in patients with QT interval <360 msec presenting with syncope, sudden cardiac death, or atrial fibrillation and a family history of the same.

AUTHOR: **JOYDEEP GHOSH, M.D., F.A.C.C.**

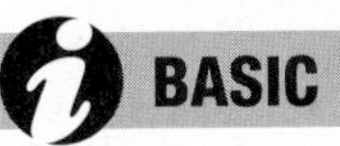

BASIC INFORMATION

DEFINITION

Sialadenitis is an inflammation of the salivary glands.

ICD-9CM CODES
527.2 Sialadenitis
ICD-10CM CODES
K11.20 Sialadenitis, unspecified

EPIDEMIOLOGY & DEMOGRAPHICS

Parotid or submandibular glands are most frequently affected (Fig. 1-855).

PHYSICAL FINDINGS & CLINICAL PRESENTATION

- Pain and swelling of the affected salivary gland
- Increased pain with meals
- Erythema, tenderness at the duct opening
- Purulent discharge from duct orifice
- Induration and pitting of the skin, with involvement of the masseteric and submandibular spatial planes in severe cases

ETIOLOGY

- Ductal obstruction is generally from a mucus plug caused by stasis of saliva with increased viscosity with subsequent stasis and infection.
- Most frequent infecting organisms are *Staphylococcus aureus, Pseudomonas, Enterobacter, Klebsiella, Enterococcus, Proteus,* and *Candida* spp.
- Sjögren's syndrome, trauma, radiation therapy, chemotherapy, dehydration, and chronic illness are predisposing factors.

DIAGNOSIS

DIFFERENTIAL DIAGNOSIS

- Salivary gland neoplasm
- Ductal stricture
- Sialolithiasis
- Decreased salivary secretion as a result of medications (e.g., amitriptyline, diphenhydramine, anticholinergics)

WORKUP

- Generally not necessary
- Ultrasound or CT scan in patients not responding to medical treatment

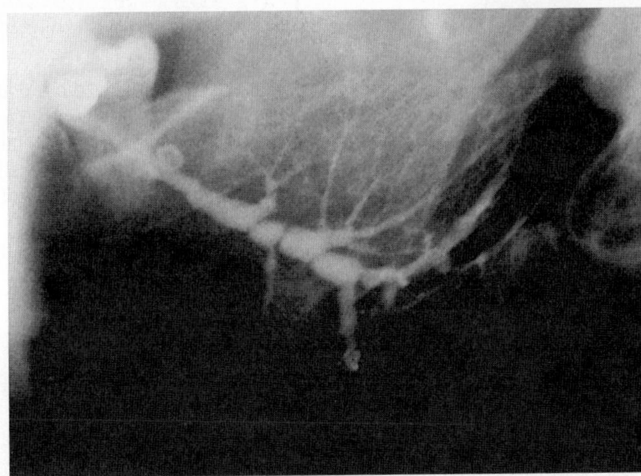

FIGURE 1-855 Sialogram of patient with chronic sialadenitis showing sausage link–like patterns and massive duct dilation. (From Blitzer CE et al: Sialadenitis. In Johnson JT, Yu VL [eds]: *Infectious diseases and antimicrobial therapy of the ears, nose, and throat,* Philadelphia, 1997, Saunders.)

LABORATORY TESTS

- Generally not indicated
- Complete blood count with differential to possibly reveal leukocytosis with left shift

IMAGING STUDIES

- Ultrasound or CT scan may be needed in patients not responding to medical therapy.
- Sialography should not be performed during the acute phase.

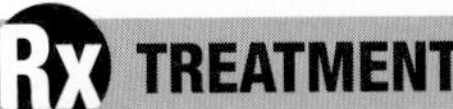

TREATMENT

NONPHARMACOLOGIC THERAPY

- Massage of the gland: may express pus and relieve some of the pressure
- Rehydration
- Warm compresses
- Oral cavity irrigations

ACUTE GENERAL Rx

- Amoxicillin-clavulanate 500 to 875 mg or cefuroxime 250 to 500 mg bid should be given for 10 days. Clindamycin is an alternative choice in patients allergic to penicillin.
- IV antibiotics (e.g., cefoxitin, nafcillin) can be given in severe cases.

DISPOSITION

Complete recovery unless the patient has underlying obstruction (e.g., ductal stricture, tumor, or stone)

REFERRAL

- To ear-nose-throat specialist for nonresolving cases despite appropriate antibiotic therapy
- For salivary gland incision and drainage, which may be necessary in resistant cases

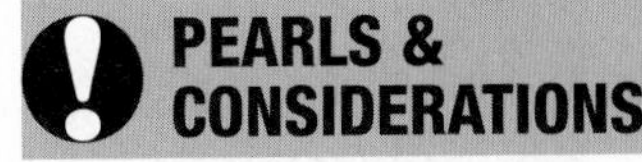

PEARLS & CONSIDERATIONS

COMMENTS

Prevention of dehydration will decrease the risk of sialadenitis.

RELATED CONTENT

Salivary Gland Inflammation (Patient Information)

AUTHOR: **FRED F. FERRI, M.D.**

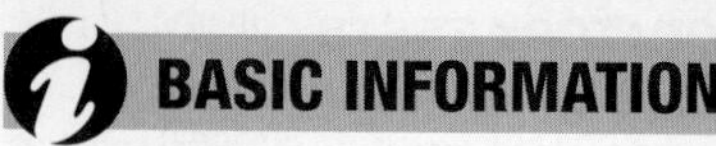

BASIC INFORMATION

DEFINITION

Sialolithiasis is the existence of hardened intraluminal deposits in the ductal system of a salivary gland.

SYNONYMS

Salivary gland stone
Salivary calculus

ICD-9CM CODES
527.5 Sialolithiasis
ICD-10CM CODES
K11.5 Sialolithiasis

EPIDEMIOLOGY & DEMOGRAPHICS

Affects patients mostly in the fifth to eighth decades and occurs most commonly in the submandibular gland (80%); only 14% are located in a parotid gland.

PHYSICAL FINDINGS & CLINICAL PRESENTATION

- Symptoms: colicky postprandial pain and swelling of a salivary gland. Tends to have a remitting/relapsing course.
- Signs: swelling and tenderness of a salivary gland. The stone may be felt by palpation of the floor of the mouth (Fig. 1-856).

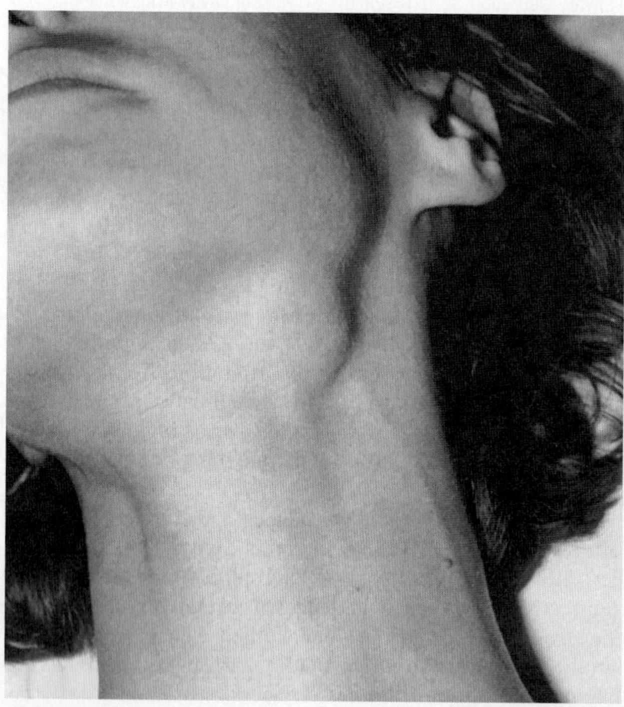

FIGURE 1-856 Patient with large calculus and obstruction of the left submandibular gland. (From Blitzer CE et al: Sialadenitis. In Johnson JT, Yu VL [eds]: *Infectious diseases and antimicrobial therapy of the ears, nose, and throat,* Philadelphia, 1997, Saunders.)

ETIOLOGY

- The cause is unknown. Contributing factors include saliva stagnation, sialadenitis (inflammation of a salivary gland), ductal inflammation, or injury.
- Salivary calculus composition is mainly calcium phosphate and carbonate, often combined with small proportions of magnesium, zinc, ammonium salts, and organic materials or debris.

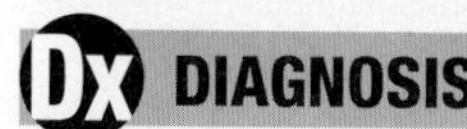

DIAGNOSIS

DIFFERENTIAL DIAGNOSIS

- Lymphadenitis
- Salivary gland tumor
- Salivary gland bacterial (*Staphylococcus* or *Streptococcus*), viral (mumps), or fungal infection (sialadenitis)
- Noninfectious salivary gland inflammation (e.g., Sjögren's syndrome, sarcoidosis, lymphoma)
- Salivary duct stricture
- Dental abscess

IMAGING STUDIES

- Plain radiograph
- Sialography

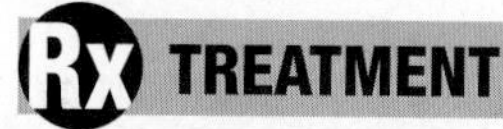

TREATMENT

- Warm soaks to area
- Antibiotics if associated bacterial sialadenitis is present
- Bland diet; avoid citrus fruit and spices
- Manual stone extraction sometimes associated with incisional enlargement of the ductal orifice
- Surgical salivary gland removal for retained hilar calculi

REFERRAL

To otorhinolaryngologist

RELATED CONTENT

Salivary Gland Stones (Patient Information)

AUTHOR: **FRED F. FERRI, M.D.**

BASIC INFORMATION

DEFINITION

Sickle cell disease is a hemoglobinopathy characterized by the production of hemoglobin S caused by substitution of the amino acid valine for glutamic acid in the sixth position of the gamma-globin chain. When exposed to lower oxygen tension, red blood cells (RBCs) assume a sickle shape, resulting in stasis of RBCs in capillaries. Painful crises are caused by ischemic tissue injury resulting from obstruction of blood flow produced by sickled erythrocytes. Vasoocclusive crises are the main reason for hospital admission of children with sickle cell disease.

SYNONYMS

Sickle cell anemia
SCA
SCD
Hemoglobin S disease

ICD-9CM CODES
286.60 Sickle cell anemia
ICD-10CM CODES
D57.1 Sickle-cell disease without crisis
D57.2 Double heterozygous sickling disorders
D57.3 Sickle-cell trait
D57.8 Other sickle-cell disorders

EPIDEMIOLOGY & DEMOGRAPHICS

- Sickle cell hemoglobin S is transmitted by an autosomal-recessive gene. In African Americans, the incidence of sickle cell anemia at birth is 1 in 600 and the incidence of all genotypes of sickle cell disease is 1 in 300.
- Sickle cell trait occurs in approximately 300 million people worldwide, with the highest prevalence of approximately 30% to 40% in sub-Saharan Africa. In the United States, it is found in nearly 10% of black Americans.
- It is estimated that 2000 babies are born with sickle cell disease in the U.S. each year.
- There is no predominant sex.

PHYSICAL FINDINGS & CLINICAL PRESENTATION

- Physical examination is variable depending on the degree of anemia and presence of acute vasoocclusive syndromes or neurologic, cardiovascular, genitourinary, and musculoskeletal complications. Pain in adults with sickle cell disease is the rule rather than the exception and is far more prevalent and severe than reported in older large-scale surveys.
- There is no clinical laboratory finding that is pathognomonic of painful crisis of sickle cell disease. The diagnosis of a painful episode is made solely on the basis of the medical therapy and physical examination.
- Bones are the most common site of pain. Dactylitis, or hand-foot syndrome (acute, painful swelling of the hands and feet), is the first manifestation of sickle cell disease in many infants. Irritability and refusal to walk are other common symptoms. After infancy, musculoskeletal pain can be symmetric, asymmetric, or migratory, and it may or may not be associated with swelling, low-grade fever, redness, or warmth.
- In both children and adults, sickle vasoocclusive episodes are difficult to distinguish from osteomyelitis, septic arthritis, synovitis, rheumatic fever, or gout.
- When abdominal or visceral pain is present, care should be taken to exclude sequestration syndromes (spleen, liver) or the possibility of an acute condition such as appendicitis, pancreatitis, cholecystitis, urinary tract infection, pelvic inflammatory disease, or malignancy.
- Pneumonia develops during the course of 20% of painful events and can present as chest and abdominal pain. In adults chest pain may be a result of vasoocclusion in the ribs and often precedes a pulmonary event. The lower back is also a frequent site of painful crisis in adults.
- The acute chest syndrome manifests with chest pain, fever, wheezing, tachypnea, and cough. Chest radiograph may reveal pulmonary infiltrates. Common causes include infection (*Mycoplasma, Chlamydia,* viruses), infarction, and fat embolism.
- Musculoskeletal and skin abnormalities seen in sickle cell anemia include leg ulcers (particularly on the malleoli) and limb-girdle deformities caused by avascular necrosis of the femoral and humeral heads. Osteonecrosis of the heads of the femur and humerus is found in nearly 50% of adults with sickle cell disease.
- Endocrine abnormalities include delayed sexual maturation and late physical maturation, especially evident in boys.
- Neurologic abnormalities on examination may include seizures and altered mental status. Strokes occur in about 10% of children and adults with sickle cell anemia.
- Infections, particularly involving *Salmonella, Mycoplasma,* and *Streptococcus,* are relatively common.
- Severe splenomegaly as a result of sequestration often occurs in children before splenic atrophy.

Dx DIAGNOSIS

DIFFERENTIAL DIAGNOSIS

- Thalassemia
- Iron-deficiency anemia, leukemia
- The differential diagnosis of patients presenting with a painful crisis is discussed in "Physical Findings"

WORKUP

- Screening of all newborns regardless of racial background is performed in the United States. Screening can be performed with sodium metabisulfite reduction test (Sickledex test).
- Hemoglobin electrophoresis will also confirm the diagnosis and is useful to identify hemoglobin variants such as fetal hemoglobin and hemoglobin A_2.
- Sickle cell disease encompasses genotypes associated with hemolysis and vasoocclusive crisis. Hemoglobin electrophoresis results, mean corpuscular volume, erythrocyte morphology, and degree of anemia can be used to differentiate among the sickle cell syndromes.
- For prenatal diagnosis, initial step is identification of parenteral globin gene mutation by DNA-based testing. If positive, then DNA-based testing of chorionic villus sampling or amniotic fluid cells is performed.

LABORATORY TESTS

- Anemia (resulting from chronic hemolysis), reticulocytosis, leukocytosis, and thrombocytosis are common.
- Elevations of bilirubin and lactate dehydrogenase are also common.
- Peripheral blood smear may reveal sickle cells, target cells, poikilocytosis, and hypochromia (Fig. 1-857).
- Elevated blood urea nitrogen and creatinine may be present in patients with progressive renal insufficiency.
- Urinalysis may reveal hematuria and proteinuria.

IMAGING STUDIES

- Chest x-ray is useful in patients presenting with chest syndrome. Cardiomegaly may be present on chest x-ray.
- MRI or bone scan is useful to rule out osteomyelitis (usually the result of *Salmonella*).
- CT scan or MRI of brain is often needed in patients with neurologic complications such as transient ischemic attack, cerebrovascular accident, seizures, or altered mental status.
- Transcranial Doppler ultrasonograhy (TCD) is a useful commodity to identify children with sickle cell anemia who are at risk for stroke. There should be an initial screening starting at age 2. Patients determined to be at risk should be enrolled in long-term transfusion programs. These are effective in reducing risk of stroke by >90%. In adults magnetic resonance angiography (MRA) can be used instead of TCD to identify those at risk for stroke.
- Doppler echocardiography may be helpful in diagnosing pulmonary hypertension but has a low positive predictive value. Screening for vasculopathy is done by estimating the tricuspid regurgitant jet velocity (TRV). Elevated

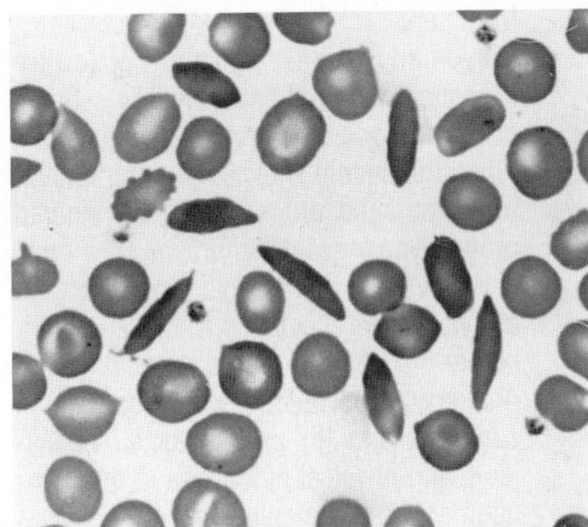

FIGURE 1-857 Photomicrograph of peripheral blood smear with sickle cells, typical of sickle cell anemia. (From Andreoli TE [ed]: *Cecil essentials of medicine,* ed 4, Philadelphia, 1997, Saunders.)

values are predictive of early mortality. The prevalence of pulmonary hypertension when right heart catheterization is performed is approximately 6% in adults with sickle cell disease.

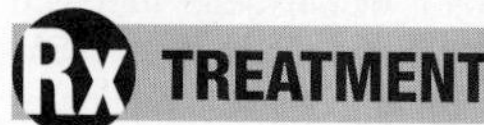

TREATMENT

NONPHARMACOLOGIC THERAPY

- Patients should be instructed to avoid conditions that may precipitate sickling crisis, such as hypoxia, infections, acidosis, and dehydration.
- Maintain adequate hydration (PO or IV).
- Correct hypoxia.

ACUTE GENERAL Rx

- Aggressively diagnose and treat suspected infections (*Salmonella* osteomyelitis and pneumococcal infections occur more often in patients with sickle cell anemia because of splenic infarcts and atrophy). Combination therapy with a cephalosporin and erythromycin plus incentive spirometry and bronchodilators is useful in patients with acute chest syndrome.
- Provide pain relief during the vasoocclusive crisis. The fear of creating or perpetuating addiction or being deceived by patients often causes physicians to prescribe subtherapeutic dosages of opioids. However, available evidence suggests that the prevalence of drug addiction among patients with sickle cell anemia is no higher than in the overall U.S. population. Medications should be administered on a fixed time schedule with a dosing interval that does not extend beyond the duration of the desired pharmacologic effect.
    1. Meperidine is contraindicated in patients with renal dysfunction or central nervous system disease because its metabolite, normeperidine (which is excreted by the kidneys), can cause seizures.
    2. Narcotics (e.g., morphine 0.1 mg/kg IV q3-4h or 0.3 mg/kg PO q4h) should be given on a fixed schedule (not prn for pain), with rescue dosing for breakthrough pain as needed.
    3. Except when contraindications exist, concomitant use of nonsteroidal anti-inflammatory drugs should be standard treatment.
    4. Nurses should be instructed not to give narcotics if the patient is heavily sedated or respirations are depressed.
    5. When the patient shows signs of improvement, narcotic drugs should be tapered gradually to prevent withdrawal syndrome. It is advisable to observe the patient on oral pain relief medications for 12 to 24 hr before discharge from the hospital.
    6. Analgesic medications should be used in combination with psychological, behavioral, and physical modalities in the management of sickle cell disease.
- Aggressively diagnose and treat any potential complications (e.g., septic necrosis of the femoral head, priapism, bony infarcts, and acute chest syndrome).
- Overall strategies for the management of acute chest syndrome are described in Table 1-452.
- Hydroxyurea (15 mg/kg body weight per day in patients with normal creatinine clearance) increases hemoglobin F levels and reduces the incidence of vasoocclusive complications. It is generally well tolerated. Side effects consist primarily of mild, reversible neutropenia. It should be avoided in patients with existing leukopenia, thrombocytopenia, or severe hypoplastic anemia. It is indicated for adults with sickle cell anemia who have moderate to severe disease, typically those with three or more acute painful crises or episodes of the acute chest syndrome in the previous year.
- Replace folic acid (1 mg PO qd) due to loss from increased utilization of folic acid stores due to chronic hemolysis. Sickle cell patients also often have mineral and vitamin deficiencies (calcium, zinc, and vitamins A, C, D, and E) and may need vitamin and nutritional supplementation.

CHRONIC Rx

- Guidelines for prompt management of fever, infections, pain, and specific complications should be reviewed.
- Genetic counseling is recommended in all cases.
- Avoid unnecessary transfusions. Exchange transfusions may be necessary for patients with acute neurologic signs, in aplastic crisis, or undergoing surgery. The target hemoglobin level is 10 to 11 g/dl (hematocrit 30%). Transfusing to a higher Hb/Hct should be avoided due to associated hyperviscosity if there is a substantial portion of HbS in the blood. Indications for transfusion in sickle cell disease are described in Table 1-453. Iron overload due to blood transfusions (transfusional hemosiderosis) can be treated with chelating agents (deferoxamine [SC infusion], deferasirox [PO], and deferiprone [PO]).
- Allogeneic stem cell transplantation can be curative in young patients with symptomatic sickle cell disease; however, the death rate from the procedure is nearly 10%, the marrow recipients are likely to be infertile, and there is an undefined risk of chemotherapy-induced malignancy. Myeloablative stem cell transplantation is generally limited to children under age 16 with severe disease.
- Penicillin V 125 mg PO bid should be administered by age 2 mo and increased to 250 mg bid by age 3 yr. Penicillin prophylaxis can be discontinued after age 5 yr except in children who have had splenectomy.

REFERRAL

- Hospitalization is generally recommended for most crises and complications.
- Psychosocial counseling and support structures should be developed.
- At least yearly evaluation by a hematologist competent in sickle cell anemia is recommended in all patients with sickle cell anemia.

TABLE 1-452 Overall Strategies for the Management of Acute Chest Syndrome

Prevention
Incentive spirometry and periodic ambulation in patients admitted for vasoocclusive crises, surgery, or febrile episodes
Watchful waiting in any hospitalized child or adult with sickle cell disease (pulse oximetry monitoring and frequent respiratory assessments)
Avoidance of overhydration
Intense education and optimum care of patients who have sickle cell anemia and asthma
Diagnostic Testing and Laboratory Monitoring
Blood cultures
Nasopharyngeal samples for viral culture (respiratory syncytial virus, influenza)
Blood counts every day and appropriate chemistries
Continuous pulse oximetry
Chest radiographs
Treatment
Blood transfusion (simple or exchange)
Supplemental O_2 for drop in pulse oximetry by 4% over baseline, or values <90%
Empirical antibiotics (cephalosporin and macrolide)
Continued respiratory therapy (incentive spirometry and chest physiotherapy as necessary)
Bronchodilators and steroids for patients with asthma
Optimum pain control and fluid management

From Kliegman RM et al: *Nelson textbook of pediatrics,* ed 19, Philadelphia, 2011, Saunders.

- Patients with pulmonary hypertension should follow up with a cardiologist and a pulmonologist.

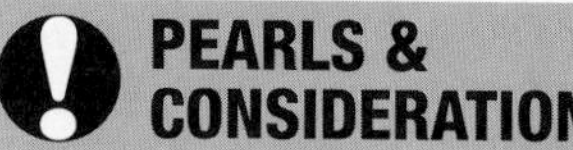

PEARLS & CONSIDERATIONS

COMMENTS

- Pain in adults with sickle cell disease is the rule rather than the exception and needs to be treated appropriately.
- Patients and their families should receive genetic counseling and should be made aware of the difference between sickle cell trait and sickle cell disease.
- Regular immunizations and pneumococcal vaccination are recommended. The prophylactic administration of penicillin soon after birth and the timely administration of pneumococcal and *Haemophilus influenzae* type b vaccines have resulted in a significant decline in the incidence of these infections. The heptavalent conjugated pneumococcal vaccine (Prevan) should be administered from 2 mo of age. The 23-valent unconjugated pneumococcal vaccine is given from age 2 yr and can be boosted once 3 yr later. Influenza vaccination can be given after 6 mo of age.

TABLE 1-453 Indications for Transfusion in Sickle Cell Disease

	Duration	Consensus	Method	Goal*
Stroke, acute	Single	+	Ex	HbS < 30%
Stroke, ongoing care	Chronic	+	Either	HbS < 30%
High-velocity transcranial Doppler	Chronic	+	Either	HbS < 30%
ACS, initial episode	Single	+	Dir > Ex	Hgb 10
ACS, recurrent	6-12 mo	+	Either	
Pulmonary hypertension	Chronic	+	Either	
Multiorgan failure	Single	+	Ex	
Major surgery	Single	+	Dir	Hgb 10
Acute anemia	Single	+	Dir	
Recurrent spleen sequestration	Chronic	+		
Sepsis/meningitis	Single	+	Dir	
Severe chronic pain	6-12 mo	+		
Congestive heart failure	Chronic	+		
Silent infarct with abnormal neuropsychology	Chronic	–		
Pregnancy		–		
Anemia/renal failure	Chronic	–		
Leg ulcers	6-12 mo	–		
Severe growth delay		–		
Severe eye disease		–		
Priapism		–		

ACS, Acute chest syndrome; *Dir,* direct; *Ex,* exchange; *Hb,* hemoglobin type; *Hgb,* hemoglobin concentration; +, consensus reached; -, consensus not reached.
*Goal of transfusion if a consensus has been reached.
From Fuhrman BP et al: *Pediatric critical care,* ed 4, Philadelphia, 2011, Saunders.

- Patients should be instructed on a well-balanced diet and appropriate folic acid supplementation.
- The presence of dactylitis, Hb 7, or leukocytosis in the absence of infection during the first 2 yr of life indicates a higher risk of severe sickle cell disease later in life.
- Among patients with sickle cell disease, acute chest syndrome is commonly precipitated by fat embolism and infection, especially community-acquired pneumonia. Among older patients and those with neurologic symptoms, the syndrome often progresses to respiratory failure.
- Poloxamer 188, a nonionic surfactant with hemorrheologic and antithrombotic properties, has been reported to produce a significant but relatively small decrease in the duration of painful episodes and an increase in the proportion of patients who achieved resolution of the symptoms. A more significant effect was observed in patients who received concomitant hydroxyurea.
- Pulmonary hypertension is a complication of chronic hemolysis and is associated with a high risk of death. It can be detected by Doppler echocardiography in more than 30% of adult patients with sickle cell disease. Cardiac catheterization will confirm the diagnosis. It is resistant to hydroxyurea therapy.
- Neurocognitive brain dysfunction is common in sickle cell disease. Trials have shown that compared with healthy controls, adults with sickle cell disease have a poorer cognitive performance, which is associated with anemia and age.
- Among patients with sickle cell disease hospitalized with vasoocclusive pain crisis, the use of inhaled nitric oxide compared with placebo did not improve time to crisis resolution.
- The average life span of individuals with sickle cell trait is similar to that of the general population. However, it is associated with a higher incidence of renal medullary cancer.

SUGGESTED READINGS

available at www.expertconsult.com

RELATED CONTENT

Sickle Cell Anemia (Patient Information)

AUTHOR: **FRED F. FERRI, M.D.**

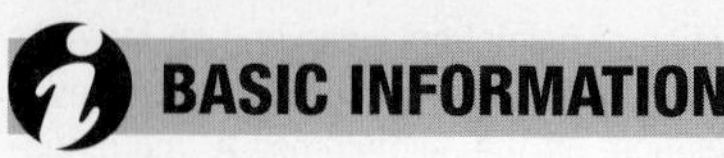

BASIC INFORMATION

DEFINITION

Sinus node dysfunction is a group of cardiac rhythm disturbances characterized by abnormalities of the sinus node, including (1) chronic, inappropriate bradycardia; (2) sinus pauses, arrest, or exit block; (3) sinoatrial exit block; and (4) alternating sinus bradycardia with paroxysmal supraventricular tachyarrhythmias known as tachycardia-bradycardia syndrome. When sinus node dysfunction is associated with symptoms, it is called sick sinus syndrome (SSS).

SYNONYMS

Sinus pause
Sinus arrest
Tachycardia- bradycardia syndrome
Sinoatrial exit block
SSS

ICD-9CM CODES
427.81 Sick sinus syndrome
ICD-10CM CODES
I49.5 Sick sinus syndrome

EPIDEMIOLOGY & DEMOGRAPHICS

- In children: associated with congenital and acquired heart disease, particularly after cardiac surgery.
- In adults: it is primarily a disease of the elderly secondary to idiopathic degenerative disease.

PHYSICAL FINDINGS & CLINICAL PRESENTATION

- Light-headedness, syncope, presyncope, palpitations. Other manifestations include dyspnea on exertion and worsening angina.
- Physical examination may be normal or reveal abnormalities (e.g., heart murmurs or gallop sounds) associated with the underlying heart disease.

ETIOLOGY

- Sinus node fibrosis is the primary etiology, which may also affect the atrioventricular node, the His bundle, or its branches.
- In addition, acute coronary syndromes, diseases of the SA nodal artery, inflammatory and infiltrative diseases such as hemochromatosis, amyloidosis, collagen vascular diseases (SLE and scleroderma), epicardial and pericardial diseases, medications (beta-blockers, calcium channel blockers, methyldopa, cimetidine, clonidine, lithium and antiarrhythmics), trauma following cardiac surgery, hypothyroidism, hypothermia, hypoxia, sepsis, muscular dystrophies (myotonic dystrophy, Friedreich ataxia), infectious etiologies such as Lyme disease, increased intracranial pressure.

DIAGNOSIS

DIFFERENTIAL DIAGNOSIS

- Bradycardia: atrioventricular block
- Tachycardia: atrial fibrillation
- Atrial flutter
- Paroxysmal atrial tachycardia
- Sinus tachycardia

WORKUP

- ECG (Fig. 1-858)
- Ambulatory cardiac rhythm monitoring
- 24-hour ambulatory ECG (Holter) with diary to correlate symptoms to findings
- Event recorder or a loop recorder if symptoms are less frequent
- Exercise stress testing to evaluate the severity of chronotropic incompetence
- Electrophysiologic testing, including sinus nodal recovery time and sinoatrial conduction time

TREATMENT

- Permanent pacemaker placement is primarily indicated if bradycardia is symptomatic. Indications for permanent pacemaker in sinus node dysfunction are described in Table 1-454.
- In tachycardia-bradycardia syndrome, drug treatment is indicated for tachycardia, primarily with AV node blocking agents after placement of the permanent pacemaker.

REFERRAL

To cardiologist

SUGGESTED READINGS
available at www.expertconsult.com

AUTHOR: **AMANDA C. DORAN, M.D., Ph.D.**

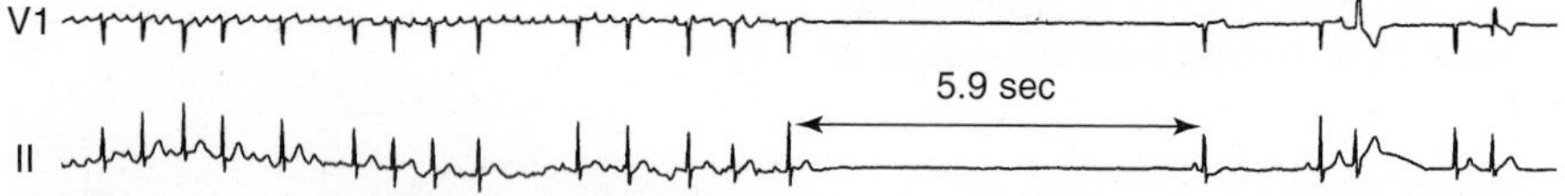

FIGURE 1-858 Tachycardia-bradycardia syndrome. Two surface ECG leads show atrial fibrillation that spontaneously terminates followed by a 5.9-second pause before sinus rhythm resumes. The patient became light-headed during this period. (From Issa Z et al: *Clinical arrhythmology and electrophysiology,* ed 2, Philadelphia, 2012, Saunders.)

TABLE 1-454 Indications for Permanent Pacing in Sinus Node Dysfunction

Class	Indications
I	• Sinus node dysfunction with documented symptomatic bradycardia or sinus pauses • Symptomatic sinus bradycardia that is iatrogenic and will occur as a consequence of essential long-term therapy of a type and dose of drugs for which there are no acceptable alternatives. • Symptomatic chronotropic incompetence.
IIa	• Sinus node dysfunction, occurring spontaneously or as a result of necessary drug therapy, with a heart rate of less than 40 beats/min when a clear association between significant symptoms consistent with bradycardia has not been documented. • Unexplained syncope when sinus abnormalities are observed or provoked with electrophysiologic study.
IIb	• A chronic heart rate of less than 40 beats/min, while awake, in the minimally symptomatic patient.
III	• Sinus node dysfunction in asymptomatic patients, including those in whom substantial sinus bradycardia (heart rate of less than 40 beats/min) is a consequence of long-term drug treatment. • Sinus node dysfunction in which symptoms suggestive of bradycardia are clearly documented as not associated with a slow heart rate. • Symptomatic bradycardia associated with non-essential drug therapy.

ACC, American College of Cardiology; *AHA,* American Heart Association; *HRA,* Heart Rhythm Society.
Adapted from ACC/AHA/HRS 2008 revised guidelines.

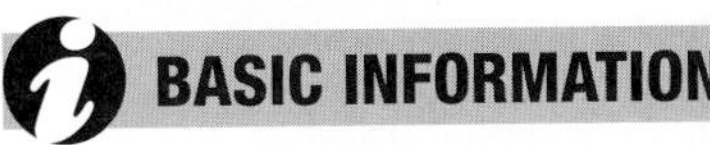

BASIC INFORMATION

DEFINITION

Silicosis is a lung disease attributable to the inhalation of silica (silicon dioxide) in crystalline form (quartz) or in cristobalite or tridymite forms.

SYNONYMS

Pneumoconiosis caused by silica

ICD-9CM CODES
502 Silicosis, occupational
ICD-10CM CODES
J62.8 Pneumoconiosis due to other dust containing silica

EPIDEMIOLOGY & DEMOGRAPHICS

- Occupational disease affecting men and women involved in gathering, milling, processing, or using silica-containing rock or sand. Jobs that can lead to silicosis are described in Box 1-76.
- An estimated 1 million Americans are exposed.

PHYSICAL FINDINGS & CLINICAL PRESENTATION

- Dyspnea
- Cough
- Wheezing
- Abnormal chest radiograph in an asymptomatic person

ETIOLOGY

- Silica particles are ingested by alveolar macrophages, which in turn release oxidants causing cell injury and cell death, attract fibroblasts, and activate lymphocytes, increasing immunoglobulins in the alveolar space.
- Hyperplasia of alveolar epithelial cells occurs.
- Collagen accumulates in the interstitium.
- Neutrophils also accumulate and secrete proteolytic enzymes, which leads to tissue destruction and emphysema.
- Silica dust may be carcinogenic (not proven).
- Exposure to silicosis predisposes to tuberculosis.
- Some patients develop rheumatoid silicotic pulmonary nodules and may have arthritic symptoms of rheumatoid arthritis (Caplan's syndrome). Scleroderma has also been associated with silicosis.

Dx DIAGNOSIS

DIFFERENTIAL DIAGNOSIS

- Other pneumoconiosis, berylliosis, hard metal disease, asbestosis
- Sarcoidosis
- Tuberculosis
- Interstitial lung disease
- Hypersensitivity pneumonitis
- Lung cancer
- Langerhans' cell granulomatosis (histiocytosis X)
- Granulomatous pulmonary vasculitis

WORKUP

- History of occupational exposure
- Chest radiograph (Fig. 1-859)

Chronic silicosis:
- Most common clinical presentation. Onset is after decades of repeated exposure.
- Characteristic finding: small, rounded lung parenchymal opacities
- Hilar lymphadenopathy with "eggshell" calcifications
- Pleural plaques (uncommon)

Accelerated silicosis (progressive massive fibrosis):
- Develops <10 years after initial exposure.
- Large parenchymal lesions resulting from coalesced small nodules
- Higher risk for progressive massive fibrosis

Acute silicosis:
- Develops several weeks to <5 years after silica exposure.
- Ground-glass appearance of the lung fields
- Chest CT scan
- Pulmonary function tests
- Combination of obstructive and restrictive changes with or without reduction in diffusing capacity
- Bronchoscopy with lung biopsy in uncertain cases

COURSE

Chronic silicosis:
- May not progress with absence of further exposure
- Accelerated silicosis: progressive respiratory failure and cor pulmonale

Acute silicosis:
- Fatal course from respiratory failure over several months to a few years

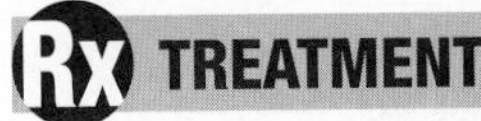

Rx TREATMENT

- Treatment is symptomatic (supplemental O_2 for hypoxemia, bronchodilators, antibiotics for infections).
- Prevention (industrial hygiene)
- Treatment of associated tuberculosis if present
- Supportive measures (oxygen, bronchodilators)
- Consider lung transplant for patients who develop chronic respiratory failure.

RELATED CONTENT

Silicosis (Patient Information)

AUTHOR: **FRED F. FERRI, M.D.**

BOX 1-76 Jobs That Can Lead to Silicosis

Mining: surface or underground mining (tunneling)
Milling: ground silica for abrasives and filler
Quarrying
Sandblasting (e.g., of buildings, preparing steel for painting)
Pottery; ceramic or clay work
Grinding, polishing using silica wheels
Stone work
Foundry work: grinding, molding, chipping
Refractory brick work
Glass making: to polish and as an abrasive
Boiler work: cleaning boilers
Manufacture of abrasives

From Goldman L, Schafer AI: *Goldman's Cecil medicine,* ed 24, Philadelphia, 2012, Saunders.

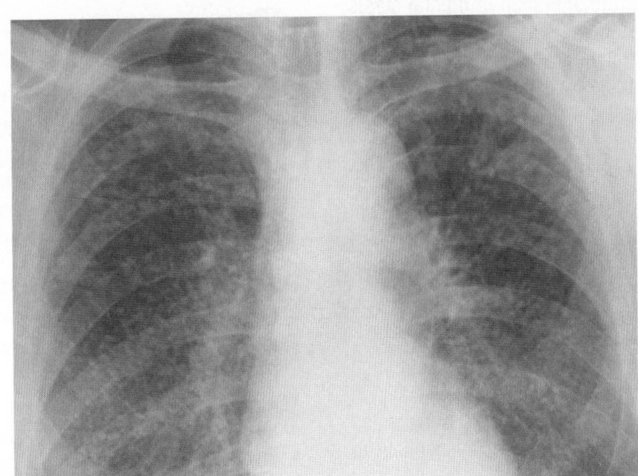

FIGURE 1-859 Simple silicosis. There are multiple small (2- to 4-mm) nodules distributed throughout the lungs, with an upper lobe predominance. (From McLoud TC: *Thoracic radiology: the requisites,* St Louis, 1998, Mosby.)

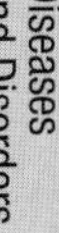

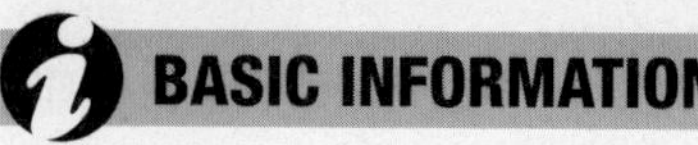

BASIC INFORMATION

DEFINITION

Cavernous sinus thrombosis (CST) is a late complication of facial or paranasal sinus infection, resulting in thrombosis of the cavernous sinus and inflammation of its surrounding anatomic structures, including cranial nerves III, IV, V (ophthalmic and maxillary branch), and VI, and the internal carotid artery.

SYNONYMS

CST
Intracranial venous sinus thrombosis or thrombophlebitis
Dural sinus thrombosis

ICD-9CM CODES
325 Phlebitis and thrombophlebitis of intracranial venous sinuses

ICD-10CM CODES
G08 Intracranial and intraspinal phlebitis and thrombophlebitis

EPIDEMIOLOGY & DEMOGRAPHICS

- CST is rare in the postantibiotic era.
- Before antibiotics the mortality rate was 80% to 100%.
- With antibiotics and early diagnosis, mortality rates have fallen to ~20%.
- Reported morbidity rates have also declined from 50%-70% to only 22% with advances in imaging modalities and aggressive medical care.

PHYSICAL FINDINGS & CLINICAL PRESENTATION

- Can be either an acute and fulminant disease or an indolent and subacute presentation.
- Septic cases of CST commonly present with high grade fever (picket fence pattern) and signs of sepsis.
- Headache, although not specific, is the most common presenting symptom and may precede fever and periorbital edema by several days. Elderly patients, however, may only demonstrate alteration in mental status without antecedent headache. The triad of unilateral or bilateral progressive chemosis, periorbital edema, and proptosis with headache is a classical presentation in patients with CST. These signs and symptoms are related to the anatomic structures affected within the cavernous sinus, notably cranial nerves III to VI, as well as impaired venous drainage from the orbit and eye.

Other common signs and symptoms include:

- Ptosis
- Cranial nerve palsies (III, IV, V, VI)
  1. Sixth nerve palsy is the most common (abducens nerve is located medially in the cavernous sinus and is surrounded by blood, making it more susceptible to inflammatory changes).
  2. Hypoesthesia or hyperesthesia of the ophthalmic and maxillary branch of the fifth nerve is common. Periorbital sensory loss and impaired corneal reflex may be noted.
- Papilledema, retinal hemorrhages, and decreased visual acuity progressing to blindness may occur from venous congestion within the retina.
- Pupil may be dilated and sluggishly reactive.
- Headache with nuchal rigidity and changes in mental status may occur if the infection spreads intracranially to the meninges and brain parenchyma.
- Infection can spread to the contralateral cavernous sinus through the intercavernous sinuses within 24 to 48 hr of initial presentation.
- Patients may also develop signs and symptoms of pituitary insufficiency.

ETIOLOGY

- CST most commonly results from contiguous spread of an infection from the sinuses (sphenoid, ethmoid, or frontal) or the medial third of the face (areas around the eyes and nose that drain to the ophthalmic vein). Nasal furuncles are the most common facial infection to produce this complication. Less-common primary sites of infection include dental abscess, tonsils, soft palate, middle ear, or orbit (orbital cellulitis).
- CST also can result from hematogenous spread of infection to the cavernous sinus by the superior and inferior ophthalmic veins or through the lateral and sigmoid sinuses. It can spread in a retrograde direction depending on the pressure gradients, because the dural sinuses are valveless.
- *Staphylococcus aureus* is the most commonly identified pathogen, found in 60% to 70% of the cases.
- *Streptococcus* is the second leading cause.
- Gram-negative rods and anaerobes may also lead to CST.
- Rarely, *Aspergillus fumigatus* and mucormycosis cause CST.
- Risk factors for dural sinus thrombosis include venous hypercoagulable disorders, infections (see above), trauma, malignancies, systemic inflammatory disorders, pregnancy, and dehydration.

Dx DIAGNOSIS

- The diagnosis of CST is made by clinical suspicion and confirmed by appropriate imaging studies.
- Proptosis, ptosis, chemosis, and cranial nerve palsy beginning in one eye and progressing to the other eye establish the diagnosis.

DIFFERENTIAL DIAGNOSIS

- Orbital or periorbital cellulitis
- Internal carotid artery aneurysm or fistula
- Cerebrovascular disease
- Migraine headache
- Allergic blepharitis
- Thyroid ophthalmopathy
- Orbital neoplasm
- Meningitis
- Epidural and subdural infections
- Epidural and subdural hematoma
- Subarachnoid hemorrhage
- Acute angle-closure glaucoma
- Trauma

WORKUP

CST is a clinical diagnosis, with laboratory tests and imaging studies confirming the clinical impression.

LABORATORY TESTS

- Complete blood count, erythrocyte sedimentation rate, blood cultures, and sinus cultures help establish and identify an infectious primary source. Metabolic panel to look for electrolyte imbalances in cases of suspected pituitary involvement (DI/SIADH).
- Lumbar puncture (LP) helps to distinguish CST from more localized processes (e.g., sinusitis, orbital cellulitis). LP reveals inflammatory cells in 75% of cases. In half of these cases, the cerebrospinal fluid profile is typical for a parameningeal focus (high white blood cells with polymorphonuclear and/or mononuclear cells, normal glucose, normal protein, culture negative), and in one third may be similar to that of a bacterial meningitis.

IMAGING STUDIES

- MRI with gadolinium, including magnetic resonance angiography and magnetic resonance venogram (Fig. 1-860), is more sensitive than CT scan and is the imaging study of choice to diagnose CST. Findings may include deformity of the internal carotid artery within the cavernous sinus and an obvious signal hyperintensity within thrombosed vascular sinuses.
- Noncontrast CT scan of the head and orbits may demonstrate increased density in the region of the cavernous sinus but has relatively low sensitivity. Contrast-enhanced CT scan may reveal underlying sinusitis, thickening of the superior ophthalmic vein, and irregular filling defects within the cavernous sinus; however, findings may be normal early in the disease course.

Rx TREATMENT

NONPHARMACOLOGIC THERAPY

Recognizing the primary source of infection (i.e., facial cellulitis, middle ear, and sinus infections) and treating the primary source expeditiously is the best way to prevent CST.

ACUTE GENERAL Rx

- Appropriate therapy should take into account the primary source of infection as well as possible associated complications such as brain abscess, meningitis, or subdural empyema.
- Broad-spectrum intravenous antibiotics are used as empiric therapy until a definite pathogen is found. Treatment should include vancomycin to cover hospital or community-acquired methicillin-resistant *Staphylococcus*

aureus or resistant *Streptococcus pneumoniae* plus a third- or fourth-generation cephalosporin:

1. Vancomycin (1 g q12h with normal renal function) plus either ceftriaxone (2 g q12h) or cefepime (2 g q8 to 12h).
2. Metronidazole 500 mg IV q6h should be added if anaerobic bacterial infection is suspected (dental or sinus infection).

- Most experts recommend anticoagulation with heparin after the diagnosis is confirmed, unless surgical intervention is planned or there is evidence of an expanding hematoma. Cerebral infarction or intracranial hemorrhage should first be ruled out before initiating heparin therapy. Early heparinization has been suggested in patients with unilateral CST to prevent clot propagation. Coumadin therapy should be avoided in the acute phase of the illness but should ultimately be instituted to achieve an INR of 2 to 3 and continued until the infection, symptoms, and signs of CST have resolved or significantly improved. Retrospective case reports and case series have demonstrated a favorable outcome in terms of decreased mortality in the anticoagulated patients.
- Steroid therapy is also controversial but may prove helpful in reducing cranial nerve dysfunction or when progression to pituitary insufficiency occurs. Corticosteroids should only be instituted after appropriate antibiotic coverage. Dexamethasone 10 mg q6h is the treatment of choice.
- Emergent surgical drainage with sphenoidotomy is indicated if the primary site of infection is believed to be the sphenoid sinus.

CHRONIC Rx

- Patients with CST are usually treated with prolonged courses (3 to 4 wk) of IV antibiotics. If there is evidence of complications such as intracranial suppuration, 6 to 8 wk of total therapy may be warranted.

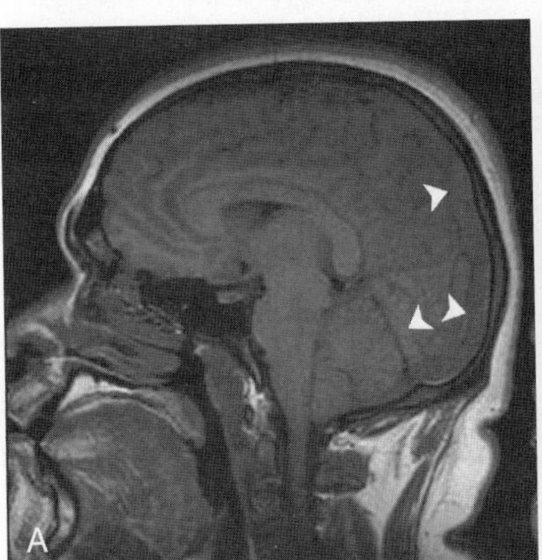

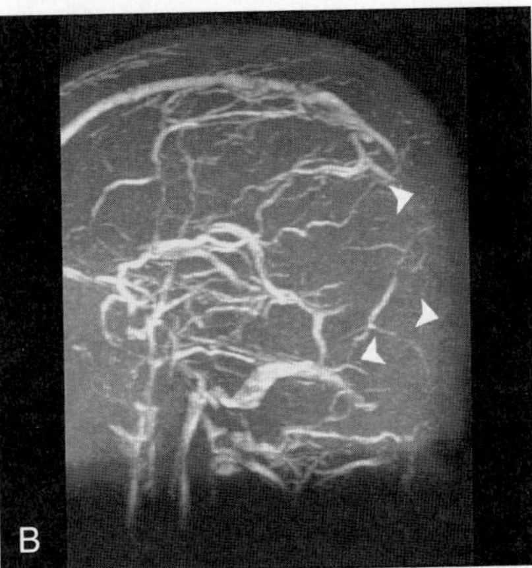

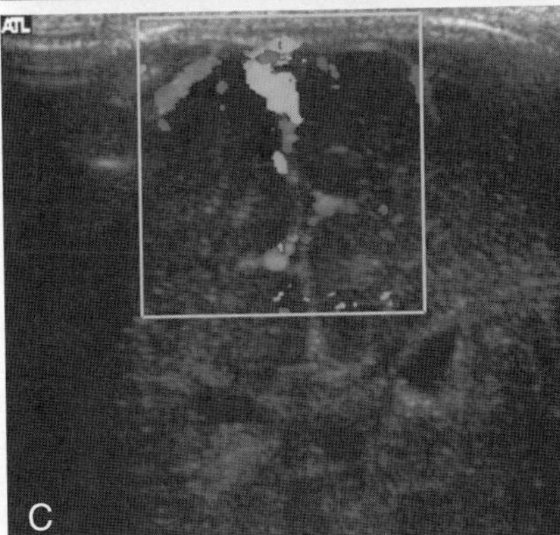

FIGURE 1-860 Superior sagittal sinus (SSS) thrombosis on magnetic resonance venogram (MRV). Sagittal T1 magnetic resonance imaging **(A)** shows intermediate signal intensity in sagittal and straight sinuses *(arrowheads).* No flow is seen on MRV **(B)** in these vessels *(arrowheads),* which is consistent with thrombosis. Color Doppler evacuation **(C)** of the SSS in another 6-mo-old patient with suspected thrombosis demonstrated a patent SSS with normal draining cortical veins. (From Fuhrman BP et al: *Pediatric critical care,* ed 4, Philadelphia, 2011, Saunders.)

- All patients should be monitored for signs of complicated infection, continued sepsis, or septic emboli while antibiotic therapy is being administered. Relapse of septic CST can occur after an initial improvement weeks after stopping antibiotic treatment.

DISPOSITION

- CST can be a life-threatening, rapidly progressive infectious disease with high morbidity and mortality rates (30%) despite antibiotic use. Morbidity and mortality rates are increased in cases of sphenoid sinus infection.
- Complications of untreated CST include extension of thrombus to other dural sinuses, carotid thrombosis with concomitant strokes, subdural empyema, brain abscess, or meningitis. Septic embolization may also occur to the lungs, resulting in acute respiratory distress syndrome, pulmonary abscess, empyema, and pneumothorax.
- Thirty percent of treated patients develop long-term sequelae, including cranial nerve palsies, blindness, pituitary insufficiency, and hemiparesis.

REFERRAL

CST if suspected, it should be considered a medical emergency. Depending on source of infection, appropriate consultation should be made (i.e., ear-nose-throat, ophthalmology, and infectious disease).

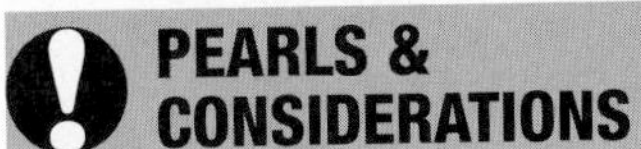

PEARLS & CONSIDERATIONS

COMMENTS

CST is a medical emergency and should be suspected with progressing chemosis, proptosis, and cranial neuropathy in a patient with headaches with or without fever.

The anatomy of the cavernous sinus explains the clinical findings: CS lies just above and lateral to the sphenoid sinus and drains the middle portion of the face by the superior and inferior ophthalmic veins; cranial nerves III, IV, V, and VI pass alongside or through the cavernous sinus.

SUGGESTED READINGS

available at www.expertconsult.com

RELATED CONTENT

Cavernous Sinus Thrombosis (Patient Information)

AUTHOR: **PRASHANTH KRISHNAMOHAN, M.B.B.S., M.D.**

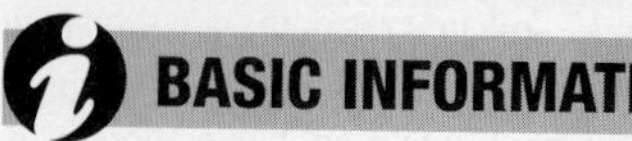

BASIC INFORMATION

DEFINITION

Sinusitis is inflammation of the mucous membranes lining one or more of the paranasal sinuses. The various presentations are:

- Acute sinusitis: infection lasting <4 wk, with complete resolution of symptoms.
- Subacute infection: lasts from 4 to 12 wk, with complete resolution of symptoms.
- Recurrent acute infection: episodes of acute infection lasting <30 days, with resolution of symptoms, which recur at intervals at least 10 days apart.
- Chronic sinusitis: inflammation lasting >12 wk, with persistent upper respiratory symptoms.
- Acute bacterial sinusitis superimposed on chronic sinusitis: new symptoms that occur in patients with residual symptoms from prior infection(s). With treatment, the new symptoms resolve but the residual ones do not.

SYNONYMS

Rhinosinusitis: sinusitis is almost always accompanied by inflammation of the nasal mucosa; thus it is now the preferred term.

ICD-9CM CODES
473.9 Sinusitis (accessory) (nasal) (hyperplastic) (nonpurulent) (purulent) (chronic)
461.9 Acute sinusitis
ICD-10CM CODES
J32.9 Chronic sinusitis, unspecified
J01.90 Acute sinusitis, unspecified

EPIDEMIOLOGY & DEMOGRAPHICS

INCIDENCE (IN U.S.): Seems to correlate with the incidence of upper respiratory tract infections and higher in women than men; 30 million cases a year in the U.S.

PEAK INCIDENCE:

- Fall, winter, spring: September through March
- In adults: greatest incidence between 45 and 74 years of age

PHYSICAL FINDINGS & CLINICAL PRESENTATION

- Patients often give a history of a recent upper respiratory illness with some improvement, then a relapse.
- Mucopurulent secretions in the nasal passage:
  1. Purulent nasal and postnasal discharge lasting 7 to 10 days
  2. Facial tightness, pressure, or pain
  3. Nasal obstruction
  4. Headache
  5. Decreased sense of smell
  6. Purulent pharyngeal secretions, brought up with cough, often worse at night
- Erythema, swelling, and tenderness over the infected sinus in a small proportion of patients:
  1. Diagnosis cannot be excluded by the absence of such findings.
  2. These findings are not common, and do not correlate with number of positive sinus aspirates.
- Intermittent low-grade fever in about half of adults with acute bacterial sinusitis.
- Toothache is a common complaint when the maxillary sinus is involved.
- Periorbital cellulitis and excessive tearing with ethmoid sinusitis:
  1. Orbital extension of infection: chemosis, proptosis, impaired extraocular movements
- Characteristics of acute sinusitis in children with upper respiratory tract infections:
  1. Persistence of symptoms
  2. Cough
  3. Bad breath
- Symptoms of chronic sinusitis (may or may not be present):
  1. Nasal or postnasal discharge
  2. Fever
  3. Facial pain or pressure
  4. Headache
- Nosocomial sinusitis is typically seen in patients with nasogastric tubes or nasotracheal intubation.

ETIOLOGY

- Each of the four paranasal sinuses is connected to the nasal cavity by narrow tubes (ostia), 1 to 3 mm in diameter; these drain directly into the nose through the turbinates. The sinuses are lined with a ciliated mucous membrane (mucoperiosteum).
- Acute viral infection:
  1. Infection with the common cold or influenza
  2. Mucosal edema and sinus inflammation
  3. Decreased drainage of thick secretions/obstruction of the sinus ostia
  4. Subsequent entrapment of bacteria
     a. Multiplication of bacteria
     b. Secondary bacterial infection
- Other predisposing factors:
  1. Tumors
  2. Polyps
  3. Foreign bodies
  4. Congenital choanal atresia
  5. Other entities that cause obstruction of sinus drainage
  6. Allergies
  7. Asthma
- Dental infections lead to maxillary sinusitis.
- Viruses recovered alone or in combination with bacteria (in 16% of cases):
  1. Rhinovirus
  2. Coronavirus
  3. Adenovirus
  4. Parainfluenza virus
  5. Respiratory syncytial virus
- The principal bacterial pathogens in sinusitis are *Streptococcus pneumoniae,* nontypeable *Haemophilus influenzae,* and *Moraxella catarrhalis.*
- In the remainder of cases *Streptococcus pyogenes, Staphylococcus aureus,* beta-hemolytic streptococci, and mixed anaerobic infections (*Peptostreptococcus, Fusobacterium, Bacteroides, Prevotella* spp.) are found.
- Infection is polymicrobial in about one third of cases.
- Anaerobic infections are seen more often in cases of chronic sinusitis and in cases associated with dental infection; anaerobes are unlikely pathogens in sinusitis in children.
- Fungal pathogens are isolated with increasing frequency in immunocompromised patients but remain uncommon pathogens in the paranasal sinuses. Fungal pathogens include: *Phaeohyphomycosis, Aspergillus, Pseudallescheria, Sporothrix,* and *Zygomycetes* spp.
- Nosocomial infections: occur in patients with nasogastric tubes, nasotracheal intubation, cystic fibrosis, and immunocompromised state.
  1. *S. aureus* (including MRSA)
  2. *Pseudomonas aeruginosa*
  3. *Klebsiella pneumoniae*
  4. *Enterobacter* spp.
  5. *Proteus mirabilis*
- Organisms typically isolated in chronic sinusitis:
  1. *S. aureus*
  2. *S. pneumoniae*
  3. *H. influenzae*
  4. *P. aeruginosa*
  5. Anaerobes

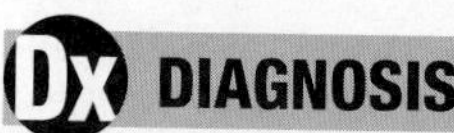

DIAGNOSIS

DIFFERENTIAL DIAGNOSIS

- Temporomandibular joint disease
- Migraine headache
- Cluster headache
- Dental infection
- Trigeminal neuralgia
- Allergic rhinitis
- Drugs (cocaine, decongestant overuse)
- Gastroesophageal reflux disease
- Wegener granulomatosis
- Cystic fibrosis

WORKUP

- The diagnosis is generally based on clinical signs and symptoms (purulent rhinorrhea and facial pain). Radiologic tests and cultures are not recommended initially and should be considered only when treatment is ineffective and sinusitis persists.
- In the normal healthy host, the paranasal sinuses should be sterile. Although the contiguous structures are colonized with bacteria and likely contaminate the sinuses, the mucociliary lining functions to remove these bacteria.
- Gold standard for diagnosis: recovery of bacteria in high-density $\geq 10^4$ colony-forming units/ml from a paranasal sinus, in the setting of a patient with history of upper respiratory infection and symptoms persisting for 7 to 10 days. Sinus aspiration is the best method for obtaining cultures; however, it must be

performed by an otorhinolaryngologist and is not practical for the primary care practitioner. Therefore, most diagnoses are based on the clinical history and presentation, possibly supported by radiologic evaluations.

1. Standard four-view sinus radiographs
    a. Complete opacification and air-fluid levels are most specific findings (average 85% and 80%, respectively)
    b. Mucosal thickening has low specificity (40% to 50%)
    c. Absence of all three of the previous findings has estimated sensitivity of 90%
    d. Overall, standard radiographs are of limited use in diagnosis, although negative films are strong evidence against the diagnosis
2. CT scans:
    a. Much more sensitive than plain radiographs in detecting acute changes and disease in the sinuses
    b. Recommended for patients requiring surgical intervention, including sinus aspiration; it is a useful adjunct to guide therapy
3. Transillumination:
    a. Used for diagnosis of frontal and maxillary sinusitis
    b. Place transilluminator in the mouth or against cheek to assess maxillary sinuses, under medial aspect of the supraorbital ridge to assess frontal sinuses
    c. Absence of light transmission indicates that sinus is filled with fluid
    d. Dullness (decreased light transmission) is less helpful in diagnosing infection
4. Endoscopy:
    a. Used to visualize secretions coming from the ostia of infected sinuses
    b. Culture collection via endoscopy often contaminated by nasal flora; not nearly as good as sinus puncture
5. Sinus puncture:
    a. Gold standard for collecting sinus cultures
    b. Generally reserved for treatment failures, suspected intracranial extension, and nosocomial sinusitis

Rx TREATMENT

NONPHARMACOLOGIC THERAPY

To help promote sinus drainage:

- Air humidification with vaporizers (for steam) or humidifiers (for a cool mist)
- Application of hot, wet towel over the face
- Sipping hot beverages
- Hydration

ACUTE GENERAL Rx

- Sinus drainage:
    1. Nasal vasoconstrictors, such as phenylephrine nose drops, 0.25% or 0.5%
    2. Topical decongestants should not be used for more than a few days because of the risk of rebound congestion
    3. Systemic decongestants
    4. Nasal or systemic corticosteroids, such as nasal beclomethasone, short-course oral prednisone
    5. Nasal irrigation, with hypertonic or normal saline (saline may act as a mild vasoconstrictor of nasal blood flow)
    6. Use of antihistamines has no proven benefit, and the drying effect on the mucous membranes may cause crusting, which blocks the ostia, thus interfering with sinus drainage
- Analgesics, antipyretics

Antimicrobial therapy:

- Most cases of acute sinusitis have a viral cause and will resolve within 2 wk without antibiotics.
- Current treatment recommendations favor symptomatic treatment for those with mild symptoms. Physicians grossly overprescribe antibiotics for presumed bacterial sinusitis despite a much higher prevalence of viral infections.
- Antibiotics should not be prescribed for mild to moderate sinusitis within the first week of illness. They should be reserved for those with severe symptoms who meet the criteria for diagnosis of sinusitis.
- Antibiotic therapy is usually empiric, targeting the common pathogens:
    1. First-line antibiotics in children include amoxicillin or amoxicillin/clavulanate. For adults amoxicillin/clavulanate or doxycycline is first-line agent, with quinolones (levofloxacin or moxifloxacin) reserved as second-line agents unless patient is penicillin allergic.
    2. Second-line antibiotics include the newer macrolides: clarithromycin, azithromycin, and oral cephalosporins: cefuroxime axetil, cefprozil, cefaclor, loracarbef, but high rate of resistance of *S. pneumoniae* is a concern with these agents as is *H. influenzae* resistance with TMP-SMX such that it is no longer used as a first-line agent.
    3. For patients with uncomplicated acute sinusitis, the less expensive first-line agents appear to be as effective as the costlier second-line agents.
- Hospitalization and IV antibiotics may be required for more severe infection and those with suspected intracranial complications. Broader-spectrum antibiotic coverage may be indicated in severe cases, to cover for MRSA, *Pseudomonas,* and fungal pathogens.
- Duration of therapy generally 5 to 7 days rather than 10 to 14 days as recommended in the past.

Surgery:

- Surgical drainage indicated
    1. If intracranial or orbital complications suspected
    2. Many cases of frontal and sphenoid sinusitis
    3. Chronic sinusitis recalcitrant to medical therapy
- Surgical debridement imperative in the treatment of fungal sinusitis

Complications:

- Untreated, sinusitis may lead to a number of serious, life-threatening complications.
- Intracranial complications include meningitis, brain abscess, and epidural and subdural empyema.
- Intracranial sequelae are more common with frontal and ethmoid infections.
- Extracranial complications include orbital cellulitis, blindness, orbital abscess, osteomyelitis.
- Extracranial sequelae are more commonly seen with ethmoid sinusitis.

CHRONIC RX

- Broad-spectrum antibiotics that cover both aerobes and anaerobes
- Duration of therapy not clearly established: range 3 to 6 wk
- Adjunctive therapy: one or more of the various options listed previously
- Surgical intervention may be necessary in nonresponders

DISPOSITION

Appropriate diagnosis and treatment are necessary to avoid the various sequelae that can occur without proper therapy.

REFERRAL

- To infectious disease specialist if failure to respond to initial therapy
- To otorhinolaryngologist for:
    1. Failure to respond to therapy
    2. Suspected fungal infection
    3. Suspected intracranial or orbital complications

PEARLS & CONSIDERATIONS

- Recurrent sinusitis is usually related to anatomic defects, poor drainage, or immunocompromised states; such patients deserve a thorough workup by an ENT specialist and/or an infectious disease specialist.
- Nosocomial sinusitis from obstruction by nasotracheal or nasogastric tubes is not uncommon and can be difficult to recognize in patients in the critical care units.

SUGGESTED READINGS

available at www.expertconsult.com

RELATED CONTENT

Sinusitis (Patient Information)

AUTHOR: **GLENN G. FORT, M.D., M.P.H.**

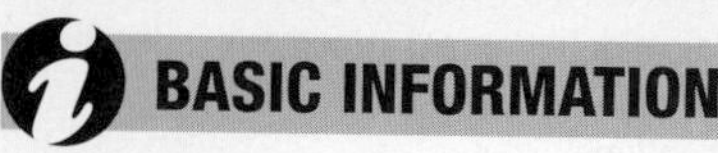

BASIC INFORMATION

DEFINITION

Sjögren's syndrome (SS) is an autoimmune disorder that targets exocrine glands. It is characterized by lymphocytic and plasma cell infiltration and destruction of salivary and lacrimal glands with subsequent diminished lacrimal and salivary gland secretions. It can occur in both primary and secondary forms.

- Primary: dry mouth (xerostomia) and dry eyes (xerophthalmia) develop as isolated entities.
- Secondary: associated with other autoimmune connective tissue diseases.

SYNONYMS

Sicca syndrome
Sicca complex

ICD-9CM CODES
710.2 Sjögren's syndrome
ICD-10CM CODES
M35.00 Sicca syndrome, unspecified

EPIDEMIOLOGY & DEMOGRAPHICS

INCIDENCE: 3.9 per 100,000
PREVALENCE: Prevalence is 0.3% to 0.6% of population; secondary SS is also common and can affect up to 15% of patients with systemic lupus erythematosus (SLE) and nearly 25% of rheumatoid arthritis (RA) and scleroderma patients.
PREDOMINANT SEX: Female predominance with a female/male ratio of approximately 9:1
PREDOMINANT AGE: Peak incidence is in the fourth and fifth decade, but SS can occur in all ages.
RISK FACTOR: Seen in all races/ethnicities, but more common in Caucasians.

PHYSICAL FINDINGS & CLINICAL PRESENTATION

- Diagnosis of SS is based on the presence of at least two of three objective diagnostic tests below:
  1. Positive serum levels of anti-SS-A/Ro and/or anti-SS-B/La or a positive rheumatoid factor and antinuclear antibody (ANA) titer of at least 1:320
  2. Salivary gland biopsy exhibiting focal sites of inflammation. One or more sites of inflammation per 4 mm^2 is considered to be positive.
  3. Keratoconjunctivitis sicca with ocular staining score of three or more (the dissipation rate of a specialized dye that is applied to the tear film that bathes the surface of the eye; a score of three or more is considered to be positive).
- Dry mouth with dry lips (cheilosis), erythema of tongue (Fig. 1-861) and other mucosal surfaces, carious teeth
- Dry eyes (conjunctival injection, corneal ulceration, blurred vision, decreased luster, enlargement of lacrimal glands, and irregularity of the corneal light reflex)
- Possible salivary gland enlargement and dysfunction, with subsequent difficulty in chewing and swallowing food and in speaking without frequent water intake, thickened saliva, and burning sensation in mouth
- Leukocytoclastic vasculitis may be present.
- Skin ulceration, photosensitivity, and allergic drug eruptions
- Extraglandular involvement occurs in 50% of patients. There are multiple systemic manifestations associated with SS, which include the following:
  - Dyspareunia can occur secondary to vaginal dryness
  - Pulmonary involvement includes chronic obstructive pulmonary disease, lymphocytic interstitial pneumonitis, fibrosis, and xerotrachea
  - Gastrointestinal conditions such as esophageal dysmotility, hepatitis, and pancreatitis can occur
  - Renal manifestations include renal tubular acidosis, Fanconi syndrome, and interstitial nephritis
  - Neurologic involvement including peripheral neuropathy and trigeminal neuropathy
  - Musculoskeletal symptoms including arthralgias and polymyopathy
  - Hematologic conditions such as lymphoma and leukopenia. Nearly 5% of patients develop B-cell lymphoma.
  - RA and other connective tissue diseases are present in secondary SS.
  - Hypothyroidism may be observed in patients with SS.

ETIOLOGY

Autoimmune disorder of unclear etiology. It is associated with certain HLA-DQ alleles. It has been postulated that viral agents (e.g., hepatitis C) may trigger the clinical presentation.

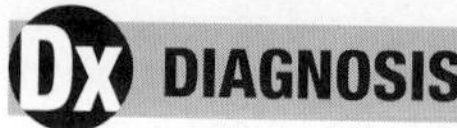

DIAGNOSIS

DIFFERENTIAL DIAGNOSIS

- Medication-related dryness (e.g., anticholinergics, antihistamines)
- Age-related exocrine gland dysfunction
- Mouth breathing
- Anxiety
- HIV infection
- Hepatitis C infection
- Diabetes mellitus
- Chronic sialadenitis
- Acromegaly
- Hyperlipidemia
- Graft-versus-host disease
- Other: sarcoidosis, primary salivary hypofunction, radiation injury, amyloidosis
- IgG4-related disease
- Ocular herpetic lesions, blepharitis, corneal abrasions
- An algorithm for the diagnosis of SS is provided in Fig. 1-862.

WORKUP

Workup involves ocular and oral examination and laboratory and radiographic testing to demonstrate the following criteria for diagnosis of primary and secondary SS.

PRIMARY:

- Symptoms and objective signs of ocular dryness:
  1. Schirmer's test (Fig. 1-863): <8 mm wetting per 5 min
  2. Positive rose bengal or fluorescein staining of cornea and conjunctiva to demonstrate keratoconjunctivitis sicca
  3. Tear breakup time and tear osmolality measured after instillation of fluorescein
- Symptoms and objective signs of dry mouth:
  1. Decreased parotid flow using Lashley cups or other methods
  2. Abnormal biopsy result of minor salivary gland (focus score >2 based on average of four assessable lobules)
  3. Assessment of rate of saliva production in which collection of ≤1.5 ml after two expectorations 15 min apart is considered positive
- Evidence of systemic autoimmune disorder:
  1. Elevated rheumatoid factor (70%-90% of patients)
  2. Elevated titer of ANA >1:320 (80% of patients)
  3. Presence of anti-SS-A (Ro) (>60% of patients) or anti-SS-B (La) antibodies (40% of patients)

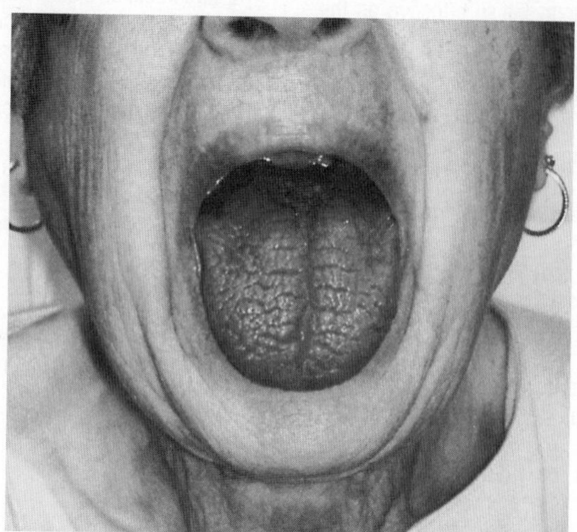

FIGURE 1-861 "Crocodile tongue" in a patient with Sjögren's syndrome. (From Noble J: *Primary care medicine*, ed 3, St Louis, 2001, Mosby.)

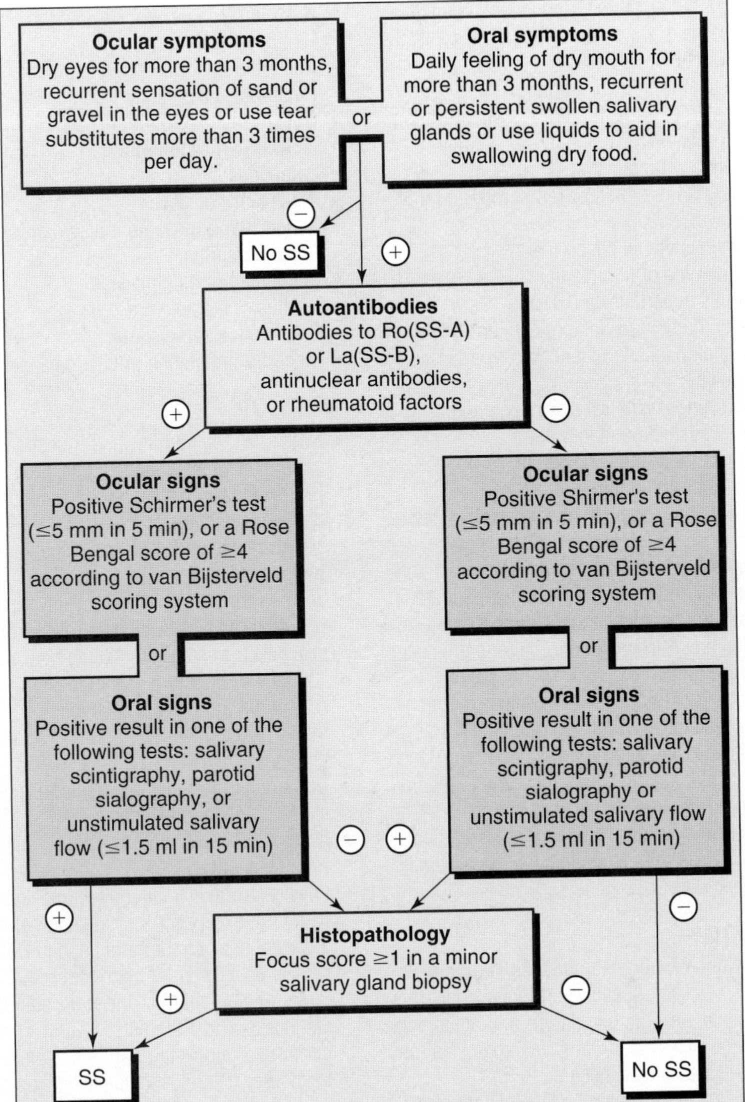

FIGURE 1-862 Suggested algorithm for the diagnosis of Sjögren's syndrome. Exclusion criteria include hepatitis C or human immunodeficiency virus infection, sarcoidosis, graft-versus-host disease, preexisting lymphoma, previous head or neck irradiation, and use of anticholinergic drugs. (From Hochberg MC et al: *Rheumatology*, ed 5, St Louis, 2011, Mosby.)

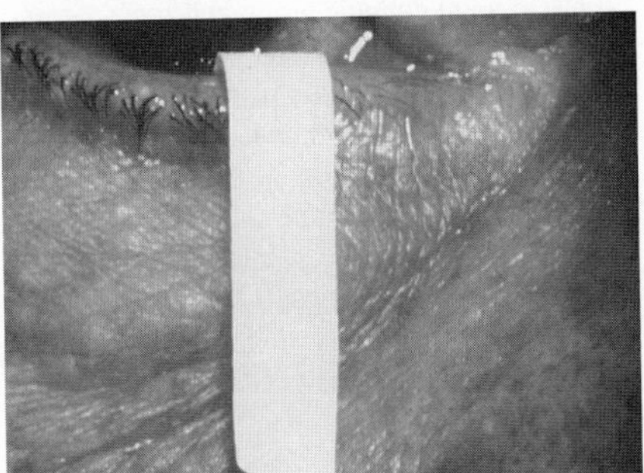

FIGURE 1-863 Schirmer test in a patient with Sjögren's syndrome. Wetting of less than 5 mm/5 min of the filter paper strip is shown. (From Hochberg MC et al: *Rheumatology*, ed 5, St Louis, 2011, Mosby.)

SECONDARY:

- Characteristic signs and symptoms of SS
- Clinical features sufficient to allow a diagnosis of RA, SLE, polymyositis, or scleroderma

LABORATORY TESTS

- Positive ANA (80% of patients) with autoantibodies anti-SS-A and anti-SS-B may be present.
- Additional laboratory abnormalities may include elevated erythrocyte sedimentation rate, anemia (normochromic, normocytic), abnormal liver function studies, elevated serum beta$_2$ microglobulin levels, rheumatoid factor, hypergammaglobulinemia, antibodies to double-stranded DNA in cases with proteinuria, serum C3 and C4, and cryoglobulins (30% of patients).
- A definite diagnosis of SS can be made with a salivary gland biopsy.

Rx TREATMENT

NONPHARMACOLOGIC THERAPY

- Adequate fluid replacement. Ameliorate skin dryness by gently blotting dry after bathing, leaving a small amount of moisture, and then applying a moisturizer.
- Increased environmental moisture by using humidifiers
- Proper oral hygiene (daily topical fluoride use and antimicrobial mouth rinses) to reduce the incidence of caries. Sugar-free chewing gum and sour lemon lozenges to stimulate salivary secretion.
- Periodic dental and ophthalmologic evaluations to screen for complications

GENERAL Rx

- Use artificial tears frequently.
- The muscarinic agonist pilocarpine (5 mg PO qid) is useful to improve dryness. A cyclosporine 0.05% ophthalmic emulsion (Restasis) may also be useful for dry eyes.
- Cevimeline (Evoxac), a cholinergic agent with muscarinic agonist activity, 30 mg PO tid is effective for the treatment of dry mouth in patients with SS.
- Hydroxychloroquine alone or in conjunction with methotrexate may be useful for arthralgias and cutaneous manifestations.
- Oral cyclosporine only improves the symptoms of subjective dryness.
- Antitumor necrosis factor agents have not shown significant clinical efficacy, and larger controlled trials are needed to establish the efficacy of rituximab for severe inflammatory manifestations.
- Propionic acid gel can be used for vaginal dryness.
- Systemic manifestations are treated according to symptoms and complications.
- Cyclophosphamide, azathioprine, and mycophenolate mofetil are generally reserved for life-threatening extraglandular manifestations.
- Fig. E1-864 describes a treatment algorithm for Sjögren's syndrome.

REFERRAL

- Rheumatology referral is generally indicated.
- Referral should be made to an oncologist when lymphoma is suspected.

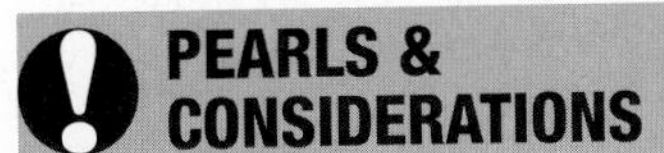

PEARLS & CONSIDERATIONS

COMMENTS

- Unusual presentations of SS may occur in association with polymyalgia rheumatica, chronic fatigue syndrome, fever of unknown origin, and inflammatory myositis.
- The most serious complication of primary SS is the development of non-Hodgkin's lymphoma and other lymphoproliferative disorders, which occur at a 44-fold increased rate as compared to age-matched controls.

SUGGESTED READINGS

available at www.expertconsult.com

RELATED CONTENT

Sjögren's Syndrome (Patient Information)

AUTHORS: **SYEDA M. SAYEED, M.D.**, and **HARALD A. HALL, M.D.**

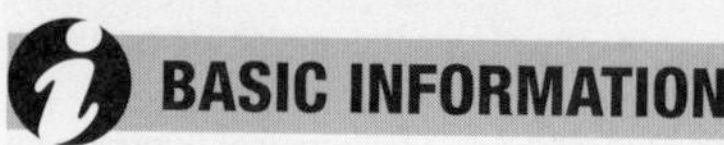

DEFINITION

The *International Classification of Sleep Disorders, Second Edition*, classifies sleep-disordered breathing disorders into three categories: central sleep apnea syndrome, obstructive sleep apnea (OSA), and sleep-related hypoventilation/hypoxic syndromes. The American Academy of Sleep Disorders defines OSA as repetitive episodes of upper airway obstruction that occur during sleep and that are typically associated with oxyhemoglobin desaturations.

SYNONYMS

Sleep apnea syndrome
Sleep-disordered breathing
Obstructive sleep apnea syndrome
Obstructive sleep apnea–hypopnea syndrome
OSA

ICD-9CM CODES
327.2 Organic sleep apnea
327.21 Organic sleep apnea, unspecified
327.23 Obstructive sleep apnea (adult) (pediatric)
ICD-10CM CODES
G47.30 Sleep apnea, unspecified
G47.31 Primary central sleep apnea
G47.33 Obstructive sleep apnea (adult) (pediatric)

EPIDEMIOLOGY & DEMOGRAPHICS

OSA is a common disease in the U.S. Data from the Wisconsin Cohort Study indicated that the prevalence of OSA in people between the ages of 30 and 60 yr is 9%-24% for men and 4%-9% for women. The estimated prevalence of OSA is 4% for men and 2% for women. The prevalence of OSA increases from 18-45 years of age, with a plateau occurring at 55-65 years of age. The prevalence is higher in obese and hypertensive patients. ~2% of children have OSA, which develops more commonly between the ages of 2-8 yr when adenotonsillar size is largest relative to upper airway. Risk factors include obesity and craniofacial and upper airway soft tissue abnormalities, and potential risk factors include heredity, current tobacco smoking, nasal congestion, and diabetes.

PHYSICAL FINDINGS & CLINICAL PRESENTATION

- Nocturnal symptoms, including nocturia and angina pectoris
- Snoring that can be loud, habitual, and bothersome to others
- Witnessed apneas that often interrupt snoring and end with a snort
- Gasping, choking, or smothering sensations that arouse the patient from sleep
- Restless sleep associated with frequent arousals
- Daytime symptoms:
  - Nonrestorative sleep
  - Not feeling refreshed upon awakening
  - Morning headache
  - Dry mouth or throat upon awakening
  - Excessive daytime sleepiness, typically during quiet activities
  - Daytime fatigue or tiredness
  - Problems with memory, concentration, and cognitive function, especially with executive functioning
  - Easily angered, short tempered, and inattentive
  - Hyperactivity in children
  - Symptoms of fibromyalgia
- Systemic hypertension (HTN)
- Obesity (body mass index >30 kg/m^2)
- History of insulin resistance or type 2 diabetes mellitus
- Mood swings, irritability, anxiety, depression
- Decreased libido and impotence
- Neck circumference of >43 cm (17 in) in men and >37 cm (15 in) in women
- Erythematous oropharynx because of snoring.
- Adenotonsillar hypertrophy, excessive soft tissue, high-arched hard palate, pendulous uvula, prominent tongue, large degree of overjet, and retrognathia or micrognathia can be present.
- Narrowing of lateral airway walls is independent predictor of OSA in men but not women.
- Craniofacial skeletal abnormalities can lead to OSA, particularly among children and nonobese adults.
- A positive family history increases an individual's risk with each additional close family member with OSA.

ETIOLOGY

- Narrowing of upper airway as a result of obesity or increased peripharyngeal fat deposition, retrognathia and/or micrognathia, adenotonsillar hypertrophy, macroglossia, or neuromuscular weakness
- Upper airway muscular weakness as a result of neuromuscular disorders, primary CNS disorders (e.g., stroke), or metabolic disorders
- Other diseases associated with the development of OSA (e.g., hypothyroidism, acromegaly)

Dx DIAGNOSIS

DIFFERENTIAL DIAGNOSIS

- Anemia
- Anxiety or panic disorder
- Behaviorally induced insufficient sleep syndrome
- Cardiac or heart disease
- Central sleep apnea
- Circadian rhythm disorder
- Depression
- Drug or alcohol abuse
- Gastroesophageal reflux
- Hypothyroidism
- Idiopathic hypersomnia with long or short sleep time
- Inadequate sleep hygiene
- Insomnia
- Medication effect
- Narcolepsy
- Nocturnal asthma
- Nocturnal gastroesophageal reflux
- Nocturnal seizures
- Obesity-hypoventilation syndrome (i.e., Pickwickian syndrome)
- Parasomnias
- Parkinson's disease
- Periodic limb movement disorder
- Primary snoring
- Pulmonary or lung disease
- Restless legs syndrome
- Shift work sleep disorder
- Sleep fragmentation (multiple causes)

WORKUP

- Evaluation should include questions about snoring, witnessed apneas, gasping or choking episodes, restless sleep, and excessive daytime sleepiness.
- Mood swings and personality changes should be addressed.
- Job performance and difficulty driving or previous motor vehicle accidents related to excessive daytime sleepiness should be discussed.
- Additional concerns include morning dry mouth/throat, morning headaches, alcohol intake, weight gain, mood or personality changes.
- A thorough drug history should include muscle relaxants and sedatives.
- A family history should target any family members with OSA.
- Physical exam is frequently normal in patients with OSA except for the presence of obesity, enlarged neck circumference, and HTN.
- OSA is confirmed by nocturnal polysomnography (PSG), which is the gold standard for diagnosis. The PSG (Fig. 1-865) should be performed during the patient's typical sleeping hours; it should include all stages of sleep as well as sleep in the supine position.
- The severity of the OSA is determined by the apnea-hypopnea index (AHI), which is derived from the total number of apneas and hypopneas divided by the total sleep time.
- Recommended severity cutoff levels for the AHI in adult patients are as follows:
  - Mild: 5-15 episodes/hr (with symptoms)
  - Moderate: 15 to 30 episodes per hr
  - Severe: >30 episodes per hr
- Criteria for the treatment of mild OSA often require symptoms, including excessive daytime sleepiness, cardiovascular disease, HTN, and mood swings.
- In-home respiratory monitoring may be effective alternative to PSG for evaluation of OSA.

LABORATORY TESTS

- Arterial blood gas testing should be performed if a patient has suspected pulmonary HTN or cor pulmonale to rule out daytime hypoxemia or hypercapnia.
- Thyroid-stimulating hormone level should be obtained if hypothyroidism is suspected.
- Fasting glucose level is recommended because OSA increases the risk of developing diabetes independent of other risk factors.

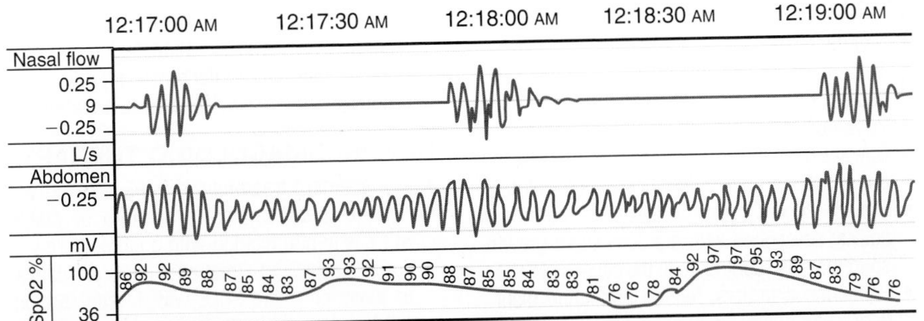

FIGURE 1-865 Polysomnographic tracing of a patient with obstructive sleep apnea during 2 minutes of non–rapid eye movement sleep. Displayed are airflow in the upper airway ("nasal flow"), recorded with a nasal pressure transducer, respiratory effort ("abdomen"), recorded by inductance plethysmography; and oxygen saturation of hemoglobin (SpO_2) recorded with pulse oximetry. (From Goldman L, Schafer AI: *Goldman's Cecil medicine,* ed 24, Philadelphia, 2012, Saunders.)

- CBC is helpful to look for anemia; iron studies if anemia is detected and ferritin level if concomitant RLS is present.
- Pulmonary function testing if pulmonary disorder is suspected or to assess severity of neuromuscular disease, if present.
- ECG or echocardiogram is indicated if a cardiac disorder (e.g., arrhythmia, pulmonary HTN) is suspected.

IMAGING STUDIES

- Plain radiography of the neck can be helpful to assess the soft tissues of patients with suspected anatomic abnormalities.
- Chest x-ray if pulmonary disease is suspected.

Rx TREATMENT

NONPHARMACOLOGIC THERAPY

- Behavioral modifications:
  - Weight loss in overweight and obese patients. Weight loss is effective for reducing the severity of OSA, and if significant, it may potentially allow some patients to discontinue continuous positive airway pressure (CPAP) therapy.
  - Weight loss with bariatric surgery may improve OSA in some patients, but its definitive role remains unclear. In a recent trial in obese patients with OSA, the use of bariatric surgery compared with conventional weight loss therapy did not result in a statistically greater reduction in AHI despite major differences in weight loss.
  - Exercise without weight loss may improve OSA.
  - Avoid alcohol for 4-6 hr before bedtime.
  - Avoid muscle relaxants and sedating medications.
  - Sleep hygiene training.
  - Avoid or eliminate supine sleeping positions.
  - Avoid medications that may worsen OSA.
- Medical treatment:
  - CPAP is the primary therapy for OSA. It delivers a constant airway pressure that acts as a pneumatic splint that relieves the upper airway obstruction.
  - Other methods of delivering positive pressure include:
    - Bilevel positive airway pressure (BiPAP), which delivers a preset inspiratory and expiratory airway pressure.
    - Autotitrating positive airway pressure (APAP), which increases or decreases the level of pressure in response to change in airflow, a vibratory snore, or change in circuit pressure.
    - Adaptive servoventilation provides a varying amount of inspiratory pressure superimposed on a low level of CPAP.
  - Oral appliance constructed by a reputable and qualified dentist may be effective for the treatment of mild OSA in certain patients, especially those with retrognathia. Mandibular advancement devices (MADs) are a good alternative to CPAP in patients who are unable to tolerate CPAP.
  - Optimal treatment of allergic rhinitis is needed; nasal irrigation with saline followed by nasal corticosteroids is often helpful.
  - Symptoms of excessive daytime sleepiness may linger and require further investigation or medical therapy.
  - Patients should be considered for surgery if multiple attempts at CPAP therapy have failed and if an oral appliance is not an option. If the patient opts for surgery, ensure that it is performed by a reputable and qualified otolaryngologist and is based on the location of airway collapse.
- Surgical treatment:
  - Adenotonsillectomy is often curative for children with OSA.
  - Nasal septoplasty should be considered for patients with nasoseptal deformities.
  - Uvulopalatopharyngoplasty, which involves resection of the uvula and the soft palate, is effective for a small number of patients. However, predicting which patients will benefit is difficult.
  - Tracheostomy is typically reserved for patients with very severe OSA who failed medical therapy or who have cor pulmonale.

DISPOSITION

- The short-term prognosis for excessive daytime sleepiness and snoring is good to excellent with the regular use of nasal CPAP, but no studies have been performed to address the long-term effects in a large population of patients.
- Residual symptoms of excessive daytime sleepiness can occur in some patients with OSA despite regular CPAP use. This has led the FDA to approve modafinil for the management of residual sleepiness.

REFERRAL

- Highly trained sleep specialists with expertise in caring for patients with OSA are recommended, especially for complex cases.
- Surgical referral to otolaryngology should be considered for children with adenotonsillar hypertrophy and for adults who are unresponsive to weight loss and CPAP therapy.
- Referral to a qualified dentist for treatment with an oral appliance may be useful for certain patients with mild OSA.

PEARLS & CONSIDERATIONS

- OSA is a common disorder that is underrecognized and underdiagnosed, so the identification of risk factors is crucial for making the correct diagnosis.
- The prevalence of OSA increases among women after menopause.
- The degree of adenotonsillar hypertrophy does not correlate with the presence of OSA in children.
- A 10% weight loss can decrease the AHI of a patient with OSA by as much as 50%.
- The single most effective therapy for OSA is nasal CPAP.
- Patients with OSA are more vulnerable than healthy persons to the effects of alcohol consumption and sleep restriction with regard to various driving performance variables.
- OSA is a risk factor for HTN. In patients with untreated HTN and OSA, the use of CPAP results in small but statistically significant reductions in blood pressure.
- OSA may also be an independent risk factor for peptic ulcer bleeding.
- Ethnic differences may exist for some populations, with South Asians having a higher prevalence and risk for cardiovascular side effects.

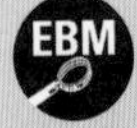

EVIDENCE

available at www.expertconsult.com

SUGGESTED READINGS

available at www.expertconsult.com

RELATED CONTENT

Sleep Apnea (Patient Information)

AUTHOR: **DON HAYES, JR., M.D., M.S.**

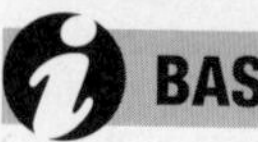

BASIC INFORMATION

DEFINITION

Slipped capital femoral epiphysis (SCFE) is defined as displacement of the capital femoral epiphysis (femoral head) posteriorly on the metaphysis (femoral neck) at the level of the physis (growth plate)

- Commonly unilateral but can present with bilateral hip involvement
- Classified as stable or unstable
- Stable SCFE: slipped capital femoral epiphysis in a child who is able to walk with minimal or no symptoms
- Unstable SCFE: slipped capital femoral epiphysis resulting in a child who cannot walk or who cannot walk without crutches and is associated with severe pain of acute onset

SYNONYMS

Slipped capital femoral epiphysis, nontraumatic
Slipped upper femoral epiphysis
Slipped upper femoral epiphysis, nontraumatic

ICD-10CM CODES
732.2 Nontraumatic slipped upper femoral epiphysis
ICD-10CM CODES
M93.003 Unspecified slipped upper femoral epiphysis (nontraumatic), unspecified hip

EPIDEMIOLOGY & DEMOGRAPHICS

INCIDENCE: Reported incidence in male children is 13.35 cases per 100,000 children, and reported incidence in female children is 8.07 cases per 100,000 children.
PEAK INCIDENCE: Average age at diagnosis is 13.5 yr for boys and 12.0 yr for girls.
PREVALENCE: 10.8 cases per 100,000 children
PREDOMINANT SEX: More common in boys than girls
GENETICS: More commonly seen in blacks and Hispanic populations; no strong evidence of genetic predisposition
RISK FACTORS: Obesity by far the greatest risk factor

PHYSICAL FINDINGS & CLINICAL PRESENTATION

- The slip occurs at the weakest part of the physeal plate and results in the head being displaced from the metaphysis.
- Typical presentation of pain in the knee, hip, groin, thigh, or all; external rotation of the extremity and limp are commonly seen. Few patients present with painless limp; <10% report inciting trauma; even fewer complain of severe hip pain and inability to bear weight.
- Important physical exam findings include limited range of motion of the affected hip on internal rotation; involved hip typically will go into obligatory external rotation if passively flexed up to 90 degrees.
- Patients with unstable SCFE are unable to bear weight, their leg is in external rotation, and any hip motion is painful.

ETIOLOGY

- Multifactorial
- The slip itself usually occurs during the preadolescent growth spurt.
- 25%-40% are bilateral slips.
- Obesity: of children diagnosed with SCFE, 63% are at the 90th percentile for weight or higher.
- Growth surges: varying levels of hormonal activity associated with the adolescent growth spurt may also contribute to the causes of SCFE.
- Endocrine disorders: related endocrine disorders include hypothyroidism, growth hormone supplementation, hypogonadism, and panhypopituitarism; consider an endocrinopathy in SCFE with unusual presentations, including patients who are younger than 8 yr, older than 15 yr, or underweight.

Dx DIAGNOSIS

DIFFERENTIAL DIAGNOSIS

- Apophyseal avulsion fracture
- Avascular necrosis
- Hip apophysitis
- Transient synovitis
- Stress fracture
- Septic arthritis
- Osteomyelitis
- Legg-Calvé-Perthes disease
- Adductor muscle strain (groin pull)

WORKUP

- Diagnosis is based on physical exam and radiologic findings.
- Laboratory testing can be done to look for secondary causes.

LABORATORY TESTS

Check renal, endocrine, growth hormone, thyroid function tests in patients <10 yr of age and body weight <50th percentile or less.

IMAGING STUDIES

- Plain radiographs are sensitive and specific to make the diagnosis of SCFE.
- B/L hip x-rays: both AP and frog-leg lateral views should be done; 60% of patients have bilateral hip involvement at presentation.
- The frog-leg lateral view is more sensitive.
- Physical blurring of the epiphysis or widening can be seen.
- Bone scans may be helpful in predicting prognosis; "cold spots" on technetium bone scan in acute SCFE may represent ischemia and/or avascular necrosis.

Rx TREATMENT

- Once diagnosis is confirmed, the patient should be placed on non–weight-bearing crutches or in a wheelchair and quickly referred to an orthopedic surgeon for surgical management.
- The initial goals of treatment are to prevent slip progression and avoid complications.
- A recent open-label observational trial suggested a potential role for intravenous bisphosphonates as adjunctive therapy for acute SCFE that has been operatively fixed but had "cold spots" on bone scan indicating ischemia or necrosis; rationale for bisphosphonate use was to decrease necrotic bone resorption and allow for revascularization.

NONPHARMACOLOGIC THERAPY

- The standard treatment of SCFE is surgery.
- The standard surgical procedure of stable SCFE is in situ fixation with a single screw.
- For unstable SCFE, treatment goals are similar to those of stable SCFE with in situ fixation, but there is controversy as to the specifics of treatment, including timing of surgery, value of reduction, and whether traction should be used.
- Prophylactic treatment of the contralateral hip in SCFE is controversial and not recommended in most patients.
- Prophylactic pinning may be indicated in high-risk patients such as those with obesity or an endocrine disorder.

DISPOSITION

- SCFE is a common preadolescent disorder with little short-term morbidity and rare long-term sequelae if diagnosed and treated before the development of a severe deformity.
- The two most feared complications of SCFE are osteonecrosis/avascular necrosis and chondrolysis.
- Osteonecrosis/avascular necrosis: occurs in up to 60% of unstable SCFE; factors associated include overreduction of unstable SCFE, reduction of stable SCFE, pin penetration of posterior quadrant, and multiplicity of pin; often leads to advanced and early degenerative osteoarthritis.
- Chondrolysis: acute dissolution of articular cartilage in association with rapid progressive joint stiffness and pain; usually as a complication of surgery but can occur in untreated SCFE as well; incidence has decreased to 1%-2% with improvement in surgical techniques.

PEARLS & CONSIDERATIONS

- Physicians should consider SCFE when a child between the ages of 10-15 yr presents with limping and groin, hip, thigh, or knee pain.
- Physical exam usually shows decreased internal rotation of the hip and obligatory external rotation.
- Radiography to rule out SCFE should include anteroposterior lateral views of the hips (frog-lateral views for stable SCFE; cross-table views for unstable SCFE).
- The standard treatment of stable SCFE is in situ fixation with a single screw.

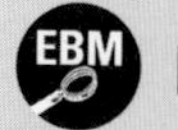

EVIDENCE

available at www.expertconsult.com

SUGGESTED READINGS

available at www.expertconsult.com

AUTHOR: **WAFFIYAH AFRIDI, M.D.**

BASIC INFORMATION

DEFINITION

- Mechanical obstruction means the blockage of the intestinal lumen, preventing the passage of luminal contents through the gut tube.
- This may be either:
  - a) Simple obstruction: in which the lumen may be *partially* or *completely blocked* but with intact intestinal blood flow
  - b) Strangulated obstruction
    - This is a surgical emergency.
    - Usually the obstruction is complete, blood flow to the obstructed segment is cut off, and tissue necrosis and gangrene may occur.

ICD 9CM CODES

560.9 Unspecified intestinal obstruction
560.1 Paralytic ileus
560.31 Gallstone ileus
560.8 Other specified intestinal obstruction
560 Intestinal obstruction

ICD-10CM CODES

K56.6 Other and unspecified intestinal obstruction
K56.9 Ileus, unspecified
K56.5 Intestinal adhesions (bands) with obstruction
K56.4 Other impaction of intestine
K56.3 Gallstone ileus
K56.2 Volvulus
K5.1 Intussusception
K56 Paralytic ileus and intestinal obstruction

EPIDEMIOLOGY & DEMOGRAPHICS

- The most frequently encountered surgical disorder of the small intestines is mechanical small bowel obstruction (SBO).
- 75% of all cases of small bowel obstruction are due to intraabdominal adhesion related to prior abdominal surgery.

PREDOMINANT SEX AND AGE: None

PHYSICAL FINDINGS & CLINICAL PRESENTATION

PHYSICAL FINDINGS

These may include:

- Abdominal distention
- Hyperactive bowel sounds (an early occurrence)
- Hypoactive bowel sounds (late finding)
- Hernia
- Rectal examination may reveal
  - Blood (suggestive of neoplasm or strangulation)
  - Masses

CLINICAL PRESENTATION

There are four key symptoms: abdominal pain, vomiting, distention, and constipation

- Abdominal pain
  - Often crampy; intermittent
  - Constant pain (that is, change in pain's character) signifies serious complication
- Nausea
- Vomiting (bilious vomiting seen in proximal obstructions)
- Diarrhea (early finding)
- Constipation (a late finding)
- Fever and/or tachycardia (these late findings may be seen with strangulation or intestinal ischemia)

ETIOLOGY

- Postoperative adhesions (may cause acute obstruction usually within one mo of surgery; or chronic obstructions can occur years later)
- Incarcerated inguinal hernia
- Malignant tumor
- IBD
- Gallstone ileus
- Stricture
- Cystic fibrosis
- Volvulus
- In children consider pyloric stenosis, intussusception, congenital atresia

DIAGNOSIS

DIFFERENTIAL DIAGNOSIS

- Cholangitis
- Cholecystitis
- Gastroenteritis
- Inflammatory bowel disease
- Endometriosis
- Mesenteric ischemia
- Pancreatitis
- Ovarian torsion

WORKUP

- During the initial evaluation of patients with suspected SBO, the primary objectives are to gauge the degree of metabolic derangement and volume depletion and to assess the need for and expediency of surgery. As with many surgical conditions, determining the correct diagnosis and management strategy hinges on a focused yet thorough history and physical examination.

LABORATORY TESTS

- Laboratory abnormalities are not diagnostic of bowel obstruction but instead may indicate complications of obstruction. Essential laboratory tests include:
  - Basic metabolic panel
  - CBC: hemoconcentration, leukocytosis
  - Urinalysis
  - Serum amylase: may be elevated
  - LDH
  - Hepatic panel
  - Type and cross-match

IMAGING STUDIES

- Initial radiographic evaluation begins with plain x-ray films of the abdomen (supine and erect) and an upright chest radiograph. An upright chest radiograph is of paramount importance to inspect for pneumoperitoneum and also for evidence of aspiration in a patient with a history of vomiting. A supine and upright plain abdominal x-ray in patients with suspected small bowel obstruction may show:
  - Ladder-like pattern of dilated small bowel loops with air-fluid levels (Fig. 1-866) indicating small bowel obstruction
  - Accumulation of air and fluid proximal and clearance of fluid and air distal to the post of obstruction
- Enteroclysis (a fluoroscopic x-ray of the small intestine) is useful in detecting obstruction and can distinguish partial from complete blockage and adhesions from metastases.
- CT scan is the study of choice if the patient has fever, tachycardia, abdominal pain, and leukocytosis. It can reveal the etiology of the obstruction: abscess, inflammatory process, extra-luminal pathology, and/or metastases.
- CT can elucidate the cause, such as the presence of a mass (Fig. 1-867) or a hernia with subsequent obstruction (Fig. 1-868). In addition, CT has high sensitivity for detecting strangulation and pneumoperitoneum indicative of a perforation and is particularly useful

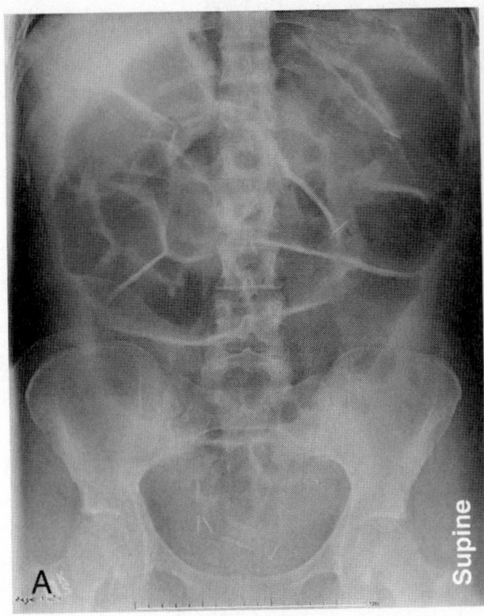

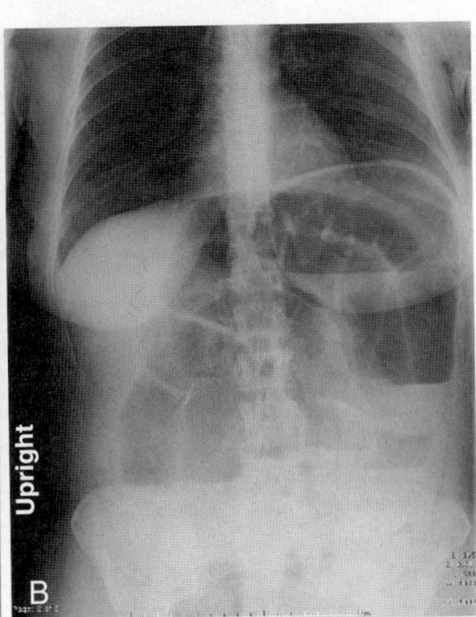

FIGURE 1-866 A, Supine film showing dilated loops of small bowel in a patient with small bowel obstruction. **B,** Upright abdominal film revealing multiple air-fluid levels and small bowel dilation, consistent with a diagnosis of small bowel obstruction. (From Marx J: *Rosen's emergency medicine: concepts and clinical practice*, ed 6, Philadelphia, 2006, Saunders.)

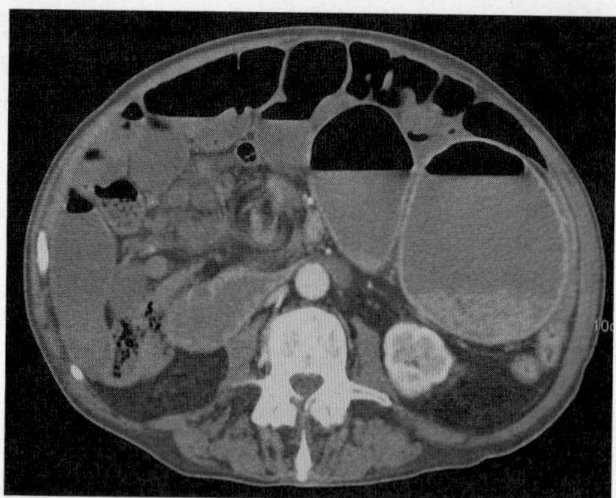

FIGURE 1-867 CT scan of small bowel volvulus with notable mesenteric torsion. (From Cameron JL, Cameron AM: *Current surgical therapy*, ed 10, Philadelphia, 2011, Saunders.)

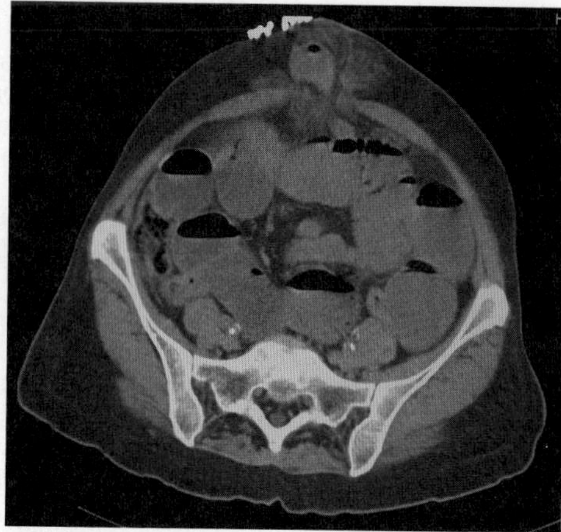

FIGURE 1-868 CT scan of complete small bowel obstruction due to incisional hernia. (From Cameron IL, Cameron AM: *Current surgical therapy*, ed 10, Philadelphia , 2011, Saunders.)

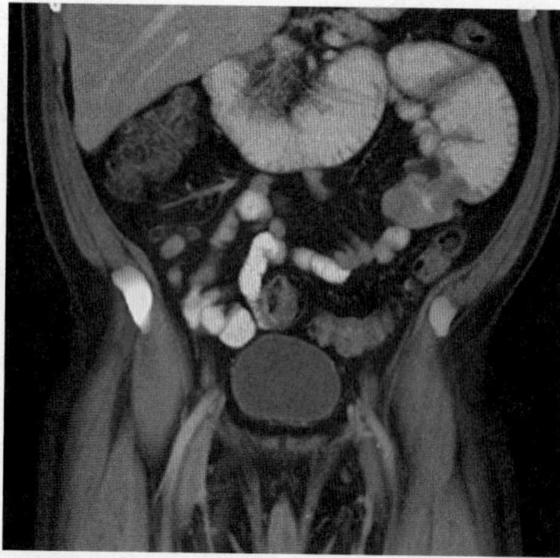

FIGURE 1-869 Coronal image of CT scan showing mass in proximal small bowel with decompressed loops of small bowel distal to obstruction. (From Cameron JL, Cameron AM: *Current surgical therapy*, ed 10, Philadelphia, 2011, Saunders.)

in the early postoperative setting to rule out ischemia, intraabdominal abscess, or morbidity as the underlying cause. It is also useful in patients with a history of malignancy to differentiate potentially recurrent disease from adhesions (Fig. 1-869).

- CT enterography, in which intraluminal distention is achieved with administration of large volumes of oral contrast such as water-methylcellulose solution, can be useful. This modality is most often used to diagnose patients with Crohn's disease–related strictures, and its benefit is high-resolution imaging of the bowel wall; however, it is impractical in the patient with gastrointestinal (GI) distress who is nauseated and vomiting.

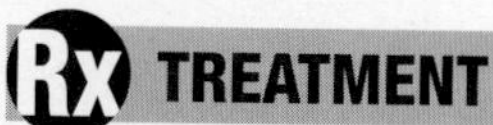

TREATMENT

EMERGENCY ROOM CARE

- Vigorous fluid resuscitation and correction of electrolyte disorders underpin the initial therapeutic goals of both nonoperative and preoperative management strategies. Placing a Foley catheter to measure urinary output, establishing adequate intravenous access, and reassessing hemodynamic and electrolyte status are all essential in the initial management.
- Initial treatment consists of:
  - Designate the patients nothing by mouth ("NPO")
  - Fluid resuscitation (with isotonic Ringer's or normal saline solution)
  - Bowel decompression (via nasogastric [NG] table placement): a standard NG tube provides symptomatic relief, prevents added gas and fluid accumulation proximally, and enables the serial assessment of antegrade fluid movement.
  - Pain management
  - Antiemetic administration
  - Surgical consultation: must be done early
  - Antibiotic administration

NONSURGICAL INPATIENT CARE:

- Continue NG suction.
- Provide adequate fluid.

Patients with low-grade partial SBOs are prone to spontaneous resolution with conservative interventions such as bowel rest, NG decompression, and appropriate fluid resuscitation. For partial or simple obstructions resolution usually occurs within 72 hr.

SURGICAL CARE

More than 25% of inpatients admitted because of SBO will require an operation. Patients with complete or high-grade partial SBO are most likely to need surgery, with less than 20% successfully managed nonoperatively. Surgery is indicated in:

- Strangulated obstruction (which is a surgical emergency)
- Simple complete obstruction: after failed nonoperative care

AUTHOR: **DANIEL K. ASIEDU, M.D., PH.D., F.A.C.P.**

BASIC INFORMATION

DEFINITION

Social anxiety disorder (SAD) is a persistent and intense fear of being embarrassed, humiliated, or negatively evaluated in social situations. SAD commonly presents as excessive anxiety or fear in situations involving social interactions (e.g., conversing with one or a group of other individuals, with sexually attractive others, with authority figures), performance situations (e.g., public speaking, acting/performing in front of an audience), or situations in which one is being observed (e.g., while eating). Individuals with SAD fear that they will behave in these situations in ways that will cause them to be embarrassed or that others will judge them negatively. Many individuals also fear that they will show anxiety symptoms that will be observed by others. The anxiety must persist in these situations for at least 6 mo, and it must occur both in peer settings and in situations with adults. The anxiety often results in avoidance of these situations, thus leading to significant occupational, academic, and/or social impairment as well as marked distress. A specifier of "performance only" should be given when the fears are confined to speaking or performing in public.

SYNONYMS

Social phobia
SAD

ICD-9CM and DSM-5 CODES
300.23
ICD-10CM CODES
F93.2 Social anxiety disorder of childhood
F40.1 Social phobias
F40.9 Phobic anxiety disorder, unspecified

EPIDEMIOLOGY & DEMOGRAPHICS

INCIDENCE (IN U.S.): Ranges from 4 to 5 to 9/1000 person-yrs; cumulative incidence of 11.0% in first three decades of life
PEAK INCIDENCE: Highest standardized incidence rates per person-yr between 10 and 19 yr of age
PREVALENCE (IN U.S.): Lifetime prevalence of 12% in epidemiologic samples, and 12-month prevalence of 7%; point prevalence of up to 30% in outpatient clinical settings
PREDOMINANT SEX: More common in women than in men (odds ratio of 1.5-2.2) in epidemiologic samples; rates are equivalent or slightly higher in males in clinical settings
PREDOMINANT AGE: Mean age at onset ~16 yr of age; median age at onset, 13 yr of age; onset rarely occurs after age 25, with 75% having an onset between 8 and 15 yr of age
GENETICS:
- Heritability ranges from 20% to 50%.
- 15% to 26% risk of SAD among first-degree relatives of those with SAD.

PHYSICAL FINDINGS & CLINICAL PRESENTATION

- Physical symptoms during social interactions such as heart palpitations, sweating, shaking, and/or blushing, which may take the form of a panic attack.
- Fear that others will observe these physical symptoms in social situations and negatively judge them; fears that they will "say something stupid," make a mistake, or offend others also are common.
- Report being "shy" most of their lives.
- Comorbid psychiatric disorders (e.g., major depression, other anxiety disorders) and substance abuse (e.g., alcohol/cannabis) are common.
- Few seek treatment specifically for SAD, and instead initially seek treatment for other psychiatric disorders (e.g., major depression, other anxiety disorders).
- The onset of SAD often precedes that of the other comorbid psychiatric conditions.

ETIOLOGY

- There is no clear etiology and likely is a combination of multiple factors.
- Research has examined developmental psychology factors (e.g., lack of modeling of socialization by parents), temperamental factors (e.g., behavioral inhibition), and occurrence of prior traumatic social experiences (e.g., significant teasing by peers, being embarrassed or humiliated in a social or performance situation).
- The risk of SAD also may be increased with family history.

DIAGNOSIS

DIFFERENTIAL DIAGNOSIS

- Other anxiety disorders (e.g., panic disorder with agoraphobia).
- As a consequence of mood disorders (e.g., avoidance of social situations associated with major depression).
- Pervasive developmental disorder (e.g., autism spectrum disorder).
- Personality disorders (e.g., schizoid personality disorder); however, in the case of avoidant personality disorder, both may be diagnosed.
- Anxiety associated with medical conditions such as stuttering or Parkinson's disease.

WORKUP

- Psychiatric history is required for a diagnosis.
- Screening measures may improve detection of SAD as it is a chronic, disabling condition for which many individuals do not seek treatment.
- Physical examination may be useful in ruling out other explanations for physical symptoms that are present, and to rule out presence of social anxiety due to a medical condition.

TREATMENT

NONPHARMACOLOGIC THERAPY

- Cognitive-behavior therapy (CBT)
- Acceptance and Commitment Therapy (ACT)
- Interpersonal Psychotherapy (IPT)
- Exposure therapy
- Social skills training

PHARMACOLOGIC THERAPY

- SSRIs/SNRIs
- Benzodiazepines (less favored)
- MAOIs (less favored)
- Beta-blockers (e.g., propranolol, atenolol: for performance-related anxiety)

ACUTE GENERAL Rx

- SAD is a chronic condition; therefore acute treatment is rarely indicated.
- However, benzodiazepines or beta-blockers may be prescribed on an as-needed basis for acute performance anxiety. Caution should be taken when prescribing benzodiazepines due to the possibility of dependence or misuse and high incidence of relapse following discontinuation, and long-term use of these medications generally is discouraged.
- Beta-blockers may also be prescribed on an as-needed basis, particularly for physical symptoms experienced during performance situations. However, evidence does not support its use for more generalized forms of SAD.

CHRONIC Rx

- CBT is effective and an appropriate first-line treatment.
- SSRIs/SNRIs (e.g., paroxetine, sertraline, venlafaxine) are also effective in the treatment of SAD and are a first-line pharmacologic treatment.
- MAOIs previously were considered gold standard treatment for SAD, but currently are less favorable due to side effects and dietary restrictions.
- Combination treatment of SSRI/SNRI and CBT is effective for SAD; however, some research has suggested that CBT alone may result in greater long-term benefit compared to combination treatment.

DISPOSITION

- SAD is a chronic condition, typically unremitting without treatment.
- Treatment may significantly improve SAD, although symptoms and impairment may continue to be present for some individuals following treatment.

REFERRAL

- If comorbid psychiatric conditions are present
- If the symptoms do not improve upon treatment or response to treatment is not optimal

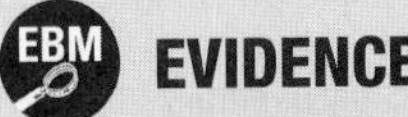

EVIDENCE

available at www.expertconsult.com

SUGGESTED READINGS

available at www.expertconsult.com

RELATED CONTENT

Anxiety (Generalized Anxiety Disorder) (Related Key Topic)

AUTHOR: **KRISTY L. DALRYMPLE, PH.D.**

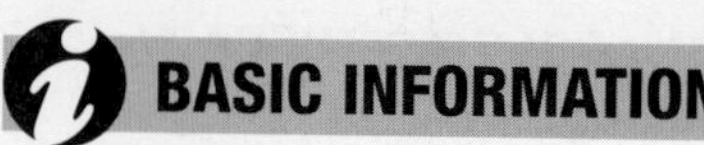

BASIC INFORMATION

DEFINITION

Somatization disorder has been replaced in DSM-5 with the diagnostic term *somatic symptom disorder*. In this condition one or more somatic symptoms are distressing or disruptive of daily life. There is often disproportionate thoughts about the seriousness of ones symptoms, persistent anxiety about one's health, and excessive time and energy devoted to the symptoms. There is often a pattern of recurring multiple somatic complaints that begin before the age of 30 yr and persist over several years. Patients complain of multiple symptoms but persistent pain is common. DSM-5 drops the term "unexplained by a medical condition" from the criteria.

SYNONYMS

Briquet's syndrome
Nonorganic physical symptoms
Medically unexplained symptoms
Functional somatic symptoms
Somatic symptom disorder

ICD-9CM and DSM-5 CODES
300.82
ICD-10CM CODES
F45.0 Somatization disorder
F45.1 Undifferentiated somatoform disease

EPIDEMIOLOGY & DEMOGRAPHICS

PREVALENCE (IN U.S.): Lifetime rates of 0.25% to 2% in women, ≤0.2% in men
PEAK INCIDENCE: Typically before age 25 yr
PREDOMINANT SEX: Women are more commonly affected in the U.S. (10:1 ratio)
PREDOMINANT AGE: Onset occurs before age 30 yr and usually in adolescence.
GENETICS: In males, there is a high risk of associated substance abuse or antisocial personality disorder.

PHYSICAL FINDINGS & CLINICAL PRESENTATION

- Onset is characteristically in the teens; course is marked by frequent, often unexplained, and frequently disabling pain symptoms and physical complaints.
- Patient frequently undergoes multiple procedures and seeks treatment from multiple physicians. Symptom focus rotates periodically with new physicians sought for new complaints.
- Patient often has a comorbid psychiatric disorder, most commonly generalized anxiety, panic disorder, or depression.

ETIOLOGY

- Believed to be the physical expression of psychological distress; there appears to be a biologic predisposition.
- May be more common in individuals without sufficient verbal or intellectual capacity to communicate psychological distress, individuals with alexithymia (inability to describe emotional states), or individuals from cultural backgrounds that consider emotional distress as an undesirable quality.
- Some aspects of somatic symptom disorder possibly learned from somatizing parents.

Dx DIAGNOSIS

DIFFERENTIAL DIAGNOSIS

- Psychological factors affecting other medical conditions (ICD-10 F45.1, DMS-5 316): psychological or behavioral factors adversely affect the medical condition in various ways, such as influencing the course of the medical condition or interfering with treatment.
- Conversion disorder: an alteration or loss of voluntary motor or sensory function without demonstrable physical cause and related to a psychological stress or a conflict. Findings provide evidence of incompatibility between the symptom and recognized neurologic or medical conditions (ICD-9 code 300.11).
- Factitious disorder (e.g., Munchausen's syndrome) and malingering: the psychologic basis of the complaints in somatization disorder is not conscious as in factitious disorder, in which the goal is to be in the patient role, and malingering, in which symptoms are also produced consciously but for some secondary gain like a monetary award in litigation or opioids.

WORKUP

- Rule out a general medical condition.
- If somatization is suspected on the basis of a history of repeated, multiple, unexplained complaints, restraint in ordering tests is recommended.

LABORATORY TESTS

No specific laboratory tests are required.

IMAGING STUDIES

No specific imaging studies are required.

Rx TREATMENT

NONPHARMACOLOGIC THERAPY

- Legitimize patient's complaints.
- Minimize diagnostic investigation and symptomatic treatment. Only do invasive testing or procedures when there are clear-cut signs, not just symptom reports.
- Set attainable treatment goals. Patients may benefit from realizing that even though they cannot be cured, that they will be cared for. This may help reassure them that they will continue to have a relationship with the caregiver.
- Treat coexisting psychiatric conditions such as depression and anxiety.

ACUTE GENERAL Rx

- At each visit do a brief physical examination focusing on the area of complaint.
- Gently praise increased functioning rather than focusing on symptoms.
- Explore recent life events and ask how the patient is handling these.
- Convey empathy with the patient's suffering and psychosocial difficulties.
- No specific pharmacologic therapy has been clearly proven effective, although a number of agents, including gabapentin and St. John's wort, have been useful in some studies.

CHRONIC Rx

- Provide one primary care practitioner to manage care.
- Avoid confronting the patient regarding the psychological origin of symptoms.
- Ensure follow-up visits at regular intervals (e.g., 2- to 4-wk intervals that are not symptom contingent; maintain the regularity even if the symptoms improve so that the patient does not need new symptoms to continue the relationship).
- Avoid invasive or expensive diagnostic procedures unless there are clear signs of new illness, not just symptoms.
- Diagnose and treat mood or anxiety disorders.
- Cognitive behavior therapy groups have been helpful for patients with unexplained somatic symptoms and can dramatically improve functioning.

DISPOSITION

A chronic condition with frequent exacerbations

REFERRAL

If the patient is open to discussing psychological issues, a referral for psychotherapy can be made.

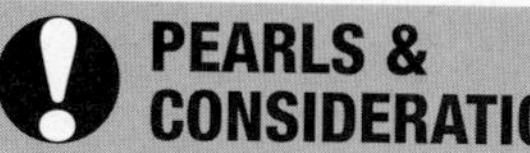

PEARLS & CONSIDERATIONS

Patients with somatization disorder respond best to establishing a regular, working relationship with a primary care provider. Avoiding confrontations about the origins of symptoms, investigating symptoms when related to actual signs of disease, and gently investigating concurrent stressors will help avoid most of the common problems with this population.

Patients with subsyndromal symptoms (i.e., failing to meet the full criteria but having three or more medically unexplained symptoms) may be just as challenging and chronic. They warrant similar approaches as utilized for the full syndrome.

SUGGESTED READINGS
available at www.expertconsult.com

RELATED CONTENT

Somatization Disorder (Patient Information)

AUTHOR: **STUART J. EISENDRATH, M.D.**

BASIC INFORMATION

DEFINITION

Spasticity is an exaggerated tone that displays a velocity-dependent increase in resistance of muscles to a passive stretch stimulus.

SYNONYMS

Hypertonicity

ICD-9CM CODES
782.85 Spasm of muscle
342.1, 343.0-344.9 Spastic paralysis
781.0 Abnormal involuntary movements/ Spasms NOS
781.2 Abnormality of gait/spastic
342.1 Spastic hemiplegia
344.0-344.9 Spastic paralysis specified as noncongenital or noninfantile
343 Infantile cerebral palsy/spastic infantile paralysis

ICD-10CM CODES
M62.838 Other muscle spasm
G81.10 Spastic hemiplegia affecting unspecified side
R25.0 Abnormal head movements
R26.0 Ataxic gait
G81.10 Spastic hemiplegia affecting unspecified side
G83.9 Paralytic syndrome, unspecified
G80.9 Cerebral palsy, unspecified

EPIDEMIOLOGY & DEMOGRAPHICS

INCIDENCE: Spasticity affects between 47% and 70% of people with multiple sclerosis, 32% to 36% of those with spinal cord injury, approximately 20% of those with stroke, more than 90% with cerebral palsy, and approximately 50% of patients with traumatic brain injury.

TABLE 1-455 Modified Ashworth Scale

0	No increase in muscle tone
1	Slight increase in muscle tone, manifested by a catch and release or by minimal resistance at the end range of motion when the part is moved in flexion or extension/abduction or adduction
1+	Slight increase in muscle tone, manifested by a catch, followed by minimal resistance throughout the remainder (less than half) of the range of motion
2	More marked increase in muscle tone through most of the range of motion, but the affected part is easily moved
3	Considerable increase in muscle tone, passive movement is difficult
4	Affected part is rigid in flexion or extension (abduction or adduction)

From Stein J: Spasticity. In Frontera WR et al (eds): *Essentials of physical medicine and rehabilitation*, ed 2, Philadelphia, 2008, Saunders.

PREDOMINANT SEX AND AGE: Spasticity is not affected by sex, race, or age group, nor is it more prevalent in any of those groups.

RISK FACTORS: Multiple sclerosis, stroke, spinal cord injury, cerebral palsy, traumatic brain injury

PHYSICAL FINDINGS & CLINICAL PRESENTATION

- Patient may present with impaired gait, impaired limb function, decreased mobility, or discomfort due to increased muscle tone.
- While increased tone may preserve strength in the affected muscles, function may be impaired, especially fine motor. Examine active and passive motion, reflexes, and functions:
  - Strength may be normal or decreased. Isometric strength is typically greater than concentric strength.
  - Tone may be variably increased to passive range of motion (modified Ashworth scale; see Table 1-455).
  - Reflexes are typically brisk.
  - Patient may have accompanying extensor plantar signs, clonus, or spontaneous flexor spasms.
  - Function may be impaired or enhanced due to increased tone.

ETIOLOGY

Upper motor neuron injury, most commonly due to multiple sclerosis, stroke, spinal cord injury, cerebral palsy, traumatic brain injury

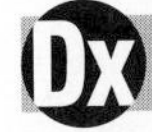

DIAGNOSIS

DIFFERENTIAL DIAGNOSIS

Rigidity, clonus, dystonia, dyskinesia, myotonia, tetanus, muscle contracture, cramps

WORKUP

- A diagnosis is established clinically.
- Investigate reversible exacerbating causes of spasticity: underlying infection, bladder distention, bowel impaction, fracture, pain.

LABORATORY TESTS

Urinalysis, complete blood count, metabolic panel

IMAGING STUDIES

Chest x-ray, abdominal x-ray series, bladder ultrasound

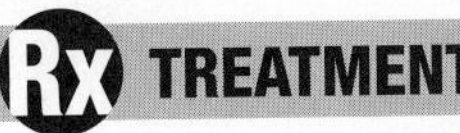

TREATMENT

First treat reversible causes of spasticity (see "Workup"), then proceed to physical and pharmacologic therapeutics. Lastly, consider surgical intervention in severe, refractory cases.

NONPHARMACOLOGIC THERAPY

- Physical therapeutics include range of motion and muscle stretching, serial casting or orthotics, muscle cooling, electrical stimulation.
- Surgical procedures include tenotomy, tendon lengthening, and tendon transfers. More invasive surgical interventions include peripheral neurectomy, myelotomy, and rhizotomy.

ACUTE GENERAL Rx

- Oral medications: baclofen, tizanidine, diazepam, dantrolene (Table E1-456)
- Other interventions: intrathecal baclofen, botulinum toxin intramuscular injections, chemical nerve blocks (with bupivacaine, phenol, or ethyl alcohol)

COMPLEMENTARY & ALTERNATIVE MEDICINE

EMG biofeedback

DISPOSITION

Typically nonprogressive, but medications may lose efficacy after long duration of use. Drug holidays (with use of alternate spasmolytic) may be beneficial.

REFERRAL

- Physicians: neurologist or physiatrist with expertise in botulinum toxin injection and/or intrathecal spasmolytic therapy is recommended when oral medications are ineffective or not tolerated.
- Physical and occupational therapy

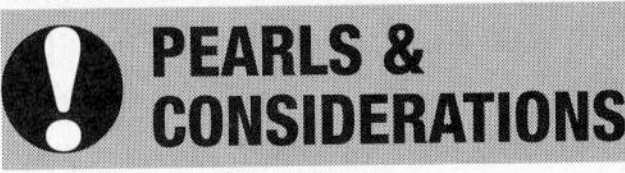

PEARLS & CONSIDERATIONS

- Assess whether the spasms recently increased in severity or intensity (as would occur with reversible exacerbating causes).
- Consider whether patient's tone is beneficial or detrimental to patient's functionality or overall health status.
- Spasticity may assist posture and mobility, as well as maintain muscle mass and bone mineralization, reduce dependent edema, and prevent deep venous thromboses.
- Spasticity may impair patient's functionality, interfere with activities of daily living, interfere with sleep, and cause discomfort.
- Monitor liver function with dantrolene and tizanidine, as these drugs may cause hepatotoxicity.

SUGGESTED READINGS

available at www.expertconsult.com

AUTHOR: **SACHIN KEDAR, M.B.B.S., M.D.**

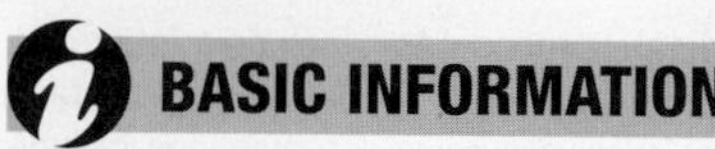

BASIC INFORMATION

DEFINITION

Spinal cord compression is the neurologic loss of function due to compression of the spinal cord or cauda equina along its course in the spinal canal. Fig. 1-874 illustrates a schematic demarcation of levels of principal dermatomes shown as distinct segments. Lesions may be complete or incomplete and develop gradually or acutely. Incomplete lesions often present as distinct syndromes, as follows:

- Central cord syndrome
- Anterior cord syndrome
- Brown-Séquard syndrome
- Conus medullaris syndrome
- Cauda equina syndrome

ICD-9CM CODES
344.89 Brown-Séquard syndrome
344.60 Cauda equina syndrome
336.8 Conus medullaris syndrome
Other lesions listed by site
ICD-10CM CODES
G83.81 Brown-Séquard syndrome
G83.4 Cauda equina syndrome
G95.81 Conus medullaris syndrome
Other lesions listed by site

EPIDEMIOLOGY

Spinal cord injury (SCI) typically occurs in males with a mean age of 38. Alcohol plays a role in at least 25% of SCI.
INCIDENCE: 11,000 new cases/yr
PREVALENCE: 171,000 persons
COST (IN U.S.): >$5 billion/yr
RISK FACTORS: underlying spinal disease can make some patients more susceptible to SCI:

- Cervical spondylosis
- Atlantoaxial instability
- Congenital conditions (tethered cord)
- Osteoporosis
- Ankylosing spondylitis or RA of the spine

PHYSICAL FINDINGS & CLINICAL PRESENTATION

Clinical features reflect the amount of spinal cord involvement:

- Motor loss and sensory abnormalities
- Babinski testing usually positive
- Clonus
- Gradual compression, often manifested by progressive difficulty walking, clonus with weight bearing, and involuntary spasm; development of sensory symptoms; bladder dysfunction (late)
- ***Central cord syndrome:*** results in a variable quadriparesis. It is described as a motor impairment greater in upper than lower extremities, bladder dysfunction, and variable degree of sensory loss below the injury level. It occurs after mild trauma in the setting of preexisting cervical spondylosis and results in variable quadriplegia.
- ***Anterior cord syndrome:*** it affects the anterior or ventral 2/3 of the spinal cord, sparing the dorsal columns. It is often a reflection of a vascular injury to the anterior spinal artery. It results in motor, pain, and temperature loss below the lesion.
- ***Brown-Séquard syndrome:***
  1. Spinal cord syndrome caused by injury to either half of the spinal cord and resulting in the loss of motor function, position, vibration, and light touch on the affected side
  2. Pain and temperature sense loss on the opposite side
- ***Conus medullaris syndrome:*** results in variable motor loss in the lower extremities with loss of bowel and bladder function
- ***Cauda equina syndrome:*** typical low back pain, weakness in both lower extremities, saddle anesthesia, and loss of voluntary bladder and bowel control

ETIOLOGY

- Trauma. Most SCIs result from high-speed motor vehicle accidents, falls, sports injuries, or violence.
- Tumor
- Infection
- Inflammatory processes
- Degenerative disk conditions with spinal stenosis
- Acute disk herniation
- Cystic abnormalities
- Ankylosing spondylitis
- Table 1-457 summarizes physical examination findings associated with vertebral fractures and spinal cord injuries

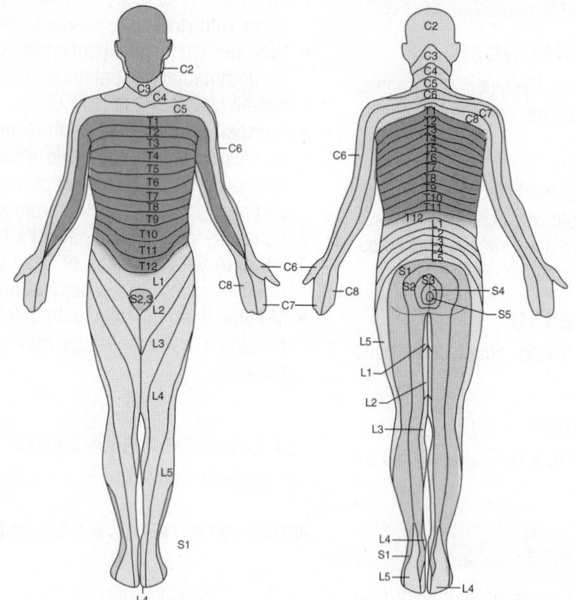

Levels of principal dermatomes

C5	Clavicles
C5,6,7	Lateral parts of upper limbs
C8, T1	Medial sides of upper limbs
C6	Thumb
C6,7,8	Hand
C8	Ring and little fingers
T4	Level of nipples
T10	Level of umbilicus
T12	Inguinal or groin regions
L1,2,3,4	Anterior and inner surfaces of lower limbs
L4,5 S1	Foot
L4	Medial side of great toe
S1,2, L5	Posterior and outer surfaces of lower limbs
S1	Lateral margin of foot and little toe
S2,3,4	Perineum

FIGURE 1-874 Schematic demarcation of levels of principal dermatomes shown as distinct segments. There is actually considerable overlap between any two adjacent dermatomes. (From Goldman L, Schafer AI: *Goldman's Cecil medicine,* ed 24, Philadelphia, 2011, Saunders.)

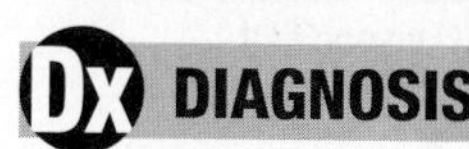

DIAGNOSIS

DIFFERENTIAL DIAGNOSIS

- See "Etiology."
- Section II describes the differential diagnosis of paraplegia.

WORKUP

- Spinal cord compression: requires an immediate referral for radiographic and neurologic assessment.
- Mental status evaluation and CNS function should be included as SCI might be associated with head injury.
- The primary assessment of a patient with an SCI in the field follows the ABCD prioritization scheme.
- With respect to airway management, suspected SCI dictates in-line immobilization of the spine at all times, so hyperextension of the neck is contraindicated. A jaw thrust must be used to open the airway, and required intubation must be done with the head/neck in a neutral position.
- Techniques to minimize spine movement include the use of log-roll movements and a back board for transfer and placement of a rigid cervical collar.
- Lab results usually unremarkable unless infectious or inflammatory causes suspected

IMAGING STUDIES

- Depend on the suspected etiology
- Neurologic signs and symptoms of SCI in the setting of normal plain x-rays should warrant further imaging studies.

TABLE 1-457 Physical Examination Findings Associated with Vertebral Fractures and Spinal Cord Injuries

Injury	Physical Examination Area	Associated Findings
Vertebral fracture	Spine	Tenderness of the neck and/or back. Examine the entire spine because vertebral fractures may occur in multiples.
	Neurologic	See spinal cord injury below.
	Chest	*Thoracic spine fractures:* check for chest tenderness, unequal breath sounds, and arrhythmia, which are suggestive of an associated intrathoracic injury or myocardial contusion.
	Abdomen/pelvis	*Thoracolumbar and lumbar spine fractures:* check for abdominal or pelvic tenderness. For instance, up to 50% of patients with a transverse process fracture and 33% of patients with a Chance fracture have concurrent intraabdominal pathology. A transverse area of ecchymosis on the lower abdominal wall (seat belt sign) increases the chance of an abdominopelvic injury.
	Extremity	*Thoracolumbar and lumbar spine fractures*: check for calcaneal tenderness because 10% of calcaneal fractures are associated with a low thoracic or lumbar fracture. Mechanistically, these areas are fractured as a result of axial loading.
Spinal cord injury	Neurologic, motor (anterior column)	Assess motor function on a scale of 0 to 5. The *motor level* is defined as the most caudal segment with at least 3/5 strength. Injuries to the first eight cervical segments result in tetraplegia (previously known as quadriplegia); lesions below the T1 level result in paraplegia.
	Neurologic, sensory (spinothalamic tract)	Assess sensory function via pinprick and light touch on the following scale: 0 = absent; 1 = impaired; 2 = normal. The *sensory level* is defined as the most caudal segment of the spinal cord with normal sensory function. The highest intact sensory level should be marked on the patient's spine to monitor for progression.
	Neurologic, sensory (dorsal column)	Assess vibratory sensory function on a scale of 0 to 2 by using a tuning fork over bony prominences. Assess position sense (proprioception) by flexing and extending the great toe.
	Neurology, deep tendon reflex	On a scale of 0 to 4, assess the deep tendon reflexes in the upper (biceps, triceps) and lower (patellar, Achilles) extremities.
	Anogenital	Assess rectal tone, sacral sensation, signs of urinary or fecal retention or incontinence, and priapism. Also check the anogenital reflexes: an *anal wink* (S2-S4) is present if the anal sphincter contracts in response to stroking the perianal skin area. The *bulbocavernosus reflex* (S3-S4) is elicited by squeezing the glans penis or clitoris (or pulling on an inserted Foley catheter), which results in reflexive contraction of the anal sphincter.
	Head-to-toe examination	A spinal cord injury may mask a patient's ability to perceive and localize pain. Imaging of high-risk areas, such as the abdomen, and areas of bruising or swelling may be required to exclude occult injuries.

From Adams JG et al: *Emergency medicine, clinical essentials,* ed 2, Philadelphia, 2013, Elsevier.

- Complete set of cervical x-rays should include anteroposterior, lateral, and open-mouth odontoid views.
- After initial resuscitative efforts, fine-cut helical CT scan with coronal and sagittal reconstructions have supplanted plain radiographs in most trauma centers as an initial evaluation in detecting spine fractures.
- MRI provides a detailed image of the spinal ligaments, intervertebral discs, and paraspinal soft tissues and is very sensitive for detecting epidural hematoma (Fig. E1-875).

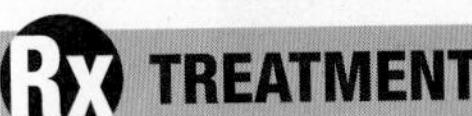

TREATMENT

- Urgent surgical decompression is usually indicated as soon as the etiology is established.
- Corticosteroids: The administration of methylprednisolone reduces the amount of secondary injury that occurs after SCI and has become an important tool in the treatment of SCI by improving outcomes. Corticosteroids should not be used in patients with associated traumatic brain injury and penetrating injuries since they might increase mortality.

DISPOSITION Important indicators regarding prognosis:

- The greater the distal motor and sensory sparing, the greater the expected recovery.
- When a plateau of recovery is reached, no further improvement is expected.
- The quicker the recovery, the greater the recovery.
- Patients with acute traumatic SCI need monitoring in the ICU and evaluation for potential life-threatening complications, including cardiovascular instability and respiratory failure.
- Prophylaxis against DVT and PE should always be provided.

REFERRAL

Immediate referral for radiographic and neurologic evaluation and treatment in all suspected cases of spinal cord compression

SUGGESTED READINGS

available at www.expertconsult.com

RELATED CONTENT

Spinal Stenosis (Patient Information)

AUTHOR: **CATHERINE ELIAS NAJEM, M.D.**

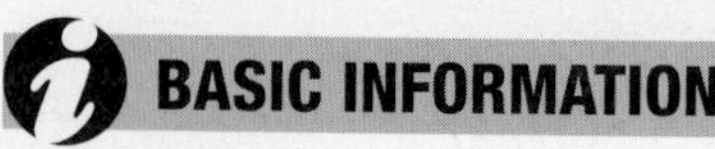

BASIC INFORMATION

DEFINITION

A spinal epidural abscess (SEA) is a focal suppurative infection occurring in the spinal epidural space.

ICD-9CM CODES
324.1 Spinal epidural abscess
ICD-10CM CODES
G06.1 Intraspinal abscess and granuloma

EPIDEMIOLOGY & DEMOGRAPHICS

INCIDENCE (IN U.S.):

- 2 to 25 cases/100,000 hospitalized patients/yr
- May be increasing over the past 3 decades

PREDOMINANT AGE:

- Median age of onset approximately 50 yr (35 yr in intravenous drug users)
- Peak incidence in seventh and eighth decades of life

PHYSICAL FINDINGS & CLINICAL PRESENTATION

- The presentation of SEA can be nonspecific.
- Fever, malaise, and back pain are the most consistent early symptoms.
- Pain is often focal. It may initially be mild but can progress to become severe.
- As the disease progresses, root pain can occur, followed by motor weakness, sensory changes, bladder and bowel dysfunction, and paralysis.
- Physical findings may be limited to fever or spinal tenderness.
- The evolution to neurologic deficits can occur as quickly as a few hours, or over weeks to months.
- Once paralysis occurs, it may quickly become irreversible without the appropriate intervention.

ETIOLOGY

- Pyogenic bacteria account for the majority of cases in the U.S. Immigrants from TB-endemic areas may present with tuberculous SEAs. Fungi and parasites can also cause this condition. The most common causative organism is *Staphylococcus aureus.* Gram-negative bacilli and anaerobes may be seen if the infection has a urinary or GI source.
- Most posterior SEAs are thought to originate from distant focus (e.g., skin and soft tissue infections), while anterior SEAs are commonly associated with diskitis or vertebral osteomyelitis. No source was found in approximately one third of cases.
- Associated predisposing conditions include diabetes mellitus, alcoholism, cancer, AIDS, and chronic renal failure, or following epidural anesthesia, spinal surgery or trauma, or IV drug use. No predisposing condition is found in approximately 20% of patients.
- Damage to the spinal cord can be caused by direct compression of the spinal cord, vascular compromise, bacterial toxins, and inflammation.

Dx DIAGNOSIS

DIFFERENTIAL DIAGNOSIS

- Herniated disk
- Vertebral osteomyelitis and diskitis
- Metastatic tumors
- Meningitis

LABORATORY TESTS

- WBC may be normal or elevated.
- ESR is usually elevated over 30 mm/hr.
- Blood cultures are positive in approximately 60% of patients with SEA.
- CSF cultures are positive in 19%, but lumbar puncture is unnecessary, and may be contraindicated.
- Once imaging is done, CT-guided aspiration or open biopsy should be done to determine causative organism. Abscess content culture is positive in 90% of patients.

IMAGING STUDIES

- MRI with gadolinium is the imaging modality of choice (Fig. 1-876); CT scan with contrast may show the abscess (Fig. 1-877) but is less sensitive than MRI.
- CT with myelography is more sensitive for cord compression.

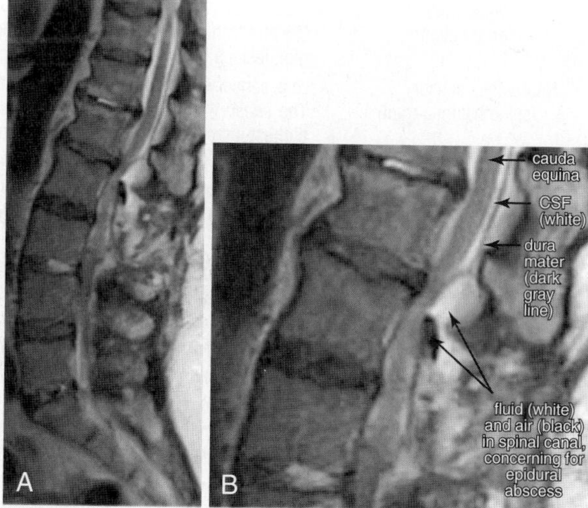

FIGURE 1-876 Same patient as in Fig. 1-877, in whom noncontrast computed tomography showed air in the spinal canal, concerning for epidural abscess. Magnetic resonance imaging (MRI) of the lumbar spine without contrast was performed, as the patient was in acute renal failure. **A,** This T_2-weighted sagittal MR image provides useful information even without gadolinium contrast. **B,** Close-up. On T_2-weighted MRI sequences, fluid including cerebrospinal fluid *(CSF)* appears white. Fat-containing tissues such as bone marrow and the spinal cord or cauda equina appear dark gray. Calcified bone appears nearly black due to an absence of resonating protons. Air appears completely black for the same reason. The midline sagittal image shows the cauda equina to be impinged upon by an epidural fluid collection containing air—an epidural abscess. The dura mater is visible as a thin, dark gray line parallel to the spinal cord. It is indented in the region of the epidural abscess. (From Broder JS: *Diagnostic imaging for the emergency physician,* Philadelphia, 2011, Saunders.)

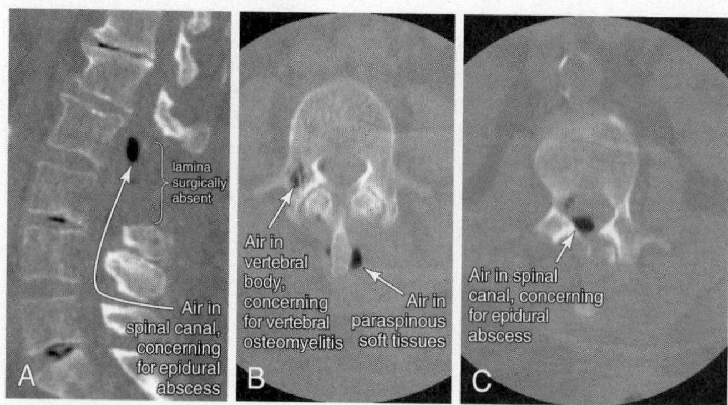

FIGURE 1-877 This 67-year-old female presented with delirium and fever. Three months prior, she had undergone lumbar laminectomy, and her wound had been treated with a wound VAC dressing. Magnetic resonance imaging was not initially available, so noncontrast computed tomography (CT) was performed. Noncontrast CT is excellent at delineating air, which appears black on bone windows. **A,** The midsagittal view demonstrates air *(black)* in the spinal canal at the L2 and L3 levels. On the axial views **(B, C),** air is visible in the spinal canal, in paraspinal soft tissues, and within the vertebral body. These findings are concerning for a paraspinal infection that has developed into an epidural abscess with vertebral osteomyelitis. (From Broder JS: *Diagnostic imaging for the emergency physician,* Philadelphia, 2011, Saunders.)

Rx TREATMENT

NONPHARMACOLOGIC THERAPY

- Surgical decompression is the mainstay of treatment. Decompression within the first 24 hr has been related to an improved prognosis.
- Nonsurgical treatment is effective in some patients, but failure rate may be excessive. This approach should not be considered and should only be attempted in the absence of signs of compressive myelopathy and with very careful follow-up.

ACUTE GENERAL Rx

- In addition to surgery, antibiotics directed at the most likely organism should be initiated. Fig. 1-878 describes an algorithm for the management of patients with SEA.
- If the organism is unknown, broad coverage against staphylococci, streptococci, and gram-negative bacilli should be initiated. Empiric antimicrobial therapy typically includes vancomycin plus an antipseudomonal cephalosporin or carbapenem. The regimen can be adjusted according to culture results. Therapy should continue for at least 4 to 6 wk.

CHRONIC Rx

Neurologic deficits may remain despite aggressive treatment.

DISPOSITION

Irreversible paralysis and death can occur in up to 25% of patients.

REFERRAL

All cases should be referred to a neurosurgeon and an infectious disease specialist.

PEARLS & CONSIDERATIONS

- It is critically important to recognize this process early; the prognosis is generally excellent if treatment is initiated while symptoms are localized and before evidence of myelopathy develops.
- The likelihood of success postsurgery is low in patients who have developed complete paralysis for longer than 36 hours.

SUGGESTED READINGS

available at www.expertconsult.com

AUTHOR: **GLENN G. FORT, M.D., M.P.H.**

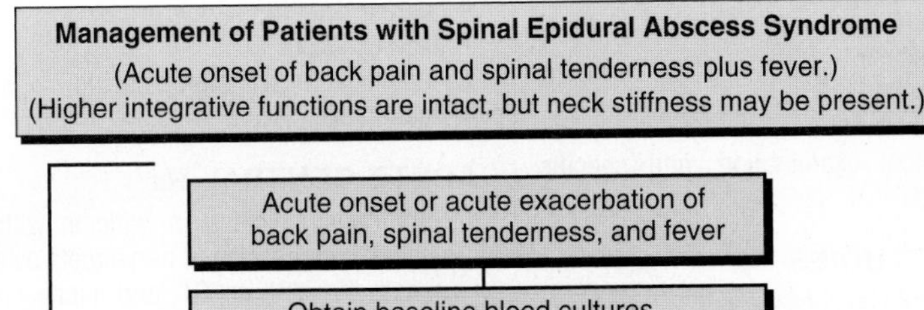

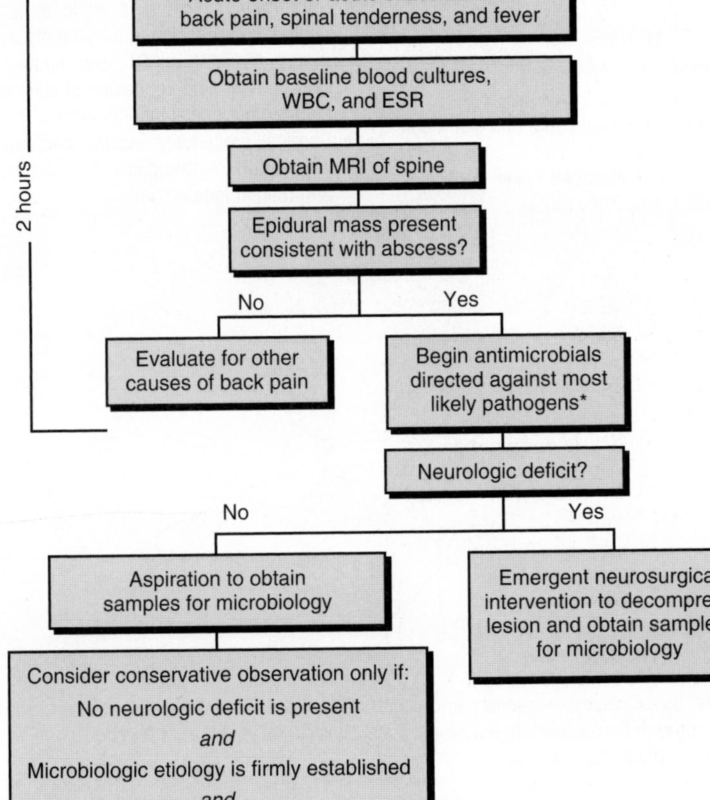

FIGURE 1-878 Algorithm for the management of patients with spinal epidural abscess syndrome. If magnetic resonance imaging *(MRI)* cannot be performed, myelography, high-contrast computed tomography (CT), or CT-myelography may be an acceptable alternative to localize an epidural abscess. *If abscess drainage can be performed promptly, antimicrobial drugs may be withheld until specimens for microbial analysis are obtained. *ESR,* Erythrocyte sedimentation rate; *WBC,* white blood cell. (From Vincent JL et al: *Textbook of critical care,* ed 6, Philadelphia, 2011, Saunders.)

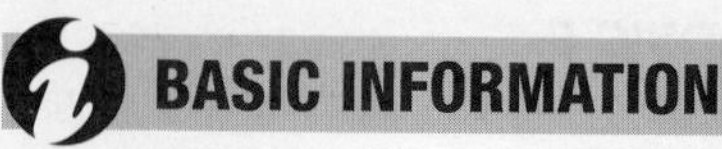

BASIC INFORMATION

DEFINITION

Spinal stenosis is the pathologic condition caused by the compressing or narrowing of the spinal canal, nerve root canal, or intervertebral foramina at the lumbar region.

SYNONYMS

Central spinal stenosis
Lateral spinal stenosis
Spondylosis

ICD-9CM CODES
724.02 Spinal stenosis lumbar, lumbosacral
ICD-10CM CODES
M48.06 Spinal stenosis, lumbar region

EPIDEMIOLOGY & DEMOGRAPHICS

More common between 50 and 60 yr of age

PHYSICAL FINDINGS & CLINICAL PRESENTATION

- Symptoms caused by direct mechanical compression or indirect vascular compression of the nerve roots or the cauda equina.
- Neurogenic claudication: leg, buttock, or back pain precipitated by walking and relieved by sitting.
- Pain may radiate down to ankles and is associated with numbness, tingling, and weakness.
- Taking a flexed posture reduces symptoms because it increases the available space in the lumbar spinal canal.
- Decreased lumbar extension.
- Normal peripheral pulses.
- Positive Romberg's sign (decreased proprioception).
- Wide-based gait.
- Reduced knee and ankle reflex.
- Urine incontinence.

ETIOLOGY

Spinal stenosis may be primary or secondary (Fig. 1-879)

- Primary stenosis (congenital or developmental narrowing)
  1. Idiopathic
  2. Achondroplasia
  3. Morquio-Ullrich syndrome
- Secondary stenosis (acquired)
  1. Degenerative (hypertrophy of the articular processes, disk degeneration, ligamentum flavum hypertrophy, spondylolisthesis)
  2. Fracture/trauma
  3. Postoperative (postlaminectomy)
  4. Paget's disease
  5. Ankylosing spondylitis
  6. Tumors
  7. Acromegaly

Dx DIAGNOSIS

DIFFERENTIAL DIAGNOSIS

- Osteoarthritis of the knee or hip
- Acute cauda equina syndrome, resulting from compression by epidural abscess or tumors
- Pain and weakness caused by multiple myeloma or osteomyelitis
- Intermittent claudication—peripheral vascular disease
- Peripheral neuropathy such as that caused by a herniated nucleus pulposus
- Scoliosis or spondylolisthesis
- Rheumatoid diseases: ankylosing spondylitis, Reiter's syndrome, fibromyalgia
- Table 1-458 compares clinical features of spinal stenosis, peripheral vascular disease, and disk disease.

WORKUP

History, physical examination, and specific imaging studies

IMAGING STUDIES

- Lumbar spine film sensitivity 66%, specificity 93%.
- Ultrasound of the spinal canal has also been used.
- CT scan of the lumbosacral spine: sensitivity (75% to 85%), specificity (80%).
- MRI of the lumbosacral spine (Fig. 1-880): sensitivity (80% to 90%), specificity (95%).
- Myelogram: sensitivity (77%), specificity (72%). Absolute stenosis is defined as the anterior-posterior (AP) diameter of the spinal canal <10 mm. Relative stenosis: 10 to 12 mm AP diameter.
- Electromyography (EMG) and nerve conduction velocity (NCV) are additional studies particularly useful in differentiating peripheral neuropathy from lumbar spinal stenosis.

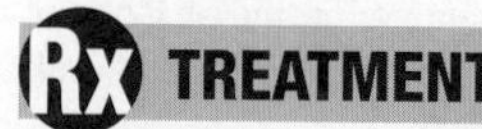

TREATMENT

NONPHARMACOLOGIC THERAPY

- Physiotherapy
- Lumbar corsets
- Back exercises
- Abdominal muscle strengthening
- Aquatic exercises

ACUTE GENERAL Rx

- Surgery is indicated in patients with significant compression of nerve roots as determined by MRI or CT and incapacitating symptoms limiting activities of daily living or bladder and bowel incontinence.
- Surgical procedures include decompressive laminectomy, arthrodesis, hemilaminectomy, and medial facetectomy.

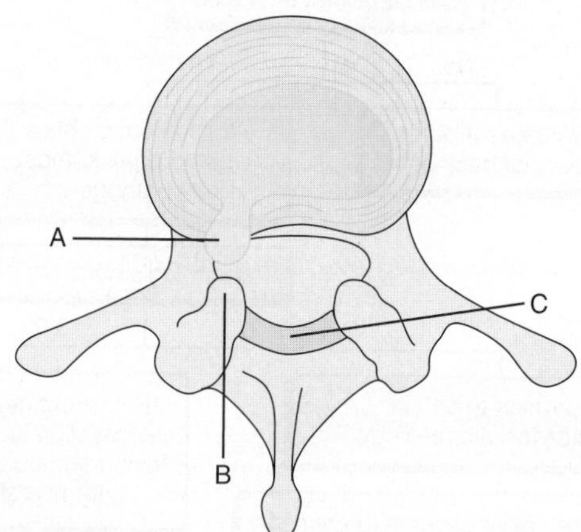

FIGURE 1-879 Spinal stenosis secondary to a combination of disk herniation *(A)*, facet joint hypertrophy *(B)*, and hypertrophy of the ligamentum flavum *(C)*. (From Firestein GS et al: *Kelly's textbook of rheumatology*, ed 9, Philadelphia, 2013, Saunders.)

TABLE 1-458 Comparative Clinical Features of Spinal Stenosis, Peripheral Vascular Disease, and Disc Disease

Feature	Spinal Stenosis	Disc Prolapse	Peripheral Vascular Disease
Reduced straight leg raise	Rarely	Usually	No
Neurologic deficit	Sometimes	Often	No
Leg pain on walking	Yes	Usually	Yes
Leg pain on sitting	No	Yes	No
Pain relief on standing still	No	No	Yes
Pain relief on sitting	Yes	No	Yes
Numbness/paresthesia	Yes	Yes	Sometimes

From Carr A, Hamilton W: *Orthopedics in primary care*, ed 2, Philadelphia, 2005, Butterworth-Heinemann.

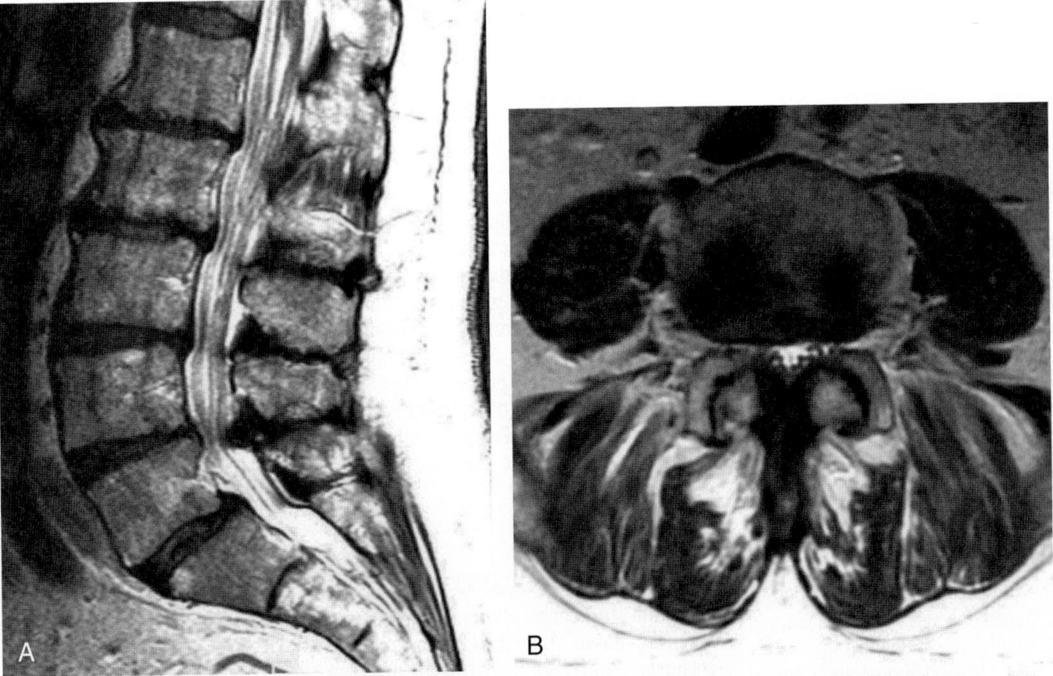

FIGURE 1-880 Degenerative spinal stenosis. A, The sagittal T2-weighted magnetic resonance image shows decreased anteroposterior diameter of the neural canal at the L4-5 level due to redundancy of the ligamentum flavum. **B,** The axial image through the L4-5 disk shows decreased cross-sectional area of the thecal sac from hypertrophic changes of the facet joints posterolateral to the thecal sac. (Courtesy Dr. John Crues, University of California, San Diego.)

- Lumbar interspinous process decompression using X-STOP device: a titanium oval spacer placed between the two adjacent spinous processes of the affected level; provides an unloading distractive force to the stenotic middle column part of the motion segment.

CHRONIC Rx

- Conservative therapy with NSAIDs (ibuprofen 800 mg PO tid, naproxen 500 mg PO bid) may be tried for symptomatic relief in addition to acetaminophen 1 g PO qid.
- Epidural steroid injections may provide temporary relief.

DISPOSITION

- Approximately 20% of patients having surgery require repeat surgery within 10 yr. Nearly one third of these patients continue to experience pain.
- The natural history of spinal stenosis is one of slow progression. Although not very common, cord compression with resultant bowel and bladder incontinence and paresis can occur.
- Operative treatment is more effective in reducing pain and disability than nonoperative treatment.

REFERRAL

- Patients who have spinal stenosis should be referred to an orthopedic surgeon specializing in back surgery or to a neurosurgeon.
- Pain clinic referrals should be made if surgery is contraindicated or if the patient does not want surgery.

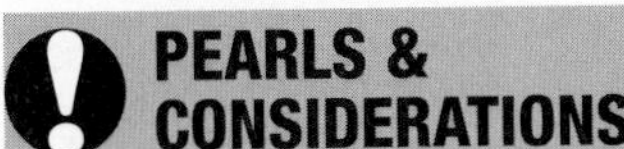

PEARLS & CONSIDERATIONS

COMMENTS

- Approximately one third of patients have coexisting peripheral vascular disease.
- The severity of cauda equina constriction is directly related to the walking ability and the pain intensity in the legs and back.
- Spinal stenosis is also a cause of chronic low back pain in the young.

SUGGESTED READINGS

available at www.expertconsult.com

RELATED CONTENT

Spinal Stenosis (Patient Information)

AUTHOR: **JORGE A. VILLAFUERTE, M.D.**

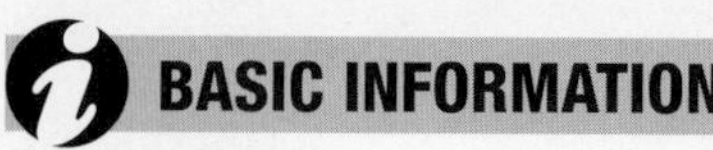

BASIC INFORMATION

DEFINITION

The spinocerebellar ataxias (SCAs) are a heterogeneous group of autosomal dominantly inherited genetic conditions that cause progressive ataxia and other neurologic symptoms.

SYNONYMS

Autosomal-dominant cerebellar ataxia (ADCA)
Machado-Joseph disease (eponym for SCA3; this may be the most common SCA)

ICD-9CM CODES
334.2 Primary cerebellar degeneration
ICD-10CM CODES
G11.9 Hereditary ataxia, unspecified
G11.8 Other hereditary ataxias

EPIDEMIOLOGY & DEMOGRAPHICS

PREVALENCE: The prevalence of the condition is approximately 3 persons per 100,000. The most common SCAs are 1, 2, 3, 6, and 7.
PREDOMINANT SEX: SCA demonstrates no gender preference.
PREDOMINANT AGE: The age of onset is often during the 30s or 40s. However, this can be highly variable, even within family groups; SCAs can occur anytime from childhood to late adulthood.
GENETICS: All SCAs are inherited in an autosomal dominant fashion; however, reduced penetrance can be present.

PHYSICAL FINDINGS & CLINICAL PRESENTATION

- Chronically progressive ataxia is the predominant symptom of all of the SCAs. It typically presents as a combination of balance and gait difficulty, limb incoordination, and dysarthria.
- More than 36 different genetic subtypes of SCA have been described to date. Although certain clinical characteristics are common to specific SCA subtypes, there is significant overlap among and variability within these conditions, so making a diagnosis on the basis of the clinical presentation alone can be challenging and sometimes impossible without genetic testing. Some of the more common SCAs and their possible distinguishing features in addition to ataxia include the following:
  - SCA1 can be characterized by nystagmus, spasticity, and neuropathy.
  - SCA2 can be characterized by slow saccades, gaze palsy, neuropathy, and sometimes parkinsonism or dementia.
  - SCA3, which is also known as *Machado-Joseph disease,* can be characterized by neuropathy, amyotrophy, parkinsonism, and dystonia.
  - SCA6 is generally felt to be a pure cerebellar syndrome with ataxia and nystagmus (gaze evoked and downbeat) as well as a frequently later age of onset.
  - SCA7 is characterized by dementia, vision loss caused by a pigmentary maculopathy, and spasticity.
  - Knowledge in this area is constantly expanding and being updated. Online sources of information (e.g., Online Mendelian Inheritance in Man [http://www.ncbi.nlm.nih.gov/omim]) can be invaluable for tracking new developments.

ETIOLOGY

Several of the SCAs are the result of polyglutamine CAG repeat expansions; this causes the accumulation of mutant proteins inside neurons, which is thought to cause dysfunction and cell death. Higher numbers of repeats are correlated with an earlier onset of symptoms, and anticipation may be present. Other types of repeat expansions and point mutations have been found with several SCAs; for others, the affected gene has not been identified.

Dx DIAGNOSIS

DIFFERENTIAL DIAGNOSIS

- Structural cerebellar abnormality: includes cerebellar tumor, inflammation (e.g., multiple sclerosis), stroke, or hemorrhage; the time course for these causes is typically more acute or subacute than chronic
- Endocrine dysfunction: hypothyroidism or hypoparathyroidism can uncommonly cause ataxia
- Alcoholic cerebellar degeneration: caused by heavy alcohol use; gait ataxia predominates
- Other toxin-induced ataxias: antiepileptic medications, lithium, and chemotherapeutic agents
- Creutzfeldt-Jakob disease: rapidly progressive ataxia, dementia, and myoclonus
- Paraneoplastic cerebellar degeneration: found in association with primary malignancies (e.g., small cell lung cancer, breast cancer); subacute-onset ataxia that progresses rapidly
- Celiac disease: gluten-sensitive enteropathy with malabsorption may be associated with ataxia; autoantibodies such as antigliadin or antiendomysial antibodies are typically present
- Multiple system atrophy: cerebellar variant of this disorder causes ataxia; there is typically associated parkinsonism with some degree of autonomic dysfunction (e.g., orthostatic hypotension, urinary incontinence)
- Friedreich's ataxia: autosomal recessive inheritance, generally younger age of onset (i.e., mean 15 yr of age), lower limb areflexia, and posterior column dysfunction
- Ataxia associated with vitamin E deficiency: can be an autosomal recessive disorder or acquired; clinically resembles Friedreich's ataxia, with areflexia and loss of position sense
- Ataxia telangiectasia: autosomal recessive inheritance, childhood onset, oculocutaneous telangiectases, and immunodeficiency
- Wilson's disease: can cause hepatic dysfunction and a variety of movement disorders, including ataxia; particularly important to screen for this in patients who are young at onset because it is treatable
- Dentatorubral-pallidoluysian atrophy: autosomal dominant like SCA but typically has ataxia with associated choreoathetosis, myoclonus, epilepsy, and dementia
- Fragile X–associated tremor/ataxia syndrome: premutation of the fragile X mutation gene; more common among males than females; late onset of ataxia (i.e., >50 yr), tremor, and sometimes parkinsonism; MRI often shows T_2 hyperintensity in the middle cerebellar peduncle
- Box 1-79 shows the classification of the various causes of ataxia.

LABORATORY TESTS

- Rule out acquired causes of ataxia, depending on the clinical scenario, with thyroid studies, toxicology screening, and the determination of the vitamin E level or presence of paraneoplastic antibodies.
- Screen for Wilson's disease with ceruloplasmin and, if indicated, a 24-hour urinary copper determination.
- Genetic testing is commercially available for many but not all of the SCAs.

IMAGING STUDIES

- MRI of the brain should be performed to exclude structural abnormalities.
- Cerebellar or brain stem atrophy can be seen with several of the SCA subtypes.

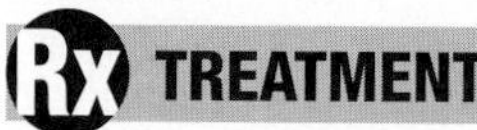

Rx TREATMENT

NONPHARMACOLOGIC THERAPY

- Speech therapy for dysarthria and dysphagia
- Physical therapy
- Occupational therapy

CHRONIC Rx

Treatment is symptomatic and supportive. In some cases, parkinsonism can respond to levodopa. Clonazepam can be helpful if tremor is prominent. Spasticity can be treated with baclofen or tizanidine. Dystonia may benefit from botulinum toxin injections.

DISPOSITION

All SCA disorders are progressive, although the speed is variable from subtype to subtype and from patient to patient. On average, patients become wheelchair bound 15 yr after the onset of ataxia, and death can occur after 20 to 25 yr.

REFERRAL

Referral to a general neurologist or to a movement disorders center is appropriate.

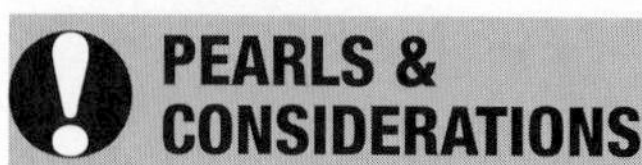

PEARLS & CONSIDERATIONS

COMMENTS

- Genetic testing can have consequences for both the patient and the family. These issues should be discussed during the informed consent process. Patients who desire asymptomatic testing as a result of a relevant family

BOX 1-79 Classification of Ataxia

Congenital Ataxias

Hereditary Ataxias

Autosomal Recessive Ataxias

- Friedreich's ataxia
- Ataxia–telangiectasia
- Ataxia with oculomotor apraxia type 1
- Ataxia with oculomotor apraxia type 2
- Autosomal recessive spastic ataxia of Charlevoix-Saguenay
- Abetalipoproteinemia
- Ataxia with isolated vitamin E deficiency
- Refsum's disease
- Cerebrotendinous xanthomatosis
- Marinesco-Sjögren syndrome
- Autosomal recessive ataxia with known gene locus
- Early-onset cerebellar ataxia

X-Linked Ataxias

- Fragile X tremor ataxia syndrome

Autosomal Dominant Ataxias

- Spinocerebellar ataxias
- Dentatorubral-pallidoluysian atrophy
- Episodic ataxias

Nonhereditary Degenerative Ataxias

- Multiple system atrophy, cerebellar type
- Sporadic adult-onset ataxia of unknown etiology

Acquired Ataxias

- Alcoholic cerebellar degeneration
- Ataxia as a result of other toxic causes (e.g., antiepileptic medications, lithium, solvents)
- Paraneoplastic cerebellar degeneration
- Other immune-mediated ataxias (e.g., gluten ataxia, ataxia associated with anti-glutamic acid decarboxylase antibodies)
- Acquired vitamin E deficiency
- Hypothyroidism
- Ataxia as a result of physical causes (e.g., heat stroke, hyperthermia)

From Goetz CG: *Textbook of clinical neurology*, ed 3, Philadelphia, 2007, Saunders.

history should undergo genetic counseling before testing.

- In symptomatic patients with a family history of dominantly inherited ataxia, the diagnostic process is relatively straightforward. Genetic testing that is directed toward likely mutations by phenotype and ethnic origin should be the first step rather than an extensive workup for other causes.

PATIENT & FAMILY EDUCATION

Patient educational materials as well as contact information for support and advocacy groups are available on the website of the National Ataxia Foundation: http://www.ataxia.org.

SUGGESTED READINGS

available at www.expertconsult.com

AUTHOR: **ANDREW DUKER, M.D.**

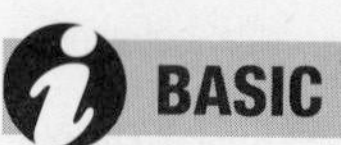

BASIC INFORMATION

DEFINITION

Spontaneous miscarriage is fetal loss before week 20 of pregnancy, calculated from the patient's last menstrual period or the delivery of a fetus weighing <500 g. Early loss is before menstrual week 12, whereas late loss refers to losses from weeks 12 to 20.

Miscarriage can also be classified as incomplete (partial passage of fetal tissue through partially dilated cervix), complete (spontaneous passage of all fetal tissue), threatened (uterine bleeding without cervical dilation or passage of tissue), inevitable (bleeding with cervical dilation without passage of fetal tissue), or missed abortion (intrauterine fetal demise without passage of tissue).

Recurrent miscarriage involves three or more spontaneous pregnancy losses before week 20 although most providers will perform an evaluation for recurrent spontaneous abortion after two losses. The definition is somewhat variable depending on the source.

SYNONYMS

Spontaneous abortion

ICD-9CM CODES
634.0 Spontaneous abortion
ICD-10CM CODES
003.9 Complete or unspecified spontaneous abortion without complication

EPIDEMIOLOGY & DEMOGRAPHICS

INCIDENCE: 5% to 20% of clinically recognized pregnancies, with 80% of miscarriages occurring in the first trimester. Recurrent miscarriage occurs in less than 1% of couples attempting to have children.

GENETICS:

- Distribution of abnormal karyotypes: autosomal trisomy (50%), monosomy 45,X (20%), triploidy (15%), tetraploidy (10%), structural chromosomal abnormalities (5%).
- With two or more spontaneous miscarriages, a karyotype should be performed to evaluate for balanced translocation, which has a substantially increased risk for abortion (depending on the actual type of translocation), and, if the pregnancy is carried to term, has 3% to 5% risk for unbalanced karyotype.

RISK FACTORS: Vaginal bleeding, especially >3 days, carries with it a 15% to 20% chance of miscarriage. Diabetes should be optimally controlled to reduce the risk.

PHYSICAL FINDINGS & CLINICAL PRESENTATION

- Profuse bleeding and cramping have a higher association with miscarriage than bleeding without cramping, which is more consistent with a threatened miscarriage.
- Cervical dilation with history or finding of fetal tissue at cervical os may be present.
- In cases of missed abortion, uterine size may be smaller than menstrual dating, in contrast to molar gestation, where size may be greater than dates.

ETIOLOGY

- In a general overview the etiology can be classified in terms of maternal (environmental) and fetal (genetic) factors, with the majority of miscarriages being related to genetic or chromosomal causes.
- Causes: uterine anomalies (unicornuate uterus risk, 50%; bicornuate or septate uterus risk, 25% to 30%); incompetent cervix (iatrogenic or congenital, associated with 20% of midtrimester losses); diethylstilbestrol exposure in utero (T-shaped uterus); submucous leiomyomas; intrauterine adhesions or synechiae; luteal phase or progesterone deficiency; autoimmune disease such as anticardiolipin antibodies; uncontrolled diabetes mellitus. Rare or controversial causes include human leukocyte antigen associations between mother and father; infections such as tuberculosis, *Chlamydia,* and *Ureaplasma;* smoking and alcohol use; irradiation; and environmental toxins. Most of the literature is observational in nature, which may skew risk factor data.

Dx DIAGNOSIS

DIFFERENTIAL DIAGNOSIS

- Normal pregnancy
- Hydatidiform molar gestation
- Ectopic pregnancy
- Dysfunctional uterine bleeding
- Pathologic endometrial or cervical lesions

WORKUP

- All patients with bleeding in the first trimester should have an evaluation for possible ectopic pregnancy.
- If there are three early, prior pregnancy losses, a workup and treatment for recurrent miscarriage should begin before next conception. If there is a strong history for second-trimester loss, consideration for cerclage should be given if the history is consistent with incompetent cervix (e.g., painless cervical dilation).
- Most providers will initiate an evaluation for couples who have had only two previous losses.
- One unexplained fetal loss beyond 10 wk or 1 birth before 34 wk because of preeclampsia should prompt an evaluation for antiphospholipid syndrome.

LABORATORY TESTS

- Type and antibody screen are used to evaluate the need for Rh immune globulin.
- During the preconception period, hemoglobin A_{1c}, anticardiolipin antibody, lupus anticoagulant, prothrombin gene 20210A, karyotyping, and anatomic evaluation to assess for uterine septum. With increasing age, oocyte quality is a factor and some practitioners will perform day 3 of the menstrual cycle FSH and anti-müllerian hormone to assess for diminished ovarian reserve.
- Progesterone level <5 mg/dl suggests nonviable gestation vs. >25 mg/dl, which suggests a good prognosis.

IMAGING STUDIES

Transvaginal sonogram (preferably) can be used in combination with menstrual dating and serum quantitative human chorionic gonadotropin to document pregnancy location, fetal heart presence, gestational sac size, and adnexal pathology.

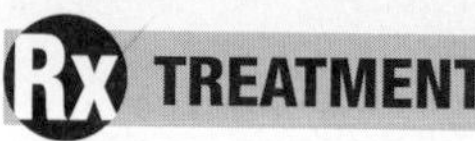

TREATMENT

NONPHARMACOLOGIC THERAPY

Depending on the patient's clinical status, desire to continue the pregnancy, and certainty of the diagnosis, expectant management can be considered. In pregnancies <6 wk or >14 wk, complete expulsion of fetal tissue usually occurs and surgical intervention such as dilation and curettage (D&C) can be avoided.

ACUTE GENERAL Rx

- Incomplete miscarriage between 6 and 14 wk can be associated with large amounts of blood loss; thus these patients should undergo D&C.
- In cases of missed abortion, if fetal demise has occurred >6 wk before or gestational age is >14 wk, there is an increased risk of hypofibrinogenemia with disseminated intravascular coagulation. Thus D&C or manual vacuum aspiration should be performed early in the disease course. Consider use of misoprostol (Cytotec) 200 mg PO q6h as an alternative approach if patient desires a less invasive approach.
- Rh-negative patients should be given RhoGAM 300 mcg IM to prevent Rh isoimmunization.

REFERRAL

Refer to obstetrician/gynecologist.

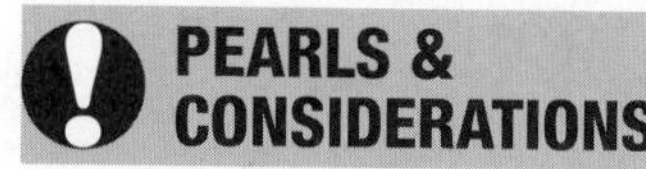

PEARLS & CONSIDERATIONS

Spontaneous pregnancy loss is recommended as a replacement for the term *abortion* and to acknowledge the emotional aspects of losing a pregnancy.

SUGGESTED READINGS

available at www.expertconsult.com

RELATED CONTENT

Miscarriage (Patient Information)
Ectopic Pregnancy (Related Key Topic)
Molar Pregnancy (Related Key Topic)
Vaginal Bleeding during Pregnancy (Related Key Topic)

AUTHOR: **RUBEN ALVERO, M.D.**

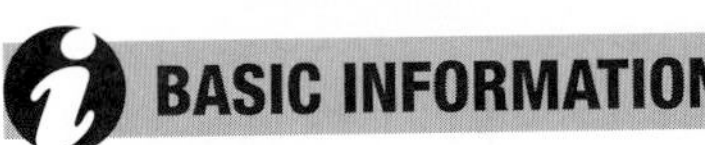

BASIC INFORMATION

DEFINITION

Squamous cell carcinoma (SCC) is a malignant tumor of the skin arising in the epithelium.

SYNONYMS

SCC
Skin cancer

ICD-9CM CODES
173.9 Skin neoplasm, site unspecified
ICD-10CM CODES
C44.5 Malignant neoplasm of skin of trunk
C44.4 Malignant neoplasm of skin of scalp and neck
D04 Carcinoma in situ of skin
C44.9 Malignant neoplasm of skin, unspecified
C44.0 Malignant neoplasm of skin of lip
C44.2 Malignant neoplasm of skin of ear and external auricular canal
C44.3 Malignant neoplasm of skin of other and unspecified parts of skin

EPIDEMIOLOGY & DEMOGRAPHICS

- SCC is the second most common cutaneous malignancy, comprising 20% of all cases of nonmelanoma skin cancer.
- Incidence is highest in lower latitudes (e.g., southern U.S., Australia).
- Male/female ratio is 2:1.
- Incidence increases with age and sun exposure.
- Average age at diagnosis is 66 yr.

PHYSICAL FINDINGS & CLINICAL PRESENTATION

- SCC commonly affects the scalp, neck region, back of hands, superior surface of the pinna, and the lip (Fig. E1-882).
- The lesion may have a scaly, erythematous macule or plaque.
- Telangiectasia, central ulceration may also be present (Fig. 1-883).
- Most SCCs present as exophytic lesions that grow over a period of months.
- Although most SCCs are relatively slow growing and nonaggressive, some (2%-5%) can exhibit rapid growth and metastases. Aggressive tumors are more common in immunocompromised patients and when arising from scars, burns, or prior injury (Marjolin's ulcer). Presence of SCC on ears, lips, or size >2 cm are high-risk features of SCC.

ETIOLOGY

Risk factors include ultraviolet B radiation, immunosuppression (kidney transplant recipients have a threefold increased risk), arsenic exposure, HPV infection, and tobacco abuse.

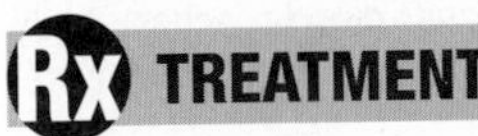

DIAGNOSIS

DIFFERENTIAL DIAGNOSIS

- Keratoacanthomas
- Actinic keratosis
- Amelanotic melanoma
- Basal cell carcinoma
- Benign tumors
- Healing traumatic wounds
- Spindle cell tumors
- Warts

WORKUP

Diagnosis is made by full-thickness skin biopsy (incisional or excisional).

Rx TREATMENT

ACUTE GENERAL Rx

- Electrodesiccation and curettage for small SCCs (<2 cm in diameter), superficial tumors, and lesions located in extremity and trunk.
- Tumors thinner than 4 mm can be managed by simple local removal.
- Lesions between 4 and 8 mm thick or those with deep dermal invasion should be excised.
- Tumors penetrating the dermis can be treated with several modalities, including excision and Mohs' surgery, radiation therapy, and chemotherapy. Mohs' surgery is commonly used for lesions on the face.
- Metastatic SCC can be treated with cryotherapy and combination of chemotherapy using 13-*cis*-retinoic acid and interferon-alpha 2A.

DISPOSITION

- Survival is related to size, location, degree of differentiation, immunologic status of the patient, depth of invasion, and presence of metastases. Risk factors for metastasis include lesions on the lip or ear, increasing lesion depth, and poor cell differentiation.
- Patients whose tumors penetrate through the dermis or exceed 8 mm in thickness are at risk of tumor recurrence.
- The most common metastatic locations are regional lymph nodes, liver, and lung.
- Tumors on the scalp, forehead, ears, nose, and lips also carry a higher risk.
- SCCs originating in the lip and pinna metastasize in 10% to 20% of cases.
- Five-year survival for metastatic SCC is 34%.

REFERRAL

Oncology referral for metastatic SCC

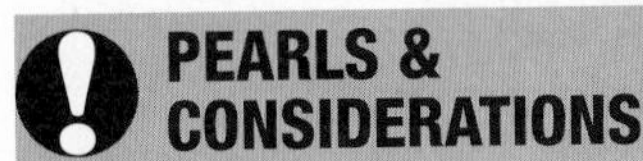

PEARLS & CONSIDERATIONS

COMMENTS

SCC arising in areas of prior radiation, thermal injury, and areas of chronic ulcers or chronic draining sinuses are more aggressive and have a higher frequency of metastasis than those originating in actinic damaged skin.

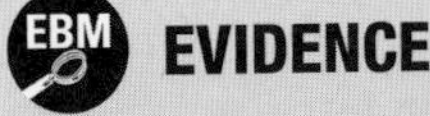

EVIDENCE

available at www.expertconsult.com

SUGGESTED READINGS

available at www.expertconsult.com

RELATED CONTENT

Squamous Cell Carcinoma (Patient Information)

AUTHOR: **FRED F. FERRI, M.D.**

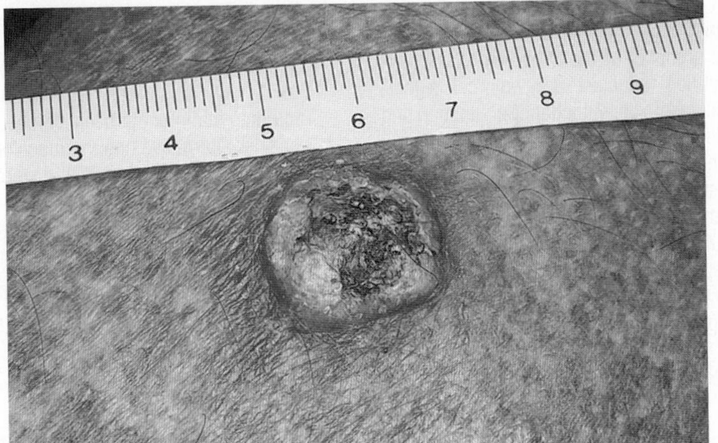

FIGURE 1-883 Squamous cell carcinoma. Nodular hyperkeratotic lesion with central erosion. (From Noble J et al: *Textbook of primary care medicine,* ed 3, St Louis, 2001, Mosby.)

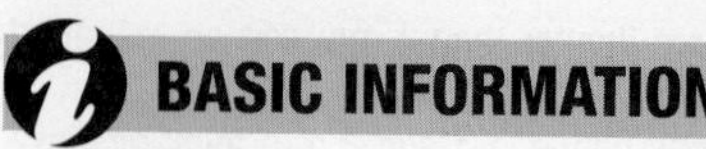

BASIC INFORMATION

DEFINITION

Statin-induced muscle syndromes (SIMS) include myopathy, myalgia, myositis, and rhabdomyolysis. Definitions for these syndromes are inconsistent in the medical literature.

- Myopathy: a general term defined as any disease of muscles.
- Myalgia: muscle weakness or pain without serum creatinine kinase elevation.
- Myositis: muscle weakness or pain with an increased serum creatinine kinase level.
- Rhabdomyolysis: muscle weakness or pain and a marked serum creatinine kinase level usually greater than 10 times the upper limit of normal and serum creatinine elevation as well as signs of brown urine and elevated urine myoglobin. A rare immune-mediated necrotizing myopathy (IMNM) has also been associated with the use of statins with symptoms persisting after discontinuation of the drug.

SYNONYMS

Statin-induced myopathies
Statin-induced myositis
Statin-induced myalgias
Statin-induced rhabdomyolysis

ICD-9CM CODES

729.1	Myalgia and myositis
728.8	Rhabdomyolysis
359.4	Toxic myopathy
359.9	Myopathy, unspecified
359.81	Critical illness myopathy
359.89	Other myopathies

ICD-10CM CODES

M60.9	Myositis, unspecified
M62.82	Rhabdomyolysis
G72.2	Myopathy due to other toxic agents
G72.9	Myopathy, unspecified
G72.81	Critical illness myopathy
G72.89	Other specified myopathies

EPIDEMIOLOGY & DEMOGRAPHICS

INCIDENCE & PREVALENCE: Risk of statin-induced rhabdomyolysis is 1.2 per 10,000 persons/yr increasing to 0.9% in patients taking high-dose statins. Rhabdomyolysis risk of death is 0.15 deaths per 1 million prescriptions. SIMS most commonly occur in people aged 51 to 75, which may reflect the pattern of statin use. The prevalence of statin-induced myalgias is about 1% to 5%, similar to placebo in clinical trials, although observational studies have suggested a prevalence of 10% or higher. Statins may cause elevated transaminases (ALT, AST) at a prevalence of 0.5% to 2.0% and rhabdomyolysis ~0.08%.

PREDOMINANT SEX AND AGE: The mean age of hospitalized patients with statin-induced myopathy or rhabdomyolysis was 64 yr. Slightly more common in women (56%).

GENETICS: Interpatient variability exists in the activity of the *CYP3A4* gene for the metabolism of simvastatin, atorvastatin, and lovastatin. Homozygous carriers of CYP2D6 (poor metabolizers) had a higher rate of discontinuation of simvastatin due to muscle syndromes compared with the CYP2D6 wild-type genotype; patients taking atorvastatin and having a muscle event were more likely to have the CYP2D6*4 allele. SLCO1B1 polymorphisms encode for the organic anion transport of statins into the liver cells. Some data exist on deficiencies in ubiquinone (coenzyme Q10) in patients with a mutation in the *COQ2* gene.

RISK FACTORS: Small body frame; age over 80 yr; women, particularly frail elderly women; patients taking multiple drugs, especially gemfibrozil, niacin, cyclosporine, itraconazole, ketoconazole, erythromycin, clarithromycin, verapamil, amiodarone; renal or liver impairment; pharmacogenetic variability; hypothyroidism; excessive alcohol intake; vigorous exercise; severe infections; excessive grapefruit juice ingestion; inherited defects of muscle metabolism such as carnitine palmityl transferase II deficiency, McArdle's disease, and myoadenylate deaminase deficiency; acquired myopathies such as postpoliomyelitis syndrome; lipophilic statins (simvastatin, atorvastatin, lovastatin); multiple conditions such as diabetes; and drugs of abuse (amphetamines, heroin, cocaine, phencyclidine).

PHYSICAL FINDINGS & CLINICAL PRESENTATION

- Myopathy can occur at any time, although it is more common within the first 4 weeks of therapy.
- Proximal generalized muscle aches, body aches, and pains, and may be mild or severe.
- Dark-colored urine
- Muscle cramps, spasms, tenderness, or stiffness
- Unusually tired or weak
- Nocturnal cramping
- Tendon pain

ETIOLOGY

- History of current statin use
- May be explained by one of three deficiencies of end products of the 3-hydroxy-3-methylglutaryl-coA reductase pathway: cell signaling and apoptosis, mitochondrial function and ubiquinone concentrations, and cholesterol concentrations and cell membrane integrity.
- The risk may be enhanced by drug interactions that interfere with hepatic metabolism and gut wall transport of interacting medications and by pharmacodynamic effects.
- Underlying metabolic muscle disorder may predispose a patient to develop myopathy.

Dx DIAGNOSIS

DIFFERENTIAL DIAGNOSIS

Bursitis, tendinitis, radiculopathy, osteoarthritis, muscle strain, myofascial pain, hypothyroidism, proton-pump inhibitor-induced polymyositis, viral illness, polymyositis, and polymyalgia rheumatica

WORKUP

Workup consists of a thorough history, including exercise history, urine color, medication history, and physical exam to palpate tenderness and obtain blood tests to evaluate muscle and kidney damage.

LABORATORY TESTS

If severe myopathy or rhabdomyolysis is suspected:

- Elevated CPK, positive serum myoglobin, elevated BUN, serum creatinine, AST, ALT, LDH, and potassium
- Urine creatinine, positive casts, and hemoglobin in urine with absence of red blood cells
- Consider electrocardiogram and assessment of calcium, phosphate, and uric acid.

If mild to moderate myopathy is suspected:

- Monitor TSH and CPK levels; CPK may only be elevated when sudden severe myopathy occurs.
- If the patient has brown or dark urine or elevated CPK, monitor BUN and serum creatinine.

IMAGING STUDIES

- Not recommended

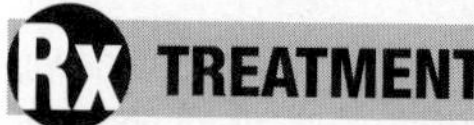

Rx TREATMENT

- Discontinue statin therapy immediately if muscle symptoms occur. An algorithm for monitoring and management of suspected statin-associated myopathy is described in Fig. E1-884.
- Depending on severity of the syndrome, consider switching to another statin once symptoms resolve, which may take up to 4 months.
- Consider alternate-day therapy or once or twice weekly therapy for long-acting statins such as atorvastatin and rosuvastatin.
- Patient willingness to rechallenge with lower dose, or if not, or if symptoms recur, consider statin such as pravastatin.
- Consider fluvastatin 80 mg extended release, which may be effective in reducing myalgia symptoms.
- Consider alternative cholesterol-lowering agents such as ezetimibe and colesevelam. Box 1-80 describes recommendations regarding statin and muscle safety.
- Consider alternative nonpharmacologic treatment such as plant stanols and sterols or red yeast rice.
- For IMNM, immunosuppressive therapy with prednisone and at least one agent have been used.

NONPHARMACOLOGIC THERAPY

- Treatment of rhabdomyolysis is generally supportive in nature (see "Rhabdomyolysis" topic).
- Use of coenzyme Q10 for mild myalgias although data are conflicting.

ACUTE GENERAL Rx

- Stop statin therapy; check history, potential drug-drug interactions, CPK, TSH, renal function, hepatic function, and urinalysis.

- If patients have suspected rhabdomyolysis, they should be hospitalized and treated with supportive therapy and monitoring of complications.
- If CPK <10× the upper limit of normal without symptoms, continue statin therapy at the same or lower dosage
- If CPK <10× the upper limit of normal with intolerable symptoms, discontinue statin.
- If CPK >10× the upper limit of normal, discontinue statin.

CHRONIC Rx

- After stopping the statin and symptom or CPK resolution, consider the same statin at a lower dosage or a different statin at an equivalent or lower dosage.
- When restarting therapy, consider statins such as low-dose rosuvastatin; long-acting fluvastatin; and alternate-day dosing of rosuvastatin, atorvastatin, or long-acting fluvastatin.
- If patient had rhabdomyolysis secondary to statin therapy, consider nonstatin treatments.
- If the patient develops myopathy after a second trial of therapy, statin treatment should be permanently discontinued and nonstatin cholesterol-lowering therapy initiated.

COMPLEMENTARY & ALTERNATIVE MEDICINE

- The effects of coenzyme Q10 on reducing or preventing SIMS remain controversial with evidence both supporting and refuting its potential benefits. Given its safety, coenzyme Q10 can be recommended if the actions listed under "Chronic Rx" are insufficient to continue the use of the statin and if the muscle symptoms have been limited to myalgias. Use coenzyme Q10 with caution in patients taking warfarin, as its anticoagulant effect may be decreased.
- Observational studies have suggested an association between vitamin D deficiency and statin-induced myopathy. Data are conflicting. The effects of supplementing vitamin D in patients with statin myopathy are limited and cannot be recommended unless a vitamin D deficiency is present.

DISPOSITION

- Usually resolves within 1 wk up to 4 mo after discontinuing statin therapy.
- Once the patient has a full recovery, an alternative statin can be tried.
- Statins should not be restarted in IMNM.

REFERRAL

- If rhabdomyolysis is suspected, immediate referral for hospitalization is suggested.

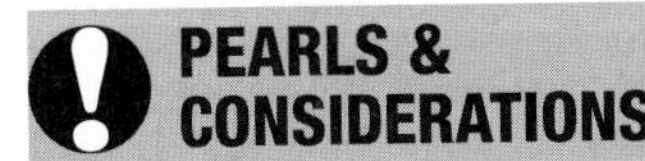

PEARLS & CONSIDERATIONS

COMMENTS

SIMS are usually mild and will resolve within a few wk after discontinuing statin therapy. However, such syndromes may progress to rhabdomyolysis.

PREVENTION

- Use the lowest statin dosage to achieve target lipid levels, and titrate dosage slowly to minimize myopathy risk.
- Avoid risk of potentiating myopathy.
- Discontinue statin therapy prior to and during surgical procedures.
- If patient requires a short-term therapy with an interacting medication such as an azole antifungal, temporarily discontinue statin therapy until interacting therapy is completed.
- If statin–fibric acid therapy is warranted, fenofibrate is preferred over gemfibrozil to decrease risk of myopathy; consider fluvastatin for a combination with gemfibrozil, if desired.
- Baseline liver function testing before initiation of statin therapy and only if clinically indicated thereafter

PATIENT & FAMILY EDUCATION

- Inform patients to promptly report muscle weakness, unexpected muscle pain, or brownish urine.
- Ensure that the pharmacist and/or primary care physician checks for drug-drug interactions with every new prescription, including those from dentists and physicians from other specialties.
- Coenzyme Q10 may lessen some of the milder muscle symptoms from statins, but patients should inform their physician and pharmacist if they decide to use this supplement.

SUGGESTED READINGS

available at www.expertconsult.com

RELATED CONTENT

Rhabdomyolysis (Related Key Topic)

AUTHORS: **LIORA FARBER, M.D., LISA COHEN, PHARM.D.,** and **ANNE L. HUME, PHARM.D.**

BOX 1-80 Recommendations to Health Care Professionals Regarding Statin and Muscle Safety

- Whenever muscle symptoms or an increased CK level is encountered in patients receiving statin therapy, health professionals should attempt to rule out other causes, because these are most likely to explain the findings. Other common causes include increased physical activity, trauma, falls, accidents, seizure, shaking chills, hypothyroidism, infections, carbon monoxide poisoning, polymyositis, dermatomyositis, alcohol abuse, and drug abuse (cocaine, amphetamines, heroin, or PCP).
- Obtaining a pretreatment, baseline CK level can be considered in patients who are at high risk of experiencing muscle toxicity (e.g., older patients or those combining a statin with an agent known to increase myotoxicity), but this is not routinely necessary in other patients.
- It is unnecessary to measure CK levels in asymptomatic patients during the course of statin therapy, because marked, clinically important CK elevations are rare and are usually related to physical exertion or other causes.
- Patients receiving statin therapy should be counseled about the increased risk of muscle symptoms, particularly if initiation of vigorous, sustained endurance exercise or a surgical operation is being contemplated; they should be advised to report such muscle symptoms to a health professional.
- Creatine kinase measurements should be obtained in symptomatic patients to help gauge the severity of muscle damage and facilitate decision of whether to continue therapy or alter doses.
- In patients who develop intolerable muscle symptoms with or without CK elevation and for whom other etiologies have been ruled out, the statin should be discontinued. Once symptoms disappear, the same or different statin at the same or a lower dose can be restarted to test the reproducibility of symptoms. Recurrence of symptoms with multiple statins and doses requires initiation of other lipid-altering therapy.
- In patients who develop tolerable muscle symptoms or have no symptoms but have a CK level <10 × ULN, statin therapy may be continued at the same or reduced doses and symptoms may be used as the clinical guide to stop or continue therapy.
- In patients who develop rhabdomyolysis (CK >10,000 IU/L or >10 × ULN with an elevation in serum creatinine or need for intravenous hydration therapy), statin therapy should be stopped. Intravenous hydration therapy in a hospital should be instituted if indicated for patients experiencing rhabdomyolysis. Once patients recover, risk vs. benefit of statin therapy should be carefully reconsidered.

CK, Creatine kinase; *PCP,* phencyclidine; *ULN,* upper limit of normal.

From McKenney JM et al: Final conclusions and recommendations of the National Lipid Association Statin Safety Assessment Task Force, *Am J Cardiol* 97(suppl 8A):89C-94C, 2006.

Status Epilepticus 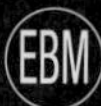 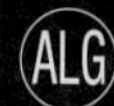 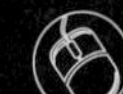

BASIC INFORMATION

DEFINITION

Status epilepticus is a medical neurologic emergency. It is historically defined as 30 min of continuous seizure activity or two or more seizures without full recovery of consciousness between seizures. However, in practice a continuous seizure that lasts >5 min should be treated as status epilepticus.

SYNONYMS

Convulsive status epilepticus
Nonconvulsive status epilepticus

ICD-9CM CODES
345.3 Grand mal status
ICD-10CM CODES
G41 Status epilepticus
G40.301 Generalized idiopathic epilepsy and epileptic syndromes, not intractable, with status epilepticus

EPIDEMIOLOGY & DEMOGRAPHICS

INCIDENCE: 40 to 100 cases per 100,000 persons

PEAK INCIDENCE: It is most common among children younger than 1 yr and adults older than 60 yr.

PREDOMINANT SEX AND AGE: No gender preference

PHYSICAL FINDINGS & CLINICAL PRESENTATION

- Patients can present with repetitive tonic clonic movements of the body (convulsive status epilepticus); other patients are comatose and nonresponsive (nonconvulsive status epilepticus).
- Patients may also present with lethargy, intermittent confusion, and involuntary movements.

ETIOLOGY

- Status epilepticus can be the result of an acute neurologic injury, such as stroke, meningitis, etc.
- In patients with epilepsy, abrupt discontinuation of antiepileptic drugs can result in status epilepticus.
- See Table 1-459 for causes of status epilepticus.

TABLE 1-459 Causes of Status Epilepticus

- Stroke (ischemic/hemorrhagic)
- CNS infections
- Traumatic head injury
- CNS toxicity: certain medications, drugs, ethanol
- Brain tumors or other mass lesions
- Metabolic disturbances: hypoglycemia, hyponatremia
- Abrupt discontinuation of antiepileptic drugs in patient with epilepsy
- Cryptogenic

CNS, Central nervous system.

DIAGNOSIS

DIFFERENTIAL DIAGNOSIS

- Convulsive syncope
- Encephalopathies: metabolic, infectious, toxic, etc.
- Nonepileptic spells

WORKUP

- ABCs
- ICU admission
- Emergent electroencephalogram (EEG)
- Continuous video EEG in refractory cases
- Investigation of the patient with status epilepticus is summarized in Box 1-81.

LABORATORY TESTS

- Routine blood workup (CBC, CMP, glucose, electrolytes)
- Urine drug screen
- Lumbar puncture and CSF analysis in patients with suspected meningitis

IMAGING STUDIES

- Immediate CT scan of the head
- MRI of the brain should be performed once the patient is in a stable condition.

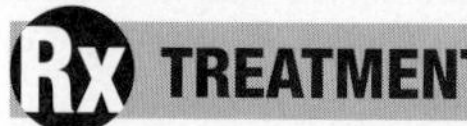

TREATMENT

- Patients with continuous seizure activity over 3 min need intravenous lorazepam 0.1 mg/kg at 2 mg/min (or diazepam 0.2 mg/kg at 5 mg/min only when lorazepam is not available).
- Lorazepam is followed by intravenous fosphenytoin 20 mg/kg (PE) at a rate not greater than 150 mg/min.
- An alternate to fosphenytoin is phenytoin 20 mg/kg IV at up to 50 mg/min as tolerated. Vital signs should be monitored during the infusion.
- If seizures continue, intravenous phenobarbital, midazolam, or propofol is an alternative. Other agents used include intravenous valproic acid and intravenous levetiracetam.
- Results of recent trials comparing intramuscular midazolam vs. intravenous lorazepam for prehospital status epilepticus show that IM midazolam may be as good as lorazepam,

BOX 1-81 Investigation of the Patient with Status Epilepticus

To Be Performed in All Patients with Status Epilepticus
- Serum glucose, electrolytes, calcium, magnesium
- Blood gas, serum osmolality
- Toxicology screen (serum and urine)
- Antiepileptic drug levels
- Complete blood count (RBC, differential WBC, platelet count)
- Liver enzymes, serum ammonium
- Blood culture
- Lumbar puncture, including:
  - Opening pressure
  - Cell count, Gram stain, smear for acid-fast bacilli
  - Viral and bacterial cultures
  - PCR for herpesvirus
- EEG, preferably continuous monitoring with video
  - To monitor for subtle or subclinical seizures
  - To guide antiepileptic drug therapy
  - To localize the epileptogenic brain region (focal slowing or epileptiform activity)

To Be Considered in Patients with Status Epilepticus
- Structural neuroimaging (CT, MRI)
  - To diagnose acute infarction, hemorrhage, vascular malformation, encephalitis, abscess, neurocysticercosis, neoplasm
  - In nonlesional cases, may localize the epileptogenic zone by evidence of focal edema in the affected cortical region
  - To assess the degree of cerebral edema and diagnose impending uncal or transtentorial herniation
  - MR angiography may identify CNS vasculitis, especially in medium or large vessel disease
- Functional neuroimaging (PET, SPECT)
  - In nonlesional cases, may identify the epileptogenic zone
- Cerebral angiography
  - To identify small vessel CNS vasculitis, which may not be visible on MR angiography
- Rheumatologic workup for vasculitides
- ESR, C-reactive protein, rheumatoid factor, serum complement levels, antineutrophil cytoplasmic antibodies
- Brain biopsy
  - To diagnose cerebral vasculitis (granulomatous compared with nongranulomatous)
  - To identify malformations of cortical development

CNS, Central nervous system; *CT,* computed tomography; *EEG,* electroencephalography; *ESR,* erythrocyte sedimentation rate; *MRI,* magnetic resonance imaging; *PCR,* polymerase chain reaction; *PET,* positron emission tomography; *RBC,* red blood cell; *SPECT,* single-photon emission computed tomography; *WBC,* white blood cell.

From Fuhrman BP et al: *Pediatric critical care,* ed 4, Philadelphia, 2011, Saunders.

with successful termination of seizures in 73% of patients in the IM midazolam group vs. 63% in the IV lorazepam group. This difference was attributed to the more rapid administration of the IM medication (1.2 min vs. 4.8 min with the IV route).

- A management algorithm for status epilepticus in adults is described in Fig. 1-885.
- Fig. E1-886 describes guidelines for the treatment of prolonged seizures and status epilepticus in infants (>1 mo), children, and adolescents and refractory status epilepticus.

NONPHARMACOLOGIC THERAPY

None

GENERAL Rx

It is important to find out the etiology of the status epilepticus (e.g., metabolic disturbance, infection). The appropriate treatment/understanding of the underlying cause of the status epilepticus will impact successful treatment.

CHRONIC Rx

- Chronic treatment of status epilepticus depends on underlying etiology.
- Patient with status epilepticus due to epilepsy will need chronic treatment.

COMPLEMENTARY & ALTERNATIVE MEDICINE

Not applicable

DISPOSITION

- Response to treatment depends on the etiology of the status epilepticus.
- When there is no CNS injury as a cause or result of the status epilepticus, the prognosis is good.
- No driving until seizure freedom in accordance with local laws and regulations.

REFERRAL

Status epilepticus is a neurologic emergency; therefore immediate neurologic consultation is warranted.

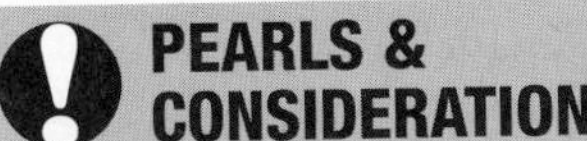

PEARLS & CONSIDERATIONS

COMMENTS

- Status epilepticus is a medical emergency that carries a high risk of mortality. Mortality among patients who present in status epilepticus is 15% to 22%. Among those who survive, functional ability will decline in 25% of cases.
- Continuous video EEG is crucial in the treatment of these patients because some of them may not be clinically seizing (convulsing) but electrographically they may still have subclinical repetitive seizures or subclinical status epilepticus.

PREVENTION

Medication compliance is crucial in patients with epilepsy.

PATIENT & FAMILY EDUCATION

- Patients with epilepsy have normal lives.
- The goal of treatment is no seizures and no side effects to medications.
- Patient education and information can be obtained at the Epilepsy Foundation: www.epilepsyfoundation.org
- Pregnant women with epilepsy should visit the Antiepileptic Drug Pregnancy Registry website for information and assistance: www2.massgeneral.org/aed
- Patients with ongoing seizures are forbidden from driving; check state regulations and laws regarding driving and epilepsy.

SUGGESTED READINGS

available at www.expertconsult.com

AUTHOR: **PATRICIO SEBASTIAN ESPINOSA, M.D., M.P.H.**

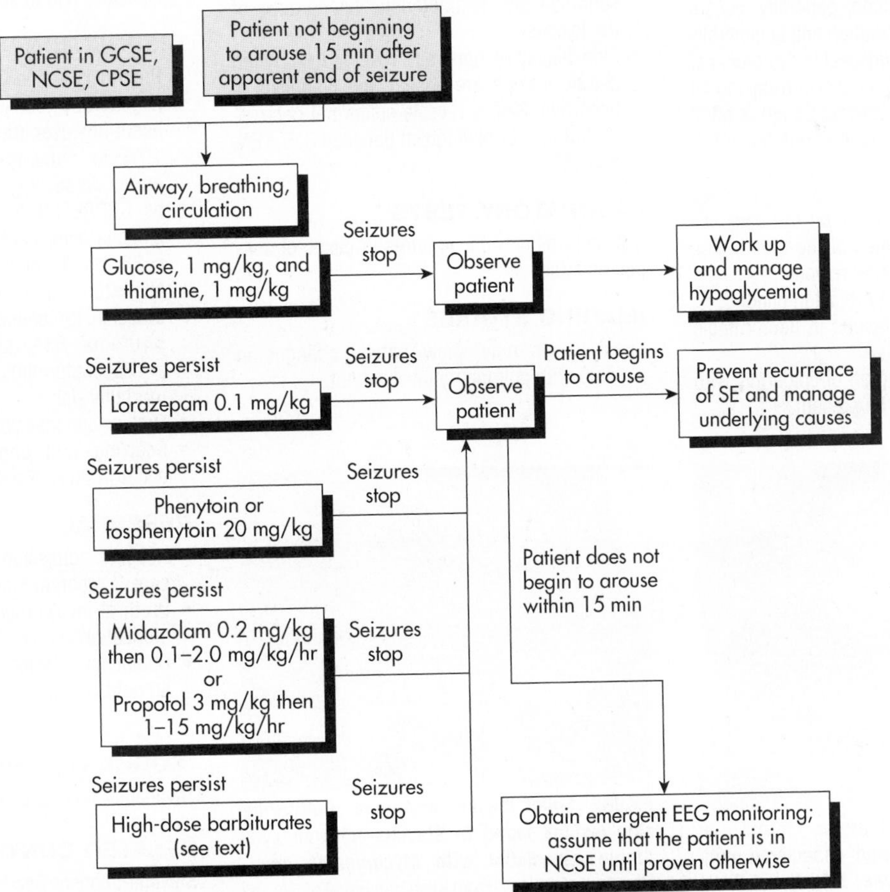

FIGURE 1-885 Management algorithm for status epilepticus. *CPSE,* Complex partial status epilepticus; *GSCE,* generalized convulsive status epilepticus; *NCSE,* nonconvulsive status epilepticus; *SE,* status epilepticus. (From Vincent JL et al: *Textbook of critical care,* ed 6, Philadelphia, 2011, Saunders.)

BASIC INFORMATION

DEFINITION

Stevens-Johnson syndrome (SJS) is a rare, severe vesiculobullous form of erythema multiforme (EM) affecting the skin, mouth, eyes, and genitalia. SJS is defined as affecting <10% of body surface area (BSA). When it affects 10%-30% of BSA, it is known as SJS–toxic epidermal necrolysis (TEN) overlap syndrome. TEN affects >30% of BSA.

SYNONYMS

SJS
Herpes iris
Febrile mucocutaneous syndrome

ICD-9CM CODES
695.1 Stevens-Johnson syndrome
ICD-10CM CODES
L51.1 Stevens-Johnson syndrome

EPIDEMIOLOGY & DEMOGRAPHICS

- SJS affects predominantly children and young adults.
- Male/female ratio is 2:1.
- Prevalence: 1:100,000 for SJS and 1:1,000,000 for TEN

PHYSICAL FINDINGS & CLINICAL PRESENTATION

- The cutaneous eruption generally occurs within 8 wk of drug initiation and is generally preceded by vague, nonspecific symptoms of low-grade fever and fatigue occurring 1 to 14 days before the skin lesions. Cough is often present. Fever may be high during the active stages.
- Enlarging red-purple macules or papules and bullae generally occur on the conjunctiva, mucous membranes of the mouth (Fig. 1-887), nares, and genital regions.
- Corneal ulcerations may result in blindness.
- Ulcerative stomatitis results in hemorrhagic crusting.
- Nikolsky sign (shearing off of epidermis with pressure on skin) can be present.
- Flat, atypical target lesions or purpuric maculae may be distributed on the trunk or be widespread (Fig. 1-888).
- The pain from oral lesions may compromise fluid intake and result in dehydration.
- Thick, mucopurulent sputum and oral lesions may interfere with breathing.

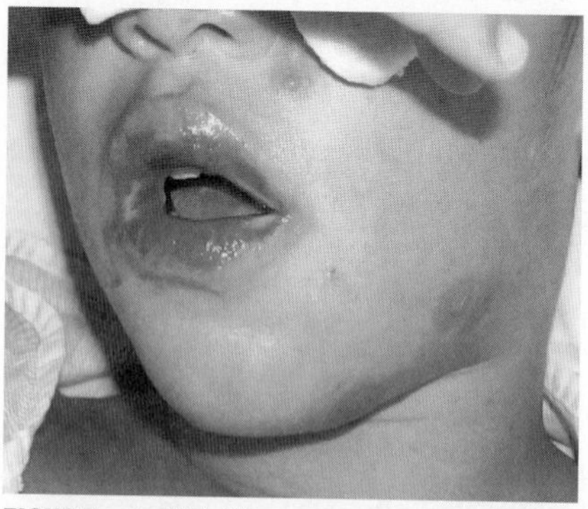

FIGURE 1-887 Lip changes found in Stevens-Johnson syndrome associated with *Mycoplasma pneumoniae* infection. (From Kliegman RM et al: *Nelson textbook of pediatrics,* ed 19, Philadelphia, 2011, Saunders.)

ETIOLOGY

- Drugs (e.g., phenytoin, sulfonamides, lamotrigine, sertraline, NSAIDs, tramadol, allopurinol, β-lactam antibiotics, phenobarbital) are the most common cause.
- Upper respiratory tract infections (e.g., *Mycoplasma pneumoniae*) and HSV infections have also been implicated.

Dx DIAGNOSIS

DIFFERENTIAL DIAGNOSIS

- Toxic erythema (drugs or infection)
- Pemphigus
- Pemphigoid
- Urticaria
- Hemorrhagic fevers
- Serum sickness
- *Staphylococcus* scalded-skin syndrome
- Behçet's syndrome

WORKUP

- Diagnosis is generally based on clinical presentation and characteristic appearance of the lesions.
- Skin biopsy is generally reserved for when classic lesions are absent and diagnosis is uncertain. Biopsy reveals epidermal necrolysis but cannot distinguish between SJS, TEN, and EM.

LABORATORY TESTS

CBC with differential, cultures in cases of suspected infection

IMAGING STUDIES

Chest x-rays may show patchy changes in patients with pulmonary involvement.

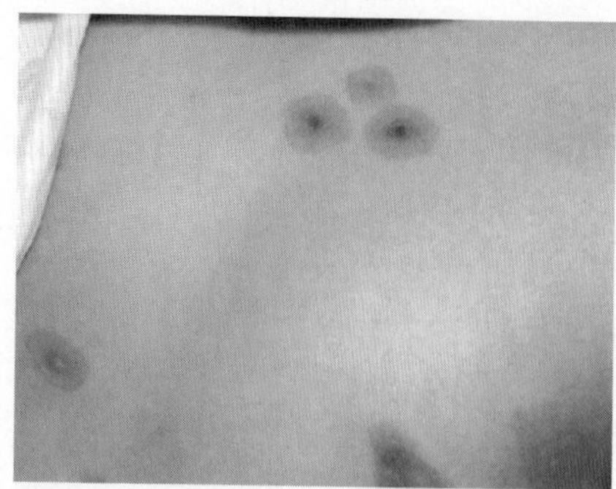

FIGURE 1-888 Classic erythema multiforme skin lesions found in Stevens-Johnson syndrome associated with *Mycoplasma pneumoniae* infection. (From Kliegman RM et al: *Nelson textbook of pediatrics,* ed 19, Philadelphia, 2011, Saunders.)

Rx TREATMENT

NONPHARMACOLOGIC THERAPY

- Withdrawal of any potential drug precipitants
- Careful skin nursing to prevent secondary infection

ACUTE GENERAL Rx

- Treatment of associated conditions (e.g., acyclovir for HSV infection, azithromycin for *Mycoplasma* infection)
- Antihistamines for pruritus
- Treatment of the cutaneous blisters with cool, wet Burow's compresses
- Relief of oral symptoms by frequent rinsing with lidocaine (Xylocaine Viscous)
- Liquid or soft diet with plenty of fluids to ensure proper hydration
- Treatment of secondary infections with antibiotics
- Corticosteroids: use remains controversial; should be used only in severe cases early in the disease; when used, prednisone 20 to 30 mg bid until new lesions no longer appear, then rapidly tapered
- Topical steroids: may use to treat papules and plaques; however, should not be applied to eroded areas
- Vitamin A: may be used for lacrimal hyposecretion
- Consider IVIG in severe cases.

DISPOSITION

- Prognosis varies with severity of disease. It is generally good in patients with limited disease; however, mortality rate may approach 10% in patients with extensive involvement. A severity of illness score known as SCORETEN that incorporates increased glucose level (>252 mg/dl), increased BUN (>28 mg/dl), electrolytes (serum bicarbonate <20 mEq/L), age (>40 yr), immunosuppression (presence of cancer), involvement >10% of BSA, and increased heart rate (>120 beats/min) can be used to calculate mortality risk.
- Oral lesions may continue for several months.
- Scarring and corneal abnormalities may occur in 20% of patients.

REFERRAL

- Hospital admission in a unit used for burn care is recommended in severe cases.
- Urethral involvement may necessitate catheterization.
- Ocular involvement should be monitored by an ophthalmologist.

SUGGESTED READINGS

available at www.expertconsult.com

RELATED CONTENT

Stevens-Johnson Syndrome (Patient Information)

AUTHOR: **FRED F. FERRI, M.D.**

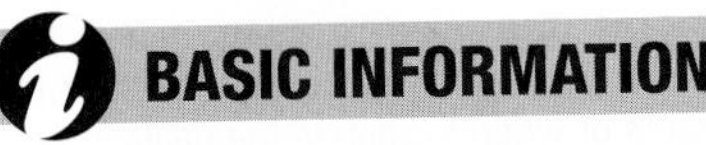

BASIC INFORMATION

DEFINITION

Stomatitis is inflammation involving the oral mucous membranes. Mucositis is inflammation and ulceration of the mucous membranes. It is most commonly seen in the mouth but can occur anywhere in the GI, genitourinary (GU), or respiratory tract. It is most often due to side effects of chemotherapy or radiation therapy (Fig. E1-889) in cancer patients.

SYNONYMS

Heterogeneous grouping of unrelated illnesses, each with its own designation(s)

ICD-9CM CODES
528.0 Stomatitis
054.2 (herpetic)
528.2 (aphthous)
112.0 (monilial)

ICD-10CM CODES
K12 Stomatitis and related lesions
K12.1 Other forms of stomatitis
K12.3 Oral mucositis (ulcerative)
K13.0 Other and unspecified lesions of oral mucosa
K12.0 Recurrent oral aphthae
B37.0 Candidal stomatitis

PHYSICAL FINDINGS & CLINICAL PRESENTATION

WHITE LESIONS:

- Candidiasis (thrush)
- Caused by yeast infection *(Candida albicans)*
- Examination: white, curdlike material that when wiped off leaves a raw bleeding surface
- Epidemiology: seen in the very young and the very old, those with immunodeficiency (AIDS, cancer), persons with diabetes, and patients treated with antibacterial agents
- Other
  1. Leukoedema: filmy opalescent-appearing mucosa, which can be reverted to normal appearance by stretching. This condition is benign.
  2. White sponge nevus: thick, white corrugated folds involving the buccal mucosa. Appears in childhood as an autosomal dominant trait. Benign condition.
  3. Darier's disease (keratosis follicularis): white papules on the gingivae, alveolar mucosa, and dorsal tongue. Skin lesions also present (erythematous papules). Inherited as an autosomal dominant trait.
  4. Chemical injury: white sloughing mucosa.
  5. Nicotine stomatitis: whitened palate with red papules.
  6. Lichen planus: linear, reticular, slightly raised striae on buccal mucosa. Skin is involved by pruritic violaceous papules on forearms and inner thighs.
  7. Discoid lupus erythematosus: lesion resembles lichen planus.
  8. Leukoplakia: white lesions that cannot be scraped off; 20% are premalignant epithelial dysplasia or squamous cell carcinoma.
  9. Hairy leukoplakia: shaggy white surface that cannot be wiped off; seen in HIV infection, caused by Epstein-Barr virus.

RED LESIONS:

- Candidiasis may present with red lesions instead of the more frequent white. Median rhomboid glossitis is a chronic variant.
- Benign migratory glossitis (geographic tongue): area of atrophic depapillated mucosa surrounded by a keratotic border. Benign lesion, no treatment required.
- Hemangiomas.
- Histoplasmosis: ill-defined, irregular patch with a granulomatous surface, sometimes ulcerated.
- Allergy.
- Anemia: atrophic reddened glossal mucosa seen with pernicious anemia.
- Erythroplakia: red patch usually caused by epithelial dysplasia or squamous cell carcinoma.
- Burning tongue (glossopyrosis): normal examination; sometimes associated with denture trauma, anemia, diabetes, vitamin B_{12} deficiency, psychogenic problems.

DARK LESIONS (BROWN, BLUE, BLACK):

- Coated tongue: accumulation of keratin; harmless condition that can be treated by scraping
- Melanotic lesions: freckles, lentigines, lentigo, melanoma, Peutz-Jeghers syndrome, Addison's disease
- Varices
- Kaposi's sarcoma: red or purple macules that enlarge to form tumors; seen in patients with AIDS

RAISED LESIONS:

- Papilloma
- Verruca vulgaris
- Condyloma acuminatum
- Fibroma
- Epulis
- Pyogenic granuloma
- Mucocele
- Retention cyst

BLISTERS:

- Primary herpetic gingivostomatitis
- Caused by herpes simplex virus type 1 or, less frequently, type 2
- Course: day 1: malaise, fever, headache, sore throat, cervical lymphadenopathy; days 2 and 3: appearance of vesicles that develop into painful ulcers of 2 to 4 mm in diameter; duration of up to 2 wk
- Recurrent intraoral herpes: rare; recurrences typically involve only the keratinized epithelium (lips)
- Pemphigus and pemphigoid
- Hand-foot-mouth disease: caused by coxsackievirus group A
- Erythema multiforme
- Herpangina: caused by echovirus
- Traumatic ulcer
- Primary syphilis
- Perlèche (or angular cheilitis)
- Recurrent aphthous stomatitis (canker sores): most common oral mucosa lesion; may be associated with many systemic diseases
- Behçet's syndrome (aphthous ulcers, uveitis, genital ulcerations, arthritis, and aseptic meningitis)
- Reiter's syndrome (conjunctivitis, urethritis, and arthritis with occasional oral ulcerations)
- Unknown cause

Course: solitary or multiple painful ulcers may develop simultaneously and heal over 10 to 14 days. The size of the lesions and the frequency of recurrences are variable.

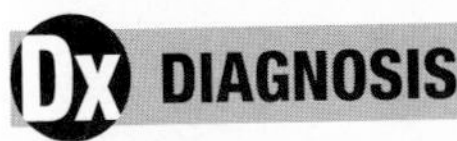

DIAGNOSIS

WORKUP

- White lesions: candidiasis (thrush) diagnosis: ovoid yeast and hyphae seen in scrapings treated with KOH culture
- Blisters:
  - Exfoliative cytology
  - Viral culture
  - Immunofluorescence for herpes antigen

Rx TREATMENT

White lesions: candidiasis (thrush) treatment:

- Topical with nystatin or clotrimazole
- Systemic with ketoconazole or fluconazole

Blisters:

- Supportive
- Consider acyclovir

Recurrent intraoral herpes/aphthous ulcerations: topical corticosteroids (dexamethasone ointment applied to the identified ulcer tid) or systemic steroids for severe cases

SUGGESTED READINGS

available at www.expertconsult.com

RELATED CONTENT

Stomatitis (Patient Information)

AUTHOR: **FRED F. FERRI, M.D.**

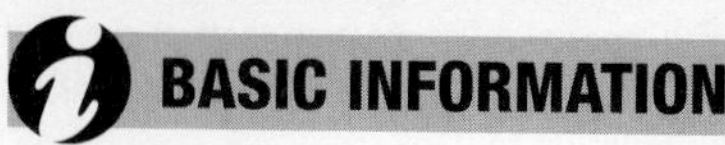

BASIC INFORMATION

DEFINITION

Strabismus is a condition of the eyes in which the visual axes of the eyes are not straight in the primary position or in which the eyes do not follow each other in the different positions of gaze.

SYNONYMS

Esotropia
Exotropia
Restrictive eye movement

ICD-9CM CODES
378.9 Strabismus
ICD-10CM CODES
H50.9 Strabismus, unspecified
H50.0 Convergent concomitant strabismus
H50.1 Divergent concomitant strabismus
H50.2 Vertical strabismus
H50.3 Intermittent heterotropia
H50.4 Other and unspecified heterotropia
H50.0 Heterophoria
H50.6 Mechanical strabismus
H50.8 Other specified strabismus
H51.9 Unspecified disorder of binocular movement

EPIDEMIOLOGY & DEMOGRAPHICS

INCIDENCE (IN U.S.): 2% of all children
PEAK INCIDENCE: Childhood
PREDOMINANT SEX: None
PREDOMINANT AGE: Birth to age 5 yr
GENETICS: None known

PHYSICAL FINDINGS & CLINICAL PRESENTATION

- Conjugate gaze loss in both eyes with the eyes focusing independently
- Amblyopia (a decrease in best-corrected visual acuity in an otherwise structurally healthy eye) may occur with untreated strabismus.

ETIOLOGY

- Many cases are congenital.
- Accommodative cases occur later with focusing.
- Rarely, there is neurologic disease or severe refractive errors.
- Hereditary form is common, with hyperopia (far-sightedness) the most common.

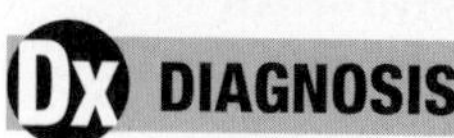

DIAGNOSIS

DIFFERENTIAL DIAGNOSIS

- Measuring eye position and movement
- Vision testing
- Refractive errors
- Central nervous system (CNS) tumors
- Orbital tumors
- Brain and CNS dysfunction

WORKUP

- Eye examination. Fig. E1-890 illustrates diagnostic tests that help differentiate between common causes of strabismus. Strabismus is classified according to the type and magnitude of misalignment. Esotropia refers to an inward deviation of the nonfixing eye and exotropia to the outward deviation of the nonfixing eye. Hypertropia is a vertical deviation in which the nonfixing eye is higher, and hypotropia is a vertical deviation in which the nonfixing eye is lower.
- Measurement of deviation: the ***Hirschberg test*** (Fig. 1-891) gives a rough estimate of the angle of a manifest strabismus and is especially useful in young or uncooperative patients or when fixation in the deviating eye is poor.
- Visual field
- MRI to rule out tumors that develop later with no apparent cause

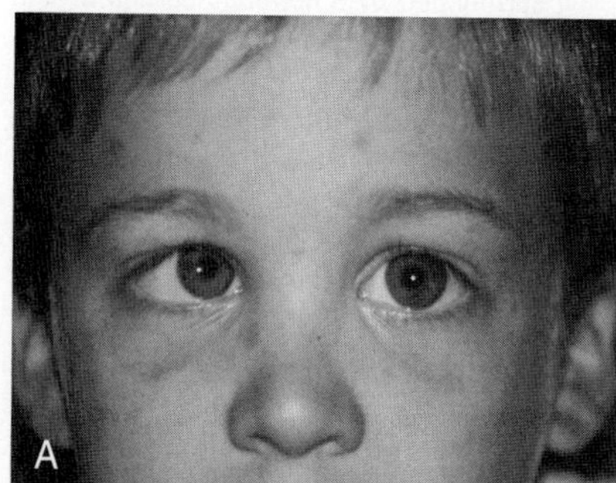

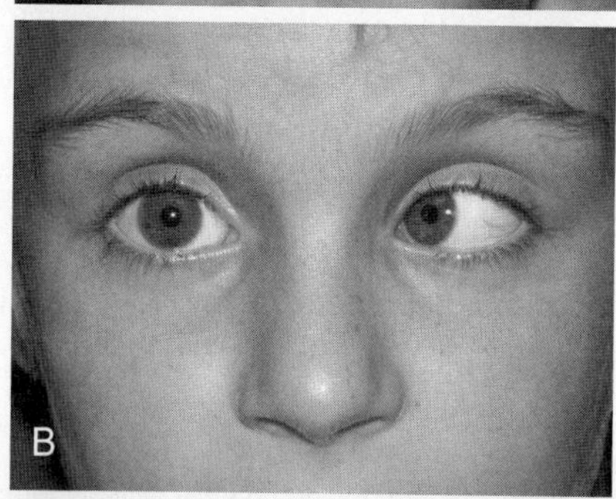

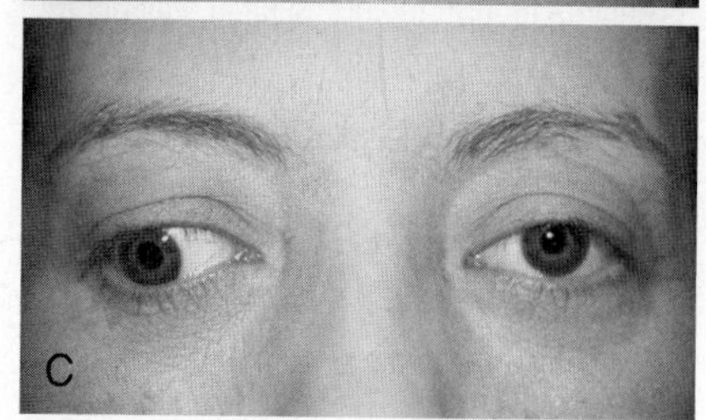

FIGURE 1-891 Hirschberg test. A, The right corneal reflex is near the temporal border of the pupil, indicating an angle of about 15°. **B,** The left corneal reflex is at the limbus, indicating an angle of about 45°. **C,** The right corneal reflex is at the limbus in a divergent squint. (**A** courtesy J. Yanguela. From Kanski JJ, Bowling B: *Clinical ophthalmology, a systematic approach*, ed 7, Philadelphia, 2010, Saunders.)

LABORATORY TESTS

Generally not needed

IMAGING STUDIES

Necessary only if other neurologic findings are found

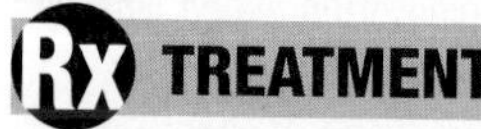

TREATMENT

NONPHARMACOLOGIC THERAPY

- Glasses
- Patching: best between age 3 and 7 yr; vision most improved by 3 to 6 mo
- Prisms
- Atropine: same as patching most of the time, although patching may give better results in resistant cases

CHRONIC Rx

- Glasses
- Alternate eye patching
- Surgery
- Prisms

DISPOSITION

- The earlier the condition is treated, the more likely the child will have normal vision in both eyes.
- After age 7 yr, visual loss is usually permanent from amblyopia.

REFERRAL

- Early for full rehabilitation of eye cosmetically and functionally
- To an ophthalmologist for management (usually)

SUGGESTED READINGS

available at www.expertconsult.com

RELATED CONTENT

Strabismus (Patient Information)

AUTHORS: **MELVYN KOBY, M.D.,** and **R. SCOTT HOFFMAN, M.D.**

BASIC INFORMATION

DEFINITION

Ischemic stroke is the sudden onset of a focal neurologic deficit as a result of ischemia. Acute ischemic stroke may be defined as relating to the first few days after onset of neurologic symptoms. However, the purpose of this chapter is to help the provider make decisions regarding the acute stroke patient within the first several hours of symptoms; this is the crucial time for definitive treatment interventions.

SYNONYMS

Stroke
Brain attack
Cerebrovascular accident (this is a nonspecific term and should not be used.)

ICD-9CM CODES

494.31 Ischemic stroke
436 Acute stroke

ICD-10CM CODES

I63 Cerebral infarction
I63.3 Cerebral infarction due to thrombosis of cerebral arteries
I63.4 Cerebral infarction due to embolism of cerebral arteries
I63.5 Cerebral infarction due to unspecified occlusion or stenosis of cerebral arteries
I63.6 Cerebral infarction due to cerebral venous thrombosis, nonpyogenic
I63.8 Other cerebral infarction
I63.9 Cerebral infarction, unspecified
I67.89 Other cerebrovascular disease

EPIDEMIOLOGY & DEMOGRAPHICS

INCIDENCE:

- ~800,000 new or recurrent strokes occur each year in the U.S.
- Stroke is the number three cause of death and the leading cause of long-term disability in the U.S.

PREVALENCE: There are ~4.5 million stroke survivors in the U.S.

RISK FACTORS: Hypertension, dyslipidemia, diabetes mellitus, and smoking are the four major risk factors. Other risk factors include atrial fibrillation, mechanical heart valve, patent foramen ovale, recent myocardial infarction, carotid stenosis, hypercoagulable states, subclinical atrial tachyarrhythmias without clinical atrial fibrillation, sickle cell disease, and obesity.

GENETICS: Multifactorial

PHYSICAL FINDINGS & CLINICAL PRESENTATION

Clinical presentation varies with the artery and region of CNS affected. Following are some common syndromic presentations. Please note that this list is not comprehensive and that all findings for a particular syndrome may not be listed here.

- Large- to medium-sized arteries:
  - Left middle cerebral artery: right face, arm, and leg weakness and sensory loss with aphasia (expressive, receptive, or both); possible hemianopia
  - Right middle cerebral artery: left face, arm, and leg weakness and sensory loss with hemineglect; possible hemianopia
  - Basilar artery: typically an acute loss of consciousness preceded by vertigo, nausea, vomiting, and diplopia; quadriparesis or quadriplegia may be seen, including "locked-in" syndrome
  - Posterior cerebral artery: unilateral hemianopia; blindness with anosognosia (Anton syndrome) if bilateral
  - Anterior cerebral artery: unilateral leg weakness and sensory loss
  - Cerebellum: ataxia (typically of the limbs), often with vertigo, nausea, and vomiting
- Small arteries (common lacunar syndromes)
  - Lateral medullary (Wallenberg's) syndrome
  - Posterior limb internal capsule

ETIOLOGY

Etiologies include atherosclerosis, cardioembolism, artery-to-artery embolism, small-vessel lipohyalinosis, arteritis, arterial dissection, and vasospasm.

DIAGNOSIS

DIFFERENTIAL DIAGNOSIS

The differential diagnosis of acute ischemic stroke includes hemorrhagic stroke (intracerebral hemorrhage), seizure with postictal paralysis, migraine with hemiparesis, syncope, hypoglycemia, hypertensive encephalopathy, and conversion disorder.

LABORATORY TESTS

- Immediate (Box 1-82): CBC, metabolic panel that includes blood glucose and renal function, PT/INR, aPTT, troponin I, and urinalysis
- National Institutes of Health Stroke Scale: a brief, focused neurologic examination aimed at providing a numeric estimate of the severity of stroke; can be performed by any health care provider trained in its use; may increase the likelihood of the correct assessment of stroke
- ECG and telemetry monitoring

BOX 1-82 Immediate Diagnostic Studies: Evaluation of a Patient with Suspected Acute Ischemic Stroke

All Patients	Selected Patients
Noncontrast brain computed tomographic scan (magnetic resonance imaging, if available)	Hepatic function tests
Blood glucose level	Toxicology screen
Serum electrolyte and renal function tests	Blood alcohol level
Electrocardiography	Pregnancy test
Markers of cardiac ischemia	Arterial blood gas tests (if hypoxia is suspected)
Complete blood count, including platelet count*	Chest radiography (if lung disease is suspected)
Prothrombin time/international normalized ratio*	Lumbar puncture (if subarachnoid hemorrhage is suspected and computed tomography scan is negative for blood)
Activated partial thromboplastin time*	Electroencephalogram (if seizures are suspected)
Oxygen saturation	

* Although it is desirable to know the results of these tests before giving a patient tissue plasminogen activator, thrombolytic therapy should not be delayed while awaiting the results unless (1) there is clinical suspicion of a bleeding abnormality or thrombocytopenia; (2) the patient has received heparin or warfarin; or (3) the patient's use of anticoagulants is not known.

From Christensen H et al: Abnormalities on ECG and telemetry predict stroke outcome at 3 months, *J Neurol Sci* 234:99-103, 2005.

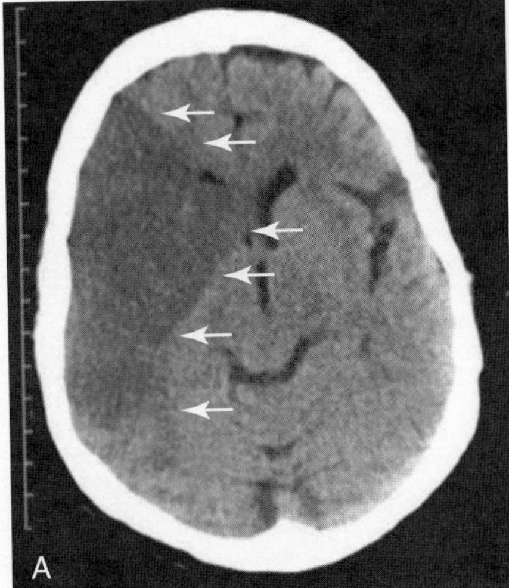

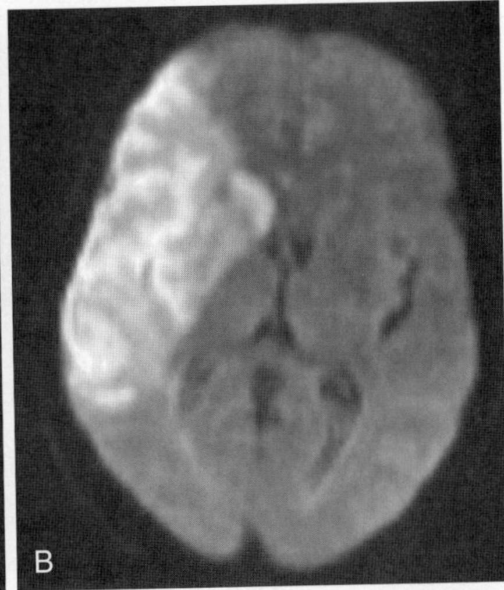

FIGURE 1-892 Large right middle cerebral artery infarct on an unenhanced computed tomographic scan **(A)** and a diffusion-weighted magnetic resonance image **(B)**. There is a mass effect, and this patient is at risk for cerebral herniation syndromes.

IMAGING STUDIES

- Immediate (Fig. 1-892): computed tomography (CT) of the head without contrast or MRI of the brain with stroke protocol to rule out hemorrhage and, if possible, to assess the extent of stroke. (Because CT typically will not show an ischemic stroke for several hours, it may also be useful to estimate how long ischemia has been present for cases in which the time of onset is unclear.)
- Several other neuroimaging studies are useful during the early stages of acute stroke to assess whether there is a thrombus that is amenable to intervention (Table 1-460).

Cross reference: see "Transient Ischemic Attack" for general workup, which is identical to that for ischemic stroke.

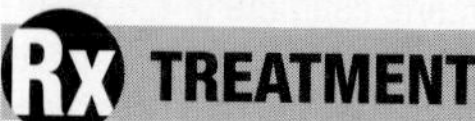

TREATMENT

NONPHARMACOLOGIC THERAPY

GENERAL CONSIDERATIONS:

- Airway and breathing should be maintained.
- Supplemental oxygen should be provided to keep the oxygen saturation at ≥92%.
- Fever is harmful during acute stroke. Ascertaining and addressing the cause while lowering an elevated temperature is strongly advised.
- Pneumatic compression devices or pharmacologic means should be applied to help prevent deep venous thromboses.
- Avoid any and all oral intake until swallowing is clearly unimpaired; this helps to avoid aspiration pneumonia.
- Early mobilization for rehabilitation is desirable.
- Consider neurosurgical intervention for craniectomy in select cases. Typical cases in which craniectomy may be performed include cerebellar ischemia with compression of the brain stem and/or the fourth ventricle as well as large right middle cerebral artery ischemia. Available evidence suggests that it may be better to perform early hemicraniectomy (<48 hr) to achieve better outcomes. Decompressive hemicraniectomy has shown good benefit in terms of mortality but not much benefit in terms of disability and functional outcomes.

IMMEDIATE CATHETER CEREBRAL ANGIOGRAPHY FOR ENDOVASCULAR INTERVENTION (Figs. 1-893 and 1-894): Methods available:

1. The Merci clot retrieval system is approved by the U.S. FDA for use up to 8 hr after the onset of symptoms.
2. The Penumbra System is also available at some centers. More recently, 2 other mechanical revascularization devices, namely the Solitaire FR (flow restoration) and Trevo, have been approved by the FDA. These devices showed better recanalization rates with fewer complications compared to the Merci device, based on SWIFT and TREVO 2 trials.
3. Intraarterial tissue plasminogen activator (TPA) is used routinely for up to 6 hr after the onset of symptoms, although it is not approved by the U.S. FDA for this purpose.

Pearls and caveats:

- Multimodal therapy (i.e., thrombectomy and intraarterial TPA) is sometimes performed.
- Endovascular treatment may be performed for select cases in which intravenous (IV) TPA has failed to recanalize an occluded artery.
- Endovascular intervention may be an option for cases in which there are systemic contraindications to IV TPA.
- Endovascular intervention is useful only for large, accessible thrombi. Therefore, if a stroke patient is a candidate for IV TPA, then he or she should probably receive IV TPA.
- One can reasonably expect an endovascular recanalization rate of 60% in appropriate patients when used alone. Combining the Solitaire device with other endovascular approaches has shown recanalization rates close to 88% in recent studies (Solitaire).
- Complications can ensue from the endovascular procedure itself, including an intracerebral hemorrhage rate that is similar to that associated with IV TPA.

TABLE 1-460 Imaging Modalities for Stroke

Imaging Modality	Advantage	Disadvantage
Cerebral catheter angiography	• Allows for the definitive assessment of cerebral circulation (gold standard) • Allows for the deployment of intra arterial thrombolysis and thrombectomy devices if a thrombus is found • Allows for the assessment of collateral circulation	• Invasive (significant risks) • High cost • Not available at all facilities
Doppler studies	• Noninvasive • May be performed at the patient's bedside	• Can be limited by the patient's body habitus • Operator dependent
Magnetic resonance angiography	• Excellent view of the large arteries of the neck and brain • No contrast material needed	• Cannot be performed in patients who are critically ill, who are unable to tolerate supine positioning, who have a pacemaker or other ferromagnetic hardware, or who are claustrophobic
Magnetic resonance perfusion	• Assesses cerebral hemodynamics • May show ischemic penumbra (i.e., the area of the brain that may be saved by timely intervention)	• Not commonly available • Not well standardized
CT angiography	• Excellent view of the large arteries of the neck and brain • Similar to magnetic resonance angiography with regard to resolution	• Requires intravenous contrast
CT perfusion	• Assesses cerebral hemodynamics • May show ischemic penumbra (i.e., the area of the brain that may be saved by timely intervention)	• Challenging to interpret in some cases • Not routinely available at many facilities • Requires intravenous contrast

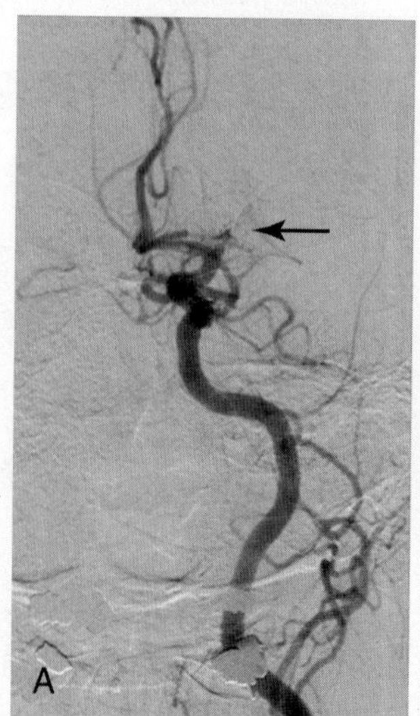

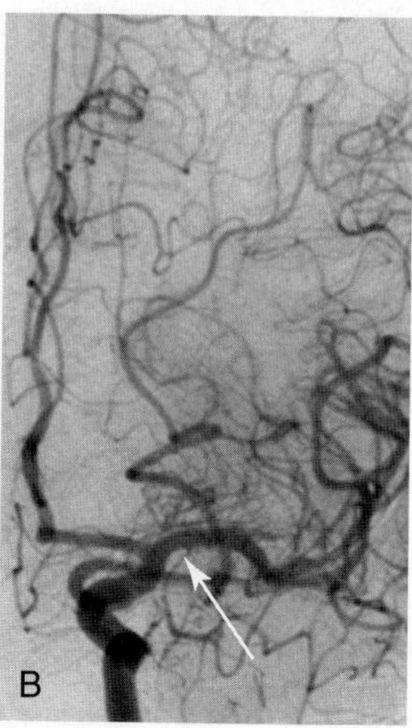

FIGURE 1-893 A, A catheter angiogram showing left middle cerebral artery occlusion, which caused severe stroke symptoms for several hours. **B,** The artery was opened with the Merci clot retrieval system, and this resulted in normal flow.

- Endovascular intervention is typically available only at select large stroke centers.
- Some practitioners are making use of perfusion imaging (i.e., CT perfusion and magnetic resonance perfusion) to assess whether there is salvageable brain tissue before performing the procedure. In some cases, this may lead to a dramatic expansion of traditional time windows; this practice is currently being studied in clinical trials.

ACUTE GENERAL Rx

INTRAVENOUS THROMBOLYSIS:

- IV TPA is the only medical therapy approved by the U.S. FDA for the treatment of acute ischemic stroke. Recent trials involving tenecteplase, a genetically engineered mutant TPA, have shown significantly better reperfusion and clinical outcomes than alteplase in patients with stroke who were selected on the basis of CT perfusion imaging.
- The time window for administration is within 3 hr of symptom onset.
- There are strict criteria for the administration of IV TPA (see Box 1-83).
- The protocol is weight based, with 90 mg being the maximum allowable dose.
- The risk of brain hemorrhage with IV TPA is about 5% in stroke patients.
- Recent data suggest that IV TPA can be administered safely and with benefit in select patients up to 4.5 hours after symptom onset. There are additional exclusion criteria if IV TPA is given beyond the 3-hr window.

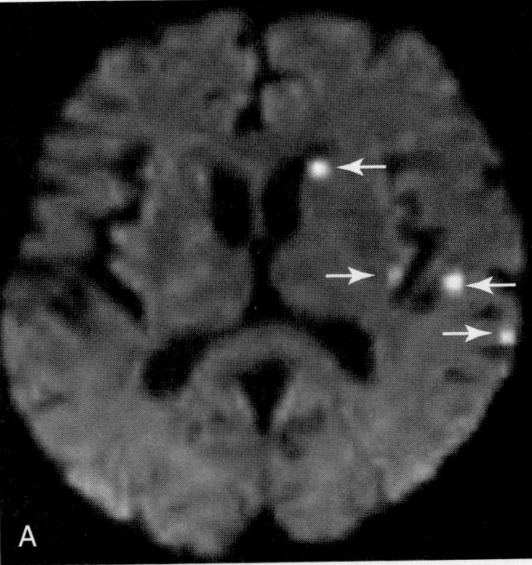

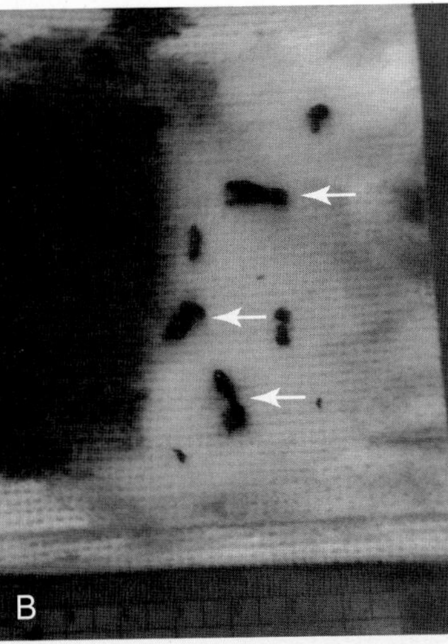

FIGURE 1-894 A, A diffusion-weighted magnetic resonance image of the same patient as shown in previous figure, this time showing only mild left cerebral ischemia after intervention. The patient was clinically normal. **B,** Thrombi removed from the middle cerebral artery with the use of the Merci clot retrieval system.

BOX 1-83 Three-Hour Criteria for Tissue Plasminogen Activator (Alteplase [Activase]) Use in Patients with Thromboembolic Stroke

Criteria for considering TPA as a treatment option:

- Noncontrast CT head without evidence of hemorrhage
- Time since onset of symptoms clearly <3 hr (3-4.5 hr with additional exclusion criteria) before TPA administration would begin

Criteria for excluding TPA as a treatment option:

- Historic and clinical findings:
  - Clinical presentation suggestive of subarachnoid hemorrhage, even if CT scan is normal
  - Sudden, severe headache, often with a loss of consciousness at onset
  - Vomiting
- Active internal bleeding, increased risk of bleeding, or known bleeding diathesis, including those resulting from:
  - Recent use of warfarin with an INR of ≥1.7
  - Use of heparin within 48 hr with a prolonged aPTT
  - Platelet count of <100,000/mm^3
  - History of intracranial hemorrhage
  - Known arteriovenous malformation or aneurysm
  - GI or GU bleeding within the past
  - 21 days
  - Arterial puncture within the past 7 days
- Recent lumbar puncture
- Stroke, intracranial surgery, or head trauma within the previous 3 mo
- Major surgery or serious trauma within the preceding 14 days
- Systolic blood pressure >185 mm Hg or diastolic blood pressure >110 mm Hg that does not decrease below that range with treatment
- Seizure at stroke onset
- Rapidly improving neurologic signs
- Isolated mild neurologic deficits
- Acute myocardial infarction
- Post–myocardial infarction pericarditis
- Blood glucose <50 mg/dl or >400 mg/dl
- Patient who is pregnant or lactating
- CT findings:
  - Evidence of intracranial hemorrhage
  - Hypodensity or effacement of the sulci in one third of the territory of the middle cerebral artery

aPTT, Activated partial thromboplastin time; *CT,* computed tomography; *GI,* gastrointestinal; *GU,* genitourinary; *INR,* international normalized ratio; *TPA,* tissue plasminogen activator.

From Rakel RE [ed]: *Principles of family practice,* ed 6, Philadelphia, 2002, Saunders.

HYPERTENSION: Elevated blood pressure is common during acute stroke, and it often subsides without specific therapy. In general, hypertension is not treated acutely unless it is extremely high (e.g., >220 mm Hg systolic blood pressure); there is evidence of organ damage caused by the hypertension; or thrombolysis is being considered, in which case the blood pressure needs to come down (if it can be safely accomplished) to <185/110 mm Hg. It is risky to severely decrease blood pressure in the presence of acute ischemic stroke as it can cause an extension of the stroke into the ischemic penumbra. A 15% to 25% decrease over the first 24 hours is recommended.

HYPOGLYCEMIA: Hypoglycemia can mimic stroke. Prompt assessment of serum glucose level and replacement as necessary are important.

HYPERGLYCEMIA: The presence of hyperglycemia worsens ischemic stroke outcome. Hyperglycemia should be managed aggressively.

HYPOTENSION: The presence of systemic hypotension in acute ischemic stroke portends a poor outcome. The cause should be sought, and volume depletion should be corrected with normal saline. Cardiac arrhythmias should be treated. Induced hypertension with vasopressor agents may be useful for select cases with an ischemic penumbra that is at risk, but caution is strongly advised.

ANTIPLATELET THERAPY: Oral or feeding tube administration of aspirin (325 mg/day) within 48 hours of stroke onset is advised to decrease the likelihood of a repeat ischemic stroke. Other oral antiplatelet regimens approved for secondary stroke prophylaxis (e.g., clopidogrel, aspirin plus extended-release dipyridamole) will also suffice and may be superior in the long term. In patients with acute ischemic stroke and atrial fibrillation, full dose anticoagulation with heparin infusion or low molecular weight heparin should be avoided in the acute setting, as this could potentially harm the patient by causing symptomatic intracranial hemorrhage and there is very little evidence to suggest any benefit.

DISPOSITION

Patients with acute ischemic stroke should be cared for in a stroke unit or an intensive care unit. Nurses with skills in stroke care and telemetry monitoring should be routine. Once the patient is stable and the workup is complete, rehabilitation should be arranged.

REFERRAL

Patients with acute ischemic stroke should be transported to a hospital in which providers are skilled in stroke care. Depending on the severity and duration of symptoms, the patient may qualify for immediate endovascular intervention at a comprehensive stroke center, even if he or she is not a candidate for IV TPA. If complications from brain edema develop, further evaluation by a neurosurgeon may be helpful during the acute phase.

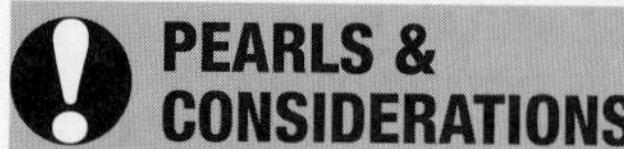

PEARLS & CONSIDERATIONS

PREVENTION

The prevention of acute ischemic stroke depends on the aggressive management of risk factors in individual patients.

Cross reference: stroke, secondary prevention

PATIENT & FAMILY EDUCATION

Patients and families need to be taught about ways to reduce the risk for recurrent stroke, including lifestyle modifications. Education about rehabilitation goals, when appropriate, should also be accomplished.

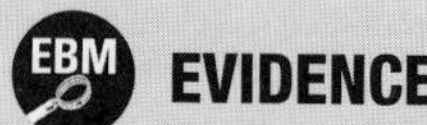

EVIDENCE

available at www.expertconsult.com

SUGGESTED READINGS

available at www.expertconsult.com

RELATED CONTENT

Fig. E3-183 Algorithm for the emergency evaluation of a patient with suspected stroke (Algorithm)

Stroke (Patient Information)

AUTHORS: **PRASHANTH KRISHNAMOHAN, M.B.B.S., M.D.,** and **MICHAEL R. DOBBS, M.D.**

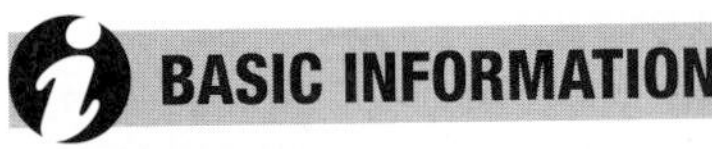

BASIC INFORMATION

DEFINITION

Hemorrhagic stroke is the sudden onset of a focal neurologic deficit caused by hemorrhage into or around the brain.

SYNONYMS

Intracerebral hemorrhage (ICH)
Intracranial hemorrhage
Cerebrovascular attack (This is a nonspecific term and should not be used.)
The term *subarachnoid hemorrhage* refers to a specific location for hemorrhage, which commonly occurs as a result of a ruptured aneurysm. Please see "Subarachnoid Hemorrhage" for additional information.

ICD-9CM CODES
431 Intracerebral hemorrhage
432.9 Unspecified intracranial hemorrhage
ICD-10CM CODES
I61 Intracerebral hemorrhage
I61.0 Intracerebral hemorrhage in hemisphere, subcortical
I61.1 Intracerebral hemorrhage in hemisphere, cortical
I61.2 Intracerebral hemorrhage in hemisphere, unspecified
I61.3 Intracerebral hemorrhage in brainstem
I61.4 Intracerebral hemorrhage in cerebellum
I61.5 Intracerebral hemorrhage, intraventricular
I61.6 Intracerebral hemorrhage, multiple localized
I61.9 Nontraumatic intracerebral hemorrhage, unspecified

EPIDEMIOLOGY & DEMOGRAPHICS

INCIDENCE: There are approximately 800~000 new or recurrent strokes per year in the United States, of which ~10% to 15% are hemorrhagic.
RISK FACTORS:
- Hypertension
- Anticoagulant use
- Thrombolysis
- Alcoholism
- Illicit drug use (e.g., cocaine)
- Cerebral amyloid angiopathy

GENETICS: Multifactorial

PHYSICAL FINDINGS & CLINICAL PRESENTATION

The presentation varies with the region of the brain that is affected. The following are common locations for hemorrhage:
- Basal ganglia
- Cerebellum
- Pons
- Lobar (i.e., amyloid angiopathy) ICH score is a widely used grading scale for risk stratification. Parameters used to calculate the ICH score include patient age, Glasgow Coma Scale (GCS) at presentation, ICH volume, intraventricular blood, and infratentorial origin of blood.

ETIOLOGY

- Rupture of vessels
- Aneurysm
- Arteriovenous malformation
- Brain tumor
- Amyloid angiopathy

Dx DIAGNOSIS

DIFFERENTIAL DIAGNOSIS

- Ischemic stroke
- Seizure with postictal paralysis
- Syncope
- Migraine with hemiparesis
- Conversion disorder

LABORATORY TESTS

- CBC, metabolic panel including blood glucose and renal function, PT/INR, aPTT, urinalysis, and toxicology screens
- ECG and telemetry monitoring

IMAGING STUDIES

- Immediate: CT scanning of the head without contrast is highly sensitive for hemorrhage (Fig. 1-895). CT spot sign on the CTA has been shown to be a reliable early predictor of hematoma expansion.
- MRI of the brain with a gradient echo sequence is also highly sensitive for hemorrhage, including intracerebral microhemorrhages that may not be visible with computed tomography scanning.

Rx TREATMENT

NONPHARMACOLOGIC THERAPY

- Surgery should be performed promptly for cases of cerebellar hemorrhage of >3 cm when the patient is deteriorating clinically, showing brain stem edema or hydrocephalus.
- Surgery for lobar or deep brain clots may be considered for select cases, although the level of evidence for efficacy is not high.
- Recent innovative surgical techniques, such as instillation of thrombolytic agents for intraventricular hemorrhage and minimally invasive surgery for hematoma evacuation, appear to be promising, although there are no large randomized controlled trials yet to prove that they are beneficial.
- Pneumatic compression devices should be applied to help prevent deep venous thromboses.
- Early mobilization for rehabilitation is desirable.

ACUTE GENERAL Rx

- Hypertension (Box 1-84): blood pressure should be quickly lowered by 15% and then gradually and safely brought to the individual patient's target range. In theory, this may diminish the expansion of the hematoma. More aggressive control of SBP to 140 or less in the acute setting has been shown to be safe, although it did not improve outcomes significantly.
- Hyperglycemia: a high blood glucose level predicts a worse outcome. Markedly elevated glucose levels should be lowered to <300 mg/dl.
- Seizures: if seizures occur, they should be treated aggressively, including with intravenous medications, if needed.
- Elevated intracranial pressure: this condition should be treated with a graded approach, which may include the elevation of the head of the bed, analgesia/sedation, hyperventilation, and osmotic therapy.
- Antipyretics should be administered for fever in addition to searching for a cause of the fever.
- Protamine sulfate is used to treat cases of heparin-induced intracerebral hemorrhage.
- Vitamin K is given for warfarin-associated intracerebral hemorrhage. In addition, recombinant factor VIIa and fresh frozen plasma are sometimes used.
- Recommendations for thrombolytic-associated intracerebral hemorrhage treatment include the consideration of the infusion of platelets and cryoprecipitate.

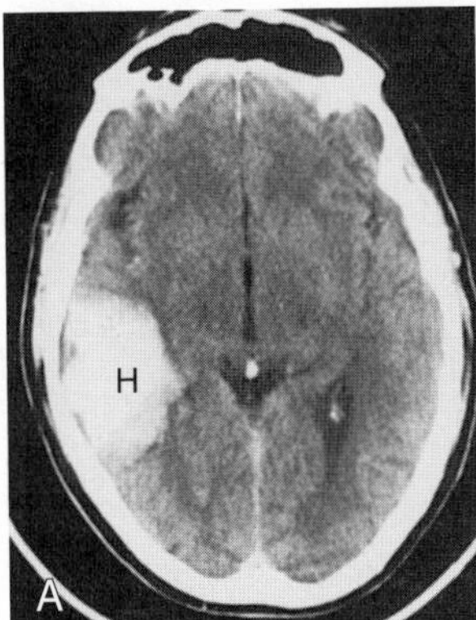

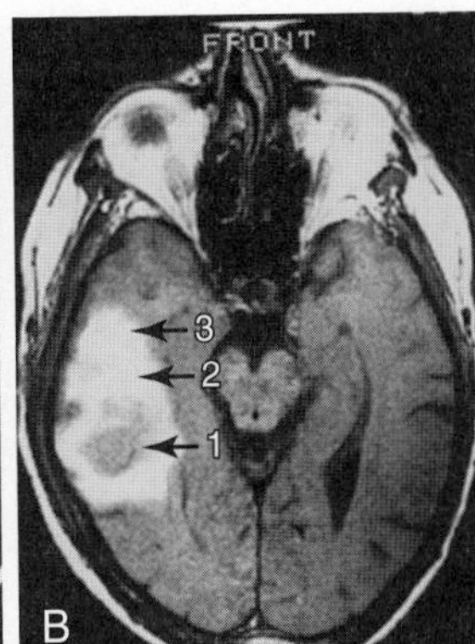

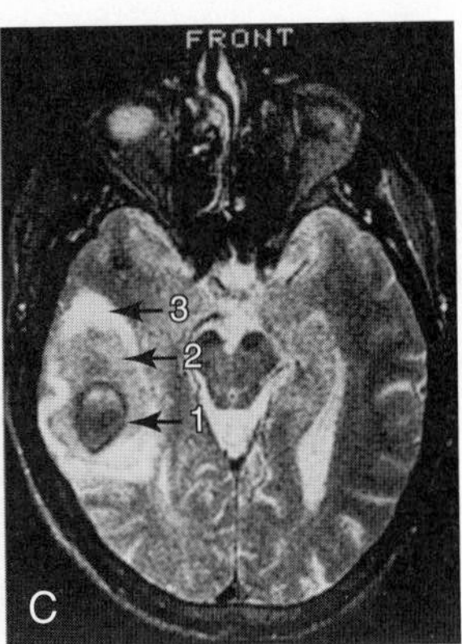

FIGURE 1-895 Hemorrhage. Axial CT image **(A)** demonstrates a large area of acute hemorrhage *(H)* in right temporal lobe. T_1-weighted **(B)** and T_2-weighted **(C)** MRI scans demonstrate the hemorrhage in various stages of breakdown. Center of lesion is dark on T_1- and T_2-weighted images, indicating oxyhemoglobin *(1)*. Intermediate zone is bright on T_1-weighted image and gray on T_2-weighted image, indicating intracellular methemoglobin *(2)*. Outer rim is bright on both T_1- and T_2-weighted images, indicating extracellular methemoglobin *(3)*. (From Vincent JL et al: *Textbook of critical care*, ed 6, Philadelphia, 2011, Saunders.)

BOX 1-84 Suggested Recommended Guidelines for the Treatment of Elevated Blood Pressure in Patients with Spontaneous Intracerebral Hemorrhage

1. SBP of >200 mm Hg or MAP of >150 mm Hg: Consider the aggressive reduction of BP with continuous intravenous infusion, with BP monitoring every 5 min.
2. SBP of >180 mm Hg or MAP of >130 mm Hg with evidence or suspicion of elevated ICP: Consider ICP monitor and reducing BP with intermittent or continuous intravenous medications to keep cerebral perfusion pressure >60 to 80 mm Hg.
3. SBP of >180 mm Hg or MAP of >130 mm Hg without evidence or suspicion of elevated ICP: Consider a modest reduction of BP (e.g., MAP of 110 mm Hg or target blood pressure of 160/90 mm Hg) with intermittent or continuous intravenous medications, and clinically reexamine the patient every 15 min.

BP, Blood pressure; *ICP,* intracranial pressure; *MAP,* mean arterial pressure; *SBP,* systolic blood pressure.
Modified from Broderick J et al: Guidelines for the management of spontaneous intracerebral hemorrhage in adults: 2007 update, *Stroke* 38:2001-2023, 2007.

- Early hematoma expansion has been associated with a poor outcome. Hemostatic therapy such as recombinant factor VII concentrates has not been shown to improve outcomes despite reducing hematoma expansion.

DISPOSITION

For large hemorrhages or unstable patients, immediate referral to a stroke center

REFERRAL

Patients with hemorrhagic stroke should be transported to a hospital where providers are skilled in the treatment of stroke and cerebrovascular diseases including the availability of neurosurgery services and neurocritical care. Depending on the severity and duration of symptoms, the patient may require neurosurgical intervention.

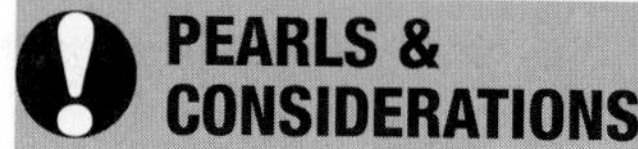

PEARLS & CONSIDERATIONS

- Outcomes are inversely correlated with hemorrhage size.
- Specific reversal agents may be useful for warfarin-, heparin-, or thrombolysis-associated hemorrhage.
- No procoagulant medications have yet been shown to be safe and effective for the mitigation of spontaneous intracerebral hemorrhage in placebo-controlled trials.

PREVENTION

Prevention depends on the aggressive management of risk factors in individual patients, including hypertension, smoking, alcohol use, and cocaine use.

PATIENT & FAMILY EDUCATION

Patients and families need to understand that most patients will not soon achieve functional independence and that rehabilitation will be a long process. Education about avoiding antithrombotic agents should be stressed as appropriate for individual circumstances.

SUGGESTED READINGS

available at www.expertconsult.com

RELATED CONTENT

Fig. E3-183 Algorithm for the emergency evaluation of a patient with suspected stroke (Algorithm)

Stroke (Patient Information)

AUTHORS: **MICHAEL R. DOBBS, M.D.,** and **PRASHANTH KRISHNAMOHAN, M.B.B.S., M.D.**

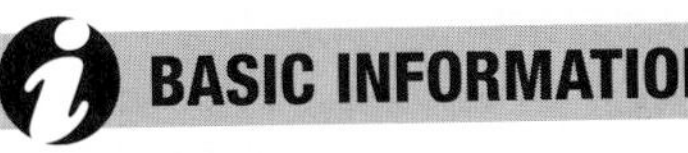

BASIC INFORMATION

DEFINITION

Secondary prevention of stroke involves preventing the recurrence of a cerebral vascular ischemic or hemorrhagic stroke after a primary event.

SYNONYMS

Brain attack
Stroke
Cerebral thrombosis
Cerebral hemorrhage
Brain infarct

ICD-9CM CODES
433 Precerebral vessel occlusion
434 Cerebral vessel thrombosis or occlusion

ICD-10CM CODES
I65.2 Occlusion and stenosis of carotid artery
I65.0 Occlusion and stenosis of vertebral artery
I65.9 Occlusion and stenosis of unspecified precerebral artery
I66 Occlusion and stenosis of cerebral artery, not resulting in cerebral infarction
I65.1 Occlusion and stenosis of basilar artery

EPIDEMIOLOGY

Stroke is the third leading cause of death in the U.S. Each year, there are a total of 800,000 strokes, of which approximately 200,000 are recurrent strokes. Thus, secondary prevention of ischemic stroke remains good treatment strategy. Secondary prevention is specifically targeted toward modifiable risk factors.

RISK FACTORS: Age is the most important nonmodifiable risk factor. Modifiable risk factors include hypertension, hyperlipidemia, cigarette smoking, excessive alcohol consumption, physical inactivity, obesity (i.e., a body mass index of >25 kg/m^2), and diabetes mellitus.

GENETICS: Multifactorial

PHYSICAL FINDINGS & CLINICAL PRESENTATION

- Stroke can have a varied presentation. Typically, the individual has a sudden definable loss of motor, sensory, visual, or cognitive functions that have a clear time of onset and that are noticed by others or by the individuals themselves.
- Physical findings such as weakness and/or numbness in one limb or on one side of the body, facial droop, visual field loss, or the inability to understand or communicate with others raises one's suspicion of a stroke event.

ETIOLOGY

- Strokes are broadly divided into ischemic or hemorrhagic (i.e., intraparenchymal or subarachnoid hemorrhage)
- Ischemic strokes can be caused by large-vessel atherosclerosis, cardioembolism such as in atrial fibrillation or cardiomyopathy, or small vessel disease such as lacunar stroke. Rare causes such as recreational drug use (e.g., cocaine abuse); arterial dissection; and hypercoagulable states need to be considered when ischemic stroke occurs in younger individuals.
- The most common cause of intracerebral hemorrhage is uncontrolled hypertension. Spontaneous rupture of a brain aneurysm causes subarachnoid hemorrhage.

Dx DIAGNOSIS

DIFFERENTIAL DIAGNOSIS

- Seizure and postictal states
- Complicated migraine
- Hypoglycemia
- Brain tumor
- Somatization disorder

WORKUP

- Blood glucose level at the bedside or in the office
- aPTT, PT/INR, CBC, and CMP
- Fasting lipid panel
- Hypercoagulability tests for young stroke patients with no obvious risk factors

IMAGING STUDIES

- Computed tomography scanning of the head without contrast can differentiate between ischemic and hemorrhagic stroke. MRI of the brain is a more specific test.
- Carotid ultrasound and transcranial Doppler are used to detect large-vessel atherosclerosis. Magnetic resonance and computed tomography angiography are good alternatives.
- Echocardiogram and ECG can be used to detect a cardioembolic source.

Rx TREATMENT

The secondary prevention of stroke is targeted toward modifiable risk factors. These include lifestyle modifications such as appropriate diet, exercise, weight loss, and smoking cessation, and risk factor modification as listed below. All patients with noncardioembolic ischemic stroke or transient ischemic attack (TIA), should be on aspirin (50 to 325 mg/day), a combination of aspirin and extended-release dipyridamole, or clopidogrel. A consultation with a neurologist should be considered for young stroke patients and for patients with no obvious cause or with stroke from unusual causes (e.g., hypercoagulable states, dissections).

PREVENTING STROKE IN SPECIFIC CONDITIONS

1. Cardioembolic strokes as a result of atrial fibrillation have two first-line drug therapies: warfarin and dabigatran. Warfarin remains a first-line therapy with an international normalized ratio (INR) between 2.0 and 3.0. Dabigatran has equal efficacy as warfarin without the need for routine monitoring of INR. Dabigatran is approved by the U.S. Food and Drug Administration at a dosing regimen of 150 mg twice a day. For patients with contraindications to anticoagulants, aspirin (325 mg/day) is recommended. The Active-A trial suggested that a combination of aspirin and clopidogrel is slightly better than aspirin alone for those unable to tolerate warfarin.
2. Cardioembolic strokes as a result of a prosthetic metallic valve: anticoagulant therapy with warfarin is recommended with a goal INR between 2.5 and 3.5.
3. Strokes as a result of large-vessel atherosclerois (i.e., symptomatic carotid stenosis): for patients with recent TIA or ischemic stroke within the last 6 months and ipsilateral severe (70% to 99%) carotid artery stenosis, carotid endarterectomy (CEA) performed by a surgeon is recommended and results in a perioperative morbidity and mortality rate of <6%. For patients with recent TIA or ischemic stroke and ipsilateral moderate (50% to 69%) carotid stenosis, CEA is recommended. When the degree of stenosis is <50%, there is no indication for CEA. Carotid stenting is not indicated except for cases in which surgery is high risk. Current trials are comparing carotid endarectomy versus carotid stenting. As of 2013, the Carotid Revascularization Endarterectomy Versus Stenting Trial (CREST) has shown no inferiority of stenting versus endarterectomy, and stenting may favor younger patients or those at higher surgical risk for complications.
4. Symptomatic intracranial atherosclerosis: treatment with aspirin has proven effective and just as efficacious as warfarin in both the WASID and WARSS studies. The utility of angioplasty and stenting in patients with symptomatic intracranial atherosclerosis is available at several stroke centers but remains investigational (Fig. 1-896). In April 2011 the NINDS stopped enrollment into the symptomatic intracranial artery stenosis stenting trial (SAMMPRIS).
5. Patent foramen ovale (PFO): the American Academy of Neurology recommends medical therapy for stroke patients with PFO. Trials are under way to evaluate if endovascular PFO closure reduces the risk of recurrent transient ischemic attacks or strokes.
6. Intracerebral hemorrhage: for immediate management, please refer to the chapter on intracerebral hemorrhage. Antiplatelet agents should be held for 3 to 4 weeks and can be restarted if there is a compelling indication such as nonvalvular atrial fibrillation. The American Stroke Association/American Heart Association 2010 guideline recommends avoiding long-term anticoagulation (e.g., warfarin, heparin) after spontaneous lobar intracerebral hemorrhage, but antiplatelet therapy (e.g., aspirin, clopidogrel, Aggrenox) may be considered in all cases of intracerebral hemorrhage where there is a definite indication. Consider a neurology consultation in these cases.

PREVENTING LONG-TERM COMPLICATIONS AFTER A STROKE

Evaluation by a physical, occupational, and speech therapist will reduce the long-term disability that can follow a stroke event. The American Stroke Association 2010 guideline

 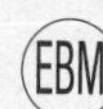

recommends a multidisciplinary approach to rehabilitation. Studies have shown an improved survival and recovery. Home-based rehabilitation can be considered after discussion with the rehabilitation specialist.

RISK FACTOR MODIFICATION

1. Hypertension: antihypertensive treatment is recommended for both the prevention of recurrent stroke and the prevention of other vascular events in persons who have had an ischemic stroke or a TIA. Absolute target blood pressure level and reduction are uncertain and should be individualized. Blood pressure should be lowered gradually over a period of months to prevent cerebral hypoperfusion and extension of stroke. Lifestyle modifications as listed above should be included as part of a comprehensive antihypertension treatment plan.
2. Diabetes: the goal for the hemoglobin A_{1c} level should be <7%. For type 2 diabetics, diet and exercise can prove very beneficial. Type 1 diabetics can also benefit from diet and compliance with their insulin regimen. Uncontrolled hyperglycemia can lead to acceleration of both intracranial and extracranial arteriosclerosis. Always consider consulting a diabetic educator.
3. Hyperlipidemia: for patients with ischemic stroke or TIA with elevated cholesterol levels, statin agents are recommended. The target goals for cholesterol lowering are an LDL-C level of <100 mg/dl and an LDL-C level of <70 mg/dl for very high-risk persons with multiple risk factors (e.g., both coronary artery disease and diabetes).
4. Cigarette smoking: absolute cessation is required. Try to offer pharmacologic therapy or counseling services to the patient. Secondhand tobacco exposure is just as dangerous, so inquire about secondhand exposure.
5. Obesity: weight reduction may be considered for all overweight ischemic stroke and TIA patients to maintain the goal of a body mass index of between 18.5 and 24.9 kg/m^2 and a waist circumference of <35 in for women and <40 in for men.
6. Excessive alcohol consumption: patients with ischemic stroke or TIA who are heavy drinkers should eliminate or reduce their consumption of alcohol. Light to moderate levels of no more than two drinks per day for men and one drink per day for nonpregnant women may be considered.

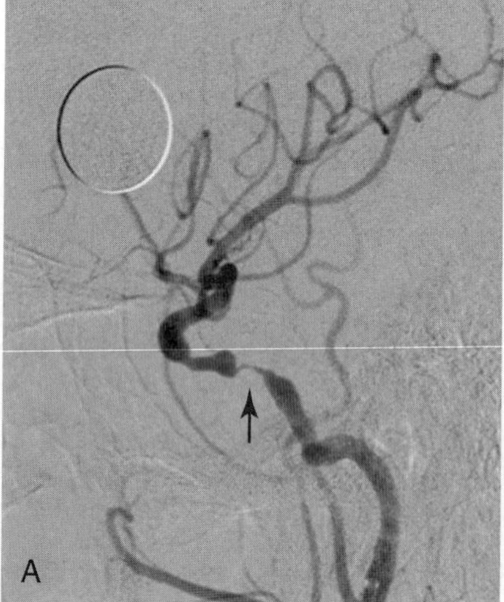

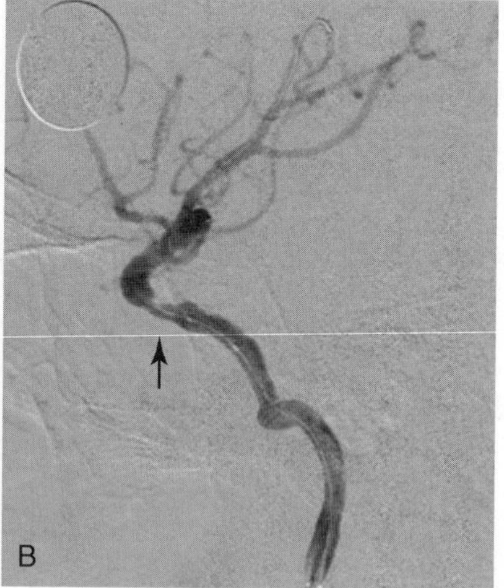

FIGURE 1-896 A, Intracranial high-grade symptomatic stenosis. **B,** This patient failed aggressive medical therapy and responded only to angioplasty and stenting.

DISPOSITION

Secondary stroke prevention is a multifaceted approach of lifestyle modification and pharmacologic intervention that is aimed at preventing or limiting disability.

REFERRAL

For complicated recurrent strokes, a referral to a neurologist who specializes in stroke is recommended.

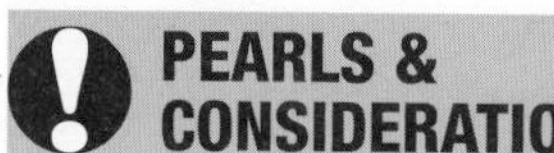

PEARLS & CONSIDERATIONS

The modification of risk factors is the best preventive measure for stroke. Lifestyle modification is a very important aspect of secondary stroke prevention. Always consider the patient's ability to afford the therapy and prescribed follow-up tests. Experience teaches us that patients sometimes will not let us know about their ability to afford therapies unless we inquire.

PREVENTION

Prevention is the goal of treatment, and compliance is the most important factor. Review risk factor reduction and pharmacologic therapy as previously discussed.

PATIENT/FAMILY EDUCATION

More information can be obtained from the following sources:

- American Heart Association, National Center, 7272 Greenville Avenue, Dallas, TX 75231
- American Stroke Association, 1-888-4-STROKE or 1-888-478-7653
- H.O.P.E. for Stroke, 250 Duck Pond Drive, Wantagh, NY 11793, 516-804-8495

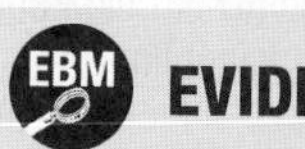

EVIDENCE

available at www.expertconsult.com

SUGGESTED READINGS

available at www.expertconsult.com

RELATED CONTENT

Stroke (Patient Information)

AUTHOR: **NAWAZ HACK, M.D.**

BASIC INFORMATION

DEFINITION

Stuttering is a problem of speech fluency, usually starting in early childhood. Stuttered speech is broken by repetitions, prolongations or abnormal stoppages of sounds, syllables, or words.

SYNONYMS

Child onset fluency disorder

ICD-9CM and DSM-5 CODES
315.35
ICD-10CM CODES
F98.5 Stuttering

EPIDEMIOLOGY & DEMOGRAPHICS

INCIDENCE: Approximately 5% of children have stuttered 6 months or more. About 1% of the population is affected by stuttering at any given time.

PREDOMINANT SEX AND AGE: During childhood, twice as many boys stutter as girls. More girls than boys outgrow stuttering, which results in four times as many men stuttering as women.

GENETICS: Studies show higher rates of stuttering within families of those who stutter and a higher concordance for stuttering in identical twins compared to fraternal twins.

RISK FACTORS: Presence of other speech or language disorder, family history of stuttering, onset after 3.5 years of age, male sex, and stuttering over 6 months in duration.

PHYSICAL FINDINGS & CLINICAL PRESENTATION

- Stuttering usually presents between the ages of 2 and 5, when normal language development begins and children are transitioning from using simple phrases to more complex sentences. Stuttered speech is characterized by at least one of the following: repetitions (for for for example), prolongations (ffffffor example), interjections, broken words, audible or silent blocking, and circumlocutions (word substitutions to bypass difficult words).
- If stuttering is left untreated, it can lead to significant impairment in academic, social, and occupational spheres. Affected individuals show fear and embarrassment around speech and may avoid speaking in some situations. Compensatory maladaptive behaviors may also develop such as eyelid closing, involuntary movements, and some physical tension around the mouth during speech.
- Differentiating stuttering from normal developmental dysfluency is important. Normal dysfluency occurs in many children, is self-limited, and does not need treatment. It is characterized by occasional stuttering events (once every 10 sentences) and brief stuttering events (<0.5 second). The child does not seem concerned about the dysfluency and the disrupted speech tends to come and go based on whether the child is tired, excited, or talking about new or complex topics. Stuttering, in comparison, is defined by more frequent (>3% to 10% of speech) and longer stuttering events (>0.5 second). Also, the repetitions are greater in number ("for for for for for example" as opposed to "for for for example") and the prolongations are longer ("Forrrrrrrrrrrrrrrrr example" as opposed to "Forrrrr example").

ETIOLOGY

- Stuttering arises from a combination of genetic and environmental influences.
- Although several specific chromosomal abnormalities have been found to explain a few cases of stuttering, the genetic causes of most cases are still being investigated. Susceptibility to nonsyndromic stuttering is associated with variations in genes governing lysosomal metabolism.
- Stuttering might be related to abnormal elevations of cerebral dopamine activity.
- Brain imaging studies show distinct differences in sensorimotor integration centers in the brains of those who stutter compared to controls.
- Although parents do not cause their child's stuttering, a critical, impatient, or interrupting speech environment can lead to worsening stuttered speech.

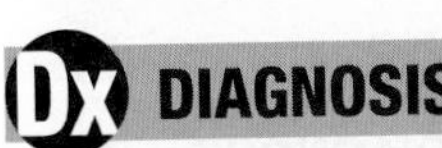

DIAGNOSIS

DIFFERENTIAL DIAGNOSIS

Stuttering is classified as neurogenic, psychogenic, or developmental. Neurogenic stuttering can result from traumatic brain injuries (TBIs) or cerebrovascular accidents. Psychogenic stuttering is usually preceded by an emotional stressor. Those affected by psychogenic stuttering are usually not overly concerned about the dysfluency and their stuttering does not improve when singing or when reciting something in a chorus, as is the case in developmental stuttering. Developmental stuttering, known simply as stuttering, is the most common form and usually presents in the preschool years.

WORKUP

- The clinical interview should include assessment of symptoms (onset, context, quality, frequency, duration, etc.) and impact on academic, social, or occupational spheres. A developmental history and family history of stuttering should be obtained, as well as assessing for family discord or recent emotional stressors. One should also try to assess parental response to the child's stuttering (intrusive/critical/anxious vs. accepting/patient/calm).
- A full physical exam should be conducted with special attention to the mental status exam and neurologic exam.
- No laboratory tests or imaging studies are indicated unless neurogenic stuttering is suspected.
- Evaluation by an audiologist for a formal hearing assessment to rule out hearing loss or discrimination disorder may be beneficial in some cases.

TREATMENT

NONPHARMACOLOGIC THERAPY

- Typically, the treatment of choice for stuttering is Speech and Language Therapy (SALT). Medications are not a first-line treatment.
- SALT consists of the following treatment modalities: fluency-shaping mechanisms, stuttering modification, delayed auditory feedback devices, and the Lidcombe approach (parental use of operant conditioning techniques).
- The above therapies help the child reduce fear about stuttering and produce speech more easily. The child is helped to speak slower and without increased physical tension and struggle. Families are encouraged to create an atmosphere of acceptance and calm for their child to speak and to model slower speech.

ACUTE GENERAL Rx

- There have been no large-scale pharmacologic treatment trials for stuttering. Smaller-scale trials and case studies have been conducted with a variety of agents, including clonidine, antipsychotics, and GABA-A partial agonists. Clonidine was found to be ineffective in reducing speech dysfluency. Weaker studies involving antipsychotic medications have found some positive effects, but almost all of these studies have serious methodologic problems and the associated side-effect profile makes using these agents for the long-term treatment of stuttering prohibitive. In some instances (e.g., a TBI patient with resulting neurogenic stuttering and psychosis), an antipsychotic might work well. A recent double-blind, randomized, placebo-controlled study of the GABA-A partial agonist pagoclone showed a modest reduction in speech dysfluency in adults.
- Case reports of deep brain stimulation of the ventral intermediate nucleus of the thalamus have shown some reduction in speech dysfluency in adults with severe stuttering.

DISPOSITION

Although adults who stutter improve in treatment, the best results occur when children are referred early. Evidence shows that treatment before age 6 decreases the chances that stuttering will continue into later life.

REFERRAL

Those with severe stuttering should be referred immediately to a speech-language pathologist for further evaluation and treatment. Those with mild stuttering should be referred if stuttering continues for longer than 6 wk or if there is significant concern by the parent or child.

SUGGESTED READINGS
available at www.expertconsult.com

AUTHOR: **JAMISON ROGERS, M.D.**

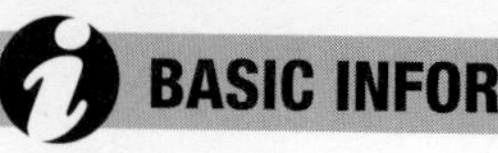

BASIC INFORMATION

DEFINITION

Subarachnoid hemorrhage (SAH) is defined as hemorrhage into the subarachnoid space. Box 1-85 describes the Hunt and Hess clinical classification of SAH.

SYNONYMS

Subarachnoid bleed

ICD-9CM CODES
430 Subarachnoid hemorrhage
ICD-10CM CODES
I60 Subarachnoid hemorrhage
I60.1 Subarachnoid hemorrhage from middle cerebral artery
I60.2 Subarachnoid hemorrhage from anterior communicating artery
I60.3 Subarachnoid hemorrhage from posterior communicating artery
I60.4 Subarachnoid hemorrhage from basilar artery
I60.5 Subarachnoid hemorrhage from vertebral artery
I60.7 Subarachnoid hemorrhage from intracranial artery, unspecified

EPIDEMIOLOGY & DEMOGRAPHICS

INCIDENCE: ~6 to 8 cases/100,000 persons per yr
PREDOMINANT SEX: Women aged >55 yr were found to have a 25% greater risk of developing SAH compared with men of the same age.
PREDOMINANT AGE: The mean age at onset is 55 yr.
PEAK INCIDENCE: Most aneurysmal SAH occurs in people who are between the ages of 55 and 60 yr.
GENETICS:
- First-degree relatives have a 5 to 12 times greater risk of developing SAH compared with the general population.
- Autosomal dominant polycystic kidney disease is known to be associated with cerebral aneurysms in 8% of cases; screening is recommended in families with this condition in which one family member has experienced a ruptured aneurysm.

RISK FACTORS: Although genetics seem to play a factor in SAH, lifestyle factors are more important for determining overall risk. These risk factors include smoking, hypertension, oral contraception, pregnancy, and amphetamine/cocaine use.

PHYSICAL FINDINGS & CLINICAL PRESENTATION

- The primary symptom is a sudden, severe headache in 97% of cases. This is classically described as the "worst headache of my life" and also called a thunderclap headache. This headache may be associated with nausea/vomiting, neck pain, seizure, or loss of consciousness.
- 30% to 60% of patients report a history of sentinel bleeds with short-lasting headaches during the weeks before the hemorrhage.
- Altered mental status and coma may result from the direct effect (hemorrhagic mass effect), but more likely is the result of acutely increased intracranial pressure.
- A posterior communication aneurysm may cause third cranial nerve palsy.
- Table E1-461 describes the World Federation of Neurologic Surgeons clinical classification of SAH.

ETIOLOGY

- Trauma is the most common cause of SAH; a ruptured aneurysm is the most common cause of spontaneous SAH (75%-80% of spontaneous SAH).
- Idiopathic SAH, also known as angiogram-negative SAH, accounts for 5% to 20% of spontaneous SAH. In these cases, no angiographic cause of the hemorrhage is found.
- Other causes of spontaneous SAH include arteriovenous malformations, bleeding into preexisting tumors, vasculitis, and cerebral artery dissection.
- Cocaine abuse, sickle cell anemia, coagulopathies, and pituitary apoplexy can also result in SAH.

DIAGNOSIS

DIFFERENTIAL DIAGNOSIS

- Intracerebral hemorrhage as a result of trauma, tumors, and stroke with hemorrhagic conversion
- Other causes: thunderclap headaches such as idiopathic thunderclap headache, migraine headache, sexual headache, cough headache, exertional headache, secondary causes including, but not limited to, pituitary apoplexy or acute hydrocephalus

WORKUP

- Computed tomography (CT) of the head: shows hemorrhage in more than 95% of cases, especially during the acute phase (i.e., 24 to 48 hr) after the onset of bleeding. Box 1-86 describes the Fisher grade of SAH on initial CT. About 3%-5% of SAH may be missed on initial CT of the head.
- Lumbar puncture should be performed in all cases of suspected SAH with "normal CT of the head." The following suggest SAH:
    - An RBC count of more than 100,000/m^3 in tubes 1 and 4.
    - Presence of xanthochromia or bilirubin in the cerebrospinal fluid.
- CT angiogram or a cerebral angiogram is imperative for determining the origin of the SAH. Angiography may also be extremely useful, because it offers a therapeutic modality via the coil embolization of the aneurysm.

LABORATORY TESTS

- Basic laboratory values, including CBC, chemistry panel, prothrombin time, partial thromboplastin time, and platelet count
- Serum troponin and sodium levels are important to guide management; elevated troponins indicate cardiac ischemia and a poor outcome. Troponin may be elevated in acute SAH, but often reflects a sympathetic side effect on the myocardium rather than an ischemic myocardial infarction.

BOX 1-85 Hunt and Hess Clinical Classification of Subarachnoid Hemorrhage

I	Asymptomatic or mild headache and neck stiffness
II	Moderate to severe headache and neck stiffness ± cranial nerve palsy
III	Mild focal deficit, lethargy, or confusion
IV	Stupor, moderate to severe hemiparesis
V	Deep coma, extensor posturing

From Vincent JL et al: *Textbook of critical care,* ed 6, Philadelphia, 2011, Saunders.

BOX 1-86 Fisher Grade of Subarachnoid Hemorrhage on Initial Computed Tomography

1	No blood detected
2	Diffuse or vertical layers <1 mm thick
3	Localized subarachnoid clot and/or vertical layers ≥1 mm thick
4	Intraparenchymal or intraventricular clot with diffuse or no SAH
Modified Fisher CT Rating Scale	
1	Minimal or diffuse thin SAH without IVH
2	Minimal or thin SAH with IVH
3	Thick cisternal clot without IVH
4	Thick cisternal clot with IVH

CT, Computed tomography; *IVH,* intraventricular hemorrhage; *SAH,* subarachnoid hemorrhage.
From Vincent JL et al: *Textbook of critical care,* ed 6, Philadelphia, 2011, Saunders.

- Sodium levels should be monitored frequently and patients should be at least normonatremic. Patients with SAH are prone to developing cerebral salt wasting, resulting in hyponatremia.

IMAGING STUDIES

- High-resolution CT scanning (Fig. 1-899) correctly identifies more than 95% of SAH cases, with blood appearing hyperdense in the subarachnoid spaces.
- Cerebral angiography is the gold standard for diagnosis.
- MRI is not a good imaging modality during the acute phase; however, its sensitivity increases after 4 to 7 days.

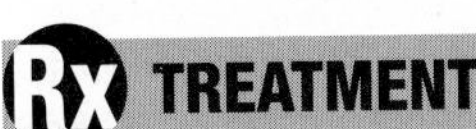

TREATMENT

NONPHARMACOLOGIC THERAPY

- Patients with a depressed level of consciousness may need to be intubated and mechanically ventilated in an intensive care unit setting.
- A lumbar drain or a ventriculostomy is required for patients who develop hydrocephalus and increased intracranial pressure. It is also recommended for patients with Hunt and Hess grade 3 or higher.

ACUTE GENERAL Rx

- Critical care management: initial management strategies are geared toward stabilizing the patient and preventing rehemorrhage and hydrocephalus.
- Blood pressure control: tight blood pressure control is paramount, before securing the aneurysm to protect against rerupture. This can be done with the use of antihypertensive infusions or as-needed medications. A systolic blood pressure of 120 to 150 mm Hg is recommended. Placement of arterial line is recommended.
- Pain control: using short-acting and less-sedating medications (e.g., codeine, low-dose morphine).
- Seizures occur in about 3% of patients during the acute phase; use of prophylactic antiepileptics is controversial.
- Vasospasm: cerebral vasospasm is a dreaded complication leading to cerebral ischemia, disability, and death after SAH. It typically develops around day 4 to 14 (but may occur up to day 21) after the hemorrhage and reaches a peak on day 6 to 8. Treatment strategies include:
  - "Triple H" therapy—*H*ypertension, *H*ypervolemia, and *H*emodilution—was originally described to maintain cerebral perfusion. However, its efficacy has been questioned in treating vasospasm. Rather, current medical therapy for vasospasm focuses upon hypertension, with typical mean arterial pressure goals of 90-100, and euvolemia instead of hypervolemia, as the latter was found to lead to significant cardiopulmonary and hemodynamic complications.
  - Nimodipine: has been shown to improve outcomes if it is administered between days 4 and 21 after the hemorrhage, even if it does not significantly reduce the amount of vasospasm detected on angiography.
- In cases of aneurysmal SAH, treatment of the aneurysm is paramount, and focuses upon occlusion/exclusion of the aneurysm to prevent rebleeding. The most common treatment methods are:
  - Microsurgical clipping: performed through a craniotomy by placing a clip around the neck of the aneurysm.
  - Endovascular coiling: performed via intra-arterial angiography; it consists of deploying platinum coils inside the aneurysm to cause thrombosis of the aneurysmal sac.

CHRONIC Rx

- Management of reversible risk factors mentioned above (smoking, hypertension)
- Management of neurologic disability through physical therapy and rehabilitation.

DISPOSITION

- SAH is often associated with a poor outcome with a death rate between 40% and 50%; 10% to 15% of patients die before they reach the hospital.
- Almost half of those who survive hospitalization have cognitive impairments that affect their lifestyles.

REFERRAL

Patients should be managed in a cerebrovascular center that maintains capacity to perform open surgical and endovascular procedures, with a critical care unit experienced in caring for neurosurgical patients.

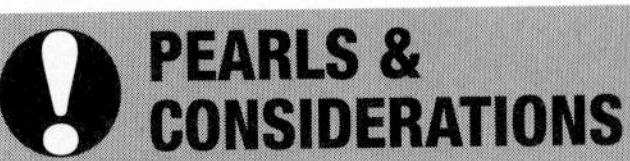

PEARLS & CONSIDERATIONS

COMMENTS

- "Thunderclap" headaches should be considered SAH till proven otherwise and evaluated by CT of the head with/without LP.
- All SAH should be managed in a critical care setting (preferably neurocritical care unit) with neurosurgical care available.
- Measures to prevent rebleeding include adequate control of blood pressure and aneurysm treatment with the use of coiling or clipping.
- A recent multicenter cohort study[1] revealed that among patients presenting to the emergency department with acute nontraumatic headache that reached maximal intensity within 2 hr and who had normal neurologic findings, the Ottawa SAH rule was highly sensitive for identifying subarachnoid hemorrhage. Additional evaluation in implementation studies is required before this rule is applied in routine clinical care.

PREVENTION

Controlling some of the modifiable risk factors, including smoking and blood pressure, may help to decrease the risk of aneurysmal rupture.

PATIENT & FAMILY EDUCATION

- SAH is a devastating condition, with most survivors developing significant cognitive deficits. A good support system and an adequate physical and cognitive rehabilitation program may prove useful to survivors.
- Screening may be useful for patients with two or three first-degree relatives with SAH.

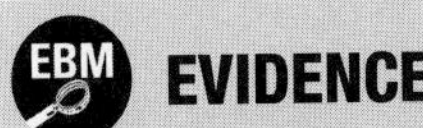

EVIDENCE

available at www.expertconsult.com

SUGGESTED READINGS

available at www.expertconsult.com

AUTHORS: **WISSAM S. Z. ASFAHANI, M.D.,** and **JUSTIN F. FRASER, M.D.**

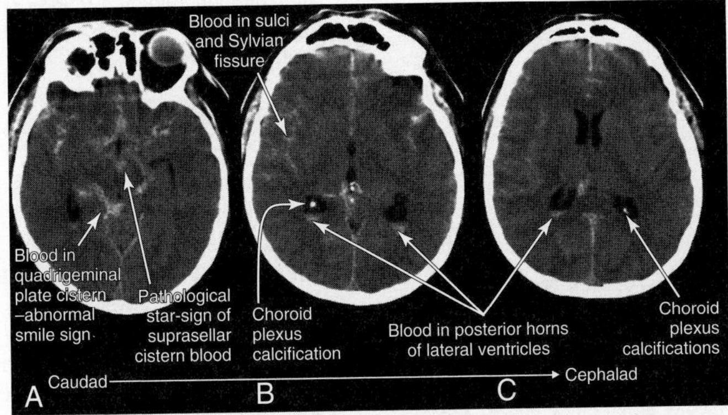

FIGURE 1-899 Subarachnoid hemorrhage (SAH), noncontrast CT, brain windows. Acute SAH appears white on noncontrast computed tomography (CT) brain windows. **A** through **C**, nonconsecutive axial slices, progressing from caudad to cephalad. In this case of diffuse SAH, note the presence of subarachnoid blood filling the sulci, as well as extending into the cisterns, Sylvian fissures, and even lateral ventricles. In **A**, blood *(white)* fills the suprasellar cistern. This star-shaped structure is normally filled with CSF *(black)*. The quadrigeminal plate cistern is normally a smile-shaped black crescent, filled with CSF, but in this case is filled with blood. Extremely bright calcifications in the choroid plexus of the posterior horns of the lateral ventricles are common, normal findings—do not mistake these for hemorrhage. Note their similarity in density to bone of the calvarium. (From Broder JS: *Diagnostic imaging for the emergency physician*, Philadelphia, 2011, Saunders.)

[1]Perry JJ et al: Clinical decision rules to rule out subarachnoid hemorrhage for acute headache, *JAMA* 310(12):1248-1255, 2013.

BASIC INFORMATION

DEFINITION

Subclavian steal syndrome is an occlusion or severe stenosis of the proximal subclavian artery leading to decreased antegrade flow or retrograde flow in the ipsilateral vertebral artery and neurologic symptoms referable to the posterior circulation.

SYNONYMS

Proximal subclavian (or innominate) artery stenosis or occlusion

ICD-9CM CODES
435.2 Subclavian steal syndrome
ICD-10CM CODES
G45.8 Other transient cerebral ischemic attacks and related syndromes

EPIDEMIOLOGY & DEMOGRAPHICS

- Similar to that of other manifestations of atherosclerosis (coronary artery disease, cerebrovascular disease, or peripheral vascular disease)
- Affects middle-aged persons (men somewhat younger than women on average) with arteriosclerotic risk factors, including family history, smoking, diabetes mellitus, hyperlipidemia, hypertension, and sedentary lifestyle

PHYSICAL FINDINGS & CLINICAL PRESENTATION

Symptoms:

- Many patients are asymptomatic.
- Upper-extremity ischemic symptoms: fatigue, exercise-related aching, coolness, numbness of the involved upper extremity.
- Neurologic symptoms are reported by 25% of patients with known unilateral subclavian steal. These include brief spells of:
  1. Vertigo
  2. Diplopia
  3. Decreased vision
  4. Oscillopsia
  5. Gait unsteadiness

These spells are only occasionally provoked by exercising the ischemic upper extremity (classic subclavian steal). Left subclavian steal is more common than right, but the latter is more serious.

- Posterior circulation stroke related to subclavian steal is rare.
- Innominate artery stenosis can cause decreased right carotid artery flow and cerebrovascular symptoms of the anterior cerebral circulation, but this is uncommon.

Physical findings:

- Delayed and smaller volume pulse (wrist or antecubital) in the affected upper extremity
- Lower blood pressure in the affected upper extremity
- Supraclavicular bruit

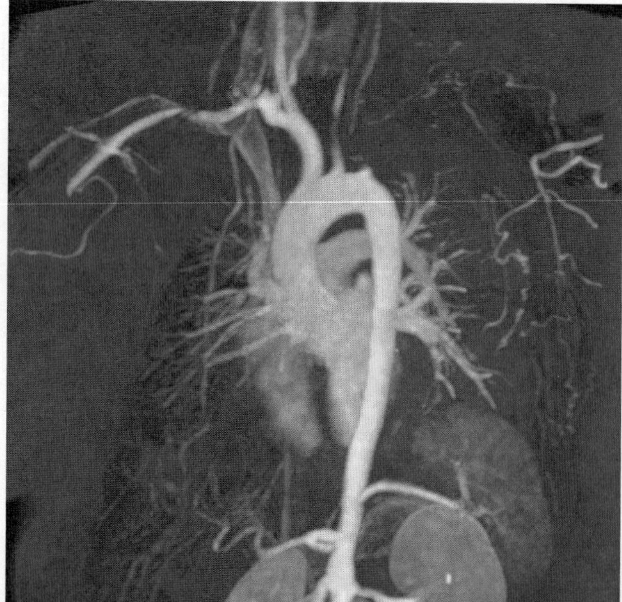

FIGURE 1-900 Magnetic resonance arteriogram demonstrating diffuse moderate stenosis of the proximal left common carotid and proximal occlusion of the left subclavian artery coming off the aortic arch with development of an extensive collateral network. (From Hochberg MC et al: *Rheumatology,* ed 5, St Louis, 2011, Mosby.)

NOTE: Inflating a blood pressure cuff will increase the bruit if it originates from a vertebral artery stenosis and decrease the bruit if it originates from a subclavian artery stenosis.

ETIOLOGY & PATHOGENESIS

Etiology:

- Atherosclerosis
- Arteritis (Takayasu's disease and temporal arteritis)
- Embolism to the subclavian or innominate artery
- Cervical rib
- Long-term use of a crutch
- Occupational (baseball pitchers and cricket bowlers)

Pathogenesis: the vertebral artery originates from the subclavian artery. For subclavian steal to occur, the occlusion must be proximal to the takeoff of the vertebral artery. On the right side, only a small distance separates the bifurcation of the innominate artery and the takeoff of the vertebral artery, explaining why the condition occurs less commonly on the right side. Occlusion of the innominate artery must affect right carotid artery flow.

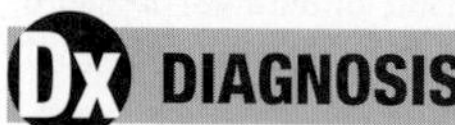

DIAGNOSIS

The carotid arteries should be evaluated at least noninvasively in all cases.

DIFFERENTIAL DIAGNOSIS

- Posterior circulation transient ischemic attack or stroke
- Upper-extremity ischemia
  1. Distal subclavian artery stenosis or occlusion
  2. Raynaud's syndrome
  3. Thoracic outlet syndrome

WORKUP

- Noninvasive upper-extremity arterial flow studies
- Doppler sonography of the vertebral, subclavian, and innominate arteries
- Arteriography, magnetic resonance arteriogram (Fig. 1-900)

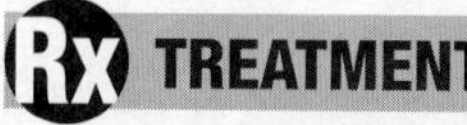

TREATMENT

- In most patients the disease is benign and requires no treatment other than atherosclerosis risk factor modification and aspirin. Symptoms tend to improve over time as collateral circulation develops.
- Vascular surgical reconstruction requires a thoracotomy; it may be indicated in innominate artery stenosis or when upper-extremity ischemia is incapacitating.

AUTHOR: **FRED F. FERRI, M.D.**

BASIC INFORMATION

DEFINITION

A subdural hematoma (SDH) is a collection of blood or blood products between the arachnoidal (superficial) layer of the brain and the dura or meningeal layer of the brain. Subdural hematomas can be acute (ASDH) or chronic (CSDH).

SYNONYMS

Subdural hemorrhage

ICD-9CM CODES
852.10 Subdural hematoma
ICD-10CM CODES
S06.5 Traumatic subdural hemorrhage

EPIDEMIOLOGY & DEMOGRAPHICS

INCIDENCE:
- The exact incidence of ASDH is unknown, but it is very common in trauma patients.
- CSDH is most common in the elderly with an incidence of 1.72 to 13.1 per 100,000.
- Patients on warfarin have a reported incidence between 21% and 36%.

PREVALENCE: Unknown
PREDOMINANT AGE AND SEX:
- Patients with cerebral atrophy such as the elderly (>70 yr) and alcoholic populations
- Infant population (e.g., shaken baby)

RISK FACTORS:
- Trauma and antithrombotic therapy are the most common risk factors for ASDH and CSDH.
- Brain atrophy secondary to advanced age and alcoholism are common risk factors, especially with the coagulopathy seen in chronic alcoholics.
- Intracranial hypotension associated with CSF shunts or leaks is uncommon but important.

PHYSICAL FINDINGS & CLINICAL PRESENTATION

Symptoms vary on the basis of acuity, size, and location. Acute traumatic SDHs are often seen in comatose patients. When associated with a midline shift (i.e., >5 mm), they can cause signs of cerebral herniation (e.g., ipsilateral pupil dilation, contralateral weakness) requiring prompt surgical evacuation.
- Patients with CSDH may present with diverse nonspecific symptoms such as headaches, confusion, aphasia, hemiparesis, TIA-like symptoms, and seizures.

ETIOLOGY

SDH is usually the result of shearing and tearing of a bridging vein between the brain parenchyma and the dura mater. Other causes of bleeding into the subdural space include contusion, extension of parenchymal hemorrhage, rarely other vascular abnormalities (e.g., AV malformation, aneurysm, dural AV fistula).

DIAGNOSIS

DIFFERENTIAL DIAGNOSIS

Other causes of subdural collections, such as hygromas, abscesses, and tumor infiltrations

WORKUP

- Clinical assessment: patient history, including medications with anticoagulant properties, alcohol abuse, trauma, cancer, and recent bacterial infections
- Physical examination, including alertness, pupil and facial symmetry, and motor weakness (i.e., pronator drift)
- Noncontrast CT scan of the head

LABORATORY TESTS

Assessment of the patient's coagulation status including CBC with platelet count, prothrombin time, partial thromboplastin time and liver function test (especially with a history of alcoholism or liver failure)

IMAGING STUDIES

CT scan of the head (Fig. 1-901): demonstrates the classic crescentic collection between the brain and inner table. For comatose and trauma patients, include a cervical spine CT scan. ASDH is usually hyperdense, whereas a CSDH is usually hypodense on noncontrast CT. Contrast is only needed if there are concerns about tumor or infection.

TREATMENT

- Correction of underlying coagulopathy, if present (e.g., Coumadin reversal)
- The majority of SDH can be managed without surgery in awake patients with normal neurologic examinations.

NONPHARMACOLOGIC THERAPY

Surgical treatment is indicated in:
- All ASDHs measuring >10 mm in thickness with a midline shift >5 mm on CT scan should be evacuated.
- CSDH with a mass effect, a clear change in the neurologic examination from baseline, or enlargement of the hematoma size, evacuation via craniotomy or burr hole should be considered.

DISPOSITION

Depending on the size and location of the SDH and the examination of the patient, observation can range from the ICU to outpatient management. When observation of the patient is considered, clinical examinations should be serially performed. Patient baseline and follow-up clinical examinations are more important than CT scan findings.

REFERRAL

Neurosurgical and operative consultation should be made available.

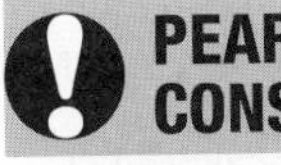

PEARLS & CONSIDERATIONS

COMMENTS

- Many elderly patients have small CSDHs or hygromas. Unless these are associated with seizures or clinical or radiographic progression, they are usually not emergent. The important thing is to recognize the cause (e.g., medication, fall risk).
- Recurrence after surgical management for CSDH is common.
- SDHs in elderly patients can have a mixed hyperdense and hypodense appearance on noncontrast CT scan; this is suggestive of acute and chronic components.

PATIENT & FAMILY EDUCATION

Individuals with SDHs are at higher risk for seizure, so surveillance is important.

RELATED CONTENT

Subdural Hematoma (Patient Information)

AUTHOR: **WISSAM S. Z. ASFAHANI, M.D.**

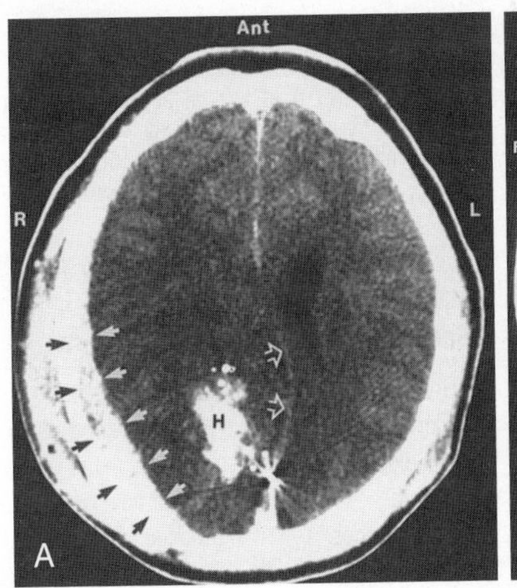

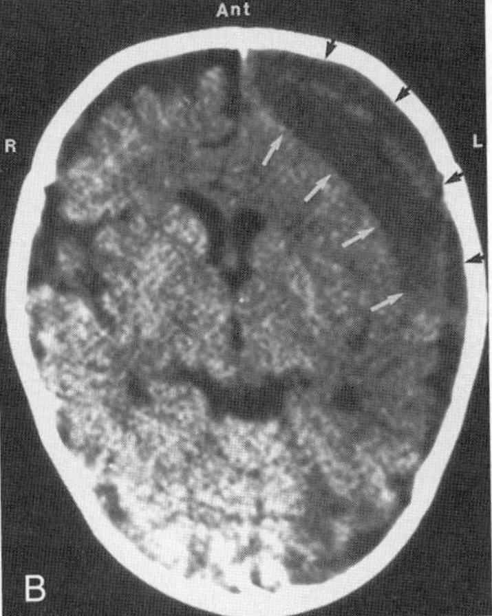

FIGURE 1-901 **A,** Noncontrast CT scan of an acute subdural hematoma shows a crescentic area of increased density in the right posterior parietal region between the brain and the skull *(black and white arrows).* An area of intraparenchymal hemorrhage *(H)* is also seen. **B,** A chronic subdural hematoma for a different patient is shown. There is an area of decreased density in the left frontoparietal region *(arrows)* that effaces the sulci, compresses the anterior horn of the left lateral ventricle, and shifts the midline somewhat to the right. (From Mettler FA [ed]: *Primary care radiology,* Philadelphia, 2000, Saunders.)

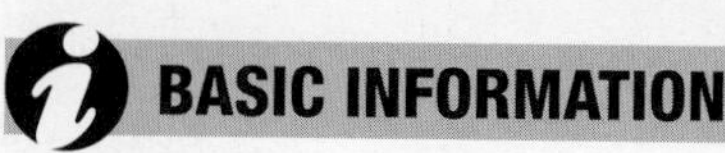

BASIC INFORMATION

DEFINITION

CDC defines suicide and suicidal behavior as:

- Suicide

Death caused by self-directed injurious behavior with any intent to die as a result of the behavior.

- Suicide attempt

A nonfatal self-directed potentially injurious behavior with any intent to die as a result of the behavior. A suicide attempt may or may not result in injury.

- Suicidal ideation

Thinking about, considering, or planning for suicide.

SYNONYMS

Self-murder

ICD-9CM CODES
Categorized by method
ICD-10CM CODES
X70 Intentional self-harm by hanging, strangulation and suffocation
X71 Intentional self-harm by drowning and submersion
X72 Intentional self-harm by handgun discharge
X75 Intentional self-harm by explosive material
X76 Intentional self-harm by smoke, fire and flames
X78 Intentional self-harm by sharp object
X81 Intentional self-harm by jumping or lying before moving object
X83 Intentional self-harm by other specific means
X64 Intentional self-poisoning by an exposure to other and unspecified drugs, medicaments, and biological substances

EPIDEMIOLOGY & DEMOGRAPHICS

INCIDENCE (IN U.S.): Mortality (CDC, 2009 data)

All suicides

- Number of deaths: 36,891 (2009, CDC)
- Deaths per 100,000 population: 11.5
- Cause of death rank: 10th leading cause of death in 2009

Firearm suicides

- Number of deaths: 17,352
- Deaths per 100,000 population: 5.8

Suffocation suicides

- Number of deaths: 8161
- Deaths per 100,000 population: 2.7

Poisoning suicides

- Number of deaths: 6358
- Deaths per 100,000 population: 2.1

Suicidal deaths are only part of the problem. More people survive suicide attempts than actually die. They are often seriously injured and need medical care.

AGE-RELATED DATA:

- Incidence of suicide increases with age (13.1 cases/100,000 persons ages 15 to 24 yr, 16.9 cases/100,000 persons ages 65 to 74 yr, and 23.5 cases/100,000 persons ages 75 to 84 yr)
- During 2002 to 2006, the greatest percentage of suicides occurred by firearm among all race/ethnicity groups for persons ages 65 yr and older. Except for Asian/Pacific Islanders, suffocation accounted for the highest percentage of suicides among those 65 yr and older (52.6%).

GENDER DIFFERENCES:

- Women attempt suicide about two to three times as often as men.
- Males succeed at taking their own lives at nearly four times the rate of females and represent 79% of all U.S. suicides.
- Suicide is the seventh leading cause of death for males and sixteenth leading cause for females.
- Firearms are the most common method of suicide among males (56%).
- Poisoning is the most common method in women (40.3%).

ENVIRONMENTAL FACTORS:

- Suicide rates traditionally decrease in times of war and increase in times of economic crises.
- After adjusting for age, suicide rates are highest in the western and northwestern regions of the United States.

MARITAL STATUS: Suicide rates are highest among the divorced, separated, and widowed and lowest among the married.

SUBSTANCE USE: CDC data: 33.3% of suicides tested positive for alcohol and 16.4% for opiates.

RISK FACTORS (Table 1-462):

- Previous suicide attempt(s).
- History of depression or other mental illness (bipolar, psychosis, PTSD, and others).
- Anxiety.
- Alcohol or drug abuse.
- Family history of suicide or violence.
- Physical illness. Patients who have recently received a cancer diagnosis have increased risk of suicide.
- Feeling alone.
- Individuals with a mental or substance use disorder account for >90% of suicides.
- Access to firearms is associated with risk for completed suicide[1]
- The concurrence of more than one condition (e.g., depression and alcohol abuse) greatly increases the risk.
- Hopelessness is a strong predictor of suicide potential.
- Rates are higher in developing countries.
- Rates vary by occupation, ethnicity, and employment status.

PROTECTIVE FACTORS (CDC):

- Effective clinical care for mental, physical, and substance abuse disorders
- Easy access to a variety of clinical interventions and support for help seeking
- Family and community support (connectedness)
- Support from ongoing medical and mental health care relationships
- Skills in problem solving, conflict resolution, and nonviolent ways of handling disputes
- Cultural and religious beliefs that discourage suicide and support instincts for self-preservation

SUICIDAL BEHAVIOR:

- All suicidal behavior should be taken seriously, as a failed attempt may lead to a completed suicide in the future.
- Nearly half of suicides are preceded by an attempt that does not end in death.
- Those with a history of attempts are 23 times more likely to eventually end their own lives than those without.

[1]Anglemyer A et al: The accessibility of firearms and risk for suicide and homicide victimization among household members, *Ann Int Med* 160:101-110, 2014.

TABLE 1-462 Suicide and Risk Factors: A Summary

Primary Diagnosis	Demographics	Personality Factors	Comorbidities	Social Factors	Other Factors
Bipolar	Male	Borderline	Substance abuse	Divorced	Means available
Schizophrenia	Older age	Narcissistic	Panic disorder	Widower	History of child abuse
Major depressive disorder	White race	Antisocial	Anxiety	Lives alone	Few reasons to live
Dysthymia	Homosexuality	Conduct disorder	Axis III dx	Isolated	Lots of adverse events
Adjustment disorder	History of attempt	Impulsive		Money worries	Change in grades
Conduct disorder	Family history			Other losses	Change in friends
Psychosis	Suicidal ideas			No religion	Giving things away
	Hopeless				Guns in the home
	Helpless				

From Sadock BJ et al: *Kaplan & Sadock's comprehensive textbook of psychiatry,* ed 9, Philadelphia, 2009, Wolters Kluwer Health/Lippincott Williams & Wilkins.

- A suicidal gesture does not have death as a goal, but can serve as a dramatic way of alerting others to some type of ongoing distress.
- Risky behaviors such as speeding or disregarding traffic laws, or abusing drugs, are considered parasuicide when the person shows total disregard for whether the actions might result in his or her death.
- Unsuccessful suicide attempts may also result from miscalculations in the plan. These people are at high risk for attempting suicide again.

EVALUATION:

- The provider must directly inquire into the presence of suicidal ideation. Approximately one half to two thirds of individuals who commit suicide visit physicians within 1 mo of taking their lives.
- Explicit suicidal intent, hopelessness, and a well-formulated plan indicate high risk. Clinicians can use the mnemonic SAL: Is the method **s**pecific? Is it **a**vailable? Is it **l**ethal?
- The concurrence of multiple psychiatric problems, substance abuse, and multiple physical problems increases the risk.
- Covert suicidal ideation occurs in patients primarily with multiple vague physical complaints, depression, anxiety, or substance abuse.
- Primary care-feasible screening tools might help to identify some adults at increased risk for suicide but have limited ability to detect suicide risk in adolescents. Psychotherapy may reduce suicide attempts in some high-risk adults, but effective interventions for high-risk adolescents are not yet proven.[2]

ACUTE INTERVENTIONS

- Place patient in a safe environment (usually hospitalization in a psychiatric unit or a medical unit with continuous observation).
- Emergency medical stabilization and clearance as required, related to severity and lethality of attempt, age, comorbid medical issues, and overall clinical presentation.

ACUTE PSYCHOPHARMACOLOGIC INTERVENTIONS

- Benzodiazepines may be useful in reducing extreme anxiety and dysphoria in an acutely suicidal patient; however, these agents should not be prescribed until the means of the suicidal attempt are known (not a benzodiazepine overdose) and patient is medically stable (i.e., respiratory system, vital signs, cognitive functioning are stable).
- Antipsychotics (typicals or atypicals) can be used if psychosis is present (e.g., voices telling patient to hurt self) and to manage acute agitation.
- If indicated, mood stabilizers and antidepressants can be started in the acute setting but may have up to a 2-wk latency period. However, awareness of increased risk of suicidal thoughts/behavior with these medications in some populations is required.

[2]O'Connor E et al: Screening for and treatment of suicide risk relevant to primary care: a systematic review for the U.S. Preventive Services Task Force, *Ann Int Med* 158:741-754, 2013.

THERAPY

- Long-term: psychotherapy aimed at factors that underlie the decision to pursue suicide or at the risk factors contributing to suicidal behavior
- Substance abuse treatment (e.g., Alcoholics Anonymous, Narcotics Anonymous) when substance use disorder is present
- Therapy should be aimed at the underlying condition (e.g., antidepressants for depression, anxiolytics or antidepressants for anxiety, substance abuse treatment, or psychotherapy for chronic low self-esteem, hopelessness).
- In elderly, loneliness and medical disability are major reasons for suicide and therefore major targets for intervention.
- Involvement of family members, spouse, loved one, caregivers if possible for therapy and management.

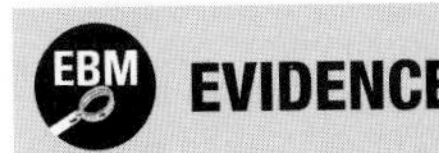

available at www.expertconsult.com

SUGGESTED READINGS

available at www.expertconsult.com

AUTHOR: **ALI KAZIM, M.D.**

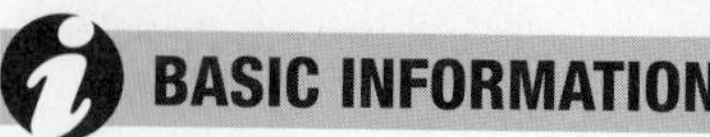

BASIC INFORMATION

DEFINITION

Superior vena cava (SVC) syndrome is a set of symptoms that results when a mediastinal mass compresses the SVC or the veins that drain into it, resulting in obstruction of blood flow from the head, neck, upper torso, or extremities to the right atrium.

ICD-9CM CODES
453.2 Vena cava thrombosis
ICD-10CM CODES
I87.1 Compression of vein

EPIDEMIOLOGY & DEMOGRAPHICS

- SVC syndrome occurs in 15,000 persons in the U.S. every year.
- More than 50% of patients present with SVC at the initial manifestation of a previously undiagnosed malignancy.
- Mirrors lung cancer (especially small cell carcinoma) and lymphoma (see "Lung Neoplasm" and "Lymphoma" in Section I).

PHYSICAL FINDINGS & CLINICAL PRESENTATION

The pathophysiology of the syndrome involves the increased pressure in the venous system draining into the SVC, producing edema of the head, neck, and upper extremities. Symptoms develop over a period of 2 wk in one third of patients and include:

- Shortness of breath
- Chest pain
- Cough
- Dysphagia, hoarseness, stridor
- Headache
- Syncope
- Visual trouble

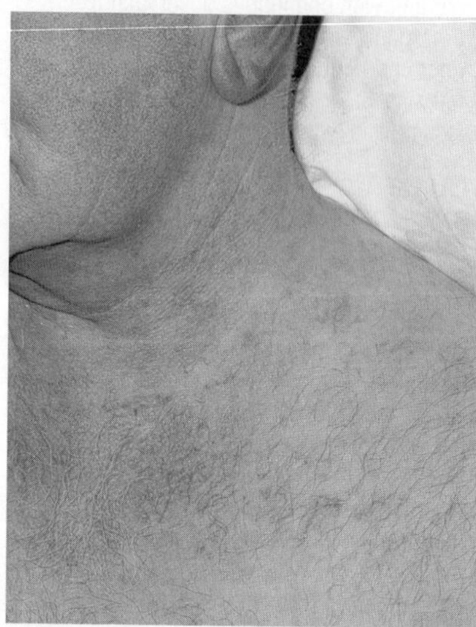

FIGURE 1-902 Superior vena cava obstruction causing dilated veins and plethora of the upper trunk and neck in a patient with bronchial carcinoma. Patients with superior vena cava obstruction are occasionally referred to dermatologists with suspected contact allergy (eyelid swelling) or angioedema (facial or hand swelling). (From White GM, Cox NH [eds]: *Diseases of the skin, a color atlas and text,* ed 2, St Louis, 2006, Mosby.)

Signs:

- Chest wall vein distention (Fig. 1-902)
- Neck vein distention
- Facial edema, facial plethora
- Upper-extremity swelling
- Cyanosis

ETIOLOGY

- Lung cancer (65% of all cases, of which half are small cell lung cancer)
- Lymphoma (15%)
- Thymoma
- Tuberculosis
- Goiter
- Aortic aneurysm (arteriosclerotic or syphilitic)
- SVC thrombosis
  1. Primary: associated with a central venous catheter
  2. Secondary: as a complication of SVC syndrome associated with one of the abovementioned causes
- Inflammatory process, fibrosing mediastinitis
- Fig. 1-903 illustrates the anatomy of superior vena cava syndrome. Table 1-463 summarizes common malignancies associated with SVC syndrome in adults.

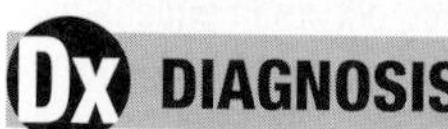

DIAGNOSIS

CT scan of the chest with contrast (Fig. 1-904) is the most useful diagnostic study. MRI is usually adequate to establish the diagnosis of SVC obstruction and to assist in the differential diagnosis of probable cause.

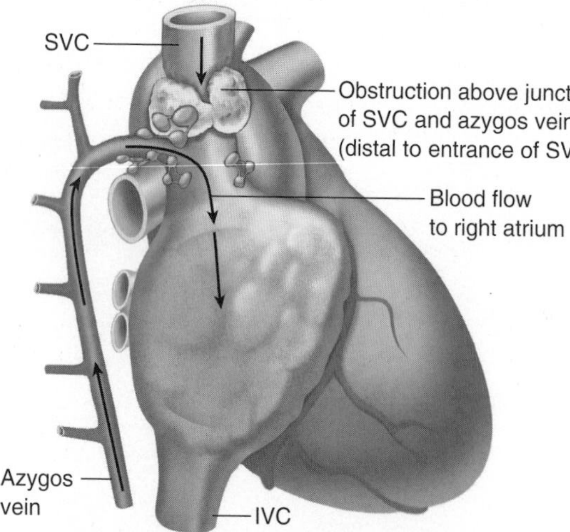

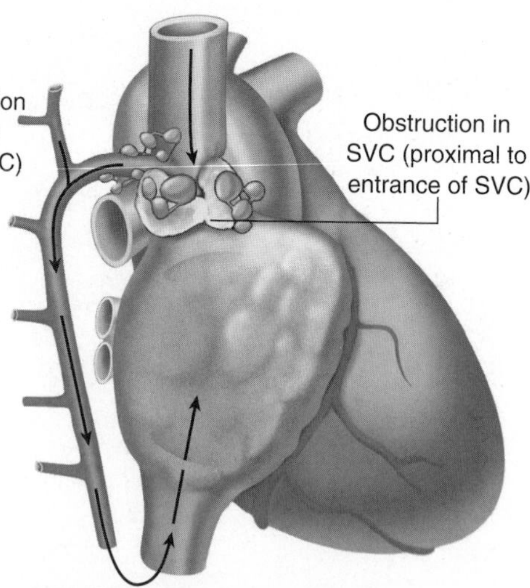

FIGURE 1-903 Anatomy of superior vena cava (SVC) syndrome. Lymph nodes may obstruct blood return above the entrance of the azygos vein **(A)**, resulting in edema of the face, neck, and arms and distended veins in the neck and arms and over the upper chest. Obstruction below the return of the azygos vein **(B)** results in retrograde flow through the azygos through collateral veins to the inferior vena cava (IVC), with all the symptoms and signs in **A** plus dilation of the veins over the abdomen as well. (Modified from Skatin AT (ed): *Atlas of diagnostic oncology,* ed 3, Philadelphia, 2003, Elsevier.)

TABLE 1-463 Malignancies Associated with Superior Vena Cava (SVC) Syndrome in Adults*

Neoplastic Diagnosis	Percentage of SVC	Percentage of Disease-Associated SVC
Lung cancer, stage 3B or 4:	48-81	
Small cell lung cancer		15-45
Squamous cell cancer		20-25
Adenocarcinoma		5-25
Large cell carcinoma		4-30
Lymphoma:	2-21	
Diffuse large cell lymphoma		64
Lymphoblastic lymphoma		33
Breast cancer	11	

*Include lung cancer, lymphomas, and metastases from other solid tumors. 75% to 85% of patients with SVC have neoplastic disease.
From Zipes DP et al (eds): *Braunwald's heart disease*, ed 7, Philadelphia, 2005, Saunders.

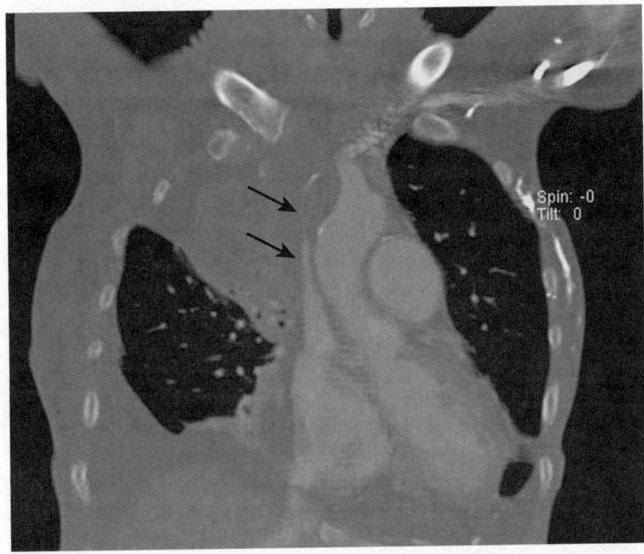

FIGURE 1-904 Computed tomography scan showing blockage of the superior vena cava *(arrows)*. (From Adams JG et al: *Emergency medicine, clinical essentials,* ed 2, Philadelphia, 2013, Elsevier.)

DIFFERENTIAL DIAGNOSIS

The syndrome is characteristic enough to exclude other diagnoses. The differential diagnosis concerns the underlying etiologies listed above.

WORKUP

- Chest radiograph (mediastinal widening, pleural effusion)
- Chest CT with contrast or MRI (in patient who cannot tolerate contrast medium)
- Venography: warranted only when an intervention (e.g., stent or surgery) is planned
- Percutaneous needle biopsy or mediastinoscopy are usually the initial diagnostic modalities used to establish a histologic diagnosis

Rx TREATMENT

- Although invasive procedures such as mediastinoscopy are associated with higher than usual risk of bleeding, a tissue diagnosis is usually needed before commencing therapy.
- Management is guided by the severity of the symptoms and the underlying etiology.
- Emergency empiric radiation is indicated in critical situations such as respiratory failure or central nervous system signs associated with increased intracranial pressure.
- Treatment of the underlying malignancy:
    1. Radiotherapy: the majority of tumors causing SVC syndrome are sensitive to radiotherapy
    2. Systemic chemotherapy
- Anticoagulant or fibrinolytic therapy in patients who do not respond to cancer treatment within a week or if an obstructing thrombus has been documented.
- Loop diuretics are often used, but their effect is limited.
- Upright positioning and fluid restriction until collateral channels develop and allow for clinical regression are useful modalities for SVC syndrome secondary to benign disease.
- Steroids (dexamethasone 4 mg q6h) may be useful in reducing the tumor burden in lymphoma and thymoma.
- Percutaneous self-expandable stents that can be placed under local anesthesia with radiologic manipulation are useful in the treatment of SVC syndrome to bypass the obstruction, especially in cases associated with malignant tumors.
- Surgical bypass grafting is infrequently used to treat SVC syndrome.

REFERRAL

To a thoracic surgeon, pulmonary specialist, or oncologist

AUTHOR: **FRED F. FERRI, M.D.**

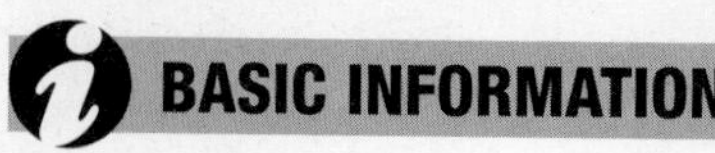

BASIC INFORMATION

DEFINITION

Syncope is the transient loss of consciousness with spontaneous recovery that results from an acute global reduction in cerebral blood flow. Syncope is a symptom, and the goal is to distinguish lethal causes from benign causes of transient loss of consciousness.

ICD-9CM CODES
780.2 Syncope
ICD-10CM CODES
R55 Syncope and collapse

EPIDEMIOLOGY & DEMOGRAPHICS

- Syncope accounts for 3% to 5% of emergency department visits.
- 30% of the adult population will experience at least one syncopal episode during their lifetimes.
- Incidence of syncope is highest in elderly men and young women.
- 15% of children and adolescents experience syncope; less than 5% have cardiac causes.

PHYSICAL FINDINGS & CLINICAL PRESENTATION

- Blood pressure: if low, consider orthostatic hypotension; if unequal in both arms (difference >20 mm Hg), consider subclavian steal or dissecting aneurysm. (NOTE: Blood pressure [BP] and heart rate should be recorded in the supine and standing positions, waiting at least 5 minutes between each position.) If there is a drop in BP but no change in heart rate (HR), the patient may be taking a beta-blocker or may have an autonomic neuropathy.
- Pulse: if patient has tachycardia, bradycardia, or irregular rhythm, consider arrhythmia.
- Heart: if there are murmurs present, consider syncope attributable to left ventricular outflow obstruction (aortic stenosis or idiopathic hypertrophic subaortic stenosis); if there are jugular venous distention and distal heart sounds, consider cardiac tamponade.
- Carotid sinus pressure: can be diagnostic if it reproduces symptoms and other causes are excluded; a pause >3 sec or a systolic BP drop >50 mm Hg without symptoms or <30 mm Hg with symptoms when sinus pressure is applied separately on each side for <5 sec is considered abnormal. This test should be avoided in patients with carotid bruits or cerebrovascular disease. ECG monitoring, IV access, and bedside atropine should be available when carotid sinus pressure is applied.

ETIOLOGY

- Neurally mediated syncope
  1. Psychophysiologic (emotional upset, panic disorders, hysteria, hyperventilation)
  2. Visceral reflex (micturition, defecation, food ingestion, coughing, ventricular contraction, glossopharyngeal neuralgia)
  3. Carotid sinus pressure
  4. Reduction of venous return caused by Valsalva maneuver
- Orthostatic hypotension
  1. Hypovolemia
  2. Vasodilator medications
  3. Autonomic neuropathy (diabetes, amyloid, Parkinson's disease, multisystem atrophy)
  4. Pheochromocytoma
  5. Carcinoid syndrome
- Cardiac
  1. Reduced cardiac output
     a. Left ventricular outflow obstruction (aortic stenosis, hypertrophic cardiomyopathy)
     b. Obstruction to pulmonary flow (pulmonary embolism, pulmonic stenosis, primary pulmonary hypertension)
     c. Myocardial infarct with pump failure
     d. Cardiac tamponade
     e. Mitral stenosis
     f. Reduction of venous return (atrial myxoma, valve thrombus)
     g. Beta-blocker therapy
  2. Arrhythmias or asystole
     a. Extreme tachycardia (>160 to 180 beats/min)
     b. Severe bradycardia (<30 to 40 beats/min)
     c. Sick sinus syndrome
     d. Atrioventricular block (second or third degree)
     e. Ventricular tachycardia or fibrillation
     f. Long QT syndrome
     g. Pacemaker malfunction
     h. Psychotropic medications and beta-blockers

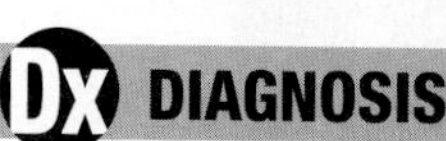

DIAGNOSIS

DIFFERENTIAL DIAGNOSIS

1. Seizure (see "Workup")
2. Vertebrobasilar transient ischemic attack (TIA) usually manifests as diplopia, vertigo, or ataxia but not loss of consciousness. Isolated episodes of transient loss of consciousness (TLOC) without accompanying neurologic symptoms are unlikely to be TIAs.
3. Recreational drugs or alcohol.
4. Functional causes, such as stress and somatoform disorders.
5. Sleep disorders, such as sleep attacks and narcolepsy, are also in the differential for TLOC.
6. Head trauma.

WORKUP

The history is crucial to diagnosing the cause of syncope and may suggest a diagnosis that can be evaluated with directed testing. History is also important to determine other etiologies for TLOC, such as seizure. Fig. E1-905 describes an algorithm for syncope evaluation.

- Sudden LOC: consider cardiac arrhythmias.
- Gradual LOC: consider orthostatic hypotension, vasodepressor syncope, hypoglycemia.
- History of aura before LOC or prolonged confusion (>1 min), amnesia, or lethargy after LOC suggests seizure rather than syncope.
- Patient's activity at the time of syncope:
  1. Micturition, coughing, defecation: consider syncope caused by decreased venous return.
  2. Turning head or while shaving: consider carotid sinus syndrome.
  3. Physical exertion in a patient with murmur: consider aortic stenosis.
  4. Arm exercise: consider subclavian steal syndrome.
  5. Assuming an upright position: consider orthostatic hypotension.
- Associated events:
  1. Chest pain: consider myocardial infarction, pulmonary embolism.
  2. Palpitations: consider arrhythmias.
  3. Incontinence (urine or fecal) and tongue biting are associated with seizure or syncope.
  4. Brief, transient shaking after LOC may represent myoclonus from global cerebral hypoperfusion and not seizures. However, sustained tonic/clonic muscle action is more suggestive of seizure.
  5. Focal neurologic symptoms or signs point to a neurologic event such as a seizure with residual deficits (e.g., Todd's paralysis) or cerebral ischemic injury.
  6. Psychological stress: syncope may be vasovagal.
- Review current medications, particularly antihypertensive and psychotropic drugs.
- All patients presenting with syncope require electrocardiography, orthostatic vital signs, and QT interval monitoring.

LABORATORY TESTS

Routine blood tests rarely yield diagnostically useful information and should be done only if they are specifically suggested by the results of the history and physical examination. Box E1-87 describes possibly useful tests. The following are commonly ordered tests:

- Pregnancy test in women of childbearing age
- Complete blood count to look for anemia and signs of infection
- Electrolytes, blood urea nitrogen, creatinine, magnesium, and calcium to look for electrolyte abnormalities and evaluate fluid status
- Serum glucose level
- Cardiac troponins, especially if the patient gives a history of chest pain before the syncopal episode
- Drug and alcohol levels with suspected toxicity

IMAGING STUDIES

- ECG to rule out arrhythmias; may be diagnostic in 5% to 10% of patients.
- Echocardiography.
- If seizure is suspected, CT scan and/or MRI of the head and electroencephalogram may be useful.
- If head trauma or neurologic signs on examination, CT or MRI may be helpful.
- If arrhythmias are suspected, a 24-hr Holter monitor or admission to a telemetry unit is appropriate. In general, Holter monitoring is rarely useful, revealing a cause for syncope in <3% of cases. Loop recorders that can be activated after syncopal episode to retrieve information about the cardiac rhythm during the preceding 4 min add considerable diagnostic yield in patients with unexplained syncope.

- Implantable cardiac monitors that function as permanent loop recorders or implantable cardioverter-defibrillators, which are placed subcutaneously in the pectoral region with the patient under local anesthesia, are useful in patients with cardiac syncope.
- Electrophysiologic studies may be indicated in patients with structural heart disease and/or recurrent syncope.

TILT-TABLE TESTING

- Useful to support a diagnosis of neurally mediated syncope. Patients age >50 yr should have stress testing before tilt-table testing. Positive results would preclude tilt-table testing.
- Indicated in patients with recurrent episodes of unexplained syncope as well as patients in high-risk occupations (e.g., pilots, bus drivers) (Fig. 1-906). The test is also useful for identifying patients with prominent bradycardic response who may benefit from implantation of a permanent pacemaker.
- It is performed by keeping the patient in an upright posture on a tilt table with footboard support. The angle of the tilt table varies from 60 to 80 degrees. The duration of upright posture during tilt-table testing varies from 25 to 45 min.
- The hallmark of neurally mediated syncope is severe hypotension associated with a paradoxic bradycardia triggered by a specific stimulus. The diagnosis of neurally mediated syncope is likely if upright tilt testing reproduces these hemodynamic changes in <15 min and causes presyncope or syncope.

PSYCHIATRIC EVALUATION

- May be indicated in young patients without heart disease who have frequently recurring transient loss of consciousness and other somatic symptoms.
- Generalized anxiety disorder, pain disorder, and major depression predispose patients to neurally mediated reactions and may result in syncope.

Rx TREATMENT

NONPHARMACOLOGIC THERAPY

- Ensure proper hydration; consider compression stockings and salt tablets in appropriate patients.
- Eliminate medications that may induce hypotension.

ACUTE GENERAL Rx

- Varies with the underlying etiology of syncope (e.g., pacemaker in patients with syncope resulting from complete heart block).
- Syncope caused by orthostatic hypotension is treated with volume replacement in patients with intravascular volume depletion. Also consider midodrine to promote venous return by adrenergic-mediated vasoconstriction and Florinef for its mineralocorticoid effects to increase intravascular volume.

DISPOSITION

Prognosis varies with the age of the patient and the etiology of the syncope. In general:

- Benign prognosis (very low 1-yr morbidity rate) in patients:
  1. Age <30 yr and having noncardiac syncope
  2. Age <70 yr and having vasovagal or psychogenic syncope or syncope of unknown cause
- Poor prognosis (high mortality and morbidity rates) in patients with cardiac syncope, with presenting systolic BP <90 mm Hg.
- Patients with the following risk factors have a higher 1-yr mortality rate: abnormal ECG, history of ventricular arrhythmia, history of congestive heart failure.

REFERRAL

Hospital admission in elderly patients without prior history of syncope or unknown etiology of their syncope and in any patients suspected of having cardiac syncope, with presenting systolic BP <90 mm Hg.

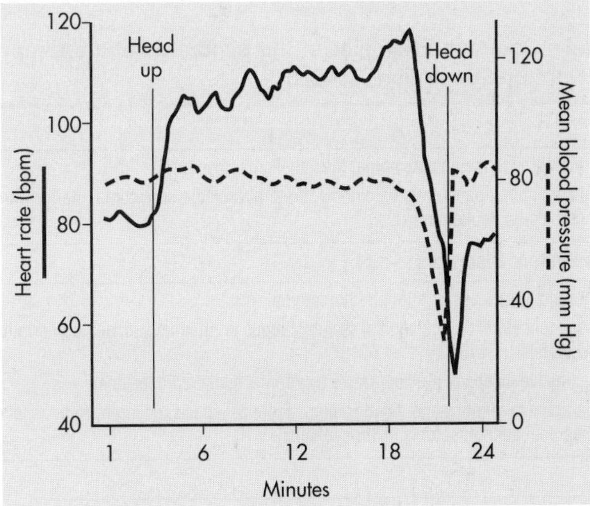

FIGURE 1-906 Head-up tilt test performed on an 18-year-old woman with a history of syncope associated with pain, preceded by a prodrome of dizziness, graying vision, and diaphoresis. A similar prodrome preceded syncope during the test. Note the precipitous and nearly simultaneous decline of heart rate and blood pressure after an initial rise in heart rate. Vital signs returned to normal rapidly after the head was lowered. (Courtesy Robert F. Sprung, University of Utah. In Goldman L, Ausiello D [eds]: *Cecil textbook of medicine,* ed 22, Philadelphia, 2004, Saunders.)

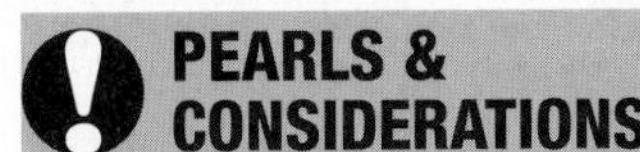

PEARLS & CONSIDERATIONS

COMMENTS

- Section III, "Palpitations, Dizziness, and/or Syncope," describes an algorithmic approach to the patient.
- The etiology of syncope is identified in <50% of cases during the initial evaluation.
- A thorough history and physical examination are the most productive means of establishing a diagnosis in patients with syncope.

SUGGESTED READINGS

available at www.expertconsult.com

RELATED CONTENT

Fig. 3-138 Algorithm for evaluating patients with symptoms of palpitation, dizziness, or syncope (Algorithm)

Syncope (Patient Information)

AUTHOR: **TZU-CHING (TEDDY) WU, M.D.**

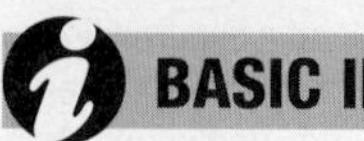

BASIC INFORMATION

DEFINITION

Syndrome of inappropriate antidiuresis (SIAD) is a syndrome characterized by excessive secretion of antidiuretic hormone (ADH) in absence of normal osmotic or physiologic stimuli (increased serum osmolarity, decreased plasma volume, hypotension).

SYNONYMS

SIAD
SIADH
Syndrome of inappropriate antidiuretic hormone secretion
Syndrome of inappropriate ADH release
Inappropriate secretion of antidiuretic hormone

ICD-9CM CODES
276.9 Inappropriate secretion of antidiuretic hormone
ICD-10CM CODES
E22 Syndrome of inappropriate secretion of antidiuretic hormone

EPIDEMIOLOGY & DEMOGRAPHICS

SIAD is the most frequent cause of hyponatremia. Nearly 50% of hyponatremia detected in the hospital setting is caused by SIAD.

PHYSICAL FINDINGS & CLINICAL PRESENTATION

- The patient is generally normovolemic or slightly hypervolemic; edema is absent.
- Delirium, lethargy, and seizures may be present if the hyponatremia is severe or of rapid onset.
- Manifestations of the underlying disease may be evident (e.g., fever from an infectious process or headaches and visual field defects from an intracranial mass).
- Diminished reflexes and extensor plantar responses may occur with severe hyponatremia.

ETIOLOGY

- Neoplasm: lung, oropharynx, stomach, duodenum, pancreas, brain, thymus, bladder, prostate, endometrium, mesothelioma, lymphoma, Ewing's sarcoma
- Pulmonary disorders: pneumonia, aspergillosis, pulmonary abscess, TB, bronchiectasis, emphysema, cystic fibrosis, status asthmaticus, respiratory failure associated with positive-pressure breathing.
- Intracranial pathology: trauma, neoplasms, infections (meningitis, encephalitis, brain abscess), hemorrhage, hydrocephalus, MS, Guillain-Barré syndrome
- Postoperative period: surgical stress, ventilators with positive pressure, anesthetic agents
- Drugs: nicotine, chlorpropamide, thiazide diuretics, vasopressin, desmopressin, oxytocin, chemotherapeutic agents (vincristine, vinblastine, cyclophosphamide), carbamazepine, phenothiazines, MAO inhibitors, tricyclic antidepressants, narcotics, nicotine, clofibrate, haloperidol, SSRIs, NSAIDs
- Other: acute intermittent porphyria, myxedema, psychosis, delirium tremens, ACTH deficiency (hypopituitarism), general anesthesia, endurance exercise
- Table 1-464 summarizes common etiologies of the syndrome of inappropriate antidiuretic hormone secretion.

DIAGNOSIS

DIFFERENTIAL DIAGNOSIS

- Hyponatremia associated with hypervolemia (congestive heart failure, cirrhosis, nephrotic syndrome)
- Factitious hyponatremia (hyperglycemia, abnormal proteins, hyperlipidemia)
- Hyponatremia associated with hypovolemia (e.g., burns, GI fluid loss)

WORKUP

- Demonstration through laboratory evaluation (see "Laboratory Tests") of excessive secretion of ADH in absence of appropriate osmotic or physiologic stimuli (abnormal result on test of water load, elevated plasma arginine vasopressin levels despite the presence of hypotonicity and clinical euvolemia)
- Demonstration of normal thyroid, adrenal, and cardiac function
- No recent or concurrent use of diuretics
- Failure to correct hyponatremia after 0.9% saline infusion
- Correction of hyponatremia through fluid restriction
- Diagnostic criteria for SIADH are decribed in Table 1-465

LABORATORY TESTS

- Hyponatremia
- Decreased effective osmolality (<275 mOsm/kg of water)
- Urine osmolality >100 mOsm/kg of water during hypotonicity
- Urinary osmolarity > serum osmolarity
- Urinary sodium usually >40 mEq/L with normal dietary salt intake
- Normal BUN, creatinine (indicative of normal renal function and absence of dehydration), normal TSH
- Decreased uric acid

IMAGING STUDIES

Chest radiograph to rule out neoplasm or infectious process

TABLE 1-464 Common Etiologies of the Syndrome of Inappropriate Antidiuretic Hormone Secretion (SIADH)

Tumors
Pulmonary/mediastinal (bronchogenic carcinoma, mesothelioma, thymoma)
Nonchest (duodenal carcinoma, pancreatic carcinoma, ureteral/prostate carcinoma, uterine carcinoma, nasopharyngeal carcinoma, leukemia)
Central Nervous System Disorders
Mass lesions (tumors, brain abscesses, subdural hematoma)
Inflammatory diseases (encephalitis, meningitis, systemic lupus erythematosus, acute intermittent porphyria, multiple sclerosis)
Degenerative/demyelinative diseases (Guillain-Barré syndrome, spinal cord lesions)
Miscellaneous (subarachnoid hemorrhage, head trauma, acute psychosis, delirium tremens, pituitary stalk section, transsphenoidal adenomectomy, hydrocephalus)
Drug-Related
Stimulated release of AVP (nicotine, phenothiazines, tricyclics)
Direct renal effects and/or potentiation of AVP antidiuretic effects (dDAVP, oxytocin, prostaglandin synthesis inhibitors)
Mixed or uncertain actions (ACE inhibitors, carbamazepine and oxcarbazepine, chlorpropamide, clofibrate, clozapine, cyclophosphamide, 3,4-methylenedioxymethamphetamine ["Ecstasy"], omeprazole; serotonin reuptake inhibitors, vincristine)
Pulmonary
Infections (tuberculosis, acute bacterial and viral pneumonia, aspergillosis, empyema)
Mechanical/ventilatory causes (acute respiratory failure, COPD, positive-pressure ventilation)
Other Causes
Acquired immunodeficiency syndrome (AIDS) and AIDS-related complex
Prolonged strenuous exercise (marathon, triathlon, ultramarathon, hot-weather hiking)
Senile atrophy
Idiopathic

ACE, Angiotensin-converting enzyme; *AVP*, arginine vasopressin; *COPD*, chronic obstructive pulmonary disease; *dDAVP*, desmopressin.
From Melmed S: *Williams textbook of endocrinology*, ed 12, Philadelphia, 2011, Saunders.

Rx TREATMENT

NONPHARMACOLOGIC THERAPY

Fluid restriction to 500 to 800 ml/day with close monitoring of levels of urinary and plasma electrolytes. Adequate intake of dietary protein and salt should be encouraged.

ACUTE GENERAL Rx

- In emergency situations (seizures, coma) SIAD can be treated with combination of:
  1. Hypertonic saline solution (slow infusion of 250 ml of 3% NaCl). Infuse 3% saline (513 mmol/L) at a rate of 1 to 2 ml/kg of body weight per hour to increase the serum sodium level by 1 to 2 mmol/L/hr.
  2. Furosemide, 20 to 40 mg IV. This combination increases the serum sodium by causing diuresis of urine that is more dilute than plasma and prevents extracellular fluid volume expansion.
- The rapidity of correction varies depending on the degree of hyponatremia and if the hyponatremia is acute or chronic; generally the serum sodium should be corrected only halfway to normal in the initial 24 hr. A prudent approach is to increase serum sodium by <0.5 mEq/L/hr and limit the total increase to 8 to 12 mmol/L during the first 24 hr.
- Close monitoring of the rate of correction (every 2 to 3 hr) is recommended to avoid overcorrection. In patients with hyponatremia of chronic duration, correction of serum sodium level by >12 mmol/L over a period of 24 hr increases the risk of osmotic demyelination.
- Conivaptan (20 to 40 mg/day IV) or tolvaptan (15 mg/day PO initially) are selective arginine-vasopressin (AVP) antagonists useful in selected hospitalized patients with moderate-to-severe hypervolemic and euvolemic hyponatremia. Their direct antagonism of the renal V_2 receptors increases urine water excretion, resulting in an increase in free water clearance (aquaresis). With these agents there is a significant increase in serum sodium concentration in as early as 8 hours and the change is maintained for several days. Potential problems associated with these agents are risk of osmotic demyelination if serum sodium levels are corrected too rapidly and are infusion-site reactions (50% of patients) with conivaptan.

TABLE 1-465 Diagnostic Criteria for the Syndrome of Inappropriate Antidiuretic Hormone Release

Essential Diagnostic Criteria
Decreased extracellular fluid effective osmolality (<270 mOsm/kg H_2O)
Inappropriate urinary concentration (>100 mOsm/kg H_2O)
Clinical euvolemia
Elevated urinary Na^+ concentration under conditions of normal salt and water intake
Absence of adrenal, thyroid, pituitary, or renal insufficiency or diuretic use
Supplemental Criteria
Abnormal water-load test (inability to excrete at least 90% of a 20-ml/kg water load in 4 hours and/or failure to dilute urine osmolality to <100 mOsm/kg)
Plasma vasopressin level inappropriately elevated relative to the plasma osmolality
No significant correction of plasma Na^+ level with volume expansion, but improvement after fluid restriction

From Floege J et al: *Comprehensive clinical nephrology*, ed 4, Philadelphia, 2010, Saunders.

CHRONIC Rx

- Depending on the underlying etiology, fluid restriction may be needed indefinitely. Monthly monitoring of electrolytes is recommended in patients with chronic SIAD.
- Demeclocycline 300 to 600 mg PO bid reduces urinary osmolality and increases serum sodium levels. It may be useful in patients with chronic SIAD (e.g., secondary to neoplasm) but use with caution in patients with hepatic disease; its side effects include nephrogenic diabetes insipidus (DI) and photosensitivity. This medication is also very expensive.
- Successful treatment of chronic nephrogenic SIAD with urea to induce osmotic diuresis has been reported in children and adults. However, oral intake of urea (30 g/day) is generally poorly tolerated.

DISPOSITION

- Prognosis varies depending on the cause. Generally, prognosis is benign when SIAD is caused by an infectious process.
- Morbidity and mortality are high (>40%) when serum sodium concentration is <110 mEq/L.

REFERRAL

Hospital admission depending on severity of symptoms and degree of hyponatremia

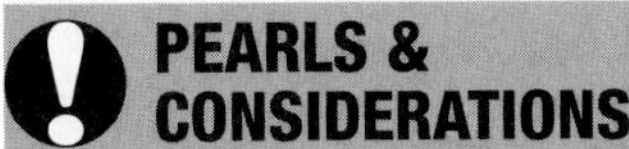

PEARLS & CONSIDERATIONS

COMMENTS

- Use of hypertonic (3%) saline is contraindicated in patients with CHF, nephrotic syndrome, or cirrhosis.
- Too rapid correction of hyponatremia can cause demyelination and permanent central nervous system damage. When considering the use of vasopressor receptor antagonists, their perceived short-term benefits of improving serum sodium need to be weighed against the risks involved with overcorrection of hyponatremia.

SUGGESTED READINGS

available at www.expertconsult.com

RELATED CONTENT

Syndrome of Inappropriate Secretion of Antidiuretic Hormone (Patient Information)

AUTHOR: **FRED F. FERRI, M.D.**

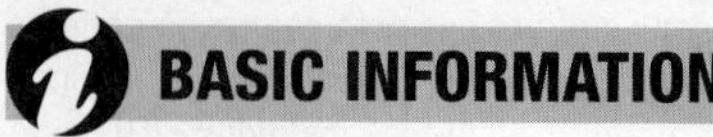

BASIC INFORMATION

DEFINITION

Syphilis is a systemic sexually transmitted treponemal disease, with acute and chronic manifestations, characterized by primary skin lesions; secondary eruption involving skin and mucous membranes; long periods of latency; and late lesions of the skin, bone, viscera, central nervous system, and cardiovascular system.

SYNONYMS

Lues

ICD-9CM CODES
097.9 Syphilis, acquired unspecified
ICD-10CM CODES
A51.0 Primary genital syphilis
A51.1 Primary anal syphilis
A51.2 Primary syphilis of other sites
A51.3 Secondary syphilis of skin and mucous membranes
A51.4 Other secondary syphilis
A51.5 Early syphilis, unspecified
A52 Late syphilis
A52.0 Cardiovascular syphilis
A52.1 Symptomatic neurosyphilis
A52.3 Asymptomatic neurosyphilis
A52.3 Neurosyphilis, unspecified
A53.9 Syphilis, unspecified

EPIDEMIOLOGY & DEMOGRAPHICS

- Widespread, primarily involving ages 20 to 35 yr. Racial differences in incidence are related to social factors. Usually more prevalent in urban areas. Estimated annual incidence of 90,000 cases in the U.S. Rates reached historic lows in the U.S. in 2000 but began increasing among males in 2001 and increase has continued. Rates are disproportionately higher among black and Hispanic men who have sex with men (MSM) compared with white MSM and among young MSM.
- Communicability is indefinite and variable. Communicable during primary, secondary, and latent mucocutaneous lesions in up to first 4 yr of latency. Most probable congenital transmission occurs in early maternal syphilis. Adequate penicillin treatment ends infectivity within 24 to 48 hr.

PHYSICAL FINDINGS & CLINICAL PRESENTATION

PRIMARY SYPHILIS: Characteristic lesion is a painless chancre on genitalia, mouth, or anus (Fig. 1-907); atypical primary lesions may occur. Usually appears 3 wk after exposure and may spontaneously involute.

SECONDARY SYPHILIS:

- Localized or diffuse mucocutaneous lesions and generalized lymphadenopathy. Common to have constitutional symptoms, flulike symptoms. May begin approximately 4 to 6 wk after appearance of primary lesion. Manifestations may resolve in 1 wk to 12 mo.
- 60% to 80% of patients have maculopapular lesions on their palms and soles.
- Condylomata lata intertriginous papules form at areas of friction and moisture, such as the vulva.
- 21% to 58% have mucocutaneous or mucosal lesions (pharyngitis, tonsillitis, "mucous patch" lesion on oral and genital mucosa).

EARLY LATENT (≤1 YR): Generally asymptomatic

LATE LATENT (>1 YR):

- Characterized by gummas (nodular, ulcerative lesions) that can involve the skin, mucous membranes, skeletal system, and viscera.
- Manifestations of cardiovascular syphilis include aortitis, aneurysm, or aortic regurgitation.
- Neurosyphilis may be asymptomatic or symptomatic. Tabes dorsalis, meningovascular syphilis, general paralysis, or insanity may occur. Iritis, choroidoretinitis, and leukoplakia may also occur.

ETIOLOGY

- *Treponema pallidum,* a spirochete
- Spread by sexual intercourse or by intrauterine transfer

Dx DIAGNOSIS

DIFFERENTIAL DIAGNOSIS

- Other genitoulcerative diseases such as herpes, chancroid (see Section II)
- See Section III for a clinical algorithm for the evaluation of genital ulcer disease

WORKUP

Confirmation is primarily through laboratory diagnosis. An algorithm for interpretation of reactive serologic tests for syphilis is described in Fig. E1-908.

LABORATORY TESTS

- Dark-field microscopy of fluid from lesion to look for treponeme is the definitive method for diagnosis of early syphilis.
- Serologic testing, both nontreponemal (VDRL, RPR) and treponemal (FTA, MHA). Many labs now screen patients for syphilis with automated treponemal antibody immunoassays and then confirm positive results with nontreponemal tests. The use of only one type of serologic test is insufficient for diagnosis because each type of test has limitations, including the possibility of false-positive test results in persons without syphilis. False-positive nontreponemal test results can be associated with various medical conditions unrelated to syphilis, including autoimmune conditions, older age, and injection-drug use; therefore, persons with a reactive nontreponemal test should receive a treponemal test to confirm the diagnosis of syphilis. Positive results on both treponemal and nontreponemal testing indicate new untreated syphilis. When the nontreponemal test is negative despite a positive screen, an additional treponemal screen may be helpful. Trials have shown that two positive treponemal screens help identify a population with likely prior or current syphilis, and treatment of these patients may be justifiable.

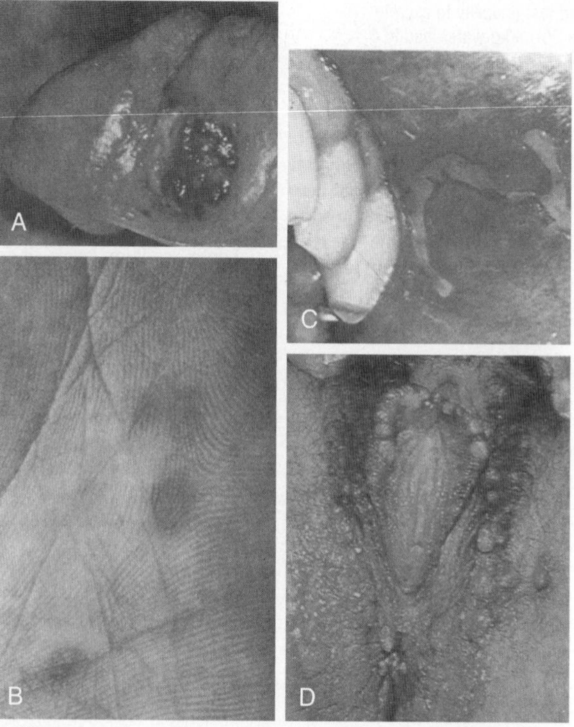

FIGURE 1-907 Syphilis lesions. A, Chancre in primary syphilis. **B,** Palmar lesions of a coppery color in secondary syphilis. **C,** Mucous patch in secondary syphilis. **D,** Condylomata lata in secondary syphilis. (**A, C,** and **D** from Forbes CD, Jackson WF: *Color atlas and text of clinical medicine,* ed 3, London, 2003, Mosby. **B** from Habif TP et al: *Skin disease: diagnosis and treatment,* St Louis, 2001, Mosby.)

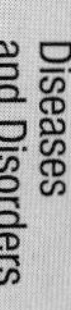

- In patients with neurosyphilis, serologic criteria for response to therapy is a fourfold or greater decrease in VDRL titer over 6 to 12 months.
- Lumbar puncture (LP) for cerebrospinal fluid VDRL (CSF-VDRL) in patients with evidence of latent syphilis. When reactive in the absence of substantial contamination of CSF with blood, it is considered diagnostic of neurosyphilis. The Centers for Disease Control and Prevention indications for LP are neurologic symptoms, treatment failure, any eye or ear involvement, or evidence of active syphilis (aortitis, gumma, iritis).

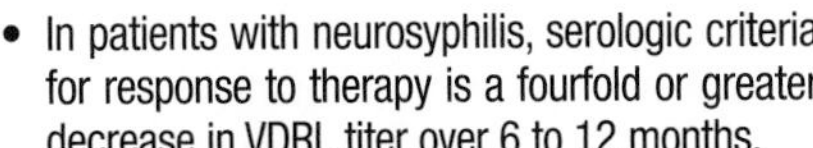

TREATMENT

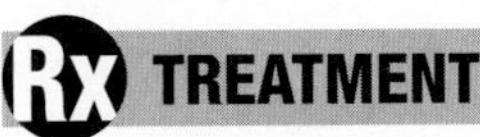

ACUTE GENERAL Rx

- Early (primary, secondary, early latent): penicillin G benzathine 2.4 million U IM × 1 *or* azithromycin 2 g PO × 1 dose
- Late (late latent, cardiovascular, gumma): penicillin G benzathine 2.4 million U IM q wk × 3 wk or doxycycline 100 mg PO bid × 4 wk
- Neurosyphilis: aqueous crystalline penicillin G 18 to 24 million U/day, administered as 3 to 4 million U IV q4h × 10 to 14 days or procaine penicillin 2.4 million U IM/day plus probenecid 500 mg PO qid, both for 10 to 14 days
- Congenital syphilis: aqueous crystalline penicillin G 50,000 U/kg/dose IV q12h × first 7 days of life and q8h after that for total of 10 days or procaine penicillin G 50,000 U/kg/dose IM/day × 10 days
- Penicillin-allergic patients with primary or secondary syphilis: doxycycline 100 mg PO bid × 14 days, or tetracycline 500 mg PO qid × 14 days, or ceftriaxone 1 g IM or IV qd × 10 to 14 days. A recent large study has shown that a single oral dose of azithromycin (2 g administered as 4 500-mg tablets) can be curative in patients with early syphilis
- Latent syphilis in penicillin-allergic patient: doxycycline 100 mg PO bid or tetracycline 500 mg qid for 28 days
- Tetracyclines are contraindicated in pregnancy. If pregnant and penicillin allergic, must be desensitized prior to treatment

DISPOSITION

- Repeat quantitative nontreponemal tests at 3, 6, and 12 mo. Pregnancy requires monthly tests until delivery.
- If a fourfold increase in titer occurs, if initial high titer fails to drop by fourfold within a year, or signs persist, retreatment may be indicated. Use treatment regimen for late syphilis.
- Pregnant women without a fourfold drop in titer in a 3-mo period need to be retreated.
- Cases should be reported to local or state health department for referral, follow-up, and partner notification.

REFERRAL

- Pregnant and possible congenital syphilis
- Pregnant and allergic to penicillin, with need to be desensitized
- Late latent syphilis with serious central nervous system, cardiovascular, or other organ system compromise

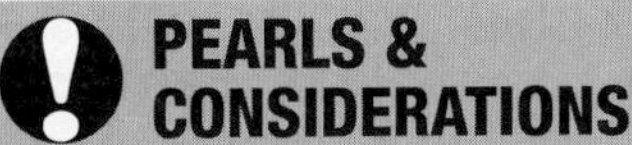

PEARLS & CONSIDERATIONS

- Jarisch-Herxheimer reaction (fever, myalgia, tachycardia, hypotension) may occur within 24 hr of treatment.
- One third of untreated patients develop central nervous system and/or cardiovascular sequelae.
- Up to 80% of those treated during late stages remain seropositive indefinitely.
- Treponemal tests remain positive even after adequate therapy.
- Male circumcision does not decrease the incidence of syphilis (unlike HIV, HSV-2, and HPV infection).
- Partner notification and treatment:
  - Persons who are exposed within 90 days preceding the diagnosis of primary, secondary, or early latent syphilis in a sex partner might be infected even if seronegative; therefore, such persons should be treated presumptively.
  - Persons who were exposed ≥90 days before the diagnosis of syphilis in a sex partner should be treated presumptively if serologic test results are not available immediately and the opportunity for follow-up is uncertain.

SUGGESTED READINGS

available at www.expertconsult.com

RELATED CONTENT

Chancroid (Related Key Topic)
Condyloma Acuminatum (Related Key Topic)
Granuloma Inguinale (Related Key Topic)
Lymphogranuloma Venereum (Related Key Topic)
Fig. 3-80 Evaluation of patients with genital lesions or ulcers (Algorithm)
Syphilis (Patient Information)

AUTHOR: **RUBEN ALVERO, M.D.**

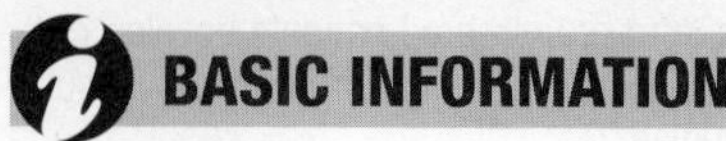

BASIC INFORMATION

DEFINITION

Syringomyelia is a condition characterized by the formation of fluid-filled tubular cavities within the cervical spinal cord, sometimes involving the medulla oblongata, in which case it will be called syringobulbia.

SYNONYMS

Syrinx

ICD-9CM CODES
336.0 Syringomyelia
ICD-10CM CODES
G95.0 Syringomyelia and syringobulbia

EPIDEMIOLOGY & DEMOGRAPHICS

INCIDENCE:

- A rare condition
- No accurate figures for the incidence of syringomyelia
- Incidence of posttraumatic syringomyelia is between 1.9% and 4.5%

PREVALENCE:

- A prevalence of 7 per 100,000 has been suggested
- About 40% to 75% of patients with Chiari malformation have syringomyelia, while in 90% of patients with syringomyelia it is associated with Chiari malformation.

PREDOMINANT SEX AND AGE:

- Symptoms commonly begin in late adolescence or early adulthood
- Both sexes are equally affected

RISK FACTORS:

- Spinal cord anomalies like spina bifida and Chiari malformations
- Base of skull anomalies like achondroplasia
- Spinal cord trauma, including birth trauma
- Intra- or extramedullary spinal tumors
- Multiple sclerosis plaques in the spine
- Spinal arteriovenous malformations
- History of meningitis

PHYSICAL FINDINGS & CLINICAL PRESENTATION

- Onset is usually insidious, often asymptomatic until the third or fourth decade.
- Cervical spine is the most commonly affected area.
  1. Neuropathic joints (Fig. 1-909), intrinsic hand atrophy, hand and/or arm weakness, and sensory loss
  2. Painless burns or other injuries in the hand
  3. Neck, back, arm, and/or leg pain
  4. Loss of pain and temperature sensation in upper extremities, but tactile sense is preserved.
  5. Sharp testing elicits no pain, but patient often perceives the sharpness of the object.
  6. A Charcot joint in the shoulder or elbow may develop.
  7. Impaired walking, toe walking in children
  8. Bowel disturbances such as constipation, and bladder disturbances, such as incontinence
- Loss of upper limb reflexes
- Hyperreflexia is present in the lower extremity.
  - Cape-like sensory loss
  - Ataxia
- Scoliosis is common, especially in children.
- Nystagmus and Horner's syndrome may also occur.
- Hemangiomas or midline tuft of hair, may also indicate underlying spine deformities

ETIOLOGY

- Cause is unknown, but condition is believed to result from obstruction of the outlet of the fourth ventricle, often associated with a Chiari I malformation, which causes fluid to be diverted down the central cord.
- A history of birth trauma often exists.
- Previous history of intramedullary tumors or meningitis leads to syrinx formation.

DIAGNOSIS

DIFFERENTIAL DIAGNOSIS

- Amyotrophic lateral sclerosis/motor neuron disease
- Multiple sclerosis
- Spinal cord tumor
- Transverse myelitis
- Tabes dorsalis
- Vitamin B_{12} deficiency
- Copper deficiency
- Progressive spinal muscular atrophy

IMAGING STUDIES

- Plain radiographs usually reveal widening of the bony canal in the region of involvement.
- Bony anomalies are often present at the base of the skull and at the C1-C2 spinal segments.
- MRI (Fig. 1-910) of the spine is the study of choice. Gadolinium contrast is necessary to rule out spinal tumors.
- CT myelography is an alternative test if MRI is contraindicated

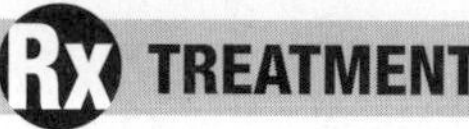

TREATMENT

- No medical treatment is available.
- Decompression laminectomy of C1 and C2.
- Syringostomy
- Insertion of a syringoperitoneal or syringopleural shunt

DISPOSITION

- Condition is slowly progressive in most cases but course may be quite variable, ranging from death in a few months to slow incapacitation over several years; progression may halt at any time.
- Surgical intervention leads to improvement in neurologic findings in 30% of patients.
- Physical and occupational therapies prevent further loss of function.

REFERRAL

Neurology and neurosurgery referral when diagnosis is suspected

SUGGESTED READINGS
available at www.expertconsult.com

RELATED CONTENT

Syringomyelia (Patient Information)

AUTHOR: **CATHERINE ELIAS NAJEM, M.D.**

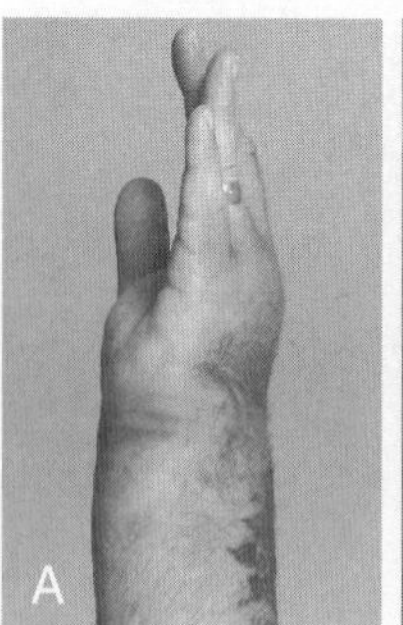

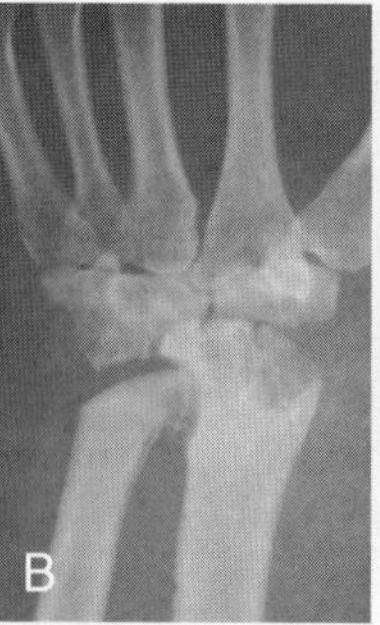

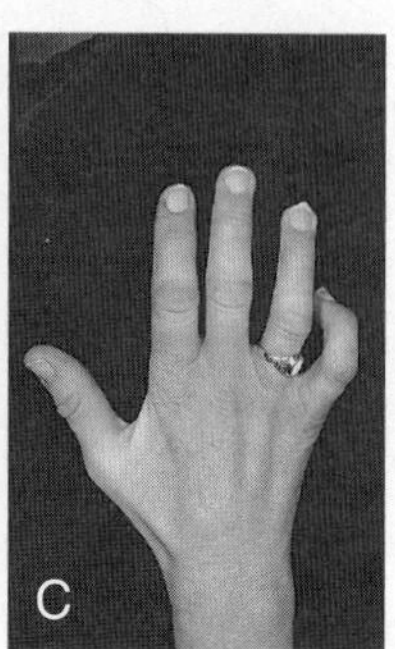

FIGURE 1-909 Syringomyelia. A, A neuropathic wrist joint in a patient with mild syringomyelia. Note the swelling and deformity of the joint. **B,** Radiograph showing the gross destruction of the proximal carpal row with attrition and simplification of the bony margins. Residual fragments of bone and considerable soft tissue swelling can also be seen. **C,** Wasting of the intrinsic muscle of the hand and "claw" deformity. (From Hochberg MC et al: *Rheumatology,* ed 5, St Louis, 2001, Mosby.)

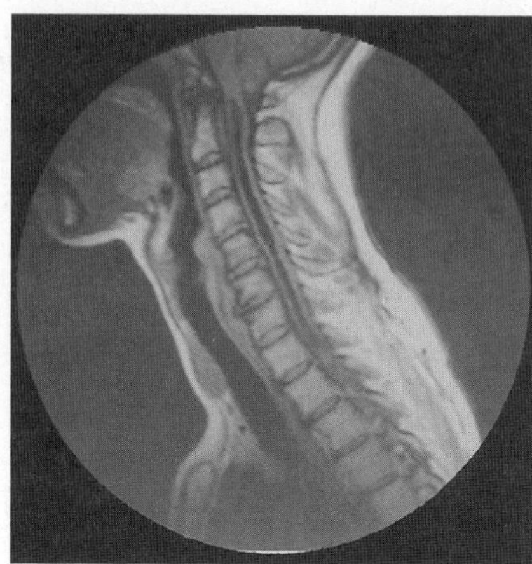

FIGURE 1-910 Magnetic resonance imaging of cervical spine in syringomyelia, showing the fluid-filled syrinx in the center of the spinal cord. (From Hochberg MC et al: *Rheumatology,* ed 5, St Louis, 2011, Mosby.)

BASIC INFORMATION

DEFINITION

Systemic lupus erythematosus (SLE) is a chronic, multisystemic disease characterized by production of autoantibodies and protean clinical manifestations.

SYNONYMS

SLE

ICD-9CM CODES

710.0 Systemic lupus erythematosus

ICD-10CM CODES

M32 Systemic lupus erythematosus
M32.0 Drug-induced systemic lupus erythematosus
M32.1+ Systemic lupus erythematosus with organ or system involvement
M32.8 Other forms of systemic lupus erythematosus
M32.9 Systemic lupus erythematosus, unspecified
M32.10 Systemic lupus erythematosus, organ or system involvement unspecified

TABLE 1-466 Potential Clinical Manifestations of Systemic Lupus Erythematosus

Target Organ	Potential Clinical Manifestations
Constitutional	Fatigue, anorexia, weight loss, fever, lymphadenopathy
Musculoskeletal	Arthritis, myositis, arthralgias, myalgias, avascular necrosis, osteoporosis
Skin	Malar rash, discoid rash, photosensitive rash, cutaneous vasculitis, livedo reticularis, periungual capillary abnormalities, Raynaud's phenomenon, alopecia, oral and nasal ulcers
Renal	Hypertension, proteinuria, hematuria, edema, nephrotic syndrome, renal failure
Cardiovascular	Pericarditis, myocarditis, conduction system abnormalities, Libman-Sacks endocarditis
Neurologic	Seizures, psychosis, cerebritis, stroke, transverse myelitis, depression, cognitive impairment, headaches, pseudotumor, peripheral neuropathy, chorea, optic neuritis, cranial nerve palsies
Pulmonary	Pleuritis, interstitial lung disease, pulmonary hemorrhage, pulmonary hypertension, pulmonary embolism
Hematologic	Immune-mediated cytopenias (hemolytic anemia, thrombocytopenia or leukopenia), anemia of chronic inflammation, hypercoagulability, thrombocytopenic thrombotic microangiopathy
Gastroenterology	Hepatosplenomegaly, pancreatitis, vasculitis affecting bowel, protein-losing enteropathy
Ocular	Retinal vasculitis, scleritis, episcleritis, papilledema

Modified from Kliegman RM et al: *Nelson textbook of pediatrics*, ed 19, Philadelphia, 2011, Saunders.

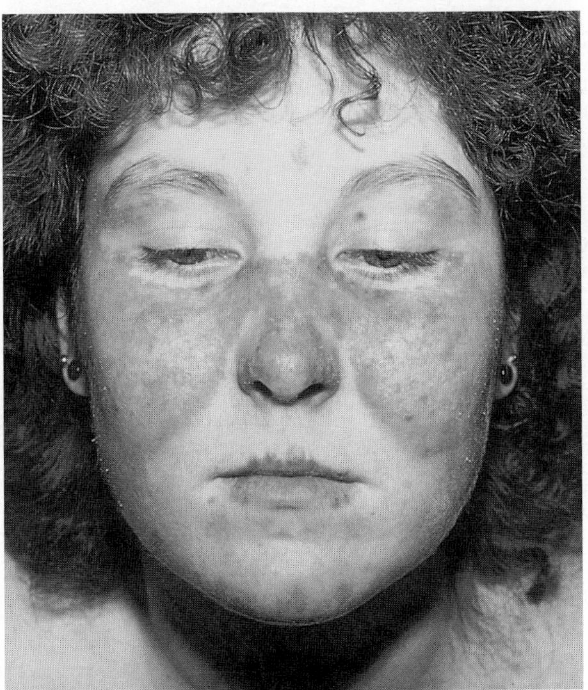

FIGURE 1-911 Acute cutaneous lupus erythematosus (LE) (systemic LE). The classic butterfly rash occurs in 10% to 50% of patients with acute LE. (From Habif TP: *Clinical dermatology: a color guide to diagnosis and therapy,* ed 3, St Louis, 1996, Mosby.)

EPIDEMIOLOGY & DEMOGRAPHICS

INCIDENCE: 20 to 70 cases per 100,000 persons. Certain ethnic groups, including those of African, Hispanic, or Asian ancestry, are at an increased risk of developing the disorder.

PREDOMINANT SEX: Female/male ratio is 9:1.

PREDOMINANT AGE: Predominant age ranges from 20 to 45 yr (childbearing age).

PHYSICAL FINDINGS & CLINICAL PRESENTATION

- Constitutional: unexplained fever, fatigue, malaise (see Table 1-466)
- Skin: malar rash sparing nasolabial folds (acute cutaneous lupus) (Fig. 1-911); annular or papulosquamous rash (subacute cutaneous lupus) (Fig. 1-912); raised erythematous patches with subsequent edematous plaques and adherent scales (discoid cutaneous lupus) (Fig. 1-913); alopecia, nasal, or oropharyngeal ulcerations; Raynaud's phenomenon; petechiae, palpable purpura, skin ulceration, or digital ischemia (vasculitis); livedo reticularis or livedo racemosa (secondary antiphospholipid antibody syndrome)
- Musculoskeletal: arthritis (tenderness, swelling, effusion) typically affecting peripheral joints; myositis
- Cardiac: pericardial rub (pericarditis), heart murmur (Libman-Sacks endocarditis and other valvular heart disease), congestive heart failure (myocarditis), premature atherosclerotic heart disease
- Pulmonary: pleuritis, pneumonitis, diffuse alveolar hemorrhage
- Gastrointestinal: abdominal pain, intestinal vasculitis, ascites
- Neurologic: headache, psychosis, seizure, acute confusional states, peripheral or cranial neuropathy, transverse myelitis, cerebral vascular accident, chronic cognitive impairment
- Hematologic: anemia (hemolytic, anemia chronic disease, aplastic anemia), thrombocytopenia, leukopenia, lymphadenopathy, secondary antiphospholipid antibody syndrome
- Renal: acute renal failure, proteinuria, nephritic syndrome, nephrotic syndrome

ETIOLOGY

Exact etiology and pathogenesis are uncertain. Genetic susceptibility to lupus is likely inherited as a polygenic trait. Multiple genetic linkages including 1q23, 2q35-37, 6p21-11, and 12q24 show strong associations with SLE. Environmental factors such as ultraviolet light exposure and Epstein-Barr virus infection may have a triggering role. Autoantibodies can be present years before the diagnosis of SLE. Evidence supports the improper processing of nuclear proteins and nucleic acid from cell death. Impairments in neutrophil cell death via a process termed NET-osis (nuclear extracellular trap) contribute to the accumulation of nuclear debris. This, in turn, can lead to the presentation of self-nuclear material to plasmacytoid dendritic cells. Plasmacytoid dendritic cells propagate antibody and immune complex production via a type I interferon-dependent mechanism.

Dx DIAGNOSIS

DIFFERENTIAL DIAGNOSIS

- Rheumatologic disorder
- Rheumatoid arthritis, mixed connective tissue disease, systemic vasculitis
- Neoplastic disorder
- Hematologic malignancy, paraneoplastic syndrome
- Systemic infection
- Other: thrombotic thrombycytopenic purpura/hemolytic uremic syndrome, primary antiphospholipid antibody syndrome

WORKUP

The diagnosis of SLE is suspected when any *four or more* of the following 1997 American College of Rheumatology criteria are present:

- Malar rash
- Discoid rash
- Photosensitivity (recurrence of unusual skin rash in sun-exposed areas)
- Oral or nasopharyngeal painless ulceration, observed by physician
- Arthritis, nonerosive
- Serositis (pleuritis, pericarditis)
- Renal disorder (persistent proteinuria >0.5 g/day, or ≥3+ on dipstick if quantitation not performed; cellular casts)
- Neurologic disorder (seizures, psychosis [in absence of offending drugs or metabolic derangement])
- Hematologic disorder:
  - Hemolytic anemia with reticulocytosis
  - Leukopenia (<4000/mm^3 total on two or more occasions)
  - Lymphopenia (<1500/mm^3 on two or more occasions)
  - Thrombocytopenia (<100,000/mm^3 in the absence of offending drugs)
- Immunologic disorder:
  - Anti–double-stranded DNA antibody (anti-dsDNA)
  - Anti-Smith antibody (anti-Sm)
  - Antiphospholipid antibodies (anticardiolipin IgM or IgG, lupus anticoagulant, anti-beta-2 glycoprotein IgM or IgG, or false-positive fluorescent treponemal antibody absorption test or *Treponema pallidum* immobilization for 6 months)
- Antinuclear antibody (ANA): an abnormal titer of ANA by immunofluorescence or equivalent assay at any time in the absence of drugs known to be associated with drug-induced lupus syndrome

LABORATORY TESTS

Suggested initial laboratory evaluation of suspected SLE:

- Complete blood count with differential, blood urea nitrogen and serum creatinine, urinalysis, ESR, PT, PTT, complements (C3, C4, CH50)
- ANA

Consider additional laboratory testing:

- Anti-dsDNA, anti-Smith, anti-SSA, anti-SSB, anti-RNP antibodies. Table 1-467 summarizes autoantibodies and clinical significance in SLE.
- Lupus anticoagulant, anticardiolipin antibodies, anti-beta-2 glycoprotein antibodies especially in patients with thrombotic events or recurrent miscarriages
- Random spot urine protein to urine creatinine ratio, 24-hour urine protein collection if proteinuria

IMAGING STUDIES

- Chest x-ray for evaluation of pulmonary involvement (pleural effusion, pulmonary infiltrates)
- Electrocardiogram for complaint of unexplained chest pain

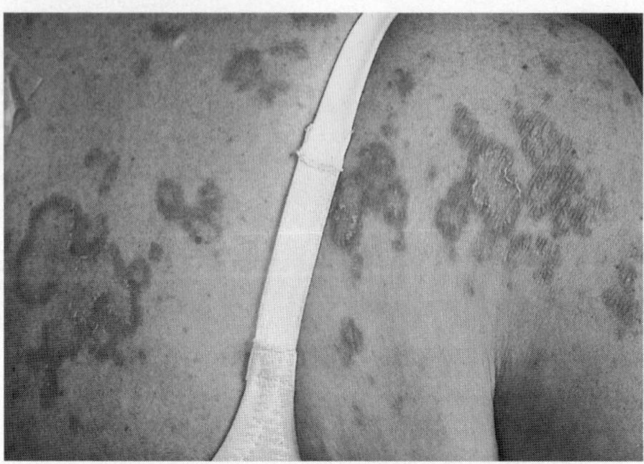

FIGURE 1-912 Subacute cutaneous lupus. (From Hochberg MC et al: *Rheumatology*, ed 4, St Louis, 2008, Mosby.)

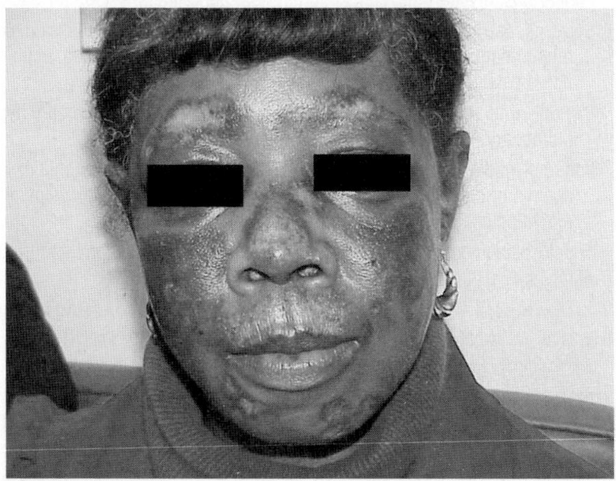

FIGURE 1-913 Discoid lupus erythematosus. (From Firestein GS et al: *Kelley's textbook of rheumatology*, ed 8, Philadelphia, 2008, Saunders.)

TABLE 1-467 Autoantibodies and Clinical Significance in Systemic Lupus Erythematosus (SLE)

Autoantibody	Prevalence in SLE	Clinical Significance
Antinuclear Antibody		
Anti-dsDNA	60%	95% specificity for SLE; fluctuates with disease activity; associated with glomerulonephritis
Anti-Smith	20%-30%	99% specificity for SLE; associated with anti-U1RNP antibodies
Anti-U1RNP	30%	Antibody associated with mixed connective tissue disease and lower frequency of glomerulonephritis
Anti-Ro/SSA	30%	Associated with Sjögren's syndrome, photosensitivity, SCLE, neonatal lupus, congenital heart block
Anti-La/SSB	20%	Associated with Sjögren's syndrome, SCLE, neonatal lupus, congenital heart block, anti-Ro/SSA
Antihistone	70%	Also associated with drug-induced lupus
Antiphospholipid	30%	Associated with arterial and venous thrombosis, pregnancy morbidity

SCLE, Subacute cutaneous lupus erythematosus.
From Firestein GS et al: *Kelly's textbook of rheumatology,* ed 9, Philadelphia, 2013, Saunders.

- Echocardiogram if unexplained murmur, evidence of new or unexplained congestive heart failure, or suspected pericarditis

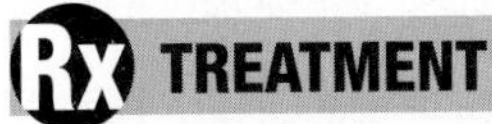

TREATMENT

NONPHARMACOLOGIC THERAPY

- Patients with SLE should avoid sunlight and use high-SPF sunscreen.
- Screening and counseling for modifiable cardiovascular risk factors like cigarette cessation are necessary for the prevention of atherosclerotic disease.
- Counseling for pregnancy planning should be performed for patients of childbearing age.
- Calcium carbonate and vitamin D_3 supplementation for prevention of early osteoporosis.

GENERAL Rx

- Defined courses of corticosteroids are useful for a variety of SLE symptoms.
- Immunosuppressive drugs such as methotrexate or azathioprine are used as steroid-sparing drugs. Indications for immunosuppressive therapy in SLE are described in Tables 1-468 and 1-469.
- Joint pain and mild serositis are generally well controlled with nonsteroidal anti-inflammatory drugs or low-dose corticosteroids. Hydroxychloroquine and methotrexate are also effective for arthritis. Leflunomide or anti-TNF agents may be considered for difficult arthritis.
- Cutaneous manifestations
  - Topical or intradermal corticosteroids are helpful for individual discoid lesions, especially in the scalp.
  - Hydroxychloroquine is efficacious. Some studies support a combination of quinacrine and hydroxychloroquine for refractory skin disease.
- Hematologic manifestations
  - Corticosteroids are first-line therapy.
  - Azathioprine can be used for thrombocytopenia or hemolytic anemia.
  - Intravenous immunoglobulin or rituximab may be considered for severe leukopenia, autoimmune hemolytic anemia, or autoimmune thrombocytopenia
- Central nervous system manifestations.
  - Headaches are treated symptomatically.
  - Anticonvulsants and antipsychotics may be indicated.
  - Standard therapy for other neuropsychiatric SLE symptoms is not established.
- Renal disease (Class III, IV, V lupus nephritis; see Table 1-470)
  - The use of high doses of intravenous cyclophosphamide with corticosteroids given at monthly intervals is more effective in preserving renal function than is treatment with glucocorticoids alone.
  - Increasingly, mycophenolate mofetil (target dose 3000 mg daily) has become the induction treatment of choice due to its improved tolerability and better fertility profile. Studies show that patients treated with mycophenolate mofetil as induction therapy had similar renal and nonrenal outcomes as compared to high-dose intravenous cyclophosphamide.
- Mycophenolate mofetil or azathioprine is used for maintenance therapy.
- Severe nonrenal organ disease
  - Evidence from systematic randomized controlled trials for nonrenal lupus treatment is comparatively limited.
  - High-dose intravenous cyclophosphamide is used as induction treatment. Azathioprine or mycophenolate mofetil may be used as maintenance drugs.
  - Intravenous immunoglobulin may be considered in severe disease when concomitant infection is present.
  - Plasmapheresis may be considered in critical situations, but efficacy is not proved in

TABLE 1-468 Indications for Immunosuppressive Therapy in Systemic Lupus Erythematosus

General Indications
Involvement of major organs or extensive involvement of nonmajor organs (skin) refractory to other agents, or both
Failure to respond to or inability to taper corticosteroids to acceptable doses for long-term use
Specific Organ Involvement
RENAL
Proliferative or membranous nephritis (nephritic or nephritic syndrome), or both
HEMATOLOGIC
Severe thrombocytopenia (platelets <20,000/mm³)
Thrombotic thrombocytopenic purpura–like syndrome
Severe hemolytic or aplastic anemia, or immune neutropenia not responding to glucocorticoids
PULMONARY
Lupus pneumonitis or alveolar hemorrhage, or both
CARDIAC
Myocarditis with depressed left ventricular function, pericarditis with impending tamponade
GASTROINTESTINAL
Abdominal vasculitis
NERVOUS SYSTEM
Transverse myelitis, cerebritis, optic neuritis, psychosis refractory to corticosteroids, mononeuritis multiplex, severe peripheral neuropathy

From Firestein GS et al: *Kelly's textbook of rheumatology,* ed 9, Philadelphia, 2013, Saunders.

TABLE 1-469 Recommended Immunosuppressive Therapy for Major Organ Involvement in Systemic Lupus Erythematosus

Disease Severity	Induction Therapy	Maintenance Therapy
Mild	High-dose GC (0.5-1 mg/kg/day prednisone ×4-6 wk, tapered to 0.125 mg/kg every other day within 3 mo) alone or in combination with AZA (1-2 mg/kg/day)	Low-dose GC (prednisone ≤0.125 mg/kg on alternative days) alone or with AZA (1-2 mg/kg/day)
	If no remission within 3 mo, treat as moderately severe	Consider further gradual tapering at the end of each year of remission
Moderate	MMF (2 g/day) (or AZA) with GC as above; if no remission after the first 6-12 mo, treat as severe	MMF tapered to 1.5 g/day for 6-12 mo and then to 1 g/day; consider further tapering at the end of each year in remission Alternative: AZA (1-2 mg/kg/day)
Severe	Pulse IV-CYC alone or in combination with pulse IV-MP for the first 6 mo (background GC 0.5 mg/kg/day for 4 wk, then taper)	Quarterly pulses of IV-CYC for at least 1 year beyond remission
	If no response, consider adding RTX or switch to MMF	Alternative: AZA (1-2 mg/kg/day), MMF (1-2 g/day)

AZA, Azathioprine; *CYC,* cyclophosphamide; *GC,* glucocorticoid; *IV,* intravenous; *MMF,* mycophenolate mofetil; *MP,* methylprednisolone; *RTX,* rituximab.
From Firestein GS et al: *Kelly's textbook of rheumatology,* ed 9, Philadelphia, 2013, Saunders.

TABLE 1-470 Severity of Lupus Nephritis*

Proliferative Disease	
Mild	Type III without severe histologic features (e.g., crescents, fibrinoid necrosis); low chronicity index (i.e., ≤3); normal renal function; nonnephrotic-range proteinuria
Moderately severe	Mild disease as defined above with partial or no response after the initial induction therapy or delayed remission (>12 months), or Focal proliferative nephritis with adverse histologic features or reproducible increase of at least 30% in serum creatinine levels, or Diffuse proliferative nephritis (class IV) without adverse histologic features
Severe	Moderately severe as defined above but not remitting after 6 to 12 months of therapy, or Proliferative disease with impaired renal function and fibrinoid necrosis or crescents in >25% of glomeruli, or Mixed membranous and proliferative nephritis, or Proliferative nephritis with high chronicity alone or in combination with high activity (chronicity index >4 or chronicity index >3 and activity index >10), or Rapidly progressive glomerulonephritis (doubling of serum creatinine within 2 to 3 months)
MEMBRANOUS NEPHROPATHY	
Mild	Nonnephrotic-range proteinuria with normal renal function
Moderate	Nephrotic-range proteinuria with normal renal function at presentation
Severe	Nephrotic-range proteinuria with impaired renal function at presentation (at least 30% increase in serum creatinine)

*Concomitant therapy with corticosteroids or other immunosuppressive drugs may modify urinary sediment and/or histologic findings and should be taken into consideration.
From Hochberg MC et al: *Rheumatology,* ed 5, St Louis, 2011, Mosby.

controlled trials and infectious complication is a substantial consideration.

- New therapy
  - Rituximab: randomized controlled trials for rituximab as an adjunct induction agent were negative in terms of both renal and nonrenal outcomes. Other clinical trials have shown an improvement in certain SLE parameters with rituximab.
  - Belimumab: in March 2011, the U.S. Food and Drug Administration approved belimumab for treatment of active SLE in adults. When used in addition to standard therapy, patients on belimumab showed increased efficacy compared to placebo based on a newly defined clinical benchmark. A majority of study patients had primary dermatologic or joint disease. Patients with CNS or serious kidney disease were excluded. Belimumab-treated patients had a reduced time to disease flare and lower glucocorticoid exposure.

DISPOSITION

- Most patients with SLE experience remissions and exacerbations.
- Five-year survival rate has improved to over 90% in patients with newly diagnosed SLE since the advent of potent immunosuppressive therapy. The 15-year survival rate is now 85%.
- African Americans, Asian Americans, and Hispanic Americans in general have a worse prognosis.
- The leading cause of death in SLE patients in developed countries is premature atherosclerosis.
- The quality of life for SLE patients is poor due to fatigue, chronic pain, and cognitive impairment.

REFERRAL

- Rheumatology consultation for all patients with SLE
- Hematology consultation for patients with significant hematologic abnormalities (e.g., severe hemolytic anemia or thrombocytopenia)
- Nephrology consultation in patients with significant renal involvement
- Dermatology consultation for patients with unexplained or unusual skin rash
- Cardiology consultation for patients with lupus carditis, arrhythmias

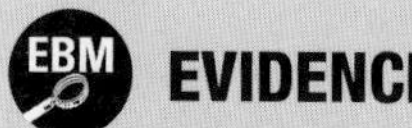

EVIDENCE

available at www.expertconsult.com

SUGGESTED READINGS

available at www.expertconsult.com

RELATED CONTENT

Systemic Lupus Erythematosus (Patient Information)

AUTHOR: **SAMUEL H. POON, M.D.**

BASIC INFORMATION

DEFINITION

Takayasu's arteritis is a chronic systemic granulomatous large-vessel vasculitis. It often presents as a pulseless disease caused by widespread arterial stenosis.

SYNONYMS

Pulseless disease
Aortitis syndrome
Aortic arch arteritis
Nonspecific aortoarteritis

ICD-9CM CODES
446.7 Takayasu disease or syndrome
ICD-10CM CODES
M31.4 Aortic arch syndrome [Takayasu]

EPIDEMIOLOGY & DEMOGRAPHICS

Takayasu's arteritis is the third most common childhood vasculitis worldwide, although it is relatively uncommon in Europe and North America. Most cases have been reported in Japan, China, India, and Mexico. There is typically a considerable delay to diagnosis in Western populations as opposed to Asian countries, owing in large part to the increased incidence in Asia.

INCIDENCE: Incidence in the U.S. is 2.6/1 million persons.

PREDOMINANT SEX AND AGE: The female/male ratio is 8:1. The age of onset is usually between 10 and 40 yr of age. The disease commonly presents between the age of 10 and 20 yr of age, with three quarters of the patients presenting during this time.

PHYSICAL FINDINGS & CLINICAL PRESENTATION

- Takayasu's arteritis is typically divided into systemic and occlusive stages, with the occlusive stage characterized by ischemia and symptoms from arterial occlusion. Table 1-471 summarizes common symptoms and signs in Takayasu's arteritis.
- The systemic stage of Takayasu's arteritis manifests as nonspecific symptoms, including the following:
  1. Low-grade fever
  2. Malaise
  3. Weight loss
  4. Fatigue
  5. Arthralgia and myalgia
  6. Carotidynia
- The occlusive stage of Takayasu's arteritis may progress to stenosis or aneurysm of the aorta and its primary branches, and may manifest as a variety of clinical signs and symptoms, such as:
  1. Arm or leg claudication, weakness, and numbness
  2. Amaurosis fugax, diplopia, headache, orthostasis, vertigo, or syncope
  3. Angina or myocardial infarction
  4. Vascular bruits of the carotid artery, subclavian artery, and aorta
  5. Discrepancy of blood pressures between the upper extremities, typically of ≥10 mm Hg
  6. Diminished or absent pulses, ischemic ulcerations, or gangrene in advanced disease
  7. Hypertension
  8. Retinopathy
  9. Aortic insufficiency as a result of aortic root dilatation and aneurysm formation
  10. Weakness of the arterial walls may give rise to localized aneurysms/dissection.

ETIOLOGY

- The cause of Takayasu's arteritis is poorly understood. Cell-mediated mechanisms are thought to be important to the pathogenesis.
- Infiltration by inflammatory cells (lymphocytes, macrophages, and multinucleated giant cells) into the vasa vasorum and media of the large elastic arteries (Fig. 1-915) leads to fibrosis, thickening, and narrowing or obliteration. Patients with Takayasu's arteritis have stenoses in ≥90% of cases, and aneurysms in ≥25% of cases. Release of metalloproteinases and reactive oxygen species may result in local aneurysms.
- Infection, in particular, tuberculosis, has been implicated in the pathogenesis of Takayasu's disease with several studies reporting an increased incidence of caseating granulomas in Takayasu patients. Additional immunologic studies lend support to a pathogenic role of CD4 and CD8 T-cells in this patient population.

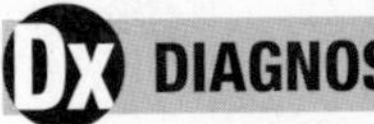

DIAGNOSIS

Diagnostic criteria for Takayasu's arteritis were established by the American College of Rheumatology in 1990. A diagnosis is made if at least three of the six criteria are present; this results in a sensitivity of 91% and specificity of 98%. The criteria are:

- Age of disease onset <40 yr
- Claudication of the extremities
- Decreased brachial artery pulse
- Systolic blood pressure difference ≥10 mm Hg between left and right arms
- Bruit over one or both of the subclavian arteries or the abdominal aorta
- Abnormal arteriogram, not related to arteriosclerosis or fibromuscular dysplasia

TABLE 1-471 Common Symptoms and Signs (%) in Takayasu's Arteritis

	STUDY					
Symptom/Sign	**Japan (n = 52)**	**India (n = 106)**	**China (n = 530)**	**Korea (n = 129)**	**USA (n = 60)**	**Mexico (n = 107)**
Fatigue/constitutional	27%	—	—	34%	43%	78%
Weight loss	—	9%	—	11%	20%	22%
Musculoskeletal	6%	5%	—	—	53%	53%
Claudication	13%	—	25%	21%	90%	29%
Headache	31%	44%	—	60%	42%	57%
Visual changes	6%	12%	10%	20%	30%	8%
Syncope/dizziness	40%	26%	14%	36%	35%	13%
Palpitations	23%	19%	—	23%	10%	43%
Dyspnea	21%	26%	11%	42%	—	72%
Carotidynia	21%	—	—	2%	32%	—
Hypertension	33%	77%	60%	40%	35%	72%
Bruit	—	35%	58%	37%	80%	94%
Decreased pulses	62%	—	37%	55%	60%	96%
Asymmetric blood pressure	—	—	—	—	47%	—

From Hochberg MC et al: *Rheumatology,* ed 5, St Louis, 2011, Mosby.

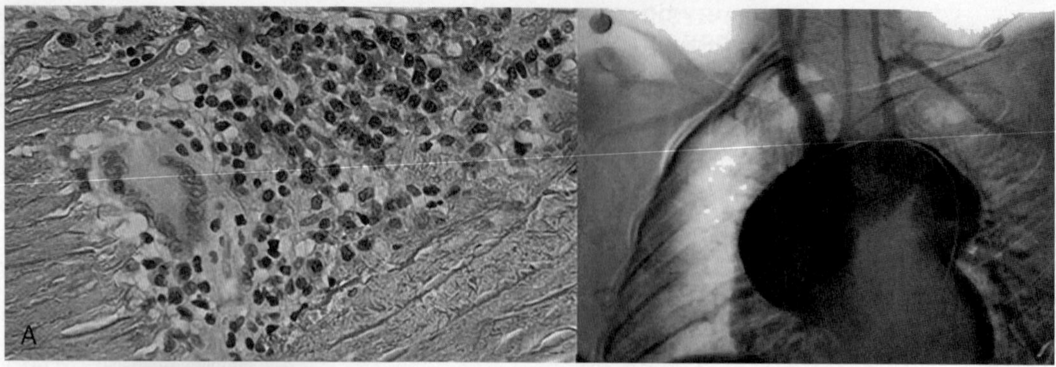

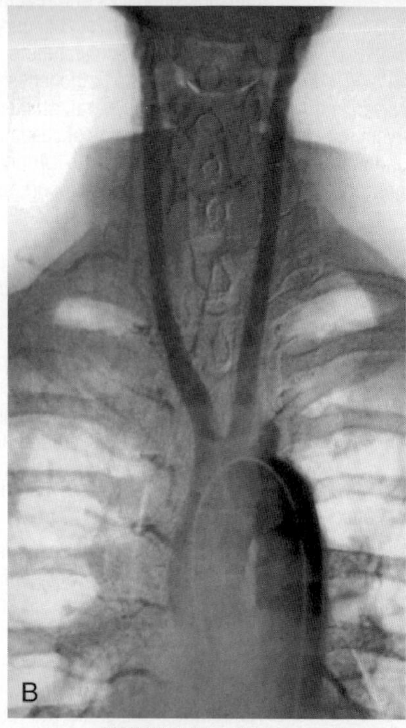

FIGURE 1-915 Takayasu disease. A, Takayasu arteritis. Granulomatous inflammation and medial destruction (left) has led to marked aortic root dilation (right) in a 17-year-old female high school student who developed symptoms of congestive heart failure and exertional angina. She also had diffuse narrowing of the left common carotid artery and irregular dilation of the innominate artery. (Hematoxylin-eosin stain; magnification ×40.) **B,** Occlusion of both subclavian arteries led to leg pressures being the only reliable measure of central aortic pressure. (Bonow RO et al: *Heart Disease*, ed 9, Philadelphia, 2012, Saunders.)

DIFFERENTIAL DIAGNOSIS

Table 1-472 describes pathologic characteristics of selected forms of vasculitis. Other causes of inflammatory arteritis must be excluded:

- Temporal arteritis (giant cell arteritis)
- Syphilis
- Tuberculosis
- Systemic lupus erythematosus
- Rheumatoid arthritis
- Buerger's disease
- Behçet's disease
- Cogan's syndrome
- Kawasaki disease
- Spondyloarthropathies

WORKUP

Any young patient with findings of absent pulses and loud bruits merits a workup for Takayasu's arteritis. The workup generally includes blood testing to look for signs of inflammation as well as imaging studies. An angiogram continues to be the diagnostic gold standard; however, due to advances in noninvasive vascular imaging, modalities such as magnetic resonance and computed tomography angiography (MRA and CTA) can be adjunctive.

LABORATORY TESTS

- Erythrocyte sedimentation rate (ESR) and serum C-reactive protein levels are usually elevated, but can be normal even in the setting of active vasculitis.
- A CBC may reveal a normal or elevated white blood cell count as well as anemia.
- Immunologic studies may include elevated immunoglobulins (IgG and IgA) and complement components (C3 and C4).
- Hypercoagulation and increase in platelet aggregation
- A positive association with HLA-B52 and HLA-B39 has been identified.
- Recent studies have attempted to establish a link between elevated levels of various interleukins and active disease.

IMAGING STUDIES

- Imaging of the entire aorta and major branch vessels using angiography, CTA or MRA
- CTA can detect changes in the vessel wall and provide an accurate representation of luminal diameters.
- Cardiovascular magnetic resonance (CMR) provides information on vessel lumen and wall thickening, cardiac morphology and function, and myocardial tissue characterization.
- Angiography (Fig. 1-916) can show the narrowing of the aorta and its branches, aneurysm formation, poststenotic dilation, and the development of any collateral circulation.

TABLE 1-472 Pathologic Characteristics of Selected Forms of Vasculitis

	Takayasu's Arteritis	Polyarteritis Nodosa	Wegener's Granulomatosis	Churg-Strauss Syndrome	Henoch-Schönlein Purpura	Cutaneous Leukocytoclastic Angiitis
Vessels involved	Elastic (large) or muscle (medium-sized) arteries	Medium-sized and small muscle arteries	Small arteries and veins; sometimes medium-sized vessels	Small arteries and veins; sometimes medium-sized vessels	Capillaries, venules, arterioles	Capillaries, venules, arterioles
Organ involvement	Aorta, aortic arch and major branches, pulmonary arteries	Skin, peripheral nerve, gastrointestinal tract, other viscera	Upper respiratory tract, lungs, kidneys, skin, eyes	Upper respiratory tract, lungs, heart, peripheral nerves	Skin, joints, gastrointestinal tract, kidneys	Skin, joints
Type of vasculitis and inflammatory cells	Granulomatous with some giant cells; fibrosis in chronic stages	Necrotizing, with mixed cellular infiltrate	Necrotizing or granulomatous (or both); mixed cellular infiltrate plus occasional eosinophils	Necrotizing or granulomatous (or both); prominent eosinophils and other mixed infiltrate	Leukocytoclastic, with some lymphocytes and variable eosinophils; IgA deposits in affected tissues	Leukocytoclastic, with occasional eosinophils

From Goldman L, Schafer AI: *Goldman's Cecil medicine*, ed 24, Philadelphia, 2012, Saunders.

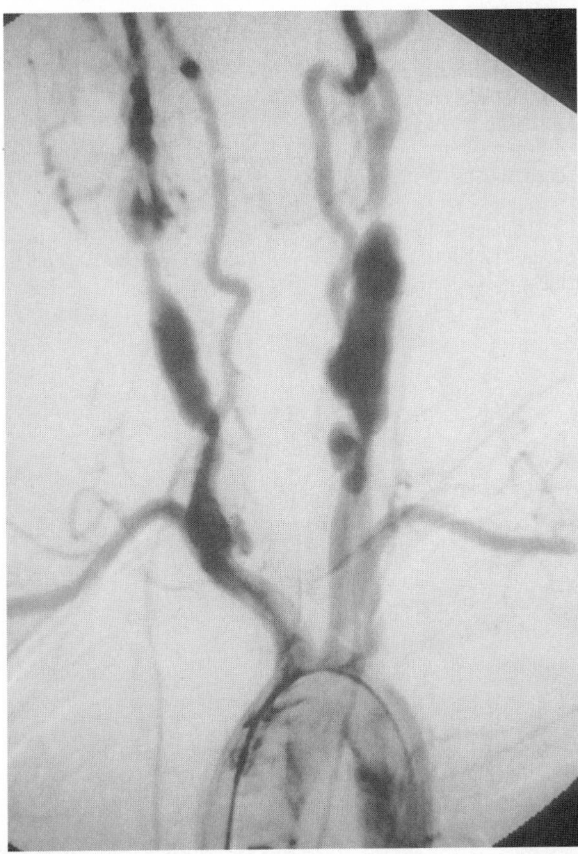

FIGURE 1-916 Angiogram of a child with Takayasu's arteritis that shows massive bilateral carotid dilation, stenosis, and poststenotic dilation. (From Behrman RE: Nelson textbook of pediatrics, ed 16, Philadelphia, 2000, Saunders.)

Angiographic findings are classified into five types:

1. Type I: lesions that involve only branches of the aortic arch
2. Type IIa: lesions that involve the ascending aorta, the aortic arch, and its branches
3. Type IIb: lesions from IIa plus the thoracic descending aorta
4. Type III: lesions that involve the thoracic descending aorta, abdominal aorta, and/or renal arteries
5. Type IV: lesions that involve the abdominal aorta and/or renal arteries
6. Type V: lesions that involve the entire aorta and its branches

- Chest radiography: pathologic changes of the aorta are often visible, with areas of alternating stenosis and dilation seen. Segmental calcification outlining areas of aortic narrowing is characteristic of Takayasu's disease.
- Ultrasound: carotid, thoracic, and abdominal ultrasound are useful adjunctive imaging studies to diagnose the occlusive disease that results from Takayasu's arteritis. The addition of Doppler is helpful to assess blood flow and absent pulses.
- Positron emission tomography using radioisotope fluorodeoxyglucose (FDG-PET) as a marker for tissue with high glucose uptake has shown promising results in terms of specificity and sensitivity.

Rx TREATMENT

ACUTE GENERAL Rx

- Glucocorticoids are effective in suppressing systemic symptoms and to stop the progression of Takayasu's arteritis. Prednisone (40 to 60 mg PO daily or 1 mg/kg/day) can be used for 3 months or intravenous steroids can be administered initially.
- Patients are monitored for symptoms and the ESR is followed. Attempts to taper prednisone can be made with resolution of constitutional symptoms, significant decline in the ESR and C-reactive protein levels, and in accordance with imaging studies. Patients often relapse when prednisone is tapered.
- Second-line agents such as cyclophosphamide, methotrexate, and azathioprine can be added if there is no response to glucocorticoids or as corticosteroid-sparing agents.
- Tumor necrosis factor (TNF)-alpha inhibitors have also shown promise as corticosteroid-sparing agents.

CHRONIC RX

- Long-term low-dose prednisone may be necessary to stop the progression of arterial stenoses, although this of course comes with the significant side effects of long-term steroid use.

- Although there have been no randomized controlled trials, use of steroid-sparing immunosuppressants is increasing. Methotrexate is the most commonly used agent, although there are also data supporting the use of azathioprine or antitumor necrosis factor as adjunctive or alternative therapy with glucocorticoids to patients who are in relapse or resistant to other treatments. There is limited experience with cyclophosphamide.
- Treatment of hypertension in these patients can be difficult, especially since typically there is concurrent glucocorticoid therapy and there is the potential for renovascular hypertension. Special monitoring should be employed when using ACE inhibitors due to the high frequency of renal artery stenosis in this population.
- Percutaneous angioplasty or bypass grafts should be considered for irreversible arterial stenoses with severe ischemia (cardiac or cerebral), severe hypertension in renal artery stenosis, or aneurysmal enlargement with risk of rupture. Five-year arterial complication rate after surgical or endovascular revascularization is 44%; the likelihood of complications increases sevenfold when inflammation is present at the time of revascularization.
- There have been positive data regarding drug-eluting stents, and in particular sirolimus-covered stents, likely related to the synergistic effect of its antiproliferative and immunosuppressive properties.
- Studies of coronary artery angioplasty and stenting in this population are limited, due to a high frequency of coronary lesions that are near the ostia; a large number of these patients have surgical interventions as opposed to percutaneous interventions.
- Aortic regurgitation may require valve replacement or repair by surgery, although the need to manipulate friable tissue can lead to complications such as valvular detachment after replacement.

DISPOSITION

- Immunosuppressant therapy may achieve clinical remission.
- No studies have proved that treatment results in regression of stenosis, although there are limited case reports describing the return of pulses with treatment.
- With the addition of a second agent for patients with treatment resistance or relapse, 50% remission has been seen.
- Quality of life is comparable to that of patients with rheumatoid arthritis or ankylosing spondylitis.
- Mortality results are mixed, with high rates in reports from Asia and lower rates in studies performed in the United States (2%). In the absence of major complications (MI, stroke, severe HTN, heart failure, aneurysm), 5-year survival rates reach 95%. In the presence of major complications, 5-year survival is 50% to 70%.
- Death can occur suddenly from a ruptured aneurysm, a myocardial infarction, or a cerebrovascular accident.

REFERRAL

Whenever the diagnosis of vasculitis is suspected, a rheumatology consultation is appropriate. Vascular surgery and cardiology consultations are recommended for any evidence of carotid, peripheral, or coronary artery disease or if a large abdominal aneurysm is found.

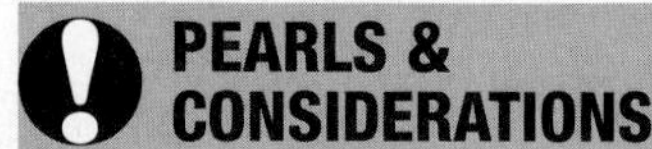

PEARLS & CONSIDERATIONS

With long-term glucocorticoid use, consider measures to protect against bone loss. Bisphosphonates have been studied prospectively with corticosteroid use in this fashion; remember to ensure adequate dietary calcium and vitamin D intake as well.

COMMENTS

The long-term prognosis of patients with treated Takayasu's disease varies by geography, and 10-yr survival ranges from 80% to 96%.

RELATED CONTENT

Vasculitis (Related Key Topic)

SUGGESTED READINGS

available at www.expertconsult.com

AUTHORS: **ELLIOTT M. GROVES, M.D., M.Eng.,** and **PRANAV M. PATEL, M.D., F.A.C.C., F.S.C.A.I.**

BASIC INFORMATION

DEFINITION

Four species of adult tapeworm (cestodes) may infect humans as the definitive host: *Taenia saginata* (beef tapeworm), *Taenia solium* (pork tapeworm), *Diphyllobothrium latum* (fish tapeworm), and *Hymenolepis nana.* In addition, several tapeworms (*T. solium, T. crassiceps, T. multiceps*) can infect human tissue in their larval form, resulting in cysticercosis, and others infect in their intermediate forms, resulting in hydatid disease (see "Echinococcosis" in Section I)

SYNONYMS

Cysticercosis (larval infection by *T. solium*)

ICD-9CM CODES
123.9 Tapeworm infestation
ICD-10CM CODES
B68.0 Taenia solium taeniasis
B68.1 Taenia saginata taeniasis
B68.9 Taeniasis unspecified
B70.0 Diphyllobothriasis
B71.9 Cestode infection, unspecified

EPIDEMIOLOGY & DEMOGRAPHICS

INCIDENCE (IN U.S.):
- Diagnosed primarily in immigrants, particularly those from Latin America and Southeast Asia
- Varies widely by country of origin and dietary practices

PREVALENCE (IN U.S.):
- *T. saginata:* <0.1%
- *D. latum:* <0.05%
- *T. solium:* <0.1%
- *H. nana:* sporadic, often in setting of outbreak

PREDOMINANT SEX: Equal sex distribution
PREDOMINANT AGE:
- *T. saginata, T. solium, D. latum:* 20 to 39 yr of age
- *H. nana* in setting of institution outbreaks: children

PHYSICAL FINDINGS & CLINICAL PRESENTATION

Adult worms
1. Attach to bowel mucosa via suckers, hooks, or grooves depending on species
2. Feed and grow, producing digestive/body/reproductive segments called proglottids
3. Cause minimal or no symptoms or sequelae but occasionally can cause nausea, anorexia, or epigastric pain.

Cysticercosis: larval infection by *T. solium*
1. Mass lesions of brain (neurocysticercosis), soft tissue, viscera
2. Neurocysticercosis may cause seizures, hydrocephalus (due to ventricle obstruction)

Prolonged infection with *D. latum*
1. Vitamin B_{12} deficiency
2. Megaloblastic anemia

ETIOLOGY

TAPEWORM:
- Adult worms consist of a head, neck, and hundreds or thousands of proglottids. Each proglottid contains male and female reproductive organs, including eggs.
- Adult worm resides in small or large bowel; proglottids and eggs are passed in stool.
- *T. saginata* may produce up to 100,000 eggs/proglottid and *T. solium* up to 50,000 eggs/proglottid.
- Eggs are ingested by the animal intermediate host.
- Eggs hatch into larvae.
- Larvae perforate the host intestinal wall and disseminate to in skeletal muscle, brain, viscera.
- Develop into cysticerci (scolex inside a cyst) over several weeks
- Humans eat infected beef *(T. saginata),* pork *(T. solium),* or fish *(D. latum).*
- Larval scolex attaches to intestinal wall and mature into adults within the GI lumen.
- *H. nana* infection is acquired by ingesting eggs in human or rodent feces.

CYSTICERCOSIS:
- Humans ingest eggs of *T. solium* in food contaminated with human feces that contain the eggs.
- Eggs hatch into larvae in gut and cross intestinal wall.
- Larvae disseminate widely through tissues (particularly soft tissue and CNS) forming cystic lesions containing either viable or nonviable larvae.

Dx DIAGNOSIS

WORKUP

- Stool examination for eggs or proglottids (tapeworm)
  1. Eggs of *Taenia* spp. cannot be differentiated by microscopy, but the species can be identified through examination of the proglottids in stool.
  2. Eggs of *Taenia* spp. are round and measure 30 to 40 micrometers.
- Cerebral CT scan (neurocysticercosis)
- Serum antibody (neurocysticercosis) with high sensitivity with multiple cysts (94%) but low with a single cyst or calcified cysts (as low as 28%)
- CBC may show eosinophilia

IMAGING STUDIES

- Tapeworm: incidental finding on upper GI series
- Neurocysticercosis:
  1. Cerebral cysts are readily demonstrated by CT scan or MRI.
  2. Calcified lesions are an incidental finding.

Rx TREATMENT

ACUTE GENERAL Rx

- All adults and children with intestinal tapeworm infections should be treated with a single oral dose of praziquantel.
  1. *T. solium:* 5-10 mg/kg
  2. *T. saginata:* 5-10 mg/kg
  3. *D. latum:* 5-10 mg/kg
  4. *H. nana:* 25 mg/kg and a repeat dose 7-10 days later if heavy infection
- Praziquantel acts by causing changes in the teguments of the worms, allowing increased permeability to calcium ions, which then accumulate inside worm and cause paralysis.
- Repeat stool screening at 1 and 3 mo to confirm cure.
- Can use purgatives adjunctively to hasten clearance of deceased worms from intestine
- An alternative therapy to praziquantel for tapeworm infections is niclosamide, 2 g PO once for adults and 1 g for children 11-34 kg and 1.5 g for children over 34 kg.
- Therapy that may be considered for symptomatic cysticercosis:
  1. May regress spontaneously (i.e., no treatment)
  2. Surgery, especially in cases of ventricular obstruction (neurocysticercosis)
  3. Albendazole 10-15 mg/kg/day PO divided in two doses for 8 days
  4. Praziquantel 50-100 mg/kg/day PO for 15-30 days divided in three doses
  5. Use of steroids in neurocysticercosis may reduce CNS inflammation and increase levels of albendazole in CNS.
- Therapy contraindicated with:
  1. Ocular infections
  2. Cerebral infections in which local inflammation caused by destruction of the parasite may cause significant damage
- Adjunctive antiepileptics may be necessary for neurocysticercosis

CHRONIC Rx

- Retreatment if required
- Avoidance of undercooked pork, meat, or fish
- Cysticercosis: proper hand washing, proper disposal of human waste

DISPOSITION

- Neurologic follow-up for patients with neurocysticercosis
- Ophthalmologic follow-up for patients with ocular involvement

REFERRAL

Patients treated for neurocysticercosis should be evaluated by a physician experienced in managing this infection, if possible.

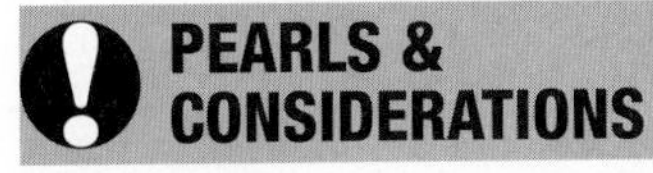

PEARLS & CONSIDERATIONS

COMMENTS

T. solium is the most dangerous of the tapeworms because of the potential for cysticercosis by means of autoinfection.

SUGGESTED READINGS

available at www.expertconsult.com

RELATED CONTENT

Cysticercosis (Related Key Topic)
Tapeworm Infection (Patient Information)

AUTHORS: **RUSSELL J. McCULLOH, M.D.,** and **GLENN G. FORT, M.D., M.P.H.**

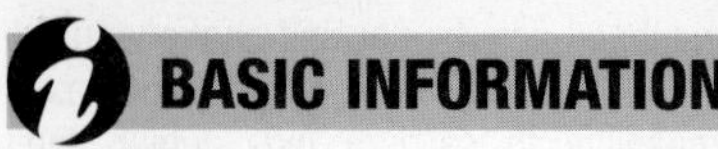

BASIC INFORMATION

DEFINITION

Tardive dyskinesia (TD) is a syndrome of involuntary movements associated with the long-term use of antipsychotic medication, particularly first-generation antipsychotics. Patients exhibit rapid, repetitive, stereotypic movements that mostly involve the oral, lingual, trunk, and limb areas.

SYNONYMS

Orofacial dyskinesia
Tardive syndrome
TD

ICD-9CM CODES DSM-5
333.72
ICD-10CM CODES
G24.0 Neuroleptic-induced tardive dyskinesia

EPIDEMIOLOGY & DEMOGRAPHICS

- The disorder is caused by dopamine-blocking antipsychotics (e.g., haloperidol) and antiemetics (e.g., metoclopramide, prochlorperazine, and promethazine).
- With first-generation antipsychotics, at least 20% of patients are affected with TD, and ~5% are expected to develop TD with each year of antipsychotic treatment.
- The incidence of TD is declining with the increased use of second-generation antipsychotics. ~0.5% to 1% of all adults develop TD yearly while taking these medications.
- Risk increases with the duration of antipsychotic treatment, in female and in elderly patients, in patients with brain damage or dementia, with concurrent anticholinergic use, and in patients with nonschizophrenia diagnoses.

PHYSICAL FINDINGS & CLINICAL PRESENTATION

- TD is classically described as a chronic condition of insidious onset, but symptoms are variable over time and may even improve despite continued antipsychotic therapy.
- The condition typically appears with the reduction or withdrawal of the antipsychotic medications.
- TD classically involves stereotypic movements of the mouth and tongue, including lip smacking and puckering, tongue twisting and protrusion, and facial grimacing.
- TD may also involve slow, writhing movements of the trunk or choreoathetotic movements of the fingers and toes.
- The involuntary mouth movements associated with TD may be suppressed by voluntary actions (e.g., putting food in the mouth, talking).
- Variants of TD with similar treatment include tardive dystonia (e.g., torticollis, blepharospasm), tardive myoclonus, tardive akathisia, and tardive tics.

ETIOLOGY

TD is caused by chronic exposure to dopamine receptor antagonists that is thought to result in the upregulation of dopamine receptors in the basal ganglia as well as damage to striatal cholinergic neurons. Dysfunction of striatal GABAergic interneurons has also been implicated. Recently, it has been proposed that dopamine receptor hypersensitivity and neurodegenerative changes might cause altered synaptic plasticity of excitatory synapses onto striatal interneurons, resulting in an imbalance between the direct and indirect basal ganglia pathways.

Dx DIAGNOSIS

DIFFERENTIAL DIAGNOSIS

- Acute extrapyramidal symptoms (e.g., short-term withdrawal dyskinesias, parkinsonism, akathisia)
- Basal ganglia movement disorders (e.g., Huntington's chorea, Tourette's syndrome, levodopa-induced dyskinesia in Parkinson's disease, Wilson's disease)
- Autoimmune diseases (Sydenham's chorea, multiple sclerosis)
- Other causes of neurologic damage (e.g., lead or mercury toxicity, HIV, neurosyphilis, head injury, neurodegeneration from illicit substances)
- Mannerisms associated with disorganized type or catatonic type schizophrenia
- Hyperthyroidism-induced choreoathetosis
- Edentulous dyskinesias and improperly fitted dentures
- Rabbit syndrome (a rare variant of extrapyramidal symptoms with rapid vertical orofacial movements without tongue involvement); may respond to anticholinergic agents

WORKUP

TD is a diagnosis of exclusion, with emphasis on a complete neuropsychiatric and medication history and a thorough physical examination.

IMAGING STUDIES

Standard brain imaging is normal in patients with TD.

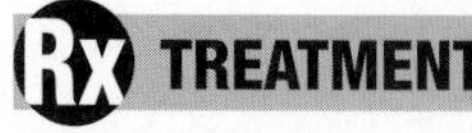

Rx TREATMENT

ACUTE GENERAL Rx

- Treatment is predicated on prevention: limit the indications for antipsychotics; use the lowest effective dose; discontinue the drugs, when feasible; and monitor patients frequently. Anticholinergic medications may worsen symptoms.
- Switch to second-generation antipsychotics, if possible.

CHRONIC Rx

- Clozapine has the best evidence for improving the symptoms of TD, although olanzapine may also be of benefit.
- Tetrabenazine, a centrally acting synaptic dopamine depleter, is becoming a first-line treatment option.
- Benzodiazepines, vitamin B_6, donepezil, piracetam, amantadine, zolpidem, propranolol, and melatonin may be helpful, although controlled trial evidence remains weak.
- For disabling TD, deep brain stimulation of the subthalamic nucleus or internal globus pallidus seems to provide significant symptom reduction without exacerbation of psychiatric symptoms.
- TD is potentially irreversible in nearly two thirds of patients; thus, patients undergoing long-term treatment with dopamine receptor–blocking medications require frequent monitoring and aggressive management at the onset of TD symptoms.

REFERRAL

Movement disorder specialist consultation if symptoms are severe

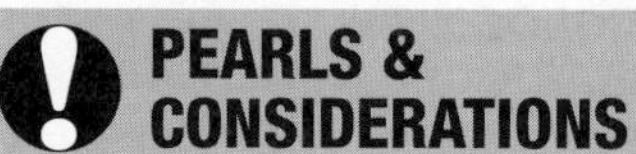

PEARLS & CONSIDERATIONS

- First-generation antipsychotics should be resumed to treat TD in the absence of active psychosis only as a last resort for persistent, disabling, and treatment-resistant TD.
- Avoid the use of anticholinergic medications (e.g., benztropine), which may exacerbate TD symptoms.
- A worsening of the overall psychopathology in patients with schizophrenia is longitudinally associated with the emergence of TD and suggestive of a worse prognosis.
- Recent evidence suggests increased overall mortality among patients with TD, which highlights the need for referral for more aggressive specialized interventions.

SUGGESTED READINGS

available at www.expertconsult.com

RELATED CONTENT

Tardive Dyskinesia (Patient Information)

AUTHOR: **JOHN A. GRAY, M.D., PH.D.**

BASIC INFORMATION

DEFINITION

Tarsal tunnel syndrome is the most common compressive neuropathy in the foot and ankle. The syndrome is secondary to a pathologic, structural, or biomechanical factor that causes compression of the posterior tibial nerve or its branches (medial calcaneal, medial plantar, lateral plantar branches), within or distal to the tarsal canal (Fig. 1-917).

ICD-9CM CODES
355.5 Tarsal tunnel syndrome
ICD-10CM CODES
G57.50 Tarsal tunnel syndrome, unspecified lower limb

EPIDEMIOLOGY & DEMOGRAPHICS

PREVALENCE: Most common entrapment neuropathy in the foot/ankle

PREDOMINANT SEX: Relatively equal

PHYSICAL FINDINGS & CLINICAL PRESENTATION

- Symptoms can vary widely in location and nature. One or many symptoms can occur.
- Common presentations: medial ankle pain, localized heel pain, distal numbness/shooting pain, and generalized foot/ankle pain that keeps the patient awake at night
- Percussion over the porta pedis resulting in Tinel's sign (distal radiation of symptoms)
- Valleix phenomenon (producing proximal symptomatology) is consistent with tarsal tunnel syndrome.
- In cases of mechanical etiology, holding the foot in a dorsiflexed and everted subtalar joint position may reproduce symptoms.
- Look for: localized edema, varicosities, palpable soft tissue masses, biomechanical abnormalities, and signs of trauma.
- Loss of motor function and permanent loss of sensation are extremely rare.

ETIOLOGY

- Inflammatory (adjacent tendonitis, recent ankle trauma)
- Compressive pathology (ganglion cyst, lipoma, varicosities)
- Structural (osseous): exostosis, severe arthritis, fracture of rearfoot/ankle
- Biomechanical: abnormal calcaneal eversion or inversion, subtalar joint pronation
- Systemic causes of neuropathy: diabetes, hypothyroidism, Reiter's syndrome, and more

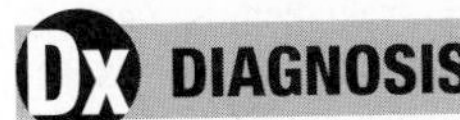

DIAGNOSIS

DIFFERENTIAL DIAGNOSIS

- Plantar fasciitis
- Calcaneal fracture/other osseous trauma.
- Ankle sprain/strain or chronic ST injury. Posterior tibial tendonitis often overlooked
- Systemic causes of peripheral neuropathy: diabetes, hypothyroidism, Reiter's syndrome
- Radiculopathy
- Peripheral vascular disease

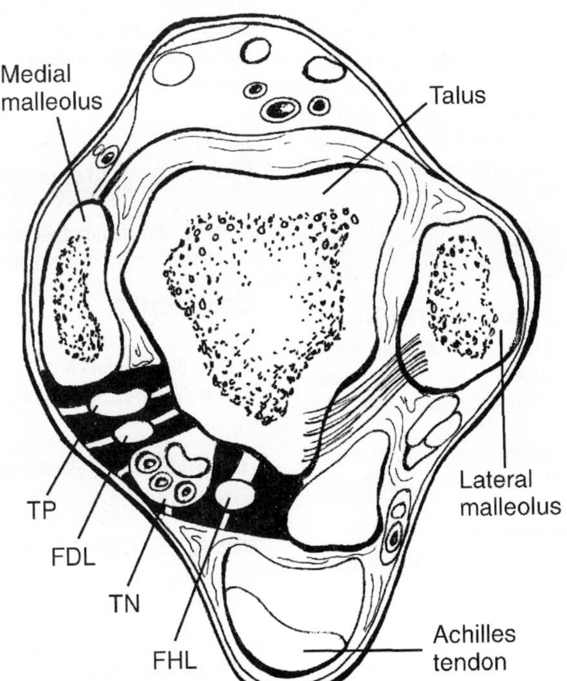

FIGURE 1-917 Anatomy of tarsal tunnel syndrome. Transverse view of ankle. Tendons and neurovascular elements are included in individual fibrous septa that connect periosteum with the deep fascia. *FDL,* Flexor digitorum longus; *FHL,* flexor hallucis longus tendon; *TN,* tibial nerve (single contour), posterior tibial artery, veins; *TP,* tibialis posterior tendon. (From Canoso J: *Rheumatology in primary care,* Philadelphia, 1997, Saunders.)

DIAGNOSTIC STUDIES

- X-rays: rule out trauma, bone tumor, structural deformity.
- Biomechanical exam
- MRI: look for soft tissue mass, edema, trauma.
- EMG/nerve conduction studies support clinical diagnosis, but false negatives are common.
- Local diagnostic injections: evaluate local versus proximal source of neuropathy.

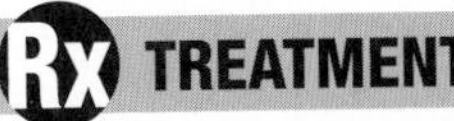

TREATMENT

- First line: rest, ice, limit aggravating activity
- Address shoegear problems: in structural cases, tight shoegear will exacerbate symptoms, while in functional cases symptoms may be aggravated by loose/unstable rearfoot fit.
- Nonsteroidal anti-inflammatory drugs
- Biomechanical: custom orthotics for optimal biomechanical function/stabilization. Heel lifts assist by promoting ankle plantar flexion, supinating the foot, and reducing pressure within the tarsal tunnel.
- Ankle bracing if ankle instability present and contributing factor
- Physical therapy (iontophoresis, other therapeutic modalities, strength/flexibility work)
- Local steroid injection
- If persistent, offloading with cast or cast walker may yield resolution in 3 to 6 wk
- Surgical: release of retinaculum, mass excision, etc.

DISPOSITION

Can yield lifelong, chronic pain with unknown specific etiology or can follow a limited course once causative factor resolved (mechanical, healed ankle sprain, soft tissue mass resection, etc.).

REFERRAL

- Physical therapy for various treatment modalities
- Podiatric or foot/ankle orthopedic surgeon for biomechanical evaluation, orthotic treatment, diagnostic/therapeutic injection, and surgery if necessary.

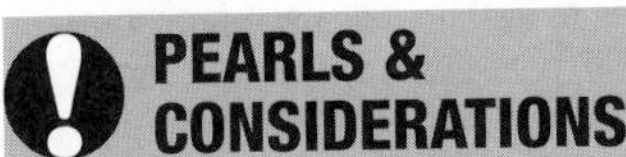

PEARLS & CONSIDERATIONS

- Be sure to rule out etiologies such as calcaneal fracture and bone or soft tissue tumor.
- Differentiation from plantar fasciitis is often difficult, yet the initial therapy can be identical (refer to "Plantar Fasciitis").

SUGGESTED READINGS

available at www.expertconsult.com

RELATED CONTENT

Tarsal Tunnel Syndrome (Patient Information)

AUTHOR: **BROOKE E. KEELEY, D.P.M.**

BASIC INFORMATION

DEFINITION

Temporomandibular joint (TMJ) syndrome refers to a group of disorders leading to symptoms of the TMJ.

SYNONYMS

Temporomandibular dysfunction
Painful temporomandibular joint
TMJ

ICD-9CM CODES
524.60 Temporomandibular joint pain-dysfunction syndrome
ICD-10CM CODES
N26.60 Temporomandibular joint disorder, unspecified

EPIDEMIOLOGY & DEMOGRAPHICS

- 15% of the population have TMJ disorders.
- Females are affected more often than males (4:1 ratio).
- Occurs between the second and fourth decades of life.
- Usually unilateral, affecting either side with equal frequency

PHYSICAL FINDINGS & CLINICAL PRESENTATION

- Often unilateral pain in the muscles of mastication, usually described as a "dull" ache
- Otalgia
- Odontalgia
- Headaches (frontal, temporal, retro-orbital)
- Tinnitus
- Dizziness
- Clicking or popping sounds with movement of the TMJ
- Joint locking
- Application of mild anterior pressure with a finger placed posteriorly to each tragus may result in tenderness, clicking, or crepitus.
- Limited range of motion of the TMJ
- Symptoms usually appear in association with a stressful life event

ETIOLOGY

- Multifactorial, encompassing local anatomic anomalies to systemic disease processes
- Myofascial pain-dysfunction syndrome: the most common cause of TMJ syndrome and results from teeth grinding and clenching the jaw (bruxism)
- Internal TMJ derangement: abnormal connection of the articular disk to the mandibular condyle
- Degenerative joint disease
- Rheumatoid arthritis
- Gouty arthritis
- Pseudogout
- Ankylosing spondylitis
- Trauma
- Prior surgery (orthodontic, intraarticular steroid injection)
- Tumors

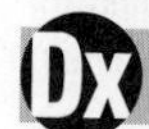

DIAGNOSIS

Can be made based on history and physical examination in most cases.

DIFFERENTIAL DIAGNOSIS

Includes the list provided above. Myofascial pain-dysfunction syndrome, internal TMJ derangement, and degenerative joint disease represent >90% of all causes of TMJ syndrome. Others not mentioned include dental problems such as loss of posterior teeth support and Eagle's syndrome (stylohyoid syndrome, carotidynia, and trigeminal neuralgia). Alternative diagnoses such as otitis, mastoiditis, salivary gland disorders, and temporal arteritis should always be excluded.

WORKUP

Radiographic imaging evaluation is used to exclude anatomic or systemic causes of disease when conservative management has failed.

LABORATORY TESTS

Laboratory examination is not very helpful.

IMAGING STUDIES

- Plain radiographs: the most common views are the panoramic, transorbital, and transpharyngeal in both opened and closed positions.
- Arthrography is helpful in looking for meniscus involvement but is seldom performed anymore.
- CT scan is highly accurate in diagnosing meniscal and osseous derangements of the TMJ.
- MRI is the procedure of choice and has replaced arthrography in cases of disabling pain or if locking occurs. It is used to determine disc position and morphology along with degenerative bony changes.

Rx TREATMENT

NONPHARMACOLOGIC THERAPY

- Soft diet to rest the muscles of mastication
- Heat 15 to 20 min four to six times per day
- Massage of the masseter and temporalis muscles
- Formed splints or bite appliances to reduce compression of retrodiscal tissue (Fig. E1-918)
- Range-of-motion exercises
- Cognitive-behavioral therapy and biofeedback have been shown to reduce pain.

ACUTE GENERAL Rx

- Nonsteroidal anti-inflammatory drugs: ibuprofen 800 PO mg tid prn, naproxen 500 mg PO bid prn, titrated to relieve symptoms
- Muscle relaxants at bedtime: diazepam 2.5 to 5 mg PO tid prn or amitriptyline 5 to 100 mg PO qd prn
- In degenerative joint disease of the TMJ, intraarticular steroid injection can be tried
- Botulism toxin injections into the masticatory muscles
- Arthrocentesis with joint lavage and lysis of adhesions (Fig. E1-919)
- In patients with pain and clicking in the TMJ that is unresponsive to nonsurgical treatment, the disc should be repositioned arthroscopically or by open surgery (discoplasty) (see "Chronic Rx")

CHRONIC Rx

- Most of the above treatments are used for myofascial pain-dysfunction syndrome; however, they can be applied to other causes of TMJ syndrome. Surgery is usually a measure of last resort in patients who do not respond to nonpharmacologic and acute general treatment.
- Surgical procedures include:
  1. Meniscoplasty
  2. Meniscectomy
  3. Subcondylar osteotomy
  4. TMJ reconstruction

DISPOSITION

The course depends on the underlying etiology; however, less than 5% of adults with temporomandibular symptoms develop chronic symptoms.

REFERRAL

All patients with TMJ syndrome refractory to conservative nonpharmacologic and acute therapy should be referred to a periodontist, oral maxillofacial surgeon, or ear-nose-throat surgeon.

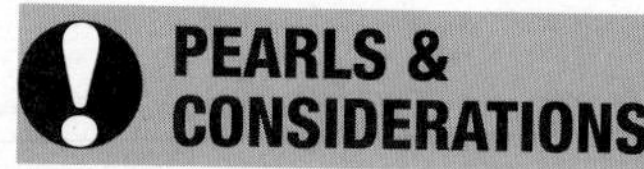

PEARLS & CONSIDERATIONS

Patients with rheumatoid arthritis involving the TMJ usually have bilateral involvement.

COMMENTS

Frequently, emotional stress initiates the myofascial pain-dysfunction, which accounts for 85% of all cases of TMJ syndrome.

SUGGESTED READINGS

available at www.expertconsult.com

RELATED CONTENT

Temporomandibular Joint (TMJ) Syndrome (Patient Information)

AUTHORS: **RYAN W. ZUZEK, M.D.,** and **DOUGLAS BURTT, M.D.**

BASIC INFORMATION

DEFINITION

Testicular neoplasms are primary cancers originating in a testis.

SYNONYMS

Testis tumor
Testicular neoplasms

ICD-9CM CODES
186.9 Testicular neoplasm
M906/3 (seminoma)
M9101/3 (embryonal carcinoma or teratoma)
M9100/3 (choriocarcinoma)
ICD-10CM CODES
C62.1 Malignant neoplasm of unspecified descended testis
C62.0 Malignant neoplasm of undescended testis

EPIDEMIOLOGY & DEMOGRAPHICS

INCIDENCE: 5.4 cases per 100,000 men annually. White men have the highest incidence at 6.3 cases/100,000 men. Testicular cancer is the most common cancer diagnosis in men between the ages of 15 and 35 yr. The incidence has been gradually increasing since 1975.
PREVALENCE: 1% to 2% of all cancers in males
PREDOMINANT AGE: Can occur in any age but most common in young adults; average age for embryonal cell carcinoma: 30 yr; average age for seminoma: 36 yr

PHYSICAL FINDINGS & CLINICAL PRESENTATION

- Testicular cancer typically presents as a painless mass in the testis. Any mass within the testicle should be considered cancer until proven otherwise. It may be found by the patient, who brings it to the attention of a physician, or it may be found by a physician on a routine examination.
- Symptoms other than scrotal or testicular swelling are typically absent unless the cancer has metastasized (10% of patients at diagnosis). Occasionally a patient may report scrotal fullness or heaviness. About 10% of patients present with acute pain. Gynecomastia from tumors that secrete beta-human chorionic gonadotropin (hCG) is found in 5% of men with testicular cancer.
- Testicular palpation should be performed with two hands. Transillumination may distinguish a solid mass (e.g., cancer) and a fluid-filled lesion (e.g., hydrocele or spermatocele). The mass is nontender; indeed, it is less sensitive than a normal testicle.

ETIOLOGY, CLASSIFICATION, & PATHOLOGY

- Cryptorchidism (undescended testes) is a major risk factor even if corrected by orchiopexy; however, treatment of undescended testis before puberty decreases the risk of testicular cancer from fivefold to twofold. Other risk factors are family history, Klinefelter's syndrome, infertility, tobacco use, and white race.
- Classification: testicular cancers can be classified as pure seminomas or nonseminomatous germ cell tumors (embryonic carcinoma, choriocarcinoma, yolk sac carcinoma, teratoma)
- Pathology: germ cell tumors account for >95% of testicular cancers

Cell Type	*Frequency (%)*
Seminoma	42
Embryonal cell carcinoma	26
Teratocarcinoma	26
Teratoma	5
Choriocarcinoma	1

- Other rare types:
  - Yolk sac carcinoma
  - Mixed germ cell tumors
  - Carcinoid tumor
  - Sertoli cell tumors
  - Leydig cell tumors
  - Lymphoma
  - Metastatic cancer to the testes
- TNM staging system for testicular cancer
  - T_0: No apparent primary
  - T_1: Testis only (excludes rete testis)
  - T_2: Beyond the tunica albuginea
  - T_3: Rete testis or epididymal involvement
  - T_4: Spermatic cord
    1. Spermatic cord
    2. Scrotum
  - N_0: No nodal involvement
  - N_1: Ipsilateral regional nodal involvement
  - N_2: Contralateral or bilateral abdominal or groin nodes
  - N_3: Palpable abdominal nodes or fixed groin nodes
  - N_4: Juxtaregional nodes
  - M_0: No distant metastases
  - M_1: Distant metastases present

The clinical stages consist of stage I, with tumor confined to the testis; stage II, with positive regional lymph nodes; and stage III, with metastases.

DIAGNOSIS

DIFFERENTIAL DIAGNOSIS

- Spermatocele
- Varicocele
- Hydrocele
- Epididymitis
- Epidermoid cyst of the testicle
- Epididymis tumors

WORKUP

Physical examination, laboratory tests, and imaging studies (see Section III, "Testicular Mass")

LABORATORY TESTS

- Serum hCG
- Serum alpha-fetoprotein (AFP): elevated in nonseminoma tumors

One or both of these tumor markers will be elevated in 70% of cases of testicular cancer.

- Serum lactate dehydrogenase (LDH) level: elevated with rapid turnover of malignant cells
- Testicular biopsy contraindicated

IMAGING STUDIES

- Testicular ultrasound
- CT scan or MRI of pelvis and abdomen
- Chest radiograph
- CT of the chest in patients with abnormal chest x-ray or in those with suspected mediastinal, hilar, or lung parenchymal disease; MRI of the brain in patients with neurologic symptoms
- PET scan is not recommended (frequent false positives).

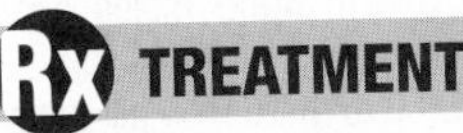

TREATMENT

- Seminoma
  1. Stage I: Radical orchiectomy plus one cycle of single agent carboplatin chemotherapy or radiation therapy (RT) to the paraaortic lymph nodes
  2. Stage IIA or IIB: RT or cisplatin-based chemotherapy (e.g., cisplatin, bleomycin, etoposide)
- Nonseminoma
  1. Stage IA: radical orchiectomy plus retroperitoneal lymph node dissection (RPLND)
  2. Stage IB: Same as stage IA plus two cycles of chemotherapy (cisplatin, bleomycin, etoposide)
  3. Advanced stages: cisplatin-based chemotherapy or RPLND
- Posttreatment surveillance for testicular cancer survivors (annually)
  1. Fertility assessment
  2. Skin examination (increased risk of dysplastic nevi)
  3. Testicular examination (3% to 4% risk of second testicular cancer)
  4. Serum tumor markers (hCG, AFP)
  5. Chest CT 4 months postoperatively

DISPOSITION

The overall cure for testicular cancer is >95% (80% for metastatic disease). Patients with pure seminomas have a better prognosis. Because treatment produces favorable outcomes even in advanced stages, the U.S. Preventive Services Task Force recommends against screening asymptomatic men for testicular cancer.

SUGGESTED READINGS

available at www.expertconsult.com

RELATED CONTENT

Testicular Cancer (Patient Information)

AUTHOR: **FRED F. FERRI, M.D.**

BASIC INFORMATION

DEFINITION

Testicular torsion is a twisting of the spermatic cord leading to cessation of testicular blood flow, ischemia, and infarction if left untreated.

SYNONYMS

Spermatic cord torsion

ICD-9CM CODES
608.2 Testicular torsion
ICD-10CM CODES
N44.03 Torsion of testis, unspecified

EPIDEMIOLOGY & DEMOGRAPHICS

INCIDENCE: Affects one in 4000 males aged <25 yr

PREDOMINANT AGE: Two thirds of all cases occur between the ages of 12 and 18 yr, but may occur at any age, including antenatally.

PHYSICAL FINDINGS & CLINICAL PRESENTATION

- Typical sequence is sudden onset of hemiscrotal pain, then swelling, nausea, and vomiting without fever or urinary symptoms.
- Physical examination may reveal a tender firm testis, high-riding testis, horizontal lie of testis, absent cremasteric reflex, and no pain with elevation of testis. Absence of the cremasteric reflex (stroking or pinching the medial thigh normally causes contraction of the cremaster muscle and elevation of the testis) is the most sensitive physical finding.
- Painless testicular swelling occurs in 10%.
- One out of three patients reports previous episodes of spontaneously remitting scrotal pain.
- In the neonate, testicular torsion should be presumed in patients with a painless, discolored hemiscrotal swelling.
- In rare cases, torsion may involve an undescended testicle. In such situations an empty hemiscrotum is palpated together with a tender lump in the inguinal area.

ETIOLOGY

- There are two types of testicular torsion: extravaginal, caused by nonadherence of the tunica vaginalis to the dartos layer, and intravaginal, caused by malrotation of the spermatic cord with the tunica vaginalis. Intravaginal torsion accounts for 90% of cases.
- Torsion usually occurs in the absence of any precipitating events. Trauma accounts for <10% of cases.

Dx DIAGNOSIS

Diagnosis is made mainly by clinical suspicion (Table E1-473). Color Doppler ultrasound evaluation or a nuclear testicular scan (Fig. E1-920) may help with the diagnosis. Ultrasonography will show absent or decreased blood flow; scintigraphy reveals decreased perfusion on symptomatic side.

DIFFERENTIAL DIAGNOSIS

See Fig. 1-921.

- Torsion of the testicular appendages (appendix testis)
- Testicular tumor
- Epididymitis
- Incarcerated inguinoscrotal hernia
- Orchitis
- Spermatocele
- Hydrocele, varicocele

WORKUP

The diagnosis is usually based on history and physical examination.

IMAGING STUDIES

- Radionuclide scrotal scanning (technetium-99m): cold testicle
- Doppler ultrasonic stethoscope (Doppler flowmetry)

Rx TREATMENT

Surgical derotation of the spermatic cord followed by bilateral testicular fixation with nonabsorbable sutures. If the affected testis is nonviable, orchiectomy of the affected testis and orchiopexy of the contralateral side are performed. Attempts at manual detorsion should not delay surgical consultation.

PROGNOSIS

- The degree of ischemia depends on the duration of torsion and the degree of rotation of the spermatic cord.
- There is an 80% testicular salvage rate if detorsion occurs within 12 hr of onset.
- After 24 hr, irreversible testicular infarction is expected.
- Because the contralateral testes can be affected (immunologic process), when treatment is delayed and return of blood flow does not occur after detorsion, some recommend orchiectomy of the infarcted testicle.

REFERRAL

To urologist

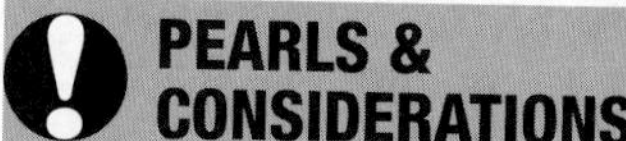

PEARLS & CONSIDERATIONS

- Manual detorsion by external rotation of the testis toward the thigh can be attempted for adolescent intravaginal torsion if an operating facility is not readily available.
- Extravaginal torsion is diagnosed in the newborn. Intravaginal torsion can occur at any age but is usually diagnosed in males ages 12 to 18 yr.

SUGGESTED READINGS

available at www.expertconsult.com

RELATED CONTENT

Testicular Torsion (Patient Information)

AUTHOR: **FRED F. FERRI, M.D.**

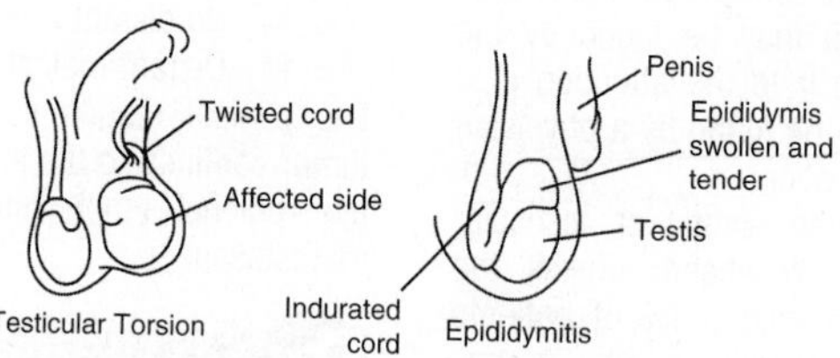

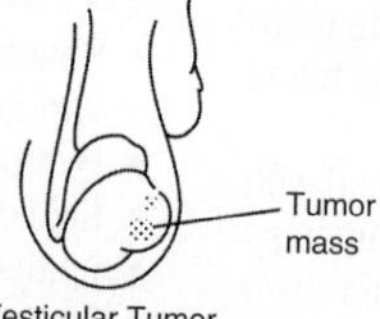

FIGURE 1-921 Physical findings in acute scrotum. Upper left, Testicular torsion. Upper right, Epididymitis. Lower, Testicular tumor. Scrotal examination, which begins with palpation of the scrotal contents, should be performed in the following order: (1) testes, (2) epididymides, (3) spermatic cord structures, and (4) inguinal ring. (From Nseyo U, Weinman E, Lamm DL: *Urology for primary care physicians*, Philadelphia, 1999, WB Saunders.)

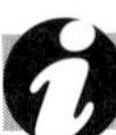

BASIC INFORMATION

DEFINITION

Tetralogy of Fallot (TOF) is a congenital heart deformity that consists of the following four features (Fig. 1-926):

1. Ventricular septal defect (VSD)
2. Infundibular stenosis that leads to the obstruction of the right ventricular (RV) outflow tract or pulmonary valve stenosis
3. An aorta that overrides the VSD by <50% of its diameter with deviation to the right
4. Concentric RV hypertrophy

SYNONYMS

TOF

ICD-9CM CODES
745.2 Tetralogy of Fallot
ICD-10CM CODES
Q21.3 Tetralogy of Fallot

EPIDEMIOLOGY & DEMOGRAPHICS

INCIDENCE:

- TOF is the most common cyanotic congenital heart malformation that is diagnosed in patients after the age of 1 yr.
- TOF accounts for nearly 7% to 10% of all cases of congenital heart disease.
- Occurs in approximately 3.9/10,000 live births in the U.S.
- It is the most common cyanotic malformation to reach adulthood without reparative surgery.

PREDOMINANT SEX: Slightly higher incidence in males than females

GENETICS: Genetic influence is suspected.

PHYSICAL FINDINGS & CLINICAL PRESENTATION

- Of the four major features of TOF, infundibular stenosis that leads to RV outflow tract obstruction and VSD are the primary defects that result in clinical manifestations. The degree of RV outflow obstruction determines the age and symptoms at presentation. RV outflow tract obstruction and the VSD result in the following:
  - Right-to-left shunting and hypoxemia
  - Altered RV hemodynamics
  - Decreased pulmonary blood flow
- The aforementioned pathophysiologic concepts result in common manifestations of TOF, including the following:
  - Cyanosis of the nail beds and lips
  - Dyspnea on exertion
  - Digital clubbing
  - The child assuming a squatting position after exercise to increase systemic vascular resistance, thereby decreasing right-to-left shunting
  - Low birth weight and growth rate
  - Palpable RV impulse
  - Systolic thrill along the left sternal border
  - Single second heart sound comprised of aortic component only
  - A grade 3 to 5 crescendo/decrescendo murmur is heard along the left mid to upper sternal border with posterior radiation
- Murmur is softened in deeply cyanotic neonates with TOF with pulmonary atresia.
- Paroxymal episodes of rapid and deep breathing (tet spells) with increased cyanosis would occur with almost complete right ventricular outflow tract obstruction.
- Tet spells, and sometimes syncope are noticed especially after feeding and defecation.
- Presentation depends on the degree of RV outflow obstruction. May present at birth with cyanosis in severe cases with insufficient pulmonary blood flow. Cases with mild to moderate obstruction and compensated pulmonary flow are usually diagnosed while patient is being evaluated for murmur or heart failure.
- After repair, patients may have a low-pitched diastolic murmur at the pulmonic area that is consistent with pulmonary regurgitation or a pansystolic murmur that is consistent with a VSD patch leak. If the patient only has a palliative shunt, a continuous murmur may be heard from the site of the shunt.

ETIOLOGY

TOF likely results from the maldevelopment of the embryologic conotruncus and is associated with some genetic disorders but the exact mechanism is unknown.

DIAGNOSIS

- The diagnosis of TOF is suspected in any neonate, infant, or child who presents with cyanosis and a heart murmur (see "Physical Findings & Clinical Presentation").
- VSD is associated with other cardiac defects:
  - Persistent foramen ovale/atrial septal defect
  - Pulmonary artery anomalies
  - Right aortic arch
  - Left superior vena cava to coronary sinus
  - Additional VSDs
  - Coronary artery anomalies
  - Aortic valve regurgitation
- Associated anomalies and syndromes include the following:
  - DiGeorge
  - de Lange
  - Goldenhar
  - Klippel-Feil
  - VACTERL
  - CHARGE
  - Pierre Robin
  - Trisomies 21, 13, and 18
  - Fetal alcohol

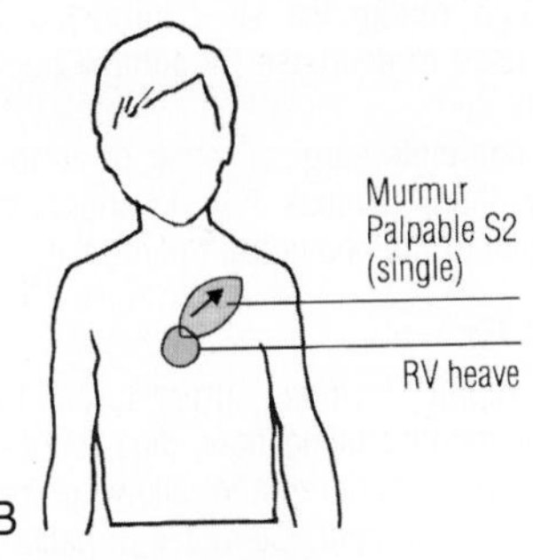

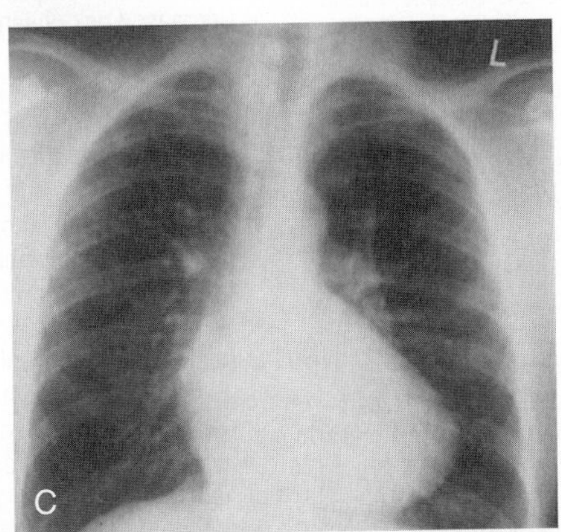

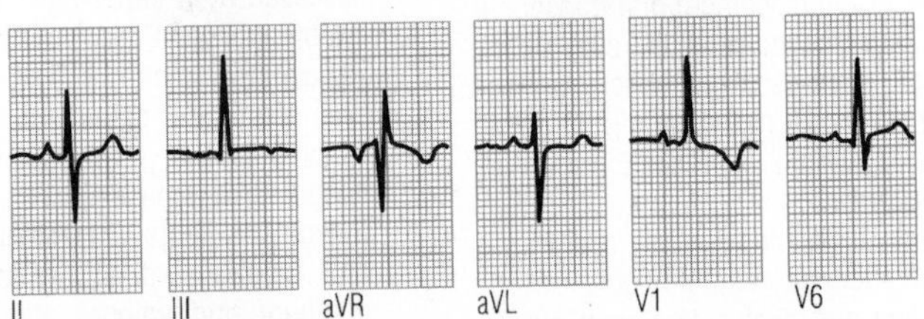

FIGURE 1-926 Features of Fallot tetralogy. A, Diagram of abnormality. *Ao,* Aorta; *PA,* pulmonary artery; *VSD,* ventricular septal defect. **B,** Physical signs. **C,** Chest x-ray showing right ventricular hypertrophy, typical "coeur en sabot." **D,** ECG showing right atrial and ventricular hypertrophy and right axis deviation. (From Souhami RL, Moxham J: *Textbook of medicine,* ed 4, London, 2002, Churchill Livingstone.)

- Alagille
- MTHFR polymorphism

DIFFERENTIAL DIAGNOSIS

- Asthma
- Isolated VSD
- Pulmonary atresia
- Patent ductus arteriosus
- Aortic stenosis
- Pneumothorax

WORKUP

- Detailed history and physical examination, including pulse oximetry
- Echocardiogram, chest radiograph, 12-lead ECG, and routine laboratory tests

LABORATORY TESTS

- Pulse oximetry to determine oxygenation.
- The CBC shows polycythemia from long-standing hypoxemia.
- Arterial blood gas levels show hypoxemia, normal pH, and pCO_2 (carbon dioxide levels).
- ECG commonly demonstrates right axis deviation, RV hypertrophy, and right atrial enlargement.
- Exercise testing may help to evaluate functional capacity and exertional arrhythmias.

IMAGING STUDIES

- Chest radiography reveals a boot-shaped heart that is commonly described as *coeur en sabot;* a prominent RV with decreased pulmonary vascularity; and a heart size that is usually normal. However, in patients with increased aortopulmonary collateral blood flow or with associated large patent ductus arteriosus, the heart size is increased with increased pulmonary vascularity.
- Echocardiography demonstrates VSD(s), anatomy and severity of right ventricular outflow tract obstruction, aortic arch anatomy, and other associated anomalies.
- Cardiac catheterization and angiography help to determine hemodynamics, the severity of right-to-left shunting, the localization of the VSD, coronary artery anatomy, right ventricular outflow obstruction, pulmonary artery stenosis, aortopulmonary collaterals.
- Cardiac MRI is used for the localization of the VSD, the anatomic assessment of the RV outflow tract, the assessment of RV function, the quantification of pulmonary regurgitation, and the detection of RV myocardial fibrosis. Magnetic resonance angiography can be a noninvasive alternative to cardiac catheterization for the evaluation of pulmonary vascular anatomy and the ascending aorta.
- Multislice spiral computed tomography can be used for diagnosis, and it is extremely important during the planning of the repair procedure. Its use may be limited by the risks associated with radiation exposure in children. It can also be used to make assessments that are similar to those usually made by MRI for patients who are unable to undergo MRI.

Rx TREATMENT

NONPHARMACOLOGIC THERAPY

- Oxygen
- Prostaglandins at time of birth to keep a patent ductus and to maintain ductal flow to the lungs
- Knee-chest position during hypoxemic spells to help reduce venous return and to increase systemic vascular resistance, thereby decreasing right-to-left shunting

ACUTE GENERAL Rx

- The acute treatment of any infant or child with TOF who is cyanotic with respiratory distress is aimed at increasing systemic vascular resistance and decreasing right-to-left shunting (e.g., phenylephrine 0.1 to 0.5 mcg/kg/min intravenously to increase systemic vascular resistance, and oxygen and morphine to decrease pulmonary vascular resistance).
- Intravenous sodium bicarbonate for metabolic acidosis and, if more is necessary, respiratory support with intubation and sedation are required to control respiratory distress in cyanotic spells.
- Intravenous b-blockers (e.g., propranolol 0.15 to 0.25 mg/kg via slow intravenous push) are used to decrease RV outflow tract contractility.
- Emergent complete surgical repair or aortopulmonary shunt (Blalock-Taussig shunt) is required if all of the above treatments fail.

CHRONIC Rx

- Palliative repair includes procedures to increase pulmonary blood flow, thus reducing right-to-left shunting and allowing for pulmonary development. Examples of palliative procedures include the Blalock-Taussig shunt, in which a shunt is made between the subclavian artery and the pulmonary artery; the Waterston shunt, which attaches the ascending aorta to the right pulmonary artery; and the Potts shunt, which attaches the descending aorta to the left pulmonary artery. These are generally performed in patients who are not candidates for complete surgical repair due to prematurity, hypoplastic pulmonary arteries, and/or other anomalies in the coronary anatomy.
- Complete surgical repair has good success and involves closing the VSD with a Dacron patch and relieving the RV outflow tract obstruction by simple resection of the infundibular stenosis, patch augmentation of the RV outflow, or the placement of a transannular patch. Patients who have the repair before the age of 2 yr are usually symptom free and can generally lead a normal life. If the repair is performed during adulthood, pulmonary valve replacement may be required.
- Postoperative issues include the following:
  - Residual pulmonic regurgitation
  - RV dilation and dysfunction from pulmonary regurgitation
  - Residual RV outflow tract obstruction
  - Branch pulmonary artery stenosis or hypoplasia
  - Sustained ventricular tachycardia
  - Sudden cardiac death
  - Atrioventricular block, atrial flutter, and atrial fibrillation
  - Progressive aortic regurgitation
  - Syndromal associations

DISPOSITION

- Almost all patients with TOF have either palliative or complete surgical repair before they reach adulthood.
- <3% of patients with TOF reach the age of 40 yr without surgery.
- Survival after the complete operative repair of TOF is excellent if the RV outflow tract obstruction has been relieved and the VSD has been closed.
- The 35-yr survival rate for patients after TOF repair is 85%.
- Adults who underwent palliative surgery during childhood can present with polycythemia, pulmonary hypertension, cyanosis, aortic regurgitation, and clubbing.
- Conduction disturbances; tricuspid, aortic, and pulmonary regurgitation; pulmonary stenosis; and cardiomegaly may present in patients who underwent complete surgical repair during childhood.
- Ventricular arrhythmia can lead to sudden cardiac death in 8.3% of surgically repaired patients by the age of 35 yr. Monomorphic ventricular tachycardia is likely the result of a reentry circuit from a scar caused by the surgery.
- A prolonged QRS duration on the preoperative ECG predicts an increased risk of postoperative supraventricular or ventricular arrhythmia. Prolongation of the QRS beyond 180 msec identifies patients who are at increased risk of ventricular tachycardia after surgery.
- Patients with signs or symptoms of arrhythmia should undergo hemodynamic and electrophysiologic testing, including pulmonic valve replacement, residual VSD closure, mapping and ablation of an arrhythmia, antiarrhythmic medication, or the placement of an implantable cardiac defibrillator.
- Reduced exercise capacity is usually the result of chronic pulmonary regurgitation or residual RV outflow tract obstruction.
- Patients with left ventricular dysfunction may benefit with angiotensin-converting enzyme inhibitors, diuretics, and digoxin.
- Women with repaired TOF should be assessed by a cardiologist before considering pregnancy to determine if pulmonic valve replacement is needed first.
- The offspring of patients with TOF are more likely than the general population to have congenital anomalies.
- Selected patients with normal RV pressures and function without evidence of residual shunt and without atrial or ventricular tachyarrhythmia are eligible to participate in competitive sports.

REFERRAL

- Infants and children with cyanotic heart disease should be referred to a pediatric cardiologist for further diagnostic evaluation. After being diagnosed with TOF, patients should be referred to centers with experience in palliative and complete surgical repair.
- Adult patients with repaired TOF should be comanaged with a cardiologist who specializes in adults with congenital heart disease on at least an annual basis.

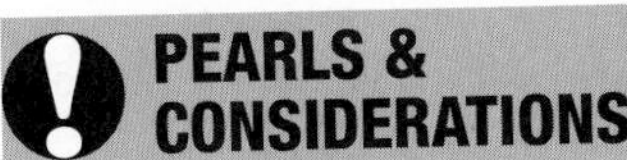

PEARLS & CONSIDERATIONS

- TOF was first described by the French physician Etienne Fallot in 1888.
- The first palliative surgical treatment for TOF was performed by Dr. Alfred Blalock at Johns Hopkins University in 1945 (i.e., the Blalock-Taussig shunt).
- The first surgical repair for TOF was performed by Dr. C. Walton Lillehei at the University of Minnesota in 1954.

COMMENTS

- The severity of RV outflow tract obstruction is the primary determinant of clinical symptoms and outcomes.
- There is a 3% increased risk of congenital heart disease in the children of parents with TOF.
- TOF requires subacute bacterial endocarditis prophylaxis before any dental work or nonsterile surgical procedures (e.g., surgery of the bowel or bladder).
- Children with TOF are at risk for neurodevelopmental delay when they reach school age.

SUGGESTED READINGS

available at www.expertconsult.com

RELATED CONTENT

Tetralogy of Fallot (Patient Information)

AUTHOR: **SYEDA M. SAYEED, M.D.**

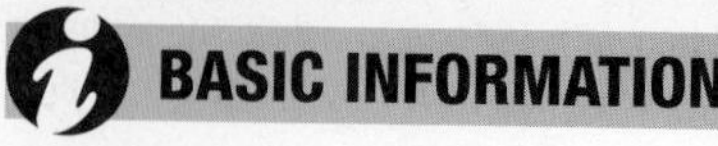

BASIC INFORMATION

DEFINITION

Thalassemias are a heterogeneous group of disorders of hemoglobin synthesis that have in common a deficient synthesis of one or more of the polypeptide chains of the normal human hemoglobin, resulting in a quantitative abnormality of the hemoglobin thus produced. Table 1-475 describes the various thalassemias. There are no qualitative changes such as those encountered in the hemoglobinopathies (e.g., sickle cell disease).

SYNONYMS

Mediterranean anemia
Cooley's anemia

ICD-9CM CODES
282.4 Thalassemia
ICD-10CM CODES
D56 Thalassemia
D56.0 Alpha thalassemia
D56.1 Beta thalassemia
D56.2 Delta-beta thalassemia
D56.3 Thalassemia trait
D56.4 Hereditary persistence of fetal hemoglobin (HPFH)
D56.8 Other thalassemias
D56.9 Thalassemia, unspecified

EPIDEMIOLOGY & DEMOGRAPHICS

- Thalassemia is among the most common genetic disorders worldwide. Approximately 4.83% of the world's population carry globin variants, including 1.67% of the population that are heterozygous for alpha-thalassemia and beta-thalassemia.
- The highest concentration of alpha-thalassemia is found in Southeast Asia and the African west coast. For example, the prevalence is 5% to 10% in Thailand. It is also common among blacks, with a prevalence of approximately 5%.
- The worldwide prevalence of beta-thalassemia is approximately 3%; in certain regions of Italy and Greece the prevalence reaches 15% to 30%. This high prevalence can be found in Americans of Italian or Greek descent.
- The distribution of thalassemia in Europe and Africa parallels that of malaria, suggesting that thalassemic persons are more resistant to the parasite, thus permitting evolutionary survival advantage.

CLASSIFICATION

Beta-thalassemia:
- Beta (+) thalassemia (suboptimal beta-globin synthesis)
- Beta (o) thalassemia (total absence of beta-globin synthesis)
- Delta-beta-thalassemia (total absence of both delta-globin and beta-globin synthesis)
- Lepore hemoglobin (synthesis of small amounts of fused delta-beta-globin and total absence of delta- and beta-globin)
- Hereditary persistence of fetal hemoglobin (HPHF) (increased hemoglobin F synthesis and reduced or absence of delta- and beta-globin)

Alpha-thalassemia:
- Silent carrier (three alpha-globin genes present)
- Alpha-thalassemia trait (two alpha-globin genes present)
- Hemoglobin H disease (one alpha-globin gene present)
- Hydrops fetalis (no alpha-globin gene)
- Hemoglobin constant sprint (elongated alpha-globin chain)

Thalassemic hemoglobinopathies:
- Hb Terre Haute, Hb Quong Sze, HbE, Hb Knossos

PHYSICAL FINDINGS & CLINICAL PRESENTATION

Beta-thalassemia:
- Heterozygous beta-thalassemia (thalassemia minor): no or mild anemia, microcytosis and hypochromia, mild hemolysis manifested by slight reticulocytosis and splenomegaly

TABLE 1-475 The Thalassemias

Thalassemia	Globin Genotype	Features	Expression	Hemoglobin Analysis
α-Thalassemia				
1 gene deletion	$-,\alpha/\alpha,\alpha$	Normal	Normal	Newborn: Bart's 1%-2%
2 gene deletion trait	$-,\alpha/-,\alpha$ -, $-/\alpha,\alpha$	Microcytosis, mild hypochromasia	Normal, mild anemia	Newborn: Bart's: 5%-10%
3 gene deletion hemoglobin H	$-,-/-,\alpha$	Microcytosis, hypochromic	Mild anemia, transfusions not required	Newborn: Bart's: 20%-30%
2 gene deletion 1 Constant Spring	$-,-/\alpha,\alpha^{Constant\ Spring}$	Microcytosis, hypochromic	Moderate to severe anemia, transfusion, splenectomy	2%-3% Constant Spring, 10%-15% hemoglobin H
4 gene deletion	$-,-/-,-$	Anisocytosis, poikilocytosis	Hydrops fetalis	Newborn: 89%-90% Bart's with Gower 1 and 2 and Portland
Nondeletional	$\alpha,\alpha/\alpha,\alpha^{variant}$	Microcytosis, mild anemia	Normal	1%-2% variant hemoglobin
β-Thalassemia				
β^0 or β^+ heterozygote: trait	β^0/A, β^+/A	Variable microcytosis	Normal	Elevated A_2, variable elevation of F
β^0-Thalassemia	β^0/β^0, β^+/β^0, E/β^0	Microcytosis, nucleated RBC	Transfusion dependent	F 98% and A_2 2% E 30%-40%
β^+-Thalassemia severe	β^+/β^+	Microcytosis, nucleated RBC	Transfusion dependent/thalassemia intermedia	F 70%-95%, A_2 2%, trace A
Silent	β^+/A	Microcytosis	Normal with only microcytosis	A_2 3.3%-3.5%
β^+/β^+	Hypochromic, microcytic	Mild to moderate anemia	A_2 2%-5%, F 10%-30%	
Dominant (rare)	B^0/A	Microcytosis, abnormal RBCs	Moderately severe anemia, splenomegaly	Elevated F and A_2
δ-Thalassemia	A/A	Normal	Normal	A_2 absent
$(\delta\beta)^0$-Thalassemia	$(\delta\beta)^0/A$	Hypochromic	Mild anemia	F 5%-20%
$(\delta\beta)^+$-Thalassemia Lepore	β^{Lepore}/A	Microcytosis	Mild anemia	Lepore 8%-20%
Lepore	$\beta^{Lepore}/\beta^{Lepore}$	Microcytic, hypochromic	Thalassemia intermedia	F 80%, Lepore 20%
γδβ-Thalassemia	$(\Upsilon^A\delta\beta)^0/A$	Microcytosis, microcytic, hypochromic	Moderate anemia, splenomegaly, homozygote: thalassemia intermedia	Decreased F and A_2 compared with δβ-thalassemia
ϒ-Thalassemia	$(\Upsilon^A\Upsilon^G)^0/A$	Microcytosis	Insignificant unless homozygote	Decreased F
Hereditary Persistence of Fetal Hemoglobin				
Deletional	A/A	Microcytic	Mild anemia	F 100% homozygotes
Nondeletional	A/A	Normal	Normal	F 20%-40%

From Kliegman RM et al: *Nelson textbook of pediatrics,* ed 19, Philadelphia, 2011, Saunders.

- Homozygous beta-thalassemia (thalassemia major): intense hemolytic anemia; transfusion dependency; bone deformities (skull and long bones); hepatomegaly; splenomegaly; iron overload leading to cardiomyopathy, diabetes mellitus, and hypogonadism; growth retardation; pigment gallstones; susceptibility to infection
- Thalassemia intermedia caused by combination of beta- and alpha-thalassemia or beta-thalassemia and Hb Lepore: resembles thalassemia major but is milder

Alpha-thalassemia:

- Silent carrier: no symptoms.
- Alpha-thalassemia trait: microcytosis only.
- Hemoglobin H disease: moderately severe hemolysis with microcytosis and splenomegaly.
- The loss of all four alpha-globin genes is incompatible with life (stillbirth of hydropic fetus). NOTE: Pregnancies with hydrops fetalis are associated with a high incidence of toxemia.

ETIOLOGY

- Beta-thalassemia: it is caused by more than 200 point mutations and, rarely, by deletions. The reduction of beta-globin synthesis results in redundant alpha-globin chains (Heinz bodies), which are cytotoxic and cause intramedullary hemolysis and ineffective erythropoiesis. The pathophysiology of beta-thalassemia is illustrated in Fig. E1-927. Fetal hemoglobin may be increased.
- Alpha-thalassemia: several mutations can result in insufficient amounts of alpha-globin available for combination with non–alpha-globins.

Dx DIAGNOSIS

LABORATORY TESTS

Beta-thalassemia:

- Microcytosis (mean cell volume: 55 to 80 fL)
- Normal red blood cell (RBC) distribution width index (RDW)
- Smear: nucleated RBCs, anisocytosis, poikilocytosis, polychromatophilia, Pappenheimer and Howell-Jolly bodies
- Hemoglobin electrophoresis: absent or reduced hemoglobin A, increased fetal hemoglobin, variable increase in the amount of hemoglobin A_2
- Markers of hemolysis: elevated indirect bilirubin and lactate dehydrogenase, decreased haptoglobin

Alpha-thalassemia:

- Microcytosis in the absence of iron deficiency
- Hemoglobin electrophoresis normal except for the presence of hemoglobin H in hemoglobin H disease

Rx TREATMENT

- Thalassemia minor: no treatment, but avoid iron administration for incorrect diagnosis of iron deficiency.
- Beta-thalassemia major (and hemoglobin H disease):
  1. Transfusion as required together with chelation of iron with desferrioxamine (by IV or subcutaneous administration, 8 to 12 hr nightly, 5 to 6 days a week at a dose of 2 to 6 g/day with a portable infusion pump). Deferiprone, an oral chelating agent, can be used as a second-line treatment of iron overload caused by blood transfusions (transfusional hemosiderosis).
  2. Splenectomy for hypersplenism if present.
  3. Bone marrow transplantation. Although hematopoietic stem cell transplantation is the only curative approach for thalassemia, it has been limited by the high cost and scarcity of human leukocyte antigen–matched donors. Before transplantation, it is necessary to administer myeloablative regimens to eradicate the endogenous thalassemic bone marrow. Commonly used agents are hydroxyurea, azathioprine, fludarabine, busulfan, and cyclophosphamide.
  4. Hydroxyurea may increase the level of hemoglobin F.

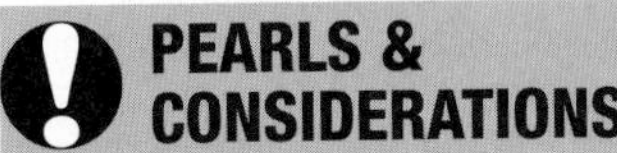

PEARLS & CONSIDERATIONS

- Polymerase chain reaction can be used to detect point mutations or deletions in chorionic villous samples, enabling first-trimester, DNA-based testing for thalassemia.
- Preimplantation genetic diagnosis can be extended to human leukocyte antigen typing on embryonic biopsies, allowing the selection of an embryo that is not affected by thalassemia and that may also serve as a stem cell donor for a previously affected child within the same family.

SUGGESTED READINGS

available at www.expertconsult.com

AUTHOR: **FRED F. FERRI, M.D.**

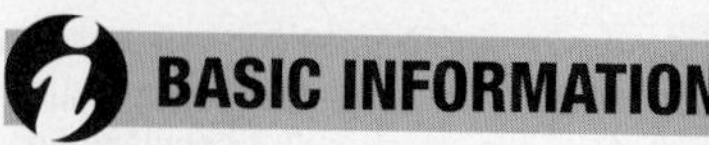

BASIC INFORMATION

DEFINITION

Thoracic outlet syndrome (TOS) describes a condition producing upper extremity symptoms believed to result from neurovascular compression at the thoracic outlet (Fig. 1-928). Three types are described on the basis of point of compression: (1) cervical rib and scalenus syndrome, in which abnormal scalene muscles or the presence of a cervical rib may cause compression; (2) costoclavicular syndrome, in which compression may occur under the clavicle; and (3) hyperabduction syndrome, in which compression may occur in the subcoracoid area. The compression occurs in three anatomical structures–arteries, veins, and nerves.

- Neurogenic TOS: Caused by compression of brachial nerve plexus
- Arterial TOS: Caused by subclavian artery compression
- Venous TOS: Caused by compression of subclavian vein

ICD-9CM CODES
353.0 Thoracic outlet syndrome
ICD-10CM CODES
G54.0 Brachial plexus disorders

EPIDEMIOLOGY & DEMOGRAPHICS

PREVALENCE: Varies from source to source; presence of cervical ribs in 0.5% to 1% of population (50% bilateral), but most are asymptomatic
PREDOMINANT SEX: Females affected more often than males (ratio of 3.5:1)
PREDOMINANT AGE: Rare in those aged <20 yr

PHYSICAL FINDINGS & CLINICAL PRESENTATION

- Symptoms and signs are related to the degree of involvement of each of the various structures at the level of the first rib.
- True venous or arterial involvement is not common.
- Diagnosis is most often used in the consideration of neural pain affecting the arm, which suggests involvement of the brachial plexus.
  1. Arterial compression: pallor, paresthesias, diminished pulses, coolness, digital gangrene, supraclavicular bruit or mass, and stroke
  2. Venous compression: edema and pain; thrombosis causing superficial venous dilation in the shoulder area
  3. "True" neural compression: lower trunk (C8, T1) findings with intrinsic weakness and diminished sensation to the ring finger and small fingers and ulnar aspect of the forearm
  4. Possible supraclavicular tenderness
  5. Provocative tests (Adson's, Wright's): may reproduce pain but are of disputed usefulness

ETIOLOGY

- Congenital cervical rib or fibrous extension of cervical rib (Fig. E1-929)
- Abnormal scalene muscle insertion
- Drooping of shoulder girdle from generalized hypotonia or trauma
- Narrowed costoclavicular interval as a result of downward and backward pressure on shoulder (sometimes seen in individuals who carry heavy backpacks), poor posturing, pregnancy
- Acute venous thrombosis with exercise (effort thrombosis)
- Bony abnormalities of first rib
- Abnormal fibromuscular bands
- Malunion of clavicle fracture

Dx DIAGNOSIS

DIFFERENTIAL DIAGNOSIS

- Carpal tunnel syndrome
- Cervical radiculopathy
- Brachial neuritis
- Ulnar nerve compression (cubital tunnel syndrome)
- Complex regional pain syndrome
- Superior sulcus tumor

WORKUP

Fig. E1-930 describes a diagnostic algorithm for thoracic outlet syndrome. Except for venous or arterial pathology, no ancillary diagnostic tests are reliable for diagnostic confirmation.

IMAGING STUDIES

- Electromyography, nerve conduction velocity studies to rule out carpal tunnel syndrome, cervical radiculopathy
- Ultrasound for initial evaluation for arterial or venous thoracic outlet syndrome
- Cervical spine radiographs to rule out cervical disk disease
- Chest radiograph to rule out lung tumor
- Computed tomography (CT) for detailed anatomical relationship of vascular structure to surrounding muscles and bones
- Arteriography or venography when vascular pathology is strongly suspected clinically

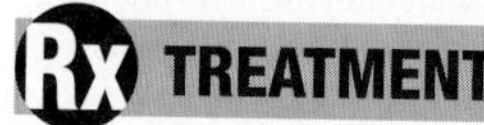

Rx TREATMENT

ACUTE GENERAL Rx

- Sling for pain relief
- Physical therapy modalities plus shoulder girdle–strengthening exercises
- Postural reeducation
- Nonsteroidal anti-inflammatory drugs

DISPOSITION

- Surgery: generally successful for vascular disorders
- Catheter-directed thrombolysis
- Nonsurgical treatment: often successful for patients with pain as the primary symptom

REFERRAL

For vascular surgery consultation when venous or arterial impairment is present

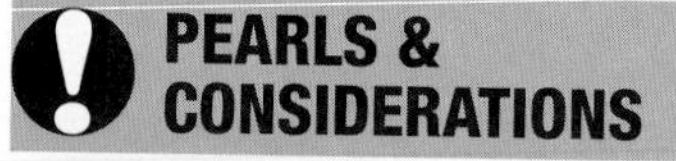

PEARLS & CONSIDERATIONS

COMMENTS

- True thoracic outlet syndrome is probably an uncommon condition.
- Diagnosis is often used to describe a wide variety of clinical symptoms.
- Considerable disagreement exists regarding the frequency of this disorder.

SUGGESTED READINGS
available at www.expertconsult.com

RELATED CONTENT

Thoracic Outlet Syndrome (Patient Information)

AUTHOR: **SYEDA M. SAYEED, M.D.**

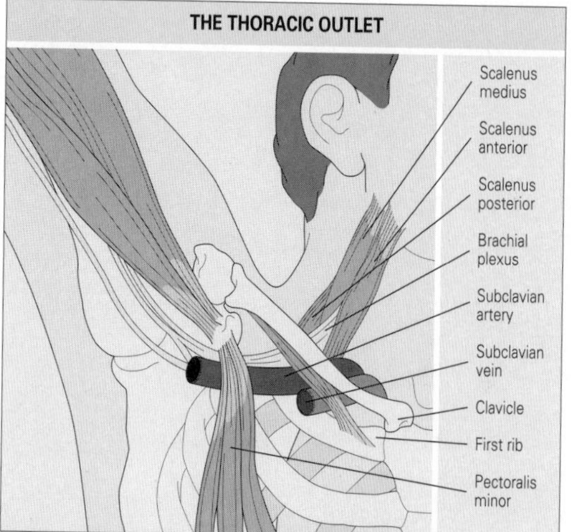

FIGURE 1-928 The thoracic outlet. Three narrow channels of the outlet include the scalene triangle, the costoclavicular passage, and the pectoralis minor attachment at the coracoid process. (Hochberg MC et al: *Rheumatology*, ed 5, St Louis, 2011, Mosby.)

BASIC INFORMATION

DEFINITION

Thrombocytosis is defined by an elevated platelet count (>450,000/mm^3) in peripheral blood. It is caused by overproduction of platelets (reactive thrombocytosis), or it may be caused by clonal expansion of megakaryocytes (autonomous thrombocytosis). Reactive thrombocytosis is driven by excessive cytokines induced by various stimuli, such as trauma or inflammation. The latter is defined as chronic myeloproliferative disorders (CMPD), of which four subgroups are well characterized: chronic myelogenous leukemia (CML), polycythemia vera (PV), primary myelofibrosis (PMF), and essential thrombocythemia (ET). In addition, platelet count can be spuriously elevated in some conditions (see differential diagnosis). Extreme thrombocytosis is defined as platelet count >1 million/mL.

SYNONYMS

Thrombocythemia

ICD-9CM CODES
289.9 Unspecified diseases of blood and blood-forming organs
238.71 Essential thrombocytosis
ICD-10CM CODES
D47.3 Essential (hemorrhagic) thrombocythemia
D75.9 Disease of blood and blood-forming organs, unspecified

EPIDEMIOLOGY & DEMOGRAPHICS

Reactive thrombocytosis is much more frequent than autonomous thrombocytosis (70% vs. 22% in one series).
Epidemiology for essential thrombocythemia:
INCIDENCE: 2.5 cases/100,000 population/yr
PREVALENCE: Estimated as 24 cases/100,000 population
PREDOMINANT SEX AND AGE: The median age at diagnosis is 60 yr. Female/male ratio is 2:1.

PHYSICAL FINDINGS & CLINICAL PRESENTATION

- Regardless of the cause, a high platelet count may be associated with vasomotor symptoms such as headache, visual disturbances, dizziness, atypical chest pain, acral dysesthesia, and erythromelalgia.
- Thrombotic and bleeding complications can occur.
- Symptoms and complications are much more likely to occur in association with autonomous thrombocytosis than reactive thrombocytosis.
- The degree of thrombocytosis does not predict the likelihood of autonomous thrombocytosis, and does not generally correlate to the risk of thrombosis.
- Splenomegaly is common with CMPD.
- Coexistent leukocytosis and erythrocytosis are common with CML and PV.
- Disease transformation from ET to PV, PMF, and acute myeloid leukemia (AML) is uncommon.

ETIOLOGY

- Etiology is unclear.
- Abnormality in Jak2-STAT pathway may play a role in pathogenesis of CMPD.

Dx DIAGNOSIS

DIFFERENTIAL DIAGNOSIS

- Spurious thrombocytosis
  - Mixed cryoglobulinemia
  - Circulating cytoplasmic fragments in patients with leukemia, lymphoma, or severe hemolysis or burns can be counted as platelets
- Reactive thrombocytosis
  - Benign hematologic disorders
  - Acute hemorrhage, iron deficiency anemia, hemolytic anemia
  - Chronic infection, such as tuberculosis
  - Acute and chronic inflammatory disorders
  - Rheumatologic disorders
  - Inflammatory bowel disease
  - Celiac disease
  - Functional and surgical asplenia
  - Tissue damage
  - Trauma, thermal burn
  - Myocardial infarction
  - Acute pancreatitis
  - Recent surgery
  - Renal failure, nephrotic syndrome
  - Exercise
  - Medications, such as vincristine, epinephrine
- Autonomous thrombocytosis
  - CML
  - PV
  - PMF
  - Myelodysplastic syndrome (5q-syndrome)
  - AML with inv(3), t(3;3)
  - Essential thrombocytosis (Box 1-90)

WORKUP

- Comprehensive history and physical examination to exclude many of the common causes of reactive thrombocytosis: history and physical examination suggestive of acute blood loss, iron deficiency, acute or chronic infection/inflammation, medication use, asplenia, malignancy, and trauma should be looked for. Fig. E1-932 describes a diagnostic algorithm for thrombocytosis. Laboratory tests are summarized in Box E1-91. The diagnosis of ET requires platelet counts >600 x 10^9/L on two separate occasions >4 weeks apart, absence of Philadelphia chromosome, and exclusion of secondary causes of thrombocytosis.
- Repeat CBC with peripheral blood smear and bone marrow biopsy (Figs. 1-933 and E1-934) to exclude spurious thrombocytosis.

LABORATORY TESTS

- CBC with peripheral blood smear: Howell-Jolly bodies and target cells are present in patients with asplenia; nucleated RBC, teardrop RBC and WBC precursors in patients with PMF
- Serum ferritin level: low ferritin level suggests iron deficiency
- Serum C-reactive protein (CRP), ESR, and plasma fibrinogen: nonspecific markers of infection or inflammation
- Philadelphia chromosome or BCR-ABL rearrangement: positive in CML
- Serum erythropoietin assay: low to normal in PV and ET
- *JAK2* mutation analysis: PV and ET; JAK2 mutation is found in 95% to 99% of patient with PV, in 40% to 60% of patients with PMF, and in about 50% of patients with ET
- Bone marrow chromosome analysis: 5q-syndrome and other myelodysplastic syndrome, CML

BOX 1-90 World Health Organization Diagnostic Criteria for Essential Thrombocythemia

Diagnosis requires that all of the following criteria be met:
- Sustained platelet count ≥450 × 10^9/L[a]
- Bone marrow biopsy specimen showing proliferation mainly of the megakaryocytic lineage, with increased numbers of enlarged, mature megakaryocytes; no significant increase or left shift of neutrophil granulopoiesis or erythropoiesis
- Failure to meet the WHO criteria for polycythemia vera,[b] primary myelofibrosis,[c] BCR-ABL1–positive chronic myelogenous leukemia,[d] myelodysplastic syndrome,[e] or other myeloid neoplasms
- Demonstration of JAK2 V617F or other clonal marker; or, in the absence of JAK2 V617F, no evidence of reactive thrombocytosis[f]

[a] Sustained during the workup process.
[b] Requires the failure of iron replacement therapy to increase the hemoglobin level to the polycythemia vera range in the presence of decreased serum ferritin. Exclusion of polycythemia vera is based on hemoglobin and hematocrit levels; red cell mass measurement is not required.
[c] Requires the absence of relevant reticulin fibrosis, collagen fibrosis, peripheral blood leukoerythroblastosis, or markedly hypercellular marrow accompanied by megakaryocyte morphology typical for primary myelofibrosis—small to large megakaryocytes with an aberrant nuclear-to-cytoplasmic ratio and hyperchromatic, bulbous, or irregularly folded nuclei and dense clustering.
[d] Requires the absence of BCR-ABL1.
[e] Requires the absence of dyserythropoiesis and dysgranulopoiesis.
[f] Causes of reactive thrombocytosis include iron deficiency, splenectomy, surgery, infection, inflammation, connective tissue disease, metastatic cancer, and lymphoproliferative disorders. However, the presence of a condition associated with reactive thrombocytosis does not exclude the possibility of essential thrombocythemia if other criteria are met.

From Swerdlow SH et al (eds): WHO classification of tumours of haematopoietic and lymphoid tissues, Lyon, France, 2008, IARC Press.

- Bone marrow exam in ET may show clusters of abnormal megakaryocytes and increased reticulin fibrosis (see Fig. E1-934).

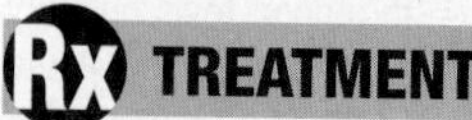

TREATMENT

Treatment for ET will be addressed in this chapter. Reactive thrombocytosis has been rarely associated with thrombosis or bleeding and generally does not require specific therapy.

ACUTE GENERAL Rx

- Vasomotor symptoms easily manageable with low-dose aspirin (<100 mg/day)
- Bleeding
  - Discontinue any platelet antiaggregating agent, such as aspirin or nonsteroidal anti-inflammatory agents.
  - Evaluate for disseminated intravascular coagulopathy and coagulation factor deficiency. Acquired factor V deficiency is occasionally present in association with autonomous thrombocytosis. In that case, treat with fresh frozen plasma infusion.
  - In case of extreme thrombocytosis, acquired von Willebrand disease may occur. Immediate platelet apheresis with definitive therapy with a platelet-lowering agent is essential in this instance.
- Thrombosis
  - Arterial or venous thrombosis occurs in 20% to 30% of patients.
  - If the platelet count is >800,000/mm^3, platelet apheresis coupled with a platelet-lowering agent should be considered with the goal of platelet count <400,000/mm^3.
  - Initial workup should include additional thrombophilic diseases, such as proteins C and S abnormality, antithrombin, anticardiolipin antibody, mutations of factor V and II, and plasma homocysteine.
  - Anticoagulant therapy for 3 to 9 mo based on the presence or absence of additional thrombophilic defects.

CHRONIC Rx

Treatment strategies for ET are based on the presence or absence of risk factors for thrombosis. Smoking cessation and obesity management should be discussed with all patients with ET. In low-risk patients (age <60 yr, no history of thrombosis or hemorrhage, platelet count <1 million/mL), observation may be adequate. The cytoreductive therapy is indicated in high-risk patients (age >60 yr and/or with previous history of thrombosis).

- Low-dose aspirin (81 mg/day) may be safe and effective in preventing vascular events. It is also effective in preventing recurrent vascular events in high-risk patients and in treating the vasomotor symptoms.
- Cytoreductive therapy
  - Hydroxyurea (HU) versus anagrelide: HU plus aspirin is suggested to be safer and more effective than anagrelide plus aspirin in regard to thrombosis, bleeding, and transformation to PMF at 5 yr in a randomized trial. Monitor liver function tests and the degree of neutropenia or anemia with HU therapy.
  - The incidence of leukemic conversion in patients with ET treated with HU alone is reported as <1%. Interferon alpha may be effective for controlling platelet count in patients failing treatment with HU.

DISPOSITION

Most patients with ET have a normal life expectancy without disease-related complications.

An International Prognostic Score for Essential thrombocythemia (IPSET) was proposed by International Working Group on Myelofibrosis Research and Treatment based on age, WBC count, and history of thromboembolism at diagnosis.

REFERRAL

Refer to hematologist/oncologist when platelet count is consistently elevated >450,000/mm^3 without causes for reactive thrombocytosis.

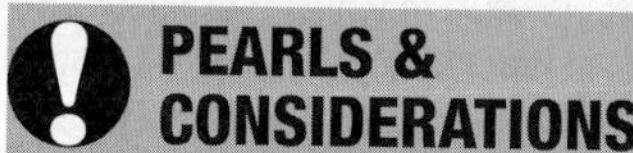

PEARLS & CONSIDERATIONS

COMMENTS

- Some patients with clinically apparent ET have Philadelphia chromosome or *BCR-ABL* rearrangement, even in the absence of other features of CML. It is suggested that it should be tested in all ET patients due to its potential therapeutic implications.
- The risk of bleeding with aspirin use in patients with ET is increased when the platelet count is >1 million/mL.

PATIENT & FAMILY EDUCATION

Smoking cessation is encouraged in both patients with ET and reactive thrombocytosis.

SUGGESTED READINGS

available at www.expertconsult.com

AUTHOR: **ETSUKO AOKI, M.D., PH.D.**

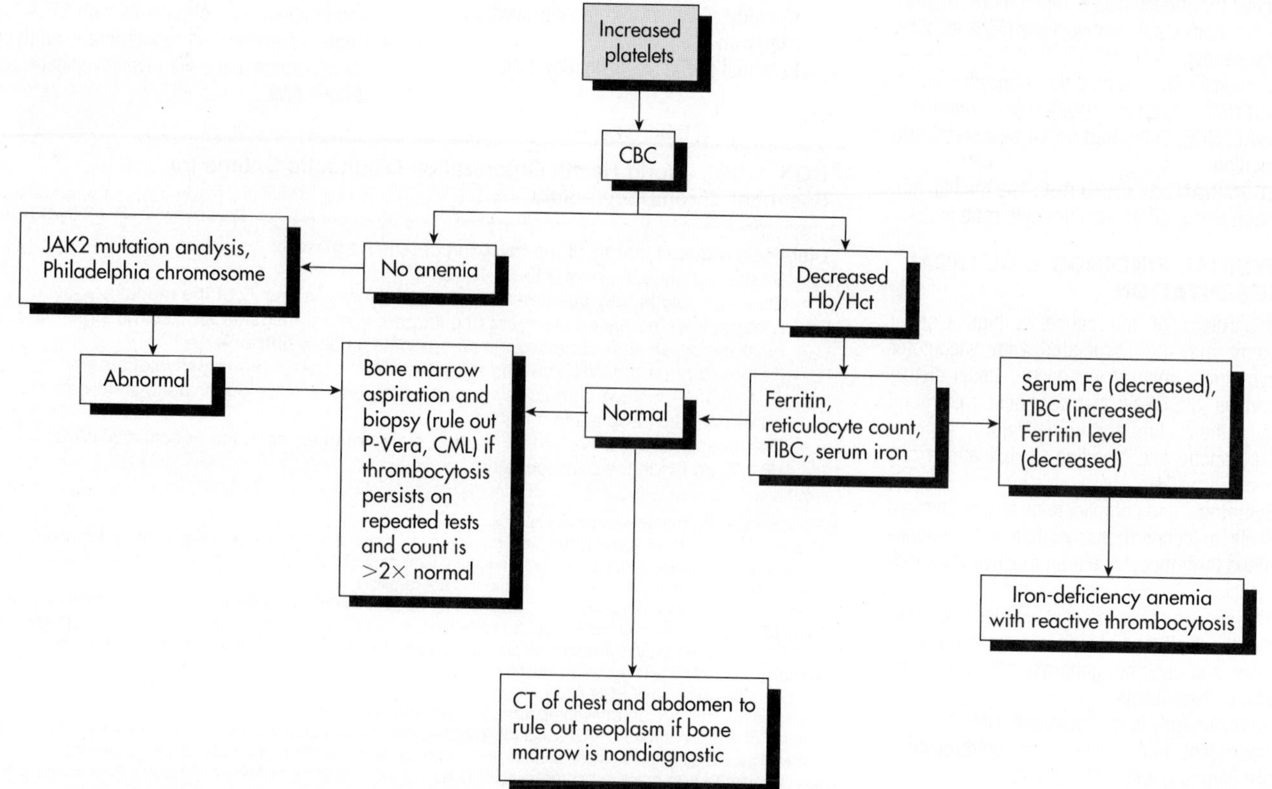

FIGURE 1-933 Essential thrombocythemia: peripheral blood smear. The peripheral blood smear in ET shows a marked thrombocytosis with anisocytosis (varying sizes) of the platelets. (From Hoffman R et al: *Hematology: basic principles and practice*, ed 5, Philadelphia, 2009, Churchill Livingstone.)

BASIC INFORMATION

DEFINITION

Superficial venous thrombophlebitis (SVT) is an inflammation of a vein with subsequent secondary thrombus formation. SVT most frequently involves superficial veins of the leg, but any superficial vein can be affected. SVT has been reported to occur in 125,000 people in the U.S. per year; however, the actual incidence is likely far greater. SVT is not always a benign condition. SVT should be regarded as the superficial venous manifestation of a systemic process known as venous thromboembolism (DVT, PE).

SYNONYMS

SVT
Superficial phlebitis
Superficial suppurative thrombophlebitis
Suppurative thrombophlebitis

ICD-9CM CODES
451.0 Thrombophlebitis, superficial
ICD-10CM CODES
I80.00 Phlebitis and thrombophlebitis of superficial vessels of unspecified lower extremity

EPIDEMIOLOGY & DEMOGRAPHICS

- Approximately 30% to 45% of patients diagnosed with SVT are men with an average age of 54 yr.
- Approximately 55% to 70% of patients diagnosed with SVT are women with an average age of 58 yr.
- The overall recurrence of SVT is 18% over an average observation period of 15 mo, equally involving varicose and nonvaricose veins.
- The lifetime incidence of SVT in those with untreated varicose veins has been estimated at 25% to 50%.

PHYSICAL FINDINGS & CLINICAL PRESENTATION

- Subcutaneous vein is palpable as a tender cord or "wormlike" mass with increased warmth and erythema.
- Induration, redness, and tenderness are localized along the course of the vein. This linear appearance rather than circular appearance is useful to distinguish thrombophlebitis from other conditions (cellulitis, erythema nodosum).
- There is some swelling of the overlying skin and subcutaneous tissue but without generalized edema of the limb.
- Low-grade fever may be present.

ETIOLOGY

- In the lower extremity, 70% of SVT occurs in patients with varicose veins, with the great saphenous vein being most commonly involved (60% to 80%).
- Intravenous catheters and infusion of caustic drugs are the most common cause of upper extremity SVT.
- Malignancy
- Pregnancy/puerperium
- Hypercoagulable states
- Previous
- DVT/SVT
- OCP (oral contraceptive pill)/HRT (hormone replacement therapy)

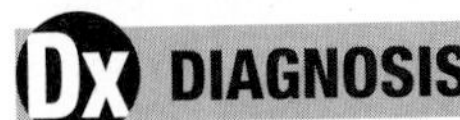

DIAGNOSIS

DIFFERENTIAL DIAGNOSIS

- Lymphangitis
- Cellulitis
- Erythema nodosum
- Panniculitis
- Acute lipodermatosclerosis

WORKUP

The clinical investigation includes not only the local findings but also the presence of varicose veins with or without the stigmata of chronic venous insufficiency. Today, duplex ultrasound is the most important additional diagnostic tool.

IMAGING STUDIES

- Duplex ultrasound offers the advantage of being inexpensive, noninvasive, and repeatable for follow-up examination.
- Ultrasonography confirms the diagnosis, shows the location of the thrombus and its location regarding the saphenofemoral and/or saphenopopliteal junctions.
- Ultrasound examination of patients with SVT has revealed that a concomitant DVT can exist in 15% to 20%.
- In up to 25% of these patients, the DVT may not be contiguous with the SVT and may be found in the contralateral leg.
- Therefore bilateral duplex exam is recommended in all cases of SVT that involve the main trunk of the great saphenous vein (GSV) or small saphenous vein (SSV).

TREATMENT

NONPHARMACOLOGIC THERAPY

- Warm, moist compresses
- Do not restrict activity. Immediate mobilization with walking exercises.

ACUTE GENERAL Rx

- Treatment guidelines for SVT are not well established because of the lack of controlled clinical trials. In general, the primary goal of management should be to prevent thrombus extension and the risk of venous thromboembolism. All other therapy is directed at patient comfort.
- In patients with migratory SVT, recurrent SVT, or SVT without varicose veins, the underlying condition should be investigated and treatment directed accordingly.
- The most common cause of upper extremity SVT is an intravenous catheter. Treatment starts with removal of the cannula and application of warm compresses. The resultant lump may persist for months. No anticoagulant therapy is required.
- In patients with lower extremity SVT in a varicose vein branch, control of pain with analgesics and the use of gradient compression stockings are usually sufficient. Patients are encouraged to continue their usual daily activities.
- Many investigators favor systemic anticoagulation when there is superficial thrombosis of 5 cm or more in length, the thrombus is within 1 cm of the saphenous junctions, or more than 5 cm of the saphenous trunk is involved, as shown by duplex ultrasonography.
- The 2012 American College of Chest Physicians guidelines recommend the use of fondaparinux (1 mg/kg/day) for 45 days over no anticoagulation in patients with lower extremity SVT within 1 cm of the saphenofemoral or saphenopopliteal junction.
- In the case of patients with varicose veins secondary to saphenous vein reflux, a catheter vein ablation procedure should be performed only after the acute SVT episode is over in order to avoid the thromboembolic complications induced by such procedures.

DISPOSITION

Clinical improvement within 10 to 14 days

REFERRAL

Referral to vascular surgeon or phlebologist with vascular lab

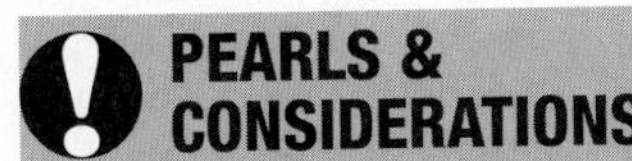

PEARLS & CONSIDERATIONS

SUPERFICIAL SUPPURATIVE THROMBOPHLEBITIS

- Superficial suppurative thrombophlebitis is associated with an intravenous catheter or multiple puncture sites secondary to IV drug abuse and is located primarily in the upper extremity.
- Clinical presentation is similar to that of nonsuppurative SVT but with associated fever, leukocytosis, and/or septicemia.
- Most cases of intravenous catheter sepsis are not complicated by suppurative thrombophlebitis; local IV catheter site infections occur in about 7% of cases and septicemia is found in only 1 of every 400 IV catheterizations.
- The incidence of peripheral vein suppurative thrombophlebitis is highest in patients with specific risk factors such as burns, steroids, and IV drug abuse.
- Treatment consists of antibiotics with adequate coverage of gram-negative rods and *Staphylococcus aureus,* including MRSA. Initial empirical treatment is with IV vancomycin 1 g q12h *plus* ceftriaxone 1 g IV q24h. Alternative regimen consists of daptomycin 6 mg/kg IV q 12h *plus* ceftriaxone 1 g IV q24h.

SUGGESTED READINGS

available at www.expertconsult.com

RELATED CONTENT

Thrombophlebitis (Patient Information)

AUTHOR: **FRANK G. FORT, M.D., F.A.C.S., R.PH.S.**

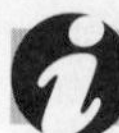

BASIC INFORMATION

DEFINITION

Thrombotic thrombocytopenic purpura (TTP) is a rare disorder characterized by thrombocytopenia (often accompanied by purpura) and microangiopathic hemolytic anemia; neurologic impairment, renal dysfunction, and fever may also be present.

SYNONYMS

TTP

ICD-9CM CODES
446.6 Thrombotic thrombocytopenic purpura
ICD-10CM CODES
M31.1 Thrombotic microangiopathy

EPIDEMIOLOGY & DEMOGRAPHICS

- TTP primarily affects females between ages 10 and 50 yr.
- Frequency is 11 cases annually per 1 million persons. There is increased incidence in HIV/AIDS and during pregnancy.

PHYSICAL FINDINGS & CLINICAL PRESENTATION

- Most patients present with nonspecific constitutional symptoms (weakness, nausea, abdominal pain, vomiting)
- Purpura (secondary to thrombocytopenia)
- Jaundice, pallor (from hemolysis)
- Mucosal bleeding
- Fever
- Fluctuating levels of consciousness (caused by thrombotic occlusion of the cerebral vessels)
- Renal failure and neurologic events are usually end-stage features

ETIOLOGY

- TTP is caused in some patients by autoantibodies or, in rare cases, by a hereditary deficiency of the protease ADAMTS13, which cleaves the high-molecular-weight multimers of von Willebrand factor. This results in abnormal platelet adhesion and activation.
- Many drugs, including clopidogrel, penicillin, antineoplastic agents (gemcitabine, mitomycin C, cyclosporine) oral contraceptives, quinine, and ticlopidine, have been associated with TTP. Other precipitating causes include infectious agents, pregnancy, malignancies, allogeneic bone marrow transplantation, and neurologic disorders.

Dx DIAGNOSIS

DIFFERENTIAL DIAGNOSIS

- Disseminated intravascular coagulation (DIC)
- Malignant hypertension
- Vasculitis
- Eclampsia or preeclampsia
- Hemolytic-uremic syndrome (typically encountered in children, often after a viral infection)
- Gastroenteritis as a result of a serotoxin-producing serotype of *Escherichia coli*
- Medications: clopidogrel, ticlopidine, penicillin, antineoplastic chemotherapeutic agents, oral contraceptives

WORKUP

- A comprehensive history, physical examination, and laboratory evaluation usually confirm the diagnosis. Fig. E1-935 is an algorithm for diagnosis of TTP.
- The disease often begins as a flulike illness ultimately followed by clinical and laboratory abnormalities.

LABORATORY TESTS

- Severe anemia and thrombocytopenia (platelet count <50,000 or >50% reduction from previous counts). Peripheral blood smear (Fig. E1-936) reveals numerous red cell fragments (schistocytes).
- Elevated blood urea nitrogen and creatinine
- Evidence of hemolysis: elevated reticulocyte count, indirect bilirubin, lactate dehydrogenase, decreased haptoglobin
- Urinalysis: hematuria (red blood cells [RBCs] and RBC casts in urine sediment) and proteinuria
- Peripheral smear: severely fragmented RBCs (schistocytes). More than 4% RBC fragments in the peripheral blood.
- No laboratory evidence of DIC (normal fibrin degradation product, fibrinogen)
- The ADAMTS13 level is not necessary and metalloproteinase deficiency need not be proved for diagnosis of TTP

Rx TREATMENT

ACUTE GENERAL Rx

- Discontinue potential offending agents.
- The American Association of Blood Banks, the American Society for Apheresis, and the British Committee for Standards in Haematology recommend daily plasma exchange with replacement of 1.0 to 1.5 times the predicted plasma volume of the patient as standard therapy for TTP. The British guidelines recommend that plasma exchange therapy be continued for a minimum of 2 days after the platelet count returns to normal (>150,000 cells/m^3).
- Corticosteroids (prednisone 1 to 2 mg/kg/day) use is controversial. They may be effective alone in patients with mild disease or may be administered concomitantly with plasmapheresis plus plasma exchange with fresh frozen plasma.
- High-dose plasma infusion (25 ml/kg/day) may be useful only if plasma exchange cannot be promptly started and for patients with very severe or refractory disease between plasma exchange sessions. High-dose plasma infusions can cause volume overload in patients with renal insufficiency.
- The monoclonal antibody rituximab has also been used for treatment of TTP.
- Platelet transfusions are contraindicated except in severely thrombocytopenic patients with documented bleeding.
- Use of antiplatelet agents (acetylsalicylic acid, dipyridamole) is controversial.
- Splenectomy is performed in refractory cases.

CHRONIC Rx

- Relapsing TTP may be treated with plasma exchange.
- Remission of chronic TTP that is unresponsive to conventional therapy has been reported after treatment with cyclophosphamide and the monoclonal antibody rituximab.
- Splenectomy done while the patients are in remission has been used in some centers to decrease the frequency of relapse in TTP.

DISPOSITION

- Survival of patients with TTP currently exceeds 80% with plasma exchange therapy.
- Relapse occurs in 20% to 40% of patients who have TTP in remission.

REFERRAL

Surgical referral for splenectomy in selected patients (see "Acute General Rx" and "Chronic Rx").

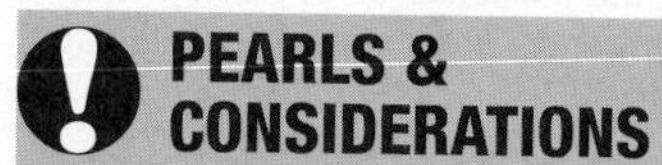

PEARLS & CONSIDERATIONS

COMMENTS

The diagnosis of TTP/hemolytic-uremic syndrome should be considered in pregnant women with vague neurologic, gastrointestinal, or renal symptoms in either the obstetric triage or emergency department areas.

SUGGESTED READINGS

available at www.expertconsult.com

RELATED CONTENT

Hemolytic Uremic Syndrome (Related Key Topic)

AUTHOR: **FRED F. FERRI, M.D.**

BASIC INFORMATION

DEFINITION

Thyroid carcinoma is a primary neoplasm of the thyroid. There are four major types of thyroid carcinoma: papillary, follicular, anaplastic, and edullary.

SYNONYMS

Papillary carcinoma of thyroid
Follicular carcinoma of thyroid
Anaplastic carcinoma of thyroid
Medullary carcinoma of thyroid

ICD-9CM CODES
193 Malignant neoplasm of thyroid
ICD-10CM CODES
C73 Malignant neoplasm of thyroid gland

EPIDEMIOLOGY & DEMOGRAPHICS

- Thyroid cancer is the most common endocrine cancer, with over 48,000 new cases in the U.S. and approximately 1100 deaths.
- Female/male ratio is 3:1.
- Median age at diagnosis: 45 to 50 yr

PHYSICAL FINDINGS & CLINICAL PRESENTATION

- Presence of thyroid nodule
- Hoarseness and cervical lymphadenopathy
- Painless swelling in the region of the thyroid

ETIOLOGY

- Risk factors: prior neck irradiation
- Multiple endocrine neoplasia II (medullary carcinoma)
- Inherited syndromes associated with thyroid cancer are described in Table 1-476.
- Exenatide, a once-weekly GLP-1 receptor agonist for the treatment of type 2 DM, can increase the risk of medullary thyroid carcinoma (MTC).

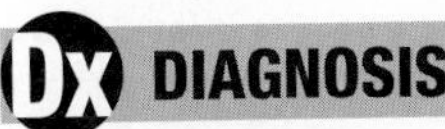

DIAGNOSIS

DIFFERENTIAL DIAGNOSIS

- Multinodular goiter
- Lymphocytic thyroiditis
- Ectopic thyroid

WORKUP

The workup of thyroid carcinoma includes laboratory evaluation and diagnostic imaging.

TABLE 1-476 Inherited Syndromes Associated with Thyroid Cancer

Multiple endocrine neoplasia (MEN) 2A and 2B
Isolated familial medullary thyroid cancer
Gardner syndrome
Familial adenomatous polyposis
Carney complex
Cowden syndrome
Familial nonmedullary thyroid cancer

From Cameron JL, Cameron AM: *Current surgical therapy*, ed 10, Philadelphia, 2011, Saunders.

However, diagnosis is confirmed with fine-needle aspiration or surgical biopsy. The characteristics of thyroid carcinoma vary with the type:

- Papillary carcinoma (85%):
  1. Most frequently occurs in women during second or third decades
  2. Histologically, psammoma bodies (calcific bodies present in papillary projections) are pathognomonic; found in 35% to 45% of papillary thyroid carcinomas
  3. Majority are not papillary lesions but mixed papillary follicular carcinomas
  4. Spread is by lymphatics and by local invasion
- Follicular carcinoma (10%):
  1. More aggressive than papillary carcinoma
  2. Incidence increases with age
  3. Tends to metastasize hematogenously to bone, producing pathologic fractures
  4. Tends to concentrate iodine (useful for radiation therapy)
- Anaplastic carcinoma (1%):
  1. Very aggressive neoplasm
  2. Two major histologic types: small cell (less aggressive, 5-yr survival approximately 20%) and giant cell (death usually within 6 mo of diagnosis)
- MTC (4%):
  1. Unifocal lesion: found sporadically in elderly patients
  2. Bilateral lesions: associated with pheochromocytoma and hyperparathyroidism; this combination is known as MEN-II and is inherited as an autosomal-dominant disorder

LABORATORY TESTS

- Thyroid function studies are generally normal. Thyroid-stimulating hormone (TSH), T_4, and serum thyroglobulin levels should be obtained before thyroidectomy in patients with confirmed thyroid carcinoma. Serum thyroglobulin levels can be useful postoperatively to monitor recurrence of thyroid carcinoma (Fig. E1-937).
- Increased plasma calcitonin assay in patients with medullary carcinoma (tumors produce thyrocalcitonin). RET proto-oncogene sequencing and measurement of plasma free metanephrine and normetanephrine levels to rule out coexistent pheochromocytoma are recommended in all patients with medullary thyroid cancer.
- Fine-needle aspiration biopsy is the best method to assess a thyroid nodule (see "Thyroid Nodule" in Section I).

IMAGING STUDIES (Fig. E1-938)

- Thyroid ultrasound can detect solitary solid nodules that have a high risk of malignancy. However, a negative ultrasound does not exclude diagnosis of thyroid carcinoma.
- Thyroid scanning with iodine-123 or technetium-99m can identify hypofunctioning (cold) nodules, which are more likely to be malignant. However, warm nodules can also be malignant.

STAGING

- Stage I: thyroid cancer of any size without distal spread in patient under age 45. In patients 45 years or older, tumor size ≤2 cm without local invasion or positive cervical lymph nodes
- Stage II: distal spread in patient younger than 45 years. In patients 45 years or older, tumors >2 cm but <4 cm without local invasion or positive cervical lymph nodes
- Stage III: tumors >4 cm in patient over 45 years of age
- Stage IV: distal spread in patient over 45 years of age

Rx TREATMENT

ACUTE GENERAL Rx

- Papillary carcinoma:
  1. Total thyroidectomy is indicated if the patient has:
     a. Extrapyramidal extension of carcinoma
     b. Papillary carcinoma limited to thyroid but a positive history of irradiation to the neck
     c. Lesion >2 cm
  2. Lobectomy with isthmectomy may be considered in patients with intrathyroid papillary carcinoma <2 cm and no history of neck or head irradiation; surgery should be followed with suppressive therapy with thyroid hormone because these tumors are TSH responsive. The accepted practice is to suppress serum TSH concentrations to <0.1 microunit/ml in patients with persistent disease, suppression to 0.1-0.5 microunit/ml in patients who are disease free but are at high risk of recurrence, and a goal TSH level of 0.3-2.0 microunits/ml in patients who are disease free and have a low risk of recurrence.
  3. Radioiodine ablation reduces rates of death and recurrence (Table 1-477). Radioiodine is administered for stages III and IV disease.
- Follicular carcinoma:
  1. Total thyroidectomy followed by TSH suppression, as previously noted
  2. Radiotherapy with iodine-131 followed by thyroid suppression therapy with triiodothyronine is useful in patients with metastasis (Table 1-477)
- Anaplastic carcinoma:
  1. At diagnosis, this neoplasm is rarely operable; palliative surgery is indicated for extremely large tumor compressing the trachea.
  2. Management is usually restricted to radiation therapy or chemotherapy (combination of doxorubicin, cisplatin, and other antineoplastic agents) (Table 1-477); these measures rarely provide significant palliation.
- Medullary carcinoma:
  1. Thyroidectomy should be performed, followed by TSH suppression.
  2. Vandetanib, an oral tyrosine kinase inhibitor, was recently FDA-approved for treatment of symptomatic or progressive, unresectable, locally advanced or metastatic medullary thyroid cancer. It is not recommended for treatment of asymptomatic or less aggressive disease due to its many serious side effects.

3. Patients and their families should be screened for pheochromocytoma and hyperparathyroidism.

DISPOSITION

Prognosis varies with the type of thyroid carcinoma: 5-yr survival approaches 80% for follicular carcinoma and is approximately 5% with anaplastic carcinoma (see Table 1-478).

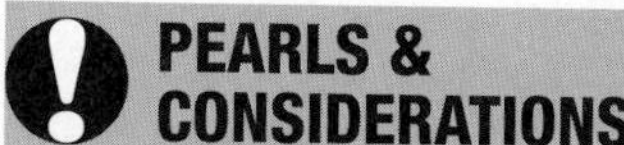

PEARLS & CONSIDERATIONS

COMMENTS

- Family members of patients with medullary carcinoma should be screened; DNA analysis for the detection of mutations in the *RET* gene structure permits the identification of *MEN IIA* gene carriers.
- Motesanib, an oral inhibitor of vascular endothelial growth factor (VEGF) receptors, has been reported effective in inducing partial responses in patients with advanced or metastatic differentiated thyroid cancer that is progressive.
- While there is little controversy regarding the benefit of radioactive iodine in iodine-avid advanced-stage well-differentiated thyroid cancer, the indications for radioactive iodine following total thyroidectomy in patients with very low risk disease is controversial. Proponents argue that its use may destroy microscopic metastases while opponents counter that the risk of secondary cancer due to radioactive iodine is not warranted in patients whose prognosis is typically excellent.
- Metastatic thyroid cancers that are refractory to radioiodine (iodine-131) are associated with a poor prognosis. Recent trials have shown that the selective mitogen-activated protein kinase (MAPK) pathway antagonist selumetinib produces clinically meaningful increases in iodine uptake and retention in some patients with thyroid cancer that is refractory to radioiodine.

SUGGESTED READINGS

available at www.expertconsult.com

RELATED CONTENT

Thyroid Cancer (Patient Information)

AUTHOR: **FRED F. FERRI, M.D.**

TABLE 1-477 Indications for Iodine-131 Treatment in Patients with Papillary, Follicular, or Hürthle Cell Thyroid Carcinoma after Initial Definitive Near-Total Thyroidectomy

No Indication
Adult patients at very low risk for cause-specific mortality or relapse: complete surgical resection, favorable histology, and limited extent of disease (e.g., PTC patients with MACIS scores <6; patients with tumor size <1 cm, N0, and M0).
Definite Indications
Distant metastasis at diagnosis
Incomplete tumor resection
Complete tumor resection but high risk for mortality or recurrence (e.g., PTC patients with MACIS scores ≥6 and pTNM stage II/III FTC or HCC)
Probable Indications
Incomplete surgery (less than near-total thyroidectomy, no lymph node dissection)
PTC or FTC in a child younger than 16 yr
If PTC, tall cell or columnar cell variant and diffuse sclerosing variant
If FTC, widely invasive or poorly differentiated tumor
Bulky nodal metastases

FTC, Follicular thyroid carcinoma; *HCC,* Hürthle cell carcinoma; *MACIS,* scoring system based on metastasis, age, completeness of resection, invasion, and size; *PTC,* papillary thyroid carcinoma; *pTNM,* pathologic tumor-node-metastasis classification.
From Melmed S et al (eds): *Williams textbook of endocrinology,* ed 12, Philadelphia, 2011, Saunders.

TABLE 1-478 Characteristics of Thyroid Cancers

Type of Cancer	Percentage of Thyroid Cancers	Age of Onset (Yr)	Treatment	Prognosis
Papillary	88	40-80	Thyroidectomy, followed by radioactive iodine ablation and TSH suppression	Good
Follicular	10	45-80	Thyroidectomy, followed by radioactive iodine ablation and TSH suppression	Fair to good
Medullary	3-4	20-50	Thyroidectomy and central compartment lymph node dissection and TSH suppression	Fair
Anaplastic	1	50-80	Isthmusectomy followed by palliative x-ray treatment	Poor
Lymphoma	<1	25-70	X-ray therapy and/or chemotherapy	Fair

From Andreoli TE et al: *Andreoli and Carpenter's Cecil essentials of medicine,* ed 8, Philadelphia, 2010, Saunders.

BASIC INFORMATION

DEFINITION

A thyroid nodule is an abnormality found on physical examination of the thyroid gland; nodules can be benign (70%) or malignant.

ICD-9CM CODES
241.0 Nodule, thyroid
ICD-10CM CODES
E04.1 Nontoxic single thyroid nodule
E05.2 Thyrotoxicosis with toxic single thyroid nodule

EPIDEMIOLOGY & DEMOGRAPHICS

- Palpable thyroid nodules occur in 4% to 7% of the population.
- Thyroid nodules can be found in 50% of autopsies; however, only one in 10 is palpable.
- Malignancy is present in 5% to 15% of all thyroid nodules and in 5% to 30% of palpable nodules.
- Incidence of thyroid nodules increases after age 45 yr. They are found more frequently in women.
- History of prior head and neck irradiation increases the risk of thyroid cancer.
- Increased likelihood that nodule is malignant: nodule increasing in size or >3 cm, regional lymphadenopathy, fixation to adjacent tissues, age <40 yr, symptoms of local invasion (dysphagia, hoarseness, neck pain, male sex, family history of thyroid cancer or polyposis [Gardner syndrome]), rapid growth during levothyroxine therapy, microcalcification within the nodule, and high intranodular vascular flow.

PHYSICAL FINDINGS & CLINICAL PRESENTATION

- Palpable, firm, and nontender nodule in the thyroid area should prompt suspicion of carcinoma. Signs of metastasis are regional lymphadenopathy and inspiratory stridor.
- Signs and symptoms of thyrotoxicosis can be found in functioning nodules.

ETIOLOGY

- History of prior head and neck irradiation
- Family history of pheochromocytoma, carcinoma of the thyroid, and hyperparathyroidism (medullary carcinoma of the thyroid is a component of MEN-II)

Dx DIAGNOSIS

DIFFERENTIAL DIAGNOSIS

- Thyroid carcinoma
- Multinodular goiter
- Thyroglossal duct cyst
- Epidermoid cyst
- Laryngocele
- Nonthyroid neck neoplasm
- Branchial cleft cyst

WORKUP

- Fine-needle aspiration (FNA) biopsy is the best diagnostic study; the accuracy can be >90%, but it is directly related to the level of experience of the physician and the cytopathologist interpreting the aspirate. FNA is not routinely recommended for thyroid nodules <1 cm in diameter unless there are significant risk factors (see above).
- FNA biopsy is less reliable with thyroid cystic lesions; surgical excision should be considered for most thyroid cysts not abolished by aspiration.
- A diagnostic approach to thyroid nodule is described in Fig. E1-939. Preoperative, ultrasonically guided FNA accurately classifies 62% to 85% of thyroid nodules as benign; however, 15% to 30% of aspirations yield indeterminate cytologic findings. Table E1-479 describes the probability of malignancy at histology based on FNA biopsy cytology.

LABORATORY TESTS

- Serum TSH should be obtained in all patients with thyroid nodules. If suppressed, obtain free T4 and free T3 and thyroid scan to rule out "hot nodule," indicative of hyperthyroid adenoma. Less than 1% of hyperfunctioning nodules are malignant.
- Thyroid-stimulating hormone (TSH), T_4, and serum thyroglobulin levels should be obtained before thyroidectomy in patients with confirmed thyroid carcinoma on FNA biopsy.
- Serum calcitonin at random or after pentagastrin stimulation is useful when suspecting medullary carcinoma of the thyroid and in anyone with a family history of medullary thyroid carcinoma.
- Serum thyroid autoantibodies (see "Thyroiditis" in Section I) are useful in patients with multinodular goiter and when suspecting thyroiditis.
- Molecular analysis of thyroid tissue for the presence of BRAF and RAS mutations and for RET/PTC and PAX8-PPAR gamma 1 gene rearrangements can be used as a diagnostic tool, since 60% to 70% of thyroid cancers harbor at least one genetic mutation. The gene expression classifier profile can be used to identify a subpopulation of patients with a low likelihood of cancer, thereby avoiding unnecessary surgery in patients with indeterminate FNA. The gene expression classifier test has a high negative predictive value for cytologically indeterminate nodules (95% for an atypical or follicular lesion of undetermined significance, 94% for a follicular neoplasm, and 85% for a lesion suggestive of cancer).

IMAGING STUDIES

- Thyroid ultrasound (Fig. E1-940) is useful to evaluate the size of the thyroid and the number, composition (solid vs. cystic), and dimensions of the thyroid nodule; solid thyroid nodules have a higher incidence of malignancy, but cystic nodules can also be malignant. The three characteristics on thyroid ultrasound most predictive of cancer are nodules >2 cm, microcalcifications, and entirely solid nodules.
- Thyroid scan can be performed with technetium-99m pertechnetate, iodine-123, or iodine-131. Iodine isotopes are preferred because up to 35% of nodules that appear functioning on pertechnetate scanning may appear nonfunctioning on radioiodine scanning. A thyroid scan:
    1. Classifies nodules as hyperfunctioning (hot), normally functioning (warm), or nonfunctioning (cold); cold nodules have a higher incidence of malignancy.
    2. Scan has difficulty evaluating nodules near the thyroid isthmus or at the periphery of the gland.
    3. Normal tissue over a nonfunctioning nodule might mask the nodule as "warm" or normally functioning.
- Both thyroid scan and ultrasound provide information about the risk of malignant neoplasia based on the characteristics of the thyroid nodule, but their value in the initial evaluation of a thyroid nodule is limited because neither provides a definite tissue diagnosis.

Rx TREATMENT

GENERAL Rx

- Evaluation of results of FNA:
    1. Normal cells: may repeat biopsy during present evaluation or reevaluate patient after 3 to 6 mo of suppressive therapy (L-thyroxine, prescribed in doses to suppress the TSH level to 0.1 to 0.5)
        a. Failure to regress indicates increased likelihood of malignancy.
        b. Reliance on repeat FNA biopsy is preferable to routine surgery for nodules not responding to thyroxine.
    2. Indeterminate: use of gene expression classifier profile. If suspicious, perform surgery; if benign, monitor with subsequent repeat FNA and gene expression classifier profile.
    3. Malignant cells: surgery

DISPOSITION

Variable with results of FNA biopsy

REFERRAL

Surgical referral for FNA biopsy

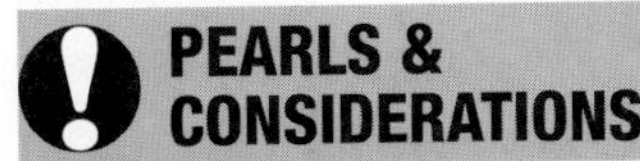

PEARLS & CONSIDERATIONS

COMMENTS

- Most solid, benign nodules grow; therefore an increase in nodule volume alone is not a reliable predictor of malignancy.
- Surgery is indicated in hard or fixed nodule, presence of dysphagia or hoarseness, and rapidly growing solid masses regardless of "benign" results on FNA.
- Suppressive therapy of malignant thyroid nodules postoperatively with thyroxine is indicated. The use of suppressive therapy for benign solitary nodules is controversial.

SUGGESTED READINGS

available at www.expertconsult.com

RELATED CONTENT

Thyroid Nodule (Patient Information)

AUTHOR: **FRED F. FERRI, M.D.**

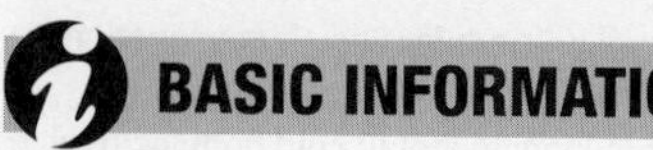

BASIC INFORMATION

DEFINITION

Thyroiditis is an inflammatory disease of the thyroid. It is a multifaceted disease with various etiologies, different clinical characteristics (depending on the stage), and distinct histopathology. Thyroiditis can be subdivided into three common types (Hashimoto's, painful, and painless) and two rare forms (suppurative and Riedel's). To add to the confusion, there are various synonyms for each form, and there is no internationally accepted classification of autoimmune thyroid disease.

SYNONYMS

Hashimoto's thyroiditis: chronic lymphocytic thyroiditis, chronic autoimmune thyroiditis, lymphadenoid goiter

Painful subacute thyroiditis: subacute thyroiditis, giant cell thyroiditis, de Quervain's thyroiditis, subacute granulomatous thyroiditis, pseudogranulomatous thyroiditis

Painless postpartum thyroiditis: subacute lymphocytic thyroiditis, postpartum thyroiditis

Painless sporadic thyroiditis: silent sporadic thyroiditis, subacute lymphocytic thyroiditis

Suppurative thyroiditis: acute suppurative thyroiditis, bacterial thyroiditis, microbial inflammatory thyroiditis, pyogenic thyroiditis

Riedel's thyroiditis: fibrous thyroiditis

ICD-9CM CODES

245.2 Hashimoto's thyroiditis
245.1 Subacute thyroiditis
245.9 Silent thyroiditis
245.0 Suppurative thyroiditis
245.3 Riedel's thyroiditis

ICD-10CM CODES

E06.3 Autoimmune thyroiditis
E06.1 Subacute thyroiditis
E06.9 Thyroiditis, unspecified
E06.0 Acute thyroiditis
E06.5 Other chronic thyroiditis

PHYSICAL FINDINGS & CLINICAL PRESENTATION

- Hashimoto's: patients may have signs of hyperthyroidism (tachycardia, diaphoresis, palpitations, weight loss) or hypothyroidism (fatigue, weight gain, delayed reflexes) depending on the stage of the disease. Usually there is diffuse, firm enlargement of the thyroid gland; the gland may also be of normal size (atrophic form with clinically manifested hypothyroidism).
- Painful subacute: exquisitely tender, enlarged thyroid, fever; signs of hyperthyroidism are initially present; signs of hypothyroidism can subsequently develop.
- Painless thyroiditis: clinical features are similar to subacute thyroiditis except for the absence of tenderness of the thyroid gland.
- Suppurative: patient is febrile with severe neck pain, focal tenderness of the involved portion of the thyroid, erythema of the overlying skin.
- Riedel's: slowly enlarging hard mass in the anterior neck; often mistaken for thyroid cancer; signs of hypothyroidism occur in advanced stages.

ETIOLOGY

- Hashimoto's: autoimmune disorder that begins with the activation of CD4 (helper) T-lymphocytes specific for thyroid antigens. The etiologic factor for the activation of these cells is unknown.
- Painful subacute: possibly postviral; usually follows a respiratory illness not considered to be a form of autoimmune thyroiditis
- Painless thyroiditis: frequently occurs postpartum
- Suppurative: infectious etiology, generally bacterial, although fungi and parasites have also been implicated; often occurs in immunocompromised hosts or after a penetrating neck injury
- Riedel's: fibrous infiltration of the thyroid; etiology unknown
- Drug induced: lithium, interferon-alfa, amiodarone, interleukin-2

DIAGNOSIS

DIFFERENTIAL DIAGNOSIS

- The hyperthyroid phase of Hashimoto's, subacute, and silent thyroiditis can be mistaken for Graves' disease.
- Riedel's thyroiditis can be mistaken for carcinoma of the thyroid.
- Painful subacute thyroiditis can be mistaken for infections of the oropharynx and trachea or for suppurative thyroiditis.
- Factitious hyperthyroidism can mimic silent thyroiditis.

WORKUP

- The diagnostic workup includes laboratory and radiologic evaluation to rule out other conditions that may mimic thyroiditis (see above) and differentiate the various forms of thyroiditis.
- The patient's medical history may be helpful in differentiating the various types of thyroiditis (e.g., presentation after childbirth is suggestive of silent [postpartum, painless] thyroiditis; occurrence after a viral respiratory infection suggests subacute thyroiditis; history of penetrating injury to the neck indicates suppurative thyroiditis).

LABORATORY TESTS

- Thyroid-stimulating hormone, free T_4: may be normal or indicative of hypothyroidism or hyperthyroidism depending on the stage of the thyroiditis.
- White blood cell (WBC) with differential: increased WBC with left shift occurs with subacute and suppurative thyroiditis.
- Antimicrosomal antibodies: detected in >90% of patients with Hashimoto's thyroiditis and 50% to 80% of patients with silent thyroiditis.
- Serum thyroglobulin levels are elevated in patients with subacute and silent thyroiditis; this test is nonspecific but may be useful in monitoring the course of subacute thyroiditis and distinguishing silent thyroiditis from factitious hyperthyroidism (low or absent serum thyroglobulin level).

IMAGING STUDIES

Twenty-four-hour radioactive iodine uptake (RAIU) is useful to distinguish Graves' disease (increased RAIU) from thyroiditis (normal or low RAIU). Table E1-480 summarizes factors that influence 24-hr thyroid iodide uptake.

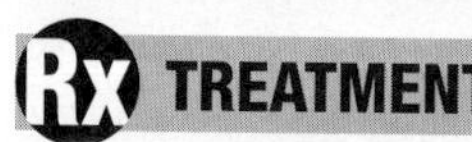

TREATMENT

ACUTE GENERAL Rx

- Treat hypothyroid phase with levothyroxine 25 to 50 mcg/day initially and monitor serum thyroid-stimulating hormone initially every 6 to 8 wk.
- Control symptoms of hyperthyroidism with beta-blockers (e.g., propranolol 20 to 40 mg PO q6h).
- Control pain in patients with subacute thyroiditis with nonsteroidal anti-inflammatory drugs. Prednisone 20 to 40 mg qd may be used if nonsteroidals are insufficient, but it should be gradually tapered off over several weeks.
- Use IV antibiotics and drain abscess (if present) in patients with suppurative thyroiditis.

DISPOSITION

- Hashimoto's thyroiditis: long-term prognosis is favorable; most patients recover their thyroid function.
- Painful subacute thyroiditis: permanent hypothyroidism occurs in 10% of patients.
- Painless thyroiditis: 6% of patients have permanent hypothyroidism.
- Suppurative thyroiditis: there is usually full recovery after treatment.
- Riedel's thyroiditis: hypothyroidism occurs when fibrous infiltration involves the entire thyroid.

REFERRAL

Surgical referral in patients with compression of adjacent neck structures and in some patients with suppurative thyroiditis

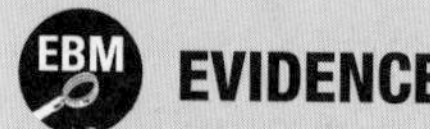

EVIDENCE

available at www.expertconsult.com

SUGGESTED READINGS

available at www.expertconsult.com

RELATED CONTENT

Thyroiditis (Patient Information)

AUTHOR: **FRED F. FERRI, M.D.**

BASIC INFORMATION

DEFINITION

Tinea capitis is a dermatophyte infection of hair shaft and follicles of the scalp, eyebrows, and eyelashes. Etiologic agents are fungal species of the genera *Microsporum* and *Trichophyton.*

SYNONYMS

Ringworm of the scalp, ringworm of the head, gray patch tinea capitis, black dot tinea capitis, tinea tonsurans, herpes tonsurans, kerion, favus

ICD-9CM CODES
110.0 Tinea capitis
ICD-10CM CODES
B35.0 Tinea barbae and tinea capitis

EPIDEMIOLOGY & DEMOGRAPHICS

Tinea capitis primarily affects prepubertal children with peak age between 3 and 7 yr old. Adult cases are rare, possibly because of the fungistatic effect of the sebum found in older persons. Urban populations, large family size, low socioeconomic status, and crowded living conditions may contribute to an increased incidence of tinea capitis. The elderly and immunocompromised individuals have an increased risk of infection. The incidence of the disease varies worldwide; however, it has been relatively low in the U.S. It is reportedly widespread in parts of central and South America, India, and Africa.

In the U.S., peak incidence occurs in school-aged children of low socioeconomic status, with African American male children accounting for the greatest proportion of cases. About 3% to 8% of American children are affected, and 34% of household contacts are asymptomatic carriers.

PHYSICAL FINDINGS & CLINICAL PRESENTATION

- Classic triad of scalp scaling, alopecia, and cervical adenopathy
- Most forms of tinea capitis begin with one or few round patches of scale or alopecia.
- Primary lesions include plaques, papules, pustules, or nodules on the scalp (usually occipital region).
- Secondary lesions include scales, alopecia (usually reversible), erythema, exudates, and edema.
- Scalp pruritus may be present.
- Fever, pain, and lymphadenopathy (commonly postcervical) may occur with inflammatory lesions.
- Different clinical patterns of tinea capitis have been described:
  - Gray patch: Lesions are scaly and well demarcated. The hairs within the patch break off a few millimeters above the scalp. One or several lesions may be present; sometimes the lesions join to form larger ones.
  - Black dot: Early lesions with erythema and scaling patch are easily overlooked until areas of alopecia develop. Hairs within the patches break at the surface of the scalp, leaving behind a pattern of swollen black dots.
  - Kerion (Fig. 1-941): inflamed, exudative, pustular, boggy, tender nodules exhibiting marked edema, and hair loss seen in severe tinea capitis. Caused by immune response to the fungus. May lead to some scarring.
  - Favus: production of scutula (hair matted together with dermatophyte hyphae and keratin debris), characterized by yellow cup-shaped crusts around hair shafts. A fetid odor may be present.

ETIOLOGY

Although most cases of tinea capitis are caused by fungi of the *Microsporum* or *Trichophyton* genera, causative species vary between geographical areas and across time. *T. tonsurans* is the predominant cause of tinea capitis, present in more than 90% of cases in North and Central America. *Microsporum canis, M. audouinii,* and *Trichophyton mentagrophytes* are less common. The most common causative species for black dot tinea capitis is *T. tonsurans*. Gray patch tinea capitis tends to be caused by *M. andouinii* and *M. canis.* Infection of the hair shaft is preceded by invasion of the stratum corneum of the scalp. Transmision of *T. tonsurans* occurs from person-to-person transmission via infected persons or asymptomatic carriers, fallen infected hairs, animal vectors, and fomites. *M. audouinii* is commonly spread by dogs and cats. Infectious fungal particles may remain viable for many months. Even though the organism remains viable on combs, hairbrushes, and other fomites for long periods of time, the role of fomites in spreading the infection may vary in different geographic areas.

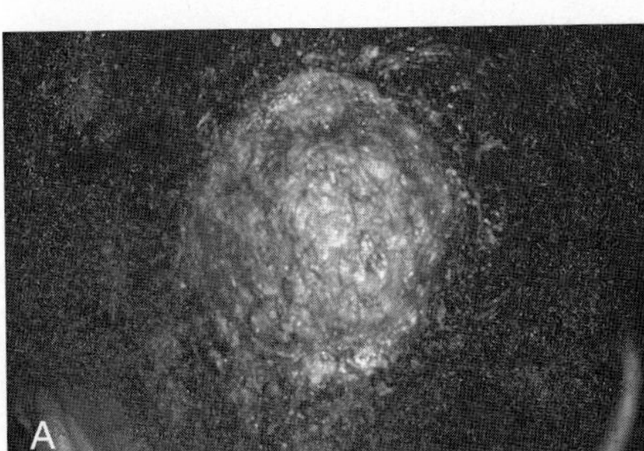

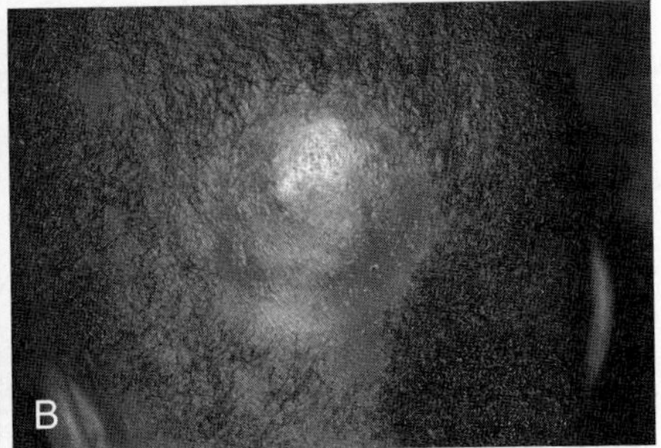

FIGURE 1-941 A, Kerion. Boggy granulomatous mass of the scalp. **B,** Scarring after kerion. (From Kliegman RM et al: *Nelson textbook of pediatrics,* ed 19, Philadelphia, 2011, Saunders.)

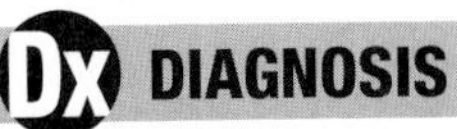

DIAGNOSIS

DIFFERENTIAL DIAGNOSIS

Seborrhea dermatitis and psoriasis may be confused with tinea of the scalp. Alopecia areata, impetigo, pediculosis, trichotillomania, traction alopecia, folliculitis, pseudopelade, seborrhea/atopic dermatitis, psoriasis, carbuncles, pyoderma, lichen ruber planus, lupus erythematosus. Table 1-481 highlights distinctive features of conditions that may be confused for tinea capitis.

WORKUP

- KOH testing of hair shaft extracted from the lesion, not the scale, because the *T. tonsurans* spores attach to or reside inside hair shafts and will rarely be found in the scales.
- Wood's ultraviolet light fluoresces blue-green on hair shafts for *Microsporum* infections but will fail to identify *T. tonsurans.*
- Fungal culture of hairs and scales on fungal medium such as Sabouraud's agar may be used to confirm the diagnosis, especially if uncertain.
- Histology of biopsies with fungal staining in cases where mycology tests are negative because of treatment initiation.

TREATMENT

- Griseofulvin is the gold standard FDA-approved treatment. It is less costly than other drug options and has an excellent long-term safety profile. Micronized and ultramicronized preparations are absorbed better, and side effects are infrequent, especially when administered with fatty meals. Periodic monitoring of hematologic, liver, and renal function may be indicated, especially in prolonged treatment over 8 wk.

  Children: Griseofulvin is approved for children older than 2 yr of age: microsize griseofulvin 10 to 25 mg/kg PO per day in one single dose or two divided doses (maximum, 1 g/day; for tinea capitis, higher doses [20-25 mg/kg/day] have been recommended) or ultramicrosize griseofulvin, 5 to 15 mg/kg PO per day (maximum, 750 mg/day), in one single dose or two divided doses. Optimally, griseofulvin is given after a meal containing fat (e.g., peanut butter or ice cream). Recommended treatment length is 6 to 8 wk and should be continued 2 wk beyond clinical resolution (until hair regrowth occurs). Some children may require higher doses to achieve clinical cure.

  Adults and elderly: microsize griseofulvin 500 mg PO per day in one single dose or divided doses. The other option is ultramicrosize griseofulvin 375 mg PO per day in one single dose or divided doses. Recommended treatment length is 4 to 6 weeks.
- New alternative treatments: oral terbinafine, itraconazole, or fluconazole are comparable in efficacy and safety to griseofulvin, with

TABLE 1-481 Differential Diagnosis of Tinea Capitis

Disorder	Differentiating Features
Psoriasis	Red skin with thick, uniform, silvery scale, sharply demarcated; often psoriasis at other body sites also
Dermatitis	Main possibility is seborrheic dermatitis: usually more diffuse and has uniform fine scaling, rather than localized areas; doesn't typically cause alopecia or significant inflammation. May also be present on the face, especially the nasolabial fold, or as otitis externa. Atopic dermatitis is generally diffuse on scalp and almost inevitably present at other sites, but may coexist with tinea capitis, especially in children.
Pityriasis amiantacea	Thick sheets of asbestos-like scale, very adherent, generally a solitary patch. This may occur in various dermatoses.
Lichen simplex	Usually nape of neck; cobblestoned or lichenified skin thickening, with broken hairs that are not coated with scale
Alopecia areata	Usually not inflamed (may be mildly so), not scaly, usually sharply defined. "Exclamation mark" hairs occur but are not coated with fungus; "cadaverized" hairs especially cause difficulty, as they mimic black dot alopecia.
Scarring alopecias	Examples: discoid lupus erythematosus, lichen planus of scalp; cause perifollicular inflammation around intact hairs; usually associated with lesions at other sites also. Dissecting cellulitis of scalp is also in this differential.
Bacterial infections	Impetigo causes crusting but little inflammation, and hairs are intact; carbuncle is deeper and very tender but may be in the differential of kerion
Trichotillomania	Broken hairs of unequal length, but hair shafts themselves and the scalp are normal
Damage from hair-dressing processes	Usually clear from the timescale
Neoplasm	May be in the differential of kerion; usually slower-growing and mainly on elderly, balding scalp, whereas kerion is in children or young adults with previously intact hair

From White GM, Cox NH (eds): *Diseases of the skin, a color atlas and text,* ed 2, St Louis, 2006, Mosby.

possibly shorter treatment and better patient compliance. Preferred when resistant or when an allergy to griseofulvin is of concern. Monitoring of CBC, liver function tests, and renal function may be indicated.
  - Terbinafine—4-wk course of therapy as effective as with griseofulvin. Dosages are 67.5 mg/day for patients weighing <20 kg; 125 mg/day for patients weighing 20 to 40 kg; and 250 mg for patients weighing >40 kg.
  - Itraconazole—3.5 mg/kg daily for 4 to 6 wk or pulse therapy of 5 mg/kg daily for 1 wk each month for 2 to 3 mo (not approved for children)
  - Fluconazole—the only oral antifungal agent approved for children <2 yr, 6 mg/kg/day for 6 wk in children (3 to 6 wk in adults) or 8 mg/kg weekly for 8 to 12 wk (cap at 150 mg weekly for adults)
- The adjuvant use of antifungal shampoos may be recommended for all patients and household contacts. Shampoo like selenium sulfide 2.5% used for 5 min or ketoconazole shampoo used 2 to 3 times/wk can help prevent infection or eradicate asymptomatic carrier state by inhibiting fungal growth.
- Severe inflammatory kerion can be managed with additional prednisone 40 mg daily (1 mg/kg/day in children) and tapering over 2 wk.
- Prompt treatment is indicated, as is examination of siblings and other household contacts for evidence of tinea capitis.
- Recommend follow-up visit every 2 to 4 wk with Wood's light, microscopic study, and fungal culture. A mycologic documented cure is the goal of treatment.
- Pets that are infected or asymptomatic carriers should be treated.
- Children receiving treatment for tinea capitis may attend school once they start therapy with griseofulvin or other effective systemic agent.

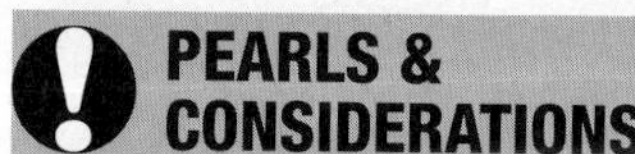

PEARLS & CONSIDERATIONS

- Systemic antifungal therapy is required for tinea capitis because topical antifungal medications are not effective.
- Shaving of the head, haircuts, or wearing a cap or scarf during treatment is unnecessary.
- Sharing of combs, hair ribbons, and hairbrushes should be discouraged.

COMMENTS

- Confirming the diagnosis of tinea capitis with a laboratory specimen is important because misdiagnosis will result in delay or improper treatment.
- Patients and their families should look for sources of infections and disinfect contaminated objects such as combs, brushes, towels, and headgear. Avoid sharing personal hygiene utensils.
- Culture of hairs and scalp dander facilitates carrier identification and prevention.

SUGGESTED READINGS

available at www.expertconsult.com

RELATED CONTENT

Tinea Capitis (Patient Information)

AUTHORS: **PRIYA SARIN GUPTA, M.D., M.P.H., NADINE MBUYI, M.D.,** and **ALVARO MENENDEZ, M.D.**

BASIC INFORMATION

DEFINITION

Tinea corporis is a dermatophyte fungal infection caused by the genera *Trichophyton* or *Microsporum.*

SYNONYMS

Ringworm
Body ringworm
Tinea circinata

ICD-9CM CODES
110.5 Tinea corporis
ICD-10CM CODES
B35.4 Tinea corporis

EPIDEMIOLOGY & DEMOGRAPHICS

- The disease is more common in warm climates.
- There is no predominant age or sex.

PHYSICAL FINDINGS & CLINICAL PRESENTATION

- Typically appears as single or multiple annular lesions with an advancing scaly border (Fig. 1-942); the margin is slightly raised, reddened, and may be pustular.
- The central area becomes hypopigmented and less scaly as the active border progresses outward (Fig. 1-943).
- The trunk and legs are primarily involved.
- Pruritus is variable.
- It is important to remember that recent topical corticosteroid use can significantly alter the appearance of the lesions.

ETIOLOGY

Trichophyton rubrum is the most common pathogen.

DIAGNOSIS

DIFFERENTIAL DIAGNOSIS

- Pityriasis rosea
- Erythema multiforme
- Psoriasis
- Cutaneous systemic lupus erythematosus
- Secondary syphilis
- Nummular eczema
- Eczema
- Granuloma annulare
- Lyme disease
- Tinea versicolor
- Contact dermatitis

WORKUP

Diagnosis is usually made on clinical grounds. It can be confirmed by direct visualization under the microscope of a small fragment of the scale using wet mount preparation and potassium hydroxide solution; dermatophytes appear as translucent branching filaments (hyphae) with lines of separation appearing at irregular intervals.

LABORATORY TESTS

- Microscopic examination of hyphae
- Mycotic culture is usually not necessary.
- Biopsy is indicated only when the diagnosis is uncertain and the patient has not responded to treatment.

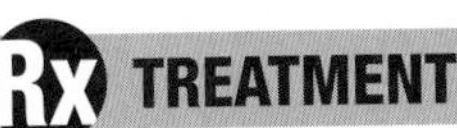

TREATMENT

NONPHARMACOLOGIC THERAPY

Affected areas should be kept clean and dry.

ACUTE GENERAL Rx

- Various creams are effective; the application area should include normal skin approximately 2 cm beyond the affected area:
  1. Butenafine cream applied qd for 14 days
  2. Terbinafine cream applied bid for 14 days
- Systemic therapy is reserved for severe cases and is usually given up to 4 wk; commonly used agents:
  1. Fluconazole, 200 mg qd
  2. Terbinafine, 250 mg qd

DISPOSITION

Majority of cases resolve without sequelae within 3 to 4 wk of therapy.

REFERRAL

Dermatology referral in patients with persistent or recurrent infections

SUGGESTED READINGS

available at www.expertconsult.com

RELATED CONTENT

Ringworm (Patient Information)

AUTHOR: **FRED F. FERRI, M.D.**

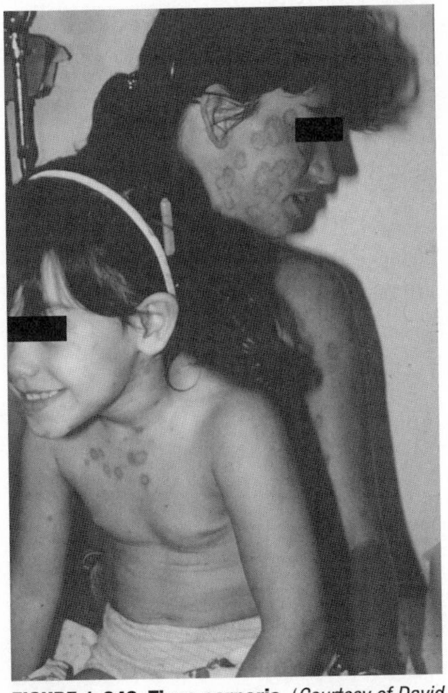

FIGURE 1-942 Tinea corporis. (*Courtesy of David Effron, MD.*)

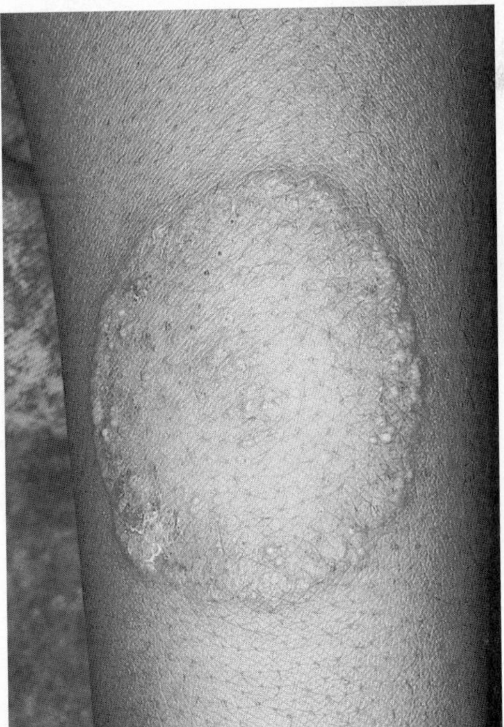

FIGURE 1-943 Annular lesion (tinea corporis). Note raised erythematous, scaling border and central clearing. (From Noble J et al: *Textbook of primary care medicine,* ed 3, St Louis, 2001, Mosby.)

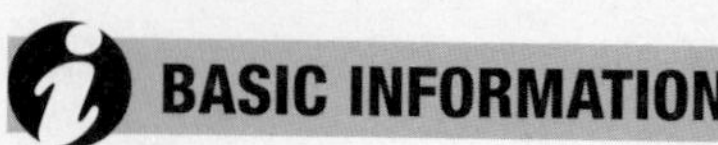

BASIC INFORMATION

DEFINITION

Tinea cruris is a dermatophyte infection of the groin.

SYNONYMS

Jock itch
Groin ringworm

ICD-9CM CODES
110.3 Tinea cruris
ICD-10CM CODES
B35.6 Tinea cruris

EPIDEMIOLOGY & DEMOGRAPHICS

- Most common during the summer in adolescent and young adult males.
- Males are affected more frequently than females; however, it has become more common in postpubertal females who are overweight or who often wear tight jeans or pantyhose.
- The infection often coexists with tinea pedis.

PHYSICAL FINDINGS & CLINICAL PRESENTATION

- Erythematous plaques have a half-moon shape and a scaling border.
- The acute inflammation tends to move down the inner thigh and usually spares the scrotum; in severe cases the fungus may spread onto the buttocks.
- Itching may be severe.
- Red papules and pustules may be present.
- An important diagnostic sign is the advancing well-defined border with a tendency toward central clearing (Fig. 1-944).

ETIOLOGY

- Dermatophytes of the genera *Trichophyton, Epidermophyton,* and *Microsporum. T. rubrum* and *E. floccosum* are the most common infecting agents.
- Transmission from direct contact (e.g., infected persons, animals). The patient's feet should be evaluated as a source of infection because tinea cruris is often associated with tinea pedis.

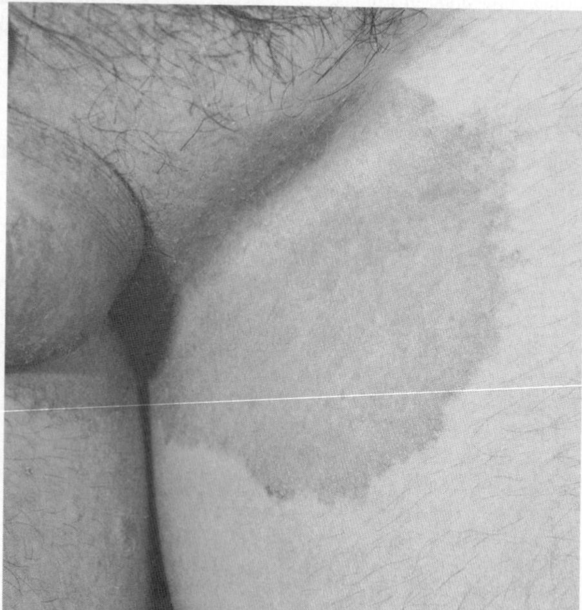

FIGURE 1-944 Tinea cruris. A half-moon–shaped plaque has a well-defined, scaling border. (From Habif TB: *Clinical dermatology: a color guide to diagnosis and therapy,* ed 3, St Louis, 1996, Mosby.)

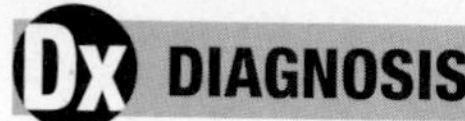

DIAGNOSIS

DIFFERENTIAL DIAGNOSIS

- Candidal intertrigo
- Psoriasis
- Seborrheic dermatitis
- Erythrasma
- Contact dermatitis
- Tinea versicolor

WORKUP

Diagnosis is based on clinical presentation and demonstration of hyphae microscopically using potassium hydroxide.

LABORATORY TESTS

- Microscopic examination
- Cultures are generally not necessary.

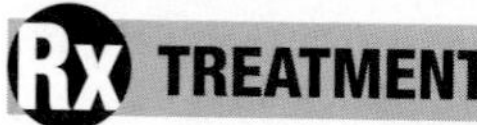

TREATMENT

NONPHARMACOLOGIC THERAPY

- Keep infected area clean and dry.
- Boxer shorts are preferred to briefs.

ACUTE GENERAL Rx

- Various topical antifungal agents are available:
  1. Butenafine cream, applied qd × 14 days
  2. Terbinafine cream, applied bid × 14 days
- Drying powders (e.g., miconazole nitrate) may be useful in patients with excessive perspiration.
- Oral antifungal therapy is generally reserved for cases unresponsive to topical agents or can be used along with topical agents in severe cases. Effective medications are fluconazole 200 mg qd × 10 days and terbinafine 250 mg qd × 30 days.

DISPOSITION

Most cases respond promptly to therapy with complete resolution within 2 to 3 wk.

SUGGESTED READINGS

available at www.expertconsult.com

RELATED CONTENT

Tinea Cruris (Patient Information)

AUTHOR: **FRED F. FERRI, M.D.**

BASIC INFORMATION

DEFINITION

Tinea pedis is a dermatophyte infection of the feet.

SYNONYMS

Athlete's foot

ICD-9CM CODES
110.4 Tinea pedis
ICD-10CM CODES
B35.3 Tinea pedis

EPIDEMIOLOGY & DEMOGRAPHICS

- Most common dermatophyte infection
- Increased incidence in hot humid weather; occlusive footwear is a contributing factor
- Occurrence is rare before adolescence
- More common in adult males

PHYSICAL FINDINGS & CLINICAL PRESENTATION

- Typical presentation is variable and ranges from erythematous scaling plaques (Fig. 1-945) and isolated blisters to interdigital maceration.
- The infection usually starts in the interdigital spaces of the foot. Most infections are found in the toe webs or on the soles.
- Fourth or fifth toes are most commonly involved.
- Pruritus is common and is most intense after removal of shoes and socks.
- Infection with *Trichophyton rubrum* often manifests with a "moccasin" distribution affecting the soles and lateral feet.

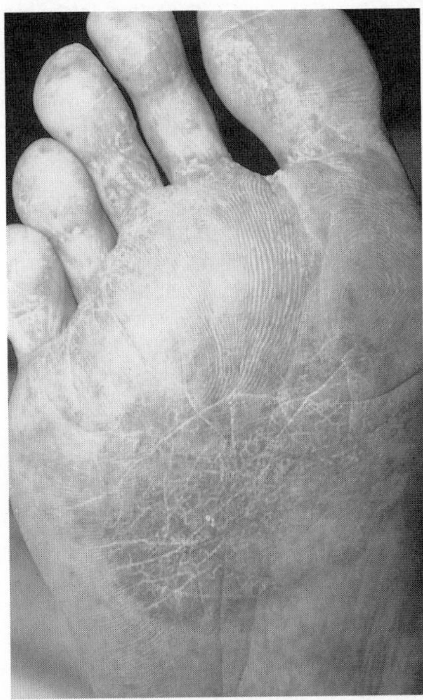

FIGURE 1-945 Tinea pedis. (From Goldstein BG, Goldstein AO: *Practical dermatology,* ed 2, St Louis, 1997, Mosby.)

ETIOLOGY

Dermatophyte infection caused by *T. rubrum, Trichophyton mentagrophytes,* or less commonly *Epidermophyton floccosum*

DIAGNOSIS

DIFFERENTIAL DIAGNOSIS

- Contact dermatitis
- Toe web infection (bacterial or candidal infection)
- Eczema
- Psoriasis
- Keratolysis exfoliativa
- Juvenile plantar dermatosis

WORKUP

- Diagnosis is usually made by clinical observation.
- Laboratory testing, when performed, generally consists of a simple potassium hydroxide preparation with mycologic examination under a light microscope to confirm the presence of dermatophytes.

LABORATORY TESTS

- Microscopic examination of a scale or the roof of a blister with 10% KOH under low or medium power will reveal hyphae.
- Mycologic culture is rarely indicated in the diagnosis of tinea pedis.
- Biopsy is reserved for when the diagnosis remains in question after testing or failure to respond to treatment.

TREATMENT

NONPHARMACOLOGIC THERAPY

- Keep infected area clean and dry. Aerate feet by using sandals when possible.
- Use 100% cotton socks rather than nylon socks to reduce moisture.
- Areas likely to become infected should be dried completely before being covered with clothes.

ACUTE GENERAL Rx

- Benzylamines: butenafine HCl 1% cream applied bid for 1 wk or qd for 4 wk is effective in interdigital tinea pedis.
- Allylamines: terbinafine cream applied bid × 14 days, or naftifine 1% cream applied qd or naftifine gel applied bid for 4 wk produces a significantly high cure rate.
- Imidazoles: econazole, ketoconazole, miconazole, and clotrimazole cream are also effective agents. Clotrimazole 1% cream is an over-the-counter treatment. It should be applied to affected and surrounding area bid for up to 4 wk.
- Ciclopirox and tolnaftate are other antifungal agents available in cream, suspension, or gel. Tolnaftate is also available as a lotion, spray, or powder.
- When using topical preparations, the application area should include normal skin approximately 2 cm beyond the affected area.
- Areas of maceration can be treated with Burow's solution soaks for 10 to 20 min bid followed by foot elevation.
- Oral agents (fluconazole 150 mg once per week for 4 wk) can be used in combination with topical agents in resistant cases.

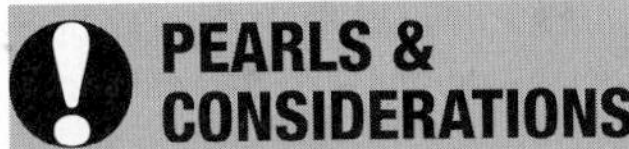

PEARLS & CONSIDERATIONS

Combination therapy of antifungal and corticosteroid (clotrimazole/betamethasone [Lotrisone]) should only be used when the diagnosis of fungal infection is confirmed and inflammation is a significant issue.

SUGGESTED READINGS

available at www.expertconsult.com

RELATED CONTENT

Athlete's Foot (Patient Information)

AUTHOR: **FRED F. FERRI, M.D.**

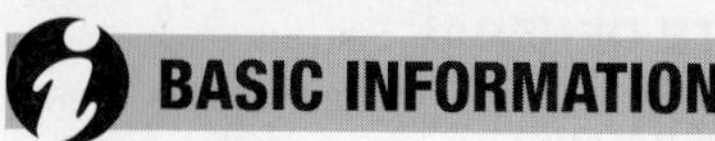

BASIC INFORMATION

DEFINITION

Tinea versicolor is a fungal infection of the skin caused by the yeast *Pityrosporum orbiculare (Malassezia furfur).*

SYNONYMS

Pityriasis versicolor

ICD-9CM CODES
111.0 Tinea versicolor
ICD-10CM CODES
B36.0 Pityriasis versicolor

EPIDEMIOLOGY & DEMOGRAPHICS

- Increased incidence in adolescence and young adulthood
- More common during the summer (hypopigmented lesions are more evident when the skin is tanned)

PHYSICAL FINDINGS & CLINICAL PRESENTATION

- Most lesions begin as multiple small, circular macules of various colors (Fig. 1-946).
- The macules may be darker or lighter than the surrounding normal skin and will scale with scraping.
- Most frequent site of distribution is trunk.
- Facial lesions are more common in children (forehead is most common facial site).
- Eruption is generally of insidious onset and asymptomatic.
- Lesions may be hyperpigmented in blacks.
- Lesions may be inconspicuous in fair-complexioned individuals, especially during the winter.
- Most patients become aware of the eruption when the involved areas do not tan (Fig. 1-947).

ETIOLOGY

The infection is caused by the lipophilic yeast *P. orbiculare* (round form) and *P. ovale* (oval form), which are normal inhabitants of the skin flora. Factors that favor proliferation are pregnancy, malnutrition, immunosuppression, oral contraceptives, and excess heat and humidity.

DIAGNOSIS

DIFFERENTIAL DIAGNOSIS

- Vitiligo
- Pityriasis alba
- Secondary syphilis
- Pityriasis rosea
- Seborrheic dermatitis
- Postinflammatory hyperpigmentation or hypopigmentation

WORKUP

Diagnosis is based on clinical appearance; identification of hyphae and budding spores ("spaghetti and meatballs" appearance) with microscopy confirms diagnosis.

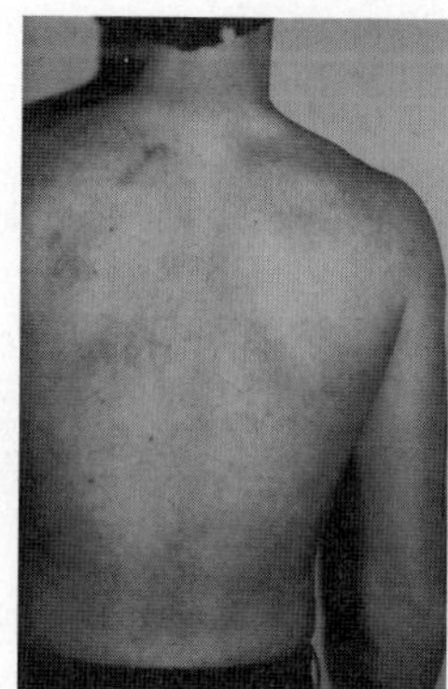

FIGURE 1-946 Tinea versicolor. (Courtesy David Effron, M.D.)

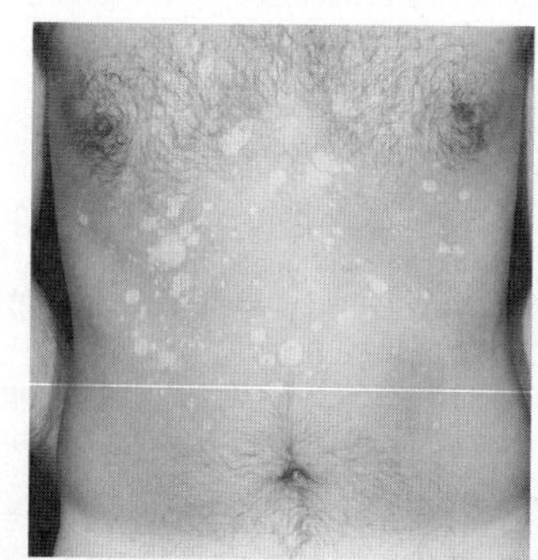

FIGURE 1-947 The classic presentation of tinea versicolor with white, oval, or circular patches on tan skin. (From Habif TB: *Clinical dermatology: a color guide to diagnosis and therapy,* ed 3, St Louis, 1996, Mosby.)

LABORATORY TESTS

Microscopic examination with potassium hydroxide confirms diagnosis.

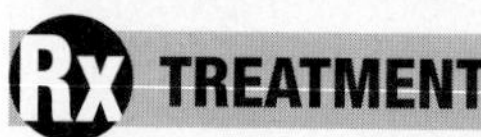

TREATMENT

NONPHARMACOLOGIC THERAPY

Sunlight accelerates repigmentation of hypopigmented areas.

ACUTE GENERAL Rx

- Topical treatment: selenium sulfide 2.5% suspension (Selsun or Exsel) applied daily for 30 min for 7 consecutive days results in a cure rate of 80% to 90%.
- Antifungal topical agents (e.g., miconazole, ciclopirox, clotrimazole) are also effective.
- Oral treatment can be given along with topical agents but is generally reserved for resistant cases. Effective agents are ketoconazole 200 mg qd for 5 days, or single 400-mg dose (cure rate >80%), fluconazole 400 mg given as a single dose (cure rate >70% at 3 wk after treatment), or itraconazole 200 mg/day for 5 days.

DISPOSITION

The prognosis is good, with death of the fungus usually occurring within 3 to 4 wk of treatment; however, recurrence is common.

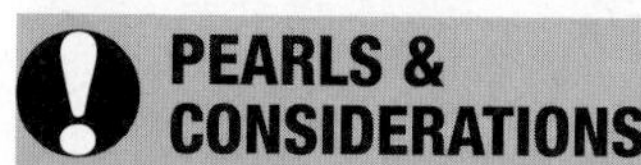

PEARLS & CONSIDERATIONS

COMMENTS

Patients should be informed that the hypopigmented areas will not disappear immediately after treatment and that several months may be necessary for the hypopigmented areas to regain their pigmentation.

RELATED CONTENT

Tinea Versicolor (Patient Information)

AUTHOR: **FRED F. FERRI, M.D.**

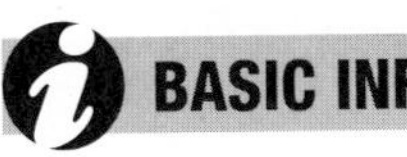

BASIC INFORMATION

DEFINITION

Tinnitus is a perceived sound in the absence of acoustic stimulus external to the head. It may be unilateral, bilateral, or lateral dominant. It is commonly described as a ringing, buzzing, roaring, hissing, whistling, humming, cricket-like, or pulsing sound. It is frequently a symptom associated with hearing loss, Meniere's disease, acoustic neuroma, drug toxicity, depression, or autoimmune inner ear disease. The sound may be internal and perceived only by the patient, called subjective or tonal tinnitus, or it may be heard by both patient and examiner, called objective or nontonal tinnitus.

SYNONYMS

Ringing in the ear(s)

ICD-9CM CODES
388.3 Tinnitus
388.30 Tinnitus, unspecified
388.31 Subjective tinnitus
388.32 Objective tinnitus
ICD-10CM CODES
H93.1 Tinnitus
H93.2 Other abnormal auditory perceptions

EPIDEMIOLOGY & DEMOGRAPHICS

PREVALENCE:

- The American Tinnitus Association reports 50 million Americans have tinnitus for >6 mo.
- Prevalence increases with age, peaking for persons aged 65-74 years.
- Prevalence in U.S. based on National Health Interview Survey (NHIS) in 1996:
    - 2.98% all ages
    - 0.26% for persons <18 yr old
    - 1.6% for persons aged 18-44 yr
    - 5.96% for persons aged 45-64 yr: 7.7% males, 4.3% females
    - 9.6% for persons aged 65-74 yr: 12% males, 7.7% females
    - 7.6% for persons >75 yr old: 11.4% males, 5.3% females
    - 2:1 South/Northeast regions
- Up to 18% of people in industrialized societies are mildly affected by chronic tinnitus, and 0.5% report tinnitus having a severe effect on their daily life.

PREDOMINANT SEX AND AGE: Persons most affected are male, Caucasian, elderly, persons with hearing impairment, persons living in southern U.S. For military veterans, tinnitus is the third most common service-related disability

RISK FACTORS: Any condition causing hearing loss or damage to the auditory system can produce tinnitus. Cochlear damage from exposure to noise is the most common cause. Exposure to ototoxic drugs is also important.

PHYSICAL FINDINGS & CLINICAL PRESENTATION

- History should focus on exposure to loud noises, evidence of hearing loss, ototoxic drugs.
- Patient should be screened for depression.
- Patient who complains of sound in ear may also complain of ear pain or fullness.
- Objective tinnitus is pulsatile and coincides with patient's pulse.
- Physical examination should focus on HEENT, neck, and neurologic exam.
- May be no significant physical findings.

ETIOLOGY

- Mechanism is poorly understood. It may originate at any point along the auditory pathway. Causes include injured cochlear hair cells, spontaneous activity in auditory nerve fibers, hyperactivity in the auditory nuclei in the brain stem, or a reduction in the suppressive activity of the central auditory cortex.
- Medications implicated in causing tinnitus: salicylates, NSAIDs, aminoglycosides, loop diuretics, valproate, quinine, chemotherapeutic agents, cisplatin, vincristine, heavy metals such as lead.

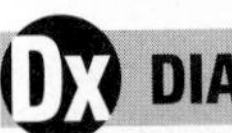

DIAGNOSIS

DIFFERENTIAL DIAGNOSIS

- Subjective/tonal tinnitus:
    - Otologic: tympanic membrane disorder, inner ear disorder (hair cells, organ of Corti), Meniere's disease
    - Ototoxic medications
    - Neurologic: multiple sclerosis, head trauma, cochlear nerve lesion, acoustic schwannoma, neurofibroma, meningioma
    - Metabolic: thyroid disorder, hyperlipidemia (leading to plaque formation), vitamin B_{12} deficiency
    - Psychogenic: depression, anxiety, fibromyalgia
    - Infectious: otitis media, Lyme disease, meningitis, syphilis
- Objective/nontonal tinnitus:
    - Vascular: arterial bruit, venous hum, arteriovenous malformation, vascular tumors
    - Neurologic: contraction of muscles of the eustachian tube, contraction of the stapedius muscle, contraction of the tensor tympani muscles, or a palatal myoclonus, glomus jugulare tumor
    - Conductive: patulous (wide-open) eustachian tube

WORKUP

- Audiometry, tympanometry
- Electronystagmography to evaluate for Meniere's disease
- Box E1-92 describes useful diagnostic tests. An algorithm for tinnitus evaluation is described in Fig. E1-948.

LABORATORY TESTS

Evaluate for metabolic abnormalities: TSH, CBC, B_{12}, lipid panel.

IMAGING STUDIES

- CT/MRI: to evaluate for subjective tinnitus
- MRI/MRA: to evaluate objective tinnitus

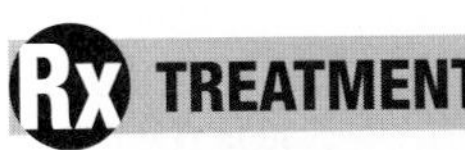

TREATMENT

NONPHARMACOLOGIC THERAPY

It is best to avoid exposure to excessive noise, ototoxic agents, wear protective equipment in noisy environments, or mask the tinnitus through amplification of normal sounds with a hearing aid. Habituation techniques include tinnitus retraining therapy. Cognitive behavioral therapy to improve coping, biofeedback to improve tinnitus distress.

ACUTE GENERAL Rx

- If the tinnitus is severe enough to cause suicidal symptoms, immediate referral to a psychiatrist and an otolaryngologist is recommended to minimize the time to diagnosis and optimize treatment.
- Patients with persistent symptoms or tinnitus accompanied by visual changes or headache should be evaluated for tumors such as acoustic neuroma.

CHRONIC Rx

There is insufficient evidence to support the use of any medication, vitamin, or nutritional supplement to treat tinnitus.

COMPLEMENTARY & ALTERNATIVE MEDICINE

Possibly effective: acupuncture, relaxation therapy, hypnosis (based on systematic review)

DISPOSITION

Clinical course is variable. ~20%-25% of patients with chronic tinnitus consider it a significant problem. Individualized tinnitus management programs can be beneficial in most patients.

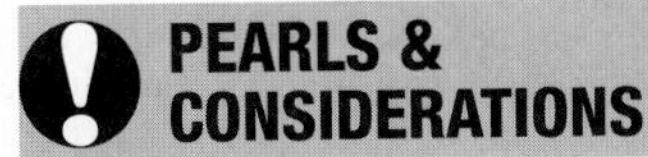

PEARLS & CONSIDERATIONS

PREVENTION

Avoid loud, chronic noise and ototoxic drugs.

PATIENT & FAMILY EDUCATION

- American Tinnitus Association: 800-634-8978, http://www.ata.org

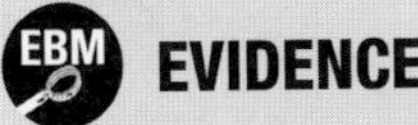

EVIDENCE

available at www.expertconsult.com

SUGGESTED READINGS

available at www.expertconsult.com

RELATED CONTENT

Tinnitus (Patient Information)

AUTHORS: **VICKY BHAGAT, M.D.**, and **DAWN HOGAN, M.D.**

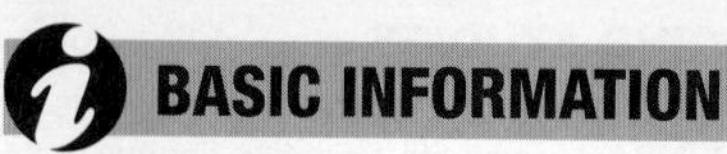

BASIC INFORMATION

DEFINITION

The term *torsades de pointes* (TdP) refers to a polymorphic ventricular tachycardia (VT) associated with a prolonged QT interval and electrocardiographically characterized by QRS complexes of changing amplitude that appear to twist around the isoelectric line, hence the name *torsades de pointes*, or "twisting of the points" (Fig. 1-949).

The torsades can be typical when initiated following short-long-short coupling intervals or can be the rarer short-coupled variant initiated by normal short coupling. Typical features of TdP include a markedly prolonged QT interval >500 msec in the beats preceding the onset of the arrhythmia, a polymorphic VT with a ventricular rate of 160 to 250 beats per minute, irregular RR intervals, and a cycling of the QRS axis through 180 degrees every 5 to 20 beats. The TdP typically starts with premature ventricular contractions (PVCs) discharging during the termination of the long T-wave and precipitate successive bursts of VT with the typical twisting appearance of progressive changes in QRS contour and amplitude. It maybe repetitive, nonsustained, or sustained, and may degenerate into ventricular fibrillation.

SYNONYM(S)

Torsades
TdP

ICD-9CM CODES
429.1 Ventricular tachycardia
ICD-10-CM CODE(S)
I47.2 Ventricular tachycardia

EPIDEMIOLOGY & DEMOGRAPHICS

INCIDENCE: In congenital long QT syndromes (LQTS), TdP may occur in up to 6% cases at rest and 9% of cases during an exercise test. Among drug-induced causes of Tdp, the incidence may vary between <1% in cases of antibiotics and antipsychotics to 2%-4% when caused by class III anti-arrhythmics such as sotalol, ibutilide, and dofetilide. The incidence during intracranial events such as subarachnoid hemorrhage may be as high as 8% if associated with hypokalemia.

PREDOMINANT SEX AND AGE: Women, perhaps due to a longer baseline QT interval, are at greater risk for torsades than men

GENETICS: If the torsades is due to underlying congenital LQTS, two patterns of inheritance have been identified: the more common autosomal-dominant Romano-Ward and Timothy syndromes, and the much rarer autosomal recessive cases. The latter are usually more severe, often but not always involving consanguineous marriages, and are often associated with congenital deafness (the Jervell Lange-Nielsen syndrome). Mutations in 8 genes have been identified.

RISK FACTORS: TdP in patients with congenital LQTS is often initiated by an external trigger (Table 1-482). Triggers can include exercise, noise, emotion, sudden waking from sleep by an alarm clock, telephone ringing, thunder, swimming, or diving. TdP in LQT1 patients is usually triggered by exercise and swimming, and noise; LQT2 by emotion, pregnancy, or noise; and LQT3 when at rest or asleep. Risk factors for drug-induced TdP are outlined in Table 1-483. Drug-induced TdP is equally common in the hospital setting vs that caused by outpatient drugs, and the risk factors for developing TdP in hospitalized patients are outlined in Table 1-484.

PATHOPHYSIOLOGY:

- The electrophysiological mechanisms responsible for torsades are not clearly understood. Most data suggest that early after depolarization are responsible for the initiation of torsades. Perpetuation may be caused by transmural entry, triggered activity, or abnormal automaticity. A distinct group of cells called the M cells, located in the mid-myocardium, have prolonged repolarization and may play a role in the genesis of TdP.
- Drugs with the potential to cause TdP most frequently inhibit the rapid potassium channels and result in prolongation of the action potential duration, producing a prolonged QT on ECG.

PHYSICAL FINDINGS & CLINICAL PRESENTATION

- Clinical features depend on whether the TdP is caused by acquired or congenital long QT syndrome. Congenital LQTS patients may have certain specific triggers, such as noise, exercise, and emotions (see "Risk Factors").
- Symptoms of the tachycardia itself include palpitations, syncope, presyncope, seizures, and sudden cardiac death (SCD).
- Patients resuscitated from SCD have an especially ominous prognosis, with a relative risk of 12.9 of experiencing another cardiac arrest.

ETIOLOGY

The etiology or triggers of TdP maybe congenital or acquired causes of QT prolongation (see Table 1-482). For a comprehensive list of drugs that can cause or have the potential to cause torsades de pointes, see "Patient/Family Education."

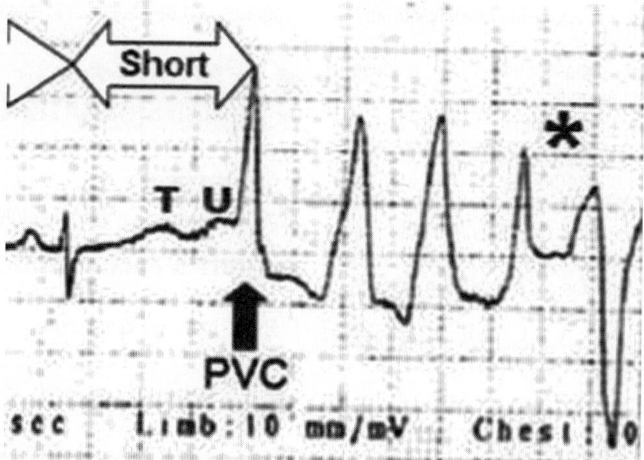

FIGURE 1-949 Onset of TdP during the recording of a standard 12-lead ECG in a young male with a history of drug addiction treated with chronic methadone therapy who presented to a hospital emergency department after ingesting an overdose of prescription and over-the-counter drugs from his parent's drug cabinet. Classic ECG features evident in this rhythm strip include a prolonged QT interval with distorted T-U complex, initiation of the arrhythmia after a short-long-short cycle sequence by a PVC that falls near the peak of the distorted T-U complex, "warm-up" phenomenon with initial R-R cycles longer than subsequent cycles, and abrupt switching of QRS morphology from predominantly positive to predominantly negative complexes *(asterisk)*. (From Drew BJ et al: Prevention of torsade de pointes in hospital settings: a scientific statement from the American Heart Association and the American College of Cardiology Foundation, *J Am Coll Cardiol* 55;934-947, 2010.)

DIAGNOSIS

DIFFERENTIAL DIAGNOSIS

Other causes of broad complex tachycardia such as:

- Polymorphic VT
- Wolff-Parkinson-White (WPW) syndrome with atrial fibrillation
- SVT with aberrancy
- ECG artifact

WORKUP

- ECG and telemetry are the mainstay of diagnosing TdP as they detect the arrhythmia, the preceding prolonged QT interval, and the long-short cycles that trigger it.
- Determination and treatment of the etiology of TdP (see Table 1-482) is key .

LABORATORY TESTS

- Electrolytes
- Thyroid function tests
- Genetic studies if suspicion of congenital LQT syndrome
- Troponin to rule out myocardial infarction

TABLE 1-482 Causes and Triggers of Torsades de Pointes

Congenital	• Romano-Ward syndrome [autosomal dominant] • Jervell Lange-Nielsen syndrome [autosomal recessive] • LQTS channelopathies
Acquired	
Metabolic syndromes	• Hypokalemia • Hypocalcemia • Hypomagnesemia • Starvation • Anorexia nervosa • Liquid protein diets • Hypothyroidism
Bradyarrhythmias	• Sinus node dysfunction • Second- or third-degree AV block
Antiarrhythmic drugs	• Quinidine • Procainamide • Disopyramide • Amiodarone and dronedarone • Sotalol • Dofetilide, ibutilide, azimilide
Antimicrobial drugs	• Erythromycin, clarithromycin, azithromycin • Pentamidine • Azole antifungals like voriconazole • Fluoroquinolones such as levofloxacin & moxifloxacin • Chloroquine
Antihistaminics	• Terfenadine • Astemizole
Psychiatric drugs	• Phenothiazines • Thioridazine • Tricyclic antidepressants • Haloperidol • Risperidone • Selective serotonin reuptake inhibitors
Antineoplastic agents	• Tyrosine kinase inhibitors such as sunitinib, dasatinib • Vorinostat • Arsenic
Gastric motility agents	• Cisapride, domperidone
Opioid dependence drugs	• Methadone
Other factors	• Myocardial ischemia • Hypothermia • Intracranial disease • HIV infection • Connective tissue disease with anti-Ro/SSA antibodies • Periodic paralysis (Andersen syndrome) • Cocaine

TABLE 1-483 Risk Factors for Drug-Induced Torsades de Pointes

- Congenital long QT
- Female gender
- Electrolyte abnormalities (hypokalemia, hypomagnesemia, hypocalcemia)
- Diuretic use
- Bradycardia
- Cardiac hypertrophy
- Myocardial fibrosis
- Congestive heart failure
- Renal and liver insufficiency
- Coadministration of drugs blocking P450 isoenzyme CYP3A4
- High doses or rapid intravenous infusion of the drug
- Baseline electrocardiographic abnormalities (prolonged QT, T-wave lability)

From Gowda RM et al: Torsades des points: the clinical considerations, *Int J Cardiol* 96(1):1-6, 2004.

TABLE 1-484 Risk Factors for Torsade de Pointes in Hospitalized Patients

- Clinically recognizable risk factors
- QTc >500 msec
- LQT2-type repolarization: notching
- Use of QT-prolonging drugs
- Concurrent use of more than one QT-prolonging drug
- Rapid infusion by intravenous route
- Heart disease
- Congestive heart failure
- Myocardial infarction
- Advanced age
- Female sex
- Hypokalemia
- Hypomagnesemia
- Hypocalcemia
- Treatment with diuretics
- Impaired hepatic drug metabolism
- Bradycardia
- Sinus bradycardia, heart block, incomplete heart block with pauses
- Premature complexes leading to short-long-short cycles
- Multiple clinically recognizable risk factors
- Clinically silent risk factors
- Occult (latent) congenital LQTS
- Genetic polymorphisms

From Drew BJ et al: Prevention of torsade de pointes in hospital settings: a scientific statement from the American Heart Association and the American College of Cardiology Foundation, *Circulation* 121(8):1047, 2010.

IMAGING STUDIES

- Echocardiography to rule out structural heart disease as a cause of VT
- Stress test to rule out myocardial ischemia. Stress ECG may sometimes unmask underlying long QT syndromes and related TdP
- CT scan of the head if intracranial disease is suspected

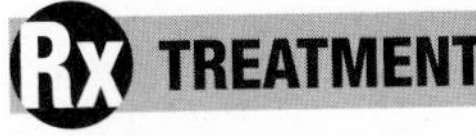

TREATMENT

The cornerstone of treatment comprises intravenous magnesium, overdrive pacing, and isoproterenol. Withdrawal of causative drugs and correction of underlying causes such as electrolyte imbalances, hypothermia, ischemia, and so on is also key

NONPHARMACOLOGIC THERAPY

- Withdrawal of any offending drugs and correction of electrolyte abnormalities are recommended in patients presenting with torsades de pointes (Class I recommendation).
- Temporary atrial or ventricular overdrive pacing is a Class I recommendation for all causes of TdP if intravenous magnesium fails.
- Acute and long-term pacing is recommended for patients presenting with TdP due to heart block and symptomatic bradycardia (Class 1) or those with recurrent pause-dependent torsades (Class IIa)
- Active internal and external rewarming if hypothermia is the etiology
- If TdP degenerates into ventricular fibrillation, defibrillation and advanced cardiac life support protocol should be followed

ACUTE GENERAL Rx

- Intravenous magnesium sulfate 1-2 g given over 1-2 min is first-line therapy for patients who present with LQTS and few episodes of torsades de pointes (Class IIa). Magnesium is not likely to be effective in patients with a normal QT interval
- Isoproterenol is reasonable as temporary treatment in patients with acute disease who present with recurrent pause-dependent TdP and who do not have congenital LQTS (Class IIa).
- Beta-blockade combined with pacing is reasonable acute therapy for patients who present with TdP and sinus bradycardia (Class IIa).
- Potassium repletion to 4.5 to 5 mmol/L may be considered for patients who present with torsades de points (Class IIb).

- Intravenous lidocaine, oral mexiletine, or phenytoin may be considered in patients who present with LQT3 and torsades de pointes (Class IIb).

CHRONIC Rx

- TdP resulting from congenital LQTS is treated with beta-blockade, pacing, and implantable cardioverter-defibrillator (ICD) in high-risk cases. For patients who continue to have syncope despite maximal drug therapy, cervical-thoracic sympathectomy may be considered.
- Long-term pacing is recommended for patients presenting with TdP due to heart block and symptomatic bradycardia.
- Avoid use of QT-prolonging drugs.
- Lifestyle modification in case of congenital LQTS.
- In patients with eating disorders, nutritional rehabilitation will correct the QT prolongation over the long term (3 to 18 mo).
- Psychiatric evaluation of patients with drug overdose and eating disorders.

DISPOSITION

Patients with TdP should be monitored in an intensive care setting.

REFERRAL

Patients should have an urgent cardiology consultation.

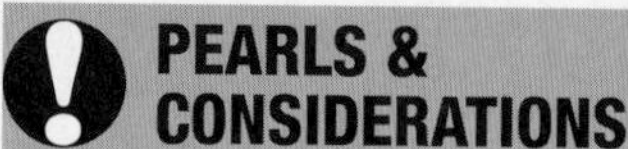

PEARLS & CONSIDERATIONS

COMMENTS

- Identification of the etiology for TdP is key in diagnosis, management, and prognosis of this condition.
- Drugs associated with TdP vary greatly in their risk for arrhythmia; an updated list can be found at www.qtdrugs.org. The risk-benefit ratio should be assessed for each individual to determine whether the potential therapeutic benefit of a drug outweighs the risk for TdP.
- Risk factors for drug-induced TdP include older age, female sex, heart disease, electrolyte disorders (especially hypokalemia and hypomagnesemia), renal or hepatic dysfunction, bradycardia or rhythms with long pauses, treatment with more than one QT-prolonging drug, and genetic predisposition.
- After initiation of a drug associated with TdP, ECG signs indicative of risk for arrhythmia include an increase in QTc from predrug baseline of >60 msec, marked QTc interval prolongation >500 msec, T-U wave distortion that becomes more exaggerated in the beat after a pause, visible T-wave alternans, new-onset ventricular ectopy, and couplets and nonsustained polymorphic ventricular tachycardia initiated in the beat after a pause.

PREVENTION

The 2011 AHA/ACC scientific statement on prevention of TdP suggests a strategy of documenting the QTc interval before and at least every 8 to 12 hr after the initiation, increased dose, or overdose of QT-prolonging drugs. If QTc prolongation is observed, documentation of more frequent measurements is recommended. The duration of QTc monitoring depends upon the duration of treatment with the QT-prolonging drug and the drug half-life.

PATIENT/FAMILY EDUCATION

- Patients should be educated about avoiding use of QT-prolonging drugs. A complete list of these drugs can be found at www.qtdrugs.org or at http://www.azcert.org/medical-pros/drug-lists/drug-lists.cfm.
- First-degree relatives of all patients with congenital LQTS should undergo genetic testing.
- Congenital LQTS patients should avoid certain specific triggers (e.g., swimming and exercise in LQTS 1 and LQTS 2 and acoustic stimuli in LQTS 2)
- It is recommended that all patients affected by LQTS avoid competitive sports activity

RELATED TOPICS

Long QT Syndrome (Related Key Topic)

AUTHOR: **GAGAN SAHNI, M.D., F.A.C.C., F.A.C.P.**

BASIC INFORMATION

DEFINITION

Torticollis is a contraction or contracture of the muscles of the neck that causes the head to be tilted to one side. It is usually accompanied by rotation of the chin to the opposite side with flexion (Fig. 1-950). Usually it is a symptom of some underlying disorder. This term is often used incorrectly in cases when the torticollis may simply be positional.

SYNONYMS

Twisted neck
"Wry neck"
Spasmodic torticollis

ICD-9CM CODES

723.5 Spastic (intermittent) torticollis
754.1 Congenital muscular (sternocleidomastoid)
333.83 Spasmodic

ICD-10CM CODES

M43.6 Torticollis
Q68.0 Congenital deformity of sternocleidomastoid muscle
G24.3 Spasmodic torticollis

PHYSICAL FINDINGS & CLINICAL PRESENTATION

- Congenital muscular torticollis:
  1. Palpable soft tissue "mass" in the sternocleidomastoid shortly after birth
  2. Mass gradually subsides, leaving a shortened, contracted sternocleidomastoid muscle
  3. Head characteristically tilted toward the side of the mass and rotated in the opposite direction
  4. Facial asymmetry and other secondary changes persisting into adulthood
- Spasmodic torticollis:
  1. "Spasms" in the cervical musculature; may be bilateral and uncontrollable
  2. Head often tilted toward the affected side
- Findings in other cases depend on etiology

ETIOLOGY

Torticollis has been found to have more than 50 different causes:

- Localized fibrous shortening of unknown cause involving the sternocleidomastoid, leading to the condition termed *congenital muscular torticollis*
- Spasmodic torticollis: of uncertain etiology, possibly a variant of dystonia musculorum deformans
- Infection, specifically pharyngitis, tonsillitis, retropharyngeal abscess
- Miscellaneous rare causes: congenital musculoskeletal deformities, trauma, inflammation from rheumatoid arthritis, vestibular disturbances, posterior fossa tumor, syringomyelia, neuritis of spinal accessory nerve, and drug reactions

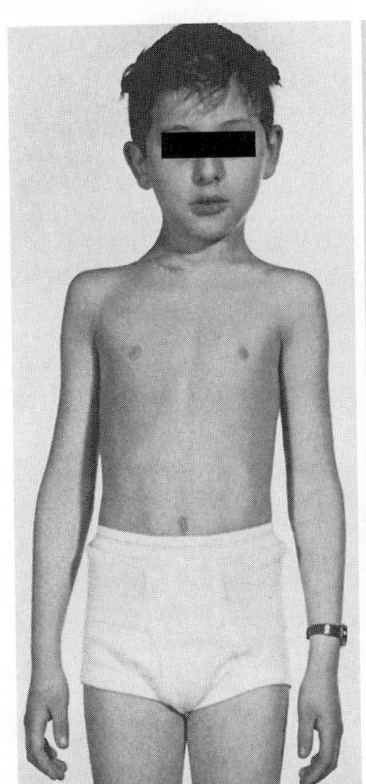

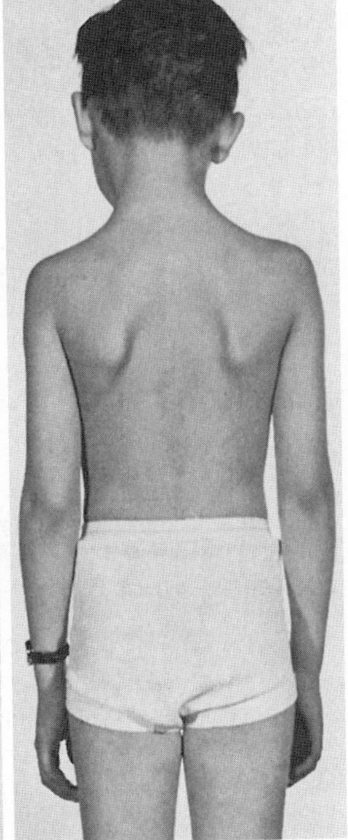

FIGURE 1-950 Torticollis. In this child, the right sternocleidomastoid muscle is contracted. (From Brinker MR, Miller MD: *Fundamentals of orthopaedics,* Philadelphia, 1999, Saunders.)

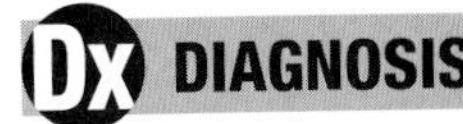

DIAGNOSIS

DIFFERENTIAL DIAGNOSIS

- Usually involves separating each disorder from the others
- Acquired positional disorders (e.g., ocular disturbances, acute disk herniation)

WORKUP

- Workup depends on the clinical situation.
- Laboratory studies are usually not helpful unless infection or rheumatoid disease is suspected.
- Section II describes a differential diagnosis for the evaluation and therapy of neck pain.
- Any child with a gradually increasing torticollis should have a complete eye examination.

IMAGING STUDIES

- Plain radiographs in cases of trauma or to rule out congenital abnormalities
- MRI in appropriate cases
- Electrodiagnostic studies: only rarely indicated to rule out neurologic causes

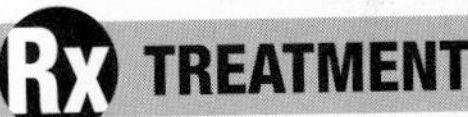

TREATMENT

- Congenital muscular torticollis: gentle stretching exercises carried out by the parent
- Spasmodic torticollis: physical therapy, psychotherapy, cervical braces, biofeedback, and pain control
- Focal dystonia responds well to injections of botulinum toxin type A or B.
- Other forms: treated according to etiology

DISPOSITION

- Most patients with congenital muscular torticollis respond well to conservative treatment.
- Spasmodic torticollis is often resistant to normal conservative treatment.
- Prognosis of other forms of torticollis depends on etiology.

REFERRAL

- Torticollis often requires a multidisciplinary approach unless the etiology is obvious.
- Children usually do not require any specific studies; however, an orthopedic consultation is recommended.
- Fixed deformity in the child; may need orthopedic referral for surgical release.

SUGGESTED READINGS

available at www.expertconsult.com

RELATED CONTENT

Torticollis (Patient Information)

AUTHOR: **LONNIE R. MERCIER, M.D.**

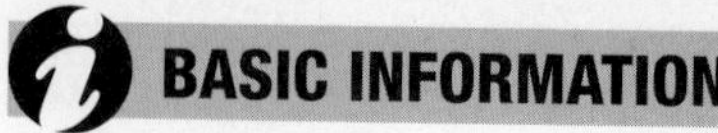

BASIC INFORMATION

DEFINITION

Tics are sudden, brief, intermittent involuntary or semi-voluntary movements (motor tics) or sounds (phonic or vocal tics) that mimic fragments of normal behavior.

Tourette's syndrome (TS) is an inherited neuropsychiatric disorder characterized by motor, vocal, and phonic tics that change during the course of illness. Onset is typically before age 18 (new-onset tics can occasionally occur after age 18 yr, but for DSM-IV criteria of TS, they must begin before this age).

SYNONYMS

Gilles de la Tourette syndrome
TS
Tourette's disorder

ICD-9CM CODES
307.23 Gilles de la Tourette disorder
ICD-10CM CODES
F95.2 Combined vocal and multiple motor tic disorder [de la Tourette]

EPIDEMIOLOGY & DEMOGRAPHICS

PREVALENCE (IN U.S.): Unknown; estimates range from 0.7% to 5%
PREDOMINANT SEX: Approximate male/female ratio of 3:1
PREDOMINANT AGE: Typical age of onset is between 2 and 15 yr (mean 5 to 7 yr)

PHYSICAL FINDINGS & CLINICAL PRESENTATION

- Neurologic examination is normal.
- Vocal and/or phonic tics could be simple (clearing of throat, sniffing, grunting or sucking sounds) or complex (repetitive short phrases, e.g., "you bet," swearing [coprolalia]).
- Motor tics can be simple (e.g., blinking, grimacing, head jerking) or complex (e.g., gesturing). Tics wax, wane, and change over time. Often they can be suppressed for short periods. Commonly they are preceded by an urge to perform the tic.
- TS is often associated with a variety of behavioral symptoms, most commonly attention deficit hyperactivity disorder (ADHD) and obsessive-compulsive disorder (OCD).

TS can be diagnosed using the DSM-5 criteria as follows:

1. Both multiple motor and one or more vocal tics must be present at some time during the illness, although not necessarily concurrent.
2. The tics may wax and wane in frequency but have persisted for more than 1 year since first tic onset
3. Age at onset is <18 yr.
4. Disturbance is not attributable to the direct physiologic effects of a substance (e.g., stimulants) or a general medical condition (e.g., Huntington's disease or postviral encephalitis).

ETIOLOGY

Exact pathogenesis is unknown. Genetic predisposition is likely as there is a strong family history of OCD or TS in patients with tics, and twin studies provide evidence for the importance of genetic factors. Recent analysis of linkage in a two-generation pedigree has led to the identification of a mutation in the HDC gene encoding l-histidine decarboxylase, the rate-limiting enzyme in histamine biosynthesis, pointing to a role for histaminergic neurotransmission in the mechanism and modulation of Tourette's syndrome and tics. Immunologic dysfunction is being explored in the pathogenesis of this complex disorder.

Dx DIAGNOSIS

DIFFERENTIAL DIAGNOSIS

- Sydenham's chorea: occurs after infection with group A *Streptococcus*
- PANDAS: pediatric autoimmune neuropsychiatric disorder associated with streptococcal infection
- Sporadic tic disorders: tend to be motor or vocal but not both
- Head trauma
- Drug intoxication: many drugs are known to induce or exacerbate tic disorder, including methylphenidate, amphetamines, pemoline, anticholinergics, and antihistamines
- Postinfectious encephalitis
- Inherited disorders: Huntington's disease, Hallervorden-Spatz disease, and neuroacanthocytosis. All these conditions should have other observed abnormalities on neurologic examination.

WORKUP

Clinical observation and history to confirm diagnosis

LABORATORY TESTS

No definitive laboratory tests

IMAGING STUDIES

CT scan and MRI of brain are normal and unnecessary in the absence of abnormal neurologic examination.

Rx TREATMENT

NONPHARMACOLOGIC THERAPY

Multidisciplinary: education of parents, teachers, psychologists, and school nurses is essential. Cognitive behavioral therapy termed habit-reversal treatment is efficacious in suppressing tics

ACUTE GENERAL Rx

Dopamine-blocking agents may be used to reduce severity of tics acutely (e.g., haloperidol 0.25 mg PO qhs initially). There are risks of side effects, such as acute dystonic reactions.

CHRONIC Rx

Tics only require treatment when they interfere with psychosocial, educational, and occupational functioning of a person.

TICS:

- Alpha-2 agonists like clonidine and guanfacine are used for treatment of motor tics and are considered by some experts as first-line medications because of their favorable adverse effect profile. However, they are more beneficial for treatment of behavioral symptoms and should be preferred for patients with predominant psychiatric problems.
- Haloperidol and pimozide are the only neuroleptics that are approved by U.S. FDA for the treatment of tics in TS. Pimozide is started as 0.5-1.0 mg at night and increased every 5 to 7 days to therapeutic dose of 2-8 mg. Haloperidol is started as 0.25-0.5 mg and can be increased to 1-4 mg depending on response and side effects. Use of neuroleptics carries a small but significant risk of tardive dyskinesia.
- Tetrabenazine: dopamine-depleting agent can be used effectively in TS patients for control of tics. It does not cause many of the typical side effects of the neuroleptics but is not readily available. Severe depression may occur with use of this medication.
- Dopamine agonists: a few small, open-label studies have found that ropinirole and pramipexole in low doses may be effective in reducing tic severity.
- Botulinum toxin local injection is effective for focal tics like eye blinking and neck and shoulder tics. The benefits are temporary, lasting 3 to 6 mo.
- Surgical treatment with deep brain stimulation has also been reported effective in some patients with disabling tics that are refractory to medications.

ADHD:
Stimulants (dextroamphetamine, methylphenidate) are useful for symptoms of ADHD but may exacerbate tics in 25% of patients, but should be used if troublesome behavioral symptoms persist.
OCD:
Selective serotonin reuptake inhibitors, such as fluoxetine, are the most effective.

DISPOSITION

- In the later teen years, intensity and frequency of tics typically diminish.
- One third of patients will achieve significant remission, although complete, lifelong remission is rare.
- One third will have mild, persistent, but "non-impairing" tics.

REFERRAL

To a neurologist to confirm initial diagnosis and for treatment in difficult cases

PEARLS & CONSIDERATIONS

- Tics do not need treatment unless they interfere with an individual's ability to function.
- Greater improvement in symptom severity among children with Tourette's and chronic tic disorder has been reported with a comprehensive behavioral intervention compared with supportive therapy and education.

- An important part of treatment is appropriate evaluation and therapy of coexisting conditions (e.g., ADHD, OCD).
- Deep brain stimulation (DBS) has shown some promising results as an alternative therapy in patients with medically refractory disease.

COMMENTS

Patient education may be obtained from the Tourette's Syndrome Association, 4240 Bell Blvd., Bayside, NY 11361-2864; 800-237-0717 or 718-224-2999; http://www.tsa-usa.org.

SUGGESTED READINGS

available at www.expertconsult.com

RELATED CONTENT

Tourette's Syndrome (Patient Information)

AUTHOR: **FARIHA ZAHEER, M.D.**

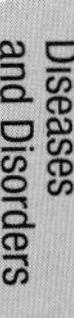

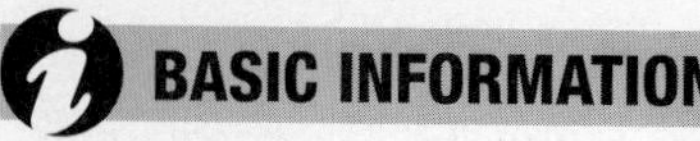

BASIC INFORMATION

DEFINITION

Toxic shock syndrome (TSS) is an acute febrile illness resulting in multiple organ system dysfunction caused most commonly by a bacterial exotoxin. Disease characteristics also include hypotension, vomiting, myalgia, watery diarrhea, vascular collapse, and an erythematous sunburnlike cutaneous rash that desquamates during recovery.

SYNONYMS

TSS

ICD-9CM CODES
040.89 Toxic shock syndrome
ICD-10CM CODES
A48.3 Toxic shock syndrome

EPIDEMIOLOGY & DEMOGRAPHICS

- Case reported incidence peak: 14 cases per 100,000 menstruating women annually in 1980; has since fallen to one case per 100,000 persons
- Occurs most commonly between ages 10 and 30 yr in healthy, young, menstruating white females
- Case fatality ratio of 3%

PHYSICAL FINDINGS & CLINICAL PRESENTATION

- Fever (>38.0° C)
- Diffuse macular erythrodermatous rash that involves both skin and mucous membranes, resembles sunburn, and also involves the palms and soles. The rash then desquamates 1 to 2 wk after disease onset in survivors
- Orthostatic hypotension
- Gastrointestinal symptoms: vomiting, diarrhea, abdominal tenderness
- Constitutional symptoms: myalgia, headache, photophobia, rigors, altered sensorium, conjunctivitis, arthralgia
- Respiratory symptoms: dysphagia, pharyngeal hyperemia, strawberry tongue
- Genitourinary symptoms: vaginal discharge, vaginal hyperemia, adnexal tenderness
- End-organ failure
- Severe hypotension and acute renal failure
- Hepatic failure
- Cardiovascular symptoms: disseminated intravascular coagulation, pulmonary edema, acute respiratory distress syndrome (ARDS), endomyocarditis, heart block

ETIOLOGY

- Menstruation-associated TSS: 45% of cases associated with tampons, diaphragm, or vaginal sponge use.
- Non–menstruation-associated TSS: 55% of cases associated with puerperal sepsis, post–cesarean section endometritis, mastitis, sinusitis, wound or skin infection, septorhinoplasty, pelvic inflammatory disease, respiratory infections following influenza, enterocolitis, and burns.
- Causative agent: *Staphylococcus aureus* infection of a susceptible individual (10% of population lacking sufficient levels of antitoxin antibodies), which liberates the disease mediator TSST-1 (exotoxin). While most cases are caused by methicillin-susceptible *S. aureus* (MSSA), cases of TSS from methicillin-resistant *S. aureus* (MRSA) have occurred, particularly those due to the more virulent community-associated MRSA strains.
- *S. aureus* exotoxins are superantigens that can activate large numbers of T cells (up to 20% at one time) resulting in a massive cytokine production: interleukin (Il-1), Il-2, TNF, and interferon gamma that then mediate the signs and symptoms of the disease.
- Other causative agents: coagulase-negative streptococci producing enterotoxins B or C, and exotoxin A–producing group A beta-hemolytic streptococci.

Dx DIAGNOSIS

DIFFERENTIAL DIAGNOSIS

- Staphylococcal food poisoning
- Septic shock
- Mucocutaneous lymph node syndrome
- Scarlet fever
- Rocky Mountain spotted fever
- Meningococcemia
- Toxic epidermal necrolysis
- Kawasaki syndrome
- Leptospirosis
- Legionnaires' disease
- Hemolytic-uremic syndrome
- Stevens-Johnson syndrome
- Scalded skin syndrome
- Erythema multiforme
- Acute rheumatic fever

WORKUP

Broad-spectrum syndrome with multiorgan system involvement and variable but acute clinical presentation, including the following:

- Fever (>38° C)
- Classic desquamating rash (1 to 2 wk)
- Hypotension/orthostatic systolic blood pressure ≤90 mm Hg
- Syncope
- Negative throat and cerebrospinal fluid cultures
- Negative serologic test for Rocky Mountain spotted fever, rubeola, and leptospirosis
- Clinical involvement of three or more of the following:
  - Cardiopulmonary: ARDS, pulmonary edema, endomyocarditis, second- or third-degree atrioventricular block
  - Central nervous system: altered sensorium without focal neurologic findings
  - Hematologic: thrombocytopenia (platelets <100,000)
  - Liver: elevated liver function test results
  - Renal: >5 cells/high-power field, negative urine cultures, azotemia, and increased creatinine (double normal)
  - Mucous membrane involvement: vagina, oropharynx, conjunctiva
  - Musculoskeletal: myalgia, creatine phosphokinase twice normal
  - Gastrointestinal: vomiting, diarrhea

LABORATORY TESTS

- Pan culture (cervix and vagina, throat, nasal passages, urine, blood, cerebrospinal fluid, wound) for *Staphylococcus, Streptococcus* (Table 1-485), and other pathogenic organisms
- Electrolytes to detect hypokalemia, hyponatremia
- Complete blood count with differential and clotting profile for anemia (normocytic or normochromic), thrombocytopenia, leukocytosis, coagulopathy, and bacteremia
- Chemistry profile to detect decreased protein, increased aspartate aminotransferase, increased alanine aminotransferase, hypocalcemia, elevated blood urea nitrogen and creatinine, hypophosphatemia, increased lactate dehydrogenase, increased creatine phosphokinase
- Urinalysis to detect white blood cells (>5 cells/high-power field), proteinemia, microhematuria
- Arterial blood gases to assess respiratory function and acid-base status
- Serologic tests considered for Rocky Mountain spotted fever, rubeola, and leptospirosis

TABLE 1-485 Staphylococcal versus Streptococcal Toxic Shock Syndrome

Feature	Staphylococcal	Streptococcal
Age	Primarily 15-35 yr	Primarily 20-50 yr
Gender	Higher frequency in women	Men and women equally affected
Severe pain	Rare	Common
Hypotension	100%	100%
Erythroderma rash	Very common	Less common
Renal failure	Common	Common
Bacteremia	Low frequency	60%
Tissue necrosis	Rare	Common
Predisposing factors	Tampons, surgery	Cuts, burns, varicella
Thrombocytopenia	Common	Common
Mortality rate	<3%	30%-70%

From Mandell GL et al: *Principles and practice in infectious diseases*, ed 7, Philadelphia, 2008, Churchill Livingstone.

IMAGING STUDIES

- Chest x-ray examination to evaluate pulmonary edema
- ECG to evaluate arrhythmia
- Sonography, CT scan, or MRI considered if pelvic abscess or tubo-ovarian abscess suspected

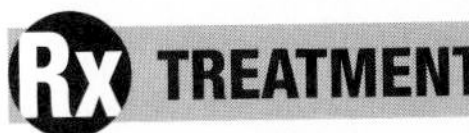

TREATMENT

NONPHARMACOLOGIC THERAPY

- For optimal outcome: high index of suspicion and early and aggressive supportive management in an ICU setting
- Aggressive fluid resuscitation (maintenance of circulating volume, cardiac output, systolic blood pressure)
- Thorough search for a localized infection or nidus: incision and drainage, debridement, removal of tampon or vaginal sponge
- Central hemodynamic monitoring, Swan-Ganz catheter, and arterial line for surveillance of hemodynamic status and response to therapy
- Foley catheter to monitor hourly urine output
- Possible military antishock trousers as temporary measure
- Acute ventilator management if severe respiratory compromise
- Renal dialysis for severe renal impairment
- Surgical intervention for indicated conditions (i.e., ruptured tubo-ovarian abscess, wound abscess, mastitis)

ACUTE GENERAL Rx

- Isotonic crystalloid (normal saline solution) for volume replacement following "7-3" rule (refers to the response in millimeters of mercury [mm Hg] of the pulmonary artery wedge pressure to volume replacement).
- Electrolyte replacement (K^+, C^+)
- Packed red blood cells, coagulation factor replacement, fresh frozen plasma to treat anemia or dilation and curettage.
- Vasopressor therapy for hypotension refractory to fluid volume replacement (e.g., dopamine beginning at 2 to 5 μg/kg/min)
- Steroids have been used but are not generally recommended due to lack of evidence of benefit.
- It is not clear whether antibiotics alter the course of acute TSS. Most authors recommend that patients receive 10 to 14 days of combination antibiotic therapy. In staphylococcal TSS, effective agents are clindamycin (900 mg IV every 8 hr in adults or 25 to 40 mg/kg per day in children) plus vancomycin (adults: 30 mg/kg per day IV in two divided doses; children: 40 mg/kg per day IV in four divided doses). Oxacillin or nafcillin sodium (2 g IV every 4 hr in adults; children: 100 to 150 mg/kg per 24 hr divided in four doses) can be used instead of vancomycin if TSS due to MSSA. An alternative to vancomycin is linezolid.
- In streptococcal TSS, effective agents are penicillin G 24 million units/day in divided doses *plus* clindamycin 900 mg IV q8h. Alternative agents are ceftriaxone 2 g IV q24h *plus* clindamycin 900 mg IV q8h.
- Broad-spectrum antibiotic including gram-negative coverage added if concurrent sepsis suspected with TSS.
- Intravenous immune globulin (IVIG): while no controlled trials exist, most authors recommend IVIG (400 mg/kg in a single dose administered over several hours) in severe cases of TSS that are not responding to fluids or vasopressors. It may neutralize superantigen and decrease tissue damage.
- Tetracycline added if considering Rocky Mountain spotted fever.

CHRONIC Rx

- Severely ill patient: may require prolonged hospitalization and supportive management with gradual recovery and/or sequelae from severe end-organ involvement (ARDS or renal failure requiring dialysis)
- Majority of patients: complete recovery
- Early-onset complications (within 2 wk):
  - Skin desquamation
  - Impaired digit sensation
  - Denuded tongue
  - Vocal cord paralysis
  - Acute tubular necrosis
  - ARDS
- Late-onset complications (after 8 wk):
  - Nail splitting and loss
  - Alopecia
  - Central nervous system sequelae
  - Renal impairment
  - Cardiac dysfunction
- Recurrent TSS:
  - More common in menstruation-related cases.
  - Less common in patients treated with beta-lactamase–resistant antistaphylococcal antibiotics.
  - Patients with history of TSS: if suspect signs and symptoms occur, have high index of suspicion and low threshold for evaluation and treatment.
  - Screen for nasal carriage of *S. aureus* in patients with *S. aureus* TSS and treat with mupirocin in those with positive cultures.

PREVENTION

- Avoidance of tampons or use of low-absorbency tampons only (<4 hr in situ) and alternate with napkins
- Education for patients concerning signs and symptoms of TSS
- Avoidance of tampons for patients with history of TSS

DISPOSITION

- Complete recovery for most patients
- Long-term management of early- and late-onset complications for minority of patients

REFERRAL

- For multidisciplinary management, involving primary physician, gynecologist, internist, infectious disease specialist, and other supportive care specialists
- To tertiary-level hospital

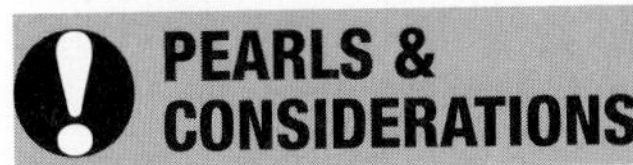

PEARLS & CONSIDERATIONS

COMMENTS

Patient information is available from American College of Gynecologists and Obstetricians.

SUGGESTED READINGS

available at www.expertconsult.com

RELATED CONTENT

Toxic Shock Syndrome (Patient Information)

AUTHOR: **GLENN G. FORT, M.D., M.P.H.**

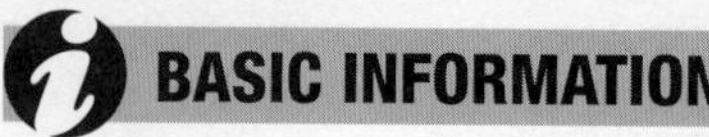

BASIC INFORMATION

DEFINITION

Toxoplasmosis is an infection caused by the protozoal parasite *Toxoplasma gondii.*

ICD-9CM CODES
130.9 Toxoplasmosis
ICD-10CM CODES
B58.9 Toxoplasmosis, unspecified

EPIDEMIOLOGY & DEMOGRAPHICS

INCIDENCE (IN U.S.):
- 3% to >50% of healthy adults (seroprevalence)
- Increases with age
- Increases with certain activities
  1. Slaughterhouse workers
  2. Cat owners
- Increases with certain geographic locations: high prevalence of cats

PREDOMINANT SEX: Equal gender distribution
PREDOMINANT AGE:
- Infancy (congenital infection)
- Prevalence increases with age

PEAK INCIDENCE: Temperate climates
GENETICS: Congenital infection: 400 to 4000 cases/yr in the U.S.
- Incidence and severity vary with the trimester of gestation during which the mother acquired infection.
  1. 10% to 25% (first trimester)
  2. 30% to 54% (second trimester)
  3. 60% to 65% (third trimester)
- Congenital infection occurring in the first trimester is the most severe.
- 89% to 100% of infections in the third trimester are asymptomatic.
- Risk to the fetus is not correlated with symptoms in the mother.

PHYSICAL FINDINGS & CLINICAL PRESENTATION

- Acquired (immunocompetent host)
  1. 80% to 90% asymptomatic
  2. Adenopathy (usually cervical)
  3. Fever
  4. Myalgias
  5. Malaise
  6. Sore throat
  7. Maculopapular rash
  8. Hepatosplenomegaly
  9. Chorioretinitis rare
- Acquired (in patients with AIDS, CD4 count <100)
  1. 89% of symptomatic cases
     a. Encephalitis
     b. Intracerebral mass lesions
  2. Pneumonitis
  3. Chorioretinitis
  4. Other end organ
- Acquired (immunocompromised patients)
  1. Encephalitis
  2. Myocarditis (especially in heart transplant patients)
  3. Pneumonitis
- Ocular infection in the immunocompetent host
  1. Congenital infection
  2. Blurred vision
  3. Photophobia
  4. Pain
  5. Loss of central vision if macula involved
  6. Focal necrotizing retinitis
  7. Typically presents in second or third decade
- Congenital
  1. Results from acute infection acquired by the mother within 6 to 8 wk before conception or during gestation
  2. Usually, asymptomatic mother
  3. No sign of disease
  4. Chorioretinitis
  5. Blindness
  6. Epilepsy
  7. Psychomotor or mental retardation
  8. Intracranial calcifications
  9. Hydrocephalus
  10. Microcephaly
  11. Encephalitis
  12. Anemia
  13. Thrombocytopenia
  14. Hepatosplenomegaly
  15. Lymphadenopathy
  16. Jaundice
  17. Rash
  18. Pneumonitis
  19. Most infected infants are asymptomatic at birth

ETIOLOGY

- *Toxoplasma gondii*
  1. Ubiquitous intracellular protozoan
  2. Present worldwide
  3. Cat is definitive host (Fig. E1-951)
- Human infection
  1. Ingestion of oocysts shed by cats in soil, litter boxes, vegetables
  2. Ingestion of inadequately cooked meat containing tissue cysts
  3. Vertical transmission

Dx DIAGNOSIS

DIFFERENTIAL DIAGNOSIS

- Lymphadenopathy
  1. Infectious mononucleosis
  2. Cytomegalovirus (CMV) mononucleosis
  3. Cat-scratch disease
  4. Sarcoidosis
  5. Tuberculosis
  6. Lymphoma
  7. Metastatic cancer
- Cerebral mass lesions in immunocompromised host
  1. Lymphoma
  2. Tuberculosis
  3. Bacterial abscess
- Pneumonitis in immunocompromised host
  1. *Pneumocystis jirovecii (carinii)* pneumonia
  2. Tuberculosis
  3. Fungal infection
- Chorioretinitis
  1. Syphilis
  2. Tuberculosis
  3. Histoplasmosis (competent host)
  4. CMV
  5. Syphilis
  6. Herpes simplex
  7. Fungal infection
  8. Tuberculosis (AIDS patient)
- Myocarditis
  1. Organ rejection in heart transplant recipients
- Congenital infection
  1. Rubella
  2. CMV
  3. Herpes simplex
  4. Syphilis
  5. Listeriosis
  6. Erythroblastosis fetalis
  7. Sepsis

WORKUP

- Acute infection, immunocompetent host
  1. CBC
  2. *Toxoplasma* serology (IgG, IgM) in serial blood specimens 3 wk apart
  3. Lymph node biopsy if diagnosis uncertain
- Immunocompromised host
  1. CNS symptoms
     a. Cerebral CT scan or MRI if CNS symptoms present
     b. Spinal tap, if safe
     c. Brain biopsy if no response to empiric therapy
  2. Ocular symptoms
     a. Funduscopic examination
     b. Serologic studies
     c. Rarely, vitreous tap
  3. Pulmonary symptoms
     a. Chest x-ray examination
     b. Bronchoalveolar lavage
     c. Transbronchial or open-lung biopsy
  4. Myocarditis
     a. Cardiac enzymes
     b. Electrocardiogram
     c. Endomyocardial biopsy for definitive diagnosis
- Toxoplasmosis in pregnancy
  1. Initial maternal screening with IgM and IgG
     a. If negative, mother at risk of acute infection and should be retested monthly
     b. If both IgG and IgM positive, obtain IgA and IgE ELISA, AC/HS test
     c. IgA and IgE ELISA, AC/HS test elevated in acute infection
     d. Ig high for 1 yr or more
     e. IgG repeated 3 to 4 wk later to determine if titer is stable
  2. Acute maternal infection not excluded or documented
     a. Fetal blood sampling (for culture, Ig, IgA, IgE)
     b. Amniotic fluid polymerase chain reaction (PCR)
  3. Fetal ultrasound every other wk if maternal infection documented
- Congenital toxoplasmosis
  1. Placental histology
  2. Specific IgM or IgA in infant's blood

LABORATORY TESTS

- Antibody studies
  1. More than one test necessary to establish diagnosis of acute toxoplasmosis
  2. IgM antibody
     a. Appears 5 days into infection
     b. Peaks at 2 wk

c. Falls to low level or disappears within 2 mo
d. May persist at low levels for 1 yr or more
3. Antibody not measurable
  a. Ocular toxoplasmosis
  b. Reactivation
  c. Immunocompromised hosts
4. IgA ELISA, IgE ELISA, and IgE ASAGA
  a. More sensitive tests
  b. Disappear more rapidly than Ig, establishing diagnosis of acute infection
5. IgG antibody
  a. Appears 1 to 2 wk after infection
  b. Peaks at 6 to 8 wk
  c. Gradually declines over months to years

IMAGING STUDIES

- Chest x-ray if pulmonary involvement suspected
- Cerebral CT scan (Fig. 1-952) or MRI if encephalitis suspected

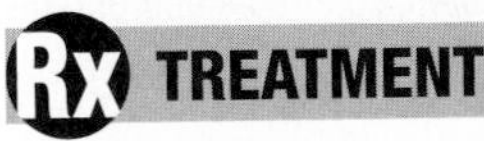

TREATMENT

NONPHARMACOLOGIC THERAPY

- Selected cases of ocular infection
  1. Photocoagulation
  2. Vitrectomy
  3. Lentectomy
- Selected cases of congenital cerebral infection
  1. Ventricular shunting

ACUTE GENERAL Rx

- Acute infection, immunocompetent host
  1. No treatment, unless severe and persistent symptoms or vital organ damage
- Acute infection, immunocompromised host, non-AIDS
  1. Treat even if asymptomatic

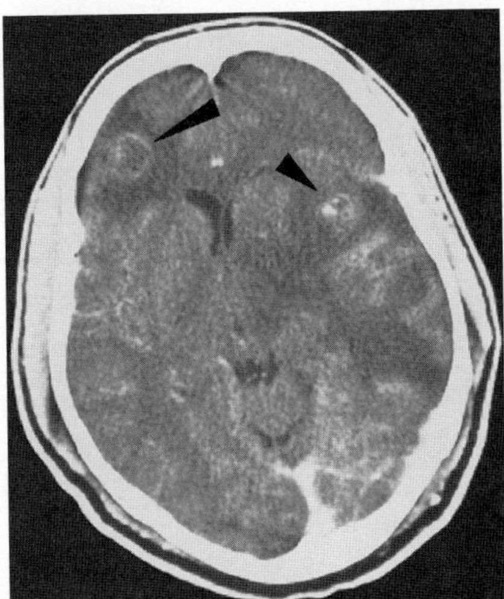

FIGURE 1-952 Toxoplasmic encephalitis in person who has AIDS. A cranial CT scan shows bilateral contrast-enhanced ring lesions with peripheral edema and mass effect. (From Cohen J, Powderly WG: *Infectious diseases,* ed 2, St Louis, 2004, Mosby.)

  2. Duration
    a. Until 4 to 6 wk after resolution of all signs and symptoms
    b. Usually 6 mo or longer
- Reactivated infection, immunocompromised host, non-AIDS
  1. Treat if symptomatic
- Acute or reactivated infection, AIDS
  1. Treat in all cases
  2. Induction course
    a. 3 to 6 wk.
    b. Maintenance therapy continued for life; consider discontinuation of suppressive therapy if the patient has a good response to antiretroviral therapy and if the CD4 count remains >200 cells/mm^3 for more than 3 mo.
  3. Empiric therapy
    a. AIDS with positive IgG
    b. Multiple ring-enhancing lesions on cerebral CT scan or MRI
    c. Response seen by day 7 in 71% and day 14 in 91%
- Ocular infection
  1. Treat in all cases
  2. Therapy continued for 1 mo or longer if needed
  3. Response seen in 70% within 10 days
  4. Retreat as needed
  5. Steroids may be indicated in patients with signs or symptoms of increased intracranial pressure
  6. Surgical treatment in selected cases
- Treatment regimens
  1. Pyrimethamine 200 mg loading dose once PO, then 50 mg (<60 kg) to 75 mg (>60 kg) q day; plus
  2. Leucovorin 10 to 20 mg PO qid, plus
  3. Sulfadiazine 1 (<60 kg) to 1.5 g (>60 kg) PO q6h

Other treatment options (if sulfa hypersensitivity or allergy is present): pyrimethamine 50 to 75 mg/day PO with leucovorin 10 to 20 mg/day PO and either (1) clindamycin 600 mg q6h PO or IV (up to 1200 mg IV) q6h, or (2) clarithromycin 1 g PO bid, or (3) dapsone 100 mg/day PO, or (4) atovaquone 750 mg PO q6h.

- Acute infection in pregnancy
  1. Treat immediately
  2. Risk of fetal infection reduced by 60% with treatment
    a. First trimester
      i. Spiramycin 3 g PO qid in two to four divided doses
      ii. Sulfadiazine 4 g PO qid in four divided doses
    b. Second and third trimester
      i. Sulfadiazine as previously described, *plus*
      ii. Pyrimethamine 25 mg PO qid, *plus*
      iii. Leucovorin 5 to 15 mg PO qid
      iv. Spiramycin as previously described
- Congenital infection
  1. Sulfadiazine 50 mg/kg PO bid, *plus*
  2. Pyrimethamine 2 mg/kg PO for 2 days, then 1 mg/kg PO, three times weekly, *plus*
  3. Leucovorin 5 to 20 mg PO three times weekly
  4. Minimum duration of treatment: 12 mo

CHRONIC Rx

Maintenance therapy in AIDS patients because of the high risk (80%) of relapse
1. Pyrimethamine 25 mg PO qid
2. Sulfadiazine 500 mg PO qid
3. Leucovorin 10 to 20 mg PO qid

DISPOSITION

- Prognosis
  1. Excellent in the immunocompetent host
  2. Good in ocular infection (although relapses are common)
- Treatment of acute infection in pregnancy
  1. Reduces incidence and severity of congenital toxoplasmosis
- Treatment of congenital infection
  1. Improvement in intellectual function
  2. Regression of retinal lesions
- AIDS
  1. 70% to 95% response to therapy

REFERRAL

- To infectious disease expert:
  1. Immunocompromised hosts
  2. Pregnant women
  3. Difficulty in making a diagnosis or deciding on treatment
- To pediatric infectious disease expert:
  1. Congenital infection
- To obstetrician:
  1. Pregnant seronegative mother
  2. Acute seroconversion
- To ophthalmologist:
  1. Congenital infection
  2. Any case of ocular infection

PEARLS & CONSIDERATIONS

COMMENTS

- Prevention of toxoplasmosis is most important in seronegative pregnant women and immunocompromised hosts.
- Patient instructions:
  1. Cook meat to 66° C.
  2. Cook eggs.
  3. Do not drink unpasteurized milk.
  4. Wash hands thoroughly after handling raw meat.
  5. Wash kitchen surfaces that come in contact with raw meat.
  6. Wash fruits and vegetables.
  7. Avoid contact with materials potentially contaminated with cat feces.

SUGGESTED READINGS

available at www.expertconsult.com

RELATED CONTENT

Toxoplasmosis (Patient Information)

AUTHOR: **PHILIP A. CHAN, M.D., M.S.**

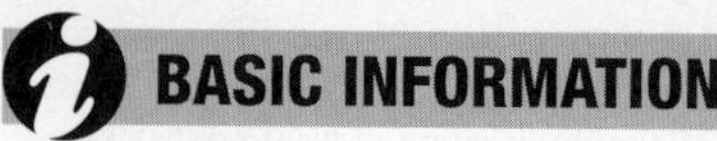

BASIC INFORMATION

DEFINITION

Acute hemolytic transfusion reaction (AHTR) is acute intravascular hemolysis caused by mismatches in the ABO system. It is caused by complement-fixing immunoglobulin (Ig) and IgG antibodies to group A and B red blood cells. Hemolytic transfusion reactions can also be caused by minor antigen systems; however, they are usually less severe. In delayed serologic transfusion reactions, hemolysis with hemoglobinemia is unusual; in delayed reactions the only manifestations may be the development of a newly positive Coombs test and fever. The clinical severity of an ABO-incompatible blood transfusion is significantly influenced by the degree of complement activation and cytokine stimulation.

SYNONYMS

AHTR

Acute hemolytic transfusion reaction

ICD-9CM CODES

999.8 Other transfusion reaction

ICD-10CM CODES

T80.9 Unspecified complication following infusion, transfusion and therapeutic injection

T80.3 ABO incompatibility reaction

T80.4 Rh incompatibility reaction

T80.8 Other complications following infusion, transfusion, and therapeutic injection

EPIDEMIOLOGY & DEMOGRAPHICS

- Acute intravascular hemolysis occurs in one to five per 50,000 transfusions.

PHYSICAL FINDINGS & CLINICAL PRESENTATION

- Hypotension
- Pain at the infusion site
- Fever, tachycardia, chest pain, dyspnea, dizziness, bronchospasm
- Lower back pain due to ischemic muscle pain or vasospasm rather than kidney pain from developing renal failure
- Severe reactions often occur in surgical patients under anesthesia who are unable to give any warning signs.

See Table 1-486.

ETIOLOGY

Most fatal hemolytic reactions are caused by clerical errors and mislabeled specimens.

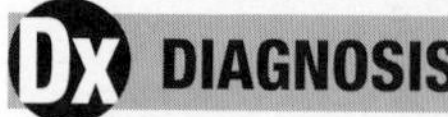

DIAGNOSIS

DIFFERENTIAL DIAGNOSIS

- Bacterial contamination of blood
- Hemoglobinopathies

WORKUP

The transfusion must be stopped immediately. The blood bank must be notified, and the donor transfusion bag must be returned to the blood bank along with a freshly drawn posttransfusion specimen.

LABORATORY TESTS

- Positive Coombs test, elevated BUN, creatinine, LDH, bilirubin (especially indirect bilirubin).
- Analyze urine for hemoglobinuria (wine-colored urine), observe plasma for hemoglobinemia (pink plasma).
- Decreased hematocrit and serum haptoglobin (haptoglobin low to 0 mg/dl).
- The direct antiglobulin test (DAT) usually becomes positive in an immune hemolytic reaction (if tested before all the incompatible RBCs are destroyed). Preparation of an antibody eluate is necessary to identify the offending antibody.
- Monitor coagulation status (PT, aPTT, fibrinogen).

TREATMENT

NONPHARMACOLOGIC THERAPY

- Stop transfusion immediately. Test anticoagulated blood from the recipient for the presence of free hemoglobin in the plasma.
- Monitor vital signs closely, and maintain IV access and adequate airway.

ACUTE GENERAL Rx

- Treatment is supportive and consists of fluid resuscitation, vasopressor support, and mannitol.
- Vigorous IV hydration (0.9% NaCl or some other suitable crystalloid solution) to maintain urine flow at >100 ml/hr until hypotension is corrected and hemoglobinuria clears. IV furosemide may be necessary to maintain adequate renal flow.
- The addition of mannitol may prevent renal damage (controversial). Mannitol, if chosen, must be used with caution; if acute tubular necrosis occurs before mannitol infusion, pulmonary edema may occur as a result of the acute increase in intravascular volume secondary to fluid expansion.
- Monitor for the presence of disseminated intravascular coagulation. PT, aPTT, and fibrinogen levels should be closely monitored.
- If sepsis is suspected, culture as appropriate.

DISPOSITION

Mortality rate exceeds 50% in severe transfusion reactions.

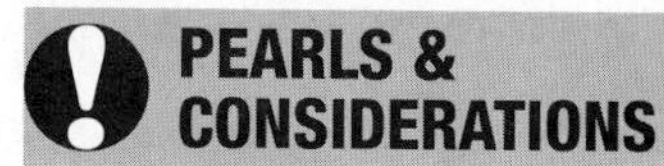

PEARLS & CONSIDERATIONS

COMMENTS

Hemolysis caused by minor antigen systems is generally less severe and may be delayed 5 to 10 days after transfusion.

SUGGESTED READINGS

available at www.expertconsult.com

AUTHOR: **FRED F. FERRI, M.D.**

TABLE 1-486 Signs and Symptoms of Acute Adverse Reactions to Blood Transfusion

Reaction	Fever	Chills/ Rigors	Nausea/ Vomiting	Chest Discomfort/ Pain	Facial Flushing	Wheezing/ Dyspnea	Back/ Lumbar Pain	Discomfort at Infusion Site	Hypotension
Acute hemolytic	X	X	X	X	X	X	X	X	X
Febrile nonhemolytic	X	X		X	X				
Nonimmune hemolysis									
Acute lung injury	X			X		X			X
Allergic									
Massive transfusion complications									
Anaphylaxis	X	X	X	X	X	X	X	X	X
Passive cytokine infusion	X	X	X			X			
Hypervolemia						X			
Bacterial sepsis	X	X	X				X	X	X
Air embolus				X		X			

From Goldman L, Bennett JC (eds): *Cecil textbook of medicine*, ed 22, Philadelphia, 2004, Saunders.

BASIC INFORMATION

DEFINITION

Transient ischemic attack (TIA) is a transient episode of neurologic dysfunction caused by focal brain, spinal cord, or retinal ischemia without acute infarction on MRI. TIA symptoms typically resolve within 60 min and almost always within 24 hr.

SYNONYMS

TIA
Amaurosis fugax
"Mini-stroke"
Pre-stroke

ICD-9CM CODES
435.9 Unspecified transient cerebral ischemia
ICD-10CM CODES
G45.9 Transient cerebral ischemic attack, unspecified

EPIDEMIOLOGY & DEMOGRAPHICS

INCIDENCE: 49 to 83 cases per 100,000 persons annually
PEAK INCIDENCE: After age 60 yr
PREVALENCE: 200,000 to 500,000 persons in the United States
PREDOMINANT SEX AND RACE: Males > females; African American > Caucasian
RISK FACTORS: Same as for ischemic stroke

PHYSICAL FINDINGS & CLINICAL PRESENTATION

TIAs often present with ipsilateral transient monocular blindness (amaurosis fugax), contralateral numbness or weakness, contralateral homonymous hemianopsia, and/or aphasia.

ETIOLOGY

Embolic (cardioembolism in 10% to 15%), large vessel atherothrombotic disease (20% to 25%), lacunar disease, hypoperfusion, hypercoagulable state, arteritis

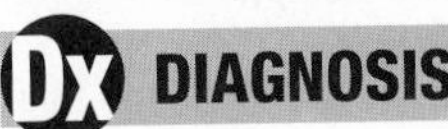

DIAGNOSIS

DIFFERENTIAL DIAGNOSIS

Seizures, hypoglycemia, complicated migraine, intracranial hemorrhage, mass lesion, vestibular disease, Bell's palsy, meningitis, multiple sclerosis, subdural hematoma, brain abscess, cervical or lumbar spine disease, conversion disorder

WORKUP

Given the high risk of stroke within the first 48 hr following TIA (up to 10%), hospital admission for workup is advised. Fig E1-953 describes a TIA algorithm. The American Heart Association recommends that the ABCD2 score be used in the evaluation of TIA. It consists of 1 point for age ≥60 years, 1 point for BP ≥140 mm Hg systolic or ≥90 mm Hg diastolic, clinical features (2 points for unilateral weakness, 1 point for speech impairment), duration of TIA (2 points for duration ≥60 min, 1 point for duration 10-59 min), presence of diabetes mellitus (1 point). According to the guidelines, it is reasonable to hospitalize patients with TIA if they present within 72 hours and have an $ABCD^2$ score ≥3. There is some debate about the usefulness of this scale since it fails to account for changes seen on echocardiogram, carotid Dopplers, or ECG that may place the patient at more imminent risk of stroke (carotid stenosis, Afib, cardiac thrombus, etc). Alternatives to this scoring system are being investigated.

LABORATORY TESTS

Complete blood count, basic metabolic panel, prothrombin time, activated partial thromboplastin time, sedimentation rate, fasting lipid panel, serum glucose and hemoglobin A_{1c} (to detect latent diabetes mellitus)

IMAGING STUDIES

- CT scan should be obtained to exclude hemorrhage; MRI with diffusion weighting if immediately available.
- Imaging of the vessels should be obtained via magnetic resonance angiography (MRA), computed tomography angiography (CTA), or carotid Dopplers/transcranial Dopplers (CD/TCD).
  - If symptoms are referable to the posterior circulation, MRA or CTA should be obtained in lieu of CD/TCD.
  - Transthoracic echocardiogram should be obtained.
  - An echocardiogram with bubble should be obtained in all patients younger than 50 yr with TIA symptoms.
- Electrocardiogram should be obtained to exclude the presence of arrhythmias, namely atrial fibrillation.
- At least 24 hr of heart rhythm monitoring should be accomplished to screen for arrhythmia.

TREATMENT

NONPHARMACOLOGIC THERAPY

- Carotid endarterectomy or carotid stenting should be considered for patients found to have carotid stenosis as the cause for TIA. Please refer to "Carotid Stenosis" chapter for more information.
- Intracranial angioplasty and stenting may be considered in cases of symptomatic intracranial atherosclerosis. Clinical trials are ongoing.

ACUTE GENERAL Rx

- In the absence of contraindications, patients who are identified to have atrial fibrillation should be considered for anticoagulation with intravenous heparin (or therapeutic lovenox) along with warfarin until target INR between 2.0 and 3.0 is achieved.
- Although no compelling evidence exists for the use of heparin in the acute treatment of TIAs without cardioembolic source, patients who develop recurrent symptoms within the same vascular territory that increase in duration, severity, and/or frequency (crescendo TIA/stuttering TIA) may benefit from its use.

CHRONIC Rx

- Chronic therapy should be aimed at modifying the four major risk factors: hypertension, dyslipidemia, diabetes mellitus, and smoking cessation.
- Antiplatelet therapy should be used to reduce the risk of recurrent TIAs or subsequent stroke. Three antiplatelet agents are commonly used in stroke prevention: aspirin, aspirin/dipyridamole, and clopidogrel. All are reasonable choices but practitioners should consider their individual patient's comorbidities when selecting an antiplatelet agent.
- Dose-adjusted warfarin (INR 2.0 to 3.0) is indicated for prevention of future strokes in atrial fibrillation patients. The direct thrombin inhibitor dabigatran and the direct factor Xa inhibitors apixaban and rivaroxaban have been approved as alternative treatments to warfarin for stroke prevention in atrial fibrillation.

PEARLS & CONSIDERATIONS

- Despite complete symptom resolution, 20% to 50% of patients with TIA have evidence of acute tissue infarction on MRI.
- Dual antiplatelet therapy in acute TIA and minor stroke is being evaluated. A recent trial revealed that among patients with TIA or minor stroke who can be treated within 24 hr after the onset of symptoms, the combination of clopidogrel and aspirin is superior to aspirin alone for reducing the risk of stroke in the first 90 days and does not increase the risk of hemorrhage.[1]

PREVENTION

A healthy lifestyle and management of cardiovascular risk factors should be encouraged.

PATIENT/FAMILY EDUCATION

Patients should be counseled on the early signs of stroke symptoms and instructed to promptly seek medical attention if they develop symptoms concerning for stroke. Patients should be encouraged to pursue a healthy lifestyle to include exercise and smoking cessation. In addition, patients should take an active role in controlling blood pressure and blood glucose. Further educational materials can be found online at http//www.strokecenter.org/education.

SUGGESTED READINGS

available at www.expertconsult.com

RELATED CONTENT

Transient Ischemic Attack (TIA) (Patient Information)

AUTHOR: **JOSEPH R. OWENS, M.D.**

[1]Wang Y et al: Clopidogrel with aspirin in acute minor stroke or transient ischemic attack, *N Engl J Med* 369:11-19, 2013.

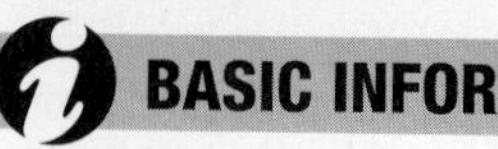

BASIC INFORMATION

DEFINITION

Demyelination in a transverse region of the spinal cord due to an inflammatory process that leads to sensory and motor changes below the lesion. The pathologic hallmark of transverse myelitis is the presence of focal collections of lymphocytes and monocytes with varying degrees of demyelination, axonal injury, and astroglial and microglial activation within the spinal cord.

SYNONYMS

None

ICD-9CM CODES

341.2 Acute (transverse) myelitis
323.82 Other causes of myelitis, transverse myelitis NOS
341.2 Acute (transverse) myelitis

ICD-10CM CODES

G37.3 Acute transverse myelitis in demyelinating disease of central nervous system
G04.89 Other myelitis

EPIDEMIOLOGY & DEMOGRAPHICS

INCIDENCE: Annual incidence ranges from 1.3 to 8 cases per million. The incidence increases to 24.6 cases per million annually if acquired demyelination causes such as multiple sclerosis (MS) are included.
PREVALENCE: Unknown
PREDOMINANT SEX: None
GENETICS: No genetic predisposition has been shown.
PEAK INCIDENCE: Bimodal peak in the incidence between 10 to 19 yr and 30 to 39 yr
RISK FACTORS: Infection, vaccination

PHYSICAL FINDINGS & CLINICAL PRESENTATION

- The clinical signs are caused by an interruption in ascending and descending neuroanatomic pathways in the transverse plane of the spinal cord, and a resulting sensory level is characteristic of transverse myelitis.
- Rapid onset of symmetric or asymmetric paraparesis or paraplegia of the lower extremities over a few days, ascending paresthesia, trunk sensory level, back pain, sphincter dysfunction, and positive Babinski with upgoing toes bilaterally. The arms may also be involved but less than the legs in most cases.
- One third to one half of patients present with localizing back pain.
- There is progression to nadir of clinical deficits between 4 hr and 21 days after symptom onset.
- Urinary incontinence or retention, GI disturbances (incontinence or constipation), and sexual dysfunction are common.

ETIOLOGY

- Demyelination due to the body's immune response to infection, post-vaccination, multiple sclerosis, or idiopathic (15% to 30% of cases).
- An autoantibody to aquaporin 4 has been identified in transverse myelitis secondary to NMO.
- About 50% of patients have had a recent upper respiratory infection.
- Epstein-Barr virus and cytomegalovirus are most common viral infections.
- Hepatitis B, varicella, enterovirus, rhinovirus, mycoplasma, syphilis, measles, Lyme disease are less common.

DIAGNOSIS

DIFFERENTIAL DIAGNOSIS

- MS
- Neuromyelitis optica (NMO)
- Tumor of spinal cord
- Herniated or slipped discs
- Spinal stenosis
- Abscess
- Vascular malformation

WORKUP

- Transverse myelitis should be suspected in patients with a history of rapid (hours to days) onset of motor weakness and sensory abnormalities with bladder or bowel dysfunction that is referable to the spinal cord. The dysfunction is bilateral (not necessarily symmetric) and there is a clearly defined sensory (dermatomal) level.
- Lumbar puncture looking for oligoclonal bands for MS or infection.
- Magnetic resonance imaging (MRI) of brain and MRI of spine at level of suspected involvement (Fig. E1-954).
- Computed tomography (CT) if MRI is unavailable; may use myelography with CT.

LABORATORY TESTS

- ANA, hepatitis B serology, Lyme disease titer, VDRL
- Cerebrospinal fluid (CSF) may show increased protein/normal protein, lymphocytes, and normal glucose.
- Serum NMO-IgG to evaluate for neuromyelitis optica.

IMAGING STUDIES

- MRI shows demyelinating lesion on T_2 with contrast enhancement.
- Chest and joint radiology
- CT or PET scan as indicated by history and examination

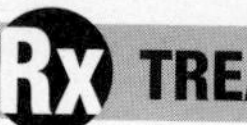

TREATMENT

Corticosteroids are the first-line treatment for transverse myelitis; IVIG and plasma exchange can be considered in intractable cases, although there is no evidence-based medicine for use of corticosteroids, plasma exchange, or IVIG. A referral to a neurologist is recommended for treatment.

NONPHARMACOLOGIC THERAPY

- Physical therapy
- Respiratory and oropharyngeal support

ACUTE GENERAL Rx

- High-dose IV corticosteroid (e.g., methylprednisolone 1000 mg/day for 3 to 5 days)
- Rescue therapy with plasma exchange may be helpful in patients who do not respond to corticosteroids
- Combination therapy with plasmapheresis and immunosuppressive agents (e.g., cyclophosphamide) may also be effective
- Naproxen, ibuprofen for pain

CHRONIC Rx

- Baclofen, tizanidine, or some other muscle relaxant for muscle spasms
- Gabapentin for pain
- Low-molecular-weight heparin for DVT prophylaxis in patients with immobility

DISPOSITION

- One third of patients with transverse myelitis will have complete recovery, one third will have fair recovery, and one third have permanent disability and do not recover. Recurrence or relapse are possible.
- Patients who need further care including urinary retention may need home nursing assistance. Some patients may benefit from a rehabilitation, either inpatient or outpatient.

REFERRAL

- Consider physical therapy.
- Consider occupational therapy.
- Consider rehab services.
- Consider psychiatric consultation (high incidence of long-term mood and anxiety disorders).

SUGGESTED READINGS

available at www.expertconsult.com

AUTHOR: **SHARLISA WALLER HUTSON, M.D.**

BASIC INFORMATION

DEFINITION

Trigeminal neuralgia is an intense, usually unilateral, paroxysmal, stabbing pain in the sensory distribution of the fifth cranial nerve.

SYNONYMS

Tic douloureux ("painful tics/spasms")

ICD-9CM CODES
350.1 Trigeminal neuralgia
ICD-10CM CODES
G50.0 Trigeminal neuralgia

EPIDEMIOLOGY & DEMOGRAPHICS

INCIDENCE: 4 per 100,000

PEAK INCIDENCE: Incidence increases with age and peaks at 67 yr; onset in 90% of patients is after age 40.

PREVALENCE: 155 in 1 million

PREDOMINANT SEX AND AGE: Male/female ratio is 1:1.5.

RISK FACTORS: Most cases are idiopathic; age and multiple sclerosis are risk factors.

PHYSICAL FINDINGS & CLINICAL PRESENTATION

- Patients present with paroxysmal, unilateral facial pain that is usually described as shock-like, stabbing, or electric (Fig. 1-959).
- Pain can be spontaneous or triggered by touch, an air current, or activities such as shaving, eating, or brushing teeth.
- In severe cases, facial spasms can accompany the pain.
- Pain is usually described in distribution of the second (V2-maxillary) and third (V3-mandibular) divisions of the trigeminal nerve.
- The pain seldom lasts more than a few seconds to a minute.
- There is usually no sensory or motor loss.

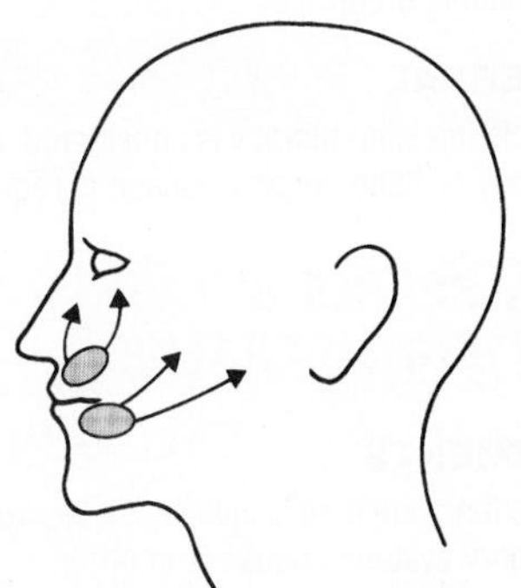

FIGURE 1-959 Trigeminal neuralgia. The two most common sites of origin and radiation of pain are shown: mouth-ear and nose-orbit. Pain usually starts in the region of the encircled area and radiates in the directions shown. (From Souhami RL, Moxham J: *Textbook of medicine,* ed 4, London, 2002, Churchill Livingstone.)

ETIOLOGY

- Idiopathic or "classic": cause usually unknown, likely an aberrant artery or vein compressing cranial nerve V at or near the pons
- Secondary: caused by nonvascular lesions such as a demyelinating plaque from multiple sclerosis, compression from meningioma, arachnoid cyst, etc.
- Box 1-93 summarizes causes of trigeminal neuralgia

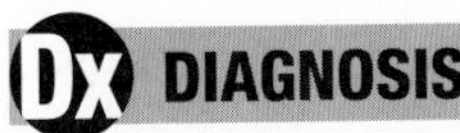

DIAGNOSIS

DIFFERENTIAL DIAGNOSIS

- Glossopharyngeal neuralgia
- Temporomandibular joint pain
- Unilateral, neuralgiform headache
- Postherpetic neuralgia
- Dental pain

WORKUP

Trigeminal neuralgia is a clinical diagnosis (see above).

IMAGING STUDIES

Neuroimaging (MRI/magnetic resonance angiogram [MRA]) should be considered in young patients with atypical symptoms (sensory loss, bilateral symptoms).

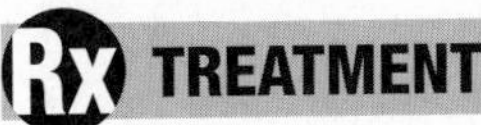

TREATMENT

NONPHARMACOLOGIC THERAPY

Patients with refractory pain eventually need secondary intervention such as nerve root decompression, selective nerve fiber destruction (rhizotomy), glycerol injection, thermal lesioning, chemical ablation, or gamma knife radiosurgery.

BOX 1-93 Causes of Tic Douloureux

Vascular compression by an artery or vein
Saccular aneurysm
Arteriovenous malformation
Vestibular schwannomas
Meningioma
Epidermoid cyst
Tumor
Primary demyelinating disorders
- Multiple sclerosis
- Charcot-Marie-Tooth disease (rare)

Infiltrative disorders
- Trigeminal amyloidoma

Nondemyelinating lesions
- Small infarct or angioma in the brainstem

Familial

From Adams JG et al: *Emergency medicine, clinical essentials*, ed 2, Philadelphia, 2013, Elsevier.

CHRONIC Rx

- Carbamazepine 100 to 200 mg bid is the recommended initial treatment. This can be titrated to pain relief by 200 mg daily to a maximum of 1200 mg divided bid.
- Oxcarbazepine can be used if carbamazepine is not tolerated due to side effects. Other medications include baclofen, gabapentin, clonazepam, levetiracetam, lamotrigine, and phenytoin.
- Drug combinations can be tried when one medication is partially effective prior to proceeding with secondary intervention.
- In the elderly population, caution should be used when initiating and titrating the above medications. Caution and extensive counseling should also be used in women of child-bearing age when initiating treatment with antiseizure medications.

DISPOSITION

- Most patients are responsive to pharmacologic treatment. Spontaneous remission is possible.
- Medical management is ineffective in 30% of patients.

REFERRAL

Referral to a neurologist is appropriate if there is uncertainty about diagnosis or if symptoms are refractory to conservative management.

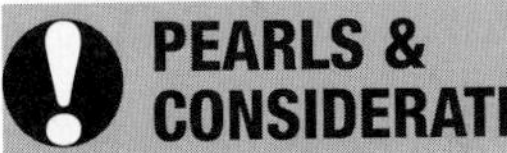

PEARLS & CONSIDERATIONS

In secondary disease, no medications have been established for treatment. Initial therapy should address underlying secondary causes. In a young patient with trigeminal neuralgia, secondary causes such as multiple sclerosis should be considered.

SUGGESTED READINGS

available at www.expertconsult.com

RELATED CONTENT

Trigeminal Neuralgia (Patient Information)

AUTHOR: **WILLIAM F. DOTSON II, M.D.**

BASIC INFORMATION

DEFINITION

Trigger finger, or digital stenosing tenosynovitis, refers to an inflammatory process of the digital flexor tendon sheath that can lead to nodule formation of the flexor tendon. These changes lead to pain and difficulty or inability to extend the digit due to inability of the flexor tendon to glide through the A1 pulley.

SYNONYMS

Digital stenosing tenosynovitis

ICD-9CM CODES
727.03 Trigger finger (acquired)
ICD-10CM CODES
M65.30 Trigger finger, unspecified finger

EPIDEMIOLOGY & DEMOGRAPHICS

In adults, the middle finger is most often affected (Fig. 1-960). In children, the thumb is most often affected.

PREDOMINANT SEX AND AGE: Female/male ratio of 4:1. Trigger finger can be found in all age groups but is commonly found in patients aged >45 yr.

RISK FACTOR: Repetitive use occupations, such as meat cutters, seamstresses, tailors, and dentists.

PHYSICAL FINDINGS & CLINICAL PRESENTATION

- Tenosynovitis of the flexor tendon always precedes the mechanical symptoms of triggering, resulting in pain over the flexor tendon with palpation, passive stretching, or resisting flexion isometrically.
- A palpable tender nodule is noted at palmar aspect of the metacarpophalangeal (MCP) joint of the affected digit.
- Painful triggering or snapping with flexion of the affected digit.
- Locking or loss of active digital extension.
- The digit can be fixed in flexion (trapped or incarcerated).
- Usually affects one digit. If more digits are involved, a systemic cause is most likely present (e.g., diabetes, rheumatoid arthritis).

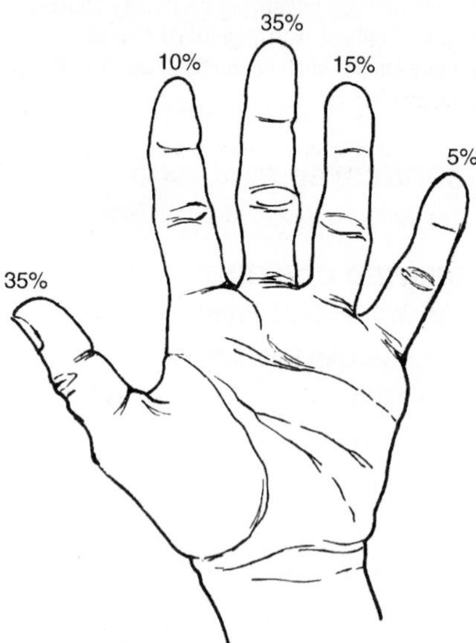

FIGURE 1-960 Trigger finger. Frequency of trigger finger according to digit in adults. In children, virtually all cases occur in the thumb. (From Canoso J: *Rheumatology in primary care,* Philadelphia, 1997, Saunders.)

ETIOLOGY

Trigger finger is described as being primary or secondary:

- Primary (idiopathic)
- Secondary
  - Diabetes
  - Rheumatoid arthritis
  - Hypothyroidism
  - Histiocytosis
  - Amyloidosis
  - Gout

DIAGNOSIS

Clinical history and physical examination

DIFFERENTIAL DIAGNOSIS

- Dupuytren's contracture
- De Quervain's tenosynovitis
- Acute digital tenosynovitis
- Proliferative tenosynovitis
- Ulnar collateral ligament injury (gamekeeper's thumb)
- Carpal tunnel syndrome
- Flexor tendon rupture
- MCP osteoarthritis

WORKUP

Pursued if a secondary cause is suspected

LABORATORY TESTS

- Complete blood count with differential
- Electrolytes, blood urea nitrogen, creatinine
- Blood glucose, Hb_{A1c}
- Thyroid function tests
- Rheumatoid factor/anti-CCP antibody
- Uric acid

IMAGING STUDIES

- Radiograph studies are not helpful unless a secondary cause has affected other organs (e.g., rheumatoid lung).
- Musculoskeletal ultrasonography can be useful in characterizing the lesion and guiding treatment.

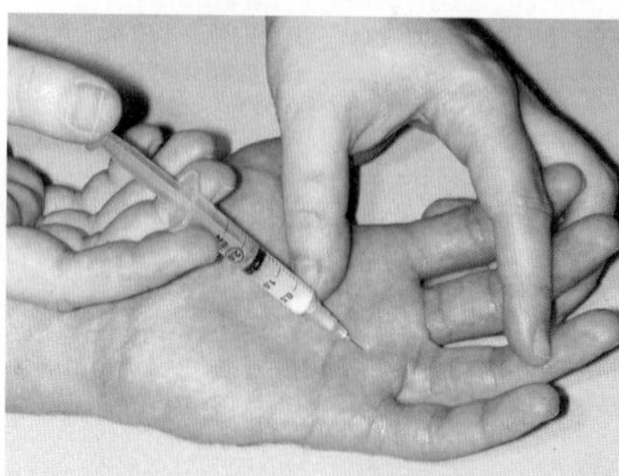

FIGURE 1-961 Injection into the palm for trigger finger. (From Carr A, Hamilton W: *Orthopedics in primary care,* ed 2, Philadelphia, 2005, Saunders.)

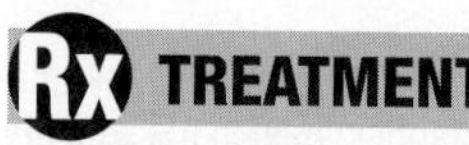

TREATMENT

The goals of treatment are to reduce swelling and inflammation in the flexor tendon sheath and allow smooth movement of the tendon under the A1 pulley of the MCP joint.

NONPHARMACOLOGIC THERAPY

- Splinting or buddy taping to the adjacent finger for 4 to 6 wk.
- Preventive measures include the use of gloves and damping tape to widen grips.
- Physiotherapy with stretching and heat.

ACUTE GENERAL Rx

- In idiopathic trigger finger, different steroid preparations with local anesthetics are used if patients have not responded to conservative treatment (Fig. 1-961).
- If symptoms do not resolve in 6 wk, a repeat injection can be tried.
- Pain control.

CHRONIC Rx

- Surgical release is indicated in patients with refractory symptoms (e.g., locked digits) despite nonpharmacologic and acute treatment.
- Surgery is also indicated in patients with recurrent symptoms despite two steroid injections.

DISPOSITION

- After steroid injection, symptoms usually resolve in 3 to 5 days, and locking resolves in 60% of the cases in 2 to 3 wk.
- If symptoms recur, a repeat steroid injection improves the symptoms in ≥80% of patients.
- Diabetic patients do not have the same success rate with steroid injections as the idiopathic group.

REFERRAL

If steroid injection therapy is considered, a rheumatology or hand surgery consult is requested.

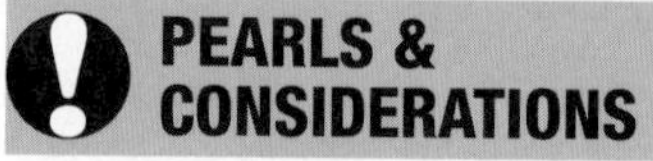

PEARLS & CONSIDERATIONS

COMMENTS

If more than one digit is involved, a workup for a secondary systemic cause is in order.

SUGGESTED READINGS

available at www.expertconsult.com

RELATED CONTENT

Trigger Finger (Patient Information)

AUTHORS: **RYAN W. ZUZEK, M.D., PAUL GORDON, M.D.,** and **DANIEL MENDEZ, M.D.**

BASIC INFORMATION

DEFINITION

Trochanteric bursitis reflects inflammation or irritation of the bursa or bursae located at the insertion of the gluteal muscles at the greater trochanter of the femur (Fig. 1-962).

SYNONYMS

Greater trochanteric pain syndrome
Greater trochanteric bursitis

ICD-9CM CODES
726.5 Bursitis trochanteric area
726.5 Enthesopathy of hip region (Bursitis of hip, Trochanteric tendinitis)
ICD-10CM CODES
M70.60 Trochanteric bursitis, unspecified hip

EPIDEMIOLOGY & DEMOGRAPHICS

- Trochanteric bursitis can be associated with other conditions, including osteoarthritis of the hip, lumbar spinal degenerative joint disease, and rheumatoid arthritis.
- Incidence peaks between the fourth and sixth decades of life but can occur at any age.
- Occurs in females more often than males (ratio of 4:1).
- Bilateral prevalence in females is 6.6% and in males is 1.9%.
- Unilateral prevalence in females is 15.0% whereas in males is 8.5%.
- Prevalence is 3200/100,000.

PHYSICAL FINDINGS & CLINICAL PRESENTATION

- Lateral hip pain is the most common symptom, though the hip joint itself is not involved. The pain is chronic, intermittent, and located over the outer lateral hip and thigh.
- Bursal swelling may be present.
- Pain is precipitated with prolonged lying or standing on the affected side.
- Walking, climbing, and running exacerbate the pain.
- Point tenderness over the greater trochanter is noted.
- Pain is reproduced with resisted hip abduction.

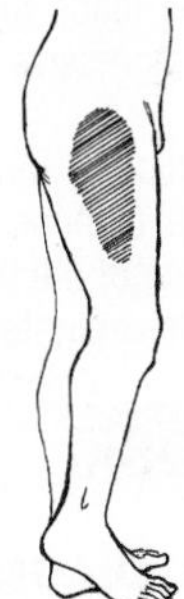

FIGURE 1-962 Typical location of pain in trochanteric bursitis syndrome. This is also a frequent pain radiation site for lumbar spine lesion, various nerve compression syndromes, and hip disease, particularly in osteonecrosis of the femoral head. (From Canoso JJ: *Rheumatology in primary care,* Philadelphia, 1997, Saunders.)

ETIOLOGY

- The specific cause of trochanteric bursitis is not known, although repetitive high-intensity use of the tensor fasciae and gluteus medius over the outer femur, trauma, infection (tuberculosis and bacterial), and crystal deposition can precipitate the disease.
- Trochanteric bursitis can occur when other conditions such as osteoarthritis of the knee and hip, sacroiliac joint disorders, leg length discrepancy, ankle sprain, and bunions of the feet cause changes in the patient's gait, placing varus stress on the hip joint.
- It can also occur as a complication resulting from arthroscopic surgery of the hip (estimated 1.4% of cases).

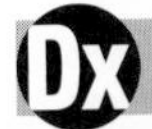

DIAGNOSIS

A detailed physical examination and clinical presentation usually make the diagnosis of trochanteric bursitis. X-ray images are helpful adjunctive studies used to exclude other conditions either associated with or mimicking trochanteric bursitis.

DIFFERENTIAL DIAGNOSIS

- Osteoarthritis of the hip
- Osteonecrosis of the hip
- Stress fracture of the hip
- Osteoarthritis of the lumbar spine
- Meralgia paresthetica
- Iliotibial band syndrome
- Fibromyalgia
- Iliopsoas bursitis
- Trochanteric tendonitis
- Trauma
- Osteomyelitis
- Tuberculosis of the greater trochanter
- Metastatic bone disease
- Septic arthritis
- Gluteal medius tendon tears

WORKUP

A workup is indicated if suspected associated conditions exist; otherwise treatment can be started on clinical grounds alone.

LABORATORY TESTS

Generally not indicated in clear cases.

IMAGING STUDIES

- Standing anterior to posterior pelvic x-rays and specific views of hip and back are used to evaluate associated symptoms such as leg length discrepancy, lumbar spondylosis, and sacroiliac joint diseases causing the bursitis. Sometimes calcifications may be seen around the greater trochanter in the areas of bursal development.
- Bone scan is usually not necessary.
- CT and MRI may show bursitis but are usually not warranted unless suspect associated conditions that would affect treatment decisions. MRI shows increased signal in bursitis.

TREATMENT

NONPHARMACOLOGIC THERAPY

- Physical therapy and iliotibial band stretching exercises can reduce irritation of the trochanteric bursa area.
- Heat application prior to exercising
- Ultrasound therapy
- Rest
- Treat gait disturbance by knee brace, shoe lift, ankle supports, foot orthotics for the specific underlying conditions

ACUTE GENERAL Rx

- NSAIDs for pain relief: ibuprofen 800 mg PO tid or naproxen 500 mg PO bid for the initial 4 wk
- Using US to enhance absorption of topical corticosteroids percutaneously (phonophoresis)
- Corticosteroid injection
- Regional anesthetic block can be used as a treatment and may also help differentiate from referred pain.

CHRONIC Rx

Although rarely done, surgical removal of the bursa or with also lengthening of iliotibial band with bursectomy is possible for patients with refractory symptoms or infection.

DISPOSITION

- Most patients respond to NSAIDs and/or nonpharmacologic therapy.
- Steroid injection: ~ 70% of patients respond after first injection and >90% respond to two injections.
- 25% of patients receiving steroid injection may develop a relapse.

REFERRAL

A rheumatology or orthopedics referral is made if steroid injection therapy is needed or if the etiology is believed to be infectious.

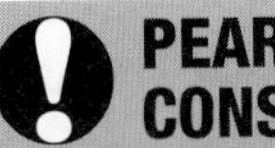

PEARLS & CONSIDERATIONS

Patients with trochanteric bursitis will commonly report "hip" pain. The physical examination readily distinguishes true hip pain from trochanteric bursitis. Relief of pain with local corticosteroid injection is helpful in differentiating trochanteric bursitis from referred pain.

COMMENTS

- The absence of pain with flexion and extension differentiates trochanteric bursitis from degenerative joint disease of the hip.
- Localization of pain over the lateral hip and thigh differentiates trochanteric bursitis from meralgia paresthetica located over the anterolateral thigh and osteoarthritis located over the inner thigh groin area.

SUGGESTED READINGS

available at www.expertconsult.com

RELATED CONTENT

Trochanteric Bursitis(Patient Information)

AUTHORS: **SYEDA M. SAYEED, M.D.,** and **UZMA NASIR, M.D.**

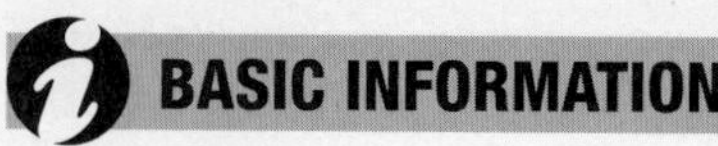

BASIC INFORMATION

DEFINITION

Miliary tuberculosis (TB) is an infection of disseminated hematogenous disease, caused by the bacterium *Mycobacterium tuberculosis* (Mtb), and is often characterized as resembling millet seeds on pathologic or radiologic examination. Extrapulmonary disease may occur in virtually every organ site.

SYNONYMS

Disseminated TB

ICD-9CM CODES
018.94 Miliary tuberculosis
ICD-10CM CODES
A19.9 Miliary tuberculosis, unspecified

EPIDEMIOLOGY & DEMOGRAPHICS

INCIDENCE (IN U.S.): >38% of AIDS patients with TB have disseminated disease, often with concurrent pulmonary and extrapulmonary active sites. (See "Tuberculosis, Pulmonary" in Section I.)

PREVALENCE (IN U.S.):

- Undetermined
- Highest prevalence
  1. AIDS patients
  2. Minorities
  3. Children
  4. Foreign-born persons
  5. Elderly

PREDOMINANT SEX:

- No specific predilection
- Male predominance in AIDS, shelters, and prisons reflected in disproportionate male TB incidence

PREDOMINANT AGE: Predominantly among 24- to 45-yr-olds

PEAK INCIDENCE: HIV-positive patients, regardless of age

PHYSICAL FINDINGS & CLINICAL PRESENTATION

- See also "Etiology"
- Common symptoms
  1. High intermittent fever (93%)
  2. Night sweats (79%)
  3. Weight loss (85%)
  4. Dyspnea (64%)
  5. Cough (82%)
- Symptoms referable to individual organ systems may predominate
  1. Meninges
  2. Pericardium
  3. Liver
  4. Kidney
  5. Bone
  6. GI tract
  7. Lymph nodes
  8. Serous spaces
     a. Pleural
     b. Pericardial
     c. Peritoneal
     d. Joint
  9. Skin
  10. Lung: cough, shortness of breath
- Adrenal insufficiency possible, caused by infection of adrenal gland
- Pancytopenia
  1. With fever and weight loss *or*
  2. Without other localizing symptoms or signs *or*
  3. With only splenomegaly
- TB hepatitis
  1. Tender liver
  2. Obstructive enzymes (alkaline phosphatase) elevated out of proportion to minimal hepatocellular enzymes (SGOT, SGPT) and bilirubin
- TB meningitis
  1. Gradual-onset headache
  2. Minimal meningeal signs
  3. Malaise
  4. Low-grade fever (may be absent)
  5. Sudden stupor or coma
  6. Cranial nerve VI palsy
- TB pericarditis
  1. Effusions resembling TB pleurisy
  2. Cardiac tamponade
- Skeletal TB
  1. Large joint arthritis (with effusions resembling TB pericarditis)
  2. Bone lesions (especially ribs)
  3. Pott's disease
     a. TB spondylitis, especially of lower thoracic spine
     b. Paraspinous TB abscess
     c. Possible psoas abscess
     d. Frequent cord compression (often relieved by steroids)
- Genitourinary TB
  1. Renal TB
     a. Papillary necrosis
     b. Destruction of renal pelvis
     c. Strictures of upper third of ureters
     d. Hematuria
     e. Pyuria with misleading bacterial cultures
     f. Preserved renal function
  2. TB orchitis or epididymitis
     a. Scrotal mass
     b. Draining abscess
  3. Chronic prostatic TB
- GI TB
  1. Diarrhea
  2. Pain
  3. Obstruction
  4. Bleeding
  5. Especially common with AIDS
  6. Bowel lesions
     a. Circumferential ulcers
     b. Short strictures
     c. Calcified granulomas
     d. TB mesenteric caseous adenitis
     e. Abscess, but rare fistula formation
     f. Often difficult to distinguish from granulomatous bowel disease (Crohn's disease)
- TB peritonitis
  1. Fluid resembles TB pleurisy
  2. PPD often negative
  3. Tender abdomen
  4. Doughy peritoneal consistency, often with ascites
  5. Peritoneal biopsy indicated for diagnosis
- TB lymphadenitis (scrofula)
  1. May involve all node groups
  2. Common adenopathies
     a. Cervical
     b. Supraclavicular
     c. Axillary
     d. Retroperitoneal
  3. Biopsy generally needed for diagnosis
  4. Surgical resection of nodes may be necessary
  5. Especially common with AIDS
- Cutaneous TB
  1. Skin infection from autoinoculation or dissemination
  2. Nodules or abscesses
  3. Tuberculids (possibly allergic reactions)
  4. Erythema nodosum
- Miscellaneous presentations
  1. TB laryngitis
  2. TB otitis
  3. Ocular TB
     a. Choroidal tubercles
     b. Iritis
     c. Uveitis
     d. Episcleritis
  4. Adrenal TB
  5. Breast TB

ETIOLOGY

- See also "Pulmonary Tuberculosis" in Section I.
- Mtb, a slow-growing, aerobic, non–spore forming, nonmotile acid-fast bacillus
- Humans are the only reservoir for Mtb.
- Pathogenesis:
  1. Acid-fast bacilli (AFB) (Mtb) are ingested by macrophages in alveoli, then transported to regional lymph nodes where spread is contained.
  2. Some AFB reach the bloodstream and disseminate widely.
  3. Immediate active disseminated disease may ensue or a latent period may develop.
  4. During latent period, T-cell immune mechanisms contain infection in granulomas until later reactivation occurs as a result of immunosuppression or other undefined factors in conjunction with reactivated pulmonary TB or alone.
- Miliary TB may occur as a consequence of the following:
  1. Primary infection: inability to contain primary infection leads to a hematogenous spread and progressive disseminated disease.
  2. In late chronic TB and in those with advanced age or poor immunity, a continuous seeding of the blood may develop and lead to disseminated disease.

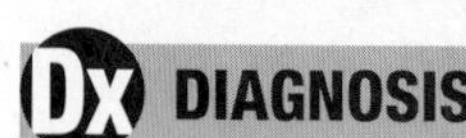

DIAGNOSIS

DIFFERENTIAL DIAGNOSIS

Widespread sites of possible dissemination associated with myriad differential diagnostic possibilities:

- Lymphoma
- Typhoid fever
- Brucellosis

- Other tumors
- Collagen-vascular disease

WORKUP

- Prompt evaluation is essential
- Sputum for AFB stain and culture and chest x-ray
- High-resolution CT is more sensitive for miliary TB than CXR
- PPD, which may be negative in immunocompromised patients
- Fluid analysis and mycobacterial culture wherever available
  1. Sputum
  2. Blood: particularly helpful in patients with AIDS
  3. Urine
  4. CSF
  5. Pleural
  6. Pericardial
  7. Peritoneal
  8. Gastric aspirates
- Biopsy of any involved tissue is advisable to make immediate diagnosis
  1. Transbronchial biopsy preferred and easily accessible
  2. Bone marrow
  3. Lymph node
  4. Scrotal mass if present
  5. Any other involved site
  6. Positive granuloma or AFB on biopsy specimen is diagnostic
- Imaging studies as needed

LABORATORY TESTS

- Culture and fluid analysis as described previously
- Smear-negative sputum often is positive weeks later on culture
- CBC is usually normal
- ESR is usually elevated

IMAGING STUDIES

- Chest x-ray examination (may or may not be positive) (see "Tuberculosis, Pulmonary" in Section I)
- CT scan or MRI of brain and spinal cord (Fig. 1-963)
  1. Tuberculoma
  2. Basilar arachnoiditis
- Barium studies of bowel

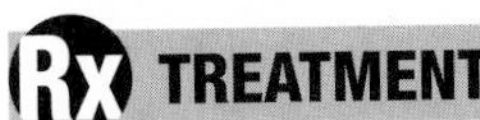

TREATMENT

NONPHARMACOLOGIC THERAPY

- Bed rest during acute phase of treatment
- High-calorie, high-protein diet to reverse malnutrition and enhance immune response to TB
- Isolation in negative-pressure rooms with high-volume air replacement and circulation (with health care provider wearing proper protective 0.5- to 1-micron filter respirators)
  1. Until three consecutive sputum AFB smears are negative, if pulmonary disease coexists
  2. Isolation not required for closed-space TB infections

ACUTE GENERAL Rx

- See "Tuberculosis, Pulmonary" in Section I.
- Therapy should be initiated immediately. Do not wait for definitive diagnosis.
- More rapid response to chemotherapy by disseminated TB foci than cavitary pulmonary TB.
- Treatment for 6 mo with INH plus rifampin plus PZA.
  1. Treatment for 12 mo often required for bone and renal TB.
  2. Prolonged treatment often required for CNS and pericardial.
  3. Prolonged treatment often required for all disseminated TB in infants.
- Compliance (rigid adherence to treatment regimen) is the chief determinant of success.
  1. Supervised directly observed therapy (DOT) is recommended for all patients.
  2. Supervised DOT is mandatory for unreliable patients.
- Steroids are often helpful additions in fulminant miliary disease with the hypoxemia and DIC.

CHRONIC Rx

- Generally not indicated beyond treatment described previously
- Prolonged treatment supervised by infectious disease expert required in a few complicated infections caused by resistant organisms

DISPOSITION

- Monthly follow-up by physician experienced in TB treatment
- Confirm sensitivity testing, and alter treatment appropriately (see "Tuberculosis, Pulmonary" in Section I)

REFERRAL

- To infectious disease expert for:
  1. HIV-positive patient
  2. Patient with suspected drug-resistant TB
  3. Patient previously treated for TB
  4. Patient whose fever has not decreased and sputum (if positive) has not converted to negative in 2 to 4 wk
  5. Patients with overwhelming pulmonary or extrapulmonary TB
- To pulmonary, orthopedic, or GI physicians for examinations or biopsy

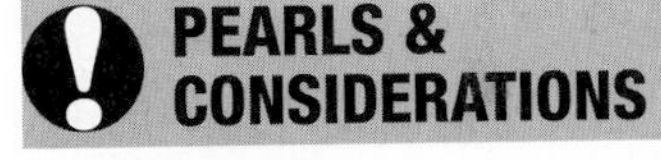

PEARLS & CONSIDERATIONS

COMMENTS

- Consider acute TB in critically ill patients with enigmatic acute respiratory distress syndrome, shock, or DIC.
- All contacts (especially close household contacts and infants) should be properly tested for PPD conversions >3 mo following exposure.
- Those with positive PPD should be evaluated for active TB and properly treated or given prophylaxis.

SUGGESTED READINGS

available at www.expertconsult.com

AUTHOR: **GLENN G. FORT, M.D., M.P.H.**

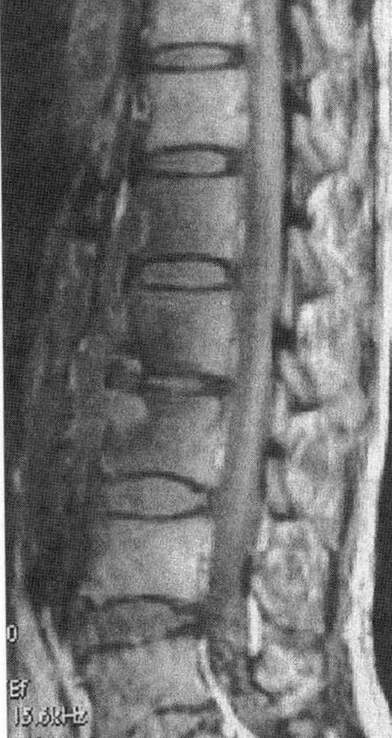

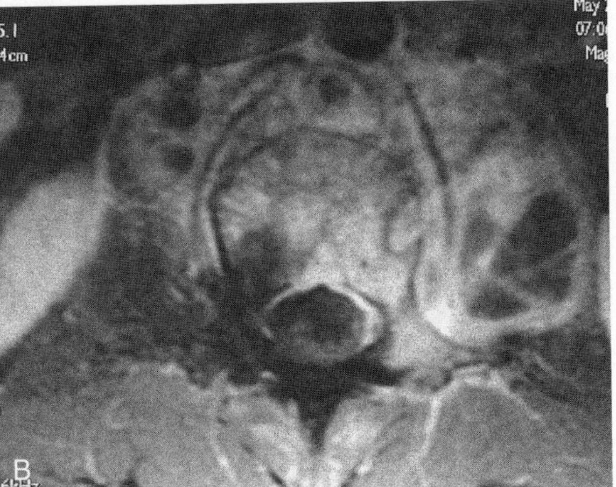

FIGURE 1-963 A and B, Magnetic resonance images of tuberculous spinal osteomyelitis with scalloping of the vertebrae (tuberculous caries) and paraspinal "cold" abscesses. (From Grainger RG, Allison D: *Grainger & Allison's diagnostic radiology, a textbook of medical imaging,* ed 4, London, 2001, Churchill Livingstone.)

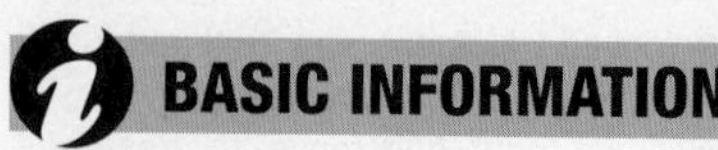

DEFINITION

Pulmonary tuberculosis (TB) is an infection of the lung and, occasionally, surrounding structures, caused by the bacterium *Mycobacterium tuberculosis* (Mtb). Multidrug-resistant (MDR) TB is defined as disease caused by strains of Mtb that are at least resistant to treatment with isoniazid and rifampin; extensively drug-resistant (XDR) TB refers to disease caused by MDR strains that are also resistant to treatment with any fluoroquinolone and any of the injectable drugs used in the treatment of second-line anti-TB drugs.

SYNONYMS

TB

ICD-9CM CODES
011.9 Pulmonary tuberculosis
ICD-10CM CODES
A15.0 Tuberculosis of lung

EPIDEMIOLOGY & DEMOGRAPHICS

INCIDENCE (WORLDWIDE):
In 2011 there were:

- 8.7 million new cases of active tuberculosis; 13% involved coinfection with HIV
- 1.4 million deaths from TB, including 430,000 among HIV-infected patients; 310,000 incident cases of multidrug-resistant TB
- Sub-Saharan Africa has the highest rates of active TB per capita.
- Absolute number of cases is highest in Asia, with India and China having the greatest burden of disease globally.

INCIDENCE (IN U.S.):

- In 2010, there were 11,181 cases of TB in the U.S. for a rate of 3.6 cases/100,000 persons—the lowest reported rate since recording began in 1953.
- >90% of new cases each yr from reactivated prior infections
- 9% newly infected
- Only 10% of patients with purified protein derivative (PPD) conversions (higher [8%/yr] in HIV-positive patients) will develop TB, most within 1 to 2 yr
- Two thirds of all new cases in racial and ethnic minorities
- 80% of new cases in children in racial and ethnic minorities
- Occurs most frequently in geographic areas and among populations with highest AIDS prevalence
  1. Urban blacks and Hispanics between 25 and 45 yr old
  2. Poor, crowded urban communities
- Nearly 36% of new cases from new immigrants
- In 2008 in the U.S., 8.2% of cases were MDR TB.

PREVALENCE (IN U.S.):

- Estimated 10 million people infected
- Varies widely among population groups

PREDOMINANT SEX:

- No specific predilection
- Male predominance in AIDS, shelters, and prisons reflected in disproportionate male incidence

PREDOMINANT AGE:

- 24 to 45 yr old
- Childhood cases common among minorities
- Nursing home outbreaks among elderly

PEAK INCIDENCE:

- Infancy
- Teenage years
- Pregnancy
- Elderly
- HIV-positive patients, regardless of age, at highest risk

GENETICS:

- Populations with widespread low native resistance have been intensely infected when initially exposed to TB.
- Following elimination of those with least native resistance, incidence and prevalence of TB tend to decline.

PHYSICAL FINDINGS & CLINICAL PRESENTATION

- See "Etiology"
- Primary pulmonary TB infection generally asymptomatic
- Reactivation pulmonary TB
  1. Fever
  2. Night sweats
  3. Cough
  4. Hemoptysis
  5. Scanty nonpurulent sputum
  6. Weight loss
- Progressive primary pulmonary TB disease: same as reactivation pulmonary TB
- TB pleurisy
  1. Pleuritic chest pain
  2. Fever
  3. Shortness of breath
- Rare massive, suffocating, fatal hemoptysis secondary to erosion of pulmonary artery within a cavity (Rasmussen's aneurysm)
- Chest examination
  1. Not specific
  2. Usually underestimates extent of disease
  3. Rales accentuated following a cough (posttussive rales)

ETIOLOGY

- Mtb, a slow-growing, aerobic, nonsporeforming, nonmotile bacillus, with a lipid-rich cell wall:
  1. Lacks pigment
  2. Produces niacin
  3. Reduces nitrate
  4. Produces heat-labile catalase
  5. Mtb staining, acid-fast and acid-alcohol fast by Ziehl-Neelsen method, appearing as red, slightly bent, beaded rods 2 to 4 microns long (acid-fast bacilli [AFB]), against a blue background
  6. Polymerase chain reaction (PCR) to detect <10 organisms/ml in sputum (compared with the requisite 10,000 organisms/ml for AFB smear detection)
  7. Culture
     a. Growth on solid media (Löwenstein-Jensen; Middlebrook 7H11) in 2 to 6 wk
     b. Growth in liquid media (BACTEC, using a radioactive carbon source for early growth detection) often in 9 to 16 days
     c. Enhanced in a 5% to 10% carbon dioxide atmosphere
  8. DNA fingerprinting (based on restriction fragment length polymorphism [RFLP])
     a. Facilitates immediate identification of Mtb strains in early growing cultures
     b. False negatives possible if growth suboptimal
  9. Humans are the only reservoir for Mtb
  10. Transmission
     a. Facilitated by close exposure to high-velocity cough (unprotected by proper mask or respirators) from patient with AFB-positive sputum and cavitary lesions, producing aerosolized droplets containing AFB, which are inhaled directly into alveoli
     b. Occurs within prisons, nursing homes, and hospitals
- Pathogenesis
  1. AFB (Mtb) ingested by macrophages in alveoli, then transported to regional lymph nodes, where spread is contained
  2. Some AFB may reach bloodstream and disseminate widely
  3. Primary TB (asymptomatic, minimal pneumonitis in lower or midlung fields, with hilar lymphadenopathy) essentially an intracellular infection, with multiplication of organisms continuing for 2 to 12 wk after primary exposure, until cell-mediated hypersensitivity (detected by positive skin test reaction to tuberculin PPD) matures, with subsequent containment of infection
  4. Local and disseminated AFB thus contained by T-cell-mediated immune responses
     a. Recruitment of monocytes
     b. Transformation of lymphocytes with secretion of lymphokines
     c. Activation of macrophages and histiocytes
     d. Organization into granulomas, where organisms may survive within macrophages (Langhans' giant cells), but within which multiplication essentially ceases (95%) and from which spread is prohibited
  5. Progressive primary pulmonary disease
     a. May immediately follow the asymptomatic phase
     b. Necrotizing pulmonary infiltrates
     c. Tuberculous bronchopneumonia
     d. Endobronchial TB
     e. Interstitial TB
     f. Widespread miliary lung lesions
  6. Postprimary TB pleurisy with pleural effusion
     a. Develops after early primary infection, although often before conversion to positive PPD

b. Results from pleural seeding from a peripheral lung lesion or rupture of lymph node into pleural space
c. May produce a large (sometimes hemorrhagic) exudative effusion (with polymorphonuclear cells early, rapidly replaced by lymphocytes), frequently without pulmonary infiltrates
d. Generally resolves without treatment
e. Portends a high risk of subsequent clinical disease, and therefore must be diagnosed and treated early (pleural biopsy and culture) to prevent future catastrophic TB illness
f. May result in disseminated extrapulmonary infection

7. Reactivation pulmonary TB
   a. Occurs months to years following primary TB
   b. Preferentially involves the apical posterior segments of the upper lobes and superior segments of the lower lobes
   c. Associated with necrosis and cavitation of involved lung, hemoptysis, chronic fever, night sweats, weight loss
   d. Spread within lung occurs via cough and inhalation
8. Reinfection TB
   a. May mimic reactivation TB
   b. Ruptured caseous foci and cavities, which may produce endobronchial spread
9. Mtb in both progressive primary and reactivation pulmonary TB
   a. Intracellular (macrophage) lesions (undergoing slow multiplication)
   b. Closed caseous lesions (undergoing slow multiplication)
   c. Extracellular, open cavities (undergoing rapid multiplication)
   d. INH and rifampin are cidal in all three sites
   e. Pyrazinamide (PZA) especially active within acidic macrophage environment
   f. Extrapulmonary reactivation disease also possible
10. Rapid local progression and dissemination in infants with devastating illness before PPD conversion occurs
11. Most symptoms (fever, weight loss, anorexia) and tissue destruction (caseous necrosis) from cytokines and cell-mediated immune responses
12. Mtb has no important endotoxins or exotoxins
13. Granuloma formation related to tumor necrosis factor (TNF) secreted by activated macrophages

Dx DIAGNOSIS

DIFFERENTIAL DIAGNOSIS

- Necrotizing pneumonia (anaerobic, gram-negative)
- Histoplasmosis
- Coccidioidomycosis
- Melioidosis
- Interstitial lung diseases (rarely)
- Cancer
- Sarcoidosis
- Silicosis
- Rare pneumonias
  1. *Rhodococcus equi* (cavitation)
  2. *Bacillus cereus* (50% hemoptysis)
  3. *Eikenella corrodens* (cavitation)

WORKUP

- Sputum for AFB stains
- Chest x-ray (Fig. E1-964)
- PPD (tuberculin skin test [TST])
  1. Recent conversion from negative to positive within 3 mo of exposure is highly suggestive of recent infection.
  2. Single positive PPD is not helpful diagnostically.
  3. Negative PPD never rules out acute TB.
  4. Be certain that positive PPD does not reflect "booster phenomenon" (prior positive PPD may become negative after several yr and return to positive only after second repeated PPD; repeat second PPD within 1 wk), which thus may mimic skin test conversion.
  5. Positive PPD reaction is determined as follows:
     a. Induration after 72 hr of intradermal injection of 0.1 ml of 5 TU-PPD
     b. 5-mm induration if HIV-positive (or other severe immunosuppressed state affecting cellular immune function), close contact of active TB, fibrotic chest lesions
     c. 10-mm induration if in high–medical risk groups (immunosuppressive disease or therapy, renal failure, gastrectomy, silicosis, diabetes), foreign-born high-risk group (Southeast Asia, Latin America, Africa, India), low socioeconomic groups, IV drug addict, prisoner, healthcare worker
     d. 15-mm induration if low risk
  6. Anergy antigen testing (using mumps, *Candida,* tetanus toxoid) may identify patients who are truly anergic to PPD and these antigens, but results are often confusing. Not recommended.
  7. Patients with TB may be selectively anergic only to PPD.
  8. Positive PPD indicates prior infection but does not itself confirm active disease.
- Interferon gamma release assays (IGRAs): diagnostic test for latent TB infection, known as the quantaferon test (QFT-G). This is a blood test that measures interferon response to specific Mtb antigens. The test is FDA approved and is available in some large TB centers and state health departments. It may assist in distinguishing true positive reactions, from individuals with latent TB, from PPD reactions related to nontuberculous mycobacteria; prior BCG vaccination; or difficult-to-interpret skin test results from people with dermatologic conditions or immediate allergic reactions to PPD. The diagnostic utility of the test as a replacement or supplement to the standard PPD is not yet fully determined. When IGRA is used for routine screening, positive results should be repeated routinely due to a high rate of false-positive results. The enzyme-linked immunospot assay (Elispot plus) incorporating a novel antigen, RV3879c, when used in combination with tuberculin testing, has been reported to enable rapid exclusion of active infection in patients with moderate to high pretest probability of TB. Other IGRAs now available for detection of TB using blood include QFT-GIT and T-spot.
- The Xpert MTB/RIF is an automated molecular test for *Mycobacterium tuberculosis* (MTB) and resistance to rifampin (RIF) that provides sensitive detection of TB and rifampin resistance directly from untreated sputum in less than 2 hr with minimal hands-on time.

LABORATORY TESTS

- Sputum for AFB stains and culture
  1. Induced sputum if patient not coughing productively
- Sputum from bronchoscopy if high suspicion of TB with negative expectorated induced sputum for AFB
  1. Positive AFB smear is essential before or shortly after treatment to ensure subsequent growth for definitive diagnosis and sensitivity testing
  2. Consider lung biopsy if sputum negative, especially if infiltrates are predominantly interstitial
- AFB stain-negative sputum may grow Mtb subsequently
- Gastric aspirates reliable, especially in HIV-negative patients
- CBC
  1. Variable values
     a. WBCs: low, normal, or elevated (including leukemoid reaction: >50,000)
     b. Normocytic, normochromic anemia often
  2. Rarely helpful diagnostically
- ESR usually elevated
- Thoracentesis
  1. Exudative effusion
     a. Elevated protein
     b. Decreased glucose
     c. Elevated WBCs (polymorphonuclear leukocytes early, replaced later by lymphocytes)
     d. May be hemorrhagic
  2. Pleural fluid usually AFB-negative
  3. Pleural biopsy often diagnostic—may need to be repeated for diagnosis
  4. Culture pleural biopsy tissue for AFB
- Bone marrow biopsy is often diagnostic in difficult-to-diagnose cases, especially miliary TB

IMAGING STUDIES

- Chest radiograph
  1. Primary infection reflected by calcified peripheral lung nodule with calcified hilar lymph node
  2. Reactivation pulmonary TB
     a. Necrosis

b. Cavitation (especially on apical lordotic views)
c. Fibrosis and hilar retraction
d. Bronchopneumonia
e. Interstitial infiltrates
f. Miliary pattern
g. Many of previous findings may also accompany progressive primary TB

3. TB pleurisy
   a. Pleural effusion, often rapidly accumulating and massive
4. TB activity not established by single chest x-ray examination
5. Serial chest x-ray examinations are excellent indicators of progression or regression

Rx TREATMENT

NONPHARMACOLOGIC THERAPY

- Increased rest during acute phase of treatment
- High-calorie, high-protein diet to reverse malnutrition and enhance immune response to TB
- Isolation in negative-pressure rooms with high-volume air replacement and circulation, with health care provider wearing proper protective 0.5- to 1-micron filter respirators, until three consecutive sputum AFB smears are negative

ACUTE GENERAL Rx

- Compliance (rigid adherence to treatment regimen) chief determinant of success.
  1. Supervised directly observed therapy (DOT) recommended for all patients and mandatory for unreliable patients
- Preferred adult regimen: DOT.
  1. Isoniazid (INH) 15 mg/kg (max 900 mg), rifampin 600 mg, ethambutol (EMB) 30 mg/kg (max 2500 mg), and pyrazinamide (PZA) (2 g [<50 kg]; 2.5 g [51 to 74 kg]; 3 g [>75 kg]) thrice weekly for 6 mo
  2. Alternative, more complicated DOT regimens
- Rifapentine, a rifampin derivative with a much longer serum half-life, was shown to be as effective when administered weekly (with weekly isoniazid) as conventional regimens for drug-sensitive pulmonary TB in non–HIV-infected patients.
- Short-course daily therapy: adult.
  1. HIV-negative patient: 6 mo total therapy (2 mo INH 300 mg, rifampin 600 mg, and EMB 15 mg/kg [max 2500 mg]) and PZA (1.5 g [<50 kg]; 2 g [51 to 74 kg]; 2.5 g [>75 kg]) daily and until smear negative and sensitivity confirmed; then INH and rifampin daily for 4 mo
  2. HIV-positive patient: 9 mo total therapy (2 mo INH, rifampin, EMB, and PZA daily until smear negative and sensitivity confirmed; then INH and rifampin qid for 7 mo)
  3. Continue treatment at least 3 mo following conversion to negative cultures
- Drug resistance (often multiple drug resistance TB [MDRTB]) increased by:
  1. Prior treatment
  2. Acquisition of TB in developing countries
  3. Homelessness, incarceration
  4. AIDS, IVDA
  5. Known contact with MDRTB
- Never add single drug to failing regimen.
- Never treat TB with fewer than two to three drugs or two to three new additional drugs.
- Other medications used in MDR or XDRTB include: moxifloxacin, cycloserine, aminoglycosides such as amikacin or kanamycin, clarithromycin, PAS, and ethionamide.
- Bedaquiline, a diarylquinoline antimycobacterial, is now FDA-approved for treatment of MDR-TB. Recommended dose is 400 mg once daily for 2 wk, followed by 200 mg 3x/wk for weeks 3-24. Bedaquiline is administered in combination with >=3 drugs to which it is susceptible.
- Monitor for clinical toxicity (especially hepatitis).
  1. Patient and physician awareness that anorexia, nausea, right upper quadrant pain, and unexplained malaise require immediate cessation of treatment
  2. Evaluation of liver function testing
     a. Minimal SGOT/SGPT elevations without symptoms generally transient and not clinically significant
- Preventive treatment for PPD conversion only (infection without disease).
  1. Must be certain that chest x-ray examination is negative and patient has no symptoms of TB
  2. Most important groups:
     a. HIV-positive and other severely immunocompromised patients
     b. Close contact with active TB
     c. Recent converter
     d. Old TB on chest x-ray examination
     e. IV drug addict
     f. Medical risk factor
     g. High-risk foreign country
     h. Homeless
  3. The traditional preventive therapy for persons with latent M. tuberculosis consists of INH 300 mg daily for 9 to 12 mo; at least 12 mo if HIV-positive patient. The CDC has issued recommendations for a new regimen consisting of isoniazid and rifapentine administered once a week for 12 weeks as directly observed therapy. Studies have demonstrated that this regimen is as effective as 9 months of isoniazid therapy for preventing tuberculosis. Patients who should not receive this regimen include children younger than 2 years, persons with HIV infection taking antiretroviral therapy, pregnant women or those who may become pregnant during the course of treatment, and patients who have latent *M. tuberculosis* infection that is presumed to be resistant to isoniazid or rifampin.
- Infants generally given prophylaxis immediately if recent contact with active TB (even if infant PPD negative), then retested with PPD in 3 mo (continuing INH if PPD becomes positive and stopping INH if PPD remains negative).
- Chronic, stable PPD (several yr) given INH prophylaxis generally only if patient is <35 yr old.
  1. INH toxicity may outweigh benefit
  2. Individualize decision
- Preventive therapy for suspected INH-resistant organisms is unclear.

CHRONIC Rx

- Generally not indicated beyond treatment described previously
- Prolonged treatment, supervised by infectious disease expert, in a few very complicated infections caused by resistant organisms

DISPOSITION

- Monthly follow-up by physician experienced in TB treatment
- Confirm sensitivity testing and alter treatment appropriately
- Frequent sputum samples until culture is negative
- Confirm chest x-ray regression at 2 to 3 mo

REFERRAL

- To infectious disease expert for:
  1. HIV-positive patient
  2. Patient with suspected drug-resistant TB
  3. Patients previously treated for TB
  4. Patients whose fever has not decreased and sputum has not converted to negative in 2 to 4 wk
  5. Patients with overwhelming pulmonary or extrapulmonary TB
- To pulmonologist for bronchoscopy or pleural biopsy

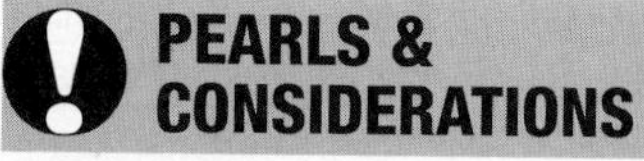

PEARLS & CONSIDERATIONS

COMMENTS

- All contacts (especially close household contacts and infants) should be properly tested for PPD conversions during 3 mo following exposure.
- Those with positive PPD should be evaluated for active TB and properly treated or given prophylaxis.
- Previous treatment is a common risk factor for XDR and MDR TB.

SUGGESTED READINGS

available at www.expertconsult.com

RELATED CONTENT

Tuberculosis (TB) (Patient Information)

AUTHOR: **GLENN G. FORT, M.D., M.P.H.**

BASIC INFORMATION

DEFINITION

Acute tubular necrosis (ATN), the most common form of acute renal failure (ARF), is a potentially reversible abrupt decline in renal function occurring over minutes to days. ATN may be secondary to ischemia or toxic insult or may be multifactorial.

SYNONYMS

ATN
Acute tubular injury
Ischemic or nephrotoxic acute renal failure (ARF)

ICD-9CM CODES
584.5 Acute renal failure with lesion of tubular necrosis
586 Renal failure, unspecified

ICD-10CM CODES
N17.0 Acute kidney failure with tubular necrosis
N19 Unspecified kidney failure

EPIDEMIOLOGY & DEMOGRAPHICS

- Most common cause of ARF among hospitalized patients.
- Patients with impaired afferent arteriolar autoregulation are most vulnerable.
- Elderly patients and patients with atherosclerotic disease, hypertension, and chronic renal failure are at an increased risk.
- Early identification of ATN is paramount as many etiologies are reversible.

PHYSICAL FINDINGS & CLINICAL PRESENTATION

- No apparent physical findings.
- Suspect ischemic ATN in the setting of hemorrhage, hypotension, recent surgery, sepsis
- Suspect nephrotoxic ATN in the setting of contrast imaging, nephrotoxic medications, rhabdomyolysis, hemolysis, or myeloma
- The classic progression of ATN includes three phases, but can be highly variable:
  1. Initiation phase (hours to days): Renal hypoperfusion, evolving ischemia. Acute decrease in glomerular filtration rate (GFR), sudden rise in BUN and serum creatinine, and decrease in urine output.
  2. Maintenance phase (1 to 2 wk): Renal cell injury established, GFR stabilizes at its nadir (5 to 10 ml/min), urine output at its lowest (usually 40 to 400 ml/day). May be complicated by hyperkalemia, metabolic acidosis, uremia, salt and water overload. Patients are at an increased risk of infection, with approximately 25% of deaths from ATN occurring during the maintenance phase.
  3. Recovery phase (>2 wk): Renal parenchymal cell repair and regeneration, gradual return of GFR to premorbid levels; may be complicated by a marked diuresis.

PATHOLOGIC FINDINGS

- Ischemic ATN: Characterized by focal necrosis of the tubular epithelium, often with associated basement membrane disruption and occlusion of the tubular lumen by casts. Eosinophilic hyaline casts and pigmented granular casts are common. Interstitial edema and leukocytic accumulation within the vasa recta may also be observed.
- Nephrotoxic ATN: Necrosis is most prominent in the proximal tubule and the basement membrane is commonly spared.

ETIOLOGY

- Diagnosis of exclusion. Pre-renal, post-renal, and other intrinsic renal causes of ARF must be ruled out.
- Ischemic processes that may contribute to ATN include hypotension, shock, prolonged prerenal azotemia, and surgery.
- Renal hypoperfusion may occur without clinically apparent hypotension.
- Medications: NSAIDs, COX-2 inhibitors, antimicrobial drugs (acyclovir, foscarnet, aminoglycosides, amphotericin B, pentamidine, cephalosporins), calcineurin inhibitors, cisplatin, ifosfamide, thiazides, anesthetics, ACE inhibitors
- Radiocontrast (contrast nephropathy)
- Hemoglobin and myoglobin (rhabdomyolysis, transfusion reactions)
- Heavy metals
- Crystals (urate, oxalate, acute phosphate nephropathy)
- Hypercalcemia
- Immunoglobulin light chain disease (amyloidosis, multiple myeloma, MGUS)

DIAGNOSIS

DIFFERENTIAL DIAGNOSIS

Rapidly progressive glomerular nephritis (RPGN), diffuse vasculitic processes such as microscopic polyangiitis, acute papillary necrosis secondary to pyelonephritis, interstitial nephritis, diffuse cortical necrosis

LABORATORY TESTS

- Urinalysis for specific gravity, U_{Na}, P_{Cr}, P_{Na}, U_{Cr}.
- Urine analysis with microscopic inspection.
- Calculate fractional excretion of sodium: $FE_{Na} = [(U_{Na} \times P_{Cr}) / (P_{Na} \times U_{Cr})] \times 100$.
- Potential biomarkers for early diagnosis of ATN are currently under investigation.

LABORATORY FINDINGS

- FE_{Na} >1%
- U_{Na} >40 mmol/L
- Urinalysis: "muddy brown" granular and epithelial cell casts
- SG <1.015

IMAGING STUDIES

Not indicated

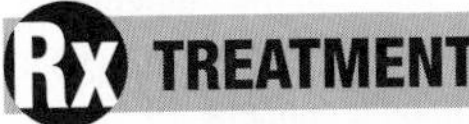

TREATMENT

ACUTE GENERAL Rx

Treatment is etiology-specific. Hemodynamic abnormalities should be corrected and potentially nephrotoxic agents discontinued. Peritoneal or hemodialysis may be required until renal function is restored. Diuretic use is not recommended.

DISPOSITION

Renal function typically recovers within 1 to 2 wk of insult. Outcomes are variable and depend upon premorbid renal function as well as the mechanism of injury. Ischemic ATN in the setting of severe multiorgan failure may carry a mortality rate exceeding 50%. However, in patients who survive the inciting incident, up to 95% will recover, with GFR approaching premorbid levels. The absence of oliguria (referred to as nonoliguric ATN) imparts a benign prognosis.

REFERRAL

Renal consultation for severe cases of ATN requiring dialysis

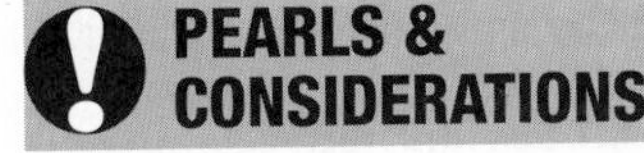

PEARLS & CONSIDERATIONS

COMMENTS

Prevention is paramount.

PREVENTION

- Aggressive restoration of intravascular volume in surgical/trauma patients to prevent ischemic ATN.
- Appropriate dosing of nephrotoxic agents in regards to body weight and GFR.
- Low-volume contrast, pre- and post-study intravenous fluids, and acetylcysteine (600 mg PO bid × 2 days or 600 to 1200 mg IV bid) to reduce the risk of contrast nephropathy.

SUGGESTED READINGS

available at www.expertconsult.com

RELATED CONTENT

Acute Kidney Injury (Related Key Topic)

AUTHOR: **BRIAN SAVOIE, M.D.**

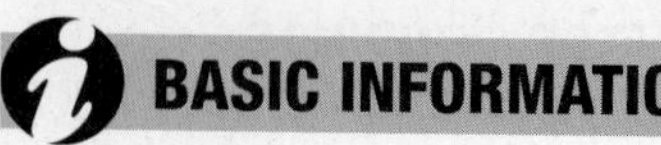

BASIC INFORMATION

DEFINITION

- Tumor lysis syndrome is a constellation of metabolic derangements that can occur after starting cancer treatment.
- It usually occurs in patients with bulky, rapidly proliferating, and treatment-responsive tumors.
- It is associated with acute leukemias, high-grade non-Hodgkin's lymphoma, solid tumors, and hematologic cancers.
- Tumor lysis syndrome occurs when large numbers of cancer cells are destroyed during cancer treatment. The result is the release of large amounts of intracellular ions and other metabolic products into the blood. This leads to:
  - Hyperkalemia
  - Hypocalcemia
  - Hyperphosphatemia
  - Hyperuricemia
  - Acute renal failure

ICD-9CM CODES
277.88 Other specified disorders of metabolism
ICD-10CM CODES
E88.3 Tumor lysis syndrome

EPIDEMIOLOGY & DEMOGRAPHICS

INCIDENCE: Unknown, but it is the most common disease-related emergency encountered by physicians caring for children or adults with hematologic cancers.

PREVALENCE:
- Varies
- Increased frequency is associated with bulky, aggressive, and treatment-sensitive tumors.

PREDOMINANT SEX AND AGE:
- No sex predilection exists.
- Occurs in all age groups. The elderly are more susceptible because of impaired renal function with age.

GENETICS: No known racial predilection

RISK FACTORS: Risk factors for developing tumor lysis syndrome include:
- Large tumor burden, as in:
  - Acute leukemias with elevated WBC count
  - Large, bulky, rapidly proliferating solid tumors
  - High-grade lymphomas
- Tumors sensitive to treatment
- Elevated pretreatment lactate dehydrogenase (LDH)
- Baseline renal insufficiency
- Older patients (due to these patients having a lower glomerular filtration rate)

PHYSICAL FINDINGS & CLINICAL PRESENTATION

CLINICAL PRESENTATION

Patients may present with a number of symptoms either before starting chemotherapy or commonly within 3 days after initiating cytotoxic treatment. Common symptoms include:
- Nausea
- Vomiting
- Edema
- Shortness of breath (from fluid overload or CHF)
- Lethargy/weakness
- Seizure
- Syncope
- Muscle cramps
- Tetany

PHYSICAL FINDINGS

Physical findings usually reflect the effects of specific metabolic derangement. Patients with tumor lysis syndrome present with hyperkalemia, hyperuremia, hypocalcemia, and hyperphosphatemia.
- Hyperkalemia causes:
  - Weakness
  - Paresthesia
  - Paralysis
  - ECG changes
  - Cardiac arrhythmias
  - Cardiac arrest
- Hyperuremia:
  - Weakness
  - Malaise
  - Vomiting
  - Pruritus
  - Restless legs
  - Ecchymoses
  - Hiccups
  - Paresthesia
  - Pericarditis
  - Dyspnea
  - Hypertension
- Hypocalcemia:
  - Paresthesia
  - Tetany
  - Bronchospasm
  - Heart block
  - Muscle twitching
- Hyperphosphatemia:
  - Oliguria
  - Anuria
  - Renal failure

ETIOLOGY

- Can occur spontaneously or after initiation of therapy in patients with:
  - Acute leukemias
  - Bulky solid tumors
  - High-grade lymphomas
- Administration of certain agents:
  - Paclitaxel
  - Hydroxyurea
  - Etoposide
  - Fludarabine
- It has been reported in some cancer patients who received:
  - Corticosteroids
  - Monoclonal antibodies
  - Radiation therapy
  - Hormonal compounds
- Intrathecal administration of chemotherapy
- Rare causes: pregnancy, fever, some patients under general anesthesia

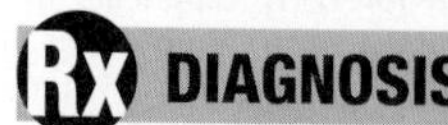

DIAGNOSIS

DIFFERENTIAL DIAGNOSIS

See "Acute Kidney Injury" topic in Section I.

LABORATORY TESTS

- Monitor BUN, creatinine phosphate, potassium, calcium, uric acid, LDH in high-risk patients before and up to 72 hr after initiating therapy. If evidence of tumor lysis syndrome develops, check these at least twice a day.
- Closely monitor urine output (for signs of oliguria).
- Perform frequent ECG or continuous cardiac monitoring to look for lethal arrhythmia (that can be caused by K or Ca abnormalities).

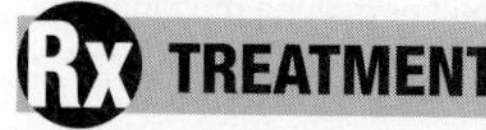

TREATMENT

GENERAL PRINCIPLES

- It is very important to identify high-risk patients (by assessing the extent of tumor burden, renal function, and pathologic findings) in order to initiate prophylactic measures before starting treatment. Delay in doing this may lead to life-threatening conditions.
- In patients with pretreatment tumor lysis syndrome:
  - Correct all metabolic derangement before starting cancer treatment, if possible.
- Careful and frequent laboratory and clinical monitoring. Check:
  - Baseline ECG/continuous cardiac monitoring
  - Renal/fluid status by checking vital signs, daily weights, fluid intake/output
  - For high-risk patients and those with overt tumor lysis syndrome, check the following at least twice daily:
    - Basic metabolic panel
    - Calcium
    - Uric acid
    - Phosphate
    - LDH

TREATMENT OPTIONS (PREVENTIVE MEASURES) FOR HIGH-RISK PATIENTS WITHOUT TUMOR LYSIS SYNDROME

- **Hydration:** prevent volume depletion and help correct electrolyte derangement
  - Start 24-48 hr before initiating cancer treatment and continue for up to 72 hr after treatment.
  - May use D_5W plus 2 amps of $NaCO_3$.
- **Control of hyperuricemia:** use allopurinol or rasburicase.
  - Allopurinol (xanthine oxidase inhibitor prevents the conversion of xanthine and hypoxanthine to uric acid)
    - Give 600 mg/day PO or IV for prophylaxis and 600-900 mg/day PO or IV to treat tumor lysis syndrome.
  - Rasburicase (recombinant urate oxidase) is used when uric acid levels cannot be lowered by standard procedures.
  - Given IV or IM at dosages from 50-100 U/kg/day for 1-5 days.
    - Do not give together with allopurinol.
    - Alkalization is not necessary.
    - Contraindicated in glucose-6-phosphate dehydrogenase deficiency and pregnancy.
- Diuretics: indicated for well-hydrated patients with poor/inadequate diuresis.

- Furosemide may be used in well-hydrated patients with elevated potassium or in patients with fluid overload.

TREATMENT OF PATIENTS WITH TUMOR LYSIS SYNDROME

- **Principles:**
  - General and preventive measures as mentioned in General Principles and Treatment Options
  - Aggressively treating electrolyte disturbances
  - Treat renal failure if above fail
- Treating electrolyte disturbances:
  - Hyperuricemia: as outlined above
  - Hyperkalemia:
    - Restrict dietary potassium
    - Stop potassium in IV fluid
    - IV infusion of glucose and insulin (to move K to intracellular space)
    - IV gluconate (cardioprotective effect)
    - PO potassium-exchange resins
    - If above measures fail, then immediate dialysis is needed.
  - Hyperphosphatemia
    - Decrease dietary intake
    - IV glucose plus insulin
    - Oral phosphate binders
  - Hypocalcemia
    - Treat only if symptomatic (e.g., neuromuscular irritability as in positive Chvostek or Trousseau sign).
    - Calcium gluconate only when symptomatic
    - Calcitrol can be used only if serum phosphate level is normal.

TREAT RENAL FAILURE

- Consider early dialysis if above methods fail.
- Dialysis prevents life-threatening complications and irreversible renal failure.
- Hemodialysis is the preferred procedure.

REFERRAL

- Nephrology
- Critical care

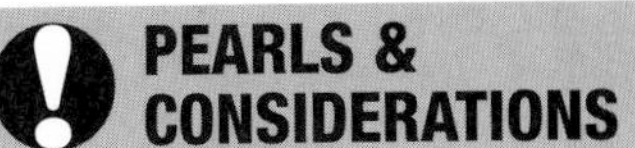

PEARLS & CONSIDERATIONS

COMMENTS

- High-risk patients should have prophylactic measures 24-48 hr before starting cytotoxic drugs. Low-intensity initial therapy is also recommended in patients at high-risk for tumor lysis syndrome.
- Prophylactic measures include:
  - IV hydration
  - Administration of allopurinol
  - Urinary alkalization
- Monitor blood chemistry and fluid status.
- Complications of tumor lysis syndrome include:
  - Uremia
  - Renal failure
  - Electrolyte disturbances
  - Cardiac arrhythmia
  - Pulmonary edema secondary to aggressive hydration
  - Metabolic alkalosis from IV bicarbonate administration

SUGGESTED READINGS

available at www.expertconsult.com

AUTHOR: **DANIEL K. ASIEDU, M.D., PH.D., F.A.C.P.**

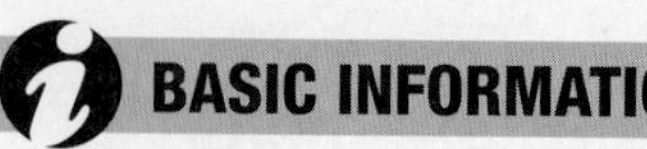

DEFINITION

Ulcerative colitis (UC) is a chronic inflammatory bowel disease of undetermined etiology. Accumulating evidence suggests that it may result from an inappropriate inflammatory response to environmental triggers and immune dysregulation involving CD4+ T-cell Th2 response in a genetically susceptible host.

SYNONYMS

UC
Inflammatory bowel disease (IBD)
Idiopathic proctocolitis
Pancolitis

ICD-9CM CODES
556.9 Ulcerative colitis
ICD-10CM Codes
K51.0 Ulcerative pancolitis
K51.2 Ulcerative proctitis
K51.3 Ulcerative rectosigmoiditis
K51.5 Left-sided colitis
K51.8 Other ulcerative colitis
K51.90 Ulcerative colitis, unspecified, without complications

EPIDEMIOLOGY & DEMOGRAPHICS

INCIDENCE: The incidence of UC is 9 to 12 cases per 100,000 persons per year; most common between ages 15 and 40 yr, with a second peak between 50 and 80 yr. The disease affects men and women at similar rates. Infection with nontyphoid salmonella or campylobacter is associated with an 8-10 time higher risk of developing ulcerative colitis in the following year.

PREVALENCE: The prevalence of UC is 7.6 to 246.0 cases per 100,000 per year. Higher prevalence in Ashkenazi Jewish descendants.

GEOGRAPHIC DISTRIBUTION: The highest incidence and prevalence of IBD are seen in northern Europe and North America, and the lowest in continental Asia.

GENETICS:
- Both specific and nonspecific gene variants are associated with UC.
- There are 47 loci associated with UC, of which 19 are specific for UC and 28 are shared with Crohn's disease.
- Abnormalities in humoral and cellular adaptive immunity are also found in UC.

PHYSICAL FINDINGS & CLINICAL PRESENTATION

- Patients with UC often present with acute onset of bloody diarrhea accompanied by tenesmus, fever, and dehydration. At presentation 40% of adults have proctitis, 40% have left-sided colitis, and 20% have pancolitis.
- Abdominal distention and tenderness may indicate the presence of complications such as toxic megacolon.
- The onset of symptoms is typically acute and is generally followed by periods of spontaneous remission and frequent relapses.
- Fever, evidence of dehydration may be present during the acute flare-up.
- Evidence of extraintestinal manifestations may be present in nearly 25% of patients: liver disease, sclerosing cholangitis, iritis, uveitis, episcleritis, arthritis, erythema nodosum, pyoderma gangrenosum, aphthous stomatitis.

Dx DIAGNOSIS

DIFFERENTIAL DIAGNOSIS

- Crohn's disease (Table 1-491)
- Bacterial infections (Table 1-492)
  1. Acute: *Campylobacter, Yersinia, Salmonella, Shigella, Chlamydia, Escherichia coli, Clostridium difficile,* gonococcal proctitis
  2. Chronic: Whipple's disease, tuberculosis, enterocolitis
- Irritable bowel syndrome
- Protozoal and parasitic infections (amebiasis, giardiasis, cryptosporidiosis)
- Neoplasm (intestinal lymphoma, carcinoma of colon)
- Ischemic bowel disease
- Diverticulitis
- Celiac sprue, lymphocytic or collagenous colitis, radiation enteritis, endometriosis
- Solitary rectal ulcer
- Acute self-limited colitis
- Medication (NSAIDs, chemotherapy)

WORKUP

An accurate diagnosis of UC should define the extent and severity of inflammation. Diagnostic workup includes:
- Comprehensive history, physical examination
- Laboratory tests (see "Laboratory Tests")
- Colonoscopy to establish the presence of mucosal inflammation; typical endoscopic findings in UC are areas of continuous friable mucosa; diffuse, uniform erythema replacing the usual mucosal vascular pattern; and pseudopolyps. The transition from abnormal to normal tissue tends to be abrupt. Rectal involvement is invariably present if the disease is active. Pathologic findings suggestive of UC include crypt abscesses and atrophy, mucin depletion, basal plasmacytosis, basal lymphoid aggregates, increased lamina propria cellularity, and Paneth cell metaplasia.

LABORATORY TESTS

- Anemia and high erythrocyte sedimentation rate (in severe colitis) are common.
- Potassium, magnesium, calcium, and albumin may be decreased.
- Antineutrophil cytoplasmic antibodies (ANCA) with a perinuclear staining pattern (pANCA) can be found in >45% of patients; there is an increased frequency in treatment-resistant left-sided colitis, suggesting a possible association between these antibodies and a relative resistance to medical therapy in patients with UC.
- Calprotectin is a protein that is measured in feces as a marker of intestinal mucosa leukocyte activity that may be useful for screening of patients with suspected IBD. Trials have shown that based on a pretest probability

TABLE 1-491 Comparison of Crohn's Disease and Ulcerative Colitis

Feature	Crohn's Disease	Ulcerative Colitis
Rectal bleeding	Sometimes	Common
Diarrhea, mucus, pus	Variable	Common
Abdominal pain	Common	Variable
Abdominal mass	Common	Not present
Growth failure	Common	Variable
Perianal disease	Common	Rare
Rectal involvement	Occasional	Universal
Pyoderma gangrenosum	Rare	Present
Erythema nodosum	Common	Less common
Mouth ulceration	Common	Rare
Thrombosis	Less common	Present
Colonic disease	50%-75%	100%
Ileal disease	Common	None except backwash ileitis
Stomach-esophageal disease	More common	Chronic gastritis can be seen
Strictures	Common	Rare
Fissures	Common	Rare
Fistulas	Common	Rare
Toxic megacolon	None	Present
Sclerosing cholangitis	Less common	Present
Risk for cancer	Increased	Greatly increased
Discontinuous (skip) lesions	Common	Not present
Transmural involvement	Common	Unusual
Crypt abscesses	Less common	Common
Granulomas	Common	None
Linear ulcerations	Uncommon	Common

From Kliegman RM et al: *Nelson textbook of pediatrics,* ed 19, Philadelphia, 2011, Saunders.

TABLE 1-492 Infectious Agents Mimicking Inflammatory Bowel Disease

Agent	Manifestations	Diagnosis	Comments
Bacterial			
Campylobacter jejuni	Acute diarrhea, fever, fecal blood, and leukocytes	Culture	Common in adolescents, may relapse
Yersinia enterocolitica	Acute → chronic diarrhea, right lower quadrant pain, mesenteric adenitis-pseudoappendicitis, fecal blood, and leukocytes Extraintestinal manifestations, mimics Crohn's disease	Culture	Common in adolescents as fever of unknown origin, weight loss, abdominal pain
Clostridium difficile	Postantibiotic onset, watery → bloody diarrhea, pseudomembrane on sigmoidoscopy	Cytotoxin assay	May be nosocomial Toxic megacolon possible
Escherichia coli 0157:H7	Colitis, fecal blood, abdominal pain	Culture and typing	Hemolytic-uremic syndrome
Salmonella	Watery → bloody diarrhea, food borne, fecal leukocytes, fever, pain, cramps	Culture	Usually acute
Shigella	Watery → bloody diarrhea, fecal leukocytes, fever, pain, cramps	Culture	Dysentery symptoms
Edwardsiella tarda	Bloody diarrhea, cramps	Culture	Ulceration on endoscopy
Aeromonas hydrophila	Cramps, diarrhea, fecal blood	Culture	May be chronic Contaminated drinking water
Plesiomonas	Diarrhea, cramps	Culture	Shellfish source
Tuberculosis	Rarely bovine, now *Mycobacterium tuberculosis* Ileocecal area, fistula formation	Culture, purified protein derivative, biopsy	Can mimic Crohn's disease
Parasites			
Entamoeba histolytica	Acute bloody diarrhea and liver abscess, colic	Trophozoite in stool, colonic mucosal flask ulceration, serologic tests	Travel to endemic area
Giardia lamblia	Foul-smelling, watery diarrhea, cramps, flatulence, weight loss; no colonic involvement	"Owl"-like trophozoite and cysts in stool; rarely duodenal intubation	May be chronic
AIDS-Associated Enteropathy			
Cryptosporidium	Chronic diarrhea, weight loss	Stool microscopy	Mucosal findings not like inflammatory bowel disease
Isospora belli	As in *Cryptosporidium*		Tropical location
Cytomegalovirus	Colonic ulceration, pain, bloody diarrhea	Culture, biopsy	More common when on immunosuppressive medications

From Kliegman RM et al: *Nelson textbook of pediatrics,* ed 19, Philadelphia, 2011, Saunders.

of IBD of 32% in adults, an abnormal fecal calprotectin test would increase the posttest probability to 91% and a normal result would reduce the probability to 3%.
- Stool examinations for ova and parasites, stool culture, and testing for *Clostridium difficile* toxin and *E. coli* 0157:H7 may be useful to eliminate other causes of diarrhea in selected patients with risk factors.

IMAGING STUDIES

Image studies (plain radiography, CT scan [Fig. 1-972]) are generally reserved for suspected complications such as perforation of bowel or toxic megacolon.

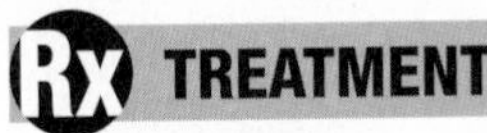

TREATMENT

NONPHARMACOLOGIC THERAPY:

- Correct nutritional deficiencies; total parenteral nutrition with bowel rest may be necessary in severe cases. Folate supplementation may reduce the incidence of dysplasia and cancer in chronic UC.
- Avoid oral feedings during acute exacerbation to decrease colonic activity; a low-roughage diet may be helpful in early relapse.
- Psychotherapy is useful in most patients. Referral to self-help groups is also important because of the chronicity of the disease and the young age of the patients.

ACUTE GENERAL Rx

The therapeutic options vary with the degree of disease (mild, severe, fulminant) and areas of involvement (distal, extensive).

- Mild disease can be treated with 5-aminosalicylate agents (mesalamine, olsalazine, balsalazide, sulfasalazine). It can be administered as an enema (40 mg once daily at bedtime for 3 to 6 wk) or suppository (500 mg bid) for patients with distal colonic disease. Oral forms in which the 5-acetyl salicylic acid is in a slow-release or pH-dependent matrix (Pentasa 1 g qid, Asacol 800 mg PO tid) can deliver therapeutic concentrations to the more proximal small bowel or distal ileum. Olsalazine can be useful for maintenance of remission of UC in patients intolerant to sulfasalazine. Usual dose is 500 mg bid taken with food. Balsalazide is indicated for mild to moderately active UC. Usual dose is three 750-mg capsules tid. Probiotics may also be helpful in inducing remission in mild-to-moderate UC.
- Mild-to-moderate UC is often treated with a combination of rectal and oral 5-aminosalicylate. Refractory patients are candidates for oral glucocorticoids or immunosuppressive agents (e.g., cyclosporine).
- Severe disease usually responds to oral corticosteroids (e.g., prednisone 40 to 60 mg/day); the FDA has recently approved an extended release formulation of the corticosteroid budesonide for induction of remission in mild to moderate ulcerative colitis. Corticosteroid suppositories or enemas are also useful for distal colitis. The immunosuppressant azathioprine also provides effective long-term treatment for Crohn's disease.
- Infliximab, a chimeric monoclonal antibody, has been shown to be effective in patients who have not responded to corticosteroid therapy. Newer therapeutic modalities include the use of adalimumab (ADA), a recombinant human monoclonal antibody against tumor necrosis factor-α (TNF-α), for the induction of clinical remission in anti–TNF-α naïve patients with moderately to severely active UC and use of tofacitinib, an oral Janus kinase inhibitor, for patients with moderately to severely active UC.

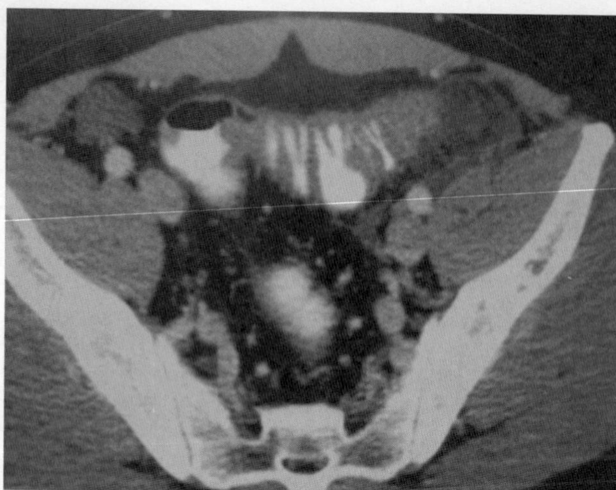

FIGURE 1-972 Computed tomography scan showing colonic wall thickening in a patient with ulcerative colitis. (From Adams JG, et al: *Emergency medicine, clinical essentials*, ed 2, Philadelphia, 2013, Elsevier.)

- Fulminant disease generally requires hospital admission and parenteral corticosteroids (e.g., IV hydrocortisone 100 mg q6h). When bowel movements have returned to normal and the patient is able to eat normally, oral prednisone is resumed. IV cyclosporine can also be used in severe refractory cases; renal toxicity is a potential complication.
- Surgery is indicated in patients who do not respond to intensive medical therapy. Proctocolectomy is usually curative in these patients and also eliminates the high risk of developing adenocarcinoma of the colon (10% to 20% of patients develop it after 10 yr with the disease). Total proctocolectomy with ileal pouch-anal anastomatosis (IPAA) is the procedure of choice for most patients who require elective surgery, since it preserves anal sphincter function. Continent ileostomy is an alternative procedure.

CHRONIC Rx

- Colonoscopic surveillance and multiple biopsies should be instituted approximately 10 yr after diagnosis because of the increased risk of colon carcinoma.
- Erythropoietin is useful in patients with anemia refractory to treatment with iron and vitamins.
- In patients on long-term steroid therapy, periodic bone density scans are recommended to screen for glucocorticoid-induced osteoporosis.

DISPOSITION

The clinical course is variable. ~66% of patients will achieve clinical remission with medical therapy, and nearly 80% of treatment compliant patients maintain remission. 15% to 20% of patients eventually require colectomy. Pouchitis is the most common long-term complication of IPAA (up to 40% of patients). >75% of patients treated medically will experience relapse.

REFERRAL

- Gastrointestinal consultation for initial diagnostic sigmoidoscopy/colonoscopy in suspected cases
- Surgical referral for patients with severe disease unresponsive to medical therapy

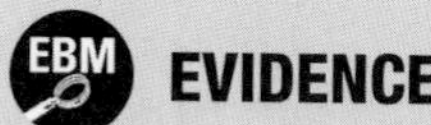

EVIDENCE

available at www.expertconsult.com

SUGGESTED READINGS

available at www.expertconsult.com

RELATED CONTENT

Ulcerative Colitis (Patient Information)

AUTHOR: **FRED F. FERRI, M.D.**

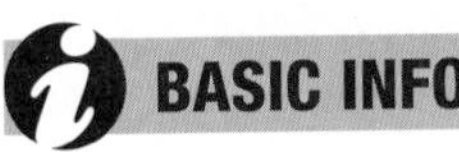

BASIC INFORMATION

DEFINITION

Urethritis is a well-defined clinical syndrome manifested by dysuria, a urethral discharge, or both.

ICD-9CM CODES
597.80 Urethritis, unspecified
098.20 Gonococcal
ICD-10CM Codes
A54.00 Gonococcal infection of lower genitourinary tract, unspecified

EPIDEMIOLOGY & DEMOGRAPHICS

- The major single specific etiology of acute urethritis is *Neisseria gonorrhoeae,* producing gonococcal urethritis (GCU). Urethritis of all other etiologies is called *nongonococcal urethritis* (NGU).
- NGU is twice as common as GCU in the U.S. NGU is the most common sexually transmitted disease (STD) syndrome occurring in men, accounting for 6 million office visits annually. NGU is more frequently encountered in higher socioeconomic groups. GCU is more common in homosexual males than heterosexual males with acute urethritis.
- *N. gonorrhoeae* is a gram-negative, kidney-shaped diplococcus with flattened opposed margins. The urethra is the most common site of infection in all men. In the United States, the rates of gonorrhea are 40 times higher in black adolescent males than in white adolescent males. In heterosexual men, the pharynx is infected in 7%, and in homosexual men the pharynx is infected in 40% and the rectum in 25%. A single episode of intercourse with an infected partner carries a transmission risk of 20% for males; female partners of an infected male will contract the disease 80% of the time.

PHYSICAL FINDINGS & CLINICAL PRESENTATION

- Symptoms of GCU: urethral discharge and dysuria are the most common symptoms. There is complaint of urethral itching. Prostatic involvement can cause frequency, urgency, and nocturia. It can involve the epididymis through spreading down the vas deferens, causing acute epididymitis.
- Incubation period: 3 to 10 days. Without treatment, urethritis persists for 3 to 7 wk, with 95% of men becoming asymptomatic after 3 mo. GCU is asymptomatic in up to 60% of contacts.
- Signs of GCU: yellow-brown discharge, meatal edema, urethral tenderness to palpation. Rectal bleeding with pus is seen with gonococcal proctitis. Periurethritis leading to urethral stenosis can occur. Disseminated infection can occur. Tenosynovitis and arthritis can occur. Rarely, hepatitis, myocarditis, endocarditis, and meningitis can occur.

Dx DIAGNOSIS

DIFFERENTIAL DIAGNOSIS

- NGU
- Herpes simplex virus

LABORATORY TESTS

- Nucleic acid amplification tests (NAATs): these tests have largely replaced culture in many settings where persons are screened for asymptomatic genital infection. They are not more sensitive than culture for detecting *N. gonorrhoeae* in cervical or urethral specimen; however, they have specificities of >99% and retain sensitivity when used to test voided urine or self-collected vaginal swabs.
- Calcium alginate or rayon swab on a metal shaft (not cotton-tipped swabs, which are bactericidal) of the urethra should be performed anywhere from 2 to 4 hr after voiding to prevent bacterial washout with voiding. Gram staining with modified Thayer-Martin media is indicated. Cultures of the pharynx and rectum when indicated.
- Concomitant serologic testing for syphilis on all patients.
- Concomitant *Chlamydia* testing on all patients.
- Offer of HIV counseling and testing to all patients.

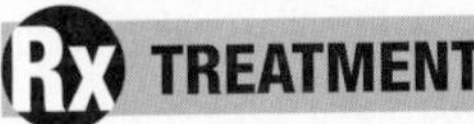

Rx TREATMENT

NONPHARMACOLOGIC THERAPY

Behavioral management: avoid intercourse until cure has been attained and sexual partners have been evaluated and treated.

ACUTE GENERAL Rx

- Ceftriaxone 250 mg IM x 1 dose *plus* azithromycin 1 g orally single dose *or* doxycycline 100 mg orally twice/day for 7 days

Alternative regimens:

- Cefixime 400 mg PO x 1 dose *plus* azithromycin 1 g orally single dose *or* doxycycline 100 mg orally twice/day for 7 days *plus* test of cure in 1 wk
- If the patient has severe cephalosporin allergy: azithromycin 2 g in a single oral dose *plus* test of cure in 1 wk
- Resistance to penicillins, fluoroquinolones, sulfonamides, and tetracyclines is now widespread.
- The use of azithromycin as the second antimicrobial is preferred over doxycycline due to the high prevalence of tetracycline resistance.
- The proportion of gonorrhea cases in heterosexual men that are fluoroquinolone resistant (QRNG) has reached 6.7%, an elevenfold increase from 0.6% in 2001. Fluoroquinolone antibiotics are no longer recommended to treat gonorrhea in the U.S.
- Dual treatment for gonococcal and chlamydial infections is based on theory and expert opinion rather than evidence from clinical trials.

CHRONIC Rx

Postgonococcal urethritis (PGU): reinfection is the most common cause of recurrence. Repeat swab and culture of the urethra, pharynx, and rectum (where applicable) are mandatory. Persistence of polymorphonuclear cells (PMNs) with the absence of gram-negative intracellular diplococci suggests a diagnosis of PGU. This occurs when GCU is treated with a regimen that is ineffective against coincident chlamydial infection; it represents NGU after GCU. The syndrome should be treated as NGU. Persistence of *N. gonorrhoeae* by smear or culture requires treatment for *N. gonorrhoeae.*

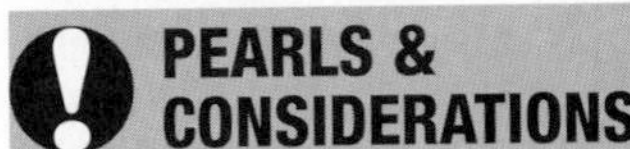

PEARLS & CONSIDERATIONS

COMMENTS

- Partner notification: the names and contact information of sexual partners should be gathered at the time of the visit and referred to the health department or the patient notifies the contact directly. Expedited partner treatment is recommended by the Centers for Disease Control and Prevention (CDC) and approved in several states. This consists of giving prescriptions to the infected patient for their partner(s) who has not been evaluated by a physician and is unlikely to seek medical care.
- On examination of the urethral smear, the presence of small numbers of PMNs provides objective evidence of urethritis. The complete absence of PMNs on a urethral smear argues against urethritis. If in addition to the PMNs there are gram-negative, intracellular diplococci, the diagnosis of gonorrhea is established.

SUGGESTED READINGS

available at www.expertconsult.com

RELATED CONTENT

Fig. 3-66 Evaluation of patients with dysuria and/or urethral/vaginal discharge (Algorithm)
Gonococcal Urethritis (Patient Information)

AUTHOR: **RUBEN ALVERO, M.D.**

BASIC INFORMATION

DEFINITION

Nongonococcal urethritis (NGU) is urethral inflammation caused by any of several organisms.

SYNONYMS

NGU

ICD-9CM CODES
099.40 Nongonococcal
099.41 Chlamydial
ICD-10CM Codes
A56.0 Chlamydial infection of lower genitourinary tract
N34.1 Nonspecific urethritis

EPIDEMIOLOGY & DEMOGRAPHICS

- Occurrence is 50% in sexually transmitted disease clinics.
- NGU most commonly affects men in a higher socioeconomic class, affecting heterosexual men more frequently than homosexual men.
- NGU carries a greater morbidity rate than gonococcal urethritis (GCU).

PHYSICAL FINDINGS & CLINICAL PRESENTATION

- Incubation period: 2 to 35 days
- Symptoms: dysuria, whitish-clear urethral discharge (Fig. 1-973), and urethral itching. The onset of symptoms in NGU is less acute than GCU.

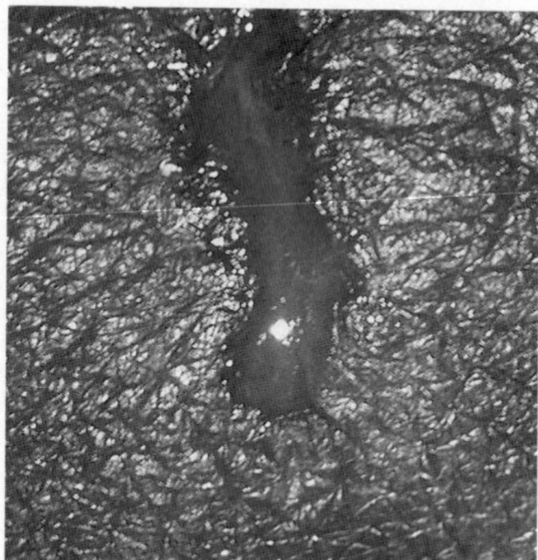

FIGURE 1-973 Urethral discharge from a man with nongonococcal urethritis. (From Mandell GL et al: *Principles and practice of infectious diseases,* ed 7, Philadelphia, 2009, Churchill Livingstone.)

- Signs: whitish-clear urethral discharge, meatal edema, and erythema. Infected women manifest pyuria, and the disease can present as acute urethral syndrome.

COMPLICATIONS

Epididymitis in heterosexual men may be linked to nonbacterial prostatitis, proctitis in homosexual men, or Reiter's syndrome.

ETIOLOGY

- Most common agent is *Chlamydia* spp., an obligate intracellular parasite possessing both DNA and RNA, which replicates by binary fission. It causes 20% to 50% of NGU cases. Two species exist:
  - *Chlamydia psittaci*
  - *Chlamydia trachomatis* with its 15 serotypes
    Serotypes A through C cause hyperendemic-blinding trachoma.
    Serotypes D through K cause genital tract infection.
    Serotypes L1 through L3 cause lymphogranuloma venereum.
- Other causes of NGU: *Mycoplasma genitalium* (found in 44% of treatment failures); *Ureaplasma urealyticum,* causing 15% to 30% of the cases of NGU; *Trichomonas vaginalis;* and herpes simplex virus. The cause of 20% of the cases of NGU has not been identified.
- Asymptomatic infection occurs in 28% of the contacts of women with chlamydial cervical infection.

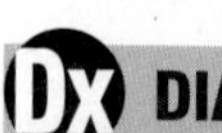

DIAGNOSIS

DIFFERENTIAL DIAGNOSIS

- GCU
- Herpes simplex virus
- Trichomoniasis

LABORATORY TESTS

- Requires demonstration of urethritis and exclusion of infection with *N. gonorrhoeae.*
- Nucleic acid amplification tests (NAATs): these tests have largely replaced culture in many settings where persons are screened for asymptomatic genital infection.
- The appearance of PMNs on urethral smear confirms the diagnosis of urethritis. Because *Chlamydia* is an intracellular parasite of the columnar epithelium, the best specimen for culture is an endourethral swab taken from an area 2 to 4 cm inside the urethra. For culture, a Dacron-tipped swab is used; avoid calcium alginate or cotton swabs. The organism can only be grown in tissue culture, which is expensive.

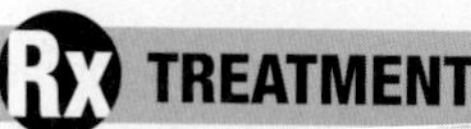

TREATMENT

Because it is impossible to differentiate among the common etiologies of NGU, the condition is treated syndromically, including in the initial treatment regimen those drugs effective against the common causative agents. In patients with isolated uncomplicated NGU, recommended regimens are azithromycin 1 g orally single dose or doxycycline 100 mg bid × 7 days. In patients with confirmed urethritis and unclear etiology, concurrent treatment for gonorrhea and *Chlamydia* is recommended. In these patients, uncomplicated infections of the urethra can be treated with combination of a single 1-g dose of oral azithromycin or 100 mg doxycycline bid × 7 days *plus*

- Cefixime 400 mg PO × 1 dose or
- Ceftriaxone 125 mg IM × 1 dose

Recommended regimen in pregnancy is azithromycin, 1 g orally as a single dose. Repeat test 3 weeks after completion of treatment to confirm cure.

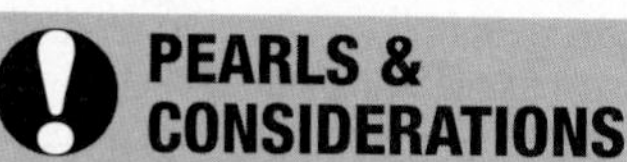

PEARLS & CONSIDERATIONS

COMMENTS

Partner notification: The names and contact information of sexual partners should be gathered at the time of the visit and referred to the health department or the patient notifies the contact directly. Expedited partner treatment is recommended by the CDC and approved in several states. This consists of giving prescriptions to the infected patient for their partner(s) who has not been evaluated by a physician and is unlikely to seek medical care.

SUGGESTED READINGS

available at www.expertconsult.com

RELATED CONTENT

Cervicitis (Related Key Topic)
Chlamydia Genital Infections (Related Key Topic)
Nongonococcal Urethritis (Patient Information)

AUTHOR: **RUBEN ALVERO, M.D.**

U

Diseases and Disorders

BASIC INFORMATION

DEFINITION

Urinary tract infection (UTI) is a term that encompasses a broad range of clinical entities that have in common a positive urine culture. A conventional threshold is growth of >100,000 colony-forming units per milliliter from a midstream-catch urine sample. In symptomatic patients, a smaller number of bacteria (between 100 and 10,000 colony-forming units per milliliter of midstream urine) is recognized as an infection.

SYNONYMS

UTI

ICD-9CM CODES
595.0 Acute cystitis
595.3 Trigonitis
595.2 Chronic cystitis
590.1 Acute pyelonephritis
590.0 Chronic pyelonephritis
590.8 Nonspecific pyelonephritis
ICD-10CM Codes
N30.00 Acute cystitis without hematuria
N30.30 Trigonitis without hematuria
N30.20 Other chronic cystitis without hematuria
N39.0 Urinary tract infection, site not specified

CLASSIFICATION

- Uncomplicated UTI: occurs in a normal urinary tract and resolves rapidly with conventional antimicrobials.
- Complicated UTI: occurs in patients with coexisting pathology (strictures, stones, comorbidities [diabetes mellitus, multiple sclerosis, spinal cord injuries]).
- First infection: the first documented UTI; tends to be uncomplicated and is easily treated.
- Unresolved bacteriuria: UTI in which the urinary tract is not sterilized during therapy. Main causes are bacterial resistance, patient noncompliance with medication, mixed bacterial infection, rapid reinfection, azotemia, infected stones, Münchausen syndrome, and papillary necrosis.
- Bacterial persistence: UTI in which the urine cultures become sterile during therapy, but a persistent source of infection from a site within the urinary tract that was excluded from the high urinary concentrations gives rise to reinfection by the same organism. Causes include infected stone, chronic bacterial prostatitis, atrophic infected kidney, vesicovaginal or enterovesical fistulas, obstructive uropathy, infected pyelocaliceal diverticula, infected ureteral stump after nephrectomy, infected necrotic papillae from papillary necrosis, infected urachal cysts, infected medullary sponge kidney, urethral diverticula, and foreign bodies.
- Reinfection: UTI in which a new infection occurs with new pathogens at variable intervals after a previous infection has been eradicated.
- Relapse: the less common form of recurrent infection; occurs within 2 wk of treatment when the same organism reappears in the same site as the previous infection. Relapsing infections of the urinary tract most commonly occur in pyelonephritis, kidney obstruction from a stone, and prostatitis.

EPIDEMIOLOGY & DEMOGRAPHICS

INCIDENCE:

- UTI is the most common bacterial infection encountered in the ambulatory care setting in the U.S. The self-reported annual incidence of UTI in women is 12%, and by age 32 half of all women report having had at least one UTI.
- In neonates: more common in boys as a result of anatomic abnormalities such as posterior urethral valves.
- In preschool children: more common in girls (4.5% vs. 0.5% for boys).
- In adulthood: more common in women, with a 1% to 3% prevalence in nonpregnant women. Table 1-493 describes factors modulating risk for acute uncomplicated UTIs in women. In pregnancy at 12 wk, the incidence of asymptomatic bacteriuria is similar to nonpregnant women, at 2% to 10%. However, 25%-30% of pregnant women with untreated asymptomatic bacteriuria develop acute pyelonephritis, especially in the second and third trimesters, and have a pyelonephritic recurrence rate of 10%. In adults aged ≥65 yr, at least 10% of men and 20% of women have bacteriuria.

PHYSICAL FINDINGS & CLINICAL PRESENTATION

- UTI presentation is inconsistent and cannot be relied on to diagnose UTI accurately or to localize the site of infection. Patients report:
  - Urinary frequency, urgency
  - Dysuria
  - Urge incontinence
  - Suprapubic pain
  - Gross or microscopic hematuria
- When negative cultures are associated with significant pyuria, vaginal discharge, or hematuria, infections with *Chlamydia trachomatis, Neisseria gonorrhoeae,* and *Trichomonas vaginalis* should be considered.
- Acute pyelonephritis presents with fever, flank or abdominal pain, chills, malaise, vomiting, and diarrhea. It is these systemic symptoms that distinguish pyelonephritis from cystitis. Complications of acute pyelonephritis are renal abscess, perinephric abscess, emphysematous pyelonephritis, and pyonephrosis.

ETIOLOGY & PATHOGENESIS

- Four major pathways:
  - Ascending from the urethra
  - Lymphatic
  - Hematogenous
  - Direct extension from another organ system
- Other risk factors: neurologic diseases, renal failure, diabetes, anatomic abnormalities, bladder outlet obstruction, urethral stricture, vesicoureteral reflux, fistula, urinary diversion, megacystis, infected stones, age, pregnancy, instrumentation, poor patient compliance, poor hygiene, infrequent voiding, diaphragm contraceptives, tampon use, douches, and catheters.
- Catheters: all patients who require a long-term Foley catheter eventually develop significant levels of bacteriuria. Treatment is reserved for individuals who become symptomatic (leukocytosis, fever, chills, malaise, loss of appetite, etc.) Using prophylactic antibiotics to treat patients who have chronic catheters is to be discouraged because of the risk of acquiring bacteria resistant to antibiotic therapy.
- Once bacteria reach the urinary tract, three factors determine whether the infection occurs (Box E1-94). These factors also determine the anatomic level of the UTI:
  - Virulence of the microorganism
  - Inoculum size
  - Adequacy of the host defense mechanisms
- Urinary pathogens: in 95% of UTIs the infecting organism is a member of the Enterobacteriaceae, enterococci, or, in young women, *Staphylococcus saprophyticus. Escherichia coli* is the most common pathogen (85% of UTI cases). In contrast, the organisms that commonly colonize the distal urethra and skin of both men and women and the vagina of women are *Staphylococcus epidermidis,* diphtheroids,

TABLE 1-493 Factors Modulating Risk for Acute Uncomplicated Urinary Tract Infections in Women

Host Determinants	Uropathogen Determinants
Behavioral: sexual intercourse, use of spermicidal products, recent antimicrobial use, suboptimal voiding habits	*Escherichia coli* virulence determinants: P, S, Dr, and type I fimbriae; hemolysin; aerobactin; serum resistance
Genetic: innate and adaptive immune response, enhanced epithelial cell adherence, antibacterial factors in urine and bladder mucosa, nonsecretor of ABO blood group antigens, P_1 blood group phenotype, reduced CXCR1 expression, previous history of recurrent cystitis	
Biologic: estrogen deficiency in postmenopausal women, micturition	

From Floege J et al: *Comprehensive clinical nephrology,* ed 4, Philadelphia, 2010, Saunders.

lactobacilli, *Gardnerella vaginalis,* and a variety of anaerobes that rarely cause UTIs. In general, the isolation of two or more bacterial species from a urine culture signifies a contaminated specimen unless the patient is being managed with an indwelling catheter or urinary diversion or has a chronic complicated infection.

- Defense mechanisms against cystitis: low pH and high osmolarity, mucopolysaccharide glycosaminoglycan protective layer, normal bladder that empties completely and has no incontinence, and the presence of estrogen.

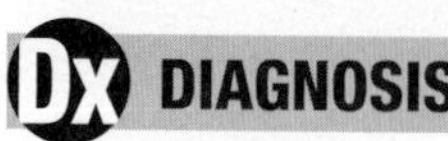

DIAGNOSIS

DIFFERENTIAL DIAGNOSIS

- Interstitial cystitis
- Vaginitis
- Urethritis (gonococcal, nongonococcal, *Trichomonas*)
- Frequency-urgency syndrome, prostatitis (acute and chronic)
- Obstructive uropathy
- Infected stones
- Fistulas
- Papillary necrosis
- Vesicoureteral reflux
- Irritation

LABORATORY TESTS

- Urinalysis with microscopic evaluation of clean-catch urine for bacteria and pyuria. The presence of ≥10 leukocytes/μl of unspun urine from a midstream catch indicates UTI. If urine dipsticks are used, the presence of positive nitrite and positive leukocyte esterase is indicative of UTI in a symptomatic patient.
- Urine culture and sensitivity are useful in complicated UTIs but generally not needed in uncomplicated UTIs.
- Complete blood count with differential (shows leukocytosis)
- Antibody-coated bacteria are seen with pyelonephritis
- An approach to the management of UTI is described in Fig. E1-974.

IMAGING STUDIES

- Warranted only if renal infection or genitourinary abnormality is suspected
- KUB (kidneys, ureter, and bladder); voiding cystourethrogram; renal sonogram; intravenous pyelogram; CT scan; nuclear scan
- Specialty examination: cystoscopy with occasional retrograde pyelography to rule out obstructive uropathy; stenting the obstruction possibly required

Rx TREATMENT

NONPHARMACOLOGIC THERAPY

- Hot sitz baths, anticholinergics, urinary analgesics
- For pyelonephritis: bed rest, analgesics, antipyretics, and IV hydration

ACUTE GENERAL Rx

- Conventional therapy of 7 days; short-term therapy of 3 or 5 days (Fig. E1-975).
- Agents of choice: nitrofurantoin, fluoroquinolones, trimethoprim plus sulfonamide (TMP-SMX), amoxicillin/clavulanate, and cephalosporins. Drug resistance needs to be considered when choosing antibiotic therapy. Currently, in the U.S., fluoroquinolone resistance exceeds 20% and TMP-SMX resistance 40% in some regions, but resistance is much lower for nitrofurantoin.
- For pyelonephritis: hospitalization until afebrile and stable, then at home by home care agency with IV antibiotic composed of aminoglycoside plus cephalosporin for 1 wk followed by oral agents (based on sensitivity) for 2 wk. Moderate forms of pyelonephritis may be successfully treated with fluoroquinolone therapy for 21 days without requiring hospitalization. Most important, complicating factors such as obstructive uropathy or infected stones must be identified and treated.
- A urinary analgesic (e.g., phenazopyridine) can also be used along with antibiotics in patients with significant dysuria.

PEARLS & CONSIDERATIONS

COMMENTS

- Asymptomatic bacteriuria: occurs in both anatomically normal and abnormal urinary tracts. This can clear spontaneously, persist, or lead to symptomatic kidney infection. Treatment is recommended in patients with vesicoureteral reflux, stones, obstructive uropathy, parenchymal renal disease, or diabetes mellitus and in pregnant or immunocompromised patients.
- Pregnancy: 25% to 30% of pregnant women with asymptomatic untreated bacteriuria develop pyelonephritis. This is associated with prematurity and low-birth-weight infants. Confirmed significant bacteriuria should be treated with an aminopenicillin and cephalosporin.
- Recurrent UTI: caused by an unresolved infection, vaginal colonization of the originally infecting organism, or reinfection with a new strain. Management of recurrent UTI includes continuous antibiotic prophylaxis, intermittent self-treatment, and postcoital prophylaxis. Prophylaxis is recommended for women who have two or more symptomatic UTIs over a 6-mo period or three or more episodes over a 12-mo period.
    - Changes after menopause: lower levels of lactobacilli, decreased estrogen, senile atrophy of the genitalia, and loss of bladder elasticity (compliance).
    - Biologic factors altering defense systems: the presence of sialosyl galactosyl globoside on the surface of the kidney acts as a powerful receptor for *Escherichia coli* and increases the risk for UTI; the presence of the blood group P_1 causes increased binding of *E. coli* that is resistant to normal infection-fighting mechanisms in the body. It is believed that some individuals are deficient in a compound called human beta-defensin-1, a naturally occurring antibiotic that fights *E. coli* within the urinary tract.
    - Cranberry juice is often used as a remedy for the prevention of UTIs, however, randomized placebo-controlled trials have shown that it is no better than placebo for preventing UTIs.

RESISTANCE

- Because of the overuse of antibiotics, organisms once sensitive to a number of antimicrobial agents are now increasingly more resistant, making effective management of UTI and pyelonephritis more difficult and potentially more dangerous. Most important has been the increasing resistance to trimethoprim plus sulfamethoxazole (TMP-SMX), the current primary care provider drug of choice for acute uncomplicated UTI in women.
- When choosing a treatment regimen, physicians should consider such factors as:
    - In vitro susceptibility
    - Adverse effects
    - Cost effectiveness
    - Resistance rates in their respective communities

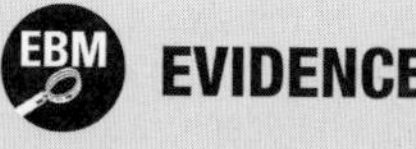

EVIDENCE

available at www.expertconsult.com

SUGGESTED READINGS

available at www.expertconsult.com

RELATED CONTENT

Pyelonephritis (Related Key Topic)
Urinary Tract Infection (Patient Information)
Urinary Tract Infection (Child) (Patient Information)

AUTHOR: **RUBEN ALVERO, M.D.**

BASIC INFORMATION

DEFINITION

Urolithiasis is the presence of calculi within the urinary tract. The five major types of urinary stones are calcium oxalate (>50%), calcium phosphate (10% to 20%), uric acid (7%), struvite (7%), and cystine (3%) (Table 1-494).

SYNONYMS

Kidney stones
Renal colic
Nephrolithiasis

ICD-9CM CODES
592.9 Urinary calculus
ICD-10CM Codes
N20.9 Urinary calculus, unspecified
N20.0 Calculus of kidney
N20.1 Calculus of ureter
N20.2 Calculus of kidney with calculus of ureter
N21.0 Calculus in bladder
N21.1 Calculus in urethra
N21.9 Calculus of lower urinary tract, unspecified

EPIDEMIOLOGY & DEMOGRAPHICS

- In the U.S., the lifetime prevalence of nephrolithiasis is 13% in men and 7% in women, annually.
- Between 1% and 1.7% of emergency department visits (1 to 2 million visits annually) are accounted for by a primary diagnosis of renal colic or renal calculus.
- The incidence of symptomatic nephrolithiasis is greatest during the summer as a result of increased humidity and temperatures with a concomitant increased risk of dehydration and concentrated urine.
- Calcium oxalate or mixed calcium oxalate/calcium phosphate stones account for nearly 70% of uroliths. Supersaturation, often expressed as the ratio of urinary calcium oxalate or calcium phosphate concentration to its solubility, is the driving force in stone formation. At levels above 1, crystals can nucleate and grow, promoting stone formation.

PHYSICAL FINDINGS & CLINICAL PRESENTATION

Stones may be asymptomatic, or they may cause the following signs and symptoms as a result of obstruction:

- Sudden onset of flank tenderness
- Nausea and vomiting
- The patient being in constant movement in an attempt to lessen the pain. (Patients with an acute abdomen are usually still because movement exacerbates the pain.)
- Pain that is referred to the testes or labium by the progression of stone down the urinary ureter
- Fever and chills that accompany the acute colic if there is superimposed infection
- Pain that may radiate anteriorly over to the abdomen and result in intestinal ileus

ETIOLOGY

- Supersaturation, often expressed as the ratio of urinary calcium oxalate or calcium phosphate concentration to its solubility, is the driving force in calcium kidney stone formation
- Increased absorption of calcium in the small bowel: type I absorptive hypercalciuria (i.e., independent of calcium intake)
- Idiopathic hypercalciuria nephrolithiasis. (This is the most common diagnosis for patients with calcium stones; the diagnosis is made only if there is no hypercalcemia and no known cause of the hypercalciuria.)
- Increased vitamin D synthesis (e.g., as a result of renal phosphate loss: type III absorptive hypercalciuria)
- Renal tubular malfunction with inadequate reabsorption of calcium and resulting hypercalciuria
- Heterozygous mutations in the NPT2a gene that result in hypophosphatemia and urinary phosphate loss
- Hyperparathyroidism with resulting hypercalcemia
- Elevated uric acid level (e.g., metabolic defects, dietary excess) (Box E1-95)
- Chronic diarrhea (e.g., inflammatory bowel disease) with increased oxalate absorption
- Type I (distal tubule) renal tubular acidosis (>1% of calcium stones)
- Long-term hydrochlorothiazide treatment
- Chronic infections with urease-producing organisms (e.g., *Proteus, Providencia, Pseudomonas, Klebsiella*). (Struvite, or magnesium ammonium phosphate crystals, is produced when the urinary tract is colonized by bacteria, thus producing elevated concentrations of ammonia [Box E1-96])
- Abnormal excretion of cystine
- Chemotherapy for malignancies
- Estrogen supplements

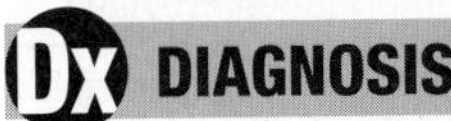

DIAGNOSIS

DIFFERENTIAL DIAGNOSIS

- Urinary tract infection
- Pyelonephritis
- Diverticulitis
- Pelvic inflammatory disease
- Ovarian pathology
- Factitious (i.e., in drug addicts)
- Appendicitis
- Small-bowel obstruction
- Ectopic pregnancy

The differential diagnosis of obstructive uropathy is described in Section II.

WORKUP

- Fig. E1-976 describes an algorithm for evaluation of suspected renal colic.
- Stone analysis should be performed on recovered stones.

TABLE 1-494 Stone Composition and Relative Occurrence

Stone Composition	Occurrence (%)
Calcium-containing stones	
Ca oxalate	60
Mixed Ca oxalate/ hydroxyapatite	20
Brushite	2
Non–calcium containing stones	
Uric acid	7
Magnesium ammonium phosphate (struvite)	7
Cystine	1-3 (10% of stones in children)
Xanthine	<1
Medication-related stones	<1

From Lipshultz LI et al: *Urology and the primary care practitioner,* ed 3, Philadelphia, 2008, Elsevier.

BOX 1-97 Components of the Medical History That Are Significant for Urolithiasis

- Diseases associated with disturbances of calcium metabolism: primary hyperparathyroidism, Wilson's disease, medullary sponge kidney, osteoporosis, immobilization, sarcoidosis, osteolytic metastases, plasmacytoma, neuroendocrine tumors, Paget's disease
- Dietary history: purine gluttony, calcium excess, milk alkali, oxalate excess, sodium excess, low citrus fruit intake
- Medications: uricosurics, diuretics, analgesics, vitamins C and D, antacids (especially phosphorus-binding agents), acetazolamide, calcium channel blockers, triamterene, estrogens, theophylline, protease inhibitors (indinavir), sulfonamides
- Diseases associated with disturbances of oxalate metabolism: primary hyperoxaluria types I and II, Crohn's disease, ulcerative colitis, intestinal bypass surgery (especially jejunoileal bypass), ileal resection
- Diseases associated with disturbances of purine metabolism
- Intrinsic metabolic disorders: anemia, neoplastic disorders (especially leukemias), intoxication, myocardial infarction, irradiation, cytotoxic chemotherapy
- Enzyme deficiency: primary gout, Lesch-Nyhan syndrome
- Altered excretion: renal insufficiency, metabolic acidosis
- Infectious history: organisms (particularly *Proteus* and *Klebsiella*), febrile, upper tract involvement, and dates (if hospitalized)

Modified from Nseyo UO (ed): *Urology for primary care physicians,* Philadelphia, 1999, Saunders.

 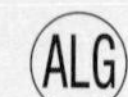

- A clinical algorithm for the evaluation of nephrolithiasis is described in Fig. E1-977.
- Box 1-97 describes events in the medical history that may be significant with regard to urolithiasis.

LABORATORY TESTS

- Urinalysis: Hematuria may be present; however, its absence does not exclude urinary stones. The evaluation of the urinary pH is of value for the identification of the type of stone: a pH of >7.5 is associated with struvite stones, whereas a pH of <5 generally is seen with uric acid or cystine stones. A low serum bicarbonate concentration with a urine pH of ≥6 is suggestive of renal tubular acidosis.
- Urine culture and sensitivity results should be obtained for all patients.
- Serum chemistries should include calcium, electrolytes, phosphate, and uric acid.
- Additional tests: 24-hr urine collection for calcium, uric acid, phosphate, oxalate, and citrate excretion is generally reserved for patients with recurrent stones.

IMAGING STUDIES

- Common diagnostic modalities for renal colic are summarized in Table 1-495.
- Plain films of the abdomen can identify radiopaque stones (e.g., calcium, uric acid) of ≥5 mm in diameter.
- Renal sonogram (Fig. 1-978) is generally not sensitive for very small calculi, but it may be helpful for identifying associated hydronephrosis. Accuracy in detecting distal ureteral stones can be high but is variable with size of the calculus and expertise of the technician and radiologist.
- Unenhanced (noncontrast) helical computed tomography scanning can be used to visualize the calculus (Fig. E1-979), which is identified by the "rim sign" or "halo" that represents the edematous ureteral wall around the stone. The test is fast and accurate (sensitivity nearly 100%; specificity, 94% to 96%), and it can be used to readily identify all stone types in all locations. This modality is being used increasingly during the initial assessment of renal colic.
- Intravenous pyelography demonstrates the size and location of the stone as well as the degree of obstruction. However, this modality is now rarely used and has largely been replaced by computed tomography.

TABLE 1-495 Common Diagnostic Imaging Modalities for Renal Colic

Modality	Information Provided	Radiation Dose	Contrast	Approximate Cost	Time
CT	Renal stones, including size and position of stones and evidence of obstruction Alternative diagnoses, such as AAA, appendicitis, and free air	4-10 mSv	No	\$750-\$1000	Less than 5 min to perform, 30 min for interpretation
CT with IV contrast	Same as noncontrast CT Delineation of renal mass lesions Additional information about vascular dissections and mesenteric ischemia	4-10 mSv	Yes	\$750-\$1000	Less than 5 min, after delay to measure creatinine
CT with IV and oral contrast	Same as CT with IV contrast Potentially improved diagnosis of bowel abnormalities	4-10 mSv	Yes	\$750-\$1000	Less than 5 min, after delay of approximately 2 hr to ingest oral contrast
Intravenous urogram	Structural and functional information about obstruction Rarely, identification of other pathology, such as AAA	1.5 mSv	Yes	\$350	Approximately 75 min
X-ray	Possible identification of stone, but not useful for hydronephrosis or most other pathology	0.5-1 mSv	No	\$250	Less than 5 min
Ultrasound	Identification of hydronephrosis or hydroureter Possible identification of stone Used to assess for AAA or biliary disease	No	No	\$150	Approximately 15-30 min—bedside ultrasound is quicker

CT, Computed tomography; *IV,* intravenous.

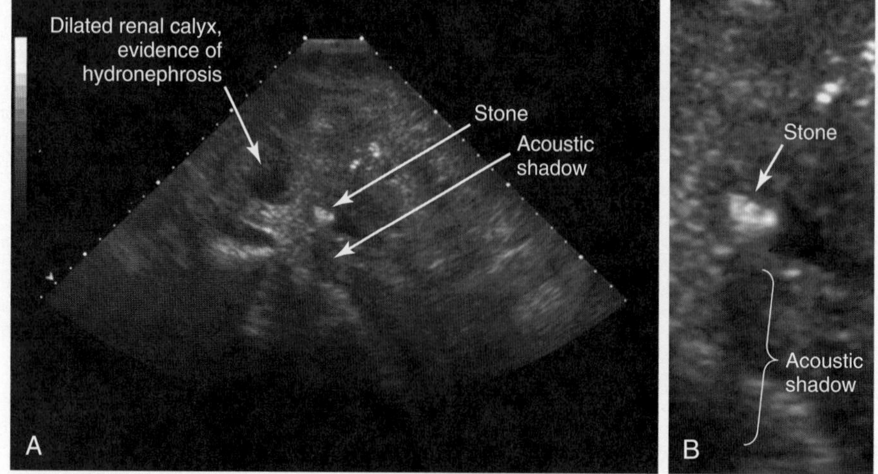

FIGURE 1-978 Ultrasound of renal stone. Ultrasound can be used to assess for renal stones and complications such as hydronephrosis. Stones can be difficult to detect, whereas hydronephrosis is usually readily observed. Because stones are dense, they reflect sound and prevent its through transmission. As a result, stones are echogenic (bright) on ultrasound, and cast an acoustic shadow (black). **A,** Short-axis view of kidney. **B,** Close-up. (From Broder JS: *Diagnostic imaging for the emergency physician*, Philadelphia, 2011, Saunders.)

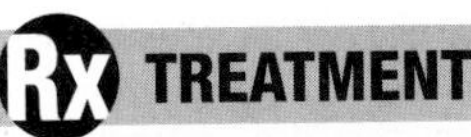

TREATMENT

NONPHARMACOLOGIC THERAPY

- An increase in water or other fluid intake is recommended; in fact, a doubling of previous fluid intake should occur unless the patient has a history of congestive heart failure or fluid overload. Generally, patients at increased risk for the development of stones should increase their fluid intake to >2 L/day (68 oz/day) to maintain a urine volume of >2 L/day.
- Normal dietary calcium intake is recommended. If one does not consume enough calcium, less is available to bind to dietary oxalate; as a result, more oxalate reaches the colon, is absorbed into the bloodstream, and excreted as calcium oxalate, thus setting the stage for calcium urolithiasis.
- Sodium restriction to decrease calcium excretion and decreased protein intake to 1 g/kg/day to decrease uric acid, calcium, and oxalate excretion should be considered.
- Increasing the amount of bran in the diet may decrease bowel transit time with an increased binding of calcium and a subsequent decrease in urinary calcium.

ACUTE GENERAL Rx

- Pain control: ketorolac (60 mg intramuscularly) can be used for moderate pain. However, the use of narcotics is generally indicated because of the severity of pain.
- Specific therapy is tailored to the stone type:
    - Uric acid calculi: control of hyperuricosuria with allopurinol 100 to 300 mg/day; increase urinary pH with potassium citrate 10-mEq tablets tid. Alkalinization of the urine may help prevent uric acid stones and cystine stones.
    - Calcium stones:
        1. Hydrochlorothiazide 25 to 50 mg qd in patients with type I absorptive hypercalciuria
        2. Decrease bowel absorption of calcium with cellulose phosphate 10 g/day in patients with type I absorptive hypercalciuria
        3. Orthophosphates to inhibit vitamin B synthesis in patients with type III absorptive hypercalciuria
        4. Potassium citrate supplementation for patients with hypocitraturic calcium nephrolithiasis
        5. Purine dietary restrictions or allopurinol for patients with hyperuricosuric calcium nephrolithiasis
        6. Paradoxically, calcium restriction is not warranted for patients who have had calcium stones and may even be harmful
    - Struvite stones:
        1. Most of these stones are large and cause obstruction and bleeding.
        2. Extracorporeal shock wave lithotripsy (ESWL) and percutaneous nephrolithotomy are generally necessary. Percutaneous nephrolithotomy is very effective for large stones in the kidney and is especially indicated for struvite stones.
        3. The prolonged use of antibiotics directed against the predominant urinary tract organism may be beneficial to prevent recurrence.
    - Cystine stones: hydration and alkalinization of the urine to pH >6.5; penicillamine and tiopronin can be used to reduce the formation of cystine; captopril is also beneficial and causes fewer side effects.
- Possibly useful medications to help with the passage of distal ureteral stones of <10 mm in diameter are tamsulosin (alpha-adrenergic antagonist) and nifedipine (calcium channel blocker used for ureteral dilatation and relaxation). Side effects may include dizziness with tamsulosin and hypotension with nifedipine.
- Administer antibiotics if fever or pyuria (>5 to 20 leukocytes/high-power field) is present.
- Surgical treatment for patients with severe pain that is unresponsive to medication and patients with persistent fever or nausea or significant impediment of urine flow:
    - Ureteroscopic stone extraction. Indications for percutaneous nephrolithotomy are described in Table E1-496.
    - ESWL for most renal stones. In 2011 the European Association of Urology recommended shock wave lithotripsy as first-line therapy for non-lower pole renal calculi <2 cm in diameter and for lower pole renal calculi <1 cm in diameter. Several types of lithotripters are in clinical use and differ from one another primarily in the way they generate shock waves. Contraindications to shock wave lithotripsy include pregnancy, active UTI, coagulopathies, and distal obstruction. Spinal or orthopedic deformities and morbid obesity may also preclude lithotripsy due to inability to properly position patient or inadequate visualization of the stone.
- Fig. E1-980 describes the management of ureteral stones.
- In 1997, the American Urological Association issued the following guidelines for the treatment of ureteral stones:
    - Proximal ureteral stones <1 cm in diameter: the options are ESWL, percutaneous nephroureterolithotomy, and ureteroscopy.
    - Proximal ureteral stones >1 cm in diameter: the options are ESWL, percutaneous nephroureterolithotomy, and ureteroscopy. The placement of a ureteral stent should be considered if the stone is causing high-grade obstruction.
    - Distal ureteral stones <1 cm in diameter: most of these stones pass spontaneously. ESWL and ureteroscopy are two accepted modes of therapy.
    - Distal ureteral stones >1 cm in diameter: the options are watchful waiting, ESWL, and ureteroscopy (after stone fragmentation).

  Fig. E1-980 describes an approach to the management of ureteral calculi.

CHRONIC Rx

The maintenance of proper hydration and dietary restrictions (see "Acute General Rx")

DISPOSITION

- >50% of patients will pass the stone within 48 hr.
- Stones will recur in approximately 50% of patients within 5 yr if no medical treatment is provided.

REFERRAL

A urology referral should be undertaken for patients with complicated or recurrent urolithiasis. Most patients with small uncomplicated ureteral or renal calculi can be followed up as outpatients, whereas patients with persistent vomiting, suspected urinary tract infection, pain that is unresponsive to oral analgesics, or obstructing calculus associated with a solitary kidney should be admitted.

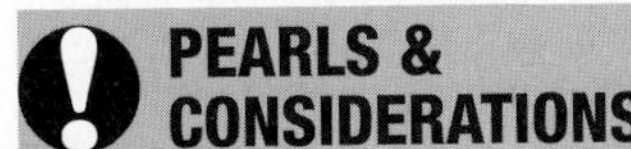

PEARLS & CONSIDERATIONS

COMMENTS

- The early identification and aggressive treatment of urinary tract infections is indicated for all patients with struvite stones.
- The alkalinization of urine (i.e., getting to a pH of >7.5 with the use of penicillamine) is useful for patients with recurrent cystine stones.
- Stones <5 mm in diameter often pass spontaneously whereas stones >10 mm generally do not.
- An algorithmic approach to the management of ureteral calculi is described in Fig. E1-980.

SUGGESTED READINGS

available at www.expertconsult.com

RELATED CONTENT

Urinary Tract Infection (Patient Information)
Kidney Stones (Patient Information)

AUTHORS: **PHILIP J. ALIOTTA, M.D., M.S.H.A.,** and **RUBEN ALVERO, M.D.**

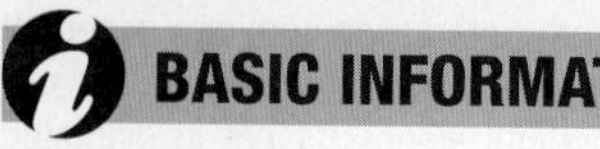

BASIC INFORMATION

DEFINITION

Urticaria is a pruritic rash involving the epidermis and the upper portions of the dermis caused by localized capillary vasodilation and followed by transudation of protein-rich fluid in the surrounding tissue and manifesting clinically with the presence of hives. Urticaria is classified according to its chronicity into acute (<6-wk duration) and chronic (>6-wk duration).

SYNONYMS

Hives
Wheals

ICD-9CM CODES
708.8 Other unspecified urticaria
ICD-10CM Codes
L50.0 Allergic urticaria
L50.1 Idiopathic urticaria
L50.2 Urticaria due to cold and heat
L50.8 Other urticaria
L50.9 Urticaria, unspecified
L50.6 Contact urticaria

EPIDEMIOLOGY & DEMOGRAPHICS

- 15% to 20% of the population will have one episode of hives during their lifetime.
- Incidence is increased in atopic patients.
- The etiology of chronic urticaria (hives lasting >6 wk) is determined in only 5% to 20% of cases.

PHYSICAL FINDINGS & CLINICAL PRESENTATION

- Presence of elevated, erythematous, or white nonpitting plaques that change in size and shape over time; they generally last a few hours and disappear without a trace.
- Annular configuration with central pallor (Fig. E1-981).
- Angioedema occurs in approximately 40% of cases of urticaria and is caused by mast cell mediator release in the subcutaneous tissue and deep dermis.

ETIOLOGY

- Foods (e.g., shellfish, eggs, strawberries, nuts)
- Drugs (e.g., penicillin, aspirin, sulfonamides)
- Systemic diseases (e.g., systemic lupus erythematosus, serum sickness, autoimmune thyroid disease, polycythemia vera)
- Food additives (e.g., salicylates, benzoates, sulfites)
- Infections (viral infections, fungal infections, chronic bacterial infections); viral upper respiratory infections are the predominant cause
- Physical stimuli (e.g., pressure urticaria, exercise-induced, solar urticaria, cold urticaria)
- Inhalants (e.g., mold spores, animal dander, pollens)
- Contact (nonimmunologic) urticaria (e.g., caterpillars, plants)
- Other: hereditary angioedema, urticaria pigmentosa, pregnancy, cryoglobulinemia, hair bleaches, chemicals, saliva, cosmetics, perfumes, pemphigoid, emotional stress, malignancy (lymphomas, endocrine tumors)
- Idiopathic urticaria is diagnosed in 50% of patients with chronic urticaria.

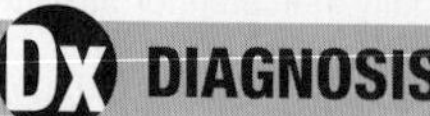

DIAGNOSIS

DIFFERENTIAL DIAGNOSIS

- Erythema multiforme
- Erythema marginatum
- Erythema infectiosum
- Urticarial vasculitis
- Herpes gestationis
- Drug eruption
- Multiple insect bites
- Bullous pemphigoid

WORKUP

- It is useful to determine whether hives are acute or chronic; a medical history focused on various etiologic factors is necessary before embarking on extensive laboratory testing.
- Most cases of acute urticaria resolve spontaneously and diagnostic testing is not required. However, in patients with acute urticaria it is crucial to rule out anaphylaxis.
- A diagnostic approach to chronic urticaria is described in Fig. E1-982.

LABORATORY TESTS

- Complete blood count with differential.
- Stool for ova and parasites in patients with chronic urticaria and suspected parasitic infestations.
- Skin testing with allergic extracts and screening for dermatographism by attempting to elicit a wheal after application of linear skin pressure should be performed only after withholding antihistamines for 36 to 72 hr to prevent false-negative results.
- Antinuclear antibody, erythrocyte sedimentation rate, thyroid-stimulating hormone, antithyroid antibodies, *Helicobacter pylori* serology, liver function tests, and eosinophil count are indicated only in patients with chronic urticaria. However, even with extensive testing, the cause of chronic urticaria is rarely established.
- Measurement of C4 may be helpful in patients who present with angioedema alone. In these patients, C1 inhibitor deficiency should be considered.
- Skin biopsy is helpful in patients with fever, arthralgias, and elevated erythrocyte sedimentation rate. Histologic evidence of leukocytoclasia (neutrophilic infiltration with fragmentation of nuclei) is indicative of urticarial vasculitis.
- When food allergy is suspected in acute urticaria, testing can be performed using skin prick, immunoCAP, and radioallergosorbent testing.

Rx TREATMENT

NONPHARMACOLOGIC THERAPY

- Remove suspected etiologic agents (e.g., stop aspirin and all nonessential drugs), and restrict diet (e.g., elimination of tomatoes, nuts, eggs, shellfish).
- Elimination of yeast should be attempted in patients with chronic urticaria (*Candida albicans* sensitivity may be a factor in patients with chronic urticaria).

ACUTE GENERAL Rx

- Oral antihistamines: use of nonsedating antihistamines (e.g., loratadine 10 mg qd, cetirizine 10 mg qd, fexofenadine 180 mg qd, levocetirizine 5 mg qd) is preferred over first-generation antihistamines (e.g., hydroxyzine, diphenhydramine).
- Doxepin (a tricyclic antidepressant that blocks both H_1 and H_2 receptors) 25 to 75 mg qhs may be effective in patients with chronic urticaria.
- Oral corticosteroids should be reserved for refractory cases (e.g., prednisone 20 mg qd or 20 mg bid).
- H_2 receptor antagonists (cimetidine, ranitidine, famotidine) can be added to H_1 antagonists in refractory cases.

CHRONIC Rx

- Use of nonsedating antihistamines, doxepin, and/or oral corticosteroids (see "Acute General Rx").
- Low dose of the immunosuppressant cyclosporine (2.5 to 3 mg/kg body weight/day) has been shown to be effective and corticosteroid sparing in chronic urticaria. Algorithms for the evaluation and management of chronic urticaria are described in Figs. E1-983 and E1-984, respectively.
- Omalizumab, a monoclonal antibody that inactivates free IgE and down-regulates surface IgE receptors, has been shown effective in trials for refractory chronic urticaria. It is, however, expensive and not currently FDA approved for this indication.
- There are insufficient data to support use of leukotriene antagonists (zafirlukast, montelukast) in patients with chronic urticaria.

DISPOSITION

- Most cases of urticaria resolve within 6 wk.
- Only 25% of patients with a history of chronic urticaria are completely cured after 5 yr.

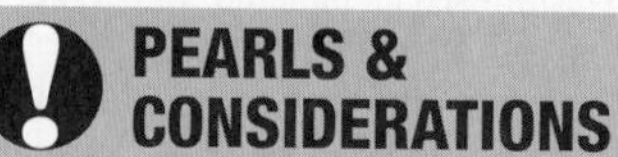

PEARLS & CONSIDERATIONS

COMMENTS

Local treatment (e.g., starch baths or oatmeal baths) may be helpful in selected patients; however, local treatment is generally not rewarding.

SUGGESTED READINGS

available at www.expertconsult.com

RELATED CONTENT

Hives (Patient Information)

AUTHOR: **FRED F. FERRI, M.D.**

BASIC INFORMATION

DEFINITION

Uterine fibroids are benign tumors of muscle cell origin. They are discrete nodular tumors that vary in size and number and that may be found as subserosal, intramural, or submucosal masses. They can also be located in the cervix, broad ligament, or on a stalk (pedunculated) (Fig. 1-985). They can also be parasitic, acquiring a blood supply from a nonuterine source.

SYNONYMS

Uterine leiomyomas
Uterine myomas

ICD-9CM CODES
218.9 Leiomyomas, fibroids
ICD-10CM Codes
D25.9 Leiomyoma of uterus, unspecified

EPIDEMIOLOGY & DEMOGRAPHICS

- Estimated prevalence of 20% to 40% of reproductive age women
- The most common benign uterine tumor
- More common in black women than white women
- Asymptomatic fibroids may be present in 40% to 50% of women aged >40 yr
- May occur singly but are often multiple
- Less than half of all fibroids are estimated to produce symptoms
- Frequently diagnosed incidentally on pelvic examination
- There is increased familial incidence
- Potential to enlarge during pregnancy as well as regress after menopause
- Symptomatic fibroids are the primary indication for approximately 30% of all hysterectomies
- Approximately 200,000 hysterectomies, 30,000 myomectomies, and thousands of selective uterine-artery embolizations and high-intensity focused ultrasound procedures are performed annually in the United States to remove or destroy uterine fibroids.[1]

PHYSICAL FINDINGS & CLINICAL PRESENTATION

- Enlarged, irregular uterus on pelvic examination
- Presenting symptoms:
  1. Menorrhagia (most common)
  2. Chronic pelvic pain (dysmenorrhea, dyspareunia, pelvic pressure)
  3. Acute pain (torsion of pedunculated fibroid, infarction, and degeneration)
  4. Urinary symptoms (frequency from bladder pressure, partial ureteral obstruction, complete ureteral obstruction)
  5. Rectosigmoid compression with constipation or intestinal obstruction
  6. Prolapse through cervix of pedunculated submucosal tumor
  7. Venous stasis of lower extremities
  8. Polycythemia
  9. Ascites

ETIOLOGY

Incompletely understood. It is suggested that fibroids arise from an original single smooth muscle cell in the myometrium. Each individual fibroid is monoclonal (all the cells are derived from one progenitor myocyte). Malignant degeneration of preexisting leiomyoma is extremely uncommon (<0.5%).

Dx DIAGNOSIS

DIFFERENTIAL DIAGNOSIS

Leiomyosarcoma, ovarian mass (neoplastic, nonneoplastic, endometrioma), inflammatory mass, pregnancy

WORKUP

- Complete pelvic examination, rectovaginal examination
- Estimation of size of mass in centimeters and location of fibroids
- Endometrial sampling may be indicated (biopsy or dilation and curettage) when abnormal bleeding and pelvic mass are present
- If urinary symptoms are prominent, cystometry, cystoscopy to rule out bladder lesions, intravenous pyelogram to rule out impingement on urinary system

LABORATORY TESTS

- Pregnancy test
- Pap smear
- Complete blood count, erythrocyte sedimentation rate
- Fecal occult blood

IMAGING STUDIES

- Pelvic ultrasound (Fig. 1-986) is useful as a primary diagnostic modality. Transvaginal ultrasound commonly has higher diagnostic accuracy.
- MRI scan is helpful in planning treatment if malignancy is strongly suspected. Also important to localize fibroids, especially if myomectomy is contemplated. Size, number, and location of fibroids are also important if a minimally invasive myomectomy is considered.
- Saline infusion sonography is helpful in determining location and degree of intrusion into uterine cavity. Important if hysteroscopic resection is contemplated. Typically at least 50% of the fibroid must be intracavitary for a hysteroscopic approach to be successful.
- Hysteroscopy may provide direct evidence of intrauterine pathology or submucosal leiomyoma that distorts uterine cavity, and surgical resection may be performed during the same procedure.

[1]Bulun SE: Uterine fibroids, *N Engl J Med* 369:1344-1355, 2013.

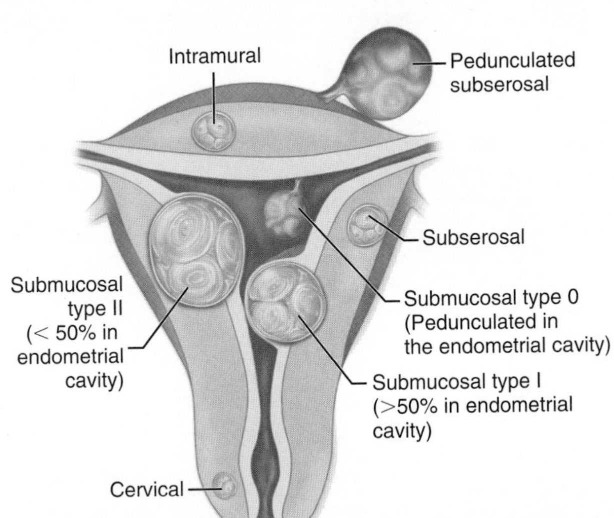

FIGURE 1-985 Drawing of uterus in the coronal plane, illustrating possible location of uterine leiomyomas. (From Fielding JR et al: *Gynecologic imaging,* Philadelphia, 2011, Saunders.)

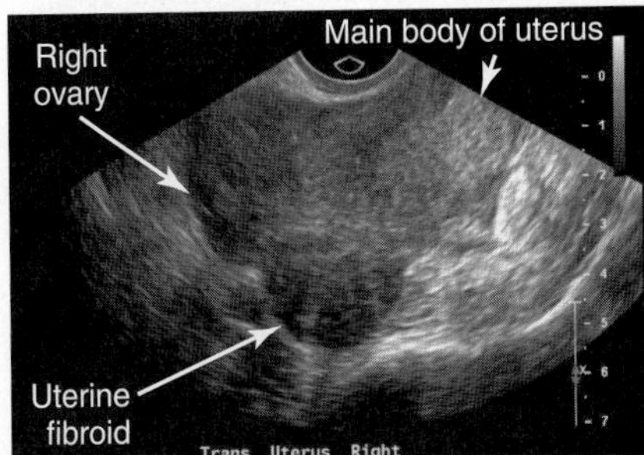

FIGURE 1-986 Fibroid uterus: endovaginal ultrasound. Ultrasound is the primary modality used for evaluation of uterine fibroids (leiomyomas). Typical features include a well-circumscribed appearance. Fibroids may be hypoechoic or hyperechoic relative to the uterus. They may be exophytic or intramural, or they may project into the uterine cavity. Malignant uterine tumors may invade adjacent structures, whereas a fibroid is contained within the uterine serosa. Uterine tumors, both benign and malignant, can show central necrosis, which usually appears hypoechoic with ultrasound. In this 38-year-old woman, the fibroid is exophytic. The right ovary lies adjacent and is difficult to distinguish in this case. (From Broder JS: *Diagnostic imaging for the emergency physician,* Philadelphia, 2011, Saunders.)

Rx TREATMENT

Management should be based on primary symptoms and may include observation with close follow-up, temporizing surgical therapies, embolization, medical management, or definitive surgical procedures. Treatment is generally indicated only when symptoms are present and are severe enough to be unacceptable to the patient.

NONSURGICAL Rx

- Patient observation and follow-up with periodic repeat pelvic examinations to ensure that tumors are not growing rapidly.
- Gonadotropin-releasing hormone (GnRH) agonist use results in 40% to 60% reduction in uterine volume. Hypoestrogenism, reversible bone loss, and hot flushes are associated with use. Limit to short-term use and consider low-dose hormonal replacement to minimize hypoestrogenic effects.
- Regrowth occurs in approximately 50% of women treated within a few months after cessation.
- Indications for GnRH:
  1. Fertility preservation in women with large myomas before attempting conception or preoperative myectomy treatment
  2. Anemia treatment to normalize hemoglobin before surgery
  3. Women approaching menopause to avoid surgery
  4. Preoperative for large myomas to make vaginal hysterectomy, hysteroscopic resection/ablation, or laparoscopic destruction more feasible
  5. Women with medical contraindications for surgery
  6. Personal or medical indications for delaying surgery
- Use of GnRH agonists may alter the consistency of the fibroid, making myomectomy more challenging.
- Progestational agents may also result in decrease in uterine size and amenorrhea, allowing iron therapy to treat anemia with limited success. Ulipristal acetate is a selective progesterone-receptor modulator that acts on progesterone receptors in myometrial and endometrial tissue and inhibits ovulation without causing large effects on estradiol levels or antiglucocorticoid activity. Recent trials have shown that treatment with ulipristal acetate for 13 wk effectively controlled excessive bleeding due to uterine fibroids and reduced the size of the fibroids.
- Other drugs used and under investigation:
  1. Danazol: androgen and multienzyme inhibitor of steroidogenesis
  2. Mifepristone: antiprogestogen shown to reduce the fibroid volume by 40% to 50% with amenorrhea
  3. Raloxifene: selective estrogen receptor modulator, either alone or with a GnRHa, shown to reduce the fibroid volume 70% up to 1 yr but only in postmenopausal women
  4. Fadrozole: aromatase inhibitor reported to have produced a 71% reduction in volume

SURGICAL Rx

- Indications
  1. Abnormal uterine bleeding with anemia refractory to hormonal therapy
  2. Chronic pain with severe dysmenorrhea, dyspareunia, or lower abdominal pressure/pain
  3. Acute pain, torsion, or prolapsing submucosal fibroid
  4. Urinary symptoms or signs such as hydronephrosis
  5. Rapid uterine enlargement premenopausal or any growth after menopause
  6. Infertility or recurrent pregnancy loss with submucous leiomyoma as only finding
  7. Enlarged uterus with compression symptoms or discomfort
- Procedures
  1. Hysterectomy (definitive procedure): Nearly 15% of women with uterine fibroids and a mean age of 45 yr require hysterectomy
  2. Abdominal myomectomy (to preserve fertility or due to patient preference)
  3. Vaginal myomectomy for prolapsed pedunculated submucous fibroid
  4. Hysteroscopic resection
  5. Laparoscopic/robotic myomectomy
  6. Uterine artery embolization (UAE): safe and effective short-term alternative to surgery, but its less invasive nature should be balanced against a higher rate for treatment failure or complications at 5 yr (32%) versus the surgery group (4%). Age 40 years and under at embolization and history of previous myomectomy are significant predictors of embolization failure.

COMPLICATIONS

- Red degeneration
- Leiomyosarcoma (<0.1%)

REFERRAL

Consultation with gynecologic oncologist if suspicion of malignancy

SUGGESTED READINGS

available at www.expertconsult.com

RELATED CONTENT

Dysfunctional Uterine Bleeding (Related Key Topic)
Uterine Fibroids (Patient Information)

AUTHORS: **ARUNDATHI G. PRASAD, M.D.,** and **RUBEN ALVERO, M.D.**

BASIC INFORMATION

DEFINITION

Uterine malignancy includes tumors from the endometrium and sarcomas. Uterine sarcoma is an abnormal proliferation of cells originating from the mesenchymal, or connective tissue, elements of the uterine wall (myometrium).

SYNONYMS

Leiomyosarcomas
Endometrial stromal sarcoma
Malignant mixed Müllerian tumors
Adenosarcomas

ICD-9CM CODES
182.0 Malignant neoplasm of body of uterus (corpus uteri), except isthmus
182.1 Malignant neoplasm of body of uterus, isthmus
182.8 Malignant neoplasm of body of uterus, other specified sites of body of uterus

ICD-10CM Codes
C54.1 Malignant neoplasm of endometrium
C54.0 Malignant neoplasm of isthmus uteri
C54.8 Malignant neoplasm of overlapping sites of corpus uteri

BOX 1-98 Risk Factors for Uterine Sarcoma

Nulliparity
Obesity
History of pelvic radiation
Exposure to tamoxifen

From Fielding JR et al: *Gynecologic imaging,* Philadelphia, 2011, Saunders.

BOX 1-99 Uterine Sarcoma Prognostic Factors

Tumor stage
Tumor grade
Tumor size
Patient age
Vascular space involvement
Mitotic count
Residual disease at surgery
Adjuvant chemotherapy

From Fielding JR et al: *Gynecologic imaging,* Philadelphia, 2011, Saunders.

EPIDEMIOLOGY & DEMOGRAPHICS

INCIDENCE: 17.1 cases per 1 million females. Endometrial cancer remains the most common gynecologic malignancy in the U.S.
PREVALENCE: Uterine sarcoma accounts for 4.3% of all cancers of the uterine corpus and is the most lethal gynecologic malignancy.
MEAN AGE AT DIAGNOSIS: 52 yr
RISK FACTORS: Box 1-98 describes risk factors for uterine sarcoma

PHYSICAL FINDINGS & CLINICAL PRESENTATION

- Abnormal vaginal bleeding is the most common symptom
- May also present as pelvic pain or pressure and pelvic mass on examination
- May appear as tumor protruding through the cervix
- Vaginal discharge may also be a presenting symptom
- Rapidly enlarging uterus or pelvic mass

ETIOLOGY

- The exact etiology is unknown.
- Prior pelvic radiation is a risk factor for sarcoma.
- Black women may be at higher risk.

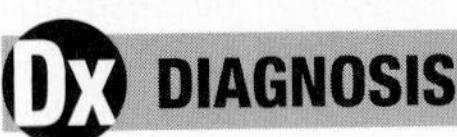

DIAGNOSIS

DIFFERENTIAL DIAGNOSIS

Leiomyoma

WORKUP

Diagnosis is made histologically by biopsy for abnormal bleeding.

BOX 1-100 Uterine Sarcoma: Key Points

The disease mainly affects postmenopausal women.
Most patients present early with postmenopausal bleeding.
The primary treatment is hysterectomy.
Adjuvant radiotherapy to the pelvis is used if poor prognosis features in stage 1 or if spread has occurred beyond the corpus.

From Greer IA et al: *Mosby's color atlas and text of obstetrics and gynecology,* London, 2001, Harcourt.

LABORATORY TESTS

Chest radiography, CT scans, and MRI are used to evaluate metastatic lesions.

IMAGING STUDIES

- Chest x-ray is usually done as routine preoperative testing.
- CT scans (Fig. E1-987) and MRI are useful for assessing tumor spread once diagnosis is made.

TREATMENT

NONPHARMACOLOGIC THERAPY

- Surgical excision is the mainstay of treatment.
- Grade and stage of tumor affect prognosis.
- The benefit of adjuvant radiotherapy in stage I endometrial adenocarcinoma to improve pelvic disease control and improve survival remains controversial despite several phase 3 trials.
- Chemotherapeutic agents have produced only partial and short-term responses.

DISPOSITION

- Survival varies with each type of sarcoma but is generally very poor. Box 1-99 describes uterine prognostic factors.
- Five-year survival for leiomyosarcoma ranges from 48% for stage I to 0% for stage IV.
- Five-year survival for malignant mixed mesodermal tumor ranges from 36% for stage I to 6% for stage IV.

REFERRAL

Uterine sarcoma should be managed by a gynecologic oncologist and radiation oncologist. Key points in the management of uterine sarcoma are described in Box 1-100.

SUGGESTED READINGS

available at www.expertconsult.com

RELATED CONTENT

Endometrial Cancer (Related Key Topic)
Uterine Cancer (Patient Information)

AUTHOR: **RUBEN ALVERO, M.D.**

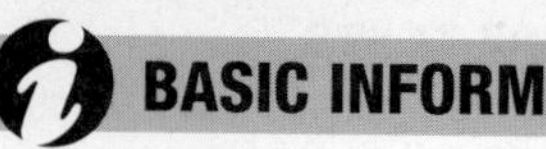

BASIC INFORMATION

DEFINITION

Uveitis is inflammation of the uveal tract, including the iris, ciliary body, and choroid. It may also involve other contiguous structures such as the sclera, cornea, retina, and vitreous humor (Fig. 1-988).

SYNONYMS

Anterior uveitis (iritis, iridocyclitis)
Intermediate uveitis (pars planitis)
Posterior uveitis (choroiditis)
Acute or chronic uveitis
Granulomatous or nongranulomatous uveitis

ICD-9CM CODES
364.3 Unspecified iridocyclitis, uveitis
ICD-10CM Codes
H20.0 Acute and subacute iridocyclitis
H20.1 Chronic iridocyclitis
H20.8 Other iridocyclitis
H20.9 Unspecified iridocyclitis

EPIDEMIOLOGY & DEMOGRAPHICS

INCIDENCE (IN U.S.): Common; busy ophthalmologist will see two or more cases per week.
PEAK INCIDENCE: Middle age or older.
PREVALENCE (IN U.S.): 17 cases per 100,000 persons
PREDOMINANT SEX: None
PREDOMINANT AGE: 38 yr. Although uveitis is less common in children than adults, it is believed to be more severe with an increased risk for vision-threatening complications.

PHYSICAL FINDINGS & CLINICAL PRESENTATION

- Symptoms of uveitis depend on the site of involvement and whether process is acute or insidious:
  - Acute anterior uveitis: pain and photophobia. Vision may not be affected initially.
  - Posterior uveitis: floaters, hazy vision. Involvement of the retina may produce blind spots or flashing lights.
  - Insidious anterior uveitis: symptoms may not be present until scarring cataracts and loss of vision occur.
- Photophobia
- Blurred visual acuity
- Irregular pupil
- Hazy cornea
- Abnormal cells and flare in anterior chamber or vitreous humor ("flare cells") noted with slit lamp examination
- Retinal hemorrhage, vascular sheathing
- Conjunctival injection
- Ciliary flush
- Keratitic precipitates (white precipitates on the posterior surface of the cornea)
- Hazy vitreous
- Retinal inflammation
- Iris nodules

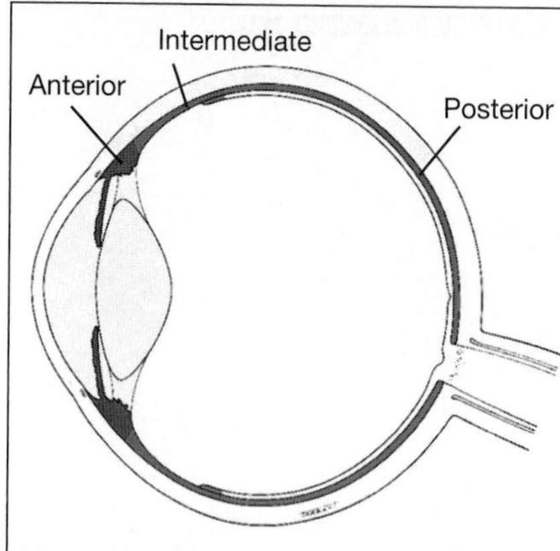

FIGURE 1-988 Anatomic classification of uveitis. (From Kanski JJ, Bowling B: *Clinical ophthalmology, a systematic approach,* ed 7, Philadelphia, 2010, Saunders.)

ETIOLOGY

- Infections: herpes simplex virus, cytomegalovirus, toxoplasmosis, tuberculosis, syphilis, HIV
- Systemic disorders (autoimmunity): sarcoidosis, Behçet's syndrome, HLA-B27–associated diseases (e.g., ankylosing spondylitis, psoriatic arthritis), inflammatory bowel disease, juvenile idiopathic arthritis (Fig. E1-989)
- There is also an association between oral bisphosphonates and uveitis, with risk of uveitis being 50% higher among new bisphosphonate users than among nonusers.
- Idiopathic (>50% of patients)

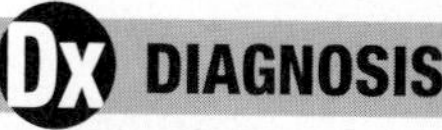

DIAGNOSIS

DIFFERENTIAL DIAGNOSIS

- Glaucoma
- Conjunctivitis
- Retinal detachment
- Retinopathy
- Keratitis
- Scleritis
- Episcleritis
- Masquerading syndromes: lymphoma, uveal melanoma, metastases (breast, lung, renal), leukemia, retinitis pigmentosa, retinoblastoma

WORKUP

- Comprehensive eye examination including slit lamp exam, dilated ophthalmoscopy

LABORATORY TESTS

- Complete blood count
- Laboratory tests for specific inflammatory causes cited previously in "Workup" (e.g., antinuclear antibody, erythrocyte sedimentation rate, syphilis (VDRL), HLA-B27, purified protein derivative, Lyme titer, angiotensin converting enzyme [ACE])

IMAGING STUDIES

- Chest radiograph in suspected sarcoidosis, tuberculosis, histoplasmosis
- Sacroiliac radiograph in suspected ankylosing spondylitis

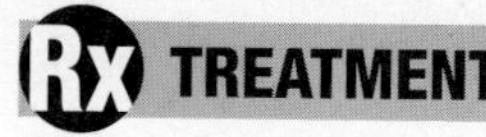

TREATMENT

ACUTE GENERAL Rx

- Corticosteroids are the mainstay of therapy for noninfectious causes. The route and dosage of medication depends on the location of inflammation, the severity, and the presence of systemic disease. Cycloplegic drops (cyclopentolate, homatropine BID to QID) and topical steroids (prednisone acetate 1% 1 gtt qh during day, prn at night until favorable response, then q4 to 6h); avoid topical corticosteroids in infectious uveitis. Periocular corticosteroid injections can be used for posterior disease; they have the advantage of achieving high intraocular levels of steroids without the systemic side effects of oral corticosteroids.
- Antibiotics for bacterial infections and antiviral agents, when infection is suspected, should be started to prevent retinal damage.
- Systemic steroids if appropriate for the underlying disease. Systemic corticosteroid therapy is generally reserved for patients with systemic disorders and those with bilateral disease that is refractory to local medication or those with major ocular disability or retinitis.
- Antimetabolites when indicated. Immunosuppressive medications used in steroid-dependent or refractory uveitis include methotrexate, sulfasalazine, azathioprine, cyclosporine, and tacrolimus. These medications can have significant toxicity and should be prescribed only by physicians experienced with their use.
- High-dose IV daclizumab has been reported as effective in reducing active inflammation in active juvenile idiopathic arthritis (JIA)-associated anterior uveitis. Additional trials are needed to better assess efficacy and safety.

REFERRAL

Urgent referral to ophthalmologist for diagnosis and treatment

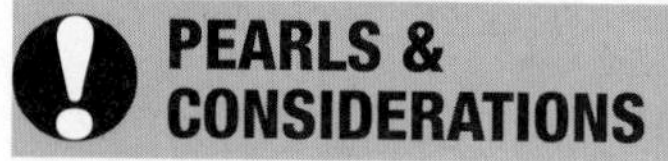

PEARLS & CONSIDERATIONS

COMMENTS

Chronic anterior uveitis is the most common form of intraocular inflammation in children. JIA is the most common cause.

SUGGESTED READINGS
available at www.expertconsult.com

AUTHORS: **MELVYN KOBY, M.D.,** and **R. SCOTT HOFFMAN, M.D.**

BASIC INFORMATION

DEFINITION

Bleeding per vagina at any time during pregnancy must be regarded as abnormal and is associated with an increased likelihood of pregnancy complications.

SYNONYMS

Hemorrhage

ICD-9CM CODES
634.9 Spontaneous abortion
640.0 Threatened abortion
641.1 Placenta previa
641.2 Placental abruption

ICD-10CM CODES
003.9 Complete or unspecified spontaneous abortion
044.10 Placenta previa with hemorrhage, unspecified trimester
045.8X9 Other premature separation of placenta, unspecified trimester

EPIDEMIOLOGY & DEMOGRAPHICS

- Common in U.S.; 20% to 25% of patients have vaginal spotting/bleeding in first trimester; of those, miscarriage occurs in 50%.
- Occurs in women of childbearing age.
- Between 1% and 2% of all pregnancies in the U.S. are ectopic.
- After one ectopic pregnancy, the chance of another is 7% to 15%.
- Ectopic pregnancy is the leading cause of maternal mortality in the first trimester.
- Average reported frequency for placental abruption is about 1 in 150 deliveries (0.3%).
- Incidence of placenta previa is 1 in 200 deliveries (0.5%).

PHYSICAL FINDINGS & CLINICAL PRESENTATION

- Bleeding: ranges from scant to life-threatening with hemodynamic instability
- Color: brown to bright red
- Can be painless or painful (cramps, back pain, severe abdominal pain)
- Fetal compromise: ranges from none to fetal demise

ETIOLOGY

- Influenced by gestational age
- Vaginal
- Cervical
- Uterine

DIAGNOSIS

DIFFERENTIAL DIAGNOSIS

- Any gestational age:
  1. Cervical lesions: polyps, decidual reaction, neoplasia
  2. Vaginal trauma
  3. Cervicitis/vulvovaginitis
  4. Postcoital trauma
  5. Bleeding dyscrasias
- Gestation <20 wk:
  1. Spontaneous abortion
  2. Presence of intrauterine device
  3. Ectopic pregnancy
  4. Molar pregnancy
  5. Implantation bleeding
  6. Low-lying placenta
- Gestation >20 wk:
  1. Molar pregnancy
  2. Placenta previa
  3. Placental abruption
  4. Vasa previa
  5. Marginal separation of the placenta
  6. Bloody show at term
  7. Preterm labor
- Section II describes the differential diagnosis of vaginal bleeding in pregnancy.

WORKUP

- Gestation <20 wk (Section III, "Bleeding, Early Pregnancy")
  1. Pelvic examination
  2. Laparoscopy
  3. Laparotomy
  4. Ultrasound to verify viable intrauterine pregnancy
- Gestation >20 wk:
  1. Ultrasound to locate placenta before pelvic examination
  2. If placenta previa, no speculum or bimanual examination
  3. If preterm labor, appropriate evaluation done

LABORATORY TESTS

- Urine pregnancy test: if positive, get quantitative beta human chorionic gonadotropin (βhCG). The following are typical although not entirely exclusive patterns:
  1. Early pregnancy: follow serially every 48 hr
  2. Normal pregnancy: βhCG doubles approximately every 48 hr
  3. Spontaneous abortion: βhCG level will fall
  4. Ectopic pregnancy: βhCG level will rise inappropriately
  5. Molar pregnancy: βhCG level is extremely high
- CBC
- Blood type and screen (Rh-negative patients need RhoGAM)
- Coagulation profile (useful in missed abortion and abruption)
- Cervical cultures/wet mount
- Pap smear for cervical malignancy; caution with biopsy, because cervix can bleed extensively

IMAGING STUDIES

Ultrasound:

- 5 to 6 wk: gestational sac (transvaginally); βhCG >1500 mIU/ml is discriminatory level for seeing a singleton gestation
- 6 to 7 wk: fetal cardiac activity
- Molar pregnancy: characteristic cluster of cysts
- Location of placenta
- Degree of placental separation: difficult to assess
- Evidence of subchorionic hemorrhage

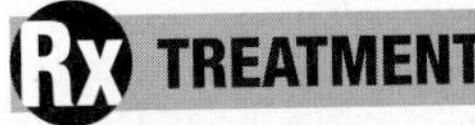

TREATMENT

NONPHARMACOLOGIC THERAPY

- Pelvic rest: no coitus, douching, or tampons
- Bed rest, if >20 wk
- Counseling: genetic, bereavement

ACUTE GENERAL Rx

- Hemodynamic stabilization
- Emergency D&C, laparotomy, or cesarean section as necessary

CHRONIC Rx

Depends on diagnosis

DISPOSITION

Depends on diagnosis

REFERRAL

- If patient is unstable and needs emergency ob/gyn management and/or surgery
- If patient has diagnosis of ectopic or molar pregnancy, because immediate surgical treatment or medical intervention is indicated
- Perinatal consultation for high-risk pregnancy

SUGGESTED READINGS

available at www.expertconsult.com

RELATED CONTENT

Abruptio Placentae (Related Key Topic)
Ectopic Pregnancy (Related Key Topic)
Molar Pregnancy (Related Key Topic)
Placenta Previa (Related Key Topic)
Sheehan's Syndrome (Related Key Topic)
Spontaneous Miscarriage (Related Key Topic)

AUTHOR: **RUBEN ALVERO, M.D.**

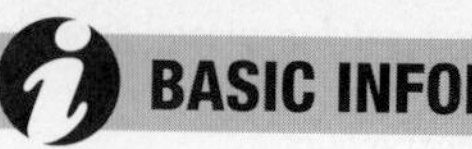

BASIC INFORMATION

DEFINITION

An abnormal passageway between the vagina and another epithelialized surface (Fig. 1-990)

SYNONYMS

Vaginal sinus

ICD-9CM CODES
619 Fistula involving female genital tract
ICD-10CM CODES
N82 Fistulae involving the female genital tract

EPIDEMIOLOGY & DEMOGRAPHICS

INCIDENCE: After benign hysterectomy: <1% (0.08%-0.26%); after radical hysterectomy: 1%-4%. Incidence difficult to estimate in developing countries because of lack of medical care and medical follow-up after obstetric care.

PREVALENCE: Rare in the developed world from obstetric complications, but in developing countries the best estimate of prevalence is as high as 124 in 100,000.

RISK FACTORS

In developing countries

- Obstetric trauma
- Prolonged labor
- Cephalopelvic disproportion causing ischemia and necrosis of the tissue between the fetal head and maternal pubic bone

In developed countries

- Fistula resulting from obstetric trauma are primarily related to vaginal lacerations, for which the risk factors include:
  - Primiparity
  - Midline episiotomies
  - Increasing birth weights
  - Use of vaginal forceps
- Abdominal hysterectomy, especially with the following:
  - Extensive bladder dissection
  - Iatrogenic injury of the bowel or bladder
  - Prolonged operating times
  - Large blood loss
  - Large volume uterus
  - Coexisting pelvic adhesions distorting the normal pelvic anatomy
- Invasive cancer
- Pelvic radiation, reported to be dependent on dosimetry
- Chronic inflammatory disease
  - Crohn disease
  - Diverticulitis
- Pelvic infection
  - Tuberculosis
  - Syphilis
  - Lymphogranuloma venereum
- Trauma
- Previous pelvic surgery
- Diabetes mellitus
- Age >50, likely as a result of poor tissue quality from menopausal estrogen deficiency, although some studies have refuted this.
- Tobacco usage
- Foreign bodies

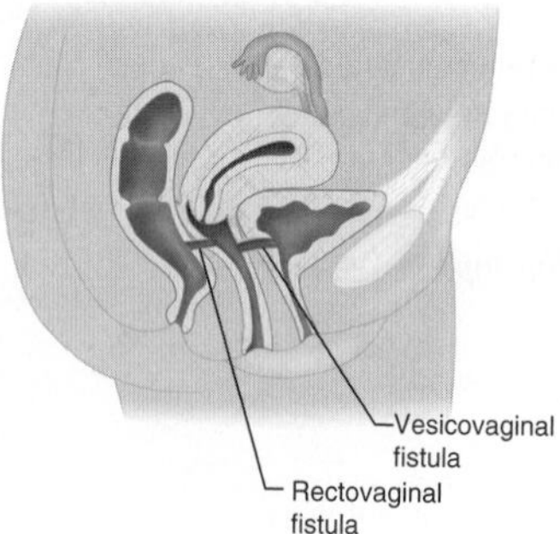

FIGURE 1-990 The two most common types of vaginal fistulas are vesicovaginal and rectovaginal. (From Fielding JR et al: *Gynecologic imaging*, Philadelphia, 2011, Saunders.)

PHYSICAL FINDINGS & CLINICAL PRESENTATION

- Flatus, stool, or urine per vaginum
- Frequent urinary tract infections
- Mucopurulent malodorous discharge per vaginum
- Dyspareunia
- Perineal pain
- Recurrent vaginal infections

ETIOLOGY

- Obstetric
  - Incompletely repaired or unidentified vaginal lacerations
  - Prolonged pressure between the fetal head and the maternal pubic bone, causing tissue necrosis
- Gynecologic
  - Poor-quality tissue with prolonged healing as a result of estrogen deficiency, infection, malignancy, or prior radiation therapy

DIAGNOSIS

DIFFERENTIAL DIAGNOSIS

- Rectal or urinary incontinence
- Pelvic inflammatory disease
- Vaginal infection
- Vaginal fistula
  - Vesicovaginal
  - Urethrovaginal
  - Ureterovaginal
  - Rectovaginal
- Urinary tract infection

WORKUP

- Thorough history and physical exam, specifically, questioning about Crohn disease symptomology; constitutional symptoms such as weight loss and fatigue, with malignancy in mind
- Obtaining of past medical records specific to obstetric and surgical procedures
- Evaluation of patient's rectal and urinary continence
- Physical exam, looking for extraintestinal signs consistent with Crohn disease; lymphadenopathy; inspection of perineum and perianal area for evidence of abscess, obvious fistula, or scarring; pelvic exam including lighted speculum exam for any vulvar, vaginal, or cervical anomaly, excluding PID
- Biopsy of fistula tract

LABORATORY TEST(S)

- Urinalysis
- Urine culture
- Complete blood count
- Administration of IV indigo carmine (if seen vaginally, diagnostic of vesicovaginal fistula)

IMAGING STUDIES

- Proctoscopy for suspected rectovaginal fistula
- Vaginogram (Fig. 1-991)
- Cystoscopy
- CT of the abdomen and pelvis to exclude malignancy (especially in women with no history of obstetric trauma, previous fistula, IBD, or known pelvic malignancy) (Fig. 1-991)
- Endoanal ultrasound, with or without hydrogen peroxide contrast injected into the suspected fistula tract
- Magnetic resonance imaging
- Intravenous urogram
- Retrograde ureteropyelography

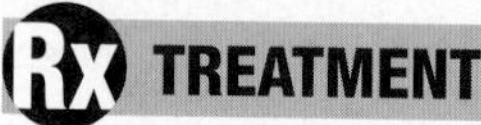

TREATMENT

NONPHARMACOLOGIC THERAPY

- Surgical repair, with multiple documented approaches
  - Transvaginal
  - Perineal
  - Abdominal
  - Laparoscopic
  - Robot assisted
  - Transrectal
- If vesicovaginal identified early
  - Prolonged urinary catheter placement, greater than 3 weeks

ACUTE GENERAL Rx

- Treatment of urinary or vaginal infection
- Estrogen replacement therapy, local vs. systemic if no contraindications
- Surgical repair of fistula with subsequent pelvic rest for 4-6 wk
- Minimizing Valsalva maneuvers

CHRONIC Rx

- If initial surgical management fails, repeat operations tailored to the cause of the fistula would be indicated, such as advancement flaps, sphincteroplasty, coloanal anastomosis (for rectovaginal fistula), gracilis flap.

DISPOSITION

- Cure rates after surgical repair vary in the literature, especially with the type of fistula repaired. With early intervention, estimated cure rates are between 84%-100% in developed countries.

REFERRAL

- If there is concern for vaginal fistula, the patient should be managed by a surgeon familiar with fistula surgery for repair and follow-up. Consider consulting with a urologist, colorectal surgeon, gynecologic oncologist, or urogynecologist.

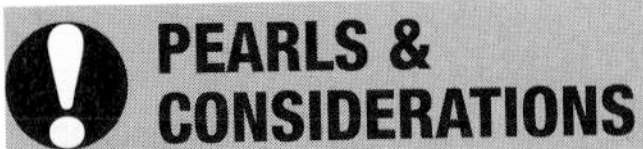

PEARLS & CONSIDERATIONS

PREVENTION

- Prompt repair of obstetric lacerations
- Screen patients most at risk before surgery
- Avoid urologic complications in surgery (e.g., injury to bladder or ureters)
- Cystoscopy with complicated hysterectomy dissections

RELATED CONTENT

Hysterectomy Complications; Obstetric Complications

AUTHOR: **AMBER N. FONTENOT FERRISS, M.D.**

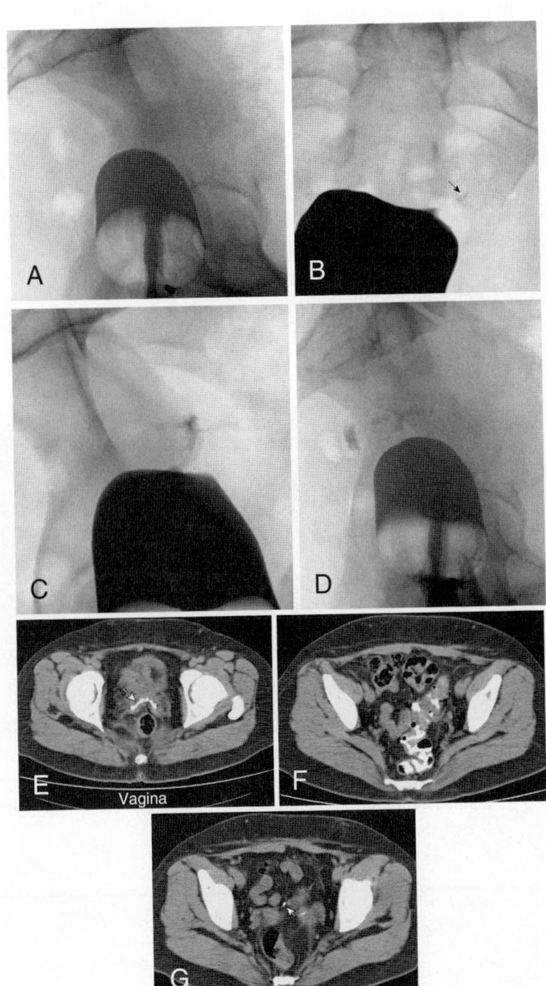

FIGURE 1-991 A 44-year-old woman with gas and stool per vaginum 1 year after hysterectomy. Vaginal fistula was treated medically. **A,** Vaginogram, patient in left lateral position. **B,** Vaginogram, patient supine. The left apical vaginal fistula has just started to fill with contrast agent (*arrow*). **C,** Contrast agent is extending horizontally, likely in a loop of bowel. **D,** Vaginogram, patient in left lateral position, demonstrates small fistula to a loop of bowel, likely the rectosigmoid colon based on its relationship to the sacrum. **E,** Unenhanced computed tomographic (CT) scan of the pelvis immediately after the vaginogram demonstrates residual contrast agent in the vagina (*arrow*). **F,** CT scan confirms contrast agent from the vagina in the rectosigmoid colon. **G,** CT scan demonstrates 3 mm diameter short fistula to the rectosigmoid (*arrow*). (From Fielding JR et al: *Gynecologic imaging*, Philadelphia, 2011, Saunders.)

BASIC INFORMATION

DEFINITION

Vaginal malignancy is an abnormal proliferation of vaginal epithelium demonstrating malignant cells below the basement membrane.

SYNONYMS

Squamous cell carcinoma of the vagina
Adenocarcinoma of the vagina
Melanoma of the vagina
Sarcoma of the vagina
Endodermal sinus tumor

ICD-9CM CODES
184.0 Vagina, vaginal neoplasm
ICD-10CM CODES
C52 Malignant neoplasm of vagina

EPIDEMIOLOGY & DEMOGRAPHICS

INCIDENCE: 0.42 cases per 100,000 persons
PREVALENCE: Vaginal cancer is the second rarest gynecologic cancer. It comprises 2% of malignancies of the female genital tract.
MEAN AGE AT DIAGNOSIS: Predominantly a disease of menopause. Mean age at diagnosis is 60 yr.

PHYSICAL FINDINGS & CLINICAL PRESENTATION

- Majority of cases are asymptomatic
- Postmenopausal vaginal bleeding and/or vaginal discharge are the most common symptoms
- May also present as pelvic pain or pressure, dyspareunia, dysuria, malodor, or postcoital bleeding
- May present as a vaginal lesion or abnormal Pap smear

ETIOLOGY

- The exact etiology is unknown.
- Vaginal intraepithelial neoplasia is believed to be a precursor for squamous cell carcinoma of the vagina.
- Long-term pessary use has been associated with vaginal malignancy.
- Prior pelvic radiation may be a risk factor.
- Clear-cell adenocarcinoma is related to in utero diethylstilbestrol exposure (DES). Treatment of pregnant women with DES ended in the early 1970s and it is anticipated that this spike in clear cell tumors will abate in the future.

Dx DIAGNOSIS

DIFFERENTIAL DIAGNOSIS

- Extension from other primary carcinoma more common than primary vaginal cancer
- Vaginitis

WORKUP

- Diagnosis is made histologically by biopsy.
- Colposcopy and biopsy should follow suspicious Pap smear.
- Cystoscopy, proctosigmoidoscopy, chest radiography, IV urography, and barium enema may be used for clinical staging.
- CT scan (Fig. 1-992), FDG, PET scan, and MRI are used to evaluate spread.
- Staging I to IV (Fig. 1-993).

IMAGING STUDIES

- Chest radiography, IV urography, and barium enema are used for staging.
- CT scan and MRI are good for assessing tumor spread.

Rx TREATMENT

NONPHARMACOLOGIC THERAPY

- Radiation therapy is the mainstay of treatment.
- Stage I tumors that are small and confined to the posterior, upper third of the vagina may be treated with radical surgery.
- Other stages require a whole-pelvis, interstitial, and/or intracavitary radiation therapy.
- Chemotherapy is used in conjunction with radiotherapy in rare select cases.

DISPOSITION

Five-year survival ranges from 80% for stage I to 17% for stage IV.

REFERRAL

Vaginal cancer should be managed by a gynecologic oncologist and radiation oncologist.

SUGGESTED READINGS
available at www.expertconsult.com

RELATED CONTENT

Vaginal Cancer (Patient Information)

AUTHOR: **RUBEN ALVERO, M.D.**

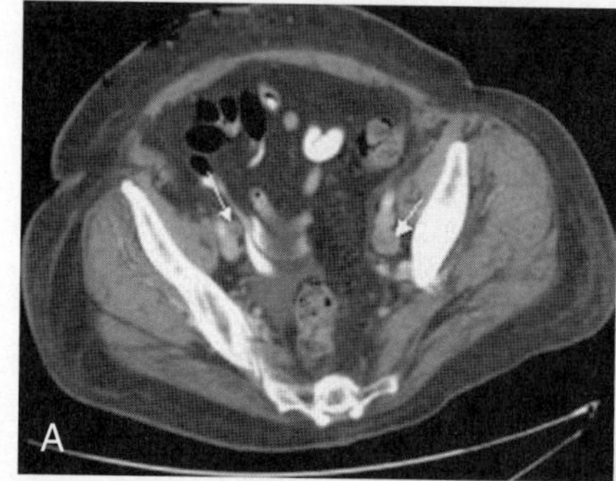

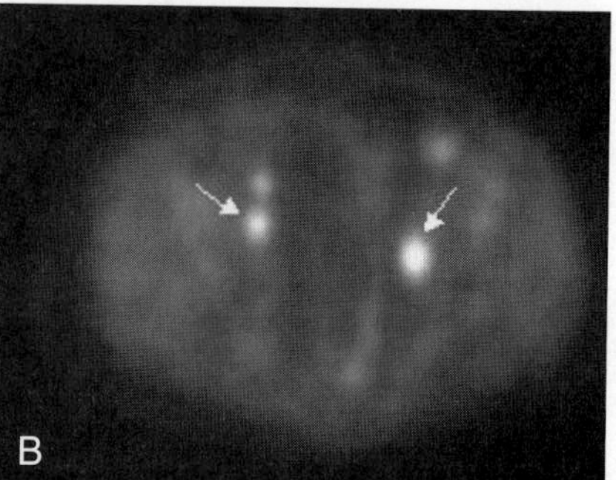

FIGURE 1-992 Vaginal cancer with lymphadenopathy. A, CT of pelvis showing mildly enlarged external iliac nodes suggestive of metastases *(arrows).* **B,** Axial FDG PET scan showing hypermetabolic nodes as hyperintense spots confirming metastases. (From Abeloff MD: *Clinical oncology,* ed 3, Philadelphia, 2004, Churchill Livingstone.)

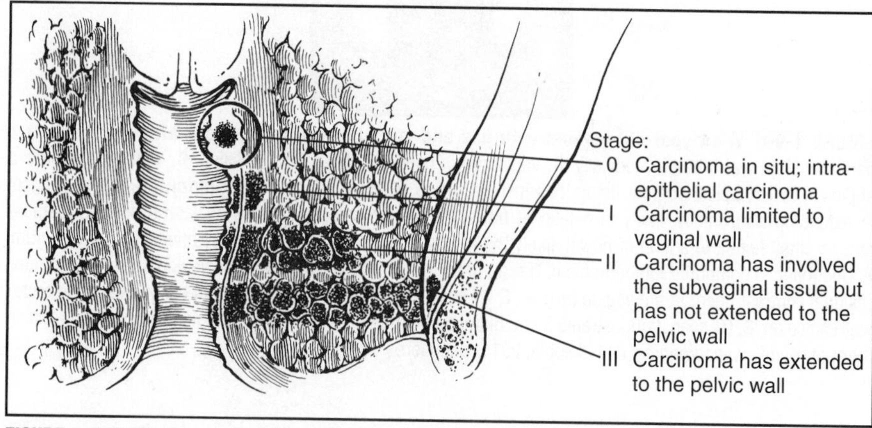

FIGURE 1-993 Staging system for vaginal cancer. Metastatic disease that involves the bladder or rectum is stage IV-a. Metastatic disease beyond the pelvis is stage IV-b. (From Copeland LJ: *Textbook of gynecology,* ed 2, Philadelphia, 2000, Saunders.)

BASIC INFORMATION

DEFINITION

Vaginismus refers to the involuntary spasm of the vaginal, introital, and/or levator ani muscles, preventing penetration or causing painful intercourse.

ICD-9CM CODES

300.11	Hysterical vaginismus
306.51	Psychogenic or functional vaginismus
625.1	Reflex vaginismus

ICD-10CM CODES

N94.1	Vaginismus
F52.5	Non-organic vaginismus
F52.5	Vaginismus not due to a substance or known physiological condition

EPIDEMIOLOGY & DEMOGRAPHICS

INCIDENCE: Estimated at 11.7% to 42% of women presenting to sexual dysfunction clinics
PREVALENCE: Affects approximately 1 in 200 women
PREDOMINANT SEX: Affects only females
RISK FACTORS: Any previous sexual trauma, including incest or rape

PHYSICAL FINDINGS & CLINICAL PRESENTATION

- Fear of pain with coitus
- Dyspareunia
- Orgasmic dysfunction

ETIOLOGY

- Learned conditioned response to real or imagined painful vaginal experience (e.g., traumatic speculum examination, incest, rape)
- Vaginitis
- Pelvic inflammatory disease
- Endometriosis
- Anatomic anomalies
- Atrophic vaginitis
- Mucosal tears
- Inadequate lubrication
- Focal vulvitis
- Painful hymenal tags
- Scarring secondary to episiotomy
- Skin disorders
- Topical allergies
- Postherpetic neuralgia

Dx DIAGNOSIS

WORKUP

- Thorough history (including sexual history)
- Careful pelvic examination
- Behavioral therapy

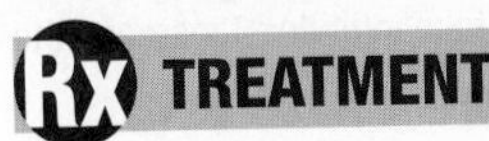

Rx TREATMENT

NONPHARMACOLOGIC THERAPY

- Deconditioning the response by systematic self-administered progressive dilation techniques using fingers or dilators
- Behavioral and/or psychosexual therapy

ACUTE GENERAL Rx

- Botulinum toxin therapy given locally has been shown to relieve the perineal muscle spasms associated with vaginismus, allowing resumption of intercourse.
  1. Acts by preventing neuromuscular transmission, causing muscle weakness
  2. Considered experimental treatment for vaginismus at this time

- Cause should be determined by history and explained to the patient so that she understands the mechanics of the muscle spasms.
- Patient must be motivated to desire painless vaginal insertion for such reasons as pleasurable coitus, tampon insertion, or gynecologic examination.
- Patient (and her partner) must be willing to patiently undergo the process of systematic desensitization and counseling.

DISPOSITION

A high percentage of successfully treated patients

REFERRAL

To a gynecologist or sex therapist

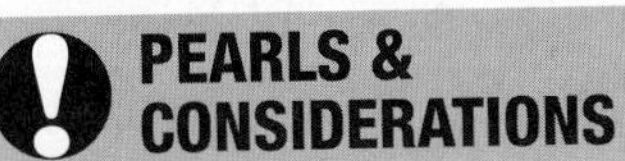

PEARLS & CONSIDERATIONS

COMMENTS

- May uncover early sexual abuse or an aversion to sexuality in general
- American Association of Sex Educators, Counselors and Therapists, 11 Dupont Circle, NW, Washington, DC, 20036.
- Sex Information and Education Council of the U.S. (SIECUS), 90 John St., New York, NY 10038.

SUGGESTED READINGS

available at www.expertconsult.com

AUTHOR: **RUBEN ALVERO, M.D.**

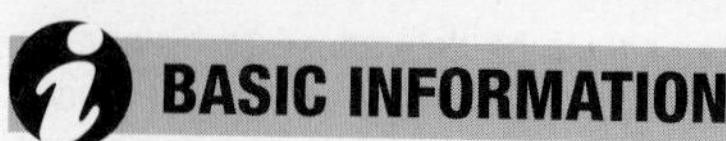

BASIC INFORMATION

DEFINITION

Estrogen-deficient vulvovaginitis is the irritation and/or inflammation of the vulva and vagina because of progressive thinning and atrophic changes secondary to estrogen deficiency (Fig. 1-994).

SYNONYMS

Atrophic vaginitis
Vulvovaginal atrophy

ICD-9CM CODES
616.10 Vulvovaginitis
ICD-10CM CODES
N95.2 Post-menopausal atrophic vaginitis

EPIDEMIOLOGY & DEMOGRAPHICS

- Seen most often in postmenopausal women
- Average age of menopause is 52 yr
- Up to half of postmenopausal women are symptomatic, but a quarter of these will not seek treatment

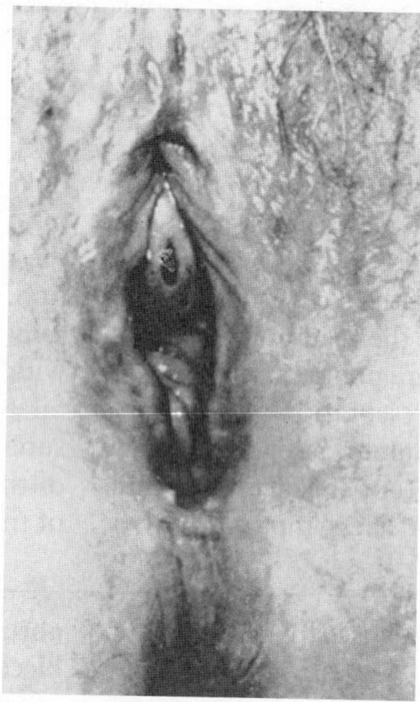

FIGURE 1-994 Advanced postmenopausal atrophy of the vulva in a 72-year-old woman. (From Symonds EM, Macpherson MBA: *Color atlas of obstetrics and gynecology,* St Louis, 1994, Mosby.)

PHYSICAL FINDINGS & CLINICAL PRESENTATION

- Thinning of pubic hair, labia minora and majora
- Decreased secretions from the vestibular glands, with vaginal dryness
- Regression of subcutaneous fat
- Vulvar and vaginal itching
- Dyspareunia
- Dysuria and urinary frequency
- Vaginal spotting

ETIOLOGY

- Estrogen deficiency. Estrogen is essential to maintaining the urogenital environment. Postmenopausal thinning of the vaginal epithelium and increase in subepithelial connective tissue results in loss of rugal folds and elasticity. Reduced blood flow also contributes to a decline in vaginal secretions.
- Smoking and use of antiestrogen medications (e.g., aromatase inhibitors) increase the risk of vulvovaginal atrophy.

Dx DIAGNOSIS

DIFFERENTIAL DIAGNOSIS

- Infectious vulvovaginitis
- Squamous cell hyperplasia
- Lichen sclerosus
- Vulvar malignancy
- Vaginal malignancy
- Cervical and endometrial malignancy
- Irritant contact dermatitis

WORKUP

- Pelvic examination
- Speculum examination
- Pap smear
- Possible endometrial biopsy if bleeding

LABORATORY TESTS

FSH and estradiol: generally after menopause, estradiol <15 pg/ml and FSH >40 mIU/ml (diagnosis of menopause usually made on a clinical basis and does not usually require FSH and/or estradiol testing)

Rx TREATMENT

NONPHARMACOLOGIC THERAPY

- Avoidance of contact irritants such as scented soaps and feminine hygiene products
- Avoidance of synthetic undergarments, tight-fitting clothing

GENERAL Rx

- Regular use of vaginal moisturizers (e.g., Replens) can decrease vaginal itching and irritation.
- Use of water or silicone-based personal lubricants (e.g., Astroglide) during intercourse is useful to reduce dyspareunia.
- Conjugated estrogen vaginal cream intravaginally. Estradiol vaginal cream (0.625 mg estrogen/gram).
  2 to 4 g/day × 2 wk then
  1 to 2 g/day × 2 wk then
  1 to 2 g × 2-3 days/wk
- Vagifem (estradiol vaginal tablets) 25 mg inserted intravaginally daily for 2 wk then twice weekly. May take up to 12 wk to feel the full benefits of the medication.
- Conjugated estrogen vaginal cream: 2 to 4 g qd (3 wk on, 1 wk off) for 3 to 5 mo.
- Hormone replacement therapy (HRT): use ultra-low doses. Estrogen use should be reviewed every 3 to 6 mo, with an attempt to taper or discontinue its use.
- Estraderm patch 0.05 mg × 2 per week.
- If uterus present:
  1. Estrogen + 2.5 mg PO Provera qd *or*
  2. Estrogen + 5 to 10 mg PO Provera × 14 days each mo

DISPOSITION

The symptoms should be improved with the therapy. Caution for vaginal bleeding if uterus present.

REFERRAL

To obstetrician/gynecologist if vaginal bleeding

SUGGESTED READINGS

available at www.expertconsult.com

RELATED CONTENT

Pruritus Vulvae (Related Key Topic)

AUTHOR: **RUBEN ALVERO, M.D.**

BASIC INFORMATION

DEFINITION

Fungal vulvovaginitis is the inflammation of vulva and vagina caused by *Candida* spp.

SYNONYMS

Candidiasis, vulvovaginal
Monilial vulvovaginitis
Vulvovaginal candidiasis
VVC

ICD-9CM CODES
112.1 Vulvovaginitis, monilial
ICD-10CM CODES
B37.3 Candidiasis of vulva and vagina

EPIDEMIOLOGY & DEMOGRAPHICS

- Second most common cause of vaginal infection
- 75% of women will have at least one episode during their childbearing years, and ~40% to 50% of these will have a second attack.
- No symptoms in 20% to 40% of women who have positive cultures

PHYSICAL FINDINGS & CLINICAL PRESENTATION

- Intense vulvar and vaginal pruritus
- Edema and erythema of vulva
- Thick, curd-like vaginal discharge ("cottage cheese" discharge)
- Adherent, dry, white, curdy patches attached to vaginal mucosa

ETIOLOGY

- *Candida albicans* is responsible for 80% to 95% of vaginal fungal infections.
- *Candida tropicalis* and *Torulopsis glabrata (Candida glabrata)* are the most common nonalbicans *Candida* species that can induce vaginitis.

PREDISPOSING HOST FACTORS

- Pregnancy
- Oral contraceptives (high-estrogen)
- Diabetes mellitus
- Antibiotics
- Immunosuppression (e.g., HIV)
- Tight, poorly ventilated, nylon underclothing, with increased local perineal moisture and temperature

DIAGNOSIS

DIFFERENTIAL DIAGNOSIS

- Bacterial vaginosis
- *Trichomonas* vaginitis
- Atrophic vaginitis

Section II describes the differential diagnosis of vaginal discharges and infections.

WORKUP

- Pelvic examination
- Speculum examination
- Hyphae or budding spores on 10% KOH preparation (positive in 50% to 70% of individuals with yeast infection)
- Normal vaginal pH

Section III, "Vaginal Discharge," describes the evaluation of discharge.

LABORATORY TESTS

Culture, especially recurrence for identification

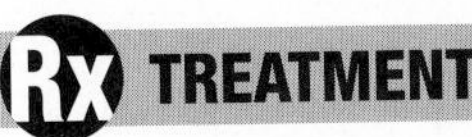

TREATMENT

ACUTE GENERAL Rx

- Cure rate of the various azole derivatives 85% to 90%; little evidence of superiority of one azole agent over another
- No significant differences in persistent symptoms with oral or vaginal treatment
- Fluconazole 150 mg PO × 1 is preferred treatment
- Cure rate of polyene cream, and suppositories: 75% to 80%
- Miconazole 200-mg suppository, one suppository × 3 days or 2% vaginal cream, one applicatorful intravaginally qhs × 7
- Clotrimazole 200-mg vaginal tablet, one tablet intravaginally qhs × 3 or 100-mg vaginal tablet one tablet intravaginally qhs × 7, or 1% vaginal cream intravaginally qhs × 7
- Butoconazole 2% cream one applicator intravaginally qhs × 3
- Terconazole 80-mg suppository or 0.8% vaginal cream, one suppository or one applicator intravaginally qhs × 3 or 0.4% vaginal cream, one applicator intravaginally qhs × 7
- Gynecazole-1 vaginal cream, one applicator intravaginally × 1
- Tioconazole 6.5% ointment (Vagi-stat), one applicator intravaginally × 1
- In pregnant patient, treat with 7-day course of topical imidazole.

CHRONIC Rx (FOUR OR MORE SYMPTOMATIC EPISODES ANNUALLY)

- Resistance or recurrence
  - 14- to 21-day course of 7-day regimens mentioned in "Acute General Rx" above
  - Fluconazole 150 mg PO × 2, 3 days apart
  - Ketoconazole 200 mg PO bid × 5 to 14 days
  - Itraconazole 200 mg PO qd × 3 days
  - Boric acid 600-mg capsule intravaginally bid × 14 days
- Prophylactic regimens
  - Clotrimazole one 500-mg vaginal tablet each month
  - Ketoconazole 200 mg PO bid × 5 days each month
  - Fluconazole 150 mg PO × 1 each month
  - Miconazole 100-mg vaginal tablet × 2 weekly

DISPOSITION

- If symptoms do not resolve completely with treatment, or if they recur within a 2- to 3-mo period, further evaluation is indicated.
- Reexamination and possibly culture are necessary.
- Positive culture in absence of symptoms should not lead to treatment. Approximately 30% of women harbor *Candida* spp. and other species in the vagina.

REFERRAL

To obstetrician/gynecologist for recurrence

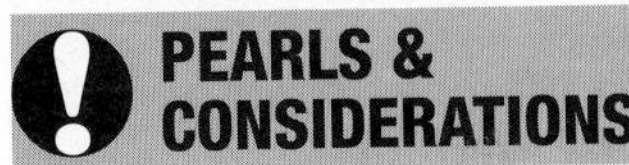

PEARLS & CONSIDERATIONS

COMMENTS

- No evidence that treating a woman's male sexual partner significantly improves woman's infection or reduces her rate of relapse.
- Many *Candida albicans* strains produce hyaluronidase, which is an enzyme that degrades hyaluronan. Elevated hyaluronan levels in vaginal secretions are associated with increased itching, burning, and discharge in women with recurrent vulvovaginal candidiasis.
- Twenty percent of cases of recurrent vulvovaginal candidiasis are due to *Candida* species other than *C. albicans*.

SUGGESTED READINGS

available at www.expertconsult.com

RELATED CONTENT

Pruritus Vulvae (Related Key Topic)
Vaginitis, Prepubescent (Related Key Topic)
Candidiasis (Patient Information)
Vaginal Yeast Infection (Patient Information)

AUTHOR: **RUBEN ALVERO, M.D.**

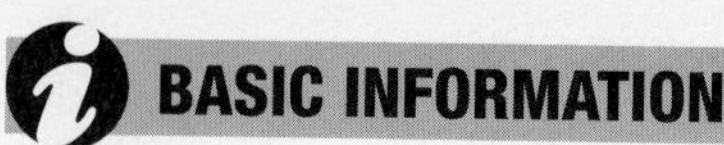

DEFINITION

Prepubescent vulvovaginitis is an inflammatory condition of the vulva and vagina.

ICD-9CM CODES
616.10 Vulvovaginitis
ICD-10CM CODES
N76.0 Acute vaginitis
N76.1 Subacute and chronic vaginitis

EPIDEMIOLOGY & DEMOGRAPHICS

- Most common gynecologic problem of the premenarchal female.
- Prepubertal girl is susceptible to irritation and trauma because of the absence of protective hair and labial fat pads and the lack of estrogenization with atrophic vaginal mucosa.
- Symptoms of vulvovaginitis and introital irritation and discharge account for 80% to 90% of gynecologic visits.
- Nonspecific etiology in approximately 75% of children with vulvovaginitis.
- Majority of vulvovaginitis in children involves a primary irritation of the vulva with secondary involvement of the lower third of the vagina.

PHYSICAL FINDINGS & CLINICAL PRESENTATION

Vulvar pain, dysuria, pruritus

1. Discharge is not a primary symptom.
2. If present, vaginal discharge may be foul smelling or bloody.

ETIOLOGY

- Infections
  1. Bacterial
  2. Protozoal
  3. Mycotic
  4. Viral
- Endocrine disorders
- Labial adhesions
- Poor hygiene
- Sexual abuse
- Allergic substance
- Trauma
- Foreign body
- Masturbation
- Constipation

Section II describes the differential diagnosis of vaginal discharge in prepubertal girls.

Dx DIAGNOSIS

DIFFERENTIAL DIAGNOSIS

- Physiologic leukorrhea
- Foreign body
- Bacterial vaginosis
- Gonorrhea
- Fungal vulvovaginitis
- *Trichomonas* vulvovaginitis
- Sexual abuse
- Pinworms

WORKUP

- Pelvic, genital examination
- Speculum examination
- Rectal examination
- Vaginoscopy if considering a foreign body
- KOH and normal saline preparation of discharge
- Knee-chest position for examination may be easier for the child to tolerate during an examination

Section III, "Vaginal Discharge," describes the evaluation of discharge.

LABORATORY TESTS

- Urinalysis to rule out urinary tract infection and diabetes
- Cultures including sexually transmitted diseases

Rx TREATMENT

NONPHARMACOLOGIC THERAPY

- Avoid tight clothing
- Perineal hygiene
- Avoid irritant chemicals
- Reassurance

ACUTE GENERAL Rx

- Group A beta *Streptococcus* and *Streptococcus pneumoniae:* penicillin V potassium 125 to 250 mg PO qid × 10 days
- *Chlamydia trachomatis:* azithromycin 1 g PO single dose
- *Neisseria gonorrhoeae:* ceftriaxone 250 mg IM × 1 day
  - Children >8 yr should also be given doxycycline 100 mg bid PO × 7 days
- *Staphylococcus aureus:* amoxicillin-clavulanate 20 to 40 mg/kg/day PO × 7 to 10 days
- *Haemophilus influenzae:* amoxicillin 20 to 40 mg/kg/day PO × 7 days
- *Trichomonas:* metronidazole 125 mg (15 mg/kg/day) tid PO × 7 to 10 days
- Pinworms: mebendazole 100-mg tablet chewable, repeat in 2 wk
- Labial agglutination: spontaneous resolution or topical estrogen cream for 7 to 10 days. High degree of efficacy with topical estrogen hormone.

CHRONIC Rx

See "Referral."

DISPOSITION

Further education:

- Young child: hygiene
- Adolescent: pregnancy prevention and safe sexual practices

REFERRAL

- To obstetrician/gynecologist
- To pediatrician

SUGGESTED READINGS
available at www.expertconsult.com

RELATED CONTENT

Pruritus Vulvae (Related Key Topic)
Vaginitis, Fungal (Related Key Topic)
Vaginitis, *Trichomonas* (Related Key Topic)
Vaginosis, Bacterial (Related Key Topic)

AUTHOR: **RUBEN ALVERO, M.D.**

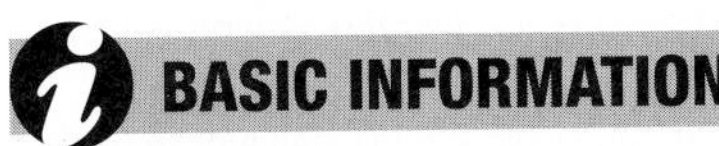

BASIC INFORMATION

DEFINITION

Trichomonas vulvovaginitis is the inflammation of vulva and vagina caused by *Trichomonas* spp.

SYNONYMS

Trichomonas vaginalis
Trichomoniasis
TV

ICD-9CM CODES
131.01 Vulvovaginitis, trichomonal
ICD-10CM CODES
A59.01 Trichomonal vulvovaginitis

EPIDEMIOLOGY & DEMOGRAPHICS

- Acquired through sexual contact
- Diagnosed in
  - 50% to 75% of prostitutes
  - 5% to 15% of women visiting gynecology clinics
  - 7% to 32% of women in sexually transmitted disease (STD) clinics
  - 5% of women in family planning clinics

PHYSICAL FINDINGS & CLINICAL PRESENTATION

- Profuse, yellow, malodorous vaginal discharge and severe vaginal itching
- Vulvar itching
- Dysuria
- Dyspareunia
- Intense erythema of the vaginal mucosa
- Cervical petechiae ("strawberry cervix")
- Asymptomatic in ~50% of women and 90% of men

ETIOLOGY

Single-cell protozoan *Trichomonas vaginalis*

RISK FACTORS

- Multiple sexual partners
- History of previous STDs

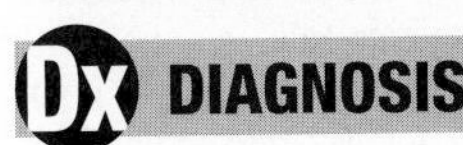

DIAGNOSIS

DIFFERENTIAL DIAGNOSIS

(Table 1-497)

- Bacterial vaginosis
- Fungal vulvovaginitis
- Cervicitis
- Atrophic vulvovaginitis

WORKUP

- Pelvic examination
- Speculum examination
- Mobile trichomonads seen on normal saline preparation (Fig. 1-995): 70% sensitivity
- Elevated pH (>5) of vaginal discharge
- Culture is considered the traditional gold standard laboratory test for diagnosis of TV.
- Nucleic acid amplification tests (NAATs) have been developed that combine excellent performance characteristics with a more rapid turnaround time compared with culture.
- APTIMA assays utilize target capture and transcription-mediated amplification (TMA) to selectively purify, amplify, and detect species-specific 16 S ribosomal RNA. APTIMA *Trichomonas vaginalis* transcription-mediated amplification may be a better laboratory test than culture based on sensitivity and time frame for results.

LABORATORY TESTS

- Culture (modified Diamond media): 90% sensitivity
- Direct enzyme immunoassay
- Fluorescein-conjugated monoclonal antibody test
- Pap test 40% detected

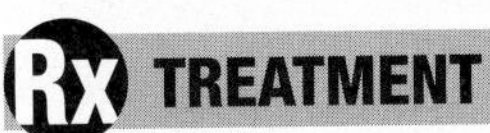

TREATMENT

NONPHARMACOLOGIC THERAPY

Condom use

ACUTE GENERAL Rx

Metronidazole 2 g PO × 1 *or* Tindamax (tinidazole) single 2-g oral dose in both sexes. Treatment of the sexual partner is essential to prevent reinfection.

CHRONIC Rx

- Metronidazole gel: less likely to achieve therapeutic levels; therefore not recommended.
- Metronidazole (retreat): 500 mg PO bid × 7 days.
- Treatment of future recurrences: metronidazole 2 g PO qd × 3 to 5 days.
- Allergy, intolerance, or adverse reactions: alternatives to metronidazole are not available. Patients who are allergic to metronidazole can be managed by desensitization.
- Pregnancy:
  - Associated with adverse outcomes (i.e., premature rupture of membranes)
  - Metronidazole 2 g PO × 1 day

DISPOSITION

Trichomonas infection is considered an STD; therefore treatment of the sexual partner is necessary.

REFERRAL

To obstetrician/gynecologist for recurrence and pregnancy

SUGGESTED READINGS
available at www.expertconsult.com

RELATED CONTENT

Pruritus Vulvae (Related Key Topic)
Vaginitis, Prepubescent (Related Key Topic)
Trichomoniasis (Patient Information)

AUTHOR: **RUBEN ALVERO, M.D.**

TABLE 1-497 Differential Diagnosis of Vaginitis

Characteristics of Vaginal Discharge	*C. Aalbicans* Vaginitis	*T. vaginalis* Vaginitis	Bacterial Vaginosis
pH	4.5	>5.0	>5.0
White curd	Usually	No	No
Odor with KOH	No	Yes	Yes
Clue cells	No	No	Usually
Motile trichomonads	No	Usually	No
Yeast cells	Yes	No	No

From Goldman L, Ausiello D (eds): *Cecil textbook of medicine,* ed 22, Philadelphia, 2004, Saunders.

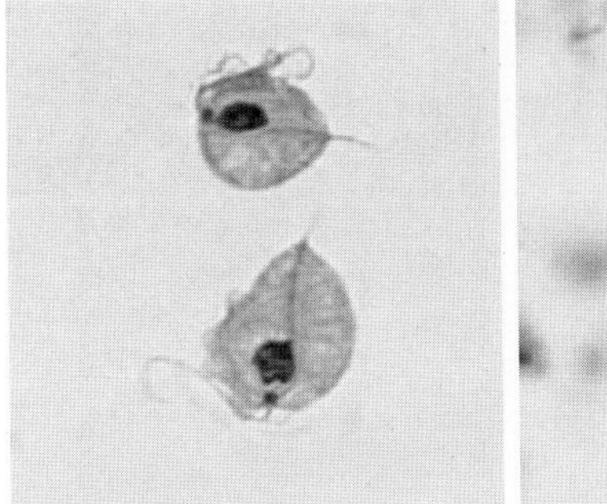

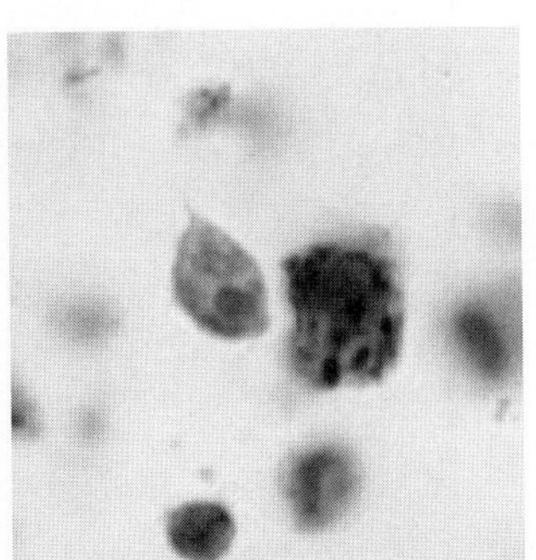

FIGURE 1-995 ***Trichomonas vaginalis*** **trophozoites stained with Giemsa *(left)* and iron hematoxylin *(right).*** (From the Centers for Disease Control and Prevention: *Laboratory identification of parasites of public health concern, Trichomoniasis.* www.dpd.cdc.gov/dpdx/HTML/ImageLibrary/Trichomoniasis_il.htm. Accessed August 30, 2010.)

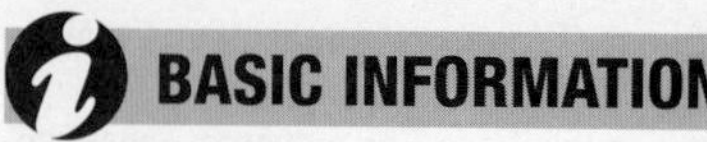

BASIC INFORMATION

DEFINITION

Bacterial vaginosis (BV) is a thin, gray, homogeneous, malodorous vaginal discharge that results from a shift in the vaginal flora from a predominance of lactobacilli to high concentrations of anaerobic bacteria.

SYNONYMS

Before 1955: nonspecific vaginitis
1955: *Haemophilus vaginalis* vaginitis
1963: *Corynebacterium vaginalis* vaginitis
1980: *Gardnerella vaginalis* vaginitis
1990: Bacterial vaginosis

ICD-9CM CODES
616.10 Vaginitis, bacterial
ICD-10 CODES
A59.01 Trichomonal vulvovaginitis

EPIDEMIOLOGY & DEMOGRAPHICS

- Most common vaginal infection
- *Gardnerella, Mycoplasma,* and *Mobiluncus* are harbored in the urethra of male partners; however:
  1. Male partners are asymptomatic.
  2. There is no improved cure rate or lower reinfection rate if the infected patient's male partner is treated.
  3. Abstinence from intercourse or condom use while the patient completes her treatment regimen may improve cure rates and lessen recurrences.

PHYSICAL FINDINGS & CLINICAL PRESENTATION

- 50% of patients are asymptomatic
- A thin, dark, or dull gray homogeneous discharge that adheres to the vaginal walls
- An offensive, "fishy" odor that is accentuated after intercourse or menses
- Pruritus (only in 13%)

ETIOLOGY

- *Gardnerella vaginalis* is detected in 40% to 50% of vaginal secretions.
  1. Increase in vaginal pH caused by decrease in hydrogen peroxide–producing lactobacilli
  2. Anaerobes predominate and produce amines
- Amines, when alkalinized by semen, menstrual blood, the use of alkaline douches, or the addition of 10% potassium hydroxide, volatilize and cause the unpleasant "fishy" odor. This amine-whiff test is one of the diagnostic approaches used for BV.
- In BV:
  1. *Bacteroides* (anaerobes) species are increased 1000× the usual concentration.
  2. *G. vaginalis* are 100× normal.
  3. *Peptostreptococcus* are 10× normal.
  4. *Mycoplasma hominis* and Enterobacteriaceae members are present in increased concentrations.

DIAGNOSIS

WORKUP

Seattle Group criteria:

- The presence of three of the four following signs will diagnose 90% correctly, with <10% false-positive results:
  1. Thin, gray, homogeneous, malodorous discharge that adheres to the vaginal walls
  2. Elevated pH >4.5
  3. Positive potassium hydroxide whiff test
  4. Clue cells present on wet mount
- Cultures are unnecessary.
- Pap smear will not identify *G. vaginalis.*
- Gram stain of vaginal secretions will reveal clue cells and abnormal mixed bacteria (Fig. 1-996).

TREATMENT

ACUTE GENERAL Rx

- Recommended regimens (equal efficacy):
  1. Metronidazole 500 mg PO bid for 7 days
  2. 0.75% metronidazole gel in vagina bid for 5 days
  3. 2% clindamycin cream qd for 7 days
- Alternate regimens (lower efficacy for BV):
  1. Clindamycin ovules 100 g intravaginally qhs for 3 days
  2. Clindamycin 300 mg PO bid for 7 days (increased incidence of diarrhea)
  3. Metronidazole ER 750 mg PO qd for 7 days
  4. Metronidazole 2 g PO single dose (higher relapse rate)
- Patients should be advised to avoid alcohol while taking metronidazole and for 24 hr thereafter due to disulfiram-type (antabuse) reaction when taken concurrently with alcohol.
- Treatment in pregnancy:
  - All pregnant patients proved to have BV should be treated because of its association with preterm labor, chorioamnionitis, and premature rupture of membranes (PROM).
- Recommended regimens:
  1. Metronidazole 250 mg PO tid for 7 days
  2. Clindamycin 300 mg PO bid for 7 days
- Existing data do not support the use of topical agents during pregnancy.
- Multiple studies and meta-analyses have not demonstrated associations between metronidazole use during pregnancy and teratogenic effects in newborns.
  3. Tinidazole, an oral antiprotozoal drug, is now FDA approved for treatment of BV. Dosage is 2 g once/day for 2 days or 1 g qd × 5 days
- Recurrent BV:
  1. Condom use may help reduce the risk of recurrence.
  2. Concurrent treatment of male partner is controversial. Consider treating the male partner if there is recurrent vaginitis or any suspicion of associated upper genital tract infection.

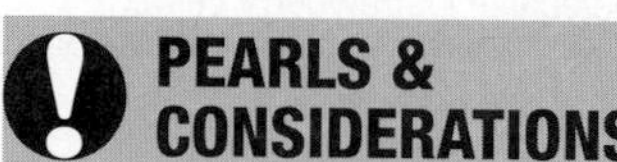

PEARLS & CONSIDERATIONS

- BV has been associated with pelvic inflammatory disease, cystitis, posthysterectomy vaginal cuff cellulitis, postabortal infection, preterm delivery, PROM, amnionitis, chorioamnionitis, and postpartum endometritis. New evidence also shows BV increases women's risk of acquiring HIV.
- Higher cumulative cure rates have been found at 3 to 4 wk for a 7-day regimen of metronidazole (500 mg twice daily) than with a single dose (2 g).
- Persistent BV is associated with several bacteria in the Clostridiales order, *Megasphaera* phylotype 2, and *P. lacrimalis.*

SUGGESTED READINGS
available at www.expertconsult.com

RELATED CONTENT

Bacterial Vaginal Infections (Patient Information)

AUTHOR: **RUBEN ALVERO, M.D.**

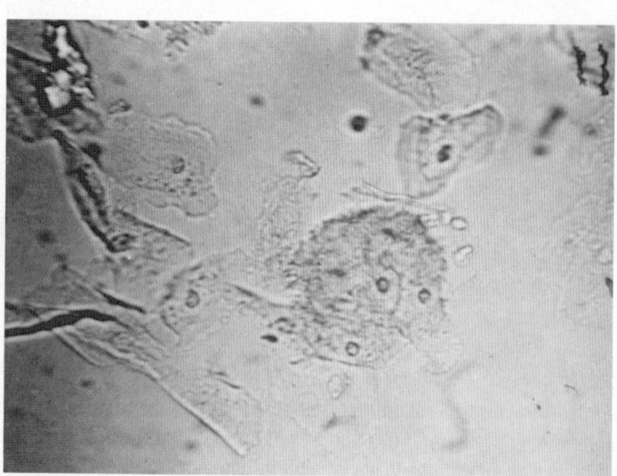

FIGURE 1-996 Clue cells characteristic of bacterial vaginosis, squamous epithelial cells whose borders are obscured by bacteria. (From Carlson K [ed]: *Primary care of women,* St Louis, 1995, Mosby.)

BASIC INFORMATION

DEFINITION

Enterococci are gram-positive, facultative, anaerobic organisms usually oval in shape and can be seen as single cells, pairs, or chains. Vancomycin-resistant *Enterococcus* (VRE) are enterococci that have become resistant to vancomycin and several antibiotics normally used to treat enterococcal infections.

SYNONYMS

VRE

ICD-9CM CODES
V09.8 Infection with microorganisms resistant to other specified drugs
ICD-10CM CODES
Z16.39 Resistance to other specified antimicrobial drug

EPIDEMIOLOGY & DEMOGRAPHICS

INCIDENCE: VRE may be associated with the use of specific classes of antibiotics.
PEAK INCIDENCE: VRE was first reported in Europe in 1986, and there has been a steady rise in the incidence of enterococcal strains resistant to vancomycin. In 2007, 80% of *E. faecium* isolates and 7% of *E. faecalis* isolates were resistant to vancomycin.
PREVALENCE: 80% of *E. faecium* are VRE; 69% of *E. faecalis* are VRE.
RISK FACTORS:
- Prior antimicrobial therapy, especially vancomycin
- Prolonged hospitalization
- Chronic medical conditions, renal failure
- Invasive devices
- ICU stay
- Colonization: VRE colonize the gastrointestinal tract; can be found on skin or perirectal swab culture or stool culture

PHYSICAL FINDINGS & CLINICAL PRESENTATION

Patients may be asymptomatic and have gastrointestinal colonization; it can be associated with diarrhea. In hospitalized patients, infection is associated with colonization and can cause wound infections, bacteremia, abscesses (intra-abdominal), and, rarely, pneumonia and urinary tract infections.

ETIOLOGY

- Enterococci are primarily found in the human digestive tract and female genital tract, where they make up a significant portion of the normal bacterial population in healthy people. Enterococci can cause urinary tract, wound, bloodstream, heart valve, and brain infections. In the great majority of cases, VRE infections occur in hospitalized patients who have compromised immune systems. Most cases of VRE are caused by the *E. faecium* strains that have acquired resistance when they came in contact with other bacteria and shared genetic information.
- VRE is most commonly transmitted from one patient to another by healthcare workers whose hands have become contaminated inadvertently with feces or fluids of a person carrying the organism. VRE are not airborne but can survive on surfaces for several weeks.

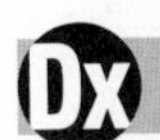

DIAGNOSIS

DIFFERENTIAL DIAGNOSIS

- Other bacterial pathogens in blood, wounds, or urine
- Once colonized, increased incidence to become infected

LABORATORY TESTS

- VRE rectal culture
- VRE stool culture
- Blood, urine, and wound cultures

Rx TREATMENT

- For rectal or stool colonization, therapy is not recommended
- Therapy is complicated by the fact that strains exhibit inherent resistance to many commonly used antibiotics.
- More than 80% of vancomycin-resistant *E. faecium* strains are also resistant to ampicillin.
- In symptomatic patients, if VRE strains are known to be susceptible, potential therapeutic agents include
  1. Linezolid: 600 mg IV or PO q12h
  2. Daptomycin: 4 mg/kg/day IV
  3. Quinupristin-dalfopristin (Synercid) only effective for *E. faecium* strains with no activity for *E. faecalis* strains: 7.5 mg/kg q8-12h. Can cause severe myalgias and arthralgias and venous irritation that often requires use of a central line, which has limited the use of this antibiotic.

REFERRAL

To infectious disease specialist

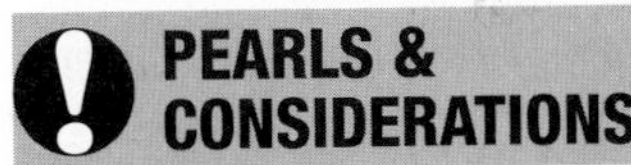

PEARLS & CONSIDERATIONS

COMMENTS

- Incidence increases with comorbidity and hospitalization.
- The number of patients already colonized with VRE in a defined geographic area (colonization pressure) is the most significant factor for predicting new acquisition of VRE.
- An association between VRE colonization and *Clostridium difficile* infection has been reported in patients with hematologic malignancies.

PREVENTION

Hand hygiene–isolation techniques, cleaning contaminated objects or surfaces, gowns and gloves, antibiotic management (prudent vancomycin use), surveillance

SUGGESTED READINGS
available at www.expertconsult.com

AUTHOR: **GLENN G. FORT, M.D., M.P.H.**

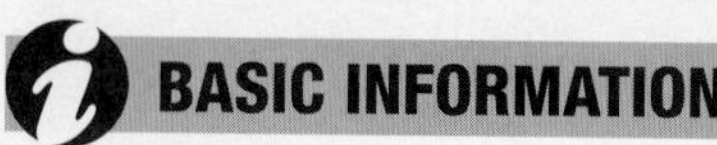

DEFINITION

Varicella is a common viral illness that is characterized by the acute onset of a generalized vesicular rash and fever.

SYNONYMS

Chickenpox

ICD-9CM CODES
052.9 Varicella
ICD-10CM CODES
B01.9 Varicella without complication
B01.0+ Varicella meningitis (G02.0)
B01.1+ Varicella encephalitis (G05.1)
B01.2+ Varicella pneumonia (J17.1)
B01.8 Varicella with other complications

EPIDEMIOLOGY & DEMOGRAPHICS

- Varicella is extremely contagious. More than 90% of unvaccinated contacts become infected.
- The incubation period of chickenpox ranges from 9 to 21 days.
- The peak incidence is during the springtime.
- The predominant age is 5 to 10 yr.
- The infectious period begins 2 days before the onset of clinical symptoms and lasts until all of the lesions have crusted.
- Most patients will have lifelong immunity after an attack of chickenpox; protection from the virus after a varicella vaccine is approximately 6 yr.

PHYSICAL FINDINGS & CLINICAL PRESENTATION

- Findings vary with the clinical course. Initial symptoms consist of fever, chills, backache, generalized malaise, and headache.
- Symptoms are generally more severe in adults.
- Initial lesions generally occur on the trunk (centripetal distribution) and occasionally on the face; these lesions consist primarily of 3- to 4-mm red papules with an irregular outline and a clear vesicle on the surface (i.e., the appearance of dewdrops on a rose petal).
- Intense pruritus generally accompanies the initial stage.
- New lesion development generally ceases by the fourth day, with subsequent crusting by the sixth day.
- Lesions generally spread to the face and the extremities (i.e., centrifugal spread).
- Patients generally present with lesions that are in different stages at the same time.
- Crusts generally fall off within 5 to 14 days.
- The fever is usually highest during the eruption of the vesicles; the patient's temperature generally returns to normal after the disappearance of vesicles.
- Signs of potential complications (e.g., bacterial skin infections, neurologic complications, pneumonia, hepatitis) may be present on physical examination.
- Mild constitutional symptoms (e.g., anorexia, myalgias, headaches, restlessness) may be present; these are most common among adults.
- Excoriations may be present if scratching is prominent.

ETIOLOGY

Varicella-zoster virus is a human herpes virus III that can manifest with either varicella or herpes zoster (i.e., shingles, which is a reactivation of varicella).

Dx DIAGNOSIS

DIFFERENTIAL DIAGNOSIS

- Other viral infection
- Impetigo
- Scabies
- Drug rash
- Urticaria
- Dermatitis herpetiformis
- Smallpox

WORKUP

The diagnosis is usually made on the basis of the patient's history and clinical presentation.

LABORATORY TESTS

- Laboratory evaluation is generally not necessary.
- The CBC may reveal leukopenia and thrombocytopenia.
- Serum varicella titers (i.e., a significant rise in the serum varicella immunoglobulin G antibody level), skin biopsies, or Tzanck smears are used only when diagnosis is in question.

Rx TREATMENT

NONPHARMACOLOGIC THERAPY

- Use antipruritic lotions for symptomatic relief.
- Avoid scratching to prevent excoriations and superficial skin infections.
- Use a mild soap for bathing.
- Hands should be washed often.

ACUTE GENERAL Rx

- Use acetaminophen for fever and myalgias; aspirin should be avoided because of the associated increased risk for Reye's syndrome.
- Oral acyclovir (20 mg/kg qid for 5 days) initiated at the earliest sign (i.e., within 24 hr of illness) is useful for healthy, nonpregnant individuals 13 yr old or older to decrease the duration and severity of signs and symptoms. Immunocompromised hosts should be treated with intravenous acyclovir 500 mg/m^2 or 10 mg/kg q8h for 7 to 10 days.
- Varicella is most contagious from 2 days before to a few days after the onset of the rash. Varicella vaccine is available for children and adults; protection lasts at least 6 yr. Healthy, nonimmune adults and children exposed to varicella-zoster virus should receive prophylaxis with live attenuated varicella vaccine (Varivax). Patients with HIV or other immunocompromised patients should not receive the live attenuated vaccine.
- Exposed patients with contraindications to varicella vaccine can be treated with varicella-zoster immunoglobulin (VariZIG), which effectively prevents varicella in susceptible individuals. The dose is 12.5 U/kg IM up to a maximum of 625 U. VariZIG must be administered as early as possible after presumed exposure (i.e., within 10 days) for postexposure prophylaxis of varicella.
- Pruritus from chickenpox can be controlled with antihistamines (e.g., hydroxyzine 25 mg q6h) and oral antipruritic lotions (e.g., calamine).
- Oral antibiotics are not routinely indicated and should be used only in patients with secondary infection and infected lesions; the most common infective organisms are *Streptococcus* sp. and *Staphylococcus* sp.

DISPOSITION

- The course is generally benign in immunocompetent adults and children.
- Infants who develop chickenpox are incapable of controlling the infection and should be given varicella-zoster immunoglobulin or gamma globulin if VariZIG is not available.

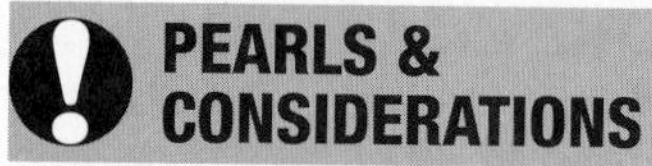

COMMENTS

- VariZIG can be obtained from the nearest regional Red Cross Blood Center or the Centers for Disease Control and Prevention in Atlanta.
- Varicella immunization is recommended for all who have not had chickenpox; the dosage for adults and adolescents (>13 yr old) is two 0.5-ml doses 4 to 8 wk apart.

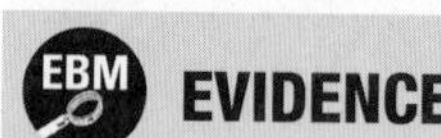

available at www.expertconsult.com

RELATED CONTENT

Chickenpox (Patient Information)

AUTHOR: **FRED F. FERRI, M.D.**

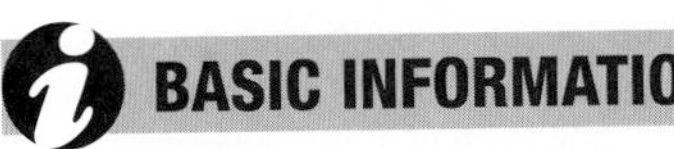

BASIC INFORMATION

DEFINITION

A varicocele is a dilation of the testicular vein and pampiniform plexus within the scrotum.

SYNONYMS

Sometimes referred to as "bag of worms" (Fig. 1-997)

ICD-9CM CODES
456.4
ICD-10CM CODES
I86.1 Scrotal varices

EPIDEMIOLOGY & DEMOGRAPHICS

PREVALENCE: A varicocele is present in up to 20% of all males. It occurs in approximately 40% of infertile men. However, only 10% to 15% of males with varicoceles have fertility problems.

RISK FACTORS: There are no reliable data on epidemiologic risk factors for varicocele, such as a family history or environmental exposures.

PHYSICAL FINDINGS & CLINICAL PRESENTATION

- While most varicoceles are painless, patients may complain of dull, aching pain that is relieved with lying down. They may also complain of testicular atrophy, one testicle being heavier than the other, a swollen testicle, or decreased fertility.
- Patients may report a mass lying posterior to and above the testis. When the patient is supine, dilation of the veins is generally decreased. Dilation and tortuosity of the veins are increased when the patient is upright and when the patient performs a Valsalva maneuver.
- The majority of cases (90%) occur more commonly on the left side because the left spermatic vein enters the left renal vein at a 90-degree angle, whereas the right testicular vein drains directly into the vena cava. Bilateral varicoceles occur in 33% of patients. A unilateral right-sided varicocele is very rare and should raise suspicion for an underlying disease causing obstruction of the vena cava.
- Physical examination reveals a soft scrotal mass that increases in size when standing and is typically described as a "bag of worms."
- Varicoceles can be graded based on physical exam. Grade one is small and is palpable only with Valsalva maneuver. Grade two is moderate and nonvisible on inspection but is palpable on standing. Grade three is large and visible on gross inspection.

ETIOLOGY

Varicoceles are caused by dysfunction of the valves in the spermatic vein, which allows pooling of blood in the pampiniform plexus.

Dx DIAGNOSIS

DIFFERENTIAL DIAGNOSIS

- Hydrocele
- Spermatocele
- Epididymal orchitis
- Testicular tumor
- Table E1-498 describes the differential diagnosis of pediatric scrotal masses and pain.

WORKUP

Patient should undergo a testicular exam in the upright and supine position.

LABORATORY TESTS

- Laboratory evaluation is generally not indicated
- Semen analysis may be performed if a varicocele is detected and the patient is infertile.

IMAGING

Usually varicoceles are diagnosed clinically. However, if there is suspicion for underlying malignancy, ultrasound may be used.

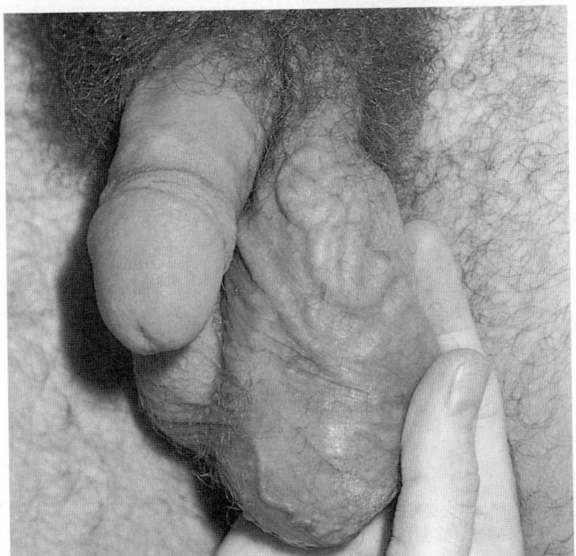

FIGURE 1-997 Varicocele. (From Swartz MH: *Textbook of physical diagnosis,* ed 5, Philadelphia, 2006, Saunders.)

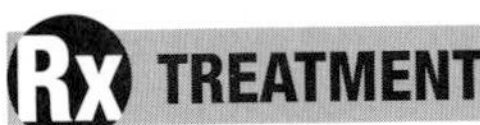

TREATMENT

There are no clear guidelines or solid evidence for treatment. Once a varicocele is identified, providers must document bilateral testicular size at regular intervals. Older men who do not want children and are asymptomatic can be treated conservatively. Surgical treatment is indicated for young men with retarded growth of a testis or abnormal sperm counts who want children.

MEDICAL MANAGEMENT

- NSAIDs are beneficial for pain relief.
- Scrotal support can reduce the feeling of "heaviness."

SURGERY

- Should surgery be advisable, varicocelectomy is performed by ligation of the veins of the pampiniform plexus through an inguinal incision or by ligating the internal spermatic vein in the retroperitoneum. This is generally performed as an ambulatory surgery.
- Although surgery will reverse abnormal sperm counts, it will not necessarily reverse fertility.
- Postoperatively the involved testis typically enlarges and catches up to the uninvolved side in 1 to 2 yr.
- The success rate of surgical repair is close to 98%; that of percutaneous repair is significantly lower.
- Sclerotherapy represents a less invasive option but is less effective in symptom reduction.

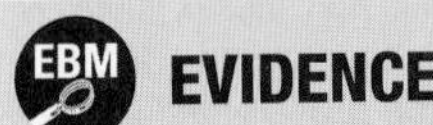

PEARLS & CONSIDERATIONS

- A varicocele in a 10-year-old boy or on the right side may be indicative of an abdominal or retroperitoneal mass. Ultrasound should be performed.
- The sudden occurrence of a left-sided varicocele in an older man indicates occlusion of the spermatic vein and should prompt evaluation for a renal tumor.

EBM EVIDENCE

available at www.expertconsult.com

SUGGESTED READINGS

available at www.expertconsult.com

RELATED CONTENT

Varicocele (Patient Information)

AUTHOR: **EMILY VAN KIRK, M.D.**

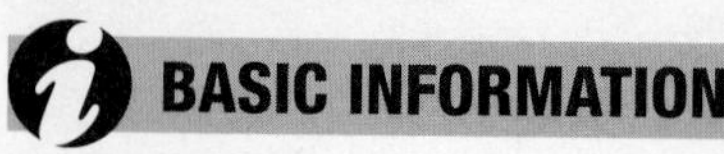

BASIC INFORMATION

DEFINITION

Veins in the leg are soft, thin-walled tubes that return blood back to the heart. This is accomplished by the presence of one-way valves and the action of the calf pump. Superficial venous insufficiency develops when venous return is impaired by valvular incompetence, obstruction, or calf muscle pump failure.

Varicose veins, the most common clinical manifestation of chronic venous disease, are bulging (>3 mm in diameter), tortuous conduits (Fig. 1-998). Reticular veins, often called "feeder veins," are bluish subdermal veins about 1 to 3 mm in diameter that give rise to telangiectasia. Spider veins or telangiectasias are very small (≤1 mm in diameter) thread veins found commonly in clusters on the surface of the skin.

SYNONYMS

Chronic venous disorder

ICD-9CM CODES
454.9 Varicose veins
454.8 Varicose veins with symptoms
ICD-10CM CODES
I83.90 Asymptomatic varicose veins of unspecified lower extremity
I83.899 Varicose veins of unspecified lower extremities with other complications

EPIDEMIOLOGY

PREVALENCE: One large U.S. cohort study found the biannual incidence of varicose veins was 3% in women and 2% in men.

The prevalence of varicose veins in Western populations was estimated in one study to be about 25% to 30% in women and 10% to 20% in men.

RISK FACTORS:
Gender: female
Genetics: family history of varicose veins
Increasing age
Multiple pregnancies

SYMPTOMS AND PHYSICAL FINDINGS

Leg complaints consistent with chronic venous disease include aching, heaviness, subjective swelling, cramps, itching, tingling, and pain. These symptoms can be exacerbated by menses, heat, and prolonged standing.

CLINICAL PRESENTATION

- Chronic vein disease is the result of the introduction of high pressures into a normal low-pressure superficial venous system.
- This increased pressure or venous hypertension causes superficial veins to distend to such a degree that vein valves fail to close, causing reflux and pooling of blood in surface veins.
- Manifested clinically by two syndromes:
  - Junctional: failure of the terminal valve at the intersection between the saphenous vein trunks and the deep system. If the great saphenous vein is involved, large varicose veins are found mainly above medial knee or calf. When the small saphenous vein is involved, large varicose veins are found in posterior knee or calf area. If the anterior accessory of great saphenous vein is involved, large varicose veins are found mainly in anterior or lateral thigh.
  - Perforator: failure of valves located in perforating vein. Large varicose veins are found most commonly in medial calf and proximal thigh region.

CLASSIFICATION

Chronic venous disease can now be classified using the Clinical-Etiology-Anatomy-Pathophysiology (CEAP) criteria to allow a precise description of the type of venous disease being discussed and provide an orderly framework for decision making (Table 1-499).

ETIOLOGY

- The underlying etiology of varicose veins remains uncertain.
- Important structural changes that occur: failure of vein valve function and vein wall dilation from fragmentation of the muscle layer.

COMPLICATIONS

- Superficial venous thrombophlebitis (SVT): a very common disorder with an incidence of 125,000 new cases per year in the U.S. The most frequent predisposing risk factors are varicose veins. The clinical findings include the presence of erythema, tenderness, and a palpable cord. Pain, increased warmth, and swelling are also present. Diagnosis is made by ultrasonography, which is useful to identify associated deep vein thrombosis that can occur in approximately 15% of patients. The location of the SVT determines the course of treatment; if the proximal great saphenous vein (GSV) is involved, a 1-mo course of low-molecular-weight heparin plus compression stockings has been found to be more effective than vein ligation. If SVT involves branch varicosities, treatment is usually symptomatic (control of pain).
- Bleeding is a more common complication than traditionally suspected. It is associated with thin-walled ectatic veins known as "blue blebs" that are found predominantly in the medial lower calf and ankle region. The best emergency treatment consists of pressure wrapping and not suture ligation, which results in delayed healing of the bleeding site. Sclerotherapy of these veins is the definitive treatment to prevent further bleeding.
- Dermal pathology of prolonged chronic venous disease (CEAP classes 4, 5, and 6).
  - Varicose eczema: see "Venous Ulcers" section.
  - Atrophie blanche: see "Venous Ulcers" section.
  - Lipodermosclerosis: see "Venous Ulcers" section.
  - Venous stasis ulcer: see "Venous Ulcers" section.

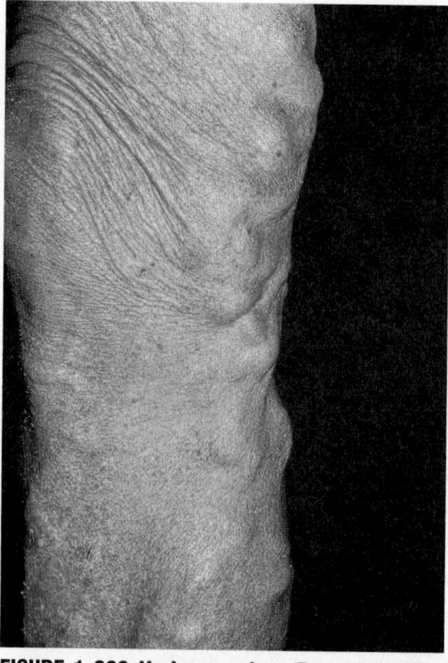

FIGURE 1-998 Varicose veins. (From White GM, Cox NH [eds]: *Diseases of the skin, a color atlas and text*, ed 2, St Louis, 2006, Mosby.)

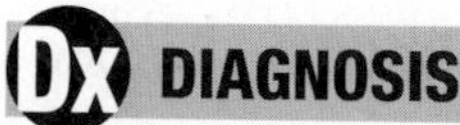

DIAGNOSIS

DIFFERENTIAL DIAGNOSIS

Other conditions that cause leg pain:
- Stress fracture
- Arthritis hip/knee joint
- Gout
- Degenerative disk disease of lower back
- Intermittent claudication secondary to peripheral arterial disease (PAD)
- Medications such as allopurinol and statins

TABLE 1-499 CEAP Classification of Chronic Venous Disease

C: Clinical
C_0: no visible or palpable signs of venous disease C_1: telangiectasias or reticular veins C_2: varicose veins C_3: edema C_4: pigmentation or eczema C_5: healed venous ulcer C_6: active venous ulcer
E: Etiology
c: congenital p: primary s: secondary or post thrombotic n: no venous cause identified
A: Anatomy
s: superficial veins p: perforator veins d: deep veins n: no venous location identified
P: Pathophysiology
r: reflux o: obstruction r,o: reflux and obstruction n: no venous pathophysiology identified

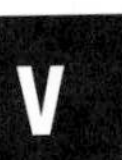

Other conditions that cause leg swelling:
- Cellulitis
- Soft tissue injury to leg/ankle/foot
- Obesity
- Diabetes
- Advancing age
- Medications such as calcium channel blockers, steroids, MAO inhibitors, and tricyclics

WORKUP

The diagnosis of chronic venous disorders is predominantly clinical. Initial evaluation consists of a thorough history and physical exam with classification of disease according to the CEAP criteria.

LABORATORY TESTS

Laboratory tests are not useful in patients with varicose veins.

IMAGING STUDIES

Duplex ultrasonography:
- Gold-standard imaging modality for the diagnosis, prognostic evaluation, pretreatment mapping, and posttreatment assessment of therapeutic intervention.
- Duplex ultrasound is used to identify and quantify points of valvular reflux within the superficial venous system.
- Assessment of valvular reflux is done with patient in the upright position, which physiologically approximates the condition in which valvular reflux occurs.
- Reverse flow of greater than 0.5 sec after distal compression is considered abnormal.

Other tests:
- Air plethysmography: may be useful in patients who have reflux in both superficial and deep venous systems or in patients with an unusual presentation of leg pain.
- Venography: has been largely replaced by duplex ultrasonography but still retains a critical role in the evaluation of chronic venous insufficiency prior to venous reconstruction.

Rx TREATMENT

CONSERVATIVE THERAPY:
- Aerobic exercise regularly for 30 min a day.
- Elevate legs above heart level to reduce swelling.
- Flex ankles frequently at work and during air travel or long car travel.
- Maintain proper weight.
- Graduated compression stockings (below knee) to alleviate symptoms in patients who are not candidates or do not desire to undergo treatment of their varicose veins.

SCLEROTHERAPY:
- Small- to medium-sized varicose veins such as spider veins and reticular varices in the absence of reflux in saphenous trunks are best treated with liquid sclerotherapy.
- The three principal sclerosants used in the U.S. are hypertonic saline, sodium tetradecylsulfate, and the newly FDA-approved solution, polidocanol.
- These agents are injected into vessels using 27-gauge or 30-gauge needles at concentrations of 23.4%, 0.1%, or 0.5%, respectively, causing injury to the endothelium with the resultant disappearance of the vein over period of time (usually 8 to 12 wk).

AMBULATORY PHLEBECTOMY:
- A procedure in which large varicose vein branches are removed with special hook instruments through a small puncture—incisions are made with an 18-gauge needle or No. 11 blade
- Performed safely under local anesthesia in an office setting and offers excellent cosmetic results and relief of symptoms:
- Most commonly performed in conjunction with endovenous ablation procedures

ENDOVENOUS ABLATION:
- Ablation of diseased saphenous vein trunks, large incompetent tributaries, or perforating veins can be achieved by using:
  - Radiofrequency energy
  - Laser energy
  - Ultrasound-guided foam sclerotherapy.
- The first two accomplish thermal injury to the vein in situ via an intraluminal catheter or bare-tipped laser wire. Chemical ablation uses a solution (polidocanol or sodium tetradecylsulfate) that is injected directly into the vein in the form of foam.
- Endovenous ablation can be performed in an office setting using local anesthesia. Patients can return to their normal daily activities immediately.
- The efficacy of these endovenous ablation procedures has been borne out by numerous published reports with occlusion rates over 95% and reflux free rates over 5-yr follow-up of 86%.

DISPOSITION

- It is important that the physician educate the patient to understand that varicose veins are a chronic and progressive disease.
- Any treatment is at best palliative, as patients in time will develop varicose veins in other areas.

REFERRAL

To either a phlebologist, preferably board certified by the newly created American Board of Phlebology, or a residency-trained vascular surgeon

SUGGESTED READINGS

available at www.expertconsult.com

RELATED CONTENT

Varicose Veins (Patient Information)

AUTHOR: **FRANK G. FORT, M.D., F.A.C.S., R.P.H.S**

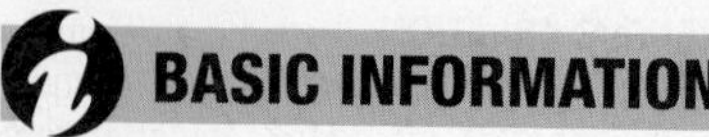

DEFINITION

Vasculitis refers generically to inflammation occurring within the walls of blood vessels. Blood vessel inflammation can result in either perforation of affected vessels with hemorrhage into adjacent structures or thrombosis with subsequent ischemia and infarction of supplied tissues. Vasculitis can occur as a primary process or secondary to another connective tissue disease, infection, or drug exposure. The systemic vasculitides are a heterogeneous group of disorders (Table E1-500). characterized by blood vessel inflammation affecting vessels of varying size and location resulting in a wide range of clinical manifestations dictated largely by which vessels are affected (Fig. E1-999). They are traditionally classified according to the size of the blood vessels predominantly affected (Table 1-501). Several of these are covered in individual chapters including chapters on granulomatosis with polyangiitis (GPA), polyarteritis nodosa (PAN), giant cell arteritis (GCA), Takayasu's arteritis, and Henoch-Schönlein purpura (HSP). Severity varies between and within specific vasculitides from a relatively benign, self-limited process to severe, life-threatening multisystem organ involvement with significant morbidity and mortality.

TABLE 1-501 Classification Scheme of Vasculitides According to Size of Predominant Blood Vessels Involved

Primary vasculitides
Predominantly large vessel vasculitides
Takayasu's arteritis
Giant cell arteritis (temporal arteritis)
Cogan's syndrome
Behçet's disease*
Predominantly medium-sized vessel vasculitides
Polyarteritis nodosa
Cutaneous polyarteritis nodosa
Buerger's disease
Kawasaki disease
Primary angiitis of the central nervous system
Predominantly small vessel vasculitides
Immune complex mediated
Goodpasture's disease (anti–glomerular basement membrane disease)†
  Cutaneous leukocytoclastic angiitis ("hypersensitivity vasculitis")
  Henoch-Schönlein purpura
  Hypocomplementemic urticarial vasculitis
  Essential cryoglobulinemia‡
  Erythema elevatum diutinum
ANCA-associated disorders§
  Wegener's granulomatosis‡
  Microscopic polyangiitis‡
  Churg-Strauss syndrome‡
  Renal-limited vasculitis
Secondary forms of vasculitis
Miscellaneous small vessel vasculitides
Connective tissue disorders‡ (rheumatoid vasculitis, lupus erythematosus, Sjögren's syndrome, inflammatory myopathies)
Inflammatory bowel disease
Paraneoplastic
Infection
Drug-induced vasculitis: ANCA-associated, other

*May involve small, medium-sized, and large blood vessels.
†Immune complexes formed in situ, in contrast to other forms of immune complex–mediated vasculitis.
‡Frequent overlap of small and medium-sized blood vessel involvement.
§Not all forms of these disorders are always associated with ANCA.
ANCA, Antineutrophil cytoplasmic antibody.
From Firestein G et al: *Kelley's textbook of rheumatology,* ed 8, Philadelphia, 2008, Saunders.

SYNONYMS

None

ICD-9CM CODES
446.0 Polyarteritis nodosa
446.1 Kawasaki disease
446.4 Wegener's granulomatosis, Churg-Strauss syndrome
446.5 Giant cell arteritis
446.7 Takayasu's arteritis
ICD-10CM CODES
M30.0 Polyarteritis nodosa
M30.3 Mucocutaneous lymph node syndrome [Kawasaki]
M31.30 Wegener's granulomatosis without renal involvement
M31.6 Other giant cell arteritis
M31.4 Aortic arch syndrome [Takayasu]

EPIDEMIOLOGY & DEMOGRAPHICS

- The epidemiology and demographics of the various vasculitides vary by the individual disease and where applicable are covered under the relevant disease chapters.
- The most common form of systemic vasculitis in the United States is giant cell arteritis, with an approximate incidence of 170 cases per 1 million per year in individuals older than 50 years.
- Antineutrophil cytoplasmic antibodies (ANCA)-associated vasculitis is significantly less common with aggregate incidence estimated at approximately 20 per million in the U.S.
- Age distribution can demonstrate significant variability between the vasculitides as demonstrated by the fact that GCA generally does not occur before age 50, while 90% of cases of HSP occur in the pediatric population and 80% of patients with Kawasaki disease are under age 5.
- While genetics clearly plays a role in disease susceptibility, familial cases of vasculitis are rare.

PHYSICAL FINDINGS & CLINICAL PRESENTATION

- Clinical presentation often includes nonspecific constitutional symptoms including fever, malaise, headache, and weight loss.
- Signs and symptoms are generally dictated by the tropism of involved vessels.
- Skin manifestations of vasculitis include petechiae, palpable purpura (Fig. 1-1000), subcutaneous nodules, livedo reticularis, ulcerations, and digital ischemia.
- Kidney involvement of medium-sized and large vessel vasculitis is often in the form of renovascular hypertension, as opposed to glomerulonephritis in small vessel vasculitis.
- Pulmonary small vessel involvement can cause alveolar hemorrhage, which can present with cough, dyspnea, and alveolar hemorrhage.
- Mononeuritis multiplex is the characteristic finding of vasculitis affecting the vasa nervorum of the peripheral nervous system.
- Gastrointestinal involvement of the mesenteric vasculature can cause postprandial pain, bleeding, and perforation.
- Arthritis, while nonspecific, can be present.
- Significant clinical variability exists between the various vasculitides, although overlapping symptoms may be seen.

ETIOLOGY

Most forms of systemic vasculitis are of unknown etiology. Cryoglobulinemic vasculitis is often secondary to hepatitis C infection, and cutaneous leukocytoclastic vasculitis can often be related to a drug exposure.

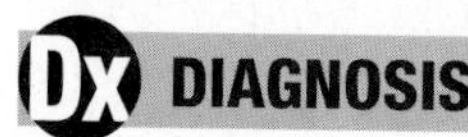

DIFFERENTIAL DIAGNOSIS

- Infective endocarditis
- Atrial myxoma
- Cholesterol emboli
- Malignancy

WORKUP

- The diagnosis of most forms of systemic vasculitis relies on the history and physical examination as well as supportive laboratory testing. Table 1-502 describes differential diagnostic features of selected forms of small vessel vasculitis.

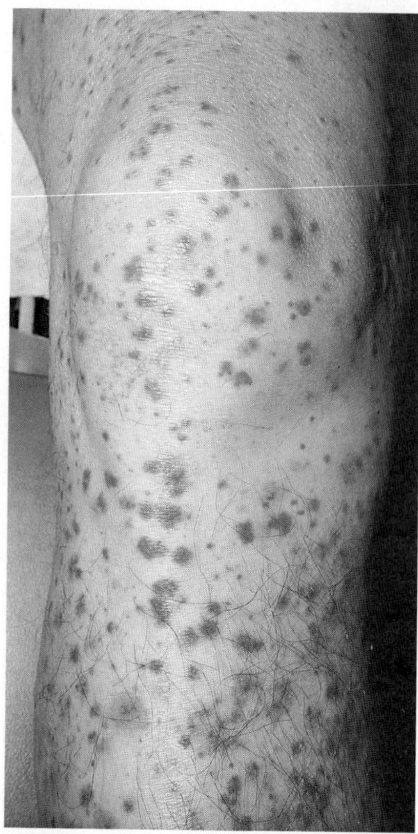

FIGURE 1-1000 Leukocytoclastic vasculitis, palpable purpura. (From James W et al: *Andrews' diseases of the skin, clinical dermatology,* ed 10, Philadelphia, 2005, Saunders.)

TABLE 1-502 Differential Diagnostic Features of Selected Forms of Small Vessel Vasculitis

Features	Microscopic Polyangiitis	Wegener's Granulomatosis	Churg-Strauss Syndrome	Henoch-Schönlein Purpura	Cryoglobulinemic Vasculitis
Vasculitic signs and symptoms	+	+	+	+	+
IgA-dominant immune deposits	–	–	–	+	–
Cryoglobulins in blood and vessels	–	–	–	–	–
Antineutrophil cytoplasmic antibodies in blood	+	+	+	–	–
Necrotizing granulomas	–	+	+	–	–
Asthma and eosinophils	–	–	+	–	–

From Floege J et al: *Comprehensive clinical nephrology*, ed 4, Philadelphia, 2010, Saunders.

- Tissue biopsy is important in establishing an accurate diagnosis; biopsy sites should target affected tissues.
- Imaging such as mesenteric angiography in the setting of PAN affecting the mesenteric vasculature can be supportive and can at times obviate the need for tissue biopsy.

LABORATORY TESTS

- Generic laboratory markers of systemic inflammation include an elevated erythrocyte sedimentation rate (ESR), C-reactive protein (CRP), and an anemia of chronic disease.
- ANCA targeting myeloperoxidase (MPO) and proteinase 3 (PR3) are frequently found in several small vessel vasculitides, including GPA (Wegener's), microscopic polyangiitis (MPA), and Churg-Strauss syndrome (CSS).
- Hepatitis C antibodies and rheumatoid factor are often present in cryoglobulinemic vasculitis.
- Urinalysis in patients with glomerulonephritis due to small vessel ANCA-associated vasculitis will generally demonstrate hematuria with an active urinary sediment with red blood cell casts and proteinuria without significant immune deposits (pauci-immune) on biopsy.

IMAGING STUDIES

- Angiography can demonstrate vascular narrowing and aneurysm formation in suspected medium-size and large vessel vasculitis.
- Pulmonary and sinus CT scans can demonstrate active pulmonary and upper airway disease in ANCA-associated vasculitis.

Rx TREATMENT

Treatment of vasculitis depends on the specific type of vasculitis and is tailored to the severity of disease activity.

ACUTE GENERAL Rx

- Systemic corticosteroids are generally required to gain initial control of active disease although mild cases of drug-induced cutaneous leukocytoclastic vasculitis can often be treated with NSAIDs and cessation of the offending medication.
- GCA, HSP, and vasculitis limited to the skin including cutaneous PAN can often be managed without further immunosuppression.
- Major organ-threatening disease in systemic vasculitis has traditionally been treated with oral or intravenous cyclophosphamide.
- Recent studies have demonstrated noninferiority of rituximab compared to cyclophosphamide in ANCA-associated vasculitis with major organ involvement.
- Less severe disease such as granulomatosis with polyangiitis (Wegener's) limited to the upper airways can be managed with methotrexate rather than cyclophosphamide.
- The goal of acute therapy is to induce remission of disease activity and is generally continued for 1 to 2 months once this is achieved, at which point chronic therapy is used to prevent disease relapse.

CHRONIC Rx

- The goal of chronic therapy is to prevent disease relapse and minimize medication side effects.
- Steroids are gradually tapered as allowed by disease activity.
- Immunomodulatory agents such as methotrexate or azathioprine are used for maintenance therapy in place of cyclophosphamide to reduce side effects.
- Cryoglobulinemic vasculitis due to chronic hepatitis C will often improve with treatment of the underlying viral infection.
- The role and dosing of rituximab for maintenance therapy following remission induction are not yet established.

DISPOSITION

Varies widely among the various vasculitides

REFERRAL

Systemic vasculitis care is generally coordinated by a rheumatologist. Renal, pulmonary, neurologic, and gastrointestinal consultation is often needed when vasculitis involves these organ systems. Isolated cutaneous leukocytoclastic vasculitis is often managed by dermatology.

SUGGESTED READINGS

available at www.expertconsult.com

RELATED CONTENT

Churg-Strauss Syndrome (Related Key Topic)
Cogan's Syndrome (Related Key Topic)
Giant Cell Arteritis (Related Key Topic)
Henoch-Schönlein Purpura (Related Key Topic)
Kawasaki Disease (Related Key Topic)
Takayasu's Arteritis (Related Key Topic)
Granulomatosis with Polyangiitis (Related Key Topic)
Polyarteritis Nodosa (Related Key Topic)

AUTHOR: **HARALD A. HALL, M.D.**

BASIC INFORMATION

DEFINITION

The spectrum of chronic venous disease (CVD) ranges from varicose veins to leg edema and skin manifestations consisting of hyperpigmentation, eczema, lipodermatosclerosis, and venous ulcer. These latter venous specific skin changes constitute an advanced form of CVD known as chronic venous insufficiency (CVI).

SYNONYMS

Stasis dermatitis
Post-thrombotic syndrome (PTS)

ICD-9CM CODES
454.1 Varicose veins of lower extremities with inflammation
ICD-10CM CODES
I87.2 Venous insufficiency (chronic) (peripheral)
I87.8 Other specified disorders of veins
I87.9 Disorder of vein, unspecified
I83.10 Varicose veins of unspecified lower extremity with inflammation

EPIDEMIOLOGY & DEMOGRAPHICS

- From 10% to 35% of adults in the U.S. have some form of CVI.
- Venous ulcers are the complication of CVI that results in the greatest morbidity and affects 4% of people over the age of 65
- The population-based costs to the U.S. government for CVI treatment and venous ulcer care have been estimated at >$1 billion a year.
- In addition, 4.6 million workdays per year are lost to chronic venous-related diseases.

PHYSICAL FINDINGS & CLINICAL PRESENTATION

The spectrum of cutaneous changes of CVI in the affected leg include:

- Varicose eczema: the most common and earliest sign, this involves the skin above the medial ankle and consists of pruritic, red, and scaly eczematous patches and plaques (Fig. 1-1001).
- Hyperpigmentation: caused by the breakdown of red blood cells and leads to hemosiderin deposition and dark staining of the skin (Fig. 1-1002).
- Atrophie blanche: usually presents as hypopigmented white patches with focal red punctate dots or telangiectasia surrounded by hyperpigmentation. Skin in this condition is avascular and prone to ulceration (Fig. 1-1003).
- Lipodermatosclerosis: a chronic, brawny induration of the skin and underlying fat that usually involves the skin from medial malleolus up to the lower border of the calf. Progression of the disease leads to an "inverted champagne bottle" appearance. The induration and lack of perfusion of the skin in this area make it susceptible to ulcer formation (Fig. 1-1004).

ETIOLOGY

- CVI occurs as a result of sustained venous hypertension in the leg, which can be caused by the following:
  1. Primary: vein valve failure with reflux in the superficial venous system or perforating veins (most common cause of CVI)
  2. Secondary: post-thrombotic syndrome in which a deep vein thrombosis causes outflow obstruction or
  3. Combination of the two above processes
- This sustained elevation in venous pressure or venous hypertension results in pathologic effects in the skin and subcutaneous tissues such as edema, eczema, hyperpigmentation, fibrosis, and ultimately venous ulceration.

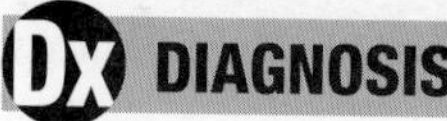

DIAGNOSIS

The diagnosis and evaluation of CVI are directed primarily by a detailed history and physical examination.

DIFFERENTIAL DIAGNOSIS

- Contact dermatitis
- Atopic dermatitis
- Cellulitis
- Dermatophyte infection
- Pretibial myxedema
- Nummular eczema
- Xerosis
- Asteatotic eczema

WORKUP

The primary goal is to identify the cause of sustained venous hypertension.

LABORATORY TESTS

Generally not indicated

IMAGING STUDIES

- Evaluation of the patient is performed in the standing position with duplex ultrasonography to identify reflux in the superficial, deep,

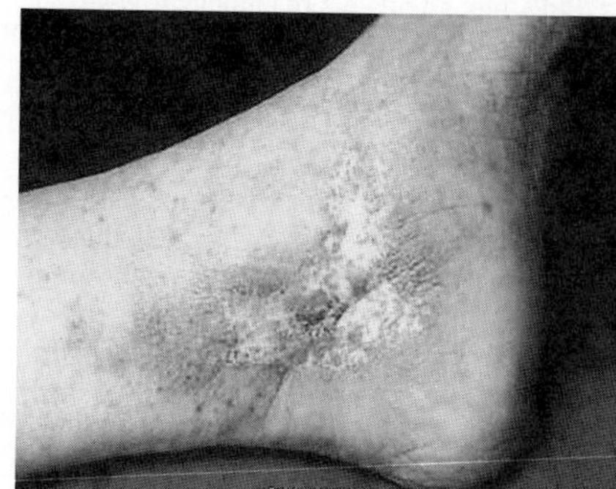

FIGURE 1-1003 Atrophie blanche.

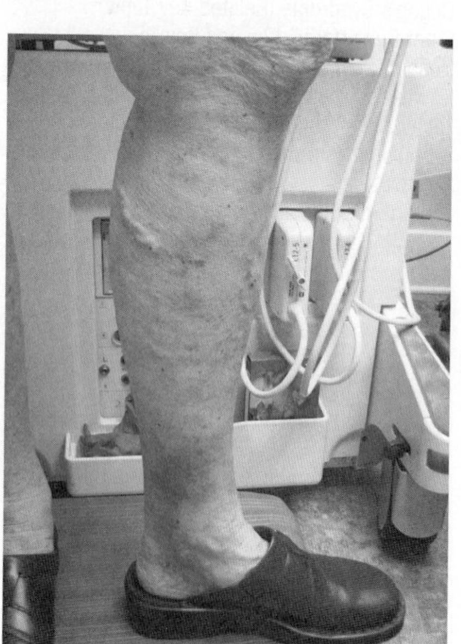

FIGURE 1-1001 Varicose eczema.

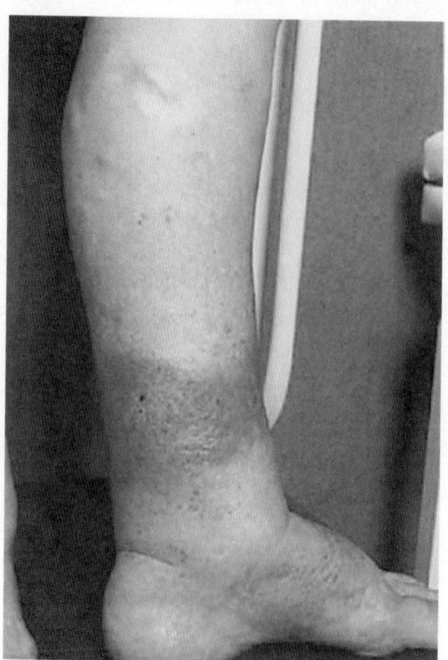

FIGURE 1-1002 Hyperpigmentation.

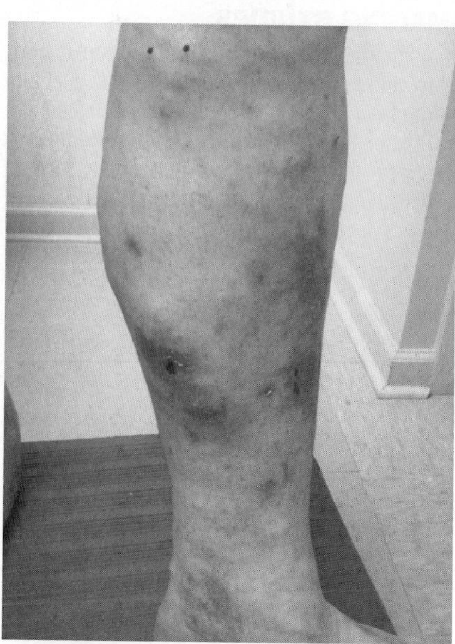

FIGURE 1-1004 Lipodermosclerosis.

and perforating veins as well as obstruction of the deep veins.
- No exam of a leg with CVI is complete without palpation of pulses and/or determination of ankle-brachial index (ABI).

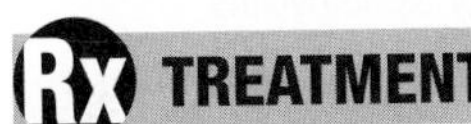

TREATMENT

NONPHARMACOLOGIC THERAPY

- Leg elevation above heart level for 30 min 3 to 4 times a day
- Weight reduction because obesity is a risk factor for DVT and CVI
- Walking exercises to improve calf function
- Physical therapy to improve ankle joint mobility
- For weeping skin lesions, wet-to-dry dressing changes

ACUTE GENERAL Rx

- The fundamental role of compression in the treatment of CVI is well recognized and has been validated by randomized controlled trials (RCTs).
- The beneficial effects of gradient compression stockings (decrease in edema and control of discomfort) are due to their effect on microvascular hemodynamics and Starling forces.
- Below-knee compression stocking with a gradient of at least 20 to 30 mm Hg will control edema, alleviate pain, and improve the quality of life in CVI patients.
- Compression stockings are contraindicated in patients with an ABI of <0.6.
- Some patients (acute lipodermatosclerosis) may benefit from nonelastic compression with the Unna gel paste gauze boot to alleviate their symptoms and acute increase in their swelling. The Unna boot is changed once a week.
- Topical corticosteroid creams or ointments (e.g., triamcinolone 0.12% bid) may be used to help reduce inflammation and itching. Steroids should never be applied to ulcer.
- Antibiotics should only be used when treating a clinically apparent, culture-proved infection. Most secondary infections are the result of *Staphylococcus* or *Streptococcus* organisms.
- Diuretics have no role in the treatment of CVI-related edema.

CHRONIC Rx

- While conservative care is fundamental, patients with CVI should be considered for correction of their underlying venous hypertension.
- The majority of patients with CVI have superficial vein or perforator vein reflux as their underlying pathology and would benefit from the newer vein ablation procedures listed below.
  - Endovenous ablation of superficial (saphenous) or perforator vein reflux
  - RF ablation with VNUS closure
  - Endovenous laser therapy (EVLT)
  - Ultrasound-guided foam sclerotherapy

COMPLEMENTARY & ALTERNATIVE MEDICINE

Several groups of drugs have been evaluated in the treatment of CVI, including coumarins, flavinoids, and saponosides (horse chestnut extracts). These drugs have venoactive properties and are widely used in Europe but are not approved for use in the U.S. The precise mechanism of action is not known. Horse chestnut seed extract has been found, in the short term, to be as effective as compression stockings in reducing pain and edema, but long-term efficacy has not been established.

REFERRAL

- Phlebology
- Vascular surgery
- Indications for referral
  - Skin and subcutaneous changes consistent with CVI
  - Associated peripheral arterial insufficiency (PAD)
  - Longstanding varicose vein disease
  - Consideration for vein ablation procedure

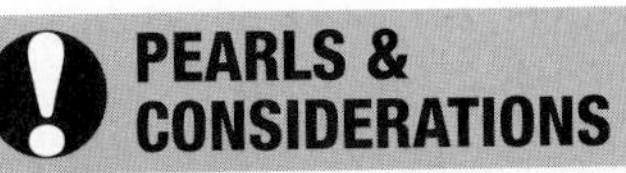

PEARLS & CONSIDERATIONS

COMMENTS

- Inflammatory skin changes from CVI are irreversible. The goal of therapy is to eliminate venous hypertension and prevent progression.
- Venous ulcers are often an end-stage manifestation of CVI. Refer to section on "Venous Ulcers" for more information.

SUGGESTED READINGS

available at www.expertconsult.com

RELATED CONTENT

Stasis Dermatitis (Patient Information)

AUTHOR: **FRANK G. FORT, M.D., F.A.C.S., R.PH.S.**

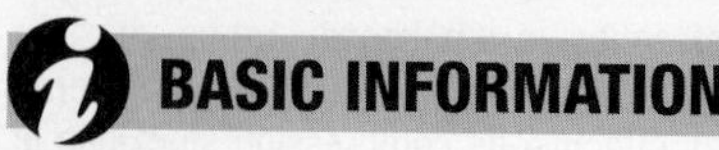

BASIC INFORMATION

DEFINITION

Venous ulcers are defined as chronic defects of the skin that fail to heal spontaneously and persist for longer than 4 weeks. Venous ulcers account for about 70% of all lower extremity ulcerations. They are usually located in the "gaiter" region and can be accompanied by varicose veins, edema, hyperpigmentation, and lipodermatosclerosis. Venous ulceration develops in patients as a result of sustained venous hypertension.

SYNONYMS

Stasis ulcers

ICD-9CM CODES

459.81 Peripheral venous insufficiency
707.1 Ulcer of the lower limb (calf: 2, ankle: 3)

ICD-10CM CODES

I87.2 Venous insufficiency (chronic) (peripheral)
L97.909 Non-pressure chronic ulcer of unspecified part of unspecified lower leg with unspecified severity

EPIDEMIOLOGY & DEMOGRAPHICS

In industrialized nations, up to 1.5% of the population will suffer from venous ulcers. In patients ≥65 yr old, the incidence increases to 4%. In the U.S., more than 500,000 people suffer from stasis ulcers.

RISK FACTORS

- Obesity
- Increasing age
- Family history of chronic venous insufficiency
- History of deep venous thromboembolism

PHYSICAL FINDINGS & CLINICAL PRESENTATION

Venous ulcers are most commonly located in the lower leg just above the ankle (gaiter region). They are a partial-thickness, irregularly shaped wound with well-defined borders with granulation tissue and fibrin present in the ulcer base (Fig. 1-1005). Venous ulcers are relatively painless and are surrounded by brown-stained skin and/or dry, itchy, and reddened skin. In about 50% of patients, there are visible varicose veins in an aching, swollen leg.

ETIOLOGY

The exact mechanism of the role of venous hypertension in the etiology of venous ulcers is not certain. Hemodynamic forces such as venous hypertension, circulatory stasis, and modified conditions of shear stress appear to play an important role in an inflammatory reaction accompanied by leukocyte activation that clinically leads to fibrosclerotic remodeling of the skin and then to ulceration.

Dx DIAGNOSIS

DIFFERENTIAL DIAGNOSIS

- Arterial ulcer
- Neurotrophic ulcers (located predominantly in the foot)
- Vasculitis
- Pyoderma gangrenosum
- Ulcerated skin tumors like basal cell or squamous cell carcinoma (Marjolin's ulcer)
- Rheumatoid arthritis

WORKUP

- The history and clinical signs and symptoms of leg ulcers are often misleading and may not differentiate venous ulcers from other leg ulcers; about 30% of leg ulcers are not of venous origin.
- Measurement of the ankle-brachial index (ABI) is essential in excluding peripheral arterial disease (PAD), which can be present in 20% of patients and is required before starting compression therapy. Arterial insufficiency is suggested by an ABI <0.9.
- Patients with lower-extremity ulcers should also be evaluated for diabetes.
- Coagulation defects have been found in 40% of patients with leg ulcers. This finding suggests that many patients with leg ulcers have a known or suspected history of deep venous thrombosis and a thrombophilia workup is indicated.
- If vasculitis is suspected, a biopsy of the edge of the ulcer can confirm the diagnosis.
- Any wound that has failed to improve after therapy of 4 wk should have a biopsy to rule out malignancy.

IMAGING STUDIES

- Evaluation of patients with venous leg ulcer should include duplex sonography to identify reflux in the superficial, deep, and perforating veins as well as possible obstruction of the deep veins.
- If the ulcer appears to be infected, consider tissue for culture, plain x-ray films, and bone scan to evaluate for osteomyelitis.

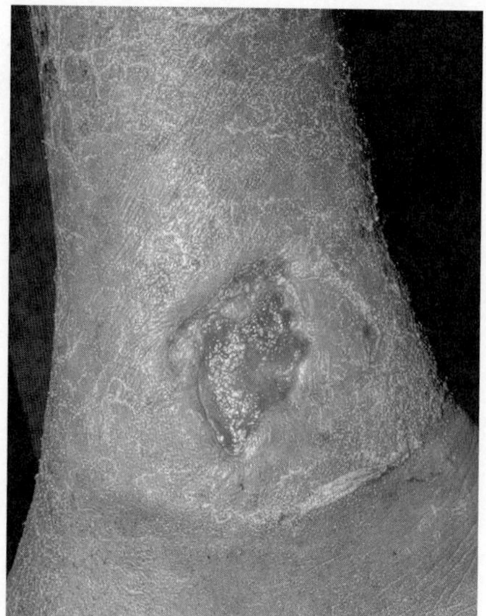

FIGURE 1-1005 Stasis ulcer. Any ulcer in this location with surrounding edema, redness, and scale is typical of a stasis ulcer. (From White GM, Cox NH [eds]: *Diseases of the skin, a color atlas and text,* ed 2, St Louis, 2006, Mosby.)

Rx TREATMENT

NONPHARMACOLOGIC THERAPY

- Surgical debridement to remove all nonviable material can be accomplished in the office setting with the use of a topical Xylocaine gel. Debridement produces the release of growth factors that allow the development of healthy granulation tissue and the initiation of the healing process.
- The first-line treatment of ulcers includes below-knee compression stockings to improve venous return to the heart, thereby decreasing edema, inflammation, and tissue ischemia (used only if the ABI is between 0.6 and 0.85 because compression can cause limb ischemia).
- There is Level A evidence that graduated compression stockings alone can lead to healing of a venous ulcer. The stockings should be worn during the day and removed at night.
- Regular, brisk walking 30 min a day, five times a week is recommended.
- Elevate leg above heart level and raise the foot of bed with 3-in blocks to reduce edema.
- Role of surgery: in a randomized controlled trial, endovenous catheter ablation of superficial reflux showed no improvement in the healing rate of ulcers but did demonstrate a reduction of ulcer recurrence from 28% to 12% at 12 mo.

ACUTE GENERAL Rx

- Dressings are used under compression stockings to provide a clean, moist environment to promote healing.
- Modern, more complex dressings have been developed and include occlusive and semi-occlusive dressings, classified according to their physical composition and ability to control wound drainage.
- Semiocclusive dressings have varying ability to absorb wound drainage. Some examples of this type are hydrocolloids (DuoDerm), hydrogels (Duoderm hydrogel), foam dressings (Allevyn), and alginates.
- Biologic wound dressings (Apligraf) and tissue-engineered products (Oasis) have been developed, and these products can either directly provide growth factors or indirectly stimulate growth factors in the ulcer bed.
- Pentoxifylline (800 mg tid) has been shown to be an effective adjuvant to compression therapy as reported in a meta-analysis of nine clinical trials.
- Skin grafting should be considered for large or refractory ulcers as long as the wound is clean and there is healthy granulation tissue.

- Published randomized clinical trials on the value of the different types of dressings in the management of leg ulcers have not shown effects on ulcer healing. Despite the lack of evidence to support their use, modern dressings remain a part of the standard of care. Decisions regarding their use should be based on local cost of the dressings and the physician's clinical experience.
- Trials involving the use of weekly, low-dose, high-frequency ultrasound for hard-to-heal venous leg ulcers do not support adding therapeutic ultrasound to standard care for venous leg ulcers.

DISPOSITION

The overall prognosis for this condition is poor; the healing rate depends on the initial size of the ulcer. Although 65% to 70% of venous ulcers are healed within 6 mo, the 5-yr recurrence rate of healed venous ulcers can be as high as 40%. Maintenance of lifelong compression therapy is recommended.

REFERRAL

All patients should be evaluated weekly during the first month of therapy. Nonhealing ulcers with little to no improvement should also be referred to a wound care clinic.

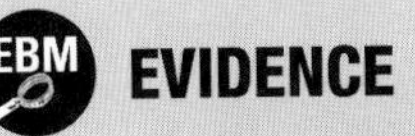

EVIDENCE

available at www.expertconsult.com

SUGGESTED READINGS

available at www.expertconsult.com

AUTHOR: **FRANK G. FORT, M.D., F.A.C.S., R.PH.S.**

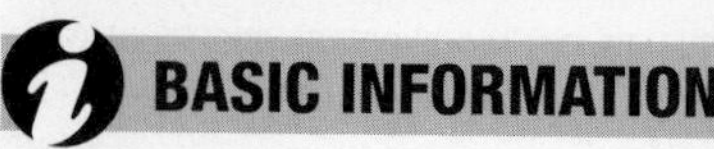

BASIC INFORMATION

DEFINITION

- *Ventricular septal defect* (VSD) refers to an abnormal communication through the septum that separates the right and left ventricles of the heart.
- VSDs may be large or small, single or multiple.
- VSDs are located at various anatomic regions of the septum and classified as follows:
  - Membranous (75% to 80%): This is the most common type of defect, and it extends into the membranous portion of the interventricular septum. The septal leaflet of the tricuspid valve may become adherent and form a "pouch" of the septum that can limit the left-to-right shunting and lead to self-closure.
  - Muscular or trabecular (5% to 20%): This defect is entirely surrounded by muscular tissue. Spontaneous closure is common.
  - Canal or inlet (8%): This defect commonly lies beneath the septal leaflet of the tricuspid valve; associated with Down syndrome.
  - Subarterial, outlet, infundibular, or supracristal (5% to 7%): This is the least common type of defect. It is usually found beneath the aortic valve, and it may lead to aortic regurgitation. High prevalence in Asian population.

SYNONYMS

VSD

ICD-9CM CODES
745.4 Ventricular septal defect
ICD-10 CODES
Q21.0 Ventricular septal defect

EPIDEMIOLOGY & DEMOGRAPHICS

- VSDs are one of the most common congenital heart abnormalities, accounting for 30% of all congenital cardiac defects.
- VSD accounts for ~25% of all congenital heart defects in children and for approximately 10% of defects in adults (the decrease is a result of spontaneous closure that occurs by adulthood).
- The prevalence of VSD is 3 to 3.5 infants per 1000 live births and 0.5/1000 adults.
- VSD is found with equal frequency among both males and females.
- VSD may be associated with the following conditions:
  - Atrial septal defect (35%)
  - Patent ductus arteriosus (22%)
  - Coarctation of the aorta (17%)
  - Subvalvular aortic stenosis (4%)
  - Subpulmonic stenosis, usually associated with progressive aortic regurgitation caused by prolapse of the aortic cusp through the defect
- Multiple VSDs are more prevalent among patients with tetralogy of Fallot and double-outlet right ventricular defects.

PHYSICAL FINDINGS & CLINICAL PRESENTATION

- Clinical presentation depends on the direction and volume of the VSD shunt, which is dictated by the size of the defect and the ratio of the pulmonary vascular resistance. Fig. 1-1006 illustrates the physiology of VSD.
  - Defects of ≤25% of the aortic annulus diameter are small defects. These typically involve small left-to-right shunts, no left ventricular volume overload, and no pulmonary artery hypertension (PAH).
  - Defects that are 25% to 75% of aortic annulus diameter are considered to be moderate in size. Small to moderate left-to-right shunting, mild to moderate left ventricular volume overload, and mild or no pulmonary artery hypertension are seen. Patients may have symptoms of congestive heart failure that may improve with medical therapy or with age as the defect decreases in size relative to increasing body size.
  - Defects of ≥75% of the aortic annulus diameter usually have moderate to large left-to-right shunting, left ventricular volume overload, and pulmonary artery hypertension. These patients usually have a history of congestive heart failure, or they may possibly develop right-to-left shunting in the setting of Eisenmenger's syndrome during late childhood, adolescence, or young adulthood.
- Infants may be asymptomatic at birth because of elevated pulmonary artery resistance. During the first few weeks of life, pulmonary arterial resistance decreases, thereby allowing for more left-to-right shunting through the VSD. This results in a subsequent increase in flow into the lungs, the left atrium, and the left ventricle, which can potentially cause left ventricular volume overload. Tachypnea, failure to thrive, and congestive heart failure may then ensue.
- In adults with VSD, the shunt is left to right in the absence of pulmonary stenosis and pulmonary hypertension. Patients typically manifest symptoms of left-sided heart failure from left ventricular volume overload (e.g., shortness of breath, orthopnea, dyspnea on exertion).
- A spectrum of physical findings may be seen, including the following:
  - Machinelike holosystolic murmur that is heard best along the left sternal border
  - Murmur becomes shorter as right heart pressures increase
  - Systolic thrill
  - Mid-diastolic rumble heard at the apex
  - S_3 heart sound
  - Rales
- With the development of pulmonary hypertension, the following occur:
  - An augmented pulmonic component of the S_2 heart sound
  - Cyanosis, clubbing, right ventricular heave, and signs of right heart failure (i.e., as seen with Eisenmenger's complex, with a reversal of the shunt in a right-to-left direction)

ETIOLOGY

- VSD is usually congenital but can be acquired.
- Acquired VSD may result from postsurgical residual leak, trauma, or myocardial infarction.
- Postinfarct ventricular septal defect (PIVSD) typically occurs 1 to 5 days after the event in 0.2% of patients in the current fibrinolytic, primary angioplasty era.

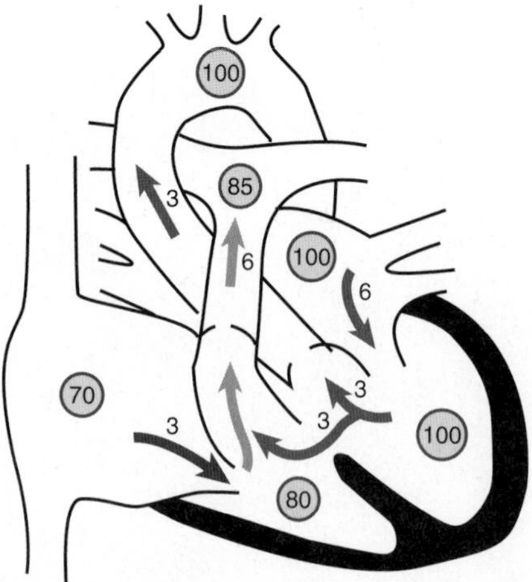

FIGURE 1-1006 Physiology of a large ventricular septal defect (VSD). Circled numbers represent oxygen saturation values. The numbers next to the arrows represent volumes of blood flow (in L/min/m²). This illustration shows a hypothetical patient with a pulmonary-to-systemic blood flow ratio (Qp:Qs) of 2:1. Desaturated blood enters the right atrium from the vena cava at a volume of 3 L/min/m² and flows across the tricuspid valve. An additional 3 L of blood shunts left to right across the VSD, the result being an increase in oxygen saturation in the right ventricle. Six liters of blood is ejected into the lungs. Pulmonary arterial saturation may be further increased because of incomplete mixing at right ventricular level. Six liters returns to the left atrium, crosses the mitral valve, and causes a mid-diastolic flow rumble. Three liters of this volume shunts left to right across the VSD, and 3 L is ejected into the ascending aorta (normal cardiac output). (From Kliegman RM et al: *Nelson textbook of pediatrics,* ed 19, Philadelphia, 2011, Saunders.)

Dx DIAGNOSIS

The diagnosis of VSD can be suspected during a physical examination. Imaging studies—particularly transthoracic echocardiography with color Doppler—establish the diagnosis.

DIFFERENTIAL DIAGNOSIS

On the basis of the physical examination alone, the diagnosis of VSD may be confused with other causes of systolic murmurs, such as mitral regurgitation, tricuspid regurgitation, aortic stenosis, pulmonary stenosis, and hypertrophic cardiomyopathy.

WORKUP

Any person who is suspected of having a VSD should undergo an ECG, a chest radiograph, and an echocardiogram.

LABORATORY TESTS

- Laboratory tests are not specific but may offer insight into the severity of the disease.
- The CBC may show polycythemia, especially in patients with Eisenmenger's complex.
- Arterial blood gas results may demonstrate hypoxemia.

IMAGING STUDIES

- ECG findings vary in accordance with the size of the VSD and depending on whether pulmonary hypertension is present. With large VSDs with pulmonary hypertension, right-axis deviation is seen, along with evidence of right ventricular hypertrophy.
- Chest x-ray findings in patients with VSD include the following:
  - Cardiomegaly that results from left ventricular volume overload that directly relates to the magnitude of the shunt
  - The enlargement of the proximal pulmonary arteries along with the redistribution and pruning of the distal pulmonary vessels as a result of sustained pulmonary hypertension (Fig. 1-1007, *A*)
- Echocardiography is the imaging modality of choice for the diagnosis of VSD:
  - Two-dimensional echocardiography and color Doppler display the size and location of the VSD (Fig. 1-1007, *B*), the chamber sizes, ventricular function, the presence of aortic valve prolapse or regurgitation, outflow tract obstruction, and the presence of tricuspid regurgitation.
  - Continuous-wave Doppler approximates the gradient between the left and right ventricles and estimates the pulmonary artery pressure.
  - The magnitude of the shunt can be determined by the calculation of the pulmonary-to-systemic flow ratio with the use of echocardiography.
- Heart catheterization is primarily indicated to assess operability of VSD patients with PAH, and in patients in whom the noninvasive testing was inconclusive, and further information, such as quantification of shunting and assessment of pulmonary pressures, is required.
- Ventriculography may help to locate the VSD:
  - MRI and computed tomography scanning can be useful to assess the pulmonary artery, the pulmonary vein, and the aortic anatomy and to confirm the anatomy of unusual VSDs (e.g., inlet or apical defects) that are not seen well with echocardiography.

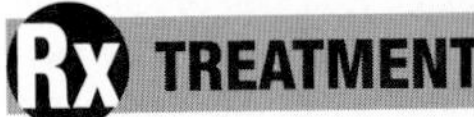

Rx TREATMENT

The decision to close a VSD depends on the type, size, and shunt severity as well as the patient's pulmonary vascular resistance, functional capacity, and associated valvular abnormalities.

NONPHARMACOLOGIC THERAPY

- Young children and adults with a small, asymptomatic VSD with a large left-to-right ventricular pressure gradient, a pulmonary-to-systemic blood flow ratio of less than 1.5:1, and no evidence of pulmonary hypertension can be observed (i.e., restrictive defect).
- Oxygen for hypoxemia and a low-salt diet are recommended for patients with congestive heart failure.

ACUTE GENERAL & CHRONIC Rx

Closure of the VSD is indicated for the following patients:

- Infants with congestive heart failure. Unrestrictive VSDs require surgical intervention within the first 2 yr of life to prevent pulmonary hypertension.

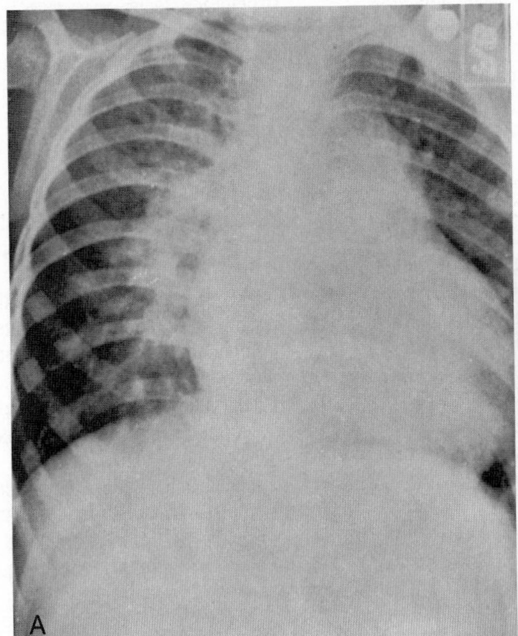

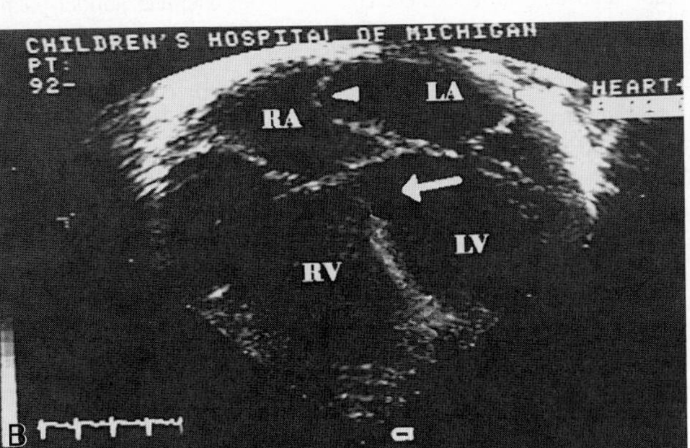

FIGURE 1-1007 A, Chest roentgenogram of a child with a large ventricular septal defect, large pulmonary blood flow, and pulmonary hypertension but only mild elevation of peripheral vascular resistance. This is reflected in the evidence of left and right ventricular enlargement, the enlargement of the main pulmonary artery, and a marked increase in pulmonary blood flow. **B,** Apical four-chamber echocardiographic view of ventricular septal defect *(large arrow)*. The small arrow points to the interatrial septum. *LA,* Left atrium; *LV,* left ventricle; *RA,* right atrium; *RV,* right ventricle. (**A** from Pacifico AD et al: Surgical treatment of ventricular septal defect. In Sabiston DC Jr, Spencer FC [eds]: *Surgery of the chest,* ed 5, Philadelphia, 1990, Saunders. **B** courtesy of Richard Humes, M.D., Children's Hospital of Michigan, Detroit.)

- Children between the ages of 1 and 6 yr with persistent VSD and a pulmonary-to-systemic blood flow ratio (Qp/Qs) of >2:1
- Adults with a Qp/Qs of ≥2 and clinical evidence of left ventricular volume overload (class I):
  - Positive history of infective endocarditis (IE) (class I)
  - Adults with a Qp/Qs of >1.5 with pulmonary artery pressure that is less than two thirds of the systemic pressure and pulmonary vascular resistance that is less than two thirds of the systemic vascular resistance (class IIa)
  - Adults with a Qp/Qs of >1.5 in the presence of left ventricular systolic or diastolic failure (class IIa)
  - Surgical closure is not indicated for VSD with severe irreversible PAH.

Surgical closure with Dacron or Gore-Tex patches or primary surgical closure has long been the gold standard of therapy. It has low operative mortality (<2%) at experienced centers. However, surgery still carries a small risk of complete heart block (CHB), postpericardiotomy syndrome, wound infection, and neurologic sequelae related to cardiopulmonary bypass. Over the last two decades, the transcatheter approach to VSD closure has improved considerably and is becoming an increasingly accepted modality of treatment for appropriately selected patients. Some studies have shown similar success rates for both surgical and percutaneous closures, and there are significantly fewer complications, days in the hospital, and blood transfusions after percutaneous closures.

Catheter-based closure in muscular VSD may be considered, especially if the VSD is remote from the tricuspid valve and the aorta, if the VSD is associated with severe left-sided heart chamber enlargement, or if there is PAH (class IIb). Device closure is indicated in residual defects after prior attempts at surgical closure, restrictive VSDs with either a significant left-to-right shunt (Qp/Qs >1.5:1) or hx of IE, trauma, or iatrogenic artifacts after surgical replacement of the aortic valve.

Surgery still remains the treatment of choice in patients with large defects, coexistent congenital anomalies requiring surgical correction, and defects with close proximity to the aortic valve. Sub-pulmonic VSDs may require surgery due to the increased risk of aortic valve prolapse. Perimembranous VSD with more than trivial aortic regurgitation should be referred to surgery. PIVSDs usually carry a high mortality rate, and surgical closure remains the gold standard in the acute setting or for large (>15 mm) septal ruptures. In the subacute or chronic setting, small or medium PIVSD (<15 mm) can be treated with percutaneous closure with comparable mortality to surgery. VSDs post myocardial infarction generally arise within 1 wk of the acute event. Surgical management within 10 d has better outcomes than waiting for cardiac stabilization.

DISPOSITION

- The natural history of an isolated VSD depends on the type of defect, its size, and any associated abnormalities.
- ~75% to 80% of small VSDs close spontaneously by the time the patient reaches the age of 10 yr.
- Only 10% to 15% of large VSDs will close spontaneously.
- Large VSDs that are left untreated may lead to arrhythmias, congestive heart failure, pulmonary hypertension, and Eisenmenger's complex.
- Eisenmenger's complex carries a poor prognosis, with most patients dying before the age of 40 yr.
- Issues to monitor in adults with unrepaired or repaired and catheter-closed VSDs include the following:
  - Development of aortic regurgitation
  - Assessment of associated coronary artery disease
  - Development of tricuspid regurgitation
  - Assessment of the degree of left-to-right shunting (in unrepaired or residual VSD after repair)
  - Ventricular dysfunction
  - Assessment of pulmonary pressure
  - Development of subpulmonary stenosis (usually as a result of a double-chambered right ventricle)
  - Development of discrete subaortic stenosis
  - Development of arrhythmia or heart block
  - Thromboembolic complications
  - Infective endocarditis
- After closure, late survival is excellent when ventricular function is normal. Pulmonary artery hypertension may improve, progress, or remain the same. Late operations may be required for tricuspid or aortic regurgitation.

REFERRAL

All infants and children diagnosed with VSD should be referred to a pediatric cardiologist. Adults with VSD should be referred to an adult cardiologist. Cardiothoracic surgeons who have experience with congenital heart disease surgery should be consulted if surgery is indicated.

FOLLOW-UP

- Adults with no residual VSD, no associated lesions, and normal pulmonary artery pressure do not require continued follow-up at a regional adult congenital heart disease (ACHD) center except on referral from the patient's cardiologist or physician.
- Adults with VSD with residual heart failure, shunts, PAH, AR, or RV outflow tract (RVOT) or LV outflow tract (LVOT) obstruction should be seen at least annually at an ACHD regional center (level of evidence: C).
- Adults with a small residual VSD and no other lesions should be seen every 3 to 5 yr at an ACHD regional center (level of evidence: C).
- Adults with device closure of a VSD should be followed up every 1 to 2 yr at an ACHD center depending on the location of the VSD and other factors.
- Patients who develop bifascicular block or transient trifascicular block after VSD closure are at risk in later years for the development of complete heart block and should be followed up yearly by history and ECG and have periodic ambulatory monitoring and/or exercise testing.

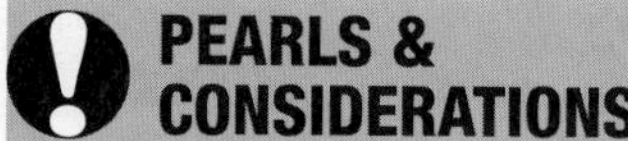

PEARLS & CONSIDERATIONS

COMMENTS

- A loud murmur does not imply a large VSD. Small, hemodynamically insignificant VSDs can cause loud murmurs.
- In patients with Eisenmenger's complex, the right-to-left shunting across the VSD is usually not associated with an audible murmur.
- The risk of patients with unrepaired VSD developing infective endocarditis is 4%. The risk is higher if aortic insufficiency is present.
- For patients with endocarditis, routine antibiotic prophylaxis for dental or surgical procedures is no longer indicated for isolated VSDs, except in the following circumstances:
  - In the presence of complex congenital heart disease with cyanosis
  - In the presence of a residual VSD after surgical closure
  - During the first 6 mo after surgical patch or percutaneous transcatheter closure
- Any patient with a newly diagnosed murmur or hemodynamic compromise after a myocardial infarction should undergo evaluation for possible VSD.
- Pregnancy with a VSD is generally well tolerated in women with small VSDs, no pulmonary artery hypertension, and no associated lesions. Women with large shunts may experience arrhythmias, ventricular dysfunction, and the progression of pulmonary hypertension.
  - Maternal use of valproic acid and phenytoin has also been suggested to cause structural defects.
- Women with VSDs and severe pulmonary artery hypertension or Eisenmenger's physiology should be counseled against pregnancy because of associated excessive maternal and fetal mortality.
  - Small perimembranous VSDs (without left heart dilatation) and corrected VSDs have a good prognosis during pregnancy, when LV function is preserved. Prepregnancy evaluation of the presence of a (residual) defect, cardiac dimensions, and an estimation of pulmonary pressures is recommended. Pre-eclampsia may occur more often than in the normal population. Usually follow-up twice during pregnancy is sufficient, and spontaneous vaginal delivery is appropriate.
- Minimally invasive periventricular device closure of VSD without cardiopulmonary bypass under guidance of transesophageal echocardiography is a promising technique, but it needs long-term follow-up.

SUGGESTED READINGS

available at www.expertconsult.com

RELATED CONTENT

Ventricular Septal Defect (VSD) (Patient Information)

AUTHOR: **RABIA ARSHAD, M.D.**

BASIC INFORMATION

DEFINITION

Vertebral compression fractures (VCFs) are defined as fractures of spinal vertebrae in which a bony surface is driven toward another bony surface. These fractures are classified as radiographic reductions in vertebral body height of more than 15% to 20%.

SYNONYMS

Thoracolumbar vertebral compression fractures
Osteoporotic fractures

ICD-9CM CODES

805.8	Compression fracture, spine
805.4N	Compression fracture, lumbar vertebra
805.2	Compression fracture, thoracic vertebra
733.13	Pathologic vertebral compression fracture; vertebral collapse; collapse of vertebra

ICD-10 CODES

M80.0	Post-menopausal osteoporosis with pathologic fracture
M80.4	Drug-induced osteoporosis with pathological fracture
M80.5	Idiopathic osteoporosis with pathological fracture
M80.8	Other osteoporosis with pathological fracture
M80.9	Unspecified osteoporosis with pathological fracture
S32.009A	Unspecified fracture of unspecified lumbar vertebra, initial encounter for closed fracture
S22.009A	Unspecified fracture of unspecified thoracic vertebra, initial encounter for closed fracture

EPIDEMIOLOGY & DEMOGRAPHICS

~700,000 VCFs occur in the United States each year, and they affect up to 25% of postmenopausal women. The prevalence increases with age, reaching a peak of 40% to 50% among women aged >80 yr. Compression fractures are also a major concern among men, although their rates of VCF are lower.

RISK FACTORS:

- Modifiable: tobacco or alcohol use, osteoporosis, estrogen deficiency (i.e., early menopause, bilateral ovariectomy, premenopausal amenorrhea for >1 yr), frailty, impaired vision, abusive situations, inadequate physical activity, low body mass index, and dietary deficiency of vitamin D or calcium
- Nonmodifiable: advanced age, female gender, dementia, Caucasian, history of fractures in adulthood and among first-degree relatives, and falls

PHYSICAL FINDINGS & CLINICAL PRESENTATION

- Asymptomatic: Most VCFs are asymptomatic, except for height loss or kyphosis (i.e., dowager's hump [Fig. 1-1008]), which is often a sign of multiple VCFs and height loss of >6 cm has a sensitivity/specificity of 94% and 30%, respectively, for VCF.
- Symptomatic: When symptomatic, VCFs usually present as acute back pain after activity (e.g., bending, lifting) or coughing; neck strain and radicular rib pain may also be present.

ETIOLOGY

- VCFs take place when the combination of bending and the axial load on the spine exceed the strength of the vertebral body.
- The primary etiology of VCF is osteoporosis.

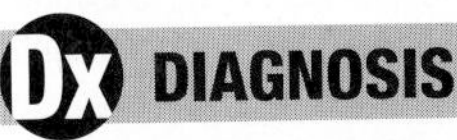

DIAGNOSIS

DIFFERENTIAL DIAGNOSIS

- Hyperparathyroidism
- Osteomalacia
- Granulomatous diseases (e.g., tuberculosis)
- Hematologic/oncologic diseases (e.g., multiple myeloma, malignancy)

WORKUP

- Only one third of VCFs are diagnosed. Guidelines for patient selection for vertebral fractural assessment are described in Box 1-101.
- VCF can be clinically suspected from the history and physical alone, though they are often diagnosed incidentally by imaging performed for another indication.
- There may or may not be a specific injury or a remembered event that led to the VCF.

LABORATORY TESTS

Tests to rule out infection or cancer may be helpful, such as a CBC, an erythrocyte sedimentation rate, an alkaline phosphatase level, and a C-reactive protein level; these tests can be reserved for individuals for whom there is clinical suspicion.

IMAGING STUDIES

- Plain frontal and lateral radiographs (x-rays) are the initial imaging method (Fig. 1-1008) and may be sufficient, particularly when no neurologic abnormalities are present. MRI and computed tomography (CT) scans may be uncomfortable or painful for the patient, especially during the acute phase.
- Although CT scans are not routinely necessary for the diagnosis, they can be helpful for visualizing fractures that are not seen on plain films, for evaluating the integrity of the posterior vertebral wall, for ruling out other causes of back pain, for detecting spinal canal narrowing, and for assessing instability.
- MRI may be useful when spinal cord compression is suspected, if neurologic symptoms are present, or to distinguish malignancy from osteoporosis (e.g., in patients <55 yr with VCF after minimal or no trauma).
- Bone density studies may be helpful to determine the severity of osteoporosis, which is a key risk factor for future fractures.

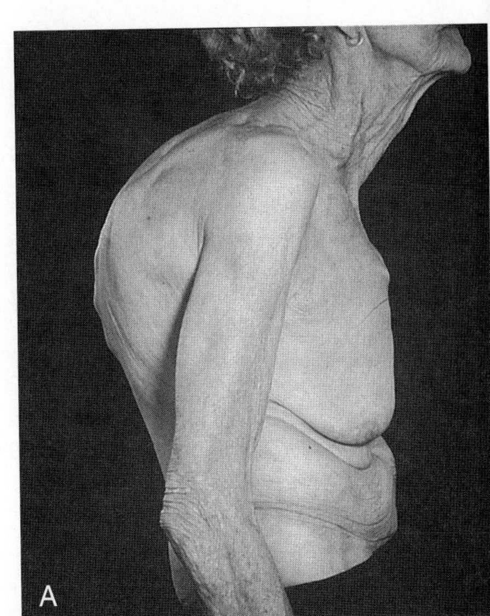

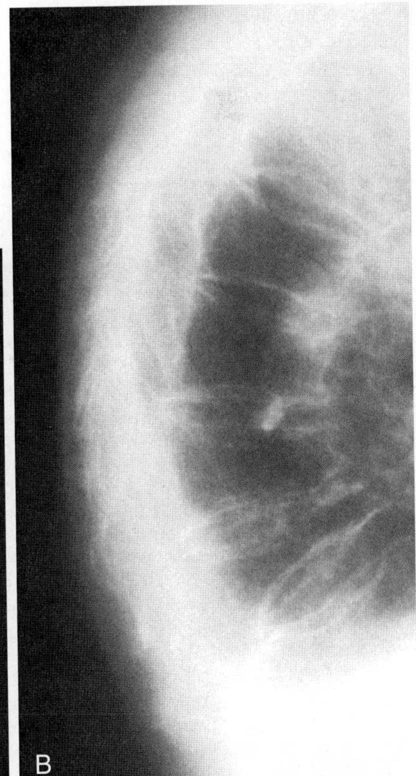

FIGURE 1-1008 Dowager's hump. A, Marked thoracic kyphosis due to multiple osteoporotic fractures in an elderly woman with corresponding radiograph (**B**). (From Hochberg MC et al [eds]: *Rheumatology,* ed 3, St Louis, 2003, Mosby.)

 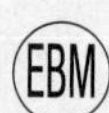

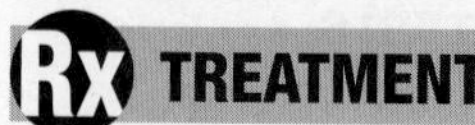

TREATMENT

NONPHARMACOLOGIC THERAPY

- Physical therapy
- External back braces
- Exercise programs: Getting the person active as soon as possible is extremely important for both short -and long-term recovery.

ACUTE GENERAL Rx

- Analgesics are first line for pain control, including acetaminophen and opioids (oral or parenteral), and pain can be expected to diminish over 4 to 6 wk.
- Nonsteroidal anti-inflammatory drugs are helpful but must be used with caution among elderly patients or when contraindicated.
- Muscle relaxants should be used judiciously because they have significant side effects, particularly in the elderly.
- Intranasal calcitonin (200 units once daily, alternating nostrils) has been shown in some small trials to hasten relief from pain when used as an adjunct to oral analgesics, and a 2- to 4-wk course may be useful for patients who do not achieve adequate control with oral analgesics alone.
- Early mobilization with physical therapy is important for recovery and prevention of subsequent fractures.
- The efficacy of vertebroplasty versus kyphoplasty versus conservative treatment remains controversial.
- Percutaneous vertebroplasty involves the injection of acrylic bone cement into the affected vertebral body in an effort to stabilize the fracture and reduce pain, whereas in kyphoplasty, a high-pressure inflatable bone tamp or balloon is expanded within the body of the affected vertebra to restore prefracture vertebral height before the injection of bone cement. These two procedures were thought to be helpful in patients who did not respond to conservative therapy; however, further studies showed them to be no more effective than sham procedures (Buchbinder et al., 2009; Kallmes et al., 2009). Nonetheless, Klazen et al. (2010) demonstrated in an open-label prospective randomized trial that for the subgroup of patients with acute osteoporotic VCFs fractures and persistent pain, percutaneous vertebroplasty may provide immediate pain relief, sustained for at least a year, which may be significantly greater than that achieved with conservative treatment. Zampiri (2011) showed in a nonrandomized cohort study that elderly patients who underwent kyphoplasty were more likely to be discharged home. McCullough et al. (2013) analyzed Medicare claims of patients with VCF treated with kyphoplasty or vertebroplasty compared with medical management and found no difference in mortality or major medical outcomes but decreased health care utilization in the conservatively managed group. These procedures are still in their infancy, and more answers should be forthcoming as to their efficacy, as well as questions regarding the amount of time that conservative therapy alone should be pursued and which procedure, if any, should be advised. Most current guidelines recommend 4 to 6 wk of medical therapy before pursuing surgical intervention in neurologically intact VCF.

CHRONIC Rx

Osteoporosis should be treated with the reduction of risk factors (e.g., smoking, alcohol), diet, exercise, calcium and vitamin D supplements, and with medications used to treat osteoporosis (e.g., bisphosphonates).

BOX 1-101 2007 ISCD Guidelines for Patient Selection for Vertebral Fractural Assessment

- Postmenopausal women with low bone mass (osteopenia) by BMD criteria, *plus* any one of the following: age >70 yr, historical height loss >4 cm (1.6 in), or prospective height loss >2 cm (0.8 in), self-reported vertebral fracture (not previously documented)
- Two or more of the following: age 60 to 69 yr, self-reported prior non-vertebral fracture, historical height loss of 2 to 4 cm, or chronic systemic diseases associated with increased risk of vertebral fractures (e.g., moderate to severe COPD or COAD, seropositive rheumatoid arthritis, Crohn's disease)
- Men with low bone mass (osteopenia) by BMD criteria, *plus* any one of the following: age >80 yr, historical height loss >6 cm (2.4 in), prospective height loss >3 cm (1.2 in), self-reported vertebral fracture (not previously documented)
- Two or more of the following: age 70 to 79 yr, self-reported prior non-vertebral fracture, historical height loss of 3 to 6 cm, on pharmacologic androgen deprivation therapy or following orchiectomy, chronic systemic diseases associated with increased risk of vertebral fractures (e.g., moderate to severe COPD or COAD, seropositive rheumatoid arthritis, Crohn's disease)
- Women or men on chronic glucocorticoid therapy (equivalent to 5 mg or more of prednisone daily for 3 mo or longer)
- Postmenopausal women or men with osteoporosis by BMD criteria, if documentation of one or more vertebral fractures will alter clinical management

BMD, Bone mineral density; *COAD,* chronic obstructive airways disease; *COPD,* chronic obstructive pulmonary disease; *ISCD,* International Society for Clinical Densitometry.

Reproduced with permission from the International Society for Clinical Densitometry.

From Hochberg MC et al: *Rheumatology,* ed 5, St Louis, 2011, Mosby.

REFERRAL

Referral is indicated for neurologic abnormalities, unremitting pain, instability, continued disability, or when the investigation of the cause of the fracture reveals serious underlying pathology.

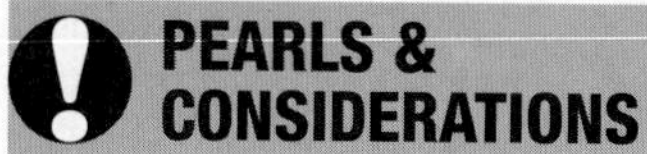

PEARLS & CONSIDERATIONS

Prevention of osteoporosis and conservative therapy remain the mainstays of treatment.

COMMENTS

- VCFs should be suspected in anyone aged >50 yr with the acute onset of low back pain. There are many opportunities for diagnosis and treatment that are easy to miss, especially for males.
- Solitary vertebral fractures higher than T7 are unusual and should raise suspicion for other pathologic causes.
- Diagnosing and treating osteoporosis reduce the incidence of VCFs.
- Getting people with VCF physically active as soon as possible will be efficacious both acutely and in the long term.
- In general, VCF will be best managed through a partnership of the patient, the primary care physician, an orthopedist, a physical therapist, a dietitian, and a social worker.

PREVENTION

Reducing the effects of modifiable risk factors is key.

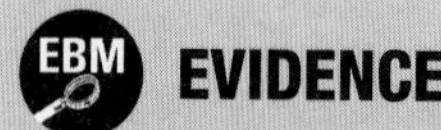

EVIDENCE

available at www.expertconsult.com

SUGGESTED READINGS

available at www.expertconsult.com

AUTHOR: **THOMAS J.T. ANDERSON, M.D.**

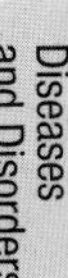

BASIC INFORMATION

DEFINITION

Vestibular neuronitis is a syndrome of sudden-onset dysfunction of the peripheral vestibular system, often severe, with prolonged vertigo, nausea, and vomiting.

SYNONYMS

Vestibular neuritis
Acute neuritis
Neurolabyrinthitis
Vestibular neuropathy

ICD-9CM CODES

078.81 Vestibular neuronitis
386.12 Neuronitis, vestibular

ICD-10 CODES

H81.2 Vestibular neuronitis
H81.8 Other disorders of vestibular function
H81.9 Disorder of vestibular function, unspecified
H81.23 Vestibular neuronitis, bilateral

EPIDEMIOLOGY & DEMOGRAPHICS

Vestibular neuritis is the second most common cause of peripheral vestibular vertigo with an incidence of about 3.5:100,000 population. Although etiology remains uncertain, thought to result from selective inflammation of the vestibular nerve, the etiology is presumed to be viral. Viral origin is supported by the fact that it occurs in epidemics, may affect several family members, and occurs more commonly in spring and early summer. The male-to-female ratio is nearly 1:1. There is selective damage to the superior part of the vestibular labyrinth, supplied by the superior vestibular portion of the eighth cranial nerve.

PHYSICAL FINDINGS & CLINICAL PRESENTATION

Course: develops, acutely, over period of hours and resolves over periods of days or weeks, although long-term sequelae may occur, such as residual imbalance and nonspecific dizziness persisting for months. Symptoms include vertigo, spontaneous peripheral nystagmus, positive head-thrust test, and imbalance. Patient reports intense sensation of rotation and difficulty standing and walking and tends to veer toward affected side; autonomic symptoms occur with pallor, sweating, nausea, and vomiting.

ETIOLOGY

Etiology remains uncertain. It is thought to be viral, or secondary to a post-viral inflammatory disorder, in origin, possibly due to herpes zoster, reactivation of herpes simplex, or other viruses, but evidence is circumstantial.

DIAGNOSIS

DIFFERENTIAL DIAGNOSIS

- Labyrinthitis: similar symptoms of vertigo, with the addition of unilateral hearing loss
- Labyrinthine infarction
- Acoustic neuroma
- Perilymph fistula
- Brain stem and cerebellar infarction
- Migraine-associated vertigo
- Meniere disease
- Multiple sclerosis

WORKUP

- Patient may fall toward affected side when attempting ambulation or during Romberg tests.
- Hallpike maneuver: checking for nystagmus and asking about recreation of vertigo symptoms
- Head-thrust test: grasp patient's head, apply brief small-amplitude rapid head turn, first to one side and then the other; patient fixates on examiner's nose: positive test is lack of corrective eye movements ("saccades") on affected side. A postive test supports the diagnosis of vestibular neuronitis.
- Laboratory testing and imaging are generally not indicated but may help rule out other etiologies

LABORATORY TESTS

- Electronystagmography (ENG): a battery of eye movement tests that may provide an objective assessment of the vestibular and oculomotor systems and may help localize the lesion's site
- Audiogram: normal

IMAGING STUDIES

Brain imaging: CT or MRI—normal

TREATMENT

NONPHARMACOLOGIC THERAPY

Vestibular exercises, when tolerated, will accelerate recovery.

ACUTE GENERAL Rx

Most treatments are empirical and related to symptoms. Further studies are needed.

- Corticosteroids: corticosteroids are often prescribed, although a recent Cochrane Review finds that there is insufficient evidence for administration. Some studies have shown that glucocorticoids administered within 3 days after onset of vestibular neuronitis may improve long-time recovery of vestibular function and reduce the length of hospital stay and may improve the caloric extent and recovery of canal paresis.
- Antihistamines: e.g., meclizine, dimenhydrinate, promethazine
- Anticholinergics: scopolamine
- Antiemetics: droperidol, prochlorperazine
- Benzodiazepines: e.g., diazepam, valium, lorazepam
- Valacyclovir, either alone or in combination, is likely ineffective in treating vestibular neuronitis.

CHRONIC Rx

- Vestibular rehabilitation exercises
- Anti-GABA agents
- Antihistamines

DISPOSITION

Most patients can be treated as outpatients, but inpatient care may be required in cases where vomiting is uncontrollable. If dehydrated because of severe vomiting, sufferers may require brief parenteral therapy.

REFERRAL

- ENT: if diagnosis uncertain, and if these patients are at risk for benign paroxysmal positional vertigo (BPPV) subsequently; also if symptoms linger
- Neurology: if question of central origin or migraine

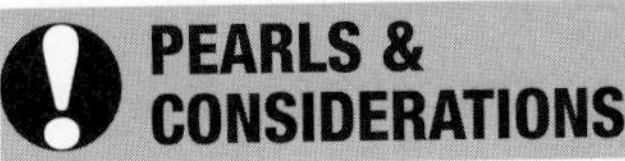

PEARLS & CONSIDERATIONS

COMMENTS

- Diagnosis unlikely to be vestibular neuronitis if hearing is impaired or other neurologic signs and symptoms are present.
- Although patients may recover from dramatic acute symptoms, subtle vestibular deficits may linger for prolonged period, if not indefinitely (i.e., residual imbalance and nonspecific dizziness).
- Program of vestibular habituation head movement exercises can reduce imbalance symptoms.

PATIENT & FAMILY EDUCATION

Vestibular Disorders Association: http://www.vestibular.org

SUGGESTED READINGS

available at www.expertconsult.com

AUTHOR: **ROCCO J. RICHARDS, M.D.**

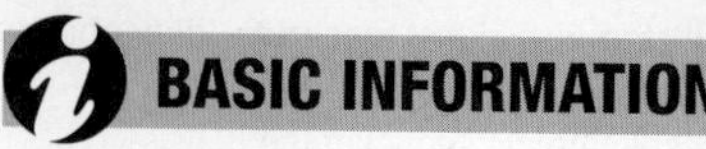

BASIC INFORMATION

DEFINITION

Vitamins are organic compounds that cannot be synthesized by humans but are required as nutrients in minute amounts. Vitamins have several different functions: They may regulate cell growth and differentiation, as catalysts, as antioxidants, and as co-enzymes. Vitamins are classified as either fat soluble (vitamins A, D, E, K) or water soluble (B group of vitamins and C). Deficiency of most vitamins is rare in Western countries. Certain groups may be prone to vitamin deficiency, and these are discussed here. Vitamin D deficiency is discussed in a separate topic.

SYNONYMS

Vitamin A: retinol
Vitamin E: alpha tocopherol
Vitamin K: phytonadione or menadiol
Vitamin B_1: thiamine
Vitamin B_2: riboflavin
Niacin: vitamin B_3; nicotinic acid
Vitamin B_5: pantothenic acid
Vitamin B_6: pyridoxine; pyridoxal phosphate
Folic acid: vitamin B_9; folate
Vitamin B_{12}: cyanocobalamin
Vitamin C: ascorbic acid

ICD-9CM CODES

264.8 Vitamin A deficiency
269.1 Vitamin E deficiency
260.0 Vitamin K deficiency
265.1 Vitamin B_1 deficiency
266.0 Vitamin B_2 deficiency
265.2 Niacin deficiency
266.1 Pyridoxine deficiency
266.2 Folic acid deficiency
266.2 Cyanocobalamin deficiency
267 Ascorbic acid deficiency

ICD-10CM CODES

E50 Vitamin A deficiency
E51 Thiamine deficiency
E53 Deficiency of other B group vitamins
E55 Vitamin D deficiency
E56 Other vitamin deficiencies
E56.0 Deficiency of vitamin E
E56.1 Deficiency of vitamin K
E53.0 Riboflavin deficiency
E52 Niacin deficiency [pellagra]
E53.1 Pyridoxine deficiency
E53.8 Deficiency of other specified B group vitamins
E54 Ascorbic acid deficiency

EPIDEMIOLOGY & DEMOGRAPHICS

Deficiency can occur in all age groups but is most common in the elderly.

Vitamin A deficiency: Affects 250 million preschool children worldwide.

Vitamin K deficiency: Varies by geographic regions; no race predilection; affects both sexes equally.

Vitamin B_1 (thiamine) deficiency: Incidence is unknown; no sex, race, or age predilection.

Vitamin B_5 (pantothenic acid) deficiency: Rare, as it is present in all foods.

Vitamin B_{12} (cobalamin) deficiency: Relatively common. Occurs in all age groups but more common in the elderly.

Vitamin B_9 (folic acid) deficiency: Mandatory fortification started in 1998. Prevalence before fortification 16% and after 0.5%. Neural tube defect associated with low maternal folate status during pregnancy. Pregnant women and the elderly are at greatest risk of folic acid deficiency.

Vitamin C (ascorbic acid) deficiency: Smokers and low-income persons are at increased risk.

PHYSICAL FINDINGS & CLINICAL PRESENTATION

- **Vitamin A:** xerophthalmia; xerosis of the cornea; keratomalacia; Bitot's spots (abnormal squamous cell proliferation and keratinization of the conjunctiva); nyctalopia (poor adaptation to darkness)/night blindness; poor bone growth; dry skin and hair
- **Vitamin E:** nerve dysfunction (ataxia; hyporeflexia, peripheral neuropathy); bone weakness.
- **Vitamin B_1 (thiamine)**:
  - Nervous system (dry beriberi): peripheral neuropathy, Wernicke encephalopathy, Korsakoff syndrome.
  - Cardiovascular (wet beriberi): edema, chest pain, increased heart rate (HR), lowered blood pressure (BP).
  - Gastrointestinal (GI): anorexia; constipation.
- **Vitamin B_2 (riboflavin)**:
  - Cheilosis (chapping and fissure of the lip)
  - Glossitis (sore red tongue)
  - Oily, scaly rashes on nasolabial folds, eyelids, scrotum, labia majoris
  - Red itchy eyes
  - Anemia
  - Peripheral neuropathy
- **Vitamin B_3 (niacin)**:
  - Pellagra (4 *Ds*—diarrhea, dermatitis, dementia, and ultimately death).
  - Hyperpigmentation of sun-exposed skin.
  - "Raw beef" swollen and painful tongue.
- **Vitamin B_6**: seborrheic dermatitis; glossitis, cheilosis, impaired proprioception; sensory ataxia, seizure.
- **Vitamin B_{12}**: Neurologic symptoms including peripheral neuropathy, ataxia, paresthesia; subacute degeneration of the spinal cord (demyelination of the dorsal column). Patients may also have dementia, depression, and weakness. Glossitis and GI symptoms such as nausea, vomiting, and anorexia are also common.
- **Vitamin B_9 (folic acid)**:
  - Patchy hyperpigmentation of skin (especially between fingers and toes) and mucous membranes
  - Moderate fever (temp <102° F) despite the absence of infection
  - Neural tube defect
  - Angular stomatitis
  - Red, beefy, smooth, and shiny tongue.
- **Vitamin C**: scurvy (poor wound healing, petechiae, follicular hyperkeratosis, fatigue, bleeding gums, weight loss).

ETIOLOGY

- Fat-soluble vitamins (vitamins A, D, E, K):
  1. Decreased ingestion, malnutrition, eating disorders.
  2. Diseases that affect fat absorption decrease the absorption of fat-soluble vitamins—for example, cystic fibrosis, celiac sprue, inflammatory bowel disease, cholestasis, hepatobiliary disease, small bowel surgery.
  3. Change in vitamin metabolism:
     - Alcoholism
     - Drugs such as cholestyramine, Coumadin
  4. Increased risk in:
     - Vegans
     - Recent immigrants
     - Refugees
     - Toddlers/preschoolers living below the poverty line
- Water-soluble vitamins (the B group of vitamins and viitamin C)—there are several etiologic factors, including:
  - Inadequate intake
  - Decreased absorption
  - Alcoholism
  - Pregnancy/lactation
  - Peritoneal dialysis
  - Medications (e.g., isoniazide, phenothiazides, tricyclic antidepressants)
  - Malabsorption
  - Low income
  - Advanced age
- Vitamin B_{12} deficiency—caused by:
  - Insufficient dietary intake, as in strict vegans
  - Decreased absorption secondary to intrinsic factor deficiency, decreased intrinsic factor secretion, gastric atrophy, gastrectomy
  - Terminal ileum disease such as celiac disease, enteritis, tropical sprue
- Folic acid deficiency—increased needs can lead to deficiency (e.g., pregnancy, lactation, malignancy).
- Derangement of folate metabolism by:
  - Medication (e.g., methotrexate)
  - Disease (e.g., hypothyroidism)
  - Increased excretion: as seen in alcoholics

Dx DIAGNOSIS

WORKUP/LABORATORY TESTS

- General initial laboratory tests include:
  1. Complete blood cell count (CBC).
     Liver function tests (LFTs).
     Basic metabolic panel (BMP).
     Albumin.
  2. Measurement of serum levels of the specific vitamin in question.
- Specific tests may be considered in the following cases:
  - Vitamin A:
    Retinol binding protein.
    Dark-adaptation threshold test.
  - Vitamin K:
    Prothrombin time/partial thromboplastin time (PT/PTT).
    Prothrombin.

Des-gamma-carboxy prothrombin (most sensitive test).
- Niacin: urine-*N*-methylnicotinamide (level <0.8 mg/day indicates niacin deficiency).
- Vitamin B_{12}:
  Serum vitamin B_{12} <100 pg/ml is diagnostic of vitamin B_{12} deficiency.
  Serum methylmalonic acid, which is elevated in B_{12} deficiency.
  Antiparietal antibody.
  Intrinsic factor antibody is decreased.
  Blood smear shows macrocytosis and hypersegmentation of megaloblasts.
  CBC shows increased mean corpuscle volume (MCV).
  Megaloblastic anemia.
- Folic acid:
  Check serum folate level
  Additional testing includes checking for serum homocysteine level, which will be elevated.
  Red cell folate level shows chronic folate status.

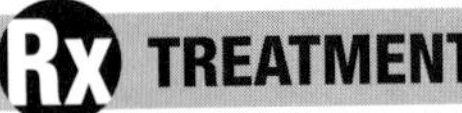

TREATMENT

Most of the vitamins are available over the counter individually or in different multivitamin formulations.

Specific vitamins:

- Vitamin A deficiency: treat with oral supplementation 10,000 IU daily.
  - Consume vitamin A–rich foods such as liver, beef, carrots, oranges, mangoes.
  - 5 servings of fruit and vegetables give enough carotenoids for a day.
- Vitamin K deficiency: treatment depends on the severity of bleeding, administered subcutaneously (SQ) or intramuscularly (IM).
- Vitamin B_1 (thiamine) deficiency: give intramuscular thiamine 50 mg for several days.
  - If B_1 deficiency is suspected and patient needs intravenous glucose, give thiamine first before intravenous glucose. This prevents the development of Korsakoff psychosis.
- Vitamin B_{12} deficiency: give 1000 mcg IM daily for 7 days, then once a week for 1 month, then once a month indefinitely.
  - A potential option is oral supplementation.
- Folic acid deficiency: daily requirement is 400 to 1000 mcg (1 mg) daily.
  - Centers for Disease Control and Prevention (CDC) recommend that women of childbearing age take 400 mcg of folic acid daily.

SUGGESTED READINGS

available at www.expertconsult.com

RELATED CONTENT

Anemia, Pernicious (Related Key Topic)
Rickets (Related Key Topic)
Vitamin D Deficiency (Related Key Topic)
Wernicke Syndrome (Related Key Topic)

AUTHOR: **DANIEL K. ASIEDU, M.D., PH.D., F.A.C.P.**

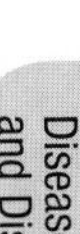

BASIC INFORMATION

- Vitamin D is a hormone and a steroid and, by definition, not a vitamin. There are two forms of vitamin D: vitamin D_2 and vitamin D_3.
- Vitamin D_2 is mainly found in some plant foods.
- Vitamin D_3 is produced in skin exposed to ultraviolet (UV) B radiation from sunlight (Fig. 1-1009). Gloson, Whistler, and DeBoot independently described rickets in the mid-seventeenth century. Sniadecki first reported the association of rickets with inadequate exposure to sunlight in 1822.
- The major functions of vitamin D include:
  - Increasing calcium and phosphorus absorption from the small intestines
  - Promoting the maturation of osteoclast to resorb calcium from bones

DEFINITION

Vitamin D deficiency is characterized by impaired bone mineralization. It is classified as a serum 25-hydroxyvitamin D (25[OH]D) level of <20 ng/ml (50 nmol/L).

SYNONYMS

The sunshine vitamin
The antirachitic factor
Cholecalciferol

ICD-9CM CODES
268.9 Vitamin D deficiency unspecified
ICD-10CM CODES
E55.9 Vitamin D deficiency, unspecified

EPIDEMIOLOGY & DEMOGRAPHICS

INCIDENCE:

- Worldwide deficiency and insufficiency affect about 1 billion people.
- Children and young adults: 40% to 50% of preadolescent Caucasian girls, and Hispanic and African American adolescents, are vitamin D deficient.

PEAK INCIDENCE: In the United States, 40% to 100% of the elderly are vitamin D deficient.

PREVALENCE: 42% of African American girls and women 15 to 49 yr old have 25(OH)D levels <20 ng/dl.

PREDOMINANT SEX AND AGE:

- Decreased skin production of vitamin D with age
- Increased prevalence among darker-skinned individuals

RISK FACTORS:

1. Age (due to decreased ability to produce D_3)
2. Sunshine-deficient areas (geographic location, living in higher latitudes)
3. Dark-skinned individuals (melanin competes with vitamin D_3 precursors for UV photons and thus decreases pre-D_3 formation)
4. Institutionalized individuals
5. Use of sunscreen (sun radiation that causes skin cancer also produces pre-vitamin D_3 in skin)
6. Patients on certain medications that antagonize vitamin D action (phenobarbital, phenytoin)
7. Intestinal resection
8. Severe chronic liver diseases (such as cirrhosis)
9. Kidney disease (e.g., nephritic syndrome).
10. Sarcoidosis and lymphomas (increased catabolism of 25[OH]D to 1,25[OH]$_2$D)
11. Intestinal malabsorption disease (caused by celiac sprue, cystic fibrosis, Whipple's disease)

PHYSICAL FINDINGS & CLINICAL PRESENTATION

- Rickets—seen in children; caused by defective mineralization in the skeleton (Fig. 1-1010)
  - Bowing of the legs
  - Leg bone pain
  - Delayed growth
  - Seizure due to hypocalcemia

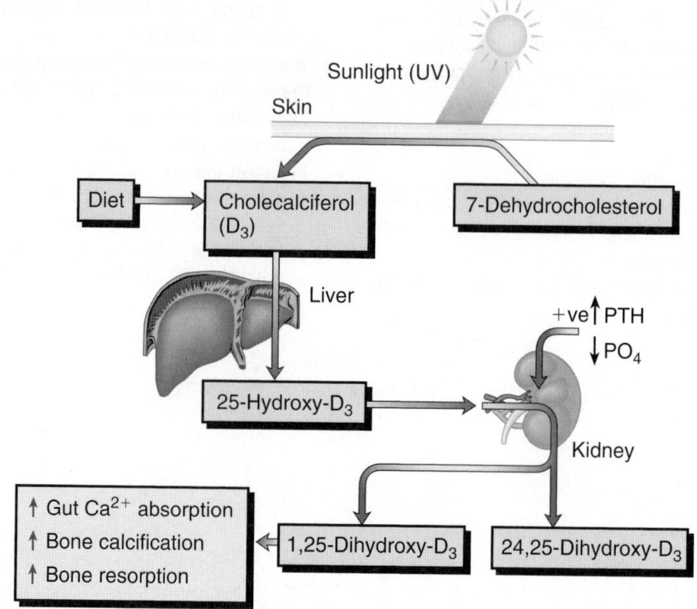

FIGURE 1-1009 The metabolism and actions of vitamin D. The primary source of vitamin D in humans is photoactivation in the skin of 7-dehydrocholesterol to cholecalciferol, which is then converted first in the liver to 25-hydroxyvitamin D and subsequently in the kidney to the much more active form, 1,25-dihydroxycholecalciferol (1,25[OH]$_2$,D_3). Regulation of the latter step is by PTH, phosphate, and feedback inhibition by 1,25(OH)$_2$,D_3. This step can also occur in lymphomatous and sarcoid tissue, resulting in the hypercalcemia that may complicate these diseases. (From Ballinger A: *Kumar & Clark's essentials of clinical medicine,* ed 6, Edinburgh, 2012, Saunders.)

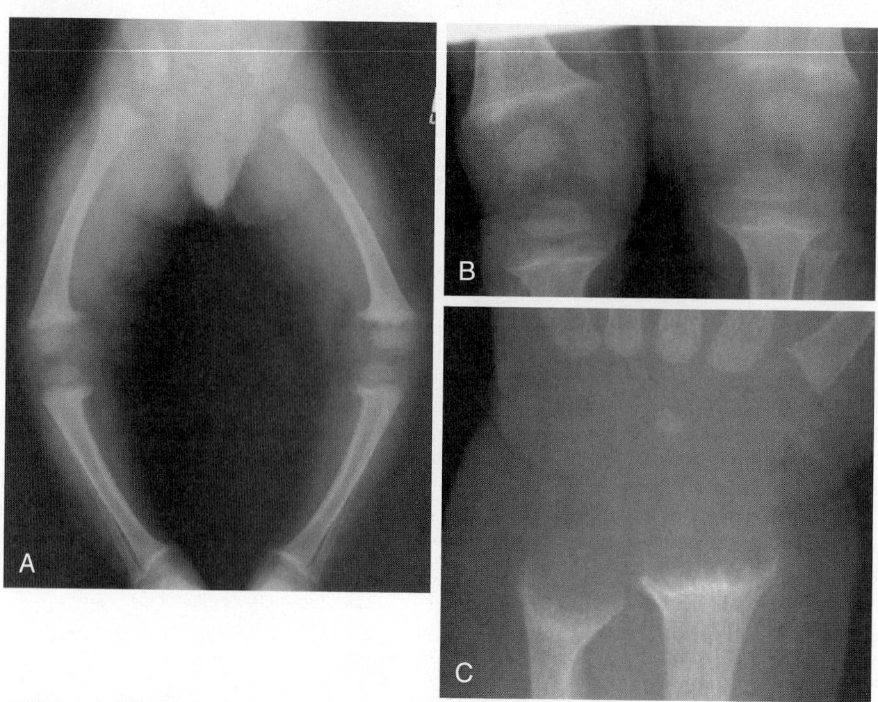

FIGURE 1-1010 Radiographs of a child with vitamin D–deficiency rickets demonstrating bowing of the femurs and tibias **(A)** and widened, frayed, demineralized epiphyseal plates **(B** and **C).** (From Hochberg MC et al: *Rheumatology,* ed 5, St Louis, 2011, Mosby.)

- Osteomalacia—seen in adults
  - Periosteal bone pain (best detected by putting a firm pressure on tibia or sternal bones)
  - Proximal muscle weakness
  - Chronic muscle aches/pain
- Fracture with very minimal trauma (brittle and easily broken bones)
- Severe hypocalcemia—especially in late vitamin D deficiency leading to seizure tetany
- Hypophosphatemia
- Neuromuscular
  - Paresthesia
  - Tetany
  - Muscle cramps

ETIOLOGY

- Inadequate exposure to sunlight, such as:
  - During winter
  - In nursing home and health care institution residents
  - With excessive use of sunscreen
- Medications:
  - Individuals on certain medications, such as phenobarbital, phenytoin, and rifampin (antagonize vitamin D action/increase vitamin D catabolism)
- Diseases and disease states:
  - Diseases causing vitamin D malabsorption:
    Cystic fibrosis
    Whipple's disease
    Celiac sprue
  - Diseases increasing vitamin D catabolism:
    Lymphoma
    Sarcoidosis
  - Intestinal resection
  - Decreased 25(OH)D production:
    Kidney disease
    Liver cirrhosis

Dx DIAGNOSIS

DIFFERENTIAL DIAGNOSIS

- Arthritis
- Fibromyalgia

WORKUP

- Population-wide screening for vitamin D deficiency is not recommended because evidence to support this practice is lacking.
- Screening is needed for individuals at risk (osteoporosis, history of falls, obese persons, pregnant and lactating women, diseases causing vitamin D malabsorption, African Americans). Workup involves blood and urine tests as well as radiography, as outlined in the next section.

LABORATORY TESTS

- Serum 25(OH)D: this is the best test to determine vitamin D status.
- Parathyroid hormone (PTH): increased levels in vitamin D insufficiency. It is a marker of vitamin D insufficiency.
- Increased (serum or bone) alkaline phosphatase
- Decreased 24-hour urine calcium (patient should not be on a thiazide)

IMAGING STUDIES

- Radiographs may show:
  - Pseudofractures of the pelvis, femur, metatarsals.
  - Nontraumatic fractures.
- Bone density:
  - Decreased bone mineral density (osteopenia or osteoporosis)

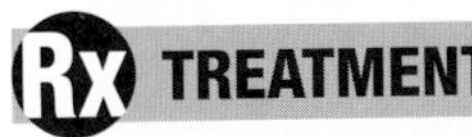

Rx TREATMENT

NONPHARMACOLOGIC THERAPY

- Natural sources of vitamin D. These include:
  - Exposure to sunlight
  - Dietary sources are not enough to meet daily requirements. Oily fish such as salmon, cod, and mackerel are rich sources of vitamin D_3.
- Foods fortified with vitamin D
  - Mainly fortified dairy products
  - Fortified orange juice

ACUTE GENERAL Rx

- Treating deficiency (general population):
  - 50,000 IU of vitamin D every week for 8 weeks, or
  - 6000 IU daily to achieve a serum level of 25(OH)D of at least 30 ng/ml
- Maintenance measures after treatment (general population): 1500 to 2000 IU daily
- Treating deficiency (obese patients, patients with malabsorption syndromes, or those taking certain medications, as indicated earlier)
  - 6000 to 10,000 IU daily
- Maintenance measures after treatment (obese patients, patients with malabsorption syndromes, or those taking certain medications, as indicated earlier):
  - 3000 to 6000 IU daily
- After treating deficiency, recheck 25(OH)D in 12 to 14 weeks.

REFERRAL

Referral to an endocrinologist is recommended if there is no response to treatment.

PREVENTION

- Food fortification with vitamin D_2 or vitamin D_3
- Adequate sun exposure
- Vitamin D supplementation (per the Endocrine Society):
  - Infants (age range 1-12 mo) require at least 400 IU/day of vitamin D.
  - Children (age range 1-18 yr) require 600 IU/day of vitamin D.
  - Adult supplementation (adults age 19 to 70 yr): 600 IU of vitamin D daily
  - Adult supplementation (persons 70 yr and older): 800 IU of vitamin D daily
  - Exceptions: pregnant or lactating women, obese persons, and patients on antiseizure medications, steroids, antifungals, and AIDS medications should be given 2× to 3× more vitamin D.
- Screening: recommended only for individuals at high risk for vitamin D deficiency such as blacks and Hispanics, obese individuals (BMI >30 kg/m^2), patients with osteoporosis, the elderly, and patients with certain chronic diseases (see "Risk Factors").

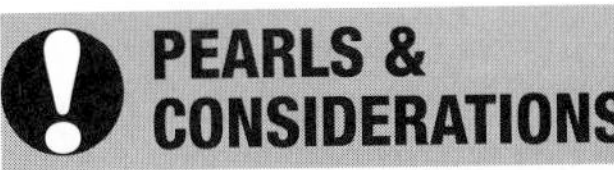

PEARLS & CONSIDERATIONS

- In the U.S., vitamin D supplements are available by prescription as vitamin D_2 (ergocalciferol) or over the counter as vitamin D_3 (cholecalciferol, usually in 400-1000 IU doses). Both vitamin D_2 and vitamin D_3 are acceptable as supplements. On average, oral vitamin D_3 raises blood levels more than does vitamin D_2.
- Upper limit of maintenance tolerability in healthy adults is 4000 IU a day. More than 4000 IU of vitamin D daily in nondeficient individuals increases the risk of harm. High-level supplements (more than 10,000 IU daily) are associated with kidney and tissue damage.
- Vitamin D supplementation is recommended for fall prevention. High-dose vitamin D supplementation (≥800 IU daily) has been shown to be favorable in the prevention of hip fracture and any nonvertebral fracture in persons 65 years of age or older.
- Prescribing more than the recommended daily amount to improve quality of life or prevent cardiovascular disease or death is not advised.
- Trials have shown that low vitamin D levels are associated with depressive symptoms, especially in persons with a history of depression. These findings suggest that vitamin D levels may be useful in patients with a history of depression.
- Vitamin D supplementation, administered with calcium, has been shown to lower the risk for falling and improve muscle strength in the elderly, especially in older vitamin D–deficient women who are at high baseline risk for falling.
- The treatment of vitamin D insufficiency decreases the risk of nonvertebral and hip fractures.
- Recent data suggest that vitamin D deficiency is associated with the risk of developing certain cancers (including breast, colon, and prostate).
- Vitamin D deficiency is associated with some autoimmune diseases (types 1 and 2 diabetes, metabolic syndrome, multiple sclerosis).

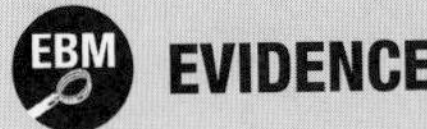

EVIDENCE

available at www.expertconsult.com

SUGGESTED READINGS

available at www.expertconsult.com

RELATED CONTENT

Vitamin D Deficiency (Patient Information)

AUTHOR: **DANIEL K. ASIEDU, M.D., PH.D., F.A.C.P.**

BASIC INFORMATION

DEFINITION

Vitiligo is the acquired loss of epidermal pigmentation that is characterized histologically by the absence of epidermal melanocytes. There are two major forms: nonsegmental (generalized) vitiligo, which accounts for >80% of cases, and segmental vitiligo, which accounts for 30% of childhood cases.

ICD-9CM CODES
709.1 Vitiligo
ICD-10CM CODES
L80 Vitiligo

EPIDEMIOLOGY & DEMOGRAPHICS

PREVALENCE: Vitiligo affects 0.5% to 1% of the population; it is the most common depigmenting disorder.

PREDOMINANT AGE: Vitiligo can begin at any age, but the age at onset is <20 yr for half of patients.

GENETICS: A positive family history is present in 25% to 30% of patients, and both sexes are equally affected. There are no differences in the rates of occurrence with regard to skin type or race.

PHYSICAL FINDINGS & CLINICAL PRESENTATION

- Hypopigmented and depigmented lesions (Fig. 1-1011) favor sun-exposed regions, intertriginous areas, genitalia, and sites over bony prominences (i.e., nonsegmental or type A vitiligo).
- Areas around the body orifices are also frequently involved.
- The lesions tend to be symmetric.
- Occasionally the lesions are linear or pseudodermatomal (i.e., segmental or type B vitiligo).
- Vitiligo lesions may occur at trauma sites (i.e., Koebner's phenomenon).
- The hair in affected areas may be white.
- The margins of the lesions are usually well demarcated; when a ring of hyperpigmentation is seen, the term *trichrome vitiligo* is used.

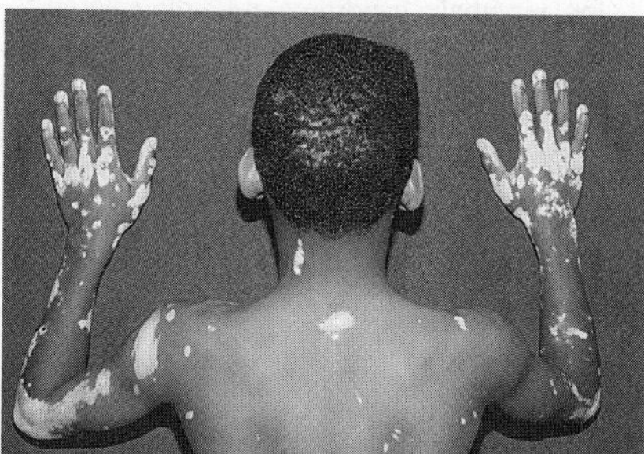

FIGURE 1-1011 Multiple, sharply demarcated, symmetric, depigmented areas of vitiligo. (From Behrman RE: *Nelson textbook of pediatrics,* Philadelphia, 2006, Saunders.)

- The term *marginal inflammatory vitiligo* is used to describe lesions with raised borders.
- Initially the disease is limited, but the lesions tend to become more extensive over time.
- Type B vitiligo is more common among children.
- Vitiligo may begin around pigmented nevi and produce a halo (i.e., Sutton's nevus); in such cases, the central nevus often regresses and disappears over time.

ETIOLOGY & PATHOGENESIS

- Three pathophysiologic theories:
  1. Autoimmune theory (i.e., autoantibodies against melanocytes)
  2. Neural theory (i.e., neurochemical mediators selectively destroy melanocytes)
  3. Self-destructive process in which melanocytes fail to protect themselves against cytotoxic melanin precursors
- Although vitiligo is considered to be an acquired disease, 25% to 30% of cases are familial. The mode of transmission is unknown; the condition seems to be polygenic or autosomal dominant with incomplete penetrance and variable expression.
- Associated disorders:
  - Alopecia areata
  - Type 1 diabetes mellitus
  - Adrenal insufficiency
  - Hyperthyroidism and hypothyroidism
  - Mucocutaneous candidiasis
  - Pernicious anemia
  - Polyglandular autoimmune syndromes
  - Melanoma

Dx DIAGNOSIS

DIFFERENTIAL DIAGNOSIS

- Acquired hypopigmentation disorders:
  - Chemical-induced (e.g., chloroquine, imatinib, phenolic-catecholic derivatives [e.g., adhesives, deodorants, latex gloves, lacquer resins, varnish, soap antioxidants, insecticides, printing ink, paints, motor oil additives, disinfectants])
  - Halo nevus
  - Idiopathic guttate hypomelanosis
  - Leprosy
  - Leukoderma associated with melanoma
  - Pityriasis alba
  - Postinflammatory hypopigmentation
  - Tinea versicolor
  - Vogt-Koyanagi syndrome (i.e., vitiligo, uveitis, and deafness)
  - Melasma
  - Mycosis fungoides
- Congenital hypopigmentation disorders:
  - Albinism, partial (piebaldism)
  - Albinism, total
  - Nevus anemicus
  - Nevus depigmentosus
  - Tuberous sclerosis
  - Ito's hypomelanosis

WORKUP

- Inquire about a personal and family history of autoimmune disease.
- Perform a physical examination.
- A Wood's light examination may enhance the lesions of light-skinned individuals.

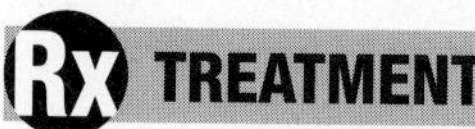

Rx TREATMENT

Treatment is indicated primarily for cosmetic purposes when depigmentation causes emotional or social distress. Depigmentation is more noticeable among patients with darker complexions.

- Cosmetic masking agents (e.g., Dermablend, Covermark) or stains (e.g., DY-O-Derm, Vitadye)
- Sunless tanning lotions (e.g., dihydroxyacetone)
- Repigmentation (This is achieved by the activation and migration of melanocytes from hair follicles; therefore, skin with little or no hair responds poorly to treatment.)
- Narrow-band ultraviolet B radiation (This is the preferred treatment for nonsegmental vitiligo. It is given twice weekly [not on successive days] during sessions that last from 5 to 10 min. The best results are achieved on the face, trunk, and limbs.)
- Psoralens and sunlight (e.g., PUVAsol)
- Topical mid-potency steroids (e.g., triamcinolone 0.1% or desonide 0.05% cream qd for 3 to 4 mo)
- Topical calcineurin inhibitors for face and neck lesions
- Intralesional steroid injection
- Systemic steroids (e.g., betamethasone 5 mg qd on two consecutive days per wk for 2 to 4 mo)
- Total depigmentation in cases of extensive vitiligo with 20% monobenzyl ether or hydroquinone (This is a permanent procedure, and patients will require lifelong protection from sun exposure.)
- Topical immunomodulators (e.g., tacrolimus, pimecrolimus) (These substances can also induce the repigmentation of vitiliginous skin lesions. However, their potential for systemic immunosuppression or for increasing the risk of skin or other malignancies remains to be defined.)
- Calcipotriol, which is a synthetic analog of vitamin D_3 (This has also been used in combination with ultraviolet light or clobetasol, with limited results.)
- Surgical techniques

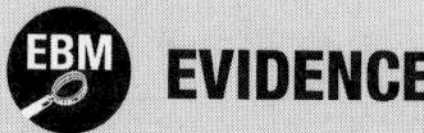

EBM EVIDENCE

available at www.expertconsult.com

SUGGESTED READING

available at www.expertconsult.com

RELATED CONTENT

Vitiligo (Patient Information)

AUTHOR: **FRED F. FERRI, M.D.**

BASIC INFORMATION

DEFINITION

Von Willebrand's disease is a congenital disorder of hemostasis characterized by defective or deficient von Willebrand factor (vWF). There are several subtypes of von Willebrand's disease. The most common type (80% of cases) is type I, which is caused by a quantitative decrease in vWF; type IIA and type IIB are results of qualitative protein abnormalities; and type III is a rare, autosomal recessive disorder characterized by a near-complete quantitative deficiency of vWF. Acquired von Willebrand's disease is a rare disorder that usually occurs in elderly patients and usually presents with mucocutaneous bleeding abnormalities and no clinically meaningful family history. It is often accompanied by a hematoproliferative or autoimmune disorder. Successful treatment of the associated illness can reverse the clinical and laboratory manifestations.

SYNONYMS

Pseudohemophilia
vWD

ICD-9CM CODES
286.4 von Willebrand's disease
ICD-10CM CODES
D68.0 von Willebrand's disease

EPIDEMIOLOGY & DEMOGRAPHICS

- Autosomal-dominant disorder
- Most common inherited bleeding disorder
- Prevalence is 1% to 2% in general population, according to screening studies; estimates based on referral for symptoms of bleeding suggest a prevalence of 30 to 100 cases per million

PHYSICAL FINDINGS & CLINICAL PRESENTATION

- Generally normal physical examination
- Mucosal bleeding (gingival bleeding, epistaxis) and gastrointestinal bleeding may occur
- Easy bruising
- Postpartum bleeding, bleeding after surgery or dental extraction, menorrhagia

ETIOLOGY

Quantitative or qualitative deficiency of vWF (see "Definition")

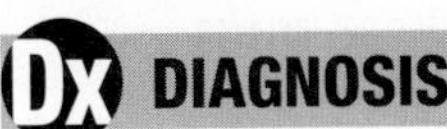

DIAGNOSIS

The diagnosis of von Willebrand's disease generally requires two criteria: (1) a personal history, family history, or physical evidence of mucocutaneous bleeding and (2) a qualitative or quantitative decrease in functional activity of von Willebrand's disease. The American Society of Hematology states that a definitive diagnosis of vWD may be made if vWF antigen levels are less than 30 IU/dl. It also describes a gray zone of 30 to 50 IU/dl, designated as "low vWF."

DIFFERENTIAL DIAGNOSIS

Platelet function disorders, clotting factor deficiencies

WORKUP

- Laboratory evaluation (see "Laboratory Tests")
- Initial testing includes partial thromboplastin time (increased), platelet count (normal), and bleeding time (prolonged)
- Subsequent tests include vWF level (decreased), factor VIII:C (decreased), and ristocetin agglutination (increased in type IIB) (Table 1-505)

LABORATORY TESTS

- Decreased factor VIII coagulant activity
- Decreased vWF antigen or ristocetin cofactor
- Normal platelet number and morphology
- Prolonged bleeding time
- Normal platelet aggregation studies
- Type IIA von Willebrand's disease can be distinguished from type I by absence of ristocetin cofactor activity and abnormal multimer
- Type IIB von Willebrand's disease is distinguished from type I by abnormal multimer

Rx TREATMENT

NONPHARMACOLOGIC THERAPY

- Avoidance of aspirin and other nonsteroidal anti-inflammatory drugs
- Evaluation for likelihood of bleeding (with measurement of bleeding time) before surgical procedures. When a patient undergoes surgery or receives repeated therapeutic doses of concentrates, factor VIII activity should be assayed every 12 hr on the day a dose is administered and every 24 hr thereafter.

GENERAL Rx

- The mainstay of treatment in von Willebrand's disease is the replacement of the deficient protein at the time of spontaneous bleeding or before invasive procedures are performed.
- Desmopressin acetate (DDAVP) is useful to release stored vWF from endothelial cells. It is used to cover minor procedures and traumatic bleeding in mild type I von Willebrand's disease. Dose is 0.3 mcg/kg in 100 ml of normal saline solution IV infused >20 min. DDAVP is also available as a nasal spray (dose of 150 mcg spray administered to each nostril) as a preparation for minor surgery and management of minor bleeding episodes. DDAVP is not effective in type IIA von Willebrand's disease and is potentially dangerous in type IIB (increased risk of bleeding and thrombocytopenia).
- In patients with severe disease, replacement therapy in the form of cryoprecipitate is the method of choice. The standard dose is 1 bag of cryoprecipitate per 10 kg of body weight.
- Factor VIII concentrate rich in vWF (Humate-P) is useful to correct bleeding abnormalities in type IIA, IIB, and type III von Willebrand's disease without alloantibodies. Alloantibodies that inactivate vWF and form circulating immune complexes develop in 15% of patients with type III von Willebrand's disease who have received multiple transfusions. In these patients, recombinant factor VIII is preferred because autoantibodies can elicit life-threatening anaphylactic reactions because of complement activation by immune complexes.
- Life-threatening hemorrhage unresponsive to therapy with cryoprecipitate or factor VIII concentrate may require transfusion of normal platelets.

SUGGESTED READINGS

available at www.expertconsult.com

RELATED CONTENT

von Willebrand's Disease (Patient Information)

AUTHOR: **FRED F. FERRI, M.D.**

TABLE 1-505 Genetic and Laboratory Findings in von Willebrand's Disease

Parameter Type	BT	VIII-C	vW-Ag	R-Cof	RIPA	Multimer Structure	Mode of Inheritance
I (classic)	P	R	R	R	R	Normal	AD
II							
A	P	N/R	N/R	R	R	Abnormal	AD
B	P	N/R	N/R	N/R	I	Abnormal	AD
III	P	R	R	R	R	Variable	AR

AD, Autosomal dominant; *AR,* autosomal recessive; *BT,* bleeding time; *I,* increased; *N/R,* normal or reduced; *P,* prolonged; *R,* reduced; *R-Cof,* ristocetin cofactor; *RIPA,* ristocetin-induced platelet aggregation (agglutination); *vW-Ag,* von Willebrand antigen (protein); *VIII-C,* factor VIII coagulant activity.

From Behrman RE: *Nelson textbook of pediatrics,* ed 17, Philadelphia, 2004, Saunders.

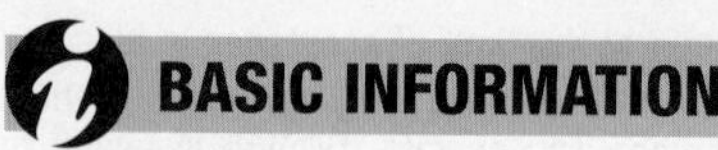

BASIC INFORMATION

DEFINITION

Vulvar cancer is an abnormal cell proliferation arising on the vulva and exhibiting malignant potential. The majority are of squamous cell origin; however, other types include adenocarcinoma, basal cell carcinoma, sarcoma, and melanoma.

SYNONYMS

Squamous cell carcinoma of the vulva (90%)
Basal cell carcinoma of the vulva
Adenocarcinoma of the vulva
Melanoma of the vulva
Bartholin gland carcinoma
Verrucous carcinoma of the vulva
Vulvar sarcoma

ICD-9CM CODES
184.4 Vulvar neoplasm
ICD-10 CODES
C51.9 Malignant neoplasm of vulva, unspecified

EPIDEMIOLOGY & DEMOGRAPHICS

INCIDENCE: 2.2 cases per 100,000 persons
PREVALENCE: Vulvar cancer is uncommon. It comprises 4% of malignancies of the female genital tract. It is the fourth most common gynecologic malignancy.
MEAN AGE AT DIAGNOSIS: Predominantly a disease of menopause. Mean age at diagnosis is 65 yr.

PHYSICAL FINDINGS & CLINICAL PRESENTATION

- Vulvar pruritus or pain is present.
- May produce a malodorous discharge or present as bleeding.
- Raised lesion that may have fleshy (Fig. 1-1013), ulcerated, leukoplakic, or warty appearance; may have multifocal lesions.
- Lesions are usually located on labia majora but may be seen on labia minora, clitoris, and perineum.
- The lymph nodes of groin may be palpable.

ETIOLOGY

- The exact etiology is unknown.
- Vulvar intraepithelial neoplasia has been reported in 20% to 30% of invasive squamous cell carcinoma of the vulva, but the malignant potential is unknown.
- Human papillomavirus is found in 30% to 50% of vulvar carcinoma, but its exact role is unclear.
- Chronic pruritus, wetness, industrial wastes, arsenicals, hygienic agents, and vulvar dystrophies have been implicated as causative agents.
- Vulvar cancer in younger women is more directly dependent on HPV infection, vulvar dysplasia, and tobacco use.

Dx DIAGNOSIS

DIFFERENTIAL DIAGNOSIS

- Lymphogranuloma inguinale
- Tuberculosis
- Vulvar dystrophies
- Vulvar atrophy
- Paget's disease

WORKUP

- Diagnosis is made histologically by biopsy
- Thorough examination of the lesion and assessment of spread. Table 1-506 describes FIGO staging of vulvar cancer
- Possible colposcopy of adjacent areas
- Cytologic smear of vagina and cervix
- Cystoscopy and proctosigmoidoscopy may be necessary

IMAGING STUDIES

- Chest radiography
- CT scan and MRI for assessing local tumor spread

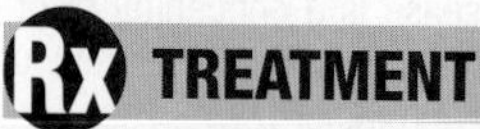

TREATMENT

NONPHARMACOLOGIC THERAPY

- Treatment is individualized depending on the stage of the tumor. Fig. 1-1014 describes a treatment algorithm for management of patients with vulvar cancer.
- Stage I tumors with <1 mm stromal invasion are treated with complete local excision without groin node dissection. Imiquimod 5% cream, a topical immune response modulator, is also effective in the treatment of vulvar intraepithelial neoplasia.

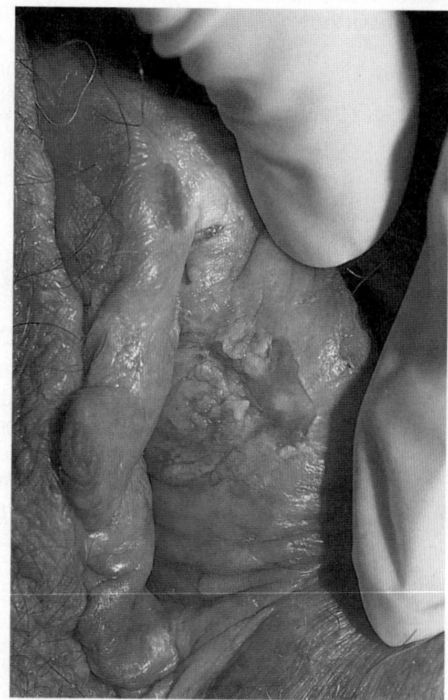

FIGURE 1-1013 Squamous cell carcinoma of the vulva. (From White GM, Cox NH [eds]: *Diseases of the skin, a color atlas and text,* ed 2, St Louis, 2006, Mosby.)

TABLE 1-506 FIGO Staging of Vulval Cancer

Stage I	Tumor confined to the vulva—2 cm or less in diameter. Nodes are not involved.
	A. Lesions less than 1 mm depth invasion
	B. Other lesions less than 2 cm in diameter
Stage II	Tumor confined to the vulva—more than 2 cm in diameter. Nodes are not involved.
Stage III	Tumor of any size with: Adjacent spread to the lower urethra and/or the vagina, the perineum and the anus, and/or unilateral lymph node involvement.
Stage IV	Tumor of any size with bilateral groin lymph node involvement:
	A. Infiltrating the bladder mucosa or the rectal mucosa, or both, including the upper part of the urethral mucosa
	B. Fixed to the bone or other distant metastases. Fixed or ulcerated nodes in either one or both groins.

From Symonds EM, Symonds IM: *Essential obstetrics and gynecology,* ed 4, London, 2004, Churchill Livingstone.

- Stage I tumors with >1 mm stromal invasion are treated with complete local excision with groin node dissection.
- Stage II tumors require radical vulvectomy with bilateral groin node dissection.
- Advanced-stage disease may require the addition of radiation and chemotherapy to the surgical regimen.
- Fig. 1-1014 describes a treatment algorithm for management of vulvar cancer.

DISPOSITION

Five-year survival ranges from 90% for stage I to 15% for stage IV.

REFERRAL

Vulvar cancer should be managed by a gynecologic oncologist and radiation oncologist.

SUGGESTED READINGS

available at www.expertconsult.com

RELATED CONTENT

Vulvar Cancer (Patient Information)

AUTHOR: **RUBEN ALVERO, M.D.**

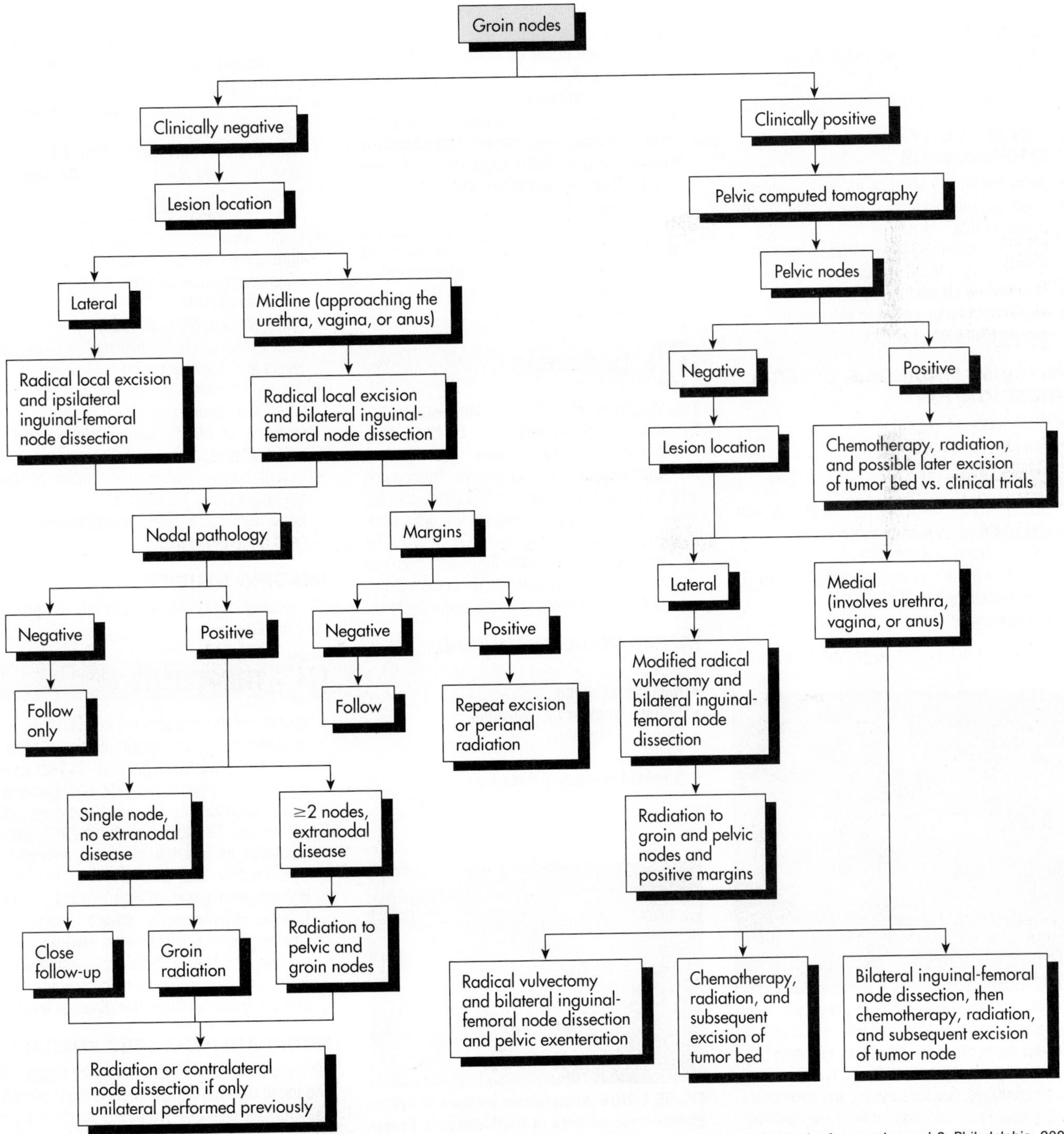

- Groin nodes
  - Clinically negative
    - Lesion location
      - Lateral
        - Radical local excision and ipsilateral inguinal-femoral node dissection → Nodal pathology
      - Midline (approaching the urethra, vagina, or anus)
        - Radical local excision and bilateral inguinal-femoral node dissection → Nodal pathology; Margins
      - Nodal pathology
        - Negative
          - Follow only
        - Positive
          - Single node, no extranodal disease
            - Close follow-up
            - Groin radiation
          - ≥2 nodes, extranodal disease
            - Radiation to pelvic and groin nodes
          - Radiation or contralateral node dissection if only unilateral performed previously
      - Margins
        - Negative
          - Follow
        - Positive
          - Repeat excision or perianal radiation
  - Clinically positive
    - Pelvic computed tomography
      - Pelvic nodes
        - Negative
          - Lesion location
            - Lateral
              - Modified radical vulvectomy and bilateral inguinal-femoral node dissection
                - Radiation to groin and pelvic nodes and positive margins
            - Medial (involves urethra, vagina, or anus)
              - Radical vulvectomy and bilateral inguinal-femoral node dissection and pelvic exenteration
              - Chemotherapy, radiation, and subsequent excision of tumor bed
              - Bilateral inguinal-femoral node dissection, then chemotherapy, radiation, and subsequent excision of tumor node
        - Positive
          - Chemotherapy, radiation, and possible later excision of tumor bed vs. clinical trials

FIGURE 1-1014 Treatment algorithm for management of patients with vulvar cancer. (From Copeland LJ: *Textbook of gynecology,* ed 2, Philadelphia, 2000, Saunders.)

BASIC INFORMATION

DEFINITION

Waldenström's macroglobulinemia (WM) is a plasma cell dyscrasia (B-cell malignancy) characterized by lymphoplasmacytic infiltration in the bone marrow or lymphatic tissue and a monoclonal immunoglobulin M protein (IgM) in the serum.

SYNONYMS

WM
Monoclonal macroglobulinemia
Lymphoplasmacytic lymphoma

ICD-9CM CODES
273.3 Waldenström's macroglobulinemia
ICD-10CM CODES
C88.0 Waldenström macroglobulinemia

EPIDEMIOLOGY & DEMOGRAPHICS

- Accounts for 2% of all hematologic cancers
- 1500 people diagnosed every year in the United States
- Overall incidence: 3.4 per million person-yr in men, 1.7 per million person-yr in women
- Median age approximately 63 yr
- More common among men than women and among whites than blacks

PHYSICAL FINDINGS & CLINICAL PRESENTATION

- Weakness
- Fatigue
- Weight loss
- Pallor
- Headache, dizziness, vertigo, deafness, and seizures (hyperviscosity syndrome)
- Easy bleeding (e.g., epistaxis)
- Retinal vein link-sausage shaped (Fig. 1-1015)
- Lymphadenopathy (15%)
- Hepatomegaly (20%)
- Most commonly encountered neurologic presentation is symmetric polyneuropathy (5%)
- Splenomegaly (15%)
- Purpura (Fig. 1-1016)
- Fever and night sweats

ETIOLOGY

- WM is an IgM-secreting lymphoplasmacytic lymphoma (LPL). The underlying mutation in this disorder has not been delineated.
- Multiple reports suggest familial clustering, which indicates a genetic predisposition. In one study, chromosomal deletions in 6q21–22.1 were confirmed in 42% of WM patients, regardless of family history. In another study, the strongest evidence of linkage was found on chromosomes 1q and 4q.
- The main risk factor for development of WM is having IgM monoclonal gammopathy of unknown significance (MGUS).
- Radiation exposure, occupational chemicals, viral infection, and chronic inflammatory stimulation have been suggested, but there is insufficient evidence to substantiate these hypotheses.
- There is a twofold to threefold increased risk of WM in people with a personal history of autoimmune diseases with autoantibodies. There is also increased risk with HIV, hepatitis, and rickettsiosis.

Dx DIAGNOSIS

The diagnosis of WM is usually established by laboratory blood tests and by bone marrow biopsy. Diagnosis requires demonstration of lymphoplasmacytic lymphoma comprising ≥10% of the bone marrow cellularity and the presence of an IgM M protein. MYD88 L265P is a commonly recurring mutation in WM that can be useful in differentiating it and non-IgM lymphoplasmacytic lymphoma (LPL) from B-cell disorders that have some of the same features.

DIFFERENTIAL DIAGNOSIS

- MGUS
- Multiple myeloma
- Chronic lymphocytic leukemia
- Hairy-cell leukemia
- Lymphoma
- Smoldering macroglobulinemia

WORKUP

In any patient suspected of having WM, specific blood tests (CBC, erythrocyte sedimentation rate [ESR], serum or urine protein electrophoresis [SPEP or UPEP, respectively], IgM level, beta 2-microglobulin, serum viscosity) should be ordered. Bone marrow biopsy confirms the diagnosis.

LABORATORY TESTS

- CBC with differential:
  - Anemia is a common finding, with a median hemoglobin value of approximately 10 g/dl. WBC count is usually normal; thrombocytopenia can occur.
  - Peripheral smear may reveal "stacked coin" rouleaux formations and malignant lymphoid cells in terminal patients.
- Elevated ESR.
- SPEP: homogeneous M spike (monoclonal gammopathy).
- Immunoelectrophoresis: confirms IgM responsible for the M spike. Table 1-507 describes physicochemical and immunologic properties of the monoclonal IgM protein in WM.
- Urine immunoelectrophoresis: monoclonal light chains are usually kappa chains. Bence Jones protein can be seen, but is not the typical finding in WM.
- IgM levels are high, generally >3 g/dl.
- Beta 2-microglobulin: elevated in 55%; high levels are associated with poor prognosis.
- Serum viscosity: symptoms usually occur when the serum viscosity is four times the viscosity of normal serum; classic feature although present in only 15% of cases.
- Cryoglobulins, rheumatoid factor, or cold agglutinins may be present.
- Bone marrow biopsy: lymphoplasmacytoid cells are characteristic.

IMAGING STUDIES

Chest x-ray can be obtained to rule out pulmonary involvement.

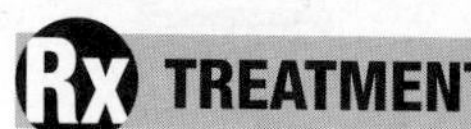

Rx TREATMENT

- Because of the incurable nature of WM, the aim of treatment is to relieve symptoms and reduce the risk of organ damage. Patients with smoldering or asymptomatic WM and preserved hematologic function should be observed without therapy. Considerations for the initiation of treatment include the following: hemoglobin concentration less than 100×10^9/L, significant adenopathy or organomegaly, symptomatic hyperviscosity, severe neuropathy, amyloidosis, cryoglobulinemia, cold-agglutinin disease, or evidence of disease transformation.
- Treatment is directed at both hyperviscocity and the lymphoproliferative disorder itself.

NONPHARMACOLOGIC THERAPY

Asymptomatic patients do not require treatment, and these patients should be monitored periodically for the onset of symptoms or changes in blood tests (e.g., worsening anemia, thrombocytopenia, rising IgM, and serum viscosity).

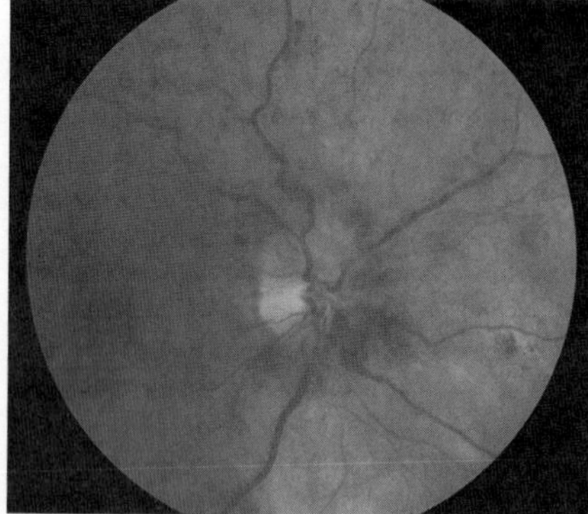

FIGURE 1-1015 Hyperviscosity syndrome. Right eye retinal image in a patient with Waldenström's macroglobulinemia and hyperviscosity syndrome showing sausaging (focal venular dilations), intraretinal hemorrhages, microaneurysms, and peripapillary cotton wool spots and disc swelling (papilledema). (From Goldman L, Schafer AI: *Goldman's Cecil medicine,* ed 24, Philadelphia, 2011, Saunders.)

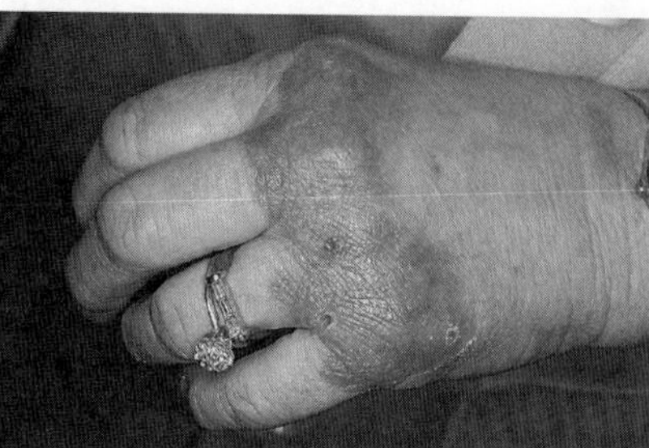

FIGURE 1-1016 Nonpalpable purpura of hyperglobulinemic purpura of Waldenström's hypergammaglobulinemia. (From Hochberg MC et al: *Rheumatology,* ed 5, St Louis, 2011, Mosby.)

TABLE 1-507 Physicochemical and Immunologic Properties of Monoclonal Immunoglobulin Protein in Waldenström's Macroglobulinemia

Properties of Monoclonal Immunoglobulin Protein	Diagnostic Condition	Clinical Manifestations
Pentameric structure	Hyperviscosity	Headaches, blurred vision, epistaxis, retinal hemorrhages, leg cramps, impaired mentation, and intracranial hemorrhage
Prescription on cooling	Cryoglobulinemia (type I)	Raynaud's phenomenon, acrocyanosis, ulcers, purpura, and cold urticaria
Autoantibody activity to myelin-associated glycoprotein, ganglioside M1, and sulfatide moieties on peripheral nerve sheaths	Peripheral neuropathies	Sensorimotor neuropathies, painful neuropathies, ataxic gait, and bilateral foot drop
Autoantibody activity to immunoglobulin G	Cryoglobulinemia (type II)	Purpura, arthralgias, renal failure, and sensorimotor neuropathies
Autoantibody activity to red blood cell antigens	Cold agglutinins	Hemolytic anemia, Raynaud's phenomenon, acrocyanosis, and livedo reticularis
Tissue deposition as amorphous aggregates	Organ dysfunction	Skin: bullous skin disease, papules, and Schnitzler syndrome Gastrointestinal: diarrhea, malabsorption, and bleeding Kidney: proteinuria and renal failure (light-chain component)
Tissue deposition as amyloid fibrils (light-chain fibrils commonly the largest component)	Organ dysfunction	Fatigue, weight loss, edema, periorbital purpura, hepatomegaly, macroglossia, and organ dysfunction of the involved organs: heart, kidney, liver, and peripheral sensory and autonomic nerves

From Hoffman R et al: *Hematology, basic principles and practice,* ed 5, Philadelphia, 2009, Churchill Livingstone.

ACUTE GENERAL Rx

- Treatment of the lymphoproliferative disorder includes single or combination therapy; although guidance has been suggested in the Mayo Stratification of Macroglobulinemia and Risk-Adapted Therapy (mSMART) Guidelines, there is no universally agreed upon standard of care:
  - Rituximab, a monoclonal anti-CD20 antibody, can be used in symptomatic patients with modest hematologic compromise, IgM-related neuropathy, or hemolytic anemia unresponsive to corticosteroids.
  - Plasmapheresis should be initial treatment in patients with symptoms of hyperviscosity.
  - DRC regimen (dexamethasone, rituximab, cyclophosphamide) in patients with severe constitutional symptoms, symptomatic bulky disease, hyperviscosity, or profound hematologic compromise.

CHRONIC Rx

- Refractory patients can be retried on original therapy if length of response from initial therapy is >2 yr. If the response from the initial therapy was <2 yr, alternative first-line agents such as fludarabine or cladribine can be used.
- Other treatment options: interferon alpha, thalidomide, and autologous stem cell transplantation.

DISPOSITION

- The onset of WM is slow and insidious. Most patients die from progression of the disease with hyperviscosity, hemorrhage, and infection, or from congestive heart failure.
- Some patients develop acute myelogenous leukemia, immunoblastic sarcoma, or chronic myelogenous leukemia as a preterminal event.
- Median survival in patients with WM is about 4 to 5 yr.
- ~10% of patients will achieve complete remission, with prognosis being more favorable (median survival 11 yr).
- A staging system using serum beta 2-microglobulin concentration, hemoglobin concentration, and serum IgM concentration before treatment provides insight into prognosis and survival.
- Other factors can negatively affect the survival: age >65, male gender, the presence of organomegaly, and the presence of cytopenias.

REFERRAL

If WM is suspected, a hematology consultation is helpful in guiding future workup, treatment, and monitoring. Autologous stem cell transplantation should be considered in all eligible patients with relapsed disease.

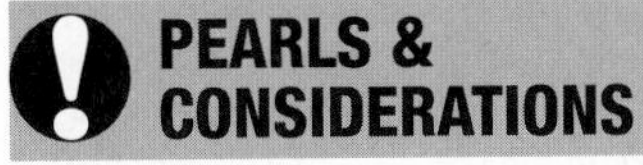

PEARLS & CONSIDERATIONS

COMMENTS

- WM was first described in 1944 by the Swedish physician Jan Gosta Waldenström.
- Amyloidosis is rare, occurring in 5% of patients with WM.

SUGGESTED READINGS

available at www.expertconsult.com

AUTHOR: **MARK F. BRADY, M.D., M.P.H., M.M.S.**

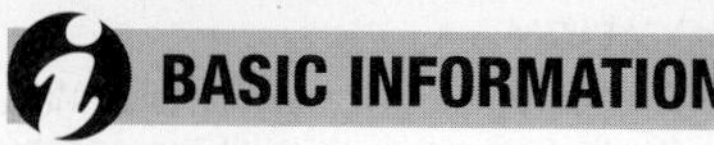

BASIC INFORMATION

DEFINITION

Warts are benign epidermal lesions caused by human papillomavirus (HPV).

SYNONYMS

Verruca vulgaris (common warts)
Verruca plana (flat warts)
Condyloma acuminatum (venereal warts)
Verruca plantaris (plantar warts)
Mosaic warts (cluster of many warts)
HPV infection

ICD-9CM CODES
078.10 Viral warts
078.19 Venereal wart (external genital organs)
ICD10CM CODES
B07.9 Viral wart, unspecified
B07.8 Other viral warts

EPIDEMIOLOGY & DEMOGRAPHICS

- Risk factors include use of communal showers, occupational handling of meat, and immunosuppression. Common warts occur most frequently in children and young adults.
- Anogenital warts are most common in young, sexually active patients. Genital warts are the most common viral sexually transmitted disease in the United States, with up to 79 million Americans carrying the causative virus, and 14 million persons are newly infected each year in the U.S.
- 66% of cervical cancers, 55% of vaginal cancers, 79% of anal cancers, and 62% of oropharyngeal cancers are attributable to HPV types 16 or 18.
- Common warts are longer lasting and more frequent in immunocompromised patients (e.g., lymphoma, AIDS, immunosuppressive drugs).
- Plantar warts occur most frequently at points of maximal pressure (over the heads of the metatarsal bones or on the heels).

PHYSICAL FINDINGS & CLINICAL PRESENTATION

- Common warts (Fig. E1-1017) have an initial appearance of a flesh-colored papule with a rough surface; they subsequently develop a hyperkeratotic appearance with black dots on the surface (thrombosed capillaries). They may be single or multiple and are most common on the hands.
- Warts obscure normal skin lines (important diagnostic feature). Cylindrical projections from the wart may become fused, forming a mosaic pattern.
- Flat warts generally are pink or light yellow, slightly elevated, and often found on the forehead, back of hands, mouth, and beard area. They often occur in lines corresponding to trauma (e.g., a scratch), are often misdiagnosed (particularly when present on the face), and are inappropriately treated with topical corticosteroids.
- Filiform warts have a fingerlike appearance with various projections; they are generally found near the mouth, beard, or periorbital and paranasal regions.
- Plantar warts are slightly raised and have a roughened surface; they may cause pain when walking; as they involute, small hemorrhages (caused by thrombosed capillaries) may be noted.
- Genital warts (Fig. E1-1018) are generally pale pink with several projections and a broad base. They may coalesce in the perineal area to form masses with a cauliflower-like appearance. Intraanal warts occur predominantly in patients who have had receptive anal intercourse, in contrast with perianal warts (Fig. 1-1019), which may occur in men and women without a history of anal sex.
- Genital warts on the cervical epithelium can produce subclinical changes that may be noted on Pap smear or colposcopy.

ETIOLOGY

- HPV infection; >150 types of viral DNA have been identified. Transmission of warts is by direct contact. Approximately 40 different types of HPV are transmitted through sexual contact.
- Genital warts: 90% are caused by HPV types 6 or 11. HPV types 16, 18, 31, 33, and 35 are found occasionally in visible genital warts (usually as coinfections with HPV 6 or 11) and can be associated with foci of high-grade, intraepithelial neoplasia, particularly in persons who are infected with HIV infection. In addition to warts on genital areas, HPV types 6 and 11 have been associated with conjunctival, nasal, oral, and laryngeal warts.

DIAGNOSIS

DIFFERENTIAL DIAGNOSIS

- Molluscum contagiosum
- Condyloma latum
- Acrochordon (skin tags) or seborrheic keratosis
- Epidermal nevi
- Hypertrophic actinic keratosis
- Squamous cell carcinomas
- Acquired digital fibrokeratoma
- Varicella-zoster virus in patients with AIDS
- Recurrent infantile digital fibroma
- Plantar corns (may be mistaken for plantar warts)

WORKUP

- Diagnosis is generally based on clinical findings.
- Suspect lesions should be biopsied.
- The application of 3% to 5% acetic acid, which causes skin color to turn white, has been used by some providers to detect HPV-infected genital mucosa. However, acetic acid application is not a specific test for HPV infection. Therefore, the routine use of this procedure for screening to detect mucosal changes attributed to HPV infection is not recommended.

LABORATORY TESTS

- Screening for cervical cancer with cytology, which is performed by either Pap smear or liquid-based cytology. Screening guidelines recommend starting screening at age 21. Annual cytology is recommended until at least three normal cytology results are obtained.
- Colposcopy with biopsy is recommended in patients with cervical squamous cell changes.

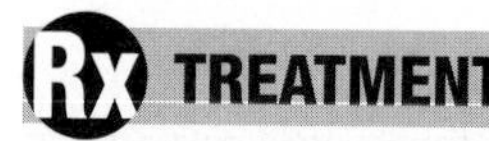

TREATMENT

NONPHARMACOLOGIC THERAPY

- Importance of use of condoms to reduce transmission of genital warts should be emphasized.
- Watchful waiting is an acceptable option in the treatment of nongenital cutaneous warts because many warts will disappear without intervention over time. However, many patients often request treatment because of social stigma or discomfort.

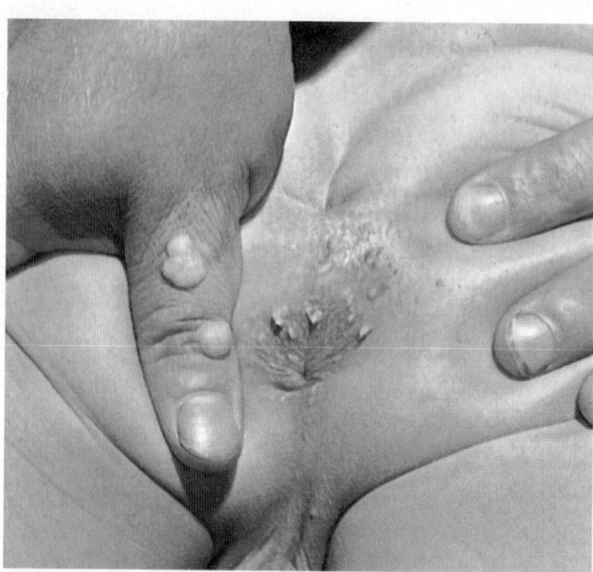

FIGURE 1-1019 Common warts of the hand in a mother and perianal condylomata acuminata in her son. (From Meneghini CL, Bonifaz E: *An atlas of pediatric dermatology,* Chicago, 1986, Year Book Medical Publishers.)

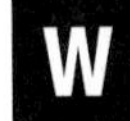

- Plantar warts that are not painful do not need treatment.
- Factors that influence selection of treatment include wart size, wart number, anatomic site of the wart, wart morphology, patient preference, cost of treatment, convenience, adverse effects, and provider experience. Factors that might affect response to therapy include the presence of immunosuppression and compliance with therapy.

GENERAL Rx

- Common warts:
  - Application of topical salicylic acid 17%. Soak area for 5 min in warm water and dry. Apply thin layer once or twice daily for up to 12 wk, avoiding normal skin. Bandage.
  - Liquid nitrogen and electrocautery are also common methods of removal. Cure rates for cryotherapy are 50% to 70% after three to four treatments.
  - Blunt dissection can be used in large lesions or resistant lesions.
  - Duct tape occlusion is also effective for treating common warts. It is cut to cover warts and left in place for 6 days. It is removed after 6 days and the warts are soaked in water and then filed with pumice stones. New tape is applied 12 hr later. This treatment can be repeated until warts resolve.
  - Recalcitrant warts can be treated with injection of *Candida* or mumps skin antigen into the wart every 3 to 4 wk for up to three treatments, photodynamic therapy with aminolevulinic acid, pulsed dye laser, and intralesional bleomycin.
- Filiform warts: surgical removal is necessary.
- Flat warts: generally more difficult to treat.
  - Tretinoin cream applied at bedtime over the involved area for several weeks may be effective.
  - Application of liquid nitrogen.
  - Electrocautery.
  - 5-Fluorouracil cream applied once or twice a day for 3 to 5 wk is also effective. Persistent hyperpigmentation may occur after Efudex use.
- Plantar warts:
  - Salicylic acid therapy (e.g., Occlusal-HP). Soak wart in warm water for 5 min, remove loose tissue, dry. Apply to area, allow to dry, reapply. Use once or twice daily; maximum 12 wk. Use of 40% salicylic acid plasters (Mediplast) is also a safe, nonscarring treatment; it is particularly useful in treating mosaic warts covering a large area.
  - Blunt dissection is also a fast and effective treatment modality.
  - Laser therapy can be used for plantar warts and recurrent warts; however, it leaves open wounds that require 4 to 6 wk to fill with granulation tissue.
  - Interlesional bleomycin is also effective but generally used when all other treatments fail.
- Genital warts:
  - Can be effectively treated with 20% podophyllin resin in compound tincture of benzoin applied with a cotton tip applicator by the treating physician and allowed to air dry. The treatment can be repeated weekly if necessary.
  - Podofilox (Condylox 0.5% gel) is available for application by the patient. Local adverse effects include pain, burning, and inflammation at the site.
  - Cryosurgery with liquid nitrogen delivered with a probe or as a spray is effective for treating smaller genital warts.
  - Carbon dioxide laser can also be used for treating primary or recurrent genital warts (cure rate >90%).
  - Imiquimod cream, 5%, is a patient-applied immune response modifier effective in the treatment of external genital and perianal warts (complete clearing of genital warts in >70% of females and >30% of males in 4 to 16 wk). Sexual contact should be avoided while the cream is on the skin. It is applied 3 times per wk before normal sleeping hours and is left on the skin for 6 to 10 hr.
  - Sinecatechins (Veregen), a botanical drug product, is also effective for treatment of external genital and perianal warts. Formulation is a 15% ointment applied to affected area tid for up to 16 wk.
- Application of trichloroacetic acid or bichloracetic acid 80% to 90% is also effective for external genital warts. A small amount should be applied only to warts and allowed to dry, at which time a white "frosting" develops. This treatment can be repeated weekly if necessary.

DISPOSITION

- Warts can be effectively treated with the previous modalities with complete resolution in the majority of patients; however, the recurrence rate is high.
- Cervical carcinomas and precancerous lesions in women are associated with genital papillomavirus infection.
- Squamous cell anal cancer is also associated with a history of genital warts.

REFERRAL

- Dermatology referral for warts resistant to conservative therapy
- Surgical referral in selected cases
- Sexually transmitted disease counseling for patients with anogenital warts

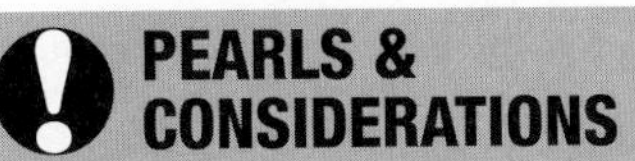

PEARLS & CONSIDERATIONS

COMMENTS

- Subungual and periungual warts are generally more resistant to treatment. Dermatology referral for cryosurgery is recommended in resistant cases.
- Examination of sex partners is not necessary for the management of genital warts because no data indicate that reinfection plays a role.
- Sexually transmitted HPV infections contribute to nearly 20,000 cases of invasive cancer in the U.S. affecting cervix, anus, vagina, penis, and oral cavity. HPV vaccination is available for females aged 11 to 26 and males aged 9 to 26.

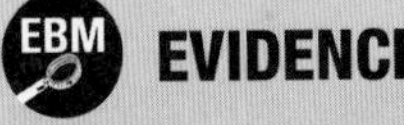

EVIDENCE

available at www.expertconsult.com

SUGGESTED READINGS

available at www.expertconsult.com

RELATED CONTENT

Warts (Patient Information)

AUTHOR: **FRED F. FERRI, M.D.**

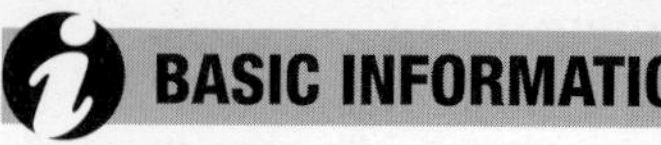

BASIC INFORMATION

DEFINITION

Wernicke syndrome is an acute neuropsychiatric disorder characterized by the classic triad of ophthalmoplegia, ataxia, and disturbances of mental activity or consciousness due to a deficiency of thiamine often associated with chronic alcoholism.

SYNONYMS

Wernicke encephalopathy (WE)
Gayet-Wernicke encephalopathy
Cerebral beriberi
Wernicke's superior hemorrhagic polioencephalitis

ICD-9CM CODES

265.1 Wernicke's encephalopathy, disease, or syndrome (superior hemorrhagic polioencephalitis)
294.0 Wernicke-Korsakoff's syndrome or psychosis, non-alcoholic
291.1 Wernicke-Korsakoff's syndrome or psychosis, alcoholic

ICD-10CM CODES

E51.2 Wernicke encephalopathy
E51.8 Other manifestations of thiamine deficiency
F04 Amnestic disorder due to known physiological condition
F10.96 Alcohol use, unspecified with alcohol-induced persisting amnestic disorder

EPIDEMIOLOGY & DEMOGRAPHICS

- A higher prevalence of WE noted on autopsy studies (0.8% to 2.8%) compared to clinical studies (0.04% to 0.13%)
  - WE lesions on autopsy of alcohol abusers: 12.5%
  - WE lesions on autopsy patients with alcohol-related deaths: 29% to 59%

PREDOMINANT SEX AND AGE:

- Male-to-female ratio of 1.7 to 1
- Estimated mortality: 17%

GENETICS:

- Biochemical studies in fibroblasts from patients with WE show thiamine-dependent enzyme, transketolase, to have a decreased affinity for thiamine pyrophosphate.
- Thiamine deficiency causes wet (cardiovascular) beriberi more commonly in the Asian population and dry beriberi (polyneuropathy and WE) in the European population.

RISK FACTORS:

- Alcohol abuse/misuse
- Diet
  - Malnutrition/unbalanced nutrition/infant formulas
  - Intravenous hyperalimentation without thiamine supplementation
  - Magnesium depletion–cofactor required by enzymes: transketolase and thiamine pyrophosphokinase
- Gastrointestinal disorders including recurrent vomiting or chronic diarrhea such as hyperemesis gravidarum
- Gastrointestinal surgical procedures (gastrointestinal resection) that cause malabsorption secondary to reduced surface area of gastric and duodenal mucosa such as bariatric surgery
- Systemic cancers
  - Most common underlying disorder onset for WE in children
  - Consumption of thiamine by fast-growing neoplastic cells
- Chemical compounds/drugs or chemotherapeutic treatments
- Systemic diseases
  - Peritoneal or hemodialysis
  - HIV/AIDS
  - Prolonged infectious febrile disease
  - Hypermetabolic states
  - Thyrotoxicosis

PHYSICAL FINDINGS & CLINICAL PRESENTATION

- WE is a clinical diagnosis with a classic triad of ophthalmoplegia, ataxia, and disturbances of mental activity or consciousness—although this triad is only seen in 16% of all patients.
- Eye movement abnormalities include nystagmus, external rectus palsies, and reduced conjugate gaze.
- Ophthalmoscopic findings include swelling of the optic discs and retinal hemorrhages.
- Clinical suspicion must remain high in patients with risk factors listed above, especially in the setting of poor nutrition.
- Diagnosis is confirmed by improvement of neurologic signs after administration of parenteral thiamine.
- Labs and radiologic studies may aid diagnosis, but these should not delay a trial of parenteral administration of thiamine.

ETIOLOGY

- The biologically active form of vitamin B_1, thiamine pyrophosphate (TP), a coenzyme for several important biochemical pathways involved in energy production, lipid metabolism, and production of amino acids and glucose-derived neurotransmitters.
- Body's reserve for thiamine is sufficient for 18 days.
- Malnutrition for 2 to 3 wk or a diet disproportionately high in carbohydrates and low in thiamine intake can lead to an impaired function of enzymes requiring TP.

DIAGNOSIS

DIFFERENTIAL DIAGNOSIS

- Other acute encephalopathies (Table 1-508)
- Paramedian thalamic infarction
- Ventriculoencephalitis, paraneoplastic encephalitis, herpes simplex encephalitis
- Miller-Fisher syndrome
- Primary cerebral lymphoma
- Multiple sclerosis, Behcet's disease, Leigh's disease
- Variant Creutzfeldt-Jakob disease

WORKUP

- WE is a clinical diagnosis based on the triad of features listed above.
- Laboratory tests and radiologic studies as listed below may be obtained to confirm diagnosis.

LABORATORY TESTS

- Blood thiamine concentration.
- Functional measurement of erythrocyte thiamine transketolase (ETKA) before and after administration of parenteral thiamine. A diagnosis may be confirmed if ETKA is low followed by a 25% increase after thiamine supplementation.
- High-performance liquid chromatography for assessment of thiamine, thiamine mono- and di-phosphate in human erythrocytes.
- Serum magnesium concentration (depletion of magnesium may mimic features of WE).

IMAGING STUDIES

MRI of brain may show bilaterally symmetric increase in T2 signal at the paraventricular regions of the thalamus and mammillary bodies. Other areas include hypothalamus, periaqueductal region, floor of the fourth ventricle, and midline cerebellum.

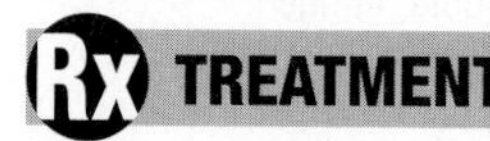

TREATMENT

ACUTE GENERAL Rx

- Treatment should be initiated in all patients with clinical suspicion of WE. Thiamine supplementation should precede glucose administration in all patients at risk for WE.
- Alcoholics with WE: treat with 500 mg of thiamine hydrochloride (dissolved in 100 ml of normal saline) infused intravenously over 30 min, 3 times daily for 2 to 3 days.

TABLE 1-508 Acute and Subacute Presentation of Nutritional Deficiency Syndromes

Syndrome	Clinical Setting
Wernicke-Korsakoff syndrome	Administration of intravenous glucose to a thiamine-deficient alcoholic patient
Wernicke-Korsakoff syndrome	Intractable vomiting due to hyperemesis gravidarum or gastroplasty
Postgastroplasty neuropathy	Intractable vomiting and severe weight loss in patients following weight reduction surgical procedures
Vitamin B_{12} myeloneuropathy	Nitrous oxide administration in cobalamin-deficient patients
Central pontine myelinolysis	Sudden change in tissue osmolarity in critically ill patients or alcoholics

From Goetz CG: *Textbook of clinical neurology*, ed 3, Philadelphia, 2007, Saunders.

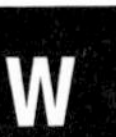

- If a response is observed, continue with 250 mg of thiamine hydrochloride intravenously or intramuscularly daily until clinical improvement ceases.
- Nonalcoholics with WE: treat with 200 mg of thiamine hydrochloride (dissolved in 100 ml of normal saline) infused intravenously over 30 min, 3 times daily for 2 to 3 days.
- Parenteral side effects may include generalized pruritus, transient local irritation, or rarely, anaphylactic or anaphylactoid reactions.
- Parenteral magnesium must be infused concurrently with thiamine.

CHRONIC Rx

Recommended oral dose after treatment for WE: thiamine 30 to 100 mg twice daily

DISPOSITION

- If prompt treatment with thiamine is not administered during the potential reversible stages of WE, Korsakoff's syndrome may develop consisting of a typical pattern of memory loss emerging after the acute global confusional state of WE resolves.
- Approximately 80% who survive WE develop Korsakoff's syndrome.

REFERRAL

In cases of altered mental status, ophthalmoplegia or ataxia of gait, consider neurology consultation. Treatment should be initiated as soon as WE is suspected.

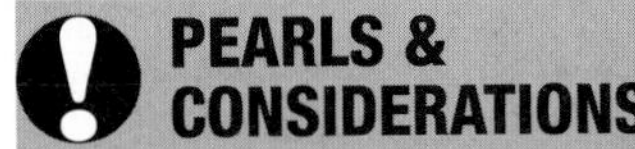

PEARLS & CONSIDERATIONS

COMMENTS

- WE should be suspected in all patients with poor nutrition.
- WE is a clinical diagnosis composed of a triad of confusion, ataxia, and ophthalmoplegia.
- Thiamine infusion should be initiated upon clinical suspicion of WE.
- Thiamine infusion should precede infusion of fluids with glucose in all patients with poor nutrition or clinical suspicion of WE.

PREVENTION

- Prophylactic treatment for patient with severe alcohol withdrawal, poor nourishment, or signs of malnutrition: thiamine 250 mg intramuscular daily for 3 to 5 days.
- In individuals susceptible to WE, 100 mg of intravenous thiamine should precede any glucose infusion.
- Recommended daily dose of thiamine for an average, healthy adult: 1.4 mg or 0.5 mg per 1000 kcal of carbohydrates consumed.
- Higher dose recommended for children, in critically ill conditions, and during pregnancy and lactation.

PATIENT & FAMILY EDUCATION

In cases of known alcohol abuse or severe illness, the patient and family should be counseled on the importance of proper nutrition, including vitamin supplementation.

SUGGESTED READINGS

available at www.expertconsult.com

RELATED CONTENT

Alcoholism (Related Key Topic)
Korsakoff's Psychosis (Related Key Topic)
Vitamin Deficiency (Related Key Topic)

AUTHOR: **D. BRANDON BURTIS, D.O.**

BASIC INFORMATION

DEFINITION

West Nile virus (WNV) infection is an illness affecting the central nervous system (CNS) caused by the mosquito-borne WNV.

SYNONYMS

West Nile virus fever
West Nile virus encephalitis
Neuroinvasive West Nile virus infection
Nonneuroinvasive West Nile virus infection

ICD-9CM CODES
066.4 West Nile virus infection
ICD-10CM CODES
A92.30 West Nile virus infection, unspecified

EPIDEMIOLOGY & DEMOGRAPHICS

- Before 1999, WNV infection was confined to areas in the Middle East, with occasional outbreaks in Europe. The infection began being diagnosed in the Western Hemisphere in 1999. First seen in the northeast and mid-Atlantic states, WNV virus infection has spread steadily each year to new regions of the U.S., with a general westward migration pattern. In 2003, a record number of cases were reported from the U.S., with over 7000 cases reported, resulting in several hundred deaths. Most deaths occur in elderly patients with WNV encephalitis. In 2003, Illinois, Ohio, Michigan, and Louisiana were hardest hit. Since 2004 the incidence of WNV infection diminished gradually as it spread to the western states. Human cases of WNV infection have now been reported across all the contiguous continental U.S. (sparing only Hawaii and Alaska). Since 1999, an estimated 780,000 cases of WNV infection have occurred in the US, with 16,196 cases of neuroinvasive disease and 1549 deaths attributable to WNV. The virus has now become endemic in North America and is likely to remain for decades to come.
- The virus is carried by a number of species of birds, as well as horses and several other animals. It is transmitted to humans through the bite of an infected mosquito. For this reason, WNV infection is seen primarily from mid-summer to mid-autumn, the period of maximum mosquito intensity.
- The majority of severe cases have been reported among individuals >50 yr of age. There is no gender predilection. Certain HLA haplotypes appear to predispose to severe disease (e.g., HLA-A68 and HLA-C08).
- Person-to-person transmission is fortunately rare but has been reported to occur by blood transfusion, organ transplantation, breast-feeding, and perhaps perinatal transmission; the blood supply is now routinely tested by nucleic acid testing methods to reduce the risk of transmission-acquired WNV in the U.S.

PHYSICAL FINDINGS & CLINICAL PRESENTATION

- Less than 20% of infected individuals develop symptomatic disease. The initial phase of illness is nonspecific, with abrupt onset of fever (West Nile fever) accompanied by malaise, eye pain, anorexia, headache, and, occasionally, rash and lymphadenopathy. Less commonly, myocarditis, hepatitis, or pancreatitis may occur.
- Encephalitis is the most common neurologic manifestation of West Nile virus infection. Aseptic meningitis may also occur.
- In approximately 1 in 150 cases, especially among elderly patients, severe neurologic sequelae will occur (West Nile neuroinvasive disease [WNND]). Most common among these are ataxia, cranial nerve palsies, optic neuritis, seizures, myelitis, and polyradiculitis.

ETIOLOGY

The WNV is a member of the flavivirus group, along with the yellow fever, dengue, St. Louis, and Japanese encephalitis viruses. It has a large reservoir in nature, infecting many species of birds, as well as certain mammals, and is spread to humans primarily by the bite of an infected *Culex* mosquito or other various species of mosquito with a peak incidence in the late summer and early fall. Neurologic disease is caused by direct invasion of the CNS.

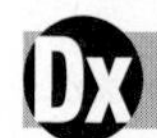

DIAGNOSIS

DIFFERENTIAL DIAGNOSIS

- Meningitis or encephalitis caused by more common viruses (e.g., enteroviruses, herpes simplex)
- Bacterial meningitis
- Vasculitis
- Fungal meningitis (e.g., cryptococcal infection)
- Tuberculous meningitis

LABORATORY TESTS

- CBC, electrolytes (hyponatremia common)
- Spinal tap and CSF examination: typically demonstrates lymphocytic pleocytosis with normal level of glucose and elevated level of protein
- CSF WNV IgM antibody level: detection in symptomatic patients is diagnostic of West Nile neuronivasive disease. The antibody can be detected within 9 days of fever onset and can persist for several months. There can be rare false-positive results in people recently vaccinated against Japanese encephalitis or yellow fever viruses.

IMAGING STUDIES

MRI of the brain to exclude mass lesions and cerebral edema

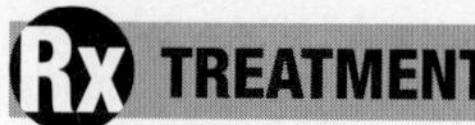

TREATMENT

NONPHARMACOLOGIC THERAPY

Hospitalization, IV hydration, ventilator support may be necessary.

ACUTE GENERAL Rx

No specific therapy has been established in clinical trials. Ribavirin and interferon alfa-2b have been shown to have in vitro activity against the virus. IV immunoglobulin (IVIG) from convalescent patient plasma is under study but no controlled trials have been reported as yet.

CHRONIC Rx

Chronic rehabilitation therapy usually necessary for patients with severe neurologic impairment. Mental status defects following WNV neuroinvasive disease appear to be more common and severe than initially recognized.

DISPOSITION

Chronic rehabilitation as needed following recovery from acute infection. Physical and mental outcome measures seem to normalize within approximately 1 yr in patients with WNV. The presence of preexisting comorbid conditions is associated with longer recovery.

REFERRAL

- Infectious disease consultant
- Public health authorities

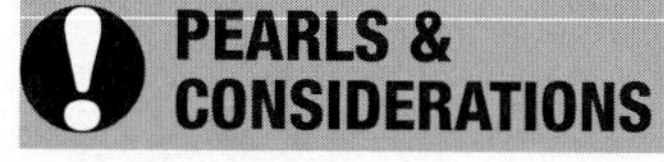

PEARLS & CONSIDERATIONS

COMMENTS

- Diagnosis requires a high index of suspicion, because disease course may be nonspecific and may mimic other, more common disorders.
- Specific laboratory diagnostic studies are available only through public-health laboratories.

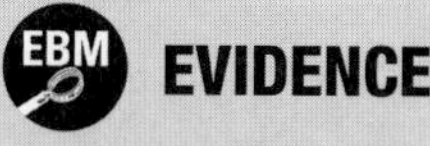

EVIDENCE

available at www.expertconsult.com

SUGGESTED READINGS

available at www.expertconsult.com

RELATED CONTENT

West Nile Virus Infection (Patient Information)

AUTHOR: **STEVEN M. OPAL, M.D.**

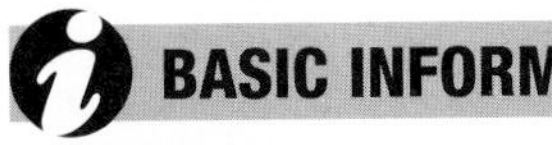

BASIC INFORMATION

DEFINITION

Whiplash refers to a hyperextension injury to the neck, often the result of being struck from behind by a fast-moving vehicle.

SYNONYMS

Acceleration flexion-extension neck injury

ICD-9CM CODES
847.0 Whiplash injury or syndrome
ICD-10CM CODES
S13.4 Sprain and strain of cervical spine

EPIDEMIOLOGY & DEMOGRAPHICS

- Whiplash occurs in more than 1 million people each year.
- Most injuries (40%) are the result of rear-end motor vehicle accidents.
- Whiplash occurs at all ages, in both sexes, and at all socioeconomic levels.
- Incidence is 4 per 1000 persons and is higher in women than men.
- Nearly 50% of patients with whiplash seek legal advice.
- Whiplash is also seen in shaken baby syndrome.

PHYSICAL FINDINGS & CLINICAL PRESENTATION

- Most present with a history of being involved in a motor vehicle accident and being rear-ended by another vehicle
- Pain not present initially but usually develops hr to a few days later
- Neck tightness and stiffness
- Occipital headache
- Shoulder, arm, and back pain
- Numbness in the arms
- Tinnitus
- Temporomandibular joint (TMJ) pain
- Dysphagia (retropharyngeal hematoma)
- Decreased range of motion of the neck
- Depressive symptoms

ETIOLOGY

- The mechanism of injury is the result of the sudden acceleration of the body forward, forcing the neck to hyperextend backward, causing injury to ligaments, muscles, bone, and/or intervertebral disk. At the end of the accident the head is thrust forward in a flexion position, sometimes causing injury to the cervical spine: C5-C6-C7.
- Motor vehicle accidents, trauma from falls, contact sports, physical abuse, and altercations are all possible causes of whiplash.
- The incidence of whiplash injury following polytrauma is low.
- Low-velocity crashes constitute a major cause of whiplash injury.

Dx DIAGNOSIS

DIFFERENTIAL DIAGNOSIS

- Osteoarthritis
- Cervical disk disease
- Fibrositis
- Neuritis
- Torticollis
- Spinal cord tumor
- TMJ syndrome
- Tension headache
- Migraine headache

WORKUP

Any patient who presents with symptoms of whiplash and musculoskeletal or neurologic signs merits a workup to exclude cervical spine fractures or herniated disk disease.

LABORATORY TESTS

Laboratory studies are not helpful.

IMAGING STUDIES

- Plain C-spine films (anteroposterior, lateral, and odontoid views)
- Flexion/extension x-rays
- CT scan to exclude fracture
- MRI as alternative or in addition to CT in selected cases

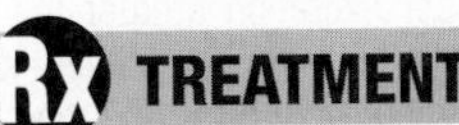

TREATMENT

NONPHARMACOLOGIC THERAPY

- Soft cervical collar for no longer than 72 hr
- Moist heat 15 to 20 min four to six times per day.
- Continue with usual activities.

TABLE 1-509 Factors Associated with Persistent and Severe Whiplash Injuries

Severe Whiplash Injury
High-speed injury
Intense and rapid onset of pain
Severe restriction of movement at presentation
Abnormal neurology
Bony injuries
Persistent Whiplash Injury
High-speed injury
Intense and rapid onset of pain
Severe restriction of movement at presentation
Abnormal neurology
Bony injuries
Increasing age
Upper limb paresthesias
Cervical spondylosis

From Carr A, Hamilton W: *Orthopedics in primary care,* ed 2, Philadelphia, 2005, Saunders.

ACUTE GENERAL Rx

- Analgesics
  1. NSAIDS
  2. Acetaminophen up to a maximum of 1 g tid
- Muscle relaxants (short-term use)

CHRONIC Rx

NSAIDs and Tylenol can be used on a long-term basis, as needed.

DISPOSITION

- Most patients recover from the acute whiplash injury within weeks.
- Factors associated with persistent and severe whiplash injuries are described in Table 1-509.
- 20% to 40% may develop chronic whiplash syndrome (symptoms of headache, neck pain, and psychiatric complaints that persist for 6 mo).
- Older age, female gender, lawyer involvement, and work status (employed at time of entry to the clinic) were found to be prognostic factors associated with a negative outcome.

REFERRAL

Orthopedic, physical therapy

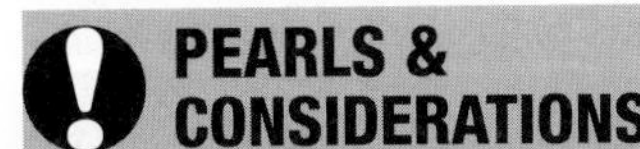

PEARLS & CONSIDERATIONS

- Nearly one third of all personal injury cases involve cervical injuries.
- There is no dose-response relationship between trauma severity and incidence of whiplash injury.

COMMENTS

The entity of chronic whiplash syndrome remains elusive. Some authorities argue that financial motivation is a factor leading to persistent neck symptoms. Other studies do not substantiate this, showing a true chronic injury to the soft tissues of the neck.

SUGGESTED READINGS

available at www.expertconsult.com

RELATED CONTENT

Whiplash (Patient Information)

AUTHOR: **JORGE A. VILLAFUERTE, M.D.**

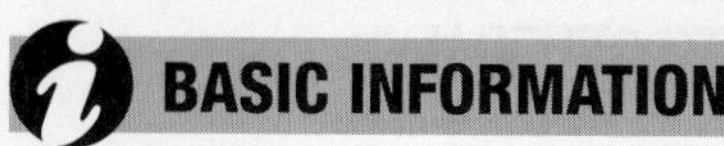

BASIC INFORMATION

DEFINITION

Wilson's disease is an autosomal recessive disorder of copper transport with inadequate biliary copper excretion, leading to an accumulation of the metal in liver, brain, kidneys, and corneas.

SYNONYMS

Progressive hepatolenticular degeneration

ICD-9CM CODES
275.1 Wilson's disease
ICD-10CM CODES
E83.00 Disorder of copper metabolism

EPIDEMIOLOGY & DEMOGRAPHICS

PREVALENCE: One case in 30,000
PREDOMINANT SEX: Affects men and women equally (autosomal recessive gene)
ONSET OF SYMPTOMS: Ages 3 to 40 yr

PHYSICAL FINDINGS & CLINICAL PRESENTATION

Hepatic presentation:
- Acute hepatitis with malaise, anorexia, nausea, jaundice, elevated transaminase, prolonged prothrombin time; rarely fulminant hepatic failure
- Chronic active (or autoimmune) hepatitis with fatigue, malaise, rashes, arthralgia, elevated transaminase, elevated serum immunoglobulin G, positive antinuclear antibody and antismooth muscle antibody
- Chronic liver disease/cirrhosis with hepatosplenomegaly, ascites, low serum albumin, prolonged prothrombin time, portal hypertension

Neurologic presentation:
- Movement disorder: tremors, ataxia
- Spastic dystonia: masklike facies, rigidity, gait disturbance, dysarthria, drooling, dysphagia
- The most common neurologic presentation in a young adult is parkinsonism.

Ophthalmic:
- Kayser-Fleischer ring; indicates copper deposition in the Descemet's membrane of the iris
- Sunflower cataracts

Psychiatric presentation:
- Depression, obsessive-compulsive disorder, psychopathic behaviors, neuroses

Other organs:
- Hemolytic anemia
- Renal disease (i.e., Fanconi's syndrome with hematuria, phosphaturia, renal tubular acidosis, vitamin D–resistant rickets)
- Cardiomyopathy
- Arthritis
- Hypoparathyroidism
- Hypogonadism

PHYSICAL FINDINGS:
- Ocular: the Kayser-Fleischer ring is a gold-yellow ring seen at the periphery of the iris (Fig. 1-1020); It is present in virtually all persons with neurologic involvement. These should be sought with slit-lamp examination by a skilled examiner.
- Stigmata of acute or chronic liver disease.
- Neurologic abnormalities: see previous.

ETIOLOGY & PATHOGENESIS

- Dietary copper is transported from the intestine to the liver, where normally it is metabolized into ceruloplasmin. In Wilson's disease, defective incorporation of copper into ceruloplasmin and a decrease of biliary copper excretion lead to accumulation of this mineral.
- The disease results from an autosomal recessive inborn error of metabolism caused by a mutation of the copper P-type adenosine triphosphatase encoded on chromosome *13q14.3.*

DIAGNOSIS

DIFFERENTIAL DIAGNOSIS

- Hereditary hypoceruloplasminemia
- Menkes' disease
- Consider the diagnosis of Wilson's disease in all cases of acute or chronic liver disease for which another cause has not been established.
- Consider Wilson's disease in patients with movement disorders or dystonia even without symptomatic liver disease.

LABORATORY TESTS

- Low serum ceruloplasmin level (<200 mg/L) present in 95% of affected patients
- 24-hr urinary copper excretion greater than 100 mcg (normal <30 mcg); increases to greater than 1200 mcg/24 hr after 500 mg of D-penicillamine (normal <500 mcg/24 hr)
- Low serum copper (<65 mcg/L)
- Abnormal liver function tests (note that aspartate aminotransferase may be higher than alanine aminotransferase)
- Low serum uric acid and phosphorus
- Abnormal urinalysis (hematuria)

BIOPSY

- Early:
  - Steatosis, focal necrosis, glycogenated hepatocyte nuclei
  - May reveal inflammation and piecemeal necrosis
- Late: cirrhosis
- Hepatic copper content (>250 mcg/g of dry weight) (normal is 20 to 50 mcg) gold standard for diagnosis
- Histochemical confirmation of excess copper can be helpful in diagnosis, but if absent, does not exclude Wilson's disease. The lack of immunoreactivity to copper-binding protein can occur because of the diffuse presence of copper in the cytoplasm and because of the assay's low sensitivity. Rhodamine and rubeanic acid stains can show dense granular lysosomal copper deposition in hepatocytes at the stage of cirrhotic nodular regeneration.

TREATMENT

- Penicillamine: (chelator therapy)
  - 0.75 to 1.5 g/day divided bid (with pyridoxine 25 mg/day)
  - Monitor complete blood count (CBC) and urinalysis weekly
- Trientine (triethylene tetramine): (chelator therapy)
  - 1 to 2 g/day divided tid
  - Monitor CBC
- Zinc: (inhibits intestinal copper absorption)
  - 50 mg tid
  - Monitor zinc level
- Ammonium tetrathiomolybdate for neurologic symptoms
- Antioxidants
- Liver transplantation (for severe hepatic failure unresponsive to chelation); liver transplantation corrects the underlying pathophysiology and can be lifesaving

PROGNOSIS

Good with early chelation treatment

REFERRAL

To gastroenterologist, neurologist

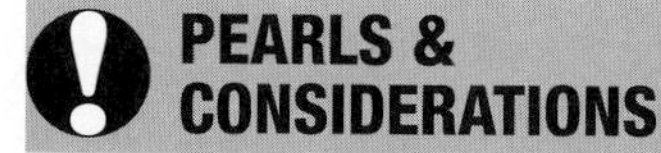

PEARLS & CONSIDERATIONS

COMMENTS

Family screening of first-degree relatives must be undertaken. Genetic diagnosis is also useful in patients with indeterminate clinical and biochemical features.

SUGGESTED READINGS

available at www.expertconsult.com

RELATED CONTENT

Wilson's Disease (Patient Information)

AUTHOR: **FRED F. FERRI, M.D.**

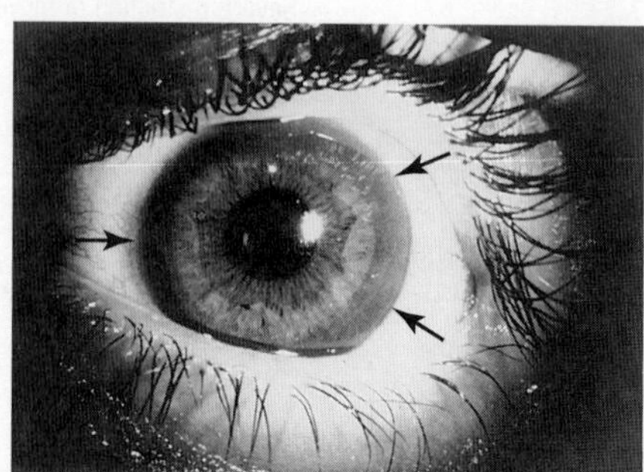

FIGURE 1-1020 Deposition of copper (Kayser-Fleischer ring, arrows) in the periphery of the cornea as seen in hepatolenticular degeneration (Wilson's disease). (From Haines DE: *Fundamental neuroscience for basic and clinical applications,* ed 3, Philadelphia, 2005, Churchill Livingstone.)

BASIC INFORMATION

DEFINITION

Wolff-Parkinson-White (WPW) syndrome is defined as the presence of preexcitation of the ventricles of the heart due to an abnormal electrical communication from the atria to the ventricles through an accessory pathway. Patients with WPW syndrome have both ventricular preexcitation and arrhythmias, which may be atrial fibrillation (AF), atrioventricular (AV) reentrant tachycardia, or both. Patients with WPW pattern have characteristic ECG findings of preexcitation: short PR interval <120 ms and the presence of a delta wave but no subjective or objective evidence of arrhythmia.

SYNONYMS

Preexcitation syndrome
WPW

ICD-9CM CODES
426.7 Wolff-Parkinson-White syndrome
ICD-10CM CODES
I45.6 Pre-excitation syndrome

EPIDEMIOLOGY & DEMOGRAPHICS

- The prevalence of a WPW pattern on the surface ECG is 0.15% to 0.25% in the general population. The prevalence is increased to 0.55% in first-degree relatives of affected patients.
- In a study of a presumed healthy population of more than 20,000 patients, the WPW pattern was recognized in 0.25%. Of these patients, only 1.8% had documented arrhythmias that were consistent with the WPW syndrome.
- The prevalence of WPW is higher among males and decreases with age.
- Most patients with WPW syndrome have structurally normal hearts, but associations with mitral valve prolapse, cardiomyopathies, and Ebstein's anomaly have been reported.

PHYSICAL FINDINGS & CLINICAL PRESENTATION

- The physical examination may be entirely normal.
- Symptoms are typically related to tachyarrhythmias, including the following:
  - Palpitations, anxiety dyspnea, chest pain or tightness
  - Syncope or near syncope
  - Sudden cardiac death (rarely; <0.4%)
- Over time, 25% of cases become asymptomatic and remain symptom free if past age 40.
- The type of tachycardia can be any of the following:
  - Supraventricular tachycardia: AV reentrant tachycardia (AVRT) most common arrhythmia, further classified as orthodromic (narrow complex and occurs in 70% of symptomatic patients), or antidromic (wide complex, in 4%-5% of patients)
  - AF (~10% to 38%), the second most common tachycardia, can be complicated by a very rapid ventricular response via conduction over the accessory pathway (AP), which can lead to ventricular fibrillation and sudden death. This risk is dependent on the antegrade refractory period of AP during AF.
  - Atrial flutter (<5%)
- Presence of WPW can be associated with other congenital cardiac defects.
- Incidence of sudden cardiac death in WPW syndrome is estimated at 0.15%-0.39% per patient per yr. The risk of death is lower in asymptomatic patients.
- Left free wall accessory pathways are most common, followed by posteroseptal, right free wall, and anteroseptal locations.

ETIOLOGY & PATHOGENESIS

- The existence of an accessory pathway allows for conduction from the atria to the ventricles while bypassing the AV node.
- If the accessory pathway is capable of anterograde conduction, two parallel routes of AV conduction are possible: one is subject to delay through the AV node, and the other occurs without delay through the accessory pathway and results in preexcitation of the ventricle. The resulting QRS complex is a fusion beat, as a portion of the ventricle is activated via the accessory pathway giving rise to the delta wave, and the remainder of the ventricle is activated by the normal activation pathway (Fig. 1-1021).
- Tachycardias occur when conduction is anterograde in one pathway (usually the normal AV pathway) and retrograde in the other (usually the accessory pathway) as a result of different refractory periods. This is usually initiated by a premature atrial or ventricular depolarization. Some patients (~5% to 10%) with WPW syndrome have multiple accessory pathways.

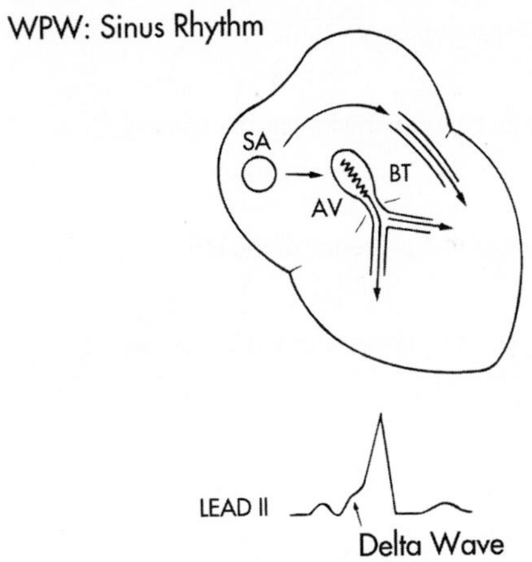

FIGURE 1-1021 With Wolff-Parkinson-White *(WPW)* syndrome, an abnormal accessory conduction pathway called a *bypass tract (BT)* connects the atria and the ventricles. (From Goldberger AL [ed]: *Clinical electrocardiography: a simplified approach,* ed 6, St Louis, 1999, Mosby.)

- Because of the involvement of usually a significant portion of the ventricle, the tachycardia circuit can be long and thus AVRT is known as a long R-P tachycardia, as opposed to AVNRT, which is usually a short R-P tachycardia.

DIAGNOSIS

- Three basic features characterize the ECG abnormalities associated with WPW pattern (Fig. 1-1022):
  1. PR interval <120 msec
  2. QRS complex >120 msec with a slurred, slowly rising onset of QRS in some leads (delta wave) and a normal terminal QRS portion
  3. Secondary ST-T wave changes directed in an opposite direction to the major delta and QRS vectors.
- ECG patterns with abnormal QRS complexes and ST and T changes can mask or mimic myocardial infarction, bundle branch block, or ventricular hypertrophy.
- Most commonly seen tachycardia is characterized by a normal QRS with a regular rate of 150-250 bpm. Onset and termination are abrupt.
- Variants of preexcitation:
  - Lown-Ganong-Levine syndrome: fibers from the atrium to the His bundle bypass the physiologic delay of the AV node (atriohisian pathways) with a short PR interval and a normal QRS complex on ECG (no delta wave)
  - Atriofascicular accessory pathways: duplication of the AV node and distal conducting system with normal baseline ECG
  - The only way to be certain of the accessory pathways' properties and propensity for rapid conduction is via an electrophysiology (EP) study.

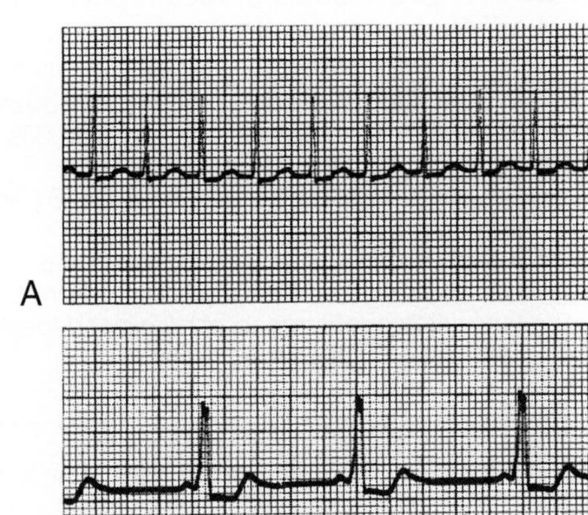

FIGURE 1-1022 A, Supraventricular tachycardia in a child with Wolff-Parkinson-White syndrome. Note the normal QRS complexes during the tachycardia. **B,** Later, the typical features of Wolff-Parkinson-White syndrome are apparent: a short P-R interval, a delta wave, and a wide QRS. (From Behrman RE: *Nelson textbook of pediatrics,* ed 18, Philadelphia, 2007, Saunders.)

RISK STRATIFICATION

- Intermittent loss or appearance of preexcitation on a beat-to-beat basis is indicative of lower risk, assessed with Holter monitoring or with exercise testing. The loss of preexcitation after administration of the antiarrhythmic drug procainamide has also been used to indicate a low-risk subgroup
- In patients with a persistent preexcitation pattern, EP study is the procedure of choice for risk stratification by inducing AF, indicating high risk.

Rx TREATMENT

- Goals of electrophysiologic evaluation in patients with WPW syndrome are described in Box 1-102.
- Urgent cardioversion, for an acute tachycardia episode with hemodynamic instability
- Stable patients treated medically
  - Narrow QRS width tachycardias:
    1. Carotid sinus massage or vagal maneuvers
    2. Atrial pacing (transvenous or transesophageal)
    3. Adenosine and verapamil are usually contraindicated given the prevalence of underlying atrial fibrillation in this population and the risk of causing ventricular fibrillation by direct ventricular stimulation through the accessory pathway when the AV node is completely blocked.
    4. AF is potentially life threatening
  - Wide QRS complex tachycardias (WCTs):
    1. Because atrial arrhythmias (Aflutter/AF) with antegrade conduction down an AP are *not* AV node dependent, AV nodal blocking therapies are ineffective and potentially dangerous.
    2. Beta-blockers, calcium channel blockers, digoxin, and adenosine should be avoided. Can try procainamide. If tachycardia persists, synchronized DCCV is the treatment of choice.
- Long-term management:
  - Priority of therapy:
    1. Asymptomatic: no therapy unless high risk or family history of sudden death, competitive athletes, high-risk occupation (pilots)
    2. Symptomatic, prior AF, aborted sudden death: further study/therapy
  - Medical therapy (asymptomatic high risk):
    1. Single drug: amiodarone, sotalol, flecainide, propafenone
    2. Combination AV nodal blocker (beta-blocker/calcium channel blocker) and drugs that exclusively work on AP (class IA arrhythmics [quinidine, procainamide, and disopyramide])
  - Recommendations for radiofrequency catheter ablation of accessory pathways:
    1. Class 1: patients with symptomatic AVRT and AF (or other atrial tachyarrhythmia) with rapid ventricular rates (RVR) via the AP when the tachycardia is drug resistant or the patient is intolerant or does not desire long-term drug therapy.
- For patients with a rapid ventricular response with hemodynamic compromise, urgent electrical cardioversion is warranted.
- Digitalis should not be used as a single drug in patients who have atrial flutter or AF, because it can reduce refractoriness in the accessory pathway and accelerate the tachycardia.
- Drug therapy for the chronic prevention of narrow complex regular tachyarrhythmias includes class IC antiarrhythmics, β-blockers, calcium channel blockers, amiodarone, or sotalol.
- For the treatment of AF in patients with WPW, the administration of AV nodal–blocking agents may not slow the ventricular rate, because the accessory pathways capable of rapid conduction do not respond to AV-blocking agents. Procainamide is the drug of choice for controlling the ventricular rate and restoring the sinus rhythm in patients with WPW who have AF.
- For long-term therapy to prevent recurrence, radiofrequency catheter ablation has become the first-line therapy for most patients. When medical therapy fails or patients are drug intolerant, or for those patients who do not wish to take drugs, or cannot tolerate the tachyarrythmias, radiofrequency ablation should be performed (class 1 indication).
- Most patients with asymptomatic preexcitation have a good prognosis; cardiac arrest is rarely the first manifestation of the disease. Usually no intervention or EP testing is indicated, as the 2% risk of catheter ablation is usually not justified considering the low risk of sudden cardiac death in asymptomatic individuals.

BOX 1-102 Goals of Electrophysiologic Evaluation in Patients with Wolff-Parkinson-White Syndrome

- Confirmation of the presence of an atrioventricular bypass tract (BT)
- Evaluation for the presence of multiple BTs
- Localization of the BT(s)
- Evaluation of the refractoriness of the BT and its implications for life-threatening arrhythmias
- Induction and evaluation of tachycardias
- Demonstration of the BT role in the tachycardia
- Evaluation of other tachycardias not dependent on the presence of the BT
- Termination of the tachycardias

From Issa Z et al: *Clinical arrhythmology and electrophysiology,* ed 2, Philadelphia, 2012, Saunders.

SUGGESTED READINGS

available at www.expertconsult.com

RELATED CONTENT

Wolff-Parkinson-White Syndrome (Patient Information)

AUTHOR: **BARRY FINE, M.D., PH.D.**

Differential Diagnosis*

*Please note that the implementation of the ICD-10CM codes has been delayed until at least 2015; therefore, for billing purposes please use the ICD-9CM codes until the ICD-10CM codes are officially implemented.

ABDOMINAL DISTENTION

ICD-9CM # 787.3
ICD-10CM # R14.0 Abdominal Distension (Gaseous)

NONMECHANICAL OBSTRUCTION

Excessive intraluminal gas.
Intraabdominal infection.
Trauma.
Retroperitoneal irritation (renal colic, neoplasms, infections, hemorrhage).
Vascular insufficiency (thrombosis, embolism).
Mechanical ventilation.
Extraabdominal infection (sepsis, pneumonia, empyema, osteomyelitis of spine).
Metabolic/toxic abnormalities (hypokalemia, uremia, lead poisoning).
Chemical irritation (perforated ulcer, bile, pancreatitis).
Peritoneal inflammation.
Severe pain, pain medications.

MECHANICAL OBSTRUCTION

Neoplasm (intraluminal, extraluminal).
Adhesions, endometriosis.
Infection (intraabdominal abscess, diverticulitis).
Gallstones.
Foreign body, bezoars.
Pregnancy.
Hernias.
Volvulus.
Stenosis at surgical anastomosis, radiation stenosis.
Fecaliths.
Inflammatory bowel disease.
Gastric outlet obstruction.
Hematoma.
Other: parasites, superior mesenteric artery (SMA) syndrome, pneumatosis intestinalis, annular pancreas, Hirschsprung's disease, intussusception, meconium.

ABDOMINAL PAIN, ADOLESCENCE[26]

ICD-9CM # 789.67
ICD-10CM # R10.817 Generalized Abdominal Tenderness
R10.827 Generalized Rebound Abdominal Tenderness

Acute gastroenteritis.
Irritable bowel syndrome (IBS).
Anxiety.
Mittelschmerz.
Appendicitis.
Inflammatory bowel disease.
Peptic ulcer disease (PUD).
Cholecystitis.
Neoplasm.
Diabetic ketoacidosis.
Functional abdominal pain.
Pelvic inflammatory disease (PID).
Pregnancy.
Pyelonephritis.
Renal stone.
Trauma.

ABDOMINAL PAIN, CHILDHOOD[26]

ICD-9CM # 789.67
ICD-10CM # R10.817 Generalized Abdominal Tenderness
R10.827 Generalized Rebound Abdominal Tenderness

Acute gastroenteritis.
Appendicitis.
Constipation.
Cholecystitis, acute.
Intestinal obstruction.
Pancreatitis.
Neoplasm.
Inflammatory bowel disease.
Other:
- Functional abdominal pain.
- Pyelonephritis.
- Pneumonia.
- Diabetic ketoacidosis.
- Heavy metal poisoning.
- Sickle cell crisis.
- Trauma.
- Anxiety.
- Sexual abuse.

ABDOMINAL PAIN, CHRONIC LOWER[38]

ICD-9CM # 789.64 Abdominal Pain, Left Lower Quadrant
789.63 Abdominal Pain, Right Lower Quadrant
789.85 Abdominal Pain, Suprapubic
ICD-10CM # R10.814 Left Lower Quadrant Abdominal Tenderness
R10.824 Left Lower Quadrant Rebound Abdominal Tenderness
R10.813 Right Lower Quadrant Abdominal Tenderness
R10.823 Right Lower Quadrant Rebound Abdominal Tenderness
R10.30 Lower Abdominal Pain, Unspecified

ORGANIC DISORDERS

Common
Gynecologic disease.
Lactase deficiency.
Diverticulitis/diverticulosis.
Crohn's disease.
Intestinal obstruction.
Uncommon
Chronic intestinal pseudoobstruction.
Mesenteric ischemia.
Malignancy (e.g., ovarian carcinoma).
Abdominal wall pain.
Spinal disease.
Testicular disease.
Metabolic diseases (e.g., diabetes mellitus, familial Mediterranean fever, C1 esterase deficiency [angioneurotic edema], porphyria, lead poisoning, tabes dorsalis, renal failure).

FUNCTIONAL DISORDERS

Common
Irritable bowel syndrome.
Functional abdominal bloating.
Uncommon
Functional abdominal pain.

ABDOMINAL PAIN, DIFFUSE

ICD-9CM # 789.67
ICD-10CM # R10.817 Generalized Abdominal Tenderness
R10.827 Generalized Rebound Abdominal Tenderness

Early appendicitis.
Aortic aneurysm.
Gastroenteritis.
Intestinal obstruction.
Diverticulitis.
Peritonitis.
Mesenteric insufficiency or infarction.
Pancreatitis.
Inflammatory bowel disease.
Irritable bowel.
Mesenteric adenitis.
Metabolic: toxins, lead poisoning, uremia, drug overdose, diabetic ketoacidosis (DKA), heavy metal poisoning.
Sickle cell crisis.
Pneumonia (rare).
Trauma.
Urinary tract infection, PID.
Other: anxiety, acute intermittent porphyria, tabes dorsalis, periarteritis nodosa, Henoch-Schönlein purpura, adrenal insufficiency.

ABDOMINAL PAIN, EPIGASTRIC

ICD-9CM # 789.66
ICD-10CM # R10.816 Epigastric Abdominal Tenderness
R10.826 Epigastric Rebound Abdominal Tenderness

Gastric: PUD, gastric outlet obstruction, gastric ulcer.
Duodenal: PUD, duodenitis.
Biliary: cholecystitis, cholangitis, biliary dyskinesia.
Hepatic: hepatitis.
Pancreatic: pancreatitis.

Intestinal: high small bowel obstruction, early appendicitis.
Cardiac: angina, MI, pericarditis.
Pulmonary: pneumonia, pleurisy, pneumothorax.
Subphrenic abscess.
Vascular: dissecting aneurysm, mesenteric ischemia.
Psychiatric: anxiety.

ABDOMINAL PAIN, INFANCY[26]

ICD-9CM # 789.67
ICD-10CM # R10.817 Generalized Abdominal Tenderness
R10.827 Generalized Rebound Abdominal Tenderness

Acute gastroenteritis.
Appendicitis.
Intussusception.
Volvulus.
Meckel diverticulum.
Other: colic, trauma.

ABDOMINAL PAIN, LEFT LOWER QUADRANT

ICD-9CM # 789.64
ICD-10CM # R10.814 Left Lower Quadrant Abdominal Tenderness
R10.824 Left Lower Quadrant Rebound Abdominal Tenderness

Intestinal: diverticulitis, diverticulosis, intestinal obstruction, perforated ulcer, inflammatory bowel disease, perforated descending colon, inguinal hernia, neoplasm, appendicitis.
Reproductive: ectopic pregnancy, ovarian cyst, torsion of ovarian cyst, tuboovarian abscess, mittelschmerz, endometriosis, seminal vesiculitis.
Renal: renal or ureteral calculi, pyelonephritis, neoplasm.
Vascular: leaking aortic aneurysm.
Psoas abscess.
Trauma.

ABDOMINAL PAIN, LEFT UPPER QUADRANT

ICD-9CM # 789.32
ICD-10CM # R19.02 Left Upper Quadrant Abdominal Swelling, Mass, and Lump

Gastric: PUD, gastritis, pyloric stenosis, hiatal hernia.
Pancreatic: pancreatitis, neoplasm, stone in pancreatic duct or ampulla.
Cardiac: MI, angina pectoris.
Splenic: splenomegaly, ruptured spleen, splenic abscess, splenic infarction.
Renal: calculi, pyelonephritis, neoplasm.
Pulmonary: pneumonia, empyema, pulmonary infarction.
Vascular: ruptured aortic aneurysm.
Cutaneous: herpes zoster.
Trauma.
Intestinal: high fecal impaction, perforated colon, diverticulitis.

ABDOMINAL PAIN, NONSURGICAL CAUSES

ICD-9CM # 789.9
ICD-10CM # R19.8 Other Specified Symptoms and Signs Involving the Digestive System and Abdomen
R10.817 Generalized abdominal tenderness

Irritable bowel syndrome.
Urinary tract infection, pyelonephritis, salpingitis, PID.
Gastroenteritis, gastritis, peptic ulcer.
Diverticular spasm.
Hepatitis, mononucleosis.
Pancreatitis.
Inferior wall myocardial infarction.
Basilar pneumonia, pulmonary embolism.
Diabetic ketoacidosis.
Strain or hematoma of rectus muscle.
Ruptured Graafian follicle.
Herpes zoster.
Nerve root compression.
Sickle cell crisis.
Acute adrenal insufficiency.
Other: acute porphyria, familial Mediterranean fever, tabes dorsalis, anxiety, sexual abuse.

ABDOMINAL PAIN, PERIUMBILICAL

ICD-9CM # 789.65
ICD-10CM # R10.815 Periumbilic Abdominal Tenderness
R10.825 Periumbilic Rebound Abdominal Tenderness

Intestinal: small bowel obstruction or gangrene, early appendicitis.
Vascular: mesenteric thrombosis, dissecting aortic aneurysm.
Pancreatic: pancreatitis.
Metabolic: uremia, DKA.
Trauma.

ABDOMINAL PAIN, POORLY LOCALIZED[26]

ICD-9CM # 789.60
ICD-10CM # R10.819 Abdominal Tenderness, Unspecified Site

EXTRAABDOMINAL

Metabolic
DKA, acute intermittent porphyria, hyperthyroidism, hypothyroidism, hypercalcemia, hypokalemia, uremia, hyperlipidemia, hyperparathyroidism.
Hematologic
Sickle cell crisis, leukemia or lymphoma, Henoch-Schönlein purpura.
Infectious
Infectious mononucleosis, Rocky Mountain spotted fever, acquired immunodeficiency syndrome (AIDS), streptococcal pharyngitis (in children), herpes zoster.
Drugs and Toxins
Heavy metal poisoning, black widow spider bites, withdrawal syndromes, mushroom ingestion.
Referred Pain
Pulmonary: pneumonia, pulmonary embolism, pneumothorax.
Cardiac: angina, MI, pericarditis, myocarditis.
Genitourinary: prostatitis, epididymitis, orchitis, testicular torsion.
Musculoskeletal: rectus sheath hematoma.
Functional
Somatization disorder, malingering, hypochondriasis, Münchausen syndrome.

INTRAABDOMINAL

Early appendicitis, gastroenteritis, peritonitis, pancreatitis, abdominal aortic aneurysm, mesenteric insufficiency or infarction, intestinal obstruction, volvulus, ulcerative colitis.

ABDOMINAL PAIN, PREGNANCY

ICD-9CM # 789.67
ICD-10CM # R10.817 Generalized Abdominal Tenderness
R10.827 Generalized Rebound Abdominal Tenderness

GYNECOLOGIC (GESTATIONAL AGE IN PARENTHESES)

Miscarriage	(<20 wk; 80% <12 wk)
Septic abortion	(<20 wk)
Ectopic pregnancy	(<14 wk)
Corpus luteum cyst rupture	(<12 wk)
Ovarian torsion	(especially <24 wk)
Pelvic inflammatory disease	(<12 wk)
Chorioamnionitis	(>16 wk)
Abruptio placentae	(>16 wk)

NONGYNECOLOGIC

Appendicitis	(Throughout)
Cholecystitis	(Throughout)
Hepatitis	(Throughout)
Pyelonephritis	(Throughout)
Preeclampsia	(>20 wk)

ABDOMINAL PAIN, RIGHT LOWER QUADRANT

ICD-9CM # 789.63
ICD-10CM # R10.813 Right Lower Quadrant Abdominal Tenderness
R10.823 Right Lower Quadrant Rebound Abdominal Tenderness

Intestinal: acute appendicitis, regional enteritis, incarcerated hernia, cecal diverticulitis,

intestinal obstruction, perforated ulcer, perforated cecum, Meckel diverticulitis.
Reproductive: ectopic pregnancy, ovarian cyst, torsion of ovarian cyst, salpingitis, tuboovarian abscess, mittelschmerz, endometriosis, seminal vesiculitis.
Renal: renal and ureteral calculi, neoplasms, pyelonephritis.
Vascular: leaking aortic aneurysm.
Cutaneous: herpes zoster.
Psoas abscess.
Trauma.
Cholecystitis.

ABDOMINAL PAIN, RIGHT UPPER QUADRANT

ICD-9CM # 789.61
ICD-10CM # R10.811 Right Upper Quadrant Abdominal Tenderness
R10.821 Right Upper Quadrant Rebound Abdominal Tenderness

Biliary: calculi, infection, inflammation, neoplasm.
Hepatic: hepatitis, abscess, hepatic congestion, neoplasm, trauma.
Gastric: PUD, pyloric stenosis, neoplasm, alcoholic gastritis, hiatal hernia.
Pancreatic: pancreatitis, neoplasm, stone in pancreatic duct or ampulla.
Renal: calculi, infection, inflammation, neoplasm, rupture of kidney.
Pulmonary: pneumonia, pulmonary infarction, right-sided pleurisy.
Intestinal: retrocecal appendicitis, intestinal obstruction, high fecal impaction, diverticulitis.
Cardiac: myocardial ischemia (particularly involving the inferior wall), pericarditis.
Cutaneous: herpes zoster.
Trauma.
Fitz-Hugh-Curtis syndrome (perihepatitis).

ABDOMINAL PAIN, SUPRAPUBIC

ICD-9CM # 789.85
ICD-10CM # R10.30 Lower Abdominal Pain, Unspecified

Intestinal: colon obstruction or gangrene, diverticulitis, appendicitis.
Reproductive system: ectopic pregnancy, mittelschmerz, torsion of ovarian cyst, PID, salpingitis, endometriosis, rupture of endometrioma.
Cystitis, rupture of urinary bladder.

ABDOMINAL WALL MASSES[38]

ICD-9CM # varies with specific diagnosis
ICD-10CM # R19.00 Intra-abdominal and Pelvic Swelling, Mass and Lump, Unspecified Site

LUMPS ARISING IN THE SKIN AND SUBCUTANEOUS FAT (THAT COULD OCCUR ANYWHERE ON THE BODY)

Lipoma.
Sebaceous cyst.

LUMPS ARISING IN THE SKIN AND SUBCUTANEOUS FAT (SPECIFIC TO THE ANTERIOR ABDOMINAL WALL)

Tumor nodule of the umbilicus (secondary to the intraperitoneal malignancy, also called *Sister Mary Joseph nodule*).

LUMPS ARISING IN THE FASCIA AND MUSCLE

Rectus sheath hematoma (usually painful).
Desmoid tumor (associated with Gardner's syndrome).

HERNIA

Incisional: It has an overlying scar. The sac may be very much larger than the neck of the hernia.
Umbilical: The hernia is through the umbilical scar. Those presenting at birth commonly resolve in the first years of life.
Paraumbilical: The neck is just lateral to the umbilical scar. Patients usually present later in life.
Epigastric: It occurs in the midline between the xiphoid process and the umbilicus. They are usually small (<2 cm). They result when a knuckle of extraperitoneal fat extrudes through a small defect in the linea alba. Commonly irreducible and without an expansile cough impulse.
Spigelian: A rare hernia found along the linea semilunaris at the lateral edge of the rectus sheath, most commonly a third of the way between the umbilicus and the pubis.

DIVARICATION OF THE RECTI

Supraumbilical elliptical swelling of the attenuated linea alba (no cough impulse).

ABORTION, RECURRENT

ICD-9CM # 761.8
ICD-10CM # P01.8 Newborn (Suspected to Be) Affected by Other Maternal Complications of Pregnancy

Congenital anatomic abnormalities.
Adhesions (uterine synechiae).
Uterine fibroids.
Endometriosis.
Endocrine abnormalities (luteal phase insufficiency, hypothyroidism, uncontrolled diabetes mellitus [DM]).
Parenteral chromosome abnormalities.
Maternal infections (cervical mycoplasma, ureaplasma, chlamydia).
DES exposure, heavy metal exposure.
Thrombocytosis.
Allogenic immunity, autoimmunity, lupus anticoagulant.

ACHES AND PAINS, DIFFUSE[24]

ICD-9CM # 719.49
ICD-10CM # M25.50 Pain in Unspecified Joint

Postviral arthralgias/myalgias.
Bilateral soft tissue rheumatism.
Overuse syndromes.
Fibrositis.
Hypothyroidism.
Metabolic bone disease.
Paraneoplastic syndrome.
Myopathy (polymyositis, dermatomyositis).
Rheumatoid arthritis (RA).
Sjögren's syndrome.
Polymyalgia rheumatica.
Hypermobility.
Benign arthralgias/myalgias.
Chronic fatigue syndrome.
Hypophosphatemia.

ACIDOSIS, HYPERCHLORIC METABOLIC[38b]

ICD-9CM # 276.2
ICD-10CM # E87.2 Acidosis

GASTROINTESTINAL BICARBONATE LOSS

Diarrhea.
External pancreatic or small bowel drainage.
Ureterosigmoidostomy, jejunal loop.
Drugs:
  Calcium chloride (acidifying agent).
  Magnesium sulfate (diarrhea).
  Cholestyramine (bile acid diarrhea).

RENAL ACIDOSIS

Hypokalemic:
Proximal RTA (type 2).
Distal (classic) RTA (type 1).
Drug-induced hypokalemia:
- Acetazolamide (proximal RTA).
- Amphotericin B (distal RTA).

Hyperkalemic:
Generalized distal nephron dysfunction (type 4 RTA).
Mineralocorticoid deficiency or resistance (pseudohypoaldosteronism type 1) PHA-I, PHA-II.
↓ Na^+ delivery to distal nephron.
Tubulointerstitial disease.
Ammonium excretion defect.
Drug-induced hyperkalemia:
- Potassium-sparing diuretics (amiloride, triamterene, spironolactone).
- Trimethoprim.
- Pentamidine.
- Angiotensin-converting enzyme inhibitors and angiotensin II receptor blockers.
- Nonsteroidal anti-inflammatory drugs.
- Cyclosporine, tacrolimus.

Differential Diagnosis II

Normokalemic:
Early renal insufficiency.

OTHER

Acid loads (ammonium chloride, hyperalimentation).
Loss of potential bicarbonate: ketosis with ketone excretion.
Dilution acidosis (rapid saline administration).
Hippurate.
Cation-exchange resins.

ACIDOSIS, LACTIC[38b]

ICD-9CM # 276.2
ICD-10CM # E87.2 Acidosis

CAUSES OF LACTIC ACIDOSIS

L-Lactic Acidosis

Conditions associated with type A lactic acidosis:
Poor tissue perfusion.
Shock:
- Cardiogenic.
- Hemorrhagic.
- Septic.

Profound hypoxemia:
- Severe asthma.
- Carbon monoxide poisoning.

Conditions associated with type B lactic acidosis:
Liver disease.
Diabetes mellitus.
Catecholamine excess:
- Endogenous
- Exogenous

Thiamine deficiency.
Ketoacidosis.
Seizure.
Malignancy.
Intracellular inorganic phosphate depletion.
Intravenous (IV) fructose.
IV xylose.
IV sorbitol.
Alcohols metabolized by alcohol dehydrogenase:
- Ethanol.
- Methanol.
- Ethylene.
- Propylene glycol.

Mitochondrial toxins:
- Salicylate intoxication.
- Cyanide poisoning.
- 2,4-Dinitrophenol ingestion.
- Nonnucleoside antireverse transcriptase drugs.

Metformin.
Inborn errors of metabolism.
Pyroglutamic acidosis.
Kombucha tea.

d-Lactic Acidosis

Short bowel syndrome.
Ischemic bowel.
Small bowel obstruction.

ACIDOSIS, METABOLIC

ICD-9CM # 276.2
ICD-10CM # E87.2 Acidosis

METABOLIC ACIDOSIS WITH INCREASED ANION GAP (AG ACIDOSIS)

Lactic acidosis.
Ketoacidosis (DM, alcoholic ketoacidosis).
Uremia (chronic renal failure).
Ingestion of toxins (paraldehyde, methanol, salicylate, ethylene glycol).
High-fat diet (mild acidosis).

METABOLIC ACIDOSIS WITH NORMAL AG (HYPERCHLOREMIC ACIDOSIS)

Renal tubular acidosis (including acidosis of aldosterone deficiency).
Intestinal loss of HCO_3^- (diarrhea, pancreatic fistula).
Carbonic anhydrase inhibitors (e.g., acetazolamide).
Dilutional acidosis (as a result of rapid infusion of bicarbonate-free isotonic saline).
Ingestion of exogenous acids (ammonium chloride, methionine, cystine, calcium chloride).
Ileostomy.
Ureterosigmoidostomy.
Drugs: amiloride, triamterene, spironolactone, β-blockers.

ACIDOSIS, RESPIRATORY

ICD-9CM # 276.2
ICD-10CM # E87.2 Acidosis

Pulmonary disease (COPD, severe pneumonia, pulmonary edema, interstitial fibrosis).
Airway obstruction (foreign body, severe bronchospasm, laryngospasm).
Thoracic cage disorders (pneumothorax, flail chest, kyphoscoliosis).
Defects in muscles of respiration (myasthenia gravis, hypokalemia, muscular dystrophy).
Defects in peripheral nervous system (amyotrophic lateral sclerosis, poliomyelitis, Guillain-Barré syndrome, botulism, tetanus, organophosphate poisoning, spinal cord injury).
Depression of respiratory center (anesthesia, narcotics, sedatives, vertebral artery embolism or thrombosis, increased intracranial pressure).
Failure of mechanical ventilator.

ACUTE KIDNEY INJURY AND LIVER DISEASE, CAUSES[12ab]

ICD-9CM # varies with specific diagnosis
ICD-10CM # S37.009A Unspecified Injury of Unspecified Kidney, Initial Encounter
K76.89 Other Specified Diseases of Liver

Prerenal uremia:	Diuretic use, gastrointestinal loss, peritoneal aspiration, hypoalbuminemia
Hepatorenal syndrome	
Acute tubular necrosis:	Hyperbilirubinemia, sepsis, toxic shock syndrome
Drugs:	Acetaminophen (paracetamol), NSAIDs, tetracycline, rifampicin, isoniazid, anesthetic agents, sulfonamides, allopurinol, methotrexate
Infections:	Hepatitis C and cryoglobulinemia, hepatitis B and polyarteritis nodosa, leptospirosis, hantavirus, Epstein-Barr virus, gram-negative sepsis, spontaneous bacterial peritonitis
Other:	Papillary necrosis and obstruction, inhalation of chlorinated hydrocarbons, mushroom poisoning *(Amanita phalloides)*

ACUTE KIDNEY INJURY, HIV PATIENT, CAUSES[12ab]

ICD-9CM # varies with specific diagnosis
ICD-10CM # S37.009A Unspecified Injury of Unspecified Kidney, Initial Encounter with B20 Human Immunodeficiency Virus [HIV] Disease

Prerenal:	Diarrhea, nausea and vomiting, cirrhosis and hepatorenal syndrome, sepsis
Vascular:	Thrombotic microangiopathy
Glomerular:	Immune complex glomerulonephritis (MPGN secondary to hepatitis C virus, postinfectious glomerulonephritis), HIVAN
Acute tubular necrosis:	Sepsis, hypotension, nephrotoxins (aminoglycosides, amphotericin, acyclovir, cidofovir, tenofovir, pentamidine)
Acute interstitial nephritis:	Drug-induced (co-trimoxazole), rifampicin, foscarnet, nevirapine), CMV infection, DILS
Drug-induced intratubular obstruction:	Sulfadiazine, indinavir, foscarnet, acyclovir
Postrenal obstruction:	Stones, tuberculosis, fungal ball, tumor
Associated with IV drug use:	Sepsis, endocarditis, heroin-associated nephropathy (FSGS), rhabdomyolysis

CMV, Cytomegalovirus; *DILS,* diffusive infiltrative lymphocytosis syndrome; *FSGS,* focal segmental glomerulosclerosis; *HIVAN,* HIV-associated nephropathy; *MPGN,* membranoproliferative glomerulonephritis

ACUTE SCROTUM

ICD-9CM # 608.9
ICD-10CM # R10.2 Pelvic and Perineal Pain

Testicular torsion.
Epididymitis.
Testicular neoplasm.
Orchitis.
Trauma.

ADNEXAL MASS[26]

ICD-9CM # varies with specific disorder
ICD-10CM # R19.00 Intra-abdominal and Pelvic Swelling, Mass and Lump, Unspecified Site

Ovary (neoplasm, endometriosis, functional cyst).
Fallopian tube (ectopic pregnancy, neoplasm, tubo-ovarian abscess, hydrosalpinx, paratubal cyst).
Uterus (fibroid, neoplasm).
Retroperitoneum (neoplasm, abdominal wall hematoma or abscess).
Urinary tract (pelvic kidney, distended bladder, urachal cyst).
Inflammatory bowel disease.
GI tract neoplasm.
Diverticular disease.
Appendicitis.
Bowel loop with feces.

ADRENAL MASSES[36]

ICD-9CM # 194.0 Adrenocortical Carcinoma
255.8 Adrenal Hyperplasia
ICD-10CM # C74.90 Malignant Neoplasm of Unspecified Part of Unspecified Adrenal Gland
E27.8 Other Specified Disorders of Adrenal Gland

UNILATERAL ADRENAL MASSES

Functional Lesions
Adrenal adenoma.
Adrenal carcinoma.
Pheochromocytoma.
Primary aldosteronism, adenomatous type.
Nonfunctional Lesions
Incidentaloma of adrenal.
Ganglioneuroma.
Myelolipoma.
Hematoma.
Adenolipoma.
Metastasis.

BILATERAL ADRENAL MASSES

Functional Lesions
ACTH-dependent Cushing's syndrome.
Congenital adrenal hyperplasia.
Pheochromocytoma.
Conn's syndrome, hyperplastic variety.
Micronodular adrenal disease.
Idiopathic bilateral adrenal hypertrophy.
Nonfunctional Lesions
Infection (tuberculosis, fungi).
Infiltration (leukemia, lymphoma).
Replacement (amyloidosis).
Hemorrhage.
Bilateral metastases.

ADRENOCORTICAL HYPERFUNCTION[1a]

ICD-9CM # 255.1
ICD-10CM # E26.9 Hyperaldosteronism, Unspecified

SYNDROMES OF ADRENOCORTICAL HYPERFUNCTION

States of Glucocorticoid Excess
Physiologic states
Stress.
Strenuous exercise.
Last trimester of pregnancy.
Pathologic states
Psychiatric conditions (pseudo-Cushing's disorders):
- Depression.
- Alcoholism.
- Anorexia nervosa.
- Panic disorders.
- Alcohol and drug withdrawal.

ACTH-dependent states:
- Pituitary adenoma (Cushing's disease).
- Ectopic ACTH syndrome.
  - Bronchial carcinoid.
  - Thymic carcinoid.
  - Islet cell tumor.
  - Small cell lung carcinoma.
- Ectopic CRH secretion.

ACTH-independent states:
- Adrenal adenoma.
- Adrenal carcinoma.
- Micronodular adrenal disease.

Exogenous sources
Glucocorticoid intake.
ACTH intake.
States of Mineralocorticoid Excess
Primary aldosteronism
Aldosterone-secreting adenoma.
Bilateral adrenal hyperplasia.
Aldosterone-secreting carcinoma.
Glucocorticoid-suppressible hyperaldosteronism.
Adrenal Enzyme Deficiencies
11b-Hydroxylase deficiency.
17a-Hydroxylase deficiency.
11b-Hydroxysteroid dehydrogenase, type II.
Exogenous Mineralocorticoids
Licorice.
Carbenoxolone.
Fludrocortisone.
Secondary hyperaldosteronism
Associated with hypertension:
- Accelerated hypertension.
- Renovascular hypertension.
- Estrogen administration.
- Renin-secreting tumors.

Without hypertension:
- Bartter syndrome.
- Sodium-wasting nephropathy.
- Renal tubular acidosis.
- Diuretic and laxative abuse.
- Edematous states (cirrhosis, nephrosis, congestive heart failure).

ACTH, Adrenocorticotropin hormone; *CRH,* corticotropin-releasing hormone.

ADRENOCORTICAL HYPOFUNCTION

ICD-9CM # 255.4
ICD-10CM # E27.49 Other Adrenocortical Insufficiency

SYNDROMES OF ADRENOCORTICAL HYPOFUNCTION

Primary Adrenal Disorders
Combined glucocorticoid and mineralocorticoid deficiency
Autoimmune:
- Isolated autoimmune disease (Addison disease).
- Polyglandular autoimmune syndrome, type I.
- Polyglandular autoimmune syndrome, type II.

Infectious:
- Tuberculosis.
- Fungal.
- Cytomegalovirus.
- Human immunodeficiency virus.

Vascular:
- Bilateral adrenal hemorrhage.
- Sepsis.
- Coagulopathy.
- Thrombosis; embolism.
- Adrenal infarction.

Infiltration:
- Metastatic carcinoma and lymphoma.
- Sarcoidosis.
- Amyloidosis.
- Hemochromatosis.

Congenital:
- Congenital adrenal hyperplasia.
  - 21-Hydroxylase deficiency.
  - 3b-ol Dehydrogenase deficiency.
  - 20,22-Desmolase deficiency.
- Adrenal unresponsiveness to ACTH.
- Congenital adrenal hypoplasia.
- Adrenoleukodystrophy.
- Adrenomyeloneuropathy.

Iatrogenic
Bilateral adrenalectomy.
Drugs:
Metyrapone, aminoglutethimide, trilostane, ketoconazole, o,p¢-DDD, mifepristone.
Mineralocorticoid deficiency without glucocorticoid deficiency:
Cortiscosterone methyl oxidase deficiency.
Isolated zona glomerulosa defect.
Heparin therapy.
Critical illness.
Converting-enzyme inhibitors.
Secondary Adrenal Disorders
Secondary adrenal insufficiency
Hypothalamic-pituitary dysfunction.
Exogenous glucocorticoids.
After removal of an ACTH-secreting tumor.
Hyporeninemic Hypoaldosteronism
Diabetic nephropathy.
Tubulointerstitial diseases.
Obstructive uropathy.
Autonomic neuropathy.
Nonsteroidal anti-inflammatory drugs.
b-Adrenergic drugs.

ACTH, Adrenocorticotropic hormone.

ADVERSE FOOD REACTIONS, DIFFERENTIAL DIAGNOSIS[22a]

ICD-9CM # varies with specific diagnosis

ICD-10CM # T78.1XXA Other Adverse Food Reactions, Not Elsewhere Classified, Initial Encounter

GASTROINTESTINAL DISORDERS (WITH VOMITING AND/OR DIARRHEA)

Structural abnormalities (pyloric stenosis, Hirschsprung's disease).
Enzyme deficiencies (primary or secondary):
Disaccharidase deficiency—lactase, fructase, sucrase-isomaltase.
Galactosemia.
Other: pancreatic insufficiency (cystic fibrosis), peptic disease.

CONTAMINANTS AND ADDITIVES

Flavorings and preservatives—rarely cause symptoms: Sodium metabisulfite, monosodium glutamate, nitrites.
Dyes and colorings—very rarely cause symptoms (urticaria, eczema): Tartrazine.
Toxins: Bacterial, fungal (aflatoxin), fish-related (scombroid, ciguatera).
Infectious organisms:
Bacteria *(Salmonella, Escherichia coli, Shigella).*
Virus (rotavirus, enterovirus).
Parasites (*Giardia, Akis simplex* [in fish]).
Accidental contaminants: Heavy metals, pesticides.
Pharmacologic agents: Caffeine, glycosidal alkaloid solanine (potato spuds), histamine (fish), serotonin (banana, tomato), tryptamine (tomato), tyramine (cheese).

PSYCHOLOGIC REACTIONS

Food phobias.

ADYNAMIC ILEUS[26]

ICD-9CM # 560.1

ICD-10CM # K56.0 Paralytic Ileus
K56.7 Ileus, Unspecified

Abdominal trauma.
Infection (retroperitoneal, pelvic, intrathoracic).
Laparotomy.
Metabolic disease (hypokalemia).
Renal colic.
Skeletal injury (rib fracture, vertebral fracture).
Medications (e.g., narcotics).

AEROPHAGIA (BELCHING, ERUCTATION)

ICD-9CM # 787.3

ICD-10CM # R14.0 Abdominal Distension (Gaseous)
R14.1 Gas Pain
R14.2 Eructation
R14.3 Flatulence

Anxiety disorders.
Rapid food ingestion.
Carbonated beverages.
Nursing infants (especially when nursing in horizontal position).
Eating or drinking in supine position.
Gum chewing.
Poorly fitting dentures, orthodontic appliances.
Hiatal hernia, gastritis, nonulcer dyspepsia.
Cholelithiasis, cholecystitis.
Ingestion of legumes, onions, peppers.

AIR-SPACE OPACIFICATION ON X-RAY[16a]

ICD-9CM # varies with specific diagnosis

ICD-10CM # R91.8 Other nonspecific abnormal finding of lung field

CAUSES OF AIR-SPACE OPACIFICATION

Edema
Cardiogenic.
Non-cardiogenic.

Inflammation/Infection
Wegener's granulomatosis.
Cryptogenic organizing pneumonia.

Blood
Idiopathic pulmonary hemosiderosis.
Antibasement membrane antibody disease.
Systemic lupus erythematosus.

Miscellaneous Causes
Eosinophilic pneumonia.
Alveolar proteinosis.
Alveolar cell carcinoma.
Alveolar microlithiasis.
Lymphoma (MALToma).
Sarcoidosis.

AIRWAY OBSTRUCTION, PEDIATRIC AGE[19]

ICD-9CM # 496 Obstruction Due to Bronchospasm
934.9 Obstruction Due to Foreign Body
478.75 Obstruction Due to Laryngospasm
506.9 Obstruction Due to Inhalation of Fumes or Vapors

ICD-10CM # J44.9 Chronic Obstructive Pulmonary Disease, Unspecified
T17.900A Unspecified Foreign Body in Respiratory Tract, Part Unspecified Causing Asphyxiation, Initial Encounter
T17.908A Unspecified Foreign Body in Respiratory Tract, Part Unspecified Causing Other Injury, Initial Encounter
T17.910A Gastric Contents in Respiratory Tract, Part Unspecified Causing Asphyxiation, Initial Encounter
T17.918A Gastric Contents in Respiratory Tract, Part Unspecified Causing Other Injury, Initial Encounter
T17.920A Food in Respiratory Tract, Part Unspecified Causing Asphyxiation, Initial Encounter
T17.928A Food in Respiratory Tract, Part Unspecified Causing Other Injury, Initial Encounter
T17.990A Other Foreign Object in Respiratory Tract, Part Unspecified in Causing Asphyxiation, Initial Encounter
T17.998A Other Foreign Object in Respiratory Tract, Part Unspecified Causing Other Injury, Initial Encounter
J38.5 Laryngeal Spasm
J68.9 Unspecified Respiratory Condition Due To Chemicals, Gases, Fumes, and Vapors

CONGENITAL CAUSES

Craniofacial dysmorphism.
Hemangioma.
Laryngeal cleft/web.
Laryngoceles, cysts.
Laryngomalacia.
Macroglossia.
Tracheal stenosis.
Vascular ring.
Vocal cord paralysis.

ACQUIRED INFECTIOUS CAUSES

Acute laryngotracheobronchitis.
Epiglottitis.
Laryngeal papillomatosis.
Membranous croup (bacterial tracheitis).
Mononucleosis.
Retropharyngeal abscess.
Spasmodic croup.
Diphtheria.

Degenerative diseases (e.g., Alzheimer's, Huntington's disease).
CVA (especially when involving thalamus, basal forebrain, and hippocampus).
Head trauma.
Postsurgical (e.g., mammillary body surgery, bilateral temporal lobectomy).
Infections (herpes simplex encephalitis, meningitis).
Wernicke-Korsakoff syndrome.
Cerebral hypoxia.
Hypoglycemia.
CNS neoplasms.
Creutzfeldt-Jakob disease.
Medications (e.g., midazolam and other benzodiazepines).
Psychosis.
Malingering.

AMNIOTIC FLUID ALPHA-FETOPROTEIN ELEVATION[16a]

ICD-9CM # V28.1
ICD-10CM # Z36 Encounter for Antenatal Screening of Mother

CAUSES OF ELEVATED AMNIOTIC FLUID α-FETOPROTEIN

Craniospinal defect (open neural tube defect).
Omphalocele.
Gastroschisis.
Duodenal atresia.
Congenital nephrosis.
Cystic hygroma.
Unbalanced D/G dislocation.
Down, Tay-Sachs, Klinefelter's, Turner's syndromes.
Fetal tumors.
Epidermolysis bullosa.
Pilonidal sinus.
Rhesus disease.
Fetal demise.
Incorrect dates.
Multiple pregnancy.

ANAL ABSCESS AND FISTULA[38]

ICD-9CM # 566
ICD-10CM # K61.0 Anal Abscess
K61.1 Rectal Abscess
K61.3 Ischiorectal Abscess
K60.3 Anal fistula

Primary anal gland infection.
Secondary abscess:
Inflammatory bowel disease:
- Crohn's disease.
- Ulcerative colitis.

Infection:
- Tuberculosis.
- Actinomycosis.
- Threadworm.

Trauma.
Leukopenia.
Immunosuppression:
- HIV.
- Drugs.

Rectal cancer.
Diabetes mellitus.

ANAL INCONTINENCE[26]

ICD-9CM # 787.6
ICD-10CM # R15.9 Full Incontinence of Feces

TRAUMATIC

Nerve injured in surgery.
Spinal cord injury.
Obstetric trauma.
Sphincter injury.

NEUROLOGIC

Spinal cord lesions.
Dementia.
Autonomic neuropathy (e.g., DM).
Obstetrics: pudendal nerve stretched during surgery.
Hirschsprung's disease.

MASS EFFECT

Carcinoma of anal canal.
Carcinoma of rectum.
Foreign body.
Fecal impaction.
Hemorrhoids.

MEDICAL

Procidentia.
Inflammatory disease.
Diarrhea.
Laxative abuse.

PEDIATRIC

Congenital.
Meningocele.
Myelomeningocele.
Spina bifida.
After corrective surgery for imperforate anus.
Sexual abuse.
Encopresis.

ANAPHYLAXIS[21]

ICD-9CM # 995.0
ICD-10CM # T78.2 Anaphylactic Shock, Unspecified, Initial Encounter

PULMONARY

Laryngeal edema.
Epiglottitis.
Foreign body aspiration.
Pulmonary embolus.
Asphyxiation.
Hyperventilation.

CARDIOVASCULAR

Myocardial infarction.
Arrhythmia.
Hypovolemic shock.
Cardiac arrest.

CNS

Vasovagal reaction.
CVA.
Seizure disorder.
Drug overdose.

ENDOCRINE

Hypoglycemia.
Pheochromocytoma.
Carcinoid syndrome.
Catamenial (progesterone-induced anaphylaxis).

PSYCHIATRIC

Vocal cord dysfunction syndrome.
Münchausen syndrome.
Panic attack/globus hystericus.

OTHER

Hereditary angioedema.
Cord urticaria.
Idiopathic urticaria.
Mastocytosis.
Serum sickness.
Idiopathic capillary leak syndrome.
Sulfite exposure.
Scombroid poisoning (tuna, blue fish, mackerel).

ANAPHYLACTOID SYNDROME OF PREGNANCY[1]

ICD-9CM # 673.11
ICD-10CM # 088.113

CARDIOVASCULAR COLLAPSE, HYPOTENSION

Acute coronary syndromes, myocardial infarction.
Cardiomyopathy.
Pulmonary embolism.
Anesthesia complications, transfusion reaction.
Sepsis, systemic inflammatory response syndrome.

RESPIRATORY ARREST

Pulmonary embolism, air embolism.
Anesthesia complications, transfusion reaction.
Aspiration.

ALTERED MENTAL STATUS, SEIZURE

Eclampsia.
Cerebrovascular accident.
Hypoglycemia.

COAGULOPATHY

Disseminated intravascular coagulation.
Consumptive coagulopathy from hemorrhage.

ANDROGEN EXCESS, REPRODUCTIVE-AGE WOMAN

ICD-9CM # varies with specific disorder
ICD-10CM # E28.1 Androgen Excess

Polycystic ovary syndrome.
Idiopathic.
Medications (e.g., anabolizing agents, testosterone, danazol).
Pregnancy (luteoma, hyperreaction luteinalis).
Sertoli-Leydig ovarian neoplasm.
Adrenal adenoma or hyperplasia.
Cushing's syndrome.
Glucocorticoid resistance.
Hypothyroidism.
Hyperprolactinemia.

ANDROGEN RESISTANCE[25]

ICD-9CM # 257.2
ICD-10CM # E34.5 Androgen resistance syndrome

CONGENITAL OR DEVELOPMENTAL DISORDERS

Uncommon causes:
- Kennedy disease (spinal and bulbar muscular atrophy).
- Partial androgen insensitivity syndrome (AR mutations).
- 5α-reductase type 2 deficiency.
- Complete androgen insensitivity syndrome (female phenotype).

ACQUIRED DISORDERS

Common causes:
- AR antagonists (bicalutamide, nilutamide).
- Drugs (spironolactone, cyproterone acetate, marijuana, histamine 2 receptor antagonists).

Uncommon causes:
- Celiac disease.

ANEMIA, APLASTIC[20]

ICD-9CM # 284
ICD-10CM # D61.09 Other Constitutional Aplastic Anemia

ACQUIRED APLASTIC ANEMIA

Secondary aplastic anemia.
Irradiation.
Drugs and chemicals.
Regular effects.
Cytotoxic agents.
Benzene.
Idiosyncratic reactions.
Chloramphenicol.
Nonsteroidal anti-inflammatory drugs.
Antiepileptics.
Gold.
Other drugs and chemicals.
Viruses.
Epstein-Barr virus (infectious mononucleosis).
Hepatitis virus (non-A, non-B, non-C, non-G hepatitis).
Parvovirus (transient aplastic crisis, some pure red cell aplasia).
Human immunodeficiency virus (acquired immunodeficiency syndrome).
Immune diseases.
Eosinophilic fasciitis.
Hyperimmunoglobulinemia.
Thymoma and thymic carcinoma.
Graft-versus-host disease in immunodeficiency.
Paroxysmal nocturnal hemoglobinuria.
Pregnancy.
Idiopathic aplastic anemia.

INHERITED APLASTIC ANEMIA

Fanconi anemia.
Dyskeratosis congenita.
Shwachman-Diamond syndrome.
Reticular dysgenesis.
Amegakaryocytic thrombocytopenia.
Familial aplastic anemias.
Preleukemia (e.g., monosomy 7).
Nonhematologic syndromes (e.g., Down, Dubowitz, Seckel).

ANEMIA, APLASTIC, DUE TO DRUGS AND CHEMICALS[1]

ICD-9CM # 284.89
ICD-10CM # D61.1 Drug-Induced Aplastic Anemia
D61.2 Aplastic Anemia Due to Other External Agents
D61.89 Other Specified Aplastic Anemias and Other Bone Marrow Failure Syndromes

Agents that regularly produce marrow depression as a major toxic effect when used in commonly employed doses or normal exposures:
Cytotoxic drugs used in cancer chemotherapy.
Alkylating agents (busulfan, melphalan, cyclophosphamide).
Antimetabolites (antifolic compounds, nucleotide analogs), antimitotics (vincristine, vinblastine, colchicine).
Some antibiotics (daunorubicin, doxorubicin [Adriamycin]).
Benzene (and less often benzene-containing chemicals; kerosene, carbon tetrachloride, Stoddard's solvent, chlorophenols).
Agents probably associated with aplastic anemia but with a relatively low probability relative to their use:
Chloramphenicol.
Insecticides.
Antiprotozoals (quinacrine and chloroquine).
Nonsteroidal anti-inflammatory drugs (including phenylbutazone, indomethacin, ibuprofen, sulindac, diclofenac, naproxen, piroxicam, fenoprofen, fenbufen, aspirin).
Anticonvulsants (hydantoins, carbamazepine, phenacemide, ethosuximide).
Gold, arsenic, and other heavy metals such as bismuth and mercury.
Sulfonamides as a class.
Antithyroid medications (methimazole, methylthiouracil, propylthiouracil).
Antidiabetes drugs (tolbutamide, carbutamide, chlorpropamide).
Carbonic anhydrase inhibitors (acetazolamide, methazolamide, mesalazine).
D-Penicillamine.
2-Chlorodeoxyadenosine.
Agents more rarely associated with aplastic anemia:
Antibiotics (streptomycin, tetracycline, methicillin, ampicillin, mebendazole and albendazole, sulfonamides, flucytosine, mefloquine, dapsone).
Antihistamines (cimetidine, ranitidine, chlorpheniramine).
Sedatives and tranquilizers (chlorpromazine, prochlorperazine, piperacetazine, chlordiazepoxide, meprobamate, methyprylon, remoxipride).
Antiarrhythmics (tocainide, amiodarone).
Allopurinol (can potentiate marrow suppression by cytotoxic drugs).
Ticlopidine.
Methyldopa.
Quinidine.
Lithium.
Guanidine.
Canthaxanthin.
Thiocyanate.
Carbimazole.
Cyanamide.
Deferoxamine.
Amphetamines.

ANEMIA, DRUG-INDUCED[17]

ICD-9CM # 283.0
ICD-10CM # D61.1 Drug-Induced Aplastic Anemia

DRUGS THAT MAY INTERFERE WITH RED CELL PRODUCTION BY INDUCING MARROW SUPPRESSION OR APLASIA

Alcohol.
Antineoplastic drugs.
Antithyroid drugs.
Antibiotics.
Oral hypoglycemic agents.
Phenylbutazone.
Azidothymidine (AZT).

DRUGS THAT INTERFERE WITH VITAMIN B_{12}, FOLATE, OR IRON ABSORPTION OR UTILIZATION

Nitrous oxide.
Anticonvulsant drugs.
Antineoplastic drugs.
Isoniazid
Cycloserine A.

DRUGS CAPABLE OF PROMOTING HEMOLYSIS

Immune Mediated
Penicillins.
Quinine.
Alpha-methyldopa.
Procainamide.
Mitomycin C.
Oxidative Stress
Antimalarials.
Sulfonamide drugs.
Nalidixic acid.

DRUGS THAT MAY PRODUCE OR PROMOTE BLOOD LOSS

Aspirin.
Alcohol.
Nonsteroidal anti-inflammatory agents.
Corticosteroids.
Anticoagulants.

ANEMIA, HYPOCHROMIC[20]

ICD-9CM # varies with specific diagnosis
280.9 Iron Deficiency
285.0 Sideroblastic
ICD-10CM # D50.8 Other Iron Deficiency Anemias
D50.9 Iron Deficiency Anemia, Unspecified
D64.0 Hereditary Sideroblastic Anemia
D64.1 Secondary Sideroblastic Anemia Due to Disease

D64.2 Secondary Sideroblastic Anemia Due to Drugs and Toxins
D64.3 Other Sideroblastic Anemias

DECREASED BODY IRON STORES

Iron-deficiency anemia.

NORMAL OR INCREASED BODY IRON STORES

Impaired iron metabolism.
Anemia of chronic disease.
Defective absorption, transport, or use of iron.
Disorders of globin synthesis:

- Thalassemia.
- Other microcytic hemoglobinopathies.

Disorders of heme synthesis: sideroblastic anemias:

- Hereditary.
- Acquired.

ANEMIA, LOW RETICULOCYTE COUNT[1a]

ICD-9CM # 285.9
ICD-10CM # D64.9 Anemia, Unspecified

MICROCYTIC ANEMIA (MCV <80)

Iron deficiency.
Thalassemia minor.
Sideroblastic anemia.
Lead poisoning.

MACROCYTIC ANEMIA (MCV >100)

Megaloblastic anemias.
Folate deficiency.
Vitamin B_{12} deficiency.
Drug-induced megaloblastic anemia.
Nonmegaloblastic macrocytosis.
Liver disease.
Hypothyroidism.

NORMOCYTIC ANEMIA (MCV 80-100)

Early iron deficiency.
Aplastic anemia.
Myelophthisic disorders.
Endocrinopathies.
Anemia of chronic disease.
Uremia.
Mixed nutritional deficiency.

ANEMIA, MEGALOBLASTIC[36]

ICD-9CM # 281.0 Pernicious Anemia
281.1 B_{12} Deficiency
281.2 Folate Deficiency
281.3 B_{12} with Folate Deficiency
281.4 Protein or Amino Acid Deficiency
281.8 Nutritional
281.9 NOS
ICD-10CM # D51.0 Vitamin B12 Deficiency Anemia Due to Intrinsic Factor Deficiency
D51.1 Vitamin B12 Deficiency Anemia Due to Selective Vitamin B12 Malabsorption with Proteinuria
D51.3 Other Dietary Vitamin B12 Deficiency Anemia
D51.8 Other Vitamin B12 Deficiency Anemias
D52.0 Dietary Folate Deficiency Anemia
D52.1 Drug-Induced Folate Deficiency Anemia
D52.8 Other Folate Deficiency Anemias
D52.9 Folate Deficiency Anemia, Unspecified
D53.1 Other Megaloblastic Anemias, Not Elsewhere Classified
D53.0 Protein Deficiency Anemia
D53.2 Scorbutic Anemia
D53.8 Other Specified Nutritional Anemias
D53.9 Nutritional Anemia, Unspecified

COBALAMIN (CBL) DEFICIENCY

Nutritional CBL Deficiency (Insufficient CBL Intake)

Vegetarians, vegans, breastfed infants of mothers with pernicious anemia.

Abnormal Intragastric Events (Inadequate Proteolysis of Food CBL)

Atrophic gastritis, partial gastrectomy with hypochlorhydria.

Loss/Atrophy of Gastric Oxyntic Mucosa (Deficient Intrinsic Factor [If] Molecules)

Total or partial gastrectomy, pernicious anemia (PA), caustic destruction (lye).

Abnormal Events in Small Bowel Lumen

Inadequate pancreatic protease (R-CBL not degraded, CBL not transferred to IF).

- Insufficiency of pancreatic protease—pancreatic insufficiency.
- Inactivation of pancreatic protease—Zollinger-Ellison syndrome.

Usurping of luminal CBL (inadequate CBL binding to IF).

- By bacteria—stasis syndromes (blind loops, pouches of diverticulosis, strictures, fistulas, anastomoses); impaired bowel motility (scleroderma, pseudoobstruction), hypogammaglobulinemia.
- By *Diphyllobothrium latum.*

Disorders of Ileal Mucosa/If Receptors (If-CBL Not Bound to if Receptors)

Diminished or absent IF receptors—ileal bypass/resection/fistula.
Abnormal mucosal architecture/function—tropical/nontropical sprue, Crohn's disease, TB ileitis, infiltration by lymphomas, amyloidosis.
IF-/post IF-receptor defects—Imerslund-Graesbeck syndrome, TC II deficiency.
Drug-induced effects (slow K, biguanides, cholestyramine, colchicine, neomycin, PAS).

DISORDERS OF PLASMA CBL TRANSPORT (TC II-CBL NOT DELIVERED TO TC II RECEPTORS)

Congenital TC II deficiency, defective binding of TC II-CBL to TC II receptors (rare).

METABOLIC DISORDERS (CBL NOT UTILIZED BY CELL)

Inborn enzyme errors (rare).
Acquired disorders: (CBL oxidized to cob[III] alamin)—N_2O inhalation.

FOLATE DEFICIENCY

Nutritional Causes

Decreased dietary intake—poverty and famine (associated with kwashiorkor, marasmus), institutionalized individuals (psychiatric/nursing homes), chronic debilitating disease/goats' milk (low in folate), special diets (slimming), cultural/ethnic cooking techniques (food folate destroyed) or habits (folate-rich foods not consumed).
Decreased diet and increased requirements:

- Physiologic: pregnancy and lactation, prematurity, infancy.
- Pathologic: intrinsic hematologic disease (autoimmune hemolytic disease), drugs, malaria; hemoglobinopathies (SS, thalassemia), RBC membrane defects (hereditary spherocytosis, paroxysmal nocturnal hemoglobinopathy); abnormal hematopoiesis (leukemia/lymphoma, myelodysplastic syndrome, agnogenic myeloid metaplasia with myelofibrosis); infiltration with malignant disease; dermatologic (psoriasis).

Folate Malabsorption

With normal intestinal mucosa:

- Some drugs (controversial).
- Congenital folate malabsorption (rare).

With mucosal abnormalities—tropical and nontropical sprue, regional enteritis.

Defective Cellular Folate Uptake—Familial Aplastic Anemia (Rare), Inadequate Cellular Utilization

Folate antagonists (methotrexate).
Hereditary enzyme deficiencies involving folate.

Drugs (Multiple Effects on Folate Metabolism)

Alcohol, sulfasalazine, triamterene, pyrimethamine, trimethoprim-sulfamethoxazole, diphenylhydantoin, barbiturates.

MISCELLANEOUS MEGALOBLASTIC ANEMIAS (NOT CAUSED BY CBL OR FOLATE DEFICIENCY)

Congenital Disorders of DNA Synthesis (Rare)

Orotic aciduria, Lesch-Nyhan syndrome, congenital dyserythropoietic anemia.

Acquired Disorders of DNA Synthesis

Thiamine-responsive megaloblastosis (rare).
Malignancy—erythroleukemia—refractory sideroblastic anemias—all antineoplastic drugs that inhibit DNA synthesis.
Toxins—alcohol.

ANERGY, CUTANEOUS[36]

ICD-9CM # 279.9
ICD-10CM # D89.9 Disorder Involving the Immune Mechanism, Unspecified

IMMUNOLOGIC

Acquired (AIDS, acute leukemia, carcinoma, CLL, Hodgkin's lymphoma, NHL).
Congenital (ataxia-telangiectasia, Di George's syndrome, severe combined immunodeficiency, Wiskott-Aldrich syndrome).

INFECTIONS

Bacterial (bacterial pneumonia, brucellosis).
Disseminated mycotic infections.
Mycobacterial (lepromatous leprosy, TB).
Viral (varicella, hepatitis, influenza, mononucleosis, measles, mumps).

IMMUNOSUPPRESSIVE MEDICATIONS

Systemic corticosteroids.
Methotrexate, cyclophosphamide.
Rifampin.

OTHER

Alcoholic cirrhosis, biliary cirrhosis, sarcoidosis, rheumatic disease.
Diabetes, Crohn's disease, uremia.
Anemia, pyridoxine deficiency, sickle cell anemia.
Burns, malnutrition, pregnancy, old age, surgery.

ANEURYSMS, THORACIC AORTA

ICD-9CM # 441.2
ICD-10CM # I71.2 Thoracic Aortic Aneurysm, Without Rupture

Trauma.
Infection.
Inflammatory (syphilis, Takayasu's disease).
Collagen vascular disease (RA, ankylosing spondylitis).
Annuloaortic ectasia (Marfan's syndrome, Ehlers-Danlos syndrome).
Congenital.
Coarctation.
Cystic medial necrosis.

ANHIDROSIS

ICD-9CM # 705.1
ICD-10CM # L74.0 Miliaria Rubra
L74.1 Miliaria Crystallina
L74.2 Miliaria Profunda

Drugs (anticholinergics).
Dehydration.
Hysteria.
Obstruction of sweat ducts (e.g., inflammation, miliaria).
Local radiant heat or pressure.
CNS lesions (medulla, hypothalamus, pons).
Spinal cord lesions.
Lesions of sympathetic nerves.
Congenital sweat gland disturbances.

ANION GAP ACIDOSIS[38b]

ICD-9CM # 276.9
ICD-10CM # E87.2 Acidosis

CLINICAL CAUSES OF HIGH ANION GAP AND NORMAL ANION GAP ACIDOSIS

High Anion Gap

Ketoacidosis:
- Diabetic ketoacidosis (acetoacetate).
- Alcoholic (β-hydroxybutyrate).
- Starvation.

Lactic acid acidosis:
- L-Lactic acid acidosis (types A and B).
- D-Lactic acid acidosis.
- Renal failure: sulfate, phosphate, urate, hippurate.

Ingestions (toxins and their metabolites):
- Ethylene glycol → glycolate, oxalate.
- Methyl alcohol → formate.
- Salicylate → ketones, lactate, salicylate.
- Paraldehyde → organic anions.
- Toluene → hippurate (commonly presents with normal anion gap).
- Propylene glycol → lactate.
- Pyroglutamic acidosis (acetaminophen use) → 5-oxoproline.

Normal Anion Gap

Gastrointestinal loss of HCO_3^- (negative urine anion gap):
- Diarrhea.
- Fistula, external.

Renal loss of HCO_3^- or failure to excrete NH_4^+ (positive urine anion gap):
- Proximal renal tubular acidosis (RTA type 2).
- Acetazolamide.
- Classic distal renal tubular acidosis (low serum K^+) RTA type 1.
- Generalized distal renal tubular defect (high serum K^+) RTA type 4.

Miscellaneous:
- NH_4Cl ingestion.
- Sulfur ingestion.
- Dilutional acidosis.
- Late stages in treatment of diabetic ketoacidosis.

ANION GAP INCREASE

ICD-9CM # 276.9
ICD-10CM # E87.8 Other Disorders of Electrolyte and Fluid Balance, Not Elsewhere Classified

Uremia.
Ketoacidosis (diabetic, starvation, alcoholic).
Lactic acidosis.
Ethylene glycol poisoning.
Salicylate overdose.
Methanol poisoning.

ANISOCORIA

ICD-9CM # 379.41
ICD-10CM # H57.02 Anisocoria

Mydriatic or miotic drugs.
Prosthetic eye.
Inflammation (keratitis, iridocyclitis).
Infections (herpes zoster, syphilis, meningitis, encephalitis, TB, diphtheria, botulism).
Subdural hemorrhage.
Cavernous sinus thrombosis.
Intracranial neoplasm.
Cerebral aneurysm.
Glaucoma.
CNS degenerative diseases.
Internal carotid ischemia.
Toxic polyneuritis (alcohol, lead).
Adie's syndrome.
Horner's syndrome.
DM.
Trauma.
Congenital.

ANOREXIA[38]

ICD-9CM # 783.0
ICD-10CM # R63.0 Anorexia

SELECTED CAUSES OF ANOREXIA

Gastrointestinal Tract/Liver

Gastric outlet obstruction or small bowel obstruction.
Gastric cancer.
Hepatic metastases.
Acute viral hepatitis.

Metabolic

Addison's disease.
Hypopituitarism.
Hyperparathyroidism.

Functional

Extremely unpleasant sight/smell.

Systemic

Chronic pain.
Renal failure.
Severe congestive heart failure.
Respiratory failure.

Psychiatric

Depression.
Anorexia nervosa.

Medications

Digoxin.
Narcotic analgesics.
Diuretics.
Antihypertensives.
Chemotherapeutic agents.
Amphetamines.

Miscellaneous

Excessive smoking.
Excessive alcohol intake.
Oral cavity disease.
Thiamine deficiency.
Early pregnancy.
Hypogeusia or dysgeusia.

ANOVULATION

ICD-9CM # 628.0
ICD-10CM # N97.0 Female Infertility Associated With Anovulation

Anorexia and bulimia.
Strenuous exercise.
Weight loss/malnutrition.
Empty sella syndrome.
Pituitary disorders (infarction, infection, trauma, irradiation, surgery, microadenomas, macroadenomas).

Idiopathic hypopituitarism.
Drug induced.
Thyroid dysfunction (hypothyroidism, hyperthyroidism).
Systemic diseases (e.g., liver disease).
Adrenal hyperfunction (Cushing's syndrome, congenital adrenal hyperplasia).
Polycystic ovarian syndrome.
Isolated gonadotropin deficiency.

APPETITE LOSS IN INFANTS AND CHILDREN[19]

ICD-9CM #	783.0	Appetite Loss
	307.59	Appetite Loss, Psychogenic Origin
ICD-10CM #	R63.0	Anorexia
	F50.8	Other Eating Disorders
	F98.29	Other Feeding Disorders of Infancy and Early Childhood

ORGANIC DISEASE

Infection (Acute or Chronic) Neurologic
Congenital degenerative disease.
Hypothalamic lesion.
Increased intracranial pressure (including a brain tumor).
Swallowing disorders (neuromuscular).
Gastrointestinal
Oral lesions (e.g., thrush or herpes simplex).
Gastroesophageal reflux.
Obstruction (especially with gastric or intestinal distention).
Inflammatory bowel disease.
Celiac disease.
Constipation.
Cardiac
Congestive heart failure (especially associated with cyanotic lesions).
Metabolic
Renal failure and/or renal tubule acidosis.
Liver failure.
Congenital metabolic disease.
Lead poisoning.
Nutritional
Marasmus.
Iron deficiency.
Zinc deficiency.
Fever
RA.
Rheumatic fever.
Drugs
Morphine.
Digitalis.
Antimetabolites.
Methylphenidate.
Amphetamines.
Miscellaneous
Prolonged restriction of oral feedings, beginning in the neonatal period.
Systemic lupus erythematosus (SLE).
Tumor.

PSYCHOLOGIC FACTORS

Anxiety, fear, depression, mania (limbic influence on the hypothalamus).
Avoidance of symptoms associated with meals (abdominal pain, diarrhea, bloating, urgency, dumping syndrome).
Anorexia nervosa.
Excessive weight loss and food aversion in athletes, simulating anorexia nervosa.

ARTERIAL OCCLUSION[15]

ICD-9CM #	444.22	Arterial Occlusion, Lower Extremities
	444.21	Arterial Occlusion, Upper Extremities
ICD-10CM #	I74.3	Embolism and Thrombosis of Arteries of the Lower Extremities
	I74.2	Embolism and Thrombosis of Arteries of the Upper Extremities

Thromboembolism (post-MI, mitral stenosis, rheumatic valve disease, atrial fibrillation, atrial myxoma, marantic endocarditis, bacterial endocarditis, Libman-Sacks endocarditis).
Atheroembolism (microemboli composed of cholesterol, calcium, and platelets from proximal atherosclerotic plaques).
Arterial thrombosis (endothelial injury, altered arterial blood flow, trauma, severe atherosclerosis, acute vasculitis).
Vasospasm.
Trauma.
Hypercoagulable states.
Miscellaneous (irradiation, drugs, infections, necrotizing).

ARTHRITIS AND ABDOMINAL PAIN

ICD-9CM #	varies with specific disorder	
ICD-10CM #	M00.9	Pyogenic Arthritis, Unspecified
	R10.817	Generalized Abdominal Tenderness
	M02.9	Reactive arthropathy

Viral syndrome.
Inflammatory bowel disease.
Celiac disease.
Vasculitis.
SLE.
RA.
Scleroderma.
Amyloidosis.
Chronic hepatitis C.
Whipple's disease.
Polyarteritis nodosa.
Behçet's disease.
Familial Mediterranean fever.
Blind loop syndrome.
Babesiosis.
Lyme disease.
Ehrlichiosis.

ARTHRITIS AND DIARRHEA

ICD-9CM #	varies with specific disorder	
ICD-10CM #	M00.9	Pyogenic Arthritis, Unspecified
	R19.7	Diarrhea, Unspecified

Viral syndrome.
Inflammatory bowel disease.
Celiac disease.
Whipple's disease.
Enterogenic (bacterial) reactive arthritis.
Collagenous colitis.
Behçet's disease.
Hyperthyroidism.
Spondyloarthropathy.
Blind loop syndrome.

ARTHRITIS AND EYE LESIONS[6]

ICD-9CM #	varies with specific diagnosis	
ICD-10CM #	M00.9	Pyogenic Arthritis, Unspecified
	M02.3	Reiter disease
	M02.9	Reactive arthropathy

SLE.
Sjögren's syndrome.
Behçet's syndrome.
Sarcoidosis.
Subacute bacterial endocarditis (SBE).
Lyme disease.
Granulomatosis with polyangiitis (Wegener's granulomatosis).
Giant cell arteritis.
Takayasu's arteritis.
RA, JRA.
Scleroderma.
Inflammatory bowel disease.
Whipple's disease.
Ankylosing spondylitis.
Reactive arthritis.
Psoriatic arthritis.

ARTHRITIS AND HEART MURMUR[6]

ICD-9CM #	varies with specific diagnosis	
ICD-10CM #	M00.9	Pyogenic Arthritis, Unspecified
	I01.8	Other Acute Rheumatic Heart Disease
	M02.9	Reactive arthropathy

SBE.
Cardiac myxoma.
Ankylosing spondylitis.
Reactive arthritis.
Acute rheumatic fever.
RA.
SLE with Libman-Sacks endocarditis.
Relapsing polychondritis.

ARTHRITIS AND MUSCLE WEAKNESS[8]

ICD-9CM #	varies with specific diagnosis	
ICD-10CM #	M00.9	Pyogenic Arthritis, Unspecified
	M62.9	Disorder of Muscle, Unspecified
	M02.9	Reactive arthropathy

RA.
Ankylosing spondylitis.
Polymyositis.
Dermatomyositis.
SLE, scleroderma, mixed connective tissue disease.
Sarcoidosis.
HIV-associated arthritis.
Whipple's disease.

ARTHRITIS AND RASH[6]

ICD-9CM #	varies with specific diagnosis	
ICD-10CM #	M00.9	Pyogenic Arthritis, Unspecified
	R21	Rash and Other Nonspecific Skin Eruption
	M02.9	Reactive arthropathy

Chronic urticaria.
Vasculitic urticaria.
SLE.
Dermatomyositis.
Polymyositis.
Psoriatic arthritis.
Reactive arthritis.
Chronic sarcoidosis.
Serum sickness.
Sweet's syndrome.
Leprosy.

ARTHRITIS AND SUBCUTANEOUS NODULES[6]

ICD-9CM #	varies with specific diagnosis	
ICD-10CM #	M00.9	Pyogenic Arthritis, Unspecified
	A18.4	Tuberculosis of Skin and Subcutaneous Tissue
	M02.9	Reactive arthropathy

RA.
Gout.
Pseudogout (rare).
Sarcoidosis.
Light chain (LA) amyloidosis (primary, multiple myeloma).
Acute rheumatic fever (ARF).
Hemochromatosis.
Whipple's disease.
Multicentric reticulohistiocytosis.

ARTHRITIS AND WEIGHT LOSS[6]

ICD-9CM #	varies with specific diagnosis	
ICD-10CM #	M00.9	Pyogenic Arthritis, Unspecified
	R63.4	Abnormal Weight Loss
	M02.9	Reactive arthropathy

Severe RA.
RA with vasculitis.
Reactive arthritis.
RA or psoriatic arthritis or ankylosing spondylitis with amyloidosis.
Cancer.
Enteropathic arthritis (Crohn's, ulcerative colitis).
HIV infection.
Whipple's disease.
Blind loop syndrome.
Scleroderma with intestinal bacterial overgrowth.

ARTHRITIS OR EXTREMITY PAIN, IN CHILDREN AND ADOLESCENTS[22a]

ICD-9CM #	varies with specific diagnosis
ICD-10CM #	M02.9 Reactive arthropathy

CAUSES OF ARTHRITIS OR EXTREMITY PAIN IN CHILDREN AND ADOLESCENTS

Rheumatic and Inflammatory Diseases
Juvenile idiopathic arthritis.
Systemic lupus erythematosus.
Juvenile dermatomyositis.
Polyarteritis.
Vasculitis.
Scleroderma.
Sjögren syndrome.
Behçet disease.
Overlap syndromes.
Granulomatosis with polyangiitis (Wegener granulomatosis).
Sarcoidosis.
Kawasaki syndrome.
Henoch-Schönlein purpura.
Chronic recurrent multifocal osteomyelitis.

Seronegative Spondyloarthropathies
Juvenile ankylosing spondylitis.
Inflammatory bowel disease.
Psoriatic arthritis.
Reactive arthritis associated with urethritis, iridocyclitis, and mucocutaneous lesions.

Infectious Illnesses
Bacterial arthritis (septic arthritis, *Staphylococcus aureus*, pneumococcus, gonococcus, *Haemophilus influenzae*).
Lyme disease.
Viral illness (parvovirus, rubella, mumps, Epstein-Barr virus, hepatitis B).
Fungal arthritis.
Mycobacterial infection.
Spirochetal infection.
Endocarditis.

Reactive Arthritis
Acute rheumatic fever.
Reactive arthritis (postinfectious due to *Shigella, Salmonella, Yersinia, Chlamydia,* or meningococcus).
Serum sickness.
Toxic synovitis of the hip.
Postimmunization.

Immunodeficiencies
Hypogammaglobulinemia.
Immunoglobulin A deficiency.
Human immunodeficiency virus.

Congenital and Metabolic Disorders
Gout.
Pseudogout.
Mucopolysaccharidoses.
Thyroid disease (hypothyroidism, hyperthyroidism).
Hyperparathyroidism.
Vitamin C deficiency (scurvy).
Hereditary connective tissue disease (Marfan syndrome, Ehlers-Danlos syndrome).
Fabry disease.
Farber disease.
Amyloidosis (familial Mediterranean fever).

Bone and Cartilage Disorders
Trauma.
Patellofemoral syndrome.
Hypermobility syndrome.
Osteochondritis dissecans.
Avascular necrosis (including Legg-Calvé-Perthes disease).
Hypertrophic osteoarthropathy.
Slipped capital femoral epiphysis.
Osteolysis.
Benign bone tumors (including osteoid osteoma).
Histiocytosis.
Rickets.

Neuropathic Disorders
Peripheral neuropathies.
Carpal tunnel syndrome.
Charcot joints.

Neoplastic Disorders
Leukemia.
Neuroblastoma.
Lymphoma.
Bone tumors (osteosarcoma, Ewing sarcoma).
Histiocytic syndromes.
Synovial tumors.

Hematologic Disorders
Hemophilia.
Hemoglobinopathies (including sickle cell disease).

Miscellaneous Disorders
Pigmented villonodular synovitis.
Plant-thorn synovitis (foreign body arthritis).
Myositis ossificans.
Eosinophilic fasciitis.
Tendinitis (overuse injury).
Raynaud phenomenon.

Pain Syndromes
Fibromyalgia.
Growing pains.
Depression (with somatization).
Reflex sympathetic dystrophy.
Regional myofascial pain syndromes.

ARTHRITIS, AXIAL SKELETON

ICD-9CM #	720.0	Arthritis, Rheumatoid, Spine
	696.0	Arthritis, Psoriatic
	715.9	Arthritis, Degenerative, NOS
	720.0	Ankylosing Spondylitis
ICD-10CM #	M45.9	Ankylosing Spondylitis of Unspecified Sites in Spine
	L40.54	Psoriatic Juvenile Arthropathy
	L40.59	Other Psoriatic Arthropathy
	M15.9	Polyosteoarthritis, Unspecified
	M45.9	Ankylosing Spondylitis of Unspecified Sites in Spine

RA.
Psoriatic arthritis.
Reiter's syndrome (reactive arthritis).
Ankylosing spondylitis.

Juvenile RA.
Degenerative disease of the nucleus pulposus.
Spondylosis deformans.
Diffuse idiopathic skeletal hyperostosis (DISH).
Alkaptonuria.
Infection.

ARTHRITIS, FEVER, AND RASH[6]

ICD-9CM #	varies with specific diagnosis	
ICD-10CM #	M00.9	Pyogenic Arthritis, Unspecified
	M02.9	Reactive arthropathy
	R21	Rash and Other Nonspecific Skin Eruption
	R50.9	Fever, Unspecified

Rubella, parvovirus B19.
Gonococcemia, meningococcemia.
Secondary syphilis, Lyme borreliosis.
Adult acute rheumatic fever, adult Still's disease, adult Kawasaki disease.
Vasculitic urticaria.
Acute sarcoidosis.
Familial Mediterranean fever.
Hyperimmunoglobulinemia D and periodic fever syndrome.

ARTHRITIS, MONOARTICULAR AND OLIGOARTICULAR[2]

ICD-9CM #	715.3	Osteoarthritis, Localized
	711.9	Infectious Arthritis
	716.6	Monoarticular Arthritis; 5th digit to be added to the above depending on site of arthritis 0. Site Unspecified 1. Shoulder Region 2. Upper Arm 3. Forearm 4. Hand 5. Pelvic Region and Thigh 6. Lower Leg 7. Ankle and/or Foot 8. Other Specified Except Spine
ICD-10CM #	M19.90	Unspecified Osteoarthritis, Unspecified Site
	M01.X0	Direct Infection of Unspecified Joint in Infectious and Parasitic Diseases Classified Elsewhere
	M13.10	Monoarthritis, Not Elsewhere Classified, Unspecified Site

Septic arthritis (*S. aureus, Neisseria gonorrhoeae,* meningococci, streptococci, *Streptococcus pneumoniae,* enteric gram-negative bacilli).
Crystalline-induced arthritis (gout, pseudogout, calcium oxalate, hydroxyapatite and other basic calcium/phosphate crystals).
Traumatic joint injury.
Hemarthrosis.
Monoarticular or oligoarticular flare of an inflammatory polyarticular rheumatic disease (RA, psoriatic arthritis, Reiter's syndrome [reactive arthritis], SLE).

ARTHRITIS, PEDIATRIC AGE[19]

ICD-9CM #	711.9	Infectious Arthritis
	714.30	Juvenile Chronic or Unspecified
	714.31	Juvenile Rheumatoid Polyarticular Acute
	714.32	Juvenile Rheumatoid Pauciarticular
	714.33	Juvenile Rheumatoid Monoarticular
ICD-10CM #	M01.X0	Direct Infection of Unspecified Joint in Infectious and Parasitic Diseases Classified Elsewhere
	M08.00	Unspecified Juvenile Rheumatoid Arthritis of Unspecified Site
	M08.3	Juvenile Rheumatoid Polyarthritis (Seronegative)
	M08.40	Pauciarticular Juvenile Rheumatoid Arthritis, Unspecified Site

RHEUMATIC DISEASES OF CHILDHOOD

Acute rheumatic fever.
SLE.
Juvenile ankylosing spondylitis.
Polymyositis and dermatomyositis.
Vasculitis.
Scleroderma.
Psoriatic arthritis.
Mixed connective tissue disease and overlap syndromes.
Kawasaki disease.
Behçet's syndrome.
Familial Mediterranean fever.
Reiter's syndrome (reactive arthritis).
Reflex sympathetic dystrophy.
Fibromyalgia (fibrositis).

INFECTIOUS DISEASES

Bacterial arthritis.
Viral or postviral arthritis.
Fungal arthritis.
Osteomyelitis.
Reactive arthritis.

NEOPLASTIC DISEASES

Leukemia.
Lymphoma.
Neuroblastoma.
Primary bone tumors.

NONINFLAMMATORY DISORDERS

Trauma.
Avascular necrosis syndromes.
Osteochondroses.
Slipped capital femoral epiphysis.
Diskitis.
Patellofemoral dysfunction (chondromalacia patellae).
Toxic synovitis of the hip.
Overuse syndromes.

GENETIC OR CONGENITAL SYNDROMES

Hematologic Disorders

Sickle cell disease.
Hemophilia.

INFLAMMATORY BOWEL DISEASE

Miscellaneous

Growing pains.
Psychogenic arthralgias (conversion reactions).
Hypermobility syndrome.
Villonodular synovitis.
Foreign body arthritis.

ARTHRITIS, POLYARTICULAR

ICD-9CM #	715.09	Generalized Osteoarthritis, Multiple Sites
	716.89	Arthritis, Multiple Sites
	714.31	Juvenile Rheumatoid, Polyarticular, Acute
ICD-10CM #	M15.0	Primary Generalized (Osteo)Arthritis
	M12.89	Other Specific Arthropathies, Not Elsewhere Classified, Multiple Sites
	M08.3	Juvenile Rheumatoid Polyarthritis (Seronegative)

RA, juvenile (rheumatoid) polyarthritis.
SLE, other connective tissue diseases, erythema nodosum, palindromic rheumatism, relapsing polychondritis.
Psoriatic arthritis, ankylosing spondylitis.
Sarcoidosis.
Lyme arthritis, bacterial endocarditis, *Neisseria gonorrhoeae* infection, rheumatic fever, Reiter's disease (reactive arthritis).
Crystal deposition disease.
Hypersensitivity to serum or drugs.
Hepatitis B, HIV, rubella, mumps.
Other: serum sickness, leukemias, lymphomas, enteropathic arthropathy, Whipple's disease, Behçet's syndrome, Henoch-Schönlein purpura, familial Mediterranean fever, hypertrophic pulmonary osteoarthropathy.

ASCITES

ICD-9CM #	789.5	Ascites NOS
	197.6	Ascites, Cancerous (Malignant)
	457.8	Ascites, Chylous

ICD-10CM #	R18.0	Malignant Ascites
	C78.6	Secondary Malignant Neoplasm of Retroperitoneum and Peritoneum
	I89.8	Other Specified Noninfective Disorders of Lymphatic Vessels and Lymph Nodes

Hypoalbuminemia: nephrotic syndrome, protein-losing gastroenteropathy, starvation.
Cirrhosis.
Hepatic congestion: CHF, constrictive pericarditis, tricuspid insufficiency, hepatic vein obstruction (Budd-Chiari syndrome), inferior vena cava or portal vein obstruction.
Peritoneal infections: TB and other bacterial infections, fungal diseases, parasites.
Neoplasms: primary hepatic neoplasms, metastases to liver or peritoneum, lymphomas, leukemias, myeloid metaplasia.
Lymphatic obstruction: mediastinal tumors, trauma to the thoracic duct, filariasis.
Ovarian disease: Meigs' syndrome, struma ovarii.
Chronic pancreatitis or pseudocyst: pancreatic ascites.
Leakage of bile: bile ascites.
Urinary obstruction or trauma: urine ascites.
Myxedema.
Chylous ascites.

ASPIRATION LUNG INJURY, CHILDREN[22a]

ICD-9CM #	507.0	
ICD-10CM #	P24.8	Neonatal aspiration syndromes

CONDITIONS PREDISPOSING TO ASPIRATION LUNG INJURY IN CHILDREN

Anatomic and Mechanical

Tracheoesophageal fistula.
Laryngeal cleft.
Vascular ring.
Cleft palate.
Micrognathia.
Macroglossia.
Achalasia.
Esophageal foreign body.
Tracheostomy.
Endotracheal tube.
Nasoenteric tube.
Collagen vascular disease (scleroderma, dermatomyositises).
Gastroesophageal reflux disease.
Obesity.

Neuromuscular

Altered consciousness.
Immaturity of swallowing/prematurity.
Dysautonomia.
Increased intracranial pressure.
Hydrocephalus.
Vocal cord paralysis.
Cerebral palsy.
Muscular dystrophy.
Myasthenia gravis.
Guillain-Barré syndrome.
Werdnig-Hoffmann disease.
Ataxia-telangiectasia.
Cerebral vascular accident.

Miscellaneous

Poor oral hygiene.
Gingivitis.
Prolonged hospitalization.
Gastric outlet or intestinal obstruction.
Poor feeding techniques (bottle propping, overfeeding, inappropriate foods for toddlers).
Bronchopulmonary dysplasia.
Viral infection.

ASTHENIA

ICD-9CM #	780.79	
ICD-10CM #	G93.3	Postviral Fatigue syndrome
	R53.1	Weakness
	R53.81	Other Malaise
	R53.83	Other Fatigue

Depression.
Chronic fatigue syndrome.
Sleep disorders.
Anemia.
Hypothyroidism.
Sedentary lifestyle.
Medications (e.g., narcotics, sedatives).
Infections.
Dehydration/electrolyte disorders.
COPD and other pulmonary disorders.
Renal failure.
CHF.
Diabetes.
Addison's disease.
Paraneoplastic syndrome.

ASTHMA, CHILDHOOD[4]

ICD-9CM #	493.0	use 5th digit
	0	Without Mention of Status Asthmaticus
	1	With Status Asthmaticus
ICD-10CM #	J45.20	Mild Intermittent Asthma, Uncomplicated
	J45.22	Mild Intermittent Asthma with Status Asthmaticus

INFECTIONS

Bronchiolitis (RSV).
Pneumonia.
Croup.
Tuberculosis, histoplasmosis.
Bronchiectasis.
Bronchiolitis obliterans.
Bronchitis.
Sinusitis.

ANATOMIC, CONGENITAL

Cystic fibrosis.
Vascular rings.
Ciliary dyskinesia.
B-lymphocyte immune defect.
Congestive heart failure.
Laryngotracheomalacia.
Tumor, lymphoma.
H-type tracheoesophageal fistula.
Repaired tracheoesophageal fistula.
Gastroesophageal reflux.

VASCULITIS, HYPERSENSITIVITY

Allergic bronchopulmonary aspergillosis.
Allergic alveolitis, hypersensitivity pneumonitis.
Churg-Strauss syndrome.
Periarteritis nodosa.

OTHER

Foreign body aspiration.
Pulmonary thromboembolism.
Psychogenic cough.
Sarcoidosis.
Bronchopulmonary dysplasia.
Vocal cord dysfunction.

ATAXIA

ICD-9CM #	781.3	Ataxia NOS
	303.0	Alcoholic, Acute
	303.9	Alcoholic, Chronic
	334.3	Cerebellar
	331.89	Cerebral
	334.0	Friedreich's
	300.11	Hysterical
ICD-10CM #	R27.0	Ataxia, Unspecified
	R27.8	Other Lack of Coordination
	R27.9	Unspecified Lack of Coordination
	F10.229	Alcohol Dependence with Intoxication, Unspecified
	F10.20	Alcohol Dependence, Uncomplicated
	G11.1	Early-Onset Cerebellar Ataxia
	G31.89	Other Specified Degenerative Diseases of Nervous System
	F44.4	Conversion Disorder with Motor Symptom or Deficit
	F44.6	Conversion Disorder with Sensory Symptom or Deficit

Vertebral-basilar artery ischemia.
Diabetic neuropathy.
Tabes dorsalis.
Vitamin B_{12} deficiency.
Multiple sclerosis and other demyelinating diseases.
Meningomyelopathy.
Cerebellar neoplasms, hemorrhage, abscess, infarct.
Nutritional (Wernicke's encephalopathy).
Paraneoplastic syndromes.
Parainfectious: Guillain-Barré syndrome, acute ataxia of childhood and young adults.
Toxins: phenytoin, alcohol, sedatives, organophosphates.
Wilson's disease (hepatolenticular degeneration).
Hypothyroidism.
Myopathy.
Cerebellar and spinocerebellar degeneration: ataxia/telangiectasia, Friedreich's ataxia.
Frontal lobe lesions: tumors, thrombosis of anterior cerebral artery, hydrocephalus.
Labyrinthine destruction: neoplasm, injury, inflammation, compression.
Hysteria.
AIDS.

ATAXIA, ACUTE OR RECURRENT[11]

ICD-9CM #
781.3 Ataxia NOS
303.0 Alcoholic, Acute
303.9 Alcoholic, Chronic
334.3 Cerebellar
331.89 Cerebral
334.0 Friedreich's
300.11 Hysterical

ICD-10CM #
R27.0 Ataxia, Unspecified
R27.8 Other Lack of Coordination
R27.9 Unspecified Lack of Coordination
F10.229 Alcohol Dependence with Intoxication, Unspecified
F10.20 Alcohol Dependence, Uncomplicated
G11.1 Early-Onset Cerebellar Ataxia
G31.89 Other Specified Degenerative Diseases of Nervous System
F44.4 Conversion Disorder with Motor Symptom or Deficit
F44.6 Conversion Disorder with Sensory Symptom or Deficit

Drug ingestion (e.g., phenytoin, carbamazepine, sedatives, hypnotics, and phencyclidine) or intoxication (e.g., alcohol, ethylene glycol, hydrocarbon fumes, lead, mercury, or thallium).
Postinfectious (cerebellitis [e.g., varicella], acute disseminated encephalomyelitis).
Head trauma.
Basilar migraine.
Benign paroxysmal vertigo (migraine equivalent).
Brain tumor or neuroblastoma (if accompanied by opsoclonus or myoclonus [i.e., "dancing eyes, dancing feet"]).
Hydrocephalus.
Infection (e.g., labyrinthitis, abscess).
Seizure (ictal or postictal).
Vascular events (e.g., cerebellar hemorrhage or stroke).
Miller-Fisher variant of Guillain-Barré syndrome (ataxia, ophthalmoplegia, and areflexia). Warning: If bulbar signs present, disease is likely progressive; patient may lose ability to protect airway and/or ability to breathe.
Inherited ataxias.
Inborn errors of metabolism (e.g., mitochondrial disorders, amino-acidopathies, urea cycle defects).
Conversion reaction.
Multiple sclerosis.

ATAXIA, CEREBELLAR, ADULT ONSET[34a]

ICD-9CM # 334.2

ICD-10CM #
G11.0 Congenital Nonprogressive Ataxia
G11.2 Late-Onset Cerebellar Ataxia

CAUSES OF ADULT ONSET CEREBELLAR ATAXIA

Inherited
Later onset SCA syndromes.
Rarely Friedreich's ataxia.
Congenital
Arnold–Chiari malformation (cerebellar ectopia).
Inflammatory
Multiple sclerosis.
Sarcoidosis.
Infections (TB, viral).
Neoplastic
Often metastatic in adults.
Meningioma, neurofibroma.
Hemangioblastoma.
Paraneoplastic
Usually with small cell bronchial carcinoma.
Vascular
Infarction, hemorrhage.
Arteriovenous malformations.
Trauma
Head injury.
Postsurgical.
Toxic
Alcohol, phenytoin, solvent abuse.
Endocrine
Hypothyroidism (very rare).
Degenerative
Multiple system atrophy (MSA).

ATAXIA, CEREBELLAR, CHILDREN[34a]

ICD-9CM # 334.2

ICD-10CM #
G11.0 Congenital Nonprogressive Ataxia
G11.2 Late-Onset Cerebellar Ataxia

CAUSES OF CEREBELLAR ATAXIA IN CHILDREN

Congenital Malformations
Cerebellar agenesis/hypoplasia.
Dandy–Walker syndrome.*
Arnold–Chiari malformation.**
Hereditary Ataxias
Friedreich's ataxia.
Trauma
Birth trauma.*
Head injury in childhood.*
Infectious
Secondary to bacterial meningitis.
Secondary to encephalitis.
Hydrocephalus*
Tumors
Medulloblastoma.
Astrocytoma.
Hemangioblastoma.

*May persist into adult life.
**May present in adult life.

ATAXIA, CHRONIC OR PROGRESSIVE[11]

ICD-9CM # varies with specific diagnosis
781.3 Ataxia NOS
0.94 Locomotor Ataxia
334.0 Friedreich's Ataxia
334.2 Cerebellar Ataxia, Primary
334.3 Other Cerebellar Ataxia
334.8 Ataxia-telangiectasia

ICD-10CM #
R27.0 Ataxia, Unspecified
R27.8 Other Lack of Coordination
R27.9 Unspecified Lack of Coordination
G11.1 Early-Onset Cerebellar Ataxia
G11.0 Congenital Nonprogressive Ataxia
G11.2 Late-Onset Cerebellar Ataxia
G11.3 Cerebellar Ataxia with Defective DNA Repair
G11.8 Other Hereditary Ataxia

Hydrocephalus.
Hypothyroidism.
Tumor or paraneoplastic syndrome.
Low vitamin E levels (e.g., cystic fibrosis).
Wilson disease.
Inborn errors of metabolism.
Inherited ataxias (e.g., ataxia-telangiectasia, Friedreich's ataxia).

ATELECTASIS

ICD-9CM # 518.0
ICD-10CM # J98.11 Atelectasis

Lung neoplasm (primary or metastatic).
Infection (pneumonia, TB, fungal, histoplasmosis).
Postoperative (lower lobes).
Sarcoidosis.
Mucoid impaction.
Foreign body.
Postinflammatory (middle lobe syndrome).
Pneumothorax.
Pleural effusion.
Pneumoconiosis.
Interstitial fibrosis.
Bulla.
Mediastinal or adjacent mass.

ATRIAL ENLARGEMENT, LEFT ATRIUM[16a]

ICD-9CM # varies with specific diagnosis
ICD-10CM # I51.7 Cardiomegaly

CAUSES OF LARGE LEFT ATRIUM

Causes Due to Volume Overload
Mitral regurgitation (often with left ventricular failure).
Ventricular septal defect.
Patent ductus arteriosus.
Atrial septal defect with shunt reversal (i.e., pulmonary hypertension).

ASD with tricuspid atresia (obligatory shunt reversal).
Aortopulmonary window.

Causes Due to Pressure Overload

Mitral stenosis.
Noncompliant left ventricle: hypertension, hypertrophic cardiomyopathy, aortic stenosis.
Left ventricular failure (often with secondary mitral regurgitation).
Left atrial myxoma.

Other Causes (Both Rare)

Atrial fibrillation.
Isolated/idiopathic.

ATRIAL ENLARGEMENT, RIGHT ATRIUM

ICD-9CM #	varies with specific disorder	
ICD-10CM #	I51.7	Cardiomegaly

Right ventricular failure.
Atrial septal defect.
Tricuspid regurgitation.
Tricuspid stenosis.
Pulmonary hypertension.
Restrictive cardiomyopathy.
Right atrial myxoma.
Ebstein's anomaly.
Anomalous pulmonary venous drainage to the right atrium.
Endomyocardial fibrosis.
Sinus of Valsalva fistula.
Arrhythmogenic right ventricular dysplasia.

ATYPICAL LYMPHOCYTOSIS, HETEROPHIL NEGATIVE, INFECTIOUS CAUSES[1a]

ICD-9CM #	288.61	
ICD-10CM #	D72.820	Lymphocytosis (Symptomatic)

MOST COMMON INFECTIOUS CAUSES OF HETEROPHIL-NEGATIVE ATYPICAL LYMPHOCYTOSIS

Babesiosis.
Cytomegalovirus.
Epstein-Barr virus (particularly in children).
Human herpesvirus 6.
Human immunodeficiency virus (especially during acute seroconversion).
Infectious mononucleosis.
Malaria.
Measles.
Toxoplasmosis.
Varicella.
Infectious hepatitis.

AV NODAL BLOCK[15]

ICD-9CM #	426.10	AV Block (Incomplete, Partial)
	426.0	AV Block, Complete
ICD-10CM #	I44.30	Unspecified Atrioventricular Block
	I44.2	Atrioventricular Block, Complete

Idiopathic fibrosis (Lenègre's disease).
Sclerodegenerative processes (e.g., Lev's disease with calcification of the mitral and aortic annuli).
AV node radiofrequency ablation procedure.
Medications (e.g., digoxin, beta-blockers, calcium channel blockers, class III antiarrhythmics).
Acute inferior wall MI.
Myocarditis.
Infections (endocarditis, Lyme disease).
Infiltrative diseases (e.g., hemochromatosis, sarcoidosis, amyloidosis).
Trauma (including cardiac surgical procedures).
Collagen vascular diseases.
Aortic root diseases (e.g., spondylitis).
Electrolyte abnormalities (e.g., hyperkalemia).

BACK PAIN

ICD-9CM #	724.5	Back Pain (Postural)
	724.2	Low Back Pain
	307.89	Back Pain Psychogenic
	724.8	Stiff Back
	847.9	Back Strain
	724.6	Backache, Sacroiliac
ICD-10CM #	M54.89	Other Dorsalgia
	M54.9	Dorsalgia, Unspecified
	M54.5	Low Back Pain
	F45.42	Pain Disorder with Related Psychological Factors
	M54.08	Panniculitis Affecting Regions of Neck and Back, Sacral and Sacrococcygeal Region
	S23.9XXA	Sprain of Unspecified Parts of Thorax, Initial Encounter
	M43.27	Fusion of Spine, Lumbosacral Region
	M43.28	Fusion of Spine, Sacral and Sacrococcygeal Region
	M53.2X7	Spinal Instabilities, Lumbosacral Region
	M53.3	Sacrococcygeal Disorders, Not Elsewhere Classified

Trauma: injury to bone, joint, or ligament.
Mechanical: pregnancy, obesity, fatigue, scoliosis.
Degenerative: osteoarthritis.
Infections: osteomyelitis, subarachnoid or spinal abscess, TB, meningitis, basilar pneumonia.
Metabolic: osteoporosis, osteomalacia.
Vascular: leaking aortic aneurysm, subarachnoid or spinal hemorrhage/infarction.
Neoplastic: myeloma, Hodgkin's disease, carcinoma of pancreas, metastatic neoplasm from breast, prostate, lung.
GI: penetrating ulcer, pancreatitis, cholelithiasis, inflammatory bowel disease.
Renal: hydronephrosis, calculus, neoplasm, renal infarction, pyelonephritis.
Hematologic: sickle cell crisis, acute hemolysis.
Gynecologic: neoplasm of uterus or ovary, dysmenorrhea, salpingitis, uterine prolapse.
Inflammatory: ankylosing spondylitis, psoriatic arthritis, Reiter's syndrome (reactive arthritis).
Lumbosacral strain.
Psychogenic: malingering, hysteria, anxiety.
Endocrine: adrenal hemorrhage or infarction.

BACK PAIN, CHILDREN AND ADOLESCENTS[22a]

ICD-9CM #	724.2	
ICD-10CM #	M54.5	Low Back Pain
	M54.9	Dorsalgia

INFLAMMATORY OR INFECTIOUS

Diskitis.
Vertebral osteomyelitis (pyogenic, tuberculous).
Spinal epidural abscess.
Pyelonephritis.
Pancreatitis.

RHEUMATOLOGIC

Pauciarticular juvenile rheumatoid arthritis.
Reiter syndrome (reactive arthritis).
Ankylosing spondylitis.
Psoriatic arthritis.

DEVELOPMENTAL

Spondylolysis.
Spondylolisthesis.
Scheuermann disease.
Scoliosis.

TRAUMATICZ (ACUTE VERSUS REPETITIVE)

Hip-pelvis anomalies.
Herniated disk.
Overuse syndromes.
Vertebral stress fractures.
Upper cervical spine instability.

NEOPLASTIC

Vertebral Tumors

Benign

Eosinophilic granuloma.
Aneurysmal bone cyst.
Osteoid osteoma.
Osteoblastoma.

Malignant

Osteogenic sarcoma.
Leukemia.
Lymphoma.
Metastatic tumors.

Spinal Cord, Ganglia, and Nerve Roots
Intramedullary spinal cord tumor.
Sympathetic chain.
Ganglioneuroma.
Ganglioneuroblastoma.
Neuroblastoma.

OTHER

Intraabdominal or pelvic pathology.
Following lumbar puncture.
Conversion reaction.
Juvenile osteoporosis.

BACK PAIN, LOW, ACUTE[2]

ICD-9CM # 724.2
ICD-10CM # M54.5 Low Back Pain

DIFFERENTIAL CONSIDERATIONS IN ACUTE LOW BACK PAIN

Emergent
Aortic dissection.
Cauda equina syndrome.
Epidural abscess or hematoma.
Meningitis.
Ruptured/expanding aortic aneurysm.
Spinal fracture or subluxation with cord or root impingement.

Urgent
Back pain with neurologic deficits.
Disk herniation causing neurologic compromise.
Malignancy.
Sciatica with motor nerve root compression.
Spinal fractures without cord impingement.
Spinal stenosis.
Transverse myelitis.
Vertebral osteomyelitis.

Common or Stable
Acute ligamentous injury.
Acute muscle strain.
Ankylosing spondylitis.
Degenerative joint disease.
Intervertebral disk disease without impingement.
Pathologic fracture without impingement.
Seropositive arthritis.
Spondylolisthesis.

Referred or Visceral
Cholecystitis.
Esophageal disease.
Nephrolithiasis.
Ovarian torsion, mass, or tumor.
Pancreatitis.
Peptic ulcer disease.
Pleural effusion.
Pneumonia.
Pulmonary embolism.
Pyelonephritis.
Retroperitoneal hemorrhage or mass.

BACK PAIN, VISCEROGENIC ORIGIN

ICD-9CM # varies with specific disorder
ICD-10CM # F45.41 Pain Disorder Exclusively Related to Psychological Factors
M54 Dorsalgia
M54.5 Low back pain

Urolithiasis.
Aortic aneurysm.
Colorectal carcinoma.
Endometriosis.
Tubal pregnancy.
Prostatitis.
Peptic ulcer.
Pancreatitis.
Diverticular spasm.
Metastatic neoplasm (e.g., bladder, uterus, ovary, kidney).

BACTERIAL OVERGROWTH, SMALL INTESTINE[38]

ICD-9CM # varies with specific diagnosis
ICD-10CM # A04.9 Bacterial intestinal infection, unspecified

Gastric surgery—Billroth II.
Small bowel diverticula.
Small bowel stricture:
- Crohn's disease.
- Radiation enteritis.

Impaired small intestinal motility:
- Scleroderma.
- Diabetes mellitus.
- Chronic intestinal pseudoobstruction.

Miscellaneous/multifactorial
- Elderly.
- Immune deficiency syndromes.
- Chronic pancreatitis.
- Cirrhosis.

BALLISM*

ICD-9CM # 333.5
ICD-10CM # G25.4 Drug-Induced Chorea
G25.5 Other Chorea

Cerebral infarction or hemorrhage.
Medications (e.g., dopamine agonists, phenytoin).
CNS neoplasm (primary or metastatic).
Nonketotic hyperosmolar state.

*Violent, flinging, nonpatterned rapid movements

BILE DUCT, DILATED[38]

ICD-9CM # varies with specific diagnosis
ICD-10CM # K83.1 Obstruction of bile duct

Normal variant.
Post-cholecystectomy.
Unsuspected bile duct stone.
Sphincter of Oddi stenosis.
Occult bile duct stricture.
Previous bile duct injury.
Early carcinoma of the pancreas, carcinoma of the bile duct, or carcinoma of the ampulla.
Extrinsic compression of the bile duct by a primary or secondary neoplasm.

BLEEDING, LOWER GI

ICD-9CM # 578.9
ICD-10CM # K92.2 Gastrointestinal Hemorrhage, Unspecified

(ORIGINATING BELOW THE LIGAMENT OF TREITZ)

Small Intestine
Ischemic bowel disease (mesenteric thrombosis, embolism, vasculitis, trauma).
Small bowel neoplasm: leiomyomas, carcinoids.
Hereditary hemorrhagic telangiectasia (Rendu-Osler-Weber syndrome).
Meckel diverticulum and other small intestine diverticula.
Aortoenteric fistula.
Intestinal hemangiomas: blue rubber-bleb nevi, intestinal hemangiomas, cutaneous vascular nevi.
Hamartomatous polyps: Peutz-Jeghers syndrome (intestinal polyps, mucocutaneous pigmentation).
Infections of small bowel: tuberculous enteritis, enteritis necroticans.
Volvulus.
Intussusception.
Lymphoma of small bowel, sarcoma, Kaposi's sarcoma.
Irradiation ileitis.
AV malformation of small intestine.
Inflammatory bowel disease.
Polyarteritis nodosa.
Other: pancreatoenteric fistulas, Henoch-Schönlein purpura, Ehlers-Danlos syndrome, SLE, amyloidosis, metastatic melanoma.

Colon
Carcinoma (particularly left colon).
Diverticular disease.
Inflammatory bowel disease.
Ischemic colitis.
Colonic polyps.
Vascular abnormalities: angiodysplasia, vascular ectasia.
Radiation colitis.
Infectious colitis.
Uremic colitis.
Aortoenteric fistula.
Lymphoma of large bowel.
Hemorrhoids.
Anal fissure.
Trauma, foreign body.
Solitary rectal/cecal ulcers.
Long-distance running.

BLEEDING, LOWER GI, PEDIATRIC[2]

ICD-9CM # 578.9
ICD-10CM # K92.2 Gastrointestinal Hemorrhage, Unspecified

<3 MO

Swallowed maternal blood.
Infectious colitis.
Milk allergy.
Bleeding diathesis.
Intussusception.
Midgut volvulus.
Meckel diverticulum.
Necrotizing enterocolitis.

<2 YR

Anal fissure.
Infectious colitis.
Milk allergy.
Colitis.
Intussusception.
Meckel diverticulum.
Polyp.
Duplication.
Hemolytic-uremic syndrome.
Inflammatory bowel disease.
Pseudomembranous enterocolitis.

<5 YR

Infectious colitis.
Anal fissure.
Polyp.
Intussusception.
Meckel diverticulum.
Henoch-Schönlein purpura.
Hemolytic-uremic syndrome.
Inflammatory bowel disease.
Pseudomembranous enterocolitis.

5 TO 18 YR

Infectious colitis.
Inflammatory bowel disease.
Pseudomembranous enterocolitis.
Polyp.
Hemolytic-uremic syndrome.
Hemorrhoids.

BLEEDING, RECTAL[38]

ICD-9CM # 578.9
ICD-10CM # K92.2 Gastrointestinal Hemorrhage, Unspecified

IN PATIENTS <40 YR

Very Common:
Hemorrhoids.
Anal fissure.
Inflammatory bowel disease (mainly proctitis).
Less Common:
Polyps (hamartomatous or adenomatous).
Infective colitis.
Meckel's diverticulum.
Intussusception.
Rare:
Colorectal cancer.

IN PATIENTS >40 YR

Hemorrhoids.
Anal fissure.
Colorectal cancer.
Colorectal polyps (mostly adenomas).
Angiodysplasia.
Diverticular disease.
Inflammatory bowel disease.
Ischemic colitis.
Infective colitis.

BLEEDING, THIRD TRIMESTER[1]

ICD-9CM # 623.8
ICD-10CM # N93.9 Abnormal uterine and vaginal bleeding, unspecified

Placental abruption.
Placenta previa.
Bloody show (extrusion of cervical mucus).
Vasa previa.
Disseminated intravascular coagulopathy.
Uterine rupture.
Cervicitis, cervical cancer, or other cervical abnormality.
Vaginal laceration.

BLEEDING, UPPER GI

ICD-9CM # 578.9
ICD-10CM # K92.2 Gastrointestinal Hemorrhage, Unspecified

(ORIGINATING ABOVE THE LIGAMENT OF TREITZ)

Swallowed Hemoptysis
Oral or pharyngeal lesions: swallowed blood from nose or oropharynx.
Esophageal: varices, ulceration, esophagitis, Mallory-Weiss tear, carcinoma, trauma.
Gastric: peptic ulcer (including Cushing and Curling's ulcers), gastritis, angiodysplasia, gastric neoplasms, hiatal hernia, gastric diverticulum, pseudoxanthoma elasticum, Rendu-Osler-Weber syndrome.
Duodenal: peptic ulcer, duodenitis, angiodysplasia, aortoduodenal fistula, duodenal diverticulum, duodenal tumors, carcinoma of ampulla of Vater, parasites (e.g., hookworm), Crohn's disease.
Biliary: hematobilia (e.g., penetrating injury to liver, hepatobiliary malignancy, endoscopic papillotomy).

BLEEDING, UPPER GI, PEDIATRIC[2]

ICD-9CM # 578.9
ICD-10CM # K92.2 Gastrointestinal Hemorrhage, Unspecified

<3 MO

Swallowed maternal blood.
Gastritis.
Ulcer, stress.
Bleeding diathesis.
Foreign body (NG tube).
Vascular malformation.
Duplication.

<2 YR

Esophagitis.
Gastritis.
Ulcer.
Pyloric stenosis.
Mallory-Weiss syndrome.
Vascular malformation.
Duplication.

<5 YR

Esophagitis.
Gastritis.
Ulcer.
Esophageal varices.
Foreign body.
Mallory-Weiss syndrome.
Hemophilia.
Vascular malformations.

5 TO 18 YR

Esophagitis.
Gastritis.
Ulcer.
Esophageal varices.
Mallory-Weiss syndrome.
Inflammatory bowel disease.
Hemophilia.
Vascular malformation.

BLEEDING, VAGINAL, NON-PREGNANT FEMALE[1]

ICD-9CM # 623.8
ICD-10CM # N93.9 Abnormal uterine and vaginal bleeding, unspecified

TRAUMA

Blunt force.
Penetrating force.
Foreign bodies.

INFECTIOUS

Vaginitis.
Cervicitis.
Endometritis.

DYSFUNCTIONAL UTERINE BLEEDING

Ovulatory.
Anovulatory.
Adenomyosis.

BENIGN GROWTHS

Uterine leiomyomas.
Cervical polyps.

MALIGNANCY

Vulvar.
Cervical.
Uterine.
Ovarian.

SYSTEMIC DISEASE

Medications
Anticoagulation (warfarin [Coumadin], low-molecular-weight heparin, clopidogrel [Plavix]).
Antipsychotics.
Corticosteroids.
Tamoxifen.
Selective serotonin reuptake inhibitors.
Contraceptives (oral, intrauterine devices, intramuscular).

BLINDNESS, GERIATRIC AGE

ICD-9CM # 369.4
ICD-10CM # H54.8 Legal Blindness, as Defined in USA

Cataracts.
Glaucoma.
Diabetic retinopathy.
Macular degeneration.

Trauma.
CVA.
Corneal scarring.
Giant cell arteritis.
Ocular herpes zoster.

BLINDNESS, MONOCULAR, TRANSIENT

ICD-9CM # 369.67
ICD-10CM # H54.41 Blindness, Right Eye, Normal Vision Left Eye
H54.42 Blindness, Left Eye, Normal Vision Right Eye

Migraine (vasospasm).
Embolic cerebrovascular disease.
Intermittent angle-closure glaucoma.
Partial retinal vein occlusion.
Hyphema.
Optic disc edema.
Giant cell arteritis.
Psychogenic.
Hypotension.
Hypercoagulopathy disorders.
Multiple sclerosis.

BLINDNESS, PEDIATRIC AGE[23]

ICD-9CM # varies with specific disorder
ICD-10CM # H54.41 Blindness, Right Eye, Normal Vision Left Eye
H54.42 Blindness, Left Eye, Normal Vision Right Eye

CONGENITAL

Optic nerve hypoplasia or aplasia.
Optic coloboma.
Congenital hydrocephalus.
Hydranencephaly.
Porencephaly.
Microencephaly.
Encephalocele, particularly occipital type.
Morning glory disc.
Aniridia.
Anterior microphthalmia.
Peter's anomaly.
Persistent pupillary membrane.
Glaucoma.
Cataracts.
Persistent hyperplastic primary vitreous.

PHAKOMATOSES

Tuberous sclerosis.
Neurofibromatosis (special association with optic glioma).
Sturge-Weber syndrome.
von Hippel–Lindau disease.

TUMORS

Retinoblastoma.
Optic glioma.
Perioptic meningioma.
Craniopharyngioma.
Cerebral glioma.
Posterior and intraventricular tumors when complicated by hydrocephalus.
Pseudotumor cerebri.

NEURODEGENERATIVE DISEASES

Cerebral storage disease.
Gangliosidoses, particularly Tay-Sachs disease (infantile amaurotic familial idiocy), Sandhoff's variant, generalized gangliosidosis.
Other lipidoses and ceroid lipofuscinoses, particularly the late-onset amaurotic familial idiocies such as those of Jansky-Bielschowsky and of Batten-Mayou-Spielmeyer-Vogt.
Mucopolysaccharidoses, particularly Hurler's syndrome and Hunter's syndrome.
Leukodystrophies (dysmyelination disorders), particularly metachromatic leukodystrophy and Canavan's disease.
Demyelinating sclerosis (myelinoclastic diseases), especially Schilder's disease and Devic's neuromyelitis optica.
Special types: Dawson's disease, Leigh's disease, Bassen-Kornzweig syndrome, Refsum's disease.
Retinal degenerations: retinitis pigmentosa and its variants, Leber's congenital type.
Optic atrophies: congenital autosomal recessive type, infantile and congenital autosomal dominant types, Leber's disease, and atrophies associated with hereditary ataxias—the types of Behr, of Marie, and of Sanger-Brown.

INFECTIOUS PROCESSES

Encephalitis, especially in the prenatal infection syndromes caused by *Toxoplasma gondii,* cytomegalovirus, rubella virus, *Treponema pallidum,* herpes simplex.
Meningitis, arachnoiditis.
Chorioretinitis.
Endophthalmitis.
Keratitis.

HEMATOLOGIC DISORDERS

Leukemia with central nervous system involvement.

VASCULAR AND CIRCULATORY DISORDERS

Collagen vascular diseases.
Arteriovenous malformations—intracerebral hemorrhage, subarachnoid hemorrhage.
Central retinal occlusion.

TRAUMA

Contusion or avulsion of optic nerves, chiasm, globe, cornea.
Cerebral contusion or laceration.
Intracerebral, subarachnoid, or subdural hemorrhage.

DRUGS AND TOXINS OTHER

Retinopathy of prematurity.
Sclerocornea.
Conversion reaction.
Optic neuritis.
Osteopetrosis.

BLISTERS, SUBEPIDERMAL

ICD-9CM # 919.2
ICD-10CM # T07 Unspecified Multiple Injuries

Burns.
Porphyria cutanea tarda.
Bullous pemphigoid.
Bullous drug reaction.
Arthropod bite reaction.
Toxic epidermal necrosis.
Dermatitis herpetiformis.
Polymorphous light eruption.
Variegate porphyria.
SLE.
Epidermolysis bullosa.
Pseudoporphyria.
Acute graft-versus-host reaction.
Linear IgA disease.
Leukocytoclastic vasculitis.
Pressure necrosis.
Urticaria pigmentosa.
Amyloidosis.

BONE DENSITY, DECREASED, GENERALIZED[16a]

ICD-9CM # 733.00
ICD-10CM # M85.80 Other Specified Disorders of Bone Density and Structure, Unspecified Site

DISORDERS ASSOCIATED WITH GENERALIZED LOSS OF BONE DENSITY

Disorders of Multiple or Uncertain Cause

Senile osteoporosis.*
Juvenile osteoporosis.
Osteogenesis imperfecta.†

Secondary Bone Disorders

Endocrine

Adrenal cortex.†
  Cushing's disease.
  Addison's disease.
Gonadal disorders.
  Postmenopausal osteoporosis.*
  Hypogonadism.†
Pituitary.
  Acromegaly.
  Hypopituitarism.
Pancreas.
  Diabetes mellitus.*
Thyroid.
  Hyperthyroidism.
  Hypothyroidism.
Parathyroid.
  Hyperparathyroidism.*

Marrow Replacement and Expansion

Myeloma.
Leukemia.
Lymphoma.
Metastatic disease.*
Gaucher's disease.
Anemias (sickle cell, thalassaemia, hemophilia).†

Drugs and Other Substances

Steroids.*†
Heparin (osteoporosis).
Anticonvulsants (osteomalacia).
Immunosuppressants.
Alcohol.*

Chronic Disease

Chronic renal disease.†
Hepatic insufficiency.†
GI malabsorption syndromes.
Chronic inflammatory polyarthropathies.
Chronic debility or immobilization.

*Common cause of decrease in bone density in adults.
†Common cause of decrease in bone density in children.

BONE DENSITY, DECREASED, LOCALIZED[16A]

ICD-9CM # V17.81
ICD-10CM # Z82.62 Family History of Osteoporosis
M85.80 Other specified disorders of bone density and structure, unspecified site

DISORDERS ASSOCIATED WITH LOCALIZED LOSS OF BONE DENSITY

Disuse osteoporosis.*
Reflex sympathetic dystrophy (Sudeck's).*
Osteolytic syndromes.
- Acro-osteolysis, primary and secondary.
- Massive osteolysis of Gorham.
- Carpotarsal osteolysis.

Transient regional osteoporosis.
Neuromuscular disorders.
Infection.*
Arthropathies.*
Tumors, primary and secondary, myelomatosis.

*Common causes.

BONE LESIONS, PREFERENTIAL SITE OF ORIGIN[35]

ICD-9CM #
170.0 Skull and Face
170.1 Mandible
170.2 Vertebral Column
170.3 Ribs, Sternum, Clavicle
170.4 Scapula, Long Bones, Upper Limb
170.5 Short Bones and Upper Limb
170.6 Pelvic Bones, Sacrum, Coccyx
170.7 Long Bones, Lower Limb
170.8 Short Bones, Lower Limb
170.9 Bone Cancer NOS
198.5 Bone Cancer, Metastatic

ICD-10CM #
C41.0 Malignant Neoplasm of Bones of Skull and Face
C41.1 Malignant Neoplasm of Mandible
C41.2 Malignant Neoplasm of Vertebral Column
C41.3 Malignant Neoplasm of Ribs, Sternum and Clavicle
C40.00 Malignant Neoplasm of Scapula and Long Bones of Unspecified Upper Limb
C40.10 malignant neoplasm of Short Bones of Unspecified Upper Limb
C41.4 Malignant Neoplasm of Pelvic Bones, Sacrum and Coccyx
C40.20 Malignant Neoplasm of Long Bones of Unspecified Lower Limb
C40.30 Malignant Neoplasm of Short Bones of Unspecified Lower Limb
C41.9 Malignant Neoplasm of Bone and Articular Cartilage, Unspecified
C79.51 Secondary Malignant Neoplasm of Bone
C79.52 Secondary Malignant Neoplasm of Bone Marrow

EPIPHYSIS

Chondroblastoma.
Giant cell tumor—after fusion of growth plate.
Langerhans' cell histiocytosis.
Clear cell chondrosarcoma.
Osteosarcoma.

METAPHYSIS

Parosteal sarcoma.
Chondrosarcoma.
Fibrosarcoma.
Nonossifying fibroma.
Giant cell tumor—before fusion of growth plate.
Unicameral bone cyst.
Aneurysmal bone cyst.

DIAPHYSIS

Myeloma.
Ewing's tumor.
Reticulum cell sarcoma.

METADIAPHYSEAL

Fibrosarcoma.
Fibrous dysplasia.
Enchondroma.
Osteoid osteoma.
Chondromyofibroma.

BONE MARROW FAILURE SYNDROMES, INHERITED[20]

ICD-9CM # 284
ICD-10CM # D61.89 Other Specified Aplastic Anemias and Other Bone Marrow Failure Syndromes

BI-LINEAGE AND TRI-LINEAGE CYTOPENIAS

Fanconi anemia.
Shwachman-Diamond syndrome.
Dyskeratosis congenita.
Amegakaryocytic thrombocytopenia:
- Other inherited thrombocytopenia disorders.

Other genetic syndromes:
- Down syndrome.
- Dubowitz syndrome.
- Seckel syndrome.
- Reticular dysgenesis.
- Schimke immunoosseous dysplasia.
- Noonan syndrome.
- Cartilage-hair hypoplasia.
- Familial marrow failure (non-Fanconi).

UNI-LINEAGE CYTOPENIA

Diamond-Blackfan anemia.
Kostmann syndrome/Congenital neutropenia:
- *ELA2* mutations.
- *HAX1* mutations.
- *GFI1* mutations.
- *WASP* mutations.
- Constitutive cell surface G-CSF-R mutations.

Other inherited neutropenia syndromes:
- Barth syndrome.
- Glycogen storage disease 1b.
- Miscellaneous.

Thrombocytopenia with absent radii.
Congenital dyserythropoietic anemias (CDAs):
- Types I, II, III, IV.
- Variants.
- Nonclassifiable CDAs.
- Groups IV, V, VI, VII.

BONE MARROW FIBROSIS[14]

ICD-9CM # 289.9
ICD-10CM # D75.9 Disease of Blood and Blood-Forming Organs, Unspecified

MYELOID DISORDERS

Myelofibrosis with myeloid metaplasia.
Metastatic cancer.
Chronic myeloid leukemia.
Myelodysplastic syndrome.
Atypical myeloid disorder.
Acute megakaryocytic leukemia.
Other acute myeloid leukemias.
Gray platelet syndrome.

LYMPHOID DISORDERS

Hairy cell leukemia.
Multiple myeloma.
Lymphoma.

NONHEMATOLOGIC DISORDERS

Connective tissue disorder.
Infections (tuberculosis, kala-azar).
Vitamin D–deficiency rickets.
Renal osteodystrophy.

BONE MASS, LOW[1a]

ICD-9CM # varies with specific diagnosis
ICD-10CM # M85.80 Other specified disorders of bone density and structure, unspecified site

SECONDARY CAUSES OF LOW BONE MASS

Endocrine Diseases

Female hypogonadism.
Hyperprolactinemia.
Hypothalamic amenorrhea.
Anorexia nervosa.
Premature and primary ovarian failure.
Female athlete triad.
Male hypogonadism.
Primary gonadal failure (e.g., Klinefelter's syndrome).
Secondary gonadal failure (e.g., idiopathic hypogonadotropic hypogonadism, androgen deprivation therapy for prostate cancer).
Hyperthyroidism.
Hyperparathyroidism.
Hypercortisolism.
Vitamin D insufficiency or deficiency.

Gastrointestinal Diseases

Subtotal gastrectomy.
Gastric bypass surgery.
Malabsorption syndromes.
Chronic obstructive jaundice.
Primary biliary cirrhosis and other cirrhoses.

Bone Marrow Disorders

Multiple myeloma.
Monoclonal gammopathy of unknown significance (MGUS).
Lymphoma.
Leukemia.
Hemolytic anemias.
Systemic mastocytosis.
Disseminated carcinoma.

Connective Tissue Diseases

Osteogenesis imperfecta.
Ehlers-Danlos syndrome.
Marfan's syndrome.
Homocystinuria.

Drugs

Alcohol.
Antiseizure medications.
Aromatase inhibitors.
Chemotherapy.
Cyclosporine.
Depo-medroxyprogesterone.
Excess thyroid hormone.
Glucocorticoids.
Gonadotropin-releasing hormone agonists.
Heparin.

Miscellaneous Causes

Immobilization.
Rheumatoid arthritis.
Chronic obstructive pulmonary disease.
Weight loss.

BONE MINERAL DENSITY, INCREASED

ICD-9CM #	733.99	
ICD-10CM #	M89.30	Hypertrophy of Bone, Unspecified Site
	M89.8X9	Other Specified Disorders of Bone, Unspecified Site
	M94.8X9	Other Specified Disorders of Cartilage, Unspecified Sites

Paget's disease of bone.
Skeletal metastases.
DISH.
Osteonecrosis.
Sarcoidosis.
Hypoparathyroidism, pseudohypoparathyroidism.
Milk-alkali syndrome.
Osteopetrosis.
Hypervitaminosis A or D.
Dysplasias (craniodiaphyseal, craniometaphyseal, frontometaphyseal).
Endosteal hyperostosis.
Fluorosis.
Heavy metal poisoning.
Ionizing radiation.
Other: lymphoma, leukemia, mastocytosis, multiple myeloma, polycythemia vera.

BONE PAIN

ICD-9CM #	varies with specific diagnosis	
ICD-10CM #	M89.8	Pain, bone

Trauma.
Neoplasm (primary or metastatic).
Osteoporosis with compression fracture.
Paget's disease of bone.
Infection (osteomyelitis, septic arthritis).
Osteomalacia.
Viral syndrome.
Sickle cell disease.
Anxiety.

BONE RESORPTION[35]

ICD-9CM #	733.90	Bone Disorder
ICD-10CM #	M89.9	Disorder of Bone, Unspecified
	M94.9	Disorder of Cartilage, Unspecified

DISTAL CLAVICLE

Hyperparathyroidism.
RA.
Scleroderma.
Posttraumatic osteolysis.
Progeria.
Pycnodysostosis.
Cleidocranial dysplasia.

INFERIOR ASPECT OF RIBS

Vascular impression, associated with but not limited to coarctation of the aorta.
Hyperparathyroidism.
Neurofibromatosis.

TERMINAL PHALANGEAL TUFTS

Scleroderma.
Raynaud's phenomenon.
Vascular disease.
Frostbite, electrical burns.
Psoriasis.
Tabes dorsalis.
Hyperparathyroidism.

GENERALIZED RESORPTION

Paraplegia.
Myositis ossificans.
Osteoporosis.

BOW LEGS (GENU VARUM), CLASSIFICATION[22a]

ICD-9CM #	736.42	Bow Legs (Genu Varum)
ICD-10CM #	E64.3	Genu varum, acquired
	Q74.1	Congenital malformation of knee

PHYSIOLOGIC

ASYMMETRIC GROWTH

Tibia vara (Blount disease).
- Infantile.
- Juvenile.
- Adolescent.

Focal fibrocartilaginous dysplasia.
Physeal injury.
Trauma.
Infection.
Tumor.

METABOLIC DISORDERS

Vitamin D deficiency (nutritional rickets).
Vitamin D–resistant rickets.
Hypophosphatasia.

SKELETAL DYSPLASIA

Metaphyseal dysplasia.
Achondroplasia.
Enchondromatosis.

BRADYCARDIA, SINUS[15]

ICD-9CM #	427.89	
ICD-10CM #	I49.8	Other Specified Cardiac Arrhythmias
	R00.1	Bradycardia, Unspecified

Idiopathic.
Degenerative processes (e.g., Lev's disease, Lenègre's disease).

Medications

β-Blockers.
Some calcium channel blockers (diltiazem, verapamil).
Digoxin (when vagal tone is high).
Class I antiarrhythmic agents (e.g., procainamide).
Class III antiarrhythmic agents (amiodarone, sotalol).
Clonidine.
Lithium carbonate.

Acute Myocardial Ischemia and Infarction

Right or left circumflex coronary artery occlusion or spasm.
High vagal tone (e.g., athletes).

BRAIN MASS[1]

ICD-9CM #	varies with specific diagnosis	
ICD-10CM #	C71	Malignant neoplasm of brain
	D33	Benign neoplasm of brain
	I61.9	Intracranial hemorrhage, unspecified

METASTATIC BRAIN TUMOR

Primary brain tumor

- Meningioma.
- Glioma.

- Pituitary adenoma.
- Vestibular schwannoma.
- Primary or secondary central nervous system lymphoma.

Infections

- Abscess.
- Toxoplasmosis.
- Neurocysticercosis.
- Tuberculoma.
- Progressive multifocal leukoencephalopathy.

VASCULAR DISEASE

Hemorrhage

- Anomalies (arteriovenous malformation).
- Intratumoral.
- Hypertensive.

Infarct

- Embolism.
- Thrombosis (sinus venous).

Inflammatory

- Multiple sclerosis.
- Encephalomyelitis.

BREAST INFLAMMATORY LESION[12]

ICD-9CM #	611.0	Acute Mastitis
	610.1	Chronic Cystic Mastitis
	771.5	Neonatal Infective Mastitis
	778.7	Neonatal Noninfective Mastitis
ICD-10CM #	N61	Inflammatory Disorders of Breast
	N60.19	Diffuse Cystic Mastopathy of Unspecified Breast
	P39.0	Neonatal Infective Mastitis
	P83.4	Breast Engorgement of Newborn

Mastitis (*S. aureus*, β-hemolytic *Streptococcus*).
Trauma.
Foreign body (sutures, breast implants).
Granuloma (TB, fungal).
Fat necrosis post biopsy.
Necrosis or infarction (anticoagulant therapy, pregnancy).
Breast malignancy.

BREAST MASS

ICD-9CM #	611.72	
ICD-10CM #	N63	Unspecified Lump in Breast

Fibrocystic breasts.
Benign tumors (fibroadenoma, papilloma).
Mastitis (acute bacterial mastitis, chronic mastitis).
Malignant neoplasm.
Fat necrosis.
Hematoma.
Duct ectasia.
Mammary adenosis.

BREATH ODOR[34]

ICD-9CM #	784.9	Halitosis
ICD-10CM #	R19.6	Halitosis

Sweet, fruity: DKA, starvation ketosis.
Fishy, stale: uremia (trimethylamines).
Ammonia-like: uremia (ammonia).
Musty fish, clover: fetor hepaticus (hepatic failure).
Foul, feculent: intestinal obstruction/diverticulum.
Foul, putrid: nasal/sinus pathology (infection, foreign body, cancer), respiratory infections (empyema, lung abscess, bronchiectasis).
Halitosis: tonsillitis, gingivitis, respiratory infections, Vincent's angina, gastroesophageal reflux, achalasia, certain foods (garlic, onions, protein drinks, etc.)
Cinnamon: pulmonary TB.

BREATHING, NOISY[34]

ICD-9CM #	786.09	Breathing, Labored
	786.1	Stridor
ICD-10CM #	R06.00	Dyspnea, Unspecified
	R06.09	Other Forms of Dyspnea
	R06.3	Periodic Breathing
	R06.83	Snoring
	R06.89	Other Abnormalities of Breathing
	R06.1	Stridor

Infection: upper respiratory infection, peritonsillar abscess, retropharyngeal abscess, epiglottitis, laryngitis, tracheitis, bronchitis, bronchiolitis.
Irritants and allergens: hyperactive airway, asthma (reactive airway disease), rhinitis, angioneurotic edema.
Compression from outside of the airway: esophageal cysts or foreign body, neoplasms, lymphadenopathy.
Congenital malformation and abnormality: vascular rings, laryngeal webs, laryngomalacia, tracheomalacia, hemangiomas within the upper airway, stenoses within the upper airway, cystic fibrosis.
Acquired abnormality (at every level of the airway): nasal polyps, hypertrophied adenoids and/or tonsils, foreign body, intraluminal tumors, bronchiectasis.
Neurogenic disorder: vocal cord paralysis.

BRONCHIAL OBSTRUCTION[16a]

ICD-9CM #	varies with specific diagnosis	
ICD-10CM #	J98.0	Tracheobronchial collapse

CAUSES OF BRONCHIAL OBSTRUCTION

Outside the Bronchus

Lymph nodes and other masses.

In the Wall of the Bronchus

Tumors

Lung carcinoma (commonly squamous cell).
Bronchial carcinoid.
Metastasis.
Hamartoma.

Inflammation

Tuberculosis.
Sarcoidosis.
Granulomatosis with polyangiitis (Wegener's granulomatosis).
Inflammatory bowel disease.

Bronchomalacia

Broncholith.

Inside the Bronchus

Mucus plug.
Inhaled foreign body.

BRONCHOPLEURAL FISTULA[16a]

ICD-9CM #	510.0	
ICD-10CM #	J86.0	Bronchopleural fistula

CAUSES OF BRONCHOPLEURAL FISTULA

Trauma

Penetrating.
Iatrogenic (especially post-pneumonectomy, post-lobectomy, post-biopsy).

Infection

Necrotizing pneumonia.
Empyema.
Tuberculosis.
Septic embolus.
Infected pulmonary infarct.

BROWN URINE

ICD-9CM #	788.69	
ICD-10CM #	R82	Other abnormal findings in urine

Bile pigments.
Myoglobin.
Concentrated urine.
Use of multivitamin supplements.
Medications (antimalarials, metronidazole, nitrofurantoin, levodopa, methyldopa, phenazopyridine).
Diet rich in fava beans.
Urinary tract infection.

BRUISING

ICD-9CM #	459.89	
ICD-10CM #	I99.8	Other Disorder of Circulatory System

Medication-induced (warfarin, aspirin, NSAIDs, prednisone).
Alcohol abuse.
Senile purpura.
Purpura simplex.
Physical abuse.
Vasculitis.
Platelet disorders.
Coagulation factor deficiencies.
Cushing's disease.
Vitamin C deficiency.
Marfan's syndrome.
Ehlers-Danlos syndrome.

Disseminated intravascular coagulation.
Leukemia.
Hereditary hemorrhagic telangiectasia.

BULLOUS DISEASES

ICD-9CM #	694.9	Bullous Dermatoses
	694.5	Bullous Pemphigoid
	694.4	Pemphigus Vulgaris
	694.4	Pemphigus Foliaceus
ICD-10CM #	L13.9	Bullous Disorder, Unspecified
	L12.0	Bullous Pemphigoid
	L12.8	Other Pemphigoid
	L10.0	Pemphigus Vulgaris
	L10.1	Pemphigus Vegetans
	L10.2	Pemphigus Foliaceous
	L10.4	Pemphigus Erythematosus
	L10.9	Pemphigus, Unspecified
	L10.0	Pemphigus Vulgaris
	L10.1	Pemphigus Vegetans
	L10.2	Pemphigus Foliaceous
	L10.4	Pemphigus Erythematosus
	L10.9	Pemphigus, Unspecified

Bullous pemphigoid.
Pemphigus vulgaris.
Pemphigus foliaceus.
Paraneoplastic pemphigus.
Cicatricial pemphigoid.
Erythema multiforme.
Dermatitis herpetiformis.
Herpes gestationis.
Impetigo.
Erosive lichen planus.
Linear IgA bullous dermatosis.
Epidermolysis bullosa acquisita.

CAFÉ-AU-LAIT SPOTS[22a]

ICD-9CM #	709	
ICD-10CM #	L81.3	Cafe au lait spots

Neurofibromatosis types 1 and 2.
McCune-Albright syndrome.
Russell-Silver syndrome.
Ataxia-telangiectasia.
Fanconi anemia.
Tuberous sclerosis.
Bloom syndrome.
Basal cell nevus syndrome.
Gaucher disease.
Chédiak-Higashi syndrome.
Hunter syndrome.
Maffucci syndrome.
Multiple mucosal neuroma syndrome.
Watson syndrome.
Proteus syndrome.
Turner syndrome.
Ring chromosome syndrome.
Jaffe-Campanacci syndrome.

CALCIFICATION ON CHEST X-RAY

ICD-9CM #	722.92	
ICD-10CM #	J98.4	Calcification of lung
	M51.84	Other Intervertebral Disc Disorders, Thoracic Region
	M51.85	Other Intervertebral Disc Disorders, Thoracolumbar Region

Lung neoplasm (primary or metastatic).
Silicosis.
Idiopathic pulmonary fibrosis.
Tuberculosis.
Histoplasmosis.
Disseminated varicella infection.
Mitral stenosis (end-stage).
Secondary hyperparathyroidism.

CALCIFICATIONS, ABDOMINAL, NONVISCERAL ON X-RAY[16a]

ICD-9CM #	728.10	
ICD-10CM #	M61.9	Calcification and Ossification of Muscle, Unspecified

NONVISCERAL ABDOMINAL CALCIFICATION

Common

Atherosclerosis.
Mesenteric lymph nodes.
Phleboliths.
Aneurysm.
Dermoid cyst.

Differentiate

Rib cartilage.
Injections in the buttocks.

Uncommon

Infestations.
- *Armillifer armillatus.*
- Cysticercosis.
- Guinea worm.
- Hydatid.

Tumors.
- Lipoma.
- Hemangioma.
- Neuroblastoma.
- Osteo/chondrosarcoma of soft tissues.
- Retroperitoneal sarcoma of soft tissues.
- Peritoneal metastases.
- Pheochromocytoma.

Tuberculosis.
- Peritonitis.
- Psoas abscess.

Meconium peritonitis.

Pseudomyxoma Peritonei

Mesenteric cyst.
Pancreatitis with saponification.
Lithopedion.

Appendices Epiploicae

Ligaments.
Foreign bodies.
Posttraumatic buttock cysts.

CALCIFICATIONS, ADRENAL GLAND ON X-RAY[16a]

ICD-9CM #	275.49	
ICD-10CM #	E27.4	Calcification, adrenal gland

ADRENAL GLAND CALCIFICATION

Common

Idiopathic.
Hemorrhage.
Tuberculosis.
Neuroblastoma/ganglioneuroma.
Pheochromocytoma.

Uncommon

Other tumors:
- Adenoma.
- Carcinoma.
- Dermoid.

Addison's disease.
Cyst.
Histoplasmosis.

CALCIFICATIONS, CARDIAC ON X-RAY[16a]

ICD-9CM #	275.49	
ICD-10CM #	I51.5	Calcification, myocardium
	I25.1	Calcification, ateriosclerotic

CAUSES OF VISIBLE CALCIFICATION WITHIN THE HEART

Coronary Artery

Atherosclerosis.

Aortic Root

Atherosclerotic aorta.
Thrombus.
Syphilis.
Ankylosing spondylitis.
Homograft calcification.

Pericardium

Chronic pericarditis, tuberculosis, hemopericardium, pyogenic or viral pericarditis.
Posttraumatic.
Postoperative.
Uremic pericarditis.
Asbestosis (may be pleural calcification applied to pericardium).

Myocardium

Ventricular aneurysm (may mimic pericardial calcification).
Calcified myocardial infarction.
Postmyocarditis.

Endocardium

Endomyocardial fibrosis.
Thrombus.

Valve Cusps

Calcified valves (particularly mitral and aortic valves).
Mitral annulus calcification.
Homograft calcification.
Old vegetation.

Valve Annulus
Submitral.
Mitral.
Aortic.
Left Atrium
Wall.
Thrombus.
Atrial myxoma.
Pulmonary Artery
Pulmonary hypertension.
Postoperative.
Postoperative Serumoma
Calcified Hydatid Cyst

CALCIFICATIONS, CUTANEOUS

ICD-9CM # 709.3
ICD-10CM # L94.2 Calcinosis Cutis
L98.8 Other Specified Disorders of the Skin and Subcutaneous Tissue

Calcification, Raynaud's phenomenon, esophageal dysmotility, sclerodactyly, and telangiectasia (CREST) syndrome.
Trauma.
Pancreatitis or pancreatic cancer.
Chronic renal failure.
Sarcoidosis.
Hyperparathyroidism.
Milk-alkali syndrome.
Hypervitaminosis D.
Panniculitis.
Idiopathic.
Iatrogenic (e.g., application of calcium alginate dressing to skin).
Multiple myeloma.
Dermatomyositis.
Parasitic infections.
Leukemia.
Lymphoma.

CALCIFICATIONS, GENITAL TRACT, FEMALE ON X-RAY[16a]

ICD-9CM # 275.49
ICD-10CM # E83.59 Other Disorders of Calcium Metabolism

FEMALE GENITAL TRACT CALCIFICATION

Uterus
Leiomyomas.
Squamous cell carcinoma.
Adenocarcinoma of endometrium.
Leiomyosarcoma.
Lithopedion.
Fallopian Tubes
Ovary.
Dermoid cyst.
Serous cystadenoma/carcinoma.
Tuberculosis.
Cysts.
Autoamputation.

CALCIFICATIONS, LIVER ON X-RAY[16a]

ICD-9CM # 573
ICD-10CM # K76.89 Other Specified Diseases of Liver
NEC K75.3 Granuloma, hepatic

LIVER CALCIFICATION

Common
Granuloma (tuberculosis, histoplasmosis, brucellosis).
- Multiple scattered round densities.

Hydatid cyst.
- Fine curvilinear in wall, or dense and irregular if contracted.

Primary liver tumor (hemangioma, hepatoblastoma, hepatoma, cholangiocarcinoma).
- Irregular patterns or multiple nodules.

Metastases (mucinous primary of colon or breast, cystadenocarcinoma of ovary).
- Finely stippled, may be extensive.

Uncommon
Hepatic artery aneurysm.
Armillifer armillatus infestation.
Chronic granulomatous disease of childhood.
Cyst (congenital or acquired).
Hematoma.
Intrahepatic gallstones.
Old liver abscess.
Portal vein thrombosis.
Differentiate
Hemochromatosis.
Thorotrast, thallium, iron.

CALCIFICATIONS, PANCREAS ON X-RAY[16A]

ICD-9CM # 275.49
ICD-10CM # K86.8 Calcification, pancreas

PANCREATIC CALCIFICATION

Common
Chronic pancreatitis.
Uncommon
Acute pancreatitis (saponification).
Tumors.
Cystadenoma.
Cystadenocarcinoma.
Islet cell tumor.
Metastases.
Hereditary pancreatitis (large clumps).
Hemorrhage.
Hyperparathyroidism.
Pseudocyst.
Cavernous lymphangioma.
Mucoviscidosis.
Kwashiorkor.

CALCIFICATIONS, SPLEEN ON X-RAY[16A]

ICD-9CM # 275.49
ICD-10CM # D73.8 Calcification, spleen

SPLENIC CALCIFICATION

Larger than 10 mm
Splenic artery aneurysm.
Splenic artery atheroma.
Cyst.
Posttraumatic.
Dermoid.
Epidermoid.
Hydatid.
Hematoma.
Infarct.
Abscess.
Tuberculosis.
Smaller than 10 mm
Histoplasmosis.
Tuberculosis.
Phleboliths.
Armillifer armillatus infestation.
Brucellosis.
Infarcts.

CALCIFICATIONS, VALVULAR ON X-RAY[16a]

ICD-9CM # 275.49
ICD-10CM # I51.5 Calcification, heart

CAUSES OF RADIOGRAPHICALLY VISIBLE VALVE CALCIFICATION

Aortic Valve
Rheumatic aortic valve disease.
Bicuspid aortic valve.
Age/degenerate aortic valve.
Syphilis.
Ankylosing spondylitis.
Homograft calcification.
Mitral Valve
Rheumatic mitral valve disease.
Mitral annulus calcification.
Old vegetation (may only be visible on CT).
Homograft calcification.
Pulmonary Valve
Congenital pulmonary valve stenosis.
Rheumatic pulmonary valve disease (rare).
Fallot's tetralogy (usually after repair).
Pulmonary hypertension.
Homograft calcification.
Tricuspid Valve
Rheumatic tricuspid valve disease.
Old vegetation (may only be visible on ultrafast CT).

CALCIUM STONES

ICD-9CM # 592.9
ICD-10CM # N20.9 Urinary Calculus, Unspecified

Medications (e.g., antacids, loop diuretics, vitamin D, acetazolamide, glucocorticoids).
Primary hyperparathyroidism.
Hypercalcemia from malignancy.
Sarcoidosis.
Prolonged immobilization.
Hyperoxaluria (e.g., Crohn's disease, celiac disease, chronic pancreatitis).
Hyperuricosuria (e.g., hyperuricemia, excessive dietary purine, allopurinol, probenecid).

Renal tubular acidosis.
Milk-alkali syndrome.
Thyrotoxicosis.
Hypocitraturia (e.g., metabolic acidosis, hypomagnesemia, hypokalemia).

CARDIAC ARREST, NONTRAUMATIC[26]

ICD-9CM # 427.5 Cardiac Arrest NOS
ICD-10CM # I46.9 Cardiac Arrest, Cause Unspecified

Cardiac (coronary artery disease, cardiomyopathies, structural abnormalities, valve dysfunction, arrhythmias).
Respiratory (upper airway obstruction, hypoventilation, pulmonary embolism, asthma, COPD exacerbation, pulmonary edema).
Circulatory (tension pneumothorax, pericardial tamponade, PE, hemorrhage, sepsis).
Electrolyte abnormalities (hypokalemia or hyperkalemia, hypomagnesemia or hypermagnesemia, hypocalcemia).
Medications (tricyclic antidepressants, digoxin, theophylline, calcium channel blockers).
Drug abuse (cocaine, heroin, amphetamines).
Toxins (carbon monoxide, cyanide).
Environmental (drowning/near-drowning, electrocution, lightning, hypothermia or hyperthermia, venomous snakes).

CARDIAC DEATH, SUDDEN[1a]

ICD-9CM # varies with specific disorder
ICD-10CM # Z86.74 Personal History of Sudden Cardiac Arrest

Ventricular tachycardia.
Bradyarrhythmia, sick sinus syndrome.
Aortic stenosis.
Tetralogy of Fallot.
Pericardial tamponade.
Cardiac tumors.
Complications of infective endocarditis.
Hypertrophic cardiomyopathy (arrhythmia or obstruction).
Myocardial ischemia.
Atherosclerosis.
Prinzmetal's angina.
Kawasaki's arteritis.

CARDIAC ENLARGEMENT[15]

ICD-9CM # 429.3 Cardiomegaly, Idiopathic
746.89 Cardiomegaly, Congenital
402.0 Cardiomegaly, Malignant
402.1 Cardiomegaly, Benign
ICD-10CM # I51.7 Cardiomegaly
Q23.8 Other Congenital Malformations of Aortic and Mitral Valves
Q24.8 Other Specified Congenital Malformations of Heart
I11.9 Hypertensive Heart Disease Without Heart Failure
I11.9 Hypertensive Heart Disease Without Heart Failure

CARDIAC CHAMBER ENLARGEMENT

Chronic Volume Overload
Mitral or aortic regurgitation.
Left-to-right shunt (PDA, VSD, AV fistula).
Cardiomyopathy
Ischemic.
Nonischemic.
Decompensated Pressure Overload
Aortic stenosis.
Hypertension.
High-Output States
Severe anemia.
Thyrotoxicosis.
Bradycardia
Severe sinus bradycardia.
Complete heart block.

LEFT ATRIUM

LV failure of any cause.
Mitral valve disease.
Myxoma.

RIGHT VENTRICLE

Chronic volume overload.
Tricuspid or pulmonic regurgitation.
Left-to-right shunt (ASD).
Decompensated pressure overload:
 Pulmonic stenosis.
 Pulmonary artery hypertension:
 - Primary.
 - Secondary (PE, COPD).
 Pulmonary venoocclusive disease.

RIGHT ATRIUM

RV failure of any cause.
Tricuspid valve disease.
Myxoma.
Ebstein's anomaly.

MULTICHAMBER ENLARGEMENT

Hypertrophic cardiomyopathy.
Acromegaly.
Severe obesity.

PERICARDIAL DISEASE

Pericardial effusion with or without tamponade.
Effusive constrictive disease.
Pericardial cyst, loculated effusion.

PSEUDOCARDIOMEGALY

Epicardial fat.
Chest wall deformity (pectus excavatum, straight back syndrome).
Low lung volumes.
AP chest x-ray.
Mediastinal tumor, cyst.

CARDIAC MURMURS

ICD-9CM # varies with specific disorder
ICD-10CM # R01.0 Benign and Innocent Cardiac Murmurs
R01.1 Cardiac murmur, unspecified

SYSTOLIC

Mitral regurgitation (MR).
Tricuspid regurgitation (TR).
Ventricular septal defect (VSD).
Aortic stenosis (AS).
Idiopathic hypertrophic subaortic stenosis (IHSS).
Pulmonic stenosis (PS).
Innocent murmur of childhood.
Coarctation of aorta.
Mitral valve prolapse (MVP).

DIASTOLIC

Aortic regurgitation (AR).
Atrial myxoma.
Mitral stenosis (MS).
Pulmonary artery branch stenosis.
Tricuspid stenosis (TS).
Graham Steell murmur (diastolic decrescendo murmur heard in severe pulmonary hypertension).
Pulmonic regurgitation (PR).
Severe mitral regurgitation (MR).
Austin Flint murmur (diastolic rumble heard in severe AR).
Severe VSD and patent ductus arteriosus.

CONTINUOUS

Patent ductus arteriosus.
Pulmonary AV fistula.

CARDIAC TUMORS[14A]

ICD-9CM # 164 Cardiac Tumors
ICD-10CM # C38.0 Malignant Neoplasm of Heart
D15.7 Benign neoplasm of other specified intrathoracic origin

PRIMARY

Benign.
 Myxoma.
 Lipoma.
 Fibroma.
 Rhabdomyoma.
 Fibroelastoma.
Malignant.
 Sarcoma.
 Mesothelioma.
 Lymphoma.

SECONDARY

Direct Extension
Lung cancer.
Breast cancer.
Mediastinal tumors.
Metastatic Tumors
Malignant melanoma.
Leukemia.
Lymphoma.
Venous Extension
Renal cell cancer.
Adrenal cancer.
Liver cancer.

CARDIOEMBOLISM

ICD-9CM # 410.9
ICD-10CM # I21.3 ST Elevation (STEMI) Myocardial Infarction of Unspecified Site
I21.9 Acute myocardial infarction, unspecified

Acute MI.
Atrial fibrillation.
Left ventricular aneurysm.
Valvular heart disease (e.g., rheumatic mitral valve disease, mitral valve prolapse).
Dilated cardiomyopathy.
Atrial septal defect.
Patent foramen ovale.
Cardioversion for atrial fibrillation.
Infective endocarditis.
Atrial septal aneurysm.
Sick sinus syndrome and cardiac arrhythmias.
Nonbacterial thrombotic endocarditis.
Prosthetic heart valves.
Atrial myxoma and other intracardiac tumors.
Cyanotic heart disease.
Balloon angioplasty.
Coronary artery bypass grafting.
Aneurysms of sinus of Valsalva.
Other: VVI pacing, ventricular support devices, heart transplantation, intracardiac defects with paradoxical embolism.

CARDIOGENIC SHOCK

ICD-9CM # 785.51
ICD-10CM # R57.0 Cardiogenic Shock

Myocardial infarction.
Arrhythmias.
Pericardial effusion/tamponade.
Chest trauma.
Valvular heart disease.
Myocarditis.
Cardiomyopathy.
CHF, end-stage.

CATARACTS, PEDIATRIC AGE

ICD-9CM # 366
ICD-10CM # H26.0 Infantile, juvenile and presenile cataracts

DEVELOPMENTAL VARIANTS

Prematurity (Y-suture vacuoles) with or without retinopathy of prematurity.

GENETIC DISORDERS

Simple Mendelian Inheritance
Autosomal dominant (most common).
Autosomal recessive.
X-linked.
Major Chromosomal Defects
Trisomy disorders (13, 18, 21).
Turner syndrome (45X).
Deletion syndromes (11p13, 18p, 18q).
Duplication syndromes (3q, 20p, 10q).
Multisystem Genetic Disorders
Alport syndrome (hearing loss, renal disease).
Alström syndrome (nerve deafness, diabetes mellitus).
Apert disease (craniosynostosis, syndactyly).
Cockayne syndrome (premature senility, skin photosensitivity).
Conradi disease (chondrodysplasia punctata).
Crouzon disease (dysostosis craniofacialis).
Hallermann-Streiff syndrome (microphthalmia, small pinched nose, skin atrophy, hypotrichosis).
Hypohidrotic ectodermal dysplasia (anomalous dentition, hypohidrosis, hypotrichosis).
Ichthyosis (keratinizing disorder with thick, scaly skin).
Incontinentia pigmenti (dental anomalies, mental retardation, cutaneous lesions).
Lowe syndrome (oculocerebrorenal syndrome: hypotonia, renal disease).
Marfan syndrome.
Marinesco-Sjögren syndrome (cerebellar ataxia, hypotonia).
Meckel-Gruber syndrome (renal dysplasia, encephalocele).
Myotonic dystrophy.
Nail-patella syndrome (renal dysfunction, dysplastic nails, hypoplastic patella).
Nevoid basal cell carcinoma syndrome (autosomal dominant, basal cell carcinoma erupts in childhood).
Peters anomaly (corneal opacifications with iris-corneal dysgenesis).
Reiger syndrome (iris dysplasia, myotonic dystrophy).
Rothmund-Thomson syndrome (poikiloderma: skin atrophy).
Rubinstein-Taybi syndrome (broad great toe, mental retardation).
Smith-Lemli-Opitz syndrome (toe syndactyly, hypospadias, mental retardation).
Sotos syndrome (cerebral gigantism).
Spondyloepiphyseal dysplasia (dwarfism, short trunk).
Werner syndrome (premature aging in 2nd decade of life).
Inborn Errors of Metabolism
Abetalipoproteinemia (absent chylomicrons, retinal degeneration).
Fabry disease (α-galactosidase A deficiency).
Galactokinase deficiency.
Galactosemia (galactose-1-phosphate uridyl transferase deficiency).
Homocystinemia (subluxation of lens, mental retardation).
Mannosidosis (acid α-mannosidase deficiency).
Niemann-Pick disease (sphingomyelinase deficiency).
Refsum disease (phytanic acid α-hydrolase deficiency).
Wilson disease (accumulation of copper leads to cirrhosis and neurologic symptoms).

ENDOCRINOPATHIES

Hypocalcemia (hypoparathyroidism).
Hypoglycemia.
Diabetes mellitus.

CONGENITAL INFECTIONS

Toxoplasmosis.
Cytomegalovirus infection.
Syphilis.
Rubella.
Perinatal herpes simplex infection.
Measles (rubeola).
Poliomyelitis.
Influenza.
Varicella-zoster.

OCULAR ANOMALIES

Microphthalmia.
Coloboma.
Aniridia.
Mesodermal dysgenesis.
Persistent papillary membrane.
Posterior lenticonus.
Persistent hyperplastic primary vitreous.
Primitive hyaloid vascular system.

MISCELLANEOUS DISORDERS

Atopic dermatitis.
Drugs (corticosteroids).
Radiation.
Trauma.

IDIOPATHIC

CAVITARY LESION ON CHEST X-RAY[16]

ICD-9CM # 793.1 Chest X-Ray Lung Shadow
ICD-10CM # R91.8 Other Nonspecific Abnormal Finding of Lung Field

NECROTIZING INFECTIONS

Bacteria: anaerobes, *Staphylococcus aureus,* enteric gram-negative bacteria, *Pseudomonas aeruginosa, Legionella* species, *Haemophilus in fluenzae, Streptococcus pyogenes, Streptococcus pneumoniae* (?), *Rhodococcus, Actinomyces.*
Mycobacteria: *Mycobacterium tuberculosis, Mycobacterium kansasii,* MAI.
Bacteria-like: *Nocardia* species.
Fungi: *Coccidioides immitis, Histoplasma capsulatum, Blastomyces hominis, Aspergillus* species, *Mucor* species.
Parasitic: *Entamoeba histolytica, Echinococcus, Paragonimus westermani.*

CAVITARY INFARCTION

Bland infarction (with or without superimposed infection).
Lung contusion.

SEPTIC EMBOLISM

S. aureus, anaerobes, others.

VASCULITIS

Wegener's granulomatosis, periarteritis.

NEOPLASMS

Bronchogenic carcinoma, metastatic carcinoma, lymphoma.

MISCELLANEOUS LESIONS

Cysts, blebs, bullae, or pneumatocele with or without fluid collections.
Sequestration.
Empyema with air-fluid level.
Bronchiectasis.

CEREBRAL INFARCTION SECONDARY TO INHERITED DISORDERS

ICD-9CM # 434.91
ICD-10CM # I63.50 Cerebral Infarction Due to Unspecified Occlusion or Stenosis of Unspecified Cerebral Artery

Homocystinuria.
Marfan's syndrome.
Ehlers-Danlos syndrome.
Rendu-Osler-Weber syndrome.
Pseudoxanthoma elasticum.
Fabry's disease.

CEREBRAL VASCULITIS, CAUSES[12c]

ICD-9CM # varies with specific diagnosis
ICD-10CM # varies with specific diagnosis

PRIMARY CEREBRAL VASCULITIDES

Takayasu arteritis.
Primary cerebral vasculitis.
Polyarteritis nodosa.

SECONDARY VASCULITIDES

Immune Disorders
Systemic lupus erythematosus.
Wegner granulomatosis.
Kawasaki syndrome.
Sarcoidosis.
Henoch-Schönlein purpura.
Primary Intracranial Infections
Bacterial meningitis (especially *Diplococcus pneumoniae*).
Tuberculous meningitis.
Mycotic infections.
Cat-scratch disease.
Human immunodeficiency virus/acquired immunodeficiency syndrome.
Malaria.
Lyme disease.
Rickettsial infections.
Brucellosis.

CEREBROVASCULAR DISEASE, ISCHEMIC[40]

ICD-9CM # 437.9
ICD-10CM # I67.9 Cerebrovascular Disease, Unspecified

VASCULAR DISORDERS

Large-vessel atherothrombotic disease.
Lacunar disease.
Arterial-to-arterial embolization.
Carotid or vertebral artery dissection.
Fibromuscular dysplasia.
Migraine.
Venous thrombosis.
Radiation.
Complications of arteriography.
Multiple, progressive intracranial arterial occlusions.

INFLAMMATORY DISORDERS

Giant cell arteritis.
Polyarteritis nodosa.
SLE.
Granulomatous angiitis.
Takayasu's disease.
Arteritis associated with amphetamine, cocaine, or phenylpropanolamine.
Syphilis, mucormycosis.
Sjögren's syndrome.
Behçet's syndrome.

CARDIAC DISORDERS

Rheumatic heart disease.
Mural thrombus.
Arrhythmias.
Mitral valve prolapse.
Prosthetic heart valve.
Endocarditis.
Myxoma.
Paradoxical embolus.

HEMATOLOGIC DISORDERS

Thrombotic thrombocytopenic purpura.
Sickle cell disease.
Hypercoagulable states.
Polycythemia.
Thrombocytosis.
Leukocytosis.
Lupus anticoagulant.

CERVICAL INSTABILITY, PEDIATRIC

ICD-9CM # 722.2
ICD-10CM # M50 Cervical disc disorders

CONGENITAL

Vertebral (Bony Anomalies)
Cranio-occipital defects (occipital vertebrae, basilar impression, occipital dysplasias, condylar hypoplasia, occipitalized atlas).
Atlantoaxial defects (aplasia of atlas arch, aplasia of odontoid process).
Subaxial anomalies (failure of segmentation and/or fusion, spina bifida, spondylolisthesis).
Ligamentous or Combined Anomalies
Found at birth as an element of somatogenic aberration.
Syndromic Disorders
Down syndrome.
Klippel-Feil syndrome.
22q11.2 deletion syndrome.
Larsen syndrome.
Marfan syndrome.
Ehlers-Danlos syndrome.

ACQUIRED

Trauma.
Infection (pyogenic, granulomatous).
Tumor (including neurofibromatosis).
Inflammatory conditions (e.g., juvenile rheumatoid arthritis).
Osteochondrodysplasias (e.g., achondroplasia, diastrophic dysplasia, metatropic dysplasia, spondyloepiphyseal dysplasia).
Storage disorders (e.g., mucopolysaccharidoses).
Metabolic disorders (rickets).
Miscellaneous (including osteogenesis imperfecta, sequela of surgery).

CHEST PAIN, CHILDREN[4]

ICD-9CM # 786.50 Chest Pain NOS
786.59 Chest Pressure
786.52 Chest Pain, Pleuritic
ICD-10CM # R07.9 Chest Pain, Unspecified
R07.82 Intercostal Pain
R07.89 Other Chest Pain
R07.1 Chest Pain on Breathing
R07.81 Pleurodynia

MUSCULOSKELETAL (COMMON)

Trauma (accidental, abuse).
Exercise, overuse injury (strain, bursitis).
Costochondritis (Tietze's syndrome).
Herpes zoster (cutaneous).
Pleurodynia.
Fibrositis.
Slipping rib.
Sickle cell anemia vasoocclusive crisis.
Osteomyelitis (rare).
Primary or metastatic tumor (rare).

PULMONARY (COMMON)

Pneumonia.
Pleurisy.
Asthma.
Chronic cough.
Pneumothorax.
Infarction (sickle cell anemia).
Foreign body.
Embolism (rare).
Pulmonary hypertension (rare).
Tumor (rare).

GASTROINTESTINAL (LESS COMMON)

Esophagitis (gastroesophageal reflux).
Esophageal foreign body.
Esophageal spasm.
Cholecystitis.
Subdiaphragmatic abscess.
Perihepatitis (Fitz-Hugh-Curtis syndrome).
Peptic ulcer disease.

CARDIAC (LESS COMMON)

Pericarditis.
Postpericardiotomy syndrome.
Endocarditis.
Mitral valve prolapse.
Aortic or subaortic stenosis.
Arrhythmias.
Marfan's syndrome (dissecting aortic aneurysm).
Anomalous coronary artery.
Kawasaki disease.
Cocaine, sympathomimetic ingestion.
Angina (familial hypercholesterolemia).

IDIOPATHIC (COMMON)

Anxiety, hyperventilation.
Panic disorder.

OTHER (LESS COMMON)

Spinal cord or nerve root compression.

Breast-related pathologic condition.
Castleman's disease (lymph node neoplasm).

CHEST PAIN (NONPLEURITIC)[9]

ICD-9CM # 786.50 Chest Pain NOS
786.59 Chest Discomfort
ICD-10CM # R07.9 Chest Pain, Unspecified
R07.82 Intercostal Pain
R07.89 Other Chest Pain

Cardiac: myocardial ischemia/infarction, myocarditis.
Esophageal: spasm, esophagitis, ulceration, neoplasm, achalasia, diverticula, foreign body.
Referred pain from subdiaphragmatic GI structures.
Gastric and duodenal: hiatal hernia, neoplasm, PUD.
Gallbladder and biliary: cholecystitis, cholelithiasis, impacted stone, neoplasm.
Pancreatic: pancreatitis, neoplasm.
Dissecting aortic aneurysm.
Pain originating from skin, breasts, and musculoskeletal structures: herpes zoster, mastitis, cervical spondylosis.
Mediastinal tumors: lymphoma, thymoma.
Pulmonary: neoplasm, pneumonia, pulmonary embolism/infarction.
Psychoneurosis.
Chest pain associated with mitral valve prolapse.

CHEST PAIN (PLEURITIC)

ICD-9CM # 786.52 Chest Pain, Pleuritic
ICD-10CM # R07.1 Chest Pain on Breathing
R07.81 Pleurodynia

Cardiac: pericarditis, postpericardiotomy/Dressler's syndrome.
Pulmonary: pneumothorax, hemothorax, embolism/infarction, pneumonia, empyema, neoplasm, bronchiectasis, pneumomediastinum, TB, carcinomatous effusion.
GI: liver abscess, pancreatitis, esophageal rupture, Whipple's disease with associated pericarditis or pleuritis.
Subdiaphragmatic abscess.
Pain originating from skin and musculoskeletal tissues: costochondritis, chest wall trauma, fractured rib, interstitial fibrositis, myositis, strain of pectoralis muscle, herpes zoster, soft tissue and bone tumors.
Collagen vascular diseases with pleuritis.
Psychoneurosis.
Familial Mediterranean fever.

CHEST WALL TUMORS, PRIMARY[5a]

ICD-9CM # varies with specific diagnosis
ICD-10CM # varies with specific diagnosis

SOFT TISSUE

Benign
Lipoma
Hemangioma
Lymphangioma
Fibroma
Rhabdomyoma
Neurofibroma
Desmoid tumor
Malignant
Malignant fibrous histiocytoma
Rhabdosarcoma
Liposarcoma
Neurofibrosarcoma
Leiomyosarcoma

BONY AND CARTILAGINOUS

Benign
Fibrous dysplasia
Osteochondroma
Chondroma
Askin tumor
Plasmacytoma
Malignant
Chondrosarcoma
Osteogenic sarcoma
Ewing sarcoma

CHILDHOOD EOSINOPHILIA

ICD-9CM # 288.3
ICD-10CM # D72.1 Eosinophilia

PHYSIOLOGIC

Prematurity.
Infants receiving hyperalimentation.
Familial.

INFECTIOUS

Parasitic (with tissue-invasive helminths, e.g., trichinosis, strongyloidiasis, pneumocystosis, filariasis, cysticercosis, cutaneous and visceral larva migrans, echinococcosis).
Bacterial (brucellosis, tularemia, cat-scratch disease, *Chlamydia*).
Fungal (histoplasmosis, blastomycosis, coccidioidomycosis, allergic bronchopulmonary aspergillosis).
Mycobacterial (tuberculosis, leprosy).
Viral (hepatitis A, hepatitis B, hepatitis C, Epstein-Barr virus).

PULMONARY

Allergic (rhinitis, asthma).
Loeffler syndrome.
Hypersensitivity pneumonitis.
Eosinophilic pneumonia.
Pulmonary interstitial eosinophilia.

DERMATOLOGIC

Atopic dermatitis.
Pemphigus.
Dermatitis herpetiformis.
Infantile eosinophilic pustular folliculitis.
Episodic angioedema and urticaria.
Eosinophilic fasciitis (Schulman syndrome).
Eosinophilic cellulitis (Wells syndrome).
Kimura disease.

ONCOLOGIC

Neoplasm (lung, gastrointestinal, uterine).
Hodgkin disease.
Leukemia.
Myelofibrosis.

IMMUNOLOGIC

T-cell immunodeficiencies.
Hyperimmunoglobulin E (Job) syndrome.
Wiskott-Aldrich syndrome.
Graft-versus-host disease.
Drug hypersensitivity.
Post-irradiation.
Post-splenectomy.

ENDOCRINE

Post-adrenalectomy.
Addison disease.
Panhypopituitarism.

CARDIOVASCULAR

Loeffler disease (fibroplastic endocarditis).
Congenital heart disease.
Hypersensitivity vasculitis.

GASTROINTESTINAL

Milk protein allergy.
Inflammatory bowel disease.
Eosinophilic esophagitis.
Eosinophilic gastroenteritis.

CHOLANGITIS, ACUTE[5a]

ICD-9CM # 576.1 Cholangitis
ICD-10CM # K83.0 Cholangitis

NONIATROGENIC

Benign Conditions
Choledocholithiasis.
Primary.
Secondary.
Pancreatitis (chronic/acute), including pancreatic pseudocyst.
Papillary stenosis.
Mirizzi syndrome.
Choledochal cysts (type V, Caroli disease).
Primary sclerosing cholangitis.
Malignancies
Pancreatic cancer.
Cholangiocarcinoma.
Porta hepatis tumor/metastasis.

IATROGENIC

Obstructed biliary endoprosthesis.
Iatrogenic biliary stricture.
Direct surgical trauma.
Ischemia-induced stricture.
Anastomotic stricture (biliobiliary/bilioenteric anastomosis).

CHOLESTASIS[14]

ICD-9CM # 574.71
ICD-10CM # K80.65 Calculus of Gallbladder and Bile Duct with Chronic Cholecystitis with Obstruction

EXTRAHEPATIC

Choledocholithiasis.
Bile duct stricture.
Cholangiocarcinoma.
Pancreatic carcinoma.
Chronic pancreatitis.

Papillary stenosis.
Ampullary cancer.
Primary sclerosing cholangitis.
Choledochal cysts.
Parasites (e.g., ascaris, clonorchis).
AIDS.
Cholangiography.
Biliary atresia.
Portal lymphadenopathy.
Mirizzi's syndrome.

INTRAHEPATIC

Viral hepatitis.
Alcoholic hepatitis.
Drug induced.
Ductopenia syndromes.
Primary biliary cirrhosis.
Benign recurrent intrahepatic cholestasis.
Byler's disease.
Primary sclerosing cholangitis.
Alagille's syndrome.
Sarcoid.
Lymphoma.
Postoperative.
Total parenteral nutrition.
Alpha-1-antitrypsin deficiency.

CHOLESTASIS, NEONATAL AND INFANTILE, DIFFERENTIAL DIAGNOSIS[22A]

ICD-9CM #	varies with specific diagnosis	
ICD-10CM #	O26.6	Liver disorders in pregnancy, childbirth and the puerperium

INFECTIOUS

Generalized bacterial sepsis.
Viral hepatitis.
- Hepatitis A, B, C, D.
- Cytomegalovirus.
- Rubella virus.
- Herpesvirus: herpes simplex, human herpesvirus 6 and 7.
- Varicella virus.
- Coxsackievirus.
- Echovirus.
- Reovirus type 3.
- Parvovirus B19.
- HIV.
- Adenovirus.

Others.
- Toxoplasmosis.
- Syphilis.
- Tuberculosis.
- Listeriosis.
- Urinary tract infection.

TOXIC

Sepsis.
Parenteral nutrition related.
Drug related.

METABOLIC

Disorders of amino acid metabolism.
- Tyrosinemia.

Disorders of lipid metabolism.
- Wolman disease.
- Niemann-Pick disease (type C).
- Gaucher disease.

Cholesterol ester storage disease.
Disorders of carbohydrate metabolism.
- Galactosemia.
- Fructosemia.
- Glycogenosis IV.

Disorders of bile acid biosynthesis.
Other metabolic defects.
- α1-Antitrypsin deficiency.
- Cystic fibrosis.
- Hypopituitarism.
- Hypothyroidism.
- Zellweger (cerebrohepatorenal) syndrome.
- Neonatal iron storage disease.
- Indian childhood cirrhosis/infantile copper overload.
- Congenital disorders of glycosylation.
- Mitochondrial hepatopathies.
- Citrin deficiency.

GENETIC OR CHROMOSOMAL

Trisomy 17, 18, 21.
Donahue syndrome.

INTRAHEPATIC CHOLESTASIS SYNDROMES

"Idiopathic" neonatal hepatitis.
Alagille syndrome (arteriohepatic dysplasia).
Nonsyndromic bile duct paucity syndrome.
Intrahepatic cholestasis (PFIC):
- FIC-1 deficiency.
- BSEP deficiency.
- MDR3 deficiency.

Familial benign recurrent cholestasis associated with lymphedema (Aagenaes).
Congenital hepatic fibrosis.
Caroli disease (cystic dilatation of intrahepatic ducts).

EXTRAHEPATIC DISEASES

Biliary atresia.
Sclerosing cholangitis.
Bile duct stricture/stenosis.
Choledochal-pancreaticoductal junction anomaly.
Spontaneous perforation of the bile duct.
Choledochal cyst.
Mass (neoplasia, stone).
Bile/mucous plug ("inspissated bile").

MISCELLANEOUS

Shock and hypoperfusion.
Associated with enteritis.
Associated with intestinal obstruction.
Neonatal lupus erythematosus.
Myeloproliferative disease (trisomy 21).
Hemophagocytic lymphohistiocytosis (HLH).
Arthrogryposis cholestatic pigmentary (ARC) syndrome.

CHOREA

ICD-9CM #	333.5	
ICD-10CM #	G25.4	Drug-Induced Chorea
	G25.5	Other Chorea

Medications (e.g., neuroleptics, tricyclics, antiparkinsonian drugs).
Cerebral palsy.
Huntington's disease.
Benign hereditary chorea.
Thyroid disorder (hyperthyroidism, hypothyroidism).
Friedreich's ataxia.
Ataxia-telangiectasia.
Hypoglycemia, hyperglycemia.
Electrolyte abnormalities (hyponatremia, hypocalcemia, hypomagnesemia, hypernatremia).
Vitamin B_{12} deficiency.
SLE.
Wilson's disease.
Alcohol.
Cocaine.
Carbon monoxide poisoning.
Mercury poisoning.

CHOREOATHETOSIS[28]

ICD-9CM #	275.1	Choreoathetosis-Agitans Syndrome
	33.5	Choreoathetosis, Paroxysmal
ICD-10CM #	G25.5	Choreoathetosis

SYSTEMIC DISEASES

SLE.
Polycythemia.
Thyrotoxicosis.
Rheumatic fever.
Cirrhosis of the liver (acquired hepatocerebral degeneration).
DM.
Wilson's disease.

PRIMARY DEGENERATIVE BRAIN DISEASES

Huntington's chorea.
Olivopontocerebellar atrophies.
Neuroacanthocytosis.

FOCAL BRAIN DISEASES

Hemichorea.
Stroke.
Tumor.
Arteriovenous malformation.

DRUG-INDUCED CHOREOATHETOSIS

Parkinson's Disease Drugs
Levodopa.
Epilepsy Drugs
Phenytoin.
Carbamazepine.
Phenobarbital.
Gabapentin.
Valproate.
Psychostimulant Drugs
Cocaine.
Amphetamine.
Methamphetamine.
Dextroamphetamine.
Methylphenidate.
Pemoline.

Psychotropic Drugs
Lithium.
Tricyclic antidepressant drugs.
Oral Contraceptive Drugs Cimetidine

CHYLOTHORAX

ICD-9CM # 457.8
ICD-10CM # I89.8 Other Specified Noninfective Disorders of Lymphatic Vessels and Lymph Nodes

Post lymph node dissection of neck or chest.
Subclavian venous catheterization.
Thoracic aneurysm repair.
Trauma to chest and neck.
Mediastinal tumor resection.
Esophagectomy, pneumonectomy.
Lymphangitis, mediastinitis.
Neoplasms (lymphoma, carcinoma of esophagus, lung, mediastinal malignancies).
Sympathectomy.
Venous thrombosis.
Congenital.

CLOUDY URINE

ICD-9CM # 788.69
ICD-10CM # R82 Other abnormal findings in urine

Concentrated urine.
Use of multivitamin supplements.
Diet high in purine-rich foods.
Pyuria.
Phosphaturia.
Urinary tract infection.
Lipiduria.
Chyluria.
Hyperoxaluria.

CLUBBING

ICD-9CM # 781.5 Clubbing Finger
ICD-10CM # R68.3 Clubbing of Fingers

Pulmonary neoplasm (lung, pleura).
Other neoplasm (GI, liver, Hodgkin's, thymus, osteogenic sarcoma).
Pulmonary infectious process (empyema, abscess, bronchiectasis, TB, chronic pneumonitis).
Extrapulmonary infectious process (subacute bacterial endocarditis, intestinal TB, bacterial or amebic dysentery, arterial graft sepsis).
Pneumoconiosis.
Cystic fibrosis.
Sarcoidosis.
Cyanotic congenital heart disease.
Endocrine (Graves' disease, hyperparathyroidism).
Inflammatory bowel disease.
Celiac disease.
Chronic liver disease, cirrhosis (particularly biliary and juvenile).
Pulmonary AV malformations.
Idiopathic.
Thyroid acropachy.
Hereditary (pachydermoperiostosis).
Chronic trauma (jackhammer operators, machine workers).

COBALAMIN DEFICIENCY[20]

ICD-9CM # 266.2
ICD-10CM # E53.8 Deficiency of Other Specified B Group Vitamins

ETIOPATHOPHYSIOLOGIC CLASSIFICATION OF COBALAMIN DEFICIENCY

Nutritional cobalamin deficiency (i.e., insufficient cobalamin intake):
Vegetarians, poverty-imposed near-vegetarians, breastfed infants of mothers with pernicious anemia.
Abnormal intragastric events (i.e., inadequate proteolysis of food cobalamin):
Atrophic gastritis, partial gastritis with hypochlorhydria, proton-pump inhibitors, H_2 blockers.
Loss or atrophy of gastric oxyntic mucosa (i.e., deficient intrinsic factor [IF] molecules):
Total or partial gastrectomy, pernicious anemia, caustic destruction (lye).
Abnormal events in small bowel lumen:
Inadequate pancreatic protease (e.g., R-cobalamin not degraded, cobalamin not transferred to IF):
- Insufficient pancreatic protease (i.e., pancreatic insufficiency).
- Inactivation of pancreatic protease (i.e., Zollinger–Ellison syndrome).

Usurping of luminal cobalamin (i.e., inadequate cobalamin binding to IF):
- By bacteria, during stasis syndromes (e.g., blind loops, pouches of diverticulosis, strictures, fistulas, anastomosis), impaired bowel motility (e.g., scleroderma), hypogammaglobulinemia.
- By *Diphyllobothrium latum* (fish tapeworm).

Disorders of ileal mucosa/IF–cobalamin receptors (i.e., IF–cobalamin not bound to IF–cobalamin receptors):
Diminished or absent IF–cobalamin receptors (e.g., ileal bypass, resection, fistula).
Abnormal mucosal architecture/function (e.g., tropical or nontropical sprue, Crohn's disease, tuberculosis ileitis, infiltration by lymphomas, amyloidosis).
IF-/post-IF–cobalamin receptor defects (e.g., Imerslund–Gräsbeck syndrome, transcobalamin II [TC II] deficiency).
Drug effects (e.g., slow K, metformin, cholestyramine, colchicine, neomycin).
Disorders of plasma cobalamin transport (i.e., TC II–cobalamin not delivered to TC II receptors):
Congenital TC II deficiency, defective binding of TC II–cobalamin to TC II receptors (rare).
Metabolic disorders (i.e., cobalamin not used by cells):
Inborn enzyme errors (rare).
Acquired disorders (e.g., cobalamin functionally inactivated by irreversible oxidation, N_2O inhalation).

COLIC, ACUTE ABDOMINAL[38]

ICD-9CM # 789.0
ICD-10CM # R10.0 Acute Abdomen

Acute gastroenteritis.
Food poisoning.
Nonspecific causes.
Constipation.
Gastric outlet obstruction:
- Chronic peptic ulceration.
- Gastric cancer.

Small bowel obstruction:
Adhesions:
- Postsurgical.
- Inflammatory (e.g., diverticular).
- Radiation.
- Meckel's diverticulum.
- Metastatic.

Stricture:
- Ischemic.
- Radiation.
- Inflammatory (e.g., Crohn's disease).

Volvulus intussusception:
- Tumor (e.g., Peutz-Jeghers syndrome).
- Superior mesenteric artery syndrome.

Intraluminal bolus:
- Gallstone.
- Bezoar.

Hernia:
- Abdominal wall.
- Internal.

Neoplasm:
- Benign (e.g., leiomyoma).
- Malignant (e.g., carcinoid tumor, adenocarcinoma).

Large bowel obstruction:
- Colon cancer.
- Diverticular disease.
- Volvulus.

Uterine:
- Missed abortion.
- Parturition.
- Period pain.

COLOR CHANGES, CUTANEOUS[34]

ICD-9CM # 709.00 Pigmentation Anomaly
ICD-10CM # L81.9 Disorder of Pigmentation, Unspecified

BROWN

Generalized: pituitary, adrenal, liver disease, ACTH-producing tumor (e.g., oat cell lung carcinoma).
Localized: nevi, neurofibromatosis.

WHITE

Generalized: albinism.
Localized: vitiligo, Raynaud's syndrome.

RED (ERYTHEMA)

Generalized: fever, polycythemia, urticaria, viral exanthems.
Localized: inflammation, infection, Raynaud's syndrome.

YELLOW

Generalized: liver disease, chronic renal disease, anemia.

Generalized (except sclera): hypothyroidism, increased intake of vegetables containing carotene.
Localized: resolving hematoma, infection, peripheral vascular insufficiency.

BLUE

Lips, mouth, nail beds: cardiovascular and pulmonary diseases, Raynaud's.

COMA

ICD-9CM # 780.01
ICD-10CM # R40.20 Unspecified Coma

Vascular: hemorrhage, thrombosis, embolism.
CNS infections: meningitis, encephalitis, cerebral abscess.
Cerebral neoplasms with herniation.
Head injury: subdural hematoma, cerebral concussion, cerebral contusion.
Drugs: narcotics, sedatives, hypnotics.
Ingestion or inhalation of toxins: CO, alcohol, lead.
Metabolic disturbances.
Hypoxia.
Acid-base disorders.
Hypoglycemia, hyperglycemia.
Hepatic failure.
Electrol yte disorders.
Uremia.
Hypothyroidism.
Hypothermia, hyperthermia.
Hypotension, malignant hypertension.
Postictal.

COMA, NORMAL COMPUTED TOMOGRAPHY[1a]

ICD-9CM # 780.01
ICD-10CM # R40.20 Unspecified coma

MENINGEAL DISORDERS

Subarachnoid hemorrhage (uncommon).
Bacterial meningitis.
Encephalitis.
Subdural empyema.

EXOGENOUS TOXINS

Sedative drugs and barbiturates.
Anesthetics and g-hydroxybutyrate.*
Alcohols.
Stimulants:
- Phencyclidines.†
- Cocaine and amphetamines.‡

Psychotropic drugs:
- Cyclic antidepressants.
- Phenothiazines.
- Lithium.

Anticonvulsants.
Opioids.
Clonidine.§
Penicillins.
Salicylates.
Anticholinergics.
Carbon monoxide, cyanide, and methemoglobinemia.

ENDOGENOUS TOXINS/ DEFICIENCIES/DERANGEMENTS

Hypoxia and ischemia.
Hypoglycemia.
Hypercalcemia.
Osmolar:
- Hyperglycemia.
- Hyponatremia.
- Hypernatremia.

Organ system failure:
- Hepatic encephalopathy.
- Uremic encephalopathy.
- Pulmonary insufficiency (carbon dioxide narcosis).

SEIZURES

Prolonged postictal state.
Spike-wave stupor.

HYPOTHERMIA OR HYPERTHERMIA

Brain stem ischemia.
Basilar artery stroke.
Brain stem or cerebellar hemorrhage.
Conversion or malingering.

---

*General anesthetic, similar to g-aminobutyric acid; recreational drug and body building aid. Rapid onset, rapid recovery often with myoclonic jerking and confusion. Deep coma (2-3 hr; Glasgow Coma Scale = 3) with maintenance of vital signs.

†Coma associated with cholinergic signs: lacrimation, salivation, bronchorrhea, and hyperthermia.

‡Coma after seizures or status (i.e., a prolonged postictal state).

§An antihypertensive agent active through the opiate receptor system; frequent overdose when used to treat narcotic withdrawal.

COMA, PEDIATRIC POPULATION[31]

ICD-9CM # 780.01
ICD-10CM # R40.20 Unspecified coma

ANOXIA

Birth asphyxia.
Carbon monoxide poisoning.
Croup/epiglottitis.
Meconium aspiration.

INFECTION

Hemolysis.
Blood loss.
Hydrops fetalis.
Infection.
Meningoencephalitis.
Sepsis.
Postimmunization encephalitis.

INCREASED INTRACRANIAL PRESSURE

Anoxia.
Inborn metabolic errors.
Toxic encephalopathy.
Reye's syndrome.
Head trauma/intracranial bleed.
Hydrocephalus.
Posterior fossa tumors.

HYPERTENSIVE ENCEPHALOPATHY

Coarctation of aorta.
Nephritis.
Vasculitis.
Pheochromocytoma.

ISCHEMIA

Hypoplastic left heart.
Shunting lesions.
Aortic stenosis.
Cardiovascular collapse (any cause).

PURPURIC CAUSES

Disseminated intravascular coagulation.
Hemolytic-uremic syndrome.
Leukemia.
Thrombotic purpura.

HYPERCAPNIA

Cystic fibrosis.
Bronchopulmonary dysplasia.
Congenital lung anomalies.

NEOPLASM

Medulloblastoma.
Glioma of brain stem.
Posterior fossa tumors.

DRUGS/TOXINS

Maternal sedation.
Alcohol.
Any drug.
Lead.
Salicylism.
Arsenic.
Pesticides.

ELECTROLYTE ABNORMALITIES

Hypernatremia (diarrhea, dehydration, salt poisoning).
Hyponatremia (SIADH, androgenital syndrome, gastroenteritis).
Hyperkalemia (renal failure, salicylism, androgenitalism).
Hypokalemia (diarrhea, hyperaldosteronism, salicylism, DKA).
Hypocalcemia (vitamin D deficiency, hyperparathyroidism).
Severe acidosis (sepsis, cold injury, salicylism, DKA).

HYPOGLYCEMIA

Birth injury or stress.
Diabetes.
Alcohol.
Salicylism.
Hyperinsulinemia.
Iatrogenic.

POSTSEIZURE

Renal Causes

Nephritis.
Hypoplastic kidneys.

Hepatic Causes

Acute hepatitis.
Fulminant hepatic failure.
Inborn metabolic errors.
Bile duct atresia.

CONGESTIVE HEART FAILURE AND CARDIOMYOPATHY[1a]

ICD-9CM # 428.0 Congestive Heart Failure
425.9 Cardiomyopathy, Secondary, Unspecified
ICD-10CM # I50.9 Heart failure, unspecified
I42.7 Cardiomyopathy due to drug and external agent

CAUSES OF CONGESTIVE HEART FAILURE AND CARDIOMYOPATHY

Coronary Artery Disease
Acute ischemia.
Myocardial infarction.
Ischemic cardiomyopathy with hibernating myocardium.
Idiopathic
Idiopathic dilated cardiomyopathy.
Idiopathic restrictive cardiomyopathy.
Peripartum.
Pressure Overload
Hypertension.
Aortic stenosis.
Volume Overload
Mitral regurgitation.
Aortic insufficiency.
Anemia.
Atrioventricular fistula.
Toxins
Ethanol.
Cocaine.
Doxorubicin (Adriamycin).
Methamphetamine.
Metabolic-Endocrine
Thiamine deficiency.
Diabetes.
Hemochromatosis.
Thyrotoxicosis.
Obesity.
Infiltrative
Amyloidosis.
Inflammatory
Viral myocarditis.
Hereditary
Hypertrophic.
Dilated.

*Genetic bases for these cardiomyopathies have been identified in a large number of individual patients and families. Most of the mutations have been found in cardiac contractile or structural proteins.

CONGESTIVE HEART FAILURE, INFANT[1]

ICD-9CM # 428.9
ICD-10CM # I05.9 Heart failure, unspecified

Critical coarctation of the aorta.
Interrupted aortic arch.
Congenital aortic stenosis.
Hypoplastic left heart syndrome.
Large ventricular septal defect.
Truncus arteriosus.
Unrecognized supraventricular tachycardia.
Cardiac tamponade.
Myocarditis.

CONJUNCTIVAL NEOPLASM

ICD-9CM # varies with specific disorder
ICD-10CM # varies with specific diagnosis

MALIGNANT

Squamous cell carcinoma.
Melanoma.
Sebaceous carcinoma.
Kaposi's sarcoma.
Metastatic neoplasms.

BENIGN

Melanocytic nevus.
Squamous papilloma.
Hemangioma.
Lymphangioma.
Myxoma.

CONSCIOUSNESS IMPAIRMENT, ACUTE, IN CRITICALLY ILL PATIENT

ICD-9CM # 293.1
ICD-10CM # F05.9 Delirium, unspecified

GENERAL CAUSES OF ACUTELY IMPAIRED CONSCIOUSNESS IN THE CRITICALLY ILL

Infection
Sepsis encephalopathy.
Central nervous system infection.
Drugs
Narcotics.
Benzodiazepines.
Anticholinergics.
Anticonvulsants.
Tricyclic antidepressants.
Selective serotonin uptake inhibitors.
Phenothiazines.
Steroids.
Immunosuppressants (cyclosporine, FK-506, OKT3).
Anesthetics.
Electrolyte and Acid-Base Disturbances
Hyponatremia.
Hypernatremia.
Hypercalcemia.
Hypermagnesemia.
Severe acidemia and alkalemia.
Organ System Failure
Shock.
Renal failure.
Hepatic failure.
Pancreatitis.
Respiratory failure (hypoxia, hypercapnia).
Endocrine Disorders
Hypoglycemia.
Hyperglycemia.
Hypothyroidism.
Hyperthyroidism.
Pituitary apoplexy.
Drug Withdrawal
Alcohol.
Opiates.
Barbiturates.
Benzodiazepines.
Vascular Causes
Shock.
Hypotension.
Hypertensive encephalopathy.
Central nervous system vasculitis.
Cerebral venous sinus thrombosis.
Central Nervous System Disorders
Hemorrhage.
Stroke.
Brain edema.
Hydrocephalus.
Increased intracranial pressure.
Meningitis.
Ventriculitis.
Brain abscess.
Subdural empyema.
Seizures.
Vasculitis.
Seizures
Convulsive and nonconvulsive status epilepticus.
Miscellaneous
Fat embolism syndrome.
Neuroleptic malignant syndrome.
Thiamine deficiency (Wernicke encephalopathy).
Psychogenic unresponsiveness.

CONSTIPATION

ICD-9CM # 564.0
ICD-10CM # K59.00 Constipation, unspecified

Intestinal obstruction.
Fecal impaction.
Diverticular disease.
GI neoplasm.
Strangulated femoral hernia.
Gallstone ileus.
Tuberculous stricture.
Adhesions.
Ameboma.
Volvulus.
Intussusception.
Inflammatory bowel disease.
Hematoma of bowel wall, secondary to trauma or anticoagulants.
Poor dietary habits: insufficient bulk in diet, inadequate fluid intake.
Change from daily routine: travel, hospital admission, physical inactivity.
Acute abdominal conditions: renal colic, salpingitis, biliary colic, appendicitis, ischemia.
Hypercalcemia or hypokalemia, uremia.
Irritable bowel syndrome, pregnancy, anorexia nervosa, depression.
Painful anal conditions: hemorrhoids, fissure, stricture.
Decreased intestinal peristalsis: old age, spinal cord injuries, myxedema, diabetes, multiple sclerosis, Parkinsonism and other neurologic diseases.
Drugs: codeine, morphine, antacids with aluminum, verapamil, anticonvulsants, anticholinergics, disopyramide, cholestyramine, alosetron, iron supplements.
Hirschsprung's disease, meconium ileus, congenital atresia in infants.

CONSTIPATION, ADULT PATIENT[38]

ICD-9CM # 564
ICD-10CM # K59.00 Constipation, unspecified

NO GROSS STRUCTURAL ABNORMALITY

Inadequate fiber intake.
Irritable bowel syndrome (associated with abdominal pain) or functional constipation.
Idiopathic slow-transit constipation.
"Obstructed defecation"—pelvic floor dysfunction (or dyssynergia).

STRUCTURAL DISORDERS

Anal fissure, infection, or stenosis.
Colon cancer or stricture.
Aganglionosis and/or abnormal myenteric plexus:
- Hirschsprung's disease.
- Chagas' disease.
- Neuropathic pseudoobstruction.

Abnormal colonic muscle:
- Myopathy.
- Dystrophia myotonica.
- Systemic sclerosis.

Idiopathic megarectum and/or megacolon.
Proximal megacolon.

NEUROLOGIC CAUSES

Diabetic autonomic neuropathy.
Damage to the sacral parasympathetic outflow.
Spinal cord damage or disease (e.g., multiple sclerosis).
Parkinson's disease.
Blunting of consciousness, mental retardation, psychosis.
Pain induced by straining (e.g., sciatic nerve compression).

ENDOCRINE OR METABOLIC CAUSES

Hypothyroidism.
Hypercalcemia.
Porphyria.
Pregnancy.

PSYCHOLOGIC DISORDERS

Depression.
Anorexia nervosa.
Denied bowel habit.

DRUG SIDE EFFECTS

CORNEAL SENSATION, DECREASED

ICD-9CM # 371.89
ICD-10CM # H18.899 Other specified disorders of cornea, unspecified eye

Herpes (simplex, zoster).
Contact lens wear.
Topical agents (NSAIDs, anesthetics, beta-blockers).
Diabetes.
Eye trauma.
Postsurgery.

COUGH

ICD-9CM # 786.2
ICD-10CM # R05 Cough

Infectious process (viral, bacterial).
Postinfectious.
"Smoker's cough."
Rhinitis (allergic, vasomotor, postinfectious).
Asthma.
Exposure to irritants (noxious fumes, smoke, cold air).
Drug-induced (especially ACE inhibitors, beta-blockers).
GERD.
Interstitial lung disease.
Lung neoplasms.
Lymphomas, mediastinal neoplasms.
Bronchiectasis.
Cardiac (CHF, pulmonary edema, mitral stenosis, pericardial inflammation).
Recurrent aspiration.
Inflammation of larynx, pleura, diaphragm, mediastinum.
Cystic fibrosis.
Anxiety.
Other: pulmonary embolism, foreign body inhalation, aortic aneurysm, Zenker's diverticulum, osteophytes, substernal thyroid, thyroiditis, PMR.

CUTANEOUS INFECTIONS, ATHLETES

ICD-9CM # 686.9
ICD-10CM # L08.9 Local infection of the skin and subcutaneous tissue, unspecified

Tinea pedis.
Tinea cruris.
Molluscum contagiosum.
Herpes simplex.
Verruca vulgaris.
Folliculitis.
Impetigo.
Furuncles.
Otitis externa.
Erythrasma.

CYANOSIS[2]

ICD-9CM # 782.5
ICD-10CM # R23.0 Cyanosis

DIFFERENTIAL DIAGNOSIS OF CYANOSIS

Peripheral Cyanosis

Low cardiac output states
Shock.
Left ventricular failure.
Hypovolemia.
Environmental exposure (cold)
Air or water.
Arterial occlusion
Thrombosis.
Embolism.
Vasospasm (Raynaud's phenomenon).
Peripheral vascular disease.
Venous obstruction
Redistribution of blood flow from extremities

Central Cyanosis

Decreased arterial oxygen saturation
High altitude (>8000 ft).
Impaired pulmonary function.
Hypoventilation.
Impaired oxygen diffusion.
Ventilation-perfusion mismatching.
- Pulmonary embolism.
- Acture respiratory distress syndrome.
- Pulmonary hypertension.

Respiratory compromise.
- Upper airway obstruction.
- Pneumonia.
- Diaphragmatic hernia.
- Tension pneumothorax.
- Polycythemia.

Anatomic Shunts

Pulmonary arteriovenous fistulae and intrapulmonary shunts.
Cerebral, hepatic, peripheral arteriovenous fistulae.
Cyanotic congenital heart disease.
Endocardial cushion defects.
Ventricular septal defects.
Coarctation of aorta.
Tetralogy of Fallot.
Total anomalous pulmonary venous drainage.
Hypoplastic left ventricle.
Pulmonary vein stenosis.
Tricuspid atresia and anomalies.
Premature closure of foramen ovale.
Dextrocardia.
Pulmonary stenosis of atrial septal defect.
Patent ductus arteriosus with reversed shunt.

Abnormal Hemoglobin

Methemoglobinemia.
Hereditary.
Acquired.
Sulfhemoglobinemia.
Mutant hemoglobin with low oxygen affinity (e.g., hemoglobin Kansas).

CYANOSIS, NEONATAL[1]

ICD-9CM # 782.5
ICD-10CM # R23.0 Cyanosis

RESPIRATORY

Upper Airway

Choanal atresia.
Macroglossia.
Glossoptosis (secondary to micrognathia).
Laryngomalacia.
Laryngeal web or cyst.
Vascular anomalies (e.g., cystic hygromas, rings).
Subglottic stenosis (commonly secondary to intubation).
Foreign body.

Lower Airway

Pneumonia.
Bronchiolitis.
Pulmonary edema.
Atelectasis.
Bronchopulmonary dysplasia.

SYSTEMIC

Sepsis.
Trauma.
Poisons.

CARDIAC

Cyanotic congenital heart diseases.
Transposition of the great vessels (most common neonatal).
Tetralogy of Fallot.
Truncus arteriosus.
Tricuspid atresia.
Total anomalous pulmonary venous return.
Ebstein anomaly.
Gastrointestinal.
Gastroesophageal reflux.

NEUROLOGIC

Seizures.
Central hypoventilation syndrome (Ondine curse).
Spinal muscular atrophy type I (Werdnig-Hoffmann).
Botulism.
Congenital myopathies.

HEMATOLOGIC

Methemoglobinemia.

DAYTIME SLEEPINESS

ICD-9CM #	varies with specific disorder	
ICD-10CM #	R53.82	Chronic fatigue, unspecified

Sleep deprivation.
Medication induced (e.g., benzodiazepines, beta-blockers, narcotics, sedative antidepressants, gabapentin).
Depression.
Obstructive sleep apnea.
Medical illness (e.g., severe anemia, hypothyroidism, COPD, hepatic failure, renal insufficiency, CHF, electrolyte disturbances).
Circadian rhythm abnormalities (e.g., jet lag, shift work sleep disorder).
Restless legs syndrome.
Posttrauma.
Narcolepsy.
Neurologic disorders (e.g., neurodegenerative disorders; parkinsonism; multiple sclerosis; lesions affecting thalamus, hypothalamus, or brain stem).

DELAYED PASSAGE OF MECONIUM[16a]

ICD-9CM #	777.1	
ICD-10CM #	P76.0	Meconium plug syndrome

Ileal atresia.
Meconium ileus.
Functional immaturity of the colon.
Colon atresia.
Anorectal malformations.
Hirschsprung's disease.
Megacystis-microcolon-intestinal hypoperistalsis syndrome.
Extrinsic compression of the distal bowel by a mass lesion.
Mesenteric cyst.
Enteric duplication cyst.
Paralytic ileus, sepsis, drugs, and metabolic upset.

DELIRIUM[26]

ICD-9CM #	780.09	Delirium NOS
	293.0	Acute Delirium
ICD-10CM #	R40.0	Somnolence
	R40.1	Stupor
	F05	Delirium due to known physiological condition

PHARMACOLOGIC AGENTS

Anxiolytics (benzodiazepines).
Antidepressants (e.g., amitriptyline, doxepin, imipramine).
Cardiovascular agents (e.g., methyldopa, digitalis, reserpine, propranolol, procainamide, captopril, disopyramide).
Antihistamine.
Cimetidine.
Corticosteroids.
Antineoplastics.
Drugs of abuse (alcohol, cannabis, amphetamines, cocaine, hallucinogens, opioids, sedative-hypnotics, phencyclidine).

METABOLIC DISORDERS

Hypercalcemia.
Hypercarbia.
Hypoglycemia.
Hyponatremia.
Hypoxia.

INFLAMMATORY DISORDERS

Sarcoidosis.
SLE.
Giant cell arteritis.

ORGAN FAILURE

Hepatic encephalopathy.
Uremia.

NEUROLOGIC DISORDERS

Alzheimer's disease.
CVA.
Encephalitis (including HIV).
Encephalopathies.
Epilepsy.
Huntington's disease.
Multiple sclerosis.
Neoplasms.
Normal-pressure hydrocephalus.
Parkinson's disease.
Pick's disease.
Wilson's disease.

ENDOCRINE DISORDERS

Addison's disease.
Cushing's disease.
Panhypopituitarism.
Parathyroid disease.
Postpartum psychosis.
Recurrent menstrual psychosis.
Sydenham's chorea.
Thyroid disease.

DEFICIENCY STATES

Niacin.
Thiamine, vitamin B_{12}, and folate.

DELIRIUM AND AGITATION, DRUG-INDUCED

ICD-9CM #	293.1	
ICD-10CM #	F05.9	Delirium, unspecified

COMMONLY USED DRUGS ASSOCIATED WITH DELIRIUM AND AGITATION

Benzodiazepines.
Opiates (especially meperidine).
Anticholinergics.
Antihistamines.
H_2 blockers.
Antibiotics.
Corticosteroids.
Metoclopramide.

DELIRUM, AGITATED[2]

ICD-9CM #	293.1	
ICD-10CM #	F05	Delirium due to known physiological condition

Metabolic causes:
- Electrolyte abnormalities.
- Hypoglycemia.
- Hypoxia.
- Uremia/hyperammonemia.

Structural lesions of the CNS:
- Trauma.
- Stroke.
- Hemorrhage.
- Mass.

Endocrine disease:
- Thyrotoxicosis.

Infections:
- Bacterial/viral meningitis/encephalitis.

Toxicologic causes:
- Sympathomimetic/stimulants.
  - Cocaine.
  - Amphetamines and derivatives.
  - Caffeine.
  - Phencyclidine/ketamine.
- Anticholinergics.
- Serotonin syndrome.
- Sedative-hypnotic withdrawal.

Heatstroke.
Postictal state.

CNS, Central nervous system.

DELIRIUM, DIALYSIS PATIENT[26]

ICD-9CM #	293.0	Acute Delirium
	293.9	Encephalopathy from Dialysis
ICD-10CM #	F05	Delirium due to known physiological condition
	F06.8	Other specified mental disorders due to known physiological condition

STRUCTURAL

Cerebrovascular accident (particularly hemorrhage).
Subdural hematoma.
Intracerebral abscess.
Brain tumor.

METABOLIC

Disequilibrium syndrome.
Uremia.
Drug effects.
Meningitis.
Hypertensive encephalopathy.
Hypotension.
Postictal state.
Hypernatremia or hyponatremia.
Hypercalcemia.
Hypermagnesemia.
Hypoglycemia.
Severe hyperglycemia.
Hypoxemia.
Dialysis dementia.

DEMYELINATING DISEASES[40]

ICD-9CM #	341.9	
ICD-10CM #	G37.9	Demyelinating disease of central nervous system, unspecified

MULTIPLE SCLEROSIS

Relapsing and chronic progressive forms.
Acute multiple sclerosis.
Neuromyelitis optica (Devic's disease).

DIFFUSE CEREBRAL SCLEROSIS

Schilder's encephalitis periaxialis diffusa.
Baló's concentric sclerosis.

ACUTE DISSEMINATED ENCEPHALOMYELITIS

After measles, chickenpox, rubella, influenza, mumps.
After rabies or smallpox vaccination.

NECROTIZING HEMORRHAGIC ENCEPHALITIS

Hemorrhagic leukoencephalitis.

LEUKODYSTROPHIES

Krabbe's globoid leukodystrophy.
Metachromatic leukodystrophy.
Adrenoleukodystrophy.
Adrenomyeloneuropathy.
Pelizaeus-Merzbacher leukodystrophy.
Canavan's disease.
Alexander's disease.

DIAPHRAGM ELEVATION, BILATERAL, SYMMETRICAL[16a]

ICD-9CM #	519.4	
ICD-10CM #	J98.6	Disorders of diaphragm

CAUSES OF BILATERAL SYMMETRICAL ELEVATION OF THE DIAPHRAGM

Supine position.
Poor inspiration.
Obesity.
Pregnancy.
Abdominal distention (ascites, intestinal obstruction, abdominal mass).
Diffuse pulmonary fibrosis.
Lymphangitis carcinomatosa.
Disseminated lupus erythematosus.
Bilateral basal pulmonary emboli.
Painful conditions (after abdominal surgery).
Bilateral diaphragmatic paralysis.

DIAPHRAGM ELEVATION, UNILATERAL[16a]

ICD-9CM #	519.4	
ICD-10CM #	J98.6	Disorders of diaphragm

CAUSES OF UNILATERAL ELEVATION OF THE DIAPHRAGM

Posture—lateral decubitus position (dependent side).
Gaseous distention of stomach or colon.
Dorsal scoliosis.
Pulmonary hypoplasia.
Pulmonary collapse.
Phrenic nerve palsy.
Eventration.
Pneumonia or pleurisy.
Pulmonary thromboembolism.
Rib fracture and other painful conditions.
Subphrenic infection.
Subphrenic mass.

DIARRHEA, ACUTE WATERY AND BLOODY[38]

ICD-9CM #		varies with specific diagnosis
	009.3	Infectious Diarrhea
	558.9	Non-infectious Diarrhea
	564.5	Functional Diarrhea
	787.91	Diarrhea
ICD-10CM #	K52.2	Allergic and dietetic gastroenteritis and colitis
	K52.89	Other specified noninfective gastroenteritis and colitis
	R19.7	Diarrhea, unspecified

ACUTE WATERY DIARRHEA

Gastrointestinal infections:

- Protozoal (e.g., *Giardia*).
- Bacterial (e.g., enterotoxigenic *Escherichia coli,* cholera).
- Viral (e.g., rotavirus, Norwalk virus).

Drugs.
Toxins.
Dietary constituents (e.g., lactose intolerance).
Onset of chronic diarrheal illness.

ACUTE BLOODY DIARRHEA

Infectious colitis:

- Confluent proctocolitis (e.g., *Shigella, Campylobacter, Salmonella, Entamoeba histolytica*).
- Segmental colitis (e.g., *Campylobacter, Salmonella,* enteroinvasive *E. coli, Aeromonas, E. histolytica*).

Drug-induced colitis (e.g., nonsteroidal anti-inflammatory drugs [NSAIDs]).
Inflammatory bowel disease.
Ischemic colitis (usually elderly patient with underlying heart disease or arrhythmias).
Antibiotic-associated colitis.

DIARRHEA, INFECTIOUS[2]

ICD-9CM #	009.2	
ICD-10CM #	A09	Infectious gastroenteritis and colitis, unspecified

ETIOLOGIC AGENTS OF INFECTIOUS DIARRHEA

Viral (60% of Cases)

Astrovirus.
Calicivirus.
Coronavirus.
Cytomegalovirus.*
Enteric adenovirus.
Hepatitis A through G.
Herpes simplex virus.
HIV enteropathy.
Norwalk-like agents.
Pararotavirus.
Norwalk virus.
Picomavirus.
Rotavirus.
Small round viruses.

Bacterial (20% of Cases)

Invasive*

Aeromonas spp.
Campylobacter spp.
Clostridium difficile.
Enteroinvasive *E. coli.*
Mycobacterium spp.
Plesiomonas shigelloides.
Salmonella spp.
Shigella spp.
Vibrio fluvialis.
Vibrio parahaemolyticus.
Vibrio vulnificus.
Yersinia enterocolitica.
Yersinia pseudotuberculosis.

Toxigenic

Food poisoning with preformed toxins.
Bacillus cereus.
Clostridium botulinum.
Staphylococcus aureus.
Toxin formation after colonization.
Aeromonas hydrophila.
Clostridium perfringens.
Enterohemorrhagic *E. coli* 0157:H7.*
Enterotoxigenic *E. coli.*
Klebsiella pneumoniae.
Shigella spp.
Vibrio cholerae.

Other bacteria

Parasitic (5% of Cases)

Protozoa

*Balantidium coli.**
Blastocystis hominis.
Cryptosporidium.
Cyclospora.
Dientamoeba fragilis.
*Entamoeba histolytica.**
Entamoeba polecki.
Enteromonas hominis.

Giardia lamblia.
Isospora belli.
Microsporidia.
Sarcocystis hominis.
Helminths
Angiostrongylus costaricense.
Anisakiasis.
Ascaris lumbricoides.
Diphyllobothrium latum.
Enterobius vermicularis.
Hookworms.
Schistosoma spp.
Strongyloides stercoralis.
Taenia spp.
Trichinella spiralis.
Trichuris trichiura.

*Associated with fever, abdominal pain, and fecal red blood cells or white blood cells. % indicates the estimated contribution to total cases.

DIARRHEA, NONINFECTIOUS[2]

ICD-9CM # 564.5
ICD-10CM # K59.1 Functional diarrhea

CAUSES OF NONINFECTIOUS DIARRHEA

Toxins

Drugs
ACE inhibitors.
Alprazolam.
Antacids (Mg).
Antibiotics.
Antidepressants.
Antiepileptic drugs.
Antihypertensives.
Antiparkinson drugs.
Beta-blockers.
Caffeine.
Cardiac antiarrhythmics.
Chemotherapy agents.
Cholesterol-lowering drugs.
Cholinergic agents.
Cholinesterase inhibitors.
Colchicine.
Digitalis.
Diuretics.
Flurouracil.
Fluoxetine.
Histamine H_2-receptor antagonists.
Hydralazine.
Lactulose.
Laxatives/cathartics.
Levodopa.
Lithium.
NSAIDs.
Neomycin.
Podophyllin.
Procainamide.
Prostaglandins.
Quinidine.
Ricinoleic acid.
Theophylline.
Thyroid hormone.
Valproic acid.

Dietetic foods
Mannitol.
Sorbitol.
Xylitol.

Fish-associated toxins
Amnestic shellfish poisoning.
Ciguatera.
Echinoderms.
Neurotoxic shellfish poisoning.
Paralytic shellfish poisoning.
Scombroid.
Tetroton.

Plant-associated toxins
Herbal preparations.
Horse chestnut.
Mushrooms—*Amanita* spp.
Nicotine.
Other plant toxins:
- Pesticides—organophosphates.
- Pokeweed.
- Rhubarb.

Miscellaneous:
- Allergic reactions.
- Carbon monoxide poisoning.
- Ethanol.
- Heavy metals.
- Monosodium glutamate (MSG).
- Opiate withdrawal.

Gastrointestinal Pathology
Appendicitis.
Autonomic dysfunction.
Bile acid malabsorption.
Blind loop.
Bowel obstruction.
Celiac disease.
Cirrhosis.
Defects in amino acid transport.
Diverticular disease.
Familial dysautonomia.
Fecal impaction.
Fecal incontinence.
GI bleed.
GI cancer.
Hirschsprung's disease.
Inflammatory bowel disease (ulcerative colitis, Crohn's disease).
Intussusception.
Irritable bowel syndrome.
Ischemic bowel.
Lactose/fructose intolerance.
Malabsorption syndromes.
Malrotation.
Postsurgical.
Postvagotomy.
Radiation therapy.
Short gut syndrome.
Small bowel resection.
Strictures.
Toxic megacolon.
Tropical sprue.
Volvulus.
Whipple's disease.

Endocrine-related
Carcinoid syndrome (serotonin).
Hormonal hypersecretion.
Hyperthyroidism (thyroid hormone).
Medullary carcinoma of the thyroid (calcitonin).
Pancreatic cholera (VIP).
Somatostatinoma (somatostatin).
Systemic mastocytosis (histamine).
Zollinger-Ellison syndrome (gastrin).

Endocrine pathology
Adrenal insufficiency.
Diabetes enteropathy.
Hypoparathyroidism.
Pancreatic insufficiency.

Systemic Illness/Other
Alcoholism.
Amyloidosis.
Connective tissue disease.
Cystic fibrosis.
Ectopic pregnancy.
Hemolytic-uremic syndrome.
Henoch-Schönlein purpura.
Lymphoma.
Otitis media—infants.
Pelvic inflammatory disease.
Pneumonia/sepsis.
Pyelonephritis.
Scleroderma/SLE.
Severe malnutrition.
Stevens-Johnson syndrome.
Toxic shock syndrome.
Wilson's disease.
Miscellaneous:
- Factitious diarrhea.
- Runner's diarrhea.

ACE, Angiotensin-converting enzyme; *GI,* gastrointestinal; *NSAIDs,* nonsteroidal anti-inflammatory drugs; *SLE,* systemic lupus erythematosus; *VIP,* vasoactive intestinal polypeptide.

DIARRHEA, TUBE-FED PATIENT[14]

ICD-9CM # 564.4
ICD-10CM # K91.89 Other postprocedural complications and disorders of digestive system

COMMON CAUSES UNRELATED TO TUBE FEEDING

Elixir medications containing sorbitol.
Magnesium-containing antacids.
Antibiotic-induced sterile gut.
Pseudomembranous colitis.

POSSIBLE CAUSES RELATED TO TUBE FEEDING

Inadequate fiber to form stool bulk.
High fat content of formula (in the presence of fat malabsorption syndrome).
Bacterial contamination of enteral products and delivery systems (causal association with diarrhea not documented).
Rapid advancement in rate (after the GI tract is unused for prolonged periods).

UNLIKELY CAUSES RELATED TO TUBE FEEDING

Formula hyperosmolality (proven not to be the cause of diarrhea).
Lactose (absent from nearly all enteral feeding formulas).

DIPLOPIA, BINOCULAR

ICD-9CM # 368.2
ICD-10CM # H53.2 Diplopia

Cranial nerve palsy (3rd, 4th, 6th).
Thyroid eye disease.
Myasthenia gravis.
Decompensated strabismus.
Orbital trauma with blowout fracture.
Orbital pseudotumor.
Cavernous sinus thrombosis.

DIPLOPIA, MONOCULAR

ICD-9CM # 368.2
ICD-10CM # H53.2 Diplopia

Postoperative corrected longstanding tropia.
Defective contact lenses.
Poorly fitting bifocals.
Trauma to iris.
Corneal disorder (e.g., dry eye, astigmatism).
Cataracts.
Lens subluxation.
Nystagmus.
Eyelid twitching.
Foreign body in aqueous or vitreous media.
Migraine.
Lesions of occipital cortex.
Psychogenic.

DIPLOPIA, VERTICAL

ICD-9CM # 368.2
ICD-10CM # H53.2 Diplopia

Myasthenia.
Superior oblique palsy.
Myositis or pseudotumor with orbital involvement.
Lymphoma or metastases affecting the orbits.
Brain stem or cerebellar lesions.
Hydrocephalus.
Third nerve palsy.
Botulism.
Wernicke's encephalopathy.
Dysthyroid orbitopathy (muscle infiltration).

DIZZINESS

ICD-9CM # 780.4
ICD-10CM # R42 Dizziness and giddiness

Viral syndrome.
Anxiety, hyperventilation.
Benign positional paroxysmal vertigo.
Medications (e.g., sedatives, antihypertensives, analgesics).
Withdrawal from medications (e.g., benzodiazepines, SSRIs).
Alcohol or drug abuse.
Postural hypotension.
Hypoglycemia, hyperglycemia.
Hematologic disorders (e.g., anemia, polycythemia, leukemia).
Head trauma.
Menière's disease.
Vertebrobasilar ischemia.
Cervical osteoarthritis.
Cardiac abnormalities (arrhythmias, cardiomyopathy, CHF, pericarditis).
Multiple sclerosis.
Peripheral vestibulopathy.
Air or sea travel.
Electrolyte abnormalities.
Eye problems (cornea, lens, retina).
Migraine.
Brain stem infarct.
Autonomic neuropathy.
Chronic otomastoiditis.
Complex partial seizures.
Ramsey Hunt syndrome.
Arteritis.
Syncope and presyncope.
Perilymph fistula.
Cerebellopontine tumor.
Hepatic or renal disease.

DRY EYE

ICD-9CM # 375.15
ICD-10CM # H04.129 Dry eye syndrome of unspecified lacrimal gland

Contacts.
Medications (antihistamines, clonidine, beta-blockers, ibuprofen, scopolamine).
Keratoconjunctivitis sicca.
Trauma.
Environmental causes (air conditioning in patient with contacts).

DYSLIPOPROTEINEMIAS, SECONDARY CAUSES[4a]

ICD-9CM # 272.4
ICD-10CM # E78.4 Other hyperlipidemia

CAUSE	*DISORDER*
Metabolic	Diabetes Lipodystrophy Glycogen storage disorders
Renal	Chronic renal failure Glomerulonephritis with nephritic syndrome
Hepatic	Cirrhosis Biliary obstruction Porphyria
Hormonal	Estrogens Progesterones Growth hormone Thyroid disorders (hypothyroidism) Corticosteroids
Lifestyle	Physical inactivity Obesity Diet rich in fats, saturated fats Alcohol intake Smoking
Medications	Retinoic acid derivatives Glucocorticoids Exogenous estrogens Thiazide diuretics Beta-adrenergic blockers (non-selective) Testosterone and other anabolic steroids Immunosuppressive medications (cyclosporine) Antiviral medications (human immunodeficiency virus protease inhibitors) Antischizophrenic agents

DYSPAREUNIA[12]

ICD-9CM # 625.0 Dyspareunia
608.89 Dyspareunia, Male
302.76 Dyspareunia, Psychogenic
ICD-10CM # N94.1 Dyspareunia
N44.8 Other noninflammatory disorders of the testis
N50.8 Other specified disorders of male genital organs
N53.12 Painful ejaculation
F52.6 Dyspareunia not due to a substance or known physiological condition

INTROITAL

Vaginismus.
Intact or rigid hymen.
Clitoral problems.
Vulvovaginitis.
Vaginal atrophy: hypoestrogen.
Vulvar dystrophy.
Bartholin or Skene gland infection.
Inadequate lubrication.
Operative scarring.

MIDVAGINAL

Urethritis.
Trigonitis.
Cystitis.
Short vagina.
Operative scarring.
Inadequate lubrication.

DEEP

Endometriosis.
Pelvic infection.
Uterine retroversion.
Ovarian pathology.
GI.
Orthopedic.
Abnormal penile size or shape.

DYSPHAGIA

ICD-9CM # 787.2
ICD-10CM # R13.10 Dysphagia, unspecified

Esophageal obstruction: neoplasm, foreign body, achalasia, stricture, spasm, esophageal web, diverticulum, Schatzki's ring.
Peptic esophagitis with stricture, Barrett's stricture.
External esophageal compression: neoplasms (thyroid neoplasm, lymphoma, mediastinal tumors), thyroid enlargement, aortic aneurysm, vertebral spurs, aberrant right subclavian artery (dysphagia lusoria).
Hiatal hernia, GERD.
Oropharyngeal lesions: pharyngitis, glossitis, stomatitis, neoplasms.
Hysteria: globus hystericus.
Neurologic and/or neuromuscular disturbances: bulbar paralysis, myasthenia gravis, ALS, multiple sclerosis, Parkinsonism, CVA, diabetic neuropathy.

Toxins: poisoning, botulism, tetanus, postdiphtheritic dysphagia.
Systemic diseases: scleroderma, amyloidosis, dermatomyositis.
Candida and herpes esophagitis.
Presbyesophagus.

DYSPHAGIA, OROPHARYNGEAL[38]

ICD-9CM # 787.22
ICD-10CM # R13.12 Dysphagia, oropharyngeal phase

FUNCTIONAL DISORDERS

Central Nervous System
Stroke.
Head injury.
Parkinson's disease.
Motor neuron disease.
Multiple sclerosis.
Tumor.
Drugs (e.g., phenothiazines).
Malformations (e.g., syrinx, Arnold–Chiari).
Neural
Motor neuron disease.
Myasthenia gravis.
Radiotherapy.
Poliomyelitis.
Familial dysautonomia.
Muscle
Autoimmune myopathy (polymyositis, dermatomyositis, systemic lupus erythematosus).
Thyrotoxic myopathy.
Guillain-Barré motor neuropathy.
Muscular dystrophies.

STRUCTURAL DISORDERS

Head/neck surgery.
Stricture.
Radiotherapy.
Tumor.
Pharyngeal pouch.
Web.
Extrinsic (e.g., osteophytes).

MISCELLANEOUS

Xerostomia.

DYSPNEA

ICD-9CM # 786.00
ICD-10CM # R06.9 Unspecified abnormalities of breathing

Upper airway obstruction: trauma, neoplasm, epiglottitis, laryngeal edema, tongue retraction, laryngospasm, abductor paralysis of vocal cords, aspiration of foreign body.
Lower airway obstruction: neoplasm, COPD, asthma, aspiration of foreign body.
Pulmonary infection: pneumonia, abscess, empyema, TB, bronchiectasis.
Pulmonary hypertension.
Pulmonary embolism/infarction.
Parenchymal lung disease.
Pulmonary vascular congestion.
Cardiac disease: ASHD, valvular lesions, cardiac dysrhythmias, cardiomyopathy, pericardial effusion, cardiac shunts.
Space-occupying lesions: neoplasm, large hiatal hernia, pleural effusions.
Disease of chest wall: severe kyphoscoliosis, fractured ribs, sternal compression, morbid obesity.
Neurologic dysfunction: Guillain-Barré syndrome, botulism, polio, spinal cord injury.
Interstitial pulmonary disease: sarcoidosis, collagen vascular diseases, DIP, Hamman-Rich pneumonitis, etc.
Pneumoconioses: silicosis, berylliosis, etc.
Mesothelioma.
Pneumothorax, hemothorax, pleural effusion.
Inhalation of toxins.
Cholinergic drug intoxication.
Carcinoid syndrome.
Hematologic: anemia, polycythemia, hemoglobinopathies.
Thyrotoxicosis, myxedema.
Diaphragmatic compression caused by abdominal distention, subphrenic abscess, ascites.
Lung resection.
Metabolic abnormalities: uremia, hepatic coma, DKA.
Sepsis.
Atelectasis.
Psychoneurosis.
Diaphragmatic paralysis.
Pregnancy.

DYSURIA

ICD-9CM # 788.1 Dysuria
306.53 Dysuria, Psychogenic
ICD-10CM # R30.0 Dysuria
R30.9 Painful micturition, unspecified

Urinary tract infection.
Estrogen deficiency (in postmenopausal female).
Vaginitis.
Genital infection (e.g., herpes, condyloma).
Interstitial cystitis.
Chemical irritation (e.g., deodorant aerosols, douches).
Meatal stenosis or stricture.
Reiter's syndrome.
Bladder neoplasm.
GI etiology (diverticulitis, Crohn's disease).
Impaired bladder or sphincter action.
Urethral carbuncle.
Chronic fibrosis posttrauma.
Radiation therapy.
Prostatitis.
Urethritis (gonococcal, *Chlamydia*).
Behçet's syndrome.
Stevens-Johnson syndrome.

EARACHE[33]

ICD-9CM # 388.70 Earache
388.72 Ear Pain, Referred
ICD-10CM # H92.09 Otalgia, unspecified ear

Otitis media.
Serous otitis media.
Eustachitis.
Otitis externa.
Otitic barotrauma.
Mastoiditis.
Foreign body.
Impacted cerumen.
Referred otalgia, as with TMJ dysfunction, dental problems, and tumors.

ECTOPIC ACTH SECRETION[14]

ICD-9CM # 255.0
ICD-10CM # E34.2 Ectopic hormone secretion, not elsewhere classified

Small cell carcinoma of lung.
Endocrine tumors of foregut origin.
- Thymic carcinoid.
- Islet cell tumor.
- Medullary carcinoid, thyroid.
- Bronchial carcinoid.

Pheochromocytoma.
Ovarian tumors.

EDEMA, CHILDREN[19]

ICD-9CM # 782.3 Edema NOS
ICD-10CM # R60.0 Localized edema
R60.1 Generalized edema
R60.9 Edema, unspecified

CARDIOVASCULAR

Congestive heart failure.
Acute thrombi or emboli.
Vasculitis of many types.

RENAL

Nephrotic syndrome.
Glomerulonephritis of many types.
End-stage renal failure.

ENDOCRINE OR METABOLIC

Thyroid disease.
Starvation.
Hereditary angioedema.

IATROGENIC

Drugs (diuretics and steroids).
Water or salt overload.

HEMATOLOGIC

Hemolytic disease of the newborn.

GASTROINTESTINAL

Hepatic cirrhosis.
Protein-losing enteritis.
Lymphangiectasis.
Cystic fibrosis.

Celiac disease.
Enteritis of many types.

LYMPHATIC ABNORMALITIES

Congenital (gonadal dysgenesis).
Acquired.

EDEMA, GENERALIZED

ICD-9CM # 782.3 Edema NOS
ICD-10CM # R60.0 Localized edema
R60.1 Generalized edema
R60.9 Edema, unspecified

Congestive heart failure (CHF).
Cirrhosis.
Nephrotic syndrome.
Pregnancy.
Idiopathic.
Acute nephritic syndrome.
Myxedema.
Medications (NSAIDs, estrogens, vasodilators).

EDEMA, LEG, UNILATERAL[26]

ICD-9CM # 782.3
ICD-10CM # R60.0 Localized edema
R60.9 Edema, unspecified

WITH PAIN

DVT.
Postphlebitic syndrome.
Popliteal cyst rupture.
Gastrocnemius rupture.
Cellulitis.
Psoas or other abscess.

WITHOUT PAIN

DVT.
Postphlebitic syndrome.
Other venous insufficiency (after saphenous vein harvest, varicosities).
Lymphatic obstruction/lymphedema (carcinoma, lymphoma, sarcoidosis, filariasis, retroperitoneal fibrosis).

EDEMA OF LOWER EXTREMITIES

ICD-9CM # 782.3
ICD-10CM # R60.0 Localized edema
R60.9 Edema, unspecified

CHF (right-sided).
Hepatic cirrhosis.
Nephrosis.
Myxedema.
Lymphedema.
Pregnancy.
Abdominal mass: neoplasm, cyst.
Venous compression from abdominal aneurysm.
Varicose veins.
Bilateral cellulitis.
Bilateral thrombophlebitis.
Vena cava thrombosis, venous thrombosis.
Retroperitoneal fibrosis.

EJECTION SOUND OR CLICK

ICD-9CM # 785.3
ICD-10CM # R01.2 Other cardiac sounds

Aortic regurgitation.
Aortic root dilatation.
Systemic hypertension.
Chronic pulmonary hypertension.
Tetralogy of Fallot.
Atrial septal defect.
Pulmonary valve stenosis.
Aortic aneurysm.

ELBOW PAIN

ICD-9CM # 719.42
ICD-10CM # M25.529 Pain in unspecified elbow

Trauma.
Infection.
Inflammatory arthritis.
Lateral or medial epicondylitis.
Entrapment neuropathy.
Olecranon bursitis.
Osteoarthritis.
Gout.
Cervical disease (referred pain).
Shoulder disease (referred pain).
Partial subluxation.
Synovial osteochondromatosis.
Loose body.

ELEVATED HEMIDIAPHRAGM

ICD-9CM # 519.4 Diaphragm Disorder
519.4 Diaphragm Paralysis
756.6 Diaphragm Eventration, Congenital
ICD-10CM # J98.6 Disorders of diaphragm
Q79.0 Congenital diaphragmatic hernia
Q79.1 Other congenital malformations of diaphragm

Neoplasm (bronchogenic carcinoma, mediastinal neoplasm, intrahepatic lesion).
Substernal thyroid.
Infectious process (pneumonia, empyema, TB, subphrenic abscess, hepatic abscess).
Atelectasis.
Idiopathic.
Eventration.
Phrenic nerve dysfunction (myelitis, myotonia, herpes zoster).
Trauma to phrenic nerve or diaphragm (e.g., surgery).
Aortic aneurysm.
Intraabdominal mass.
Pulmonary infarction.
Pleurisy.
Radiation therapy.
Rib fracture.

EMBOLI, ARTERIAL[26]

ICD-9CM # 444.22 Embolism, Artery, Lower Extremity
444.21 Embolism, Artery, Upper Extremity
ICD-10CM # I74.3 Embolism and thrombosis of arteries of the lower extremities
I74.2 Embolism and thrombosis of arteries of the upper extremities

Myocardial infarction with mural thrombi.
Atrial fibrillation.
Cardiomyopathies.
Prosthetic heart valves.
CHF.
Endocarditis.
Left ventricular aneurysm.
Left atrial myxoma.
Sick sinus syndrome.
Paradoxical embolus from venous thrombosis.
Aneurysms of large blood vessels.
Atheromatous ulcers of large blood vessels.

EMESIS, PEDIATRIC AGE[19]

ICD-9CM # 787.03
ICD-10CM # R11.10 Vomiting, unspecified
R11.11 Vomiting without nausea
R11.12 Projectile vomiting

INFANCY

Gastrointestinal Tract

Congenital:

Regurgitation—chalasia, gastroesophageal reflux.
Atresia—stenosis (tracheoesophageal fistula, prepyloric diaphragm, intestinal atresia).
Duplication.
Volvulus (errors in rotation and fixation, Meckel diverticulum).
Congenital bands.
Hirschsprung's disease.
Meconium ileus (cystic fibrosis), meconium plug.

Acquired:

Acute infectious gastroenteritis, food poisoning (staphylococcal, clostridial).
Pyloric stenosis.
Gastritis, duodenitis.
Intussusception.
Incarcerated hernia—inguinal, internal secondary to old adhesions.
Cow's milk protein intolerance, food allergy, eosinophilic gastroenteritis.
Disaccharidase deficiency.
Celiac disease—presents after introduction of gluten in diet; inherited risk.
Adynamic ileus—the mediator for many nongastrointestinal causes.
Neonatal necrotizing enterocolitis.
Chronic granulomatous disease with gastric outlet obstruction.

Nongastrointestinal Tract

Infectious—otitis, urinary tract infection, pneumonia, upper respiratory tract infection, sepsis, meningitis.

Metabolic—aminoaciduria and organic aciduria, galactosemia, fructosemia, adrenogenital syndrome, renal tubular acidosis, diabetic ketoacidosis, Reye's syndrome.

Central nervous system—trauma, tumor, infection, diencephalic syndrome, rumination, autonomic responses (pain, shock).

Medications—anticholinergics, aspirin, alcohol, idiosyncratic reaction (e.g., codeine).

CHILDHOOD

Gastrointestinal Tract

Peptic ulcer—vomiting is a common presentation in children younger than 6 yr old.

Trauma—duodenal hematoma, traumatic pancreatitis, perforated bowel.

Pancreatitis—mumps, trauma, cystic fibrosis, hyperparathyroidism, hyperlipidemia, organic acidemias.

Crohn's disease.

Idiopathic intestinal pseudoobstruction.

Superior mesenteric artery syndrome.

Nongastrointestinal Tract

Central nervous system—cyclic vomiting, migraine, anorexia nervosa, bulimia.

ENCEPHALOMYELITIS, NONVIRAL CAUSES[25a]

ICD-9CM # varies with specific disorder
ICD-10CM # G04.81 Other encephalitis and encephalomyelitis

Subacute bacterial endocarditis.
Rocky Mountain spotted fever.
Typhus.
Ehrlichia.
Q fever.
Chlamydia.
Mycoplasma.
Legionella.
Brucellosis.
Listeria.
Whipple's disease.
Cat-scratch disease.
Syphilis (meningovascular).
Relapsing fever.
Lyme disease.
Leptospirosis.
Nocardia.
Actinomycosis.
Tuberculosis.
Cryptococcus.
Histoplasma.
Toxoplasma.
Plasmodium falciparum.
Trypanosomiasis.
Behçet's disease.
Vasculitis.
Carcinoma.
Drug reactions.

ENCEPHALOPATHY, HYPERTENSIVE[38b]

ICD-9CM # 293.9

Cerebral infarction.
Subarachnoid hemorrhage.
Intracerebral hemorrhage.
Subdural or epidural hematoma.
Brain tumor or other mass lesion.
Seizure disorder.
Central nervous system vasculitis.
Encephalitis/meningitis.
Drug ingestion.
Drug withdrawal.

ENCEPHALOPATHY, METABOLIC[36]

ICD-9CM #	291.2	Alcoholic Encephalopathy
	572.2	Hepatic Encephalopathy
	251.2	Hypoglycemic Encephalopathy
	349.82	Toxic Encephalopathy
	984.9	Lead Encephalopathy
	293.9	Encephalopathy
ICD-10CM #	F10.27	Alcohol dependence with alcohol-induced persisting dementia
	K72.90	Hepatic failure, unspecified without coma
	K72.91	Hepatic failure, unspecified with coma
	G92	Toxic encephalopathy
	T56.0X1A	Toxic effect of lead and its compounds, accidental (unintentional), initial encounter
	T56.0X2A	Toxic effect of lead and its compounds, intentional self-harm, initial encounter

Substrate deficiency: hypoxia/ischemia, carbon monoxide poisoning, hypoglycemia.

Cofactor deficiency: thiamine, vitamin B_{12}, pyridoxine (INH administration).

Electrolyte disorders: hyponatremia, hypercalcemia, carbon dioxide narcosis, dialysis, hypermagnesemia, disequilibrium syndrome.

Endocrinopathies: DKA, hyperosmolar coma, hypothyroidism, hyperadrenocorticism, hyperparathyroidism.

Endogenous toxins: liver disease, uremia, porphyria.

Exogenous toxins: drug overdose (sedative/hypnotics, ethanol, narcotics, salicylates, tricyclic antidepressants), drug withdrawal, toxicity of therapeutic medications, industrial toxins (e.g., organophosphates, heavy metals), sepsis.

Heat stroke.

Epilepsy (postictal).

ENTHESOPATHY

ICD-9CM # code not available
ICD-10CM # M46.00 Spinal enthesopathy, site unspecified

Viremia or bacteremia.
Ankylosing spondylitis.
Psoriatic arthritis.
Drug-induced (quinolones, etretinate).
Reactive arthritis.
DISH.
Reiter's syndrome.

EOSINOPHILIC LUNG DISEASE[16a]

ICD-9CM # 495.8
ICD-10CM # J67.8 Hypersensitivity pneumonitis due to other organic dusts

IDIOPATHIC

Simple pulmonary eosinophilia (Löffler's syndrome).
Acute eosinophilic pneumonia.
Chronic eosinophilic pneumonia.
Hypereosinophilic syndrome.

DRUG-INDUCED

Aminosalicylic acid.
Para-arminosalicylic acid.
NSAIDs.
Captopril.
Cocaine.
Minocycline.
Nitrofurantoin.
Phenytoin.

INFECTION

Parasitic (ascariasis, paragonimiasis. tropical eosinophilia).
Fungal (aspergillus).
Bacterial (TB, atypical mycobacterial infection, brucella).
Viral (respiratory syncytial virus).

IMMUNOLOGIC DISEASES

Wegener's granulomatosis.
Churg–Strauss syndrome.
Rheumatoid disease.
Sarcoidosis.

NEOPLASMS

Bronchogenic carcinoma.
Bronchial carcinoid.
Lymphoma (Hodgkin's, non-Hodgkin's).

EPIGASTRIC PAIN[38]

ICD-9CM # 789.66
ICD-10CM # R10.816 Epigastric abdominal tenderness
R10.826 Epigastric rebound abdominal tenderness

Peptic ulceration (uncomplicated).*
Peptic ulceration (perforated).*
Biliary colic.*
Acute pancreatitis.*
Abdominal aortic aneurysm.
Anxiety.
Inferior wall MI.

*Conditions that also cause right upper quadrant pain.

EPILEPSY

ICD-9CM # 345.9 Epilepsy NOS
ICD-10CM # G40.909 Epilepsy, unspecified, not intractable, without status epilepticus

Psychogenic spells.
Transient ischemic attack.
Hypoglycemia.
Syncope.
Narcolepsy.
Migraine.
Paroxysmal vertigo.
Arrhythmias.
Drug reaction.

EPISTAXIS

ICD-9CM # 784.7
ICD-10CM # R04.0 Epistaxis

Trauma.
Medications (nasal sprays, NSAIDs, anticoagulants, antiplatelets).
Nasal polyps.
Cocaine use.
Coagulopathy (hemophilia, liver disease, DIC, thrombocytopenia).
Systemic disorders (hypertension, uremia).
Infections.
Anatomic malformations.
Rhinitis.
Nasal polyps.
Local neoplasms (benign and malignant).
Desiccation.
Foreign body.

ERECTILE DYSFUNCTION, ORGANIC[31]

ICD-9CM # 607.84
ICD-10CM # N52.9 Male erectile dysfunction, unspecified

Neurogenic abnormalities: Somatic nerve neuropathy, central nervous system abnormalities.
Psychogenic causes: Depression, performance anxiety, marital conflict.
Endocrine causes: Hyperprolactinemia, hypogonadotropic hypogonadism, testicular failure, estrogen excess.
Trauma: Pelvic fracture, prostate surgery, penile fracture.
Systemic disease: DM, renal failure, hepatic cirrhosis.
Medications: Diuretics, antidepressants, H_2 blockers, exogenous hormones, alcohol, antihypertensives, nicotine abuse, finasteride, etc.
Structural abnormalities: Peyronie's disease.

EROSIONS, GENITALIA

ICD-9CM # 599.84
ICD-10CM # N36.8 Other specified disorders of urethra

Candidiasis.
Intraepithelial neoplasia.
Squamous cell carcinoma.
Lichen planus.
Pemphigus vulgaris.
Erythema multiforme.
Lichen sclerosus.
Bullous pemphigoid.
Extramammary Paget's disease.
Impetigo.

ERYTHEMATOUS ANNULAR SKIN LESIONS

ICD-9CM # varies with diagnosis
ICD-10CM # L53.8 Other specified erythematous conditions

Tinea corporis.
Warfarin plaques.
Erythema multiforme.
Erythema annulare.
Cutaneous lupus.
Cutaneous sarcoidosis.
Trauma.
Acute febrile neutrophilic dermatosis (Sweet's syndrome).

ERYTHROCYTOSIS[20]

ICD-9CM # 289.6
ICD-10CM # D75.0 Familial erythrocytosis

CAUSES OF ERYTHROCYTOSIS

Relative or Spurious Erythrocytosis (Normal Red Cell Mass)

Hemoconcentration secondary to dehydration (diarrhea, diaphoresis, diuretics, water deprivation, emesis, ethanol, hypertension, preeclampsia, pheochromocytoma, carbon monoxide intoxication).

True or Absolute Erythrocytosis

Polycythemia vera.
Primary congenital polycythemia.
Secondary erythrocytosis caused by:
Congenital causes (e.g., activating mutation of erythropoietin receptor).
Hypoxia caused by carbon monoxide poisoning, high oxygen affinity hemoglobin, high-altitude residence, chronic pulmonary disease, hypoventilation syndromes such as sleep apnea, right to left cardiac shunt, neurologic defects involving the respiratory center.
Nonhypoxic causes with pathologic erythropoietin production.
- Renal disease (cysts, hydronephrosis, renal artery stenosis, focal glomerulonephritis, renal transplantation).
- Tumors (renal cell cancer, hepatocellular carcinoma, cerebellar hemangioblastoma, uterine fibromyoma, adrenal tumors, meningioma, pheochromocytoma).

Drug-associated causes:
- Androgen therapy.
- Exogenous erythropoietin growth factor therapy.

ERYTHRODERMA

ICD-9CM # 695.9 Secondary
696.2 Maculopapular
696.1 Psoriaticum
695.89 Exfoliative
778.8 Neonatorum
ICD-10CM # L53.9 Erythematous condition, unspecified

Drug reaction (e.g., allopurinol, ampicillin, phenytoin, vancomycin, dapsone, omeprazole, carbamazepine).
Atopic dermatitis.
Psoriasis.
Contact dermatitis.
Idiopathic.
Pityriasis rubra.
Chronic actinic dermatitis.
Bullous pemphigoid.
Paraneoplastic.
Cutaneous T-cell lymphoma.
Connective tissue disease.
Hypereosinophilia syndrome.

ESOPHAGEAL PERFORATION[26]

ICD-9CM # 530.4 Perforation, Nontraumatic
862.22 Injury, Traumatic
ICD-10CM # K22.3 Perforation of esophagus
S27.819A Unspecified injury of esophagus (thoracic part), initial encounter

Trauma.
Caustic burns.
Iatrogenic.
Foreign bodies.
Spontaneous rupture (Boerhaave's syndrome).
Postoperative breakdown of anastomosis.

ESOPHAGITIS[25a]

ICD-9CM # 530.12
ICD-10CM # K20.9 Esophagitis, unspecified

INFECTIOUS

Candidiasis.
Cytomegalovirus.
Herpes simplex virus.
HIV infection, acute.

NONINFECTIOUS

Gastroesophageal reflux.
Mucositis from cancer chemotherapy.
Mucositis from radiation therapy.
Aphthous ulcers.

ESOTROPIA

ICD-9CM # 378.00 Nonaccommodative
378.35 Accommodative
378.05 Alternating
ICD-10CM # H50.00 Unspecified esotropia
H50.43 Accommodative component in esotropia
H50.05 Alternating esotropia

Congenital.
Accommodative esotropia.
Myasthenia gravis.
Abducens palsy.
Pseudo-sixth nerve palsy.
Medial rectus entrapment (e.g., blowout fracture).
Posterior internuclear ophthalmoplegia.
Wernicke's encephalopathy.
Thyroid myopathy.
Chiari malformation.

EXANTHEMS[28]

ICD-9CM # 782.1
ICD-10CM # R21 Rash and other nonspecific skin eruption

Measles.
Rubella.
Erythema infectiosum (fifth disease).
Roseola exanthema.
Varicella.
Enterovirus.
Adenovirus.
Epstein-Barr virus.
Kawasaki disease.
Staphylococcal scalded skin.
Scarlet fever.
Meningococcemia.
Rocky Mountain spotted fever.

EYELID NEOPLASM

ICD-9CM # varies with specific disorder
ICD-10CM # C44.101 Unspecified malignant neoplasm of skin of unspecified eyelid, including canthus

MALIGNANT

Melanoma.
Basal cell carcinoma.
Squamous cell carcinoma.
Bowen's disease.
Sebaceous cell carcinoma.
Metastatic lymphoma/leukemia.

BENIGN

Melanocytic nevus.
Pilar, eccrine, or apocrine tumor.
Neurofibroma.
Keratosis.
Squamous papilloma.
Keratoacanthoma.

EYELID RETRACTION

ICD-9CM # 374.89
ICD-10CM # H02.89 Other specified disorders of eyelid

Congenital.
Graves' ophthalmopathy.
Myasthenia gravis.
Postsurgical.
Guillain-Barré syndrome.
Cerebellar disease.
Horizontal gaze palsy.
Partial palsy of superior rectus muscle.
Encephalitis.
Closed head injury.
Disseminated sclerosis.
Eye trauma.
Contact lens wear.
Proptosis.
Eyelid neoplasm.
Atopic dermatitis.
Herpes zoster ophthalmicus.
Botulinum toxin injection.
Cyclic oculomotor paralysis.
Spheroid wing meningioma.
Hepatic cirrhosis.
Down syndrome.
Essential hypertension.
Meningitis.
Paget's disease of bone.

EYE PAIN

ICD-9CM # 379.91
ICD-10CM # H57.13 Ocular pain, bilateral

Foreign body.
Herpes zoster.
Trauma.
Conjunctivitis.
Iritis.
Iridocyclitis.
Uveitis.
Blepharitis.
Ingrown lashes.
Orbital or periorbital cellulitis/abscess.
Sinusitis.
Headache.
Glaucoma.
Inflammation of lacrimal gland.
Tic douloureux.
Cerebral aneurysm.
Cerebral neoplasm.
Entropion.
Retrobulbar neuritis.
UV light.
Dry eyes.
Irritation or inflammation from eye drops, dust, cosmetics, etc.

FACIAL PAIN

ICD-9CM # 784.0
ICD-10CM # G50.1 Atypical facial pain

Infection, abscess.
Postherpetic neuralgia.
Trauma, posttraumatic neuralgia.
Tic douloureux.
Cluster headache, "lower-half headache."
Geniculate neuralgia.
Anxiety, somatization syndrome.
Glossopharyngeal neuralgia.
Carotidynia.

FACIAL PARALYSIS[28]

ICD-9CM # 351.0 Facial (7th Nerve) Palsy
ICD-10CM # G51.0 Bell's palsy

INFECTION

Bacterial: otitis media, mastoiditis, meningitis, Lyme disease.
Viral: herpes zoster, mononucleosis, varicella, rubella, mumps, Bell's palsy.
Mycobacterial: TB, meningitis, leprosy.
Miscellaneous: syphilis, malaria.

TRAUMA

Temporal bone fracture, facial laceration.
Surgery.

NEOPLASM

Malignant: squamous cell carcinoma, basal cell and adenocystic tumors, leukemia, parotid neoplasms, metastatic tumors.
Benign: facial nerve neuroma, vestibular schwannoma, congenital cholesteatoma.

IMMUNOLOGIC

Guillain-Barré syndrome, periarteritis nodosa.
Reaction to tetanus antiserum.

METABOLIC

Pregnancy.
Hypothyroidism.
DM.

FAILURE TO THRIVE

ICD-9CM #	783.4	
ICD-10CM #	R62.50	Unspecified lack of expected normal physiological development in childhood

PSYCHOSOCIAL/BEHAVIORAL

Inadequate diet because of poverty/food insufficiency, errors in food preparation.
Poor parenting skills (lack of knowledge of sufficient diet).
Child/parent interaction problems (autonomy struggles, coercive feeding, maternal depression).
Food refusal.
Rumination.
Parental cognitive or mental health problems.
Child abuse or neglect; emotional deprivation.

NEUROLOGIC

Cerebral palsy.
Hypothalamic and other CNS tumors (diencephalic syndrome).
Neuromuscular disorders.
Neurodegenerative disorders.

RENAL

Recurrent urinary tract infection.
Renal tubular acidosis.
Renal failure.

ENDOCRINE

Diabetes mellitus.
Diabetes insipidus.
Hypothyroidism/hyperthyroidism.
Growth hormone deficiency.
Adrenal insufficiency.

GENETIC/METABOLIC/ CONGENITAL

Sickle cell disease.
Inborn errors of metabolism (organic acidosis, hyperammonemia, storage disease).
Fetal alcohol syndrome.
Skeletal dysplasias.
Chromosomal disorders.
Multiple congenital anomaly syndromes (VATER [vertebral defects, imperforate anus, tracheoesophageal fistula, radial and renal dysplasia], CHARGE [coloboma, heart disease, atresia choanae, retarded growth and retarded development and/or central nervous system anomalies, genital hypoplasia, ear anomalies and/or deafness]).

GASTROINTESTINAL

Pyloric stenosis.
Gastroesophageal reflux.
Repair of tracheoesophageal fistula.
Malrotation.
Malabsorption syndromes.
Celiac disease.
Milk intolerance: lactose, protein.
Pancreatic insufficiency syndromes (cystic fibrosis).
Chronic cholestasis.
Inflammatory bowel disease.
Chronic congenital diarrhea states.
Short bowel syndrome.
Pseudoobstruction.
Hirschsprung disease.
Food allergy.

CARDIAC

Cyanotic heart lesions.
Congestive heart failure.
Vascular rings.

PULMONARY/RESPIRATORY

Severe asthma.
Cystic fibrosis; bronchiectasis.
Chronic respiratory failure.
Bronchopulmonary dysplasia.
Adenoid/tonsillar hypertrophy.
Obstructive sleep apnea.

MISCELLANEOUS

Collagen vascular disease.
Malignancy.
Primary immunodeficiency.
Transplantation.

INFECTIONS

Perinatal infection (TORCHES [toxoplasma, other, rubella, cytomegalovirus, herpes simplex]).
Occult/chronic infections.
Parasitic infestation.
Tuberculosis.
HIV.

FATIGUE

ICD-9CM #	780.7	Fatigue NOS
	300.5	Fatigue Psychogenic
	780.7	Chronic Fatigue Syndrome
ICD-10CM #	R53.83	Other fatigue
	F48.0	Neurasthenia

Depression.
Anxiety, emotional stress.
Inadequate sleep.
Chronic fatigue syndrome.
Prolonged physical activity.
Pregnancy and postpartum period.
Anemia.
Hypothyroidism.
Medications (beta-blockers, anxiolytics, antidepressants, sedating antihistamines, clonidine, methyldopa).
Viral or bacterial infections.
Sleep apnea syndrome.
Dieting.
Renal failure, CHF, COPD, liver disease.

FATIGUE, CHRONIC

ICD-9CM #	780.7	
ICD-10CM #	R53.83	Other fatigue
	F48.0	Neurasthenia

CHRONIC INFECTIONS

Hepatitis C.
Lyme disease.
Parasitic and fungal infections.
Tuberculosis.
Human immunodeficiency virus.
Xenotropic murine leukemia retrovirus.

SLEEP DISORDERS

Obstructive sleep apnea.
Restless leg syndrome.
Circadian rhythm disorder.
Upper airway resistance syndrome.
Narcolepsy/parasomnias.
Alpha-delta sleep disorder.

ENDOCRINE/METABOLIC DISORDERS

Addison's disease.
Cushing's syndrome.
Poorly controlled diabetes.
Thyroid disorders.
Hemochromatosis.
Hypopituitarism.
Diabetes insipidus.

GENERAL MEDICAL DISORDERS

Anemia (any cause).
Chronic renal/hepatic failure.
Malnutrition.
Medication side effects.
Chronic pain disorders.

PSYCHOLOGICAL

Mood disorders (depression, anxiety, bipolar).
Schizophrenia.
Posttraumatic stress disorder.
Anorexia nervosa/bulimia.
Childhood abuse and/or neglect.

CHRONIC INFLAMMATION

Rheumatoid arthritis.
Systemic lupus erythematosus.
Sjögren's syndrome.
Polymyositis/dermatomyositis.
Vasculitis.
Sarcoidosis.

CARDIOPULMONARY

Congestive heart failure.
Neurally mediated hypotension.
Postural orthostatic tachycardia syndrome.
Pulmonary hypertension.
Chronic obstructive pulmonary disease.
Mitral valve prolapse.

GASTROINTESTINAL

Celiac disease.
Inflammatory bowel disease.
Autoimmune hepatitis.
Hepatic cirrhosis.

MALIGNANCY

Lymphoma and occult malignancies.
Postchemotherapy syndrome.

NEUROLOGIC DISORDERS

Multiple sclerosis.
Myasthenia gravis.
Muscular dystrophies.
Parkinson's disease.
Early dementia.

LIFESTYLE FACTORS

Chronic overwork.
Persistent unresolved stress.
Inadequate exercise.
Morbid obesity (body mass index >40).
Alcoholism/drug abuse.

FATTY LIVER

ICD-9CM # 571.8
ICD-10CM # K76.0 Fatty (change of) liver, not elsewhere classified
K76.89 Other specified diseases of liver

Obesity.
Alcohol abuse.
DM.
Acute fatty liver of pregnancy.
Medications (tetracycline, valproic acid, glucocorticoids, amiodarone, estrogen, methotrexate).
Reye's syndrome.
Wilson's disease.
Nonalcoholic steatosis.

FEVER AND JAUNDICE

ICD-9CM # 789.6 Fever
782.4 Jaundice
ICD-10CM # R50.9 Fever, unspecified
R17 Unspecified jaundice

Bacterial sepsis.
Cholangitis.
Hepatic abscess.
Leptospirosis.
Malaria.
Viral hepatitis.
Yellow fever.

FEVER AND LYMPHADENOPATHY

ICD-9CM # 780.60

Regional
Cervical
Streptococci.
Tuberculosis.
Viral upper respiratory infection.
Peripheral
Bartonella henselae.
Herpesviruses.
Lymphoma.
Metastatic cancer.
Sporotrichosis.
Streptococci.
Inguinal
Chancroid.
Herpes.
Lymphogranuloma venereum.
Syphilis (primary).
GENERALIZED
Cytomegalovirus.
Epstein-Barr virus.
HIV.
Lymphoma.
Sarcoidosis.
Syphilis (secondary).
Toxoplasmosis.
Viral hepatitis.

FEVER AND RASH

ICD-9CM # 782.1 Exanthem
57.9 Exanthem, Viral
789.6 Fever
ICD-10CM # R21 Rash and other nonspecific skin eruption
R21 Rash and other nonspecific skin eruption
R50.9 Fever, unspecified

Drug hypersensitivity: penicillin, sulfonamides, thiazides, anticonvulsants, allopurinol.
Viral infection: measles, rubella, varicella, erythema infectiosum, roseola, enterovirus infection, viral hepatitis, infectious mononucleosis, acute HIV.
Other infections: meningococcemia, staphylococcemia, scarlet fever, typhoid fever, *Pseudomonas* bacteremia, Rocky Mountain spotted fever, Lyme disease, secondary syphilis, bacterial endocarditis, babesiosis, brucellosis, listeriosis.
Serum sickness.
Erythema multiforme.
Erythema marginatum.
Erythema nodosum.
SLE.
Dermatomyositis.
Allergic vasculitis.
Pityriasis rosea.
Herpes zoster.

FEVER AND RASH IN ICU[38]

ICD-9CM # 782.1 Exanthem
789.6 Fever
ICD-10CM # R21 Rash and other nonspecific skin eruption
R50.9 Fever, unspecified

DIFFERENTIAL DIAGNOSTIC CLINICAL FEATURES OF FEVER AND RASH IN THE ICU

Rash with Shock
Infectious causes: toxic shock syndrome, meningococcemia, postsplenectomy sepsis, overwhelming *Staphylococcus aureus* bacteremia/acute bacterial endocarditis, arboviral hemorrhagic fevers, hemorrhagic smallpox, *Vibrio vulnificus,* gas gangrene, dengue fever.
Noninfectious cause: systemic lupus erythematosus (on steroids).
Rash with Mental Changes
Infectious causes: Rocky Mountain spotted fever, meningococcemia (with meningitis), *S. aureus* acute bacterial endocarditis, Chikungunya fever, typhus.
Noninfectious cause: systemic lupus erythematosus.
Rash with Conjunctival Suffusion
Infectious causes: Rocky Mountain spotted fever, dengue fever, arboviral hemorrhagic fevers, toxic shock syndrome.
Noninfectious cause: adult Kawasaki's disease.
Rash with Relative Bradycardia
Infectious causes: Rocky Mountain spotted fever, typhus, dengue fever, typhoid, arboviral hemorrhagic fevers.
Noninfectious cause: drug rash.
Rash with Abdominal Pain
Infectious causes: *V. vulnificus,* gas gangrene, *Clostridium sordelli,* scarlet fever.
Noninfectious causes: cholesterol emboli syndrome, systemic lupus erythematosus.
Rash on Palms and Soles
Infectious causes: Rocky Mountain spotted fever, toxic shock syndrome, chickenpox, smallpox, monkeypox, scarlet fever.
Noninfectious cause: drug rash.
Rash with Diarrhea
Infectious causes: *V. vulnificus,* gas gangrene, toxic shock syndrome, dengue fever, arboviral hemorrhagic fevers.
Noninfectious cause: none.
Rash with Edema of Dorsum of Hands/Feet
Infectious causes: Rocky Mountain spotted fever, toxic shock syndrome.
Noninfectious cause: adult Kawasaki's disease.
Rash with Bullae
Infectious causes: *V. vulnificus, S. aureus* complicated skin/skin structure infection, gas gangrene.
Noninfectious cause: none.
Rash with Heart Murmur
Infectious cause: acute bacterial endocarditis.
Noninfectious cause: systemic lupus erythematosus.
Rash with Gangrene of Nose Tip
Infectious cause: *S. aureus* acute bacterial endocarditis.
Noninfectious causes: systemic lupus erythematosus, vasculitis.
Rash with Cerebrovascular Accident
Infectious causes: cholesterol emboli syndrome, *S. aureus* acute bacterial endocarditis.
Noninfectious cause: none.
Rash with Splenomegaly
Infectious causes: Rocky Mountain spotted fever, typhus.
Noninfectious causes: systemic lupus erythematosus, adult Kawasaki's disease.
Rash with Deafness
Infectious causes: Rocky Mountain spotted fever, typhus, meningococcal meningitis.
Noninfectious cause: none.
Rash with Hepatosplenomegaly
Infectious causes: Rocky Mountain spotted fever, typhus.
Noninfectious cause: atypical measles.
Rash with Hepatomegaly
Infectious cause: typhus.
Noninfectious cause: none.

FEVER, AFTER TRAVEL TO THE TROPICS[1a]

ICD-9CM # 789.6
ICD-10CM # R50.81 Fever presenting with conditions classified elsewhere

CAUSES OF FEVER AFTER TRAVEL TO THE TROPICS

80% of Specific Infections Causing Fever (Includes Respiratory and Urinary Tract Infection)

Malaria.
Viral hepatitis.
Febrile illness unrelated to foreign travel.
Dengue fever.
Enteric fever (typhoid and paratyphoid fevers).

Other Causes

Gastroenteritis.
Rickettsia.
Leptospirosis.
Schistosomiasis.
Amebic liver abscess.
Tuberculosis.
Acute HIV infection.
Others.

FEVER, DRUG-INDUCED[14a]

ICD-9CM # 789.6

SELECTED AGENTS ASSOCIATED WITH DRUG-INDUCED FEVER

Common

Antimicrobial:
- Amphotericin B.
- β-Lactams.
- Sulfonamides.

Cardiovascular:
- Procainamide.
- Quinidine.

Central nervous system:
- Carbamazepine.
- Phenytoin.

Miscellaneous:
- Bleomycin.
- Interferon-α.
- Interleukin-2.

Less Common

Antimicrobial:
- Clindamycin.
- Fluoroquinolones.
- Rifampin.

Cardiovascular:
- Diltiazem.
- Hydralazine.

Central nervous system:
- Haloperidol.
- Serotonin reuptake inhibitors.

Miscellaneous:
- Allopurinol.
- Cimetidine.
- Tacrolimus.

FEVER, HOSPITAL ASSOCIATED[14a]

ICD-9CM # 780.60 Fever
ICD-10CM # R50.2 Drug induced fever
R50.9 Fever, unspecified

SELECTED CAUSES OF HOSPITAL-ASSOCIATED FEVER

Common

Infectious:
- *Clostridium difficile* enterocolitis.
- Pneumonia.
- Surgical wound.
- Urinary tract.
- Vascular catheter.

Noninfectious:
- Drug-induced fever.
- Hematoma.
- Immediate postoperative state.
- Transfusion reaction.
- Venous thromboembolism.

Less Common

Infectious:
- Biliary tract disease.
- Endometritis.
- Intraabdominal abscess.
- Mediastinitis.
- Sinusitis.

Noninfectious:
- Adrenal insufficiency.
- Gout.
- Myocardial infarction.
- Organ infarction.
- Pancreatitis.

FEVER IN RETURNING TRAVELERS AND IMMIGRANTS[28]

ICD-9CM # varies with specific disorder
ICD-10CM # R50.81 Fever presenting with conditions classified elsewhere

Differential diagnosis of some selected systemic febrile illnesses to consider in returned travelers and immigrants.*

COMMON

Acute respiratory tract infection (worldwide).
Gastroenteritis (worldwide) [foodborne, waterborne, fecal-oral].
Enteric fever, including typhoid (worldwide) [food, water].
Urinary tract infection (worldwide) [sexual contact].
Drug reactions [antibiotics, prophylactic agents, other] {rash frequent}.
Malaria (tropics, limited areas of temperate zones) [mosquitoes].
Arboviruses (Africa; tropics) [mosquitoes, ticks, mites].
Dengue (Asia, Caribbean, Africa) [mosquitoes].
Viral hepatitis (worldwide).
Hepatitis A (worldwide) [food, fecal-oral].
Hepatitis B (worldwide, especially Asia, sub-Saharan Africa) [sexual contact] {long incubation period}.
Hepatitis C (worldwide) [blood or sexual contact].
Hepatitis E (Asia, North Africa, Mexico, others) [food, water].
Tuberculosis (worldwide) [airborne, milk] {long period to symptomatic infection}.
Sexually transmitted diseases (worldwide) [sexual contact].

LESS COMMON

Filariasis (Asia, Africa, South America) [biting insects] {long incubation period, eosinophilia}.
Measles (developing world) [airborne] {in susceptible individual}.
Amebic abscess (worldwide) [food].
Brucellosis (worldwide) [milk, cheese, food, animal contact].
Listeriosis (worldwide) [foodborne] {meningitis}.
Leptospirosis (worldwide) [animal contact, open fresh water] {jaundice, meningitis}.
Strongyloidiasis (warm and tropical areas) [soil contact] {eosinophilia}.
Toxoplasmosis (worldwide) [undercooked meat].

RARE

Relapsing fever (western Americas, Asia, northern Africa) [ticks, lice].
Hemorrhagic fevers (worldwide) [arthropod and nonarthropod transmitted].
Yellow fever (tropics) [mosquitoes] {hepatitis}.
Hemorrhagic fever with renal syndrome (Europe, Asia, North America) [rodent urine] {renal impairment}.
Hantavirus pulmonary syndrome (western North America, other) [rodent urine] {respiratory distress syndrome}.
Lassa fever (Africa) [rodent excreta, person to person] {high mortality rate}
Other—chikungunya, Rift Valley, Ebola-Marburg, etc. (various) [insect bites, rodent excreta, aerosols, person to person] {often severe}.
Rickettsial infections {rashes and eschars}.
Leishmaniasis, visceral (Middle East, Mediterranean, Africa, Asia, South America) [biting flies] {long incubation period}.
Acute schistosomiasis (Africa, Asia, South America, Caribbean) [fresh water].
Chagas' disease (South and Central America) [reduviid bug bites] {often asymptomatic}.
African trypanosomiasis (Africa) [tsetse fly bite] {neurologic syndromes, sleeping sickness}.
Bartonellosis (South America) [sandfly bite] {skin nodules}.
HIV infection/AIDS (worldwide) [sexual and blood contact].
Trichinosis (worldwide) [undercooked meat] {eosinophilia}.
Plague (temperate and tropical plains) [animal exposures and fleas].
Tularemia (worldwide) [animal contact, fleas, aerosols] {ulcers, lymph nodes}.
Anthrax (worldwide) [animal, animal product contact] {ulcers}.
Lyme disease (North America, Europe) [tick bites] {arthritis, meningitis, cardiac abnormalities}.

*Diagnoses for which particular symptoms are indicative are in *italics*. Exposure to regions of the world that are most likely to be significant to the diagnosis are presented in (parentheses). Vectors, risk behaviors, and sources associated with acquisition are presented in [brackets]. Special clinical characteristics are listed within {braces}.

FEVER, NONINFECTIOUS CAUSES[2]

ICD-9CM # 780.60
ICD-10CM # R50.9 Fever, unspecified

DIFFERENTIAL DIAGNOSIS—NONINFECTIOUS CAUSES OF FEVER

Critical Diagnoses

Acute myocardial infarction.
Pulmonary embolism/infarction.
Intracranial hemorrhage.
Cerebrovascular accident.
Neuroleptic-malignant syndrome.
Thyroid storm.
Acute adrenal insufficiency.
Transfusion reaction.
Pulmonary edema.

Emergent Diagnoses

Congestive heart failure.
Dehydration.
Recent seizure.
Sickle cell disease.
Transplant rejection.
Pancreatitis.
Deep vein thrombosis.

Nonemergent Diagnoses

Drug fever.
Malignancy.
Gout.
Sarcoidosis.
Crohn's disease.
Postmyocardiotomy syndrome.

FEVER, POST-PARTUM[1]

ICD-9CM # 780.60
ICD-10CM # R50.9 Fever, unspecified

MOST COMMON

Metritis.
Urinary tract infection.
Pneumonia.
Wound infection.
Mastitis.
Superficial or deep vein thrombosis.

MOST THREATENING

Toxic shock syndrome.
Necrotizing fasciitis.
Pelvic phlegmon.
Pelvic abscess.
Peritonitis.
Septic pelvic thrombosis.
Breast abscess.

FEVER, PERIODIC[12c]

ICD-9CM # 780.60
ICD-10CM # R50.9 Fever, unspecified

HEREDITARY

NONHEREDITARY

Infectious

Hidden infectious focus (e.g., aortoenteric fistula, Caroli's disease).
Recurrent reinfection (e.g., chronic meningococcemia, host defense defect).
Specific infection (e.g., Whipple's disease, malaria).
Noninfectious inflammatory disorder, e.g.:
- Adult-onset Still's disease.
- Juvenile chronic rheumatoid arthritis.
- Periodic fever, aphthous stomatitis, pharyngitis, and adenitis.
- Schnitzler syndrome.
- Behçet's syndrome.
- Crohn's disease.
- Sarcoidosis.
- Extrinsic alveolitis.
- Humidifier lung, polymer fume fever.
- Neoplastic.

Lymphoma (e.g., Hodgkin's disease, angioimmunoblastic lymphoma).
Solid tumor (e.g., pheochromocytoma, myxoma, colon carcinoma).

Vascular (e.g., recurrent pulmonary embolism)

Hypothalamic

Psychogenic periodic fever.
Factitious or fraudulent.

FEVER, PEDIATRIC, ACUTE[1]

ICD-9CM # 780.60
ICD-10CM # R50.9 Fever, unspecified

COMMON VIRAL INFECTIONS

Central Nervous System

Meningitis.
Encephalitis.
Tumor.
Brain abscess.

Head, Ears, Eyes, Nose, and Throat

Otitis media.
Pharyngitis.
Retropharyngeal abscess.
Peritonsillar abscess.
Lateral pharyngeal wall abscess.
Stomatitis.
Influenza.
Sinusitis.
Parotitis.
Cervical adenitis.
Periorbital cellulitis.
Orbital cellulitis or abscess.

Respiratory System

Bronchiolitis.
Croup.
Epiglottitis.
Pneumonia.
Upper respiratory infection.

Cardiovascular System

Myocarditis.
Pericarditis.
Endocarditis.

Genitourinary System

Urinary tract infection.
Tuboovarian abscess.

Gastrointestinal Tract

Acute viral gastroenteritis.
Bacterial enteritis.
Appendicitis.

Focal Soft Tissue Infections

Cellulitis.

Musculoskeletal System

Osteomyelitis.
Septic arthritis.

Rheumatologic Disorders

Acute rheumatic fever.
Juvenile rheumatoid arthritis.
Henoch-Schönlein purpura.

Vasculitis

Behçet syndrome.

Malignancy

Leukemia.
Lymphoma.
Sarcoma.

Systemic Illness

Bacteremia.
Viremia.
Sepsis.
Kawasaki disease.
Toxic shock syndrome.
Rocky Mountain spotted fever.
Meningococcemia.

MISCELLANEOUS DISORDERS

Toxicologic

Anticholinergic toxidromes.
Salicylate overdose.
Amphetamine.
Cocaine.

Endocrine

Thyrotoxicosis.

FEVER, RECURRENT OR PERIODIC, IN CHILDREN[22a]

ICD-9CM # 780.60 Fever
ICD-10CM # R50.2 Drug induced fever
R50.9 Fever, unspecified

INFECTIOUS DISEASES

Brucellosis.
Rat-bite fever.
Relapsing fever.

RHEUMATIC DISEASES

Juvenile idiopathic arthritis (systemic onset).
Behçet disease.
Systemic lupus erythematosus.
Relapsing polychondritis.
Crohn's disease.

HEREDITARY AUTOINFLAMMATORY SYNDROMES

Familial Mediterranean fever (FMF).
Cryopyrinopathies:
- Familial cold autoinflammatory syndrome (FCAS).
- Muckle-Wells syndrome (MWS).
- Chronic infantile neurologic cutaneous and articular (CINCA) syndrome, also called neonatal-onset multisystem inflammatory disease (NOMID).

Tumor necrosis factor receptor–associated periodic syndrome (TRAPS).
Hyperimmunoglobulinemia D with periodic fever syndrome (HIDS).

CYCLIC HEMATOPOIESIS

Hereditary form.
Acquired form.

IDIOPATHIC CONDITIONS

Periodic fever with aphthous stomatitis, pharyngitis, and adenitis (PFAPA).

FINGER LESIONS, INFLAMMATORY

ICD-9CM # varies with specific disorder
ICD-10CM # B08.8 Other specified viral infections characterized by skin and mucous membrane lesions
L03.0 Cellulitis of finger and toe

Paronychia.
Herpes simplex type 1 (herpetic whitlow).
Dyshidrotic eczema (pompholyx).
Herpes zoster.
Bacterial endocarditis (Osler's nodes).
Psoriatic arthritis.

FLACCID PARALYSIS, ACUTE, DIFFERENTIAL DIAGNOSIS[22a]

ICD-9CM # 344.9 Flaccid Paralysis
ICD-10CM # G83.9 Paralytic syndrome, unspecified

Brain stem stroke.
Brain stem encephalitis.
Acute anterior poliomyelitis.
- Caused by poliovirus.
- Caused by other neurotropic viruses.

Acute myelopathy.
- Space-occupying lesions.
- Acute transverse myelitis.

Peripheral neuropathy.
- Guillain-Barré syndrome.
- Post-rabies vaccine neuropathy.
- Diphtheritic neuropathy.
- Heavy metals, biologic toxins, or drug intoxication.
- Acute intermittent porphyria.
- Vasculitic neuropathy.
- Critical illness neuropathy.
- Lymphomatous neuropathy.

Disorders of neuromuscular transmission.
- Myasthenia gravis.
- Biologic or industrial toxins.
- Tic paralysis.

Disorders of muscle.
- Hypokalemia.
- Hypophosphatemia.
- Inflammatory myopathy.
- Acute rhabdomyolysis.
- Trichinosis.
- Periodic paralyses.

FLATULENCE AND BLOATING[33]

ICD-9CM # 787.3
ICD-10CM # R14.0 Abdominal distension (gaseous)
R14.1 Gas pain
R14.2 Eructation
R14.3 Flatulence

Ingestion of nonabsorbable carbohydrates.
Ingestion of carbonated beverages.
Malabsorption: pancreatic insufficiency, biliary disease, celiac disease, bacterial overgrowth in small intestine.
Lactase deficiency.
Irritable bowel syndrome.
Anxiety disorders.
Food poisoning, giardiasis.

FLUSHING[27]

ICD-9CM # 782.62
ICD-10CM # R23.2 Flushing

Physiologic flushing: menopause, ingestion of monosodium glutamate (Chinese restaurant syndrome), ingestion of hot drinks.
Drugs: alcohol (with or without disulfiram, metronidazole, or chlorpropamide), nicotinic acid, diltiazem, nifedipine, levodopa, bromocriptine, vancomycin, amyl nitrate.
Neoplastic disorders: carcinoid syndrome, VIPoma syndrome, medullary carcinoma of thyroid, systemic mastocytosis, basophilic chronic myelocytic leukemia, renal cell carcinoma.
Anxiety.
Agnogenic flushing.

FOLATE DEFICIENCY[20]

ICD-9CM # 281.2
ICD-10CM # D52.0 Dietary folate deficiency anemia
D52.1 Drug-induced folate deficiency anemia
D52.8 Other folate deficiency anemias
D52.9 Folate deficiency anemia, unspecified

ETIOPATHOPHYSIOLOGIC CLASSIFICATION OF FOLATE DEFICIENCY

Nutritional causes:
Decreased dietary intake:
- Poverty and famine.
- Institutionalized individuals (e.g., psychiatric, nursing homes), chronic debilitating disease.
- Prolonged feeding of infants with goat's milk, special slimming diets or food fads (i.e., folate-rich foods not consumed), cultural or ethnic cooking techniques (i.e., food folate destroyed).

Decreased diet and increased requirements:
- Physiologic (e.g., pregnancy and lactation, prematurity, hyperemesis gravidarum, infancy).
- Pathologic (e.g., intrinsic hematologic diseases involving hemolysis with compensatory erythropoiesis, abnormal hematopoiesis, or bone marrow infiltration with malignant disease and dermatologic disease such as psoriasis).

Folate malabsorption:
With normal intestinal mucosa:
- Some drugs (controversial).
- Congenital folate malabsorption (rare).

With mucosal abnormalities (e.g., tropical and nontropical sprue, regional enteritis).
Defective cellular folate uptake:
Familial aplastic anemia (rare).
Acute cerebral folate deficiency.
Inadequate cellular use:
Folate antagonists (e.g., methotrexate).
Hereditary enzyme deficiencies involving folate.
Drugs:
Multiple effects on folate metabolism (e.g., alcohol, sulfasalazine, triamterene, pyrimethamine, trimethoprim-sulfamethoxazole, diphenylhydantoin, barbiturates).
Acute folate deficiency:
Intensive care unit setting.
Uncertain origin.

FOOT AND ANKLE PAIN[12a]

ICD-9CM # varies with specific disorder
ICD-10CM # M25.5 Pain in joint
M25.9 Joint disorder, unspecified

TENDON, LIGAMENT, AND MUSCLE

Gastrocnemius-soleus strain.
Plantaris rupture.
Anterior talofibular ligament tear.
Calcaneofibular ligament tear.
Deltoid ligament tear.
Anterolateral impingement due to complete tear of anterior talofibular ligament and anterior inferior tibiofibular ligament.
Syndesmotic impingement due to tear of syndesmosis.
Sinus tarsi syndrome (lateral hindfoot pain and instability due to injury of contents of the sinus and tarsal tunnel).
Achilles tendinitis.
Achilles rupture.
Plantar fasciitis.
Posterior tibial tendon dysfunction.
Flexor hallucis longus dysfunction.
Tibialis anterior tendon tear.
Peroneus brevis tendon tear.

BONE

Fracture of talus.
Calcaneal fracture.
Navicular fractures.
Lisfranc fracture-dislocation (fracture of the first metatarsal base with dislocation of medial cuneiform).
Metatarsal stress fracture.
Freiberg's infraction (sclerosis and flattening of the second metatarsal head due to trauma or microtrauma).
Avascular necrosis of the talus.
Fracture of the phalanges.
Fracture of the sesamoids.
Sesamoiditis.
Metatarsalgia.

JOINT

Osteoarthritis.
Gout.
Rheumatoid arthritis.
Other inflammatory arthritides.

Charcot's joint.
Osteochondral lesion of the talus.

PERIARTICULAR STRUCTURES

Shin splint (periosteal avulsion and periostitis at the insertion of the medial soleus due to repetitive overuse, such as in running and hiking).
Hallux rigidus.
Hallux valgus.
Ingrown toenail.
Toe deformities.
Turf toe (sprain of the first metatarsophalangeal joint due to hyperextension forces).
Plantar fasciitis.
Plantar fibromatosis.

NERVES

Anterior tarsal tunnel syndrome (involvement of deep peroneal nerve under the superficial fascia of the ankle).
Morton's neuroma.

VESSELS

Atherosclerosis.
Compartment syndrome.

REFERRED PAIN

Complex regional pain syndrome.

FOOT AND ANKLE PAIN, IN DIFFERENT AGE GROUPS[8]

ICD-9CM # varies with specific diagnosis
ICD-10CM # M25.579 Pain in unspecified ankle and joints of unspecified foot

COMMON CAUSES OF FOOT AND ANKLE PAIN IN DIFFERENT AGE GROUPS

Childhood (2-10 yr)
Intraarticular:
Club foot.
Congenital midfoot and forefoot deformities.
Septic arthritis.
Periarticular:
Osteomyelitis.
Adolescence (10-18 yr)
Intraarticular:
Arch disorders (pes cavus, pes planus).
Periarticular:
Osteomyelitis.
Tumors.
Early Adulthood (18-30 yr)
Intraarticular:
Metatarsalgia.
Hallux valgus.
Hallux rigidus.
Osteochondritis.
Accessory ossicles.
Periarticular:
Achilles tendonitis.
Achilles tendon rupture.
Fasciitis.
Referred:
Lumbar spine.
Knee.
Adulthood (30-50 yr)
Intraarticular:
Osteoarthritis.
Inflammatory arthritis.
Gout.
Metatarsalgia.
Hallux valgus.
Hallux rigidus.
Osteochondritis.
Accessory ossicles.
Periarticular:
Ischemic foot pain.
Diabetes.
Bursitis.
Tendonitis.
Plantar fasciitis.
Corns.
Referred:
Lumbar spine.
Knee.
Old Age (>50 yr)
Intraarticular:
Osteoarthritis.
Inflammatory arthritis.
Gout.
Metatarsalgia.
Hallux valgus.
Hallux rigidus.
Periarticular:
Ischemic foot pain.
Diabetes.
Bursitis.
Tendonitis.
Plantar fasciitis.
Corns.
Referred:
Lumbar spine.
Knee.

FOOT DERMATITIS

ICD-9CM # varies with specific disorder
ICD-10CM # B35.3 Tinea pedis
K25 Unspecified contact dermatitis

Tinea pedis.
Dyshidrotic eczema.
Tylosis (mechanically induced hyperkeratosis, fissuring, and dryness).
Allergic contact dermatitis.
Psoriasis.
Peripheral vascular insufficiency.
Neuropathic foot ulcers (DM, poorly fitting shoes).
Acquired plantar keratoderma.
Sézary's syndrome.

FOOTDROP

ICD-9CM # varies with specific disorder
ICD-10CM # M21.379 Foot drop, unspecified foot

Peripheral neuropathy.
L5 radiculopathy.
Peroneal nerve compression.
Sciatic nerve palsy.
Scapuloperoneal syndromes.
Spasticity.
Peroneal nerve compression.
Myopathy.
Dystonia.

FOOT LESION, ULCERATING

ICD-9CM # 917.9
ICD-10CM # S90.929A Unspecified superficial injury of unspecified foot, initial encounter
S90.933A Unspecified superficial injury of unspecified great toe, initial encounter
S90.936A Unspecified superficial injury of unspecified lesser toe(s), initial encounter
L08.89 Other specified local infections of the skin and subcutaneous tissue

Cellulitis.
Plantar wart.
Squamous cell carcinoma.
Actinomycosis (Madura foot).
Plantar fibromatosis.
Pseudoepitheliomatous hyperplasia.

FOOT PAIN

ICD-9CM # varies with specific diagnosis
ICD-10CM # M25.579 Pain in unspecified ankle and joints of unspecified foot

Trauma (fractures, musculoskeletal and ligamentous strain).
Inflammation (plantar fasciitis, Achilles tendonitis or bursitis, calcaneal apophysitis).
Arterial insufficiency, Raynaud's phenomenon, thromboangiitis obliterans.
Gout, pseudogout.
Calcaneal spur.
Infection (cellulitis, abscess, lymphangitis, gangrene).
Decubitus ulcer.
Paronychia, ingrown toenail.
Thrombophlebitis, postphlebitic syndrome.

FOOT PAIN BY AGE[22a]

ICD-9CM # varies with specific diagnosis
ICD-10CM # M25.579 Pain in unspecified ankle and joints of unspecified foot

0-6 YEARS

Poorly fitting shoes.
Foreign body.
Fracture.
Osteomyelitis.
Leukemia.
Puncture wound.
Drawing of blood.
Dactylitis.
Juvenile rheumatoid arthritis (JRA).

6-12 YEARS

Poorly fitting shoes.
Sever disease.
Enthesopathy (JRA).
Foreign body.
Accessory navicular.
Tarsal coalition.
Ewing sarcoma.
Hypermobile flatfoot.
Trauma (sprains, fractures).
Puncture wound.

12-20 YEARS

Poorly fitting shoes.
Stress fracture.
Foreign body.
Ingrown toenail.
Metatarsalgia.
Plantar fasciitis.
Osteochondroses (avascular necrosis).
Freiberg.
Köhler.
Achilles tendinitis.
Trauma (sprains).
Plantar warts.
Tarsal coalition.

FOREARM AND HAND PAIN

ICD-9CM #	959.3	Forearm Injury
	959.4	Hand Injury
ICD-10CM #	S59.809A	Other specified injuries of unspecified elbow, initial encounter
	S59.919A	Unspecified injury of unspecified forearm, initial encounter
	S69.80XA	Other specified injuries of unspecified wrist, hand and finger(s), initial encounter
	S69.90XA	Unspecified injury of unspecified wrist, hand and finger(s), initial encounter

Epicondylitis.
Tenosynovitis.
Osteoarthritis.
Cubital tunnel syndrome.
Carpal tunnel syndrome.
Trauma.
Herpes zoster.
Peripheral vascular insufficiency.
Infection (cellulitis, abscess).

FOREARM FRACTURES[1aa]

ICD-9CM #	759.33
ICD-10CM #	S52 Fracture of forearm

TRAUMATIC

Wrist sprain, elbow sprain.
Ligamentous injuries, forearm contusions, hematomas.
Dislocations of the elbow or wrist (including nursemaid's elbow).

INFECTIOUS

Cellulitis of the forearm, abscesses.
Necrotizing fasciitis.

VASCULAR

Acute arterial occlusion.
Venous thrombosis.

NEUROLOGIC

Neurapraxias, carpal tunnel syndrome.
Systemic neurologic syndromes involving the nerves of the upper extremities.

ARTHRITIS

Septic joint, gonococcal arthritis, rheumatoid arthritis, osteoarthritis.
Pseudogout, gout.
Systemic lupus erythematosus, rheumatic fever, viral syndrome.
Reiter syndrome, Lyme disease, serum sickness.

OTHER

Olecranon bursitis, soft tissue masses.
Normal growth plates, nutrient vessels.

GAIT ABNORMALITY

ICD-9CM #	781.2	Gait Abnormality
ICD-10CM #	R26.0	Ataxic gait
	R26.1	Paralytic gait
	R26.89	Other abnormalities of gait and mobility
	R26.9	Unspecified abnormalities of gait and mobility

Parkinsonism.
Degenerative joint disease (hips, back, knees).
Multiple sclerosis.
Trauma, foot pain.
CVA.
Cerebellar lesions.
Infections (tabes, encephalitis, meningitis).
Sensory ataxia.
Dystonia, cerebral palsy, neuromuscular disorders.
Metabolic abnormalities.

GALACTORRHEA[28]

ICD-9CM #	611.6	
ICD-10CM #	N64.3	Galactorrhea not associated with childbirth

Prolonged suckling.
Drugs (INH, phenothiazines, reserpine derivatives, amphetamines, spironolactone and tricyclic antidepressants).
Major stressors (surgery, trauma).
Hypothyroidism.
Pituitary tumors.

GASTRIC DILATATION[16a]

ICD-9CM #	536.1	
ICD-10CM #	K31.0	Acute dilatation of stomach

CAUSES OF A MASSIVELY DILATED STOMACH

Mechanical Gastric Outlet Obstruction
Duodenal or pyloric canal ulceration.
Carcinoma of pyloric antrum.
Extrinsic compression.
Paralytic Ileus
Surgery.
Trauma.
Peritonitis.
Pancreatitis.
Cholecystitis.
Diabetes.
Hepatic coma.
Drugs.
Gastric Volvulus
Intubation.
Air swallowing.

GASTRIC EMPTYING, DELAYED[1a]

ICD-9CM #	578.89	
ICD-10CM #	K30	Functional dyspepsia

CAUSES OF DELAYED GASTRIC EMPTYING

Mechanical Causes
Peptic ulcer disease, scarred pylorus.
Malignancy: gastric cancer, gastric lymphoma, pancreatic cancer.
Gastric surgery: vagotomy, gastric resection, Roux-en-Y anastomosis.
Crohn's disease.
Endocrine and Metabolic Causes
Diabetes mellitus.
Hypothyroidism.
Hypoadrenal states.
Electrolyte abnormalities.
Chronic renal failure.
Medications.
Anticholinergics.
Opiates.
Dopamine agonists.
Tricyclic antidepressants.
Abnormalities of Gastric Smooth Muscle
Scleroderma.
Polymyositis, dermatomyositis.
Amyloidosis.
Pseudo-obstruction.
Myotonic dystrophy.
Neuropathy.
Scleroderma.
Amyloidosis.
Autonomic neuropathy.
Central Nervous System or Psychiatric Disorders
Brain stem tumors.
Spinal cord injury.
Anorexia nervosa.
Stress.
Miscellaneous
Idiopathic gastroparesis.
Gastroesophageal reflux disease.
Nonulcer (functional) dyspepsia.
Cancer cachexia or anorexia.

GASTRIC EMPTYING, RAPID

ICD-9CM # 536.8 Gastric Motility Disorder
ICD-10CM # K30 Functional dyspepsia

Pancreatic insufficiency.
Dumping syndrome.
Peptic ulcer.
Celiac disease.
Promotility agents.
Zollinger-Ellison disease.

GENITAL DISCHARGE, FEMALE[12]

ICD-9CM # 629.9
ICD-10CM # N94.9 Unspecified condition associated with female genital organs and menstrual cycle

Physiologic discharge: cervical mucus, vaginal transudation, bacteria, squamous epithelial cells.
Individual variation.
Pregnancy.
Sexual response.
Menstrual cycle variation.
Infection.
Foreign body: tampon, cervical cap, other.
Neoplasm.
Fistula.
IUD.
Cervical ectropion.
Spermicide.
Nongenital causes: urinary incontinence, urinary tract fistula, Crohn's disease, rectovaginal fistula.

GENITAL SORES[1a]

ICD-9CM #	054.10	Genital Herpes
	91.0	Genital Syphilis
	078.11	Condyloma Acuminatum
	099.0	Chancroid
	099.2	Granuloma Inguinale
	099.1	Lymphogranuloma Venereum
	629.8	Ulcer, Genital Site, Female
	608.89	Ulcer, Genital Site, Male
ICD-10CM #	A60.9	Anogenital herpesviral infection, unspecified
	A51.0	Primary genital syphilis
	A63.0	Anogenital (venereal) warts
	A57	Chancroid
	A58	Granuloma inguinale
	A55	Chlamydial lymphogranuloma (venereum)
	N94.89	Other specified conditions associated with female genital organs and menstrual cycle
	N50.8	Other specified disorders of male genital organs

Herpes genitalis.
Syphilis.
Chancroid.
Lymphogranuloma venereum.
Granuloma inguinale.
Condyloma acuminatum.
Neoplastic lesion.
Trauma.

GLOMERULONEPHRITIS, RAPIDLY PROGRESSIVE[1a]

ICD-9CM # 583.4
ICD-10CM # N05.9 Unspecified nephritic syndrome with unspecified morphologic changes

DIFFERENTIAL DIAGNOSIS OF RAPIDLY PROGRESSIVE GLOMERULONEPHRITIS

Linear Immune Staining
Anti-GBM disease.
Goodpasture's syndrome.
Rarely membranous glomerulonephritis.

Granular Immune Staining
Subacute bacterial endocarditis (past infectious).
Lupus nephritis.
Cryoglobulinemia.
Membranoproliferative glomerulonephritis (type II more than type I).
Immunoglobulin A nephropathy, Henoch-Schönlein purpura.
Idiopathic.

No Immune Staining (Pauci-immune)
Antineutrophil cytoplasmic antibody-associated vasculitis (Wegener granulomatosis, microscopic polyangiitis, Churg-Strauss syndrome).
Idiopathic.

GLOMERULOPATHIES, THROMBOTIC, MICROANGIOPATHIC[1a]

ICD-9CM # 446.6
ICD-10CM # M31.1 Thrombotic microangiopathy

THROMBOTIC MICROANGIOPATHIC GLOMERULOPATHIES

Thrombotic thrombocytopenic purpura.
Hemolytic-uremic syndrome.
Malignant hypertension.
Scleroderma renal crisis.
Preeclampsia, eclampsia.
HELLP syndrome (hemolysis, elevated liver enzymes, low platelets).
Antiphospholipid antibody syndrome.
Drugs: oral contraceptives, quinine, cyclosporine, tacrolimus, ticlopidine, clopidogrel.

GLOMERULOSCLEROSIS, FOCAL SEGMENTAL[1a]

ICD-9CM # 582.1
ICD-10CM # N03.3 Chronic nephritic syndrome with diffuse mesangial proliferative glomerulonephritis

ETIOLOGY OF FOCAL SEGMENTAL GLOMERULOSCLEROSIS (FSGS)

Primary idiopathic FSGS.
Secondary FSGS.
HIV (usually collapsing variant).
Reflux nephropathy.
Heroin abuse.
Sickle cell disease.
Oligomeganephronia.
Renal dysgenesis or agenesis (low nephron mass).
Radiation nephritis.
Familial podocytopathies.
NPHS1 (nephrin) mutation.
NPHS2 (podocin) mutation.
TRPC6 (cation channel) mutation.
ACTN4 (a-actinin 4 mutation).

GLOSSODYNIA[38]

ICD-9CM # 529.6
ICD-10CM # K14.6 Glossodynia

DENTURE-RELATED

Dentures (ill-fitting, monomer from denture base).
Dental plaque.
Oral parafunction.

INFECTIVE/DERMATOLOGIC

Candidiasis.
Lichen planus.

DEFICIENCY STATES

Iron, B_{12}, folate, B_2 (riboflavin), B_6 (pyridoxine), zinc.

ENDOCRINE

Diabetes.
Myxedema.*
Hormonal changes occurring during menopause.*

NEUROLOGICALLY MEDIATED

Referred from tonsils, teeth.
Lingual nerve neuropathy.
Glossopharyngeal neuralgia.
Esophageal reflux.*

IATROGENIC

Mouthwash.

XEROSTOMIA

PSYCHOGENIC

IDIOPATHIC

*Unproven associations

GLUCOCORTICOID DEFICIENCY[14]

ICD-9CM # 255.4
ICD-10CM # E27.1 Primary adrenocortical insufficiency
E27.3 Drug-induced adrenocortical insufficiency

ACTH-independent causes.
TB.
Autoimmune (idiopathic).
Other rare causes:
- Fungal infection.
- Adrenal hemorrhage.
- Metastases.
- Sarcoidosis.
- Amyloidosis.
- Adrenoleukodystrophy.
- Adrenomyeloneuropathy.
- HIV infection.
- Congenital adrenal hyperplasia.
- Medications (e.g., ketoconazole).

ACTH-dependent causes:
Hypothalamic-pituitary-adrenal suppression.
- Exogenous.
- Glucocorticoid.
- ACTH.
- Endogenous—cure of Cushing's syndrome.

Hypothalamic-pituitary lesions.
- Neoplasm:
  - Primary pituitary tumor.
  - Metastatic tumor.
  - Craniopharyngioma.
- Infection:
  - Tuberculosis.
  - Actinomycosis.
  - Nocardiosis.
- Sarcoid.
- Head trauma.
- Isolated ACTH deficiency.

GOITER

ICD-9CM #	240.9	Goiter, Unspecified
	241.9	Goiter, Adenomatous
	246.1	Goiter, Congenital
	240.9	Goiter, Nontoxic Diffuse
	241.1	Goiter, Nontoxic Multinodular
	240.0	Simple Goiter
	242.1	Thyrotoxic Goiter
ICD-10CM #	E01.2	Iodine-deficiency related (endemic) goiter, unspecified
	E04.9	Nontoxic goiter, unspecified
	E04.9	Nontoxic goiter, unspecified
	E07.1	Dyshormogenetic goiter
	E01.2	Iodine-deficiency related (endemic) goiter, unspecified
	E04.9	Nontoxic goiter, unspecified
	E04.2	Nontoxic multinodular goiter
	E04.0	Nontoxic diffuse goiter
	E05.10	Thyrotoxicosis with toxic single thyroid nodule without thyrotoxic crisis or storm

Thyroiditis.
Toxic multinodular goiter.
Graves' disease.
Medications (PTU, methimazole, sulfonamides, sulfonylureas, ethionamide, amiodarone, lithium, etc.).
Iodine deficiency.
Sarcoidosis, amyloidosis.
Defective thyroid hormone synthesis.
Resistance to thyroid hormone.

GRANULOMATOUS DERMATITIDES

ICD-9CM #	varies with specific disorder	
ICD-10CM #	L92.9	Granulomatous disorder of the skin and subcutaneous tissue, unspecified

Granuloma annulare.
Sarcoidosis.
Necrobiosis lipoidica diabeticorum.
Cutaneous Crohn's disease.
Rheumatoid nodules.
Annular elastolytic giant cell granuloma (actinic granuloma).
Foreign body granuloma.

GRANULOMATOUS DISORDERS[32]

ICD-9CM #	446.4	Granulomatosis
	288.1	Granulomatous Disease
ICD-10CM #	M31.30	Wegener's granulomatosis without renal involvement
	K75.3	Granulomatous hepatitis
	L92.9	Granulomatous disorder of skin and subcutaneous tissue, unspecified

INFECTIONS

Fungi
Histoplasma.
Coccidioides.
Blastomyces.
Sporothrix.
Aspergillus.
Cryptococcus.
Protozoa
Toxoplasma.
Leishmania.
Metazoa
Toxocara.
Schistosoma.
Spirochetes
Treponema pallidum.
T. pertenue.
T. carateum.
Mycobacteria
M. tuberculosis.
M. leprae.
M. kansasii.
M. marinum.
M. avian.
Bacille Calmette-Guérin (BCG) vaccine.
Bacteria
Brucella.
Yersinia.
Other Infections
Cat scratch.
Lymphogranuloma.

NEOPLASIA

Carcinoma.
Reticulosis.
Pinealoma.
Dysgerminoma.
Seminoma.
Reticulum cell sarcoma.
Malignant nasal granuloma.

CHEMICALS

Beryllium.
Zirconium.
Silica.
Starch.

IMMUNOLOGIC ABERRATIONS

Sarcoidosis.
Crohn's disease.
Primary biliary cirrhosis.
Wegener's granulomatosis.
Giant cell arteritis.
Peyronie's disease.
Hypogammaglobulinemia.
SLE.
Lymphomatoid granulomatosis.
Histiocytosis X.
Hepatic granulomatous disease.
Immune complex disease.
Rosenthal-Melkersson syndrome.
Churg-Strauss allergic granulomatosis.

LEUKOCYTE OXIDASE DEFECT

Chronic granulomatous disease of childhood.

EXTRINSIC ALLERGIC ALVEOLITIS

Farmer's lung.
Bird fancier's.
Mushroom worker's.
Suberosis (cork dust).
Bagassosis.
Maple bark stripper's.
Paprika splitter's.
Coffee bean.
Spatlese lung.

OTHER DISORDERS

Whipple's disease.
Pyrexia of unknown origin.
Radiotherapy.
Cancer chemotherapy.
Panniculitis.
Chalazion.
Sebaceous cyst.
Dermoid.
Sea urchin spine injury.

GRANULOMATOUS LIVER DISEASE

ICD-9CM # 572.8
ICD-10CM # K75.3 Granulomatous hepatitis

Sarcoidosis.
Wegener's granulomatosis.
Vasculitis.
Inflammatory bowel disease.
Allergic granulomatosis.
Erythema nodosum.
Infections (fungal, viral, parasitic).
Primary biliary cirrhosis.
Lymphoma.
Hodgkin's disease.
Drugs (e.g., allopurinol, hydralazine, sulfonamides, penicillins).
Toxins (copper sulfate, beryllium).

GREEN OR BLUE URINE

ICD-9CM # 788.69
ICD-10CM # R82 Other abnormal findings in urine

Pseudomonal urinary tract infection
Medications: triamterene, amitriptyline, IV cimetidine, IV promethazine.
Biliverdin.
Dyes (methylene blue, indigo carmine).

GROIN LUMP[38]

ICD-9CM # varies with specific diagnosis
ICD-10CM # R19.09 Other intra-abdominal and pelvic swelling, mass and lump
R22.9 Localized swelling, mass and lump, unspecified

COMMON CAUSES

Inguinal hernia.
Femoral hernia.
Lymph node.

OTHER CAUSES

Saphena varix.
Femoral artery aneurysm/pseudoaneurysm.
Psoas abscess.
Lipoma of the cord.
Encysted hydrocele of the cord (male).
Testicular maldescent (male).
Hydrocele of canal of Nuck (female).

GROIN MASSES

ICD-9CM # 959.1
ICD-10CM # R22.9 Localized swelling, mass and lump, unspecified
S39.848A Other specified injuries of external genitals, initial encounter

Hernia (inguinal, femoral).
Hydrocele.
Varicocele.
Sebaceous cyst.
Hidradenitis of inguinal apocrine glands.
Neoplasm: lymphoma, metastases.
Lipoma.
Hematoma.
Reactive inguinal adenopathy, femoral adenitis.
Folliculitis, psoas abscess.
Epididymitis, testicular torsion, ectopic testes.
Aneurysm or pseudoaneurysm of femoral artery.

GROIN PAIN[5a]

ICD-9CM # 338 Groin Pain
ICD-10CM # R52 Pain, unspecified

DIFFERENTIAL DIAGNOSIS OF GROIN PAIN

Surgery
Workers' Compensation.
Hernia.
Recurrent hernia.
Posthernia.
Orthopedic
Hip disorders.
Acetabular labral tears.
Avascular necrosis.
Chondritis dissecans.
Legg-Calvé-Perthes disease.
Osteoarthritis.
Pelvic stress fractures.
Slipped femoral capital epiphysis.
Synovitis.
Urology
Cystitis.
Epididymitis.
Nephrolithiasis.
Prostate cancer.
Prostatitis.
Torsion of testes.
Urethral extravasation.
Urinary tract infection.
Vas granuloma/fibrosis.
Dermatology
Lymphadenitis.
Psoriasis/burn.
Sebaceous cyst/hidradenitis.
Thrombophlebitis/cellulitis.
Neurosurgery
Disk disease.
Spinal injuries, inflammation, tumors.
Spondylolisthesis.
Spondylolysis.
Rheumatology
Connective tissue disorders.
Iliopsoas bursitis.
Osteitis pubis.
Systemic lupus erythematosus.
Neurology
Lumbosacral disorders.
Neurofibromatosis.
Infectious Disease
Herpes zoster.
HIV/tuberculosis.
Lyme disease.
Psoas abscess.
Sports Medicine
"Sports hernia" (adductor strains).
Gilmore's groin.
Vascular
Abscess hematoma.
Post-vein stripping.
Pseudoaneurysm.
Vascular graft.
Gastroenterology
Appendicitis/adhesions.
Diverticulitis.
Inflammatory retroperitoneal phlegmon (pancreatitis).
Meckel diverticulum.
Granulomatous colitis.
Gynecology
Cesarean section.
Cervical cancer.
Endometriosis.
Tubal/ovarian disorders.

GROIN PAIN, ACTIVE PATIENT[37]

ICD-9CM # 959.1 Groin Injury
848.8 Groin Pain
ICD-10CM # S39.848 A Other specified injuries of external genitals, initial encounter
R52 Pain, unspecified

MUSCULOSKELETAL

Avascular necrosis of the femoral head.
Avulsion fracture (lesser trochanter, anterior superior iliac spine, anterior inferior iliac spine).
Bursitis (iliopectineal, trochanteric).
Entrapment of the ilioinguinal or iliofemoral nerve.
Gracilis syndrome.
Muscle tear (adductors, iliopsoas, rectus abdominis, gracilis, sartorius, rectus femoris).
Myositis ossificans of the hip muscles.
Osteitis pubis.
Osteoarthritis of the femoral head.
Slipped capital femoral epiphysis.
Stress fracture of the femoral head or neck and pubis.
Synovitis.

HERNIA-RELATED

Avulsion of the internal oblique muscle in the conjoined tendon.
Defect at the insertion of the rectus abdominis muscle.
Direct inguinal hernia.
Femoral ring hernia.
Indirect inguinal hernia.
Inguinal canal weakness.

UROLOGIC

Epididymitis.
Fracture of the testis.
Hydrocele.
Kidney stone.
Posterior urethritis.

Prostatitis.
Testicular cancer.
Torsion of the testis.
Urinary tract infection.
Varicocele.

GYNECOLOGIC

Ectopic pregnancy.
Ovarian cyst.
Pelvic inflammatory disease.
Torsion of the ovary.
Vaginitis.

LYMPHATIC ENLARGEMENT IN GROIN

GYNECOMASTIA

ICD-9CM # 611.1 Gynecomastia, Nonpuerperal
ICD-10CM # N62 Hypertrophy of breast

Physiologic (puberty, newborns, aging).
Drugs (estrogen and estrogen precursors, 5-alpha reductase inhibitors, digitalis, testosterone and exogenous androgens, clomiphene, cimetidine, spironolactone, ketoconazole, amiodarone, ACE inhibitors, isoniazid, phenytoin, methyldopa, metoclopramide, phenothiazine).
Increased prolactin level (prolactinoma).
Liver disease.
Adrenal disease.
Thyrotoxicosis.
Increased estrogen production (hCG-producing tumor, testicular tumor, bronchogenic carcinoma).
Secondary hypogonadism.
Primary gonadal failure (trauma, castration, viral orchitis, granulomatous disease).
Defects in androgen synthesis.
Testosterone deficiency.
Klinefelter's syndrome.

HALITOSIS

ICD-9CM # 784.9
ICD-10CM # R19.6 Halitosis

Tobacco use.
Alcohol use.
Dry mouth (mouth breathing, inadequate fluid intake).
Foods (onion, garlic, meats, nuts, protein drinks).
Disease of mouth or nose (infections, cancer, inflammation).
Medications (antihistamines, antidepressants).
Systemic disorders (diabetes, uremia).
GI disorders (esophageal diverticula, hiatal hernia, GERD, achalasia).
Sinusitis.
Pulmonary disorders (bronchiectasis, pneumonia, neoplasms, TB).

HAND PAIN AND SWELLING[6]

ICD-9CM # varies with specific diagnosis
ICD-10CM # 729.5 Pain in limb

Trauma.
Gout.
Pseudogout.
Cellulitis.
Lymphangitis.
DVT of upper extremity.
Thrombophlebitis.
RA.
Remitting seronegative symmetrical synovitis with pitting edema (RS3PE).
Polymyalgia rheumatica.
Mixed connective tissue disease.
Scleroderma.
Rupture of the olecranon bursa.
Metzger's syndrome (neoplasia).
The puffy hand of drug addiction.
Reflex sympathetic dystrophy.
Eosinophilic fasciitis.
Sickle cell (hand-foot syndrome).
Leprosy.
Factitial (the rubber band syndrome).

HEADACHE[13]

ICD-9CM # 784.0 Headache NOS
307.81 Headache, Tension
346.2 Headache, Cluster
346.9 Headache, Migraine
784.0 Headache, Vascular
ICD-10CM # G44.1 Vascular headache, not elsewhere classified
R51 Headache
G44.209 Tension-type headache, unspecified, not intractable
G44.009 Cluster headache syndrome, unspecified, not intractable
G43.909 Migraine, unspecified, not intractable, without status migrainosus
G44.1 Vascular headache, not elsewhere classified

Vascular: migraine, cluster headaches, temporal arteritis, hypertension, cavernous sinus thrombosis.
Musculoskeletal: neck and shoulder muscle contraction, strain of extraocular and/or intraocular muscles, cervical spondylosis, temporomandibular arthritis.
Infections: meningitis, encephalitis, brain abscess, sepsis, sinusitis, osteomyelitis, parotitis, mastoiditis.
Cerebral neoplasm.
Subdural hematoma.
Cerebral hemorrhage/infarct.
Pseudotumor cerebri.
Normal-pressure hydrocephalus (NPH).
Postlumbar puncture.
Cerebral aneurysm, arteriovenous malformations.
Posttrauma.
Dental problems: abscess, periodontitis, poorly fitting dentures.
Trigeminal neuralgia, glossopharyngeal neuralgia.
Otitis and other ear diseases.
Glaucoma and other eye diseases.
Metabolic: uremia, carbon monoxide inhalation, hypoxia.
Pheochromocytoma, hypoglycemia, hypothyroidism.
Effort induced: benign exertional headache, cough, headache, coital cephalalgia.
Drugs: alcohol, nitrates, histamine antagonists.
Paget's disease of the skull.
Emotional, psychiatric.

HEADACHE, ACUTE[11]

ICD-9CM # 784.0
ICD-10CM # R51 Headache

DIFFERENTIAL DIAGNOSIS OF ACUTE HEADACHE

Evaluation of the first acute headache should exclude pathologic causes listed here before consideration of more common etiologies.
Increased intracranial pressure (ICP): Trauma, hemorrhage, tumor, hydrocephalus, pseudotumor cerebri, abscess, arachnoid cyst, cerebral edema.
Decreased ICP: After ventriculoperitoneal shunt, lumbar puncture, cerebrospinal fluid leak from basilar skull fracture.
Meningeal inflammation: Meningitis, leukemia, subarachnoid or subdural hemorrhage.
Vascular: Vasculitis, arteriovenous malformation, hypertension, cerebrovascular accident.
Bone, soft tissue: Referred pain from scalp, eyes, ears, sinuses, nose, teeth, pharynx, cervical spine, temporomandibular joint.
Infection: Systemic infection, encephalitis, sinusitis, etc.
First migraine.

HEADACHE AND FACIAL PAIN[36]

ICD-9CM # 784.0 Headache NOS
784.0 Facial Pain
ICD-10CM # R51 Headache
G44.1 Vascular headache, not elsewhere classified

VASCULAR HEADACHES

Migraine

Migraine with headaches and inconspicuous neurologic features:
- Migraine without aura ("common migraine").

Migraine with headaches and conspicuous neurologic features:
- With transient neurologic symptoms:
  Migraine with typical aura ("classic migraine").
  Sensory, basilar, and hemiplegic migraine.
- With prolonged or permanent neurologic features ("complicated migraine"):
  Ophthalmoplegic migraine.
  Migrainous infarction.

Migraine without headaches but with conspicuous neurologic features ("migraine equivalents"):
- Abdominal migraine.
- Benign paroxysmal vertigo of childhood.
- Migraine aura without headache ("isolated auras," transient migrainous accompaniments).

Cluster Headaches

Episodic cluster headache ("cyclic cluster headaches").

Chronic cluster headaches.

Chronic paroxysmal hemicrania.

Other Vascular Headaches

Headaches of reactive vasodilation (fever, drug-induced, postictal, hypoglycemia, hypoxia, hypercarbia, hyperthyroidism).

Headaches associated with arterial hypertension:
- Chronic severe hypertension (diastolic 120 mm Hg).
- Paroxysmal severe hypertension (pheochromocytoma, some coital headaches).

Headaches caused by cranial arteritis:
- Giant cell arteritis ("temporal arteritis").
- Other vasculitides.

HEADACHES ASSOCIATED WITH DEMONSTRABLE MUSCLE SPASM

Headache caused by posturally induced or perilesional muscle spasm:
- Headaches of sustained or impaired posture (e.g., prolonged close work, driving).
- Headaches associated with cervical spondylosis and other diseases of cervical spine.
- Myofascial pain dysfunction syndrome (headache or facial pain associated with disorders of teeth, jaws, and related structures, or "TMJ syndrome").

Headaches caused by psychophysiologic muscular contraction ("muscle contraction headaches," or tension-type headache associated with disorder of pericranial muscles).

HEADACHES AND FACIAL PAIN WITHOUT DEMONSTRABLE PHYSICAL SUBSTRATE

Headaches of uncertain etiology:
- "Tension headaches" (tension-type headache unassociated with disorder of pericranial muscles).
- Some forms of posttraumatic headache.

Psychogenic headaches (e.g., hypochondriacal, conversional, delusional, malingered).

Facial pain of uncertain etiology ("atypical facial pain").

COMBINED TENSION-MIGRAINE HEADACHES

Episodic migraine superimposed on chronic tension headaches.

Chronic daily headaches:
- Associated with analgesic and/or ergotamine overuse ("rebound headaches").
- Not associated with drug overuse.

HEADACHES AND HEAD PAINS CAUSED BY DISEASES OF EYES, EARS, NOSE, SINUSES, TEETH, OR SKULL

HEADACHES CAUSED BY MENINGEAL INFLAMMATION

Subarachnoid hemorrhage.

Meningitis and meningoencephalitis.

Others (e.g., meningeal carcinomatosis).

HEADACHES ASSOCIATED WITH ALTERED INTRACRANIAL PRESSURE ("TRACTION HEADACHES")

Increased Intracranial Pressure

Intracranial mass lesions (neoplasm, hematoma, abscess, etc.).

Hydrocephalus.

Benign intracranial hypertension.

Venous sinus thrombosis.

Decreased Intracranial Pressure

Post–lumbar puncture headaches.

Spontaneous hypoliquorrheic headaches.

HEADACHES AND HEAD PAINS CAUSED BY CRANIAL NEURALGIAS

Presumed Irritation of Superficial Nerves

Occipital neuralgia.

Supraorbital neuralgia.

Presumed Irritation of Intracranial Nerves

Trigeminal neuralgia ("tic douloureux").

Glossopharyngeal neuralgia.

HEADACHE, CHRONIC[11]

ICD-9CM # 784.0
ICD-10CM # R51 Headache

DIFFERENTIAL DIAGNOSIS OF RECURRENT OR CHRONIC HEADACHES

Migraine (with or without aura).

Tension.

Analgesic rebound.

Caffeine withdrawal.

Sleep deprivation (e.g., in children with sleep apnea) or chronic hypoxia.

Tumor.

Psychogenic: Conversion disorder, malingering.

Cluster headache.

HEAD AND NECK, SOFT TISSUE MASSES

ICD-9CM # varies with specific diagnosis
ICD-10CM # R22.0 Localized swelling, mass and lump, head
R22.1 Localized swelling, mass and lump, neck

Lipoma.

Pilar cyst.

Epidermal inclusion cyst.

Dermoid cyst.

Bone cyst.

Hemangioma.

Eosinophilic granuloma.

Other: facial nerve neuroma, teratoma, rhabdomyoma, rhabdomyosarcoma, branchial cleft cyst.

HEARING LOSS, ACUTE[26]

ICD-9CM # 388.2
ICD-10CM # H91.23 Sudden idiopathic hearing loss, bilateral

Infectious: mumps, measles, influenza, herpes simplex, herpes zoster, CMV, mononucleosis, syphilis.

Vascular: macroglobulinemia, sickle cell disease, Berger's disease, leukemia, polycythemia, fat emboli, hypercoagulable states.

Metabolic: diabetes, pregnancy, hyperlipoproteinemia.

Conductive: cerumen impaction, foreign bodies, otitis media, otitis externa, barotrauma, trauma.

Medications: aminoglycosides, loop diuretics, antineoplastics, salicylates, vancomycin.

Neoplasm: acoustic neuroma, metastatic neoplasm.

HEARTBURN AND INDIGESTION[33]

ICD-9CM # 787.1 Heartburn
536.8 Indigestion
ICD-10CM # R12 Heartburn
K30 Functional dyspepsia

Reflux esophagitis.

Gastritis.

Nonulcer dyspepsia.

Functional GI disorder (anxiety disorder, social/environmental stresses).

Excessive intestinal gas (ingestion of flatulogenic foods, GI stasis, constipation).

Gas entrapment (hepatitis or splenic flexure syndrome).

Neoplasm (adenocarcinoma of stomach or esophagus, lymphoma).

Gallbladder disease.

HEART FAILURE WITH PRESERVED LEFT VENTRICULAR EJECTION FRACTION[14A]

ICD-9CM # 428.9
ICD-10CM # I50.9 Heart failure, unspecified

CAUSES OF (AND ALTERNATIVE EXPLANATIONS FOR) HEART FAILURE WITH PRESERVED LEFT VENTRICULAR EJECTION FRACTION (>45%-50%)

Inaccurate diagnosis of heart failure (e.g., pulmonary disease, obesity).

Inaccurate measurements of ejection fraction.

Systolic function overestimated by ejection fraction (e.g., mitral regurgitation).

Episodic, unrecognized systolic dysfunction.

Intermittent ischemia.

Arrhythmia.

Severe hypertension.
Alcohol abuse.
Diastolic dysfunction.
Abnormalities of myocardial relaxation:
- Ischemia.
- Hypertrophy.

Abnormalities of myocardial compliance:
- Hypertrophy.
- Aging.
- Fibrosis.
- Diabetes.
- Infiltrative disease (amyloidosis, sarcoidosis).
- Storage disease (hemochromatosis).
- Endomyocardial disease (endomyocardial fibrosis, radiation, anthracyclines).

Pericardial disease (constriction, tamponade).

HEART FAILURE, ACUTE[2]

ICD-9CM # 428.9
ICD-10CM # I50.9 Heart failure, unspecified

COMMON PRECIPITATING CAUSES OF ACUTE HF

Systemic hypertension.
Myocardial infarction or ischemia.
Dysrhythmia.
Systemic infection.
Anemia.
Dietary, physical, environmental, and emotional excesses.
Pregnancy.
Thyrotoxicosis or hypothyroidism.
Acute myocarditis.
Acute valvular dysfunction.
Pulmonary embolus.
Pharmacologic complications.

HEART FAILURE, CHRONIC[4a]

ICD-9CM # 428.0
ICD-10CM # I50.9 Heart failure, unspecified

Myocardial disease.
Coronary artery disease.
- Myocardial infarction.*
- Myocardial ischemia.*

Chronic pressure overload.
- Hypertension.*
- Obstructive valvular disease.*

Chronic volume overload.
- Regurgitant valvular disease.
- Intracardiac (left-to-right) shunting.
- Extracardiac shunting.

Nonischemic dilated cardiomyopathy.
- Familial or genetic disorders.
- Infiltrative disorders.*
- Toxic or drug-induced damage.
- Metabolic disorder.*
- Viral or other infectious agents.

Disorders of rate and rhythm.
- Chronic bradyarrhythmias.
- Chronic tachyarrhythmias.

Pulmonary heart disease
- Cor pulmonale.
- Pulmonary vascular disorders.

High-output states.
Metabolic disorders.
- Thyrotoxicosis.
- Nutritional disorders (beriberi).

Excessive blood flow requirements.
- Systemic arteriovenous shunting.
- Chronic anemia.

*Indicates conditions that can also lead to HF with a preserved EF.

HEART FAILURE, PATHOGENIC CAUSES[14a]

ICD-9CM # 428.9
ICD-10CM # I50.9 Heart failure, unspecified

IMPAIRED SYSTOLIC (CONTRACTILE) FUNCTION

Ischemic damage or dysfunction:
- Myocardial infarction.
- Persistent or intermittent myocardial ischemia.
- Hypoperfusion (shock).

Chronic pressure overloading:
- Hypertension.
- Obstructive valvular disease.

Chronic volume overload:
- Regurgitant valvular disease.
- Intracardiac left-to-right shunting.
- Extracardiac shunting.

Nonischemic dilated cardiomyopathy:
- Familial/genetic disorders.
- Toxic/drug-induced damage
- Immunologically mediated necrosis.
- Infectious agents.
- Metabolic disorders.
- Infiltrative processes.
- Idiopathic conditions.

IMPAIRED DIASTOLIC FUNCTION (RESTRICTED FILLING, INCREASED STIFFNESS)

Pathologic myocardial hypertrophy:
- Primary (hypertrophic cardiomyopathies).
- Secondary (hypertension).

Aging.
Ischemic fibrosis.
Restrictive cardiomyopathy:
- Infiltrative disorders (amyloidosis, sarcoidosis).
- Storage diseases (hemochromatosis, genetic abnormalities).

Endomyocardial disorders.

MECHANICAL ABNORMALITIES

Intracardiac:
- Obstructive valvular disease.
- Regurgitant valvular disease.
- Intracardiac shunts.
- Other congenital abnormalities.

Extracardiac:
- Obstructive (coarctation, supravalvular aortic stenosis).
- Left-to-right shunting (patent ductus arteriosus).

DISORDERS OF RATE AND RHYTHM

Bradyarrhythmias (sinus node dysfunction, conduction abnormalities).
Tachyarrhythmias (ineffective rhythms, chronic tachycardia).

PULMONARY HEART DISEASE

Cor pulmonale.
Pulmonary vascular disorders.

HIGH-OUTPUT STATES

Metabolic disorders:
Thyrotoxicosis.
Nutritional disorders (beriberi).
Excessive blood flow requirements:
- Chronic anemia.
- Systemic arteriovenous shunting.

HEART FAILURE, PREGNANCY

ICD-9CM # 428.90
ICD-10CM # I50.9 Heart failure, unspecified

Congenital valvular heart disease exacerbated by pregnancy.
Peripartum cardiomyopathy.
Untreated thyrotoxicosis.
Hypothyroidism.
Pulmonary hypertension.
Myocardial infarction.

HEAT STROKE[1]

ICD-9CM # 992
ICD-10CM # T67.0 Heatstroke and sunstroke

Sepsis.
Encephalitis.
Meningitis.
Brain abscess.
Malaria (cerebral falciparum).
Typhoid fever.
Tetanus.
Alcohol withdrawal syndrome.
Neuroleptic malignant syndrome (see Tips and Tricks box).
Anticholinergic toxicity.
Salicylate toxicity.
Phencyclidine hydrochloride (PCP), cocaine, or amphetamine toxicity.
Status epilepticus.
Cerebral hemorrhage.
Diabetic ketoacidosis.
Thyroid storm.

HEEL PAIN

ICD-9CM # varies with specific diagnosis
ICD-10CM # M25.50 Pain in unspecified joint

Achilles tendonitis/tendinopathy (insertional, noninsertional).
Retrocalcaneal bursitis (superficial, deep).
Plantar fasciopathy.
Neuropathy (tarsal tunnel, posterior tibial nerve [medial calcaneal branch], abductor digiti quinti).
Calcaneal stress fracture.
Puncture wound, foreign body.
Cellulitis.
Spondyloarthropathy.
Fat pad atrophy.
Soft tissue tumor.

S1 radiculopathy.
Paget's disease of bone.
Haglund deformity.
Primary or metastatic bone tumor.

HEEL PAIN, PLANTAR[24]

ICD-9CM # 729.5
ICD-10CM # M79.609 Pain in unspecified limb

SKIN

Keratoses.
Verruca.
Ulcer.
Fissure.

CONNECTIVE TISSUE

Fat
Atrophy.
Panniculitis.
Dense Connective Tissue
Inflammatory fasciitis.
Fibromatosis.
Enthesopathy.
Bursitis.
Bone (Calcaneus)
Stress fracture.
Paget's disease.
Benign bone cyst/tumor.
Malignant bone tumor.
Metabolic bone disease (osteopenia).
Nerve
Tarsal tunnel.
Plantar nerve entrapment.
S1 nerve root radiculopathy.
Painful peripheral neuropathy.

INFECTION

Dermatomycoses.
Acute osteomyelitis.
Plantar abscess.

MISCELLANEOUS

Foreign body.
Nonunion calcaneus fracture.
Psychogenic.
Idiopathic.

HEMARTHROSIS

ICD-9CM # 848.9 Hemarthrosis (Sprain) NOS
ICD-10CM # T14.90 Injury, unspecified

Trauma.
Anticoagulant therapy.
Thrombocytopenia, thrombocytosis.
Bleeding disorders (e.g., von Willebrand's disease).
Charcot's joint.
Idiopathic.
Other: pigmented villonodular synovitis, hemangioma, synovioma, AV fistula, ruptured aneurysm.

HEMATEMESIS[38]

ICD-9CM # 578.0
ICD-10CM # K92.0 Hematemesis

CAUSES OF HEMATEMESIS

Very Common
Gastric or duodenal ulcer or erosions.
Common
Mallory-Weiss tear (a laceration at the gastroesophageal junction).
Ulcerative esophagitis.
Esophageal varices.
Uncommon
Vascular malformations.
Ulcerated gastrointestinal stromal tumor.
Carcinoma of esophagus or stomach.
Aortoenteric fistula.

HEMATURIA

ICD-9CM # 599.7 Hematuria, Benign (Essential)
ICD-10CM # R31.9 Hematuria, unspecified

Use the mnemonic TICS:
T (trauma): blow to kidney, insertion of Foley catheter or foreign body in urethra, prolonged and severe exercise, very rapid emptying of overdistended bladder.
(tumor): hypernephroma, Wilms' tumor, papillary carcinoma of the bladder, prostatic and urethral neoplasms.
(toxins): turpentine, phenols, sulfonamides and other antibiotics, cyclophosphamide, NSAIDs.
I (infections): glomerulonephritis, TB, cystitis, prostatitis, urethritis, *Schistosoma haematobium,* yellow fever, blackwater fever.
(inflammatory processes): Goodpasture's syndrome, periarteritis, postirradiation.
C (calculi): renal, ureteral, bladder, urethra.
(cysts): simple cysts, polycystic disease.
(congenital anomalies): hemangiomas, aneurysms, AVM.
S (surgery): invasive procedures, prostatic resection, cystoscopy.
(sickle cell disease and other hematologic disturbances): hemophilia, thrombocytopenia, anticoagulants.
(somewhere else): bleeding genitals, factitious (drug addicts).

HEMATURIA, DIFFERENTIAL BASED ON AGE AND SEX

ICD-9CM # 599.7 Hematuria Benign (Essential) other codes vary with cause
ICD-10CM # R31.9 Hematuria, unspecified

0 TO 20 YR

Acute urinary tract infections.
Acute glomerulonephritis.
Congenital urinary tract anomalies with obstruction.
Trauma to genitals.

20 TO 40 YR

Acute urinary tract infection.
Trauma to genitals.
Urolithiasis.
Bladder cancer.

40 TO 60 YR (WOMEN)

Acute urinary tract infection.
Bladder cancer.
Urolithiasis.

40 TO 60 YR (MEN)

Acute urinary tract infection.
Bladder cancer.
Urolithiasis.

60 YR AND OLDER (WOMEN)

Acute urinary tract infection.
Bladder cancer.
Vaginal trauma or irritation.
Urolithiasis.

60 YR AND OLDER (MEN)

Acute urinary tract infection.
Benign prostatic hyperplasia.
Bladder cancer.
Urolithiasis.
Trauma.

HEMATURIA, IN CHILDREN[2]

ICD-9CM # 599.7
ICD-10CM # R31.9 Hematuria, unspecified

EXTRARENAL

Trauma.
Meatal stenosis or posterior urethral valves.
Exercise.
Menstruation or rectal bleeding.
Foreign bodies.
Cystitis, urethritis, or epididymitis.

INTRARENAL

Pyelonephritis.
Renal or bladder stones or tumors.
Poststrepotococcal or idiopathic glomerulonephritis.
Acute interstitial nephritis.
Acute tubular necrosis.
Basement membrane glomerular disease.
Renal vein or arterial thrombosis.
Recurrent familial hematuria.
Polycystic kidney disease.

SYSTEMIC

Henoch-Schönlein purpura.
Systemic lupus erythematosus.
Hemolytic-uremic syndrome.
Infectious mononucleosis.
Sickle cell disease or other hemoglobinopathies.
Bacterial endocarditis or artificial cardiac valves.
Bleeding disorders, warfarin, or aspirin.
Medications such as amitriptyline or chlorpromazine, radiocontrast dyes.
Munchausen syndrome or factitious.

HEMIPARESIS/HEMIPLEGIA

ICD-9CM # 436.0 Acquired Due to Acute CVA, Flaccid
436.1 Acquired Due to CVA, Acute, Spastic

ICD-10CM # G81.00 Flaccid hemiplegia affecting unspecified side
G81.10 Spastic hemiplegia affecting unspecified side

CVA.
Transient ischemic attack.
Cerebral neoplasm.
Multiple sclerosis or other demyelinating disorder.
CNS infection.
Migraine.
Hypoglycemia
Subdural hematoma.
Vasculitis.
Todd's paralysis.
Epidural hematoma.
Metabolic (hyperosmolar state, electrolyte imbalance).
Psychiatric disorders.
Congenital disorders.
Leukodystrophies.

HEMOLYSIS AND HEMOGLOBINURIA

ICD-9CM # 773.2 Hemolysis
791.2 Hemoglobinuria
ICD-10CM # P55.8 Other hemolytic diseases of newborn
P55.9 Hemolytic disease of newborn, unspecified
R82.3 Hemoglobinuria

Erythrocyte trauma (prosthetic cardiac valves, marching and severe trauma, extensive burns).
Infections (malaria, *Bartonella, Clostridium welchii*).
Brown recluse spider bite.
Incompatible blood transfusions.
Hemolytic-uremic syndrome.
Thrombotic thrombocytopenic purpura (TTP).
Paroxysmal nocturnal hemoglobinuria (PNH).
Drugs (penicillins, quinidine, methyldopa, sulfonamides, nitrofurantoin).
Erythrocyte enzyme deficiencies (e.g., exposure to fava beans in patients with glucose-6-phosphate dehydrogenase deficiency).

HEMOLYSIS, INTRAVASCULAR

ICD-9CM # 283.2
ICD-10CM # D59.6 Hemoglobinuria due to hemolysis from other external causes
D59.8 Other acquired hemolytic anemias

Infections.
Exertional hemolysis (e.g., prolonged march).
Valve hemolysis.
Microangiopathic hemolytic anemia.
Osmotic and chemical agents.
Thermal injury.
Cold agglutinins.
Venoms (snakes, spiders).
Paroxysmal nocturnal hemoglobinuria (PNH).

HEMOLYSIS, MECHANICAL

ICD-9CM # 283.19
ICD-10CM # D59.4 Other nonautoimmune hemolytic anemias

Prosthetic heart valves.
Aortic stenosis.
Malignant hypertension.
Metastatic adenocarcinoma.
Traumatic exercise.
Renal transplants.
Renal cortical necrosis.
Glomerulonephritis.
Thrombotic thrombocytopenic purpura (TTP), hemolytic-uremic syndrome (HUS).
Renal vasculitis.
Scleroderma.
Diabetes.

HEMOPERITONEUM

ICD-9CM # 568.81
ICD-10CM # K66.1 Hemoperitoneum

Ruptured Graafian follicle.
Ruptured spleen.
Ectopic pregnancy.
Traumatic laceration of liver.
Ruptured aneurysm.
Ruptured bladder.
Traumatic laceration of bowel, pancreas, uterus.

HEMOPTYSIS

ICD-9CM # 786.3
ICD-10CM # R04.2 Hemoptysis

CARDIOVASCULAR

Pulmonary embolism/infarction.
Left ventricular failure.
Mitral stenosis.
AV fistula.
Severe hypertension.
Erosion of aortic aneurysm.

PULMONARY

Neoplasm (primary or metastatic).
Infection.
Pneumonia: *Streptococcus pneumoniae, Klebsiella pneumoniae, Staphylococcus aureus, Legionella pneumophila.*
Bronchiectasis.
Abscess.
TB.
Bronchitis.
Fungal infections (aspergillosis, coccidioidomycosis).
Parasitic infections (amebiasis, ascariasis, paragonimiasis).
Vasculitis: Wegener's granulomatosis, Churg-Strauss syndrome, Henoch-Schönlein purpura.
Goodpasture's syndrome.
Trauma (needle biopsy, foreign body, right-sided heart catheterization, prolonged and severe cough).
Cystic fibrosis, bullous emphysema.
Pulmonary sequestration.
Pulmonary AV fistula.
SLE.
Idiopathic pulmonary hemosiderosis.
Drugs: aspirin, anticoagulants, penicillamine.
Pulmonary hypertension.
Mediastinal fibrosis.

OTHER

Epistaxis, trauma.
Laryngeal bleeding (laryngitis, laryngeal neoplasm).
Hematologic disorders (clotting abnormalities, DIC, thrombocytopenia).

HEPATIC CYSTS[36]

ICD-9CM # 751.62 Hepatic Cyst, Congenital
122.8 *Echinococcus* Infection, Liver
ICD-10CM # Q44.6 Cystic disease of liver
B67.8 Echinococcosis, unspecified, of liver

CONGENITAL HEPATIC CYSTS

Parenchymal: solitary cyst, polycystic disease.
Ductal: localized dilatation, multiple cystic dilatations of intrahepatic ducts (Caroli's disease).

ACQUIRED HEPATIC CYSTS

Inflammatory cysts: retention cysts, echinococcal cyst, amebic cyst.
Neoplastic cyst.
Peliosis hepatis.

HEPATIC GRANULOMAS[1a]

ICD-9CM # 572.8
ICD-10CM # K75.3 Granulomatous hepatitis

INFECTIONS

Bacterial, spirochetal: TB and atypical mycobacterial infections, tularemia, brucellosis, leprosy, syphilis, Whipple's disease, listeriosis.
Viral: mononucleosis, CMV.
Rickettsial: Q fever.
Fungal: coccidioidomycosis, histoplasmosis, cryptococcal infections, actinomycosis, aspergillosis, nocardiosis.
Parasitic: schistosomiasis, clonorchiasis, toxocariasis, ascariasis, toxoplasmosis, amebiasis.

HEPATOBILIARY DISORDERS

Primary biliary cirrhosis, granulomatous hepatitis, jejunoileal bypass.

SYSTEMIC DISORDERS

Sarcoidosis, Wegener's granulomatosis, inflammatory bowel disease, Hodgkin's disease, lymphoma.

DRUGS/TOXINS

Beryllium, parenteral foreign material (starch, talc, silicone, etc.), phenylbutazone, a-methyldopa, procainamide, allopurinol, phenytoin, nitrofurantoin, hydralazine.

HEPATITIS, ACUTE[25a]

ICD-9CM # varies with specific disorder
ICD-10CM # B17.8 Acute viral hepatitis, unspecified
B15 Acute hepatitis A

B16	Acute hepatitis B
B17.1	Acute hepatitis C
B17.2	Acute hepatitis E

Infectious:
- Hepatitis A, B, C, D, G.
- Epstein-Barr virus.
- Cytomegalovirus.
- Herpes simplex virus.
- Yellow fever.
- Leptospirosis.
- Q fever.
- HIV.
- Brucellosis.
- Lyme disease.
- Syphilis.

Noninfectious:
- Drug induced.
- Autoimmune.
- Ischemic.
- Acute fatty liver of pregnancy.
- Acute Budd-Chiari syndrome.
- Wilson's disease.

HEPATITIS, CHRONIC[25a]

ICD-9CM #	571.40	Hepatitis, Noninfectious, Chronic
	072.22	Hepatitis B, Chronic
	070.44	Hepatitis C, Chronic
ICD-10CM #	K73.9	Chronic hepatitis, unspecified
	B18.0	Chronic viral hepatitis B with delta-agent
	B18.2	Chronic viral hepatitis C

Chronic viral hepatitis:
- Hepatitis B.
- Hepatitis C.
- Hepatitis D.

Autoimmune hepatitis and variant syndromes.
Hereditary hemochromatosis.
Wilson's disease.
α_1-Antitrypsin deficiency.
Fatty liver and nonalcoholic steatohepatitis.
Alcoholic liver disease.
Drug-induced liver disease.
Hepatic granulomas:
- Infectious.
- Drug induced.
- Neoplastic.
- Idiopathic.

HEPATITIS, IN CHILDREN[22a]

ICD-9CM #	varies with specific diagnosis	
ICD-10CM #	B17.9	Acute viral hepatitis, unspecified
	K73.9	Chronic hepatitis, unspecified

CAUSES AND DIFFERENTIAL DIAGNOSIS OF HEPATITIS IN CHILDREN

Infectious

Hepatotropic viruses:
- HAV.
- HBV.
- HCV.
- HDV.
- HEV.
- Hepatitis non–A-E viruses.

Systemic infection that can include hepatitis:
- Adenovirus.
- Arbovirus.
- Coxsackievirus.
- Cytomegalovirus.
- Enterovirus.
- Epstein-Barr virus.
- "Exotic" viruses (e.g., yellow fever).
- Herpes simplex virus.
- Human immunodeficiency virus.
- Paramyxovirus.
- Rubella.
- Varicella zoster.

Other.

Nonviral liver infections

Abscess.
Amebiasis.
Bacterial sepsis.
Brucellosis.
Fitz-Hugh-Curtis syndrome.
Histoplasmosis.
Leptospirosis.
Tuberculosis.
Other.

Autoimmune

Autoimmune hepatitis.
Sclerosing cholangitis.
Other (e.g., systemic lupus erythematosus, juvenile rheumatoid arthritis).

Metabolic

α1-Antitrypsin deficiency.
Tyrosinemia.
Wilson disease.
Other.

Toxic

Iatrogenic or drug induced (e.g., acetaminophen).
Environmental (e.g., pesticides).

Anatomic

Choledochal cyst.
Biliary atresia.
Other.

Hemodynamic

Shock.
Congestive heart failure.
Budd-Chiari syndrome.
Other.

Nonalcoholic Fatty Liver Disease

Idiopathic.
Reye syndrome.
Other.

HEPATOMEGALY

ICD-9CM #	789.1	
ICD-10CM #	R16.0	Hepatomegaly, not elsewhere classified

FREQUENT JAUNDICE

Infectious hepatitis.
Toxic hepatitis.
Carcinoma: liver, pancreas, bile ducts, metastatic neoplasm to liver.
Cirrhosis.
Obstruction of common bile duct.
Alcoholic hepatitis.
Biliary cirrhosis.
Cholangitis.
Hemochromatosis with cirrhosis.

INFREQUENT JAUNDICE

CHF.
Amyloidosis.
Liver abscess.
Sarcoidosis.
Infectious mononucleosis.
Alcoholic fatty infiltration.
Nonalcoholic steatohepatitis.
Lymphoma.
Leukemia.
Budd-Chiari syndrome.
Myelofibrosis with myeloid metaplasia.
Familial hyperlipoproteinemia type 1.
Other: amebiasis, hydatid disease of liver, schistosomiasis, kala-azar *(Leishmania donovani),* Hurler's syndrome, Gaucher's disease, kwashiorkor.

HEPATOMEGALY, BY SHAPE OF LIVER[38]

ICD-9CM #	789.1	
ICD-10CM #	R16.0	Hepatomegaly, not elsewhere classified

DIFFUSELY ENLARGED AND SMOOTH

Massive

Metastatic disease.
Alcoholic liver disease with fatty infiltration.
Myeloproliferative diseases (e.g., polycythemia rubra vera, myelofibrosis).

Moderate

The above causes.
Hemochromatosis.
Hematologic disease (e.g., chronic myeloid leukemia, lymphoma).
Fatty liver (e.g., diabetes mellitus, obesity).
Infiltrative disorders (e.g., amyloid).

Mild

The above causes.
Hepatitis (viral, drugs).
Cirrhosis.
Biliary obstruction.
Granulomatous disorders (e.g., sarcoid).
HIV infection.

DIFFUSELY ENLARGED AND IRREGULAR

Metastatic disease.
Cirrhosis.
Hydatid disease.
Polycystic liver disease.

LOCALIZED SWELLINGS

Riedel's lobe (a normal variant—the lobe may be palpable in the right lumbar region).
Metastasis.
Large simple hepatic cyst.
Hydatid cyst.
Hepatoma.
Liver abscess (e.g., amebic abscess).

HERMAPHRODITISM[4]

ICD-9CM # 752.7 Hermaphroditism, Congenital
ICD-10CM # Q56.3 Pseudohermaphroditism, unspecified
Q56.4 Indeterminate sex, unspecified

FEMALE PSEUDOHERMAPHRODITISM

Androgen exposure:
- Fetal source:
  - 21-Hydroxylase (P450 c21) deficiency.
  - 11β-Hydroxylase (P450 c11) deficiency.
  - 3β-Hydroxysteroid dehydrogenase II (3β-HSD II) deficiency.
  - Aromatase (P450arom) deficiency.
- Maternal source.
- Virilizing ovarian tumor.
- Virilizing adrenal tumor.
- Androgenic drugs.

Undetermined origin:
- Associated with genitourinary and GI tract defects.

MALE PSEUDOHERMAPHRODITISM

Defects in testicular differentiation:
- Denys-Drash syndrome (mutation in WT1 gene).
- WAGR syndrome (*W*ilms tumor, *a*niridia, *g*enitourinary malformation, *r*etardation).
- Deletion of 11p13.
- Camptomelic syndrome (autosomal gene at 17q24.3-q25.1) and SOX 9 mutation.
- XY pure gonadal dysgenesis (Swyer syndrome).
  - Mutation in SRY gene.
  - Unknown cause.
- XY gonadal agenesis.

Deficiency of testicular hormones:
- Leydig cell aplasia.
- Mutation in LH receptor.
- Lipoid adrenal hyperplasia (P450 scc) deficiency; mutation in StAR (steroidogenic acute regulatory protein).
- 3α-HSD II deficiency.
- 17-Hydroxylase/17, 20-lyase (P450 c17) deficiency.
- Persistent Müllerian duct syndrome.
  - Gene mutations, Müllerian-inhibiting substance (MIS).
  - Receptor defects for MIS.

Defect in androgen action:
- 5α-Reductase II mutations.
- Androgen receptor defects:
  - Complete androgen insensitivity syndrome.
  - Partial androgen insensitivity syndrome.
  - Reifenstein and other syndromes.
  - Smith-Lemli-Opitz syndrome.

Defect in conversion of 7-dehydrocholesterol to cholesterol.

TRUE HERMAPHRODITISM

XX.
XY.
XX/XY chimeras.

HICCUPS[21]

ICD-9CM # 786.8
ICD-10CM # R06.6 Hiccough

TRANSIENT HICCUPS

Sudden excitement, emotion.
Gastric distention.
Esophageal obstruction.
Alcohol ingestion.
Sudden change in temperature.

PERSISTENT OR CHRONIC HICCUPS

Toxic/metabolic: uremia, DM, hyperventilation, hypocalcemia, hypokalemia, hyponatremia, gout, fever.
Drugs: benzodiazepines, steroids, α-methyldopa, barbiturates.
Surgery/general anesthesia.
Thoracic/diaphragmatic disorders: pneumonia, lung cancer, asthma, pleuritis, pericarditis, myocardial infarction, aortic aneurysm, esophagitis, esophageal obstruction, diaphragmatic hernia or irritation.
Abdominal disorders: gastric ulcer or cancer, hepatobiliary or pancreatic disease, IBD, bowel obstruction, intraabdominal or subphrenic abscess, prostatic infection or cancer.
Central nervous system disorders: traumatic, infectious, vascular, structural.
Ear, nose, and throat disorders: pharyngitis, laryngitis, tumor, irritation of auditory canal.
Psychogenic disorders.
Idiopathic disorders.

HILAR AND MEDIASTINAL LYMPH NODE ENLARGEMENT[14a]

ICD-9CM # 85.6
ICD-10CM # R59.0 Mediastinal adenopathy

DISORDERS ASSOCIATED WITH HILAR AND MEDIASTINAL LYMPH NODE ENLARGEMENT

Sarcoidosis.
Lymphoma.
Fungal disease.
Tuberculosis.
Metastatic cancer.
Silicosis, coal worker's pneumoconiosis, beryllium lung.

HIP PAIN, CHILDREN[26]

ICD-9CM # 959.6 Hip Injury
719.95 Hip Joint Disorder
843.9 Hip Strain
ICD-10CM # S79.819A Other specified injuries of unspecified hip, initial encounter
S79.829A Other specified injuries of unspecified thigh, initial encounter
S79.919A Unspecified injury of unspecified hip, initial encounter

TRAUMA

Hip or pelvis fractures.
Overuse injuries.

INFECTION

Septic arthritis.
Osteomyelitis.

INFLAMMATION

Transient synovitis.
Juvenile RA.
Rheumatic fever.

NEOPLASM

Leukemia.
Osteogenic or Ewing's sarcoma.
Metastatic disease.

HEMATOLOGIC DISORDERS

Hemophilia.
Sickle cell anemia.

MISCELLANEOUS

Legg-Calvé-Perthes disease.
Slipped capital femoral epiphysis.

HIP PAIN, DIFFERENTIAL DIAGNOSIS[18b]

ICD-9CM # varies with specific diagnosis
ICD-10CM # M25.559 Pain in unspecified hip

ARTICULAR

Inflammatory joint diseases.
- Rheumatoid arthritis.
- Spondyloarthropathies.
- Polymyalgia rheumatica.

Degenerative joint disease.
- Primary osteoarthritis.
- Secondary osteoarthritis.

Metabolic joint diseases.
- Gout.
- Pseudogout.
- Ochronosis.
- Hemochromatosis.
- Wilson's disease.
- Acromegaly.

Femoroacetabular impingement.
Acetabular labral tear.
Infections.
Tumors.
- Benign.
  - Pigmented villonodular sclerosis.
  - Osteochondromatosis.
- Malignant.
  - Synovial sarcoma.
  - Synovial metastasis.

Hemarthrosis.
In children:
- Toxic synovitis.
- Juvenile chronic arthritis.

REFERRED PAIN

Thoracolumbar spine.
Intraabdominal structures.
Retroperitoneal structures.

PERIARTICULAR

Bursitis.
- Trochanteric.
- Iliopsoas.
- Ischiogluteal.

Tendinitis.
- Trochanteric.
- Adductor.

Acute calcific periarthritis.
Heterotropic ossification.

OSSEOUS

Bone lesions.
Fractures.
Neoplasms.
Infection.
Osteonecrosis of the femoral head.
Paget's disease.
Metabolic bone disease.
Stress fracture.
Transient osteoporosis.
In children:
- Congenital dislocation of the hip.
- Acetabular dysplasia.
- Coxa vara.
- Slipped capital femoral epiphysis.
- Legg-Calvé-Perthes disease.
- Rickets.

NEUROLOGIC

Entrapment neuropathies.
Lateral femoral cutaneous nerve (meralgia paresthetica).
Lumbar nerve root compression.
L2, L3, and L4.

VASCULAR

Atherosclerosis of aorta, iliac vessels.

HIP PAIN, IN DIFFERENT AGE GROUPS[8]

ICD-9CM # 719.45
ICD-10CM # M25.559 Pain in unspecified hip

COMMON CAUSES OF HIP PAIN IN DIFFERENT AGE GROUPS

Childhood (2-10 yr)
Intraarticular:
Developmental dislocation of the hip.
Perthes' disease.
Irritable hip.
Rickets.
Periarticular:
Osteomyelitis.
Referred:
Abdominal.

Adolescence (10-18 yr)
Intraarticular:
Slipped upper femoral epiphysis.
Torn labrum.
Periarticular:
Trochanteric bursitis.
Snapping hip.
Osteomyelitis.
Tumors.
Referred:
Abdominal.
Lumbar spine.

Early Adulthood (18-30 yr)
Intraarticular:
Inflammatory arthritis.
Torn labrum.
Periarticular:
Bursitis.
Referred:
Abdominal.
Lumbar spine.

Adulthood (30-50 yr)
Intraarticular:
Osteoarthritis.
Inflammatory arthritis.
Osteonecrosis.
Transient osteoporosis.
Periarticular:
Bursitis.
Referred:
Abdominal.
Lumbar spine.

Old Age (>50 yr)
Intraarticular:
Osteoarthritis.
Inflammatory arthritis.
Referred:
Abdominal.
Lumbar spine.

HIP PAIN WITHOUT OBVIOUS FRACTURE[2]

ICD-9CM # 338
ICD-10CM # R52 Pain, unspecified
M25.559 Pain in unspecified hip

DIFFERENTIAL DIAGNOSIS OF A PAINFUL HIP WITHOUT OBVIOUS FRACTURE

Referred pain (lumbar spine, hip, or knee).
Avascular necrosis of the femoral head.
Degenerative joint disease or osteoarthritis.
Herniation of a lumbar disk.
Diskitis.
Toxic synovitis of the hip.
Septic arthritis.
Bursitis.
Tendonitis.
Ligamentous injuries of the knee or hip.
Occult fracture.
Slipped capital femoral epiphysis.
Perthes' disease.
Tumor (lymphoma).
Deep venous thrombosis.
Arterial insufficiency.
Osteomyelitis.
Iliopsoas abscess.
Retroperitoneal hematoma.
Inguinal hernia.
Inguinal lymphadenopathy.
Genitourinary complaints.
Sports-related hernia.

HIRSUTISM

ICD-9CM # 704.1
ICD-10CM # L68.0 Hirsutism

Idiopathic: familial, possibly increased sensitivity to androgens.
Menopause.
Polycystic ovarian syndrome.
Drugs: androgens, anabolic steroids, methyltestosterone, minoxidil, diazoxide, phenytoin, glucocorticoids, cyclosporine.
Congenital adrenal hyperplasia.
Adrenal virilizing tumor.
Ovarian virilizing tumor: arrhenoblastoma, hilus cell tumor.
Pituitary adenoma.
Cushing's syndrome.
Hypothyroidism (congenital and juvenile).
Acromegaly.
Testicular feminization.

HIV INFECTION, ANORECTAL LESIONS[26]

ICD-9CM # 042 HIV Infection, Symptomatic
V08 HIV Infection, Asymptomatic
ICD-10CM # B20 Human immunodeficiency virus [HIV] disease
Z21 Asymptomatic human immunodeficiency virus [HIV] infection status

COMMON CONDITIONS

Anal fissure.
Abscess and fistula.
Hemorrhoids.
Pruritus ani.
Pilonidal disease.

COMMON STDs

Gonorrhea.
Chlamydia.
Herpes.
Chancroid.
Syphilis.
Condylomata acuminata.

ATYPICAL CONDITIONS

Infectious: TB, CMV, actinomycosis, cryptococcus.
Neoplastic: lymphoma, Kaposi's sarcoma, squamous cell carcinoma.
Other: idiopathic and ulcer.

HIV INFECTION, CHEST RADIOGRAPHIC ABNORMALITIES[26]

ICD-9CM # 042 HIV Infection, Symptomatic
V08 HIV Infection, Asymptomatic
ICD-10CM # B20 Human immunodeficiency virus [HIV] disease
Z21 Asymptomatic human immunodeficiency virus [HIV] infection status

DIFFUSE INTERSTITIAL INFILTRATION

Pneumocystis jiroveci.
Cytomegalovirus.
Mycobacterium tuberculosis.
Mycobacterium avium complex.
Histoplasmosis.
Coccidioidomycosis.
Lymphoid interstitial pneumonitis.

FOCAL CONSOLIDATION

Bacterial pneumonia.
Mycoplasma pneumoniae.
Pneumocystis jiroveci.
Mycobacterium tuberculosis.
Mycobacterium avium complex.

NODULAR LESIONS

Kaposi's sarcoma.
Mycobacterium tuberculosis.
Mycobacterium avium complex.
Fungal lesions.
Toxoplasmosis.

CAVITARY LESIONS

Pneumocystis jiroveci.
Mycobacterium tuberculosis.
Bacterial infection.

PLEURAL EFFUSION

Kaposi's sarcoma.
(Small effusion may be associated with any infection).

ADENOPATHY

Kaposi's sarcoma.
Lymphoma.
Mycobacterium tuberculosis.
Cryptococcus.

PNEUMOTHORAX

Kaposi's sarcoma.

HIV INFECTION, COGNITIVE IMPAIRMENT[25a]

ICD-9CM # 042 HIV Infection, Symptomatic
ICD-10CM # B20 Human immunodeficiency virus [HIV] disease

EARLY TO MID-STAGE HIV DISEASE

Depression.
Alcohol and substance abuse.
Medication-induced cognitive impairment.
Metabolic encephalopathies.
HIV-related cognitive impairment.

ADVANCED HIV DISEASE (CD4+ <100/MM^3)

Opportunistic infection of CNS.
Neurosyphilis.
CNS lymphoma.
Progressive multifocal leukoencephalopathy.
Depression.
Metabolic encephalopathies.
Medication-induced cognitive impairment.
Stroke.
HIV dementia.

HIV INFECTION, CUTANEOUS MANIFESTATIONS[21]

ICD-9CM # 042 HIV Infection, Symptomatic
V08 HIV Infection, Asymptomatic
ICD-10CM # B20 Human immunodeficiency virus [HIV] disease
Z21 Asymptomatic human immunodeficiency virus [HIV] infection status

BACTERIAL INFECTION

Bacillary angiomatosis: Numerous angiomatous nodules associated with fever, chills, weight loss.
Staphylococcus aureus: Folliculitis, ecthyma, impetigo, bullous impetigo, furuncles, carbuncles.
Syphilis: May occur in different forms (primary, secondary, tertiary); chancre may become painful because of secondary infection.

FUNGAL INFECTION

Candidiasis: Mucous membranes (oral, vulvovaginal), less commonly candida intertrigo or paronychia.
Cryptococcoses: Papules or nodules that strongly resemble molluscum contagiosum; other forms include pustules, purpuric papules, and vegetating plaques.
Seborrheic dermatitis: Scaling and erythema in the hair-bearing areas (eyebrows, scalp, chest, and pubic area).

ARTHROPOD INFESTATIONS

Scabies: Pruritus with or without rash, usually generalized but can be limited to a single digit.

VIRAL INFECTION

Herpes simplex: Vesicular lesion in clusters; perianal, genital, orofacial, or digital; can be disseminated.
Herpes zoster: Painful dermatomal vesicles that may ulcerate or disseminate.
HIV: Discrete erythematous macules and papules on the upper trunk, palms, and soles are the most characteristic cutaneous finding of acute HIV infection.
Human papillomavirus: Genital warts (may become unusually extensive).
Kaposi's sarcoma (herpesvirus): Erythematous macules or papules; enlarge at varying rates; violaceous nodules or plaques; occasionally painful.
Molluscum contagiosum: Discrete umbilicated papules commonly on the face, neck, and intertriginous sites (axilla, groin, or buttocks).

NONINFECTIOUS

Drug reactions: More frequent and severe in HIV patients.
Nutritional deficiencies: Mainly seen in children and patients with chronic diarrhea; diffuse skin manifestations, depending upon the deficiency.
Psoriasis: Scaly lesions; diffuse or localized; can be associated with arthritis.
Vasculitis: Palpable purpuric eruption (can resemble septic emboli).

HIV INFECTION, ESOPHAGEAL DISEASE

ICD-9CM # varies with specific diagnosis
ICD-10CM # B20 Human immunodeficiency virus [HIV] disease
K21.9 Gastro-esophageal reflux disease without esophagitis

Candida infection.
Cytomegalovirus infection.
Aphthous ulcer.
Herpes simplex.

HIV INFECTION, HEPATIC DISEASE[25a]

ICD-9CM # 042 HIV Infection, Symptomatic
ICD-10CM # B20 Human immunodeficiency virus [HIV] disease

VIRUSES

Hepatitis A.
Hepatitis B.
Hepatitis C.
Hepatitis D (with HBV).
Epstein-Barr virus.
Cytomegalovirus.
Herpes simplex virus.
Adenovirus.
Varicella-zoster virus.

MYCOBACTERIA

Mycobacterium avium complex.
Mycobacterium tuberculosis.

FUNGI

Histoplasma capsulatum.
Cryptococcus neoformans.

Coccidioides immitis.
Candida albicans.
Pneumocystis jiroveci.
Penicillium marneffei.

PROTOZOA

Toxoplasma gondii.
Cryptosporidium parvum.
Microsporida.
Schistosoma.

BACTERIA

Bartonella henselae (peliosis hepatis).

MALIGNANCY

Kaposi's sarcoma (HHV-8).
Non-Hodgkin's lymphoma.
Hepatocellular carcinoma.

MEDICATIONS

Zidovudine.
Didanosine.
Ritonavir.
Other HIV-1 protease inhibitors.
Fluconazole.
Macrolide antibiotics.
Isoniazid.
Rifampin.
Trimethoprim-sulfamethoxazole.

HIV INFECTION, LOWER GI TRACT DISEASE[25a]

ICD-9CM #	042	HIV Infection, Symptomatic
ICD-10CM #	B20	Human immunodeficiency virus [HIV] disease

CAUSES OF ENTEROCOLITIS

Bacteria
Campylobacter jejuni and other spp.
Salmonella spp.
Shigella flexneri.
Aeromonas hydrophila.
Plesiomonas shigelloides.
Yersinia enterocolitica.
Vibrio spp.
Mycobacterium avium complex.
Mycobacterium tuberculosis.
Escherichia coli (enterotoxigenic, enteroadherent).
Bacterial overgrowth.
Clostridium difficile (toxin).
Parasites
Cryptosporidium parvum.
Microsporida (*Enterocytozoon bieneusi, Septata intestinalis*).
Isospora belli.
Entamoeba histolytica.
Giardia lamblia.
Cyclospora cayetanensis.
Viruses
Cytomegalovirus.
Adenovirus.
Calicivirus.
Astrovirus.
Picobirnavirus.
Human immunodeficiency virus.
Fungi
Histoplasma capsulatum.

CAUSES OF PROCTITIS

Bacteria
Chlamydia trachomatis.
Neisseria gonorrhoeae.
Treponema pallidum.
Viruses
Herpes simplex.
Cytomegalovirus.

HIV INFECTION, OCULAR MANIFESTATIONS[36]

ICD-9CM #	042	HIV Infection, Symptomatic
	V08	HIV Infection, Asymptomatic
ICD-10CM #	B20	Human immunodeficiency virus [HIV] disease
	Z21	Asymptomatic human immunodeficiency virus [HIV] infection status

EYELIDS

Molluscum contagiosum.
Kaposi's sarcoma.

CORNEA/CONJUNCTIVA

Keratoconjunctivitis sicca.
Bacterial/fungal ulcerative keratitis.
Herpes simplex.
Herpes zoster ophthalmicus.
Conjunctival microvasculopathy.
Kaposi's sarcoma.

RETINA, CHOROID, AND VITREOUS

Microvasculopathy.
Endophthalmitis.
Cytomegalovirus retinitis.
Acute retinal necrosis.
Syphilis.
Toxoplasmosis.
Pneumocystis choroidopathy.
Cryptococcosis.
Mycobacterial infection.
Intraocular lymphoma.
Candidiasis.
Histoplasmosis.

DRUGS ASSOCIATED WITH OCULAR TOXICITY

Rifabutin.
Didanosine.

NEUROOPHTHALMIC

Disc edema.
Primary or secondary optic neuropathy.
Cranial nerve palsies.

ORBITAL

Lymphoma.
Infection.
Pseudotumor.

HIV INFECTION, PULMONARY DISEASE[25a]

ICD-9CM #	042	HIV Infection, Symptomatic
ICD-10CM #	B20	Human immunodeficiency virus [HIV] disease
	I28.8	Other diseases of pulmonary vessels

MYCOBACTERIAL

M. tuberculosis.
M. kansasii.
M. avium complex.
Other nontuberculous mycobacteria.

OTHER BACTERIAL

Streptococcus pneumoniae.
Staphylococcus aureus.
Haemophilus influenzae.
Enterobacteriaceae.
Pseudomonas aeruginosa.
Moraxella catarrhalis.
Group A *Streptococcus.*
Nocardia spp.
Rhodococcus equi.
Chlamydia pneumoniae.

FUNGAL

Pneumocystis carinii.
Cryptococcus neoformans.
Histoplasma capsulatum.
Coccidioides immitis.
Aspergillus spp.
Blastomyces dermatitidis.
Penicillium marneffei.

VIRAL

Cytomegalovirus.
Herpes simplex virus.
Adenovirus.
Respiratory syncytial virus.
Influenza viruses.
Parainfluenza virus.

OTHER

Toxoplasma gondii.
Strongyloides stercoralis.
Kaposi's sarcoma.
Lymphoma.
Lung cancer.
Lymphocytic interstitial pneumonitis.
Nonspecific interstitial pneumonitis.
Bronchiolitis obliterans with organizing pneumonia.
Pulmonary hypertension.
Emphysema-like or bullous disease.
Pneumothorax.
Congestive heart failure.
Diffuse alveolar damage.
Pulmonary embolus.

HOARSENESS

ICD-9CM #	784.49	
ICD-10CM #	R49.8	Other voice and resonance disorders

Allergic rhinitis.
Infections (laryngitis, epiglottitis, tracheitis, croup).
Vocal cord polyps.
Voice strain.
Irritants (tobacco smoke).
Vocal cord trauma (intubation, surgery).
Neoplastic involvement of vocal cord (primary or metastatic).
Neurologic abnormalities (multiple sclerosis, ALS, parkinsonism).
Endocrine abnormalities (puberty, menopause, hypothyroidism).
Other (laryngeal webs or cysts, psychogenic, muscle tension abnormalities).

HYDROCEPHALUS

ICD-9CM # 331.4
ICD-10CM # G91.1 Obstructive hydrocephalus

Head trauma.
Brain neoplasm (primary or metastatic).
Spinal cord tumor.
Cerebellar infarction.
Exudative or granulomatous meningitis.
Cerebellar hemorrhage.
Subarachnoid hemorrhage.
Aqueductal stenosis.
Third ventricle colloid cyst.
Hindbrain malformation.
Viral encephalitis.
Metastases to leptomeninges.

HYPERCALCEMIA

ICD-9CM # 275.42 Hypercalcemia Disorder
ICD-10CM # E83.52 Hypercalcemia

Malignancy: increased bone resorption via osteoclast-activating factors, secretion of PTH-like substances, prostaglandin E_2, direct erosion by tumor cells, transforming growth factors, colony-stimulating activity. Hypercalcemia is common in the following neoplasms:
- Solid tumors: breast, lung, pancreas, kidneys, ovary.
- Hematologic cancers: myeloma, lymphosarcoma, adult T-cell lymphoma, Burkitt's lymphoma.

Hyperparathyroidism: increased bone resorption, GI absorption, and renal absorption; etiology: Parathyroid hyperplasia, adenoma.
- Hyperparathyroidism or renal failure with secondary hyperparathyroidism.

Granulomatous disorders: increased GI absorption (e.g., sarcoidosis).
Paget's disease: increased bone resorption, seen only during periods of immobilization.
Vitamin D intoxication, milk-alkali syndrome; increased GI absorption.
Thiazides: increased renal absorption.
Other causes: familial hypocalciuric hypercalcemia, thyrotoxicosis, adrenal insufficiency, prolonged immobilization, vitamin A intoxication, recovery from acute renal failure, lithium administration, pheochromocytoma, disseminated SLE.

HYPERCALCEMIA, MALIGNANCY-INDUCED

ICD-9CM # 275.42
ICD-10CM # E83.52 Hypercalcemia

Lung carcinoma	(6% frequency, 35% of hypercalcemic cases)
Breast carcinoma	(10% frequency, 25% of hypercalcemic cases)
Multiple myeloma	(33% frequency, 10% of hypercalcemic cases)
Lymphoma	(4% of hypercalcemic cases)
Genitourinary cancer	(6% of hypercalcemic cases)

HYPERCAPNIA, PERSISTENT[36]

ICD-9CM # 786.09
ICD-10CM # R06.00 Dyspnea, unspecified
R06.09 Other forms of dyspnea
R06.89 Other abnormalities of breathing

Hypercapnia with normal lungs: CNS disturbances (CVA, parkinsonism, encephalitis), metabolic alkalosis, myxedema, primary alveolar hypoventilation, spinal cord lesions.
Diseases of the chest wall (e.g., kyphoscoliosis, ankylosing spondylitis).
Neuromuscular disorders (e.g., myasthenia gravis, Guillain-Barré syndrome, amyotrophic lateral sclerosis, muscular dystrophy, poliomyelitis).
COPD.

HYPERCOAGULABLE STATE, ASSOCIATED DISORDERS[20]

ICD-9CM # 289.82
ICD-10CM # D68.69 Other thrombophilia

Systemic lupus erythematosus in association with the presence of a lupus anticoagulant or antiphospholipid antibodies.
Malignancy:
- Disease-related: includes migratory superficial thrombophlebitis (Trousseau syndrome), nonbacterial thrombotic endocarditis, thrombosis associated with chronic DIC, thrombotic microangiopathy.
- Treatment-related: associated with the administration of various chemotherapeutic agents (L-asparaginase, mitomycin, some adjuvant chemotherapeutic agents for treatment of breast cancer, thalidomide or lenalidomide in conjunction with high doses of dexamethasone).

Infusion of prothrombin complex concentrates.
Nephrotic syndrome.
Heparin-induced thrombocytopenia.
Myeloproliferative disorders.
Paroxysmal nocturnal hemoglobinuria.

DIC, Disseminated intravascular coagulopathy.

HYPERGASTRINEMIA

ICD-9CM # varies with specific disorder
ICD-10CM # E16.4 Abnormal secretion of gastrin

Decreased gastrin release inhibition from medications (proton pump inhibitors [PPIs], H_2 receptor antagonists), vagotomy.
Chronic renal failure.
Hypochlorhydria due to atrophic gastritis, gastric carcinoma, pernicious anemia.
Gastrinoma (Zollinger-Ellison syndrome).
Pyloric obstruction.
Hyperplasia of antral G cells.
RA.

HYPERHIDROSIS[4]

ICD-9CM # 780.8 Hyperhidrosis
ICD-10CM # R61 Generalized hyperhidrosis

CORTICAL

Emotional.
Familial dysautonomia.
Congenital ichthyosiform erythroderma.
Epidermolysis bullosa.
Nail-patella syndrome.
Jadassohn-Lewandowsky syndrome.
Pachyonychia congenita.
Palmoplantar keratoderma.

HYPOTHALAMIC

Drugs
Antipyretics.
Emetics.
Insulin.
Meperidine.
Exercise Infection
Defervescence.
Chronic illness.
Metabolic
Debility.
DM.
Hyperpituitarism.
Hyperthyroidism.
Hypoglycemia.
Obesity.
Porphyria.
Pregnancy.
Rickets.
Infantile scurvy.
Cardiovascular
Heart failure.
Shock.
Vasomotor
Cold injury.
Raynaud phenomenon.
RA.
Neurologic
Abscess.
Familial dysautonomia.
Postencephalitic.
Tumor.
Miscellaneous
Chédiak-Higashi syndrome.
Compensatory.
Phenylketonuria.

Pheochromocytoma.
Vitiligo.
Medullary
Physiologic gustatory sweating.
Encephalitis.
Granulosis rubra nasi.
Syringomyelia.
Thoracic sympathetic trunk injury.
Spinal
Cord transection.
Syringomyelia.
Changes in Blood Flow
Mallucci syndrome.
Arteriovenous fistula.
Klippel-Trenaunay syndrome.
Glomus tumor.
Blue rubber bleb nevus syndrome.

HYPERKALEMIA

ICD-9CM # 276.7
ICD-10CM # E87.5 Hyperkalemia

Pseudohyperkalemia.
- Hemolyzed specimen.
- Severe thrombocytosis (platelet count 0.106 ml).
- Severe leukocytosis (white blood cell count 0.105 ml).
- Fist clenching during phlebotomy.

Excessive potassium intake (often in setting of impaired excretion).
- Potassium replacement therapy.
- High-potassium diet.
- Salt substitutes with potassium.
- Potassium salts of antibiotics.

Decreased renal excretion.
- Potassium-sparing diuretics (e.g., spironolactone, triamterene, amiloride).
- Renal insufficiency.
- Mineralocorticoid deficiency.
- Hyporeninemic hypoaldosteronism (DM).
- Tubular unresponsiveness to aldosterone (e.g., SLE, multiple myeloma, sickle cell disease).
- Type 4 RTA.
- ACE inhibitors.
- Heparin administration.
- NSAIDs.
- Trimethoprim-sulfamethoxazole.
- Beta-blockers.
- Pentamidine.

Redistribution (excessive cellular release).
- Acidemia (each 0.1 decrease in pH increases the serum potassium by 0.4 to 0.6 mEq/L). Lactic acidosis and ketoacidosis cause minimal redistribution.
- Insulin deficiency.
- Drugs (e.g., succinylcholine, markedly increased digitalis level, arginine, beta-adrenergic blockers).
- Hypertonicity.
- Hemolysis.
- Tissue necrosis, rhabdomyolysis, burns.
- Hyperkalemic periodic paralysis.

HYPERKALEMIA, DRUG-INDUCED[38b]

ICD-9CM # 276.7
ICD-10CM # E87.5 Hyperkalemia

IMPAIRED RENIN-ALDOSTERONE ELABORATION/FUNCTION

Cyclooxygenase inhibitors (NSAIDs).
β-Adrenergic antagonists.
Spironolactone.
Angiotensin-converting enzyme inhibitors and angiotensin II receptor blockers.
Heparin.

INHIBITORS OF RENAL POTASSIUM SECRETION

Potassium-sparing diuretics (amiloride, triamterene).
Trimethoprim.
Pentamidine.
Cyclosporine.
Digitalis overdose.
Lithium.

ALTERED POTASSIUM DISTRIBUTION

Insulin antagonists (somatostatin, diazoxide).
β-Adrenergic antagonists.
α-Adrenergic agonists.
Hypertonic solutions.
Digitalis.
Succinylcholine.
Arginine hydrochloride, lysine hydrochloride.

HYPERKINETIC MOVEMENT DISORDERS[30]

ICD-9CM # 314.8 Hyperkinetic Syndrome
275.1 Choreoathetosis
335.5 Hemiballism
333.7 Dystonia Due to Drugs
333.6 Dystonia, Idiopathic
ICD-10CM # F90.8 Attention-deficit hyperactivity disorder, other type
E83.00 Disorder of copper metabolism, unspecified
E83.01 Wilson's disease
E83.09 Other disorders of copper metabolism
G24.02 Drug induced acute dystonia
G24.1 Genetic torsion dystonia

Chorea, choreoathetosis: drug-induced, Huntington's chorea, Sydenham's chorea.
Tardive dyskinesia (e.g., phenothiazines).
Hemiballismus (lacunar CVA near subthalamic nuclei in basal ganglia, metastatic lesions, toxoplasmosis [in AIDS]).
Dystonia (idiopathic, familial, drug-induced [prochlorperazine, metoclopramide]), Wilson's disease.
Liver failure.
Thyrotoxicosis.
SLE, polycythemia.

HYPERMAGNESEMIA

ICD-9CM # 275.2
ICD-10CM # E83.40 Disorders of magnesium metabolism, unspecified
E83.41 Hypermagnesemia
E83.42 Hypomagnesemia
E83.49 Other disorders of magnesium metabolism

Renal failure (decreased GFR).
Decreased renal excretion secondary to salt depletion.
Abuse of antacids and laxatives containing magnesium in patients with renal insufficiency.
Endocrinopathies (deficiency of mineralocorticoid or thyroid hormone).
Increased tissue breakdown (rhabdomyolysis).
Redistribution: acute DKA, pheochromocytoma.
Other: lithium, volume depletion, familial hypocalciuric hypercalcemia.

HYPEROSTOSIS, CORTICAL BONE[16a]

ICD-9CM # varies with specific diagnosis
ICD-10CM # M48.19 Ankylosing hyperostosis [Forestier], multiple sites in spine

DISORDERS ASSOCIATED WITH HYPEROSTOSIS OF CORTICAL BONE

Progressive diaphyseal dysplasia.
Endosteal hyperostosis.
Pachydermoperiostosis.
Hypertrophic oseoarthropathy.
Thyroid acropachy.
Hypervitaminosis A.
Paget's disease.
Infantile cortical hyperostosis.

HYPERPHOSPHATEMIA

ICD-9CM # 275.3
ICD-10CM # E83.30 Disorder of phosphorus metabolism, unspecified

Excessive phosphate administration.
Excessive oral intake or IV administration.
Laxatives containing phosphate (phosphate tablets, phosphate enemas).
Decreased renal phosphate excretion.
Acute or chronic renal failure.
Hypoparathyroidism or pseudohypoparathyroidism.
Acromegaly, thyrotoxicosis.
Bisphosphonate therapy.
Tumor calcinosis.
Sickle cell anemia.
Transcellular shift out of cells.
Chemotherapy of lymphoma or leukemia, tumor lysis syndrome, hemolysis.
Acidosis.
Rhabdomyolysis, malignant hyperthermia.

Artifact: in vitro hemolysis.
Pseudohyperphosphatemia: hyperlipidemia, paraproteinemia, hyperbilirubinemia.

HYPERPIGMENTATION[5]

ICD-9CM # 709.00
ICD-10CM # L81.4 Other melanin hyperpigmentation

Addison's disease.*
Arsenic ingestion.
ACTH- or MSH-producing tumors (e.g., oat cell carcinoma of the lung).*
Drug induced (i.e., antimalarials, some cytotoxic agents).
Hemochromatosis ("bronze" diabetes).
Malabsorption syndrome (Whipple's disease and celiac sprue).
Melanoma.
Melanotropic hormone injection.*
Pheochromocytoma.
Porphyrias (porphyria cutanea tarda and variegate porphyria).
Pregnancy.
Progressive systemic sclerosis and related conditions.
PUVA therapy (psoralen administration) for psoriasis and vitiligo.*

ACTH, Adrenocorticotropic hormone; *MSH,* melanocyte-stimulating hormone; *PUVA,* psoralen plus ultraviolet A.
*Accentuation on sun-exposed surfaces.

HYPERPROLACTINEMIA[26a]

ICD-9CM # 253.1
ICD-10CM # E22.1 Hyperprolactinemia

PHYSIOLOGIC

Pregnancy.
Lactation.
Stress.
Sleep.
Coitus.
Exercise.

PATHOLOGIC

Hypothalamic-Pituitary Stalk Damage
Tumors: craniopharyngioma, suprasellar pituitary mass extension, meningioma, dysgerminoma, hypothalamic metastases.
Granulomas.
Infiltrations.
Rathke's cyst.
Irradiation.
Trauma: pituitary stalk section, sellar surgery, head trauma.
Pituitary
Prolactinoma.
Acromegaly.
Macroadenoma (compressive).
Idiopathic.
Plurihormonal adenoma.
Lymphocytic hypophysitis or parasellar mass.
Macroprolactinemia.
Systemic Disorders
Chronic renal failure.
Polycystic ovary syndrome.
Cirrhosis.
Pseudocyesis.
Epileptic seizures.
Cranial irradiation.
Chest: neurogenic chest wall trauma, surgery, herpes zoster.

PHARMACOLOGIC

Neuropeptide
Thyrotropin-releasing hormone.
Drug-Induced Hypersecretion
Dopamine receptor blockers:
Phenothiazines: chlorpromazine, perphenazine.
Butyrophenones: haloperidol.
Thioxanthenes.
Metoclopramide.
Dopamine synthesis inhibitors:
α-Methyldopa.
Catecholamine depleters:
Reserpine.
Cholinergic Agonist
Physostigmine.
Antihypertensives
Labetalol.
Reserpine.
Verapamil.
H_2 Antihistamines
Cimetidine.
Ranitidine.
Estrogens
Oral contraceptives.
Oral contraceptive withdrawal.
Anticonvulsant
Phenytoin.
Anesthetics

Neuroleptics
Chlorpromazine.
Risperidone.
Promazine.
Promethazine.
Trifluoperazine.
Fluphenazine.
Butaperazine.
Perphenazine.
Thiethylperazine.
Thioridazine.
Haloperidol.
Pimozide.
Thiothixene.
Molindone.
Opiates and Opiate Antagonists
Heroin.
Methadone.
Apomorphine.
Morphine.
Antidepressants
Tricyclic antidepressants: chlorimipramine, amitriptyline.
Selective serotonin reuptake inhibitors: fluoxetine.

HYPERSPLENISM, ASSOCIATED CONDITIONS

ICD-9CM # 289.4
ICD-10CM # D73.1 Hypersplenism

Cirrhosis.
Portal vein thrombosis.
Myeloproliferative diseases.
Lymphomas.
Leukemias.
Splenic vein thrombosis.
Autoimmune disease.
Sickle cell disease.
Thalassemias.
Gaucher's disease.
Niemann-Pick disease.

HYPERTENSION, ADRENOCORTICAL CAUSES[26a]

ICD-9CM # 401
ICD-10CM # I15.8 Other secondary hypertension

LOW RENIN AND HIGH ALDOSTERONE

Primary Aldosteronism

Aldosterone-producing adenoma (APA)	35% of cases
Bilateral idiopathic hyperplasia (IHA)	60% of cases
Primary (unilateral) adrenal hyperplasia	2% of cases
Aldosterone-producing adrenocortical carcinoma	<1% of cases
Familial hyperaldosteronism (FH)	
Glucocorticoid-remediable aldosteronism (FH type I)	<1% of cases
FH type II (APA or IHA)—<2% of cases	
Ectopic aldosterone-producing adenoma or carcinoma	<0.1% of cases

LOW RENIN AND LOW ALDOSTERONE

Hyperdeoxycorticosteronism
Congenital adrenal hyperplasia.
11β-Hydroxylase deficiency.
17α-Hydroxylase deficiency.
Deoxycorticosterone-producing tumor.
Primary cortisol resistance.
Apparent mineralocorticoid excess (AME)/11β-HSD* deficiency.
Genetic: Type 1 AME.
Acquired: Licorice or carbenoxolone ingestion (type 1 AME), Cushing's syndrome (type 2 AME).
Cushing's Syndrome
Exogenous glucocorticoid administration—most common cause.
Endogenous.
ACTH[†]-dependent—85% of cases: Pituitary, ectopic.
ACTH-independent—15% of cases: Unilateral adrenal disease (adenoma or carcinoma), bilateral adrenal disease (massive macronodular hyperplasia [rare], primary pigmented nodular adrenal disease [rare]).

*HSD, hydroxysteroid dehydrogenase
†ACTH, corticotropin

Differential Diagnosis II

HYPERTENSION, ENDOCRINE CAUSES[26a]

ICD-9CM # 401
ICD-10CM # I15.8 Other secondary hypertension

ADRENAL-DEPENDENT CAUSES

Pheochromocytoma.
Primary aldosteronism.
Hyperdeoxycorticosteronism.
Congenital adrenal hyperplasia: 11β-Hydroxylase deficiency, 17α-hydroxylase deficiency.
Deoxycorticosterone-producing tumor.
Primary cortisol resistance.
Cushing's syndrome.

AME/11β-HSD (HYDROXYSTEROID DEHYDROGENASE) DEFICIENCY

Genetic.
Type 1 apparent mineralocorticoid excess (AME).
Acquired.
Licorice or carbenoxolone ingestion (type 1 AME).
Cushing's syndrome (type 2 AME).

THYROID-DEPENDENT CAUSES

Hypothyroidism.
Hyperthyroidism.

PARATHYROID-DEPENDENT CAUSES

Hyperparathyroidism.

PITUITARY-DEPENDENT CAUSES

Acromegaly.
Cushing's syndrome.

HYPERTENSION, IN CHILDREN[2]

ICD-9CM # 401
ICD-10CM # I10 Essential (primary) hypertension

PRIMARY

Essential hypertension.

SECONDARY

Renal
Glomerulonephritis.
Henoch-Schönlein purpura.
Pyelonephritis.
Obstruction of reflux.
Polycystic kidney disease.
Diabetic nephropathy.
Trauma.
Renal transplant or hemodialysis.
Tuberous sclerosis.
Systemic lupus nephritis.
Endocrine
Pheochromocytoma.
Cushing's syndrome.
Congenital adrenal hyperplasia.
Corticosteroid treatment.
Hyperthyroidism.
Neuroblastoma.
Ovarian tumor.
Cardiac
Congestive heart failure.
Coarctation of the aorta.
Vascular
Hemolytic-uremic syndrome.
Kawasaki syndrome.
Renal artery thrombosis or stenosis.
Neurologic
Central nervous system tumor or infection.
Central nervous system trauma or abuse.
Increased intracranial pressure.
Guillain-Barré syndrome.
Neoplastic
Neuroblastoma.
Wilms' tumor.
Pheochromocytoma.
Adrenal carcinoma.
Drugs
Corticosteroids.
Cocaine.
Sympathomimetics.
Oral contraceptives.
Phencyclidine.
Beta-blocker or clonidine withdrawal.
Lead, mercury.
Others
Iatrogenic fluid overload.
Volume overload from end-stage renal disease.

HYPERTENSIVE CRISIS SYNDROMES[38b]

ICD-9CM # 997.91
ICD-10CM # I13 Hypertensive heart and renal disease
I15 Secondary hypertension

Malignant hypertension.
Nonmalignant hypertension with target organ disorders:
Patient requiring emergency surgery with poorly controlled hypertension.
Hyperviscosity syndrome.
Postoperative patient.
Renal transplant patient: acute rejection, transplant renal artery stenosis.
Quadriplegic patient with autonomic hyperreflexia.
Severe burns.
Acute aortic dissection.
Intracranial hemorrhage, ischemic stroke, or subarachnoid hemorrhage.
Hypertensive encephalopathy.
Myocardial ischemia/acute left ventricular failure.
Preeclampsia/eclampsia.
Antiphospholipid antibody syndrome.
Acute renal failure:
- Scleroderma renal crisis.
- Chronic glomerulonephritis.
- Reflux nephropathy.
- Analgesic nephropathy.
- Acute glomerulonephritis.
- Radiation nephritis.
- Ask-Upmark kidney.
- Chronic lead intoxication.

Renovascular hypertension:
- Fibromuscular dysplasia.
- Atherosclerosis.

Endocrine hypertension:
- Congenital adrenal hyperplasia.
- Pheochromocytoma.
- Oral contraceptives.
- Aldosteronism.
- Cushing disease/syndrome.

Systemic vasculitis.
Atheroembolic renal crisis.
Drugs:
- Oral contraceptives.
- Nonsteroidal antiinflammatory agents.
- Atropine.
- Corticosteroids.
- Sympathomimetics.
- Erythropoietin.
- Lead intoxication.
- Cyclosporine.

Catecholamine excess states:
- Pheochromocytoma.
- MAO/tyramine interaction.
- Antihypertensive withdrawal.
- Cocaine intoxication, sympathomimetic overdose.

HYPERTRICHOSIS[7]

ICD-9CM # 704.1 Hypertrichosis NOS
757.4 Hypertrichosis, Congenital
ICD-10CM # L68.0 Hirsutism
L68.1 Acquired hypertrichosis lanuginosa
L68.3 Polytrichia
L68.9 Hypertrichosis, unspecified
Q84.1 Congenital morphological disturbances of hair, not elsewhere classified

DRUGS

Dilantin.
Streptomycin.
Hexachlorobenzene.
Penicillamine.
Diazoxide.
Minoxidil.
Cyclosporine.

SYSTEMIC ILLNESS

Hypothyroidism.
Anorexia nervosa.
Malnutrition.
Porphyria.
Dermatomyositis.

IDIOPATHIC

HYPERTROPHIC OSTEOARTHROPATHY

ICD-9CM # 731.2
ICD-10CM # M89.40 Other hypertrophic osteoarthropathy, unspecified site

Idiopathic.
Pulmonary disease (e.g., pulmonary fibrosis, cystic fibrosis, sarcoidosis).
Bronchogenic carcinoma.
AIDS.
GI neoplasm (e.g., esophagus, colon).
Hepatic neoplasm, cirrhosis.
Cardiovascular diseases, aortic aneurysm, aortic prosthesis.
Congenital cyanotic heart disease, patent ductus arteriosus.
Pulmonary infections, bacterial endocarditis, amebic dysentery.
Inflammatory bowel disease.
Connective tissue diseases.
Lymphomas.
Thyroid acropachy.

HYPERVENTILATION, PERSISTENT[36]

ICD-9CM # 786.01
ICD-10CM # R06.4 Hyperventilation

Fibrotic lung disease.
Metabolic acidosis (e.g., diabetes, uremia).
CNS disorders (midbrain and pontine lesions).
Hepatic coma.
Salicylate intoxication.
Fever.
Sepsis.
Psychogenic (e.g., anxiety).

HYPOCALCEMIA

ICD-9CM # 275.41
ICD-10CM # E83.51 Hypocalcemia

Renal insufficiency: hypocalcemia caused by:
- Increased calcium deposits in bone and soft tissue secondary to increased serum phosphate level.
- Decreased production of 1,25-dihydroxyvitamin D.
- Excessive loss of 25-OHD (nephrotic syndrome).

Hypoalbuminemia: each decrease in serum albumin (g/L) will decrease serum calcium by 0.8 mg/dl but will not change free (ionized) calcium.
Vitamin D deficiency:
- Malabsorption (most common cause).
- Inadequate intake.
- Decreased production of 1,25-dihydroxyvitamin D (vitamin D–dependent rickets, renal failure).
- Decreased production of 25-OHD (parenchymal liver disease).
- Accelerated 25-OHD catabolism (phenytoin, phenobarbital).
- End-organ resistance to 1,25-dihydroxyvitamin D.

Hypomagnesemia: hypocalcemia caused by:
- Decreased PTH secretion.
- Inhibition of PTH effect on bone.

Pancreatitis, hyperphosphatemia, osteoblastic metastases: hypocalcemia is secondary to increased calcium deposits (bone, abdomen).
Pseudohypoparathyroidism (PHP): autosomal recessive disorder characterized by short stature, shortening of metacarpal bones, obesity, and mental retardation; the hypocalcemia is secondary to congenital end-organ resistance to PTH.
Idiopathic hypoparathyroidism, surgical removal of parathyroids (e.g., neck surgery).
"Hungry bones syndrome": rapid transfer of calcium from plasma into bones after removal of a parathyroid tumor.
Sepsis.
Massive blood transfusion (as a result of EDTA in blood).

HYPOCAPNIA

ICD-9CM # 786.01
ICD-10CM # R06.8 Hypoventilation

Hyperventilation.
Pneumonia, pneumonitis.
Fever, sepsis.
Medications (salicylates, beta-adrenergic agonists, progesterone, methylxanthines).
Pulmonary disease (asthma, interstitial fibrosis).
Pulmonary embolism.
Hepatic failure.
Metabolic acidosis.
High altitude.
CHF.
Pregnancy.
Pain.
CNS lesions.

HYPOGLYCEMIA

ICD-9CM #	251.2	Spontaneous
	250.3	Diabetic
	251.0	Due to Insulin
	579.3	Postoperative
	251.2	Reactive
ICD-10CM #	E16.2	Hypoglycemia, unspecified
	E10.65	Type 1 diabetes mellitus with hyperglycemia
	E15	Nondiabetic hypoglycemic coma
	K91.2	Postsurgical malabsorption, not elsewhere classified
	E16.2	Hypoglycemia, unspecified

Oral hypoglycemics (therapeutic, factitious).
Exogenous insulin (therapeutic, factitious).
Postoperative gastric emptying (alimentary hyperinsulinism).
Severe malnutrition.
Liver disease.
Hypermetabolic state (sepsis).
Ketotic hypoglycemia.
Insulinoma.
Antibodies to endogenous insulin.
Hormone deficiencies (glucagon, growth hormone, hypoadrenalism).
Enzyme disorders in metabolism of glycogen, hexose, glycolysis, and Krebs cycle.
Idiopathic.

HYPOGLYCEMIA, IN INFANTS AND CHILDREN[22a]

ICD-9CM # 251.2 Hypoglycemia
ICD-10CM # E16.2 Hypoglycemia, unspecified

CLASSIFICATION OF HYPOGLYCEMIA IN INFANTS AND CHILDREN

NEONATAL TRANSIENT HYPOGLYCEMIA

Associated with Inadequate Substrate or Immature Enzyme Function in Otherwise Normal Neonates
Prematurity.
Small for gestational age.
Normal newborn.
Transient Neonatal Hyperinsulinism Also Present in:
Infant of diabetic mother.
Discordant twin.
Birth asphyxia.
Infant of toxemic mother.

NEONATAL, INFANTILE, OR CHILDHOOD PERSISTENT HYPOGLYCEMIAS

Hormonal Disorders
Hyperinsulinism.
Recessive K_{ATP} channel HI.
Recessive HADH (hydroxyl acyl CoA dehydrogenase) mutation HI.
Recessive UCP2 (mitochondrial uncoupling protein 2) mutation HI.
Focal K_{ATP} channel HI.
Dominant K_{ATP} channel HI.
Dominant glucokinase HI.
Dominant glutamate dehydrogenase HI (hyperinsulinism/hyperammonemia syndrome).
Dominant mutation in HNF4A (hepatic nuclear factor 4 alpha) HI with MODY later in life.
Dominant mutation in SLC16A1 (the pyruvate transporter)-exercise-induced hypoglycemia.
Acquired islet adenoma.
Beckwith-Wiedemann syndrome.
Insulin administration (Munchausen syndrome by proxy).
Oral sulfonylurea drugs.
Congenital disorders of glycosylation.
Counter-Regulatory Hormone Deficiency
Panhypopituitarism.
Isolated growth hormone deficiency.
Addison disease.
Epinephrine deficiency.
Glycogenolysis and Gluconeogenesis Disorders
Glucose-6-phosphatase deficiency (GSD 1a).
Glucose-6-phosphate translocase deficiency (GSD 1b).
Amylo-1,6-glucosidase (debranching enzyme) deficiency (GSD 3).
Liver phosphorylase deficiency (GSD 6).
Phosphorylase kinase deficiency (GSD 9).
Glycogen synthetase deficiency (GSD 0).
Fructose-1,6-diphosphatase deficiency.
Pyruvate carboxylase deficiency.
Galactosemia.
Hereditary fructose intolerance.
Lipolysis Disorders
Fatty Acid Oxidation Disorders
Carnitine transporter deficiency (primary carnitine deficiency).
Carnitine palmitoyltransferase-1 deficiency.
Carnitine translocase deficiency.

Carnitine palmitoyltransferase-2 deficiency.
Secondary carnitine deficiencies.
Very long, long-, medium-, short-chain acyl-CoA dehydrogenase deficiency.

OTHER ETIOLOGIES

Substrate-Limited

Ketotic hypoglycemia.
Poisoning—drugs.
Salicylates.
Alcohol.
Oral hypoglycemic agents.
Insulin.
Propranolol.
Pentamidine.
Quinine.
Disopyramide.
Ackee fruit (unripe)—hypoglycin.
Vacor (rat poison).
Trimethoprim-sulfamethoxazole (with renal failure).

Liver Disease

Reye syndrome.
Hepatitis.
Cirrhosis.
Hepatoma.

Amino Acid and Organic Acid Disorders

Maple syrup urine disease.
Propionic acidemia.
Methylmalonic acidemia.
Tyrosinosis.
Glutaric aciduria.
3-Hydroxy-3-methylglutaric aciduria.

Systemic Disorders

Sepsis.
Carcinoma/sarcoma (secreting—insulin-like growth factor II).
Heart failure.
Malnutrition.
Malabsorption.
Anti-insulin receptor antibodies.
Anti-insulin antibodies.
Neonatal hyperviscosity.
Renal failure.
Diarrhea.
Burns.
Shock.
Postsurgical.
Pseudohypoglycemia (leukocytosis, polycythemia).
Excessive insulin therapy of insulin-dependent diabetes mellitus.
Factitious.
Nissen fundoplication (dumping syndrome).
Falciparum malaria.

GSD, Glycogen storage disease; *HI,* hyperinsulinemia; K_{ATP}, regulated potassium channel.

HYPOGONADISM

ICD-9CM #	256.3	Female
	257.2	Male
	256.3	Ovarian
	253.4	Pituitary
	257.2	Testicular
ICD-10CM #	E28.310	Symptomatic premature menopause
	E29.1	Testicular hypofunction
	E28.39	Other primary ovarian failure
	E23.6	Other disorders of pituitary gland

HYPERGONADOTROPIC HYPOGONADISM

Hormone resistance (androgen, LH insensitivity).
Gonadal defects (e.g., Klinefelter's syndrome, myotonic dystrophy).
Drug-induced (e.g., spironolactone, cytotoxins).
Alcoholism, radiation-induced.
Mumps orchitis.
Anatomic defects, castration.

HYPOGONADOTROPIC HYPOGONADISM

Pituitary lesions (neoplasms, granulomas, infarction, hemochromatosis, vasculitis).
Drug-induced (e.g., glucocorticoids).
Hyperprolactinemia.
Genetic disorders (Laurence-Moon-Biedl syndrome, Prader-Willi).
Delayed puberty.
Other: chronic disease, nutritional deficiency, Kallmann's syndrome, idiopathic isolated LH or FSH deficiency.

HYPOKALEMIA

ICD-9CM #	276.8
ICD-10CM #	E87.6 Hypokalemia

Cellular shift (redistribution) and undetermined mechanisms.
Alkalosis (each 0.1 increase in pH decreases serum potassium by 0.4 to 0.6 mEq/L).
Insulin administration.
Vitamin B_{12} therapy for megaloblastic anemias, acute leukemias.
Hypokalemic periodic paralysis: rare familial disorder manifested by recurrent attacks of flaccid paralysis and hypokalemia.
Beta-adrenergic agonists (e.g., terbutaline), decongestants, bronchodilators, theophylline, caffeine.
Barium poisoning, toluene intoxication, verapamil intoxication, chloroquine intoxication.
Correction of digoxin intoxication with digoxin antibody fragments (Digibind).
Increased renal excretion.
Drugs:
- Diuretics, including carbonic anhydrase inhibitors (e.g., acetazolamide).
- Amphotericin B.
- High-dose sodium penicillin, nafcillin, ampicillin, or carbenicillin.
- Cisplatin.
- Aminoglycosides.
- Corticosteroids, mineralocorticoids.
- Foscarnet sodium.

RTA: distal (type 1) or proximal (type 2).
Diabetic ketoacidosis (DKA), ureteroenterostomy.
Magnesium deficiency.
Postobstruction diuresis, diuretic phase of ATN.
Osmotic diuresis (e.g., mannitol).
Bartter's syndrome: hyperplasia of juxtaglomerular cells leading to increased renin and aldosterone, metabolic alkalosis, hypokalemia, muscle weakness, and tetany (seen in young adults).
Increased mineralocorticoid activity (primary or secondary aldosteronism), Cushing's syndrome.
Chronic metabolic alkalosis from loss of gastric fluid (increased renal potassium secretion).
GI loss:
- Vomiting, nasogastric suction.
- Diarrhea.
- Laxative abuse.
- Villous adenoma.
- Fistulas.
- Inadequate dietary intake (e.g., anorexia nervosa).
- Cutaneous loss (excessive sweating).
- High dietary sodium intake, excessive use of licorice.

HYPOMAGNESEMIA

ICD-9CM #	275.2	
ICD-10CM #	E83.40	Disorders of magnesium metabolism, unspecified
	E83.41	Hypermagnesemia
	E83.42	Hypomagnesemia
	E83.49	Other disorders of magnesium metabolism

GASTROINTESTINAL AND NUTRITIONAL

Defective GI absorption (malabsorption).
Inadequate dietary intake (e.g., alcoholics).
Parenteral therapy without magnesium.
Chronic diarrhea, villous adenoma, prolonged nasogastric suction, fistulas (small bowel, biliary).

EXCESSIVE RENAL LOSSES

Diuretics.
RTA.
Diuretic phase of ATN.
Endocrine disturbances (DKA, hyperaldosteronism, hyperthyroidism, hyperparathyroidism), SIADH, Bartter's syndrome, hypercalciuria, hypokalemia.
Cisplatin, alcohol, cyclosporine, digoxin, pentamidine, mannitol, amphotericin B, foscarnet, methotrexate.
Antibiotics (gentamicin, ticarcillin, carbenicillin).
Redistribution: hypoalbuminemia, cirrhosis, administration of insulin and glucose, theophylline, epinephrine, acute pancreatitis, cardiopulmonary bypass.
Miscellaneous: sweating, burns, prolonged exercise, lactation, "hungry-bones" syndrome.

HYPONATREMIA

ICD-9CM # 276.1
ICD-10CM # E87.1 Hypo-osmolality and hyponatremia

Renal loss from renal disease, diuretics.
GI loss (diarrhea, vomiting, suction).
Hypertonic hyponatremia (e.g., increased serum osmolality from hyperglycemia).
Transcutaneous loss (extensive burns, excessive sweating).
Fluid sequestration (e.g., ascites).
Osmotic diuresis (e.g., mannitol, glucose).
Dilutional (psychogenic polydipsia, iatrogenic).
Syndrome of inappropriate antidiuretic hormone secretion.
Edema with water and sodium retention.
Artifact (e.g., severe hyperlipidemia).
Laboratory error.
Adrenal insufficiency.

HYPOPHOSPHATEMIA

ICD-9CM # 275.3
ICD-10CM # E83.30 Disorder of phosphorus metabolism, unspecified
E83.31 Familial hypophosphatemia

Decreased intake (prolonged starvation [alcoholics], hyperalimentation, or IV infusion without phosphate).
Malabsorption.
Phosphate-binding antacids.
Renal loss:
  RTA.
  Fanconi syndrome, vitamin D–resistant rickets.
  ATN (diuretic phase).
  Hyperparathyroidism (primary or secondary).
  Familial hypophosphatemia.
  Hypokalemia, hypomagnesemia.
  Acute volume expansion.
  Glycosuria, idiopathic hypercalciuria.
  Acetazolamide.
Transcellular shift into cells:
  Alcohol withdrawal.
  DKA (recovery phase).
  Glucose-insulin or catecholamine infusion.
  Anabolic steroids.
  Total parenteral nutrition.
  Theophylline overdose.
  Severe hyperthermia; recovery from hypothermia.
  "Hungry bones" syndrome.

HYPOPIGMENTATION

ICD-9CM # 709.00
ICD-10CM # L81.9 Disorder of pigmentation, unspecified

Vitiligo.
Tinea versicolor.
Atopic dermatitis.
Chemical leukoderma.
Idiopathic hypomelanosis.
Sarcoidosis.
SLE.
Scleroderma.
Oculocutaneous albinism.
Phenylketonuria.
Nevoid hypopigmentation.

HYPOTENSION, POSTURAL

ICD-9CM # 458.0
ICD-10CM # I95.89 Other hypotension

Antihypertensive medications (especially a-blockers, diuretics, ACE inhibitors).
Volume depletion (hemorrhage, dehydration).
Impaired cardiac output (constrictive pericarditis, aortic stenosis).
Peripheral autonomic dysfunction (DM, Guillain-Barré).
Idiopathic orthostatic hypotension.
Central autonomic dysfunction (Shy-Drager syndrome).
Peripheral venous disease.
Adrenal insufficiency.

HYPOTHYROIDISM, CONGENITAL[22a]

ICD-9CM # 243
ICD-10CM # E03.0 Congenital hypothyroidism with diffuse goiter
E03.1 Congenital hypothyroidism without goiter

ETIOLOGIC CLASSIFICATION OF CONGENITAL HYPOTHYROIDISM

PRIMARY HYPOTHYROIDISM

Defect of fetal thyroid development (dysgenesis):
  Aplasia.
  Hypoplasia.
  Ectopia.
Defect in thyroid hormone synthesis (dyshormonogenesis):
  Iodide transport defect: mutation in thyroglobulin gene.
  Thyroid organification, or coupling defect: mutation in thyroid peroxidase gene.
  Defects in H_2O_2 generation: mutations in DUOXA2 maturation factor or *DUOX2* gene.
  Thyroglobulin synthesis defect: mutation in thyroglobulin gene.
  Deiodination defect: mutation in *DEHAL1* gene.
TSH unresponsiveness:
  $G_s\alpha$ mutation (e.g., type 1A pseudohypothyroidism).
  Mutation in TSH receptor.
Defect in thyroid hormone transport: mutation in monocarboxylate transporter 8 *(MCT8)* gene.
Iodine deficiency (endemic goiter).
Maternal antibodies: thyrotropin receptor–blocking antibody (TRBAb, also termed *thyrotropin-binding inhibitor immunoglobulin*).
Maternal medications:
  Iodides, amiodarone.
  Propylthiouracil, methimazole.
  Radioiodine.

CENTRAL (HYPOPITUITARY) HYPOTHYROIDISM

PIT-1 mutations:
  Deficiency of thyroid-stimulating hormone (TSH).
  Deficiency of growth hormone.
  Deficiency of prolactin.
PROP-1 mutations:
  Deficiency of TSH.
  Deficiency of growth hormone.
  Deficiency of prolactin.
  Deficiency of luteinizing hormone.
  Deficiency of follicle-stimulating hormone.
  ±Deficiency of adrenocorticotropic hormone.
TSH deficiency: mutation in TSH β subunit gene (manifests as primary hypothyroidism with elevated TSH level).
Multiple pituitary deficiencies (e.g., craniopharyngioma).
Thyroid-releasing hormone (TRH) deficiency:
  Isolated.
  Multiple hypothalamic deficiencies (e.g., septooptic dysplasia).
TRH unresponsiveness.
Mutations in TRH receptor.

HYPOTONIA, INFANTILE, DIFFERENTIAL DIAGNOSIS[22a]

ICD-9CM # 360.30 Hypotonia
ICD-10CM # H44.40 Unspecified hypotony of eye

Cerebral hypotonia.
  Benign congenital hypotonia.
  Chromosome disorders.
  - Prader-Willi syndrome.
  - Trisomy.
  Chronic nonprogressive encephalopathy.
  - Cerebral malformation.
  - Perinatal distress.
  - Postnatal disorders.
  Peroxisomal disorders.
  - Cerebrohepatorenal syndrome (Zellweger syndrome).
  - Neonatal adrenoleukodystrophy.
  Other genetic defects.
  - Familial dysautonomia.
  - Oculocerebrorenal syndrome (Lowe syndrome).
  Other metabolic defects.
  - Acid maltase deficiency (see "Metabolic Myopathies").
  - Infantile G_M, gangliosidosis.
Spinal cord disorders.
Spinal muscular atrophies.
  Acute infantile.
  - Autosomal dominant.
  - Autosomal recessive.
  - Cytochrome-*c* oxidase deficiency.
  - X-linked.
  Chronic infantile.
  - Autosomal dominant.
  - Autosomal recessive.
  - Congenital cervical spinal muscular atrophy.
  - Infantile neuronal degeneration.
  - Neurogenic arthrogryposis.

Polyneuropathies.
- Congenital hypomyelinating neuropathy.
- Giant axonal neuropathy.
- Hereditary motor-sensory neuropathies.

Disorders of neuromuscular transmission.
- Familial infantile myasthenia.
- Infantile botulism.
- Transitory myasthenia gravis.

Fiber-type disproportion myopathies.
- Central core disease.
- Congenital fiber-type disproportion myopathy.
- Myotubular (centronuclear) myopathy.
  - Acute.
  - Chronic.
- Nemaline (rod) myopathy.
  - Autosomal dominant.
  - Autosomal recessive.

Metabolic myopathies.
- Acid maltase deficiency.
- Cytochrome-*c* oxidase deficiency.

Muscular dystrophies.
- Bethlem myopathy.
- Congenital dystrophinopathy.
- Congenital muscular dystrophy.
  - Merosin deficiency, primary.
  - Merosin deficiency, secondary.
  - Merosin positive.
- Congenital myotonic dystrophy.

HYPOVOLEMIC SHOCK, PEDIATRIC POPULATION[12c]

ICD-9CM #	785.59	Hypovolemic Shock
ICD-10CM #	R57.1	Hypovolemic shock
	R57.8	Other shock

ETIOLOGIES OF HYPOVOLEMIC SHOCK

Whole blood loss.
- Absolute loss: hemorrhage.
  - External bleeding.
  - Internal bleeding.
    - Gastrointestinal.
    - Intraabdominal (spleen, liver).
    - Major vessel injury.
    - Intracranial (in infants).
    - Fractures.
- Relative loss.
  - Pharmacologic (barbiturates, vasodilators).
  - Positive pressure ventilation.
  - Spinal cord injury.
  - Sepsis.
  - Anaphylaxis.

Plasma loss.
- Burns.
- Capillary leak syndromes.
  - Inflammation, sepsis.
  - Anaphylaxis.
  - Protein-losing syndromes.

Fluid and electrolyte loss.
- Vomiting and diarrhea.
- Excessive diuretic use.
- Endocrine:
  - Adrenal insufficiency.
  - Diabetes insipidus.
  - Diabetes mellitus.

ILIAC FOSSA PAIN, LEFT SIDED[38]

ICD-9CM #	varies with specific diagnosis
ICD-10CM #	M25.5 Pain in joint

GASTROINTESTINAL CAUSES OF ACUTE LEFT ILIAC FOSSA PAIN

Nonspecific left iliac fossa pain including constipation.
Acute gastroenteritis.
Acute diverticulitis.
Colonic carcinoma.
Colonic ischemia.
Localized small bowel perforation.

ILIAC FOSSA PAIN, RIGHT SIDED[38]

ICD-9CM #	varies with specific diagnosis
ICD-10CM #	M25.5 Pain in joint

DIFFERENTIAL DIAGNOSIS OF RIGHT ILIAC FOSSA PAIN

Gastrointestinal Causes

Nonspecific right iliac fossa pain.
Acute appendicitis.
Mesenteric adenitis.
Terminal ileitis.
Acute inflammation of Meckel's diverticulum.
Crohn's disease of the terminal ileum.
Cecal carcinoma.
Inflammatory cecal lesion (e.g., diverticulitis in a solitary cecal diverticulum).
Inflammatory lesion of the terminal ileum (e.g., foreign body perforation).

Non-Gastrointestinal Causes

Ruptured ovarian follicle (mittelschmerz).
Acute salpingitis (pelvic inflammatory disease).
Rupture/torsion or hemorrhage of an ovarian cyst.
Endometriosis.
Ectopic pregnancy.
Urinary tract infection.

IMMUNODEFICIENCY, CONGENITAL (PRIMARY)

ICD-9CM #	279.2	
ICD-10CM #	D80.0	Hereditary hyopgammaglobulinemia
	D80.1	Nonfamilial hypogammaglobulinemia
	D80.2	Selective deficiency of IgA
	D80.3	Selective deficiency of IgG
	D80.4	Selective deficiency of IgM

CONGENITAL (PRIMARY) CAUSES OF IMMUNODEFIENCY

T-lymphocyte Deficiencies

DiGeorge syndrome (thymic aplasia with reduced CD4 and CD3 cells).
Purine nucleoside phosphorylase deficiency (marked T-cell depletion).

B-lymphocyte Deficiencies

Bruton X-linked agammaglobulinemia (absence of B cells, plasma cells, and antibody).
Selective immunoglobulin G (IgG) subclass deficiencies.
Selective IgA deficiency.
Hyper-IgM immunodeficiency (elevated IgM but reduced IgG and IgA).

Mixed T- and B-lymphocyte Deficiencies

Common variable immunodeficiency (leads to various B-cell activation or differentiation defects and gradual deterioration of T-cell number and function).
Severe combined immunodeficiency (severe reduction in IgG and absence of T cells).
Wiskott-Aldrich syndrome (decreased T-cell number and function, low IgM, occasionally low IgG).
Ataxia-telangiectasia (decreased T-cell number and function; IgA, IgE, IgG_2, and IgG_4 deficiency).

Disorders of Complement

C3 deficiency (congenital absence of C3 or consumption of C3 due to deficiency of C3b inactivator).

Phagocyte Defects

Chronic granulomatous disease (defect in nicotinamide adenine dinucleotide phosphate oxidase in phagocytic cells).
Chédiak-Higashi syndrome (impaired microbicidal activity of phagocytes).
Kostmann syndrome, Shwachman-Diamond syndrome, cyclic neutropenia (low neutrophil count).

IMPOTENCE[27]

ICD-9CM #	302.72	Psychosexual
	607.84	Organic
	997.99	Organic Postprostatectomy
ICD-10CM #	F52.21	Male erectile disorder
	F52.8	Other sexual dysfunction not due to a substance or known physiological condition
	N52.9	Male erectile dysfunction, unspecified

Psychogenic.
Endocrine: hyperprolactinemia, DM, Cushing's syndrome, hypothyroidism or hyperthyroidism, abnormality of hypothalamic-pituitary-testicular axis.
Vascular: arterial insufficiency, venous leakage, AV malformation, local trauma.
Medications.
Neurogenic: autonomic or sensory neuropathy, spinal cord trauma or tumor, CVA, multiple sclerosis, temporal lobe epilepsy.
Systemic illness: renal failure, COPD, cirrhosis of liver, myotonic dystrophy.
Peyronie's disease.
Prostatectomy.

INCONTINENCE, FECAL[38]

ICD-9CM #	787.6	
ICD-10CM #	R15.9	Full incontinence of feces

NORMAL SPHINCTER

Diarrhea.
Anorectal conditions:

- Rectal carcinoma.
- Inflammatory bowel disease.
- Hemorrhoids.
- Mucosal prolapse.
- Fissure-in-ano.
- Abnormal rectal sensation.

ABNORMAL SPHINCTER

Congenital abnormalities.
Anal sepsis.
Neurologic conditions.
Rectal prolapse.
Sphincter trauma.
Neurogenic (idiopathic) incontinence.

INFERTILITY, FEMALE[14]

ICD-9CM # 628.9
ICD-10CM # N97.9 Female infertility, unspecified

FALLOPIAN TUBE PATHOLOGY

PID or puerperal infection.
Congenital anomalies.
Endometriosis.
Secondary to past peritonitis of nongenital origin.
Amenorrhea and anovulation.
Minor anovulatory disturbances.

CERVICAL AND UTERINE FACTORS

Leiomyomas and polyps.
Uterine anomalies.
Intrauterine synechiae (Asherman's syndrome).
Destroyed endocervical glands (postsurgery or postinfection).

VAGINAL FACTORS

Congenital absence of vagina.
Imperforate hymen.
Vaginismus.
Vaginitis.

IMMUNOLOGIC FACTORS

Sperm-immobilizing antibodies.
Sperm-agglutinating antibodies.

NUTRITIONAL AND METABOLIC FACTORS

Thyroid disorders.
DM.
Severe nutritional disturbances.

INFERTILITY, MALE[14]

ICD-9CM # 606.9
ICD-10CM # N46.9 Male infertility, unspecified

DECREASED PRODUCTION OF SPERMATOZOA

Varicocele.
Testicular failure.
Endocrine disorders.
Cryptorchidism.
Stress, smoking, caffeine, nicotine, recreational drugs.

DUCTAL OBSTRUCTION

Epididymal (postinfection).
Congenital absence of vas deferens.
Ejaculatory duct (postinfection).
Postvasectomy.

INABILITY TO DELIVER SPERM INTO VAGINA

Ejaculatory disturbances.
Hypospadias.
Sexual problems (i.e., impotence), medical or psychological.

ABNORMAL SEMEN

Infection.
Abnormal volume.
Abnormal viscosity.
Abnormal sperm motion.

IMMUNOLOGIC FACTORS

Sperm-immobilizing antibodies.
Sperm-agglutinating antibodies.

INSOMNIA[33]

ICD-9CM # 780.52 Insomnia NOS
307.42 Insomnia, Chronic Associated with Anxiety or Depression
780.51 Insomnia with Sleep Apnea
ICD-10CM # G47.00 Insomnia, unspecified
F51.01 Primary insomnia
F51.03 Paradoxical insomnia
F51.09 Other insomnia not due to a substance or known physiological condition

Anxiety disorder, psychophysiologic insomnia.
Depression.
Drugs (e.g., caffeine, amphetamines, cocaine), hypnotic-dependent sleep disorder.
Pain, fibromyalgia.
Inadequate sleep hygiene.
Restless leg syndrome.
Obstructive sleep apnea.
Sleep bruxism.
Medical illness (e.g., GERD, sleep-related asthma, parkinsonism and movement disorders).
Narcolepsy.
Other: periodic leg movement of sleep, central sleep apnea, REM behavioral disorder.

INTESTINAL PSEUDOOBSTRUCTION[36]

ICD-9CM # 560.1 Adynamic Intestinal Obstruction
564.9 Intestinal Disorder, Functional
ICD-10CM # K56.0 Paralytic ileus
K56.7 Ileus, unspecified
K59.9 Functional intestinal disorder, unspecified

"PRIMARY" (IDIOPATHIC INTESTINAL PSEUDOOBSTRUCTION)

Hollow visceral myopathy:
  Familial.
  Sporadic.
Neuropathic:
  Abnormal myenteric plexus.
  Normal myenteric plexus.

SECONDARY

Scleroderma.
Myxedema.
Amyloidosis.
Muscular dystrophy.
Hypokalemia.
Chronic renal failure.
DM.
Drug toxicity caused by:
  Anticholinergics.
  Opiate narcotics.
Ogilvie's syndrome.

INTRAABDOMINAL MASS LESION, NEONATAL[16a]

ICD-9CM # 789.3
ICD-10CM # R19.00 Intra-abdominal and pelvic swelling, mass and lump, unspecified site

CAUSES OF A NEONATAL INTRA-ABDOMINAL MASS LESION

Complicated meconium ileus.
Dilated bowel proximal to an obstruction.
Mesenteric or duplication cyst.
Abscess.
GU causes:
  Hydronephrosis.
  Renal cystic disease.
  Mesoblastic nephroma.
  Wilms' tumor.
  Adrenal hemorrhage.
  Neuroblastoma.
  Retroperitoneal teratoma.
  Ovarian cyst.
  Hydrometrocolpos.
Hemangioendothelioma.
Hepatoblastoma.
Choledochal, hepatic, or splenic cysts.

INTRACEREBRAL HEMORRHAGE, NONHYPERTENSIVE CAUSES

ICD-9CM # 431
ICD-10CM # I61.9 Nontraumatic intracerebral hemorrhage, unspecified

Trauma.
Anticoagulation.
Intracranial tumors.
Vascular malformations.
Bleeding disorders.
Vasculitides (e.g., polyarteritis nodosa, granulomatous angiitis).

Cocaine and other sympathomimetic agents.
Cerebral amyloid angiopathy.

INTRACRANIAL LESION

ICD-9CM # 348.8
ICD-10CM # G93.89 Other specified disorders of brain

Tumor (primary or metastatic).
Abscess.
Stroke.
Intracranial hemorrhage.
Angioma.
Multiple sclerosis (initial single lesion).
Granuloma.
Herpes encephalitis.
Artifact.

INTRAOCULAR NEOPLASM

ICD-9CM # varies with specific disorder
ICD-10CM # C69.9 Malignant disorder of eye, unspecified

MALIGNANT

Retinoblastoma.
Melanoma.
Reticulum cell sarcoma.
Metastatic tumor.

BENIGN

Melanocytic nevus.
Hemangioma.
Reactive lymphoid hyperplasia.

IRON OVERLOAD[20]

ICD-9CM # 275.0
ICD-10CM # E83.10 Disorder of iron metabolism, unspecified

HEREDITARY IRON OVERLOAD

Hereditary hemochromatosis:
- HFE-associated (type 1).
- Non–HFE-associated:
  - Transferrin receptor 2–associated (type 3).

Juvenile hemochromatosis (type 2):
- Hemojuvelin-associated (type 2A).
- Hepcidin-associated (type 2B).

Autosomal dominant hemochromatosis:
- Ferroportin-associated (type 4).

DMT1-associated hemochromatosis.
Atransferrinemia.
Aceruloplasminemia.

ACQUIRED IRON OVERLOAD

Iron-loading anemias (refractory anemias with hypercellular erythroid marrow).
Chronic liver disease.
Porphyria cutanea tarda.
Insulin resistance–associated hepatic iron overload.
African dietary iron overload.[a]
Medical iron ingestion.[a]
Parenteral iron overload:
- Transfusional iron overload.
- Inadvertent iron overload from therapeutic injections.

PERINATAL IRON OVERLOAD

Neonatal hemochromatosis.
Trichohepatoenteric syndrome.
Cerebrohepatorenal syndrome.
GRACILE[b] (Fellman) syndrome.

FOCAL SEQUESTRATION OF IRON

Idiopathic pulmonary hemosiderosis.
Renal hemosiderosis.
Associated with neurologic abnormalities:
- Pantothenate kinase–associated neurodegeneration (formerly called Hallervorden-Spatz syndrome).
- Neuroferritinopathy.
- Friedreich's ataxia.

---

[a] May have a genetic component.
[b] *GRACILE,* Growth retardation, aminoaciduria, cholestasis, iron overload, lactic acidosis, and early death.

ISCHEMIA, UPPER EXTREMITY, CAUSES[5a]

ICD-9CM # 903.8 Ischemia, Upper Extremity
ICD-10CM # S45.809A Unspecified injury of other specified blood vessels at shoulder and upper arm level, unspecified arm, initial encounter

VASOSPASM

Raynaud disease.
Medication induced: vasopressors, b-blockers.
Ergot poisoning.

INTRINSIC ARTERIAL DISEASE

Atherosclerosis.
Radiation arteritis.
Azotemic arteriopathy.
Spontaneous dissection.
Fibromuscular dysplasia.

INFLAMMATORY DISEASES

Connective tissue disorders.
Buerger disease.
Takayasu arteritis.
Temporal (giant cell) arteritis.
Hypersensitivity angiitis.

NONINFLAMMATORY MEDICAL DISEASE

Thrombophilic states.
Myeloproliferative disorders.
Cold injury.
Hepatitis-associated vasculitis.
Cryoglobulinemia.
Vinyl chloride exposure.

EMBOLISM

Cardiac (most common).
Proximal aneurysm.
Arterial thoracic outlet syndrome.
Atheroembolism.
Paradoxic embolus (with accompanying septal defect).

TRAUMA

Iatrogenic.
Blunt arterial injury.
Penetrating arterial injury.
Hypothenar hammer syndrome.
Vibration.

ISCHEMIC BOWEL DISEASE[1]

ICD 9CM # 557.1
ICD 10CM # K55.1 Vascular disorder of intestine
I99 Other and unspecified disorders of circulatory system

Abdominal aortic aneurysm: rupture or expansion.
Perforated ulcer or viscus.
Ruptured ectopic pregnancy (woman of child-bearing age).
Incarcerated or strangulated hernia.
Septic shock.
Intussusception.
Volvulus.
Salpingitis or tuboovarian abscess.
Torsion of the ovary or testicle.
Appendicitis.
Pelvic mass or torsion.
Pancreatitis.
Diverticulitis.
Ruptured ovarian cyst.
Renal colic.
Biliary colic.
Also consider atypical manifestations of:
- Inferior wall myocardial infarction.
- Pulmonary embolism.
- Pneumonia.
- Diabetic ketoacidosis.
- Acute glaucoma.

Differential diagnoses are listed in order of urgency.

ISCHEMIC COLITIS, NONOCCLUSIVE[21]

ICD-9CM # 557.1
ICD-10CM # K55.1 Chronic vascular disorders of intestine

ACUTE DIMINUTION OF COLONIC INTRAMURAL BLOOD FLOW

Small Vessel Obstruction

Collagen-vascular disease.
Vasculitis, diabetes.
Oral contraceptives.

Nonocclusive Hypoperfusion

Hemorrhage.
CHF, MI, arrhythmias.
Sepsis.
Vasoconstricting agents: vasopressin, ergot.
Increased viscosity: polycythemia, sickle cell disease, thrombocytosis.

INCREASED DEMAND ON MARGINAL BLOOD FLOW

Increased Motility

Mass lesion, stricture.
Constipation.

Increased Intraluminal Pressure

Bowel obstruction.
Colonoscopy.
Barium enema.

ISCHEMIC NECROSIS OF CARTILAGE AND BONE[14]

ICD-9CM # 733.90
ICD-10CM # M89.9 Disorder of bone, unspecified
M94.9 Disorder of cartilage, unspecified

ENDOCRINE/METABOLIC

Ethanol abuse.
Glucocorticoid therapy.
Cushing's disease.
DM.
Hyperuricemia.
Osteomalacia.
Hyperlipidemia.

STORAGE DISEASES (E.G., GAUCHER'S DISEASE)

Hemoglobinopathies (e.g., sickle cell disease).
Trauma (e.g., dislocation, fracture).
HIV infection.
Dysbaric conditions (e.g., caisson disease).
Collagen-vascular disorders.
Irradiation.
Pancreatitis.
Organ transplantation.
Hemodialysis.
Burns.
Intravascular coagulation.
Idiopathic, familial.

JAUNDICE

ICD-9CM # 782.4 Jaundice NOS
576.8 Jaundice, Obstructive
277.4 Bilirubin Excretion Disorders
ICD-10CM # R17 Unspecified jaundice
K83.8 Other specified diseases of biliary tract
E80.7 Disorder of bilirubin metabolism, unspecified

PREDOMINANCE OF DIRECT (CONJUGATED) BILIRUBIN

Extrahepatic obstruction.
Common duct abnormalities: calculi, neoplasm, stricture, cyst, sclerosing cholangitis.
Metastatic carcinoma.
Pancreatic carcinoma, pseudocyst.
Ampullary carcinoma.
Hepatocellular disease: hepatitis, cirrhosis.
Drugs: estrogens, phenothiazines, captopril, methyltestosterone, labetalol.
Cholestatic jaundice of pregnancy.
Hereditary disorders: Dubin-Johnson syndrome, Rotor's syndrome.
Recurrent benign intrahepatic cholestasis.

PREDOMINANCE OF INDIRECT (UNCONJUGATED) BILIRUBIN

Hemolysis: hereditary and acquired hemolytic anemias.
Inefficient marrow production.
Impaired hepatic conjugation: chloramphenicol.
Neonatal jaundice.
Hereditary disorders: Gilbert's syndrome, Crigler-Najjar syndrome.

JAUNDICE, CLASSIFICATION[1a]

ICD-9CM # 782.4
ICD-10CM # R17 Unspecified jaundice

PREHEPATIC (PREDOMINANTLY UNCONJUGATED HYPERBILIRUBINEMIA)

Overproduction

Hemolysis (e.g., spherocytosis, sickle cell disease, hemolysis of the newborn, autoimmune disorders).
Ineffective erythropoiesis (e.g., megaloblastic anemias).
Hematomas.
Pulmonary emboli.

HEPATIC (UNCONJUGATED HYPERBILIRUBINEMIA)

Decreased Hepatic Uptake

Gilbert syndrome.
Drugs (e.g., rifampin, radiographic contrast agents).
Neonatal jaundice.
Posthepatitis.
Decreased cystolic binding proteins (e.g., newborn or premature infants).
Portacaval shunt.
Prolonged fasting.

Decreased Conjugation Due to Limited Glucuronyl Transferase Activity

Gilbert's disease.
Crigler-Najjar syndrome, types I and II.
Neonatal jaundice.
Breast-milk jaundice.
Chronic persistent hepatitis.
Wilson's disease.
Noncirrhotic portal fibrosis.
Drug inhibition (e.g., chloramphenicol).

PREDOMINANTLY CONJUGATED HYPERBILIRUBINEMIA

Impaired Hepatic Excretion

Familial disorders (Dubin-Johnson syndrome, Rotor syndrome, benign recurrent cholestasis, cholestasis of pregnancy).
Hepatocellular infiltrative disorders.
Liver metastasis.
Liver cirrhosis.
Hepatitis (viral, bacterial, parasitic, autoimmune, ethanol, and drug-induced).
Drug-induced cholestasis (especially chlorpromazine, erythromycin estolate, isoniazid, halothane).
Primary biliary cirrhosis.
Primary sclerosing cholangitis.
Pericholangitis.
Congestive heart failure.
Shock.
Toxemia of pregnancy.
Sarcoidosis.
Hepatic trauma.
Amyloidosis.
Autoimmune cholangiopathy.
Vanishing bile duct syndrome.
Sepsis.
Postoperative complications.

EXTRAHEPATIC

Extrahepatic Biliary Obstruction

Gallstones, choledocholithiasis.
Cholecystitis.
Tumors of the head of the pancreas (adenocarcinoma, mucinous duct ectasia, neuroendocrine tumors, metastasis).
Tumors of bile ducts (cholangiocarcinoma, Klatskin tumor: cholangiocarcinoma at the bifurcation).
Gallbladder cancer.
Tumors of the ampulla of Vater (adenoma, adenocarcinoma).
Tumors of the duodenum (adenocarcinoma, lymphoma).
Hemobilia (blood in the biliary tree).
Biliary strictures (postcholecystectomy, post-liver transplantation, primary sclerosing cholangitis).
Congential disorders (biliary atresia, idiopathic dilation of common bile duct, cystic fibrosis).
Metastasis to the hepatic hilum.
Primary bile duct lymphoma.
Cholangiopathy of acquired immunodeficiency syndrome.
Choledochal cysts.
Infectious cholangiopathy (*Clonorchis sinensis, Ascaris lumbricoides, Fasciola hepatica).*
Chronic pancreatitis (fibrosis of the head of the pancreas).

JAUNDICE, NEONATAL[1a]

ICD-9CM # 774.6
ICD-10CM # P59.9 Neonatal jaundice, unspecified

PREHEPATIC

Hereditary spherocytosis.
Nonspherocytic hemolytic anemia (glucose-6-phosphate dehydrogenase deficiency, α-thalassemia, vitamin K_3–induced hemolysis, pyruvate kinase deficiency).

HEPATIC

Crigler-Najjar syndrome, types I and II.
α_1-Antitrypsin deficiency.
Sepsis.
Drug-induced.
Hypothyroidism.
Breast-milk jaundice.
Fetomaternal blood group incompatibility (Rhesus, Landsteiner groups ABO).

POSTHEPATIC

Extrahepatic biliary obstruction.
Biliary atresia.
Bile duct paucity.
Alagille syndrome.

JOINT AND PERIARTICULAR PAIN, ACUTE[12a]

ICD-9CM # 719.40
ICD-10CM # M25.50 Joint pain

COMMON ACUTE MONOARTHRITIS

Septic arthritis (nongonococcal, gonococcal).
Crystal arthritis (gout, pseudogout).
Reactive arthritides.
Lyme disease.
Plant thorn synovitis.
Other infections (mycobacterial, viral, soft tissue).

TRAUMA OR INTERNAL DERANGEMENT

Loose bodies.
Stress fractures.
Ischemic necrosis.
Hemarthrosis.

ACUTE MONOARTHRITIS OF POLYARTHRITIS

Psoriatic arthritis.
Enteropathic arthritis.
Rheumatoid arthritis/palindromic rheumatism.
Juvenile inflammatory arthritides.

MONOARTHROPATHIES FROM NONINFLAMMATORY DISEASE

Osteoarthritis.
Charcot's joints.
Storage diseases (hemochromatosis, ochronosis).

SYNOVIAL DISEASES

Pigmented villonodular synovitis.
Lipoma arborescens.
Synovial osteochondromatosis.
Reflex sympathetic dystrophy.
Sarcoidosis.
Amyloid.

ACUTE MONOARTHRITIS OF SYSTEMIC DISEASE

Systemic lupus erythematosus.
Vasculitides (antineutrophil cytoplasmic antibody positive and negative).
Henoch-Schönlein purpura.
Behçet's disease.
Bacterial endocarditis.
Familial Mediterranean fever.
Relapsing polychondritis.

SOFT TISSUE LESIONS

BONE DISEASES

Paget's disease.
Osteomyelitis (Brodie's abscess).
Osteogenic/osteoid tumors.
Metastatic disease.
Pulmonary hypertrophic osteoarthropathy.

This table shows the causes of inflammation in any one joint (monoarthritis) and pain around the joint that presents without inflammation (monoarthropathy).

JOINT PAIN, ANTERIOR HIP, MEDIAL THIGH, KNEE[28]

ICD-9CM # 719.4 add 5th digit

0 Site NOS
1 Shoulder Region
2 Upper Arm (Elbow, Humerus)
3 Forearm (Radius, Wrist, Ulna)
4 Hand
5 Pelvic Region and Thigh
6 Lower Leg (Fibula, Patella, Tibia)
7 Ankle and/or Foot

ICD-10CM # M25.50 Pain in unspecified joint
M25.559 Pain in unspecified hip
M25.569 Pain in unspecified knee

ACUTE

Acute rheumatic fever.
Adductor muscle strain.
Avascular necrosis.
Crystal arthritis.
Femoral artery (pseudo) aneurysm.
Fracture (femoral neck or intertrochanteric).
Hemarthrosis.
Hernia.
Herpes zoster.
Iliopectineal bursitis.
Iliopsoas tendinitis.
Inguinal lymphadenitis.
Osteomalacia.
Painful transient osteoporosis of hip.
Septic arthritis.

SUBACUTE AND CHRONIC

Adductory muscle strain.
Amyloidosis.
Acute rheumatic fever.
Femoral artery aneurysm.
Hernia (inguinal or femoral).
Iliopectineal bursitis.
Iliopsoas tendinitis.
Inguinal lymphadenopathy.
Osteochondromatosis.
Osteomyelitis.
Osteitis deformans (Paget's disease).
Osteomalacia (pseudofracture).
Postherpetic neuralgia.
Sterile synovitis (e.g., RA, psoriatic, SLE).

JOINT PAIN, HIP, LATERAL THIGH[28]

ICD-9CM # 959.6 Hip Injury
719.95 Hip Joint Disorder
843.9 Hip Strain
ICD-10CM # S79.919A Unspecified injury of unspecified hip, initial encounter
S79.929A Unspecified injury of unspecified thigh, initial encounter
M25.9 Joint disorder, unspecified

ACUTE

Herpes zoster.
Iliotibial tendinitis.
Impacted fracture of femoral neck.
Lateral femoral cutaneous neuropathy (meralgia paresthetica).
Radiculopathy: L4-5.
Trochanteric avulsion fracture (greater trochanter).
Trochanteric bursitis.
Trochanteric fracture.

SUBACUTE AND CHRONIC

Lateral femoral cutaneous neuropathy (meralgia paresthetica).
Osteomyelitis.
Postherpetic neuralgia.
Radiculopathy: L4-5.
Tumors.

JOINT PAIN, POLYARTICULAR

ICD-9CM # 719.40
ICD-10CM # M25.50 Pain in unspecified join

Osteoarthritis.
RA.
Fibromyalgia.
Viral syndrome (e.g., human parvovirus B19 infection).
SLE.
Psoriatic arthritis.
Ankylosing spondylitis.

JOINT PAIN, POSTERIOR HIPS, THIGH, BUTTOCKS[28]

ICD-9CM # 719.4 add 5th digit

0 Site NOS
1 Shoulder Region
2 Upper Arm (Elbow, Humerus)
3 Forearm (Radius, Wrist, Ulna)
4 Hand
5 Pelvic Region and Thigh
6 Lower Leg (Fibula, Patella, Tibia)
7 Ankle and/or Foot

ICD-10CM # M25.50 Pain in unspecified joint
M25.559 Pain in unspecified hip
M25.569 Pain in unspecified knee

ACUTE

Gluteal muscle strain.
Herpes zoster.
Ischial bursitis.
Ischial or sacral fracture.
Osteomalacia (pseudofracture).
Sciatic neuropathy.
Radiculopathy: L5-S1.

SUBACUTE AND CHRONIC

Gluteal muscle strain.
Ischial bursitis.
Lumbar spinal stenosis.
Osteoarthritis of hip.
Osteitis deformans (Paget's disease).
Osteomyelitis.
Osteochondromatosis.
Osteomalacia (pseudofracture).
Postherpetic neuralgia.
Radiculopathy: L5-S1.
Tumors.

JOINT SWELLING

ICD-9CM # 719.0 add 5th digit

0 Site NOS
1 Shoulder Region
2 Upper Arm (Elbow, Humerus)
3 Forearm (Radius, Wrist, Ulna)
4 Hand
5 Pelvic Region and Thigh
6 Lower Leg (Fibula, Patella, Tibia)
7 Ankle and/or Foot

ICD-10CM # M25.40 Effusion, unspecified joint

Trauma.
Osteoarthritis.
Gout.
Pyogenic arthritis.
Pseudogout.
RA.
Viral syndrome.

JUGULAR VENOUS DISTENTION

ICD-9CM # 459.89 Increased Venous Pressure
ICD-10CM # I99.8 Other disorder of circulatory system

Right-sided heart failure.
Cardiac tamponade.
Constrictive pericarditis.
Goiter.
Tension pneumothorax.
Pulmonary hypertension.
Cardiomyopathy (restrictive).
Superior vena cava syndrome.
Valsalva maneuver.
Right atrial myxoma.
COPD.

KERATITIS, NONINFECTIOUS

ICD-9CM # 370.9
ICD-10CM # H16.9 Unspecified keratitis

Collagen vascular disease.
Atopic keratoconjunctivitis.
Chemical injury.
Thermal injury.
Ectropion/entropion.
Lid defects.
Exophthalmos.
Keratoconjunctivitis sicca.
Erythema multiforme.
Mucous membrane pemphigoid.
DM (delayed epithelial healing).
Neuroparalytic (cranial nerve VII).
Neurotrophic (diabetes, cranial nerve V).

KIDNEY ENLARGEMENT, UNILATERAL[38]

ICD-9CM # 591
ICD-10CM # N13.30 Unspecified hydronephrosis

Hydronephrosis (may be bilateral).
Polycystic kidney (may be bilateral).
Simple cyst of kidney.
Renal cell carcinoma.
Pyonephrosis (may be bilateral).
Acute renal vein thrombosis.

KNEE PAIN[28]

ICD-9CM #	844.1	Collateral Ligament Sprain, Medial
	844.2	Cruciate Ligament Sprain
	716.96	Knee Inflammation
	959.7	Knee Injury
	718.86	Knee Instability
	836.1	Lateral Meniscus Tear
	836.0	Medial Meniscus Tear
	844.8	Patellar Sprain
	719.56	Knee Stiffness
	719.06	Knee Swelling
ICD-10CM #	S83.419A	Sprain of medial collateral ligament of unspecified knee, initial encounter
	S83.509A	Sprain of unspecified cruciate ligament of unspecified knee, initial encounter
	M23.50	Chronic instability of knee, unspecified knee
	M23.8X9	Other internal derangements of unspecified knee
	S83.289A	Other tear of lateral meniscus, current injury, unspecified knee, initial encounter
	S83.249A	Other tear of medial meniscus, current injury, unspecified knee, initial encounter
	M25.669	Stiffness of unspecified knee, not elsewhere classified

DIFFUSE

Articular.
Anterior.
Prepatellar bursitis.
Patellar tendon enthesopathy.
Chondromalacia patellae.
Patellofemoral osteoarthritis.
Cruciate ligament injury.
Medial plica syndrome.

MEDIAL

Anserine bursitis.
Spontaneous osteonecrosis.
Osteoarthritis.
Medial meniscal tear.
Medial collateral ligament bursitis.
Referred pain from hip and L3.
Fibromyalgia.

LATERAL

Iliotibial band syndrome.
Meniscal cyst.
Lateral meniscal tear.
Collateral ligament.
Peroneal tenosynovitis.

POSTERIOR

Popliteal cyst (Baker's cyst).
Tendinitis.
Aneurysms, ganglions, sarcoma.

KNEE PAIN, IN DIFFERENT AGE GROUPS[8]

ICD-9CM # 719.46
ICD-10CM # M25.569 Pain in unspecified knee

COMMON CAUSES OF KNEE PAIN IN DIFFERENT AGE GROUPS

CHILDHOOD (2-10 YR)

Intraarticular:
Juvenile arthritis.
Osteochondritis dissecans.
Infection.
Torn discoid meniscus.
Periarticular:
Osteomyelitis.
Referred:
Perthes' disease.
Irritable hip.

ADOLESCENCE (10-18 YR)

Intraarticular:
Osteochondritis dissecans.
Torn meniscus.
Anterior knee pain syndrome.
Patellar instability.
Periarticular:
Osgood–Schlatter disease.
Sinding–Larsen–Johansson syndrome.
Osteomyelitis.
Bone tumors.
Referred:
Slipped upper femoral epiphysis.

EARLY ADULTHOOD (18-30 YR)

Intraarticular:
Torn meniscus.
Patellar instability.

Anterior knee pain syndrome.
Inflammatory arthritis.
Periarticular:
Ligament injuries.
Bursitis.
ADULTHOOD (30-50 YR)
Intraarticular:
Degenerate meniscal tears.
Osteoarthritis.
Inflammatory arthritis.
Periarticular:
Bursitis.
Referred:
Osteoarthritis of hip.
Spinal disorders.
OLD AGE (>50 YR)
Intraarticular:
Osteoarthritis.
Inflammatory arthritis.
Periarticular:
Bursitis.
Referred:
Osteoarthritis of hip.
Spinal disorders.

LARGE BOWEL STRICTURE[16a]

ICD-9CM # 751.2
ICD-10CM # S36.5 Injury of colon

CAUSES OF LARGE BOWEL STRICTURES

Physiologic:
- Spasm.
- Distended bladder.

Maligant:
- Annular carcinoma.
- Scirrhous carcinoma.
- Lymphoma.

Diverticular disease:
- Muscle thickening.
- Pericolic abscess.
- Superimposed malignancy.

Ischemia.
Radiation colitis.
Inflammatory bowel disease:
- Ulcerative colitis.
- Crohn's disease.
- Tuberculosis.
- Lymphogranuloma venereum.
- Amebiasis.

Extrinsic disease:
- Intraabdominal masses.
- Melastatic carcinoma.
- Endometriosis.
- Pelvic lipomatosis.
- Cholecystitis.
- Pancreatitis.

Miscellaneous:
- Postoperative anastomosis.
- Trauma.
- Hirschsprung's disease.

LEFT AXIS DEVIATION[22]

ICD-9CM # 426.3 Left Bundle Branch Block
426.2 Left Bundle Branch Hemiblock
429.3 Left Ventricular Hypertrophy
ICD-10CM # I44.7 Left bundle-branch block, unspecified
I44.4 Left anterior fascicular block
I44.5 Left posterior fascicular block
I44.60 Unspecified fascicular block
I44.69 Other fascicular block

Normal variation.
Left anterior fascicular block (hemiblock).
Left bundle branch block.
Left ventricular hypertrophy.
Mechanical shifts causing a horizontal heart, high diaphragm, pregnancy, ascites.
Some forms of ventricular tachycardia.
Endocardial cushion defects and other congenital heart disease.

LEFT BUNDLE BRANCH BLOCK

ICD-9CM # 426.3
ICD-10CM # I44.7 Left bundle-branch block, unspecified

Ischemic heart disease.
Electrolyte abnormalities (e.g., hyperkalemia).
Cardiomyopathy.
Idiopathic.
LVH.
Pulmonary embolism.
Cardiac trauma.
Bacterial endocarditis.

LEG CRAMPS, NOCTURNAL

ICD-9CM # 729.82 Muscle Cramps
ICD-10CM # R25.2 Cramp and spasm

Diabetic neuropathy.
Medications.
Electrolyte abnormalities (hypokalemia, hyponatremia, hypocalcemia, hyperkalemia, hypophosphatemia).
Respiratory alkalosis.
Uremia.
Hemodialysis.
Peripheral nerve injury.
ALS.
Alcohol use.
Heat cramps.
Vitamin B_{12} deficiency.
Hyperthyroidism.
Contractures.
DVT.
Hypoglycemia.
Peripheral vascular insufficiency.
Baker's cyst.

LEG LENGTH DISCREPANCIES[23]

ICD-9CM # 736.81 Leg Length Discrepancy, Acquired
755.30 Leg Length Discrepancy, Congenital
ICD-10CM # M21.759 Unequal limb length (acquired), unspecified femur
M21.769 Unequal limb length (acquired), unspecified tibia and fibula
Q72.899 Other reduction defects of unspecified lower limb

CONGENITAL

Proximal femoral local deficiency.
Coxa vara.
Hemiatrophy-hemihypertrophy (anisomelia).
Developmental dysplasia of the hip.

DEVELOPMENTAL

Legg-Calvé-Perthes disease.

NEUROMUSCULAR

Polio.
Cerebral palsy (hemiplegia).

INFECTIOUS

Pyogenic osteomyelitis with physeal damage.

TRAUMA

Physeal injury with premature closure.
Overgrowth.
Malunion (shortening).

TUMOR

Physeal destruction.
Radiation-induced physeal injury.
Overgrowth.

LEG MOVEMENT WHEN STANDING, INVOLUNTARY

ICD-9CM # varies with specific disorder
ICD-10CM # R25.8 Other abnormal involuntary movements

Benign essential tremor.
Orthostatic tremor.
Spastic ataxia.
Cerebellar truncal tremor.
Postanoxic myoclonus.

LEG PAIN WITH EXERCISE

ICD-9CM # 729.82 Muscle Cramps
ICD-10CM # R25.2 Cramp and spasm

Shin splints.
Arteriosclerosis obliterans.
Neurogenic (spinal cord compression or ischemia).
Venous claudication.
Popliteal cyst.
DVT.
Thromboangiitis obliterans.
Adventitial cysts.
Popliteal artery entrapment syndrome.
McArdle syndrome.

LEG SWELLING[1]

ICD-9CM # 782.3
ICD-10CM # R60.0

Deep vein thrombosis.
Cellulitis.
Baker cyst rupture or inflammation.
Congestive heart failure.
Renal failure.
Liver failure.
Inferior vena cava compression.
Musculoskeletal trauma.
Polyarteritis nodosa.
Erythema nodosum.
Myositis.
Tendinitis.
Lymphedema.
Superficial thrombophlebitis.
Compartment syndrome.

LEG ULCERS[28]

ICD-9CM #	440.23	Lower Limb, Arteriosclerotic
	707.1	Lower Limb, Chronic
	707.1	Lower Limb, Neurogenic
	250.70	Lower Limb, Chronic DM Type 2
	250.71	Lower Limb, Chronic DM Type 1
ICD-10CM #	I70.25	Atherosclerosis of native arteries of other extremities with ulceration
	L97.909	Non-pressure chronic ulcer of unspecified part of unspecified lower leg with unspecified severity

VASCULAR

Arterial: arteriosclerosis, thromboangiitis obliterans, AV malformation, cholesterol emboli.
Venous: superficial varicosities, incompetent perforators, DVT, lymphatic abnormalities.

VASCULITIS HEMATOLOGIC

Sickle cell anemia, thalassemia, polycythemia vera, leukemia, cold agglutinin disease.
Macroglobulinemia, protein C and protein S deficiency, cryoglobulinemia, lupus anticoagulant, antiphospholipid syndrome.

INFECTIOUS

Fungal: Blastomycosis, coccidioidomycosis, histoplasmosis, sporotrichosis.
Bacterial: Furuncle, ecthyma, septic emboli.
Protozoal: leishmaniasis.

METABOLIC

Necrobiosis lipoidica diabeticorum.
Localized bullous pemphigoid.
Gout, calcinosis cutis, Gaucher's disease.

TUMORS

Basal cell carcinoma, squamous cell carcinoma, melanoma.
Mycosis fungoides, Kaposi's sarcoma, metastatic neoplasms.

TRAUMA

Burns, cold injury, radiation dermatitis.
Insect bites.
Factitial, excessive pressure.

NEUROPATHIC

Diabetic trophic ulcers.
Tabes dorsalis, syringomyelia.

DRUGS

Warfarin, IV colchicine extravasation, methotrexate, halogens, ergotism, hydroxyurea.

PANNICULITIS

Weber-Christian disease.
Pancreatic fat necrosis, alpha-antitrypsinase deficiency.

LEPTOMENINGEAL LESIONS

ICD-9CM # varies with specific disorder
ICD-10CM # G03.9 Leptomeningitis

Metastases.
Multiple sclerosis.
Bacterial or viral meningitis.
Vasculitis.
Lyme disease.
Tuberculosis.
Fungal infections (e.g., *Cryptococcus*).
Sarcoidosis.
Wegener's granulomatosis.
Neurocysticercosis.
Rheumatoid nodules.
Histiocytosis.

LEUKOCORIA

ICD-9CM # 379.90
ICD-10CM # H57.9 Unspecified disorder of eye and adnexa

Cataract.
Retinal detachment.
Retinoblastoma.
Retinal telangiectasia.
Retrolenticular vascularized membrane.
Familial exudative vitreoretinopathy.

LID RETRACTION, CAUSES[20a]

ICD-9CM # 374.41 Lid Retraction
ICD-10CM # H02.539 Eyelid retraction unspecified eye, unspecified lid

Thyroid eye disease.
Neurogenic.
- Contralateral unilateral ptosis.
- Unopposed levator action due to facial palsy.
- 3rd nerve misdirection.
- Marcus Gunn jaw-winking syndrome.
- Collier sign of the dorsal midbrain (Parinaud syndrome).
- Infantile hydrocephalus (setting sun sign).
- Parkinsonism.
- Sympathomimetic drops.

Mechanical.
- Surgical over-correction of ptosis.
- Scarring of upper lid skin.

Congenital.
- Isolated.
- Duane retraction syndrome.
- Down syndrome.
- Transient "eye popping" reflex in normal infants.

Miscellaneous.
- Prominent globe (pseudo-lid retraction).
- Uremia (Summerskill sign).
- Idiopathic.

LIMB ISCHEMIA, ACUTE, NONTRAUMATIC[5a]

ICD-9CM # 903.8
ICD-10CM # Atherosclerosis of arteries of extremities

CAUSES OF NONTRAUMATIC ACUTE LIMB ISCHEMIA

Atherosclerotic

In situ thrombosis.
Atheroembolism from thoracic aortic aneurysm/abdominal aortic aneurysm.
Femoral/popliteal aneurysm with or without compression.
Dissection.

Nonatherosclerotic

Embolism from cardiac thrombosis (atrial fibrillation, post–myocardial infarction akinesis).
Graft thrombosis, graft aneurysm.
Mycotic emboli.
Raynaud syndrome.
Arteritis with thrombosis.
Inherited and acquired hypercoagulable states.
Drug-induced vasospasm.
External compression (Baker cyst, popliteal entrapment).

Mimics

Phlegmasia cerulea dolens.
Acute neuropathy.
Hypovolemia.
Systemic shock.

LIMP

ICD-9CM #	781.2	Gait Abnormality
	719.75	Gait Disorder Due to Joint Abnormality in Hip, Buttock, or Femur
	719.76	Gait Disorder Due to Joint Abnormality in Lower Leg
	719.77	Gait Disorder Due to Joint Abnormality in Ankle and/or Foot
	300.11	Hysterical Gait Disorder
ICD-10CM #	R26.0	Ataxic gait
	R26.1	Paralytic gait
	R26.89	Other abnormalities of gait and mobility

Differential Diagnosis II

R26.9	Unspecified abnormalities of gait and mobility
M25.80	Other specified joint disorders, unspecified joint
F44.4	Conversion disorder with motor symptom or deficit
F44.6	Conversion disorder with sensory symptom or deficit

Degenerative joint disease, osteochondritis dissecans, chondromalacia patellae.
Trauma to extremities, vertebral disk, hips.
Poorly fitting shoes, foreign body in shoe, unequal leg length.
Splinter in foot.
Joint infection (septic arthritis, osteomyelitis), viral arthritis.
Abdominal pain (e.g., appendicitis, incarcerated hernia), testicular torsion.
Polio, neuromuscular disorders, Guillain-Barré syndrome, multiple sclerosis.
Osgood-Schlatter disease.
Legg-Calvé-Perthes disease.
Factitious, somatization syndrome.
Neoplasm (local or metastatic).
Other: diskitis, periostitis, sickle cell disease, hemophilia.

LIMPING, PEDIATRIC AGE[23]

ICD-9CM # 781.2 Gait Abnormality
ICD-10CM # R26.0 Ataxic gait
R26.1 Paralytic gait
R26.89 Other abnormalities of gait and mobility
R26.9 Unspecified abnormalities of gait and mobility

TODDLER (1-3 YR)

Infection:
- Septic arthritis:
  - Hip.
  - Knee.
- Osteomyelitis.
- Diskitis.

Occult trauma:
- Toddler's fracture.

Neoplasia.

CHILDHOOD (4-10 YR)

Infection:
- Septic arthritis:
  - Hip.
  - Knee.
- Osteomyelitis.
- Diskitis.
- Transient synovitis, hip.

LCPD.
Tarsal coalition.
Rheumatologic disorder:
- JRA.

Trauma.
Neoplasia.

ADOLESCENCE (11 + YR)

SCFE.
Rheumatologic disorder:
- JRA.

Trauma.
Tarsal coalition.
Hip dislocation (DDH).
Neoplasia.

DDH, Developmental dysplasia of the hip; *JRA,* juvenile RA; *LCPD,* Legg-Calvé-Perthes disease; *SCFE,* slipped capital femoral epiphysis.

LIVEDO RETICULARIS

ICD-9CM # code not available
ICD-10CM # L95.0 Livedoid vasculitis

Emboli (SBE, left atrial myxoma, cholesterol emboli).
Thrombocythemia or polycythemia.
Antiphospholipid antibody syndrome.
Cryoglobulinemia, cryofibrinogenemia.
Leukocytoclastic vasculitis.
SLE, RA, dermatomyositis.
Pancreatitis.
Drugs (quinine, quinidine, amantadine, catecholamines).
Physiologic (cutis marmorata).
Congenital.

LIVER DISEASE, PREGNANCY[38]

ICD-9CM # varies with specific diagnosis
ICD-10CM # K75.89 Other specified inflammatory liver diseases

INCIDENTAL TO PREGNANCY

Viral hepatitis.
Alcohol related.
Autoimmune chronic active hepatitis.

RELATED TO PREGNANCY (POSSIBLY INFLUENCED BY HORMONES PRESENT IN PREGNANCY)

Complicated gallstone disease.
Hepatic adenoma.
Focal nodular hyperplasia.
Budd-Chiari syndrome.

SPECIFIC TO PREGNANCY

Severe hyperemesis gravidarum.
Benign intrahepatic cholestasis.
Acute fatty liver of pregnancy.
Preeclampsia (HELLP).

LIVER LESIONS, BENIGN, OFTEN CONFUSED WITH MALIGNANCY

ICD-9CM # 573.8
ICD-10CM # K76.1 Chronic passive congestion of liver
K76.89 Other specified diseases of liver

Fatty infiltration.
Adenoma.
Hemangioma.
Cysts.
Flow artifacts.
Focal nodular hyperplasia.
Nonenhanced vessels.

LOW-VOLTAGE ECG

ICD-9CM # 794.31
ICD-10CM # R94.31 Abnormal electrocardiogram [ECG] [EKG]

Hypothyroidism.
Obesity.
Pericardial effusion.
Anasarca.
Pleural effusion.
Pneumothorax.
Amyloidosis.
Aortic stenosis.

LUNG CANCER, OCCUPATIONAL CAUSES[16a]

ICD-9CM # 162.9
ICD-10CM # C34.90 Malignant neoplasm of unspecified part of unspecified bronchus or lung

CAUSES OF OCCUPATIONAL LUNG CANCER

Asbestos	Lagging, insulation
Arsenic	Metal smelting, pesticide manufacture
Beryllium	Electronics, dental prosthetic manufacture
Chromium	Coloring pigment production, electroplating
Nickel	Electroplating
Silica	Grinding, quarrying, sandblasting
Radon	Mining
Uranium	Mining

LUNG VOLUMES IN DIFFUSE LUNG DISEASE[14a]

ICD-9CM # varies with specific disorder
ICD-10CM # varies with specific disorder

LARGE LUNG VOLUMES

Emphysema.
Chonic asthma.
Diffuse bronchiolitis obliterans.
Highly trained athletes.
Lymphangioleiomyomatosis.

SMALL LUNG VOLUMES

End-stage lung fibrosis.
Bilateral diaphragmatic paralysis.
Massive ascites.

NORMAL LUNG VOLUMES

Sarcoidosis.
Langerhans cell histiocytosis.

Neurofibromatosis.
Emphysema with pulmonary fibrosis.

LYMPHADENOPATHY[14]

ICD-9CM # 785.6
ICD-10CM # R59.9 Enlarged lymph nodes, unspecified

GENERALIZED

AIDS.
Lymphoma: Hodgkin's disease, non-Hodgkin's lymphoma.
Leukemias, reticuloendotheliosis.
Infectious mononucleosis, CMV, and other viral infections.
Diffuse skin infection: generalized furunculosis, multiple tick bites.
Parasitic infections: toxoplasmosis, filariasis, leishmaniasis, Chagas' disease.
Serum sickness.
Collagen vascular diseases (RA, SLE).
Dengue (arbovirus infection).
Sarcoidosis and other granulomatous diseases.
Drugs: INH, hydantoin derivatives, antithyroid and antileprosy drugs.
Secondary syphilis.
Hyperthyroidism, lipid-storage diseases.

LOCALIZED

Cervical Nodes
Infections of the head, neck, ears, sinuses, scalp, pharynx.
Mononucleosis.
Lymphoma.
TB.
Malignancy of head and neck.
Rubella.
Scalene/Supraclavicular Nodes
Lymphoma.
Lung neoplasm.
Bacterial or fungal infection of thorax or retroperitoneum.
GI malignancy.
Axillary Nodes
Infections of hands and arms.
Cat-scratch disease.
Neoplasm (lymphoma, melanoma, breast carcinoma).
Brucellosis.
Epitrochlear Nodes
Infections of the hand.
Lymphoma.
Tularemia.
Sarcoidosis, secondary syphilis (usually bilateral).
Inguinal Nodes
Infections of leg or foot, folliculitis (pubic hair).
LGV, syphilis.
Lymphoma.
Pelvic malignancy.
Pasteurella pestis.
Hilar Nodes
Sarcoidosis.
TB.
Lung carcinoma.
Fungal infections, systemic.
Mediastinal Nodes
Sarcoidosis.
Lymphoma.
Lung neoplasm.
TB.
Mononucleosis.
Histoplasmosis.
Abdominal/Retroperitoneal Nodes
Lymphoma.
TB.
Neoplasm (ovary, testes, prostate, and other malignancies).

LYMPHANGITIS[25a]

ICD-9CM # 457.2
ICD-10CM # I89.1 Lymphangitis

Acute:
Group A streptococci.
Staphylococcus aureus.
Pasteurella multocida.
Chronic:
Sporothrix schenckii (sporotrichosis).
Mycobacterium marinum (swimming pool granuloma).
Mycobacterium kansasii.
Nocardia brasiliensis.
W.bancrofti.

LYMPHOCYTOSIS, ATYPICAL[25a]

ICD-9CM # 288.8
ICD-10CM # D72.89 Other specified disorders of white blood cells

Epstein-Barr virus primary infection (infectious mononucleosis).
Cytomegalovirus primary infection (heterophile-negative mono).
Human herpesvirus 6 primary infection (roseola).
Primary HIV infection.
Toxoplasmosis.
Acute viral hepatitis.
Rubella, mumps.
Drug reactions (e.g., phenytoin, sulfa).

MACROTHROMBOCYTOPENIA, INHERITED[20]

ICD-9CM # varies with specific diagnosis
ICD-10CM # varies with specific disorder

Bernard-Soulier syndrome.
MHY9-related disorders:
- May-Hegglin anomaly.
- Sebastian syndrome.
- Fechtner syndrome.
- Epstein syndrome.

Gray platelet syndrome.
Montreal platelet syndrome.
Mediterranean macrothrombocytopenia.
Mediterranean stomatocytosis/macrothrombocytemia.
GATA1 mutations.
Sialyl-Lewis-S antigen deficiency.
Paris-Trousseau syndrome.
Platelet-type von Willebrand's disease.

MALABSORPTION[38]

ICD-9CM # 579
ICD-10CM # K90.89 Other intestinal malabsorption

CAUSES OF MALABSORPTION

More Common
Celiac disease.
Chronic pancreatitis.
Post gastrectomy.
Crohn's disease.
Small bowel resection.
Small intestinal bacterial overgrowth.
Lactase deficiency.
Less Common
AIDS (*Myobacterium avium* intracellulare, AIDS enteropathy).
Whipple's disease.
Intestinal lymphoma.
Immunoproliferative small intestinal disease (alpha heavy chain disease).
Radiation enteritis.
Collagenous sprue.
Tropical sprue.
Non-granulomatous ulcerative jejunoileitis.
Eosinophilic gastroenteritis.
Amyloidosis.
Zollinger-Ellison syndrome.
Intestinal lymphangiectasia.
Systemic mastocytosis.
Chronic mesenteric ischemia.
Abetalipoproteinemia (autosomal recessive).

MALNUTRITION, CAUSES IN EARLY LIFE[22a]

ICD-9CM # V77.2
ICD-10CM # E46 Unspecified protein-energy malnutrition

0-6 MO

Breastfeeding difficulties.
Improper formula preparation.
Impaired parent/child interaction.
Congenital syndromes.
Prenatal infections or teratogenic exposures.
Poor feeding (sucking, swallowing) or feeding refusal (aversion).
Maternal psychological disorder (depression or attachment disorder).
Congenital heart disease.
Cystic fibrosis.
Neurologic abnormalities.
Child neglect.
Recurrent infections.

6-12 MO

Celiac disease.
Food intolerance.
Child neglect.
Delayed introduction of age-appropriate foods or poor transition to food.
Recurrent infections.
Food allergy.

AFTER INFANCY

Acquired chronic diseases.
Highly distractible child.
Inappropriate mealtime environment.
Inappropriate diet (e.g., excessive juice consumption, avoidance of high-calorie foods).
Recurrent infections.

MEDIASTINAL COMPARTMENTS, ANATOMY AND PATHOLOGY[39]

ICD-9CM # varies with specific diagnosis
ICD-10CM # varies with specific disorder

ANTERIOR

Normal Structures

Lymph nodes.
Connective tissue.
Thymus (remnant in adults).

Masses

Thymoma.
Germ cell neoplasm.
Lymphoma.
Thyroid enlargement (intrathoracic goiter).
Other tumors.

MIDDLE

Normal Structures

Pericardium.
Heart.
Vessels: Ascending aorta, venae cavae, main pulmonary arteries.
Trachea.
Lymph nodes.
Nerves: Phrenic, upper vagus.

Masses

Carcinoma.
Lymphoma.
Pericardial cyst.
Bronchogenic cyst.
Benign lymph node enlargement (granulomatous disease).

POSTERIOR

Normal Structures

Vessels: Descending aorta.
Esophagus.
Vertebral column.
Nerves: Sympathetic chain, lower vagus.
Lymph nodes.
Connective tissue.

Masses

Neurogenic tumor.
Diaphragmatic hernia.

MEDIASTINAL MASSES OR WIDENING ON CHEST X-RAY

ICD-9CM # 785.6 Adenopathy
519.3 Disease NEC
793.2 Shift (CXR)
ICD-10CM # R59.9 Enlarged lymph nodes, unspecified
J98.5 Diseases of mediastinum, not elsewhere classified

Lymphoma: Hodgkin's disease and non-Hodgkin's lymphoma.
Sarcoidosis.
Vascular: aortic aneurysm, ectasia, or tortuosity of aorta or bronchocephalic vessels.
Carcinoma: lungs, esophagus.
Esophageal diverticula.
Hiatal hernia.
Achalasia.
Prominent pulmonary outflow tract: pulmonary hypertension, pulmonary embolism, right-to-left shunts.
Trauma: mediastinal hemorrhage.
Pneumomediastinum.
Lymphadenopathy caused by silicosis and other pneumoconioses.
Leukemias.
Infections: TB, viral (rare), *Mycoplasma* (rare), fungal, tularemia.
Substernal thyroid.
Thymoma.
Teratoma.
Bronchogenic cyst.
Pericardial cyst.
Neurofibroma, neurosarcoma, ganglioneuroma.

MEDIASTINITIS, ACUTE[25a]

ICD-9CM # 519.2
ICD-10CM # J98.5 Diseases of mediastinum, not elsewhere classified

Esophageal perforation.
Iatrogenic.
EGD, esophageal dilation, esophageal variceal sclerotherapy, nasogastric tube, Sengstaken-Blackmore tube, endotracheal intubation, esophageal surgery, paraesophageal surgery, transesophageal echocardiography, anterior stabilization of cervical vertebral bodies.
Swallowed foreign bodies.
Trauma.
Spontaneous perforation (e.g., emesis, carcinoma).
Head and neck infections (e.g., tonsillitis, pharyngitis, parotitis, epiglottitis, odontogenic).
Infections originating at another site (e.g., TB, pneumonia, pancreatitis, osteomyelitis of sternum, clavicle, ribs).
Cardiothoracic surgery (median sternotomy) (e.g., CABG, valve replacement, other types of cardiothoracic surgery).

MELANONYCHIA

ICD-9CM # varies with specific disorder
ICD-10CM # NEC L81.4 Melanin hyperpigmentation

Pregnancy.
Trauma.
Medications (e.g., AZT, 5-fluorouracil, doxorubicin, psoralens).
Nail matrix nevus.
HIV infection.
Onychomycosis.
Melanocyte hyperplasia.
Verrucae.
Pustular psoriasis.
Lichen planus.
Basal cell carcinoma.
Nail matrix melanoma.
Subungual keratosis.
Addison's disease.
Bowen's disease.

MEMORY LOSS SYMPTOMS, ELDERLY PATIENTS

ICD-9CM # varies with specific disorder
ICD-10CM # R41.2 Retrograde amnesia

Age-related mild cognitive impairment.
Depression (pseudodementia).
Medications (e.g., anticholinergics, sedatives).
Hypothyroidism.
Chronic hypoxia.
Cerebrovascular infarcts.
Alzheimer's disease.
Hepatic disease.
Chronic renal failure.
Hyperthyroidism.
Frontotemporal dementia.
Lewy body dementia.

MENINGITIS, CHRONIC[26]

ICD-9CM # 322.2
ICD-10CM # G03.1 Chronic meningitis

TB.
Fungal CNS infection.
Tertiary syphilis.
CNS neoplasm.
Metabolic encephalopathies.
Multiple sclerosis.
Chronic subdural hematoma.
SLE cerebritis.
Encephalitides.
Sarcoidosis.
NSAIDs.
Behçet's syndrome.
Anatomic defects (traumatic, congenital, postoperative).
Granulomatous angiitis.

MENINGITIS, RECURRENT[25a]

ICD-9CM # varies with specific disorder
ICD-10CM # G03.2 Benign recurrent meningitis [Mollaret]

Drug induced (with rechallenge).
Parameningeal focus.
Infection (sinusitis, mastoiditis, osteomyelitis, brain abscess).
Tumor (epidermoid cyst, craniopharyngioma).
Posttraumatic (bacterial).
Mollaret's meningitis.
SLE.
Herpes simplex virus.

MENTAL STATUS CHANGES AND COMA[2]

ICD-9CM # 780.97
ICD-10CM # R41.82 Altered mental status, unspecified

METABOLIC/SYSTEMIC ETIOLOGY OF ALTERED MENTAL STATUS AND COMA

Hypoxia

Severe pulmonary disease (hypoventilation).
Severe anemia.
Environmental/toxin:
- Methemoglobinemia.
- Cyanide.
- Carbon monoxide.
- Decreased atmospheric oxygen (high altitude).
- Near-drowning.

Disorders of Glucose

Hypoglycemia:
- Chronic alcohol abuse and liver disease.
- Excessive use of insulin or other hypoglycemic agents.
- Insulinoma.

Hyperglycemia:
- Diabetic ketoacidosis.
- Nonketotic hyperosmolar coma.

Decreased Cerebral Blood Flow

Hypovolemic shock.
Cardiac:
- Vasovagal syncope.
- Arrhythmias.
- Myocardial infarction.
- Valvular disorders.
- Congestive heart failure.
- Pericardial effusion/tamponade.
- Myocarditis.

Infectious:
- Septic shock.
- Bacterial meningitis.

Vascular/hematologic:
- Hypertensive encephalopathy.
- Pseudotumor cerebri.
- Hyperviscosity (sickle cell, polycythemia).
- Hyperventilation.
- Cerebral lupus vasculitis.
- Thrombotic thrombocytopenic purpura.
- Disseminated intravascular coagulation.

Metabolic Cofactor Deficiency

Thiamine (Wernicke-Korsakoff syndrome).
Pyridoxine (isoniazid overdose).
Folic acid (chronic alcohol abuse).
Cyanocobalamin.
Niacin.

Electrolye/pH Disturbances

Acidosis/alkalosis.
Hypernatremia/hyponatremia.*
Hypercalcemia/hypocalcemia.
Hypophosphatemia.
Hypermagnesemia/hypomagnesemia.

Endocrine Disorders

Myxedema coma, thyrotoxicosis.
Hypopituitarism.
Addison's disease (primary or secondary).
Cushing's disease.
Pheochromocytoma.
Hyperparathyroidism/hypoparathyroidism.

Endogenous Toxins

Hyperammonemia (liver failure).
Uremia (renal disease).
Carbon dioxide narcosis (pulmonary disease).
Porphyria.

Exogenous Toxins

Alcohols:
- Ethanol, isopropyl alcohol, methanol, ethylene glycol.

Acid poisons:
- Salicylates.
- Paraldehyde.
- Ammonium chloride.

Antidepressant medications:
- Lithium.
- Tricyclic antidepressants (TCAs).
- Selective serotonin reuptake inhibitors (SSRIs).
- Monamine oxidase inhibitors (MAOIs).

Stimulants:
- Amphetamines/methamphetamines.
- Cocaine.
- Over-the-counter sympathomimetics.

Narcotics/opiates:
- Morphine.
- Heroin.
- Codeine, oxycodone, meperidine, hydrocodone.
- Methadone.
- Fentanyl.
- Propoxyphene.

Sedative-hypnotics:
- Benzodiazepines.
- Barbiturates.
- Rohypnol.
- Bromide.

Hallucinogens:
- Lysergic acid diethylamide (LSD).
- Marijuana.
- Mescaline, peyote.
- Mushrooms.
- Phencyclidine (PCP).

Herbs/plants
- Aconite.
- Jimson weed.
- Morning glory.

Volatile substances:
- Hydrocarbons (gasoline, butane, toluene, benzene, chloroform).
- Nitrites.
- Anesthetic agents (nitrous oxide, ether).

Other:
- γ-Hydroxybutyrate (GHB).
- Ketamine.
- Penicillin.
- Cardiac glycosides.
- Anticonvulsants.
- Steroids.
- Heavy metals.
- Cimetidine.
- Organophosphates.

Disorders of Temperature Regulation/ Environmental

Hypothermia.
Heat stroke.
Malignant hyperthermia.
Neuroleptic malignant syndrome.
High-altitude cerebral edema (HACE).
Dysbarism.

Primary Glial or Neuronal Disorders

Adrenoleukodystrophy.
Creutzfeldt-Jakob disease.
Progressive multifocal leukoencephalopathy.
Marchiava-Bignami disease.
Gliomatosis cerebri.
Central pontine myelinolysis.

Other Disorders of Unknown Etiology

Seizures.
Postictal states.
Reye's syndrome.†
Intussusception.†

---

*Can be associated with dilution of formula in infant feeding.
†Prominent in the pediatric population.

MENTAL STATUS CHANGES AND COMA, STRUCTURAL CAUSES[1]

ICD-9CM # 780.09
ICD-10CM # R40.1

COMMON AGE-RELATED CAUSES OF ALTERED MENTAL STATUS AND COMA

Infant

Infection.
Trauma, abuse.
Metabolic.

Child

Toxic ingestion.

Adolescent, Young Adult

Toxic ingestion.
Recreational drug use.
Trauma.

Elderly

Medication changes.
Over-the-counter medications.
Infection.
Alterations in living environment.
Stroke.
Trauma.

MENTAL STATUS CHANGES AND COMA, METABOLIC AND SYSTEMIC CAUSES[1]

ICD-9CM # 780.09
ICD-10CM # CM40.1

METABOLIC AND SYSTEMIC CAUSES OF ALTERED MENTAL STATUS AND COMA

Hypoxia, Hypercapnia

Severe pulmonary disease (hypoventilation).
Severe anemia.
Environmental, toxic.
Methemoglobinemia.
Cyanide.
Carbon monoxide.
Decreased atmospheric oxygen (high altitude).
Near-drowning.

Glucose Disorders

Hypoglycemia:

- Chronic alcohol abuse and liver disease.
- Excessive dosage of insulin or other hypoglycemic agents.
- Insulinoma.

Hyperglycemia:

- Diabetic ketoacidosis.
- Nonketotic hyperosmolar coma.

Decreased Cerebral Blood Flow

Hypovolemic shock.

Cardiac:

- Vasovagal syncope.
- Arrhythmias.
- Myocardial infarction.
- Valvular disorders.
- Congestive heart failure.
- Pericardial effusion, tamponade.
- Myocarditis.

Infectious

- Septic shock.
- Bacterial meningitis.

Vascular, hematologic

- Hypertensive encephalopathy.
- Pseudotumor cerebri.
- Hyperviscosity (sickle cell, polycythemia).
- Hyperventilation.
- Cerebral vasculitis as a manifestation of systemic lupus erythematosus.
- Thrombotic thrombocytopenic purpura.
- Disseminated intravascular coagulation.

Metabolic Cofactor Deficiency

Thiamine (Wernicke-Korsakoff syndrome).
Pyridoxine (isoniazid overdose).
Folic acid (chronic alcohol abuse).
Cyanocobalamin.
Niacin.

Electrolyte, pH Disturbances

Acidosis, alkalosis.
Hypernatremia, hyponatremia.*
Hypercalcemia, hypocalcemia.
Hypophosphatemia.
Hypermagnesemia, hypomagnesemia.

Endocrine Disorders

Myxedema coma, thyrotoxicosis.
Hypopituitarism.
Addison disease (primary or secondary).
Cushing disease.
Pheochromocytoma.
Hyperparathyroidism, hypoparathyroidism.

Endogenous Toxins

Hyperammonemia (liver failure).
Uremia (renal disease).
Carbon dioxide narcosis (pulmonary disease).
Porphyria.

Exogenous Toxins

Alcohols:

- Ethanol, isopropyl alcohol, methanol, ethylene glycol.

Acid poisons:

- Salicylates.
- Paraldehyde.
- Ammonium chloride.

Antidepressant medications:

- Lithium.
- Tricyclic antidepressants.
- Selective serotonin reuptake inhibitors.
- Monoamine oxidase inhibitors.

Stimulants:

1. Amphetamines, methamphetamines.
2. Cocaine.
3. Over-the-counter sympathomimetics.

Narcotics, opiates:

- Morphine.
- Heroin.
- Codeine, oxycodone, meperidine, hydrocodone.
- Methadone.
- Fentanyl.
- Propoxyphene.

Sedative-hypnotics:

- Benzodiazepines.
- Barbiturates.
- Rohypnol.
- Bromide.

Hallucinogens:

- Lysergic acid diethylamide.
- Marijuana.
- Mescaline, peyote.
- Mushrooms.
- Phencyclidine.

Herbs, plants:

- Aconite.
- Jimsonweed.
- Morning glory.

Volatile substances:

- Hydrocarbons (gasoline, butane, toluene, benzene, chloroform).
- Nitrites.
- Anesthetic agents (nitrous oxide, ether).

Other:

- γ-Hydroxybutyrate.
- Ketamine.
- Penicillin.
- Cardiac glycosides.
- Anticonvulsants.
- Steroids.
- Heavy metals.
- Cimetidine.
- Organophosphates.

Disorders of Temperature Regulation, Environmental

Hypothermia.
Heat stroke.
Malignant hyperthermia.
Neuroleptic malignant syndrome.
High-altitude cerebral edema.
Dysbarism.

Primary Glial or Neuronal Disorders

Adrenoleukodystrophy.
Creutzfeldt-Jakob disease.
Progressive multifocal leukoencephalopathy.
Marchiafava-Bignami disease.
Gliomatosis cerebri.
Central pontine myelinolysis.

Other Disorders with Unknown Etiology

Seizures.
Postictal states.
Reye syndrome.†
Intussusception.†

*Can be associated with dilution of formula in infant feeding.

†Prominent in the pediatric population.

MESENTERIC ARTERIAL EMBOLISM, ASSOCIATED FACTORS[2]

ICD-9CM # 557.0
ICD-10CM # I74.09 Other arterial embolism and thrombosis of abdominal aorta

FACTORS ASSOCIATED WITH MESENTERIC ARTERIAL EMBOLISM

Coronary artery disease.
Post-myocardial infarction mural thrombi.
Congestive heart failure.
Valvular heart disease.
Rheumatic mitral valve disease.
Nonbacterial endocarditis.
Arrhythmias.
Chronic atrial fibrillation.
Aortic aneurysms or dissections.
Coronary angiography.

MESENTERIC ISCHEMIA, NONOCCLUSIVE[26]

ICD-9CM #	557.0	Mesenteric Artery Embolism or Infarction
	557.1	Mesenteric Artery Insufficiency, Chronic
	902.39	Mesenteric Vein Injury
ICD-10CM #	K55.0	Acute vascular disorders of intestine
	K55.1	Chronic vascular disorders of intestine
	S35.8X9A	Unspecified injury of other blood vessels at abdomen, lower back and pelvis level, initial encounter

Cardiovascular disease resulting in low-flow states (CHF, cardiogenic shock, post cardiopulmonary bypass, dysrhythmias).
Septic shock.
Drug induced (cocaine, vasopressors, ergot alkaloid poisoning).

MESENTERIC VENOUS THROMBOSIS[26]

ICD-9CM # 557.0
ICD-10CM # I82.91 Chronic embolism and thrombosis of unspecified vein

Hypercoagulable states (protein C or S deficiency, antithrombin III deficiency, Factor V Leyden, malignancy, polycythemia vera, sickle cell disease, homocystinemia, lupus anticoagulant, cardiolipin antibody).

Trauma (operative venous injury, abdominal trauma, postsplenectomy).
Inflammatory conditions (pancreatitis, diverticulitis, appendicitis, cholangitis).
Other: CHF, renal failure, portal hypertension, decompression sickness.

METASTATIC NEOPLASMS

ICD-9CM #	198.5	Bone and Bone Marrow
	198.3	Brain and Spinal Cord
	197.7	Liver
	197.0	Lung
ICD-10CM #	C79.51	Secondary malignant neoplasm of bone
	C79.52	Secondary malignant neoplasm of bone marrow
	C79.31	Secondary malignant neoplasm of brain
	C78.7	Secondary malignant neoplasm of liver and intrahepatic bile duct
	C78.00	Secondary malignant neoplasm of unspecified lung

To: Bone
Breast
Lung
Prostate
Thyroid
Kidney
Bladder
Endometrium
Cervix
Melanoma

To: Liver
Colon
Stomach
Pancreas
Breast
Lymphomas
Bronchus
Lung
Sarcoma
Choriocarcinoma
Kidney

To: Brain
Lung
Breast
Melanoma
GU tract
Colon
Sinuses
Sarcoma
Skin
Thyroid

To: Lung
Breast
Colon
Kidney
Testis
Stomach
Thyroid
Melanoma

MICROCEPHALY[4]

ICD-9CM #	742.1	Microcephalus
ICD-10CM #	Q02	Microcephaly

PRIMARY (GENETIC)

Familial (autosomal recessive).
Autosomal dominant.
Syndromes:
- Down (21-trisomy).
- Edward (18-trisomy).
- Cri-du-chat (5 p-).
- Cornelia de Lange.
- Rubinstein-Taybi.
- Smith-Lemli-Opitz.

SECONDARY (NONGENETIC)

Radiation.
Congenital infections:
- Cytomegalovirus.
- Rubella.
- Toxoplasmosis.

Drugs:
- Fetal alcohol.
- Fetal hydantoin.

Meningitis/encephalitis.
Malnutrition.
Metabolic.
Hyperthermia.
Hypoxic-ischemic encephalopathy.

MICROPENIS[27]

ICD-9CM #	752.69	Penile Agenesis or Atresia
	607.89	Penile Atrophy
	752.64	Micropenis (Congenital)
ICD-10CM #	N48.89	Other specified disorders of penis
	Q55.62	Hypoplasia of penis

HYPOGONADOTROPIC HYPOGONADISM (HYPOTHALAMIC OR PITUITARY DEFICIENCIES)

Kallmann's syndrome: autosomal dominant; associated with hyposmia.
Prader-Willi syndrome: hypotonia, mental retardation, obesity, small hands and feet.
Rud syndrome: hyposomia, ichthyosis, mental retardation.
De Morsier's syndrome (septooptic dysplasia): hypopituitarism, hypoplastic optic discs, absent septum pellucidum.

HYPERGONADOTROPIC HYPOGONADISM

Primary testicular defect: disorders of testicular differentiation or inborn errors of testosterone synthesis.
Klinefelter's syndrome.
Other X polysomies (i.e., XXXXY, XXXY).
Robinow's syndrome: brachymesomelic dwarfism, dysmorphic facies.

PARTIAL ANDROGEN INSENSITIVITY

Idiopathic

Defective morphogenesis of the penis.

MIOSIS

ICD-9CM #	379.42	Miosis, Persistent Not Due to Miotics
ICD-10CM #	H57.03	Miosis

Medications (e.g., morphine, pilocarpine).
Neurosyphilis.
Congenital.
Iritis.
CNS pontine lesion.
CNS infections.
Cavernous sinus thrombosis.
Inflammation/irritation of cornea or conjunctiva.

MONOARTHRITIS, ACUTE

ICD-9CM #	716.60	
ICD-10CM #	M13.10	Monoarthritis, not elsewhere classified, unspecified site

Overuse.
Trauma.
Gout.
Pseudogout.
Osteoarthritis.
Infectious arthritis (e.g., gonococcal, Lyme disease, viral, mycobacteria, fungi).
Osteomyelitis.
Avascular necrosis of bone.
Hemarthrosis.
Bowel disease–associated arthritis.
Bone malignancy.
Psoriatic arthritis.
Juvenile RA.
Sarcoidosis.
Hemoglobinopathies.
Vasculitic syndromes.
Behçet's syndrome.
Foreign body synovitis.
Hypertrophic pulmonary osteoarthropathy.
Amyloidosis, familial Mediterranean fever.

MONOCYTOSIS[20]

ICD-9CM #	288.63	
ICD-10CM #	D72.821	Monocytosis (symptomatic)

Inflammatory diseases:
- Infectious diseases:
  - Tuberculosis.
  - Syphilis.
  - Subacute bacterial endocarditis.
  - Fever of unknown origin.
- Autoimmune/granulomatous.
- Systemic lupus erythematosus.
- Rheumatoid arthritis.
- Temporal arteritis.
- Myositis.
- Polyarteritis.
- Ulcerative colitis.
- Regional enteritis.
- Sarcoidosis.

Malignant disorders:
- Preleukemia.
- Nonlymphocytic leukemia.
- Histiocytoses.
- Hodgkin's disease.
- Non-Hodgkin's lymphoma.
- Carcinomas.

Miscellaneous:
- Chronic neutropenia.
- Post splenectomy.

MONONEUROPATHY

ICD-9CM #	355.9	
ICD-10CM #	G58.9	Mononeuropathy, unspecified

Herpes zoster.
Herpes simplex.
Vasculitis.
Trauma, compression.
Diabetes.
Postinfectious or inflammatory.

MONONEUROPATHY, ISOLATED[2]

ICD-9CM # varies with specific diagnosis
ICD-10CM # G56.90 Unspecified mononeuropathy of unspecified upper limb

UPPER EXTREMITY

Radial nerve.
- Axilla.
- Humerus.
- Elbow (posterior interosseous neuropathy).
- Wrist (superficial cutaneous radial neuropathy).

Ulnar nerve.
- Axilla.
- Humerus.
- Elbow.
- Condylar groove.
- Cubital tunnel.

Wrist (Guyon's canal).
Hand.
- Superficial terminal ulnar neuropathy.
- Deep terminal ulnar neuropathy.
  - Proximal hypothenar.
  - Distal hypothenar.

Median nerve.
Axilla.
Humerus (musculocutaneous mononeuropathy).
Forearm.
- Anterior interosseus.
- Pronator syndrome (?).

Wrist (carpal tunnel).
Hand (recurrent motor branch).
Suprascapular mononeuropathy.
- Axillary mononeuropathy.

LOWER EXTREMITY

Sciatic nerve.
Femoral nerve.
- Iliacus compartment (proximal).
- Saphenous mononeuropathy (distal).

Lateral femoral cutaneous (meralgia paresthetica).
Peroneal nerve.
- Common peroneal mononeuropathy (fibular head, popliteal fossa).
- Deep peroneal mononeuropathy (anterior compartment).

Tibial nerve.
- Popliteal fossa (proximal).
- Tarsal tunnel (distal).

Sural nerve.
- Popliteal fossa, calf (proximal).
- Fifth metatarsal base (distal).

Plantar nerve.
- Distal to tarsal tunnel.
- Interdigital neuropathies (Morton's neuroma).

Obturator mononeuropathy.

MONONUCLEOSIS, MONOSPOT NEGATIVE[1a]

ICD-9CM # 075
ICD-10CM # B27.90 Infectious mononucleosis, unspecified without complication

DIFFERENTIAL DIAGNOSIS OF MONOSPOT-NEGATIVE MONONUCLEOSIS

Acute HIV infection.
EBV mononucleosis (particularly in children).
Cytomegalovirus.
Acute toxoplasmosis.
Streptococcal pharyngitis.
Acute hepatitis B infection.

EBV, Epstein-Barr virus; *HIV,* human immunodeficiency virus.

MUSCLE DISEASE[34a]

ICD-9CM # 728
ICD-10CM # M60.009 Infective myositis, unspecified site

CLASSIFICATION OF MUSCLE DISEASE

Muscular Dystrophies
Duchenne.
Becker.
Limb girdle.
Childhood.
Facioscapulohumeral.

Myotonic Disorders
Dystrophia myotonica.
Myotonica congenita.

Inflammatory
Infective: bacterial, viral, parasitic.
Unknown cause: polymyositis, dermatomyositis, sarcoidosis.

Endocrine
Thyroid disease—hyper- and hypothyroidism.
Cushing's disease.
Addison's disease.
Hyperparathyroidism.

Metabolic
Glycogen storage diseases.
Periodic paralyses.
Mitochondrial diseases.

Drug-induced
Corticosteroids.
Chloroquine.
Amiodarone.
Penicillamine.
Alcohol.
Zidovudine.
Clofibrate.

Other
Inclusion body myositis.

MUSCLE WEAKNESS

ICD-9CM # 728.9
ICD-10CM # M62.9 Disorder of muscle, unspecified

Physical deconditioning.
Impaired cardiac output (e.g., mitral stenosis, mitral regurgitation).
Uremia, liver failure.
Electrolyte abnormalities (hypokalemia, hyperkalemia, hypophosphatemia, hypercalcemia), hypoglycemia.
Drug induced (e.g., statin myopathy).
Muscular dystrophies.
Steroid myopathy.
Alcoholic myopathy.
Myasthenia gravis, Lambert-Eaton syndrome.
Infections (polio, botulism, HIV, hepatitis, diphtheria, tick paralysis, neurosyphilis, brucellosis, TB, trichinosis).
Pernicious anemia, other anemias, beriberi.
Psychiatric illness (depression, somatization syndrome).
Organophosphate or arsenic poisoning.
Inflammatory myopathies (e.g., collagen vascular disease, RA, sarcoidosis).
Endocrinopathies (e.g., adrenal insufficiency, hypothyroidism), diabetic neuropathy.
Other: motor neuron disease, mitochondrial myopathy, l-tryptophan (eosinophilia-myalgia), rhabdomyolysis, glycogen storage disease, lipid storage disease.

MUSCLE WEAKNESS, LOWER MOTOR NEURON VERSUS UPPER MOTOR NEURON[40]

ICD-9CM # 728.9
ICD-10CM # M62.9 Disorder of muscle, unspecified

LOWER MOTOR NEURON

Weakness, usually severe.
Marked muscle atrophy.
Fasciculations.
Decreased muscle stretch reflexes.
Clonus not present.
Flaccidity.
No Babinski sign.
Asymmetric and may involve one limb only in the beginning to become generalized as the disease progresses.

UPPER MOTOR NEURON

Weakness, usually less severe.
Minimal disuse muscle atrophy.
No fasciculations.
Increased muscle stretch reflexes.
Clonus may be present.
Spasticity.
Babinski sign.
Often initial impairment of only skilled movements.
In the limbs the following muscles may be the only ones weak or weaker than the others: triceps; wrist and finger extensors; interossei; iliopsoas; hamstrings; and foot dorsiflexors, inverters, and extroverters.

MYDRIASIS

ICD-9CM # 379.43 Mydriasis, Persistent Not Due to Mydriatics
ICD-10CM # H57.04 Mydriasis

Coma.
Medications (cocaine, atropine, epinephrine, etc.).
Glaucoma.
Cerebral aneurysm.
Ocular trauma.
Head trauma.
Optic atrophy.
Cerebral neoplasm.
Iridocyclitis.

MYELIN DISORDERS

ICD-9CM # varies with specific disorder
ICD-10CM # varies with specific diagnosis

Multiple sclerosis.
Vitamin B_{12} deficiency.
Radiation.
Hypoxia.
Toxicity from carbon monoxide, alcohol, mercury.
Progressive multifocal encephalopathy.
Acute disseminated encephalomyelitis.
Acute hemorrhagic leukoencephalopathy.
Phenylketonuria.
Adrenoleukodystrophy.
Krabbe's disease.

MYELOPATHY AND MYELITIS[36]

ICD-9CM #	722.70	Myelopathy, Discogenic Intervertebral NOS
	336.9	Myelopathy, Nondiscogenic Unspecified
ICD-10CM #	M51.9	Unspecified thoracic, thoracolumbar and lumbosacral intervertebral disc disorder
	G95.9	Disease of spinal cord, unspecified

INFLAMMATORY

Infectious: spirochetal TB, zoster, rabies, HIV, polio, rickettsial, fungal, parasitic.
Noninfectious: idiopathic transverse myelitis, multiple sclerosis.

TOXIC/METABOLIC

DM, pernicious anemia, chronic liver disease, pellagra, arsenic.

TRAUMA COMPRESSION

Spinal neoplasm, cervical spondylosis, epidural abscess, epidural hematoma.

VASCULAR

AV malformation, SLE, periarteritis nodosa, dissecting aortic aneurysm.

PHYSICAL AGENTS

Electrical injury, irradiation.

NEOPLASTIC

Spinal cord tumors, paraneoplastic myelopathy.

MYOCARDIAL ISCHEMIA[36]

ICD-9CM #	414.8	Ischemia (Chronic)
	411.89	Ischemia, Acute without MI
ICD-10CM #	I25.5	Ischemic cardiomyopathy
	I25.89	Other forms of chronic ischemic heart disease
	I25.9	Chronic ischemic heart disease, unspecified
	I24.8	Other forms of acute ischemic heart disease

Atherosclerotic obstructive coronary artery disease.
Nonatherosclerotic coronary artery disease:
Coronary artery spasm.
Congenital coronary artery anomalies:
- Anomalous origin of coronary artery from pulmonary artery.
- Aberrant origin of coronary artery from aorta or another coronary artery.
- Coronary arteriovenous fistula.
- Coronary artery aneurysm.

Acquired disorders of coronary arteries:
- Coronary artery embolism.
- Dissection:
  - Surgical.
  - During percutaneous coronary angioplasty.
  - Aortic dissection.
  - Spontaneous (e.g., during pregnancy).
- Extrinsic compression:
  - Tumors.
  - Granulomas.
  - Amyloidosis.
- Collagen-vascular disease:
  - Polyarteritis nodosa.
  - Temporal arteritis.
  - RA.
  - SLE.
  - Scleroderma.
- Miscellaneous disorders:
  - Irradiation.
  - Trauma.
  - Kawasaki disease.

Syphilis.
Hereditary disorders:
- Pseudoxanthoma elasticum.
- Gargoylism.
- Progeria.
- Homocystinuria.
- Primary oxaluria.

"Functional" causes of myocardial ischemia in absence of anatomic coronary artery disease:
- Syndrome X.
- Hypertrophic cardiomyopathy.
- Dilated cardiomyopathy.
- Muscle bridge.
- Hypertensive heart disease.
- Pulmonary hypertension.
- Valvular heart disease; aortic stenosis, aortic regurgitation.

MYOCLONUS

ICD-9CM # 333.2
ICD-10CM # G25.3 Myoclonus

Physiologic (e.g., exercise or anxiety induced).
Renal failure.
Hepatic failure.
Hyponatremia.
Hypoglycemia or severe hyperglycemia.
Postdialysis.
Epileptic myoclonus.
Postencephalitis.
CNS lesion (stroke, neoplasm).
CNS trauma.
Parkinson's disease.
Medications (e.g., tricyclics, L-dopa).
Friedreich's ataxia.
Ataxia-telangiectasia.
Wilson's disease.
Huntington's disease.
Progressive supranuclear palsy.
Heavy metal poisoning.
Benign familial.

MYOPATHIC SYNDROMES, DRUG-INDUCED[18b]

ICD-9CM # 359.9 Myopathic Syndromes
ICD-10CM # G72.9 Myopathy, unspecified

TYPE OF MYOPATHY

Necrotizing myopathy
Inflammatory myopathy
Mitochondrial myopathy
Hypokalemic myopathy
Antimicrotubular myopathy
Lysosomal storage myopathy
Corticosteroid myopathy
Others

DRUGS

HMG-CoA reductase inhibitors (statins), fibrates, alcohol
Penicillamine, interferon-a, procainamide
Zidovudine
Diuretics, laxatives, licorice, amphotericin B, alcohol
Colchicine, vincristine
Chloroquine, hydroxychloroquine, quinacrine, amiodarone, perhexiline
Corticosteroids, especially fluorinated
Ipecac syrup, emetine

Differential Diagnosis II

MYOPATHIES ASSOCIATED WITH REST PAIN[18b]

ICD-9CM # 359.9 Myopathies
ICD-10CM # G72.9 Myopathy, unspecified

Childhood dermatomyositis.
Hypothyroid myopathy.
Acute alcoholic myopathy.
Drug-induced myopathies.
Infectious myopathies.
Myopathies associated with metabolic bone disease.
Carnitine palmitoyl transferase deficiency.
Rhabdomyolysis from any cause.

MYOPATHIES, HIV ASSOCIATED[12a]

ICD-9CM # 729.82
ICD-10CM # R25.2

HIV-Associated Myopathies	Myopathies Secondary to Antiretrovirals	Others
HIV polymyositis	Zidovudine myopathy	Opportunistic infections involving muscle (toxoplasmosis)
Inclusion body myositis	Toxic mitochondrial myopathies related to other NRTIs[a]	
Nemaline myopathy		Tumor infiltrations of skeletal muscle
Diffuse infiltrative lymphocytosis syndrome	HIV-associated lipodystrophy syndrome	Rhabdomyolysis

HIV-Associated Myopathies	Myopathies Secondary to Antiretrovirals	Others
HIV wasting syndrome Vasculitic processes Myasthenia gravis and other myasthenic syndromes Chronic fatigue and fibromyalgia	Immune reconstitution syndrome related to HAART[b]	

[a]NRTIs, nucleoside reverse transcriptase inhibitors.
[b]HAART, highly active antiretroviral therapy

MYOPATHIES, INFECTIOUS

ICD-9CM # 359.8
ICD-10CM # G72.9 Myopathy, unspecified

HIV.
Viral myositis.
Trichinosis.
Toxoplasmosis.
Cysticercosis.

MYOPATHIES, INFLAMMATORY

ICD-9CM # 359.9
ICD-10CM # G72.9 Myopathy, unspecified

SLE, RA.
Sarcoidosis.
Paraneoplastic syndrome.
Polymyositis, dermatomyositis.
Polyarteritis nodosa.
Mixed connective tissue disease.
Scleroderma.
Inclusion body myositis.
Sjögren's syndrome.
Cimetidine, D-penicillamine.

MYOPATHIES, METABOLIC[18b]

ICD-9CM # 359.9 Myopathies
ICD-10CM # G72.9 Myopathy, unspecified

DISORDERED GLYCOGEN METABOLISM

- Myophosphorylase deficiency (McArdle disease).
- Phosphorylase b kinase deficiency.
- Phosphofructokinase deficiency.
- Debrancher enzyme deficiency.
- Brancher enzyme deficiency.
- Phosphoglycerate kinase deficiency.
- Phosphoglycerate mutase deficiency.
- Lactate dehydrogenase deficiency.
- Acid maltase deficiency.
- Aldolase deficiency.
- b-Enolase deficiency.

DISORDERED LIPID METABOLISM

- Carnitine deficiencies.
- Carnitine palmitoyltransferase deficiency.
- Fatty acid acyl-CoA dehydrogenase deficiencies.

MITOCHONDRIAL MYOPATHIES

- Coenzyme Q10 deficiency.
- Respiratory chain complex deficiencies.

ENDOCRINE

- Acromegaly.
- Hypothyroidism.
- Hyperthyroidism.
- Hyperparathyroidism.
- Cushing disease.
- Addison disease.
- Hyperaldosteronism.

METABOLIC-NUTRITIONAL

- Uremia.
- Hepatic failure.
- Malabsorption.
- Periodic paralysis.
- Vitamin D deficiency.
- Vitamin E deficiency.

ELECTROLYTE DISORDERS

- Sodium: hypernatremia and hyponatremia.
- Potassium: hyperkalemia and hypokalemia.
- Calcium: hypercalcemia and hypocalcemia.
- Phosphate: hypophosphatemia.
- Magnesium: hypomagnesemia.

MYOPATHIES, TOXIC[1a]

ICD-9CM # 359.4
ICD-10CM # G72.2 Myopathy due to other toxic agents

Inflammatory: cimetidine, D-penicillamine.
Noninflammatory necrotizing or vacuolar: cholesterol-lowering agents, chloroquine, colchicine.
Acute muscle necrosis and myoglobinuria: cholesterol-lowering drugs, alcohol, cocaine.
Malignant hyperthermia: halothane, ethylene, others; succinylcholine.
Mitochondrial: zidovudine.
Myosin loss: nondepolarizing neuromuscular blocking agents; glucocorticoids.

MYOSITIS, INFECTIOUS CAUSES[18b]

ICD-9CM # 728.0 Myositis

VIRAL

Influenza A and B viruses.
Enteroviruses (coxsackieviruses, echoviruses).
Human immunodeficiency virus.
Human T-cell lymphotrophic virus type 1.
Hepatitis B and C viruses.
Cytomegalovirus.
Epstein-Barr virus.
Adenovirus.
Varicella-zoster virus.
Parainfluenza.

PARASITIC

Trichinella species.
Echinococcus species.
Schistosoma species.
Toxoplasma gondii.
Trypanosoma cruzi.
Sarcocystis species.

BACTERIAL

Staphylococcus aureus.
Streptococcus, groups A and B.
Aeromonas hydrophila.
Borrelia burgdorferi.
Clostridium perfringens.
Anaerobic streptococci.
Mycobacterium species.
Rickettsia species.

FUNGAL

Candida species.
Cryptococcus neoformans.
Microsporida.

MYOSITIS, INFLAMMATORY[1a]

ICD-9CM # 729.1
ICD-10CM # M60.009 Infective myositis, unspecified site

INFECTIOUS

Viral myositis:
Retroviruses (HIV, HTLV-I).
Enteroviruses (echovirus, Coxsackievirus).
Other viruses (influenza, hepatitis A and B, Epstein-Barr virus).
Bacterial: pyomyositis.
Parasites: trichinosis, cysticercosis.
Fungi: candidiasis.

IDIOPATHIC

Granulomatous myositis (sarcoid, giant cell).
Eosinophilic myositis.
Eosinophilia-myalgia syndrome.

ENDOCRINE/METABOLIC DISORDERS

Hypothyroidism.
Hyperthyroidism.
Hypercortisolism.
Hyperparathyroidism.
Hypoparathyroidism.
Hypocalcemia.
Hypokalemia.

METABOLIC MYOPATHIES

Myophosphorylase deficiency (McArdle's disease).
Phosphofructokinase deficiency.
Myoadenylate deaminase deficiency.
Acid maltase deficiency.
Lipid storage diseases.
Acute rhabdomyolysis.

DRUG-INDUCED MYOPATHIES

Alcohol.
D-Penicillamine.
Zidovudine.
Colchicine.
Chloroquine, hydroxychloroquine.
Lipid-lowering agents.
Cyclosporine.
Cocaine, heroin, barbiturates.
Corticosteroids.

NEUROLOGIC DISORDERS
Muscular dystrophies.
Congenital myopathies.
Motor neuron disease.
Guillain-Barré syndrome.
Myasthenia gravis.

NAIL CLUBBING

ICD-9CM # 729.1
ICD-10CM # R68.3 Clubbing of nails

COPD.
Pulmonary malignancy.
Cirrhosis.
Inflammatory bowel disease.
Chronic bronchitis.
Congenital heart disease.
Endocarditis.
AV malformations.
Asbestosis.
Trauma.
Idiopathic.

NAIL, HORIZONTAL WHITE LINES (BEAU'S LINES)

ICD-9CM # 703.9
ICD-10CM # L60.4 Beau's lines

Malnutrition.
Idiopathic.
Trauma.
Prolonged systemic illnesses.
Pemphigus.
Raynaud's disease.

NAIL KOILONYCHIA

ICD-9CM # 703.8
ICD-10CM # L60.8 Other nail disorders

Trauma.
Iron deficiency.
SLE.
Hemochromatosis.
Raynaud's disease.
Nail-patella syndrome.
Idiopathic.

NAIL ONYCHOLYSIS

ICD-9CM # 703.8
ICD-10CM # L60.1 Onycholysis

Infection.
Trauma.
Psoriasis.
Connective tissue disorders.
Sarcoidosis.
Hyperthyroidism.
Amyloidosis.
Nutritional deficiencies.

NAIL PITTING

ICD-9CM # 703.8
ICD-10CM # L60.8 Other nail disorders

Psoriasis.
Alopecia areata.
Reiter's syndrome.
Trauma.
Idiopathic.

NAIL SPLINTER HEMORRHAGE

ICD-9CM # 703.8
ICD-10CM # L60.8 Other nail disorders

SBE.
Trauma.
Malignancies.
Oral contraceptives.
Pregnancy.
SLE.
Antiphospholipid syndrome.
Psoriasis.
RA.
Peptic ulcer disease.

NAIL STRIATIONS

ICD-9CM # 703.8
ICD-10CM # L60.8 Other nail disorders

Psoriasis.
Alopecia areata.
Trauma.
Atopic dermatitis.
Vitiligo.

NAIL TELANGIECTASIA

ICD-9CM # 703.8
ICD-10CM # L60.8 Other nail disorders

RA.
Scleroderma.
Trauma.
SLE.
Dermatomyositis.

NAIL WHITENING (TERRY'S NAILS)

ICD-9CM # 703.8
ICD-10CM # L60.8 Other nail disorders

Malnutrition.
Trauma.
Liver disease (cirrhosis, hepatic failure).
DM.
Hyperthyroidism.
Idiopathic.

NAIL YELLOWING

ICD-9CM # 703.8
ICD-10CM # L60.8 Other nail disorders

Tobacco abuse.
Nephrotic syndrome.
Chronic infections (TB, sinusitis).
Bronchiectasis.
Lymphedema.
Raynaud's disease.
RA.
Pleural effusions.
Thyroiditis.
Immunodeficiency.

NASAL AND PARANASAL SINUS TUMORS[16a]

ICD-9CM # 873.23
ICD-10CM # C30.0 Malignant neoplasm of nasal cavity

BENIGN AND MALIGNANT NASAL AND PARANASAL SINUS TUMORS
Epithelial Tumors

BENIGN
Papilloma.
Adenoma.
Inverting papilloma.

MALIGNANT
Squamous carcinoma.
Adenocarcinoma.
Melanoma.
Adenoid cystic carcinoma.
Malignant salivary tumors.

MESENCHYMAL TUMORS
Benign
Osteoma.
Ossifying fibroma complex.
Angiofibroma.
Chondroma.
Malignant
Osteogenic sarcoma.
Fibrosarcoma.
Angiosarcoma.
Chondrosarcoma.
Lymphoma.
Rhabdomyosarcoma.

NASAL MASSES, CONGENITAL[16a]

ICD-9CM # 478.19
ICD-10CM # J34.1 Cyst and mucocele of nose and nasal sinus
J34.89 Other specified disorders of nose and nasal sinuses

Dermoid.
Nasal cerebral heterotopia (glioma).
Frontal meningoencephalocele.
Nasolacrimal duct mucocele.
Nasal hamartoma.
Nasal hemangioma.

NAUSEA AND VOMITING

ICD-9CM # 787.01
ICD-10CM # R11.2 Nausea with vomiting, unspecified

Infections (viral, bacterial).
Intestinal obstruction.
Metabolic (uremia, electrolyte abnormalities, DKA, acidosis, etc.).
Severe pain.
Anxiety, fear.
Psychiatric disorders (bulimia, anorexia nervosa).
Pregnancy.

Medications (NSAIDs, erythromycin, morphine, codeine, aminophylline, chemotherapeutic agents, etc.).
Withdrawal from substance abuse (drugs, alcohol).
Head trauma.
Vestibular or middle ear disease.
Migraine headache.
CNS neoplasms.
Radiation sickness.
PUD.
Carcinoma of GI tract.
Reye's syndrome.
Eye disorders.
Abdominal trauma.

NECK AND ARM PAIN

ICD-9CM #	723.1	Neck Pain
	847.0	Neck Strain
	959.09	Neck Injury
	959.2	Arm Injury
	840.9	Arm Strain
ICD-10CM #	M54.2	Cervicalgia
	S46.919A	Strain of unspecified muscle, fascia and tendon at shoulder and upper arm level, unspecified arm, initial encounter

Cervical disk syndrome.
Trauma, musculoskeletal strain.
Rotator cuff syndrome.
Bicipital tendonitis.
Glenohumeral arthritis.
Acromioclavicular arthritis.
Thoracic outlet syndrome.
Pancoast tumor.
Infection (cellulitis, abscess).
Angina pectoris.

NECK MASS[28]

ICD-9CM #	784.2	
ICD-10CM #	R22.1	Localized swelling, mass and lump, neck

CONGENITAL ANOMALIES

Thyroglossal duct cyst.
Bronchial apparatus anomalies.
Teratomas.
Ranula.
Dermoid cysts.
Hemangioma.
Laryngoceles.
Cystic hygroma.

NONNEOPLASTIC INFLAMMATORY ETIOLOGIES

Folliculitis.
Adenopathy secondary to peritonsillar abscess.
Retropharyngeal or parapharyngeal abscess.
Salivary gland infections.
Viral infections (mononucleosis, HIV, CMV).
TB.
Cat-scratch disease.
Toxoplasmosis.
Actinomyces.
Atypical mycobacterium.
Jugular vein thrombus.

NEOPLASM (PRIMARY OR METASTATIC)

Lipoma.

NECK PAIN[28]

ICD-9CM #	723.1	Neck Pain (Nondiscogenic)
	959.09	Neck Injury
ICD-10CM #	M54.2	Cervicalgia

INFLAMMATORY DISEASES

RA.
Spondyloarthropathies.
Juvenile RA.

NONINFLAMMATORY DISEASE

Cervical osteoarthritis.
Diskogenic neck pain.
Diffuse idiopathic skeletal hyperostosis.
Fibromyalgia or myofascial pain.

INFECTIOUS CAUSES

Meningitis.
Osteomyelitis.
Infectious diskitis.

NEOPLASMS

Primary.
Metastatic.

REFERRED PAIN

Temporomandibular joint pain.
Cardiac pain.
Diaphragmatic irritation.
GI sources (gastric ulcer, gallbladder, pancreas).

NECK PAIN FROM RHEUMATOLOGIC DISORDERS[12a]

ICD-9CM #	723.1	
ICD-10CM #	M54.2	Cervicalgia

Rheumatoid arthritis
- Without disease of the C1-C2 joint.
- With structural cervical abnormalities: C1-C2 subluxation, C1-C2 facet involvement.

Spondyloarthropathies.
Reactive arthritis.
Psoriatic arthritis.
Enteropathic arthritis.
Polymyalgia rheumatica.
Osteoarthritis.
Fibromyalgia.
Nonspecific musculoskeletal pain.
Miscellaneous spondyloarthropathies.
- Whipple's disease.
- Behçet's disease.
- Paget's disease.
- Acromegaly.
- Ossification of the posterior longitudinal ligament.
- Diffuse idiopathic skeletal hyperostosis.

NECROTIZING PNEUMONIAS[1a]

ICD-9CM #	482.8	
ICD-10CM #	J15.8	Pneumonia due to other specified bacteria

COMMON

Tuberculosis.
Staphylococcus.
Gram-negative bacilli.
Anaerobes.
Fungi.
Pneumocystis jirovecii.

RARE

Streptococcus pneumoniae.
Legionella.
Viruses.
Mycoplasma pneumoniae.

NEPHRITIC SYNDROME, ACUTE[1a]

ICD-9CM #	580.89	
ICD-10CM #	N00.8	Acute nephritic syndrome with other morphologic changes

LOW SERUM COMPLEMENT LEVEL

Acute postinfectious glomerulonephritis.
Membranoproliferative glomerulonephritis.
SLE.
Subacute bacterial endocarditis.
Visceral abscess "shunt" nephritis.
Cryoglobulinemia.

NORMAL SERUM COMPLEMENT LEVEL

IgA nephropathy.
Antiglomerular basement membrane disease.
Polyarteritis nodosa.
Wegener's glomerulonephritis.
Henoch-Schönlein purpura.
Goodpasture's syndrome.

NEPHROCALCINOSIS

ICD-9CM #	275.49	
ICD-10CM #	E83.59	Other disorders of calcium metabolism

Sarcoidosis.
Hyperparathyroidism.
Chronic glomerulonephritis.
Milk-alkali syndrome.
Distal renal tubular acidosis.
Medullary sponge kidney.
Bartter's syndrome.
Hypervitaminosis D.
Idiopathic hypercalciuria.
Hyperoxaluria.
Cortical necrosis.
Tuberculosis.
Idiopathic hypercalciuria.
Rapidly progressive osteoporosis.

NEUROGENIC BLADDER[29]

ICD-9CM # 396.54
ICD-10CM # N31.9 Neuromuscular dysfunction of bladder, unspecified

SUPRATENTORIAL

CVA.
Parkinson's disease.
Alzheimer's disease.
Cerebral palsy.

SPINAL CORD

Spinal cord injury.
Spinal stenosis.
Central cord syndrome.
ALS.
Multiple sclerosis.
Myelodysplasia.

PERIPHERAL NEUROPATHY

Diabetes.
Alcohol.
Shingles.
Syphilis.

OTHER

Migraine.
Bell's palsy.
Psychogenic.

NEUROLOGIC DEFICIT, FOCAL[26]

ICD-9CM # 436 CVA
435.9 TIA
ICD-10CM # G45.9 Transient cerebral ischemic attack, unspecified
I67.848 Other cerebrovascular vasospasm and vasoconstriction

TRAUMATIC: INTRACRANIAL, INTRASPINAL

Subdural hematoma.
Intraparenchymal hemorrhage.
Epidural hematoma.
Traumatic hemorrhagic necrosis.

INFECTIOUS

Brain abscess.
Epidural and subdural abscesses.
Meningitis.

NEOPLASTIC

Primary central nervous system tumors.
Metastatic tumors.
Syringomyelia.
Vascular.
Thrombosis.
Embolism.
Spontaneous hemorrhage: arteriovenous malformation, aneurysm, hypertensive.

METABOLIC

Hypoglycemia.
B_{12} deficiency.
Postseizure.
Hyperosmolar nonketotic.

NEUROLOGIC DEFICIT, MULTIFOCAL[26]

ICD-9CM # 436 CVA
435.9 TIA
ICD-10CM # I67.89 Other cerebrovascular disease
G45.9 Transient cerebral ischemic attack, unspecified
I67.848 Other cerebrovascular vasospasm and vasoconstriction

Acute disseminated encephalomyelitis: postviral or postimmunization.
Infectious encephalomyelitis: poliovirus, enteroviruses, arbovirus, herpes zoster, Epstein-Barr virus.
Granulomatous encephalomyelitis: sarcoid.
Autoimmune: SLE.
Other: familial spinocerebellar degenerations.

NEUROMUSCULAR JUNCTION DYSFUNCTION[1a]

ICD-9CM # varies with specific diagnosis
ICD-10CM # N31.9 Neuromuscular dysfunction of bladder, unspecified

DISORDERS OF THE NEUROMUSCULAR JUNCTION

Autoimmune
Myasthenia gravis.
Lambert-Eaton myasthenic syndrome.
Congenital
Presynaptic defects in ACh resynthesis, packaging, or release.
Synaptic defect: congenital end plate AChE deficiency.
Postsynaptic defects: slow-channel syndromes.
Postsynaptic defects: decreased response to ACh.
Fast-channel syndromes.
AChR deficiency without kinetic abnormality.
Familial limb-girdle myasthenia.
Toxic
Botulism.
Drug-induced disorders.
Organophosphate intoxication.

Ach, Acetylcholine; *AChE,* acetylcholinesterase; *AChR,* acetylcholine receptor.

NEURONOPATHIES, SENSORY (GANGLIONOPATHIES)[2]

ICD-9CM # varies with specific diagnosis
ICD-10CM # G60.0 Hereditary motor and sensory neuropathy

Herpes:
Herpes simplex I and II.
Varicella zoster (shingles).
Inflammatory sensory polyganglionopathy (ISP).
Paraneoplastic.
Primary biliary cirrhosis.
Sjögren's syndrome (keratoconjunctivitis sicca).
Toxin-induced:
Pyridoxine (vitamin B_6) overdose.
Metals:
- Platinum (cisplatin).
- Methyl mercury.

Vitamin E deficiency.

NEUROPATHIC BLADDER

ICD-9CM # 596.59
ICD-10CM # N31.9 Neuromuscular dysfunction of bladder, unspecified

Diabetes.
Stroke.
Multiple sclerosis.
Parkinson's disease.
Dementia.
Encephalopathy.
Brain trauma.
Spinal cord trauma.
Pelvic surgery.
Spina bifida.

NEUROPATHIES WITH FACIAL NERVE INVOLVEMENT

ICD-9CM # varies with specific disorder
ICD-10CM # G51.8 Other disorders of facial nerve

Sarcoidosis.
HIV.
Lyme disease.
Guillain-Barré.
Others: chronic inflammatory polyneuropathy, Tangier disease, amyloidosis.

NEUROPATHIES, AUTONOMIC[22a]

ICD-9CM # 357 Neuropathies
ICD-10CM # G63 Polyneuropathy in diseases classified elsewhere

GUILLAIN-BARRÉ SYNDROME

Non–Gullain-Barré syndrome autoimmunity.
- Paraneoplastic (type I antineuronal nuclear antibody).
- Lambert-Eaton syndrome.
- Antibodies to neuronal nicotinc acetylcholine receptors.
- Antibodies to P/Q type calcium channels.
- Other autoantibodies.
- Systemic lupus erythematosus.

HEREDITARY

- Type I autosomal dominant.
- Type II autosomal recessive (Morvan disease).
- Type III autosomal recessive (Riley-Day).
- Type IV autosomal recessive (congenital insensitivity to pain with anhidrosis).
- Type V absence of pain.

METABOLIC
- Fabry disease.
- Diabetes mellitus.
- Tangier disease.
- Porphyria.

INFECTIOUS
- HIV.
- Chagas' disease.
- Botulism.
- Leprosy.
- Diphtheria.

OTHER
- Triple A (Allgrove) syndrome.
- Navajo Indian neuropathy.
- Multiple endocrine neoplasia type 2b.

TOXINS

NEUROPATHIES, AUTONOMIC, PERIPHERAL, CAUSES[14a]

ICD-9CM #	337.00	Neuropathies
ICD-10CM #	G90.09	Other idiopathic peripheral autonomic neuropathy

METABOLIC
Diabetes mellitus.
Alcohol.
Acute intermittent porphyria.
Uremia.

AUTOIMMUNE
Autoimmune autonomic ganglionopathy.
Guillain-Barré syndrome.
Morvan's syndrome.
Lambert-Eaton myasthenic syndrome.
Chronic inflammatory demyelinating polyradiculoneuropathy.
Sjögren syndrome.
Systemic lupus erythematosus.
Mixed connective tissue diseases.

PARAPROTEINEMIC
Amyloidosis.

NUTRITIONAL
Cyanocobalamin deficiency.
Thiamine deficiency.
Gluten-sensitive neuropathy.

TOXIC
Heavy metals.
Organic solvents.
Organophosphates.
Vacor.
Acrylamide.

DRUG INDUCED
Cisplatin.
Vincristine.
Amiodarone.
Metronidazole.
Perhexiline.
Paclitaxel.

INFECTIOUS
Human immunodeficiency virus.
Leprosy.
Chagas' disease.
Botulism.
Diphtheria.
Lyme disease.

GENETIC
Hereditary sensory and autonomic neuropathies.
- Types I and II.
- Type III (familial dysautonomia).
- Type IV (congenital insensitivity to pain).
- Type V.

Fabry disease.

IDIOPATHIC
Adie's syndrome.
Ross' syndrome.
Acute cholinergic neuropathy.
Chronic idiopathic anhidrosis.
Amyotrophic lateral sclerosis.

NEUROPATHIES, PAINFUL[40]

ICD-9CM #	355.9	Neuropathy NOS
	357.5	Alcoholic
	357.8	Chronic Progressive or Relapsing
	356.2	Congenital Sensory
	356.0	Dejerine-Sottas
	356.60	Diabetic Polyneuropathy, Type II
	356.61	Diabetic Polyneuropathy Type I
ICD-10CM #	G58.9	Mononeuropathy, unspecified
	G62.1	Alcoholic polyneuropathy
	G61.89	Other inflammatory polyneuropathies
	G60.0	Hereditary motor and sensory neuropathy
	G60.0	Hereditary motor and sensory neuropathy
	E11.42	Type 2 diabetes mellitus with diabetic polyneuropathy
	E10.42	Type 1 diabetes mellitus with diabetic polyneuropathy

MONONEUROPATHIES
Compressive neuropathy (carpal tunnel, meralgia paresthetica).
Trigeminal neuralgia.
Ischemic neuropathy.
Polyarteritis nodosa.
Diabetic mononeuropathy.
Herpes zoster.
Idiopathic and familial brachial plexopathy.

POLYNEUROPATHIES
DM.
Paraneoplastic sensory neuropathy.
Nutritional neuropathy.
Multiple myeloma.
Amyloid.
Dominantly inherited sensory neuropathy.
Toxic (arsenic, thallium, metronidazole).
AIDS-associated neuropathy.
Tangier disease.
Fabry's disease.

NEUROPATHIES, PERIPHERAL, ASYMMETRICAL PROXIMAL/DISTAL[2]

ICD-9CM #	varies with specific diagnosis	
ICD-10CM #	G99.0	Autonomic neuropathy in diseases classified elsewhere

BRACHIAL PLEXOPATHY
Open
Direct plexus injury (knife or gunshot wound).
Neurovascular (plexus ischemia).
Iatrogenic (central line insertion).
Closed
Traction injuries:
 "Stingers."
 Traction neurapraxia.
 Partial or complete nerve root avulsion.
Radiation.
Neoplastic.
Idiopathic brachial plexitis.
Throracic outlet.

LUMBOSACRAL PLEXOPATHIES
Open
Closed
Traction injuries:
 Pelvic double vertical shearing fracture.
 Posterior hip dislocation.
 Retroperitoneal hemorrhage.
Vasospastic (deep buttock injection).
Neoplastic.
Radiation.
Idiopathic lumbosacral plexitis.
Infectious:
 Herpesvirus (sacrococcygeal).
 Herpes simplex II.
 Herpes zoster.
Cytomegalovirus (CMV) polyradiculopathy (HIV).

NEUROPATHIES, TOXIC AND METABOLIC[22a]

ICD-9CM #	337.00	Neuropathies
ICD-10CM #	NEC G62.2	Toxic neuropathy

METALS
Arsenic (insecticide, herbicide).
Lead (paint, batteries, pottery).
Mercury (metallic, vapor).
Thallium (rodenticides).
Gold.

OCCUPATIONAL OR INDUSTRIAL CHEMICALS
Acrylamide (grouting, flocculation).
Carbon disulfide (solvent).
Cyanide.

Dichlorophenoxyacetate.
Dimethylaminopropionitrite.
Ethylene oxide (gas sterilization).
Hexacarbons (glue, solvents).
Organophosphates (insecticides, petroleum additive).
Polychlorinated biphenyls.
Tetrachlorbiphenyl.
Trichloroethylene.

DRUGS

Amiodarone.
Chloramphenicol.
Chloroquine.
Cisplatin.
Colchicine.
Dapsone.
Ethambutol.
Ethanol.
Gold.
Hydralazine.
Isoniazid.
Metronidazole.
Nitrofurantoin.
Nitrous oxide.
Nucleosides (antiretroviral agents ddC, ddl, d4T, others).
Penicillamine.
Pentamidine.
Phenytoin.
Pyridoxine (excessive).
Statins.
Stilbamidine.
Suramin.
Taxanes (paclitaxel, docetaxel).
Thalidomide.
Tryptophan (eosinophilia-myalgia syndrome).
Vincristine.

METABOLIC DISORDERS

Fabry disease.
Krabbe disease.
Leukodystrophies.
Porphyria.
Tangier disease.
Tyrosinemia.
Uremia.

NEUTROPENIA WITH DECREASED MARROW RESERVE[20]

ICD-9CM # 288.09
ICD-10CM # D70.8 Other neutropenia

PRIMARY

Severe congenital neutropenia.
Shwachman–Diamond syndrome.
Cyclic neutropenia.

SECONDARY

Lymphoproliferative disorder of granular lymphocytes.
Chemotherapy.
Drug induced (nonimmune).
Nutritional.
Viral infection (varicella, EBV, measles, CMV, hepatitis, HIV).

NEUTROPENIA WITH NORMAL MARROW RESERVE[20]

ICD-9CM # 288.0
ICD-10CM # D70.9 Neutropenia, unspecified

Chronic benign neutropenia of infancy and childhood.
Ethnic or benign familial neutropenia.
Autoimmune neutropenia.
Alloimmune neutropenia.
Drug-induced neutropenia.
Infection-related neutropenia.
Hypersplenism.

NEUTROPENIA, IN CHILDHOOD[38a]

ICD-9CM # 288.09
ICD-10CM # D70.8 Other neutropenia
D70.9 Neutropenia unspecified

ACQUIRED

Infection.
Immune mediated.
Hypersplenism.
Vitamin B_{12}, folate, copper deficiency.
Drugs or toxic substances.
Aplastic anemia.
Malignancies or preleukemic disorders.
Ionizing radiation.

CONGENITAL

Cyclic neutropenia.
Severe congenital neutropenia (Kostmann syndrome).
Chronic benign neutropenia of childhood.
Shwachman-Diamond syndrome.
Fanconi anemia.
Metabolic disorders (amino acidopathies, Barth syndrome, glycogen storage disorders).
Osteopetrosis.
Neutropenia with pigmentation abnormalities, e.g., Chédiak-Higashi.

NEUTROPHILIA[20]

ICD-9CM # 288.60
ICD-10CM # D72.0 Neutrophilia, hereditary giant
D71 Functional disorders of polymorphonuclear neutrophils

CLASSIFICATION OF NEUTROPHILIA

Primary (No Other Evident Associated Disease)

Hereditary neutrophilia.
Chronic idiopathic neutrophilia.
Chronic myelogenous leukemia (CML) and other myeloproliferative diseases.
Familial myeloproliferative disease.
Congenital anomalies and leukemoid reaction.
Leukocyte adhesion factor deficiency (LAD).
Familial cold urticaria and leukocytosis.

Secondary

Infection.
Stress neutrophilia.
Chronic inflammation.
Drug induced.
Nonhematologic malignancy.
Generalized marrow stimulation as in hemolysis.
Asplenia and hyposplenism.

NIPPLE LESIONS

ICD-9CM # varies with specific disorder
ICD-10CM # varies with specific diagnosis

Contact dermatitis.
Trauma.
Paget's disease.
Sebaceous hyperplasia.
Neurofibroma.
Accessory nipple.
Papillary adenoma.
Nevoid hyperkeratosis.
Cellulitis.

NODULAR LESIONS, SKIN

ICD-9CM # 782.2
ICD-10CM # R22.9 Localized swelling, mass and lump, unspecified

Lipoma.
Cherry angioma.
Angiokeratoma.
Hemangioma.
Classic Kaposi's sarcoma.
Nodular melanoma.
Pyogenic granuloma.
Angiosarcoma.
Eccrine poroma.

NODULES, PAINFUL

ICD-9CM # varies with specific disorder
ICD-10CM # R22.9 Localized swelling, mass and lump, unspecified

Arthropod bite or sting.
Erythema nodosum.
Glomus tumor.
Neuroma.
Leiomyoma.
Angiolipoma.
Dermatofibroma.
Osler's node.
Blue rubber bleb nevus.
Vasculitis.
Sweet's syndrome.

NYSTAGMUS

ICD-9CM # 379.50 Nystagmus NOS
386.11 Benign Positional
386.2 Central Positional
379.59 Congenital
ICD-10CM # H55.00 Unspecified nystagmus
H55.89 Other irregular eye movements

Medications (meperidine, barbiturates, phenytoin, phenothiazines, etc.).
Multiple sclerosis.
Congenital.
Neoplasm (cerebellar, brain stem, cerebral).
Labyrinthine or vestibular lesions.
CNS infections.
Optic atrophy.
Other: Arnold–Chiari malformation, syringobulbia, chorioretinitis, meningeal cysts.

NYSTAGMUS, MONOCULAR

ICD-9CM # 379.50
ICD-10CM # H55.09 Other forms of nystagmus
H55.00 Unspecified nystagmus

Amblyopia.
Strabismus.
Multiple sclerosis.
Monocular blindness.
Internuclear ophthalmoplegia.
Lid fasciculations.
Brain stem infarct.

ODYNOPHAGIA[38]

ICD-9CM # varies with specific diagnosis
ICD-10CM # varies with specific diagnosis

CAUSES OF ODYNOPHAGIA

Infections
Herpes simplex virus.
Cytomegalovirus.
Candidiasis.
Chemical, Inflammatory
Gastroesophageal reflux.
Drug induced (Slow-K, tetracyclines, quinidine).
Radiation.
Graft-versus-host disease.
Crohn's disease.
Dermatologic diseases (pemphigus and pemphigoid).

OPACIFICATION OF HEMIDIAPHRAGM ON X-RAY[16a]

ICD-9CM # 419.4
ICD-10CM # varies with specific diagnosis

CAUSES OF OPACIFICATION OF A HEMITHORAX

Pleural effusion.
Consolidation.
Collapse.
Massive tumor.
Fibrothorax.
Combination of above lesions.
Pneumonectomy.
Lung agenesis.

OPHTHALMOPLEGIA[1a]

ICD-9CM # 378.9 Ophthalmoplegia NOS
378.52 Cerebellar Ataxia Syndrome
376.22 Exophthalmic
ICD-10CM # H51.9 Unspecified disorder of binocular movement
H49.00 Third [oculomotor] nerve palsy, unspecified eye

BILATERAL

Botulism.
Myasthenia gravis.
Wernicke's encephalopathy.
Acute cranial polyneuropathy.
Brain stem stroke.

UNILATERAL

Carotid-posterior (3rd cranial nerve, pupil involved communicating aneurysm).
Diabetic-idiopathic (3rd or 6th cranial nerve, pupil spared).
Myasthenia gravis.
Brain stem stroke.

OPSOCLONUS*

ICD-9CM # 379.59
ICD-10CM # H55.89 Other irregular eye movements

Multiple sclerosis.
Encephalitis.
CNS lymphoma.
Hydrocephalus.
Pontine hemorrhage.
Thalamic disorder (glioma, hemorrhage).
Hyperosmolar coma.
Carcinoma, paraneoplastic.
Cocaine.
Medications (e.g., phenytoin, haloperidol, amitriptyline, diazepam, vidarabine).

*Spontaneous, multivector, chaotic eye movement

OPTIC ATROPHY[34a]

ICD-9CM # 377.1
ICD-10CM # H47.20 Unspecified optic atrophy

CAUSES OF OPTIC ATROPHY

Optic Nerve Compression
Pituitary tumor.
Carotid aneurysm.
Glaucoma.
Optic nerve tumor.
Sphenoid meningioma.
Olfactory groove meningioma.
Optic Neuritis Following Longstanding Papilledema Central Retinal Artery Occlusion Toxic/Metabolic
Diabetes.
Methyl alcohol.
Tobacco.
Quinine.
Ethambutol.
Lead and arsenic.
Anemia.
Secondary to Retinal Disease
Senile macular degeneration.
Retinitis pigmentosa.
Severe chorioretinitis.
Secondary to Trauma
Orbital fracture.
Hereditary
Leber's optic atrophy.
Hereditary ataxias.
Spinocerebellar degeneration.

ORAL MUCOSA, ERYTHEMATOUS LESIONS[9]

ICD-9CM # 528.3 Oral Abscess
528.9 Oral Disease (Soft Tissue)
528.8 Hyperplasia (Tongue)
ICD-10CM # K12.2 Cellulitis and abscess of mouth
K13.70 Unspecified lesions of oral mucosa
K13.79 Other lesions of oral mucosa

Allergy.
Erythroplakia.
Candidiasis.
Geographic tongue.
Stomatitis areata migrans.
Plasma cell gingivitis.
Pemphigus vulgaris.

ORAL MUCOSA, PIGMENTED LESIONS[9]

ICD-9CM # 528.3 Oral Abscess
528.9 Oral Disease (Soft Tissue)
528.8 Hyperplasia (Tongue)
ICD-10CM # K12.2 Cellulitis and abscess of mouth
K13.70 Unspecified lesions of oral mucosa
K13.79 Other lesions of oral mucosa
K13.5 Oral submucous fibrosis

Racial pigmentation.
Oral melanotic macule.
Peutz-Jeghers syndrome.
Neurofibromatosis.
Albright's syndrome.
Addison's disease.
Chloasma.
Drug reaction: quinacrine, Minocin, chlorpromazine, Myleran.
Amalgam tattoo.
Lead line.
Smoker's melanosis.
Nevi.
Melanoma.

ORAL MUCOSA, PUNCTATE EROSIVE LESIONS[9]

ICD-9CM # 528.3 Oral Abscess
528.9 Oral Disease (Soft Tissue)
528.8 Hyperplasia (Tongue)
ICD-10CM # K12.2 Cellulitis and abscess of mouth

K13.70 Unspecified lesions of oral mucosa
K13.79 Other lesions of oral mucosa

Viral lesion: Herpes simplex, coxsackievirus (A, B, A16), herpes zoster.
Aphthous stomatitis.
Sutton's disease (giant aphthae).
Behçet's syndrome.
Reiter's syndrome.
Neutropenia.
Acute necrotizing ulcerative gingivostomatitis (ANUG).
Drug reaction.
Inflammatory bowel disease.
Contact allergy.

ORAL MUCOSA, WHITE LESIONS[9]

ICD-9CM # 528.3 Oral Abscess
528.9 Oral Disease (Soft Tissue)
528.8 Hyperplasia (Tongue)
ICD-10CM # K12.2 Cellulitis and abscess of mouth
K13.70 Unspecified lesions of oral mucosa
K13.79 Other lesions of oral mucosa
K13.5 Oral submucous fibrosis

Leukoplakia.
White, hairy leukoplakia.
Squamous cell carcinoma.
Lichen planus.
Stomatitis nicotinica.
Benign intraepithelial dyskeratosis.
White spongy nevus.
Leukoedema.
Darier-White disease.
Pachyonychia congenital.
Candidiasis.
Allergy.
SLE.

ORAL ULCERS, ACUTE

ICD-9CM # varies with diagnosis
528.9 Traumatic Ulcer of Oral Mucosa
ICD-10CM # K13.70 Unspecified lesions of oral mucosa
K13.79 Other lesions of oral mucosa

Trauma (including thermal trauma).
Aphthous stomatitis.
Syphilis.
Herpes simplex infection.
Herpes zoster.

ORAL VESICLES AND ULCERS[1a]

ICD-9CM # 528.9
ICD-10CM # K13.70 Unspecified lesions of oral mucosa
K13.79 Other lesions of oral mucosa

Aphthous stomatitis.
Primary herpes simplex infection.
Vincent's stomatitis.
Syphilis.
Coxsackievirus A (herpangina).
Fungi (histoplasmosis).
Behçet's syndrome.
SLE.
Reiter's syndrome.
Crohn's disease.
Erythema multiforme.
Pemphigus.
Pemphigoid.

ORBITAL LESIONS, CALCIFIED

ICD-9CM # 376.89
ICD-10CM # H05.89 Other disorders of orbit

Chronic inflammation.
Phlebolith.
Dermoid cyst.
Mucocele walls.
Tumors (lacrimal gland, fibro-osseous).
Meningioma (optic sheath).
Lymphangioma.
Orbital varix.

ORBITAL LESIONS, CYSTIC

ICD-9CM # 376.9
ICD-10CM # H05.9 Unspecified disorder of orbit

Sweat gland cyst.
Dermoid cyst.
Lacrimal gland cyst.
Abscess.
Conjunctival cyst.
Lymphangioma.
Schwannoma.

ORGASM DYSFUNCTION[12]

ICD-9CM # 302.73 Orgasm Inhibited, Female Psychosexual
302.74 Orgasm Inhibited, Male Psychosexual
ICD-10CM # F52.31 Female orgasmic disorder
F52.32 Male orgasmic disorder

Anorgasmia: inadequate stimulation or learning.
Spinal cord lesion or injury.
Multiple sclerosis.
Alcoholic neuropathy.
Amyotrophic lateral sclerosis.
Spinal cord accident.
Spinal cord trauma.
Peripheral nerve damage.
Radical pelvic surgery.
Herniated lumbar disk.
Hypothyroidism.
Addison's disease.
Cushing's disease.
Acromegaly.
Hypopituitarism.
Pharmacologic agents (e.g., SSRIs, beta-blockers).
Psychogenic.

OROFACIAL PAIN

ICD-9CM # 784.0
ICD-10CM # R51 Facial pain

Dental abscess.
Sinusitis.
Otitis media.
Otitis externa.
Wisdom tooth eruption.
Sialoadenitis.
Herpes zoster.
Trigeminal neuralgia.
Parotitis.
Anxiety disorder.
Malingering.

OSTEOPOROSIS, SECONDARY CAUSES

ICD-9CM # 733.00
ICD-10CM # M81.0 Age-related osteoporosis without current pathological fracture

Medication induced (e.g., glucocorticoids, anticonvulsants, heparin, LHRH agonists or antagonists).
Hyperparathyroidism.
Hyperthyroidism.
Prolonged immobilization.
Chronic renal failure.
Sickle cell disease.
Multiple myeloma.
Myeloproliferative diseases.
Leukemias and lymphomas.
Acromegaly.
Prolactinoma.
DM.
Total parenteral nutrition.
Malabsorption.
Chronic hypophosphatemia.
Connective tissue disorders (e.g., osteogenesis imperfecta, Marfan's syndrome, Ehlers-Danlos).
Hepatobiliary disease.
Postgastrectomy.
Aluminum-containing antacids.
Systemic mastocytosis.
Homocystinuria.

OSTEOSCLEROSIS, DIFFUSE[16a]

ICD-9CM # varies with specific diagnosis
ICD-10CM # Q77.4 Congenital osteosclerosis

DISORDERS ASSOCIATED WITH DIFFUSE OSTEOSCLEROSIS

Neoplastic Causes*

Prostate carcinoma, breast carcinoma, gastrointestinal adenocarcinoma, carcinoid tumors, transitional cell carcinoma of the bladder, myeloma, lymphoma, leukemia.

Hematologic Causes*

Sickle cell disorders, mastocytosis, myelofibrosis, polycythemia vera.

Metabolic Causes*

Renal osteodystrophy, primary hyperparathyroidism, familial hypophosphatemic osteomalacia, hypervitaminosis D, fluorosis, hypoparathyroidism, pseudohypoparathyroidism.

***Primary Osseous Disorders*†**

Osteoporosis.
Pyknodysostosis.
Paget's disease.

* Involvement principally of cancellous bone
† Involvement of cancellous and cortical bone

OVULATORY DYSFUNCTION[21]

ICD-9CM #	628.0	Anovulatory Cycle
	626.5	Ovulation Pain
ICD-10CM #	N97.0	Female infertility associated with anovulation
	N92.3	Ovulation bleeding

HYPERANDROGENIC ANOVULATION

Polycystic ovarian syndrome.
Late-onset congenital adrenal hyperplasias.
Ovarian hyperthecosis.
Androgen-producing ovarian tumors.
Androgen-producing adrenal tumors.
Cushing's syndrome.

HYPOESTROGENIC ANOVULATION (HYPOTHALAMIC OR PITUITARY ETIOLOGY)

Hypogonadotropic Hypoestrogenic States

Reversible:
- Functional hypothalamic amenorrheas:
  - Eating disorders (anorexia nervosa, excessive weight loss).
  - Excessive athletic training.

Neoplastic:
- Craniopharyngioma.
- Pituitary stalk compression.

Infiltrative diseases:
- Histiocytosis-X.
- Sarcoidosis.

Hypophysitis.

Pituitary adenomas:
- Hyperprolactinemia.
- Euprolactinemic galactorrhea.

Endocrinopathies:
- Hypothyroidism/hyperthyroidism.
- Cushing's disease.

Irreversible:
- Kallmann's syndrome.
- Isolated gonadotropin deficiency (hypothalamic or pituitary origin).
- Panhypopituitarism/pituitary insufficiency:
  - Sheehan's syndrome, pituitary apoplexy.
  - Pituitary irradiation or ablation.

Hypergonadotropic Hypoestrogenic States

Physiologic states:
- Menopause.
- Perimenopause.

Premature ovarian failure.

Immune-related:
- Radiation/chemotherapy-induced.
- Ovarian dysgenesis.
- Turner's syndrome.
- 46XX with mutations of X.
- Androgen insensitivity syndrome.

MISCELLANEOUS

Endometriosis.
Luteal phase defect.

PAIN, MIDFOOT

ICD-9CM #	719.47	
ICD-10CM #	M25.579	Pain in unspecified ankle and joints of unspecified foot

MEDIAL ASPECT

Tendonitis of posterior tibialis.
Tendonitis of flexor digitorum longus.
Tendonitis of flexor hallucis longus.
Infection (osteomyelitis, septic arthritis, cellulitis) of foot.
Peripheral vascular insufficiency.
Fracture.
Osteoarthritis.
Gout, pseudogout.
Neuropathy.
Tumor.

LATERAL ASPECT

Peroneus longus tendonitis.
Peroneus brevis tendonitis.
Infection (osteomyelitis, septic arthritis, cellulitis) of foot.
Peripheral vascular insufficiency.
Fracture.
Osteoarthritis.
Gout, pseudogout.
Neuropathy.
Tumor.

PAIN, PLANTAR ASPECT, HEEL

ICD-9CM #	719.47	
ICD-10CM #	M25.579	Pain in unspecified ankle and joints of unspecified foot

Plantar fasciitis.
Tarsal tunnel syndrome.
Neuroma.
Infection (osteomyelitis, septic arthritis, cellulitis) of foot.
Peripheral vascular insufficiency.
Fracture.
Bone cyst.
Osteoarthritis.
Gout, pseudogout.
Neuropathy.
Tumor.
Heel pad atrophy.
Plantar fascia rupture.

PAIN, POSTERIOR HEEL

ICD-9CM #	729.5	
ICD-10CM #	M79.609	Pain in unspecified limb

Achilles tendonitis.
Retrocalcaneal bursitis.
Retroachilles bursitis.
Infection (osteomyelitis, septic arthritis, cellulitis) of foot.
Peripheral vascular insufficiency.
Fracture.
Osteoarthritis.
Gout, pseudogout.
Neuropathy.
Tumor.

PALINDROMIC RHEUMATISM[6]

ICD-9CM #	719.3	use 5th digit
		0 Site Unspecified
		1 Shoulder Region
		2 Upper Arm (Elbow, Humerus)
		3 Forearm (Radius, Wrist, Ulna)
		4 Hand (Carpal, Metacarpal, Fingers)
		5 Pelvic Region and Thigh
		6 Lower Leg
		7 Ankle and Foot
		8 Other
		9 Multiple
ICD-10CM #	M12.30	Palindromic rheumatism, unspecified site
	M12.319	Palindromic rheumatism, unspecified shoulder
	M12.329	Palindromic rheumatism, unspecified elbow
	M12.339	Palindromic rheumatism, unspecified wrist
	M12.349	Palindromic rheumatism, unspecified hand
	M12.359	Palindromic rheumatism, unspecified hip
	M12.369	Palindromic rheumatism, unspecified knee
	M12.379	Palindromic rheumatism, unspecified ankle and foot
	M12.38	Palindromic rheumatism, vertebrae
	M12.39	Palindromic rheumatism, multiple sites

Palindromic RA.
Essential palindromic rheumatism.
Crystal synovitis (gout, CPPD, pseudogout, calcific periarthritis).
Lyme borreliosis, stages 2 and 3.
Sarcoidosis.
Whipple's disease.
Acute rheumatic fever.
Reactive arthritis (rare).

PALMOPLANTAR HYPERKERATOSIS

ICD-9CM # 701.1
ICD-10CM # L85.1 Acquired keratosis [keratoderma] palmaris et plantaris
L85.2 Keratosis punctata (palmaris et plantaris)
L87.0 Keratosis follicularis et parafollicularis in cutem penetrans

Superficial skin infection.
Chronic eczema.
Repeated trauma.
Psoriasis.
Reiter's syndrome.
Paraneoplastic acrokeratosis.

PALPITATIONS[33]

ICD-9CM # 785.1 Palpitations
ICD-10CM # R00.2 Palpitations

Anxiety.
Electrolyte abnormalities (hypokalemia, hypomagnesemia).
Exercise.
Hyperthyroidism.
Ischemic heart disease.
Ingestion of stimulant drugs (cocaine, amphetamines, caffeine).
Medications (digoxin, beta-blockers, calcium channel antagonists, hydralazines, diuretics, minoxidil).
Hypoglycemia in type 1 DM.
Mitral valve prolapse.
Wolff-Parkinson-White (WPW) syndrome.
Sick sinus syndrome.

PANCREATIC CALCIFICATIONS

ICD-9CM # 577.8
ICD-10CM # K86.1 Other chronic pancreatitis
K86.8 Other specified diseases of pancreas

Chronic pancreatitis.
Hyperparathyroidism.
Metastatic neoplasm.
Pseudocyst.
Hereditary pancreatitis.
Cystoadenoma.
Cystoadenocarcinoma.
Cavernous lymphangioma.
Hemorrhage.
Acute pancreatitis (saponification).

PANCREATITIS, ACUTE, IN CHILDREN[22a]

ICD-9CM # 577.0
ICD-10CM # K85 Acute pancreatitis

CAUSES OF ACUTE PANCREATITIS IN CHILDREN

Drugs and Toxins
Acetaminophen overdose.
Alcohol.
L-Asparaginase.
Azathioprine.
Carbamazepine.
Cimetidine.
Corticosteroids.
Enalapril.
Erythromycin.
Estrogen.
Furosemide.
Isoniazid.
Lisinopril.
6-Mercaptopurine.
Methyldopa.
Metronidazole.
Organophosphate poisoning.
Pentamidine.
Retrovirals: DDC, DDI, tenofovir.
Sulfonamides: mesalamine, 5-aminosalicylates, sulfasalazine, trimethoprim/sulfamethoxazole.
Sulindac.
Tetracycline.
Thiazides.
Valproic acid.
Venom (spider, scorpion, Gila monster lizard).
Vincristine.

Genetic
Cationic trypsinogen gene (*PRSS1*).
Chymotrypsin C gene (*CTRC*).
Cystic fibrosis gene (*CFTR*).
Trypsin inhibitor gene (*SPINK1*).

Infectious
Ascariasis.
Coxsackie B virus.
Epstein-Barr virus.
Hepatitis A, B.
Influenza A, B.
Leptospirosis.
Malaria.
Measles.
Mumps.
Mycoplasma.
Reye syndrome: varicella, influenza B.
Rubella.
Rubeola.
Septic shock.

Obstructive
Ampullary disease.
Ascariasis.
Biliary tract malformations.
Choledochal cyst.
Choledochocele.
Cholelithiasis, microlithiasis, and choledocholithiasis (stones or sludge).
Duplication cyst.
Endoscopic retrograde cholangiopancreatography (ERCP) complication.
Pancreas divisum.
Pancreatic ductal abnormalities.
Postoperative.
Sphincter of Oddi dysfunction.
Tumor.

Systemic Disease
Autoimmune pancreatitis.
Brain tumor.
Collagen vascular diseases.
Crohn disease.
Diabetes mellitus.
Head trauma.
Hemochromatosis.
Hemolytic-uremic syndrome.
Hyperlipidemia: type I, IV, V.
Hyperparathyroidism/Hypercalcemia.
Kawasaki disease.
Malnutrition.
Organic acidemia.
Peptic ulcer.
Periarteritis nodosa.
Renal failure.
Systemic lupus erythematosus.
Transplantation: bone marrow, heart, liver, kidney, pancreas.
Vasculitis.

Traumatic
Blunt injury.
Burns.
Child abuse.
Hypothermia.
Surgical trauma.
Total body cast.

PANCREATITIS, DRUG-INDUCED[2]

ICD-9CM # 577.0
ICD-10CM # K85.3 Drug induced acute pancreatitis

DEFINITE

Acetaminophen.
Azathioprine.
Cimetidine.
Cisplatin.
Corticosteroids.
Didanosine.
Erythromycin.
Estrogens.
Ethyl alcohol.
Furosemide.
l-Asparaginase.
Mercaptopurine.
Metronidazole.
Methyldopa.
Nitrofurantoin.
Octreotide.
Organophosphates.
Pentamidine.
Ranitidine.
Tetracycline.
Salicylates.
Sulfonamides, trimethoprim-sulfamethoxazole, sulfasalazine.
Sulindac.
Valproic acid.

Differential Diagnosis II

POSSIBLE

Bumetanide.
Carbamazepine.
Chlorthalidone.
Clonidine.
Colchicine.
Cyclosporine.
Cytarabine.
Diazoxide.
Enalapril.
Ergotamine.
Ethacrynic acid.
Indomethacin.
Isoniazid.
Isotretinoin.
Mefenamic acid.
Opiates.
Phenformin.
Piroxicam.
Procainamide.
Rifampin.
Thiazides.

PANCYTOPENIA[20]

ICD-9CM # 284.1
ICD-10CM # D61.818 Other pancytopenia

PANCYTOPENIA WITH HYPOCELLULAR BONE MARROW

Acquired aplastic anemia.
Inherited aplastic anemia (Fanconi anemia and others).
Some myelodysplasia syndromes.
Rare aleukemic leukemia (acute myelogenous leukemia).
Some acute lymphoblastic leukemias.
Some lymphomas of bone marrow.

PANCYTOPENIA WITH CELLULAR BONE MARROW

Primary bone marrow diseases.
Myelodysplasia syndromes.
Paroxysmal nocturnal hemoglobinuria.
Myelofibrosis.
Some aleukemic leukemias.
Myelophthisis.
Bone marrow lymphoma.
Hairy cell leukemia.
Secondary to systemic diseases.
Systemic lupus erythematosus, Sjögren syndrome.
Hypersplenism.
Vitamin B_{12}, folate deficiency (familial defect).
Overwhelming infection.
Alcohol.
Brucellosis.
Ehrlichiosis.
Sarcoidosis.
Tuberculosis and atypical mycobacteria.

HYPOCELLULAR BONE MARROW ± CYTOPENIA

Q fever.
Legionnaires disease.
Mycobacteria.
Tuberculosis.*
Anorexia nervosa, starvation.
Hypothyroidism.

*Pancytopenia in tuberculosis only rarely is associated with a hypocellular bone marrow at biopsy or autopsy. Marrow failure in the setting of tuberculosis is almost always fatal; exceptional patients probably had underlying myelodysplasia or acute leukemia.

PANCYTOPENIA SYNDROME, INHERITED[22a]

ICD-9CM # 284.1
ICD-10CM # D61.818 Other pancytopenia

Fanconi anemia.
Shwachman-Diamond syndrome.
Dyskeratosis congenita.
Congenital amegakaryocytic thrombocytopenia.
Unclassified inherited bone marrow failure syndromes.
Other genetic syndromes:
- Down syndrome.
- Dubowitz syndrome.
- Seckel syndrome.
- Reticular dysgenesis.
- Schimke immunoosseous dysplasia.
- Familial aplastic anemia (non-Fanconi).
- Cartilage-hair hypoplasia.
- Noonan syndrome.

PAPILLEDEMA

ICD-9CM # 377.00 Papilledema NOS
377.02 With Decreased Ocular Pressure
377.01 With Increased Intracranial Pressure
377.03 With Retinal Disorder
ICD-10CM # H47.10 Unspecified papilledema

CNS infections (viral, bacterial, fungal).
Medications (lithium, cisplatin, corticosteroids, tetracycline, etc.).
Head trauma.
CNS neoplasm (primary or metastatic).
Pseudotumor cerebri.
Cavernous sinus thrombosis.
SLE.
Sarcoidosis.
Subarachnoid hemorrhage.
Carbon dioxide retention.
Arnold–Chiari malformation and other developmental or congenital malformations.
Orbital lesions.
Central retinal vein occlusion.
Hypertensive encephalopathy.
Metabolic abnormalities.

PAPULOSQUAMOUS DISEASES[14]

ICD-9CM # 709.8
L98.8 Other specified disorders of the skin and subcutaneous tissue
ICD-10CM #

Psoriasis.
Pityriasis rubra pilaris.
Pityriasis rosea.
Lichen planus.
Lichen nitidus.
Secondary syphilis.
Pityriasis lichenoides.
Parapsoriasis.
Mycosis fungoides.
Dermatophytosis.
Tinea versicolor.

PARANEOPLASTIC NEUROLOGIC SYNDROMES

ICD-9CM # varies with specific disorder
ICD-10CM # G13.0 Paraneoplastic neuromyopathy and neuropathy

Lambert-Eaton myasthenic syndrome.
Myasthenia gravis.
Guillain-Barré syndrome.
Amyotrophic lateral sclerosis.
Dermatomyositis.
Carcinoid myopathy.
Cerebellar degeneration.
Encephalomyelitis.
Optic neuritis, uveitis, retinopathy.
Stiff-man syndrome.
Autonomic neuropathy.
Brachial neuritis.
Sensory neuropathy.
Progressive multifocal leukoencephalopathy.

PARANEOPLASTIC SYNDROMES, ENDOCRINE[36]

ICD-9CM # varies specific disorder
ICD-10CM # G13.0 Paraneoplastic neuromyopathy and neuropathy

Hypercalcemia.
Syndrome of inappropriate secretion of antidiuretic hormone.
Hypoglycemia.
Zollinger-Ellison syndrome.
Ectopic secretion of human chorionic gonadotropin.
Cushing's syndrome.

PARANEOPLASTIC SYNDROMES, NONENDOCRINE[36]

ICD-9CM # varies with specific disorder
ICD-10CM # G13.0 Paraneoplastic neuromyopathy and neuropathy

CUTANEOUS

Dermatomyositis.
Acanthosis nigricans.
Sweet's syndrome.
Erythema gyratum repens.
Systemic nodular panniculitis (Weber-Christian disease).

RENAL

Nephrotic syndrome.
Nephrogenic diabetes insipidus.

NEUROLOGIC

Subacute cerebellar degeneration.
Progressive multifocal leukoencephalopathy.

Subacute motor neuropathy.
Sensory neuropathy.
Ascending acute polyneuropathy (Guillain-Barré syndrome).
Myasthenic syndrome (Eaton-Lambert syndrome).

HEMATOLOGIC

Microangiopathic hemolytic anemia.
Migratory thrombophlebitis (Trousseau's syndrome).
Anemia of chronic disease.

RHEUMATOLOGIC

Polymyalgia rheumatica.
Hypertrophic pulmonary osteoarthropathy.

PARAPARESIS, ACUTE OR SUBACUTE[34a]

ICD-9CM # varies with specific diagnosis
ICD-10CM # G82.2 Paraparesis

CAUSES OF ACUTE OR SUBACUTE PARAPARESIS

Trauma to a Previously Normal Spine

Vertebral Disease

Metastatic carcinoma.
Cervical spondylosis.
Dorsal disk prolapse.
Paget's disease.
Rheumatoid arthritis.
Pott's disease of spine.

Tumors

Extradural or intradural carcinoma, lymphoma, myeloma, leukemia.
Dorsal meningioma.
Neurofibroma.

Hematologic Disease

Any cause of thrombocytopenia.
Other clotting disorders.
Leukemia.
Anticoagulant treatment.
Epidural or intramedullary hemorrhage.

Infection

Epidural abscess.
TB abscess.
Syphilitic myelitis.
HIV infection.
Vascular myelopathy.

Vascular

Anterior spinal artery occlusion.
Infarction secondary to hypotension.
Embolic infarction.
Infarction secondary to aortic dissection.
Arteriovenous malformation: infarction or hemorrhage.
Primary intramedullary hemorrhage.
Vasculitis—polyarteritis nodosa (PAN).

Inflammatory

Myelitis of unknown cause.
Multiple sclerosis.
Systemic lupus erythematosus.
Sarcoidosis.

Metabolic

Subacute degeneration of the cord.

PARAPARESIS, CHRONIC PROGRESSIVE[34a]

ICD-9CM # varies with specific diagnosis
ICD-10CM # G82.2 Paraparesis

CAUSES OF CHRONIC PROGRESSIVE PARAPARESIS

Vertebral Disease
Cervical spondylosis.
Dorsal disk prolapse.
Rheumatoid arthritis.
Pott's disease of spine.
Ankylosing spondylitis.
Tumors
Meningioma.
Neurofibroma.
Glioma.
Ependymoma.
Chordoma.
Lipoma.
Syringomyelia
With Arnold–Chiari malformation.
With tumor.
Posttraumatic.
Infection
Tropical spastic paraparesis (HTLV 1 infection).
Syphilitic myelitis.
Vascular
Arteriovenous malformation.
Inflammatory
Multiple sclerosis.
Sarcoidosis.
Radiation myelopathy.
Arachnoiditis.
Metabolic
Subacute combined degeneration of the cord.
Paget's disease.
Degenerative
Motor neuron disease.
Hereditary
Hereditary spastic paraplegia.

PARAPLEGIA

ICD-9CM #	344.1	Paraplegia, Acquired
	343.0	Paraplegia, Congenital
	438.50	Paraplegia, Late Effect of CVA
ICD-10CM #	G82.20	Paraplegia, unspecified
	G80.1	Spastic diplegic cerebral palsy
	I69.969	Other paralytic syndrome following unspecified cerebrovascular disease affecting unspecified side

Trauma: penetrating wounds to motor cortex, fracture-dislocation of vertebral column with compression of spinal cord or cauda equina, prolapsed disk, electrical injuries.
Neoplasm: parasagittal region, vertebrae, meninges, spinal cord, cauda equina, Hodgkin's disease, NHL, leukemic deposits, pelvic neoplasms.
Multiple sclerosis and other demyelinating disorders.
Mechanical compression of spinal cord, cauda equina, or lumbosacral plexus: Paget's disease, kyphoscoliosis, herniation of intervertebral disk, spondylosis, ankylosing spondylitis, RA, aortic aneurysm.
Infections: spinal abscess, syphilis, TB, poliomyelitis, leprosy.
Thrombosis of superior sagittal sinus.
Polyneuritis: Guillain-Barré syndrome, diabetes, alcohol, beriberi, heavy metals.
Heredofamilial muscular dystrophies.
ALS.
Congenital and familial conditions: syringomyelia, myelomeningocele, myelodysplasia.
Hysteria.

PARASELLAR MASSES[26a]

ICD-9CM # code varies with specific diagnosis
ICD-10CM # code varies with specific diagnosis

GENETIC

Transcription factor mutations (e.g., PROP1[a]).

CYSTS

Rathke's.
Arachnoid.
Epidermoid.
Dermoid.

TUMORS

Hormone-secreting or nonfunctional pituitary adenoma.
Granular cell tumor.
Craniopharyngioma (cystic components).
Chordoma.
Meningioma.
Sarcoma.
Glioma.
Schwannoma.
Germ cell tumor.
Vascular tumor.
Solid or hematological metastasis.

MALFORMATION AND HAMARTOMAS

Ectopic pituitary, neurohypophyseal, or salivary tissue.
Hypothalamic hamartoma.
Gangliocytoma.

MISCELLANEOUS LESIONS

Aneurysms.
Hypophysitis.
Infections.
Sarcoidosis.
Giant cell granuloma.
Histiocytosis X.

[a] PROP1, prophet of Pit1 (paired-like homeodomain transcription factor).

PARESTHESIAS

ICD-9CM # 782.0
ICD-10CM # R20.2 Paresthesia of skin
G54.8 Other nerve root and plexus disorders

Multiple sclerosis.
Nutritional deficiencies (thiamin, vitamin B_{12}, folic acid).
Compression of spinal cord or peripheral nerves.
Medications (e.g., INH, lithium, nitrofurantoin, gold, cisplatin, hydralazine, amitriptyline, sulfonamides, amiodarone, metronidazole, dapsone, disulfiram, chloramphenicol).
Toxic chemicals (e.g., lead, arsenic, cyanide, mercury, organophosphates).
DM.
Myxedema.
Alcohol.
Sarcoidosis.
Neoplasms.
Infections (HIV, Lyme disease, herpes zoster, leprosy, diphtheria).
Charcot-Marie-Tooth syndrome and other hereditary neuropathies.
Guillain-Barré neuropathy.

PARKINSONISM-PLUS SYNDROMES

ICD-9CM # varies with specific disorder
ICD-10CM # G21.8 Other secondary parkinsonism

Parkinson's disease.
Shy-Drager syndrome.
Corticobasal degeneration.
Olivo-ponto-cerebellar atrophy.
Dementia with Lewy bodies.
Progressive supranuclear palsy.
Striatonigral degeneration.

PAROTID SWELLING[3]

ICD-9CM # 527.2 Allergic Parotitis
72.9 Infectious Parotitis
527.8 Salivary Gland Obstruction
527.5 Salivary Gland Obstruction with Calculus
527.8 Salivary Gland Stricture
527.3 Salivary Gland Abscess
235.1 Salivary Gland Neoplasm
ICD-10CM # K11.20 Sialoadenitis, unspecified
B26.9 Mumps without complication
K11.8 Other diseases of salivary glands
K11.5 Sialolithiasis
K11.3 Abscess of salivary gland

INFECTIOUS

Mumps.
Parainfluenza.
Influenza.
Cytomegalovirus infection.
Coxsackievirus infection.
Lymphocytic choriomeningitis.
Echovirus infection.
Suppuration (bacterial).
Actinomyces infection.
Mycobacterial infection.
Cat-scratch disease.

NONINFECTIOUS

Drug hypersensitivity (thiouracil, phenothiazines, thiocyanate, iodides, copper, isoprenaline, lead, mercury, phenylbutazone).
Sarcoidosis.
Tumors, mixed.
Hemangioma, lymphangioma.
Sialectasis.
Sjögren's syndrome.
Mikulicz's syndrome (scleroderma, mixed connective tissue disease, SLE).
Recurrent idiopathic parotitis.
Pneumoparotitis.
Trauma.
Sialolithiasis.
Foreign body.
Cystic fibrosis.
Malnutrition (marasmus, alcohol cirrhosis).
Dehydration.
DM.
Waldenström's macroglobulinemia.
Reiter's syndrome (reactive arthritis).
Amyloidosis.

NONPAROTID SWELLING

Hypertrophy of masseter muscle.
Lymphadenopathy.
Rheumatoid mandibular joint swelling.
Tumors of jaw.
Infantile cortical hyperostosis.

PELVIC MASS

ICD-9CM # 789.39
ICD-10CM # R19.09 Other intra-abdominal and pelvic swelling, mass and lump

Hemorrhagic ovarian cyst.
Simple ovarian cyst (follicle or corpus luteum).
Ovarian carcinoma, carcinoma of fallopian tube, colorectal carcinoma, metastatic carcinoma, prostate carcinoma, bladder carcinoma, lymphoma, Hodgkin's disease.
Cystadenoma, teratoma, endometrioma.
Leiomyoma.
Leiomyosarcoma.
Diverticulitis, diverticular abscess.
Appendiceal abscess, tuboovarian abscess.
Ectopic pregnancy, intrauterine pregnancy.
Paraovarian cyst.
Hydrosalpinx.

PELVIC PAIN, CAUSES IN WOMEN[2]

ICD-9CM # 338.4
ICD-10CM # N94 Pain and other conditions associated with female genital organs and menstrual cycle
G10.2 Pelvic and perineal pain
G89.4 Chronic pain syndrome

POTENTIAL CAUSES OF PELVIC PAIN IN WOMEN

Reproductive Tract
Ovarian torsion.
Ovarian cyst.
Salpingitis/tubo-ovarian abscess.
Septic pelvic thrombophlebitis.
Endometritis.
Endometriosis.
Uterine perforation.
Uterine fibroids.
Dysmenorrhea.
Pregnancy-related

First trimester

Ectopic pregnancy.
Threatened abortion.
Nonviable pregnancy.
Ovarian hyperstimulation syndrome.

Second and third trimesters

Placenta previa.
Placental abruption.
Round ligament pain.
Intestinal Tract
Appendicitis.
Diverticulitis.
Ischemic bowel.
Perforated viscus.
Bowel obstruction.
Incarcerated/strangulated hernia.
Inflammatory bowel disease.
Gastroenteritis.
Urinary Tract
Pyelonephritis.
Cystitis.
Ureteral stone.

PELVIC PAIN, CHRONIC[7]

ICD-9CM # 625.9 Pelvic Pain, Female
789.09 Pelvic Pain, Male
ICD-10CM # N94.89 Other specified conditions associated with female genital organs and menstrual cycle
R10.2 Pelvic and perineal pain
R10.10 Upper abdominal pain, unspecified
R10.2 Pelvic and perineal pain
R10.30 Lower abdominal pain, unspecified

GYNECOLOGIC DISORDERS

Primary dysmenorrhea.
Endometriosis.
Adenomyosis.
Adhesions.
Fibroids.
Retained ovary syndrome after hysterectomy.
Previous tubal ligation.
Chronic pelvic infection.

MUSCULOSKELETAL DISORDERS

Myofascial pain syndrome.

GASTROINTESTINAL DISORDERS

Irritable bowel syndrome.
Inflammatory bowel disease.

URINARY TRACT DISORDERS

Interstitial cystitis.
Nonbacterial urethritis.

PELVIC PAIN, GENITAL ORIGIN[26]

ICD-9CM #	625.9	Pelvic Pain, Female
	789.09	Pelvic Pain, Male
ICD-10CM #	N94.89	Other specified conditions associated with female genital organs and menstrual cycle
	R10.2	Pelvic and perineal pain
	R10.10	Upper abdominal pain, unspecified
	R10.2	Pelvic and perineal pain
	R10.30	Lower abdominal pain, unspecified

PERITONEAL IRRITATION

Ruptured ectopic pregnancy.
Ovarian cyst rupture.
Ruptured tuboovarian abscess.
Uterine perforation.

TORSION

Ovarian cyst or tumor.
Pedunculated fibroid.

INTRATUMOR HEMORRHAGE OR INFARCTION

Ovarian cyst.
Solid ovarian tumor.
Uterine leiomyoma.

INFECTION

Endometritis.
Pelvic inflammatory disease.
Trichomonas cervicitis or vaginitis.
Tuboovarian abscess.

PREGNANCY-RELATED

First Trimester

Ectopic pregnancy.
Abortion.
Corpus luteum hematoma.

Late Pregnancy

Placental problems.
Preeclampsia.
Premature labor.

MISCELLANEOUS

Endometriosis.
Foreign objects.
Pelvic adhesions.
Pelvic neoplasm.
Primary dysmenorrhea.

PELVIC PAIN, NON-PREGNANT FEMALE[1]

ICD-9CM #	625.9	
ICD-10CM #	N94.89	Other specified conditions associated with female genital organs and menstrual cycle
	R10.2	Pelvic and perineal pain
	R10.10	Upper abdominal pain, unspecified
	R10.30	Lower abdominal pain, unspecified

DIFFERENTIAL DIAGNOSIS OF PELVIC PAIN IN NONPREGNANT FEMALES

Gynecologic Diagnoses

Infectious:
- Vaginitis.
- Cervicitis.
- Endometritis.
- Tuboovarian abscess.
- Pelvic inflammatory disease.

Ovarian:
- Ovarian torsion.
- Ruptured ovarian cyst.
- Ovarian tumor.
- Degenerating ovarian tumor.
- Mittelschmerz.

Cervical:
- Cervical polyps.
- Cervical stenosis.
- Cervical cancer.

Uterine:
- Uterine fibroids.
- Degenerating uterine fibroids.
- Adenomyosis.
- Endometrial carcinoma.

Extrauterine:
- Endometriosis.
- Adhesions.
- Residual accessory ovary.

Nongynecologic Diagnoses

Gastrointestinal:
- Acute appendicitis.
- Mesenteric lymphadenitis.
- Diverticulitis.
- Inflammatory bowel disease.
- Irritable bowel syndrome.
- Bowel obstruction.
- Intraabdominal abscess.
- Colorectal carcinoma.

Urinary:
- Cystitis.
- Renal colic.
- Bladder cancer.

Musculoskeletal:
- Abdominal wall pain.
- Lumbar back pain.
- Fibromyalgia.
- Muscular strain.
- Piriformis syndrome.

Neurologic:
- Lumbar radiculopathy.
- Shingles.
- Spondylosis.

Psychologic:
- Personality disorders.
- Major depressive disorder.

PENILE RASH

ICD-9CM #	782.1	
ICD-10CM #	R21	Rash and other nonspecific skin eruption

Herpes simplex 2.
Balanitis (Candida).
Condyloma acuminatum.
Molluscum contagiosum.
Scabies.
Pediculosis pubis.
Pearly penile papules.
Lichen nitidus.
Fox-Fordyce disease (follicular papules).
Trauma.

PERIANAL PAIN[38]

ICD-9CM #	569.42	
ICD-10CM #	K62.89	Other specified diseases of anus and rectum

Fissure-in-ano
Anal sepsis
- Anal abscess
- Anal fistula

Hemorrhoids
- Internal hemorrhoids
- External hemorrhoids

Pruritus ani
Proctalgia fugax
Chronic perianal pain syndromes
- Coccygodynia
- Descending perineum syndrome
- Levator ani syndrome
- Idiopathic perineal pain

PERICARDIAL EFFUSION

ICD-9CM #	420.90	
ICD-10CM #	I30.9	Acute pericarditis, unspecified
	I31.3	Pericardial effusion

Pericarditis.
Uremia.
Myxedema.
Neoplasm (leukemia, lymphoma, metastatic).
Hemorrhage (trauma, leakage of thoracic aneurysm).
SLE, rheumatoid disease.
Myocardial infarction.

PERIODIC PARALYSIS, HYPERKALEMIC

ICD-9CM # 344.9
ICD-10CM # G83.9 Paralytic syndrome, unspecified

Chronic renal failure.
Renal insufficiency with excessive potassium supplementation.
Potassium-sparing diuretics.
Endocrinopathies (hypoaldosteronism, adrenal insufficiency).

PERIODIC PARALYSIS, HYPOKALEMIC

ICD-9CM # 344.9
ICD-10CM # G83.9 Paralytic syndrome, unspecified

Chronic diarrhea (laxative abuse, sprue, villous adenoma).
Potassium-depleting diuretics.
Medications (amphotericin B, corticosteroids).
Chronic licorice ingestion.
Thyrotoxicosis.
Renal tubular acidosis.
Conn's syndrome.
Barter's syndrome.
Barium intoxication.

PERITONEAL CARCINOMATOSIS[14]

ICD-9CM # 197.6
ICD-10CM # C78.6 Secondary malignant neoplasm of retroperitoneum and peritoneum

PRIMARY DISORDERS OF THE PERITONEUM: MESOTHELIOMA

Metastatic spread from:
Stomach.
Colon.
Pancreas.
Carcinoid.

Other Intraabdominal Organs

Ovary.
Pseudomyxoma peritonei.

Extraabdominal Primary Tumors

Breast.
Lung.

Hematologic Malignancy

Lymphoma.

PERITONEAL EFFUSION[18]

ICD-9CM # 792.9
ICD-10CM # R18 Ascites
R85.9 Unspecified abnormal finding in specimens from digestive organs and abdominal cavity
R88.8 Abnormal findings in other body fluids and substances

TRANSUDATES

Increased hydrostatic pressure or decreased plasma oncotic pressure.
Congestive heart failure.
Hepatic cirrhosis.
Hypoproteinemia.

EXUDATES

Increased capillary permeability or decreased lymphatic resorption.
Infections (TB, spontaneous bacterial peritonitis, secondary bacterial peritonitis).
Neoplasms (hepatoma, metastatic carcinoma, lymphoma, mesothelioma).
Trauma.
Pancreatitis.
Bile peritonitis (e.g., ruptured gallbladder).

CHYLOUS EFFUSION

Damage or obstruction to thoracic duct.
Trauma.
Lymphoma.
Carcinoma.
Tuberculosis.
Parasitic infection.

PERIUMBILICAL SWELLING

ICD-9CM # 789.3
ICD-10CM # R19.00 Intra-abdominal and pelvic swelling, mass and lump, unspecified site

Umbilical hernia.
Lipoma.
Epigastric hernia.
Umbilical granuloma.
Omphalocele.
Gastroschisis.
Caput medusae.

PHEOCHROMOCYTOMA-TYPE SPELLS[26a]

ICD-9CM # 255.6
ICD-10CM # I15.2 Hypertension due to pheochromocytoma

DIFFERENTIAL DIAGNOSIS OF PHEOCHROMOCYTOMA-TYPE SPELLS

Endocrine Causes

Carbohydrate intolerance.
Hyperadrenergic spells.
Hypoglycemia.
Pancreatic tumors (e.g., insulinoma).
Pheochromocytoma.
Primary hypogonadism (menopausal syndrome).
Thyrotoxicosis.

Cardiovascular Causes

Angina.
Cardiovascular deconditioning.
Labile essential hypertension.
Orthostatic hypotension.
Paroxysmal cardiac arrhythmia.
Pulmonary edema.
Renovascular disease.
Syncope (e.g., vasovagal reaction).

Psychologic Causes

Factitious (e.g., drugs, Valsalva).
Hyperventilation.
Severe anxiety and panic disorders.
Somatization disorder.

Pharmacologic Causes

Chlorpropamide-alcohol flush.
Combination of a monoamine oxidase inhibitor and a decongestant.
Illegal drug ingestion (cocaine, phencyclidine, lysergic acid diethylamide).
Sympathomimetic drug ingestion.
Vancomycin ("red man syndrome").
Withdrawal of adrenergic-inhibitor.

Neurologic Causes

Autonomic neuropathy.
Cerebrovascular insufficiency.
Diencephalic epilepsy (autonomic seizures).
Migraine headache.
Postural orthostatic tachycardia syndrome.
Stroke.

Other Causes

Carcinoid syndrome.
Mast cell disease.
Recurrent idiopathic anaphylaxis.
Unexplained flushing spells.

PHOTODERMATOSES[14]

ICD-9CM # 692.72
ICD-10CM # L56.0 Drug phototoxic response
L56.1 Drug photoallergic response
L56.2 Photocontact dermatitis [berloque dermatitis]

Polymorphous light eruption.
Chronic actinic dermatitis.
Solar urticaria.
Phototoxicity and photoallergy.
Porphyrias.

PHOTOSENSITIVITY

ICD-9CM # 692.72
ICD-10CM # L56.0 Drug phototoxic response
L56.1 Drug photoallergic response
L56.2 Photocontact dermatitis [berloque dermatitis]

Solar urticaria.
Photoallergic reaction.
Phototoxic reaction.
Polymorphous light eruption.
Porphyria cutanea tarda.
SLE.
Drug induced (e.g., tetracyclines).

PIGMENTURIA[2]

ICD-9CM # varies with specific diagnosis
ICD-10CM # R82 Other abnormal findings in urine

HEMOGLOBINURIA

Hemolysis.

HEMATURIA

Renal causes.
Trauma.

ACUTE INTERMITTENT PORPHYRIA

BILIRUBINURIA

Food

Beets.

Drugs

Vitamin B_{12}.
Rifampin.
Phenytoin.
Laxatives.

PITUITARY REGION TUMORS[16a]

ICD-9CM # varies with specific diagnosis
ICD-10CM # varies with specific diagnosis

PRIMARY TUMORS IN THE SELLAR AND PARASELLAR REGION

Tumor

Pituitary macroadenoma.
Meningioma.
Schwannoma (e.g., of fifth nerve).
Chordoma.
Chondrosarcoma.
Crangiopharyngioma.
Rathke's cleft cyst.
Dermoid.
Epidermoid.
Tuber cinerum hamartoma.
Optic glioma.
Germ cell tumors.

PLEURAL EFFUSIONS

ICD-9CM # 511.9 Pleural Effusion, Unspecified
ICD-10CM # J91.8 Pleural effusion in other conditions classified elsewhere

EXUDATIVE

Neoplasm: bronchogenic carcinoma, breast carcinoma, mesothelioma, lymphoma, ovarian carcinoma, multiple myeloma, leukemia, Meigs' syndrome.
Infections: viral pneumonia, bacterial pneumonia, *Mycoplasma,* TB, fungal and parasitic diseases, extension from subphrenic abscess.
Trauma.
Collagen vascular diseases: SLE, RA, scleroderma, polyarteritis, granulomatosis with polyangiitis (Wegener's granulomatosis).
Pulmonary infarction.
Pancreatitis.
Postcardiotomy/Dressler's syndrome.
Drug-induced SLE (hydralazine, procainamide).
Postabdominal surgery.
Ruptured esophagus.
Chronic effusion secondary to congestive failure.

TRANSUDATIVE

CHF.
Hepatic cirrhosis.
Nephrotic syndrome.
Hypoproteinemia from any cause.
Meigs' syndrome.

PLEURAL EFFUSIONS, MALIGNANCY-ASSOCIATED

ICD-9CM # 197.2
ICD-10CM # C78.2 Secondary malignant neoplasm of pleura

Lung cancer	(30% to 40%)
Breast cancer	(20% to 25%)
Lymphoma	(10% to 15%)
Leukemia	(5% to 10%)
GI tract	(5%)
GU tract	(5%)
Reproductive	(3%)

PNEUMATOSIS INTESTINALIS IN NEONATE AND OLDER CHILD[16A]

ICD-9CM # varies with specific diagnosis
ICD-10CM # varies with specific diagnosis

CAUSES OF PNEUMATOSIS INTESTINALIS IN THE NEONATE AND THE OLDER CHILD

Necrotizing enterocolitis.
Bowel ischemia, inflammation, and obstruction.
Cyanotic congenital heart disease.
Hirschsprung's disease.
Gastroschisis.
Anorectal atresia.
Inflammatory bowel disease.
Lymphoma.
Leukemia.
CMV and rotavirus gastroenteritis.
Colonoscopy.
Caustic ingestion.
Short bowel syndrome.
Congenital immune deficiency states.
Clostridium infection.
Chronic steroid use.
Posthepatic, renal, or bone marrow transplant.
Collagen vascular disease.
Graft-versus-host disease.
AIDS.

PNEUMONIA, RECURRENT

ICD-9CM # 482.9 Bacterial Pneumonia
480.9 Viral Pneumonia
484.1 Fungal Pneumonia
485 Segmental Pneumonia
ICD-10CM # J15.9 Unspecified bacterial pneumonia
J12.9 Viral pneumonia, unspecified
B25.0 Cytomegaloviral pneumonitis
J18.0 Bronchopneumonia, unspecified organism

Mechanical obstruction from neoplasm.
Chronic aspiration (tube feeding, alcoholism, CVA, neuromuscular disorders, seizure disorder, inability to cough).
Bronchiectasis.
Kyphoscoliosis.
COPD, CHF, asthma, silicosis, pulmonary fibrosis, cystic fibrosis.
Pulmonary TB, chronic sinusitis.
Immunosuppression (HIV, corticosteroids, leukemia, chemotherapy, splenectomy).

PNEUMOPERITONEUM, NEONATAL[16a]

ICD-9CM # varies with specific diagnosis
ICD-10CM # varies with specific diagnosis

CAUSES OF NEONATAL PNEUMOPERITONEUM

Necrotizing enterocolitis.
Spontaneous perforation of a hollow viscus.
- Stomach.
- Duodenum.
- Ileum.
- Colon.

Malrotation and volvulus.
Distal obstruction.
Perforation of Meckel's diverticulum.
Anterior abdominal wall defects.
- Pentalogy of Cantrell.
- Omphalocele.
- Gastroschisis.
- Cloacal exstrophy.

Stress and peptic ulcers.
Mechanical ventilation (air leak) or resuscitation ("bagging").
Post-laparotomy.
Iatrogenic gastric perforation with an orogastric tube.
Iatrogenic colon perforation.
- Thermometer.
- During an enema.

Indomethacin.
Dexamethasone treatment.

PNEUMOTHORAX, IN CHILDREN[22a]

ICD-9CM # 512 Pneumothorax
ICD-10CM # J93.0 Spontaneous tension pneumothorax
J93 Pneumothorax
J93.9 Pneumothorax unspecified

SPONTANEOUS

Primary idiopathic—usually resulting from ruptured subpleural blebs.
Secondary blebs.
Congenital lung disease:
- Congenital cystic adenomatoid malformation.
- Bronchogenic cysts.
- Pulmonary hypoplasia.

Conditions associated with increased intrathoracic pressure:
- Asthma.
- Bronchiolitis.

Differential Diagnosis II

- Air-block syndrome in neonates.
- Cystic fibrosis.
- Airway foreign body.

Infection:
- Pneumatocele.
- Lung abscess.
- Bronchopleural fistula.

Diffuse lung disease:
- Langerhans cell histiocytosis.
- Tuberous sclerosis.
- Marfan syndrome.
- Ehlers-Danlos syndrome.

Metastatic neoplasm—usually osteosarcoma (rare).

TRAUMATIC

Noniatrogenic.
- Penetrating trauma.
- Blunt trauma.
- Loud music (air pressure).

Iatrogenic.
- Thoracotomy.
- Thoracoscopy, thoracentesis.
- Tracheostomy.
- Tube or needle puncture.

Mechanical ventilation.

POLYCYTHEMIA

ICD-9CM # 790.0
ICD-10CM # D45 Polycythemia primary
D75.1 Polycythemia secondary

Tobacco abuse.
Chronic lung disease.
High altitude.
Sleep apnea.
Right-to-left cardiac shunts.
Erythropoietin administration.
Androgens/anabolic steroids.
Polycystic kidney disease.
Renal cell carcinoma.
Hepatocellular carcinoma.
Polycythemia vera.
Carbon monoxide exposure.
Primary familial and congenital polycythemia.
High-oxygen–affinity hemoglobins.
Uterine leiomyoma, meningioma, pheochromocytoma, parathyroid carcinoma.
Cobalt exposure.

POLYCYTHEMIA, RELATIVE VERSUS ABSOLUTE[20]

ICD-9CM # 790.0
ICD-10CM # D75.1 Secondary polycythemia

RELATIVE OR SPURIOUS POLYCYTHEMIA

Decreased plasma volume—reduced fluid intake, marked loss of body fluids (diaphoresis, vomiting, diarrhea, "third-spacing").
Gaisböck syndrome.
Overfilling of blood in collection vacuum tubes.

ABSOLUTE POLYCYTHEMIA

Primary Congenital and Familial Polycythemia

Secondary Polycythemia:

Acquired:
Hypoxia:
- Pulmonary disease.
- Cyanotic congenital heart disease.
- Hypoventilation syndromes—sleep apnea, Pickwickian syndrome.

High altitude.
Smokers' polycythemia, carbon monoxide intoxication due to industrial exposure.
Postrenal transplantation erythrocytosis.
Aberrant erythropoietin production:
- Tumors—renal cell carcinoma, Wilms' tumor, hepatic carcinoma, uterine leiomyomata, virilizing ovarian tumors, vascular cerebellar tumors.
- Miscellaneous renal and hepatic disorders—solitary renal cysts, polycystic kidney disease, renal artery stenosis, hydronephrosis, viral hepatitis.

Endocrine disorders—Cushing's syndrome, primary aldosteronism.
Androgen use.
Erythropoietin use.

Congenital:
Abnormal high-affinity hemoglobin variants.
Bisphosphoglycerate deficiency.
Congenital methemoglobinemia.
Chuvash polycythemia (von Hippel–Lindau mutations).
Prolyl hydroxylase mutations.

Polycythemia Vera

POLYMYALGIAS[18b]

ICD-9CM # varies with specific diagnosis
ICD-10CM # M35.3 Polymyalgia rheumatic

DISEASE ENTITIES WITH POLYMYALGIAS

Rheumatoid arthritis.
Rotator cuff syndrome.
Osteoarthritis of shoulder and hip joints.
Fibromyalgia.
Polymyositis/dermatomyositis.
Spondyloarthritis.
Systemic lupus erythematosus.
Vasculitides.
Paraneoplastic myalgias.
Infection-associated myalgias.
Statin therapy.
RS3PE (remitting seronegative symmetric synovitis and pitting edema).
Parkinson's disease.
Hypothyroidism.

POLYNEUROPATHY[40]

ICD-9CM # 357.9
ICD-10CM # G61.9 Inflammatory polyneuropathy, unspecified

PREDOMINANTLY MOTOR

Guillain-Barré syndrome.
Porphyria.
Diphtheria.
Lead.
Hereditary sensorimotor neuropathy, types I and II.
Paraneoplastic neuropathy.

PREDOMINANTLY SENSORY

Diabetes.
Amyloidosis.
Leprosy.
Lyme disease.
Paraneoplastic neuropathy.
Vitamin B_{12} deficiency.
Hereditary sensory neuropathy, types I-IV.

PREDOMINANTLY AUTONOMIC

Diabetes.
Amyloidosis.
Alcoholic neuropathy.
Familial dysautonomias.

MIXED SENSORIMOTOR

Systemic diseases: renal failure, hypothyroidism, acromegaly, RA, periarteritis nodosa, SLE, multiple myeloma, macroglobulinemia, remote effect of malignancy.
Medications: isoniazid, nitrofurantoin, ethambutol, chloramphenicol, chloroquine, vincristine, vinblastine, dapsone, disulfiram, diphenylhydantoin, cisplatin, 1-tryptophan.
Environmental toxins: *N*-hexane, methyl *N*-butyl ketone, acrylamide, carbon disulfide, carbon monoxide, hexachlorophene, organophosphates.
Deficiency disorders: malabsorption, alcoholism, vitamin B_1 deficiency, Refsum's disease, metachromatic leukodystrophy.

POLYNEUROPATHY, DEMYELINATING[2]

ICD-9CM # varies with specific diagnosis
ICD-10CM # G37.9 Demyelinating disease of central nervous system, unspecified

Guillain-Barré syndrome.
Acute inflammatory demyelinating polyradiculoneuropathy (AIDP).
Acute motor axonal neuropathy (AMAN).
Acute motor and sensory axonal neuropathy (AMSAN).
Miller Fisher syndrome.
Chronic inflammatory demyelinating polyradiculoplexo-neuropathy.
Malignancy.
HIV.
Hepatitis B.
Buckthorn.
Diphtheria.

POLYNEUROPATHY, DISTAL SENSORIMOTOR[2]

ICD-9CM # varies with specific diagnosis
ICD-10CM # G63 Polyneuropathy in diseases classified elsewhere

Diabetes mellitus.
Alcoholism.
Neoplastic or paraneoplastic.

Hereditary motor and sensory neuropathies (Charcot-Marie-Tooth).
Cryptogenic sensorimotor polyneuropathies (CSPN).
HIV.
Toxins:
Organic or industrial agents:
- Acrylamide.
- Allyl chloride.
- Carbon disulfide.
- Ethylene oxide.
- Hexacarbons.
- Methyl bromide.
- Organophosphate-induced delayed polyneuropathy (OPIDP).
- Polychlorinated biphenyls (PCBs).
- Trichloroethylene.
- Vacor.

Metals:
- Arsenic.
- Gold.
- Mercury (inorganic).
- Thallium.

Therapeutic agents:
- Amiodarone.
- Antiretrovirals.
- Dapsone.
- Disulfiram.
- Isoniazid.
- Metronidazole.
- Nitrofurantoin.
- Paclitaxel (Taxol).
- Phenytoin.
- Statins (HMG-CoA reductase inhibitors).
- Thalidomide.
- Vinca alkaloids (vincristine, vinblastine).

Nutritional:
- Beriberi (thiamine or vitamin B1).
- Pellagra (niacin, B vitamins).
- Pernicious anemia (vitamin B12).
- Pyridoxine deficiency (vitamin B6).

End-organ dysfunction:
- Acromegaly.
- Chronic pulmonary disease.
- Hypothyroidism.
- Renal failure (uremic neuropathy).

Paraproteinemias:
- Amyloidosis.
- Monoclonal gammopathy of unknown significance (MGUS).
- Multiple myeloma.
- Waldenström's macroglobulinemia.

Porphyria.

HMG-CoA, Hydroxymethylglutaryl coenzyme A.

POLYNEUROPATHY, DRUG-INDUCED[40]

ICD-9CM # 357.6
ICD-10CM # G62.0 Drug-induced polyneuropathy

DRUGS IN ONCOLOGY

Vincristine.
Procarbazine.
Cisplatin.
Misonidazole.
Metronidazole (Flagyl).
Taxol.

DRUGS IN INFECTIOUS DISEASES

Isoniazid.
Nitrofurantoin.
Dapsone.
ddC (dideoxycytidine).
ddI (dideoxyinosine).

DRUGS IN CARDIOLOGY

Hydralazine.
Perhexiline maleate.
Procainamide.
Disopyramide.

DRUGS IN RHEUMATOLOGY

Gold salts.
Chloroquine.

DRUGS IN NEUROLOGY AND PSYCHIATRY

Diphenylhydantoin.
Glutethimide.
Methaqualone.

MISCELLANEOUS

Disulfiram (Antabuse).
Vitamin: (pyridoxine in megadoses).

POLYNEUROPATHY, SYMMETRIC[40]

ICD-9CM # 357.9
ICD-10CM # G61.9 Inflammatory polyneuropathy, unspecified

ACQUIRED NEUROPATHIES

Toxic:
- Drugs.
- Industrial toxins.
- Heavy metals.
- Abused substances.

Metabolic/endocrine:
- Diabetes.
- Chronic renal failure.
- Hypothyroidism.
- Polyneuropathy of critical illness.

Nutritional deficiency:
- Vitamin B_{12} deficiency.
- Alcoholism.
- Vitamin E deficiency.

Paraneoplastic:
- Carcinoma.
- Lymphoma.

Plasma cell dyscrasia:
- Myeloma, typical, atypical, and solitary forms.
- Primary systemic amyloidosis.

Idiopathic chronic inflammatory demyelinating polyneuropathies.
Polyneuropathies associated with peripheral nerve autoantibodies.
Acquired immunodeficiency syndrome.

INHERITED NEUROPATHIES

Neuropathies with Biochemical Markers

Refsum's disease.
Bassen-Kornzweig disease.
Tangier disease.
Metachromatic leukodystrophy.
Krabbe's disease.
Adrenomyeloneuropathy.
Fabry's disease.

Neuropathies without Biochemical Markers or Systemic Involvement

Hereditary motor neuropathy.
Hereditary sensory neuropathy.
Hereditary sensorimotor neuropathy.

POLYURIA

ICD-9CM # 788.42
ICD-10CM # R35.8 Other polyuria

DM.
Diabetes insipidus.
Primary polydipsia (compulsive water drinking).
Hypercalcemia.
Hypokalemia.
Postobstructive uropathy.
Diuretic phase of renal failure.
Drugs: diuretics, caffeine, alcohol, lithium.
Sickle cell trait or disease, chronic pyelonephritis (failure to concentrate urine).
Anxiety, cold weather.

POPLITEAL SWELLING

ICD-9CM #	459.2	Venous Obstruction
	747.4	Vein Anomaly, Lower Limb Vessel
	442.3	Artery Aneurysm
	904.41	Artery Injury
	447.8	Entrapment Syndrome
	727.51	Baker's Cyst
	451.2	Phlebitis, Lower Extremity
	727.67	Rupture of Achilles Tendon
ICD-10CM #	I87.1	Compression of vein
	I72.4	Aneurysm of artery of lower extremity
	S85.009A	Unspecified injury of popliteal artery, unspecified leg, initial encounter
	I77.3	Arterial fibromuscular dysplasia
	M71.20	Synovial cyst of popliteal space [Baker], unspecified knee
	I80.3	Phlebitis and thrombophlebitis of lower extremities, unspecified
	M66.369	Spontaneous rupture of flexor tendons, unspecified lower leg

Phlebitis (superficial).
Lymphadenitis.
Trauma: fractured tibia or fibula, contusion, traumatic neuroma.

DVT.
Ruptured varicose vein.
Baker's cyst.
Popliteal abscess.
Osteomyelitis.
Ruptured tendon.
Aneurysm of popliteal artery.
Neoplasm: lipoma, osteogenic sarcoma, neurofibroma, fibrosarcoma.

PORTAL HYPERTENSION[1a]

ICD-9CM # 572.3
ICD-10CM # K76.6 Portal hypertension

INCREASED RESISTANCE TO FLOW

Presinusoidal
Portal or splenic vein occlusion (thrombosis, tumor).
Schistosomiasis.
Congenital hepatic fibrosis.
Sarcoidosis.
Sinusoidal
Cirrhosis (all causes).
Alcoholic hepatitis.
Postsinusoidal
Venoocclusive disease.
Budd-Chiari syndrome.
Constrictive pericarditis.

INCREASED PORTAL BLOOD FLOW

Splenomegaly not caused by liver disease.
Arterioportal fistula.

POSTMENOPAUSAL BLEEDING

ICD-9CM # 627.1
ICD-10CM # N95.0 Postmenopausal bleeding

Hormone replacement therapy.
Neoplasm (uterine, ovarian, cervical, vaginal, vulvar).
Atrophic vaginitis.
Vaginal infection.
Polyp.
Extragenital (GI, urinary).
Tamoxifen.
Trauma.

POSTURAL HYPOTENSION, NONNEUROLOGIC CAUSES

ICD-9CM # 458.0
ICD-10CM # I95.1 Orthostatic hypotension

Diuretics and hypertensive agents.
GI hemorrhage.
Alcohol.
Excessive heat.
Rapid volume loss from diarrhea, vomiting.
Hemodialysis.
Extensive burns.
Pyrexia.
Aortic stenosis (impaired output).
Constrictive pericarditis, atrial myxoma (impaired cardiac filling).
Adrenal insufficiency.
Diabetes insipidus.
Vasodilatory agents (e.g., nitrates).

PREMATURE GRAYING, SCALP HAIR

ICD-9CM # varies with specific disorder
ICD-10CM # varies with specific diagnosis

Chemical exposure (e.g., phenol/catechol derivatives, sulfhydryls, arsenic).
Physical agents (e.g., ionizing radiation, lasers).
Hyperthyroidism.
Vitamin B_{12} deficiency.
Down's syndrome.
Chronic and severe protein deficiency.
Vitiligo.
Idiopathic.
Myotonic dystrophy.
Ataxia-telangiectasia.
Progeria.
Werner's syndrome.

PREMATURE VENTRICULAR CONTRACTIONS AND VENTRICULAR TACHYCARDIA[2]

ICD-9CM # 427.6
ICD-10CM # I49.40 Unspecified premature depolarization
I47.2 Ventricular tachycardia

CAUSES OF PREMATURE VENTRICULAR CONTRACTIONS AND VENTRICULAR TACHYCARDIA

Acute or previous myocardial infarction/ischemia.
Hypokalemia.
Hypoxemia.
Ischemic heart disease.
Valvular disease.
Catecholamine excess.*
Other drug intoxications (especially cyclic antidepressants).
Idiopathic causes.†
Digitalis toxicity.
Hypomagnesemia.
Hypercapnia.
Class I antidysrhythmic agents.
Ethanol.
Myocardial contusion.
Cardiomyopathy.
Acidosis.
Alkalosis.
Methylxanthine toxicity.

*Relative increase in sympathetic tone from drugs (direct or indirect) or conditions that augment catecholamine release or decrease parasympathetic tone.

†Isolated premature ventricular contractions (PVCs) can occur in up to 50% of young subjects without obvious cardiac or noncardiac disease; however, multiform and repetitive PVCs and ventricular tachycardia are rarely seen in this population.

PROPTOSIS[30]

ICD-9CM # 376.30
ICD-10CM # H05.20 Unspecified exophthalmos
H05.2 Ocular proptosis

Thyrotoxicosis.
Orbital pseudotumor.
Optic nerve tumor.
Cavernous sinus AV fistula, cavernous sinus thrombosis.
Cellulitis.
Metastatic tumor to orbit.

PROPTOSIS AND PALATAL NECROTIC ULCERS

ICD-9CM # 528.9 Ulcer of Palate
376.30 Proptosis
ICD-10CM # K13.70 Unspecified lesions of oral mucosa
K13.79 Other lesions of oral mucosa
H05.20 Unspecified exophthalmos

Cavernous sinus thrombosis.
Bacterial orbital cellulitis.
Metastatic neoplasm.
Rhinocerebral mucormycosis.
Ecthyma gangrenosum.
CNS aspergillosis.

PROTEIN-LOSING ENTEROPATHY, PEDIATRIC AGE[22a]

ICD-9CM # 579.8
ICD-10CM # E44.0 Moderate protein-energy malnutrition

CAUSES OF PROTEIN-LOSING ENTEROPATHY

Mucosal inflammation:
- Infection:
  - Cytomegalovirus.
  - Bacterial overgrowth.
  - Invasive bacterial infection.
- Gastric inflammation:
  - Ménétrier disease.
  - Eosinophilic gastroenteropathy.
- Intestinal inflammation:
  - Celiac disease.
  - Crohn disease.
- Eosinophilic gastroenteropathy:
  - Tropical sprue.
  - Radiation enteritis.

Primary intestinal lymphangiectasia.
Secondary intestinal lymphangiectasia:
- Constrictive pericarditis.
- Congestive heart failure.
- Post–Fontan procedure.
- Malrotation.
- Lymphoma.
- Sarcoidosis.
- Radiation therapy.

Colonic inflammation:
- Inflammatory bowel diseases.
- Necrotizing enterocolitis.

Congenital disorders of glycosylation.

PROTEINURIA

ICD-9CM # 791.0
ICD-10CM # R80.9 Proteinuria, unspecified

Nephrotic syndrome as a result of primary renal diseases.
Malignant hypertension.
Malignancies: multiple myeloma, leukemias, Hodgkin's disease.
CHF.
DM.
SLE, RA.
Sickle cell disease.
Goodpasture's syndrome.
Malaria.
Amyloidosis, sarcoidosis.
Tubular lesions: cystinosis.
Functional (after heavy exercise).
Pyelonephritis.
Pregnancy.
Constrictive pericarditis.
Renal vein thrombosis.
Toxic nephropathies: heavy metals, drugs.
Radiation nephritis.
Orthostatic (postural) proteinuria.
Benign proteinuria: fever, heat, or cold exposure.

PRURITUS

ICD-9CM # 698.9 Pruritus NOS
697.0 Pruritus Ani
698.1 Pruritus, Genital Organs
ICD-10CM # L29.9 Pruritus, unspecified
L29.3 Anogenital pruritus, unspecified

Dry skin.
Drug-induced eruption, fiberglass exposure.
Scabies.
Skin diseases.
Myeloproliferative disorders: mycosis fungoides, Hodgkin's lymphoma, multiple myeloma, polycythemia vera.
Cholestatic liver disease.
Endocrine disorders: DM, thyroid disease, carcinoid, pregnancy.
Carcinoma: breast, lung, gastric.
Chronic renal failure.
Iron deficiency.
AIDS.
Neurosis.
Sjögren's syndrome.

PRURITUS ANI[26]

ICD-9CM # 697.0
ICD-10CM # L29.0 Pruritus ani

FECAL IRRITATION

Poor hygiene.
Anorectal conditions (fissure, fistula, hemorrhoids, skin tags, perianal clefts).
Spicy foods, citrus foods, caffeine, colchicine, quinidine.

CONTACT DERMATITIS

Anesthetic agents, topical corticosteroids, perfumed soap.

DERMATOLOGIC DISORDERS

Psoriasis, seborrhea, lichen simplex or sclerosus.

SYSTEMIC DISORDERS

Chronic renal failure, myxedema, DM, thyrotoxicosis, polycythemia vera, Hodgkin's disease.

SEXUALLY TRANSMITTED DISEASES

Syphilis, herpes simplex virus, human papillomavirus.

OTHER INFECTIOUS AGENTS

Pinworms.
Scabies.
Bacterial infection, viral infection.

PRURITUS VULVAE[34a]

ICD-9CM # 698.1
ICD-10CM # L29.3 Anogenital pruritus, unspecified

CAUSES OF PRURITUS VULVAE

Diseases Special to Vulval Skin
Lichen sclerosus et atrophicus.
Leukoplakia.
Carcinoma.
Skin Disease
Psoriasis.
Atopic dermatitis.
Irritant and allergic contact dermatitis (especially medicaments).
Infection
Candidiasis.
Trichomonas.
Infestation
Pediculosis.
Psychogenic
Anxiety.
Depression.
Unknown

PSEUDOCYANOSIS, ETIOLOGY

ICD-9CM # varies with etiology
ICD-10CM # varies with etiology

Medications: amiodarone, minocycline, chlorpromazine.
Heavy metals:
Gold (systemic absorption).
Silver (systemic absorption).
Local contact with color dyes, gold, silver.

PSEUDOHERMAPHRODITISM, FEMALE

ICD-9CM # 255.2 Adrenal
752.7 Without Adrenocortical Disorder
ICD-10CM # E25.0 Congenital adrenogenital disorders associated with enzyme deficiency
E25.8 Other adrenogenital disorders
E25.9 Adrenogenital disorder, unspecified
Q56.3 Pseudohermaphroditism, unspecified
Q56.4 Indeterminate sex, unspecified

Congenital adrenal hyperplasia.
Maternal use of testosterone or related steroids.
Virilizing ovarian or adrenal tumor.
Virilizing luteoma of pregnancy.
Disturbances in differentiation of urogenital structures, non-androgen related.
Maternal virilizing adrenal hyperplasia.
Fetal P450 aromatase deficiency.

PSEUDOHERMAPHRODITISM, MALE

ICD-9CM # 255.2 Adrenal
752.7 Without Adrenocortical Disorder
ICD-10CM # E25.0 Congenital adrenogenital disorders associated with enzyme deficiency
E25.8 Other adrenogenital disorders
E25.9 Adrenogenital disorder, unspecified
Q56.3 Pseudohermaphroditism, unspecified
Q56.4 Indeterminate sex, unspecified

Maternal ingestion of progestogens.
End-organ resistance to androgenic hormones.
5-Alpha-reductase-2 deficiency.
XY gonadal dysgenesis.
Testicular regression syndrome.
Defects in testosterone metabolism by peripheral tissues.
Testosterone biosynthesis defects.

PSEUDOINFARCTION[22]

ICD-9CM # code varies with specific diagnosis
ICD-10CM # varies with specific diagnosis

Cardiac tumors, primary and secondary.
Cardiomyopathy (particularly hypertrophic and dilated).
Chagas' disease.
Chest deformity.
COPD (particularly emphysema).
HIV infection.
Hyperkalemia.
Left anterior fascicular block.
Left bundle branch block.
Left ventricular hypertrophy.
Myocarditis and pericarditis.
Normal variant.
Pneumothorax.
Poor R wave progression, rotational changes, and lead placement.
Pulmonary embolism.

Trauma to chest (nonpenetrating).
Wolff-Parkinson-White syndrome.
Rare causes: pancreatitis, amyloidosis, sarcoidosis, scleroderma.

PSYCHOSIS[28]

ICD-9CM #	298.9	Psychosis NOS
	298.90	Psychosis, Affective
	291.0	Psychosis, Alcoholic
	290.41	Psychosis, Acute Arteriosclerotic
ICD-10CM #	# F29	Unspecified psychosis not due to a substance or known physiological condition
	F29	Unspecified psychosis not due to a substance or known physiological condition
	F10.231	Alcohol dependence with withdrawal delirium
	F01.51	Vascular dementia with behavioral disturbance

PRIMARY

Schizophrenia related.*
Major depression.
Dementia.
Bipolar disorder.

SECONDARY

Drug use.†
Drug withdrawal.‡
Drug toxicity.§
Charles Bonnet syndrome.
Infections (pneumonia).
Electrolyte imbalance.
Syphilis.
Congestive heart failure.
Parkinson's disease.
Trauma to temporal lobe.
Postpartum psychosis.
Hypothyroidism/hyperthyroidism.
Hypomagnesemia.
Epilepsy.
Meningitis.
Encephalitis.
Brain abscess.
Herpes encephalopathy.
Hypoxia.
Hypercarbia.
Hypoglycemia.
Thiamine deficiency.
Postoperative states.

*Includes schizophrenia, schizophreniform disorder, brief reactive psychosis.
†Includes hypnotics, glucocorticoids, marijuana, phencyclidine, atropine, dopaminergic agents (e.g., amantadine, bromocriptine, l-dopa), immunosuppressants.
‡Includes alcohol, barbiturates, benzodiazepines.
§Includes digitalis, theophylline, cimetidine, anticholinergics, glucocorticoids, catecholaminergic agents.

PTOSIS

ICD-9CM #	374.30	Ptosis NOS
	743.61	Congenital
	374.33	Mechanical
	374.32	Myogenic
	374.31	Paralytic
ICD-10CM #	H02.409	Unspecified ptosis of unspecified eyelid
	Q10.0	Congenital ptosis
	H02.419	Mechanical ptosis of unspecified eyelid
	H02.429	Myogenic ptosis of unspecified eyelid
	H02.439	Paralytic ptosis unspecified eyelid

Third nerve palsy.
Myasthenia gravis.
Horner's syndrome.
Senile ptosis.

PUBERTY, DELAYED[27]

ICD-9CM #	259.0	
ICD-10CM #	E30.0	Delayed puberty

NORMAL OR LOW SERUM GONADOTROPIN LEVELS

Constitutional delay in growth and development.
Hypothalamic and/or pituitary disorders:
- Isolated deficiency of growth hormone.
- Isolated deficiency of Gn-RH.
- Isolated deficiency of LH and/or FSH.
- Multiple anterior pituitary hormone deficiencies.
- Associated with congenital anomalies: Kallmann's syndrome; Prader-Willi syndrome; Laurence-Moon-Biedl syndrome; Friedreich's ataxia.
- Trauma.
- Postinfection.
- Hyperprolactinemia.
- Postirradiation.
- Infiltrative disease (histiocytosis).
- Tumor.
- Autoimmune hypophysitis.
- Idiopathic.

Functional:
- Chronic endocrinologic or systemic disorders.
- Emotional disorders.
- Drugs: cannabis.

INCREASED SERUM GONADOTROPIN LEVELS

Gonadal abnormalities:

Congenital:
- Gonadal dysgenesis.
- Klinefelter's syndrome.
- Bilateral anorchism.
- Resistant ovary syndrome.
- Myotonic dystrophy in males.
- 17-Hydroxylase deficiency in females.
- Galactosemia.

Acquired:
- Bilateral gonadal failure resulting from trauma or infection or after surgery, irradiation, or chemotherapy.
- Oophoritis: isolated or with other autoimmune disorders.

Uterine or vaginal disorders:
- Absence of uterus and/or vagina.
- Testicular feminization: complete or incomplete androgen insensitivity.

PUBERTY, PRECOCIOUS

ICD-9CM #	255.2	
ICD-10CM #	E25.0	Congenital adrenogenital disorders associated with enzyme deficiency
	E25.8	Other adrenogenital disorders
	E25.9	Adrenogenital disorder, unspecified

Idiopathic.
Congenital virilizing adrenal hyperplasia.
Hypothalamic tumors.
Head trauma.
Hydrocephalus.
Degenerative CNS disease.
Arachnoid cyst.
Sex chromosome abnormalities (e.g., 47, XXY, 48, XXXY).
Perinatal asphyxia.
CNS infection (e.g., meningitis, encephalitis).

PULMONARY CRACKLES

ICD-9CM #	code not available	
ICD-10CM #	R09.8	Friction sounds, chest

Pneumonia.
Left ventricular failure.
Asbestosis, silicosis, interstitial lung disease.
Chronic bronchitis.
Alveolitis (allergic, fibrosing).
Neoplasm.

PULMONARY CYSTS ON X-RAY[16a]

ICD-9CM #	793.1	
ICD-10CM #	Q33.0	Polycystic lungs, congenital
	J98.4	Pulmonary manifestations

CAUSES OF CYSTS IN THE LUNG ON CHEST RADIOGRAPH

Cystic fibrosis.
Cystic bronchiectasis.
Bronchopulmonary dysplasia (neonate and older).
Tuberculosis (apical thick walled).
Pulmonary abscess (thick wall, fluid level).
Empyema.
Streptococcal pneumatocele (thin wall, postinfective).
Cavitating pneumonia.
Mycetoma (apical cyst with contents).
Cystic congenital adenomatoid malformation (basal cysts of varying size).
Diaphragmatic hernia (cysts of similar size).
Hiatal hernia (posterior).
Morgagni hernia (midline anterior).
Bronchopulmonary sequestration (basal).
Congenital lobar emphysema.
Hydatid disease (in endemic areas).

Kerosene inhalation (pneumatocele).
Histiocytosis and other causes of interstitial disease.

PULMONARY EDEMA, NONCARDIOGENIC[16a]

ICD-9CM # 518.4
ICD-10CM # J81.0 Acute pulmonary edema

CAUSES OF NONCARDIOGENIC PULMONARY EDEMA

Adult respiratory distress syndrome.
Drowning.
Asphyxia.
Upper airway obstruction (usually with cardiomegaly).
High altitude.
Increased intracranial pressure.
Postictal.
Noxious gases:
- Smoke.
- Nitrous dioxide (silo filler's disease).
- Sulfur dioxide.
- Nitrogen mustard.

Drugs:
- Asprin.
- Diazepam, chlordiazepoxide, barbiturates.
- Narcotics (heroin, methadone, morphine).
- Beta-adrenergic drugs (terbutaline).
- Contrast media.
- Colchicine.
- Fluorescein.
- Hydrochlorothiazide.
- Nitrofurantoin.
- Propoxyphene.

Poisons:
- Parathion.

Transfusion reactions.
Renal failure: transplantation.
Bone marrow transplantation.
Fat embolism.
Pancreatitis.

PULMONARY HEMORRHAGE, PEDIATRIC AGE

ICD-9CM # 770.3
ICD-10CM # P26.9 Pulmonary hemorrhage newborn

CAUSES OF PULMONARY HEMORRHAGE (HEMOPTYSIS)

Focal Hemorrhage

Bronchitis and bronchiectasis (especially cystic fibrosis related).
Infection (acute or chronic), pneumonia, abscess.
Tuberculosis.
Trauma.
Pulmonary arteriovenous malformation.
Foreign body (chronic).
Neoplasm including hemangioma.
Pulmonary embolus with or without infarction.
Bronchogenic cysts.

Diffuse Hemorrhage

Idiopathic of infancy.
Congenital heart disease (including pulmonary hypertension, venoocclusive disease, congestive heart failure).
Prematurity.
Cow's milk hyperreactivity (Heiner syndrome).
Goodpasture syndrome.
Collagen vascular diseases (systemic lupus erythematosus, rheumatoid arthritis).
Henoch-Schönlein purpura and vasculitic disorders.
Granulomatous disease (Wegener granulomatosis).
Celiac disease.
Coagulopathy (congenital or acquired).
Malignancy.
Immunodeficiency.
Exogenous toxins.
Hyperammonemia.
Pulmonary hypertension.
Pulmonary alveolar hemosiderosis.
Tuberous sclerosis.
Lymphangiomyomatosis or lymphangioleiomyomatosis.
Physical injury or abuse.

PULMONARY HEMORRHAGIC SYNDROMES, DIFFUSE[16a]

ICD-9CM # 770.3
ICD-10CM # P26.1 Massive pulmonary hemorrhage originating in the perinatal period
R04.8 Pulmonary hemorrhage

CLASSIFICATION OF DIFFUSE PULMONARY HEMORRHAGE SYNDROMES

Non-immunocompromised patients

Antibasement membrane antibody disease/Goodpasture's syndrome.
Diseases of presumed immune etiology, with or without nephropathy:
- Systemic lupus erythematosus.
- Rheumatoid arthritis.
- Systemic sclerosis.
- Systemic necrotizing vasculitis.
- Granulomatosis with polyangiitis (Wegener's granulomatosis).
- Microscopic polyarteritis.

Diseases with no known immune etiology:
- Idiopathic pulmonary hemosiderosis.
- Rapidly progressive glomerulonephritis without immune complexes.
- Fibrillary glomerulonephritis.
- Drug-induced (anticoagulants, trimellitic anhydride, cocaine, lymphangiography).
- Valvular heart disease.
- Disseminated intravascular coagulation.
- Acute lung injury.
- Tumors.

Immunocompromised Patients

Blood dyscrasias.
Infection.
Tumors.

PULMONARY INFILTRATES, IMMUNOCOMPROMISED HOST[39]

ICD-9CM # 518.3
ICD-10CM # J82 Pulmonary eosinophilia, not elsewhere classified
J98.4 Other disorders of lung

CAUSES OF PULMONARY INFILTRATES IN THE IMMUNOCOMPROMISED HOST

Infections:
- Bacteria:
  - Gram-positive cocci, especially *Staphylococcus.*
  - Gram-negative bacilli.
  - *Mycobacterium tuberculosis.*
  - Nontuberculous mycobacteria.
  - *Nocardia.*
- Viruses:
  - Cytomegalovirus.
  - Herpesvirus.
- Fungi:
  - *Aspergillus.*
  - *Cryptococcus.*
  - *Candida.*
  - *Mucor.*
  - *Pneumocystis jiroveci.*
- Protozoa:
  - *Toxoplasma gondii* (rare).

Pulmonary effects of therapy:
- Chemotherapeutic agents.
- Radiation therapy.

Pulmonary hemorrhage.
Congestive heart failure.
Disseminated malignancy.
Nonspecified interstitial pneumonitis (no defined etiology).

PULMONARY LESIONS

ICD-9CM # 518.3 Pulmonary Infiltrate
518.89 Pulmonary Nodule
508.9 Pulmonary Disorder Due to Unspecified External Agent
861.20 Pulmonary Injury NOS
ICD-10CM # J82 Pulmonary eosinophilia, not elsewhere classified
J98.4 Other disorders of lung
J70.9 Respiratory conditions due to unspecified external agent
S27.309A Unspecified injury of lung, unspecified, initial encounter

TB.
Legionella pneumonia.
Mycoplasma pneumonia.

Differential Diagnosis II

Viral pneumonia.
Pneumocystis carinii.
Hypersensitivity pneumonitis.
Aspiration pneumonia.
Fungal disease (aspergillosis, histoplasmosis).
ARDS associated with pneumonia.
Psittacosis.
Sarcoidosis.
Septic emboli.
Metastatic cancer.
Multiple pulmonary emboli.
Rheumatoid nodules.

PULMONARY MASS, SOLITARY, CAUSES[16a]

ICD-9CM # 793.1
ICD-10CM # R91.1 Solitary pulmonary nodule

CAUSES OF A SOLITARY PULMONARY MASS

Bronchial carcinoma.
Bronchial carcinoid.
Granuloma.
Hamartoma.
Metastasis.
Chronic pneumonia or abscess.
Hydatid cyst.
Pulmonary hematoma.
Bronchocele.
Fungus ball.
Massive fibrosis in coal workers.
Bronchogenic cyst.
Sequestration.
Arteriovenous malformation.
Pulmonary infarct.
Round atelectasis.

PULMONARY MASS, SOLITARY, MIMICS[16a]

ICD-9CM # varies with specific diagnosis
ICD-10CM # varies with specific diagnosis

SIMULANTS OF A SOLITARY PULMONARY MASS

Extrathoracic artifacts.
Cutaneous masses.
Bony lesions.
Pleural tumors or plaques.
Encysted pleural fluid.
Pulmonary vessels.

PULMONARY NODULE, SOLITARY

ICD-9CM # 518.89
ICD-10CM # J98.4 Other disorders of lung

Bronchogenic carcinoma.
Granuloma from histoplasmosis.
TB granuloma.
Granuloma from coccidioidomycosis.
Metastatic carcinoma.
Bronchial adenoma.
Bronchogenic cyst.
Hamartoma.
AV malformation.
Other: fibroma, intrapulmonary lymph node, sclerosing hemangioma, bronchopulmonary sequestration.

PULMONARY–RENAL SYNDROMES, CAUSES[12b]

ICD-9CM # varies with specific diagnosis
ICD-10CM # varies with specific diagnosis

Systemic vasculitis	Anti-GBM disease (Goodpasture's) ANCA associated • Granulomatosis with polyangiitis (Wegener's granulomatosis) • Microscopic polyarteritis • Churg-Strauss syndrome • Drugs (penicillamine, hydralazine, propylthiouracil) Immune complex disease • Lupus erythematosus • Henoch-Schönlein purpura • Mixed cryoglobulinemia • Rheumatoid vasculitis
Infection	Severe bacterial pneumonia; postinfectious glomerulonephritis; *Legionella;* hantavirus; opportunistic infection in immunocompromised patients; infective endocarditis
Pulmonary edema and AKI	Volume overload; severe left ventricular failure
Multiorgan failure	Acute respiratory distress syndrome and AKI
Other	Paraquat poisoning; renal vein or IVC thrombosis with pulmonary emboli

AKI, Acute kidney injury; *ANCA,* anti-neutrophil cytoplasmic antibody; *GBM,* glomerular basement membrane; *IVC,* inferior vena cava.

PULSELESS ELECTRICAL ACTIVITY

ICD-9CM # 427.5
ICD-10CM # I46.9 Cardiac arrest, cause unspecified

Hypovolemia.
Hypoxia.
Hyperkalemia.
Acidosis.
Cardiac tamponade.
Tension pneumothorax.
Pulmonary embolus.
Drug overdose.
Hypothermia.

PUPILLARY DILATATION, POOR RESPONSE TO DARKNESS

ICD-9CM # varies with specific disorder
ICD-10CM # H21.569 Pupillary abnormality, unspecified eye

Drugs (narcotics, general anesthetics, cholinergics).
Acute trauma (spasm from prostaglandin release).
Inflammation, infection (interruption of inhibitory fibers to the Edinger-Westphal nucleus).
Old age (loss of inhibition at midbrain from reticular activating formation).
Horner's syndrome (sympathetic neuron interruption).
Adie's syndrome tonic pupil.
Lymphoma.
Congenital miosis.

PURPURA

ICD-9CM # 287.2 Purpura NOS
287.0 Autoimmune
287.0 Henoch-Schönlein
287.3 Idiopathic Thrombocytopenic
446.6 Thrombocytopenic
ICD-10CM # D69.2 Other nonthrombocytopenic purpura
D69.0 Allergic purpura
D69.49 Other primary thrombocytopenia
M31.1 Thrombotic microangiopathy

THROMBOTIC

Trauma.
Septic emboli, atheromatous emboli.
DIC.
Thrombocytopenia.
Meningococcemia.
Rocky Mountain spotted fever.
Hemolytic-uremic syndrome.
Viral infection: echo, coxsackie.
Scurvy.
Other: left atrial myxoma, cryoglobulinemia, vasculitis, hyperglobulinemic purpura.

PURPURA, NONPALPABLE[20]

ICD-9CM # 287.2
ICD-10CM # D69.2 Other nonthrombocytopenic purpura

INCREASED TRANSMURAL PRESSURE GRADIENT

Acute (Valsalva, coughing, vomiting, high altitude, weight lifting).
Chronic—Venous stasis.

DECREASED MECHANICAL INTEGRITY OF MICROCIRCULATION AND SUPPORTING TISSUES

Age related (infancy and actinic purpura).
Glucocorticoid excess—Cushing syndrome and glucocorticoid therapy.
Vitamin C deficiency (scurvy).
Abnormal connective tissue—Ehlers-Danlos syndrome.
Amyloid infiltration of blood vessels.
Colloid milium.
Hormonal—Female easy bruising syndrome (purpura simplex).
Lorenzo's oil.
MELAS syndrome.

TRAUMA TO BLOOD VESSELS

Physical:
- Injuries.
- Child abuse.
- Factitial purpura.

Ultraviolet purpura:
- Purpuric sunburn.
- Solar purpura.

Infectious:
- Bacterial.
- Rickettsial.
- Fungal.
- Viral.
- Parasitic.

Embolic:
- Infectious organisms.
- Atheroemboli (cholesterol crystal emboli).
- Fat emboli.

Allergic and/or inflammatory:
- Serum sickness.
- Pigmented purpuric eruptions.
- Pyoderma gangrenosum.
- Contact dermatitis.
- Familial Mediterranean fever.

Neoplastic.
Metabolic:
- Erythropoietic porphyria.
- Calciphylaxis.

Immunoglobulin related (hyperglobulinemic purpura of Waldenström and light-chain vasculitis).
Drug related.
Thrombotic:
- Disseminated intravascular coagulation.
- Warfarin (Coumadin)-induced skin necrosis.
- Protein C or protein S deficiency, factor V Leiden, prothrombin G20201A.
- Purpura fulminans.
- Paroxysmal nocturnal hemoglobinuria.
- Antiphospholipid antibody syndrome.
- Hemangioma with thrombocytopenia and consumptive coagulopathy (Kasabach-Merritt syndrome).

UNKNOWN CAUSE—PSYCHOGENIC PURPURA

PURPURA, NONPURPURIC DISORDERS SIMULATING PURPURA[1A]

ICD-9CM # varies with specific diagnosis
ICD-10CM # varies with specific diagnosis

Disorders with telangiectasias:
- Cherry angiomas.
- Hereditary hemorrhagic telangiectasia.
- Chronic actinic telangiectasia.
- Scleroderma.
- CREST syndrome.
- Ataxia-telangiectasia.
- Chronic liver disease.
- Pregnancy-related telangiectasia.

Kaposi sarcoma and other vascular sarcomas.
Fabry disease.
Neonatal extramedullary hematopoiesis.
Angioma serpiginosum.

PURPURA, PALPABLE[20]

ICD-9CM # 287.2
ICD-10CM # D69.2 Other nonthrombocytopenic purpura

Cutaneous vasculitis:
- Systemic vasculitides.
- Paraneoplastic vasculitis.
- Henoch-Schönlein purpura.
- Acute hemorrhagic edema of infancy.
- Livedoid vasculitis.
- Idiopathic.
- Urticarial.

Cryoglobulinemia.
Cryofibrinogenemia.
Primary cutaneous diseases.

QT INTERVAL PROLONGATION[22]

ICD-9CM # 794.31
ICD-10CM # R94.31 Abnormal electrocardiogram [ECG] [EKG]

Drugs:
- Class I antiarrhythmics (e.g., disopyramide, procainamide, quinidine).
- Class III antiarrhythmics.
- Tricyclic antidepressants.
- Phenothiazines.
- Astemizole.
- Terfenadine.
- Adenosine.
- Antibiotics (e.g., erythromycin and other macrolides).
- Antifungal agents.
- Pentamidine, chloroquine.

Ischemic heart disease.
Cerebrovascular disease.
Rheumatic fever.
Myocarditis.
Mitral valve prolapse.
Electrolyte abnormalities.
Hypocalcemia.
Hypothyroidism.
Liquid protein diets.
Organophosphate insecticides.
Congenital prolonged QT syndrome.

RECTAL MASS, PALPABLE[38]

ICD-9CM # varies with specific diagnosis
ICD-10CM # R22.9 Localized swelling, mass and lump, unspecified

Rectal carcinoma.
Rectal polyp.
Hypertrophied anal papilla.
Diverticular phlegmon (prolapsing into the pouch of Douglas).
Sigmoid colon carcinoma (prolapsing into the pouch of Douglas).
Metastatic deposits at the pelvic reflection (Blumer's shelf).
Primary pelvic malignancy (uterine, ovarian, prostatic, or cervical).
Mesorectal lymph nodes.
Endometriosis.
Solitary rectal ulcer syndrome.
Foreign body.
Feces.
Presacral cyst.
Amebic granuloma.
Vaginal tampon and even the pubic bone may be mistaken for a rectal mass.

RECTAL PAIN

ICD-9CM # 569.42
ICD-10CM # K62.89 Other specified diseases of anus and rectum

Anal fissure.
Thrombosed hemorrhoid.
Anorectal abscess.
Foreign bodies.
Fecal impaction.
Endometriosis.
Neoplasms (primary or metastatic).
Pelvic inflammatory disease.
Inflammation of sacral nerves.
Compression of sacral nerves.
Prostatitis.
Other: proctalgia fugax, uterine abnormalities, myopathies, coccygodynia.

RED BLOOD CELL APLASIA, ACQUIRED, ETIOLOGY

ICD-9CM # 284.0
ICD-10CM # D61.01 Constitutional (pure) red blood cell aplasia

Idiopathic (>50% of cases).
Medications (most frequent with phenytoin).
Non-Hodgkin's lymphoma.
Viral infections (parvovirus B19, EB virus, mumps, hepatitis).
Myelodysplastic syndromes.
Thymoma.
Autoimmune diseases.
Allogenic bone marrow transplant from ABO incompatible donor.
Pregnancy.

RED EYE

ICD-9CM # 379.93
ICD-10CM # H57.8 Other specified disorders of eye and adnexa

Infectious conjunctivitis (bacterial, viral).
Allergic conjunctivitis.
Acute glaucoma.
Keratitis (bacterial, viral).
Iritis.
Trauma.

RED EYE, ACUTE[1b]

ICD-9CM # 379.93
ICD-10CM # H57.8

Obvious open globe.
Corneal abrasion.
Corneal ulcer.
Subconjunctival hemorrhage.
Hyphema.
Occult open globe.
Herpes simplex virus glaucoma.
Iritis, traumatic iritis.
Scleritis.
Conjunctivitis.
Blepharitis.
Ultraviolet keratitis.
Episcleritis.
Conjunctival foreign body.
Dry eye.
Contact lens overwear syndrome.

RED HOT JOINT

ICD-9CM # varies with specific disorder
ICD-10CM # varies with specific diagnosis

Trauma.
Gout.
Infection (septic joint).
Pseudogout (calcium pyrophosphate dehydrate crystal deposition).
Psoriatic arthropathy.
Reactive arthritis.
Palindromic rheumatism.

RED URINE

ICD-9CM # 788.69
ICD-10CM # R39.19 Other difficulties with micturition

Hematuria.
Porphyrins.
Hemoglobinuria.
Myoglobinuria.
Medications (phenazopyridine, aminosalicylic acid, deferoxamine, phenazopyridine, phenolphthalein, NSAIDs, rifampin, phenytoin, methyldopa, doxorubicin, phenacetin).
Foods (beets, berries, maize).
Urate crystalluria.

RENAL ALLOGRAFT DYSFUNCTION[14a]

ICD-9CM # 593.9
ICD-10CM # T86.1 Complications of renal allograft

IMMEDIATE/DELAYED GRAFT FUNCTION (1-3 DAYS)

Acute tubular necrosis.
Hyperacute humoral rejection.
Urinary leak or obstruction.
Renal artery or vein thrombosis.
Recurrence of disease (e.g., focal segmental glomerulosclerosis).

EARLY POSTTRANSPLANTATION PERIOD (FIRST MONTH)

Acute cellular rejection.
Acute humoral rejection.
Calcineurin inhibitor toxicity.
Urinary tract obstruction.
Volume depletion.
Recurrence of disease.

Late Acute dysfunction

Acute rejection.
Cyclosporine or tacrolimus toxicity.
Recurrence of primary disease.
Tubulointerstitial nephritis, drug-induced.
Renal artery stenosis.
Infection (bacterial urinary tract infection [UTI], cytomegalovirus, BK virus).
Hemodynamic (volume; use of angiotensin-converting enzyme inhibitor, angiotensin II receptor blocker).

Chronic Dysfunction

Chronic rejection.
Cyclosporine or tacrolimus toxicity.
Recurrent renal disease.
De novo renal disease.
Urinary tract obstruction.
Bacterial UTI.
Hypertensive nephrosclerosis.

RENAL ARTERY OCCLUSION, CAUSES

ICD-9CM # 593.81
ICD-10CM # N28.0 Ischemia and infarction of kidney

Atrial fibrillation.
Angiography or stent placement.
Abdominal aortic surgery.
Trauma.
Renal artery aneurysm/dissection.
Vasculitis.
Thrombosis in patient with fibromuscular dysplasia.
Atherosclerosis.
Septic embolism.
Mural thrombus thromboembolism.
Atrial myxoma thromboembolism.
Mitral stenosis thromboembolism.
Prosthetic valve thromboembolism.
Renal cell carcinoma.

RENAL COLIC[1b]

ICD-9CM # 788.0
ICD-10CM # N23

Vascular:
- Abdominal aortic aneurysm.
- Aortic dissection.
- Renal artery dissection.
- Renal artery stenosis.
- Renal vein thrombosis.
- Renal infarct.
- Mesenteric ischemia.
- Retroperitoneal hemorrhage.

Gastrointestinal:
- Incarcerated hernia.
- Appendicitis.
- Cholecystitis.
- Biliary colic.
- Pancreatitis.
- Bowel obstruction.
- Diverticulitis.

Gynecologic:
- Ectopic pregnancy.
- Ovarian torsion.
- Tuboovarian abscess.
- Pelvic inflammatory disease.
- Endometriosis.

Genitourinary:
- Testicular torsion.
- Pyelonephritis.
- Perinephric abscess.
- Urinary tract tumor.
- Renal papillary necrosis.
- Upper urinary tract hemorrhage.

Musculoskeletal:
- Lumbar strain.
- Radiculopathy.
- Disk herniation.
- Vertebral compression fracture.

Dermatologic:
- Herpes zoster.

Miscellaneous:
- Factitious.

RENAL CYSTIC DISORDERS

ICD-9CM # varies with specific disorder
ICD-10CM # Q61.01 Congenital single renal cyst

Simple cysts.
Acquired cystic kidney disease.
Autosomal dominant polycystic kidney disease.
Autosomal recessive polycystic kidney disease.
Medullary cystic disease.
Medullary sponge kidney.

RENAL FAILURE, ACUTE, PIGMENT-INDUCED[2]

ICD-9CM # 586
ICD-10CM # N19 Unspecified kidney failure

CAUSES OF PIGMENT-INDUCED ACUTE RENAL FAILURE

Rhabdomyolysis and myoglobinuria.
Vigorous exercise.

Arterial embolization.
Status epilepticus.
Status asthmaticus.
Coma-induced and pressure-induced myonecrosis.
Heat stress.
Diabetic ketoacidosis.
Myopathy.
Alcoholism.
Hypokalemia.
Hypophosphatemia.
Hemoglobinuria.
Transfusion reactions.
Snake envenomation.
Malaria.
Mechanical destruction of RBCs by prosthetic valves.
G6PD deficiency.

G6PD, Glucose-6-phosphate dehydrogenase; *RBCs,* red blood cells.

RENAL FAILURE, CHRONIC[14a]

ICD-9CM # 585.9

CAUSES OF CHRONIC RENAL FAILURE

Diabetic glomerulosclerosis (systemic disease involving the kidney).
Hypertensive nephrosclerosis.
Glomerular disease:
- Glomerulonephritis.
- Amyloidosis, light chain disease (systemic disease involving the kidney).
- Systemic lupus erythematosus, Wegener granulomatosis (systemic disease involving the kidney).

Tubulointerstitial disease:
- Reflux nephropathy (chronic pyelonephritis).
- Analgesic nephropathy.
- Obstructive nephropathy (stones, benign prostatic hypertrophy).
- Myeloma kidney (systemic disease involving the kidney).

Vascular disease:
- Scleroderma (systemic disease involving the kidney).
- Vasculitis (systemic disease involving the kidney).
- Renovascular renal failure (ischemic nephropathy).
- Atheroembolic renal disease (systemic disease involving the kidney).

Cystic disease:
- Autosomal dominant polycystic kidney disease.
- Medullary cystic kidney disease.

RENAL FAILURE, INTRINSIC OR PARENCHYMAL CAUSES[36]

ICD-9CM #	584	Acute, use 4th digit
	5	With Acute Tubular Necrosis
	6	With Cortical Necrosis
	7	With Medullary Necrosis
	8	With Other Unspecified Pathologic Condition in Kidney
	9	Renal Failure Unspecified
	585	Renal Failure, Chronic
ICD-10CM #	N17.0	Acute kidney failure with tubular necrosis
	N17.1	Acute kidney failure with acute cortical necrosis
	N17.2	Acute kidney failure with medullary necrosis
	N17.8	Other acute kidney failure
	N17.9	Acute kidney failure, unspecified
	N18.9	Chronic kidney disease, unspecified

ABNORMALITIES OF THE VASCULATURE

Renal arteries: atherosclerosis, thromboembolism, arteritis.
Renal veins: thrombosis.
Microvasculature: vasculitis, thrombotic microangiopathy.

ABNORMALITIES OF GLOMERULI (ACUTE GLOMERULONEPHRITIS)

Antiglomerular membrane disease (Goodpasture's syndrome).
Immune complex glomerulonephritis: SLE, postinfectious, idiopathic, membranoproliferative.

ABNORMALITIES OF INTERSTITIUM (ACUTE INTERSTITIAL NEPHRITIS)

Drugs (e.g., antibiotics, NSAIDs, diuretics, anticonvulsants, allopurinol).
Infectious pyelonephritis.
Infiltrative: lymphoma, leukemia, sarcoidosis.

ABNORMALITIES OF TUBULES

Physical obstruction (uric acid, oxalate, light chains).
Acute tubular necrosis:
- Ischemic.
- Toxic (antibiotics, chemotherapy, immunosuppressives, radiocontrast dyes, heavy metals, myoglobin, hemolysed RBCs).

RENAL FAILURE, POSTRENAL CAUSES[36]

ICD-9CM #	584	Acute, use 4th digit
	5	With Acute Tubular Necrosis
	6	With Cortical Necrosis
	7	With Medullary Necrosis
	8	With Other Unspecified Pathologic Condition in Kidney
	9	Renal Failure Unspecified
	585	Renal Failure, Chronic
ICD-10CM #	N17.0	Acute kidney failure with tubular necrosis
	N17.1	Acute kidney failure with acute cortical necrosis
	N17.2	Acute kidney failure with medullary necrosis
	N17.8	Other acute kidney failure
	N17.9	Acute kidney failure, unspecified
	N18.9	Chronic kidney disease, unspecified

URETER AND RENAL PELVIS

Intrinsic obstruction:
- Blood clots.
- Stones.
- Sloughed papillae: diabetes, sickle cell disease, analgesic nephropathy.
- Inflammatory: fungus ball.

Extrinsic obstruction:
- Malignancy.
- Retroperitoneal fibrosis.
- Iatrogenic: inadvertent ligation of ureters.

BLADDER

Prostatic hypertrophy or malignancy.
Neuropathic bladder.
Blood clots.
Bladder cancer.
Stones.

URETHRAL

Strictures.
Congenital valves.

RENAL FAILURE, PRERENAL CAUSES[36]

ICD-9CM #	584	Acute, use 4th digit
	5	With Acute Tubular Necrosis
	6	With Cortical Necrosis
	7	With Medullary Necrosis
	8	With Other Unspecified Pathologic Condition in Kidney
	9	Renal Failure Unspecified
	585	Renal Failure, Chronic
ICD-10CM #	N17.0	Acute kidney failure with tubular necrosis
	N17.1	Acute kidney failure with acute cortical necrosis
	N17.2	Acute kidney failure with medullary necrosis
	N17.8	Other acute kidney failure
	N17.9	Acute kidney failure, unspecified
	N18.9	Chronic kidney disease, unspecified

DECREASED CARDIAC OUTPUT

CHF.
Arrhythmias.
Pericardial constriction or tamponade.
Pulmonary embolism.

HYPOVOLEMIA

GI tract loss (vomiting, diarrhea, nasogastric suction).
Blood losses (trauma, GI tract surgery).
Renal losses (diuretics, mineralocorticoid deficiency, postobstructive diuresis).
Skin losses (burns).

VOLUME REDISTRIBUTION (DECREASE IN EFFECTIVE BLOOD VOLUME)

Hypoalbuminemic states (cirrhosis, nephrosis).
Sequestration of fluid in "third" space (ischemic bowel, peritonitis, pancreatitis).
Peripheral vasodilation (sepsis, vasodilators, anaphylaxis).

ALTERED RENAL VASCULAR RESISTANCE

Increase in afferent vascular resistance (NSAIDs, liver disease, sepsis, hypercalcemia, cyclosporine).
Decrease in efferent arteriolar tone (ACE inhibitors).

RENAL INFARCTION[12b]

ICD-9CM # 593.81 Renal Infarction
ICD-10CM # N28.0 Ischemia and infarction of kidney

CAUSES OF RENAL INFARCTION

Thrombosis: Spontaneous
Atherosclerotic disease of aorta and renal artery.
Fibromuscular dysplasia of renal artery.
Aneurysms of aorta or renal artery.
Dissection of aorta or renal artery.
- Marfan's syndrome.
- Ehlers-Danlos syndrome.

Vasculitis involving renal artery.
- Polyarteritis nodosa.
- Takayasu's arteritis.
- Kawasaki disease.
- Thromboangiitis obliterans.
- Other necrotizing vasculitides.

Inflammatory disease of the aorta or renal artery.
- Syphilis.
- Tuberculosis.
- Mycoses.

Hypercoagulable states.
- Nephrotic syndrome.
- Antiphospholipid syndrome.
- Antithrombin III deficiency.
- Homocystinuria.

Thrombotic microangiopathies.
- Hemolytic-uremic syndrome.
- Thrombotic thrombocytopenic purpura.
- Antiphospholipid syndrome.
- Malignant hypertension.
- Scleroderma.
- Sickle cell nephropathy.
- Polycythemia vera.
- Postpartum hemolytic-uremic syndrome.
- Hyperacute vascular allograft rejection.

Thrombosis: Induced
Traumatic.
Following endovascular intervention.
Post renal transplantation.

Embolism
Cardiac source.
- Atrial fibrillation or other arrhythmias.
- Native and prosthetic valvular heart disease.
- Infective endocarditis.
- Marantic endocarditis.

Myocardial infarction with mural thrombi.
- Left atrial myxoma or other tumor.

Noncardiac sources.
- Atheromatous embolic disease.
- Paradoxical emboli.
- Fat emboli.
- Tumor emboli.

Therapeutic renal embolization.
Segmental renal infarction of childhood.
Cisplatinum and gemcitabine.
Sickle cell disease or sickle cell trait.

RENAL PARENCHYMAL DISEASE, CHRONIC[16a]

ICD-9CM # 593.9
ICD-10CM # N28.9 Disorder of kidney and ureter, unspecified

DIFFERENTIAL DIAGNOSIS OF CHRONIC RENAL PARENCHYMAL DISEASE

No Papillary/Caliceal Abnormality

Diffuse parenchymal loss

Bilateral:
- Chronic glomerulonephritis.
- Diffuse small-vessel disease.
- Hereditary nephropathies.

Unilateral:
- Renal artery stenosis.
- Postirradiation.
- Rare:
  - Hypoplastic kidney.
  - Postobstructive atrophy.

FOCAL PARENCHYMAL LOSS

Infarct.
Previous trauma.

Papillary/Caliceal Abnormality

Diffuse parenchymal loss
Obstructive nephropathy.
Generalized reflux nephropathy.

No Parenchymal Loss
Papillary necrosis.
TB.
Medullary sponge kidney.
Megacalices.
Pelvicaliceal cyst.

Focal Parenchymal Loss
Focal reflux nephropathy (chronic atrophic pyelonephritis).
TB.
Calculus disease.

RENAL VEIN THROMBOSIS, CAUSES

ICD-9CM # 453.3
ICD-10CM # I82.3 Embolism and thrombosis of renal vein

Nephrotic syndrome.
Renal cell carcinoma.
Aortic aneurysm causing compression.
Lymphadenopathy.
Retroperitoneal fibrosis.
Estrogen therapy.
Pregnancy.
Renal cell carcinoma with vein invasion.
Severe dehydration.

RESPIRATORY FAILURE, HYPOVENTILATORY[28]

ICD-9CM # 518.81 Respiratory Failure
ICD-10CM # J96.00 Acute respiratory failure, unspecified whether with hypoxia or hypercapnia
J96.90 Respiratory failure, unspecified, unspecified whether with hypoxia or hypercapnia

ABNORMAL RESPIRATORY CAPACITY (NORMAL RESPIRATORY WORKLOADS)

Acute depression of central nervous system:
- Various causes.

Chronic central hypoventilation syndromes:
- Obesity-hypoventilation syndrome.
- Sleep apnea syndrome.
- Hypothyroidism.
- Shy-Drager syndrome (multisystem atrophy syndrome).

Acute toxic paralysis syndromes:
- Botulism.
- Tetanus.
- Toxic ingestion or bites.
- Organophosphate poisoning.

Neuromuscular disorders (acute and chronic):
- Myasthenia gravis.
- Guillain-Barré syndrome.
- Drugs.
- Amyotrophic lateral sclerosis.
- Muscular dystrophies.
- Polymyositis.
- Spinal cord injury.
- Traumatic phrenic nerve paralysis.

ABNORMAL PULMONARY WORKLOADS

Chronic obstructive pulmonary disease:
- Chronic bronchitis.
- Asthmatic bronchitis.
- Emphysema.

Asthma and acute bronchial hyperreactivity syndromes.
Upper airway obstruction.
Interstitial lung diseases.

ABNORMAL EXTRAPULMONARY WORKLOADS

Chronic thoracic cage disorders:
- Severe kyphoscoliosis.
- After thoracoplasty.
- After thoracic cage injury.

Acute thoracic cage trauma and burns.
Pneumothorax.
Pleural fibrosis and effusions.
Abdominal processes.

RETINOPATHY, HYPERTENSIVE

ICD-9CM # 362.11
ICD-10CM # H35.039 Hypertensive retinopathy, unspecified eye

Retinal venous obstruction.
Diabetic retinopathy.
Ocular ischemic syndrome.
Hyperviscosity.
Tortuosity of retinal artery.

RHINITIS

ICD-9CM # 472.0
ICD-10CM # J31.0 Chronic rhinitis

Allergic rhinitis.
Infectious rhinitis.
Vasomotor rhinitis.
Exercise-induced rhinitis.
Emotional rhinitis.
Rhinitis medicamentosa.
Hormone-mediated rhinitis (menses, pregnancy, oral contraceptives, hypothyroidism).
GERD.
Chemical- or irritant-induced rhinitis.
Rhinitis mimics:
- Deviated septum.
- Enlarged adenoids.
- Nasal polyps/tumors.
- Foreign bodies.
- CSF rhinorrhea.
- Sarcoidosis.
- Midline granuloma.
- Granulomatosis with polyangiitis (Wegener's granulomatosis).
- SLE.
- Sjögren's syndrome.

RIB DEFECTS ON X-RAY[16a]

ICD-9CM # varies with specific diagnosis
ICD-10CM # varies with specific diagnosis

CAUSES OF SUPERIOR MARGINAL RIB DEFECTS

Normal
Isolated defects.
Projectional artifacts (due to lordosis).

Neurologic
Paralytic poliomyelitis.
Quadriparesis.

Collagen Vascular Disease
Rheumatoid arthritis.
SLE.
Systemic sclerosis.

Local Pressure
Chest drainage tube.
Osteochondroma.
Neural tumor.
Coarctation of aorta.

Hyperparathyroidism Miscellaneous
Osteogenesis imperfecta.
Marfan's syndrome.

RIB NOTCHING ON X-RAY[16a]

ICD-9CM # varies with specific diagnosis
ICD-10CM # varies with specific diagnosis

CAUSES OF INFERIOR RIB NOTCHING

ARTERIAL

Aortic obstruction

Aortic coarctation.
Aortic thrombosis.
Aortitis.

Subclavian artery obstruction

Blalock-Taussig operation.
Arteritis.
Atherosclerotic occlusion.

Pulmonary oligemia

Pulmonary atresia.
Tetralogy of Fallot.
Multiple pulmonary arterial stenoses.

VENOUS

Chronic superior vena caval obstruction

Arteriovenous

Arteriovenous malformation
Pulmonary.
Chest wall.

Neural

Neurofibromas

RIGHT AXIS DEVIATION[22]

ICD-9CM # varies with specific diagnosis
ICD-10CM # varies with specific diagnosis

Normal variation.
Right ventricular hypertrophy.
Left posterior fascicular block.
Lateral myocardial infarction.
Pulmonary embolism.
Dextrocardia.
Mechanical shifts or emphysema causing a vertical heart.

SALIVARY GLAND ENLARGEMENT

ICD-9CM # 527.1
ICD-10CM # K11.1 Hypertrophy of salivary gland

Neoplasm.
Sialolithiasis.
Infection (mumps, bacterial infection, HIV, TB).
Sarcoidosis.
Idiopathic.
Acromegaly.
Anorexia/bulimia.
Chronic pancreatitis.
Medications (e.g., phenylbutazone).
Cirrhosis.
DM.

SALIVARY GLAND SECRETION, DECREASED

ICD-9CM # 527.7
ICD-10CM # K11.7 Disturbances of salivary secretion
R68.2 Dry mouth, unspecified

Medications (antihistamines, antidepressants, neuroleptics, antihypertensives).
Dehydration.
Anxiety.
Sjögren's syndrome.
Sarcoidosis.
Mumps.
Amyloidosis.
CNS disorders.
Head and neck radiation.

SCLERODERMA-LIKE SYNDROMES[1a]

ICD-9CM # varies with specific diagnosis
ICD-10CM # varies with specific diagnosis

OTHER DISEASES

Morphea.
Eosinophilic fasciitis.
Scleredema (of Buschke).
Scleromyxedema.
Graft-versus-host disease.
Nephrogenic-fibrosing dermopathy.

ENVIRONMENTAL AGENTS AND DRUGS

Bleomycin.
L-Tryptophan.
Organic solvents.
Pentazocine.
Toxic oil syndrome.
Vinyl chloride disease.
Gadolinium.

SCROTAL MASSES, BOYS AND ADOLESCENTS[22a]

ICD-9CM # varies with specific diagnosis
ICD-10CM # R22.9 Localized swelling, mass and lump, unspecified

PAINFUL

Testicular torsion.
Torsion of appendix testis.
Epididymitis.
Trauma: ruptured testis, hematocele.
Inguinal hernia (incarcerated).
Mumps orchitis.

PAINLESS

Hydrocele.
Inguinal hernia.*

Varicocele.*
Spermatocele.*
Testicular tumor.*
Henoch-Schönlein purpura.*
Idiopathic scrotal edema.

*May be associated with discomfort.

SCROTAL PAIN[28]

ICD-9CM #	878.2	Scrotal Injury, Traumatic
	608.9	Scrotal Disorder NOS
	608.4	Scrotal Cellulitis
	608.83	Scrotal Hemorrhage, Nontraumatic
	608.4	Scrotal Nodule, Inflammatory
ICD-10CM #	S31.30XA	Unspecified open wound of scrotum and testes, initial encounter
	N50.9	Disorder of male genital organs, unspecified
	R10.2	Pelvic and perineal pain
	N49.9	Inflammatory disorder of unspecified male genital organ
	N50.1	Vascular disorders of male genital organs
	N49.9	Inflammatory disorder of unspecified male genital organ

Torsion:
- Appendages.
- Spermatic cord.

Infection:
- Orchitis.
- Abscess.
- Epididymitis.

Neoplasia:
- Benign.
- Malignant.

Incarcerated hernia.
Trauma.
Hydrocele.
Spermatocele.
Varicocele.

SCROTAL SWELLING

ICD-9CM #	608.86	
ICD-10CM #	N50.8	Other specified disorders of male genital organs

Hydrocele.
Varicocele.
Neoplasm.
Acute epididymitis.
Orchitis.
Trauma.
Hernia.
Torsion of spermatic cord.
Torsion of epididymis.
Torsion of testis.
Insect bite.
Folliculitis.
Sebaceous cyst.
Thrombosis of spermatic vein.
Other: lymphedema, dermatitis, fat necrosis, Henoch-Schönlein purpura, idiopathic scrotal edema.

SEIZURE

ICD-9CM #	780.39	
ICD-10CM #	R56.9	Unspecified convulsions

Syncope.
Alcohol abuse/withdrawal.
TIA.
Hemiparetic migraine.
Psychiatric disorders.
Carotid sinus hypersensitivity.
Hyperventilation, prolonged breath holding.
Hypoglycemia.
Narcolepsy.
Movement disorders (tics, hemiballismus).
Hyponatremia.
Brain tumor (primary or metastatic).
Tetanus.
Strychnine, phencyclidine poisoning.

SEIZURE, PEDIATRIC[2]

ICD-9CM #	780.39	Infantile Seizures
	779.0	Seizures, Newborn
ICD-10CM #	R56.9	Unspecified convulsions
	P90	Convulsions of newborn

FIRST MONTH OF LIFE

First Day
Hypoxia.
Drugs.
Trauma.
Infection.
Hyperglycemia.
Hypoglycemia.
Pyridoxine deficiency.

Day 2-3
Infection.
Drug withdrawal.
Hypoglycemia.
Hypocalcemia.
Developmental malformation.
Intracranial hemorrhage.
Inborn error of metabolism.
Hyponatremia or hypernatremia.

Day >4
Infection.
Hypocalcemia.
Hyperphosphatemia.
Hyponatremia.
Developmental malformation.
Drug withdrawal.
Inborn error of metabolism.

1 TO 6 MO

As above.

6 MO TO 3 YR

Febrile seizures.
Birth injury.
Infection.
Toxin.
Trauma.
Metabolic disorder.
Cerebral degenerative disease.

>3 YR

Idiopathic.
Infection.
Trauma.
Cerebral degenerative disease.

SEIZURE MIMICS[1a]

ICD-9CM #	varies with specific diagnosis
ICD-10CM #	varies with specific diagnosis

NON-EPILEPTIC EPISODIC DISORDERS THAT MAY RESEMBLE SEIZURES

Movement disorders: myoclonus, paroxysmal choreoathetosis, episodic ataxias, hyperexplexia (startle disease).
Migraine: confusional, vertebrobasilar, visual auras.
Syncope.
Behavioral and psychiatric: psychogenic nonepileptic attacks (pseudoseizures), hyperventilation syndrome, panic or anxiety disorder, dissociative states.
Cataplexy (usually associated with narcolepsy).
Transient ischemic attack.
Alcoholic blackouts.
Hypoglycemia.

SEXUAL DYSFUNCTION, FEMALE[1a]

ICD-9CM #	302.7	
ICD-10CM #	R37	Sexual dysfunction, unspecified

FACTORS THAT MAY INFLUENCE SEXUAL FUNCTIONING IN WOMEN

Biological
Medications (e.g., antidepressants, antihypertensives).
Vaginal atrophy, pain with intercourse.
Low testosterone levels (e.g., bilateral oophorectomy).
Illness (e.g., diabetes, hypothyroidism, cerebrovascular accident).
Sleep disturbances, fatigue.
Disability or pain from illness (e.g., arthritis).
Incontinence.

Psychological
Depression.
Body image.

Interpersonal
Marital issues.
Poor communication.
Partner's sexual problems (e.g., erectile dysfunction).
Partner's health problems (e.g., myocardial infarction).

Sociocultural
Ageism ("too old" to want sex).
Multiple other obligations and commitments.
Lack of partner.

SEXUALLY TRANSMITTED DISEASES, ANORECTAL REGION[26]

ICD-9CM #	569.49	Infection and Region
ICD-10CM #	K62.89	Other specified diseases of anus and rectum

ULCERATIVE

Lymphogranuloma venereum.
Herpes simplex virus.
Early (primary) syphilis.
Chancroid *(Haemophilus ducreyi).*
Cytomegalovirus.
Idiopathic (usually HIV positive).

NONULCERATIVE

Condyloma acuminatum.
Gonorrhea.
Chlamydia *(Chlamydia trachomatis).*
Syphilis.

SEXUAL PRECOCITY[41]

ICD-9CM #	259.1	
ICD-10CM #	E30.1	Precocious puberty
	E30.8	Other disorders of puberty

TRUE PRECOCIOUS PUBERTY

Premature reactivation of LHRH pulse generator.

INCOMPLETE SEXUAL PRECOCITY

(Pituitary gonadotropin independent).
Males
Chorionic gonadotropin-secreting tumor.
Leydig cell tumor.
Familial testotoxicosis.
Virilizing congenital adrenal hyperplasia.
Virilizing adrenal tumor.
Premature adrenarche.
Females
Granulosa cell tumor (follicular cysts may be manifested similarly).
Follicular cyst.
Feminizing adrenal tumor.
Premature thelarche.
Premature adrenarche.
Late-onset virilizing congenital adrenal hyperplasia.
In Both Sexes
McCune-Albright syndrome.
Primary hypothyroidism.

SHOULDER PAIN

ICD-9CM #	952.2	Shoulder Injury
	718.81	Shoulder Instability
	726.19	Shoulder Ligament or Muscle Instability
	840.9	Shoulder Strain, Site Unspecified
ICD-10CM #	M24.819	Other specific joint derangements of unspecified shoulder, not elsewhere classified
	M75.80	Other shoulder lesions, unspecified shoulder
	S43.409A	Unspecified sprain of unspecified shoulder joint, initial encounter
	S46.919A	Strain of unspecified muscle, fascia and tendon at shoulder and upper arm level, unspecified arm, initial encounter
	S43.499A	Other sprain of unspecified shoulder joint, initial encounter
	S46.019A	Strain of muscle(s) and tendon(s) of the rotator cuff of unspecified shoulder, initial encounter
	S46.819A	Strain of other muscles, fascia and tendons at shoulder and upper arm level, unspecified arm, initial encounter

WITH LOCAL FINDINGS IN SHOULDER

Trauma: contusion, fracture, muscle strain, trauma to spinal cord.
Arthrosis, arthritis, RA, ankylosing spondylitis.
Bursitis, synovitis, tendinitis, tenosynovitis.
Aseptic (avascular) necrosis.
Local infection: septic arthritis, osteomyelitis, abscess, herpes zoster, TB.

WITHOUT LOCAL FINDINGS IN SHOULDER

Cardiovascular disorders: ischemic heart disease, pericarditis, aortic aneurysm.
Subdiaphragmatic abscess, liver abscess.
Cholelithiasis, cholecystitis.
Pulmonary lesions: apical bronchial carcinoma, pleurisy, pneumothorax, pneumonia.
GI lesions: PUD, gastric neoplasm, peptic esophagitis.
Pancreatic lesions: carcinoma, calculi, pancreatitis.
CNS abnormalities: neoplasm, vascular abnormalities.
Multiple sclerosis.
Syringomyelia.
Polymyositis/dermatomyositis.
Psychogenic.
Polymyalgia rheumatica.
Ectopic pregnancy.

SHOULDER PAIN BY LOCATION

ICD-9CM #	952.2	Shoulder Injury
	726.19	Shoulder Ligament or Muscle Instability
	840.8	Shoulder Separation
ICD-10CM #	M75.80	Other shoulder lesions, unspecified shoulder

TOP OF SHOULDER (C4)

Cervical source.
Acromioclavicular.
Sternoclavicular.
Diaphragmatic.

SUPEROLATERAL (C5)

Rotator cuff tendinitis.
Impingement.
Adhesive capsulitis.
Glenohumeral arthritis.

ANTERIOR

Bicipital tendinitis and rupture.
Glenoid labral tear.
Adhesive capsulitis.
Glenohumeral arthritis.
Osteonecrosis.

AXILLARY

Neoplasm (Pancoast's, mediastinal).
Herpes zoster.

SHOULDER PAIN, IN DIFFERENT AGE GROUPS[8]

ICD-9CM #	719.41	
ICD-10CM #	M25.519	Pain in unspecified shoulder

COMMON CAUSES OF SHOULDER PAIN IN DIFFERENT AGE GROUPS

Childhood (2-10 yr)
Intraarticular:
Instability.
Periarticular:
Osteochondromas.
Adolescence (10-18 yr)
Intraarticular:
Instability.
Early Adulthood (18-30 yr)
Intraarticular:
Instability.
Acromioclavicular joint sprain.
Periarticular:
Calcific tendonitis.
Impingement.
Referred:
Cervical.

Adulthood (30-60 yr)
Intraarticular:
Osteochondritis.
Osteoarthritis.
Frozen shoulder.
Inflammatory arthritis.
Periarticular:
Calcific tendonitis.
Impingement.
Rotator cuff tear.
Bicipital tendonitis.
Referred:
Cervical.
Old Age (>60 yr)
Intraarticular:
Osteochondritis.
Osteoarthritis.
Frozen shoulder.
Inflammatory arthritis.
Periarticular:
Impingement.
Rotator cuff tear.
Referred:
Cervical.

SINUS NODE DYSFUNCTION[14a]

ICD-9CM # 427.81
ICD-10CM # varies with specific diagnosis

CAUSES OF SINUS NODE DYSFUNCTION

Intrinsic
Hypothyroidism.
Fibrocalcific degeneration.
Increased vagal tone, especially in sleep apnea.
Congenital mutations.
Scleroderma.
Amyloidosis.
Chagas disease.
Extrinsic
Trauma, including cardiac surgery.
Drugs:
- Calcium-channel blockers.
- β-Blockers.
- Digoxin.
- Antiarrhythmic medications (amiodarone, dronedarone, sotalol, flecainide, propafenone).
- Lithium.

SKIN INDURATION, CHRONIC[18b]

ICD-9CM # varies with specific diagnosis
ICD-10CM # varies with specific diagnosis

CONDITIONS ASSOCIATED WITH CHRONIC SKIN INDURATION

Systemic sclerosis.
Localized scleroderma.
Scleroderma variants.
Scleredema.
- Scleredema adultorum of Buschke.
- Scleredema diabeticorum.
- Scleredema neonatorum.

Scleromyxedema.
Nephrogenic fibrosing dermopathy.
Eosinophilic syndromes.
- Eosinophilic fasciitis (diffuse fasciitis with eosinophilia, Schulman disease).
- Eosinophilia-myalgia syndrome.
- Toxic oil syndrome.

Chronic graft-versus-host disease.
Pseudoscleroderma (local injection of vitamin K, bleomycin, pentazocine).
Metabolic diseases.
- Porphyria cutanea tarda.
- Phenylketonuria.
- Werner syndrome.
- Acromegaly.

Pachydermoperiostitis.
Polyneuropathy, organomegaly, endocrinopathy, monoclonal gammopathy (POEMS).
Stiff skin syndrome.
Reflex sympathetic dystrophy.
Hemiplegia.

SMALL BOWEL MASSES[38]

ICD-9CM # varies with specific diagnosis
ICD-10CM # varies with specific diagnosis

Cyst:
- Mesenteric cyst.

Tumor:
- Benign.
- Malignant.

Intussusception.
Inflammation:
- Crohn's disease.

SMALL BOWEL OBSTRUCTION[26]

ICD-9CM #	751.1	Small Intestine Obstruction, Congenital
	560.81	Small Intestine Obstruction Due to Adhesion
ICD-10CM #	K56.5	Intestinal adhesions [bands] with obstruction (postprocedural) (postinfection)
	Q41.9	Congenital absence, atresia and stenosis of small intestine, part unspecified

INTRINSIC

Congenital (atresia, stenosis).
Inflammatory (Crohn's, radiation enteritis).
Neoplasms (metastatic or primary).
Intussusception.
Traumatic (hematoma).

EXTRINSIC

Hernias (internal and external).
Adhesions.
Volvulus.
Compressing masses (tumors, abscesses, hematomas).

INTRALUMINAL

Foreign body.
Gallstones.
Bezoars.
Barium.
Ascaris infestation.

SMALL INTESTINE ULCERATION

ICD-9CM # 569.82
ICD-10CM # K63.3 Ulcer of intestine

Inflammatory bowel disease.
Celiac disease.
Vasculitis, SLE, Behçet's syndrome.
Uremia.
Infections (*Campylobacter,* TB, *Yersinia,* parasites, typhoid, cytomegalovirus [CMV], *Clostridium).*
Mesenteric insufficiency.
Neoplasms.
Radiation.
Drugs (salicylates, potassium, indomethacin, antimetabolites).
Meckel diverticulum.
Zollinger-Ellison syndrome.
Lymphocytic enterocolitis.
Stomal ulceration.

SMELL DISTURBANCE

ICD-9CM # varies with specific disorder
ICD-10CM # R43.8 Other disturbances of smell and taste

Upper respiratory tract infection.
Nasal or paranasal sinus disease.
Exposure to noxious vapors.
Head trauma.
Idiopathic.
Dental caries, periodontal disease.
Medications.

SORE THROAT[2]

ICD-9CM # 484.1
ICD-10CM # J02 Acute pharyngitis

DIFFERENTIAL DIAGNOSIS FOR SORE THROAT

Infectious Causes

Aerobes

Common:
- *Streptococcus pyogenes* (GABHS).
- GABHS.
- *Peptostreptococcus* spp.
- Non–group A streptococcus.
- *Neisseria gonorrhoeae.*
- *Neisseria meningitides.*
- *Mycoplasma pneumoniae.*
- *Arcanobacterium hemolyticum.*
- *Chlamydia trachomatis.*
- *Staphylococcus aureus.*

Uncommon:
- *Haemophilus influenzae.*
- *Haemophilus parainfluenzae.*
- *Coccidioides* spp.
- *Corynebacterium diphtheriae.*
- *Streptococcus pneumoniae.*
- *Yersinia enterocolitica.*
- *Treponema pallidum.*
- *Francisella tularensis.*
- *Legionella pneumophila.*
- *Mycobacterium* spp.

Anaerobes

Bacteroides spp.
Peptococcus spp.

Clostridium spp.
Fusobacterium spp.
Prevotella spp.

Other

Candida spp.

Viral

Rhinovirus.
Adenovirus.
Coronavirus.
Herpes simplex 1, 2.
Influenza A, B.
Parainfluenza.
Cytomegalovirus.
Epstein-Barr.
Varicella-zoster.
Hepatitis virus.

Noninfectious Causes

Systemic

Kawasaki disease.
Stevens-Johnson syndrome.
Cyclic neutropenia.
Thyroiditis.
Connective tissue disease.

Trauma, miscellaneous

Penetrating injury.
Angioneurotic edema.
Retained foreign body.
Anomalous aortic arch.
Laryngeal fracture.
Calcific retropharyngeal tendinitis.
Retropharyngeal hematoma.
Caustic exposure.

Tumor

Tongue.
Larynx.
Thyroid.
Leukemia.

SPASTIC PARAPLEGIAS

ICD-9CM # 344.1
ICD-10CM # G82.20 Paraplegia, unspecified

Cervical spondylosis.
Friedreich's ataxia.
Multiple sclerosis.
Spinal cord tumor.
HIV.
Tertiary syphilis.
Vitamin B_{12} deficiency.
Spinocerebellar ataxias.
Syringomyelia.
Spinal cord AV malformations.
Adrenoleukodystrophy.

SPINAL CORD COMPRESSION, EPIDURAL

ICD-9CM # varies with specific disorder
ICD-10CM # varies with specific diagnosis

Osteoarthritis.
Meningioma.
Spinal epidural abscess.
Spinal epidural hematoma.
Spinal epidural vascular malformations.
RA.
Metastatic cancer (vertebral, intramedullary, leptomeninges).
Radiation myelopathy.
Neurofibroma.
Sarcoidosis.
Paraneoplastic myelopathy.
Histiocytosis.

SPINAL CORD DYSFUNCTION

ICD-9CM # 336.9 Spinal Cord Compression
336.9 Spinal Cord Disease NOS
742.9 Spinal Cord Disease, Congenital
281.1 Spinal Cord Degeneration, B_{12} Deficiency Anemia
336.8 Spinal Cord Atrophy, Acute
336.10 Spinal Cord Atrophy, Adult
ICD-10CM # G95.9 Disease of spinal cord, unspecified
G95.9 Disease of spinal cord, unspecified
Q07.9 Congenital malformation of nervous system, unspecified
D51.1 Vitamin B12 deficiency anemia due to selective vitamin B12 malabsorption with proteinuria
D51.3 Other dietary vitamin B12 deficiency anemia
D51.8 Other vitamin B12 deficiency anemias
G95.89 Other specified diseases of spinal cord
G95.19 Other vascular myelopathies

Trauma.
Multiple sclerosis.
Transverse myelitis.
Neoplasm (primary, metastatic).
Syringomyelia.
Spinal epidural abscess.
HIV myelopathy.
Diskitis.
Spinal epidural hematoma.
Spinal cord infarction.
Spinal AV malformation.
Subarachnoid hemorrhage.

SPINAL CORD DYSFUNCTION, NONTRAUMATIC[2]

ICD-9CM # 742.9
ICD-10CM # Q07.9 Congenital malformation of nervous system, unspecified

NONTRAUMATIC ETIOLOGIES OF SPINAL CORD DYSFUNCTION

Processes Affecting the Spinal Cord or Blood Supply Directly

Multiple sclerosis.
Transverse myelitis.
Spinal arteriovenous malformation/subarachnoid hemorrhage.
Syringomyelia.
HIV myelopathy.
Other myelopathies.
Spinal cord infarction.

Compressive Lesions Affecting the Spinal Cord

Spinal epidural abscess.
Spinal epidural hematoma.
Diskitis.
Neoplasm.
Metastatic.
Primary CNS.

HIV, Human immunodeficiency virus; *CNS,* central nervous system.

SPINAL CORD ISCHEMIC SYNDROMES

ICD-9CM # varies with specific disorder
ICD-10CM # varies with specific diagnosis

Systemic hypotension.
Venous or arterial occlusion.
Arterial dissection.
Thromboembolism.
Endovascular procedures.
Vasculitis.
Fibrocartilaginous embolism.
Regional hemodynamic compromise.

SPINAL TUMORS[14]

ICD-9CM # 299.7
ICD-10CM # varies with specific diagnosis

EXTRADURAL

Metastases.
Primary bone tumors arising in spine.

INTRADURAL EXTRAMEDULLARY

Meningiomas.
Neurofibromas.
Schwannomas.
Lipomas.
Arachnoid cysts.
Epidermoid cysts.
Metastasis.

INTRAMEDULLARY

Ependymoma.
Glioma.
Hemangioblastoma.
Lipoma.
Metastases.

SPLENIC CYSTS, CLASSIFICATION[5a]

ICD-9CM # 289.59 Splenic Cysts
ICD-10CM # D73.4 Cyst of spleen

Primary (true).
Parasitic.

Nonparasitic.
Congenital.
Epidermoid.
Dermoid.
Mesothelial (serous).
Transitional.
Neoplastic.
Secondary (false): pseudocysts.
Traumatic.
Degenerative.
Inflammatory.
Hemorrhagic.

SPLENIC TUMORS, CLASSIFICATION[5A]

ICD-9CM # 159.1 Splenic Tumors
ICD-10CM # C26.1 Malignant neoplasm of spleen

Malignant.
Lymphoproliferative disease.
Non-Hodgkin lymphoma.
Hodgkin disease.
Hairy cell leukemia.
Chronic lymphocytic leukemia.
Myeloproliferative disease.
Chronic myelogenous leukemia.
Myelofibrosis.
Primary tumors.
Angiosarcoma.
Metastatic tumors.
Benign.
Hemangiomas.
Hamartomas.
Lymphangiomas.
Sclerosing angiomatoid nodular transformation (SANT).

SPLENOMEGALY

ICD-9CM # 789.2 Splenomegaly Unspecified
289.51 Chronic Congestive
759.0 Congenital
789.2 Unknown Origin
ICD-10CM # R16.1 Splenomegaly, not elsewhere classified
D73.2 Chronic congestive splenomegaly
R16.1 Splenomegaly, not elsewhere classified

Hepatic cirrhosis.
Neoplastic involvement: CML, CLL, lymphoma, multiple myeloma.
Bacterial infections: TB, infectious endocarditis, typhoid fever, splenic abscess.
Viral infections: infectious mononucleosis, viral hepatitis, HIV.
Gaucher's disease and other lipid storage diseases.
Sarcoidosis.
Parasitic infections (malaria, kala-azar, histoplasmosis).
Hereditary and acquired hemolytic anemias.
Idiopathic thrombocytopenic purpura (ITP).
Collagen vascular disorders: SLE, RA (Felty's syndrome), polyarteritis nodosa.
Serum sickness, drug hypersensitivity reaction.
Splenic cysts and benign tumors: hemangioma, lymphangioma.
Thrombosis of splenic or portal vein.
Polycythemia vera, myeloid metaplasia.

SPLENOMEGALY AND HEPATOMEGALY[38]

ICD-9CM # 789.2 Splenomegaly
789.1 Hepatomegaly
ICD-10CM # R16.1 Splenomegaly, not elsewhere classified
R16.0 Hepatomegaly, not elsewhere classified

CAUSES OF SPLENOMEGALY AND HEPATOSPLENOMEGALY

Massive Splenomegaly

Hematologic disease (e.g., chronic myeloid leukemia, myelofibrosis).

Moderate Splenomegaly

The above causes.
Portal hypertension.
Hematologic disease (e.g., lymphoma, leukemia, thalassemia).
Storage disease (e.g., Gaucher's disease).

Small Splenomegaly

The above causes.
Infective (hepatitis, leptospirosis, malaria, bacterial endocarditis).
Hematologic disease (e.g., hemolytic anemias, essential thrombocythemia, polycythemia rubra vera).
Connective tissue diseases or vasculitis (e.g., rheumatoid arthritis, systemic lupus erythematosus, polyarteritis nodosa).
Solitary cyst, polycystic syndrome, hydatid cyst.
Infiltration (amyloid, sarcoid).

Hepatosplenomegaly

Chronic liver disease with portal hypertension.
Hematologic disease (e.g., myeloproliferative disease, lymphoma).
Infection (e.g., amyloid, sarcoid).
Connective tissue disease (e.g., systemic lupus erythematosus).

SPLENOMEGALY, CHILDREN[20]

ICD-9CM # 782.2
ICD-10CM # R16.1 Splenomegaly, not elsewhere classified

DISORDERS OF THE BLOOD

Hemolytic anemia: congenital/acquired.
Thalassemia.
Sickle cell disease.
Leukemia.
Osteopetrosis.
Myelofibrosis/myeloid metaplasia/thrombocythemia.

INFECTIONS: ACUTE AND CHRONIC

Viral:
Congenital (e.g., TORCH association).
Mononucleosis (e.g., EBV, CMV infection).
Virus-associated hemophagocytic syndrome.
Human immunodeficiency virus.
Bacterial:
Sepsis/abscess.
Brucellosis.
Salmonellosis.
Tularemia.
Tuberculosis.
Subacute bacterial endocarditis.
Syphilis.
Lyme disease.
Fungal:
Histoplasmosis (disseminated).
Rickettsial:
Rocky Mountain spotted fever.
Cat scratch disease.
Parasitic:
Toxoplasmosis.
Malaria.
Leishmaniasis (kala-azar).
Schistosomiasis.
Echinococcosis.

HEPATIC/PORTAL SYSTEM DISORDERS

Acute/chronic active hepatitis.
Cirrhosis/hepatic fibrosis/biliary atresia.
Portal or splenic venous obstruction (Banti syndrome).

AUTOIMMUNE DISEASE

Juvenile rheumatoid arthritis.
Systemic lupus erythematosus.
Autoimmune lymphoproliferative syndrome (Canale–Smith syndrome).

NEOPLASMS/CYSTS

Lymphomas (Hodgkin and non-Hodgkin).
Hemangiomas/lymphangiomas.
Hamartomas.
Congenital or acquired (posttraumatic) cysts.

STORAGE DISEASES/INBORN ERRORS OF METABOLISM

Lipidoses: Gaucher disease, Niemann–Pick disease, others.
Mucopolysaccharidoses.
Defects in carbohydrate metabolism: galactosemia, fructose intolerance.
Sea-blue histiocyte syndrome.

MISCELLANEOUS DISORDERS

Histiocytoses:
Reactive.
Langerhans cell.
Malignant.
Sarcoidosis.
Congestive heart failure.
Familial Mediterranean fever.

CMV, Cytomegalovirus; *EBV,* Epstein-Barr virus; *TORCH,* toxoplasmosis, other infections, rubella, cytomegalovirus infection, herpes simplex.

STATURAL OVERGROWTH[26A]

ICD-9CM # 253.0
ICD-10CM # E34.4

FETAL OVERGROWTH

Maternal diabetes mellitus.

Cerebral gigantism (Sotos syndrome).
Weaver's syndrome.
Beckwith-Wiedemann syndrome.
Other insulin-like growth factor 2 (IGF2) excess syndromes.

POSTNATAL OVERGROWTH LEADING TO CHILDHOOD TALL STATURE

Familial (constitutional) tall stature.
Cerebral gigantism.
Beckwith-Wiedemann syndrome.
Exogenous obesity.
Excess growth hormone (GH) secretion (pituitary gigantism).
McCune-Albright syndrome or multiple endocrine neoplasia (MEN) associated with excess GH secretion.
Precocious puberty.
Marfan's syndrome.
Klinefelter's syndrome (XXY).
Weaver's syndrome.
Fragile X syndrome.
Homocystinuria.
XYY.
Hyperthyroidism.

POSTNATAL OVERGROWTH LEADING TO ADULT TALL STATURE

Familial (constitutional) tall stature.
Androgen or estrogen deficiency/estrogen resistance (in males).
Testicular feminization.
Excess GH secretion.
Marfan's syndrome.
Klinefelter's syndrome (XXY).
XYY.

STEATOHEPATITIS

ICD-9CM #	571.8	
ICD-10CM #	K76.0	Fatty (change of) liver, not elsewhere classified
	K76.89	Other specified diseases of liver

Alcohol abuse.
Obesity.
DM.
Parenteral nutrition.
Medications (high-dose estrogen, amiodarone, corticosteroids, methotrexate, nifedipine).
Jejunoileal bypass.
Abetalipoproteinemia.
Wilson's disease, Weber-Christian disease.

STOMATITIS, BULLOUS

ICD-9CM #	528.0	
ICD-10CM #	K12.30	Oral mucositis (ulcerative), unspecified

Erythema multiforme.
Erosive lichen planus.
Bullous pemphigoid.
SLE.
Pemphigus vulgaris.
Mucous membrane pemphigoid.

STRIDOR IN NEONATES[1]

ICD-9CM #	786.1	
ICD-10CM #	R06.1	Stridor

INTRINSIC LESIONS

Larynx
Laryngomalacia.
Infection (laryngitis).
Vocal cord paralysis.
Laryngeal web.
Laryngocele or laryngeal cyst.
Laryngotracheal esophageal cleft.
Foreign body.
Trachea
Tracheomalacia.
Tracheal stenosis.
Tracheoesophageal fistula.
Subglottic hemangioma.
Tracheal web.
Extrinsic Compression
Vascular ring.
Anomalous innominate artery.
Mediastinal mass.
Esophageal foreign body.
Other
Macroglossia.
Gastroesophageal reflux.

STRIDOR, PEDIATRIC AGE[4]

ICD-9CM #	786.1	Stridor
	748.3	Stridor, Laryngeal, Congenital
ICD-10CM #	R06.1	Stridor

RECURRENT

Allergic (spasmodic) croup.
Respiratory infections in a child with otherwise asymptomatic anatomic narrowing of the large airways.
Laryngomalacia.

PERSISTENT

Laryngeal obstruction:
- Laryngomalacia.
- Papillomas, other tumors.
- Cysts and laryngoceles.
- Laryngeal webs.
- Bilateral abductor paralysis of the cords.
- Foreign body.

Tracheobronchial disease:
- Tracheomalacia.
- Subglottic tracheal webs.

Endotracheal, endobronchial tumors.
Subglottic tracheal stenosis.
Congenital.
Acquired.
Extrinsic masses.
Mediastinal masses.
Vascular ring.
Lobar emphysema.
Bronchogenic cysts.
Thyroid enlargement.
Esophageal foreign body.
Tracheoesophageal fistulas.
Other.
Gastroesophageal reflux.
Macroglossia, Pierre Robin syndrome.
Cri-du-chat syndrome.
Hysterical stridor.
Hypocalcemia.

STROKE[36]

ICD-9CM #	436	Acute Stroke
ICD-10CM #	I64	Stroke
	I67.89	Other cerebrovascular disease

Hypoglycemia.
Drug overdose or intoxication.
Hysterical conversion reaction.
Hyperventilation.
Metabolic encephalopathy.
Migraine.
Syncope.
Transient global amnesia.
Seizures.
Vestibular vertigo.

STROKE, PEDIATRIC AGE[23]

ICD-9CM #	436	Stroke, Acute
ICD-10CM #	I67.89	Other cerebrovascular disease

CARDIAC DISEASE

Congenital:
- Aortic stenosis.
- Mitral stenosis; mitral prolapse.
- Ventricular septal defects.
- Patent ductus arteriosus.
- Cyanotic congenital heart disease involving right-to-left shunt.

Acquired:
- Endocarditis (bacterial, SLE).
- Kawasaki disease.
- Cardiomyopathy.
- Atrial myxoma.
- Arrhythmia.
- Paradoxical emboli through patent foramen ovale.
- Rheumatic fever.
- Prosthetic heart valve.

HEMATOLOGIC ABNORMALITIES

Hemoglobinopathies:
- Sickle cell (SS) disease.
- Sickle (SC) disease.

Polycythemia.
Leukemia/lymphoma.
Thrombocytopenia.
Thrombocytosis.
Disorders of coagulation:
- Protein C deficiency.
- Protein S deficiency.
- Factor V Leiden.
- Antithrombin III deficiency.
- Lupus anticoagulant.

Oral contraceptive pill use.
Pregnancy and the postpartum state.
Disseminated intravascular coagulation.
Paroxysmal nocturnal hemoglobinuria.
Inflammatory bowel disease (thrombosis).

INFLAMMATORY DISORDERS

Meningitis:
- Viral.
- Bacterial.
- Tuberculosis.

Systemic infection:
- Viremia.
- Bacteremia.
- Local head and neck infections.

Drug-induced inflammation:
- Amphetamine.
- Cocaine.

Autoimmune disease:
- SLE.
- Juvenile RA.
- Takayasu's arteritis.
- Mixed connective tissue disease.
- Polyarteritis nodosum.
- Primary CNS vasculitis.
- Sarcoidosis.
- Behçet's syndrome.
- Granulomatosis with polyangiitis (Wegener's granulomatosis).

METABOLIC DISEASE ASSOCIATED WITH STROKE

Homocystinuria.
Pseudoxanthoma elasticum.
Fabry's disease.
Sulfite oxidase deficiency.
Mitochondrial disorders:
- MELAS.
- Leigh syndrome.

Ornithine transcarbamylase deficiency.

INTRACEREBRAL VASCULAR PROCESSES

Ruptured aneurysm.
Arteriovenous malformation.
Fibromuscular dysplasia.
Moyamoya disease.
Migraine headache.
Postsubarachnoid hemorrhage vasospasm.
Hereditary hemorrhagic telangiectasia.
Sturge-Weber syndrome.
Carotid artery dissection.
Postvaricella.

TRAUMA AND OTHER EXTERNAL CAUSES

Child abuse.
Head trauma/neck trauma.
Oral trauma.
Placental embolism.
ECMO therapy.

CNS, Central nervous system; *ECMO,* extracorporeal membrane oxygenation; *MELAS,* mitochondrial encephalomyopathy, lactic acidosis, and stroke.

STROKE, YOUNG ADULT, CAUSES[1a]

ICD-9CM # 436
ICD-10CM # I64 Stroke
I67.89 Other cerebrovascular disease

Cardiac factors (ASD, MVP, patent foramen ovale).
Inflammatory factors (SLE, polyarteritis nodosa).
Infections (endocarditis, neurosyphilis).
Drugs (cocaine, heroin, oral contraceptives, decongestants).
Arterial dissection.
Hematolic factors (DIC, TTP, deficiency of protein S, protein C, antithrombin III).
Migraine.
Postpartum angiopathy.
Other: premature atherosclerosis, fibromuscular dysplasia.

ST-SEGMENT DEPRESSION, NON-CORONARY CAUSES[4a]

ICD-9CM # 794.31
ICD-10CM # R94.31

NONCORONARY CAUSES OF ST-SEGMENT DEPRESSION

Anemia.
Cardiomyopathy.
Digitalis use.
Glucose load.
Hyperventilation.
Hypokalemia.
Intraventricular conduction disturbance.
Left ventricular hypertrophy.
Mitral valve prolapse.
Preexcitation syndrome.
Severe aortic stenosis.
Severe hypertension.
Severe hypoxia.
Severe volume overload (aortic, mitral regurgitation).
Sudden excessive exercise.
Supraventricular tachyarrhythmias.

ST-SEGMENT ELEVATION[1]

ICD-9CM # 794.31
ICD-10CM # R94.31 Abnormal ECG

DIFFERENTIAL DIAGNOSIS OF ST-SEGMENT ELEVATION ON ELECTROCARDIOGRAPHY

ST-segment elevation myocardial infarction.
Pericarditis.
Benign early repolarization.
Left bundle branch block.
Left ventricular hypertrophy.
Left ventricular aneurysm.
Paced ventricular rhythms.
Prinzmetal angina.
Hyperkalemia.
Hypothermia with Osborne waves.
Intracranial hemorrhage.
Brugada syndrome.
Normal variant.

ST SEGMENT ELEVATIONS, NONISCHEMIC

ICD-9CM # 794.31
ICD-10CM # R94.31 Abnormal electrocardiogram [ECG] [EKG]

Early repolarization.
Acute pericarditis.
LVH.
Normal pattern variant.
LBBB.
Pulmonary embolism.
Hyperkalemia.
Postcardioversion.

SUDDEN DEATH, PEDIATRIC AGE[4]

ICD-9CM # varies with specific disorder
ICD-10CM # R99 Ill-defined and unknown cause of mortality

SIDS AND SIDS "MIMICS"

SIDS.
Long QT syndromes.
Inborn errors of metabolism.
Child abuse.
Myocarditis.
Duct-dependent congenital heart disease.

CORRECTED OR UNOPERATED CONGENITAL HEART DISEASE

Aortic stenosis.
Tetralogy of Fallot.
Transposition of great vessels (postoperative atrial switch).
Mitral valve prolapse.
Hematologic left heart syndrome.
Eisenmenger's syndrome.

CORONARY ARTERIAL DISEASE

Anomalous origin.
Anomalous tract.
Kawasaki disease.
Periarteritis.
Arterial dissection.
Marfan's syndrome.
Myocardial infarction.

MYOCARDIAL DISEASE

Myocarditis.
Hypertrophic cardiomyopathy.
Dilated cardiomyopathy.
Arrhythmogenic right ventricular dysplasia.

CONDUCTION SYSTEM ABNORMALITY/ARRHYTHMIA

Long Q-T syndromes.
Proarrhythmic drugs.
Preexcitation syndromes.
Heart block.
Commotio cordis.
Idiopathic ventricular fibrillation.
Heart tumor.

MISCELLANEOUS

Pulmonary hypertension.
Pulmonary embolism.
Heat stroke.
Cocaine.
Anorexia nervosa.
Electrolyte disturbances.

SIDS, Sudden infant death syndrome.

SUDDEN DEATH, YOUNG ATHLETE

ICD-9CM # varies with specific diagnosis
ICD-10CM # R99 Ill-defined and unknown cause of mortality

Hypertrophic cardiomyopathy.
Coronary artery anomalies.
Myocarditis.
Ruptured aortic aneurysm (Marfan's syndrome).
Arrhythmias.
Aortic valve stenosis.
Asthma.
Trauma (cerebral, cardiac).
Drug and alcohol abuse.
Heat stroke.
Cardiac sarcoidosis.
Atherosclerotic coronary artery disease.
Dilated cardiomyopathy.

SWOLLEN LIMB

ICD-9CM # 729.81 Swollen Arm or Hand
729.81 Swollen Leg or Foot
ICD-10CM # M79.89 Other specified soft tissue disorders

Trauma.
Insect bite.
Abscess.
Lymphedema.
Thrombophlebitis.
Lipoma.
Neurofibroma.
Postphlebitic syndrome.
Myositis ossificans.
Nephrosis, cirrhosis, CHF.
Hypoalbuminemia.
Varicose veins.

TALL STATURE[27]

ICD-9CM # 253.0 Growth Hormone Overproduction, Gigantism
ICD-10CM # E22.0 Acromegaly and pituitary gigantism

Constitutional (familial or genetic)—most common cause

ENDOCRINE CAUSES

Growth hormone excess—gigantism.
Sexual precocity (tall as children, short as adults):
- True sexual precocity.
- Pseudosexual precocity.

Androgen deficiency:
- Klinefelter's syndrome.
- Bilateral anorchism.

GENETIC CAUSES

Klinefelter's syndrome.
Syndromes of XYY, XXYY.

MISCELLANEOUS SYNDROMES AND DISORDERS

Cerebral gigantism or Sotos' syndrome: prominent forehead, hypertelorism, high arched palate, dolichocephaly, mental retardation, large hands and feet, and premature eruption of teeth. Large at birth, with most rapid growth in first 4 yr of life.
Marfan's syndrome: disorder of mesodermal tissues, subluxation of the lenses, arachnodactyly, and aortic aneurysm.
Homocystinuria: same phenotype as Marfan's syndrome.
Obesity: tall as infants, children, and adolescents.
Total lipodystrophy: large hands and feet, generalized loss of subcutaneous fat, insulin-resistant DM, and hepatomegaly.
Beckwith-Wiedemann syndrome: neonatal tallness, omphalocele, macroglossia, and neonatal hypoglycemia.
Weaver-Smith syndrome: excessive intrauterine growth, mental retardation, megalocephaly, widened bifrontal diameter, hypertelorism, large ears, micrognathia, camptodactyly, broad thumbs, and limited extension of elbows and knees.
Marshall-Smith syndrome: excessive intrauterine growth, mental retardation, blue sclerae, failure to thrive, and early death.

TARDIVE DYSKINESIA[13]

ICD-9CM # 781.3 Dyskinesia
300.11 Hysterical Dyskinesia
333.82 Orofacial Dyskinesia
307.9 Psychogenic Dyskinesia
ICD-10CM # R27.9 Unspecified lack of coordination
F44.4 Conversion disorder with motor symptom or deficit
F44.6 Conversion disorder with sensory symptom or deficit
G24.4 Idiopathic orofacial dystonia

DIFFERENTIAL DIAGNOSIS

Medications (antidepressants, anticholinergics, amphetamines, lithium, l-dopa, phenytoin).
Brain neoplasms.
Ill-fitting dentures.
Huntington's disease.
Idiopathic dystonias (tics, blepharospasm, aging).
Wilson's disease.
Extrapyramidal syndrome (postanoxic or postencephalitic).
Torsion dystonia.

TASTE AND SMELL LOSS[1a]

ICD-9CM # 781.1 Smell and Taste Disturbance of Sensation
ICD-10CM # R43.0 Anosmia
R43.1 Parosmia
R43.2 Parageusia

TASTE

Local: radiation therapy.
Systemic: cancer, renal failure, hepatic failure, nutritional deficiency (vitamin B_{12}, zinc), Cushing's syndrome, hypothyroidism, DM, infection (influenza), drugs (antirheumatic and antiproliferative).
Neurologic: Bell's palsy, familial dysautonomia, multiple sclerosis.

SMELL

Local: allergic rhinitis, sinusitis, nasal polyposis, bronchial asthma.
Systemic: renal failure, hepatic failure, nutritional deficiency (vitamin B_{12}), Cushing's syndrome, hypothyroidism, DM, infection (viral hepatitis, influenza), drugs (nasal sprays, antibiotics).
Neurologic: head trauma, multiple sclerosis, Parkinson's disease, frontal brain tumor.

TELANGIECTASIA

ICD-9CM # 448.9
ICD-10CM # I78.8 Other diseases of capillaries
I78.9 Disease of capillaries, unspecified

Oral contraceptive agents.
Pregnancy.
Rosacea.
Varicose veins.
Trauma.
Drug induced (corticosteroids, systemic or topical).
Spider telangiectases.
Hepatic cirrhosis.
Mastocytosis.
SLE, dermatomyositis, systemic sclerosis.

TENDINOPATHY[26]

ICD-9CM # 727.9
ICD-10CM # M67.90 Unspecified disorder of synovium and tendon, unspecified site
M71.9 Bursopathy, unspecified

INTRINSIC FACTORS

Anatomic Factors
Malalignment.
Muscle weakness or imbalance.
Muscle inflexibility.
Decreased vascularity.

Systemic Factors
Inflammatory conditions (e.g., SLE).
Pregnancy.
Quinolone-induced tendinopathy.

Age-Related Factors
Tendon degeneration.
Increased tendon stiffness.
Tendon calcification.
Decreased vascularity.

EXTRINSIC FACTORS

Repetitive Mechanical Load
Excessive duration.
Excessive frequency.

Excessive intensity.
Poor technique.
Workplace factors.

Equipment Problems

Footwear.
Athletic field surface.
Equipment factors (e.g., racquet size).
Protective gear.

TESTICULAR FAILURE[10]

ICD-9CM # 257.1 Testicular Failure
ICD-10CM # E29 Testicular dysfunction

PRIMARY

Klinefelter's syndrome (XXY).
XYY.
Vanishing testes syndrome (in utero or early postnatal torsion).
Noonan's syndrome.
Varicocele.
Myotonic dystrophy.
Orchitis (mumps, gonorrhea).
Cryptorchidism.
Chemical exposure.
Irradiation to testes.
Spinal cord injury.
Polyglandular failure.
Idiopathic oligospermia or azoospermia.
Germinal cell aplasia (Sertoli cell–only syndrome).
Idiopathic testicular failure.
Testicular torsion.
Testicular trauma.
Diethylstilbestrol (maternal use during pregnancy leading to in utero estrogen exposure).
Testicular tumor with subsequent irradiation therapy, chemotherapy, or surgery (retroperitoneal lymph node dissection or orchiectomy).

SECONDARY

Delayed puberty.
Kallmann's syndrome.
Isolated gonadotropin deficiency.
Prader-Labhart-Willi syndrome.
Lawrence-Moon-Biedl syndrome.
Central nervous system irradiation.
Prepubertal panhypopituitarism.
Postpubertal panhypopituitarism.
Hypogonadism secondary to hyperprolactinemia.
Adrenogenital syndrome.
Chronic liver disease.
Chronic renal failure/uremia.
Hemochromatosis.
Cushing's syndrome.
Malnutrition.
Massive obesity.
Sickle cell anemia.
Hyper/hypothyroidism.
Anabolic steroid use.

TESTICULAR PAIN

ICD-9CM #	608.9	
ICD-10CM #	N50.9	Disorder of male genital organs, unspecified
	R10.2	Pelvic and perineal pain

Testicular torsion.
Trauma.
Epididymitis.
Orchitis.
Neoplasm.
Urolithiasis.
Inguinal hernia.
Infection (cellulitis, abscess, folliculitis).
Anxiety.

TESTICULAR SIZE VARIATIONS[10]

ICD-9CM #	608.3	Testicular Atrophy
	608.89	Testicular Mass
	257.2	Hypogonadism
ICD-10CM #	N50.0	Atrophy of testis
	N44.2	Benign cyst of testis
	N44.8	Other noninflammatory disorders of the testis
	N50.3	Cyst of epididymis
	N50.8	Other specified disorders of male genital organs
	N53.12	Painful ejaculation
	E29.1	Testicular hypofunction

SMALL TESTES

Hypothalamic-pituitary dysfunction.
Gonadotropin deficiency.
Growth hormone deficiency.
Normal variant.
Primary hypogonadism.
Autoimmune destruction.
Chemotherapy.
Cryptorchidism.
Irradiation.
Klinefelter's syndrome.
Orchiditis.
Testicular regression syndrome.
Torsion.
Trauma.

LARGE TESTES

Adrenal rest tissue.
Compensatory.
Fragile X syndrome.
Idiopathic.
Tumor.

TETANUS[26]

ICD-9CM # 037
ICD-10CM # A35 Other tetanus

Acute abdomen.
Black widow spider bite.
Dental abscess.
Dislocated mandible.
Dystonic reaction.
Encephalitis.
Head trauma.
Hyperventilation syndrome.
Hypocalcemia.
Meningitis.
Peritonsillar abscess.
Progressive fluctuating muscular rigidity (stiff-man syndrome).
Psychogenic.
Rabies.
Sepsis.
Subarachnoid hemorrhage.
Status epilepticus.
Strychnine poisoning.
Temporomandibular joint syndrome.

THROMBOCYTOPENIA

ICD-9CM #	287.3	Congenital or Primary
	287.4	Secondary
	287.5	Thrombocytopenia NOS
ICD-10CM #	D47.3	Essential (hemorrhagic) thrombocythemia
	D69.59	Other secondary thrombocytopenia
	D69.6	Thrombocytopenia, unspecified

INCREASED DESTRUCTION

Immunologic

Drugs: quinine, quinidine, digitalis, procainamide, thiazide diuretics, sulfonamides, phenytoin, aspirin, penicillin, heparin, gold, meprobamate, sulfa drugs, phenylbutazone, nonsteroidal anti-inflammatory drugs (NSAIDs), methyldopa, cimetidine, furosemide, INH, cephalosporins, chlorpropamide, organic arsenicals, chloroquine, platelet glycoprotein IIb/IIIa receptor inhibitors, ranitidine, indomethacin, carboplatin, ticlopidine, clopidogrel.
Idiopathic thrombocytopenic purpura (ITP).
Transfusion reaction: transfusion of platelets with plasminogen activator (PLA) in recipients without PLA-1.
Fetal/maternal incompatibility.
Collagen vascular diseases (e.g., SLE).
Autoimmune hemolytic anemia.
Lymphoreticular disorders (e.g., CLL).

Nonimmunologic

Prosthetic heart valves.
Thrombotic thrombocytopenic purpura (TTP).
Sepsis.
DIC.
Hemolytic-uremic syndrome (HUS).
Giant cavernous hemangioma.

DECREASED PRODUCTION

Abnormal marrow.
Marrow infiltration (e.g., leukemia, lymphoma, fibrosis).
Marrow suppression (e.g., chemotherapy, alcohol, radiation).
Hereditary disorders.
Wiskott-Aldrich syndrome: X-linked disorder characterized by thrombocytopenia, eczema, and repeated infections.
May-Hegglin anomaly: increased megakaryocytes but ineffective thrombopoiesis.
Vitamin deficiencies (e.g., vitamin B_{12}, folic acid).

SPLENIC SEQUESTRATION, HYPERSPLENISM

DILUTIONAL, AS A RESULT OF MASSIVE TRANSFUSION

THROMBOCYTOPENIA, IN PREGNANCY[20]

ICD-9CM # 287.4
ICD-10CM # D69.59 Other secondary thrombocytopenia

Incidental thrombocytopenia of pregnancy (gestational thrombocytopenia).
Preeclampsia/eclampsia.*
Peripartum/postpartum thrombotic microangiopathy.
Disseminated intravascular coagulation (DIC) secondary to:
- Abruptio placentae.
- Endometritis.
- Amniotic fluid embolism.
- Retained fetus.

Thrombotic thrombocytopenic purpura.
Hemolytic-uremic syndrome.

*Preeclampsia/eclampsia usually is not associated with overt DIC.

THROMBOCYTOPENIA, INHERITED DISORDERS[1a]

ICD-9CM # 287.3
ICD-10CM # D47.3 Essential (hemorrhagic) thrombocythemia

Amegakaryocytic thrombocytopenia.
Thrombocytopenia–absent radii.
MYH9-related thrombocytopenia:
- May-Hegglin anomaly.
- Fechtner syndrome.
- Epstein syndrome.
- Sebastian syndrome.

X-linked macrothrombocytopenia.
Wiskott-Aldrich syndrome.
X-linked thrombocytopenia.
Thrombocytopenia and radioulnar synostosis.
Familial platelet disorder—AML.
Familial dominant thrombocytopenia.
Paris-Trousseau thrombocytopenia.
Bernard-Soulier syndrome.
Bernard-Soulier carrier/Mediterranean macrothrombocytopenia.

THROMBOCYTOSIS

ICD-9CM # 289.9 Thrombocytosis, Essential
ICD-10CM # D75.9 Disease of blood and blood-forming organs, unspecified

Iron deficiency.
Posthemorrhage.
Neoplasms (GI tract).
CML.
Polycythemia vera.
Myelofibrosis with myeloid metaplasia.
Infections.
After splenectomy.
Postpartum.
Hemophilia.
Pancreatitis.
Cirrhosis.
Idiopathic.

THROMBOSIS OR THROMBOTIC DIATHESIS[1a]

ICD-9CM # 444
ICD-10CM # I74.09 Other arterial embolism and thrombosis of abdominal aorta

DIFFERENTIAL DIAGNOSIS OF THE PATIENT PRESENTING WITH THROMBOSIS OR THROMBOTIC DIATHESIS

Inherited (Primary) Hypercoagulable States

Activated protein C resistance caused by factor V Leiden mutation.
Prothrombin gene mutation (G to A transition at position 20210 in the 3-untranslated region).
Antithrombin III deficiency.
Protein C deficiency.
Protein S deficiency.
Dysfibrinogenemias (rare).

Acquired (Secondary) Hypercoagulable States

In association with physiologic or thrombogenic stimuli:
- Pregnancy (especially the postpartum period).
- Estrogen use (oral contraceptives, hormone replacement therapy).
- Immobilization.
- Trauma.
- Postoperative state.

Advancing age.
Obesity.
Prolonged air travel.
Lupus anticoagulant or antiphospholipid antibody syndrome.
In association with other clinical disorders.

Mixed/Unknown

Activated protein C resistance in the absence of factor V Leiden.
Elevated factor VIII level.
Elevated factor XI level.
Elevated factor IX level.
Elevated thrombin activatable fibrinolysis inhibitor (TAFI) level.
Decreased free tissue factor pathway inhibitor (TFPI) level.
Decreased plasma fibrinolytic activity.

THYROMEGALY

ICD-9CM # varies with specific diagnosis
ICD-10CM # varies with specific diagnosis

Goiter.
Graves' disease.
Thyroiditis (lymphocytic, granulomatous, suppurative).
Toxic adenoma.
Neoplasm (primary, metastatic).

THYROTOXICOSIS[26a]

ICD-9CM # 242.8
ICD-10CM # E05.80

CAUSES OF THYROTOXICOSIS

Sustained Hormone Overproduction (Hyperthyroidism)

Low TSH, High RAIU:
- Graves' disease (von Basedow's disease).
- Toxic multinodular goiter.
- Toxic adenoma.
- Chorionic gonadotropin-induced.
  - Gestational hyperthyroidism: physiologic hyperthyroidism of pregnancy, familial gestational hyperthyroidism due to TSH receptor mutations.
  - Trophoblastic tumors
- Inherited nonimmune hyperthyroidism associated with TSH receptor or G protein mutations.

Low TSH, Low RAIU:
- Iodide-induced hyperthyroidism (Jod-Basedow effect).
- Amiodarone-associated hyperthyroidism due to iodide release.

Struma Ovarii:
- Metastatic functioning thyroid carcinoma.

Normal or Elevated TSH:
- TSH-secreting pituitary tumors.
- Thyroid hormone resistance with pituitary predominance.

Transient Hormone Excess (Thyrotoxicosis)

Low TSH, Low RAIU
- Thyroiditis.
  - Autoimmune: lymphocytic thyroiditis (silent thyroiditis, painless thyroiditis, postpartum thyroiditis), acute exacerbation of Hashimoto's disease.
- Viral or postviral.
  - Subacute (granulomatous, painful, postviral) thyroiditis.
- Drug-induced or associated thyroiditis.
  - Amiodarone.
  - Lithium, interferon-α, interleukin-2, GM-CSF.
- Infectious thyroiditis.

Exogenous Thyroid Hormone.
- Iatrogenic overreplacement.
- Thyrotoxicosis factitia.
- Ingestion of natural products containing thyroid hormone.
  - "Hamburger" thyrotoxicosis.
  - Natural foodstuffs.
  - Thyromimetic compounds (e.g., tiratricol PLB).
  - Occupational exposure to thyroid hormone (e.g., pill manufacturing, veterinary occupations).

GM-CSF, granulocyte-macrophage colony-stimulating factor; *RAIU*, radioactive iodine uptake; *TSH*, thyroid-stimulating hormone.

TICK-RELATED INFECTIONS

ICD-9CM #	082.0	Rocky Mountain Spotted Fever
	066.1	Colorado Tick Fever
	088.82	Babesiosis
	082.8	Ehrlichiosis
	088.81	Lyme Disease
ICD-10CM #	A77.0	Spotted fever due to Rickettsia rickettsii
	A93.2	Colorado tick fever
	B60.0	Babesiosis
	A77.8	Other spotted fevers
	A69.20	Lyme disease, unspecified

Lyme disease.
Rocky Mountain spotted fever.
Babesiosis.
Tularemia.
Q fever.
Colorado tick fever.
Ehrlichiosis.
Relapsing fever.

TICS

ICD-9CM #	307.20	
ICD-10CM #	F95.9	Tic disorder, unspecified

Tourette's syndrome.
Physiologic tic.
Anxiety disorder.
Huntington's disease.
Medications (e.g., antipsychotics, carbamazepine, phenytoin, phenobarbital).
Encephalitis.
Head trauma.
Schizophrenia.
Carbon monoxide poisoning.
Stroke.
Sydenham's chorea.
Creutzfeldt-Jakob disease.

TORSADES DE POINTES[22]

ICD-9CM #	code not available	
ICD-10CM #	I47.2	Ventricular tachycardia

Antiarrhythmics known to increase the QT interval (e.g., quinidine, procainamide, amiodarone, disopyramide, sotalol).
Tricyclic antidepressants and phenothiazines.
Histamine (H_1) antagonists (e.g., astemizole, terfenadine).
Antiviral and antifungal agents and antibiotics.
Hypokinemia.
Hypomagnesemia.
Insecticide poisoning.
Bradyarrhythmias.
Congenital long QT syndrome.
Subarachnoid hemorrhage.
Chloroquinine, pentamidine.
Cocaine abuse.

TOXIC MEGACOLON, CAUSES[5a]

ICD-9CM #	564.7	Toxic Megacolon
ICD-10CM #	K59.3	Megacolon, not elsewhere classified

INFLAMMATORY

Ulcerative colitis.
Crohn's disease.

INFECTIOUS

Bacterial.

- *Clostridium difficile* pseudomembranous colitis.
- *Salmonella* (typhoid and nontyphoid).
- *Shigella.*
- *Campylobacter.*
- *Yersinia.*

Parasitic.

- *Entamoeba histolytica.*
- *Cryptosporidium.*

Viral.

- Cytomegalovirus colitis.

OTHER

- Ischemia.
- Kaposi sarcoma.

TRACHEOBRONCHIAL NARROWING ON X-RAY[16a]

ICD-9CM #	varies with specific diagnosis
ICD-10CM #	varies with specific diagnosis

CAUSES OF TRACHEOBRONCHIAL NARROWING

Long-segment/Diffuse Narrowing

Sarcoidosis.
Amyloidosis.
Granulomatosis with polyangiitis (Wegener's granulomatosis).
Relapsing polychondritis.
Tracheobronchopathia osteochondroplastica.
Pemphigoid.

Short-segment Narrowing

Previous intubation or tracheostomy.
Congenital stenosis or web.
Extrinsic compression (from thyroid).
Adenoid cystic carcinoma.
Squamous carcinoma.

TREMOR

ICD-9CM #	781.0	Tremor NOS
	333.1	Benign Essential Tremor
	333.1	Familial Tremor
ICD-10CM #	R25.0	Abnormal head movements
	R25.1	Tremor, unspecified
	R25.2	Cramp and spasm
	R25.3	Fasciculation
	R25.9	Unspecified abnormal involuntary movements
	G25.0	Essential tremor
	G25.1	Drug-induced tremor
	G25.2	Other specified forms of tremor

REST TREMORS

Parkinson's disease.
Other parkinsonian syndromes (less commonly).
Midbrain (rubral) tremor: rest < postural < kinetic.
Wilson's disease (also acquired hepatocerebral degeneration).
Essential tremor—only if severe: rest < postural and action.

POSTURAL AND ACTION (TERMINAL) TREMORS

Physiologic tremor.
Exaggerated physiologic tremor (these factors can also aggravate other forms of tremor).
Stress, fatigue, anxiety, emotion.
Endocrine: hypoglycemia, thyrotoxicosis, pheochromocytoma, adrenocorticosteroids.
Drugs and toxins: b-agonists, dopamine agonists, amphetamines, lithium, tricyclic antidepressants, neuroleptics, theophylline, caffeine, valproic acid, alcohol withdrawal, mercury (Hatter's shakes), lead, arsenic, others.
Essential tremor (familial or sporadic)
Primary writing tremor.
With other CNS disorders.
Parkinson's disease.
Other akinetic-rigid syndromes.
Idiopathic dystonia, including focal dystonias.
With peripheral neuropathy.
Charcot-Marie-Tooth syndrome (controversial whether to call this the Roussy-Levy syndrome).
Variety of other peripheral neuropathies (especially dysgammaglobulinemia).
Cerebellar tremor.

KINETIC (INTENTION) TREMOR

Disease of cerebellar outflow (dentate nucleus and superior cerebellar peduncle): multiple sclerosis, trauma, tumor, vascular disease, Wilson's acquired hepatocerebral degeneration, drugs, toxins (e.g., mercury), others.

MISCELLANEOUS RHYTHMICAL MOVEMENT DISORDERS

Psychogenic tremor.
Orthostatic tremor.
Rhythmical movements in dystonia (dystonic tremor).
Rhythmical myoclonus (segmental myoclonus—e.g., palatal or branchial myoclonus, spinal myoclonus, limb myorhythmia).
Oscillatory myoclonus.
Asterixis.
Clonus.
Epilepsia partialis continua.
Hereditary chin quivering.
Spasmus nutans.
Head bobbing with third ventricular cysts.
Nystagmus.

TREMOR, IN CHILDREN, CAUSES[22a]

ICD-9CM #	781.0	Tremor
ICD-10CM #	R25.0	Abnormal head movements
	R25.1	Tremor, unspecified
	R25.2	Cramp and spasm
	R25.3	Fasciculation
	R25.9	Unspecified abnormal involuntary movements

BENIGN

Enhanced physiologic tremor.
Shuddering attacks.
Jitteriness.
Spasmus nutans.

STATIC INJURY/STRUCTURAL

Cerebellar malformation.
Stroke (particularly in the midbrain or cerebellum).
Multiple sclerosis.

HEREDITARY/DEGENERATIVE

Familial essential tremor.
Fragile X premutation.
Wilson disease.
Huntington disease.
Juvenile parkinsonism (tremor is rare).
Pallidonigral degeneration.

METABOLIC

Hyperthyroidism.
Hyperadrenergic state (including pheochromocytoma and neuroblastoma).
Hypomagnesemia.
Hypocalcemia.
Hypoglycemia.
Hepatic encephalopathy.
Vitamin B_{12} deficiency.
Inborn errors of metabolism.
Mitochondrial disorders.

DRUGS/TOXINS

Valproate, phenytoin, carbamazepine, lamotrigine, gabapentin, lithium, tricyclic antidepressants, stimulants (cocaine, amphetamine, caffeine, thyroxine, bronchodilators), neuroleptics, cyclosporin, toluene, mercury, thallium, amiodarone, nicotine, lead, manganese, arsenic, cyanide, naphthalene, ethanol, lindane, serotonin reuptake inhibitors.

PERIPHERAL NEUROPATHIES

PSYCHOGENIC

TUBULOINTERSTITIAL DISEASE, ACUTE[14]

ICD-9CM # 584.5
ICD-10CM # N17.0 Acute kidney failure with tubular necrosis

DRUGS

Antibiotics, penicillins, cephalosporins, rifampin.
Sulfonamides: cotrimoxazole, sulfamethoxazole.
NSAIDs: propionic acid derivatives.
Miscellaneous: phenytoin, thiazides, allopurinol, cimetidine, ifosfamide.

INFECTIONS

Invasion of renal parenchyma.
Reaction to systemic infections: streptococcal, diphtheria, hantavirus.

SYSTEMIC DISEASES

Immune mediated: SLE, transplanted kidney, cryoglobulinemias.
Metabolic: Urate, oxalate.
Neoplastic: Lymphoproliferative diseases.

IDIOPATHIC

TUBULOINTERSTITIAL KIDNEY DISEASE[14]

ICD-9CM # 584.5
ICD-10CM # N17.0 Acute kidney failure with tubular necrosis

Ischemic and toxic acute tubular necrosis.
Allergic interstitial nephritis.
Interstitial nephritis secondary to immune complex-related collagen vascular disease (e.g., SLE, Sjögren's).
Granulomatous diseases (sarcoidosis, uveitis).
Pigment-related tubular injury (myoglobinuria, hemoglobinuria).
Hypercalcemia with nephrocalcinosis.
Tubular obstruction (drugs such as indinavir, uric acid in tumor lysis syndrome).
Myeloma kidney or cast nephropathy.
Infection-related interstitial nephritis: *Legionella, Leptospira.*
Infiltrative diseases (e.g., lymphoma).

TUMOR MARKERS ELEVATION[38]

ICD-9CM # 795.8
ICD-10CM # R97.8 Other abnormal tumor markers

CAUSES OF ELEVATED LEVELS OF TUMOR MARKERS

Carcinoembryonic Antigen (CEA)

Colonic cancer (higher levels if the tumor is more differentiated or is extensive or has spread to the liver).
Lung or breast cancer; seminoma.
Cigarette smokers.
Cirrhosis, inflammatory bowel disease, rectal polyps, pancreatitis.
Advanced age.

Alpha-Fetoprotein

Hepatocellular cancer: very high titers or a rising titer is strongly suggestive, but >10% of patients do not have an elevated level.
Hepatic regeneration (e.g., cirrhosis, alcoholic or viral hepatitis).
Cancer of the stomach, colon, pancreas, or lung.
Teratocarcinoma or embryonal cell carcinoma (testis, ovary, extragonadal).
Pregnancy.
Ataxia-telangiectasia.
Normal variant.

Prostate-Specific Antigen

Prostate carcinoma (localized disease).
Prostatic hyperplasia.
Prostatitis.
Prostatic infarction.

Cancer-Associated Antigen (CA-19-9) *

Pancreatic carcinoma (80% with advanced, well-differentiated cancer have an elevated level).
Other gastrointestinal cancers: colon, stomach, bile duct.
Acute or chronic pancreatitis.
Chronic liver disease.
Biliary tract disease.

*Patients who cannot synthesize Lewis blood group antigens (~5% of the population) do not produce CA-19-9 antigen.

UREMIC ENCEPHALOPATHY, DIFFERENTIAL DIAGNOSIS[12b]

ICD-9CM # 348.30 Uremic Encephalopathy
ICD-10CM # G93.40 Encephalopathy, unspecified

Differential Diagnosis	*Comment*
Hypertensive encephalopathy	
Systemic inflammatory response syndrome (SIRS):	Observed in septic patients
Systemic vasculitis:	Vasculitis or lupus with cerebral involvement
Drug-induced neurotoxicity	
Analgesics:	Meperidine, codeine, morphine, gabapentin
Antibiotics:	High-dose penicillins (may cause seizures), acyclovir, ethambutol (optic nerve damage), erythromycin and aminoglycosides (may cause ototoxicity), nitrofurantoin and isoniazid (peripheral neuropathy)
Psychotropics:	Lithium, haloperidol, clonazepam, diazepam, chlorpromazine
Immunosuppressants:	Cyclosporine, tacrolimus
Chemotherapeutics:	Cisplatinum, ifosfamide
Others:	High doses of loop diuretics (ototoxic), ephedrine, methyldopa, aluminum
Cerebral atheroembolic disease:	Follows recent aortic or cardiac angiography; associated with peripheral manifestations, including lower extremity cyanosis, livedo reticularis, and eosinophilia
Subdural hematoma	
Posterior leukoencephalopathy:	• Observed particularly following renal transplantation due to reversible, abnormal permeability of the blood-brain barrier • Often manifests as headache followed by mental depression, visual loss, and seizures in the context of volume expansion, acute hypertension, and often treatment with corticosteroids or calcineurin inhibitors • Lesions in the parietal, temporal, and occipital lobes may be seen on imaging studies

URETERAL COLIC[24a]

ICD-9CM # 788.0
ICD-10CM # R33.8 Other retention of urine
N13.8 Other obstructive and reflux uropathy

DIAGNOSTIC DIFFERENTIALS OF RENAL OR URETERAL COLIC

Acute cholecystitis, acute cholelithiasis.
Acute appendicitis.
Pelvic inflammatory disease.
Diverticulosis and/or diverticulitis.
Intestinal obstruction.
Leaking abdominal aortic aneurysm.
Musculoskeletal sprains.
Herniated disk.
Hepes zoster (shingles).
Gastrointestinal dysfunction with ileus and/or toxic colonic dilatation.

URETERIC OBSTRUCTION, CONGENITAL[16a]

ICD-9CM # 593.4
ICD-10CM # N13.8 Other obstructive and reflux uropathy
N20.9 Urolithiasis

CONGENITAL CAUSES OF URETERIC OBSTRUCTION

Primary megaureter.
Ureterocele (ectopic and orthotopic).
Ureteric valve.
Distal ureteric stenosis.
Ureteric atresia.
Circumcaval ureter and variants.
Bladder diverticulum.

URETHRAL DISCHARGE AND DYSURIA

ICD-9CM # 788.7 Urethral Discharge
599.9 Urethral Discharge, Bloody
788.1 Dysuria
ICD-10CM # R36.0 Urethral discharge without blood
R36.9 Urethral discharge, unspecified
N36.9 Urethral disorder, unspecified
N39.9 Disorder of urinary system, unspecified
R30.0 Dysuria
R30.9 Painful micturition, unspecified

Urethritis (gonococcal, chlamydial, trichomonal).
Cystitis.
Prostatitis.
Vaginitis (candidiasis, chemical).
Meatal stenosis.
Interstitial cystitis.
Trauma (foreign body, masturbation, horseback or bike riding).

URETHRAL OBSTRUCTION, CHILDREN[16a]

ICD-9CM # 593.4
ICD-10CM # N13.8 Other obstructive and reflux uropathy

CAUSES OF URETHRAL OBSTRUCTION IN CHILDREN

Intrinsic Lesions

Valve (posterior, anterior, saccular diverticulum).
Stenosis, atresia.
Inflammatory stricture.
Traumatic stricture:
External trauma (saddle injury, and so on).
Iatrogenic trauma (catheter, cystoscopy, surgery).
Urethral "tumors":
Girls: leiomyoma.
Boys: polyp, rhabdomyosarcoma.
Miscellaneous (epidemolysis bullosa).

Extrinsic Lesions

Presacral mass dissecting inferiorly (tumor, cyst).
Fecal impaction (Hirschsprung's, postrepair anal atresia, habitual constipation, neuropathy).
Mass originating in genital organs:
Boys: utricle cyst, prostate rhabdomyosarcoma, seminal vesicle cyst, Cowper's duct cyst.
Girls: hydrometrocolpos, hydrocolpos, fused labia.

URIC ACID STONES

ICD-9CM # 792.9
ICD-10CM # N20.9 Urolithiasis

Hyperuricemia.
Excessive dietary purine.
Medications (salicylates, allopurinol, probenecid).
Urine pH <5.5 (e.g., diarrhea, high animal protein diet).
Decreased urine output (dehydration, malabsorption, diarrhea, inadequate fluid intake).
Tumor lysis.
Hemolytic anemia.
Myeloproliferative disorders.

URINARY INCONTINENCE, CHILDREN[22a]

ICD-9CM # 788.3 Urinary Incontinence
ICD-10CM # R32 Unspecified urinary incontinence

CAUSES OF URINARY INCONTINENCE IN CHILDHOOD

Overactive bladder.
Infrequent voiding.
Detrusor-sphincter dyssynergia.
Non-neurogenic neurogenic bladder (Hinman syndrome).
Vaginal voiding.
Giggle incontinence.
Cystitis.
Bladder outlet obstruction (posterior urethral valves).
Ectopic ureter and fistula.
Sphincter abnormality (epispadias, exstrophy; urogenital sinus abnormality).
Neuropathic.
Overflow incontinence.
Traumatic.
Iatrogenic.
Behavioral.
Combination.

URINARY RETENTION[24a]

ICD-9CM # 788.20
ICD-10CM # R33.9 Retention of urine, unspecified

COMMON CAUSES OF URINARY RETENTION

Obstructive Cause

Urethral stricture.
Enlarged prostate.
Lower genitourinary tract malignancy.
Pelvic malignancy.
Bladder stones.
Foreign body.
Blood clot.
Posterior urethral valves.
Ureterocele.

Primary Detrusor Insufficiency

Detrusor areflexia.
Multiple sclerosis.
Iatrogenic injury during abdominal or back surgery.
Spinal cord injury.
Myelomeningocele.

URINARY RETENTION, ACUTE

ICD-9CM # 788.20
ICD-10CM # R33.9 Retention of urine, unspecified

Mechanical obstruction: urethral stone, foreign body, urethral stricture, BPH, prostate carcinoma, prostatitis, trauma with hematoma formation.
Neurogenic bladder.
Neurologic disease (MS, parkinsonism, tabes dorsalis, CVA).
Spinal cord injury.
CNS neoplasm (primary or metastatic).
Spinal anesthesia.
Lower urinary tract instrumentation.
Medications (antihistamines, antidepressants, narcotics, anticholinergics).
Abdominal or pelvic surgery.
Alcohol toxicity.
Pregnancy.
Anxiety.
Encephalitis.
Postoperative pain.
Spina bifida occulta.

URINARY TRACT OBSTRUCTION[14a]

ICD-9CM # varies with specific diagnosis
ICD-10CM # N21.8 Other lower urinary tract calculus
N20.9 Urolithiasis

INTRARENAL

Uric acid nephropathy.
Sulfonamide precipitates.
Acyclovir, indinavir precipitates.
Multiple myeloma.

URETERAL

Intrinsic

Intraluminal.
- Nephrolithiasis.
- Papillary necrosis.
- Blood clots.
- Fungus balls.

Intramural.
- Ureteropelvic junction dysfunction.
- Ureterovesical junction dysfunction.
- Ureteral valve, polyp, or tumor.
- Ureteral stricture.
  - Schistosomiasis.
  - Tuberculosis.
  - Scarring from instrumentation.
  - Drugs (e.g., nonsteroidal anti-inflammatory agents [NSAIDs]).

Extrinsic

Vascular system.
- Aneurysm: abdominal aorta or iliac vessels.
- Aberrant vessels: ureteropelvic junction.
- Venous: retrocaval ureter.

Gastrointestinal tract.
- Crohn's disease.
- Diverticulitis.
- Appendiceal abscess.
- Colon cancer.
- Pancreatic tumor, abscess, or cyst.

Reproductive system.
- Uterus: pregnancy, prolapse, tumor, endometriosis.
- Ovary: abscess, tumor, ovarian remnants.
- Gartner's duct cyst, tubo-ovarian abscess.

Retroperitoneal disease.
- Retroperitoneal fibrosis: radiation, drugs, idiopathic.
- Inflammatory: tuberculosis, sarcoidosis.
- Hematoma.
- Primary tumor (e.g., lymphoma, sarcoma).
- Metastatic tumor (e.g., cervix, ovarian, bladder, colon).
- Lymphocele.
- Pelvic lipomatosis.

BLADDER

Neurogenic bladder.
- Diabetes mellitus.
- Spinal cord defect.
- Trauma.
- Multiple sclerosis.
- Stroke.
- Parkinson's disease.
- Spinal anesthesia.
- Anticholinergics.

Bladder neck dysfunction.
Bladder calculus.
Bladder cancer.

URETHRA

Urethral stricture.
Prostate hypertrophy or cancer.
Obstruction from instrumentation.

URINE CASTS

ICD-9CM # 791.7
ICD-10CM # R82.99 Other abnormal findings in urine

Normal finding.
Pyelonephritis.
Chronic renal disease.
Nephrotic syndrome.
Acute tubular necrosis.
Interstitial nephritis.
Nephritic syndrome.
Glomerulonephritis.
Eclampsia.
Heavy metal ingestion.
Allograft rejection.
Hypothyroidism.

URINE COLOR ABNORMALITIES[24a]

ICD-9CM # 791.9
ICD-10CM # R82.5 Elevated urine levels of drugs, medicaments and biological substances
R82.99 Other abnormal findings in urine

COMMON CAUSES OF ABNORMAL URINE COLOR

Colorless

Disease
- Diabetes mellitus.
- Diabetes insipidus.

Drug
- Ethyl alcohol.
- Diuretics.

Miscellaneous
- Overhydration.

Yellow-orange

Drug
- Tetracycline.
- Flutamide.
- Pyridium.
- Azo Gantrisin (Roche Labs, Nutley, NJ).
- Sulfasalazine.
- Vitamin B.

Miscellaneous
- Dehydration.

Milky White

Disease
- Urinary tract infection/pyuria.

Blue-green

Disease
- *Pseudomonas* urinary tract infection.

Drug
- Methylene blue.
- Urised (Polymedica Pharmaceuticals, Woburn, MA).
- Indigo carmine.
- Doan's pills (Novartis Consumer Health, Parsippany, NJ).
- Clorets (Cadbury Adams, Parsippany, NJ).
- Amitriptyline.

Red-brown

Disease
- Hematuria.
- Hemolytic anemia.
- Hemoglobinuria.
- Lead poisoning.
- Mercury poisoning.
- Porphyria.

Drug
- Rifampin.
- Ex-Lax (Novartis Consumer Health, Parsippany, NJ).
- Phenolphthalein.
- Phenothiazines.
- Nitrofurantoin.
- Doxorubicin.

Miscellaneous
- Beets.
- Blackberries.
- Rhubarb.

Brown-black

DISEASE
- Fecaluria.
- Methemoglobinuria.
- Melaninuria.

DRUG
- Metronidazole.
- Methyldopa.
- Methocarbamol.

MISCELLANEOUS
- Fava beans.
- Aloe.

URINE, RED[29]

ICD-9CM # varies with specific diagnosis
ICD-10CM # varies with specific diagnosis

WITH A POSITIVE DIPSTICK

Hematuria.
Hemoglobinuria: negative urinalysis.
Myoglobinuria: negative urinalysis.

WITH A NEGATIVE DIPSTICK

Drugs

Aminosalicylic acid.
Deferoxamine mesylate.
Ibuprofen.
Phenacetin.
Phenolphthalein.
Phensuximide.
Rifampin.
Anthraquinone laxatives.
Doxorubicin.
Methyldopa.
Phenazopyridine.
Phenothiazine.
Phenytoin.

Differential Diagnosis II

Dyes
Azo dyes.
Eosin.
Foods
Beets, berries, maize.
Rhodamine B.
Metabolic
Porphyrins.
Serratia marcescens (red diaper syndrome).
Urate crystalluria.

UROPATHY, OBSTRUCTIVE[36]

ICD-9CM # 599.6
ICD-10CM # N13.9 Obstructive and reflux uropathy, unspecified
N20.9 Urolithiasis

INTRINSIC CAUSES

Intraluminal
Intratubular deposition of crystals (uric acid, sulfas).
Stones.
Papillary tissue.
Blood clots.
Intramural
Functional.
Ureter (ureteropelvic or ureterovesical dysfunction).
Bladder (neurogenic): spinal cord defect or trauma, diabetes, multiple sclerosis, Parkinson's disease, cerebrovascular accidents.
Bladder neck dysfunction.
Anatomic
Tumors.
Infection, granuloma.
Strictures.

EXTRINSIC CAUSES

Originating in the Reproductive System
Prostate: benign hypertrophy or cancer.
Uterus: pregnancy, tumors, prolapse, endometriosis.
Ovary: abscess, tumor, cysts.
Originating in the Vascular System
Aneurysms (aorta, iliac vessels).
Aberrant arteries (ureteropelvic junction).
Venous (ovarian veins, retrocaval ureter).
Originating in the Gastrointestinal Tract
Crohn's disease.
Pancreatitis.
Appendicitis.
Tumors.
Originating in the Retroperitoneal Space
Inflammations.
Fibrosis.
Tumor, hematomas.

UROSEPSIS[24a]

ICD-9CM # 995.91
ICD-10CM # A41.9 Sepsis, unspecified organism

COMMON CAUSES OF UROSEPSIS

Obstructing ureteral stone with pyonephrosis.
Staghorn calculus with urinary tract infection.
Ureteral obstruction with proximal urinary tract infection.
Urinary retention with urinary tract infection.
Acute prostatitis with prostatic abscess.
Perinephric abscess or renal carbuncle.
Urethral stricture with periurethral abscess.
Fournier gangrene.
Foreign body within urinary tract (e.g., Foley catheter).

UTERINE BLEEDING, ABNORMAL[12]

ICD-9CM # 626.9
ICD-10CM # N92.6 Irregular menstruation, unspecified
N93.9 Abnormal uterine and vaginal bleeding, unspecified

PREGNANCY

Threatened abortion.
Incomplete abortion.
Complete abortion.
Molar pregnancy.
Ectopic pregnancy.
Retained products of conception.

OVULATORY

Vulva: infection, laceration, tumor.
Vagina: infection, laceration, tumor, foreign body.
Cervix: polyps, cervical erosion, cervicitis, carcinoma.
Uterus: fibroids (submucous fibroids most likely to cause abnormal bleeding), polyps, adenomyosis, endometritis, intrauterine device, atrophic endometrium.
Pregnancy complications: ectopic pregnancy; threatened, incomplete, complete abortion; retained products of conception.
Abnormality of clotting system.
Midcycle bleeding.
Halban's disease (persistent corpus luteum).
Menorrhagia.
Pelvic inflammatory disease.

ANOVULATORY

Physiologic causes:
- Puberty.
- Perimenopausal.

Pathologic causes:
- Ovarian failure (FSH over 40 IU/ml).
- Hyperandrogenism.
- Hyperprolactinemia.
- Obesity.
- Hypothalamic dysfunction (polycystic ovaries); LH/FSH ratio greater than 2:1.
- Hyperplasia.
- Endometrial carcinoma.
- Estrogen-producing tumors.
- Hypothyroidism.

UVEITIS, PEDIATRIC AGE

ICD-9CM # 364.3
ICD-10CM # H20.9 Anterior uveitis

ANTERIOR UVEITIS

Juvenile rheumatoid arthritis (pauciarticular).
Sarcoidosis.
Trauma.
Tuberculosis.
Kawasaki disease.
Ulcerative colitis.
Postinfectious (enteric or genital) with arthritis and rash.
Spirochetal (syphilis, leptospiral).
Heterochromic iridocyclitis (Fuchs).
Viral (herpes simplex, herpes zoster).
Ankylosing spondylitis.
Stevens-Johnson syndrome.
Idiopathic.
Drugs.

POSTERIOR UVEITIS (CHOROIDITIS—MAY INVOLVE RETINA)

Toxoplasmosis.
Parasites (toxocariasis).
Sarcoidosis.
Tuberculosis.
Viral (rubella, herpes simplex, HIV, cytomegalovirus).
Subacute sclerosing panencephalitis.
Idiopathic.

ANTERIOR AND/OR POSTERIOR UVEITIS

Sympathetic ophthalmia (trauma to other eye).
Vogt-Koyanagi-Harada syndrome (uveo-otocutaneous syndrome: poliosis, vitiligo, deafness, tinnitus, uveitis, aseptic meningitis, retinitis).
Behçet syndrome.
Lyme disease.

VAGINAL BLEEDING, PREGNANCY[7]

ICD-9CM # 626.6 Irregular Vaginal Bleeding
ICD-10CM # N93.9 Abnormal uterine and vaginal bleeding, unspecified

FIRST TRIMESTER

Implantation bleeding.
Abortion.
- Threatened.
- Complete.
- Incomplete.
- Missed.

Ectopic pregnancy.
Neoplasia.
Hydatidiform mole.
Cervix.

THIRD TRIMESTER

Placenta previa.
Placental abruption.
Premature labor.
Choriocarcinoma.

VAGINAL DISCHARGE, PREPUBERTAL GIRLS[19]

ICD-9CM # 623.5 Vaginal Discharge
ICD-10CM # N89.8 Other specified noninflammatory disorders of vagina

Irritative (bubble baths, sand).
Poor perineal hygiene.
Foreign body.
Associated systemic illness (group A streptococci, chickenpox).
Infections.
Escherichia coli with foreign body.
Shigella organisms.
Yersinia organisms.
Infections (consider sexual abuse).
Chlamydia trachomatis.
Neisseria gonorrhoeae.
Trichomonas vaginalis.
Tumor (rare).

VALVULAR HEART DISEASE[1a]

ICD-9CM # varies with specific diagnosis
ICD-10CM # varies with specific diagnosis

MAJOR CAUSES OF VALVULAR HEART DISEASE IN ADULTS

Aortic Stenosis
Bicuspid aortic valve.
Rheumatic fever.
Degenerative stenosis.
Aortic Regurgitation
Bicuspid aortic valve.
Aortic dissection.
Endocarditis.
Rheumatic fever.
Aortic root dilation.
Mitral Stenosis
Rheumatic fever.
Mitral Regurgitation

Chronic

Mitral valve prolapse.
Left ventricular dilation.
Posterior wall myocardial infarction.
Rheumatic fever.
Endocarditis.

Acute

Posterior wall or papillary muscle ischemia.
Papillary muscle or chordal rupture.
Endocarditis.
Prosthetic valve dysfunction.
Systolic anterior motion of mitral valve.

TRICUSPID REGURGITATION

Functional (annular) dilation.
Tricuspid valve prolapse.
Endocarditis.
Carcinoid heart disease.

VASCULITIS, CLASSIFICATION[26]

ICD-9CM # 447.6
ICD-10CM # I77.6 Arteritis, unspecified

LARGE VESSEL DISEASE

Arteritis
Giant cell arteritis.
Takayasu's arteritis.
Arteritis associated with Reiter's syndrome (reactive arthritis), ankylosing spondylitis.

MEDIUM AND SMALL VESSEL DISEASE

Polyarteritis Nodosa
Primary (idiopathic).
Associated with viruses (hepatitis B or C, CMV, HIV, herpes zoster).
Associated with malignancy (hairy cell leukemia).
Familial Mediterranean fever.
Granulomatous Vasculitis
Granulomatosis with polyangiitis (Wegener's granulomatosis).
Lymphomatoid granulomatosis.
Behçet's Disease

Kawasaki Disease (Mucocutaneous Lymph Node Syndrome)

PREDOMINANTLY SMALL VESSEL DISEASE

Hypersensitivity Vasculitis (Leukocytoclastic Vasculitis)
Henoch-Schönlein purpura.
Mixed cryoglobulinemia.
Serum sickness.
Vasculitis associated with connective tissue diseases (SLE, Sjögren's syndrome).
Vasculitis associated with specific syndromes:
Primary biliary cirrhosis.
Lyme disease.
Chronic active hepatitis.
Drug-induced vasculitis.
Churg-Strauss Syndrome
Goodpasture's Syndrome
Erythema Nodosum
Panniculitis
Buerger's Disease (Thrombophlebitis Obliterans)

VASCULITIS (DISEASES THAT MIMIC VASCULITIS)[28]

ICD-9CM # varies with specific disease
ICD-10CM # varies with specific diagnosis

EMBOLIC DISEASE

Infectious or marantic endocarditis.
Cardiac mural thrombus.
Atrial myxoma.
Cholesterol embolization syndrome.

NONINFLAMMATORY VESSEL WALL DISRUPTION

Atherosclerosis.
Arterial fibromuscular dysplasia.
Drug effects (vasoconstrictors, anticoagulants).
Radiation.
Genetic disease (neurofibromatosis, Ehlers-Danlos syndrome).
Amyloidosis.
Intravascular malignant lymphoma.

DIFFUSE COAGULATION

Disseminated intravascular coagulation.
Thrombotic thrombocytopenic purpura.
Hemolytic-uremic syndrome.
Protein C and S deficiencies, factor V/Leiden mutation.
Antiphospholipid syndrome.

VEGETATIVE STATE, PERSISTENT[1a]

ICD-9CM # 780.03
ICD-10CM # R40.3 Persistent vegetative state

PERSISTENT VEGETATIVE STATE: COMMON CAUSES*

Trauma (diffuse axonal injury).
Cardiac arrest and hypoperfusion (laminar necrosis of cortical mantle and/or thalamic necrosis).
Bihemispheric infarctions.
Purulent meningitis or encephalitis (cortical injury).
Carbon monoxide.
Prolonged hypoglycemic coma.

*A vegetative state may not necessarily begin with coma but can also develop as the end stage of neurodegenerative diseases (e.g., Alzheimer's disease) of adults or children and can accompany severe congenital developmental abnormalities of the brain such as anencephaly.

VENTILATION–PERFUSION MISMATCH ON LUNG SCAN

ICD-9CM # varies with specific disorder
ICD-10CM # varies with specific diagnosis

Pulmonary embolism.
Emphysema.
Irradiation.
Pulmonary hypertension.
AV malformations.
Pulmonary thrombosis.
External compression of pulmonary artery (neoplasm, cysts, fibrosing mediastinitis).
Vasculitis.
Tuberculosis.
Pulmonary thrombosis.
Congenital (pulmonary artery hypoplasia, congenital heart disease with upper lobe diversion).
Sequestered segment.
Parasitic lung disease.
Intraluminal obstruction from catheter fragments.

VENTRICULAR FAILURE

ICD-9CM # 429.9 Ventricular Dysfunction
ICD-10CM # I51.9 Heart disease, unspecified

LEFT VENTRICULAR FAILURE

Systemic hypertension.
Valvular heart disease (AS, AR, MR).
Cardiomyopathy, myocarditis.
Bacterial endocarditis.
Myocardial infarction.
Idiopathic hypertrophic subaortic stenosis.

RIGHT VENTRICULAR FAILURE

Valvular heart disease (mitral stenosis).
Pulmonary hypertension.
Bacterial endocarditis (right-sided).
Right ventricular infarction.

BIVENTRICULAR FAILURE

Left ventricular failure.
Cardiomyopathy.
Myocarditis
Arrhythmias.
Anemia.
Thyrotoxicosis.
Arteriovenous fistula.
Paget's disease.
Beriberi.

VERRUCOUS LESIONS

ICD-9CM #	varies with specific disorder
ICD-10CM #	varies with specific diagnosis

Warts.
Seborrheic keratosis.
Lichen simplex.
Acanthosis nigricans.
Scabies (Norwegian, crusted).
Verrucous carcinoma.
Nevus sebaceous.
Deep fungal infection.

VERTIGO

ICD-9CM #	780.4	Vertigo NOS
	386.11	Benign Paroxysmal Positional
	386.2	Central Origin
	386.10	Peripheral
	386.12	Vestibular (Neuronitis)
ICD-10CM #	R42	Dizziness and giddiness
	H81.13	Benign paroxysmal vertigo, bilateral
	H81.49	Vertigo of central origin, unspecified ear
	H81.399	Other peripheral vertigo, unspecified ear
	H81.23	Vestibular neuronitis, bilateral

PERIPHERAL

Otitis media.
Acute labyrinthitis.
Vestibular neuronitis.
Benign positional vertigo.
Meniere's disease.
Ototoxic drugs: streptomycin, gentamicin.
Lesions of the eighth nerve: acoustic neuroma, meningioma, mononeuropathy, metastatic carcinoma.
Mastoiditis.

CNS OR SYSTEMIC

Vertebrobasilar artery insufficiency.
Posterior fossa tumor or other brain tumors.
Infarction/hemorrhage of cerebral cortex, cerebellum, or brain stem.
Basilar migraine.
Metabolic: drugs, hypoxia, anemia, fever.
Hypotension/severe hypertension.
Multiple sclerosis.
CNS infections: viral, bacterial.
Temporal lobe epilepsy.
Arnold–Chiari malformation, syringobulbia.
Psychogenic: ventilation, hysteria.

VERTIGO, CENTRAL[1]

ICD-9CM #	780.4
ICD-10CM #	R42

MAJOR CAUSES OF CENTRAL VERTIGO

Demyelination.
- Acquired.
- Leukodystrophies.
- Multiple sclerosis.

Familial disorders.
- Friedreich ataxia.
- Spinocerebellar ataxia.
- Familial episodic ataxia (type 1 and type 2).
- Olivopontocerebellar atrophy.

Central nervous system infections.
- Lyme neuroborreliosis.
- Meningitis.
- Tuberculosis.

Intrinsic brainstem lesion.
- Tumor.
- Arteriovenous malformation.
- Trauma.

Migraine.
- Basilar.
- Benign paroxysmal positional vertigo of childhood.

Toxins.
- Drugs, alcohol.
- Analgesics.
- Anticonvulsants.
- Antihypertensives.
- Hypnotics.
- Tranquilizers.

Metabolic and endocrine disorders.
- Hyperinsulinism.
- Impaired glucose tolerance.
- Diabetes mellitus.
- Hypertriglyceridemia.
- Hypothyroidism.

Systemic conditions.
- Paget disease.

Stroke/ischemia.
- Vertebrobasilar.
- Cerebellar.
- Posterior inferior cerebellar artery syndrome.
- Lateral medullary syndrome.
- Medial medullary infarct.
- Basilar artery syndrome.
- Anterior inferior cerebellar artery.

Other causes of posterior ischemia.
- Subclavian steal syndrome.
- Rotational vertebral artery occlusion syndrome.
- Vertebral artery dissection.
- Vertebral or basilar artery dolichoectasia.
- Neoplasm of the fourth ventricle.
- Chiari malformation.

Superficial siderosis of the central nervous system.
Vestibular epilepsy.

VESICULOBULLOUS DISEASES[14]

ICD-9CM #	709.8	
ICD-10CM #	L94.2	Calcinosis cutis
	L98.8	Other specified disorders of the skin and subcutaneous tissue

IMMUNOLOGICALLY MEDIATED DISEASES

Bullous pemphigoid.
Herpes gestationis.
Mucous membrane pemphigoid.
Epidermolysis bullosa acquisita.
Dermatitis herpetiformis.
Pemphigus (vulgaris, foliaceus, paraneoplastic).

HYPERSENSITIVITY DISEASES

Erythema multiforme minor.
Erythema multiforme major (Stevens-Johnson syndrome).
Toxic epidermal necrolysis.

METABOLIC DISEASES

Porphyria cutanea tarda.
Pseudoporphyria.
Diabetic blisters.

INHERITED GENETIC DISORDERS

Epidermolysis bullosa.
Simplex.
Junctional.
Dystrophic.

INFECTIOUS DISEASES

Impetigo.
Staphylococcal scalded skin syndrome.
Herpes simplex.
Varicella.
Herpes zoster.

VISION LOSS, ACUTE, PAINFUL

ICD-9CM #	368.11	Vision Loss, Sudden
ICD-10CM #	H53.139	Sudden visual loss, unspecified eye

Acute angle-closure glaucoma.
Corneal ulcer.
Uveitis.
Endophthalmitis.
Factitious.
Somatization syndrome.
Trauma.

VISION LOSS, ACUTE, PAINLESS

ICD-9CM #	368.11	Vision Loss, Sudden
ICD-10CM #	H53.139	Sudden visual loss, unspecified eye

Retinal artery occlusion.
Optic neuritis.
Retinal vein occlusion.
Vitreous hemorrhage.
Retinal detachment.
Exudative macular degeneration.
CVA.
Ischemic optic neuropathy.
Factitious.
Somatization syndrome, anxiety reaction.

VISION LOSS AFTER DIVING[1b]

ICD-9CM # 368.11
ICD-10CM # H53.139

DIFFERENTIAL DIAGNOSIS OF DECREASED VISION AFTER DIVING

Decompression sickness.
Arterial gas embolism.
Bubbles under contact lenses.
Displaced contact lens.
Antifog agent keratopathy.
Contact lens adherence syndrome.
Transdermal scopolamine
Hyperoxic myopia.
Oxymetazoline optic neuropathy.
Diving-induced migraine phenomena.
Eye disorders not related to diving.

VISION LOSS, CHILDREN

ICD-9CM # 368.9
ICD-10CM # H53.9 Unspecified visual disturbance

Craniopharyngioma.
Hereditary optic atrophy.
Optic nerve glioma.
Glioma of chiasm.
Albinism.
Optic nerve hypoplasia.

VISION LOSS, CHRONIC, PROGRESSIVE

ICD-9CM # 369.9 Vision Loss NOS
ICD-10CM # H54.7 Unspecified visual loss

Cataract.
Macular degeneration.
Cerebral neoplasm.
Refractive error.
Open-angle glaucoma.

VISION LOSS, MONOCULAR, TRANSIENT

ICD-9CM # 369.9
ICD-10CM # H54.7 Unspecified visual loss

Thromboembolism.
Vasculitis.
Migraine (vasospasm).
Anxiety reaction.
CNS tumor.
Temporal arteritis.
Multiple sclerosis.

VITREOUS HEMORRHAGE[20a]

ICD-9CM # 379.23 Vitreous Hemorrhage
ICD-10CM # H43.13 Vitreous hemorrhage, bilateral

CAUSES OF VITREOUS HEMORRHAGE

Acute posterior vitreous detachment associated either with a retinal tear or avulsion of a peripheral vessel.
Proliferative retinopathies.
- Diabetic.
- Following retinal vein occlusion.
- Sickle cell disease.
- Eales disease.
- Vasculitis.

Miscellaneous retinal disorders.
- Macroaneurysm.
- Telangiectasis.
- Capillary hemangioma.

Trauma.
- Blunt.
- Penetrating.
- Iatrogenic.

Systemic.
- Bleeding disorders.
- Terson syndrome.

VOCAL CORD PARALYSIS

ICD-9CM # 478.30 Unspecified
478.31 Unilateral Partial
478.32 Unilateral Complete
478.33 Bilateral Partial
478.34 Bilateral Complete
ICD-10CM # J38.00 Paralysis of vocal cords and larynx, unspecified
J38.01 Paralysis of vocal cords and larynx, unilateral
J38.02 Paralysis of vocal cords and larynx, bilateral

Neoplasm: primary or metastatic (e.g., lung, thyroid, parathyroid, mediastinum).
Neck surgery (parathyroid, thyroid, carotid endarterectomy, cervical spine).
Idiopathic.
Viral, bacterial, or fungal infection.
Trauma (intubation, penetrating neck injury).
Cardiac surgery.
RA.
Multiple sclerosis.
Parkinsonism.
Toxic neuropathy.
CVA.
CNS abnormalities: hydrocephalus, Arnold–Chiari malformation, meningomyelocele.

VOLUME DEPLETION[1a]

ICD-9CM # 276.5
ICD-10CM # E86.9 Volume depletion, unspecified

GI losses:
Upper: bleeding, nasogastric suction, vomiting.
Lower: bleeding, diarrhea, enteric or pancreatic fistula, tube drainage.
Renal losses:
Salt and water: diuretics, osmotic diuresis, postobstructive diuresis, acute tubular necrosis (recovery phase), salt-losing nephropathy, adrenal insufficiency, renal tubular acidosis.
Water loss: diabetes insipidus.
Skin and respiratory losses:
Sweat, burns, insensible losses.
Sequestration without external fluid loss:
Intestinal obstruction, peritonitis, pancreatitis, rhabdomyolysis, internal bleeding.

VOLUME EXCESS[1a]

ICD-9CM # varies with specific diagnosis
ICD-10CM # varies with specific diagnosis

PRIMARY RENAL SODIUM RETENTION (INCREASED EFFECTIVE CIRCULATING VOLUME)

Renal failure, nephritic syndrome, acute glomerulonephritis.
Primary hyperaldosteronism.
Cushing's syndrome.
Liver disease.

SECONDARY RENAL SODIUM RETENTION (DECREASED EFFECTIVE CIRCULATING VOLUME)

Heart failure.
Liver disease.
Nephrotic syndrome (minimal change disease).
Pregnancy.

VOMITING

ICD-9CM # 787.03
ICD-10CM # R11.10 Vomiting, unspecified
R11.11 Vomiting without nausea
R11.12 Projectile vomiting

GI disturbances:
Obstruction: esophageal, pyloric, intestinal.
Infections: viral or bacterial enteritis, viral hepatitis, food poisoning, gastroenteritis.
Pancreatitis.
Appendicitis.
Biliary colic.
Peritonitis.
Perforated bowel.
Diabetic gastroparesis.

Other: gastritis, PUD, IBD, GI tract neoplasms.
Drugs: morphine, digitalis, cytotoxic agents, bromocriptine.
Severe pain: MI, renal colic.
Metabolic disorders: uremia, acidosis/alkalosis, hyperglycemia, DKA, thyrotoxicosis.
Trauma: blows to the testicles, epigastrium.
Vertigo.
Reye's syndrome.
Increased intracranial pressure.
CNS disturbances: trauma, hemorrhage, infarction, neoplasm, infection, hypertensive encephalopathy, migraine.
Radiation sickness.
Nausea and vomiting of pregnancy, hyperemesis gravidarum.
Motion sickness.
Bulimia, anorexia nervosa.
Psychogenic: emotional disturbances, offensive sights or smells.
Severe coughing.
Pyelonephritis.
Boerhaave's syndrome.
Carbon monoxide poisoning.

VOMITING, NEONATAL[1]

ICD-9CM # 787.03
ICD-10CM # R11.10

CAUSES OF NEONATAL VOMITING

Anatomic Causes

Esophagus, trachea, great vessels:
- Stricture.
- Web.
- Tracheoesophageal fistula.
- Laryngeal cleft.
- Double aortic arch.

Stomach and duodenum:
- Pyloric stenosis.
- Duodenal atresia (usually noted on the first day of life)

Small and large intestine:
- Volvulus secondary to malrotation.
- Incarcerated hernia.
- Hirschsprung disease (secondary to obstipation).
- Necrotizing enterocolitis.

Genitourinary:
- Testicular torsion.

Nonanatomic Causes

Infection:
- Septicemia.
- Meningitis.
- Urinary tract infection.
- Gastroenteritis.
- Otitis media

Increased intracranial pressure:
- Cerebral edema.
- Subdural hematoma.
- Hydrocephalus.
- Brain tumor.

Congenital adrenal hyperplasia (salt-losing variety).
Inborn errors of metabolism.
Renal disease.

VULVAR LESIONS[12]

ICD-9CM #	625.8	Vulvar Mass
	098.0	Vulvar Ulcer, Gonococcal
	091.0	Vulvar Ulcer, Syphilitic
	616.51	Behçet's
	624.0	Leukoplakia
	624.8	Dysplasia
	233.3	Carcinoma
	616.9	Inflammatory Lesion
	624.4	Vulvar Scar (Old)
	624.1	Vulvar Atrophy
ICD-10CM #	N77.0	Ulceration of vulva in diseases classified elsewhere
	N90.7	Vulvar cyst
	N90.89	Other specified noninflammatory disorders of vulva and perineum
	D07.1	Carcinoma in situ of vulva
	N90.89	Other specified noninflammatory disorders of vulva and perineum
	N90.5	Atrophy of vulva

RED LESION

Infection/Infestation

Fungal infection:
 Candida.
 Tinea cruris.
 Intertrigo.
 Pityriasis versicolor.
Sarcoptes scabiei.
Erythrasma: *Corynebacterium minutissimum.*
Granuloma inguinale: Calymmatobacterium granulomatis.
Folliculitis: *Staphylococcus aureus.*
Hidradenitis suppurativa.
Behçet's syndrome.

Inflammation

Reactive vulvitis.
Chemical irritation:
 Detergent.
 Dyes.
 Perfume.
 Spermicide.
 Lubricants.
 Hygiene sprays.
 Podophyllum.
 Topical 5-FU.
 Saliva.
 Gentian violet.
 Semen.
Mechanical trauma: scratching.
Vestibular adenitis.
Essential vulvodynia.
Psoriasis.
Seborrheic dermatitis.

Neoplasm

Vulvar intraepithelial neoplasia (VIN):
 Mild dysplasia.
 Moderate dysplasia.
 Severe dysplasia.
 Carcinoma-in-situ.
Vulvar dystrophy.
Bowen's disease.
Invasive cancer:
 Squamous cell carcinoma.
 Malignant melanoma.
 Sarcoma.
 Basal cell carcinoma.
 Adenocarcinoma.
 Paget's disease.
 Undifferentiated.

WHITE LESION

Vulvar dystrophy:
 Lichen sclerosus.
 Vulvar dystrophy.
 Vulvar hyperplasia.
 Mixed dystrophy.
VIN.
Vitiligo.
Partial albinism.
Intertrigo.
Radiation treatment.

DARK LESION

Lentigo.
Nevi (mole).
Neoplasm (see "Neoplasm, Vulvar," below).
Reactive hyperpigmentation.
Seborrheic keratosis.
Pubic lice.

ULCERATIVE LESION

Infection

Herpes simplex.
Vaccinia.
Treponema pallidum.
Granuloma inguinale.
Pyoderma.
Tuberculosis.

Noninfectious

Behçet's disease.
Crohn's disease.
Pemphigus.
Pemphigoid.
Hidradenitis suppurativa (see "Neoplasm, Vulvar," below).

Neoplasm

Basal cell carcinoma.
Squamous cell carcinoma.
Vulvar tumor <1 cm:
 Condyloma acuminatum.
 Molluscum contagiosum.
 Epidermal inclusion.
 Vestibular cyst.
 Mesonephric duct.
 VIN.
 Hemangioma.
 Hidradenoma.
 Neurofibroma.
 Syringoma.
 Accessory breast tissue.
 Acrochordon.
 Endometriosis.
 Fox-Fordyce disease.
 Pilonidal sinus.
Vulvar tumor >1 cm:
 Bartholin cyst or abscess.
 Lymphogranuloma venereum.
 Fibroma.

Lipoma.
Verrucous carcinoma.
Squamous cell carcinoma.
Hernia.
Edema.
Hematoma.
Acrochordon.
Epidermal cysts.
Neurofibromatosis.
Accessory breast tissue.

WEAKNESS, ACUTE, EMERGENT[26]

ICD-9CM # 780.7
ICD-10CM # M62.81 Muscle weakness (generalized)

Demyelinating disorders (Guillain-Barré, chronic inflammatory demyelinating polyneuropathy [CIDP]).
Myasthenia gravis.
Infectious (poliomyelitis, diphtheria).
Toxic (botulism, tick paralysis, paralytic shellfish toxin, puffer fish, newts).
Metabolic (acquired or familial hypokalemia, hypophosphatemia, hypermagnesemia).
Metal poisoning (arsenic, thallium).
Porphyria.

WEAKNESS, GRADUAL ONSET

ICD-9CM # 780.7
ICD-10CM # M62.81 Muscle weakness (generalized)

Depression.
Malingering.
Anemia.
Hypothyroidism.
Medications (e.g., sedatives, antidepressants, narcotics).
CHF.
Renal failure.
Liver failure.
Respiratory insufficiency.
Alcoholism.
Nutritional deficiencies.
Disorders of motor unit.
Basal ganglia disorders.
Upper motor neuron lesions.

WEAKNESS, NONNEUROMUSCULAR CAUSES

ICD-9CM # 780.79
ICD-10CM # G93.3 Postviral fatigue syndrome
R53.1 Weakness
R53.81 Other malaise
R53.83 Other fatigue

Anxiety disorder.
Infectious process.
Anemia.
Renal insufficiency.
Hyperventilation.
Malignancy.
Hypothyroidism.
Hypotension.
Hypercapnia.
Hypoglycemia.
Cardiac arrhythmias.
Hepatic insufficiency.
Electrolyte imbalance.
Malnutrition.
Cerebrovascular insufficiency.

WEIGHT GAIN

ICD-9CM # 783.1 Abnormal Weight Gain
278.00 Obesity
ICD-10CM # R63.5 Abnormal weight gain
E66.9 Obesity, unspecified

Sedentary lifestyle.
Fluid overload.
Discontinuation of tobacco abuse.
Endocrine disorders (hypothyroidism, hyperinsulinism associated with maturity-onset DM, Cushing's syndrome, hypogonadism, insulinoma, hyperprolactinemia, acromegaly).
Medications (nutritional supplements, oral contraceptives, glucocorticoids, etc.).
Anxiety disorders with compulsive eating.
Laurence-Moon-Biedl syndrome, Prader-Willi syndrome, other congenital diseases.
Hypothalamic injury (rare; <100 cases reported in medical literature).

WEIGHT LOSS

ICD-9CM # 783.2 Abnormal Weight Loss
ICD-10CM # R63.4 Abnormal weight loss

Malignancy.
Psychiatric disorders (depression, anorexia nervosa).
New-onset DM.
Malabsorption.
COPD.
AIDS.
Uremia, liver disease.
Thyrotoxicosis, pheochromocytoma, carcinoid syndrome.
Addison's disease.
Intestinal parasites.
Peptic ulcer disease.
Inflammatory bowel disease.
Food faddism.
Postgastrectomy syndrome.

WHEEZING

ICD-9CM # 786.09
ICD-10CM # R06.2 Wheezing

Asthma.
COPD.
Interstitial lung disease.
Infections (pneumonia, bronchitis, bronchiolitis, epiglottitis).
Cardiac asthma.
GERD with aspiration.
Foreign body aspiration.
Pulmonary embolism.
Anaphylaxis.
Obstruction of airway (neoplasm, goiter, edema or hemorrhage from trauma, aneurysm, congenital abnormalities, strictures, spasm).
Carcinoid syndrome.

WHEEZING, PEDIATRIC AGE[4]

ICD-9CM # 786.09 Wheezing
ICD-10CM # R06.2 Wheezing

Reactive airways disease.
Atopic asthma.
Infection-associated airway reactivity.
Exercise-induced asthma.
Salicylate-induced asthma and nasal polyposis.
Asthmatic bronchitis.
Other hypersensitivity reactions:
- Hypersensitivity pneumonitis.
- Tropical eosinophilia.
- Visceral larva migrans.
- Allergic bronchopulmonary aspergillosis.

Aspiration:
- Foreign body.
- Food, saliva, gastric contents.
- Laryngotracheoesophageal cleft.
- Tracheoesophageal fistula, H-type.
- Pharyngeal incoordination or neuromuscular weakness.

Cystic fibrosis.
Primary ciliary dyskinesia.
Cardiac failure.
Bronchiolitis obliterans.
Extrinsic compression of airways:
- Vascular ring.
- Enlarged lymph node.
- Mediastinal tumor.
- Lung cysts.

Tracheobronchomalacia.
Endobronchial masses.
Gastroesophageal reflux.
Pulmonary hemosiderosis.
Sequelae of bronchopulmonary dysplasia.
"Hysterical" glottic closure.
Cigarette smoke, other environmental insults.

WRIST AND HAND PAIN, IN DIFFERENT AGE GROUPS[8]

ICD-9CM # 959.3
ICD-10CM # S69.80XA Other specified injuries of unspecified wrist, hand and finger(s), initial encounter
S69.90XA Unspecified injury of unspecified wrist, hand and finger(s), initial encounter

COMMON CAUSES OF WRIST AND HAND PAIN IN DIFFERENT AGE GROUPS

CHILDHOOD (2-10 YR)

Intraarticular:
Infection.

Periarticular:
Fracture.
Osteomyelitis.

ADOLESCENCE (10-18 YR)
Intraarticular:
Infection.
Periarticular:
Trauma.
Osteomyelitis.
Tumors.
Ganglion.
Idiopathic wrist pain.
EARLY ADULTHOOD (18-30 YR)
Intraarticular:
Inflammatory arthritis.
Infection.
Osteoarthritis.
Periarticular:
Peripheral nerve entrapment.
Tendonitis.
Referred:
Cervical.
ADULTHOOD (30-50 YR)
Intraarticular:
Inflammatory arthritis.
Infection.
Osteoarthritis.
Periarticular:
Peripheral nerve entrapment.
Tendonitis.
Referred:
Cervical.
Chest.
Cardiac.
OLD AGE (>50 YR)
Intraarticular:
Inflammatory arthritis.
Osteoarthritis.
Periarticular:
Peripheral nerve entrapment.
Tendonitis.
Referred:
Cervical.
Chest.
Cardiac.

WRIST PAIN

ICD-9CM #	959.3	
ICD-10CM #	S69.80XA	Other specified injuries of unspecified wrist, hand and finger(s), initial encounter
	S69.90XA	Unspecified injury of unspecified wrist, hand and finger(s), initial encounter

MECHANICAL

Osteoarthritis.
Ligament tear.
Fracture.
Ganglion.
De Quervain's tenosynovitis.
Avascular necrosis (scaphoid, lunate).
Nonunion of scaphoid or lunate.
Neoplasm.

METABOLIC

Pregnancy.
Diabetes.
Gout.
Pseudogout.
Paget's disease.
Acromegaly.
Hypothyroidism.
Hyperparathyroidism.

INFECTIOUS

Osteomyelitis.
Septic arthritis.
Cat-scratch disease.
Tick bite (Lyme disease, babesiosis).
Tuberculosis.

NEUROLOGIC

Peripheral neuropathy.
Nerve injury (median, ulnar, radial nerve).
Thoracic outlet compression syndrome.
Distal posterior interosseous nerve syndrome.

RHEUMATOLOGIC

Psoriasis.
RA.
SLE, mixed connective tissue disorder (MCTD).
Scleroderma.

MISCELLANEOUS

Granulomatous (sarcoidosis).
Amyloidosis.
Multiple myeloma.
Leukemia.

XEROPHTHALMIA[28]

ICD-9CM #	372.53	Xerophthalmia
ICD-10CM #	H11.149	Conjunctival xerosis, unspecified, unspecified eye

MEDICATIONS

Tricyclic antidepressants: amitriptyline (Elavil), doxepin (Sinequan).
Antihistamines: diphenhydramine (Benadryl), chlorpheniramine (Chlor-Trimeton), promethazine (Phenergan), and many cold and decongestant preparations.
Anticholinergic agents: antiemetics such as scopolamine, antispasmodic agents such as oxybutynin chloride (Ditropan).

ABNORMALITIES OF EYELID FUNCTION

Neuromuscular disorders.
Aging.
Thyrotoxicosis.

ABNORMALITIES OF TEAR PRODUCTION

Hypovitaminosis A.
Stevens-Johnson syndrome.
Familial diseases affecting sebaceous secretions.

ABNORMALITIES OF CORNEAL SURFACES

Scarring from past injuries and herpes simplex infection.

XEROSTOMIA[28]

ICD-9CM #	527.7	
ICD-10CM #	K11.7	Disturbances of salivary secretion
	R68.2	Dry mouth, unspecified

MEDICATIONS

Tricyclic antidepressants: amitriptyline (Elavil), doxepin (Sinequan).
Antihistamines: diphenhydramine (Benadryl), chlorpheniramine (Chlor-Trimeton), promethazine (Phenergan), and many cold and decongestant preparations.
Anticholinergic agents: antiemetics such as scopolamine, antispasmodic agents such as oxybutynin chloride (Ditropan).

DEHYDRATION

Debility.
Fever.

POLYURIA

Alcohol intake.
Arrhythmia.
Diabetes.

PREVIOUS HEAD AND NECK IRRADIATION SYSTEMIC DISEASES

Sjögren's syndrome.
Sarcoidosis.
Amyloidosis.
Human immunodeficiency virus (HIV) infection.
Graft-versus-host disease.

YELLOW URINE

ICD-9CM #	788.69	
ICD-10CM #	R82	Other abnormal findings in urine

Normal coloration.
Concentrated urine.
Use of multivitamin supplements.
Diet rich in carrots.
Use of Cascara.
Urinary tract infection

REFERENCES

1. From Adams JG, et al: *Emergency medicine, clinical essentials*, ed 2, Philadelphia, 2013, Elsevier.

1a. Andreoli TE, editor: *Cecil essentials of medicine*, ed 5, Philadelphia, 2001, Saunders.

1b. Auerbach P: *Wilderness medicine*, Philadelphia, 2012, Saunders.

1c. *Ballinger A: Kumar & Clark's essentials of clinical medicine*, ed 6, Edinburgh, 2012, Saunders.

2. Barkin RM, Rosen P: *Emergency pediatrics: a guide to ambulatory care*, ed 5, St Louis, 1998, Mosby.

3. Baude AI: *Infectious diseases and medical microbiology*, ed 2, Philadelphia, 1986, Saunders.

4. Behrman RE: *Nelson textbook of pediatrics*, ed 16, Philadelphia, 2000, Saunders.

4a. Bonow RO, et al.: *Braunwauld's heart disease*, ed 9, Philadelphia, 2012, Elsevier.

5. Callen JP: *Color atlas of dermatology*, ed 2, Philadelphia, 2000, WB Saunders.

5a. Cameron JL, Cameron AM: *Current surgical therapy*, ed 10, Philadelphia, 2011, Saunders.

6. Canoso J: *Rheumatology in primary care*, Philadelphia, 1997, Saunders.

7. Carlson KJ: *Primary care of women*, ed 2, St Louis, 2000, Mosby.

8. Carr A, Hamilton W: *Orthopedics in primary care*, ed 2, Philadelphia, 2005, Saunders.

9. Conn R: *Current diagnosis*, ed 9, Philadelphia, 1997, Saunders.

10. Copeland LJ: *Textbook of gynecology*, ed 2, Philadelphia, 2000, Saunders.

11. Custer JW, Rau RE: *The Harriet Lane handbook*, ed 18, St Louis, 2009, Mosby.

12. Danakas G (ed): *Practical guide to the care of the gynecologic/obstetric patient*, St Louis, 1997, Mosby.

12a. Firestein GS, Budd RC, Gabriel SE, et al.: *Kelly's textbook of rheumatology*, ed 9, Philadelphia, 2013, Saunders.

12b. Floege J, et al: *Comprehensive clinical nephrology*, ed 4, Philadelphia, 2010, Saunders.

12C. Fuhrman BP, et al.: *Pediatric critical care*, ed 4, Philadelphia, 2011, Saunders.

13. Goldberg RJ: *The care of the psychiatric patient*, ed 3, St Louis, 2006, Mosby.

14. Goldman L, Ausiello D: *Cecil textbook of medicine*, ed 21, Philadelphia, 2004, Saunders.

14a. Goldman L, Schafer AI: *Goldman's Cecil medicine*, ed 24, Philadelphia, 2012, Saunders.

15. Goldman L, Braunwauld E, editors: *Primary cardiology*, Philadelphia, 1998, Saunders.

16. Gorbach SL: *Infectious diseases*, ed 2, Philadelphia, 1998, Saunders.

16a. Grainger RG, Allison D: *Grainger & Allison's diagnostic radiology, a textbook of medical imaging*, ed 4, London, 2001, Churchill Livingstone.

17. Harrington J: *Consultation in internal medicine*, ed 2, St Louis, 1997, Mosby.

18. Henry JB: *Clinical diagnosis and management by laboratory methods*, ed 20, Philadelphia, 2001, Saunders.

18b. Hochberg MC, et al.: *Rheumatology*, ed 5, St. Louis, 2011, Mosby.

19. Hoekelman R: *Primary pediatric care*, ed 3, St Louis, 1997, Mosby.

20. Hoffmann R, et al.: *Hematology: basic principles and practice*, ed 5, Philadelphia, 2009, Churchill Livingstone.

20a. Kanski JJ, Bowling B: *Clinical ophthalmology, a systematic approach*, ed 7, Philadelphia, 2011, Saunders.

21. Kassirer J, (ed): *Current therapy in adult medicine*, ed 4, St Louis, 1998, Mosby.

22. Khan MG: *Rapid ECG interpretation*, Philadelphia, 2003, Saunders.

22a. Kliegman RM, et al.: *Nelson textbook of pediatrics*, ed 19, Philadelphia, 2011, Saunders.

23. Kliegman R: *Practical strategies in pediatric diagnosis and therapy*, Philadelphia, 1996, Saunders.

24. Klippel J, (ed): *Practical rheumatology*, London, 1995, Mosby.

24a. Lipshultz LI, Khera M, Atwal DT: *Urology and the primary care practitioner*, ed 3, Philadelphia, 2008, Elsevier.

25. Melmed S, Polonsky KS, Larsen PR, Kronenberg HM: *Williams textbook of endocrinology*, ed 12, Philadelphia, 2011, Saunders.

25a. Mandell GL: *Mandell, Douglas, and Bennett's principles and practice of infectious diseases*, ed 6, New York, 2005, Churchill Livingstone.

26. Marx J, (ed): *Rosen's emergency medicine: concepts and clinical practice*, ed 5, St Louis, 2002, Mosby.

26a. Melmed S, Polonsky KS, Larsen PR, Kronenberg HM: *Williams textbook of endocrinology*, ed 12, Philadelphia, 2011, Saunders.

27. Moore WT, Eastman RC: *Diagnostic endocrinology*, ed 2, St Louis, 1996, Mosby.

28. Noble J, (ed): *Primary care medicine*, ed 3, St Louis, 2001, Mosby.

29. Nseyo UO: *Urology for primary care physicians*, Philadelphia, 1999, Saunders.

30. Palay D (ed): *Ophthalmology for the primary care physician*, St Louis, 1997, Mosby.

31. Rakel RE: *Principles of family practice*, ed 6, Philadelphia, 2002, Saunders.

32. Schwarz MI: *Interstitial lung disease*, ed 2, St Louis, 1993, Mosby.

33. Seller RH: *Differential diagnosis of common complaints*, ed 4, Philadelphia, 2000, Saunders.

34. Siedel HM (ed): *Mosby's guide to physical examination*, ed 4, St Louis, 1999, Mosby.

34a. Souhami RL, Moxham J: *Textbook of medicine*, ed 4, London, 2002, Churchill Livingstone.

35. Specht N: *Practical guide to diagnostic imaging*, St Louis, 1998, Mosby.

36. Stein JH (ed): *Internal medicine*, ed 5, St Louis, 1998, Mosby.

37. Swain R, Snodgrass JG: Managing groin pain, *Phys Sportmed* 23:56, 1995.

38. Talley NJ, Martin CJ: *Clinical gastroenterology*, ed 2, Sydney, 2006, Churchill Livingstone.

38a. Tschudy MM, Arcara KM: *The Harriet Lane handbook*, ed 19, Philadelphia, 2012, Mosby.

38b. Vincent JL, et al.: *Textbook of critical care*, ed 6, Philadelphia, 2011, Saunders.

39. Weinberg SE, et al.: *Principles of pulmonary medicine*, ed 5, Philadelphia, 2008, Saunders.

40. Wiederholt WC: *Neurology for non-neurologists*, ed 4, Philadelphia, 2000, Saunders.

41. Wilson JD: *Williams textbook of endocrinology*, ed 9, Philadelphia, 1998, Saunders.

Clinical Algorithms*

*Please note that the implementation of the ICD-10CM codes has been delayed until at least 2015; therefore, for billing purposes please use the ICD-9CM codes until the ICD-10CM codes are officially implemented.

PLEASE NOTE: These algorithms are designed to assist clinicians in the evaluation and treatment of patients. They may not apply to all patients with a particular disorder and are not intended to replace the clinician's individual judgment.

Additional algorithms available at www.expertconsult.com

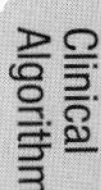

ICD-9CM # 789.61
ICD-10CM # R10.1 Abdominal pain, upper abdomen

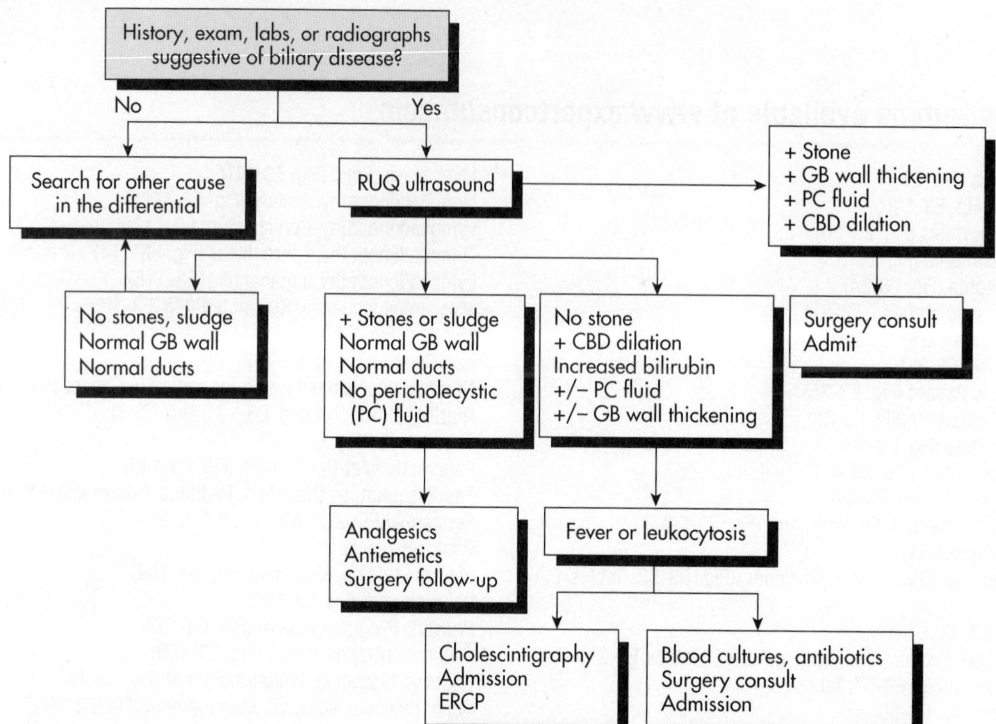

FIGURE 3-1 Treatment algorithm for right upper quadrant (RUQ) pain. *CBD*, Common bile duct; *ERCP*, endoscopic retrograde cholangiopancreatography; *GB*, gallbladder; *RUQ*, right upper quadrant; +, with; −, without; ±, with or without. (From Adams JG et al: *Emergency medicine, clinical essentials,* ed 2, Philadelphia, 2013, Elsevier.)

ICD-9CM # 276.2 Lactic acidosis
276.2 Metabolic acidosis
276.2 Respiratory acidosis
276.3 Respiratory alkalosis
276.3 Metabolic alkalosis
ICD-10CM # E87.2 Acidosis
E87.3 Alkalosis

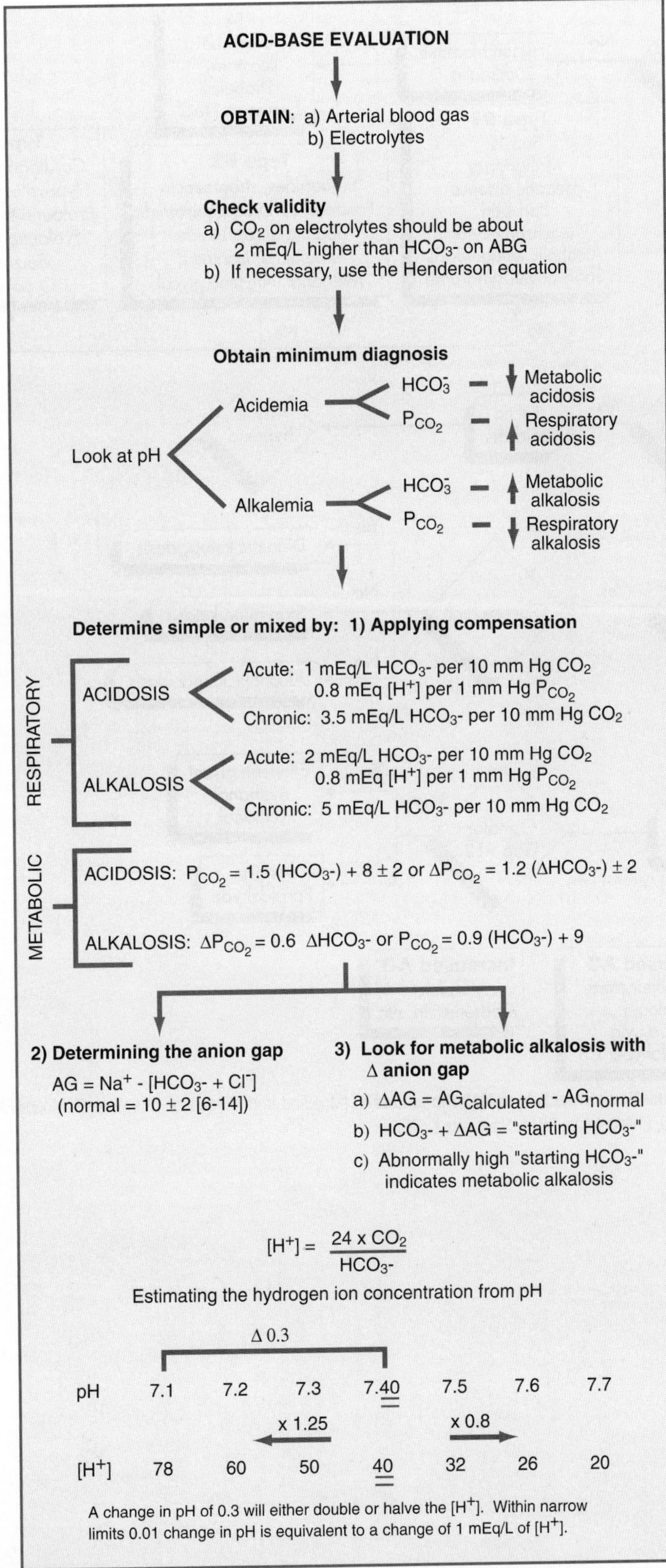

FIGURE 3-2 Scheme for assessing acid-base homeostasis. (From Andreoli TE [ed]: *Cecil essentials of medicine*, ed 7, Philadelphia, 2008, Saunders.)

ICD-9CM # 276.2
ICD-10CM # E87.2 Acidosis

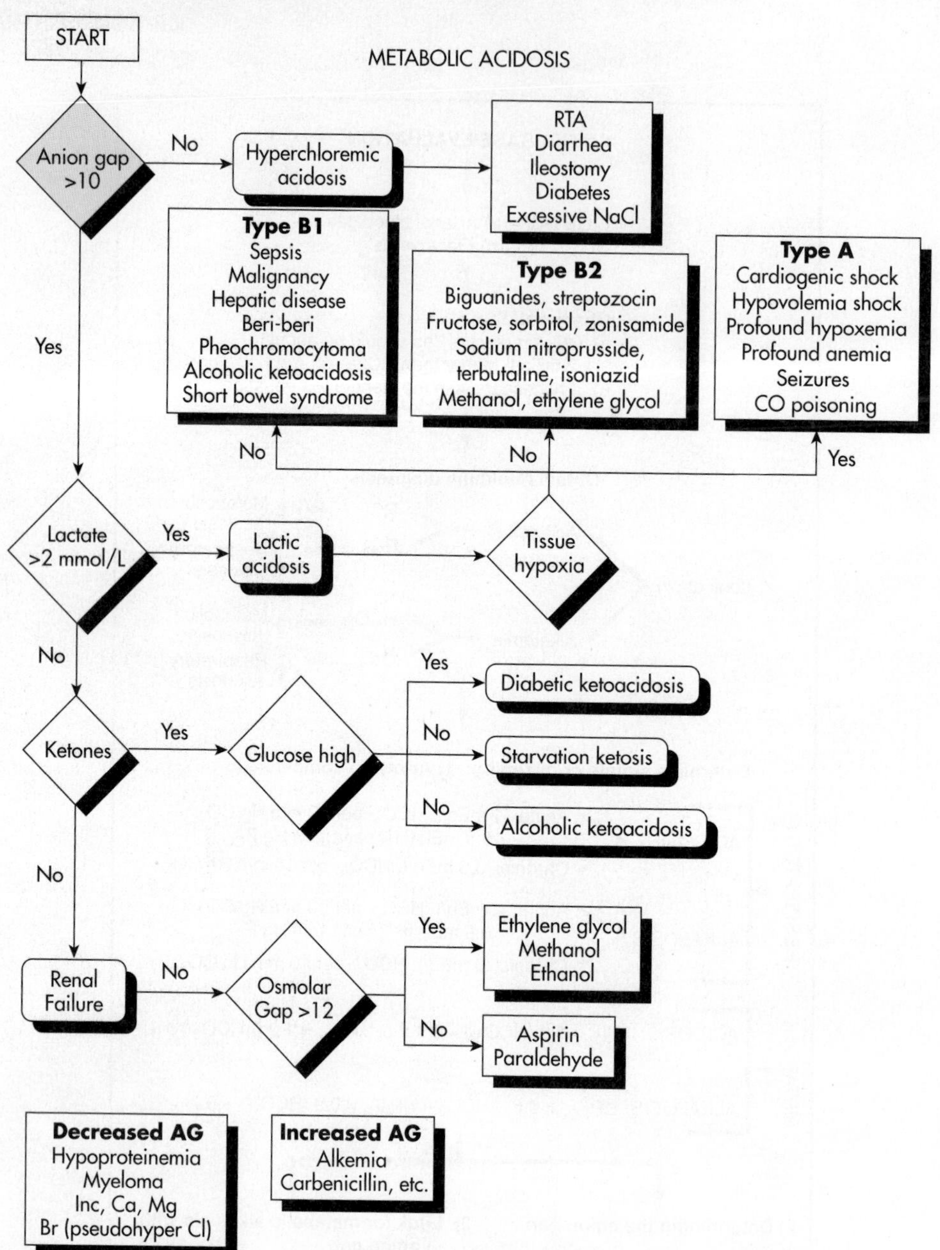

FIGURE 3-3 Diagnostic approach to metabolic acidosis. (Modified from Vincent JL, Ahraham E, Moore FA, et al: *Textbook of critical care*, ed 6, Philadelphia, 2011, Saunders.)

ACIDOSIS, RESPIRATORY, ACUTE

ICD-9CM # 276.2
ICD-10CM # E87.2 Acidosis

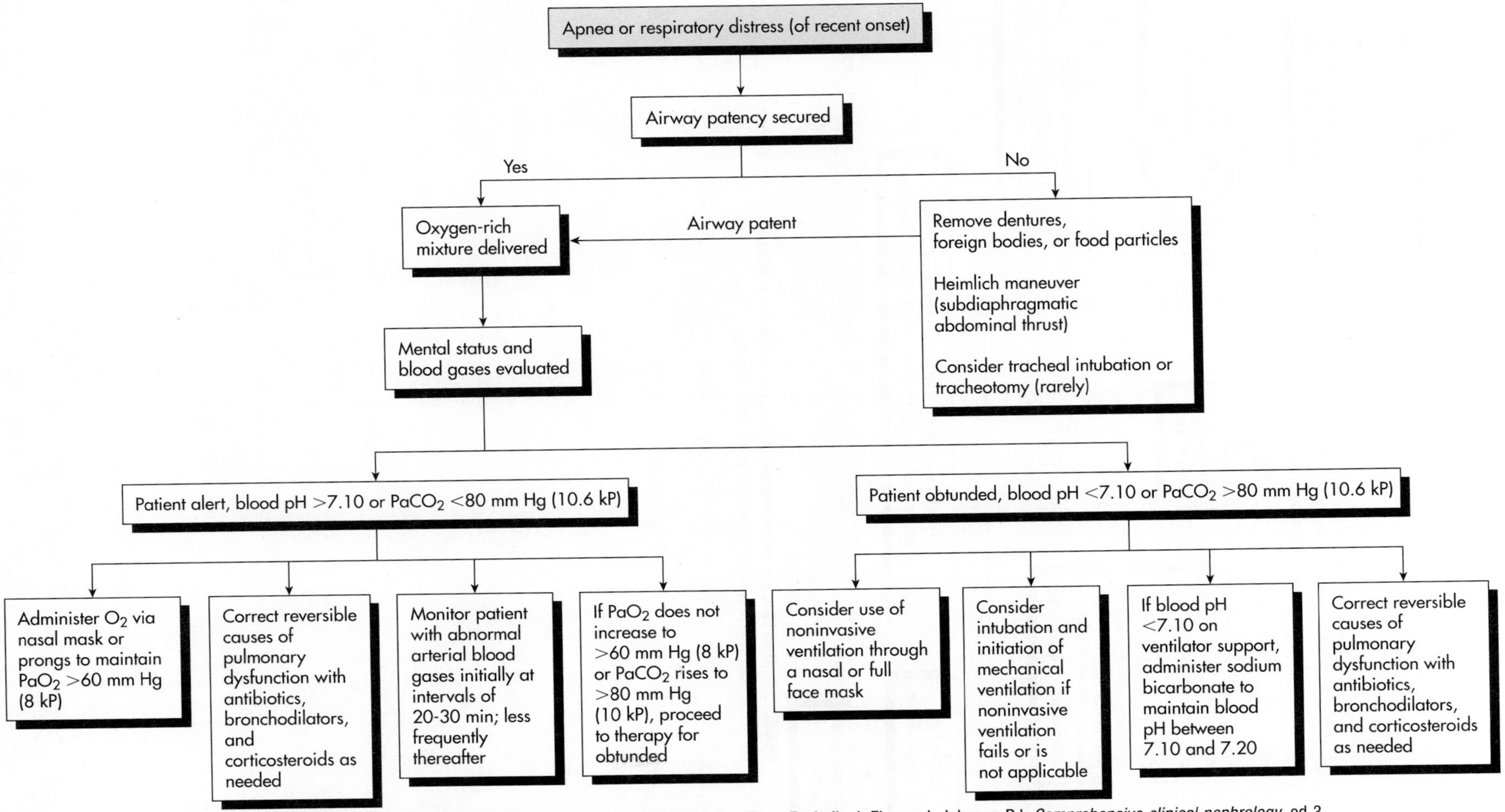

- Apnea or respiratory distress (of recent onset)
  - Airway patency secured
    - **Yes** → Oxygen-rich mixture delivered
    - **No** → Remove dentures, foreign bodies, or food particles. Heimlich maneuver (subdiaphragmatic abdominal thrust). Consider tracheal intubation or tracheotomy (rarely)
      - Airway patent → Oxygen-rich mixture delivered
- Oxygen-rich mixture delivered → Mental status and blood gases evaluated
  - Patient alert, blood pH >7.10 or $PaCO_2 < 80$ mm Hg (10.6 kP)
    - Administer O_2 via nasal mask or prongs to maintain $PaO_2 > 60$ mm Hg (8 kP)
    - Correct reversible causes of pulmonary dysfunction with antibiotics, bronchodilators, and corticosteroids as needed
    - Monitor patient with abnormal arterial blood gases initially at intervals of 20-30 min; less frequently thereafter
    - If PaO_2 does not increase to >60 mm Hg (8 kP) or $PaCO_2$ rises to >80 mm Hg (10 kP), proceed to therapy for obtunded
  - Patient obtunded, blood pH <7.10 or $PaCO_2 > 80$ mm Hg (10.6 kP)
    - Consider use of noninvasive ventilation through a nasal or full face mask
    - Consider intubation and initiation of mechanical ventilation if noninvasive ventilation fails or is not applicable
    - If blood pH <7.10 on ventilator support, administer sodium bicarbonate to maintain blood pH between 7.10 and 7.20
    - Correct reversible causes of pulmonary dysfunction with antibiotics, bronchodilators, and corticosteroids as needed

FIGURE 3-4 Algorithm for management of acute respiratory acidosis. (From Feehally J, Floege J, Johnson RJ: *Comprehensive clinical nephrology*, ed 3, St Louis, 2007, Mosby.)

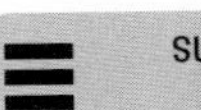

ICD-9CM # 276.2
ICD-10CM # E87.2 Acidosis

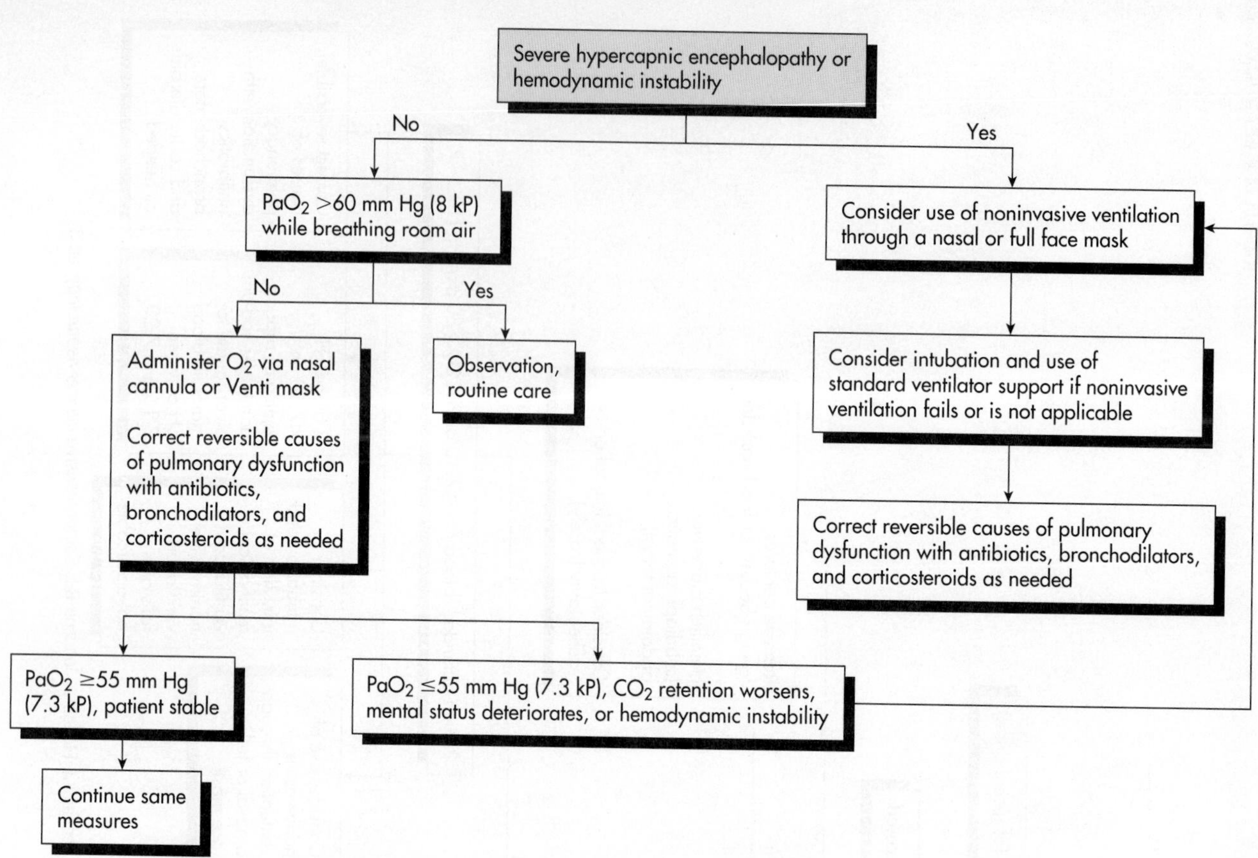

FIGURE 3-5 Algorithm for management of chronic respiratory acidosis. (From Feehally J, Floege J, Johnson RJ: *Comprehensive clinical nephrology*, ed 3, St Louis, 2007, Mosby.)

ADRENAL MASS

ICD-9CM # 194.0 Adrenal cortical carcinoma site NOS M8370/3
255.8 Adrenal hyperplasia
ICD-10CM # C74.90 Malignant neoplasm of unspecified part of unspecified adrenal gland
E27.8 Other specified disorders of adrenal gland

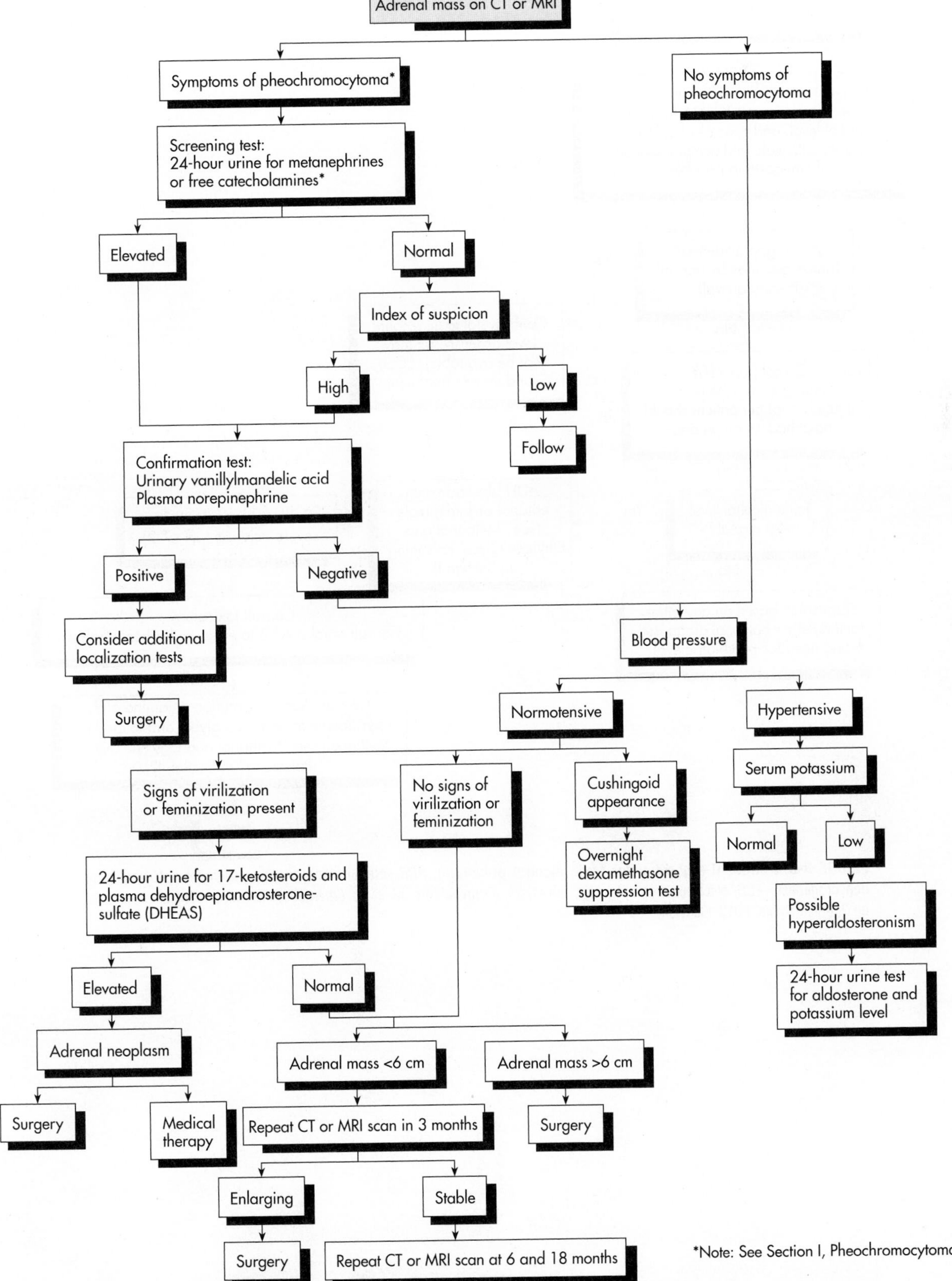

*Note: See Section I, Pheochromocytoma.

FIGURE 3-7 Evaluation of adrenal mass. *CT,* Computed tomography; *MRI,* magnetic resonance imaging. (Modified from Greene HL, Johnson WP, Lemcke D [eds]: *Decision making in medicine,* ed 2, St Louis, 1998, Mosby.)

ICD-9CM # E 860
ICD-10CM # T51.1 Methanol poisoning
T51.8 Ethylene glycol poisoning

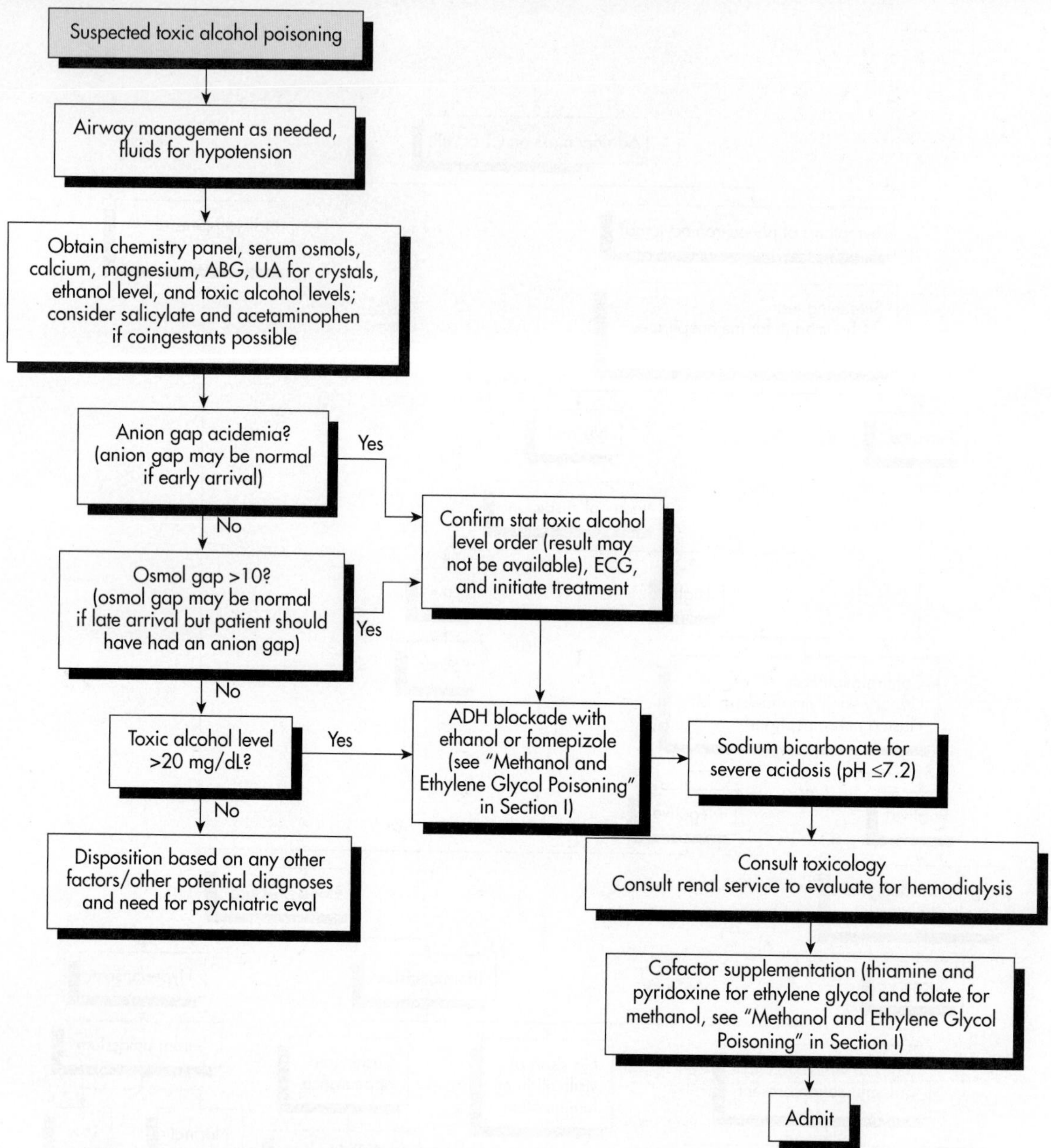

FIGURE 3-8 Treatment algorithm for toxic alcohol poisoning. *ABG,* arterial blood gas measurements; *ADH,* alcohol dehydrogenase; *ECG,* electrocardiography; *UA,* urinalysis. (From Adams JG et al: *Emergency medicine, clinical essentials,* ed 2, Philadelphia, 2013, Elsevier.)

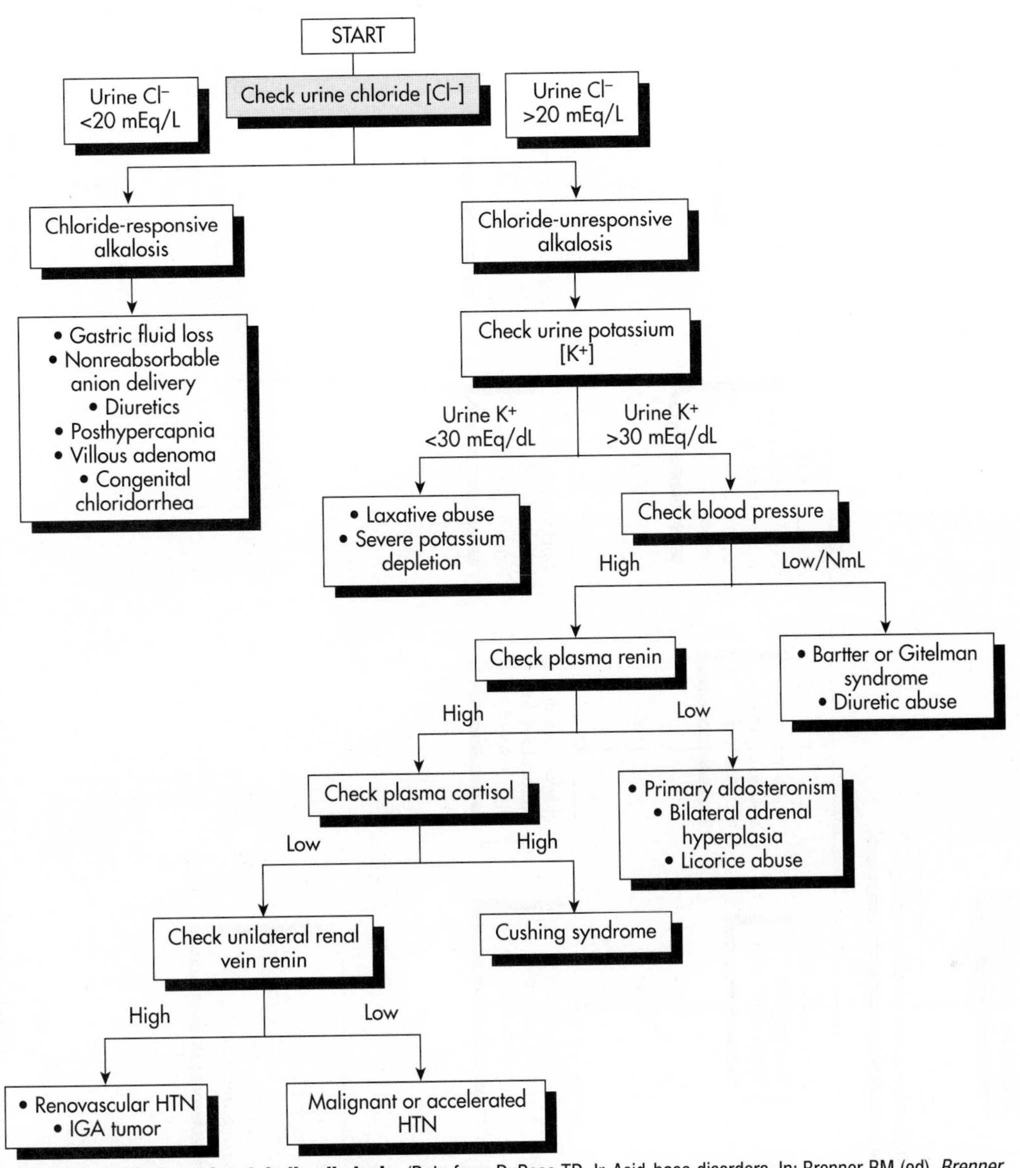

FIGURE 3-9 Workup of metabolic alkalosis. (Data from DuBose TD Jr. Acid-base disorders. In: Brenner BM (ed). *Brenner and Rector's the kidney*, ed 8, Philadelphia, 2008, Saunders, p. 513.)

ALKALOSIS, RESPIRATORY TREATMENT

ICD-9CM # 276.3
ICD-10CM # E87.3 Alkalosis

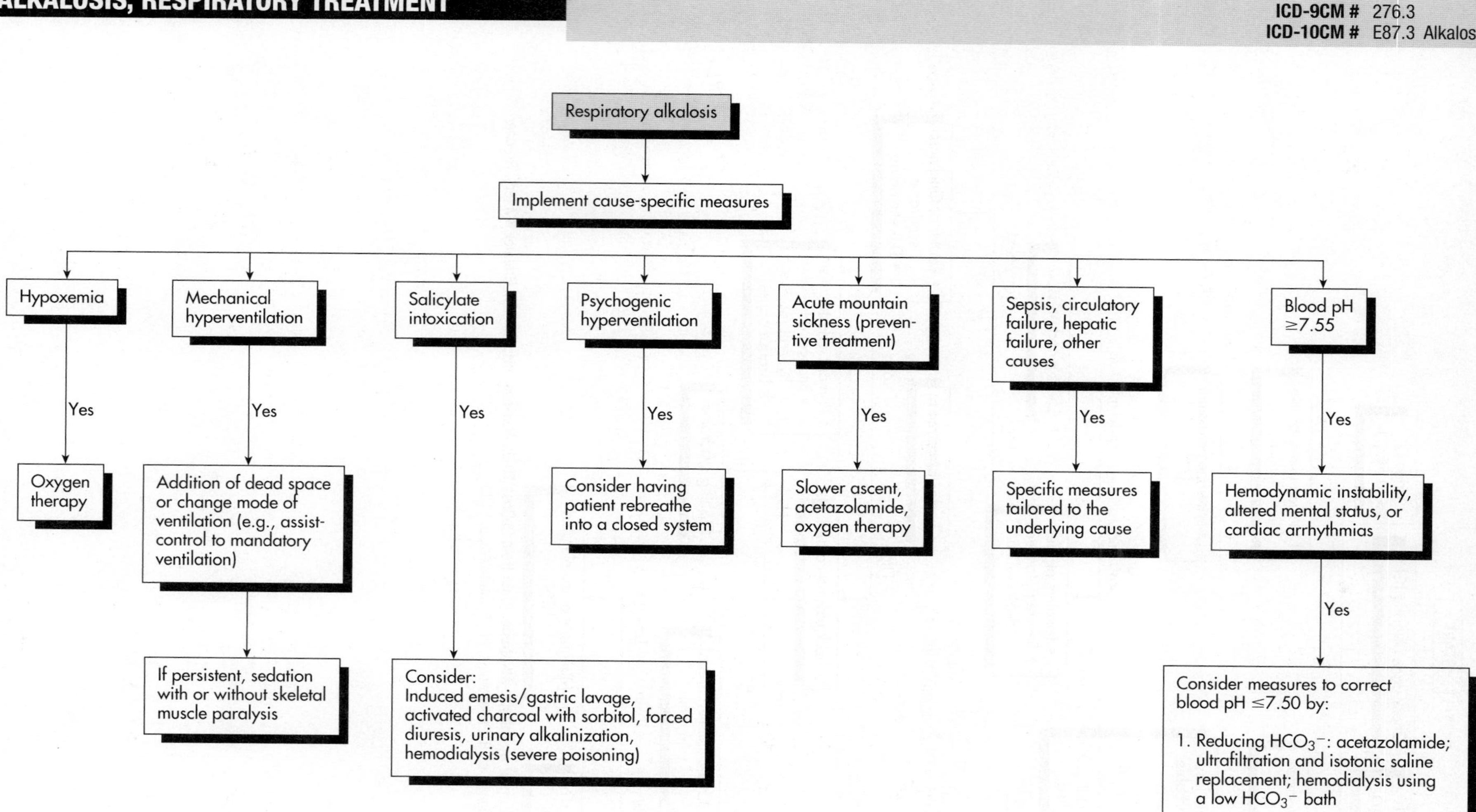

FIGURE 3-10 Recommended treatment of respiratory alkalosis. (From Feehally J, Floege J, Johnson RJ: *Comprehensive clinical nephrology,* ed 3, St Louis, 2007, Mosby.)

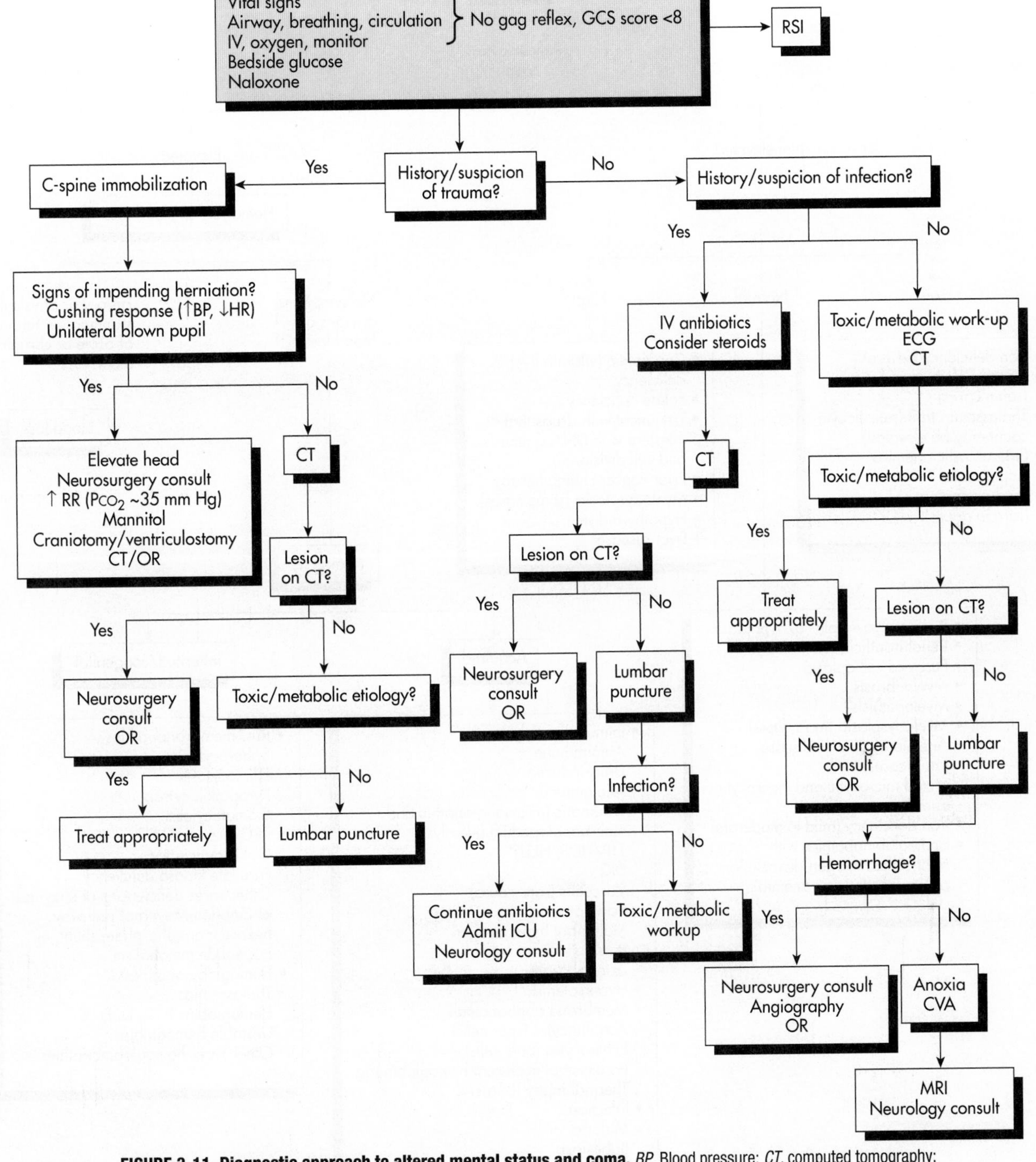

FIGURE 3-11 Diagnostic approach to altered mental status and coma. *BP*, Blood pressure; *CT*, computed tomography; *CVA*, cerebrovascular accident; *ECG*, electrocardiography; *GCS*, Glasgow Coma Scale; *HR*, heart rate; *ICU*, intensive care unit; *MRI*, magnetic resonance imaging; *OR*, operating room; *RR*, respiratory rate; *RSI*, rapid-sequence intubation. (From Adams JG et al: *Emergency medicine, clinical essentials*, ed 2, Philadelphia, 2013, Elsevier.)

ICD-9CM # 285.9 Anemia NOS
ICD-10CM # D63.9 Anemia, unspecified

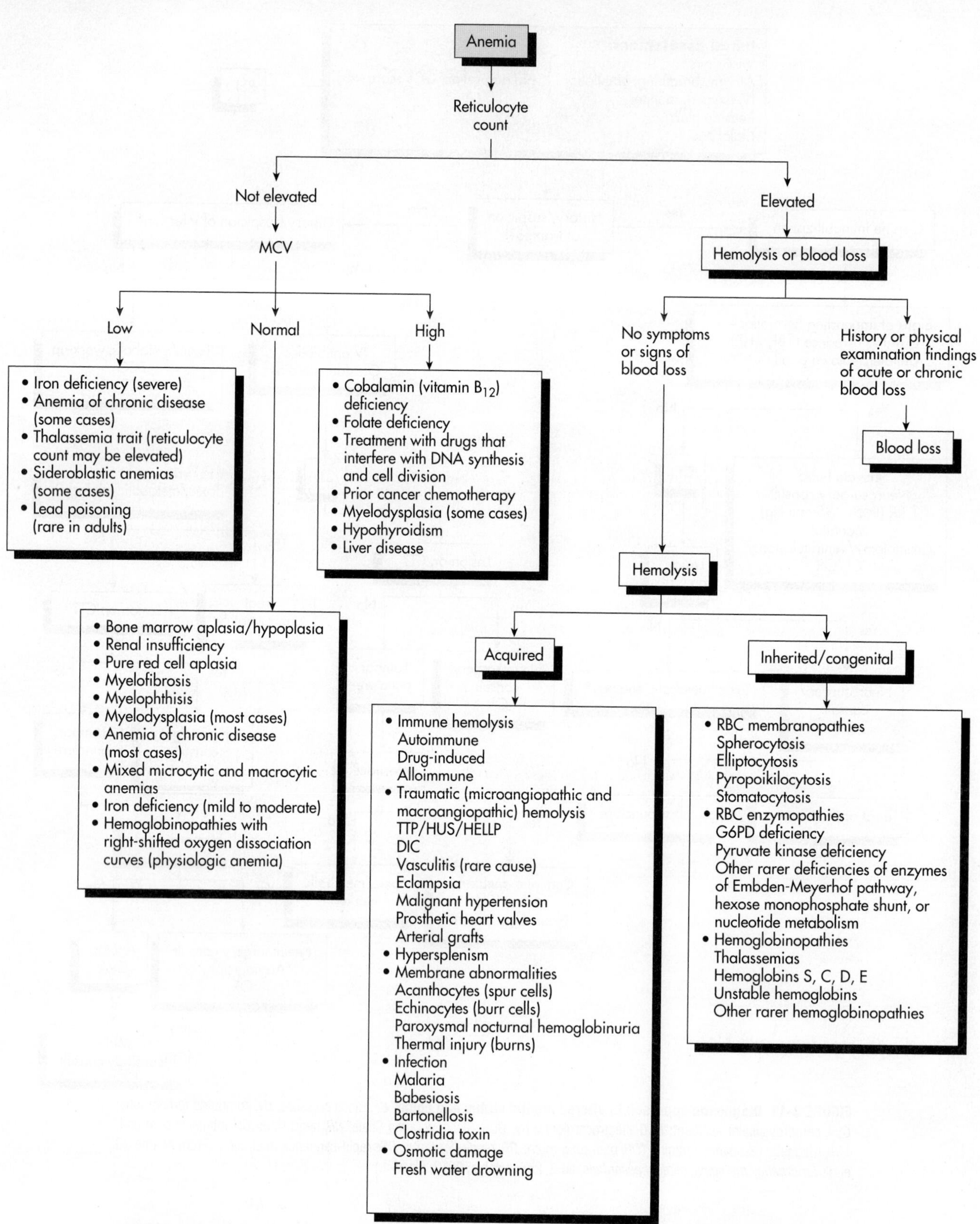

FIGURE 3-12 Algorithm for diagnosis of anemias. *DIC,* Disseminated intravascular coagulation; *G6PD,* glucose-6-phosphate-dehydrogenase; *HELLP, h*epatomegaly-*e*levated *l*iver (function tests)-*l*ow *p*latelets; *HUS,* hemolytic-uremic syndrome; *MCV,* mean corpuscular volume; *RBC,* red blood cell; *TTP,* thrombotic thrombocytopenic purpura. (From Goldman L, Ausiello D [eds]: *Cecil textbook of medicine,* ed 23, Philadelphia, 2008, Saunders.)

ANEMIA, MACROCYTIC

ICD-9CM # 281.9
ICD-10CM # D53.9 Macrocytic anemia

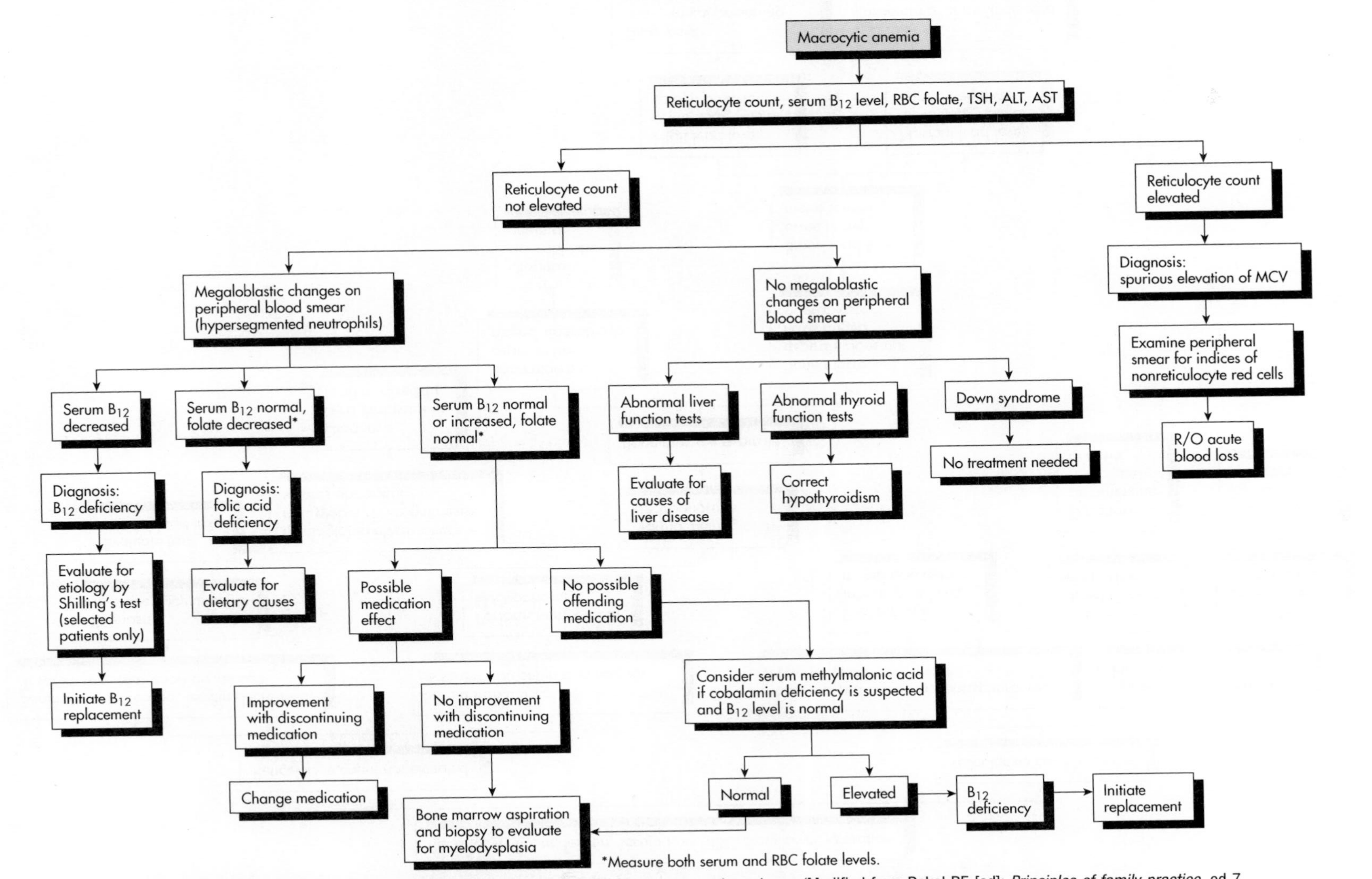

FIGURE 3-14 Differential diagnosis of macrocytic anemia. *MCV,* Mean corpuscular volume. (Modified from Rakel RE [ed]: *Principles of family practice,* ed 7, Philadelphia, 2007, Saunders.)

ANEMIA, MICROCYTIC

ICD-9CM # 282.4
ICD-10CM # D50.9 Microcytic (hypochromic) anemia

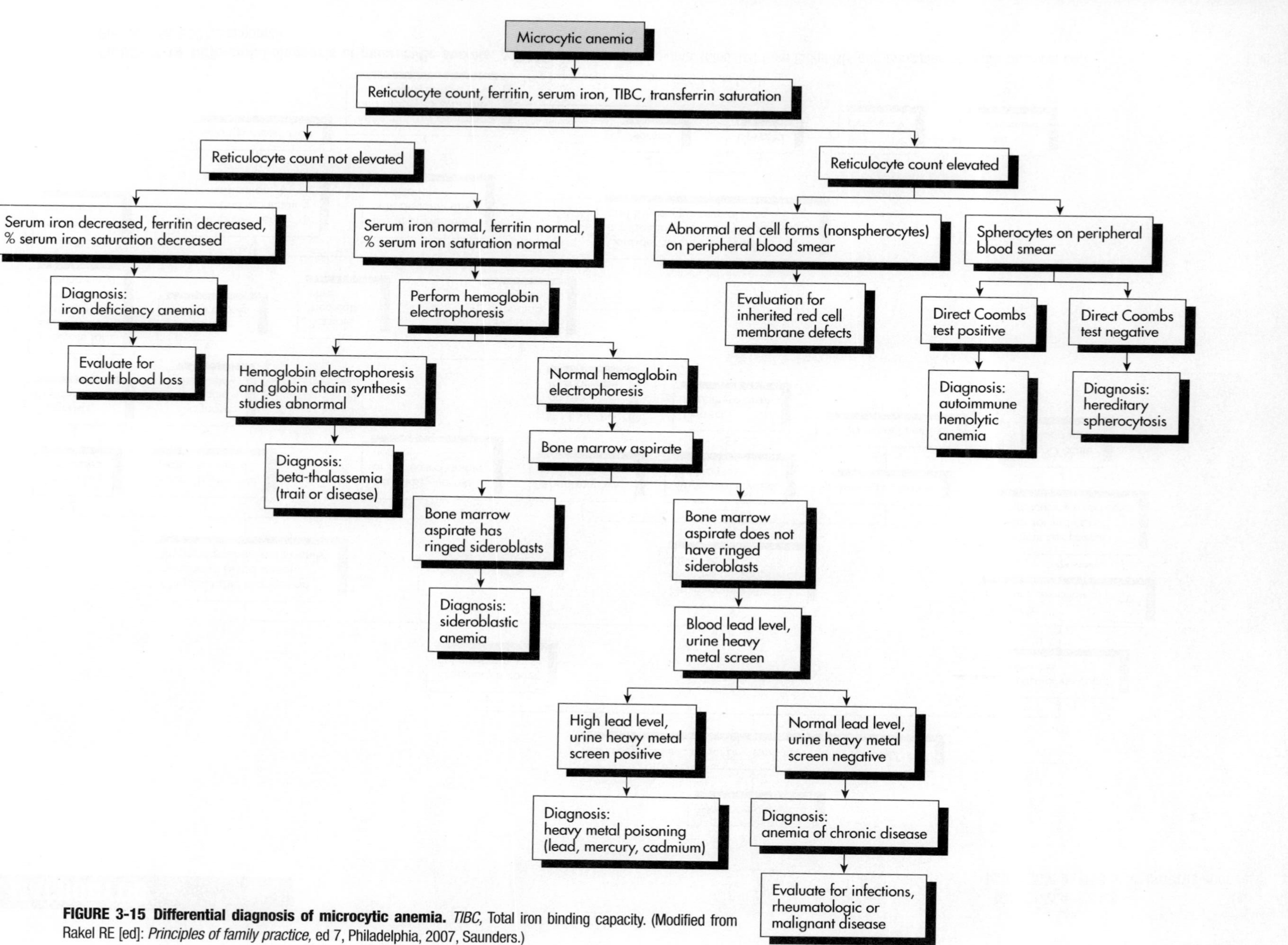

FIGURE 3-15 Differential diagnosis of microcytic anemia. *TIBC,* Total iron binding capacity. (Modified from Rakel RE [ed]: *Principles of family practice,* ed 7, Philadelphia, 2007, Saunders.)

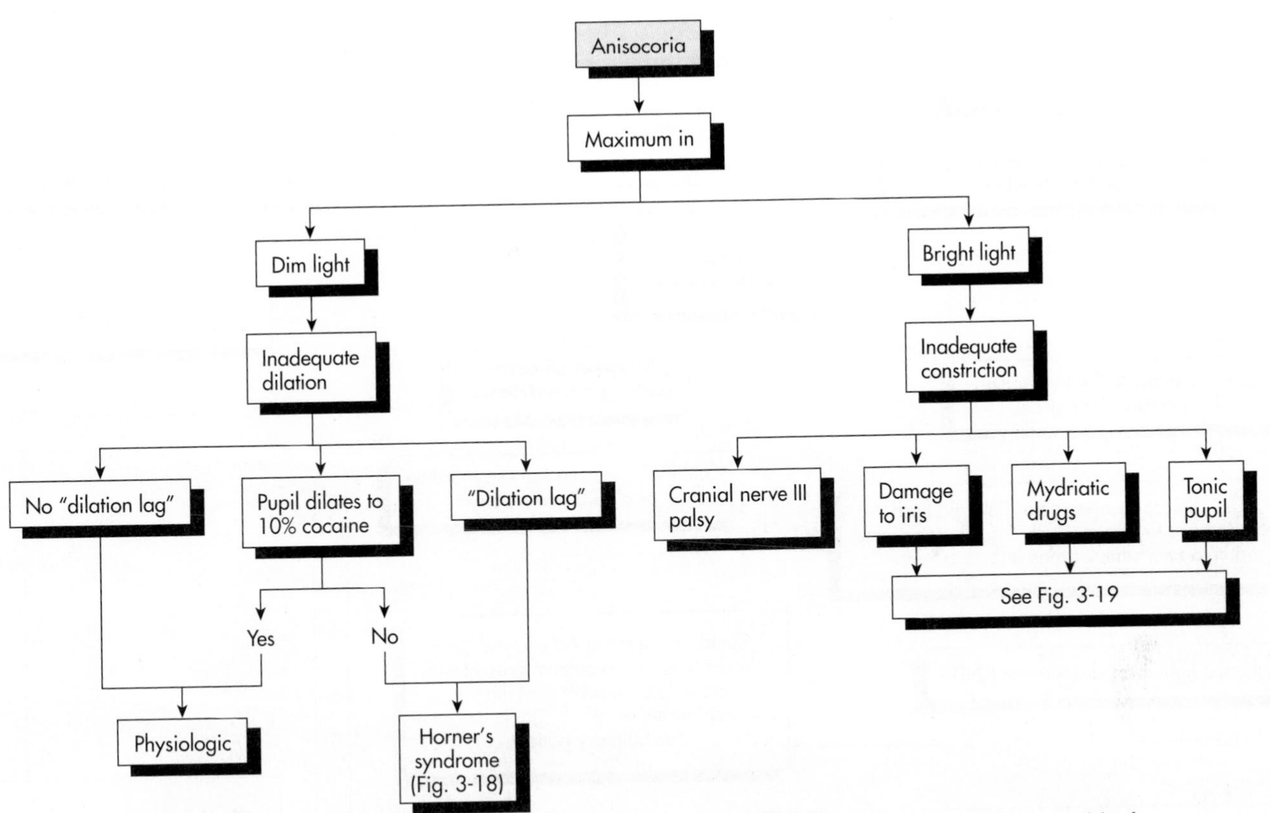

FIGURE 3-17 Algorithm for the approach to unequal pupils (anisocoria). (From Andreoli TE [ed]: *Cecil essentials of medicine,* ed 7, Philadelphia, 2008, Saunders.)

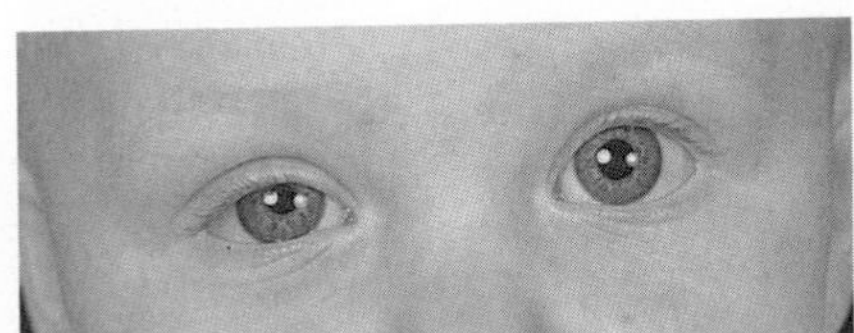

FIGURE 3-18 Horner's syndrome clearly acquired in infancy must be evaluated for neuroblastoma, a treatable tumor. This baby, with a right ptosis and miosis, developed a flush during cycloplegia that made the vasomotor abnormality very clear—the Horner's side remained pale. The baby had no sign of Horner's syndrome during her first 8 months, but at 16 months Horner's syndrome is obvious (ptosis, miosis, and upside-down ptosis). Because the syndrome was acquired, a chest radiograph was ordered; it showed a mass in the pulmonary apex. Magnetic resonance imaging confirmed the lesion. Surgery showed it to be a neuroblastoma. (From Yanoff M, Duker JS: *Ophthalmology,* ed 2, St Louis, 2004, Mosby.)

ICD-9CM # 379.41
ICD-10CM # H57.02 Anisocoria

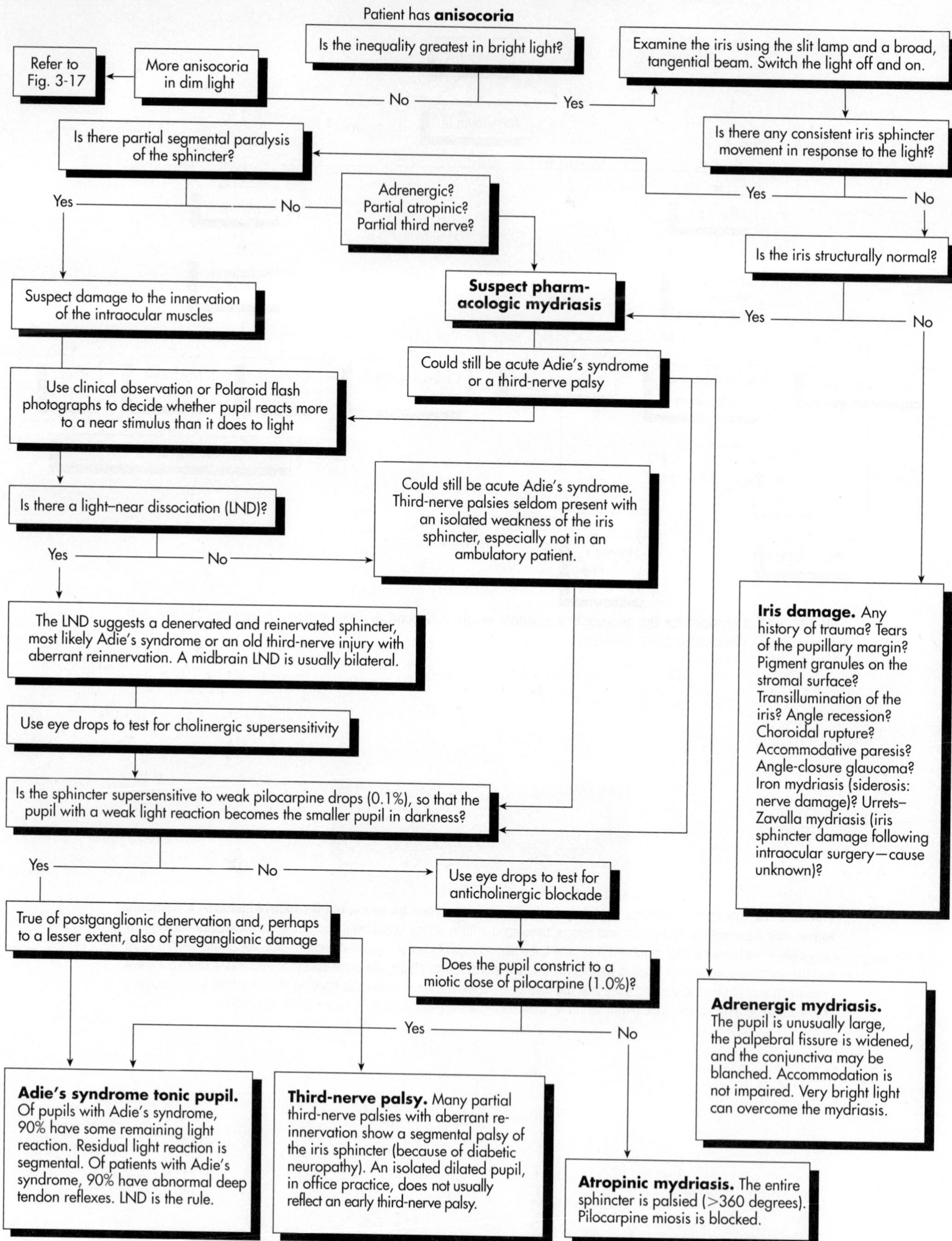

FIGURE 3-19 Diagnosis of pupillary abnormalities in which anisocoria increases in bright light. Initial pupillary inequality is greater in bright light than in darkness, which indicates that the sphincter of the large pupil is weak or that a parasympathetic lesion is present on that side. (From Yanoff M, Duker JS: *Ophthalmology,* ed 2, St Louis, 2004, Mosby.)

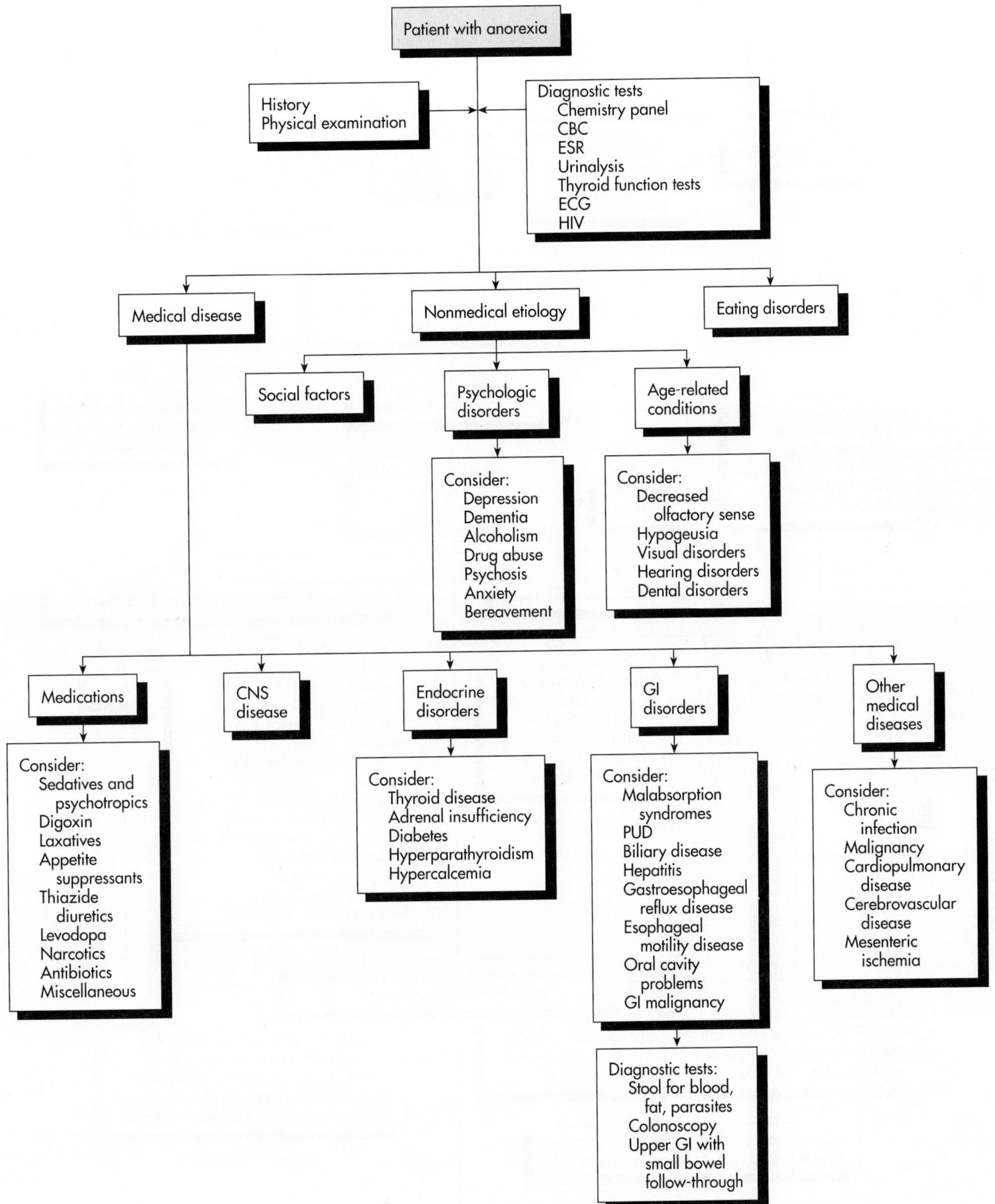

FIGURE 3-20 Evaluation of anorexia. *CBC,* Complete blood count; *CNS,* central nervous system; *ECG,* electrocardiogram; *ESR,* erythrocyte sedimentation rate; *GI,* gastrointestinal; *PUD,* peptic ulcer disease. (Modified from Greene HL, Johnson WP, Lemcke D [eds]: *Decision making in medicine,* ed 2, St Louis, 1998, Mosby.)

ICD-9CM # V82.5
ICD-10CM # X43 Accidental poisoning by an exposure to other drugs acting on the autonomic nervous system

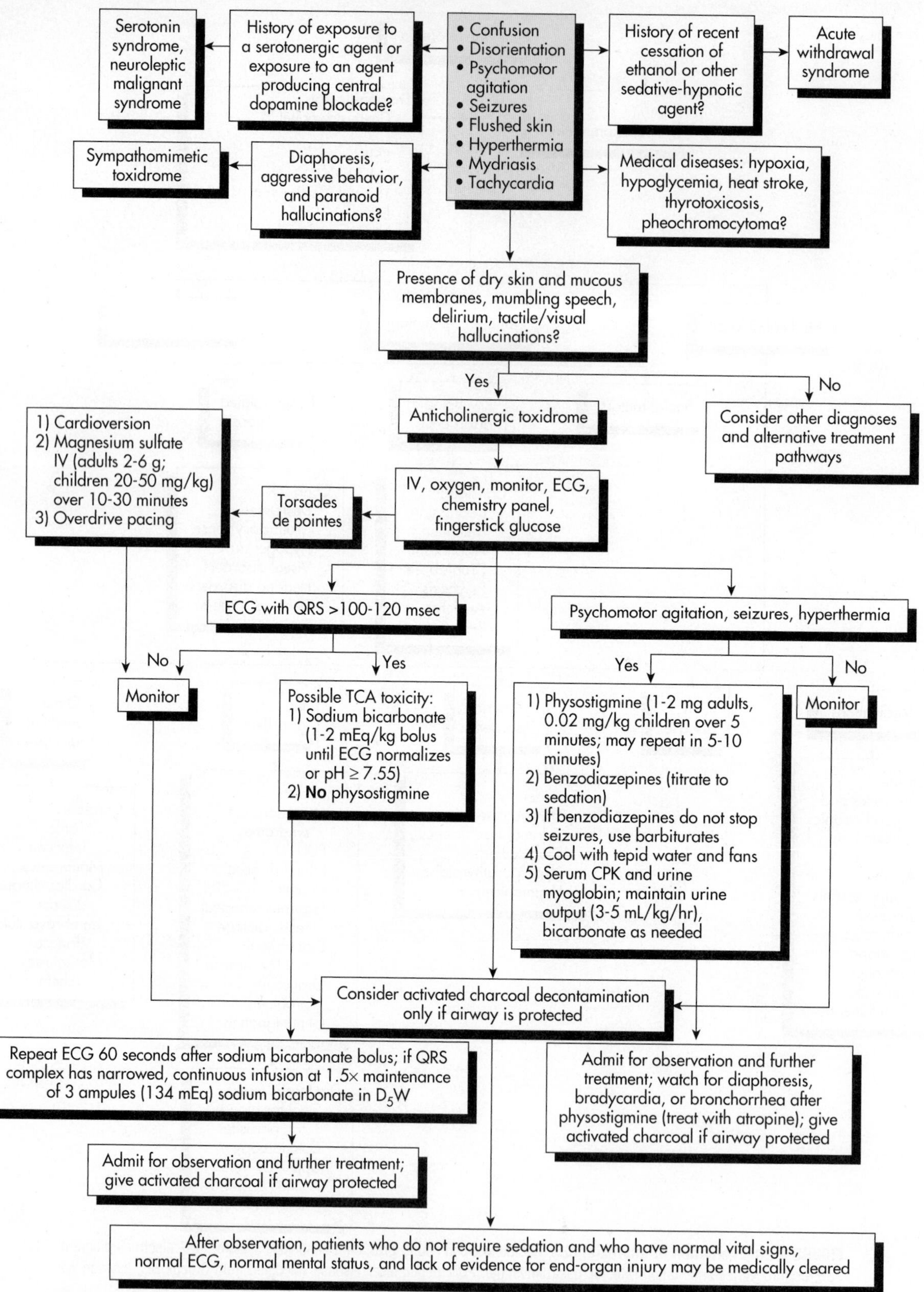

FIGURE 3-21 Algorithm for the recognition and treatment of anticholinergic toxicity. *CPK*, Creatine phosphokinase; *D_5W*, 5% dextrose in water; *ECG*, electrocardiogram; *IV*, intravenous line; *TCA*, tricyclic antidepressant. (From Adams JG et al: *Emergency medicine, clinical essentials*, ed 2, Philadelphia, 2013, Elsevier.)

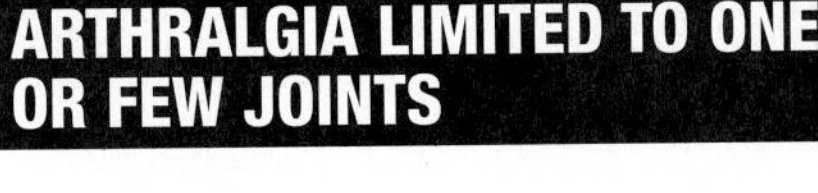

ARTHRALGIA LIMITED TO ONE OR FEW JOINTS

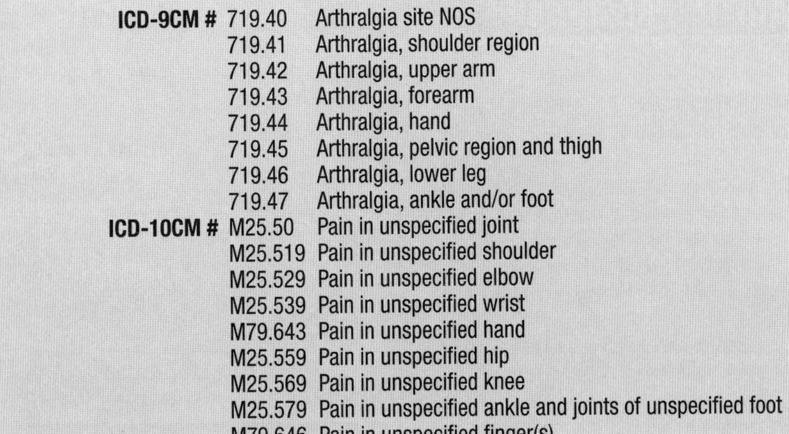

ICD-9CM # 719.40 Arthralgia site NOS
719.41 Arthralgia, shoulder region
719.42 Arthralgia, upper arm
719.43 Arthralgia, forearm
719.44 Arthralgia, hand
719.45 Arthralgia, pelvic region and thigh
719.46 Arthralgia, lower leg
719.47 Arthralgia, ankle and/or foot

ICD-10CM # M25.50 Pain in unspecified joint
M25.519 Pain in unspecified shoulder
M25.529 Pain in unspecified elbow
M25.539 Pain in unspecified wrist
M79.643 Pain in unspecified hand
M25.559 Pain in unspecified hip
M25.569 Pain in unspecified knee
M25.579 Pain in unspecified ankle and joints of unspecified foot
M79.646 Pain in unspecified finger(s)

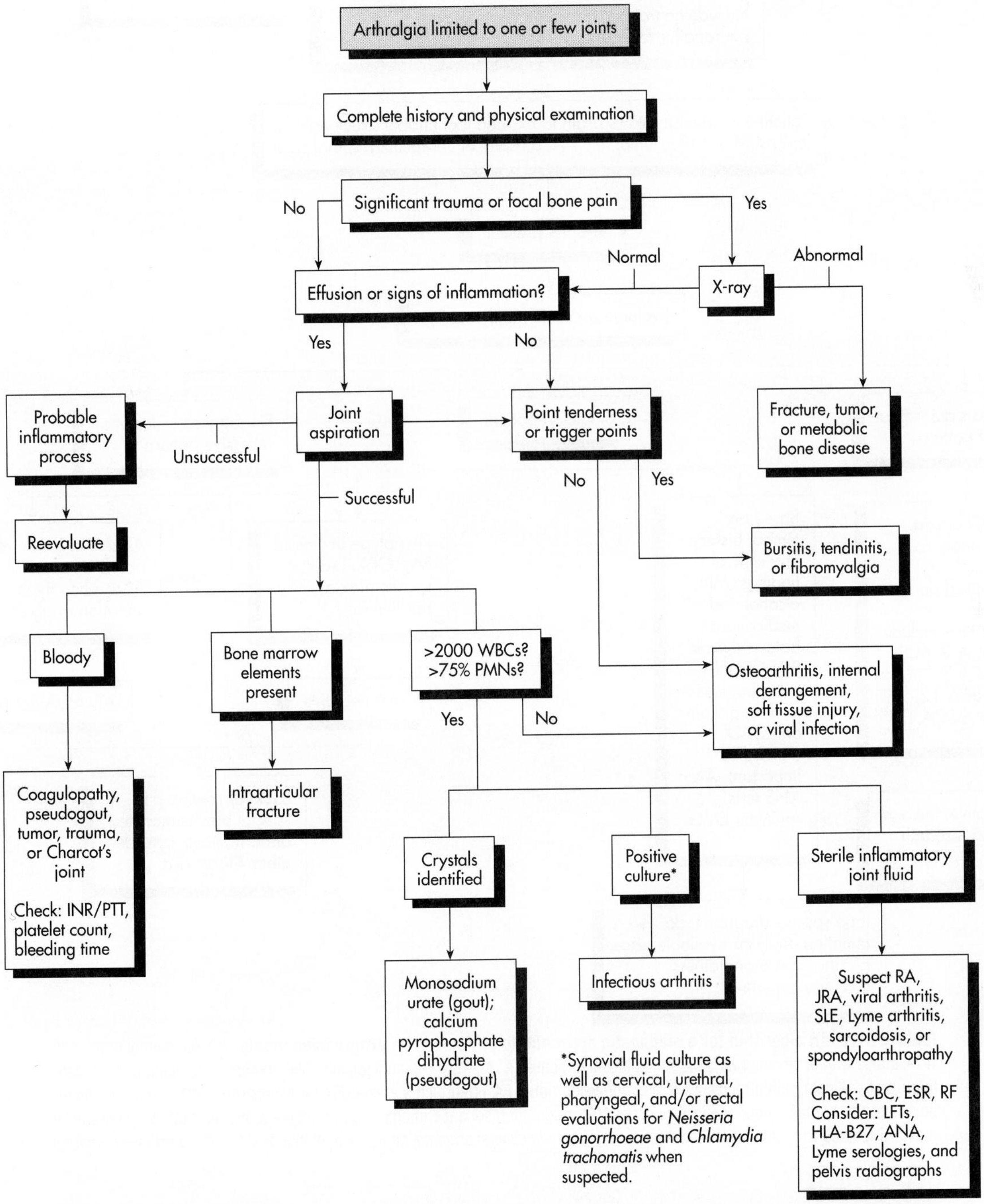

Arthralgia limited to one or few joints
Complete history and physical examination
Significant trauma or focal bone pain
No
Yes
Effusion or signs of inflammation?
X-ray
Normal
Abnormal
Yes
No
Probable inflammatory process
Unsuccessful
Joint aspiration
Point tenderness or trigger points
Fracture, tumor, or metabolic bone disease
Reevaluate
Successful
No
Yes
Bursitis, tendinitis, or fibromyalgia
Bloody
Bone marrow elements present
>2000 WBCs? >75% PMNs?
Osteoarthritis, internal derangement, soft tissue injury, or viral infection
Yes
No
Coagulopathy, pseudogout, tumor, trauma, or Charcot's joint

Check: INR/PTT, platelet count, bleeding time
Intraarticular fracture
Crystals identified
Positive culture*
Sterile inflammatory joint fluid
Monosodium urate (gout); calcium pyrophosphate dihydrate (pseudogout)
Infectious arthritis
Suspect RA, JRA, viral arthritis, SLE, Lyme arthritis, sarcoidosis, or spondyloarthropathy

Check: CBC, ESR, RF
Consider: LFTs, HLA-B27, ANA, Lyme serologies, and pelvis radiographs

*Synovial fluid culture as well as cervical, urethral, pharyngeal, and/or rectal evaluations for *Neisseria gonorrhoeae* and *Chlamydia trachomatis* when suspected.

FIGURE 3-22 A diagnostic approach to arthralgia in a few joints. *ANA*, Antinuclear antibodies; *CBC*, complete blood count; *ESR*, erythrocyte sedimentation rate; *JRA*, juvenile rheumatoid arthritis; *LFTs*, liver function tests; *PMNs*, polymorphonuclear neutrophils; *PT*, prothrombin time; *PTT*, partial thromboplastin time; *RA*, rheumatoid arthritis; *RF*, rheumatoid factor; *SLE*, systemic lupus erythematosus; *WBCs*, white blood cells. (Modified from American College of Rheumatology Ad Hoc Committee on Clinical Guidelines: *Arthritis Rheum* 39:1, 1996.)

ICD-9CM #	781.3	Ataxia NOS
	303.9	Alcoholic, chronic
	334.3	Cerebellar
	331.89	Cerebral
	334.0	Friedreich's
ICD-10CM #	A52.11	Tabes dorsalis
	G11.1	Early-onset cerebellar ataxia
	G31.89	Other specified degenerative diseases of nervous system
	G11.1	Early-onset cerebellar ataxia
	R27.0	Ataxia, unspecified
	R27.8	Other lack of coordination
	R27.9	Unspecified lack of coordination

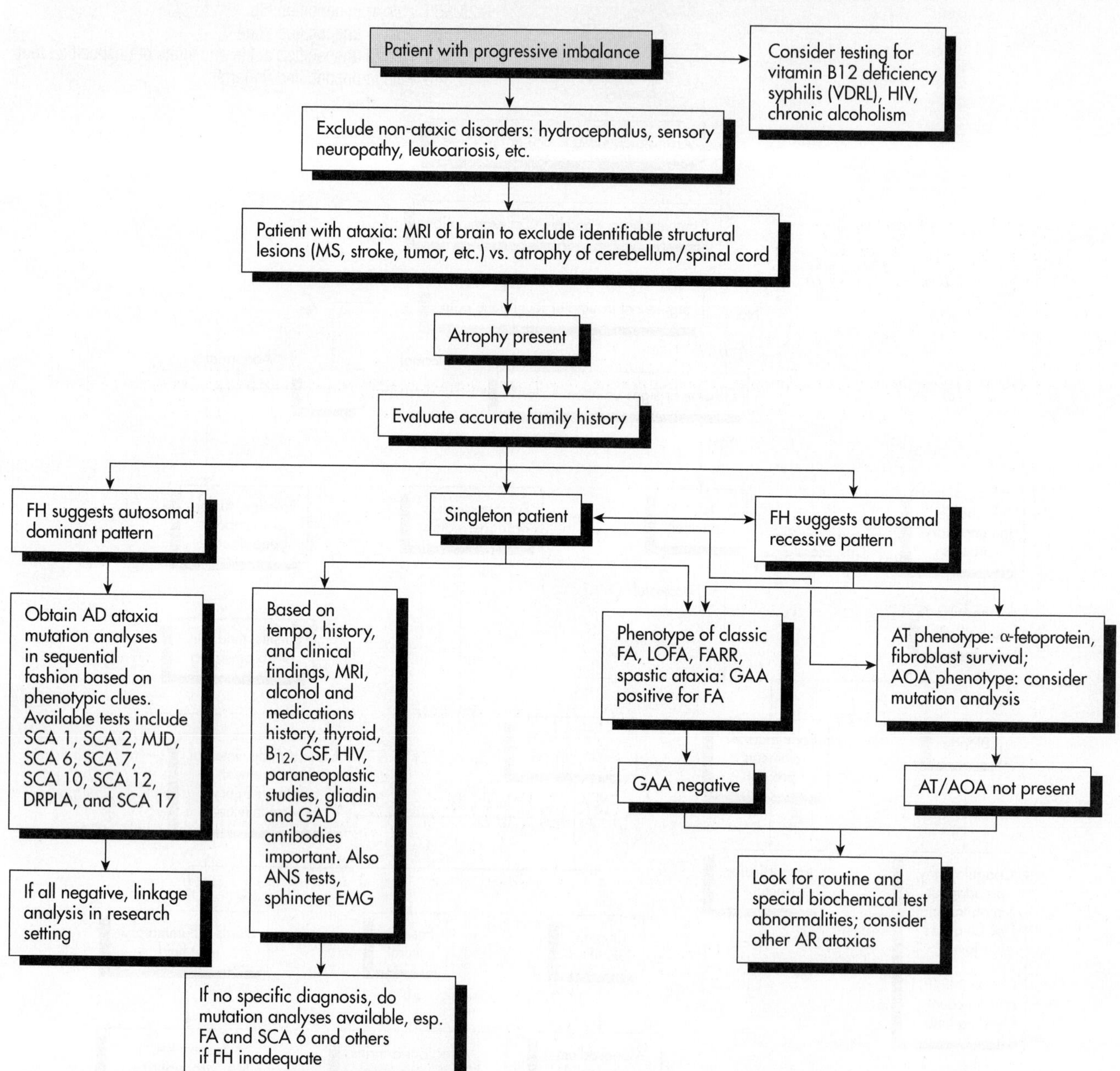

FIGURE 3-25 An algorithm for a diagnostic approach to patients with progressive ataxia. *AD,* Autosomal dominant; *AOA,* ataxia with oculomotor apraxia; *AR,* autosomal recessive; *AT,* ataxia-telangiectasia; *CSF,* cerebrospinal fluid; *DRPLA,* dentatorubral-pallidoluysian atrophy; *EMG,* electromyelography; *FA,* Friedreich's ataxia; *FH,* family history; *GAD,* glutamate decarboxylase; *HIV,* human immunodeficiency virus; *MRI,* magnetic resonance imaging; *MS,* multiple sclerosis; *SCA,* spinocerebellar ataxia. (Modified from Bradley WG et al [eds]: *Neurology in clinical practice,* ed 4, Philadelphia, 2004, Butterworth Heinemann.)

BACK PAIN

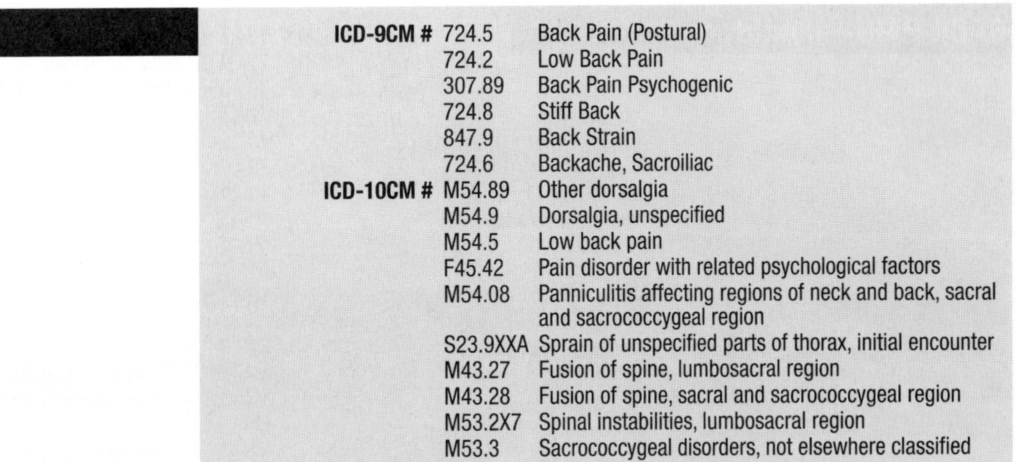

ICD-9CM #	724.5	Back Pain (Postural)
	724.2	Low Back Pain
	307.89	Back Pain Psychogenic
	724.8	Stiff Back
	847.9	Back Strain
	724.6	Backache, Sacroiliac
ICD-10CM #	M54.89	Other dorsalgia
	M54.9	Dorsalgia, unspecified
	M54.5	Low back pain
	F45.42	Pain disorder with related psychological factors
	M54.08	Panniculitis affecting regions of neck and back, sacral and sacrococcygeal region
	S23.9XXA	Sprain of unspecified parts of thorax, initial encounter
	M43.27	Fusion of spine, lumbosacral region
	M43.28	Fusion of spine, sacral and sacrococcygeal region
	M53.2X7	Spinal instabilities, lumbosacral region
	M53.3	Sacrococcygeal disorders, not elsewhere classified

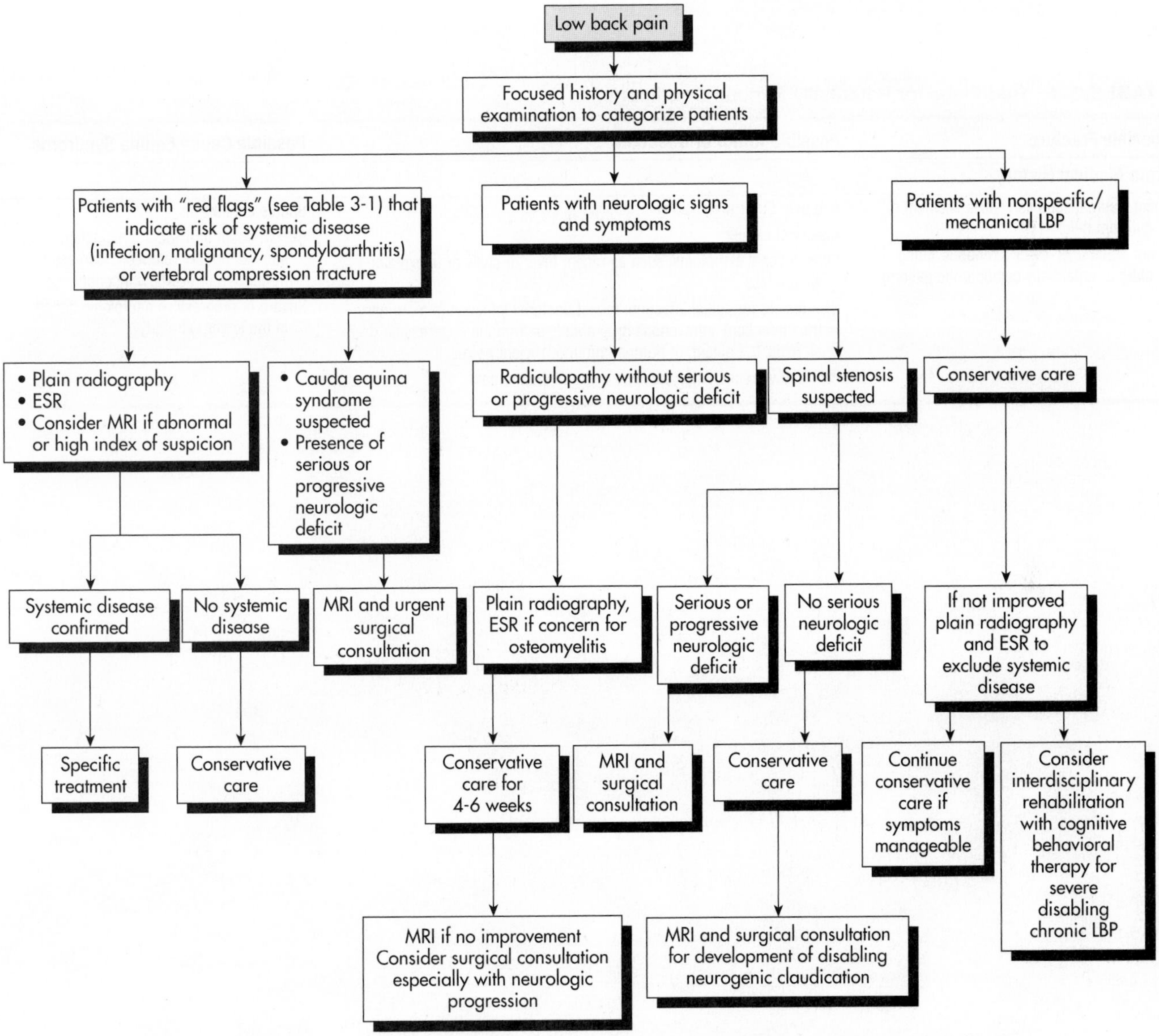

Low back pain

Focused history and physical examination to categorize patients

Patients with "red flags" (see Table 3-1) that indicate risk of systemic disease (infection, malignancy, spondyloarthritis) or vertebral compression fracture

Patients with neurologic signs and symptoms

Patients with nonspecific/ mechanical LBP

- Plain radiography
- ESR
- Consider MRI if abnormal or high index of suspicion

- Cauda equina syndrome suspected
- Presence of serious or progressive neurologic deficit

Radiculopathy without serious or progressive neurologic deficit

Spinal stenosis suspected

Conservative care

Systemic disease confirmed

No systemic disease

MRI and urgent surgical consultation

Plain radiography, ESR if concern for osteomyelitis

Serious or progressive neurologic deficit

No serious neurologic deficit

If not improved plain radiography and ESR to exclude systemic disease

Specific treatment

Conservative care

Conservative care for 4-6 weeks

MRI and surgical consultation

Conservative care

Continue conservative care if symptoms manageable

Consider interdisciplinary rehabilitation with cognitive behavioral therapy for severe disabling chronic LBP

MRI if no improvement Consider surgical consultation especially with neurologic progression

MRI and surgical consultation for development of disabling neurogenic claudication

FIGURE 3-26 Algorithm for the differential diagnosis and treatment of low back pain. *ESR,* erythrocyte sedimentation rate; *LBP,* low back pain; *MRI,* magnetic resonance imaging. (Rom Firestein GS, Budd RC, Gabriel SE, et al: *Kelly's textbook of rheumatology,* ed 9, Philadelphia, 2013, Saunders.)

ICD-9CM #	724.5	Back Pain (Postural)
	724.2	Low Back Pain
	307.89	Back Pain Psychogenic
	724.8	Stiff Back
	847.9	Back Strain
	724.6	Backache, Sacroiliac
ICD-10CM #	M54.89	Other dorsalgia
	M54.9	Dorsalgia, unspecified
	M54.5	Low back pain
	F45.42	Pain disorder with related psychological factors
	M54.08	Panniculitis affecting regions of neck and back, sacral and sacrococcygeal region
	S23.9XXA	Sprain of unspecified parts of thorax, initial encounter
	M43.27	Fusion of spine, lumbosacral region
	M43.28	Fusion of spine, sacral and sacrococcygeal region
	M53.2X7	Spinal instabilities, lumbosacral region
	M53.3	Sacrococcygeal disorders, not elsewhere classified

TABLE 3-1 Red Flags for Potentially Serious Conditions

Possible Fracture	Possible Tumor or Infection	Possible Cauda Equina Syndrome
From Medical History		
Major trauma, such as vehicle accident or fall from height Minor trauma or even strenuous lifting (in older or potentially osteoporotic patient)	Age over 50 or under 20 yr History of cancer Constitutional symptoms, such as recent fever or chills or unexplained weight loss Risk factors for spinal infection: recent bacterial infection (e.g., urinary tract infection), intravenous drug abuse, or immune suppression (from steroids, transplant, or human immunodeficiency virus) Pain that worsens when supine; severe nighttime pain	Saddle anesthesia Recent onset of bladder dysfunction, such as urinary retention, increased frequency, or overflow incontinence Severe or progressive neurologic deficit in the lower extremity

BLEEDING DISORDERS

ICD-9CM # 286.9
ICD-10CM # D68.8 Other specified coagulation defects
D68.9 Coagulation defect, unspecified

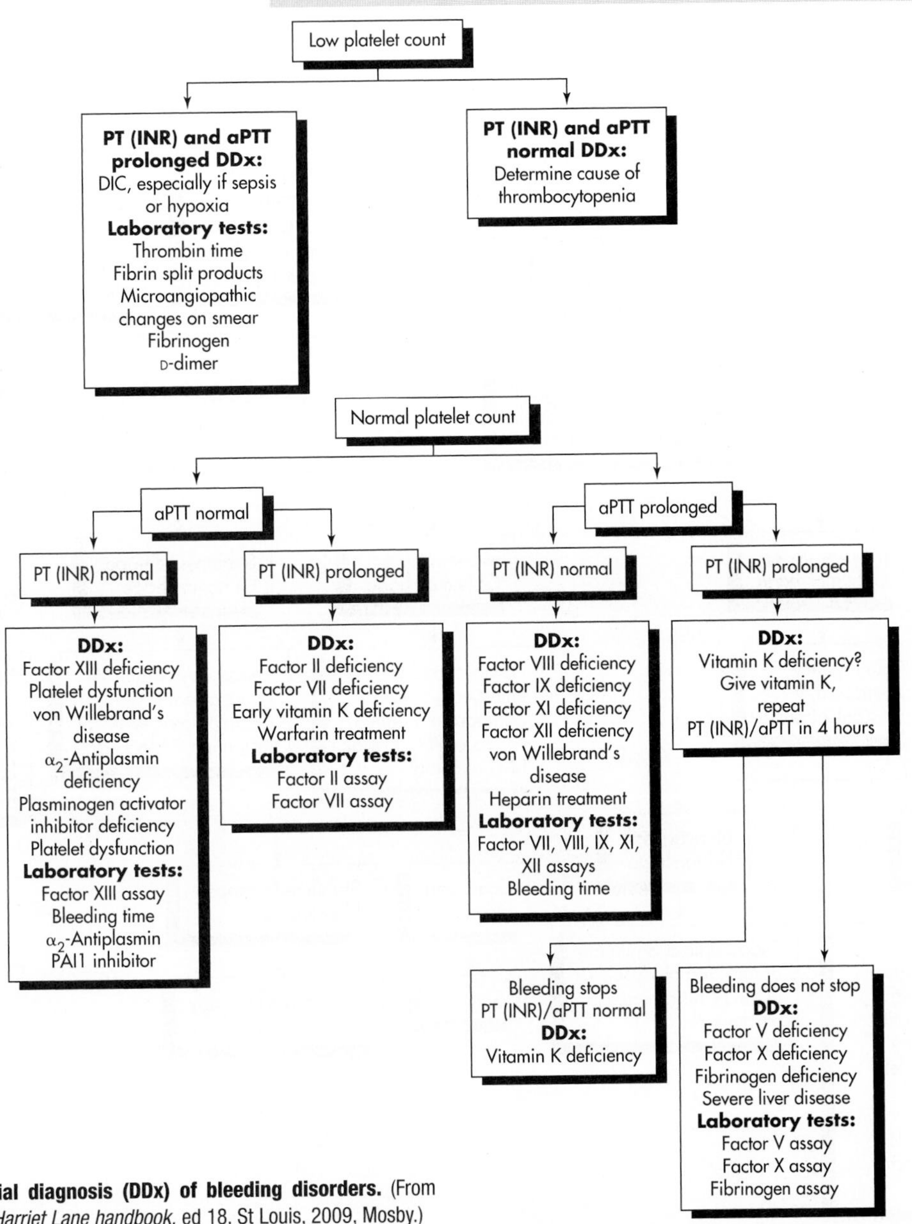

FIGURE 3-28 Differential diagnosis (DDx) of bleeding disorders. (From Cluster JW, Rau RE: *The Harriet Lane handbook*, ed 18, St Louis, 2009, Mosby.)

BOX 3-1 Bleeding Disorders

Congenital

Disorder of platelet number or function

Thrombocytopenia: Secondary to bone marrow disease or defective megakaryocyte maturation

Disorders of platelet function: Bernard-Soulier syndrome, Glanzmann thrombasthenia, storage pool diseases

Factor VIII deficiency: See text (Section I)

Factor IX deficiency: See text (Section I)

von Willebrand's disease: See text (Section I)

Acquired

Disseminated intravascular coagulation: Characterized by prolonged PT and aPTT, decreased fibrinogen and platelets, increased fibrin degradation products, and elevated D-dimers. Treatment includes identifying and treating underlying disorder. Replacement of depleted coagulation factors with FFP may be necessary in severe cases, especially when bleeding is present; 10-15 ml/kg will raise clotting factors 20%. Fibrinogen, if depleted, can be given as cryoprecipitate. Platelet transfusions may also be necessary.

Liver disease: The liver is the major site of synthesis of factors V, VII, IX, X, XI, XII, XIII, prothrombin, plasminogen, fibrinogen, protein C and S, and ATIII. Treatment with FFP and platelets may be needed, but this will increase hepatic protein load. Vitamin K should be given to patients with liver disease and clotting abnormalities.

Vitamin K deficiency: Factors II, VII, IX, X, protein C, and protein S are vitamin K dependent. Early vitamin K deficiency may present with isolated prolonged PT because factor VII has the shortest half-life. Fibrinogen should be normal.

Hemolytic-uremic syndrome/thrombotic thrombocytopenic purpura (HUS/TTP): Characterized by the triad of microangiopathic hemolytic anemia, uremia, and thrombocytopenia. HUS/TTP is often triggered by bacterial enteritis, especially caused by *Escherichia coli* O157:H7, although there are a variety of causes. HUS does not typically include coagulation abnormalities, such as those seen in DIC. Avoid blood products in patients with HUS thought to be secondary to pneumococcal infection. TTP includes the triad of HUS in addition to fever and CNS changes and is more common in older adolescents and adults.

From Custer JW, Rau RE: *The Harriet Lane handbook*, ed 18, St Louis, 2009, Mosby.

ICD-9CM # 578.9
ICD-10CM # K92.2 Gastrointestinal bleeding

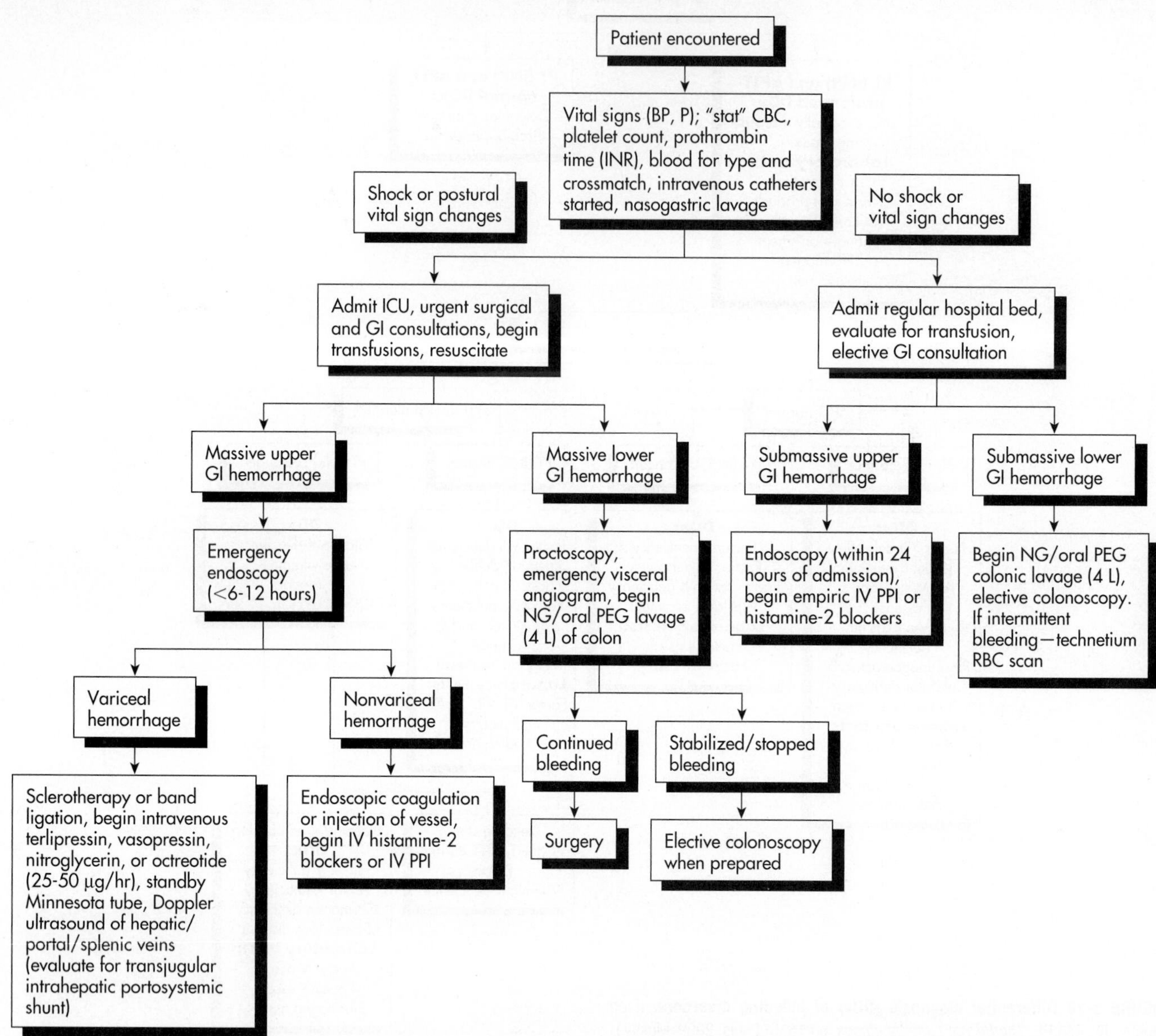

FIGURE 3-30 Approach to the patient with gastrointestinal hemorrhage. *BP,* Blood pressure; *CBC,* complete blood count; *GI,* gastrointestinal; *ICU,* intensive care unit; *IV,* intravenous; *INR,* International Normalized Ratio; *NG,* nasogastric; *P,* weight; *PEG,* percutaneous endoscopic gastrostomy; *PPI,* proton pump inhibitor; *RBC,* red blood cell. (Modified from Goldman L, Ausiello D [eds]: *Cecil textbook of medicine,* ed 23, Philadelphia, 2008, Saunders.)

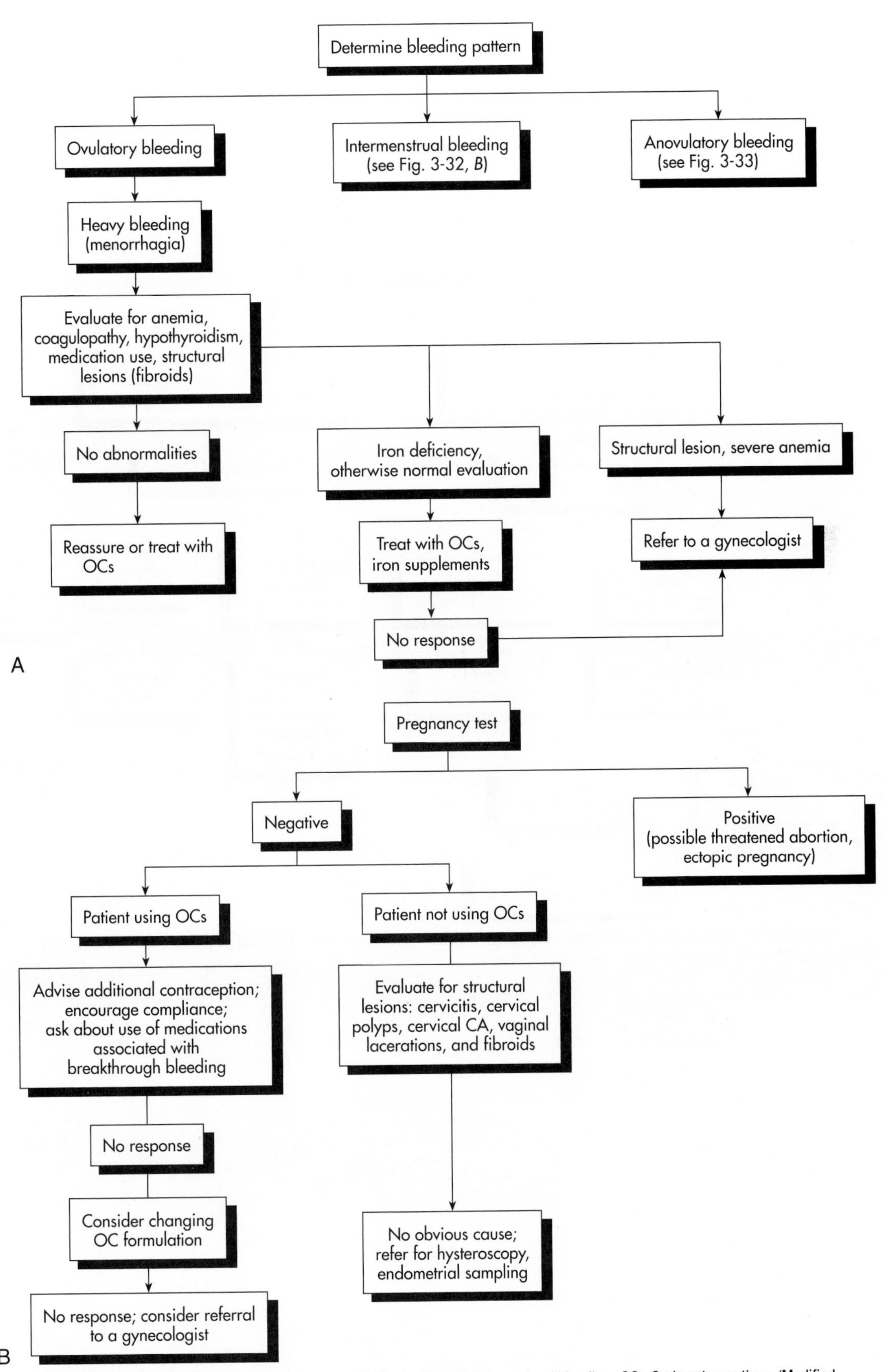

FIGURE 3-32 **A,** Evaluation of ovulatory bleeding. **B,** Evaluation of intermenstrual bleeding. *OCs,* Oral contraceptives. (Modified from Appleby J, Henderson M, Wathen PI: *Intern Med* Sept:17, 1996.)

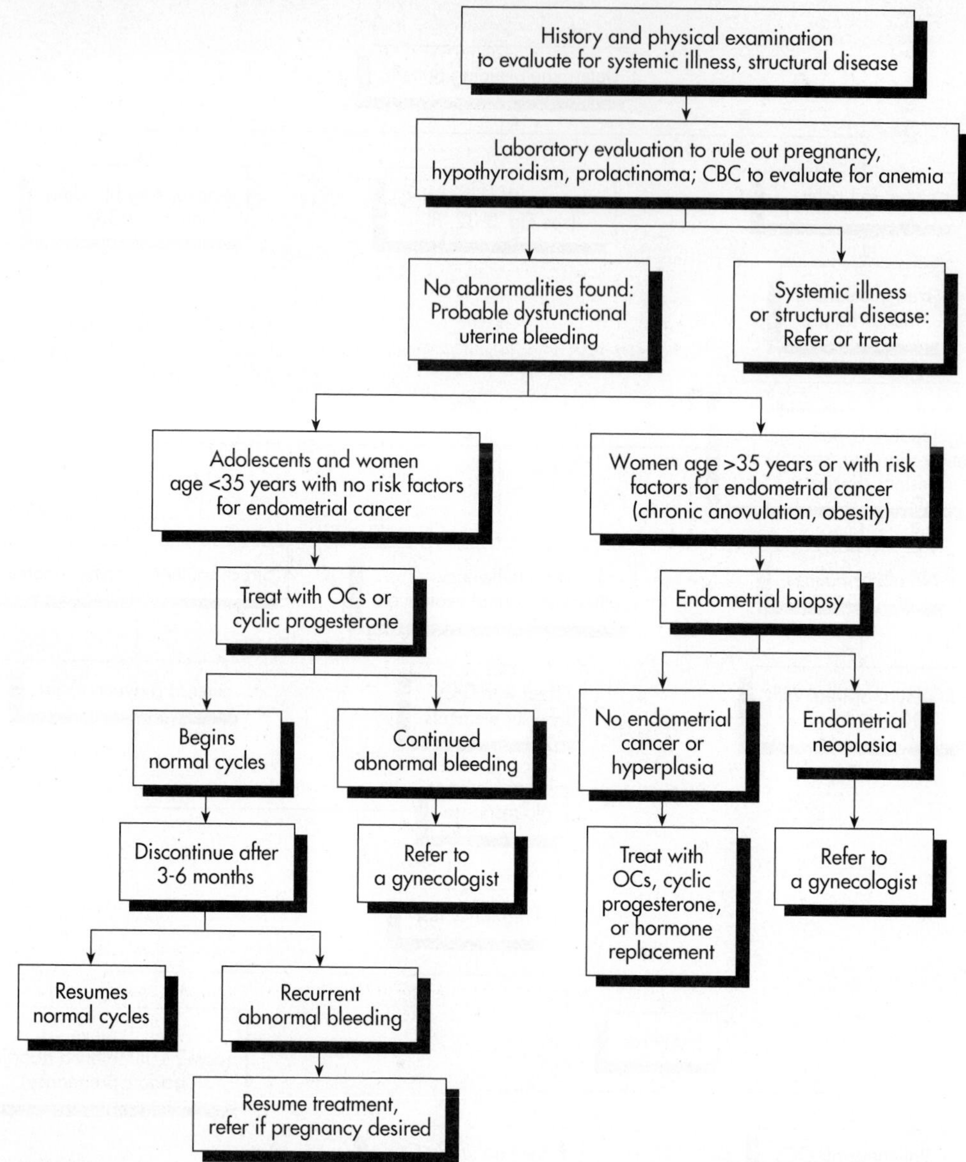

FIGURE 3-33 Evaluation of anovulatory bleeding. *CBC,* Complete blood count; *OCs,* oral contraceptives. (From Appleby J, Henderson M, Wathen PI: *Intern Med,* Sept:17, 1996.)

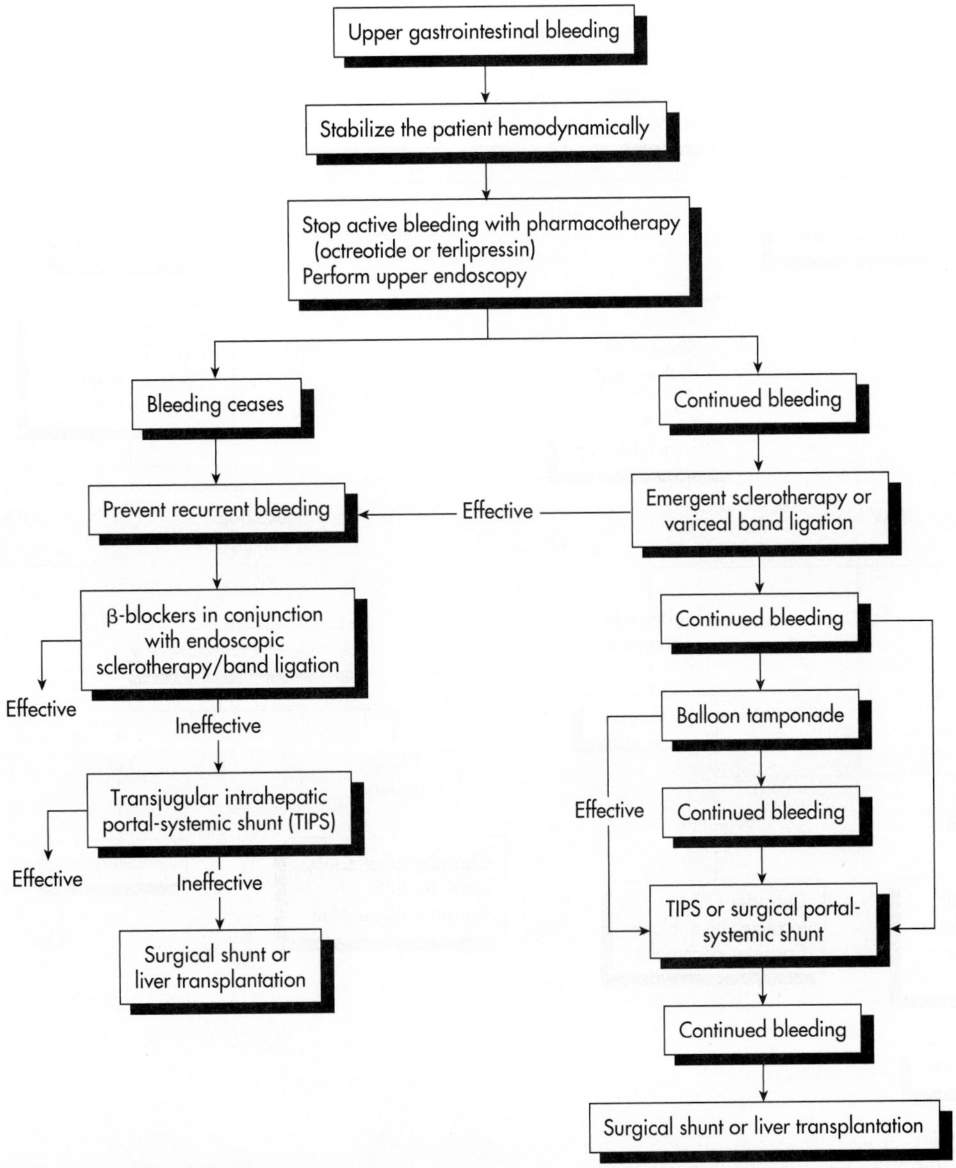

Upper gastrointestinal bleeding

Stabilize the patient hemodynamically

Stop active bleeding with pharmacotherapy
(octreotide or terlipressin)
Perform upper endoscopy

Bleeding ceases

Continued bleeding

Prevent recurrent bleeding

Effective

Emergent sclerotherapy or variceal band ligation

β-blockers in conjunction with endoscopic sclerotherapy/band ligation

Continued bleeding

Effective

Ineffective

Balloon tamponade

Transjugular intrahepatic portal-systemic shunt (TIPS)

Effective

Continued bleeding

Effective

Ineffective

TIPS or surgical portal-systemic shunt

Surgical shunt or liver transplantation

Continued bleeding

Surgical shunt or liver transplantation

FIGURE 3-34 Management algorithm for variceal bleeding. (From Goldman L, Schafer AL [eds]: *Cecil textbook of medicine,* ed 24, Philadelphia, 2012, Saunders.)

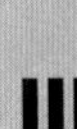

ICD-9CM #	427.89	Unspecified bradycardia
	427.81	Chronic bradycardia
	770.8	Newborn bradycardia
	337	Reflex bradycardia
ICD-10CM #	R00.1	Bradycardia
	I49.8	Other specified cardiac arrhythmias
	I49.5	Sick sinus syndrome

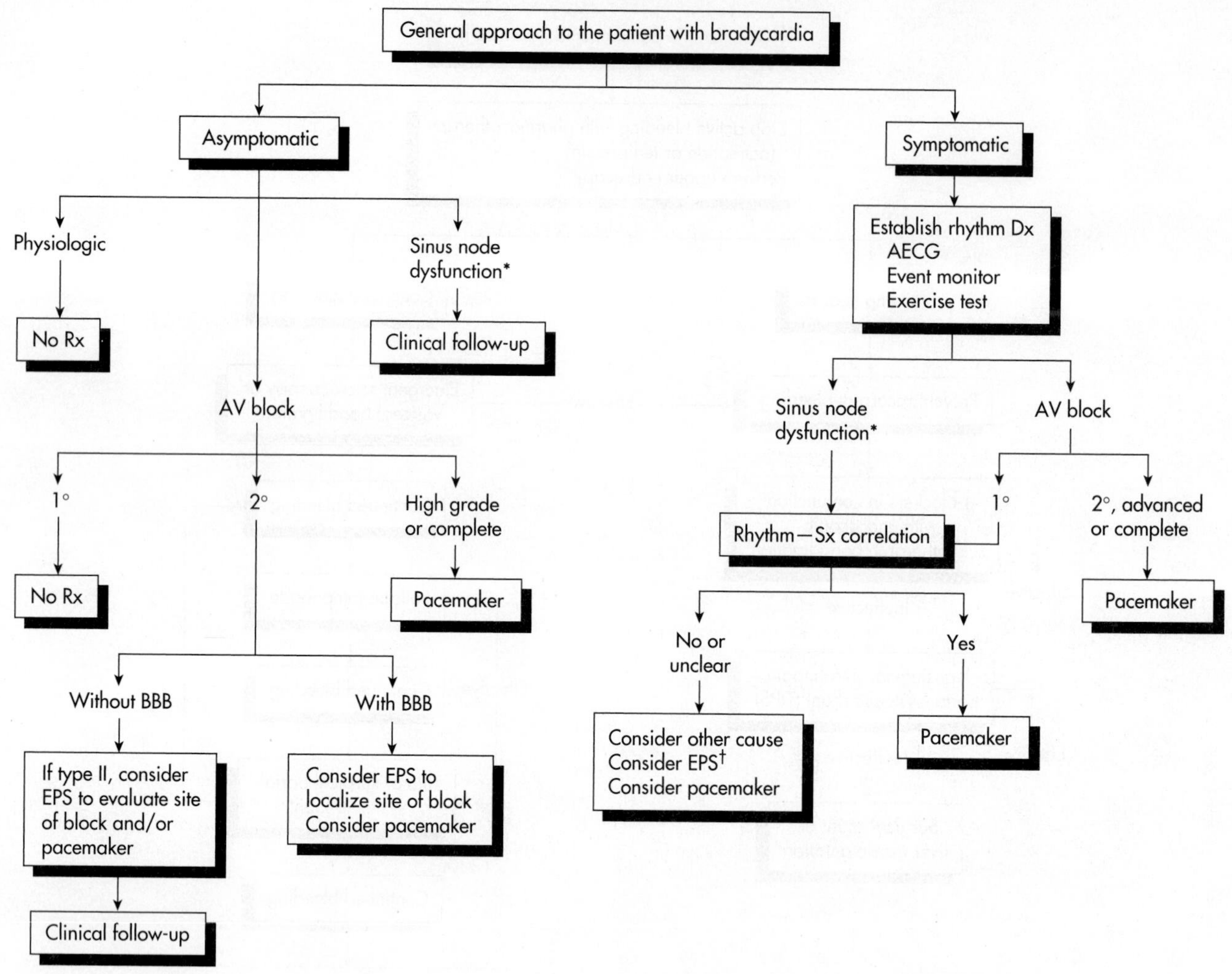

*Includes bradycardia-tachycardia syndrome.
†EPS includes sinus node function and ventricular arrhythmia induction studies.

FIGURE 3-35 General approach to the patient with bradycardia. *AECG,* Ambulatory electrocardiography; *AV,* atrioventricular; *BBB,* bundle branch block; *Dx,* diagnostic; *EPS,* electrophysiologic study; *Rx,* treatment; *Sx,* symptoms; *1°,* first-degree; *2°,* second-degree. (From Goldman L, Braunwald E [eds]: *Primary cardiology,* ed 2, Philadelphia, 2003, Saunders.)

BREAST, NIPPLE DISCHARGE EVALUATION

ICD-9CM # 611.79
ICD-10CM # N64.52 Nipple discharge
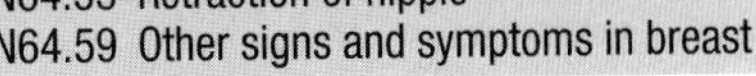
N64.51 Induration of breast
N64.53 Retraction of nipple
N64.59 Other signs and symptoms in breast

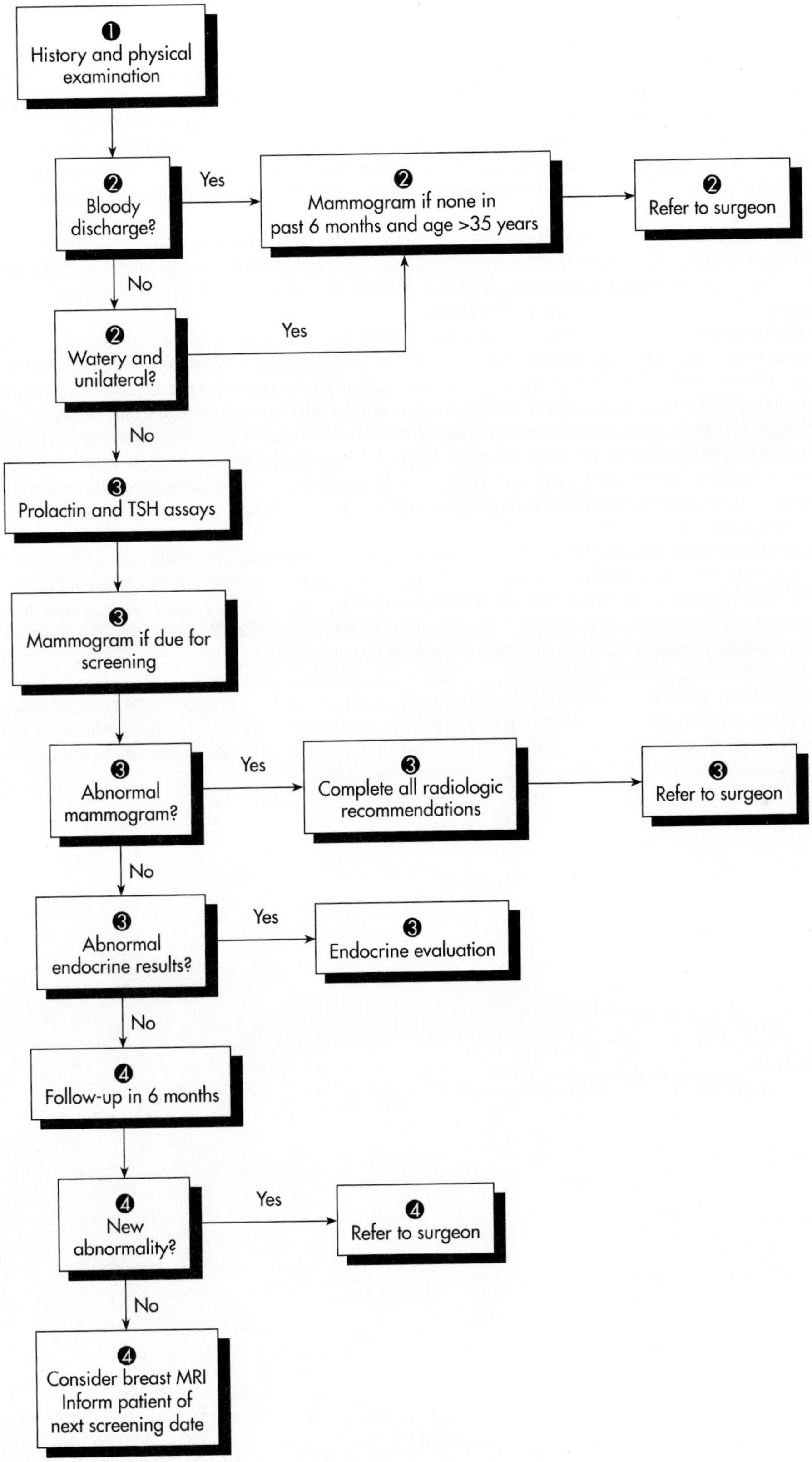

1. History and physical examination → 2
2. Bloody discharge?
   - Yes → 2 Mammogram if none in past 6 months and age >35 years → 2 Refer to surgeon
   - No → 2 Watery and unilateral?
     - Yes → 2 Mammogram if none in past 6 months and age >35 years
     - No → 3 Prolactin and TSH assays
3. Prolactin and TSH assays → 3 Mammogram if due for screening → 3 Abnormal mammogram?
   - Yes → 3 Complete all radiologic recommendations → 3 Refer to surgeon
   - No → 3 Abnormal endocrine results?
     - Yes → 3 Endocrine evaluation
     - No → 4 Follow-up in 6 months
4. Follow-up in 6 months → 4 New abnormality?
   - Yes → 4 Refer to surgeon
   - No → 4 Consider breast MRI; Inform patient of next screening date

*Without palpable mass.

FIGURE 3-37 Breast cancer screening and evaluation. (Modified from Institute for Clinical Systems Integration, Minneapolis: *Postgrad Med* 100:182, 1996.)

ICD-9CM # 611.79
ICD-10CM # N64.52 Nipple discharge
N64.51 Induration of breast
N64.53 Retraction of nipple
N64.59 Other signs and symptoms in breast

FIGURE 3-37 (Continued)

1. **History and physical examination.*** Patients who present with a complaint of nipple discharge should be evaluated with breast-related history taking and a physical examination. History taking is aimed at uncovering and characterizing any other breast-related symptom. A risk assessment should also be undertaken for identified risk factors, including patient age over 50 years, any past personal history of breast cancer, history of hyperplasia on previous breast biopsies, and family history of breast cancer in first-degree relatives (mother, sister, daughter). Physical examination should include inspection of the breast for any evidence of ulceration or contour changes and inspection of the nipple for Paget's disease. Palpation should be performed with the patient in both the upright and the supine positions to determine the presence of any palpable mass.
2. **Bloody discharge?** If the discharge appears frankly bloody, the patient should be referred to a surgeon for evaluation. At the time of referral, a mammogram of the involved breast should be obtained if the patient is over 35 years of age and has not had a mammogram within the preceding 6 months. Similarly, patients with a watery, unilateral discharge should be referred to a surgeon for evaluation and possible biopsy.
3. **Endocrine tests. Mammogram.** If the discharge appears frankly milky or is bilateral, serum prolactin and serum thyroid-stimulating hormone *(TSH)* assays should be performed to rule out the presence of an endocrinologic basis for the symptoms. At the time of that visit, a mammogram should also be performed if the patient is due for routine mammographic screening according to the recommended intervals. A patient with an abnormal mammogram should be further evaluated radiologically to better characterize the lesion and then be referred to a surgeon if appropriate. Make certain that all recommended additional views, ultrasound examinations, and follow-up studies have been obtained before referral to a surgeon. Should the mammogram appear normal, results of the assays for TSH and prolactin should be reviewed. If the results are abnormal, the patient should undergo appropriate evaluation for etiology, either by a primary care physician or by an endocrinologist.
4. **Six-month follow-up results.** If results of the mammogram and the endocrinologic screening studies are normal, the patient should return for a follow-up visit in 6 months to ensure that there has been no specific change in the character of the discharge, such as development of frank bleeding or Paget's disease, that would warrant surgical evaluation. If the evaluation at that follow-up visit fails to reveal any palpable or visible abnormalities, the patient should be returned to the routine screening process with studies performed at the recommended intervals.

---

*ICSI health care guidelines are designed to assist clinicians by providing an analytic framework for the evaluation and treatment of patients. They are not intended either to replace a clinician's judgment or to establish a protocol for all patients with a particular condition. A guideline will rarely establish the only approach to a problem. In addition, guidelines are "living documents" that are expected to be imperfect and are subject to annual review and revision.

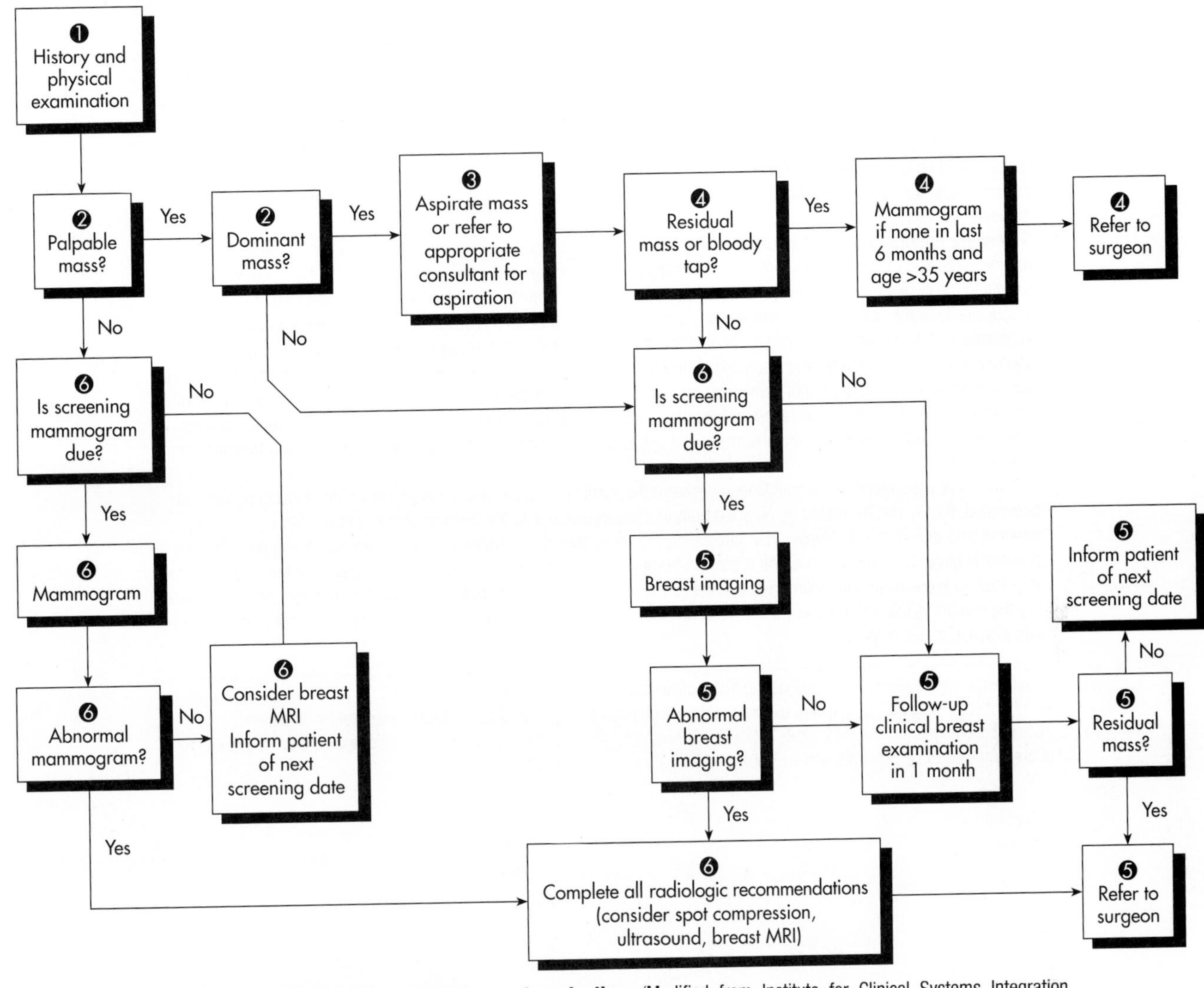

FIGURE 3-39 Breast cancer screening and evaluation. (Modified from Institute for Clinical Systems Integration, Minneapolis: *Postgrad Med* 100:182, 1996.)

1. **History and physical examination.*** Primary care evaluation is initiated with history taking aimed at uncovering and characterizing any breast-related symptom. A risk assessment should also be undertaken for identified risk factors, including patient age over 50 years, any past personal history of breast cancer, history of hyperplasia on previous breast biopsies, and family history of breast cancer in first-degree relatives (mother, sister, daughter). Physical examination should include inspection of the breast for any evidence of ulceration or contour changes and inspection of the nipple for Paget's disease. Palpation should be performed with the patient in both the upright and supine positions to determine the presence of any palpable mass.
2. **Palpable mass? Dominant mass?** A dominant mass is a palpable finding that is discrete and clearly different from the surrounding parenchyma. If a palpable mass is identified, it should be determined whether it represents a dominant (i.e., discrete) mass, which requires immediate evaluation. The primary care physician or appropriate consultant should attempt to aspirate any dominant mass because a simple cyst may be uncovered, in which case aspiration completes the evaluation process.
3. **Aspirate mass or refer for aspiration.** Aspiration of a dominant palpable mass should be performed by the primary care physician or by the appropriate consultant. The breast skin is prepped with alcohol. Then, with the lesion immobilized by the nonoperating hand, an 18- to 25-gauge needle mounted on a 10-ml syringe is directed to the central portion of the mass for a single attempt at aspiration. Successful aspiration of a simple cyst would yield a nonbloody fluid with complete resolution of the dominant mass. Typical watery fluid may be discarded. However, cyst fluid that is bloody or unusually tenacious should be examined cytologically.
4. **Residual mass or bloody tap?** Mammogram if none in past 6 months. Refer to surgeon. Should the mass remain after the attempt at aspiration or should frank blood be aspirated during the process, the presence of a malignant process cannot be ruled out. Patients with a residual mass or bloody tap should be referred to a surgeon for possible biopsy. Before the referral, a mammogram should be obtained for any patient over age 35 years who has not had a mammogram within the preceding 6 months. In patients 35 years and under, obtaining any other breast-imaging studies should be left to the discretion of the surgeon or radiologist.
5. **Is screening mammogram due?** Breast imaging. Follow-up clinical breast examination. Refer to surgeon. Should physical examination demonstrate a palpable mass that is not clearly a discrete and dominant mass, its size, location, and character should be documented in anticipation of a follow-up examination. A screening mammogram should be obtained if one has not been done within the recommended interval. If no mammogram is required or if a required

Continued on following page

FIGURE 3-39 (Continued)

mammogram demonstrates no abnormality, a follow-up examination in 1 month is indicated. Breast MRI should be considered. Should any residual mass be identified, the patient should be referred to a surgeon for possible biopsy. Patients with a persisting nondominant palpable mass that does not resolve within 1 month and those with any recurring cystic mass should be referred for surgical evaluation. If no mass is apparent at the time of the follow-up examination, the patient should then be informed of the appropriate date for her next screening examination, according to the recommended intervals.

6. **Screening mammogram and results.** After completion of the physical examination, the appropriateness of a routine screening mammogram should be determined. If a mammogram is done, the radiologist should provide the results to the primary care physician for reporting to the patient. Should any abnormalities be uncovered, it will be the responsibility of the radiologist to complete any additional imaging studies required for the complete radiographic characterization of the lesion. The radiologist should make certain that all recommended additional views, follow-up studies, and ultrasound examinations have been completed before referral to a surgeon. However, it is important that the primary care physician who ordered the mammogram review the results of these studies to understand fully the opinion of the radiologist and to ensure that all recommendations of the radiologist have been completed. Should the radiologist recommend that surgical consultation is warranted, it will be the responsibility of the primary care physician to establish this referral.

   NOTE: The importance of communication between the surgical consultant and the primary care physician cannot be overstated. Biopsy results should be reported both to the surgeon and to the primary care physician. More important, patients who do not require biopsy after surgical consultation should be returned to the routine screening process. This process is under the supervision of the primary care physician. Therefore it is absolutely necessary for the primary care physician to know when the patient reenters the routine screening population. In the event that new symptoms arise during the screening interval, the patient should be evaluated by the primary care physician using the primary care evaluation process of this guideline.

---

*CSI health care guidelines are designed to assist clinicians by providing an analytic framework for the evaluation and treatment of patients. They are not intended either to replace a clinician's judgment or to establish a protocol for all patients with a particular condition. A guideline will rarely establish the only approach to a problem. In addition, guidelines are living documents that are expected to be imperfect and are subject to annual review and revision.

CARDIOMEGALY ON CHEST X-RAY

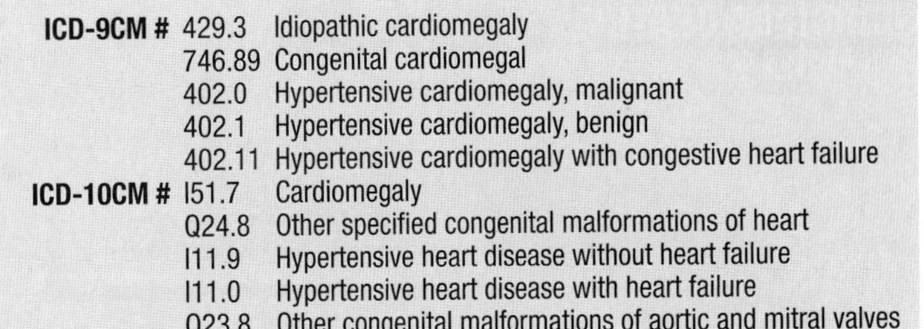

ICD-9CM #	429.3	Idiopathic cardiomegaly
	746.89	Congenital cardiomegal
	402.0	Hypertensive cardiomegaly, malignant
	402.1	Hypertensive cardiomegaly, benign
	402.11	Hypertensive cardiomegaly with congestive heart failure
ICD-10CM #	I51.7	Cardiomegaly
	Q24.8	Other specified congenital malformations of heart
	I11.9	Hypertensive heart disease without heart failure
	I11.0	Hypertensive heart disease with heart failure
	Q23.8	Other congenital malformations of aortic and mitral valves

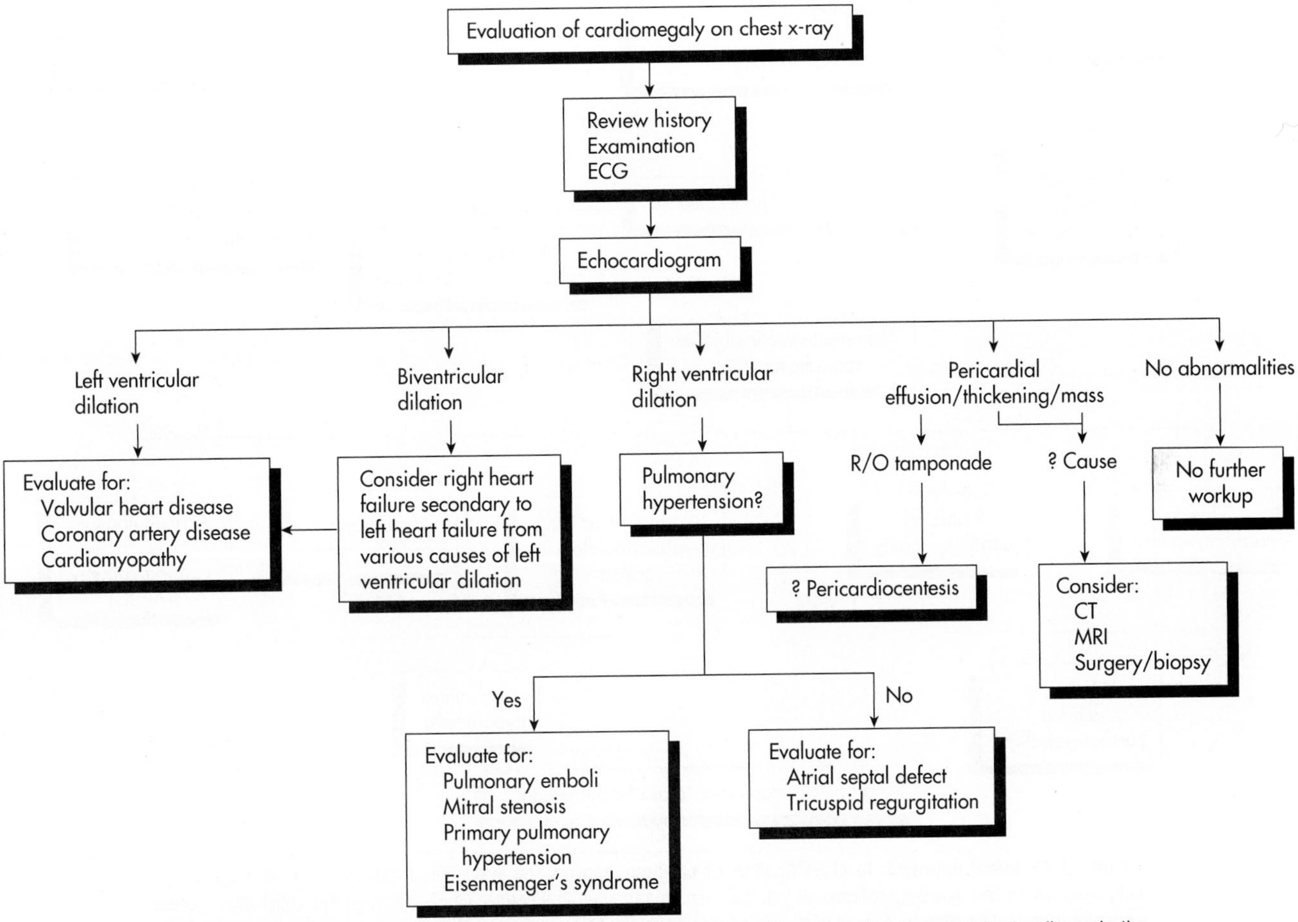

Evaluation of cardiomegaly on chest x-ray

Review history
Examination
ECG

Echocardiogram

Left ventricular dilation

Evaluate for:
Valvular heart disease
Coronary artery disease
Cardiomyopathy

Biventricular dilation

Consider right heart failure secondary to left heart failure from various causes of left ventricular dilation

Right ventricular dilation

Pulmonary hypertension?

Yes

Evaluate for:
Pulmonary emboli
Mitral stenosis
Primary pulmonary hypertension
Eisenmenger's syndrome

No

Evaluate for:
Atrial septal defect
Tricuspid regurgitation

Pericardial effusion/thickening/mass

R/O tamponade

? Pericardiocentesis

? Cause

Consider:
CT
MRI
Surgery/biopsy

No abnormalities

No further workup

FIGURE 3-42 Approach to the patient with cardiomegaly. When cardiomegaly is found on the chest radiograph, the history and physical examination should be reviewed and an electrocardiogram *(ECG)* performed before obtaining a two-dimensional Doppler echocardiographic study. Cardiomegaly may be explained by left ventricular dilation, biventricular dilation, right ventricular dilation, or pericardial abnormalities, or it may be found to be spurious on the echocardiogram. Rarely, isolated abnormalities of the atrium, particularly the left atrium, may cause abnormalities on the chest radiograph but will not cause true cardiomegaly. Depending on the echocardiographic findings, further tests can help elucidate the cause of echocardiographically confirmed cardiomegaly. *CT,* Computed tomography; *MRI,* magnetic resonance imaging; *R/O,* rule out. (From Goldman L, Braunwald E [eds]: *Primary cardiology,* ed 2, Philadelphia, 2003, Saunders.)

ICD-9CM # 425.4
ICD-10CM # I42.5 Other restrictive cardiomyopathy
I42.8 Other cardiomyopathies

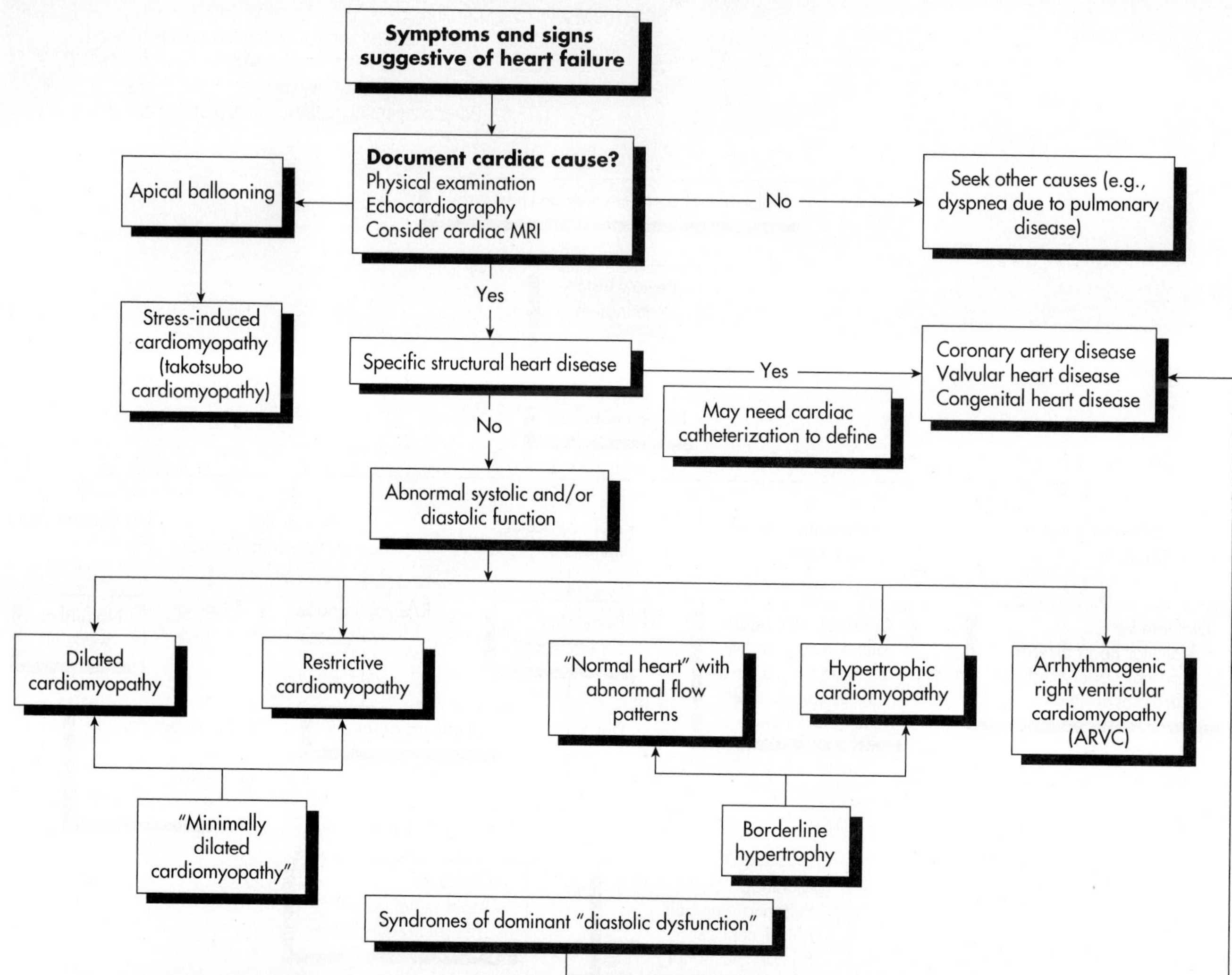

FIGURE 3-43 Initial approach to classification of cardiomyopathy. The evaluation of symptoms or signs consistent with heart failure first includes confirmation that they can be attributed to a cardiac cause. Although this conclusion is often apparent from routine physical examination, echocardiography serves to confirm cardiac disease and provides clues to the presence of other cardiac disease, such as focal abnormalities, suggesting primary valve disease or congenital heart disease. Having excluded these conditions, cardiomyopathy is generally considered to be dilated, restrictive, or hypertrophic. Patients with apparently normal cardiac structure and contraction are occasionally found to demonstrate abnormal intracardiac flow patterns consistent with diastolic dysfunction but should also be evaluated carefully for other causes of their symptoms. Most patients with so-called diastolic dysfunction also demonstrate at least borderline criteria for left ventricular hypertrophy, frequently in the setting of chronic hypertension and diabetes. A moderately decreased ejection fraction without marked dilation or a pattern of restrictive cardiomyopathy is sometimes referred to as "minimally dilated cardiomyopathy," which may represent either a distinct entity or a transition between acute and chronic disease. (From Goldman L, Ausiello D [eds]: *Cecil textbook of medicine,* ed 23, Philadelphia, 2008, Saunders.)

ICD-9CM # 425.4
ICD-10CM # I42.5 Other restrictive cardiomyopathy
I42.8 Other cardiomyopathies

TABLE 3-2 Profiles of Myocardial Disease

	Hypertrophic	Dilated	Restrictive	ARVC
Causes	Genetic	Myocarditis Metabolic/endocrine Genetic	Infiltrative or storage diseases Endomyocardial (e.g., Löffler's, carcinoid) Genetic	Genetic
Ejection fraction	Increased	Reduced	25%-50%	Normal until end stage 30% regional LV disease
Left ventricular End-diastolic dimension	Usually decreased	Increased	Normal	Normal until end stage Right ventricle dilated
Left ventricular wall thickness	Increased	Normal	Normal or mildly increased	Normal
Atrial size	Increased	Increased	Increased; may be massive	Left atrium normal; right dilated in severe disease
Valvular disease	Mitral regurgitation (SAM)	Mitral (functional); tricuspid regurgitation in late stages	Mitral and tricuspid regurgitation, rarely severe	Tricuspid regurgitation in severe disease
Common symptoms	Dyspnea; chest pain, syncope Late: orthopnea, PND	Dyspnea, fatigue Late: orthopnea, PND	Dyspnea Late: orthopnea, PND, right heart failure	Palpitations, syncope Late: right heart failure
Arrhythmia	Atrial fibrillation, ventricular tachycardia; conduction block in PRKAG2, mitochondrial; Fabry's disease	Ventricular tachyarrhythmias; heart block in Chagas' disease, giant cell myocarditis, laminopathies	Atrial fibrillation; conduction block in sarcoid, amyloidosis, desminopathy	Ventricular ectopy and tachycardia

From Goldman L, Schafer AI: *Goldman's Cecil medicine,* ed 24, Philadelphia, 2012, Saunders.
ARVC, Arrhythmogenic right ventricular cardiomyopathy; *LV,* left ventricular; *SAM,* systolic anterior motion of mitral valve; *PND,* paroxysmal nocturnal dyspnea.

ICD-9CM #	437.1	Cerebral ischemia (chronic)
	435.9	Cerebral ischemia intermittent (transient)
ICD-10CM #	I67.82	Cerebral ischemia
	I67.81	Acute cerebrovascular insufficiency
	I67.89	Other cerebrovascular disease
	I67.848	Other cerebrovascular vasospasm and vasoconstriction
	G45.9	Transient cerebral ischemic attack, unspecified

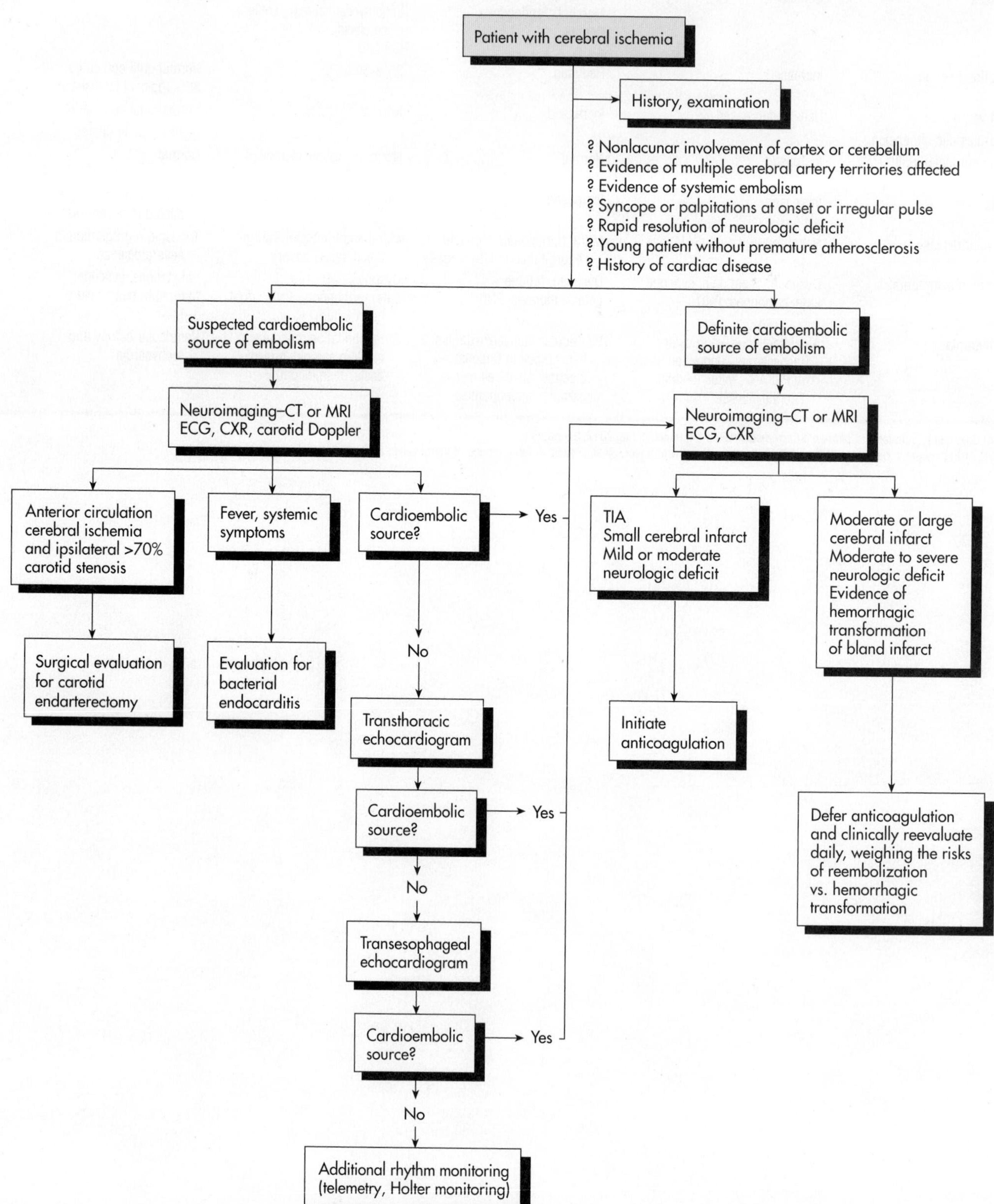

FIGURE 3-45 Evaluation of patients with cerebral ischemia for a cardioembolic source. *CT,* Computed tomography; *CXR,* chest radiograph; *ECG,* electrocardiogram; *MRI,* magnetic resonance imaging; *TIA,* transient ischemic attack. (Modified from Johnson R [ed]: *Current therapy in neurologic disease,* ed 5, St Louis, 1997, Mosby.)

ICD-9CM # 786.50
ICD-10CM # R07.2 Pain(s) heart
R07.3 Pain(s) chest anterior wall
R07.4 Pain(s) chest

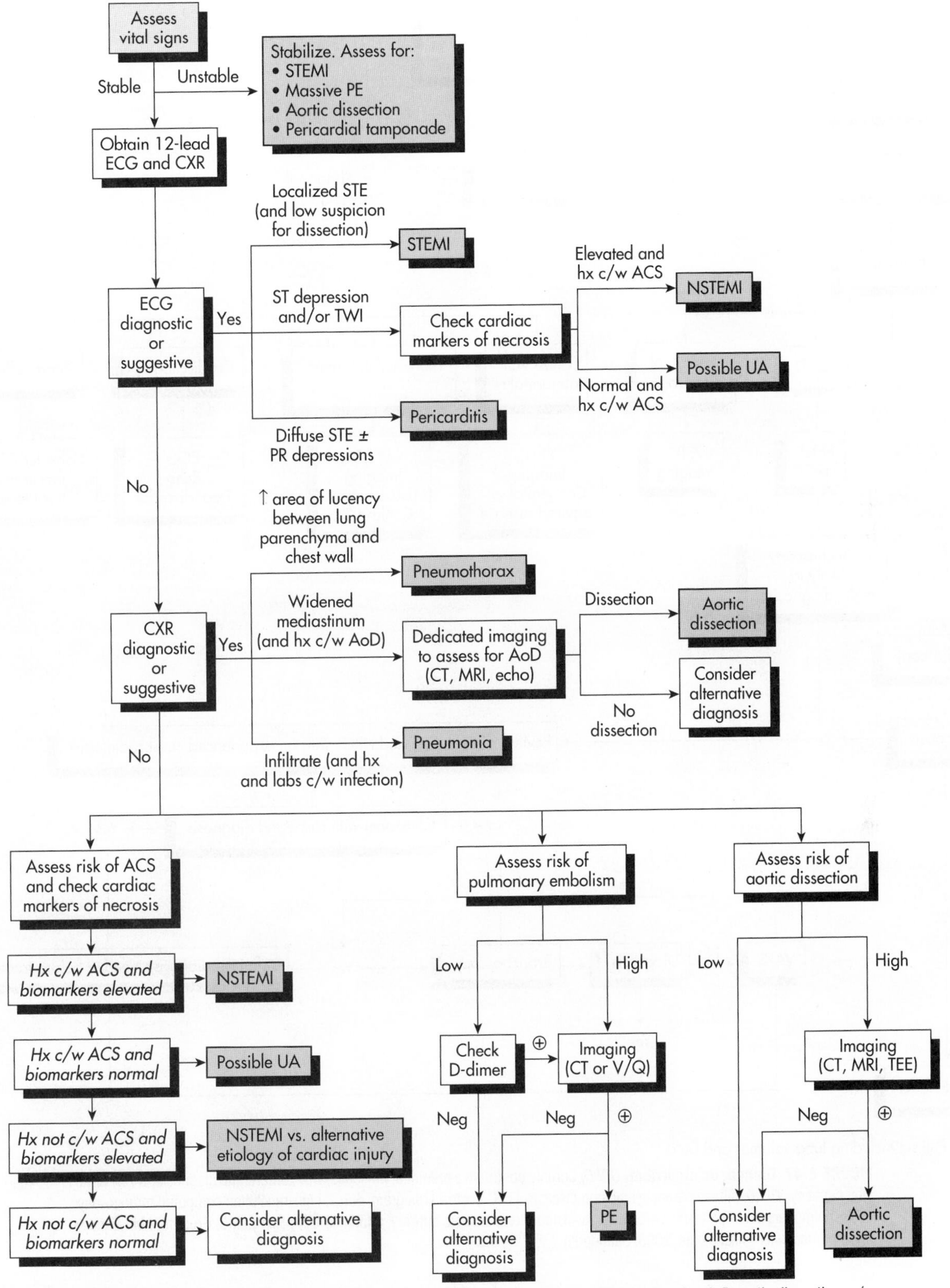

FIGURE 3-46 Algorithm for the initial diagnostic approach to a patient with chest pain. *AoD*, aortic dissection; *c/w*, consistent with; *CXR*, chest x-ray; *hx*, history; *NSTEMI*, non–ST-segment myocardial infarction; *PE*, pulmonary embolism; *STE*, ST elevation; *STEMI*, ST-segment myocardial infarction; *TEE*, transesophageal echocardiography; *UA*, unstable angina; *V/Q*, ventilation-perfusion scan. (From Bonow RO et al: *Braunwauld's heart disease*, ed 9, Philadelphia, 2012, Elsevier.)

ICD-9CM # 793.1
ICD-10CM # R91.8 Other nonspecific abnormal finding of lung field

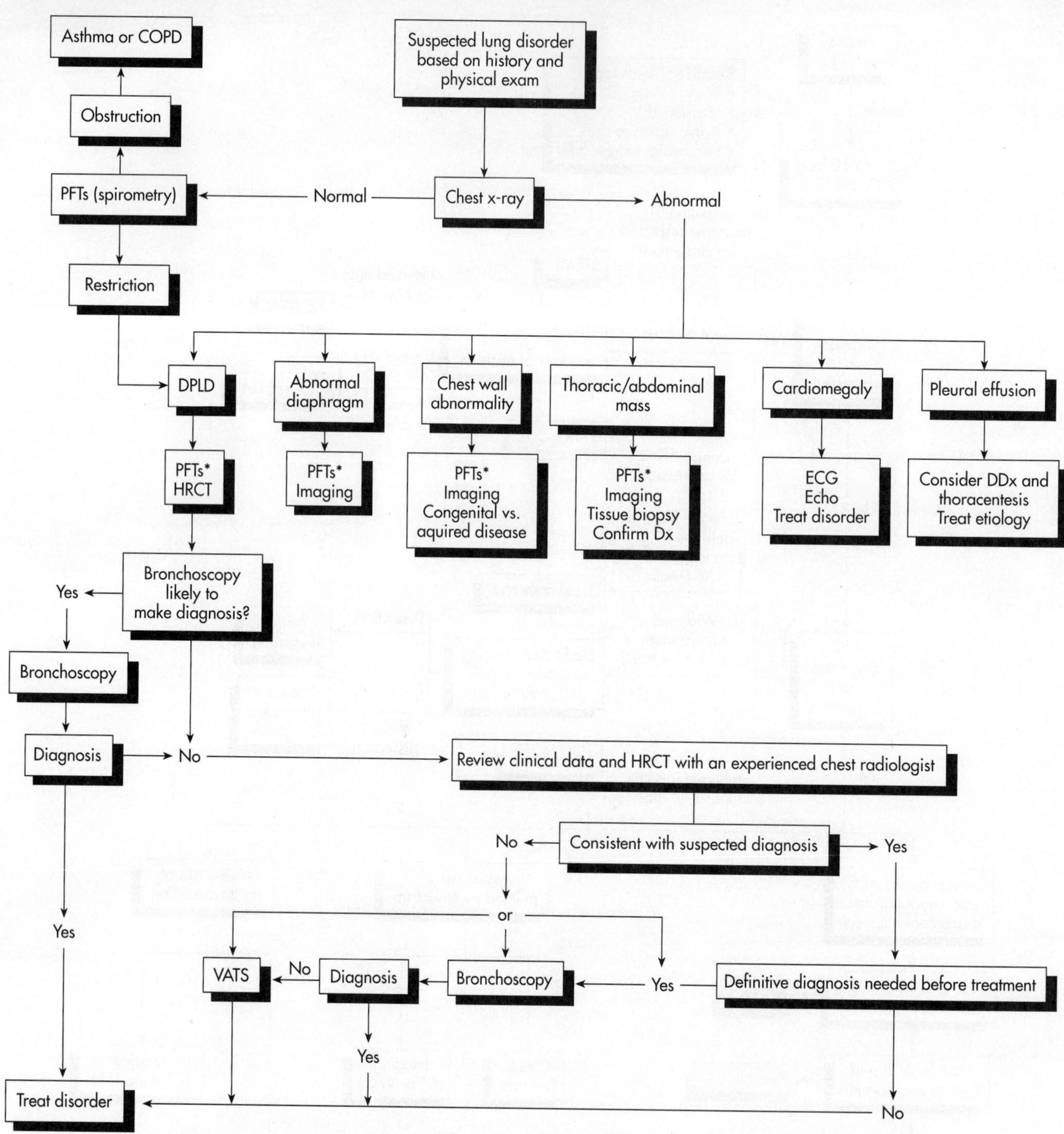

FIGURE 3-47 Diagnostic algorithm. *COPD,* Chronic obstructive pulmonary disease; *DDx,* differential diagnosis; *D LCO,* diffusion capacity; *DPLD,* diffuse parenchymal lung disease; *ECG,* electrocardiogram; *HRCT,* high-resolution computed tomography; *PFTs,* pulmonary function tests; *VATS,* video-assisted thoracoscopic surgery. (Modified from Runge MS, Greganti MA: *Netter's internal medicine,* Philadelphia, 2008, Saunders.)

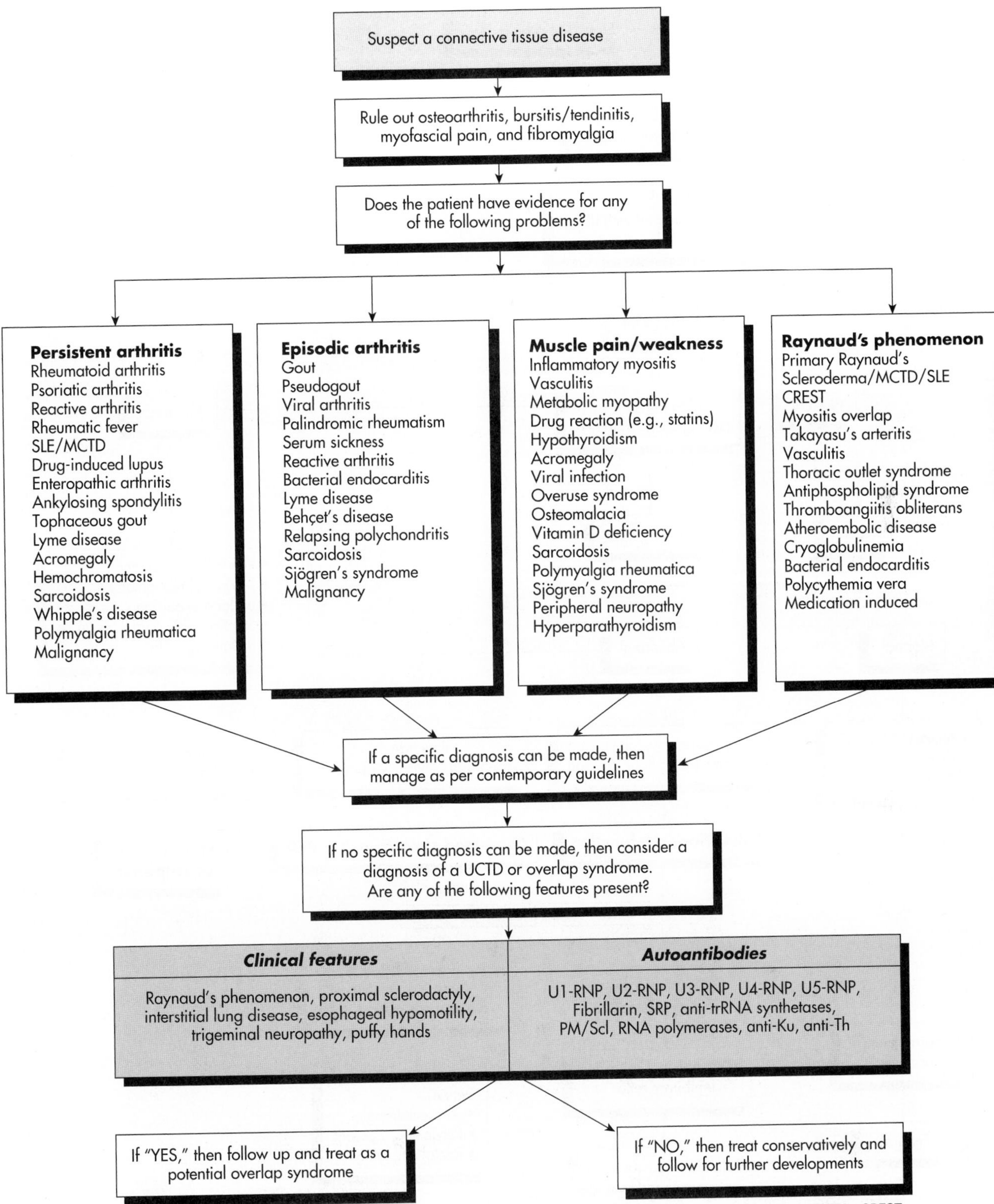

FIGURE 3-48 Algorithm for evaluating patients with undifferentiated connective tissue disease (UCTD). *CREST,* calcinosis, Raynaud's phenomenon, esophageal dysmotility, sclerodactyly, and telangiectasia; *MCTD,* mixed connective tissue disease; *SLE,* systemic lupus erythematosus. (From Firestein GS, Budd RC, Gabriel SE, et al: *Kelly's textbook of rheumatology,* ed 9, Philadelphia, 2013, Saunders. [Original credit: Courtesy Dr. George Raj, Non Surgical Spine and Joint Clinic PS, Bellingham, Wash.])

ICD-9CM # 564.0
ICD-10CM # K59.00 Constipation, unspecified

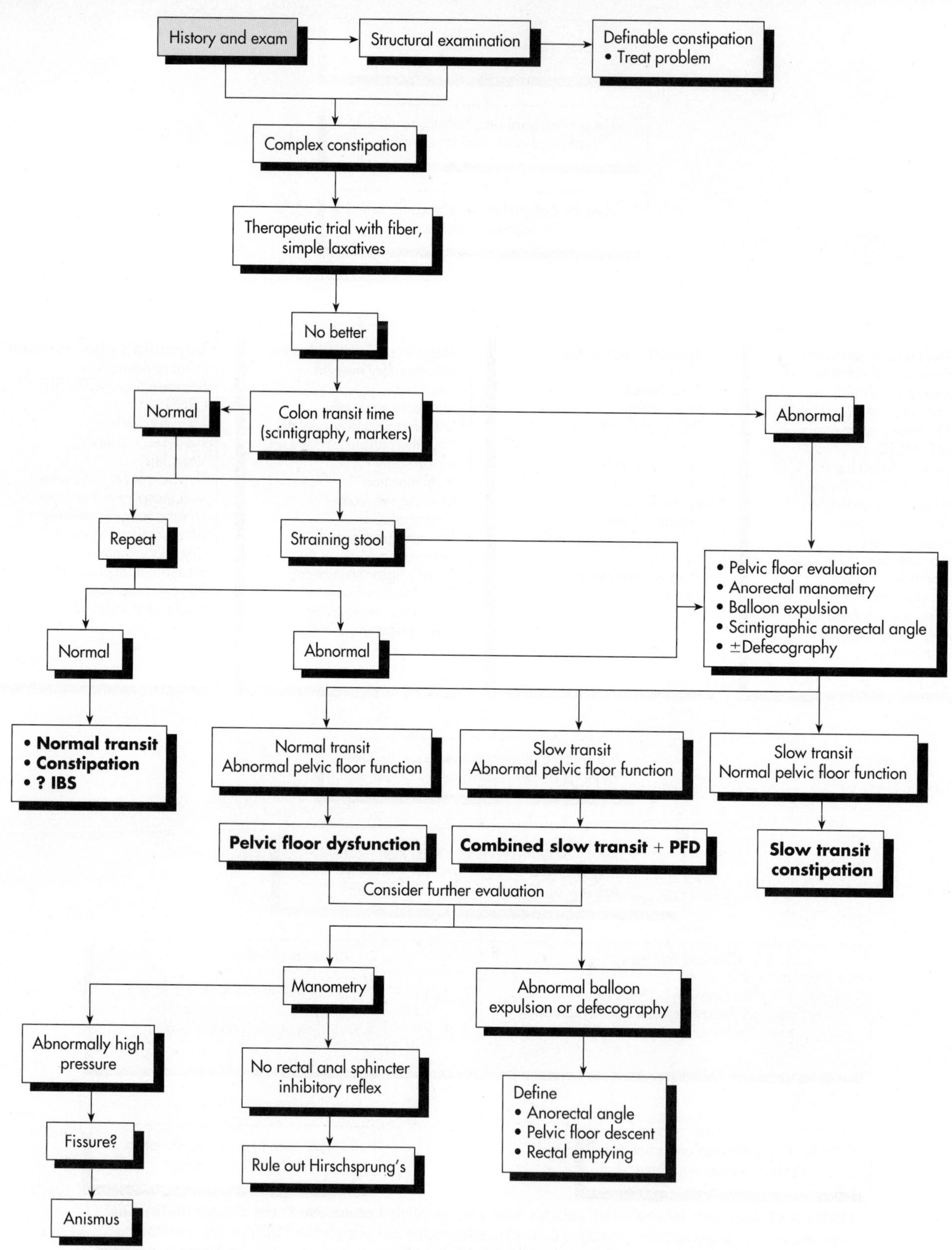

FIGURE 3-49 Evaluation of constipation. *IBS,* Irritable bowel syndrome; *PFD,* pelvic floor dysfunction. (From Pemberton JH et al: *The pelvic floor: its functions and disorders,* Philadelphia, 2001, Saunders.)

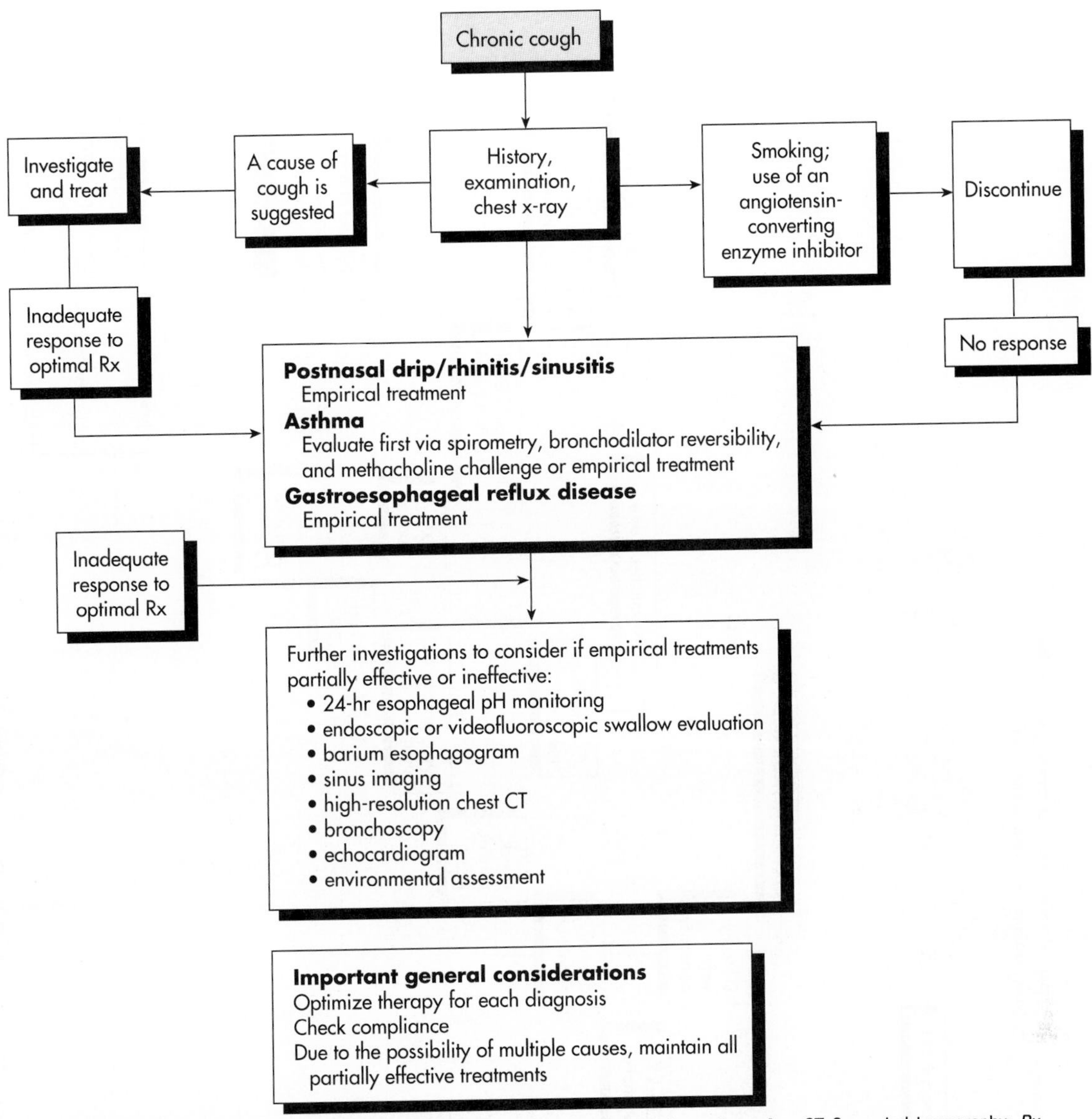

FIGURE 3-52 Algorithm for the management of chronic cough lasting >8 weeks. *CT,* Computed tomography; *Rx,* prescription. (From Goldman L, Schafer AI: *Goldman's Cecil medicine,* ed 24, Philadelphia, 2012, Saunders.)

TABLE 3-3 Testing Characteristics of Diagnostic Protocol for Evaluation of Chronic Cough

Tests	Diagnosis	Positive Predictive Value (%)	Negative Predictive Value (%)
Sinus radiograph	Sinusitis	57-81	95-100
Methacholine inhalation challenge	Asthma	60-82	100
Modified barium esophagography	GERD, esophageal stricture	38-63	63-93
Esophageal pH*	GERD	89-100	>100
Bronchoscopy	Endobronchial mass/lesion	50-89	100

From Goldman L, Schafer AI: *Goldman's Cecil medicine,* ed 24, Philadelphia, 2012, Saunders.
*24-Hour esophageal pH monitoring. *GERD,* Gastroesophageal reflux disease.

CYANOSIS

ICD-9CM # 782.5 Cyanosis NOS
ICD-10CM # R23.0 Cyanosis

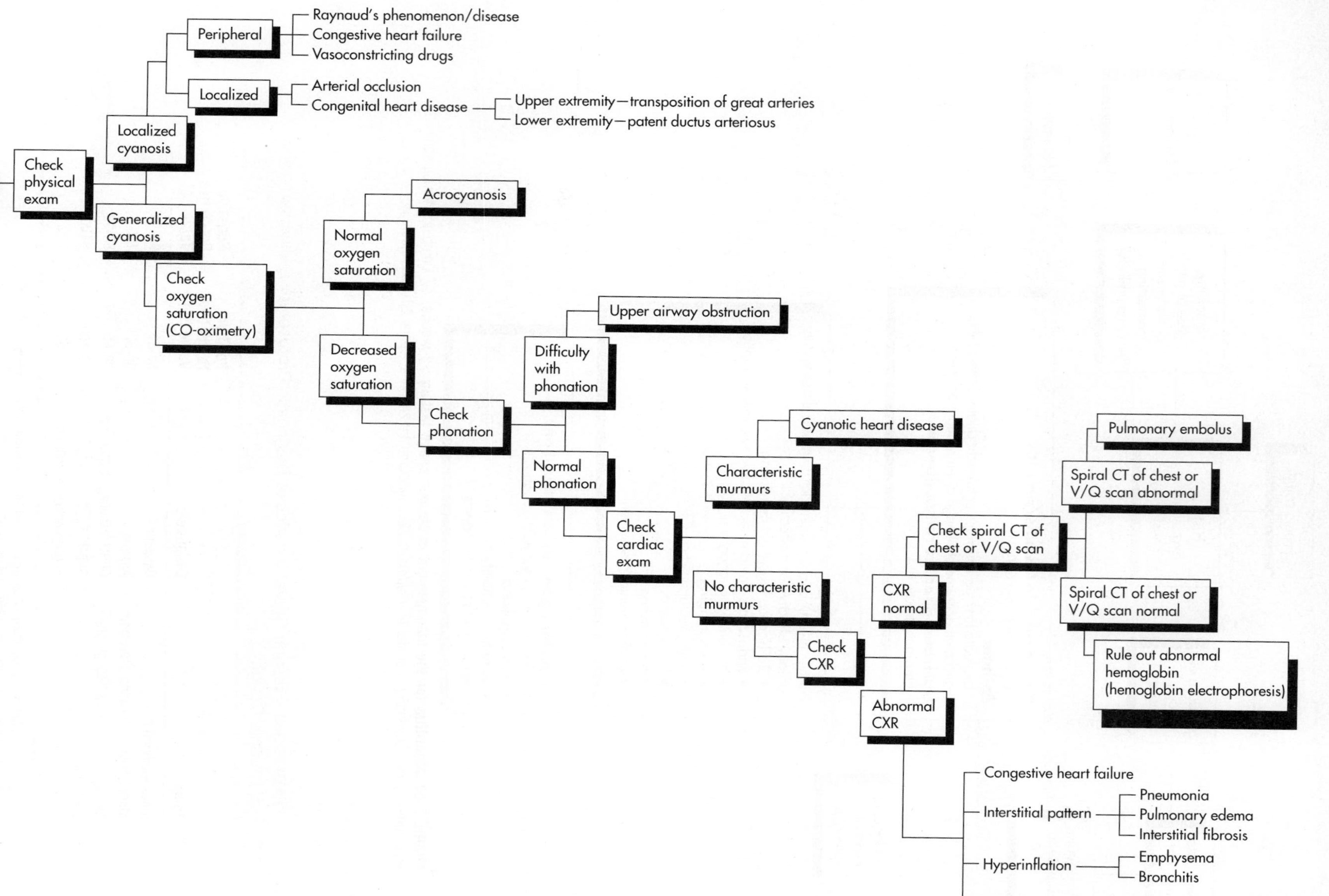

FIGURE 3-54 Cyanosis. *A-V,* Arteriovenous; *CXR,* chest x-ray; *V/Q,* ventilation-perfusion. (From Healey PM: *Common medical diagnosis: an algorithmic approach,* ed 3, Philadelphia, 2000, Saunders.)

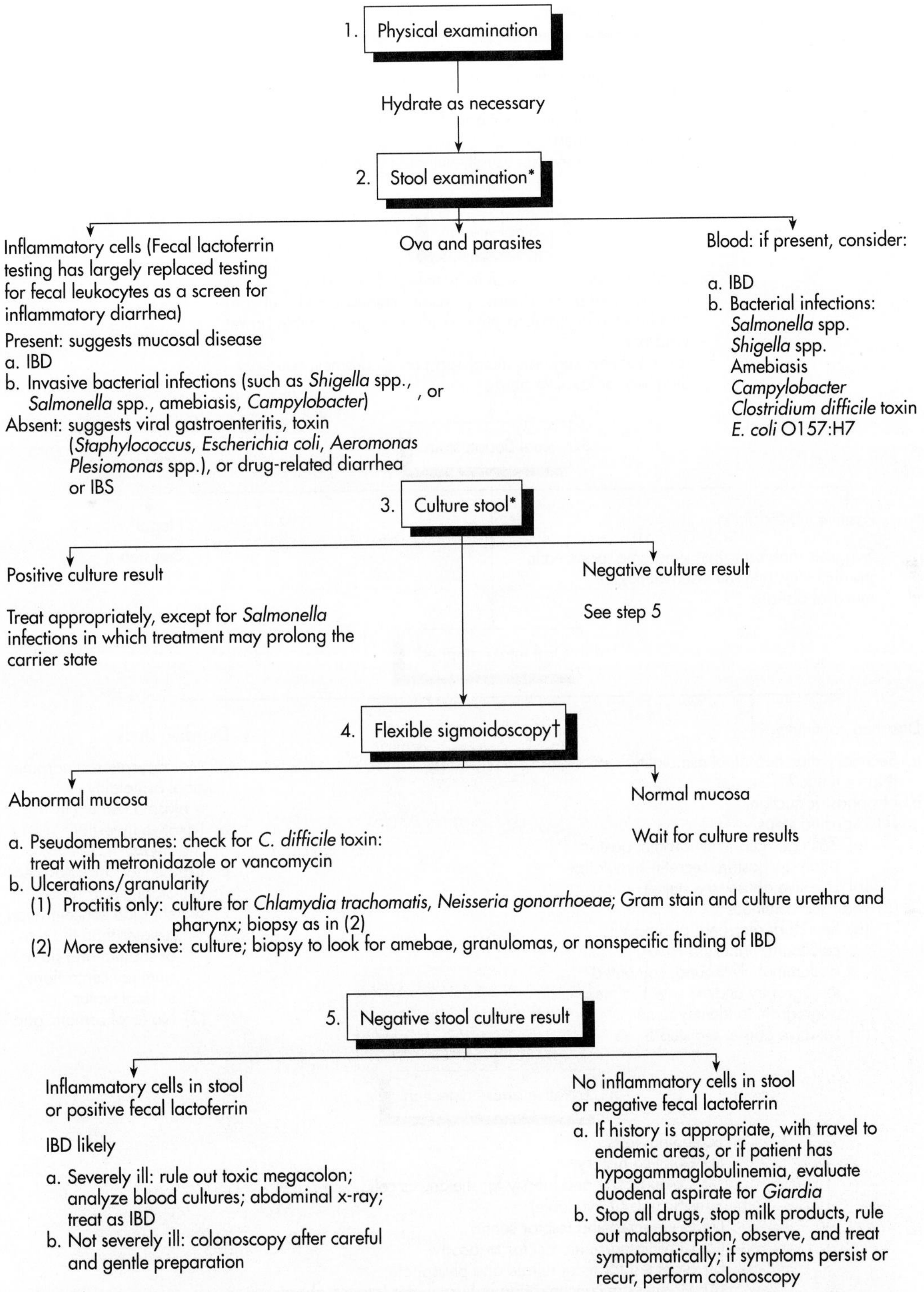

1. Physical examination

Hydrate as necessary

2. Stool examination*

Inflammatory cells (Fecal lactoferrin testing has largely replaced testing for fecal leukocytes as a screen for inflammatory diarrhea)

Present: suggests mucosal disease
a. IBD
b. Invasive bacterial infections (such as *Shigella* spp., *Salmonella* spp., amebiasis, *Campylobacter*), or

Absent: suggests viral gastroenteritis, toxin (*Staphylococcus, Escherichia coli, Aeromonas Plesiomonas* spp.), or drug-related diarrhea or IBS

Ova and parasites

Blood: if present, consider:

a. IBD
b. Bacterial infections:
Salmonella spp.
Shigella spp.
Amebiasis
Campylobacter
Clostridium difficile toxin
E. coli O157:H7

3. Culture stool*

Positive culture result

Treat appropriately, except for *Salmonella* infections in which treatment may prolong the carrier state

Negative culture result

See step 5

4. Flexible sigmoidoscopy†

Abnormal mucosa

a. Pseudomembranes: check for *C. difficile* toxin: treat with metronidazole or vancomycin
b. Ulcerations/granularity
(1) Proctitis only: culture for *Chlamydia trachomatis, Neisseria gonorrhoeae;* Gram stain and culture urethra and pharynx; biopsy as in (2)
(2) More extensive: culture; biopsy to look for amebae, granulomas, or nonspecific finding of IBD

Normal mucosa

Wait for culture results

5. Negative stool culture result

Inflammatory cells in stool or positive fecal lactoferrin

IBD likely

a. Severely ill: rule out toxic megacolon; analyze blood cultures; abdominal x-ray; treat as IBD
b. Not severely ill: colonoscopy after careful and gentle preparation

No inflammatory cells in stool or negative fecal lactoferrin
a. If history is appropriate, with travel to endemic areas, or if patient has hypogammaglobulinemia, evaluate duodenal aspirate for *Giardia*
b. Stop all drugs, stop milk products, rule out malabsorption, observe, and treat symptomatically; if symptoms persist or recur, perform colonoscopy

FIGURE 3-59 Diagnostic steps in the assessment of acute diarrhea. *For most uses of acute diarrhea, testing is not indicated. Stool examination and culture should be reserved for patients with severe illness, bloody stool, severe dehydration, immunosuppression, and for suspected nosocomial infection. †The role of lower endoscopy in acute diarrhea is limited. It should be considered only if the diagnosis is unclear after blood and stool tests in severely symptomatic patients. ‡Acute diarrhea is defined as stool with increased water content, volume, or frequency that lasts less than 14 days. *IBD,* Inflammatory bowel disease; *IBS,* irritable bowel syndrome. (Modified from Stein JH [ed]: *Internal medicine,* ed 5, St Louis, 1998, Mosby.)

ICD-9CM # 787.91
ICD-10CM # R19.7 Diarrhea, unspecified

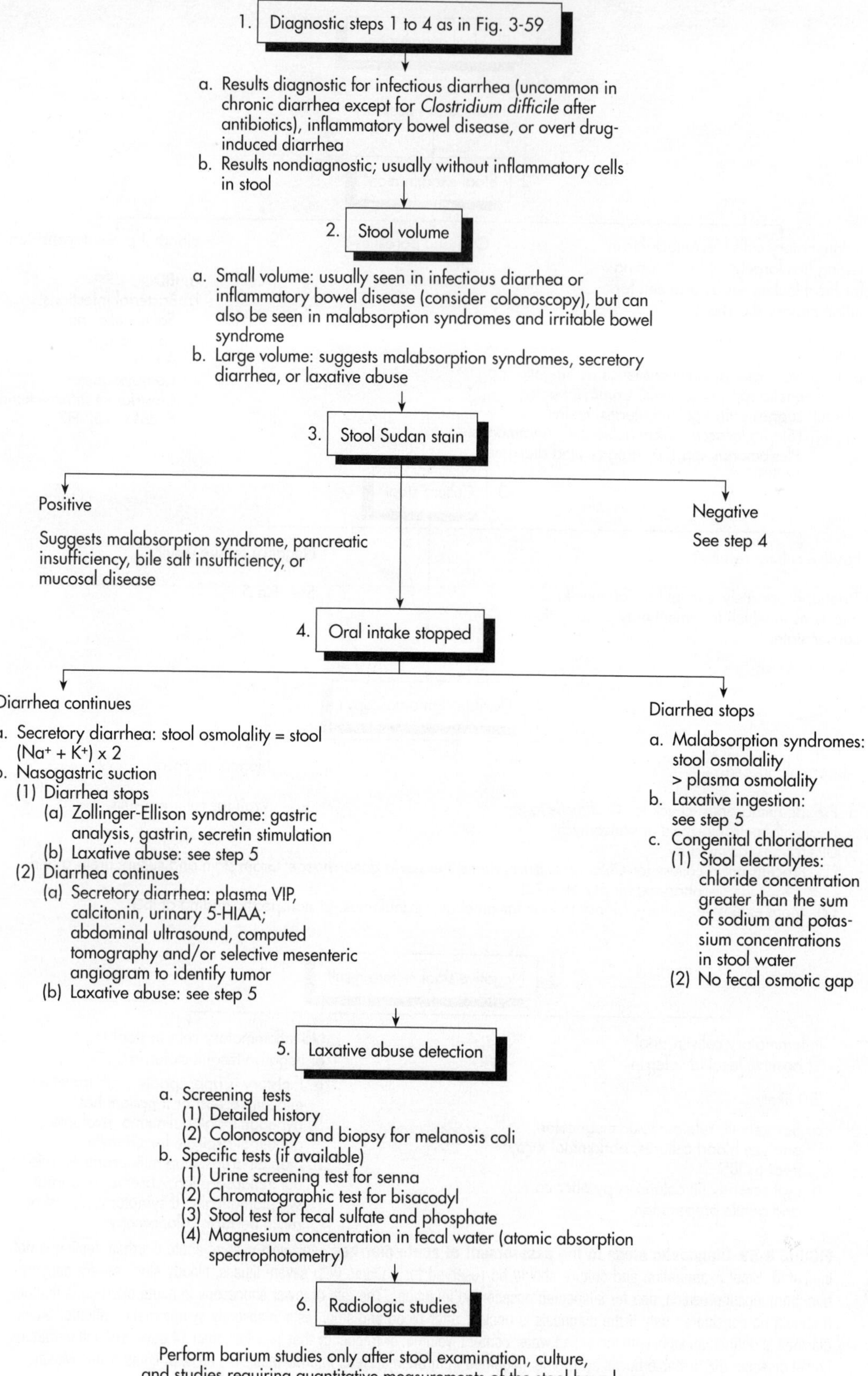

FIGURE 3-60 Diagnostic approach to the patient with chronic diarrhea (patients who are HIV negative). *5-HIAA,* 5-Hydroxyindoleacetic acid; *VIP,* vasoactive intestinal polypeptide. (Modified from Stein JH [ed]: *Internal medicine,* ed 5, St Louis, 1998, Mosby.)

DILATED PUPIL

ICD-9CM # 379.43 Pupil dilation
ICD-10CM # H57.04 Mydriasis

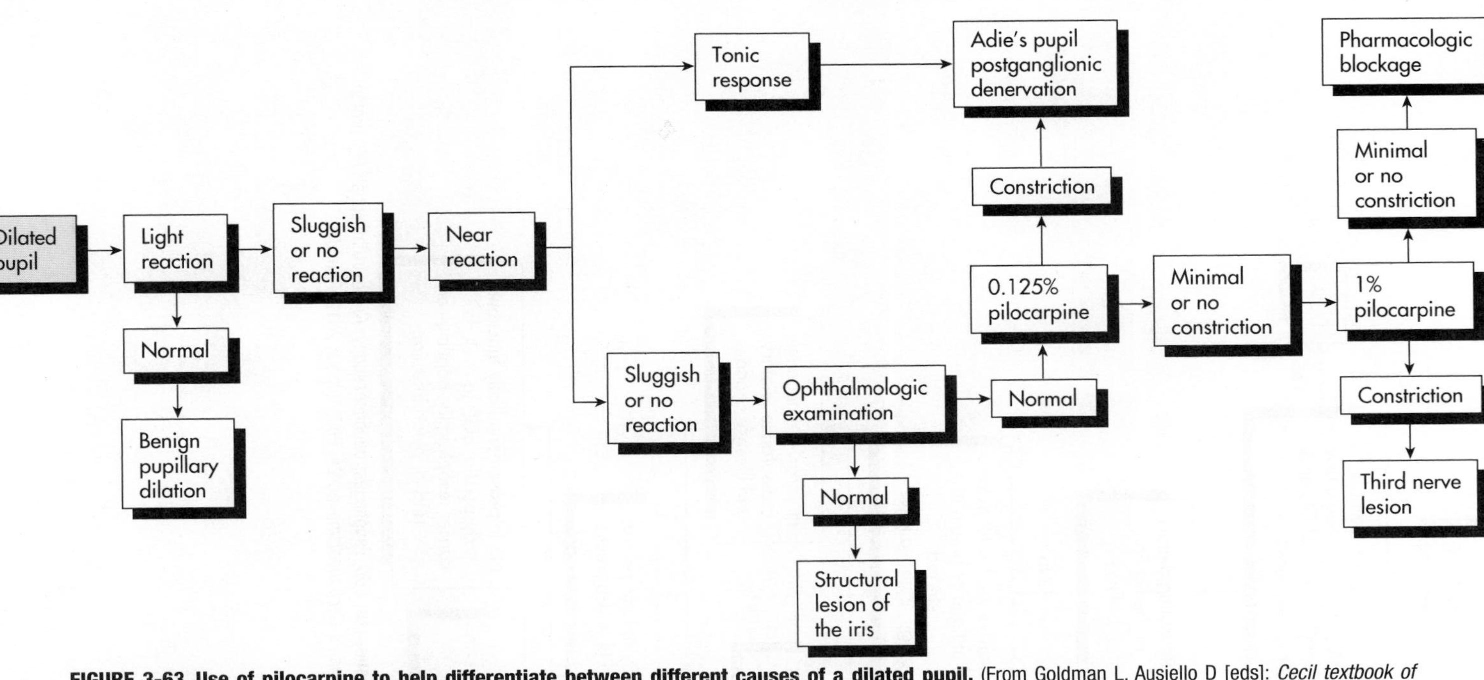

FIGURE 3-63 Use of pilocarpine to help differentiate between different causes of a dilated pupil. (From Goldman L, Ausiello D [eds]: *Cecil textbook of medicine,* ed 23, Philadephia, 2008, Saunders.)

ICD-9CM #	563.3	Dyspepsia atonic
	536.8	Dyspepsia disorders other unspecified function of stomach
	306.4	Dyspepsia, psychogenic
ICD-10CM #	K30	Functional dyspepsia
	F45.8	Other somatoform disorders

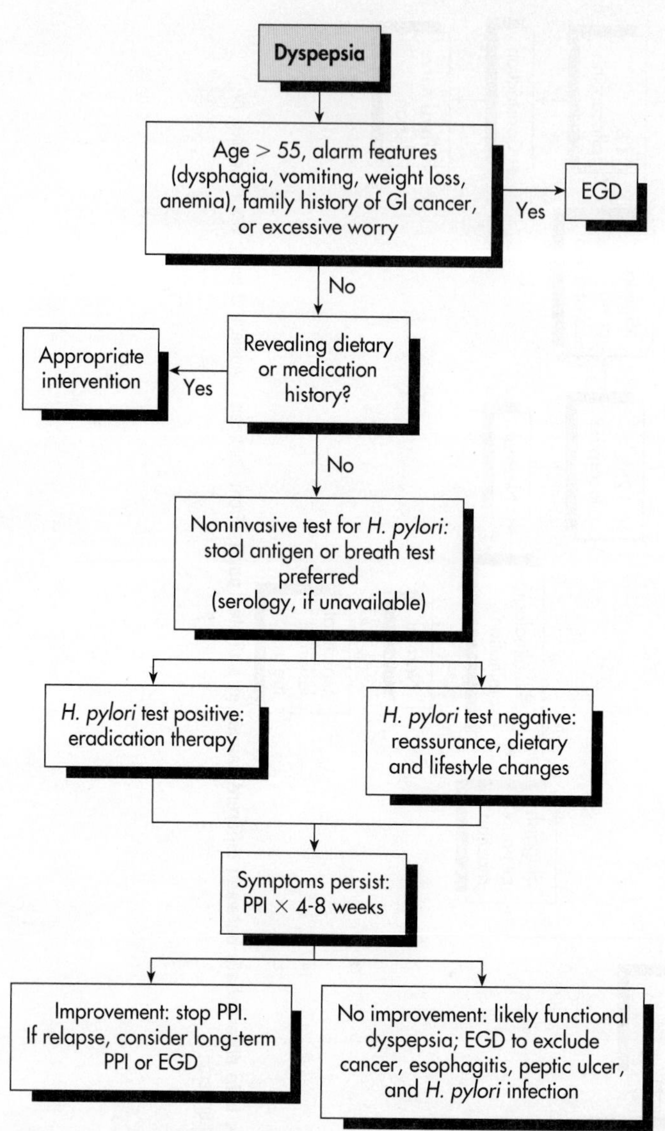

FIGURE 3-64 Approach to the patient with dyspepsia. *EGD,* Esophagastroduodenoscopy; *GI,* gastrointestinal; *PPI,* proton pump inhibitor. (From Goldman L, Schafer AI: *Goldman's Cecil medicine,* ed 24, Philadelphia, 2012, Saunders.)

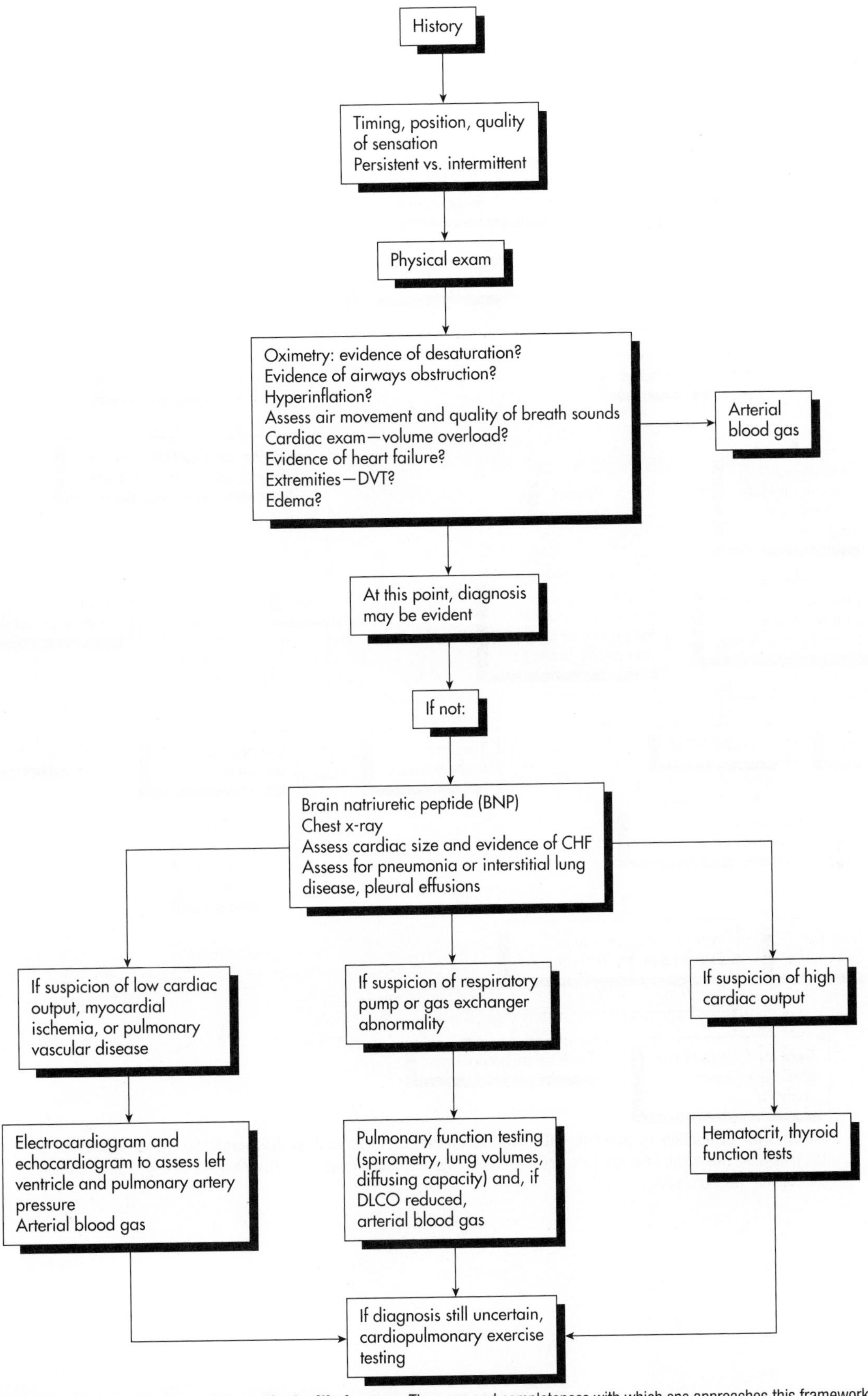

FIGURE 3-65 Algorithm for the evaluation of the patient with dyspnea. The pace and completeness with which one approaches this framework depends on the intensity and acuity of the patient's symptoms. In a patient with severe, acute dyspnea, for example, an arterial blood gas measurement may be one of the first laboratory evaluations, whereas this measurement might not be obtained until much later in the workup in a patient with chronic breathlessness of unclear cause. A therapeutic trial of a medication, for example, a bronchodilator, may be instituted at any point if one is fairly confident of the diagnosis based on the data available at that time. *CHF,* Congestive heart failure; *DLCO,* diffusing capacity of the lung for carbon monoxide; *DVT,* deep venous thrombosis. (Modified from Schwartzstein RM, Feller-Kopman D: Approach to the patient with dyspnea. In Braunwald E, Goldman L [eds]: *Primary cardiology,* ed 2, Philadelphia, 2003, Saunders.)

DYSURIA AND/OR URETHRAL/ VAGINAL DISCHARGE

ICD-9CM #	788.1	Dysuria
	788.7	Urethral discharge
	623.5	Vaginal discharge
ICD-10CM #	R30.0	Dysuria
	R30.9	Painful micturition, unspecified
	R36.0	Urethral discharge without blood
	R36.9	Urethral discharge, unspecified
	N89.8	Other specified noninflammatory disorders of vagina

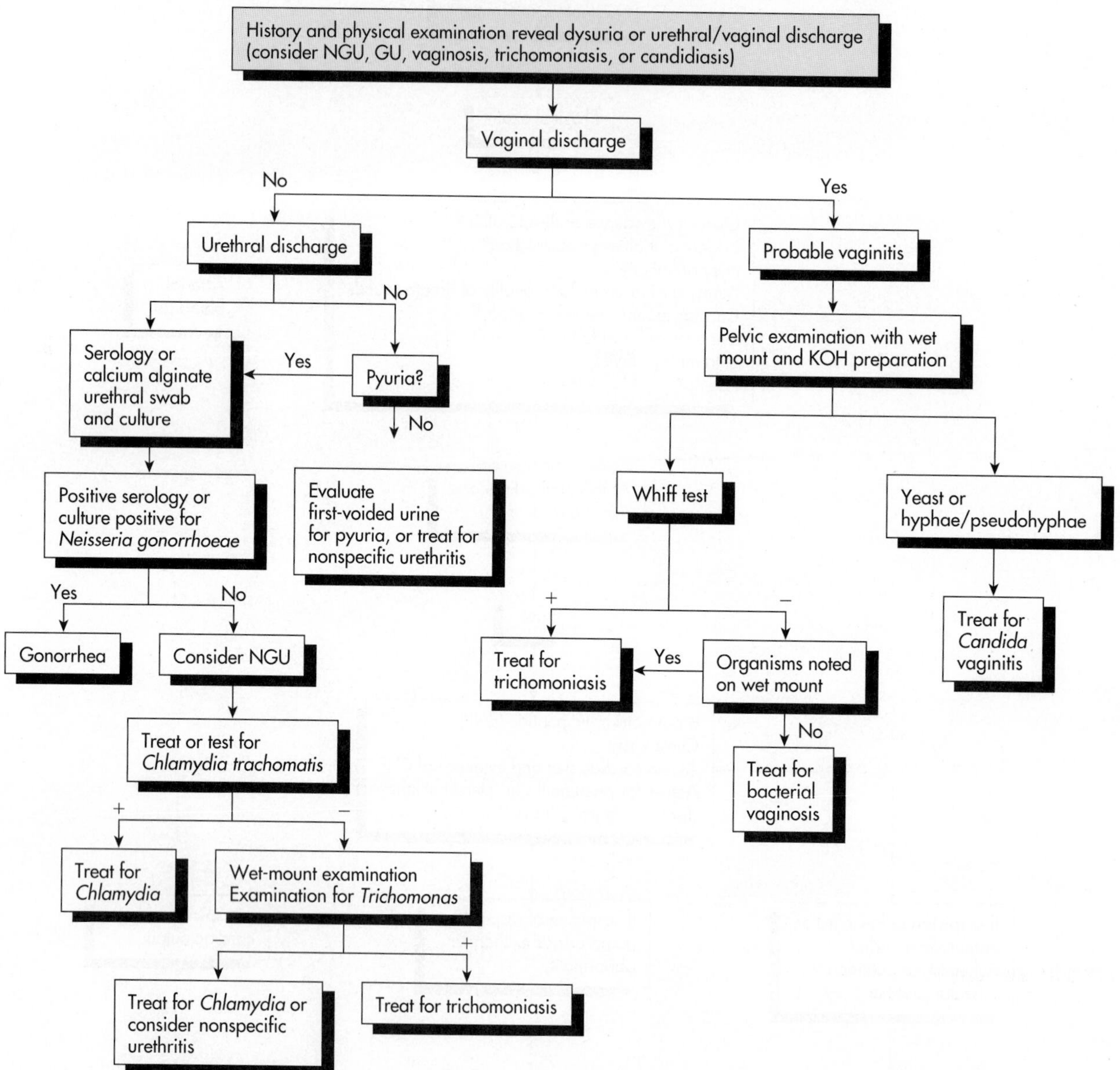

FIGURE 3-66 Evaluation of patients with dysuria and/or urethral/vaginal discharge. *GU,* Gonococcal urethritis; *KOH,* potassium hydroxide; *NGU,* nongonococcal urethritis. (Modified from Nseyo UO [ed]: Urology for primary care physicians, Philadelphia, 1999, Saunders.)

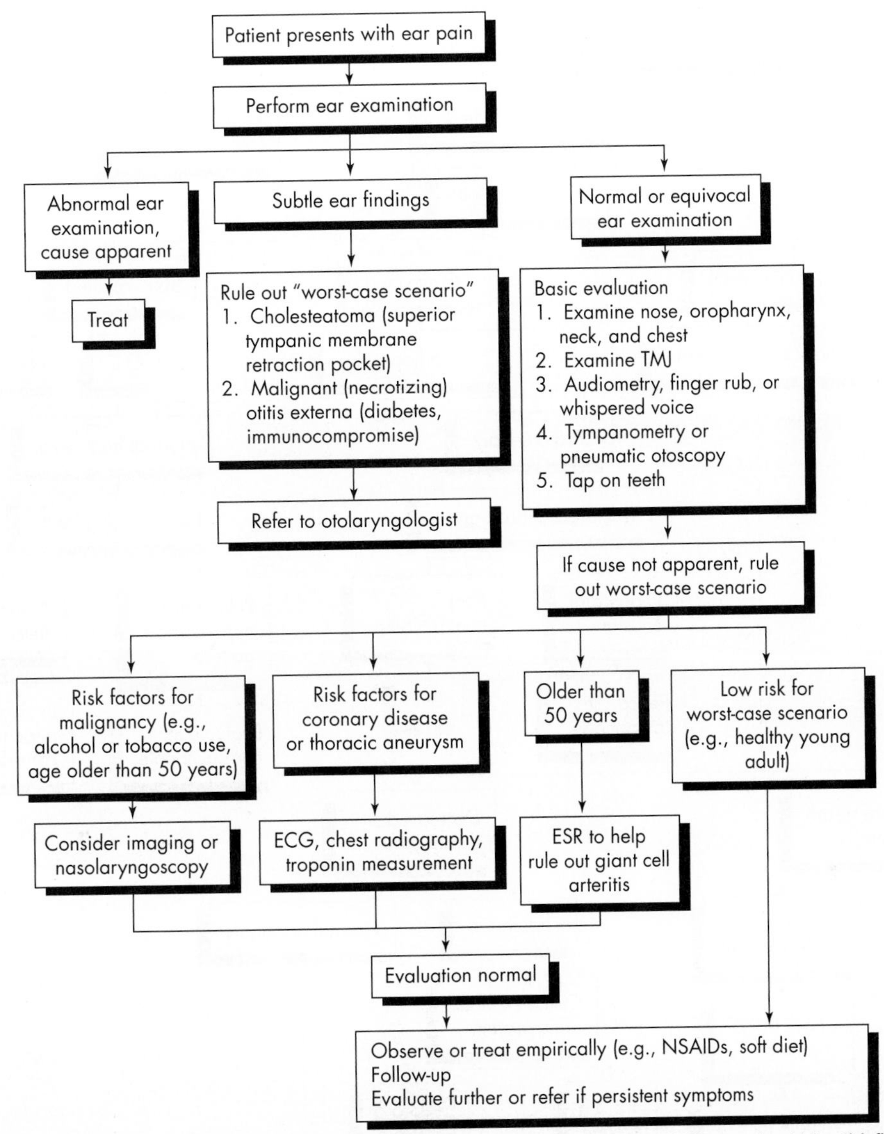

FIGURE 3-67 Management of ear pain. *ECG*, Electrocardiography; *ESR*, erythrocyte sedimentation rate; *NSAIDs*, nonsteroidal anti-inflammatory drugs; *TMJ*, temporomandibular joint. (Modified from Ely JW et al: Diagnosis of ear pain, *Am Fam Physician* 77[5]:622, 2008.)

ICD-9CM #	782.3	Edema NOS
	782.3	Edema, lower extremities
ICD-10CM #	R60.0	Localized edema
	R60.1	Generalized edema
	R60.9	Edema, unspecified

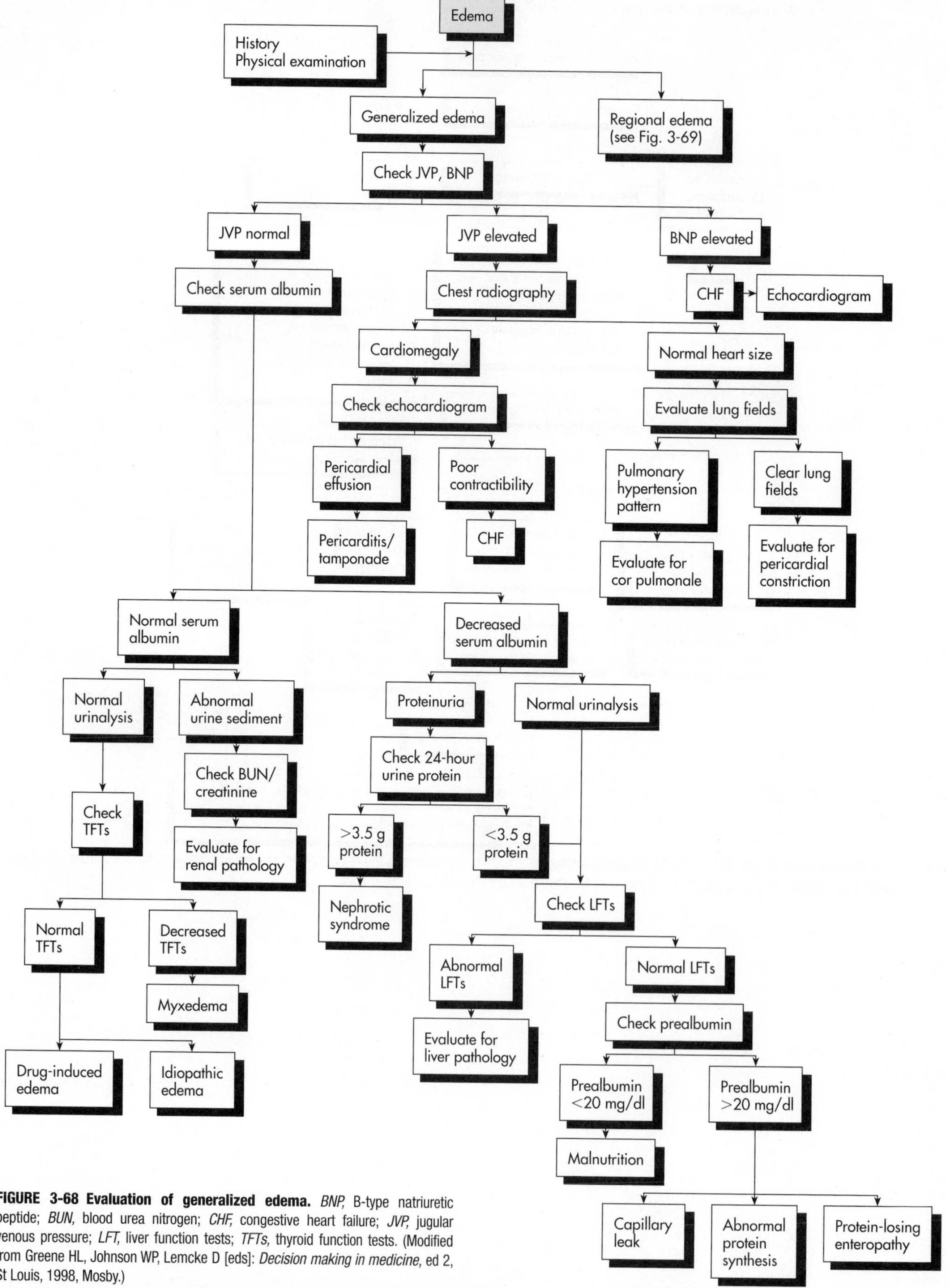

Edema
History
Physical examination
Generalized edema
Regional edema
(see Fig. 3-69)
Check JVP, BNP
JVP normal
JVP elevated
BNP elevated
Check serum albumin
Chest radiography
CHF
Echocardiogram
Cardiomegaly
Normal heart size
Check echocardiogram
Evaluate lung fields
Pericardial effusion
Poor contractibility
Pulmonary hypertension pattern
Clear lung fields
Pericarditis/ tamponade
CHF
Evaluate for cor pulmonale
Evaluate for pericardial constriction
Normal serum albumin
Decreased serum albumin
Normal urinalysis
Abnormal urine sediment
Proteinuria
Normal urinalysis
Check BUN/ creatinine
Check 24-hour urine protein
Check TFTs
Evaluate for renal pathology
>3.5 g protein
<3.5 g protein
Nephrotic syndrome
Check LFTs
Normal TFTs
Decreased TFTs
Abnormal LFTs
Normal LFTs
Myxedema
Evaluate for liver pathology
Check prealbumin
Drug-induced edema
Idiopathic edema
Prealbumin <20 mg/dl
Prealbumin >20 mg/dl
Malnutrition
Capillary leak
Abnormal protein synthesis
Protein-losing enteropathy

FIGURE 3-68 Evaluation of generalized edema. *BNP,* B-type natriuretic peptide; *BUN,* blood urea nitrogen; *CHF,* congestive heart failure; *JVP,* jugular venous pressure; *LFT,* liver function tests; *TFTs,* thyroid function tests. (Modified from Greene HL, Johnson WP, Lemcke D [eds]: *Decision making in medicine,* ed 2, St Louis, 1998, Mosby.)

EDEMA, REGIONAL

ICD-9CM # 250.6
ICD-10CM # T78.3 Edema, essential, acute

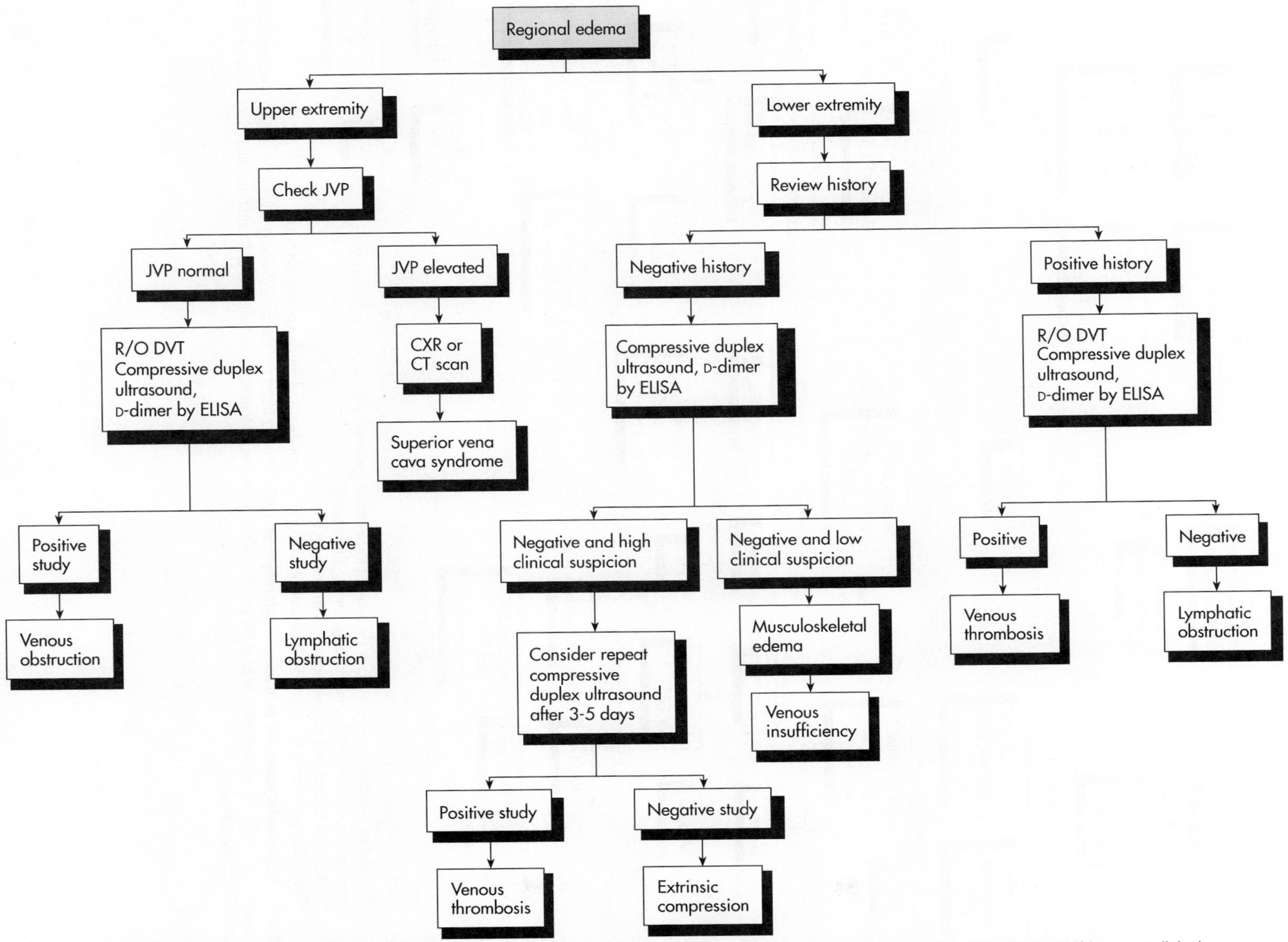

- Regional edema
  - Upper extremity → Check JVP
    - JVP normal → R/O DVT Compressive duplex ultrasound, D-dimer by ELISA
      - Positive study → Venous obstruction
      - Negative study → Lymphatic obstruction
    - JVP elevated → CXR or CT scan → Superior vena cava syndrome
  - Lower extremity → Review history
    - Negative history → Compressive duplex ultrasound, D-dimer by ELISA
      - Negative and high clinical suspicion → Consider repeat compressive duplex ultrasound after 3-5 days
        - Positive study → Venous thrombosis
        - Negative study → Extrinsic compression
      - Negative and low clinical suspicion → Musculoskeletal edema → Venous insufficiency
    - Positive history → R/O DVT Compressive duplex ultrasound, D-dimer by ELISA
      - Positive → Venous thrombosis
      - Negative → Lymphatic obstruction

FIGURE 3-69 Evaluation of regional edema. *CT,* Computed tomography; *CXR,* chest x-ray examination; *DVT,* deep venous thrombosis; *ELISA,* enzyme-linked immunosorbent assay; *JVP,* jugular venous pressure. (Modified from Greene HL, Johnson WP, Lemcke D [eds]: *Decision making in medicine,* ed 2, St Louis, 1998, Mosby.)

ICD-9CM # 289.0 Polycythemia, acquired
ICD-10CM # D75.0 Familial erythrocytosis

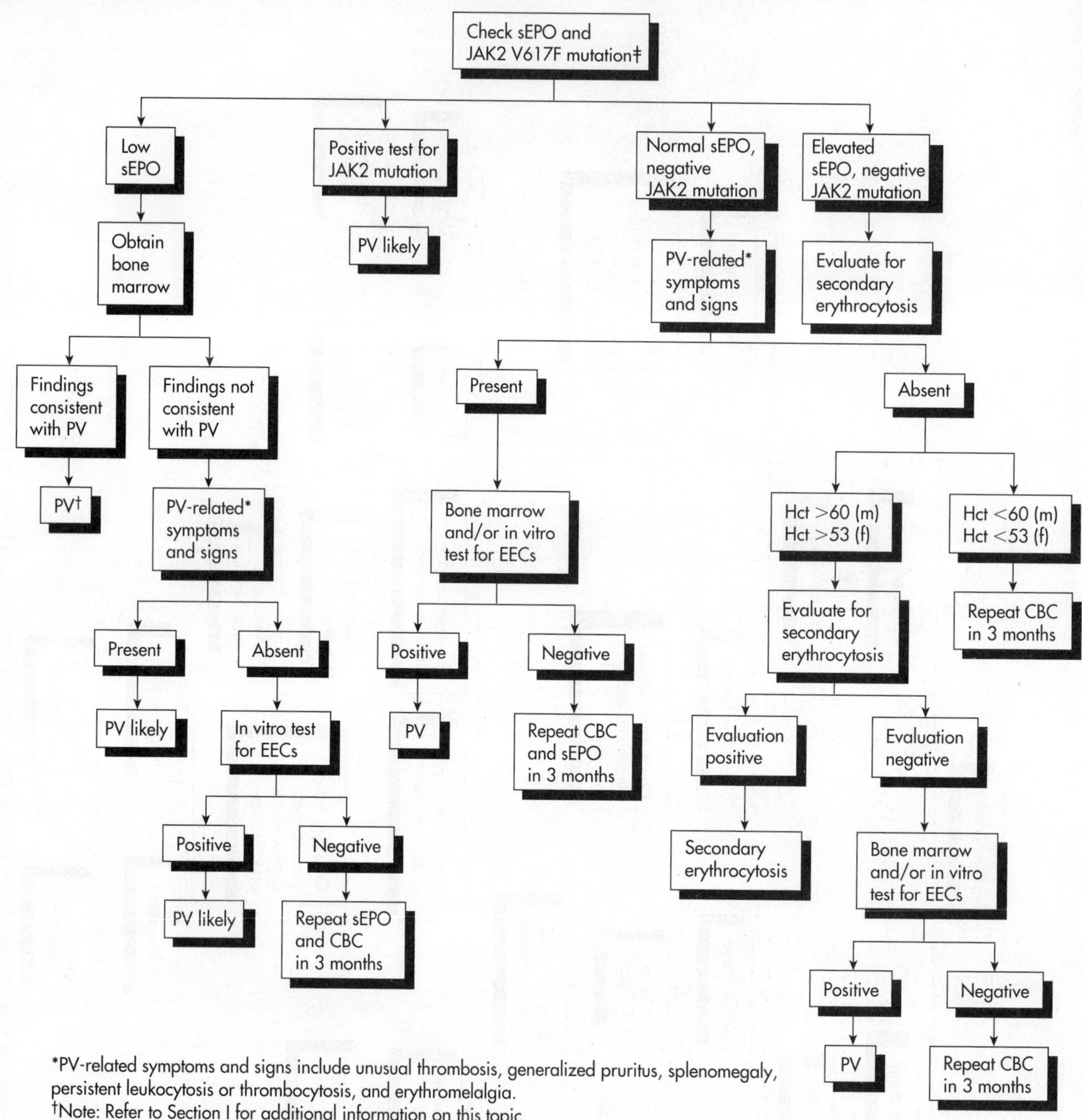

*PV-related symptoms and signs include unusual thrombosis, generalized pruritus, splenomegaly, persistent leukocytosis or thrombocytosis, and erythromelalgia.
†Note: Refer to Section I for additional information on this topic.
‡The JAK2 mutation is found in >95% of patients with PV and can be used for diagnostic purposes.

FIGURE 3-71 A diagnostic approach to acquired erythrocytosis. *CBC,* Complete blood cell count; *EEC,* endogenous (spontaneous) erythroid colonies; *f,* female; *Hct,* hematocrit; *m,* male; *PV,* polycythemia vera; *sEPO,* serum erythropoietin level. (Modified from Goldman L, Schafer AL [eds]: *Cecil textbook of medicine,* ed 24, Philadelphia, 2012, Saunders.)

ERYTHRODERMA

ICD-9CM #	695.9	Secondary
	695.89	Exfoliative
	696.2	Maculopapular
	696.1	Psoriaticum
	778.8	Neonatorum
ICD-10CM #	L53.9	Erythematous condition, unspecified
	L41.0	Pityriasis lichenoides et varioliformis acuta
	L41.1	Pityriasis lichenoides chronica
	L41.8	Other parapsoriasis
	L40.0	Psoriasis vulgaris
	L40.1	Generalized pustular psoriasis
	L40.2	Acrodermatitis continua
	L40.3	Pustulosis palmaris et plantaris
	L40.4	Guttate psoriasis
	L40.8	Other psoriasis
	L26	Exfoliative dermatitis
	L30.4	Erythema intertrigo
	L53.8	Other specified erythematous conditions
	L92.0	Granuloma annulare
	L95.1	Erythema elevatum diutinum
	L98.2	Febrile neutrophilic dermatosis [Sweet]
	P83.8	Other specified conditions of integument specific to newborn

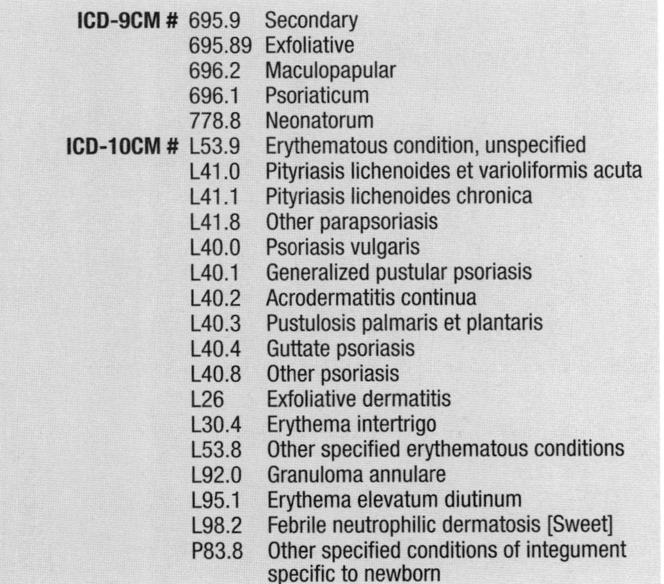

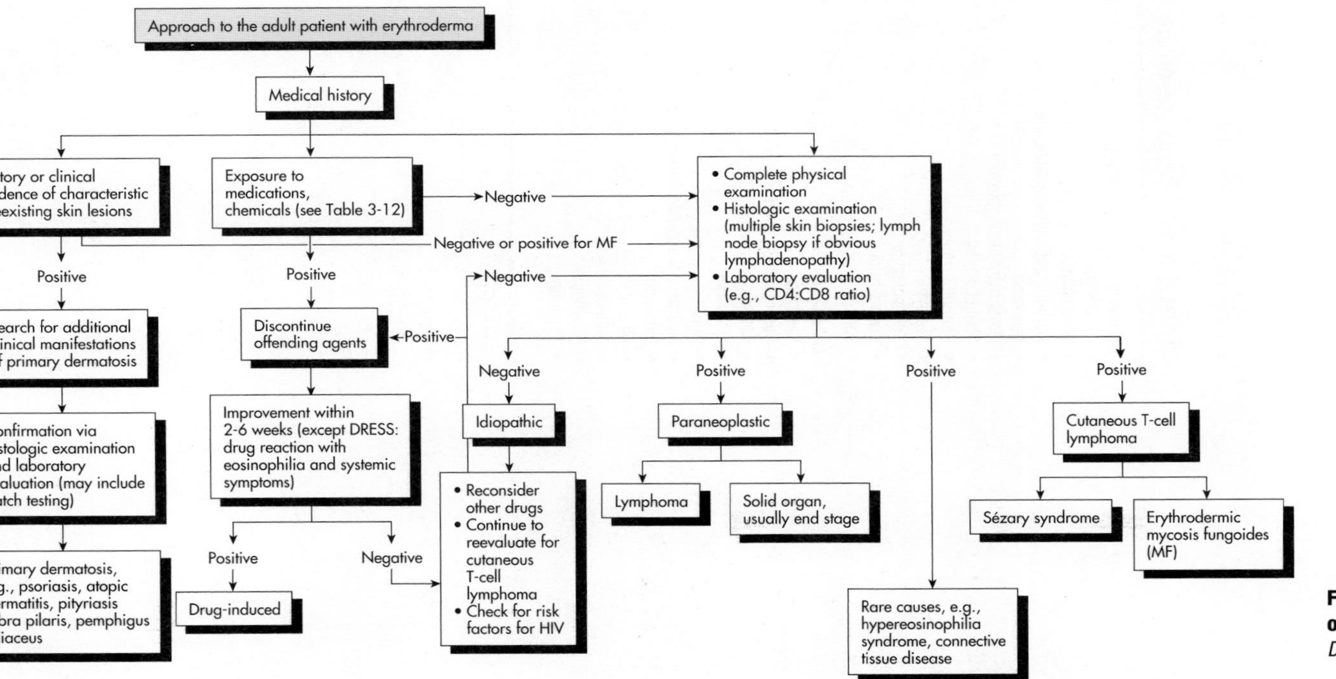

FIGURE 3-72 Approach to the differential diagnosis of adult erythroderma. (From Bolognia JL et al [eds]: *Dermatology,* ed 2, St Louis, 2008, Mosby.)

ICD-9CM #	695.9	Secondary
	695.89	Exfoliative
	696.2	Maculopapular
	696.1	Psoriaticum
	778.8	Neonatorum
ICD-10CM #	L53.9	Erythematous condition, unspecified
	L41.0	Pityriasis lichenoides et varioliformis acuta
	L41.1	Pityriasis lichenoides chronica
	L41.8	Other parapsoriasis
	L40.0	Psoriasis vulgaris
	L40.1	Generalized pustular psoriasis
	L40.2	Acrodermatitis continua
	L40.3	Pustulosis palmaris et plantaris
	L40.4	Guttate psoriasis
	L40.8	Other psoriasis
	L26	Exfoliative dermatitis
	L30.4	Erythema intertrigo
	L53.8	Other specified erythematous conditions
	L92.0	Granuloma annulare
	L95.1	Erythema elevatum diutinum
	L98.2	Febrile neutrophilic dermatosis [Sweet]
	P83.8	Other specified conditions of integument specific to newborn

TABLE 3-12 Drugs Associated with Erythroderma

Common
- Allopurinol
- Ampicillin/amoxicillin/penicillin G
- Carbamazepine/oxcarbazepine
- Dapsone
- Omeprazole/lansoprazole
- Phenobarbital
- Phenothiazines
- Phenytoin
- Sulfasalazine
- Sulfonamides
- Vancomycin

Less Common
- Captopril
- Carboplatin/cisplatin
- Cytokines (IL-2/GM-CSF)
- Diflunisal
- Gold
- Hydroxychloroquine/mefloquine
- Isoniazid
- Mercury
- Minocycline
- Nifedipine
- Thalidomide

Rare
- Amiodarone
- Aztreonam
- Cimetidine
- Chlorpromazine
- Clofazimine
- Codeine
- Diltiazem
- Erythropoietin
- Fluorouracil
- Indinavir sulfate
- Lithium
- Mitomycin C
- Pentostatin
- Piroxicam
- Practolol
- Ranitidine
- Rifampin (rifampicin)
- Tear gas (CS gas)
- Teicoplanin
- Terbinafine
- Tobramycin
- Tramadol
- Vinca alkaloids
- Zidovudine

ESOPHAGEAL FOREIGN BODY

ICD-9CM # 938
ICD-10CM # T18.8 Foreign body entering through orifice, gastrointestinal tract, specified part

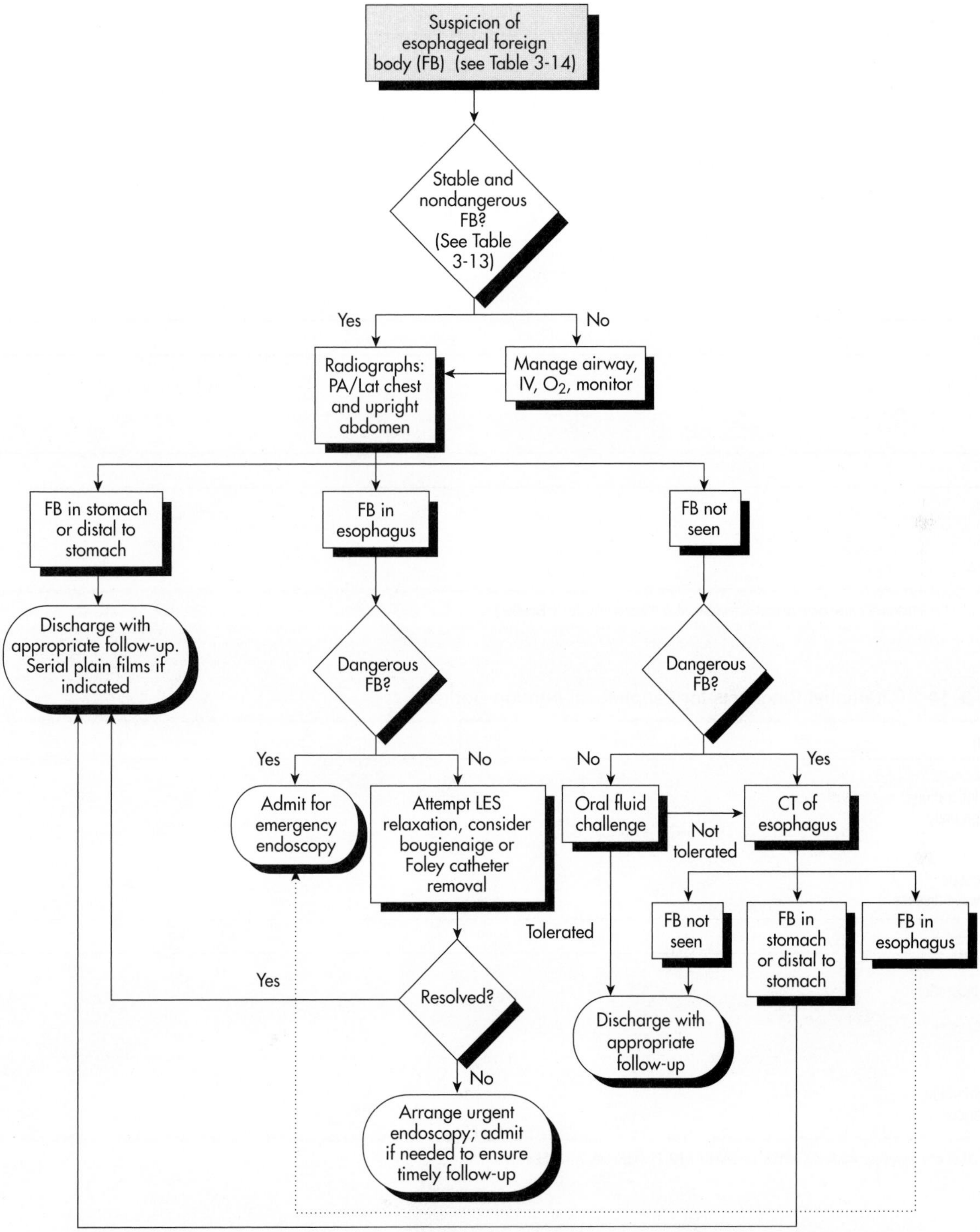

Suspicion of esophageal foreign body (FB) (see Table 3-14)

Stable and nondangerous FB? (See Table 3-13)

Yes

No

Radiographs: PA/Lat chest and upright abdomen

Manage airway, IV, O_2, monitor

FB in stomach or distal to stomach

FB in esophagus

FB not seen

Discharge with appropriate follow-up. Serial plain films if indicated

Dangerous FB?

Dangerous FB?

Yes

No

No

Yes

Admit for emergency endoscopy

Attempt LES relaxation, consider bougienaige or Foley catheter removal

Oral fluid challenge

Not tolerated

CT of esophagus

Tolerated

FB not seen

FB in stomach or distal to stomach

FB in esophagus

Yes

Resolved?

Discharge with appropriate follow-up

No

Arrange urgent endoscopy; admit if needed to ensure timely follow-up

FIGURE 3-73 Diagnostic algorithm for the evaluation of a suspected esophageal foreign body. *CT*, Computed tomography; *IV*, intravenous line; *Lat*, lateral; *LES*, lower esophageal sphincter; *PA*, posteroanterior. (From Adams JG et al: *Emergency medicine, clinical essentials*, ed 2, Philadelphia, 2013, Elsevier.)

TABLE 3-13 Most Threatening and Most Common Esophageal Foreign Bodies

Most Threatening
In Children
Disc batteries Bones Needles Other sharp objects
In Adults
Disc batteries Bones Packets of illicit drugs Toothpicks
Most Common
In Children
Coins Marbles Buttons Toys
In Adults
Food boluses Bones Dentures Oral piercings

(From Adams JG, et al: *Emergency medicine, clinical essentials*, ed 2, Philadelphia, 2013, Elsevier.)

TABLE 3-14 Differential Diagnosis for Esophageal Foreign Bodies

In Children
Perforation Abrasion or laceration Airway foreign body Esophagitis Epiglottitis Globus hystericus Reactive airways disease
In Adults
Perforation Abrasion or laceration Spasm Esophagitis Diverticulum Malignancy Myocardial infarction Globus hystericus

(From Adams JG et al: *Emergency medicine, clinical essentials*, ed 2, Philadelphia, 2013, Elsevier.)

FATIGUE

ICD-9CM #	780.7	Fatigue NOS
	300.5	Fatigue Psychogenic
	780.7	Chronic Fatigue Syndrome
ICD-10CM #	R53.83	Other fatigue
	F48.8	Other specified nonpsychotic mental disorders
	R53.83	Other fatigue

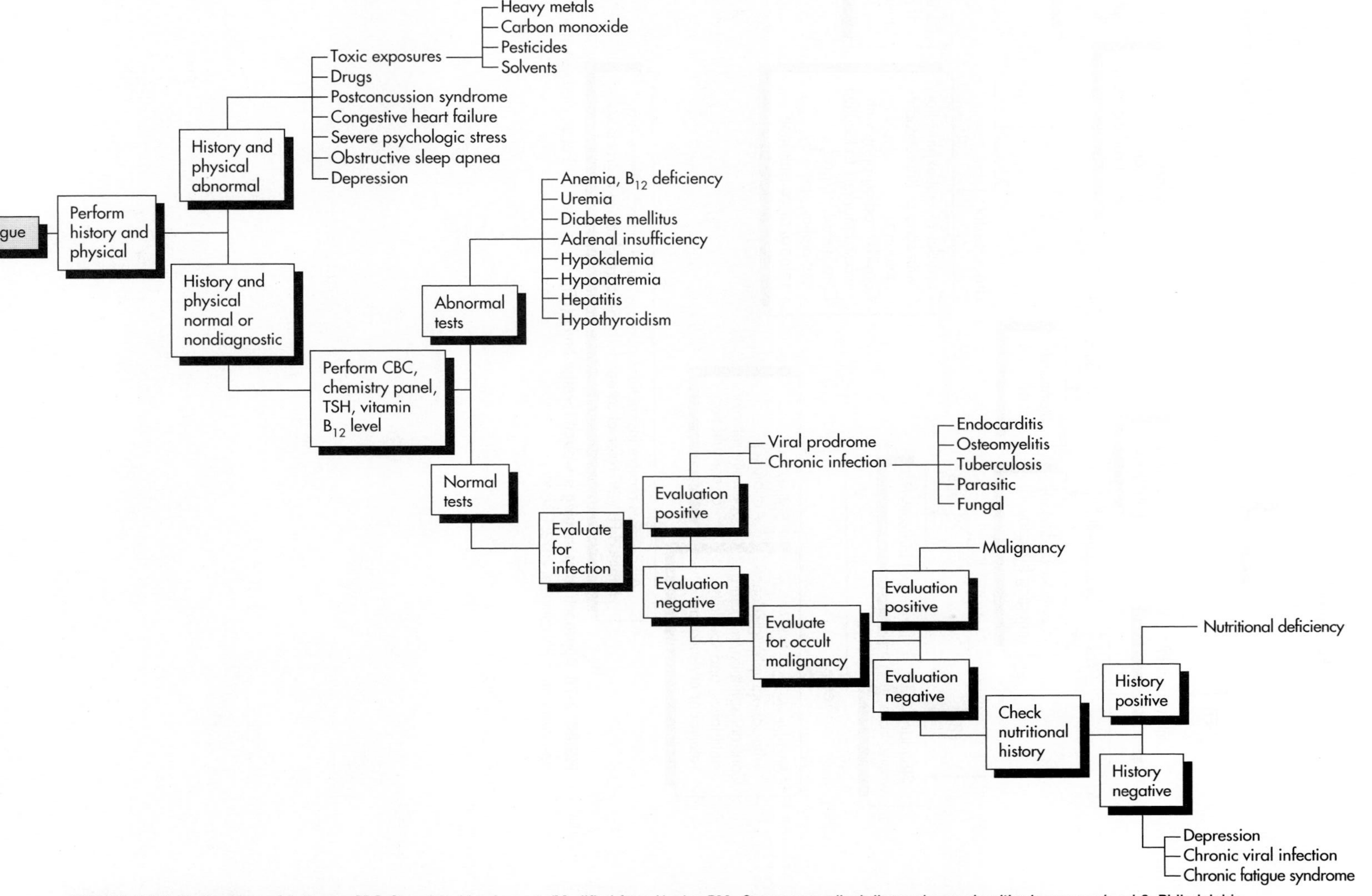

FIGURE 3-74 Evaluation of fatigue. *CBC*, Complete blood count. (Modified from Healey PM: *Common medical diagnosis: an algorithmic approach*, ed 3, Philadelphia, 2000, Saunders.)

ICD-9CM # 729.6
ICD-10CM # M79.5 Residual foreign body in soft tissue

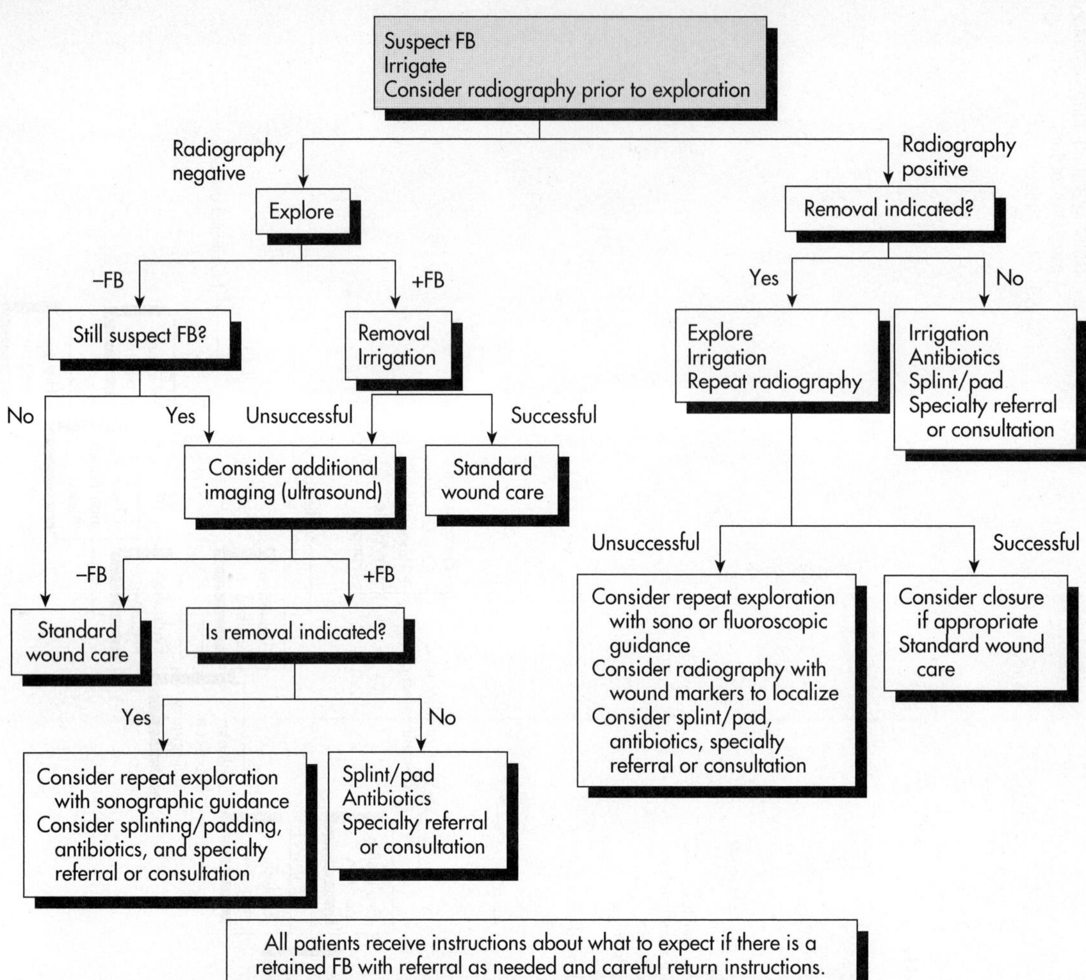

FIGURE 3-78 Approach to managing a wound foreign body (FB). (From Adams JG et al: *Emergency medicine, clinical essentials*, ed 2, Philadelphia, 2013, Elsevier.)

GENITAL LESIONS OR ULCERS

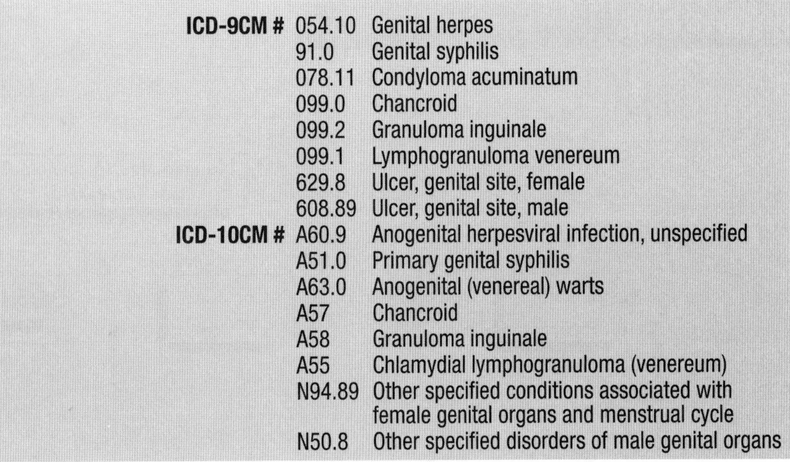

ICD-9CM #	054.10	Genital herpes
	91.0	Genital syphilis
	078.11	Condyloma acuminatum
	099.0	Chancroid
	099.2	Granuloma inguinale
	099.1	Lymphogranuloma venereum
	629.8	Ulcer, genital site, female
	608.89	Ulcer, genital site, male
ICD-10CM #	A60.9	Anogenital herpesviral infection, unspecified
	A51.0	Primary genital syphilis
	A63.0	Anogenital (venereal) warts
	A57	Chancroid
	A58	Granuloma inguinale
	A55	Chlamydial lymphogranuloma (venereum)
	N94.89	Other specified conditions associated with female genital organs and menstrual cycle
	N50.8	Other specified disorders of male genital organs

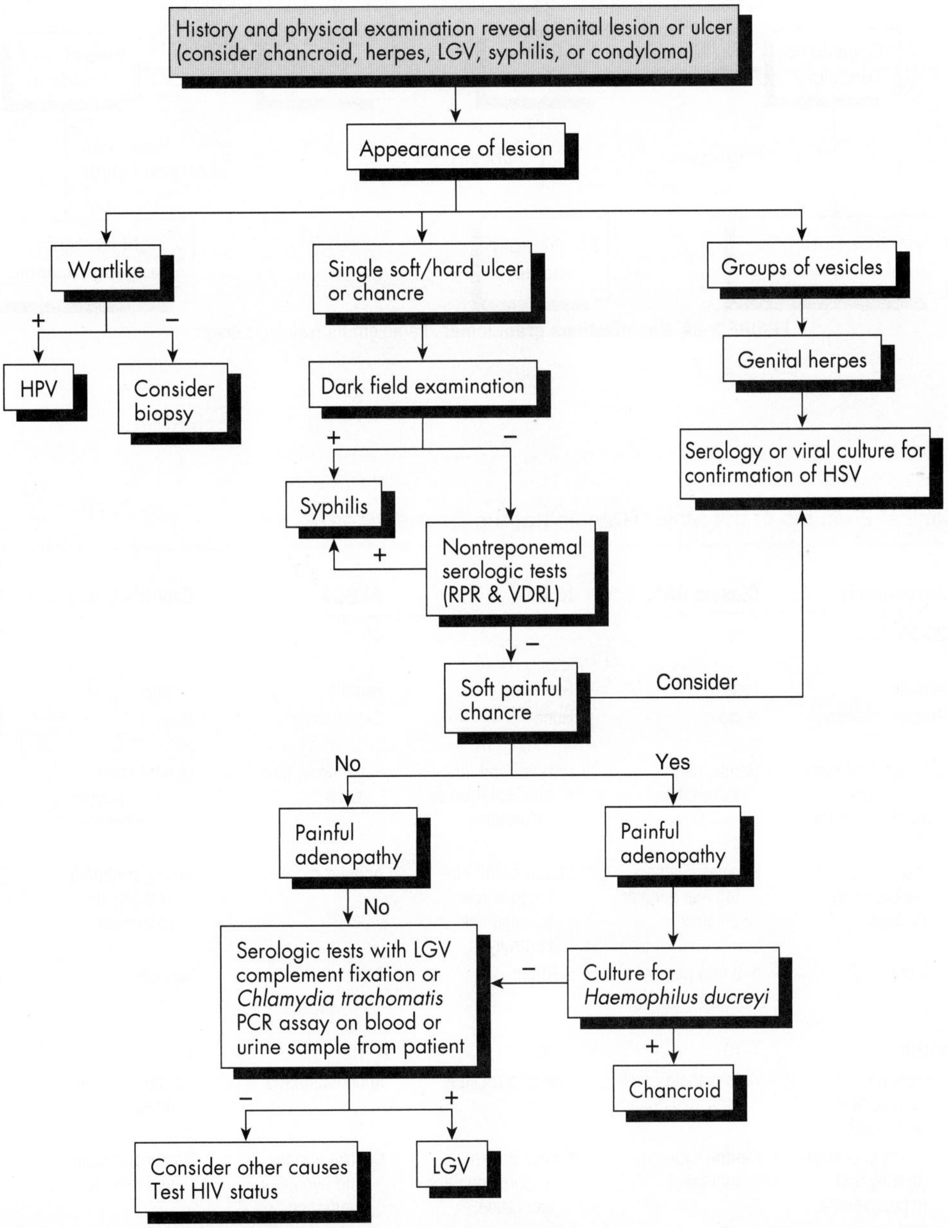

History and physical examination reveal genital lesion or ulcer (consider chancroid, herpes, LGV, syphilis, or condyloma)

Appearance of lesion

Wartlike

+

–

HPV

Consider biopsy

Single soft/hard ulcer or chancre

Dark field examination

+

–

Syphilis

Nontreponemal serologic tests (RPR & VDRL)

+

–

Soft painful chancre

Consider

No

Yes

Painful adenopathy

No

Painful adenopathy

Serologic tests with LGV complement fixation or *Chlamydia trachomatis* PCR assay on blood or urine sample from patient

Culture for *Haemophilus ducreyi*

–

+

Chancroid

–

+

Consider other causes Test HIV status

LGV

Groups of vesicles

Genital herpes

Serology or viral culture for confirmation of HSV

FIGURE 3-80 Evaluation of patients with genital lesions or ulcers. *HIV,* Human immunodeficiency virus; *HPV,* human papillomavirus; *HSV,* herpes simplex virus; *LGV,* lymphogranuloma venereum; *RPR,* rapid plasma reagin; *VDRL,* Venereal Disease Research Laboratory. (Modified from Nseyo UO [ed]: *Urology for primary care physicians,* Philadelphia, 1999, Saunders.)

ICD-9CM # variable with specific diagnosis
ICD-10CM # A58 Granuloma inguinale

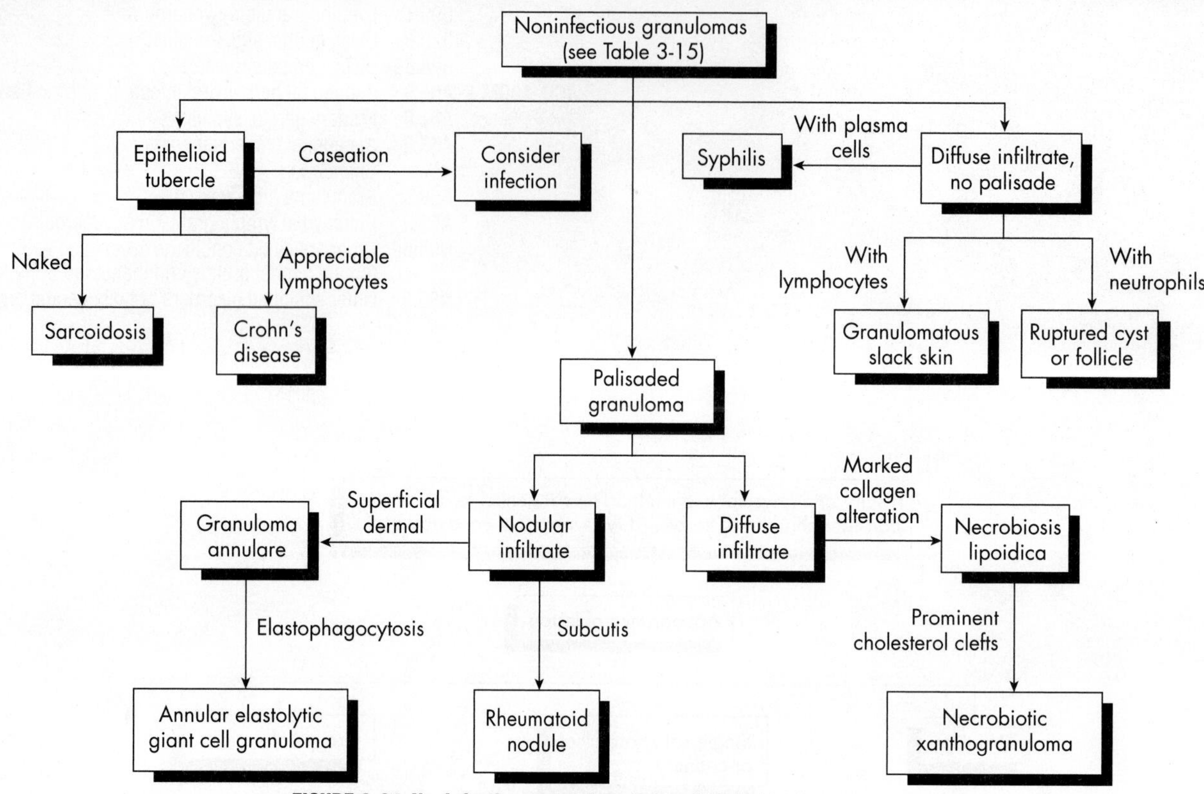

FIGURE 3-84 Noninfectious granulomas. Paradigm for histologic diagnosis.

TABLE 3-15 Clinical Features of the Major Granulomatous Dermatitides

	Sarcoidosis	Classic GA*	NLD	AEGCG	Crohn's Disease	Rheumatoid Nodule
Average age (years)	25-35, 45-65	<30		40	35	30-40
Sex	Female	Female	Female	Female	Female	Female
Racial predilection in United States	African American	None	None	Caucasian	None	None
Site	Symmetric on face, neck, upper trunk, extremities	Hands, feet, extremities	Anterior and lateral distal lower extremities	Face, neck, forearms	Genital areas, lower >upper extremities	Juxtaarticular areas, elbows, hands, ankles, feet
Appearance	Red to red-brown papules and plaques	Papules coalescing into annular plaques	Plaques with elevated borders, telangiectasias centrally	Annular plaques	Dusky erythema and swelling, ulceration	Skin-colored, firm, mobile subcutaneous nodules
Size of lesions	1-5 cm	1-2 mm papules, <5 cm annular plaques	>10 cm	1-6 cm	Variable	1-3 cm
Number of lesions	Variable	1-10	1-10	1-10	1-5	1-10
Associations	Systemic manifestations of sarcoidosis	Rare diabetes mellitus, malignancy	Diabetes mellitus	Actinic damage	Intestinal Crohn's disease	Rheumatoid arthritis
Special clinical characteristics	Occasional central atrophy and hypopigmentation	Central hyperpigmentation	Yellow-brown atrophic centers, ulceration	Central atrophy and hypopigmentation	Draining sinuses and fistulae	Occasional ulceration, especially at site of trauma

From Bolognia JL et al: *Dermatology,* ed 2, St Louis, 2008, Mosby.
AEGCG, Annular elastolytic giant cell granuloma; *GA,* granuloma annulare; *NLD,* necrobiosis lipoidica diabeticorum.
*Clinical variants include generalized, micropapular, nodular, perforating, subcutaneous, and patch GA.

ICD-9CM # 389.00 Hearing loss, conductive
389.10 Hearing loss, sensorineural
ICD-10CM # H90.2 Conductive hearing loss, unspecified
H90.5 Unspecified sensorineural hearing loss

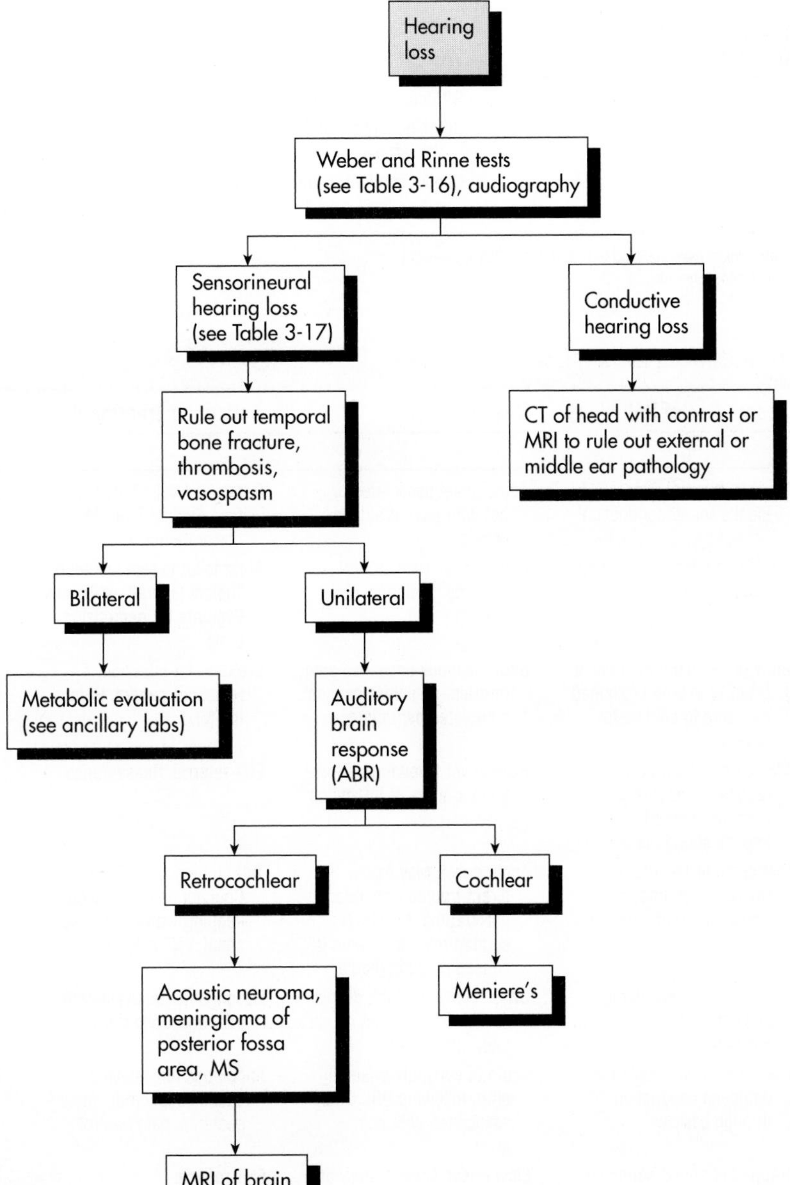

FIGURE 3-85 Evaluation of hearing loss. *CT,* Computed tomography; *MRI,* magnetic resonance imaging; *MS,* multiple sclerosis. (From Ferri FF: *Ferri's best test: a practical guide to clinical laboratory medicine and diagnostic imaging,* ed 3, Philadelphia, 2014, Mosby.)

BOX 3-2 Hearing Loss

Diagnostic imaging
Best test
None

Ancillary tests
CT of head with contrast or MRI with contrast
CT of temporal bone without contrast

Lab evaluation
Best test
None

Ancillary tests
CBC
ALT, AST
ANA, VDRL
TSH

From Ferri FF: *Ferri's best test: a practical guide to clinical laboratory medicine and diagnostic imaging,* ed 3, Philadelphia, 2014, Mosby.
ALT, Alanine aminotransferase; *ANA,* antibody to nuclear antigens; *AST,* angiotensin sensitivity test; *CBC,* complete blood count; *CT,* computed tomography; *TSH,* thyroid-stimulating hormone; *VDRL,* Venereal Disease Research Laboratory.

ICD-9CM # 389.00 Hearing loss, conductive
389.10 Hearing loss, sensorineural
ICD-10CM # H90.2 Conductive hearing loss, unspecified
H90.5 Unspecified sensorineural hearing loss

TABLE 3-16 Interpretation of the Weber and Rinne Tests

	WEBER WITHOUT LATERALIZATION	WEBER LATERALIZES RIGHT	WEBER LATERALIZES LEFT
Rinne both ears: AC >BC	Normal	S/N loss in the left ear	S/N loss in the right ear
Rinne left ear: BC >AC	–	Combined loss: conduction and S/N loss in the left ear	Conduction loss in the left ear
Rinne right ear: BC >AC	–	Conduction loss in the right ear	Combined loss: conduction and S/N loss in the right ear

(From Adams JG et al: *Emergency medicine, clinical essentials*, ed 2, Philadelphia, 2013, Elsevier.)
AC, Air conduction; *BC*, bone conduction; *S/N*, sensorineural.

TABLE 3-17 Lesions That Cause Hearing Loss

	Description of Pathology	Onset/Course	Actions or Treatment	Prognosis
Conductive Lesion				
Foreign body	Mass in external canal blocks sound conduction	Acute onset associated or not with pain, drainage, or odor	Removal. Evaluate for infection. Evaluate for TM perforation	Excellent
Otitis externa	Edema and detritus obstruct external canal	Rapid onset. Pain, edema, swelling. Drainage, odor often present	Aural toilet to remove debris. Topical (± oral) antibiotics. Evaluate for necrotizing otitis	Excellent if treated appropriately
Exostosis	Bony growths obstruct canal. Often seen with prolonged exposure to cold water (divers)	Slow insidious onset. No pain or drainage unless causes complete obstruction	Evaluate for infection. Reassure patient. Refer to ENT	Good
Tympanosclerosis	TM scarring from perforations or infections. Decreased mobility impairs sound conduction	Slow onset following perforations, trauma or infections	ENT referral. Reassurance	Variable
Perforated TM	Disruption of TM integrity results in impaired transmission of sound to ossicle	Acute onset. May follow direct trauma or sudden barotrauma. May have sudden relief from pain if caused by otitis media	Treat infectious causes. Counsel on importance of keeping water out of ear canal. ENT referral	Good
Sterile effusion (barotrauma)	Fluid in middle ear dampens conduction through ossicles	Often following flight, diving, or URI. Bubbles can cause intermittent pain	Decongestants. Evaluate for infection. Follow-up	Excellent
Acute otitis media	Pus (or fluid) in middle ear dampens conduction through ossicles	Acute to subacute onset, often following URI. Often associated with pain ± fever	Antibiotics (unless viral cause suspected), decongestants, pain control	Excellent if treated appropriately
Cholesteatoma	Trapped stratified squamous epithelial mass in middle ear. Interferes with ossicle conduction	Slow onset. Often history of previous perforations or chronic infections	ENT referral	Variable. May destroy ossicles or erode into surrounding structures
Glomus tumor	Vascular tumor occupies middle ear space. Interferes with ossicle conduction	Slow onset. May be associated with rushing pulsatile sensation	ENT referral	Variable
Cancer	Squamous cell most common. Obstructs external canal	Slow onset. Often noticed first by others. Painless unless occlusion causes otitis externa	ENT referral. Evaluate for secondary infection	Variable
Sensorineural Lesion				
Perilymph fistula (inner ear barotrauma)	Disruption of round or oval window allows leakage of perilymph into middle ear	Sudden onset of hearing loss often with tinnitus and vertigo. Frequently follows straining or abrupt change in pressure. Turning in direction of fistula exacerbates symptoms	Complete bed rest. Elevate head of bed and avoid increases in CSF pressure. Severe symptoms or noncompliance may require hospitalization. ENT consultation for possible oval or round window patch	Variable

TABLE 3-17 Lesions That Cause Hearing Loss—cont'd

	Description of Pathology	Onset/Course	Actions or Treatment	Prognosis
Conductive Lesion				
Viral cochleitis	Cochlear inflammation. Often following URI	Rapid onset. Often following URI	Steroids often used (no good data)	Variable
Presbycusis	Age-related hearing loss. May be related to previous chronic noise exposure	Slow onset. Usually symmetric. High frequencies most affected. Tinnitus may occur	Hearing aid may help with both hearing loss and tinnitus	Variable
Acoustic neuroma	Benign schwannoma of 8th cranial nerve	Slow onset. Usually unilateral. May exhibit tinnitus, vertigo. May exhibit facial hyperesthesias or twitching	May require surgical excision if symptoms debilitating	Variable
Ototoxic agents	Direct toxicity to inner ear structures	Variable onset. High frequency most affected. Exposure to ototoxic drugs. May have associated tinnitus	Stop use of offending agent	Variable. Hearing loss at time of stopping offending agent is usually permanent
Multiple sclerosis	Multiple demyelinating lesions interfere with nerve conduction	Often other associated neurologic findings. May wax and wane	Standard multiple sclerosis treatment (steroids, cytotoxic agents)	Variable
Stroke/CVA	Focal ischemic lesion of auditory nerve or auditory cortex	Sudden onset. Often associated with other neurologic deficits	Treat CVA risk factors (ASA, anticoagulants, glycemic control, BP control)	Variable
Meningitis	Infection enters inner ear through CNS-perilymph connection. Damages organ of Corti	Follows clinical picture of meningitis	Treat infection. Steroids may limit inflammation and damage	Variable
Meniere disease (endolymphatic hydrops)	Abnormal homeostasis of inner ear fluids (clinical diagnosis; definitive diagnosis made histologically)	Episodic spells of vertigo. Associated sensation of fullness, tinnitus, and SNHL or auditory distortion. Low-frequency ranges most affected	Reduce salt, caffeine, nicotine (vasoconstrictors) intake. Consider diuretics, antihistamines, anticholinergics. ENT referral	Variable
Chronic noise exposure	Direct mechanical damage to cochlear structures and hair cells	Slow onset. Usually high frequency most affected	Prevention measures (earplugs). Stop exposure	Usually permanent
Skull trauma	Interruption of cranial nerve VIII, ossicle disruption, or shearing effects on organ of Corti	Sudden onset after trauma	ENT consultation for possible surgical repair	Variable: ossicle disruption has better prognosis than nerve or organ of Corti damage
Autoimmune causes	Vascular or neuronal inflammatory changes	Bilateral asymmetric SNHL. May be fluctuating or progressive. Often other systemic autoimmune findings	Outpatient autoimmune evaluation. Steroids and cytotoxic agents may slow progression	Variable

(From Adams JG et al: *Emergency medicine, clinical essentials*, ed 2, Philadelphia, 2013, Elsevier.)

ASA, Acetylsalicylic acid; *BP*, blood pressure; *CNS*, central nervous system; *CSF*, cerebrospinal fluid; *CVA*, cerebrovascular accident; *ENT*, ear, nose, and throat; *SNHL*, sensorineural hearing loss; *TM*, tympanic membrane; *URI*, upper respiratory infection.

ICD-9CM # 599.7
ICD-10CM # R31.9 Hematuria, unspecified

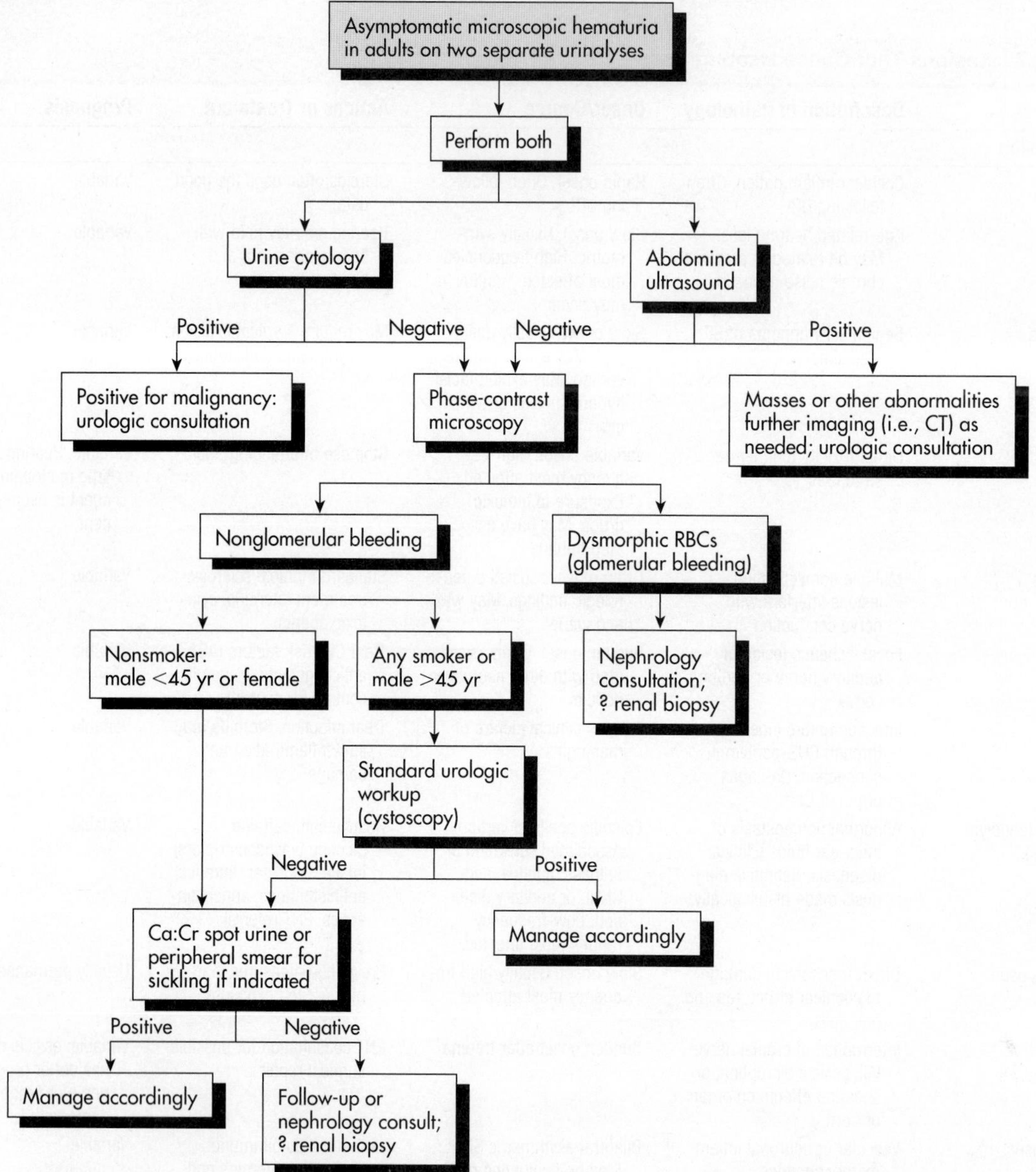

FIGURE 3-87 Suggested algorithm for the evaluation of adult asymptomatic microscopic hematuria. These patients must have no symptoms referable to the hematuria and a negative urinalysis except for red blood cells *(RBCs)*. Adults with gross hematuria require a full urologic evaluation. *Ca:Cr,* Calcium:creatinine ratio. (Modified from Nseyo UO [ed]: *Urology for primary care physicians,* Philadelphia, 1999, Saunders.)

HEMOPTYSIS

ICD-9CM # 786.3
ICD-10CM # R04.2 Hemoptysis

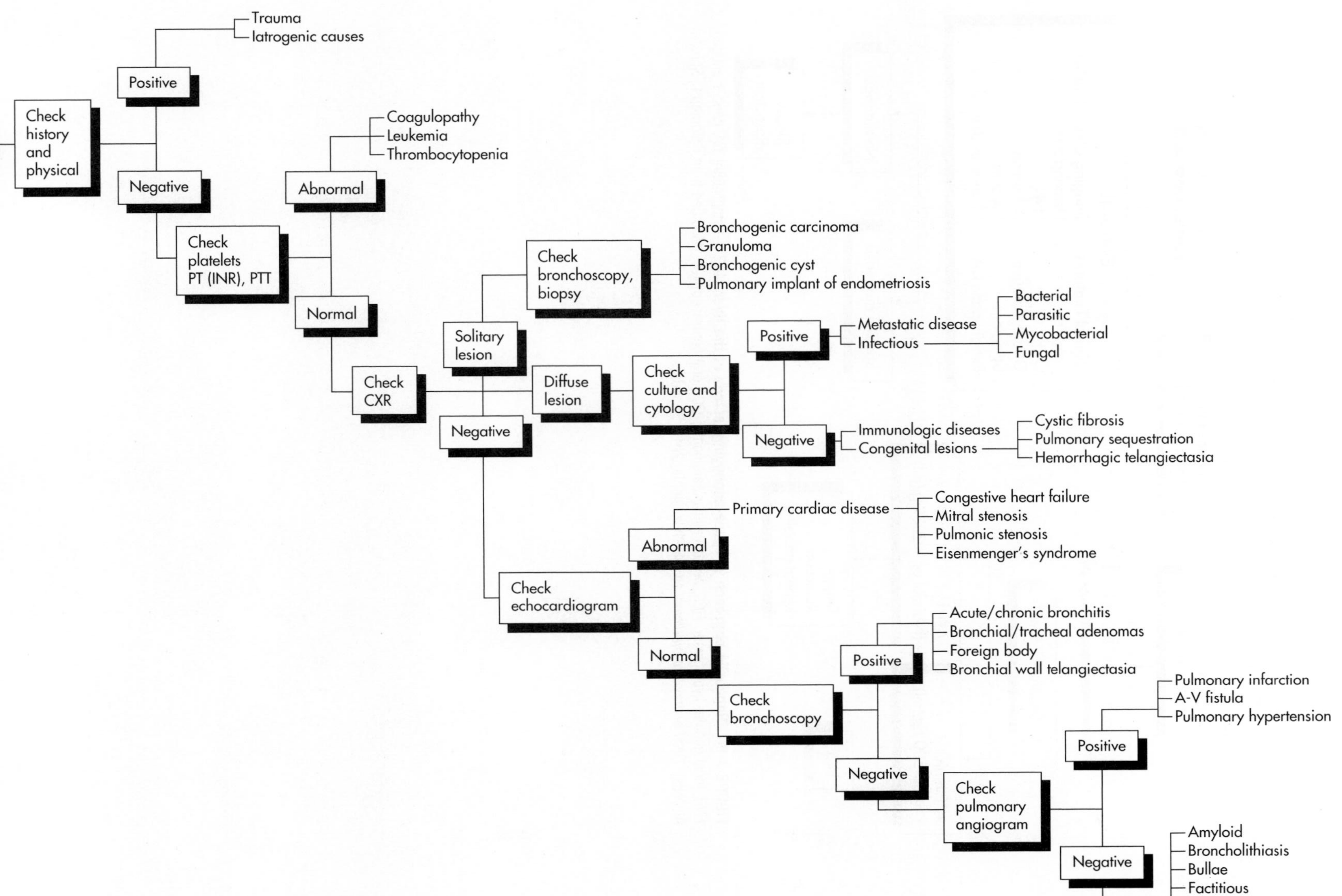

FIGURE 3-89 Evaluation of hemoptysis. *A-V,* Arteriovenous; *CXR,* chest x-ray; *INR,* International Normalized Ratio; *PT,* prothrombin time; *PTT,* partial thromboplastin time. (From Healey PM: *Common medical diagnosis: an algorithmic approach,* ed 3, Philadelphia, 2000, Saunders.)

ICD-9CM # 751.60
ICD-10CM # Q44.7 Other congenital malformations of liver

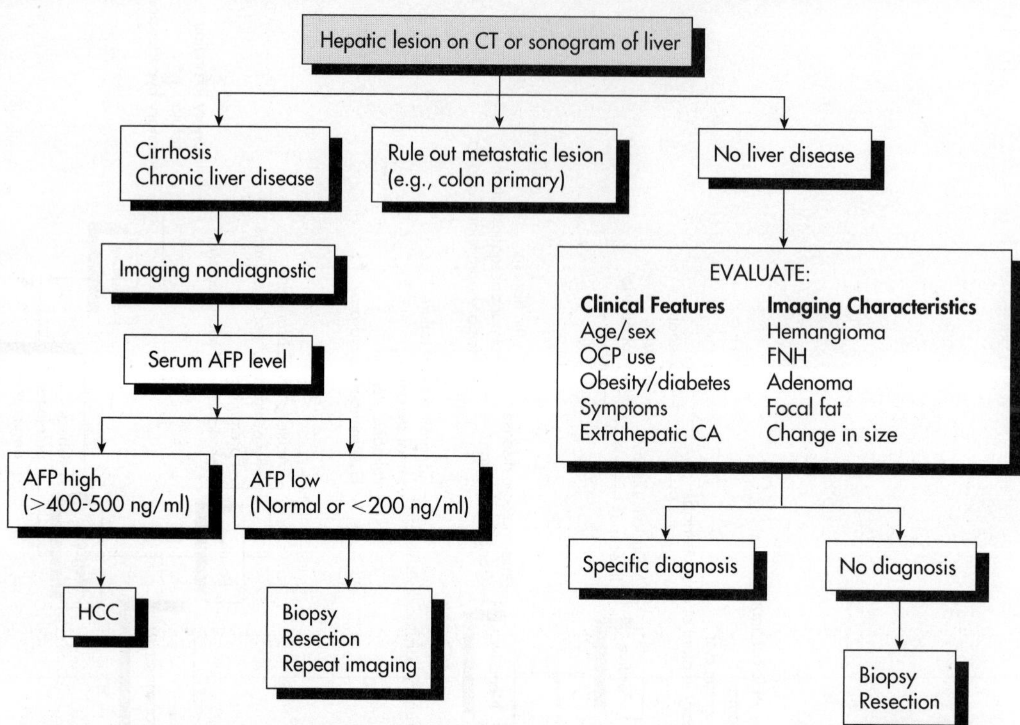

FIGURE 3-90 Diagnostic approach to space-occupying lesions of the liver. *AFP,* α-Fetoprotein; *CA,* cancer antigen; *FNH,* focal nodular hyperplasia; *HCC,* hepatocellular carcinoma; *OCP,* oral contraceptives. (Modified from Goldman L, Schafer AL [eds]: *Cecil textbook of medicine,* ed 24, Philadelphia, 2012, Saunders.)

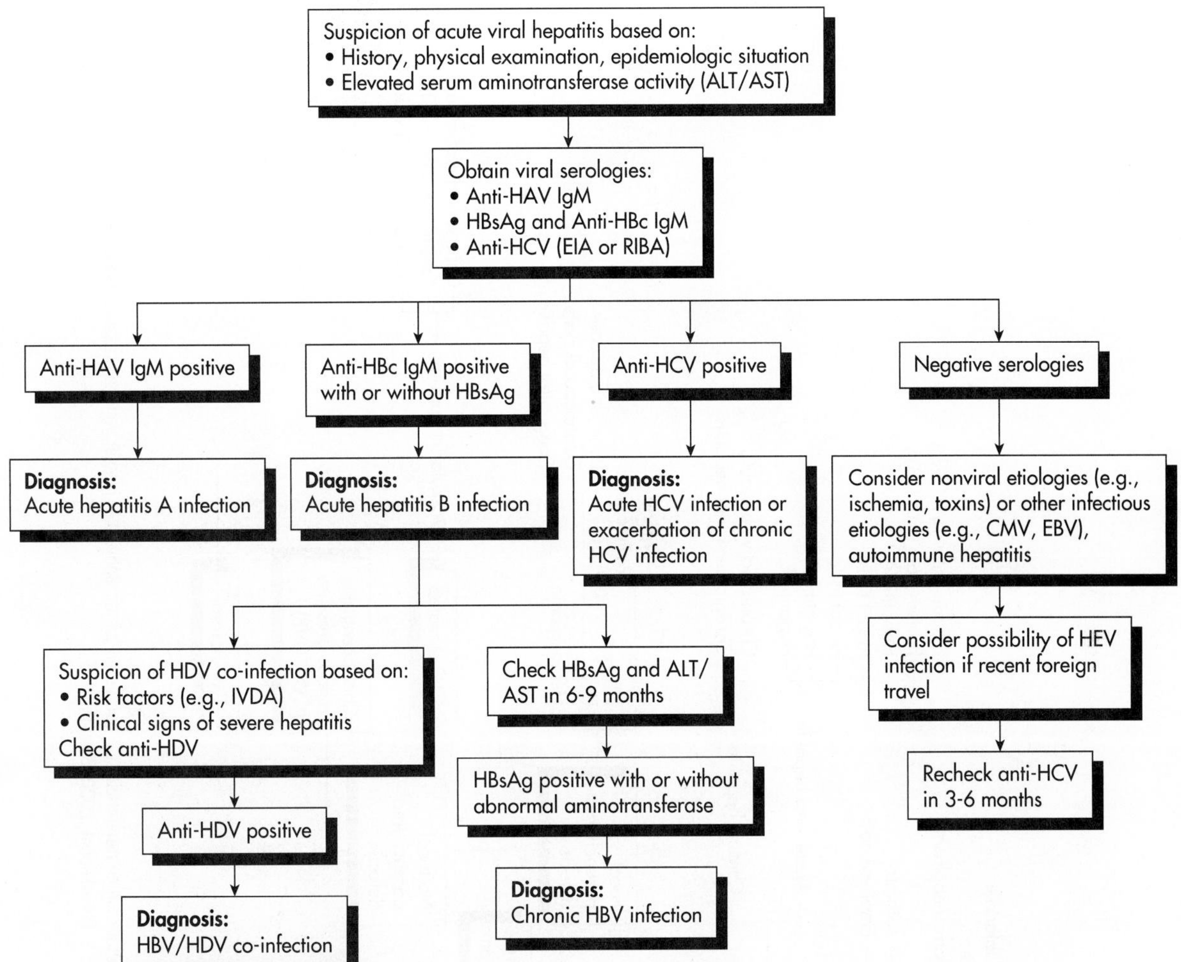

FIGURE 3-91 A flow diagram showing the use of specific serologic tests for the diagnosis of acute viral hepatitis in relation to the clinical and epidemiologic setting. Co-infections and superinfections of chronic hepatitis B or C patients should always be considered in cases that do not fit well with the clinical or serologic picture. *CMV,* Cytomegalovirus; *EBV,* Epstein-Barr virus; *EIA,* enzyme immunoassay; *HBV,* hepatitis B virus; *HCV,* hepatitis C virus; *HDV,* hepatitis D virus; *HEV,* hepatoencephalomyelitis virus; *IVDA,* intravenous drug abuse; *RIBA,* recombinant immunoblot assay. (Modified from Mandell GL: *Mandell, Douglas, and Bennett's principles and practice of infectious diseases,* ed 7, New York, 2008, Churchill Livingstone.)

HEPATOMEGALY

ICD-9CM # 789.1
ICD-10CM # R16.0 Hepatomegaly, not elsewhere classified

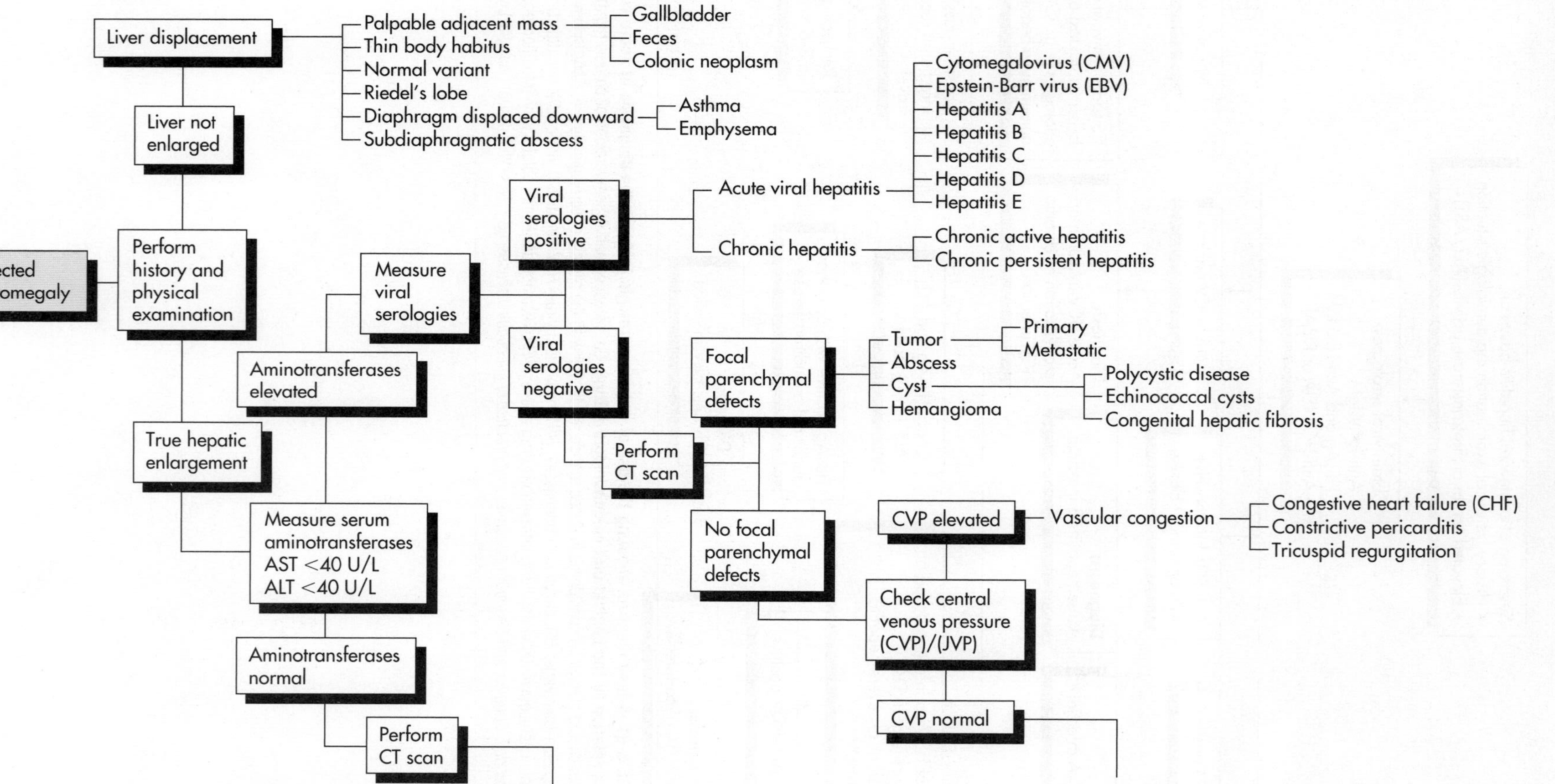

FIGURE 3-92 Hepatomegaly. *ALT,* Alanine aminotransferase; *AST,* aspartate aminotransferase; *CT,* computed tomography; *JVP,* jugular venous pressure. (Modified from Healey PM: *Common medical diagnosis: an algorithmic approach,* ed 3, Philadelphia, 2000, Saunders.)

ICD-9CM # 789.1
ICD-10CM # R16.0 Hepatomegaly, not elsewhere classified

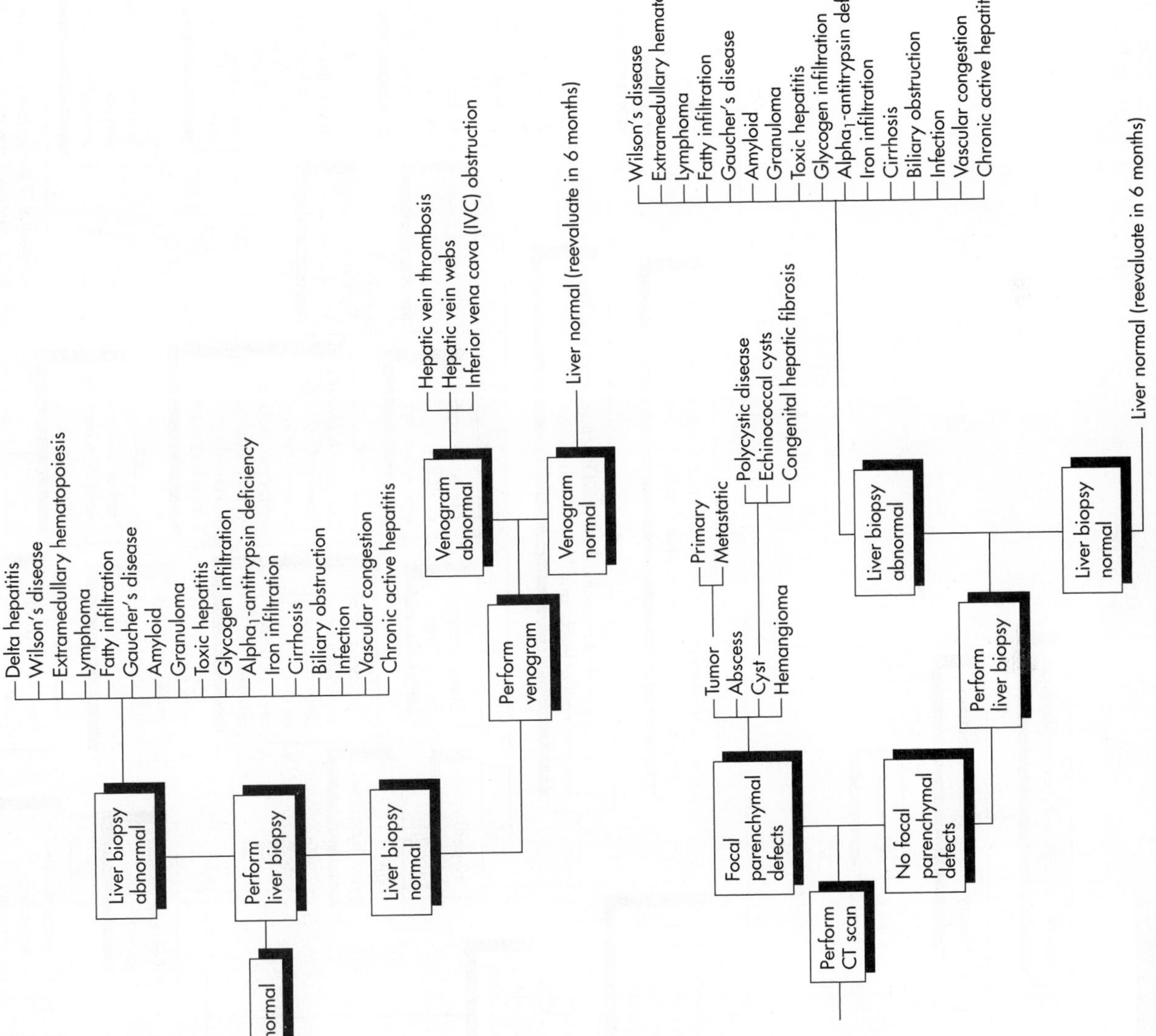

FIGURE 3-92 (Continued)

HYPERPIGMENTATION

ICD-9CM # 709.00
ICD-10CM # L81.4 Other melanin hyperpigmentation

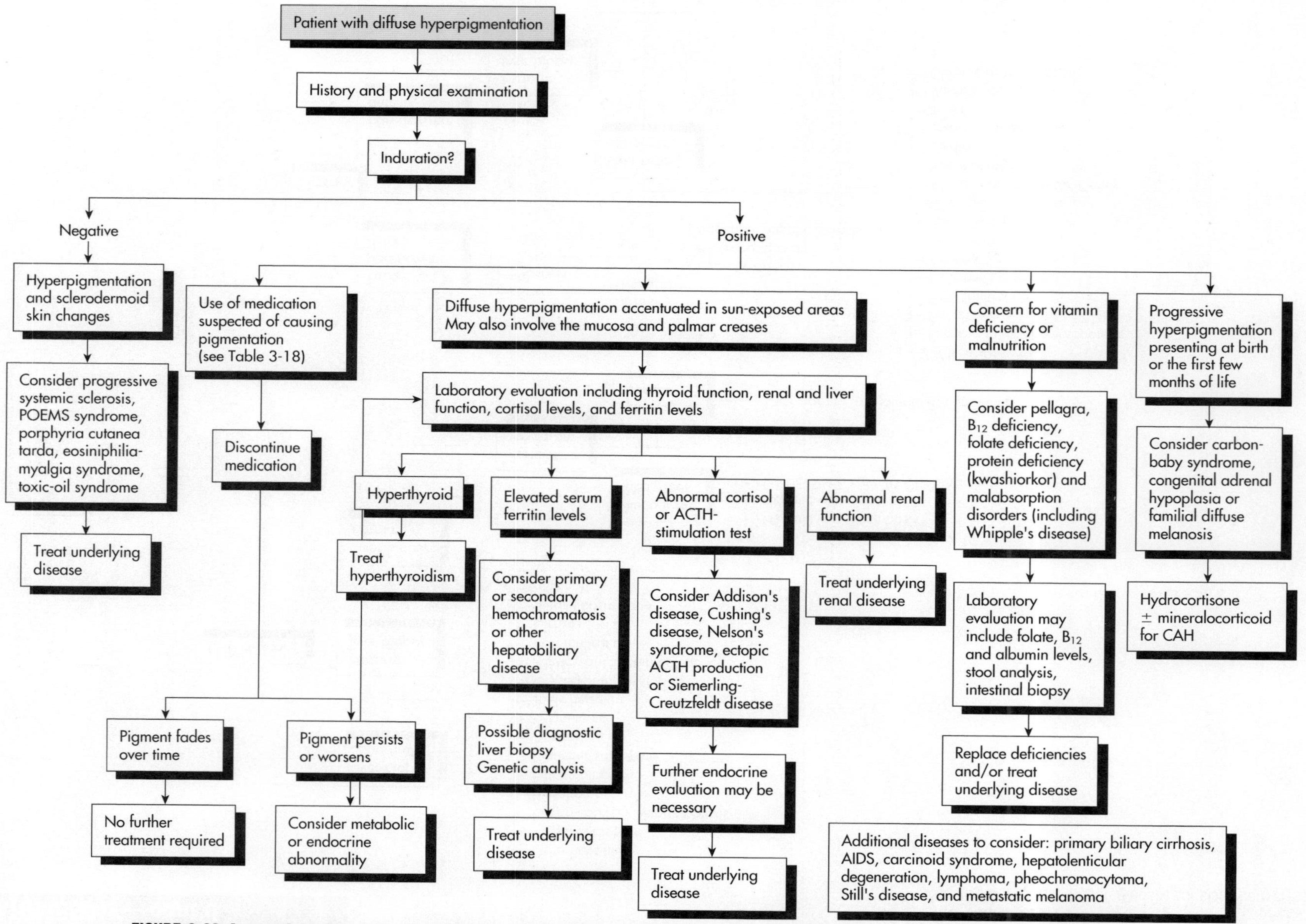

Patient with diffuse hyperpigmentation
→ History and physical examination
→ Induration?

- Negative
  - Hyperpigmentation and sclerodermoid skin changes
  - → Consider progressive systemic sclerosis, POEMS syndrome, porphyria cutanea tarda, eosiniphilia-myalgia syndrome, toxic-oil syndrome
  - → Treat underlying disease
- Positive
  - Use of medication suspected of causing pigmentation (see Table 3-18)
    - → Discontinue medication
      - → Pigment fades over time → No further treatment required
      - → Pigment persists or worsens → Consider metabolic or endocrine abnormality
  - Diffuse hyperpigmentation accentuated in sun-exposed areas May also involve the mucosa and palmar creases
    - → Laboratory evaluation including thyroid function, renal and liver function, cortisol levels, and ferritin levels
      - Hyperthyroid → Treat hyperthyroidism (→ Pigment persists or worsens; → Laboratory evaluation)
      - Elevated serum ferritin levels → Consider primary or secondary hemochromatosis or other hepatobiliary disease → Possible diagnostic liver biopsy Genetic analysis → Treat underlying disease
      - Abnormal cortisol or ACTH-stimulation test → Consider Addison's disease, Cushing's disease, Nelson's syndrome, ectopic ACTH production or Siemerling-Creutzfeldt disease → Further endocrine evaluation may be necessary → Treat underlying disease
      - Abnormal renal function → Treat underlying renal disease
  - Concern for vitamin deficiency or malnutrition
    - → Consider pellagra, B_{12} deficiency, folate deficiency, protein deficiency (kwashiorkor) and malabsorption disorders (including Whipple's disease)
    - → Laboratory evaluation may include folate, B_{12} and albumin levels, stool analysis, intestinal biopsy
    - → Replace deficiencies and/or treat underlying disease
  - Progressive hyperpigmentation presenting at birth or the first few months of life
    - → Consider carbon-baby syndrome, congenital adrenal hypoplasia or familial diffuse melanosis
    - → Hydrocortisone ± mineralocorticoid for CAH

Additional diseases to consider: primary biliary cirrhosis, AIDS, carcinoid syndrome, hepatolenticular degeneration, lymphoma, pheochromocytoma, Still's disease, and metastatic melanoma

FIGURE 3-93 Approach to the adult patient with diffuse hyperpigmentation. *ACTH,* Adrenocorticotropic hormone; *AIDS,* acquired immunodeficiency syndrome; *CAH,* congenital adrenal hyperplasia; POEMS, polyneuropathy, organomegaly, endocrinopathies, monoclonal gammopathy, skin changes. (From Bolognia JL et al [eds]: *Dermatology,* ed 2, St Louis, 2008, Mosby.)

TABLE 3-18 Drugs and Chemicals Associated with Hyperpigmentation

Drug or Chemical	Clinical Features	Histopathology/Comment
Cancer Chemotherapeutic Agents		
BCNU (Topical)	• Hyperpigmentation at site of application (no reaction seen with parenteral administration)	• Hyperplasia of basal melanocytes consistent with postinflammatory hyperpigmentation
Bleomycin	• Linear, flagellate bands, associated with minor trauma • Nails may be involved • Hyperpigmentation overlying joints	• Increased epidermal melanin • Little dermal pigment incontinence • No increase in epidermal melanocytes
Busulfan	• Generalized hyperpigmentation resembling Addison's disease; sometimes seen in association with drug-induced pulmonary fibrosis	• Increased melanin in basal keratinocytes and in dermal macrophages
Cyclophosphamide	• Diffuse hyperpigmentation of the skin and mucous membranes • Localized pigment of the nails (transverse or longitudinal bands), palms and soles, or teeth	• Pigmentation usually regresses within 6 to 12 months after therapy is discontinued
Dactinomycin	• Generalized hyperpigmentation, most prominent on the face	• Pigmentation fades after treatment discontinued
Daunorubicin	• Hyperpigmentation of light-exposed areas • Transverse brown-black nail bands	• Structurally similar to doxorubicin
Doxorubicin	• Pigmentation of the nails; hyperpigmentation of the palmar creases, palms, soles, buccal mucosa, dorsae of the knuckles and tongue	• Increased epidermal melanin • Increased number of melanocytes
5-Fluorouracil	• Hyperpigmentation in sun-exposed areas • Increased pigmentation of skin overlying veins used for infusion, dorsae of the hands and trunk	• Synergistic hyperpigmentation of irradiation portal sites
Hydroxyurea	• Reversible hyperpigmentation over pressure points and the back • Nails may be involved	• Lichenoid eruption with secondary hyperpigmentation
Mechlorethamine (nitrogen mustard)	• Topical use for cutaneous lymphoma may result in generalized hyperpigmentation • More intense in lesional skin	• Disaggregation of melanosomes within keratinocytes • Increased number of melanocytes
Methotrexate	• Uniform hyperpigmentation in sun-exposed areas	• Uncommon • May be postinflammatory hyperpigmentation secondary to photosensitivity reaction
Antimalarials		
Amino quinolones (chloroquine, hydroxychloroquine, amodiaquine)	• Yellow-brown or gray to blue-black pigment, usually in pretibial areas; face, hard palate, and subungual areas may be involved	• Dyspigmentation in up to 25% of patients • Dermal deposition of melanin-drug complexes; hemosiderin around capillaries • May fade, but rarely resolves, upon discontinuation of drug
Heavy Metals		
Arsenic	• Areas of bronze hyperpigmentation ± superimposed raindrops • Keratoses on the palms and soles associated with pigmentation	• May appear 1-20 years after exposure • Dermal and epidermal deposition of arsenic • Increased epidermal melanin synthesis
Bismuth	• Generalized blue-gray discoloration of face, neck, dorsal hands • Oral mucosa and gingivae may be involved	• Bismuth granules in the papillary and reticular dermis
Gold	• Permanent blue-gray discoloration in sun-exposed areas, mostly around the eyes (chrysiasis)	• Gold particles within macrophage lysosomes in the dermis
Iron	• Permanent brown pigment at injection or application sites	• Pigment coats collagen fibers and is deposited in dermal macrophages
Lead	• "Lead line" in gingival margin • Nail pigmentation	• Lead line is due to subepithelial deposition of lead granules
Mercury	• Slate-gray pigmentation, particularly in skin folds	• Brown-black granules free in dermis, in association with elastic fibers, and within macrophages
Silver	• Generalized slate-gray pigmentation, increased in sun-exposed areas • Nails and sclerae may also be involved • Localized at sites of application	• Silver granules in the basement membrane and on the membrana propria of eccrine glands
Hormones		
Oral contraceptives	• Melasma; increased pigment of nipples and nevi	• Increased melanocytes and increased melanin synthesis
ACTH/MSH	• Diffuse brown or bronze pigmentation; seen in Addison's disease and Cushing's syndrome	• Increased melanin synthesis

From Bolognia JL et al [eds]: *Dermatology,* ed 2, St Louis, 2008, Mosby.

ICD-9CM # 709.00
ICD-10CM # L81.4 Other melanin hyperpigmentation

TABLE 3-18 Drugs and Chemicals Associated with Hyperpigmentation—cont'd

Drug or Chemical	Clinical Features	Histopathology/Comment
Miscellaneous Compounds		
Amiodarone	• Slate-gray to violaceous discoloration of sun-exposed skin	• Yellow-brown granules in dermis, mostly perivascular • Lysosomal inclusions with a lipid-like substance
Azidothymidine (zidovudine, AZT)	• Nail and mucocutaneous hyperpigmentation	• Skin biopsy shows increased epidermal and dermal melanin
Clofazimine	• Diffuse red to red-brown discoloration of skin • Violet-brown to bluish discoloration, especially lesional skin	• Redness secondary to drug in fat • Phagolysosomes with lipofuscin material
Dioxins	• Chloracne most common skin finding • Hyperpigmentation may occur in sun-exposed areas	• Rare, except in accidental exposure
Hydroquinone	• Hyperpigmentation in areas of application due to exogenous ochronosis	• Yellow-brown banana-shaped fibers in papillary dermis
Minocycline	• Blue-black discoloration in old acne scars or sites of inflammation as well as lower extremities • May also involve nails, sclerae, oral mucosa, bones, and teeth • Generalized "muddy brown" pigmentation pattern in some patients	• Iron-containing granules and/or increased melanin, depending on clinical type
Psoralens	• Increased pigmentation after exposure to UVA light (PUVA)	• Proliferation of follicular melanocytes • Increased synthesis and transfer of melanin
Psychotropic drugs (phenothiazine, chlorpromazine, imipramine, desipramine)	• Slate-gray discoloration in sun-exposed areas	• Golden-brown granules in the upper dermis • Electron-dense inclusion bodies

HYPOGLYCEMIA

ICD-9CM # 251.2
ICD-10CM # E16.2 Hypoglycemia, spontaneous
E16.0 Hypoglycemia, drug-induced
E16.1 Hypoglycemia, reactive
E16.3 Hypersecretion, glucagon

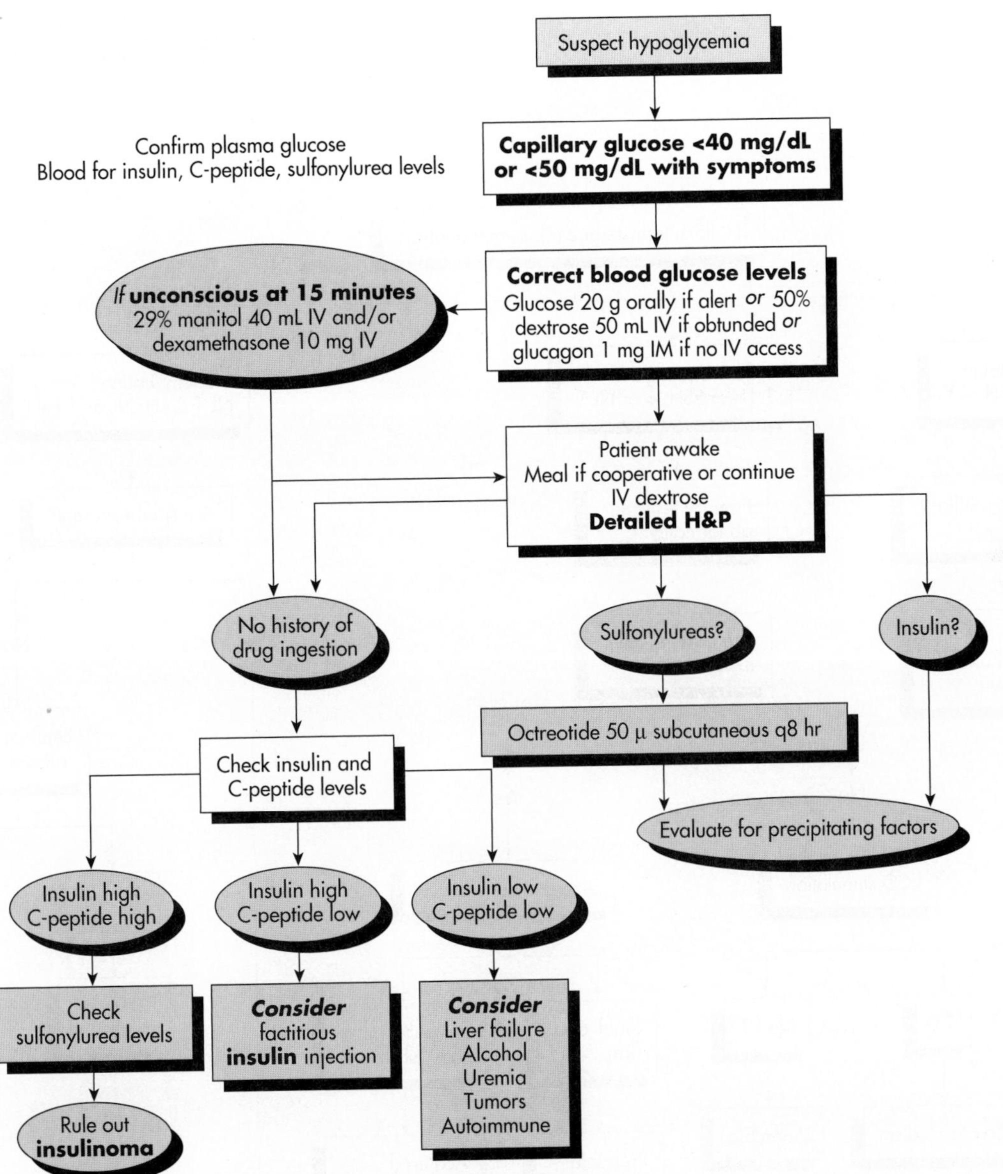

FIGURE 3-94 Decision tree for suspected hypoglycemia in adults. (From Vincent JL, Ahraham E, Moore FA, et al: *Textbook of critical care*, ed 6, Philadelphia, 2011, Saunders.)

ICD-9CM #	256.3	Female
	257.2	Male
	256.3	Ovarian
	253.4	Pituitary
	257.2	Testicular
ICD-10CM #	E28.310	Symptomatic premature menopause
	E29.1	Testicular hypofunction
	E28.39	Other primary ovarian failure
	E23.6	Other disorders of pituitary gland
	E29.1	Testicular hypofunction

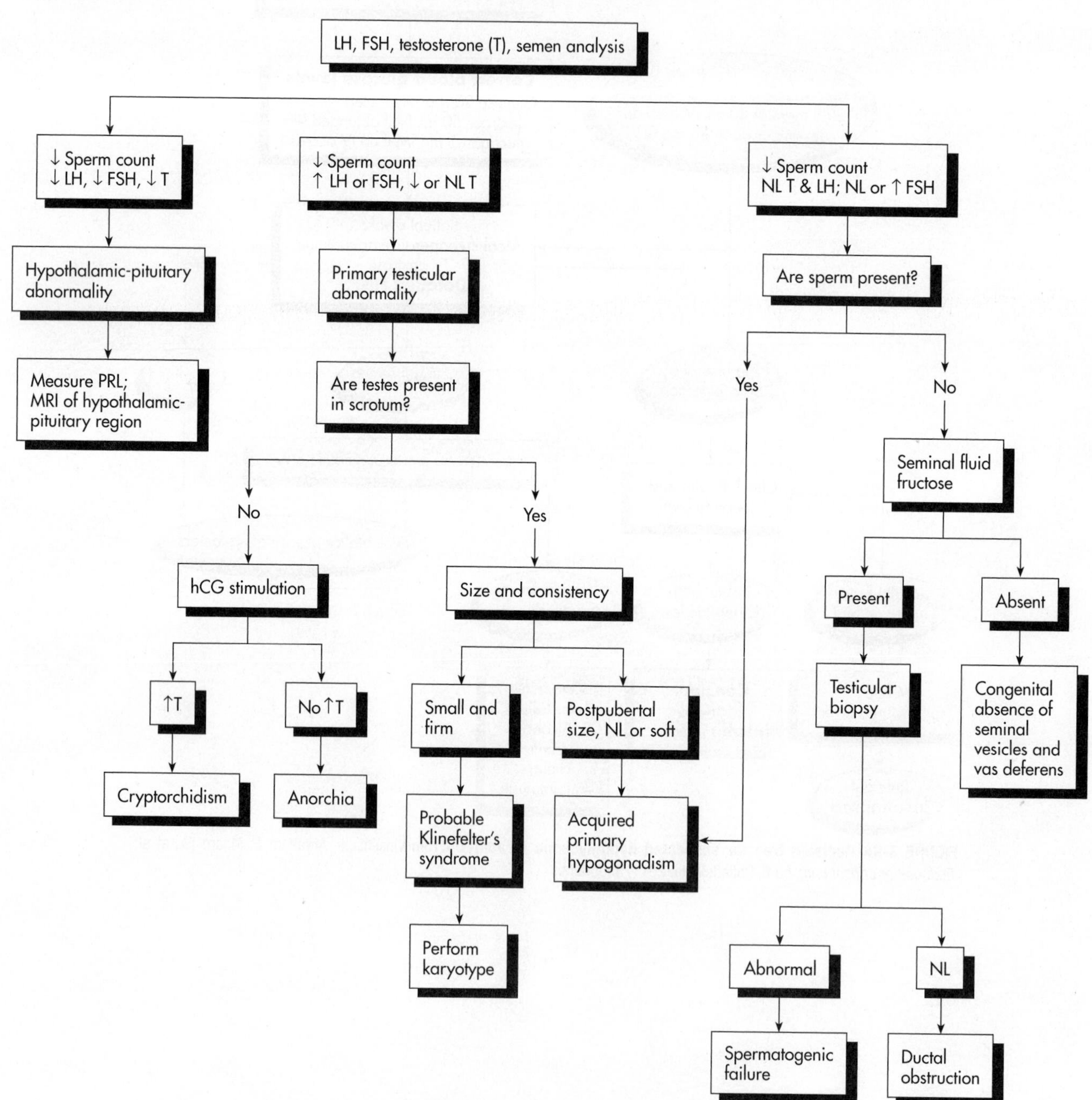

FIGURE 3-95 Laboratory evaluation of hypogonadism in men. *FSH,* Follicle-stimulating hormone; *hCG,* human chorionic gonadotropin; *LH,* luteinizing hormone; *MRI,* magnetic resonance imaging; *NL,* normal; *PRL,* prolactin; ↑, elevated; ↓, decreased or low. (From Andreoli TE [ed]: *Cecil essentials of medicine,* ed 7, Philadelphia, 2008, Saunders.)

HYPOTENSION

ICD-9CM #	458.9	Hypotension, NOS
	458.1	Hypotension, chronic
	458.2	Hypotension, iatrogenic
	458.0	Hypotension, orthostatic or postural
ICD-10CM#	I95.9	Hypotension, unspecified
	I95.89	Other hypotension
	I95.3	Hypotension of hemodialysis
	I95.1	Orthostatic hypotension

- Hypotension
  - Check for orthostatic changes
    - Orthostatic hypotension only
      - Check intravascular volume
        - Decreased volume
          - Blood loss
          - Dehydration
          - Third spacing of fluid
            - Ascites
            - Pleural effusions
            - Edema
          - Adrenal insufficiency
        - Normal volume
          - Check drug history
            - Drug history positive
              - Antihypertensives
              - Nitrates
              - Phenothiazines
              - Minor tranquilizers
              - Tricyclic antidepressants
            - Drug history negative
              - Autonomic dysfunction
                - Idiopathic postural hypotension
                - Shy-Drager syndrome
                - Spinal cord lesions
                - Peripheral neuropathy
    - Nonorthostatic hypotension
      - Check tissue perfusion
        - Perfusion normal
          - Vasovagal hypotension
        - Decreased perfusion
          - Check intravascular volume
            - Decreased volume
              - Toxic shock syndrome
              - Hypovolemia
              - Sepsis
              - Neuropathic
              - Anaphylactic
              - Drug-induced
              - Addisonian crisis
              - Metabolic acidosis
            - Volume normal or increased
              - Cardiovascular hypotension
                - Heart failure
                - Valvular dysfunction
                - Pericardial tamponade
                - Arrhythmia
                - Pulmonary embolus

FIGURE 3-96 Hypotension. (From Healey PM: *Common medical diagnosis: an algorithmic approach,* ed 3, Philadelphia, 2000, Saunders.)

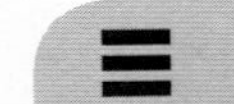

IMMUNODEFICIENCY DISEASES, PRIMARY

ICD-9CM # 279.9
ICD-10CM # D89.9 Disorder involving the immune mechanism, unspecified

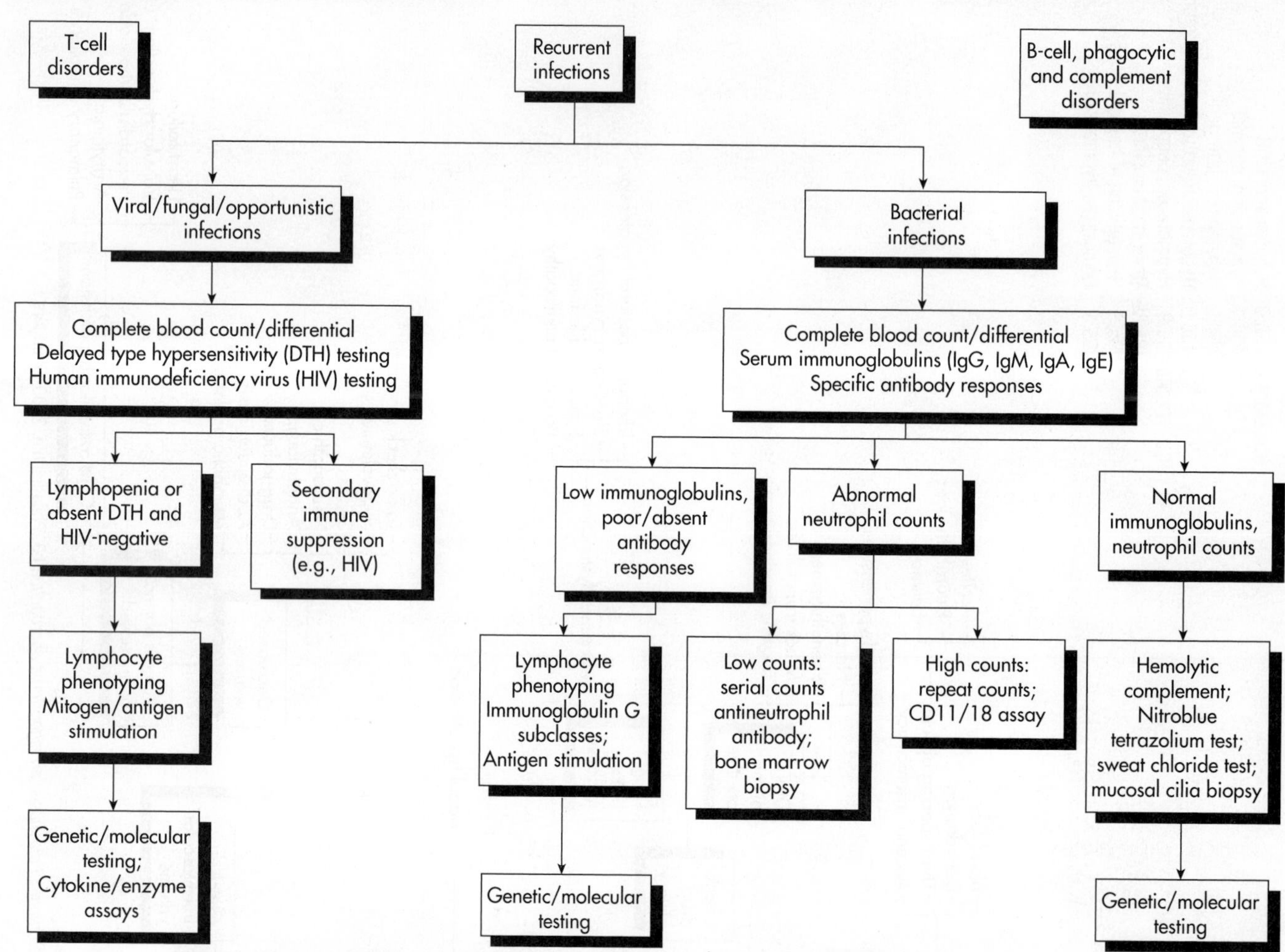

FIGURE 3-97 A diagnostic testing algorithm for primary immunodeficiency diseases. (From Lindegren ML et al: Applying public health strategies to primary immunodeficiency diseases: a potential approach to genetic disorders, *MMWR Recomm Rep* 53[RR-1]:1-29, 2004.)

INFECTIONS OF SOFT TISSUE, JOINTS, AND BONE

ICD-9CM # variable with specific disorder
ICD-10CM # M00.9 Pyogenic arthritis, unspecified
M86.9 Osteomyelitis unspecified
T84.3 Infection and inflammatory reaction
M79.9 Soft tissue disorder, unspecified

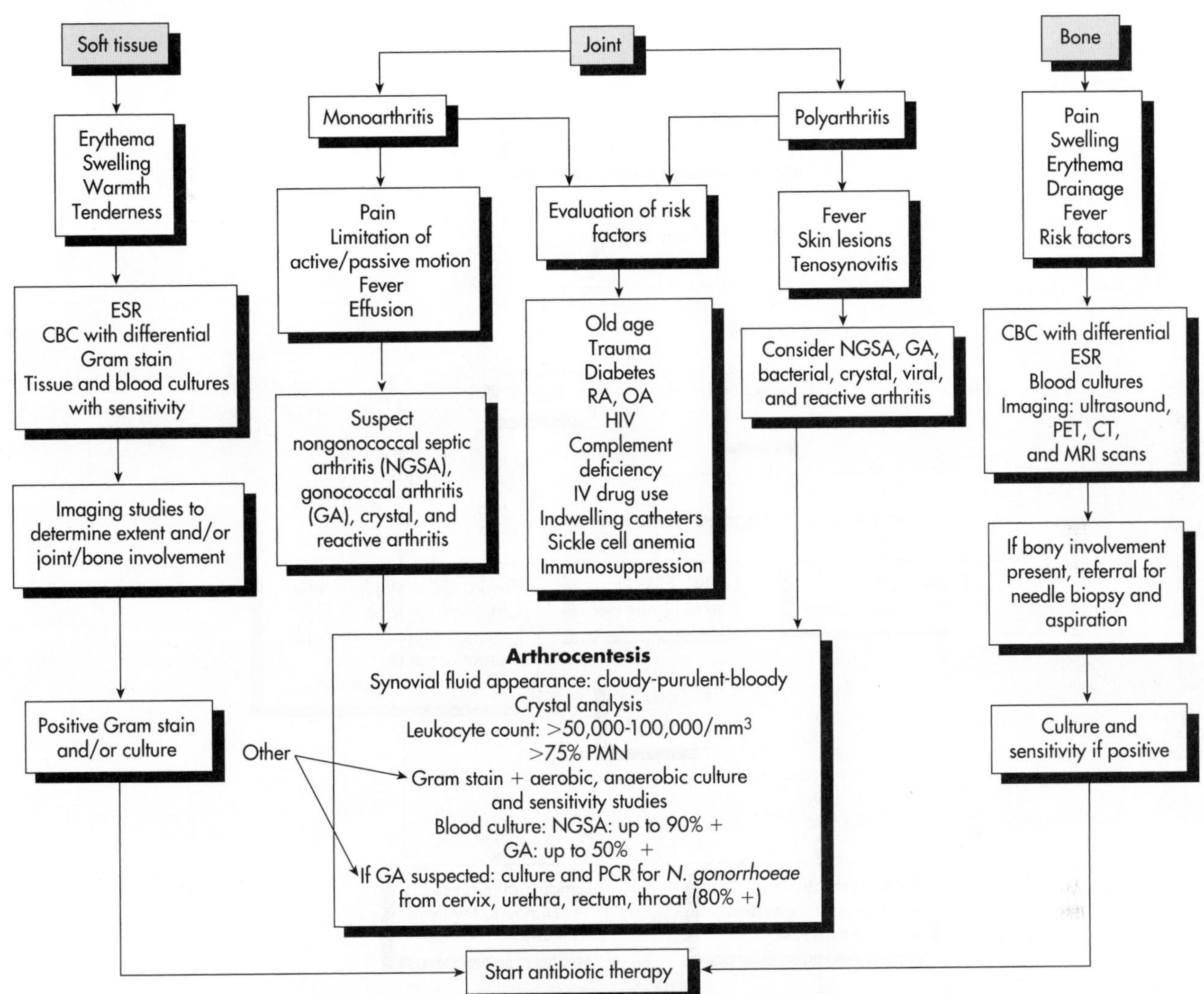

FIGURE 3-98 Clinical evaluation of infections of soft tissues, joints, and bone. *CBC,* Complete blood count; *CT,* computed tomography; *ESR,* erythrocyte sedimentation rate; *GA,* gonococcal arthritis; *HIV,* human immunodeficiency virus; *IV,* intravenous; *MRI,* magnetic resonance imaging; *NGSA,* nongonococcal septic arthritis; *OA,* osteoarthritis; *PCR,* polymerase chain reaction; *PET,* positron emission tomography; *PMN,* polymorphonuclear leukocyte; *RA,* rheumatoid arthritis. (From Goldman L, Schafer AI: *Goldman's Cecil medicine,* ed 24, Philadelphia, 2012, Saunders.)

ICD-9CM # variable with specific disorder
ICD-10CM # M00.9 Pyogenic arthritis, unspecified
M01.1 Tuberculous arthritis
M01.2 Arthritis in Lyme disease
M01.5 Arthritis in viral disease
M02.9 Reactive arthropathy, unspecified
M08.9 Juvenile arthritis, unspecified
M10.9 Gout, unspecified

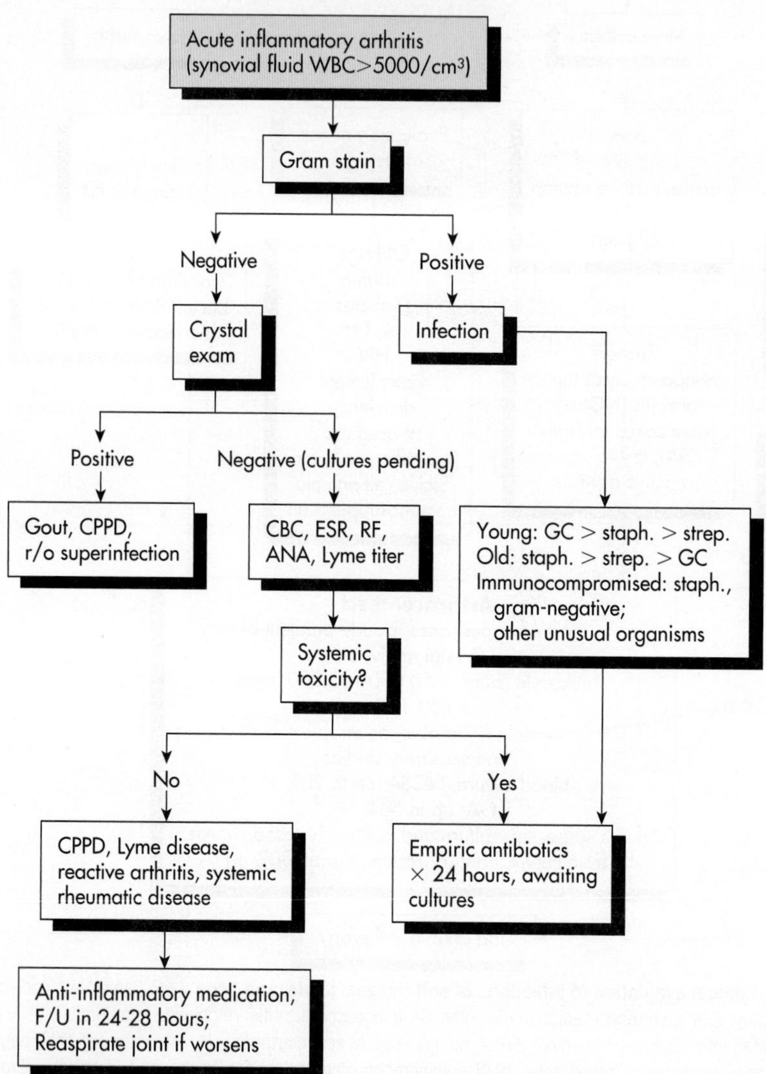

FIGURE 3-99 Approach to acute inflammatory arthritis. *ANA,* Antinuclear antibody test; *CBC,* complete blood count; *CPPD;* calcium pyrophosphate deposition disease; *ESR,* erythrocyte sedimentation rate; *F/U,* follow-up; *GC,* gonococcal infection; *RF,* rheumatoid factor; *r/o,* rule out; *staph.,* staphylococcal infection; *strep.,* streptococcal infection; *WBC,* white blood cell count. (From Harris ED et al [eds]: *Kelley's textbook of rheumatology,* ed 7, Philadelphia, 2005, Saunders.)

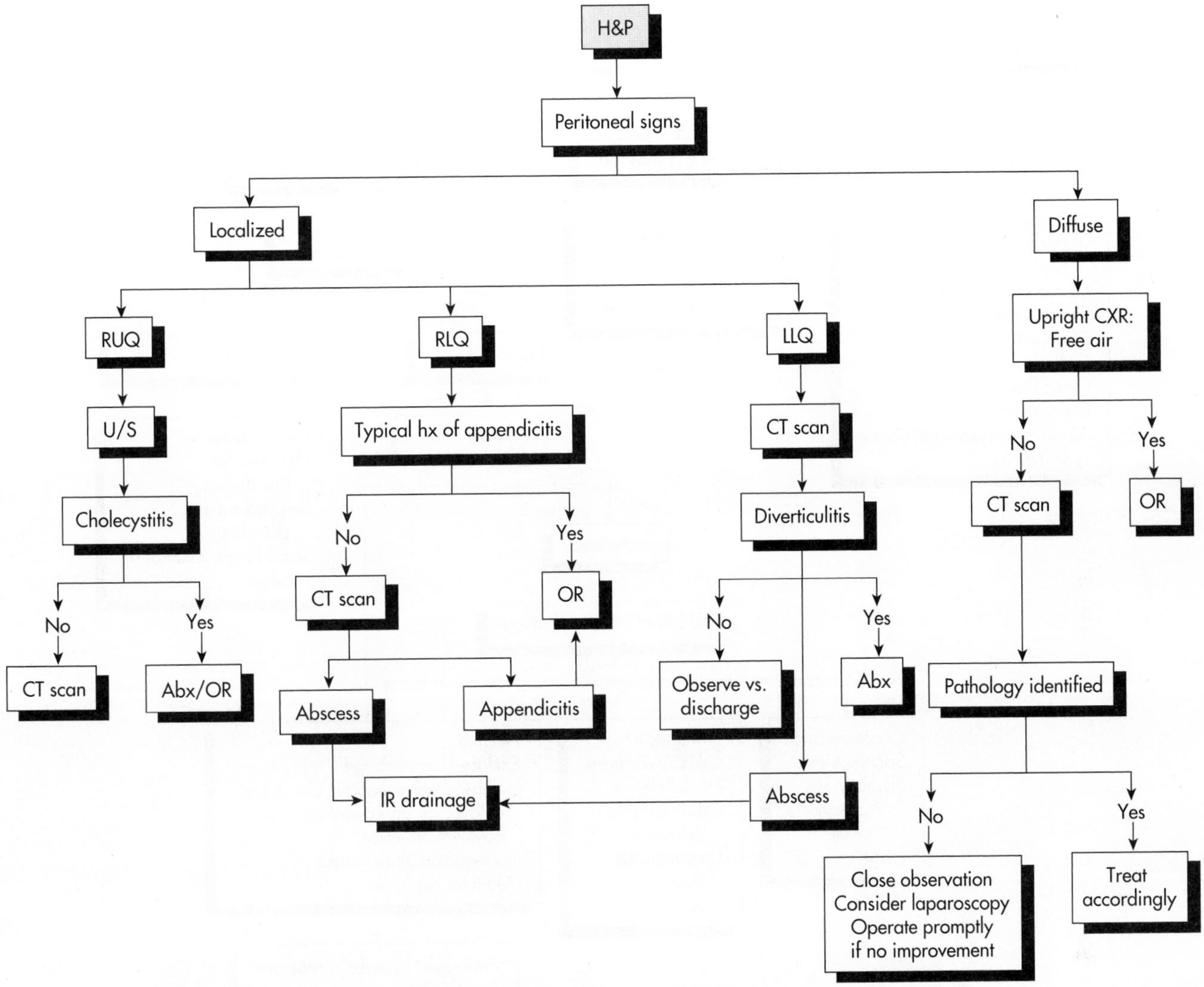

- H&P
  - Peritoneal signs
    - Localized
      - RUQ
        - U/S
          - Cholecystitis
            - No → CT scan
            - Yes → Abx/OR
      - RLQ
        - Typical hx of appendicitis
          - No → CT scan
            - Abscess → IR drainage
            - Appendicitis → OR
          - Yes → OR
      - LLQ
        - CT scan
          - Diverticulitis
            - No → Observe vs. discharge
            - Yes → Abx
            - Abscess → IR drainage
    - Diffuse
      - Upright CXR: Free air
        - No → CT scan
          - Pathology identified
            - No → Close observation / Consider laparoscopy / Operate promptly if no improvement
            - Yes → Treat accordingly
        - Yes → OR

FIGURE 3-100 Algorithm for the diagnosis and management of patients with suspected IAI. *H&P,* History and physical exam; *RUQ,* right upper quadrant; *RLQ,* right lower quadrant; *LLQ,* left lower quadrant; *U/S,* ultrasound; *Abx,* antibiotics; *hx,* history; *IR,* interventional radiology; *CXR,* chest radiograph. (From Cameron JL, Cameron AM: *Current surgical therapy,* ed 10, Philadelphia, 2011, Saunders.)

ICD-9CM # 774.6 Jaundice neonatal, NOS
ICD-10CM # P59.9 Neonatal jaundice, unspecified

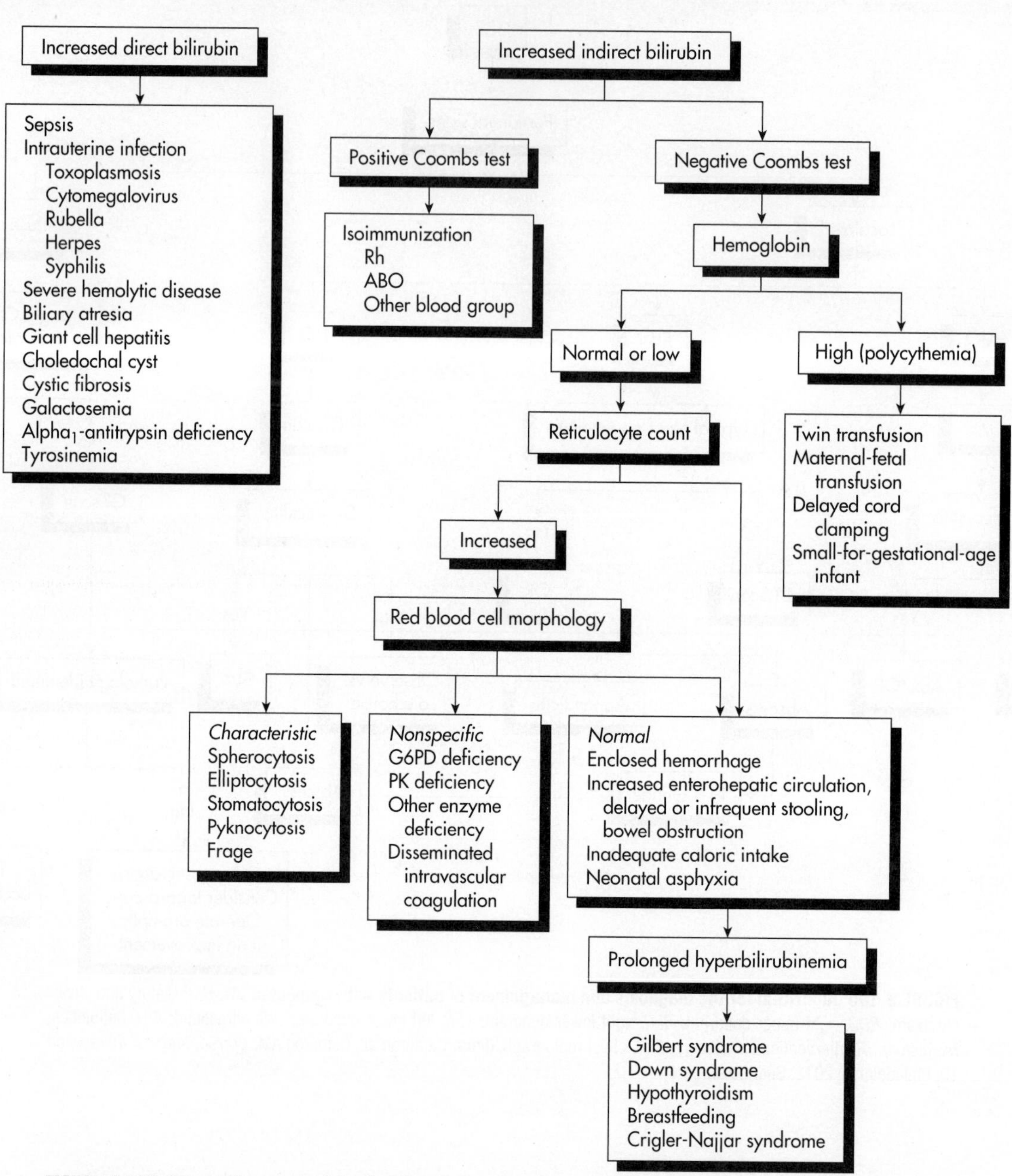

FIGURE 3-103 Schematic approach to the diagnosis of neonatal jaundice. *G6PD,* Glucose-6-phosphate dehydrogenase; *PK,* pyruvate kinase. (From Oski FA: Differential diagnosis of jaundice. In Taeusch HW, Ballard RA, Avery MA [eds]: *Schaffer and Avery's diseases of the newborn,* ed 6, Philadelphia, 1991, Saunders.)

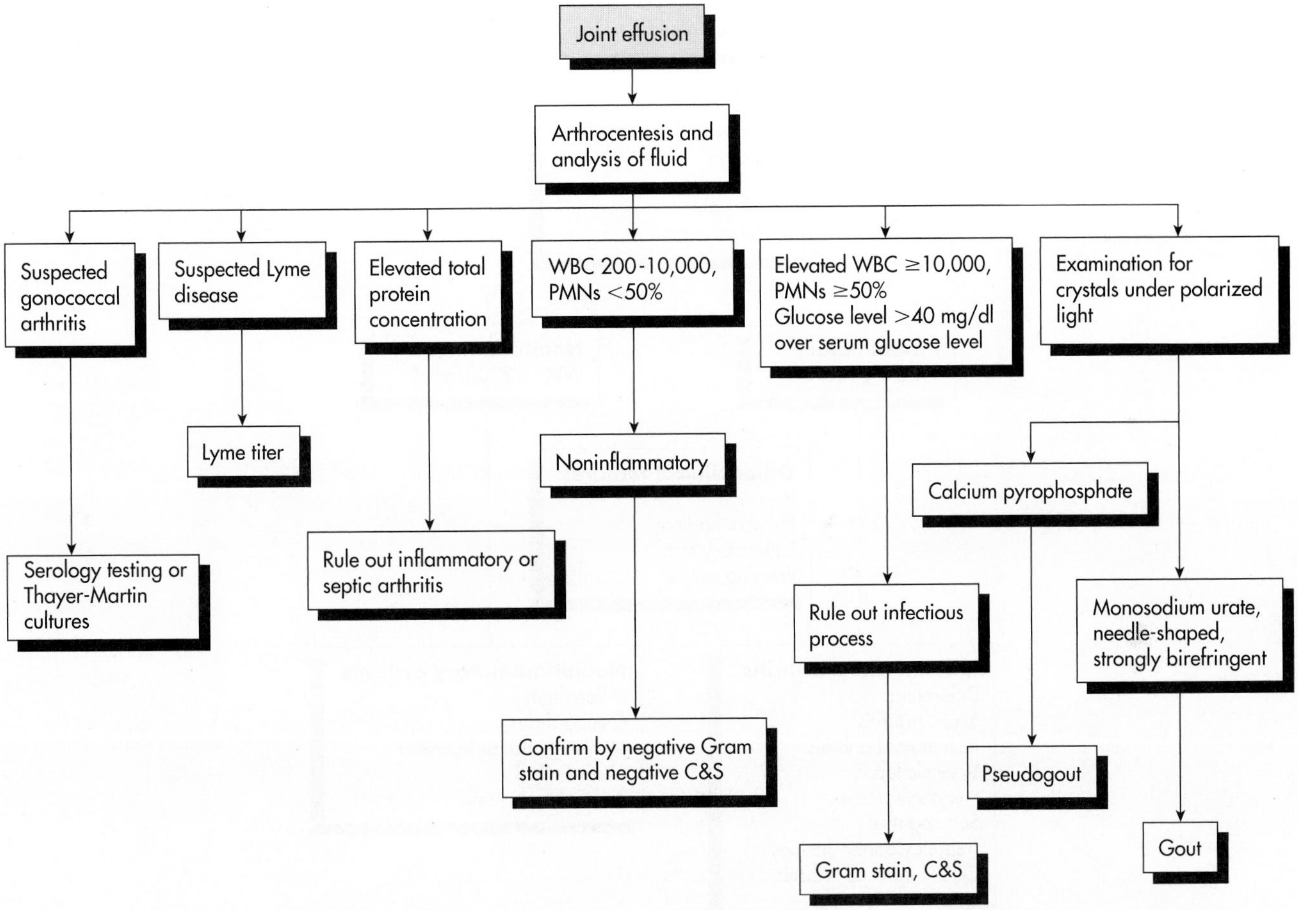

JOINT EFFUSION

ICD-9CM # 719.00
ICD-10CM # M25.40 Effusion, unspecified joint

- Joint effusion
  - Arthrocentesis and analysis of fluid
    - Suspected gonococcal arthritis
      - Serology testing or Thayer-Martin cultures
    - Suspected Lyme disease
      - Lyme titer
    - Elevated total protein concentration
      - Rule out inflammatory or septic arthritis
    - WBC 200-10,000, PMNs $<50\%$
      - Noninflammatory
        - Confirm by negative Gram stain and negative C&S
    - Elevated WBC $\geq 10{,}000$, PMNs $\geq 50\%$, Glucose level >40 mg/dl over serum glucose level
      - Rule out infectious process
        - Gram stain, C&S
    - Examination for crystals under polarized light
      - Calcium pyrophosphate
        - Pseudogout
      - Monosodium urate, needle-shaped, strongly birefringent
        - Gout

FIGURE 3-104 Joint effusion. *C&S,* Culture and sensitivity; *PMNs,* polymorphonuclear leukocytes; *WBC,* white blood cell count.

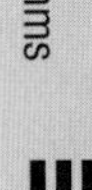

ICD-9CM # 719.00
ICD-10CM # M25.40 Effusion, unspecified joint

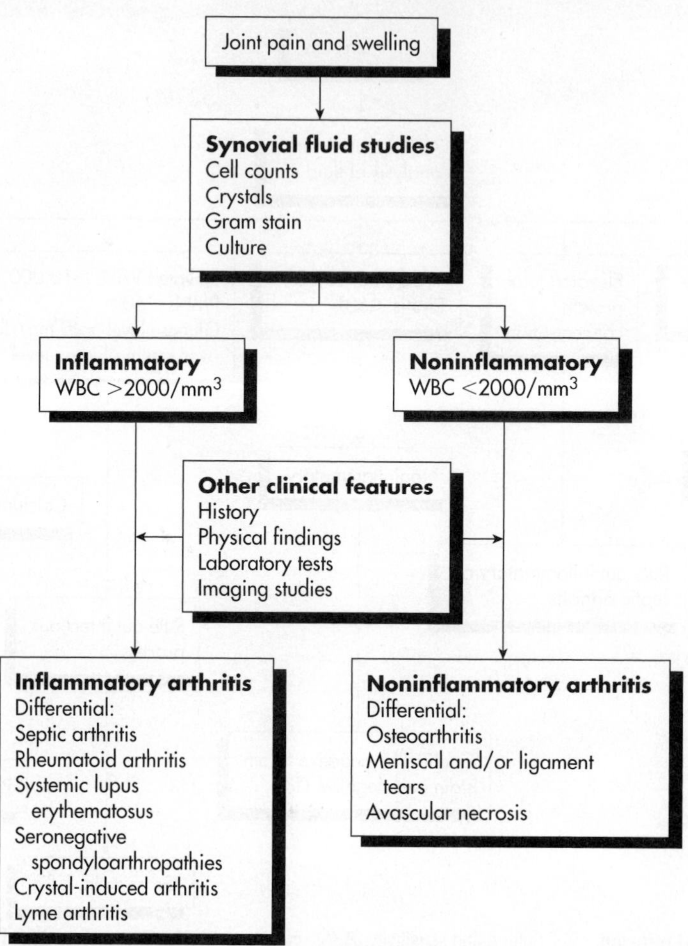

FIGURE 3-105 Diagnostic approach for swollen joints. *WBC,* White blood cell count. (From Goldman L, Schafer AL [eds]: *Cecil textbook of medicine,* ed 24, Philadelphia, 2012, Saunders.)

KNEE PAIN, ANTERIOR

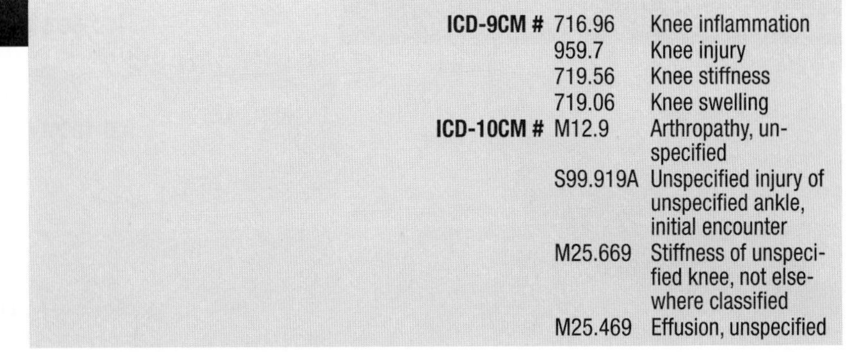

ICD-9CM #	716.96	Knee inflammation
	959.7	Knee injury
	719.56	Knee stiffness
	719.06	Knee swelling
ICD-10CM #	M12.9	Arthropathy, unspecified
	S99.919A	Unspecified injury of unspecified ankle, initial encounter
	M25.669	Stiffness of unspecified knee, not elsewhere classified
	M25.469	Effusion, unspecified

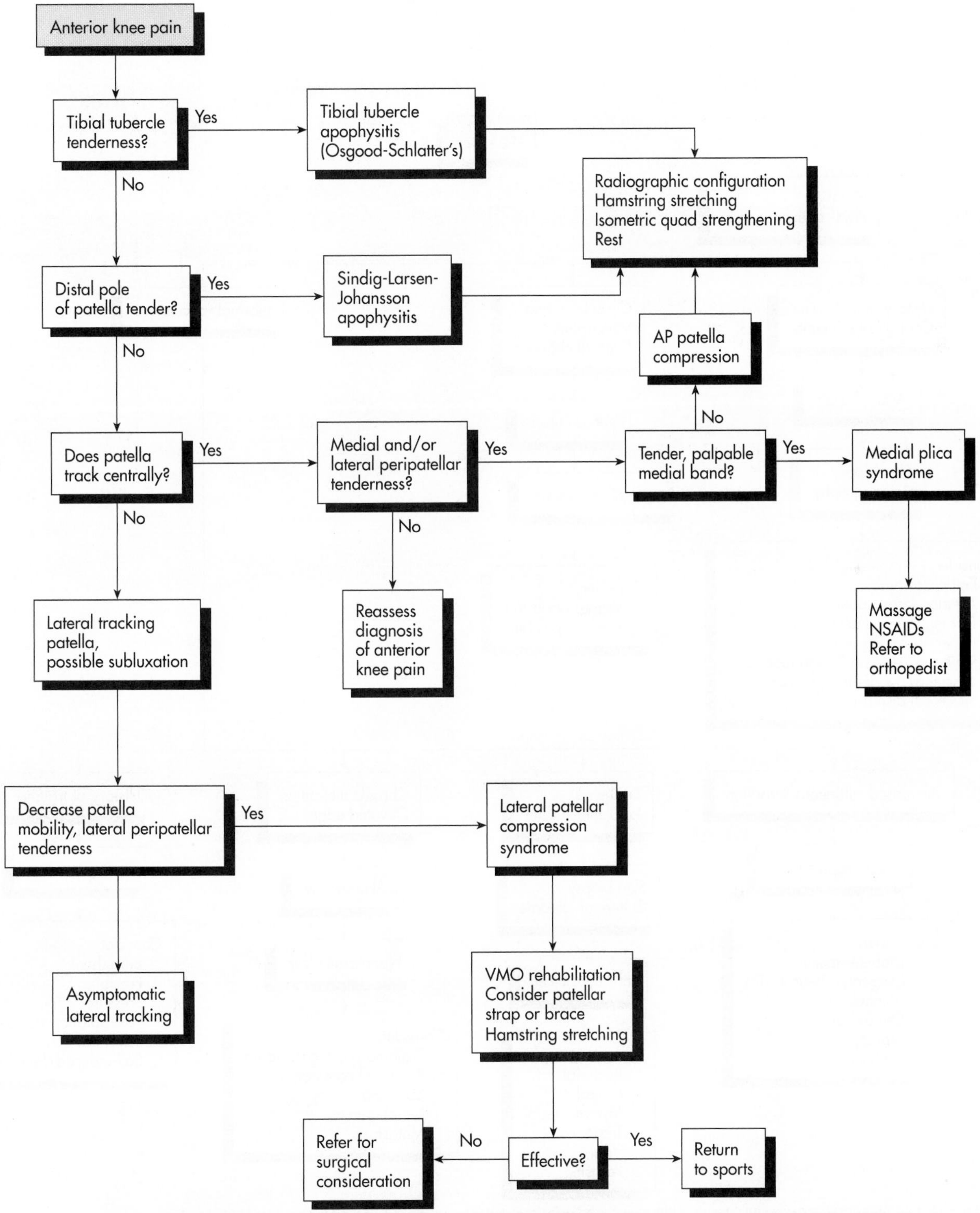

Anterior knee pain

Tibial tubercle tenderness? — Yes → Tibial tubercle apophysitis (Osgood-Schlatter's) → Radiographic configuration / Hamstring stretching / Isometric quad strengthening / Rest

No ↓

Distal pole of patella tender? — Yes → Sindig-Larsen-Johansson apophysitis → Radiographic configuration / Hamstring stretching / Isometric quad strengthening / Rest

No ↓

Does patella track centrally? — Yes → Medial and/or lateral peripatellar tenderness?

- Medial and/or lateral peripatellar tenderness? — No → Reassess diagnosis of anterior knee pain
- Medial and/or lateral peripatellar tenderness? — Yes → Tender, palpable medial band?
  - Tender, palpable medial band? — Yes → Medial plica syndrome → Massage / NSAIDs / Refer to orthopedist
  - Tender, palpable medial band? — No → AP patella compression → Radiographic configuration / Hamstring stretching / Isometric quad strengthening / Rest

No ↓

Lateral tracking patella, possible subluxation

Decrease patella mobility, lateral peripatellar tenderness — Yes → Lateral patellar compression syndrome → VMO rehabilitation / Consider patellar strap or brace / Hamstring stretching → Effective?

- Effective? — Yes → Return to sports
- Effective? — No → Refer for surgical consideration

Decrease patella mobility, lateral peripatellar tenderness ↓ Asymptomatic lateral tracking

FIGURE 3-107 Evaluation and management of knee extensor mechanism pain. Focused treatment based on specific etiology will prevent recurrence. *AP,* Anteroposterior; *NSAIDs,* nonsteroidal anti-inflammatory drugs; *VMO,* vastus medialis obliquus muscle. (From Scudieri G [ed]: *Sports medicine, principles of primary care,* St Louis, 1997, Mosby.)

ICD-9CM #	440.23	Ulcer, lower limb, arteriosclerotic
	707.1	Ulcer, lower limb, chronic
	707.9	Ulcer, non-healing
	707.0	Pressure ulcer
ICD-10CM #	I70.25	Atherosclerosis of native arteries of other extremities with ulceration
	L97.909	Non-pressure chronic ulcer of unspecified part of unspecified lower leg with unspecified severity
	L98.499	Non-pressure chronic ulcer of skin of other sites with unspecified severity
	L89.90	Pressure ulcer of unspecified site, unspecified stage

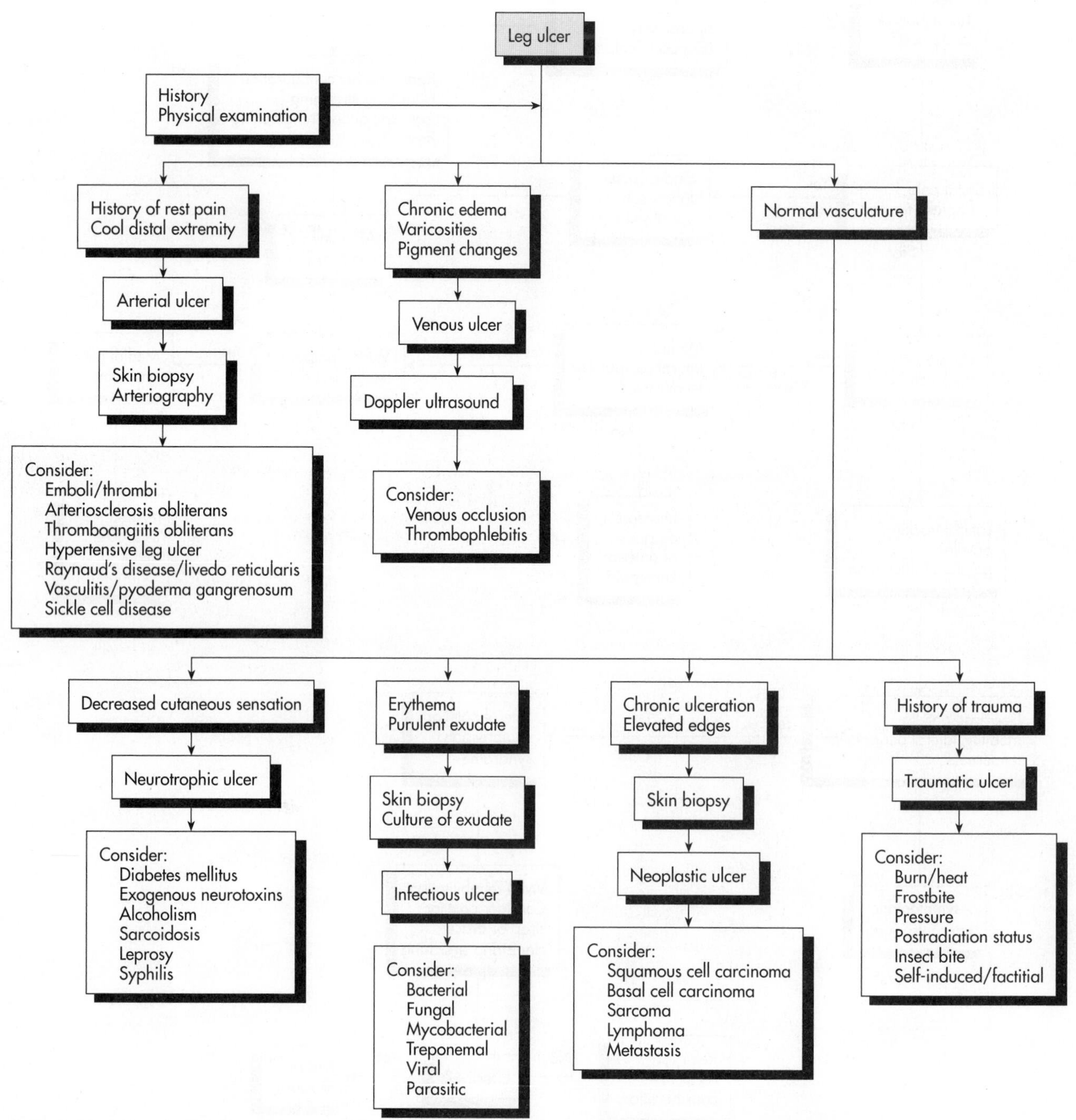

FIGURE 3-108 Leg ulcer. (From Greene HL, Johnson WP, Lemcke D [eds]: *Decision making in medicine,* ed 2, St Louis, 1998, Mosby.)

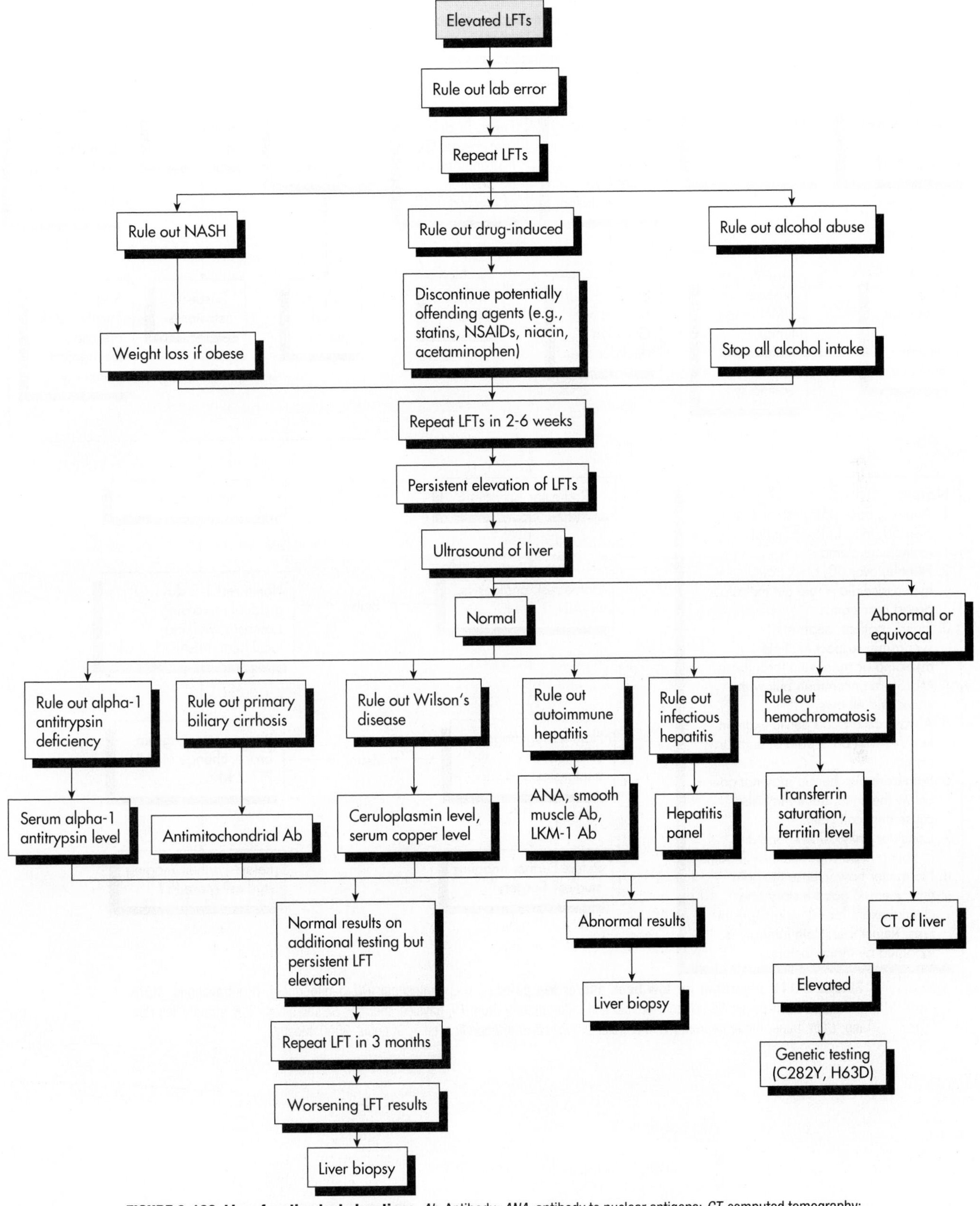

FIGURE 3-109 Liver function test elevations. *Ab,* Antibody; *ANA,* antibody to nuclear antigens; *CT,* computed tomography; *IEP,* immuno-electrophoresis; *LFTs,* liver function tests; *LKM,* liver-kidney microsome; *NASH,* nonalcoholic steatohepatitis; *NSAIDs,* nonsteroidal anti-inflammatory drugs.

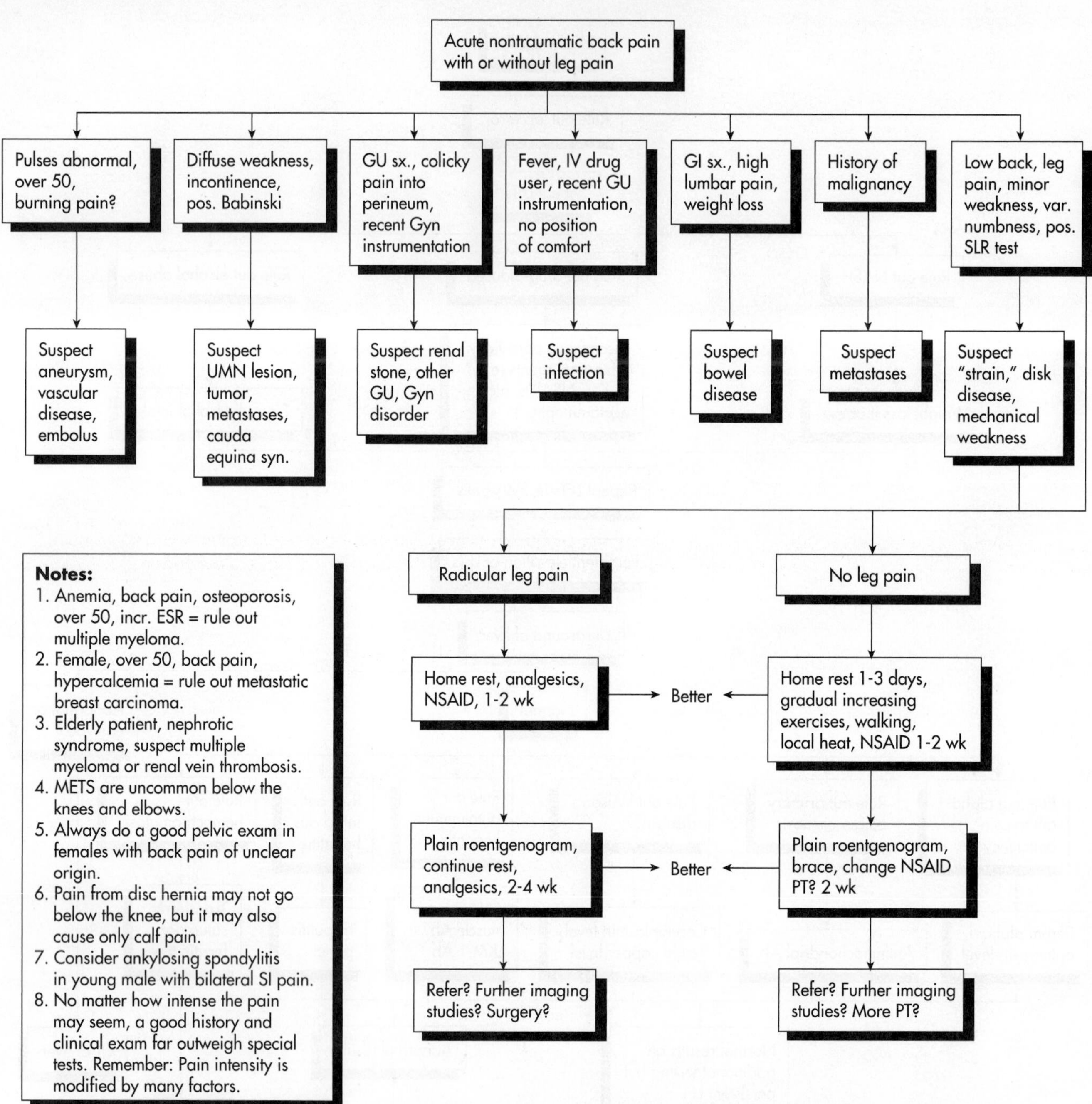

FIGURE 3-111 Algorithm for low back and/or leg pain. *GI,* Gastrointestinal; *GU,* genitourinary; *IV,* intravenous; *METS,* metabolic equivalents; *NSAID,* nonsteroidal anti-inflammatory drug; *PT,* physical therapy; *SI,* sacroiliac; *SLR,* straight-leg raising; *UMN,* upper motor neuron. (From Mercier LR: *Practical orthopedics,* ed 2, St Louis, 2000, Mosby.)

LYMPHADENOPATHY, GENERALIZED

ICD-9CM # 785.6 Lymphadenopathy, unknown etiology
ICD-10CM # I88.9 Lymphadenitis
R59.9 Enlarged lymph nodes

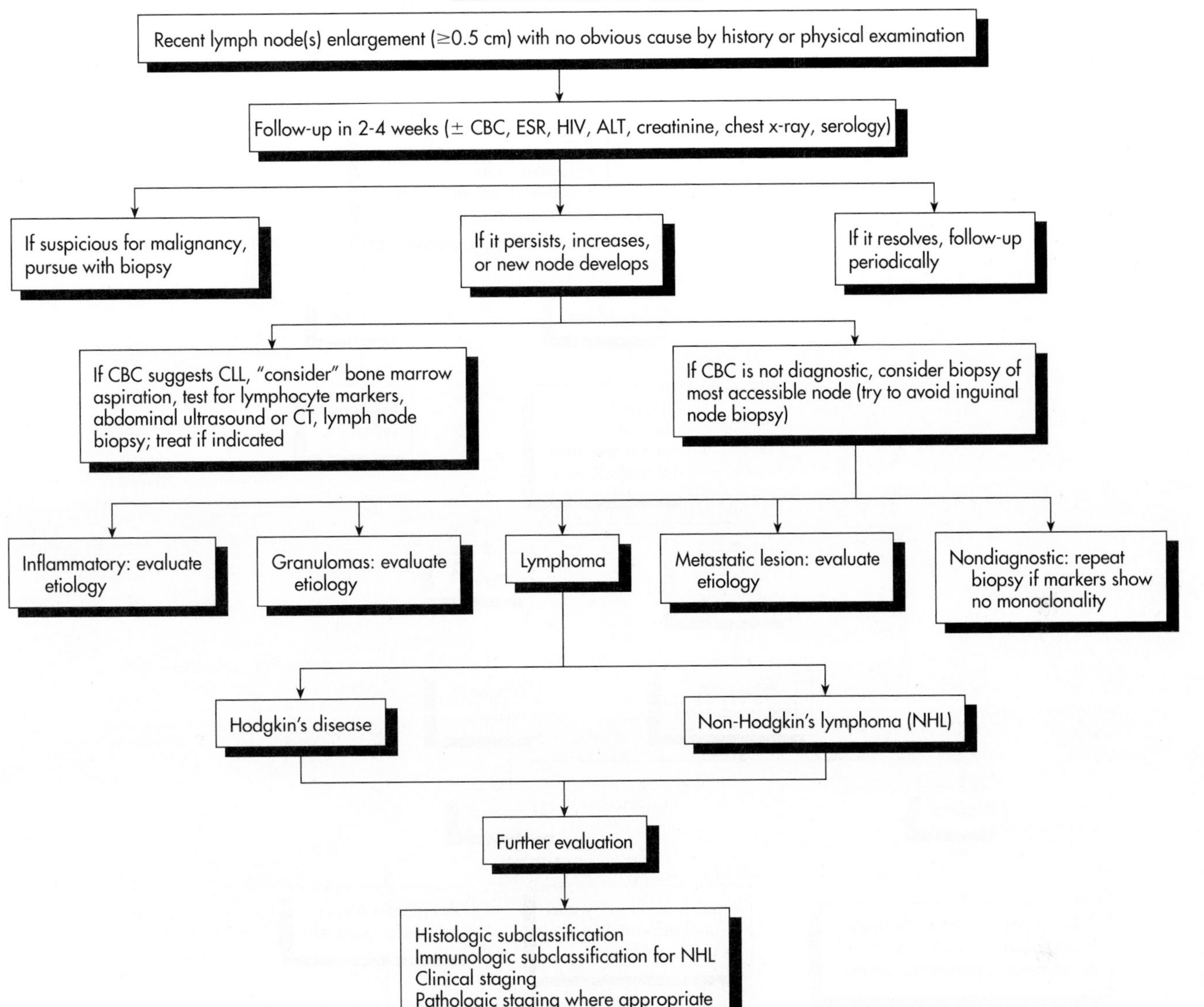

FIGURE 3-115 Workup of lymphadenopathy. *ALT,* Alanine aminotransferase; *CBC,* complete blood count; *CLL,* chronic lymphocytic leukemia; *CT,* computed tomography; *ESR,* erythrocyte sedimentation rate. (Modified from Noble J [ed]: *Primary care medicine*, ed 3, St Louis, 2001, Mosby.)

ICD-9CM # 579.9
ICD-10CM # K90.89 Other intestinal malabsorption

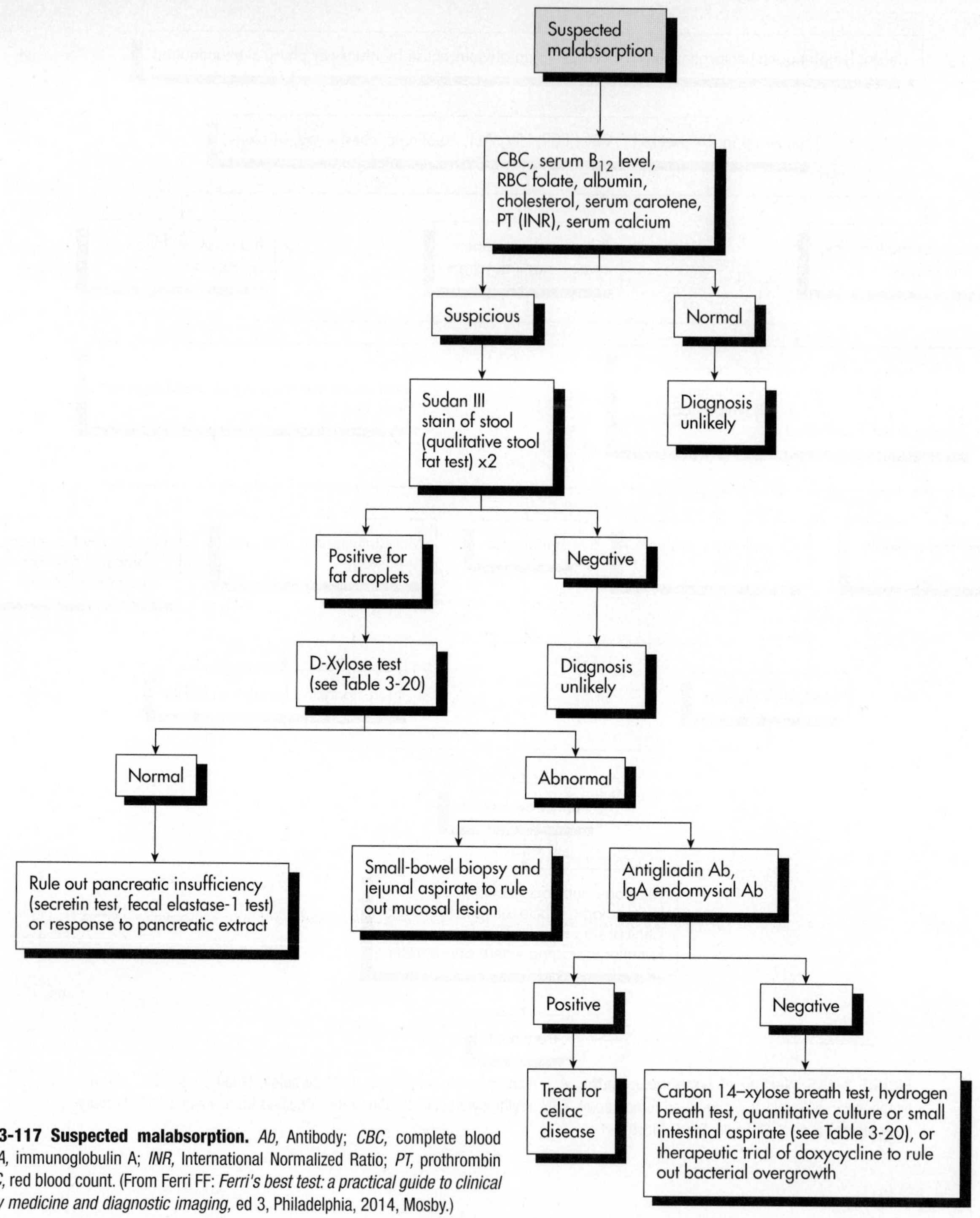

FIGURE 3-117 Suspected malabsorption. *Ab,* Antibody; *CBC,* complete blood count; *IgA,* immunoglobulin A; *INR,* International Normalized Ratio; *PT,* prothrombin time; *RBC,* red blood count. (From Ferri FF: *Ferri's best test: a practical guide to clinical laboratory medicine and diagnostic imaging,* ed 3, Philadelphia, 2014, Mosby.)

BOX 3-3 Malabsorption, Suspected

Diagnostic Imaging
Best Test
Small-bowel series
Ancillary Test
CT of pancreas with IV contrast

Lab Evaluation
Best Test
Biopsy of small bowel

Ancillary Tests
Albumin, total protein
ALT, AST, PT
Serum lytes, BUN, creatinine
Sudan III stain of stool for fecal leukocytes
CBC, RBC folate, serum iron, serum carotene, cholesterol, serum calcium
Hydrogen 14-C xylose breath test
D-Xylose test, secretin test
Quantitative fecal test
Antigliadin antibody, IgA endomysial antibody

From Ferri FF: *Ferri's best test: a practical guide to clinical laboratory medicine and diagnostic imaging,* ed 3, Philadelphia, 2014, Elsevier Mosby.
ALT, Alanine aminotransferase; AST, aspartate aminotransferase; BUN, blood urea nitrogen; CBC, complete blood count; CT, computed tomography; IgA, immunoglobulin A; IV, intravenous; PT, prothrombin time; RBC, red blood count.

TABLE 3-20 Tests for the Evaluation of Malabsorption*

Test	Comments
General Tests of Absorption	
Quantitative stool fat test	Gold standard test of fat malabsorption, with which all other tests are compared. Requires ingestion of a high-fat diet (100 g) for 2 days before and during the collection. Stool is collected for 3 days. Normally, <7 g/24 hr is excreted on a high-fat diet. Borderline abnormalities of 8-14 g/24 hr may be seen in secretory or osmotic diarrheas that are not caused by malabsorption. There are false-negative findings if fat intake is inadequate. False-positive results can occur if mineral oil laxatives or rectal suppositories (e.g., cocoa butter) are given to the patient before stool collection.
Qualitative stool fat test	Sudan stain of a stool sample for fat. Many fat droplets per medium-power field (×40) constitute a positive test result. The nuclear magnetic resonance method determines the percentage of fat in the stool (normal, <20%). The test depends on an adequate fat intake (100 g/day). There is high sensitivity (90%) and specificity (90%) with fat malabsorption of >10 g/24 hr. Sensitivity drops with stool fat in the range of 6-10 g/24 hr.
D-Xylose test	A test of small intestinal mucosal absorption, used to distinguish mucosal malabsorption from malabsorption due to pancreatic insufficiency. An oral dose of D-xylose (24 g/500 ml water) is administered, and D-xylose excretion is measured in a 5-hr urine collection. Normally, >4 g of D-xylose is excreted in the urine over 5 hr. The test also may be positive in bacterial overgrowth owing to metabolism of D-xylose by bacteria in the intestinal lumen. False-positive test results occur with renal failure, ascites, and an incomplete urine collection. Blood levels at 1 and 3 hr improve sensitivity. May be normal with mild or limited mucosal disease.
Hydrogen breath test	Most useful in the diagnosis of lactase deficiency. An oral dose of lactose (1 g/kg body weight) is administered after measurement of basal breath H_2 levels. The sole source of H_2 in the mammal is bacterial fermentation; unabsorbed lactose makes its way to colonic bacteria, resulting in excess breath H_2. A *late peak* (within 3-6 hr) of >20 ppm of exhaled H_2 after lactose ingestion suggests lactose malabsorption. Absorption of other carbohydrates (e.g., sucrose, glucose, fructose) also can be tested.
Specific Tests for Malabsorption	
TESTS FOR PANCREATIC FUNCTION	
Secretin stimulation test	The gold standard test of pancreatic function. Requires duodenal test intubation with a double-lumen tube and collection of pancreatic juice in response to IV secretin. Allows measurement of bicarbonate (HCO_3–) and pancreatic enzymes. A sensitive test of pancreatic function, but labor intensive and invasive.
Fecal elastase-1 test	Stool test for pancreatic function. Equal sensitivity to the secretin stimulation test for the diagnosis of moderate-to-severe pancreatic insufficiency. More specific than the fecal chymotrypsin test. Unreliable with mild insufficiency. False-positive results occur with increased stool volume and intestinal mucosal diseases.
TESTS FOR BACTERIAL OVERGROWTH	
Quantitative culture of small intestinal aspirate	Gold standard test for bacterial overgrowth. Greater than 10^5 colony-forming units (CFU)/ml in the jejunum suggests bacterial overgrowth. Requires special anaerobic sample collection, rapid anaerobic and aerobic plating, and care to avoid oropharyngeal contamination. False-negative results occur with focal jejunal diverticula and when overgrowth is distal to the site aspirated.
Hydrogen breath test	The 50-g glucose breath test has a sensitivity of 90% for growth of 10^5 colonic-type bacteria in the small intestine. If bacterial overgrowth is present, increased H_2 is excreted in the breath. A hydrogen level (within 2 hr) of >20 ppm suggests bacterial overgrowth. False-negative results occur with non-hydrogen-producing organisms.
^{14}C-D-xylose breath test	This test uses 1 g of carbon 14–labeled D-xylose. It has a sensitivity and specificity >90% for growth of 10^5 test colonic-type bacteria in the small intestine. Bacteria metabolize D-xylose with release of $^{14}CO_2$, which is absorbed and exhaled. Non-degraded D-xylose is absorbed in the small bowel and does not reach the colon, yielding a greater specificity than the lactulose H_2 breath test. A nonradioactive ^{13}C-D-xylose breath test is suitable for children and pregnant women.
TESTS FOR MUCOSAL DISEASE	
Small bowel biopsy	Obtained for a specific diagnosis when there is a high index of suspicion for small intestinal disease. Several biopsy specimens (4-5) must be obtained to maximize the diagnostic yield. Distal duodenal biopsy specimens are usually adequate for diagnosis, but occasionally enteroscopy with jejunal biopsy specimens is necessary. Small intestinal biopsy provides a specific diagnosis in some diseases (e.g., intestinal infection, Whipple's disease, abetalipoproteinemia, agammaglobulinemia, lymphangiectasia, lymphoma, amyloidosis). In other conditions, such as celiac disease and tropical sprue, the biopsy specimens show characteristic findings, but the diagnosis is made on improvement after treatment.
TESTS OF ILEAL FUNCTION	
Schilling test	A test of vitamin B_{12} absorption
^{75}SeHCAT test	This is a test of bile acid absorption. Seven days after ingestion of radiolabeled synthetic selenium-homocholic acid conjugated with taurine (^{75}SeHCAT), whole body retention is measured by a gamma-counting device. The result is expressed as a fraction of baseline ingestion. Retention values of less than 10% are abnormal and indicate bile acid malabsorption with a sensitivity of 80-90% and specificity of 70%-100%. The radiation dose is equivalent to a plain chest x-ray. Liver disease and bacterial overgrowth may give false results. Not approved for use in the United States.

From Goldman L, Schafer AI: *Goldman's Cecil Medicine*, ed 24, Philadelphia, 2012, Saunders.

*Not all these tests are readily available. A strong suspicion for any disease may warrant foregoing an extensive work-up and obtaining the test with highest diagnostic yield. In some cases, empirical treatment, such as removing lactose from the diet of an otherwise healthy individual with lactose intolerance, is warranted without any testing.

ICD-9CM # 782.1
ICD-10CM # R21 Rash and other nonspecific skin eruption

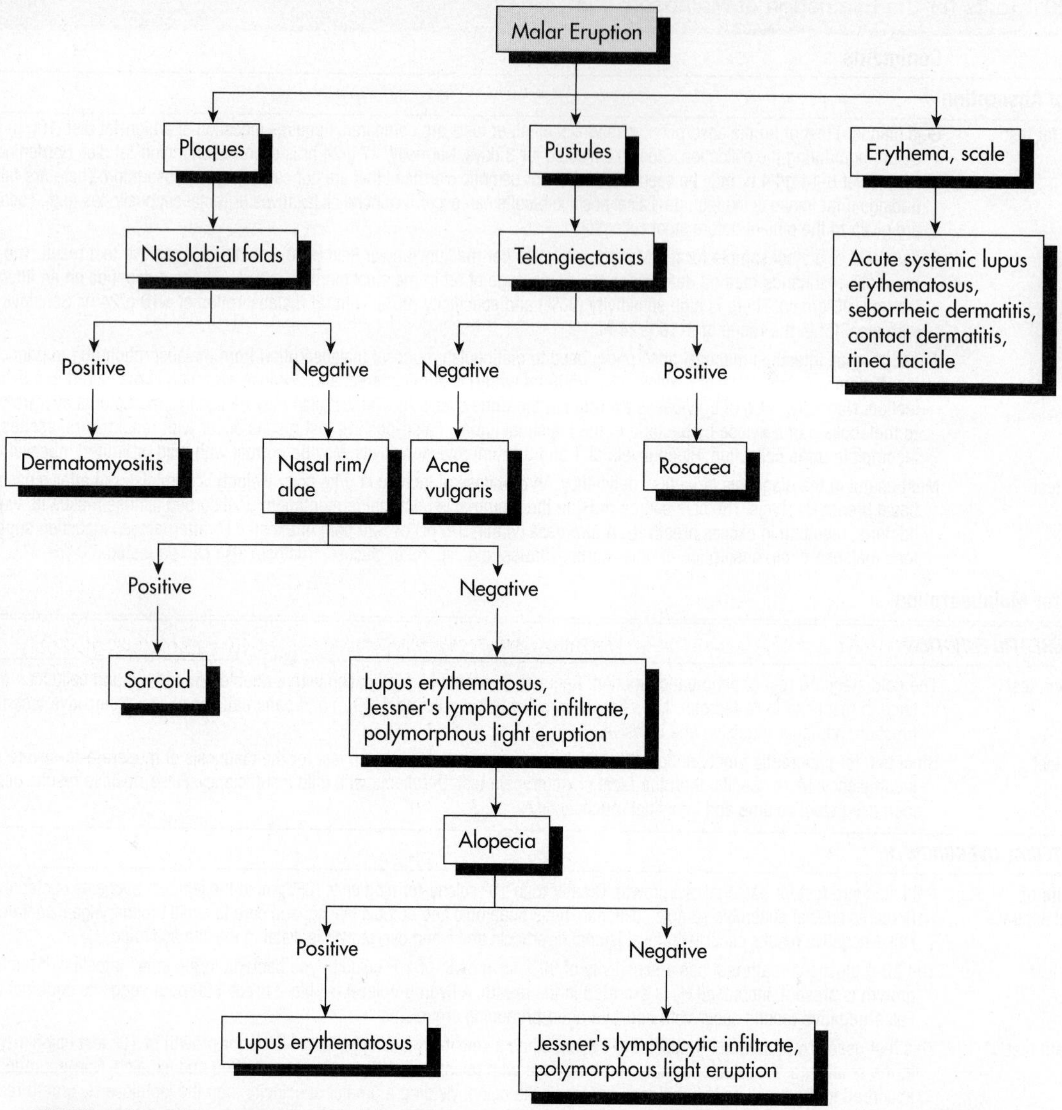

Malar Eruption
- Plaques
  - Nasolabial folds
    - Positive → Dermatomyositis
    - Negative → Nasal rim/alae
      - Positive → Sarcoid
      - Negative → Lupus erythematosus, Jessner's lymphocytic infiltrate, polymorphous light eruption
        - Alopecia
          - Positive → Lupus erythematosus
          - Negative → Jessner's lymphocytic infiltrate, polymorphous light eruption
- Pustules
  - Telangiectasias
    - Negative → Acne vulgaris
    - Positive → Rosacea
- Erythema, scale
  - Acute systemic lupus erythematosus, seborrheic dermatitis, contact dermatitis, tinea faciale

FIGURE 3-118 Clinical algorithm for diagnosis of a malar eruption, which must be confirmed by appropriate cultures, serology, and biopsy. (From Harris ED et al [eds]: *Kelley's textbook of rheumatology*, ed 7, Philadelphia, 2005, Saunders.)

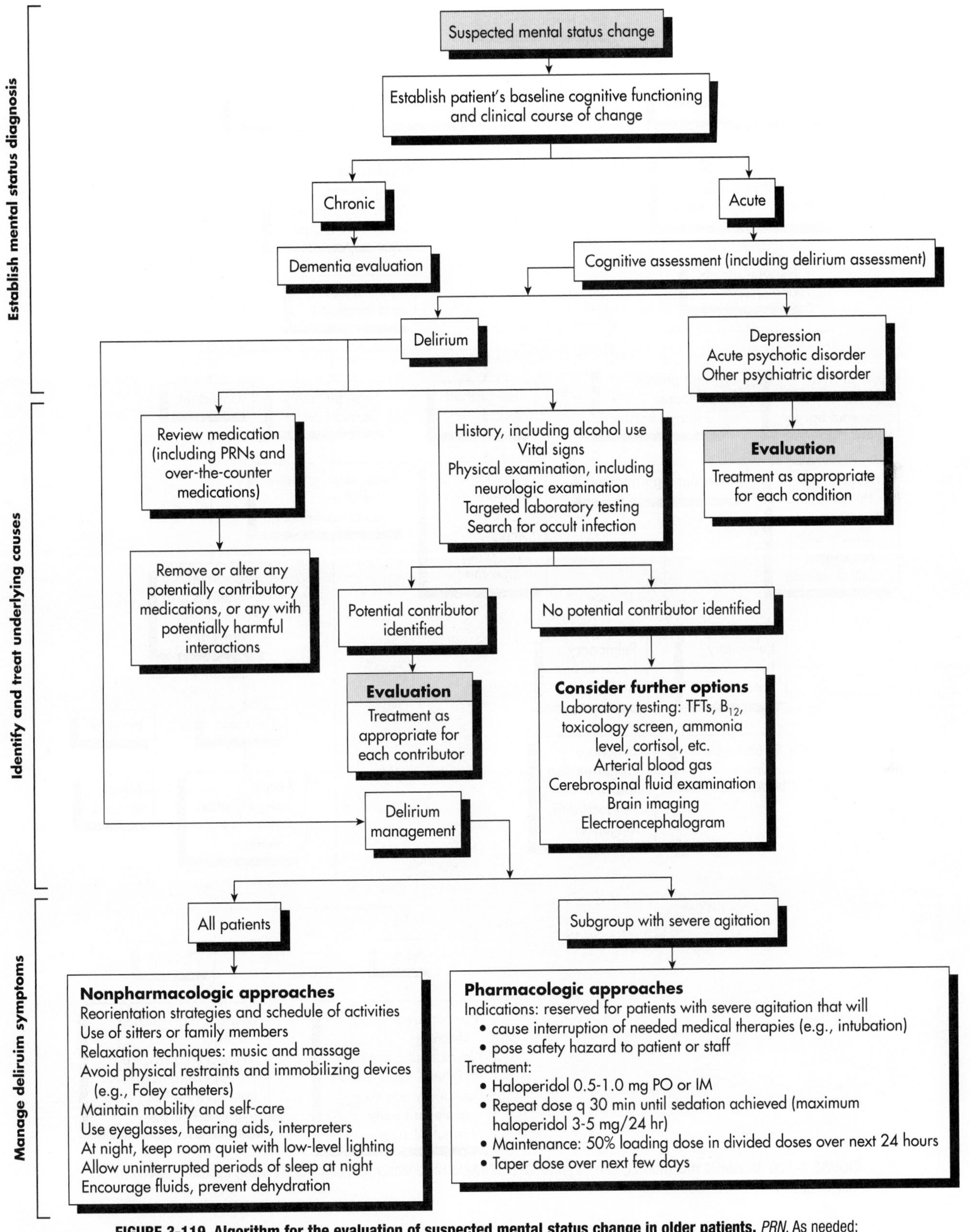

FIGURE 3-119 Algorithm for the evaluation of suspected mental status change in older patients. *PRN,* As needed; *TFTs,* thyroid function tests. (From Goldman L, Schafer AI: *Goldman's Cecil medicine,* ed 24, Philadelphia, 2012, Saunders.)

ICD-9CM # 785.2 Murmur, heart
ICD-10CM # R01.1 Cardiac murmur, unspecified

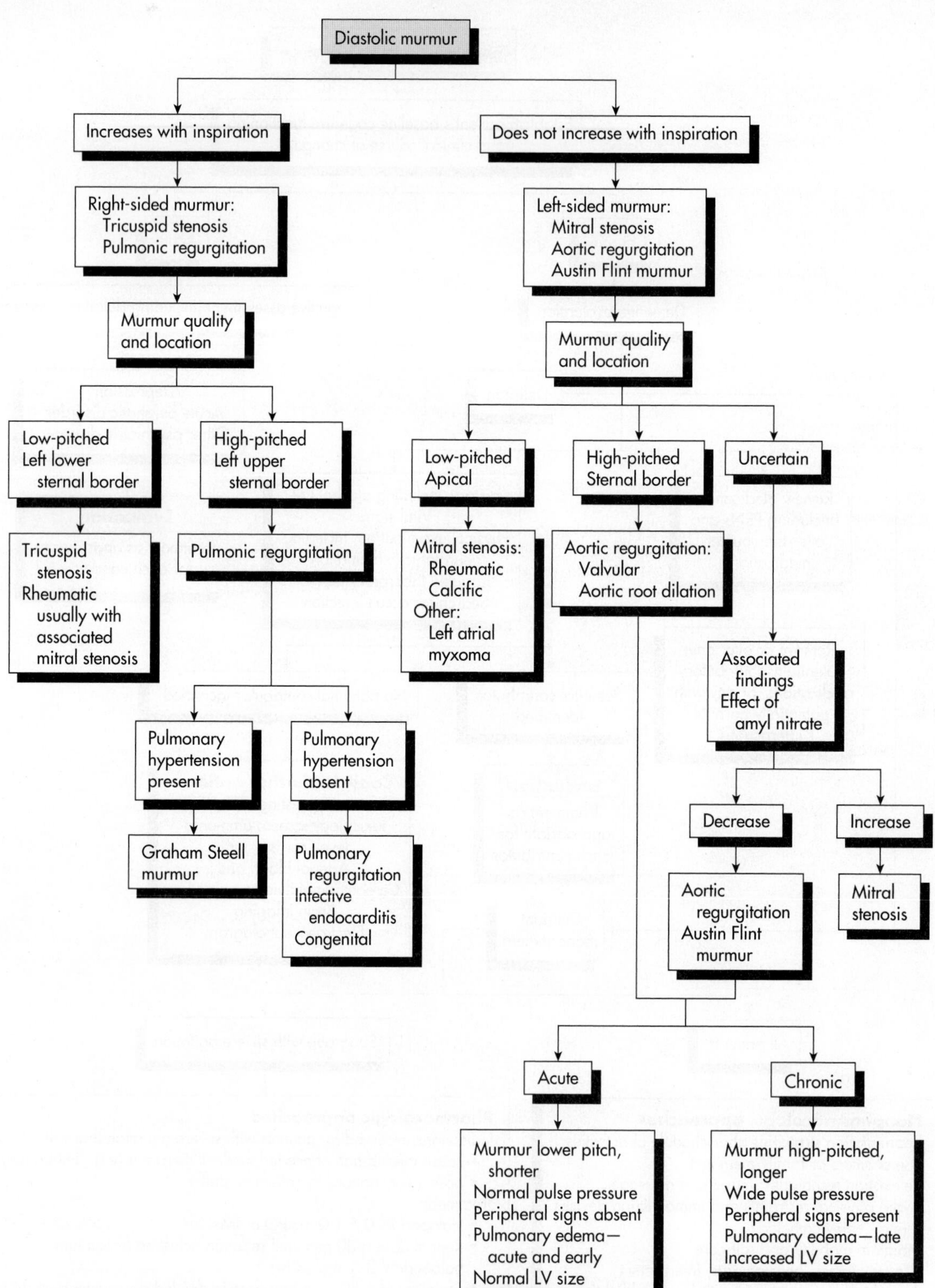

FIGURE 3-120 Diastolic murmur. *LV,* Left ventricle. (From Greene HL, Johnson WP, Lemcke DL [eds]: *Decision making in medicine,* ed 2, St Louis, 1998, Mosby.)

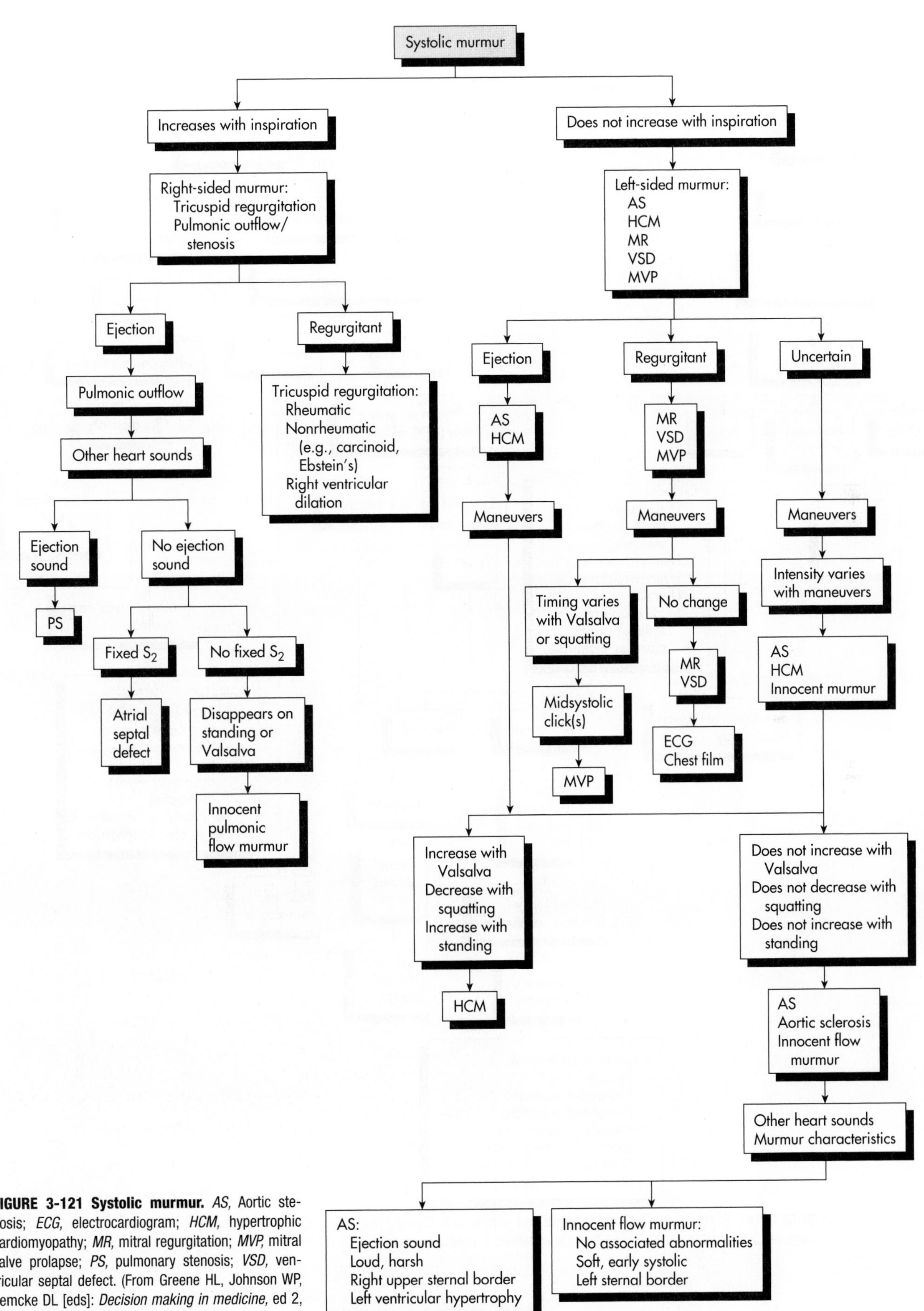

FIGURE 3-121 Systolic murmur. *AS,* Aortic stenosis; *ECG,* electrocardiogram; *HCM,* hypertrophic cardiomyopathy; *MR,* mitral regurgitation; *MVP,* mitral valve prolapse; *PS,* pulmonary stenosis; *VSD,* ventricular septal defect. (From Greene HL, Johnson WP, Lemcke DL [eds]: *Decision making in medicine,* ed 2, St Louis, 1998, Mosby.)

ICD-9CM # 729.82
ICD-10CM # R25.2 Cramp and spasm

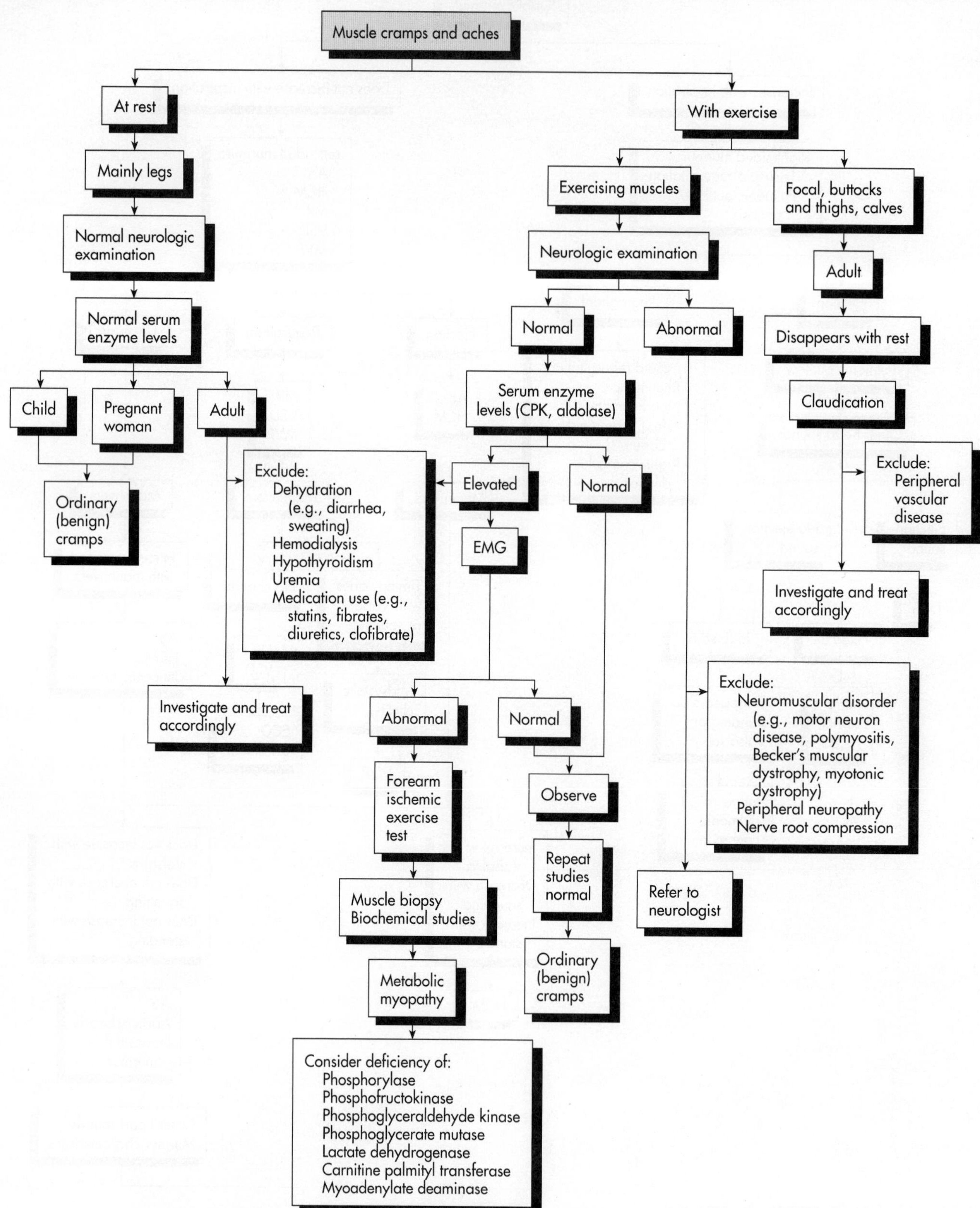

FIGURE 3-122 Evaluation of muscle cramps and aches. *CPK,* Creatine phosphokinase; *EMG,* electromyography. (From Greene HL, Johnson WP, Lemcke D [eds]: *Decision making in medicine,* ed 2, St Louis, 1998, Mosby.)

MUSCLE WEAKNESS

ICD-9CM # 728.9
ICD-10CM # M62.9 Disorder of muscle, unspecified

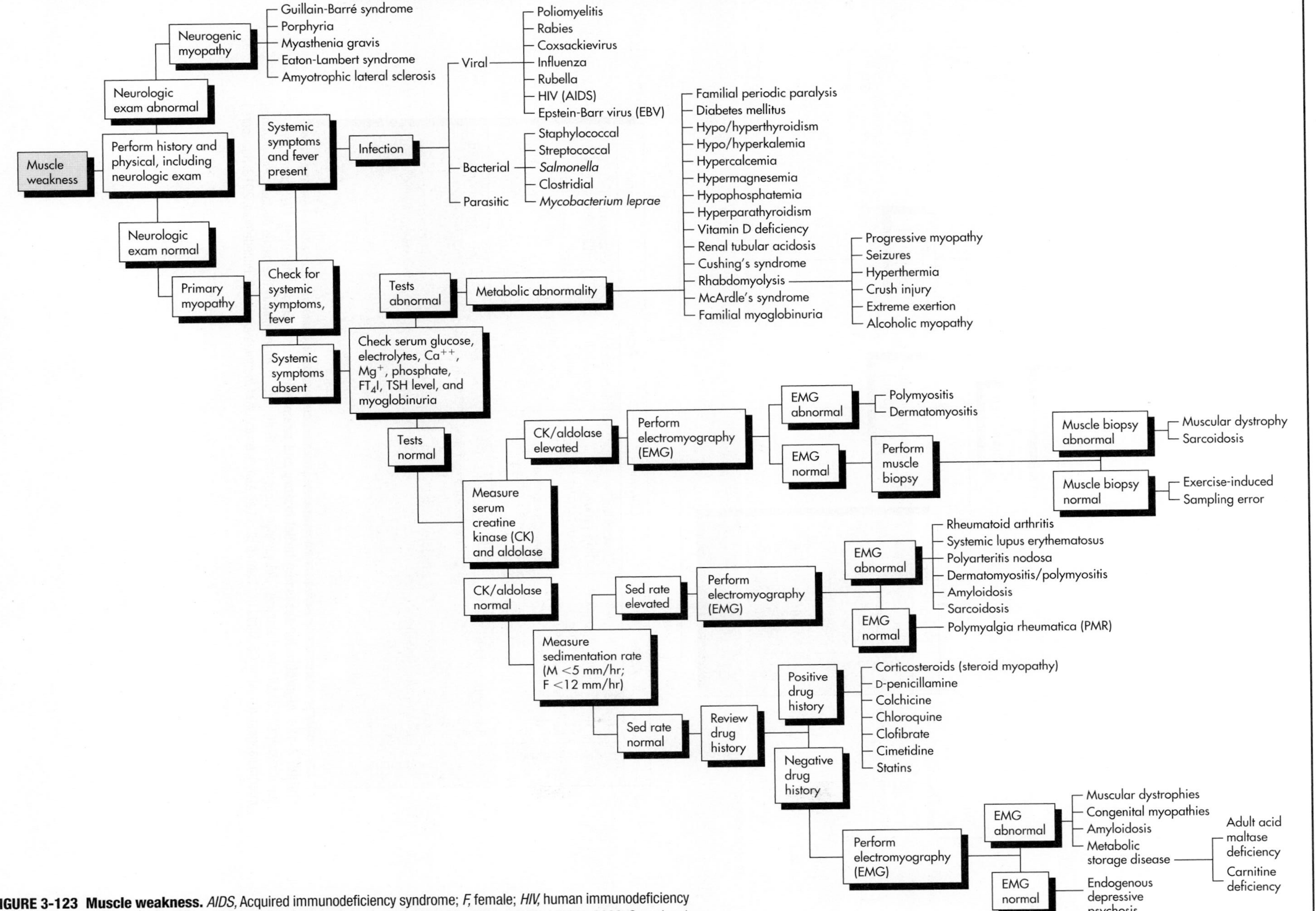

FIGURE 3-123 Muscle weakness. *AIDS,* Acquired immunodeficiency syndrome; *F,* female; *HIV,* human immunodeficiency virus; *M,* male. (From Healey PM: *Common medical diagnosis: an algorithmic approach,* ed 3, Philadelphia, 2000, Saunders.)

ICD-9CM # 719.40
ICD-10CM # M25.50 -Pain(s) joint
-Arthralgia (allergic)
-Arthrodynia
-Polyarthralgia

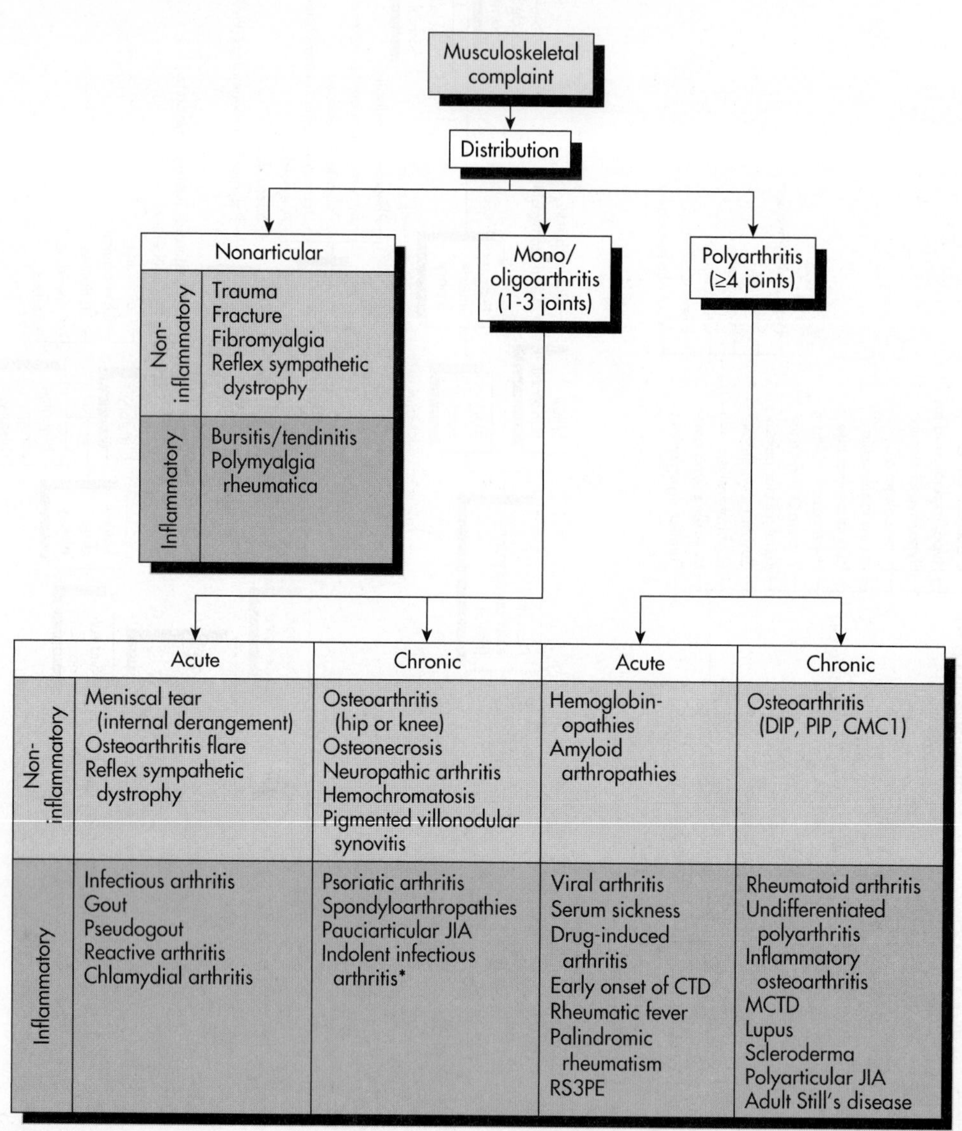

FIGURE 3-124 Algorithm for assessing initial history and examination. *CMC*, carpometacarpal; *CTD*, connective tissue disease; *DIP*, distal interphalangeal; *JIA*, juvenile idiopathic arthritis; *MCTD*, mixed connective tissue disease; *PIP*, proximal interphalangeal. (Firestein GS, Budd RC, Gabriel SE, et al: *Kelly's textbook of rheumatology*, ed 9, Philadelphia, 2013, Saunders.)

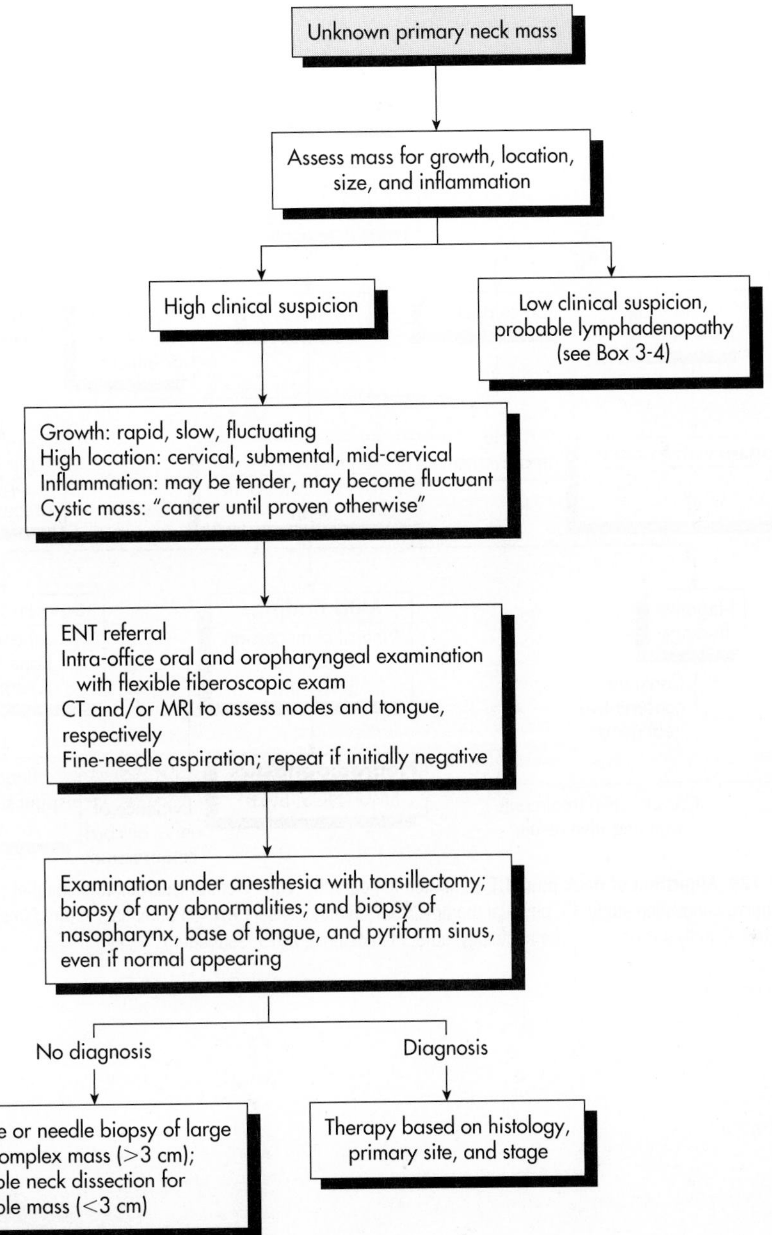

FIGURE 3-128 Evaluation of an unknown primary neck mass. *CT,* Computed tomography; *ENT,* ear, nose, and throat; *MRI,* magnetic resonance imaging. (From Goldman L, Schafer AL [eds]: *Cecil textbook of medicine,* ed 24, Philadelphia, 2012, Saunders.)

BOX 3-4 An Approach to the Patient with Lymphadenopathy

1. Does the patient have a known illness that causes lymphadenopathy? Treat and monitor for resolution.
2. Is there an obvious infection to explain the lymphadenopathy (e.g., infectious mononucleosis)? Treat and monitor for resolution.
3. Are the nodes very large and/or very firm and thus suggestive of malignancy? Perform a biopsy.
4. Is the patient very concerned about malignancy and unable to be reassured that malignancy is unlikely? Perform a biopsy.
5. If none of the preceding are true, perform a complete blood cell count and if it is unrevealing, monitor for a predetermined period (usually 2 to 6 weeks). If the nodes do not regress or if they increase in size, perform a biopsy.

From Goldman L, Ausiello D (eds): *Cecil textbook of medicine,* ed 23, Philadelphia, 2008, Saunders.

ICD-9CM #	723.1	Neck Pain (Nondiscogenic)
	959.09	Neck Injury
ICD-10CM #	M54.2	Cervicalgia
	S19.9XXA	Unspecified injury of neck, initial encounter

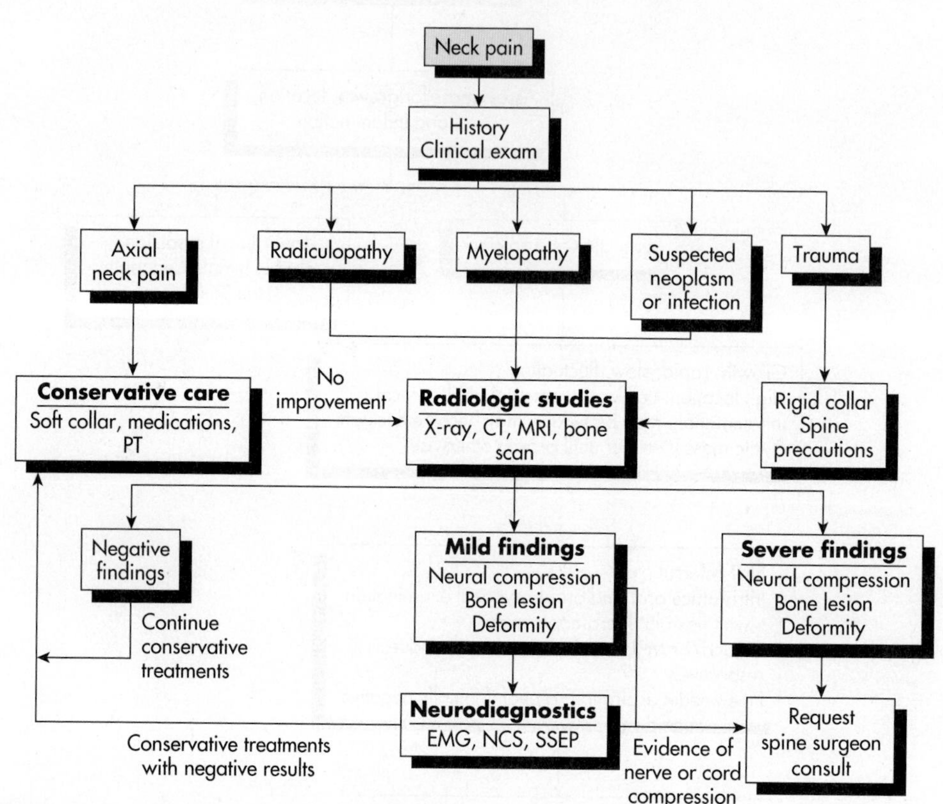

FIGURE 3-129 Algorithm of neck pain. CT, computed tomography; EMG, electromyogram; MRI, magnetic resonance imaging; NCS, nerve conduction study; PT, physical therapy; SSEP, somatosensory evoked potentials. (From Firestein GS, Budd RC, Gabriel SE, et al: Kelly's textbook of rheumatology, ed 9, Philadelphia, 2013, Saunders.)

NYSTAGMUS

ICD-9CM # 379.50 Nystagmus NOS
386.11 Benign Positional
386.2 Central Positional
379.59 Congenital
ICD-10CM # H55.00 Unspecified nystagmus
H81.13 Benign paroxysmal vertigo, bilateral
H81.49 Vertigo of central origin, unspecified ear
H55.89 Other irregular eye movements

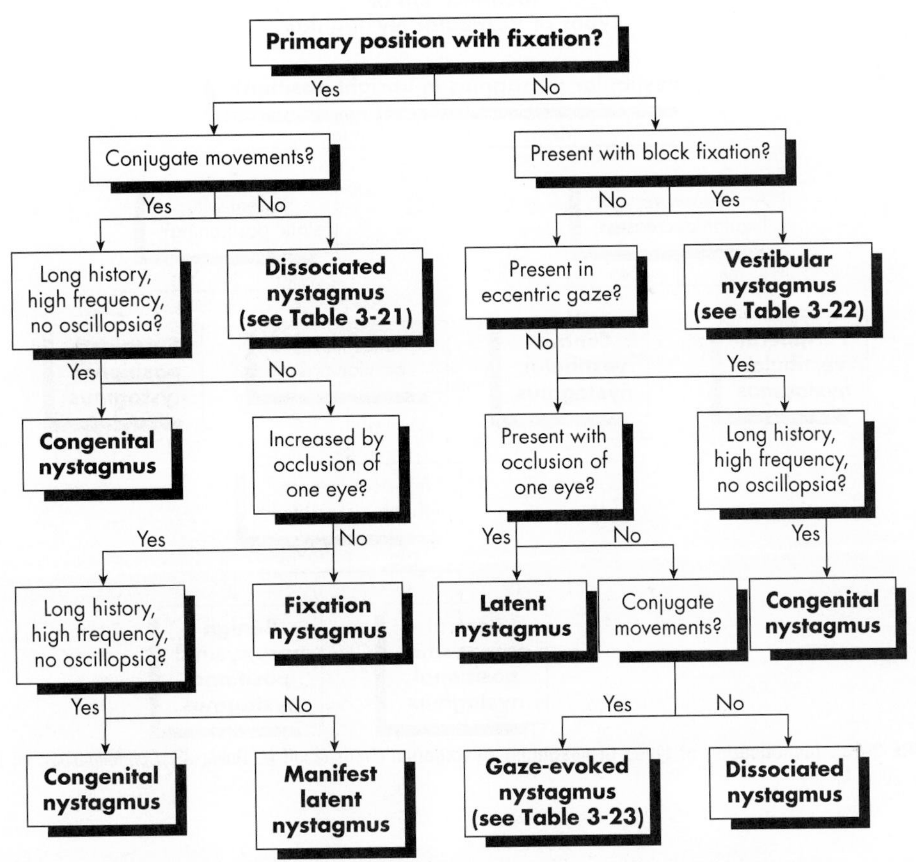

FIGURE 3-132 Identification of types of nystagmus. (From Yanoff M, Duker JS: *Ophthalmology,* ed 2, St Louis, 2004, Mosby.)

TABLE 3-21 Characteristics and Localizations of Dissociated Nystagmus

Nystagmus	Characteristics	Localization
Acquired pendular in adults	Pendular, horizontal, vertical, torsional, disconjugate (coexisting palatal myoclonus)	Brain stem, cerebellum
Superior oblique myokymia	Pendular, jerk, torsional, vertical, high frequency, small amplitude, monocular	Trochlear nucleus
See-saw	Pendular, vertical, torsional, rising eye intorts, falling eye extorts; rarely jerk	Midbrain (interstitial nucleus of Cajal)
Abducting "nystagmus" of internuclear ophthalmoplegia	Jerk, horizontal, decreasing velocity slow components, larger in abducting eye	Medial longitudinal fasciculus in pons, midbrain horizontal gaze
Abducting nystagmus of myasthenia gravis	Gaze-paretic nystagmus in horizontal gaze, greater paresis of medial rectus muscle	Myoneural junction—myasthenia gravis

From Yanoff M, Duker JS: *Ophthalmology,* ed 2, St Louis, 2004, Mosby.

ICD-9CM #	379.50	Nystagmus NOS
	386.11	Benign Positional
	386.2	Central Positional
	379.59	Congenital
ICD-10CM #	H55.00	Unspecified nystagmus
	H81.13	Benign paroxysmal vertigo, bilateral
	H81.49	Vertigo of central origin, unspecified ear
	H55.89	Other irregular eye movements

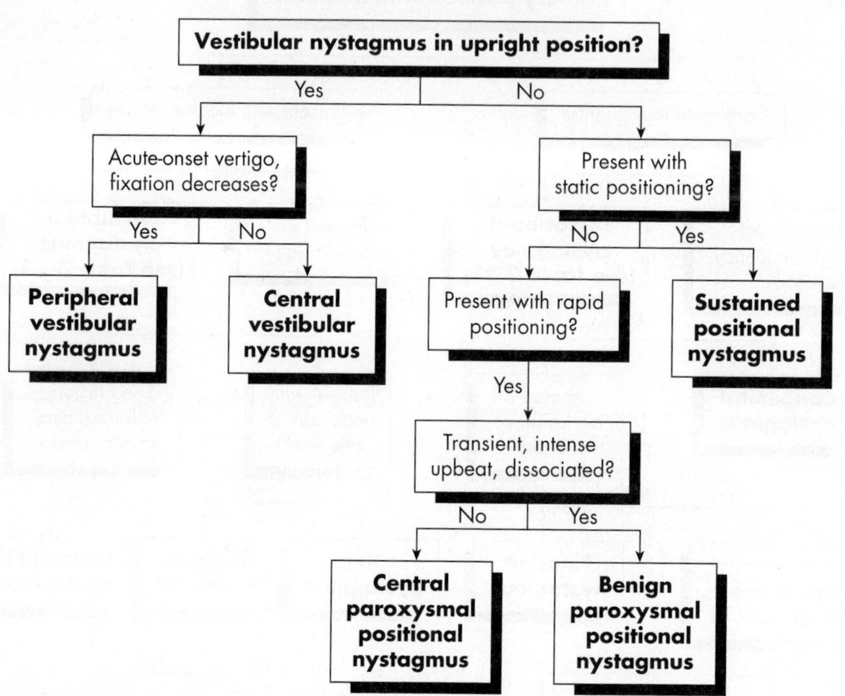

FIGURE 3-133 Identification of types of vestibular nystagmus. (From Yanoff M, Duker JS: *Ophthalmology,* ed 2, St Louis, 2004, Mosby.)

TABLE 3-22 Characteristics and Localizations of Vestibular Nystagmus

Nystagmus	Characteristics	Localization
Spontaneous peripheral vestibular	Jerk, horizontal, small torsional, inhibited by fixation	Labyrinth, eighth nerve (acute)
Central vestibular (fixation) nystagmus	Jerk, pendular, horizontal, vertical, torsional, not inhibited by fixation	Brain stem, cerebellum
Sustained positional vestibular	Jerk, horizontal, small torsional, direction fixed, direction changing (static positioning)	Labyrinth, eighth nerve or brain stem, cerebellum
Benign paroxysmal positional	Jerk, dissociated upbeat, latency, not inhibited by fixation, fatigue (Nylen–Barany maneuver)	Posterior vertical canal
Central paroxysmal positional	Jerk, symmetric, upbeat, downbeat	Brain stem, cerebellum

From Yanoff M, Duker JS: *Ophthalmology,* ed 2, St Louis, 2004, Mosby.

ICD-9CM # 379.50 Nystagmus NOS
386.11 Benign Positional
386.2 Central Positional
379.59 Congenital
ICD-10CM # H55.00 Unspecified nystagmus
H81.13 Benign paroxysmal vertigo, bilateral
H81.49 Vertigo of central origin, unspecified ear
H55.89 Other irregular eye movements

TABLE 3-23 Characteristics and Localizations of Gaze-Evoked Nystagmus

Nystagmus	Characteristics	Localization
Physiologic, endpoint	Jerk, small amplitude, intermittent, extremes of horizontal and up gaze	Physiologic
Gaze-paretic (symmetric)	Jerk (decreasing velocity slow components) at 30° eccentric gaze	Nonlocalizing (drugs, mental fatigue)
Gaze-paretic (asymmetric)	Jerk (decreasing velocity slow components), horizontal, at 30° eccentric gaze, larger amplitude toward side of lesion	Lesions of brain stem, cerebellum, cerebral hemisphere
Rebound	Jerk, horizontal, decreases and direction can reverse in eccentric gaze, transient jerk nystagmus on return to primary gaze, fast components beating toward eccentric gaze	Cerebellum
Myasthenia gravis	Jerk, horizontal or vertical, gradual onset in prolonged eccentric gaze	Myoneural junction (fatigue—increasing transmission block)

From Yanoff M, Duker JS: *Ophthalmology,* ed 2, St Louis, 2004, Mosby.

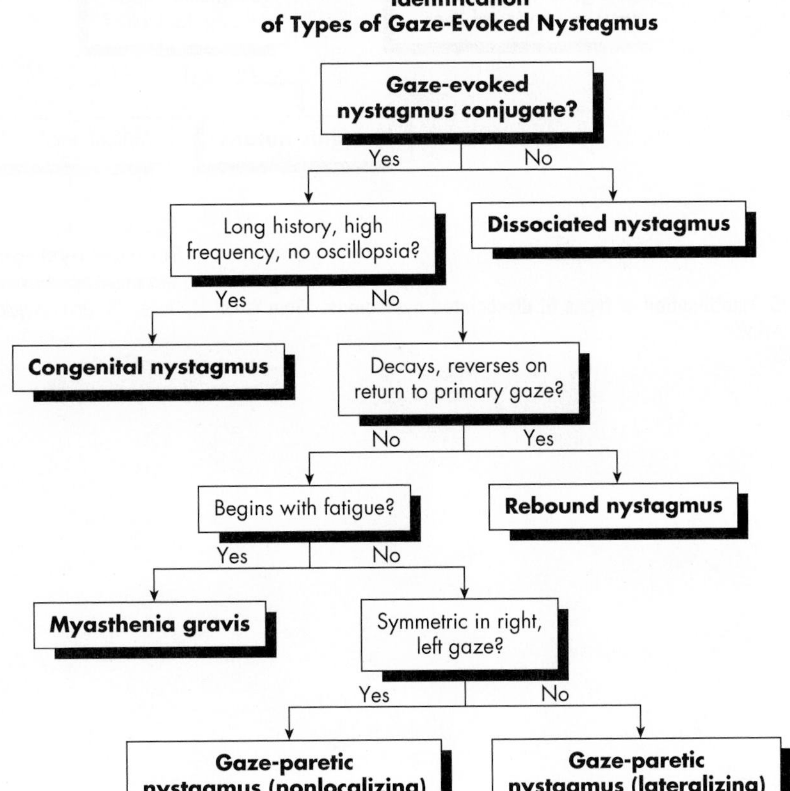

FIGURE 3-134 Identification of types of gaze-evoked nystagmus. (From Yanoff M, Duker JS: *Ophthalmology,* ed 2, St Louis, 2004, Mosby.)

ICD-9CM #	379.50	Nystagmus NOS
	386.11	Benign Positional
	386.2	Central Positional
	379.59	Congenital
ICD-10CM #	H55.00	Unspecified nystagmus
	H81.13	Benign paroxysmal vertigo, bilateral
	H81.49	Vertigo of central origin, unspecified ear
	H55.89	Other irregular eye movements

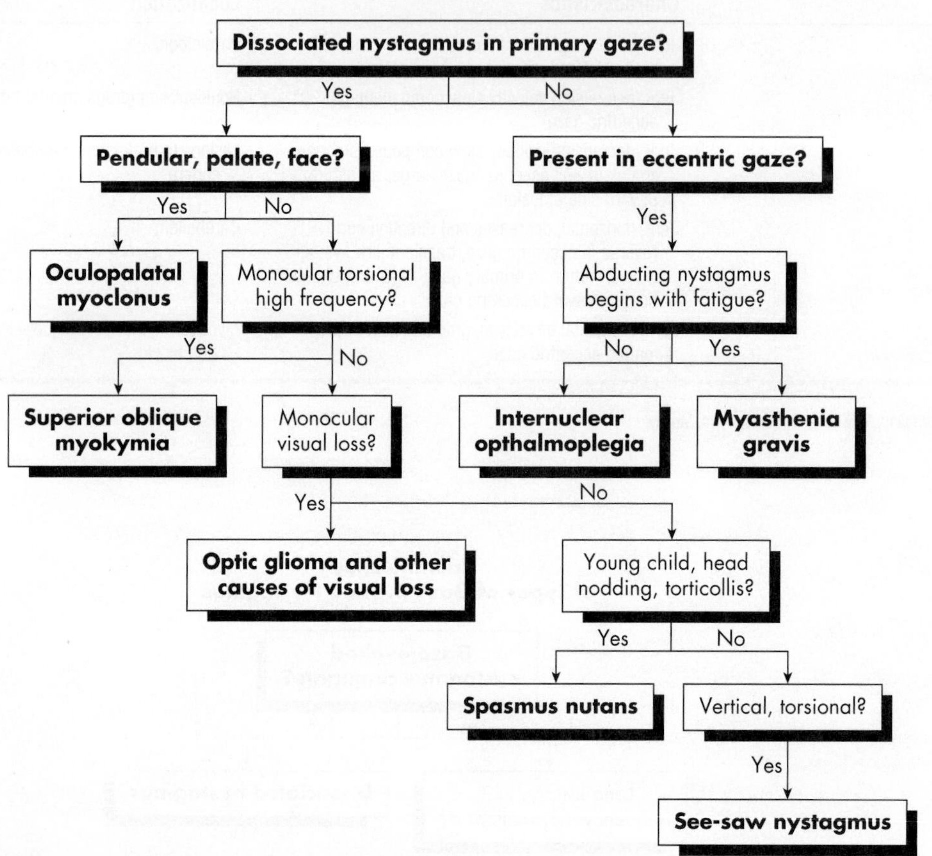

FIGURE 3-135 Identification of types of dissociated nystagmus. (From Yanoff M, Duker JS: *Ophthalmology,* ed 2, St Louis, 2004, Mosby.)

OLIGURIA

ICD-9CM # 788.5
ICD-10CM # R34 Anuria and oliguria

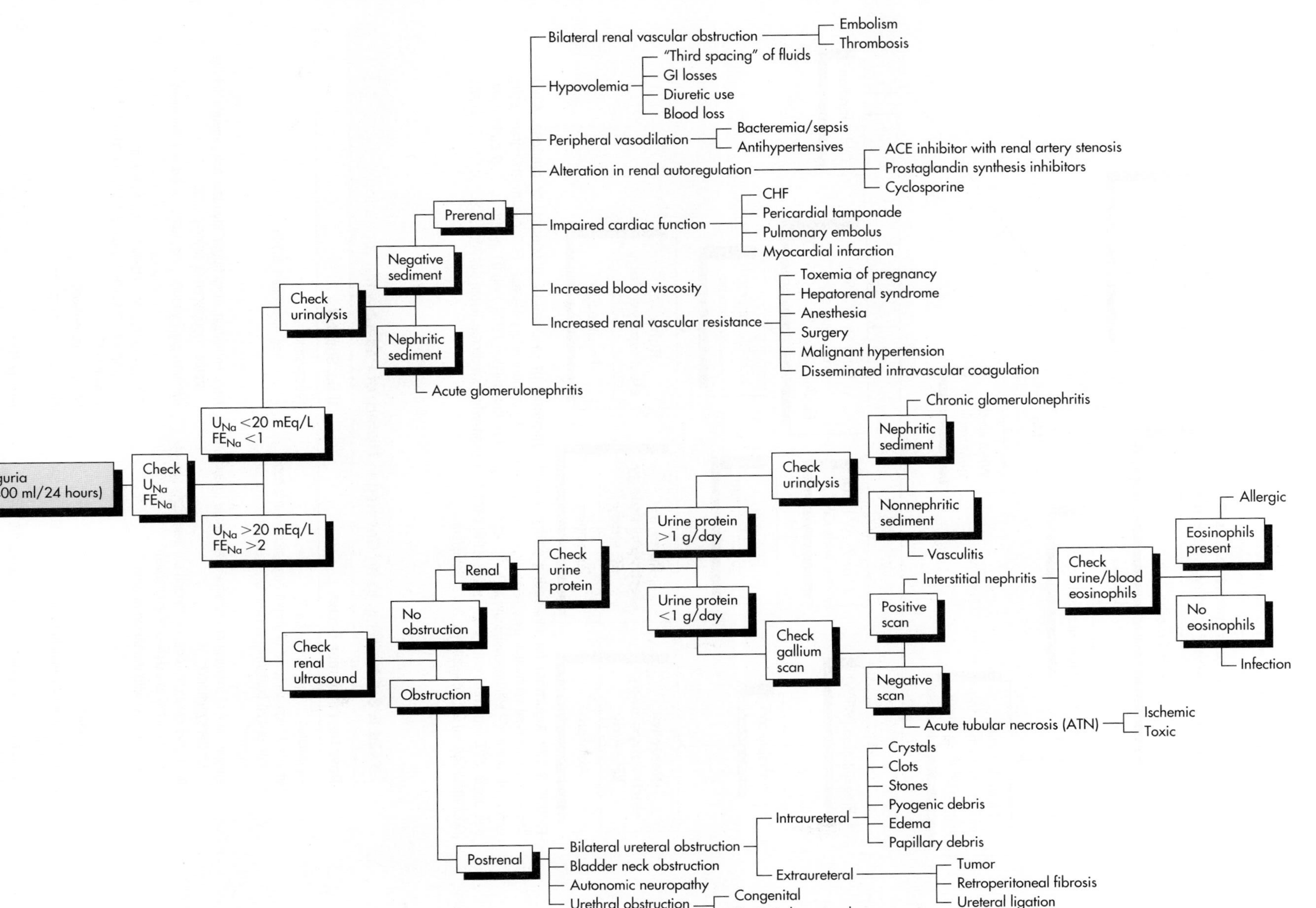

FIGURE 3-136 Evaluation of oliguria. *ACE,* Angiotensin-converting enzyme; *CHF,* congestive heart failure; *GI,* gastrointestinal. (From Healey PM: *Common medical diagnosis: an algorithmic approach,* ed 3, Philadelphia, 2000, Saunders.)

PALPITATIONS, DIZZINESS, AND/OR SYNCOPE

ICD-9CM # 780.4 Dizziness
780.2 Syncope
ICD-10CM # R42 Dizziness and giddiness
R55 Syncope and collapse

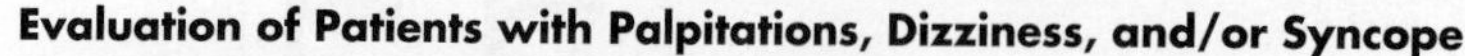

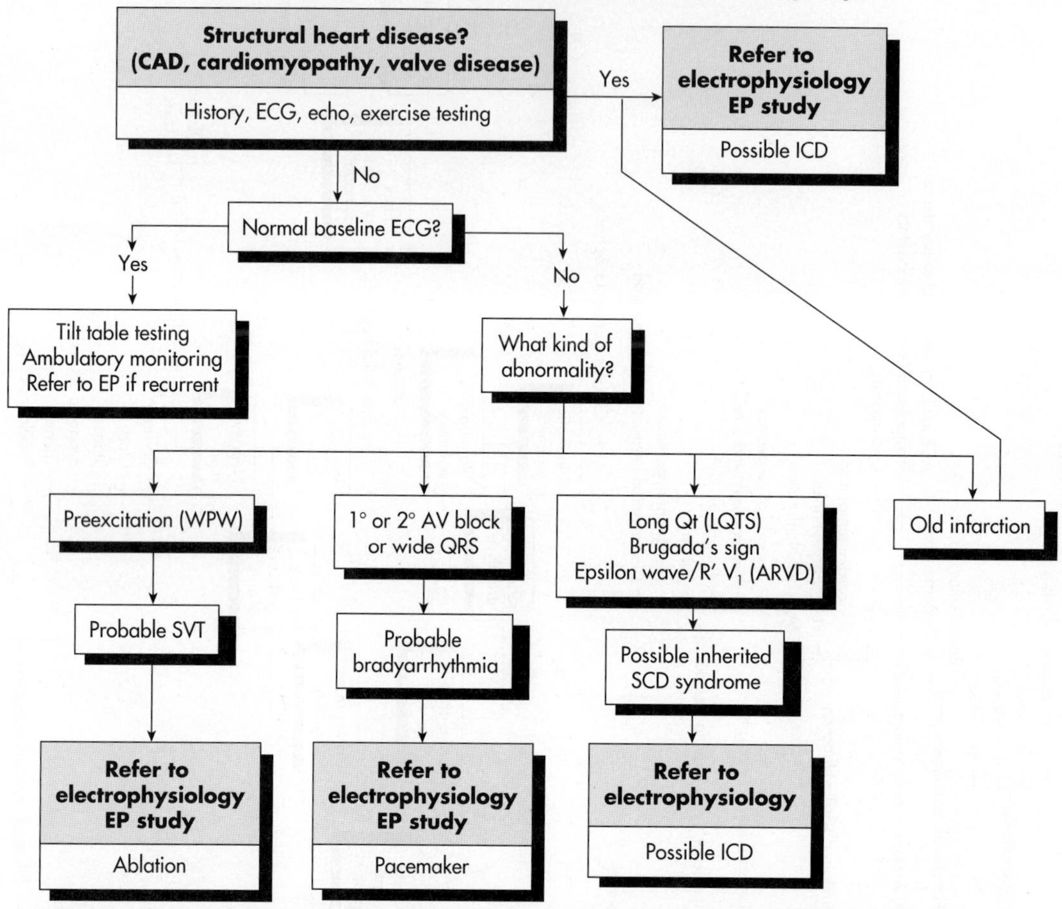

FIGURE 3-138 Algorithm for evaluating patients with symptoms of palpitation, dizziness, or syncope. *ARVD,* Arrhythmogenic right ventricular dysplasia; *AV,* atrioventricular; *CAD,* coronary artery disease; *ECG,* electrocardiogram; *echo,* echocardiogram; *EP,* electrophysiology; *ICD,* implantable cardioverter-defibrillator; *LQTS,* long QT syndrome; *SCD,* sudden cardiac death; *SVT,* supraventricular tachycardia; *WPW,* Wolff-Parkinson-White syndrome. (From Goldman L, Schafer AI: *Goldman's Cecil medicine,* ed 24, Philadelphia, 2012, Saunders.)

TABLE 3-24 Items to be Covered in History of Patient with Palpitation

Does the Palpitation Occur:	If So, Suspect:
As isolated "jumps" or "skips"?	Extrasystoles
In attacks known to be of abrupt beginning, with a heart rate of 120 beats/min or over, with regular or irregular rhythm?	Paroxysmal rapid heart action
Independent of exercise or excitement adequate to account for the symptom?	Atrial fibrillation, atrial flutter, thyrotoxicosis, anemia, febrile states, hypoglycemia, anxiety state
In attacks developing rapidly though not absolutely abruptly, unrelated to exertion or excitement?	Hemorrhage, hypoglycemia, tumor of the adrenal medulla
In conjunction with the taking of drugs?	Tobacco, coffee, tea, alcohol, epinephrine, ephedrine, aminophylline, atropine, thyroid extract, monoamine oxidase inhibitors
On standing?	Postural hypotension
In middle-aged women, in conjunction with flushes and sweats?	Menopausal syndrome
When the rate is known to be normal and the rhythm regular?	Anxiety state

From Goldman L, Braunwald E: Chest discomfort and palpitation. In Isselbacher KJ, Braunwald E et al [eds]: *Harrison's principles of internal medicine,* ed 13, New York, 1994, McGraw-Hill.

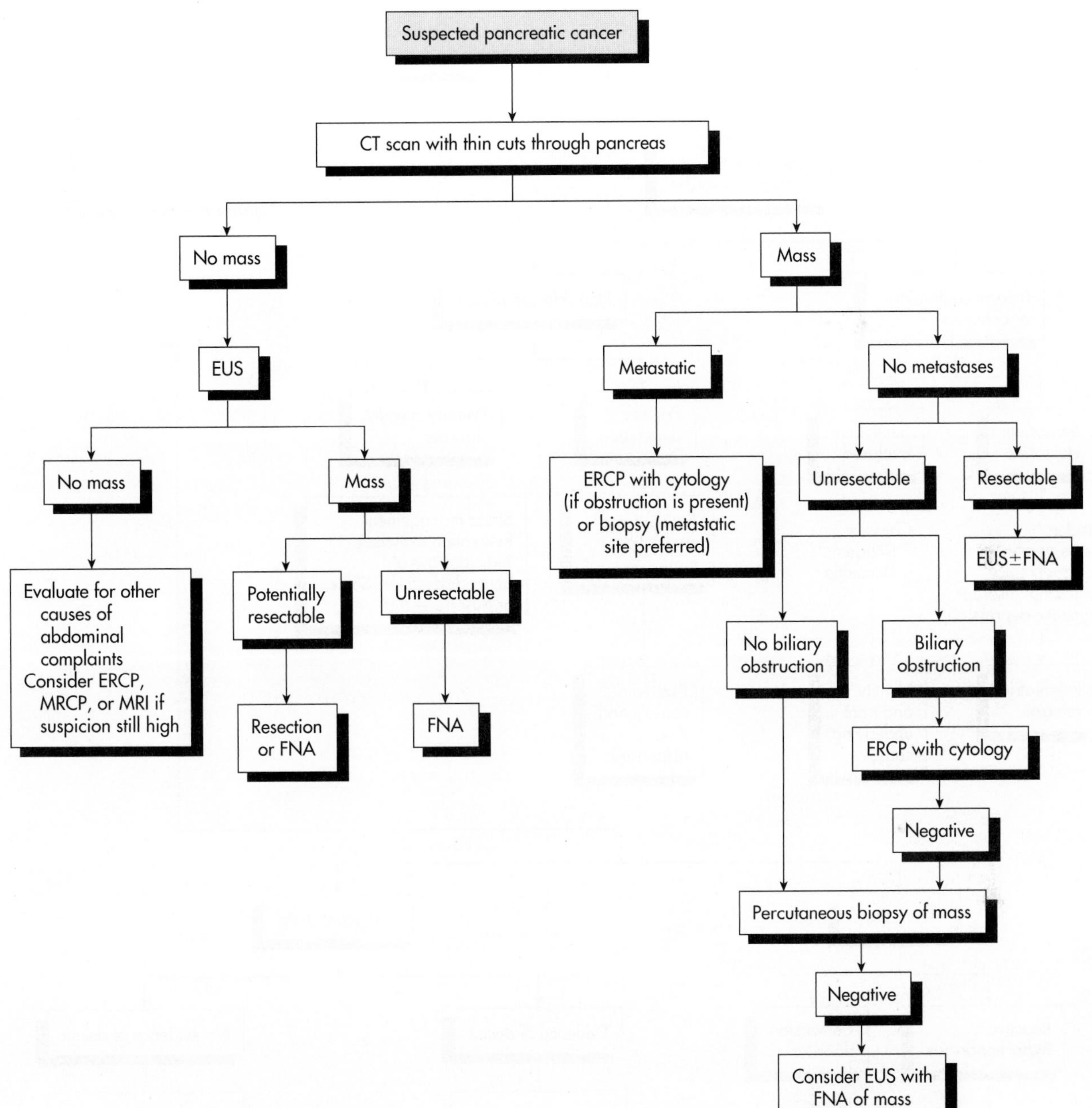
Suspected pancreatic cancer
CT scan with thin cuts through pancreas
No mass
Mass
EUS
Metastatic
No metastases
No mass
Mass
ERCP with cytology (if obstruction is present) or biopsy (metastatic site preferred)
Unresectable
Resectable
EUS±FNA
Evaluate for other causes of abdominal complaints
Consider ERCP, MRCP, or MRI if suspicion still high
Potentially resectable
Unresectable
No biliary obstruction
Biliary obstruction
Resection or FNA
FNA
ERCP with cytology
Negative
Percutaneous biopsy of mass
Negative
Consider EUS with FNA of mass

FIGURE 3-140 Diagnostic algorithm for pancreatic cancer. Intraoperative fine-needle aspiration (FNA) if found inoperable during surgery. *CT,* Computed tomography; *ERCP,* endoscopic retrograde cholangiopancreatography; *EUS,* endoscopic ultrasonography; *MRI,* magnetic resonance imaging. (From Goldman L, Schafer AL [eds]: *Cecil textbook of medicine,* ed 24, Philadelphia, 2012, Saunders.)

PATIENT WITH ILL-DEFINED PHYSICAL COMPLAINTS

ICD-9CM # 301.9 Personality disorder NOS
301.51 Munchausen syndrome
ICD-10CM # F68.12 Factitious disorder with predominantly physical signs and symptoms

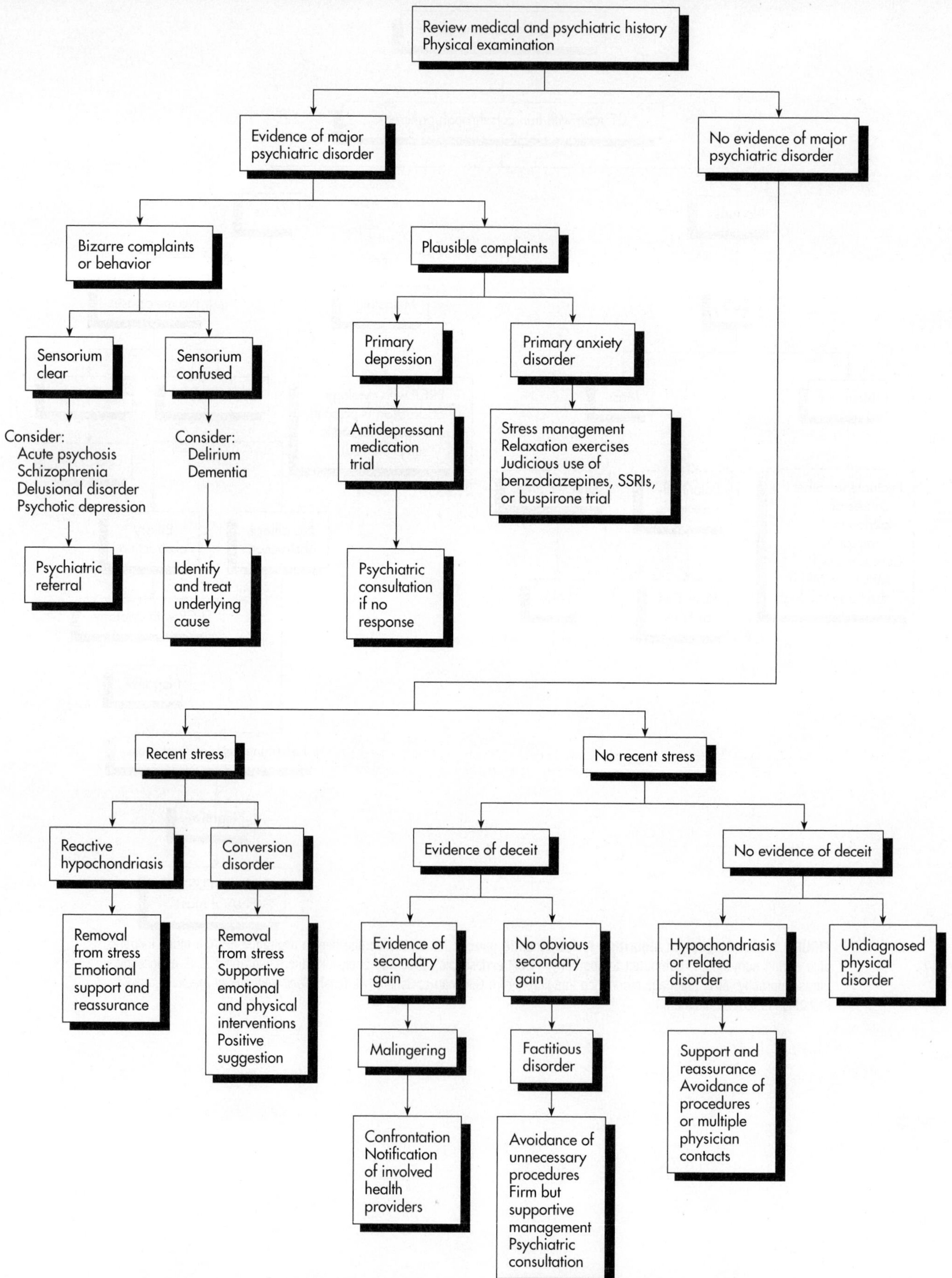

FIGURE 3-142 Patient with ill-defined physical complaints. Previous or recent evaluations are noncontributory. *SSRIs,* Selective serotonin reuptake inhibitors. (From Greene H, Johnson WP, Lemcke D [eds]: *Decision making in medicine,* ed 2, St Louis, 1998, Mosby.)

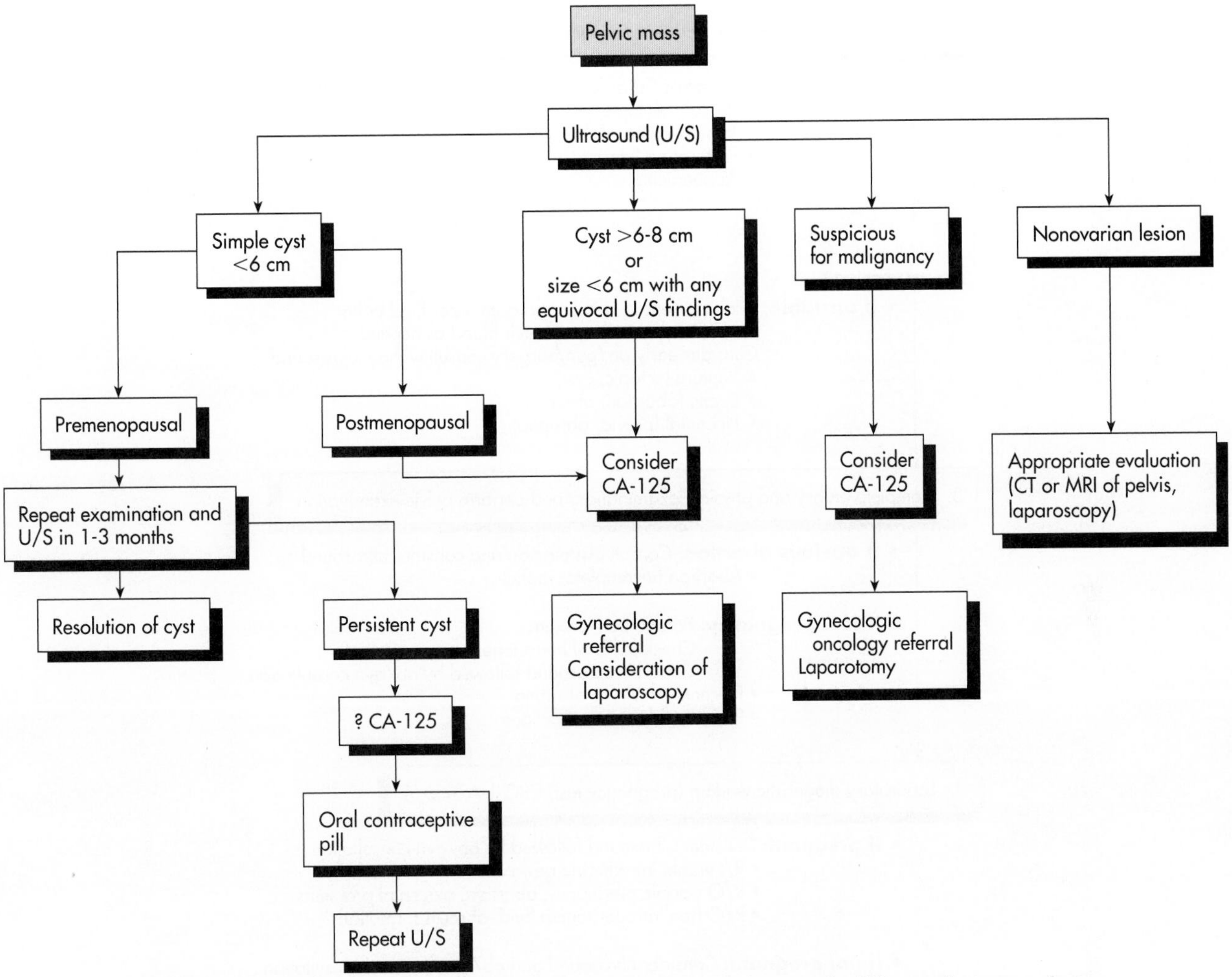

Pelvic mass

Ultrasound (U/S)

Simple cyst <6 cm

Cyst >6-8 cm or size <6 cm with any equivocal U/S findings

Suspicious for malignancy

Nonovarian lesion

Premenopausal

Postmenopausal

Consider CA-125

Consider CA-125

Appropriate evaluation (CT or MRI of pelvis, laparoscopy)

Repeat examination and U/S in 1-3 months

Resolution of cyst

Persistent cyst

Gynecologic referral Consideration of laparoscopy

Gynecologic oncology referral Laparotomy

? CA-125

Oral contraceptive pill

Repeat U/S

FIGURE 3-143 Approach to the patient with a pelvic mass. *CT,* Computed tomography; *MRI,* magnetic resonance imaging. (Modified from Carlson KJ et al: *Primary care of women,* ed 2, St Louis, 2002, Mosby.)

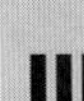

PELVIC PAIN, REPRODUCTIVE-AGE WOMEN

ICD-9CM # 625.9
ICD-10CM # N94.89 Other specified conditions associated with female genital organs and menstrual cycle
R10.2 Pelvic and perineal pain

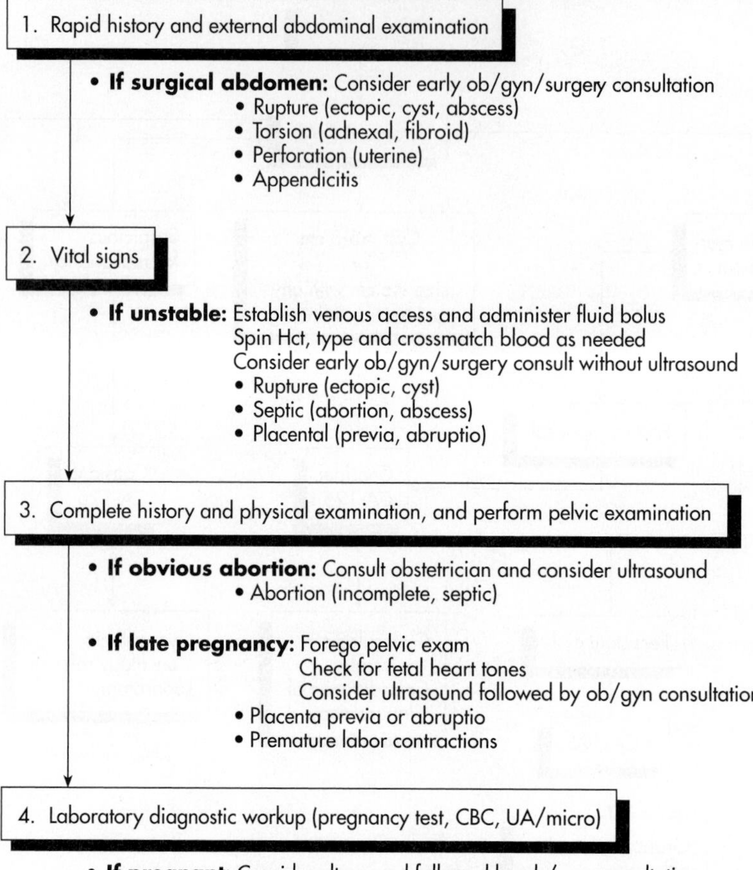

FIGURE 3-144 Evaluation and management of reproductive-age women with acute pelvic pain. *CBC,* Complete blood count; *GI,* gastrointestinal; *GU,* genitourinary; *Hct,* hematocrit; *PID,* pelvic inflammatory disease; *UA/micro,* urinalysis with microscopy. (From Marx JA [ed]: *Rosen's emergency medicine,* ed 6, St Louis, 2006, Mosby.)

ICD-9CM # 356.9 Peripheral nerve neuropathy
355.10 Lower extremity neuropathy
354.11 Upper extremity neuropathy
ICD-10CM # G60.9 Hereditary and idiopathic neuropathy, unspecified
G57.10 Meralgia paresthetica, unspecified lower limb
G90.09 Other idiopathic peripheral autonomic neuropathy

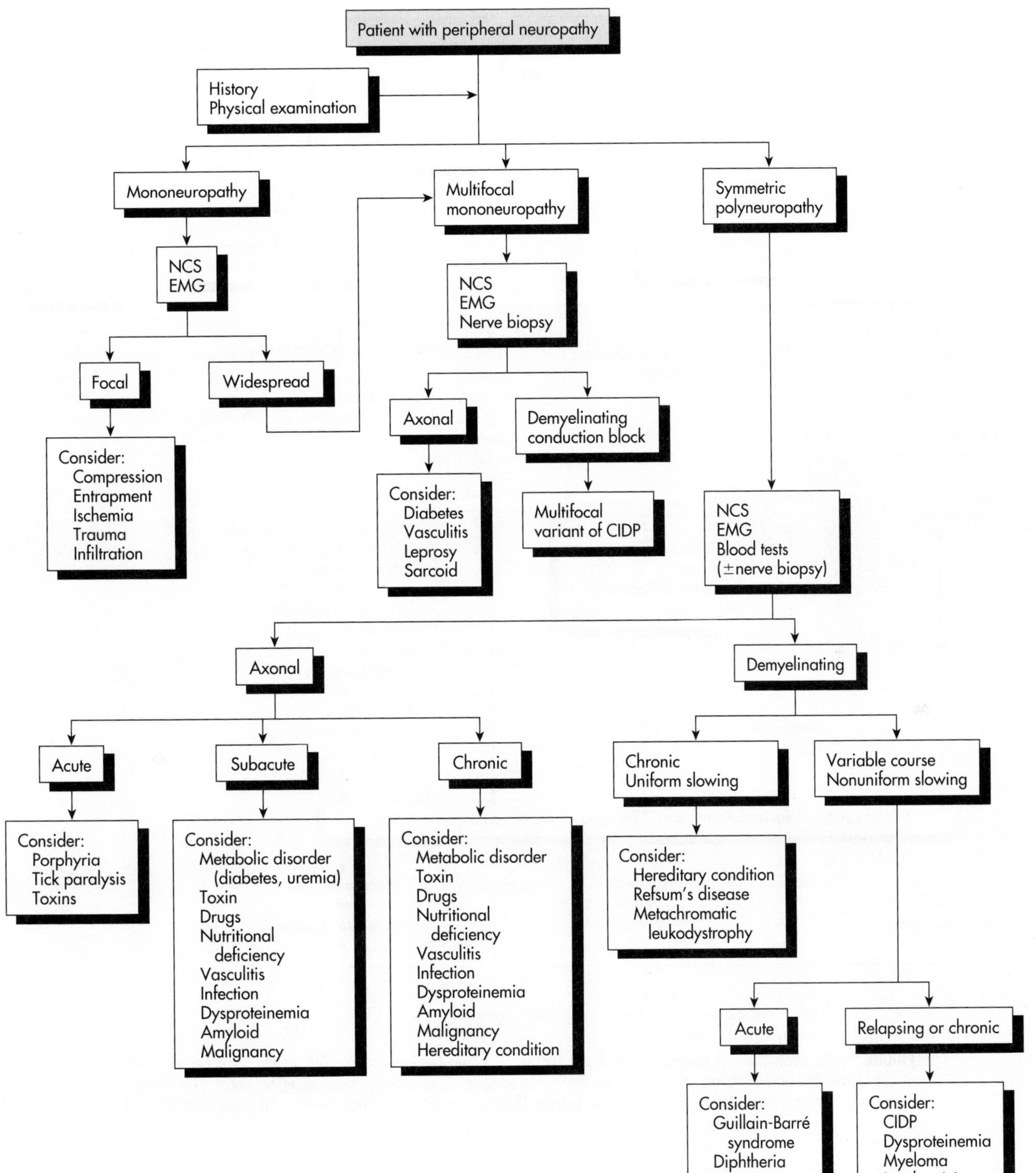

FIGURE 3-146 Approach to the patient with peripheral neuropathy. *CIDP,* Chronic inflammatory demyelinating polyradiculopathy; *EMG,* electromyogram; *NCS,* nerve conduction studies. (From Greene HL, Johnson WP, Lemcke DL: *Decision making in medicine,* ed 2, St Louis, 1988, Mosby.)

ICD-9CM # 253 Pituitary adenoma
253.0 Acromegaly
253.1 Prolactinoma
ICD-10CM # D44.3 Neoplasm of uncertain behavior of pituitary gland
E22.8 Other hyperfunction of pituitary gland
E22.0 Acromegaly and pituitary gigantism

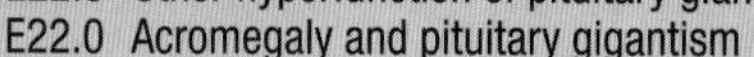

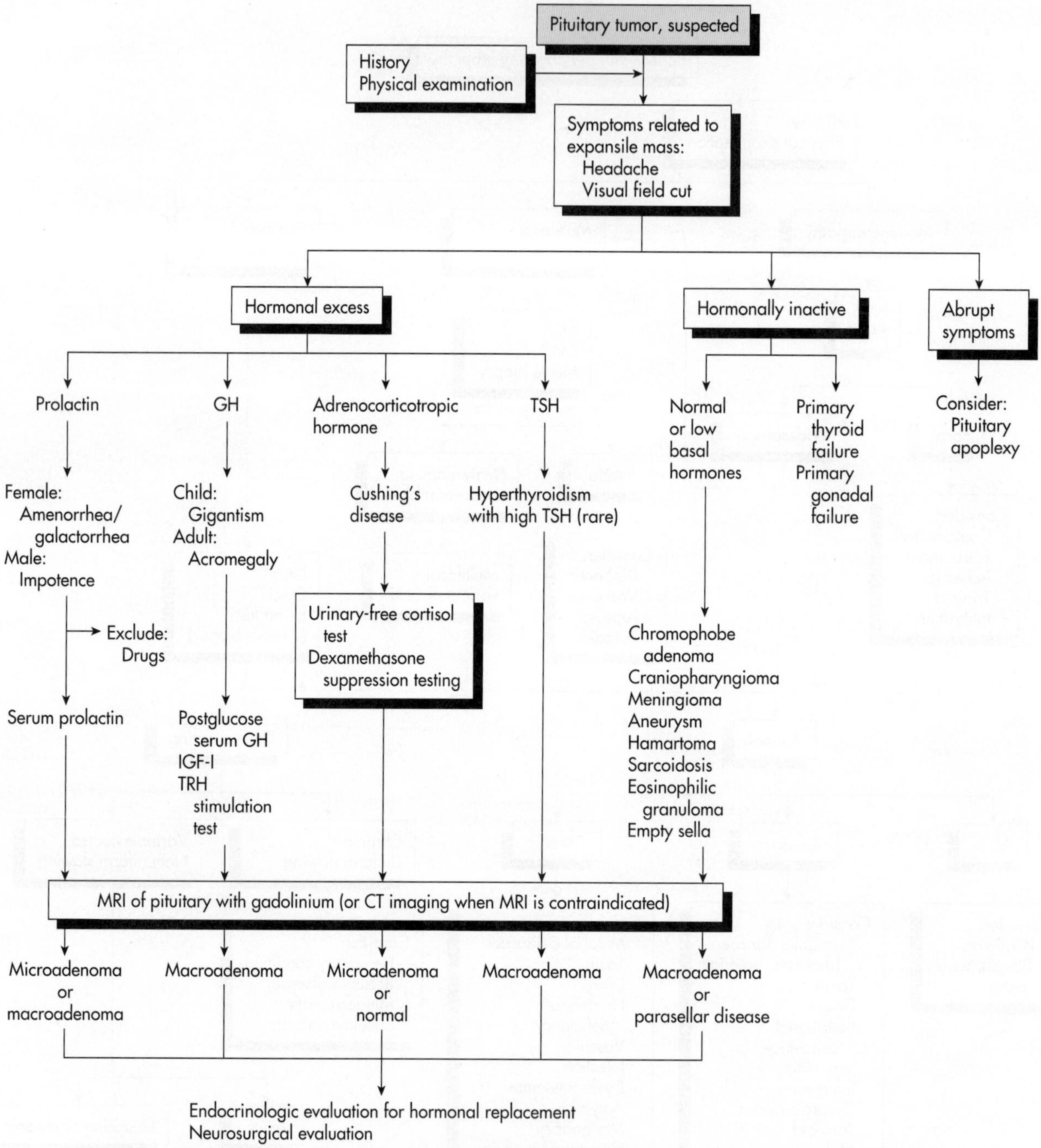

Pituitary tumor, suspected

History
Physical examination

Symptoms related to expansile mass:
Headache
Visual field cut

Hormonal excess

Prolactin
Female:
Amenorrhea/galactorrhea
Male:
Impotence
Exclude:
Drugs
Serum prolactin

GH
Child:
Gigantism
Adult:
Acromegaly
Postglucose serum GH
IGF-I
TRH stimulation test

Adrenocorticotropic hormone
Cushing's disease
Urinary-free cortisol test
Dexamethasone suppression testing

TSH
Hyperthyroidism with high TSH (rare)

Hormonally inactive

Normal or low basal hormones
Chromophobe adenoma
Craniopharyngioma
Meningioma
Aneurysm
Hamartoma
Sarcoidosis
Eosinophilic granuloma
Empty sella

Primary thyroid failure
Primary gonadal failure

Abrupt symptoms
Consider:
Pituitary apoplexy

MRI of pituitary with gadolinium (or CT imaging when MRI is contraindicated)

Microadenoma or macroadenoma
Macroadenoma
Microadenoma or normal
Macroadenoma
Macroadenoma or parasellar disease

Endocrinologic evaluation for hormonal replacement
Neurosurgical evaluation

FIGURE 3-148 Evaluation of suspected pituitary tumor. *CT,* Computed tomography; *GH,* growth hormone; *IGF-I,* one of the insulin-like growth factors; *MRI,* magnetic resonance imaging; *TRH,* thyrotropin-releasing hormone; *TSH,* thyroid-stimulating hormone. (From Greene HL, Johnson WP, Lemcke DL: *Decision making in medicine,* ed 2, St Louis, 1998, Mosby.)

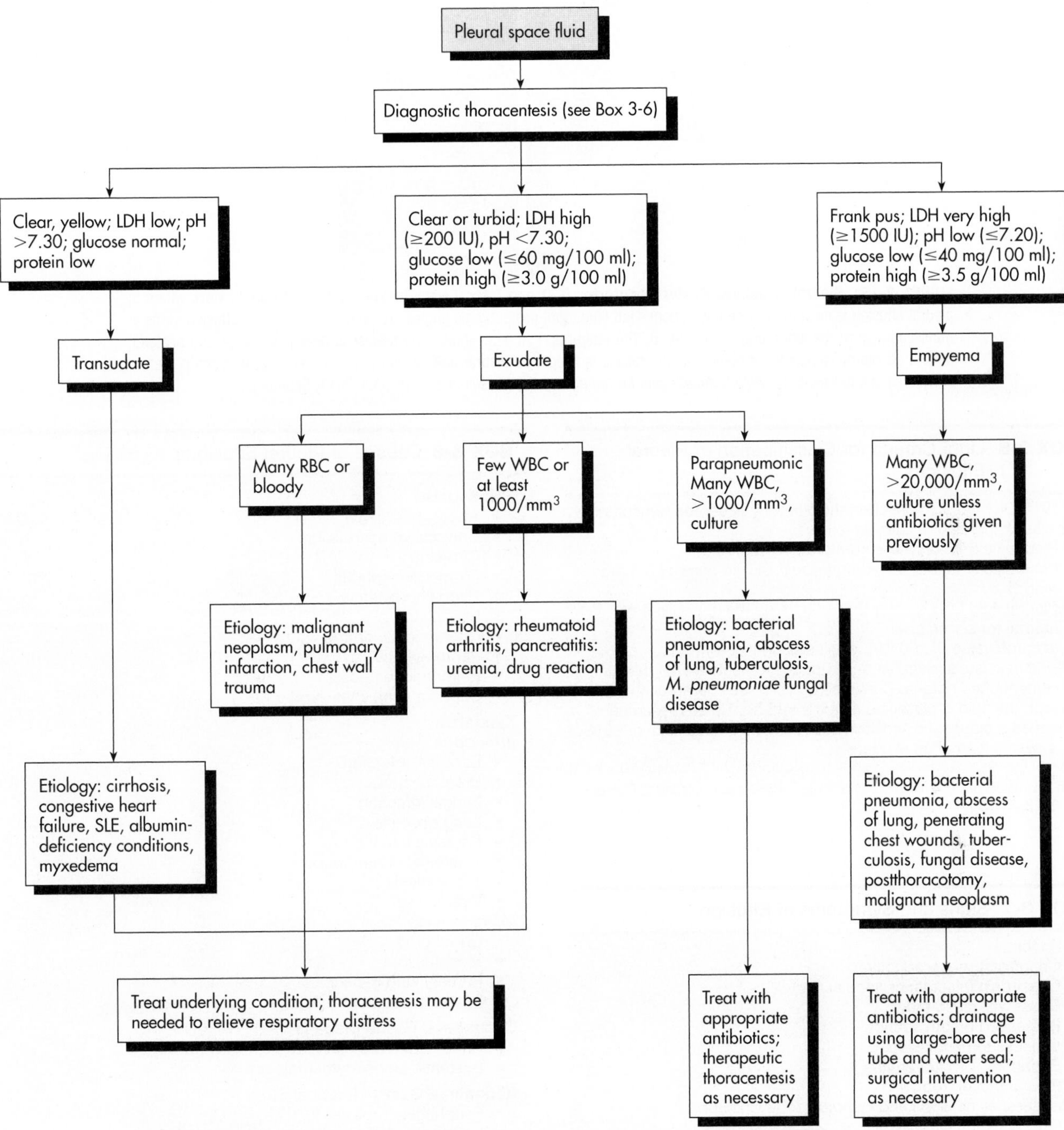

FIGURE 3-150 Evaluation, common etiologies, and management of pleural effusion and empyema. *LDH,* Lactate dehydrogenase; *RBC,* red blood cells; *SLE,* systemic lupus erythematosus; *WBC,* white blood cells. (From Kassirer J [ed]: *Current therapy in adult medicine,* ed 4, St Louis, 1998, Mosby.)

ICD-9CM # 511.9 Pleural effusion, unspecified
ICD-10CM# J91.8 Pleural effusion in other conditions classified elsewhere

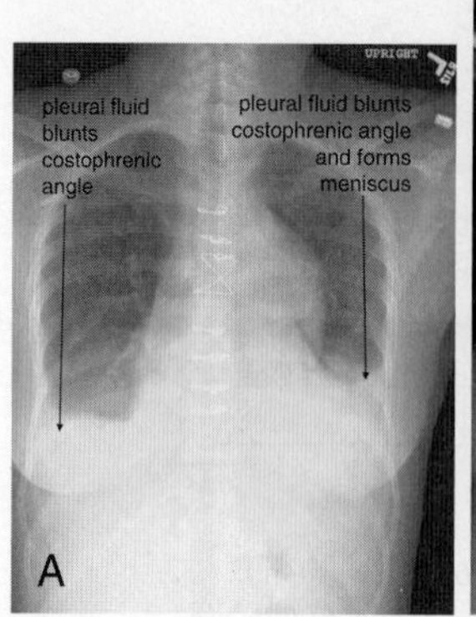

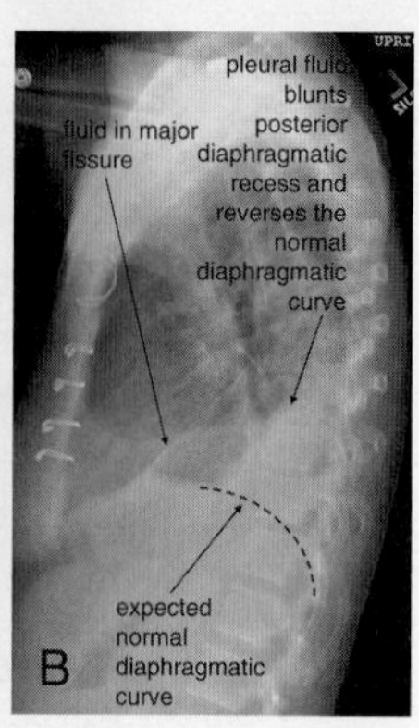

FIGURE 3-151 Pleural effusions: Posterior-anterior (PA) and lateral upright views. A, A PA upright view, where a pleural effusion is most evident on this patient's left side. Both costophrenic angles are blunted. The pleural effusion forms a meniscus against the left lateral chest wall. **B,** The lateral upright view shows two meniscus densities, suggesting bilateral pleural effusions. The posterior diaphragmatic recess is filled with pleural fluid, which forms a meniscus with the posterior chest wall. (From Broder JS: *Diagnostic imaging for the emergency physician*, Philadelphia, 2011, Saunders.)

BOX 3-6 Light Criteria for Classification of Pleural Effusions

In 1972, Light et al. developed the currently accepted benchmark for classifying pleural fluid, as follows:

- Pleural fluid protein-to-serum protein ratio >0.5 : 1
- Pleural fluid lactate dehydrogenase (LDH)-to-serum LDH ratio >0.6 : 1
- Pleural fluid LDH greater than two thirds the upper limit of normal for serum LDH
  (a cutoff value of 200 IU/L was used previously)

Pleural fluid is classified as an exudate if it meets any of the aforementioned criteria. Conversely, if all three characteristics are absent, the fluid is classified as a transudate. These researchers achieved a diagnostic sensitivity of 99% and a specificity of 98% for classification of an exudate.

(From Adams JG, et al: *Emergency medicine, clinical essentials*, ed 2, Philadelphia, 2013, Elsevier.)

BOX 3-7 Signs and Symptoms of Effusion*

- Dyspnea
- Cough (dry, nonproductive)
- Chest pain (pleuritic or nonpleuritic)
- Chest wall discomfort
- Decreased breath sounds
- Dullness to percussion
- Egophony, tactile fremitus
- Pleural friction rub

Disease-specific signs and symptoms may include:

- Orthopnea
- Paroxysmal nocturnal dyspnea
- Fever
- Night sweats

(From Adams JG, et al: *Emergency medicine, clinical essentials*, ed 2, Philadelphia, 2013, Elsevier.)
*A detailed past medical history may uncover the cause of the effusion.

BOX 3-8 Causes of Pleural Effusions

Transudates

- Atelectasis (early)
- Congestive heart failure
- Cirrhosis
- Glomerulonephritis
- Hypoalbuminemia
- Myxedema
- Nephrotic syndrome
- Peritoneal dialysis
- Pulmonary embolism
- Superior vena cava syndrome

Exudates

Infectious

- Bacterial infection
- Bronchiectasis
- Fungal infection
- Lung abscess
- Parasitic infection
- Traumatic hemothorax
- Tuberculosis
- Viral illness

Malignancies

- Lymphoma
- Mesothelioma
- Primary lung cancer
- Pulmonary metastasis

Connective Tissue Disease

- Rheumatoid arthritis
- Systemic lupus erythematosus

Abdominal/Gastrointestinal

- Esophageal rupture
- Pancreatic disorders
- Subphrenic abscess

Other

- Atelectasis (chronic)
- Chylothorax
- Drug reactions (amiodarone)
- Postpartum state
- Pulmonary infarction or embolism
- Uremia

(From Adams JG, et al: *Emergency medicine, clinical essentials*, ed 2, Philadelphia, 2013, Elsevier.)

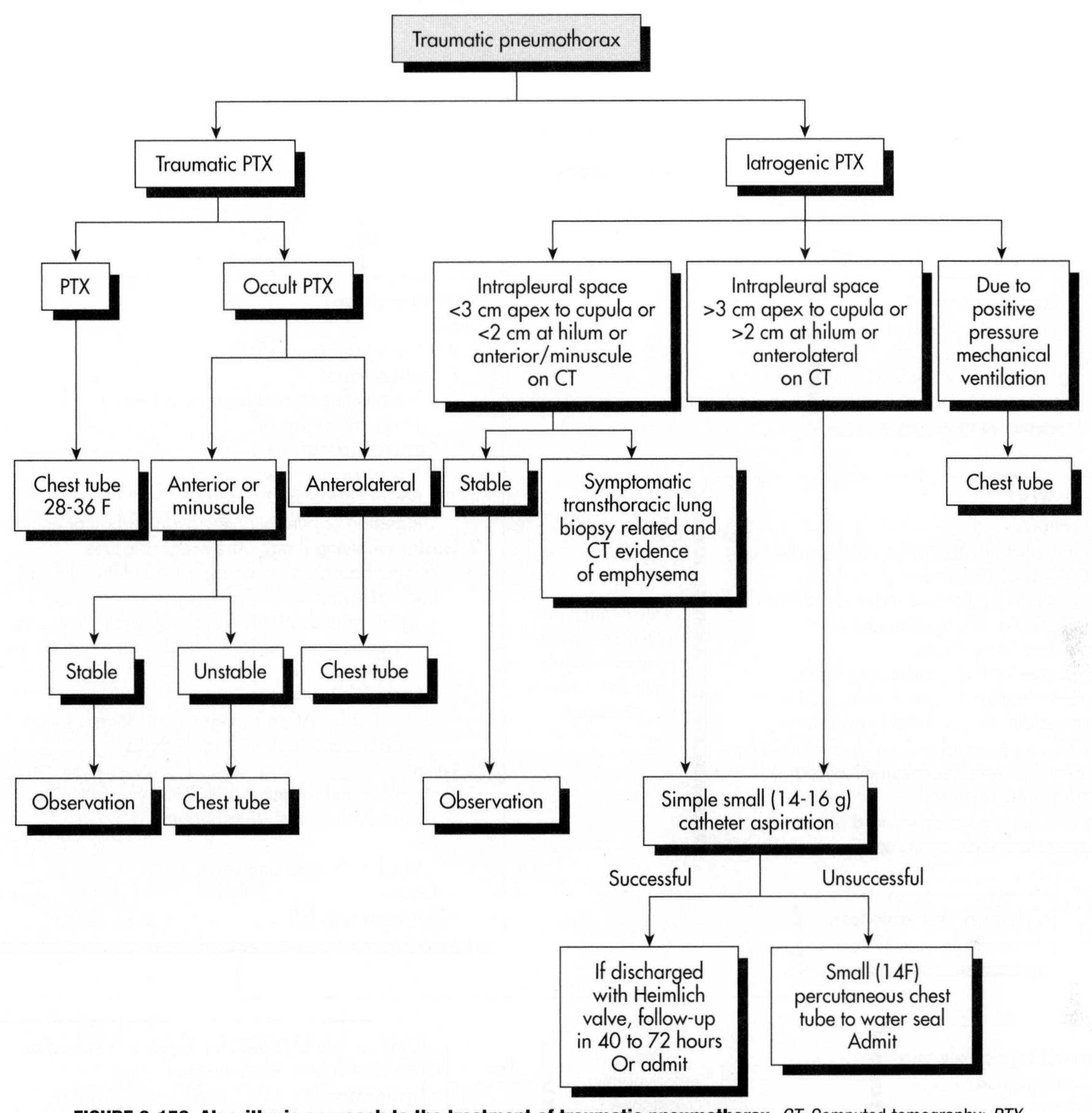

FIGURE 3-152 Algorithmic approach to the treatment of traumatic pneumothorax. *CT*, Computed tomography; *PTX*, pneumothorax. (From Adams JG, et al: *Emergency medicine, clinical essentials*, ed 2, Philadelphia, 2013, Elsevier.)

ICD-9CM #	V82.5	Chemical poisoning
	E 865	Accidental poisoning from foodstuffs and poisonous plants
ICD-10CM #	Z13.88	Encounter for screening for disorder due to exposure to contaminants
	E865.8	Accidental poisoning from other specified foods

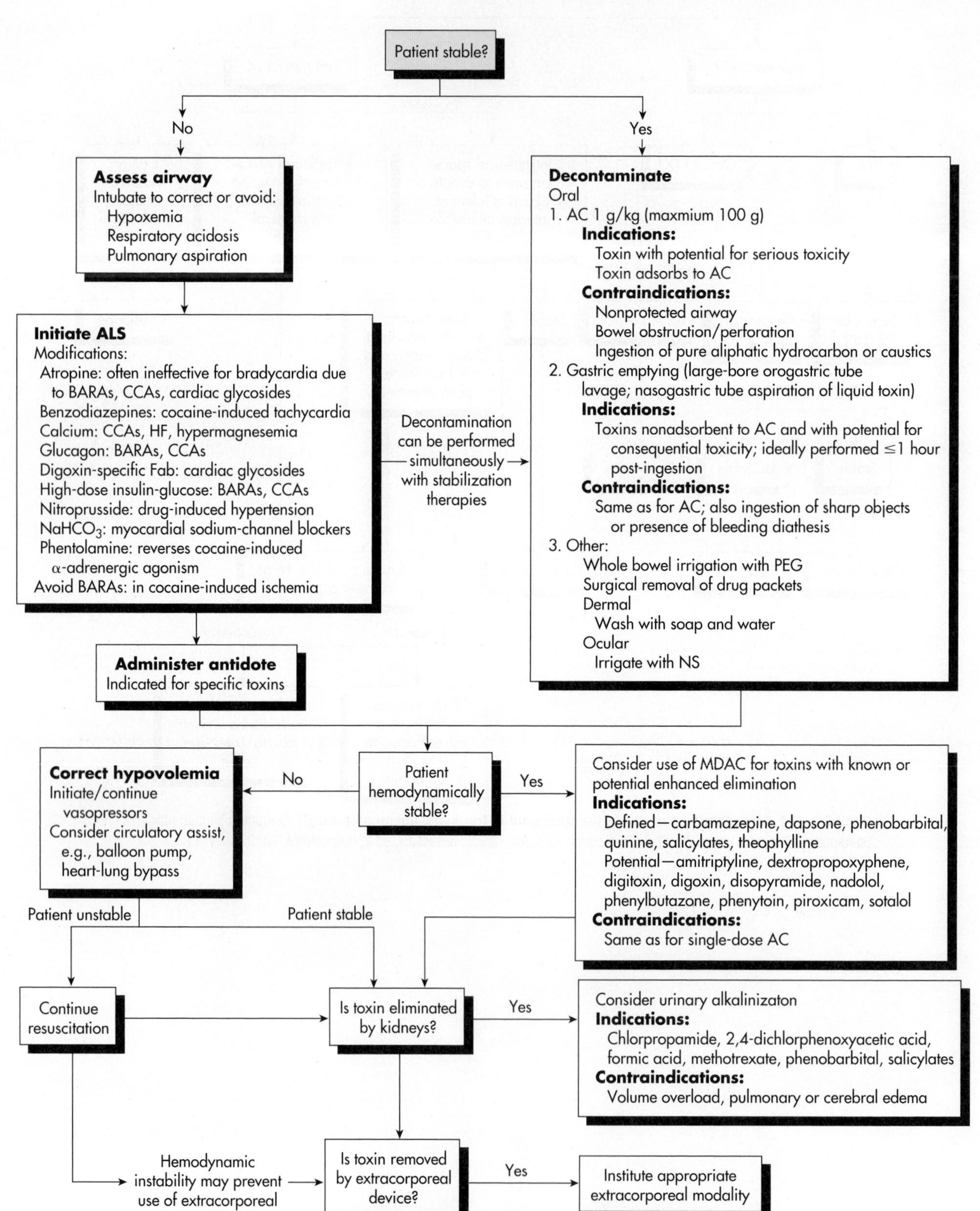

FIGURE 3-153 Algorithm for the management of acute poisoning. See also Table 3-25. *AC,* Activated charcoal; *ALS,* advanced life support; *BARAs,* β-adrenergic receptor antagonists; *CCAs,* L-type calcium-channel antagonists; *HF,* hydrofluoric acid; *MDAC,* multidose activated charcoal; *NS,* 0.9% saline solution; *PEG,* nonabsorbable polyethylene glycol solution. (From Goldman L, Schafer AI: *Goldman's Cecil medicine,* ed 24, Philadelphia, 2012, Saunders.)

ICD-9CM # V82.5 Chemical poisoning
E 865 Accidental poisoning from foodstuffs and poisonous plants
ICD-10CM # Z13.88 Encounter for screening for disorder due to exposure to contaminants
E865.8 Accidental poisoning from other specified foods

TABLE 3-25 Pathophysiology, Clinical Effects, and Management of Specific Drugs and Toxicants

Drug or Toxicant	Pathophysiology	Clinical Effects	Laboratory	Specific Therapy
Acetaminophen	NAPQI (toxic metabolite) binds hepatic and renal tubular cells; acetaminophen itself induces transient decrease in functional factor VII	Initial: nausea, vomiting, coma, lactic acidosis in severe cases Days 1-3: elevated INR, aminotransferase, and bilirubin levels; RUQ tenderness; increased creatinine level in severe cases Days 4-14: gradual recovery or continued increase in INR and creatinine, lactic acidosis, coma, cerebral edema, death	Potentially toxic level ≥150 µg/ml 4 hr after ingestion* INR may be transiently elevated in first 24 hr because of decrease in functional factor VII; further increases indicate hepatic necrosis; elevated aminotransferase and bilirubin levels not predictive of hepatic failure Creatinine elevated in severe cases	NAC can increase INR but not aPTT†
Amphetamines	Increased release of presynaptic norepinephrine and dopamine Increased serotonin release (especially MDMA, PMA, DOB, other synthetic amphetamines)	Mild: euphoria, decreased appetite, repetitive behavior Moderate: vomiting, agitation, hypertension, tachycardia, mydriasis, bruxism, diaphoresis Severe: hypertension or hypotension, arrhythmias, hyperthermia, seizures, coma, hepatotoxicity, rhabdomyolysis, DIC, hyponatremia (SIADH), renal failure, cerebral infarction or hemorrhage	Not helpful; many false-positives and false-negatives on screening tests	IV crystalloids External cooling Benzodiazepines or barbiturates to control agitation or seizures Benzodiazepines or nitroprusside for hypertension See SSRIs/SRIs for features and treatment of serotonin syndrome
β-Adrenergic receptor antagonists	Blocks catecholamines from β-adrenergic receptors α- and β-adrenergic receptor antagonism: carvedilol, labetalol Delayed rectifier potassium-channel blockade: sotalol	Bradyarrhythmias, decreased myocardial contractility, hypotension, respiratory depression, decreased consciousness with seizures or coma (lipophilic agents, e.g., propranolol), prolonged QT interval (sotalol)	ECG No specific tests	IV glucagon, 3.5-5 mg over 2-min period; if no increase in BP or HR, can repeat up to 10 mg; if effective, immediately start continuous infusion at 2-10 mg/hr; if still unstable, options include (1) regular insulin, 1 U/kg by IV bolus, followed by 1 U/kg/hr, plus dextrose to maintain euglycemia; (2) norepinephrine or dobutamine infusion titrated to desirable BP and HR; (3) IV milrinone, 50 µg/kg over 10-min period, then 0.375-0.75 µg/kg/min based on hemodynamic status‡ Electrical pacing and IABP in refractory cases
L-type calcium-channel antagonists	Blocks L-type voltage-sensitive calcium channels, thereby decreasing calcium entry into myocardial and vascular smooth muscle cells Decreases pancreatic insulin release and increases insulin resistance	Bradyarrhythmias (verapamil, diltiazem), hypotension, hyperglycemia	ECG No specific tests	IV 10% calcium chloride, 10-20 mg/kg (0.1-0.2 ml/kg); can repeat once; if BP improves, continuous infusion at 0.2-0.5 ml/kg/hr (20-50 mg/kg/hr) Ionized Ca2+ levels should not exceed 2× normal (severe cases will be refractory to calcium therapy) Glucagon, high-dose insulin and dextrose, catecholamines, and milrinone (as for β-adrenergic antagonists)

From Goldman L, Schafer AI: *Goldman's Cecil medicine,* ed 24, Philadelphia, 2012, Saunders.

*A nomogram to evaluate the potential toxicity of levels drawn more than 4 hours after ingestion is provided in Fig. 3-3, from Rumack BH, Matthew H: Acetaminophen poisoning and toxicity, *Pediatrics* 1975(55):871-876. The nomogram is valid only for levels drawn after a single acute ingestion.

†NAC can be discontinued in patients with uncomplicated disease after a loading dose plus six maintenance doses if hepatic aminotransferase levels are normal and acetaminophen is not detected; otherwise, the full regimen should be administered.

‡Adjust infusion for reduced renal function.

ICD-9CM # V82.5 Chemical poisoning
E 865 Accidental poisoning from foodstuffs and poisonous plants
ICD-10CM # Z13.88 Encounter for screening for disorder due to exposure to contaminants
E865.8 Accidental poisoning from other specified foods

TABLE 3-25 Pathophysiology, Clinical Effects, and Management of Specific Drugs and Toxicants—cont'd

Drug or Toxicant	Pathophysiology	Clinical Effects	Laboratory	Specific Therapy
Cardiac glycosides, including digoxin, bufadienolides (toxic toad venom), or cardenolides (e.g., oleander, lily of the valley, dogbane)	Inhibits Na+, K+-ATPase Decreased CNS sympathetic output Decreased baroreceptor sensitivity Increased vagal acetylcholine discharge	Bradyarrhythmias, including second- and third-degree AV block and asystole Ventricular ectopy, tachycardia, fibrillation Junctional tachycardia, paroxysmal atrial tachycardia with block Weakness, visual disturbances, nausea, vomiting	Serum digoxin level Serum potassium (hyperkalemia occurs in acute poisoning; hypokalemia may be present in chronic poisoning), magnesium, and creatinine levels	Correct hypokalemia and hypomagnesemia; do not give calcium Digoxin-specific antibody fragments (Fab) indicated if patient has hemodynamically significant arrhythmias, serum potassium ≥5 mg/L, Mobitz II or third-degree AV block, ingestion of bufadienolide- or cardenolide-containing agents, or renal insufficiency Empirical dose Chronic: 2-5 vials Acute: 10-20 vials Calculated dose Chronic: number of vials = 2 × serum digoxin level (ng/ml) × 5.6 × weight (kg)/1000 Acute: number of vials = 2 × oral digoxin dose (mg) × 0.8
Cyclic antidepressants	Myocardial sodium- and potassium-channel blockade Blockade of α-adrenergic and cholinergic muscarinic receptors Inhibition of norepinephrine re-uptake	Decreased level of consciousness (can develop rapidly), myoclonus, seizures, coma Anticholinergic toxidrome Sinus tachycardia, ventricular conduction delays, ventricular arrhythmias, asystole Hypotension	Serum levels not helpful in management	Intermittent IV boluses of NaHCO3 (1 mEq/kg) to maintain arterial pH at 7.5 because acidemia can worsen cardiovascular complications Intubation and neuroparalytic drugs may be useful to ameliorate acidemia from muscular hyperactivity while seizures are being treated Contraindicated drugs: types IA and IC antiarrhythmic agents; physostigmine, flumazenil
Ethylene glycol, methanol (e.g., antifreeze, window cleaners, camping stove fuels)	Ethylene glycol: toxic metabolites produce cytotoxicity in CNS, kidneys, lungs, heart, liver, muscles; metabolic acidosis is due to glycolate accumulation; oxalate complexes with calcium, so hypocalcemia can develop Methanol: metabolized to formic acid, which is responsible for metabolic acidosis and inhibition of cytochrome aa3; target organs include retina, optic nerve, CNS	Ethylene glycol: CNS depression, cerebral edema, seizures, anion gap metabolic acidosis, renal failure with acute tubular necrosis, pulmonary edema, myositis Methanol: nausea, vomiting; cerebral edema, hemorrhage, infarcts; necrosis of thalamus and putamen; anion gap metabolic acidosis; visual disturbances, papilledema, hyperemic optic disc, nonreactive pupils	Serum ethylene glycol and methanol levels; levels may be low or undetectable if significant metabolism has occurred Ethylene glycol: serum calcium, creatinine, BUN levels; examine urine for calcium oxalate crystals; false hyperlactatemia occurs with certain analyzers using l-lactate oxidase, which cross-reacts with glycolic and glyoxylic acids	For both: fomepizole (which inhibits alcohol dehydrogenase and blocks formation of toxic metabolites), 15 mg/kg IV loading dose, then 10 mg/kg IV for 4 doses during the next 48 hr, then 15 mg/kg for subsequent doses; interval dosing is q12h (q4h during hemodialysis, with dosing interval adjustments at start and finish); continue until ethylene glycol or methanol is no longer detectable Use of ethanol is no longer recommended Hemodialysis: initiate if level is ≥50 mg/dl or metabolic acidosis with end-organ toxicity; continue until acidosis resolves and serum level of ethylene glycol or methanol is undetectable Monitor for cerebral edema with possible herniation Ethylene glycol: IV calcium for symptomatic hypocalcemia Methanol: folinic acid, 50 mg IV q4h until methanol not detectable and acidosis cleared

ICD-9CM #	V82.5	Chemical poisoning
	E 865	Accidental poisoning from foodstuffs and poisonous plants
ICD-10CM #	Z13.88	Encounter for screening for disorder due to exposure to contaminants
	E865.8	Accidental poisoning from other specified foods

TABLE 3-25 Pathophysiology, Clinical Effects, and Management of Specific Drugs and Toxicants—cont'd

Drug or Toxicant	Pathophysiology	Clinical Effects	Laboratory	Specific Therapy
γ-Hydroxybutyrate (GHB) and its precursors (γ-butyrolactone and 1,4-butanediol [1,4-BD])	Agonist effect on CNS GHB receptors; indirect action with opioid receptors (may increase proenkephalins); metabolized to GABA, interacts with GABAB receptors; decreases dopamine release	CNS: rapid loss of consciousness, with recovery typical within 2-4 hr; myoclonus (possible seizures) Respiratory depression; bradycardia; nausea, vomiting	No specific tests	Supportive care, including respiratory support as needed Withdrawal resembles sedative-hypnotic withdrawal and can be treated with benzodiazepines or pentobarbital
Lithium	Decreases brain inositol; alters CNS serotonin, dopamine, and norepinephrine; inhibits adenylate cyclases, including those that mediate vasopressin-induced renal concentration and thyroid function	Chronic toxicity usually more severe than acute toxicity: tremor, hyperreflexia, drowsiness, incoordination, clonus, confusion, ataxia; in severe cases, seizures, coma, death; recovery may take weeks, and CNS deficits may persist Sinus node dysfunction, QT prolongation, T wave abnormalities, U waves Nephrogenic diabetes insipidus, hypothyroidism, hyperthyroidism, hypercalcemia, pseudotumor cerebri Acute toxicity: nausea, vomiting, diarrhea, and milder neurologic findings	Peak serum levels: Normal dose 2-3 hr; up to 5 hr for sustained-release lithium Acute overdose: peak may be delayed ≥4-12 hr	Replenish intravascular volume, maintain urinary output at 1-2 ml/kg/hr Consider GI decontamination with oral polyethylene glycol electrolyte solution within 1-2 hr after acute overdose of sustained-release drug Hemodialysis§ in patients with altered mental status, ataxia, seizures, or coma or in patients with mild symptoms in the setting of acute overdose or renal insufficiency Ineffective or contraindicated therapies include oral activated charcoal, diuretics, and aminophylline
Opioids (e.g., heroin, morphine, oxycodone, fentanyl)	Agonist effect at CNS μ, κ, and δ opioid receptors; result is cell hyperpolarization and decreased neurotransmitter release	CNS depression, respiratory depression, miosis Dextromethorphan increases CNS serotonin and inhibits NMDA receptors, which causes hallucinations Propoxyphene and its metabolite norpropoxyphene block sodium channels and can cause seizures and wide-complex arrhythmias similar to cyclic antidepressants; NaHCO3 treats arrhythmias Seizure risk with tramadol, meperidine, propoxyphene Rapid, powerful heroin-like effect when sustained-release oxycodone is crushed before ingestion, snorting, or smoking QTc prolongation and torsades de pointes with methadone	Rapid urine drug screens detect morphine and codeine but may not detect semisynthetic and synthetic opioids; some interferents/irrelevants	IV naloxone, 0.4-2 mg; can repeat up to 10 mg if no response Continuous infusion for recurrent symptoms or sustained-release opioid ingestion; give 50% of dose that produces desired effect 15 min after initial effect is obtained, then infuse two thirds of this dose every hr; infusion rate can be increased or decreased to maintain normal respiration and avoid withdrawal symptoms Contraindicated therapies: nalmefene and naltrexone should not be used for acute opioid reversal

§Continue hemodialysis until the serum lithium level is less than 1 mEq/L. Recheck the level 8 hr after dialysis, and restart hemodialysis if the level is higher than 1 mEq/L. Repeat this cycle until the serum lithium level remains lower than 1 mEq/L.

‖A double-blind, randomized, placebo-controlled trial of pralidoxime in acute organophosphorus poisoning found no significant difference in mortality rates or need for intubation.

Continued on following page

ICD-9CM # V82.5 Chemical poisoning
E 865 Accidental poisoning from foodstuffs and poisonous plants
ICD-10CM # Z13.88 Encounter for screening for disorder due to exposure to contaminants
E865.8 Accidental poisoning from other specified foods

TABLE 3-25 Pathophysiology, Clinical Effects, and Management of Specific Drugs and Toxicants—cont'd

Drug or Toxicant	Pathophysiology	Clinical Effects	Laboratory	Specific Therapy
Organophosphorus compounds and carbamates (e.g., diazinon, mevinphos, fenthion, aldicarb)	Inhibits acetylcholinesterase, resulting in excessive acetylcholine stimulation of nicotinic and muscarinic receptors in autonomic and somatic motor nervous systems and CNS	Nicotinic-mediated effects: tachycardia, mydriasis, hypertension, delirium, coma, seizures, muscle weakness, fasciculations Muscarinic-mediated effects: salivation, lacrimation, urination, vomiting, defecation, miosis, bronchorrhea, bronchospasm, bradycardia	Serum (butyrylcholinesterase) or RBC (acetylcholinesterase) activity <50% of normal Clinical recovery occurs before serum cholinesterase levels normalize	Atropine, 1-2 mg by initial IV bolus; double the dose every 5 min (2 mg, 4 mg, 8 mg, 16 mg, etc.) until drying of bronchial secretions, adequate oxygenation, pulse >80 bpm, systolic blood pressure >80 mm Hg achieved; continuous infusion at 10%-20% of total stabilizing dose per hr; stop infusion if patient develops any signs or symptoms of anticholinergic toxidrome; restart infusion at lower rate when signs or symptoms abate Pralidoxime[I] chloride 30 mg/kg (maximum 2 g) IV bolus over 30 min, then 8-10 mg/kg/hr (maximum 650 mg/hr) continuous infusion; administer as soon as possible after poisoning; continue 12-24 hr after atropine no longer required and symptoms resolve
Salicylates	Inhibits cyclooxygenase; decreases formation of prostaglandins and thromboxane A2; stimulates CNS medullary respiratory receptor and chemoreceptor trigger zone; impairs platelet function; disrupts carbohydrate metabolism; uncouples oxidative phosphorylation; increases vascular permeability	Acute toxicity Mild: nausea, vomiting, diaphoresis, tinnitus, decreased hearing, hyperpnea, tachypnea Moderate–severe: confusion, delirium, coma, seizures, hyperthermia, ALI; death can occur within hours of overdose Chronic toxicity: same as acute, but may not have diaphoresis or vomiting Consider diagnosis in patients with new-onset confusion, anion gap metabolic acidosis, or ALI	Serum salicylate level: toxic ≥30 mg/dl; level ≥100 mg/dL indicates life-threatening toxicity with possible sudden, rapid clinical deterioration; in chronic toxicity, levels may be minimally elevated (>30 mg/dl), and clinical evaluation is more reliable for gauging degree of toxicity Arterial blood gases: respiratory alkalosis with metabolic acidosis Anion gap metabolic acidosis Prolonged PT and PTT, ketonuria, ketonemia	Multidose activated charcoal q2-3h in acute overdose with progressive symptoms or rising salicylate level
SSRIs/SRIs	Inhibits re-uptake of serotonin SRIs have additional effects (e.g., duloxetine inhibits norepinephrine re-uptake, nefazodone inhibits serotonergic 5-HT2 receptors, trazodone inhibits peripheral α-adrenergic receptors, venlafaxine inhibits norepinephrine and dopamine re-uptake)	Vomiting, blurred vision, CNS depression, tachycardia Seizures and coma rare Torsades de pointes reported with citalopram Serotonin syndrome: clonus, agitation, tremor, diaphoresis, hyperreflexia; hyperthermia and hypertonicity in severe cases	No specific tests If serotonin syndrome suspected: electrolytes, BUN, glucose, liver enzymes, coagulation panel, blood gases, chest radiograph	Respiratory support as needed Benzodiazepines for agitation or seizures Serotonin syndrome: consider cyproheptadine, 12 mg PO initial dose then 2 mg PO q2h (to a maximum of 32 mg/day) until symptoms resolve Critical care therapies for hyperthermia, rhabdomyolysis, DIC, ARDS, renal and hepatic dysfunction, torsades de pointes

ALI, Acute lung injury; aPTT, activated partial thromboplastin time; ARDS, acute respiratory distress syndrome; AV, atrioventricular; BP, blood pressure; bpm, beats per minute; BUN, blood urea nitrogen; CNS, central nervous system; DIC, disseminated intravascular coagulation; DOB, 4-bromo-2,5-dimethoxyamphetamine; ECG, electrocardiogram; GABA, α-aminobutyric acid; GI, gastrointestinal; HR, heart rate; IABP, intra-aortic balloon counterpulsation; INR, international normalized ratio; IV, intravenous; MDMA, 3,4-methylenedioxymethamphetamine; Na^1,K^1-ATPase, sodium, potassium adenosine triphosphatase; NAC, N-acetylcysteine; NAPQI, N-acetyl-p-benzoquinone imine; NMDA, N-methyl-D-aspartate; PMA, paramethoxyamphetamine; PT, prothrombin time; PTT, partial thromboplastin time; RBC, red blood cell; RUQ, upper right quadrant (abdomen); SIADH, syndrome of inappropriate antidiuretic secretion; SRI, serotonin re-uptake inhibitor; SSRI, selective serotonin re-uptake inhibitor.

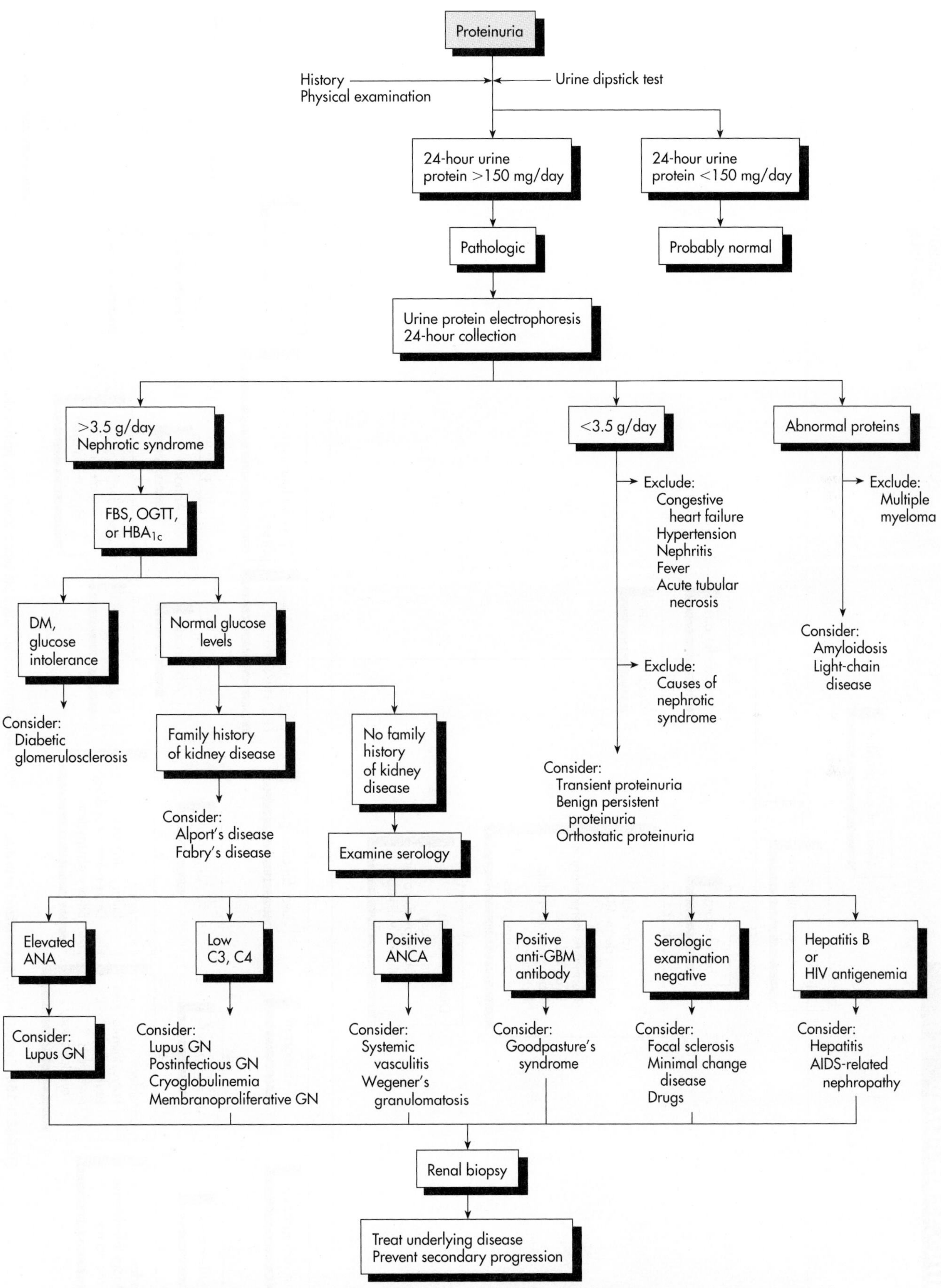

FIGURE 3-155 Proteinuria. *AIDS,* Acquired immunodeficiency syndrome; *ANA,* antinuclear antibody; *ANCA,* antineutrophil cytoplasmic autoantibody; *anti-GBM,* anti-glomerular basement membrane; *FBS,* fasting blood sugar; *GN,* glomerulonephritis; *OGTT,* oral glucose tolerance test. (Modified from Greene HL, Johnson WP, Lemcke DL [eds]: *Decision making in medicine,* ed 2, St Louis, 1998, Mosby.)

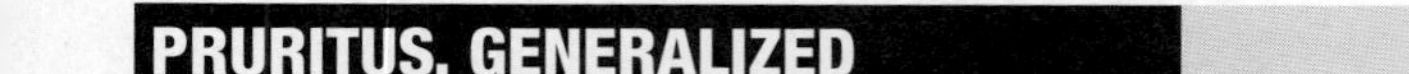

PRURITUS, GENERALIZED

ICD-9CM # 698.9 Pruritus NOS
ICD-10CM # L29.9 Pruritus, unspecified

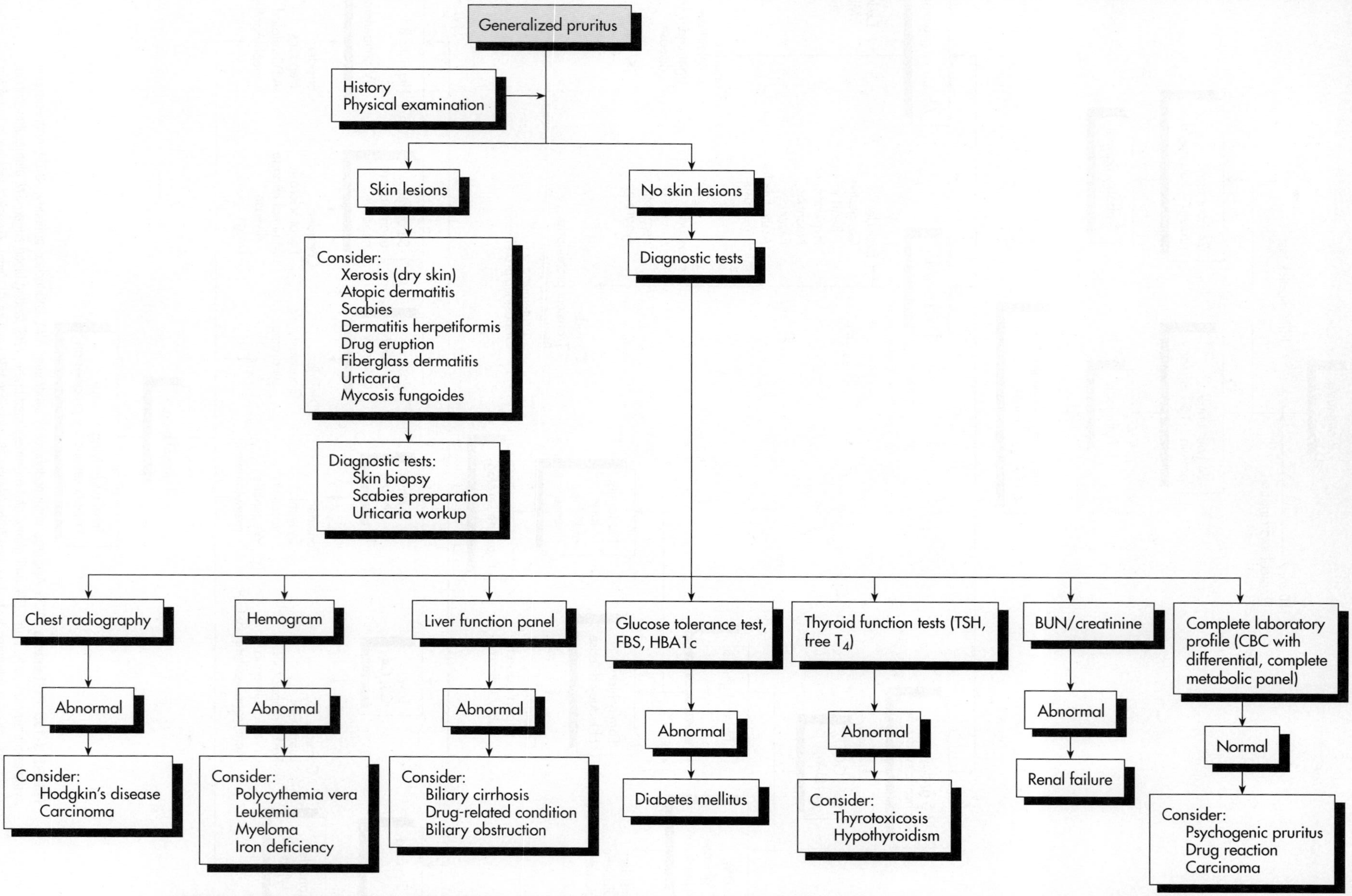

Generalized pruritus
- History / Physical examination
- Skin lesions
  - Consider: Xerosis (dry skin), Atopic dermatitis, Scabies, Dermatitis herpetiformis, Drug eruption, Fiberglass dermatitis, Urticaria, Mycosis fungoides
    - Diagnostic tests: Skin biopsy, Scabies preparation, Urticaria workup
- No skin lesions
  - Diagnostic tests
    - Chest radiography → Abnormal → Consider: Hodgkin's disease, Carcinoma
    - Hemogram → Abnormal → Consider: Polycythemia vera, Leukemia, Myeloma, Iron deficiency
    - Liver function panel → Abnormal → Consider: Biliary cirrhosis, Drug-related condition, Biliary obstruction
    - Glucose tolerance test, FBS, HBA1c → Abnormal → Diabetes mellitus
    - Thyroid function tests (TSH, free T_4) → Abnormal → Consider: Thyrotoxicosis, Hypothyroidism
    - BUN/creatinine → Abnormal → Renal failure
    - Complete laboratory profile (CBC with differential, complete metabolic panel) → Normal → Consider: Psychogenic pruritus, Drug reaction, Carcinoma

FIGURE 3-156 Evaluation of generalized pruritus. *BUN,* Blood urea nitrogen; *CBC,* complete blood count; *FBS,* fasting blood sugar; *HBA1c,* hemoglobin A1c; T_4, thyroxine; *TSH,* thyroid-stimulating hormone. (From Greene HL, Johnson WP, Lemcke DL [eds]: *Decision making in medicine*, ed 2, St Louis, 1998, Mosby.)

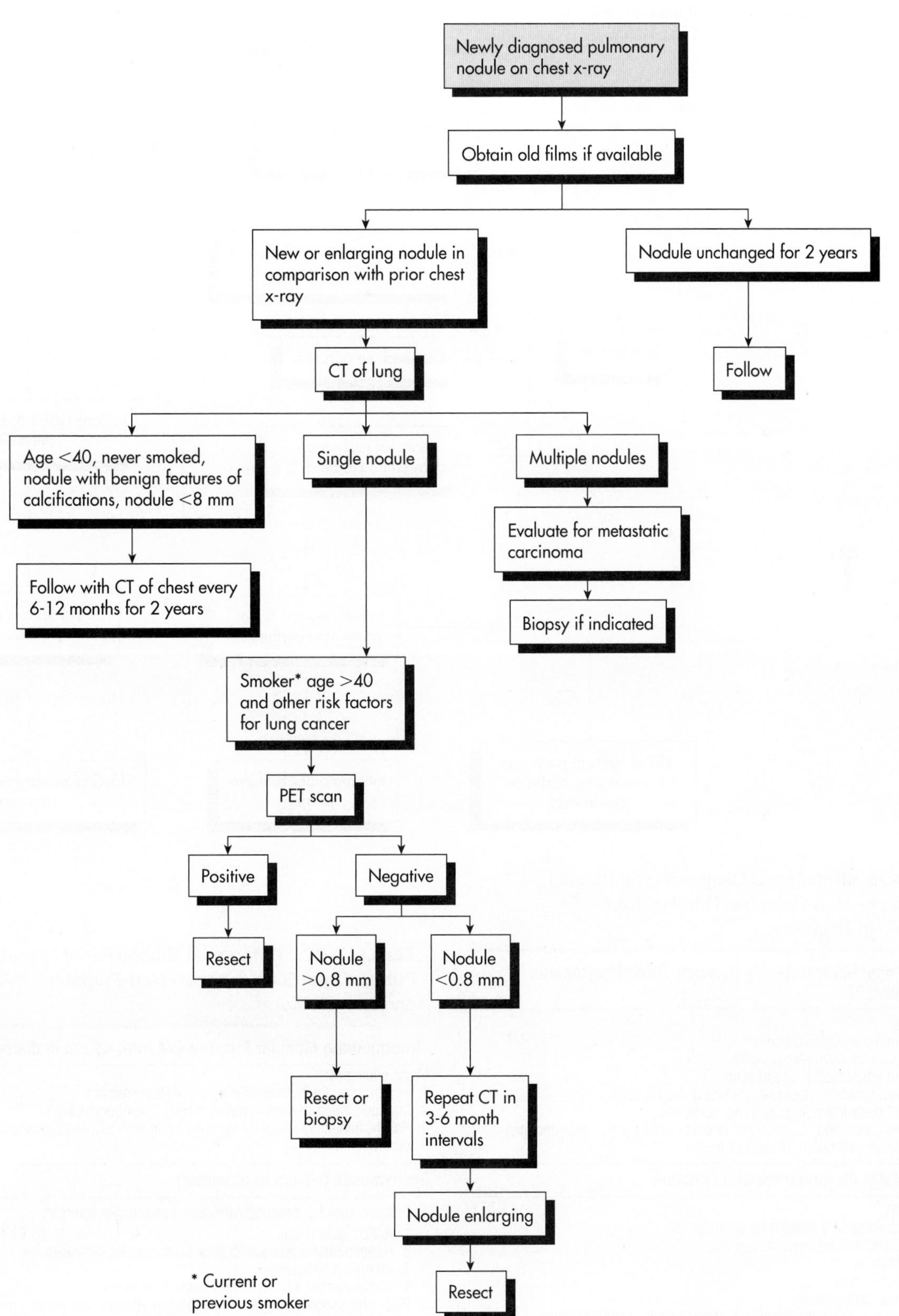

FIGURE 3-159 Pulmonary nodule. *CT,* Computed tomography; *PET,* positron emission tomography.

PURPURA, PALPABLE

ICD-9CM # 287.2
ICD-10CM # D69.2 Other nonthrombocytopenic purpura

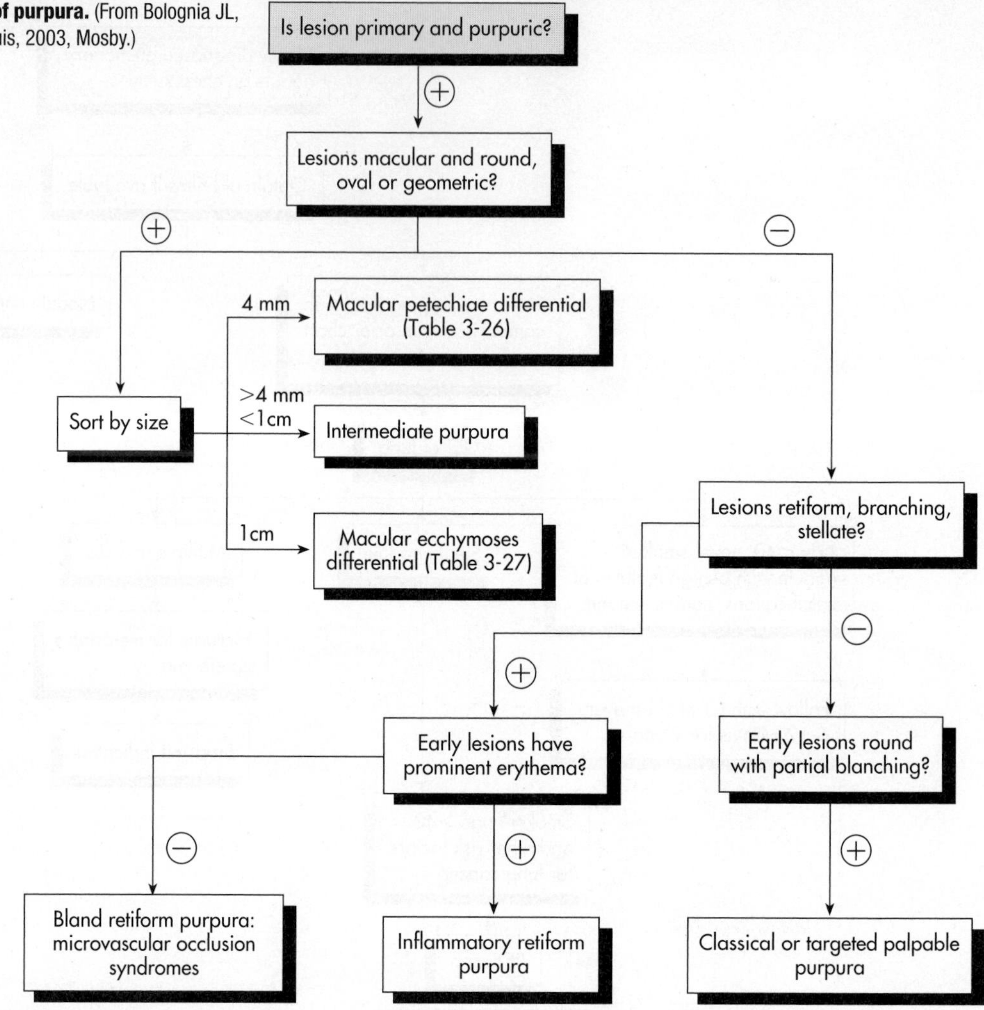

FIGURE 3-160 Differential diagnosis of purpura. (From Bolognia JL, Jorizzo JL, Rapini RP: *Dermatology,* St Louis, 2003, Mosby.)

TABLE 3-26 Differential Diagnosis of Petechial Hemorrhage—Non-Palpable, Non-Retiform and ≤4 mm in Diameter

Pathophysiology: Hemostatically Relevant Thrombocytopenia (<550,000/mm^3) **

Major etiologies*
1. Idiopathic thrombocytopenic purpura
2. Thrombotic thrombocytopenic purpura
3. Disseminated intravascular coagulation
4. Other acquired thrombocytopenias, including drug-related
   a. Peripheral destruction (e.g., quinine, quinidine)
   b. Decreased production, idiosyncratic or dose-related (e.g., chemotherapy)
   c. Bone marrow infiltration, fibrosis or failure

Pathophysiology: Abnormal Platelet Function

Major etiologies*
1. Congenital or hereditary platelet function defects
2. Acquired platelet function defects
   a. Aspirin, NSAIDs
   b. Renal insufficiency
   c. Monoclonal gammopathy
3. Thrombocytosis in myeloproliferative disease (often >1,000,000/mm^3)

Pathophysiology: Non-Platelet Etiologies

Major etiologies*
1. Spiking elevations of intravascular venous pressure (Valsalva maneuver-like, e.g., repetitive vomiting, childbirth, paroxysmal coughing, seizure)
2. Fixed increased pressure (e.g., stasis, ligatures)
3. Trauma (often linear)
4. Perifollicular (vitamin C deficiency)
5. Mildly inflammatory conditions
   a. Chronic pigmented purpura
   b. Hypergammaglobulinemic purpura of Waldenström

TABLE 3-27 Differential Diagnosis for Macular Purpura and Ecchymoses—Non-Palpable and Non-Retiform

Intermediate Macular Purpura (>4 mm, <1 cm in diameter)

Major etiologies*
1. Hypergammaglobulinemic purpura of Waldenström
2. Infection/inflammation in patients with thrombocytopenia
3. Rarely, minimally inflamed immune complex vasculitis (usually dependent distribution)

Ecchymoses (≥1 cm in diameter)

A. Pathophysiology: procoagulant defect plus minor trauma*
   1. Anticoagulant use
   2. Hepatic insufficiency with poor procoagulant synthesis
   3. Vitamin K deficiency
   4. Disseminated intravascular coagulation (some)
B. Pathophysiology: poor dermal support of vessels plus minor trauma*
   1. Actinic (solar, senile) purpura
   2. Corticosteroid therapy, topical or systemic
   3. Vitamin C deficiency (scurvy)
   4. Systemic amyloidosis (light chain-related, some familial types)
   5. Ehlers-Danlos syndrome (primarily type IV)
C. Pathophysiology: other causes plus minor trauma*
   1. Hypergammaglobulinemic purpura of Waldenström
   2. Platelet function defects, including von Willebrand disease, medications, metabolic diseases
   3. Acquired or congenital thrombocytopenia

**Most patients do not have petechiae until platelets ≤20,000/mm^3.
*Partial list.

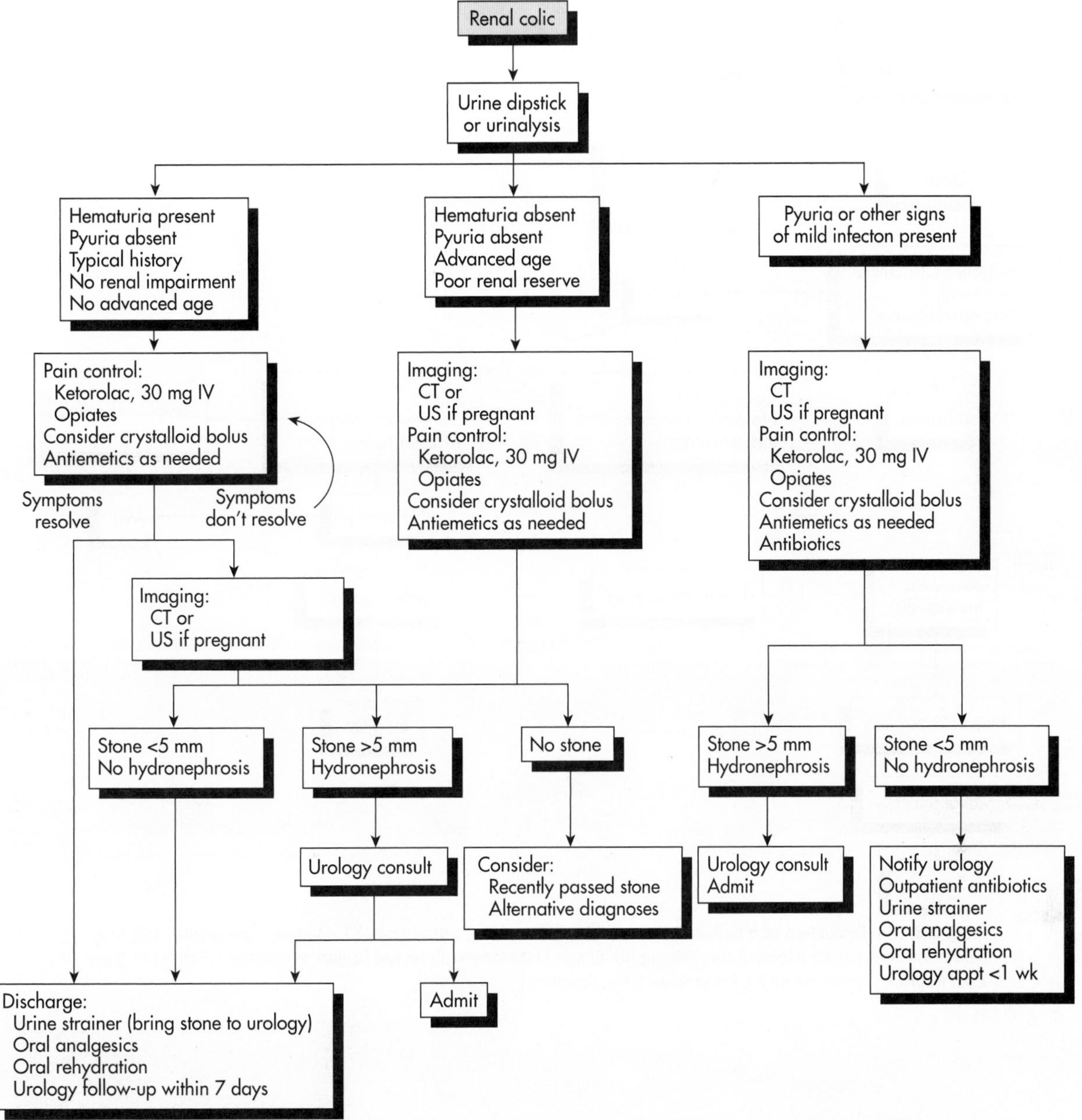

FIGURE 3-162 Guideline algorithm for the evaluation, treatment, and disposition of patients with presumed renal colic. *CT*, Computed tomography; *IV*, intravenously; *US*, ultrasonography. (From Adams JG, et al: *Emergency medicine, clinical essentials*, ed 2, Philadelphia, 2013, Elsevier.)

ICD-9CM # 236.91 Neoplasm of uncertain behavior of kidney and ureter
ICD-10CM # D41.10 Neoplasm of uncertain behavior of unspecified renal pelvis

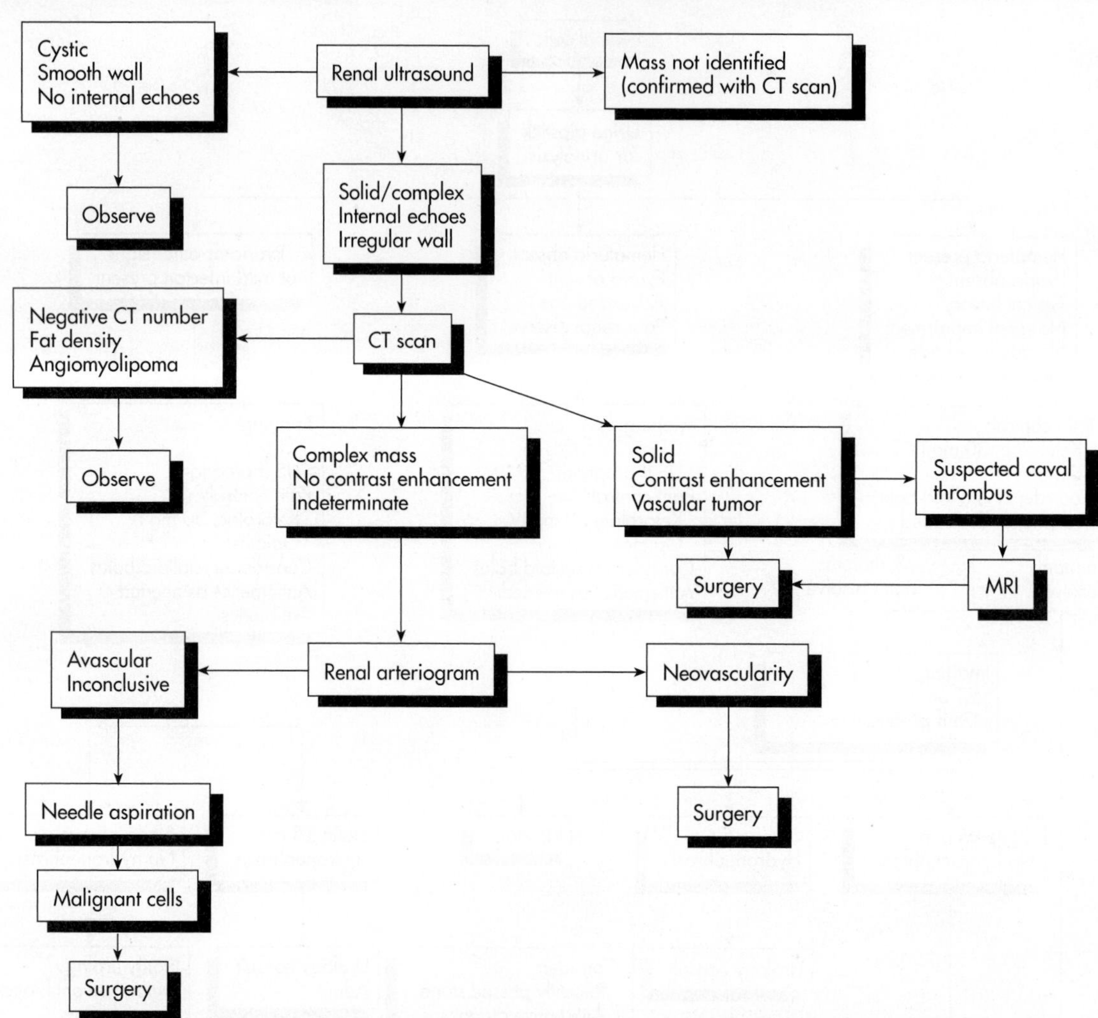

FIGURE 3-164 Evaluation of a patient with a renal mass on renal ultrasound. *CT,* Computed tomography; *MRI,* magnetic resonance imaging. (Modified from Williams RD: Tumors of the kidney, ureter, and bladder. In Goldman L, Schafer AL [eds]: *Cecil textbook of medicine,* ed 23, Philadelphia, 2008, Saunders.)

RESPIRATORY DISTRESS

ICD-9CM #	786.09	Respiratory distress NOS
	518.82	Respiratory distress, acute
ICD-10CM #	R06.00	Dyspnea, unspecified
	R06.09	Other forms of dyspnea
	R06.3	Periodic breathing
	R06.89	Other abnormalities of breathing
	J80	Acute respiratory distress syndrome

- Stridor
  - Yes → History of fever, voice change
    - Yes → Visualize pharynx, larynx, glottis*
      - Abn → Epiglottitis, Abscess, Foreign body, Bacterial tracheitis
      - WNL → Croup
    - No → Wheezing
      - No → Visualize pharnyx, larynx, glottis
        - Abn → Foreign body, Neck injury, Cord paralysis, Extrinsic/intrinsic mass, Laryngomalacia
        - WNL → Visualize trachea (elective bronchoscopy)
          - WNL → Spasmodic croup
          - Abn → Tracheomalacia, Extrinsic/intrinsic mass, Congenital abnormality
      - Yes → Inspir/expir film
        - WNL → Asthma, Bronchiolitis, Congenital abnormality
        - Abn → Foreign body, Extrinsic/intrinsic mass
  - No → Acute onset
    - Yes → Trauma
      - Yes → Chest x-ray
        - Abn → Pneumothorax, Contusion, Hemothorax, Flail chest, Rib fracture
        - WNL → Musculoskeletal
      - No → Heart, liver, renal disease
        - No → Wheezing
          - Yes → Response to β-agonist
            - Yes → Asthma, Bronchiolitis
            - No → Chest x-ray, ABG, if needed
          - No → Chest x-ray, ABG, if needed
            - Abn → Pneumonia, Bronchiolitis, Empyema, Effusion, Pulmonary embolism, Pulmonary edema
            - WNL → Pulmonary embolism; Other: Acidosis, Salicylism, Shock, ↓ FiO_2
        - Yes → Chest x-ray
          - WNL → Wheezing
          - Abn → Effusion, CHF, Pulmonary edema
            - Yes → Treat with diuretics
            - No → Wheezing
    - No → Asthma, Psychogenic, Congenital abnormality, Degenerative, CF, Bronchiectasis, Foreign body, CHF, Pneumonia

*Do not visualize without immediate capability of airway intervention. If epiglottitis is suspected, procedure should be performed under controlled conditions, often in the operating room.

FIGURE 3-165 Respiratory distress in a pediatric patient. *ABG,* Arterial blood gas; *Abn,* abnormal; *CF,* cystic fibrosis; *CHF,* congestive heart failure; *WNL,* within normal limits. (From Barkin RM, Rosen P: *Emergency pediatrics,* St Louis, 1999, Mosby.)

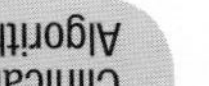
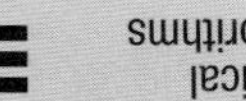

SCROTAL MASS

ICD-9CM # 608.89
ICD-10CM # N44.2 Benign cyst of testis
N44.8 Other noninflammatory disorders of the testis
N50.3 Cyst of epididymis
N50.8 Other specified disorders of male genital organs

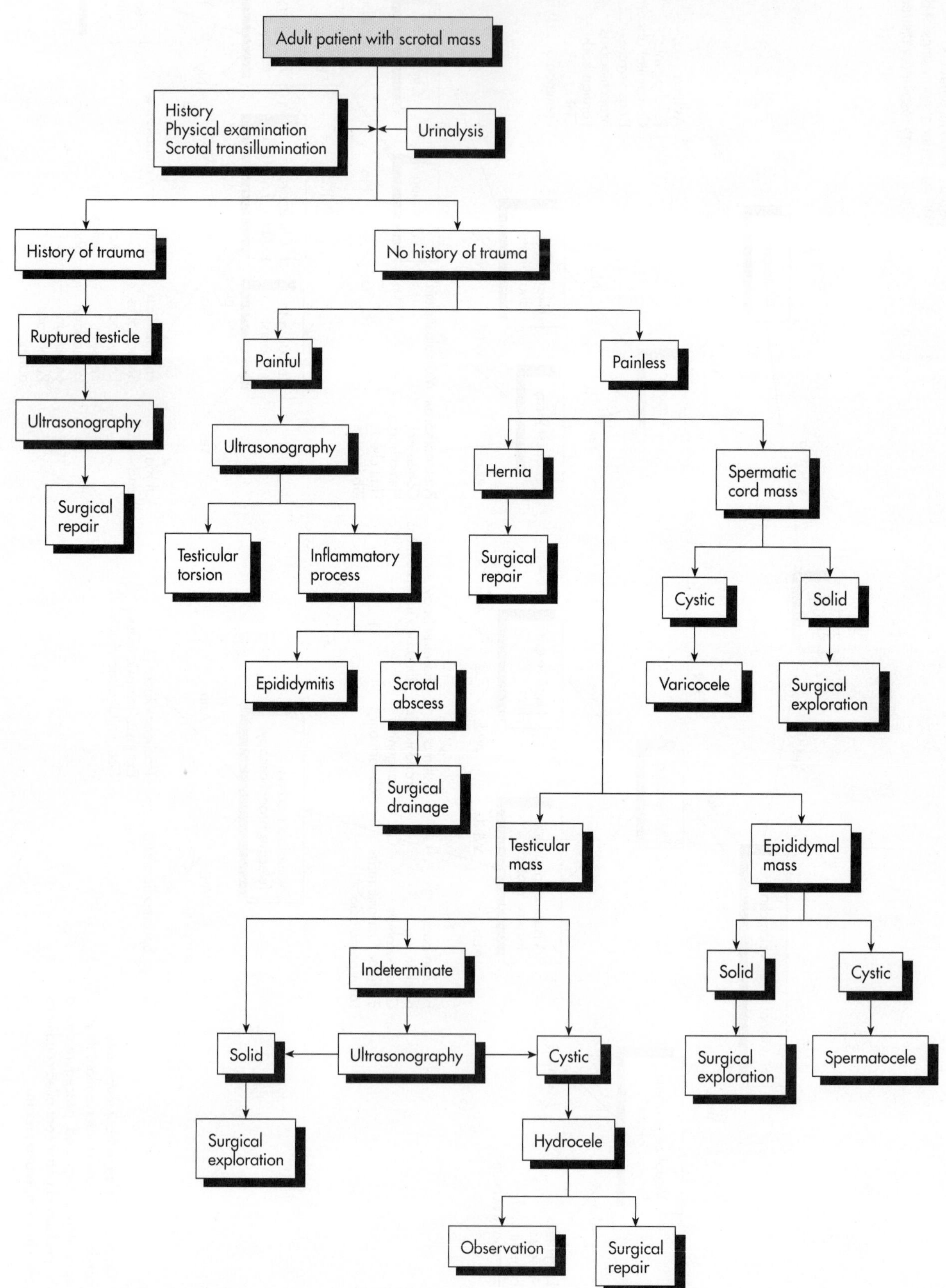

FIGURE 3-167 Evaluation of scrotal mass. (From Greene HL, Johnson WP, Lemcke DL [eds]: *Decision making in medicine,* ed 2, St Louis, 1998, Mosby.)

SHOCK

ICD-9CM # 785.50 Shock NOS
995.0 Shock anaphylactic
785.51 Shock cardiogenic
785.59 Shock septic
958.4 Shock traumatic
977.9 Shock due to drug, medicine incorrectly administered
ICD-10CM # R57.9 Shock, unspecified
R57.0 Cardiogenic shock
R57.1 Hypovolemic shock
R57.8 Other shock

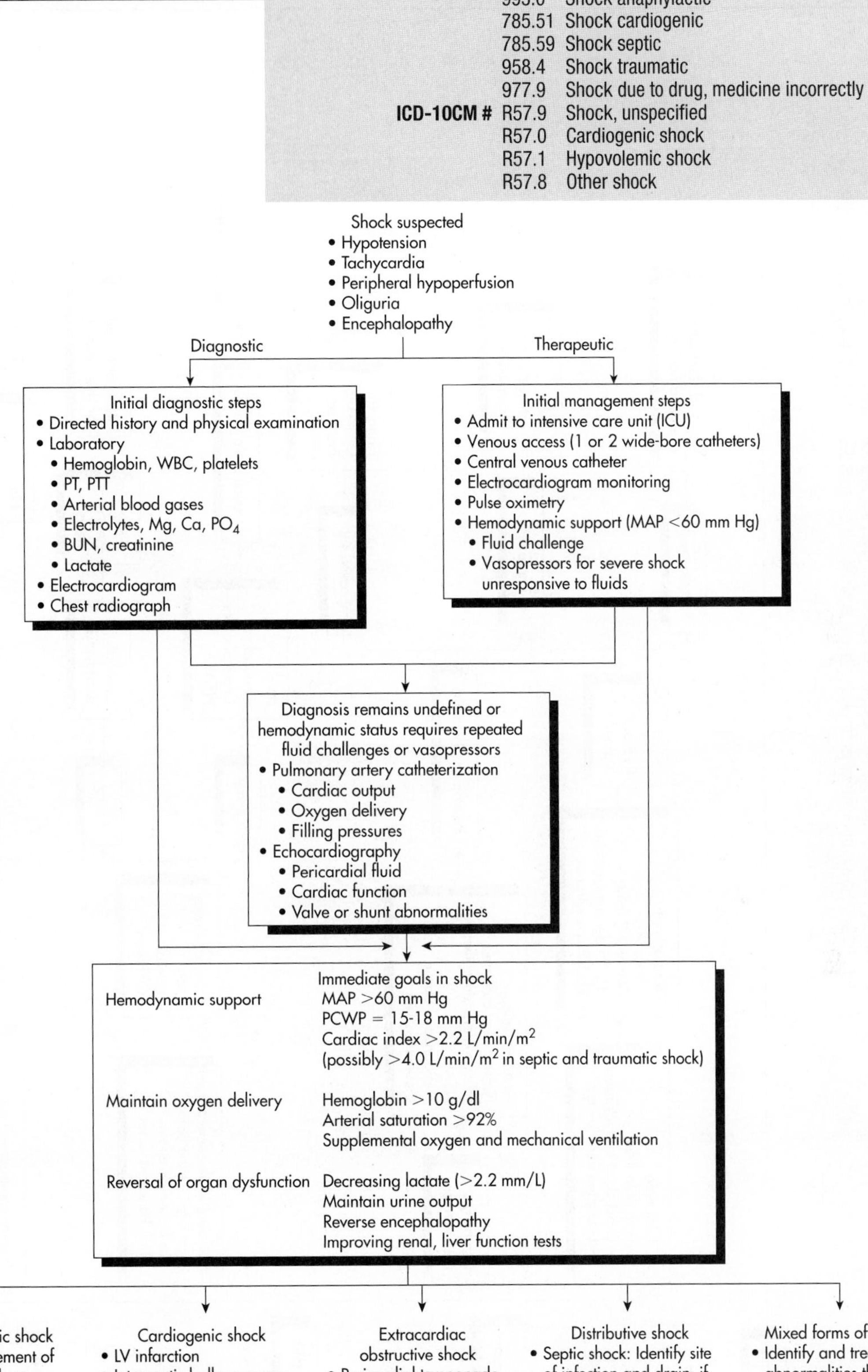

FIGURE 3-173 An approach to the diagnosis and treatment of shock. *BUN,* Blood urea nitrogen; *CT,* computed tomography; *LV,* left ventricular; *MAP,* mean arterial pressure; *MRI,* magnetic resonance imaging; *PA,* pulmonary arterial; *PCWP,* pulmonary capillary wedge pressure; *PT,* prothrombin time; *PTT,* partial thromboplastin time; *RV,* right ventricular; *WBC,* white blood cell count. (From Goldman L, Ausiello D [eds]: *Cecil textbook of medicine,* ed 24, Philadelphia, 2012, Saunders.)

SHOULDER PAIN

ICD-9CM #	variable with specific disorder
ICD-10CM #	S34.109A Unspecified injury to unspecified level of lumbar spinal cord, initial encounter
	M24.819 Other specific joint derangements of unspecified shoulder, not elsewhere classified
	M75.80 Other shoulder lesions, unspecified shoulder
	S43.409A Unspecified sprain of unspecified shoulder joint, initial encounter
	S46.919A Strain of unspecified muscle, fascia and tendon at shoulder and upper arm level, unspecified arm, initial encounter

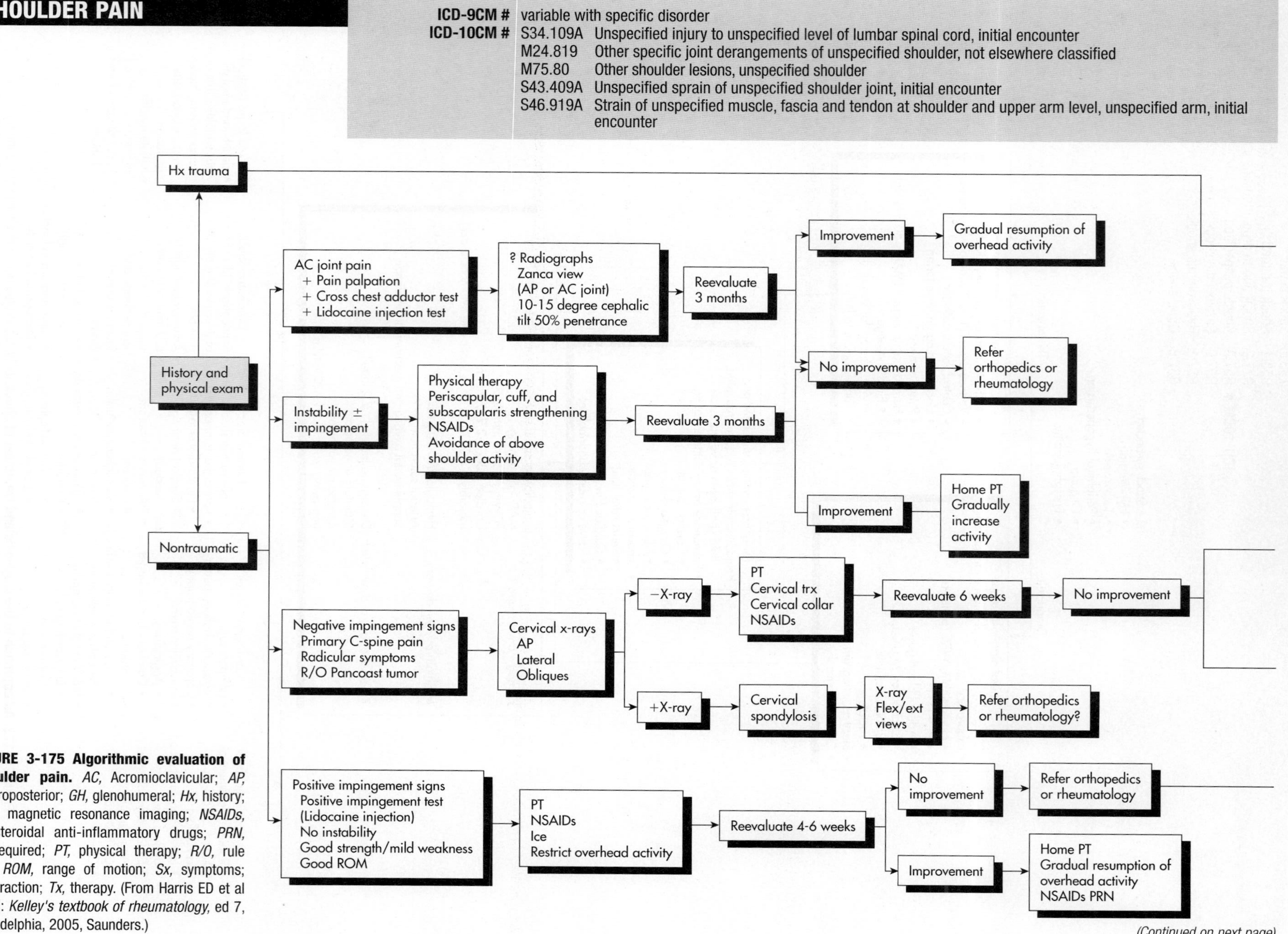

FIGURE 3-175 Algorithmic evaluation of shoulder pain. *AC,* Acromioclavicular; *AP,* anteroposterior; *GH,* glenohumeral; *Hx,* history; *MRI,* magnetic resonance imaging; *NSAIDs,* nonsteroidal anti-inflammatory drugs; *PRN,* as required; *PT,* physical therapy; *R/O,* rule out; *ROM,* range of motion; *Sx,* symptoms; *trx,* traction; *Tx,* therapy. (From Harris ED et al [eds]: *Kelley's textbook of rheumatology,* ed 7, Philadelphia, 2005, Saunders.)

(Continued on next page)

SHOULDER PAIN—cont'd

ICD-9CM # variable with specific disorder

ICD-10CM #
S34.109A Unspecified injury to unspecified level of lumbar spinal cord, initial encounter
M24.819 Other specific joint derangements of unspecified shoulder, not elsewhere classified
M75.80 Other shoulder lesions, unspecified shoulder
S43.409A Unspecified sprain of unspecified shoulder joint, initial encounter
S46.919A Strain of unspecified muscle, fascia and tendon at shoulder and upper arm level, unspecified arm, initial encounter

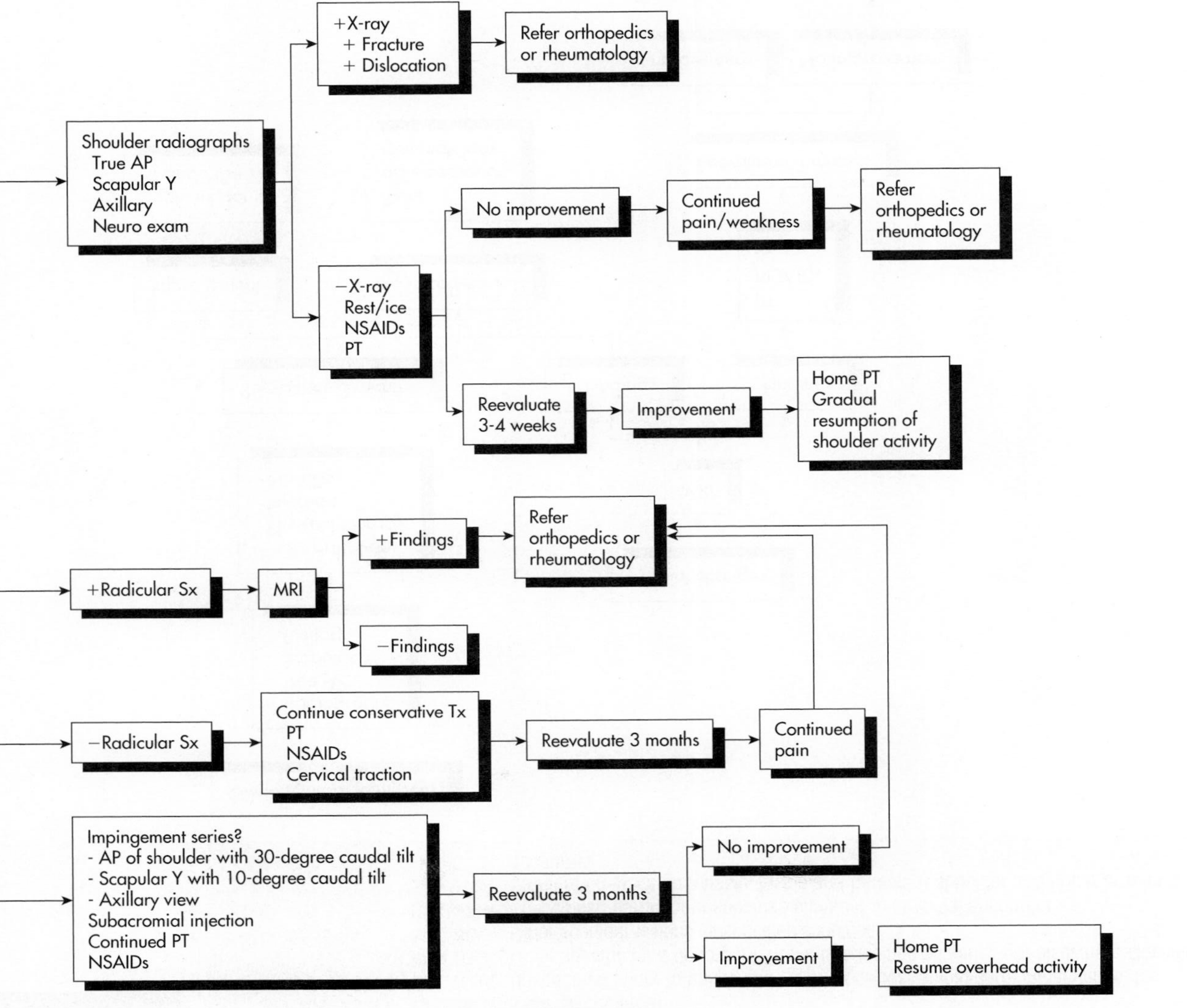

FIGURE 3-175 (Continued)

SHOULDER PAIN—cont'd

ICD-9CM #	variable with specific disorder	
ICD-10CM #	S34.109A	Unspecified injury to unspecified level of lumbar spinal cord, initial encounter
	M24.819	Other specific joint derangements of unspecified shoulder, not elsewhere classified
	M75.80	Other shoulder lesions, unspecified shoulder
	S43.409A	Unspecified sprain of unspecified shoulder joint, initial encounter
	S46.919A	Strain of unspecified muscle, fascia and tendon at shoulder and upper arm level, unspecified arm, initial encounter

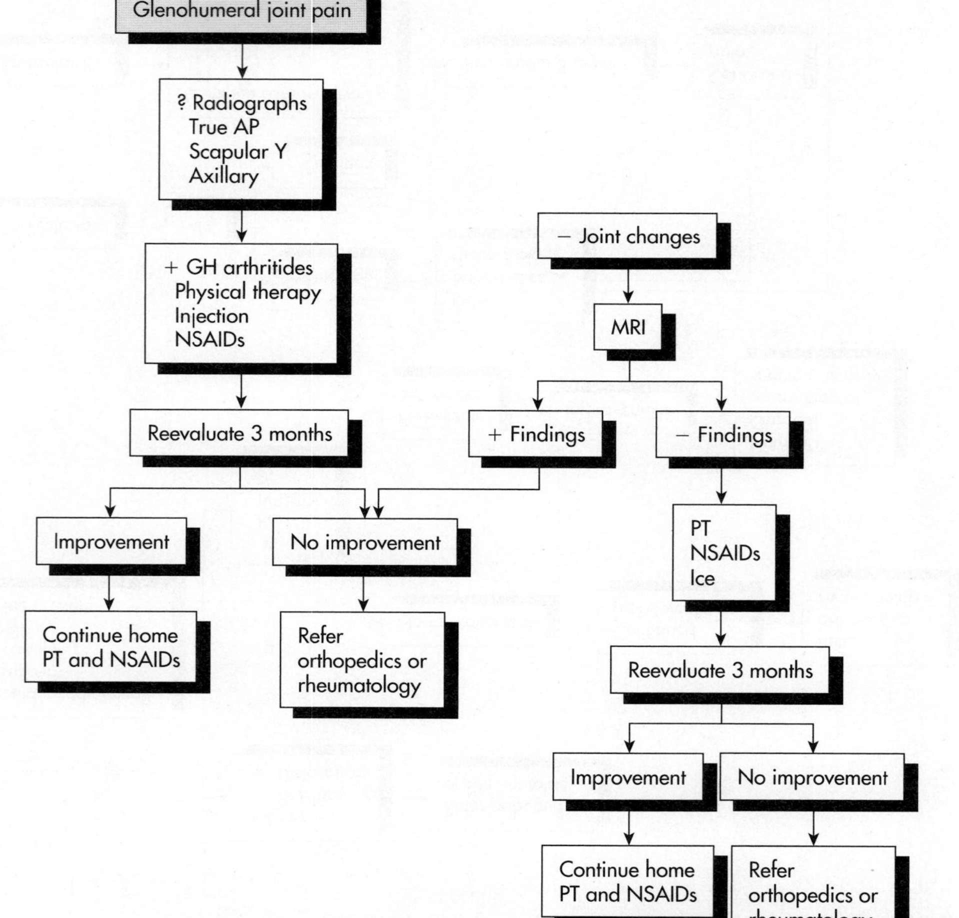

FIGURE 3-175 (Continued)

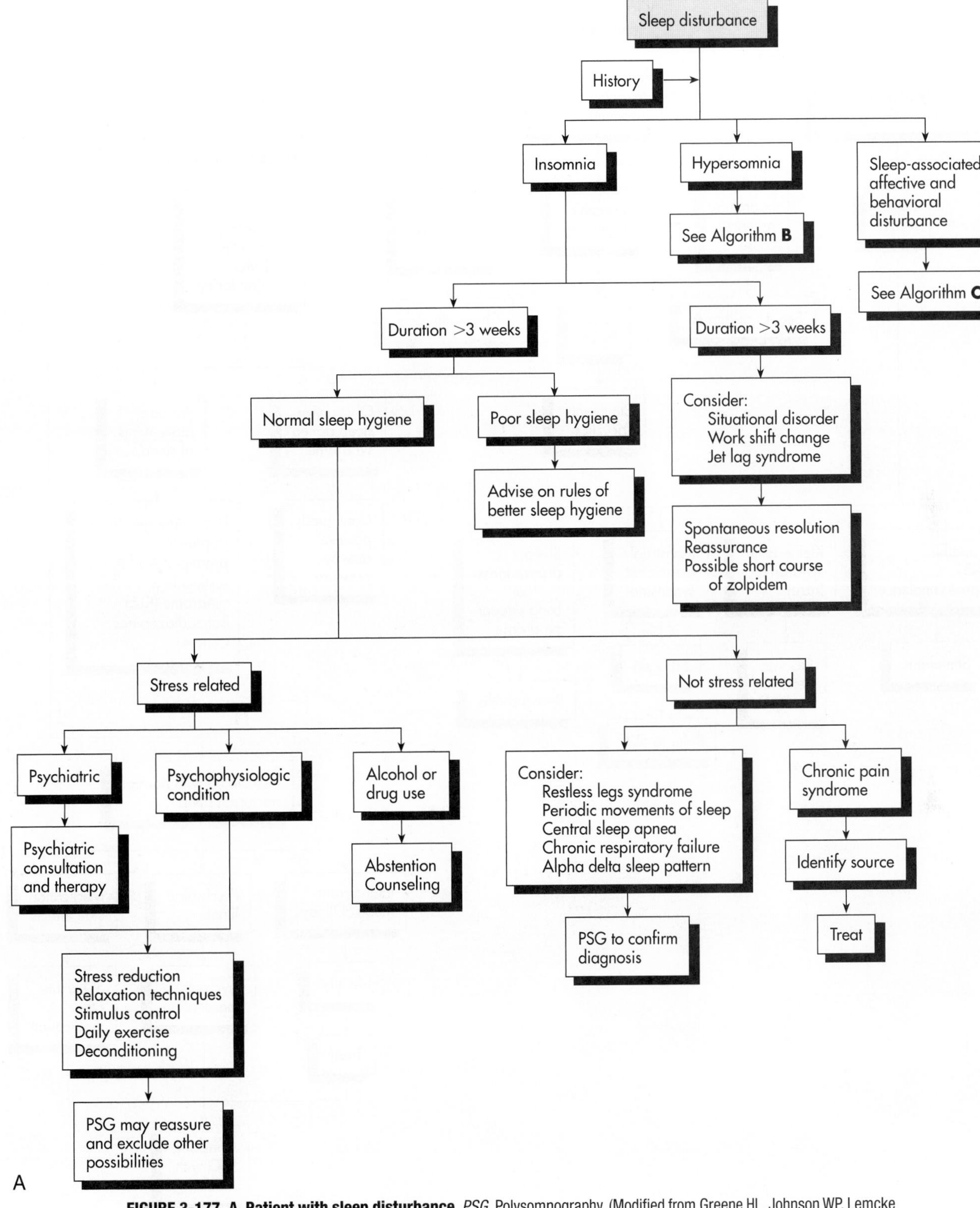

FIGURE 3-177 A, Patient with sleep disturbance. *PSG,* Polysomnography. (Modified from Greene HL, Johnson WP, Lemcke DL [eds]: *Decision making in medicine,* ed 2, St Louis, 1998, Mosby.)

Continued on following page

ICD-9CM # 780.50 Sleep disorder, unspecified cause
ICD-10CM # G47.9 Sleep disorder, unspecified

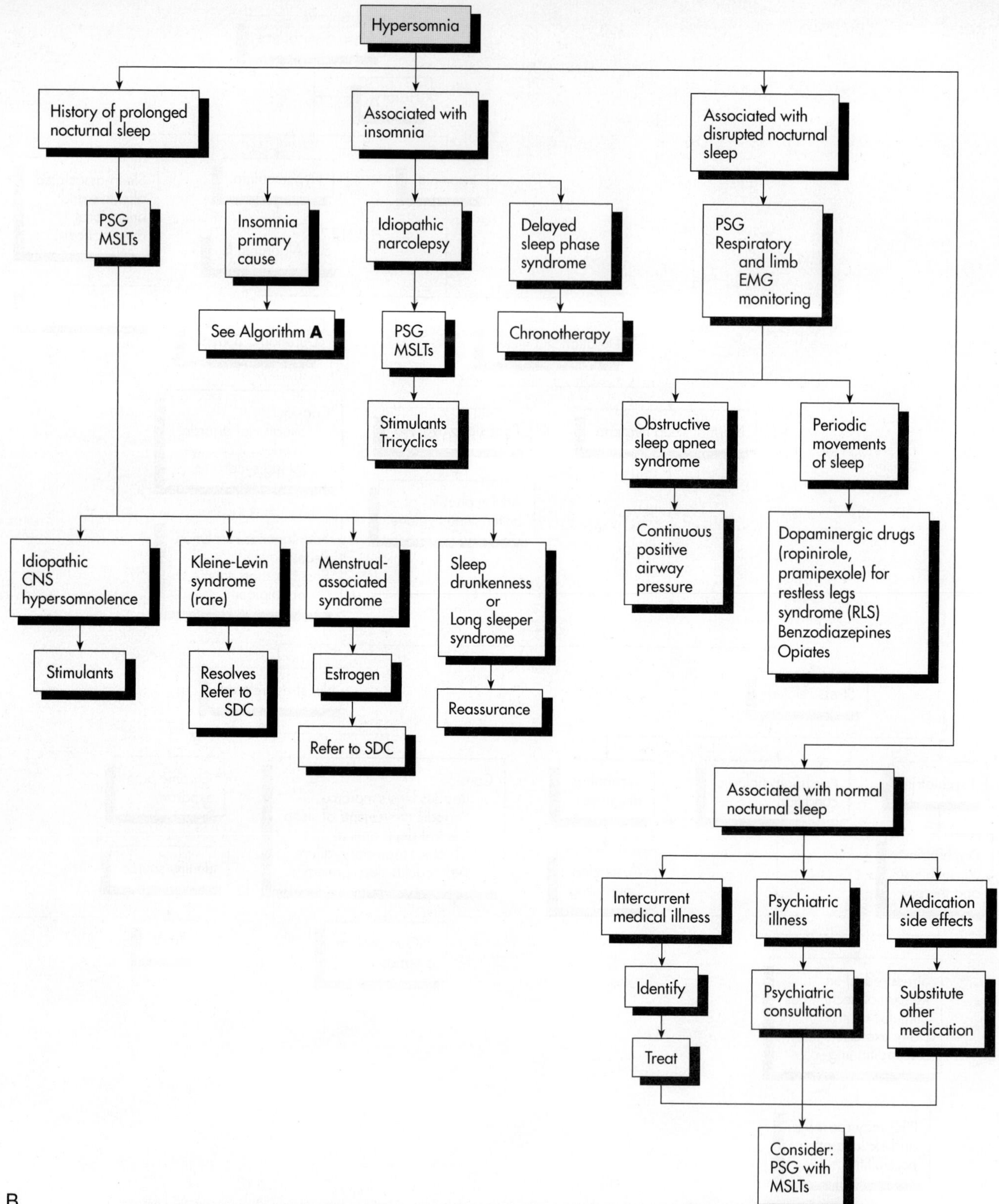

FIGURE 3-177 (Continued) **B, Hypersomnia.** *CNS,* Central nervous system; *EMG,* electromyelogram; *MSLTs,* multiple sleep latency tests; *PSG,* polysomnography; *SDC,* sleep disorders clinic. (Modified from Greene HL, Johnson WP, Lemcke DL [eds]: *Decision making in medicine,* ed 2, St Louis, 1998, Mosby.)

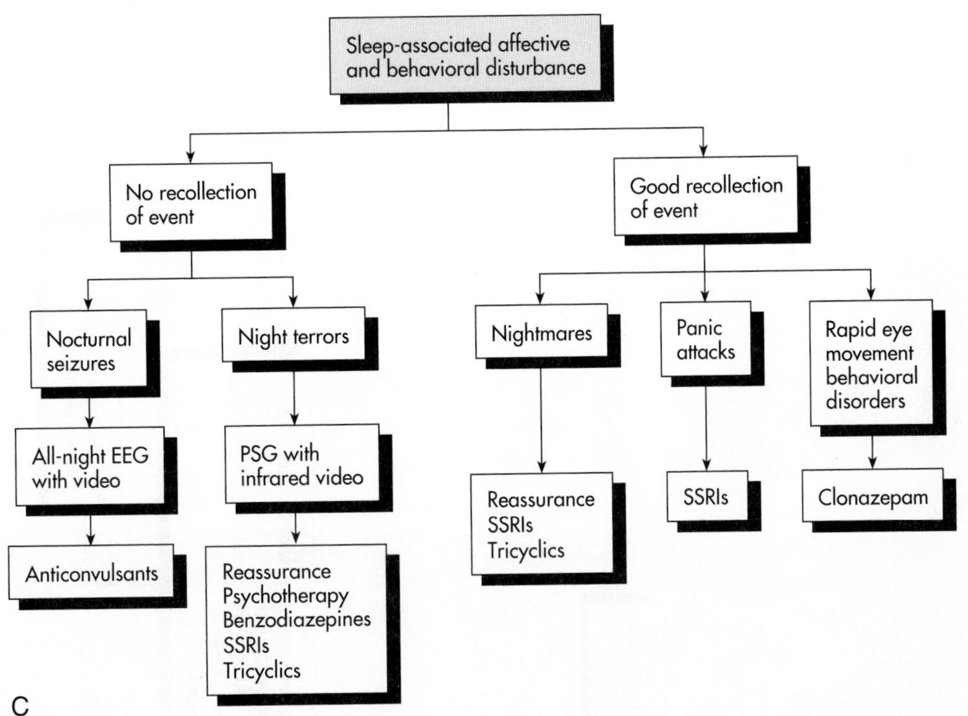

FIGURE 3-177 (Continued) **C, Sleep-associated affective and behavioral disturbance.** *EEG,* Electroencephalogram; *PSG,* polysomnography; *SSRIs,* selective serotonin reuptake inhibitors. (Modified from Greene HL, Johnson WP, Lemcke DL [eds]: *Decision making in medicine,*ed 2, St Louis, 1998, Mosby.)

SPLENOMEGALY

ICD-9CM #	789.2	Splenomegaly, unspecified
	289.51	Splenomegaly, chronic congestive
	759.0	Splenomegaly, congenital
	789.2	Splenomegaly, unknown etiology
ICD-10CM #	R16.1	Splenomegaly, not elsewhere classified
	D73.2	Chronic congestive splenomegaly
	Q89.01	Asplenia (congenital)
	Q89.09	Congenital malformations of spleen
	R16.1	Splenomegaly, not elsewhere classified

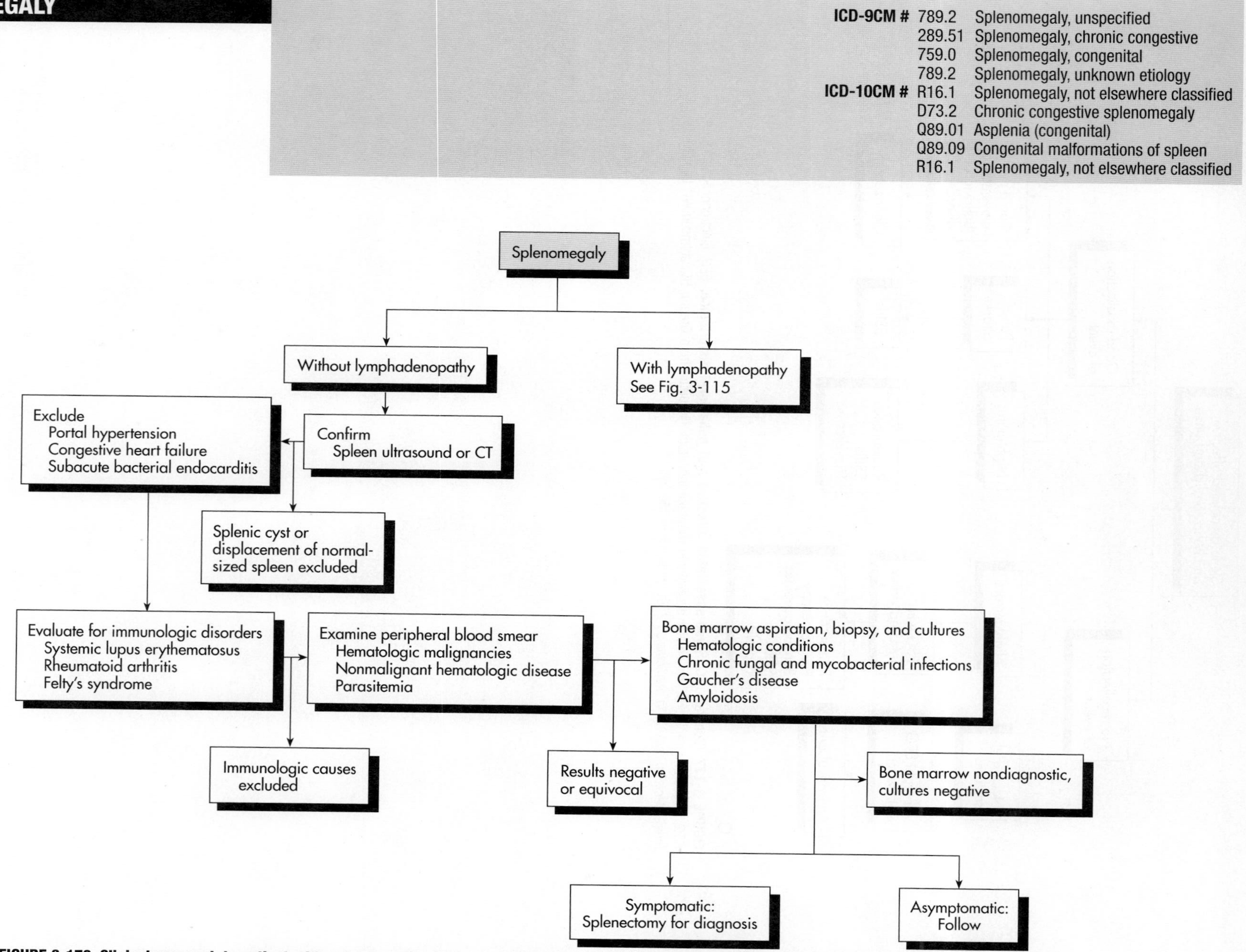

FIGURE 3-179 Clinical approach to patient with splenomegaly. *CT,* Computed tomography. (Modified from Stein JH [ed]: *Internal medicine,* ed 5, St Louis, 1998, Mosby.)

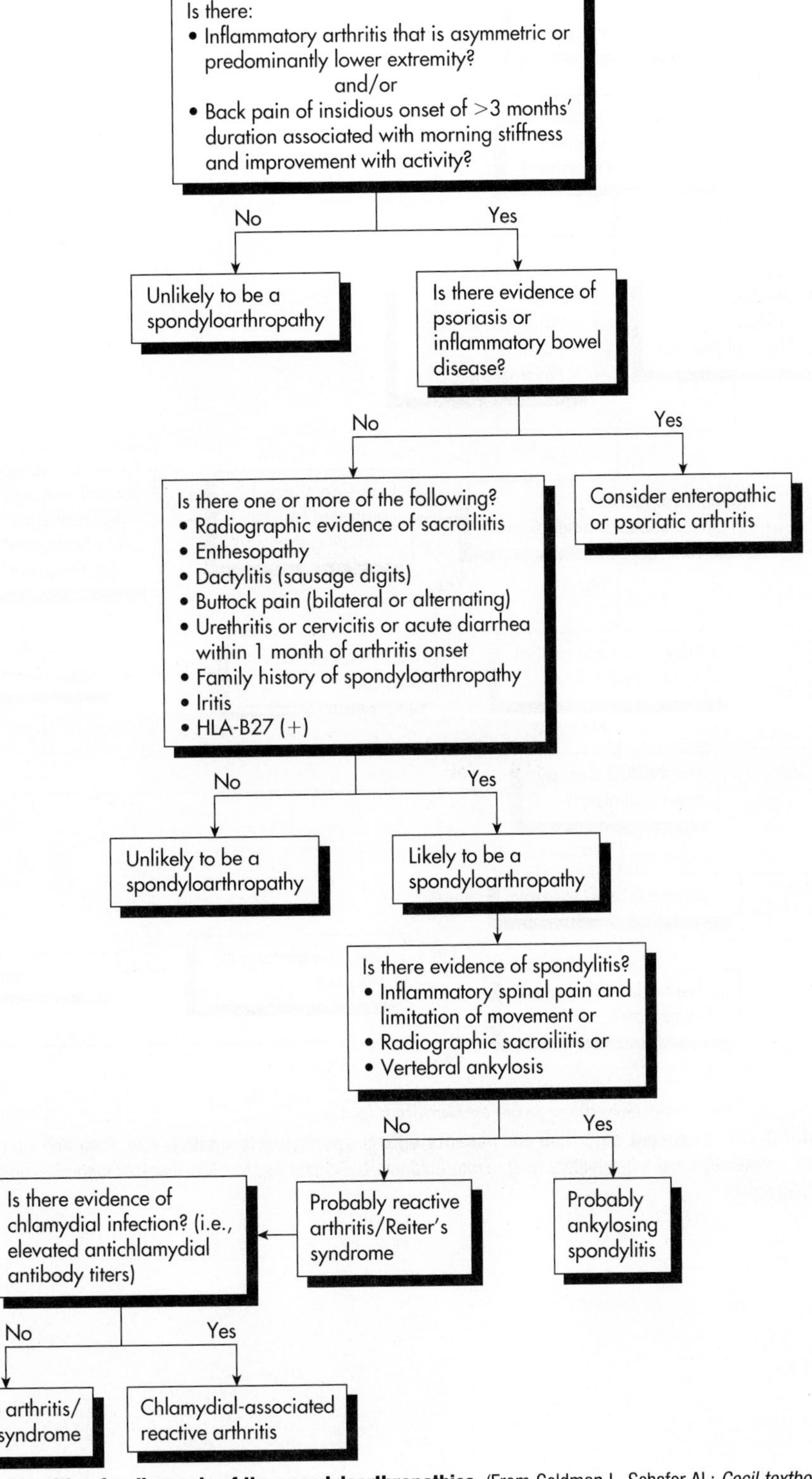

FIGURE 3-180 Algorithm for diagnosis of the spondyloarthropathies. (From Goldman L, Schafer AL: *Cecil textbook of medicine,* ed 24, Philadelphia, 2012, Saunders.)

ICD-9CM # 720.7
ICD-10CM # M46.90 Unspecified inflammatory spondylopathy, site unspecified

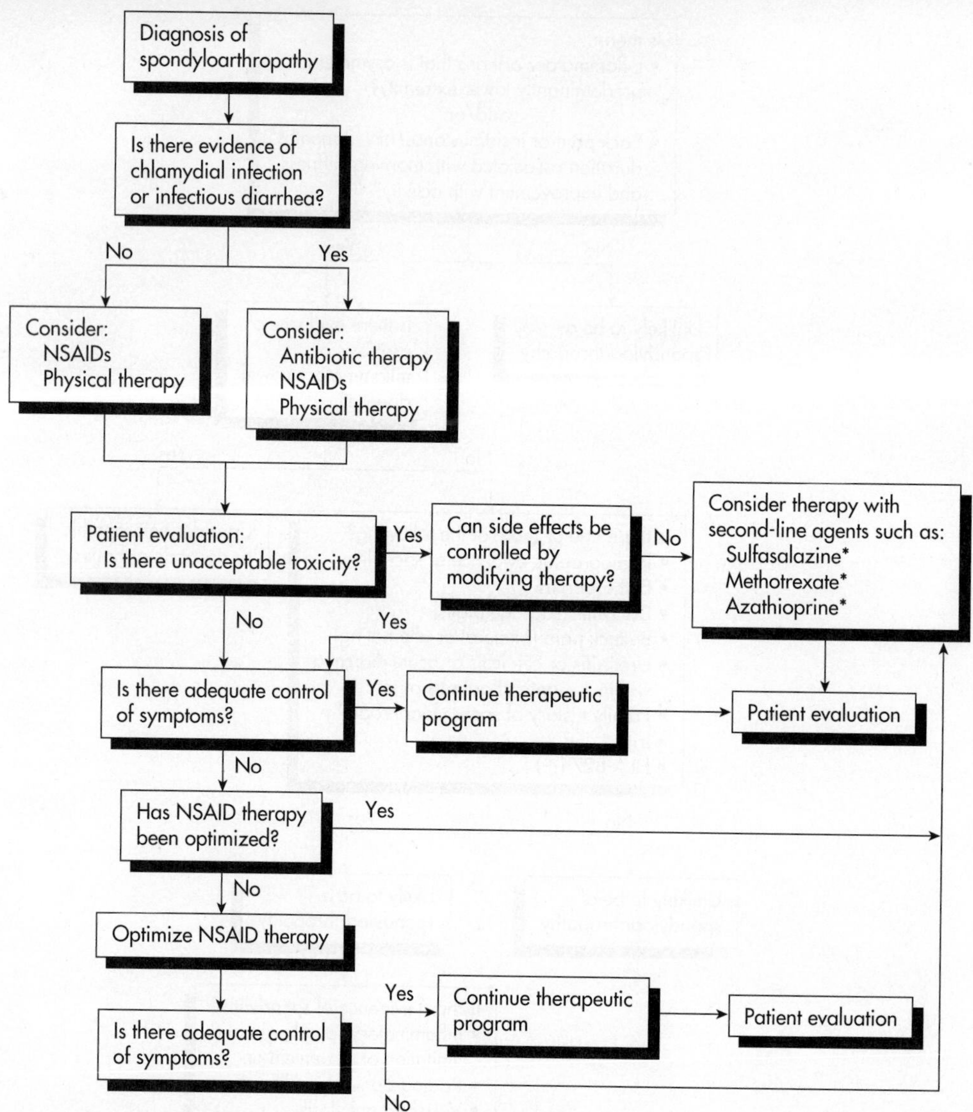

FIGURE 3-181 Treatment algorithm for patients with a spondyloarthropathy. *FDA,* Food and Drug Administration; *NSAID,* nonsteroidal anti-inflammatory drug. (From Goldman L, Schafer AL: *Cecil textbook of medicine,* ed 24, Philadelphia, 2012, Saunders.)

TACHYCARDIA, DIAGNOSTIC APPROACH

ICD-9CM # 785.0
ICD-10CM # R00.0 Tachycardia, unspecified

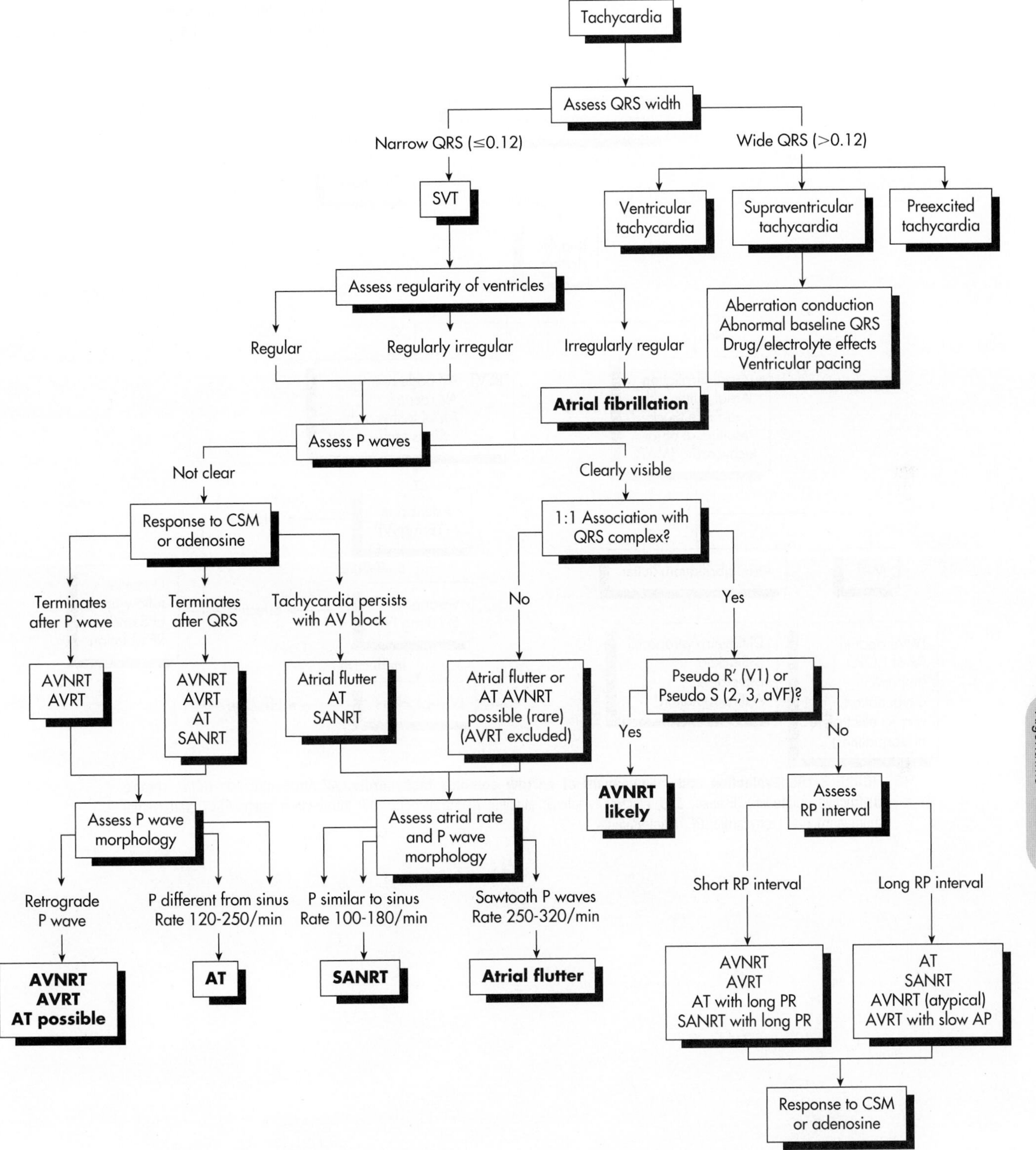

FIGURE 3-185 Stepwise approach to the diagnosis of type of tachycardia based on 12-lead electrocardiogram during the episode. The initial step is to determine whether the tachycardia has a wide or narrow QRS complex (see Fig. 3-186). For wide complex tachycardia, see Figure 3-188; the remainder of the algorithm is helpful in diagnosing the type of narrow-complex tachycardia. *AP,* Accessory pathway; *AT,* atrial tachycardia; *AV,* atrioventricular; *AVNRT,* AV nodal reentrant tachycardia; *AVRT,* AV reciprocating tachycardia; *CSM,* carotid sinus massage; *SANRT,* sinoatrial nodal reentry tachycardia; *SVT,* supraventricular tachycardia. (From Zipes DP, Libby P, Bonow RO, Braunwald E [eds]: *Braunwald's heart disease,* ed 7, Philadelphia, 2005, Saunders.)

ICD-9CM #	427.2	Paroxysmal tachycardia
	427.0	Supraventricular paroxysmal tachycardia
	427.42	Ventricular flutter
	427.1	Ventricular paroxysmal tachycardia
	427.89	Atrial tachycardia
ICD-10CM #	I49.02	Ventricular flutter
	I49.8	Other specified cardiac arrhythmias
	R00.1	Bradycardia, unspecified

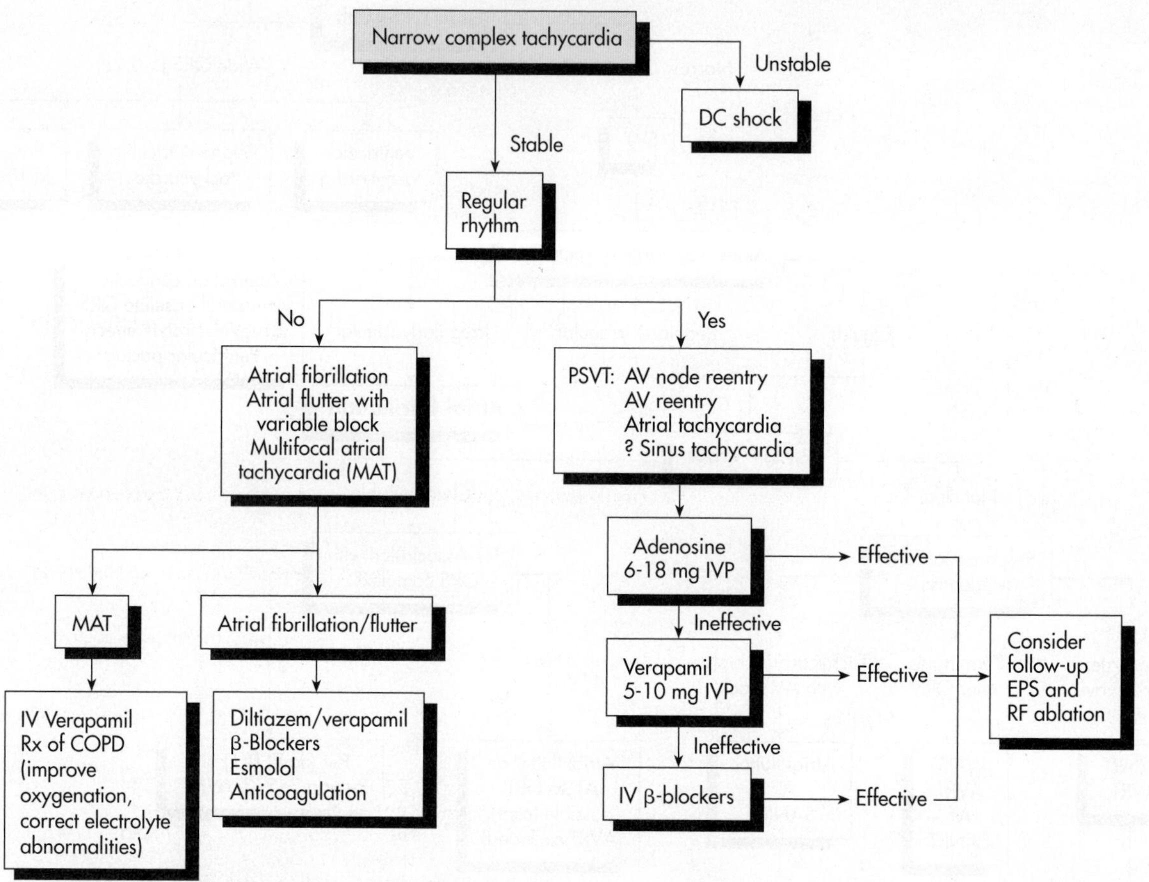

FIGURE 3-186 Evaluation and management of narrow complex tachycardia. *AV,* Atrioventricular; *COPD,* chronic obstructive pulmonary disease; *EPS,* electrophysiologic studies; *IV,* intravenous; *IVP,* intravenous push; *PSVT,* paroxysmal supraventricular tachycardia; *RF,* radiofrequency.

TACHYCARDIA, WIDE COMPLEX

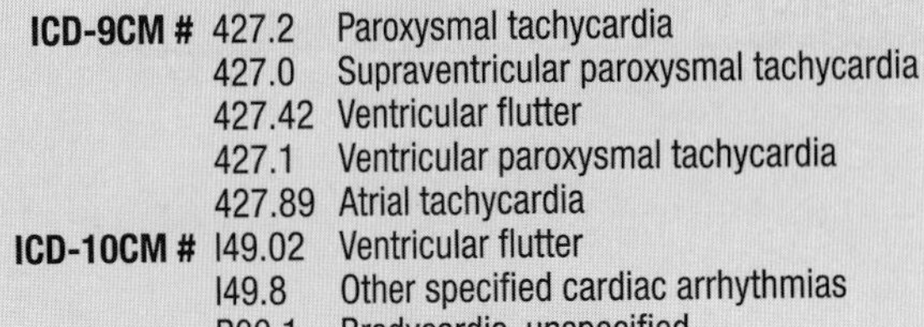

ICD-9CM #	427.2	Paroxysmal tachycardia
	427.0	Supraventricular paroxysmal tachycardia
	427.42	Ventricular flutter
	427.1	Ventricular paroxysmal tachycardia
	427.89	Atrial tachycardia
ICD-10CM #	I49.02	Ventricular flutter
	I49.8	Other specified cardiac arrhythmias
	R00.1	Bradycardia, unspecified

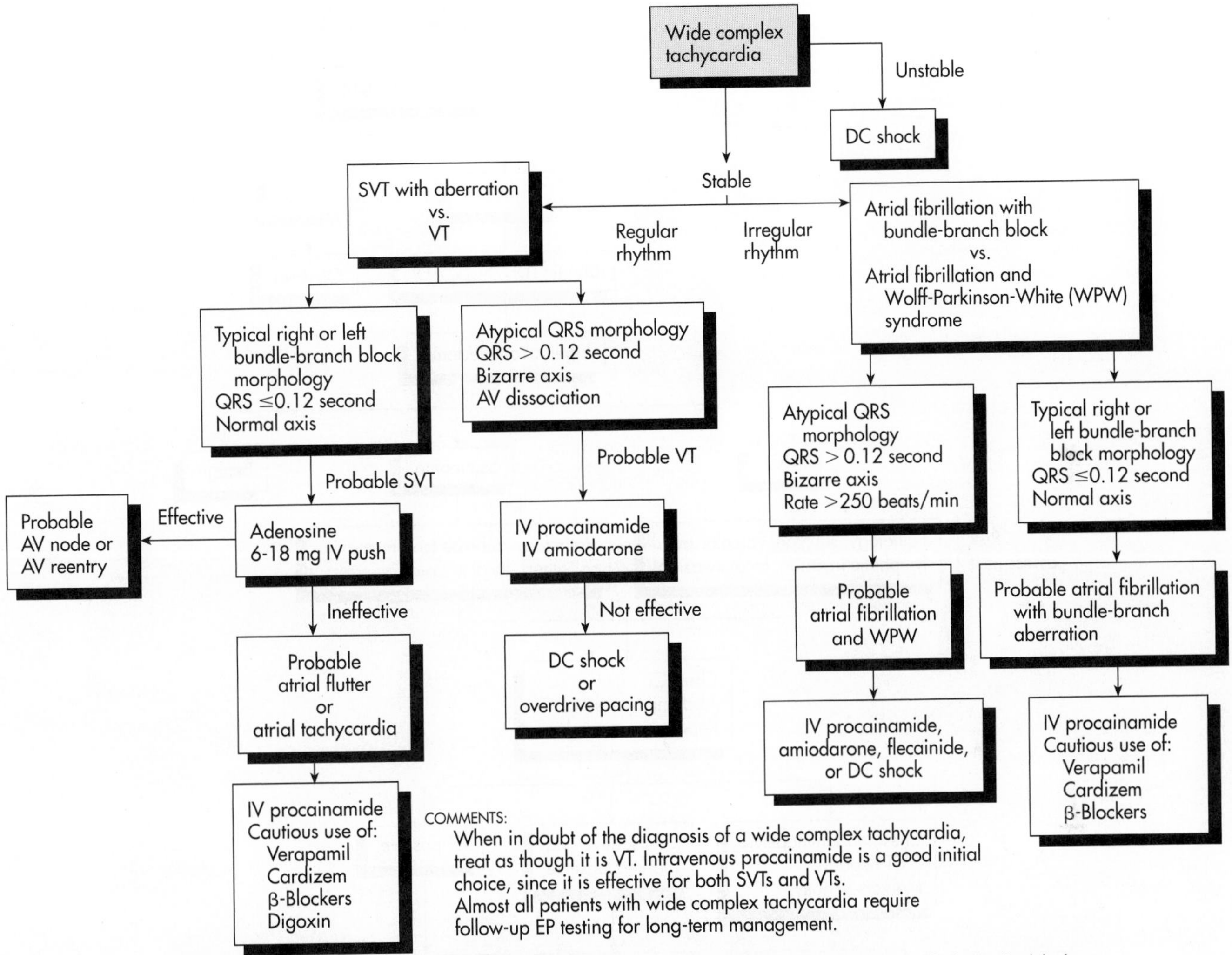

Wide complex tachycardia

Unstable

DC shock

Stable

Regular rhythm

Irregular rhythm

SVT with aberration vs. VT

Typical right or left bundle-branch block morphology
QRS ≤0.12 second
Normal axis

Probable SVT

Adenosine 6-18 mg IV push

Effective

Probable AV node or AV reentry

Ineffective

Probable atrial flutter or atrial tachycardia

IV procainamide
Cautious use of:
Verapamil
Cardizem
β-Blockers
Digoxin

Atypical QRS morphology
QRS > 0.12 second
Bizarre axis
AV dissociation

Probable VT

IV procainamide
IV amiodarone

Not effective

DC shock or overdrive pacing

Atrial fibrillation with bundle-branch block vs. Atrial fibrillation and Wolff-Parkinson-White (WPW) syndrome

Atypical QRS morphology
QRS > 0.12 second
Bizarre axis
Rate >250 beats/min

Probable atrial fibrillation and WPW

IV procainamide, amiodarone, flecainide, or DC shock

Typical right or left bundle-branch block morphology
QRS ≤0.12 second
Normal axis

Probable atrial fibrillation with bundle-branch aberration

IV procainamide
Cautious use of:
Verapamil
Cardizem
β-Blockers

COMMENTS:
When in doubt of the diagnosis of a wide complex tachycardia, treat as though it is VT. Intravenous procainamide is a good initial choice, since it is effective for both SVTs and VTs.
Almost all patients with wide complex tachycardia require follow-up EP testing for long-term management.

FIGURE 3-188 Evaluation and management of wide complex tachycardia. *AV,* Atrioventricular; *EP,* electrophysiologic; *IV,* intravenous; *SVT,* supraventricular tachycardia; *VT,* ventricular tachycardia. (From Driscoll CE et al: *The family practice desk reference,* ed 3, St Louis, 1996, Mosby.)

TABLE 3-31 Major Features in the Differential Diagnosis of Wide QRS Beats

Supports SVT	Supports VT
Slowing or termination by vagal tone	Fusion beats
Onset with premature P wave	Capture beats
RP interval <100 msec	AV dissociation
P and QRS rate and rhythm linked to suggest that ventricular activation depends on atrial discharge, e.g., 2:1 AV block rSR′ V1	P and QRS rate and rhythm linked to suggest that atrial activation depends on ventricular discharge, e.g., 2:1 VA block
Long-short cycle sequence	"Compensatory" pause
	Left axis deviation; QRS duration >140 msec
	Specific QRS contours (see text)

From Zipes DP et al [eds]: *Braunwauld's heart disease,* ed 7, Philadelphia, 2005, Saunders.
SVT, Supraventricular tachycardia; *VT,* ventricular tachycardia.

ICD-9CM #	186.9	Testicular neoplasm
	M906/3	(seminoma)
	M9101/3	(embryonal carcinoma or teratoma)
	M9100/3	(choriocarcinoma)
ICD-10CM #	C62.90	Malignant neoplasm of unspecified testis, unspecified whether descended or undescended

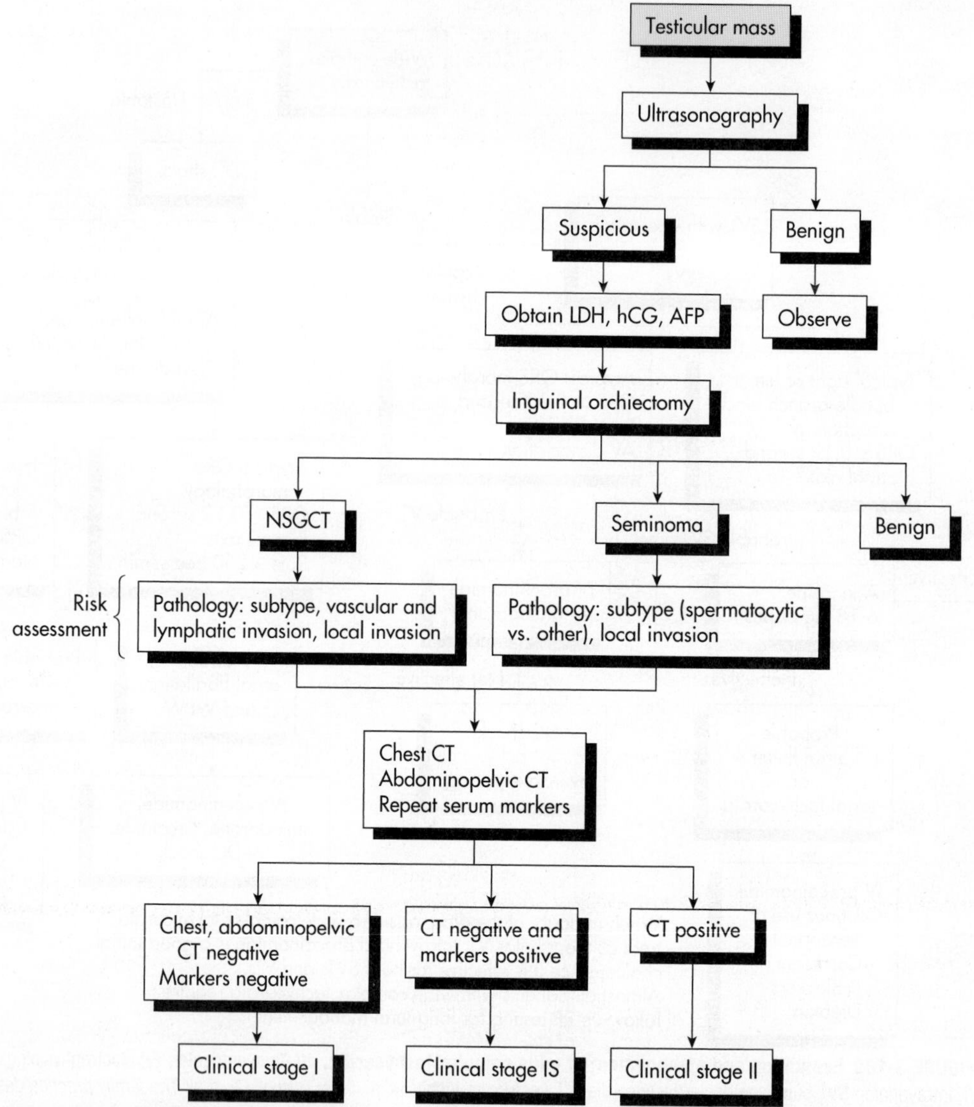

FIGURE 3-189 Diagnosis, staging, and risk assessment of patients with testicular germ cell tumor. *AFP,* α-fetoprotein; *CT,* computed tomography; *hCG,* human chorionic gonadotropin; *LDH,* lactic dehydrogenase; *NSGCT,* nonseminoma germ cell tumor. (From Abeloff MD: *Clinical oncology,* ed 4, New York, 2007, Churchill Livingstone.)

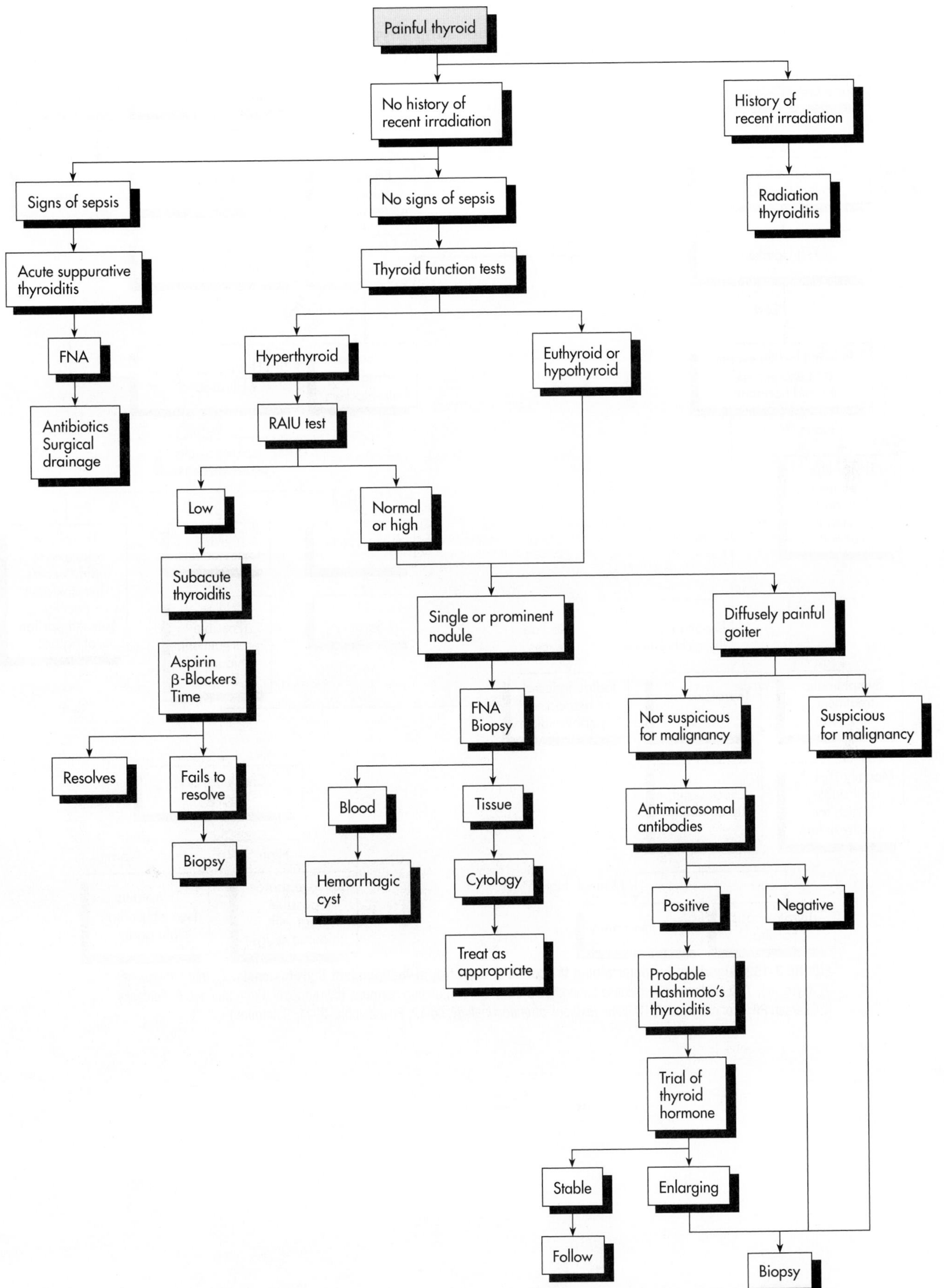
Painful thyroid
No history of recent irradiation
History of recent irradiation
Radiation thyroiditis
Signs of sepsis
No signs of sepsis
Acute suppurative thyroiditis
FNA
Antibiotics Surgical drainage
Thyroid function tests
Hyperthyroid
Euthyroid or hypothyroid
RAIU test
Low
Normal or high
Subacute thyroiditis
Aspirin β-Blockers Time
Resolves
Fails to resolve
Biopsy
Single or prominent nodule
Diffusely painful goiter
FNA Biopsy
Blood
Tissue
Hemorrhagic cyst
Cytology
Treat as appropriate
Not suspicious for malignancy
Suspicious for malignancy
Antimicrosomal antibodies
Positive
Negative
Probable Hashimoto's thyroiditis
Trial of thyroid hormone
Stable
Enlarging
Follow
Biopsy

FIGURE 3-191 Painful thyroid. *FNA,* Fine-needle aspiration; *RAIU,* radioactive iodine uptake. (From Greene HL, Johnson WP, Lemcke DL [eds]: *Decision making in medicine,* ed 2, St Louis, 1998, Mosby.)

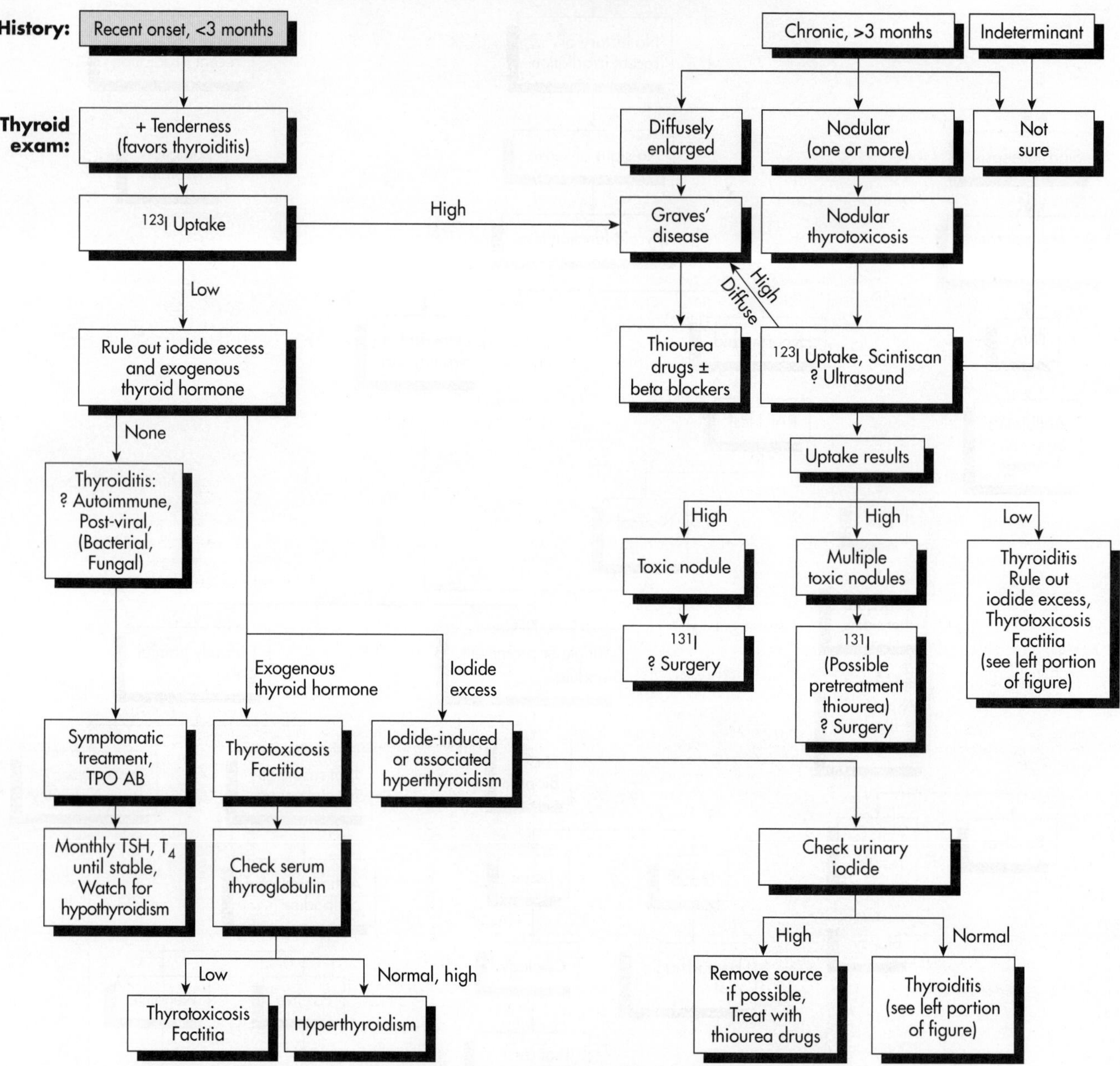

FIGURE 3-192 Algorithm for determining the cause of thyrotropin-independent thyrotoxicosis. *T_3*, triiodothyronine; *T_4*, thyroxine; *TPO AB*, thyroid peroxidase antibody; *TSH*, thyroid-stimulating hormone (thyrotropin). (From Melmed S, Polonsky KS, Larsen PR, Kronenberg HM, *Williams textbook of endocrinology*, ed 12, Philadelphia, 2011, Saunders.)

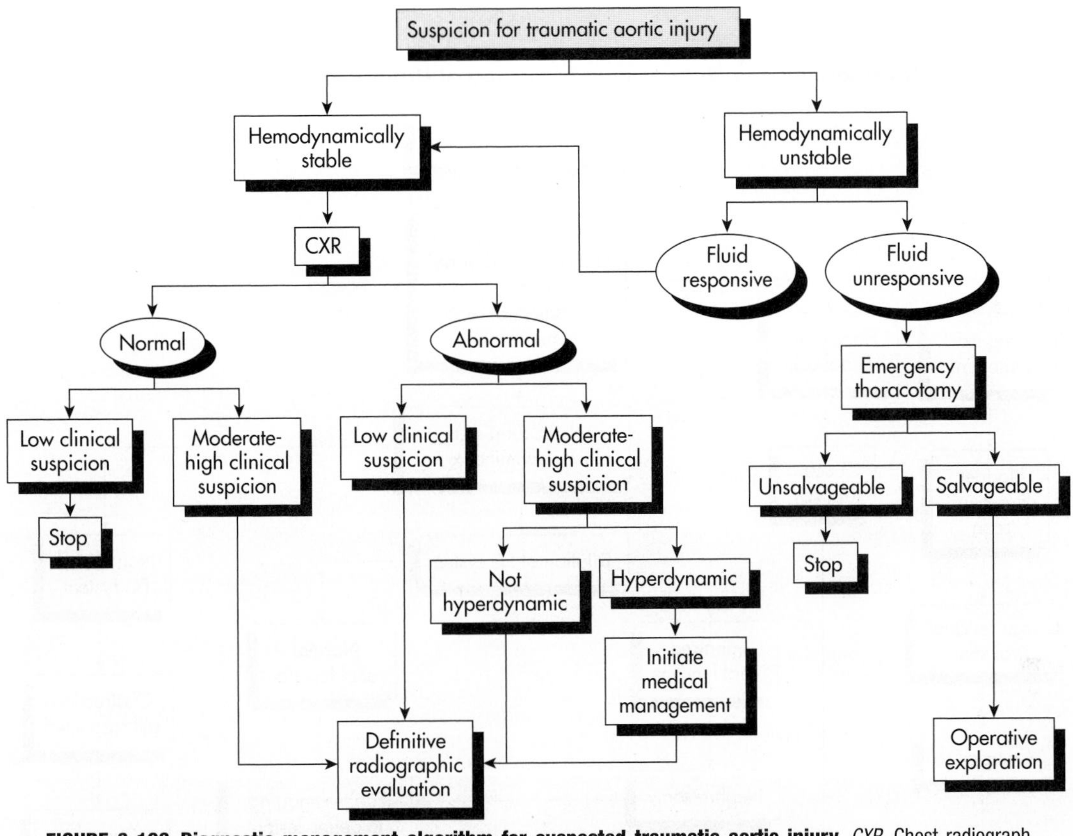

FIGURE 3-193 Diagnostic management algorithm for suspected traumatic aortic injury. *CXR*, Chest radiograph. (From Adams JG, et al: *Emergency medicine, clinical essentials*, ed 2, Philadelphia, 2013, Elsevier.)

BOX 3-9 Pros and Cons of Imaging Modalities for Great Vessel Injury

Chest Radiography

Pros
- Inexpensive
- Performed at the bedside
- Easy to interpret

Cons
- Nonspecific
- False-negative rate of 7% to 10% for traumatic aortic injury

Computed Tomographic Angiography

Pros
- Identifies mediastinal hematoma and differentiates its causes
- Identifies aortic injury, including intimal tears
- Sensitivity and specificity approaching 100% for traumatic aortic injury

Cons
- Poor delineation of nonaortic vascular injuries
- Requires relative hemodynamic stability to obtain

Aortography

Pros
- Traditional “gold standard”
- Beneficial in the diagnosis of branch vessel injuries
- Delineates equivocal computed tomographic angiographic findings

Cons
- Difficult to obtain on an emergency basis
- Requires relative hemodynamic stability

Transesophageal Echocardiography

Pros
- May be performed at the bedside
- Not limited by body habitus

Cons
- Poor availability on an emergency basis
- Contraindicated in patients with an unstable cervical spine or suspected esophageal trauma

(From Adams JG, et al: *Emergency medicine, clinical essentials*, ed 2, Philadelphia, 2013, Elsevier.)

ICD-9CM # varies with specific diagnosis
ICD-10CM # N21.8 Other lower urinary tract calculus

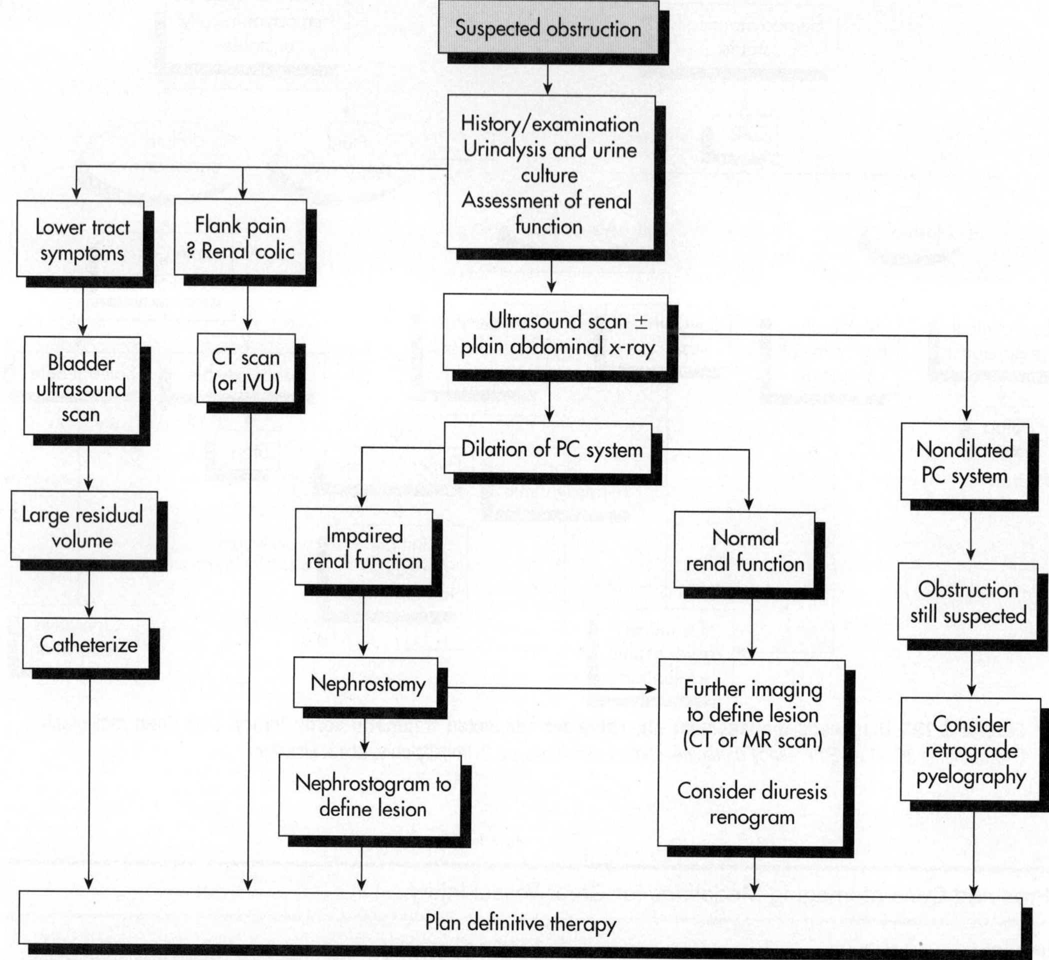

FIGURE 3-195 Investigation and management of suspected urinary tract obstruction. A full history and examination should be performed together with urinalysis, urine microscopy and culture, and measurement of renal function and serum electrolytes. Ultrasound is a useful first-line investigation for any patient with suspected urinary tract obstruction. Helical (spiral) computed tomography (CT) is now the preferred imaging technique when renal calculi are suspected. Either CT or magnetic resonance (MRI) urography can accurately diagnose both the site and the cause of obstruction in most cases. If there is renal impairment, insertion of a nephrostomy allows the effective relief of the obstruction and time for renal function to recover while definitive therapy is planned. *IVU,* Intravenous urography; *PC,* pelvicalyceal. (From Floege J et al: *Comprehensive clinical nephrology,* ed 4, Philadelphia, 2010, Saunders.)

BOX 3-10 Diagnostic Tests Used in Obstructive Uropathy

Upper Urinary Tract Obstruction	Lower Urinary Tract Obstruction
Sonography (ultrasound)	Some of the tests listed at left
Plain films of the abdomen (KUB)	Cystoscopy
Excretory or intravenous pyelography (very rarely needed)	Voiding cystourethrogram
Retrograde pyelography	Retrograde urethrography
Isotopic renography	Urodynamic tests
Computed tomography (helical CT)	Debimetry
Magnetic resonance imaging	Cystometrography
Pressure flow studies (the Whitaker test)	Electromyography
	Urethral pressure profile

KUB, Kidneys, ureter, bladder.

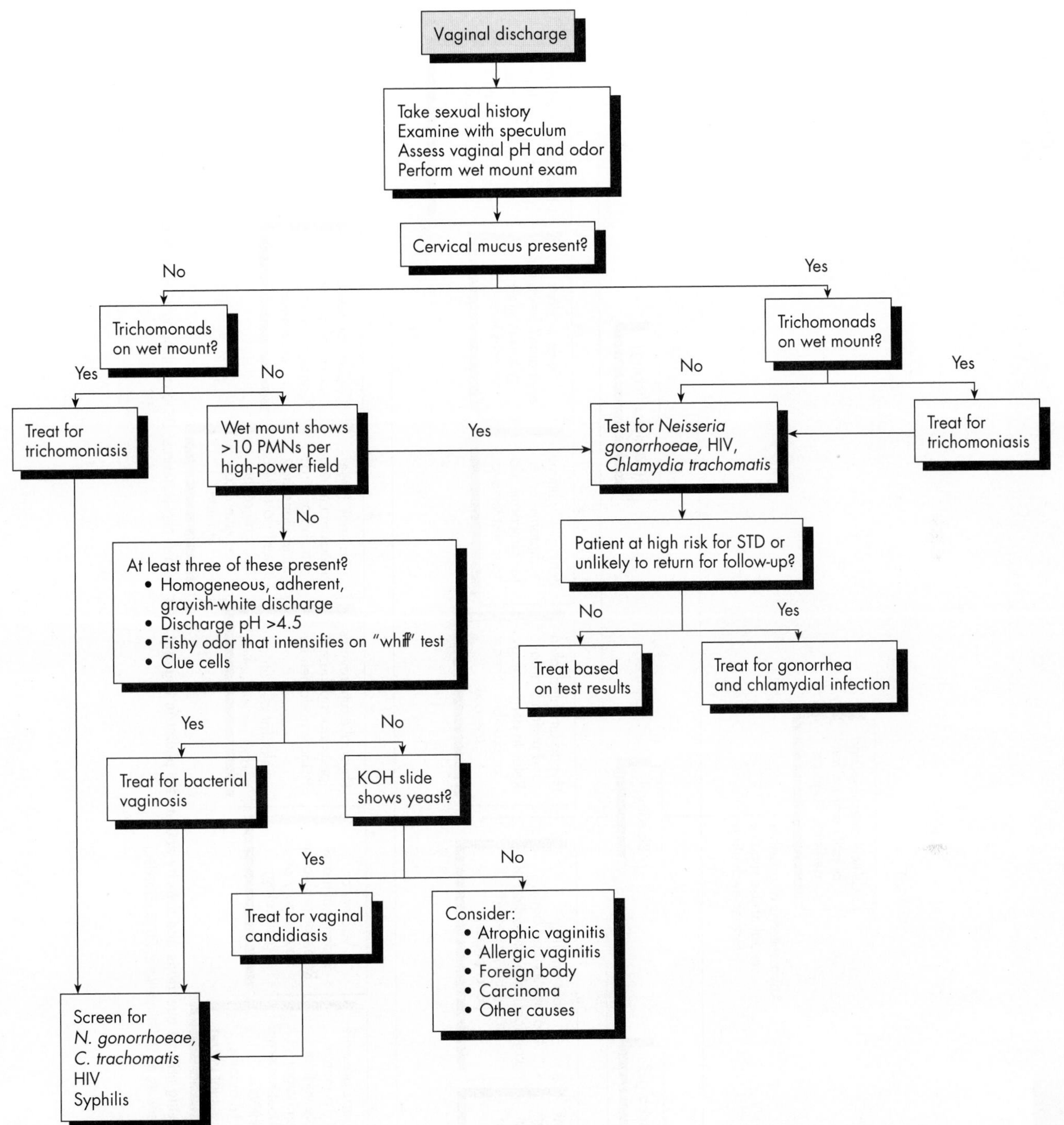

FIGURE 3-196 Evaluation of vaginal discharge. *HIV*, Human immunodeficiency virus; *KOH*, potassium hydroxide; *PMN*, polymorphonuclear leukocyte; *STD*, sexually transmitted disease.

ICD-9CM # 616.10
ICD-10CM # N76.0

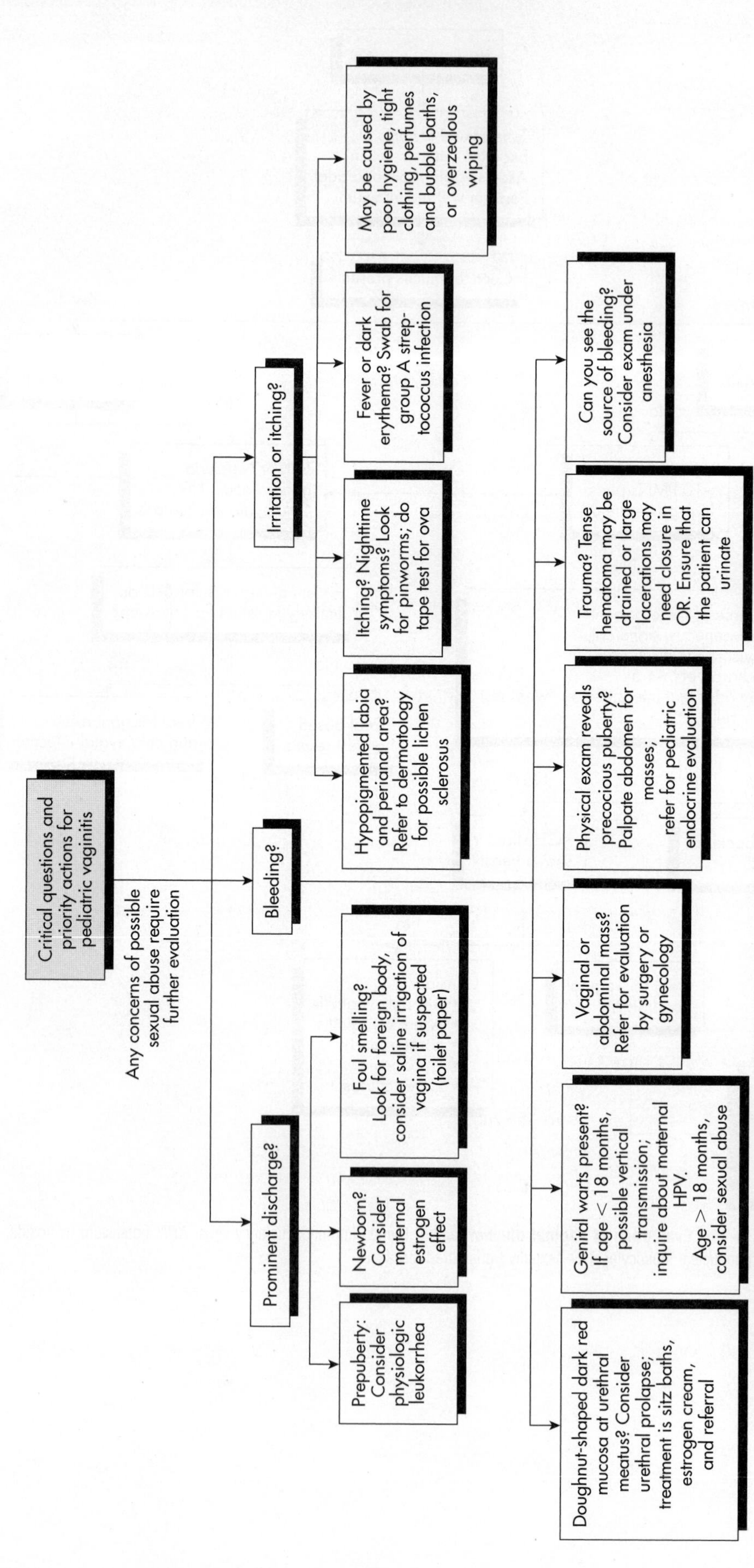

FIGURE 3-198 Algorithm showing critical questions and priority actions for pediatric vaginitis. *HPV*, Human papillomavirus; *OR*, operating room. (From Adams JG, et al: *Emergency medicine, clinical essentials*, ed 2, Philadelphia, 2013, Elsevier.)

VENTRICULAR FIBRILLATION OR PULSELESS VENTRICULAR TACHYCARDIA

ICD-9CM # 427.41 Ventricular fibrillation
427.1 Ventricular tachycardia
ICD-10CM # I49.01 Ventricular fibrillation

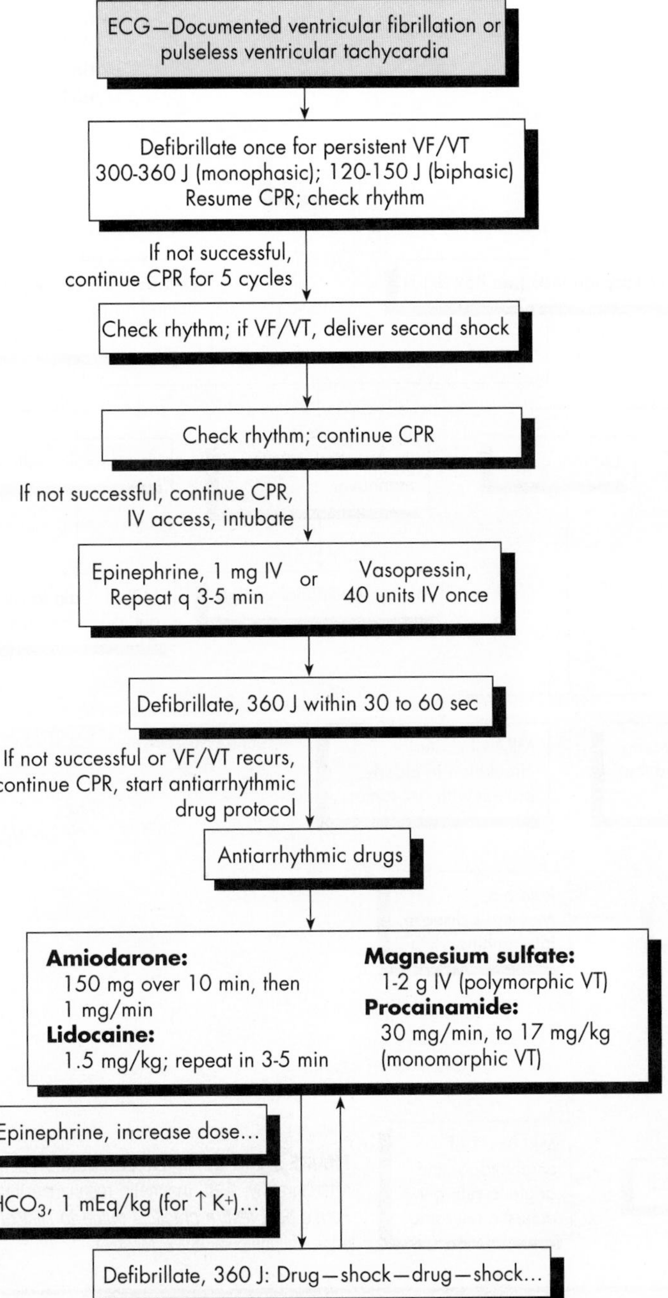

FIGURE 3-199 General algorithm for advanced cardiac life support (ACLS) response to ventricular fibrillation (VF) or pulseless ventricular tachycardia (VT). *Note:* In a 2008 advisory, 200 compression-only sequences were suggested as an alternative to standard CPR cycles between shocks, and this approach is under consideration for future guidelines. *CPR,* Cardiopulmonary resuscitation; *ECG,* electrocardiogram. (From Goldman L, Schafer AI: *Goldman's Cecil medicine,* ed 24, Philadelphia, 2012, Saunders.)

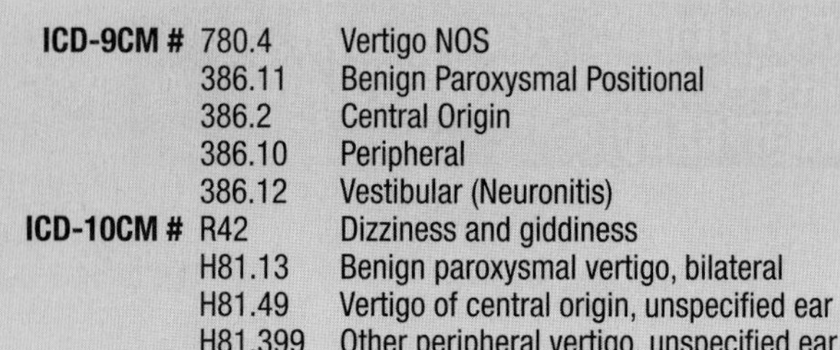

ICD-9CM #	780.4	Vertigo NOS
	386.11	Benign Paroxysmal Positional
	386.2	Central Origin
	386.10	Peripheral
	386.12	Vestibular (Neuronitis)
ICD-10CM #	R42	Dizziness and giddiness
	H81.13	Benign paroxysmal vertigo, bilateral
	H81.49	Vertigo of central origin, unspecified ear
	H81.399	Other peripheral vertigo, unspecified ear
	H81.23	Vestibular neuronitis, bilateral

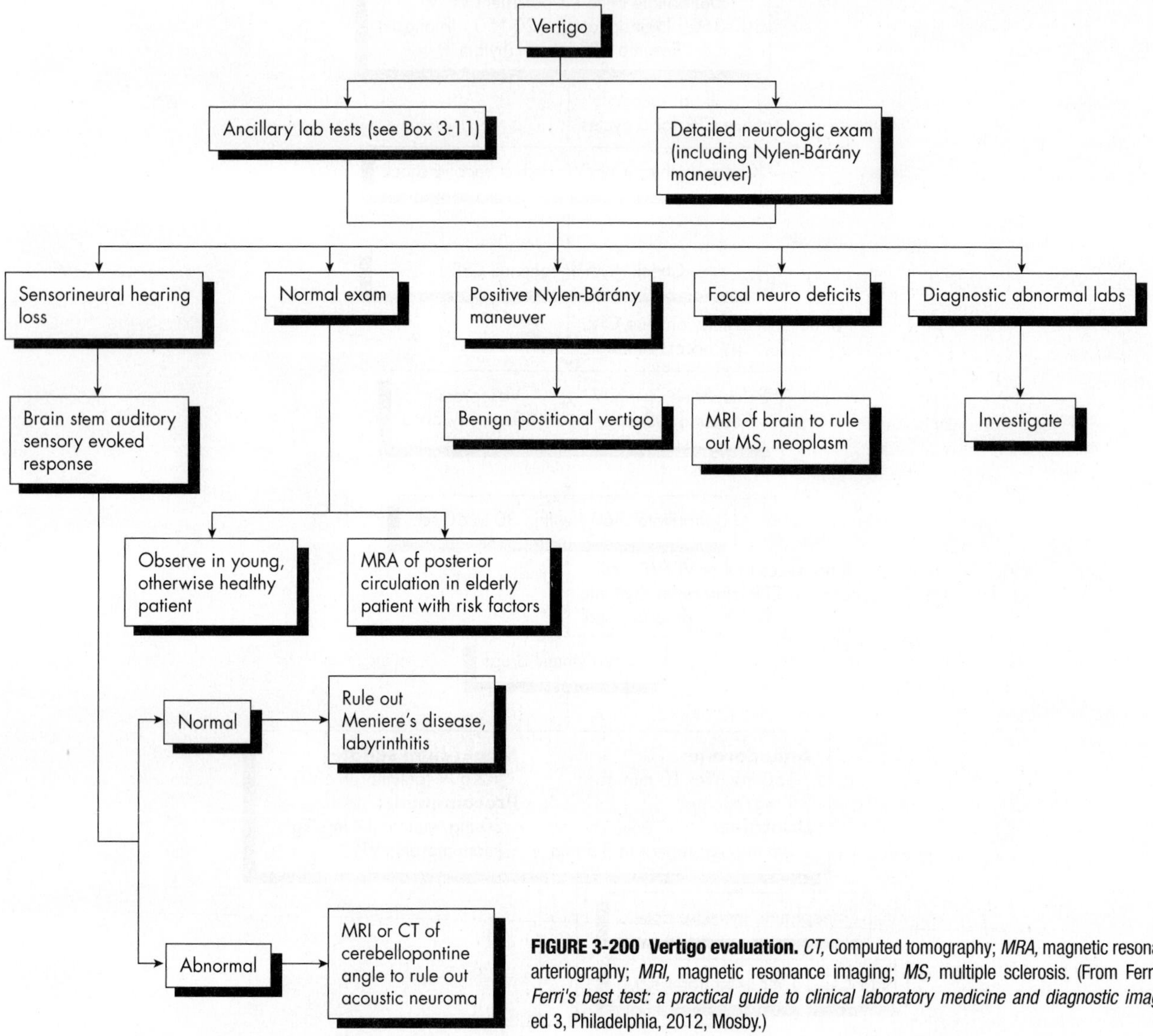

Vertigo

Ancillary lab tests (see Box 3-11)

Detailed neurologic exam (including Nylen-Bárány maneuver)

Sensorineural hearing loss

Normal exam

Positive Nylen-Bárány maneuver

Focal neuro deficits

Diagnostic abnormal labs

Brain stem auditory sensory evoked response

Benign positional vertigo

MRI of brain to rule out MS, neoplasm

Investigate

Observe in young, otherwise healthy patient

MRA of posterior circulation in elderly patient with risk factors

Normal

Rule out Meniere's disease, labyrinthitis

Abnormal

MRI or CT of cerebellopontine angle to rule out acoustic neuroma

FIGURE 3-200 Vertigo evaluation. *CT,* Computed tomography; *MRA,* magnetic resonance arteriography; *MRI,* magnetic resonance imaging; *MS,* multiple sclerosis. (From Ferri FF: *Ferri's best test: a practical guide to clinical laboratory medicine and diagnostic imaging,* ed 3, Philadelphia, 2012, Mosby.)

BOX 3-11 Vertigo

Diagnostic Imaging
Best Test
MRI of brain

Ancillary Tests
MRA of posterior circulation
CT of cerebellopontine region if MRI is contraindicated

Lab evaluation
Best test
None

Ancillary Tests
CBC with differential
Serum glucose, creatinine, ALT, electrolytes

From Ferri FF: *Ferri's best test: a practical guide to clinical laboratory medicine and diagnostic imaging,* ed 2, Philadelphia, 2009, Elsevier Mosby.

ALT, Alanine aminotransferase; *CBC,* complete blood count; *CT,* computed tomography; *MRA,* magnetic resonance angiography; *MRI,* magnetic resonance imaging.

ICD-9CM # 787.03 Vomiting
ICD-10CM # R11.10 Vomiting, unspecified
R11.11 Vomiting without nausea
R11.12 Projectile vomiting

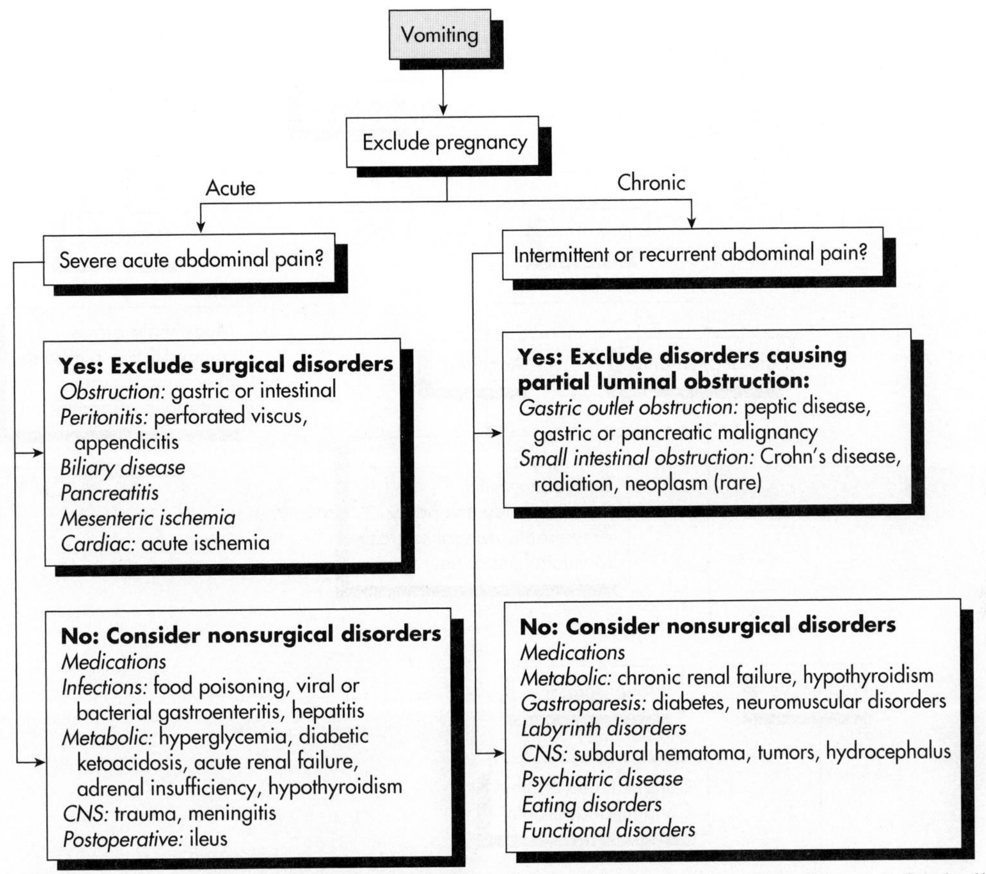

FIGURE 3-201 Approach to the patient with vomiting. *CNS,* Central nervous system. (From Goldman L, Schafer AI: *Goldman's Cecil medicine,* ed 24, Philadelphia, 2012, Saunders.)

ICD-9CM # 780.79
ICD-10CM # G93.3 Postviral fatigue syndrome
R53.1 Weakness
R53.81 Other malaise
R53.83 Other fatigue

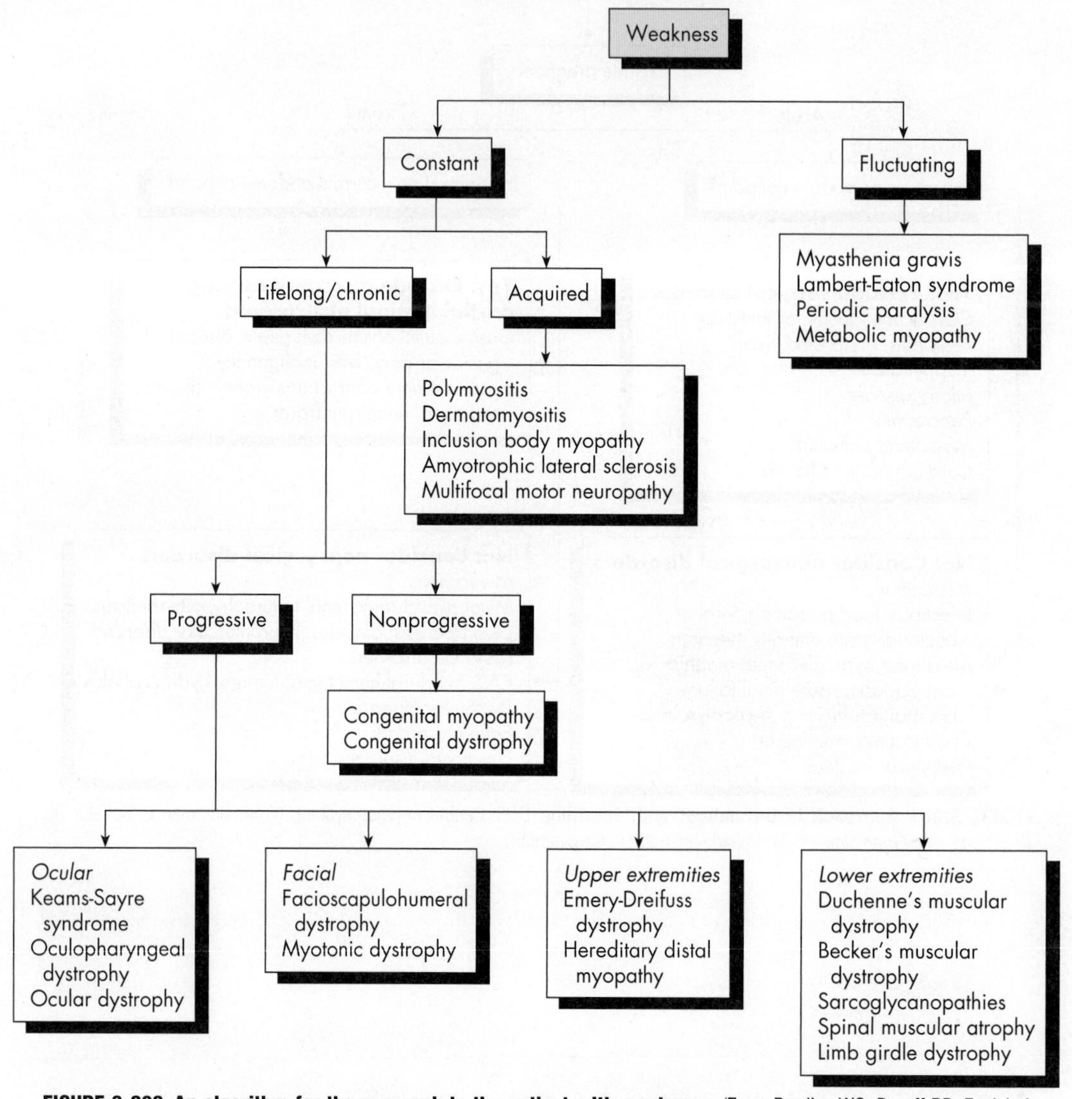

FIGURE 3-202 An algorithm for the approach to the patient with weakness. (From Bradley WG, Daroff RB, Fenichel GM, Jankovic J [eds]: *Neurology in clinical practice,* ed 4, Philadelphia, 2004, Butterworth Heinemann.)

WEIGHT GAIN

ICD-9CM #	783.1	Abnormal weight gain
	278.00	Obesity
ICD-10CM #	R63.5	Abnormal weight gain
	E66.9	Obesity, unspecified

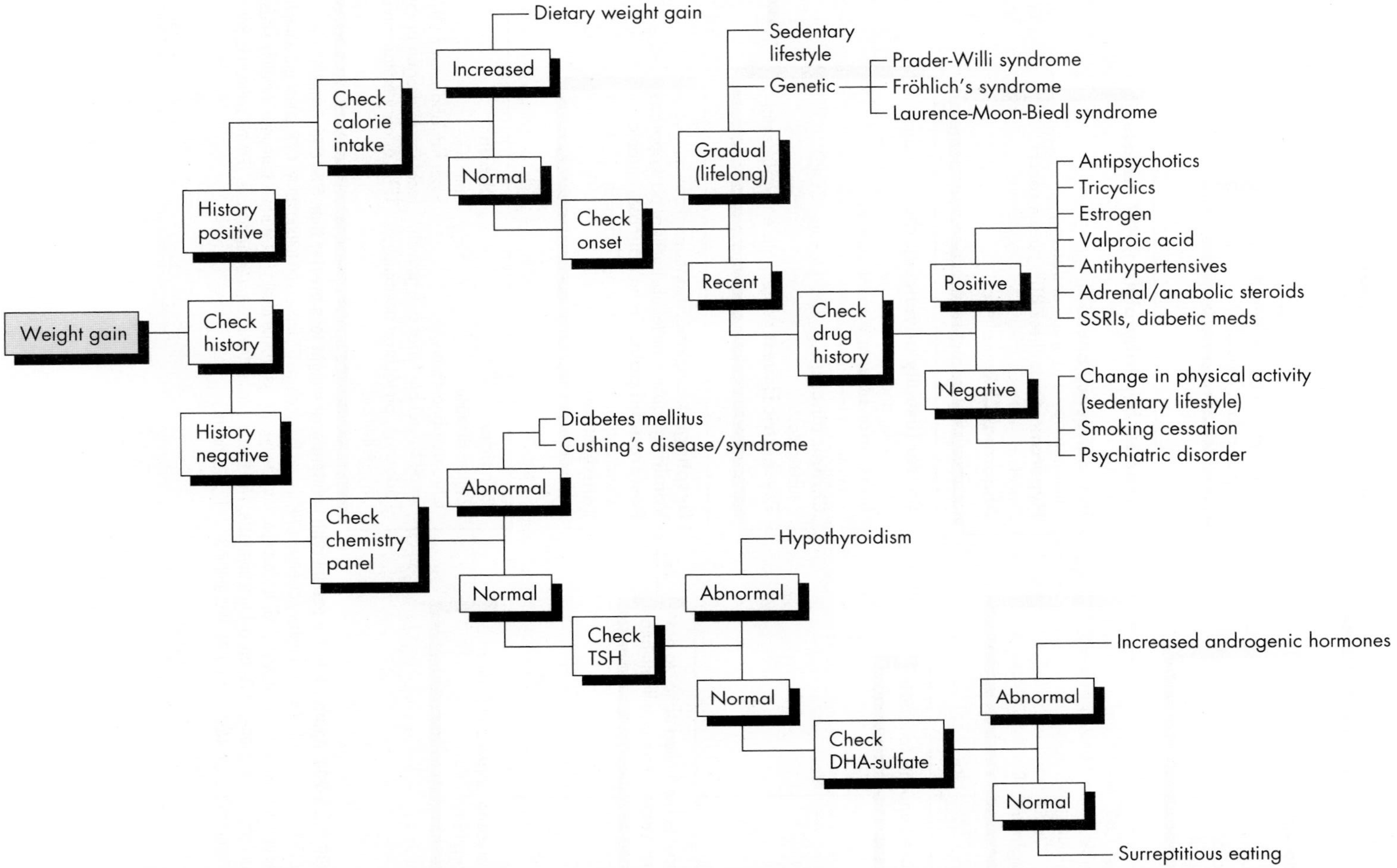

- Weight gain
  - Check history
    - History positive
      - Check calorie intake
        - Increased
          - Dietary weight gain
        - Normal
          - Check onset
            - Gradual (lifelong)
              - Sedentary lifestyle
              - Genetic
                - Prader-Willi syndrome
                - Fröhlich's syndrome
                - Laurence-Moon-Biedl syndrome
            - Recent
              - Check drug history
                - Positive
                  - Antipsychotics
                  - Tricyclics
                  - Estrogen
                  - Valproic acid
                  - Antihypertensives
                  - Adrenal/anabolic steroids
                  - SSRIs, diabetic meds
                - Negative
                  - Change in physical activity (sedentary lifestyle)
                  - Smoking cessation
                  - Psychiatric disorder
    - History negative
      - Check chemistry panel
        - Abnormal
          - Diabetes mellitus
          - Cushing's disease/syndrome
        - Normal
          - Check TSH
            - Abnormal
              - Hypothyroidism
            - Normal
              - Check DHA-sulfate
                - Abnormal
                  - Increased androgenic hormones
                - Normal
                  - Surreptitious eating

FIGURE 3-203 Weight gain. *DHA,* Dehydroepiandrosterone; *SSRIs,* serotonin reuptake inhibitors; *TSH,* thyroid-stimulating hormone. (Modified from Healey PM: *Common medical diagnosis: an algorithmic approach,* ed 3, Philadelphia, 2000, Saunders.)

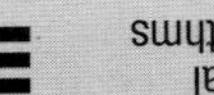
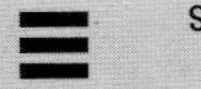

ICD-9CM # 783.2 Weight loss
ICD-10CM # R63.4 Abnormal weight loss

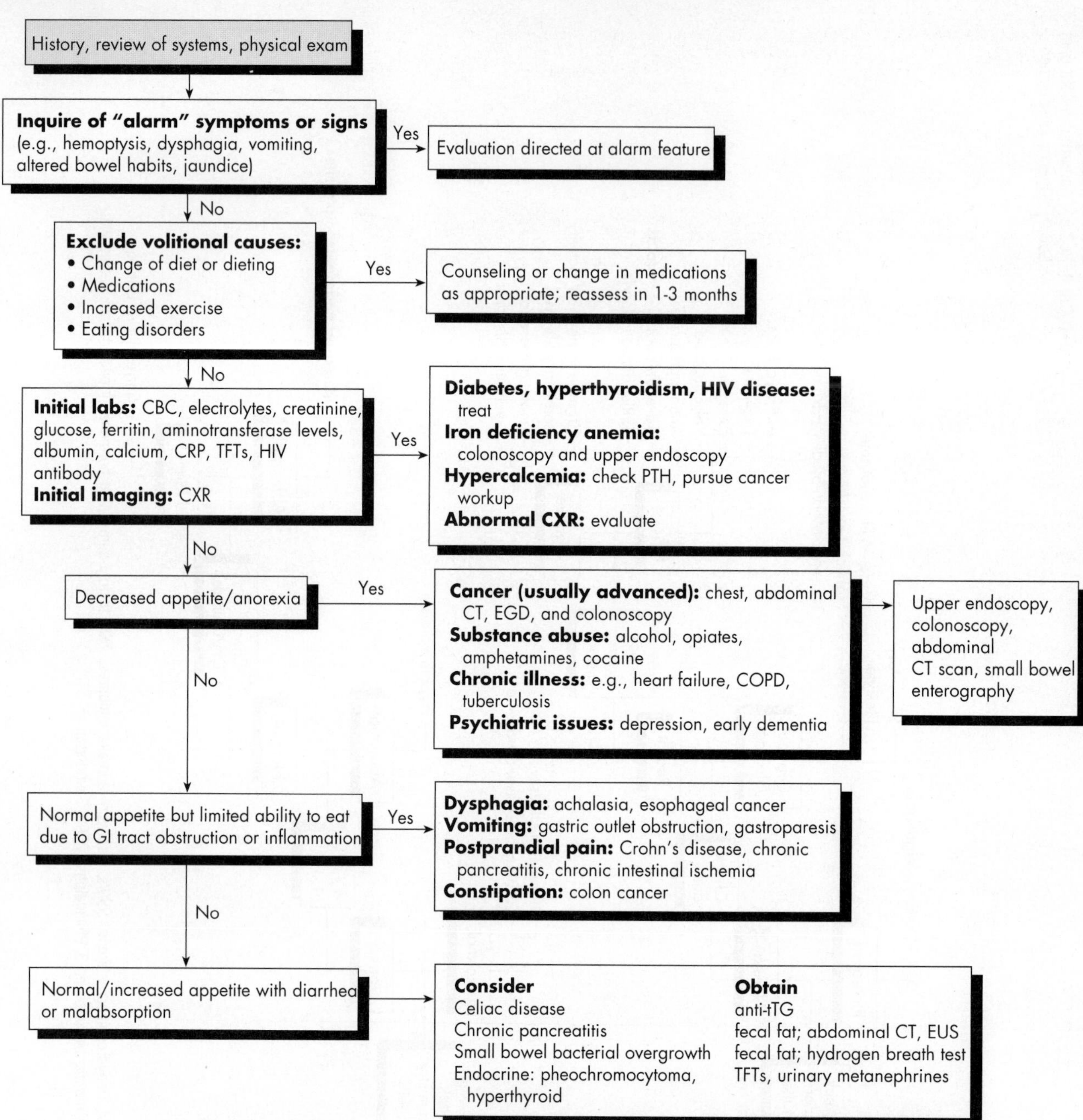

FIGURE 3-204 Approach to the patient with unintentional weight loss greater than 5%. *CBC,* Complete blood count; *COPD,* chronic obstructive pulmonary disease; *CRP,* C-reactive protein; *CT,* computed tomography; *CXR,* chest radiograph; *EGD,* esophagogastroduodenoscopy; *EUS,* endoscopic ultrasound; *GI,* gastrointestinal; *HIV,* human immunodeficiency virus; *PTH,* parathyroid hormone; *TFTs,* thyroid function tests; *tTG,* tissue transglutaminase; *U/A,* urinalysis. (From Goldman L, Schafer AI: *Goldman's Cecil Medicine,* ed 24, Philadelphia, 2012, Saunders.)

Laboratory Tests and Interpretation of Results

This section contains more than 300 commonly performed laboratory tests. In general, the tests are discussed in the following format:

1. Laboratory test.
2. Normal range in adult patients. Normal values are given using the present (traditional) reference interval, followed by the Système Internationale (SI) reference interval, the conversion factor (CF), and the suggested minimum increment (SMI).
3. Common abnormalities, such as positive test, increased or decreased value.
4. Causes of abnormal result.

The normal ranges may differ slightly, depending on the laboratory. The reader should be aware of the "normal range" of the particular laboratory performing the test. Every attempt has been made to present current laboratory test data, with emphasis on practical considerations.

ACE LEVEL

See ANGIOTENSIN-CONVERTING ENZYME

ACETONE (serum or plasma)

Normal: Negative
Elevated In: DKA, starvation, isopropanol ingestion

ACETYLCHOLINE RECEPTOR (AChR) ANTIBODY

Normal: <0.03 nmol/L
Elevated in: Myasthenia gravis. Changes in AChR concentration correlate with the clinical severity of myasthenia gravis following therapy and during therapy with prednisone and immunosuppressants. False-positive AChR antibody results may be found in patients with Eaton-Lambert syndrome.

ACID-BASE REFERENCE VALUES

See Tables 4-1 and 4-2.

ACID PHOSPHATASE (serum)

Normal range: 0-5.5 U/L (0-90 nkat/L [CF: 16.67; SMI:2 nkat/L])
Elevated in: Carcinoma of prostate, other neoplasms (breast, bone), Paget's disease, osteogenesis imperfecta, malignant invasion of bone, Gaucher's disease, multiple myeloma, myeloproliferative disorders, benign prostatic hypertrophy, prostatic palpation or surgery, hyperparathyroidism, liver disease, chronic renal failure, idiopathic thrombocytopenic purpura, bronchitis

ACID SERUM TEST

See HAM TEST

ACTIVATED CLOTTING TIME (ACT)

Normal: This test is used to determine the dose of protamine sulfate to reverse the effect of heparin as an anticoagulant during angioplasty, cardiac surgery, and hemodialysis. The accepted goal during cardiopulmonary bypass surgery is usually 400-500 sec.

ACTIVATED PARTIAL THROMBOPLASTIN TIME (APTT, APTT)

See PARTIAL THROMBOPLASTIN TIME

ADRENOCORTICOTROPIC HORMONE

Normal: 9-52 pg/ml
Elevated in: Addison's disease, ectopic ACTH-producing tumors, congenital adrenal hyperplasia, Nelson's syndrome, pituitary-dependent Cushing's disease
Decreased in: Secondary adrenocortical insufficiency, hypopituitarism, adrenal adenoma or adrenal carcinoma

ALANINE AMINOPEPTIDASE

Normal:
Male: 1.11-1.71 mcg/ml
Female: 0.96-1.52 mcg/ml
Elevated in: Liver or pancreatic disease, ethanol use, oral contraceptives use, malignancy, tobacco use, pregnancy
Decreased in: Abortion

ALANINE AMINOTRANSFERASE (ALT, SGPT)

See Fig. E4-1, an algorithm for evaluation of elevated ALT.
Normal range: 0-35 U/L (0.058 μkat/L [CF: 0.02 μkat/L])
Elevated in: Liver disease (hepatitis, cirrhosis, Reye's syndrome), hepatic congestion, infectious mononucleosis, myocardial infarction, myocarditis, severe muscle trauma, dermatomyositis/polymyositis, muscular dystrophy, drugs (antibiotics, narcotics, antihypertensive agents, heparin,

TABLE 4-1 Commonly Used Acid-Base Reference Values for Arterial and Venous Plasma or Serum (Averaged from Various Sources)

	ARTERIAL		VENOUS	
	Conventional Units	**SI Units***	**Conventional Units**	**SI Units***
pH	7.40 (7.35-7.45)	7.40 (7.35-7.45)	7.37 (7.32-7.42)	7.37 (7.32-7.42)
Pco_2	40 mm Hg (35-45)	5.33 kPa (4.67-6.10)	45 mm Hg (45-50)	6.10 kPa (5.33-6.67)
Po_2	80-100 mm Hg	10.66-13.33 kPa	40 mm Hg (37-43)	5.33 kPa (4.93-5.73)
HCO_3 (CO_2 combining power)	24 mEq/L (20-28)	24 mmol/L (20-28)	26 mEq/L (22-30)	26 mmol/L (22-30)
CO_2 content	25 mEq/L (22-28)	25 mmol/L (22-28)	27 mEq/L (24-30)	27 mmol/L(24-30)

From Ravel R: *Clinical laboratory medicine,* ed 6, St Louis, 1995, Mosby.
*International system.

TABLE 4-2 Summary of Laboratory Findings in Primary Uncomplicated Respiratory and Metabolic Acid-Base Disorders*

Disorder	Pco_2	pH	Base Excess
Acute primary respiratory hypoactivity (respiratory acidosis)	Increase	Decrease	Normal/positive
Acute primary respiratory hyperactivity (respiratory alkalosis)	Decrease	Increase	Normal/negative
Uncompensated metabolic acidosis	Normal	Decrease	Negative
Uncompensated metabolic alkalosis	Normal	Increase	Positive
Partially compensated metabolic acidosis	Decrease	Decrease	Negative
Partially compensated metabolic alkalosis	Increase	Increase	Positive
Chronic primary respiratory hypoactivity (compensated respiratory acidosis)	Increase	Normal	Positive
Fully compensated metabolic alkalosis	Increase	Normal	Positive
Chronic primary respiratory hyperactivity (compensated respiratory alkalosis)	Decrease	Normal	Negative
Fully compensated metabolic acidosis	Decrease	Normal	Negative

From Ravel R: *Clinical laboratory medicine,* ed 6, St Louis, 1995, Mosby.
*Base excess results refer to negative (−) values more than 22 and positive (+) values more than 12.

labetalol, statins, NSAIDs, amiodarone, chlorpromazine, phenytoin), malignancy, renal and pulmonary infarction, convulsions, eclampsia, shock liver

ALBUMIN (serum)

Normal range: 4-6 g/dl (40-60 g/L [CF:10; SMI: 1 g/L])
Elevated in: Dehydration (relative increase)
Decreased in: Liver disease, nephrotic syndrome, poor nutritional status, rapid IV hydration, protein-losing enteropathies (e.g., inflammatory bowel disease), severe burns, neoplasia, chronic inflammatory diseases, pregnancy, oral contraceptives, prolonged immobilization, lymphomas, hypervitaminosis A, chronic glomerulonephritis

ALCOHOL DEHYDROGENASE

Normal: 0-7 U/L
Elevated in: Drug-induced hepatocellular damage, obstructive jaundice, malignancy, inflammation, infection

ALDOLASE (serum)

Normal range: 0-6 U/L (0-100 nkat/L [CF: 16.67; SMI: 20 nkat/L])
Elevated in: Muscular dystrophy, rhabdomyolysis, dermatomyositis/polymyositis, trichinosis, acute hepatitis and other liver diseases, myocardial infarction, prostatic carcinoma, hemorrhagic pancreatitis, gangrene, delirium tremens, burns
Decreased in: Loss of muscle mass, late stages of muscular dystrophy

ALDOSTERONE

Normal range:
Recumbent: 50-150 ng/L
Upright: 150-300 ng/L
(Highest levels in neonates, decreasing over time to adult levels)
Elevated in: Primary aldosteronism, secondary aldosteronism, pseudoprimary aldosteronism
Decreased in:
Patient with hypertension: diabetes mellitus, Turner's syndrome, acute alcohol intoxication, excess secretion of deoxycorticosterone, corticosterone, and 18-hydroxycorticosterone
Patient without hypertension: Addison's disease, hypoaldosteronism resulting from renin deficiency, isolated aldosterone deficiency

ALKALINE PHOSPHATASE (ALP) (serum)

See Fig. E4-2 for approach to elevated ALP.
Normal range: 30-120 U/L (0.5-2 μkat/L [CF:0.01667; SMI: 0.1 μkat/L])
Elevated in:
LIVER AND BILIARY TRACT ORIGIN
Extrahepatic bile duct obstruction
Intrahepatic biliary obstruction
Liver cell acute injury
Liver passive congestion
Drug-induced liver cell dysfunction
Space-occupying lesions
Primary biliary cirrhosis
Sepsis
BONE ORIGIN (OSTEOBLAST HYPERACTIVITY)
Physiologic (rapid) bone growth (childhood and adolescence)
Metastatic tumor with osteoblastic reaction
Fracture healing
Paget's disease of bone
CAPILLARY ENDOTHELIAL ORIGIN
Granulation tissue formation (active)
PLACENTAL ORIGIN
Pregnancy
Some parenteral albumin preparations
OTHER
Thyrotoxicosis
Benign transient hyperphosphatasemia
Primary hyperparathyroidism
Decreased in: Hypothyroidism, pernicious anemia, hypophosphatemia, hypervitaminosis D, malnutrition

ALPHA-1-ANTITRYPSIN (serum)

Normal range: 110-140 mg/dl
Decreased in: Homozygous or heterozygous deficiency

ALPHA-1-FETOPROTEIN (serum)

See α-1 FETOPROTEIN

ALT

See ALANINE AMINOTRANSFERASE

ALUMINUM (serum)

Normal range: 0-6 ng/ml
Elevated in: Chronic renal failure on dialysis, parenteral nutrition, industrial exposure

AMA

See ANTIMITOCHONDRIAL ANTIBODY

AMEBIASIS SEROLOGIC TEST

Test description: Test is used to support diagnosis of amebiasis caused by *Entamoeba histolytica*. Serum acute and convalescent titers are drawn 1-3 weeks apart. A fourfold increase in titer is the most indicative result.

AMINOLEVULINIC ACID (δ-ALA) (24-hr urine collection)

Normal: 1.5-7.5 mg/day
Elevated in: Acute porphyrias, lead poisoning, DKA, pregnancy, anticonvulsant drugs, hereditary tyrosinemia
Decreased in: Alcoholic liver disease

AMMONIA (serum)

See Fig. E4-3 for approach to hyperammonemia in pediatric patients.
Normal range: 10-80 μg/dl (5-50 μmol/L [CF: 0.5872; SMI:5 μmol/L])
Elevated in: Hepatic failure, hepatic encephalopathy, Reye's syndrome, portacaval shunt, drugs (diuretics, polymyxin B, methicillin)
Decreased in: Drugs (neomycin, lactulose, tetracycline), renal failure

AMYLASE (serum)

Normal range: 0-130 U/L (0-2.17 μkat/L [CF: 0.01667; SMI: 0.01 μkat/L])
Elevated in: Acute pancreatitis, pancreatic neoplasm, abscess, pseudocyst, ascites, macroamylasemia, perforated peptic ulcer, intestinal obstruction, intestinal infarction, acute cholecystitis, appendicitis, ruptured ectopic pregnancy, salivary gland inflammation, peritonitis, burns, diabetic ketoacidosis, renal insufficiency, drugs (morphine), carcinomatosis (of lung, esophagus, ovary), acute ethanol ingestion, mumps, prostate tumors, post–endoscopic retrograde cholangiopancreatography, bulimia, anorexia nervosa
Decreased in: Advanced chronic pancreatitis, hepatic necrosis, cystic fibrosis

AMYLASE, URINE

See URINE AMYLASE

AMYLOID A PROTEIN (serum)

Normal: <10 mcg/ml
Elevated in: Inflammatory disorders (acute phase–reacting protein), infections, acute coronary syndrome, malignancies

ANA

See ANTINUCLEAR ANTIBODY

ANCA

See ANTINEUTROPHIL CYTOPLASMIC ANTIBODY

ANDROSTENEDIONE (serum)

Normal:
Male: 75-205 ng/dl
Female: 85-275 ng/dl
Elevated in: Congenital adrenal hyperplasia, polycystic ovary syndrome, ectopic ACTH-producing tumor, Cushing's syndrome, hirsutism, hyperplasia of ovarian stroma, ovarian neoplasm
Decreased in: Ovarian failure, adrenal failure, sickle cell anemia

ANGIOTENSIN II

Normal: 10-60 pg/ml
Elevated in: Hypertension, CHF, cirrhosis, renin-secreting renal tumor, volume depletion
Decreased in: ACE inhibitor drugs, ARB drugs, primary aldosteronism, Cushing's syndrome

ANGIOTENSIN-CONVERTING ENZYME (ACE level)

Normal range: <40 nmol/ml/min (<670 nkat/L [CF: 16.67; SMI: 10 nkat/L])
Elevated in: Sarcoidosis, primary biliary cirrhosis, alcoholic liver disease, hyperthyroidism, hyperparathyroidism, diabetes mellitus, amyloidosis, multiple myeloma, lung disease (asbestosis, silicosis, berylliosis, allergic alveolitis, coccidioidomycosis), Gaucher's disease, leprosy

ANH

See ATRIAL NATRIURETIC HORMONE

ANION GAP

Normal range: 9-14 mEq/L
Elevated in: Lactic acidosis, ketoacidosis (diabetes, alcoholic starvation), uremia (chronic renal failure), ingestion of toxins (paraldehyde, methanol, salicylates, ethylene glycol), hyperosmolar nonketotic coma, antibiotics (carbenicillin)
Decreased in: Hypoalbuminemia, severe hypermagnesemia, IgG myeloma, lithium toxicity, laboratory error (falsely decreased sodium or overestimation of bicarbonate or chloride), hypercalcemia of parathyroid origin, antibiotics (e.g., polymyxin)

ANTICARDIOLIPIN ANTIBODY (ACA)

Normal range: Negative. Test includes detection of IgG, IgM, and IgA antibodies to phospholipid, cardiolipin
Present In: Antiphospholipid antibody syndrome, chronic hepatitis C

ANTICOAGULANT

See CIRCULATING ANTICOAGULANT

ANTIDIURETIC HORMONE

Normal range: mOsm/kg 295-300 (4-12 pg/ml)
Elevated in: SIADH, antipsychotic medications, ectopic ADH from systemic neoplasm, Guillain-Barré syndrome, CNS infections, brain tumors, nephrogenic diabetes insipidus
Decreased in: Central diabetes insipidus, nephritic syndrome, psychogenic polydipsias, demeclocycline, lithium, phenytoin, alcohol

ANTI-DNA

Normal range: Absent
Present in: Systemic lupus erythematosus, chronic active hepatitis, infectious mononucleosis, biliary cirrhosis

ANTI-DS DNA

Normal: <25 U
Elevated in: Systemic lupus erythematosus

ANTIGLOMERULAR BASEMENT ANTIBODY

See GLOMERULAR BASEMENT MEMBRANE ANTIBODY

ANTIHISTONE

Normal: <1 U
Elevated in: Drug-induced lupus erythematosus

ANTIMITOCHONDRIAL ANTIBODY (AMA, MITOCHONDRIAL ANTIBODY)

Normal range: <1:20 titer
Elevated in: Primary biliary cirrhosis (85%-95%), chronic active hepatitis (25%-30%), cryptogenic cirrhosis (25%-30%)

ANTINEUTROPHIL CYTOPLASMIC ANTIBODY (ANCA)

Positive test: Cytoplasmic pattern (cANCA): positive in Wegener's granulomatosis (see Fig. E4-4 and Table E4-3 for approach to patient with positive c-ANCA)
Perinuclear pattern (pANCA): positive in inflammatory bowel disease, primary biliary cirrhosis, primary sclerosing cholangitis, autoimmune chronic active hepatitis, crescentic glomerulonephritis (see Fig. E4-5 and Table E4-3 for approach to patient with positive P-ANCA)

ANTINUCLEAR ANTIBODY (ANA)

See Fig. E4-6 for approach to positive ANA pattern
Normal range: <1:20 titer
Positive test: Systemic lupus erythematosus (more significant if titer >1:160), drugs (phenytoin, ethosuximide, primidone, methyldopa, hydralazine, carbamazepine, penicillin, procainamide, chlorpromazine, griseofulvin, thiazides), chronic active hepatitis, age over 60 years (particularly age over 80 years), rheumatoid arthritis, scleroderma, mixed connective tissue disease, necrotizing vasculitis, Sjögren's syndrome, tuberculosis, pulmonary interstitial fibrosis. Table 4-4 describes diseases associated with ANA subtypes. Fig. 4-7 illustrates various fluorescent ANA test patterns.

TABLE 4-4 Disease-Associated ANA Subtypes

Nuclear Location	Disease(s)
"Native" DNA (dsDNA, or dsDNA/ssDNA complex)	SLE (60%-70%; range, 35%-75%) Also PSS (5%-55%), MCTD (11%-25%), RA (5%-40%), DM (5%-25%), SS (5%)
sNP	SLE (50%) Also other collagen diseases
DNP (DNA-histone complex)	SLE (52%) Also MCTD (8%), RA (3%)
Histones	Drug-induced SLE (95%) Also SLE (30%), RA (15%-24%)
ENA Sm	SLE (30%-40%; range, 28%-40%) Also MCTD (0%-8%); RNP (U1-RNP) MCTD (in high titer without any other ANA subtype present: 95%-100%) Also SLE (26%-50%), PSS (11%-22%), RA (10%), SS (3%)
SS-A (Ro)*	SS without RA (60%-70%) Also SLE (26%-50%), neonatal SLE (over 95%), PSS (30%), MCTD (50%), SS with RA (9%), PBC (15%-19%)
SS-B (La)	SS without RA (40%-60%) Also SLE (5%-15%), SS with RA (5%)
Scl-70*	PSS (15%-43%)
Centromere*	CREST syndrome (70%-90%; range, 57%-96%) Also PSS (4%-20%), PBC (12%)
Nucleolar	PSS (scleroderma) (54%-90%) Also SLE (25%-26%), RA (9%)
RAP (RANA)	SS with RA (60%-76%) Also SS without RA (5%)
Jo-1	Polymyositis (30%)
PM-1	Polymyositis or PMS/PSS overlap syndrome (60%-90%) Also DM (17%)
ssDNA	SLE (60%-70%) Also CAH, infectious mononucleosis, RA, chronic GN, chronic infections, PBC
Cytoplasmic Location	**Disease(s)**
Mitochondrial	Primary biliary cirrhosis (90%-100%) Also CAH (7%-30%), cryptogenic cirrhosis (30%), acute hepatitis, viral hepatitis (3%), other liver diseases (0%-20%), SLE (5%), SS and PSS (8%)
Microsomal†	Chronic active hepatitis (60%-80%), Hashimoto's thyroiditis (97%)
Ribosomal	SLE (5%-12%)
Smooth muscle‡	Chronic active hepatitis (60%-91%) Also cryptogenic cirrhosis (28%), acute hepatitis, viral hepatitis (5%-87%), infectious mononucleosis (81%), MS (40%-50%), malignancy (67%), PBC (10%-50%)

From Ravel R: *Clinical laboratory medicine,* ed 6, St Louis, 1995, Mosby.
CAH, Chronic active hepatitis; *DM,* dermatomyositis; *GN,* glomerulonephritis; *MS,* multiple sclerosis; *PBC,* primary biliary cirrhosis; *SS,* Sjögren's syndrome.
*Not detected using rat or mouse liver or kidney tissue method.
†Not detected by cultured cell method.
‡Detected by cultured cells but better with rat or mouse tissue.

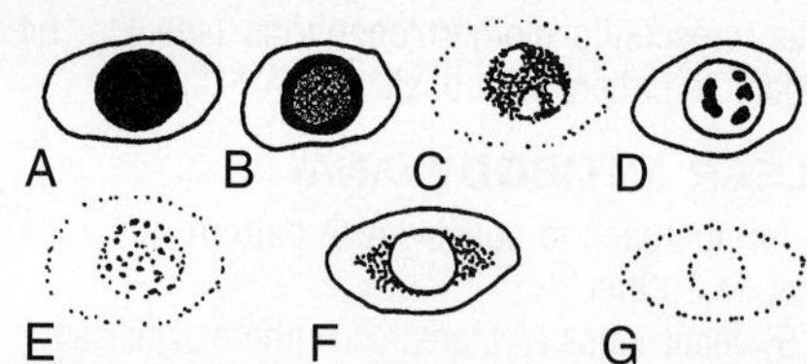

FIGURE 4-7 Fluorescent antinuclear antibody test patterns (HEP-2 cells). A, Solid (homogeneous). **B,** Peripheral (rim). **C,** Speckled. **D,** Nucleolar. **E,** Anticentromere. **F,** Antimitochondrial. **G,** Normal (nonreactive). (From Ravel R [ed]: *Clinical laboratory medicine*, ed 6, St Louis, 1995, Mosby.)

ANTI-RNP ANTIBODY

See EXTRACTABLE NUCLEAR ANTIGEN

ANTI-Scl-70

Normal: Absent
Elevated in: Scleroderma

ANTI-Sm (anti-Smith) ANTIBODY

See EXTRACTABLE NUCLEAR ANTIGEN

ANTI-SMOOTH MUSCLE ANTIBODY

See SMOOTH MUSCLE ANTIBODY

ANTISTREPTOLYSIN O TITER (Streptozyme, ASLO titer)

Normal range for adults: <160 Todd units
Elevated in: Streptococcal upper airway infection, acute rheumatic fever, acute glomerulonephritis, increased levels of β-lipoprotein

NOTE: A fourfold increase in titer between acute and convalescent specimens is diagnostic of streptococcal upper airway infection regardless of the initial titer.

ANTITHROMBIN III

See Table 4-5.

TABLE 4-5 Assay Measurements in Heterozygous Antithrombin (ATIII) Deficiency for Diagnosis

	ACTIVITY		
Type	**Antigen**	**Heparin Cofactor**	**Progressive ATIII**
I	Low	Low	Low
II			
Active site defect	Normal	Low	Low
Heparin-binding site defect	Normal	Low	Normal

From Hoffman R et al: *Hematology: basic principles and practice,* ed 5, Philadelphia, 2009, Churchill Livingstone.

Normal range: 81%-120% of normal activity; 17-30 mg/dl
Decreased in: Hereditary deficiency of antithrombin III, disseminated intravascular coagulation, pulmonary embolism, cirrhosis, thrombolytic therapy, chronic liver failure, postsurgery, third trimester of pregnancy, oral contraceptives, nephrotic syndrome, IV heparin >3 days, sepsis, acute leukemia, carcinoma, thrombophlebitis
Elevated in: Warfarin drugs, post–myocardial infarction

APOLIPOPROTEIN A-1 (Apo A-1)

Normal: Desirable >120 mg/dl
Elevated in: Familial hyperalphalipoproteinemia, statins, niacin, estrogens, weight loss, familial cholesteryl ester transfer protein (CETP) deficiency
Decreased in: Familial hypoalphalipoproteinemia, Tangier disease, diuretics, androgens, cigarette smoking, hepatocellular disorders, chronic renal failure, nephritic syndrome, coronary heart disease, cholestasis

APOLIPOPROTEIN B (Apo B)

Normal: Desirable <100 mg/dl; high risk >120 mg/dl
Elevated in: High saturated fat diet, high-cholesterol diet, hyperapobetalipoproteinemia, familial combined hyperlipidemia, anabolic steroids, diuretics, beta-blockers, corticosteroids, progestins, diabetes, hypothyroidism, chronic renal failure, liver disease, Cushing's syndrome, coronary heart disease
Decreased in: Statins, niacin, low-cholesterol diet, malnutrition, abetalipoproteinemia, hypobetalipoproteinemia, hyperthyroidism

ARTERIAL BLOOD GASES

Normal range:
Po_2: 75-100 mm Hg
Pco_2: 35-45 mm Hg
HCO_3: 24-28 mEq/L
pH: 7.35-7.45
Abnormal values: Acid-base disturbances (see the following)

METABOLIC ACIDOSIS
Metabolic acidosis with increased AG (AG acidosis)
Lactic acidosis
Ketoacidosis (diabetes mellitus, alcoholic ketoacidosis)
Uremia (chronic renal failure)
Ingestion of toxins (paraldehyde, methanol, salicylate, ethylene glycol)
High-fat diet (mild acidosis)
Metabolic acidosis with normal AG (hyperchloremic acidosis)
Renal tubular acidosis (including acidosis of aldosterone deficiency)
Intestinal loss of HCO_3^- (diarrhea, pancreatic fistula)
Carbonic anhydrase inhibitors (e.g., acetazolamide)
Dilutional acidosis (as a result of rapid infusion of bicarbonate-free isotonic saline)
Ingestion of exogenous acids (ammonium chloride, methionine, cystine, calcium chloride)
Ileostomy
Ureterosigmoidostomy
Drugs: amiloride, triamterene, spironolactone, β-blockers

RESPIRATORY ACIDOSIS
Pulmonary disease (COPD, severe pneumonia, pulmonary edema, interstitial fibrosis)
Airway obstruction (foreign body, severe bronchospasm, laryngospasm)
Thoracic cage disorders (pneumothorax, flail chest, kyphoscoliosis)
Defects in muscles of respiration (myasthenia gravis, hypokalemia, muscular dystrophy)
Defects in peripheral nervous system (amyotrophic lateral sclerosis, poliomyelitis, Guillain-Barré syndrome, botulism, tetanus, organophosphate poisoning, spinal cord injury)
Depression of respiratory center (anesthesia, narcotics, sedatives, vertebral artery embolism or thrombosis, increased intracranial pressure)
Failure of mechanical ventilator

METABOLIC ALKALOSIS
Divided into chloride-responsive (urinary chloride <15 mEq/L) and chloride-resistant forms (urinary chloride level >15 mEq/L)
Chloride-responsive
Vomiting
Nasogastric (NG) suction
Diuretics
Posthypercapnic alkalosis
Stool losses (laxative abuse, cystic fibrosis, villous adenoma)
Massive blood transfusion
Exogenous alkali administration
Chloride-resistant
Hyperadrenocorticoid states (Cushing's syndrome, primary hyperaldosteronism, secondary mineralocorticoidism [licorice, chewing tobacco])
Hypomagnesemia
Hypokalemia
Bartter's syndrome

RESPIRATORY ALKALOSIS
Hypoxemia (pneumonia, pulmonary embolism, atelectasis, high-altitude living)
Drugs (salicylates, xanthines, progesterone, epinephrine, thyroxine, nicotine)
Central nervous system (CNS) disorders (tumor, cerebrovascular accident [CVA], trauma, infections)

Psychogenic hyperventilation (anxiety, hysteria)
Hepatic encephalopathy
Gram-negative sepsis
Hyponatremia
Sudden recovery from metabolic acidosis
Assisted ventilation

ARTHROCENTESIS FLUID

***Interpretation of results*:**

1. **Color:** Normally it is clear or pale yellow; cloudiness indicates inflammatory process or presence of crystals, cell debris, fibrin, or triglycerides.
2. **Viscosity:** Normally it has a high viscosity because of hyaluronate; when fluid is placed on a slide, it can be stretched to a string >2 cm in length before separating (low viscosity indicates breakdown of hyaluronate [lysosomal enzymes from leukocytes] or the presence of edema fluid).
3. **Mucin clot:** Add 1 ml of fluid to 5 ml of a 5% acetic acid solution and allow 1 minute for the clot to form; a firm clot (does not fragment on shaking) is normal and indicates the presence of large molecules of hyaluronic acid (this test is nonspecific and infrequently done).
4. **Glucose:** Normally it approximately equals serum glucose level; a difference of more than 40 mg/dl is suggestive of infection.
5. **Protein:** Total protein concentration is <2.5 g/dl in the normal synovial fluid; it is elevated in inflammatory and septic arthritis.
6. **Microscopic examination for crystals**
   a. **Gout:** Monosodium urate crystals
   b. **Pseudogout:** Calcium pyrophosphate dihydrate crystals

ASLO TITER

See ANTISTREPTOLYSIN O TITER

ASPARTATE AMINOTRANSFERASE (AST, SGOT)

Normal range: 0-35 U/L (0-0.58 μkat/L [CF: 0.01667, SMI: 0.01 μkat/L])
Elevated in:
HEART
Acute myocardial infarction
Pericarditis (active: some cases)
LIVER
Hepatitis virus, Epstein-Barr, or cytomegalovirus infection
Active cirrhosis
Liver passive congestion or hypoxia
Alcohol- or drug-induced liver dysfunction
Space-occupying lesions (active)
Fatty liver (severe)
Extrahepatic biliary obstruction (early)
Drug-induced
SKELETAL MUSCLE
Acute skeletal muscle injury
Muscle inflammation (infectious or noninfectious)
Muscular dystrophy (active)
Recent surgery
Delirium tremens
KIDNEY
Acute injury or damage
Renal infarct
OTHER
Intestinal infarction
Shock
Cholecystitis
Acute pancreatitis
Hypothyroidism
Heparin therapy (60%-80% of cases)
Fig. E4-1 describes an approach to the evaluation of AST elevation.

ATRIAL NATRIURETIC HORMONE (ANH)

Normal: 20-77 pg/ml
Elevated in: CHF, volume overload, cardiovascular disease with high filling pressure
Decreased with: Prazosin and other alpha-blockers

B-TYPE NATRIURETIC PEPTIDE (BNP)

Normal range: up to 100 mcg/L. Natriuretic peptides are secreted to regulate fluid volume, blood pressure, and electrolyte balance. They have activity in both the central and peripheral nervous systems. In humans the main source of circulatory BNP is the heart ventricles.
Elevated in: Heart failure. This test is useful to differentiate heart failure patients from those with chronic obstructive pulmonary disease presenting with dyspnea. Levels are also increased in asymptomatic left ventricular dysfunction, arterial and pulmonary hypertension, cardiac hypertrophy, valvular heart disease, arrhythmia, and acute coronary syndrome. See Figure 4-8.

BASOPHIL COUNT

Normal range: 0.4%-1% of total WBC; 40-100/mm^3
Elevated in: Leukemia, inflammatory processes, polycythemia vera, Hodgkin's lymphoma, hemolytic anemia, after splenectomy, myeloid metaplasia, myxedema
Decreased in: Stress, hypersensitivity reaction, steroids, pregnancy, hyperthyroidism, postirradiation

BICARBONATE

Normal: Arterial: 21-28 mEq/L
Venous: 22-29 mEq/L

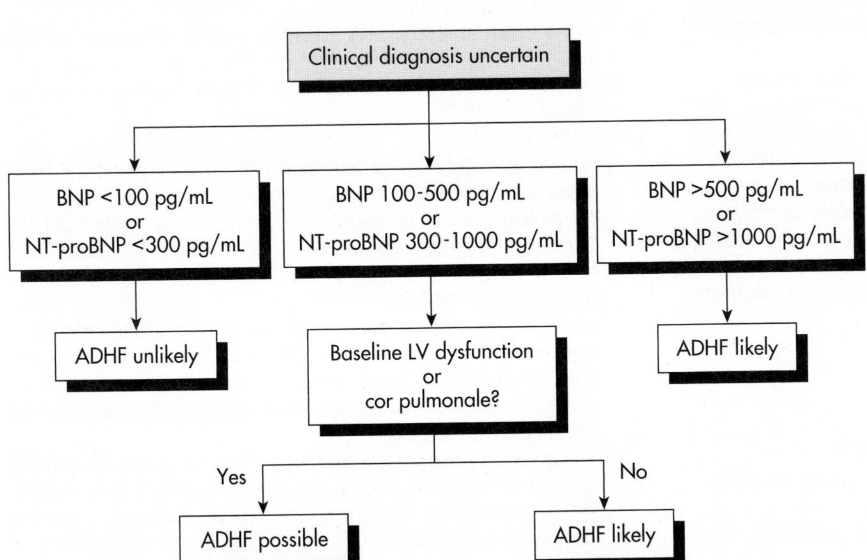

FIGURE 4-8 Interpretation of natriuretic peptide levels. *ADHF,* Acute decompensated heart failure; *BNP,* B-type natriuretic peptide; *NT-proBNP,* inactive N-terminal fragment of BNP. (From Adams JG, et al: *Emergency medicine, clinical essentials,* ed 2, Philadelphia, 2013, Elsevier.)

Elevated in: Metabolic alkalosis, compensated respiratory acidosis, diuretics, corticosteroids, laxative abuse
Decreased in: Metabolic acidosis, compensated respiratory alkalosis, acetazolamide, cyclosporine, cholestyramine, methanol or ethylene glycol poisoning

BILE ACID BREATH TEST (breath test, hydrogen breath test)

Normal: The test determines the radioactivity of $_{14}CO_2$ in breath samples at 2 and 4 hr.

2 hr after dose: 0.11 ± 0.14
4 hr after dose: 0.52 ± 0.09

Elevated in: GI bacterial overgrowth, disease or resection of terminal ileum and other H_2 blocker USF cimetidine

BILE, URINE

See URINE BILE

BILIRUBIN, DIRECT (conjugated bilirubin)

Normal range: 0-0.2 mg/dl (0-4 μmol/L [CF: 17.10; SMI: 2 μmol/L])
Elevated in: Hepatocellular disease, biliary obstruction, drug-induced cholestasis, hereditary disorders (Dubin-Johnson syndrome, Rotor's syndrome)

BILIRUBIN, INDIRECT (unconjugated bilirubin)

Normal range: 0-1.0 mg/dl (2-18 μmol/L [CF: 17.10; SMI: 2 μmol/L])
Elevated in:

A. Increased bilirubin production (if normal liver, serum unconjugated bilirubin is usually less than 4 mg/100 ml)
   1. Hemolytic anemia
      a. Acquired
      b. Congenital
   2. Resorption from extravascular sources
      a. Hematomas
      b. Pulmonary infarcts
   3. Excessive ineffective erythropoiesis
      a. Congenital (congenital dyserythropoietic anemias)
      b. Acquired (pernicious anemia, severe lead poisoning; if present, bilirubinemia is usually mild)
B. Defective hepatic unconjugated bilirubin clearance (defective uptake or conjugation)
   1. Severe liver disease
   2. Gilbert's syndrome
   3. Crigler-Najjar type I or II
   4. Drug-induced inhibition
   5. Portacaval shunt
   6. Congestive heart failure
   7. Hyperthyroidism (uncommon)

BILIRUBIN, TOTAL

See Fig. E4-9 and Table E4-6, for evaluation of hyperbilirubinemia and liver disease.
Normal range: 0-1.0 mg/dl (2-18 μmol/L [CF: 17.10, SMI: 2 μmol/L])
Elevated in: Liver disease (hepatitis, cirrhosis, cholangitis, neoplasm, biliary obstruction, infectious mononucleosis), hereditary disorders (Gilbert's disease, Dubin-Johnson syndrome), drugs (steroids, statins, niacin, acetaminophen, diphenylhydantoin, phenothiazines, penicillin, erythromycin, clindamycin, captopril, amphotericin B, sulfonamides, azathioprine, isoniazid, 5-aminosalicylic acid, allopurinol, methyldopa, indomethacin, halothane, oral contraceptives, procainamide, tolbutamide, labetalol), hemolysis, pulmonary embolism or infarct, hepatic congestion secondary to congestive heart failure

BILIRUBIN, URINE

See URINE BILE

BLADDER TUMOR ASSOCIATED ANTIGEN

Normal: ≤14 U/ml. Test is used to detect bladder cancer recurrence. Sensitivity 57%-83% and specificity 68%-72%.
Elevated in: Bladder cancer, renal stones, nephritis, UTI, hematuria, renal cancer, cystitis, recent bladder or urinary tract trauma

BLEEDING TIME (modified Ivy method)

See Fig. E4-10 for evaluation of patients with prolonged bleeding time.
Normal range: 2 to 9.5 min
Elevated in: Thrombocytopenia, capillary wall abnormalities, platelet abnormalities (Bernard-Soulier disease, Glanzmann's disease), drugs (aspirin, warfarin, anti-inflammatory medications, streptokinase, urokinase, dextran, β-lactam antibiotics, moxalactam), disseminated intravascular coagulation, cirrhosis, uremia, myeloproliferative disorders, von Willebrand's disease.
Bleeding time tests are no longer performed at many hospitals and have been replaced by the platelet function analyzer (PFA-100) assay.

BLOOD VOLUME, TOTAL

Normal: 60-80 ml/kg
Elevated in: Polycythemia vera, pulmonary disease, CHF, renal insufficiency, pregnancy, acidosis, thyrotoxicosis
Decreased in: Anemia, hemorrhage, vomiting, diarrhea, dehydration, burns, starvation

BNP

See B-TYPE NATRIURETIC PEPTIDE

BORDETELLA PERTUSSIS SEROLOGY

Test description: PCR of nasopharyngeal aspirates or secretions is used to identify *Bordetella pertussis,* the organism responsible for whooping cough.

BRCA ANALYSIS

DESCRIPTION OF ANALYSIS

Comprehensive BRCA analysis:

BRCA1: Full sequence determination in both forward and reverse directions of approximately 5500 base pairs comprising 22 coding exons and one noncoding exon (exon 4) and approximately 800 adjacent base pairs in the noncoding intervening sequence (intron). Exon 1, which is noncoding, is not analyzed. The wild-type *BRCA1* gene encodes a protein comprising 1863 amino acids.

BRCA2: Full sequence determination in both forward and reverse directions of approximately 10,200 base pairs comprising 26 coding exons and approximately 900 adjacent base pairs in the noncoding intervening sequence (intron). Exon 1, which is noncoding, is not analyzed. The wild-type *BRCA2* gene encodes a protein comprising 3418 amino acids.

The noncoding intronic regions of *BRCA1* and *BRCA2* that are analyzed do not extend more than 20 base pairs proximal to the 5' end and 10 base pairs distal to the 3' end of each exon.

Single-site BRCA analysis: DNA sequence analysis for a specified mutation in *BRCA1* and/or *BRCA2.*

Multisite 3 BRCA analysis: DNA sequence analysis of specific portions of *BRCA1* exon 2, *BRCA1* exon 20, and *BRCA2* exon 11 designed to detect only mutations 187delAG and 5385insC in *BRCA1* and 6174delT in *BRCA2.*

Interpretive Criteria:

"Positive for a deleterious mutation": Includes all mutations (nonsense, insertions, deletions) that prematurely terminate ("truncate") the protein product of *BRCA1* at least 10 amino acids from the C-terminus, or the protein product of *BRCA2* at least 110 amino acids from the C-terminus (based on documentation of deleterious mutations in *BRCA1* and *BRCA2*).

In addition, specific missense mutations and noncoding intervening sequence (IVS) mutations are recognized as deleterious on the basis of data derived from linkage analysis of high-risk families, functional assays, biochemical evidence, and/or demonstration of abnormal mRNA transcript processing.

"Genetic variant, suspected deleterious": Includes genetic variants for which the available evidence indicates a likelihood, but not proof, that the mutation is deleterious. The specific evidence supporting such an interpretation will be summarized for individual variants on each such report.

"Genetic variant, favor polymorphism": Includes genetic variants for which available evidence indicates that the variant is highly unlikely to contribute substantially to cancer risk. The specific evidence supporting such an interpretation will be summarized for individual variants on each such report.

"Genetic variant of uncertain significance": Includes missense mutations and mutations that occur in analyzed intronic regions whose clinical significance has not yet been determined, as well as chain-terminating mutations that truncate *BRCA1* and *BRCA2* distal to amino acid positions 1853 and 3308, respectively.

"No deleterious mutation detected": Includes nontruncating genetic variants observed at an allele frequency of approximately 1% of a suitable control population (providing that no data suggest clinical significance), as well as all genetic variants for which published data demonstrate absence of substantial clinical significance. Also includes mutations in the protein-coding region that neither alter the amino acid sequence nor are predicted to significantly affect exon splicing, and base pair alterations in noncoding portions of the gene that have been demonstrated to have no deleterious effect on the length or stability of the mRNA transcript.

There may be uncommon genetic abnormalities in *BRCA1* and *BRCA2* that will not be detected by *BRCA* analysis. This analysis, however, is believed to rule out the majority of abnormalities in these genes, which are believed responsible for most hereditary susceptibility to breast and ovarian cancer.

"Specific variant/mutation not identified": Specific and designated deleterious mutations or variants of uncertain clinical significance are not present in the individual being tested. If one (or rarely two) specific deleterious mutations have been identified in a family member, a negative analysis for the specific mutation(s) indicates that the tested individual is at the general population risk of developing breast or ovarian cancer.

BREATH HYDROGEN TEST (Hydrogen breath test)

Normal: This test is for bacterial overgrowth. H_2 excretion fasting: 4.6±5.1, after lactulose, early increase <12. Lactulose usually results in a colonic response >30 min after ingestion.

Elevated in: A high fasting breath H_2 level and an increase of at least 12 ppm within 30 min after lactulose challenge are indicative of bacterial overgrowth in the small intestine. The increase must precede the colonic response.

False positives in: Accelerated gastric emptying, laxative use

False negatives in: Use of antibiotics and patients who are nonhydrogen producers

BUN

See UREA NITROGEN, BLOOD

C282Y AND H63D MUTATION ANALYSIS

Procedure: Detection of the C282Y and H63D mutations is accomplished by amplification of exons 2 and 4 of the *HFE* gene on chromosome 6 by polymerase chain reaction (PCR) followed by allele-specific hybridization and chemiluminescent detection of hybridized probes. H63D is viewed by some as a polymorphism rather than a mutation because of its prevalence in the population, because 15% of the individuals affected with hereditary hemochromatosis (HH) are compound heterozygotes for C282Y and H63D and about 1% of patients are H63D homozygotes, which suggests that H63D may be causative in the development of the disorder at reduced penetrance.

Interpretation: Homozygosity for the C282Y mutation has been associated with an increased risk of being affected with HH compared with the general population. The genotype is observed in 60%-90% of individuals affected with HH and occurs in less than 1% of the general population. However, approximately 25% of asymptomatic individuals with this genotype do not develop the disorder.

C3

See COMPLEMENT

C4

See COMPLEMENT

CALCITONIN (serum)

Normal range: <100 pg/ml (<100 ng/L [CF: 1; SMI: 10 ng/L])

Elevated in: Medullary carcinoma of the thyroid (particularly if level >1500 pg/ml), carcinoma of the breast, apudomas, carcinoids, renal failure, thyroiditis

CALCIUM (serum)

See Fig. 4-11 for evaluation of hypercalcemia.

Normal range: 8.8-10.3 mg/dl (2.2-2.58 μmol/L [CF: 0.2495; SMI: 0.02 μmol/L])

ELEVATED

Relatively common:

Neoplasia
Bone primary
Myeloma
Acute leukemia
Nonbone solid tumors
Breast
Lung
Squamous nonpulmonary
Kidney
Neoplasm secretion of parathyroid hormone-related protein (PTHrP, "ectopic PTH")
Primary hyperparathyroidism
Thiazide diuretics
Tertiary (renal) hyperparathyroidism
Idiopathic
Spurious (artifactual) hypercalcemia
Dehydration
Serum protein elevation
Laboratory technical problem (lab error)

Relatively uncommon:

Sarcoidosis
Hyperthyroidism
Immobilization (mostly seen in children and adolescents)
Diuretic phase of acute renal tubular necrosis
Vitamin D intoxication
Milk-alkali syndrome
Addison's disease
Lithium therapy
Idiopathic hypercalcemia of infancy
Acromegaly
Theophylline toxicity

Table 4-7 describes the laboratory differential diagnosis of hypercalcemia.

DECREASED

Artifactual
Hypoalbuminemia
Hemodilution
Primary hypoparathyroidism
Pseudohypoparathyroidism
Vitamin D–related
Vitamin D deficiency
Malabsorption
Renal failure
Magnesium deficiency
Sepsis
Chronic alcoholism
Tumor lysis syndrome
Rhabdomyolysis
Alkalosis (respiratory or metabolic)
Acute pancreatitis
Drug-induced hypocalcemia
Large doses of magnesium sulfate
Anticonvulsants

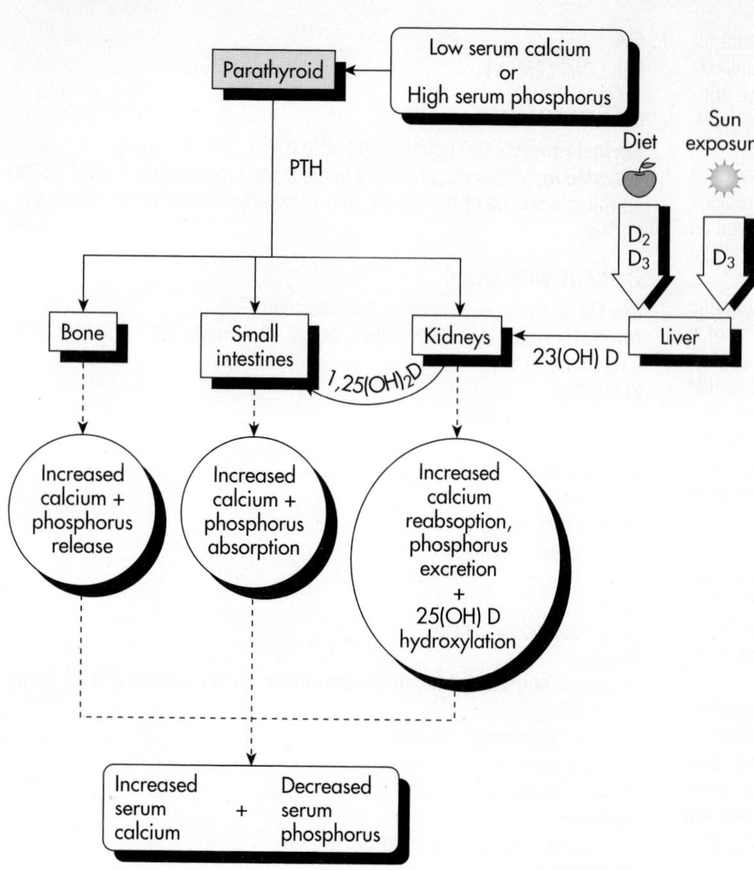

FIGURE 4-11 Calcium homeostasis. Parathyroid hormone (PTH) is released from the parathyroid glands in response to hypocalcemia and hyperphosphatemia. PTH acts on bone, the small intestines, and the kidneys to effect a rise in serum calcium and a net decrease in serum phosphorus. Hydroxylation of inactive forms of vitamin D occurs in the liver and kidneys. 1,25(OH)2D facilitates intestinal absorption of calcium and phosphorus. *1,25(OH)2D,* 1,25-Dihydroxyvitamin D; *25(OH) D,* 25-hydroxyvitamin D; *D2,* vitamin D2; *D3,* vitamin D3. (From Adams JG, et al: *Emergency medicine, clinical essentials,* ed 2, Philadelphia, 2013, Elsevier.)

TABLE 4-7 Laboratory Differential Diagnosis of Hypercalcemia

	PLASMA TESTS					URINE TESTS			
Diagnosis	**Ca**	**PO_4**	**PTH**	**25(OH)D**	**$1,25(OH)_2D$**	**cAMP**	**TmP/GFR**	**Ca**	**Comments**
Primary hyperparathyroidism	↑	N/↓	↑	N	N/↑	↑	↓	↑	Parathyroid adenoma most common
MEN I									Parathyroid hyperplasia; also includes pituitary and pancreatic neoplasms
MEN IIa									Parathyroid hyperplasia; also includes medullary thyroid carcinoma and pheochromocytoma
MEN IIb									Parathyroid disease uncommon, primarily medullary thyroid carcinoma and pheochromocytoma
FHH	↑	N	N/↑	N	N	N/↑	N/↓	↓↓	Autosomal dominant inheritance; hypercalcemia present within first decade; benign
Malignancy									
Solid tumor, humoral	↑	N/↓	↓	N	N	↑	↓	↑↑	Primarily epidermoid tumors; PTH-related protein(s) is mediator
Solid tumor, osteolytic	↑	N/↑	↓	N	N	↓	↑	↑↑	
Lymphoma	↑	N/↑	↓	N/↓	↑	↓	↑	↑↑	
Granulomatous disease	↑	N/↑	↓	N/↓	↑↑	↓	↑	↑↑	Sarcoid most common etiology
Vitamin D intoxication	↑	N/↑	↓	↑↑	N	↓	↑	↑↑	
Hyperthyroidism	↑	N	↓	N	N	N	N	↑↑	Plasma concentrations of T_4 and/or T_3 are elevated

Ca, Calcium; *cAMP,* cyclic adenosine monophosphate; *FHH,* familial hypocalciuric hypercalcemia; *GFR,* glomerular filtration rate; *MEN,* multiple endocrine neoplasia; *25(OH)D,* 25 hydroxyvitamin D; *PO_4,* phosphate; *PTH,* parathyroid hormone; *T_3,* triiodothyronine; *T_4,* thyroxine; *TmP,* renal threshold for phosphorus.
From Moore WT, Eastman RC: *Diagnostic endocrinology,* ed 2, St Louis, 1996, Mosby.

TABLE 4-8 Laboratory Differential Diagnosis of Hypocalcemia

	PLASMA TESTS					URINE TESTS					
Diagnosis	**Ca**	**PO_4**	**PTH**	**25(OH)D**	**$1,25(OH)_2D$**	**cAMP**	**cAMP after PTH**	**TmP/GFR**	**TmP/GFR after PTH**	**Ca**	**Comments**
Hypopara-thyroidism	↓	↑	N/↓	N	↓	↓	↑↑	↑	↓↓	N/↓	Deficiency of PTH
Pseudohypoparathyroidism											
Type I	↓	↑	↑↑	N	↓	↓	NC	↑	↑	N/↓	Resistance to PTH; patients may have Albright's hereditary osteodystrophy and resistance to multiple hormones
Type II	↓	N	↑↑	N	↓	↓	↑	↑	↑	N/↓	Renal resistance to cAMP
Vitamin D deficiency	↓	N/↓	↑↑	↓↓	N/↓	↑	↑	↓	↓	↓↓	Deficient supply (e.g., nutrition) or absorption (e.g., pancreatic insufficiency) of vitamin D
Vitamin D–dependent Rickets											
Type I	↓	N/↓	↑↑	N	↓	↑↑		↓		↓↓	Deficient activity of renal 25(OH) D-1α-hydroxylase
Type II	↓	N/↓	↑↑	N	↑↑	↑		↓		↓↓	Resistance to $1,25(OH)_2D$

From Moore WT, Eastman RC: *Diagnostic endocrinology,* ed 2, St Louis, 1996, Mosby.
Ca, Calcium; *cAMP,* cyclic adenosine monophosphate; *FHH,* familial hypocalciuric hypercalcemia; *GFR,* glomerular filtration rate; *MEN,* multiple endocrine neoplasia; *NC,* no change or small increase; *(OH)D,* hydroxycalciferol D; *PO_4,* phosphate; *PTH,* parathyroid hormone; *T_3,* triiodothyronine; *T_4,* thyroxine; *TmP,* renal threshold for phosphorus.

Mithramycin
Gentamicin
Cimetidine

Table 4-8 describes the laboratory differential diagnosis of hypocalcemia.

CALCIUM, URINE

See URINE CALCIUM

CANCER ANTIGEN 15-3 (CA 15-3)

Normal: <30 U/ml

Elevated in: Approximately 80% of women with metastatic breast cancer. Clinical sensitivity is 0.60, specificity 0.87, positive predictive value 0.91. This test is generally used to predict recurrence of breast cancer and evaluate response to therapy. May also be elevated in liver cancer, pancreatic cancer, ovarian cancer, colorectal cancer. Elevations can also occur with benign breast and liver disease.

CANCER ANTIGEN 27-29 (CA 27-29)

Normal: <38 U/ml

Elevated in: Approximately 75% of women with metastatic breast cancer. Clinical sensitivity is 0.57, specificity 0.97, positive predictive value 0.83, negative predictive value 0.92. This test is generally used to predict recurrence of breast cancer and evaluate response to therapy. May also be elevated in liver cancer, pancreatic cancer, ovarian cancer, colorectal cancer. Elevations can also occur with benign breast and liver disease.

CANCER ANTIGEN 72-4 (CA 72-4)

Normal: <4.0 ng/ml

Elevated in: Gastric cancer (elevated in >50% of patients). Often used in combination with CA 72-4, CA 19-9, and CEA to monitor gastric cancer after treatment.

CANCER ANTIGEN 125 (CA 125)

Normal range: <1.4%

This test uses an antibody against antigen from tissue culture of an ovarian tumor cell line. Various published evaluations report sensitivity of about 75%-80% in patients with ovarian carcinoma. There is also an appreciable incidence of elevated values in nonovarian malignancies and in certain benign conditions (see below). Test values may transiently increase during chemotherapy.

MALIGNANT

Epithelial ovarian carcinoma, 75%-80% (range, 25%-92%; better in serous than mucinous cystadenocarcinoma)
Endometrial carcinoma, 25%-48% (2%-90%)
Pancreatic carcinoma, 59%
Colorectal carcinoma, 20% (15%-56%)
Endocervical adenocarcinoma, 83%
Squamous cervical or vaginal carcinoma, 7%-14%
Lung carcinoma, 32%
Breast carcinoma, 12%-40%
Lymphoma, 35%

BENIGN

Cirrhosis, 40%-80%
Acute pancreatitis, 38%
Acute peritonitis, 75%
Endometriosis, 88%
Acute pelvic inflammatory disease, 33%
Pregnancy first trimester, 2%-24%
During menstruation (occasionally)
Renal failure (?frequency)
Normal persons, 0.6%-1.4%

CAPTOPRIL STIMULATION TEST

Normal: Test performed by giving 25 mg captopril orally after overnight fast. Patient should be seated during test. After captopril, aldosterone <15 ng/dl, renin >2 ng angiotensin I/ml/hr.

Interpretation: In patients with primary aldosteronism, plasma aldosterone remains high and plasma renin activity remains low after captopril.

CARBAMAZEPINE (Tegretol)

Normal therapeutic range: 4-12 mcg/ml

CARBOHYDRATE ANTIGEN 19-9

Normal: <37.0 U/ml

Elevated in: GI cancer, most frequently pancreatic cancer. Amount of elevation has no relation to tumor mass. Elevations can also occur with cirrhosis, cholangitis, and chronic or acute pancreatitis.

CARBON DIOXIDE, PARTIAL PRESSURE

Normal:
Male: 35-48 mm Hg
Female: 32-45 mm Hg
Elevated in: Respiratory acidosis
Decreased in: Respiratory alkalosis

CARBON MONOXIDE

See CARBOXYHEMOGLOBIN

CARBOXYHEMOGLOBIN

Normal range: Saturation of hemoglobin <2%; smokers <9%
Elevated in: Smoking, exposure to smoking, exposure to automobile exhaust fumes, malfunctioning gas-burning appliances

CARCINOEMBRYONIC ANTIGEN (CEA)

Normal range:
Nonsmokers: 0-2.5 ng/ml (0-2.5 μg/L [CF: 1; SMI: 0.1 μg/L])
Smokers: 0-5 ng/ml (0-5 μg/L [CF: 1; SMI: 0.1 μg/L])
Elevated in:
Colorectal carcinomas, pancreatic carcinomas, and metastatic disease (usually produce higher elevations: >20 ng/ml)
Carcinomas of the esophagus, stomach, small intestine, liver, breast, ovary, lung, and thyroid (usually produce lesser elevations)
Benign conditions (smoking, inflammatory bowel disease, hypothyroidism, cirrhosis, pancreatitis, infections) (usually produce levels <10 ng/ml)

CAROTENE (serum)

Normal range: 50-250 μg/dl (0.9-4.6 μmol/L [CF: 0.01863; SMI: 0.1 μmol/L])
Elevated in: Carotenemia, chronic nephritis, diabetes mellitus, hypothyroidism, nephrotic syndrome, hyperlipidemia
Decreased in: Fat malabsorption, steatorrhea, pancreatic insufficiency, lack of carotenoids in diet, high fever, liver disease

CATECHOLAMINES, URINE

See URINE CATECHOLAMINES

CBC

See COMPLETE BLOOD COUNT

CD40 LIGAND

Normal: <5 mcg/L. CD40 ligand is a soluble protein that is shed from activated leukocytes and platelets and used in risk stratification for acute coronary syndrome.
Elevated in: Acute coronary syndrome. Increased CD40 ligand is associated with higher incidence of death or nonfatal MI.

CD4+ T-LYMPHOCYTE COUNT (CD4+ T-cells)

Calculated as total WBC × % lymphocytes × % lymphocytes stained with CD4.

This test is used primarily to evaluate immune dysfunction in HIV infection. It is useful as a prognostic indicator and as a criterion for initiating prophylaxis for several opportunistic infections that are sequelae of HIV infection. Progressive depletion of CD4+ T-lymphocytes is associated with an increased likelihood of clinical complications (Table 4-9).

TABLE 4-9 Relation of CD4 Lymphocyte Counts to the Onset of Certain HIV-Associated Infections and Neoplasms in North America

CD4 Count (Cells/mm³)*	Opportunistic Infection or Neoplasm	Frequency (%)†
>500	Herpes zoster, polydermatomal	5-10
200-500	*Mycobacterium tuberculosis* infection, pulmonary and extrapulmonary	2-20
	Oral hairy leukoplakia	40-70
	Candida pharyngitis (thrush)	40-70
	Recurrent *Candida* vaginitis	15-30 (F)
	Kaposi's sarcoma, mucocutaneous	15-30 (M)
	Bacterial pneumonia, recurrent	15-20
	Cervical neoplasia	1-2 (F)
100-200	*Pneumocystis carinii* pneumonia	15-60
	Herpes simplex, chronic, ulcerative	5-10
	Histoplasma capsulatum infection, disseminated	0-20
	Kaposi's sarcoma, visceral	3-8 (M)
	Progressive multifocal leukoencephalopathy	2-3
	Lymphoma, non-Hodgkin's	2-5
<100	*Candida* esophagitis	15-20
	Mycobacterium avium-intracellulare, disseminated	25-40
	Toxoplasma gondii encephalitis	5-25
	Cryptosporidium enteritis	2-10
	CMV retinitis	20-35
	Cryptococcus neoformans encephalitis	2-5
	CMV esophagitis or colitis	6-12
	Lymphoma, central nervous system	4-8

From Andreoli TE (ed): *Cecil essentials of medicine,* ed 5, Philadelphia, 2000, Saunders.
CMV, Cytomegalovirus; *F,* exclusively in women; *HIV,* human immunodeficiency virus; *M,* almost exclusively in men.
*Table indicates CD4 count at which specific infections or neoplasms generally begin to appear. Each infection may recur or progress during the subsequent course of HIV disease.
†Even within the United States, great regional differences in the incidence of specific opportunistic infections are apparent. For example, disseminated histoplasmosis is common in the Mississippi River drainage area but very rare in individuals who have lived exclusively on the East or West Coast.

CEA

See CARCINOEMBRYONIC ANTIGEN

CEREBROSPINAL FLUID (CSF)

Interpretation of results:

1. Appearance of the fluid
   a. Clear: normal.
   b. Yellow color (xanthochromia) in the supernatant of centrifuged CSF within 1 hour or less after collection is usually the result of previous bleeding (subarachnoid hemorrhage); it may also be caused by increased CSF protein, melanin from meningeal melanosarcomas, or carotenoids.
   c. Pinkish color is usually the result of a bloody tap; the color generally clears progressively from tubes 1 to 4 (the supernatant is usually crystal clear in traumatic taps).
   d. Turbidity usually indicates the presence of leukocytes (bleeding introduces approximately 1 WBC/500 RBCs into the CSF).
2. CSF pressure: elevated pressure can be seen with meningitis, meningoencephalitis, pseudotumor cerebri, mass lesions, and intracerebral bleeding.
3. Cell count: in the adult the CSF is normally free of cells (although up to 5 mononuclear cells/mm³ is considered normal); the presence of granulocytes is never normal.
   a. Neutrophils: seen in bacterial meningitis, early viral meningoencephalitis, and early tuberculosis (TB) meningitis.
   b. Increased lymphocytes: TB meningitis, viral meningoencephalitis, syphilitic meningoencephalitis, fungal meningitis.
4. Protein: serum proteins are generally too large to cross the normal blood–CSF barrier; however, increased CSF protein is seen with meningeal inflammation, traumatic tap, increased CNS synthesis, tissue degeneration, obstruction to CSF circulation, and Guillain-Barré syndrome.
5. Glucose
   a. Decreased glucose is seen with bacterial meningitis, TB meningitis, fungal meningitis, subarachnoid hemorrhage, and some cases of viral meningitis.
   b. A mild increase in CSF glucose can be seen in patients with very elevated serum glucose levels.

Table 4-10 describes CSF findings in central nervous system disorders.

CERULOPLASMIN (serum)

Normal range: 20-35 mg/dl (200-350 mg/L [CF: 10; SMI: 10 mg/L])
Elevated in: Pregnancy, estrogens, oral contraceptives, neoplastic diseases (leukemias, Hodgkin's lymphoma, carcinomas), inflammatory states, systemic lupus erythematosus, primary biliary cirrhosis, rheumatoid arthritis
Decreased in: Wilson's disease (values often <10 mg/dl), nephrotic syndrome, advanced liver disease, malabsorption, total parenteral nutrition, Menkes' syndrome

CHLAMYDIA GROUP ANTIBODY SEROLOGIC TEST

Test description: Acute and convalescent sera is drawn 2-4 weeks apart. A fourfold increase in titer between acute and convalescent sera is necessary for confirmation. A single titer ≥1:64 is considered indicative of psittacosis or LGV.

CHLAMYDIA TRACHOMATIS PCR

Test description: Test is performed on endocervical swab, urine, and intraurethral swab
Normal: Negative

CHLORIDE (serum)

Normal range: 95-105 mEq/L (95-105 mmol/L [CF: 1; SMI: 1 mmol/L])
Elevated in: Dehydration, excessive infusion of normal saline solution, cystic fibrosis (sweat test), hyperparathyroidism, renal tubular disease, metabolic acidosis, prolonged diarrhea, drugs (ammonium chloride administration, acetazolamide, boric acid, triamterene)
Decreased in: Congestive heart failure, syndrome of inappropriate antidiuretic hormone secretion, Addison's disease, vomiting, gastric suction, salt-losing nephritis, continuous infusion of D_5W, thiazide diuretic administration, diaphoresis, diarrhea, burns, diabetic ketoacidosis

CHLORIDE (sweat)

Normal: 0-40 mmol/L
Borderline/indeterminate: 41-60 mmol/L
Consistent with cystic fibrosis: >60 mmol/L
False low results can occur with edema, excessive sweating, and hypoproteinemia.

CHLORIDE, URINE

See URINE CHLORIDE

TABLE 4-10 Cerebrospinal Fluid Findings in Central Nervous System Disorders

Condition	Pressure (mm H_2O)	Leukocytes (mm^3)	Protein (mg/dl)	Glucose (mg/dl)	Comments
Normal	50-80	<5, ≥75% lymphocytes	20-45	>50 (or 75% serum glucose)	
Common Forms of Meningitis					
Acute bacterial meningitis	Usually elevated (100-300)	100-10,000 or more; usually 300-2000; PMNs predominate	Usually 100-500	Decreased, usually <40 (or <66% serum glucose)	Organisms usually seen on Gram stain and recovered by culture; latex agglutination of CSF usually positive
Partially treated bacterial meningitis	Normal or elevated	5-10,000; PMNs usual but mononuclear cells may predominate if pretreated for extended period	Usually 100-500	Normal or decreased	Organisms may be seen on Gram stain; latex agglutination CSF may be positive; pretreatment may render CSF sterile
Viral meningitis or meningoencephalitis	Normal or slightly elevated (80-150)	Rarely >1000 cells; eastern equine encephalitis and lymphocytic choriomeningitis may have cell counts of several thousand; PMNs early but mononuclear cells predominate through most of the course	Usually 50-200	Generally normal; may be decreased to <40 in some viral diseases, particularly mumps (15%-20% of cases)	HSV encephalitis is suggested by focal seizures or by focal findings on CT or MRI scans or EEG. Enteroviruses and HSV infrequently recovered from CSF. HSV and enteroviruses may be detected by PCR of CSF.
Uncommon Forms of Meningitis					
Tuberculous meningitis	Usually elevated	10-500; PMNs early but lymphocytes predominate through most of the course	100-3000; may be higher in presence of block	<50 in most cases; decreases with time if treatment is not provided	Acid-fast organisms almost never seen on smear; organisms may be recovered in culture of large volumes of CSF; *Mycobacterium tuberculosis* may be detected by PCR of CSF
Fungal meningitis	Usually elevated	5-500; PMNs early but mononuclear cells predominate through most of the course; cryptococcal meningitis may have no cellular inflammatory response	25-500	<50; decreases with time if treatment is not provided	Budding yeast may be seen; organisms may be recovered in culture; cryptococcal antigen (CSF and serum) may be positive in cryptococcal infection
Syphilis (acute) and leptospirosis	Usually elevated	50-500; lymphocytes predominate	50-200	Usually normal	Positive CSF serology; spirochetes not demonstrable by usual techniques of smear or culture; darkfield examination may be positive
Amebic *(Naegleria)* meningoencephalitis	Elevated	1000-10,000 or more; PMNs predominate	50-500	Normal or slightly decreased	Mobile amebae may be seen by hanging-drop examination of CSF at room temperature

TABLE 4-10 Cerebrospinal Fluid Findings in Central Nervous System Disorders, (Continued)

Condition	Pressure (mm H_2O)	Leukocytes (mm³)	Protein (mg/dl)	Glucose (mg/dl)	Comments
Brain and Parameningeal Abscesses					
Brain abscess	Usually elevated (100-300)	5-200; CSF rarely acellular; lymphocytes predominate; if abscess ruptures into ventricle, PMNs predominate and cell count may reach >100,000	75-500	Normal unless abscess ruptures into ventricular system	No organisms on smear or culture unless abscess ruptures into ventricular system
Subdural empyema	Usually elevated (100-300)	100-5000; PMNs predominate	100-500	Normal	No organisms on smear or culture of CSF unless meningitis also present; organisms found on tap of subdural fluid
Cerebral epidural abscess	Normal to slightly elevated	10-500; lymphocytes predominate	50-200	Normal	No organisms on smear or culture of CSF
Spinal epidural abscess	Usually low, with spinal block	10-100; lymphocytes predominate	50-400	Normal	No organisms on smear or culture of CSF
Chemical (drugs, dermoid cysts, myelography dye)	Usually elevated	100-1000 or more; PMNs predominate	50-100	Normal or slightly decreased	Epithelial cells may be seen within CSF by use of polarized light in some children with dermoids
Noninfectious Causes					
Sarcoidosis	Normal or elevated slightly	0-100; mononuclear	40-100	Normal	No specific findings
Systemic lupus erythematosus with CNS involvement	Slightly elevated	0-500; PMNs usually predominate; lymphocytes may be present	100	Normal or slightly decreased	No organisms on smear or culture; LE preparation may be positive; positive neuronal and ribosomal P protein antibodies in CSF
Tumor, leukemia	Slightly elevated to very high	0-100 or more; mononuclear or blast cells	50-1000	Normal to decreased (20-40)	Cytology may be positive

From Behrman RE: *Nelson textbook of pediatrics*, ed 17, Philadelphia, 2004, Saunders.
CNS, Central nervous system; *CSF*, cerebrospinal fluid; *CT*, computed tomography; *EEG*, electroencephalogram; *HSV*, herpes simplex virus; *MRI*, magnetic resonance imaging; *PCR*, polymerase chain reaction; *PMN*, polymorphonuclear neutrophils.

CHOLECYSTOKININ-PANCREOZYMIN (CCK, CCK-PZ)

Normal: <80 pg/ml
Elevated in: Pancreatic disease, celiac disease, gastric ulcer, postgastrectomy, IBS, fatty food intolerance

CHOLESTEROL, HIGH-DENSITY LIPOPROTEIN

See HIGH-DENSITY LIPOPROTEIN CHOLESTEROL

CHOLESTEROL, LOW-DENSITY LIPOPROTEIN

See LOW-DENSITY LIPOPROTEIN CHOLESTEROL

CHOLESTEROL, TOTAL

Normal range: Varies with age
Generally <200 mg/dl (<5.20 mmol/L [CF: 0.02586; SMI: 0.05 mmol/L])
Elevated in: Primary hypercholesterolemia, biliary obstruction, diabetes mellitus, nephrotic syndrome, hypothyroidism, primary biliary cirrhosis, high-cholesterol diet, pregnancy third trimester, myocardial infarction, drugs (steroids, phenothiazines, oral contraceptives)
Decreased in: Medications (statins, niacin), starvation, malabsorption, sideroblastic anemia, thalassemia, abetalipoproteinemia, hyperthyroidism, Cushing's syndrome, hepatic failure, multiple myeloma, polycythemia vera, chronic myelocytic leukemia, myeloid metaplasia, Waldenström's macroglobulinemia, myelofibrosis

CHORIONIC GONADOTROPINS, HUMAN (serum) (HCG)

Normal range, serum: Female, premenopausal: <0.8 IU/L; postmenopausal <3.3 IU/L
Male: <0.7 IU/L

Elevated in:
Pregnancy, choriocarcinoma, gestational trophoblastic neoplasia (including molar gestations), placental site trophoblastic tumors; human antimouse antibodies (HAMA) can produce false serum assay for hCG.
The principal use of this test is to diagnose pregnancy. The concentration of hCG increases significantly during the initial 6 weeks of pregnancy.
Normal range: Varies with gestational stage:
1 wk: 5-50 mU/ml
1-2 wk: 50-550 mU/ml
2-3 wk: up to 5000 mU/ml
3-4 wk: up to 10,000 mU/ml
4-5 wk: up to 50,000 mU/ml
2-3 mo: 10,000-100,000 mU/ml
Peak values approaching 100,000 IU/L occur 60-70 days following implantation.
hCG levels generally double every 1-3 days. In patients with concentration <2000 IU/L, an increase of serum hCG <66% after 2 days is suggestive of spontaneous abortion or ruptured ectopic gestation.

CHYMOTRYPSIN

Normal: <10 mcg/L
Elevated in: Acute pancreatitis, chronic renal failure, oral enzyme preparations, gastric cancer, pancreatic cancer
Decreased in: Chronic pancreatitis, late cystic fibrosis

CIRCULATING ANTICOAGULANT (lupus anticoagulant)

Normal: Negative
Detected in: Systemic lupus erythematosus, drug-induced lupus, long-term phenothiazine therapy, multiple myeloma, ulcerative colitis, rheumatoid arthritis, postpartum, hemophilia, neoplasms, chronic inflammatory states, AIDS, nephrotic syndrome

NOTE: The name is a misnomer because these patients are prone to hypercoagulability and thrombosis.

CK

See CREATINE KINASE

CLONIDINE SUPPRESSION TEST

Interpretation: Clonidine inhibits neurogenic catecholamine release and will cause a decrease in plasma norepinephrine into the reference interval in hypertensive subjects without pheochromocytoma.Test is performed by giving 4.3 mcg clonidine/kg orally after overnight fast. Norepinephrine is measured at 3 hr. Result should be within established reference range and decrease to <50% of baseline concentration. Lack of decrease in norepinephrine is suggestive of pheochromocytoma.

CLOSTRIDIUM DIFFICILE TOXIN ASSAY (stool)

Normal: Negative
Detected in: Antibiotic-associated diarrhea and pseudomembranous colitis

CO

See CARBOXYHEMOGLOBIN

COAGULATION FACTORS

See Table 4-11 for characteristics of coagulation factors.
Factor reference ranges:
V: >10%
VII: >10%
VIII: 50%-170%
IX: 60%-136%
X: >10%
XI: 50%-150%
XII: >30%

Table 4-12 describes screening laboratory results in coagulation factor deficiencies.

TABLE 4-12 Screening Laboratory Results in Coagulation Factor Deficiencies

Deficient Factor	Frequency	PT	PTT	TT
I (fibrinogen)	Rare	↑	↑	↑
II (prothrombin)	Very rare	↑	↑	↑
V 1:1,000,000	↑	↑	NL	
VII	1:500,000	↑	NL	NL
VIII	1:5000 (male)	NL	↑	NL
IX	1:30,000 (male)	NL	↑	NL
X 1:500,000	↑	↑	NL	
XI	Rare*	NL	↑	NL
XII or HMWK or PK†	Rare	NL	↑	NL
XIII	Rare	NL	NL	↑

From Andreoli TE (ed): *Cecil essentials of medicine,* ed 5, Philadelphia, 2001, Saunders.
↑Increased over normal range; *HMWK,* high-molecular-weight kininogen; *NL,* normal; *PK,* prekallikrein; *PT,* prothrombin time; *PTT,* partial thromboplastin time; *TT,* thrombin time.
*Except in those of Ashkenazi Jewish descent (approximately 4% are heterozygous for factor XI deficiency).
†Not associated with clinical bleeding.

COLD AGGLUTININS TITER

Normal range: <1:32
Elevated in:
Primary atypical pneumonia (*Mycoplasma* pneumonia), infectious mononucleosis, CMV infection
Others: hepatic cirrhosis, acquired hemolytic anemia, frostbite, multiple myeloma, lymphoma, malaria

COMPLEMENT

Normal range:
C3: 70-160 mg/dl (0.7-1.6 g/L [CF: 0.01; SMI: 0.1 g/L])
C4: 20-40 mg/dl (0.2-0.4 g/L [CF: 0.01; SMI: 0.1 g/L])
Abnormal values:
Decreased C3: Active SLE, immune complex disease, acute glomerulonephritis, inborn C3 deficiency, membranoproliferative glomerulonephritis, infective endocarditis, serum sickness, autoimmune/chronic active hepatitis

TABLE 4-11 Characteristics of Coagulation Factors

Factor	Descriptive Name	Source	Approximate Half-Life (hr)	Function
I	Fibrinogen	Liver	120	Substrate for fibrin clot (CP)
II	Prothrombin	Liver (VKD)	60	Serine protease (CP)
V	Proaccelerin, labile factor	Liver	12-36	Cofactor (CP)
VII	Serum prothrombin conversion accelerator, proconvertin	Liver (VKD)	6	(?) Serine protease (EP)
VIII	Antihemophilic factor or globulin	Endothelial cells and (?) elsewhere	12	Cofactor (IP)
IX	Plasma thromboplastin component, Christmas factor	Liver (VKD)	24	Serine protease (IP)
X	Stuart-Prower factor	Liver (VKD)	36	Serine protease (CP)
XI	Plasma thromboplastin antecedent	(?) Liver	40-84	Serine protease (IP)
XII	Hageman factor	(?) Liver	50	Serine protease contact activation (IP)
XIII	Fibrin-stabilizing factor	(?) Liver	96-180	Transglutaminase (CP)
Prekallikrein	Fletcher factor	(?) Liver	?	Serine protease contact activation (IP)
High-molecular-weight kininogen	Fitzgerald factor, Flaujeac or Williams factor	(?) Liver	?	Cofactor, contact activation (IP)

From Noble J (ed): *Primary care medicine,* ed 3, St Louis, 2001, Mosby.
CP, Common pathway; *EP,* extrinsic pathway; *IP,* intrinsic pathway; *VKD,* vitamin K dependent.

Decreased C4: Immune complex disease, active SLE, infective endocarditis, inborn C4 deficiency, hereditary angioedema, hypergammaglobulinemic states, cryoglobulinemic vasculitis

COMPLEMENT DEFICIENCY

Table 4-13 describes complement deficiency states.

COMPLETE BLOOD COUNT (CBC)

See Fig. E4-13, which describes an algorithm for the evaluation of patients with neutropenia.

White blood cells 3200-9800/mm^3 (3.2-9.8 × 10^9/L [CF: 0.001; SMI: 0.1 × 10^9/L])

Red blood cells
- Male: 4.3-5.9 × 10^6/mm^3 (4.3-5.9 × 10^{12}/L [CF: 0.001; SMI: 0.1 × 10^{12}/L])
- Female: 3.5-5 × 10^6/mm^3 (3.5-5 × 10^{12}/L [CF: 0.001; SMI: 0.1 × 10^{12}/L])

Hemoglobin
- Male: 13.6-17.7 g/dl (136-172 g/L [CF: 10; SMI: 1 g/L])
- Female: 12-15 g/dl (120-150 g/L [CF: 10; SMI: 1 g/L])

Hematocrit
- Male: 39%-49% (0.39-0.49 [CF: 0.01; SMI: 0.01])
- Female: 33%-43% (0.33-0.43 [CF: 0.01; SMI: 0.01])

Mean corpuscular volume (MCV): 76-100 μm^3 (76-100 fL [CF: 1; SMI: 1 fL])

Mean corpuscular hemoglobin (MCH): 27-33 pg (27-33 pg [CF: 1; SMI: 1 pg])

TABLE 4-13 Complement Deficiency States

Component	No. of Reported Patients	Mode of Inheritance	Functional Defects	Disease Associations
Classic Pathway				
C1qrs	31	ACD	Impaired IC handling, delayed C' activation, impaired immune response	CVD, 48%; infection (encapsulated bacteria), 22%; both, 18%; healthy, 12%
C4	21	ACD	Impaired C' activation in absence of specific antibody	Infection (meningococcal), 74%; healthy, 26%
C2	109	ACD		
Alternative Pathway				
D	3	ACD	Impaired IC handling, opson/phag; granulocytosis, CTX, immune response and absent SBA	CVD, 79%; recurrent infection (encapsulated bacteria), 71%
P	70	XL		
Junction of Classic and Alternative Pathways				
C3	19	ACD	Impaired CTX; absent SBA	Infection (*Neisseria,* primarily meningococcal), 58%; CVD, 4%
Terminal Components				
C5	27	ACD	Absent SBA	Both, 1%
C6	77	ACD		Healthy, 25%
C7	73	ACD		
C8	73	ACD		
C9	165	ACD	Impaired SBA	Healthy, 91%; infection, 9%
Plasma Proteins Regulating C' Activation				
C1-INH	Many	AD	Uncontrolled generation of an inflammatory mediator on C' activation	Hereditary angioedema
H	13	Acq	Uncontrolled AP activation → low C3	CVD, 40%; CVD plus infection (encapsulated bacteria), 40%; healthy, 20%
I	14	ACD	Uncontrolled AP activation → low C3	Infection (encapsulated bacteria), 100%
Membrane proteins regulating C' activation	Many	Acq	Impaired regulation of C3b and C8 deposited on host RBCs; PMN, platelets → cell lysis	Paroxysmal nocturnal hemoglobinuria
Decay-accelerating factor				
Homologous restriction factor				
CD59	>20	ACD	Impaired PMN adhesive functions (i.e., margination), CTX, C3bi-mediated opson/phag	Infection (*Staphylococcus aureus, Pseudomonas* spp.), 100%
CR3 autoantibodies				
C3 nephritic factors	>59	Acq	Stabilize AP, convertase → low C3	MPGN, 41%; PLD, 25%; infection (encapsulated bacteria), 16%; MPGN plus PLD, 10%; PLD plus infection, 5%; MPGN plus PLD plus infection, 3%; MPGN plus infection, 2%
C4 nephritic factor		Acq	Stabilize CP, C3 convertase → low C3	Glomerulonephritis, 50%; CVD, 50%

From Mandell GL: *Mandell, Douglas, and Bennett's principles and practice of infectious diseases,* ed 6, New York, 2005, Churchill Livingstone.

ACD, Autosomal codominant; *Acq,* acquired; *AD,* autosomal dominant; *AP,* alternative pathway; *C',* complement; *CP,* classic pathway; *CTX,* chemotaxis; *CVD,* collagen-vascular disease; *IC,* immune complex, *MPGN,* membranoproliferative glomerulonephritis; *PLD,* partial lipodystrophy; *PMN,* polymorphonuclear neutrophil; *RBCs,* red blood cells; *SBA,* serum bactericidal activity; *XL,* X-linked.

Mean corpuscular hemoglobin concentration (MCHC): 33-37 g/dl (330-370 g/L [CF: 10; SMI: 10 g/L])
Red blood cell distribution width index (RDW): 11.5%-14.5%
Platelet count: 130-400 × 10^3/mm^3 (130-400 × 10^9/L [CF: 1; SMI: 5 × 10^9/L])
Differential:
- 2-6 stabs (bands, early mature neutrophils)
- 60-70 segs (mature neutrophils)
- 1-4 eosinophils
- 0-1 basophils
- 2-8 monocytes
- 25-40 lymphocytes

CONJUGATED BILIRUBIN

See BILIRUBIN, DIRECT

COOMBS, DIRECT

Normal: Negative
Positive: Autoimmune hemolytic anemia, erythroblastosis fetalis, transfusion reactions, drugs (α-methyldopa, penicillins, tetracycline, sulfonamides, levodopa, cephalosporins, quinidine, insulin)
False-positive: May be seen with cold agglutinins

COOMBS, INDIRECT

Normal: Negative
Positive: Acquired hemolytic anemia, incompatible cross-matched blood, anti-Rh antibodies, drugs (methyldopa, mefenamic acid, levodopa)

COPPER (serum)

Normal range: 70-140 μg/dl (11-22 μmol/L [CF: 0.1574, SMI: 0.2 μmol/L])
Decreased in: Wilson's disease, Menkes' syndrome, malabsorption, malnutrition, nephrosis, total parenteral nutrition, acute leukemia in remission
Elevated in: Aplastic anemia, biliary cirrhosis, systemic lupus erythematosus, hemochromatosis, hyperthyroidism, hypothyroidism, infection, iron deficiency anemia, leukemia, lymphoma, oral contraceptives, pernicious anemia, rheumatoid arthritis

COPPER, URINE

See URINE COPPER

CORTICOTROPIN RELEASING HORMONE (CRH) STIMULATION TEST

Normal: A dose of 0.5 mg of dexamethasone is given every 6 hours for 2 days; 2 hours after last dose 1 mcg/kg CRH is given IV. Samples are drawn after 15 min. Normally there is a twofold to fourfold increase in mean baseline concentration of ACTH or cortisol. Cortisol >1.4 mcg/L is virtually 100% specific and 100% diagnostic.
Interpretation:
Normal or exaggerated response: Pituitary Cushing's disease
No response: Ectopic ACTH-secreting tumor
A positive response to CRH or a suppressed response to high-dose dexamethasone has a 97% positive predictive value for Cushing's disease. However, a lack of response to either test excludes Cushing's disease in only 64%-78% of patients. When the tests are considered together, negative responses from both have a 100% predictive value for ectopic ACTH secretion.

CORTISOL, PLASMA

Normal range: Varies with time of collection (circadian variation):
8 AM: 4-19 μg/dl (110-520 nmol/L [CF: 27.59; SMI: 10 nmol/L])
4 PM: 2-15 μg/dl (50-410 nmol/L [CF: 27.59; SMI: 10 nmol/L])
Elevated in: Ectopic adrenocorticotropic hormone production (i.e., oat cell carcinoma of lung), loss of normal diurnal variation, pregnancy, chronic renal failure, iatrogenic, stress, adrenal or pituitary hyperplasia, or adenomas
Decreased in: Primary adrenocortical insufficiency, anterior pituitary hypofunction, secondary adrenocortical insufficiency, adrenogenital syndromes

C-PEPTIDE

Elevated in: Insulinoma, sulfonylurea administration
Decreased in: Insulin-dependent diabetes mellitus, factitious insulin administration

CPK

See CREATINE KINASE

C-REACTIVE PROTEIN

Normal range: 6.8-820 μg/dl (68-8200 μg/L [CF: 10; SMI: 10 μg/L])
Elevated in: Rheumatoid arthritis, rheumatic fever, inflammatory bowel disease, bacterial infections, myocardial infarction, oral contraceptives, third trimester of pregnancy (acute phase reactant), inflammatory and neoplastic diseases Table 4-14 shows a comparison of erythrocyte sedimentation rate and C-reactive protein, and Table 4-15 shows conditions associated with elevated C-reactive protein levels.

C-REACTIVE PROTEIN, HIGH SENSITIVITY (Hs-CRP, cardio-CRP)

This is a cardiac risk marker. It is increased in patients with silent atherosclerosis years before a cardiovascular event and is independent of cholesterol level and other lipoproteins. It can be used to help stratify cardiac risk.

INTERPRETATION OF RESULTS

Cardio-CRP result (mg/L)	*Risk*
0.6	Lowest risk
0.7-1.1	Low risk
1.2-1.9	Moderate risk
2.0-3.8	High risk
3.9-4.9	Highest risk
≥5.0	Results may be confounded by acute inflammatory disease. If clinically indicated, a repeat test should be performed in 2 or more weeks.

CREATINE KINASE (CK, CPK)

Fig. E4-14 describes a diagnostic approach to creatine kinase elevation.
Normal range: 0-130 U/L (0-2.16 μkat/L [CF: 0.01667; SMI: 0.01 μkat/L])
Elevated in: Myocardial infarction, myocarditis, rhabdomyolysis, myositis, crush injury/trauma, polymyositis, dermatomyositis, vigorous exercise, muscular dystrophy, myxedema, seizures, malignant hyperthermia syndrome, IM injections, cerebrovascular accident, pulmonary embolism and infarction, acute dissection of aorta
Decreased in: Steroids, decreased muscle mass, connective tissue disorders, alcoholic liver disease, metastatic neoplasms

CREATINE KINASE ISOENZYMES

CK-BB

Elevated in: Cerebrovascular accident, subarachnoid hemorrhage, neoplasms (prostate, gastrointestinal tract, brain, ovary, breast, lung), severe shock, bowel infarction, hypothermia, meningitis

CK-MB

Elevated in: Myocardial infarction (MI), myocarditis, pericarditis, muscular dystrophy, cardiac defibrillation, cardiac surgery, extensive rhabdomyolysis, strenuous exercise (marathon runners), mixed connective tissue disease, cardiomyopathy, hypothermia

NOTE: CK-MB exists in the blood in two subforms. MB_2 is released from cardiac cells and converted in the blood to MB_1. Rapid assay of CK-MB subforms can detect MI (CK-MB_2 ≥1.0 U/L, with a ratio of CK-MB_2/CK-MB_1 ≥1.5) within 6 hours of onset of symptoms.

Fig. 4-15 illustrates the time course of CK, AST, troponins, and LDH activity after acute MI.

CK-MM

Elevated in: Crush injury, seizures, malignant hyperthermia syndrome, rhabdomyolysis, myositis, polymyositis, dermatomyositis, vigorous exercise, muscular dystrophy, IM injections, acute dissection of aorta

CREATININE (serum)

See Fig. 4-16.

TABLE 4-14 Comparison of Erythrocyte Sedimentation Rate and C-Reactive Protein

	Erythrocyte Sedimentation Rate	C-Reactive Protein
Advantages	• Much clinical information in the literature • May reflect overall health status	• Rapid response to inflammatory stimuli • Wide range of clinically relevant values are detectable • Unaffected by age and gender • Reflects value of a single acute phase protein • Can be measured on stored sera • Quantitation is precise and reproducible
Disadvantages	• Affected by age and gender • Affected by red blood cell morphology • Affected by anemia and polycythemia • Reflects levels of many plasma proteins, not all of which are acute phase proteins • Responds slowly to inflammatory stimuli • Requires fresh sample • May be affected by drugs	• None

From Firestein GS, Budd RC, Gabriel SE, et al: *Kelly's textbook of rheumatology*, ed 9, Philadelphia, 2013, Saunders.

TABLE 4-15 Conditions Associated with Elevated C-Reactive Protein Levels

Normal or Minor Elevation (<1 mg/dL)	Moderate Elevation (1-10 mg/dL)	Marked Elevation (>10 mg/dL)
• Vigorous exercise • Common cold • Pregnancy • Gingivitis • Seizures • Depression • Insulin resistance and diabetes • Several genetic polymorphisms • Obesity	• Myocardial infarction • Malignancies • Pancreatitis • Mucosal infection (bronchitis, cystitis) • Most connective tissue diseases • Rheumatoid arthritis	• Acute bacterial infection (80%-85%) • Major trauma • Systemic vasculitis

From Firestein GS, Budd RC, Gabriel SE, et al: *Kelly's textbook of rheumatology*, ed 9, Philadelphia, 2013, Saunders.

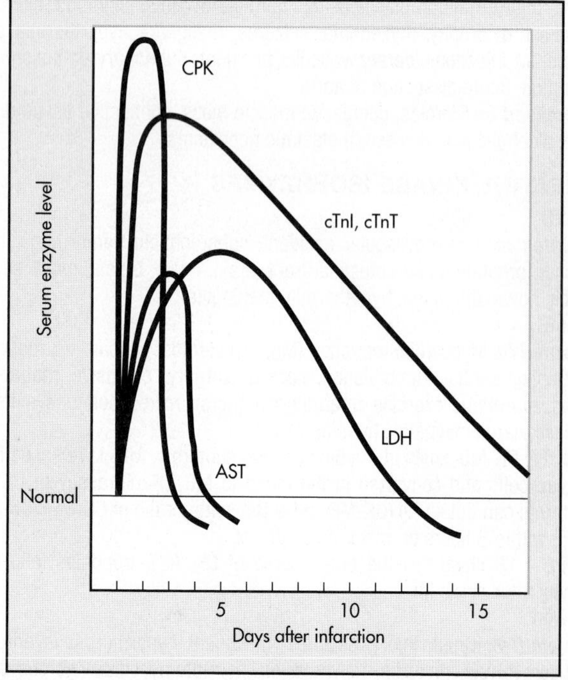

FIGURE 4-15 Evaluation of creatine kinase elevation. *CPK,* Creatine kinase; *cTnI,* cardiac troponin I; *cTnT,* cardiac troponin T; *AST,* aspartate aminotransferase; *LDH,* lactate dehydrogenase. (From Greene HL, Johnson WP, Lemcke D [eds]: *Decision making in medicine,* ed 2, St Louis, 1998, Mosby.)

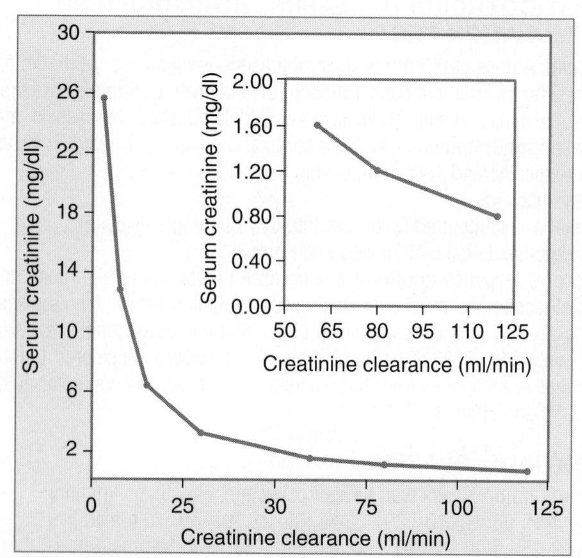

FIGURE 4-16 Relationship between creatinine clearance and serum creatinine. In steady state, serum creatinine should increase twofold for each 50% reduction in creatinine clearance. *Inset* represents enlarged view of changes in serum creatinine as creatinine clearance decreases from 120 to 60 ml/min. If serum creatinine is 0.8 mg/dl when creatinine clearance is 120 ml/min, creatinine clearance can decrease by 33% such that increased serum creatinine is still within normal range. (From Vincent JL et al: *Textbook of critical care,* ed 6, Philadelphia, 2011, Saunders.)

BOX 4-1 Calculation of the Creatinine Clearance

$C_{cr} = U_{cr} \times V/P_{cr}$
where C_{cr}= clearance of creatinine (ml/min)
U_{cr} = urine creatinine (mg/dl)
V = volume of urine (ml/min) (for 24-hr volume: divide by 1440)
P_{cr} = plasma creatinine (mg/dl)
Normal range: 95 to 105 ml/min/1.75m^2

BOX 4-2 Cockcroft-Gault Formula to Calculate Creatinine Clearance (C_{cr})

$$C_{cr} = \frac{(140 - \text{age in year}) \times (\text{lean body weight in kg})}{S_{cr}\text{in mg/dl} - 72}$$

Normal range: 0.6-1.2 mg/dl (50-110 μmol/L [CF: 88.4; SMI: 10 μmol/L])
Elevated in: Renal insufficiency (acute and chronic), decreased renal perfusion (hypotension, dehydration, congestive heart failure), urinary tract infection, rhabdomyolysis, ketonemia

Drugs (antibiotics [aminoglycosides, cephalosporins], hydantoin, diuretics, methyldopa)
Falsely elevated in: Diabetic ketoacidosis, administration of some cephalosporins (e.g., cefoxitin, cephalothin)
Decreased in: Decreased muscle mass (including amputees and older persons), pregnancy, prolonged debilitation

CREATININE CLEARANCE

Normal range: 75-124 ml/min (1.24-2.08 ml/sec [CF: 0.01667; SMI: 0.02 ml/sec])

Box 4-1 describes a formula for calculation of creatinine clearance.

The Cockcroft-Gault formula to calculate creatinine clearance is described in Box 4-2.
Elevated in: Pregnancy, exercise
Decreased in: Renal insufficiency, drugs (cimetidine, procainamide, antibiotics, quinidine)

CREATININE, URINE

See URINE CREATININE

CRYOGLOBULINS (serum)

Normal range: Not detectable
Present in: Collagen vascular diseases, chronic lymphocytic leukemia, hemolytic anemias, multiple myeloma, Waldenström's macroglobulinemia, chronic active hepatitis, Hodgkin's disease

CRYPTOSPORIDIUM ANTIGEN BY EIA (stool)

Normal range: Not detected
Present in: Cryptosporidiosis

CSF

See CEREBROSPINAL FLUID

CYSTATIN C

Normal: Cystatin C is a cysteine protease inhibitor that is produced at a constant rate by all nucleated cells. It is freely filtered by the glomerulus and reabsorbed (but not secreted) by the renal tubules with no extrarenal excretion. Its concentration is not affected by diet, muscle mass, or acute inflammation. Normal range when measured by particle-enhanced nephelometric immunoassay (PENIA) is <0.28 mg/L.
Elevated in: Renal disorders. Good predictor of the severity of acute tubular necrosis. Cystatin C increases more rapidly than creatinine in the early stages of GFR impairment. The cystatin C concentration is an independent risk factor for heart failure in older adults and appears to provide a better measure of risk assessment than the serum creatinine concentration.

CYSTIC FIBROSIS PCR

Test description: Test can be performed on whole blood or tissue. Common mutations in the cystic fibrosis transmembrane regulator (CFTR) gene can be used to detect 75%-80% of mutant alleles.

CYTOMEGALOVIRUS BY PCR

Test description: Test can be performed on whole blood, plasma, or tissue. Qualitative PCR is highly sensitive but may not be able to differentiate between latent and active infection.

D-DIMER

Normal range: <0.5 mcg/ml
Elevated in:
DVT, pulmonary embolism, high levels of rheumatoid factor, activation of coagulation and fibrolytic system from any cause
D-dimer assay by ELISA assists in the diagnosis of DVT and pulmonary embolism. This test has significant limitations because it can be elevated whenever the coagulation and fibrinolytic systems are activated and can also be falsely elevated with high rheumatoid factor levels.

DEHYDROEPIANDROSTERONE SULFATE

Normal:
Males:

Ages 19-30:	125-619 mcg/dl
31-50:	59-452 mcg/dl
51-60:	20-413 mcg/dl
61-83:	10-285 mcg/dl

Females:

Ages 19-30:	29-781 mcg/dl
31-50:	12-379 mcg/dl
Postmenopausal:	30-260 mcg/dl

Elevated in: Hirsutism, congenital adrenal hyperplasia, adrenal carcinomas, adrenal adenomas, polycystic ovary syndrome, ectopic ACTH-producing tumors, Cushing's disease, spironolactone

DEHYDROTESTOSTERONE (serum, urine)

Normal:
Serum: Males: 30-85 ng/dl; females: 4-22 ng/dl
Urine, 24 h: Males: 20-50 mcg/day; females: <8 mcg/day
Elevated in: Hirsutism
Decreased in: 5-α-reductase deficiency, hypogonadism

DEOXYCORTICOSTERONE (11-deoxycorticosterone, DOC) (serum)

Normal: 2-19 ng/dl. Normal secretion depends on ACTH and is suppressible by dexamethasone.
Elevated in: Adrenogenital syndromes due to 17- and 11-hydroxylase deficiencies, pregnancy
Decreased in: Preeclampsia

DEXAMETHASONE SUPPRESSION TEST, OVERNIGHT

Normal: Test is performed by giving 1 mg dexamethasone orally at 11 PM and measuring serum cortisol at 8 AM the following morning. Normal response is cortisol suppression to <3 mcg/dl; If dose of 4 mg dexamethasone is given, cortisol suppression will be to <50% of baseline.
Interpretation: Cushing's syndrome (<10 mcg/dl), endogenous depression (half of patients suppress test values <5 mcg/dl). Most patients with pituitary Cushing's disease demonstrate suppression, whereas patients with adrenal adenoma, carcinoma, and ectopic ACTH-producing tumors do not.

DIGOXIN

Normal therapeutic range: 0.5-2 ng/ml
Elevated in: Impaired renal function, excessive dosing, concomitant use of quinidine, amiodarone, verapamil, fluoxetine, nifedipine. Toxicity may occur at a lower blood concentration in the presence of hypokalemia, hypomagnesemia, and hypercalcemia.

DILANTIN

See PHENYTOIN

DISACCHARIDE ABSORPTION TESTS

Normal: Test is used to diagnose malabsorption due to disaccharide deficiency. It is performed by giving disaccharide orally 1 g/kg body weight to a total of 25 g. Blood is drawn at 0, 30, 60, 90, and 120 min. Normal response is a change in glucose from fasting value >30 mg/dl, inconclusive when increase is 20-30 mg/dl, abnormal when increase is >20 mg/dl. Test can also be performed by measuring air at 0, 30, 60, 90, and 120 min. Normal is H_2 >20 ppm above baseline level before a colonic response.
Decreased in: Disaccharide deficiency (lactose, fructose, sorbitol), celiac disease, sprue, acute gastroenetetitis

DOC

See DEOXYCORTICOSTERONE

DONATH-LANDSTEINER (D-L) TEST FOR PAROXYSMAL COLD HEMOGLOBINURIA

Normal: No hemolysis
Interpretation: Hemolysis indicates presence of bithermic cold hemolysins or Donath-Landsteiner antibodies (D-L Ab)

DOPAMINE

Normal range: 175 pg/ml
Elevated in: Pheochromocytomas, neuroblastomas, stress, vigorous exercise, certain foods (bananas, chocolate, coffee, tea, vanilla)

D-XYLOSE ABSORPTION

Normal range: 21%-31% excreted in 5 hours
Decreased in: Malabsorption syndrome

D-XYLOSE ABSORPTION TEST

Normal range:
URINE: ≥4 g/5 hours (5-hour urine collection in adults >12 years [25-g dose])
SERUM: ≥25 mg/dl (adult, 1 hour, 25-g dose, normal renal function)
Normal results: In patients with malabsorption, normal results suggest pancreatic disease as an etiology of the malabsorption.
Abnormal results: Celiac disease, Crohn's disease, tropical sprue, surgical bowel resection, AIDS. False-positives can occur with decreased renal function, dehydration/hypovolemia, surgical blind loops, decreased gastric emptying, vomiting.

ELECTROPHORESIS, HEMOGLOBIN

See HEMOGLOBIN ELECTROPHORESIS

ELECTROPHORESIS, PROTEIN

See PROTEIN ELECTROPHORESIS

ENA COMPLEX

See EXTRACTABLE NUCLEAR ANTIGEN

ENDOMYSIAL ANTIBODIES

Normal: Not detected
Present in: Celiac disease, dermatitis herpetiformis

EOSINOPHIL COUNT

Normal range: 1%-4% eosinophils (0-440/mm^3)
Elevated in
HELMINTHIC PARASITES:
Ascaris lumbricoides (invasive larval stage)
Hookworms (invasive larval stage)
Strongyloides stercoralis (initial infection and autoinfection)
Trichinosis
Filariasis
Echinococcus granulosus and *E. multilocularis*
Toxocara species
Animal hookworms
Angiostrongylus cantonensis and *A. costaricensis*
Schistosomiasis
Liver flukes
Fasciolopsis buski
Anisakiasis
Capillaria philippinensis
Paragonimus westermani
"Tropical eosinophilia" (unidentified microfilariae)
OTHER INFECTIONS/INFESTATIONS
Pulmonary aspergillosis
Severe scabies
ALLERGIES
Asthma
Hay fever
Drug reactions
Atopic dermatitis
AUTOIMMUNE AND RELATED DISORDERS
Polyarteritis nodosa
Necrotizing vasculitis
Eosinophilic fasciitis
Pemphigus
NEOPLASTIC DISEASES
Hodgkin's disease
Mycosis fungoides
Chronic myelocytic leukemia
Eosinophilic leukemia
Polycythemia vera
Mucin-secreting adenocarcinomas
IMMUNODEFICIENCY STATES
Hyperimmunoglobulin E with recurrent infection
Wiskott-Aldrich syndrome
OTHER
Addison's disease
Inflammatory bowel disease
Dermatitis herpetiformis
Toxic/chemical syndrome
Eosinophilic myalgia syndrome, tryptophan, toxic oil syndrome
Hypereosinophilic syndrome (unknown etiology)

EPINEPHRINE, PLASMA

Normal range: 0-90 pg/ml
Elevated in: Pheochromocytomas, neuroblastomas, stress, vigorous exercise, certain foods (bananas, chocolate, coffee, tea, vanilla), hypoglycemia

EPSTEIN-BARR VIRUS SEROLOGY

Normal range: IgG anti-VCA <1:10 or negative
Abnormal:
IgG anti-VCA >1:10 or positive indicates either current or previous infection
IgM anti-VCA >1:10 or positive indicates current or recent infection
Anti-EBNA ≥ 1.5 or positive indicates previous infection
Table 4-16 and Fig. 4-17 describe test interpretation.

ERYTHROCYTE SEDIMENTATION RATE (ESR, sed rate, sedimentation rate)

Normal range:
Male: 0-15 mm/hr
Female: 0-20 mm/hr
Elevated in: Collagen vascular diseases, infections, myocardial infarction, neoplasms, inflammatory states (acute phase reactant), hyperthyroidism, hypothyroidism, rouleaux formation
Decreased in: Sickle cell disease, polycythemia, corticosteroids, spherocytosis, anisocytosis, hypofibrinogenemia, increased serum viscosity

ERYTHROPOIETIN (EP)

Normal: 3.7-16.0 IU/L by radioimmunoassay
Erythropoietin is a glycoprotein secreted by the kidneys that stimulates RBC production by acting on erythroid-committed stem cells.

TABLE 4-16 Antibody Tests in Epstein-Barr Viral Infection

	Appearance	Peak	Disappears
Heterophil Ab	3-5 days after onset of Sx (range, 0-21 days)	During second wk after onset of Sx (1-4 wk)	2-3 mo after onset of Sx (still found at 1 yr in 20% of cases)
VCA-IgM	Beginning of Sx (1 wk before to 1 wk after Sx begin)	During first wk after onset of Sx (0-21 days)	2-3 mo after onset of Sx (1-6 mo)
VCA-IgG	3 days after onset of Sx (0-2 wk)	During second wk after onset of Sx (1-3 wk)	Decline to lower level, then persists for life
EBNA-IgG	3 wk after onset of Sx (1-4 wk)	8 mo after appearance (3-12 mo)	Lifelong
EA-D	5 days after onset of Sx (during first 1-2 wk after onset of Sx)	14-21 days after onset of Sx (1-4 wk)	9 wk after appearance (2-6 mo)
EBNA-IgM	Same as VCA-IgM	Same as VCA-IgM	Same as VCA-IgM

From Ravel R: *Clinical laboratory medicine*, ed 6, St Louis, 1995, Mosby.
Ab, Antibody; *EA*, early antigen; *EBNA*, Epstein-Barr virus nuclear antigen; *Sx*, symptoms; *VCA*, viral capsid antigen.

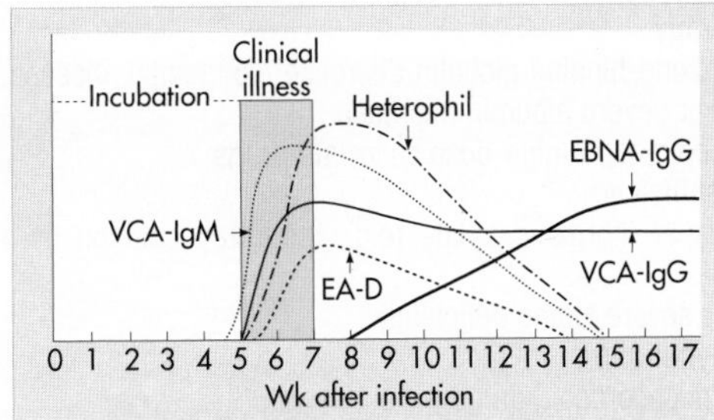

FIGURE 4-17 Tests in Epstein-Barr viral infection. See Table 4-16 for abbreviations. (From Ravel R [ed]: *Clinical laboratory medicine*, ed 6, St Louis, 1995, Mosby.)

Increased in:

Extremely high: Generally seen in patients with severe anemia (Hct <25, Hb, >7) such as in cases of aplastic anemia, severe hemolytic anemia, hematologic cancers

Very high: Patients with mild to moderate anemia (Hct, 25-35; Hb, 7-10)

High: Patients with mild anemia (e.g., AIDS, myelodysplasia)

Erythropoietin can be inappropriately elevated in patients with malignant neoplasms, renal cysts, postrenal transplant, meningioma, hemangioblastoma, and leiomyoma.

Decreased in: Renal failure, polycythemia vera, autonomic neuropathy

ESTRADIOL (serum)

Normal range:

Female, premenopausal: 30-400 pg/ml, depending on phase of menstrual cycle

Female, postmenopausal: 0-30 pg/ml

Male, adult: 10-50 pg/ml

Decreased in: Ovarian failure

Elevated in: Tumors of ovary, testis, adrenal, or nonendocrine sites (rare)

ESTROGEN

Normal range (serum):

Males:	20-80 pg/ml
Females:	
Follicular:	60-200 pg/ml
Luteal:	160-400 pg/ml
Postmenopausal:	<130 pg/ml

Normal range (urine):

Males:	4-23 μg/g creatinine
Females:	
Follicular:	7-65 μg/g creatinine
Midcycle:	32-104 μg/g creatinine
Luteal:	8-135 μg/g creatinine

Elevated in: Hyperplasia of adrenal cortex, ovarian tumors producing estrogen, granulosa and thecal cell tumors, testicular tumors

Decreased in: Menopause, hypopituitarism, primary ovarian malfunction, anorexia nervosa, hypofunction of adrenal cortex, ovarian agenesis, psychogenic stress, gonadotropin-releasing hormone deficiency

ETHANOL (blood)

Normal range:

Negative (values <10 mg/dl are considered negative)

Ethanol is metabolized at 10-25 mg/dl/hr. Levels ≥80 mg/dl are considered evidence of impairment for driving. Fatal blood concentration is considered to be >400 mg/dl.

EXTRACTABLE NUCLEAR ANTIGEN (ENA complex, anti-RNP antibody, anti-SM, anti-Smith)

Normal: Negative

Present in: Systemic lupus erythematosus, rheumatoid arthritis, Sjögren's syndrome, mixed connective tissue disease

FACTOR V LEIDEN

Test description: PCR test performed on whole blood or tissue. This single mutation, found in 2%-8% of the general Caucasian population, is the single most common cause of hereditary thrombophilia.

FASTING BLOOD SUGAR

See GLUCOSE, FASTING

FBS

See GLUCOSE, FASTING

FDP

See FIBRIN DEGRADATION PRODUCT

FECAL FAT, QUANTITATIVE (72-hr collection)

Normal range: 2-6 g/24 hr (7-21 mmol/dl [CF: 3.515; SMI: 1 mmol/dl])

Elevated in: Malabsorption syndrome

FECAL GLOBIN IMMUNOCHEMICAL TEST

Normal: Negative. This test is performed by immunochromatography on a cellulose strip that has been impregnated with various antibodies. The test uses a small amount of toilet water as the specimen and is placed onto absorbent pads of card similar to traditional OB card. There is no direct handling of stool. This test is specific for the globin portion of the hemoglobin molecule, which confers lower GI bleeding specificity. It specifically detects blood from the lower GI tract; guaic tests are not lower GI specific. It is more sensitive than typical Hemoccult test (detection limit 50 mcg Hb/g feces versus >500 mcg Hb/g feces for Hemoccult). It has no dietary restrictions and gives no false-positives due to plant peroxidases and red meats. It has no medication restrictions. Iron supplements and NSAIDs do not cause false-positives. Vitamin C does not cause false-negatives.

Positive in: Lower GI bleeding

FERRITIN (serum)

Normal range: 18-300 ng/ml (18-300 μg/L [CF: 1; SMI: 10 μg/L])
Elevated in: Hyperthyroidism, inflammatory states, liver disease (ferritin elevated from necrotic hepatocytes), neoplasms (neuroblastomas, lymphomas, leukemia, breast carcinoma), iron replacement therapy, hemochromatosis, hemosiderosis
Decreased in: Iron deficiency anemia

α-1 FETOPROTEIN

Normal range: 0-20 ng/ml (0-20 μg/L [CF: 1; SMI: 1 μg/L])
Elevated in: Hepatocellular carcinoma (usually values >1000 ng/ml), germinal neoplasms (testis, ovary, mediastinum, retroperitoneum), liver disease (alcoholic cirrhosis, acute hepatitis, chronic active hepatitis), fetal anencephaly, spina bifida, basal cell carcinoma, breast carcinoma, pancreatic carcinoma, gastric carcinoma, retinoblastoma, esophageal atresia

FIBRIN DEGRADATION PRODUCT (FDP)

Normal range: <10 μg/ml
Elevated in: Disseminated intravascular coagulation, primary fibrinolysis, pulmonary embolism, severe liver disease

NOTE: The presence of rheumatoid factor may cause falsely elevated FDP.

FIBRINOGEN

Normal range: 200-400 mg/dl (2-4 g/L [CF: 0.01; SMI: 0.1 g/L])
Elevated in: Tissue inflammation or damage (acute phase protein reactant), oral contraceptives, pregnancy, acute infection, myocardial infarction
Decreased in: Disseminated intravascular coagulation, hereditary afibrinogenemia, liver disease, primary or secondary fibrinolysis, cachexia

FOLATE (folic acid)

Normal range:
Plasma: 2-10 ng/ml (4-22 nmol/L [CF: 2.266; SMI: 2 nmol/L])
Red blood cells: 140-960 ng/ml (550-2200 nmol/L [CF: 2.266; SMI: 10 nmol/L])
Decreased in: Folic acid deficiency (inadequate intake, malabsorption), alcoholism, drugs (methotrexate, trimethoprim, phenytoin, oral contraceptives, Azulfidine), vitamin B_{12} deficiency (defective red cell folate absorption), hemolytic anemia
Elevated in: Folic acid therapy

FOLLICLE-STIMULATING HORMONE (FSH)

Normal range: 5-20 mIU/ml
Elevated in: Menopause, primary gonadal failure, alcoholism, castration, Klinefelter's syndrome, gonadotropin-secreting pituitary hormones
Decreased in: Pregnancy, polycystic ovary disease, anorexia nervosa, anterior pituitary hypofunction

FREE T_4

See T_4, FREE

FREE THYROXINE INDEX

Normal range: 1.1-4.3

INCREASED THYROXINE OR FREE THYROXINE VALUES

Laboratory error
Primary hyperthyroidism (T_4/T_3 type)
Severe thyroxine-binding globulin elevation
Excess therapy of hypothyroidism
Excessive dose of levothyroxine
Active thyroiditis (subacute, painless, early active Hashimoto's disease)
Familial dysalbuminemic hyperthyroxinemia (some FT_4 kits, especially analog types)
Peripheral resistance to T_4 syndrome
Amiodarone or propranolol
Postpartum transient toxicosis
Factitious hyperthyroidism
Jod-Basedow (iodine-induced) hyperthyroidism
Severe nonthyroid illness
Acute psychosis (especially paranoid schizophrenia)
T_4 sample drawn 2-4 hr after levothyroxine dose
Struma ovarii
Pituitary thyroid-stimulating hormone–secreting tumor
Certain x-ray contrast media (Telepaque and Oragrafin)
Acute porphyria
Heparin effect (some T_4 and FT_4 kits)
Amphetamine, heroin, methadone, and phencyclidine abuse
Perphenazine or 5-fluorouracil
Antithyroid or anti-IgG heterophil (HAMA) autoantibodies
"T_4" hyperthyroidism
Hyperemesis gravidarum; about 50% of patients
High altitudes

DECREASED THYROXINE OR FREE THYROXINE VALUES

Laboratory error
Primary hypothyroidism
Severe nonthyroid illness
Lithium therapy
Severe thyroxine-binding globulin decrease (congenital, disease, or drug-induced) or severe albumin decrease
Dilantin, Depakene, or high-dose salicylate drugs
Pituitary insufficiency
Large doses of inorganic iodide (e.g., saturated solution of potassium iodide)
Moderate or severe iodine deficiency
Cushing's syndrome
High-dose glucocorticoid drugs
Pregnancy, third trimester (low normal or small decrease)
Addison's disease; some patients (30%)
Heparin effect (a few FT_4 kits)
Desipramine or amiodarone drugs
Acute psychiatric illness

FTA-ABS (serum)

Normal: Nonreactive
Reactive in: Syphilis, other treponemal diseases (yaws, pinta, bejel), SLE, pregnancy

FUROSEMIDE STIMULATION TEST

Normal: Test is performed by giving 60 mg furosemide orally after overnight fast. Patient should be on a normal diet without medications the week before the test. Normal results: renin 1-6 ng angiotensin L/ml/hr.
Elevated in: Renovascular hypertension, Barrter's syndrome, high-renin essential hypertension, pheochromocytoma
No response in: Primary aldosteronism, low-renin essential hypertension, hyporeninemic hypoaldosteronism

GAMMA-GLUTAMYL TRANSFERASE (GGT)

See γ-GLUTAMYL TRANSFERASE

GASTRIN (serum)

Normal range: 0-180 pg/ml (0-180 ng/L [CF: 1; SMI: 10 ng/L])
Elevated in: Zollinger-Ellison syndrome (gastrinoma), pernicious anemia, hyperparathyroidism, retained gastric antrum, chronic renal failure, gastric ulcer, chronic atrophic gastritis, pyloric obstruction, malignant neoplasms of the stomach, H_2-blockers, omeprazole, calcium therapy, ulcerative colitis, rheumatoid arthritis

GASTRIN STIMULATION TEST

Normal: Gastrin stimulation test after calcium infusion is performed by giving a calcium infusion (15 mg Ca/kg in 500 ml normal saline over 4 hours). Serum is drawn in fasting state before infusion and at 1, 2, 3, and 4 hr. Normal response is little or no increase over baseline gastrin level.
Elevated in: Gastrinoma (gastrin >400 pg/ml), duodenal ulcer (gastrin level increase <400 ng/L)
Decreased in: Pernicious anemia, atrophic gastritis

GLIADIN ANTIBODIES, IgA AND IgG

Normal: <25 U, equivocal 20-25 U, positive >25 U. Test is useful to monitor compliance with gluten-free diet in patients with celiac disease.
Elevated in: Celiac disease with dietary noncompliance

GLOMERULAR BASEMENT MEMBRANE (gBm) ANTIBODY

Normal: Negative
Present in: Goodpasture's syndrome

GLOMERULAR FILTRATION RATE

See Box 4-3.

BOX 4-3 Common Equations for Estimating Glomerular Filtration Rate or Creatinine Clearance

Cockcoft-Gault ($C_{Cr} \cdot BSA/1.73\,m^2$)
For men: $C_{Cr} = [(140 - age) \cdot weight\ (kg)]/S_{Cr} \cdot 72$
For women: $C_{Cr} = ([(140 - age) \cdot weight\ (kg)]/S_{Cr} \cdot 72) \cdot 0.85$

MDRD (1)
$GFR = 170 \cdot [S_{Cr}]^{-0.999} \cdot [age]^{-0.176} \cdot$ [0.762 if patient is female] $\cdot$ [1.18 if patient is black] $\cdot [BUN]^{-0170} \cdot [Alb]^{0.318}$

MDRD (2)
$GFR = 186 \cdot [S_{Cr}]^{-1.154} \cdot [age]^{-0.203} \cdot$ [0.742 if patient is female] $\cdot$ [1.212 if patient is black]

Jellife (1) ($C_{Cr} \cdot BSA/1.73\,m^2$)
For men: $(98 - [0.8 \cdot (age - 20)])/S_{Cr}$
For women: $(98 - [0.8 \cdot (age - 20)])S_{Cr} \cdot 0.90$

Jellife (2)
For men: $(100/S_{Cr}) - 12$
For women: $(80/S_{Cr}) - 7$

Mawer
For men: $weight \cdot [29.3 - (0.203 \cdot age)] \cdot [1 - (0.03 \cdot S_{Cr})]$
For women: $weight \cdot [25.3 - (0.175 \cdot age)] \cdot [1 - (0.03 \cdot S_{Cr})]$

Bjornsson
For men: $[27 - (0.173 \cdot age)] \cdot weight \cdot 0/S_{Cr}$
For women: $[25 - (0.175 \cdot age)] \cdot weight \cdot 0.07/S_{Cr}$

Gates
For men: $(89.4 \cdot S_{Cr}^{-1.2}) + (55 - age) \cdot (0.447 \cdot S_{Cr}^{-1.1})$
For women: $(89.4 \cdot S_{Cr}^{-1.2}) + (55 - age) \cdot (0.447 \cdot S_{Cr}^{-1.1})$

Salazar-Corcoran
For men: $[137 - age] \cdot [(0.285 \cdot weight) + (12.1 \cdot height^2)]/(51 \cdot S_{Cr})$
For women: $[146 - age] \cdot [(0.287 \cdot weight) + (9.74 \cdot height^2)]/(60 \cdot S_{Cr})$

From Vincent JL et al: *Textbook of critical care,* ed 6, Philadelphia, 2011, Saunders.

Normal:

Ages 20-29	116 ml/min/1.73 m²
Ages 30-39	107 ml/min/1.73 m²
Ages 40-49	99 ml/min/1.73 m²
Ages 50-59	93 ml/min/1.73 m²
Ages 60-69	85 ml/min/1.73 m²
Ages >75	75 ml/min/1.73 m²

Decreased in: Renal insufficiency, decreased renal blood flow

GLUCAGON

Normal: 20-100 pg/ml
Elevated in: Glucagonoma (900-7800 pg/ml), chronic renal failure, diabetes mellitus, glucocorticoids, insulin, nifedipine, danazol, sympathomimetic amines
Decreased in: Hyperlipoproteinemia (types III, IV), beta-blockers, secretin

GLUCOSE, FASTING (FBS, fasting blood sugar)

Fig. E4-18 describes the approach to hypoglycemia. An algorithm for evaluation of hypoglycemia in children is described in Fig. E4-19.
Normal range: 60-99 mg/dl (3.8-6.0 mmol/L [CF: 0.05551; SMI: 0.1 mmol/L])
Elevated in: Diabetes mellitus, stress, infections, myocardial infarction, cerebrovascular accident, Cushing's syndrome, acromegaly, acute pancreatitis, glucagonoma, hemochromatosis, drugs (glucocorticoids, diuretics [thiazides, loop diuretics]), glucose intolerance, impaired fasting glucose
Decreased in: Sulfonylurea therapy, insulin therapy, reactive hypoglycemia (e.g., subtotal gastrectomy), starvation, insulinoma, glycogen storage disorders, severe liver disease or renal disease, ethanol-induced hypoglycemia, mesenchymal tumors that secrete insulin-like hormones

GLUCOSE, POSTPRANDIAL

Normal range: <140 mg/dl (<7.8 mmol/L [CF: 0.05551; SMI: 0.1 mmol/L])
Elevated in: Diabetes mellitus, glucose intolerance
Decreased in: Post–gastrointestinal resection, reactive hypoglycemia, hereditary fructose intolerance, galactosemia, leucine sensitivity

GLUCOSE TOLERANCE TEST

Normal values above fasting:
30 min: 30-60 mg/dl (1.65-3.3 mmol/L [CF: 0.05551; SMI: 0.1 mmol/L])
60 min: 20-50 mg/dl (1.1-2.75 mmol/L [CF: 0.05551; SMI: 0.1 mmol/L])
120 min: 5-15 mg/dl (0.28-0.83 mmol/L [CF: 0.05551; SMI: 0.1 mmol/L])
180 min: fasting level or below
Abnormal in: Glucose intolerance, diabetes mellitus, Cushing's syndrome, acromegaly, pheochromocytoma, gestational diabetes

GLUCOSE-6-PHOSPHATE DEHYDROGENASE (G6PD) SCREEN (blood)

Normal: G6PD enzyme activity detected
Abnormal: If a deficiency is detected, quantitation of G6PD is necessary; a G6PD screen may be falsely interpreted as "normal" after an episode of hemolysis because most G6PD-deficient cells have been destroyed.

γ-GLUTAMYL TRANSFERASE (GGT)

Normal range: 0-30 U/L (0.050 μkat/L [CF: 0.01667; SMI: 0.01 μkat/L])
Elevated in: Chronic alcoholic liver disease, neoplasms (hepatoma, metastatic disease to the liver, carcinoma of the pancreas), systemic lupus erythematosus, congestive heart failure, trauma, nephrotic syndrome, sepsis, cholestasis, drugs (phenytoin, barbiturates)

GLYCOHEMOGLOBIN (glycated glycosylated] hemoglobin), (HbA_{1C})

Normal range: 4.0%-5.9%
Elevated in: Uncontrolled diabetes mellitus (glycated hemoglobin levels reflect the level of glucose control over the preceding 120 days), lead toxicity, alcoholism, iron deficiency anemia, hypertriglyceridemia
Decreased in: Hemolytic anemias, decreased red blood cell survival, pregnancy, acute or chronic blood loss, chronic renal failure, insulinoma, congenital spherocytosis, hemoglobin S, C, and D diseases

GROWTH HORMONE

Normal: Male: 1-9 ng/ml; female: 1-16 ng/ml
Elevated in: Pituitary gigantism, acromegaly, ectopic GH secretion, cirrhosis, renal failure, anorexia nervosa, stress, exercise, prolonged fasting, amphetamines, beta-blockers, insulin, levodopa, metoclopramide, clonidine, vasopressin, human growth hormone (HGH) supplementation
Decreased in: Hypopituitarism, pituitary dwarfism, adrenocortical hyperfunction, bromocriptine, corticosteroids, glucose

GROWTH HORMONE RELEASING HORMONE (GHRH)

Normal: <50 pg/ml
Elevated in: Acromegaly caused by GHRH secretion by neoplasms

GROWTH HORMONE SUPPRESSION TEST (after glucose)

Normal: Test is done by giving 1.75 g glucose/kg orally after overnight fast. Blood is drawn at baseline, after 60 min, and after 120 min of glucose load. Normal response is growth hormone suppression to <2 ng/ml or undetectable levels.
Abnormal: There is no or incomplete suppression from the high basal level in gigantism or acromegaly.

HAM TEST (acid serum test)

Normal: Negative
Positive in: Paroxysmal nocturnal hemoglobinuria
False-positive in: Hereditary or acquired spherocytosis, recent transfusion with aged red blood cells, aplastic anemia, myeloproliferative syndromes, leukemia, hereditary dyserythropoietic anemia type II

HAPTOGLOBIN (serum)

Normal range: 50-220 mg/dl (0.50-2.2 g/L [CF: 0.01; SMI: 0.01 g/L])
Elevated in: Inflammation (acute phase reactant), collagen vascular diseases, infections (acute phase reactant), drugs (androgens), obstructive liver disease
Decreased in: Hemolysis (intravascular more than extravascular), megaloblastic anemia, severe liver disease, large tissue hematomas, infectious mononucleosis, drugs (oral contraceptives)

HBA_{1C}

See GLYCOHEMOGLOBIN

HDL

See HIGH-DENSITY LIPOPROTEIN CHOLESTEROL

HELICOBACTER PYLORI (serology, stool antigen)

Normal range: Not detected
Detected in: *H. pylori* infection. Positive serology can indicate current or past infection. Positive stool antigen test indicates acute infection (sensitivity and specificity >90%). Stool testing should be delayed at least 4 weeks after eradication therapy.

HEMATOCRIT

Normal range:
Male: 39%-49% (0.39-0.49 [CF: 0.01; SMI: 0.01])
Female: 33%-43% (0.33-0.43 [CF: 0.01; SMI: 0.01])
Elevated in: Polycythemia vera, smoking, chronic obstructive pulmonary disease, high altitudes, dehydration, hypovolemia
Decreased in: Blood loss (gastrointestinal, genitourinary) anemia

HEMOGLOBIN

Normal range:
Male: 13.6-17.7 g/dl (136-172 g/L [CF: 10; SMI: 1 g/L])
Female: 12.0-15.0 g/dl (120-150 g/L [CF: 10; SMI: 1 g/L])
Elevated in: Hemoconcentration, dehydration, polycythemia vera, chronic obstructive pulmonary disease, high altitudes, false elevations (hyperlipemic plasma, white blood cells >50,000/mm^3), stress
Decreased in: Hemorrhagic (gastrointestinal, genitourinary) anemia

HEMOGLOBIN A_{1C}

See GLYCATED HEMOGLOBIN

HEMOGLOBIN ELECTROPHORESIS

Table 4-17 describes neonatal hemoglobin electrophoresis patterns, and Table 4-18 summarizes types of hemoglobin.
Normal range: HbA_1: 95%-98%
HbA_2: 1.5%-3.5%
HbF: <2%
HbC: absent
HbS: absent

HEMOGLOBIN, GLYCATED

See GLYCOHEMOGLOBIN

HEMOGLOBIN, GLYCOSYLATED

See GLYCOHEMOGLOBIN

HEMOGLOBIN H

See Table 4-18.
Normal: Negative
Present in: Hemoglobin H disease, alpha-thalassemia trait, unstable hemoglobin disorders

TABLE 4-17 Neonatal Hemoglobin (Hb) Electrophoresis Patterns*

FA	Fetal Hb and adult normal Hb; the normal newborn pattern.
FAV	Indicates the presence of both HbF and HbA. However, an anomalous band (V) is present, which does not appear to be any of the common Hb variants.
FAS	Indicates fetal Hb, adult normal HbA, and HbS, consistent with benign sickle cell trait.
FS	Fetal and sickle HbS without detectable adult normal HbA. Consistent with clinically significant homozygous sickle Hb genotype (S/S) or sickle β-thalassemia, with manifestations of sickle cell anemia during childhood.
FC†	Designates the presence of HbC without adult normal HbA. Consistent with clinically significant homozygous HbC genotype (C/C), resulting in a mild hematologic disorder presenting during childhood.
FSC	HbS and HbC present. This heterozygous condition could lead to the manifestations of sickle cell disease during childhood.
FAC	HbC and adult normal HbA present, consistent with benign HbC trait.
FSA	Heterozygous HbS/β-thalassemia, a clinically significant sickling disorder.
F†	Fetal HbF is present without adult normal HbA. Although this may indicate a delayed appearance of HbA, it is also consistent with homozygous β-thalassemia major, or homozygous hereditary persistence of fetal HbF.
FV†	Fetal HbF and an anomalous Hb variant (V) are present.
AF	May indicate prior blood transfusion. Submit another filter paper blood specimen when the infant is 4 mo of age, at which time the transfused blood cells should have been cleared.

From Tschudy MM, Arcara KM: *The Harriet Lane handbook,* ed 19, Philadelphia, 2012, Mosby.
NOTE: HbA: $\alpha2\beta2$; HbF: $\alpha2\gamma2$; HbA2: $\alpha2\delta2$.
*Hemoglobin variants are reported in order of decreasing abundance; for example, FA indicates more fetal than adult hemoglobin.
†Repeat blood specimen should be submitted to confirm the original interpretation.

TABLE 4-18 Types of Hemoglobin

	Hemoglobin	Structure	Comment
Normal	A	$\alpha_2\beta_2$	97% of adult hemoglobin
	A_2	$\alpha_2\delta_2$	2% of adult Hb; elevated in β-thalassemia
	F	$\alpha_2\gamma_2$	Normal Hb in fetus from 3rd to 9th month; increased in β-thalassemia
Abnormal chain production	H	β_4	Found in α-thalassemia, biologically useless
	Barts	γ_4	Found in α-thalassemia, biologically useless
Abnormal chain structure	S	$\alpha_2\beta_2$	Substitution of valine for glutamic acid in position 6 of β chain
	C	$\alpha_2\beta_2$	Substitution of lysine for glutamic acid in position 6 of β chain

From Ballinger A: *Kumar & Clark's essentials of clinical medicine,* ed 6, Edinburgh, 2012, Saunders.

HEMOGLOBIN, URINE

See URINE HEMOGLOBIN, FREE

HEMOSIDERIN, URINE

See URINE HEMOGLOBIN, FREE

HEPARIN-INDUCED THROMBOCYTOPENIA ANTIBODIES

Normal: Antigen assay: Negative, <0.45; weak, 0.45-1.0; strong, >1.0
Elevated in: Heparin-induced thrombocytopenia

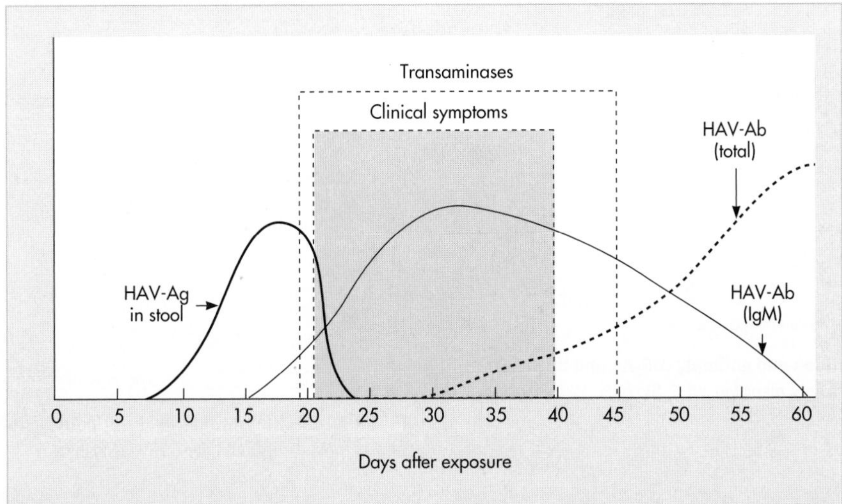

FIGURE 4-20 Serologic tests in HAV infection. (From Ravel R [ed]: *Clinical laboratory medicine,* ed 6, St Louis, 1995, Mosby.)

HEPATITIS A ANTIBODY

Normal: Negative
Present in: Viral hepatitis A; can be IgM or IgG (if IgM, acute hepatitis A; if IgG, previous infection with hepatitis A)
See Fig. 4-20 for serologic tests in HAV infection.

HAV-IGM ANTIBODY

Appearance: About the same time as clinical symptoms (3-4 weeks after exposure; range, 14-60 days), or just before beginning of AST/ALT elevation (range, 10 days before to 7 days after)
Peak: About 3-4 weeks after onset of symptoms (1-6 weeks)
Becomes nondetectable: 3-4 months after onset of symptoms (1-6 months). In a few cases HAV-IgM antibody can persist as long as 12-14 months.

HAV TOTAL ANTIBODY

Appearance: About 3 weeks after IgM becomes detectable (therefore about the middle of clinical symptom period to early convalescence)
Peak: About 1-2 months after onset
Becomes nondetectable: Remains elevated for life but can somewhat slowly fall

HEPATITIS A VIRAL INFECTION

Best all-purpose test(s) to diagnose acute HAV infection = HAV-Ab (IgM)
Best all-purpose test(s) to demonstrate past HAV infection/immunity = HAV-Ab (total)

HEPATITIS B SURFACE ANTIGEN (HBsAg)

Normal: Not detected
Detected in: Acute viral hepatitis type B, chronic hepatitis B
Appearance: 2-6 weeks after exposure (range, 6 days to 6 months); 5%-15% of patients are negative at onset of jaundice
Peak: 1-2 weeks before to 1-2 weeks after onset of symptoms
Becomes nondetectable: 1-3 months after peak (range, 1 week to 5 months)

HEPATITIS B VIRAL INFECTION

See Table 4-19
Figs. 4-21, 4-22, and 4-23 illustrate antigens and antibodies in hepatitis B infection.

HB_S
-Ag
HB_SAg: shows current active HBV infection.
Persistence over 6 months indicates carrier/chronic HBV infection.
HBV nucleic acid probe: present before and longer than HB_SAg.
More reliable marker for increased infectivity than HB_SAg and/or HB_eAg.
-Ab
HB_SAb-total: shows previous healed HBV infection and evidence of immunity.

TABLE 4-19 Serologic Markers of Hepatitis B Infection

	HBsAg	anti-HBc	anti-HBs	IgM anti-HBc
Susceptible to infection	Negative	Negative	Negative	Negative
Immune due to natural infection	Negative	Positive	Positive	Negative
Immune due to hepatitis B vaccination	Negative	Negative	Positive	Negative
Acutely infected	Positive	Positive	Negative	Positive
Chronically infected	Positive	Positive	Negative	Negative

From Ballinger A: *Kumar & Clark's essentials of clinical medicine,* ed 6, Edinburgh, 2012, Saunders.

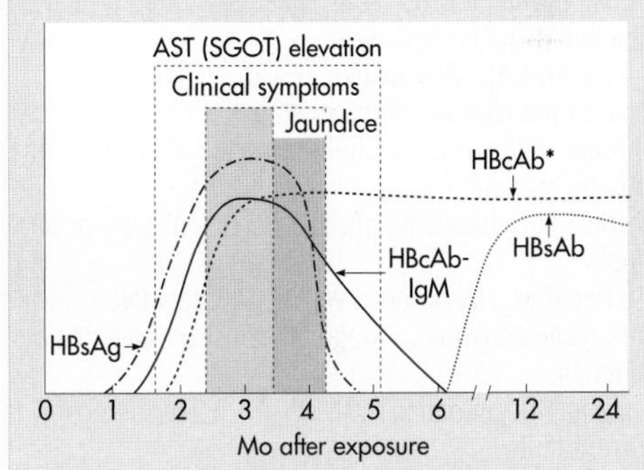

FIGURE 4-21 HBV surface antigen-antibody and core antibodies. Note "core window." *HB_CAb = HB_CAb-IgM + HBCAb-IgG (combined). (From Ravel R [ed]: *Clinical laboratory medicine,* ed 6, St Louis, 1995, Mosby.)

HB_C
-Ab
HB_CAb-IgM: shows either acute or very recent infection by HBV.
In convalescent phase of acute HBV, may be elevated when HB_SAg has disappeared (core window).
Negative HB_CAb-IgM with positive HB_SAg suggests either very early acute HBV or carrier/chronic HBV.
HB_CAb-total: only useful to show past HBV infection if HB_SAg and HB_CAb-IgM are both negative.

HB_E
-Ag
HB_e-AbAg: when present, especially without HB_eAb, suggests increased patient infectivity.

FIGURE 4-22 HBV surface antigen and antibody (HB$_{S}$Ag and HB$_{S}$Ab-total). (From Ravel R [ed]: *Clinical laboratory medicine,* ed 6, St Louis, 1995, Mosby.)

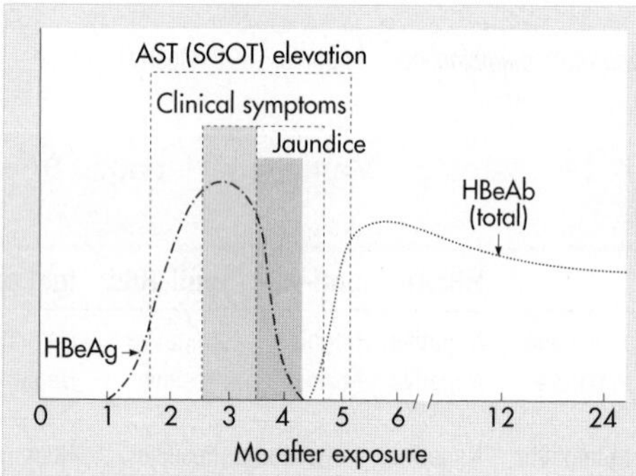

FIGURE 4-23 HBVe antigen and antibody. (From Ravel R [ed]: *Clinical laboratory medicine,* ed 6, St Louis, 1995, Mosby.)

HB$_{e}$Ab-total: when present, suggests less patient infectivity.

I. HB$_{S}$Ag positive, HB$_{C}$Ab negative
   About 5% (range, 0%-17%) of patients with early-stage HBV acute infection (HB$_{C}$Ab rises later)

II. HB$_{S}$Ag positive, HB$_{C}$Ab positive, HB$_{S}$Ab negative
   a. Most of the clinical symptom stage
   b. Chronic HBV carriers without evidence of liver disease ("asymptomatic carriers")
   c. Chronic HBV hepatitis (chronic persistent type or chronic active type)

III. HB$_{S}$Ag negative, HB$_{C}$Ab positive,* HB$_{S}$Ab negative
   a. Late clinical symptom stage or early convalescence stage (core window)
   b. Chronic HBV infection with HB$_{S}$Ag below detection levels with current tests
   c. Old previous HBV infection

IV. HB$_{S}$Ag negative, HB$_{C}$Ab positive, HB$_{S}$Ab positive
   a. Late convalescence to complete recovery
   b. Old infection

HEPATITIS C VIRAL INFECTION

Fig. 4-24 illustrates antigens and antibodies in hepatitis C infection.

HEPATITIS C RNA

Normal: Negative
Elevated in: Hepatitis C. Detection of hepatitis C-RNA is used to confirm current infection and to monitor treatment. Quantitative assays (viral load) are needed before treatment to assess response (<2 log decrease after 12-week treatment indicates lack of response).

HCV

-Ag

HCV nucleic acid probe: shows current infection by HCV (especially with PCR amplification).

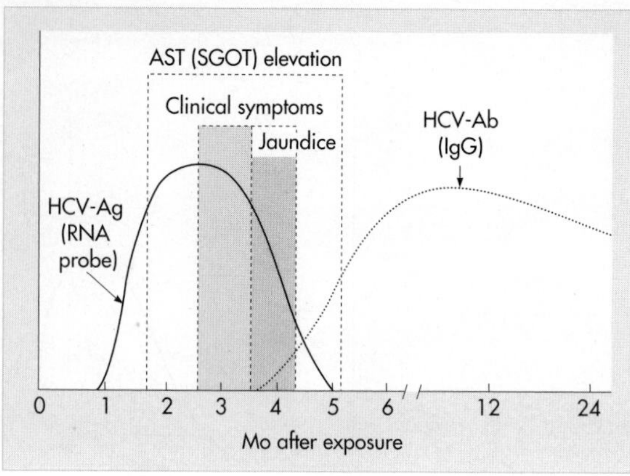

FIGURE 4-24 HCV antigen and antibody. (From Ravel R [ed]: *Clinical laboratory medicine,* ed 6, St Louis, 1995, Mosby.)

-Ab

HCV-Ab (IgG): current, convalescent, or old HCV infection.

HAV

-Ag

HAV-Ag by EM: shows presence of virus in stool early in infection.

-Ab

HAV-Ab (IgM): current or recent HAV infection.
HAV-Ab (total): convalescent or old HAV infection.

HEPATITIS D VIRAL INFECTION

Fig. 4-25 illustrates antigens and antibodies in hepatitis D infection.
Best current all-purpose screening test = HDV-Ab (total)
Best test to differentiate acute from chronic infection = HDV-Ab (IgM)

DELTA HEPATITIS COINFECTION (acute HDV1 acute HBV) OR SUPERINFECTION (acute HDV1 chronic HBV)

HDV

-Ag

HDV-Ag: shows current infection (acute or chronic) by HDV.
HDV nucleic acid probe: detects antigen before and longer than HDV-Ag by EIA.

-Ab

HDV-Ab (IgM): high elevation in acute HDV; does not persist.
Low or moderate elevation in convalescent HDV; does not persist.
Low to high persistent elevation in chronic HDV (depends on degree of cell injury and sensitivity of the assay).
HDV-Ab (total): high elevation in acute HDV; does not persist.
High persistent elevation in chronic HDV.

HDV-Ag

Detected by DNA probe, less often by immunoassay
Appearance: Prodromal stage (before symptoms); just at or after initial rise in ALT (about a week after appearance of HB$_{S}$Ag and about the time HB$_{C}$Ab-IgM level begins to rise)
Peak: 2-3 days after onset
Becomes nondetectable: 1-4 days (may persist until shortly after symptoms appear)

HDV-Ab (IgM)

Appearance: About 10 days after symptoms begin (range, 1-28 days)
Peak: About 2 weeks after first detection
Becomes nondetectable: About 35 days (range, 10-80 days) after first detection (most other IgM antibodies take 3-6 months to become nondetectable)

HDV-Ab (total)

Appearance: About 50 days after symptoms begin (range, 14-80 days); about 5 weeks after HDV-Ag (range, 3-11 weeks)
Peak: About 2 weeks after first detection
Becomes nondetectable: About 7 months after first detection (range, 4-14 months)

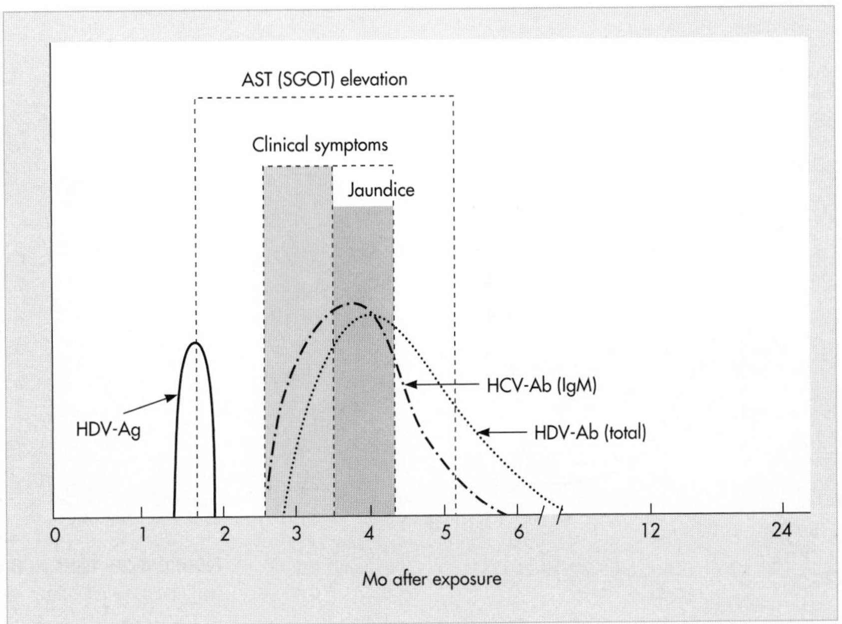

FIGURE 4-25 HDV antigen and antibodies. (From Ravel R [ed]: *Clinical laboratory medicine,* ed 6, St Louis, 1995, Mosby.)

HER-2/*NEU*

Normal: Negative
Present in: 25%-30% of primary breast cancers. It can also be found in other epithelial tumors, including lung, hepatocellular, pancreatic, colon, stomach, ovarian, cervical, and bladder cancer. Trastuzumab (Herceptin) is a humanized monoclonal antibody against Her-2/*neu.* This test is useful to identify patients with metastatic; recurrent; and/or treatment refractory, unresectable, locally advanced breast cancer for trastuzumab treatment.

HERPES SIMPLEX VIRUS (HSV)

Test description: The PCR test can be performed on serum biopsy samples, CSF, vitreous humor.

HFE SCREEN FOR HEREDITARY HEMOCHROMATOSIS

Test description: PCR test can be performed on whole blood or tissue. One mutation (C282Y) and two polymorphisms (H63D, S65C) account for the majority of alleles associated with this disease.

HETEROPHIL ANTIBODY

Normal: Negative
Positive in: Infectious mononucleosis

HIGH-DENSITY LIPOPROTEIN (HDL) CHOLESTEROL

Normal range:
Male: 40-70 mg/dl (0.8-1.8 mmol/L [CF: 0.02586; SMI: 0.05 mmol/L])
Female: 50-90 mg/dl (1.1-2.35 mmol/L [CF: 0.02586; SMI: 0.05 mmol/L])
Increased in: Use of gemfibrozil, statins, fenofibrate, nicotinic acid, estrogens, regular aerobic exercise, small (1 oz) daily alcohol intake
Decreased in: Deficiency of apoproteins, liver disease, probucol ingestion, Tangier disease

NOTE: A cholesterol/HDL ratio >4.0 is associated with increased risk of coronary artery disease.

HLA ANTIGENS

Associated disorders: see Table 4-20.

HOMOCYSTEINE (plasma)

Normal range:
0-30 years: 4.6-8.1 mcmol/L
30-59 years: 6.3-11.2 mcmol/L (males), 4.5-7.9 mcmol/L (females)
>59 years: 5.8-11.9 mcmol/L
Increased: Thrombophilic states, B_6, B_{12}, folic acid, riboflavin deficiency, pregnancy, homocystinuria

NOTE: An increased homocysteine level is an independent risk factor for atherosclerosis.

HUMAN CHORIONIC GONADOTROPIN (hCG)

Normal range: Varies with gestational stage:
1 wk: 5-50 mU/ml
1-2 wk: 50-550 mU/ml
2-3 wk: up to 5000 mU/ml
3-4 wk: up to 10,000 mU/ml
4-5 wk: up to 50,000 mU/ml
2-3 mo: 10,000-100,000 mU/ml

TABLE 4-20 HLA Antigens Associated with Specific Diseases

Antigen	Condition	Antigen	Condition
HLA-B27	Ankylosing spondylitis	HLA-B8, Dw3	Celiac disease
Reiter's syndrome	HLA-B8, Dw3	Dermatitis herpetiformis	
Psoriatic arthritis	HLA-B8	Myasthenia gravis	
HLA-A10, B18, Dw2	C2 deficiency	HLA-B8	Chronic active hepatitis in children
HLA-A2, B40, Cw3	C4 deficiency	HLA-Drw4	Active chronic hepatitis in adults
HLA-B7, Dw2	Multiple sclerosis	HLA-B13, Bw17	Psoriasis
HLA-A3	Hemochromatosis		

From Cerra FB: *Manual of critical care,* St Louis, 1987, Mosby.
HLA, Human leukocyte antigen.

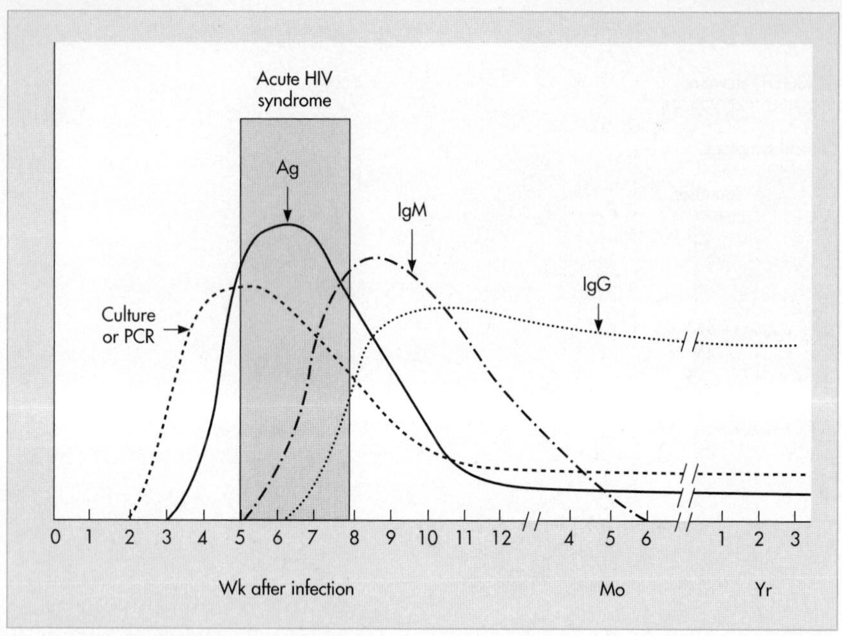

FIGURE 4-26 Tests in HIV-1 infection. (From Ravel R [ed]: *Clinical laboratory medicine,* ed 6, St Louis, 1995, Mosby.)

TABLE 4-21 Indications for Plasma HIV RNA Testing*

Clinical Indication	Information	Use
Syndrome consistent with acute HIV infection	Establishes diagnosis when HIV antibody test is negative or indeterminate	Diagnosis†
Initial evaluation of newly diagnosed HIV infection	Baseline viral load set point	Decision to start or defer therapy
Every 3-4 mo in patients not on therapy	Changes in viral load	Decision to start therapy
4-8 wk after initiation of antiretroviral therapy	Initial assessment of drug efficacy	Decision to continue or change therapy
3-4 mo after start of therapy	Maximal effect of therapy	Decision to continue or change therapy
Every 3-4 mo in patients on therapy	Durability of antiretroviral effect	Decision to continue or change therapy
Clinical event or significant decline in CD4+ T cells	Association with changing or stable	Decision to continue, initiate, or change

From Report of the NIH Panel to Define Principles of Therapy of HIV Infection, *MMWR Recomm Rep* 47(RR-5):1-41, 1998.
*Acute illness (e.g., bacterial pneumonia, tuberculosis, HSV, PCP) and immunizations can cause increase in plasma HIV RNA for 2-4 wk; viral load testing should not be performed during this time. Plasma HIV RNA results should usually be verified with a repeat determination before starting or making changes in therapy. HIV RNA should be measured using the same laboratory and the same assay.
†Diagnosis of HIV infection determined by HIV RNA testing should be confirmed by standard methods (e.g., Western blot serology) performed 2-4 mo after the initial indeterminate or negative test.

Elevated in: Normal pregnancy, hydatidiform mole, choriocarcinoma, germ cell tumors of testicle, some nontrophoblastic neoplasms (e.g., neoplasms of cervix, gastrointestinal tract, ovary, lung, breast)

HUMAN HERPES VIRUS 8 (HHV8)

Test description: PCR test can be performed on whole blood, tissue, bone marrow, and urine. HHV8 is found in all forms of Kaposi's sarcoma.

HUMAN IMMUNODEFICIENCY VIRUS ANTIBODY, TYPE 1 (HIV-1)

Normal range: Not detected

Abnormal result: HIV antibodies usually appear in the blood 1-4 months after infection.

Testing sequence:

1. ELISA is the recommended initial screening test. Sensitivity and specificity are >99%. False-positive ELISA may occur with autoimmune disorders, administration of immune globulin manufactured before 1985, within 6 weeks of testing, in the presence of rheumatoid factor, in the presence of DLA-DR antibodies in multigravida female, with administration of influenza vaccine within 3 months of testing, with hemodialysis, with positive plasma reagin test, and with certain medical disorders (hemophilia, hypergammaglobulinemia, alcoholic hepatitis).
2. A positive ELISA is confirmed with Western blot. False-positive Western blot may result from connective tissue disorders, human leukocyte antigen antibodies, polyclonal gammopathies, hyperbilirubinemia, presence of antibody to another human retrovirus, or cross-reaction with other non-virus-derived proteins in healthy persons. Undetermined Western blot may occur in AIDS patients with advanced immunodeficiency (caused by loss of antibodies) and in recent HIV infections.
3. PCR is used to confirm indeterminate Western blot results or negative results in persons with suspected HIV infection.

Fig. 4-26 describes tests in HIV infection; indications for plasma HIV RNA testing are described in Table 4-21.

HUMAN IMMUNODEFICIENCY VIRUS TYPE 1 (HIV-1) ANTIGEN (p24), QUALITATIVE (p24 ANTIGEN)

Normal range: Negative. This test detects uncomplexed HIV-1 p24 antigen. The core protein p24 is the first detectable protein encoded by the group-specific antigen *(gag)* gene. This protein is a marker for viremia. This test should not be used in place of HIV-1 antibody testing as a screen for HIV-1 infection. HIV-1 p24 may be detectable in the first month of acute HIV-1 infection and generally falls to undetectable levels during the asymptomatic stage of HIV-1 infection. A negative result does not exclude the possibility of infection or exposure to HIV-1. It is recommended that a negative result be followed with repeat testing at least 8 weeks after the original test. This test is used primarily for screening of donated blood and plasma and as an aid for the prognosis of HIV-1 infection.

HUMAN IMMUNODEFICIENCY VIRUS TYPE 1 (HIV-1) **VIRAL LOAD**

Normal range: HIV-1 RNA, quant. bDNA 3: less than 50 copies/ml or less than 1.7 log copies/ml

This test should be used only in individuals with documented HIV-1 infection for monitoring the progression of infection, response to antiretroviral therapy, and disease prognosis. It is not indicated for diagnosis of HIV infection.

HUMAN PAPILLOMA VIRUS (HPV)

Test description: PCR test can be performed on cervical smears, biopsies, scrapings, liquid cytology specimen, and anogenital tissues.

HUNTINGTON'S DISEASE PCR

Test description: PCR can be performed on whole blood. Huntington's disease is caused by the expansion of the trinucleotide repeat CAG within IT 15 (huntingtin). Pre- and post-test counseling should be performed when ordering this test.

HYDROGEN BREATH TEST

See BREATH HYDROGEN TEST

5-HYDROXYINDOLE-ACETIC ACID, URINE

See URINE 5-HYDROXYINDOLE-ACETIC ACID

IMMUNE COMPLEX ASSAY

Normal: Negative

Detected in: Collagen vascular disorders, glomerulonephritis, neoplastic diseases, malaria, primary biliary cirrhosis, chronic acute hepatitis, bacterial endocarditis, vasculitis

IMMUNOGLOBULINS

Normal range:

IgA: 50-350 mg/dl (0.5-3.5 g/L [CF: 0.01; SMI: 0.01 g/L])
IgD: <6 mg/dl (<60 mg/L [CF: 0.01; SMI: 0.01 g/L])
IgE: <25 μg/dl (<0.00025 g/L [CF: 0.01; SMI: 0.01 g/L])
IgG: 800-1500 mg/dl (8-15 g/L [CF: 0.01; SMI: 0.01 g/L])
IgM: 45-150 mg/dl (0.45-1.5 g/L [CF: 0.01; SMI: 0.01 g/L])

Elevated in:

IgA: Lymphoproliferative disorders, Berger's nephropathy, chronic infections, autoimmune disorders, liver disease

IgE: Allergic disorders, parasitic infections, immunologic disorders, IgE myeloma

IgG: Chronic granulomatous infections, infectious diseases, inflammation, myeloma, liver disease

IgM: Primary biliary cirrhosis, infectious diseases (brucellosis, malaria), Waldenström's macroglobulinemia, liver disease

Decreased in:

IgA: Nephrotic syndrome, protein-losing enteropathy, congenital deficiency, lymphocytic leukemia, ataxia-telangiectasia, chronic sinopulmonary disease

IgE: Hypogammaglobulinemia, neoplasms (breast, bronchial, cervical), ataxia-telangiectasia

IgG: Congenital or acquired deficiency, lymphocytic leukemia, phenytoin, methylprednisolone, nephrotic syndrome, protein-losing enteropathy

IgM: Congenital deficiency, lymphocytic leukemia, nephrotic syndrome

INFLUENZA A AND B TESTS

Test description: PCR can be performed on nasopharyngeal swab, wash, or aspirate

Normal: Negative

INSULIN AUTOANTIBODIES

Normal: Negative

Present in: Exogenous insulin from insulin therapy. The presence of islet cell antibodies indicates ongoing beta cell destruction. This test is useful in the early diagnosis of type 1a diabetes mellitus and in the identification of patients at high risk for type 1a diabetes.

INSULIN, FREE

Normal: <17 mcU/ml

Elevated in: Insulin overdose, insulin resistance syndromes, endogenous hyperinsulinemia

Decreased in: Inadequately treated type 1 DM

INSULIN-LIKE GROWTH FACTOR-1 (IGF-1) (serum)

Normal range:

Ages 16-24: 182-780 ng/ml
Ages 25-39: 114-492 ng/ml
Ages 40-54: 90-360 ng/ml
Ages >55: 71-290 ng/ml

Elevated in: Adolescence, acromegaly, pregnancy, precocious puberty, obesity

Decreased in: Malnutrition, delayed puberty, diabetes mellitus, hypopituitarism, cirrhosis, old age

INSULIN-LIKE GROWTH FACTOR-II

Normal range: 288-736 ng/ml

Elevated in: Hypoglycemia associated with non–islet cell tumors, hepatoma, and Wilms' tumor

Decreased in: Growth hormone deficiency

INTERNATIONAL NORMALIZED RATIO (INR)

The INR is a comparative rating of prothrombin time (PT) ratios. The INR represents the observed PT ratio adjusted by the International Reference Thromboplastin. It provides a universal result indicative of what the patient's PT result would have been if measured using the primary World Health Organization International Reference reagent. For proper interpretation of INR values, the patient should be on stable anticoagulant therapy.

RECOMMENDED INR RANGES:

Proximal deep vein thrombosis:	2-3
Pulmonary embolism:	2-3
Transient ischemic attacks:	2-3
Atrial fibrillation:	2-3
Mechanical prosthetic valves:	2.5-3.5
Recurrent venous thromboembolic disease:	2.5-3.5

INTRINSIC FACTOR ANTIBODIES

Normal: Negative

Present in: Pernicious anemia (>50% of patients). Cyanocobalamin may give false-positive results.

IRON (serum)

Normal: Male: 65-175 mcg/dl; female: 50-1170 mcg/dl

Elevated in: Hemochromatosis, excessive iron therapy, repeated transfusions, lead poisoning, hemolytic anemia, aplastic anemia, pernicious anemia

Decreased in: Iron deficiency anemia, hypothyroidism, chronic infection

IRON-BINDING CAPACITY, TOTAL (TIBC)

Normal range: 250-460 μg/dl (45-82 μmol/L [CF: 0.1791; SMI: 1 μmol/L])

Elevated in: Iron deficiency anemia, pregnancy, polycythemia, hepatitis, weight loss

Decreased in: Anemia of chronic disease, hemochromatosis, chronic liver disease, hemolytic anemias, malnutrition (protein depletion)

Table 4-22 describes TIBC and serum iron abnormalities.

IRON SATURATION (% TRANSFERRIN SATURATION)

Normal:

Male: 20%-50%
Female: 15%-50%

Elevated in: Hemochromatosis, excessive iron intake, aplastic anemia, thalassemia, vitamin B_6 deficiency

Decreased in: hypochromic anemias, GI malignancy

LACTATE (blood)

Normal range: 0.5-2.0 mEq/L

Elevated in: Tissue hypoxia (shock, respiratory failure, severe CHF, severe anemia, carbon monoxide or cyanide poisoning), systemic disorders (liver or renal failure, seizures), abnormal intestinal flora (d-lactic acidosis), drugs or toxins (salicylates, ethanol, methanol, ethylene glycol), G6PD deficiency

TABLE 4-22 Serum Iron and Total Iron-Binding Capacity Patterns

SI↓	TIBC↓	Chronic diseases
		Uremia
SI↓	TIBC	Chronic iron deficiency anemia
		Pregnancy in third trimester
SI	TIBC↓	Hemachromatosis
		Iron therapy overload (TIBC may be normal)
		Hemolytic anemia; thalassemia; lead poisoning; megaloblastic anemia; aplastic, pyridoxine deficiency, or other sideroblastic anemias
SI	TIBC	Oral contraceptives
		Acute hepatitis (some report TIBC is low normal)
		Chronic hepatitis (some patients)
SI	TIBC NL	B_{12} or folate deficiency
SI↓	TIBC	Chronic iron deficiency (some patients)
	NL	Acute infection, surgery, tissue damage
SI NL	TIBC	B_{12}/folate deficiency plus iron deficiency

NL, Normal; *SI,* serum iron; *TIBC,* total iron-binding capacity.
From Ravel R: *Clinical laboratory medicine,* ed 6, St Louis, 1995, Mosby.

LACTATE DEHYDROGENASE (LDH)

Normal range: 50-150 U/L (0.82-2.66 μkat/L [CF: 0.01667; SMI: 0.02 μkat/L])
Elevated in:
Infarction of myocardium, lung, kidney
Diseases of cardiopulmonary system, liver, collagen, central nervous system
Hemolytic anemias, megaloblastic anemias, transfusions, seizures, muscle trauma, muscular dystrophy, acute pancreatitis, hypotension, shock, infectious mononucleosis, inflammation, neoplasia, intestinal obstruction, hypothyroidism

LACTATE DEHYDROGENASE ISOENZYMES

Normal range:
LDH_1: 22%-36% (cardiac, red blood cell) (0.22-0.36 [CF: 0.01, SMI: 0.01])
LDH_2: 35%-46% (cardiac, red blood cell) (0.35-0.46)
LDH_3: 13%-26% (pulmonary) (0.15-0.26)
LDH_4: 3%-10% (striated muscle, liver) (0.03-0.1)
LDH_5: 2%-9% (striated muscle, liver) (0.02-0.09)

Normal ratios:
$LDH_1 < LDH_2$
$LDH_5 < LDH_4$
Abnormal values:
$LDH_1 > LDH_2$: Myocardial infarction (can also be seen with hemolytic anemias, pernicious anemia, folate deficiency, renal infarct)
$LDH_5 > LDH_4$: Liver disease (cirrhosis, hepatitis, hepatic congestion)

LACTOSE TOLERANCE TEST (serum)

Normal: Test is performed by giving 2 g/kg body weight lactose orally and drawing glucose level at 0, 30, 45, 60, and 90 min. Normal response is change in glucose from fasting value to >30 mg/dl. Inconclusive response is increase of 20-30 mg/dl, abnormal response is increase <20 mg/dl.
Abnormal in: Lactase deficiency

LAP SCORE

See LEUKOCYTE ALKALINE PHOSPHATASE

LEAD

Normal: Child, <10 mcg/dl; adult, <25 mcg/dl; acceptable for industrial exposure, <50 mcg/dl
Elevated in: Lead exposure, lead poisoning

LDH

See LACTATE DEHYDROGENASE

LDL

See LOW-DENSITY LIPOPROTEIN CHOLESTEROL

LEGIONELLA PNEUMOPHILA PCR

Test description: PCR can be performed on lung tissue, water sputum, bronchoalveolar lavage, and other respiratory fluids.

LEGIONELLA TITER

Normal: Negative
Positive in: Legionnaire's disease (presumptive: ≥1:256 titer; definitive: fourfold titer increase to ≥1:128)

LEUKOCYTE ALKALINE PHOSPHATASE (LAP)

Normal range: 13-100 (33-188 U)
Elevated in: Leukemoid reactions, neutrophilia secondary to infections (except in sickle cell crisis—no significant increase in LAP score), Hodgkin's disease, polycythemia vera, hairy cell leukemia, aplastic anemia, Down's syndrome, myelofibrosis
Decreased in: Acute and chronic granulocytic leukemia, thrombocytopenic purpura, paroxysmal nocturnal hemoglobinuria, hypophosphatemia, collagen disorders

LEUKOCYTE COUNT

See COMPLETE BLOOD COUNT

LIPASE

Normal range: 0-160 U/L (0-2.66 μkat/L [CF: 0.01667; SMI: 0.02 μkat/L])
Elevated in: Acute pancreatitis, perforated peptic ulcer, carcinoma of pancreas (early stage), pancreatic duct obstruction, bowel infarction, intestinal obstruction

LIPOPROTEIN(a)

Normal: Male: 1.35-19.6 mg/dl; female: 1.24-20.1 mg/dl
Elevated in: Coronary artery disease, uncontrolled diabetes, hypothyroidism, chronic renal failure, pregnancy, tobacco use, infections, nephritic syndrome
Decreased in: Niacin, omega-3 fatty acids, estrogens, tamoxifen, statins

LIPOPROTEIN CHOLESTEROL, HIGH-DENSITY

See HIGH-DENSITY LIPOPROTEIN CHOLESTEROL

LIPOPROTEIN CHOLESTEROL, LOW-DENSITY

See LOW-DENSITY LIPOPROTEIN CHOLESTEROL

LIVER KIDNEY MICROSOME TYPE 1 ANTIBODIES (LKM1)

Normal: <20 U
Elevated in: Autoimmune hepatitis type 2

LKM1

See LIVER KIDNEY MICROSOME TYPE 1 ANTIBODIES

LOW-DENSITY LIPOPROTEIN (LDL) CHOLESTEROL

Normal range: 50-130 mg/dl (1.30-1.68 mmol/L [CF: 0.02586; SMI: 0.05 mmol/L])

<70	Optimal in diabetics, prior MI, and patients with cardiac risk factors
100-129	Near or above optimal
130-159	Borderline high
160-189	High
≥190	Very high

LUPUS ANTICOAGULANT

See CIRCULATING ANTICOAGULANT

LUTEINIZING HORMONE

Normal range: 5-25 mIU/ml
Elevated in: Postmenopause, pituitary adenoma, primary gonadal dysfunction, polycystic ovary syndrome
Decreased in: Severe illness, anorexia nervosa, malnutrition, pituitary or hypothalamic impairment, severe stress

LYME DISEASE ANTIBODY TITER

Normal range: Negative

Positive result: Fig. 4-27 illustrates the usual serologic response in Lyme disease.

A serologic test is not necessary or helpful for several days after a tick bite because it is only 40%-50% sensitive in this stage, and a negative test does not rule out the diagnosis.

LYMPHOCYTES

Normal range: 15%-40%

Total lymphocyte count = 800-2600/mm^3

Total T lymphocyte = 800-2200/mm^3

CD4 lymphocytes = ≥ 400/mm^3

CD8 lymphocytes = 200-800/mm^3

Normal CD4/CD8 ratio is 2.0.

Elevated in: Chronic infections, infectious mononucleosis and other viral infections, chronic lymphocytic leukemia, Hodgkin's disease, ulcerative colitis, hypoadrenalism, idiopathic thrombocytopenia

Decreased in:

AIDS, bone marrow suppression from chemotherapeutic agents or chemotherapy, aplastic anemia, neoplasms, steroids, adrenocortical hyperfunction, neurologic disorders (multiple sclerosis, myasthenia gravis, Guillain-Barré syndrome)

CD4 lymphocytes are calculated as total white blood cells × % lymphocytes × % lymphocytes stained with CD4. They are decreased in AIDS and other immune dysfunction.

Table 4-23 describes various lymphocyte abnormalities in peripheral blood.

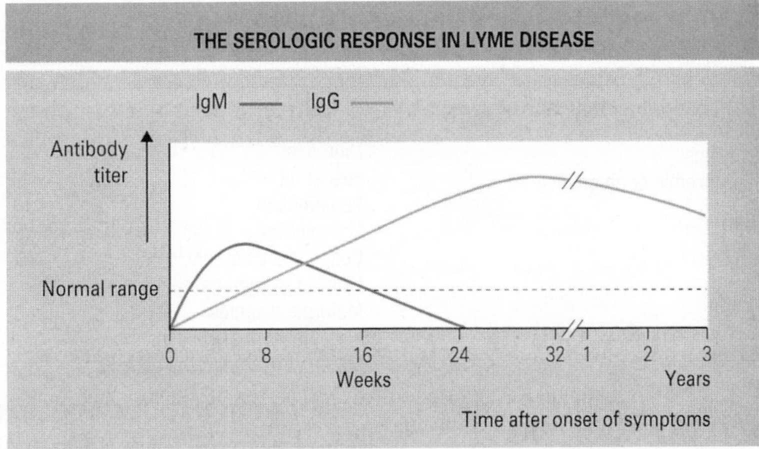

FIGURE 4-27 IgM and IgG responses in Lyme disease.

TABLE 4-23 Differential Diagnosis of Abnormal Lymphocytes in Peripheral Blood

Lymphocyte Type	Usual Disease Association	Cytologic Features	Laboratory Features	Clinical Features
Small lymphocyte	Chronic lymphocytic leukemia	B-cell surface markers with low concentration of surface immunoglobulin, CD5 antigen	Hypogammaglobulinemia in 50%; positive direct Coombs test in 15%; on node biopsy, diffuse, well-differentiated lymphocytic infiltrate	Elderly adults; presentation runs gamut from asymptomatic with lymphocytosis only to bulky disease with adenopathy, splenomegaly, and "packed" bone marrow
Atypical lymphocyte	Infectious mononucleosis, other viral illnesses	Suppressor T-cell markers	Heterophil agglutinin; positive serology for Epstein-Barr virus, cytomegalovirus, Toxoplasma, HBsAg	Pharyngitis, fever, adenopathy, rash, splenomegaly, palatal petechiae, jaundice
Plasmacytoid lymphocyte	Waldenström's macroglobulin anemia	Cytoplasmic IgM, periodic acid-Schiff positivity	IgM paraprotein, rouleaux, cryoglobulins	Adenopathy, splenomegaly, absence of bone lesions, hyperviscosity syndrome, cryopathic phenomena
Lymphoblast	ALL	Terminal transferase positivity, common ALL antigen, B- or T-precursor markers	Anemia, granulocytopenia, thrombocytopenia, hyperuricemia, diffuse bone marrow infiltration	Peak incidence in childhood, acute onset, bone pain frequent
Lymphosarcoma cell	Lymphocytic lymphoma	B-cell surface markers with high concentration of monoclonal surface immunoglobulin	Nodular or diffuse, poorly differentiated lymphocytic lymphoma on node biopsy, patchy, peritrabecular bone marrow involvement	Middle-aged to older adults, generalized adenopathy, constitutional symptoms
Sézary cell	Cutaneous lymphomas	T-lymphocyte surface markers	Skin biopsy is diagnostic	Exfoliative erythroderma, cutaneous plaques or tumors
Hairy cell	Hairy cell leukemia	B-lymphocyte markers, cytoplasmic projections, tartrate-resistant acid phosphatase, interleukin-2 receptors, CD11 antigen	Pancytopenia	Middle-aged males, moderate to marked splenomegaly without adenopathy
Prolymphocyte	Prolymphocytic leukemia	B-cell surface markers with high concentration of surface immunoglobulin, CD5 negative	Marked lymphocytosis (frequently >100 × 10^9/L)	Elderly adults, massive splenomegaly, minimum adenopathy, poor response to therapy

From Stein JH (ed): *Internal medicine,* ed 5, St Louis, 1998, Mosby.
ALL, Acute lymphoblastic leukemia.

Laboratory Tests IV

MAGNESIUM (serum)

See Fig. E4-28 for evaluation of hypermagnesemia and Fig. E4-29 for evaluation of hypomagnesemia.

Normal range: 1.8-3.0 mg/dl (0.80-1.20 mmol/L [CF: 0.4114; SMI: 0.02 mmol/L])

CAUSES OF HYPERMAGNESEMIA

I. Decreased renal excretion
   A. Renal failure—glomerular filtration rate less than 30 ml/min
   B. Hyperparathyroidism
   C. Hypothyroidism
   D. Addison's disease
   E. Lithium intoxication
   F. Familial hypocalciuric hypercalcemia
II. Other causes: usually in association with decrease in glomerular filtration rate
   A. Endogenous loads
      1. Diabetic ketoacidosis
      2. Severe tissue injury—burns
   B. Exogenous loads
      1. Gastrointestinal
         a. Magnesium-containing laxatives and antacids
         b. High-dose vitamin D analogs
      2. Parenteral: management of toxemia of pregnancy

CAUSES OF HYPOMAGNESEMIA

Alcoholic abuse
Diuretic use
Renal losses
Acute and chronic renal failure
Postobstructive diuresis
Acute tubular necrosis
Chronic glomerulonephritis
Chronic pyelonephritis
Interstitial nephropathy
Renal transplantation
Gastrointestinal losses
Chronic diarrhea
Nasogastric suctioning
Short bowel syndrome
Protein-calorie malnutrition
Bowel fistula
Total parenteral nutrition
Acute pancreatitis
Endocrine
Diabetes mellitus
Hyperaldosteronism
Hyperthyroidism
Hyperparathyroidism
Acute intermittent porphyria
Pregnancy
Drugs
Aminoglycosides
Amphotericin
β-agonists
Cisplatin
Cyclosporine
Diuretics
Foscarnet
Pentamidine
Theophylline
Congenital disorders
Familial hypomagnesemia
Maternal diabetes
Maternal hypothyroidism
Maternal hyperparathyroidism

MEAN CORPUSCULAR VOLUME (MCV)

Normal range: 76-100 μm^3 (76-100 fL) (76-100 fL [CF: 1; SMI: 1 fL])

See Tables 4-24 and 4-25 for descriptions of MCV abnormalities.

TABLE 4-24 Some Causes of Increased Mean Corpuscular Volume (Macrocytosis)

Causes	% of all Macrocytosis Patients*	% of Macrocytosis in Each Disease†
Common		
Folate or B_{12} deficiency	20-30 (5-50)‡	80-90 (4-100)
Chronic liver disease	15-20 (6-28)	25-30 (8-65)
Chronic alcoholism	10-12 (3-15)	60 (26-90)
Cytotoxic chemotherapy	10-15 (2-20)	30-40 (13-82)
Cardiorespiratory abnormality	8 (7-9.5)	?
Reticulocytosis	6-7 (0-15)	Depends on severity
Myelodysplastic syndromes	Frequent over age 40 yr	>60 in RAEB and RARS
Unexplained	25 (22.5-27)	—
Normal newborn		
Less Common	**<4%**	
Noncytotoxic drugs		
Zidovudine		
Phenytoin		30 (14-50)
Azathioprine		
Hypothyroidism		20-30 (8-55)
Chronic leukemia/myelofibrosis		
Radiotherapy for malignancy		
Chronic renal disease (occasional patients)		
Distance-runner macrocytosis (some persons)		
Down syndrome		
Artifactual (e.g., cold agglutinins)		

From Ravel R: *Clinical laboratory medicine,* ed 6, St Louis, 1995, Mosby.
RAEB, Refractory anemia with excessive blasts; *RARS,* refractory anemia with ring sideroblasts (formerly called "IASA," or idiopathic acquired sideroblastic anemia).
*Percentage of all patients with macrocytosis.
†Percentage of patients with each condition listed who have macrocytosis.
‡Numbers in parentheses are literature range.

TABLE 4-25 Some Causes of Decreased Mean Corpuscular Volume (Microcytosis)

Common	Less Common
Chronic iron deficiency	Some cases of polycythemia
α- or β-thalassemia (minor)	Some cases of lead poisoning
Anemia of chronic disease	Some cases of congenital spherocytosis
	Some cases of sideroblastic anemia
	Certain abnormal hemoglobins (HbE, Hb Lepore)

From Ravel R: *Clinical laboratory medicine,* ed 6, St Louis, 1995, Mosby.

METANEPHRINES, URINE

See URINE METANEPHRINES

METHYLMALONIC ACID (serum)

Normal: <0.2 mcmol/L
Elevated in: Vitamin B_{12} deficiency, pregnancy, methylmalonic acidemia

MITOCHONDRIAL ANTIBODY (AMA)

Normal: Negative
Present in: Primary biliary cirrhosis (>90% of patients)

MONOCYTE COUNT

Normal range: 2%-8%
Elevated in: Viral diseases, parasites, infections, neoplasms, inflammatory bowel disease, monocytic leukemia, lymphomas, myeloma, sarcoidosis
Decreased in: Aplastic anemia, lymphocytic leukemia, glucocorticoid administration

MYCOPLASMA PNEUMONIAE PCR

Test description: PCR can be performed on sputum, bronchoalveolar lavage, nasopharyngeal and throat swabs, other respiratory fluids, and lung tissue

MYELIN BASIC PROTEIN, CEREBROSPINAL FLUID

Normal: <2.5 ng/ml
Elevated in: Multiple sclerosis, CNS trauma, stroke, encephalitis

MYOGLOBIN, URINE

See URINE MYOGLOBIN

NEISSERIA GONORRHOEAE PCR

Test description: Test can be performed on endocervical swab, urine, and intraurethral swab
Normal: Negative

NEUTROPHIL COUNT

Normal range: 50%-70%
Subsets:
Stabs (bands, early mature neutrophils): 2%-6%
Segs (mature neutrophils): 60%-70%
Elevated in: Acute bacterial infections, acute myocardial infarction, stress, neoplasms, myelocytic leukemia
Decreased in: Viral infections, aplastic anemias, immunosuppressive drugs, radiation therapy to bone marrow, agranulocytosis, drugs (antibiotics, antithyroidals, clopidogrel), lymphocytic and monocytic leukemias

Box 4-4 describes various drugs that can cause neutropenia.

NOREPINEPHRINE

Normal range: 0-600 pg/ml
Elevated in: Pheochromocytomas, neuroblastomas, stress, vigorous exercise, certain foods (bananas, chocolate, coffee, tea, vanilla)

5′-NUCLEOTIDASE

Normal range: 2-16 IU/L (3-27 × 10^8 kat/L [CF: 1.67 × 10^8; SMI: 1 × 10^8 kat/L])
Elevated in: Biliary obstruction, metastatic neoplasms to liver, primary biliary cirrhosis, renal failure, pancreatic carcinoma, chronic active hepatitis

BOX 4-4 Drugs That Cause Neutropenia

Antiarrhythmics: tocainide, procainamide, propranolol, quinidine
Antibiotics: chloramphenicol, penicillins, sulfonamides, *p*-aminosalicylic acid (PAS), rifampin, vancomycin, isoniazid, nitrofurantoin
Antimalarials: dapsone, quinine, pyrimethamine
Anticonvulsants: phenytoin, mephenytoin, trimethadione, ethosuximide, carbamazepine
Hypoglycemic agents: tolbutamide, chlorpropamide
Antihistamines: cimetidine, brompheniramine, tripelennamine
Antihypertensives: methyldopa, captopril
Anti-inflammatory agents: aminopyrine, phenylbutazone, gold salts, ibuprofen, indomethacin
Antithyroid agents: propylthiouracil, methimazole, thiouracil
Diuretics: acetazolamide, hydrochlorothiazide, chlorthalidone
Phenothiazines: chlorpromazine, promazine, prochlorperazine
Immunosuppressive agents: antimetabolites
Cytotoxic agents: alkylating agents, antimetabolites, anthracyclines, *Vinca* alkaloids, cisplatin, hydroxyurea, dactinomycin
Other agents: recombinant interferons, allopurinol, ethanol, levamisole, penicillamine, zidovudine, streptokinase, carbamazepine, clopidogrel, ticlopidine

Modified from Goldman L, Ausiello D (eds): *Cecil textbook of medicine,* ed 22, Philadelphia, 2004, Saunders.

OSMOLALITY (serum)

Normal range: 280-300 mOsm/kg (280-300 mmol/kg [CF: 1; SMI: 1 mmol/kg])

It can also be estimated by the following formula:

$$2\,([Na] + [K] + glucose/18 + BUN/2.8)$$

Elevated in: Dehydration, hypernatremia, diabetes insipidus, uremia, hyperglycemia, mannitol therapy, ingestion of toxins (ethylene glycol, methanol, ethanol), hypercalcemia, diuretics
Decreased in: Syndrome of inappropriate diuretic hormone secretion, hyponatremia, overhydration, Addison's disease, hypothyroidism

OSMOLALITY, URINE

See URINE OSMOLALITY

OSMOTIC FRAGILITY TEST

Normal: Hemolysis begins at 0.50, w/v [5.0 g/L] and is complete at 0.30, w/v [3.0 g/L] NaCl.
Elevated in: Hereditary spherocytosis, hereditary stomatocytosis, spherocytosis associated with acquired immune hemolytic anemia
Decreased in: Iron deficiency anemia, thalassemias, liver disease, leptocytosis associated with asplenia

PARACENTESIS FLUID

Testing and evaluation of results:

1. Process the fluid as follows:
   a. Tube 1: LDH, glucose, albumin
   b. Tube 2: protein, specific gravity
   c. Tube 3: cell count and differential
   d. Tube 4: save until further notice
2. Draw serum LDH, protein, albumin.
3. Gram stain, AFB stain, bacterial and fungal cultures, amylase, and triglycerides should be ordered only when clearly indicated; bedside inoculation of blood-culture bottles with ascitic fluid improves sensitivity in detecting bacterial growth.
4. If malignant ascites is suspected, consider a carcinoembryonic antigen level on the paracentesis fluid and cytologic evaluation.
5. In suspected spontaneous bacterial peritonitis (SBP) the incidence of positive cultures can be increased by injecting 10 to 20 ml of ascitic fluid into blood culture bottles.
6. Peritoneal effusion can be subdivided as exudative or transudative based on its characteristics (see Section II).
7. The serum-ascites albumin gradient (serum albumin level–ascitic fluid albumin level [SAAG]) correlates directly with portal pressure and can

also be used to classify ascites. Patients with gradients ≥1.1 g/dl have portal hypertension, and those with gradients ≤1.1 g/dl do not; the accuracy of this method is >95%.

8. For the differential diagnosis of ascites, refer to Section II.
9. An ascitic fluid polymorphonuclear leukocyte count >500/μl is suggestive of SBP.
10. A blood-ascitic fluid albumin gradient.

PARATHYROID HORMONE (PTH)

Normal:
Serum, intact molecule 10-65 pg/ml
Plasma 1.0-5.0 pmol/L
Elevated in: Hyperparathyroidism (primary or secondary), pseudohypoparathyroidism, anticonvulsants, corticosteroids, lithium, INH, rifampin, phosphates, Zollinger-Ellison syndrome, hereditary vitamin D deficiency
Decreased in: Hypoparathyroidism, sarcoidosis, cimetidine, beta-blockers, hyperthyroidism, hypomagnesemia

PARIETAL CELL ANTIBODIES

Normal: Negative
Present in: Pernicious anemia (>90%), atrophic gastritis (up to 50%), thyroiditis (30%), Addison's disease, myasthenia gravis, Sjögren's syndrome, type 1 DM

PARTIAL THROMBOPLASTIN TIME (PTT), ACTIVATED PARTIAL THROMBOPLASTIN TIME (APTT)

See Table 4-26.

TABLE 4-26 Clinical Peculiarities of Coagulation Protein Screening Tests

Long aPTT, normal or long PT, no bleeding	Normal aPTT, PT, *with bleeding*
Long APTT Only	
Factor XII deficiency	Factor XIII deficiency or inhibitor
Prekallikrein deficiency	α_2-Antiplasmin deficiency or defect
High-molecular-weight kininogen	Plasminogen activator inhibitor defiency or defect
Lupus anticoagulant	α_1-Antitrypsin Pittsburgh defect
Long APTT and PT	
Dysfibrinogenemia with fibrinopeptide B release	
Lupus anticoagulant	

From Hoffman R et al: *Hematology: basic principles and practice,* ed 5, Philadelphia, 2009, Churchill Livingstone.

Normal range: 25-41 sec
Elevated in: Heparin therapy, coagulation factor deficiency (I, II, V, VIII, IX, X, XI, XII), liver disease, vitamin K deficiency, disseminated intravascular coagulation, circulating anticoagulant, warfarin therapy, specific factor inhibition (PCN reaction, rheumatoid arthritis), thrombolytic therapy, nephrotic syndrome
NOTE: Useful to evaluate the intrinsic coagulation system.

PEPSINOGEN I

Normal: 124-142 ng/ml
Elevated in: ZE syndrome, duodenal ulcer, acute gastritis
Decreased in: Atrophic gastritis, gastric carcinoma, myxedema, pernicious anemia, Addison's disease

pH, BLOOD

Normal values:
Arterial: 7.35-7.45
Venous: 7.32-7.42
For abnormal values, refer to ARTERIAL BLOOD GASES.

pH, URINE

See URINE pH

PHENOBARBITAL

Normal therapeutic range: 15-30 mcg/ml for epilepsy control

PHENYTOIN (Dilantin)

Normal therapeutic range: 10-20 mcg/ml

PHOSPHATASE, ACID

See ACID PHOSPHATASE

PHOSPHATASE, ALKALINE

See ALKALINE PHOSPHATASE

PHOSPHATE (serum)

See Fig. E4-30 for approach to hyperphosphatemia and Fig. E4-31 for diagnostic evaluation of hypophosphatemia.
Normal range: 2.5-5 mg/dl (0.8-1.6 mmol/L [CF: 0.3229; SMI: 0.05 mmol/L])
DECREASED
Parenteral hyperalimentation
Diabetic acidosis
Alcohol withdrawal
Severe metabolic or respiratory alkalosis
Antacids that bind phosphorus
Malnutrition with refeeding using low-phosphorus nutrients
Renal tubule failure to reabsorb phosphate (Fanconi's syndrome; congenital disorder; vitamin D deficiency)
Glucose administration
Nasogastric suction
Malabsorption
Gram-negative sepsis
Primary hyperthyroidism
Chlorothiazide diuretics
Therapy of acute severe asthma
Acute respiratory failure with mechanical ventilation
INCREASED
Renal failure
Severe muscle injury
Phosphate-containing antacids
Hypoparathyroidism
Tumor lysis syndrome

PLASMINOGEN

Normal: Immunoassay (antigen): <20 mg/dl
Elevated in: Infection, trauma, neoplasm, myocardial infarction (acute phase reactant), pregnancy, bilirubinemia
Decreased in: DIC, severe liver disease, thrombolytic therapy with streptokinase or urokinase, alteplase

PLATELET AGGREGATION

Normal: Full aggregation (generally >60%) in response to epinephrine, thrombin, ristocetin, ADP, collagen
Elevated in: Heparin, hemolysis, lipemia, nicotine, hereditary and acquired disorders of platelet adhesion, activation, and aggregation
Decreased in: Aspirin, some penicillins, chloroquine, chlorpromazine, clofibrate, captopril, Glanzmann's thrombasthenia, Bernard-Soulier syndrome, Wiskott-Aldrich syndrome, cyclooxygenase deficiency. In von Willebrand's disease there is normal aggregation with ADP, collagen, and epinephrine but abnormal agglutination with ristocetin.

PLATELET ANTIBODIES

Normal: Absent
Present in: ITP (>90% of patients with chronic ITP). Patients with nonimmune thrombocytopenias may have false-positive results.

PLATELET COUNT

See Fig. E4-32 for evaluation of thrombocytosis. Box E4-5 describes testing for thrombocytopenia.
Normal range: 130-400 × 10^3/mm^3 (130-400 × 10^9/L [CF: 1; SMI: 5 × 10^9/L])
Elevated in.
Reactive Thrombocytosis.
Infections or inflammatory states—vasculitis, allergic reactions, etc.
Surgery and tissue damage—myocardial infarction, pancreatitis, etc.
Postsplenectomy state
Malignancy—solid tumors, lymphoma

Iron deficiency anemia, hemolytic anemia, acute blood loss
Uncertain etiology
Rebound effect after chemotherapy or immune thrombocytopenia
Renal disorders—renal failure, nephrotic syndrome

MYELOPROLIFERATIVE DISORDERS

Chronic myeloid leukemia
Primary thrombocythemia
Polycythemia vera
Idiopathic myelofibrosis

Decreased:

A. Increased destruction
    1. Immunologic
        a. Drugs: quinine, quinidine, digitalis, procainamide, thiazide diuretics, sulfonamides, phenytoin, aspirin, penicillin, heparin, gold, meprobamate, sulfa drugs, phenylbutazone, NSAIDs, methyldopa, cimetidine, furosemide, INH, cephalosporins, chlorpropamide, organic arsenicals, chloroquine
        b. Idiopathic thrombocytopenic purpura
        c. Transfusion reaction: transfusion of platelets with platelet antigen HPA-1a (PL^{A1}) in recipients without PL^{A1}
        d. Fetal/maternal incompatibility
        e. Vasculitis (e.g., systemic lupus erythematosus)
        f. Autoimmune hemolytic anemia
        g. Lymphoreticular disorders (e.g., chronic lymphocytic leukemia)
    2. Nonimmunologic
        a. Prosthetic heart valves
        b. Thrombotic thrombocytopenic purpura
        c. Sepsis
        d. Disseminated intravascular coagulation
        e. Hemolytic-uremic syndrome
        f. Giant cavernous hemangioma
B. Decreased production
    1. Abnormal marrow
        a. Marrow infiltration (e.g., leukemia, lymphoma, fibrosis)
        b. Marrow suppression (e.g., chemotherapy, alcohol, radiation)
    2. Hereditary disorders
        a. Wiskott-Aldrich syndrome: X-linked disorder characterized by thrombocytopenia, eczema, and repeated infections
        b. May-Hegglin anomaly: increased megakaryocytes but ineffective thrombopoiesis
    3. Vitamin deficiencies (e.g., vitamin B_{12}, folic acid)
C. Splenic sequestration, hypersplenism
D. Dilutional, secondary to massive transfusion

PLATELET FUNCTION ANALYSIS 100 ASSAY (PFA)

Normal: This test is a two-component assay where blood is aspirated through two capillary tubes, one of which is coated with collagen and ADP (COL/ADP) and the other with collagen and epinephrine (COL/EPI). The test measures the ability of platelets to occlude an aperture in a biologically active membrane treated with COL/ADP and COL/EPI. During the test, the platelets adhere to the surface of the tube and cause blood flow to cease. The closing time refers to the cessation of blood flow and is reported in conjunction with the hematocrit and platelet count. Hematocrit count must be >25% and platelet count >50 K/microliter for the test to be performed

COL/ADP: 70-120 sec
COL/EPI: 75-120 sec

Elevated in: Acquired platelet dysfunction, von Willebrand's disease, anemia, thrombocytopenia, use of aspirin and NSAIDs

POTASSIUM (serum)

Normal range: 3.5-5 mEq/L (3.5-5 mmol/L [CF: 1; SMI: 0.1 mmol/L])

CAUSES OF HYPERKALEMIA

(see Fig. E4-33 for diagnostic approach to hyperkalemia, Fig. E4-34 for evaluation and treatment of hyperkalemia, and Fig. E4-35 for electrocardiographic changes in hyperkalemia.)

I. Pseudohyperkalemia
    A. Hemolysis of sample
    B. Thrombocytosis
    C. Leukocytosis
    D. Laboratory error
II. Increased potassium intake and absorption
    A. Potassium supplements (oral and parenteral)
    B. Dietary—salt substitutes
    C. Stored blood
    D. Potassium-containing medications
III. Impaired renal excretion
    A. Acute renal failure
    B. Chronic renal failure
    C. Tubular defect in potassium secretion
        1. Renal allograft
        2. Analgesic nephropathy
        3. Sickle cell disease
        4. Obstructive uropathy
        5. Interstitial nephritis
        6. Chronic pyelonephritis
        7. Potassium-sparing diuretics
        8. Miscellaneous (lead, systemic lupus erythematosus, pseudohypoaldosteronism)
    D. Hypoaldosteronism
        1. Primary (Addison's disease)
        2. Secondary
            a. Hyporeninemic hypoaldosteronism (type IV RTA)
            b. Congenital adrenal hyperplasia
            c. Drug-induced
                (1) NSAIDs
                (2) ACE inhibitors
                (3) Heparin
                (4) Cyclosporine
IV. Transcellular shifts
    A. Acidosis
    B. Hypertonicity
    C. Insulin deficiency
    D. Drugs
        1. β-blockers
        2. Digitalis toxicity
        3. Succinylcholine
    E. Exercise
    F. Hyperkalemic periodic paralysis
V. Cellular injury
    A. Rhabdomyolysis
    B. Severe intravascular hemolysis
    C. Acute tumor lysis syndrome
    D. Burns and crush injuries

CAUSES OF HYPOKALEMIA

See Fig. E4-36 for diagnostic evaluation of hypokalemia.

I. Decreased intake
    A. Decreased dietary potassium
    B. Impaired absorption of potassium
    C. Clay ingestion
    D. Kayexalate
II. Increased loss
    A. Renal
        1. Hyperaldosteronism
            a. Primary
                (1) Conn's syndrome
                (2) Adrenal hyperplasia
            b. Secondary
                (1) Congestive heart failure
                (2) Cirrhosis
                (3) Nephrotic syndrome
                (4) Dehydration
            c. Bartter's syndrome
        2. Glycyrrhizic acid (licorice, chewing tobacco)
        3. Excessive adrenal corticosteroids
            a. Cushing's syndrome
            b. Steroid therapy
            c. Adrenogenital syndrome
        4. Renal tubular defects
            a. Renal tubular acidosis
            b. Obstructive uropathy

c. Salt-wasting nephropathy
5. Drugs
a. Diuretics
b. Aminoglycosides
c. Mannitol
d. Amphotericin
e. Cisplatin
f. Carbenicillin
B. Gastrointestinal
1. Vomiting
2. Nasogastric suction
3. Diarrhea
4. Malabsorption
5. Ileostomy
6. Villous adenoma
7. Laxative abuse
C. Increased losses from the skin
1. Excessive sweating
2. Burns
III. Transcellular shifts
A. Alkalosis
1. Vomiting
2. Diuretics
3. Hyperventilation
4. Bicarbonate therapy
B. Insulin
1. Exogenous
2. Endogenous response to glucose
C. β_2-Agonists (albuterol, terbutaline, epinephrine)
D. Hypokalemia periodic paralysis
1. Familial
2. Thyrotoxic
IV. Miscellaneous
A. Anabolic state
B. Intravenous hyperalimentation
C. Treatment of megaloblastic anemia
D. Acute mountain sickness

POTASSIUM, URINE

See URINE POTASSIUM

PROCAINAMIDE

Normal therapeutic range: 4-10 mcg/ml

PROGESTERONE (serum)

Normal:
Female: Follicular phase: 15-70 ng/dl
Luteal phase: 200-2500 ng/dl
Male: 15-70 ng/dl
Elevated in: Congenital adrenal hyperplasia, clomiphene, corticosterone, 11-deoxycortisol, dihydroprogesterone, molar pregnancy, lipoid ovarian tumor
Decreased in: Primary or secondary hypogonadism, oral contraceptives, ampicillin, threatened abortion

PROLACTIN

See Fig. E4-37 for the evaluation of hyperprolactinemia.
Normal range: <20 ng/ml (<20 μg/L [CF: 1; SMI: 1 μg/L])
Elevated in: Prolactinomas (level >200 highly suggestive), drugs (phenothiazines, cimetidine, tricyclic antidepressants, metoclopramide, estrogens, antihypertensives [methyldopa], verapamil, haloperidol), postpartum, stress, hypoglycemia, hypothyroidism

PROSTATE-SPECIFIC ANTIGEN (PSA)

Normal range: 0-4 ng/ml

Table 4-27 describes age-specific reference ranges for PSA.

Elevated in: Benign prostatic hypertrophy, carcinoma of prostate, prostatitis, postrectal examination, prostate trauma.

Factors affecting serum PSA are described in Table 4-28.

TABLE 4-27 Age-Specific Reference Ranges for PSA

	Serum PSA (ng/ml)		
Age (yr)	**Whites**	**Japanese**	**African Americans**
40-49	0-2.5	0-2.0	0-2.0
50-59	0-3.5	0-3.0	0-4.0
60-69	0-4.5	0-4.0	0-4.5
70-79	0-6.5	0-5.0	0-5.5

From Nseyo UO (ed): *Urology for primary care physicians,* Philadelphia, 1999, Saunders.
PSA, Prostate-specific antigen.

TABLE 4-28 Factors Affecting Serum PSA

Factors Affecting Serum PSA	Duration of Effect
Prostate cell number	NA
Prostate size	NA
Recent ejaculation	6-48 hours
Prostate manipulation	
Vigorous massage	1 week
Cystoscopy	1 week
Prostate biopsy	4-6 weeks
Prostatitis	
Acute	3-6 months
Chronic	Unknown
Prostate cancer	NA
Drugs: finasteride*	3-6 months

From Nseyo UO (ed): *Urology for primary care physicians,* Philadelphia, 1999, Saunders.
NA, Not applicable; *PSA,* prostate-specific antigen.
*Lowers PSA for as long as patient is on the medication.

NOTE: Measurement of free PSA is useful to assess the probability of prostate cancer in patients with normal digital rectal examination and total PSA between 4 and 10 ng/ml. In these patients, the global risk of prostate cancer is 25%; however, if the free PSA is >25%, the risk of prostate cancer decreases to 8%, whereas if the free PSA is <10%, the risk of cancer increases to 56%. Free PSA is also useful to evaluate the aggressiveness of prostate cancer. A low free PSA percentage generally indicates a high-grade cancer, whereas a high free PSA percentage is generally associated with a slower-growing tumor.
Decreased in: 5-Alpha reductase inhibitors (finasteride, dutasteride), saw palmetto use, antiandrogens

PROSTATIC ACID PHOSPHATASE

Normal: 0-0.8 U/L
Elevated in: Prostate cancer (especially in metastatic prostate cancer), BPH, prostatitis, post–prostate surgery or manipulation, hemolysis, androgens, clofibrate
Decreased in: Ketoconazole

PROTEIN (serum)

Normal range: 6-8 g/dl (60-80 g/L [CF: 10; SMI: 1 g/L])
Elevated in: Dehydration, multiple myeloma, Waldenström's macroglobulinemia, sarcoidosis, collagen vascular diseases
Decreased in: Malnutrition, low-protein diet, overhydration, malabsorption, pregnancy, severe burns, neoplasms, chronic diseases, cirrhosis, nephrosis

PROTEIN C ASSAY

See Table 4-29.
Normal: 70%-140%
Elevated in: Oral contraceptives, stanozol

Decreased in: Congenital protein C deficiency, warfarin therapy, Vitamin K deficiency, renal insufficiency, consumptive coagulopathies

TABLE 4-29 Assay Measurement in Heterozygote Protein C Deficiency

	ACTIVITY		
Type	**Antigen**	**Amidolytic**	**Coagulant**
I	Low	Low	Low
II	Normal	Low	Low
	Normal	Normal	Low

From Hoffman R et al: *Hematology: basic principles and practice,* ed 5, Philadelphia, 2009, Churchill Livingstone.

PROTEIN ELECTROPHORESIS (serum)

Normal range:

Albumin: 60%-75% (0.6-0.75 [CF: 0.01; SMI: 0.01])
α-1: 1.7%-5% (0.02-0.05)
α-2: 6.7%-12.5% (0.07-0.13)
β: 8.3%-16.3% (0.08-0.16)
γ: 10.7%-20% (0.11-0.2)

Albumin: 3.6-5.2 g/dl (36-52 g/L [CF: 0.01; SMI: 1 g/L])
α-1: 0.1-0.4 g/dl (1-4 g/L)
α-2: 0.4-1 g/dl (4-10 g/L)
β: 0.5-1.2 g/dl (5-12 g/L)
γ: 0.6-1.6 g/dl (6-16 g/L)

Elevated in:

Albumin: dehydration
α-1: neoplastic diseases, inflammation
α-2: neoplasms, inflammation, infection, nephrotic syndrome
β: hypothyroidism, biliary cirrhosis, diabetes mellitus
γ: See IMMUNOGLOBULINS

Decreased in:

Albumin: malnutrition, chronic liver disease, malabsorption, nephrotic syndrome, burns, systemic lupus erythematosus
α-1: emphysema (α-1 antitrypsin deficiency), nephrosis
α-2: hemolytic anemias (decreased haptoglobin), severe hepatocellular damage
β: hypocholesterolemia, nephrosis
γ: See IMMUNOGLOBULINS

Fig. 4-38 describes serum protein electrophoretic patterns.

PROTEIN S ASSAY

See Table 4-30.
Normal: 65%-140%
Elevated in: Presence of lupus anticoagulant

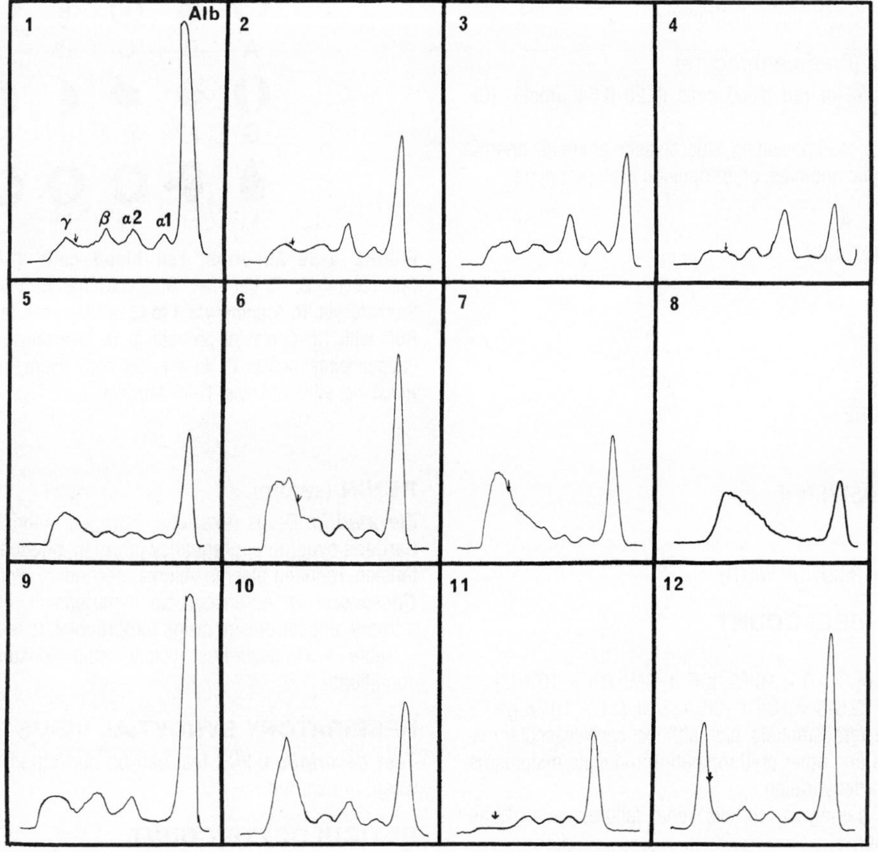

FIGURE 4-38 Typical serum protein electrophoretic patterns. *1,* Normal (*arrow* near γ region indicates serum application point). *2,* Acute reaction pattern. *3,* Acute reaction or nephrotic syndrome. *4,* Nephrotic syndrome. *5,* Chronic inflammation, cirrhosis, granulomatous diseases, rheumatoid-collagen group. *6,* Same as 5, but γ elevation is more pronounced. There is also partial (but not complete) β-γ fusion. *7,* Suggestive of cirrhosis but could be found in the granulomatous diseases or the rheumatoid-collagen group. *8,* Characteristic pattern of cirrhosis. *9,* α-1 Antitrypsin deficiency with mild γ elevation suggesting concurrent chronic disease. *10,* Same as 5, but the γ elevation is marked. The configuration of the γ peak superficially mimics that of myeloma, but is more broad-based. There are superimposed acute reaction changes. *11,* Hypogammaglobulinemia or light-chain myeloma. *12,* Myeloma, Waldenström's macroglobulinemia, idiopathic or secondary monoclonal gammopathy. (From Ravel R [ed]: *Clinical laboratory medicine,* ed 6, St Louis, 1995, Mosby.)

Laboratory Tests IV

TABLE 4-30 Assay Measurements in Heterozygote Protein S Deficiency

	ACTIVITY		
Type	**Protein S Total Antigen**	**Protein S Free Antigen**	**Protein S Activity**
I (classic)	Low	Low	Low
II	Normal	Normal	Low
III	Normal	Low	Low

From Hoffman R et al: *Hematology: basic principles and practice,* ed 5, Philadelphia, 2009, Churchill Livingstone.

Decreased in: Hereditary deficiency, acute thrombotic events, DIC, surgery, oral contraceptives, pregnancy, hormone replacement therapy, l-asparaginase treatment

PROTHROMBIN TIME (PT)

Normal range: 10-12 sec
Elevated in: Liver disease, oral anticoagulants (warfarin), heparin, factor deficiency (I, II, V, VII, X), disseminated intravascular coagulation, vitamin K deficiency, afibrinogenemia, dysfibrinogenemia, drugs (salicylate, chloral hydrate, diphenylhydantoin, estrogens, antacids, phenylbutazone, quinidine, antibiotics, allopurinol, anabolic steroids)
Decreased in: Vitamin K supplementation, thrombophlebitis, drugs (glutethimide, estrogens, griseofulvin, diphenhydramine)

PROTOPORPHYRIN (Free erythrocyte)

Normal range: 16-36 μg/dl of red blood cells (0.28-0.64 μmol/L [CF: 0.0177; SMI: 0.02 μmol/L])
Elevated in: Iron deficiency, lead poisoning, sideroblastic anemias, anemia of chronic disease, hemolytic anemias, erythropoietic protoporphyria

PSA

See PROSTATE-SPECIFIC ANTIGEN

PT

See PROTHROMBIN TIME

PTH

See PARATHYROID HORMONE

PTT

See PARTIAL THROMBOPLASTIN TIME

RDW

See RED BLOOD CELL DISTRIBUTION WIDTH

RED BLOOD CELL (RBC) COUNT

Normal range:
Male: 4.3-5.9 × 10^6/mm^3 (4.3-5.9 × 10^{12}/L [CF: 1; SMI: 0.1 × 10^{12}/L])
Female: 3.5-5 × 10^6/mm^3 (3.5-5 × 10^{12}/L [CF: 1; SMI: 0.1 × 10^{12}/L])
Elevated in: Polycythemia vera, smokers, high altitude, cardiovascular disease, renal cell carcinoma and other erythropoietin-producing neoplasms, stress, hemoconcentration/dehydration
Decreased in: Anemias, hemolysis, chronic renal failure, hemorrhage, failure of marrow production

RED BLOOD CELL DISTRIBUTION WIDTH (RDW)

Measures variability of red cell size (anisocytosis)
Normal range: 11.5-14.5
Normal RDW and elevated mean corpuscular volume (MCV): Aplastic anemia, preleukemia
Normal MCV: Normal, anemia of chronic disease, acute blood loss or hemolysis, chronic lymphocytic leukemia (CLL), chronic myelocytic leukemia, nonanemic enzymopathy or hemoglobinopathy
Decreased MCV: Anemia of chronic disease, heterozygous thalassemia
Elevated RDW and elevated MCV: Vitamin B_{12} deficiency, folate deficiency, immune hemolytic anemia, cold agglutinins, CLL with high count, liver disease
Normal MCV: Early iron deficiency, early vitamin B_{12} deficiency, early folate deficiency, anemic globinopathy
Decreased MCV: Iron deficiency, red blood cell fragmentation, HbH disease, thalassemia intermedia

RED BLOOD CELL FOLATE

See FOLATE

RED BLOOD CELL MASS (Volume)

Normal range:
Male: 20-36 ml/kg body weight (1.15-1.21 L/m^2 body surface area)
Female: 19-31 ml/kg body weight (0.95-1.00 L/m^2 body surface area)
Elevated in: Polycythemia vera, hypoxia (smokers, high altitude, cardiovascular disease), hemoglobinopathies with high oxygen affinity, erythropoietin-producing tumors (renal cell carcinoma)
Decreased in: Hemorrhage, chronic disease, failure of marrow production, anemias, hemolysis

RED BLOOD CELL MORPHOLOGY

See Fig. 4-39.

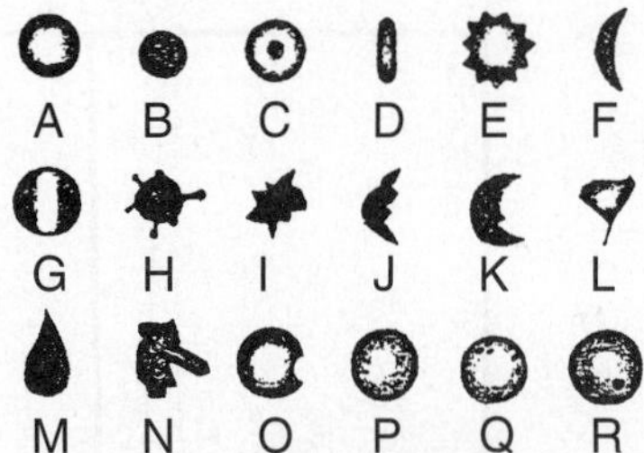

FIGURE 4-39 Abnormal red blood cells (RBCs). A, Normal RBC. **B,** Spherocyte. **C,** Target cell. **D,** Elliptocyte. **E,** Echinocyte. **F,** Sickle cell. **G,** Stomatocyte. **H,** Acanthocyte. **I** to **L,** Schistocytes. **M,** Teardrop RBC. **N,** Distorted RBC with Hb C crystal protruding. **O,** Degmacyte. **P,** Basophilic stippling. **Q,** Pappenheimer bodies. **R,** Howell-Jolly body. (From Ravel R [ed]: *Clinical laboratory medicine,* ed 6, St Louis, 1995, Mosby.)

RENIN (serum)

Elevated in: Drugs (thiazides, estrogen, minoxidil), chronic renal failure, Bartter's syndrome, pregnancy (normal), pheochromocytoma, renal hypertension, reduced plasma volume, secondary aldosteronism
Decreased in: Adrenocortical hypertension, increased plasma volume, primary aldosteronism, drugs (propranolol, reserpine, clonidine)

Table 4-31 describes typical renin-aldosterone patterns in various conditions.

RESPIRATORY SYNCYTIAL VIRUS (RSV) SCREEN

Test description: PCR test can be performed on nasopharyngeal swab, wash, or aspirate

RETICULOCYTE COUNT

See Fig. E4-40 and Table 4-32.
Normal range: 0.5%-1.5%
Elevated in: Hemolytic anemia (sickle cell crisis, thalassemia major, autoimmune hemolysis), hemorrhage, postanemia therapy (folic acid, ferrous sulfate, vitamin B_{12}), chronic renal failure
Decreased in: Aplastic anemia, marrow suppression (sepsis, chemotherapeutic agents, radiation), hepatic cirrhosis, blood transfusion, anemias of disordered maturation (iron deficiency anemia, megaloblastic anemia, sideroblastic anemia, anemia of chronic disease)

TABLE 4-31 Typical Renin-Aldosterone Patterns in Various Conditions

	Plasma Renin	Aldosterone
Primary aldosteronism	Low	High
"Low-renin" essential hypertension	Low	Normal
Cushing's syndrome	Low	Low-normal
Licorice ingestion syndrome	Low	Low
High-salt diet	Low	Low
Oral contraceptives	High	Normal
Cirrhosis	High	High
Malignant hypertension	High	High
Unilateral renal disease	High	High
"High-renin" essential hypertension	High	High
Pregnancy	High	High
Diuretic overuse	High	High
Juxtaglomerular tumor (Bartter's syndrome)	High	High
Low-salt diet	High	High
Addison's disease	High	Low
Hypokalemia	High	Low

From Ravel R: *Clinical laboratory medicine,* ed 6, St Louis, 1995, Mosby.

TABLE 4-32 Combining the Reticulocyte Count and Red Blood Cell Parameters for Diagnosis

MCV, RDW	Reticulocyte Count <75,000/μL	Reticulocyte Count >100,000/μL
Low, Normal	Anemia of chronic disease	
Normal, Normal	Anemia of chronic disease	
High, Normal	Chemotherapy/antivirals/alcohol	Chronic liver disease
	Aplastic anemia	
Low, High	Iron deficiency anemia	Sickle cell-β-thalassemia
Normal, High	Early iron, folate, vitamin B_{12} deficiency	Sickle cell anemia, sickle cell disease
	Myelodysplasia	
High, High	Folate or vitamin B_{12} deficiency	Immune hemolytic anemia
	Myelodysplasia	Chronic liver disease

From Hoffman R et al: *Hematology: basic principles and practice,* ed 5, Philadelphia, 2009, Churchill Livingstone.
MCV, Mean corpuscular volume; *RDW,* red blood cell distribution width.

RHEUMATOID FACTOR

Normal: Negative. Present in titer >1:20

RHEUMATIC DISEASES

Rheumatoid arthritis
Sjögren's syndrome
Systemic lupus erythematosus
Polymyositis/dermatomyositis
Mixed connective tissue disease
Scleroderma

INFECTIOUS DISEASES

Subacute bacterial endocarditis
Tuberculosis
Infectious mononucleosis
Hepatitis
Syphilis
Leprosy
Influenza

MALIGNANCIES

Lymphoma
Multiple myeloma
Waldenström's macroglobulinemia
Postradiation or postchemotherapy

MISCELLANEOUS

Normal adults, especially the elderly
Sarcoidosis
Chronic pulmonary disease (interstitial fibrosis)
Chronic liver disease (chronic active hepatitis, cirrhosis)
Mixed essential cryoglobulinemia
Hypergammaglobulinemic purpura

RNP

See EXTRACTABLE NUCLEAR ANTIGEN

ROTAVIRUS SEROLOGY

Test description: PCR test is performed on stool specimen
Normal: Negative

SED RATE

See ERYTHROCYTE SEDIMENTATION RATE

SEDIMENTATION RATE

See ERYTHROCYTE SEDIMENTATION RATE

SEMEN ANALYSIS

Table 4-33 describes semen analysis reference ranges.

TABLE 4-33 Semen Analysis Reference Ranges

Color	Grayish white
pH	7.3-7.8 (literature range, 7.0-7.8)
Volume	2.0-5.0 ml (literature range, 1.5-6.0 ml)
Sperm count	20-250 million/ml (literature range for upper limit varies from 100-250 million/ml)
Motility	>60% motile <3 hours after specimen is obtained (literature range, >40% to >70%)
% Normal sperm	>60% (literature range, >60% to >70%)
Viscosity	Can be poured from a pipet in droplets rather than a thick strand

From Ravel R (ed): *Clinical laboratory medicine,* ed 6, St Louis, 1995, Mosby.

SGOT

See ASPARTATE AMINOTRANSFERASE

SGPT

See ALANINE AMINOTRANSFERASE

SICKLE CELL TEST

Normal: Negative
Positive in: Sickle cell anemia, sickle cell trait, combination of *Hb S* gene with other disorders such as alpha-thalassemia, beta-thalassemia.

SMOOTH MUSCLE ANTIBODY

Normal: Negative
Present in: Chronic acute hepatitis, primary sclerosing cholangitis, primary biliary cirrhosis, autoimmune hepatitis, infectious mononucleosis

SODIUM (serum)

Normal range: 135-147 mEq/L (135-147 mmol/L [CF: 1; SMI: 1 mmol/L])

HYPONATREMIA

See Fig. E4-42 for the evaluation and treatment of hyponatremia. Table E4-34 describes drugs associated with hyponatremia.

A. Sodium and water depletion (deficit hyponatremia)
   1. Loss of gastrointestinal secretions with replacement of fluid but not electrolytes
      a. Vomiting
      b. Diarrhea
      c. Tube drainage

2. Loss from skin with replacement of fluids but not electrolytes
   a. Excessive sweating
   b. Extensive burns
3. Loss from kidney
   a. Diuretics
   b. Chronic renal insufficiency (uremia) with acidosis
4. Metabolic loss
   a. Starvation with acidosis
   b. Diabetic acidosis
5. Endocrine loss
   a. Addison's disease
   b. Sudden withdrawal of long-term steroid therapy
6. Iatrogenic loss from serous cavities
   a. Paracentesis or thoracentesis

B. Excessive water (dilution hyponatremia)
1. Excessive water administration
2. Congestive heart failure
3. Cirrhosis
4. Nephrotic syndrome
5. Hypoalbuminemia (severe)
6. Acute renal failure with oliguria

C. Inappropriate antidiuretic hormone (IADH) syndrome
D. Intracellular loss (reset osmostat syndrome)
E. False hyponatremia (actually a dilutional effect)
1. Marked hypertriglyceridemia
2. Marked hyperproteinemia
3. Severe hyperglycemia

HYPERNATREMIA
See Fig. E4-41 for evaluation and treatment of hypernatremia. Dehydration is the most frequent overall clinical finding in hypernatremia.
1. Deficient water intake (either orally or intravenously)
2. Excess kidney water output (diabetes insipidus, osmotic diuresis)
3. Excess skin water output (excess sweating, loss from burns)
4. Excess gastrointestinal tract output (severe protracted vomiting or diarrhea without fluid therapy)
5. Accidental sodium overdose
6. High-protein tube feedings

STREPTOZYME

See ANTISTREPTOLYSIN O TITER

SUCROSE HEMOLYSIS TEST (sugar water test)

Normal: Absence of hemolysis
Positive in:
Paroxysmal nocturnal hemoglobinuria
False-positive: autoimmune hemolytic anemia, megaloblastic anemias
False-negative: may occur with use of heparin or EDTA

SUDAN III STAIN (qualitative screening for fecal fat)

Normal: Negative. Test should be preceded by diet containing 100-150 g of dietary fat/day for 1 week, avoidance of high-fiber diet, and avoidance of suppositories or oily material before specimen collection.
Positive in: Steatorrhea, use of castor oil or mineral oil droplets

SYNOVIAL FLUID ANALYSIS

Table 4-35 describes the classification and interpretation of synovial fluid analysis.

T_3 (TRIIODOTHYRONINE)

See Table 4-36 for T_3 abnormalities.
Normal range: 75-220 ng/dl (1.2-3.4 nmol/L [CF: 0.01536; SMI: 0.1 nmol/L])

TABLE 4-35 Classification and Interpretation of Synovial Fluid Analysis

Group	Diseases	Appearance	Viscosity	Mucin Clot	WBC/mm³	% PMN	Glucose (mg/dl) (Blood-Synovial Fluid)	Protein (g/dl)
Normal	—	Clear	↑	Firm	<200	<25	<10	<2.5
I (noninflammatory)	Osteoarthritis, aseptic necrosis, traumatic arthritis, erythema nodosum, osteochondritis dissecans	Clear, yellow (may be xanthochromic if traumatic arthritis)	↑	Firm	↑ Up to 10,000	<25	<10	<2.5
II (inflammatory)	Crystal-induced arthritis, rheumatoid arthritis, Reiter's syndrome, collagen vascular disease, psoriatic arthritis, serum sickness, rheumatic fever	Clear, yellow, turbid	↓	Friable	↑↑ Up to 100,000	40-90	<40	<2.5
III (septic)	Bacterial (staphylococcal, gonococcal, tuberculosis)	Turbid	↓/↑	Friable	↑↑↑ Up to 5 million	40-100	20-100	>2.5

↑, Elevated; ↑↑ >markedly high; ↓, decreased; *PMN,* polymorphonuclear leukocytes. Note that there is considerable overlap in the numbers listed above.

TABLE 4-36 Findings in Thyroid Function Tests in Various Clinical Conditions

Condition	T_4	FT_4I	T_3	FT_3I	TSH	TSI	TRH Stimulation
Hyperthyroidism							
Graves' disease	↑	↑	↑	↑	↓	+	↓
Toxic nodular goiter	↑	↑	↑	↑	↓	–	↓
Pituitary TSH-secreting tumors	↑	↑	↑	↑	↑	–	↓
T_3 thyrotoxicosis	N	N	↑	↑	↓	+, –	↓
T_4 thyrotoxicosis	↑	↑	N	N	↓	+, –	↓
Hypothyroidism							
Primary	↓	↓	↓	↓	↑	+, –	↑
Secondary	↓	↓	↓	↓	↓ N	–	↓
Tertiary	↓	↓	↓	↓	↓, N	–	N
Peripheral unresponsiveness	↑, N	↑, N	↑, N	↑	↑, N	–	N,↑

From Tilton RC, Barrows A: *Clinical laboratory medicine,* St Louis, 1992, Mosby.
↑, Increased; ↓, decreased; +, – variable; *N,* normal.

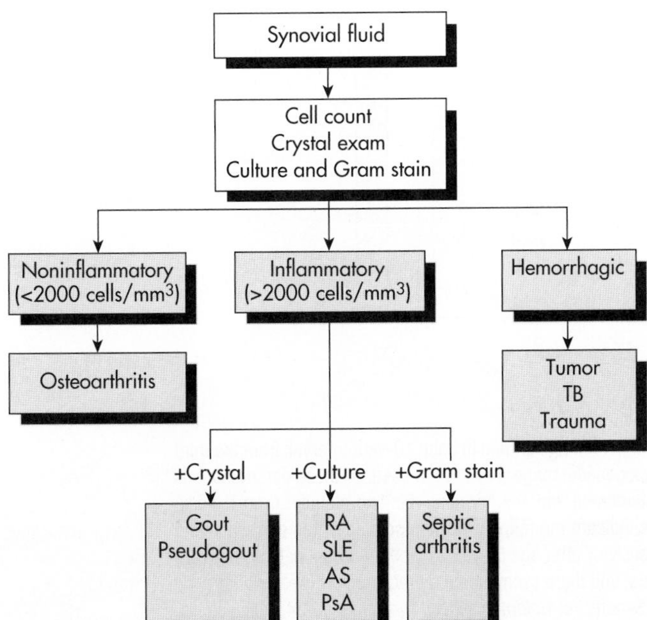

FIGURE 4-43 Algorithm for analysis of joint fluid. Examples of inflammatory arthritis are indicated, although many conditions can produce these findings. *AS,* ankylosing spondylitis; *PsA,* psoriatic arthritis; *RA,* rheumatoid arthritis; *SLE,* systemic lupus erythematosus; *TB,* tuberculosis. (From Goldman L, Schafer AI: *Goldman's Cecil medicine,* ed 24, Philadelphia, 2012, Saunders.)

Abnormal values:

A. Elevated in hyperthyroidism (usually earlier and to a greater extent than serum T_4).
B. Useful in diagnosing:
   1. T_3 hyperthyroidism (thyrotoxicosis): increased T_3, normal FTI.
   2. Toxic nodular goiter: increased T_3, normal or increased T_4. See Figure 4-43.
   3. Iodine deficiency: normal T_3, possibly decreased T_4.
   4. Thyroid replacement therapy with liothyronine (Cytomel): normal T_4, increased T_3 if patient is symptomatically hyperthyroid.

Not ordered routinely but indicated when hyperthyroidism is suspected and serum-free T_4 or FTI inconclusive.

T_3 RESIN UPTAKE (T3RU)

Normal range: 25%-35%

Abnormal values: Increased in hyperthyroidism. T_3 resin uptake (T_3RU or RT_3U) measures the percentage of free T_4 (not bound to protein); it does not measure serum T_3 concentration; T_3RU and other tests that reflect thyroid hormone binding to plasma protein are also known as *thyroid hormone-binding ratios* (THBR).

T_4, FREE (free thyroxine)

Normal range: 0.8-2.8 ng/dl

Elevated in:

Graves' disease, toxic multinodular goiter, toxic adenoma, iatrogenic and factitious causes, transient hyperthyroidism

Serum-free T_4 directly measures unbound thyroxine. Free T_4 can be measured by equilibrium dialysis (gold standard of free T_4 assays) or by immunometric techniques (influenced by serum levels of lipids, proteins, and certain drugs). The free thyroxine index (FTI) can also be easily calculated by multiplying T_4 times T_3RU and dividing the result by 100; the FTI corrects for any abnormal T_4 values secondary to protein binding: FTI = $T_4 \times T_3$RU/100.

Normal values equal 1.1 to 4.3.

T_4, SERUM T_4

Normal range: 0.8-2.8 ng/dl (10-36 pmol/L [CF: 12.87; SMI: 1 pmol/L])

Abnormal values: Serum thyroxine (T_4)

Elevated in:

1. Graves' disease
2. Toxic multinodular goiter
3. Toxic adenoma
4. Iatrogenic and factitious
5. Transient hyperthyroidism
   a. Subacute thyroiditis
   b. Hashimoto's thyroiditis
   c. Silent thyroiditis
6. Rare causes: hypersecretion of TSH (e.g., pituitary neoplasms), struma ovarii, ingestion of large amounts of iodine in a patient with preexisting thyroid hyperplasia or adenoma (Jod-Basedow phenomenon), hydatidiform mole, carcinoma of thyroid, amiodarone therapy of arrhythmias.

Serum thyroxine test measures both circulating thyroxine bound to protein (represents >99% of circulating T_4) and unbound (free) thyroxine. Values vary with protein binding; changes in the concentration of T_4 secondary to changes in thyroxine-binding globulin (TBG) can be caused by the following:

Increased TBG (↑T_4)	*Decreased TBG (↓T_4)*
Pregnancy	Androgens, glucocorticoids
Estrogens	Nephrotic syndrome, cirrhosis
Acute infectious hepatitis	Acromegaly
Oral contraceptives	Hypoproteinemia
Familial	Familial
Fluorouracil, clofibrate	Phenytoin, ASA and other NSAIDs, heroin, methadone, high-dose penicillin, asparaginase
	Chronic debilitating illness

To eliminate the suspected influence of protein binding on thyroxine values, two additional tests are available: T_3 resin uptake and serum free thyroxine. See Table 4-37.

TABLE 4-37 Effects of Pregnancy on Thyroid Physiology

Physiologic Change	Thyroid-Related Consequences
↑ Serum thyroxine-binding globulin	↑ Total T_4 and T_3; ↑ T_4 production
↑ Plasma volume	↑ T_4 and T_3 pool size; ↑ T_4 production; ↑ cardiac output
D3 expression in placenta and (?) uterus	↑ T_4 production
First-trimester ↑ in hCG	↑ Free T_4; ↓ basal thyrotropin; ↑ T_4 production
↑ Renal I^- clearance	↑ Iodine requirements
↑ T_4 production; fetal T_4 synthesis during second and third trimesters	
↑ Oxygen consumption by fetoplacental unit, gravid uterus, and mother	↑ Basal metabolic rate; ↑ cardiac output

From Melmed S, Polonsky KS, Larsen PR, Kronenberg HM: *Williams textbook of endocrinology,* ed 12, Philadelphia, 2011, Saunders.

D3, type 3 iodothyronine deiodinase; *I^-,* plasma iodide; *hCG,* human chorionic gonadotropin; *T_3,* triiodothyronine; *T_4,* thyroxine.

TEGRETOL

See CARBAMAZEPINE.

TESTOSTERONE (total testosterone)

Normal range: Variable with age and sex.

Serum/plasma

Males: 280-1100 ng/dl   Females: 15-70 ng/dl

Urine

Males: 50-135 μg/day   Females: 2-12 μg/day

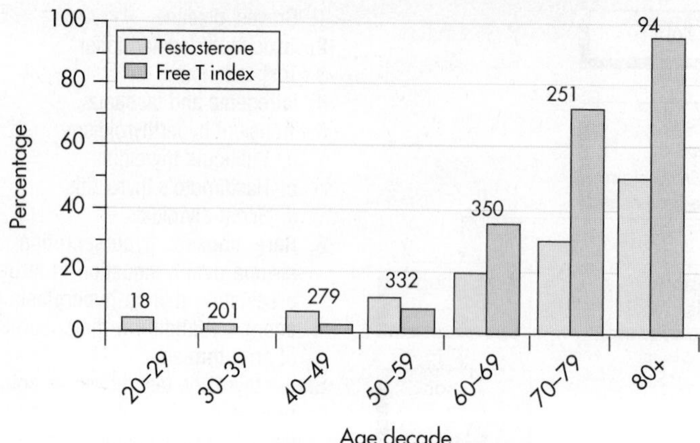

FIGURE 4-44 Hypogonadism in aging men. Bar height indicates the percentage of men in each 10-year interval, from the third to the ninth decades, with at least one testosterone value in the hypogonadal range. The criteria used for these determinations are total testosterone less than 11.3 nmol/L (325 ng/dL) and testosterone and sex hormone–binding globulin (free T index) less than 0.153 nmol/nmol. The numbers above each pair of bars indicate the number of men studied in the corresponding decade. The fraction of men who are hypogonadal increases progressively after age 50 years by either criterion. More men are hypogonadal by free T index than by total testosterone after 50 years, and there seems to be a progressively greater difference with increasing age between the two criteria. (From Goldman L, Schafer AI: *Goldman's Cecil medicine*, ed 24, Philadelphia, 2012, Saunders.)

Elevated in: Testicular tumors, ovarian masculinizing tumors, testosterone replacement therapy
Decreased in: Hypogonadism, sleep apnea. See Figure 4-44.

THEOPHYLLINE

Normal therapeutic range: 10-20 mcg/ml

THORACENTESIS FLUID

Testing and evaluation of results:

1. Pleural effusion fluid should be differentiated in exudate or transudate. The initial laboratory studies should be aimed only at distinguishing an exudate from a transudate.
   a. Tube 1: protein, LDH, albumin.
   b. Tubes 2, 3, 4: save the fluid until further notice. In selected patients with suspected empyema, a pH level may be useful (generally ≤7.0). See following for proper procedure to obtain a pH level from pleural fluid.
   NOTE: Do not order further tests until the presence of an exudate is confirmed on the basis of protein and LDH determinations; however, if the results of protein and LDH determinations cannot be obtained within a reasonable time (resulting in unnecessary delay), additional laboratory tests should be ordered at the time of thoracentesis.
2. A serum/effusion albumin gradient of ≤1.2 g/dl is indicative of exudative effusions, especially in patients with congestive heart failure (CHF) treated with diuretics.
3. Note the appearance of the fluid:
   a. A grossly hemorrhagic effusion can be a result of a traumatic tap, neoplasm, or an embolus with infarction.
   b. A milky appearance indicates either of the following:
      (1) Chylous effusion: caused by trauma or tumor invasion of the thoracic duct; lipoprotein electrophoresis of the effusion reveals chylomicrons and triglyceride levels >115 mg/dl.
      (2) Pseudochylous effusion: often seen with chronic inflammation of the pleural space (e.g., TB, connective tissue diseases).
4. If transudate, consider CHF, cirrhosis, chronic renal failure, and other hypoproteinemic states and perform subsequent workup accordingly.
5. If exudate, consider ordering these tests on the pleural fluid:
   a. Cytologic examination for malignant cells (for suspected neoplasm).
   b. Gram stain, cultures (aerobic and anaerobic), and sensitivities (for suspected infectious process).
   c. AFB stain and cultures (for suspected TB).
   d. pH: a value <7.0 suggests parapneumonic effusion or empyema; a pleural fluid pH must be drawn anaerobically and iced immediately; the syringe should be prerinsed with 0.2 ml of 1:1000 heparin.
   e. Glucose: a low glucose level suggests parapneumonic effusions and rheumatoid arthritis.
   f. Amylase: a high amylase level suggests pancreatitis or ruptured esophagus.
   g. Perplexing pleural effusions are often a result of malignancy (e.g., lymphoma, malignant mesothelioma, ovarian carcinoma), TB, subdiaphragmatic processes, prior asbestos exposure, and postcardiac injury syndrome.

THROMBIN TIME (TT)

Normal range: 11.3-18.5 sec
Elevated in: Thrombolytic and heparin therapy, disseminated intravascular coagulation, hypofibrinogenemia, dysfibrinogenemia

THYROGLOBULIN

Normal: 3-40 ng/ml. Thyroglobulin is a tumor marker for monitoring the status of patients with papillary or follicular thyroid cancer following resection.
Elevated in: Papillary or follicular thyroid cancer, Hashimoto's thyroiditis, Graves' disease, subacute thyroiditis

THYROID MICROSOMAL ANTIBODIES

Normal: Undetectable. Low titers may be present in 5%-10% of normal individuals
Elevated in: Hashimoto's disease, thyroid carcinoma, early hypothyroidism, pernicious anemia

THYROID-STIMULATING HORMONE (TSH)

See Fig. E4-45 for an algorithmic approach to thyroid testing.
Normal range: 2-11 μU/ml (2-11 mU/L [CF: 1; SMI: 1 mU/L])

CONDITIONS THAT INCREASE SERUM THYROID-STIMULATING HORMONE VALUES

Laboratory error
Primary hypothyroidism
Synthroid therapy with insufficient dose
Lithium or amiodarone; some patients
Hashimoto's thyroiditis in later stage
Large doses of inorganic iodide (e.g., SSKI)
Severe nonthyroid illness in recovery phase
Iodine deficiency (moderate or severe)
Addison's disease
TSH specimen drawn in evening (peak of diurnal variation)
Pituitary TSH-secreting tumor
Therapy of hypothyroidism (3-6 wk after beginning therapy [range, 1-8 wk]; sometimes longer when pretherapy TSH is over 100 μU/ml)

Acute psychiatric illness
Peripheral resistance to T_4 syndrome
Antibodies (e.g., HAMA) interfering with monoclonal sandwich method of TSH assay
Telepaque (iopanoic acid) and Oragrafin (ipodate) x-ray contrast media
Amphetamines
High altitudes

CONDITIONS THAT DECREASE SERUM THYROID-STIMULATING HORMONE VALUES

Laboratory error
T_4/T_3 toxicosis (diffuse or nodular etiology)
Excessive therapy for hypothyroidism
Active thyroiditis (subacute, painless, or early active Hashimoto's disease)
Multinodular goiter containing areas of autonomy
Severe nonthyroid illness (especially acute trauma, dopamine, or glucocorticoid)
T_3 toxicosis
Pituitary insufficiency
Cushing's syndrome (and some patients on high-dose glucocorticoid)
Jod-Basedow (iodine-induced) hyperthyroidism
Thyroid-stimulating hormone drawn 2-4 hr after levothyroxine dose
Postpartum transient toxicosis
Factitious hyperthyroidism
Struma ovarii
Radioimmunoassay, surgery, or antithyroid drug therapy for hyperthyroidism 4-6 weeks (range, 2 wk to 2 yr) after the treatment
Interleukin-2 drugs (3%-6% of cases) or α-interferon therapy (1% of cases)
Hyperemesis gravidarum
Amiodarone therapy.

See Table 4-38 for changes in thyroid hormone levels during illness.

TABLE 4-38 Changes in Thyroid Hormone Levels during Illness

Severity of Illness	Free T_3	Free T_4	Reverse T_3	TSH	Probable Cause
Mild	↓	N	↑	N	↓ D2, D1
Moderate	↓↓	N, ↑↓	↑↑	N, ↓	↓↓ D2, D1,?↑ D3
Severe	↓↓↓	↓	↑	↓↓	↓↓ D2, D1, ↑D3
Recovery	↓	↓	↑	↑	?

From Melmed S, Polonsky KS, Larsen PR, Kronenberg HM: *Williams textbook of endocrinology*, ed 12, Philadelphia, 2011, Saunders.
D1 through *D3*, iodothyronine deiodinases; *N*, no change; T_3, triiodothyronine; T_4, thyroxine; *TSH*, thyroid-stimulating hormone.

THYROTROPIN (TSH) RECEPTOR ANTIBODIES

Normal: <130% of basal activity
Elevated in: Values between 1.3 and 2.0 are found in 10% of patients with thyroid disease other than Graves' disease. Values >2.8 have been found only in patients with Graves' disease.

THYROTROPIN RELEASING HORMONE (TRH) STIMULATION TEST

Normal: Baseline TSH <11 microU/ml; Stimulated TSH: more than double the baseline.

In primary hypothyroidism the TSH increase is 2× to 3× the normal result. In secondary hypothyroidism no TSH response occurs. In tertiary hypothyroidism (hypothalamic failure) there is a delayed rise in the TSH level.

THYROXINE (T_4)

Normal range: 4-11 μg/dl (51-142 nmol/L [CF: 12.87; SMI: 1 nmol/L])

TIBC

See IRON-BINDING CAPACITY, TOTAL

TISSUE TRANSGLUTAMINASE ANTIBODY

Normal: Negative
Present in: Celiac disease (specificity; 94%-97%, sensitivity, 90%-98%), dermatitis herpetiformis

TRANSFERRIN

Normal range: 170-370 mg/dl (1.7-3.7 g/L [CF: 0.01; SMI: 0.01 g/L])
Elevated in: Iron deficiency anemia, oral contraceptive administration, viral hepatitis, late pregnancy
Decreased in: Nephrotic syndrome, liver disease, hereditary deficiency, protein malnutrition, neoplasms, chronic inflammatory states, chronic illness, thalassemia, hemochromatosis, hemolytic anemia

TRIGLYCERIDES

Normal range: <150 mg/dl (<1.80 mmol/L [CF: 0.01129; SMI: 0.02 mmol/L])
Elevated in: Hyperlipoproteinemias (types I, IIb, III, IV, V), hypothyroidism, pregnancy, estrogens, acute myocardial infarction, pancreatitis, alcohol intake, nephrotic syndrome, diabetes mellitus, glycogen storage disease
Decreased in: Malnutrition, congenital abetalipoproteinemias, drugs (e.g., gemfibrozil, fenofibrate, nicotinic acid, clofibrate)

TRIIODOTHYRONINE

See T_3

TROPONINS (serum)

See Box 4-6 for causes of troponin elevations.

BOX 4-6 Causes of Serum Troponin T and I Elevations, Including Both Acute Coronary Syndromes, Noncoronary Cardiac Events, and Noncardiac Ailments

Acute coronary syndrome/acute myocardial infarction
Shock of any form (cardiogenic, obstructive, distributive)
Myocarditis and myopericarditis
Cardiomyopathies
Acute congestive heart failure (pulmonary edema)
Sepsis
Pulmonary embolism
Renal failure
Sympathomimetic ingestions
Polytrauma
Burns
Acute CNS event
Rhabdomyolysis
Cardiac neoplasm, inflammatory syndromes, and infiltrative diseases
Congenital coronary anomalies
Extreme physical exertion

From Vincent JL et al: *Textbook of critical care*, ed 6, Philadelphia, 2011, Saunders.

Normal range: 0-0.4 ng/ml (negative). If there is clinical suspicion of evolving acute MI or ischemic episode, repeat testing in 5-6 hours is recommended.
Indeterminate: 0.05-0.49 ng/ml. Suggest further tests. In a patient with unstable angina and this troponin I level, there is an increased risk of a cardiac event in the near future.
Strong probability of acute MI:
≥ 0.05 ng/ml

Cardiac troponin T (cTnT) is a highly sensitive marker for myocardial injury for the first 48 hours after MI and for up to 5-7 days (see Fig. 4-15, under "Creatine Kinase Isoenzymes"). It may also be elevated in renal failure, chronic muscle disease, and trauma.

Cardiac troponin I (cTnI) is highly sensitive and specific for myocardial injury (≥CK-MB) in the initial 8 hours, peaks within 24 hours and lasts up to 7 days. With progressively higher levels of cTnI, the risk of mortality increases because the amount of necrosis increases.

TSH

See THYROID-STIMULATING HORMONE

TT

See THROMBIN TIME

TUBERCULIN TEST (PPD)

Abnormal results: see Box 4-7. Box 4-8 describes factors associated with false-negative tuberculin tests.

BOX 4-7 PPD Reaction Size Considered "Positive" (Intracutaneous 5 TU Mantoux Test at 48 hr)

5 mm or More
- HIV infection or risk factors for HIV
- Close recent contact with active TB case
- Persons with chest x-ray consistent with healed TB

10 mm or More
- Foreign-born persons from countries with high TB prevalence in Asia, Africa, and Latin America
- IV drug users
- Medically underserved low-income population groups (including Native Americans, Hispanics, and blacks)
- Residents of long-term care facilities (nursing homes, mental institutions)
- Medical conditions that increase risk for TB (silicosis, gastrectomy, undernourishment, diabetes mellitus, high-dose corticosteroids or immunosuppression Rx, leukemia or lymphoma, other malignancies)
- Employees of long-term care facilities, schools, child-care facilities, health care facilities

15 mm or More
- All others not already listed

TB, Tuberculosis; *TU,* tuberculin units.

BOX 4-8 Factors Associated with False-Negative Tuberculin Tests

Technical Errors
- Improper administration
- Inaccurate reading
- Loss of potency of antigen

Patient-Related Factors (Anergy)
- Age (elderly)
- Nutritional status
- Medications: corticosteroids, immunosuppressive agents
- Severe tuberculosis
- Coexisting diseases
  - HIV infection
  - Viral illness or vaccination
  - Lymphoreticular malignancies
  - Sarcoidosis
  - Solid tumors
  - Lepromatous leprosy
  - Sjögren's syndrome
  - Ataxia telangiectasia
  - Uremia
  - Primary biliary cirrhosis
  - Systemic lupus erythematosus
- Severe systemic disease of any etiology

From Stein JH (ed): *Internal medicine,* ed 4, St Louis, 1994, Mosby.

UNCONJUGATED BILIRUBIN

See BILIRUBIN, DIRECT

UREA NITROGEN, BLOOD (BUN)

Normal range: 8-18 mg/dl (3-6.5 mmol/L [CF: 0.357; SMI: 0.5 mmol/L])

Box 4-9 describes factors affecting BUN level independent of renal function.

Elevated in: Drugs (aminoglycosides and other antibiotics, diuretics, lithium, corticosteroids), dehydration, gastrointestinal bleeding, decreased renal blood flow (shock, congestive heart failure, myocardial infarction), renal disease (glomerulonephritis, pyelonephritis, diabetic nephropathy), urinary tract obstruction (prostatic hypertrophy)

Decreased in: Liver disease, malnutrition, third trimester of pregnancy, overhydration, acromegaly, celiac disease

BOX 4-9 Factors Affecting Blood Urea Nitrogen Level Independent of Renal Function

Disproportionate Increase in Blood Urea Nitrogen
- Volume depletion ("prerenal azotemia")
- Gastrointestinal hemorrhage
- Corticosteroid or cytotoxic agents
- High-protein diet
- Obstructive uropathy
- Sepsis
- Catabolic states, tissue breakdown

Disproportionate Decrease in Blood Urea Nitrogen
- Low-protein diet
- Liver disease

From Andreoli TE (ed): *Cecil essentials of medicine,* ed 5, Philadelphia, 2001, Saunders.

URIC ACID (serum)

Normal range: 2-7 mg/dl

Elevated in: Renal failure, gout, excessive cell lysis (chemotherapeutic agents, radiation therapy, leukemia, lymphoma, hemolytic anemia), hereditary enzyme deficiency (hypoxanthine-guanine-phosphoribosyl transferase), acidosis, myeloproliferative disorders, diet high in purines or protein, drugs (diuretics, low doses of ASA, ethambutol, nicotinic acid), lead poisoning, hypothyroidism, Addison's disease, nephrogenic diabetes insipidus, active psoriasis, polycystic kidneys

Decreased in: Drugs (allopurinol, febuxostat, high doses of ASA, probenecid, warfarin, corticosteroid), deficiency of xanthine oxidase, syndrome of inappropriate antidiuretic hormone secretion, renal tubular deficits (Fanconi's syndrome), alcoholism, liver disease, diet deficient in protein or purines, Wilson's disease, hemochromatosis

URINALYSIS

Normal range:

Color: light straw
Appearance: clear
Ketones: absent
pH: 4.5-8 (average, 6)
Protein: absent
Glucose: absent
Specific gravity: 1.005-1.030
Occult blood absent
Microscopic examination:
  Red blood cells: 0-5 (high-power field)
  White blood cells: 0-5 (high-power field)
  Bacteria (spun specimen): absent
  Casts: 0-4 hyaline (low-power field)

Abnormalities in the microscopic examination of urine are described in Table 4-39.

TABLE 4-39 Microscopic Examination of the Urine

Finding	Associations
Casts	
Red blood cell	Glomerulonephritis, vasculitis
White blood cell	Interstitial nephritis, pyelonephritis
Epithelial cell	Acute tubular necrosis, interstitial nephritis, glomerulonephritis
Granular	Renal parenchymal disease (nonspecific)
Waxy, broad	Advanced renal failure
Hyaline	Normal finding in concentrated urine
Fatty	Heavy proteinuria
Cells	
Red blood cell	Urinary tract infection, urinary tract inflammation
White blood cell	Urinary tract infection, urinary tract inflammation
Eosinophil	Acute interstitial nephritis
(Squamous) epithelial cell	Contaminants
Crystals	
Uric acid	Acid urine, acute uric acid nephropathy, hyperuricosuria
Calcium phosphate	Alkaline urine
Calcium oxalate	Acid urine, hyperoxaluria, ethylene glycol poisoning
Cystine	Cystinuria
Sulfur	Sulfa-containing antibiotics

From Andreoli TE (ed): *Cecil essentials of medicine,* ed 5, Philadelphia, 2001, Saunders.

URINE AMYLASE

Normal range: 35-260 U Somogyi/hr (6.5-48.1 U/hr [CF: 0.185; SMI: 1 U/hr])
Elevated in: Pancreatitis, carcinoma of the pancreas

URINE BILE

Normal: Absent
Abnormal:
Urine bilirubin: hepatitis (viral, toxic, drug-induced), biliary obstruction
Urine urobilinogen: hepatitis (viral, toxic, drug-induced), hemolytic jaundice, liver cell dysfunction (cirrhosis, infection, metastases)

URINE CALCIUM

Normal range: <250 mg/24 hr (<6.2 mmol/dl [CF: 0.02495; SMI: 0.1 mmol/dl])
Elevated in: Primary hyperparathyroidism, hypervitaminosis D, bone metastases, multiple myeloma, increased calcium intake, steroids, prolonged immobilization, sarcoidosis, Paget's disease, idiopathic hypercalciuria, renal tubular acidosis
Decreased in: Hypoparathyroidism, pseudohypoparathyroidism, vitamin D deficiency, vitamin D–resistant rickets, diet low in calcium, drugs (thiazide diuretics, oral contraceptives), familial hypocalciuric hypercalcemia, renal osteodystrophy, potassium citrate therapy

URINE cAMP

Elevated in: Hypercalciuria, familial hypocalciuric hypercalcemia, primary hyperparathyroidism, pseudohypoparathyroidism, rickets
Decreased in: Vitamin D intoxication, sarcoidosis

URINE CATECHOLAMINES

Normal range:
Norepinephrine: <100 μg/24 hr (<590 nmol/day [CF: 5.911; SMI: 10 nmol/day])
Epinephrine: <10 μg/24 hr (55 nmol/day [CF: 5.458; SMI: 5 nmol/day])
Elevated in: Pheochromocytoma, neuroblastoma, severe stress

URINE CHLORIDE

Normal range: 110-250 mEq/day (110-250 mmol/day [CF: 1; SMI: 1 mmol/day])
Elevated in: Corticosteroids, Bartter's syndrome, diuretics, metabolic acidosis, severe hypokalemia
Decreased in: Chloride depletion (vomiting), colonic villous adenoma, chronic renal failure, renal tubular acidosis

URINE COPPER

Normal range: <40 μg/24 hr (<0.6 μmol/day [CF: 0.01574; SMI: 0.2 μmol/day])

URINE CORTISOL, FREE

Normal range: 10-110 μg/24 hr (30-300 nmol/day [CF: 2.759; SMI: 10 nmol/day])
Elevated: See CORTISOL, PLASMA

URINE CREATININE (24 HR)

Normal range:
Male: 0.8-1.8 g/day (7-16 mmol/day [CF: 8.840; SMI: 0.1 mmol/day])
Female: 0.6-1.6 g/day (5.3-14 mmol/day)
NOTE: Useful test as an indicator of completeness of 24-hr urine collection.

URINE CRYSTALS

Uric acid: acid urine, hyperuricosuria, uric acid nephropathy
Sulfur: antibiotics containing sulfa
Calcium oxalate: ethylene glycol poisoning, acid urine, hyperoxaluria
Calcium phosphate: alkaline urine
Cystine: cystinuria

URINE EOSINOPHILS

Normal: Absent
Present in: Interstitial nephritis, acute tubular necrosis, urinary tract infection, kidney transplant rejection, hepatorenal syndrome

URINE GLUCOSE (qualitative)

Normal: Absent
Present in: Diabetes mellitus, renal glycosuria (decreased renal threshold for glucose), glucose intolerance

URINE HEMOGLOBIN, FREE

Normal: Absent
Present in: Hemolysis (with saturation of serum haptoglobin binding capacity and renal threshold for tubular absorption of hemoglobin)

URINE HEMOSIDERIN

Normal: Absent
Present in: Paroxysmal nocturnal hemoglobinuria, chronic hemolytic anemia, hemochromatosis, blood transfusion, thalassemias

URINE 5-HYDROXYINDOLE-ACETIC ACID (URINE 5-HIAA)

Normal range: 2-8 mg/24 hr (10-40 μmol/day [CF: 5.23; SMI: 5 μmol/day])
Elevated in: Carcinoid tumors, after ingestion of certain foods (bananas, plums, tomatoes, avocados, pineapples, eggplant, walnuts), drugs (monoamine oxidase inhibitors, phenacetin, methyldopa, glycerol guaiacolate, acetaminophen, salicylates, phenothiazines, imipramine, methocarbamol, reserpine, methamphetamine). See Table 4-40.

URINE INDICAN

Normal: Absent
Present in: Malabsorption secondary to intestinal bacterial overgrowth

URINE KETONES (semiquantitative)

Normal: Absent
Present in: Diabetic ketoacidosis, alcoholic ketoacidosis, starvation, isopropanol ingestion

URINE METANEPHRINES

Normal range: 0-2.0 mg/24 hr (0-11.0 μmol/day [CF: 5.458; SMI: 0.5 μmol/day])

TABLE 4-40 Factors That Interfere with Determination of Urinary 5-HIAA

Foods	Drugs
Factors That Produce False-Positive Results	
Avocado	Acetaminophen
Banana	Acetanilid
Chocolate	Caffeine
Coffee	Fluorouracil
Eggplant	Guaifenesin
Pecan	l-Dopa
Pineapple	Melphalan
Plum	Mephenesin
Tea	Methamphetamine
Walnuts	Methocarbamol
	Methysergide maleate
	Phenmetrazine
	Reserpine
	Salicylates
Factors That Cause False-Negative Results	
None	Corticotropin
	p-Chlorophenylalanine
	Chlorpromazine
	Heparin
	Imipramine
	Isoniazid
	Methenamine mandelate
	Methyldopa
	Monoamine oxidase inhibitors
	Phenothiazine
	Promethazine

From Melmed S, Polonsky KS, Larsen PR, Kronenberg HM: *Williams textbook of endocrinology*, ed 12, Philadelphia, 2011, Saunders.
5-HIAA, 5-hydroxyindoleacetic acid.

Elevated in: Pheochromocytoma, neuroblastoma, drugs (caffeine, phenothiazines, monoamine oxidase inhibitors), stress See Table E4-41.

URINE MYOGLOBIN

Normal: Absent
Present in: Severe trauma, hyperthermia, polymyositis/dermatomyositis, carbon monoxide poisoning, drugs (narcotic and amphetamine toxicity), hypothyroidism, muscle ischemia

URINE NITRITE

Normal: Absent
Present in: Urinary tract infections

URINE OCCULT BLOOD

Normal: Negative
Positive in: Trauma to urinary tract, renal disease (glomerulonephritis, pyelonephritis), renal or ureteral calculi, bladder lesions (carcinoma, cystitis), prostatitis, prostatic carcinoma, menstrual contamination, hematopoietic disorders (hemophilia, thrombocytopenia), anticoagulants, ASA

URINE OSMOLALITY

Normal range: 50-1200 mOsm/kg (50-1200 mmol/kg [CF: 1; SMI: 1 mmol/kg])
Elevated in: Syndrome of inappropriate antidiuretic hormone secretion, dehydration, glycosuria, adrenal insufficiency, high-protein diet
Decreased in: Diabetes insipidus, excessive water intake, IV hydration with D_5W, acute renal insufficiency, glomerulonephritis

URINE pH

Normal range: 4.6-8 (average, 6)
Elevated in: Bacteriuria, vegetarian diet, renal failure with inability to form ammonia, drugs (antibiotics, sodium bicarbonate, acetazolamide)
Decreased in: Acidosis (metabolic, respiratory), drugs (ammonium chloride, methenamine mandelate), diabetes mellitus, starvation, diarrhea

URINE PHOSPHATE

Normal range: 0.8-2.0 g/24 hr
Elevated in: Acute tubular necrosis (diuretic phase), chronic renal disease, uncontrolled diabetes mellitus, hyperparathyroidism, hypomagnesemia, metabolic acidosis, metabolic alkalosis, neurofibromatosis, adult-onset vitamin D–resistant hypophosphatemic osteomalacia
Decreased in: Acromegaly, acute renal failure, decreased dietary intake, hypoparathyroidism, respiratory acidosis

URINE POTASSIUM

Normal range: 25-100 mEq/24 hr (25-100 mmol/day [CF: 1; SMI: 1 mmol/day])
Elevated in: Aldosteronism (primary, secondary), glucocorticoids, alkalosis, renal tubular acidosis, excessive dietary potassium intake
Decreased in: Acute renal failure, potassium-sparing diuretics, diarrhea, hypokalemia

URINE PROTEIN (quantitative)

Normal range: <150 mg/24 hr (<0.15 g/day [CF: 0.001; SMI: 0.01 g/day])
Elevated in:
Nephrotic syndrome as a result of primary renal diseases
Malignant hypertension
Malignancies: multiple myeloma, leukemias, Hodgkin's disease
Congestive heart failure
Diabetes mellitus
Systemic lupus erythematosus, rheumatoid arthritis
Sickle cell disease
Goodpasture's syndrome
Malaria
Amyloidosis, sarcoidosis
Tubular lesions: cystinosis
Functional (after heavy exercise)
Pyelonephritis
Pregnancy
Constrictive pericarditis
Renal vein thrombosis
Toxic nephropathies: heavy metals, drugs
Radiation nephritis
Orthostatic (postural) proteinuria
Benign proteinuria: fever, heat or cold exposure

URINE SEDIMENT

See Fig. 4-46 for evaluation of common abnormalities.

URINE SODIUM (QUANTITATIVE)

See Table 4-42 for use of urine electrolytes in the differential diagnosis of hypokalemia.
Normal range: 40-220 mEq/day (40-220 mmol/day [CF: 1; SMI: 1 mmol/day])
Elevated in: Diuretic administration, high sodium intake, salt-losing nephritis, acute tubular necrosis, vomiting, Addison's disease, syndrome of inappropriate antidiuretic hormone secretion, hypothyroidism, congestive heart failure, hepatic failure, chronic renal failure, Bartter's syndrome, glucocorticoid deficiency, interstitial nephritis caused by analgesic abuse, mannitol, dextran, or glycerol therapy, milk-alkali syndrome, decreased renin secretion, postobstructive diuresis
Decreased in: Increased aldosterone, glucocorticoid excess, hyponatremia, prerenal azotemia, decreased salt intake

URINE SPECIFIC GRAVITY

Normal range: 1.005-1.030

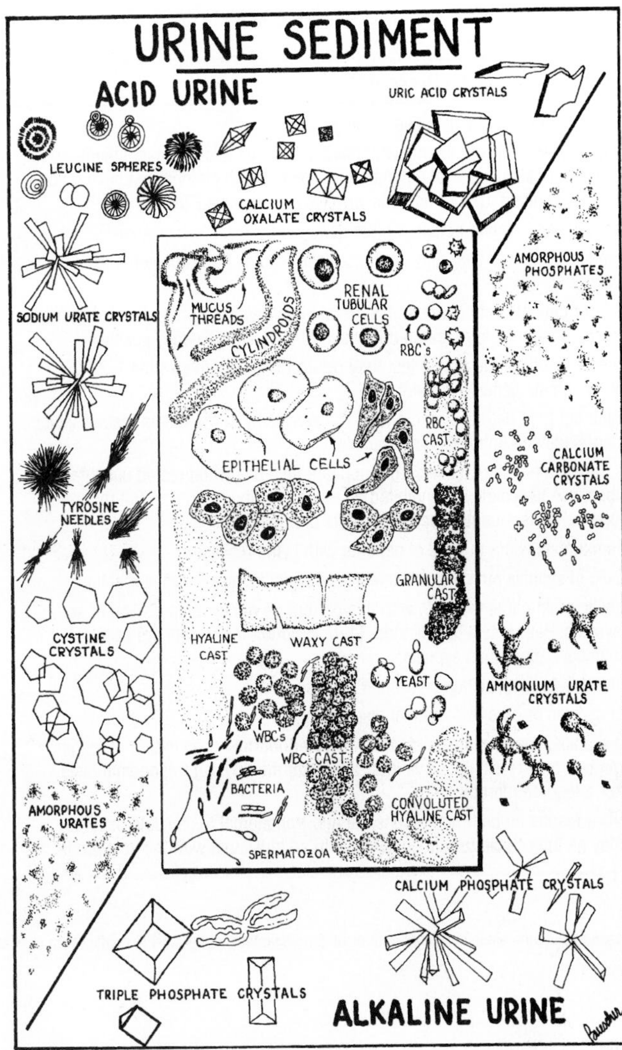

FIGURE 4-46 Microscopic examination of urinary sediment. (From Grigorian Greene M: *The Harriet Lane handbook: a manual for pediatric house officers*, ed 17, St Louis, 2007, Mosby.)

TABLE 4-42 Urine Electrolytes* in the Differential Diagnosis of Hypokalemia

Condition	Urine Electrolyte	
	Na^+	Cl^-
Vomiting		
Recent	High†	Low‡
Remote	Low	Low
Diuretics		
Recent	High	High
Remote	Low	Low
Diarrhea or Laxative Abuse	Low	High
Bartter's or Gitelman's Syndrome	High	High

From Vincent JL et al: *Textbook of Critical Care*, ed 6, Philadelphia, 2011, Saunders.
*Do not use the urine electolytes in this fashion during polyuric states.
†High = urine concentration >15 mmol/L.
‡Low = urine concentration <15 mmol/L.

Elevated in: Dehydration, excessive fluid losses (vomiting, diarrhea, fever), x-ray contrast media, diabetes mellitus, congestive heart failure, syndrome of inappropriate antidiuretic hormone secretion, adrenal insufficiency, decreased fluid intake
Decreased in: Diabetes insipidus, renal disease (glomerulonephritis, pyelonephritis), excessive fluid intake or IV hydration

URINE VANILLYLMANDELIC ACID (VMA)

Normal range: <6.8 mg/24 hr (<35 μmol/day [CF: 5.046; SMI: 1 μmol/day])
Elevated in: Pheochromocytoma, neuroblastoma, ganglioblastoma, drugs (isoproterenol, methocarbamol, levodopa, sulfonamides, chlorpromazine), severe stress, after ingestion of bananas, chocolate, vanilla, tea, coffee
Decreased in: Drugs (monoamine oxidase inhibitors, reserpine, guanethidine, methyldopa)

VARICELLA-ZOSTER VIRUS (VZV) SEROLOGY

Test description: Test can be performed on whole blood, tissue, skin lesions, and CSF

VASOACTIVE INTESTINAL PEPTIDE (VIP)

Normal: <50 pg/ml
Elevated in: Pancreatic VIP-omas, neuroblastoma, pancreatic islet call hyperplasia, liver disease, MEN I, ganglioneuroma, ganglioneuroblastoma

VDRL

Normal range: Negative
Positive test: Syphilis, other treponemal diseases (yaws, pinta, bejel)

NOTE: A false-positive test may be seen in patients with systemic lupus erythematosus and other autoimmune diseases, infectious mononucleosis, HIV, atypical pneumonia, malaria, leprosy, typhus fever, rat-bite fever, relapsing fever.

NOTE: See Table 4-43 for interpretation of serologic tests for syphilis.

VISCOSITY (serum)

Normal range: 1.4-1.8 relative to water (1.10-1.22 centipoise)
Elevated in: Monoclonal gammopathies (Waldenström's macroglobulinemia, multiple myeloma), hyperfibrinogenemia, systemic lupus erythematosus, rheumatoid arthritis, polycythemia, leukemia

VITAMIN B_{12}

See Fig. E4-47 for the Schilling test.
Normal:
190-900 ng/ml
Causes of vitamin B_{12} deficiency:
1. Pernicious anemia (antibodies against intrinsic factor and gastric parietal cells)
2. Dietary (strict lacto-ovovegetarians, food faddists)
3. Malabsorption (achlorhydria, gastrectomy, ileal resection, pancreatic insufficiency, drugs [omeprazole, cholestyramine])

Falsely low levels occur in patients with severe folate deficiency, in patients using high doses of ascorbic acid, and when cobalamin levels are measured after nuclear medicine studies (radioactivity interferes with cobalamin radioimmunoassay).
Falsely high or normal levels in patients with cobalamin deficiency can occur in severe liver disease and chronic granulocytic leukemia.
The absence of anemia or macrocytosis does not exclude the diagnosis of cobalamin deficiency.

VITAMIN D, 1,25 DIHYDROXY CALCIFEROL

Normal: 16-65 pg/ml
Elevated in: Tumor calcinosis, primary hyperparathyroidism, sarcoidosis, tuberculosis, idiopathic hypercalciuria
Decreased in: Postmenopausal osteoporosis, chronic renal failure, hypoparathyroidism, tumor-induced osteomalacia, rickets, elevated blood lead levels

VITAMIN K

Normal: 0.10-2.20 ng/ml

TABLE 4-43 Interpretation of Serologic Tests for Syphilis*

Nontreponemal Tests	Treponemal Tests	Interpretation of Finding: Is Syphilis Present?*
Nonreactive	Nonreactive	Early primary syphilis is not ruled out by negative serologic tests.
		Early syphilis is present in 13%-30% of patients who have a negative microhemagglutination *Treponema pallidum* test; in about 30% of patients who present with chancre but have a nonreactive reagin test; and in about 10% of patients who have a negative FTA-ABS test.
		Late syphilis is present in a very small fraction of patients.
		Adequately treated syphilis in remote past may produce these results, but treponemal tests usually remain reactive.
	Reactive	Observed in about 10% of patients with chancre. The treponemal tests may turn positive shortly before the reagin tests. Reagin tests repeated after several days are generally positive.
		In adequately treated early syphilis, the reagin test may return to nonreactive within 1-2 yr, whereas the treponemal tests generally do not.
		Late syphilis is not ruled out by a negative reagin test. The sensitivity of the reagin tests is lower than that of treponemal tests in untreated late syphilis.
		In secondary syphilis, rarely, a highly reactive serum appears negative when tested undiluted with a reagin test because flocculation is inhibited by relative antibody excess. Not reported to occur with treponemal tests. Quantitative reagin tests are positive.
		False-positive treponemal tests occur in 40% of patients with Lyme disease.
Reactive	Nonreactive borderline (FTA-ABS)	Finding is not diagnostic of syphilis but constitutes a classic biologic false-positive reaction.
		Not diagnostic of syphilis; most patients (90%) with this pattern do not develop clinical or serologic evidence of syphilis. Repeat test is indicated. Chronic borderline results are associated with a variety of conditions other than syphilis.
	Beaded (FTA-ABS)	Not diagnostic of syphilis. Seen with collagen vascular disease.
	Reactive	Findings diagnostic of syphilis or other treponemal disease.
		In adequately treated syphilis, one would expect (1) a sustained fourfold drop in titer of reagin test, although reagin test may remain positive after adequate therapy; (2) treponemal tests remain positive after adequate therapy.
		Concurrent false-positive results on both nontreponemal and treponemal tests could occur in rare instances. It may be impossible to rule out syphilis in an individual with this test profile.

From Stein JH (ed): *Internal medicine,* ed 4, St Louis, 1994, Mosby.
FTA-ABS, Fluorescent treponemal antibody, absorbed.
*Serologic data must always be interpreted in the light of a total clinical evaluation. Diagnosis based on serologic criteria alone is fraught with error. Serologic tests apparently in conflict with clinical diagnosis should be confirmed by repetition or possibly referral to a reference laboratory.

Decreased in: Primary biliary cirrhosis, anticoagulants, antibiotics, cholestyramine, GI disease, pancreatic disease, cystic fibrosis, obstructive jaundice, hypoprothrombinemia, hemorrhagic disease of the newborn

VON WILLEBRAND FACTOR

Normal: Levels vary according to blood type; blood type O: 50-150 U/dl; blood type non-O: 90-200 U/dl
Decreased in: von Willebrand's disease (however, in type II von Willebrand's disease the antigen may be normal but the function is impaired)

WBC

See COMPLETE BLOOD COUNT

WESTERGREN

See ERYTHROCYTE SEDIMENTATION RATE

WHITE BLOOD COUNT

See COMPLETE BLOOD COUNT

Clinical Practice Guidelines

PART A
THE PERIODIC HEALTH EXAMINATION*

Age-Specific Charts, 1605

PART B
IMMUNIZATIONS AND CHEMOPROPHYLAXIS

Childhood and Adolescent Immunizations, 1615

General Recommendations on Immunization, 1621

Immunizations for Adults, 1633

*Data modified from U.S. Preventive Services Task Force: *Guide to clinical preventive services: report of the U.S. Preventive Services Task Force*, ed 2, Washington, DC, 1996 (revised 2001), U.S. Department of Health and Human Services. Text downloaded from http://text.nlm.nih.gov

PART A • THE PERIODIC HEALTH EXAMINATION

Age-Specific Charts

TABLE 5-1 Birth to 10 Years

Interventions considered and recommended for the Periodic Health Examination	Leading causes of death
	Conditions originating in perinatal period Congenital anomalies Sudden infant death syndrome Unintentional injuries (non–motor vehicle) Motor vehicle injuries

INTERVENTIONS FOR THE GENERAL POPULATION

Screening

Height and weight
Blood pressure
Vision screen (ages 3-4 yr)
Hemoglobinopathy screen (birth)[1]
Phenylalanine level (birth)[2]
Thyroxine and/or thyroid-stimulating hormone (birth)[3]
Lead level

Counseling

Injury prevention

Child safety car seats (age <5 yr)
Lap/shoulder belts (age ≥5 yr)
Bicycle helmet; avoid bicycling near traffic
Smoke detector, flame-retardant sleepwear
Hot water heater temperature <120°-130° F
Window/stair guards, pool fence
Safe storage of drugs, toxic substances, firearms, and matches
Syrup of ipecac, poison control phone number
CPR training for parents/caretakers

Diet and exercise

Breastfeeding, iron-enriched formula and foods (infants and toddlers)
Limit fat and cholesterol; maintain caloric balance; emphasize grains, fruits, vegetables (age ≥2 yr)
Regular physical activity*

Substance use

Effects of passive smoking*
Antitobacco message*

Dental health

Regular visits to dental care provider*
Floss, brush with fluoride toothpaste daily*
Advice about baby bottle tooth decay*

Immunizations

Diphtheria-tetanus-pertussis (DTaP)[4]
Inactivated poliovirus vaccine (IPV)[5]
Measles-mumps-rubella (MMR)[6]
Haemophilus influenzae type b (Hib) conjugate[7]
Hepatitis A vaccine (HR4)
Hepatitis B[8]
Varicella[9]
Pneumococcal vaccine[10]
Influenza[11]
Meningococcal conjugate vaccine (MCV)[12]
Rotavirus (RV)[13]
Human papillomavirus vaccine (HPV)[14]

Chemoprophylaxis

Ocular prophylaxis (birth)

INTERVENTIONS FOR HIGH-RISK POPULATIONS

Population	***Potential Interventions (see detailed high-risk definitions)***
Preterm or low birth weight	Hemoglobin/hematocrit (HR1)
Infants of mothers at risk for HIV	HIV testing (HR2)
Low income; immigrants	Hemoglobin/hematocrit (HR1); PPD (HR3)
TB contacts	PPD (HR3)
Native American/Alaska Native	Hemoglobin/hematocrit (HR1); PPD (HR3); pneumococcal vaccine (HR5)
Residents of long-term care facilities	PPD (HR3); hepatitis A vaccine (HR4); influenza vaccine (HR6)
Certain chronic medical conditions	PPD (HR3); pneumococcal vaccine (HR5); influenza vaccine (HR6)
Increased individual or community lead exposure	Blood lead level (HR7)
Inadequate water fluoridation	Daily fluoride supplement (HR8)
Family history of skin cancer; nevi; fair skin, eyes, hair	Avoid excess/midday sun, use protective clothing* (HR9)

CPR, Cardiopulmonary resuscitation; *HR,* high risk; *PPD,* purified protein derivative; *STDs,* sexually transmitted diseases; *TB,* tuberculosis.

[1]Whether screening should be universal or targeted to high-risk groups depends on the proportion of high-risk individuals in the screening area and other considerations. [2]If done during first 24 hr of life, repeat by age 2 wk. [3]Optimally between day 2 and 6, but in all cases before newborn nursery discharge. [4]2, 4, 6, and 12-18 mo; once between age 4-6 yr. [5]2, 4, 6-18 mo; once between age 4-6 yr. [6]12-15 mo and 4-6 yr. [7]2, 4, 6 and 12-15 mo; no dose needed at 6 mo if PRP-OMP vaccine is used for first 2 doses. [8]Birth, 1 mo, 6 mo; or, 0-2 mo, 1-2 mo later, and 6-18 mo. If not done in infancy: current visit, and 1 and 6 mo later. [9]12-18 mo; or any child without history of chickenpox or previous immunization. Include information on risk in adulthood, duration of immunity, and potential need for booster doses. Administer a second dose of varicella vaccine at age 4-6 yr. [10]Pneumococcal polysaccharide vaccine (PPSV) can be administered at the same time as the other childhood vaccines at a separate site. [11]Influenza vaccine is recommended in children 6 mo-18 yr of age. [12]Administer meningococcal conjugate vaccine (MCV) to children aged 2 through 10 yr with terminal complement component deficiency, anatomic or functional asplenia, and certain other high risk groups (see *MMWR* 54[RR-7], 2005). Persons who received MPSV 3 or more years previously and who remain at increased risk for meningococcal disease should be revaccinated with MCV. [13]Administer first dose at 2 mo. If Rotarix® is administered at ages 2 and 4 mo, a dose at 6 mo is not indicated. [14]HPV4 may be administered in a 3-dose series to males aged 9 through 26 yr and females aged 11 to 26 yr to reduce the likelihood of acquiring genital warts.

*The ability of clinician counseling to influence this behavior is unproven.

HR1: Infants aged 6-12 mo who are living in poverty, black, Native American or Alaska Native, immigrants from developing countries, preterm and low-birth-weight infants, infants whose principal dietary intake is unfortified cow's milk.

HR2: Infants born to high-risk mothers whose HIV status is unknown. Women at high risk include past or present injection drug users; persons who exchange sex for money or drugs and their sex partners; injection drug–using, bisexual, or HIV-positive sex partners currently or in past; persons seeking treatment for STDs; persons who received a blood transfusion between 1978 and 1985.

HR3: Persons infected with HIV, close contacts of persons with known or suspected TB, persons with medical risk factors associated with TB, immigrants from countries with high TB prevalence, medically underserved low-income populations (including homeless), residents of long-term care facilities.

HR4: Hepatitis A vaccine (Hep A) is recommended for all children at 1 yr of age (i.e., 12-23 mo). The two doses in the series should be administered at least 6 mo apart. Children who are not vaccinated by 2 yr of age can be vaccinated at subsequent visits.

HR5: Immunocompetent persons ≥2 yr with certain medical conditions, including chronic cardiac or pulmonary disease, diabetes mellitus, and anatomic asplenia, as well as cochlear implant candidates and recipients. Immunocompetent persons ≥2 yr living in high-risk environments or social settings (e.g., certain Native American and Alaska Native populations).

HR6: Annual vaccinations of children ≥6 mo who are residents of chronic care facilities or who have chronic cardiopulmonary disorders, metabolic diseases (including diabetes mellitus), hemoglobinopathies, immunosuppression, or renal dysfunction.

HR7: Children approximately age 12 mo who (1) live in communities in which the prevalence of lead levels requiring individual intervention, including residential lead hazard control or chelation, is high or undefined; (2) live in or frequently visit a home built before 1950 with dilapidated paint or with recent or ongoing renovation or remodeling; (3) have close contact with a person who has an elevated lead level; (4) live near lead industry or heavy traffic; (5) live with someone whose job or hobby involves lead exposure; (6) use lead-based pottery; or (7) take traditional ethnic remedies that contain lead.

HR8: Children living in areas with inadequate water fluoridation (<0.6 ppm).

HR9: Persons with a family history of skin cancer; a large number of moles; atypical moles; poor tanning ability; or light skin, hair, and eye color.

TABLE 5-2 Ages 11 to 24 Years

Interventions considered and recommended for the Periodic Health Examination	Leading causes of death
	Motor vehicle accidents/other unintentional injuries
	Homicide
	Suicide
	Malignant neoplasms
	Heart diseases

INTERVENTIONS FOR THE GENERAL POPULATION

Screening	**Diet and exercise**
Height and weight	Limit fat and cholesterol; maintain caloric balance; emphasize grains, fruits, vegetables
Blood pressure[1]	Adequate calcium intake (females)
Papanicolaou (Pap) test[2] (females)	Regular physical activity*
Chlamydia screen[3] (females <25 yr)	**Dental health**
HIV screening	Regular visits to dental care provider*
Lipid panel (in high-risk young adults only)	Floss, brush with fluoride toothpaste daily
Rubella serology or vaccination history[4] (females >12 yr)	***Immunizations***
Assess for problem drinking	Tetanus, diphtheria, pertussis†
Lead level	Hepatitis B[5]
Counseling	Measles-mumps-rubella (MMR) (11-12 yr)[6]
Injury prevention	Varicella (11-12 yr)[7]
Lap/shoulder belts	Rubella (females >12 yr)[4]
Bicycle/motorcycle/ATV helmets*	Meningococcal[8]
Smoke detector*	Human papilloma virus (females 11-26 yr, males 9-26 yr)[9]
Safe storage/removal of firearms*	Influenza[10]
Substance use	Pneumococcal polysaccharide vaccine (PPSV)[11]
Avoid tobacco use	***Chemoprophylaxis***
Avoid underage drinking and illicit drug use*	Multivitamin with folic acid (females)
Avoid alcohol/drug use while driving, swimming, boating, etc.*	
Sexual behavior	
STD prevention: abstinence*; avoid high-risk behavior*; condoms/female barrier with spermicide*	
Unintended pregnancy: contraception	

INTERVENTIONS FOR HIGH-RISK POPULATIONS

Population	***Potential Interventions (see detailed high-risk definitions)***
High-risk sexual behavior	RPR/VDRL (HR1); screen for gonorrhea (female) (HR2), HIV (HR3), chlamydia (female) (HR4); hepatitis A vaccine (HR5)
Injection or street drug use	RPR/VDRL (HR1); HIV screen (HR3); hepatitis A vaccine (HR5); PPD (HR6); advice to reduce infection risk (HR7)
TB contacts; immigrants; low income	PPD (HR6)
Native Americans/Alaska Natives	Hepatitis A vaccine (HR5); PPD (HR6); pneumococcal vaccine (HR8)
Travelers to developing countries	Hepatitis A vaccine (HR5)
Certain chronic medical conditions	PPD (HR6); pneumococcal vaccine (HR8); influenza vaccine (HR9)
Settings where adolescents and young adults congregate	Second MMR (HR10)
Susceptible to varicella, measles, mumps	Varicella vaccine (HR11); MMR (HR12)
Institutionalized persons; health care/lab workers	Hepatitis A vaccine (HR5); PPD (HR6); influenza vaccine (HR9)
Family history of skin cancer; nevi; fair skin, eyes, hair	Avoid excess/midday sun, use protective clothing* (HR13)
Prior pregnancy with neural tube defect	Folic acid 4.0 mg (HR14)
Inadequate water fluoridation	Daily fluoride supplement (HR15)
Pregnancy	HIV screen, Tdap vaccine (given in second or early third trimester of pregnancy)
Infants 6-11 mo of age travelling internationally	MMR

ATV, All-terrain vehicle; *HR,* high risk; *PPD,* purified protein derivative; *RPR,* rapid plasmin reagin; *STD,* sexually transmitted disease; *TB,* tuberculosis; *VDRL,* Venereal Disease Research Laboratory.

[1]Periodic blood pressure for persons aged ≥21 yr. [2]If sexually active at present or in the past: q ≤3 yr. If sexual history is unreliable, begin Pap tests at age 21 yr. [3]If sexually active, Table 5-6 summarizes cervical cancer screening guidelines. [4]Serologic testing, documented vaccination history, and routine vaccination against rubella (preferably with MMR) are equally acceptable alternatives. [5]If not previously immunized: current visit and 1 and 6 mo later. [6]If no previous second dose of MMR. [7]If susceptible to chickenpox. [8]Meningococcal conjugate vaccine (MCV) can be administered at 11-12 yr visit, at high school entry, or at beginning of college (especially indicated in students living in college dormitories). [9]Quadrivalent human papillomavirus (types 6, 11, 16, 18) recombinant vaccine (Gardasil) should be given to all females aged 11-26 yr who have not been previously vaccinated. The vaccine is indicated for the prevention of cervical cancer and genital warts caused by the human papilloma virus (HPV) 6, 11, 16, or 18. Gardasil is an intramuscular injection for administration to the thigh or upper arm. The schedule consists of three 0.5-ml doses, with the second dose given 2 mo after the first, and the final dose administered 6 mo after the initial dose. HPV4 may also be administered in a 3-dose series to males aged 9 through 26 years to reduce their likelihood of acquiring genital warts. A bivalent HPV vaccine is available for prevention of cervical dysplasia in females. [10]Influenza vaccine is recommended for children 6 mo to 18 yr of age. [11]Administer to children with certain underlying medical conditions (see *MMWR* 46[RR-8], 1997), including a cochlear implant. A single revaccination should be administered to children with functional or anatomic asplenia or other immunocompromising condition after 5 yr.

*The ability of clinician counseling to influence this behavior is unproven.

†Tdap vaccine is recommended for adolescents aged 11-12 yr who have completed the recommended childhood DTP/DTaP vaccination series and have not received a Td booster dose. Adolescents aged 13-18 yr who missed the 11-12-yr Td/Tdap booster dose should also receive a single dose of Tdap if they have completed the recommended childhood DTP/DTaP vaccination series. A 5-yr interval from the last Td dose is encouraged when Tdap is used as a booster drug; however, a shorter interval may be used if pertussis immunity is needed.

HR1: Persons who exchange sex for money or drugs and their sex partners, persons with other STDs (including HIV), and sexual contacts of persons with active syphilis. Clinicians should also consider local epidemiology.

HR2: Females who have had two or more sex partners in the last year or a sex partner with multiple sexual contacts; exchanged sex for money or drugs; or have a history of repeated episodes of gonorrhea. Clinicians should also consider local epidemiology.

HR3: Males who had sex with males after 1975; past or present injection drug users; persons who exchange sex for money or drugs and their sex partners; injection drug–using, bisexual, or HIV-positive sex partner currently or in the past; recipients of a blood transfusion between 1978 and 1985; persons seeking treatment for STDs. Clinicians should also consider screening for HIV in general population.

HR4: Sexually active females with multiple risk factors, including history of prior STD, new or multiple sex partners, age <25 yr, nonuse or inconsistent use of barrier contraceptives, or cervical ectopy. Clinicians should consider local epidemiology of the disease in identifying other high-risk groups.

HR5: Persons living in, traveling to, or working in areas where the disease is endemic and where periodic outbreaks occur (e.g., countries with high or intermediate endemicity; certain Alaska Native, Pacific Island, Native American, and religious communities); men who have sex with men; injection or street drug users; persons with clotting factor disorders or chronic liver disease, diabetics. Vaccine may be considered for institutionalized persons and workers in these institutions; military personnel; and day-care, hospital, and laboratory workers. Clinicians should also consider local epidemiology.

HR6: HIV-positive, close contacts of persons with known or suspected TB, health care workers, persons with medical risk factors associated with TB, immigrants from countries with high TB prevalence, medically underserved low-income populations (including homeless), alcoholics, injection drug users, and residents of long-term care facilities.

HR7: Persons who continue to inject drugs.

HR8: Immunocompetent persons with certain medical conditions, including chronic cardiac, renal, or pulmonary disease; diabetes mellitus; cochlear implant candidates and recipients; and anatomic asplenia. Immunocompetent persons who live in high-risk environments or social settings (e.g., certain Native American and Alaska Native populations). Adults who smoke cigarettes, persons with asymptomatic or symptomatic HIV infection.

HR9: Annual vaccination of residents of chronic care facilities; persons with chronic cardiopulmonary disorders, metabolic diseases (including diabetes mellitus), hemoglobinopathies, immunosuppression, or renal dysfunction; and health care providers for high-risk patients.

HR10: Adolescents and young adults in settings where such individuals congregate (e.g., high schools and colleges) if they have not previously received a second dose.

HR11: Healthy persons aged ≥13 yr without a history of chickenpox or previous immunization. Consider serologic testing for presumed susceptible persons aged ≥13 yr.

HR12: Persons born after 1956 who lack evidence of immunity to measles or mumps (e.g., documented receipt of live vaccine on or after the first birthday, laboratory evidence of immunity, or a history of physician-diagnosed measles or mumps).

HR13: Persons with a family or personal history of skin cancer; a large number of moles; atypical moles; poor tanning ability; or light skin, hair, and eye color.

HR14: Women with prior pregnancy affected by neural tube defect who are planning pregnancy.

HR15: Persons aged <17 yr living in areas with inadequate water fluoridation (<0.6 ppm).

TABLE 5-3 Ages 25 to 64 Years

Interventions considered and recommended for the Periodic Health Examination	Leading causes of death Malignant neoplasms Heart diseases Motor vehicle and other unintentional injuries HIV infection Suicide and homicide
INTERVENTIONS FOR THE GENERAL POPULATION	
Screening	**Injury prevention**
Blood pressure	Lap/shoulder belts
Height and weight	Motorcycle/bicycle/ATV helmets*
Lipid panel (men aged 35-64 yr, women aged 45-64 yr)	Smoke detector*
HIV screening	Safe storage/removal of firearms*
Papanicolaou (Pap) test (women)[1]	**Sexual behavior**
Fecal occult blood test[2] and/or colonoscopy (≥50 yr)	STD prevention: avoid high-risk behavior*; condoms/female barrier with spermicide*
Mammogram ± clinical breast examination[3] (women 40-69 yr)	Unintended pregnancy: contraception
Bone density scan in postmenopausal women	**Dental health**
Assess for problem drinking	Regular visits to dental care provider*
Rubella serology or vaccination history[4] (women of childbearing age)	Floss, brush with fluoride toothpaste daily*
Counseling	***Immunizations***
Substance use	Tetanus-diphtheria-pertussis (Tdap) booster
Tobacco cessation	Rubella[4] (women of childbearing age)
Avoid alcohol/drug use while driving, swimming, boating, etc.*	Influenza vaccine†
Diet and exercise	Human papillomavirus[5]
Limit fat and cholesterol; maintain caloric balance; emphasize grains, fruits, vegetables	Herpes zoster (≥60 yr)[6]
Adequate calcium intake (women)	***Chemoprophylaxis***
Regular physical activity*	Multivitamin with folic acid (women planning or capable of pregnancy)
INTERVENTIONS FOR HIGH-RISK POPULATIONS	
Population	***Potential Interventions (see detailed high-risk definitions)***
High-risk sexual behavior	RPR/VDRL (HR1); screen for gonorrhea (female) (HR2), HIV (HR3), chlamydia (female) (HR4); hepatitis B vaccine (HR5); hepatitis A vaccine (HR6)
Injection or street drug use	RPR/VDRL (HR1); HIV screen (HR3); hepatitis B vaccine (HR5); hepatitis A vaccine (HR6); PPD (HR7); advice to reduce infection risk (HR8)
Low income; TB contacts; immigrants; alcoholics	PPD (HR7)
Native Americans/Alaska Natives	Hepatitis A vaccine (HR6); PPD (HR7); pneumococcal vaccine (HR9)
Travelers to developing countries	Hepatitis B vaccine (HR5); hepatitis A vaccine (HR6)
Certain chronic medical conditions	PPD (HR7); pneumococcal vaccine (HR9); influenza vaccine (HR10)
Blood product recipients	HIV screen (HR3); hepatitis B vaccine (HR5); hepatitis C screen
Susceptible to measles, mumps, or varicella	MMR (HR11); varicella vaccine (HR12)
Institutionalized persons	Hepatitis A vaccine (HR6); PPD (HR7); pneumococcal vaccine (HR9); influenza vaccine (HR10)
Health care/lab workers	Hepatitis B vaccine (HR5); hepatitis A vaccine (HR6); PPD (HR7); influenza vaccine (HR10)
Family history of skin cancer; fair skin, eyes, hair	Avoid excess/midday sun, use protective clothing* (HR13)
Previous pregnancy with neural tube defect	Folic acid 4.0 mg (HR14)
Cardiovascular risk factors	Lipid panel (HR 15)
Pregnancy	HIV screen, Tdap vaccine (in second or early third trimester of pregnancy)
Diabetes mellitus	Hepatitis B vaccine (HR5)

ATV, All-terrain vehicle; *HPV,* human papillomavirus; *HR,* high risk; *MMR,* measles-mumps-rubella; *PPD,* purified protein derivative; *RPR,* rapid plasma reagin; *STD,* sexually transmitted disease; *TB,* tuberculosis; *Tdap,* tetanus and diphtheria toxoids and acellular pertussis; *VDRL,* Venereal Disease Research Laboratory.

[1]Women who are or have been sexually active and who have a cervix: q ≤3 yr. Routine Pap smear screening is unnecessary for women who have undergone a complete hysterectomy for benign disease. The American College of Obstetricians and Gynecologists (ACOG) recommends that routine Pap smears should start at age 21. Women 30 and older should wait 3 yrs between paps once they have had three consecutive clear tests. [2]Annually. [3]Mammogram q1-2 yr, or mammogram q1-2 yr with annual clinical breast examination. [4]Serologic testing, documented vaccination history, and routine vaccination (preferably with MMR) are equally acceptable. [5]Quadrivalent human papillomavirus (types 6, 11, 16, 18) recombinant vaccine (Gardasil) should be given to all females aged 9-26 yr who have not been previously vaccinated. The vaccine is indicated for the prevention of cervical cancer and genital warts caused by the human papillomavirus (HPV) 6, 11, 16, or 18. Gardasil is an intramuscular injection for administration to the thigh or upper arm. The schedule consists of three 0.5-ml doses, with the second dose given 2 mo after the first, and the final dose administered 6 mo after the initial dose. Gardasil is also indicated in males aged 9 to 26 yr for prevention of genital warts. A bivalent HPV vaccine is available for prevention of cervical dysplasia in females. [6]Herpes zoster vaccine (Zostavax) is indicated for prevention of herpes zoster (shingles) in individuals 60 yr or older. Zostavax is administered as a single dose subcutaneously. It is a lyophilic preparation of the Oka/Merck strain of live, attenuated varicella-zoster virus (VZV). It should not be administered to individuals with a history of primary or acquired immunodeficiency states, persons on immunosuppressive therapy (including high-dose corticosteroids), those with active untreated tuberculosis, and those who may be pregnant.

*The ability of clinician counseling to influence this behavior is unproven.

†A live attenuated influenza vaccine (LAIV, Flumist) administered intranasally is available for healthy persons aged 2 to 49 yr.

HR1: Persons who exchange sex for money or drugs and their sex partners, persons with other STDs (including HIV), and sexual contacts of persons with active syphilis. Clinicians should also consider local epidemiology.

HR2: Women who exchange sex for money or drugs or who have had repeated episodes of gonorrhea. Clinicians should also consider local epidemiology.

HR3: Men who had sex with men after 1975; past or present injection drug users; persons who exchange sex for money or drugs and their sex partners; persons with current or past injection drug–using, bisexual, or HIV-positive sex partners; recipients of a blood transfusion between 1978 and 1985; persons seeking treatment for STDs. Clinicians should also consider local epidemiology and HIV screening in the general population.

HR4: Sexually active women with multiple risk factors, including history of STD, new or multiple sex partners, nonuse or inconsistent use of barrier contraceptives, or cervical ectopy. Clinicians should also consider local epidemiology.

HR5: Blood product recipients (including hemodialysis patients), persons with frequent occupational exposure to blood or blood products, men who have sex with men, injection drug users and their sex partners, persons with multiple recent sex partners, persons with other STDs (including HIV), travelers to countries with endemic hepatitis B, all diabetics age 19 to 59.

HR6: Persons living in, traveling to, or working in areas where the disease is endemic and where periodic outbreaks occur (e.g., countries with high or intermediate endemicity; certain Alaska Native, Pacific Island, Native American, and religious communities); men who have sex with men; injection or street drug users; patients with clotting factor disorders or chronic liver disease. Consider for institutionalized persons and workers in these institutions; military personnel; and day-care, hospital, and laboratory workers. Clinicians should also consider local epidemiology.

HR7: HIV-positive, close contacts of persons with known or suspected TB, health care workers, persons with medical risk factors associated with TB, immigrants from countries with high TB prevalence, medically underserved low-income populations (including homeless), alcoholics, injection drug users, and residents of long-term care facilities.

HR8: Persons who continue to inject drugs.

HR9: Immunocompetent institutionalized persons and immunocompetent persons with certain medical conditions, including chronic cardiac, renal, or pulmonary disease; anatomic asplenia; diabetes mellitus; or cochlear implant candidates and recipients. Immunocompetent persons who live in high-risk environments or social settings (e.g., certain Native American and Alaska Native populations), adults who smoke cigarettes, persons with asymptomatic or symptomatic HIV infection.

HR10: Annual vaccination of residents of long-term care facilities; persons with chronic cardiopulmonary disorders, metabolic diseases (including diabetes mellitus), hemoglobinopathies, immunosuppression, or renal dysfunction; and health care providers of high-risk patients.

HR11: Persons born after 1956 who lack evidence of immunity to measles or mumps (e.g., documented receipt of live vaccine on or after the first birthday, laboratory evidence of immunity, or a history of physician-diagnosed measles or mumps).

HR12: Healthy adults without a history of chickenpox or previous immunization. Consider serologic testing for presumed susceptible adults.

HR13: Persons with a family or personal history of skin cancer; a large number of moles; atypical moles; poor tanning ability; or light skin, hair, and eye color.

HR14: Women with previous pregnancy affected by neural tube disorder who are planning pregnancy.

HR15: Clinicians should consider a fasting serum lipid panel on a case-by-case basis.

TABLE 5-4 Ages 65 and Older

Interventions considered and recommended for the Periodic Health Examination	Leading causes of death Heart diseases Malignant neoplasms (lung, colorectal, breast) Cerebrovascular disease Chronic obstructive pulmonary disease Pneumonia and influenza
INTERVENTIONS FOR THE GENERAL POPULATION	
Screening	**Injury prevention**
Blood pressure	Lap/shoulder belts
Height and weight	Motorcycle and bicycle helmets*
Fecal occult blood test[1] and/or colonoscopy	Fall prevention*
Mammogram ± clinical breast examination[2] (women ≤69 yr)	Safe storage/removal of firearms*
Papanicolaou (Pap) test (women)[3]	Smoke detector*
Bone density scan in postmenopausal patients	Set hot water heater to <120°-130° F
Vision screening	CPR training for household members
Assess for hearing impairment	**Dental health**
Assess for problem drinking	Regular visits to dental care provider*
Offer HIV screen	Floss, brush with fluoride toothpaste daily*
Counseling	**Sexual behavior**
Substance use	STD prevention: avoid high-risk sexual behavior*; use condoms
Tobacco cessation	***Immunizations***
Avoid alcohol/drug use while driving, swimming, boating, etc.*	Pneumococcal vaccine
Diet and exercise	Influenza[1]
Limit fat and cholesterol; maintain caloric balance; emphasize grains, fruits, vegetables	Tetanus-diphtheria (Td) boosters every 10 years, with 1 substitute Tdap dose
Adequate calcium intake (women)	Herpes zoster[4]
Regular physical activity*	
INTERVENTIONS FOR HIGH-RISK POPULATIONS	
Population	***Potential Interventions (see detailed high-risk definitions)***
Institutionalized persons	PPD (HR1); hepatitis A vaccine (HR2); amantadine/rimantadine (HR4)
Chronic medical conditions; TB contacts; low income; immigrants; alcoholics	PPD (HR1)
Persons ≥75 yr or ≥70 yr with risk factors for falls	Fall prevention intervention (HR5)
Cardiovascular disease risk factors	Consider lipid screening (HR6)
Family history of skin cancer; nevi; fair skin, eyes, hair	Avoid excess/midday sun, use protective clothing* (HR7)
Native Americans/Alaska Natives	PPD (HR1); hepatitis A vaccine (HR2)
Travelers to developing countries	Hepatitis A vaccine (HR2); hepatitis B vaccine (HR8)
Blood product recipients	HIV screen (HR3); hepatitis B vaccine (HR8)
High-risk sexual behavior	Hepatitis A vaccine (HR2); HIV screen (HR3); hepatitis B vaccine (HR8); RPR/VDRL (HR9)
Injection or street drug use	PPD (HR1); hepatitis A vaccine (HR2); HIV screen (HR3); hepatitis B vaccine (HR8); RPR/VDRL (HR9); advice to reduce infection risk (HR10)
Health care/lab workers	PPD (HR1); hepatitis A vaccine (HR2); amantadine/rimantadine (HR4); hepatitis B vaccine (HR8)
Persons susceptible to varicella	Varicella vaccine (HR11)
Men aged 65 to 75 who have ever smoked	Ultrasound of abdominal aorta (HR12)

HR, High risk; *PPD,* purified protein derivative; *RPR,* rapid plasma reagin; *STD,* sexually transmitted disease; *TB,* tuberculosis; *VDRL,* Venereal Disease Research Laboratory.

[1]Annually. [2]Mammogram q1-2 yr, or mammogram q1-2 yr with annual clinical breast exam. [3]The American Cancer Society (ACS) recommends that Pap testing can be discontinued at age 65 after three negative Pap tests or two negative HPV tests in past three years. ACOG (American College of Obstetricians and Gynecologists) recommends discontinuing Pap testing at age 65 to 70 after three negative tests in preceding 10 years. [4]Herpes zoster vaccine (Zostavax) is indicated for prevention of herpes zoster (shingles) in individuals age ≥60 yr. Zostavax is administered as a single dose subcutaneously. It is a lyophilic preparation of the Oka/Merck strain of live, attenuated varicella zoster virus (VZV). It should not be administered to individuals with a history of primary or acquired immunodeficiency states, persons on immunosuppressive therapy (including high-dose corticosteroids), those with active untreated tuberculosis, and those who may be pregnant.

*The ability of clinician counseling to influence this behavior is unproven.

HR1: HIV-positive, close contacts of persons with known or suspected TB, health care workers, persons with medical risk factors associated with TB, immigrants from countries with high TB prevalence, medically underserved low-income populations (including homeless), alcoholics, injection drug users, and residents of long-term care facilities.

HR2: Persons living in, traveling to, or working in areas where the disease is endemic and where periodic outbreaks occur (e.g., countries with high or intermediate endemicity; certain Alaska Native, Pacific Island, Native American, and religious communities); men who have sex with men; injection or street drug users; persons with clotting factor disorders or chronic liver disease. Consider for institutionalized persons and workers in these institutions and day-care, hospital, and laboratory workers. Clinicians should also consider local epidemiology and HIV screening in the general population.

HR3: Men who had sex with men after 1975; past or present injection drug users; persons who exchange sex for money or drugs and their sex partners; persons with current or past injection drug–using, bisexual, or HIV-positive sex partners; recipients of a blood transfusion between 1978 and 1985; persons seeking treatment for STDs. Clinicians should also consider local epidemiology.

HR4: Consider for persons who have not received influenza vaccine or are vaccinated late, when the vaccine may be ineffective because of major antigenic changes in the virus; for unvaccinated persons who provide home care for high-risk persons; as supplemental protection in persons who are expected to have a poor antibody response; and for high-risk persons in whom the vaccine is contraindicated.

HR5: Persons aged ≥75 yr or 70-74 yr with one or more additional risk factors, including use of certain psychoactive and cardiac medications (e.g., benzodiazepines, antihypertensives); use of four or more prescription medications; impaired cognition, strength, balance, or gait. Intensive individualized, home-based multifactorial fall prevention intervention is recommended in settings where adequate resources are available to deliver such services.

HR6: Clinicians should consider fasting lipid panel screening on a case-by-case basis for persons aged 65 to 75 yr, especially in those with additional risk factors (e.g., smoking, diabetes, or hypertension).

HR7: Persons with a family or personal history of skin cancer; a large number of moles; atypical moles; poor tanning ability; or light skin, hair, and eye color.

HR8: Blood product recipients (including hemodialysis patients), persons with frequent occupational exposure to blood or blood products, men who have sex with men, injection drug users and their sex partners, persons with multiple recent sex partners, persons with other STDs (including HIV), travelers to countries with endemic hepatitis B.

HR9: Persons who exchange sex for money or drugs and their sex partners, persons with other STDs (including HIV), and sexual contacts of persons with active syphilis. Clinicians should also consider local epidemiology.

HR10: Persons who continue to inject drugs.

HR11: Healthy adults without a history of chickenpox or previous immunization. Consider serologic testing for presumed susceptible adults.

HR12: Consider ultrasound of abdominal aorta to screen for abdominal aortic aneurysm in all men aged 65 to 75 yr who have ever smoked.

TABLE 5-5 Pregnant Women*

Interventions considered and recommended for the Periodic Health Examination

INTERVENTIONS FOR THE GENERAL POPULATION	
Screening	Offer amniocentesis (15-18 wk)[1] (age ≥35 yr)
First visit	Offer multiple marker testing[1] (15-18 wk)
Blood pressure	Offer serum α-fetoprotein[1] (16-18 wk)
Hemoglobin/hematocrit	***Counseling***
Hepatitis B surface antigen (HBsAg)	Tobacco cessation; effects of passive smoking
RPR/VDRL	Alcohol/other drug use
Chlamydia screen (<25 yr)	Nutrition, including adequate calcium intake
Rubella serology or vaccination history	Encourage breastfeeding
D(Rh) typing, antibody screen	Lap/shoulder belts
Offer CVS (<13 wk)[1] or amniocentesis (15-18 wk)[1] (age ≥35 yr)	Infant safety car seats
Offer hemoglobinopathy screening	STD prevention: avoid high-risk sexual behavior†; use condoms†
Assess for problem or risk drinking	***Chemoprophylaxis***
Offer HIV screening[2]	Multivitamin with folic acid[3]
Follow-up visits	
Blood pressure	
Urine culture (12-16 wk)	

INTERVENTIONS FOR HIGH-RISK POPULATIONS	
Population	***Potential Interventions (see detailed high-risk definitions)***
High-risk sexual behavior	Screen for chlamydia (first visit) (HR1), gonorrhea (first visit) (HR2), HIV (first visit) (HR3); HBsAg (third trimester) (HR4); RPR/VDRL (third trimester) (HR5)
Blood transfusion between 1978 and 1985	HIV screen (first visit) (HR3)
Injection drug use	HIV screen (HR3); HBsAg (third trimester) (HR4); advice to reduce infection risk (HR6)
Unsensitized D-negative women	D(Rh) antibody testing (24-28 wk) (HR7)
Risk factors for Down syndrome	Offer CVS (first trimester), amniocentesis (15-18 wk)[1] (HR8)
Prior pregnancy with neural tube defect	Offer amniocentesis (15-18 wk),[1] folic acid 4.0 mg[3] (HR9)

CVS, Chorionic villus sampling; *HR,* high risk; *RPR,* rapid plasma reagin; *VDRL,* Venereal Disease Research Laboratory.
[1]Women with access to counseling and follow-up services, reliable standardized laboratories, skilled high-resolution ultrasound and, for those receiving serum marker testing, amniocentesis capabilities. [2]Universal screening is recommended. [3]Beginning at least 1 mo before conception and continuing through the first trimester.
*See Tables 5-2 and 5-3 for other preventive services recommended for women of this age group.
†The ability of clinician counseling to influence this behavior is unproven.

HR1: Women with history of STD or new or multiple sex partners. Clinicians should also consider local epidemiology. Chlamydia screen should be repeated in third trimester if at continued risk.

HR2: Women younger than 25 yr with two or more sex partners in the last year or whose sex partner has multiple sexual contacts, women who exchange sex for money or drugs, and women with a history of repeated episodes of gonorrhea. Clinicians should also consider local epidemiology. Gonorrhea screen should be repeated in the third trimester if at continued risk.

HR3: Universal screening for HIV infection is recommended for all pregnant women. It is especially important in women with the following individual risk factors: past or present injection drug use; history of exchanging sex for money or drugs; injection drug–using, bisexual, or HIV-positive sex partner currently or in the past; recipients of a blood transfusion between 1978 and 1985; persons seeking treatment for STDs.

HR4: Women who are initially HBsAg negative who are at high risk because of injection drug use, who have suspected exposure to hepatitis B during pregnancy, and who have had multiple sex partners.

HR5: Women who exchange sex for money or drugs, women with other STDs (including HIV), and sexual contacts of persons with active syphilis. Clinicians should also consider local epidemiology.

HR6: Women who continue to inject drugs.

HR7: Unsensitized D-negative women.

HR8: Prior pregnancy affected by Down syndrome, advanced maternal age (≥35 yr), known carriage of chromosome rearrangement.

HR9: Women with previous pregnancy affected by neural tube defect.

TABLE 5-6 Cervical Cancer Screening Guidelines

Group	ACOG 2009	USPSTF 2012	ACS 2012
Women age <21	No screening	No screening	No screening
Women age 21-29	Cytology every 2 years; HPV testing not recommended	Cytology every 3 years; HPV testing not recommended	Cytology every 3 years; HPV testing not recommended
Women age 30-65	Cytology every 3 years if three consecutive normal results; addition of HPV testing also appropriate	Cytology every 3 years or cytology plus HPV testing every 5 years	Cytology plus HPV every 5 years (preferred) or cytology alone every 3 years; both are regardless of screening history
Women age <65	Following three normal screening results and no abnormal results in the last 10 years, screening may be discontinued	If adequately screened in the past, screening should be discontinued	If adequately screened in the past, screening should be discontinued
Women with total hysterectomy and no prior history of high-grade CIN	No need to continue screening if hysterectomy was for benign indication	Screening should be discontinued	Screening should be discontinued

ACOG, American College of Obstetricians and Gynecologists; *ACS,* American Cancer Society; *CIN,* Cervical intraepithelial neoplasia; *HPV,* human papillomavirus; *USPSTF,* U.S. Preventive Services Task Force.

PART B • IMMUNIZATIONS AND CHEMOPROPHYLAXIS

Childhood and Adolescent Immunizations

TABLE 5-7 Recommended Immunization Schedule for Persons Aged 0 Through 18 Years: United States, 2014 (For those who fall behind or start late, see the schedule below and the catch-up schedule [Table 5-8])

These recommendations must be read with the footnotes that follow. For those who fall behind or start late, provide catch-up vaccination at the earliest opportunity as indicated by the divided bars. To determine minimum intervals between doses, see the catch-up schedule (Table 5-8). School entry and adolescent vaccine age groups are in bold.

Vaccines	Birth	1 mo	2 mos	4 mos	6 mos	9 mos	12 mos	15 mos	18 mos	19-23 mos	2-3 yrs	**4-6 yrs**	7-10 yrs	**11-12 yrs**	13-15 yrs	16-18 yrs
Hepatitis B[1] (HepB)	1st dose	← 2nd dose →					← 3rd dose →									
Rotavirus[2] (RV) RV1 (2-dose series); RV5 (3-dose series)			1st dose	2nd dose	See footnote 2											
Diphtheria, tetanus, & acellular pertussis[3] (DTaP: <7 yrs)			1st dose	2nd dose	3rd dose			← 4th dose →				5th dose				
Tetanus, diphtheria, & acellular pertussis[4] (Tdap: ≥7 yrs)														(Tdap)		
Haemophilus influenzae type b[5] (Hib)			1st dose	2nd dose	See footnote 5		← 3rd or 4th dose → see footnote 5									
Pneumococcal conjugate[6] (PCV13)			1st dose	2nd dose	3rd dose		← 4th dose →									
Pneumococcal polysaccharide[6] (PPSV23)																
Inactivated poliovirus[7] (IPV) (<18 yrs)			1st dose	2nd dose			← 3rd dose →					4th dose				
Influenza[8] (IIV; LAIV) 2 doses for some: see footnote 8							Annual vaccination (IIV only)							Annual vaccination (IIV or LAIV)		
Measles, mumps, rubella[9] (MMR)							← 1st dose →					2nd dose				
Varicella[10] (VAR)							← 1st dose →					2nd dose				
Hepatitis A[11] (HepA)								← 2-dose series see footnote 11 →								
Human papillomavirus[12] (HPV2: females only; HPV4: males and females)														(3-dose series)		
Meningococcal[13] (Hib-MenCY ≥ 6 wks; MenACWY-D ≥ 9 mos; MenACWY-CRM ≥ 2 mos)							see footnote 13							1st dose		booster

Range of recommended ages for all children

Range of recommended ages for catch-up immunization

Range of recommended ages for certain high-risk groups

Range of recommended ages during which catch-up is encouraged and for certain high-risk groups

Not routinely recommended

This schedule includes recommendations in effect as of January 1, 2014. Any dose not administered at the recommended age should be administered at a subsequent visit, when indicated and feasible. The use of a combination vaccine generally is preferred over separate injections of its equivalent component vaccines. Vaccination providers should consult the relevant Advisory Committee on Immunization Practices (ACIP) statement for detailed recommendations, available online at http://www.cdc.gov/vaccines/hcp/acip-recs/index.html. Clinically significant adverse events that follow vaccination should be reported to the Vaccine Adverse Event Reporting System (VAERS) online (http://www.vaers.hhs.gov) or by telephone (800-822-7967). Suspected cases of vaccine-preventable diseases should be reported to the state or local health department. Additional information, including precautions and contraindications for vaccination, is available from CDC online (http://www.cdc.gov/vaccines/recs/vac-admin/contraindications.htm) or by telephone (800-CDC-INFO [800-232-4636]).

This schedule is approved by the Advisory Committee on Immunization Practices (http://www.cdc.gov/vaccines/acip), the American Academy of Pediatrics (http://www.aap.org), the American Academy of Family Physicians (http://www.aafp.org), and the American College of Obstetricians and Gynecologists (http://www.acog.org).

NOTE: The above recommendations must be read along with the footnotes for Table 5-8.

TABLE 5-8 Catch-up Immunization Schedule for Persons Aged 4 Months Through 18 Years Who Start Late or Who Are More Than 1 Month Behind: United States

The table below provides catch-up schedules and minimum intervals between doses for children whose vaccinations have been delayed. A vaccine series does not need to be restarted, regardless of the time that has elapsed between doses. Use the section appropriate for the child's age. Always use this table in conjunction with Table 5-7 and the footnotes that follow.

Persons aged 4 months through 6 years					
Vaccine	Minimum Age for Dose 1	Minimum Interval Between Doses			
		Dose 1 to dose 2	Dose 2 to dose 3	Dose 3 to dose 4	Dose 4 to dose 5
Hepatitis B[1]	Birth	4 weeks	8 weeks and at least 16 weeks after first dose; minimum age for the final dose is 24 weeks		
Rotavirus[2]	6 weeks	4 weeks	4 weeks[2]		
Diphtheria, tetanus, pertussis[3]	6 weeks	4 weeks	4 weeks	6 months	6 months[3]
Haemophilus influenzae type b[5]	6 weeks	4 weeks if first dose administered at younger than age 12 months 8 weeks (as final dose) if first dose administered at age 12 through 14 months No further doses needed if first dose administered at age 15 months or older	4 weeks[5] if current age is younger than 12 months and first dose administered at <7 months old 8 weeks and age 12 months through 59 months (as final dose)[5] if current age is younger than 12 months and first dose administered between 7 through 11 months (regardless of Hib vaccine [PRP-T or PRP-OMP] used for first dose); OR if current age is 12 through 59 months and first dose administered at younger than age 12 months; OR first 2 doses were PRP-OMP and administered at younger than 12 months. No further doses needed if previous dose administered at age 15 months or older	8 weeks (as final dose) This dose only necessary for children aged 12 through 59 months who received 3 (PRP-T) doses before age12 months and started the primary series before age 7 months	
Pneumococcal[6]	6 weeks	4 weeks if first dose administered at younger than age 12 months 8 weeks (as final dose for healthy children) if first dose administered at age 12 months or older No further doses needed for healthy children if first dose administered at age 24 months or older	4 weeks if current age is younger than 12 months 8 weeks (as final dose for healthy children) if current age is 12 months or older No further doses needed for healthy children if previous dose administered at age 24 months or older	8 weeks (as final dose) This dose only necessary for children aged 12 through 59 months who received 3 doses before age 12 months or for children at high risk who received 3 doses at any age	
Inactivated poliovirus[7]	6 weeks	4 weeks[7]	4 weeks	6 months[7] minimum age 4 years for final dose	
Meningococcal[13]	6 weeks	8 weeks[13]	see footnote 13	see footnote 13	
Measles, mumps, rubella[9]	12 months	4 weeks			
Varicella[10]	12 months	3 months			
Hepatitis A[11]	12 months	6 months			
Persons aged 7 through 18 years					
Tetanus, diphtheria; tetanus, diphtheria, & acellular pertussis[4]	7 years[4]	4 weeks	4 weeks if first dose administered at younger than age 12 months 6 months if first dose administered at 12 months or older	6 months if first dose of DTaP/DT administered at younger than age 12 months	
Human papillomavirus[12]	9 years	Routine dosing intervals are recommended[12]			
Hepatitis A[11]	12 months	6 months			
Hepatitis B[1]	Birth	4 weeks	8 weeks (and at least 16 weeks after first dose)		
Inactivated poliovirus[7]	6 weeks	4 weeks	4 weeks[7]	6 months[7]	
Meningococcal[13]	6 weeks	8 weeks[13]			
Measles, mumps, rubella[9]	12 months	4 weeks			
Varicella[10]	12 months	3 months if person is younger than age 13 years 4 weeks if person is aged 13 years or older			

NOTE: The above recommendations must be read along with the footnotes on the following pages.

Footnotes — Recommended immunization schedule for persons aged 0 through 18 years—United States, 2014

For further guidance on the use of the vaccines mentioned below, see: http://www.cdc.gov/vaccines/hcp/acip-recs/index.html.
For vaccine recommendations for persons 19 years of age and older, see the adult immunization schedule.

Additional information

- For contraindications and precautions to use of a vaccine and for additional information regarding that vaccine, vaccination providers should consult the relevant ACIP statement available online at http://www.cdc.gov/vaccines/hcp/acip-recs/index.html.
- For purposes of calculating intervals between doses, 4 weeks = 28 days. Intervals of 4 months or greater are determined by calendar months. Vaccine doses administered 4 days or less before the minimum interval are considered valid. Doses of any vaccine administered ≥5 days earlier than the minimum interval or minimum age details, see *MMWR, General Recommendations on Immunization and Reports* / Vol. 60 / No. 2; Table 1. *Recommended and minimum ages and intervals between vaccine doses* available online at http://www.cdc.gov/mmwr/pdf/rr/rr6002.pdf.
- Information on travel vaccine requirements and recommendations is available at http://wwwnc.cdc.gov/travel/destinations/list.
- For vaccination of persons with primary and secondary immunodeficiences, see Table 13, "Vaccination of persons with primary and secondary immundeficienc," in General Recommendations on Immunization (ACIP), available at http://www.cdc.gov/mmwr/pdf/rr/rr6002.pdf.; and American Academy of Pediatrics. Immunization in Special Clinical Circumstances, in Pickering LK, Baker CJ, Kimberlin DW, Long SS eds. *Red Book: 2012 report of the Committee on Infectious Diseases. 29th ed.* Elk Grove Village, IL: American Academy of Pediatrics.

1. **Hepatitis B (HepB) vaccine. (Minimum age: birth)**
Routine vaccination:
At birth:
- Administer monovalent HepB vaccine to all newborns before hospital discharge.
- For infants born to hepatitis B surface antigen (HBsAg)-positive mothers, administer HepB vaccine and 0.5 mL of hepatitis B immune globulin (HBIG) within 12 hours of birth. These infants should be tested for HBsAg and antibody to HBsAg (anti-HBs) 1 to 2 months after completion of the HepB series, at age 9 through 18 months (preferably at the next well-child visit).
- If mother's HBsAg status is unknown, within 12 hours of birth administer HepB vaccine regardless of birth weight. For infants weighing less than 2,000 grams, administer HBIG in addition to HepB vaccine within 12 hours of birth. Determine mother's HBsAg status as soon as possible and, if mother is HBsAg-positive, also administer HBIG for infants weighing 2,000 grams or more as soon as possible, but no later than age 7 days.

Doses following the birth dose:
- The second dose should be administered at age 1 or 2 months. Monovalent HepB vaccine should be used for doses administered before age 6 weeks.
- Infants who did not receive a birth dose should receive 3 doses of a HepB-containing vaccine on a schedule of 0, 1 to 2 months, and 6 months starting as soon as feasible. See Table 5-8.
- Administer the second dose 1 to 2 months after the first dose (minimum interval of 4 weeks), administer the third dose at least 8 weeks after the second dose AND at least 16 weeks after the **first** dose. The final (third or fourth) dose in the HepB vaccine series should be administered no earlier than age 24 weeks.
- Administration of a total of 4 doses of HepB vaccine is permitted when a combination vaccine containing HepB is administered after the birth dose.

Catch-up vaccination:
- Unvaccinated persons should complete a 3-dose series.
- A 2-dose series (doses separated by at least 4 months) of adult formulation Recombivax HB is licensed for use in children aged 11 through 15 years.
- For other catch-up guidance, see Table 5-8.

2. **Rotavirus (RV) vaccines. (Minimum age: 6 weeks for both RV1 [Rotarix] and RV5 [RotaTeq])**
Routine vaccination:
- Administer a series of RV vaccine to all infants as follows:
  1. If Rotarix is used, administer a 2-dose series at 2 and 4 months of age.
  2. If RotaTeq is used, administer a 3-dose series at ages 2, 4, and 6 months.
  3. If any dose in the series was RotaTeq or vaccine product is unknown for any dose in the series, a total of 3 doses of RV vaccine should be administered.

Catch-up vaccination:
- The maximum age for the first dose in the series is 14 weeks, 6 days.
- Vaccination should not be initiated for infants aged 15 weeks, 0 days or older.
- The maximum age for the final dose i n the series is 8 months, 0 days.
- If RV-1(Rotraix) is adminitered for the first and second doses, a third dose is not indicted.
- For other catch-up guidance, see Table 5-8.

3. **Diphtheria and tetanus toxoids and acellular pertussis (DTaP) vaccine. (Minimum age: 6 weeks. Exception: DTaP-IPV [Kinrix]: 4 years)**
Routine vaccination:
- Administer a 5-dose series of DTaP vaccine at ages 2, 4, 6, 15 through 18 months, and 4 through 6 years. The fourth dose may be admintered as early as age 12 months, provided at least 6 months have elapsed since the third dose.

Catch-up vaccination:
- The fifth dose of DTaP vaccine is not necessary if the fourth dose was administered at age 4 years or older.
- For other catch-up guidance, see Table 5-8.

4. **Tetanus and diphtheria toxoids and acellular pertussis (Tdap) vaccine. (Minimum age: 10 years for Boostrix, 11 years for Adacel)**
Routine vaccination:
- Administer 1 dose of Tdap vaccine to all adolescents aged 11 through 12 years.
- Tdap may be administered regardless of the interval since the last tetanus and diphtheria toxoid-containing vaccine.
- Administer 1 dose of Tdap vaccine to pregnant adolescents during each pregnancy (preferred during 27 through 36 weeks gestation) regardless of time since prior Td or Tdap vaccination.

Catch-up vaccination:
- Persons aged 7 through 10 years who are not fully immunized with DTaP vaccine should receive Tdap vaccine as 1 (preferably the first) dose in the catch-up series; if additional doses are needed, use Td vaccine.
For children 7 through 10 years who receive a dose of Tdap as part of the catch-up series, an adolescent Tdap vaccine dose at age 11 through 12 years should NOT be administered. Td should be
- administered instead 10 years after the Tdap dose.
Persons aged 11 through 18 years who have not received Tdap vaccine should receive a dose followed by tetanus and diphtheria
- toxoids (Td) booster doses every 10 years thereafter.
Inadvertent doses of DTaP vaccine:
  - If administered inadvertently to a child aged 7 through 10 years may count as part of the catch-up series. This dose may count as the adolescent Tdap dose, or the child can later receive a Tdap booster dose at age 11 through 12 years.
  - If administered inadvertently to an adolescent aged 11 through 18 years, the dose should be counted as the adolescent Tdap booster.
- For other catch-up guidance, see Table 5-8.

5. ***Haemophilus influenzae*** **type b (Hib) conjugate vaccine. (Minimum age: 6 weeks for PRP-T [ACTHIB, DTaP-IPV/Hib (Pentacel) and Hib-Men CY (MenHibrix)], PRP-OMP [PedvaxHIB or COMVAX], 12 months for PRP-T [Hiberix])**
   Routine vaccination:
   - Administer a 2- or 3-dose Hib vaccine primary series and a booster dose (dose 3 or 4 depending on vaccine used in primary series) at age 12 through 15 months to complete a full Hib vaccine series.
   - The primary series with ActHIB, MenHibrix, or Pentacel consists of 3 doses and should be administered at 2, 4, and 6 months of age. The primary series with PedvaxHib or COMVAX consists of 2 doses and should be administered at 2 and 4 months of age; a dose at age 6 months is not indicated.
   - One booster dose (dose 3 or 4 depending on vaccine used in primary series) of any Hib vaccine should be administered at age 12 through 15 months. An exception is Hiberix vaccine. Hiberix should only be used for the booster (final) dose in children aged 12 months through 4 years who have received at least 1 prior dose of Hib-containing vaccine.
   - For recommendations on the use of MenHibrix in patients at increased risk for meningococcal disease, please refer to the meningococcal vaccine footnotes and also to *MMWR* March 22, 2013; 62(RR02);1-22, available at http://www.cdc.gov/mmwr/pdf/rr/rr6202.pdf.

   Catch-up vaccination:
   - If dose1 was administered at ages 12 through 14 months, administer a second (final) dose at least 8 weeks after dose 1, regardless of Hib vaccine used in the primary series.
   - If the first 2 dose were PRP-OMP (PedvaxHIB or COMVAX), and were administered at age 11 months or younger, the third (and final) dose should be administered at age 12 through 15 months and at least 8 weeks after the second dose.
   - If the first dose was administered at age 7 through 11 months, administer the second dose at least 4 weeks later and a third (and final) dose at age 12 through 15 months or 8 weeks after second dose, whichever is later, regardless of Hib vaccine used for first dose.
   - If first dose is administered at younger than 12 months of age and second dose is given between 12 through 14 months of age, a third (and final) dose should be given 8 weeks later.
   - For unvaccinated children aged 15 months or older, administer only 1 dose.
   - For other catch-up guidance, see Table 5-8. For catch-up guidance related to MenHibrix, please see the meningococcal vaccine footnotes and also *MMWR* March 22, 2013; 62(RR02);1-22, available at http://www.cdc.gov/mmwr/pdf/rr/rr6202.pdf.

   Vaccination of persons with high-risk conditions:
   - Children aged 12 through 59 months who are at increased risk for Hib disease, including chemotherapy recipients and those with anatomic or functional asplenia (including sickle cell disease), human immunodeficiency virus (HIV) infection, immunoglobulin deficiency, or early component complement defiency, who have either no doses or only 1 dose of Hib vaccine before 12 months of age, should receive 2 additional doses of Hib vaccine 8 weeks apart; children who received 2 or more doses of Hib vaccine before 12 months of age should receive 1 additional dose.
   - For patients younger than 5 years of age undergoing chemotherapy or radiation treatment who received a Hib vaccine dose(s) within 14 days of starting therapy or during therapy, repeat the dose(s) at least 3 months following therapy completion.
   - Recipients of hematopoietic stem cell transplant (HSCT) should be revaccinated with a 3-dose regimen of Hib vaccine starting 6 to 12 months after successful transplant, regardless of vaccination history; doses should be administered at least 4 weeks apart.
   - A single dose of any Hib-containing vaccine should be administered to unimmunized* children and adolescents 15 months of age and older undergoing an elective splenectomy; if possible, vaccine should be administered at least 14 days before procedure.
   - Hib vaccine is not routinely recommended for patients 5 years or older. However, 1 dose of Hib vaccine should be administered to unimmunized* persons aged 5 years or older who have anatomic or functional asplenia (including sickle cell disease) and unvaccinated persons 5 through 18 years of age with human immunodeficiency virus (HIV) infection.

   ** Patients who have not received a primary series and booster dose or at least 1 dose of Hib vaccine after 14 months of age are considered un immunized.*

6. **Pneumococcal vaccines. (Minimum age: 6 weeks for PCV13, 2 years for PPSV23) Routine vaccination with PCV13:**
   - Administer a 4-dose series of PCV13 vaccine at ages 2, 4, and 6 months and at age 12 through 15 months.
   - For children aged 14 through 59 months who have received an age-appropriate series of 7-valent PCV (PCV7), administer a single supplemental dose of 13-valent PCV (PCV13).

   Catch-up vaccination with PCV13:
   - Administer 1 dose of PCV13 to all healthy children aged 24 through 59 months who are not completely vaccinated for their age.
   - For other catch-up guidance, see Table 5-8.

   Vaccination of persons with high-risk conditions with PCV13 and PPSV23:
   - All recommended PCV13 doses should be administered prior to PPSV23 vaccination if possible.
   - For children 2 through 5 years of age with any of the following conditions: chronic heart disease (particularly cyanotic congenital heart disease and cardiac failure); chronic lung disease (including asthama if treated with high-dose oral corticosteroid therapy); diabetes mellitus; cerebrospinal fluid leak; cochlear implant; sickle cell disease and other hemoglobinopathies; anatomic or functional asplenia; HIV infection; chronic renal failure; nephrotic syndrome; diseases associated with treatment with immunosuppressive drugs or radiation therapy, including malignant neoplasms, leukemias, lymphomas, and Hodgkin disease; solid organ transplantation; or cngenital immunodeficiency:
     1. Administer 1 dose of PCV13 if 3 doses of PCV (PCV7 and/or PCV13) were received previously.
     2. Administer 2 doses of PCV13 at least 8 weeks apart if fewer than 3 doses of PCV (PCV7 and/or PCV13) were received previously.
     3. Administer 1 supplemental dose of PCV13 if 4 doses of PCV7 or other age-appropriate complete PCV7 series was received previously.
     4. The minimum interval between doses of PCV (PCV7 or PCV13) is 8 weeks.
     5. For children with no history of PPSV23 vaccination, administer PPSV23 at least 8 weeks after the most recent dose of PCV13.
   - For children aged 6 through 18 years who have cerebrospinal fluid leak; cochlear implant; sickle cell disease and other hemoglobinopathies; anatomic or functional asplenia; congential or acquired immunodeficiencies; HIV infection; chronic renal failure; nephrotic syndrome; diseases associated with treatment with immunosuppressive drugs or radiation therapy, including malignant neoplasms, leukemias, lymphomas, and Hodgkin disease; generalized malignancy; solid organ transplantation; or multiple myeloma:
     1. If neither PCV13 nor PPSV23 has been received previously, administer 1 dose of PCV13 now and 1 dose of PPSV23 at least 8 weeks later.
     2. If PCV13 has been received previously but PPSV23 has not, administer 1 dose of PPSV23 at least 8 weeks after the most recent dose of PCV13.
     3. If PPSV23 has been received but PCV13 has not, administer 1 dose of PCV13 at least 8 weeks after the most recent dose of PPSV23.
   - For children aged 6 through 18 years with chronic heart disease (particularly cyanotic congenital heart disease and cardiac failure), chronic lung disease (including asthma if treated with high-dose oral corticosteroid therapy), diabetes mellitus, alcoholism, or chronic liver disease, who have not received PPSV23, administer 1 dose of PPSV23. If PCV13 has been received previously, then PPSV23 should be administered at least 8 weeks after any prior PCV13 dose.
   - A single revaccination with PPSV23 should be administered 5 years after the first dose to children with sickle cell disease or other hemoglobinopathies; anatomic or functional asplenia; congenital or acquired immunodeficiencies; HIV infection; chronic renal failure; nephrotic syndrome; diseases associated with treatment with immunosuppressive drugs or radiation therapy, including malignant neoplasms, leukemias, lymphomas, and Hodgkin disease; generalized malignancy; solid organ transplantation; or multiple myeloma.

7. **Inactivated poliovirus vaccine (IPV). (Minimum age: 6 weeks)**
   Routine vaccination:
   - Administer a 4-dose series of IPV at ages 2, 4, 6 through 18 months, and 4 through 6 years. The final dose in the series should be administered on or after the fourth birthday and at least 6 months after the previous dose.

   Catch-up vaccination:
   - In the first 6 month of life, minimum age and minimum intervals are only recommended if the person is at risk for imminent exposure to circulating poliovirus (i.e., travel to a polio-endemic region or during an outbreak).
   - If 4 or more doses are administered before age 4 years, an additional dose should be administered at age 4 through 6 years and at least 6 months after the previous dose.
   - A fourth dose is not necessary if the third dose was administered at age 4 years or older and at least 6 months after the previous dose.
   - If both OPV and IPV were administered as part of a series, a total of 4 doses should be administered, regardless of the child's current age. IPV is not routinely recommended for U.S. residents aged 18 years or older.
   - For other catch-up guidance, see Table 5-8.
8. **Influenza vaccines. (Minimum age:6 months for inactivated influenza) vaccine [IIV], 2 years for live, attenuated influenza vaccine [LAIV])**
   Routine vaccination:
   - Administer influenza vaccine annually to all children beginning at age 6 months. For most healthy, nonpregnant persons aged 2 through 49 years, either LAIV or IIV may be used. However, LAIV should NOT be administered to some persons, including 1) those with asthma, 2) children 2 through 4 years who had wheezing in the past 12 months, or 3) those who have any other underlying medical conditions that predispose them to influenza complications. For all other contraindications to use of LAIV see *MMWR* 2013; 62 (No. RR-7):1-43, available at http://www.cdc.gov/mmwr/pdf/rr/rr6207.pdf.

   For children aged 6 months through 8 years:
   - For the 2013–14 season, administer 2 doses (separated by at least 4 weeks) to children who are receiving influenza vaccine for the first time. Some children in this age group who have been vaccinated previously will also need 2 doses. For additional guidance, follow dosing guidelines in the 2013-14 ACIP influenza vaccine recommendations, *MMWR* 2013; 62 (No. RR-7):1-43, available at http://www.cdc.gov/mmwr/pdf/rr/rr6207.pdf.
   - For the 2014-15 season, follow dosing guidlines in the 2014 ACIP influenza vaccine recommendations.

   For persons aged 9 years and older:
   - Administer 1 dose.
9. **Measles, mumps, and rubella (MMR) vaccine. (Minimum age: 12 months for routine vaccination)**
   Routine vaccination:
   - Administer a 2-dose series of MMR vaccine at ages12 through 15 months and 4 through 6 years. The second dose may be administered before age 4 years, provided at least 4 weeks have elapsed since the first dose.
   - Administer 1 dose of MMR vaccine to infants aged 6 through 11 months before departure from the United States for international travel. These children should be revaccinated with 2 doses of MMR vaccine, the fist at age 12 through 15 months (12 months if the child remains in an area where disease risk is high), and the second dose at least 4 weeks later.
   - Administer 2 doses of MMR vaccine to children aged 12 months and older before departure from the United States for international travel. The first dose should be administered on or after age 12 months and the second dose at least 4 weeks later.

   Catch-up vaccination:
   - Ensure that all school-aged children and adolescents have had 2 doses of MMR vaccine; the minimum interval between the 2 doses is 4 weeks.
10. **Varicella (VAR) vaccine. (Minimum age: 12 months)**
    Routine vaccination:
    - Administer a 2-dose series of VAR vaccine at ages 12 through 15 months and 4 through 6 years. The second dose may be administered before age 4 years, provided at least 3 months have elapsed since the first dose. If the second dose was administered at least 4 weeks after the first dose, it can be accepted as valid.

    Catch-up vaccination:
    - Ensure that all persons aged 7 through 18 years without evidence of immunity (see *MMWR* 2007; 56 [No. RR-4], available at http://www.cdc.gov/mmwr/pdf/rr/rr5604.pdf) have 2 doses of varicella vaccine. For children aged 7 through 12 years, the recommended minimum interval between doses is 3 months (if the second dose was administered at least 4 weeks after the first dose, it can be accepted as valid); for persons aged 13 years and older, the minimum interval between doses is 4 weeks.
11. **Hepatitis A vaccine (HepA). (Minimum age: 12 months)**
    Routine vaccination:
    - Initiate the 2-dose HepA vaccine series at 12 through 23 months; separate the 2 doses by 6 to 18 months.
    - Children who have received 1 dose of HepA vaccine before age 24 months should receive a second dose 6 to 18 months after the first dose.
    - For any person aged 2 years and older who has not already received the HepA vaccine series, 2 doses of HepA vaccine separated by 6 to 18 months may be administered if immunity against hepatitis A virus infection is desired.

    Catch-up vaccination:
    - The minimum interval between the two doses is 6 months.

    Special populations:
    - Administer 2 doses of HepA vaccine at least 6 months apart to previously unvaccinated persons who live in areas where vaccination programs target older children, or who are at increased risk for infection. This includes persons traveling to or working in countries that have high or intermediate endemicity of infection; men having sex with men; users of injection and non-injection illicit drugs; persons who work with HAV-infected primates or with HAV in a research laboratory; persons with clotting-factor disorders; persons with chronic liver disease; and persons who anticipate close, personal contact (e.g., household or regular babysitting) with an international adoptee during the first 60 days after arrival in the United States frm a country with high or intermediate endemicity. The first should be administered as soon as the adoption is planned, ideally 2 or more weeks before the arrival of the adoptee.
12. **Human papillomavirus (HPV) vaccines. (Minimum age: 9 years for HPV2 [Cervarix] and HPV4 [Gardisil])**
    Routine vaccination:
    - Administer a 3-dose series of HPV vaccine on a schedule of 0, 1-2, and 6 months to all adolescents aged 11 through 12 years. Either HPV4 or HPV2 may be used for females, and only HPV4 may be used for males.
    - The vaccine series may be started at age 9 years.
    - Administer the second dose 1 to 2 months after the first dose (minimum interval of 4 weeks), administer the third dose 24 weeks after the first dose and 16 weeks after the second dose (minimum interval of 12 weeks).

    Catch-up vaccination:
    - Administer the vaccine series to females (either HPV2 or HPV4) and males (HPV4) at age 13 through 18 years if not previously vaccinated.
    - Use recommended routine dosing intervals (see above) for vaccine series catch-up.
13. **Meningococcal conjugate vaccines. (Minimum age: 6 weeks for Hib-MenCY [MenHibrix], 9 months for MenACWY-D [Menactra], 2 years for MenACWY-CRM [Menveo])**
    Routine vaccination:
    - Administer a single dose of Menactra or Menveo vaccine at age 11 through 12 years, with a booster dose at age 16 years.

- Adolescents aged 11 through 18 years with human immunodeficiency virus (HIV) infection should receive a 2-dose primary series of Menactra or Menveo with at least 8 weeks between doses.
- For children aged 2 months through 18 years with high-risk conditions, see below.

Catch-up vaccination:

- Administer Menactra or Menveo vaccine at age 13 through 18 years if not previously vaccinated.
- If the first dose is administered at age 13 through 15 years, a booster dose should be administered at age 16 through 18 years with a minimum interval of at least 8 weeks between doses.
- If the first dose is administered at age 16 years or older, a booster dose is not needed.
- For other catch-up guidance, see Table 5-8.

Vaccination of persons with high-risk conditions and other persons at increased risk of disease:

- Children with anatomic or functional asplenia (including sickle cell disease):
  1. For children younger than 19 months of age, administer a 4-dose infant series of MenHibrix or Menveo at 2, 4, 6, and 12 through 15 months of age.
  2. For children aged 19 through 23 months who have not completed a series of MenHibrix or Menveo, administer 2 primary doses of Menveo at least 3 months apart.
  3. For children aged 24 months and older who have not received a complete series of MenHibrix or Menveo or Menactra, administer 2 primary doses of either Menactra or Menveo at least 2 months apart. If Menactra is administered to a child with asplenia (including sickle cell disease), do not administer Menactra until 2 years of age and at least 4 weeks after the completion of all PCV13 doses.
- Children with persistent complement component deficiency:
  1. For children younger than 19 months of age, administer a 4-dose infant series of either MenHibrix or Menveo at 2, 4, 6, and 12 through 15 months of age.
  2. For children 7 through 23 months who have not initiated vaccination, two options exist depending on age and vaccine brand:
     a. For children who initiate vaccination with Menveo at 7 months through 23 months of age, a 2-dose series should be administered with the second dose after 12 months of age and at least 3 months after the first dose.
     b. For children who initiate vaccination with Menactra at 9 months through 23 months of age, a 2-dose series of Menactra should be administered at least 3 months apart.
     c. For children aged 24 months and older who have not received a complete series of MenHibrix, Menveo, or Menactra, administer 2 primary doses of either Menactra or Menveo at least 2 months apart.
- For children who travel to or reside in countries in which meningococcal disease is hyperendemic or epidemic, including countries in the African meningitis belt or the Hajj, administer an age- appropriate formulation and series of Menactra or Menveo for protection against serogroups A and W menigococcal disease. Prior receipt of MenHibrix is not sufficiant for children traveling to the meningitis belt or the Hajj because it does not contain serogroups A or W.
- For children at risk during a community outbreak attributable to a vaccine serogroup, administer or complete an age- and formulation-appropriate series of MenHibrix, Menactra, or Menveo.
- For booster doses among persons with high-risk conditions, refer to *MMWR* 2013; 62(RR02);1-22, available at http://www.cdc.gov/mmwr/preview/mmwrhtml/rr6202a1.htm.

Catch-up recommendations for persons with high-risk conditions:

1. If MenHibrix is administered to achieve protection against meningococcal disease, a complete age-appropriate series of MenHibrix should be administered.
2. If the first dose of MenHibrix is given at or after 12 months of age, a total of 2 doses should be given at least 8 weeks apart to ensure protection against serogroups C and Y meningococcal disease.
3. For children who initiate vaccination with Menveo at 7 months through 9 months of age, a 2-dose series should be administered with the second dose after 12 months of age and at least 3 months after the first dose.
4. For other catch-up recommendations for these persons, refer to *MMWR* 2013; 62(RR02);1-22, available at http://www.cdc.gov/mmwr/preview/mmwrhtml/rr6202a1.htm.

For complete information on use of meningococcal vaccines, including guidance related to vaccination of persons at increased risk of infection, see *MMWR* March 22, 2013; 62(RR02);1-22, available at http://www.cdc.gov/mmwr/pdf/rr/rr6202.pdf.

General Recommendations on Immunization

TABLE 5-9 Recommended and Minimum Ages and Intervals between Vaccine Doses*†

Vaccine and Dose Number	Recommended Age for this Dose	Minimum Age for this Dose	Recommended Interval to Next Dose	Minimum Interval to Next Dose
HepB-1[§]	Birth	Birth	1-4 months	4 weeks
HepB-2	1-2 months	4 weeks	2-17 months	8 weeks
HepB-3[¶]	6-18 months	24 weeks	—	—
DTaP-1[§]	2 months	6 weeks	2 months	4 weeks
DTaP-2	4 months	10 weeks	2 months	4 weeks
DTaP-3	6 months	14 weeks	6-12 months	6 months**,††
DTaP-4	15-18 months	12 months	3 years	6 months**
DTaP-5	4-6 years	4 years	—	—
Hib-1[§§§]	2 months	6 weeks	2 months	4 weeks
Hib-2	4 months	10 weeks	2 months	4 weeks
Hib-3[¶¶]	6 months	14 weeks	6-9 months	8 weeks
Hib-4	12-15 months	12 months	—	—
IPV-1[§]	2 months	6 weeks	2 months	4 weeks
IPV-2	4 months	10 weeks	2-14 months	4 weeks
IPV-3	6-18 months	14 weeks	3-5 years	6 months
IPV-4***	4-6 years	4 years	—	—
PCV-1[§§]	2 months	6 weeks	8 weeks	4 weeks
PCV-2	4 months	10 weeks	8 weeks	4 weeks
PCV-3	6 months	14 weeks	6 months	8 weeks
PCV-4	12-15 months	12 months	—	—
MMR-1[†††]	12-15 months	12 months	3-5 years	4 weeks
MMR-2[†††]	4-6 years	13 months	—	—
Varicella-1[†††]	12-15 months	12 months	3-5 years	12 weeks[§§§]
Varicella-2[†††]	4-6 years	15 months	—	—
HepA-1	12-23 months	12 months	6-18 months**	6 months**
HepA-2	≥18 months	18 months	—	—
Influenza inactivated[¶¶¶]	≥6 months	6 months****	1 month	4 weeks
LAIV (intranasal)[¶¶¶]	2-49 years	2 years	1 month	4 weeks
MCV4-1[††††]	11-12 years	2 years	5 years	8 weeks
MCV4-2	16 years	11 years (+8 weeks)	—	—
MPSV4-1[††††]	—	2 years	5 years	5 years
MPSV4-2	—	7 years	—	—
Td	11-12 years	7 years	10 years	5 years
Tdap[§§§§]	≥11 years	7 years	—	—
PPSV-1	—	2 years	5 years	5 years
PPSV-2[¶¶¶¶]	—	7 years	—	—
HPV-1*****	11-12 years	9 years	2 months	4 weeks
HPV-2	11-12 years (+2 months)	9 years (+4 weeks)	4 months	12 weeks[†††††]
HPV-3[†††††]	11-12 years (+6 months)	9 years (+24 weeks)	—	—
Rotavirus-1[§§§§§]	2 months	6 weeks	2 months	4 weeks
Rotavirus-2	4 months	10 weeks	2 months	4 weeks
Rotavirus-3[¶¶¶¶¶]	6 months	14 weeks	—	—
Herpes zoster******	≥60 years	60 years	—	—

DTaP, Diphtheria and tetanus toxoids and acellular pertussis; *HepA,* hepatitis A; *HepB,* hepatitis B; *Hib, Haemophilus influenzae* type b; *HPV,* human papillomavirus; *IPV,* inactivated poliovirus; *LAIV,* live, attenuated influenza vaccine; *MCV4,* quadrivalent meningococcal conjugate vaccine; *MMR,* measles, mumps, and rubella; *MMRV,* measles, mumps, rubella, and varicella; *MPSV4,* quadrivalent meningococcal polysaccharide vaccine; *PCV,* pneumococcal conjugate vaccine; *PPSV,* pneumococcal polysaccharide vaccine; *PRP-OMB,* polyribosylribitol phosphate-meningococcal outer membrane protein conjugate; *Td,* tetanus and diphtheria toxoids; *Tdap,* tetanus toxoid, reduced diphtheria toxoid, and acellular pertussis.

*Combination vaccines are available. Use of licensed combination vaccines is generally preferred to separate injections of their equivalent component vaccines. When administering combination vaccines, the minimum age for administration is the oldest age for any of the individual components; the minimum interval between doses is equal to the greatest interval of any of the individual components.

†Information on travel vaccines, including typhoid, Japanese encephalitis, and yellow fever, is available at http://www.cdc.gov/travel. Information on other vaccines that are licensed in the United States but not distributed, including anthrax and smallpox, is available at http://www.bt.cdc.gov.

§Combination vaccines containing the hepatitis B component are available. These vaccines should not be administered to infants aged <6 weeks because of the other components (i.e., Hib, DTaP, HepA, and IPV).

¶HepB-3 should be administered at least 8 weeks after HepB-2 and at least 16 weeks after HepB-1 and should not be administered before age 24 weeks.

**Calendar months.

††The minimum recommended interval between DTaP-3 and DTaP-4 is 6 months. However, DTaP-4 need not be repeated if administered at least 4 months after DTaP-3.

§§For Hib and PCV, children receiving the first dose of vaccine at age ≥7 months require fewer doses to complete the series.

¶¶If PRP-OMP (Pedvax-Hib, Merck Vaccine Division) was administered at ages 2 and 4 months, a dose at age 6 months is not necessary.

***A fourth dose is not needed if the third dose was administered at ≥4 years and at least 6 months after the previous dose.

†††Combination MMRV vaccine can be used for children aged 12 months to 12 years.

TABLE 5-9 Recommended and Minimum Ages and Intervals between Vaccine Doses—cont'd

§§§The minimum interval from Varicella-1 to Varicella-2 for persons beginning the series at age ≥13 years is 4 weeks.

¶¶¶One dose of influenza vaccine per season is recommended for most persons. Children aged <9 years who are receiving influenza vaccine for the first time or who received only 1 dose the previous season (if it was their first vaccination season) should receive 2 doses this season.

****The minimum age for inactivated influenza vaccine varies by vaccine manufacturer. See package insert for vaccine-specific minimum ages.

††††Revaccination with meningococcal vaccine is recommended for previously vaccinated persons who remain at high risk for meningococcal disease. (Source: CDC. Updated recommendations from the Advisory Committee on Immunization Practices (ACIP) for revaccination of persons at prolonged increased risk for meningococcal disease. *MMWR* 2009;58:[1042-3]).

§§§§Only 1 dose of Tdap is recommended. Subsequent doses should be given as Td. For one brand of Tdap, the minimum age is 11 years. For management of a tetanus-prone wound in persons who have received a primary series of tetanus-toxoid–containing vaccine, the minimum interval after a previous dose of any tetanus-containing vaccine is 5 years.

¶¶¶¶A second dose of PPSV 5 years after the first dose is recommended for persons aged ≤65 years at highest risk for serious pneumococcal infection and those who are likely to have a rapid decline in pneumococcal antibody concentration. (Source: CDC. Prevention of pneumococcal disease: recommendations of the Advisory Committee on Immunization Practices [ACIP]. *MMWR* 1997;46[No. RR-8]).

*****Bivalent HPV vaccine is approved for females aged 10-25 years. Quadrivalent HPV vaccine is approved for males and females aged 9-26 years.

†††††The minimum age for HPV-3 is based on the baseline minimum age for the first dose (i.e., 108 months) and the minimum interval of 24 weeks between the first and third dose. Dose 3 need not be repeated if it is administered at least 16 weeks after the first dose.

§§§§§The first dose of rotavirus must be administered at age 6 weeks through 14 weeks and 6 days. The vaccine series should not be started for infants aged ≥15 weeks, 0 days. Rotavirus should not be administered to children older than 8 months, 0 days of age regardless of the number of doses received between 6 weeks and 8 months, 0 days of age.

¶¶¶¶¶If 2 doses of Rotarix (GlaxoSmithKline) are administered as age appropriate, a third dose is not necessary.

******Herpes zoster vaccine is recommended as a single dose for persons aged ≥60 years.

TABLE 5-10 Guidelines for Spacing of Live and Inactivated Antigens

Antigen Combination	Recommended Minimum Interval between Doses
Two or more inactivated*	May be administered simultaneously or at any interval between doses
Inactivated and live	May be administered simultaneously or at any interval between doses
Two or more live intranasal or injectable†	28 days minimum interval, if not administered simultaneously

From Centers for Disease Control and Prevention: General recommendations on immunization: recommendations of the Advisory Committee on Immunization Practices (ACIP), *MMWR* 60(2):38, 2011.

*Certain experts suggest a 28-day interval between tetanus toxoid, reduced diphtheria toxoid, and acellular pertussis (Tdap) vaccine and tetravalent meningococcal conjugate vaccine if they are not administered simultaneously.

†Live oral vaccines (e.g., Ty21a typhoid vaccine and rotavirus vaccine) may be administered simultaneously or at any interval before or after inactivated or live injectable vaccines.

TABLE 5-11 Guidelines for Administering Antibody-Containing Products* and Vaccines

Type of Administration	Products Administered		Recommended Minimum Interval Between Doses
Simultaneous (during the same office visit)	Antibody-containing products and inactivated antigen		Can be administered simultaneously at different anatomic sites or at any time interval between doses
	Antibody-containing products and live antigen		Should not be administered simultaneously.† If simultaneous administration of measles-containing vaccine or varicella vaccine is unavoidable, administer at different sites and revaccinate or test for seroconversion after the recommended interval
Nonsimultaneous	**Administered First**	**Administered Second**	
	Antibody-containing products	Inactivated antigen	No interval necessary
	Inactivated antigen	Antibody-containing products	No interval necessary
	Antibody-containing products	Live antigen	Dose related†,‡
	Live antigen	Antibody-containing products	2 weeks†

From Centers for Disease Control and Prevention: General recommendations on immunization: recommendations of the Advisory Committee on Immunization Practices (ACIP), *MMWR* 60:(RR-2), 2011.

*Blood products containing substantial amounts of immune globulin include intramuscular and intravenous immune globulin, specific hyperimmune globulin (e.g., hepatitis B immune globulin, tetanus immune globulin, varicella zoster immune globulin, and rabies immune globulin), whole blood, packed red blood cells, plasma, and platelet products.

†Yellow fever vaccine; rotavirus vaccine; oral Ty21a typhoid vaccine; live, attenuated influenza vaccine; and zoster vaccine are exceptions to these recommendations. These live, attenuated vaccines can be administered at any time before or after or simultaneously with an antibody-containing product.

‡The duration of interference of antibody-containing products with the immune response to the measles component of measles-containing vaccine, and possibly varicella vaccine, is dose related.

TABLE 5-12 Recommended Intervals between Administration of Antibody-Containing Products and Measles- or Varicella-Containing Vaccine, by Product and Indication for Vaccination

Product/Indication	Dose (mg IgG/kg) and Route*	Recommended Interval before Measles- or Varicella-Containing Vaccine† Administration (months)
Tetanus IG	250 units (10 mg IgG/kg) IM	3
Hepatitis A IG		
Contact prophylaxis	0.02 ml/kg (33 mg IgG/kg) IM	3
International travel	0.06 ml/kg (10 mg IgG/kg) IM	3
Hepatitis B IG	0.06 ml/kg (10 mg IgG/kg) IM	3
Rabies IG	20 IU/kg (22 mg IgG/kg) IM	4
Varicella IG	125 units/10 kg (60–200 mg IgG/kg) IM, maximum 625 units	5
Measles prophylaxis IG		
Standard (i.e., nonimmunocompromised) contact	0.25 ml/kg (40 mg IgG/kg) IM	5
Immunocompromised contact	0.50 ml/kg (80 mg IgG/kg) IM	6
Blood transfusion		
RBCs, washed	10 ml/kg negligible IgG/kg IV	None
RBCs, adenine-saline added	10 ml/kg (10 mg IgG/kg) IV	3
Packed RBCs (hematocrit 65%)§	10 ml/kg (60 mg IgG/kg) IV	6
Whole blood (hematocrit 35%-50%)§	10 ml/kg (80-100 mg IgG/kg) IV	6
Plasma/platelet products	10 ml/kg (160 mg IgG/kg) IV	7
Cytomegalovirus IGIV	150 mg/kg maximum	6
IGIV		
Replacement therapy for immune deficiencies¶	300-400 mg/kg IV¶	8
Immune thrombocytopenic purpura treatment	400 mg/kg IV	8
Postexposure varicella prophylaxis**	400 mg/kg IV	8
Immune thrombocytopenic purpura treatment	1000 mg/kg IV	10
Kawasaki disease	2 g/kg IV	11
Monoclonal antibody to respiratory syncytial virus F protein (Synagis [MedImmune])††	15 mg/kg IM	None

From Centers for Disease Control and Prevention: General recommendations on immunization: recommendations of the Advisory Committee on Immunization Practices (ACIP), *MMWR* 60:(RR-2), 2011.

HIV, human immunodeficiency virus; *IG,* immune globulin; *IgG,* immune globulin G; *IGIV,* intravenous immune globulin; *mg IgG/kg,* milligrams of immune globulin G per kilogram of body weight; *IM,* intramuscular; *IV,* intravenous; *RBCs,* red blood cells.

*This table is not intended for determining the correct indications and dosages for using antibody-containing products. Unvaccinated persons might not be protected fully against measles during the entire recommended interval, and additional doses of IG or measles vaccine might be indicated after measles exposure. Concentrations of measles antibody in an IG preparation can vary by manufacturer's lot. Rates of antibody clearance after receipt of an IG preparation also might vary. Recommended intervals are extrapolated from an estimated half-life of 30 days for passively acquired antibody and an observed interference with the immune response to measles vaccine for 5 months after a dose of 80 mg IgG/kg.

†Does not include zoster vaccine. Zoster vaccine may be given with antibody-containing blood products.

§Assumes a serum IgG concentration of 16 mg/mL.

¶Measles and varicella vaccinations are recommended for children with asymptomatic or mildly symptomatic HIV infection but are contraindicated for persons with severe immunosuppression from HIV or any other immunosuppressive disorder.

**The investigational VariZIG, similar to licensed varicella-zoster IG (VZIG), is a purified human IG preparation made from plasma containing high levels of antivaricella antibodies (IgG). The interval between VariZIG and varicella vaccine (Var or MMRV) is 5 months.

††Contains antibody only to respiratory syncytial virus.

TABLE 5-13 Contraindications and Precautions* to Commonly Used Vaccines

Vaccine	Contraindications	Precautions
DTaP	Severe allergic reaction (e.g., anaphylaxis) after a previous dose or to a vaccine component Encephalopathy (e.g., coma, decreased level of consciousness, or prolonged seizures), not attributable to another identifiable cause, within 7 days of administration of previous dose of DTP or DTaP	Progressive neurologic disorder, including infantile spasms, uncontrolled epilepsy, progressive encephalopathy; defer DTaP until neurologic status clarified and stabilized Temperature of ≥105° F (≥40° C) within 48 hours after vaccination with a previous dose of DTP or DTaP Collapse or shock-like state (i.e., hypotonic hyporesponsive episode) within 48 hours after receiving a previous dose of DTP/DTaP Seizure ≤3 days after receiving a previous dose of DTP/DTaP Persistent, inconsolable crying lasting ≥3 hours within 48 hours after receiving a previous dose of DTP/DTaP GBS <6 weeks after previous dose of tetanus toxoid-containing vaccine History of arthus-type hypersensitivity reactions after a previous dose of tetanus toxoid-containing vaccine; defer vaccination until at least 10 years have elapsed since the last tetanus-toxoid–containing vaccine Moderate or severe acute illness with or without fever
DT, Td	Severe allergic reaction (e.g., anaphylaxis) after a previous dose or to a vaccine component	GBS <6 weeks after previous dose of tetanus toxoid-containing vaccine History of Arthus-type hypersensitivity reactions after a previous dose of tetanus toxoid-containing vaccine; defer vaccination until at least 10 years have elapsed since the last tetanus-toxoid–containing vaccine Moderate or severe acute illness with or without fever
Tdap	Severe allergic reaction (e.g., anaphylaxis) after a previous dose or to a vaccine component Encephalopathy (e.g., coma, decreased level of consciousness, or prolonged seizures), not attributable to another identifiable cause, within 7 days of administration of previous dose of DTP, DTaP, or Tdap	GBS <6 weeks after a previous dose of tetanus toxoid-containing vaccine Progressive or unstable neurologic disorder, uncontrolled seizures, or progressive encephalopathy until a treatment regimen has been established and the condition has stabilized History of Arthus-type hypersensitivity reactions after a previous dose of tetanus toxoid-containing vaccine; defer vaccination until at least 10 years have elapsed since the last tetanus toxoid-containing vaccine Moderate or severe acute illness with or without fever
IPV	Severe allergic reaction (e.g., anaphylaxis) after a previous dose or to a vaccine component	Pregnancy Moderate or severe acute illness with or without fever
MMR[†§]	Severe allergic reaction (e.g., anaphylaxis) after a previous dose or to a vaccine component Pregnancy Known severe immunodeficiency (e.g., from hematologic and solid tumors, receipt of chemotherapy, congenital immunodeficiency, or long-term immunosuppressive therapy[¶] or patients with HIV infection who are severely immunocompromised)[§]	Recent (≤11 months) receipt of antibody-containing blood product (specific interval depends on product) History of thrombocytopenia or thrombocytopenic purpura Need for tuberculin skin testing[††] Moderate or severe acute illness with or without fever
Hib	Severe allergic reaction (e.g., anaphylaxis) after a previous dose or to a vaccine component Age <6 weeks	Moderate or severe acute illness with or without fever
Hepatitis B	Severe allergic reaction (e.g., anaphylaxis) after a previous dose or to a vaccine component	Infant weight <2000 g[§§] Moderate or severe acute illness with or without fever
Hepatitis A	Severe allergic reaction (e.g., anaphylaxis) after a previous dose or to a vaccine component	Pregnancy Moderate or severe acute illness with or without fever
Varicella	Severe allergic reaction (e.g., anaphylaxis) after a previous dose or to a vaccine component Known severe immunodeficiency (e.g., from hematologic and solid tumors, receipt of chemotherapy, congenital immunodeficiency, or long-term immunosuppressive therapy[¶] or patients with HIV infection who are severely immunocompromised)[§] Pregnancy	Recent (≤11 months) receipt of antibody-containing blood product (specific interval depends on product)[¶¶] Moderate or severe acute illness with or without fever
PCV	Severe allergic reaction (e.g., anaphylaxis) after a previous dose (of PCV7, PCV13, or any diphtheria toxoid-containing vaccine) or to a component of a vaccine (PCV7, PCV13, or any diphtheria toxoid-containing vaccine)	Moderate or severe acute illness with or without fever
TIV	Severe allergic reaction (e.g., anaphylaxis) after a previous dose or to vaccine component, including egg protein	GBS <6 weeks after a previous dose of influenza vaccine Moderate or severe acute illness with or without fever
LAIV	Severe allergic reaction (e.g., anaphylaxis) after a previous dose or to vaccine component, including egg protein Pregnancy Immunosuppression Certain chronic medical conditions***	GBS <6 weeks after a previous dose of influenza vaccine Moderate or severe acute illness with or without fever
PPSV	Severe allergic reaction (e.g., anaphylaxis) after a previous dose or to a vaccine component	Moderate or severe acute illness with or without fever
MCV4	Severe allergic reaction (e.g., anaphylaxis) after a previous dose or to a vaccine component	Moderate or severe acute illness with or without fever

TABLE 5-13 Contraindications and Precautions* to Commonly Used Vaccines—cont'd

Vaccine	Contraindications	Precautions
MPSV4	Severe allergic reaction (e.g., anaphylaxis) after a previous dose or to a vaccine component	Moderate or severe acute illness with or without fever
HPV	Severe allergic reaction (e.g., anaphylaxis) after a previous dose or to a vaccine component	Pregnancy Moderate or severe acute illness with or without fever
Rotavirus	Severe allergic reaction (e.g., anaphylaxis) after a previous dose or to a vaccine component SCID	Altered immunocompetence other than SCID History of intussusception Chronic gastrointestinal disease††† Spina bifida or bladder exstrophy††† Moderate or severe acute illness with or without fever
Zoster	Severe allergic reaction (e.g., anaphylaxis) after a previous dose or to a vaccine component Substantial suppression of cellular immunity Pregnancy	Moderate or severe acute illness with or without fever

From Centers for Disease Control and Prevention: General recommendations on immunization: recommendations of the Advisory Committee on Immunization Practices (ACIP), *MMWR* 60:(RR-2), 2011.

DT, diphtheria and tetanus toxoids; *DTaP,* diphtheria and tetanus toxoids and acellular pertussis; *GBS,* Guillian-Barré syndrome; *HBsAg,* hepatitis B surface antigen; *Hib, Haemophilus influenzae* type b; *HIV,* human immunodeficiency virus; *HPV,* human papillomavirus; *IPV,* inactivated poliovirus; *LAIV,* live, attenuated influenza vaccine; *MCV4,* quadrivalent meningococcal conjugate vaccine; *MMRV* measles, mumps, rubella; *MPSV4,* quadrivalent meningococcal polysaccharide vaccine; *PCV,* pneumococcal conjugate vaccine; *PPSV,* pneumococcal polysaccharide vaccine; *SCID,* severe combined immunodeficiency; *Td,* tetanus and diphtheria toxoids; *Tdap,* tetanus toxoid, reduced diphtheria toxoid, and acellular pertussis; *TIV,* trivalent inactivated influenza vaccine.

*Events or conditions listed as precautions should be reviewed carefully. Benefits of and risks for administering a specific vaccine to a person under these circumstances should be considered. If the risk from the vaccine is believed to outweigh the benefit, the vaccine should not be administered. If the benefit of vaccination is believed to outweigh the risk, the vaccine should be administered. Whether and when to administer DTaP to children with proven or suspected underlying neurologic disorders should be decided on a case-by-case basis.

†HIV-infected children may receive varicella and measles vaccine if $CD4^+$ T-lymphocyte count is <15%. (Source: Adapted from American Academy of Pediatrics. Passive immunization. In: Pickering LK, ed. Red book: 2009 report of the committee on infectious diseases. 28th ed. Elk Grove Village. IL: American Academy of Pediatrics: 2009.)

§MMR and varicella vaccines can be administered on the same day. If not administered on the same day, these vaccines should be separated by at least 28 days.

¶Substantially immunosuppressive steroid dose is considered to be ≥2 weeks of daily receipt of 20 mg or 2 mg/kg body weight of prednisone or equivalent.

††Measles vaccination might suppress tuberculin reactivity temporarily. Measles-containing vaccine can be administered on the same day as tuberculin skin testing. If testing cannot be performed until after the day of MMR vaccination, the test should be postponed for ≥4 weeks after the vaccination. If an urgent need exists to skin test, do so with the understanding that reactivity might be reduced by the vaccine.

§§Hepatitis B vaccination should be deferred for infants weighing <2000 g if the mother is documented to be HBsAg-negative at the time of the infant's birth. Vaccination can commence at chronological age 1 month or at hospital discharge. For infants born to HBsAg-positive women, hepatitis B immune globulin and hepatitis B vaccine should be administered within 12 hours after birth, regardless of weight.

¶¶Vaccine should be deferred for the appropriate interval if replacement immune globulin products are being administered.

***Source: CDC. Prevention and control of seasonal influenza with vaccines: recommendations of the Advisory Committee on Immunization Practices (ACIP), 2010. *MMWR* 2010;59(No. RR-8).

†††For details see CDC. Prevention of rotavirus gastroenteritis among infants and children: recommendations of the Advisory Committee on Immunization Practices. *MMWR* 2009;58(No. RR-2).

TABLE 5-14 Conditions Commonly Misperceived as Contraindications to Vaccination

Vaccine	Conditions Commonly Misperceived as Contraindications (i.e., Vaccination May be Administered under These Conditions)
General for all vaccines, including DTaP, pediatric DT, adult Td, adolescent-adult Tdap, IPV, MMR, Hib, hepatitis A, hepatitis B, varicella, rotavirus, PCV, TIV, LAIV, PPSV, MCV4, MPSV4, HPV, and herpes zoster	Mild acute illness with or without fever Mild-to-moderate local reaction (i.e., swelling, redness, soreness); low-grade or moderate fever after previous dose Lack of previous physical examination in well-appearing person Current antimicrobial therapy* Convalescent phase of illness Preterm birth (hepatitis B vaccine is an exception in certain circumstances)† Recent exposure to an infectious disease History of penicillin allergy, other nonvaccine allergies, relatives with allergies, or receiving allergen extract immunotherapy
DTaP	Fever of <105° F (<40° C), fussiness or mild drowsiness after a previous dose of DTP/DTaP Family history of seizures Family history of sudden infant death syndrome Family history of an adverse event after DTP or DTaP administration Stable neurologic conditions (e.g., cerebral palsy, well-controlled seizures, or developmental delay)
Tdap	Fever of ≥105° F (≥40° C) for <48 hours after vaccination with a previous dose of DTP or DTaP Collapse or shock-like state (i.e., hypotonic hyporesponsive episode) within 48 hours after receiving a previous dose of DTaP Seizure <3 days after receiving a previous dose of DTP/DTaP Persistent, inconsolable crying lasting <3 hours within 48 hours after receiving a previous dose of DTP/DTaP History of extensive limb swelling after DTP/DTaP/Td that is not an arthus-type reaction Stable neurologic disorder History of brachial neuritis Latex allergy that is not anaphylactic Breastfeeding Immunosuppression
IPV	Previous receipt of ≥1 dose of oral polio vaccine
MMR§,¶	Positive tuberculin skin test Simultaneous tuberculin skin testing** Breastfeeding Pregnancy of recipient's mother or other close or household contact Recipient is female of childbearing age Immunodeficient family member or household contact Asymptomatic or mildly symptomatic HIV infection Allergy to eggs
Hepatitis B	Pregnancy Autoimmune disease (e.g., systemic lupus erythematosus or rheumatoid arthritis)
Varicella	Pregnancy of recipient's mother or other close or household contact Immunodeficient family member or household contact†† Asymptomatic or mildly symptomatic HIV infection Humoral immunodeficiency (e.g., agammaglobulinemia)
TIV	Nonsevere (e.g., contact) allergy to latex, thimerosal, or egg Concurrent administration of Coumadin or aminophylline
LAIV	Health care providers that see patients with chronic diseases or altered immunocompetence (an exception is providers for severely immunocompromised patients requiring care in a protected environment) Breastfeeding Contacts of persons with chronic disease or altered immunocompetence (an exception is contacts of severely immunocompromised patients requiring care in a protected environment)
PPSV	History of invasive pneumococcal disease or pneumonia
HPV	Immunosuppression Previous equivocal or abnormal Papanicolaou test Known HPV infection Breastfeeding History of genital warts
Rotavirus	Prematurity Immunosuppressed household contacts Pregnant household contacts
Zoster	Therapy with low-dose methotrexate (≤0.4 mg/kg/week), azathioprine (≤3.0 mg/kg/day), or 6-mercaptopurine (≤1.5 mg/kg/day) for treatment of rheumatoid arthritis, psoriasis, polymyositis, sarcoidosis, inflammatory bowel disease, or other conditions Health care providers of patients with chronic diseases or altered immunocompetence Contacts of patients with chronic diseases or altered immunocompetence Unknown or uncertain history of varicella in a U.S.-born person

From Centers for Disease Control and Prevention: General recommendations on immunization: recommendations of the Advisory Committee on Immunization Practices (ACIP), *MMWR* 60:(RR-2), 2011.

DT, Diphtheria and tetanus toxoids; *DTP,* diphtheria toxoid, tetanus toxoid, and pertussis; *DTaP,* diphtheria and tetanus toxoids and acellular pertussis; *HBsAg,* hepatitis B surface antigen; *Hib, Haemophilus influenzae* type b; *HPV,* human papillomavirus; *IPV,* inactivated poliovirus; *LAIV,* live, attenuated influenza vaccine; *MCV4,* quadrivalent meningococcal conjugate vaccine; *MMR,* measles, mumps, and rubella; *MPSV4,* quadrivalent meningococcal polysaccharide vaccine; *PCV,* pneumococcal conjugate vaccine; *PPSV,* pneumococcal polysaccharide vaccine; *Td,* tetanus and diphtheria toxoids; *Tdap,* tetanus toxoid, reduced diphtheria toxoid, and acellular pertussis; *TIV,* trivalent inactivated influenza vaccine.

TABLE 5-14 Conditions Commonly Misperceived as Contraindications to Vaccination—cont'd

*Antibacterial drugs might interfere with Ty21a oral typhoid vaccine, and certain antiviral drugs might interfere with varicella-containing vaccines and LAIV.

†Hepatitis B vaccination should be deferred for infants weighing <2000 g if the mother is documented to be HBsAg-negative at the time of the infant's birth. Vaccination can commence at chronologic age 1 month or at hospital discharge. For infants born to HBsAg-positive women, hepatitis B immune globulin and hepatitis B vaccine should be administered within 12 hours after birth, regardless of weight.

§MMR and varicella vaccines can be administered on the same day. If not administered on the same day, these vaccines should be separated by at least 28 days.

¶HIV-infected children should receive immune globulin after exposure to measles. HIV-infected children can receive varicella and measles vaccine if $CD4^{+}$ T-lymphocyte count is >15%. (Source: Adapted from American Academy of Pediatrics. Passive immunization. In: Pickering LK, ed. Red book: 2009 report of the Committee on Infectious Diseases, 28th ed. Elk Grove Village, IL: American Academy of Pediatrics; 2009.)

**Measles vaccination might suppress tuberculin reactivity temporarily. Measles-containing vaccine can be administered on the same day as tuberculin skin testing. If testing cannot be performed until after the day of MMR vaccination, the test should be postponed for at least 4 weeks after the vaccination. If an urgent need exists to skin test, do so with the understanding that reactivity might be reduced by the vaccine.

††If a vaccinee experiences a presumed vaccine-related rash 7–25 days after vaccination, the person should avoid direct contact with immunocompromised persons for the duration of the rash.

VACCINE ADMINISTRATION*

INFECTION CONTROL AND STERILE TECHNIQUE

Persons administering vaccines should follow appropriate precautions to minimize risk for spread of disease. Hands should be cleansed with an alcohol-based, waterless antiseptic hand rub or washed with soap and water between each patient contact. Occupational Safety and Health Administration (OSHA) regulations do not require that gloves be worn when administering vaccinations unless persons administering vaccinations are likely to come into contact with potentially infectious body fluids or have open lesions on their hands. Needles used for injections must be sterile and disposable to minimize the risk for contamination. A separate needle and syringe should be used for each injection. Changing needles between drawing vaccine from a vial and injecting it into a recipient is not necessary. Different vaccines should never be mixed in the same syringe unless specifically licensed for such use, and no attempt should be made to transfer between syringes.

For all intramuscular injections, the needle should be long enough to reach the muscle mass and prevent vaccine from seeping into subcutaneous tissue but not so long as to involve underlying nerves, blood vessels, or bone. Vaccinators should be familiar with the anatomy of the area where they are injecting vaccine. Intramuscular injections are administered at a 90-degree angle to the skin, preferably into the anterolateral aspect of the thigh or the deltoid muscle of the upper arm depending on the age of the patient.

Decision on needle size and site of injection must be made for each person on the basis of the size of the muscle, the thickness of adipose tissue at the injection site, the volume of the material to be administered, injection technique, and the depth below the muscle surface into which the material is to be injected (Fig. 5-1). Aspiration before injection of vaccines or toxoids (i.e., pulling back on the syringe plunger after needle insertion before injection) is not required because no large blood vessel exists at the recommended injection sites.

INFANTS (AGED <12 MONTHS)

For the majority of infants, the anterolateral aspect of the thigh is the recommended site for injection because it provides a large muscle mass (Fig. 5-2). The muscles of the buttock have not been used for administration of vaccines in infants and children because of concern about potential injury to the sciatic nerve, which is well documented after injection of antimicrobial agents into the buttock. If the gluteal muscle must be used, care should be taken to define the anatomic landmarks.[†] Injection technique is the most important parameter to ensure efficient intramuscular vaccine delivery. If the subcutaneous and muscle tissue are bunched to minimize the chance of striking bone, a 1-inch needle is required to ensure intramuscular administration in infants. For the majority of infants, a 1-inch, 22- to 25-gauge needle is sufficient to penetrate muscle in an infant's thigh. For newborn (first 28 days of life) and premature infants, a ⅝-inch-long needle usually is adequate if the skin is stretched flat between thumb and forefinger and the needle inserted at a 90-degree angle to the skin.

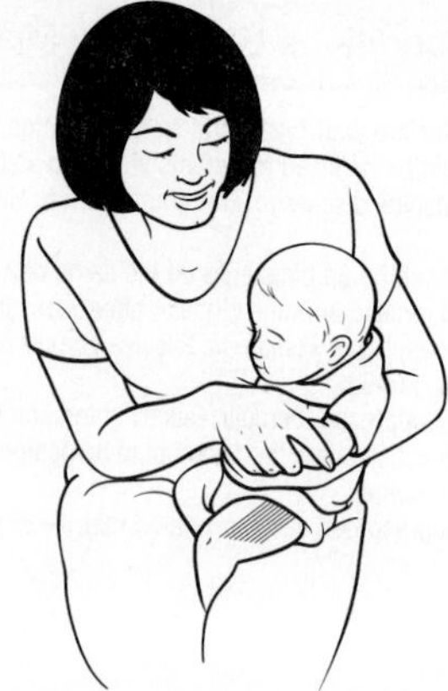

FIGURE 5-2 Intramuscular/subcutaneous site of administration: anterolateral thigh. (Adapted from Minnesota Department of Health. In Centers for Disease Control and Prevention: General recommendations on immunization: recommendations of the Advisory Committee on Immunization Practices [ACIP], *MMWR* 55[RR-15]:6, 2006.)

TODDLERS AND OLDER CHILDREN (AGED 12 MONTHS TO 10 YEARS)

The deltoid muscle should be used if the muscle mass is adequate. The needle size for deltoid site injections can range from 22 to 25 gauge and from ⅝ to 1 inch on the basis of the size of the muscle and the thickness of adipose tissue at the injection site (Fig. 5-3). A ⅝-inch needle is adequate

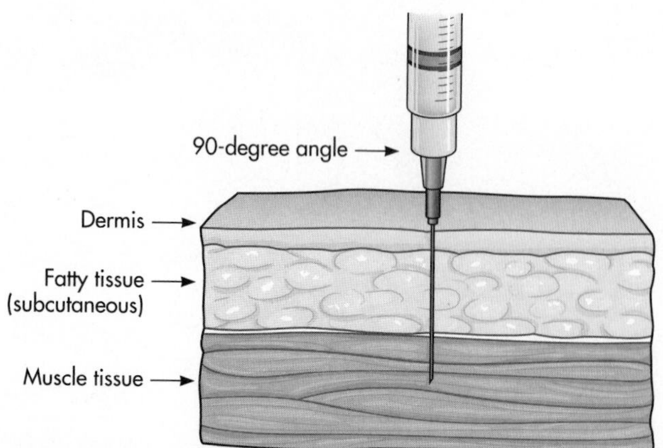

FIGURE 5-1 Intramuscular needle insertion. (Adapted from California Immunization Branch. In Centers for Disease Control and Prevention: General recommendations on immunization: recommendations of the Advisory Committee on Immunization Practices [ACIP], *MMWR* 55[RR-15]:16, 2006.)

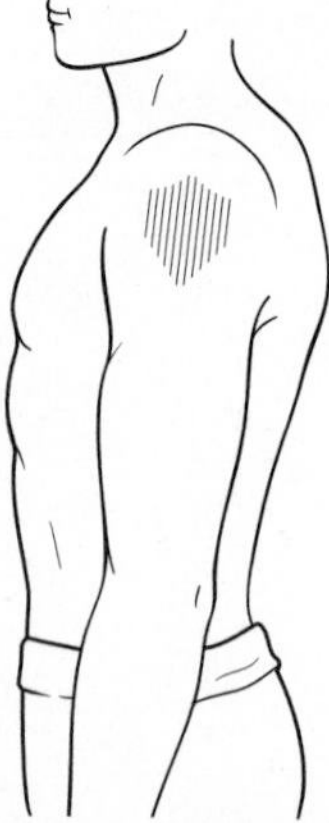

FIGURE 5-3 Intramuscular site of administration: deltoid. (Adapted from Minnesota Department of Health. In Centers for Disease Control and Prevention: General recommendations on immunization: recommendations of the Advisory Committee on Immunization Practices [ACIP], *MMWR* 55[RR-15]:17, 2006.)

*From Centers for Disease Control and Prevention: General recommendations on immunization: recommendations of the Advisory Committee on Immunization Practices (ACIP), *MMWR* 55(RR-15):14-16, 2006.

†If the gluteal muscle is chosen, injection should be administered lateral and superior to a line between the posterior superior iliac spine and the greater trochanter or in the ventrogluteal site, the center of a triangle bounded by the anterior superior iliac spine, the tubercle of the iliac crest, and the upper border of the greater trochanter.

only for the deltoid muscle and only if the skin is stretched flat between the thumb and forefinger and the needle inserted at a 90-degree angle to the skin. For toddlers, the anterolateral thigh can be used, but the needle should be at least 1 inch in length.

ADOLESCENTS AND ADULTS (AGED >11 YEARS)

For adults and adolescents, the deltoid muscle is recommended for routine intramuscular vaccinations. The anterolateral thigh also can be used. For men and women weighing <130 lb (<60 kg) a ⅝- to 1-inch needle is sufficient to ensure intramuscular injection. For women weighing 130 to 200 lb (60 to 90 kg) and men 130 to 260 lb (60 to 118 kg), a 1- to 1½-inch needle is needed. For women weighing >200 lb (>90 kg) or men weighing >260 lb (>118 kg), a 1½-inch needle is required.

SUBCUTANEOUS INJECTIONS

Subcutaneous injections are administered at a 45-degree angle, usually into the thigh for infants younger than 12 months and in the upper-outer triceps area of persons aged 12 months and older. Subcutaneous injections can be administered into the upper-outer triceps area of an infant if necessary. A ⅝-inch, 23- to 25-gauge needle should be inserted into the subcutaneous tissue (Figs. 5-4 and 5-5).

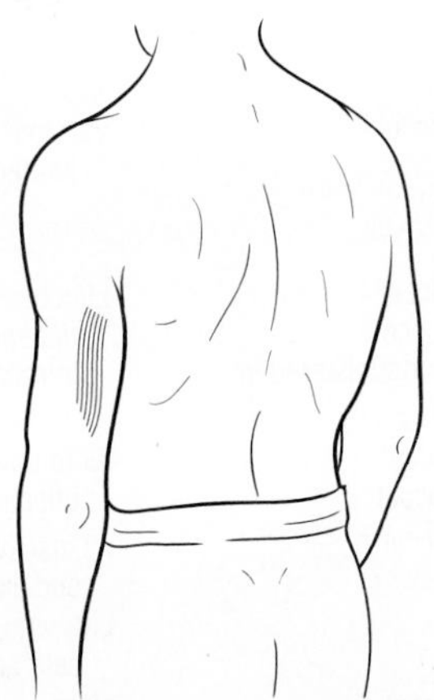

FIGURE 5-4 Subcutaneous site of administration: triceps. (Adapted from Minnesota Department of Health. In Centers for Disease Control and Prevention: General recommendations on immunization: recommendations of the Advisory Committee on Immunization Practices [ACIP], *MMWR* 55[RR-15]:17, 2006.)

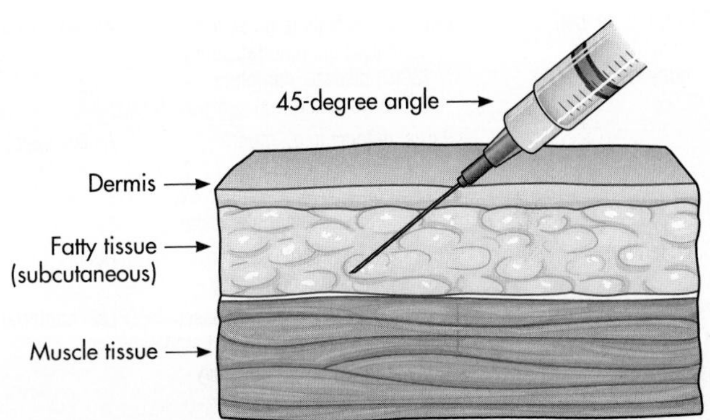

FIGURE 5-5 Subcutaneous needle insertion. (Adapted from California Administration Branch. In Centers for Disease Control and Prevention: General recommendations on immunization: recommendations of the Advisory Committee on Immunization Practices [ACIP], *MMWR* 55[RR-15]:17, 2006.)

TABLE 5-15 Treatment of Anaphylaxis in Children and Adults with Drugs Administered Intramuscularly or Orally

Drug	Dosage
Children	
Primary Regimen	
Epinephrine 1:1000 (aqueous) (1 mg/ml)*	0.01 mg/kg up to 0.5 mg (administer 0.01 ml/kg/dose up to 0.5 mL) IM repeated every 10–20 minutes up to 3 doses
Secondary Regimen	
Diphenhydramine	1–2 mg/kg oral, IM, or IV, every 4–6 hours (100 mg, maximum single dose)
Hydroxyzine	0.5–1 mg/kg oral, IM, every 4–6 hours (100 mg, maximum single dose)
Prednisone	1.5–2 mg/kg oral (60 mg, maximum single dose); use corticosteroids as long as needed
Adults	
Primary Regimen	
Epinephrine 1:1000 (aqueous)*	0.01 mg/kg up to 0.5 mg (administer 0.01 ml/kg/dose up to 0.5 ml) IM repeated every 10–20 minutes up to 3 doses
Secondary Regimen	
Diphenhydramine	1–2 mg/kg up to l00 mg IM or oral, every 4–6 hours

From Centers for Disease Control and Prevention: General recommendations on immunization: recommendations of the Advisory Committee on Immunization Practices (ACIP), *MMWR* 60:(RR-2), 2011. Adapted from American Academy of Pediatrics. Passive immunization. In: Pickering LK, Baker CJ, Kimberlin DW, Long SS, eds: *Red book: 2009 report of the Committee on Infectious Diseases,* 28th ed. Elk Grove Village, IL: American Academy of Pediatrics, 2009:66-7; Immunization Action Coalition. Medical management of vaccine reactions in adult patients (available at www.immunize.org/catg.d/p3082.pdf); and *Mosby's drug consult,* St Louis, 2005, Mosby.

IM, Intramuscular; *IV,* intravenous.

*If the agent causing the anaphylactic reaction was administered by injection, epinephrine may be injected into the same site to slow absorption.

TABLE 5-16 Vaccination of Persons with Primary and Secondary Immunodeficiencies

Primary	Specific Immunodeficiency	Contraindicated Vaccines*	Risk-Specific Recommended Vaccines*	Effectiveness and Comments
B-lymphocyte (humoral)	Severe antibody deficiencies (e.g., X-linked agammaglobulinemia and common variable immunodeficiency)	OPV† Smallpox LAIV BCG Ty21a (live typhoid) Yellow fever	Pneumococcal Consider measles and varicella vaccination	The effectiveness of any vaccine is uncertain if it depends only on the humoral response (e.g., PPSV or MPSV4). IGIV interferes with the immune response to measles vaccine and possibly varicella vaccine.
	Less severe antibody deficiencies (e.g., selective IgA deficiency and IgG subclass deficiency	OPV† BCG Yellow fever Other live vaccines appear to be safe.	Pneumococcal	All vaccines likely effective; immune response might be attenuated.
T-lymphocyte (cell-mediated and humoral)	Complete deficits (e.g., severe combined immunodeficiency [SCID] disease, complete DiGeorge syndrome)	All live vaccines§,¶,**	Pneumococcal	Vaccines might be ineffective.
	Partial defects (e.g., most patients with DiGeorge syndrome, Wiskott-Aldrich syndrome, ataxia-telangiectasia)	All live vaccines§,¶,**	Pneumococcal Meningococcal Hib (if not administered in infancy)	Effectiveness of any vaccine depends on degree of immune suppression.
Complement	Persistent complement, properdin, or factor B deficiency	None	Pneumococcal Meningococcal	All routine vaccines likely effective.
Phagocytic function	Chronic granulomatous disease, leukocyte adhesion defect, and myeloperoxidase deficiency	Live bacterial vaccines§	Pneumococcal††	All inactivated vaccines safe and likely effective. Live viral vaccines likely safe and effective.
Secondary	HIV/AIDS	OPV† Smallpox BCG LAIV Withhold MMR and varicella in severely immunocompromised persons. Yellow fever vaccine might have a contraindication or a precaution depending on clinical parameters of immune function***	Pneumococcal Consider Hib (if not administered in infancy) and meningococcal vaccination.	MMR, varicella, rotavirus, and all inactivated vaccines, including inactivated influenza, might be effective.§§
	Malignant neoplasm, transplantation, immunosuppressive or radiation therapy	Live viral and bacterial, depending on immune status§,¶	Pneumococcal	Effectiveness of any vaccine depends on degree of immune suppression.
	Asplenia	None	Pneumococcal Meningococcal Hib (if not administered in infancy)	All routine vaccines likely effective.
	Chronic renal disease	LAIV	Pneumococcal Hepatitis B¶¶	All routine vaccines likely effective.

From Centers for Disease Control and Prevention: General recommendations on immunization: recommendations of the Advisory Committee on Immunization Practices (ACIP), *MMWR* 60:(RR-2), 2011. Adapted from American Academy of Pediatrics. Passive immunization. In: Pickering LK, Baker CJ, Kimberlin DW, Long SS, eds: *Red book: 2009 report of the Committee on Infectious Diseases,* 28th ed. Elk Grove Village, IL: American Academy of Pediatrics; 2009:74–5.

AIDS, acquired immunodeficiency syndrome; *BCG,* bacille Calmette-Guérin; *Hib, Haemophilus influenzae* type b; *HIV,* human immunodeficiency virus; *IG,* immunoglobulin; *IGIV,* immune globulin intravenous; *LAIV,* live, attenuated influenza vaccine; *MMR,* measles, mumps, and rubella; *MPSV4,* quadrivalent meningococcal polysaccharide vaccine; *OPV,* oral poliovirus polysaccharide vaccine; *PPSV,* pneumococcal polysaccharide vaccine.

*Other vaccines that are universally or routinely recommended should be given if not contraindicated.

†OPV is no longer available in the United States.

§Live bacterial vaccines: BCG and oral Ty21a *Salmonella typhi* vaccine.

¶Live viral vaccines: MMR, MMRV, OPV, LAIV, yellow fever, zoster, rotavirus, varicella, and vaccinia (smallpox). Smallpox vaccine is not recommended for children or the general public.

**Regarding T-lymphocyte immunodeficiency as a contraindication for rotavirus vaccine, data exist only for severe combined immunodeficiency.

††Pneumococcal vaccine is not indicated for children with chronic granulomatous disease beyond age-based universal recommendations for PCV. Children with chronic granulomatous disease are not at increased risk for pneumococcal disease.

§§HIV-infected children should receive IG after exposure to measles and may receive varicella and measles vaccine if CD4+ T-lymphocyte count is ≥15%.

¶¶Indicated based on the risk from dialysis-based bloodborne transmission.

***Symptomatic HIV infection or CD4+ T-lymphocyte count of <200/mm³ or <15% of total lymphocytes for children aged <6 years is a contraindication to yellow fever vaccine administration. Asymptomatic HIV infection with CD4+ T-lymphocyte count of 200–499/mm³ for persons aged ≥6 years or 15%–24% of total lymphocytes for children aged <6 years is a precaution for yellow fever vaccine administration. Details of yellow fever vaccine recommendations are available from CDC. (CDC. Yellow fever vaccine recommendations of the Advisory Committee on Immunization Practices [ACIP]. *MMWR* 2010;59[No. RR-7].)

TABLE 5-17 Immunizations for Pediatric Oncology Patients

Vaccine	Indications and Comments
DtaP	Indicated for incompletely immunized children <7 yr, even during active chemotherapy
Td	Indicated 1 yr after completion of therapy in children 7 yr
Hib	Indicated for incompletely immunized children if <7 yr
HBV	Indicated for incompletely immunized children
23PS	Indicated for asplenic patients
PCV13	Indicated for incompletely immunized children <5 yr
Meningococcus	Consider in asplenic patients
IPV	Indicated for incompletely immunized children; also recommended for all household contacts requiring immunization to reduce the risk of vaccine-associated polio
MMR	Contraindicated until child is in remission and finished with all chemotherapy for 3-6 mo; may need to reimmunize after chemotherapy if titers have fallen below protective levels
Influenza	Defer in active chemotherapy; may give as early as 3-4 wk after remission and off chemotherapy if during influenza season; peripheral granulocyte and lymphocyte counts should be >1000/μL; should also be given to household contact of children with cancer
Varicella	Consider immunizing children who have remained in remission and have finished chemotherapy for >1 yr; with absolute lymphocyte count of >700/μl and platelet count of >100,000/μL within 24 hr of immunization; check titers of previously immunized children to verify protective levels of antibodies

From *MMWR* 49(RR-10):1-147, 2000.
DtaP, Diphtheria, tetanus, and pertussis; *HBV,* hepatitis B virus; *Hib, Haemophilus influenzae* type b; *IPV,* inactivated polio vaccine; *MMR,* measles, mumps, rubella; *PCV13,* pneumococcal conjugate vaccine; *23PS,* 23-valent pneumococcal polysaccharide vaccine; *Td,* tetanus, diphtheria.

TABLE 5-18 Approaches to the Evaluation and Vaccination of Persons Vaccinated Outside the United States Who Have No (or Questionable) Vaccination Records

Vaccine	Recommended Approach	Alternative Approach*
MMR	Revaccination with MMR	Serologic testing for IgG antibodies to measles, mumps, and rubella
Hib	Age-appropriate revaccination	—
Hepatitis A	Age-appropriate revaccination	Serologic testing for IgG antibodies to hepatitis A
Hepatitis B	Age-appropriate revaccination and serologic testing for HBsAg†	—
Poliovirus	Revaccinate with inactivated poliovirus vaccine	Serologic testing for neutralizing antibody to poliovirus types 1, 2, and 3 (limited availability)
DTaP	Revaccination with DTaP, with serologic testing for specific IgG antibody to tetanus and diphtheria toxins in the event of a severe local reaction	Persons whose records indicate receipt of ≥3 doses: serologic testing for specific IgG antibody to diphtheria and tetanus toxins before administering additional doses, or administer a single booster dose of DTaP, followed by serologic testing after 1 month for specific IgG antibody to diphtheria and tetanus toxins with revaccination as appropriate
Tdap	Age-appropriate vaccination of persons who are candidates for Tdap vaccine on the basis of time since last diphtheria and tetanus-toxoid–containing vaccines.	—
Varicella	Age-appropriate vaccination of persons who lack evidence of varicella immunity	—
Pneumococcal conjugate	Age-appropriate vaccination	—
Rotavirus	Age-appropriate vaccination	—
HPV	Age-appropriate vaccination	—
Zoster	Age-appropriate vaccination	—

From Centers for Disease Control and Prevention: General recommendations on immunization: recommendations of the Advisory Committee on Immunization Practices (ACIP), *MMWR* 60:(RR-2), 2011.

DTaP, Diphtheria and tetanus toxoids and acellular pertussis; *HBsAg,* hepatitis B surface antigen; *Hib, Haemophilus influenzae* type b; *HPV,* human papillomavirus; *IgG,* immune globulin G; *MMR,* measles, mumps, and rubella; *Tdap,* tetanus toxoid, reduced diphtheria toxoid, and acellular pertussis.

*There is a recommended approach for all vaccines and an alternative approach for some vaccines.

†In rare instances, hepatitis B vaccine can give a false-positive HBsAg result up to 18 days after vaccination; therefore, blood should be drawn to test for HBsAg before vaccinating. (Source: CDC. A comprehensive immunization strategy to eliminate transmission of hepatitis B virus infection in the United States: recommendations of the Advisory Committee on Immunization Practices [ACIP]; Part I: Immunization in infants, children, and adolescents, *MMWR* 2005;54(No. RR-16.])

Immunizations for Adults

TABLE 5-19 Recommended Adult Immunization Schedule, by Vaccine and Age Group[1]

These recommendations must be read with the footnotes that follow.

<table>
<tr><th>VACCINE ▼ AGE GROUP ▶</th><th>19-21 years</th><th>22-26 years</th><th>27-49 years</th><th>50-59 years</th><th>60-64 years</th><th>≥ 65 years</th></tr>
<tr><td>Influenza [2,*]</td><td colspan="6">1 dose annually</td></tr>
<tr><td>Tetanus, diphtheria, pertussis (Td/Tdap) [3,*]</td><td colspan="6">Substitute 1-time dose of Tdap for Td booster; then boost with Td every 10 yrs</td></tr>
<tr><td>Varicella [4,*]</td><td colspan="6">2 doses</td></tr>
<tr><td>Human papillomavirus (HPV) Female [5,*]</td><td colspan="2">3 doses</td><td></td><td></td><td></td><td></td></tr>
<tr><td>Human papillomavirus (HPV) Male [5,*]</td><td colspan="2">3 doses</td><td></td><td></td><td></td><td></td></tr>
<tr><td>Zoster [6]</td><td></td><td></td><td></td><td></td><td colspan="2">1 dose</td></tr>
<tr><td>Measles, mumps, rubella (MMR) [7,*]</td><td colspan="4">1 or 2 doses</td><td></td><td></td></tr>
<tr><td>Pneumococcal 13-valent conjugate (PCV13) [8,*]</td><td colspan="5">1 or 2 doses</td><td>1 dose</td></tr>
<tr><td>Pneumococcal polysaccharide (PPSV23) [9,10]</td><td colspan="6">1 dose</td></tr>
<tr><td>Meningococcal [11,*]</td><td colspan="6">1 or more doses</td></tr>
<tr><td>Hepatitis A [12,*]</td><td colspan="6">2 doses</td></tr>
<tr><td>Hepatitis B [13,*]</td><td colspan="6">3 doses</td></tr>
<tr><td>Haemophilus influenzae type b (Hib) [14,*]</td><td colspan="6">1 or 3 doses</td></tr>
</table>

*Covered by the Vaccine Injury Compensation Program

- **For all persons in this category who meet the age requirements and who lack documentation of vaccination or have no evidence of previous infection; zoster vaccine recommended regardless of prior episode of zoster**
- **Recommended if some other risk factor is present (e.g., on the basis of medical, occupational, lifestyle, or other indication)**
- No recommendation

Report all clinically significant postvaccination reactions to the Vaccine Adverse Event Reporting System (VAERS). Reporting forms and instructions on filing a VAERS report are available at www.vaers.hhs.gov or by telephone, 800-822-7967.

Information on how to file a Vaccine Injury Compensation Program claim is available at www.hrsa.gov/vaccinecompensation or by telephone, 800-338-2382. To file a claim for vaccine injury, contact the U.S. Court of Federal Claims, 717 Madison Place, N.W., Washington, D.C. 20005; telephone, 202-357-6400.

Additional information about the vaccines in this schedule, extent of available data, and contraindications for vaccination is also available at www.cdc.gov/vaccines or from the CDC-INFO Contact Center at 800-CDC-INFO (800-232-4636) in English and Spanish, 8:00 a.m. - 8:00 p.m. Eastern Time, Monday - Friday, excluding holidays.

Use of trade names and commercial sources is for identification only and does not imply endorsement by the U.S. Department of Health and Human Services.

The recommendations in this schedule were approved by the Centers for Disease Control and Prevention's (CDC) Advisory Committee on Immunization Practices (ACIP), the American Academy of Family Physicians (AAFP), the American College of Physicians (ACP), American College of Obstetricians and Gynecologists and American College of Nurse-Midwives (ACNM).

TABLE 5-20A Vaccines That Might Be Indicated for Adults Based on Medical and Other Indications: United States[1]

Note: These recommendations *must* be read with the footnotes that follow containing number of doses, intervals between doses, and other important information.

VACCINE ▼ INDICATION ►	Pregnancy	Immuno-compromising conditions (excluding human immunodeficiency virus [HIV])[4,6,7,10,15]	HIV infection CD4+ T lymphocyte count[4,6,7,10,14,15] < 200 cells/μL	HIV infection ≥ 200 cells/μL	Men who have sex with men (MSM)	Heart disease, chronic lung disease, chronic alcoholism	Asplenia (including elective splenectomy and persistent complement component deficiencies)[10,14]	Chronic liver disease	Kidney failure, end-stage renal disease, receipt of hemodialysis	Diabetes	Healthcare personnel
Influenza[2,*]	1 dose IIV annually				1 dose IIV or LAIV annually	1 dose IIV annually					1 dose IIV or LAIV annually
Tetanus, diphtheria, pertussis (Td/Tdap)[3,*]	1 dose Tdap each pregnancy	Substitute 1-time dose of Tdap for Td booster; then boost with Td every 10 yrs									
Varicella[4,*]	Contraindicated			2 doses							
Human papillomavirus (HPV) Female[5,*]		3 doses through age 26 yrs				3 doses through age 26 yrs					
Human papillomavirus (HPV) Male[5,*]		3 doses through age 26 yrs				3 doses through age 21 yrs					
Zoster[6]	Contraindicated				1 dose						
Measles, mumps, rubella (MMR)[7,*]	Contraindicated			1 or 2 doses							
Pneumococcal 13-valent conjugate (PCV13)[8,*]	1 or 2 doses										
Pneumococcal polysaccharide (PPSV23)[9,10]		1 dose									
Meningococcal[11,*]	1 or more doses										
Hepatitis A[12,*]	2 doses										
Hepatitis B[13,*]	3 doses										
Haemophilus influenzae type b (Hib)[14,*]		post-HSCT recipients only	1 or 3 doses								

*Covered by the Vaccine Injury Compensation Program

- (light shading) For all persons in this category who meet the age requirements and who lack documentation of vaccination or have no evidence of previous infection; zoster vaccine recommended regardless of prior episode of zoster
- (dark shading) Recommended if some other risk factor is present (e.g., on the basis of medical, occupational, lifestyle, or other indications)
- (no shading) No recommendation

These schedules indicate the recommended age groups and medical indications for which administration of currently licensed vaccines is commonly indicated for adults ages 19 years and older, as of February 1, 2014. For all vaccines being recommended on the Adult Immunization Schedule: a vaccine series does not need to be restarted, regardless of the time that has elapsed between doses. Licensed combination vaccines may be used whenever any components of the combination are indicated and when the vaccine's other components are not contraindicated. For detailed recommendations on all vaccines, including those used primarily for travelers or that are issued during the year, consult the manufacturers' package inserts and the complete statements from the Advisory Committee on Immunization Practices (www.cdc.gov/vaccines/hcp/acip-recs/index.html.) Use of trade names and commercial sources is for identification only and does not imply endorsement by the U.S. Department of Health and Human Services.

Footnotes: Recommended Immunization Schedule for Adults Aged 19 Years or Older — United States, 2014

1. **Additional information**
   - Additional guidance for the use of the vaccines described in this supplement is available at http://www.cdc.gov/vaccines/hcp/acip-recs/index.html.
   - Information on vaccination recommendations when vaccination status is unknown and other general immunization information can be found in the General Recommendations on Immunization at www.cdc.gov/mmwr/preview/mmwrhtml/rr6002a1.htm.
   - Information on travel vaccine requirements and recommendations (e.g., for hepatitis A and B, meningococcal, and other vaccines) is available at wwwnc.cdc.gov/travel/destinations.list.
   - Additional information and resources regarding vaccination of pregnant women can be found at http://www.cdc.gov/vaccines/adults/rec-vac/pregnant.html.
2. **Influenza vaccination**
   - Annual vaccination against influenza is recommended for all persons aged 6 months or older.
   - Persons aged 6 months or older, including pregnant women and persons with hives-only allergy to eggs, can receive the inactivated influenza vaccine (IIV). An age-appropriate IIV formulation should be used.
   - Adults aged 18 to 49 years can receive the recombinant influenza vaccine (RIV) (FluBlok). RIV does not contain any egg protein.
   - Healthy, nonpregnant persons aged 2 to 49 years without high-risk medical conditions can receive either intranasally administered live, attenuated influenza vaccine (LAIV) (FluMist), or IIV. Health care personnel who care for severely immunocompromised persons (i.e., those who require care in a protected environment) should receive IIV or RIV rather than LAIV.
   - The intramuscularly or intradermally administered IIV are options for adults aged 18 to 64 years.
   - Adults aged 65 years or older can receive the standard-dose IIV or the high-dose IIV (Fluzone High-Dose).
3. **Tetanus, diphtheria, and acellular pertussis (Td/Tdap) vaccination**
   - Administer 1 dose of Tdap vaccine to pregnant women during each pregnancy (preferred during 27 to 36 weeks' gestation) regardless of number of years since prior Td or Tdap vaccination.
   - Persons aged 11 years or older who have not received Tdap vaccine or for whom vaccine status is unknown should receive a dose of Tdap followed by tetanus and diphtheria toxoids (Td) booster doses every 10 years thereafter. Tdap can be administered regardless of interval since the most recent tetanus or diphtheria-toxoid containing vaccine.
   - Adults with an unknown or incomplete history of completing a 3-dose primary vaccination series with Td-containing vaccines should begin or complete a primary vaccination series including a Tdap dose.
   - For unvaccinated adults, administer the first 2 doses at least 4 weeks apart and the third dose 6 to 12 months after the second.
   - For incompletely vaccinated (i.e., less than 3 doses) adults, administer remaining doses.
   - Refer to the Advisory Commitee on Immunization Practices (ACIP) statement for recommendations for administering Td/Tdap as prophylaxis in wound management (see footnote #1).
4. **Varicella vaccination**
   - All adults without evidence of immunity to varicella (as defined below) should receive 2 doses of single-antigen varicella vaccine or a second dose if they have received only 1 dose.
   - Vaccination should be emphasized for those who have close contact with persons at high risk for severe disease (e.g., health care personnel and family contacts of persons with immunocompromising conditions) or are at high risk for exposure or transmission (e.g., teachers; child care employees; residents and staff members of institutional settings, including correctional institutions; college students; military personnel; adolescents and adults living in households with children; nonpregnant women of childbearing age; and international travelers).
   - Pregnant women should be assessed for evidence of varicella immunity. Women who do not have evidence of immunity should receive the first dose of varicella vaccine upon completion or termination of pregnancy and before discharge from the health care facility. The second dose should be administered 4 to 8 weeks after the first dose.
   - Evidence of immunity to varicella in adults includes any of the following:
     — documentation of 2 doses of varicella vaccine at least 4 weeks apart;
     — U.S.-born before 1980, except health care personnel and pregnant women;
     — history of varicella based on diagnosis or verification of varicella disease by a health care provider;
     — history of herpes zoster based on diagnosis or verification of herpes zoster disease by a health care provider; or
     — laboratory evidence of immunity or laboratory confirmation of disease.

5. **Human papillomavirus (HPV) vaccination**
   - Two vaccines are licensed for use in females, bivalent HPV vaccine (HPV2) and quadrivalent HPV vaccine (HPV4), and one HPV vaccine for use in males (HPV4).
   - For females, either HPV4 or HPV2 is recommended in a 3-dose series for routine vaccination at age 11 or 12 years and for those aged 13 through 26 years, if not previously vaccinated.
   - For males, HPV4 is recommended in a 3-dose series for routine vaccination at age 11 or 12 years and for those aged 13 through 21 years, if not previously vaccinated. Males aged 22 through 26 years may be vaccinated.
   - HPV4 is recommended for men who have sex with men through age 26 years for those who did not get any or all doses when they were younger.
   - Vaccination is recommended for immunocompromised persons (including those with HIV infection) through age 26 years for those who did not get any or all doses when they were younger.
   - A complete series for either HPV4 or HPV2 consists of 3 doses. The second dose should be administered 4 to 8 weeks (minimum interval of 4 weeks) after the first dose; the third dose should be administered 24 weeks after the first dose and 16 weeks after the second dose (minimum interval of at least 12 weeks).
   - HPV vaccines are not recommended for use in pregnant women. However, pregnancy testing is not needed before vaccination. If a woman is found to be pregnant after initiating the vaccination series, no intervention is needed; the remainder of the 3-dose series should be delayed until completion of pregnancy.
6. **Zoster vaccination**
   - A single dose of zoster vaccine is recommended for adults aged 60 years and older regardless of whether they report a prior episode of herpes zoster. Although the vaccine is licensed by the U.S. Food and Drug Administration for use among and can be administered to persons aged 50 years and older, ACIP recommends that vaccination begin at age 60 years.
   - Persons aged 60 years and older with chronic medical conditions may be vaccinated unless their condition constitutes a contraindication, such as pregnancy or severe immunodeficiency.
7. **Measles, mumps, rubella (MMR) vaccination**
   - Adults born before 1957 are generally considered immune to measles and mumps. All adults born in 1957 or later should have documentation of 1 or more doses of MMR vaccine unless they have a medical contraindication to the vaccine or laboratory evidence of immunity to each of the 3 diseases. Documentation of provider-diagnosed disease is not considered acceptable evidence of immunity for measles, mumps, or rubella.

   Measles component:
   - A routine second dose of MMR vaccine, administered a minimum of 28 days after the first dose, is recommended for adults who:
     —are students in postsecondary educational institutions;
     —work in a health care facility; or
     —plan to travel internationally.
   - Persons who received inactivated (killed) measles vaccine or measles vaccine of unknown type during 1963–1967 should be revaccinated with 2 doses of MMR vaccine.

   Mumps component:
   - A routine second dose of MMR vaccine, administered a minimum of 28 days after the first dose, is recommended for adults who:
     —are students in a postsecondary educational institution;
     —work in a health care facility; or
     —plan to travel internationally.
   - Persons vaccinated before 1979 with either killed mumps vaccine or mumps vaccine of unknown type who are at high risk for mumps infection (e.g., persons who are working in a health care facility) should be considered for revaccination with 2 doses of MMR vaccine.

   Rubella component:
   - For women of childbearing age, regardless of birth year, rubella immunity should be determined. If there is no evidence of immunity, women who are not pregnant should be vaccinated. Pregnant women who do not have evidence of immunity should receive MMR vaccine upon completion or termination of pregnancy and before discharge from the health care facility.

   Health care personnel born before 1957:
   - For unvaccinated health care personnel born before 1957 who lack laboratory evidence of measles, mumps, and/or rubella immunity or laboratory confirmation of disease, health care facilities should consider vaccinating personnel with 2 doses of MMR vaccine at the appropriate interval for measles and mumps or 1 dose of MMR vaccine for rubella.
8. **Pneumococcal conjugate (PCV13) vaccination**
   - Adults aged 19 years or older with immunocompromising conditions (including chronic renal failure and nephrotic syndrome), functional or anatomic asplenia, cerebrospinal fluid leaks, or cochlear implants who have not previously received PCV13 or PPSV23 should receive a single dose of PCV13 followed by a dose of PPSV23 at least 8 weeks later.
   - Adults aged 19 years or older with the aforementioned conditions who have previously received 1 or more doses of PPSV23 should receive a dose of PCV13 one or more years after the last PPSV23 dose was received. For adults who require additional doses of PPSV23, the first such dose should be given no sooner than 8 weeks after PCV13 and at least 5 years after the most recent dose of PPSV23.
   - When indicated, PCV13 should be administered to patients who are uncertain of their vaccination status history and have no record of previous vaccination.
   - Although PCV13 is licensed by the U.S. Food and Drug Administration for use among and can be administered to persons aged 50 years and older, ACIP recommends PCV13 for adults aged 19 years or older with the specific medical conditions noted above.
9. **Pneumococcal polysaccharide (PPSV23) vaccination**
   - When PCV13 is also indicated, PCV13 should be given first (see footnote 8).
   - Vaccinate all persons with the following indications:
     —all adults aged 65 years or older;
     —adults younger than 65 years with chronic lung disease (including chronic obstructive pulmonary disease, emphysema, and asthma), chronic cardiovascular diseases, diabetes mellitus, chronic renal failure, nephrotic syndrome, chronic liver disease (including cirrhosis), alcoholism, cochlear implants, cerebrospinal fluid leaks, immunocompromising conditions, and functional or anatomic asplenia (e.g., sickle cell disease and other hemoglobinopathies, congenital or acquired asplenia, splenic dysfunction, or splenectomy [if elective splenectomy is planned, vaccinate at least 2 weeks before surgery]);
     —residents of nursing homes or long-term care facilities; and
     —adults who smoke cigarettes.
   - Persons with immunocompromising conditions and other selected conditions are recommended to receive PCV13 and PPSV23 vaccines. See footnote # 10 for information on timing of PCV13 and PPSV23 vaccinations.
   - Persons with asymptomatic or symptomatic HIV infection should be vaccinated as soon as possible after their diagnosis.
   - When cancer chemotherapy or other immunosuppressive therapy is being considered, the interval between vaccination and initiation of immunosuppressive therapy should be at least 2 weeks. Vaccination during chemotherapy or radiation therapy should be avoided.
   - Routine use of PPSV23 vaccine is not recommended for American Indians/Alaska Natives or other persons younger than 65 years unless they have underlying medical conditions that are PPSV23 indications. However, public health authorities may consider recommending PPSV23 for American Indians/Alaska Natives who are living in areas where the risk for invasive pneumococcal disease is increased.
   - When indicated, PPSV23 should be administered to patients who are uncertain of their vaccination status and have no record of previous vaccination.
10. **Revaccination with PPSV23**
    - One-time revaccination 5 years after the first dose of PPSV23 is recommended for persons aged 19 through 64 years with chronic renal failure or nephrotic syndrome, functional or anatomic asplenia (e.g., sickle cell disease or splenectomy), or immunocompromising conditions.
    - Persons who received 1 or 2 doses of PPSV23 before age 65 years for any indication should receive another dose of the vaccine at age 65 years or later if at least 5 years have passed since their previous dose.
    - No further doses of PPSV23 are needed for persons vaccinated with PPSV23 at or after age 65 years.
11. **Meningococcal vaccination**
    - Administer 2 doses of quadrivalent meningococcal conjugate vaccine (MenACWY-D [Menactra]) at least 2 months apart to adults of all ages with functional asplenia or persistent complement component deficiencies. HIV infection is not an indication for routine indication with MenACWY-D. If an HIV-infected person of any age is vaccinated, 2 doses of MenACWY-D should be administered at least 2 months apart.
    - Administer a single dose of meningococcal vaccine to microbiologists routinely exposed to isolates of *Neisseria meningitidis*, military recruits, persons at risk during an outbreak attributable to a vaccine serogroup, and persons who travel to or live in countries in which meningococcal disease is hyperendemic or epidemic.
    - First-year college students up through age 21 years who are living in residence halls should be vaccinated if they have not received a dose on or after their 16th birthday.
    - MenACWY-D is preffered for adults wuth any of the preceding indicatins who are aged 55 years or younger as well as for adults aged 56 years or older who a) were vaccinated previously with MenACWY-D and are recommended for revaccination, or b) for whom multiple doses are anticipated. Meningococcal polysaccharide vaccine (MenACWY-CRM [Menveo] is preferred for adults aged 56 years or older who have not received Men ACWY-D previously and who require a single dose only (e.g., travelers.)
    - Revaccination with MenACWY-D every 5years is recommended for adults previously vaccinated with MenACWY-D or MenACWY-CRM who remain at increased risk for infection (e.g., adults with anatomic or functional asplenia, those with persistent complement component deficiencies, or microbiologists).

12. **Hepatitis A vaccination**
 - Vaccinate any person seeking protection from hepatitis A virus (HAV) infection and persons with any of the following indications:
   - —men who have sex with men and persons who use injection or noninjection illicit drugs;
   - —persons working with HAV-infected primates or with HAV in a research laboratory setting;
   - —persons with chronic liver disease and persons who receive clotting factor concentrates;
   - —persons traveling to or working in countries that have high or intermediate endemicity of hepatitis A; and
   - —unvaccinated persons who anticipate close personal contact (e.g., household or regular babysitting) with an international adoptee during the first 60 days after arrival in the United States from a country with high or intermediate endemicity. (See footnote #1 for more information on travel recommendations). The first dose of the 2-dose hepatitis A vaccine series should be administered as soon as adoption is planned, ideally 2 or more weeks before the arrival of the adoptee.
 - Single-antigen vaccine formulations should be administered in a 2-dose schedule at either 0 and 6 to 12 months (Havrix), or 0 and 6 to 18 months (Vaqta). If the combined hepatitis A and hepatitis B vaccine (Twinrix) is used, administer 3 doses at 0, 1, and 6 months; alternatively, a 4-dose schedule may be used, administered on days 0, 7, and 21 to 30 followed by a booster dose at month 12.

13. **Hepatitis B vaccination**
 - Vaccinate persons with any of the following indications and any person seeking protection from hepatitis B virus (HBV) infection:
   - — sexually active persons who are not in a long-term, mutually monogamous relationship (e.g., persons with more than 1 sex partner during the previous 6 months); persons seeking evaluation or treatment for a sexually transmitted disease (STD); current or recent injection drug users; and men who have sex with men;
   - — health care personnel and public safety workers who are potentially exposed to blood or other infectious body fluids;
   - — persons with diabetes who are younger than age 60 years as soon as feasible after diagnosis; persons with diabetes who are age 60 years or older at the discretion of the treating clinician based on the likelihood of acquiring HBV infection, including the risk posed by an increased need for assisted blood glucose monitoring in long-term care facilities, the likelihood of experiencing chronic sequelae if infected with HBV, and the likelihood of immune response to vaccination;
   - — persons with end-stage renal disease, including patients receiving hemodialysis, persons with HIV infection, and persons with chronic liver disease;
   - — household contacts and sex partners of hepatitis B surface antigen–positive persons, clients and staff members of institutions for persons with developmental disabilities, and international travelers to countries with high or intermediate prevalence of chronic HBV infection; and
   - —all adults in the following settings: STD treatment facilities, HIV testing and treatment facilities, facilities providing drug abuse treatment and prevention services, health care settings targeting services to injection drug users or men who have sex with men, correctional facilities, end-stage renal disease programs and facilities for chronic hemodialysis patients, and institutions and nonresidential day care facilities for persons with developmental disabilities.
 - Administer missing doses to complete a 3-dose series of hepatitis B vaccine to those persons not vaccinated or not completely vaccinated. The second dose should be administered 1 month after the first dose; the third dose should be given at least 2 months after the second dose (and at least 4 months after the first dose). If the combined hepatitis A and hepatitis B vaccine (Twinrix) is used, give 3 doses at 0, 1, and 6 months; alternatively, a 4-dose Twinrix schedule, administered on days 0, 7, and 21 to 30 followed by a booster dose at month 12 may be used.
 - Adult patients receiving hemodialysis or with other immunocompromising conditions should receive 1 dose of 40 mcg/mL (Recombivax HB) administered on a 3-dose schedule at 0, 1, and 6 months or 2 doses of 20 mcg/mL (Engerix-B) administered simultaneously on a 4-dose schedule at 0, 1, 2, and 6 months.

14. ***Haemophilus influenzae* type b (Hib) vaccination**
 - One dose of Hib vaccine should be administered to persons who have functional or anatomic asplenia or sickle cell disease or are undergoing elective splenectomy if they have not previously received Hib vaccine. Hib vaccination 14 or more days before splenectomy is suggested.
 - Recipients of a hematopoietic stem cell transplant should be vaccinated with a 3-dose regimen 6 to 12 months after a successful transplant, regardless of vaccination history; at least 4 weeks should separate doses.
 - Hib vaccine is not recommended for adults with HIV infection since their risk for Hib infection is low.

15. **Immunocompromising conditions**
 - Inactivated vaccines generally are acceptable (e.g., pneumococcal, meningococcal, and inactivated influenza vaccine) and live vaccines generally are avoided in persons with immune deficiencies or immunocompromising conditions. Information on specific conditions is available at http://www.cdc.gov/vaccines/pubs/acip-list.htm.

TABLE 5-20B Contraindications and Precautions to Commonly Used Vaccines in Adults[1*†]

Vaccine	Contraindications	Precautions
Influenza, inactivated vaccine (IIV)	Severe allergic reaction (e.g., anaphylaxis) after previous dose of any influenza vaccine or to a vaccine component, including egg protein.	Moderate or severe acute illness with or without fever. History of Guillain-Barré Syndrome (GBS) within 6 weeks of previous influenza vaccination. Persons who experience only hives with exposure to eggs should receive IIV with additional safety precautions.[2]
Influenza, live attenuated (LAIV)[3]	Severe allergic reaction (e.g., anaphylaxis) after previous dose of any influenza vaccine or to a vaccine component, including egg protein. Conditions for which the Advisory Committee on Immunization Practices (ACIP) recommends against use, but which are not contraindications in vaccine package insert: immune suppression, certain chronic medical conditions such as asthma, diabetes, heart or kidney disease. and pregnancy.[4]	Moderate or severe acute illness with or without fever. History of GBS within 6 weeks of previous influenza vaccination. Receipt of specific antivirals (i.e., amantadine, rimantadine, zanamivir, or oseltamivir) 48 hours before vaccination. Avoid use of these antiviral drugs for 14 days after vaccination.
Tetanus, diphtheria, pertussis (Tdap); tetanus, diphtheria (Td)	Severe allergic reaction (e.g., anaphylaxis) after a previous dose or to a vaccine component. For pertussis-containing vaccines: encephalopathy (e.g., coma, decreased level of consciousness, or prolonged seizures) not attributable to another identifiable cause within 7 days of administration of a previous dose of Tdap or diphtheria and tetanus toxoids and pertussis (DTP) or diphtheria and tetanus toxoids and acellular pertussis (DTaP) vaccine.	Moderate or severe acute illness with or without fever. GBS within 6 weeks after a previous dose of tetanus toxoid–containing vaccine. History of arthus-type hypersensitivity reactions after a previous dose of tetanus or diptheria toxoid–containing vaccine; defer vaccination until at least 10 years have elapsed since the last tetanus toxoid-containing vaccine. For pertussis-containing vaccines: progressive or unstable neurologic disorder, uncontrolled seizures, or progressive encephalopathy until a treatment regimen has been established and the condition has stabilized.
Varicella[2]	Severe allergic reaction (e.g., anaphylaxis) after a previous dose or to a vaccine component. Known severe immunodeficiency (e.g., from hematologic and solid tumors, receipt of chemotherapy, congenital immunodeficiency, or long-term immunosuppressive therapy[5] or patients with human immunodeficiency virus (HIV) infection who are severely immunocompromised). Pregnancy.	Recent (within 11 months) receipt of antibody-containing blood product (specific interval depends on product).[6,7] Moderate or severe acute illness with or without fever. Receipt of specific antivirals (i.e., acyclovir, famciclovir, or valacyclovir) 24 hours before vaccination; avoid use of these antiviral drugs for 14 days after vaccination.
Human papillomavirus (HPV)	Severe allergic reaction (e.g., anaphylaxis) after a previous dose or to a vaccine component.	Moderate or severe acute illness with or without fever. Pregnancy.
Zoster	Severe allergic reaction (e.g., anaphylaxis) to a vaccine component. Known severe immunodeficiency (e.g., from hematologic and solid tumors, receipt of chemotherapy, or long-term immunosuppressive therapy[5] or patients with HIV infection who are severely immunocompromised). Pregnancy.	Moderate or severe acute illness with or without fever. Receipt of specific antivirals (i.e., acyclovir, famciclovir, or valacyclovir) 24 hours before vaccination; avoid use of these antiviral drugs for 14 days after vaccination.
Measles, mumps, rubella (MMR)[3]	Severe allergic reaction (e.g., anaphylaxis) after a previous dose or to a vaccine component. Known severe immunodeficiency (e.g., from hematologic and solid tumors, receipt of chemotherapy, congenital immunodeficiency, or long-term immunosuppressive therapy[5] or patients with HIV infection who are severely immunocompromised). Pregnancy.	Moderate or severe acute illness with or without fever. Recent (within 11 months) receipt of antibody-containing blood product (specific interval depends on product).[6,7] History of thrombocytopenia or thrombocytopenic purpura. Need for tuberculin skin testing.[8]

TABLE 5-20B Contraindications and Precautions to Commonly Used Vaccines in Adults[1*†]—cont'd

Vaccine	Contraindications	Precautions
Pneumococcal polysaccharide (PPSV)	Severe allergic reaction (e.g., anaphylaxis) after a previous dose or to a vaccine component.	Moderate or severe acute illness with or without fever.
Pneumococcal conjugate (PCV13)	Severe allergic reaction (e.g., anaphylaxis) after a previous dose or to a vaccine component, including to any vaccine containing diphtheria toxoid.	Moderate or severe acute illness with or without fever.
Meningococcal, conjugate, (MCV4); meningococcal, polysaccharide (MPSV4)	Severe allergic reaction (e.g., anaphylaxis) after a previous dose or to a vaccine component.	Moderate or severe acute illness with or without fever.
Hepatitis A (HepA)	Severe allergic reaction (e.g., anaphylaxis) after a previous dose or to a vaccine component.	Moderate or severe acute illness with or without fever.
Hepatitis B (HepB)	Severe allergic reaction (e.g., anaphylaxis) after a previous dose or to a vaccine component.	Moderate or severe acute illness with or without fever.

1. Vaccine package inserts and the full ACIP recommendations for these vaccines should be consulted for additional information on vaccine-related contraindications and precautions and for more information on vaccine excipients. Events or conditions listed as precautions should be reviewed carefully. Benefits of and risks for administering a specific vaccine to a person under these circumstances should be considered. If the risk from the vaccine is believed to outweigh the benefit, the vaccine should not be administered. If the benefit of vaccination is believed to outweigh the risk, the vaccine should be administered. A contraindication is a condition in a recipient that increases the chance of a serious adverse reaction. Therefore, a vaccine should not be administered when a contraindication is present.
2. CDC. Prevention and control of influenza with vaccines: recommendations of the Advisory Committee on Immunization Practices (ACIP) — United States, 2012–13 influenza season. MMWR 2012;61:613-8.
3. LAIV, MMR, and varicella vaccines can be administered on the same day. If not administered on the same day, these live vaccines should be separated by at least 28 days.
4. For a complete list of conditions that CDC considers to be reasons to avoid getting LAIV, see CDC. Prevention and control of influenza with vaccines: recommendations of the Advisory Committee on Immunization Practices (ACIP), 2010. MMWR 2010;59(No. RR-8). Available at http://www.cdc.gov/vaccines/pubs/acip-list.htm.
5. Immunosuppressive steroid dose is considered to be 2 or more weeks of daily receipt of 20 mg prednisone or the equivalent. Vaccination should be deferred for at least 1 month after discontinuation of such therapy. Providers should consult ACIP recommendations for complete information on the use of specific live vaccines among persons on immune-suppressing medications or with immune suppression because of other reasons.
6. Vaccine should be deferred for the appropriate interval if replacement immune globulin products are being administered.
7. See CDC. General recommendations on immunization: recommendations of the Advisory Committee on Immunization Practices (ACIP). MMWR 2011;60(No. RR-2). Available at http://www.cdc.gov/vaccines/pubs/acip-list.htm.
8. Measles vaccination might suppress tuberculin reactivity temporarily. Measles-containing vaccine may be administered on the same day as tuberculin skin testing. If testing cannot be performed until after the day of MMR vaccination, the test should be postponed for at least 4 weeks after the vaccination. If an urgent need exists to skin test, do so with the understanding that reactivity might be reduced by the vaccine.

* Adapted from CDC. Table 6. Contraindications and precautions to commonly used vaccines. General recommendations on immunization: recommendations of the Advisory Committee on Immunization Practices. MMWR 2011;60(No. RR-2):40–41 and from Atkinson W, Wolfe S, Hamborsky J, eds. Appendix A. Epidemiology and prevention of vaccine preventable diseases. 12th ed. Washington, DC: Public Health Foundation, 2011. Available at http://www.cdc.gov/vaccines/pubs/pinkbook/index.html.

† Regarding latex allergy. Consult the package insert for any vaccine administered.

TABLE 5-21 Immunization and Pregnancy

Vaccine	Before Pregnancy	During Pregnancy	After Pregnancy	Type of Vaccine	Route
Hepatitis A	If at high risk for disease	If at high risk for disease	If at high risk for disease	Inactivated	IM
Hepatitis B	Yes, if at risk	Yes, if at risk	Yes, if at risk	Inactivated	IM
Human papillomavirus (HPV)	Yes, if 9 to 26 years of age	No, under study	Yes, if 9 to 26 years of age	Inactivated	IM
Influenza TIV	Yes	Yes	Yes	Inactivated	IM
Influenza LAIV	Yes, if <50 years and healthy; avoid conception for 4 weeks	No	Yes, if <50 years and healthy; avoid conception for 4 weeks	Live	Nasal spray
MMR	Yes, avoid conception for 4 weeks	No	Yes, give immediately post-partum if susceptible to rubella	Live	SC
Meningococcal:	If indicated	If indicated	If indicated		
• Polysaccharide				Inactivated	SC
• Conjugate				Inactivated	IM
Pneumococcal polysaccharide	If indicated	If indicated	If indicated	Inactivated	IM or SC
Tetanus/diphtheria Td	Yes, Tdap preferred	If indicated	Yes, Tdap preferred	Toxoid	IM
Tdap, one dose only	Yes, preferred	If high risk of pertussis; otherwise, Td preferred	Yes, preferred	Toxoid/inactivated	IM
Varicella	Yes, avoid conception for 4 weeks	No	Yes, give immediately post-partum if susceptible	Live	SC

IM, Intramuscular; *LAIV,* live, attenuated influenza vaccine; *SC,* subcutaneous; *Tdap,* tetanus and diphtheria toxoids and acellular pertussis; *TIV,* trivalent inactivated influenza vaccine.

TABLE 5-22 Immunizing Agents and Immunization Schedules for Health Care Workers (HCWs)*

Generic Name	Primary Schedule and Booster(s)	Indications	Major Precautions and Contraindications	Special Considerations
Immunizing Agents Strongly Recommended for Health Care Workers				
Hepatitis B (HB) recombinant vaccine	Two doses IM 4 wk apart; third dose 5 mo after second; booster doses not necessary	**Preexposure:** HCWs at risk for exposure to blood or body fluids	Based on limited data no risk of adverse effects to developing fetuses is apparent. Pregnancy should *not* be considered a contraindication to vaccination of women. Previous anaphylactic reaction to common baker's yeast is a contraindication to vaccination.	The vaccine produces neither therapeutic nor adverse effects on HB-infected persons. Prevaccination serologic screening is not indicated for persons being vaccinated because of occupational risk. HCWs who have contact with patients or blood should be tested 1-2 mo after vaccination to determine serologic response.
Hepatitis B immune globulin (HBIG)	0.06 ml/kg IM as soon as possible after exposure. A second dose of HBIG should be administered 1 mo later if the HB vaccine series has not been started.	**Postexposure prophylaxis:** For persons exposed to blood or body fluids containing HBsAg and who are not immune to HBV infection—0.06 ml/kg IM as soon as possible (but no later than 7 days after exposure)		
Influenza vaccine (inactivated whole-virus and split-virus vaccines)	Annual vaccination with current vaccine Administered IM	HCWs who have contact with patients at high risk for influenza or its complications; HCWs who work in long-term care facilities; HCWs with high-risk medical conditions or who are aged ≥65 yr	History of anaphylactic hypersensitivity to egg ingestion	No evidence exists of risk to mother or fetus when the vaccine is administered to a pregnant woman with an underlying high-risk condition. Influenza vaccination is recommended during second and third trimesters of pregnancy because of increased risk for hospitalization.
Measles live-virus vaccine	One dose SC; second dose at least 1 mo later	HCWs† born during or after 1957 who do not have documentation of having received two doses of live vaccine on or after the first birthday **or** a history of physician-diagnosed measles or serologic evidence of immunity. Vaccination should be considered for all HCWs who lack proof of immunity, including those born before 1957.	Pregnancy; immunocompromised persons,‡ including HIV-infected persons who have evidence of severe immunosuppression; anaphylaxis after gelatin ingestion or administration of neomycin; recent administration of immune globulin.	MMR is the vaccine of choice if recipients are likely to be susceptible to rubella and/or mumps as well as measles. Persons vaccinated between 1963 and 1967 with a killed measles vaccine alone, killed vaccine followed by live vaccine, or with a vaccine of unknown type should be revaccinated with two doses of live measles virus vaccine.
Mumps live-virus vaccine	One dose SC; second dose at least 1 mo later	HCWs† believed to be susceptible can be vaccinated. Adults born before 1957 can be considered immune.	Pregnancy; immunocompromised persons,‡ history of anaphylactic reaction after gelatin ingestion or administration of neomycin	MMR is the vaccine of choice if recipients are likely to be susceptible to measles and rubella, as well as mumps.
Hepatitis A virus (HAV) vaccine	Two doses of vaccine either 6-12 mo apart (HAVRIX), or 6 mo apart (VAQTA)	Not routinely indicated for HCWs in the United States. Persons who work with HAV-infected primates or with HAV in a research laboratory setting should be vaccinated.	History of anaphylactic hypersensitivity to alum or, for HAVRIX, the preservative 2-phenoxyethanol. The safety of the vaccine in pregnant women has not been determined; the risk associated with vaccination should be weighed against the risk for hepatitis A in women who may be at high risk for exposure to HAV.	
Meningococcal vaccine	One dose in volume and by route specified by manufacturer; single booster for adults 19 to 21 years of age if the first dose was given before age 16	Laboratory personnel and others with exposure risk.	The safety of the vaccine in pregnant women has not been evaluated; it should not be administered during pregnancy unless the risk for infection is high.	

TABLE 5-22 Immunizing Agents and Immunization Schedules for Health Care Workers (HCWs)—cont'd

Generic Name	Primary Schedule and Booster(s)	Indications	Major Precautions and Contraindications	Special Considerations
Typhoid vaccine, IM, SC, and oral	IM vaccine: One 0.5-ml/dose, booster 0.5 ml every 2 yr SC vaccine: Two 0.5-ml doses, ≥4 wk apart, booster 0.5 ml SC or 0.1 ID every 3 yr if exposure continues Oral vaccine: Four doses on alternate days. The manufacturer recommends revaccination with the entire 4-dose series every 5 yr	Workers in microbiology laboratories who frequently work with *Salmonella typhi*	Severe local or systemic reaction to a previous dose. Ty21a (oral) vaccine should not be administered to immunocompromised persons† or to persons receiving antimicrobial agents.	Vaccination should not be considered an alternative to the use of proper procedures when handling specimens and cultures in the laboratory.
Vaccinia vaccine (smallpox)	One dose administered with a bifurcated needle; boosters administered every 10 yr	Laboratory workers who directly handle cultures with vaccinia, recombinant vaccinia viruses, or orthopox viruses that infect human beings	The vaccine is contraindicated in pregnancy, in persons with eczema or a history of eczema, and in immunocompromised persons† and their household contacts.	Vaccination may be considered for HCWs who have direct contact with contaminated dressings or other infectious material from volunteers in clinical studies involving recombinant vaccinia virus.
Other Vaccine-Preventable Diseases				
Tetanus and diphtheria and pertussis (Tdap)	Two IM doses 4 wk apart or tetanus and diphtheria toxoid for adults with uncertain or incomplete primary vaccination; third dose 6-12 mo after second dose; booster every 10 yr. Substitute a one-time dose of Tdap for one of the doses of Td, either in the primary series or for the routine booster, whichever comes first.	All adults	Except in the first trimester, pregnancy is not a precaution. History of a neurologic reaction or immediate hypersensitivity reaction after a previous dose. History of severe local (Arthus-type) reaction after a previous dose. Such persons should not receive further routine or emergency doses of Td for 10 yr.	Tetanus prophylaxis in wound management‡
Pneumococcal polysaccharide vaccine (23 valent)	One dose, 0.5 ml, IM or SC; revaccination recommended for those at highest risk ≥5 yr after the first dose	Adults who are at increased risk of pneumococcal disease and its complications because of underlying health conditions; older adults, especially those age ≥65 who are healthy	The safety of vaccine in pregnant women has not been evaluated; it should not be administered during pregnancy unless the risk for infection is high. Previous recipients of any type of pneumococcal polysaccharide vaccine who are at highest risk for fatal infection or antibody loss may be revaccinated ≥5 yr after the first dose.	
Rubella live-virus vaccine	One dose SC; second dose at least 1 mo later	Indicated for HCWs,† both men and women, who do not have documentation of having received live vaccine on or after their first birthday **or** laboratory evidence of immunity. Adults born before 1957, **except women who can become pregnant,** can be considered immune.	Pregnancy; immunocompromised persons†; history of anaphylactic reaction after administration of neomycin	The risk for rubella vaccine–associated malformations in the offspring of women pregnant when vaccinated or who become pregnant within 3 mo after vaccination is negligible. Such women should be counseled regarding the theoretic basis of concern for the fetus. MMR is the vaccine of choice if recipients are likely to be susceptible to measles or mumps as well as rubella.
Varicella-zoster live-virus vaccine	Two 0.5-ml doses SC 4-8 wk apart if ≥13 yr	Indicated for HCWs† who do not have either a reliable history of varicella or serologic evidence of immunity	Pregnancy, immunocompromised persons,‡ history of anaphylactic reaction after receipt of neomycin or gelatin. Avoid salicylate use for 6 wk after vaccination.	Vaccine is available from the manufacturer for certain patients with acute lymphocytic leukemia in remission. Because 71%-93% of persons without a history of varicella are immune, serologic testing before vaccination is likely to be cost effective.

TABLE 5-22 Immunizing Agents and Immunization Schedules for Health Care Workers (HCWs)—cont'd

Generic Name	Primary Schedule and Booster(s)	Indications	Major Precautions and Contraindications	Special Considerations
Varicella-zoster immune globulin (VZIG)	Persons <50 kg: 125 μg/10 kg IM; persons ≥50 kg: 625 μg§	Persons known or likely to be susceptible (particularly those at high risk for complications, e.g., pregnant women) who have close and prolonged exposure to a contact case or to an infectious hospital staff worker or patient		Serologic testing may help in assessing whether to administer VZIG. If use of VZIG prevents varicella disease, patient should be vaccinated subsequently.
BCG Vaccination				
Bacille Calmette-Guérin (BCG) vaccine (TB)	One percutaneous dose of 0.3 ml; no booster dose recommended	Should be considered only for HCWs in areas where multidrug TB is prevalent, a strong likelihood of infection exists, and where comprehensive infection control precautions have failed to prevent TB transmission to HCWs	Should not be administered to immunocompromised persons,‡ pregnant women	In the United States TB-control efforts are directed toward early identification, treatment of cases, and preventive therapy with isoniazid.
Other Immunobiologics That Are or May Be Indicated for HCWs				
Immune globulin (hepatitis A)	**Postexposure**—One IM dose of 0.02 ml/kg administered ≤2 wk after exposure	Indicated for HCWs exposed to feces of infectious patients	Contraindicated in persons with IgA deficiency; do not administer within 2 wk after MMR vaccine or 3 wk after varicella vaccine. Delay administration of MMR vaccine for ≥3 mo and varicella vaccine ≥5 mo after administration of immune globulin	Administer in large muscle mass (deltoid, gluteal).

Modified from *MMWR* 46(RR-18), 1998.

HBsAg, Hepatitis B surface antigen; *HBV,* hepatitis B virus; *HIV,* human immunodeficiency virus; *IM,* intramuscular; *MMR,* measles, mumps, rubella vaccine; *SC,* subcutaneous; *TB,* tuberculosis.

*Persons who provide health care to patients or work in institutions that provide patient care (e.g., physicians, nurses, emergency medical personnel, dental professionals and students, medical and nursing students, laboratory technicians, hospital volunteers, and administrative and support staff in health care institutions).

†All HCWs (i.e., medical or nonmedical, paid or volunteer, full time or part time, student or nonstudent, with or without patient-care responsibilities) who work in health care institutions (e.g., inpatient and outpatient, public and private) should be immune to measles, rubella, and varicella.

‡Persons immunocompromised because of immune deficiency diseases, HIV infection, leukemia, lymphoma or generalized malignancy, or immunosuppressed as a result of therapy with corticosteroids, alkylating drugs, antimetabolites, or radiation.

§Some experts recommend 125 μg/10 kg regardless of total body weight.

TABLE 5-23 Recommendations for Persons with Medical Conditions Requiring Special Vaccination Considerations

Condition	Tdap	MMR	Varicella	HBV	HAV	Pneumovax[a]	Influenza[b]	HbCV	Meningococcal	IPV	Other Live Vaccines[c]	Other Killed Vaccines[d]
HIV infection	Rou	Rou/Contr[e]	Contr[f]	Rou[g]	Rou	Rec	Rec	Cons	Rou	Rou	Contr	Rou
Severe immunocompromise[h]	Rou	Contr	Contr[f]	Rou[g]	Rou	Rec	Rec	Rou[i]	Rou	Rou	Contr	Rou
Renal failure	Rou	Rou	Rou	Rec[g]	Rou	Rec	Rec	Rou	Rou	Rou	Rou	Rou
Diabetes	Rou	Rou	Rou	Rou	Rou	Rec	Rec	Rou	Rou	Rou	Rou	Rou
Chronic liver disease	Rou	Rou	Rou	Rou	Rec	Rec	Rec	Rou	Rou	Rou	Rou	Rou
Cardiac disease	Rou	Rou	Rou	Rou	Rou	Rec	Rec	Rou	Rou	Rou	Rou	Rou
Pulmonary disease	Rou	Rou	Rou	Rou	Rou	Rec	Rec	Rou	Rou	Rou	Rou	Rou
Alcoholism	Rou	Rou	Rou	Rou	Rou	Rec	Rec	Rou	Rou	Rou	Rou	Rou
Functional/anatomic asplenia	Rou	Rou	Rou	Rou	Rou	Rec[j]	Rec	Rec[j]	Rec[j]	Rou	Rou	Rou
Terminal complement deficiency	Rou	Rou	Rou	Rou	Rou	Rou	Rou	Rou	Rec	Rou	Rou	
Clotting factor disorders	Rou	Rou	Rou	Rec	Rec	Rou	Rou	Rou	Rou	Rou	Rou	Rou

Modified and updated from *MMWR* 42(RR-4):16, 1993.

Cons, Consider vaccination; *Contr,* contraindicated; *HAV,* hepatitis A virus; *HbCV, Haemophilus influenzae* conjugate vaccine; *HBV,* hepatitis B virus; *IPV,* inactivated poliomyelitis vaccine; *MMR,* measles-mumps-rubella; *Rec,* recommended; *Rou,* routine as outlined for all adults; *Tdap,* tetanus and diphtheria toxoids and acellular pertussis.

[a]Pneumovax should be repeated in 5 yr for patients in whom vaccine is recommended. Asthma without chronic obstructive pulmonary disease is not an indication for the vaccine.

[b]Influenza vaccine should also be given to caregivers and household members.

[c]Includes bacille Calmette-Guérin, vaccinia, oral typhoid, yellow fever (if exposure cannot be avoided, persons with HIV can be given yellow fever vaccine; see text).

[d]Includes rabies (check postvaccination titers in HIV or severely immunocompromised persons), Lyme disease, inactivated typhoid, cholera, plague, and anthrax.

[e]For asymptomatic, nonseverely immunocompromised persons with HIV, MMR can be used; it is contraindicated in severely immunocompromised persons. MMR can be considered in symptomatic HIV patients without severe immunocompromise.

[f]Varicella can be given to household members and caregivers, but if varicella-like rash develops after vaccination, contact should be avoided.

[g]Recommended for persons with severe chronic renal failure approaching or already receiving dialysis, and higher doses should be given. Antibody titers should be measured after vaccination in these patients and in those with HIV or severe immunocompromise (who may require higher doses) to ensure adequate response. Yearly titers should be measured in dialysis patients.

[h]Severe immunocompromise can result from congenital immunodeficiency, leukemia, lymphoma, malignancy, organ transplant, chemotherapy, radiation therapy, or high-dose corticosteroids.

[i]Only for persons with Hodgkin's disease.

[j]Give at least 2 wk in advance of elective splenectomy.

TABLE 5-24 Vaccinations for International Travel

Disease*	Areas Affected†	Prophylaxis Recommended	Ideal Time between Last Vaccine Dose and Travel
Tetanus	All	All travelers; vaccine series/booster	Probably 30 days for series; anamnestic response to booster
Measles	All	If born after 1956; ensure immunity by antibody titer, diagnosed measles, or two doses of vaccine	As MMR, 7-14 days
Rubella	All	If born after 1956 and any female of childbearing age; rubella titer or one dose of vaccine	As MMR, 7-14 days
Mumps	All	If born after 1956; ensure immunity by antibody titer, diagnosed mumps, or one dose of vaccine	As MMR, 7-14 days
Varicella	All	All travelers; antibody titer, reported illness, or vaccine series	7-14 days
Hepatitis B	5%-20% of population are carriers in Africa, Middle East except Israel, all Southeast Asia, Amazon basin, Haiti, and Dominican Republic; 1%-5% of population are carriers in south-central and southwest Asia, Israel, Japan, Americas, Russia, and eastern and southern Europe	Travelers for more than 6 mo in close contact with population or for less time but with high-risk activities (close household contact, seeking dental or medical care, sex); vaccine series	Probably 30 days
Hepatitis A	Developing countries	Travelers to rural areas; eating and drinking in settings of poor sanitation; vaccine or pooled immune globulin	Vaccine, 30 days Pooled IG, 2 days
Influenza	Tropics throughout the year; southern hemisphere from April to September	Travelers for whom vaccine is otherwise indicated; give current vaccine and revaccinate in fall as usual	7-14 days
Meningococcus*	Sub-Saharan Africa "belt" (Senegal to Ethiopia) from December to June; required for pilgrims to Saudi Arabia during Hajj; epidemics reported in other African nations, India, Nepal, and Mongolia	All travelers; vaccine	7-10 days
Rabies	Endemic dog rabies exists in Mexico, El Salvador, Guatemala, Peru, Colombia, Ecuador, India, Nepal, Philippines, Sri Lanka, Thailand, and Vietnam	Travelers staying for more than 30 days or at high risk of exposure to domestic or wild animals; vaccine series/booster	7-14 days
Poliomyelitis	Developing countries not in western hemisphere; at risk all year in tropics; in temperate zones, incidence increases in summer and fall	All travelers; vaccine series/booster	Parenteral vaccine series, 28 day
Typhoid fever	Many countries in Asia, Africa, Central America, and South America	Travelers with prolonged stay in rural areas with poor sanitation; vaccine series/booster	Oral vaccine, 7 days Parenteral vaccine, probably 14 days
Yellow fever*	North and central South America, forest-savannah zones of Africa; some countries in Africa, Asia, and Middle East require travelers from endemic areas to be vaccinated	All travelers; vaccine/booster at approved yellow fever vaccination center.	10 days
Japanese encephalitis	Seasonally in most areas of Asia, Indian subcontinent, and western Pacific islands; in temperate zones, incidence increases in summer and early fall; in tropics, year-round incidence	Travelers staying for more than 30 days in high-risk rural areas; staying outdoors during transmission season; vaccine series	10 days
Cholera*	Certain undeveloped countries	If required by local authorities, one dose usually suffices; primary series only for those living in high-risk areas under poor sanitary conditions or those with compromised gastric defense mechanisms (achlorhydria, antacid therapy, previous ulcer surgery); booster every 6 mo	Probably 30 days
Plague	Africa, Asia, and Americas in rural mountainous or upland areas	Travelers whose research or field activities bring them in contact with rodents; vaccine series/booster; consider taking tetracycline (500 mg four times a day) for chemoprophylaxis (inferred from clinical experience in treating plague)	Probably 30 days

From Noble J: *Primary care medicine,* ed 3, St Louis, 2001, Mosby.

IG, Immune globulin; *MMR,* measles-mumps-rubella.

*Only yellow fever vaccine is required for entry by any country; cholera vaccine may be required by some local authorities. Meningococcus vaccine is required for pilgrims to Mecca, in Saudia Arabia, during Hajj. However, it is important to follow Centers for Disease Control and Prevention (CDC) recommendations for all vaccines to prevent disease. If a required vaccine is contraindicated or withheld for any reason, attempts should be made to obtain a waiver from the country's consulate or embassy.

†Because areas affected can change, and for more specific details, consult the CDC's traveler's hotline.

Recommendations and Implementation Strategies for Hepatitis B Vaccination of Adults

BOX 5-1 Adults Recommended to Receive Hepatitis B Vaccination

Persons at Risk for Infection by Sexual Exposure
- Sex partners of persons who are HBsAg positive
- Sexually active persons who are not in a long-term, mutually monogamous relationship (e.g., persons who have had more than one sex partner during the previous 6 months)
- Persons seeking evaluation or treatment for a sexually transmitted disease
- Men who have sex with men

Persons at Risk for Infection by Percutaneous or Mucosal Exposure to Blood
- Current or recent users of injection drugs
- Household contacts of persons who are HBsAg positive
- Residents and staff of facilities for developmentally disabled persons
- Health care and public safety workers with reasonably anticipated risk for exposure to blood or blood-contaminated body fluids
- Persons with end-stage renal disease, including predialysis, hemodialysis, peritoneal dialysis, and home dialysis patients

Others
- International travelers to regions with high or intermediate levels (HBsAg prevalence of ≥2%) of endemic HBV infection
- Persons with chronic liver disease
- Persons with HIV infection
- All other persons seeking protection from HBV infection

From CDC: A comprehensive immunization strategy to eliminate transmission of hepatitis B virus infection in the United States: recommendations of the Advisory Committee on Immunization Practices (ACIP), *MMWR* 55(RR-16):15, 2006.

HbsAg, Hepatitis B surface antigen; *HBV,* hepatitis B virus.

BOX 5-2 Hepatitis B Vaccine Schedules for Adults (Aged ≥20 yr)*

0, 1, and 6 months
0, 1, and 4 months
0, 2, and 4 months
0, 1, 2, and 12 months†

From CDC: A comprehensive immunization strategy to eliminate transmission of hepatitis B virus infection in the United States: recommendations of the Advisory Committee on Immunization Practices (ACIP), *MMWR* 55(RR-16):15, 2006.

*All schedules are applicable to single-antigen hepatitis B vaccines; Twinrix (combined hepatitis A and hepatitis B vaccine) may be administered at 0, 1, and 6 months.

†A 4-dose schedule of Engerix-B is licensed for all age groups.

TABLE 5-25 Recommended Doses of Currently Licensed Formulations of Adult Hepatitis B Vaccine by Group and Vaccine Type

	SINGLE-ANTIGEN VACCINE				COMBINATION VACCINE	
	Recombivax HB[a]		Engerix-B[b]		Twinrix[b,c]	
Group	Dose (μg)[d]	Vol. (ml)	Dose (μg)[d]	Vol. (ml)	Dose (μg)[d]	Vol. (ml)
Adults (aged ≥20 yr)	10	1.0	20	1.0	20	1.0
Hemodialysis patients and other immunocompromised persons aged ≥20 yr	40[e]	1.0	40[f]	2.0	—[g]	—

From Centers for Disease Control and Prevention: A comprehensive immunization strategy to eliminate transmission of hepatitis B virus infection in the United States: recommendations of the Advisory Committee on Immunization Practices (ACIP), *MMWR* 55(RR-16):10, 2006.
HB, Hepatitis B.
[a]Merck & Co., Inc., Whitehouse Station, New Jersey.
[b]GlaxoSmithKline Biologicals, Rixensart, Belgium.
[c]Combined hepatitis A and hepatitis B vaccine, recommended for persons aged >18 yr who are at increased risk for both hepatitis B virus and hepatitis A virus infections.
[d]Recombinant hepatitis B surface antigen protein dose.
[e]Dialysis formulation administered on a 3-dose schedule at 0, 1, and 6 mo.
[f]Two 1.0-ml doses administered in 1 or 2 injections on a 4-dose schedule at 0, 1, 2, and 6 mo.
[g]Not applicable.

TABLE 5-26 Recommended HIV/AIDS, Sexually Transmitted Disease (STD), and Viral Hepatitis Prevention Services by Risk Population

Risk Population[a]	Recommended Services
High-Risk Heterosexuals	
Persons seeking sexually transmitted disease evaluation or treatment	Hepatitis B vaccination Testing for HIV infection[b] Testing for syphilis, gonorrhea, and chlamydia, as clinically indicated[c]
Sexually active men not in a long-term, mutually monogamous relationship	Hepatitis B vaccination Annual testing for HIV infection[b,d]
Sexually active women not in a long-term, mutually monogamous relationship	Hepatitis B vaccination[e] Annual testing for HIV infection[b,d] Annual testing for chlamydia (NOTE: Also recommended for all sexually active females aged <25 yr)[c]
Men Who Have Sex with Men (MSM)	
All MSM	Hepatitis A vaccination Hepatitis B vaccination[e]
Sexually active MSM not in a long-term, mutually monogamous relationship	Hepatitis A vaccination Hepatitis B vaccination[e] Annual testing for HIV infection[b] Annual testing for syphilis, gonorrhea, and chlamydia[c]
Injection-Drug Users	
	Hepatitis A vaccination[f] Hepatitis B vaccination Testing for hepatitis C virus infection[g] Annual testing for HIV infection[b] Substance-abuse treatment[h]

From Centers for Disease Control and Prevention (CDC): A comprehensive immunization strategy to eliminate transmission of hepatitis B virus infection in the United States: recommendations of the Advisory Committee on Immunization Practices (ACIP), *MMWR* 55(RR-16):17, 2006.
[a]Testing for HIV infection, chlamydia, gonorrhea, syphilis, and hepatitis B surface antigen also is recommended for pregnant women. (CDC: Revised recommendations for HIV testing of adults, adolescents, and pregnant women in health care settings, *MMWR* 55[RR-14], 2006; CDC: Sexually transmitted diseases treatment guidelines, *MMWR* 55[RR-11], 2006; CDC: A comprehensive immunization strategy to eliminate transmission of hepatitis B virus infection in the United States: recommendations of the Advisory Committee on Immunization Practices [ACIP]. Part 1: immunization of infants, children, and adolescents, *MMWR* 54[RR-16], 2005.)
[b]CDC: Revised recommendations for HIV testing of adults, adolescents, and pregnant women in health care settings, *MMWR* 55(RR-14), 2006.
[c]CDC: Sexually transmitted diseases treatment guidelines 2006, *MMWR* 55(RR-11), 2006.
[d]HIV screening is recommended for all persons aged 13-64 yr. Repeat screening is recommended at least annually for persons likely to be at high risk for HIV infection, including MSM or heterosexuals who themselves or whose sex partners have had more than one partner since their most recent HIV test.
[e]Hepatitis B vaccination is recommended for persons who have had more than one sex partner during the previous 6 mo.
[f]CDC: Prevention of hepatitis A through active or passive immunization: recommendations of the Advisory Committee on Immunization Practices (ACIP), *MMWR* 55(RR-7), 2006.
[g]CDC: Recommendations for prevention and control of hepatitis C virus (HCV) infection and HCV-related chronic disease, *MMWR* 47(RR-19), 1998. Recommended frequency of testing for hepatitis C virus infection has not been determined.
[h]CDC: *Substance abuse treatment for injection drug users: a strategy with many benefits,* Atlanta, 2002, U.S. Department of Health and Human Services, CDC. Available at http://www.cdc.gov/idu/facts/treatment.htm.

TABLE 5-27 Guidelines for Postexposure Prophylaxis* of Persons with Nonoccupational Exposures† to Blood or Body Fluids That Contain Blood by Exposure Type and Vaccination Status

	TREATMENT	
Exposure	**Unvaccinated Person‡**	**Previously Vaccinated Person§**
HBsAg-Positive Source		
Percutaneous (e.g., bite or needlestick) or mucosal exposure to HBsAg-positive blood or body fluids	Administer hepatitis B vaccine series and hepatitis B immune globulin (HBIG)	Administer hepatitis B vaccine booster dose
Sex or needle-sharing contact with a person who is HBsAg positive	Administer hepatitis B vaccine series and HBIG	Administer hepatitis B vaccine booster dose
Victim of sexual assault/abuse by a perpetrator who is HBsAg positive	Administer hepatitis B vaccine series and HBIG	Administer hepatitis B vaccine booster dose
Source with Unknown HBsAg Status		
Victim of sexual assault/abuse by a perpetrator with unknown HBsAg status	Administer hepatitis B vaccine series	No treatment
Percutaneous (e.g., bite or needlestick) or mucosal exposure to potentially infectious blood or body fluids from a source with unknown HBsAg status	Administer hepatitis B vaccine series	No treatment
Sexual or needle-sharing contact with person with unknown HBsAg status	Administer hepatitis B vaccine series	No treatment

From Centers for Disease Control and Prevention: A comprehensive immunization strategy to eliminate transmission of hepatitis B virus infection in the United States: recommendations of the Advisory Committee on Immunization Practices (ACIP), *MMWR* 55(RR-16):30, 2006.

HBsAg, Hepatitis B surface antigen.

*When indicated, immunoprophylaxis should be initiated as soon as possible, preferably within 24 hours. Studies are limited on the maximum interval after exposure during which postexposure prophylaxis is effective, but the interval is unlikely to exceed 7 days for percutaneous exposures or 14 days for sexual exposures. The hepatitis B vaccine series should be completed.

†These guidelines apply to nonoccupational exposures. Guidelines for management of occupational exposures have been published separately and also can be used for management of nonoccupational exposures if feasible.

‡A person who is in the process of being vaccinated but has not completed the vaccine series should complete the series and receive treatment as indicated.

§A person who has written documentation of a complete hepatitis B vaccine series and did not receive postvaccination testing.

TABLE 5-28 Typical Interpretation of Serologic Test Results for Hepatitis B Virus Infection

SEROLOGIC MARKER				
HBsAg	**Total Anti-HBc**	**IgM Anti-HBc**	**Anti-HBs**	**Interpretation**
–*	–	–	–	Never infected
+†‡	–	–	–	Early acute infection; transient (up to 18 days) after vaccination
+	+	+	–	Acute infection
–	+	+	+ or –	Acute resolving infection
–	+	–	+	Recovered from past infection and immune
+	+	–	–	Chronic infection
–	+	–	–	False-positive (i.e., susceptible), past infection, "low-level" chronic infection,§ or passive transfer of anti-HBc to infant born to mother who is HBsAg positive
–	–	–	+	Immune if concentration is >10 mIU/ml after vaccine series completion‖; passive transfer after hepatitis B immune globulin administration

From Centers for Disease Control and Prevention: A comprehensive immunization strategy to eliminate transmission of hepatitis B virus infection in the United States: recommendations of the Advisory Committee on Immunization Practices (ACIP), *MMWR* 55(RR-16):4, 2006.

HBc, Antibody to hepatitis B core antigen; *HBs,* antibody to HBsAg; *HBsAg,* hepatitis B surface antigen; *Ig,* immunoglobulin.

*Negative test result.

†Positive test result.

‡To ensure that an HBsAg-positive test result is not a false-positive, samples with reactive HBsAg results should be tested with a licensed neutralizing confirmatory test if recommended in the manufacturer's package insert.

§Persons positive only for anti-HBc are unlikely to be infectious except under unusual circumstances in which they are the source for direct percutaneous exposure of susceptible recipients to large quantities of virus (e.g., blood transfusion or organ transplant).

‖Milliinternational units per milliliter.

Hepatitis A Prophylaxis

TABLE 5-29 Recommended Dosages of Hepatitis A Immune Globulin

Setting	Duration of Coverage	Dose
Preexposure prophylaxis	Short term (<3 mo)	0.02 ml/kg
	Long term (3-5 mo)*	0.06 ml/kg
Postexposure prophylaxis	—	0.02 ml/kg

Modified from Centers for Disease Control and Prevention: Prevention of hepatitis A through active or passive immunization: recommendations of the Advisory Committee on Immunization Practices (ACIP), *MMWR* 55(RR-07):9, 2006.

NOTE: Immune globulin should be administered intramuscularly into the deltoid or gluteal muscle in children younger than 24 mo; it may be administered in the anterolateral thigh muscle.

*Repeat every 5 mo if continued exposure to hepatitis A virus occurs.

TABLE 5-30 Licensed Dosages of Hepatitis A Vaccines

Vaccine	Patient's Age	Dose	Volume (ml)	Number of Doses	Schedule (mo)*
Hepatitis A vaccine, inactivated (Havrix)	12 mo to 18 yr	720 EL.U.	0.5	2	0, 6-12
	≥19 yr	1440 EL.U.	1.0	2	0, 6-12
Hepatitis A vaccine, inactivated (Vaqta)	12 mo to 18 yr	25 U	0.5	2	0, 6-18
	≥19 yr	50 U	1.0	2	0, 6-18
Combined hepatitis A and hepatitis B vaccine (Twinrix)	≥18 yr	720 EL.U. of hepatitis A antigen and 20 mcg of hepatitis B surface antigen protein	1.0	3	0, 1, and 6

Modified from Centers for Disease Control and Prevention: Prevention of hepatitis A through active or passive immunization: recommendations of the Advisory Committee on Immunization Practices (ACIP), *MMWR* 55(RR-07):10, 2006.

*Zero represents the timing of the initial dose; subsequent numbers represent months after the initial dose.

Influenza Treatment and Prophylaxis

BOX 5-3 Summary of Seasonal Influenza Vaccination Recommendations

Children

All children aged 6 months-18 years should be vaccinated annually.

Children and adolescents at higher risk for influenza complications should continue to be a focus for vaccination efforts as providers and programs transition to routinely vaccinating all children and adolescents, including those who:

- are aged 6 months-4 years (59 months)
- have chronic pulmonary (including asthma), cardiovascular (except hypertension), renal, hepatic, cognitive, neurologic/neuromuscular, hematologic, or metabolic disorders (including diabetes mellitus)
- are immunosuppressed (including immunosuppression caused by medications or by human immunodeficiency virus)
- are receiving long-term aspirin therapy and therefore might be at risk for experiencing Reye's syndrome after influenza virus infection
- are residents of long-term care facilities
- will be pregnant during the influenza season

Note: Children aged <6 months cannot receive influenza vaccination. Household and other close contacts (e.g., day-care providers) of children aged <6 months, including older children and adolescents, should be vaccinated.

Adults

Annual vaccination against influenza is recommended for any adult who wants to reduce the risk of becoming ill with influenza or of transmitting it to others. Vaccination is recommended for all adults without contraindications in the following groups, because these persons either are at higher risk for influenza complications, or are close contacts of the persons at higher risk:

- persons aged ≥50 years
- women who will be pregnant during the influenza season
- persons who have chronic pulmonary (including asthma), cardiovascular (except hypertension), renal, hepatic, cognitive, neurologic/neuromuscular, hematologic, or metabolic disorders (including diabetes mellitus)
- persons who have immunosuppression (including immunosuppression caused by medications or by human immunodeficiency virus)
- residents of nursing homes and other long-term care facilities
- health-care personnel
- household contacts and caregivers of children aged <5 years and adults aged ≥50 years, with particular emphasis on vaccinating contacts of children aged <6 months
- household contacts and caregivers of persons with medical conditions that put them at higher risk for severe complications from influenza

Modified from *MMWR* 58:(RR-8), 2009.

RECOMMENDED VACCINES FOR DIFFERENT AGE GROUPS

When vaccinating children aged 6 to 35 months with TIV, health care providers should use TIV that has been licensed by the FDA for this age group (i.e., TIV manufactured by Sanofi Pasteur [FluZone]). TIV from Novartis (Fluvirin) is FDA approved in the United States for use among persons aged 4 years and older. TIV from GlaxoSmithKline (Fluarix and FluLaval) or CSL Biotherapies (Afluria) is labeled for use in persons aged 18 years and older because data to demonstrate efficacy among younger persons have not been provided to the FDA. LAIV from MedImmune (FluMist) is licensed for use by healthy, nonpregnant persons aged 2 to 49 years. A vaccine dose does not need to be repeated if inadvertently administered to a person who does not have an age indication for the vaccine formulation given. Expanded age and risk group indications for licensed vaccines are likely over the next several years, and vaccination providers should be alert to these changes. In addition, several new vaccine formulations are being evaluated in immunogenicity and efficacy trials; when licensed, these new products will increase the influenza vaccine supply and provide additional vaccine choices for practitioners and their patients.

INFLUENZA VACCINES AND USE OF INFLUENZA ANTIVIRAL MEDICATIONS

Administration of TIV and influenza antivirals during the same medical visit is acceptable. The effect on safety and effectiveness of LAIV coadministration with influenza antiviral medications has not been studied. However, because influenza antivirals reduce replication of influenza viruses, LAIV should not be administered until 48 hours after cessation of influenza antiviral therapy, and influenza antiviral medications should not be administered for 2 weeks after receipt of LAIV. Persons receiving antivirals within the period 2 days before to 14 days after vaccination with LAIV should be revaccinated at a later date.

PERSONS WHO SHOULD NOT BE VACCINATED WITH TIV

TIV should not be administered to persons known to have anaphylactic hypersensitivity to eggs or other components of the influenza vaccine. Prophylactic use of antiviral agents is an option for preventing influenza among such persons. Information about vaccine components is located in package inserts from each manufacturer. Persons with moderate to severe acute febrile illness usually should not be vaccinated until their symptoms have abated. However, minor illnesses with or without fever do not contraindicate use of influenza vaccine. Guillain-Barré syndrome within 6 weeks after a previous dose of TIV is considered a precaution for use of TIV.

CONSIDERATIONS WHEN USING LAIV

LAIV is an option for vaccination of healthy, nonpregnant persons aged 2 to 49 years, including health care providers and other close contacts of high-risk persons (except severely immunocompromised persons who require care in a protected environment). No preference is indicated for LAIV or TIV when considering vaccination of healthy, nonpregnant persons aged 2 to 49 years. Use of the term *healthy* in this recommendation refers to persons who do not have any of the underlying medical conditions that confer high risk for severe complications (see "Persons Who Should Not Be Vaccinated with LAIV"). However, during periods when inactivated vaccine is in short supply, use of LAIV is encouraged when feasible for eligible persons (including health care providers) because use of LAIV by these persons might increase availability of TIV for persons in groups targeted for vaccination but who cannot receive LAIV. Possible advantages of LAIV include its potential to induce a broad mucosal and systemic immune response in children, its ease of administration, and possibly increased acceptability of an intranasal rather than intramuscular route of administration.

If the vaccine recipient sneezes after administration, the dose should not be repeated. However, if nasal congestion is present that might impede delivery of the vaccine to the nasopharyngeal mucosa, deferral of administration should be considered until resolution of the illness, or TIV should be administered instead. No data exist about concomitant use of nasal corticosteroids or other intranasal medications.

Although FDA licensure of LAIV excludes children aged 2 to 4 years with a history of asthma or recurrent wheezing, the precise risk, if any, of wheezing caused by LAIV among these children is unknown because experience with LAIV among these young children is limited. Young children might not have a history of recurrent wheezing if their exposure to respiratory viruses has been limited because of their age. Certain children might have a history of wheezing with respiratory illnesses but have not had asthma diagnosed. The following screening recommendations should be used to assist persons who administer influenza vaccines in providing the appropriate vaccine for children aged 2 to 4 years.

Clinicians and vaccination programs should screen for possible reactive airways diseases when considering use of LAIV for children aged 2 to 4 years and should avoid use of this vaccine in children with asthma or a recent wheezing episode. Health care providers should consult the medical record, when available, to identify children aged 2 to 4 years with asthma or recurrent wheezing that might indicate asthma. In addition, to identify children who might be at greater risk for asthma and possibly at increased risk for wheezing after receiving LAIV, parents or caregivers of children aged 2 to 4 years should be asked, "In the past 12 months, has a health care provider ever told you that your child had wheezing or asthma?" Children whose parents or caregivers answer "yes" to this question and children who have asthma or who had a wheezing episode noted in the medical record during the preceding 12 months should not receive LAIV. TIV is available for use in children with asthma or possible reactive airways diseases.

LAIV can be administered to persons with minor acute illnesses (e.g., diarrhea or mild upper respiratory tract infection with or without fever). However, if nasal congestion is present that might impede delivery of the vaccine to the nasopharyngeal mucosa, deferral of administration should be considered until resolution of the illness.

PERSONS WHO SHOULD NOT BE VACCINATED WITH LAIV

The effectiveness or safety of LAIV is not known for the following groups, who should not be vaccinated with LAIV:

- Persons with a history of hypersensitivity, including anaphylaxis, to any of the components of LAIV or eggs
- Persons younger than 2 years or aged 50 years or older
- Persons with any of the underlying medical conditions that serve as an indication for routine influenza vaccination, including asthma, reactive airways disease, or other chronic disorders of the pulmonary or cardiovascular systems; other underlying medical conditions, including metabolic diseases such as diabetes, renal dysfunction, and hemoglobinopathies; or known or suspected immunodeficiency diseases or immunosuppressed states
- Children aged 2 to 4 years whose parents or caregivers report that a health care provider has told them during the preceding 12 months that their child had wheezing or asthma, or whose medical record indicates a wheezing episode has occurred during the preceding 12 months
- Children or adolescents receiving aspirin or other salicylates (because of the association of Reye syndrome with wild-type influenza virus infection)
- Persons with a history of Guillain-Barré syndrome after influenza vaccination
- Pregnant women

CONCURRENT ADMINISTRATION OF INFLUENZA VACCINE WITH OTHER VACCINES

Use of LAIV concurrently with measles, mumps, rubella (MMR) alone, and MMR and varicella vaccine among children aged 12 to 15 months has been studied, and no interference with immunogenicity to antigens in any of the vaccines was observed. Among adults aged 50 years or older, the safety and immunogenicity of zoster vaccine and TIV were similar whether administered simultaneously or spaced 4 weeks apart. In the absence of specific data indicating interference, following ACIP's general recommendations for vaccination is prudent. Inactivated vaccines do not interfere with the immune response to other inactivated vaccines or to live vaccines. Inactivated or live vaccines can be administered simultaneously with LAIV. However, after administration of a live vaccine, at least 4 weeks should pass before another live vaccine is administered.

TABLE 5-31 Live, Attenuated Influenza Vaccine (LAIV) Compared with Inactivated Influenza Vaccine (TIV) for Seasonal Influenza, United States Formulations

Factor	LAIV	TIV
Route of administration	Intranasal spray	Intramuscular injection
Type of vaccine	Live virus	Noninfectious virus (i.e.,inactivated)
Number of included virus strains	3 (2 influenza A, 1 influenza B)	3 (2 influenza A, 1 influenza B)
Vaccine virus strains updated	Annually	Annually
Frequency of administration	Annually*	Annually*
Approved age	Persons aged 2-49 yr	Persons aged ≥6 mo
Interval between 2 doses recommended for children aged ≥6 mo to 8 yr who are receiving influenza vaccine for the first time	4 wk	4 wk
Can be administered to persons with medical risk factors for influenza-related complications†	No	Yes
Can be administered to children with asthma or children aged 2-4 yr with wheezing during the preceding year§	No	Yes
Can be administered to family members or close contacts of immunosuppressed persons not requiring a protected environment	Yes	Yes
Can be administered to family members or close contacts of immunosuppressed persons requiring a protected environment (e.g., hematopoietic stem cell transplant recipient)	No	Yes
Can be administered to family members or close contacts of persons at high risk but not severely immunosuppressed	Yes	Yes
Can be simultaneously administered with other vaccines	Yes¶	Yes**
If not simultaneously administered, can be administered within 4 wk of another live vaccine	Prudent to space 4 wk apart	Yes
If not simultaneously administered, can be administered within 4 wk of an inactivated vaccine	Yes	Yes

Modified from *MMWR* 56(RR-6), 2007.

*Children aged 6 months-8 years who have never received influenza vaccine before should receive 2 doses. Those who only receive 1 dose in their first year of vaccination should receive 2 doses in the following year, spaced 4 weeks apart.

†Persons at higher risk for complications of influenza infection because of underlying medical conditions should not receive LAIV. Persons at higher risk for complications of influenza infection because of underlying medical conditions include adults and children with chronic disorders of the pulmonary or cardiovascular systems; adults and children with chronic metabolic diseases (including diabetes mellitus), renal dysfunction, hemoglobinopathies, or immunosuppression; children and adolescents receiving long-term aspirin therapy (at risk for developing Reye's syndrome after wild-type influenza infection); persons who have any condition (e.g., cognitive dysfunction, spinal cord injuries, seizure disorders, or other neuromuscular disorders) that can compromise respiratory function or the handling of respiratory secretions or that can increase the risk for aspiration; pregnant women; and residents of nursing homes and other chronic-care facilities that house persons with chronic medical conditions.

§Clinicians and immunization programs should screen for possible reactive airways diseases when considering use of LAIV for children aged 2-4 years and should avoid use of this vaccine in children with asthma or a recent wheezing episode. Health care providers should consult the medical record, when available, to identify children aged 2-4 years with asthma or recurrent wheezing that might indicate asthma. In addition, to identify children who might be at greater risk for asthma and possibly at increased risk for wheezing after receiving LAIV, parents or caregivers of children aged 2-4 years should be asked: "In the past 12 months, has a health care provider ever told you that your child had wheezing or asthma?" Children whose parents or caregivers answer "yes" to this question and children who have asthma or who had a wheezing episode noted in the medical record during the preceding 12 months should not receive LAIV.

¶LAIV coadministration has been evaluated systematically only among children aged 12–15 months who received measles, mumps, and rubella vaccine or varicella vaccine.

**TIV coadministration has been evaluated systematically only among adults who received pneumococcal polysaccharide or zoster vaccine.

INDICATIONS FOR USE OF ANTIVIRALS

PERSONS FOR WHOM ANTIVIRAL TREATMENT SHOULD BE CONSIDERED

If possible, antiviral treatment should be started within 48 hours of influenza illness onset. The effectiveness of initiating antiviral treatment more than 48 hours after illness onset has not been established. Persons for whom antiviral treatment should be considered include:

- Persons hospitalized with laboratory-confirmed influenza (limited data suggest benefit even for persons whose antiviral treatment is initiated more than 48 hours after illness onset)
- Persons with laboratory-confirmed influenza pneumonia
- Persons with laboratory-confirmed influenza and bacterial coinfection
- Persons with laboratory-confirmed influenza infection who are at higher risk for influenza complications
- Persons presenting to medical care with laboratory-confirmed influenza within 48 hours of influenza illness onset who want to decrease the duration or severity of their symptoms and transmission of influenza to others at higher risk for complications

PERSONS FOR WHOM ANTIVIRAL CHEMOPROPHYLAXIS SHOULD BE CONSIDERED DURING PERIODS OF INCREASED INFLUENZA ACTIVITY IN THE COMMUNITY

- Persons at high risk during the 2 weeks after influenza vaccination (after the second dose for children younger than 9 years who have not previously been vaccinated) if influenza viruses are circulating in the community
- Persons at high risk for whom influenza vaccine is contraindicated
- Family members or health care providers who are unvaccinated and are likely to have ongoing, close exposure to persons at high risk or unvaccinated persons or infants younger than 6 months
- Persons and their family members and close contacts and health care workers when circulating strains of influenza virus in the community are not matched with vaccine strains
- Persons with immune deficiencies or those who might not respond to vaccination (e.g., persons infected with HIV or other immunosuppressed conditions or who are receiving immunosuppressive medications)
- Unvaccinated staff and persons during response to an outbreak in a closed institutional setting with residents at high risk (e.g., extended-care facilities)

Modified from *MMWR* 57(RR-7), 2008.

Note: Recommended antiviral medications (neuraminidase inhibitors) are not licensed for chemoprophylaxis of children younger than 1 year (oseltamivir) or younger than 5 years (zanamivir). Updates or supplements to these recommendations (e.g., expanded age or risk group indications for licensed vaccines) might be required. Health care providers should be alert to announcements of recommendation updates and should check the CDC influenza website periodically for additional information (http://www.cdc.gov/flu).

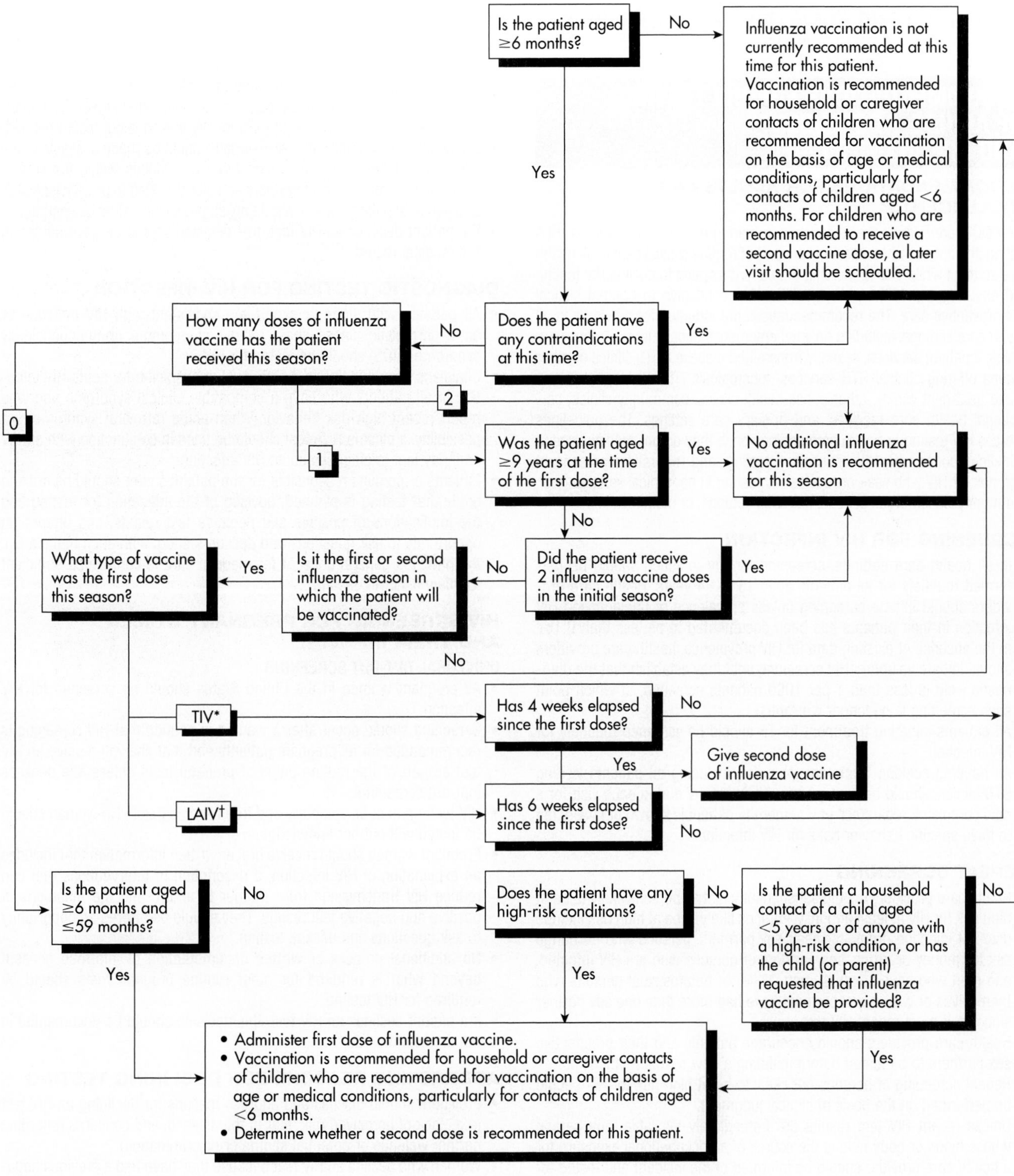

Is the patient aged ≥6 months?

No → Influenza vaccination is not currently recommended at this time for this patient. Vaccination is recommended for household or caregiver contacts of children who are recommended for vaccination on the basis of age or medical conditions, particularly for contacts of children aged <6 months. For children who are recommended to receive a second vaccine dose, a later visit should be scheduled.

Yes → Does the patient have any contraindications at this time?

Yes → (Influenza vaccination is not currently recommended at this time for this patient.)

No → How many doses of influenza vaccine has the patient received this season?

0 → Is the patient aged ≥6 months and ≤59 months?

1 → Was the patient aged ≥9 years at the time of the first dose?

2 → No additional influenza vaccination is recommended for this season

Was the patient aged ≥9 years at the time of the first dose? Yes → No additional influenza vaccination is recommended for this season

No → Did the patient receive 2 influenza vaccine doses in the initial season?

Yes → No additional influenza vaccination is recommended for this season

No → Is it the first or second influenza season in which the patient will be vaccinated?

No → No additional influenza vaccination is recommended for this season

Yes → What type of vaccine was the first dose this season?

TIV* → Has 4 weeks elapsed since the first dose?

LAIV† → Has 6 weeks elapsed since the first dose?

Yes → Give second dose of influenza vaccine

No → (later visit should be scheduled)

Is the patient aged ≥6 months and ≤59 months?

Yes → Administer first dose (see below)

No → Does the patient have any high-risk conditions?

Yes → Administer first dose (see below)

No → Is the patient a household contact of a child aged <5 years or of anyone with a high-risk condition, or has the child (or parent) requested that influenza vaccine be provided?

No → (Influenza vaccination is not currently recommended at this time for this patient.)

Yes →

- Administer first dose of influenza vaccine.
- Vaccination is recommended for household or caregiver contacts of children who are recommended for vaccination on the basis of age or medical conditions, particularly for contacts of children aged <6 months.
- Determine whether a second dose is recommended for this patient.

*Trivalent inactivated influenza vaccine.
†Live, attenuated influenza vaccine.

FIGURE 5-6 Algorithm for determining recommended influenza immunization actions for children. (Modified with permission from the American Academy of Pediatrics' Committee on Infectious Diseases: Prevention of influenza: recommendations for influenza immunization of children, 2006-2007, *Pediatrics* 119:846-51.315, 2007.)

HIV Testing and Postexposure Prophylaxis

RECOMMENDATIONS FOR HIV TESTING OF ADULTS, ADOLESCENTS, AND PREGNANT WOMEN

RECOMMENDATIONS FOR ADULTS AND ADOLESCENTS*

The CDC recommends that diagnostic human immunodeficiency virus (HIV) testing and opt-out HIV screening be a part of routine clinical care in all health care settings while also preserving the patient's option to decline HIV testing and ensuring a provider-patient relationship conducive to optimal clinical and preventive care. The recommendations are intended for providers in all health care settings, including hospital emergency departments, urgent-care clinics, inpatient services, sexually transmitted disease (STD) clinics or other venues offering clinical STD services, tuberculosis (TB) clinics, substance abuse treatment clinics, other public health clinics, community clinics, correctional health care facilities, and primary care settings. The guidelines address HIV testing in health care settings only; they do not modify existing guidelines concerning HIV counseling, testing, and referral for persons at high risk for HIV who seek or receive HIV testing in nonclinical settings (e.g., community-based organizations, outreach settings, or mobile vans).

SCREENING FOR HIV INFECTION

- In all health care settings, screening for HIV infection should be performed routinely for all patients aged 13 to 64 years. Health care providers should initiate screening unless prevalence of undiagnosed HIV infection in their patients has been documented to be less than 0.1%. In the absence of existing data for HIV prevalence, health care providers should initiate voluntary HIV screening until they establish that the diagnostic yield is less than 1 per 1000 patients screened, at which point such screening is no longer warranted.
- All patients initiating treatment for TB should be screened routinely for HIV infection.
- All patients seeking treatment for STDs, including all patients visiting STD clinics, should be screened routinely for HIV during each visit for a new complaint, regardless of whether the patient is known or suspected to have specific behavior risks for HIV infection.

REPEAT SCREENING

- Health care providers should subsequently test all persons likely to be at high risk for HIV at least annually. Persons likely to be at high risk include users of injection drugs and their sex partners, persons who exchange sex for money or drugs, sex partners of persons who are HIV infected, and men who have sex with men (MSM) or heterosexual persons who themselves or whose sex partners have had more than one sex partner since their most recent HIV test.
- Health care providers should encourage patients and their prospective sex partners to be tested before initiating a new sexual relationship.
- Repeat screening of persons not likely to be at high risk for HIV should be performed on the basis of clinical judgment.
- Unless recent HIV test results are immediately available, any person whose blood or body fluid is the source of an occupational exposure for a health care provider should be informed of the incident and tested for HIV infection at the time the exposure occurs.

CONSENT AND PRETEST INFORMATION

- Screening should be voluntary and undertaken only with the patient's knowledge and understanding that HIV testing is planned.
- Patients should be informed orally or in writing that HIV testing will be performed unless they decline (opt-out screening). Oral or written information should include an explanation of HIV infection and the meanings of positive and negative test results, and the patient should be offered an opportunity to ask questions and decline testing. With such notification, consent for HIV screening should be incorporated into the patient's general informed consent for medical care on the same basis as are other screening or diagnostic tests; a separate consent form for HIV testing is not recommended.
- Easily understood informational materials should be made available in the languages of the commonly encountered populations within the service area. The competence of interpreters and bilingual staff to provide language assistance to patients with limited English proficiency must be ensured.
- If a patient declines an HIV test, this decision should be documented in the medical record.

DIAGNOSTIC TESTING FOR HIV INFECTION

- All patients with signs or symptoms consistent with HIV infection or an opportunistic illness characteristic of acquired immunodeficiency syndrome (AIDS) should be tested for HIV.
- Clinicians should maintain a high level of suspicion for acute HIV infection in all patients who have a compatible clinical syndrome and who report recent high-risk behavior. When acute retroviral syndrome is a possibility, a plasma RNA test should be used in conjunction with an HIV antibody test to diagnose acute HIV infection.
- Patients or persons responsible for the patient's care should be notified orally that testing is planned, advised of the indication for testing and the implications of positive and negative test results, and offered an opportunity to ask questions and decline testing. With such notification, the patient's general consent for medical care is considered sufficient for diagnostic HIV testing.

HIV SCREENING FOR PREGNANT WOMEN AND THEIR INFANTS*

UNIVERSAL OPT-OUT SCREENING

- All pregnant women in the United States should be screened for HIV infection.
- Screening should occur after a woman is notified that HIV screening is recommended for all pregnant patients and that she will receive an HIV test as part of the routine panel of prenatal tests unless she declines (opt-out screening).
- HIV testing must be voluntary and free from coercion. No woman should be tested without her knowledge.
- Pregnant women should receive oral or written information that includes an explanation of HIV infection, a description of interventions that can reduce HIV transmission from mother to infant, and the meanings of positive and negative test results. They should be offered an opportunity to ask questions and decline testing.
- No additional process or written documentation of informed consent beyond what is required for other routine prenatal tests should be required for HIV testing.
- If a patient declines an HIV test, this decision should be documented in the medical record.

ADDRESSING REASONS FOR DECLINING TESTING

- Providers should discuss and address reasons for declining an HIV test (e.g., lack of perceived risk, fear of the disease, and concerns regarding partner violence or potential stigma or discrimination).
- Women who decline an HIV test because they have had a previous negative test result should be informed of the importance of retesting during each pregnancy.
- Logistical reasons for not testing (e.g., scheduling) should be resolved.
- Certain women who initially decline an HIV test might accept at a later date, especially if their concerns are discussed. Certain women will continue to decline testing, and their decisions should be respected and documented in the medical record.

TIMING OF HIV TESTING

- To promote informed and timely therapeutic decisions, health care providers should test women for HIV as early as possible during each pregnancy. Women who decline the test early in prenatal care should be encouraged to be tested at a subsequent visit.

*Data from *MMWR* 57(RR-10), 2008.

- A second HIV test during the third trimester, preferably less than 36 weeks of gestation, is cost effective even in areas of low HIV prevalence and may be considered for all pregnant women. A second HIV test during the third trimester is recommended for women who meet one or more of the following criteria:
  - Women who receive health care in jurisdictions with elevated incidence of HIV or AIDS among women aged 15 to 45 years. In 2004, these jurisdictions included Alabama, Connecticut, Delaware, the District of Columbia, Florida, Georgia, Illinois, Louisiana, Maryland, Massachusetts, Mississippi, Nevada, New Jersey, New York, North Carolina, Pennsylvania, Puerto Rico, Rhode Island, South Carolina, Tennessee, Texas, and Virginia.[†]
  - Women who receive health care in facilities in which prenatal screening identifies at least one pregnant woman who is infected with HIV per 1000 women screened.
  - Women who are known to be at high risk for acquiring HIV (e.g., users of injection drugs and their sex partners, women who exchange sex for money or drugs, women who are sex partners of persons who are infected with HIV, and women who have had a new or more than one sex partner during this pregnancy).
  - Women who have signs or symptoms consistent with acute HIV infection. When acute retroviral syndrome is a possibility, a plasma RNA test should be used in conjunction with an HIV antibody test to diagnose acute HIV infection.

[†]A second HIV test in the third trimester is as cost effective as other common health interventions when HIV incidence among women of childbearing age is ≥17 HIV cases per 100,000 person-years. In 2004, in jurisdictions with available data on HIV case rates, a rate of 17 new HIV diagnoses per year per 100,000 women aged 15 to 45 years was associated with an AIDS case rate of at least nine AIDS diagnoses per year per 100,000 women aged 15 to 45 years (CDC, unpublished data, 2005). As of 2004, the jurisdictions listed above exceeded these thresholds. The list of specific jurisdictions where a second test in the third trimester is recommended will be updated periodically based on surveillance data.

RAPID TESTING DURING LABOR

- Any woman with undocumented HIV status at the time of labor should be screened with a rapid HIV test unless she declines (opt-out screening).
- Reasons for declining a rapid test should be explored (see "Addressing Reasons for Declining Testing").
- Immediate initiation of appropriate antiretroviral prophylaxis should be recommended to women on the basis of a reactive rapid test result without waiting for the result of a confirmatory test.

POSTPARTUM/NEWBORN TESTING

- When a woman's HIV status is still unknown at the time of delivery, she should be screened immediately postpartum with a rapid HIV test unless she declines (opt-out screening).
- When the mother's HIV status is unknown postpartum, rapid testing of the newborn as soon as possible after birth is recommended so that antiretroviral prophylaxis can be offered to infants exposed to HIV. Women should be informed that identifying HIV antibodies in the newborn indicates that the mother is infected.
- For infants whose HIV exposure status is unknown and who are in foster care, the person legally authorized to provide consent should be informed that rapid HIV testing is recommended for infants whose biologic mothers have not been tested.
- The benefits of neonatal antiretroviral prophylaxis are best realized when it is initiated within 12 hours after birth.

CONFIRMATORY TESTING

- Whenever possible, uncertainties regarding laboratory test results indicating HIV infection status should be resolved before final decisions are made regarding reproductive options, antiretroviral therapy, cesarean delivery, or other interventions.
- If the confirmatory test result is not available before delivery, immediate initiation of appropriate antiretroviral prophylaxis should be recommended to any pregnant patient whose HIV screening test result is reactive to reduce the risk for perinatal transmission.

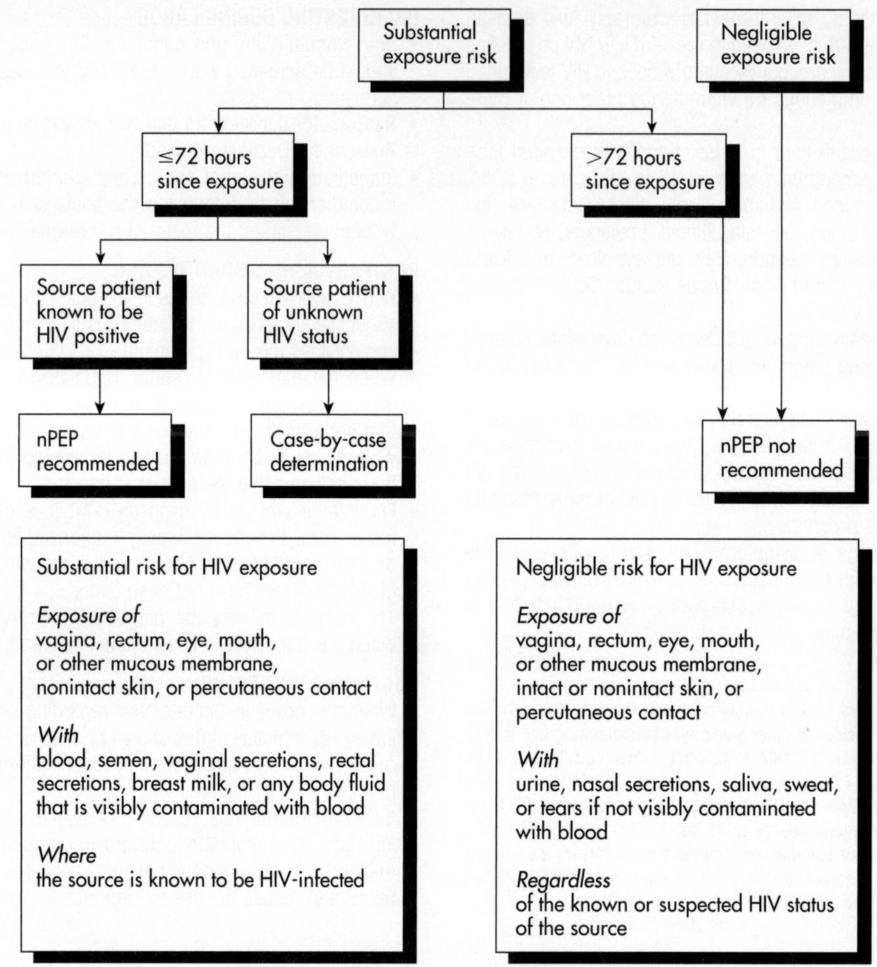

FIGURE 5-7 Algorithm for evaluation and treatment of possible nonoccupational HIV exposure. *nPEP,* Nonoccupational postexposure prophylaxis. (Modified from *MMWR* 54[RR-2], 2005.)

TABLE 5-32 HIV Exposure, Estimated Per-Act Risk

Exposure Route	Risk per 10,000 Exposures to an Infected Source
Blood transfusion	9000
Needle-sharing injection drug use	67
Receptive anal intercourse	50
Percutaneous needle stick	30
Receptive penile-vaginal intercourse	10
Insertive anal intercourse	6.5
Insertive penile-vaginal intercourse	5
Receptive oral intercourse	1
Insertive oral intercourse	0.5

Modified from *MMWR* 54(RR-2), 2005.
Estimates of risk for transmission from sexual exposures assume no condom use.
Source refers to oral intercourse performed on a man.

TABLE 5-33 Regimens for 28-Day Postexposure Prophylaxis for HIV Infection*

Regimen	Dose	Daily Pill Burden† *no.*	Advantages	Disadvantages
Two-Drug Regimens				
Tenofovir–emtricitabine (Truvada)‡	One tablet (300 mg of tenofovir with 200 mg of emtricitabine) once daily	1	Well-tolerated; once-daily dosing	Potential nephrotoxicity
Zidovudine–lamivudine (Combivir)§	One tablet (300 mg of zidovudine with 150 mg of lamivudine) twice daily	2	Preferred in pregnancy	Twice-daily dosing; less well-tolerated than tenofovir–emtricitabine (nausea, asthenia, neutropenia, anemia, abnormal liver-enzyme levels)
Three-Drug Regimens¶				
Ritonavir–lopinavir (Kaletra) (plus either tenofovir–emtricitabine or zidovudine–lamivudine)	Two tablets (50 mg of ritonavir with 200 mg of lopinavir per tablet) twice daily, or four tablets once daily	5 or 6	Either once-daily or twice-daily dosing; one copayment; no refrigeration required; most experience in pregnancy; high genetic barrier to resistance	Gastrointestinal side effects such as diarrhea; may cause elevated liver-enzyme levels or hepatitis
Ritonavir plus atazanavir (plus either tenofovir–emtricitabine or zidovudine–lamivudine)	100 mg of ritonavir plus 300 mg of atazanavir once daily	3 or 4	Once-daily dosing; well tolerated	Ritonavir must be refrigerated; potential for asymptomatic jaundice, renal stones; may cause elevated liver-enzyme levels or hepatitis
Ritonavir plus darunavir (plus either tenofovir–emtricitabine or zidovudine–lamivudine)	100 mg of ritonavir plus two tablets, each containing 400 mg of darunavir, once daily	4 or 5	Once-daily dosing; high genetic barrier to resistance	Ritonavir must be refrigerated; gastrointestinal side effects; may cause elevated liver-enzyme levels or hepatitis

From Landovitz RJ, Currier JS: Postexposure prophylaxis for HIV infection, *N Engl J Med* 361:1768-75, 2009.

*Tenofovir, emtricitabine, and lamivudine all have activity against hepatitis B. Patients with chronic active hepatitis B (i.e., patients who are positive for hepatitis B surface antigen) may have flares of hepatitis on withdrawal of these agents at the completion of postexposure prophylaxis treatment. Referral to a hepatitis specialist or serial monthly monitoring of liver-enzyme levels for up to 6 months after treatment should be considered.

†The daily pill burden in the three-drug regimens depends on which two-drug regimen is chosen.

‡The dose of tenofovir–emtricitabine should be reduced to one tablet every 48 hours in patients with a creatinine clearance of 30 to 49 ml per minute. Tenofovir–emtricitabine is not recommended in patients with a creatinine clearance of less than 30 ml per minute or in patients who are undergoing hemodialysis; see the guidelines from the Department of Health and Human Services for considerations regarding doses of individual agents in patients with advanced renal dysfunction.

§Zidovudine–lamivudine is not recommended in patients with a creatinine clearance of less than 50 ml per minute; see the guidelines from the Department of Health and Human Services for considerations regarding doses of individual agents in patients with renal dysfunction.

¶The boosting agent ritonavir is not considered to be an active drug in tabulating the number of agents in the three-drug regimen.

TABLE 5-34 Antiretroviral Therapy Medications, Adult Dosage, and Side Effects

Medication	Adult Dosage*	Side Effects and Toxicities
Combination Tablets		
Lopinavir/ritonavir (Kaletra)‡	3 tablets twice daily 400 mg lopinavir/100 mg ritonavir	Diarrhea, nausea, vomiting; asthenia; elevated transaminases; hyperglycemia; fat redistribution; lipid abnormalities; possible increased bleeding in persons with hemophilia; pancreatitis
Zidovudine/lamivudine (Combivir)	1 tablet twice daily 300 mg zidovudine/150 mg lamivudine	See following individual medications
Zidovudine/lamivudine/abacavir (Trizivir)	1 tablet twice daily 300 mg zidovudine/150 mg lamivudine/300 mg abacavir	See following individual medications
Lamivudine/abacavir (Epzicom)	1 tablet once daily 300 mg lamivudine/600 mg abacavir	See following individual medications
Emtricitabine/tenofovir (Truvada)	1 tablet once daily 200 mg emtricitabine/300 mg tenofovir	See following individual medications
Single Agents		
Nucleoside and nucleotide reverse transcriptase inhibitors (side effects as a class: lactic acidosis, severe hepatomegaly with steatosis, including some fatal cases)		
Abacavir (Ziagen, ABC)‡	300 mg twice daily or 600 mg once daily	Severe hypersensitivity reaction (can be fatal); nausea; vomiting
Didanosine (Videx, ddI)‡	>60 kg (132 lb) body weight: 200 mg twice daily or 400 mg daily; if with tenofovir, 250 mg/daily <60 kg (132 lb): 125 mg twice daily or 250 mg daily; if with tenofovir, dose not established Do not use with stavudine (d4T, Zerit) during pregnancy; avoid ddI/d4T combination in general because of increased risk for adverse events (e.g., neuropathy, pancreatitis, and hyperlactatemia)	Pancreatitis; nausea, diarrhea; peripheral neuropathy
Emtricitabine (Emtriva, FTC)	200 mg once daily	Minimal toxicity; lactic acidosis and hepatic steatosis a rare but possibly life-threatening event
Lamivudine (Epivir, 3TC)‡	150 mg twice daily or 300 mg once daily	Minimal toxicity; lactic acidosis and hepatic steatosis a rare but possibly life-threatening event
Stavudine (Zerit, d4T)‡	>60 kg (132 lb) body weight: 40 mg twice daily <60 kg (132 lb) body weight: 30 mg twice daily Do not use with didanosine (ddI, Videx) during pregnancy; avoid ddI/d4T combination in general because of increased risk of adverse events (e.g., neuropathy, pancreatitis, and hyperlactatemia)	Pancreatitis; peripheral neuropathy; rapidly progressive ascending neuromuscular weakness (rare)
Tenofovir (Viread)	300 mg daily	Nausea, vomiting, diarrhea; headache; asthenia; flatulence; renal impairment
Zidovudine (Retrovir, AZT)‡	200 mg three times daily or 300 mg twice daily	Bone marrow suppression (anemia, neutropenia); gastrointestinal intolerance; headache; insomnia; asthenia; and myopathy
Nonnucleoside reverse transcriptase inhibitors (side effects as a class: Stevens-Johnson syndrome)		
Efavirenz (Sustiva)	600 mg daily at bedtime	Rash; central nervous system symptoms (e.g., dizziness, impaired concentration, insomnia, and abnormal dreams); transaminase elevation; false-positive cannabinoid test
Protease inhibitors (side effects as a class: gastrointestinal intolerance, hyperlipidemia, hyperglycemia, diabetes, fat redistribution, and possible increased bleeding in hemophiliacs; do not use during known or possible pregnancy)		
Atazanavir (Reyataz)	400 mg once daily; if administered with tenofovir plus ritonavir, 300 mg once daily	Indirect hyperbilirubinemia; prolonged PR interval (use caution in patients with underlying cardiac conduction defects or on concomitant medications that can cause PR prolongation)
Fosamprenavir (Lexiva)‡	1400 mg twice daily	Gastrointestinal intolerance, nausea, vomiting, diarrhea; rash; elevated transaminases; headache
Indinavir (Crixivan)	800 mg q8h With ritonavir (might increase risk for renal adverse events): 800 mg indinavir and 100 mg ritonavir q12h or 800 mg indinavir and 200 mg ritonavir every q12h	Gastrointestinal intolerance, nausea; nephrolithiasis; headache; asthenia; blurred vision; metallic taste; thrombocytopenia; hemolytic anemia; indirect hyperbilirubinemia (inconsequential)
Nelfinavir (Viracept)‡	750 mg three times daily or one 250 mg twice daily	Diarrhea; elevated transaminases
Ritonavir (Norvir)‡	See doses used in combination with other specific protease inhibitors	Gastrointestinal intolerance; nausea, vomiting, diarrhea; paresthesias; hepatitis; pancreatitis; asthenia; taste perversion; many drug interactions
Saquinavir (hard-gel capsule) (Invirase)	With ritonavir: 400 mg saquinavir and 400 mg ritonavir twice daily or 1000 mg saquinavir and 100 mg ritonavir twice daily	Gastrointestinal intolerance; nausea, diarrhea; headache; elevated transaminases
Saquinavir (soft-gel capsule) (Fortavase)	With ritonavir: 400 mg saquinavir and 400 mg ritonavir twice daily or 1000 mg saquinavir and 100 mg ritonavir twice daily	Gastrointestinal intolerance; nausea, diarrhea; abdominal pain; dyspepsia; headache; elevated transaminases

*For pediatric dosing information, see *Guidelines for use of antiretroviral agents in pediatric HIV infection.* Available at http://www.aidsinfo.nih.gov/guidelines/default_db2.asp?id=51.
‡Pediatric formulation available.
Sources: Modified from U.S. Department of Health and Human Services and the Henry J. Kaiser Family Foundation: *Guidelines for the use of antiretroviral agents in HIV-infected adults and adolescents.* Available at http://www.aidsinfo.nih.gov/guidelines/default_db2.asp?id=50 (refer to website for updated versions); Bartlett JG, Finkbeiner AK: HIV drugs: the guide to living with HIV infection, 2001. Available at http://www.thebody.com/jh/bartlett/drugs.html.

TABLE 5-35 Laboratory Tests Generally Recommended for Persons after Exposure to HIV*

Test	RECOMMENDED DURING TREATMENT		RECOMMENDED AT FOLLOW-UP		
	Baseline	Symptom-Directed†	4-6 wk	12 wk	24 wk
ELISA for HIV antibodies	Yes	Yes	Yes	Yes	Yes
Creatinine, liver function, and complete blood count with differential count	Yes	Yes	No	No	No
HIV viral load	No	Yes	No	No	No
Anti-HBs antibodies	Yes‡	No	No	No	No
HBsAg	Yes‡§	No	No	No	No
HCV antibodies	Yes	No	Yes	Yes	Yes
HCV RNA¶	No	Yes	Yes	Yes	Yes
Screening, including rapid plasma reagin test, for other sexually transmitted infections‖	Yes	Yes	No	Yes	No

From Landovitz RJ, Currier JS: Postexposure prophylaxis for HIV infection, *N Engl J Med* 361:1768-1775, 2009.

Anti-HBs antibodies, Hepatitis B virus surface antibodies; *ELISA,* enzyme-linked immunosorbent assay; *HBsAg,* hepatitis B surface antigen; *HCV,* hepatitis C virus.

*Patients who receive zidovudine plus lamivudine–based regimens should have a complete blood count and measurement of liver-enzyme levels at 2 weeks of treatment, irrespective of the presence or absence of clinical symptoms. Tenofovir plus emtricitabine–based regimens generally involve few side effects, and symptom-directed assessment of serum creatinine or liver-enzyme levels should be considered. The addition of a ritonavir-boosted protease inhibitor should be followed by symptom-directed assessment of liver-enzyme levels, serum glucose levels, or both.

†Symptom-directed tests are for signs or symptoms of toxic effects (rash, nausea, vomiting, or abdominal pain) or HIV seroconversion (fever, fatigue, lymphadenopathy, rash, or oral or genital ulcers).

‡If tests for anti-HBs antibodies and HBsAg are both negative, a vaccination series against HBV infection should be initiated and completed.

§If the patient is HBsAg-positive, he or she should have monthly follow-up of liver function tests after discontinuation of postexposure prophylactic regimens containing tenofovir, lamivudine, or emtricitabine; referral to a specialist in viral hepatitis should be considered.

¶HCV RNA testing may identify early HCV seroconversion; early detection and treatment during acute HCV infection may avert or ameliorate chronic disease. Data are from Dienstag and McHutchison.

‖Rapid plasma reagin testing and testing of urethral-swab and rectal-swab specimens for gonorrhea and chlamydia and of pharyngeal-swab specimens for gonorrhea should be performed as appropriate, according to the patient's sexual risk-taking behaviors and the type of exposure to HIV.

BOX 5-4 Situations for Which Expert Consultation for HIV Postexposure Prophylaxis Is Advised*

- Delayed (i.e., later than 24-36 hours) exposure report
  - The interval after which there is no benefit from postexposure prophylaxis (PEP) is undefined
- Unknown source (e.g., needle in sharps disposal container or laundry)
  - Decide use of PEP on a case-by-case basis
  - Consider the severity of the exposure and the epidemiologic likelihood of HIV exposure
  - Do not test needles or other sharp instruments for HIV
- Known or suspected pregnancy in the exposed person
  - Does not preclude the use of optimal PEP regimens
  - Do not deny PEP solely on the basis of pregnancy
- Resistance of the source virus to antiretroviral agents
  - Influence of drug resistance on transmission risk is unknown
  - Selection of drugs to which the source person's virus is unlikely to be resistant is recommended if the source person's virus is known or suspected to be resistant to one or more of the drugs considered for the PEP regimen
  - Resistance testing of the source person's virus at the time of the exposure is not recommended
- Toxicity of the initial PEP regimen
  - Adverse symptoms such as nausea and diarrhea are common with PEP
  - Symptoms often can be managed without changing the PEP regimen by prescribing antimotility and/or antiemetic agents
  - Modification of dose intervals (i.e., administering a lower dose of drug more frequently throughout the day, as recommended by the manufacturer) in other situations might help alleviate symptoms

*Local experts and/or the National Clinicians' Postexposure Prophylaxis Hotline (PEPline [888-448-4911]).

BOX 5-5 Occupational Exposure Management Resources

National Clinicians' Postexposure Prophylaxis Hotline (PEPline) Run by University of California–San Francisco/San Francisco General Hospital staff; supported by the Health Resources and Services Administration, Ryan White CARE Act, HIV/AIDS Bureau, AIDS Education and Training Centers, and CDC	Phone: 888-448-4911 Internet: http://www.ucsf.edu/hivcntr
Needlestick! A website to help clinicians manage and document occupational blood and body fluid exposures. Developed and maintained by the University of California, Los Angeles (UCLA), Emergency Medicine Center, UCLA School of Medicine, and funded in part by CDC and the Agency for Healthcare Research and Quality	Internet: http://www.needlestick.mednet.ucla.edu
Hepatitis Hotline	Phone: 888-443-7232 Internet: http://www.cdc.gov/ncidod/diseases/hepatitis/index.htm
Reporting to CDC: Occupationally acquired HIV infections and failures of PEP	Phone: 800-893-0485
HIV Antiretroviral Pregnancy Registry	Phone: 800-258-4263 Fax: 800-800-1052 Address: 1410 Commonwealth Dr., Suite 215, Wilmington, NC 28405 Internet: http://www.glaxowellcome.com/preg_reg/antiretroviral
Food and Drug Administration Report unusual or severe toxicity to antiretroviral agents	Phone: 800-332-1088 Address: MedWatch, HF-2, FDA, 5600 Fishers Lane, Rockville, MD 20857 Internet: http://www.fda.gov/medwatch
HIV/AIDS Treatment Information Service	Internet: http://www.hivatis.org

BOX 5-6 Management of Occupational Blood Exposures

Provide Immediate Care to the Exposure Site
- Wash wounds and skin with soap and water
- Flush mucous membranes with water

Determine Risk Associated with Exposure
- Type of fluid (e.g., blood, visibly bloody fluid, other potentially infectious fluid or tissue, and concentrated virus)
- Type of exposure (e.g., percutaneous injury, mucous membrane or nonintact skin exposure, and bites resulting in blood exposure)

Evaluate Exposure Source
- Assess the risk of infection using available information
- Test known sources for HBsAg, anti-HCV, and HIV antibodies (consider using rapid testing)
- For unknown sources, assess risk of exposure to HBV, HCV, or HIV infection
- Do not test discarded needles or syringes for virus contamination

Evaluate the Exposed Person
- Assess immune status for HBV infection (i.e., by history of hepatitis B vaccination and vaccine response)

Give PEP for Exposures Posing Risk of Infection Transmission
- HBV: See Table 5-27
- HCV: PEP not recommended
- HIV: See Tables 5-33, 5-34, and 5-35 and Figure 5-7
  - Initiate PEP as soon as possible, preferably within hours of exposure
  - Offer pregnancy testing to all women of childbearing age not known to be pregnant
  - Seek expert consultation if viral resistance is suspected
  - Administer PEP for 4 weeks if tolerated

Perform Follow-up Testing and Provide Counseling
- Advise exposed persons to seek medical evaluation for any acute illness occurring during follow-up

HBV Exposures
- Perform follow-up anti-HBs testing in persons who receive hepatitis B vaccine
  - Test for anti-HBs 1 to 2 months after last dose of vaccine
  - Anti-HBs response to vaccine cannot be ascertained if HBIG was received in the previous 3 to 4 months

HCV Exposures
- Perform baseline and follow-up testing for anti-HCV and alanine aminotransferase 4 to 6 months after exposures
- Perform HCV RNA at 4 to 6 weeks if earlier diagnosis of HCV infection desired
- Confirm repeatedly reactive anti-HCV enzyme immunoassays with supplemental tests

HIV Exposures
- Perform HIV-antibody testing for at least 6 months after exposure (e.g., at baseline, 6 weeks, 3 months, and 6 months)
- Perform HIV-antibody testing if illness compatible with an acute retroviral syndrome occurs
- Advise exposed persons to use precautions to prevent secondary transmission during the follow-up period
- Evaluate exposed persons taking PEP within 72 hr after exposure and monitor for drug toxicity for at least 2 weeks

HBIG, Hepatitis B immune globulin; *HBsAg,* hepatitis B surface antigen; *HBV,* hepatitis B virus; *HCV,* hepatitis C virus; *HIV,* human immunodeficiency virus; *PEP,* postexposure prophylaxis; *RNA,* ribonucleic acid.

Endocarditis Prophylaxis*

TABLE 5-36 Cardiac Conditions Associated with the Highest Risk of Adverse Outcome from Endocarditis for Which Prophylaxis with Dental Procedures Is Recommended

Prosthetic cardiac valve
Previous infective endocarditis
CHD*
Unrepaired cyanotic CHD, including palliative shunts and conduits
Completely repaired congenital heart defect with prosthetic material or device, whether placed by surgery or by catheter intervention, during the first 6 mo after the procedure†
Repaired CHD with residual defects at the site or adjacent to the site of a prosthetic patch or prosthetic device (that inhibit endothelialization)
Cardiac transplant recipients who develop cardiac valvulopathy

CHD, Congenital heart disease.
*Except for the conditions listed above, antibiotic prophylaxis is no longer recommended for any other form of CHD.
†Prophylaxis is recommended because endothelialization of prosthetic material occurs within 6 mo after the procedure.

TABLE 5-37 Dental Procedures for Which Endocarditis Prophylaxis Is Recommended for Patients in Table 5-36

All dental procedures that involve manipulation of gingival tissue or the periapical region of teeth or perforation of the oral mucosa*

*The following procedures and events do not need prophylaxis: routine anesthetic injections through noninfected tissue, taking dental radiographs, placement of removable prosthodontic or orthodontic appliances, adjustment of orthodontic appliances, placement of orthodontic brackets, shedding of deciduous teeth, and bleeding from trauma to the lips or oral mucosa.

TABLE 5-38 Regimens for a Dental Procedure

	REGIMEN: SINGLE DOSE 30-60 MIN BEFORE PROCEDURE		
Situation	**Agent**	**Adults**	**Children**
Oral	Amoxicillin	2 g	50 mg/kg
Unable to take oral medication	Ampicillin	2 g IM or IV	50 mg/kg IM or IV
	OR		
	Cefazolin or ceftriaxone*	1 g IM or IV	50 mg/kg IM or IV
Allergic to penicillins or ampicillin, oral	Cephalexin*†	2 g	50 mg/kg
	OR		
	Clindamycin	600 mg	20 mg/kg
	OR		
	Azithromycin or clarithromycin	500 mg	15 mg/kg
Allergic to penicillins or ampicillin and unable to take oral medicine	Cefazolin or ceftriaxone†	1 g IM or IV	50 mg/kg IM or IV
	OR		
	Clindamycin	600 mg IM or IV	20 mg/kg IM or IV

IM, Intramuscular; *IV,* intravenous.
*Or other first-generation or second-generation oral cephalosporin in equivalent adult or pediatric dosage.
†Cephalosporins should not be used in an individual with a history of anaphylaxis, angioedema, or urticaria with penicillins or ampicillin.

*From Prevention of infective endocarditis. A guideline from the American Heart Association Rheumatic Fever, Endocarditis, and Kawasaki Disease Committee, Council on Cardiovascular Disease in the Young, and the Council on Clinical Cardiology, Council on Cardiovascular Surgery and Anesthesia, and the Quality of Care and Outcomes Research Interdisciplinary Working Group. *Circulation* published online Apr 19, 2007, DOI: 10.1161/CIRCULATIONAHA.106.183095. Print ISSN: 0009-7322. Online ISSN: 1524-4539.

TABLE 5-39 Summary of Major Changes in Updated Recommendations

We concluded that bacteremia resulting from daily activities is much more likely to cause IE than bacteremia associated with a dental procedure.

We concluded that only an extremely small number of cases of IE might be prevented by antibiotic prophylaxis even if prophylaxis is 100% effective.

Antibiotic prophylaxis is not recommended based solely on an increased lifetime risk of acquisition of IE.

Limit recommendations for IE prophylaxis only to those conditions listed in Table 5-36.

Antibiotic prophylaxis is no longer recommended for any other form of CHD, except for the conditions listed in Table 5-36.

Antibiotic prophylaxis is recommended for all dental procedures that involve manipulation of gingival tissues or periapical region of teeth or perforation of oral mucosa only for patients with underlying cardiac conditions associated with the highest risk of adverse outcome from IE (see Table 5-36).

Antibiotic prophylaxis is recommended for procedures on respiratory tract or infected skin, skin structures, or musculoskeletal tissue only for patients with underlying cardiac conditions associated with the highest risk of adverse outcome from IE (see Table 5-36).

Antibiotic prophylaxis solely to prevent IE is not recommended for GU or GI tract procedures.

The writing group reaffirms the procedures noted in the 1997 prophylaxis guidelines for which endocarditis prophylaxis is not recommended and extends this to other common procedures, including ear and body piercing, tattooing, and vaginal delivery and hysterectomy.

A guide to the clinical preventive services described is available online at http://www.ahrq.gov/clinic/pocketgd07/.
CHD, Congenital heart disease; *GI,* gastrointestinal; *GU,* genitourinary; *IE,* infective endocarditis.

I. Complementary and Alternative Medicine

II. Nutrition

III. Acute Poisoning

IV. Impairment and Disability Issues

V. Primary Care Procedures (available online)

VI. Patient Teaching Guides (available online)

Definitions of Complementary and Alternative Medicine Terms

Acupuncture Thin needles are inserted superficially on the skin at locations throughout the body. These points are located along "channels" of energy. Heat can be applied by burning (moxibustion), electric current (electroacupuncture), or pressure (acupressure). Healing is proposed by the restoration of a balance of energy flow called *Qi.* Another explanation suggests that, possibly, the stimulation activates endorphin receptors.

Alexander Technique A bodywork technique in which rebalancing of "postural sets" (i.e., physical alignment) is taught by mentally focusing on the way correct alignments should look and feel and through verbal and tactile guidance by the practitioner.

Applied Kinesiology A form of treatment that uses nutrition, physical manipulation, vitamins, diets, and exercise to restore and energize the body. Weak muscles are proposed as a source of dysfunctional health.

Aromatherapy A form of herbal medicine that uses various oils from plants. Route of administration can be through absorption in the skin or inhalation. The aromatic biochemical structures of certain herbs are thought to act in areas of the brain related to past experiences and emotions (e.g., limbic system).

Ayurveda A major health system that originated in India and incorporates the body, mind, and spirit to prevent and treat disease. Includes special types of diets, herbs, and minerals.

Biofeedback A mind-body therapy procedure in which sensors are placed on the body to measure muscle tension, heart rate, and sweat responses or neural activity. Information is provided by visual, auditory, or body-muscle cell activation so as to teach either to increase or decrease physiologic activity, which, when reconstituted, is proposed to improve health problems (e.g., pain, anxiety, or high blood pressure). In some cases, relaxation exercises complement this procedure.

Chelation Therapy Involves the removal—through intravenous infusion of a chelating agent (synthetic amino acid ethylenediamine tetraacetic acid [EDTA])—of heavy metals, including lead, nickel, and cadmium, as a way to treat certain diseases. Ancillary treatments include the use of vitamins, changes in diet, and exercise.

Cognitive Therapy Psychological therapy in which the major focus is altering and changing irrational beliefs through a type of Socratic dialogue and self-evaluation of certain illogical thoughts. Conditioning and learning are important components of this therapy.

Craniosacral Therapy A form of gentle manual manipulation used for diagnosis and for making corrections in a system made up of cerebrospinal fluid, cranial and dural membranes, cranial bones, and sacrum. This system is proposed to be dynamic, with its own physiologic frequency. Through touch and pressure, tension is proposed to be reduced and cranial rhythms normalized, leading to improvement in health and disease.

Modified from Spencer JW: *Complementary/alternative medicine: an evidence-based approach*, St Louis, 1999, Mosby.

Diathermy The use of high-frequency electrical currents as a form of physical therapy and in surgical procedures. The term *diathermy,* derived from the Greek words *dia* and *therma,* literally means "heating through." The three forms of diathermy used by physical therapists are short wave, ultrasound, and microwave.

Eye Movement Desensitization and Reprocessing (EMDR) A technique that proposes to remove painful memories by behavioral techniques. Rhythmic, multisaccadic eye movements are produced by allowing the patient to track and follow a moving object while imagining a stressful memory or event. By using deconditioning, including verbal interaction with the therapist, the painful memory is extinguished and health improved.

Feldenkrais Method A bodywork technique that integrates physics, judo, and yoga. The practitioner directs sequences of movement using verbal or hands-on techniques or teaches a system of self-directed exercise to treat physical impairments through the learning of new movement patterns.

Hatha Yoga The branch of yoga practice that involves physical exercise, breathing practices, and movement. These exercises are designed to have a salutary effect on posture, flexibility, and strength and are intended ultimately to prepare the body to remain still for long periods of meditation.

Hellerwork A bodywork technique that treats and improves proper body alignment through the development of a more complete awareness of the physical body. The goal is to realign fascia for improvement of standing, sitting, and breathing using "body energy," verbal feedback, and changing emotions and attitudes.

Homeopathy A form of treatment in which substances (minerals, plant extracts, chemicals, or disease-producing germs), which in sufficient doses would produce a set of illness symptoms in healthy individuals, are given in microdoses to produce a "cure" of those same symptoms. The *symptom* is not thought to be part of the illness but part of a curative process.

Hyperbaric Oxygen A therapy in which 100% oxygen is given at or above atmospheric pressure. An increase in oxygen in the tissue is proposed to increase blood circulation and improve healing and health and influence the course of disease.

Jin Shin Jyutsu An ancient bodywork technique to harmonize body, mind, and spirit by gentle touch that uses specific "healing points" at the body surface. The points are proposed to overlie flowing energy (Qi). The therapist's fingers are used to "redirect, balance, and provide a more efficient energy flow" to and throughout the body.

Light Therapy Natural light or light of specified wavelengths is used to treat disease. This may include ultraviolet light, colored light, or low-intensity laser light. Generally, the eye is the initial entry point for the light because of its direct connection to the brain.

Magnetic Therapy Magnets are placed directly on the skin, theoretically stimulating living cells and increasing blood flow by ionic currents that are created from polarities on the magnets.

Mediterranean Diet A diet that is thought to provide optimal distribution of daily caloric intake of different nutrients and includes 50% to 60% carbohydrates, 30% fats, and 10% proteins. The diet is derived from the eating habits of people in the Mediterranean area, who were shown to have reduced rates of cardiovascular disease.

Mind-Body Therapies A group of therapies that emphasize using the mind or brain in conjunction with the body to assist healing. Mind-body therapies can involve varying degrees of levels of consciousness, including *hypnosis,* in which selective attention is used to induce a specific altered state (trance) for memory retrieval, relaxation, or suggestion; *visual imagery,* in which the focus is on a target visual stimulus; *yoga,* which involves integration of posture and controlled breathing, relaxation, and/or meditation; *relaxation,* which includes lighter levels of altered states of consciousness through indirect or direct focus; and *meditation,* in which there is an intentional use of posture, concentration, contemplation, and visualization.

Muscle Energy Technique A manual therapy in osteopathic medicine that includes both passive mobilization and muscle reeducation. Diagnosis of somatic dysfunction is performed by the practitioner, after which the patient is guided to provide corrective muscle contraction.

Music Therapy The use of music in an either active or passive mode. Used mainly to reduce stress, anxiety, and pain.

Naturopathy A major health system that includes practices that emphasize diet, nutrition, homeopathy, acupuncture, herbal medicine, manipulation, and various mind-body therapies. Focal points include self-healing and treatment through changes in lifestyle and emphasis on health prevention.

Ornish Diet A life-choice program based on eating a vegetarian diet containing less than 10% fat. The diet is high in complex carbohydrates and fiber. Meat and fish are generally avoided.

Oslo Diet An eating plan that emphasizes increased intake of fish and reduced total fat intake. Diet is combined with regular endurance exercise.

Pilates An educational and exercise approach using the proper body mechanics, movements, truncal and pelvic stabilization, coordinated breathing, and muscle contractions to promote strengthening. Attention is paid to the entire musculoskeletal system.

Prayer The use of prayer(s) that are offered to "some higher being" or authority to heal and/or arrest disease. May be practiced by the individual patient, by groups, or by other(s) with or without the patient's knowledge (e.g., intercessory).

Pritikin Diet A weight management plan that is based on a vegetarian framework. Meals are low in fat, high in fiber, and high in complex carbohydrates.

Qi Gong A form of Chinese exercise-stimulation therapy that proposes to improve health by redirecting mental focus, breathing, coordination, and relaxation. The goal is to "rebalance" the body's own healing capacities by activating proposed electrical or energetic currents that flow along meridians located throughout the body. These meridians, however, do not follow conventional nerve or muscle pathways. In Chinese medical training and practice this therapy includes "external Qi," which is energy transmitted from one person to another so as to heal.

Raja Yoga Yoga practice that includes all of the other forms of yoga. The practitioner is instructed to follow moral directives, physical exercises, breathing exercises, meditation, devotion, and service to others to facilitate religious awakening.

Reflexology A bodywork technique that uses reflex points on the hands and feet. Pressure is applied at points that correspond to various body parts, to eliminate blockages thought to produce pain or disease.

Reiki Comes from the Japanese word meaning "universal life force energy." The practitioner serves as a conduit for healing energy directed into the body or energy field of the recipient without physical contact with the body.

Rolfing A bodywork technique that involves the myofascia. The body is realigned by using the hands to apply deep pressure and friction that allow more sufficient posture, movement, and the "release" of emotions from the body.

Shiatsu A Japanese bodywork technique involving finger pressure at specific points on the body mainly to balance "energy" in the body. The major focus is on prevention by keeping the body healthy. The therapy uses more than 600 points on the skin that are proposed to be connected to pathways through which energy flows.

T'ai Chi A technique that uses slow, purposeful motor-physical movements of the body to control and achieve a more balanced physiologic and psychological state.

Therapeutic Touch A body energy field technique in which hands are passed over the body without actually touching to recreate and change proposed "energy imbalances" for restoring innate healing forces. Verbal interaction between patient and therapist helps maximize effects.

Traditional Chinese Medicine An ancient form of medicine that focuses on prevention and secondarily treats disease with an emphasis on maintaining balance through the body by stimulating a constant, smooth-flowing Qi energy. Herbs, acupuncture, massage, diet, and exercise are also used.

Trager Psychophysical Integration A bodywork technique in which the practitioner enters a meditative state and guides the client through gentle, light, rhythmic, nonintrusive movements. "Mentastics" exercises using self-healing movements are taught to the clients.

AUTHOR: **ANNE L. HUME, PHARM.D.**

Relaxation Techniques

Relaxation Techniques

Relaxation Technique	Summary	Further Resources
Breathing exercise	This is the foundation of most relaxation techniques. Have patients place one hand on the chest and the other on the abdomen. Instruct them to take a slow, deep breath, as if they were sucking in all the air in the room. While doing this, the hand on the abdomen should rise higher than the hand on the chest. This promotes diaphragmatic breathing that increases alveolar expansion in the bases of the lungs. Have them hold the breath for a count of 7 and then exhale. Exhalation should take twice as long as inhalation. Repeat this for a total of five breaths, and encourage patients to do this three times a day.	*Conscious Breathing* by Gay Hendricks is one of many good resources on using breathing for relaxation and health.
Meditation		
Transcendental/The relaxation response	To prevent distracting thoughts, the subject repeats a mantra (a word or sound) over and over again while sitting in a comfortable position. If a distracting thought comes to mind, it is accepted and let go, with the mind focusing again on the mantra.	www.mindbody.harvard.edu or *The Relaxation Response* by Herbert Benson; www.tm.org for information on transcendental meditation.
Mindful meditation	This represents the philosophy of living in the present or in the moment. The *body scan* is one technique where the subject uses breathing to obtain a relaxed state while lying or sitting. The mind progressively focuses on different parts of the body, where it feels any and all sensations intentionally but nonjudgmentally before moving on to another part of the body. A patient with back pain may focus on the quality and characteristics of the pain as if to better understand it and bring it under control.	*Full Catastrophe Living* by Jon Kabat-Zinn describes this technique in full and the program for stress reduction at the University of Massachusetts Medical Center.
Centering prayer	This is a form similar to transcendental meditation that has a more religious foundation. The subject repeats a "sacred word" similar to a mantra. As thoughts come to mind, they are accepted and let go, clearing the mind to become more centered on the spirit within, as if the mind's preoccupied thoughts are the layers of an onion that are peeled away, allowing better understanding of the spirit at the core.	www.Centeringprayer.com; look under "method of centering prayer" for a nondenominational discussion.
Progressive muscle relaxation (PMR)	A form of relaxation in which the subject is attuned to the difference in feeling when the muscles are tensed and then relaxed. In a comfortable position, start by tensing the whole body from head to toe. While doing this, notice the feelings of tightness. Take a deep breath in and as you let it out, let the tension release and the muscles relax. This is then followed by progressive tension and relaxation throughout the body. One may start by clenching the fists and then tensing the arms, shoulders, chest, abdomen, hips, legs, and so on, with each step followed by relaxation.	www.uaex.edu/publications/pub/fshei28.htm is a good review of PMR as well as other relaxation exercises. It is sponsored by the University of Arkansas. *You Must Relax* is a book by the founder of this technique, Edmund Jacobson.
Visualization/Self-hypnosis	The subject uses visualization to recruit images that create a relaxed state. For example, if a person is anxious, visualizing images of a place and a time that were peaceful and comforting would help induce relaxation. This is best used in conjunction with a breathing exercise.	There are many CDs, MP3s, and DVDs that can guide people through a visualization "script" that can result in relaxation. Emmett Miller is one well-known author.
Autogenic training	This induces a physiologic response by using simple phrases. For example, "My legs are heavy and warm" is meant to increase the blood flow to this area, resulting in relaxation. This is done progressively from head to toe with the use of deep breathing and repetition of the phrase. After completing this, focus attention on any body part that may still be tense, and then focus the breath and phrase to that area until the whole body is relaxed.	The British Autogenic Society at www.autogenictherapy.org.uk is a good resource for more information.

Continued on following page

Relaxation Techniques—cont'd

Relaxation Technique	Summary	Further Resources
Exercise/Movement		
Aerobic	While performing an aerobic exercise, focus attention on a phrase, sound, word, or prayer and passively disregard other thoughts that may enter the mind. Some may focus on their breathing, saying to themselves, "In" with inhalation and "Out" with exhalation, or repeating "one-two, one-two" with each step they take with jogging. Doing this will help the mind focus, preventing other thoughts that may cause tension.	*Beyond the Relaxation Response* by Herbert Benson includes discussion of his research on inducing the relaxation response while exercising.
Yoga	This has been practiced for thousands of years in India. In America, it has been divided into three aspects: breathing (pranayama yoga), bodily postures or asanas (hatha yoga), and meditation to maintain balance and health. Regular practice induces relaxation.	For the following therapies, it is best to encourage patients to take a class at a local community center or gym and to pick up an introductory book at a library or bookstore.
T'ai chi	An ancient Chinese martial art that uses slow, graceful movements combined with inner mindfulness and breathing techniques to help bring balance between the mind and body.	See above.
Qi gong	A traditional Chinese practice that uses movement, meditation, and controlled breathing to balance the body's vital energy force, Qi.	See above.

From Rakel RE (ed): *Principles of family practice,* ed 6, Philadelphia, 2002, Saunders.

Overview of Selected Natural Products

This table includes a few of the common uses and side effects of selected natural products. The evidence supporting the uses and side effects of these products varies considerably and may be based on anecdotal information or theoretical concerns with the natural products.

Natural Products	Common Use(s)	Adverse Effects/Potential Concerns
African plum (Pygeum)	Benign prostatic hyperplasia	Nausea and abdominal pain have been reported, but pygeum is generally well tolerated. Pygeum does not decrease prostate size or influence PSA concentrations.
Andrographis	Prevention and treatment of viral respiratory infections	Headache, fatigue, rash, diarrhea, and vomiting. Products are standardized to 4%-6% andrographolide; this botanical is commonly used in combination products.
Black cohosh	Menopausal symptoms (hot flashes), induction of labor in pregnant women, premenstrual syndrome	Dyspepsia, rash, weight gain, headache, and cramping have been reported. Concern exists that black cohosh causes liver toxicity. The potential development of mild estrogen-like adverse effects, especially endometrial hyperplasia, is of concern.
Butterbur	Prevention of migraine headaches; allergic rhinitis; urinary tract spasms; pain	Diarrhea, stomach upset, fatigue, belching, headache, and drowsiness may occur. Due to concern about hepatotoxicity, butterbur products should be free of pyrrolizidine alkaloids. Products should be standardized to 15% petasin and isopetasin.
Chamomile (German)	Motion sickness, anxiety, insomnia; gastrointestinal spasms; mucositis	Allergic reactions occur on rare occasion. Patients with a ragweed allergy should use chamomile with caution.
Chasteberry	Premenstrual dysphoric disorder, premenstrual syndrome, menopausal symptoms, female infertility, mastalgia	Gastrointestinal upset, headache, rash, acne, weight gain, and menstrual bleeding have been reported.
Chitosan	Weight loss, Crohn's disease, hypercholesterolemia, anemia	Gastrointestinal upset, nausea, flatulence, and constipation have been reported. Patients with a shellfish allergy should avoid the use of chitosan.
Chondroitin sulfate	Osteoarthritis, osteoporosis, hyperlipidemia	Gastrointestinal upset, nausea, diarrhea, constipation, and alopecia. Concern exists that chondroitin may have anticoagulant activity due to its structural similarity to part of heparin.
Cinnamon	Type 2 diabetes mellitus, flatulence, gastrointestinal spasms, anorexia, menopausal symptoms, impotence	Cassia cinnamon is one of three types of cinnamon in commercial food products; this is the only type that may have minor effects to improve blood glucose concentrations.
Coenzyme Q10	Congestive heart failure, angina, dilated cardiomyopathy, statin-induced myopathy, Parkinson's disease, chronic fatigue syndrome, HIV/AIDS	Nausea, vomiting, diarrhea, anorexia, heartburn, and rash have been reported. Coenzyme Q10 is structurally similar to vitamin K; concern exists about potential interaction with warfarin.
Cranberry	Prevention and treatment of urinary tract infections; type 2 diabetes mellitus; chronic fatigue syndrome; pleurisy	Gastrointestinal upset and diarrhea have been reported with large doses of cranberry. Uric acid kidney stone formation is also possible with large doses of cranberry over prolonged periods of time.
Dehydroepiandrosterone (DHEA)	Slow or reverse aging, weight loss, metabolic syndrome, erectile dysfunction, immune stimulant, osteoporosis, systemic lupus erythematosus, multiple sclerosis, depression, schizophrenia	Acne and other androgenic effects commonly occur in women. Alopecia, insulin resistance, hepatic dysfunction, and hypertension have been reported. Ingested wild yam and soy cannot be converted into DHEA by humans.
Devil's claw	Osteoarthritis, atherosclerosis, gout, myalgias, fever, migraines	Diarrhea, nausea, and vomiting, as well as allergic reactions, have been reported.
Echinacea	Prevention and treatment of viral respiratory infections; urinary tract infections; chronic fatigue syndrome; attention deficit hyperactivity disorder	Nausea, vomiting, diarrhea, heartburn, headaches, dizziness, arthralgias, and allergic reactions have been reported with echinacea. Patients with a ragweed allergy should use echinacea with caution because the risk of allergic reactions may be increased.

Continued on following page

Natural Products	Common Use(s)	Adverse Effects/Potential Concerns
Eleuthero (Siberian ginseng)	Maintenance of a normal blood pressure; atherosclerosis; Alzheimer's disease; chronic fatigue syndrome; diabetes; herpes simplex infections	Drowsiness, anxiety, and irritability have been reported.
Evening primrose oil (EPO)	Premenstrual syndrome, mastalgia, osteoporosis, asthma, menopausal symptoms, eczema, chronic fatigue syndrome	EPO is well tolerated.
Fenugreek	Type 2 diabetes mellitus, anorexia, atherosclerosis; also used as galactogogue	Gastrointestinal upset, flatulence, and hypoglycemia are possible side effects. Patients with a peanut allergy (and an allergy to related plants) should use fenugreek with caution. Nursing mothers who use fenugreek may notice a "maple syrup" smell in their sweat and in the urine of their infants. This may be mistaken to be maple syrup urine disease in the infant.
Feverfew	Prevention of migraines; fever; menstrual-related problems; arthritis; infertility; asthma	Gastrointestinal side effects are the most common with feverfew. A "post-feverfew syndrome" has been reported in individuals who have taken feverfew for prolonged periods of time and then have abruptly stopped the herbal.
Fish oil	Hypertriglyceridemia, coronary heart disease, hypertension, asthma, depression, rheumatoid arthritis, osteoporosis, psoriasis	Heartburn, nausea, rash, and a "fishy" aftertaste can occur. Contamination with pesticides (as well as with mercury and other heavy metals) is a potential concern, although this is unlikely.
Garlic	Hyperlipidemia, hypertension, peripheral arterial disease, type 2 diabetes mellitus	Nausea, vomiting, heartburn, and body odor are most common. "Deodorized" garlic products may lack the active ingredient, allicin.
Ginger	Nausea and vomiting secondary to pregnancy, chemotherapy, motion sickness, surgery	Heartburn, belching, and dermatitis have been reported. In overdoses, ginger has been associated with central nervous system depression and arrhythmias. Efficacy for hyperemesis gravidarum is unknown, and use is not recommended.
Ginkgo	Alzheimer's disease, vascular dementias, tinnitus, acute mountain sickness, intermittent claudication	Gastrointestinal side effects, headaches, dizziness, and allergic skin reactions. Seizures have been reported in several case reports. Products should contain 24% ginkgo flavone glycosides and 6% terpenoids.
Ginseng (Panax)	Increased resistance to stress and improved well-being; increased physical stamina; depression; diabetes; erectile dysfunction	Insomnia has been reported with ginseng. Vaginal bleeding, mastalgia, and amenorrhea have also been reported.
Glucosamine sulfate	Osteoarthritis	Nausea, heartburn, skin reactions, and headache have been reported. Increased glucose concentrations have been a concern but have not been well documented. Patients with a shellfish allergy should use glucosamine with caution.
Green tea	Improve cognitive performance; prevention of breast, prostate, and colon cancer; hyperlipidemia; Parkinson's disease; obesity; diabetes; cardiovascular disease	Nausea, vomiting, dyspepsia, dizziness, insomnia, and nervousness have been reported. Side effects may be a result of the large amount of caffeine in green tea products. Hepatotoxicity has been a potential concern with green tea.
Hawthorn	Mild heart failure, angina, arrhythmias, hypertension	Mild gastrointestinal effects, dizziness, rash, palpitations, and nervousness have been reported.
Hoodia	Obesity	Side effects have not been reported. Many products lack the actual ingredient.
Horse chestnut	Chronic venous insufficiency, including varicose veins; benign prostate hyperplasia; diarrhea	Mild nausea, vomiting, dizziness, headache, and itching. Products are standardized to 16%-20% aescin.
Huperzine	Alzheimer's disease, increased alertness and energy, myasthenia gravis, memory enhancement	Nausea, vomiting, diarrhea, sweating, and blurred vision as a result of the cholinergic effects of huperzine have been reported.
Kava	Anxiety, insomnia, restlessness, seizure disorders, depression, chronic fatigue syndrome	Gastrointestinal upset, headache, dizziness, "kava" dermopathy, and allergic skin reactions. Hepatotoxicity is the primary concern with kava; some countries have banned the use of kava.
Melatonin	Jet lag, insomnia, migraine, chronic fatigue syndrome, breast cancer, osteoporosis; also used for insomnia in children with ADHD	Daytime drowsiness, headache, and dizziness have been reported. Vaginal bleeding has occurred in perimenopausal women. Melatonin from animal sources should be avoided.
Melissa	Cold sores (topically), anxiety, insomnia, Alzheimer's disease, hypertension, dyspepsia	Nausea, vomiting, dizziness, and wheezing have occurred with oral melissa.
Methylsulfonylmethane (MSM)	Chronic pain, arthritis, diabetes, osteoporosis, allergies, obesity, premenstrual syndrome	Nausea, bloating, diarrhea, fatigue, and insomnia have been associated with MSM. This substance is used frequently in combination with glucosamine and chondroitin.
Milk thistle	Protective agent against liver damage due to alcohol, acetaminophen, and carbon tetrachloride; hepatitis C	Nausea, abdominal fullness, diarrhea, and allergic reactions. Patients with a ragweed allergy should use milk thistle with caution.
Peppermint	Irritable bowel syndrome, sinusitis, morning sickness, dysmenorrhea	Heartburn has been reported, as well as laryngeal and bronchial spasm in infants and children.
Policosanol	Hyperlipidemia, intermittent claudication, atherosclerosis	Migraines, insomnia, dizziness, skin rash, and bleeding have been reported with policosanol. The product has antiplatelet effects.
Probiotics	Treatment and prevention of diarrhea including antibiotic-associated diarrhea; irritable bowel syndrome; atopic dermatitis; Crohn's disease	Theoretically, probiotic products may increase risk of infections in immunocompromised individuals.
Red clover phytoestrogens	Menopausal symptoms, premenstrual syndrome, asthma	Rash, myalgias, headaches, and vaginal bleeding have been reported. Theoretically, endometrial hyperplasia is an adverse effect from the use of these compounds.
Red yeast rice	Hyperlipidemia, indigestion, diarrhea, circulatory conditions, HIV/AIDS	Gastrointestinal upset and dizziness may occur. Red yeast rice may contain lovastatin-like compounds and potentially cause rhabdomyolysis.

Natural Products	Common Use(s)	Adverse Effects/Potential Concerns
S-adenosylmethionine (SAM-e)	Depression, anxiety, dementia, osteoarthritis, heart disease	Nausea, vomiting, diarrhea, headache, and nervousness have been reported. Concern exists that SAM-e raises homocysteine levels.
St. John's wort	Depression, anxiety, chronic fatigue syndrome, HIV/AIDS	Anxiety, gastrointestinal upset, vaginal bleeding, neuropathy, and rash can occur. Hypomania has been induced by St. John's wort.
Tea tree oil	Topical use for acne, fungal infections, lice, scabies	Local inflammation and contact dermatitis may occur.
Valerian	Insomnia, depression, chronic fatigue syndrome, menstrual cramps	Headaches, gastrointestinal upset, and drowsiness can occur. Hepatotoxicity is a potential concern with valerian.

AIDS, Acquired immune deficiency syndrome; *HIV,* human immunodeficiency virus.

AUTHOR: **ANNE L. HUME, PHARM.D.**

Natural Products and Drug Interactions

This table lists interactions between selected natural products and prescription and nonprescription drugs. Although many of the listed interactions are theoretical in nature and have not been documented to occur in humans, those involving St. John's wort are potentially life threatening in nature, depending on the individual drug. Other interactions are based on small studies of healthy volunteers and use pharmaceutical-quality natural products that may or may not be commercially available.

Natural Products	Drugs	Interactions
Andrographis	Immune suppressants	Andrographis may stimulate immune function, potentially decreasing the effectiveness of drugs such as cyclosporine, tacrolimus, and prednisone.
	Antihypertensive agents	Andrographis may lower blood pressure, potentiating the hypotensive effects of antihypertensive agents.
	Antiplatelet and anticoagulant agents	Andrographis may have antiplatelet activity, potentially increasing the risk of bleeding.
Black cohosh	Hepatotoxic drugs	Concern exists that the risk of hepatotoxicity with black cohosh is increased in the presence of hepatotoxic drugs such as acetaminophen.
	Cisplatin	Animal studies suggest that the efficacy of cisplatin against breast cancer cells may be decreased by black cohosh.
	CYP2D6 substrates	Black cohosh may modestly inhibit CYP2D6 enzyme activity to result in higher drug concentrations.
Butterbur	CYP3A4 inducers (rifampin, carbamazepine, etc.)	Drugs that induce the activity of CYP3A4 increase the risk of the formation of hepatotoxic metabolites from pyrrolizidine alkaloids from some butterbur products.
Chamomile	CNS depressants (benzodiazepines, opiates, barbiturates, etc.)	Chamomile may have additive CNS depressant effects.
	CYP1A2 substrates	Chamomile may inhibit CYP1A2 enzyme activity to result in higher drug concentrations.
	CYP3A4 substrates	Chamomile may inhibit CYP3A4 enzyme activity to result in higher drug concentrations.
	Estrogens	Chamomile may compete for estrogen receptors.
	Tamoxifen	Chamomile may interfere with the effects of tamoxifen because of its estrogenic effects.
Chaste tree berry	Antipsychotic agents	Chaste tree berry may antagonize the effects of antipsychotic agents through its dopaminergic activity.
	Metoclopramide	Chaste tree berry may antagonize the effects of metoclopramide through its dopaminergic activity.
	Dopamine agonists	Chaste tree berry may possess additive effects to drugs such as levodopa and ropinirole through its dopaminergic activity.
	Oral contraceptives/estrogens	Chaste tree berry may possess additive hormonal effects.
Chondroitin	Warfarin	High-dose chondroitin has structural similarity to a heparinoid and may possess weak anticoagulant effects.
Cinnamon	Hypoglycemic agents	Cinnamon may possess additive effects on blood glucose to those of hypoglycemic agents.
Coenzyme Q10	Antihypertensive agents	Coenzyme Q10 may possess additive effects on blood pressure to those of antihypertensive agents.
	Warfarin	Coenzyme Q10 may lessen the anticoagulant effects of warfarin because of its structural similarity to vitamin K.
	Chemotherapy	The antioxidant effects of coenzyme Q10 may blunt the efficacy of certain chemotherapeutic agents that depend on the formation of free radicals.
Cranberry	CYP2C9 substrates (warfarin)	Cranberry may inhibit CYP2C9 enzyme activity to result in higher drug concentrations; evidence with warfarin is contradictory.
Dehydroepiandrosterone (DHEA)	Tamoxifen and aromatase inhibitors such as anastrozole and exemestane	DHEA may interfere with the antiestrogenic effects of these drugs.
	CYP3A4 substrates	DHEA may slightly inhibit CYP3A4 enzyme activity to result in higher drug concentrations.

Continued on following page

Natural Products	Drugs	Interactions
Devil's claw	Antihypertensive agents	Devil's claw may possess additive effects on blood pressure to those of antihypertensive agents.
	Hypoglycemic agents	Devil's claw may possess additive effects on blood glucose to those of hypoglycemic agents.
	H_2 antagonists and PPIs	Devil's claw may raise gastric pH and blunt the efficacy of H_2 antagonists and PPIs.
	CYP3A4 substrates	Devil's claw may inhibit CYP3A4 enzyme activity to result in higher drug concentrations.
	CYP2C9 substrates	Devil's claw may inhibit CYP2C9 enzyme activity to result in higher drug concentrations.
	CYP2C19 substrates	Devil's claw may inhibit CYP2C19 enzyme activity to result in higher drug concentrations.
	Warfarin	Devil's claw may inhibit CYP2C9 enzyme activity to result in higher concentrations of warfarin; purpura has been reported.
Echinacea	Immune suppressants	Echinacea may stimulate immune function, potentially decreasing the effectiveness of drugs such as cyclosporine, tacrolimus, and prednisone.
	CYP3A4 substrates	Echinacea may modestly induce hepatic CYP3A4 enzyme activity to result in lower drug concentrations.
	CYP1A2 substrates	Echinacea may inhibit CYP1A2 enzyme activity to result in higher drug concentrations.
Eleuthero (Siberian ginseng)	CNS depressants (benzodiazepines, opiates, barbiturates, etc.)	Eleuthero may have additive CNS depressant effects.
	Antiplatelet and anticoagulant agents	Eleuthero may have antiplatelet activity, potentially increasing the risk of bleeding.
	CYP3A4 substrates	Eleuthero may inhibit CYP3A4 enzyme activity to result in higher drug concentrations.
	CYP1A2 substrates	Eleuthero may modestly inhibit CYP1A2 enzyme activity to result in higher drug concentrations.
	CYP2C9 substrates	Eleuthero may modestly inhibit CYP2C9 enzyme activity to result in higher drug concentrations.
	CYP2D6 substrates	Eleuthero may inhibit CYP2D6 enzyme activity to result in higher drug concentrations.
	Digoxin	Concentration of digoxin has been reported to increase but without evidence of toxicity.
Evening primrose oil (EPO)	Antiplatelet and anticoagulant agents	EPO may have anticoagulant activity, potentially increasing the risk of bleeding.
Fenugreek	Antiplatelet and anticoagulant agents	Fenugreek may have antiplatelet activity, potentially increasing the risk of bleeding.
	Hypoglycemic agents	Fenugreek may potentially lower blood glucose concentrations and have additive effects with hypoglycemic agents.
Feverfew	Antiplatelet and anticoagulant agents	Feverfew may have antiplatelet activity, potentially increasing the risk of bleeding.
	CYP3A4 substrates	Feverfew may inhibit CYP3A4 enzyme activity to result in higher drug concentrations.
	CYP1A2 substrates	Feverfew may inhibit CYP1A2 enzyme activity to result in higher drug concentrations.
	CYP2C9 substrates	Feverfew may inhibit CYP2C9 enzyme activity to result in higher drug concentrations.
	CYP2C19 substrates	Feverfew may inhibit CYP2C19 enzyme activity to result in higher drug concentrations.
Fish oils (omega-3 fatty acids)	Antiplatelet and anticoagulant agents	Fish oils may have antiplatelet activity, potentially increasing the risk of bleeding, although this has not been documented in humans.
	Antihypertensive agents	Fish oils may possess additive effects on blood pressure to those of antihypertensive agents.
	Oral contraceptives	Oral contraceptives may potentially interfere with the triglyceride-lowering effects of fish oil.
Garlic	Antiplatelet and anticoagulant agents	Garlic may have antiplatelet activity, potentially increasing the risk of bleeding.
	CYP3A4 substrates	Garlic may potentially induce CYP3A4 enzyme activity to result in lower drug concentrations; evidence is contradictory.
	CYP2E1 substrates	Garlic may modestly inhibit CYP2E1 enzyme activity to result in higher drug concentrations.
Ginger	Antiplatelet and anticoagulant agents	Ginger may have antiplatelet activity, potentially increasing the risk of bleeding.
	Hypoglycemic agents	Ginger may potentially lower blood glucose concentrations and have additive effects with hypoglycemic agents.
Ginkgo	Antiplatelet and anticoagulant agents	Ginkgo may have antiplatelet activity, potentially increasing the risk of bleeding.
	CYP2C19 substrates	Ginkgo may induce CYP2C19 enzyme activity to result in lower drug concentrations.
	CYP1A2 substrates	Ginkgo may modestly inhibit CYP1A2 enzyme activity to result in higher drug levels.
	CYP2C9 substrates	Ginkgo may modestly inhibit CYP2C9 enzyme activity to result in higher drug concentrations.
	CYP2D6 substrates	Ginkgo may inhibit CYP2D6 enzyme activity to result in higher drug concentrations.
Ginseng (Panax)	Antiplatelet and anticoagulant agents	Panax ginseng may have antiplatelet properties; American ginseng may decrease the effectiveness (international normalized ration [INR]) of warfarin.
	CYP2D6 substrates	Panax ginseng may modestly inhibit CYP2D6 enzyme activity to result in higher drug concentrations.
	Immune suppressants	Panax ginseng may stimulate immune function, potentially decreasing the effectiveness of drugs such as cyclosporine, tacrolimus, and prednisone.
	Hypoglycemic agents	Panax ginseng may potentially lower blood glucose levels and have additive effects with hypoglycemic agents.
Glucosamine	Warfarin	High-dose glucosamine (along with high-dose chondroitin) may have additive effects to those of warfarin because of structural similarity to heparin.

Natural Products	Drugs	Interactions
Green tea extract	Antiplatelet agents	Green tea possesses compounds that may have antiplatelet activity, potentially increasing the risk of bleeding.
	Amphetamines	Caffeine in green tea may increase the risk of CNS toxicity.
	Cocaine	Caffeine in green tea may increase the risk of CNS toxicity.
	Oral contraceptives	Oral contraceptives may decrease the clearance of caffeine in green tea.
	Warfarin	Small amounts of vitamin K have been reported to be present in green tea, potentially decreasing the effectiveness of warfarin.
	Theophylline	Caffeine potentially decreases theophylline clearance.
	Verapamil	Verapamil decreases caffeine clearance, resulting in increased concentrations.
	Quinolone antibiotics	Some quinolone antibiotics decrease the clearance of caffeine.
	Hepatotoxic drugs	Concern exists that the risk of hepatotoxicity with green tea is increased in the presence of hepatotoxic drugs such as acetaminophen.
Hawthorn	β-Blockers	Hawthorn and β-blockers may have additive effects on blood pressure and heart rate.
	CCBs, nitrates	Hawthorn and CCBs (or nitrates) may have additive effects due to coronary vasodilation.
	Digoxin	Hawthorn may have additive effects to those of digoxin.
	Phosphodiesterase inhibitors	Hawthorn may have additive vasodilatory and hypotensive effects with sildenafil, tadalafil, and vardenafil.
Horse chestnut seed extract (HCSE)	Antiplatelet and anticoagulant agents	HCSE may have antiplatelet activity, potentially increasing the risk of bleeding.
	Hypoglycemic agents	HCSE may potentially lower blood glucose concentrations and have additive effects with hypoglycemic agents.
Huperzine	AChE inhibitors (donepezil, etc.)	Huperzine may have additive effects when combined with AChE inhibitors.
	Anticholinergic drugs	The effectiveness of huperzine and/or the anticholinergic drug may be decreased by their concomitant administration.
	Cholinergic drugs (bethanechol, neostigmine, etc.)	Huperzine may have additive effects when combined with cholinergic drugs.
Kava	CYP3A4 substrates	Kava may inhibit CYP3A4 enzyme activity to result in higher drug concentrations.
	CYP1A2 substrates	Kava may inhibit CYP1A2 enzyme activity to result in higher drug concentrations.
	CYP2C9 substrates, CYP2C19 substrates	Kava may inhibit CYP2C9 and CYP2C19 enzyme activity to result in higher drug concentrations.
	CYP2D6 substrates	Kava may inhibit CYP2D6 enzyme activity to result in higher drug concentrations.
	P-glycoprotein substrates (digoxin; etoposide, paclitaxel, vinblastine, vincristine; itraconazole; diltiazem, verapamil; and many other drugs)	Kava may inhibit P-glycoprotein transporter systems.
	Hepatotoxic drugs	Concern exists that the risk of hepatotoxicity from kava is increased in the presence of hepatotoxic drugs such as acetaminophen.
Melatonin	Antiplatelet and anticoagulant agents	Melatonin may potentiate the effects of antiplatelets and anticoagulants, although the mechanism is unknown.
	CNS depressants	Melatonin may have additive CNS depressant effects.
	Fluvoxamine	Fluvoxamine may increase levels of melatonin.
	Immune suppressants	Melatonin may stimulate immune function, potentially decreasing the effectiveness of drugs such as cyclosporine, tacrolimus, and prednisone.
	Hypoglycemic agents	Melatonin may impair glucose utilization and may decrease the efficacy of hypoglycemic agents.
Milk thistle	Estrogens (and other drugs that undergo glucuronidation)	Silymarin may increase the clearance of estrogens.
	CYP2C9 substrates	Milk thistle may modestly inhibit CYP2C9 enzyme activity to result in higher drug concentrations.
Peppermint oil	H_2 antagonists and proton pump inhibitors	Peppermint oil may raise gastric pH and blunt efficacy of H_2 antagonists and PPIs.
	CYP3A4 substrates	Peppermint oil may modestly inhibit CYP3A4 enzyme activity to result in higher drug concentrations.
	CYP1A2 substrates	Peppermint oil may modestly inhibit CYP1A2 enzyme activity to result in higher drug concentrations.
	CYP2C9 substrates, CYP2C19 substrates	Peppermint oil may modestly inhibit CYP2C9 and CYP2C19 enzyme activity to result in higher drug concentrations.
Policosanol	Antiplatelet and anticoagulant agents	Policosanol may have antiplatelet activity, potentially increasing the risk of bleeding.
Probiotics	Antibiotics	Antibiotics may kill the live organisms in different probiotic preparations.
	Immune suppressants	Theoretically, probiotics may cause bacterial or fungal infections in patients who are taking immune suppressants chronically.

Continued on following page

Natural Products	Drugs	Interactions
Red clover phytoestrogens	Antiplatelet and anticoagulant agents	Theoretically, red clover may possess coumarins, which increase the risk of bleeding with antiplatelet and anticoagulants.
	CYP3A4 substrates	Red clover may inhibit CYP3A4 enzyme activity to result in higher drug concentrations.
	CYP2C9 substrates, CYP2C19 substrates	Red clover may inhibit CYP2C9 and CYP2C19 enzyme activity to result in higher drug concentrations.
	CYP1A2 substrates	Red clover may inhibit CYP1A2 enzyme activity to result in higher drug concentrations.
Red yeast rice	CYP3A4 inhibitors	Drugs that inhibit CYP3A4 may decrease the metabolism of lovastatin in red yeast rice.
	Statins	Red yeast rice contains lovastatin and increases the risk of myopathy (and hepatotoxicity).
	Fibrates and niacin	Fibrates and niacin may increase concentrations of lovastatin in red yeast rice.
S-adenosylmethionine (SAM-e)	Antidepressants (including MAOIs)	Additive effects are possible, and there is potential for toxicity.
	Serotonergic drugs (triptans, SSRIs, tramadol, meperidine, dextromethorphan, etc.)	SAM-e may increase the risk of development of serotonin syndrome when used concomitantly.
Soy phytoestrogens	Antibiotics	Antibiotics may decrease the efficacy of soy because intestinal bacteria convert isoflavones into more active forms.
	Estrogens	Soy potentially may inhibit the effects of estrogen.
	Tamoxifen/aromatase inhibitors	Soy's estrogenic effects may antagonize the antitumor effects of tamoxifen/aromatase inhibitors.
	MAOIs	Fermented soy products may contain tyramine.
St. John's wort	CYP3A4 substrates	St. John's wort strongly induces CYP3A4 enzyme activity to result in lower drug concentrations.
	CYP1A2 substrates	St. John's wort modestly induces CYP1A2 enzyme activity to result in lower drug levels.
	CYP2C9 substrates	St. John's wort induces CYP2C9 enzyme activity to result in lower drug concentrations.
	P-glycoprotein substrates (digoxin; etoposide, paclitaxel, vinblastine, vincristine; itraconazole; diltiazem, verapamil; and other drugs)	St. John's wort induces P-glycoprotein transporter systems.
	Serotonergic drugs (triptans, SSRIs, tramadol, meperidine, dextromethorphan, etc.)	St. John's wort may increase the risk of development of serotonin syndrome when used concomitantly.
Valerian	CNS depressants (benzodiazepines, opiates, barbiturates, alcohol, etc.)	Valerian may increase the sedative effects of CNS depressants.
	CYP3A4 substrates	Valerian may modestly inhibit the CYP3A4 enzyme activity.

AChE, Acetylcholinesterase; *CCBs,* calcium channel blockers; *CNS,* central nervous system; *MAOIs,* monoamine oxidase inhibitor; *PPIs,* proton pump inhibitors; *SSRIs,* selective serotonin reuptake inhibitors.

EXAMPLES OF DRUGS METABOLIZED BY CYP ENZYMES

The following are examples of drugs that are metabolized through the different cytochrome P450 isoenzymes:

CYP1A2 substrates: theophylline, imipramine, clozapine, naproxen

CYP2C9 substrates: warfarin, tamoxifen, irbesartan, ibuprofen, glipizide

CYP2C19 substrates: omeprazole and other proton pump inhibitors, phenytoin, phenobarbital, cyclophosphamide

CYP2D6 substrates: S-metoprolol, propafenone, paroxetine, risperidone, tramadol

CYP2E1 substrates: acetaminophen, alcohol

CYP3A4 substrates: most statins, indinavir, amlodipine, verapamil, alprazolam, buspirone

(For a complete list of drugs and their respective metabolic pathways through the cytochrome P450 isoenzyme systems go to http://medicine.iupui.edu/flockhart.)

AUTHOR: **ANNE L. HUME, PHARM.D.**

Commonly Ingested Plants with Significant Toxic Potential

Plant	Symptoms	Management
Autumn crocus *(Colchicum autumnale)*	Vomiting Diarrhea Initial leukocytosis followed by bone marrow failure Multisystem organ failure	Activated charcoal decontamination Aggressive fluid resuscitation and supportive care
Belladonna alkaloids: jimson weed *(Datura stramonium)* Belladonna ("deadly nightshade"; *Atropa belladonna*)	Anticholinergic toxidrome Seizures	Supportive care, benzodiazepines Consider physostigmine if patient is a threat to self or others; only use if no conduction delays on ECG
Cardiac glycoside–containing plants (foxglove, lily of the valley, oleander, yellow oleander, etc.)	Nausea Vomiting Bradycardia Dysrhythmias (AV block, ventricular ectopy) Hyperkalemia	Digoxin-specific Fab fragments
Jequirity bean and other abrin-containing species (e.g., rosary pea, precatory bean)	Oral pain Vomiting Diarrhea Shock Hemolysis Renal failure	Supportive care, including aggressive volume resuscitation and correction of electrolyte abnormalities
Monkshood (*Aconitum* species)	Numbness and tingling of lips/tongue Vomiting Bradycardia	Atropine for bradycardia Supportive care
Oxalate-containing plants: *Philodendron, Diffenbachia, Colocasia* ("elephant ear")	Local tissue injury Oral pain Vomiting	Supportive care, pain control
Poison hemlock *(Conium maculatum)*	Vomiting Agitation followed by CNS depression Paralysis Respiratory failure	Supportive care
Pokeweed	Hemorrhagic gastroenteritis Burning of mouth and throat	Supportive care
Rhododendron	Vomiting Diarrhea Bradycardia	Atropine for symptomatic bradycardia Supportive care
Tobacco	Vomiting Agitation Diaphoresis Fasciculations Seizures	Supportive care
Water hemlock (*Cicuta* species)	Abdominal pain Vomiting Delirium Seizures	Supportive care, including benzodiazepines for seizures
Yew (*Taxus* species)	GI symptoms QRS widening Hypotension CV collapse	Supportive care Atropine for bradycardia Sodium bicarbonate does not appear to be effective

AV, Atrioventricular; *CNS,* central nervous system; *CV,* cardiovascular; *ECG,* electrocardiogram; *Fab,* fragment, antigen binding; *GI,* gastrointestinal.
From Kliegman RM et al: *Nelson textbook of pediatrics,* ed 19, Philadelphia, 2011, Saunders.

Appendix If

Herbs Associated with Toxicity

Herbal Product	Toxic Chemicals	Toxic Effects
Aconite (*Aconitum* spp.)	Aconitine alkaloids	Nausea, vomiting, paresthesias, weakness, hypotension, asystole, arrhythmias, bradycardia
Chamomile (*Matricaria chamomilla, Anthemis nobilis*)	Allergens	Anaphylaxis, contact dermatitis
Chapparal (*Larrea divaricate, Larrea tridentate*)	Nordihydroguaiaretic acid	Nausea, vomiting, lethargy, hepatitis
Cinnamon oil (*Cinnamomum* spp.)	Cinnamaldehyde	Dermatitis, abuse syndrome
Coltsfoot (*Tussilago farfara*)	Pyrrolizidines	HVOD
Comfrey (*Symphytum officinale*)	Pyrrolizidines	HVOD
Crotalaria spp.	Pyrrolizidines	HVOD
Echinacea (*Echinacea angustifolia*, Compositae spp.)	Polysaccharides	Asthma, atopy, angioedema, anaphylaxis, urticaria
Eucalyptus (*Eucalyptus globulus*)	1,8-cineole	Drowsiness, ataxia, nausea, vomiting, seizures, coma, respiratory failure
Garlic (*Allium sativum*)	Allicin	Dermatitis, chemical burns, oxidizing agent
Germander (*Teucrium chamaedrys*)		Hepatotoxicity
Ginseng (*Panax ginseng*)	Ginsenoside	Ginseng abuse, diarrhea, anxiety, insomnia, hypertension
Glycerated asafetida	Oxidants	Methemoglobinemia
Groundsel (*Senecio longilobus*)	Pyrrolizidines	HVOD
Heliotrope, turnsole (*Crotalaria fulva, Heliotropium, Cynoglossum officinale*)	Pyrrolizidines	HVOD
Jin bu huan (*Stephania* spp., *Corydalis* spp.)	L-Tetrahydropalmitine	Hepatitis, lethargy, coma
Kava-kava (*Piper methysticum*)	Kawain, methysticin	Hepatic failure, "kavaism," neurotoxicity
Kelp	Iodine	Thyroid dysfunction
Laetrile	Cyanide	Coma, seizures, death
Licorice (*Glycyrrhiza glabra*)	Glycyrrhetic acid	Hypertension, cardiac arrhythmias, hypokalemia
Ma huang (*Ephedra sinica*)	Ephedrine	Cardiac arrhythmias, seizures, stroke, hypertension
Monkshood (*Aconitum napellus, A. columbianum*)	Aconite	Cardiac arrhythmias, weakness, coma, shock, paresthesias, vomiting, seizures
Nutmeg (*Myristica fragrans*)	Myristicin, eugenol	Hallucinations, emesis, headache
Nux vomica	Strychnine	Seizures, abdominal pain, respiratory arrest
Pennyroyal (*Mentha pulegium* or *Hedeoma* spp.)	Pulegone	Centrilobular liver necrosis, fetotoxicity, seizures, shock
Ragwort (golden) (*Senecio aureus, Echium*)	Pyrrolizidines	HVOD
Wormwood (*Artemisia* spp.)	Thujone	Seizures, dementia, tremors, headache

HVOD, Hepatic veno-occlusive disease.
From Fuhrman BP et al: *Pediatric critical care,* ed 4, Philadelphia, 2011, Saunders.

Websites Providing Data on Herbal Therapy Hazards

Web Address	Website
http://www.fda.gov or http://www.vmcfsan.fda.gov/-dms/aems/html	On the U.S. Food and Drug Administration website under the title "Medwatch," some herb warnings can be found ("special adverse event monitoring system" link)
http://www.faseb.org/aspet/H&MIG3.htm#top	ASPET Herbal and Medicinal Plant Interest Group: a site for an herb discussion group with pharmacologists
http://www.nnlm.nlm.nih.gov/pnr/uwmhg/	University of Washington Medicinal Herb Garden
http://www.nim.nih.gov/medlineplus/herbalmedicine.html	Provides an update on ongoing clinical studies involving herbal products, news, and many links
http://www.update-software.com/abstracts/mainindex.html	The Cochrane Collaboration maintains an updated international database of clinical trials involving complementary and alternative medicine
http://www.amfoundation.org/	Providing consumers and professionals with responsible evidence-based information on the integration of alternative and conventional medicine
http://www.herbmed.org/	An interactive electronic herbal database provides hyperlinked access to scientific data underlying the use of herbs for health; an evidence-based information resource for professionals, researchers, and general public
http://nccam.nih.gov/	The National Center for Complementary and Alternative Medicine is 1 of 27 institutes and centers that make up the U.S. National Institutes of Health; their mission is to support rigorous research on complementary and alternative medicine, train researchers, and disseminate information to the public and professionals
http://toxnet.nlm.nih.gov/	A cluster of databases on toxicology, hazardous chemicals, and related areas

From Floege J et al: *Comprehensive clinical nephrology,* ed 4, Philadelphia, 2010, Saunders.

Dietary Supplements: What Every Primary Care Provider Should Know

Primary care providers must be knowledgeable regarding the safety, efficacy, and drug interactions associated with common dietary supplements because of the following:

- An estimated 38% of adults ages 18 years and older reported the use of at least one form of complementary and alternative medicine (CAM) according to the National Health Interview Survey in 2007.
- Almost 17.8% of adults specifically reported the use of dietary supplements, with fish oil, glucosamine, echinacea, flaxseed, and ginseng most frequently used.
- Although the use of dietary supplements has plateaued as a result of consumer concerns about effectiveness and potential adverse effects, usage remains common and potentially dangerous.

COMMON TERMINOLOGY

- A *dietary supplement* is defined as an oral product containing vitamins, minerals, herbs, or other botanicals; amino acids; dietary substances used to supplement the diet by increasing the total dietary intake; or a concentrate, metabolite, constituent, extract, or combination.
- *CAM* refers to the broad domain of healing practices that include diverse health systems, modalities, and practices and their accompanying theories and beliefs (see glossary of terms in Appendix Ia).
- *Complementary therapies* are those that are used *in addition to* conventional therapies, whereas *alternative therapies* are those that are used *instead of* conventional therapies. Most consumers in the United States use dietary supplements as a complementary therapy.
- *Standardization* refers to the practice of producing dietary supplements with a specific amount of a given compound that may or may not include the actual active ingredient. For example, feverfew has been standardized to its parthenolide content.

LEGISLATION

The U.S. Food and Drug Administration (FDA) is frequently criticized for not closely regulating dietary supplements and monitoring their safety. However, although the agency regulates prescription drugs and over-the-counter (OTC) products, the FDA has limited regulatory authority over dietary supplements. This is because the Dietary Supplement and Health Education Act (DSHEA) of 1994 and its resulting regulations limit the FDA's authority. As a result of DSHEA, the FDA is able to act only when a dietary supplement has been documented to contain a prescription drug, as was the case with glyburide in a natural treatment for diabetes and diazepam in an osteoarthritis preparation. In addition, the FDA can act when safety issues related to a product have been clearly documented, although these cases are frequently challenged in the courts.

HEALTH CLAIMS

Dietary supplements generally are marketed under three types of health claims. The first category is the "nutrient content" claim, in which the product is identified as an excellent source of, typically, a mineral such as calcium, based on recommended daily values. The second type is the "significant scientific agreement" claim; these claims are used when some evidence of the product's efficacy exists (e.g., fish oil supplements). The third and most common type of health claim is called a "structure/function" claim; these claims state that the product has some effect on health—for example, "helps to maintain a healthy heart." However, dietary supplements are not permitted to carry claims stating that they are effective in preventing, treating, or curing diseases.

INFORMATION RESOURCES

Appendix Ic provides a brief overview of common dietary supplements. Until recently, few evidence-based resources on dietary supplements were available. Clinical studies and systematic reviews on dietary supplements are now widely available through PubMed, EMBASE, and the Cochrane Database of Systematic Reviews. Although more information is available, references on specific products vary in their interpretation of the available evidence and may exhibit an unintentional bias, either pro or con, regarding the safety and efficacy of dietary supplements.

"Gold standard" evidence-based databases on dietary supplements (subscription required) include the following:

- Natural Medicines Comprehensive Database (http://www.naturaldatabase.com): This database includes listings for many dietary supplements and is organized in a clinician-friendly manner. Monographs include the different common and scientific names; uses and likely effectiveness for different uses; chemical constituents; interactions with drugs, diseases, foods, and laboratory tests; adverse effects; and cautions. The information is extensively referenced and is updated on a daily basis. The primary limitation is that the evaluation of data on clinical effectiveness could be more rigorous.
- Natural Standard (http://www.naturalstandard.com): This database includes listings for dietary supplements and other forms of complementary and alternative medicine. The evidence supporting the assessments in this database is critically evaluated and rigorous in nature. The primary limitation is that many fewer dietary supplements are included in this database.

Evidence-based free websites on dietary supplements include the following:

- National Center for Complementary and Alternative Medicine (NCCAM) (http://nccam.nih.gov)
- Office of Dietary Supplements International Bibliographic Information on Dietary Supplements (http://dietary-supplements.info.nih.gov/Health_Information/IBIDS.aspx)
- Memorial Sloan-Kettering Cancer Center (http://www.mskcc.org/mskcc/html/11570.cfm)

DRUG INTERACTIONS

Clinically significant interactions have been documented between dietary supplements and prescription or OTC drugs. The challenge for primary care providers is to identify real, clinically relevant interactions versus potential or theoretical interactions. Data on interactions with dietary supplements are usually based on isolated case reports or on studies enrolling healthy volunteers. As with drug-drug interactions, the likelihood of an interaction and its severity are influenced especially by concomitant medical conditions, such as heart failure and presence or absence of impaired kidney and liver function.

Appendix Id lists interactions between selected natural products and prescription and nonprescription drugs. The following two broad interactions are particularly important in primary care practice:

- St. John's wort, commonly used for depression, is a potent inducer of cytochrome P450 3A4 isoenzymes and has been documented to increase the clearance of many drugs that are metabolized through this (and other) pathways. (For a list of common drugs cleared in this manner, readers should consult http://medicine.iupui.edu/flockhart/clinlist.htm.) In addition, St. John's wort may induce P-glycoprotein transporter systems that are important for digoxin and some chemotherapeutic agents. St. John's wort has also been associated with the development of serotonin syndrome when used with drugs that have significant serotonergic activity.
- Dietary supplements such as garlic, ginkgo, and feverfew, as well as many others, have been purported to either have antiplatelet activity or have effects on the clotting cascade. This may be important for adults also taking aspirin (and other platelet-active agents) or warfarin.

COUNSELING POINTS

The single most important counseling point related to dietary supplements is always to ask patients about their use of these products and to do so in an open, nonjudgmental manner. The approach should emphasize that many consumers have been interested in vitamins, minerals, herbs, teas, and so on, to maintain their health or to treat illness. If the clinician is unaware of the safety, efficacy, and interactions of a specific product, several websites are available to quickly scan for information. Also, access to drug information centers at colleges of pharmacy is almost always available, and some hospitals now offer programs in integrative medicine.

Patients should be asked about their goals in using the product, as well as how long they have taken it and in what dosage. Allergies to plants should be documented because cross-allergies are common. Clinicians should appreciate that individuals who use dietary supplements may be interested in making lifestyle changes and potentially decreasing their use of prescription drugs. In addition, if an individual is also consulting an alternative medicine practitioner, clinicians should recognize that some alternative health systems discourage the use of established therapies such as vaccines.

Although problems with safety and efficacy have been identified, many dietary supplements are benign except for their cost. Some patients are at higher risk for adverse outcomes from the use of dietary supplements (e.g., those with chronic kidney and liver disease). Patients should be counseled specifically to avoid purchasing dietary supplements over the Internet.

RESEARCH ISSUES

Many clinical and observational studies of dietary supplements have been published. In the past, clinicians frequently stated either that published studies of dietary supplements did not exist or that only a few were available. The reason for this finding was that until recently the National Library of Medicine did not abstract from the peer-reviewed alternative medicine literature. Fortunately, much more research is now readily available. As with all research, the more rigorous the study methodology, the less likely the dietary supplement is to demonstrate clinical benefit.

In evaluating published studies of dietary supplements, the following should be considered:

- Has the correct plant and part of the plant (root, stem, leaf) been used? This critical information may not be known to many clinicians. Consulting a resource such as the National Medicines Comprehensive Database can usually provide the needed information to judge this component of the study.
- Has the content of active ingredients been verified throughout the study? In a recent review of 81 major randomized controlled trials of herbal products, only 12 (15%) reported performing tests to quantify actual contents, and 3 (4%) provided adequate data to compare actual with expected content values of at least one chemical constituent.
- Is the severity of the disease appropriate for study? Negative studies with dietary supplements sometimes inappropriately enroll participants who have moderate-to-severe disease (e.g., those with depression or benign prostatic hyperplasia) when only mild disease would be appropriate.
- Is the duration of the study appropriate? Early studies comparing glucosamine and nonsteroidal anti-inflammatory agents (NSAIAs) demonstrated greater efficacy with the NSAIAs because of an inadequate study duration for glucosamine to show any benefit.
- Is a placebo group included? Recent studies with dietary supplements for menopausal symptoms and osteoarthritis have demonstrated placebo responses over 40% to 50%.
- Was the blinding maintained throughout the study? Some dietary supplements, such as saw palmetto, have distinctive odors and tastes that are not easily masked.
- Is the preparation commercially available? Most important, when a study with dietary supplements does show benefit, it frequently is difficult to use the product in practice because the specific formulation studied is not commercially available.

AUTHOR: **ANNE L. HUME, PHARM.D.**

Vitamins and Their Functions

	Biochemistry and Physiology	Deficiency [RDA*]	Toxicity [TUL†]	Assessment of Status
Fat-Soluble Vitamins				
Vitamin A	A family of the retinoid compounds, each member having biologic activity qualitatively similar to retinol. Carotenoids are structurally related to retinoids. Some carotenoids, most notably β-carotene, are metabolized into compounds with vitamin A activity and are therefore considered to be provitamin A compounds. Vitamin A is an integral component of rhodopsin and iodopsins, light-sensitive proteins in rod and cone cells in the retina. *Additional functions:* induction and maintenance of cellular differentiation in certain tissues; signal for appropriate morphogenesis in the developing embryo; maintenance of cell-mediated immunity. One microgram of retinol = 3.33 IU of vitamin A.	Follicular hyperkeratosis and night blindness are early indicators. Conjunctival xerosis, degeneration of the cornea (keratomalacia), and de-differentiation of rapidly proliferating epithelia are later indications of deficiency. *Bitot spots* (focal areas of the conjunctiva or cornea with foamy appearance) are an indication of xerosis. Blindness, due to corneal destruction and retinal dysfunction, ensues if left uncorrected. Increased susceptibility to infection is also a consequence. [F: 700 μg; M: 900 μg]	In adults, >150,000 μg may cause acute toxicity: fatal intracranial hypertension, skin exfoliation, and hepatocellular necrosis. *Chronic* toxicity may occur with habitual daily intake of >10,000 μg: alopecia, ataxia, bone and muscle pain, dermatitis, cheilitis, conjunctivitis, pseudotumor cerebri, hepatocellular necrosis, hyperlipidemia, and hyperostosis are common. Single, large doses of vitamin A (30,000 μg), or habitual intake of >4500 μg/day in early pregnancy can be teratogenic. Excessive intake of carotenoids causes a benign condition characterized by yellowish discoloration of the skin. Habitually large doses of canthaxanthin, a carotenoid, have the additional capability of inducing a retinopathy. [3000 μg]	Retinol concentration in the plasma and vitamin A concentrations in the milk and tears are reasonably accurate measures of adequate status. Toxicity is best assessed by elevated levels of retinyl esters in plasma. A quantitative measure of dark adaptation for night vision or an electroretinogram are useful functional tests.
Vitamin D	A group of sterol compounds whose parent structure is cholecalciferol (vitamin D_3). Cholecalciferol is formed in the skin from 7-dehydrocholesterol (provitamin D_3) by exposure to UVB radiation. A plant sterol, ergocalciferol (provitamin D_2) can be similarly converted into vitamin D_2 and has similar vitamin D activity. The vitamin undergoes sequential hydroxylations in the liver and kidney at the 25 and 1 positions, respectively, producing the most bioactive form of the vitamin, 1,25-dihydroxy vitamin D. Maintains intracellular and extracellular concentrations of calcium and phosphate by enhancing intestinal absorption of the two ions and, in conjunction with PTH, promoting their mobilization from bone mineral. Retards proliferation and promotes differentiation in certain epithelia. One microgram = 40 IU.	Deficiency results in disordered bone modeling called *rickets* in childhood and *osteomalacia* in adults. Expansion of the epiphyseal growth plates and replacement of normal bone with unmineralized bone matrix are the cardinal features of rickets; the latter feature also characterizes osteomalacia. Deformity of bone and pathologic fractures occur. Decreased serum concentrations of calcium and phosphate may occur. [15 μg, ages 19-70 yr; 20 μg, age >70 yr]	Excess amounts result in abnormally high concentrations of calcium and phosphate in the serum: metastatic calcifications, renal damage, and altered mentation may occur. [50 μg]	The serum concentration of the major circulating metabolite, 25-hydroxyvitamin D, is an excellent indicator of systemic status except in chronic renal failure, in which the impairment of renal L-hydroxylation results in disassociation of the mono- and dihydroxyvitamin concentrations. Measuring the serum concentration of 1,25-dihydroxyvitamin D is then necessary.

Continued on following page

	Biochemistry and Physiology	Deficiency [RDA*]	Toxicity [TUL†]	Assessment of Status
Vitamin E	A group of at least 8 naturally occurring compounds, some of which are tocopherols and some of which are tocotrienols. At present, the only dietary form that is thought to be biologically active in humans is α-tocopherol. Acts as an antioxidant and free radical scavenger in lipophilic environments, most notably in cell membranes. Acts in conjunction with other antioxidants such as selenium.	Deficiency due to dietary inadequacy rare. Usually seen in (1) premature infants, (2) individuals with fat malabsorption, and (3) individuals with abetalipoproteinemia. Red blood cell fragility occurs and can produce a hemolytic anemia. Neuronal degeneration produces peripheral neuropathies, ophthalmoplegia, and destruction of posterior columns of spinal cord. Neurologic disease is frequently irreversible if deficiency is not corrected early enough. May contribute to the hemolytic anemia and retrolental fibroplasia seen in premature infants. Reported to suppress cell-mediated immunity. [15 mg]	Depressed levels of vitamin K-dependent procoagulants and potentiation of oral anticoagulants have been reported, as has impaired WBC function. Doses of 800 mg/day have been reported to increase slightly the incidence of hemorrhagic stroke. [1000 mg]	Plasma or serum concentration of α-tocopherol is most commonly used. Additional accuracy is obtained by expressing this value per mg of total plasma lipid. RBC peroxide hemolysis test is not entirely specific but is a useful functional measure of the antioxidant potential of cell membranes.
Vitamin K	A family of naphthoquinone compounds with similar biologic activity. Phylloquinone (vitamin K_1) is derived from plants; a variety of menaquinones (vitamin K_2) is derived from bacterial sources. Serves as an essential cofactor in the post-translational γ-carboxylation of glutamic acid residues in many proteins. These proteins include several circulating procoagulants and anticoagulants as well as proteins in a variety of tissues.	Deficiency syndrome, uncommon except in (1) breast-fed newborns, in whom it may cause "hemorrhagic disease of the newborn," (2) adults with fat malabsorption or who are taking drugs that interfere with vitamin K metabolism (e.g., coumarin, phenytoin, broad-spectrum antibiotics), and (3) individuals taking large doses of vitamin E and anticoagulant drugs. Excessive hemorrhage is the usual manifestation. [F: 90 μg; M: 120 μg]	Rapid intravenous infusion of K_1 has been associated with dyspnea, flushing, and cardiovascular collapse; this is likely related to the dispersing agents in the solution. Supplementation may interfere with coumarin-based anticoagulation. Pregnant women taking large amounts of the provitamin menadione may deliver infants with hemolytic anemia, hyperbilirubinemia, and kernicterus. [no TUL established]	Prothrombin time is typically used as a measure of functional K status; it is neither sensitive nor specific for vitamin K deficiency. Determination of undercarboxylated prothrombin in the plasma is more accurate but less widely available.
Water-Soluble Vitamins				
Thiamine (vitamin B_1)	A water-soluble compound containing substituted pyrimidine and thiazole rings and a hydroxyethyl side chain. The coenzyme form is thiamine pyrophosphate (TPP). Serves as a coenzyme in many α-ketoacid decarboxylation and transketolation reactions. Inadequate thiamine availability leads to impairments of above reactions, resulting in inadequate adenosine triphosphate synthesis and abnormal carbohydrate metabolism, respectively. May have an additional role in neuronal conduction independent of aforementioned actions.	Classic deficiency syndrome ("beriberi") described in Asian populations consuming polished rice diet. Alcoholism and chronic renal dialysis are also common precipitants. High carbohydrate intake increases need for B_1. *Mild deficiency:* irritability, fatigue, and headaches. *More severe deficiency:* combinations of peripheral neuropathy, cardiovascular dysfunction, and cerebral dysfunction. Cardiovascular involvement ("wet beriberi"): congestive heart failure and low peripheral vascular resistance. Cerebral disease: nystagmus, ophthalmoplegia, and ataxia (Wernicke's encephalopathy); hallucinations, impaired short-term memory, and confabulation ("Korsakoff's psychosis"). Deficiency syndrome responds within 24 hr to parenteral thiamine but is partially or wholly irreversible after a certain stage. [F: 1.1 mg; M: 1.2 mg]	Excess intake is largely excreted in the urine, although parenteral doses of > 400 mg/day are reported to cause lethargy, ataxia, and reduced tone of the gastrointestinal tract. [TUL not established]	The most effective measure of B_1 status is the erythrocyte transketolase activity coefficient, which measures enzyme activity before and after addition of exogenous TPP: RBCs from a deficient individual express a substantial increase in enzyme activity with addition of TPP. Thiamine concentrations in blood or urine are also used.
Riboflavin (vitamin B_2)	Consists of a substituted isoalloxazine ring with a ribitol side chain. Serves as a coenzyme for a diverse array of biochemical reactions. The primary coenzymatic forms are flavin mononucleotide (FMN) and flavin adenine dinucleotide (FAD). Riboflavin holoenzymes participate in oxidation-reduction reactions in a myriad of metabolic pathways.	Deficiency is usually seen in conjunction with deficiencies of other B vitamins. Isolated deficiency of riboflavin produces hyperemia and edema of nasopharyngeal mucosa, cheilosis, angular stomatitis, glossitis, seborrheic dermatitis, and a normochromic, normocytic anemia. [F: 1.1; M: 1.3]	Toxicity not reported in humans. [TUL not established]	The most common method of assessment is determining the activity coefficient of glutathione reductase in RBCs (the test is invalid for individuals with glucose-6-phosphate dehydrogenase [G6PD] deficiency). Measurements of blood and urine concentrations are less desirable methods.

	Biochemistry and Physiology	Deficiency [RDA*]	Toxicity [TUL†]	Assessment of Status
Niacin (vitamin B_3)	Refers to nicotinic acid and the corresponding amide, nicotinamide. The active coenzymatic forms are composed of nicotinamide affixed to adenine dinucleotide, forming NAD or NADP. More than 200 apoenzymes use these compounds as electron acceptors or hydrogen donors, either as a coenzyme or as a co-substrate. The essential amino acid tryptophan is a precursor of niacin; 60 mg of dietary tryptophan yields approximately 1 mg of niacin. Dietary requirements thus depend partly on tryptophan intake. Requirement is often determined on basis of caloric intake (i.e., niacin equivalents/1000 kcal). Large doses of nicotinic acid (1.5-3 g/day) effectively lower low-density lipoprotein cholesterol and elevate high-density lipoprotein cholesterol.	Pellagra is the classic deficiency syndrome and is often seen in populations in which corn is the major source of energy. Still endemic in parts of China, Africa, and India. Diarrhea, dementia (or associated symptoms of anxiety or insomnia), and a pigmented dermatitis that develops in sun-exposed areas are typical features. Glossitis, stomatitis, vaginitis, vertigo, and burning dysesthesias are early signs. Reported to occasionally occur in carcinoid syndrome because tryptophan is diverted to other synthetic pathways. [F: 14 mg; M: 16 mg]	Human toxicity known largely through studies examining hypolipidemic effects. Includes vasomotor phenomenon (flushing), hyperglycemia, parenchymal liver damage, and hyperuricemia. [35 mg]	Assessment of status is problematic: blood levels of vitamin not reliable. Measurement of urinary excretion of the niacin metabolites, N-methylnicotinamide and 2-pyridone, is thought to be the most effective means of assessment at present.
Vitamin B_6	Refers to several derivatives of pyridine, including pyridoxine (PN), pyridoxal (PL), and pyridoxamine (PM), which are interconvertible in the body. The coenzymatic forms are pyridoxal-5-phosphate (PLP) and pyridoxamine-5-phosphate (PMP). As a coenzyme, B_6 is involved in many transamination reactions (and thereby in gluconeogenesis), in the synthesis of niacin from tryptophan, in the synthesis of several neurotransmitters, and in the synthesis of δ-aminolevulinic acid (and therefore in heme synthesis). It also has functions unrelated to coenzymatic activity: PL and PLP bind to hemoglobin and alter O_2 affinity; PLP also binds to steroid receptors, inhibiting receptor affinity to DNA and thereby modulating steroid activity.	Deficiency usually seen in conjunction with other water-soluble vitamin deficiencies. Stomatitis, angular cheilosis, glossitis, irritability, depression, and confusion occur in moderate to severe depletion; normochromic, normocytic anemia has been reported in severe deficiency. Abnormal electroencephalograms and, in infants, convulsions have also been observed. Some sideroblastic anemias respond to B_6 administration. Isoniazid, cycloserine, penicillamine, ethanol, and theophylline can inhibit B_6 metabolism. [Ages 19-50 yr: 1.3 mg; >50 yr: 1.5 mg for women, 1.7 mg for men]	Long-term use with doses exceeding 200 mg/day (in adults) may cause peripheral neuropathies and photosensitivity. [100 mg]	Many useful laboratory methods of assessment exist. The plasma or erythrocyte PLP levels are most common. Urinary excretion of xanthurenic acid after an oral tryptophan load or activity indices of RBC alanine or aspartic acid transaminases (ALT and AST, respectively) are all functional measures of B_6-dependent enzyme activity.
Folate	A group of related pterin compounds. More than 35 forms of the vitamin are found naturally. The fully oxidized form, folic acid, is not found in nature but is the pharmacologic form of the vitamin. All folate functions relate to its ability to transfer one-carbon groups. It is essential in the de novo synthesis of nucleotides and in the metabolism of several amino acids, and is an integral component for the regeneration of the "universal" methyl donor, S-adenosylmethionine. Inhibition of bacterial and cancer cell folate metabolism is the basis for the sulfonamide antibiotics and chemotherapeutic agents such as methotrexate and 5-fluorouracil, respectively.	Women of childbearing age are most likely to be deficient. *Classic deficiency syndrome:* megaloblastic anemia, diarrhea. The hematopoietic cells in bone marrow become enlarged and have immature nuclei, reflecting ineffective DNA synthesis. The peripheral blood smear demonstrates macro-ovalocytes and polymorphonuclear leukocytes with an average of more than 3.5 nuclear lobes. Megaloblastic changes also occur in other epithelia that proliferate rapidly (e.g., oral mucosa, gastrointestinal tract), producing glossitis and diarrhea, respectively. Sulfasalazine and diphenytoin inhibit absorption and predispose to deficiency. [400 μg of dietary folate equivalents (DFE); 1 DFE = 1 μg food folate = 0.6 μg folic acid]	Doses >1000 μg/day may partially correct the anemia of B_{12} deficiency and may therefore mask (and perhaps exacerbate) the associated neuropathy. Large doses also reported to lower seizure threshold in individuals prone to seizures. Parenteral administration is rarely reported to cause allergic phenomena, which is probably due to dispersion agents. [1000 μg]	Serum folate measures short-term folate balance, whereas RBC folate is a better reflection of tissue status. Serum homocysteine rises early in deficiency but is nonspecific because B_{12} or B_6 deficiency, renal insufficiency, and older age may also cause elevations.

Continued on following page

	Biochemistry and Physiology	Deficiency [RDA*]	Toxicity [TUL†]	Assessment of Status
Vitamin C (ascorbic and dehydroascorbic acid)	Ascorbic acid readily oxidizes to dehydroascorbic acid in aqueous solution. The latter can be reduced in vivo, so it possesses vitamin C activity. Total vitamin C is therefore the sum of ascorbic and dehydroascorbic acid content. It serves primarily as a biologic antioxidant in aqueous environments. Biosyntheses of collagen, carnitine, bile acids, and norepinephrine, as well as proper functioning of the hepatic mixed-function oxygenase system, depend on this property. Vitamin C in foodstuffs increases the intestinal absorption of nonheme iron.	Overt deficiency is uncommon in developed countries. The classic deficiency syndrome is scurvy: fatigue, depression, and widespread abnormalities in connective tissues, such as inflamed gingivae, petechiae, perifollicular hemorrhages, impaired wound healing, coiled hairs, hyperkeratosis, bleeding into body cavities. In infants, defects in ossification and bone growth may occur. Tobacco smoking lowers plasma and leukocyte vitamin C levels. [F: 75 mg; M: 90 mg; increase requirement for cigarette smokers by 35 mg/day]	≥500 mg/day (in adults) may cause nausea and diarrhea. >1 g/day modestly increases risk for oxalate kidney stones. Supplementation may interfere with laboratory tests based on redox potential (e.g., fecal occult blood testing, serum cholesterol, and glucose). Withdrawal from chronic ingestion of high doses of vitamin C supplements should be done gradually because accommodation appears to occur, raising a concern of "rebound scurvy." [2 g]	Plasma ascorbic acid concentration reflects recent dietary intake, whereas WBC levels more closely reflect tissue stores. Women's plasma levels are approximately 20% higher than men's for any given dietary intake.
Vitamin B_{12}	A group of closely related cobalamin compounds composed of a corrin ring (with a cobalt atom in its center) connected to a ribonucleotide through an aminopropanol bridge. Microorganisms are the ultimate source of all naturally occurring B_{12}. The two active coenzyme forms are deoxyadenosylcobalamin and methylcobalamin. These coenzymes are needed for the synthesis of succinyl coenzyme A (CoA), which is essential in lipid and carbohydrate metabolism, and for the synthesis of methionine. The latter reaction is essential for amino acid metabolism, for purine and pyrimidine synthesis, for many methylation reactions, and for the intracellular retention of folates.	Dietary inadequacy is a rare cause of deficiency except in strict vegetarians. Most deficiencies arise from loss of intestinal absorption, which may occur with pernicious anemia, pancreatic insufficiency, atrophic gastritis, small bowel bacterial overgrowth, or ileal disease. Megaloblastic anemia and megaloblastic changes in other epithelia (see "Folate") are the result of sustained depletion. Demyelination of peripheral nerves, posterior and lateral columns of spinal cord, and nerves within the brain may occur. Altered mentation, depression, and psychoses occur. Hematologic and neurologic complications may occur independently. Folate supplementation, in doses of 1000 μg/day, may partly correct the anemia, thereby masking (or perhaps exacerbating) the neuropathic complication. [2.4 μg]	A few allergic reactions have been reported to crystalline B_{12} preparations and are probably due to impurities, not the vitamin. [TUL not established]	Serum, or plasma, concentrations are generally accurate. Subtle deficiency with neurologic complications, as described in the "Deficiency" column, can best be established by concurrently measuring the concentration of plasma B_{12} and serum methylmalonic acid because the latter is a sensitive indicator of cellular deficiency.
Biotin	A bi-cyclic compound consisting of a ureido ring fused to a substituted tetrahydrothiophene ring. Endogenous synthesis by intestinal flora may contribute significantly to biotin nutriture. Most dietary biotin is linked to lysine, a compound called biotinyl lysine, or biocytin. The lysine must be hydrolyzed by an intestinal enzyme called biotinidase before intestinal absorption occurs. Acts primarily as a coenzyme for several carboxylases; each holoenzyme catalyzes an ATP-dependent CO_2 transfer. The carboxylases are critical enzymes in carbohydrate and lipid metabolism.	Isolated deficiency is rare. Deficiency in humans has been produced by prolonged total parenteral nutrition lacking the vitamin and by ingestion of large quantities of raw egg white, which contains avidin, a protein that binds biotin with such high affinity that it renders it bio-unavailable. Alterations in mental status, myalgias, hyperesthesias, and anorexia occur. Later, a seborrheic dermatitis and alopecia develop. Deficiency is usually accompanied by lactic acidosis and organic aciduria. [30 μg]	Toxicity has not been reported in humans with doses as high as 60 mg/day in children. [TUL not established]	Plasma and urine concentrations of biotin are diminished in the deficient state. Elevated urine concentrations of methyl citrate, 3-methylcrotonylglycine, and 3-hydroxyisovalerate are also observed in deficiency.

	Biochemistry and Physiology	Deficiency [RDA*]	Toxicity [TUL†]	Assessment of Status
Pantothenic acid	Consists of pantoic acid linked to β-alanine through an amide bond. An essential component of CoA and phosphopantetheine, which are essential for synthesis and β-oxidation of fatty acids, as well as synthesis of cholesterol, steroid hormones, vitamins A and D, and other isoprenoid derivatives. CoA is also involved in the synthesis of several amino acids and δ-aminolevulinic acid, a precursor for the corrin ring of vitamin B_{12}, the porphyrin ring of heme, and of cytochromes. CoA is also necessary for the acetylation and fatty acid acylation of a variety of proteins.	Deficiency rare: only reported as a result of feeding semisynthetic diets or an antagonist to the vitamin. Experimental, isolated deficiency in humans produces fatigue, abdominal pain, vomiting, insomnia, and paresthesias of the extremities. [5 mg]	In doses of 10 g/day, diarrhea is reported to occur. [TUL not established]	Whole blood and urine concentrations of pantothenate are indicators of status; serum levels are not thought to be accurate.

PTH, Parathyroid hormone; *UVB,* ultraviolet B.

*Recommended daily allowance (RDA) established for female (F) and male (M) adults by the U.S. Food and Nutrition Board, 1999-2001. In some instances, insufficient data exist to establish an RDA, in which case the adequate intake (AI) established by the board is listed.

†Tolerated upper intake (TUL) established for adults by the U.S. Food and Nutrition Board, 1999-2001.

From Goldman L, Schafer AI: *Goldman's Cecil medicine,* ed 24, Philadelphia, 2012, Saunders.

Nutritional Trace Elements and Their Clinical Implications

	Biochemistry and Physiology	Deficiency [RDA*]	Toxicity [TUL†]	Assessment of Status
Chromium	Dietary chromium consists of both inorganic and organic forms. Its primary function in humans is to potentiate insulin action. It accomplishes this function as a circulating complex called *glucose tolerance factor,* thereby affecting carbohydrate, fat, and protein metabolism.	Deficiency in humans only described in long-term total parenteral nutrition (TPN) patients receiving insufficient chromium. Hyperglycemia or impaired glucose tolerance occurs. Elevated plasma free fatty acid concentrations, neuropathy, encephalopathy, and abnormalities in nitrogen metabolism are also reported. Whether supplemental chromium may improve glucose tolerance in glucose-intolerant individuals remains controversial. [F: 25 μg; M: 35 μg]	Toxicity after oral ingestion is uncommon and seems confined to gastric irritation. Airborne exposure may cause contact dermatitis, eczema, skin ulcers, and bronchogenic carcinoma. [no TUL established]	Plasma or serum concentration of chromium is a crude indicator of chromium status; it appears to be meaningful when the value is markedly above or below the normal range.
Copper	Copper is absorbed by a specific intestinal transport mechanism. It is carried to the liver where it is bound to ceruloplasmin, which circulates systemically and delivers copper to target tissues in the body. Excretion of copper is largely through bile, and then into the feces. Absorptive and excretory processes vary with the levels of dietary copper, providing a means of copper homeostasis. Copper serves as a component of many enzymes, including amine oxidases, ferroxidases, cytochrome c oxidase, dopamine β-hydroxylase, superoxide dismutase, and tyrosinase.	Dietary deficiency is rare; it has been observed in premature and low-birthweight infants fed exclusively a cow's milk diet and in individuals on long-term TPN without copper. Clinical manifestations include depigmentation of skin and hair, neurologic disturbances, leukopenia, hypochromic microcytic anemia, and skeletal abnormalities. Anemia arises from impaired utilization of iron and is therefore a conditioned form of iron deficiency anemia. The deficiency syndrome, except the anemia and leukopenia, is also observed in Menkes' disease, a rare inherited condition associated with impaired copper utilization. [900 μg]	Acute copper toxicity has been described after excessive oral intake and with absorption of copper salts applied to burned skin. Milder manifestations include nausea, vomiting, epigastric pain, and diarrhea; coma and hepatic necrosis may ensue in severe cases. Toxicity may be seen with doses as low as 70 μg/kg/day. Chronic toxicity is also described. Wilson's disease is a rare, inherited disease associated with abnormally low ceruloplasmin levels and accumulation of copper in the liver and brain, eventually leading to damage to these two organs. [10 mg]	Practical methods for detecting marginal deficiency are not available. Marked deficiency is reliably detected by diminished serum copper and ceruloplasmin concentrations as well as low red blood cell (RBC) superoxide dismutase activity.
Fluorine	Known more commonly by its ionic form, fluoride. It is incorporated into the crystalline structure of bone, thereby altering its physical characteristics.	Intake of <0.1 mg/day in infants and <0.5 mg/day in children is associated with an increased incidence of dental caries. Optimal intake in adults is between 1.5 and 4 mg/day. [F: 3 mg; M: 4 mg]	Acute ingestion of >30 mg/kg body weight is likely to cause death. Excessive chronic intake (0.1 mg/kg/day) leads to mottling of teeth (dental fluorosis), calcification of tendons and ligaments, and exostoses and may increase the brittleness of bones. [10 mg]	Estimates of intake or clinical assessment are used because no good laboratory test exists.

Continued on following page

	Biochemistry and Physiology	Deficiency [RDA*]	Toxicity [TUL†]	Assessment of Status
Iodine	Readily absorbed from the diet, concentrated in the thyroid, and integrated into the thyroid hormones, thyroxine (T_4) and triiodothyronine (T_3). These hormones circulate largely bound to thyroxine-binding globulin. They modulate resting energy expenditure and, in the developing human, growth and development.	In the absence of supplementation, populations relying primarily on food from soils with low iodine content have endemic iodine deficiency. Maternal iodine deficiency leads to fetal deficiency, which produces spontaneous abortions, stillbirths, hypothyroidism, cretinism, and dwarfism. Permanent cognitive deficits may result from iodine deficiency during first 2 years of life. In the adult, compensatory hypertrophy of the thyroid goiter occurs along with varying degrees of hypothyroidism. [150 μg]	Large doses (>2 mg/day in adults) may induce hypothyroidism by blocking thyroid hormone synthesis. Supplementation with >100 mg/day to an individual who was formerly deficient occasionally induces hyperthyroidism. [1.1 mg]	Iodine status of a population can be estimated by the prevalence of goiter. Urinary excretion of iodine is an effective laboratory means of assessment. Thyroid-stimulating hormone (TSH) blood level is an indirect, and therefore not entirely specific, means of assessment.
Iron	Conveys the capacity to participate in redox reactions to a number of metalloproteins such as hemoglobin, myoglobin, cytochrome enzymes, and many oxidases and oxygenases. Primary storage form is ferritin and, to a lesser degree, hemosiderin. Intestinal absorption is 15%-20% for "heme" iron and 1%-8% for iron contained in vegetables. Absorption of the latter form is enhanced by the ascorbic acid in foodstuffs; by poultry, fish, or beef; and by an iron-deficient state. It is decreased by phytate and tannins.	The most common micronutrient deficiency in the world. Women of childbearing age are the highest-risk group because of menstrual blood losses, pregnancy, and lactation. The classic deficiency syndrome is hypochromic, microcytic anemia. Glossitis and koilonychia ("spoon" nails) are also observed. Easy fatigability often is an early symptom, before anemia appears. In children, mild deficiency of insufficient severity to cause anemia is associated with behavioral disturbances and poor school performance. [postmenopausal F and M: 8 mg; premenopausal F: 18 mg]	Iron overload typically occurs when habitual dietary intake is extremely high, intestinal absorption is excessive, repeated parenteral administration occurs, or a combination of these factors exists. Excessive iron stores usually accumulate in the reticuloendothelial tissues and cause little damage ("hemosiderosis"). If overload continues, iron eventually begins to accumulate in tissues such as the hepatic parenchyma, pancreas, heart, and synovium, causing hemochromatosis. Hereditary hemochromatosis results from homozygosity of a common recessive trait. Excessive intestinal absorption of iron is seen in homozygotes. [45 mg]	Negative iron balance initially leads to depletion of iron stores in the bone marrow: a bone marrow biopsy and the concentration of serum ferritin are accurate indicators of early depletion. As the severity of deficiency proceeds, serum iron (SI) decreases and total iron-binding capacity (TIBC) increases: an iron saturation (SI/TIBC) of <16% suggests iron deficiency. Microcytosis, hypochromia, and anemia ensue. Elevated levels of serum ferritin or an iron saturation of >60% suggest iron overload, although systemic inflammation elevates serum ferritin regardless of iron status.
Manganese	A component of several metalloenzymes. Most manganese is in mitochondria, where it is a component of manganese superoxide dismutase.	Manganese deficiency in the human has not been conclusively demonstrated. It is said to cause hypocholesterolemia, weight loss, hair and nail changes, dermatitis, and impaired synthesis of vitamin K–dependent proteins. [F: 1.8 mg; M: 2.3 mg]	Toxicity by oral ingestion is unknown in humans. Toxic inhalation causes hallucinations, other alterations in mentation, and extrapyramidal movement disorders. [11 mg]	Until the deficiency syndrome is better defined, an appropriate measure of status will be difficult to develop.
Molybdenum	A cofactor in several enzymes, most prominently xanthine oxidase and sulfite oxidase.	A probable case of human deficiency is described as being secondary to parenteral administration of sulfite and resulted in hyperoxypurinemia, hypouricemia, and low sulfate excretion. [45 μg]	Toxicity not well described in humans, although it may interfere with copper metabolism at high doses. [2 mg]	Laboratory means of assessment not meaningful until deficiency syndrome is better described.
Selenium	Most dietary selenium is in the form of an amino acid complex. Nearly complete absorption of such forms occurs. Homeostasis is largely performed by the kidney, which regulates urinary excretion as a function of selenium status. Selenium is a component of several enzymes, most notably glutathione peroxidase and superoxide dismutase. These enzymes protect against oxidative and free radical damage of various cell structures. The antioxidant protection conveyed by selenium apparently operates in conjunction with vitamin E because deficiency of one seems to potentiate damage induced by a deficiency of the other. Selenium also participates in the enzymatic conversion of thyroxine to its more active metabolite, triiodothyronine.	Deficiency is rare in North America but has been observed in individuals on long-term TPN lacking selenium. Such individuals have myalgias and/or cardiomyopathies. Populations in some regions of the world, most notably some parts of China, have marginal intake of selenium. In these regions Keshan's disease, a condition characterized by cardiomyopathy, is endemic; it can be prevented (but not treated) by selenium supplementation. [55 μg]	Toxicity is associated with nausea, diarrhea, alterations in mental status, peripheral neuropathy, loss of hair and nails: such symptoms were observed in adults who inadvertently consumed 27-2400 mg. [400 μg]	Erythrocyte glutathione peroxidase activity and plasma, or whole blood, selenium concentrations are the most commonly used methods of assessment. They are moderately accurate indicators of status.

	Biochemistry and Physiology	Deficiency [RDA*]	Toxicity [TUL†]	Assessment of Status
Zinc	Intestinal absorption occurs by a specific process that is enhanced by pregnancy and corticosteroids and diminished by coingestion of phytates, phosphates, iron, copper, lead, or calcium. Diminished intake of zinc leads to an increased efficiency of absorption and decreased fecal excretion, providing a means of zinc homeostasis. Zinc is a component of more than 100 enzymes, among which are DNA polymerase, RNA polymerase, and transfer RNA synthetase.	Zinc deficiency has its most profound effect on rapidly proliferating tissues. *Mild deficiency:* growth retardation in children. *More severe deficiency:* growth arrest, teratogenicity, hypogonadism and infertility, dysgeusia, poor wound healing, diarrhea, dermatitis on the extremities and around orifices, glossitis, alopecia, corneal clouding, loss of dark adaptation, and behavioral changes. Impaired cellular immunity is observed. Excessive loss of gastrointestinal secretions through chronic diarrhea and fistulas may precipitate deficiency. Acrodermatitis enteropathica is a rare, recessively inherited disease in which intestinal absorption of zinc is impaired. [F: 8 mg; M: 11 mg]	Acute zinc toxicity can usually be induced by ingestion of >200 mg of zinc in a single day (in adults). It is manifested as epigastric pain, nausea, vomiting, and diarrhea. Hyperpnea, diaphoresis, and weakness may follow inhalation of zinc fumes. Copper and zinc compete for intestinal absorption: long-term ingestion of >25 mg/day of zinc may lead to copper deficiency. Long-term ingestion of >150 mg/day has been reported to cause gastric erosions, low high-density lipoprotein cholesterol levels, and impaired cellular immunity. [40 mg]	No accurate indicators of zinc status exist for routine clinical use. Plasma, RBC, and hair zinc concentrations are often misleading. Acute illness, in particular, is known to diminish plasma zinc levels, in part by inducing a shift of zinc out of the plasma compartment and into the liver. Functional tests that determine dark adaptation, taste acuity, and rate of wound healing lack specificity.

*Recommended daily allowance (RDA) established for female (F) and male (M) adults by the U.S. Food and Nutrition Board, 1999-2001. In some instances, insufficient data exist to establish an RDA, in which case the adequate intake (AI) established by the board is listed.

†Tolerated upper limit (TUL) established for adults by the U.S. Food and Nutrition Board, 1999-2001.

From Goldman L, Schafer AI: *Goldman's Cecil medicine,* ed 24, Philadelphia, 2012, Saunders.

Summary of Vitamin and Mineral Deficiencies

Vitamin and Mineral Deficiencies	Neurologic Syndrome or Syndromes	Supporting Tests	Treatment	Causes (Other Than Malnutrition)
A (retinol)	Blindness from retinal or corneal damage	Visual fields, visual acuity Serum level <30-65 μg/dl	30,000 IU vitamin A daily × 1 wk	Hypothyroidism, diabetes, renal or liver failure
B_1 (thiamine)	Wernicke's encephalopathy: ataxia, nystagmus, ophthalmoparesis, confusion, delirium Korsakoff's syndrome: amnesia, confabulation Beriberi: axonal neuropathy	MRI: symmetric lesions of midbrain (periaqueductal area), pons, hypothalamus, thalamus, cerebellum MRI: necrosis of mammillary bodies, dorsomedial and anterior thalamus Nerve conduction tests: decreased amplitude Serum thiamine level <20 ng/dl Erythrocyte transketolase	Prevent by 100 mg PO daily before and 1 year after bariatric surgery, 100 mg IV before glucose administration or refeeding Treat Wernicke's encephalopathy with 5 days of thiamine, 100-500 mg IV or IM daily, then PO 100 mg daily Antioxidants (*N*-acetylcysteine)	Alcoholism, bariatric or other major GI surgery, prolonged vomiting, hemodialysis, diuretic treatment of heart failure, cachexia, 5-fluorouracil, other blockers of thiamine phosphate production
B_3 (niacin)	Pellagra: confusion, dementia, weakness, ataxia, spasticity, myoclonus, glossitis, dermatitis, photosensitivity	Erythrocyte NAD, plasma niacin, urinary N_1-methylnicotinamide	Nicotinic acid, 50 mg PO tid or 25 mg IV tid; nicotinamide, 50-100 mg IM or PO tid	Alcoholism, corn- or cereal-based diet, Hartnup's syndrome, carcinoid syndrome
B_5 (pantothenic acid)	Dysesthesias, foot paresthesias	Deficient coenzyme A	5 mg PO daily	Severe malnutrition
B_6 (pyridoxine)	Neuropathy, sensory ataxia, depression Infantile pyridoxine-deficient epilepsy	Plasma PLP <27 nmol/L; urinary 4-pyridoxic acid, <3 nmol ↑ Homocysteine after methionine loading challenge ↑ α-AASA in urine, plasma, CSF	50-100 mg PO daily for neuropathy (preventive use if taking B_6 antagonist) 100-200 mg daily for adult epilepsy	Diverticulosis, isoniazid, cycloserine, other antagonists Genetic defects in antiquitin (aldehyde dehydrogenase), pyridoxal synthesis
B_{12} (cobalamin)	Myelopathy with spastic paraparesis and sensory ataxia, peripheral neuropathy, optic neuropathy, memory loss, dementia; indirect contributor to stroke	Blood level <200 pg/ml ↑ Methylmalonic acid >145 nmol/L Intrinsic factor antibodies Schilling test, megaloblastic anemia Delayed somatosensory evoked potentials ↑ Homocysteine, total >12.5 μmol/L	IM B_{12}, 1000 μg daily for 1 week, then weekly for 1 month, then monthly or oral B_{12}, 1000 μg daily, or nasal B_{12}, 500 μg weekly for lifetime if abnormal absorption, 50-100 μg daily if normal absorption	Achlorhydria, gastric or ileal resection, blind loop syndrome, sprue, HIV infection, nitrous oxide anesthesia (especially abuse), fish tapeworm, vegan diet
D (calciferol)	Proximal myopathy, often painful; cognitive impairment Secondary compression of spinal cord, plexus, or peripheral nerves from rickets or osteomalacia	25-(OH) vitamin D_3 level <10 ng/ml in urine Serum calcium ↑ PTH >54 pg/ml Osteopenia/porosis on bone densitometry	Daily supplementation with 400 IU, >50,000 IU 3 times per wk if malabsorption; use blood level or urine calcium excretion to guide (should be >100 mg/day)	Lack of exposure to sunlight, including sunblock protection; chronic antiepileptic drug use
E (tocopherol)	Spinal and cerebellar ataxia, Babinski's sign, ophthalmoplegia, peripheral neuropathy, retinitis pigmentosa	Vitamin E level <2.5 mg/L (normal, 6-15 with normal lipid level) ↑ A-β-lipoprotein levels, antigliadin antibodies Genetic analysis to rule out other spinocerebellar ataxias such as Friedreich's ataxia	Supplement with 6-800 IU, 5-10 mg/kg twice daily, for ataxia of genetic causes, water-soluble 200 mg/kg/day or IM α-tocopherol for malabsorption	Biliary atresia, celiac sprue, Genetic: ↓ α-tocopherol transport protein (8q13), microsomal triglyceride transfer protein

Continued on following page

Vitamin and Mineral Deficiencies	Neurologic Syndrome or Syndromes	Supporting Tests	Treatment	Causes (Other Than Malnutrition)
Folate	Dementia, B_{12} deficiency, stroke	↑ Homocysteine, plasma level <2.5 μg/L	1 mg 3 times per day until normal level, then maintenance of 1 mg/day Pregnancy: additional 0.4 mg/day if taking a folate antagonist	Malabsorption or use of antagonist (methotrexate) or antiepileptic medication
K (phytonadione)	Intracranial hemorrhage	INR or PT elevation	IM phytonadione at birth, maternal vitamin K for last month of pregnancy	Medication use that increases metabolism, such as phenytoin
Copper	Myelopathy, neuropathy	Serum Cu <75 μg/dl, ↓ urinary Cu, ceruloplasmin <23 mg/dl MRI: ↑ T_2 signal in cervical cord, dorsal column Mutation in ATP7A gene (Menkes' disease)	Elemental Cu, 8 mg/day PO week 1, 6 mg/day week 2, 4 mg/day week 3, 2 mg/day ongoing malabsorption Menkes' disease: 250 mg SC bid	Wilson's disease, Menkes' disease, alcoholism, malabsorption, gastric bypass, zinc toxicity
Magnesium	Seizures, encephalopathy	Serum magnesium <1.5 mg/ dl, correct for low albumin	Magnesium sulfate IV or PO Avoid magnesium-wasting drugs	Alcoholism, especially beer
Potassium	Muscle weakness, chronic, acute	Serum potassium <3.5 mEq/L, ECG	IV or PO KCl until normalized	Diuretic use, bulimia

AASA, Aminoadipic semialdehyde; *CSF,* cerebrospinal fluid; *ECG,* electrocardiography; *GI,* gastrointestinal; *HIV,* human immunodeficiency virus; *INR,* international normalized ratio; *MRI,* magnetic resonance imaging; *NAD,* nicotinamide adenine dinucleotide; *PLP,* pyridoxal-5-phosphate (active coenzyme of pyridoxine); *PT,* prothrombin time; *PTH,* parathyroid hormone.
From Goldman L, Schafer AI: *Goldman's Cecil medicine,* ed 24, Philadelphia, 2012, Saunders.

Historical and Physical Findings in Poisoning

Sign	Toxin
Odor	
Bitter almonds	Cyanide
Acetone	Isopropyl alcohol, methanol, paraldehyde, salicylates
Alcohol	Ethanol
Wintergreen	Methyl salicylate
Garlic	Arsenic, thallium, organophosphates, selenium
Ocular Signs	
Miosis	Opioids (except propoxyphene, meperidine, and pentazocine), organophosphates and other cholinergics, clonidine, phenothiazines, sedative-hypnotics, olanzapine
Mydriasis	Atropine, cocaine, amphetamines, antihistamines, TCAs, carbamazepine, serotonin syndrome, PCP, LSD, postanoxic encephalopathy
Nystagmus	Phenytoin, barbiturates, sedative-hypnotics, alcohols, carbamazepine, PCP, ketamine, dextromethorphan
Lacrimation	Organophosphates, irritant gas or vapors
Retinal hyperemia	Methanol
Cutaneous Signs	
Diaphoresis	Organophosphates, salicylates, cocaine and other sympathomimetics, serotonin syndrome, withdrawal syndromes
Alopecia	Thallium, arsenic
Erythema	Boric acid, elemental mercury, cyanide, carbon monoxide, disulfuram, scombroid, anticholinergics
Cyanosis (unresponsive to oxygen)	Methemoglobinemia (e.g., benzocaine, dapsone, nitrites, phenazopyridine), amiodarone, silver
Oral Signs	
Salivation	Organophosphates, salicylates, corrosives, ketamine, PCP, strychnine
Oral burns	Corrosives, oxalate-containing plants
Gum lines	Lead, mercury, arsenic, bismuth
Gastrointestinal Signs	
Diarrhea	Antimicrobials, arsenic, iron, boric acid, cholinergics, colchicine, withdrawal
Hematemesis	Arsenic, iron, caustics, NSAIDs, salicylates
Cardiac Signs	
Tachycardia	Sympathomimetics (e.g., amphetamines, cocaine), anticholinergics, antidepressants, theophylline, caffeine, antipsychotics, atropine, salicylates, cellular asphyxiants (cyanide, carbon monoxide, hydrogen sulfide), withdrawal
Bradycardia	β-Blockers, calcium channel blockers, digoxin, clonidine and other central α_2 agonists, organophosphates, opioids, sedative-hypnotics
Hypertension	Sympathomimetics (amphetamines, cocaine, LSD), anticholinergics, clonidine (early), monoamine oxidase inhibitors
Hypotension	β-Blockers, calcium channel blockers, cyclic antidepressants, iron, phenothiazines, barbiturates, clonidine, theophylline, opioids, arsenic, amatoxin mushrooms, cellular asphyxiants (cyanide, carbon monoxide, hydrogen sulfide), snake envenomation
Respiratory Signs	
Depressed respirations	Opioids, sedative-hypnotics, alcohol, clonidine, barbiturates
Tachypnea	Salicylates, amphetamines, caffeine, metabolic acidosis (ethylene glycol, methanol, cyanide), carbon monoxide, hydrocarbons

Continued on following page

Historical and Physical Findings in Poisoning

Sign	Toxin
Central Nervous System Signs	
Ataxia	Alcohol, anticonvulsants, benzodiazepines, barbiturates, lithium, dextromethorphan, carbon monoxide, inhalants
Coma	Opioids, sedative-hypnotics, anticonvulsants, cyclic antidepressants, antipsychotics, ethanol, anticholinergics, clonidine, GHB, alcohols, salicylates, barbiturates
Seizures	Sympathomimetics, anticholinergics, antidepressants (especially TCAs, bupropion, venlafaxine), isoniazid, camphor, lindane, salicylates, lead, organophosphates, carbamazepine, tramadol, lithium, ginkgo seeds, water hemlock, withdrawal
Delirium/psychosis	Sympathomimetics, anticholinergics, LSD, PCP, hallucinogens, lithium, dextromethorphan, steroids, withdrawal
Peripheral neuropathy	Lead, arsenic, mercury, organophosphates

GHB, Gamma hydroxybutyrate; *LSD,* lysergic acid diethylamide; *NSAID,* nonsteroidal anti-inflammatory drug; *PCP,* phencyclidine; *TCA,* tricylic antidepressant.
From Goldman L, Schafer AI: *Goldman's Cecil medicine,* ed 24, Philadelphia, 2012, Saunders.

Recognizable Poison Syndromes

Poison Syndrome	SIGNS Vital	Mental Status	Pupils	Skin	Bowel Sounds	Other	Possible Toxins
Sympathomimetic	Hypertension, tachycardia, hyperthermia	Agitated, psychosis, delirium	Dilated	Diaphoretic	Normal to increased		Amphetamines, cocaine, Ecstasy, pseudoephedrine, caffeine, theophylline
Anticholinergic	Hypertension, tachycardia, hyperthermia	Agitation, delirium, mumbling speech	Dilated	Dry	Decreased		Antihistamines, tricyclic antidepressants, atropine, jimson weed, phenothiazines
Cholinergic	Bradycardia (although may show tachycardia), BP and temp typically normal	Confusion, coma, fasciculations	Small	Diaphoretic	Hyperactive	Diarrhea, urination, bronchorrhea, bronchospasm, emesis, lacrimation, salivation	Organophosphates, nerve gases, Alzheimer medications
Opioids	Respiratory depression (hallmark of toxicity), bradycardia, hypotension, hypothermia	Depression, coma	Pinpoint	Normal	Normal to decreased		Methadone, suboxone, morphine, oxycodone, heroin, etc.
Sedative-hypnotics	Respiratory depression, HR normal to decreased, BP normal to decreased, temp normal to decreased	Somnolence, coma	Small	Normal	Normal		Barbiturates, benzodiazepines, ethanol
Serotonin syndrome	Hyperthermia, tachycardia, hypertension or hypotension (autonomic instability)	Agitation, confusion, coma	Dilated	Diaphoretic	Increased	Neuromuscular hyperexcitability: clonus, hyperreflexia (lower extremities > upper extremities)	SSRIs, lithium, MAOIs, linezolid, tramadol, meperidine, dextromethorphan
Salicylates	Tachypnea, hyperpnea, tachycardia, hyperthermia	Agitation, confusion, coma	Normal	Diaphoretic	Normal	Nausea, vomiting, tinnitus, ABG with primary respiratory alkalosis and primary metabolic acidosis	Aspirin, bismuth subsalicylate (Pepto-Bismol), methylsalicylates
Withdrawal	Tachycardia, tachypnea, hyperthermia	Lethargy, confusion, delirium	Dilated	Diaphoretic	Increased		Withdrawal from opioids, sedative-hypnotics, ethanol

ABG, Arterial blood gas; *BP,* blood pressure; *HR,* heart rate; *MAOI,* monoamine oxidase inhibitor; *SSRI,* selective serotonin reuptake inhibitor; *temp,* temperature.
From Kliegman RM et al: *Nelson textbook of pediatrics,* ed 19, Philadelphia, 2011, Saunders.

Antidotes and Indications for Use

Antidote	Indication for Use	Dose*	Treatment End Point	Comments
Antivenom (Fab)[†]	Crotalines	4-6 vials; repeat for persistent or worsening clinical condition; repeat doses of 2 vials at 6, 12, and 18 hr after initial antivenom dose(s) are recommended	Halt in progression of circumferential and proximal swelling Resolving systemic effects	Better safety profile than equine-derived antivenom Repetitive dosing indicated for recurrent soft tissue swelling
Antivenom, *Latrodectus* (equine)[†]	Black widow spider (*Latrodectus* sp.)	1 vial diluted in 100 ml NS, infused over 1 hr; can repeat	Resolution of symptoms, vital signs normal	Dilution and slow infusion rate are critical to avoid anaphylactoid reaction Indications include severe pain unresponsive to opioids and severe hypertension Serum sickness can occur IV calcium is ineffective
Atropine	Carbamates Nerve agents Organophosphorus compounds	2 mg IV; double the dose every 5 min to achieve atropinization and hemodynamic stability; then start continuous infusion of 10%-20% of total stabilizing dose per hr	Cessation of excessive oral and pulmonary secretions, >80 bpm, systolic blood pressure >80 mm Hg	Doubling of the dose every 5 min (e.g., 2 mg, 4 mg, 8 mg, 16 mg) estimated to achieve atropinization within 30 min Stop infusion if patient develops any signs or symptoms of anticholinergic toxidrome; restart infusion at lower rate when signs or symptoms abate
Calcium[‡]	Calcium-channel antagonists	Calcium chloride 10%, 20-50 mg (0.2-0.5 ml)/kg/hr	Reversal of hypotension; may not reverse bradycardia	All indications: Monitor ionized calcium levels IV extravasation causes tissue necrosis, especially with calcium chloride Can administer at faster than stated rates for immediate life-threatening conditions Taper infusions and monitor for relapse of toxicity when discontinuing therapy Calcium chloride contains three times more elemental calcium than calcium gluconate does Calcium-channel antagonists may be ineffective in severe toxicity
	Hydrofluoric acid	Systemic toxicity: calcium gluconate 10%, 1-3 g (10-30 ml) per dose IV over 10-min period; repeat as needed every 5-10 min	Reversal of life-threatening manifestations of hypocalcemia and hyperkalemia	Can dilute and give intraarterially or IV with a Bier block for extremity exposures and burns
	Hyperkalemia (except cardiac glycosides)	Calcium gluconate 10%, 1 g (10 ml) per dose IV over 10-min period; repeat as needed every 5-10 min	Reversal of myocardial depression and conduction delays	May precipitate ventricular arrhythmias
	Hypermagnesemia	Calcium gluconate 10%, 1-2 g (10-20 ml) per dose IV over 10-min period; repeat as needed every 5-10 min	Reversal of respiratory depression, hypotension, and cardiac conduction blocks	Simultaneous therapies to increase magnesium elimination should be instituted
	Hypocalcemia (e.g., ethylene glycol)	Calcium gluconate 10%, 0.5-1.0 g (5-10 ml) per dose over 10-min period; repeat as needed every 10 min	Reversal of tetany	Correct symptomatic hypocalcemia; avoid excessive administration that may increase production of calcium oxalate crystals in ethylene glycol poisoning

Continued on following page

Antidote	Indication for Use	Dose*	Treatment End Point	Comments
L-Carnitine	Valproate-induced hyperammonemia or hepatotoxicity	100 mg/kg (maximum 6 g) IV over 30 min, then 15 mg/kg IV over 30-min period q4h (max 6 g/day)	Treat until clinical improvement occurs	Levocarnitine is active form Adjust dose for end-stage renal disease
Cyanide antidote kit	Cyanide		Resolution of lactic acidosis and moderate to severe clinical signs and symptoms: seizures, coma, dyspnea, apnea, hypotension, bradycardia	
Amyl nitrate		Amyl nitrite: 0.3-ml pearls, crush and inhale over 30-sec period		Coordinate amyl nitrite with continued oxygenation and give only until sodium nitrite infusion is begun; nitrites may produce hypotension and excess methemoglobinemia
Sodium nitrite		Sodium nitrite 3%: 10 ml IV over 10-min period		Sodium nitrite dose must be adjusted if patient has hemoglobin <12 g/dl
Sodium thiosulfate		Sodium thiosulfate 25%: 50 ml (12.5 g) IV over 10-min period		Sodium thiosulfate dosing can be repeated
Deferoxamine	Iron	15 ml/kg/hr IV (max 8 g/day) Mild to moderate: administer for 6-12 hr Severe toxicity: administer 24 hr	Resolution of clinical signs and symptoms Do not use urine color, which is an unreliable marker for iron clearance	Indications: symptomatic patients with lethargy, severe abdominal pain, hypovolemia, acidosis, shock; any symptomatic patient with peak serum iron level >350 g/dl Prolonged therapy can cause pulmonary toxicity
Digoxin-specific antibody fragments (Fab)	Digoxin Digitalis Other cardiac glycosides (e.g., bufodienalides [*Bufo toads*], oleander)	Unknown digoxin dose or serum level or for plant or toad source: acute toxicity—10-20 vials; chronic toxicity—3-6 vials Digoxin dose known: number of vials = (mg ingested × 0.8) ÷ 0.5 Digoxin serum level known: number of vials = [serum level (ng/ml) × weight (kg)] ÷ 100	Resolution of hyperkalemia, symptomatic bradydysrhythmias, ventricular arrhythmias, Mobitz II or third-degree heart block	Each vial binds 0.5 mg of digoxin or digitoxin Monitor ECG and potassium levels Digoxin serum levels unreliable after antidote administered unless test is specific for free serum digoxin
Dimercaprol (BAL)	Arsenic Lead Mercury, elemental and inorganic salts	Arsenic: 3-5 mg/kg IM q4h Lead: 75 mg/m^2 (4 mg/kg) IM q4h for 5 days Inorganic mercury: 5 mg/kg IM, then 2.5 mg/kg IM q12h for 10 days or until patient clinically improved	Arsenic: 24-hr urinary arsenic <50 μg/L Lead: encephalopathy resolved, blood lead level <100 μg/dl, and succimer therapy can be started Mercury, elemental and inorganic: 24-hr urinary mercury <20 μg/L	Maximum adult dose is 3 g/day BAL started 4 hr before initiation of concomitant $CaNa_2EDTA$ for lead encephalopathy Dosing not well established for arsenic and elemental or inorganic mercury toxicity; not used for organic mercury poisoning Adverse effects: painful injections, fever, diaphoresis, agitation, headache, salivation, nausea and vomiting, hemolysis in G6PD-deficient patients, chelation of essential metals Check essential metal levels if chelation is prolonged Succimer is replacing BAL for many indications except lead encephalopathy Treatment end points for arsenic and mercury include improving clinical condition
Edetate calcium disodium ($CaNa_2EDTA$)	Lead	1500 mg/m^2/24 hr (max 3 g) by continuous infusion	Treat for 5 days, followed by 2-day hiatus; repeat until encephalopathy resolved, lead level <100 μg/dl, and succimer therapy can be started	Use in patients with lead encephalopathy or lead level >100 g/dl Administer BAL 4 hr before initiating $CaNa_2EDTA$ Hydrate patient and establish good urinary output before starting therapy Avoid thrombophlebitis by diluting in NS or D_5W to a concentration ≤0.5% Substitution of Na_2EDTA can cause fatal hypocalcemia
Flumazenil	Benzodiazepines Venlafaxine	0.1 mg/min IV to a total dose of 1 mg	Reversal of respiratory depression	Limit use to reversal of inadequate respiration in benzodiazepine-toxic patients Increases intracranial pressure and risk for seizures in presence of underlying seizure disorder or ingestion of seizure-producing toxicants Monitor for resedation up to 2 hr after last dose

Antidote	Indication for Use	Dose*	Treatment End Point	Comments
Folinate (tetrahydrofolic acid [leucovorin])	Methanol Methotrexate	Methanol: 50 mg IV q4h Methotrexate: 100 mg/m^2 IV q3-6h	Methanol: methanol undetectable, metabolic acidosis cleared Methotrexate: serum level $<1 \times 10^{-8}$ mol/L	Essential therapy for both toxicants Methotrexate: large ingestions may require increased dose Glucarpidase administered 2-4 hr before or after folinate
Fomepizole	Ethylene glycol Methanol	Dose 1: 15 mg/kg IV Doses over next 48 hr: 10 mg/kg IV All subsequent doses: 15 mg/kg IV Administer q12h, except when HD performed: HD initiation: ½ next dose if >6 hr since last dose HD ongoing: q4h End of HD (based on time of last dose): <1 hr, no dose; 1-3 hr, ½ next dose; >3 hr, next dose	For both: serum level <20 mg/dl and metabolic acidosis resolved	Start immediately if toxic alcohol suspected, without waiting for confirmatory levels Dose amount is not affected by interval timing of doses
Glucagon	β-Adrenergic receptor antagonists Calcium-channel antagonists	Bolus of 3.5-5 mg IV; can repeat to achieve clinical effect, then infusion of 2-10 mg/hr	Reversal of hypotension and bradycardia; taper infusion	Can precipitate vomiting; be prepared to protect airway Mild hyperglycemia occurs Maximum dosing amounts unknown; bolus doses up to 30 mg reported Duration of effect is 15 min; thus infusion must be started immediately
Hydroxocobalamin	Cyanide	Initial: 5 g IV over 15-min period Second dose: 5 g IV over 15 min–2 hr; maximum total dose is 10 g Follow each hydroxocobalamin dose with sodium thiosulfate 25%: 50 ml (12.5 g) IV over 10-min period	Resolution of lactic acidosis and moderate to severe clinical signs and symptoms: seizures, coma, dyspnea, apnea, hypotension, bradycardia	Can be administered IV push if patient is in cardiac arrest Do not give hydroxocobalamin and sodium thiosulfate through the same IV line Adverse effects: red discoloration of plasma, urine, mucous membranes, skin; transient hypertension Interference with laboratory colorometric assays: Levels increased: bilirubin; creatinine; glucose; hemoglobin; magnesium; co-oximetry total Hb, COHb%, MetHb% Levels decreased: AST, ALT, creatinine, co-oximetry O_2Hb%
Hyperbaric oxygen (HBO)	Carbon monoxide Experimental: carbon tetrachloride, cyanide, hydrogen sulfide	3.0 atm pressure for 60 min (25 min O_2, 5 min air, 25 min O_2, 5 min air), then 2.0 atm for 65 min (30 min O_2, 5 min air, 30 min O_2), then "surface" to 1.0 atm	One treatment Second treatment rarely administered (controversial)	Carbon monoxide: treatment protocols may vary HBO indicated for loss of consciousness; seizures; cerebellar dysfunction; impaired cognition; headache, nausea/vomiting persisting after 4 hr O_2 therapy regardless of carboxyhemoglobin level Experimental indications: treatment protocols not established
Insulin-glucose	Calcium-channel antagonists β-Adrenergic receptor antagonists	Regular insulin, 1 U/kg bolus, followed by 0.5-1 U/kg/hr Titrate 50% dextrose IV to avoid hypoglycemia	Reversal of myocardial depression	Beneficial in case series and reports Initiate if glucagon and vasopressor or inotropic drugs fail to reverse myocardial depression; more effective if used before onset of cardiogenic shock Monitor glucose and potassium; hypoglycemia can occur during and after therapy Hyperglycemia results from toxicant-induced insulin resistance, and initial dextrose requirements may be less than anticipated. Recovery may be heralded by normalization of glucose levels, with increased dextrose required to avoid hypoglycemia
Intralipid	Cardiac toxicity from local anesthetics (e.g., bupivacaine, ropivacaine) Experimental: verapamil, diltiazem, tricyclic antidepressants, bupropion, propranolol	Use 20% formulation Initial bolus: 1.5 ml/kg IV over 1 min, followed immediately by infusion of 0.25 ml/kg/min for 30-60 min Can repeat bolus for asystole	Return of hemodynamic stability	Use based on animal experiments and human case reports; numerous dosing regimens have been used Use if advanced life support measures fail; continue CPR as needed during drug administration

Continued on following page

Antidote	Indication for Use	Dose*	Treatment End Point	Comments
Methylene blue	Methemoglobin-producing agents	1-2 mg/kg body weight (0.1-0.2 ml/kg) of 1% methylene blue is administered over 5-min period; repeat dose for persistent or recurrent symptoms or signs	Resolution of dyspnea and altered mental status	Use if patient is symptomatic (i.e., dyspneic, altered mental status) Maximum dose should not exceed 7 mg/kg (0.7 ml/kg) Contraindicated in G6PD-deficient patients; may cause hemolysis Some toxicants (e.g., dapsone) may require prolonged therapy
N-Acetylcysteine (NAC)	Acetaminophen Experimental: carbon tetrachloride, chloroform, pennyroyal oil	Oral: Load—140 mg/kg Maintenance (starting 4 hr after load)—70 mg/kg q4h IV: Load—150 mg/kg over 1-hr period Maintenance infusion—12.5 mg/kg over 4-hr period, then 6.25 mg/kg per hour as continuous infusion	Administer 24 hr of NAC and repeat AST and APAP levels: if AST normal and APAP not detected, stop NAC; if AST normal and APAP detected, continue NAC for 12 hr, then reassess AST and APAP levels; if AST elevated, continue NAC for total of 72 hr of therapy After 72 hr of therapy, if INR <2.0, stop NAC After patient has received 72 hr of therapy, if INR ≥2.0 or severe hepatotoxicity present, continue NAC until INR <2.0	Most effective if initiated within 8 hr after ingestion; may be started any time after ingestion and is beneficial in severe hepatotoxic states Use IV in patients unable to tolerate PO or with severe hepatotoxicity; the dose and timing differ from the oral regimen Dosage and administration of FDA-approved IV formulation assume early treatment of acute overdose without hepatotoxicity; longer duration of treatment required in patients with hepatotoxicity Treatment end points simplified for ease of use INR result not valid indicator if FFP recently administered
Naloxone	Opioids	Bolus: 0.4-2 mg via IV, sublingual injection, or endotracheal instillation; 0.4-0.8 mg SC Continuous infusion: establish bolus dose required to reverse respiratory depression Begin infusing two thirds of reversal dose every hour, and titrate to maintain adequate respirations Rebolus with half of reversal dose 15 min after reversing respiratory depression	Initial: reversal of respiratory depression with resolution of hypoxia and hypercapnia Final: resolution of CNS and respiratory depression	Preventilate patients with respiratory depression by bag-valve mask or intubation before administration Use smaller doses in opioid-dependent patients; some opioids (e.g., propoxyphene, pentazocine, fentanyls) may require larger doses of naloxone; use continuous infusion for recurrent symptoms and prolonged action of some formulations (e.g., sustained-release morphine, methadone) Resedation can occur Do not use nalmefene or naltrexone to reverse acute toxicity
Octreotide	Sulfonylureas	50 mg SC q6h	Resolution of hypoglycemia and dextrose not required	Maintain dextrose infusion as needed
Physostigmine	Anticholinergic agents (e.g., diphenhydramine, jimsonweed [*Datura* sp.], scopolamine)	1-2 mg IV over 5-min period; can repeat once after 10-15 min if no effect	Reversal of anticholinergic effects	Duration of effect is 60-90 min Benzodiazepine used for subsequent treatment of agitation and seizures; additional physostigmine used rarely (e.g., refractory seizures or agitation) Adverse effects include seizures, excessive oral secretions, bradyarrhythmias; contraindicated in cyclic antidepressant toxicity
Pralidoxime chloride	Organophosphorus compounds Nerve agents—sarin, VX	30 mg/kg IV bolus (max 2 g) over 30 min, followed by continuous infusion of 8-10 mg/kg/hr (max 650 mg/hr)	Resolution of signs and symptoms, atropine no longer required	Can give initial dose over 2-min period for life-threatening clinical effects Administer early when diagnosis known or strongly suspected Efficacy variable, depending on the organophosphate Fat-soluble organophosphates may require prolonged treatment
Pyridoxine	Ethylene glycol (theoretical efficacy)	100 mg IV	One dose	Efficacy theoretical Pyridoxine may stop seizures, but patient can remain comatose (isoniazid, mushrooms); use benzodiazepines and phenobarbital concomitantly to manage seizures Excessive dosing can cause neuropathy
	Isoniazid Monomethylhydrazine mushrooms	5 g IV, repeat for refractory seizures	Resolution of seizures	

Antidote	Indication for Use	Dose*	Treatment End Point	Comments
Sodium bicarbonate ($NaHCO_3$)	Reversal of myocardial sodium-channel blockers (e.g., cyclic antidepressants, cocaine, propoxyphene, sodium-channel-blocking antiarrhythmics with $\tau_{recovery}$ >1 sec, piperidine phenothiazines (thioridazine, mesoridazine)	1-2 mEq $NaHCO_3$/kg via intermittent bolus; repeat as needed	Narrowing of prolonged QRS, resolution of ventricular arrhythmias, reversal of hypotension	Monitor blood pH (optimal pH approximately 7.50); avoid pH >7.55
	Altered tissue distribution or enhanced elimination of salicylates; may be used in chlorophenoxy herbicides, chlorpropamide, formic acid, methotrexate, phenobarbital	1-2 mEq $NaHCO_3$/kg, followed by 3 ampules (150 ml) $NaHCO_3$ (44 mEq per 50 ml) in 850 ml of D_5W, infused at 2-3 times normal maintenance fluid rate	Serum salicylate <30 mg/dl and patient clinically stable	Monitor urinary pH hourly; adjust infusion to maintain urine pH of 7.5-8.0 (avoid blood pH >7.55) Monitor ABGs Maintain normokalemia
Succimer (DMSA)	All forms: Arsenic Lead Mercury	10 mg/kg/dose q8h for 5 days, followed by q12h for 14 days Drug holiday for 2 wk; repeat if treatment end point not reached	Arsenic: 24-hr urinary arsenic <50 μg/L Lead: resolution of encephalopathy, gastrointestinal symptoms, neuropathy, nephropathy, arthralgias, myalgias, and blood lead level <70 μg/dl Mercury, elemental and inorganic: 24-hr urinary mercury <20 μg/L Mercury, organic: end point not well established	Oral chelator; adverse effects include rash, transient AST and alkaline phosphatase elevations, and gastrointestinal distress; minimal chelation of essential metals occurs Dosing for arsenic and mercury not well established Therapeutic end point for organic mercury not established; neurotoxicity not responsive to chelation therapy; suggest chelation until blood mercury level within normal value range for reference laboratory
Vitamin K	Anticoagulants (e.g., warfarin, long-acting anticoagulant rodenticides [LAARs])	Subcutaneous: AquaMEPHYTON (K_1), 10-25 mg, repeat every 6-12 hr until oral vitamin K_1 started Oral: 25-50 mg q6h; larger doses may be required	INR is normal 48-72 hr after stopping vitamin K_1 therapy Can also monitor factor VII activity	Anaphylactoid reaction can occur with IV administration Severe bleeding may also require FFP or factor concentrates Base decision to treat on finding of elevated INR; do not administer prophylactic vitamin K_1 Oral therapy has been required for months with LAAR poisoning because of lipophilicity of toxicant, with slow body clearance

ABG, Arterial blood gas; *ALT,* alanine aminotransferase; *APAP,* acetyl-para-aminophenol (acetaminophen); *AST,* aspartate aminotransferase; *BAL,* British antilewisite; bpm, beats per minute; *CNS,* central nervous system; *COHb%,* percent carboxyhemoglobin; *CPR,* cardiopulmonary resuscitation; *D_5W,* 5% dextrose in water; *DMSA,* 2,3-dimercaptosuccinic acid; *ECG,* electrocardiogram; *FDA,* Food and Drug Administration; *FFP,* fresh-frozen plasma; *G6PD,* glucose-6-phosphate dehydrogenase; *Hb,* hemoglobin; *HD,* hemodialysis; *IM,* intramuscular; *INR,* international normalized ratio; *IV,* intravenous; *MetHb%,* percent methemoglobinemia; *NS,* normal saline; *$O_2Hb\%$,* percent oxyhemoglobin; *PO,* per os (by mouth); *SC,* subcutaneous; $\tau_{recovery}$, drug blockade recovery rate.

*Dose concentrations and infusion times are not given. Drug dosages may require adjustment in patients with renal or hepatic failure.

†Administer antivenom in a monitored setting; antivenom must be reconstituted and then diluted; initially infuse at a rate of 2 to 5 ml/hr, and double the infusion rate every 5 minutes as tolerated to administer antivenom over a 1-hour period.

‡Ten percent calcium chloride solution = 100 mg/ml (27.2 mg/ml elemental calcium); 10% calcium gluconate solution = 100 mg/ml (9 mg/ml elemental calcium).

From Goldman L, Schafer AI: *Goldman's Cecil medicine,* ed 24, Philadelphia, 2012, Saunders.

Impairment and Disability Issues

Impairment describes harm to anatomy and physiology, whereas *disability* denotes the difficulty a person has performing a function. Reporting disability for different sectors of society has its own nuances. Proper evaluation of impairment/disability starts with knowing who is asking for what. It is an area of practice in which an understanding of some basic concepts can make it rewarding rather than distressing.

- Ultimately, disability is a measure of function. Functional outcomes are becoming increasingly important in medicine, mirroring the shift towards patient-centeredness. All practitioners should have some facility with documenting the effects of an intervention on a patient's physical, psychological, and social functioning. For example, the continuation of an opioid analgesic should be predicated on meeting functional goals negotiated between the patient and physician before initiation of the treatment. Even a brief comment on walking distance or work tolerance is better than nothing.
- Some concepts apply to all venues of disability. Primary care providers should rarely be in the position to determine whether a patient can be on or off a specific job. Rather, their task is to give general parameters about which physical exertions are medically dangerous. Try to be specific and use objective criteria where appropriate, but don't be intimidated by a form. Ballpark estimates can often suffice. For example, many chronic low back pain patients may conservatively and safely be described as being able to lift/carry up 10 lbs, push/pull 25 lbs, and change positions as needed to keep comfortable. Have thorough medical records and be consistent; lawyers may focus on contradictions in your documentation to help their clients.
- Rehabilitation centers across the country are required to monitor function using a standardized set of criteria called the "Functional Independence Measure (FIM)," which categorizes activities of daily living into divisions such as mobility, transfers, feeding, grooming/hygiene, dressing, and bathing and toileting. In therapy notes, you may come across scores in these categories rating patients on a seven-point scale from totally dependent to moderate-assistance (mod A; patient can perform 50% of task) to modified-independent (patient requires an assistive device) to independent.
- Psychosocial contributing factors such medicolegal issues can profoundly influence patients' presentations through somatization from secondary gain. However, it is important to differentiate this from malingering, Munchausen's syndrome, or "gaming the system," which are remarkably less prevalent.
- The number of stakeholders expands in the disability system to include the employer, the government, the legal system, and the payer. Each sector has its own regulations. You may be required to fill out disability questionnaires as a condition of accepting payment for clinical services from a payer, such as in the workers' compensation system. Much more commonly, you will be seeing patients for clinical services paid for by an evaluation and management code. In these cases, you are not obligated to provide free medicolegal assessments. Settling payment issues in advance can avoid misunderstanding. Again, before assessing disability, understand who is asking and why.

GOVERNMENT-ADMINISTERED DISABILITY

State Temporary Disability Insurance (TDI) programs, the Family Medical Leave Act of 1993 (FMLA), the Social Security Administration (SSA), and the Department of Veterans Affairs offer disability benefits through the state and federal government.

- State TDI forms must be filled out for the patient to receive any income. They are generally very basic and just engage the social support network for a patient. This may not be the best venue to stipulate partial disability.
- The FMLA provides unpaid leave for qualified medical and family reasons. Because it is a federal program, the forms involved are standard across states and employers. They can be intimidating at first, but are reasonably easy to complete once the basic definitions used are understood. It is recommended that you familiarize yourself with this paperwork the first few times it is encountered. Completing the form for subsequent patients should not be overly burdensome.
- The SSA and the Department of Veterans Affairs have their own internal mechanisms for quantifying disability, but they may subpoena your records or request a summary narrative as part of their processes. If you've kept good clinical notes, your existing documentation should satisfy their requirements. Many patients choose to apply for Social Security Disability Insurance (SSDI) and/or Supplemental Security Income (SSI) through a legal representative. These lawyers may send you a lengthy questionnaire to prepare their case. There are physicians whose practices perform these services and who can be hired by attorneys to facilitate patients' applications. If this nonclinical work appeals to you, consider affiliating with the SSA or contracting your time to lawyers under separate indenture. If not, you may want to recommend the law office contact a suitable practice.

WORKERS' COMPENSATION

In workers' compensation, the payer and employer join the provider in trying to rehabilitate the injured worker. Confidentially issues are handled differently because these stakeholders may have a right to protected health information.

- Each state has their own laws regarding reporting requirements, and the federal Department of Labor governs injured federal employees. If you plan on accepting workers' compensation patients, you must familiarize yourself with the necessary paperwork. Typically, this is a standard, short form that includes measures of function. It may make sense to copy your state's parameters and create a "work note" to be used uniformly in your practice for cases both inside and outside of the workers' compensation system. Functional limitations should pertain to any task, not just to the employee's vocation. In general, employees should not be labeled "on" or "off."
- A notification that an employee has reached "maximal medical improvement" should be made once an employee's condition is expected to change over months/years rather than days/weeks. At this juncture, they will transition from temporary disability benefits to permanent disability benefits, possibly including vocational rehabilitation. If ongoing sequelae exist, a permanent impairment rating may be needed to resolve an employee's claim and allow them to progress to the next stage of their life. These are more sophisticated determinations, usually directed by the American Medical Association's (AMA) *Guides to the Evaluation of Permanent Impairment*, now in its sixth edition. Analysis of permanent impairment, causation, and apportionment generally fall

outside of workers' compensation reporting requirements. Someone with appropriate training may be best suited to complete this task. Consider providing these more detailed services under a separate indenture, such as a consultation arrangement with the employee's attorney. Your state workers' compensation board may have specific guidelines governing these reports. In any case, the work should be done under a clear written agreement, not based on a verbal request by the employee. Very complex cases may also require a formal functional capacity evaluation through an appropriate rehabilitation resource.

PERSONAL INJURY

Patients hurt in car accidents or other personal injuries often are involved in legal cases covering medical care, personal damages, and pain and suffering. Most commonly, you will be helping these patients with their clinical issues under their regular medical insurance, although some providers agree to provide services under a legal lien on the claim. Regardless of your role in a personal injury case, it is helpful to document objective details about the injury and functional parameters. If you are asked to keep someone out of work, try to delineate functional limitations as you would in a workers' compensation employee.

- Similar to the workers' compensation system, it is helpful to state when a patient has reached maximal medical improvement. Personal injury claims can take longer to resolve than in the workers' compensation system, as the employer and insurance company are strongly incentivized to reach a resolution in those cases. In general, an ongoing legal case may hinder a patient from achieving a healthful balance of wellness. It is in the patient's best interest to move the claim toward completion.
- Quantifying permanent disability is a key component of resolving these cases. If a clinician is providing services under a legal lien, there may be a conflict of interest in having that provider quantify the permanent impairment. There may be financial implications to the degree of disability awarded, and this may influence whether or not the clinician will receive payment on their lien. These cases are almost always contentious, and may be best handled by providers with special training, such as an independent medical examiner. Again, the determination typically follows the AMA's *Guides to the Evaluation of Permanent Impairment.* A clinician's role is to manage the patient's injuries, not to negotiate medicolegal issues. If you are not appropriately trained, consider deferring questions regarding disability to someone who is.

PRIVATE DISABILITY

Some patients purchase private insurance plans to provide income in addition to that offered through the government in the case of long-term disability. These forms vary by insurance carrier and change over time. They may need to be filled out periodically to maintain benefits. Many providers opt to charge a separate fee for the completion of this type of paperwork.

CONCLUSION

In summary, impairment and disability are measures of function and should be followed by all good doctors as part of patient-centered care. Providers can be most effective interacting with the various disability systems if they know when they are acting as clinicians and when they are acting as legal consultants. Understanding the principles involved with the different sectors will help you avoid confusion between obligations and opportunities when doing this work.

SUGGESTED READINGS

Rondinelli RD: *Guides to the evaluation of permanent impairment,* ed 6, Arlington, VA, 2007, American Medical Association.

American Academy of Physical Medicine and Rehabilitation: Disability evaluation. Accessed March 7, 2014, at http://now.aapmr.org/rehab-essentials/special-assessment-mgmt-strategy/Pages/Disability-evaluation.aspx.

Holmes, EB: Impairment rating and disability determination. Accessed March 7, 2014, at http://emedicine.medscape.com/article/314195-overview#a1.

AUTHOR: **MATTHEW J. SMITH, M.D.**

A

Bolded page numbers indicate principal textual treatment.
Page numbers followed by *f* indicate figures; *t*, tables; *b*, boxes; *e*, online content.

B

F

G

H

I

J

K

L

M

N

O

P

Q

R

S

T

U

V

W